Reducing Young Children's Fears, ...
Reducing Distress from Otoscopy i...
  Children, 201
Encouraging Opening the Mouth ...
  Examination, 206
Encouraging Deep Breaths, 213
Promoting Relaxation During Abd...
  Palpation, 219
Examination of Genitalia, 221
Heel Punctures, 267
Guidelines for Pain Management ...
  Circumcision, 271
Laser Therapy, 302
Blood Glucose Testing, 317
Heel Punctures, 337
Use of Opioids and Extubation Pr...
Immunizations, 534
Dental Visits, 611
Returning to School with Visible Sk...
Lead Chelation Therapy, 682
Painless Suturing and Wound Clea...
Intramuscular Ceftriaxone (Rocep...
Norplant and Depo-Provera, 857
Hepatitis B Immunization, 865
Removal of Transparent Dressing, ...
Lumbar Puncture and Bone Marr...
Bladder Catheterization or Supra...
  Aspiration, 1146
Drawing Blood from Central Lines, ...
Guidelines for Skin/Vessel Punctures, 1149
Encouraging a Child's Acceptance of Oral
  Medication, 1151
Venipuncture, 1192
Minimizing Pain of Access for Hemodialysis, 1296
Blood Gas Monitoring, 1314
Arterial Blood Punctures, 1316
Extubation and the Use of Opioids, 1324
Intramuscular Ceftriaxone (Rocephin), 1359
Intravenous RespiGam and Intramuscular
  Palivizumab, 1368
Thoracentesis or Placement of Chest Tube, 1371
Reducing Pain of Allergy Skin Tests and "Allergy
  Shots," 1385
Abdominal Circumference Measurements, 1428
Palpating the Abdomen for Abdominal Pain, 1434
Chest Tube Removal, 1505
Noninvasive Local Anesthesia, 1672
Lumbar Puncture, 1679
Avoiding Pain of Venipuncture, 1712
Minimizing Pain of Blood Glucose
  Monitoring, 1748
Reducing the Pain of Aspiration of Synovial Fluid
  in Joints (Arthrocentesis), 1823

Living "in Step," 71
... or, 86
... 87

... Refrigerated Infant

... irst Year, 524
... hecklist, 549
... nt's First Year, 550
... of Lactose Intolerance, 570

... ash, 579
... s, 587

... s, 620
... dler Years, 624
... school Years, 646
... g with Sexual Abuse of

... School, 716
... 21
... n Vehicles, 733
... e Skate Safety, 735
... ool Years, 736
... olescence, 836
... y, 852
Supporting Siblings of Children with Special
  Needs, 930
Stuttering in Young Children, 1011
Helping a Child Learn Language, 1013
Supporting Siblings During Hospitalization, 1084
Discharge from Ambulatory Settings, 1092
The Child with Fever, 1132
House Rules for Smoking Households, 1382
"Allergy-Proofing" the Home and Commu-
  nity, 1398
Use of a Peak Expiratory Flow Meter, 1399
Use of a Metered-Dose Inhaler, 1399
Following Cardiac Catheterization, 1474
Administering Digoxin, 1482
Topics to Include in Discharge Teaching Follow-
  ing Cardiac Surgery, 1509
Orthoses, 1774
Prostheses, 1775
Cast Care, 1786

# CONGRATULATIONS

## You now have access to Mosby's "Get Connected" Bonus Package!

### Here's what's included to help you "Get Connected"

**sign on at:**

http://www.mosby.com/MERLIN/Wong/ncic/

A web site just for you as you learn pediatric nursing with the new 7th edition of Wong's Nursing Care of Infants and Children

**what you will receive:**

Whether you're a student, an instructor, or a clinician, you'll find information just for you. Things like:
- Content Updates    - Links to Related Products
- Author Information . . . and more

**plus:**

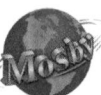 **WebLinks**

An exciting program that allows you to directly access hundreds of active web sites keyed specifically to the content of this book. The WebLinks are continually updated, with new ones added as they develop. **Go online to register for free access to this valuable resource.**

## Free CD-ROM Companion

with every copy of Wong's Nursin of Infants and Children, 7th edit

With a Strong Emphasis on Clinical and Function Relevance, this Valuable CD-ROM Features:

**Critical Thinking Exercises**
**Case Studies**
**Nursing Care Plans to Build and Individualize**
**Anatomy Reviews**
**Procedures and Guidelines to Print and Carry**

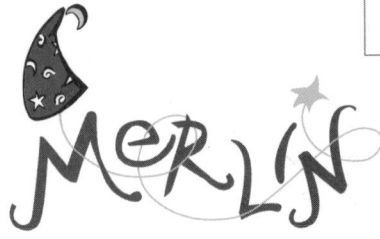

Mosby's Electronic Resource Links & Information Network

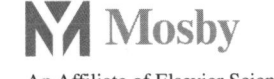 Mosby

An Affiliate of Elsevier Science

# Wong's

# Nursing Care of Infants and Children

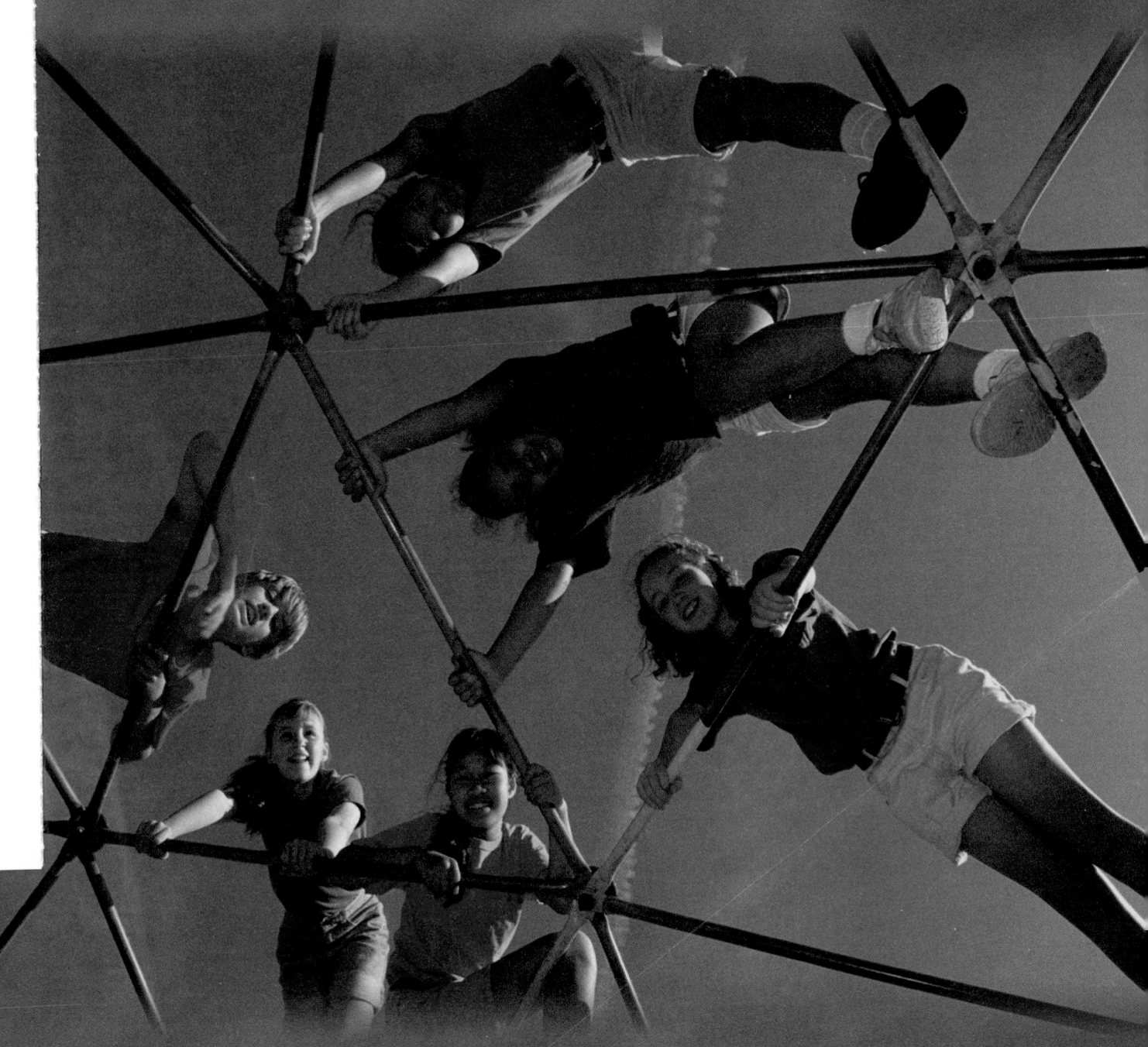

# Expand Your Knowledge

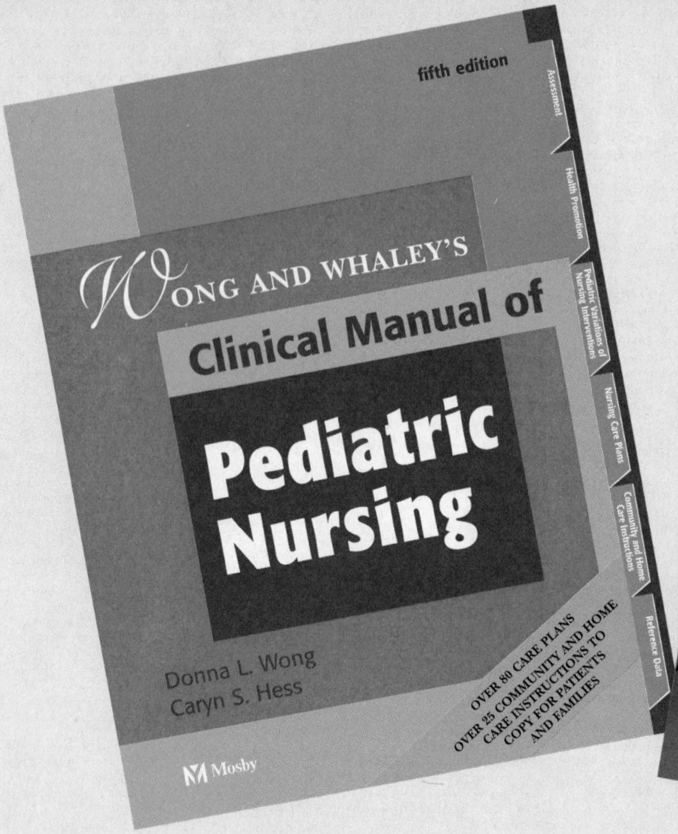

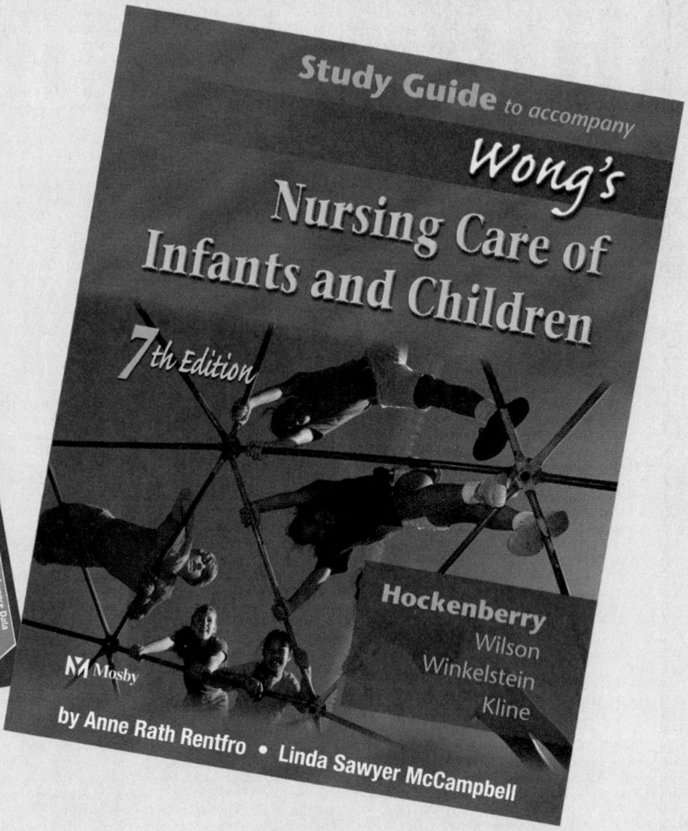

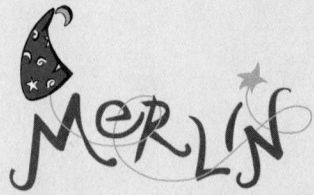

# Wong's
# Nursing Care of
# Infants and Children

### Senior Consultant

## Donna L. Wong, PhD, RN, PNP, CPN, FAAN

Adjunct Associate Professor, University of Oklahoma College of Medicine—Tulsa
Adjunct Professor, University of Oklahoma College of Nursing
Adjunct Professor/Consultant, Oral Roberts University, Anna Vaughn School of Nursing
Consultant, Children's Hospital at Saint Francis, Tulsa, Oklahoma
Consultant, Texas Children's Hospital, Houston, Texas

### Primary Author

## Marilyn J. Hockenberry, PhD, RN-CS, PNP, FAAN

Director, Center for Clinical Research
Nurse Scientist, Texas Children's Hospital
Director of Nurse Practitioners, Texas Children's Cancer Center
Professor, Department of Pediatrics, Baylor College of Medicine, Houston, Texas

### Section Editors

## David Wilson, MS, RNC

Staff Nurse, Children's Hospital at Saint Francis
Tulsa, Oklahoma

## Marilyn L. Winkelstein, PhD, RN

Associate Professor
Johns Hopkins University School of Nursing
Staff Educator
Johns Hopkins Hospital Children's Center
Baltimore, Maryland

## Nancy E. Kline, PhD, RN, CPNP

Assistant Professor of Pediatrics
Baylor College of Medicine
Pediatric Nurse Practitioner
Texas Children's Cancer Center
Houston, Texas

## Seventh Edition

*with 750 illustrations*

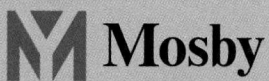

## Mosby

An Affiliate of Elsevier Science
St. Louis   London   Philadelphia   Sydney   Toronto

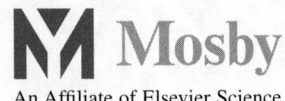

An Affiliate of Elsevier Science

11830 Westline Industrial Drive
St. Louis, Missouri 63146

---

**NOTICE**

Nursing is an ever-changing field. Standard safety precautions must be followed, but as new research and clinical experience broaden our knowledge, changes in treatment and drug therapy may become necessary or appropriate. Readers are advised to check the most current product information provided by the manufacturer of each drug to be administered to verify the recommended dose, the method and duration of administration, and contraindications. It is the responsibility of the licensed health care provider, relying on experience and knowledge of the patient, to determine dosages and the best treatment for each individual patient. Neither the publisher nor the author assumes any liability for any injury and/or damage to persons or property arising from this publication.

---

Previous editions copyrighted 1979, 1983, 1987, 1991, 1995, 1999

**International Standard Book Number 0-323-01722-3**

*Vice President and Publishing Director, Nursing:* Sally Schrefer
*Executive Editor:* Loren S. Wilson
*Senior Developmental Editor:* Michele D. Hayden
*Publishing Services Manager:* John Rogers
*Project Manager:* Helen Hudlin
*Design Manager:* Bill Drone

GW/QWV

Printed in the United States of America

Last digit is the print number:   9   8   7   6   5   4   3   2   1

This book is dedicated to Donna Wong who has been an inspiration to nurses caring for children and their families since the publication of her first nursing textbook in 1979.

Dr. Wong, with her commitment to excellence in nursing practice, has been a role model to us all. Her legacy continues in this newest edition of *Nursing Care of Infants and Children*.

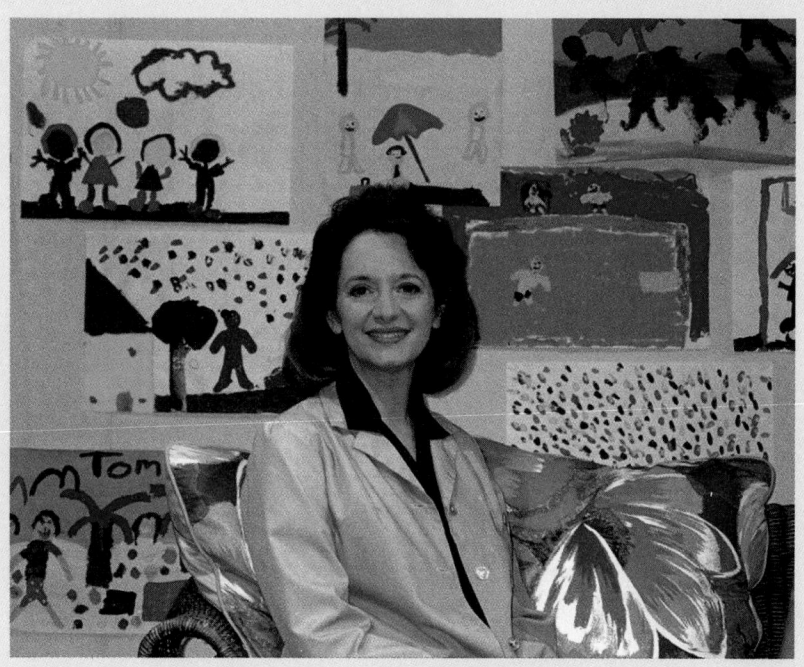

# Contributors

## CONTRIBUTING EDITOR

**Patrick Barrera, BS**

Research Program Coordinator
Clinical Research Center
Texas Children's Hospital
Houston, Texas

■ ■ ■

**Chris L. Algren, Ed, MSN, RN**

Director, Medical Center East Surgical Pavilion
Vanderbilt Children's Hospital
Nashville, Tennessee

**Debra Arnow, MSN, RN, CNA**

Manager, Patient Care Services
Vanderbilt Children's Hospital
Nashville, Tennessee

**Annette L. Baker, MSN, RN, PNP**

Pediatric Nurse Practitioner
Cardiovascular Program
Children's Hospital
Boston, Massachusetts

**Rose A. Urdiales Baker, MSN, RN, CS**

Burn Research Nurse
Children's Hospital Medical Center of Akron
Instructor
Kent State University School of Nursing
Akron, Ohio

**Douglas R. Bloom, PhD**

Pediatric Neuropsychologist
Learning Support Center
Texas Children's Hospital
Houston, Texas

**Christine A. Brosnan, DrPH, RN**

Assistant Professor
School of Nursing
University of Texas Health Science Center at Houston
Houston, Texas

**Jean Park Brown, MS, RNC**

Clinical Nurse Specialist
Shriners Hospitals for Children
Greenville, South Carolina

**Rosalind Bryant, MN, RN-CS, PNP**

Pediatric Nurse Practitioner
Texas Children's Cancer Center
Texas Children's Hospital
Instructor, Department of Pediatrics
Baylor College of Medicine
Houston, Texas

**Nancy R. Calles, BSN, RN, ACRN**

HIV Education and Research Coordinator
Baylor College of Medicine
Texas Children's Hospital
Houston, Texas

**Carol Turnage Carrier, MSN, RN, CNS**

Neonatal Clinical Nurse Specialist
Texas Children's Hospital
Houston, Texas

**Christine Chordas, MSN, RN, CPNP**

Pediatric Nurse Practitioner
Department of Pediatric Oncology
Dana-Farber Cancer Institute
Boston, Massachusetts

**Helen Currier, BSN, RN, CNN**

Clinical Program Specialist, Renal Service
Texas Children's Hospital
Houston, Texas

**Martha R. Curry, MS, RN, CPNP**

Pediatric Nurse Practitioner
Rheumatology Service
Texas Children's Hospital
Instructor, Department of Pediatrics
Baylor College of Medicine
Houston, Texas

**Carolyn V. Daigneau, MS, RN-CS, PNP**

Pediatric Nurse Practitioner
Gastroenterology and Nutrition
Texas Children's Hospital
Instructor, Department of Pediatrics
Baylor College of Medicaine
Houston, Texas

**Bogdan R. Dinu**
Research Associate, Department of Pediatrics
Baylor College of Medicine
Texas Children's Cancer Center
Texas Children's Hospital
Houston, Texas

**Susan D. Fernbach, BSN, RN**
Cardiovascular Genetics Clinic Coordinator
Texas Children's Hospital
Baylor College of Medicine
Houston, Texas

**Nancy Ohanian Gerhard, MN, RN, CNS**
Clinical Nurse Specialist
Department of Pediatric Hematology/Oncology
St. Joseph's Children's Hospital
Paterson, New Jersey

**Mikel Gray, PhD, CUNP, CCCN, FAAN**
Nurse Practitioner and Professor
Department of Urology and School of Nursing
University of Virginia
Charlottesville, Virginia

**Melody Brown Hellsten, MSN, RN, CPNP**
Pediatric Nurse Practitioner
Texas Children's Cancer Center
Texas Children's Hospital
Instructor, Department of Pediatrics
Baylor College of Medicine
Houston, Texas

**Linda M. Kollar, MSN, RN**
Associate Director for Clinical Services
Division of Adolescent Medicine
Children's Hospital Medical Center
Cincinnati, Ohio

**Kevin R. Krull, PhD, ABPP**
Head, Child Neuropsychology Program
Texas Children's Hospital
Assistant Professor, Department of Pediatrics
Baylor College of Medicine
Houston, Texas

**Rosita Y. Maley, MN, RN, CCRN**
Clinical Specialist
Cardiology and Cardiovascular Surgery
Texas Children's Hospital
Houston, Texas

**Bonnie L. Minter, MS, RN, CPNP**
Pediatric Nurse Practitioner
Grady Health System
Emory University, Pediatric ID Program
Atlanta, Georgia

**Mary Mondozzi, MSN, RN, CS**
Burn Center Education Coordinator
Children's Hospital Medical Center of Akron
Akron, Ohio

**Barbara A. Montagnino, MS, RN, CNS**
Clinical Nurse Specialist
Progressive Care Unit, Section of Critical Care
Texas Children's Hospital
Houston, Texas

**Patricia O'Brien, MSN, RN, PNP**
Pediatric Nurse Practitioner
Cardiovascular Program
Children's Hospital
Boston, Massachusetts

**Jill Brace O'Neill, MS, RN-CS, PNP**
Coordinator, Clinical Research
Hematology, Oncology, and Stem Cell Transplant
Children's Hospital
Boston, Massachusetts
Pediatric Nurse Practitioner, Jimmy Fund Clinic
    and David P. Perini Quality of Life Clinic
Dana-Farber Cancer Institute
Boston, Massachusetts

**Nancy Rabin, MN, RN**
Clinical Training and Development Specialist
Texas Children's Hospital
Houston, Texas

**Theresa E. Reed, BSN, RN**
Nutrition Support Nurse Supervisor
Texas Children's Hospital
Houston, Texas

**Amy Nadel Romanczuk, MSN, RN**
Pediatric Ambulatory Care
Medical University of South Carolina
Charleston, South Carolina

**Elizabeth M. Saewyc, PhD, RN, PHN**
Assistant Professor
Center for Adolescent Nursing
University of Minnesota School of Nursing
Minneapolis, Minnesota

**Barbara Schreiner, MN, RN, CDE, BC-ADM**
Associate Director, Diabetes Care Center
Texas Children's Hospital
Assistant Professor, Department of Pediatrics
Baylor College of Medicine
Houston, Texas

**Patricia Liberatore Schwartz, PhD, RNC, CPNP**
Lecturer
Rutgers, The State University of New Jersey
Rutgers, New Jersey
Consultant
Texas Children's Hospital
Houston, Texas

**Nicole Sevier, MSN, RN, CPNP**
Pediatric Nurse Practitioner
Texas Children's Cancer Center
Texas Children's Hospital
Instructor, Department of Pediatrics
Baylor College of Medicine
Houston, Texas

**Cara Simon, MSN, RN, CPNP, ACRN**
Pediatric Nurse Practitioner
Texas Children's Cancer Center
Texas Children's Hospital
Instructor, Department of Pediatrics
Baylor College of Medicine
Houston, Texas

**Sandra Upchurch, PhD, RN, CDE**
Assistant Professor
School of Nursing
University of Texas Health Science Center at Houston
Houston, Texas

**Lisa M. Vallino, BSN, RN**
Vice President/Clinical Director
Progressive IVs, Inc., d.b.a. I.V. House
Formerly PACTS for Life/PALS Program
Director and Emergency Services Nurse
Cardinal Glennon Children's Hospital
St. Louis, Missouri

**Marlene Walden, PhD, RNC, NNP, CCNS**
Neonatal Nurse Practitioner
Neonatal Service
Texas Children's Hospital
Assistant Professor, Department of Pediatrics
Baylor College of Medicine
Houston, Texas

# Reviewers

**Margaret M. Andrews, PhD, RN, CTN**
Chairperson and Professor
Department of Nursing
Nazareth College
Rochester, New York

**Cathy Ascher, RN, MSN**
Department of Pediatric Neurology
Schneider Children's Hospital
New Hyde Park, New York

**Debbie Fraser Askin, MN, RNC**
Assistant Professor of Nursing
University of Manitoba
Neonatal Nurse Practitioner
Neonatal Intensive Care Unit
St. Boniface Hospital
Winnipeg, Manitoba, Canada

**Susan Givens Bell, MS, RNC**
Staff Nurse
Neonatal Intensive Care Unit
All Children's Hospital
St. Petersburg, Florida

**Carol C. Bowman, MS, RD, LD**
Quality Improvement Coordinator
Department of Nutrition and Food Service
Saint Francis Hospital
Tulsa, Oklahoma

**Scott L. DeBoer, MSN, RN, CFRN**
Flight Nurse Educator
University of Chicago Aeromedical Network
University of Chicago Hospitals
Consultant, Peds-R-Us Medical Education
Chicago, Illinois

**Edith M. Eby, PharmD**
Clinical Pharmacy Specialist
Texas Children's Cancer Center
Texas Children's Hospital
Houston, Texas

**Anne Marie Frey, BSN, RN, CRNI**
Clinical Nurse, Level Four
I.V. Team
The Children's Hospital of Philadelphia
Philadelphia, Pennsylvania

**Mark A. Gilger, MD**
Associate Professor of Pediatrics
Gastroenterology and Nutrition Section
Baylor College of Medicine
Houston, Texas

**Mary Astor Gomez, MSN, RN**
Children's Memorial Medical Center
Transport Team
Chicago, Illinois

**Jacquelyn Luzader, RN, CSPI**
Division of Endocrinology
Children's Hospital Medical Center of Akron
Akron, Ohio

**Wendy Mackey, MSN, RN**
Clinical Nurse Specialist
Pediatric Surgery and Trauma
Yale New Haven Children's Hospital
Yale University
New Haven, Connecticut

**Byrthe Marit McCormick, BSN, RN**
Pediatric Surgical Nurse Clinician
Connecticut Children's Medical Center
Hartford, Connecticut

**Lynn Pittsinger-Kazimer, APRN, MSN, CPNP**
Program/Care Manager, Craniofacial Team
Connecticut Children's Medical Center
Hartford, Connecticut

**Kerstin I. West-Wilson, MS, BS, RNC**
International Board-Certified Lactation Consultant
Clinical Nurse III
Neonatal Intensive Care Unit
Children's Hospital at Saint Francis
Tulsa, Oklahoma

# Preface

The new century brings with it the seventh edition of *Nursing Care of Infants and Children.* This text has been a landmark book in pediatric nursing since it was first published over two decades ago. This kind of recognition places a unique accountability and responsibility on us to continue to strive to provide students with the latest information they need to become competent, critical thinkers and to attain the sensitivity necessary to become caring pediatric nurses.

To accomplish this, three section editors, David Wilson, Marilyn Winkelstein, and Nancy Kline, along with Patrick Barrera serving as contributing editor, have joined Marilyn Hockenberry on this edition of the book. This team has put together an expert writing staff of 54 nurses and multidisciplinary specialists who assisted in reviewing, revising, rewriting, or authoring portions of the text on areas undergoing rapid and complex change, such as immunizations, genetics, home care, high-risk newborn care, adolescent health issues, and numerous diseases. We have carefully preserved aspects of the book that have met with such universal acceptance—its state-of-the-art evidence-based information; its strong, integrated focus on the family and community; its logical and user-friendly organization; and its easy reading style.

We have tried to meet the increasing demands of faculty and students to teach and to learn in an environment characterized by rapid change, enormous amounts of information, fewer traditional clinical facilities, and less time. To help students quickly locate essential information, most of the features used in the last edition have been retained, and new ones, such as Evidence-Based Practice boxes, have been added. Most important, this text encourages students to *think critically.*

This book is about families with children, and the philosophy of family-centered care is emphasized. This book is also about providing atraumatic care—care that minimizes the psychologic and physical stress that health promotion and illness can inflict. Features such as Family Focus, Community Focus, and Atraumatic Care boxes bring these philosophies to life throughout the text. Finally, the philosophy of delivering nursing care is addressed. We believe strongly that children and families need consistent caregivers. The establishment of the therapeutic relationship with the child and family is explored as the essential foundation for providing quality nursing care.

This text serves as a reference manual for the practicing nurse. The latest recommendations have been included from authoritative organizations such as the American Academy of Pediatrics, Centers for Disease Control and Prevention, Agency for Healthcare Research and Quality, American Pain Society, American Nurses' Association, and the National Association of Pediatric Nurse Associates and Practitioners. To expand the universe of available information, web sites and e-mail addresses have been included for hundreds of organizations and other educational resources.

## ORGANIZATION OF THE BOOK

The same general approach to the presentation of content has been preserved from previous editions, although much content has been added, condensed, and rearranged within this framework to improve flow, minimize duplication, and emphasize health care trends, such as home and community care. This book is divided into two broad parts. The first part of the book, sometimes called the "age and stage" approach, considers infancy, childhood, and adolescence from a developmental context. It emphasizes the importance of the nurse's role in health promotion and maintenance and in considering the family as the focus of care. From a developmental perspective, the care of common health problems is presented, giving readers a sense of what normal problems can be expected in otherwise healthy children and demonstrating when during childhood these problems are most likely to occur. The second part of the book presents the more serious health problems not specific to any particular age group but that frequently require hospitalization or major medical and nursing intervention.

**UNIT I (Chapters 1 through 5)** provides an overview of the multitude of influences on a child who is developing as a member of a family unit, maturing within a culture, community, and a society. Chapter 1 includes a discussion of morbidity and mortality in infancy and childhood, including Canadian child mortality, and examines child health care from a historical perspective. Because unintentional injury is one of the leading causes of death in children, an overview of this topic is included. The nursing process, with emphasis on nursing diagnosis and outcomes and the importance of developing critical thinking skills, is presented. The role of the nurse as caring provider, family advocate, health promoter, teacher, counselor, and coordinator of care is discussed.

# Special Features

Much effort has been directed toward making this book easy to teach from and, more important, easy to learn from. In this edition the following features have been included to benefit educators, students, and practitioners.

□ A functional and attractive **FULL-COLOR DESIGN** visually enhances the organization of each chapter as well as the special features.

□ Many of the **COLOR PHOTOGRAPHS** are new, and anatomic drawings are easy to follow, with color appropriately used to illustrate important aspects, such as saturated and desaturated blood. As an example, the full-color heart illustrations in Chapter 34 clearly depict congenital cardiac defects and associated hemodynamic changes.

□ **FAMILY HOME CARE** boxes help nurses and students teach parents about the special needs of their infants and children.

□ **EVIDENCE-BASED PRACTICE** boxes have been added to this edition to focus the reader's attention on application of both research and critical thought processes to support and guide the outcomes of nursing care and to provide measurable outcomes that nurses can use to validate their unique role in the health care system.

□ **COMMUNITY FOCUS** boxes address issues that expand to the community, such as increasing immunization rates, preventing lead poisoning, or decreasing smoking among teens.

□ **CRITICAL THINKING EXERCISES** describe brief scenarios of the child-family-nurse interaction that depict real-life clinical situations. From the synthesis of the topical content and a critical analysis of possible options, the reader chooses the best intervention and learns to make clinical judgments. Immediately following the scenario, a rationale is offered for the correct answer and explanations are given for the incorrect options.

□ **CULTURAL AWARENESS** boxes integrate concepts of culturally sensitive care throughout the text. Their emphasis is on the clinical application of the information, whether it focuses on toilet training or on male or female circumcision.

□ **ATRAUMATIC CARE** boxes emphasize the importance of providing competent care without creating undue physical and psychologic distress. Although many of the boxes provide suggestions for managing pain, atraumatic care also considers approaches to promoting self-esteem and preventing embarrassment.

□ **NURSING CARE PLANS** include **RATIONALES** for nursing interventions that may not be immediately evident to the student. This strengthens the connection between the text and the interventions in the care plans. All care plans include patient and family goals and the most recent NANDA nursing diagnoses.

Numerous pedagogic devices that enhance student learning have been retained from previous editions:

□ **CHAPTER OUTLINES** with page numbers begin each chapter, which allows readers to quickly locate topics of interest.

□ **RELATED TOPICS** sections at the beginning of each chapter indicate the chapter or chapters where additional discussion(s) of a given topic can be found. On turning to the cross-referenced chapter(s), readers will find the topic listed in the chapter outline with a page number.

□ **NURSING ALERTS** call the reader's attention to considerations that if ignored could lead to a deteriorating or emergency situation. Key assessment data, risk factors, and danger signs are among the kinds of information included.

□ **NURSING TIPS** present handy information of a non-emergency nature that makes patients more comfortable and the nurse's job a little easier.

□ **GUIDELINES** boxes summarize important nursing interventions for a variety of situations and conditions.

□ **EMERGENCY TREATMENT** boxes are flagged by colored thumb tabs, enabling the reader to quickly locate interventions for crisis situations.

□ **FAMILY FOCUS** boxes present issues of special significance to families who have a child with a particular disorder. This feature is another method of highlighting the needs or concerns of families that should be addressed when family-centered care is provided.

□ **KEY TERMS** are highlighted throughout each chapter to reinforce student learning.

□ Hundreds of **TABLES** and **BOXES** highlight key concepts and nursing interventions.

□ **KEY POINTS,** located at the end of each chapter, help the reader summarize major points, make connections, and synthesize information

□ **APPENDICES** provide additional materials to assist with assessment, including family, developmental, growth, and laboratory evaluation. The NANDA-approved nursing diagnoses and translations of the Wong-Baker FACES Pain Rating Scale also are found here.

□ **INDEX,** detailed and cross-referenced, allows readers to quickly access discussions.

□ **PRINTED ENDPAPERS** on the inside front and back covers provide information nurses refer to often, such as vital signs and blood pressure as well as listings of some of the text's features and their page numbers.

Chapter 2 provides the opportunity to expand the discussion of social, cultural, and religious influences on child development and health promotion, including socioeconomic factors, customs, and health beliefs and practices. The content clearly describes the role of the nurse with such additions as guidelines for culturally sensitive interactions and an updated table, which includes discussion of religious beliefs that affect nursing care. Cultural Awareness boxes throughout the entire text highlight the influences of culture on children and families. Chapter 3, devoted to the family, further emphasizes the importance of this social group to the health and welfare of children. Family theories are the focus of the chapter, which includes a variety of parenting situations that reflect contemporary society. An important example is a revised section on nontraditional families. Family strengths and vulnerabilities are addressed, and current findings on adoption, divorce, single-parenting, stepfamilies, and dual-earner families have been incorporated. The child in the context of family, culture, and community has been broadened to include discussion in a new Chapter 4 of the issue of community health nursing. Chapter 4 provides important information on community-based nursing care, with emphasis on epidemiology as it applies to the detection and identification of causes of morbidity and mortality in pediatrics. Chapter 5 focuses on heredity as it relates to health promotion and the influence of the Human Genome Project on future treatment strategies for inherited diseases. The chapter is written in student-friendly terms to encourage understanding of the complex changes in the field of genetics. Family concerns and ethical issues that arise because of these advances are highlighted throughout the chapter.

**UNIT II (Chapters 6 and 7)** is concerned with the principles of nursing assessment, including communication and interviewing skills, observation, physical and behavioral assessment, and health guidance. Chapter 6 contains guidelines for communicating with children, adolescents and their families, telephone triage, and a detailed description of a health assessment, including an extensive discussion of family assessment and nutritional assessment. In conjunction with new JCAHO guidelines, assessment of pain as the sixth vital sign has been incorporated into the unit. Information on taking a sexual history has been added. Content on communication techniques is outlined to reduce reading time and provide a concise format for reference. Chapter 7 continues to provide a comprehensive approach to physical examination and developmental assessment, using the latest literature on temperature measurement and the new growth charts on how to assess a child's body mass index (BMI).

**UNIT III (Chapters 8 through 11)** stresses the importance of the neonatal period, the time of greatest risk to a child's survival, and discusses several health concerns encountered in the vulnerable first month of life. The nutrition section of Chapter 8 has been updated and revised to include the latest benefits of breast-feeding, incorporating the *Baby Friendly Hospital Initiative* and the *10 Steps to Successful Breast-Feeding*. Infant formula tables and the sections on infant abduction, newborn circumcision, and pain management have all been updated. Newborn screening guidelines now include univer-

sal newborn hearing assessment. The latest information on preparation for home discharge, newborn skin care, and umbilical cord care has been added. Chapter 9 has been revised and updated in the areas of birth trauma and hyperbilirubinemia, including management of breast-feeding jaundice. Updated management protocols and screening guidelines are included for neonatal hypoglycemia, PKU, IDM, and galactosemia. Chapter 10 includes a new expanded developmental outcomes section. Numerous updates include the latest literature on neonatal pain management (including atraumatic care guidelines for neonatal heelsticks and new neonatal pain assessment tools), retinopathy of prematurity, evidence-based neonatal skin care guidelines, and bronchopulmonary dysplasia/chronic lung disease. The most recent classifications of intraventricular/germinal matrix hemorrhage and neonatal seizures are presented in this chapter. Chapter 11 has been extensively revised, including new color photos, and discusses anorectal malformations, management of the child with spina bifida, cranial deformities including plagiocephaly, developmental dysplasia of the hip, cleft lip and cleft palate, biliary atresia, abdominal wall defects, congenital diaphragmatic hernia, and management of genitourinary tract defects. The gender assignment section has also been revised according to the latest guidelines and recommendations.

**UNITS IV through VII (Chapters 12 to 21)** present the major developmental stages, expanded to provide a broader concept of the stages and the health problems most often associated with each age group. Special emphasis is placed on the preventive aspects of care. The chapters on health promotion follow a standard approach that is used consistently for each age group.

The chapters on health problems primarily reflect more typical and age-related concerns. The information on many disorders has been revised to reflect recent changes. Examples include the latest information on communicable diseases, immunizations, cow's milk sensitivity and lactose intolerance, colic, failure to thrive, passenger safety, pacifier use and thumb sucking, lead poisoning, wound healing, sexual abuse, Lyme disease, attention deficit hyperactivity disorder, school-related violence, smoking, diet, contraception, teenage pregnancy, drug abuse, and suicide. The section on sudden infant death syndrome (SIDS) has been extensively updated to include the latest American Academy of Pediatrics considerations for co-sleeping and use of apnea monitors in infancy.

The chapters on adolescence include the latest American Medical Association (AMA) guidelines for adolescent prevention services (GAPS), rankings of body mass index percentiles, nonsmoking strategies, and current trends in suicide. All psychosocial/physiologic conditions discussed include the latest diagnostic criteria from the *Diagnostic and Statistical Manual of Mental Disorders (DSM-IV-TR)*. A new section on the gay, lesbian, and bisexual adolescent has been added to Chapter 19.

**UNIT VIII (Chapters 22 to 25)** deals with children who have the same developmental needs as growing children but who, because of congenital or acquired physical, cognitive, or sensory impairment, require alternative interventions to facilitate development. Chapter 22 reflects current trends in the care of families and children with chronic illness or disability such as home care, normalizing children's lives, focusing on developmental needs, enabling and empowering families, and providing early intervention. Extensive revisions have been made in Chapter 23 to reflect increased awareness of the need for quality nursing care at the end of life. This chapter highlights common fears experienced by the child and family and includes discussion of the nurses' reaction to caring for dying children. Pain management strategies using World Health Organization guidelines are emphasized.

The content in Chapter 24 on cognitive, sensory, and communication impairment includes important updates on the definition and classification of mental retardation. Major updates on hearing impairment, including the use of cochlear implants for sensorineural hearing loss, are presented.

Chapter 25 has been extensively revised by an expert in child home care and includes new information on home care management of children with chronic health conditions. New information includes guidelines for choosing a home health care agency, home care coordination, parent-professional collaboration in the home, and new critical thinking exercises.

**UNIT IX (Chapters 26 and 27)** is concerned with the impact of hospitalization on the child and the family and presents a comprehensive overview of the stressors imposed by hospitalization and nursing interventions available to prevent or eliminate them. Chapter 26 discusses pain assessment and management and presents new material on assessment instruments for nonverbal children and drug dosages for intravenous administration. Chapter 27 discusses safe implementation of procedures with children, including emphasis on the use of therapeutic hugging. We have tried to include as much available research as possible to base the nursing interventions on scientific findings, not just traditional practice. A new section on bladder catheterization has been added, as well as updates on peripheral and central venous access devices, injections, restraints, wound care products, special pressure-reducing devices, and infection control. Major revisions include NPO guidelines before sedation and general sedation guidelines for nursing practice.

**UNITS X through XIV (Chapters 28 to 40)** consider serious health problems of infants and children primarily from a biologic system orientation, which has the practical organizational value of permitting health care problems and nursing considerations to relate to specific pathophysiologic disturbances. Important additions and revisions include discussion of hepatitis, all blood disorders, respiratory syncytial virus (RSV), tuberculosis, the new classification for asthma, effects of passive smoking, seizures, chemotherapy, acquired immunodeficiency syndrome (AIDS), diabetes mellitus, and burns. Chapter 39 has a new section on considerations for the female athlete as well as updated sections on the management of various sports injuries. Care and management of the child with a fracture has been updated as have the sections on immobility, mobilization devices, cast care, and orthotics. Conditions such as systemic lupus erythematosis and juvenile rheumatoid arthritis have been revised and updated. Chapter 40 includes updates on Guillain-Barré syndrome, cerebral palsy, muscular dystrophy, botulism, and spinal muscular atrophy. New management therapies are presented in the section on spinal cord injuries and rehabilitation, and new drug therapy is discussed for myasthenia gravis.

Extensive **Appendices** are also included and contain information on family assessment; developmental assessment; growth measurements, including a complete set of the newly revised National Center for Health Statistics growth charts; pediatric laboratory values; NANDA-approved nursing diagnoses; and several foreign-language translations of the Wong-Baker FACES Pain Rating Scale. All of the appendices reflect the most current versions of forms, charts, and measurements.

## UNIFYING PRINCIPLES

Several unifying principles have guided the organizational structure of this book since its inception. These principles continue to strengthen the book with each revision in order to produce a text that is consistent in approach throughout each chapter.

### The Family as the Unit of Care

The child is an essential member of the family unit. Nursing care is most effective when it is delivered with the belief that *the family is the patient.* This belief permeates the book. The family is seen as a myriad of structures; each has the potential to provide a caring, supportive environment in which the child can grow, mature, and maximize his or her human potential. In addition to family-centered care being integrated into every chapter, an entire chapter is devoted to understanding the family as the core focus in children's lives. Another chapter discusses the social, cultural, and religious influences that impact family beliefs. Separate sections in yet another chapter deal in depth with family communication and family assessment. The impact of illness, hospitalization, home care, and the death of a child are covered extensively in three additional chapters. The needs of the family are emphasized throughout the text under Nursing Considerations with a separate section on family support. Numerous Family Focus and Family Home Care boxes are included to assist nurses in understanding and providing helpful information to families.

### An Integrated Approach to Development

Children are not small adults but special individuals with unique minds, bodies, and needs. No book on pediatric nursing is complete without extensive coverage of communication, nutrition, play, safety, dental care, sexuality, sleep, self-esteem, and, of course, parenting. Nurses promote the healthy expression of development and need to understand how this is observed in children at different ages and stages.

Effective parenting depends on the parent's knowledge of development, and it is often the nurse's responsibility to provide parents with a developmental awareness of their children's needs. For these reasons, coverage of the many dimensions of childhood are integrated within each developmental stage chapter, rather than being presented in a separate chapter. Safety concerns, for instance, are much different for a toddler than for an adolescent. Sleep needs change with age as do nutritional needs. As a result, the units on each stage of childhood contain complete information on all these functions as they relate to the specific age. In the unit on the school-age child, for instance, information is presented on nutritional needs; age-appropriate play and its significance; safety concerns characteristic of the age-group; appropriate dental care; sleep characteristics; and means of promoting self-esteem, a particularly significant concern for school-age children. The challenges of being the parent of a school-age child are presented, and interventions are suggested that nurses can use to promote healthy parenting. Using the integrated approach, students gain an appreciation for the unique characteristics and needs of children at every age and stage of development.

## Focus on Wellness and Illness: Child, Family, and Community

In a pediatric nursing text, a focus on illness is expected. Children become ill, and nurses typically are involved in helping children get well. However, it is not sufficient to prepare students to care primarily for sick children. First, health is more than the absence of disease. Being healthy is being whole in mind, body, and spirit. Therefore the majority of the first half of the book is devoted to discussions that promote physical, psychosocial, mental, and spiritual wellness. Much emphasis is placed on anticipatory guidance of parents to prevent injury or illness in the child. Second, health care is more than ever prevention focused. The objectives set forth in *Healthy People 2010* clearly establish a health care agenda in which solutions to medical/social problems lie in preventive strategies. Third, health care is moving from acute care settings to the community, the home, short-stay centers, and clinics. In this edition, a new chapter on community nursing has been added to stress the importance of community-based nursing care. Nurses must be prepared to function in all settings. To be successful, they must understand the pathophysiology, diagnosis, and treatment of health conditions. Competent nursing care flows from this knowledge and is enhanced by an awareness of childhood development, family dynamics, and communication skill.

## Nursing Care

Although this text incorporates information from numerous disciplines (medicine, pathophysiology, pharmacology, nutrition, psychology, sociology), its primary purpose is to provide information on the nursing care of children and families. Discussions of all disorders conclude with a section on Nursing Considerations. In addition, over 30 care plans are included. Taken together, they provide coverage of nursing care for numerous diseases, disorders, conditions, and crises of childhood.

The purpose of the care plans, like every other feature of the book, is to teach to convey information. They include all current nursing diagnoses approved by NANDA, through its Thirteenth Conference, which have a potential bearing on health problems. Although the care plans can be individualized for use with a specific patient in a clinical setting, that is not their main purpose. For every diagnosis, appropriate patient goals, extensive possible interventions with rationales, and outcomes are presented. Thus a complete range of nursing care is presented within the context of a care plan and the nursing process.

For every health problem for which a care plan is included, the surrounding narrative text is presented according to the nursing process. In these instances specific headings for assessment, nursing diagnoses, planning, implementation, and evaluation, with unifying logos for the five steps, present appropriate information that is then amplified in the care plan, presented in a standard nursing practice context. In keeping with our general purpose of providing practical as well as conceptual information on every page of this book, the care plans provide guidelines and standards for excellence in nursing practice.

## Critical Role of Research and Evidence-Based Practice

The seventh edition is the product of an extensive review of the literature published since the book was last revised. Many readers and researchers have come to rely on the copious references that reflect significant contributions from a broad audience of professionals. So that information is accurate and current, the majority of citations are less than 5 years old, and almost every chapter has entries within 1 year of publication. Examples of current "cutting-edge" information are recommendations from the American Academy of Pediatrics on immunizations and sleep position. The section on pain reflects guidelines from the Agency for Health Care Policy and Research (AHCPR) (now the Agency for Healthcare Research and Quality [AHRQ]) and the American Pain Society. The discussions on skin care reflect the AHCPR's guidelines on pressure ulcers. Lead poisoning has been completely rewritten to reflect the latest Centers for Disease Control and Prevention statements on lead poisoning prevention, diagnosis, and treatment. The American Diabetes Association's new classifications of diabetes mellitus is included as well as the most recent treatment guidelines for asthma.

This book reflects the art and science of pediatric nursing. A central goal in every revision is to base care on research, not tradition. Evidence-based practice produces measurable outcomes that nurses can use to validate their unique role in the health care system.

## CANADIAN CONTENT

The seventh edition of this text includes Canadian statistics regarding infant and child health in Chapter 1 and Canadian immunization schedules in Chapter 12. Throughout the text numerous Canadian resource organizations are also provided. These efforts have been made in an attempt to make the text as valuable as possible to Canadian readers.

◾ ◾ ◾

Just as children and their families bring with them a value system and unique background that affect their role within the health care system, so it is that each nurse brings to each child and family an individual set of characteristics and values that will affect their relationship. Although we have attempted to present a total picture of the child in each age-group both in wellness and in illness, no one child, family, or nurse will be found in this book. We hope that each page, chapter, and unit builds a foundation on which the nurse can begin to construct an ideal of comprehensive, atraumatic, and individualized nursing care for infants, children, adolescents, and their families.

# Teaching/Learning Package

For the seventh edition of this text, an extensive number of ancillary products for instructors and students to use in class and clinical settings are offered:

**MERLIN.** *Mosby's Electronic Resource Links & Information Network* is an innovative web site that provides a wealth of continually updated content, resources, and state-of-the-art information on pediatric nursing, including links to related web sites, important new content updates, Donna Wong's most recent lectures, and more! Use the web address in the text to access *MERLIN's* wide array of information, including course resources for instructors (*Instructor's Manual, Test Bank, Image Collection*) and learning resources for students (WebLinks, crossword puzzles, and more).

**CD Companion.** FREE with every text, this valuable CD-ROM contains a variety of activities to enhance learning through the use of Critical Thinking Exercises, Case Studies, Anatomy Reviews, and Guidelines and Clinical Manifestations boxes. Also included are Nursing Care Plans to build, individualize, and print out.

**Instructor's Electronic Resource.** This innovative electronic resource for the instructor is available online and on CD and contains the following components:

*Instructor's Manual,* with learning objectives, chapter outlines, and accompanying teaching strategies and learning activities.

*Test Bank,* with over 1400 multiple-choice stand-alone test items. An answer key with page references to the text is included.

*Electronic Image Collection,* containing more than 400 full-color illustrations and photos from the text, to help instructors develop presentations and explain key concepts. All images can be printed out as acetates for overhead projection.

## Available for Purchase

**Virtual Clinical Excursions: CD and Workbook Companion.** A CD-ROM and workbook have been developed as a "virtual clinical" experience to expand student opportunities for critical thinking. This package guides the student through a computer-generated virtual clinical environment and helps the user apply textbook content to "virtual patients" in that environment. Seven case studies are presented that allow students to use this textbook as a reference to assess, diagnose, plan, implement, and evaluate "real" patients using actual clinical scenarios. The state-of-the-art technologies reflected on this CD-ROM demonstrate *cutting-edge* learning opportunities for students and facilitate knowledge retention of the information found in this textbook. The clinical simulations and workbook represent the next generation of research-based learning tools that promote critical thinking and meaningful learning.

**Study Guide.** This comprehensive and challenging study aid presents a variety of questions to enhance learning of key concepts and content from the text. Multiple-choice, matching, and true-false questions are included as well as Critical Thinking Case Studies. Answers for all questions are included in the back of the book.

**Whaley and Wong's Pediatric Nursing Video Series.** Narrated by Donna Wong, this outstanding series of six videotapes provides an opportunity to see nurses, children, and families in actual clinical settings. The following topics are included in the series: *Communicating with Children and Families, Pain Assessment and Management, Growth and Development, Medications and Infections, Family-Centered Care,* and *Pediatric Assessment.*

**Wong and Whaley's Clinical Manual of Pediatric Nursing, Edition 5.** This manual contains a wealth of information for use as a reference for students and in the clinical setting. The manual includes over 80 Nursing Care Plans, home care instructions that can be copied and given to families, detailed descriptions of nursing skills and procedures, and much, much more!

**Pediatric Quick Reference.** A handy and invaluable clinical guide for pediatric nursing, the *Pediatric Quick Reference* covers physiologic assessment, pain assessment and management, fluid requirements, emergency information, and laboratory values.

# Acknowledgments

This new seventh edition of *Nursing Care of Infants and Children* brings with it the addition of a new era of authors for the book. This book, dedicated to **Donna Wong,** reflects her legacy as a pioneer for pediatric nurse education. I am grateful for her leadership and continued mentorship. To carry out her legacy, we have joined together numerous authors with diverse expert nursing backgrounds to continue the commitment to providing latest state-of-the-art information on pediatric nursing practice. I am grateful to the many nursing faculty members, practitioners, and students who have offered their comments, recommendations, and suggestions. I am grateful to my three Section Editors, **David Wilson, Marilyn Winkelstein,** and **Nancy Kline;** our contributors; and the many reviewers who brought constructive criticism, suggestions, and clinical expertise to this edition. We could not have completed this enormous task of updating and adding information without the dedication of these special people.

I am especially thankful to **Patrick Barrera,** Contributing Editor, for this book. His commitment to excellence has provided attention to detail that is essential to maintaining the text's uniqueness and quality. His extensive efforts at searching the literature have provided the book with the most up-to-date information available to pediatric nursing practice. Appreciation also goes to **Vanessa Blackstone** for her continued support and devotion. Thanks go to **Paul Kuntz** and **Jim Deleon** for their beautiful color photography and to the health care professionals, children, and parents who generously allowed us to use or take their photographs.

No book is ever a reality without the dedication and perseverance of the editorial staff. Although it is impossible to list every individual at Elsevier Science who has made exceptional efforts to produce this text, we are especially grateful to **Sally Schrefer, Loren Wilson, Shelly Hayden, Diane Todd, Helen Hudlin, John Rogers,** and **Bill Drone** for their support and commitment to excellence.

**Marilyn J. Hockenberry**

# Contents in Brief

## Part I

## Child Health Promotion and Maintenance

### UNIT I
### Children, Their Families, and the Nurse

1 Perspectives of Pediatric Nursing, 1

2 Social, Cultural, and Religious Influences on Child Health Promotion, 30

3 Family Influences on Child Health Promotion, 64

4 Community-Based Nursing Care of the Child and Family, 103

5 Hereditary Influences on Health Promotion of the Child and Family, 110

### UNIT II
### Assessment of the Child and Family

6 Communication and Health Assessment of the Child and Family, 139

7 Physical and Developmental Assessment of the Child, 170

### UNIT III
### Family-Centered Care of the Newborn

8 Health Promotion of the Newborn and Family, 240

9 Health Problems of the Newborn, 295

10 The High-Risk Newborn and Family, 333

11 Conditions Caused by Defects in Physical Development, 415

### UNIT IV
### Family-Centered Care of the Infant

12 Health Promotion of the Infant and Family, 493

13 Health Problems During Infancy, 554

### UNIT V
### Family-Centered Care of the Young Child

14 Health Promotion of the Toddler and Family, 591

15 Health Promotion of the Preschooler and Family, 628

16 Health Problems of Early Childhood, 649

### UNIT VI
### Family-Centered Care of the School-Age Child

17 Health Promotion of the School-Age Child and Family, 698

18 Health Problems of Middle Childhood, 739

### UNIT VII
### Family-Centered Care of the Adolescent

19 Health Promotion of the Adolescent and Family, 802

20 Physical Health Problems of Adolescence, 839

21 Behavioral Health Problems of Adolescence, 869

### UNIT VIII
### Family-Centered Care of the Child with Special Needs

22 Family-Centered Care of the Child with Chronic Illness or Disability, 905

23 Family-Centered End-of-Life Care, 947

24 The Child with Cognitive, Sensory, or Communication Impairment, 977

25 Family-Centered Home Care, 1016

## Part II

# Nursing Care of the Ill or Hospitalized Child

### UNIT IX

**The Child Who Is Hospitalized**

26 Family-Centered Care of the Child During Illness and Hospitalization, 1031

27 Pediatric Variations of Nursing Interventions, 1101

### UNIT X

**The Child with Disturbance of Fluid and Electrolytes**

28 Balance and Imbalance of Body Fluids, 1171

and Electrolyte

on, 1255

Related to
utrients

Oxygen
1303

function, 1343

Dysfunction, 1416

Related
ation

Dysfunction, 1464

Immunologic

### UNIT XIII

**The Child with Disturbance of Regulatory Mechanisms**

36 The Child with Cancer, 1584

37 The Child with Cerebral Dysfunction, 1641

38 The Child with Endocrine Dysfunction, 1703

### UNIT XIV

**The Child with a Problem That Interferes with Physical Mobility**

39 The Child with Musculoskeletal or Articular Dysfunction, 1757

40 The Child with Neuromuscular or Muscular Dysfunction, 1832

### APPENDICES

A Family Assessment, 1870

B Developmental/Sensory Assessment, 1874

C Growth Measurements, 1881

D Common Laboratory Tests, 1895

E NANDA-Approved Nursing Diagnoses 2001-2002, 1904

F Translations of Wong-Baker FACES Pain Rating Scale, 1905

# Contents

## PART I

## Child Health Promotion and Maintenance

### Unit I

### Children, Their Families, and the Nurse

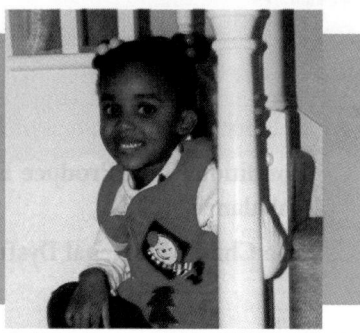

### Chapter 1

**Perspectives of Pediatric Nursing, 1**

HEALTH DURING CHILDHOOD, 1
*Healthy People 2010, 1*
Mortality, 2
  Infant Mortality, 2
  Childhood Mortality, 4
Morbidity, 6
  Childhood Morbidity, 6
  The New Morbidity, 6
Injuries—The Leading Killer, 6
  Host and Agent, 7
  Environment, 10
  Injury Prevention, 10
Evolution of Child Health Care in the
  United States, 11
PEDIATRIC NURSING, 13
Philosophy of Care, 13
  Family-Centered Care, 13
  Atraumatic Care, 15
  Case Management, 15
Role of the Pediatric Nurse, 18
  Therapeutic Relationship, 18
  Family Advocacy/Caring, 19
  Disease Prevention/Health
    Promotion, 20
  Health Teaching, 21
  Support/Counseling, 21
  Restorative Role, 21

Coordination/Collaboration, 21
Ethical Decision Making, 21
Research, 22
Health Care Planning, 22
Future Trends, 23
CRITICAL THINKING AND THE PROCESS OF
  NURSING CHILDREN AND FAMILIES, 24
Critical Thinking, 24
Nursing Process, 25
  Assessment, 25
  Nursing Diagnosis, 25
  Planning, 27
  Implementation, 27
  Evaluation, 27
  Documentation, 27

### Chapter 2

**Social, Cultural, and Religious Influences on Child Health Promotion, 30**

CULTURE, 30
The Child and Family in North
  America, 31
Social Roles, 32
  Primary- and Secondary-Group
    Influences, 32
Cultural Shock, 33
SUBCULTURAL INFLUENCES, 34

Ethnicity, 34
Minority-Group Membership, 35
Social Class/Occupation, 35
  Affluence, 35
  Middle and Upper Class, 36
  Lower and Working Class, 36
  Intellectual Skills, 36
  Communication Skills, 36
  Aspirations, 37
Schools, 37
  Socialization, 37
Peer Cultures, 37
Biculture, 38
Mass Media, 38
  Reading Materials, 39
  Movies, 39
  Television, 39
SOCIOECONOMIC INFLUENCES, 40
Poverty, 40
Homelessness, 41
Migrant Families, 42
CULTURAL INFLUENCES, 42
Cultural Relativity, 43
Relationships with Health Care
  Providers, 43
  Communication, 44
Food Customs, 45
HEALTH BELIEFS AND PRACTICES, 47
Health Beliefs, 47
  Natural Forces, 47
  Supernatural Forces, 47
  Imbalance of Forces, 48

Health Practices, 48
Folklore Related to Prenatal Influences, 49
Importance of Culture to Nurses, 50
CULTURAL AWARENESS, 51
HEREDITARY FACTORS, 51
Physical Characteristics, 57
RELIGIOUS INFLUENCES, 57
Religious Beliefs, 57

# Chapter 3

Family Influences on Child
Health Promotion, 64

GENERAL CONCEPTS, 65
Definition of Family, 65
Family Theories, 65
  Family Systems Theory, 65
  Family Stress Theory, 66
  Developmental Theory, 67
  Structural-Functional Theory, 68
Family Nursing Interventions, 69
FAMILY STRUCTURE AND FUNCTION, 70
Family Structure, 70
  Traditional Nuclear Family, 70
  Nuclear Family, 71
  Blended Family, 71
  Extended Family, 71
  Single-Parent Family, 71
  Binuclear Family, 72
  Polygamous Family, 72
  Communal Family, 72
  Gay or Lesbian Family, 72
Family Function, 73
  Family Strengths and Functioning
    Style, 73
  Vulnerable Families, 73
FAMILY ROLES AND RELATIONSHIPS, 75
Parental Roles, 75
Role Learning, 75
  Role Structuring in Children, 76
Family Size and Configuration, 77
  Family Size, 77
  Spacing of Children, 78
  Sibling Interaction, 78
  Ordinal Position, 79
  Multiple Births, 79
PARENTING, 81
Motivation for Parenthood, 81
Preparation for Parenthood, 81
Goals of Parenting, 82
Transition to Parenthood, 82
  Parental Factors Affecting Transition to
    Parenthood, 82
  Support Systems, 83

Parenting Behaviors, 84
  Attitudes Toward Childrearing, 84
  Parental Styles of Control, 84
Limit-Setting and Discipline, 85
  Minimizing Misbehavior, 85
  General Guidelines for Implementing
    Discipline, 85
  Types of Discipline, 85
Influence of the "Experts," 88
SPECIAL PARENTING SITUATIONS, 88
Parenting the Adopted Child, 89
  Motivation for Adoption, 89
  Sources of Adoptive Children, 89
  Preparation for Adoption, 90
  Parenting Adopted Children, 90
  Special Adoptive Situations, 92
Parenting and Divorce, 94
  Impact of Divorce on Children, 94
  Children's Developmental Tasks
    Related to Divorce, 96
  Custody and Parenting Partnerships, 96
Single-Parenting, 97
  Single Fathers, 98
Parenting in Reconstituted Families, 98
  Stepparenting, 98
  Effects on Children, 99
Parenting in Dual-Earner Families, 99
  Working Mothers, 99
Foster Parenting, 100
Accommodating Contemporary Parenting
  Situations, 100

# Chapter 4

Community-Based Nursing
Care of the Child and Family,
103

COMMUNITY HEALTH CONCEPTS, 103
Community, 103
Demography, 104
Epidemiology, 104
  Distribution of Disease, Injury, or
    Illness, 105
  Epidemiologic Triangle, 105
  Levels of Prevention, 105
Economics, 106
COMMUNITY NURSING PROCESS, 106
Community Needs Assessment, 107
Community Planning, 107
Community Implementation, 107
Community Evaluation, 107

# Chapter 5

Hereditary Influences
on Health Promotion
of the Child and Family, 110

GENETIC INFLUENCES ON HEALTH, 110
Heredity in Health Problems, 111
Congenital Malformations, 111
Chromosome (Cytogenetic) Disorders, 113
  Causes of Chromosome Defects, 113
  Errors in Cell Division, 114
  Autosomal Chromosome
    Abnormalities, 116
  Sex Chromosome Abnormalities, 116
Single-Gene (Monogenic) Disorders, 118
  Autosomal Inheritance Patterns, 118
  X-Linked Inheritance Patterns, 120
Gene Variation and Nontraditional
  Inheritance, 121
Mitochondrial Disorders, 122
Hereditary Cancer Genes, 122
Cytogenetic and Molecular Genetic
  Diagnosis, 123
  Cytogenetic Diagnostic Techniques, 123
  Molecular Diagnostic Techniques, 123
Multifactorial Disorders, 124
  Disorders of the Intrauterine
    Environment, 124
Therapeutic Management of Genetic
  Disease, 124
  Therapeutic Modalities, 124
  Environmental Manipulation, 125
IMPACT OF HEREDITARY DISORDERS
  ON THE FAMILY, 125
Genetic Screening, 125
  Purposes of Screening, 125
  Significance of Screening
    to Families, 127
Prenatal Diagnosis, 128
  Indications for Prenatal Testing and
    Types of Procedures, 128
Genetic Evaluation and Counseling, 130
  Clients, 130
  Counseling Services, 131
  Estimation of Risks, 131
  Interpretation of Risks, 131
Role of Nurses in Genetic Counseling
  and Referral, 132
  Taking a Family History, 133
  Follow-Up Care, 134
  Supportive Counseling, 135
  Burden of Genetic Defect, 136
  Barriers to Effective Counseling, 137

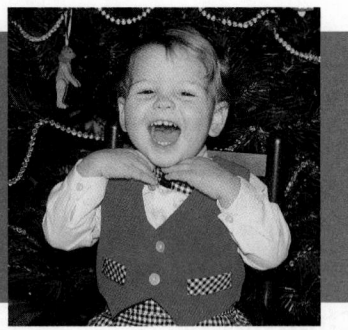

## Unit II

# Assessment of the Child and Family

## Chapter 6

### Communication and Health Assessment of the Child and Family, 139

**COMMUNICATION, 139**
**Verbal Communication—The Power of Words, 140**
　Avoidance Language, 140
　Distancing Language, 140
**Nonverbal Communication—Paralanguage, 140**
　Confirming and Disconfirming Behaviors, 140
**GUIDELINES FOR COMMUNICATION AND INTERVIEWING, 141**
**Establishing a Setting for Communication, 141**
　Appropriate Introduction, 141
　Role Clarification and Explanation of the Interview, 141
　Preliminary Acquaintance, 141
　Assurance of Privacy and Confidentiality, 141
**Computer Privacy and Applications in Nursing, 142**
**Telephone Triage and Counseling, 142**
**COMMUNICATING WITH FAMILIES, 143**
**Communicating with Parents, 143**
　Encouraging the Parent to Talk, 143
　Directing the Focus, 144
　Listening, 144
　Using Silence, 145
　Being Empathic, 145
　Defining the Problem, 145
　Solving the Problem, 146
　Providing Anticipatory Guidance, 146
　Avoiding Blocks to Communication, 146
　Communicating with Families Through an Interpreter, 146
**Communicating with Children, 147**
　Communication Related to Development of Thought Processes, 148
**Communication Techniques, 150**
**HISTORY TAKING, 153**
**Performing a Health History, 153**
　Identifying Information, 153
　Chief Complaint, 154
　Present Illness, 154

　Past History, 155
　Pain History, 157
　Family Medical History, 158
　Psychosocial History, 158
　Sexual History, 158
　Review of Systems, 159
**FAMILY ASSESSMENT, 160**
**Assessment of Family Structure, 160**
**Assessment of Family Function, 162**
**NUTRITIONAL ASSESSMENT, 164**
**Dietary Intake, 164**
　Dietary History, 164
**Clinical Examination, 165**
**Evaluation of Nutritional Assessment, 168**


## Chapter 7

### Physical and Developmental Assessment of the Child, 170

**GENERAL CONCEPTS OF A PEDIATRIC PHYSICAL ASSESSMENT, 171**
**Recommendations for Health Supervision, 171**
**Sequence of the Examination, 171**
**Preparation of the Child, 172**
**PHYSICAL EXAMINATION, 174**
**Growth Measurements, 174**
　Growth Charts, 174
　Length, 175
　Height, 176
　Weight, 177
　Skinfold Thickness and Arm Circumference, 177
　Head Circumference, 177
**Physiologic Measurements, 178**
　Temperature, 178
　Pulse, 179
　Respiration, 179
　Blood Pressure (BP), 182
**General Appearance, 186**
**Skin, 187**
　Factors Influencing Assessment, 187
　Variations in Skin Color, 188
　Texture, 189
　Temperature, 189
　Turgor, 189
　Accessory Structures, 189
**Lymph Nodes, 190**
**Head, 190**
**Neck, 191**
**Eyes, 192**

　Inspection of External Structures, 192
　Inspection of Internal Structures, 194
　Vision Testing, 195
**Ears, 200**
　Inspection of External Structures, 200
　Auditory Testing, 203
　Vestibular Testing, 204
**Nose, 204**
　Inspection of External Structures, 204
　Inspection of Internal Structures, 204
**Mouth and Throat, 206**
　Inspection of Internal Structures, 206
**Chest, 208**
**Lungs, 210**
　Inspection, 210
　Palpation, 211
　Percussion, 212
　Auscultation, 212
**Heart, 213**
　Inspection, 214
　Palpation, 214
　Auscultation, 215
**Abdomen, 217**
　Inspection, 217
　Auscultation, 218
　Percussion, 219
　Palpation, 219
**Genitalia, 220**
　Male Genitalia, 220
　Female Genitalia, 222
**Anus, 223**
**Back and Extremities, 223**
　Spine, 223
　Extremities, 224
　Joints, 225
　Muscles, 225
**Neurologic Assessment, 225**
　Behavior, 225
　Cognitive-Perceptual Development, 225
　Motor Functioning, 225
　Sensory Functioning, 225
　Cerebellar Functioning, 226
　Reflexes, 226
　Cranial Nerves, 227
　"Soft" Signs, 228
**GENERAL CONCEPTS OF MENTAL FUNCTION AND PERSONALITY DEVELOPMENT, 230**
**Theoretic Foundations of Personality Development, 230**
　Psychosexual Development (Freud), 230
　Psychosocial Development (Erikson), 231

Theoretic Foundations of Mental
  Development, 231
  Cognitive Development (Piaget), 231
  Moral Development (Kohlberg), 232
  Spiritual Development, 233

DEVELOPMENTAL ASSESSMENT, 233
Denver II, 235
Revised Prescreening Developmental
  Questionnaire (R-PDQ), 237

Developmental Screening and
  Interpretation, 237

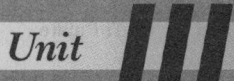

# Unit III

# Family-Centered Care of the Newborn

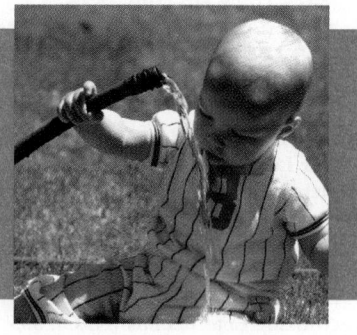

## Chapter 8

Health Promotion of the
Newborn and Family, 240

ADJUSTMENT TO EXTRAUTERINE LIFE, 240
Immediate Adjustments, 240
  Respiratory System, 240
  Circulatory System, 241
Physiologic Status of Other Systems, 241
  Thermoregulation, 241
  Hemopoietic System, 241
  Fluid and Electrolyte Balance, 242
  Gastrointestinal System, 242
  Renal System, 242
  Integumentary System, 242
  Musculoskeletal System, 243
  Defenses Against Infection, 243
  Endocrine System, 243
  Neurologic System, 243
  Sensory Functions, 243
NURSING CARE OF THE NEWBORN AND
  FAMILY, 244
Assessment, 244
  Initial Assessment: Apgar Scoring, 244
  Transitional Assessment: Periods of
    Reactivity, 245
  Behavioral Assessment, 245
  Assessment of Attachment
    Behaviors, 247
  Clinical Assessment of Gestational
    Age, 247
  Physical Assessment, 250
Nursing Diagnoses, 263
Planning, 263
Implementation, 264
  Maintain a Patent Airway, 265
  Maintain a Stable Body
    Temperature, 265
  Protect from Infection and Injury, 265
  Provide Optimum Nutrition, 273
  Promote Parent-Infant Bonding
    (Attachment), 282
  Prepare for Discharge and Home
    Care, 286
Evaluation, 288

Nursing Care Plan: The Normal Newborn
  and Family, 289

## Chapter 9

Health Problems
of the Newborn, 295

BIRTH INJURIES, 295
Soft Tissue Injury, 295
Head Trauma, 296
  Caput Succedaneum, 296
  Subgaleal Hemorrhage, 296
  Cephalhematoma, 297
Fractures, 298
Paralyses, 298
  Facial Paralysis, 298
  Brachial Palsy, 299
  Phrenic Nerve Paralysis, 299
DERMATOLOGIC PROBLEMS
  IN THE NEWBORN, 300
Erythema Toxicum Neonatorum, 300
Candidiasis, 300
Bullous Impetigo, 301
"Birthmarks," 301
PROBLEMS RELATED TO PHYSIOLOGIC
  FACTORS, 303
Hyperbilirubinemia, 303
  Pathophysiology, 304
  Physiologic Jaundice, 304
Nursing Care Plan: The Newborn
  with Hyperbilirubinemia, 313
Hemolytic Disease of the Newborn
  (HDN), 310
  Blood Incompatibility, 310
Hypoglycemia, 316
Hyperglycemia, 317
Hypocalcemia, 318
Hemorrhagic Disease of the Newborn, 319
INBORN ERRORS OF METABOLISM
  (IEMs), 319
Congenital Hypothyroidism (CH), 320
Phenylketonuria (PKU), 322
Galactosemia, 324

PROBLEMS CAUSED BY PERINATAL
  ENVIRONMENTAL FACTORS, 325
Infectious Agents, 325
Chemical Agents, 326
Fetal Alcohol Syndrome, 326
Radiation, 330

## Chapter 10

The High-Risk Newborn
and Family, 333

GENERAL MANAGEMENT OF HIGH-RISK
  NEWBORNS, 334
Identification of High-Risk
  Newborns, 334
  Classification of High-Risk
    Newborns, 334
Intensive Care Facilities, 334
  Organization of Services, 335
  Transporting High-Risk
    Newborns, 335
NURSING CARE OF HIGH-RISK
  NEWBORNS, 335
Assessment, 335
  Systematic Assessment, 336
  Monitoring Physiologic Data, 337
Nursing Diagnoses, 338
Planning, 338
Implementation, 338
  Respiratory Support, 338
  Thermoregulation, 338
  Protection from Infection, 341
  Hydration, 341
  Nutrition, 342
  Feeding Resistance, 348
  Skin Care, 349
  Administration of Medications, 350
  Neonatal Pain, 351
  Developmental Outcome, 357
  Facilitating Parent-Infant
    Relationships, 366
  Discharge Planning and Home
    Care, 368
  Neonatal Loss, 369

Evaluation, 371
*Nursing Care Plan: The High-Risk Infant, 371*
HIGH-RISK CONDITIONS RELATED
 TO DYSMATURITY, 374
Preterm Infants, 374
Postmature Infants, 376
HIGH RISK RELATED TO DISTURBED
 RESPIRATORY FUNCTION, 376
Apnea of Prematurity (AOP), 376
Respiratory Distress Syndrome (RDS), 379
Meconium Aspiration Syndrome
 (MAS), 388
Extraneous Air Syndromes
 (Air Leaks), 389
Bronchopulmonary Dysplasia (BPD), 390
HIGH RISK RELATED TO INFECTIOUS
 PROCESSES, 393
Sepsis, 393
 Sources of Infection, 393
Necrotizing Enterocolitis (NEC), 395
HIGH RISK RELATED TO
 CARDIOVASCULAR/HEMATOLOGIC
 COMPLICATIONS, 397
Patent Ductus Arteriosus (PDA), 397
Persistent Pulmonary Hypertension of the
 Newborn (PPHN), 397
Anemia, 398
Polycythemia, 399
Retinopathy of Prematurity (ROP), 399
HIGH RISK RELATED TO NEUROLOGIC
 DISTURBANCE, 400
Perinatal Hypoxic-Ischemic Brain
 Injury, 400
Germinal Matrix–Intraventricular
 Hemorrhage (GM/IVH), 401
Intracranial Hemorrhage (ICH), 403
 Subdural Hemorrhage, 403
 Subarachnoid Hemorrhage, 403

Intracerebellar Hemorrhage, 403
Neonatal Seizures, 403
HIGH RISK RELATED TO MATERNAL
 CONDITIONS, 404
Infants of Diabetic Mothers (IDMs), 404
Drug-Exposed Infants, 406
 Opiate Exposure, 406
Cocaine Exposure, 407
Infants of Mothers Who Smoke, 408

## Chapter 11

### Conditions Caused by Defects in Physical Development, 415

DEFECTS IN PHYSICAL DEVELOPMENT, 415
Prenatal Development, 416
 Fetal Growth and Differentiation, 416
 Sensitive Periods in Prenatal
 Development, 416
Birth of a Child with a Physical
 Defect, 416
Nursing Care of the Surgical Neonate, 419
MALFORMATIONS OF THE CENTRAL NERVOUS
 SYSTEM (CNS), 423
Defects of Neural Tube Closure, 423
Anencephaly, 425
Spina Bifida (SB)/Myelodysplasia, 425
Myelomeningocele
 (Meningomyelocele), 425
Latex Allergy, 433
*Nursing Care Plan: The Infant with
 Myelomeningocele, 434*
Hydrocephalus, 436
CRANIAL DEFORMITIES, 443
Microcephaly, 444
Craniosynostosis, 444

Craniofacial Abnormalities, 445
Plagiocephaly, 446
SKELETAL DEFECTS, 446
Developmental Dysplasia of the Hip
 (DDH), 446
Congenital Clubfoot, 451
Metatarsus Adductus (Varus), 453
Skeletal Limb Deficiency, 453
DISORDERS OF THE GASTROINTESTINAL (GI)
 TRACT, 454
Cleft Lip (CL) and/or Cleft Palate
 (CP), 454
*Nursing Care Plan: The Child with Cleft Lip
 and/or Cleft Palate, 461*
Esophageal Atresia (EA) and
 Tracheoesophageal Fistula (TEF), 463
*Nursing Care Plan: The Infant with Esophageal
 Atresia and Tracheoesophageal Fistula, 467*
Anorectal Malformations, 466
Biliary Atresia, 470
Abdominal Wall Defects, 472
 Omphalocele, 472
 Gastroschisis, 473
HERNIAS, 474
Umbilical Hernia, 474
Congenital Diaphragmatic Hernia
 (CDH), 475
Inguinal Hernia, 477
Femoral Hernia, 478
DEFECTS OF THE GENITOURINARY
 (GU) TRACT, 478
Phimosis, 479
Hydrocele, 479
Cryptorchidism (Cryptorchism), 480
Hypospadias, 481
Epispadias/Exstrophy Complex, 482
Obstructive Uropathy, 484
Ambiguous genitalia, 487

## Unit *IV*

## Family-Centered Care of the Infant

## Chapter 12

### Health Promotion of the Infant and Family, 493

PROMOTING OPTIMUM GROWTH
 AND DEVELOPMENT, 494
Biologic Development, 494
 Proportional Changes, 494
 Sensory Changes, 495
 Maturation of Systems, 496
 Fine Motor Development, 498
 Gross Motor Development, 498

Psychosocial Development, 501
 Developing a Sense of Trust
 (Erikson), 501
Cognitive Development, 502
 Sensorimotor Phase (Piaget), 502
Development of Body Image, 504
Development of Sexual Identity, 504
Social Development, 504
 Attachment, 504
 Language Development, 506
 Personal-Social Behavior, 506
 Play, 507

Temperament, 507
 Childrearing Practices Related to
 Temperament, 509
Coping with Concerns Related to Normal
 Growth and Development, 514
 Separation and Stranger Fear, 514
 Spoiled Child Syndrome, 515
 Limit-Setting and Discipline, 516
 Alternate Child Care
 Arrangements, 516
 Thumb Sucking and Use of
 Pacifier, 518
 Teething, 519
 Infant Shoes, 519

**PROMOTING OPTIMUM HEALTH DURING INFANCY, 520**
**Nutrition, 520**
   The First 6 Months, 520
   The Second 6 Months, 521
   Selection and Preparation of Solid Foods, 522
   Food Storage, 523
   Method of Introduction, 523
   Weaning, 524
**Sleep and Activity, 525**
   Sleep Problems, 525
**Dental Health, 527**
**Immunizations, 527**
   Schedule for Immunizations, 528
   Recommendations for Routine Immunizations, 530
   Recommendations for Selected Immunizations, 535
   Reactions, 535
   Contraindications/Precautions, 535
   Administration, 538
**Injury Prevention, 541**
   Aspiration of Foreign Objects, 541

Suffocation, 544
Motor Vehicle Injuries, 545
Falls, 546
Poisoning, 547
Burns, 547
Drowning, 548
Bodily Damage, 548
Nurse's Role in Injury Prevention, 548
**Anticipatory Guidance—Care of Families, 550**

## Chapter 13

**Health Problems During Infancy, 554**

**NUTRITIONAL DISTURBANCES, 554**
**Vitamin Disturbances, 554**
**Mineral Disturbances, 555**
**Vegetarian Diets, 560**
**Nursing Considerations, 560**

Protein and Energy Malnutrition (PEM), 566
   Kwashiorkor, 566
   Marasmus, 567
**Food Sensitivity, 568**
   Cow's Milk Allergy, 569
   Lactose Intolerance, 570
**FEEDING DIFFICULTIES, 571**
**Improper Feeding Technique, 571**
**Regurgitation and "Spitting Up," 571**
**Paroxysmal Abdominal Pain (Colic), 571**
**Rumination, 574**
**Failure to Thrive (FTT), 574**
**SKIN DISORDERS, 578**
**Diaper Dermatitis, 578**
**Seborrheic Dermatitis, 580**
**Atopic Dermatitis (AD) (Eczema), 580**
**DISORDERS OF UNKNOWN ETIOLOGY, 582**
**Sudden Infant Death Syndrome (SIDS), 582**
   Infants at Risk for SIDS, 584
**Apnea of Infancy (AOI), 585**

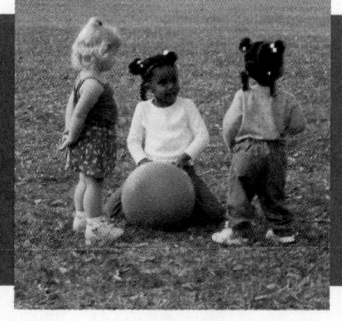

*Unit* **V**

# Family-Centered Care of the Young Child

## Chapter 14

**Health Promotion of the Toddler and Family, 591**

**PROMOTING OPTIMUM GROWTH AND DEVELOPMENT, 591**
**Biologic Development, 592**
   Proportional Changes, 592
   Sensory Changes, 592
   Maturation of Systems, 592
   Gross and Fine Motor Development, 593
**Psychosocial Development, 594**
   Developing a Sense of Autonomy (Erikson), 594
**Cognitive Development, 594**
   Sensorimotor Phase (Piaget), 594
   Preconceptual Phase (Piaget), 596
**Moral Development, 597**
   Preconventional or Premoral Level (Kohlberg), 597
**Spiritual Development, 598**
**Development of Body Image, 598**
**Development of Sexuality, 598**
**Social Development, 598**
   Individuation-Separation, 598

Language Development, 599
Personal-Social Behavior, 599
Play, 600
**Toys, 601**
   Selecting Toys, 601
   Toy Safety, 601
**Temperament, 601**
**Coping with Concerns Related to Normal Growth and Development, 603**
   Toilet Training, 603
   Sibling Rivalry, 605
   Temper Tantrums, 607
   Negativism, 608
   Coping with Stress, 608
**PROMOTING OPTIMUM HEALTH DURING TODDLERHOOD, 609**
**Nutrition, 609**
   Nutritional Counseling, 610
**Sleep and Activity, 611**
**Dental Health, 611**
   Regular Dental Examinations, 611
   Removal of Plaque, 611
   Fluoride, 613
   Low-Cariogenic Diet, 613
**Injury Prevention, 616**
   Motor Vehicle Injuries, 616

Drowning, 620
Burns, 620
Poisoning, 622
Falls, 622
Aspiration and Suffocation, 623
Bodily Damage, 623
**Anticipatory Guidance—Care of Families, 624**

## Chapter 15

**Health Promotion of the Preschooler and Family, 628**

**PROMOTING OPTIMUM GROWTH AND DEVELOPMENT, 628**
**Biologic Development, 628**
   Gross and Fine Motor Behavior, 629
**Psychosocial Development, 630**
   Developing a Sense of Initiative (Erikson), 630
   Oedipal Stage (Freud), 630
**Cognitive Development, 631**
   Preoperational Phase (Piaget), 631
**Moral Development, 631**

Preconventional or Premoral Level
  (Kohlberg), 631
Spiritual Development, 632
Development of Body Image, 632
Development of Sexuality, 632
Social Development, 632
  Language, 633
  Personal-Social Behavior, 633
  Play, 633
Temperament, 636
Coping with Concerns Related to Normal
  Growth and Development, 636
  Preschool and Kindergarten
    Experience, 636
  Sex Education, 637
  Gifted Children, 640
  Aggression, 641
  Speech Problems, 642
  Stress, 642
  Fears, 642
PROMOTING OPTIMUM HEALTH DURING THE
  PRESCHOOL YEARS, 644
Nutrition, 644
Sleep and Activity, 645
  Sleep Problems, 645
Dental Health, 646

Injury Prevention, 646
Anticipatory Guidance—Care of
  Families, 647


## Chapter 16

### Health Problems of Early Childhood, 649

INFECTIOUS DISORDERS, 649
Communicable Diseases, 649
Nursing Care Plan: The Child with
  a Communicable Disease, 662
Conjunctivitis, 662
Stomatitis, 664
INTESTINAL PARASITIC DISEASES, 665
General Nursing Considerations, 665
Giardiasis, 666
Enterobiasis (Pinworms), 667
INGESTION OF INJURIOUS AGENTS, 668
Principles of Emergency Treatment, 669
  Assessment, 669
  Gastric Decontamination, 670
  Prevention of Recurrence, 673

Heavy Metal Poisoning, 675
Lead Poisoning, 675
  Children and Lead, 676
  Causes of Lead Poisoning, 676
  Anticipatory Guidance, 679
  Screening for Lead Poisoning, 679
CHILD MALTREATMENT, 683
Child Neglect, 683
  Types of Neglect, 683
Physical Abuse, 684
  Munchausen Syndrome by Proxy
    (MSBP), 684
  Factors Predisposing to Physical
    Abuse, 684
Sexual Abuse, 685
  Characteristics of Abusers and
    Victims, 686
  Initiation and Perpetuation
    of Sexual Abuse, 686
Nursing Care of the Maltreated Child, 687
Nursing Care Plan: The Child Who
  Is Maltreated, 694

## Unit VI

## Family-Centered Care of the School-Age Child

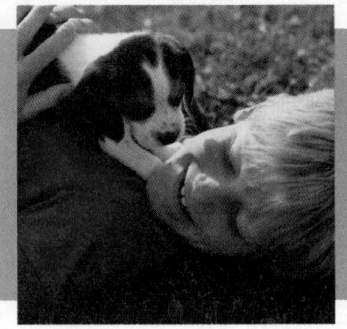

## Chapter 17

### Health Promotion of the School-Age Child and Family, 698

PROMOTING OPTIMUM GROWTH
  AND DEVELOPMENT, 698
Biologic Development, 699
  Proportional Changes, 699
  Maturation of Systems, 699
  Prepubescence, 700
Psychosocial Development, 700
  Developing a Sense of Industry
    (Erikson), 700
Temperament, 701
Cognitive Development (Piaget), 702
Moral Development (Kohlberg), 704
Spiritual Development, 705
Language Development, 705
Social Development, 706
  Social Relationships and
    Cooperation, 706
  Relationships with Families, 707

Development of Self-Concept, 707
  Body Image, 708
  Self-Esteem, 709
Development of Sexuality, 709
  Sex Education, 710
  Nurse's Role in Sex Education, 710
Play, 711
  Rules and Rituals, 711
  Quiet Games and Activities, 712
  Ego Mastery, 712
COPING WITH CONCERNS RELATED
  TO NORMAL GROWTH AND
  DEVELOPMENT, 714
School Experience, 714
  Anticipatory Socialization, 714
  Role of the Teacher, 715
  Role of the Parents, 716
Limit-Setting and Discipline, 716
  Dishonest Behavior, 717
Coping with Stress, 717
  Fears, 719
  Latchkey Children, 720
PROMOTING OPTIMUM HEALTH DURING THE
  SCHOOL YEARS, 720
Health Behaviors, 720

Nutrition, 721
  Outside Influences, 721
  School Programs, 722
Sleep and Rest, 723
  Sleep Problems, 723
Physical Activity, 724
  Physical Fitness, 724
  Acquisition of Skills, 726
  Television and Video Games, 726
Dental Health, 727
  Brushing, 727
School Health, 728
  Health Education, 728
  School Nursing Services, 729
Injury Prevention, 730
  Risk-Taking Behavior, 732
  Motor Vehicle Injury, 732
  Bicycle Injury, 733
  Other Vehicles, 734
  Injuries at School, 735
  Farm Injuries, 735
  Other Injuries, 735
  Nurse's Role in Injury Prevention, 736
Anticipatory Guidance—
  Care of Families, 736

# Chapter 18

## Health Problems of Middle Childhood, 739

DISORDERS AFFECTING THE SKIN, 740
The Skin, 740
  Purposes of the Skin, 740
  Skin Structure, 740
  Skin of Younger Children, 742
Skin Lesions, 742
Wounds, 745
  Process of Wound Healing, 745
  Factors That Influence Healing, 748
General Therapeutic Management, 749
  Dressings, 749
  Topical Therapy, 749
  Systemic Therapy, 749
Nursing Care of the Child with a Skin Disorder, 751
Nursing Care Plan: The Child with a Skin Disorder, 756
INFECTIONS OF THE SKIN, 754
Bacterial Infections, 754
Viral Infections, 755
Dermatophytoses (Fungal Infections), 759
Scabies, 760
Pediculosis Capitis, 761

SYSTEMIC DISORDERS RELATED TO SKIN LESIONS, 763
Systemic Mycotic (Fungal) Infections, 763
Rickettsial Infections, 763
Lyme Disease, 763
Cat Scratch Disease (CSD), 766
SKIN DISORDERS RELATED TO CHEMICAL OR PHYSICAL CONTACTS, 767
Contact Dermatitis, 767
Poison Ivy, Oak, and Sumac, 767
Foreign Bodies, 768
  Cactus Spines, 769
Sunburn, 769
Cold Injury, 770
Hypothermia, 771
SKIN DISORDERS RELATED TO DRUG SENSITIVITY, 772
Drug Reactions, 772
Erythema Multiforme, 772
Erythema Multiforme Exudativum (Stevens-Johnson Syndrome) (SJS), 773
Toxic Epidermal Necrolysis (TEN) (Lyell Disease), 773
MISCELLANEOUS AND CONGENITAL SKIN PROBLEMS, 773
Neurofibromatosis-1 (NF1), 773
BITES AND STINGS, 775
Arthropod Bites and Stings, 775
  Hymenoptera Stings, 775

  Arachnid Bites, 776
  Ticks, 777
Animal Bites, 778
Snakebites, 779
Human Bites, 779
DENTAL DISORDERS, 780
Dental Caries, 780
Periodontal Disease, 781
Malocclusion, 781
Trauma, 782
DISORDERS OF CONTINENCE, 783
Enuresis, 783
Encopresis, 785
DISORDERS WITH BEHAVIORAL COMPONENTS, 786
Attention Deficit Hyperactivity Disorder (ADHD), 786
Learning Disability (LD), 791
Tic Disorders, 792
Tourette Syndrome (TS), 793
Posttraumatic Stress Disorder (PTSD), 794
School Phobia, 794
Recurrent Abdominal Pain (RAP), 796
Conversion Reaction, 797
Childhood Depression, 797
Childhood Schizophrenia, 799

# Unit VII

# Family-Centered Care of the Adolescent

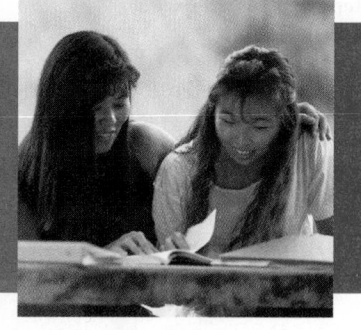

# Chapter 19

## Health Promotion of the Adolescent and Family, 802

PROMOTING OPTIMUM GROWTH AND DEVELOPMENT, 802
Biologic Development, 803
  Neuroendocrine Events of Puberty, 803
  Changes in Reproductive Hormones, 803
  Pubertal Sexual Maturation, 805
  Physical Growth During Puberty, 807
  Other Physiologic Changes, 809
Cognitive Development, 809
  Emergence of Formal Operational Thought (Piaget), 809
  Adolescent Conceptions of Self, 810
  Changes in Social Cognition, 810
Development of Value Autonomy, 811
  Moral Development, 811
  Spiritual Development, 811

Psychosocial Development, 812
  Identity Development, 812
  Development of Autonomy, 812
  Achievement, 813
  Sexuality, 814
  Intimacy, 816
Social Environments, 817
  Families, 817
  Peer Groups, 818
  Schools, 818
  Work, 819
  Community and Society, 819
PROMOTING OPTIMUM HEALTH DURING ADOLESCENCE, 820
Adolescents' Perspectives on Health, 820
Factors That Promote Adolescent Health and Well-Being, 821
  Contexts for Adolescent Health Promotion, 822
  Schools, 822
  School-Based and School-Linked Health Services, 822

  Communities, 823
  Health Care Settings, 823
  Adolescent Health Screening, 824
Health Concerns of Adolescence, 826
  Parenting and Family Adjustment, 826
  Psychosocial Adjustment, 827
  Intentional and Unintentional Injury, 828
  Dietary Habits, Eating Disorders, and Obesity, 829
  Physical Fitness, 830
  Sexual Behavior, Sexually Transmitted Diseases (STDs) and Unintended Pregnancy, 830
  Use of Tobacco, Alcohol, and Other Substances, 831
  Depression and Suicide, 832
  Physical, Sexual, and Emotional Abuse, 832
  School and Learning Problems, 833
  Hypertension, 833
  Hyperlipidemia, 833

Infectious Diseases/
    Immunizations, 833
**Health Promotion Among Special Groups**
    **of Adolescents, 834**
    Adolescents of Color, 834
    Gay, Lesbian, and Bisexual
        Adolescents, 835
    Rural Adolescents, 836
**Nursing Considerations, 837**

## Chapter 20
### Physical Health Problems of Adolescence, 839

**COMMON HEALTH CONCERNS OF**
    **ADOLESCENCE, 839**
**Acne, 839**
**Vision Changes, 842**
**HEALTH PROBLEMS OF THE MALE**
    **REPRODUCTIVE SYSTEM, 842**
**Penile Problems, 842**
**Testicular Tumors, 843**
**Varicocele, 843**
**Epididymitis, 844**
**Testicular Torsion, 844**
**Gynecomastia, 844**
**HEALTH PROBLEMS OF THE FEMALE**
    **REPRODUCTIVE SYSTEM, 844**
**Gynecologic Examination, 844**
**Menstrual Disorders, 845**
    Primary Amenorrhea, 845
    Secondary Amenorrhea, 845
    Menstrual Irregularities in the Female
        Athlete, 846
**Dysmenorrhea, 846**
**Endometriosis, 847**
**Premenstrual Syndrome (PMS), 847**
**Dysfunctional Uterine Bleeding**
    **(DUB), 848**

**Vaginitis and Vulvitis**
    **(Vulvovaginitis), 848**
**HEALTH PROBLEMS RELATED TO**
    **SEXUALITY, 849**
**Adolescent Pregnancy, 850**
    Medical Aspects, 850
    Complications of Pregnancy, 850
    Causal Factors, 851
    Social and Economic Aspects, 851
    Mother-Infant Relationship, 851
    Adolescent Fathers, 852
**Adolescent Abortion, 853**
**Contraception, 854**
    Contraceptive Methods, 854
    Use of Contraception, 855
**Rape, 858**
    Assailants, 858
**SEXUALLY TRANSMITTED DISEASES**
    **(STDs), 860**
**Gonorrhea, 861**
**Chlamydial Infection, 862**
**Pelvic Inflammatory Disease**
    **(PID), 863**
**Human Papillomavirus (HPV), 864**
**Human Immunodeficiency Virus**
    **(HIV) Infection and Acquired**
    **Immunodeficiency Syndrome**
    **(AIDS), 864**
**Hepatitis B Virus (HBV), 865**
**Other Sexually Transmitted Genital**
    **Lesions, 865**
**Nursing Considerations, 866**

## Chapter 21
### Behavioral Health Problems of Adolescence, 869

**EATING PROBLEMS/DISORDERS, 869**
**Adipose Tissue, 869**

**Obesity, 870**
    Obesity in Adolescence, 872
    Complications of Adolescent Obesity, 873
**Anorexia Nervosa (AN), 876**
*Nursing Care Plan: The Adolescent with*
    *Anorexia Nervosa, 881*
**Bulimia, 882**
**"Fear of Fat" Syndrome, 883**
**SUBSTANCE ABUSE, 884**
**Overview, 884**
    Definitions, 884
    Patterns of Drug Use, 884
    Types of Drugs Abused, 884
**Tobacco, 885**
    Process of Becoming a Smoker, 887
    Smokeless Tobacco, 887
**Alcohol, 888**
**Additional Drugs, 890**
**Therapeutic Management, 892**
**Nursing Considerations, 893**
    Long-Term Management, 894
    Prevention, 895
**SUICIDE, 895**
**Incidence, 896**
**Factors Associated with Suicide Risk, 897**
    Individual Factors, 897
    Family Factors, 899
    Social/Environmental Factors, 899
**Methods, 899**
    Completed Suicide, 899
    Suicide Attempt, 899
**Precipitating Factors, 899**
**Nursing Considerations, 899**
    Prevention, 899
    Screening for Suicidality, 901
    Care of the Suicidal Adolescent, 902

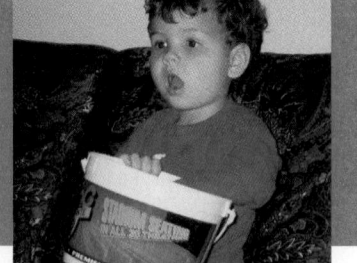

## Unit VIII
# Family-Centered Care of the Child with Special Needs

## Chapter 22
### Family-Centered Care of the Child with Chronic Illness or Disability, 905

**PERSPECTIVES IN THE CARE OF CHILDREN**
    **WITH SPECIAL NEEDS, 905**
**Scope of the Problem, 905**
**Trends in Care, 907**

Developmental Focus, 907
Family Development, 907
Family-Centered Care, 907
Normalization, 908
Home Care, 908
Mainstreaming, 908
Early Intervention, 909
Managed Care, 909
**Cultural Issues, 910**

**IMPACT OF CHRONIC ILLNESS OR DISABILITY**
    **ON THE CHILD, 910**
**Promoting Normal Development, 910**
    Infant, 910
    Toddler, 912
    Preschooler, 913
    School-Age Child, 914
    Adolescent, 916
**Helping the Child to Cope, 917**
    Coping Mechanisms, 917

Normalization, 917
Hopefulness, 918
Health Education/Self-Care, 918
Realistic Future Goals, 919
THE FAMILY OF THE CHILD WITH SPECIAL
NEEDS, 920
Assessing Family Strengths
and Adjustment, 921
Accepting the Child's Condition/Support
at the Time of Diagnosis, 921
Managing the Condition on an Ongoing
Basis, 923
Special Information Needs, 923
Family Management Styles, 924
Meeting the Child's Normal
Developmental Needs, 925
Meeting Developmental Needs of Other
Family Members, 925
Parents, 925
Sibling Issues, 928
Extended Family Members
and Friends, 929
Coping with Ongoing Stress and Periodic
Crises, 931
Concurrent Stresses Within
the Family, 931
Coping Mechanisms, 931
Parental Empowerment, 932
Assisting Family Members in Managing
Their Feelings, 933
Shock and Denial, 933
Adjustment, 933
Reintegration and
Acknowledgment, 934
Establishing a Support System, 935
Intrafamilial Resources, 935
Social Support Systems, 936
Parent-to-Parent Support, 936
Parent-Professional Partnerships, 937
Community Resources, 938
Nursing Care Plan: The Child with Chronic
Illness or Disability, 939

## Chapter 23

Family-Centered End-of-Life
Care, 947

PALLIATIVE CARE IN CHILDHOOD TERMINAL
ILLNESS, 948
Scope of the Problem, 948
Principles of Palliative Care, 948
Decision Making at the End of Life, 948
Ethical Considerations in End-of-Life
Decision Making, 949
Physician/Health Care Team Decision
Making, 949
Parental Decision Making, 950

Awareness of Dying in Children with Life-
Threatening Illness, 950
Developmental Age, 951
Previous Knowledge, 951
Honesty, 952
Children's Understanding of and
Reactions to Dying, 953
Infants and Toddlers, 953
Preschool Children, 953
School-Age Children, 954
Adolescents, 954
Delivery of Palliative Care Services, 955
Hospital, 955
Home Care, 955
Hospice Care, 955
NURSING CARE OF THE CHILD AND FAMILY AT
THE END OF LIFE, 956
Management of Pain and Suffering, 956
Pain and Symptom Management, 956
Parents' and Siblings' Need for Education
and Support Through the Caregiving
Process, 958
Educational Needs, 958
Emotional Support, 958
Religious and Spiritual Support, 958
Sibling Support, 958
Caregiver Support, 959
Care at the Time of Death, 960
Physical Changes, 960
Emotional Changes, 961
Postmortem Care, 961
Nursing Care Plan: The Child Who Is
Terminally Ill or Dying, 962
Care of the Family Experiencing
Unexpected Childhood Death, 964
Community-Based Follow-up, 965
SPECIAL DECISIONS AT THE TIME OF DYING
AND DEATH, 966
Right to Die/Do Not Resuscitate
(DNR), 966
Viewing of the Body, 966
Organ or Tissue Donation/Autopsy, 966
Siblings' Attendance at Funeral
Services, 967
CARE OF THE GRIEVING FAMILY, 968
Grief, 968
Parental Grief, 969
Sibling Grief, 969
Mourning, 970
Shock and Disbelief, 970
Expression of Grief, 970
Disorganization and Despair, 971
Reorganization, 971
Bereavement Programs, 971
THE NURSE AND THE CHILD WITH LIFE-
THREATENING ILLNESS, 972
Nurses' Reactions to Caring for Children
with Life-Threatening Illness, 972
Denial, 972
Anger and Depression, 972

Guilt, 972
Ambivalence, 972
Coping with Stress, 973
Self-Awareness, 973
Knowledge and Practice, 973
Support Systems, 973
Other Strategies, 974

## Chapter 24

The Child with Cognitive,
Sensory, or Communication
Impairment, 977

COGNITIVE IMPAIRMENT, 977
General Concepts, 977
Nursing Care of Children with Cognitive
Impairment, 979
Nursing Care Plan: The Child with Mental
Retardation, 988
Down Syndrome, 987
Fragile X Syndrome, 993
SENSORY IMPAIRMENT, 994
Hearing Impairment, 994
Visual Impairment, 1000
The Deaf-Blind Child, 1006
COMMUNICATION IMPAIRMENT, 1007
General Concepts, 1007
Language Impairment, 1007
Speech Impairment, 1007
Nonspeech Communication, 1007
Autism, 1008
Nursing Care of Children with
Communication Impairment, 1010

## Chapter 25

Family-Centered Home
Care, 1016

GENERAL CONCEPTS OF HOME CARE, 1016
Home Care Trends, 1017
Effective Home Care, 1017
Discharge Planning and Selection of a
Home Care Agency, 1018
Case Management, 1019
Role of the Nurse, Training, and
Standards of Care, 1020
FAMILY-CENTERED HOME CARE, 1021
Respect for Diversity, 1021
Parent-Professional Collaboration, 1022
The Nursing Process, 1023
Promotion of Optimum Development,
Self-Care, and Education, 1024
Safety Issues in the Home, 1028
Family-to-Family Support, 1028

# PART II

## Nursing Care of the Ill or Hospitalized Child

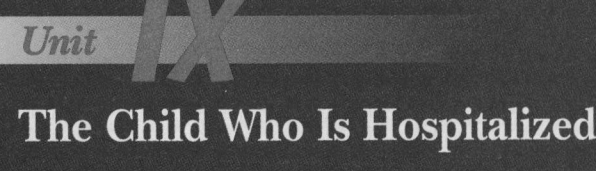

### Unit IX

### The Child Who Is Hospitalized

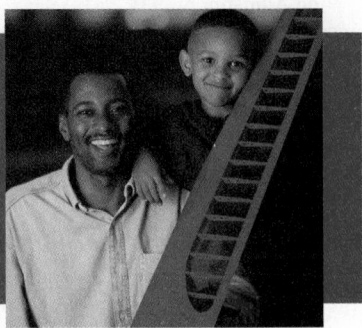

## Chapter 26

### Family-Centered Care of the Child During Illness and Hospitalization, 1031

**STRESSORS OF HOSPITALIZATION AND CHILDREN'S REACTIONS, 1032**
**Separation Anxiety, 1032**
   Early Childhood, 1033
   Later Childhood, 1033
**Loss of Control, 1034**
   Infants, 1034
   Toddlers, 1034
   Preschoolers, 1034
   School-Age Children, 1035
   Adolescents, 1035
**Bodily Injury and Pain, 1036**
   Infants, 1036
   Toddlers, 1037
   Preschoolers, 1037
   School-Age Children, 1038
   Adolescents, 1039
**Effects of Hospitalization on the Child, 1039**
   Individual Risk Factors, 1039
   Changes in the Pediatric Population, 1040
   Beneficial Effects of Hospitalization, 1040
**STRESSORS AND REACTIONS OF THE FAMILY OF THE CHILD WHO IS HOSPITALIZED, 1040**
**Parental Reactions, 1040**
**Sibling Reactions, 1041**
**Altered Family Roles, 1041**
**NURSING CARE OF THE CHILD WHO IS HOSPITALIZED, 1041**
**Preventing or Minimizing Separation, 1041**
   Parent Participation, 1042
   Strategies to Minimize the Effects of Separation, 1043
**Minimizing Loss of Control, 1044**
   Promoting Freedom of Movement, 1044
   Maintaining the Child's Routine, 1045

   Encouraging Independence, 1045
   Promoting Understanding, 1046
**Preventing or Minimizing Bodily Injury, 1046**
**Pain Assessment, 1046**
   Fallacies and Facts, 1048
   Principles of Pain Assessment in Children, 1049
**Pain Management, 1057**
   Nonpharmacologic Management, 1057
   Pharmacologic Management, 1057
**Providing Developmentally Appropriate Activities, 1068**
**Using Play/Expressive Activities to Minimize Stress, 1069**
   Diversional Activities, 1070
   Expressive Activities, 1071
**Maximizing Potential Benefits of Hospitalization, 1072**
   Fostering Parent-Child Relationships, 1072
   Providing Educational Opportunities, 1072
   Promoting Self-Mastery, 1072
   Providing Socialization, 1072
**Supporting Family Members, 1073**
   Providing Information, 1074
*Nursing Care Plan: The Child in the Hospital, 1075*
*Nursing Care Plan: The Family of the Child Who Is Ill or Hospitalized, 1080*
**PREPARATION FOR HOSPITALIZATION, 1083**
**Guidelines in Preparing for Hospitalization, 1084**
   Group Size and Timing of Preparation, 1084
   Setting of the Tour, 1085
   Preparatory Materials, 1085
   Opportunity for Discussion, 1085
   Prehospital Counseling by Parents, 1086
**Hospital Admission Procedure, 1086**
   Nursing Admission History, 1086
   Physical Assessment, 1089

   Placing the Child, 1090
   Adolescent Unit, 1090
**Nursing Care During Special Hospital Situations, 1091**
   Ambulatory/Outpatient Setting, 1091
   Isolation, 1092
   Emergency Admission, 1093
   Intensive Care Unit (ICU), 1093
**Discharge Planning and Home Care, 1095**
   Assessment, 1096
   Planning, 1096
   Transitional Care, 1097
   Evaluation and Continuing Support, 1097

## Chapter 27

### Pediatric Variations of Nursing Interventions, 1101

**GENERAL CONCEPTS RELATED TO PEDIATRIC PROCEDURES, 1102**
**Informed Consent, 1102**
   Requirements for Obtaining Informed Consent, 1102
   Eligibility for Giving Informed Consent, 1102
**Preparation for Diagnostic and Therapeutic Procedures, 1103**
   Psychologic Preparation, 1103
   Physical Preparation, 1108
   Performance of the Procedure, 1109
   Postprocedural Support, 1109
   Use of Play in Procedures, 1110
**Surgical Procedures, 1110**
   Preoperative Care, 1110
   Postoperative Care, 1113
*Nursing Care Plan: The Child Undergoing Surgery, 1114*
**Compliance, 1118**
   Assessment, 1118
   Compliance Strategies, 1120
**GENERAL HYGIENE AND CARE, 1121**
**Maintaining Healthy Skin, 1121**
**Bathing, 1125**

Oral Hygiene, 1127
Hair Care, 1128
Feeding the Sick Child, 1128
Controlling Elevated Temperatures, 1130
Family Teaching and Home Care, 1131
SAFETY, 1132
Infection Control, 1132
Environmental Factors, 1135
Toys, 1136
Limit-Setting, 1136
Transporting Infants and Children, 1136
Restraining Methods and Therapeutic
    Holding, 1136
    Mummy Restraint or Swaddle, 1138
    Jacket Restraint, 1140
    Arm and Leg Restraints, 1140
    Elbow Restraint, 1140
POSITIONING FOR PROCEDURES, 1140
Jugular Venipuncture, 1140
Femoral Venipuncture, 1141
Extremity Venipuncture, 1141
Lumbar Puncture, 1141
Bone Marrow Aspiration/Biopsy, 1142

Other Procedures, 1142
COLLECTION OF SPECIMENS, 1142
Urine Specimens, 1143
    Clean-Catch Specimens, 1144
    Twenty-Four-Hour Collection, 1144
    Bladder Catheterization and Other
        Techniques, 1144
Stool Specimens, 1146
Blood Specimens, 1147
Respiratory Secretion Specimens, 1148
ADMINISTRATION OF MEDICATION, 1149
Determination of Drug Dosage, 1149
Preparation for Safe Administration, 1150
    Checking Dosage, 1150
    Identification, 1151
    Parents, 1151
    Child, 1151
Oral Administration, 1151
    Preparation, 1151
    Administration, 1153
Intramuscular (IM) Administration, 1153

Selecting the Syringe and Needle, 1153
    Determining the Site, 1154
    Administration, 1155
Subcutaneous and Intradermal
    Administration, 1157
Intravenous (IV) Administration, 1158
Nasogastric, Orogastric, or Gastrostomy
    Administration, 1159
Rectal Administration, 1159
Optic, Otic, and Nasal
    Administration, 1160
Family Teaching and Home Care, 1161
ALTERNATIVE FEEDING TECHNIQUES, 1162
Gavage Feeding, 1162
    Preparations, 1162
    Procedure, 1162
Gastrostomy Feeding, 1164
PROCEDURES RELATED TO
    ELIMINATION, 1165
Enema, 1165
Ostomies, 1166
Family Teaching and Home Care, 1167

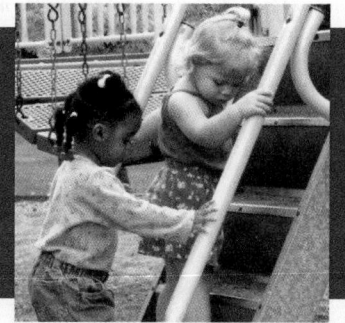

## Unit X

# The Child with Disturbance of Fluid and Electrolytes

## Chapter 28

### Balance and Imbalance of Body Fluids, 1171

DISTRIBUTION OF BODY FLUIDS, 1171
Water Balance, 1172
    Mechanisms of Fluid Movement, 1172
    Changes in Fluid Volume Related to
        Growth, 1173
    Water Balance in Infants, 1173
DISTURBANCES OF FLUID AND ELECTROLYTE
    BALANCE, 1174
Dehydration, 1174
    Types of Dehydration, 1176
    Degree of Dehydration, 1178
Water Intoxication, 1180
Edema, 1180
    Mechanisms of Edema Formation, 1180
DISTURBANCES OF ACID-BASE
    BALANCE, 1181
Acid-Base Imbalance, 1182
    Hydrogen Ion Concentration, 1182
    Compensatory Mechanisms, 1182
    Laboratory Measurements, 1183
    Associated Disturbances in Acid-Base
        Balance, 1183

Respiratory Acidosis, 1183
Respiratory Alkalosis, 1184
Metabolic Acidosis, 1184
Metabolic Alkalosis, 1184
NURSING RESPONSIBILITIES IN FLUID AND
    ELECTROLYTE DISTURBANCES, 1185
Assessment, 1185
    History, 1185
    Clinical Observations, 1185
    Intake and Output (I & O)
        Measurement, 1186
Oral Fluid Intake, 1186
    The Child Who Is NPO, 1188
Parenteral Fluid Therapy, 1188
    Intravenous Infusion, 1188
    Intraosseous Infusion, 1191
    Preparing the Child and Parents, 1192
    The Procedure, 1192
    Securing a Peripheral Intravenous
        (PIV) Line, 1194
    Removal of a Peripheral Intravenous
        Line, 1196
    Complications, 1196
Venous Access Devices (VADs), 1198
    Peripheral Intermittent Infusion
        Device, 1198

Peripherally Inserted Central Catheters
    (PICCs), 1198
Long-Term Central VADs, 1200
Complications, 1201
Parent/Child Teaching, 1202
Total Parenteral Nutrition (TPN), 1203
    Complications, 1203
    Home Total Parenteral Nutrition
        (HTPN), 1204

## Chapter 29

### Conditions That Produce Fluid and Electrolyte Imbalance, 1207

GASTROINTESTINAL (GI) DISORDERS, 1207
Diarrhea, 1207
Acute Diarrheal Disease, 1208
Nursing Care Plan: The Child with Acute
    Diarrhea (Gastroenteritis), 1215
Chronic Diarrheal Disease, 1216
Intractable Diarrhea of Infancy, 1216
Chronic Nonspecific Diarrhea
    (CNSD), 1216
Vomiting, 1217

SHOCK STATES, 1219
Shock, 1219
Septic Shock, 1222
Anaphylaxis, 1224
Toxic Shock Syndrome (TSS), 1226
BURNS, 1227
Overview, 1227
Burn Wound Characteristics, 1228
   Extent of Injury, 1228
   Depth of Injury, 1228
   Severity of Injury, 1229
Pathophysiology, 1230
   Local Response, 1230
   Systemic Responses, 1231
   Complications, 1233
Therapeutic Management, 1234
   Emergency Care, 1234
   Management of Minor Burns, 1235
   Management of Major Burns, 1236
   Management of the Burn Wound, 1238
Nursing Considerations, 1242
   Acute Phase, 1243
   Management and Rehabilitative
      Phases, 1243
   Prevention of Burn Injury, 1248
Nursing Care Plan: The Child with Burns:
   Management and Rehabilitative
   Stages, 1249
Future Research Needs, 1253

## Chapter 30

### The Child with Renal Dysfunction, 1255

RENAL STRUCTURE AND FUNCTION, 1255
RENAL PHYSIOLOGY, 1256
   Glomerular Filtration, 1256
   Tubular Function, 1257
   Renal Development and Function
      in Early Infancy, 1258
Renal Pelvis and Ureters: Structure
   and Function, 1258
Urethrovesical Unit: Structure
   and Function, 1259
GENITOURINARY TRACT DISORDERS, 1262
Urinary Tract Infection (UTI), 1262
Vesicoureteral Reflux (VUR), 1269
GLOMERULAR DISEASE, 1270
Acute Glomerulonephritis (AGN), 1270
Chronic or Progressive
   Glomerulonephritis, 1274
Nephrotic Syndrome, 1274
   Types of Nephrotic Syndrome, 1274
RENAL TUBULAR DISORDERS, 1279
Tubular Function, 1279
Renal Tubular Acidosis, 1279
   Proximal Tubular Acidosis
      (Type II), 1279
   Distal Tubular Acidosis (Type I), 1280

Nephrogenic Diabetes Insipidus
   (NDI), 1280
MISCELLANEOUS RENAL DISORDERS, 1281
Hemolytic Uremic Syndrome (HUS), 1281
Familial Nephritis (Alport
   Syndrome), 1282
Unexplained Proteinuria, 1282
Renal Trauma, 1282
RENAL FAILURE, 1283
Acute Renal Failure (ARF), 1283
Chronic Renal Failure (CRF), 1287
Nursing Care Plan: The Child with Chronic
   Renal Failure (CRF), 1294
RENAL REPLACEMENT THERAPY, 1293
Hemodialysis, 1293
   Procedure, 1294
   Home Hemodialysis, 1296
Peritoneal Dialysis (PD), 1297
   Procedure, 1297
   Home Dialysis, 1297
Continuous Venovenous Hemofiltration
   (CVVH), 1298
Transplantation, 1298
   Procedure, 1299
   Selection of Donor Tissue, 1299
   Suppression of the Immune
      Response, 1299
   Rejection, 1300

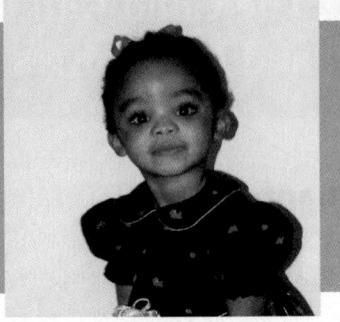

*Unit* **XI**

# The Child with Problems Related to Transfer of Oxygen and Nutrients

## Chapter 31

### The Child with Disturbance of Oxygen and Carbon Dioxide Exchange, 1303

RESPIRATORY TRACT STRUCTURE
   AND FUNCTION, 1303
Structure, 1303
   Chest, 1304
   Airways, 1305
   Respiratory Units, 1306
Function, 1306
   Gas Exchange, 1308
   Defenses of the Respiratory Tract, 1310
ASSESSMENT OF RESPIRATORY
   FUNCTION, 1310
Physical Assessment, 1310
   Respiration, 1310

   Associated Observations, 1310
Diagnostic Procedures, 1312
   Pulmonary Function Tests, 1312
   Radiology and Other Diagnostic
      Procedures, 1312
   Blood Gas Determination, 1313
RESPIRATORY THERAPY, 1317
Oxygen Therapy, 1317
   Oxygen Administration, 1317
   Oxygen Toxicity, 1319
Aerosol Therapy, 1319
Bronchial (Postural) Drainage, 1320
Chest Physiotherapy (CPT), 1320
Artificial Ventilation, 1323
   Care of the Patient, 1324
   Endotracheal Airways, 1324
Tracheostomy, 1325
   Tracheostomy Care, 1326
   Decannulation, 1329

   Home Care of the Child with a
      Tracheostomy, 1329
RESPIRATORY EMERGENCY, 1331
Respiratory Failure, 1331
   Conditions That Predispose to
      Respiratory Failure, 1331
   Recognition of Respiratory
      Failure, 1332
Management and Related Nursing
   Considerations, 1332
   Observation and Monitoring, 1332
   Family Support, 1332
Cardiopulmonary Resuscitation
   (CPR), 1333
   Resuscitation Procedure, 1334
Airway Obstruction, 1338
   Infants, 1338
   Children, 1341

## Chapter 32

### The Child with Respiratory Dysfunction, 1343

RESPIRATORY INFECTION, 1343
General Aspects of Respiratory
Infections, 1343
*Nursing Care Plan: The Child with Acute
Respiratory Infection, 1347*
UPPER RESPIRATORY TRACT INFECTIONS
(URIs), 1350
Acute Viral Nasopharyngitis, 1350
Acute Streptococcal Pharyngitis, 1351
Tonsillitis, 1352
Infectious Mononucleosis, 1354
Influenza, 1356
Otitis Media (OM), 1356
Otitis Externa, 1361
CROUP SYNDROMES, 1361
Acute Epiglottitis, 1362
Acute Laryngitis, 1363
Acute Laryngotracheobronchitis
(LTB), 1363
Acute Spasmodic Laryngitis, 1365
Bacterial Tracheitis, 1365
INFECTIONS OF THE LOWER AIRWAYS, 1365
Bronchitis, 1366
Respiratory Syncytial Virus
(RSV)/Bronchiolitis, 1366
PNEUMONIA, 1368
Viral Pneumonia, 1369
Primary Atypical Pneumonia, 1369
Bacterial Pneumonia, 1369
Chlamydial Pneumonia, 1371

OTHER INFECTIONS OF THE RESPIRATORY
TRACT, 1371
Pertussis (Whooping Cough), 1371
Tuberculosis (TB), 1372
PULMONARY DISTURBANCE CAUSED
BY NONINFECTIOUS IRRITANTS, 1376
Foreign Body (FB) Aspiration, 1376
Foreign Body (FB) in the Nose, 1378
Aspiration Pneumonia, 1378
Hydrocarbon Pneumonia, 1378
Lipoid Pneumonia, 1379
Powder, 1379
Acute (Adult) Respiratory Distress
Syndrome (ARDS), 1379
Smoke Inhalation Injury, 1380
Passive Smoking, 1382
LONG-TERM RESPIRATORY
DYSFUNCTION, 1383
Allergic Rhinitis, 1383
Asthma, 1385
*Nursing Care Plan: The Child
with Asthma, 1402*
Cystic Fibrosis (CF), 1401

## Chapter 33

### The Child with Gastrointestinal Dysfunction, 1416

GASTROINTESTINAL (GI) STRUCTURE AND
FUNCTION, 1416
DEVELOPMENT OF THE GASTROINTESTINAL
TRACT, 1416
Digestion, 1417
Absorption, 1418

Assessment of Gastrointestinal
Function, 1419
INGESTION OF FOREIGN SUBSTANCES, 1419
Pica, 1422
Foreign Bodies, 1423
DISORDERS OF MOTILITY, 1424
Constipation, 1424
Hirschsprung Disease (Congenital
Aganglionic Megacolon), 1426
Gastroesophageal Reflux (GER), 1429
Irritable Bowel Syndrome (IBS), 1432
INFLAMMATORY CONDITIONS, 1432
Acute Appendicitis, 1432
*Nursing Care Plan: The Child
with Appendicitis, 1436*
Meckel Diverticulum, 1435
Inflammatory Bowel Disease (IBD), 1437
Ulcerative Colitis (UC), 1438
Crohn Disease (CD), 1438
Peptic Ulcer Disease (PUD), 1443
OBSTRUCTIVE DISORDERS, 1446
Hypertrophic Pyloric Stenosis (HPS), 1446
Intussusception, 1448
Malrotation and Volvulus, 1449
MALABSORPTION SYNDROMES, 1450
Celiac Disease (Gluten-Sensitive
Enteropathy), 1450
Short Bowel Syndrome (SBS), 1451
GASTROINTESTINAL BLEEDING, 1454
Upper and Lower Gastrointestinal
Bleeding, 1454
HEPATIC DISORDERS, 1456
Acute Hepatitis, 1456
Cirrhosis, 1460

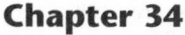
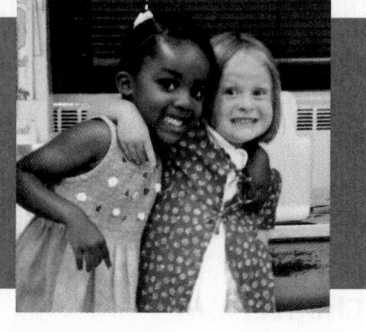

## Unit XII

# The Child with Problems Related to Production and Circulation of Blood

## Chapter 34

### The Child with Cardiovascular Dysfunction, 1464

CARDIAC STRUCTURE AND FUNCTION, 1465
Cardiac Development and Function, 1465
Embryologic Development, 1465
Postnatal Development, 1466
Basic Cardiac Physiology, 1468
Assessment of Cardiac Function, 1468
History, 1468
Physical Examination, 1469
Tests of Cardiac Function, 1469
Radiography, 1469

Electrocardiography, 1469
Echocardiography, 1471
Cardiac Catheterization, 1471
CONGENITAL HEART DISEASE (CHD), 1474
Altered Hemodynamics, 1474
Classification and Clinical
Consequences, 1475
Congestive Heart Failure (CHF), 1476
*Nursing Care Plan: The Child with Congestive
Heart Failure, 1485*
Hypoxemia, 1484
Altered Hemodynamics, 1484
Pulmonary Artery Hypertension, 1490
Defects with Increased Pulmonary Blood
Flow, 1491

Atrial Septal Defect (ASD), 1492
Ventricular Septal Defect (VSD), 1493
Atrioventricular Canal (AVC)
Defect, 1493
Patent Ductus Arteriosus (PDA), 1494
Obstructive Defects, 1491
Coarctation of the Aorta (COA), 1494
Aortic Stenosis (AS), 1495
Pulmonic Stenosis (PS), 1496
Defects with Decreased Pulmonary Blood
Flow, 1496
Tetralogy of Fallot (TOF), 1497
Tricuspid Atresia, 1497
Mixed Defects, 1498

Transposition of the Great Arteries
(TGA) or Transposition of the
Great Vessels (TGV), 1499
Total Anomalous Pulmonary Venous
Connection (TAPVC), 1499
Truncus Arteriosus (TA), 1500
Hypoplastic Left Heart Syndrome
(HLHS), 1501
**Nursing Care of the Family and Child with
Congenital Heart Disease, 1498**
Help Family Adjust to the
Disorder, 1498
Educate Family About the
Disorder, 1502
Help Family Cope with Effects of the
Disorder, 1502
Prepare Child and Family for
Surgery, 1503
Provide Postoperative Care, 1504
Provide Emotional Support, 1508
Plan for Discharge and Home
Care, 1509
**ACQUIRED CARDIOVASCULAR
DISORDERS, 1509**
**Bacterial (Infective) Endocarditis
(BE), 1509**
**Rheumatic Fever (RF), 1511**
**Kawasaki Disease (KD) (Mucocutaneous
Lymph Node Syndrome), 1514**
**Systemic Hypertension, 1516**
**Hyperlipidemia
(Hypercholesterolemia), 1519**
**Cardiomyopathy, 1522**
**Cardiac Dysrhythmias, 1523**

HEART TRANSPLANTATION, 1526

## Chapter 35

### The Child with Hematologic or Immunologic Dysfunction, 1530

**THE HEMATOLOGIC SYSTEM AND ITS
FUNCTION, 1530**
**Origin of Formed Elements, 1530**
Red Blood Cells (RBCs,
Erythrocytes), 1532
Hemoglobin (Hgb), 1532
White Blood Cells (WBCs,
Leukocytes), 1534
Platelets, 1535
**Assessment of Hematologic
Function, 1535**
**RED BLOOD CELL DISORDERS, 1535**
**Anemia, 1535**
**Blood Transfusion Therapy, 1540**
**ANEMIA CAUSED BY NUTRITIONAL
DEFICIENCIES, 1542**
**Iron Deficiency Anemia, 1542**
**ANEMIAS CAUSED BY INCREASED
DESTRUCTION OF RED BLOOD
CELLS, 1546**
**Hereditary Spherocytosis (HS), 1546**
**Sickle Cell Anemia (SCA), 1547**
*Nursing Care Plan: The Child with Sickle Cell
Anemia, 1555*
**β-Thalassemia, 1555**

**ANEMIAS CAUSED BY IMPAIRED OR
DECREASED PRODUCTION OF RED BLOOD
CELLS, 1559**
**Aplastic Anemia, 1559**
**DEFECTS IN HEMOSTASIS, 1561**
**Mechanisms Involved in Normal
Hemostasis, 1561**
Vascular Influence, 1561
Platelet Role, 1561
Clotting Factors, 1561
**Hemophilia, 1561**
**von Willebrand Disease (vWD), 1566**
**Idiopathic Thrombocytopenic Purpura
(ITP), 1566**
**Disseminated Intravascular Coagulation
(DIC), 1567**
**OTHER HEMATOLOGIC DISORDERS, 1568**
**Neutropenia, 1568**
**Henoch-Schönlein Purpura (HSP), 1569**
**IMMUNOLOGIC DEFICIENCY DISORDERS, 1570**
**Mechanisms Involved in Immunity, 1571**
Specific Immune Mechanisms, 1572
**Human Immunodeficiency Virus (HIV)
Infection and Acquired
Immunodeficiency Syndrome
(AIDS), 1572**
*Nursing Care Plan: The Child and Adolescent
with HIV Infection, 1577*
**Wiskott-Aldrich Syndrome, 1577**
**Severe Combined Immunodeficiency
Disease (SCID), 1579**

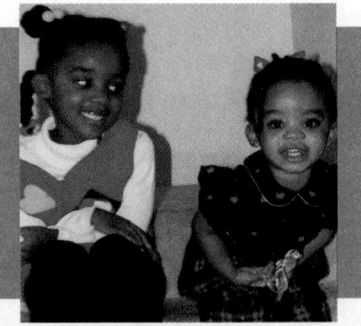

## Unit XIII

# The Child with Disturbance of Regulatory Mechanisms

## Chapter 36

### The Child with Cancer, 1584

**CANCER IN CHILDREN, 1584**
**Etiologic Factors, 1585**
Prevention, 1586
**Diagnostic Evaluation, 1587**
Complete History, 1587
Review of Symptoms, 1587
Physical Examination, 1587
Laboratory Tests, 1587
Imaging Studies, 1587
Biopsy, 1587
**Modes of Therapy, 1588**
Surgery, 1588
Chemotherapy, 1588
Radiation Therapy, 1594

Biologic Response Modifiers
(BRMs), 1594
Bone Marrow Transplantation
(BMT), 1595
**Complications of Therapy, 1596**
Pediatric Oncologic Emergencies, 1596
**NURSING CARE OF THE CHILD
WITH CANCER, 1597**
**Assessment, 1597**
Signs and Symptoms of Cancer in
Children, 1597
**Nursing Diagnoses, 1597**
**Planning, 1598**
**Implementation, 1598**
Managing Side Effects
of Treatment, 1598

Nursing Care During Bone Marrow
Transplantation (BMT), 1602
Preparation for Procedures, 1603
Pain Management, 1604
Health Promotion, 1604
Family Education, 1605
Cessation of Therapy, 1606
**Evaluation, 1606**
*Nursing Care Plan: The Child
with Cancer, 1606*
**CANCERS OF THE BLOOD AND LYMPH
SYSTEMS, 1608**
**Leukemias, 1610**
**Lymphomas, 1616**
**Hodgkin Disease, 1616**
**Non-Hodgkin Lymphoma (NHL), 1618**

NERVOUS SYSTEM TUMORS, 1619
Brain Tumors, 1619
Neuroblastoma, 1625
BONE TUMORS, 1626
General Considerations, 1626
Osteogenic Sarcoma, 1627
Ewing Sarcoma (Primitive Neuroectodermal Tumor [PNET] of the Bone), 1628
OTHER SOLID TUMORS, 1629
Wilms Tumor, 1629
Rhabdomyosarcoma, 1631
Retinoblastoma, 1632
Testicular Tumors, 1635
THE CHILDHOOD CANCER SURVIVOR, 1635
Long-Term Sequelae of Treatment, 1635

**Chapter 37**

The Child with Cerebral Dysfunction, 1641

CEREBRAL STRUCTURE AND FUNCTION, 1641
Development of the Neurologic System, 1642
Central Nervous System (CNS), 1642
Brain Coverings, 1642
The Brain, 1643
Increased Intracranial Pressure (ICP), 1645
EVALUATION OF NEUROLOGIC STATUS, 1646
Assessment: General Aspects, 1646
History, 1646
Physical Examination, 1646
Altered States of Consciousness, 1647
Level of Consciousness (LOC), 1647
Coma Assessment, 1647
Neurologic Examination, 1649
Vital Signs, 1649
Skin, 1650
Eyes, 1650

Motor Function, 1651
Posturing, 1651
Reflexes, 1651
Special Diagnostic Procedures, 1652
THE CHILD WITH CEREBRAL COMPROMISE, 1654
Nursing Care of the Unconscious Child, 1654
Respiratory Management, 1656
Intracranial Pressure Monitoring, 1656
Nutrition and Hydration, 1658
Medications, 1658
Thermoregulation, 1659
Elimination, 1659
Hygienic Care, 1659
Positioning and Exercise, 1659
Stimulation, 1659
Family Support, 1660
Nursing Care Plan: The Unconscious Child, 1662
Head Injury, 1661
Near-Drowning, 1674
INTRACRANIAL INFECTIONS, 1676
Bacterial Meningitis, 1677
Nonbacterial (Aseptic) Meningitis, 1680
Tuberculous (TB) Meningitis, 1681
Brain Abscess, 1681
Encephalitis, 1681
Rabies, 1682
Reye Syndrome (RS), 1683
Human Immunodeficiency Virus (HIV) Encephalopathy, 1684
SEIZURE DISORDERS, 1684
Epilepsy, 1684
Nursing Care Plan: The Child with Epilepsy, 1697
Febrile Seizures, 1696
HEADACHE, 1698
Assessment, 1698
Migraine Headache, 1699

**Chapter 38**

The Child with Endocrine Dysfunction, 1703

THE ENDOCRINE SYSTEM, 1703
Hormones, 1703
Control of Hormone Secretion, 1704
Neuroendocrine Interrelationships, 1705
DISORDERS OF PITUITARY FUNCTION, 1706
Hypopituitarism, 1706
Pituitary Hyperfunction, 1713
Precocious Puberty, 1714
Diabetes Insipidus (DI), 1715
Syndrome of Inappropriate Antidiuretic Hormone (SIADH), 1716
DISORDERS OF THYROID FUNCTION, 1717
Juvenile Hypothyroidism, 1717
Goiter, 1718
Lymphocytic Thyroiditis, 1718
Hyperthyroidism, 1719
DISORDERS OF PARATHYROID FUNCTION, 1721
Hypoparathyroidism, 1722
Hyperparathyroidism, 1722
DISORDERS OF ADRENAL FUNCTION, 1723
Adrenal Hormones, 1723
Adrenal Cortex, 1723
Adrenal Medulla, 1724
Acute Adrenocortical Insufficiency, 1725
Chronic Adrenocortical Insufficiency (Addison Disease), 1726
Cushing Syndrome, 1727
Congenital Adrenal Hyperplasia (CAH), 1729
Hyperaldosteronism, 1731
Pheochromocytoma, 1731
DISORDERS OF PANCREATIC HORMONE SECRETION, 1732
Diabetes Mellitus (DM), 1732
Nursing Care Plan: The Child with Diabetes Mellitus, 1752

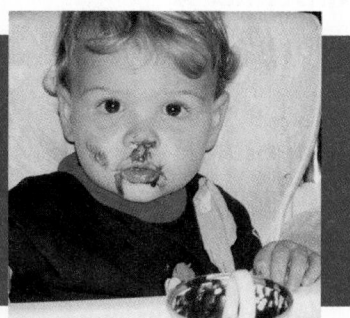

# Unit XIV

## The Child with a Problem That Interferes with Physical Mobility

**Chapter 39**

The Child with Musculoskeletal or Articular Dysfunction, 1757

THE CHILD AND TRAUMA, 1758
Trauma Management, 1758
Epidemiology of Trauma, 1758
Prevention of Injury, 1759
Assessment of Trauma, 1760

Emergency Management, 1760
Systematic Assessment, 1761
THE IMMOBILIZED CHILD, 1761
Immobilization, 1761
Physiologic Effects of Immobilization, 1762
Psychologic Effects of Immobilization, 1766
Effect on Families, 1767

Nursing Care Plan: The Child Who Is Immobilized, 1772
Mobilization Devices, 1773
Orthotics and Prosthetics, 1773
Crutches and Canes, 1775
Wheelchairs, 1776
THE CHILD WITH A FRACTURE, 1776
Fractures, 1776
Bone Healing and Remodeling, 1781

**The Child in a Cast, 1784**
The Cast, 1784
**The Child in Traction, 1787**
Purposes of Traction, 1788
Types of Traction (General), 1788
Upper Extremity Traction, 1789
Lower Extremity Traction, 1789
Cervical Traction, 1790
**Distraction, 1792**
**External Fixation, 1792**
**Internal Fixation, 1793**
**Fracture Complications, 1793**
Circulatory Impairment, 1793
Nerve Compression Syndromes, 1793
Compartment Syndromes, 1793
Epiphyseal Damage, 1794
Nonunion, 1794
Malunion, 1794
Infection, 1794
Kidney Stones, 1794
Pulmonary Emboli, 1795
**Amputation, 1795**
**INJURIES AND HEALTH PROBLEMS RELATED TO SPORTS PARTICIPATION, 1796**
**Preparation for Sports, 1796**
**Types of Injury, 1797**
**Contusions, 1798**
**Dislocations, 1798**
**Sprains and Strains, 1799**
**Overuse Syndrome, 1800**
Stress Fractures, 1801
**Heat Injury/Illness, 1801**

**Underwater Sports–Related Injuries, 1802**
Sports and Accidental Drowning, 1802
**Health Concerns Associated with Sports, 1802**
Nutrition, 1802
Considerations for the Female Athlete, 1804
Drug Misuse by Athletes, 1804
Sudden Death, 1805
**Nurse's Role in Children's Sports, 1805**
**MUSCULOSKELETAL DYSFUNCTION, 1807**
**Torticollis, 1807**
**Legg-Calvé-Perthes Disease, 1807**
**Slipped Femoral Capital Epiphysis, 1808**
**Kyphosis and Lordosis, 1809**
**Scoliosis, 1810**
*Nursing Care Plan: The Child with Structural Scoliosis, 1815*
**ORTHOPAEDIC INFECTIONS, 1817**
**Osteomyelitis, 1817**
**Septic Arthritis, 1818**
**Tuberculosis, 1818**
Skeletal Tuberculosis, 1818
**SKELETAL AND ARTICULAR DYSFUNCTION, 1819**
**Osteogenesis Imperfecta (OI), 1819**
**Juvenile Rheumatoid Arthritis, (Juvenile Idiopathic Arthritis), 1820**
*Nursing Care Plan: The Child with Juvenile Rheumatoid Arthritis, 1826*
**Systemic Lupus Erythematosus (SLE), 1825**

**Chapter 40**
The Child with Neuromuscular or Muscular Dysfunction, 1832

**NEUROMUSCULAR DYSFUNCTION, 1832**
**Classification and Diagnosis, 1832**
Classification, 1833
Diagnostic Tools, 1834
**Cerebral Palsy (CP), 1834**
*Nursing Care Plan: The Child with Cerebral Palsy, 1844*
**Hypotonia, 1843**
**Infantile Spinal Muscular Atrophy (SMA) (Werdnig-Hoffmann Disease), 1846**
**Juvenile Spinal Muscular Atrophy (Kugelberg-Welander Syndrome), 1846**
**Guillain-Barré Syndrome (GBS) (Infectious Polyneuritis), 1847**
**Tetanus, 1848**
**Botulism, 1850**
**Myasthenia Gravis (MG), 1851**
Neonatal Myasthenia Gravis, 1852
**Spinal Cord Injuries, 1852**
Review of Essential Neuromuscular Physiology, 1852
**MUSCULAR DYSFUNCTION, 1863**
**Juvenile Dermatomyositis, 1863**
**Muscular Dystrophies (MDs), 1864**
**Pseudohypertrophic (Duchenne) Muscular Dystrophy (DMD), 1864**

*Appendices*

**Appendix A**
Family Assessment, 1870

**Appendix B**
Developmental/Sensory Assessment, 1874

**Appendix C**
Growth Measurements, 1881

**Appendix D**
Common Laboratory Tests, 1895

**Appendix E**
NANDA-Approved Nursing Diagnoses 2001-2002, 1904

**Appendix F**
Translations of Wong-Baker FACES Pain Rating Scale, 1905

# Chapter 1

# Perspectives of Pediatric Nursing

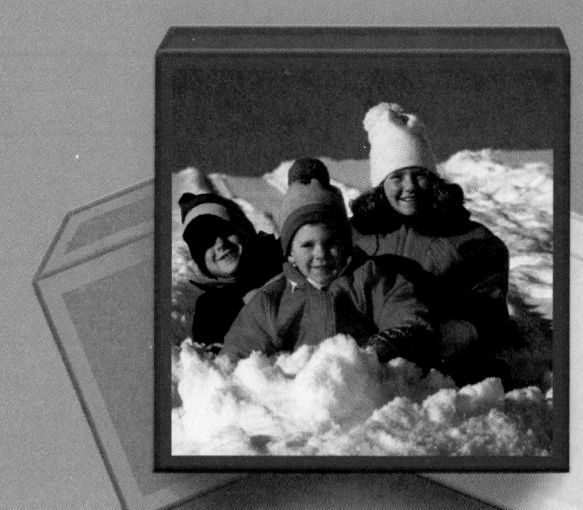

## Chapter Outline

**HEALTH DURING CHILDHOOD, 1**
*Healthy People 2010*, 1
**Mortality, 2**
 Infant Mortality, 2
 Childhood Mortality, 4
**Morbidity, 6**
 Childhood Morbidity, 6
 The New Morbidity, 6
**Injuries—The Leading Killer, 6**
 Host and Agent, 7
 Environment, 10
 Injury Prevention, 10
**Evolution of Child Health Care in the United States, 11**

**PEDIATRIC NURSING, 13**
**Philosophy of Care, 13**
 Family-Centered Care, 13
 Atraumatic Care, 15
 Case Management, 15
**Role of the Pediatric Nurse, 18**
 Therapeutic Relationship, 18
 Family Advocacy/Caring, 19
 Disease Prevention/Health
  Promotion, 20
 Health Teaching, 21
 Support/Counseling, 21
 Restorative Role, 21
 Coordination/Collaboration, 21
 Ethical Decision Making, 21

 Research, 22
 Health Care Planning, 22
**Future Trends, 23**
**CRITICAL THINKING AND THE PROCESS OF NURSING CHILDREN AND FAMILIES, 24**
**Critical Thinking, 24**
**Nursing Process, 25**
 Assessment, 25
 Nursing Diagnosis, 25
 Planning, 27
 Implementation, 27
 Evaluation, 27
 Documentation, 27

## Related Topics

Cancer in Children, Ch. 36
Case Management, Ch. 25
The Child and Trauma, Ch. 39
Classification of High-Risk Newborns, Ch. 10
Cultural/Religious Influences on Health
 Care, Ch. 2

Immunizations, Ch. 12
Injury Prevention: Infant, Ch. 12; Toddler,
 Ch. 14; Preschooler, Ch. 15; School-Age
 Child, Ch. 17; Adolescent, Ch. 19
Preschool and Kindergarten Experience,
 Ch. 15

Scope of the Problem (Chronic
 Illness/Disability), Ch. 22
Suicide, Ch. 21

## HEALTH DURING CHILDHOOD

Health is a complex phenomenon. The World Health Organization (WHO) has defined *health* as "a state of complete physical, mental, and social well-being and not merely the absence of disease." Despite this broad definition, health is traditionally assessed by observing *mortality* (death) and *morbidity* (illness) rates over time. Therefore the balance between physical, mental, and social well-being and the *presence* of disease becomes the prime indicator of health.

 Information concerning mortality and morbidity is important to nurses because this knowledge provides a rationale for

planning and delivering care. Such data provide information about (1) the causes of death and illness, (2) high-risk age-groups for disorders or hazards, (3) advances in treatment and prevention, and (4) specific areas of health counseling.

### Healthy People 2010

Although the health of people, including children, in the United States improved dramatically during the previous century, there remains cause for concern. There is a growing awareness that many serious domestic problems, such as drug abuse, violence, unwanted pregnancies, and acquired immunodeficiency syndrome (AIDS), have a direct effect on the health of the nation. However, solutions to these

---
■ Marilyn L. Winkelstein, PhD, RN, revised this chapter.

problems do not lie in better or more innovative medical treatment, but in *prevention.*

In 1979, the Surgeon General's Report, **Healthy People,** and **Healthy People 2000: National Health Promotion and Disease Prevention Objectives** established national health objectives and served as the basis for the development of state and community plans. **Healthy People 2010** was released to the public in January 2000. This document builds on initiatives pursued over the last two decades. Objectives and goals for *Healthy People 2010* were developed through a broad consultation process characterized by community collaboration and participation. The document contains two overriding goals and 10 leading health indicators (Box 1-1). The 10 leading health indicators are the priority areas for the nation's health. In addition to serving as a method to evaluate public health progress over the next decade, the leading health indicators also serve as a focal point to coordinate national health improvement efforts. Many states are currently working with community coalitions to develop their own versions of *Healthy People 2010.* The *Healthy People Toolkit*\* found on the Internet provides examples of state and national experiences in setting and using objectives. Individuals, groups, and organizations are encouraged to integrate the objectives and goals into current programs, special events, publications, and meetings. Schools, colleges, and civic and faith-based organizations can use the objectives and indicators to structure activities to improve the health of their members. Finally, health care providers can use the document to encourage their patients to pursue healthier lifestyles and to monitor their results over time.

## Mortality

Figures describing rates of occurrence for events such as death in children are referred to as *vital statistics. Mortality statistics* describe the incidence or number of individuals

\*www.health.gov/healthypeople/state/toolkit.

who have died over a specific period. They are usually presented as rates per 100,000. Mortality rates are calculated from a sample of death certificates.

In the United States the **National Center for Health Statistics (NCHS),** under the Department of Health and Human Services (DHHS), Public Health Service (PHS), is responsible for the collection, analysis, and dissemination of data on the health of the American people.

Several important changes have taken place in the reporting of health statistics over the past 10 years. For example, since 1991, figures for birth and death have been based on the person's state of residence, not on the state in which the event occurred.

The tabulation of race for live births (the denominator of infant mortality rates) has changed from race of child to race of mother. Formerly, to determine the child's race in mixed parentage in which one parent was white, the child was assigned the race of the other parent. In general, this change in assignment of race from child to mother results in more white births and fewer nonwhite births. However, infant deaths are recorded by the decedent's race, resulting in a lower infant mortality rate for whites than nonwhites. As a result of these changes in the early 1990s, figures for births, deaths, and infant mortality rates by race are not comparable to statistics reported before these changes were made.

> **NURSING ALERT** Because of the complexity of compiling such data, statistics may vary in different reports and should be interpreted cautiously. For example, figures may be *estimated* (from previously collected data), *provisional* (from temporary current data), or *final* (from complete provisional data). Final statistics are often published 2 or more years after data collection.

### Infant Mortality

The *infant mortality rate* is the number of deaths during the first year of life per 1000 live births. It may be further divided into *neonatal mortality* (<28 days of life) and *postneonatal mortality* (28 days to 11 months). In the United States there has been a dramatic decrease in infant mortality. At the beginning of the twentieth century the rate was approximately 200 infant deaths per 1000 live births. In 2000, the infant mortality rate was 6.9 deaths per 1000 live births.

The mortality rate in 2000 for white infants was 5.7 and the rate for black infants was 14.0 (Hoyert and others, 2000). These decreases resulted primarily because of improvements in perinatal care, such as treatment of respiratory distress syndrome and fewer deaths from sudden infant death syndrome (SIDS). A major challenge for the twenty-first century will be to reduce the large gap between infant mortality for white and black infants.

From a worldwide perspective the United States lags behind other nations in reducing infant mortality. In 1998, the United States ranked second-to-last among nations that have the lowest infant mortality rates, with Hong Kong having the lowest rate (Hoyert and others, 2000) (Table 1-1). The United States is behind neighboring countries such as Canada, which ranked fifteenth. Although the reason is un-

**TABLE 1-1**   Infant mortality rate (IMR) for 1998 for countries of >2,500,000 population and with IMR equal to or less than the United States rate for 1998 (rate per 100,000 live births)

| Country | IMR 1998 |
|---|---|
| Hong Kong | 3.2* |
| Sweden | 3.4*† |
| Switzerland | 3.4† |
| Japan | 3.6 |
| Norway | 4.0 |
| Singapore | 4.2* |
| Finland | 4.2 |
| Germany | 4.6* |
| Denmark | 4.7* |
| France | 4.8* |
| Austria | 4.9* |
| Australia | 5.0* |
| Netherlands | 5.2 |
| Czech Republic | 5.2* |
| Canada | 5.5‡ |
| Italy | 5.5‡ |
| Belgium | 5.5 |
| New Zealand | 5.5* |
| Israel | 5.7 |
| United Kingdom | 5.8*† |
| Greece | 6.1* |
| Ireland | 6.2* |
| United States | 7.2 |
| Portugal | 8.4* |

From Hoyert and others: Annual summary of vital statistics: 2000, *Pediatrics* 108(6):1241-1255, 2001.
Sources: *United Nations 1998 Demographic Yearbook; Population and Vital Statistics Report*, Statistical Papers, Series A, Vol L11, No 1, January 2000; *Population and Vital Statistics Report*, Statistical Papers, Series A, Vol L111, No 1, January 2001.
*Provisional data.
†1999 data, no 1998 data.
‡1997 data, no 1998 data.

**TABLE 1-2**   Death rates by age and sex: United States, preliminary 2000 (rates per 100,000 population)

| Age | All Races | | |
|---|---|---|---|
| | **Both Sexes** | **Male** | **Female** |
| All ages* | 873.6 | 874.8 | 872.3 |
| Under 1 year† | 727.4 | 797.0 | 654.7 |
| 1-4 | 32.8 | 36.4 | 29.0 |
| 5-14 | 18.6 | 21.6 | 15.5 |
| 15-24 | 81.5 | 117.3 | 43.9 |

Modified from Minino AM, Smith BL: Deaths: preliminary data for 2000, *National Vital Statistics Reports* 49(12), 2001.
*Figures for age groups >19 are included in "All ages" but not distributed among age groups.
†Death rate for "Under 1 year" (based on population estimates) differs from infant mortality rates (based on live births).

known, a major difference between the United States and these other countries is that the other countries all have national health programs.

*Birth weight* is considered the major determinant of neonatal death in technologically developed countries. There is a definite relationship between birth weight and mortality (Guyer and others, 2000). The lower the birth weight, the higher the mortality. The relatively high incidence of *low birth weight (LBW)* (<2500 g) in the United States is considered a key factor in its higher neonatal mortality rates when compared with other countries. Access to and the use of high-quality prenatal care is a promising preventive strategy to decrease early delivery and infant mortality. Other factors that increase the risk of infant mortality include black race, male gender, short or long gestation, maternal age, and lower level of maternal education (Guyer and others, 2000).

Although there has been a steady and significant decline in infant mortality, the number of deaths occurring in the first year of life is still proportionately high when compared with death rates at other ages (Table 1-2). Research indicates that serious health conditions in preterm LBW infants are most likely to occur during the first 6 months after hospital discharge. Families with LBW preterm infants weighing <2500 g are potentially eligible to take leave granted by

the *Family Medical Leave Act of 1993* to care for their infants (see p. 13). In the United States, the death rate for infants under 1 year of age is greater than the rate for individuals ages 1 through 54 years. It is not until age 55 and over that the death rate begins to exceed the rate for infants.

During the first half of the twentieth century, neonatal mortality rates had not shown the remarkable reduction observed in postnatal infant mortality. The *perinatal mortality rate* is commonly defined as the number of fetal deaths (fetuses of 28 weeks or more of gestation) and deaths in infants under 7 days per 1000 live births. However, other definitions do exist, such as deaths in infants under 28 days and fetal deaths with a gestation of 20 weeks or more. As a result of efforts to decrease neonatal deaths, neonatal mortality declined from 20.5 per 1000 births in 1950 to 4.6 per 1000 live births in 2000 (Hoyert and others, 2001). This decline has largely resulted from advances in neonatal intensive care and better treatment of perinatal illnesses, such as respiratory distress syndrome and treatment with surfactant. As Table 1-3 demonstrates, many of the leading causes of death during infancy continue to occur during the perinatal period. The first four causes—congenital anomalies, disorders relating to short gestation and unspecified LBW, sudden infant death syndrome, and newborn affected by maternal complications of pregnancy—accounted for about half (48%) of all deaths of infants under 1 year of age (Minino and Smith, 2001).

Although a number of perinatal problems have benefited from improved treatment, congenital anomalies continue to be a leading cause of infant mortality. The incidence of the majority of birth defects has remained substantially the same. The incidence of heart defects has been rising, but the increase is the result of enhanced methods of detection, not increased numbers of affected infants. With the current recommendation of folic acid supplementation for all women of childbearing age, defects such as anencephaly and spina bifida are expected to decrease by as much as 50%. (See Spina Bifida [Myelomeningocele], Chapter 11.)

LBW is a major indicator of infant health and a significant predictor of infant mortality (Hoyert and others, 2001; MacDorman and Atkinson, 1999). Many birth defects are

**TABLE 1-3**   Mortality rates for 10 leading causes of infant death, 2000, preliminary data (rates per 1000 live births)

| Rank | Cause of Death (Based on Tenth Revision, International Classification of Diseases) | Percent | Rate |
|------|-----------------------------------------------------------------------------------|---------|------|
|      | All races, all causes                                                             | 100.0   | 688.4 |
| 1    | Congenital anomalies                                                              | 20.6    | 142.2 |
| 2    | Disorders relating to short gestation and unspecified low birth weight            | 15.4    | 105.8 |
| 3    | Sudden infant death syndrome                                                      | 7.7     | 52.9 |
| 4    | Newborn affected by maternal complications of pregnancy                           | 4.9     | 33.8 |
| 5    | Newborn affected by complications of placenta, cord, and membranes                | 3.7     | 25.3 |
| 6    | Respiratory distress syndrome                                                     | 3.6     | 25.0 |
| 7    | Infections specific to the perinatal period                                       | 2.9     | 20.3 |
| 8    | Bacterial sepsis of newborn                                                       | 2.6     | 17.8 |
| 9    | Intrauterine hypoxia and birth asphyxia                                           | 2.3     | 15.8 |
| 10   | Diseases of the circulatory system                                                | 2.3     | 15.5 |

Modified from Minino AM, Smith BL: Deaths: preliminary data for 2000, *National Vital Statistics Reports* 49(12), 2001.

**TABLE 1-4**   Five leading causes of death in children in the United States: selected age intervals, 2000, preliminary data (rates per 100,000)

| Rank | Ages 1-4 | Rate | Ages 5-14 | Rate | Ages 15-24 | Rate |
|------|----------|------|-----------|------|------------|------|
|      | All causes | 32.6 | All causes | 18.5 | All causes | 80.7 |
| 1    | Accidents | 11.7 | Accidents | 7.3 | Accidents | 35.5 |
| 2    | Congenital anomalies | 3.1 | Cancer | 2.6 | Homicide | 12.5 |
| 3    | Cancer | 2.6 | Congenital anomalies | 1.0 | Suicide | 10.1 |
| 4    | Homicide | 2.1 | Homicide | 0.9 | Cancer | 4.3 |
| 5    | Heart disease | 1.1 | Suicide | 0.7 | Heart disease | 2.4 |

Modified from Minino AM, Smith BL: Deaths: preliminary data for 2000, *National Vital Statistics Reports* 49(12), 2001.

associated with LBW, and reducing LBW will prevent congenital anomalies. Infant mortality resulting from human immunodeficiency virus (HIV) infection decreased significantly during the 1990s. In 1998, HIV/AIDS accounted for less than 0.3% of all deaths in childhood (Murphy, 2000).

When infant death rates are categorized according to race, a disturbing difference is seen. Infant mortality for whites is considerably lower than for all other races in the United States, with blacks having twice the rate of whites. Although the infant mortality of both groups has declined, the gap has remained constant (Guyer and others, 2000). The LBW rate is also much higher for black infants than for any other group. Reasons for these higher rates remain unknown (Guyer and others, 2000). One encouraging note is that the gap in mortality rates between white and nonwhite races other than blacks has been narrowing in recent years. Infant mortality rates for Hispanics and Asian Pacific Islanders have decreased dramatically during the past two decades (Guyer and others, 2000).

## Childhood Mortality

Death rates for children older than 1 year of age have always been lower than those for infants (see Table 1-2). Children ages 5 to 14 years have the lowest rate of death. However, a sharp rise occurs during later adolescence, primarily from injuries, homicide, and suicide (Table 1-4). In 2000, these causes were responsible for approximately 72% of deaths in teenagers and young adults 15 to 24 years

old (Minino and Smith, 2001). The trend in racial differences that occurs in infant mortality is also apparent in childhood deaths for all ages and for both sexes. Whites have fewer deaths for all ages, and male deaths outnumber female deaths.

After 1 year of age, there is a dramatic change in the cause of death, with unintentional injuries (accidents) being the leading cause from the youngest ages to the adolescent years.

*Violent deaths* have been steadily increasing among young people ages 10 through 25 years, especially blacks and males. Homicide is the second leading cause of death in the 15- to 24-year age-group (see Table 1-4). Children 12 years of age and older tend to be killed by nonfamily members (acquaintances and gangs, typically of the same race) and most frequently by firearms. Firearm homicide is the leading cause of death among black males ages 15 to 19 years (Ikeda and others, 1997). *Suicide,* a form of self-violence, is the third leading cause of death among adolescents 15 to 24 years of age (see Table 1-4).

The causes of increased violence against children and self-inflicted violence are not fully understood. In young children the increase in homicide may represent a more accurate identification of child abuse. In all cases the problem of child homicide is an extremely complex one that involves numerous social, economic, and other influences. Prevention lies in a better understanding of the social and psychologic factors that lead to the high rates of homicide and sui-

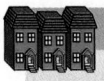

## COMMUNITY FOCUS
### Violence in Children

Community violence has reached epidemic proportions in the United States. Recently, political leaders have recognized violence as a public health emergency and a preventable problem (Fry-Bowers, 1997). The serious problem of community violence affects the lives of many children and expands throughout the family, schools, and the workplace. Nurses working with children, adolescents, and families have a critical role in reducing violence through early identification and symptom recognition of the mental-emotional stress that can result from these experiences (Jones, 1997).

During the past decade, the incidence of violent crimes has dramatically increased, making the United States the most violent country in the industrialized world. The multifaceted origins of the problem of violence include developmental factors, gang involvement, access to firearms, drugs, the media, poverty, and family conflict. Often, the silent and underrecognized groups of victims are the children who witness acts of community violence. Studies suggest that chronic exposure to violence has a negative effect on a child's cognitive, social, psychologic, and moral development. Also, multiple exposures to episodes of violence do not inoculate children against the negative effects; continued exposure can result in lasting symptoms of stress. Behaviors that may be exhibited by children living in chronic violence include difficulty concentrating in school, memory impairment, aggressive play, uncaring behaviors, and constricted activities and thinking for fear of reliving the traumatic event (Fry-Bowers, 1997).

The growing national concern about the increase in the prevalence of violent crimes has prompted nurses to actively participate in ensuring that children grow up in safe environments. Pediatric nurses are positioned to assess children and adolescents for signs of exposure to violence and well-known risk factors as well as to provide nonviolent problem-solving strategies, counseling, and referrals.* These activities will impact community practice and expand the nurses' role in the future health environment (Jones, 1997). Suggestions for professional resources include the following:

### *ORGANIZATIONS

**Administration for Children, Youth, and Families**
U.S. Department of Health and Human Services
330 C Street NW
Washington, DC 20447
(202) 205-8051

**Center to Prevent Handgun Violence**
1225 Eye Street NW, Suite 1100
Washington, DC 20005
(202) 289-7319

*From Fry-Bowers EK: Community violence: its impact on the development of children and implications for nursing practice, *Pediatr Nurs* 23(2):117-128, 1997.

**The National Congress of Parents and Teachers**
700 Rush Street
Chicago, IL 60611
(312) 670-6782

**National Institute for Violence Prevention**
One Cleveland Park
Roxbury, MA 02119
(617) 427-0692

**National Organization for Victim Assistance**
1757 Park Road NW
Washington, DC 20010
(805) 373-9977

**National School Safety Center**
4165 Thousand Oaks Boulevard
Westlake Village, CA 91362
(805) 373-9977

**Stop the Violence Movement Clearinghouse**
The National Urban League
500 East 62nd Street
New York, NY 10021
(212) 310-9000

**Targeted Outreach Program**
Boys and Girls Club of America
National Headquarters
1230 West Peachtree Street NW
Atlanta, GA 30309
(404) 487-5700

### LITERATURE AND MEDIA

American Academy of Pediatrics
Speaker's Kit: Silence the Violence
  To obtain, contact:
  American Academy of Pediatrics
  141 Northwest Point Boulevard
  Elk Grove Village, IL 60007
  (800) 433-9016

Garbarino J: *Let's talk about living in a violent world*, Chicago, 1993, Erickson Institute.
  To obtain, contact:
  Erickson Institute
  25 West Chicago Avenue
  Chicago, IL 60610

Osofsky JD, Fenichel E, editors: Caring for infants and toddlers in violent environments: hurt, healing and hope, *Zero to Three*, 14(3):entire issue, 1993-94.

Reiss AJ: *Understanding and preventing violence*, Washington, DC, 1993, National Academy Press.

---

cide. Nurses need to be especially aware of young people who are depressed, repeatedly in trouble with the criminal justice system, or associated with groups known to be violent. Prevention requires identification of these young people as well as therapeutic intervention by qualified professionals.

Pediatric nurses can assess children and adolescents for risk factors related to violence. Families who own firearms must be educated about their safe use and storage. The presence of a gun in a household increases the risk of suicide by about fivefold and the risk of homicide by about threefold. Legislative efforts may focus on preventing specific groups, such as felons and children, from having access

to firearms. Technologic changes such as a childproof safety device and loading indicator could improve the safety of firearms. (See Community Focus box.)

The major declines in death rates during childhood have occurred in deaths caused by gastrointestinal diseases, infectious diseases, perinatal conditions, neoplasms, and injuries. The absence of infectious disease as a leading cause of death is testimony to the role antibacterial agents and immunizations have played in the declining mortality rates. More effective treatment of severe infections has resulted in other disorders becoming more prominent in the list of leading killers. Most notable among these are neoplasms, although fewer children die from cancer than ever before. (For example, see Leukemias, Chapter 36.)

Deaths caused by infectious diseases have decreased in recent years. In particular, deaths from HIV infection have decreased. HIV was no longer one of the 15 leading causes of death in children in 1998 (Guyer and others, 2000).

## Morbidity

Measuring the prevalence of a specific illness in the population at a particular time is known as *morbidity statistics*. Morbidity statistics are generally presented as rates per 1000 population. Unlike mortality, morbidity is difficult to define and may denote acute illness, chronic disease, or disability. Source of data also influences the statistics. Common sources include reasons for visits to physicians, diagnoses for hospital admission, or household interviews such as the National Health Interview Survey (NHIS), Child Health Supplement. Unlike death rates, which are updated annually, morbidity statistics are revised less frequently and do not necessarily represent the general population.

### Childhood Morbidity

*Acute illness* is defined as symptoms severe enough to limit activity or require medical attention. Respiratory illness accounts for approximately 50% of all acute conditions, 11% are caused by infections and parasitic disease, and 15% are caused by injuries. The chief illness of childhood is the common cold.

The types of diseases that children contract during childhood vary according to age. For example, upper respiratory tract infections and diarrhea decrease in frequency with age, whereas other disorders, such as acne and headaches, increase. Children who have had a particular type of problem are more likely to have that problem again. Morbidity is not distributed randomly in children. Children from poor families have more health problems than children from nonpoor families. This finding suggests the need for heightened efforts to improve access to health care for low-income children.

Recent concern has focused on groups of children who have increased morbidity—homeless children, children living in poverty, children of LBW, children with chronic illnesses, foreign-born adopted children, and children in day-care centers. A number of factors place these groups at risk for poor health. A major cause is barriers to health care, especially for the homeless, the poverty stricken, and those with chronic health problems. Other factors include improved survival of children with chronic health problems, particularly infants of very LBW. Children living in or exposed to at-risk environments, such as country of origin (for adopted children) and daycare centers, are more likely to have medical conditions such as infections (Lears, Guth, and Lewandowski, 1998; Loubiala and others, 1997).

Injuries are an additional factor influencing morbidity. Each year 40,000 to 50,000 children are injured permanently, and at least 1 million children seek medical care because of unintentional injuries (Mofenson and Greensher, 1997).

The most important aspect of morbidity is the degree of disability it produces. *Disability* can be measured in days off from school or days confined to bed. It can be a result of an acute or chronic disorder. On average, a child loses 5.3 school days per year because of injury or illness. (The incidence of chronic conditions is discussed in Chapter 22).

Although childhood is a time of relative health, it is rare for a child never to become ill. Education of parents regarding the usual types of childhood illnesses and recognition of those symptoms requiring treatment are important aspects of nursing care. As with childhood mortality, future progress in decreasing childhood morbidity rests more on parent education than on medical advances. Nurses play a vital role in advancing child care through health promotion.

### The New Morbidity

In addition to disease and injury, children face behavioral, social (family), and educational problems that are referred to as the *new morbidity* or *pediatric social illness*. These problems (i.e., poverty, violence, aggression, noncompliance, school failure, and adjustment to divorce or bereavement) interfere with children's social and academic development. Estimates on the incidence of these problems vary from 5% to 30%.

The new morbidity is difficult to identify in children. For example, the proportion of children with these problems is *greater* than the number of visits children make to health care facilities with a new morbidity diagnosis. Consequently, many children seen at a health care center have another primary disorder, usually physical, and are only diagnosed with a psychosocial or psychosomatic problem at a later time. In addition, there is greater emphasis by health care professionals on organic deviations than on mental or social ones. Insurance companies generally do not reimburse counseling for psychosocial problems. Consequently there is a disincentive to spend additional time on these issues. However, nurses in primary care facilities need to be aware of these problems and of the need to investigate them. Practitioners who ask directly about specific psychosocial issues, show empathy, provide reassurance, and listen attentively are likely to hear about social problems from parents.

Although no conclusive characteristics have been identified for children with new morbidity problems, some findings appear to identify children at high risk for injuries. These include (1) children from low socioeconomic status, (2) children of the male gender, and (3) children with a sibling who has had a previous injury (Altemeier, 2000).

## Injuries—The Leading Killer

Injuries, the leading cause of death in children over age 1 year, are responsible for more deaths and disabilities in children than are all causes of disease combined (see Table 1-4). Injuries have not shown the dramatic declines seen in other areas of childhood mortality because an injury has traditionally been regarded as an unavoidable accident or a behavioral problem rather than as a health problem. The term *accident* suggests a chaotic, random event that is related to "luck" or "chance"; the term *injury* is preferred because it connotes a sense of responsibility and control. In addition, injury control has not received high priority or sufficient financial support. Research on injuries has not been based on a theoretic framework, as has that done on diseases. There is a need to view injuries and their prevention in terms of a *host* (the affected person), the *environment* (the time and place), and the *agent* (the object that is the direct cause).

## Host and Agent

The type of injury and the circumstances surrounding it are closely related to normal growth and developmental behavior (Box 1-2). As children develop, their innate curiosity impels them to investigate activities and to mimic the behavior of others. This is essential to acquire competency as an adult, but it predisposes children to numerous hazards.

The developmental stage of the child partially determines the types of injuries that are most likely to occur at a specific age and helps provide clues to preventive measures. For example, small infants are helpless in any environment. When they begin to roll over or propel themselves, they can fall from unprotected surfaces. The crawling infant who has a natural tendency to place objects in the mouth is at risk for aspiration or poisoning. The mobile toddler with the instinct to explore and investigate and the ability to run and climb may experience falls, burns, and collisions with objects. As children grow older, their absorption with play makes them oblivious to environmental hazards such as street traffic or water. The need to conform and gain acceptance compels older children and adolescents to accept challenges and dares. Although the rate of injuries is high in children less than 9 years of age, most fatal injuries occur in later childhood and adolescence.

The pattern of deaths caused by unintentional injuries, especially from motor vehicles, drowning, and burns, is remarkably consistent in most Western societies. However, the United States far exceeds other countries in the number of violent deaths. The leading causes of death from injuries for each age-group according to sex are presented in Table 1-5. Although the incidence of increasing violence is highlighted in the United States, it is important to note that accidents continue to account for more teen deaths than any other source (Annie E. Casey Foundation, 2001). Fortunately, prevention strategies such as the use of car restraints, bicycle helmets, and smoke detectors have resulted in a significant decrease in fatalities for children. Currently, all states have enacted legislation requiring young children to be properly restrained in motor vehicles. Despite safety efforts, the overwhelming cause of death in children over 1 year of age is motor vehicle (MV)–related fatalities, including occupant, pedestrian, bicycle, and motorcycle deaths (Fig. 1-1). In fact, MV-related accidents now account for more than half of all injury deaths (National Center for Health Statistics, 1997). The majority of deaths from injuries occur in males. Even though the *percentage* of infants dying from MV injuries is small compared with the total number of deaths in that age-group, children under 1 year of age still have a high death rate from MV accidents, primarily from a failure to be properly restrained.

Pedestrian injuries in children account for significant numbers of MV-related deaths. Most pedestrian injuries oc-

---

### Box 1-2
### Childhood Injuries: Risk Factors

**Sex**—Preponderance of males; difference mainly the result of behavioral characteristics, especially aggression

**Temperament**—Children with difficult temperament profile, especially persistence, high activity, and negative reactions to new situations (Nyman, 1987)

**Stress**—Predisposes to increased risk taking and self-destructive behavior; general lack of self-protection

**Alcohol and drug use**—Associated with higher incidence of motor vehicle injuries, drownings, homicides, and suicides

**History of previous injury**—Associated with increased likelihood of another injury, especially if initial injury required hospitalization

**Developmental characteristics**
  Mismatch between child's developmental level and skill required for activity (e.g., all-terrain vehicles)
  Natural curiosity to explore environment
  Desire to assert self and challenge rules
  In older child, desire for peer approval and acceptance

**Cognitive characteristics** (age specific)
  *Infancy*—Sensorimotor: explores environment through taste and touch
  *Young child*
    Object permanence: actively searches for attractive object
    Cause and effect: unaware of consequential dangers
    Transductive reasoning: may fail to learn from experiences; for example, falling from a step is not perceived as same type of danger as climbing a tree
    Magical and egocentric thinking: cannot comprehend danger to self or others; cannot take place of others to realize danger; if thinking something is safe, believes it to be so
  *School-age child*—Transitional cognitive processes: unable to fully comprehend causal relationships; attempts dangerous acts without detailed planning regarding consequences
  *Adolescent*—Formal operations: preoccupied with abstract thinking and loses sight of reality; may lead to feeling of invulnerability

**Anatomic characteristics** (especially in young children)
  *Large head*—Predisposes to cranial injury
  *Large spleen and liver with wide costal arch*—Predisposes to direct trauma to these organs
  *Small and light body*—May be thrown easily, especially inside a moving vehicle
  *Left-handedness*—Combination of environmental biases and certain neuroanatomic or biologic differences may increase susceptibility to injury (Graham and others, 1993)

**Other factors**—Poverty, family stress (i.e., maternal illness, recent environmental change), substandard alternative child care, young maternal age, low maternal education, multiple siblings

---

cur at midblock, at intersections, in driveways, and in parking lots. Driveway injuries typically involve small children and large vehicles backing up. Parents may not be alert to the dangers leading to such injuries and consequently fail to protect their children.

Bicycle injuries are another important cause of childhood deaths, especially from head injuries. Children ages 5 to 9 years are at greatest risk of bicycling fatalities. The majority of bicycling deaths are from head injuries. Helmets reduce the risk of head injury by 85%, but few children wear helmets (National Safety Council, 2000). Community-wide bicycle helmet campaigns and mandatory-use laws have resulted in significant increases in helmet use. However, even with a mandatory-use law, issues such as stylishness, comfort,

**TABLE 1-5** Mortality from leading types of unintentional injuries, United States, 1997 (rates per 100,000 population in each age-group)

| Type of Accident | Age (Years) | | | |
|---|---|---|---|---|
| | Under 1 | 1-4 | 5-14 | 15-24 |
| **Males** | | | | |
| All causes | 818.0 | 39.8 | 24.0 | 124.4 |
| Unintentional injuries (all types) | 22.3 | 15.2 | 10.6 | 52.3 |
| Motor vehicle | 4.4 (2) | 5.3 (1) | 5.8 (1) | 38.3 (1) |
| Drowning | 1.8 (4) | 3.9 (2) | 1.6 (2) | 3.2 (2) |
| Fires and burns | 1.5 (5) | 2.5 (3) | 0.8 (3) | — |
| Firearms | — | — | 0.5 (4) | 1.5 (4) |
| Ingestion of food or object | 2.5 (3) | 0.5 (5) | — | — |
| Falls | — | — | — | 1.2 (5) |
| Mechanical suffocation | 9.1 (1) | 0.6 (4) | 0.4 (5) | — |
| Poisoning | — | — | — | 2.8 (3) |
| All other unintentional injuries | 3.1 | 2.3 | 1.4 | 5.3 |
| *Accidents as a percent of all deaths | 2.7% | 38.2% | 44.3% | 42.0% |
| **Females** | | | | |
| All causes | 662.9 | 31.8 | 17.4 | 46.0 |
| Unintentional injuries (all types) | 18.1 | 10.9 | 6.7 | 20.0 |
| Motor vehicle | 4.4 (2) | 4.7 (1) | 4.3 (1) | 17.1 (1) |
| Drowning | 1.4 (4) | 2.0 (2) | 0.6 (3) | 0.4 (3) |
| Fires and burns | 1.2 (5) | 2.0 (2) | 0.7 (2) | — |
| Firearms | — | — | 0.1 (4) | 0.1 (5) |
| Ingestion of food or object | 1.5 (3) | 0.4 (4) | — | — |
| Falls | — | — | — | 0.2 (4) |
| Mechanical suffocation | 6.9 (1) | 0.3 (5) | 0.1 (4) | — |
| Poisoning | — | — | — | 0.8 (2) |
| All other unintentional injuries | 2.7 | 1.5 | 0.9 | 1.5 |
| *Accidents as a percent of all deaths | 2.7% | 34.2% | 38.2% | 43.4% |

Modified from National Safety Council: *Injury facts,* Itasca, IL, 2000, National Safety Council Data Source,
National Center for Health Statistics.
*Indicates rank among the leading types of accidents.

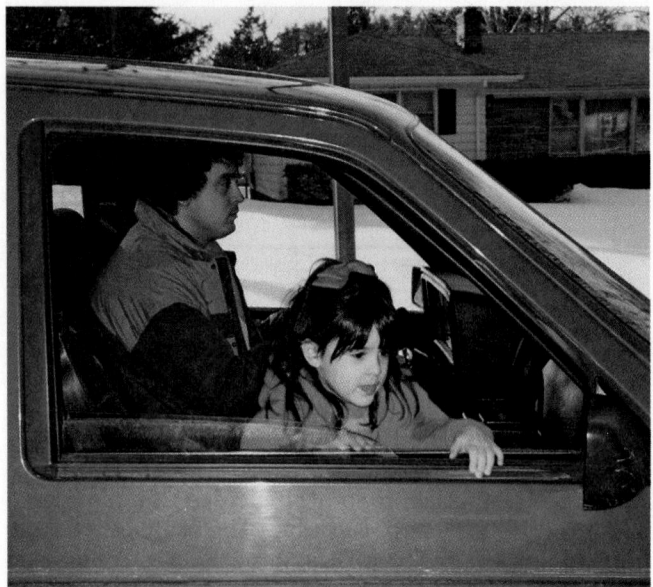

**Fig. 1-1** Motor vehicle injuries are the leading cause of death in children over 1 year of age. The majority of fatalities involve occupants who are unrestrained.

and social acceptability remain important factors in compliance. Nurses can educate children and families about pedestrian and bicycle safety. In particular, school nurses can promote helmet wearing and encourage peer leaders to act as role models.

Drowning and burns are the second and third leading causes of death in boys ages 1 to 14, but this order is reversed in girls (Fig. 1-2). Drowning continues to be a significant cause of death in older teenagers. In addition, improper use of firearms is a major cause of death among males (Fig. 1-3). During infancy, more males succumb to death from aspiration or suffocation than do females (Fig. 1-4). More than half of all poisonings occur in children under 2 years of age (Fig. 1-5). By ages 4 to 5 years, unintentional poisonings are uncommon. Another increase occurs in the 15- to 24-year age-group, where poisoning is the third leading cause of death in males and second in females. Poisoning in this age-group is typically intentional and usually represents death from suicide (especially females) or drug abuse.

Analyzing deaths from specific types of injuries by age and sex permits identification of high-risk groups. When comparing deaths from injuries with other causes of childhood mortality, it is clear that preventing injuries offers the

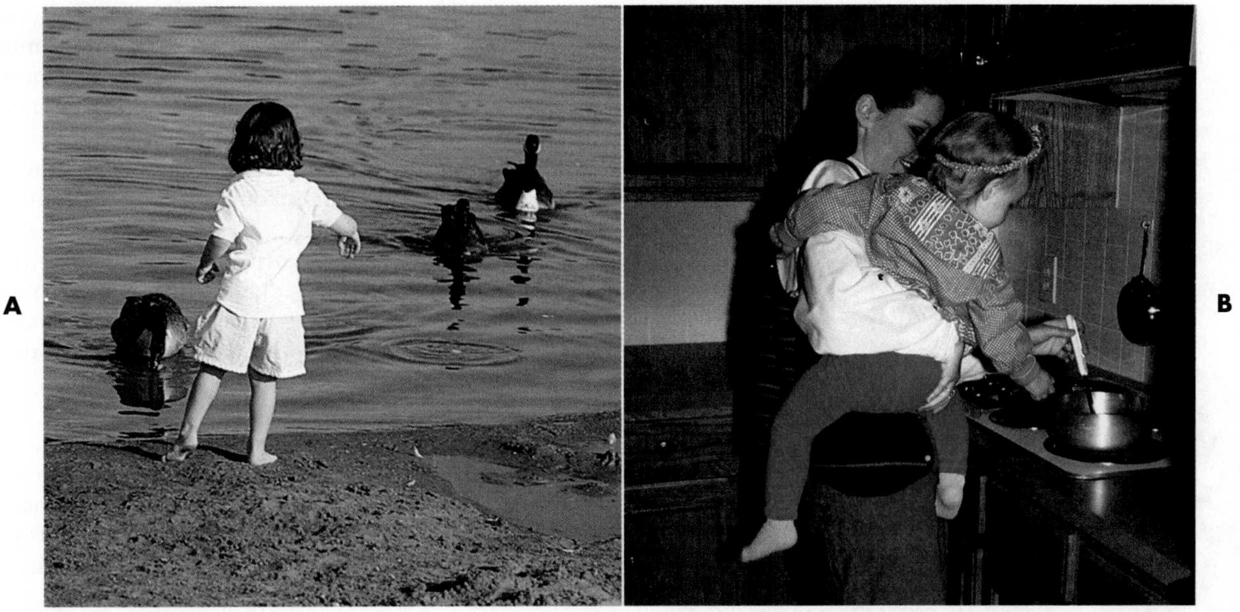

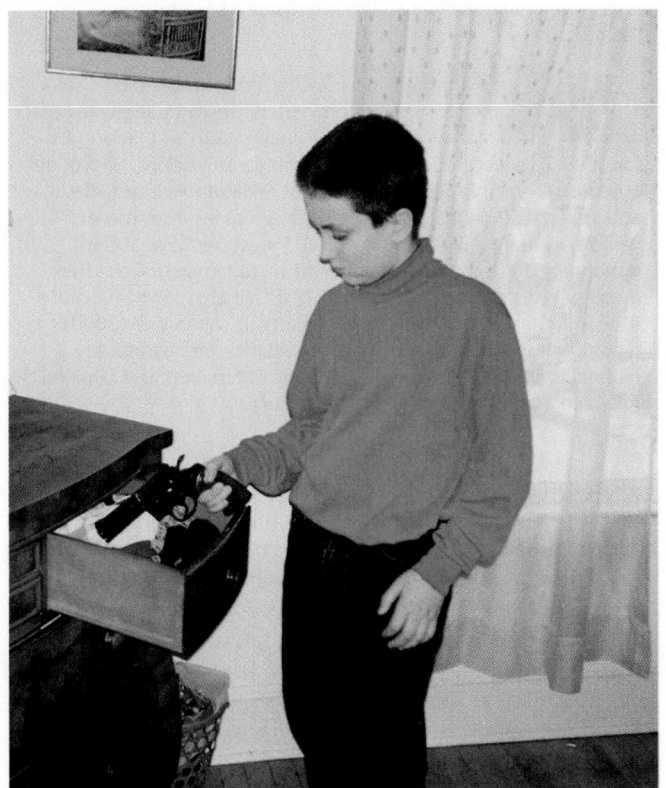

**Fig. 1-2** **A,** Drowning is the second leading cause of death from injury in boys and the third in girls ages 5 to 14 years. **B,** Burns are the second leading cause of death from injury in girls and the third in boys ages 1 to 14 years.

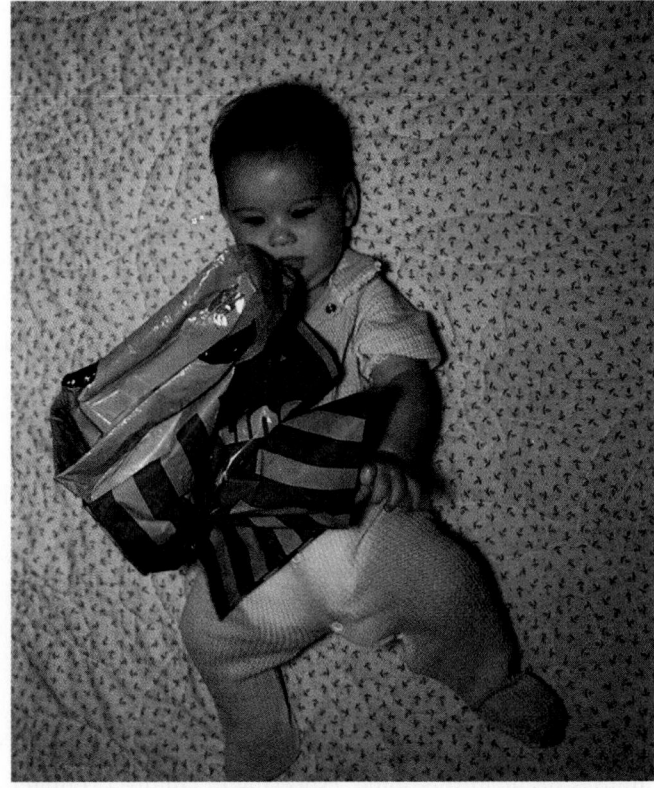

**Fig. 1-3** Improper use of firearms is the fourth leading cause of death from injury in boys 5 to 24 years and girls ages 5 to 14 years.

**Fig. 1-4** Mechanical suffocation is often the leading cause of death from injury in infants.

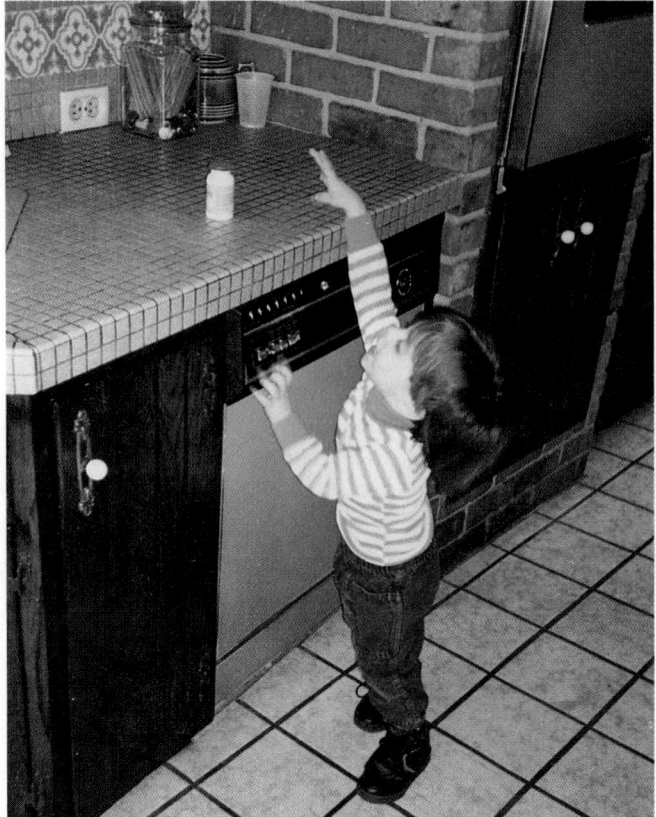

**Fig. 1-5** Poisoning causes a considerable number of injuries in children under 4 years of age, but it is the third leading cause of death from injury in males and second in females (usually from suicide) ages 15 to 24 years.

greatest promise for improving survival. Nurses play a major role in providing anticipatory guidance to parents and older children regarding the hazards during each age period.

Not all injuries are unintentional. Some may be intentional and represent abuse or suicide. An important nursing consideration when injuries do occur is to determine if they were intentional.

> **NURSING ALERT**
>
> The history of the injury is essential in assessing intentional injury from abuse or neglect. The following questions are important:
>
> **When**—Did the parent or guardian seek immediate medical attention or has there been a long delay?
>
> **Where**—Does the reported location of the accident correlate with the nature of the injury?
>
> **How**—Are the circumstances surrounding the injury logical?

## Environment

A number of environmental factors, such as place, time, and equipment, contribute to injuries. The highest number of injuries occur in the home, especially in children younger than 6 years of age. Older children experience injuries outside the home, especially at school and recreational sites. Among recreational and sports activities, football is one of the most hazardous athletic activities and accounts for 20 in-

juries per 100,000 participants per year. Serious, potentially fatal injuries result from spinal cord trauma. Among females, gymnastics poses the greatest risk. For drowning, a leading cause of death, risk factors include living in a warm climate, swimming in undesignated areas, being unable to swim, misusing or not using a personal flotation device, and using open boats. The most common cause of dental injury is falling against an object.

The identification of environmental hazards has had tremendous influence on reducing the incidence of fatal injuries. For example, placing fences around swimming pools and putting guards on windows has decreased the incidence of fatal drownings and falls.

### Injury Prevention

Theoretically, all injuries are preventable. A primary nursing responsibility is to anticipate and recognize when safety measures apply. Injury prevention necessitates protection, education, and legislation. The two major strategies for injury prevention are:

1. **Passive strategies,** which provide automatic protection by product and environmental design (e.g., the use of automatic seat belts or air bags). Such devices require no active participation by the individual and have the greatest success rate.
2. **Active strategies,** which *persuade* individuals to change their behavior for increased self-protection, such as using seat belts voluntarily, or *require* compliance with safety regulations, such as laws that mandate the use of safety restraints in young children. Persuasion through education has been much less effective than legislated change, but it remains a key strategy.

> **NURSING ALERT**
>
> Although health care professionals play a major role in injury prevention, research indicates that their counseling is incomplete and lacking in focus. A survey of 465 pediatricians, family physicians, and pediatric nurse practitioners indicated that 66% of them provided anticipatory guidance about preventing injuries from motor vehicle accidents, 59% about poison ingestion, 32% about drowning, but only 16% about firearms to families of children under 5 years of age (Barkin, Fink, and Gelberg, 1999). Because time is limited during well-child office visits, Altemeier (2000) recommends focusing anticipatory guidance on children at highest risk (boys and low socioeconomic families) and families in which a child has had a previous injury.

The preventive aspects of child care are an ongoing part of health promotion throughout childhood. To protect the child from injury, persons who are responsible for children need to be aware of normal behavioral characteristics that render children vulnerable to injuries and factors in the environment that create a hazard to safety. Parents are often surprisingly unaware of their child's developmental progress and capabilities. Anticipatory guidance regarding developmental expectations will alert parents to the types of injuries that are most likely at any given age and to environmental circumstances that precipitate an injury. For example, infants must not be left where they can fall or roll over, and toddlers must not be given objects or toys with small removable parts or sharp edges. Children should not be given unsupervised access to places where they can fall, drown, or be burned.

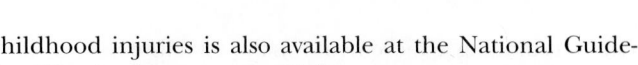

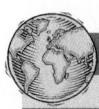
## CULTURAL AWARENESS
### Safety Counseling

Cultural factors need to be considered when instituting safety instruction because noncompliance is one of the major deterrents to injury prevention. For example, cultural characteristics, such as the lack of future orientation and resistance to changing long-standing habits, can interfere with a cultural group's acceptance of injury prevention practices (Foss, 1987). One study found that efforts regarding the use of seat belts among Mexican-American parents were more effective when the dominant decision-making male in the family and the influential older woman, often a grandmother, were included in the educational efforts (Faber, 1986).

Early in the parent-child relationship, parents need advice on how to provide a safe environment for their child, what types of behaviors they can expect at various stages of development, and their responsibility for their child's safety. This education is particularly important for first-time parents. (See Cultural Awareness box.) Safety responsibility in areas such as the purchase of an infant car restraint, should begin *before* the child is born.

It cannot be assumed that parents of one or more children are familiar with all areas of child safety. The addition of a new infant may cause sibling rivalry and the new infant may be at risk from a jealous older sibling. Parents should be cautioned against leaving the infant alone with an older child who feels threatened by the newcomer.

The American Academy of Pediatrics TIPP (The Injury Prevention Program) has developed a comprehensive system for injury prevention that provides useful information for parents. TIPP consists of three major elements*:

1. A policy statement on injury prevention by the American Academy of Pediatrics Committee on Injury and Posion Prevention
2. Childhood safety counseling schedules
3. Safety information sheets and safety surveys for use in providing anticipatory guidance to parents

Providing a safe environment for the child involves the combined efforts of family, nurses, and community. At each age there are environmental factors hazardous to the child. The specific hazards vary according to the season (drowning, injuries related to winter heating devices), geographic area (water injuries in areas with swimming pools, rivers, or lakes; heater burns in cold climates), and socioeconomic level (lead poisoning and street injuries in slum areas, bicycle injuries in middle-class areas). In an effort to decrease injuries, the United States Government has established the **Consumer Product Safety Commission (CPSC)** to protect the public against unreasonable risks and death associated with products. The CPSC provides a large number of publications that recommend various areas of safety concerns for children.† An updated summary of the priority rankings of

childhood injuries is also available at the National Guideline Clearinghouse *www.guideline.gov*.

Safety should be an intrinsic element of nursing practice. Nurses who themselves practice safety, who are alert to safety needs in the environment, and who recognize the need for safety education contribute to injury reduction. Special problems and preventive measures are discussed, as appropriate, throughout the book and are related to the various age levels and conditions that predispose a child to specific hazards.

## Evolution of Child Health Care in the United States

Children in colonial America were born into a world with many hazards to their health and survival. Epidemics were common. Control or treatment was unknown. Physicians were few, and only a small number had any formal training. Midwives were untrained, basing their practice on past experiences. Books providing information on child care and feeding were scarce and, when available, were useful only to a minority of literate parents.

Medical care by physicians was limited to wealthy families who lived in or could travel to more developed cities. Children who lived on farms were mainly cared for by another family member or by a competent neighbor. Traveling medicine men, with their various forms of quackery, were common. Children who were bought as slaves or born to slaves had only as much care as their owner was able or willing to provide. Native American children were treated according to the tradition of each tribe, which was often a mixture of medicine, magic, and religion. With the colonization of America, Native Americans were exposed to many new, often fatal, diseases.

Statistics on childhood mortality during the colonial period are largely unavailable. Epidemic diseases included smallpox, measles, mumps, chickenpox, influenza, diphtheria, yellow fever, cholera, and whooping cough. However, the disease that surpassed all others as a cause of childhood death was dysentery. Sometimes entire families succumbed to this illness. Other diseases that contributed to childhood illness were the "slow epidemics" of tuberculosis, nutritional diseases, and injuries.

Although scientific knowledge was accumulating, especially from work done in Europe, there were no organized efforts in the United States to apply that knowledge to the care of the sick. It was not until the Industrial Revolution was well under way in the nineteenth century that the consequences of childhood illness and injury and the effects of child labor, poverty, and neglect became widely recognized. The end of the nineteenth century is often regarded as the dark ages of pediatrics, and the first half of the twentieth century is regarded as the dawn of improved health care for children.

The study of pediatrics began in the late 1800s, particularly under the influence of a Prussian-born physician, *Abraham Jacobi* (1830-1919), who is referred to as the *Father of Pediatrics.* With several other physicians he broke new ground in the scientific and clinical investigation of childhood diseases.

---

*Available from **American Academy of Pediatrics,** 141 Northwest Point Blvd, PO Box 747, Elk Grove Village, IL, 60009-0747, (888) 227-1770, fax: (847) 228-1281; www.aap.org.
†For more information call (800) 638-CPSC or (800) 638-2272.

One outstanding achievement was the establishment of "milk stations," where mothers could bring sick children for treatment and learn the importance of pure milk and its proper preparation.

The crusade for pure milk helped bring the dairy industry under legal control and led to the establishment of infant welfare stations. The remarkable decline in infant mortality since 1900 has been achieved through prevention and health-promoting measures such as improved sanitation and pasteurization of milk. Before these regulations existed, the unsanitary milk supply was a chief source of infantile diarrhea and tuberculosis. Cows were often kept in filthy stables and fed garbage and distillery wastes. Milk from cows who were fed distillery wastes was reported to make infants "tipsy."

At the same time, increasing concern developed for the social welfare of children, especially those who were homeless or employed as factory laborers. The work of one such reformer, *Lillian Wald* (1867-1940), had far-reaching effects on child health and nursing. She founded the Henry Street Settlement in New York City, which eventually provided nursing services, social work, and an organized program of social, cultural, and educational activities. Wald is regarded as the *founder of public health or community nursing.* She was instrumental in establishing the role of the first full-time school nurse, *Lina Rogers.* Soon other nurses were employed to teach parents and children about the prevention or need for treatment of minor skin conditions, malnutrition, and other impairments or illnesses identified in the school. An outgrowth of nursing involvement in school health was the development of pediatric courses and specialized clinical experience in schools of nursing.

As more causes of disease were identified, there was an emphasis on isolation and asepsis. In the early 1900s children with contagious diseases were isolated from adult patients. Parents were prohibited from visiting because they might transmit disease to and from the home. Even toys and personal articles of clothing were kept from the child. It was not until the 1940s and the famous work of Spitz and Robertson on institutionalized children that the effects of isolation and maternal deprivation were recognized. This research brought forth a surge of interest in the psychologic health of children and resulted in changes for hospitalized children, such as rooming-in, sibling visitations, child life (play) programs, prehospitalization preparation, parent education, and hospital schooling.

Influenced by social reformers such as Lillian Wald, national leaders took action to improve children's living conditions. In 1909 President Theodore Roosevelt called the first *White House Conference on Children,* which focused on the care of dependent children and addressed the deplorable working conditions of youngsters. As a result of this conference, the *U.S. Children's Bureau* was established in 1912 and placed under the Department of Health, Education and Welfare (now the *Department of Health and Human Services*).

The establishment of the Children's Bureau marked the beginning of a period of studies of economic and social factors related to infant mortality, maternal deaths, and maternal and infant care in rural areas, all of which created the basis for stimulating better standards of care for mothers and children. These studies led to the first *Maternity and Infancy Act* (Sheppard-Towner Act) in 1921, which provided grants to states to develop a Division of Maternal and Child Health (MCH) as a unit of the health department. However, this bill eventually lapsed because of opposition from those (especially the American Medical Association [AMA]) who viewed it as a socialist movement.

However the passage of the Maternity and Infancy Act was a turning point for the creation of the *American Academy of Pediatrics* in 1930.

With the passage of *Title V of the Social Security Act (SSA)* in 1935, a federal-state partnership was established under the administration of the Children's Bureau. Title V included federal grants-in-aid to states (matched by state funds) for three types of work: *Maternal and Child Health (MCH), Crippled Children's Services (CCS),* and *child welfare services.* The first programs provided by Title V were prenatal, postnatal, and child health clinics and training of personnel. The early emphasis of the CCS program was on orthopaedic care. With the recognition that a child's ability to function could be limited by a chronic illness, state CCS programs became involved with children who had developmental, behavioral, and educational problems and, more recently, with home care of children with complex medical conditions. This broadened concept was reflected in 1985 by the passage of legislation that changed the name of the CCS to the *Program for Children with Special Health Needs (CSHN).*

Numerous other federal programs have been developed. Some that have had a major impact on maternal and child health include the following:

**Medicaid.** In 1965 Medicaid was created under Title XIX of the SSA to reduce financial barriers to health care for the poor. It is the largest maternal-child health program. A major project under Medicaid is the Child Health Assessment Program (CHAP), which provides services for a large number of pregnant women and children. Not all poor children are eligible for Medicaid; financial eligibility varies considerably from state to state.

**Aid to Families with Dependent Children (AFDC).** AFDC was established by the SSA of 1935 as a cash grant program to enable states to aid needy children without fathers.

**MCH Services Block Grant.** The MCH Services Block Grant provides health services to mothers and children, particularly those with low income or limited access to health services. Its primary purposes are to reduce infant mortality, reduce the incidence of preventable disease and handicapping conditions among children, and increase the availability of prenatal, delivery, and postpartum care to eligible mothers.

**Alcohol, Drug Abuse, and Mental Health Block Grant.** Established by the Omnibus Budget Reconciliation Act of 1981, this block grant provides funds to states for (1) projects to support prevention, treatment, and rehabilitation related to substance abuse and (2) grants to community mental health centers for the identification, assessment, and treatment of severely mentally disturbed children and adolescents.

**Social Services Block Grant.** Established under Title XX of the SSA, the Social Services Block Grant provides states with funds for child daycare, protective and emergency services, counseling, family planning, home-based services, information and referral, and adoption and foster care services.

**Women, Infants, and Children (WIC).** In 1974 the WIC Special Supplemental Food Program was started. This program provides nutritious food and nutrition education to low-income, pregnant, postpartum, and lactating women and to infants and children up to age 5 years. Other nutrition programs include Food Stamps, National School Lunch Program, School Breakfast Program, and Child Care Food Program. The Child Care Food Program provides financial assistance for nutritious meals to children in daycare centers, family and group daycare homes, and Head Start centers.

**Education for All Handicapped Children Act (P.L. 94-142).** In 1975 P.L. 94-142 was passed to provide free, appropriate public education to all handicapped children from ages 3 to 21 years and to provide for supportive services (such as speech and counseling) that ensure the benefit of special education.

**Education of the Handicapped Act Amendments of 1986 (P.L. 99-457).** In 1986 P.L. 99-457 was passed to allow for the provision of federal funding to states to develop and implement a statewide, comprehensive, coordinated, and multidisciplinary program of early intervention services for handicapped infants and toddlers and their families.

**Omnibus Budget Reconciliation Act of 1990.** Passage of this act required states to extend Medicaid coverage to all children ages 6 to 18 years with family incomes below 133% of the poverty level.

**Family and Medical Leave Act (FMLA).** Signed into law in 1993, FMLA allows eligible employees to take up to 12 weeks of unpaid leave from their jobs every year to care for newborn or newly adopted children; to care for children, parents, or spouses who have serious health conditions; or to recover from their own serious health conditions. After the leave, the law entitles employees to return to their previous jobs or to equivalent jobs with the same pay, benefits, and other conditions.

Despite the number of federal and state programs available to assist children and families, there are serious barriers to health care in the United States, including (1) *financial barriers,* such as not having insurance, having insurance that does not cover certain services, or being unable to pay for services; (2) *system barriers,* such as having to travel great distances for health care or state-to-state variations in Medicaid benefits; and (3) *knowledge barriers,* such as a lack of understanding about the need or value of prenatal or child health supervision or a lack of awareness of the services that are available. The current thrust in health care is to improve children's and families' access to health care.

One of the major changes in health care delivery has been the establishment of a *prospective payment system* based on *diagnosis-related groups (DRGs).* The DRG categories define *pretreatment (prospective) billing* for almost all U.S. hospitals reimbursed by Medicaid. Because hospitals are financially responsible when Medicaid patients exceed the allotted admission stay, more patients are discharged early. This has created an immense need for home care and other sources of community-based services. Health care cost containment remains a national priority, and some form of prospective payment affects almost everyone. Nurses need to be aware of changing trends in health care economics and need to be prepared to meet the challenges presented by *managed care companies* and *health maintenance organizations (HMOs).*\*

Today 85% of all employed families and many families covered by Medicaid are in managed health care plans. Children are being enrolled in these plans at a higher rate than adults, and children now represent a disproportionately larger share of all managed care members (David and Lucille Packard Foundation, 1998). However, evidence supporting managed care for children is inconclusive and contradictory. For example, although managed health care has improved access to preventive health care for some children, Medicaid-managed care has resulted in reduced access to specialty care for children with chronic conditions (Szilagy, 1998). If managed care is to work for children, the following features must be present: (1) accessible, continuous, comprehensive, coordinated, family-centered, and compassionate care; (2) a defined benefit package crafted around the changing physical and emotional needs of children; (3) access to pediatric specialists for children with chronic or disabling illnesses; (4) coordinated care both within the managed care network and encouragement for active participation of parents; (6) fair reimbursement rate, particularly for children with special health needs; and (7) rewards to plans that improve the health of children they serve (David and Lucille Packard Foundation, 1998).

## PEDIATRIC NURSING
### Philosophy of Care

Nursing of infants and children is consistent with the *definition of nursing* as "the diagnosis and treatment of human responses to actual or potential health problems." This definition incorporates the four essential features of contemporary nursing practice:

1. Attention to the full range of human experiences and responses to health and illness without restriction to a problem-focused orientation
2. Integration of objective data with knowledge gained from an understanding of the patient or group's subjective experience
3. Application of scientific knowledge to the processes of diagnosis and treatment
4. Provision of a caring relationship that facilitates health and healing (American Nurses' Association, 1995)

### Family-Centered Care\*

The philosophy of *family-centered care* recognizes the family as the constant in a child's life. Service systems and personnel must support, respect, encourage, and enhance the strength and competence of the family by developing mutuality and a partnership with parents (Newton, 2000). Families are supported in their natural caregiving and decision-making roles by building on their unique strengths and acknowledging their expertise in caring for their child both within and outside the hospital setting (Newton, 2000). Patterns of living at home and in the community are promoted. The needs of all family members, not just the child's, are

---

\*For information on managed care references and resources, contact www.nursingworld.org.

---

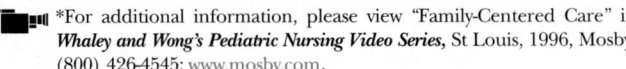 \*For additional information, please view "Family-Centered Care" in *Whaley and Wong's Pediatric Nursing Video Series,* St Louis, 1996, Mosby; (800) 426-4545; www.mosby.com.

**Box 1-3 ■ ■ □**
**The Key Elements of Family-Centered Care**

Incorporating into policy and practice the recognition that the *family is the constant* in a child's life while the service systems and support personnel within those systems fluctuate

Facilitating *family/professional collaboration* at all levels of hospital, home, and community care:

☐ Care of an individual child
☐ Program development, implementation, and evaluation
☐ Policy formation

*Exchanging complete and unbiased information* between family members and professionals in a supportive manner at all times

Incorporating into policy and practice the recognition and *honoring of cultural diversity*, strengths, and individuality within and across all families, including *ethnic, racial, spiritual, social, economic, educational, and geographic diversity*

Recognizing and respecting *different methods of coping* and implementing comprehensive policies and programs that will provide *developmental, educational, emotional, environmental, and financial support* to meet the diverse needs of families

Encouraging and facilitating *family-to-family support* and networking

Ensuring that *home, hospital, and community service and support systems* for children needing specialized health and developmental care and their families are *flexible, accessible, and comprehensive* in responding to diverse family-identified needs

*Appreciating families as families* and children as children, recognizing that they possess a wide range of strengths, concerns, emotions, and aspirations beyond their need for specialized health and developmental services and support

From Shelton TL, Stepanek JS: *Family-centered care for children needing specialized health and developmental services*, Bethesda, MD, 1994, Association for the Care of Children's Health.

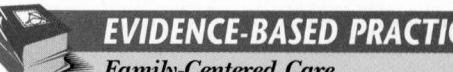

**EVIDENCE-BASED PRACTICE**
*Family-Centered Care*

Although professionals readily accept the concept of family-centered care, they have been slow to implement practices that embody the "family as the patient." This lag has occurred in part because family-centered care requires a shift in orientation regarding provision of services. The philosophy requires stretching beyond clinical practices that have become tradition to the institution and personnel.

Family-centered care requires viewing families as the center of care, with their input serving as the major determinant of the interventions provided. For example, exclusion policies are replaced with *family-based care*, such as parental and child *choice* regarding separation during procedures, open visiting hours, and no limitations on the ages or numbers of visitors, except per family request. In fact, should the word "visitors" even be used? Family members certainly are not visitors to their child; nurses and other staff are!

In your practice, what policies can be considered family-based care? How can those that are not family-based care be changed? What reasons do staff give for preferring practices that exclude families? Compare the agency's policies with its mission statement and purpose. Sadly, you may find what Hostler (1992) reported: during visits to 30 leading hospitals in the United States, not one single model of excellence in the implementation of family-centered care was found. Fortunately, models of family-centered care, such as the Nursing Mutual Participation Mode (Curley, 1988; Curley and Wallace, 1992), do exist and have documented benefits, such as the following (Curley and Wallace, 1992; Johnson, Jeppson, and Redburn, 1992):

☐ Families experience greater feelings of confidence and competence and less stress in caring for their children
☐ The dependence of families on professional caregivers decreases
☐ Costs of care decrease
☐ Professionals experience greater job satisfaction
☐ Both parents and providers are empowered to develop new skills and expertise

considered (Box 1-3). The philosophy acknowledges diversity among family structures and backgrounds; family goals, dreams, strategies, and actions; and family support, service, and information needs.

Two basic concepts in family-centered care are enabling and empowerment. Professionals *enable* families by creating opportunities and means for all family members to display their present abilities and competencies and to acquire new ones that are necessary to meet the needs of the child and family. *Empowerment* describes the interaction of professionals with families in such a way that families maintain or acquire a sense of control over their family lives and acknowledge positive changes that result from helping behaviors that foster their own strengths, abilities, and actions.

The *parent-professional partnership* is a powerful mechanism for enabling and empowering families.* Parents serve

*For information about parent-professional partnerships, a free pamphlet, *Equals in This Partnership*, is available from **The National Center for Infants, Toddlers, and Families**, 200 M St NW, Suite 200, Washington, DC 20036, (202) 638-1144.

as respected equals with professionals and have the rightful role in deciding what is important for themselves and their family; the professional's role is to support and strengthen the family's ability to nurture and promote its members' development in a way that is both enabling and empowering. Professionals must also work together as a team to benefit children and their families.

Partnerships imply the belief that partners are capable individuals who become more capable by sharing knowledge, skills, and resources in a manner that benefits all participants. Collaboration is viewed as a continuum. Families have the option of being anywhere along that continuum, depending on the strengths and needs of the child, the family, and the professionals involved. The nurse can help *every* family, including those with a history of serious personal or family problems, to identify their strengths, build on them, and assume a comfortable level of participation. (See Evidence-Based Practice box.) Recently, parents of children with special health care needs have been sharing their experiences and educating caregivers about family-centered care. In the future, health care must be based within the family system so that health beliefs and behaviors can focus on health promotion and illness prevention. Although caring for the family is strongly emphasized throughout the text, it is highlighted in features such as Cultural Awareness, Family Focus (see p. 26), and Family Home Care boxes.

## Atraumatic Care

Although tremendous advances have been made in pediatric care, much of what is done to children to cure illness and prolong life is traumatic, painful, upsetting, and frightening. Unfortunately, minimizing the trauma of medical interventions has not kept pace with the technologic advances. With knowledge of the stressors imposed on ill children and their families and armed with interventions that are safe and effective in eliminating or reducing the stressors, health professionals must direct their attention to providing atraumatic care.

*Atraumatic care* is the provision of therapeutic care in settings, by personnel, and through the use of interventions that eliminate or minimize the psychologic and physical distress experienced by children and their families in the health care system. *Therapeutic care* encompasses the prevention, diagnosis, treatment, or palliation of chronic or acute conditions. *Setting* refers to the place in which that care is given—the home, the hospital, or any other health care setting. *Personnel* include anyone directly involved in providing therapeutic care. *Interventions* range from psychologic approaches, such as preparing children for procedures, to physical interventions, such as providing space for a parent to room in with a child. *Psychologic distress* may include anxiety, fear, anger, disappointment, sadness, shame, or guilt. *Physical distress* may range from sleeplessness and immobilization to the experience of disturbing sensory stimuli such as pain, temperature extremes, loud noises, bright lights, or darkness. Atraumatic care is concerned with the who, what, when, where, why, and how of any procedure performed on a child for the purpose of preventing or minimizing psychologic and physical stress (Wong, 1989).

The overriding goal in providing atraumatic care is: **first, do no harm.** Three principles provide the framework for achieving this goal: (1) prevent or minimize the child's separation from the family; (2) promote a sense of control; and (3) prevent or minimize bodily injury and pain. Examples of providing atraumatic care include fostering the parent-child relationship during hospitalization, preparing the child before any unfamiliar treatment or procedure, controlling pain, allowing the child privacy, providing play activities for expression of fear and aggression, providing choices to children, and respecting cultural differences.

Throughout the text the concept of atraumatic care is an integral part of all discussions of nursing care. Selected examples are highlighted in Atraumatic Care boxes. Many other boxes and tables focusing on culture, family teaching, research, and critical thinking incorporate aspects of providing care as atraumatically as possible. Chapter 26, Family-Centered Care of the Child During Illness and Hospitalization, is organized according to the principles of providing atraumatic care.

## Case Management

Case management was developed as an approach to coordinate care and control costs. Although the movement began in adult care, it was quickly adapted to pediatric care. Benefits of case management, such as improved patient and family satisfaction, decreased fragmentation of care, and the ability to describe and measure outcomes for a homogenous group of patients, became apparent.

Case managers have responsibility and accountability for a particular group of patients and use a system of critical paths derived from standards of care. The model includes a timeline for care as a component of the process. These timelines have a variety of names: critical paths, guidelines for care, case management plans, Caremaps,* coordinated care plans, care paths, or other titles that are agreed on within a specific agency (Tables 1-6 and 1-7). Regardless of the name, these timelines are multidisciplinary plans that include all of the components of care for an episode or multiple episodes of illness as well as the outcomes that are expected as a result of delivering that care. They can be confined to inpatient care or can include the entire continuum of care, including home care. (See Chapter 25.) Care paths are the tools of case management. Many nursing skills that are not acknowledged are made visible by the numerous responsibilities outlined by the care path (MacPhee and Hoffenberg, 1996).

Variances from the timelines are recorded daily in an effort to determine why there are delays in providing care or why a patient's illness follows a different course than was expected. Variances are categorized as patient, system, caregiver, or community problems. Through a retrospective review process, changes are made to make care more effective and more efficient. By using case management, hospitals have reported reductions in the length of stay and in the cost of providing care. Improvements in the efficiency of hospital systems and in nurses' job satisfaction have also been noted.

Concurrent with the movement to provide care in a systematic manner have been efforts by professional and government organizations to develop *clinical practice guidelines* for the care of an illness, disease, or related problem. Although timelines for care are usually developed within an institution and reflect local practice patterns, clinical guidelines are developed on a national level to reflect the research that has been conducted relative to a specific disease or illness. One federal agency that has developed clinical guidelines is the *Agency for Health Care Policy and Research (AHCPR)* (Box 1-4), now known as the *Agency for Healthcare Research and Quality (AHRQ)*.

As the movement for providing care based on guidelines continues, institutions are challenged to incorporate clinical guidelines into the locally developed timelines for care. The result of this effort is professionally developed clinical guidelines that can be integrated into practice at the local level.

---

*Caremap is a registered trademark of the **Center for Case Management, Inc,** South Natick, MA 01760, (508) 651-2600.

**TABLE 1-6** Example of critical path for preterm infant

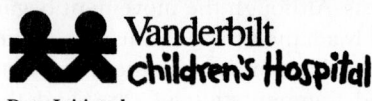 **Vanderbilt Children's Hospital**

**Preterm**
Criteria for Use: Birth Weight <1500g

Date Initiated _____
RN _____

| | Admission Day | Acute Phase | Stable Phase | Discharge Phase |
|---|---|---|---|---|
| **Labs Tests Treatments** | (Cord blood) HepB/RPR Type & Cross **Evaluate for:** CXR Surfactant PCV ABG/CBG Plts CBC/Diff | Evaluate frequency ————————————————————————————→ | | |
| | | Na/K ——————————— | | Na/K weekly |
| | | Bili T&D ——————————— | Eye exam-<30wks or <1300g- | |
| | | State Screen a Bld TF or | or <1800g w/02 exposure— | |
| | | DOL 7 ——————————— | due at 32 weeks _____ | |
| | | Phototherapy | Eye F/U ——————————————————→ | |
| | | | Immunization/permit/DOL 60 | |
| | Cultures Blood/Urine/LP | | | Audiology screen Immunization/permit |
| **RESP** | Evaluate resp status/ intervention | Evaluate resp status/intervnt Wean vent | Wean 02 as tolerated ————→ | D/C oxim 24-48 p RA |
| | | Eval need for resp meds (Methylzanthines) | D/C oxim 24-48 p RA Change to nasal cannula? | Home 02 referral ————→ Move to complex path |
| **CV** | Blood out 5/Kg—TF Direct donor info ————→ | Prop Indocin 24hr if vent Eval for murmur ———————————————————————————→ Direct donor info to family Blood out 5/kg-TF | | |
| **NEURO** | Head circum Assess comfort/pain ————→ | Head circum q mon ———————————————————————————→ Assess comfort/pain level HUS/DOL 7 _____ | HUS/R/O PVL/DOL 30 | F/U _____ |
| **MEDS** | Aqua M (0.5mg) Erythromycin Eval abx need | Day 2-3—D/C abx or cont Trough/Gent/4th dose Day 7-10—D/C abx Vit A QOD | | |
| **FEN** | D7.5 w/UAC/UVC 2.0-3.5 Fr 80-90 cc/kg/day | Advancing Glucose Trophic fdg Eval PCVC need/consent Nutritional consult ————→ Lactation consult ————→ | Advance Fdgs 5-10 kg/d ————→ Con't—Bolus at 1200g Eval Readiness to PO Nutritional consult ————→ Lactation F/U ————→ D/C IL @ 50/kg fdg D/C TPN @ 100/kg fdg | If OG ——————→ PO Nutritional consult Lactation F/U |
| **Teaching/ D/C Plan** | Orient to Unit Visit/guidelines | Teaching sheet begun Visit/call plan ID'd Introduction to Intermed ————→ | Teaching sheet progressing Visit/call plan eval Eval for Intermed status Orient to intermediate | Teaching sheet complete |
| | | BT Hosp _____ SW Screen ————→ WIC form needed  y__ n__ Est BT Date _____ Est DC Date _____ Ins _____ Parents Reaching Out info | BT info given ————→ SW F/U ———————————————————→ WIC form given  y__ n__ Circ permit y n F/U PCP _____ | BT permit obtained Circ Care Wean to Bass Car Seat/Oximeter check Appts/consults _____ _____ _____ NICU F/U _____ |
| | If infant to be discharged home w/high tech needs, advance to Complex Discharge Path | | | TEIS _____ |
| **CLINICAL TARGETS MET/DATE/INIT** | | 02<60% ×48 hr _____ Gluc/Elect wnl _____ Fdgs Init _____ Progress to stable _____ | Extubated/02<50% _____ Wt gain × 7 days _____ Tol Adv Fdgs _____ 50% Tch sheet complete ____ Progress to D/C _____ | RA >24 hr w/sats >92% ____ Wt >1800g _____ Tol full PO fdgs _____ Tol Bass × 24 _____ Tching Complete _____ |

**TABLE 1-7**   Clinical pathway: type 1 diabetes

| Aspect of Care | 1st Hour (First Labs Drawn)<br>Date:          Time start: | Hour 2-24<br>Date:          Time end: | Day 2<br>Date: |
|---|---|---|---|
| **Physiologic Standards** | | | |
| **LABS** | Blood: Glucose, pH, Lytes, hemoglobin A1c, BUN, Creatinine<br>Urine: Dip for ketones<br>Critical DKA = pH <7.2 HCO₃ <10<br>Serious DKA = pH <7.25 HCO₃ <15<br>Moderate DKA = pH <7.3 HCO₃ <17<br>Mild DKA = pH <7.35 HCO₃ <18 | Blood:<br>If Critical DKA: Glucose, pH, Lytes q hr<br>If Serious DKA: Glucose q 1 hr, pH, Lytes q 4 hr<br>If Mild DKA: Glucose premeal and bedtime, 2400, 0300, repeat Lytes × 1<br>Urine: Ketones q void until negative | Blood: Glucose premeal, bedtime, 2400, 0300<br>Urine: Ketones q void until negative |
| Outcomes | Identify level of DKA | Electrolyte and acid/base balance achieved | **Negative ketones***<br>Glucose 70-400 |
| **ASSESSMENT/ MONITORING (KEY SYSTEMS)** | Respiratory: Fruity breath, Kussmaul breathing<br>Hydration, Neuro status<br>Baseline vitals<br>Any signs of concurrent illness<br>Accurate weight in kg | If Critical DKA: Neuro checks × 24 hours, cardiac monitor, VS q hr<br>If Serious DKA: Neuro checks, VS q 1 hr × 4 then q 4 hr<br>If Mild DKA: VS q 4 hr × 1 then q shift | VS q shift<br>Accurate weight in kg<br>Accurate height in cm |
| Outcomes | | No cerebral edema, no cardiac arrhythmias, arrest | Maintains/regains weight |
| **IV FLUIDS**<br>Maintenance = 100 × 1st 10 kg + 50 × 2nd 10 kg + 25 × >20 kg | If Moderate to Critical DKA or if Mild DKA and unable to tol. PO then:<br>Bolus: 20 mL/kg LR or NS over first hour<br>Repeat if in hypovolemic shock<br>If Mild DKA and tol. PO then no IV | If Moderate to Critical DKA: 0.45NS 20 mEq Kphos 20 mEq Kacetate<br><br>Rate: $\dfrac{(85\text{mL/kg} + \text{Maint}) - \text{bolus(s)}}{23}$<br><br>Add D5 when glucose <250<br>Add K⁺ if K⁺ drops <3.0 | DC IV if tolerates adequate PO fluids |
| Outcomes | No shock | Neuro status maintained<br>No cardiac arrhythmias/arrest | Hydration maintained |
| **MEDICATIONS** | If Moderate to Critical DKA or if Mild DKA and unable to tol. PO then:<br>Insulin drip 0.1 u/kg<br>Mannitol 1 gm/kg at bedside<br>K⁺ PO/IV if K⁺ <3.0<br>If Mild DKA and able to tol. PO then insulin SQ per MD order | If Moderate to Critical DKA:<br>Insulin drip 0.1 unit/kg until Lytes WNL<br>Mannitol 1 g/kg at bedside until off insulin drip<br>Glucose falls no more than 100 mg/dL/hr | Insulin SQ per MD order (give ½ hour before insulin drip turned off) |
| Outcomes | | No cerebral edema | Electrolyte and acid/base balance maintained |
| **NUTRITION** | If Moderate to Critical DKA: NPO<br>If Mild DKA and able to tol. PO then push sugar-free fluids:<br>(Minimum per age)<br><1: 2 oz/hr × 16 hr<br>1-3: 3 oz/hr × 16 hr<br>>4: 4 oz/hr × 16 hr | If Critical DKA: NPO × 24 hr<br>If Mild to Serious DKA: NPO until Lytes corrected or per Endocrine order only<br>When able to drink: push sugar-free fluids per age guideline | Basic Meal Plan per age<br>Push sugar-free fluids |
| Outcomes | | Neuro status maintained | Nutritional status and hydration maintained |
| **Behavioral/Developmental** | | | |
| **TEACHING** | Assess family knowledge/experience with Type 1 diabetes<br>Assess best way to learn and any barriers to learning (language, literacy)<br>Begin teaching skills with 1st SQ | Once DKA at Mild level RN with:<br>1. *Real Ins and Outs* video<br>2. Family to give 1st SQ dose<br>3. Family to learn blood sugar tests<br>4. Family to learn to test urine ketones<br>5. Basic Meal Plan/Schedule reviewed | On Day 2:<br>1. *Balancing Highs and Lows* video<br>2. High and Low signs/symptoms and treatment<br>3. Continue 2-5 from day 1<br>4. Family to draw mixed insulin |
| Outcomes | Identify Individual learning needs | Parent to do skills on the 1st day: Parent to give 1st SQ | Knowledge: Treatment regimen, daily cares |

From Children's Hospital of Wisconsin. Reprinted with permission.
*Tracked outcome.

*Continued*

**TABLE 1-7** Clinical pathway: type 1 diabetes—cont'd

| Aspect of Care | 1st Hour (First Labs Drawn)<br>Date:     Time start: | Hour 2-24<br>Date:     Time end: | Day 2<br>Date: |
|---|---|---|---|
| **Family** | | | |
| **FAMILY SUPPORT/ COPING** | Prepare family for diagnosis of Type 1 diabetes<br>Consult Diabetes MSW<br>Consult Diabetes CNS | Usual coping methods assessed<br>Developmentally appropriate methods for initiating invasive procedures presented to family | Family support systems assessed<br>Plans for return to work and school assessed |
| Outcomes | Family grief acknowledged (ongoing) | Child and family able to cope with procedures | Child and family plan to return to usual activities |
| **Discharge (System)** | | | |
| **DISCHARGE PLANNING/ PLACEMENT** | If Critical DKA: Intensive care<br>If Moderate to Serious DKA: Hospitalize<br>If Mild DKA: After Lytes correct, no concurrent illness—may arrange for care outpatient | Discharge planning called to order blood sugar meter and home health nursing<br>Follow-up Diabetes Clinic appointment scheduled | Discharge orders to reflect follow up care and plans faxed to Home RN<br>Has blood sugar meter |
| **CONSULTS** | Pediatric Endocrine<br>Clinical Nurse Specialist<br>Pediatric Social Worker<br>Pediatric Dietitian<br>Discharge Planning | | |
| **Safety** | | | |
| **HEALTH AND SAFETY** | | | Up-to-date in immunizations<br>Wears well-fitting shoes<br>Wears helmet when appropriate<br>Use of seatbelts/pads<br>Good oral hygiene<br>Use of sharps container for disposal |
| Outcomes | | | General health care maintained |

It is expected that future payment for health care will be tied to clinical guidelines. This effort will provide encouragement for care to be provided in the most cost-effective manner while ensuring care that is based on guidelines that reflect current research rather than traditional practice.

# Role of the Pediatric Nurse

Pediatric nurses are involved in every aspect of a child's and family's growth and development. Nursing functions vary according to regional job structures, individual education and experience, and personal career goals. Just as clients (children and their families) have unique backgrounds, each nurse brings an individual set of variables that affects the nurse-patient relationship. No matter where pediatric nurses practice, their primary concern is the welfare of the child and family.

## Therapeutic Relationship

The establishment of a therapeutic relationship is the essential foundation for providing quality nursing care. Pediatric nurses need to be meaningfully related to children and their families and yet separate enough to distinguish their own feelings and needs. In a *therapeutic relationship,* caring, well-defined boundaries separate the nurse from the child and family. These boundaries are positive and professional and promote the family's control over the child's health care. Effective family advocacy demands that these boundaries be established (Rushton, McEnhill, and Armstrong, 1996). Both the nurse and the family are empowered, and open communication is maintained. In a

## GUIDELINES
### Exploring Your Relationships with Children and Families

To foster therapeutic relationships with children and families, you must first become aware of your caregiving style, including how effectively you take care of yourself. The following questions should help you understand the therapeutic quality of your professional relationships.

### NEGATIVE ACTIONS

Are you overinvolved with children and their families?
  Do you work overtime to care for the family?
  Do you spend off-duty time with children's families either in or out of the hospital?
  Do you call frequently (either the hospital or home) to see how the family is doing?
  Do you show favoritism toward certain patients?
  Do you buy clothes, toys, food, or other items for the child and family?
  Do you compete with other staff members for the affection of certain patients and families?
  Do other staff members comment to you about your closeness to the family?
  Do you attempt to influence families' decisions rather than facilitate their informed decision making?
Are you underinvolved with children and families?
  Do you restrict parent or visitor access to children, using excuses such as the unit is too busy?
  Do you focus on the technical aspects of care and lose sight of the person who is the patient?
Are you overinvolved with children and underinvolved with their parents?
  Do you become critical when parents don't visit their children?
  Do you compete with parents for their children's affection?

### POSITIVE ACTIONS

Do you strive to empower families?
  Do you explore families' strengths and needs in an effort to increase family involvement?
  Have you developed teaching skills to instruct families rather than doing everything for them?
  Do you work with families to find ways to decrease their dependence on health care providers?
  Can you separate families' needs from your own needs?

---

Data from Barnsteiner J, Gillis-Donovan J: Being related and separate: a standard for therapeutic relationships, *MCN* 15(4):223-228, 1990; Fochtman D: Therapeutic relationships, *J Pediatr Oncol Nurs* 8(1):1-2, 1991 (editorial); and Fochtman D: Commitment, *J Pediatr Oncol Nurs* 8(3):103-104, 1991 (editorial).

Do you strive to empower yourself?
  Are you aware of your emotional responses to different people and situations?
  Do you seek to understand how your own family experiences influence reactions to patients and families, especially as they affect tendencies toward overinvolvement or underinvolvement?
  Do you have a calming influence, not one that will amplify emotionality?
  Have you developed interpersonal skills in addition to technical skills?
  Have you learned about ethnic and religious family patterns?
  Do you communicate directly with persons with whom you are upset or take issue?
  Are you able to "step back" and withdraw emotionally, if not physically, when emotional overload occurs, yet remain committed?
  Do you take care of yourself and your needs?
  Do you maintain clear, open communication?
  Do you periodically interview family members to determine their current issues (e.g., feelings, attitudes, responses, wishes), communicate these findings to peers, and update records?
  Do you avoid relying on initial interview data, assumptions, or gossip regarding families?
  Do you ask questions if families are not participating in care?
  Do you assess families for feelings of anxiety, fear, intimidation, worry about making a mistake, a perceived lack of competence to care for their child, or fear of health care professionals' overstepping their boundaries into family territory or vice versa?
  Do you explore these issues with family members and provide encouragement and support to enable families to help themselves?
  Do you keep communication channels open among self, family, physicians, and other care providers?
  Do you resolve conflicts and misunderstandings directly with those who are involved?
  Do you clarify information for families or seek the appropriate person to do so?
Do you recognize that from time to time a therapeutic relationship can change to a social relationship or an intimate friendship?
  Are you able to acknowledge the fact when it occurs and understand why it happened?
  Can you ensure that there is someone else who is more objective and can take your place in the therapeutic relationship?

---

*nontherapeutic relationship* these boundaries are blurred, and many of the nurse's actions may serve personal needs, such as a need to feel wanted and involved, rather than the family's needs. For example, in the home care setting, several factors challenge the maintenance of clear boundaries. The informal environment, the casual social conversations among family members, the participation by family members in the care of the child, and the attempt by some families to incorporate the home care nurse into the family all present major challenges to the establishment of clear boundaries.

Exploring whether relationships with patients are therapeutic or nontherapeutic helps nurses to identify problem areas early in their interactions with children and families. (See Guidelines box.) Although questions for exploring types of involvement can be labeled negative or positive, no one action makes a relationship therapeutic or nonthera-

peutic. For example, a nurse may spend additional time with the family but still recognize his or her own needs and maintain professional separateness. An important clue to nontherapeutic relationships is the staff's concerns about their peer's actions with the family.*

### Family Advocacy/Caring

Although nurses are responsible to themselves, the profession, and the institution of employment, their primary responsibility is to the consumer of nursing services—the child and family. The nurse must work with family members, iden-

---

*For information on one hospital's guidelines for establishing therapeutic relationships between nurses and children and families, contact Jane H. Barnsteiner, PhD, RN, FAAN, Director of Nursing Practice and Research, Children's Hospital of Philadelphia, 34th and Civic Center Blvd, Philadelphia, PA 19104-4399, (215) 590-3147; e-mail: barnsteiner@email.chop/edu.

tify *their* goals and needs, and plan interventions that best meet the defined problems. As an advocate, the nurse assists children and their families in making informed choices and acting in the child's best interest. Advocacy involves ensuring that families are aware of all available health services, informed adequately of treatments and procedures, involved in the child's care, and encouraged to change or support existing health care practices. The United Nations Declaration of the Rights of the Child (Box 1-5) provides guidelines for nursing practice to ensure that every child receives optimum care. The nurse uses this knowledge to adapt care for the child's optimum physical and emotional well-being.

As nurses care for children and families, they must demonstrate *caring*, expressing compassion and empathy for others. Aspects of caring embody the concept of atraumatic care and the development of a therapeutic relationship with clients. Parents perceive caring as a sign of quality nursing care, which is often focused on the nontechnical needs of the child and family. Parents describe "personable" care as actions by the nurse that include acknowledging the parent's presence, listening, making the parent feel comfortable in the hospital environment, involving the parent and child in the nursing care, showing interest and concern for their welfare, showing affection and sensitivity to the parent and child, communicating with them, and individualizing the nursing care. Parents perceive "personable" nursing care as being integral to establishing a positive relationship.

The nurse is aware of the needs of children and works with all caregivers to ensure that these fundamental requirements are met. This often necessitates that the nurse expand the boundaries of practice to less traditional settings. The nurse may be involved in education, political or legislative change, rehabilitation, screening, administration, and even engineering and architecture. Regardless of how removed from direct patient care individual nurses become, they continue to foster health care practices that promote the well-being of children by incorporating knowledge of child growth and development into particular roles of practice. For example, as educators, nurses are responsible for helping others learn about and care for children. Their audience may be other nurses, parents, schoolteachers, other members of the health team, or the community.

## Disease Prevention/Health Promotion

Current trends in health care have focused on prevention of illness and maintenance of health rather than treatment of disease or disability. Nursing has kept pace with this change, especially in the area of child care. In 1965, specialized *pediatric nurse practitioner (PNP)* programs began to develop and have led to several specialized ambulatory or primary care roles for nurses. The thrust of these programs has been to educate nurses beyond the basic preparational stage in areas of child health maintenance so that all children can receive high-quality care. The practitioner programs have expanded to prepare numerous types of specialized PNPs in areas such as school health care, acute care, and oncology. Although the curriculum varies, the course content generally includes history taking, physical diagnosis, growth and development, health education, pharmacology, counseling, common childhood problems, and planning care for individuals and groups. Programs are now part of graduate nursing education.

The *clinical nurse specialist (CNS)* role was developed in an attempt to provide expert nursing care. In addition, the CNS serves as a role model for the staff's clinical practice, as a researcher to validate nursing observations and interventions, as a change agent within the health care system, and as a consultant and teacher to the health care team. The CNS is competent in providing nursing care during all stages of illness or wellness and functions in many settings where patients may be found—the hospital, home, community, clinic, or long-term facility. The CNS role has developed within each of the traditional specialty areas and includes subspecialties such as cardiovascular, oncologic, and neurologic pediatric CNS. The educational preparation includes a graduate degree in nursing. Several graduate programs now combine the PNP and CNS roles. Although the title for the merged roles varies, these nurses are commonly called *advanced nurse practitioners (ANPs or ARNPs)*.

Every nurse involved with child care must practice preventive health care. Regardless of the identified problem, the role of the nurse is to plan care that fosters every aspect of growth and development. Based on a thorough assessment process, problems related to nutrition, immunizations, safety, dental care, development, socialization, discipline, or schooling often become obvious. Once the problem is identified, the nurse acts to intervene directly or to refer the family to other health care providers or agencies.

The best approach to prevention is education and anticipatory guidance. In this text each chapter on health promotion includes sections on anticipatory guidance. An appreciation of the hazards or conflicts of each developmental period enables the nurse to guide parents regarding childrearing practices aimed at preventing potential problems. One of the most significant examples is safety. Because each age-group is at risk for special types of injuries, preventive teaching can help prevent most injuries, thus significantly lowering permanent disability and mortality rates from injuries.

Prevention also involves less obvious aspects of child care. Besides preventing physical disease or injury, the nurse's role is also to promote mental health. For example, it is not sufficient to administer immunizations without regard for the psychologic trauma associated with the proce-

---

**Box 1-5** ■ ■ ■
**United Nations' Declaration of the Rights of the Child**

All children need the following:
To be free from discrimination
To develop physically and mentally in freedom and dignity
To have a name and nationality
To have adequate nutrition, housing, recreation, and medical services
To receive special treatment if handicapped
To receive love, understanding, and material security
To receive an education and develop his or her abilities
To be the first to receive protection in disaster
To be protected from neglect, cruelty, and exploitation
To be brought up in a spirit of friendship among people

dure. Optimum health care involves providing care with a humane approach; the nurse and all other health care professionals must ensure that "humane care" is provided.

## Health Teaching

Health teaching is inseparable from family advocacy and prevention. Health teaching may be a direct goal of the nurse, such as during parenting classes, or may be indirect, such as helping parents and children understand a diagnosis or medical treatment, encouraging children to ask questions about their bodies, referring families to health-related professional or lay groups, supplying patients with appropriate literature, and providing anticipatory guidance.

Health teaching is often one area in which nurses need preparation and practice with competent role models because it involves transmitting information at the child's and family's level of understanding and desire for information. As an effective educator, the nurse focuses on providing the appropriate health teaching with generous feedback and evaluation to promote learning.

## Support/Counseling

Attention to emotional needs requires support and, sometimes, counseling. The role of child advocate or health teacher is supportive by the very nature of the individualized approach. Support can be offered in the following ways: listening, touching, and physical presence. Touching and physical presence are most helpful with children because they facilitate nonverbal communication.

Counseling involves a mutual exchange of ideas and opinions that provides the basis for mutual problem solving. It involves support, teaching, techniques to foster the expression of feelings or thoughts, and approaches to help the family cope with stress. Optimally, counseling not only helps resolve a crisis or problem but also enables the family to attain a higher level of functioning, greater self-esteem, and closer relationships. Although counseling is often the role of nurses in specialized areas, counseling techniques are discussed in various sections of this text to help students and nurses cope with immediate crises and refer families for additional professional assistance.

## Restorative Role

The most basic of all nursing roles is the restoration of health through caregiving activities. Nurses are intimately involved with meeting the physical and emotional needs of children, including feeding, bathing, toileting, dressing, security, and socialization. Although they are responsible for instituting physicians' orders, they are also held singularly accountable for their own actions and judgments, regardless of written orders.

A significant aspect of restoration of health is continual assessment and evaluation of physical status. Indeed, the concentrated focus throughout the text on physical assessment, pathophysiology, and scientific rationale for therapy serves to assist the nurse in decision making regarding health status. The nurse must be aware of normal findings in order to intelligently identify and document deviations. In addition, the pediatric nurse never loses sight of the emotional and developmental needs of the individual child, which can significantly influence the course of the disease process.

## Coordination/Collaboration

The nurse, as a member of the health care team, collaborates and coordinates nursing services with the activities of other professionals. Working in isolation does not serve the child's best interest. The concept of "holistic care" can be realized only through a unified interdisciplinary approach. Being aware of individual contributions and limitations to the child's care, the nurse must collaborate with other specialists to provide high-quality health services. Failure to recognize limitations can be nontherapeutic at best and destructive at worst. For example, the nurse who feels competent in counseling but who is really inadequate in this area may not only prevent the child from dealing with a crisis but may also impede future success with a qualified professional.

Even nurses who practice in isolated geographic areas widely separated from other health professionals cannot be considered independent. Every nurse works interdependently with the child and family, collaborating on needs and interventions so that the final care plan is one that truly meets the child's needs. Unfortunately, this aspect of collaboration and coordination frequently is lacking in health care planning. Numerous disciplines often work together to formulate a comprehensive approach without consulting with clients regarding their ideas or preferences. The nurse is in a vital position to include consumers in their care, either directly or indirectly, by communicating their thoughts to the health care team.

## Ethical Decision Making

Ethical dilemmas arise when competing moral considerations underlie various alternatives. Parents, nurses, physicians, and other health care team members may reach different but morally defensible decisions by assigning different weight to competing moral values. These competing moral values may include *autonomy*, the patient's right to be self-governing; *nonmaleficence*, the obligation to minimize or prevent harm; *beneficence*, the obligation to promote the patient's well-being; and *justice*, the concept of fairness (Cornelison, 1998; Salvatore and Baxter, 1998). Nurses must determine the most beneficial or least harmful action within the framework of societal mores, professional practice standards, the law, institutional rules, religious traditions, the family's value system, and the nurse's personal values.

When ethical conflicts occur, nurses may experience conflicting loyalties to their profession, colleagues, patients and families, institutions, and society. Moreover, the nurse's role in ethical decision making can be ambiguous. A nurse may be obliged to carry out procedures that are based on physician orders or hospital policy but inconsistent with the patient's best interest. At times, members of the health care team do not seek the nurse's input or involvement, leaving the nurse with incomplete information about the clinical situation or without a voice in decision making.

The role of nurses as members of the health care team justifies their participation in collaborative ethical decision making. Nurses routinely use a systematic problem-solving method known as the *nursing process* to resolve clinical problems. Each decision requires the nurse to collect pertinent physiologic and psychosocial data, assess relevant values held by the patient and family, and incorporate these data into a plan of care. Each of these activities is a crucial component of ethical decision making.

Furthermore, because nurses spend the most time directly caring for the child, they are in a unique position to provide insight about the patient's condition and response to therapy. In addition, they assist families in dealing with their grief and stress and often interpret information regarding the child's condition, prognosis, and treatment options to help families make informed decisions. Because of their relationship to families, nurses are often able to represent the child's and parents' values, beliefs, and preferences, thus serving as an important liaison for communication between the family and other health care team members.

Participation in ethical decision making requires knowledge of ethical theory and principles, as well as skills in moral reasoning, communication, and group processes. Nurses have an individual responsibility to clarify their personal values and beliefs and to be informed about contemporary ethical thinking; legal, institutional, and public policy; and professional guidelines.

The nurse also uses the professional code of ethics for guidance and as a means for professional self-regulation. The Code of Ethics for Nurses by the American Nurses' Association (ANA) focuses on the nurse's accountability and responsibility to the client and emphasizes the nursing role as an independent professional, one that upholds its own legal liability (Box 1-6).

Nurses must prepare themselves systematically for collaborative ethical decision making. This can be accomplished through formal coursework, continuing education, contemporary literature, and working to establish an environment conducive to ethical discourse. Moreover, nurses must be knowledgeable about mechanisms for dispute resolution, case review by ethics committees, procedural safeguards, state statutes, and case law.

Nurses may face ethical issues regarding patient care, such as the use of lifesaving measures for very-low-birth-weight newborns or the terminally ill child's right to refuse treatment. They may struggle with questions regarding truthfulness, balancing their rights and their responsibilities in caring for children with AIDS, whistle-blowing, or resource allocation. Throughout the text such dilemmas are addressed in boxes entitled Evidence-Based Practice. Conflicting ethical arguments are presented to help nurses clarify their value judgments when confronted with sensitive issues.

### Research

Practicing nurses should contribute to research because they are the individuals observing human responses to health and illness. Unfortunately, few nurses systematically record or analyze such observations. For example, pediatric nurses devise innovative methods to encourage children to comply with treatments. If these interventions are clinically evaluated and shared with other nurses in research publications, nursing practice can be based primarily on science, not tradition or trial and error.

The current emphasis on measurable outcomes to determine the efficacy of interventions (often in relation to the cost) demands that nurses know whether clinical interventions result in positive outcomes for their clients. This demand has influenced the current trend toward *evidence-based practice,* which implies questioning *why* something is effective and *if* there is a better approach. The concept of evidence-based practice also involves analyzing and translating published clinical research into the everyday practice of nursing. When nurses base their clinical practice on science and research and document their clinical outcomes, they will be able to validate their contributions to health, wellness, and cure, not only to their patients, third-party payers, and institutions but also to the nursing profession (Freda, 1998). Evaluation is essential to the nursing process, and research is one of the best ways to accomplish this.

### Health Care Planning

In recent years the nurse's role has expanded beyond the nucleus of the family. As a change leader with world class standards of excellence, the nursing role has expanded and

---

**Box 1-6** ◼ ◼ ◻
## Code of Ethics for Nurses: Provisions

The ANA House of Delegates approved these nine provisions of the new *Code of Ethics for Nurses* at its June 30, 2001 meeting in Washington, DC. In July, 2001, the Congress of Nursing Practice and Economics voted to accept the new language of the interpretive statements, resulting in a fully approved revised *Code of Ethics for Nurses With Interpretive Statements.*

1. The nurse, in all professional relationships, practices with compassion and respect for the inherent dignity, worth, and uniqueness of every individual, unrestricted by considerations of social or economic status, personal attributes, or the nature of health problems.
2. The nurse's primary commitment is to the patient, whether an individual, family, group, or community.
3. The nurse promotes, advocates for, and strives to protect the health, safety, and rights of the patient.
4. The nurse is responsible and accountable for individual nursing practice and determines the appropriate delegation of tasks consistent with the nurse's obligation to provide optimum patient care.
5. The nurse owes the same duties to self as to others, including the responsibility to preserve integrity and safety, to maintain competence, and to continue personal and professional growth.
6. The nurse participates in establishing, maintaining, and improving health care environments and conditions of employment conducive to the provision of quality health care and consistent with the values of the profession through individual and collective action.
7. The nurse participates in the advancement of the profession through contributions to practice, education, administration, and knowledge development.
8. The nurse collaborates with other health professionals and the public in promoting community, national, and international efforts to meet health needs.
9. The profession of nursing, as represented by associations and their members, is responsible for articulating nursing values, for maintaining the integrity of the profession and its practice, and for shaping social policy.

From American Nurses' Association/Center for Ethics and Human Rights, *www.ana.org/ethics/chcode.htm.*

now includes the *community-based health-driven system.* Traditionally, nurses have been involved in public health care either on a continuous or an episodic basis. Rarely, however, have nurses been involved in health care planning, especially on a political or legislative level. Nurses must incorporate a political component into their professional role identity and must also affect the decision-making body of government (Brown, 1996).* As the largest health care profession, nursing needs to have a voice, especially as a family and consumer advocate. This suggests a knowledge and awareness of community needs, an interest in government formulation of bills, support of politicians to ensure passage (or rejection) of significant legislation, and active involvement in groups dedicated to the welfare of children, (e.g., professional nursing societies, parent-teacher organizations, parent support groups, religious organizations, and voluntary organizations).

Health care planning involves not only providing new services but also promoting the highest quality of existing ones. Nursing needs to ensure the excellence of its own profession through each individual member, who practices according to the Code of Nurses and standards of practice. A *standard of practice* is the level of performance that is expected of a professional. Pediatric nurses are obligated to follow the Standards of Maternal and Child Health Nursing (Box 1-7) and specific standards for their specialty, such as pediatric oncology nursing or school nursing.† They should also be involved in making certain their colleagues implement these standards through education, role modeling, and supervision.

Throughout the text the highest standards of nursing practice are continually reflected in the emphasis on thorough assessment, focus on scientific rationale as the basis for care, summary of nursing care goals and responsibilities, and comprehensive discussion of growth and development. Family-centered principles are continually evident in the consideration of dynamics that affect the child, parents, siblings, and extended members. The nurse is viewed as a vital component of the health care delivery system.

## Future Trends

The present shift in focus from treatment of disease to promotion of health will expand nurses' roles in ambulatory care, with prevention and health teaching receiving a major emphasis. As prospective payment becomes more obvious in pediatric care, the need for home care and community health services will require nurses to be more independent and highly skilled beyond the traditional care settings. Both of these trends are illustrated throughout the book, with increased emphasis on prevention through anticipatory guidance, child health and family assessment, discharge planning,

and care in the home and community. As changing social policy shapes the expanding health care arena, the focus of nursing care is no longer what we *do for* families, but rather what we *do in partnership with* them (Plotnick and Presler, 1996). Therefore the philosophy of family-centered care and community care is no longer an option, but a mandate.

Technologic advances related to patient care, as well as the demand for computer knowledge in the work setting, are obvious. As more positions are created that do not require a nursing background, such as "patient care educator" and unlicensed assistive personnel, nurses will be required to continually update their knowledge and prove their unique contribution.

In an era of restructuring, reengineering, and downsizing, nurses must examine their role in relation to the health care system. Traditionally, the focus of nursing practice was *provider of care* for the purpose of promotion, maintenance, and restoration of health. Today, there is an expansion of that historical focus to *manager of care,* which requires a shift in thinking and different skills. If the profession of nursing takes the lead in the redesign of health care delivery, nurses can shift from task performance to a truly collaborative practice. This collaborative practice requires working with and through others from a broad systems perspective to delegate appropriate tasks with knowledge, understanding, and confidence (White and Begun, 1996). One aspect of collaborative practice is the use of *unlicensed assistive personnel (UAPs),* "individuals who are trained to function in an assistive role to the registered professional nurse in the provision of [student] care activities as delegated by and under the supervision of the registered professional nurse" (American Nurses' Association, 1994).

---

**Box 1-7** ■ ■ ■
**American Nurses' Association Standards of Maternal and Child Health Nursing Practice**

**Standard I:** The nurse helps children and parents attain and maintain optimum health.
**Standard II:** The nurse assists families to achieve and maintain a balance between the personal growth needs of individual family members and optimum family functioning.
**Standard III:** The nurse intervenes with vulnerable clients and families at risk to prevent potential developmental and health problems.
**Standard IV:** The nurse promotes an environment free of hazards to reproduction, growth and development, wellness, and recovery from illness.
**Standard V:** The nurse detects changes in health status and deviations from optimum development.
**Standard VI:** The nurse carries out appropriate interventions and treatment to facilitate survival and recovery from illness.
**Standard VII:** The nurse assists clients and families to understand and cope with developmental and traumatic situations during illness, childbearing, childrearing, and childhood.
**Standard VIII:** The nurse actively pursues strategies to enhance access to and utilization of adequate health care services.
**Standard IX:** The nurse improves maternal and child health nursing practice through evaluation of practice, education, and research.

From American Nurses' Association: *Standards of maternal and child health nursing practice,* Washington, DC, 1983, The Association. (As of this writing, unrevised and out of print.)

---

*The following are sources of information on government issues: White House Comment Line, (202) 456-1111, 9 am-5 pm EST; White House fax: (202) 456-2461; White House e-mail: president@whitehouse.gov.

†Available from the **Association of Pediatric Oncology Nurses,** 4700 W Lake Ave, Glenview, IL 60025-1485, (847) 375-4724, fax: (877) 734-8755, and the **National Association of School Nurses,** Lamplighter Lane, PO Box 1300, Scarborough, ME 04074, (207) 883-2117; www.nasn.org.

An essential element for the safe and effective use of UAPs is the nurses' ability to appropriately delegate activities to these individuals (Box 1-8). Future implications for nursing practice include developing strategies to improve the supervision of UAPs (Bernreuter and Cardona, 1997).

> **NURSING ALERT** When the RN determines that someone who is not licensed to practice nursing can apparently safely provide a selected nursing activity or task for a patient and delegates that activity to the individual, the RN remains legally responsible and accountable for the care provided.

Changing demographics will also impact pediatric nursing. Although the actual number of children under age 18 years will increase from 64.3 million in 1990 to an estimated 78 million in 2020, their relative importance in terms of proportion of the total population will decrease from 26% to 24%. In other words, the adult population is growing faster than the pediatric population. Accompanying this trend is a decrease in younger children and an increase in older children, as well as a decrease in the white population with an increase in minority groups. For example, white births are expected to decline, black births are projected to rise, and the largest increases will occur in Hispanic and Asian births. Such changes will impact the delivery of health care, with problems of adolescents and minority groups taking on more significance. As the elderly make up a larger percentage of the population, health care dollars will be split between the youngest and the oldest groups, with shrinking resources having to meet the needs of both. Nurses will need to keep abreast of developments in adolescent medicine and continually adapt their care to the cultural milieu in which they practice. An ever-present challenge will be cost containment without sacrificing quality care.

---

**Box 1-8** ■ ■ ■
### The Five Rights of Delegation

**RIGHT TASK**
One that is delegable for a specific patient

**RIGHT CIRCUMSTANCES**
Appropriate patient setting, available resources, and other relevant factors considered

**RIGHT PERSON**
Right person delegating the right task, to the right person, to be performed on the right person

**RIGHT DIRECTION AND COMMUNICATION**
Clear, concise description of the task, including its objective, limits, and expectations

**RIGHT SUPERVISION**
Appropriate monitoring, evaluation, intervention (as needed), and feedback

Modified from the National Council State Boards of Nursing, 1995.

---

## CRITICAL THINKING AND THE PROCESS OF NURSING CHILDREN AND FAMILIES
### Critical Thinking

A systematic thought process is essential to a profession. It assists the professional in meeting the needs of the client. *Critical thinking* is purposeful, goal-directed thinking that assists individuals to make judgments based on evidence rather than guesswork (Alfaro-LeFevre, 1995). It is based on the scientific method of inquiry, in which the nursing process also has its roots. Critical thinking and the nursing process are considered crucial to professional nursing in that they comprise a holistic approach to problem solving.

Critical thinking is a complex developmental process based on rational and deliberate thought. Becoming a critical thinker provides a common denominator for knowledge that exemplifies disciplined and self-directed thinking. The knowledge is acquired, assessed, and organized by thinking. The cognitive skills used in high-quality thinking require intellectual discipline, self-evaluation, counterthinking, opposition, challenge, and support (Paul, 1993). Critical thinking transforms the ways in which individuals view themselves, understand the world, and make decisions.

Crucial dimensions of critical thought include the perfections of thought, the elements of thought, and the domains of thought. A logical connection develops between the elements and the problem at hand when thinking is clear, precise, accurate, relevant, consistent, and fair. Self-evaluation questions that enhance the development of critical thinking are listed in Box 1-9 (Paul, 1993).

In recognition of the importance of this skill, Critical Thinking Exercises have been included in this text. These exercises present a nursing practice situation that challenges the student to use the skills of critical thinking to come to the best conclusion. The student is led by self-evaluation questions (see Box 1-9) to make a rational and deliberate response based on self-directed thinking. The critical thinking skills used in formulating the best response include intellectual discipline, self-evaluation, reflection, and counterthinking. The benefit of these thinking exercises is that they may enhance nursing performance in clinical judgment.

---

**Box 1-9** ■ ■ ■
### Critical Thinking Self-Evaluation Questions

☐ What is the purpose of my thinking?
☐ What precise questions am I trying to answer?
☐ Within what point of view am I thinking?
☐ What information am I using?
☐ How am I interpreting that information?
☐ What concepts or ideas are central to my thinking?
☐ What conclusions am I coming to?
☐ What am I taking for granted, and what assumptions am I making?
☐ If I accept the conclusions, what are the implications?
☐ What would the consequences be if I put my thoughts into action?

From Paul R: *Critical thinking: what every person needs to survive in a rapidly changing world*, Rohnert Park, CA, 1993, Foundation for Critical Thinking.

# Nursing Process

The nursing process is a method of problem identification and problem solving that describes what the nurse actually does. The five-step model that is accepted as the nursing process is as follows: assessment, diagnosis (problem identification), planning (with outcome development), implementation, and evaluation. The second step of the nursing process, nursing diagnosis, is the naming of the child's or family's problem in common nursing language. The American Nurses' Association has established Standards of Care (use of the nursing process) and Standards of Professional Performance (professional behavior) (Box 1-10). In the Standards of Care, the nursing diagnosis phase of the nursing process is separated into two steps: the nursing diagnosis and outcome identification. This model therefore represents a six-step process.

## Assessment

Assessment is a continuous process that operates at all phases of problem solving and is the foundation for decision making. It uses multiple nursing skills and consists of the purposeful collection, classification, and analysis of data from a variety of sources. To provide an accurate and comprehensive assessment, the nurse must consider information about the patient's biophysical, psychologic, sociocultural, and spiritual background.

## Nursing Diagnosis

The second stage of the nursing process is problem identification and nursing diagnosis. At this point the nurse must interpret and make decisions about the data gathered. The nurse organizes or clusters these data into categories to identify significant areas and makes one of the following decisions:

- **No dysfunctional health problems** are evident; no interventions are indicated.

- **Risk for dysfunctional health problems** exists; interventions are needed to facilitate health promotion.
- **Actual dysfunctional health problems** are evident; interventions are needed to facilitate health promotion.

The nursing diagnosis is the naming of the cue clusters that are obtained during the assessment phase. The North American Nursing Diagnosis Association's (NANDA's) currently accepted definition of the term *nursing diagnosis* is that it is a clinical judgment about individual, family, or community responses to actual and potential health problems and life processes. Nursing diagnoses provide the basis for selection of nursing interventions to achieve outcomes for which the nurse is accountable (Carroll-Johnson, 1991).

Both NANDA and Marjory Gordon (2000) have developed frameworks or classification systems for nursing diagnoses. NANDA bases its framework on 9 *human response patterns,* and Gordon bases hers on 11 *functional health patterns* (Box 1-11; see also Appendix E).

The nursing diagnosis is composed of three components: problem, etiology, and signs and symptoms (often referred to as *PES*). The first component—the *problem statement*—describes the child's response to health pattern deficits in the child, family, or community. This is the patient's response to disturbances of life processes, patterns, functions, or development, including those occurring secondary to disease.

Not all children will have actual health problems. Some will have a potential health problem, which is a risk state that requires nursing intervention to prevent the development of an actual problem. Potential health problems indicate the presence of *risk factors* (signs indicating a potential health problem), which predispose a child and family to a dysfunctional health pattern and are limited to individuals at greater risk than the population as a whole. Intervention is directed toward reducing risk factors. To differentiate actual from potential health problems, the word *risk* is included in the nursing diagnosis statement (e.g., *Risk for infection*).

---

## Box 1-10 ■ ■ ■
### American Nurses' Association Standards for Practice

**STANDARDS OF CARE (USE OF THE NURSING PROCESS)**

Standard

 I **Assessment:** The nurse collects client health data.

 II **Diagnosis:** The nurse analyzes assessment data and determines diagnoses.

 III **Outcome Identification:** The nurse identifies expected outcomes individualized to the patient.

 IV **Planning:** The nurse develops a plan of care that prescribes interventions to attain expected outcomes.

 V **Implementation:** The nurse implements the interventions identified in the plan of care.

 VI **Evaluation:** The nurse evaluates the patient's progress toward attainment of outcomes.

**STANDARDS OF PROFESSIONAL PERFORMANCE (PROFESSIONAL BEHAVIOR)**

Standard

 I **Quality of Care:** The nurse systematically evaluates the quality and effectiveness of nursing practice.

 II **Performance Appraisal:** The nurse evaluates his or her own nursing practice in relation to professional practice standards and relevant statutes and regulations.

 III **Education:** The nurse acquires and maintains current knowledge and competency in nursing practice.

 IV **Collegiality:** The nurse interacts with and contributes to the professional development of peers and other health care providers as colleagues.

 V **Ethics:** The nurse's decisions and actions on behalf of patients are determined in an ethical manner.

 VI **Collaboration:** The nurse collaborates with the patient, family, and other health care providers in providing patient care.

 VII **Research:** The nurse uses research findings in practice.

 VIII **Resource Utilization:** The nurse considers factors related to safety, effectiveness, and cost in planning and delivering client care.

From American Nurses' Association: *Standards of clinical nursing practice,* ed 2, Washington, DC, 1998, American Nurses' Publishing, American Nurses' Foundation.

---

**Box 1-11** ▪ ■ ▫
## Classification Systems
## for Nursing Diagnoses

### HUMAN RESPONSE PATTERNS*

**Exchanging**—Involves mutual giving and receiving
**Communicating**—Involves sending messages
**Relating**—Involves establishing bonds
**Valuing**—Involves the assigning of relative worth
**Choosing**—Involves the selection of alternatives
**Moving**—Involves activity
**Perceiving**—Involves the reception of information
**Knowing**—Involves the meaning associated with information
**Feeling**—Involves the subjective awareness of sensation or affect

### FUNCTIONAL HEALTH PATTERNS†

**Health perception–health management pattern**—Perceptions related to general health management and preventive practices
**Nutritional-metabolic pattern**—Intake of food and fluids related to metabolic requirements
**Elimination pattern**—Regularity and control of excretory functions: bowel, bladder, skin, and wastes
**Activity-exercise pattern**—Activity patterns that require energy expenditure and provide for rest
**Sleep-rest pattern**—Effectiveness of sleep and rest periods
**Cognitive-perceptual pattern**—Adequacy of language, cognitive skills, and perception related to required or desired activities; includes pain perception
**Self-perception–self-concept pattern**—Beliefs and evaluation of self-worth
**Role-relationship pattern**—Family and social roles, especially parent-child relationships
**Sexuality-reproductive pattern**—Problems or potential problems with sexuality or reproduction
**Coping–stress tolerance pattern**—Stress tolerance level and coping patterns, including support systems
**Value-belief pattern**—Values, goals, or beliefs that influence health-related decisions and actions

---

*Modified from the North American Nursing Diagnosis Association; *Nursing diagnoses: definitions and classifications, 1999-2000*, Philadelphia, 1999, NANDA.
†Modified from Gordon M: *Manual of nursing diagnosis*, ed 9, St Louis, 2000, Mosby.

---

## FAMILY FOCUS
### Using Defining Characteristics to Select an Appropriate Nursing Diagnosis

An 18-month-old only child is admitted with respiratory distress and a presumptive diagnosis of epiglottitis. Initial nursing actions are focused on the physiologic status of the child. As the condition stabilizes, family assessment data are gathered. The child's immunizations are current, he is clean and well nourished, and his developmental age is appropriate. The parents are present at admission. Both are employed, and the child is cared for by the maternal grandparents. The mother is distraught about the sudden onset of the respiratory distress. She states that earlier just a "runny nose" was present. She asks appropriate questions and seems to understand that epiglottitis is a sudden illness that typically follows symptoms of a cold. She asks what she can do to make her child more comfortable and less fearful, and she is able to implement the suggestions. The father supports both the child and the mother but assumes a more passive, "listening" role.

At least three nursing diagnoses that relate to family and parent situations can be considered. The first step is to review the definition and defining characteristics for each and decide which is most appropriate for this family:

**Altered parenting**—Inability of nurturing figure to create an environment that promotes optimum growth and development of another human being
*Selected defining characteristics:*
    Inattentive to infant/child needs
    Inappropriate caretaking behaviors
**Family coping: potential for growth**—Family member has effectively managed adaptive tasks involved with client's health challenge and is exhibiting desire and readiness for enhanced health and growth in regard to self and in relation to client
*Selected defining characteristics:*
    Family member attempts to describe growth impact or crisis on own values, priorities, goals, or relationships
**Altered family process**—Inability of family system (household members) to meet needs of members, carry out family functions, or maintain communication for mutual growth and maturation
*Selected defining characteristics:*
    Inability of family members to relate to each other for mutual growth and maturation
    Failure to send and receive clear messages
    Inability to accept and receive help

Among these choices, the most appropriate nursing diagnosis is *Family coping: potential for growth*. The parents are attentive to the child's needs and appear to have appropriate caregiving skills. The sudden illness of the child has disrupted the family's pattern, but the mother demonstrates effective coping and the ability to learn and implement new comforting skills. The other two diagnoses require some maladaptive feature, which is not found in this situation.

---

The second component, the *etiology,* describes the physiologic, situational, and maturational factors that cause the problem or influence its development. The etiology is written using NANDA diagnostic categories (e.g., *Noncompliance related to powerlessness*). In using the PES format, it is important that the nurse not link the problem statement and etiology with words that imply cause and effect. Etiologies are probable causes; using words that imply cause and effect can result in legal or professional difficulties. Although a direct cause-effect relationship may not be involved, the etiology does influence the problem. Therefore the phrase *related to* is used to indicate a relationship between the problem and its etiology.

Differentiating among various etiologies is critically important because *interventions to alter the health problem are directed toward the etiology*. This is a primary concept in understanding the nursing process and the PES format. For example, a problem statement of *Noncompliance in dietary restrictions* could have various causal factors, such as (1) knowledge deficit, (2) denial of illness, (3) low economic resources, or (4) cultural conflict. Interventions for a knowledge deficit would be very different from interventions for low economic resources.

The third component, *signs and symptoms,* refers to a cluster of cues and defining characteristics that are derived from patient assessment and indicate actual health problems. When a defining characteristic is essential for the diagnosis to be made, it is considered critical. These critical defining characteristics help differentiate between diagnostic categories. For example, in deciding between the diagnostic categories related to family function and coping, the defining characteristics are critical in choosing the most appropriate nursing diagnosis. (See Family Focus box.)

**TABLE 1-8**  Characteristics of standard and individualized nursing care plans

| | Standard Care Plan* | Individualized Care Plan |
|---|---|---|
| Assessment | Information is specific only to problem | Information is specific to identified problem and to child and family |
| Nursing diagnosis | All probable nursing diagnoses with general etiologic factors are considered | Only nursing diagnoses specific to child and family are considered; cause of disease directs actual plan of care |
| Planning | Goals are broad and represent patient goals | Goals are specific and reflect patient outcomes |
| Implementation | Nursing interventions are broad and are applicable to most patients with problem | Nursing interventions are specific and provide direction for nursing care of individual patient |
| Evaluation | Progress patient is *expected* to make is identified | Progress patient has actually made toward outcome is identified |

*Describes format used in care plans in the text; may differ from other types of standardized nursing care plans.

Nursing diagnoses do *not* describe everything that nursing does. Nursing practice consists of three dimensions: dependent, interdependent, and independent activities. The differences reside in the source of authority for the action. *Dependent activities* are those areas of nursing practice that hold the nurse accountable for implementing the prescribed treatment. *Interdependent activities* are those areas of nursing practice in which nursing responsibility and accountability overlap with other disciplines, such as medicine, and require collaboration between the two disciplines. *Independent activities* are those areas of nursing practice that are the direct responsibility of the nurse.

Throughout the text, Nursing Care Plans incorporate nursing diagnoses that relate to the specific condition or disorder. Because nursing diagnoses should prescribe only those interventions that nurses can perform independently or interdependently, nursing interventions related to medical management are identified by an asterisk.

### Planning

Once the nursing diagnoses have been identified, a plan of care is developed, and outcomes or goals are established. The *outcome* is the projected change in a patient's health status, clinical condition, or behavior that occurs after nursing interventions have been instituted. The ultimate goal of nursing care is to convert the nursing diagnoses into a desired health state. The plan must be established before the interventions are developed and implemented.

The end point of the planning phase is the development of the nursing plan of care. The care plans in this text provide guidelines for the care of children and families with a particular problem and are standard care plans as opposed to individualized care plans (Table 1-8). *Standard care plans* are sufficiently broad to account for situations that may develop in patients with particular problems. For this reason, the care plans often have numerous nursing diagnoses, both expected and potential. These possible nursing diagnoses guide patient observation and data collection in monitoring the development of adverse reactions.

*Individualized care plans* are concerned with only those diagnoses that apply to the particular patient situation. In actual practice not all the problems presented in a standard care plan may be relevant. When a standard nursing care plan is used to develop an individualized plan of care, problems not pertinent to the situation are eliminated, and the outcomes are individualized to the specific situation. To help the reader develop an individualized care plan, the

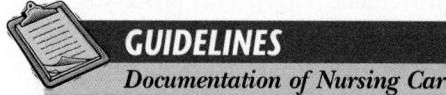

## GUIDELINES
### Documentation of Nursing Care

Initial assessments and reassessments
Nursing diagnoses and patient care needs
Interventions identified to meet the patient's nursing care needs
Nursing care provided
Patient's response to, and the outcomes of, the care provided
Abilities of patient and, as appropriate, significant other(s) to manage continuing care needs after discharge

nursing diagnoses in the text are listed in order of priority. In general, potential problems are discussed toward the end of the plan, except in instances in which nursing interventions are essential in preventing a potential problem from becoming an actual problem.

### Implementation

The implementation phase begins when the nurse puts the selected intervention into action and accumulates feedback regarding its effects. The feedback returns in the form of observation and communication and provides a database on which to evaluate the outcome of the nursing intervention. Throughout the implementation stage, the patient's physical safety and psychologic comfort in terms of atraumatic care are the main concerns.

### Evaluation

Evaluation is the last step in the decision-making process. The nurse gathers, sorts, and analyzes data to determine if (1) the goal has been met, (2) the plan requires modification, or (3) another alternative should be considered. Observation guidelines are included in the standard care plans to help the reader identify methods for evaluating whether the goals or outcomes are achieved. The evaluation stage either completes the nursing process or serves as the basis for the selection of other alternatives for intervention in solving the specific problem.

### Documentation

Although documentation is not one of the five steps of the nursing process, it is essential for evaluation. The nurse can assess and identify problems, plan, and implement without documentation; however, evaluation is best performed with written evidence of progress toward outcomes. The patient's medical record should include evidence of those elements listed in the Guidelines box.

The nursing process has become an integral part of professional practice. The **Joint Commission on Accreditation of Healthcare Organizations (JCAHO)** has incorporated the nursing process into the accreditation process. The first standard on which nursing service is evaluated states that individualized, goal-directed nursing care is provided to patients through the use of the nursing process. The JCAHO accredits many types of health care providers such as hospitals, nursing homes, ambulatory services, and home health agencies. Organizations that refuse or fail accreditation are unable to receive federal funds, such as Medicare or Medicaid.

Another focus area for JCAHO accreditation is the use of **continuous quality improvement (CQI).** This process is an ongoing review of systems, problem identification, and resolution that allows the institution to establish and maintain quality care (Sullivan and Decker, 1997). JCAHO standards change over time. In 2000, new standards addressing the issues of pain assessment and management were added.*

Currently the attention in health care is also focused on patient outcomes. Criteria have been established for changes that should occur in the patient as a result of interactions with the health care team. At discharge the care is evaluated to ensure that the outcomes were met.

---

*The **Joint Commission on Accreditation of Healthcare Organizations (JCAHO)** has established a toll-free hotline (800) 994-6610 to encourage patients, their families, caregivers, and others to share concerns regarding quality of care issues at accredited health care organizations. Complaints (may be anonymous) may be sent to the Office of Quality Mentoring, Joint Commission, One Renaissance Blvd, Oakbrook Terrace, IL, 60181; fax: (630) 792-5636; e-mail: complain@jcaho.org; www.jcaho.org

## KEY POINTS

- *Healthy People 2010* broadened the health care objectives achieved in the 1990s and focuses on prevention as the method of achieving its goals.
- Although the infant mortality rate in the United States is at an all-time low, the United States lags significantly behind most other major countries, such as Canada.
- Low birth weight, which is closely related to early gestational age, is considered the leading cause of neonatal death in the United States.
- Injuries are the leading cause of death in children over age 1 year, with the majority being MV injuries.
- Childhood morbidity encompasses acute illness, chronic disease, and disability.
- Eighty percent of childhood illnesses are attributable to infections, with respiratory infections occurring two to three times as often as all other illnesses combined.
- The "new morbidity" refers to behavioral, social, and educational problems that can significantly alter a child's health.
- Developmental stage and environment are important determinants in the prevalence of injuries at a given age and thus help to direct preventive measures.
- Two strategies for injury prevention in children are (1) *passive,* which provides automatic protection by product and environmental design; and (2) *active,* which persuades people to change their behaviors for increased self-protection.
- During the first half of the 1900s, public health initiatives, such as environmental strategies to control infection and the development of antibiotics, were the major advances leading to decreased childhood deaths.
- During the latter half of the 1900s, the advancement and application of medical knowledge and technology, specifically in the care of high-risk and low-birth-weight newborns, lowered the number of deaths in children, especially the neonatal mortality rate.
- The work of Lillian Wald, a social reformer, has had far-reaching effects on child health and nursing. She started

visiting nurse services in New York City and was instrumental in establishing the role of the full-time school nurse.
- The philosophy of family-centered care recognizes the family as the constant in a child's life and that service systems and personnel must support, respect, encourage, and enhance the strength and competence of the family.
- Atraumatic care is the provision of therapeutic care in settings, by personnel, and through the use of interventions that eliminate or minimize the psychologic and physical distress experienced by children and their families in the health care system.
- Managed care is a health care delivery system that attempts to balance cost and quality through a network of health care providers and predetermined payment for services.
- The pediatric nurse's roles include a therapeutic relationship, family advocacy, disease prevention and health promotion, health teaching, support and counseling, coordination and collaboration, ethical decision making, research, and health care planning.
- With the shift in focus from treatment of disease to promotion of health, nurses' roles are expanding outside traditional health care facilities, such as in ambulatory care centers, schools, the family's home, and the community.
- Changing demographics in the United States will result in greater significance of adolescents' and minority groups' problems and decreasing resources for health care.
- Critical thinking is purposeful, goal-directed thinking based on rational and deliberate thought.
- The process of nursing children and families includes accurate and comprehensive *assessment,* analysis and synthesis of assessment data to arrive at a *nursing diagnosis, planning* of care, *implementation* of the plan, and *evaluation* of interventions.

# REFERENCES

Alfaro-Lefevre R: *Applying nursing process,* Philadelphia, 1995, JB Lippincott.

Altemeirer WA: Prevention of pediatric injuries: so much to do, so little time, *Pediatr Ann* 29(6):324-325, 2000.

American Nurses' Association: *Registered professional nurses and unlicensed assistive personnel,* Washington, DC, 1994, American Nurses' Publishing.

American Nurses' Association: *Nursing's social policy statement,* Washington, DC, 1995, American Nurses' Publishing.

Annie E Casey Foundation: *Kids count data book: state profiles of child well-being,* Washington, DC, 2001, Center for the Study of Social Policy.

Barkin S, Fink A, Gelberg L: Predicting clinician injury prevention counseling for young children, *Arch Pediatr Adolesc Med* 153:1226-1231, 1999.

Bernreuter ME, Cardonna S: Survey and critique of studies related to unlicensed assistive personnel from 1975 to 1997, Part 2, *JONA* 27(7/8):49-55, 1997.

Brown SG: Incorporating political socialization theory into baccalaureate nursing education, *Nurs Outlook* 44(3):120-123, 1996.

Carroll-Johnson RM, editor: *Classification of nursing diagnoses: proceedings of the Ninth Conference,* North American Nursing Diagnosis Association (NANDA), Philadelphia, 1991, JB Lippincott.

Cornelison AH: A profile of ethical principles, *J Pediatr Nurs* 13(6):383-386, 1998.

Curley M: Effects of the nursing mutual participation model of care on parental stress in the pediatric intensive care unit, *Heart Lung* 17(6):682-688, 1988.

Curley M, Wallace J: Effects of the nursing mutual participation model of care on parental stress in the pediatric intensive care unit: a replication, *Pediatr Nurs* 7(6):377-385, 1992.

David and Lucille Packard Foundation: Children and managed health care, Executive Summary, *Future Child* 8(2, summer/fall):2-7, 1998.

Faber M: A review of efforts to protect children in car crashes, *Fam Community Health* 9(3):25-41, 1986.

Foss R: Sociocultural perspective on child occupant protection, *Pediatrics* 80(6):886-893, 1997.

Freda MC: Toward evidence-based practice, *MCN* 23:177, 1998.

Fry-Bowers EK: Community violence: its impact on the development of children and implications for nursing practice, *Pediatr Nurs* 23(2):117-121, 1997.

Gordon M: *Manual of nursing diagnosis,* ed 9, St Louis, 2000, Mosby.

Graham CJ and others: Left-handedness as a risk factor for unintentional injury in children, *Pediatrics* 92(6):823-826, 1993.

Guyer B and others: Annual summary of vital statistics—1998, *Pediatrics* 104(6):1229-1245, 1999.

Guyer B and others: Annual summary of vital statistics: trends in the health of Americans during the 20th century, *Pediatrics* 106(6):1307-1317, 2000.

Hostler S: Personal communication. In Johnson BH, Jeppson ES, Redburn L: *Caring for children and families: guidelines for hospitals,* Bethesda, MD, 1992, Association for the Care of Children's Health.

Hoyert DL and others: Annual summary of vital statistics: 2000, *Pediatrics* 108(6):1241-1255, 2001.

Ikeda RM and others: Trends in fatal firearm-related injuries, United States, 1962-1993, *Am J Prev Med* 13(5):396-400, 1997.

Johnson BH, Jeppson ES, Redburn L: *Caring for children and families: guidelines for hospitals,* Bethesda, MD, 1992, Association for the Care of Children's Health.

Jones FC: Community violence, children and youth: considerations for programs, policy, and nursing roles, *Pediatr Nurs* 23(2):131-137, 1997.

Lears MK, Guth KJ, Lewandowski L: International adoption: a primer for pediatric nurses, *Pediatr Nurs* 24:578-586, 1998.

Loubiala PJ and others: Day-care centers and diarrhea: a public health perspective, *J Pediatr* 131:476-179, 1997.

MacDorman MF, Atkinson JO: Infant mortality statistics from the 1997 period linked birth/infant death data set, *National Vital Statistics Reports,* vol 47, no 23, Hyattsville, MD, 1999, National Center for Health Statistics.

MacPhee M, Hoffenberg E: Nursing case management for children with failure to thrive, *J Pediatr Health Care* 10(2):63-73, 1996.

Minino AM, Smith BL: Deaths: preliminary date for 2000, *National Vital Statistics Reports* vol 49, no 12, Hyattsville, MD, 2001, National Center for Heatlh Statistics.

Mofenson HC, Greensher J: Injury prevention. In Hoekelman RA: *Primary pediatric care,* ed 3, St Louis, 1997, Mosby.

Murphy SL: Deaths: final data for 1998, *National Vital Statistics Reports,* vol 48, no 11, Hyattsville, MD, 2000, National Center for Health Statistics.

National Center for Health Statistics: *Health, United States, 1996-1997, and injury chartbook,* Hyattsville, MD, 1997, US Department of Health and Human Services.

National Safety Council: *Injury facts,* Itaska, IL, 2000, National Safety Council.

Newton MS: Family-centered care: current realities in parent participation, *Pediatr Nurs* 26(2):164-168, 2000.

Nyman G: Infant temperament, childhood accidents, and hospitalizations, *Clin Pediatr* 26(8):398-404, 1987.

Paul R: *Critical thinking: what every person needs to survive in a rapidly changing world,* Rohnert Park, CA, 1993, Foundation for Critical Thinking.

Plotnik J, Presler B: Rugged individualism and compassion: the foundation of public policy, *MCN* 21(1):20-33, 1996.

Rushton CH, McEnhill M, Armstrong L: Establishing therapeutic boundaries as patient advocates, *Pediatr Nurs* 22(3):185-189, 1996.

Salvatore T, Baxter T: *Administrative ethics: a guide for home care providers,* Springfield, PA, 1998, HCMA.

Sullivan EJ, Decker PJ: *Effective leadership and management in nursing,* ed 4, Menlo Park, CA, 1997, Addison-Wesley-Longman.

Szilagy P: Managed care for children: effect on access to care and utilization of health, *Future Child* 8(2, summer): 39-60, 1998.

White KR, Begun JW: Profession building in the new health care system, *Nurs Adm Q* 20(3):79-85, 1996.

Wong D: Principles of atraumatic care. In Feeg V, editor: *Pediatric nursing: forum on the future: looking toward the 21st century,* Pitman, NJ, 1989, Anthony J Jannetti.

Chapter **2**

# Social, Cultural, and Religious Influences on Child Health Promotion

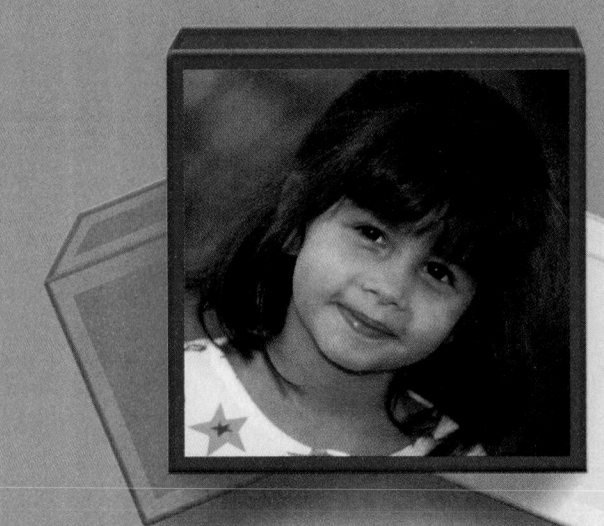

## Chapter Outline

**CULTURE, 30**
**The Child and Family in North America, 31**
**Social Roles, 32**
    Primary- and Secondary-Group
        Influences, 32
**Cultural Shock, 33**
**SUBCULTURAL INFLUENCES, 34**
**Ethnicity, 34**
**Minority-Group Membership, 35**
**Social Class/Occupation, 35**
    Affluence, 35
    Middle and Upper Class, 36
    Lower and Working Class, 36
    Intellectual Skills, 36
    Communication Skills, 36
    Aspirations, 37

Schools, 37
    Socialization, 37
**Peer Cultures, 37**
**Biculture, 38**
**Mass Media, 38**
    Reading Materials, 39
    Movies, 39
    Television, 39
**SOCIOECONOMIC INFLUENCES, 40**
**Poverty, 40**
**Homelessness, 41**
**Migrant Families, 42**
**CULTURAL INFLUENCES, 42**
**Cultural Relativity, 43**
**Relationships with Health Care Providers, 43**
    Communication, 44
**Food Customs, 45**

**HEALTH BELIEFS AND PRACTICES, 47**
**Health Beliefs, 47**
    Natural Forces, 47
    Supernatural Forces, 47
    Imbalance of Forces, 48
**Health Practices, 48**
**Folklore Related to Prenatal Influences, 49**
**Importance of Culture to Nurses, 50**
**CULTURAL AWARENESS, 51**
**HEREDITARY FACTORS, 51**
**Physical Characteristics, 57**
**RELIGIOUS INFLUENCES, 57**
**Religious Beliefs, 57**

## Related Topics

Communicating with Families Through an
    Interpreter, Ch. 6
Family Influences on Child Health
    Promotion, Ch. 3

Lactose Intolerance, Ch. 13
Nutritional Assessment, Ch. 6
Sickle Cell Anemia, Ch. 35
Skin, Ch. 7

Toddler, Ch. 14; Preschooler, Ch. 15; School-
    Age Child, Ch. 17; Adolescent, Ch. 19
Vegetarian Diets, Ch. 13

## CULTURE

The future of any society depends on its children. Therefore society must provide for their care, nurture, and socialization. Culture plays a critical role in the socialization agenda of children through particular views of parenting and child development (Yoos and others, 1995). The customs and values of the culture help to organize a society's childrearing system and are transmitted from one generation to the next through the medium of the family.

Culture is the context of the child's experience of health and illness, wellness and sickness (Talabere, 1996). A holistic view of any child requires that nurses develop some understanding of the ways that culture contributes to the development of social and emotional relationships and influences childrearing practices and attitudes toward health.

*Transcultural nursing* knowledge has become imperative because of the increased migration of people worldwide. Professional nurses are providing care to diverse populations from almost every point of the globe. This orientation to transcultural nursing includes an awareness of the nurse's own frame of reference. With a conscious effort to recognize and appreciate the views and beliefs of health care recipients, nurses can provide culturally competent nursing care (Phillips and Lobar, 1995; Yoos and others, 1997).

*Culture* is a pattern of assumptions, beliefs, and practices that unconsciously frames or guides the outlook and decisions of a group of people (Buchwald and others, 1994). Culture differs from both race and ethnicity. *Race* is defined as a division of mankind possessing traits that are transmissible by descent and that are sufficient to characterize it as a distinct human type. *Ethnicity* is the affiliation of a set of persons who share a unique cultural, social, and linguistic heritage. *Socialization* is the process by which children acquire the beliefs, values, and behaviors of a given society in order to function within that group.

Culture is a complex whole in which each part is interrelated (Spector, 2000). A culture is composed of individuals who share a set of values, beliefs, practices (language, dress, diet, health care), social relationships, law, politics, economics, and norms of behavior that are learned, integrative, social, and satisfying (Habayeb, 1995). Culture is not a surface veneer that covers a basic outlook shared by all human beings but an ingrained orientation to life that serves as a frame of reference for individual perception and judgment. People from one culture differ from those in other cultures in the ways they think, solve problems, perceive, and structure the world. Culture is, essentially, the way of life of a group of people that incorporates experiences of the past, influences thought and action in the present, and transmits these traditions to future group members. Adaptation is necessary, however, for the culture to survive in an ever-changing world. Consciously and unconsciously, the members abandon, modify, or assume new patterns to meet the needs of the group.

The observable components of a culture, such as material objects (dress, art, utensils, and other artifacts) and actions, are sometimes termed the *material overt* or *manifest culture; nonmaterial covert culture* refers to those aspects that cannot be observed directly, such as the ideas, beliefs, customs, and feelings of the culture. Related to the large culture are many *subcultures,* each with an identity of its own. Children are socialized into a particular subculture rather than into the culture as a whole. Subcultural influences, such as ethnicity and social class, are discussed in more detail later in this chapter.

The culture in which children are reared determines the type of food they will eat, the language they will speak, the ideals of behavior they will follow, and the way they will conduct themselves in social roles (Yoos and others, 1995). To be acceptable members of the culture, children must learn how the culture expects them to behave toward others in the group. In turn, they learn how they can expect others to behave toward them.

Cultures and subcultures contribute to the uniqueness of child members in such a subtle way and at such an early age that children grow up to feel that their beliefs, attitudes, values, and practices are the "correct," or "normal" ones; those of other cultures may be viewed as "deviant" or "wrong." A set of values learned in childhood is apt to characterize children's attitudes and behavior for life, guiding their long-range strivings and monitoring their short-range, impulsive inclinations. Thus every ongoing society socializes each succeeding generation to its cultural heritage.

The manner and sequence of the growth and development phenomenon are universal and fundamental features of all children; however, the variations in behavioral responses that children display to similar events are believed to be determined by their culture. Inborn temperament and modes of behavior that prompt children to behave in their own preferred and highly individual manner may be in harmony or in conflict with the culture. Such forces as heredity and maturation impose limits on the influence that parents and other social groups may bring to bear.

The culture fosters and reinforces those behaviors deemed desirable and appropriate; it attempts to depress or extinguish those at conflict with cultural norms. Some cultures encourage aggressive behaviors in their children; others favor amiability and compliance. Some foster individual resourcefulness and competition; others emphasize cooperation and submission to group interest. The child from a culture that values cooperation will not respond to a challenge such as, "I'll bet you can get dressed faster than Johnny can," whereas a child from a culture that emphasizes individual achievement will be stimulated by the challenge.

Cultures may also differ in whether status in the group is based on age or on skill. Even children's play and their types of games are culturally determined. In some cultures children play in groups composed of members of the same sex; in others they play in mixed-sex groups. In some cultures team games predominate; in others most play is limited to individual games.

Standards and norms vary from culture to culture and from location to location; a practice that is accepted in one area may meet with disapproval or create tension in another. The extent to which cultures tolerate divergence from the established norm varies among cultures and subcultural groups. Although conformity provides a degree of security, it is a decided deterrent to change.

## The Child and Family in North America

America's orientation toward homogenization—"the great melting pot"—is changing. Increased awareness of the growing proportion of ethnic minorities that make up the U.S. population, coupled with a new positive value and emphasis being placed on ethnic diversity, has resulted in a renewed interest in cultural variation.

The frontier background of the American culture has contributed to the overall orientation to life and childrearing. There has always been a basic optimistic view of the world, a belief that things can be better and that the children can and will be better off than the parents. This hopeful outlook and a general future orientation, together with the possibility of upward social mobility, have created a pervasive overall attitude of optimism. Increasing development of self-confidence and autonomy in children is fostered and encouraged. Children are generally permitted a greater degree of freedom than in more tradition-oriented cultures, where individuals remain in one social class for life.

Family life in North America is characterized by increasing geographic and economic mobility. There is less reliance on tradition, families are fragmented, and there is limited opportunity to transmit and acquire the traditional and accepted customs of a culture. Consequently, young adults rely to a greater extent on the professed experts, peers, and the mass media for acquisition of acceptable patterns of behavior, including childrearing practices. Conflicting information can be a source of confusion and frustration as parents attempt to determine the comparatively stable, essential components of the culture and transmit these to their children.

Children in North America grow up with a number of adults who differ from one another but who all provide input as role models, teachers, and standards for behavior. Most children live in some form of nuclear family located in sharply differentiated neighborhoods determined by income and ethnic status within a highly technical, largely urban society. Class differences in childrearing persist, but they are becoming less divergent as a result of the increased homogeneity of the culture.

Studies have indicated that early in life children become aware of their racial or ethnic status and of the discriminatory attitudes of the majority culture toward their group. The direct effects of discrimination are anger and low self-esteem, which become manifest in a variety of behaviors. Inner conflicts and suppressed hostility that focus children's attention inward may be factors in the failure of many children to achieve in other areas.

Evidence indicates that changes in attitudes are slowly taking place in some groups and in some places. *Cultural pluralism* supports the rights of group differences and promotes a mutual respect for the existence of cultural differences (Culley, 1996). With growing awareness, interest, and understanding by increasing numbers of the majority group, which have accompanied the recent emergence of racial and ethnic pride, minority-group children are becoming more secure and confident in their racial or ethnic identity. Individuals vary in their reactions to membership in a minority group, and much of this variation can be attributed to familial factors. As with all children, the most important influences on development of a positive self-image are warm, understanding parents who take an active interest in fostering their children's growth. Parents who accept their children and react positively and constructively rather than in a negative and self-defeating manner will help their children develop feelings of self-worth, self-esteem, and self-acceptance. The more adequate children feel, the more positive will be their attitudes toward both majority and minority children, the greater will be their ability to withstand prejudice and intolerance, and the less will be their need for counteraggressive behavior.

## Social Roles

Much of children's self-concept is derived from their ideas about their social roles. *Roles* are cultural creations; therefore the culture prescribes patterns of behavior for persons in a variety of social positions. All persons who hold similar social positions have an obligation to behave in a particular manner. A role prohibits some behaviors and allows others. Because it delineates and clarifies roles, the culture is a significant influence on the development of children's self-concept (i.e., attitudes and beliefs they have about themselves).

A social group consists of a system of roles carried out in both primary and secondary groups. A *primary group* is characterized by intimate, continued face-to-face contact, mutual support of members, and the ability to order or constrain a considerable proportion of individual members' behavior. Two such groups are the family and the peer group, both of which exert a great deal of influence on the child.

*Secondary groups* are groups that have limited, intermittent contact and in which there is generally less concern for members' behavior. These groups offer little in terms of support or pressure toward conformity except in rigidly limited areas. Examples of secondary groups are professional associations and social organizations such as church groups (also considered in relation to subgroups).

A concept of social role also depends largely on whether a child is reared in a primary- or secondary-group community. Children are subjected to perceptively different forms of parental training in these two types of environments.

### Primary- and Secondary-Group Influences

Children are reared within a primary-group environment and within a secondary-group environment. The influences, strengths, and limitations of both groups are significant. In a primary-group community (e.g., family, peer group, some contemporary rural, religious, or ethnic communities), all members know each other, most belong to the same subgroups, and all are concerned about each member's behavior. There is a high degree of material and psychologic support among the community members, and because there is one traditional set of values that the entire group agrees on and supports, there is little conflict of values. In a stable community where the members remain within comparatively defined limits and relatives are likely to live close together, young members have ample opportunity to observe and absorb the practices and customs of the culture. Any member of the community feels justified in evaluating and censuring the conduct of another member.

Children reared in the relative isolation of secondary-group environmental influences tend to learn that there is only one acceptable way to respond to any given situation. The entire group agrees, and any tendency to deviate is met with collective disapproval. It is the parents' duty to see that the children learn and adhere to social roles and modes of behavior defined and strengthened by the views of the community.

The childrearing orientation in a secondary-group environment, such as urban communities, can differ considerably from that of a primary-group environment. The interaction between primary and secondary groups may serve to reinforce values when both groups endorse that value, or create confusion or conflict when one group rejects a value accepted by the other. An urban community is dynamic and rapidly changing. Many of the traditional behaviors and values may not meet the needs of the changing society. Consequently, parents are often uncertain about what to teach their children. They may wish to rear their children with values consistent with their own, but the differences in experience between the generations are too great. As a result, they often grant their children autonomy in some areas of decision making early in the developmental process, and other secondary groups assume a greater influence. The children are exposed to an assortment of social groups with diverse sets of values and expectations. None of the groups is highly dominant in its influence; therefore the children are exposed to an eclectic set of values, some in agreement and some at conflict with the others. From these they must ultimately select those that they determine to be best for them and adopt them to form a consistent set of roles and behaviors to be incorporated into the self-concept.

Conditioning children to feel either guilt or shame for misdeeds is a technique used by a culture to control social behavior—to internalize the norms and expectations of others. Some cultural groups value a well-developed conscience (superego) and condition their children to feel *guilt* following wrongdoing. Offenders get an uncomfortable physical feeling and want to purge themselves. Because guilt is based within the individual, successful conditioning produces self-regulated persons who punish themselves without their being caught in the act of wrongdoing.

In many cultural groups guilt is lacking, and social controls are based on the use of shame. Offenders do not want anyone to see them when they have been guilty of wrongful deeds. Sometimes children in these groups learn that anything is acceptable as long as one is not caught; the shame results when the forbidden act is found out by others.

Although both techniques are used by members of both primary- and secondary-group communities, shame is apt to be more successful in a primary-group community because most behaviors are quite public. In secondary-group communities it is less effective; people are not as apt to be caught and, if caught, can withdraw and join a group that is unaware of the misdeed. Guilt probably has a greater influence on behavior in urban communities, although many authorities believe that the trend in urban North America is shifting away from a guilt orientation. Rapid changes in the North American culture leave parents unsure of their own values; therefore much of their function is abandoned to the school and peers. Peers are notorious for using shame as a disciplinary technique.

## Cultural Shock

The term *cultural shock* describes the "feelings of helplessness and discomfort and a state of disorientation experienced by an outsider attempting to comprehend or effectively adapt to a different cultural group because of differences in cultural practices, values, and beliefs" (Leininger, 1978). This state occurs in both clients and health care providers who move from one cultural setting to another. It can happen to persons who immigrate to a new country (such as Asian refugees) or to persons from a subcultural group who must adjust to the ways of an unfamiliar subgroup (such as children entering the school subculture or consumers who enter the hospital subculture). Cultural shock is characterized by the inability to respond to or function in a new or strange situation. (See Critical Thinking Exercise box.)

Numerous factors influence reactions to a new environment. Language barriers, including dialects and jargon (such as medical language) specific to a subcultural group, inhibit effective communication. Habits and customs (such as different role behaviors or etiquette) and differences in attitudes and beliefs are puzzling to the stranger in the new environment. The outsider experiences an intense sense of isolation and feelings of loneliness and nonrelatedness.

Nurses are challenged to overcome culture shock and develop the dynamics of *cultural sensitivity,* an awareness of cultural similarities and differences. In doing so, the nurse is helped to practice *culturally competent* care that goes beyond cultural sensitivity to implementation (Talabere, 1996). Becoming more culturally sensitive will enhance valuable knowledge of various cultural groups. Suggestions

---

### Critical Thinking Exercise

#### Cultural Sensitivity

A woman from the Middle East is visiting her child who is hospitalized for a serious illness. Her husband left for home a short time ago to wash and change clothes. She speaks little English. You need to obtain consent from her for an emergency procedure. She is hesitant and refuses to sign the consent form. What should you do?

FIRST, THINK ABOUT IT . . .

- Within what point of view are you thinking?
- If you accept your conclusions, what are the implications?

---

1. Document that the mother refuses to sign the consent form and inform the physician that the procedure cannot be done.
2. Realize that she may be hesitant to sign for consent without her husband present because her culture requires the man to make the decisions for the welfare of the family members.
3. Explain to her that you cannot help her child unless she signs for permission to do so.
4. Realize that she may not understand what you're saying and try to find an interpreter.

---

*The best response is two. Typically, in the Arab culture the point of view exists that men make the decisions and wives are expected to support those decisions. Trying to find an interpreter or intimidating the mother to sign does not address the main issue of the Arab cultural tradition. The implications may be that in emergency cases treatment is often approved by the institution or state if a physician documents that treatment is necessary and that any delay in treatment may jeopardize the health of the child. In this situation, contacting the father first is appropriate.*

to gain cultural insights include the following (Boyer, 1996; Sekhon, 1996):

- Set a language goal.
- Use note cards when conversing, if necessary.
- Do not be afraid to mix a little English with your new language.
- Start by asking "yes" and "no" questions.
- Tour an ethnic grocery store.
- Have dinner at an ethnic restaurant.
- Attend cultural events and celebrations in your community.

**NURSING ALERT**   Because American cultures and subcultures can be so diverse, it is essential that nurses be aware of and knowledgeable about the predominant groups in their work community and apply the knowledge in their practice.

**NURSING ALERT**   Any generalization made about an ethnic group may not apply to certain groups or individuals.

When minority groups immigrate to another country, a certain degree of cultural and ethnic blending occurs through the involuntary process of *acculturation,* those gradual changes produced in a culture by the influence of another culture that cause one or both cultures to be more similar to the other. However, the changes occur to various degrees in different families and groups. Many groups continue to identify with their traditional heritage while adapting to the ill-defined concept of the "American way." Acculturation may be referred to as *assimilation,* which is the process of developing a new cultural identity (Spector, 2000).

## SUBCULTURAL INFLUENCES

Except in rare situations, children grow and develop in a blend of cultures and subcultures. In a large, complex society such as the United States, different groups have their own set of standards, values, and expectations within the collective ways of the large culture. Most were formed when groups of people clustered together by preference, by external pressures from the majority culture, or by geographic isolation. Although many cultural differences are related to geographic boundaries, subcultures are not always restricted by location.

There are even subcultures related to the age stages of development that have traditions, games, loyalties, and rules. Age-related subcultures are easily identified in the behavior of school-age children and adolescents. The culture is handed down by word of mouth from one "generation" to the next, and its rituals and behavior standards are highly resistant to outside influence.

Children's membership in a cultural subgroup is, for the most part, involuntary. They are born into a family with a specific ethnic and/or racial heritage, socioeconomic level, and religious beliefs. Although in the complex American so-

ciety there are countless subcultures and considerable variation in the way of life, those subcultures which seem to exert the greatest influence on childrearing are ethnicity, social class, and occupational role. In addition, schools and peer-group subcultures are strong influences in the socialization of the child.

### Ethnicity

*Ethnicity* is the classification of or affiliation with any of the basic groups or divisions of mankind or any heterogeneous population differentiated by customs, characteristics, language, or similar distinguishing factors. Ethnic differences extend to many areas and include such manifestations as family structure, language, food preferences, moral codes, and expression of emotion. Some standards of behavior result from the cultural heritage of the specific ethnic group (e.g., the traditional role of the father). Others reflect the interaction between subcultures, most notably between members of the majority culture and a minority subculture. The term *ethnic* has aroused strong negative feelings and is often rejected by the general population (Spector, 2000).

To establish their place in the group, children learn how to adhere to a mode of behavior that is in accordance with standards distinctive to the group and learn how they can expect others to behave toward them. They take their cues from observing and imitating those to whom they are exposed. For example, children of a racial minority form a perception of their role as a group member by observing the manner in which role models within the subgroup respond to treatment by people outside the subgroup. When they see group members display an attitude of inferiority, they assume this to be the appropriate behavior. These perceptions are then incorporated into their own self-concept.

In the United States the cross-cultural lines are becoming blurred as subcultures are assimilated and blended into the larger culture (Fig. 2-1). Although ethnic differences in childrearing are probably diminishing, they remain important. It is particularly difficult for persons to attempt to maintain an identity with a subculture while living and conforming to the requirements of the larger culture. Universal customs and language of the dominant culture used in commercial and educational systems are different from those of the minority culture. Often the values are in conflict. Consequently, children reared in this environment are confused about roles and values, and they usually adopt those of the more influential or higher-status culture. Youth, in particular, are influenced by the locally dominant group.

*Ethnocentrism* is the emotional attitude that one's own ethnic group is superior to others; that one's values, beliefs, and perceptions are the correct ones; and that the group's ways of living and behaving are the best way (Williams and Kruse, 1999). *Ethnic stereotyping* or labeling stems from ethnocentric views of people. Ethnocentrism implies that all other groups are inferior and that their ways are not in the best interests of the group. It is a common attitude among a dominant ethnic group and strongly influences the ability of one person to evaluate the beliefs and behaviors of oth-

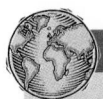

## CULTURAL AWARENESS
### Classification of Minority Groups

According to the 1990 U.S. Census Group Profiles, African-Americans are referred to as **blacks** and defined as "any persons whose lineage included ancestors who originated from any of the black racial groups of Africa." An **Asian** or **Pacific Islander** is any person with "origins in any of the original peoples of the Far East, Southeast Asia, the Indian subcontinent, or the Pacific Islands." Native Americans are referred to as **American Indians** and **Alaskan Natives** and defined "as persons having origins in the original peoples of North America, and who maintain cultural identification through tribal affiliations or community recognition." **Hispanics** are defined as "persons of Mexican, Puerto Rican, Cuban, Central or South American, or other Spanish culture or origin, regardless of race." The term **Latino** is often used to describe individuals in this group (Council of Economic Advisors, 1998).

ers objectively. This inherent viewpoint of individuals tends to bias their interpretation and understanding of the behavior of others. Nurses must overcome the natural tendency to have ethnocentric attitudes when giving care to people from different cultures (Williams and Kruse, 1999).

## Minority-Group Membership

The United States has more racial, ethnic, and religious minority groups than any other country as a result of high immigration rates and high birth rates among these groups. Ethnic minority groups are becoming increasingly important because it is anticipated that these groups will produce children at a faster rate than will the majority white population. Consequently, the minority population is increasing while the majority white population is decreasing. The term *cultural diversity* refers to the differences that exist among these various groups of people (Talabere, 1996).

Blacks are the largest minority group, followed closely by Hispanics. Currently, Hispanics are the fastest growing minority in the United States and have many health needs that are not being met (Warda, 2000). By the year 2010, Hispanics will surpass non-Hispanic African-Americans as the largest U.S. racial or ethnic group. In 2050, 22% of the U.S. population is expected to be Hispanic (Council of Economic Advisors, 1998). (See Cultural Awareness box.)

## Social Class/Occupation

Although there are exceptions, probably the greatest influence on childrearing practices and their consequences is the social class of the family into which a child is born. Differences in childrearing goals and practices, as well as attitudes toward health, have been found to be greater between social classes than between races or ethnic groups. In North America, social class and socioeconomic level are essentially synonymous and are most easily determined by occupation; for example, the upper middle class consists primarily of professional and business people, almost all with a college education. The working class includes employees in manufacturing, trades, and service occupations (such as barbers or hairdressers) who have a high

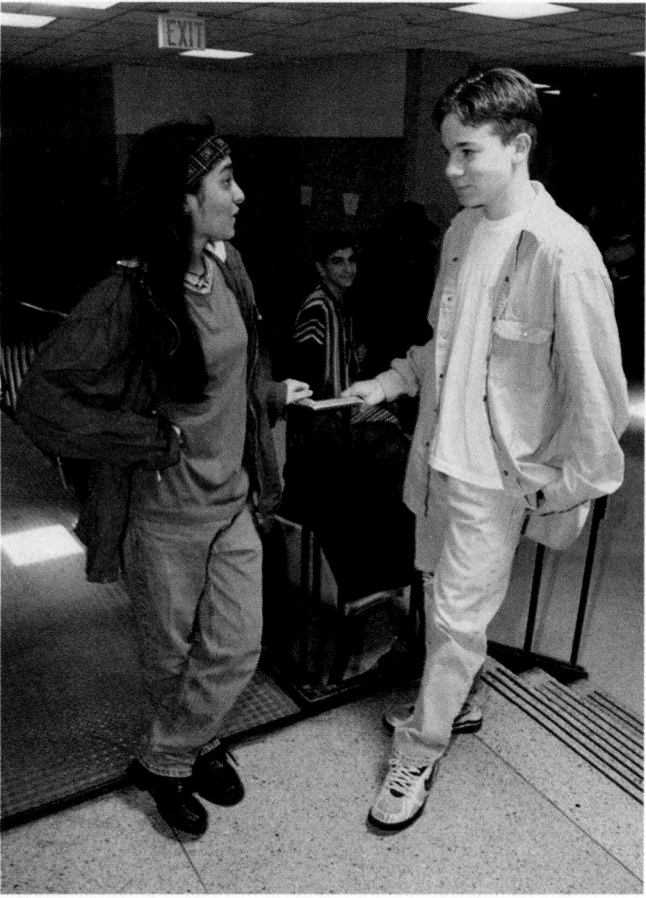

**Fig. 2-1**  Youngsters from different cultural backgrounds interact within the larger culture.

school education. In the lower class the breadwinners are typically unskilled laborers or unemployed families who may or may not be on public assistance. Children are reared differently by parents who vary in education, occupation, and income levels, so their social class can be expected to produce substantial variation in their upbringing.

### Affluence

On the far end of the socioeconomic spectrum are the children of affluent members of society. Although they can live within the warmth of a positive family relationship, many of them appear to be just as deprived as poverty-stricken children. Wealth does not provide protection against many of life's problems and disappointments, especially in the area of parent-child relationships. Like their counterparts in the poverty groups, children of the affluent may suffer from discrimination, inadequate parenting, or unsatisfactory role models.

Children of the wealthy suffer most from lack of parental contact. There may be long separations from loving, caring parents because of social or business interests. Some have a cold, sometimes hostile parent who is rarely available to them. Even their places of residence contribute to their isolation and loneliness. Paid parent surrogates, including servants, sports professionals (such as tennis or swimming instructors), and private school personnel, provide them with adult companionship and authority. During the early years many wealthy children form stronger attachments to these people than to their parents. However, as the children grow older, they become aware of class distinctions. They realize that they must separate from these early relationships to form bonds with individuals in their class. Parents may begin involving the older adolescent in the family business and in adult social activities. But for many young people a meaningful life with their family has come too late, and they feel lonely, isolated, and unloved.

Many children from wealthy families, like those from poor families, seem to thrive and flourish, making positive contributions to their families and society. However, some grow up to display a lack of motivation or self-discipline, and boredom. They are suspicious of others, finding it difficult to believe they are liked for themselves and not for their money or position, and they do not trust others enough to enter into true friendships. Affluent children may also fail to acquire skills to handle responsibility and money.

### Middle and Upper Class

Children from these classes live in an enriched environment that provides material comforts and broader opportunities. The parents are usually educated beyond high school and have occupations that require judgment, creativity, and resourcefulness. These attributes are fostered in their children. Other authority figures such as teachers with whom the children are routinely in contact are usually from a middle-class background and have activities and expectations for the children that are similar to those of the parents.

Most middle-class parents are future oriented, have higher educational and occupational aspirations for their children, and use long-range planning to meet these goals. Middle-class parents typically encourage their children to participate in activities that foster achievements, such as dancing lessons, athletics, and Scouting, in the belief that this will make them well-rounded, self-directed adults.

In the area of discipline, middle-class parents are more apt to use manipulative techniques such as reasoning or drawing on the child's sense of guilt. They tend to scold and use isolation rather than physical punishment. There is more concern regarding the *intent* of the act than the *consequence* of the act.

It is believed that upper-class parents are more permissive and foster desirable behavior through positive reinforcement. However, much of the actual child care in upper-class families is delegated to surrogates, such as housekeepers, governesses, or private schools. The parent serves as an arbitrator between the children and the servants.

### Lower and Working Class

The uncertainty of their life leads members of the lower classes to be present oriented (i.e., to take advantage of gratification when possible). This orientation is distinctly different from that of most members of the middle class, who may be more willing to delay gratification to achieve a long-term goal.

Children in lower-class families encounter major educational disadvantages, reflected in the high incidence of academic failure and attendant dropout rate. Some of the major educational disadvantages many children from the lower social class encounter are related to intellectual and communication skills:

- Parents are more likely to value the concrete and tangible rather than the abstract and are therefore less inclined to encourage the latter in their children.
- Parents are less likely to read to the child or encourage educational play because of their own educational level.
- No role models may be available to support the value of education.
- Inadequate funding and poor quality of education may exist in neighborhood schools.
- Poor health and inadequate nutrition of the children are common.
- Parents are more likely to have limited communication skill, such as simple grammar, inability to express abstractions, and ethnic dialects, which hampers interactions with teachers from middle-class backgrounds.

Parents from lower and working classes are generally tradition oriented, stressing obedience and conformity to parental values and external regulations. The most frequently used form of discipline for undesirable behavior is physical punishment. Parents are usually less concerned with the direction of children's activities than with conduct; they are more concerned that children stay out of trouble.

With better job security through unionization, unemployment compensation, and other welfare features, some segments of the lower classes are finding life more predictable. They are less apt to seize gratifications lest the opportunity vanish and are beginning to develop long-range goals, including an increased interest in education for their children.

### Intellectual Skills

There appear to be differences in intellectual skills and scholastic achievement between children in the upper and middle classes and those in the lower classes. The more apparent differences lie in the areas of abstract thinking and manipulation. Although the relative merits of testing techniques and standards are a matter of question, there is a higher incidence of academic failure in children from the lower class with its attendant dropout rate. In addition, children from the lower classes are often penalized within the school because they do not possess the symbols, attitudes, and behaviors characteristically valued by the dominant class group. There is a social class bias in educative influence. Most teachers come from the middle classes, and school board members are from middle and upper classes.

### Communication Skills

Any concept that occurs to a person can be expressed in language. However, ease of communication and use of language codes vary among the social classes. Language is much more restricted in the lower classes, and the classes are more easily differentiated by grammar than by pronunciation. Persons in the middle classes use different grammar from those in the lower classes and are able to express more complicated ideas; persons in the lower classes use very simple grammar and are less likely to offer explanations.

These communication differences are highly significant in relation to school achievement. School is constructed around the elaborate language codes of the middle class; therefore children from the lower classes must learn these language skills, which places them at a decided disadvantage. This is particularly true for bilingual children and children from ethnic groups who have developed a dialect unique to their own group.

Historically, schools have participated in devaluing Native American languages, cultures, and traditional ways of learning and knowing (Robinson-Zanartu, 1996). Unfortunately, Native American children have been deficient in their preparation for school (Dykeman, Nelson, and Appleton, 1995). Also, children of Native American nations have been "at risk" for low achievement, overrepresentation in special education, and dropping out (Robinson-Zanartu, 1996). Many regional dialects and variations in language usage must be taken into consideration when communicating with persons from these groups. English words that sound like another word in a foreign language can cause considerable misunderstanding.

### Aspirations

Middle-class parents typically are positively oriented toward change, whereas parents in the lower classes tend to remain tradition oriented. Consequently, the lower class tends to emphasize conformity to parental values and external regulations, whereas middle-class parents tend to be more concerned with producing self-directed children. This attitude difference reflects the occupation orientation of the different classes. Middle-class occupations tend to involve more self-direction and getting ahead; lower-class occupations tend to be standardized with direct supervision.

With few exceptions, parents in all classes love their children and in a broad sense have similar goals regarding childrearing. Differences lie in the parental behavior toward the children in attempting to help them to reach these goals. Parents in the lower classes tend to be more restrictive and rely on coercive techniques in child training. They stress obedience and conformity, and the most frequently used form of discipline for undesirable behavior is physical punishment. However, these more punitive strategies can be modified with early intervention.

The very poor, who consistently exist on or below the poverty level, live in a perpetual state of despair. Their limited skills give them no bargaining power in the job market, and the education needed to improve their status is beyond them. The poor desire better things for their children but are trapped in a circular pattern that perpetuates their life condition. Their powerlessness to control their fate or condition is a source of fatalism and resignation that is often characteristic of the group in general. Optimism, when it is manifested, is more likely to be expressed in terms of luck or chance. This fatalistic attitude is a significant impediment to occupational and educational aspirations and to seeking health care. It also inhibits them from seeking health care or practicing preventive health care measures. For example, if

someone is injured or killed in an automobile accident, it is more likely to be considered bad luck, not something that could have been prevented by wearing a seat belt.

## Schools

When children enter school, their radius of relationships extends to include a wider variety of peers and a new focus of authority. Although parents continue to exert the major influence on the children, in the school environment teachers have the most significant psychologic impact on their development and socialization. The function of teachers is primarily limited to teaching, but, like parents, they are concerned about the emotional welfare of the children. Both parents and teachers must constrain behavior, and both are in a position to enforce standards of conduct.

### Socialization

Next to the family the schools exert the major force in providing continuity between generations by conveying a vast amount of culture from the older members to the young. In this way children are prepared to carry out the traditional social roles they are expected to assume as adults in society. School is the center of "cultural diffusion" wherein the cultural standards of the larger group are mediated to the local community. It governs what is taught and, to a large extent, how it is taught. School rules and regulations regarding attendance, authority relationships, and the system of sanctions and rewards based on achievement transmit to the child the behavioral expectations of the adult world of employment and relationships. School is often the only institution in which children systematically learn about the negative consequences of behaviors that deviate from social expectations. In addition, the school provides an opportunity for some children to participate in the larger society in rewarding ways and often provides avenues for social mobility for both students and teachers. Through education individuals in the lower classes are offered the opportunity for further education and the capacity to move up in the social strata.

Teachers have the responsibility for transmitting the knowledge and values of the dominant culture (i.e., those values on which there is broad consensus). They are expected to stimulate and guide the intellectual development of children and their sense of esthetics and to foster their capacity for creative problem solving.

Traditionally the socialization process of school has begun when the child enters kindergarten or first grade. Today, with over 60% of mothers of preschool children working outside the home, this socialization process begins much earlier for a significant number of children in a variety of child care settings.

## Peer Cultures

Peer groups also have an impact on the socialization of children (Fig. 2-2). Peer relationships become increasingly important and influential as children proceed through school. In school, children have what can be regarded as a culture

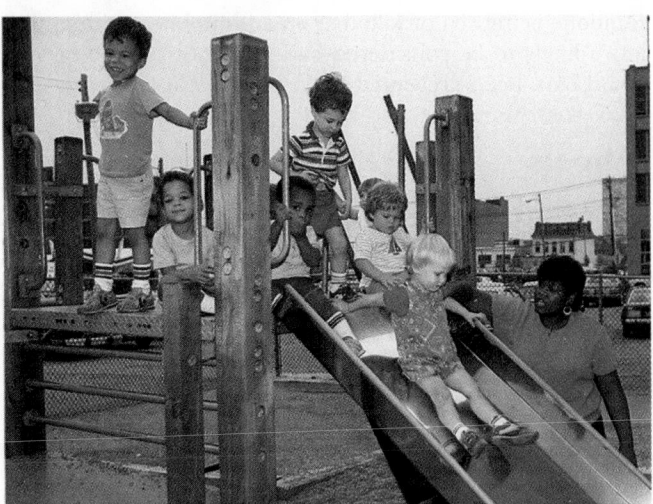

**Fig. 2-2** Children from a variety of cultural and ethnic backgrounds begin to socialize in the child care setting.

of their own. It is most apparent in the school and in the unsupervised play group. The play group presents this culture in a much purer form than does the school, in which the culture is partly produced by adults.

During their lives children are exposed to value systems such as those of the family, ethnic group, and social class. In peer-group interaction they are confronted with a variety of these sets of values. The values imposed by the peer group are especially compelling because children must accept and conform to them in order to be accepted as members of the group. When the peer values are not too different from those of family and teachers, the mild conflict created by these small differences serves to separate children from the adults in their lives and to strengthen the feeling of belonging to the peer group.

The kind of socialization provided by the peer group depends on the special subculture that develops from the background, interests, and capabilities of its members. Some groups support school achievement, others focus on athletic prowess, and still others are decidedly against educative goals. Scholastic achievement is strongly related to the value system of the peer groups. Many conflicts between teachers and students and between parents and students can be attributed to fear of rejection by peers. There is often a conflict between what is expected from parents regarding academic achievement and what is expected from the peer culture. This is especially pronounced in high school and is discussed further in Chapter 19.

Although it has neither the traditional authority of the parents nor the legal authority of the schools for teaching information, the peer group manages to convey a substantial amount of information to its members, especially about taboo subjects such as sex and drugs. Children's need for the friendship of their peers brings them into an increasingly complex social system. The world of the peer group is different from the adult world, and through peer relationships, children learn ways in which to deal with dominance

and hostility and to relate with persons in positions of leadership and authority. Other functions of the peer subculture are to relieve boredom and to provide recognition that individual members do not receive from teachers and other authority figures.

The peer-group culture has secrets, mores, and codes of ethics with which they promote feelings of group solidarity and detachment from adults. They have traditions and folkways that are transferred from "generation to generation" of schoolchildren and that have a great influence over the behavior of all members of the group. There are age-related games and other activities, and as children move from one level to the next, folkways of the younger group are discarded as those of the new are adopted. For example, a school-age child rides a bicycle to school; the high school student prefers a car. As they advance, children are forward oriented only—they look forward with anticipation but may look backward with contempt.

## Biculture

Some children are exposed to the values, role relationships, and lifestyles of two or more cultures. The virtual "straddling" of two cultures is referred to as *biculturation* and involves the ability to efficiently bridge the gap between an individual's culture of origin and the dominant culture (Rogers, 1995). This may occur because the child's parents are from two or more different cultures. In Hawaii, for example, it is common for children to be of four or more cultures. Other children straddle cultures as members of a minority culture within the dominant culture. This biculture is sometimes observed in the play group but usually is not a significant factor until children enter school. Then they must unlearn some of the established practices of one culture in order to become socialized in the other, especially in role relationships. For example, children from Hispanic and Asian cultures are taught to look away when scolded; in U.S. schools the teacher expects direct eye contact—"Look at me when I speak to you." Children learn new roles and social behavior more rapidly than their adult counterparts.

This biculture is particularly marked in language differences. The bilingual child is said to be at a disadvantage in school situations of the dominant culture, in which there is controversy over bilingual education. Those supporting bilingual education adhere to the principle that children will understand more readily and perform more realistically (especially in testing situations) if learning is directed in their own language; others contend that children living in a dominant culture should adopt the ways of that culture, including language. There is less conflict for children when their language and culture are supported by the school, even if the dominant language is used.

## Mass Media

There is no doubt that the media provide children with a means for extending their knowledge about the world in which they live and have contributed to narrowing the differences between classes. However, there is growing concern regarding the enormous influence the media can have on the developing child and on health promotion behaviors.

Links have been established between mass media and an increase in the use of tobacco, alcohol, and violent behavior in adolescents (American Academy of Pediatrics, 2001; Strasburger and Donnerstein, 1999). The images of risky behavior presented by the media may serve to establish or reinforce teenagers' perceptions of their social environment. Also, media content may directly influence risk perception; media protagonists seldom suffer adverse consequences of their behaviors despite their grossly distorted experiences with violence, illness, or crime.

Children may identify closely with people or characters portrayed in reading materials, movies, videos, and television programming and commercials. Another concern is children's unrestricted use of the Internet and electronic mail. Parental supervision of children's access to "cyberspace" is just as essential as supervision of their access to television.

## Reading Materials

The oldest form of mass media—books, newspapers, and magazines—contributes to children's competence in almost every direction and provides enjoyment. Recognition of the impact that reading matter in schools has on the value system and socialization processes has prompted reevaluation of textbook content in several areas: the stereotyped male and female role models, the sugarcoated view of life situations, and the biased history of minority groups.

Fairy tales, for generations the mainstay of young children's literature, for a time suffered condemnation as being sexist, overly violent in content, and riddled with unfavorable stereotypes, such as the wicked stepmother, dwarfs, and physical unattractiveness associated with evil. They are now believed to provide an excellent medium for explaining puzzling and important topics such as death, stepparents, and inner feelings and turmoils. To a young child the world is peopled by giants—adults who control their lives, threaten their autonomy, and want children to do something against their will. Children can see these giants overcome. The split view of parents is also portrayed in fairy tales: the "good" parents who give children whatever they want and the "mean" parents who deprive their children of things. Although they do not provide solutions, fairy tales confront children with emotional predicaments and offer suggestions for dealing with them.

Comic books and other pulp reading material have been popular in every generation, sometimes at the expense of the literature provided by schools, libraries, and parents. Many children have nothing else to read. The easy reading, quick action, and adventure in brief episodes seem to fulfill a need for children who are striving to understand both aggression in others and their own impulses. Reading ability, intelligence, and school adjustment apparently have no relationship to the number and type of comic books read. Most comic books appear to be relatively harmless to the majority of children and are in some ways even beneficial.

Comic books seem to have only a minor influence on the acquisition of beliefs, values, and behaviors of a particular culture. The popularity of this medium has prompted some educators to encourage translations of literature into comic book form in order to stimulate students' interest in the classics.

## Movies

Movies that are not closely bound to reality and often portray an assortment of socially approved behaviors perhaps make a contribution to children's value systems and do provide opportunities for desirable social learning. On the other hand, children, especially adolescents, flock to "macho" movies and those whose heroes resort to violent resolution of problems, such karate and wild automobile chases. The carryover of these influences into daily life and relationships may account in part for the increase in violent behavior of young persons.

A recent concern is the plethora of "slasher" and R-rated movies available to children and teenagers in theaters and through cable television and videocassettes. The content of movies has changed markedly during the past few years, with mutilation being a major theme. To children who are unable to distinguish between reality and fantasy, these films play on their deepest fears and result in bedtime fears, nightmares, and a fearful view of the world.

Young children can be frightened by some of the movies considered safe for family viewing. For example, *Bambi* can be frightening to young children, and the villainous witches in *Snow White* and the *Wizard of Oz* are terrifying figures. Also, certain classic Disney movies, such as *Snow White* and *Cinderella,* depict stepmothers as evil, destructive persons; such portrayals can have a deleterious effect on child-stepmother relationships or can be confusing to children who have developed a positive relationship with a stepmother.

## Television

The medium that has the most impact on children in the United States today is television; it has become one of the most significant socializing agents in the lives of young children. The content of programs and commercials provides multiple sources for acquiring information, modeling behaviors, and observing value orientations. Besides producing a leveling effect on class differences in general information and vocabulary, TV exposes children to a wider variety of topics and events than they encounter in day-to-day life. Television always has time to talk to children and is a form of access to the adult world. However, positive results occur only when viewing is relatively light. Yet the average child in the United States spends more time watching television (over 21 hours per week) than in any other activity except sleeping (Fig. 2-3) (American Academy of Pediatrics, 1999).

Most researchers have concluded that protracted television viewing can have detrimental effects on children. Increased verbal and physical aggressiveness, reduced persistence at problem solving, greater sex-role stereotyping, and reduced creativity have been reported repeatedly. In fairness, no one has yet defined the long-term effects of

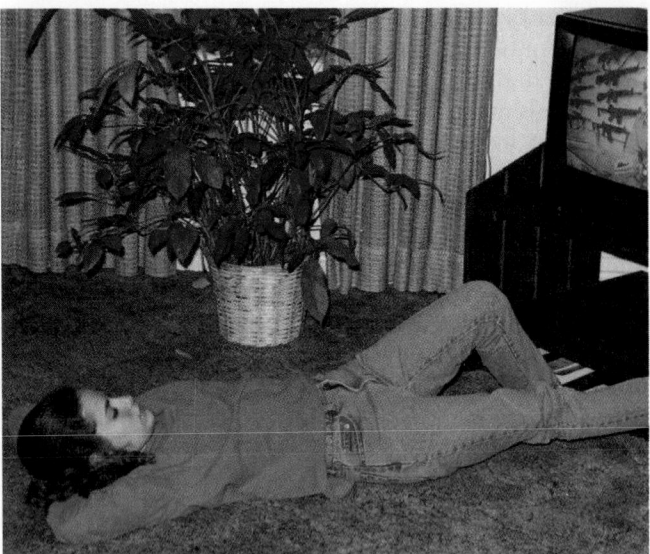

**Fig. 2-3** The average child in the United States spends more time watching television than in any other activity except sleeping.

other electronic factors such as stereo headphones vs conversation, computer games or drills vs active social play, or videotapes vs books. However, it is clear that children in the modern electronic environment are constantly stimulated from the outside, which allows them little time to reflect and develop the inner speech that feeds brain development.

Most programs are designed to attract attention by visual jolts; the child establishes the habit of ignoring language in favor of frenetic visual and auditory gimmicks. Even "educational" programming intended to teach children to read does not teach the habits of mind needed to become good readers.

Like movies, television programs and commercials contain many implicit and explicit messages that promote alcohol consumption, smoking, violence, and promiscuous or unsafe sexual activity. An area of increasing concern is Music Television (MTV), especially when it features heavy metal rock groups whose lyrics and videos sensationalize violent sex, suicide, and Satanism. Although no clear evidence documents a relationship between television viewing and sexual activity or alcohol or tobacco use, the frequency of adolescent pregnancy and sexually transmitted diseases, the prevalence of alcohol-related deaths among adolescents, and the popularity of smoking among youth represent major sources of concern and speculation.

Considerable controversy has been and continues to be generated regarding the favorable vs deleterious influence of television on child development and behavior. Derksen and Strasburger (1994) found that television has a powerful influence in the development of unhealthy behaviors and negative attitudes in children. Several factors encourage the learning or performing of television-influenced behaviors (Box 2-1).

# SOCIOECONOMIC INFLUENCES

## Poverty

A subcultural influence closely related to but different from social class is the condition known as poverty. It is a relative concept and is usually associated with the general standards of a population. The term *poverty* implies both visible and invisible impoverishment. *Visible poverty* refers to lack of money or material resources, which includes insufficient clothing, poor sanitation, and deteriorating housing. *Invisible poverty* refers to social and cultural deprivation such as limited employment opportunities, inferior educational opportunities, lack of or inferior medical services and health care facilities, and an absence of public services.

An *absolute standard* of poverty attempts to delimit some basic set of resources needed for adequate existence; a *relative standard* reflects the median standard of living in a society and is the term used in referring to childhood poverty in the United States. That is, what appears to be deprivation in one area may be a standard or norm in another.

An important development affecting the American family since the end of World War II is the widening disparity in income status among generations. Research indicates that the safety net (federal financial support) is working less effectively for children than for elderly people and poor adults (Ozawa and Yat-sang, 1996). Although general poverty rates are basically the same today as they were two decades ago, who is poor has changed. Historically, elderly Americans were more likely to be poor than children, but federal programs such as Medicare and Social Security reduced poverty rates for the elderly. Children in the United States today are nearly twice as likely to be poor as are citizens over 65 years of age (Annie E. Casey Foundation, 1999).

Despite the enormous wealth in the United States, there has been no change in the poverty rate for children between 1985 and 1994. Presently, it is estimated that 1 in 5 children (21%) lives in poverty (income of $17,960 or less for a family of four in 2001 [U.S. Census Bureau, 2002]). This rate of poverty is substantially higher than the rate in other comparable countries. Although white children saw their poverty rate increase the most during the 1980s (1 in 7 are poor), minority children are more likely to be poor. Almost 50% of African-American children and more than 33% of Hispanic children live in families with incomes below the poverty level (Annie E. Casey Foundation, 1999). Large numbers of Native American children also live in poverty, with unemployment rates on some reservations estimated at 80%.

Many Americans picture the typical child who is poor as a city dweller with unemployed parents, usually living in a single-parent home. Although chronic poverty is more concentrated in central city areas, 60% of the nation's poor children live in the suburbs or rural areas of the country (Bennett and others, 1999). The chances of being poor increase substantially when children are born to parents who have not graduated from high school. The poverty rate for children living with parents who dropped out of high school was 57% in 1995, compared with 4% for children who had at least one parent with a college degree (Annie E. Casey Foundation, 1999).

The character of American poverty is changing. Historically, most of the poor were *episodically poor* (i.e., their incomes would fall below the official poverty line from time to time, reflecting short-term fluctuations in household composition or economic circumstances). Today, increasing numbers of families are *chronically poor* (i.e., with incomes below the poverty line year after year).

Approximately one fourth of children in families with married parents would be poor if they depended on the father's income alone. Escalating health care costs and unaffordable health insurance premiums, coupled with the unavailability and unaffordability of safe housing, the expense of child care, and low-paying marginal jobs result in families with incomes twice the federal poverty level living in substandard housing, foregoing health care, and eating unbalanced meals and insufficient food. Such factors illustrate the growing inability of the American family to provide economic essentials that all children need. In 2000, 11.6% (~8.5 million) of all children in the United States were uninsured (Mills, 2001). Uninsured children are more likely to miss school, jeopardizing their education as well as their health.

Throughout the United States there are groups of people, geographically segregated, who constitute what are known as "pockets of poverty." These are seen in the dense urban areas, such as the ghettos, and many rural areas, especially those geographically isolated from the needed facilities and services. The nonurbanized regions identified as poverty areas in the United States are Appalachia, the deep South, the lower Southwest, and northern New England. Also, certain ethnic or racial groups are overrepresented in the impoverished population. The most obvious of these are blacks, Latinos, and Native Americans.

A high correlation between poverty and the prevalence of illness has long been observed. Impoverished families suffer from poor nutrition; they have little if any preventive health care, inadequate health maintenance, and very limited access to health services. One of the most significant health problems related to poverty is a high infant mortality rate (Annie E. Casey Foundation, 1999). Health care often ranks low on the list of priorities. Day-to-day needs of food, clothing, and lodging take precedence over health care as long as the ailing person feels able to perform activities of daily living.

Poor families may be denied access to some institutions for emergency or other hospital care. Frequently they must travel long distances to service centers that are willing to assume their care. In an emergency they must find money for taxi fare, borrow an automobile, or seek other means of transportation. They must find care for dependents, such as other infants and small children, or take them along when taking the ill child for care. Families tend to delay preventive care indefinitely unless health services are relatively accessible. They are more likely to consult folk practitioners or other persons within their community.

Poor nutrition accounts for many health problems in the lower classes. Lack of funds and ignorance result in a diet that may be seriously lacking in essential food substances, especially protein, vitamins, and iron. This inadequate diet often leads to nutritional deficiency disorders and growth retardation in children. In many the total intake is insufficient to support normal growth. Unstructured eating patterns and irregularly scheduled mealtimes can also contribute to erratic food intake and a proportionately larger consumption of nonnourishing snacks, which can result in excessive weight gain.

Dental problems are more prevalent because of deficient preventive care. Lack of standard immunizations together with reduced resistance from poor nutrition renders the exposed children in poor segments of the population vulnerable to communicable diseases. Poor sanitation and crowded living conditions also contribute to the higher incidence and perpetuation of illness. In general, poor people become ill more frequently and remain ill for longer periods of time than those in the general population.

## Homelessness

One of the most pressing problems in the United States is the growing number of homeless families. *Homeless individuals* are those persons who lack resources and community ties necessary to provide for their own adequate shelter. In the past the homeless population traditionally included single adults, mostly men. Currently, the fastest growing segment of the homeless consists of families, most commonly single mothers with two or three children.

Homeless children have increased in numbers as poverty has become feminized, minorities have become poorer, and low-income housing has become less accessible. Estimates on the number of homeless children in the United States are greater than 500,000, accounting for more than one third of the overall homeless population (Ensign and Santelli, 1998;

Weinreb and others, 1998). The majority of children are less than 5 years of age and are predominantly from minority groups.

Many families are becoming homeless because of physical abuse, substance abuse, disagreements with the landlord, and poor living conditions. Other reasons include job layoffs, low income, parental mental illness, domestic conflict, and unexpected family or economic crises.

Another group of homeless children are the "runaway" and "throwaway" adolescents. Many runaways are victims of physical and sexual abuse and leave home because of long-term family or school problems. Poor parent-child relationships, extreme family conflict, feelings of alienation from parents, inconsistency in supervision, and unpredictability in discipline are other factors often cited.

Lack of a permanent dwelling deprives children of the most basic necessities for proper growth and development. Homelessness disrupts a child's friendships and schooling (Strehlow and Amos-Jones, 1999). Homeless children suffer from physical and mental disorders that exceed those found in poor children who have a permanent residence. The health care needs that remain unmet for homeless children include routine immunizations, adequate nutrition, lack of screening for routine problems, and high rates of acute and chronic illnesses (Weinreb and others, 1998).

## Migrant Families

One of the most disadvantaged groups is migrant farmworkers and their children. It is currently estimated that there are between 3 and 5 million migrant farmworkers and their dependents nationwide. The exact number of children is unknown, but over 600,000 school-age children are enrolled in education programs in 47 of the 50 states (American Academy of Pediatrics, 2000). Children of migrant farmworkers are at an increased risk for health problems, with over 73% living in poverty and fewer that 20% using need-based services (American Academy of Pediatrics, 2000).

The low position of these families on the economic scale and their rootless, mobile existence subject them to inadequate sanitation, substandard housing, social isolation, and lack of educational and medical facilities. This lifestyle is especially deleterious to the children. Schooling and health care are inadequate. Children are apt to live in a number of localities and attend a variety of schools in the course of a year with no continuity in either education or health care (Box 2-2). Because both parents work in the fields, children receive little adult supervision; therefore injury rates are high and meals are erratic. Except where prohibited and enforced by law, children are even recruited to work in the fields along with the adults. Migrants generally suffer more illness, both acute and chronic, than does the general population. They are subject to unhealthy environments, poverty, and insufficient medical care; their health-seeking behavior in general is an illness- or injury-oriented recourse to medical care. Affected persons will postpone seeking care for themselves or their children until physical pain or suffering is almost unbearable. The health problems of migrant children appear to be dental caries, upper respiratory tract infections,

---

**Box 2-2** ■ ■ ■
**Strategies for Adapting Health Care to the Lifestyle of Migrant Children**

- Provide vaccinations and preventive services at the time of acute visits.
- Provide patients with copies of the medical record, including their vaccination record and growth chart.
- Stress to parents the importance of bringing all medications and immunization records to every clinic (or emergency department) visit.
- Ask parents about their planned length of stay in your area and their future travel itinerary.
- Provide the name, address, and telephone number of clinics, physicians, and schools at their next destination.

Adapted from American Academy of Pediatrics: *Guidelines for the care of migrant farmworkers' children*, Elk Grove Village, IL, 2000, The Academy.

---

tuberculosis, otitis media, scabies and lice, intestinal parasites, pesticide exposure, injuries, teenage pregnancy, and growth and development delay.

Tuberculosis rates among migrant families are high. A risk factor for the increased incidence of tuberculosis in children has been the migration of families from high-risk prevalence areas of tuberculosis, such as Asia, African, and Latin America (Castiglia, 1997). Also, farmworkers are approximately six times more likely to develop the disease than the general population of employed adults. Drug-resistant tuberculosis is an important consideration among this population; it requires altered treatment regimens, and higher rates of resistance have been found in the ethnic and social groups constituting much of the migrant farm workforce (Ampofo and Saiman, 2002).

When medical care is provided to a migrant family, follow-up care is usually impossible because of their transient lifestyle. Compliance with medical therapies is primarily related to accessibility and availability. For example, medications provided by health workers are more likely to be taken than those that must be obtained at a pharmacy. In addition, medications are often discontinued following self-perceived recovery.

## CULTURAL INFLUENCES

Nurses need to consider cultural differences in clients when providing health care. An understanding of the various beliefs regarding the causation of illness and disease, as well as traditional health practices, is essential to successful intervention. The more nurses know about the values, beliefs, and customs of other ethnic groups, the better able they are to meet the needs of these families and to gain their cooperation and compliance.

**NURSING TIP** Develop a cultural reference manual that includes a brief description of the culture; views on health, illness, diet, and other matters; and a list of interpreters, ethnic community services, or other sources for quick reference (Kuensting and Sanders, 1995).

## Cultural Relativity

Although clinical characteristics of a disease or condition are essentially the same across cultures, how a child or family interprets or experiences the disease or condition varies. Culture as an influence is one obvious explanation for variance. *Cultural relativity* is the concept that any behavior must be judged first in relation to the context of the culture in which it occurs. Nurses must first relate to the family's perceptions and interpretations of experiences from the family's background and cultural belief system before they can intervene effectively. Compliance is more likely if treatment regimens do not interfere with work or family responsibilities.

Some cultures, for example, may view a chronic illness or disability as affecting only particular aspects of a child's life, and the child as a whole is viewed as normal. In contrast, Chinese families more frequently describe the illness as having global effects on many aspects of the child's present and future life (Martinson, Armstrong, and Qiao, 1997). These contrasting views may result in a difference in the goals and expectations parents have for their children.

In some cultures the child's gender may influence a family's perception of the implications of an illness or disability. For example, in the Arabic and Asian cultures and for some families of Jewish, Italian, Greek, or Indian origin, the male child is held in higher esteem than the female child. The male child may receive better health care and the most food, because this is the child who will take care of his parents in their old age.

Defining disease or signs and symptoms of illness is also influenced by culture. Some cultures, for example, perceive diarrhea as a cleansing of the body that is essential for health maintenance and illness prevention or cure. Furthermore, signs or symptoms resulting from diarrhea and ensuing dehydration, such as malaise, fever, anorexia, and irritability, may be viewed as separate illnesses.

Nurses can often recognize a family's health-related cultural perceptions and interpretations through discussion and observation. Implications of these perceptions should be explored and considered when planning effective culturally appropriate interventions.

## Relationships with Health Care Providers

The manner of relating with health care providers differs considerably among cultural groups. One area of conflict to some nurses is the attitude toward time and waiting that is part of some cultures. The time orientation of Hispanic and black ethnic groups is in the present. For example, blacks are very flexible in their time orientation; a black family may be late for or miss appointments because other issues take precedence over the appointment, and they may not communicate this to the health agency. Hispanics, too, have a very relaxed view of time. Whereas the dominant culture in the United States says that "time flies," the Hispanic says, "time walks."

The Japanese, on the other hand, consider time to be valuable and to be used wisely. They tend to be punctual for medical appointments and persistent in following prescribed regimens. A Vietnamese family will subordinate time to values considered to be more significant, such as propriety. They may be late for an appointment because of an overextended visit by a friend in their home. In general, Asian-Americans view the American focus on time as offensive. They spend hours getting to know people and view predetermined, abrupt endings as rude. Introductory small talk is considered good manners.

Navajo Indians view time on a continuum with no beginning and no end. The present-time orientation may cause a Navajo to eat two meals a day today, four meals tomorrow, no meals the next day, and three meals the day after. This becomes an important nursing consideration if a Navajo is told to take medication with meals to ensure three doses per day.

In many cultural groups the mother assumes the responsibility for health care; in others both parents are involved equally in relationships with health workers. A somewhat different approach is apparent in some of the Asian cultures. For example, the father in Vietnamese or Filipino families, as unquestioned head of the family, is traditionally the family member who interacts with persons, including health care providers, outside the family unit. Therefore he is the one who represents the family in health matters. In the Hispanic family the father, as head of the house, makes decisions regarding illness and treatment of adult family members, but the grandmother in the extended family is consulted regarding child care. Usually the family confers with other members before reaching a decision regarding treatment or hospitalization of a child. The Arab family also relies on others to give advice and guidance in a time of crisis. A Japanese father may appear to be passive and uninvolved but actually is involved according to his own cultural standards.

> **NURSING ALERT**
>
> In working with families, it is essential for nurses to identify key members—failure to include these significant individuals in teaching can seriously hinder adherence to the plan of care.

Nurses should make themselves aware of any specific attitudes regarding the manner of approach to a child in a given culture. Navajo Indians do not like a stranger near their infants. It is feared that the stranger may "witch" the child and cause the child harm. On the other hand, if a stranger, particularly a woman, lavishes attention on a Hispanic infant but fails to touch the child, the infant will develop symptoms of the "evil eye" (see p. 47). Vietnamese and Korean families may become upset if a newborn is admired at length for fear the evil spirits will overhear and desire the infant.

Some groups, such as the Amish, consider a child's admission to the hospital a family affair, with all members gathering to support and console the child and the parents. In other groups the family is willing to relinquish the care of the child to the hospital authority without interference. Their visits with the child are short, although intense, but this behavior may be misinterpreted by the hospital staff as disinterest or abandonment.

All ethnic groups are entitled to be treated with dignity and respect. Family members should be addressed by their

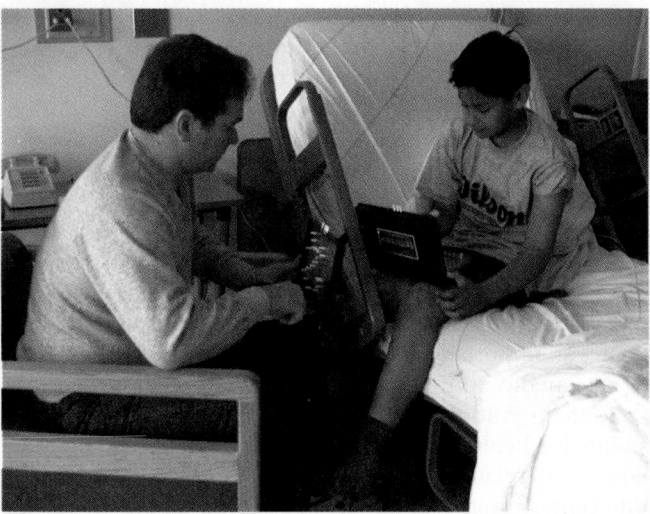

**Fig. 2-4** Fathers from many cultures assume an active parenting role.

last names; many groups consider it an affront to be called by their first names. Stereotyping is to be condemned. People are individuals who are evaluated in relation to their cultural standards, needs, and preferences (Fig. 2-4).

Nurses who are members of a majority culture may encounter tension and distrust in a child from a minority culture as a result of the child's learned conception or relationships with other persons in the majority group. Based on these perceptions, minority children often suspect that nurses may have hostile feelings toward them and fear ill treatment. When such children are hospitalized, this feeling compounds the feelings of loneliness, helplessness, and retribution that accompany fearful happenings and separation from families. The reverse situation may be encountered by a nurse from a minority culture attempting to meet the needs of a child who has been conditioned to view the nurse's cultural or ethnic group as inferior. Either situation is more likely to occur if the nurse or the child has had little or no personal contact with the other's culture. For example, a child from a minority culture from the inner city who lives in a neighborhood and attends school only with children from his or her minority culture may be more suspicious of a nurse from a different culture than may a child from the same minority group who lives in a culturally diverse neighborhood or who attends an integrated school. Taking the opportunity to become familiar with cultures different from one's own and making an effort to get to know each other as individuals can shatter myths and, with time, build the trust needed to establish rewarding relationships between children, their families, and the nurse.

## Communication

Communication is basic to all human relationships, but it may be a source of distress and misunderstanding between persons from different ethnic groups, especially if the languages are different. Prejudice has been found to be one of the biggest barriers to cross cultural communication (Taylor, 1998). Ideally, conversations with families who are unable to speak the dominant language are best conducted by a

health care worker who speaks the language of the family. If this is not possible, it may be necessary to engage the services of an interpreter. However, use of an interpreter can be a source of misunderstanding if the interpreter is unfamiliar with the medical terminology or if there are no corresponding words in the second language to express the ideas and concepts under discussion. (See Communicating with Families Through an Interpreter, Chapter 6.)

Some persons with poor or limited language comprehension may simply smile and nod in agreement if they do not understand the questions or directives. It is vital that the family members fully understand all implications of a child's care and management before they sign permits for special procedures or assume responsibility for the child's care. It is not uncommon for an Asian family to indicate "yes" when in fact they mean "no" in order to avoid social disharmony. They tend to use indirectness rather than confrontation and may become evasive when direct questioning makes them feel uncomfortable.

> **NURSING TIP** Helpful communication tools include the following:
> - Have a series of audio and audiovisual recordings in several languages designed to greet and familiarize the family with the hospital.
> - In the event an interpreter is not available, develop a multilingual booklet containing illustrations of commonly used phrases and hospital routines.
> - Have legal consent forms and explanations of common diagnostic tests available in several languages.
> - Keep cards with common greetings, phrases, and names of body parts in the family's language with the patient's chart (e.g., *miseries* [pain] and *locked bowels* [constipation] for African-Americans and *caida de la mollera* [fallen fontanel from dehydration], *susto* [fright], *dolor, duels,* or *lele* [pain], and *la diarrhea* [diarrhea] for Hispanics).

Nonverbal communication is a practiced art in many American Indian tribes, and the members are highly sensitive to body language. They emphasize periods of silence to formulate thoughts in preparation for speech and often remain silent after listening to statements by others in order to properly assimilate what has been said. Interruption, interjection, or haste to arrive at abrupt conclusions is perceived as immature behavior.

*Eye contact* is viewed differently in cultures. Although Caucasians are advised to look people straight in the eye, it is not uncommon for persons in some ethnic groups to avoid eye contact and become uncomfortable when conversing with health care workers. In non-Western cultures a patient may not look directly into the nurse's eyes as a sign of respect. Some Native Americans will make eye contact during the initial greeting, but continued, unwavering eye contact is considered insulting and disrespectful. Asians may consider eye contact a sign of hostility or impoliteness.

The level of comfort with body space or distance from others varies among cultures. Caucasians are generally comfortable at an arm's length, Hispanics tend to get closer, and Asians prefer a greater distance. Also, gestures may have different meanings. For example, some Asians consider pointing with a finger or foot disrespectful. Some Native Americans consider vigorous handshaking a sign of aggression, whereas to Caucasians the gesture is a sign of goodwill and strong character.

Families may be reluctant to question or otherwise initiate contact with health professionals. In the Asian cultures, for example, it is considered a sign of disrespect to question those who are viewed as persons of authority. A Japanese family may wait silently rather than ask or question. They believe that the health professionals know best and will meet their needs without being asked. It is also important to avoid criticism. Criticism can cause the Japanese-American to "lose face," to feel ashamed, which is highly undesirable.

Language has been considered the biggest barrier to the use of health care services by many families, especially Southeast Asians (Mattson, 1995). Often, families may have poor language comprehension, so it is necessary to speak slowly and carefully, not loudly, when conversing with them. Many persons are able to read and write English better than they can speak or understand it. Also, the dominant language usually takes over in anxiety-provoking situations, even in persons who are able to communicate satisfactorily under ordinary circumstances.

Terms of address and use of first and last names vary among cultures and can create confusion in institutions. For example, in Asian cultures, the family name is given first in respect for the family and the given names follow. Therefore all siblings in a family have the same first name (in some families it may be the middle names that are the same). Ethiopians use no last names but have a very complex system whereby women retain their last names after marriage and the paternal grandfather's name becomes a child's last name. The Mennonites refer to children as sons and daughters of a particular parent, such as "Josiah's son," rather than by the son's name.

Although all people share the basic emotions, there are decided ethnic variations in the ways emotions are expressed. In some cultures (e.g., persons of Italian, Latin, or Jewish background) emotions are expressed openly and members are accustomed to sharing their sorrows and joys with family and friends. Conversely, Nordic and Asian groups are more restrained in expressing emotion.

Health care providers generally ask questions and use handouts, booklets, and—particularly with children—dolls and pictures as communication aids. This is uncommon in some cultures. For example, Native American healers ask few questions and do not use forms. In some cultures it is considered inappropriate or taboo to look at the inside of the body, even in pictures, or to use dolls or puppets (Malach and Segel, 1990). Nurses need to consider both verbal and nonverbal communication techniques to interact effectively with children and their families from different cultures. (See Guidelines box.)

## Food Customs

Food customs and symbolism of various cultural, ethnic, and religious groups are an integral part of their lives. Although in a large country such as the United States most people have adopted the eclectic food habits that have evolved over countless generations, many ethnic and geographic food traditions and preferences are retained. Spe-

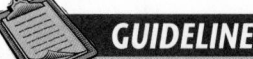

### GUIDELINES
#### Culturally Sensitive Interactions

**NONVERBAL STRATEGIES**

Invite family members to choose where they would like to sit or stand, allowing them to select a comfortable distance.
Observe interactions with others to determine which body gestures (e.g., shaking hands) are acceptable and appropriate. Ask when in doubt.
Avoid appearing rushed.
Be an active listener.
Observe for cues regarding appropriate eye contact.
Learn appropriate use of pauses or interruptions for different cultures.
Ask for clarification if nonverbal meaning is unclear.

**VERBAL STRATEGIES**

Learn proper terms of address.
Use a positive tone of voice to convey interest.
Speak slowly and carefully, not loudly, when families have poor language comprehension.
Encourage questions.
Learn basic words and sentences of family's language, if possible.
Avoid professional terms.
When asking questions, tell family why the questions are being asked, the way in which the information they provide will be used, and how it might benefit their child.
Repeat important information more than once.
Always give the reason or purpose for a treatment or prescription.
Use information written in the family's language.
Offer the services of an interpreter when necessary (see Chapter 6).
Learn from families and representatives of their culture methods of communicating information without creating discomfort.
Address intergenerational needs (e.g., family's need to consult with others).
Be sincere, open, and honest and, when appropriate, share personal experiences, beliefs, and practices to establish rapport and trust.

cial holidays, ceremonies, and life experiences such as births, birthdays, weddings, and death are often marked by special food items or feasts. In many cultures specific food practices are followed during pregnancy in the belief that certain foods damage the developing fetus.

The distinctive food customs of ethnic groups are a product of their native environment, determined by availability. Fish is a staple food of people living near the ocean, such as those from Japan, Polynesia, and Scandinavia. Fruit and vegetable preferences are also directly related to the climate in which these grow naturally or can be cultivated. The types of grain that are ethnically associated are often those that grow best in the native lands. For example, wheat and basmati rice are the staple grains of South Asians, and roti (unleavened bread) is most commonly eaten in the home (Sekhon, 1996). The diet of the Eskimo is predominantly fish and meat, depending on which is the most easily procured in the area. Even in the continental United States there are regional favorites, such as rice, hominy grits, and okra in the southern states. In some cultures food is highly spiced; in others foods tend to be bland. Table 2-1 outlines some of the foods associated with specific ethnic groups.

**TABLE 2-1** Characteristic food choices for six groups

| Vegetables | Fruits | Meats and Alternatives | Grain Products | Others |
|---|---|---|---|---|
| **African-American** | | | | |
| Broccoli, corn, greens (mustard, collard, kale, turnip, beet, etc.), lima beans, okra, peas, pumpkin | Grapefruit, grapes, nectarine, plums, watermelon | Sausage, pig's feet, ears, etc., bacon, luncheon meat, organ meats, turkey, catfish, perch, red snapper, tuna, salmon, sardines, shrimp, kidney beans, red beans, black-eyed peas, peanuts, and peanut butter | Corn bread, hominy grits, biscuits, muffins, cooked cereal, crackers | Chitterlings, salt pork, gravies, buttermilk |
| **Hispanic** | | | | |
| Avocado, chilies, corn, lettuce, peas, potato, prickly pear (cactus leaf called *nopales*), zucchini | Guava, lemon, mango, melons, prickly pear (cactus fruit called *tuna*), zapote (or sapote) | Lamb, tripe, sausage *(chorizo)*, bologna, bacon, pinto beans, pink beans, garbanzo beans, lentils, peanuts, and peanut butter | Tortillas, corn flour, oatmeal, sweet bread *(pan dulce)* | Salsa (tomato, pepper, and onion relish), chili sauce, guacamole, lard *(manteca)*, pork cracklings |
| **Japanese** | | | | |
| Bamboo shoots, broccoli, burdock root, cauliflower, celery, cucumbers, eggplant, gourd *(kampyo)*, mushrooms, napa cabbage, peas, peppers, radishes (daikon or pickles called *takuwan*), snow peas, squash, sweet potato, turnips, water chestnuts, yamaimo | Apricot, cherries, grapefruit, grapes, lemon, lime, melons, persimmon, pineapple, pomegranate, plums (dried pickled *umeboshi*), strawberries | Turkey, raw tuna or sea bass *(sashimi)*, mackerel, sardines *(mezashi)*, shrimp, abalone, squid, octopus, soybean curd *(tofu)*, soybean paste *(miso)*, soybeans, red beans *(azuki)*, lima beans, peanuts, almonds, cashews | Rice, rice crackers, noodles (wholewheat noodle called *soba* or *udon*), oatmeal | Soy sauce, Nori paste (used to season rice), bean thread *(konyaku)*, ginger *(shoga;* dried form called *denishoga)* |
| **Chinese** | | | | |
| Bamboo shoots, bean sprouts, bok choy, broccoli, celery, Chinese cabbage, corn, cucumbers, eggplant, greens (collard, Chinese, broccoli, mustard, kale), leeks, lettuce, mushrooms, peppers, scallions, snow peas, taro, water chestnuts, white turnips, white radishes, winter melon | Figs, grapes, kumquats, loquats, mangoes, melons, persimmons, pineapple, plums, pomegranates | Organ meats, duck, white fish, shrimp, lobster, oyster, sardines, soybeans, tofu, black beans, chestnuts *(kuri)* | Rice, barley, millet | Soy sauce, sweet and sour sauce, mustard sauce, ginger root, plum sauce, red bean paste |
| **Vietnamese\*** | | | | |
| Bamboo shoots, bean sprouts, cabbage, carrots, cucumbers, greens, lettuce, mushrooms, onions, peas, spinach, yams | Apples, bananas, eggfruit *(o-ma)*, grapefruit, jackfruit, lychee, mandarins, mangoes, oranges, papayas, pineapple, tangerines, watermelon | Beef, blood, brain, chicken, duck, eggs, fish, goat, kidney, lamb, liver, pork, shellfish, soybeans | French bread, rice, rice noodles, wheat noodles | Fish sauce, fresh herbs, garlic, ginger, lard, MSG, peanut oil, sesame seeds, sesame seed oil, vegetable oil |
| **Indian (East)** | | | | |
| Cauliflower, carrots, cucumbers, corn gourds, leeks, eggplant, beets, radishes, hot peppers, bell peppers, peas, French beans, okra, pumpkins, red and white cabbage, mung sprouts, bean sprouts, potatoes, tapioca root, sweet potatoes | Oranges, limes, grapes, watermelon, mangoes, guava, honeydew, chiku, cantaloupe, pineapple, green, yellow, and red bananas, berries, custard apples | Lamb, beef, duck, chicken, shrimp, catfish, buffalo, sunfish, sardines, fresh crab, lobster, peanuts, cashews, almonds, chickpeas, split peas, black-eyed peas, dry mung beans | Rice pancakes, wheat chapati, puri, mixed grain flour bread | Fresh coconut juice, curries, tomato sauce, tamarind sauce, dried grain curries *(pulses)*, yogurt-curry garnished with coriander (fresh leaves) |

From Endres JB, Rockwell RE: *Food, nutrition, and the young child*, St Louis, 1980, Mosby. Modified from *Nutrition during pregnancy and lactation*, California Department of Public Health, revised 1975.
NOTE: Foods common to all ethnic groups have been omitted.
\*Information supplied by Hanh-Trang Tran-Viet, Carbondale, IL.

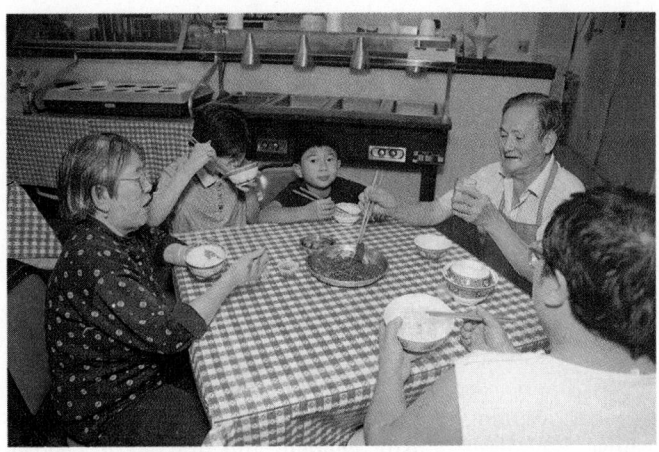

**Fig. 2-5**   Food customs outside the home can differ significantly from traditional cultural practices.

There are a number of restrictions related to food items. Some have a physiologic origin, such as lack of dairy foods in the diets of some persons of African or Asian ancestry with lactose intolerance. Others have religious restrictions, such as kosher foods and food preparation of the Orthodox Jewish faith and the vegetarian diet of Seventh Day Adventists. (See Vegetarian Diets, Chapter 13.)

Children in a strange environment, such as the hospital, feel much more comfortable when they are served familiar foods (Fig. 2-5). Hospital food often tastes strange and bland, especially to children who enjoy the highly seasoned foods of their culture. Also, the family may be concerned that the child is not receiving foods appropriate to their culture and beliefs. When possible, it is advisable to provide children's ethnic foods or allow families to bring favorite foods that are not available on the hospital menu. Concern for differences in food habits and patterns projects an attitude of respect for the family's ethnic or religious heritage.

## HEALTH BELIEFS AND PRACTICES

The nurse encounters people of many different racial and ethnic origins in the process of meeting the health needs of children and families. Some of these families have become so enculturated to the majority culture that their health beliefs and practices are consistent with those of the health care system. For many families, however, traditional practices and beliefs are an integral part of their daily lives. Health care workers should be aware that other people may live by different rules and priorities from those of the health care provider, and these rules and priorities decisively influence health-related behavior.

### Health Beliefs

The beliefs related to the cause of illness and the maintenance of health are an integral part of the cultural heritage of families. Often inseparable from religious beliefs, they influence the way that families cope with health problems and

the way that they respond to health care providers. Predominant among most cultures are beliefs related to natural forces, supernatural forces, and imbalance between forces.

### Natural Forces

The most common natural forces held responsible for ill health if the body is not adequately protected include cold air entering the body, impurities in the air, or other natural sources. For example, a Chinese parent may overdress the infant in an effort to keep cold wind from entering the child's body. The Chinese believe that cold weather, rain, or wind is responsible for "cold" conditions. They also believe that an innate energy called *chi* enters and leaves the body through the mouth, nose, and ears and flows through the body in definite pathways, or meridians, at specific times and locations. Lack of chi and blood is believed to be a cause of fatigue, low energy, and a variety of ailments.

In the African-American culture, natural phenomena such as phases of the moon, seasons of the year, and planet positions are believed to affect the body and its processes; therefore health maintenance is strongly associated with the ability to read "the signs." Some cultures consider such behavior as overeating, overwork, anxiety, and inadequate food and sleep to be natural causes of illness. Most Native Americans consider health to be a state of harmony with nature and the universe.

### Supernatural Forces

High on the list of causes of illness are forces beyond comprehension and logical explanation. Evil influences such as voodoo, witchcraft, or evil spirits are viewed in some cultures as causes of illness, especially those illnesses that cannot be explained by other means.

A health belief that is common among people from Latin American, Mediterranean, Near Eastern, some Asian, and some African societies is the concept of the "evil eye." (**Mal ojo** is the Hispanic term.) It is part of the concept of health as a state of balance; illness is a state of imbalance (see following section). Strength and power are associated with the evil eye; therefore, as long as an individual's strength and weakness remain in balance, he or she is unlikely to become a victim of the evil eye. Weaknesses are not necessarily physical. For example, an excess of some emotion, such as envy, can create a weakness. Infants and small children, because of immature development of their internal strength-weakness states, are believed to be especially vulnerable to the gaze of the evil eye. Consequently, the evil eye serves to rationalize an inexplicable onset of illness in children who display such symptoms as restlessness, crying, diarrhea, vomiting, and fever.

Although seldom expressed to health care providers, the belief that a witch can cast a spell or curse over others at the request of someone who wishes the person ill or dead is found in Hispanic, African, and Australian aboriginal cultures. The victim is often tortured in effigy by pins driven into a doll at the location where the intended victim is to be hurt. "Voodoo deaths" have occurred from the victim's belief in the curse and may result from dehydration as the victim gives up the will to live and refuses to drink (Chidester, 1990).

### Imbalance of Forces

The concept of balance or equilibrium is widespread throughout the world. One of the most common imbalances supported by the Hispanic, Filipino, Chinese, and Arab cultures is that which exists between "hot" and "cold." This belief is reputedly derived from the Hippocratic theory of humoral pathology, which states that illness is caused by an imbalance of the four humors: phlegm, blood, black bile, and yellow bile (Sekhon, 1996). "Hot" and "cold" describe certain properties and conditions completely unrelated to temperature. Diseases, areas of the body, foods, and illnesses are classified as either "hot" or "cold." In Chinese health belief the forces are termed *yin* ("cold") and *yang* ("hot") (Wang and Martinson, 1996). To maintain health and prevent illness, these forces must be kept in balance.

Illness is treated by restoring normal balance through the application of appropriate "hot" or "cold" remedies. A "cold" condition such as a respiratory disease is believed to be caused by exposure to cold weather, rain, or cold wind entering the body; it is treated by administration of "hot" foods, herbs, or drugs. Menstruation is considered to be a "hot" condition; therefore women are cautioned against ingesting "hot" foods, which might increase menstrual flow or produce cramping. Ingesting too much of either "hot" or "cold" foods can also be interpreted as a cause of illness.

Health care workers who are aware of this belief are better able to understand why some persons refuse to eat certain foods. It is often useful to discuss the diet with the family to determine their feelings and beliefs regarding food choices. It is possible to help families devise a diet that contains the necessary balance of basic food groups prescribed by the medical subculture while conforming to the beliefs of the ethnic subculture.

The "hot-cold" food classification may have adverse effects. For example, newborn infants are often started on evaporated milk formulas. Evaporated milk is considered to be a "hot" food, whereas whole milk is viewed as a "cold" food. Infants tend to develop rashes, which are believed to be caused by "hot" foods; in such cases parents may decide to switch to whole milk. However, parents fear that it is dangerous to change too rapidly, so they often feed the child some type of neutralizing substance, which may create additional health problems. Such a problem might be averted if, before discharge from the hospital, the family's preference is determined and a formula prescribed that is agreeable to both the family and the practitioner.

### Health Practices

There are numerous similarities among cultures regarding prevention and treatment of illness. All cultures have some types of home remedies that they apply before seeking help from other persons. Within the ethnic community, folk healers who are endowed with the ability to "cure"

maladies are sought for special situations and when home remedies are unsuccessful. There is the *curandero* (male) or *curandera* (female) of the Mexican-American community whose healing powers are believed to be a gift from God. The Asian consults an herbalist, knowledgeable in medicines, or perhaps an ethnic practitioner practiced in Asian therapies, including *acupuncture* (insertion of needles), *acupressure* (application of pressure), and *moxibustion* (application of heat). Native Americans consult a variety of healers with specific skills and knowledge. Specialized medicine persons diagnose illness, provide nonsacred treatments (usually by way of massage and herbs), and care for souls. Other specialists perform services or affect cures through the use of spiritual means. Native Hawaiians consult *kahunas* and practice *ho' oponopono* to heal family imbalance or disputes.

The folk healers are very powerful persons in their community and have the ability to acquire information about an illness without resorting to probing questions. They "speak the language" of the family who seeks help and often combine their rituals and potions with prayer and entreaties to God. They also are able to create an atmosphere conducive to successful management. Furthermore, they exhibit a sincere interest in the family and their problem.

Some folk remedies are compatible with the medical regimen and can be used to reinforce the treatment plan. For example, aspirin (a "hot" medication) is an appropriate therapy for "cold" diseases such as the common cold and arthritis. It is not uncommon to discover that a folk prescription has a scientific basis. In any case, practices that do no harm should be respected.

In cultures who believe in the concept, overcoming the effect of the evil eye usually requires specialized rituals conducted by the appropriate practitioner. For example, the Chicano *curandera* ascertains that the condition is truly the result of the evil eye by performing an assessment ritual and then, on a confirmed diagnosis, performing a curative ritual. Sometimes the faith in the folk practitioner delays obtaining needed medical treatment, although the practitioner will usually suggest medical care if his or her ministrations are unsuccessful.

Health practices of different cultures may also present problems of assessment and interpretation. For example, certain cultural practices or remedies can be misdiagnosed as evidence of "child abuse" by uninformed professionals (Box 2-3). It is important to explain why these and other familiar remedies may now be considered harmful. Families need to understand how such practices can place them in jeopardy with child protective services, and they need to explore alternative measures that are more acceptable to the dominant culture (Hayes and Dreher, 1991).

Other cultural health remedies that are detrimental to health include eating clay or excessive amounts of salt. A mercury compound, *azogue* (the Spanish name for quicksilver), is commonly used in Mexico and sometimes sold illegally to low-income Hispanic families in the United States as a "remedy" for diarrhea. Alert health care workers know that the drug can cause permanent central nervous system damage. A careful history can reveal these practices, but it

## Box 2-3 ■ ■ ■
### Cultural Practices Possibly Considered Abusive by the Dominant Culture

**Coining**—A Vietnamese practice that may produce weltlike lesions on the child's back when a coin, held on edge, is repeatedly rubbed lengthwise on the oiled skin to rid the body of the disease.

**Cupping**—An Old World practice (also practiced by the Vietnamese) of placing a container (e.g., tumbler, bottle, jar) containing steam against the skin surface to "draw out the poison" or other evil element. When the heated air within the container cools, a vacuum is created that produces a bruiselike blemish on the skin directly beneath the mouth of the container.

**Burning**—A practice of some Southeast Asian groups whereby small areas of skin are burned to treat enuresis and temper tantrums.

**Female genital mutilation (female circumcision)**—Removal of or injury to any part of the female genital organ; practiced in Africa, the Middle East, Latin America, India, the Far East, North America, Australia, and Western Europe.

**Forced kneeling**—A child discipline measure of some Caribbean groups in which a child is forced to kneel for a long period of time.

**Topical garlic application**—A practice of Yemenite Jews in which crushed garlic cloves or garlic-petroleum jelly plaster is applied to the wrists to treat infectious disease; the practice can result in blisters or garlic burns.

**Traditional remedies that contain lead**—*Greta* and *azarcon* (Mexico; used for digestive problems), *paylooah* (Southeast Asia; used for rash or fever), and *surma* (India; used as a cosmetic to improve eyesight).

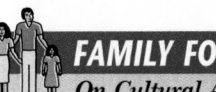

### FAMILY FOCUS
*On Cultural Awareness*

I am a pediatric emergency nurse with a high regard for cultural diversities and a respect for healing practices and beliefs. I even made a manual for my emergency department that contains some of the information needed to help us to understand and communicate with subcultures in the urban community that we serve. Although I learned a great deal putting this manual together, it doesn't come close to the lesson I learned with the following experience:

A 15-month-old Bosnian female in status epilepticus was carried in by her parents. They were very frightened and spoke very little English. I learned that the child had received a measles, mumps, and rubella (MMR) immunization the day before. As I proceeded to unwrap her from the blanket she was in, I quickly assessed the A, B, Cs (airway, breathing, and circulation). I noticed that she was very warm (probably a febrile seizure) and that a rag soaked in alcohol was tied around each thigh. Focusing on her potential airway compromise and trying to calm the parents, I proceeded to put an oxygen mask on her, undress her for a full assessment, and remove the alcohol rags. I spoke to the parents all the while in a calm, soothing voice. Once an IV was established and I gave her Ativan, the seizures stopped. So did the communication between her parents and me. I noticed that they would no longer give me eye contact, and the mother would not even speak to me after the seizures stopped. It wasn't until I was returning to the department from admitting her that I realized why they might have stopped communicating with me . . . I had removed the rags! Had I only thought to replace the rags or asked their permission to remove the rags, things may have been different.

Laura L. Kuensting, MSN(R), RN
Cardinal Glennon Children's Hospital
St. Louis, Missouri

---

may require the collaboration of a folk healer to convince a user to stop the practice.

Haitian folk medicine considers it essential to rid the newborn of meconium to ensure neonatal survival. The newborn's first food is a *lok,* or purgative, prepared by cooking a mixture of castor oil, grated nutmeg, sour orange juice, garlic, unrefined sugar, and water. It may be administered several times until the color of the newborn's bowel movement changes from black to yellow. All other oral intake may be restricted until this occurs, which may result in dehydration.

Faith healing and religious rituals are closely allied with many folk-healing practices. Wearing of amulets, medals, and other religious relics believed by the culture to protect the individual and facilitate healing is a common practice. It is important for health workers to recognize the value of this practice and keep the items where the family has placed them or nearby. It offers comfort and support and rarely impedes medical and nursing care. If an item must be removed during a procedure, it should be replaced, if possible, when the procedure is completed. The reason for its temporary removal should be explained to the family so that they are reassured that their wishes will be respected. (See Family Focus box.)

Nurses can be most effective by operating from a multicultural perspective, which means using appropriate aspects of each health cultural orientation under consideration to develop culturally acceptable health care interventions.

**NURSING ALERT** Avoid directly attacking traditional health cultural beliefs and practices as wrong or harmful, or implying that biomedical measures are uniformly correct and effective and the only way to prevent illness or treat sickness. Such attacks usually result in rejection of biomedical health care practitioners and health teaching based on biomedicine or scientific facts.

Although most subcultures in the large, developed countries have become acculturated to the Western medical system, many still maintain faith in traditional healing practices and practitioners. When the folk practices do not interfere with the welfare of the patient, they need not be discouraged. Often a compromise can be reached that accomplishes the goal of the nurse while maintaining the dignity and self-esteem of the client.

## Folklore Related to Prenatal Influences

Since ancient times the striking appearance of abnormal human development has been of concern, as evidenced by descriptions in primitive drawings and on clay tablets, and has served as the origin of numerous legendary and mythologic creatures. Consequently, the processes of pregnancy and birth have been surrounded by strongly held beliefs and superstitions that involve taboos and prescriptions for behavior directed toward ensuring the well-being of the unborn child. Even in the face of scientific advances, these superstitions and folkways have survived for generations and may persist in various forms as part of a cultural heritage. The degree to which these beliefs are expressed depends on the strength of the cultural influence, the attitudes of the individual families, and the confidence and credibility engendered by the health care providers.

One of the most universal explanations of defective development has been maternal impressions. It has been a widespread belief that the appearance of the unborn child will be improved if the pregnant woman looks at beautiful people or things. The same concept in reverse has been used to explain birth defects. For example, if a pregnant woman was frightened by a rabbit, it was believed that her child would be born with a cleft ("hare") lip; a microcephalic infant was attributed to the mother's seeing a monkey during pregnancy; and the mother's viewing a person with missing limbs would cause the unborn child to be similarly affected. Activities such as a mother reaching her arms above her head, wearing a lei, walking in circles, or tying knots were believed to cause the umbilical cord to be knotted or twisted around the neck of the fetus. Even the shape of birthmarks and other skin defects is sometimes believed to reflect maternal impressions. For example, eating strawberries by the mother is associated with nevi. Articles of apparel or adornment, food cravings, emotions such as fright and anger, undesirable thoughts, and the time and manner of announcing the pregnancy are all believed to influence the well-being of the unborn child.

Expectant mothers who are able to rationalize the illogical nature of the beliefs will, through a normal fear of having an abnormal infant, conform to the superstitions. In most instances these customs are relatively harmless and are not in conflict with sound health practices. However, there may be situations wherein conformity to cultural or subcultural beliefs may compromise the health and well-being of either the mother or the fetus (e.g., the practice of eating clay, cornstarch, chalk, or other substances). Nurses and other health care workers must be understanding and take care to explore with the mother all the ramifications of the practice without creating undue stress and guilt.

Prolonged stimulation of the autonomic nervous system caused by extreme stress or long-term anxiety produces physiologic changes in the maternal system, such as increased heart rate, vasoconstriction, and decreased gastric motility. In addition to the indirect effect produced by constriction of uterine blood flow, the stress hormones cross the placental membrane to affect the fetus directly. Assisting the expectant mother in dealing with her stresses or securing counseling services for her is part of the nursing considerations.

**NURSING ALERT** Not all of these beliefs are unfounded. There is evidence that maternal emotions may indeed affect the fetus.

## Importance of Culture to Nurses

A general consensus exists among nurses that cultural competence of professional nursing practice should be raised (Lester, 1998). To understand and deal effectively with families in a multicultural community, it is important that nurses be aware of their own attitudes and values. Nurses, too, are a product of their own cultural background and education. They are part of the "nursing culture." Nurses function within the framework of a professional culture with its own values and traditions and, as such, become socialized into that culture by educational program and later by the work environment and professional associations.

Frequently nurses and other health care workers are not aware of their own cultural values and how those values influence their thoughts and actions. Those who are aware of their own culturally founded behavior are more sensitive to cultural behavior in others (Box 2-4). To recognize that a behavior may be characteristic of a culture rather than

---

### Box 2-4 ■ ■ ■
### Exploring Your Cultural Heritage

To provide culturally sensitive care to children and their families from cultures that are different from your own, you must first become aware of your own cultural values and beliefs and recognize how they influence your attitudes and behaviors. As you begin to understand the values that culture instills, you become better prepared to assess another culture objectively. The following questions have no right or wrong answers. They should help you clarify your attitudes and beliefs and how they influence your ability to work with people from diverse cultural backgrounds.

What ethnic group, socioeconomic class, religion, age-group, and community do you belong to?
- ☐ What about these groups do you find embarrassing or would like to change? Why?
- ☐ What sociocultural factors in your background might be rejected by members of other cultures?
- ☐ What did your parents and significant others say about people who were different from your family?

What do you believe or value?
- ☐ How do you define health, disease, illness?
- ☐ Are you usually on time? Early? Late?
- ☐ How do you feel if others are late? Frustrated? Angry? Not respected?
- ☐ What are your views on childhood education?
- ☐ Are you comfortable with physical contact (touching, embracing)? How much and with whom?
- ☐ What are your religious views and biases? Do you adhere to religious rituals?
- ☐ What are your feelings on childrearing practices (including nutrition, discipline, play, roles)?

What experiences have you had with people from ethnic groups, socioeconomic classes, religions, age-groups, or communities different from your own?
- ☐ What were those experiences like?
- ☐ How did you feel about them?

What personal qualities do you have that will help you establish interpersonal relationships with persons from other cultural groups?

What personal qualities may be detrimental?

---

Data from Randall-David E: *Strategies for working with culturally diverse communities and clients,* Washington, DC, 1989, Association for the Care of Children's Health; and Niederhauser V: Health care of immigrant children: incorporating culture into practice, *Pediatr Nurs* 15(6):569-574, 1989.

being an "abnormal" behavior places nurses at an advantage in their relationships with families. When nurses respect the cultural differences of a family, they are better able to determine whether the behavior is distinctive to the individual or a characteristic of the culture. What appears to be puzzling behavior may simply be the customary response in the culture (e.g., expression of emotion).

Cultural standards and values, the family structure and function, and past experiences with health care influence a family's feelings and attitudes toward health, their children, and health care delivery systems. It is often difficult for nurses to be nonjudgmental and objective in working with families whose behaviors and attitudes differ from or conflict with their own. Being aware of one's own feelings and attitudes, as well as respecting those of the family, is essential to a helping relationship and achievement of nursing goals. Relying only on one's own values and experiences for guidance can result in frustration and disappointment. It is one thing to know what is needed to deal with a health problem; it is often quite another to implement a fruitful course of action unless nurses work within the cultural and socioeconomic framework of the family. (See Critical Thinking Exercise box.)

It is essential to make an effort to adapt ethnic practices to the health needs of the family rather than attempt to change long-standing beliefs. To aid their efforts to understand and respect the cultural beliefs of families, nurses should have a readily available resource file containing pertinent information about the cultural and subcultural characteristics of the community in which they practice (e.g., traditional practices related to infant feeding practices and the time and manner of weaning and toilet training). Bridging cultural gaps in delivery of health care to children requires the establishment of a close relationship with families and other influential persons in the community (such as the local folk healer) and periodic assessment of one's own attitudes and behaviors and those of other health workers toward persons of other racial or ethnic origins.

## CULTURAL AWARENESS

Cultural and religious rituals, such as the Jewish ceremony *Upsherenish* (inaugural haircutting ceremony), are important practices among families from various cultures. In the Upsherenish, a male child's hair is not cut until 3 years of age. Any procedure requiring haircutting, such as placement of an intravenous line in a scalp vein, must be discussed with parents to obtain their permission.

Some characteristics of selected cultures are outlined in Table 2-2. Nurses must assess the cultural and religious practices of families to identify how these practices are similar to and different from those of their own cultural and religious backgrounds. Guidelines for assessing cultural and religious practices of families are described on p. 45.

---

### Critical Thinking Exercise

#### Cultural Practices

Knowledge of cultural practices in a locality can be as important as knowledge of communicable diseases. What is true about this statement?

FIRST, THINK ABOUT IT . . .
- What is the purpose of your thinking?
- Within what point of view are you thinking?

1. It is not valuable unless the nurse uses it to assess contributing cultural factors that may aid or hinder the care of the child and family.
2. It is not helpful unless the nurse is part of the culture.
3. It is valuable only in making nurses aware of diversities in care.
4. It is learned only from reading about the traditional beliefs and practices of cultural groups.

*The best response is one. Information about a culture serves no purpose and is not valuable unless you apply the knowledge to the situation. A nurse does not need to be a part of a culture to be aware of differences and to respect its practices. Although cultural knowledge may be helpful in awareness of diversities in practices and care, putting the knowledge to use is the challenge and the goal. Information about cultures is learned from a variety of methods: observation, previous experience and interactions, television, journals, textbooks, travel, and so on. Also, it is important to remember that the nurse interprets cultural knowledge from within the nurse's own point of view.*

---

**NURSING ALERT** These generalizations are presented to help nurses learn the unique beliefs and practices of various groups and are not meant to be stereotypes of any group. It is critical to remember that no cultural group is homogeneous, every racial and ethnic group contains great diversity, and knowledge of a culture may not reflect an individual member's beliefs (Nance, 1995).

## HEREDITARY FACTORS

Some groups of people are more susceptible and others more resistant to certain illnesses than are persons from other groups. An innate susceptibility is acquired through generations of evolutionary changes that take place within constrained or segregated populations. The proximity to disease, environmental factors, and the general physical status are significant factors associated with health problems.

Historically, the increased health risks associated with ethnicity have been explained in terms of genetic differences or related factors such as socioeconomic status (Scribner, 1996). The genetic constitution of individuals as groups is known to influence the degree to which they are susceptible to a specific disorder. It may be a result of an inherent lack of resistance to a disease organism, a trait that is an advantage in one environment but places the possessor at a disadvantage in another, or it may be the consequence of intermarriage within a relatively narrow range of geographic, ethnic, or religious restrictions.

**TABLE 2-2** Cultural characteristics related to health care of children and families

| Cultural Group | Health Beliefs | Health Practices |
|---|---|---|
| **Asians**<br>**Chinese** | A healthy body viewed as gift from parents and ancestors and must be cared for<br>Health is one of the results of balance between the forces of *yin* (cold) and *yang* (hot)—energy forces that rule the world<br>Illness caused by imbalance<br>Believe blood is source of life and is not regenerated<br>*Chi* is innate energy<br>Lack of chi and blood results in deficiency that produces fatigue, poor constitution, and long illness | Goal of therapy is to restore balance of yin and yang<br>Acupuncturist applies needles to appropriate meridians identified in terms of yin and yang<br>Acupressure and *tai chi* replacing acupuncture in some areas<br>*Moxibustion* is application of heat to skin over specific meridians<br>Wide use of medicinal herbs procured and applied in prescribed ways<br>Folk healers are herbalist, spiritual healer, temple healer, fortune healer<br>Meals may or may not be planned to balance hot and cold<br>Milk intolerance relatively common<br>Use of condiments (e.g., monosodium glutamate and soy sauce) may create difficulty with some diet regimens (e.g., low-salt diets) |
| **Japanese** | Three major belief systems:<br>  *Shinto* religious influence<br>    Humans inherently good<br>    Evil caused by outside spirits<br>    Illness caused by contact with polluting agents (e.g., blood, corpses, skin diseases)<br>  Chinese and Korean influence<br>    Health achieved through harmony and balance between self and society<br>    Disease caused by disharmony with society and not caring for body<br>  Portuguese influence<br>    Upholds germ theory of disease | Believe evil removed by purification<br>Energy restored by means of acupuncture, acupressure, massage, and moxibustion along affected meridians<br>*Kampō* medicine—use of natural herbs<br>Believe in removal of diseased parts<br>Trend is to use both Western and Asian healing methods<br>Care for disabled viewed as family's responsibility<br>Take pride in child's good health<br>Seek preventive care, medical care for illness<br>May avoid some food combinations (e.g., milk and cherries, watermelon and crab) and believe pickled plums to have special properties |
| **Vietnamese** | Good health considered to be balance between yin and yang<br>Believe person's life has been predisposed toward certain phenomena by cosmic forces<br>Health believed to be result of harmony with existing universal order; harmony attained by pleasing good spirits and avoiding evil ones<br>Belief in *am duc*, the amount of good deeds accumulated by ancestors<br>Many use rituals to prevent illness<br>Practice some restrictions to prevent incurring wrath of evil spirits | Family uses all means possible before using outside agencies for health care<br>Fortune-tellers determine event that caused disturbance<br>May visit temple to procure divine instruction<br>Use astrologer to calculate cyclic changes and forces<br>Regard health as family responsibility; outside aid sought when resources run out<br>Certain illnesses considered only temporary (such as pustules, open wounds) and ignored<br>Seek generalist health healers<br>May use special diets to prevent illness and promote health<br>Lactose intolerance prevalent |
| **Filipinos** | Believe God's will and supernatural forces govern universe<br>Illness, accidents, and other misfortunes are God's punishment for violations of His will<br>Widely accept "hot" and "cold" balance and imbalance as cause of health and illness | Some use amulets as a shield from witchcraft or as good luck pieces<br>Catholics substitute religious medals and other items |
| **African-Americans** | Illness classified as:<br>  Natural—affected by forces of nature without adequate protection (e.g., cold air, pollution, food and water)<br>  Unnatural—evil influences (e.g., witchcraft, voodoo, hoodoo, hex, fix, root work); symptoms often associated with eating<br>Believe serious illness sent by God as punishment (e.g., parents punished by illness or death of child)<br>Believe serious illness can be avoided<br>May resist health care because illness is "will of God" | Self-care and folk medicine very prevalent<br>Folk therapies usually religious in origin<br>Attempt home remedies first; poorer people do not seek help until illness serious<br>Usually seek help from:<br>  "Old lady"—woman in community with a common knowledge of herbs; consulted regarding pediatric care<br>  Spiritualist—has received gift from God for healing incurable diseases or solving personal problems; strongly based in Christianity<br>  Priest (voodoo priest/priestess)—most powerful healer<br>  Root doctor—meets need for herbs, oils, candles, and ointments<br>Prayer is common means for prevention and treatment |

Sources: Anderson and Fenichel, 1989; Clark, 1981; DeSantis, 1988; Geissler, 1994; Giger and Davidhizar, 1995; Holland and Sweeney, 1985; Hollingsworth, Brown, and Brooten, 1980; Orgue, Bloch, and Monrroy, 1983; Randall-David, 1989; Sodetaini-Shibata, 1981.

| Family Relationships | Communication | Comments |
| --- | --- | --- |
| Extended family pattern common<br>Strong concept of loyalty of young to old<br>Respect for elders taught at early age—acceptance without questioning or talking back<br>Children's behavior a reflection on family<br>Family and individual honor and "face" important<br>Self-reliance and self-restraint highly valued; self-expression repressed<br>Males valued more highly than females; women submissive to men in family | Open expression of emotions unacceptable<br>Often smile when do not comprehend | Do not react well to painful diagnostic workup; are especially upset by drawing of blood<br>Deep respect for their bodies and believe it best to die with bodies intact; therefore may refuse surgery<br>Believe in reincarnation<br>Older members fear hospitals; often believe hospital is a place to go to die<br>Children sometimes breast-fed for up to 4 or 5 years* |
| Close intergenerational relationships<br>Family provides anchor<br>Family tends to keep problems to self<br>Value self-control and self-sufficiency<br>Concept of *haji* (shame) imposes strong control; unacceptable behavior of children reflects on family<br>Many adopt practices of contemporary middle class<br>Concern for child's missing school may result in sending to school before fully recovered from illness | Issei—born in Japan; usually speak Japanese only<br>Nisei, Sansei, and Yonsei have few language difficulties<br>New immigrants able to read and write English better than able to speak or understand it<br>Make significant use of nonverbal communication with subtle gestures and facial expression<br>Tend to suppress emotions<br>Will often wait silently | Generational categories:<br>  *Issei*—1st generation to live in United States<br>  *Nisei*—2nd generation<br>  *Sansei*—3rd generation<br>  *Yonsei*—4th generation<br>Issei and Nisei—tolerant and permissive child-rearing until 5 or 6, then emphasis on emotional reserve and control<br>Cleanliness highly valued<br>Time considered valuable and used wisely |
| Family is revered institution<br>Multigenerational families<br>Family is chief social network<br>Children highly valued<br>Individual needs and interests are subordinate to those of a family group<br>Father is main decision maker<br>Women taught submission to men<br>Parents expect respect and obedience from children | Many immigrants are not proficient in speaking and understanding English<br>May hesitate to ask questions<br>Questioning authority is sign of disrespect; asking questions considered impolite<br>Use indirectness rather than forthrightness in expressing disagreement<br>May avoid eye contact with health professionals as a sign of respect | Tendency to practice emotional control may make assessment of pain more difficult<br>Consider status more important than money<br>Children taught emotional control<br>Time concept more relaxed—consider punctuality less significant than other values (i.e., propriety)<br>Place high value on social harmony |
| Family is highly valued, with strong family ties<br>Multigenerational family structure common, often including collateral members<br>Personal interests are subordinated to family interests and needs<br>Members avoid any behavior that would bring shame on the family | Immigrants and older persons may not be able to speak or understand English | Tend to have a fatalistic outlook on life<br>Believe time and providence will solve all |
| Strong kinship bonds in extended family; members come to aid of others in crisis<br>Less likely to view illness as a burden<br>Augmented families common (unrelated persons living in same household)<br>Place strong emphasis on work and ambition<br>Sex-role sharing among parents<br>Elderly members respected | Alert to any evidence of discrimination<br>Place importance on nonverbal behavior<br>May use nonstandard English or "Black English"<br>Use "testing" behaviors to assess personnel in health care situations before seeking active care<br>Best to use simple, direct, but caring approach | High level of caution or distrust of majority group<br>Social anxiety related to tradition of humiliation, oppression, and loss of dignity<br>Will elect to retain dignity rather than seek care if values are compromised<br>Strong sense of peoplehood<br>High incidence of poverty<br>Black minister a strong influence in black community<br>Visits by family minister are sought, expected, and valued in helping to cope with illness and suffering |

*Most Asian cultures consider the child 1 year old at the time of birth. Traditional Chinese custom adds 1 year on January 1 regardless of the birthday—a child born in December is 2 years old the next January.

*Continued*

**TABLE 2-2** Cultural characteristics related to health care of children and families—cont'd

| Cultural Group | Health Beliefs | Health Practices |
|---|---|---|
| Haitians* | Illnesses have a supernatural or natural origin<br>Supernatural illnesses are caused by angry voodoo spirits, enemies, or the dead, especially deceased ancestors<br>Natural illnesses are based on conceptions of natural causation:<br>  Irregularities of blood volume, flow, purity, viscosity, color, and temperature (hot/cold)<br>Gas *(gaz)*<br>Movement and consistency of mother's milk<br>"Hot"/"cold" imbalance in the body<br>Bone displacement<br>Movement of diseases<br>Health is maintained by good dietary and hygienic habits | Health is a personal responsibility<br>Foods have properties of "hot"/"cold" and "light"/"heavy" and must be in harmony with one's life cycle and bodily states<br>Natural illnesses treated by home remedies first<br>Supernatural illness treated by healers: voodoo priest *(houngan)* or priestess *(mambo)*, midwife *(fam saj)*, and herbalist or leaf doctor *(dokte fey)*<br>Amulets and prayer used to protect against illness due to curses or willed by evil people |
| Hispanics<br>  Mexicans (Latinos, Chicanos, Raza-Latinos) | Health beliefs have strong religious association<br>Believe in body imbalance as a cause of illness, especially imbalance between *caliente* ("hot") and *frio* ("cold") or "wet" and "dry"<br>Some maintain good health is a result of "good luck"—a reward for good behavior<br>Illness prevented by performing properly, eating proper foods, and working proper amount of time; accomplished through prayer, wearing religious medals or amulets, and sleeping with relics at home<br>Illness is a punishment from God for wrongdoing, forces of nature, and the supernatural | Seek help from *curandero* or *curandera*, especially in rural areas<br>Curandero(a) receives position by birth, apprenticeship, or a "calling" via dream or vision<br>Treatments involve use of herbs, rituals, and religious artifacts<br>Practice for severe illness—make promises, visit shrines, offer medals and candles, offer prayers<br>Adhere to "hot" and "cold" food prescriptions and prohibitions for prevention and treatment of illness |
| Puerto Ricans | Subscribe to the "hot-cold" theory of causation of illness<br>Believe some illness caused by evil spirits and forces | Infrequent use of health care systems<br>Seek folk healers—use of herbs, rituals<br>Consult spiritualist medium for mental disorders<br>Treatments classified as "hot" or "cold" |
| Cubans† | Prevention and good nutrition related to good health | Diligent users of the medical model<br>Eclectic health-seeking practices, including preventive measures, and, in some instances, folk medicine of both religious and nonreligious origins; home remedies; in many instances seek assistance of santeros and spiritualists to complement medical treatment<br>Nutrition is important; parents show overconcern with eating habits of their children and spend a considerable part of the budget on food; traditional Cuban diet is rich in meat and starch; consumption of fresh vegetables added in United States |
| Native Americans<br>  (numerous tribes) | Believe health is state of harmony with nature and universe<br>Respect of bodies through proper management<br>All disorders believed to have aspects of supernatural<br>Violation of a restriction or prohibition thought to cause illness<br>Fear of witchcraft<br>May carry objects believed to guard against witchcraft<br>Theology and medicine strongly interwoven | Medicine persons—altruistic persons who must use powers as well as herbs and rituals in purely positive ways<br>Persons capable of both good and evil—perform negative acts against enemies<br>Diviner-diagnosticians—diagnose but do not have powers or skill to implement medical treatment<br>Specialists—use herbs and curative but nonsacred medical procedures<br>Singers—cure by the power of their song obtained from supernatural beings; effect cures by laying on of hands |

Sources: Anderson and Fenichel, 1989; Clark, 1981; DeSantis, 1988; Geissler, 1994; Giger and Davidhizar, 1995; Holland and Sweeney, 1985; Hollingsworth, Brown, and Brooten, 1980; Orgue, Bloch, and Monrroy, 1983; Randall-David, 1989; Sodetaini-Shibata, 1981.
*This section was written by Lydia DeSantis, PhD, RN.
†This section was written by Mercedes Sandaval, PhD.

| Family Relationships | Communication | Comments |
| --- | --- | --- |
| Maintenance of family reputation paramount<br>Lineal authority supreme; children in a subordinate position in family hierarchy<br>Children valued for parental social security in old age and expected to contribute to family welfare at an early age<br>Children viewed as "gifts from God" and treated with indulgence and affection | Recent immigrants and older persons may speak only Haitian creole<br>May prefer family or friends to act as translators and confidants<br>Often smile and nod in agreement when do not understand<br>Quiet and gentle communication style and lack of assertiveness lead health care providers to falsely believe they comprehend health teaching and are compliant<br>Will not ask questions if health care provider is busy or rushed | Will use biomedical and ethnomedical (folk) systems simultaneously<br>Resistant to dietary and work restrictions<br>Adherence to prescribed treatments directly related to perceived severity of illness |
| Traditionally men considered breadwinners and key decision makers in matters outside the home; women considered homemakers<br>Males considered big and strong *(macho)*<br>Strong kinship; extended families include *compadres* (godparents) established by ritual kinship<br>Children valued highly and desired, taken everywhere with family<br>Many homes contain shrines with statues and pictures of saints<br>Elderly treated with respect | May use nonstandard English<br>Some bilingual; many only speak Spanish<br>May have a strong preference for native language and revert to it in times of stress<br>May shake hands or engage in introductory embrace<br>Interpret prolonged eye contact as disrespectful | High degree of modesty—often a deterrent to seeking medical care and open discussions of sex<br>Youngsters often reluctant to share communal showers in schools<br>Relaxed concept of time—may be late for appointments<br>More concerned with present than with future and therefore may focus on immediate solutions rather than long-term goals<br>Magicoreligious practices common<br>May view hospital as place to go to die |
| Family usually large and home centered—the core of existence<br>Father has complete authority in family—family provider and decision maker<br>Wife and children subordinate to father<br>Children valued—seen as a gift from God<br>Children taught to obey and respect parents; corporal punishment to ensure obedience | May use nonstandard English<br>Spanish speaking or bilingual<br>Strong sense of family privacy—may view questions regarding family as impudent | Relaxed sense of time<br>Pay little attention to *exact* time of day<br>Suspicious and fearful of hospitals |
| Strong family ties with mother and father kinships<br>Children supported and assisted by parents long after becoming adults<br>Elderly cared for at home | Most are bilingual (English/Spanish) except for segments of the senior population | In less than 30 years Cubans have been able to obtain a higher standard of living than other Hispanic groups in the United States<br>Have been able to retain many of their former social institutions: bilingual and private schools, clinics, social clubs, the family as an extended network of support, etc.<br>Many do not feel discriminated against or harbor feelings of inferiority with respect to Anglo-Americans or "mainstream" population |
| Extended family structure—usually includes relatives from both sides of family<br>Elder members assume leadership roles | Most continue to speak their Indian language as well as English<br>Nonverbal communication | Time orientation—present<br>Respect for age<br>Going to hospital associated with illness or disease; therefore may not seek prenatal care because pregnancy viewed as natural process<br>Tend to take time to form an opinion of professionals<br>Sexual matters not openly discussed with members of opposite sex |

A geographic constraint is illustrated by the classic example of the common communicable disease rubeola. The rubeola virus, or the populations that were continually exposed to it, became altered in such a way that the disease was considered to be a universal disease of childhood from which the majority of children suffered without ill effects. When other populations (e.g., the inhabitants of the Hawaiian Islands) were exposed to the virus by explorers and missionaries, they experienced a violent response that resulted in high mortality.

Another communicable disease, tuberculosis, appears to be more prevalent in certain ethnic groups such as the Native Americans of the Southwest, Vietnamese immigrants, and Mexican-Americans. In many populations it is difficult to determine how much the increased incidence can be attributed to ethnic factors and how much is related to the lifestyles in the lower social strata.

A number of diseases show ethnic or racial differences. For example, Tay-Sachs disease, characterized by early neurologic deterioration and mental retardation, affects primarily Ashkenazi Jewish families, particularly those of Northeastern European origin, whereas Sephardic Jewish families appear to be no more at risk for the disease than other populations. The incidence of cystic fibrosis is highest in whites and almost nonexistent in Asians, and the rare affected African-Americans are usually in areas where there is apt to be mixed ancestry. Some selected genetic disorders that are more prevalent in certain populations are listed in Table 2-3. A classic disorder of blacks, especially Africans, is sickle cell disease (see Chapter 35); however, the incidence

**TABLE 2-3**   Distribution of selected genetic traits and disorders by population or ethnic group

| Ethnic or Population Group | Genetic or Multifactorial Disorder Present in Relatively High Frequency | Ethnic or Population Group | Genetic or Multifactorial Disorder Present in Relatively High Frequency |
|---|---|---|---|
| Aland Islanders | Ocular albinism (Forsius-Erikkson type) | Jews | |
| Amish | Limb-girdle muscular dystrophy (IN—Adams, Allen counties) | Ashkenazi | Tay-Sachs disease (infantile) |
| | Ellis–van Creveld syndrome (PA—Lancaster county) | | Niemann-Pick disease (infantile) |
| | Pyruvate kinase deficiency (OH—Mifflin county) | | Gaucher disease (adult type) |
| | Hemophilia B (PA—Holmes county) | | Familial dysautonomia (Riley-Day syndrome) |
| Armenians | Familial Mediterranean fever | | Bloom syndrome |
| | Familial paroxysmal polyserositis | | Torsion dystonia |
| Blacks (African) | Sickle cell disease | | Factor XI (PTA) deficiency |
| | Hemoglobin C disease | Sephardic | Familial Mediterranean fever |
| | Hereditary persistence of hemoglobin F | | Ataxia-telangiectasia (Morocco) |
| | G-6-PD deficiency, African type | | Cystinuria (Libya) |
| | Lactase deficiency, adult | | Glycogen storage disease III (Morocco) |
| | β-Thalassemia | Lebanese | Dyggve-Melchoir-Clausen syndrome |
| Burmese | Hemoglobin E disease | Mediterranean people (Italians, Greeks) | G-6-PD deficiency, Mediterranean type |
| Chinese | Alpha thalassemia | | β-Thalassemia |
| | G-6-PD deficiency, Chinese type | | Familial Mediterranean fever |
| | Lactase deficiency, adult | Middle Eastern people | Dubin-Johnson syndrome (Iran) |
| Costa Rican | Malignant osteopetrosis | | Ichthyosis vulgaris (Iraq) |
| English | Cystic fibrosis | | Werdnig-Hoffman disease (Karaite Jews) |
| | Hereditary amyloidosis, type III | | G-6-PD deficiency, Mediterranean type |
| Eskimos | Congenital adrenal hyperplasia | | Phenylketonuria (Yemen) |
| | Pseudocholinesterase deficiency | | Metachromatic leukodystrophy (Habbanite Jews, Saudi Arabia) |
| | Methemoglobinemia | Navajo Indians | Ear anomalies |
| Finns | Congenital nephrosis | Nova Scotia Acadians | Niemann-Pick disease, type D |
| | Generalized amyloidosis syndrome, V | Polish | Phenylketonuria |
| | Polycystic liver disease | Polynesians | Clubfoot |
| | Retinoschisis | Portuguese | Joseph disease |
| | Aspartylglycosaminuria | Scandinavians (Norwegians, Swedes, Danes) | Cholestasis-lymphedema (Norwegians) |
| | Diastrophic dwarfism | | Sjögren-Larsson syndrome (Swedes) |
| French Canadians (Quebec) | Tyrosinemia | | Krabbe disease |
| | Morquio syndrome | | Phenylketonuria |
| Gypsies (Czech) | Congenital glaucoma | Scots | Phenylketonuria |
| Hopi Indians | Tyrosinase-positive albinism | | Cystic fibrosis |
| Icelanders | Phenylketonuria | | Hereditary amyloidosis, type III |
| Irish | Phenylketonuria | Thai | Lactase deficiency, adult |
| | Neural tube defects | | Hemoglobin E disease |
| Japanese | Acatalasemia | Zuni Indians | Tyrosinase-positive albinism |
| | Cleft lip/palate | | |
| | Oguchi disease | | |

Sources: Cohen, 1984; Damon, 1969; Der Kaloustian, Maffah, and Loiselet, 1980; Ferak, Genčík, and Genčíkova, 1982; Goodman, 1979; McKusick, 1992; Scriver, 1989.

of cardiovascular disease, pneumonia, and diabetes is also high among African-Americans. Native Americans have particularly high rates of diabetes, tuberculosis, diarrhea, alcoholism, and suicide. Racial and ethnic differences are further considered in relation to diseases and defects as they are discussed throughout the book.

Common food items and drugs may cause health problems in certain ethnic groups. For example, people of Mediterranean, African, Near Eastern, and Asian origin frequently have glucose-6-phosphate dehydrogenase (G-6-PD) deficiency. They may develop acute hemolytic anemia after they ingest fava (horse or broad) beans or certain drugs such as aspirin preparations, sulfonamides, or primaquine. Other groups, especially southern Europeans, Jews, Arabs, African-Americans, Asians, and Native Americans, have a deficiency of lactase, the enzyme needed to metabolize lactose. Ingestion of lactose can cause abdominal distention, flatus, and diarrhea. Unknowing but well-meaning health care workers may be responsible for these symptoms in their clients when they prescribe foods or food supplements containing lactose as sources of nutrients.

## Physical Characteristics

Among racial groups there are observable differences in physical appearance. The most obvious are skin and hair coloring and texture. Skin color is determined by the amount of melanin present in the skin. People from countries located near the equator have darkly pigmented skin, which serves to protect the skin from the year-round exposure to the sun's rays; those from the northern countries have very light skin, which provides for maximum exposure to the sun's rays (necessary for vitamin D metabolism) during the short daylight hours. There can be wide variations in skin color between these two extremes in terms of geographic origin or from intermixing of persons with dark and light skin color.

As a consequence of the dark pigmentation, the detection of skin color changes can be difficult and requires modification of assessment techniques. For example, vasomotor alterations, cyanosis, and jaundice observable in the skin are not easily recognized in very dark skin. Variations in the skin color can alter the appearance of the skin in a given circumstance. (See Table 7-9.)

In the newborn, variations are often related to racial or ethnic origin. For example, newborn infants of Asian and black parents are smaller than infants of white parentage, and bluish pigmented areas (mongolian spots) on the sacral region are a common observation in Asian, African-American, Native American, and Mexican infants.

Evaluation of stature and body build reveals some racial tendencies. Children from Asian countries are commonly smaller, falling below the 10th percentile on weight and height charts used for children in the United States. This difference in stature can lead to misinterpretation of health status and capabilities. A small child may appear very intelligent for body size but be of average mental ability for age.

## RELIGIOUS INFLUENCES

Probably the most influential factor in shaping the culture of the United States is the Judeo-Christian faith. Many immigrants came to the United States for religious freedom and established a religious and moral atmosphere that persists today. However, there are individual differences that are part of the general culture.

The religious orientation of the family dictates a code of morality, as well as influencing the family's attitudes toward education, male and female role identity, and attitudes regarding their ultimate destiny (Fig. 2-6). It may also determine the school that the children attend, the companions with whom they associate, and often their mate selection. In many cultures the religious beliefs are such an integral part of the culture that it is difficult to distinguish one from the other. In a few instances, such as in the Mennonite and Amish communities, religion is the basis for a common way of life that determines where the children are reared and their lifestyle.

## Religious Beliefs

Religious and spiritual dimensions of life are among the most important influences in many people's lives. The terms *religion* and *spirituality* are often used interchangeably; however, spirituality subsumes religion. Both religion and spirituality lend meaning in life and provide a source of love and relatedness between individuals and their God (Lukoff, Lu, and Turner, 1995). Holistic nursing care is promoted through an integration of spiritual and psychosocial care. The care focuses on activities that support a person's system of beliefs and worship, such as prayer, reading religious materials, and

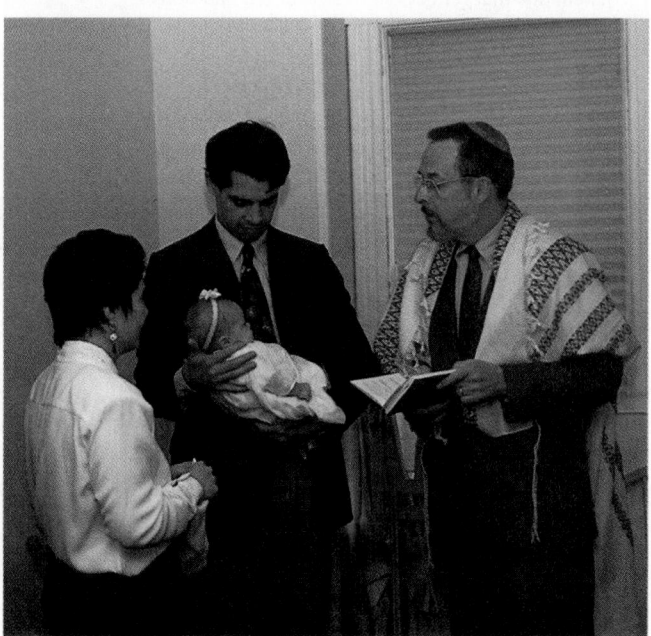

**Fig. 2-6**    Soon after an infant is born, many families have special religious ceremonies.

assisting with religious rituals. Meeting the spiritual needs of the child and family can provide strength, whereas unmet spiritual needs can result in spiritual distress and debilitation (Fulton and Moore, 1995). In practice, application of the nursing process for spiritual care (Box 2-5) can provide for the spiritual well-being of the child and family.

Religion influences the lifestyles of most cultures. Among many groups illness, injury, or death is believed to be sent by God as a punishment for sin. Some may believe that health workers will be unable to help a person whom God is punishing and may express a fatalistic attitude toward treatment, stating that it is "the will of God." Others view it as a test of strength, as the testing of Job in the Bible, and strive to remain faithful and overcome the conflicts.

Dietary restrictions are clarified, especially in denominations in which there may be many variations. When specific religious practices do not interfere with the health of the child or the therapy (such as fasting), the wishes of the family are respected. Family members are asked whether they want a clergy member present and whether they prefer hospital staff to call or prefer to do this on their own.

> **NURSING TIP** Children will rarely voice a need for spiritual support. Listen closely for indirect references.

It is important to determine the wishes of the family regarding baptism, rites or practices related to death, and other religious rituals (such as circumcision, Communion, or use of amulets or icons). Many religions have special clothing requirements, such as a cap (Keppah) for the head (Orthodox Jews) or underclothes (Mormons). Respecting these rituals is especially important during a physical examination or preparation for surgery. An important role of the nurse is to be aware of spiritual needs of families and convey an attitude of concern for this important element of the child's care. Religion, which offers families understanding and spiritual support, is a valuable asset to health care. Characteristics of selected religions with beliefs that affect health care are outlined in Table 2-4.

In some instances the rights of the family and the responsibility of the state may be in conflict. For example, Jehovah's Witnesses refuse blood transfusions for themselves and for their children. Parents, by law, have the pri-

---

## Box 2-5 ■ ■ ■
### Application of the Nursing Process for Spiritual Care

**ASSESSMENT**

Observe the environment for religious articles.
Observe if the child uses religious rituals, such as prayers or stories, or receives visits from spiritual leaders.
Ask open-ended questions to elicit the importance of religion.
Assess physical and psychosocial behaviors that are indicators of spiritual distress (anger, guilt, fear, alienation, sleeplessness, regression); assess family interactions and relationships.

**PLANNING**

Be aware of needs related to specific religious beliefs.
Consider the developmental stage of the child, particularly with regard to lack of abstract thinking and the need for a sense of accomplishment and control.
Develop a trusting relationship and include family members in the process.
Teach family interventions to promote spiritual well-being.

**IMPLEMENTATION**

Offer opportunities for religious rituals and expressions if they are part of the child's spiritual life.
Offer use of self by listening to the concerns of the child and family.
Explore the spiritual dimension through the use of therapeutic play, bibliotherapy, and other forms of artistic expression while involving family members; provide direction and choices to support management of the chronic condition.

**OUTCOMES**

Use of religious practices, if relevant
Positive statements about meaning and purpose in life
Statements that reflect forgiveness of self and others
Restored relationships with significant others

From Fulton RA, Moore CM: Spiritual care of the school-age child with a chronic condition, *J Pediatr Nurs* 10(4):224-231, 1995.

---

## TABLE 2-4 Religious beliefs that affect nursing care

| Beliefs About Birth and Death | Beliefs About Diet and Food Practices | Beliefs Regarding Medical Care | Comments |
|---|---|---|---|
| **Baptist (27 Groups)** | | | |
| **Birth:** No baptism<br>Believers are baptized by immersion as adults<br>**Death:** Clergy seeks to minister by counsel and prayer with patient and family<br>**Organ donation/transplantation:** Both organ donation and transplantation are generally approved of when they do not seriously endanger donor and when they offer medical hope for recipient | Some groups discourage coffee, tea, and alcohol | May encounter some resistance to some therapies, such as abortion<br>Some believe in predestination; may respond passively to care | Fundamentalist and conservative groups accept Bible as inspired word of God |

From Carpenito LJ: *Nursing diagnosis: application to clinical practice*, ed 4, Philadelphia, 1992, JB Lippincott; Conley L: Childbearing and childrearing practices in Mormonism, *Neonatal Network* 9(3):41-48, 1990; Kozier B, Erb G: *Fundamentals of nursing*, ed 5, Menlo Park, CA, 1995, Addison-Wesley; McQuay JE: Cross cultural customs and beliefs related to health crisis, death, and organ donation/transplantation, *Crit Care Nurs Clin North Am* 7(3):581-594, 1995; and Spector RE: *Cultural diversity in health and illness*, ed 5, Upper Saddle River, NJ, 2000, Prentice-Hall Health.

**TABLE 2-4**    Religious beliefs that affect nursing care—cont'd

| Beliefs About Birth and Death | Beliefs About Diet and Food Practices | Beliefs Regarding Medical Care | Comments |
|---|---|---|---|
| **Buddhist** | | | |
| **Birth:** No baptism<br>Infant presentation<br>**Death:** Last rite chanting is often practiced at bedside soon after death; the deceased's family or Buddhist priest should be contacted<br>**Organ donation/transplantation:** Believe that organ donation is a matter of individual conscience | No requirements or restrictions<br>Some sects are strictly vegetarian<br>Discourage use of alcohol and drugs | Illness is believed to be a trial to aid development of soul; illness due to Karmic causes<br>May be reluctant to have surgery or certain treatments on holy days<br>Cleanliness is believed to be of great importance<br>Family may request Buddhist priest for counseling | Optimistic outlook; teach ways to overcome fears, anxieties, apprehension |
| **Church of Christ Scientist (Christian Science)** | | | |
| **Birth:** No baptism<br>**Death:** No last rites; autopsy is not permitted except in cases of sudden death; it is an individual's decision to choose burial or cremation<br>**Organ donation/transplantation:** Church takes no specific position on transplantation or donation as distinct from other medical or surgical procedures | No requirements or restrictions | Oppose human intervention with drugs or other therapies; however, accept legally required immunizations<br>Many adhere to belief that disease is human mental concept that can be dispelled by spiritual truth to extent that they refuse all medical treatment | Many desire services of practitioner or reader; will sometimes refuse even emergency treatment until they have consulted a reader |
| **Church of Jesus Christ of Latter Day Saints (Mormon)** | | | |
| **Birth:** No baptism<br>Infant is blessed by church official at first opportunity after birth (in church)<br>Baptism by immersion at 8 years<br>**Death:** Believe that it is proper to bury the dead in the ground, and cremation is discouraged<br>**Organ donation/transplantation:** Question of whether one should will his or her organs to be used as transplants is left to the individual | Prohibit tea, coffee, alcohol<br>Some individuals avoid chocolate and other products that contain caffeine<br>Encourage sparing use of meats<br>Fasting for 24 hours on first Sunday of each month (from after evening meal Saturday until evening meal Sunday) | Devout adherents believe in divine healing through anointment with oil and laying on of hands by church officials (appointed church members)<br>Medical therapy is not prohibited | May request *Sacrament* on Sunday while in hospital<br>Financial support for sick is available through well-funded welfare system<br>Discourage cremation<br>Discourage use of tobacco<br>Married adults wear special undergarments |
| **Episcopal (Anglican)** | | | |
| **Birth:** Infant baptism is mandatory; urgent if poor prognosis<br>**Death:** Last rites (Rite for Anointing of the Sick) are not mandatory for all members; when death is imminent, family and pastor are gathered, and it is usually highly desirable to have Litany at the Time of Death read<br>**Organ donation/transplantation:** No objections to organ donation/transplantation as long as moral integrity of donor is not violated | Abstain from meat on fast days<br>May fast on Wednesday, Friday, during Lent, and before Christmas<br>Some fast for 6 hours before receiving Holy Communion | Some believe in spiritual healing<br>Rite for anointing of the sick is available but not mandatory | Religious icons are very important<br>Communion four times yearly: Christmas, Easter, June 30, and August 15; may be mandatory for some |
| **Friends (Quakers)** | | | |
| **Birth:** No baptism<br>Infant's name is recorded in official book<br>**Death:** Do not believe in life after this life; each individual has a divine nature<br>**Organ donation/transplantation:** No formal statement; both are permitted | No requirements or restrictions<br>Most practice moderation<br>Avoid alcohol and illicit drugs | No special rites or restrictions | Believe in plain speech and dress<br>Pacifists |

*Continued*

**TABLE 2-4** Religious beliefs that affect nursing care—cont'd

| Beliefs About Birth and Death | Beliefs About Diet and Food Practices | Beliefs Regarding Medical Care | Comments |
|---|---|---|---|
| **Hindu**<br>**Birth:** No baptism<br>**Death:** Certain prescribed rites are followed after death; priest may tie thread around neck or wrist to signify blessing; family will wash the body; are particular about who touches their dead; bodies are to be cremated<br>**Organ donation/transplantation:** No religious laws prohibiting donation; individual decision | Many dietary restrictions<br>Beef and veal are not eaten<br>Some are strict vegetarians | Illness or injury is believed to represent sins committed in previous life<br>Accept most modern medical practices | Cremation is preferred |
| **Islam (Muslim/Moslem)**<br>**Birth:** At birth, the first words said to the infant in his/her right ear are Allah-o-Akbar (Allah is great) and the remainder of the Call for Prayer is recited. An Aqeeqa (party) to celebrate the birth of the child is arranged by the parents. Circumcision of the male child is practiced.<br>**Death:** In Islam, life is seen as a test in preparation for the everlasting life in the hereafter; therefore, according to Islam, death is simply a transition. Islam teaches that God has prescribed the time of death for everyone and only He knows when, where, or how a person is going to die. Islam encourages making the best use of all of God's gifts including the precious gift of life in this world. At the time of death, there are specific rituals (e.g., bathing, wrapping the body in cloth) that must be done. Before moving and handling the body, it is preferable to contact someone from the person's Mosque or the local Islamic Society to perform these rituals<br>**Organ donation/transplantation:** Permitted; however; there are some stipulations depending on the type of transplant/donation and its effect on the donor and recipient. It is advisable to contact the individual's Mosque or the local Islamic Society for further consultation | Prohibit all pork products; fasting is practiced during the ninth month of the Islamic year (Ramadan) | Believers are encouraged in the Qu'ran to seek treatment. It is taught that only Allah cures; however, Muslims are taught not to refuse treatment in the belief that Allah will take care of them because he also chooses at times to work through the efforts of humans | Muslims do not use alcohol or mind-altering drugs |
| **Jehovah's Witness**<br>**Birth:** No baptism<br>**Death:** No official last rites practiced when death occurs<br>**Organ donation/transplantation:** No definite statement related to this issue; do not encourage organ donation but believe it is a matter for individual conscience | Eat nothing to which blood has been added; can eat animal flesh that has been drained | Adherents are generally absolutely opposed to transfusions, including banking of own blood<br>May be opposed to use of albumin, globulin, factor replacement (hemophilia), vaccines<br>Not opposed to nonblood plasma expanders | Often possible to obtain a court order appointing a hospital official as temporary guardian to consent to a child's transfusion when parents refuse consent<br>Autopsy is approved only as required by law<br>No restrictions on giving blood sample |

From Carpenito LJ: *Nursing diagnosis: application to clinical practice,* ed 4, Philadelphia, 1992, JB Lippincott; Conley L: Childbearing and childrearing practices in Mormonism, *Neonatal Network* 9(3):41-48, 1990; Kozier B, Erb G: *Fundamentals of nursing,* ed 5, Menlo Park, CA, 1995, Addison-Wesley; McQuay JE: Cross cultural customs and beliefs related to health crisis, death, and organ donation/transplantation, *Crit Care Nurs Clin North Am* 7(3):581-594, 1995; and Spector RE: *Cultural diversity in health and illness,* ed 5, Upper Saddle River, NJ, 2000, Prentice-Hall Health.

**TABLE 2-4**    Religious beliefs that affect nursing care—cont'd

| Beliefs About Birth and Death | Beliefs About Diet and Food Practices | Beliefs Regarding Medical Care | Comments |
|---|---|---|---|
| **Judaism (Orthodox and Conservative)** | | | |
| **Birth:** No baptism<br>Ritual circumcision of male infants on eighth day; performed by Mohel (ritual circumciser familiar with Jewish law and aseptic technique)<br>**Death:** According to tradition, during last moments of life, relatives and close friends remain with the deceased<br>**Organ donation/transplantation:** This is permitted and considered a Mitzuah (good deed)<br>Donation or transplantation of organs requires rabbinical consent | Numerous dietary kosher laws exist<br>Are allowed only meat from animals that are vegetable eaters and are ritually slaughtered; fish that have scales and fins<br>Milk products served first can be followed by meat in a few minutes, but milk may not be consumed for several hours after eating meat<br>Fasting for 24 hours is part of Yom Kippur observance<br>Matzo replaces leavened bread during Passover week | May resist surgical procedures during Sabbath, which extends from sundown Friday until sundown Saturday<br>Seriously ill and pregnant women are exempt from fasting<br>Illness is grounds for violating dietary laws (e.g., patient with congestive heart failure does not have to use kosher meats, which are high in sodium) | Oppose all forms of mutilation, including autopsy; amputated limbs, organs, or surgically removed tissues should be made available to family for burial<br>May oppose prolongation of life after irreversible brain damage |
| **Lutheran** | | | |
| **Birth:** Baptize infants shortly after birth<br>**Death:** Last rites optional<br>**Organ donation/transplantation:** Considered a matter of personal choice | No requirements or restrictions | Church or pastor may be notified of hospitalization<br>Communion may be given before or after surgery or similar crisis | Accept scientific developments |
| **Methodist** | | | |
| **Birth:** Infant baptism is practiced but is usually done within the community of the Church after counseling and guidance from clergy. However, in emergency situations, a request for baptism would not be seen as inappropriate.<br>**Death:** In the case of perinatal death, there are prayers within the United Methodist Book of worship that could be said by anyone. Prayer, scripture, and singing are often seen as appropriate and desirable<br>**Organ donation/transplantation:** This is supported and encouraged; It is considered a part of good stewardship | No requirements or restrictions | In the Methodist tradition, it is believed that every person has the right to death with dignity and has the right to be involved in all medical decisions. Refusal of aggressive treatment is seen as an appropriate option. | Some encourage donation of body or body parts to science |
| **Nazarene** | | | |
| **Birth:** Baptism optional<br>**Death:** No last rites | No requirements or restrictions<br>Alcohol is prohibited | Church official administers Communion and laying on of hands<br>Adherents believe in divine healing but not exclusive of medical treatment | Cremation is permitted |
| **Pentecostal (Assembly of God, Four-Square)** | | | |
| **Birth:** No baptism<br>Baptism by complete immersion after age of accountability<br>**Death:** No official last rites practices when death occurs<br>**Organ donation/transplantation:** No official position | Abstain from alcohol, eating strangled animals, or anything to which blood has been added<br>Some individuals may not consume pork | No restrictions regarding medical care<br>Deliverance from sickness is provided for in atonement; may pray for divine intervention in health matters and seek God in prayer for themselves and others when ill | Some insist illness is divine punishment; most consider it an intrusion of Satan<br>Practice glossolalia (speaking in tongues) |

*Continued*

**TABLE 2-4    Religious beliefs that affect nursing care—cont'd**

| Beliefs About Birth and Death | Beliefs About Diet and Food Practices | Beliefs Regarding Medical Care | Comments |
|---|---|---|---|
| **Presbyterian** | | | |
| **Birth:** Infant baptism by sprinkling<br>**Death:** Last rites are not a sacramental procedure; instead, they read scripture and pray<br>**Organ donation/transplantation:** Individual conscience and a person's right to make decisions regarding his or her own body | No requirements or restrictions | Communion is administered when appropriate and convenient<br>Blood transfusion is accepted<br>Believe science should be used for relief of suffering | Full forgiveness is granted for any illness connected with a sin |
| **Roman Catholic** | | | |
| **Birth:** Infant baptism is mandatory; especially urgent if poor prognosis, when it may be performed by anyone<br>**Death:** Rite for Anointing of the Sick is a sacrament for the living; if prognosis is poor while patient is alive, patient or his or her family may request it<br>**Organ donation/transplantation:** Transplantation of organs is viewed by Catholics as ethically and morally acceptable to Vatican; organ donation is viewed as an act of charity | Fasting (eating only one full meal and no eating between meals) and abstaining from meat are mandatory on Ash Wednesday and Good Friday; fasting is optional during Lent; no meat on Fridays during Lent as a general rule<br>Children and most hospital patients are exempt from fasting<br>Some older Catholics may adhere to rule of no meat on Friday | Encourage anointing of the sick<br>Traditional church teaching does not approve of contraceptives or abortion | Family may request that major amputated limb be buried in consecrated ground<br>Autopsy is acceptable<br>Religious articles are important |

From Carpenito LJ: *Nursing diagnosis: application to clinical practice,* ed 4, Philadelphia, 1992, JB Lippincott; Conley L: Childbearing and childrearing practices in Mormonism, *Neonatal Network* 9(3):41-48, 1990; Kozier B, Erb G: *Fundamentals of nursing,* ed 5, Menlo Park, CA, 1995, Addison-Wesley; McQuay JE: Cross cultural customs and beliefs related to health crisis, death, and organ donation/transplantation, *Crit Care Nurs Clin North Am* 7(3):581-594, 1995; and Spector RE: *Cultural diversity in health and illness,* ed 5, Upper Saddle River, NJ, 2000, Prentice-Hall Health.

mary obligation to care for and make decisions about their minor children. However, the legal principle of **parens patriae** says that the state has an overriding interest in the health and welfare of its citizens. Parents' refusal of medical treatment for their child that is deemed essential can be interpreted as neglect. In addition to advocating for the child and family, the nurse's role may include assuming the role of consultant to the staff and family regarding new, alternative methods to transfusion and, if necessary, coordinating with officials to petition juvenile or family court for temporary guardianship of the child.

## KEY POINTS

- Culture is the sum total of mores, traditions, and beliefs about how people function and encompasses other products of human works and thoughts specific to members of an intergenerational group, community, or population.
- Nurses have a responsibility to understand the influence of culture, race, and ethnicity on the development of social and emotional relationships, childrearing practices, and attitudes toward health.
- A child's self-concept evolves from ideas about his or her social roles.
- Primary groups are characterized by intimate contact, mutual support, and behavior constraint among members.
- Secondary groups have limited, intermittent contact, little mutual support, and no pressure for conformity.
- Guilt and shame are two behaviors commonly conditioned in children to control social behavior.

- Important subcultural influences on children include ethnicity, social class, occupation, schools, peers, biculture, and mass media.
- A trend that has significantly influenced the American family is increasing geographic and economic mobility.
- Membership in a minority group presents special challenges for children, although changes in societal attitudes are slowly taking place.
- Socioeconomic influences play a major role in the ability to seek opportunities for health promotion and wellness.
- Religious practices greatly influence health promotion beliefs in families.
- A child's physical characteristics and susceptibility to health problems are strongly related to ethnic and cultural variations of hereditary and socioeconomic forces.
- Hereditary forces play an important role in a child's susceptibility to health problems.

- Groups of children suffering from greater physical and mental health problems are those living in poverty, those who are homeless, or those who have migrant families.
- Drug response, food sensitivity, disease resistance, physical characteristics, and disease states may demonstrate ethnic or cultural variations.
- Because verbal and nonverbal communication is an important cultural consideration, nurses need to acknowledge and respect their patient's practices in order for productive interaction to occur.
- Cultural beliefs related to cause of illness and maintenance of health may focus on natural forces, supernatural forces, or imbalance of forces.
- In planning and implementing patient care, nurses need to strive to adapt ethnic practices to the family's health needs rather than attempt to change long-standing beliefs.
- No cultural group is homogeneous; every racial and ethnic group contains great diversity.

## REFERENCES

American Academy of Pediatrics, Committee on Public Education: Children, adolescents, and television, *Pediatrics* 107(2): 423-426, 2001.

American Academy of Pediatrics, Committee on Public Education: Media education, *Pediatrics* 104(2):341-343, 1999.

American Academy of Pediatrics: *Guidelines for the care of migrant farmworkers' children,* Elk Grove Village, IL, 2000, The Academy.

Ampofo KK, Saiman L: Pediatric tuberculosis, *Pediatr Ann* 31(2):98-108, 2002.

Annie E Casey Foundation: *Kids count data book: state profiles of child well-being,* Washington, DC, 1999, Center for the Study of Social Policy.

Bennett NG and others: *Young children in poverty: a statistical update,* New York, 1999, National Center for Children in Poverty, Columbia University.

Boyer K: A little Spanish goes a long way, *Nurs Spectrum* 4:13, 1996.

Buchwald D and others: Caring for patients in a multicultural society, *Patient Care* 28(11):105-120, 1994.

Castiglia PT: Tuberculosis, a pediatric concern, *J Pediatr Health Care* 11(2):75-77, 1997.

Chidester D: *Patterns of transcendence: religion, death, and dying,* Belmont, CA, 1990, Wadsworth.

Council of Economic Advisors: The President's Initiative on Race: *Changing America: indicators of social and economic well-being by race and Hispanic origin,* Washington, DC, 1998, Executive Office of the President, Council of Economic Advisors.

Cully L: A critique of multiculturalism in health care: the challenge for nurse education, *J Adv Nurs* 23:564-570, 1996.

Derksen DJ, Strasberger VC: Children and the influence of the media, *Prim Care* 21(4):747-759, 1994.

Dykeman C, Nelson JR, Appleton V: Building strong working alliances with American Indian families, *Soc Work Educ* 17(3): 148-157, 1995.

Ensign J, Santelli J: Health status and service use: comparison of adolescents at a school-based health clinic with homeless adolescents, *Arch Pediatr Adolesc Med* 152(1):20-24, 1998.

Fulton RA, Moore CM: Spiritual care of the school-age child with a chronic condition, *J Pediatr Nurs* 10(4):224-231, 1995.

Habayeb GL: Cultural diversity: a nursing concept not yet reliably defined, *Nurs Outlook* 43(5):224-227, 1995.

Hayes J, Dreher C: Providing culturally sensitive care. In Smith D, editor: *Comprehensive child and family nursing skills,* St Louis, 1991, Mosby.

Kuensting L, Sanders G, editors: *Cultural considerations,* Park Ridge, IL, 1995, Emergency Nurses Association.

Leininger M: *Transcultural nursing,* New York, 1978, Wiley.

Lester L: Cultural competence: a nursing dialogue 2, *Am J Nurs* 98(9):36-42, quiz 43, 1998.

Lukoff D, Lu FG, Turner R: Cultural considerations in the assessment and treatment of religious and spiritual problems, *Psychiatr Clin North Am* 18(3):467-485, 1995.

Malach F, Segel N: Perspectives on health care delivery systems for American Indian families, *Child Health Care* 19(4):219-228, 1990.

Martinson IM, Armstrong V, Qiao J: The experience of the family of children with chronic illness at home in China, *Pediatr Nurs* 23(4):371-375, 1997.

Mattson S: Culturally sensitive perinatal care for Southeast Asians, *J Obstet Gynecol Neonat Nurs* 24(4):335-341, 1995.

Mills RJ: *Health insurance coverage: 2000,* Washington, DC, 2001, US Census Bureau (GPO Document No P60-215).

Nance TA: Intercultural communication: finding common ground, *J Obstet Gynecol Neonat Nurs* 24(3):249-255, 1995.

Ozawa MN, Yat-sang L: How safe is the safety net for poor children? *Soc Work Res* 20(4): 238-254, 1996.

Phillips S, Lobar S: Performing a culturally competent child health assessment, *Florida Nurse* 43(6):23, 1995.

Prevention and control of tuberculosis in migrant farm workers, *MMWR* 41(RR-10): 1-15, 1992.

Robinson-Zanartu C: Serving Native American children and families: considering cultural variables, *Lang, Speech, Hearing Services Schools* 27:373-384, 1996.

Rogers G: Educating case managers for culturally competent practice, *J Case Manag* 4(2):60-65, 1995.

Scribner R: Paradox as paradigm: the health outcomes of Mexican Americans, *Am J Public Health* 86(3):303-304, 1996.

Sekhon SK: Insights into South Asian culture: food and nutritional values, *Top Clin Nutr* 11(4):47-56, 1996.

Spector RE: *Cultural diversity in health and illness,* ed 5, Upper Saddle River, NJ, 2000, Prentice-Hall Health.

Strasburger VC, Donnerstein E: Children, adolescents, and the media: issues and solutions, *Pediatrics* 103(1):129–39, 1999.

Strehlow AJ, Amos-Jones T: The homeless as a vulnerable population, *Nurs Clin North Am* 34(2):261-274, 1999.

Talabere LR: Meeting the challenge of cultural care in nursing: diversity, sensitivity, competence, and congruence, *J Cult Divers* 3(2):53-61, 1996.

Taylor R: Check your cultural competence, *Nurs Manag* 29(8):30-32, 1998.

US Census Bureau: *Preliminary estimate of poverty thresholds for 2001,* Washington, DC, 2002, The Bureau, *www.census.gov/ hhes/poverty/threshld/thresh01.html,* 2002.

Wang R, Martinson IM: Behavioral responses of healthy Chinese siblings to the stress of childhood cancer in the family, *J Pediatr Nurs* 11(6):383-391, 1996.

Warda MR: Mexican Americans' perceptions of culturally competent care, *West J Nurs Res* 22(2):203-224, 2000.

Weinreb L and others: Determinants of health and service use patterns in homeless and low income–housed children, *Pediatrics* 102(3):554-562, 1998.

Williams LA, Kruse L: A culture fair: a creative, fun, and informative method of cultural awareness education, *J Nurs Staff Dev* 15(2):71-74, 1999.

Wright J: Homeless children: two years later, *Am J Dis Child* 147(5):518-519, 1993.

Yoos HL and others: An asthma management program for urban minority children, *J Pediatr Health Care* 11(2):66-74, 1997.

Yoos HL and others: Child-rearing beliefs in the African-American community: implications for culturally competent pediatric care, *J Pediatr Nurs* 10(6): 343-353, 1995.

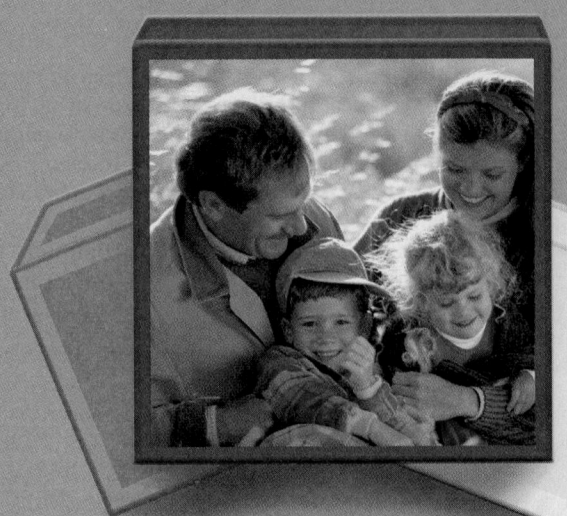

# Chapter 3

# Family Influences on Child Health Promotion

## Chapter Outline

**GENERAL CONCEPTS, 65**
**Definition of Family, 65**
**Family Theories, 65**
Family Systems Theory, 65
Family Stress Theory, 66
Developmental Theory, 67
Structural-Functional Theory, 68
**Family Nursing Interventions, 69**
**FAMILY STRUCTURE AND FUNCTION, 70**
**Family Structure, 70**
Traditional Nuclear Family, 70
Nuclear Family, 71
Blended Family, 71
Extended Family, 71
Single-Parent Family, 71
Binuclear Family, 72
Polygamous Family, 72
Communal Family, 72
Gay or Lesbian Family, 72
**Family Function, 73**
Family Strengths and Functioning Style, 73
Vulnerable Families, 73

**FAMILY ROLES AND RELATIONSHIPS, 75**
**Parental Roles, 75**
**Role Learning, 75**
Role Structuring in Children, 76
**Family Size and Configuration, 77**
Family Size, 77
Spacing of Children, 78
Sibling Interaction, 78
Ordinal Position, 79
Multiple Births, 79
**PARENTING, 81**
**Motivation for Parenthood, 81**
**Preparation for Parenthood, 81**
**Goals of Parenting, 82**
**Transition to Parenthood, 82**
Parental Factors Affecting Transition to
Parenthood, 82
Support Systems, 83
**Parenting Behaviors, 84**
Attitudes Toward Childrearing, 84
Parental Styles of Control, 84
**Limit-Setting and Discipline, 85**
Minimizing Misbehavior, 85
General Guidelines for Implementing
Discipline, 85
Types of Discipline, 85
**Influence of the "Experts," 88**

**SPECIAL PARENTING SITUATIONS, 88**
**Parenting the Adopted Child, 89**
Motivation for Adoption, 89
Sources of Adoptive Children, 89
Preparation for Adoption, 90
Parenting Adopted Children, 90
Special Adoptive Situations, 92
**Parenting and Divorce, 94**
Impact of Divorce on Children, 94
Children's Developmental Tasks Related
to Divorce, 96
Custody and Parenting Partnerships, 96
**Single-Parenting, 97**
Single Fathers, 98
**Parenting in Reconstituted Families, 98**
Stepparenting, 98
Effects on Children, 99
**Parenting in Dual-Earner Families, 99**
Working Mothers, 99
**Foster Parenting, 100**
**Accommodating Contemporary Parenting
Situations, 100**

## Related Topics

Adolescent Pregnancy, Ch. 20
Alternate Child Care Arrangements, Ch. 12
Communicating with Families, Ch. 6
Family Assessment, Ch. 6

Family-Centered Care of the Child with
Chronic Illness or Disability, Ch. 22
Preschool and Kindergarten Experience,
Ch. 15

Promotion of Parent-Infant Bonding
(Attachment), Ch. 8
Sibling Rivalry, Ch. 14
Social, Cultural, and Religious Influences on
Child Health Promotion, Ch. 2

# GENERAL CONCEPTS

## Definition of Family

The term *family* has been defined in a number of ways and for a number of purposes according to the individual's own frame of reference, value judgment, or discipline. For example, biology describes the family as fulfilling the biologic function of perpetuation of the species. Psychology emphasizes the interpersonal aspects of the family and its responsibility for personality development. Economics views the family as a productive unit providing for material needs, and sociology depicts it as the social unit that reacts with the larger society. Others define family in relation to the persons who make up the family unit; the most common type of relationships are *consanguineous* (blood relationships), *affinal* (marital relationships), and *family of origin* (family unit a person is born into).

Earlier definitions emphasized that family members were related by legal ties or genetic relationships and lived in the same household with specific roles. Later definitions have been broadened to reflect both structural and functional changes. A family can be defined as an institution where individuals, related through biology or enduring commitments, and representing similar or different generations and genders, participate in roles involving mutual socialization, nurturance, and emotional commitment (Lerner, Sparks, and McCubbin, 1999).

A great deal of emotion has been generated about some of the newer concepts of family, such as communal families, single-parent families, and homosexual families. To accommodate these and other varieties of family styles, the descriptive term **household** is being used more frequently.

**NURSING TIP**   The way that a nurse assesses a household will often determine the types of interventions used to support family members, such as counseling and health referrals (Cody, 1996).

Although the concept of household is recognized and appreciated, the term *family* is used throughout this book to indicate the relationships between dependent children and one or more protective adults. It also implies relationships among siblings. Family members share a sense of belonging to their own family that deeply affects their lives. The understanding or perception of "family" is uniquely meaningful to an individual and is based on that person's experience and interpretation. This perception is held to be accurate until an experience leads to expansion or reinterpretation of the initial concept (Cody, 1996). Whatever form the family takes, children need to feel that their family is acceptable and valuable (Visher and Visher, 1995).

Nursing of infants and children is intimately involved with care of the child *and* the family. Consequently, nurses must be aware of the functions of the family, various types of family structures, and theories that provide a foundation for understanding the changes within a family and for directing family-oriented interventions.

## Family Theories

A *family theory* can be used to describe families and how the family unit responds to events both within and outside the family. Each family theory makes certain assumptions about the family and has inherent strengths and limitations. Most nurses use a combination of theories in their work with children and families. The theories most frequently used are discussed below as well as summarized in Table 3-1. Other theories that may be used less often but continue to have relevance for nursing practice are summarized in Table 3-1 with examples of applications of these theories to specific family situations.

### Family Systems Theory

*Family systems theory* is derived from general systems theory, a science of "wholeness" that is characterized by interaction among the components of the system and between the system and the environment. *General systems theory* expanded scientific thought from a simplistic view of direct cause and effect (*A* causes *B*) to a more complex and interrelated theory (*A* influences *B*, but *B* also affects *A*). In family systems theory the family is viewed as a system that continually interacts with its members and the environment. The emphasis is on the *interaction* between the members, such that a change in one family member creates a change in other members, which in turn results in a new change in the original member. Consequently, a problem or dysfunction does not lie in any one member but rather in the type of interactions used by the family. Because it is the interactions, rather than individual members, that are viewed as the source of the problem, the family becomes the patient and the focus of care. Examples of the application of family systems theory to clinical problems include nonorganic failure to thrive and child abuse. According to family systems theory, the problem does not rest solely with the parent or child but exists in the type of interactions between the parent and child as well as in a host of other factors that affect their relationship.

Understanding family systems theory requires knowledge of numerous basic definitions and concepts that are beyond the focus of this discussion. However, some general concepts that are unique to this theory and have significance to understanding family dynamics are presented.

The family is viewed as a whole that is different from the sum of the individual members. For example, in a household of parents and one child, there are not only three individuals, but also four interactive units that characterize the family system. These include three dyads (the marital relationship, the mother-child relationship, and the father-child relationship) and a triangle (the mother-father-child relationship). To effect positive change in a family, it is necessary to work with and through the several subsystems of the family.

Another important concept, *adaptability,* views the family as a highly adaptable unit. When problems exist within the family, change can be effected by altering the interaction or feedback messages that perpetuate disruptive behavior. *Feedback* refers to processes within the family that help iden-

**TABLE 3-1**  Summary of family theories and applications

| Assumptions | Strengths | Limitations | Applications |
|---|---|---|---|
| **Family Systems Theory** | | | |
| A change in any one part of a family system affects all other parts of the family system (circular causality)<br>Family systems are characterized by periods of rapid growth and change and periods of relative stability<br>Both too little change and too much change are dysfunctional for the family system; therefore a balance between morphogenesis (change) and morphostasis (no change) is necessary<br>Family systems can initiate change, as well as react to it | Applicable for family in normal everyday life as well as for family dysfunction and pathology<br>Useful for families of varying structure and various stages of life cycle | More difficult to determine cause-and-effect relationships because of circular causality | Mate selection, courtship processes, family communication, boundary maintenance, power and control within family, parent-child relationships, adolescent pregnancy and parenthood |
| **Family Stress Theory** | | | |
| Stress is an inevitable part of family life, and any event, even if positive, can be stressful for family<br>Family encounters both normative expected stressors and unexpected situational stressors over life cycle<br>Stress has a cumulative effect on family<br>Families cope and respond to stressors with a wide range of responses and effectiveness | Potential to explain and predict family behavior in response to stressors and to develop effective interventions to promote family adaptation<br>Focuses on positive contribution of resources, coping, and social support to adaptive outcomes<br>Can be used by many disciplines in health field | Relationships between all variables in framework not yet adequately described<br>Not yet known if certain combinations of resources and coping strategies are applicable to all stressful events | Transition to parenthood and other normative transitions, single-parent families, families experiencing work-related stressors (dual-earner, unemployment), acute or chronic childhood illness or disability, infertility, death of a child, divorce, teenage pregnancy and parenthood |
| **Developmental Theory** | | | |
| Families develop and change over time in similar and consistent ways<br>Family and its members must perform certain time-specific tasks set by themselves and by persons in the broader society<br>Family role performance at one stage of family life cycle influences family's behavioral options at next stage<br>Family tends to be in stage of disequilibrium entering a new life cycle stage and strives toward homeostasis within stages | Provides a dynamic, rather than static, view of family<br>Addresses both changes within family and changes in family as a social system over its life history<br>Anticipates potential stressors that normally accompany transitions to various stages and when problems may peak because of lack of resources | Traditional model more easily applied to two-parent families with children<br>Use of age of oldest child and marital duration as marker of stage transition may be problematic (e.g., in step-families, single-parent families) | Anticipatory guidance, educational strategies, and developing and strengthening family resources for management of transition to parenthood; family adjustment to children entering school, becoming adolescents, leaving home; management of "empty nest" years and retirement |

tify strengths and needs and determine how well goals are being accomplished. Positive feedback initiates change, whereas negative feedback resists change.

When the family system is disrupted, change can occur at any point in the system. Although family systems theorists may pursue the family history in trying to understand current family interaction and problem patterns, the emphasis is on what is occurring *now* in the family and on intervening to change that pattern. This focus allows for sometimes rapid and dramatic changes.

A major factor that influences a family's adaptability is its *boundary,* an imaginary but very real line that exists between the family and its environment. This boundary, or line, may be open or closed. An ***open family*** welcomes input into its system by accepting new ideas, information, re-

sources, and opportunities. This type of family reaches out for help and uses the available support systems. In contrast, a ***closed family*** resists input by viewing change as threatening. The family is suspicious of any available support and strives to maintain the family system by avoiding outside influences. Having knowledge of the boundaries is critical when teaching or counseling families. Although open families are receptive to intervention, closed families typically resist assistance and more effort is required to gain their trust and acceptance.

### Family Stress Theory

***Family stress theory*** explains how families react to stressful events and suggests factors that promote adaptation to these events. Families encounter ***stressors*** (events that cause stress

**TABLE 3-1**   Summary of family theories and applications—cont'd

| Assumptions | Strengths | Limitations | Applications |
|---|---|---|---|
| **Structural-Functional Theory** | | | |
| Family performs at least one societal function (e.g., reproduction, socializing children, producing and consuming goods and services) while also meeting family needs<br>Family, as a social system, tends toward stability<br>Family behaviors are largely determined by norms | Considers interplay within family as well as between family and the larger social system (school, workplace)<br>Views family as both open to outside influence and transactions and as a system that tends to maintain boundaries | Strong emphasis on family stability and maintaining status quo | Dual-career or dual-worker families and management of combined work and family roles and responsibilities<br>Relationships of family unit with schools, other societal institutions |
| **Symbolic Interactional Theory** | | | |
| Family is a unit of interacting persons, with each occupying a position within the family to which a number of roles are assigned; family relationships are continually in flux<br>The definition family members make of situations partially determines the effects situations have for them<br>Family members communicate through symbols that have both meaning and value attached to them | More culture- and value-free, less normative and prescriptive<br>Views family as a living social unit and examines both behavior and perceptions | Looks more at family at one point in time<br>Focuses on internal family interactions and processes; less emphasis on family-community and society interactions and relationships<br>Complex framework with many concepts, assumptions | Family communications, decision making, problem solving |
| **Exchange Theory** | | | |
| Overall assumption is that humans, families, groups, associations, and even nations seek rewarding statuses, relationships, interactions, and feeling states so that their rewards are maximized and their costs are minimized | Breadth and versatility<br>Applicable to various family forms, to families of other cultures and countries<br>Can be applied to individuals, families, groups, organizations, societies | What constitutes a reward or cost is not clear<br>Does not directly address how individuals or families acquire meaning and value in determining what is a reward or cost | Rewards and costs associated with paid employment of mothers, decision to have children or be child-free, parenting responsibilities, kin and intergenerational relationships, marital dissolution |
| **Conflict Theory** | | | |
| Families are viewed as ongoing competitive social systems<br>The conflict inherent in family relationships can be managed by negotiation and problem solving<br>Complete suppression of conflict in a family system is likely to have negative consequences for the family unit or its members or both | Applicable to all family forms and structures<br>Appropriate for examining many situations families are facing in today's society<br>Can see how family conflict changes over time | Can be perceived as having a "negative" focus<br>Can view all conflict as power struggle, which severely limits use of this theory<br>Needs further use and testing | Divorce, remarriage, stepfamily relationships, conflict over any aspect of family life—relationships with children, in-laws, work-family issues, caretaking of dependent members (children, elders), family violence |

and have the potential to provide change in the family social system), including those that are predictable (e.g., parenthood) and those that are unpredictable (e.g., illness or unemployment). These stressors are cumulative, involving simultaneous demands from work, family, and community life. Too many stressful events occurring within a relatively short period of time—usually 1 year—can overwhelm the family's ability to cope, thus placing the family system at risk for breakdown or its members at risk for physical and emotional health problems. When the family experiences too many stressors for it to cope adequately, a state of *crisis* ensues. For adaptation to occur under these circumstances, a change in family structure and/or interaction is necessary.

The *resiliency model of family stress, adjustment, and adaptation* emphasizes the stressful situation as not necessarily

pathologic or detrimental to the family but demonstrates that the family needs to make fundamental structural or systemic changes to adapt to the situation (McCubbin and McCubbin, 1994). For example, bringing a child with special needs to a treatment facility for therapy might be considered stressful for a family without a car or money for public transportation, yet may be defined as only a minor inconvenience by another family with adequate and appropriate resources.

## Developmental Theory

*Developmental theory* is an outgrowth of several theories of development. Foremost among the developers are Duvall (1977), who described eight developmental tasks of the family throughout its life span (Box 3-1), derived from Erikson's

---

### Box 3-1 ■ ■ ■
### Duvall's Developmental Stages of the Family

**STAGE I: MARRIAGE AND AN INDEPENDENT HOME: THE JOINING OF FAMILIES**

Reestablish couple identity.
Realign relationships with extended family.
Make decisions regarding parenthood.

**STAGE II: FAMILIES WITH INFANTS**

Integrate infants into family unit.
Accommodate to new parenting and grandparenting roles.
Maintain marital bond.

**STAGE III: FAMILIES WITH PRESCHOOLERS**

Socialize children.
Parents and children adjust to separation.

**STAGE IV: FAMILIES WITH SCHOOLCHILDREN**

Children develop peer relations.
Parents adjust to their children's peer and school influences.

**STAGE V: FAMILIES WITH TEENAGERS**

Adolescents develop increasing autonomy.
Parents refocus on midlife marital and career issues.
Parents begin a shift toward concern for older generation.

**STAGE VI: FAMILIES AS LAUNCHING CENTERS**

Parents and young adults establish independent identities.
Renegotiate marital relationship.

**STAGE VII: MIDDLE-AGED FAMILIES**

Reinvest in couple identity with concurrent development of
   independent interests.
Realign relationships to include in-laws and grandchildren.
Deal with disabilities and death of older generation.

**STAGE VIII: AGING FAMILIES**

Shift from work role to leisure and semiretirement or full
   retirement.
Maintain couple and individual functioning while adapting to
   aging process.
Prepare for own death and dealing with loss of spouse, siblings,
   and other peers.

Modified from Wright LM, Leahey M: *Nurses and families: a guide to family assessment and intervention*, Philadelphia, 1984, FA Davis.

---

### Box 3-2 ■ ■ ■
### Family Development Stages for Divorce

**STAGE I: DECISION TO DIVORCE**

Accept the inability to resolve marital discord.

**STAGE II: PLANNING THE BREAKUP**

Create viable arrangements for all members of the family.

**STAGE III: SEPARATION**

Resolve attachment to spouse.
Develop cooperative co-parenting relationships.

**STAGE IV: DIVORCE**

Resolve the emotional divorce.

**STAGE V: SINGLE-PARENT FAMILY OR NONCUSTODIAL SINGLE PARENT**

Maintain parental contact with ex-spouse.
Maintain parental contact with children (noncustodial parent).
Maintain relationship with ex–in-laws (custodial parent).
Rebuild a personal social network.

Modified from Danielson C, Hamel-Bissell B, Winstead-Fry P: *Families, health, and illness,* St Louis, 1993, Mosby.

---

For example, should divorce occur, the family life cycle takes a different course (Box 3-2). New life cycle norms have also been developed for blended (step) families, low-income families, alcoholic families, and dual-career families (Friedman, 1998).

Developmental theory can be applied to nursing practice in a number of ways. For example, the nurse can assess how well new parents are accomplishing the individual and family developmental tasks associated with transition to parenthood. New applications should emerge as more is learned about developmental stages for nonnuclear and nontraditional families.

### Structural-Functional Theory

*Structural-functional theory,* one of the dominant orientations in modern sociology, focuses less on family change and more on the interrelatedness, interdependence, and integration between family members and all aspects of society and its subcultures, particularly the occupational subsystem (Friedman, 1998). *Structure* refers to the arrangement of roles that constitute a social system; *function* is the contribution made by an activity or role to the whole and the consequences of the activity for the system. The family is described as a social system with members who have specific roles and functions. The family process is directed toward maintaining an equilibrium between the complementary roles within the family (e.g., husband-wife, father-daughter, mother-son, or wife–mother-in-law).

Internal relationships involve the division of labor between family members and the functions of these divisions for family maintenance. *Expressive roles* are seen in integrative or solidifying activities, such as hugging, that bring emotional satisfaction to the family members. *Instrumental roles* are activities, such as earning an income, that occur external to the family but that also include satisfactory goal attainment of the family. Traditionally, expressive roles have

---

eight stages of psychosocial development, and Rogers (1962), who incorporated role theory into the developmental concept. The family is described as a small group, a semiclosed system of personalities that interacts with the larger cultural social system. As an interrelated system, changes do not occur in one part without a series of changes in other parts.

Developmental theory addresses family change over time by using Duvall's family life cycle stages, based on the predictable changes in the structure, function, and roles of the family, with the age of the oldest child as the marker for stage transition. Thus the arrival of the first child marks the transition from stage I to stage II. As the first child grows and develops, the family enters subsequent stages. In every stage the family is faced with certain developmental tasks. At the same time, each member of the family must achieve individual developmental tasks as part of each family life cycle stage.

Additions to family development theory reflect more inclusive and accurate versions of contemporary family life.

## Box 3-3
### Family Nursing Interventions

Behavior modification
Case management and coordination
Collaborative strategies
Contracting
Counseling, including support, cognitive reappraisal, and reframing
Empowering families through active participation
Environmental modification
Family advocacy
Family crisis intervention
Networking, including use of self-help groups and social support
Providing information and technical expertise
Role modeling
Role supplementation
Teaching strategies, including stress management, lifestyle modifications, and anticipatory guidance

From Friedman MM: *Family nursing: theory and practice*, ed 4, Norwalk, CT, 1998, Appleton & Lange.

 *Critical Thinking Exercise*

### Family Theories

As the school nurse, you are working with a family that consists of a mother, father, and their 10-year-old son and 16-year-old daughter. The daughter, Jenny, has stopped going to school this week. Although she has had many conflicts with her parents, her relationship with her father is very strained. He recently took away her driving privileges because of curfew violations. Jenny says she is quitting school if she cannot drive. Which of the following three family theories would you apply when working with this family?

FIRST, THINK ABOUT IT . . .
• What concepts or ideas are central to your thinking?
• What conclusions are you coming to?

1. Developmental theory
2. Family stress theory
3. Family system theory

*The best response is three. In family system theory the family is viewed as a system that continually interacts with its members. Family interactions rather than individual members are viewed as the source of the problems. The conclusion that developmental or family stress theory could be applied is not conceptually accurate because the family is experiencing an interaction problem more than a developmental or stress-related problem.*

been assigned to the wife-mother, whereas the husband-father has assumed the instrumental roles. However, the classic breadwinner husband, homemaker wife, and two children now make up only a small proportion of families in North America. Both expressive and instrumental roles are becoming less gender-specific.

From a structural-functional viewpoint, the major goal of the family is socialization of its members into society. Families perform certain functions ultimately directed toward this goal. Functions of the family as outlined by Friedman (1998) are:

**Affective** to meet the psychologic needs of family members
**Socialization** and **social placement** to help children become productive members of society
**Reproductive** to ensure family continuity and societal survival
**Economic** to provide and allocate sufficient resources for the family
**Health care** for the provision of physical necessities, such as food, clothing, shelter, and a high level of wellness

This framework can be applied in nursing practice to assess how well the family is accomplishing these five functions in relation to its overall goal.

Structural-functional theory focuses heavily on the integration of the family within the occupational systems. In many instances occupational roles are segregated from family roles. However, with increasing numbers of women in the workforce and greater emphasis on careers, negotiating work-family conflicts in dual-earner families has become a significant facet of family life.

## Family Nursing Interventions

In working with children, nurses must include family members in their plan of care. In essence, the *patient is the family*. To discover family dynamics and the family unit's strengths and weaknesses, a thorough family assessment is needed

(see Chapter 6). The interventions nurses use with families depend on their theoretic model of the family. For example, in family systems theory the focus is on the interactions of the members, rather than on an individual member. In this case, using group dynamics to involve all members in the intervention process and being a skillful communicator are essential.

Systems theory also presents an excellent opportunity for anticipatory guidance. Since each member of the family reacts to every stress experienced by that system, such as the birth of a child, nurses can intervene to help the family prepare for and cope with the change. Also, at each stress point there is an opportunity for change and learning because families are more open to interventions at this time (Brazelton, 1995).

In the family stress theory, crisis intervention strategies are employed, and the chief focus is on helping members cope with the challenging event. In the developmental theory a primary nursing function is to provide anticipatory guidance that prepares members for transition to the next family stage. Nurses use a variety of strategies when working with families (Box 3-3). It is important for nurses to be aware of their degree of professional competence in using family nursing interventions. An important nursing role is to recognize situations where referral to more specialized services is required. (See Critical Thinking Exercise box.)

Just as appropriate strategies differ, the level of assistance a family needs will also depend on the type of crisis, factors affecting family adjustment (see Table 22-2), and the family's level of functioning. Highly functioning families usually need informational interventions. Vulnerable families (see p. 73) benefit from a wider range of supportive and therapeutic interventions.

## FAMILY STRUCTURE AND FUNCTION

### Family Structure

The *family structure*, or *family composition*, consists of individuals, each with a socially recognized status and position, who interact with one another on a regular, recurring basis

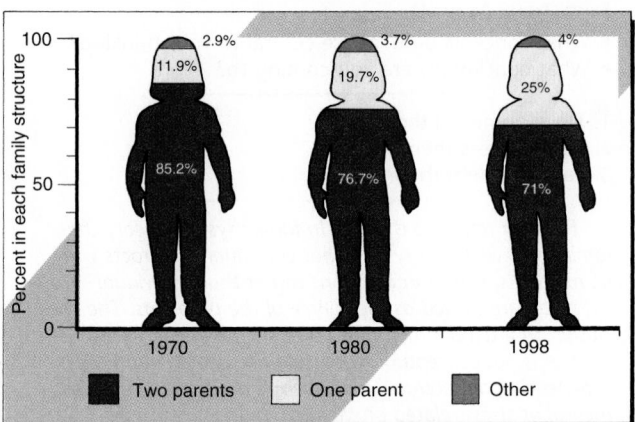

**Fig. 3-1** Percentage of children under age 18 living with one or neither parent, 1970, 1980, and 1998. (Data from US Census Bureau, 1996: *Living arrangements of children*, pp 70-74, Washington, DC, 2001, US Government Printing Office.)

in socially sanctioned ways. When members are gained or lost through events (e.g., marriage, divorce, birth, death, abandonment, incarceration), the family composition is altered and roles must be redefined or redistributed.

Traditionally, the family structure refers to either nuclear or extended families. However, family composition has assumed new configurations in recent years, with the single-parent family and blended family becoming prominent forms (Lerner, Sparks, and McCubbin, 1999; Friedman, 1998) (Fig. 3-1). In any case, the predominant structural pattern in any society depends to a large extent on the mobility of families as they pursue economic goals and as relationships change. It is not uncommon for children to belong to several different family groups during their lifetimes.

The particular family structure a child participates in impacts the direction of nursing care. A nurse must be able to meet the needs of children from many diverse family structures and home situations. The U.S. Census Bureau uses four major definitions: the traditional nuclear family, the nuclear family, the blended family or household, and the extended family or household (Furukawa, 1994) (Table 3-2). These four family types, as well as other, less common family structures, are discussed in the following paragraphs.

### Traditional Nuclear Family

A traditional nuclear family consists of a married couple and their biologic children. A child in a traditional nuclear family lives with both biologic parents and, if siblings are present, only full brothers and sisters (i.e., siblings who share the same two biologic parents). No other persons are present in the household (i.e., no steprelatives, foster or adopted children, half-siblings, other relatives, or nonrelatives).

**TABLE 3-2** Living arrangements of children by race and ethnicity: fall 1996 (in thousands)

| Living Arrangements | All Races | White | White Non-Hispanic | Black | American Indian and Alaska Native | Asian and Pacific Islander | Hispanic[1] |
|---|---|---|---|---|---|---|---|
| Children | 71,494 | 56,212 | 46,657 | 11,631 | 1,073 | 2,578 | 10,428 |
| Living with— | | | | | | | |
| Two parents[2] | 50,685 | 43,466 | 36,837 | 4,397 | 667 | 2,156 | 7,112 |
| Both married to each other | 49,186 | 42,333 | 36,110 | 4,126 | 605 | 2,123 | 6,627 |
| In a traditional nuclear family[3] | 39,746 | 34,859 | 30,132 | 2,985 | 395 | 1,507 | 5,024 |
| One parent | 18,165 | 11,131 | 8,632 | 6,320 | 345 | 369 | 2,870 |
| Mother only | 16,340 | 9,599 | 7,274 | 6,088 | 320 | 333 | 2,689 |
| Father only | 1,825 | 1,533 | 1,358 | 232 | 25 | 36 | 181 |
| Neither parent | 2,644 | 1,615 | 1,188 | 915 | 62 | 54 | 445 |
| Grandparents only | 1,266 | 637 | 501 | 571 | 34 | 24 | 143 |
| Other relatives only | 688 | 447 | 272 | 199 | 19 | 22 | 183 |
| Nonrelatives only | 622 | 622 | 383 | 122 | 9 | 8 | 105 |
| Other arrangement | 69 | 46 | 32 | 22 | — | 1 | 14 |
| At least 1 stepparent | 4,902 | 4,066 | 3,556 | 649 | 94 | 93 | 563 |
| At least 1 foster parent | 313 | 224 | 153 | 86 | 2 | 2 | 75 |

From US Census Bureau: Washington, DC, 2001, *1996 Survey of Income and Program Participation, Wave 2*, US Government Printing Office.
— Represents zero or rounds to zero.
[1]People of Hispanic origin may be of any race.
[2]In the SIPP data children identify both of their parents regardless of their marital status. This means that both married and unmarried parents are included in this category in this table. This represents a difference from the current population survey (CPS) because only married parents are recorded in two-parent households. Correspondingly, there are more children in two-parent households in the SIPP and more in single-parent households in the CPS.
[3]Children in a traditional nuclear family live with both biologic parents and, if siblings are present, with full brothers and sisters. No other household members are present.

## Nuclear Family

The nuclear family is composed of two parents and their children. The parent-child relationship may be biologic, step-, adoptive, or foster. Sibling ties may be biologic, step-, half-, or adoptive. The parents are not necessarily married. No other relatives or nonrelatives are present in the household.

## Blended Family

A blended family or household includes at least one stepparent, stepsibling, and/or half-sibling. A stepparent is the spouse of a child's biologic parent but is not the child's biologic parent. Stepsiblings do not share a common biologic parent; the biologic parent of one child is the stepparent of the other. Half-siblings share only one biologic parent. Often, nurses may have the opportunity to interact with blended families in the community. (See Family Home Care box.)

## Extended Family

An extended family or household includes at least one parent, one or more children, and one or more members (related or unrelated) other than a parent or sibling. Parent-child and sibling relationships may be biologic, step-, adoptive, or foster.

One issue that arises within the extended family is when grandparents find themselves rearing their grandchildren. Nearly 1.3 million children are being raised by their grandparents, with an additional 4.1 million children being raised by a grandparent with one of their parents present in the home (U.S. Census Bureau, 2001). Nearly 44% of the time, the grandparent takes over the parenting role because of a parent's substance abuse problem. Other issues that lead to the grandparent/parent role include child abuse, neglect, or abandonment (28%); the parent's inability to handle the child (11%); death of the parent (5%); parental unemployment (4%); and parental divorce (4%) (Woodworth, 1996) (Fig. 3-2).

Some of the issues facing grandparents as parents include financial burdens (46% are on fixed incomes). Of the 33% that are single grandparents, 96% are grandmothers. There is often no involvement with state agencies, and legal and medical issues become troublesome, with dilemmas created by situations such as school enrollment and needs for child care and special service programs (Woodworth, 1996). One resource for these families is the **Grandparent Information Center.***

## Single-Parent Family

A most striking development is the overall trend toward single-parent families as opposed to two-parent families. The *single-parent family* is not a new phenomenon, and the terms "single parent" and "two parent" leave much left unsaid because there is extensive variation within the definitions. Throughout history, deaths from disease, childbirth, and wars have resulted in many single-parent families, although frequently remarriage occurs. The contemporary single-parent family, however, has emerged partially as a consequence of women's rights movements wherein more women (and men) have established separate households because of divorce, death, desertion, or illegitimacy. In addition, a more liberal attitude in the courts has made it possible for single persons, both male and female, to adopt children, whereas previously, rigid prerequisites specified that both a father and a mother must be present in the home. Although single-parent families are usually headed by mothers, it is becoming increasingly common for fathers to be awarded custody of dependent children in divorce

---

*For information contact the local **American Association of Retired Persons** representative or office. Support for raising grandchildren is found on the American Association of Retired Persons website: www.aarp.org/confacts/grandparents/grandfacts. Also see www.grandsplace.com, a website dedicated to grandparents raising grandchildren.

---

### FAMILY HOME CARE
*Blended Families and Living "in Step"*

Blending families can pose many challenges. If parents bring concerns and questions to health care providers, the following suggestions may be helpful:

Let relationships develop slowly and naturally. Don't expect too much too soon, from the children, from your spouse, or from yourself.

Don't criticize or belittle lost (or new) parents, or try to erase or replace them. Stepparents are additional parents.

Expect confused feelings, anxieties, competition for attention, bids for loyalty. Decide on standards of discipline and behavior and stick to them.

Communicate. Don't pretend everything is fine if it isn't. Look at problems squarely and deal with them openly.

If you need help, admit it and get it. Read a book, get counseling, join a support group, call a family meeting.

From Stein B: Yours, mine, and ours: a look at stepfamilies, *Growing Parent* 12(9):1-5, 1984.

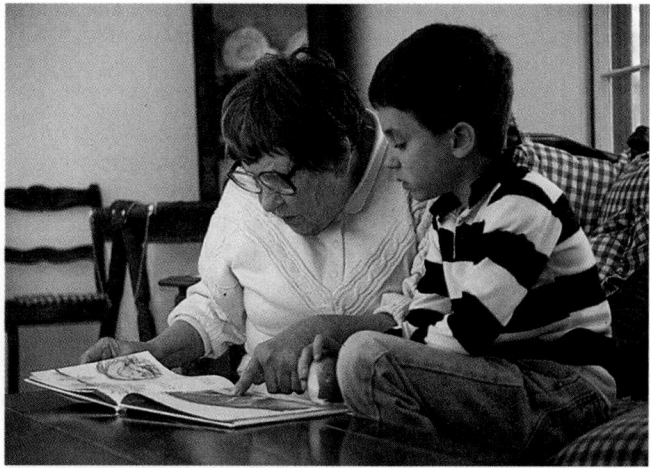
**Fig. 3-2**  Children benefit from interaction with grandparents, who sometimes assume the parenting role.

settlements. A significant number of single-parent families result from a single mother who wishes to have a child but does not choose to have a husband. Also, unmarried mothers often choose to keep and raise their children rather than place them for adoption or marry, and these mothers and children are frequently absorbed into the extended family. With the increased psychologic independence of women as a whole and the increased acceptability of illegitimacy in society, more unmarried women are deliberately choosing mother-child families. The challenges of these single-parent families are discussed on p. 97.

## Binuclear Family

The term *binuclear family* is used to describe the situation that allows parents to continue the parenting role while terminating the spousal unit. The degree of cooperation between households and the time the child spends with each can vary. In *joint custody* the court assigns divorcing parents equal rights and responsibilities to the minor child or children. These alternate family forms are efforts on the part of those concerned to view divorce as a process of reorganization and redefinition of a family rather than as a family dissolution. Joint custody and co-parenting are discussed further on p. 96 in relation to special parenting situations.

## Polygamous Family

Although it is not legally sanctioned in the United States, sometimes the conjugal unit can be extended by the addition of spouses in polygamous matings. *Polygamy* generally refers to either wives *(polygyny)* or, very rarely, husbands *(polyandry)*. Many societies practice polygyny that is further designated as *sororal,* in which the wives are sisters, or *non-sororal,* in which the wives can be unrelated. Sororal polygyny is widespread throughout the world, and although plural marriages produce problems of adjustment for the members, co-wives who are sisters are more likely to get along with each other and display less jealousy than co-wives who are not. Most often, mothers and their children share a husband and father, usually with each mother and her children maintaining a separate household, particularly when the wives are unrelated.

A special form of sororal polygyny is the *sororate,* in which a cultural rule specifies that the preferred mate for a widower is the sister of his deceased wife. In a sororate the marriages are successive rather than concurrent.

Where it exists, polygamy is usually accorded a higher status than monogamy. It may be limited to ruling families or to high-status persons and tends to be practiced by a small segment of the population. This is probably a result of economic factors and the unequal sex ratio in some areas at the time of biologic maturity.

## Communal Family

The *communal family* emerged, as have all previous experimental communities, from a disenchantment with most contemporary life choices. Although communal families may have divergent beliefs, practices, and organization, the basic impetus for formation has been dissatisfaction with social systems and life goals of the larger communities and

with the nuclear family structure, in particular, as it exists from either an ideologic or a practical perspective. Relatively uncommon today, communal groups share common ownership of property and goods; in cooperatives there is private ownership of property, but certain goods and services are shared and exchanged cooperatively without monetary consideration. There is strong reliance on group members and material interdependence. Both provide collective security for nonproductive members, share homemaking and childrearing functions, and help overcome the problem of interpersonal isolation or loneliness.

Unlike the traditional extended family, nuclear units in a commune may come and go at will. There is no consanguineous tie between the units. The mother-child tie is strong during infancy and early childhood, but many parents are happy to relinquish older children to the care of others. Although the parents maintain primary responsibility for the health and well-being of the children, the children are free to form close relationships with a number of adults in the commune and are encouraged to do so.

## Gay or Lesbian Family

A *same-sex, homosexual,* or *gay* or *lesbian family* is one in which there is a common-law tie between two persons of the same sex who have children. Estimates of the number of children of gay or lesbian parents range from 3 to 14 million (Ariel and McPherson, 2000). While most children in gay or lesbian households are biologic from a former, legal marriage, there are other means by which homosexuals acquire children. For example, they may be foster or adoptive parents, lesbian mothers may conceive through artificial fertilization, or a gay male couple may become parents through use of a surrogate mother.

There is no evidence that children growing up with one or more homosexual parents will be more dysfunctional than children raised by heterosexual parents (Ariel and McPherson, 2000). An extensive review of the published literature evaluating children whose parents were gay or lesbian compared with children whose parents were heterosexual found no differences in the development of sexual or gender identity or gender role behavior; adolescent sexual orientation; behavioral, emotional, or psychiatric difficulties; personality characteristics; locus of control beliefs; moral maturity; or intelligence (Patterson, 1992). The primary variable predicting measures of children's adjustment to living with gay or lesbian parents was their perception of satisfactory parenting arrangements between their parents (Patterson, 1995; Perrin, 2002).

Disclosure of parental homosexuality ("coming out") to children is a concern for most families. There are a number of factors to consider before disclosing their information to the children: parents should be comfortable with their own sexual preference, it should be discussed with the children before they know or suspect, the discussion should be planned and should take place in a quiet setting where interruptions are unlikely, and children should be assured that the parent relationship with them will not change as a result of the discussion (Lynch and Murray, 2000).

Gay or lesbian parents may face critical periods during their child's development. The preschool child may have difficulty understanding the family constellation and the absence of the father or mother. During the school-age years the acceptance of gay and lesbian families within the community may impact the child's adjustment. During middle school and early adolescence, issues related to sexuality and sexual behavior become significant, and the family situation may be troublesome for some children when conformity is the key to feeling normal. Later in adolescence, parents may report difficulties in supporting their children's emerging sexual identification. Adolescents may be reluctant to discuss or accept their parents' homosexuality even though they seemed to accept it at an earlier stage of development (Perrin and Kulkin, 1996).

Parents should also be prepared for questions from their children, such as "What does being gay mean?" "What makes a person gay?" "Will I be gay, too?" and "What should I tell my friends about it?" Also, the earlier children are informed, the easier it is for them to deal with the information. Although most children are accepting, during their own sexual awakening in adolescence they may have difficulty dealing with the fact of their parent's homosexuality. In addition, if the parent develops a partner relationship in which the couple live together in a spouselike relationship, the children may develop a resentment toward the partner or have other problems similar to those seen in heterosexual stepparent families.

Because this family form is more common than most people may realize, it is important for the nurse to understand that homosexual families are different from the heterosexual family form, not necessarily better or worse. The gay or lesbian family environment can be just as healthy as any other. Nurses need to be nonjudgmental and to learn how to accept differences rather than demonstrate a homophobic prejudice that can have a detrimental effect on the nurse–child-family relationship. Moreover, the more knowledge of the child's family constellation and lifestyle nurses have, the more help they can be to the gay or lesbian parent and the child. (See Critical Thinking Exercise box.)

## Family Function

Authorities agree that families serve society in many ways. They play a vital role in the economy because they produce and consume goods and services. They also are the basic unit for replacing dying members of the society. Furthermore, to maintain its continuity, society must transmit its knowledge, customs, values, and beliefs to the young. Where children are not an economic necessity, their primary function is to receive and to give love. Although goals for socialization and childrearing practices differ from one culture to another, in most societies the family appears to have three major objectives in relation to children: caregiving, nurturing, and training.

### Family Strengths and Functioning Style

*Family function* refers to the interactions of family members, especially the quality of those relationships and interactions. Researchers have become increasingly interested in family characteristics that seem to help families function ef-

**Critical Thinking Exercise**

*Family Structure*

As the nurse, you are interviewing the mother of John, a school-age boy. The mother says their family consists of herself, her son, her lesbian partner, and two foster children. John's father lives in another state and has no contact with him. John has one grandparent who lives in another city in a nursing home. When planning care for John and his family, John's family should be considered to be which of the following?

First, Think About It . . .
- Within what point of view are you thinking?
- What concepts or ideas are central to your thinking?

1. Nuclear family of mother, father, and son
2. Single-parent family of mother and son
3. Extended family of mother, father, grandparent, and son
4. Family members identified by the mother

*The best response is four. The general point of view exists that the family defines its members. In this situation, John's family consists of those people who live in his home at the present time. Traditionally, the idea is that family composition has referred to either nuclear or extended families. However, many alternative family structures such as John's occur. The nurse needs to recognize that not all families are traditional in their membership.*

fectively. Knowledge of these factors guides the nurse at each step of the nursing process. The nurse is better able to predict the ways in which families may cope and respond to a stressful event, provide individualized support that builds on family strengths and unique functioning style, and assist family members in obtaining appropriate resources.

Friedman (1998) discusses five major functions that describe family purpose as it relates to individual family members and the greater society.

**Affective function:** Meeting the psychologic needs of family members
**Socialization function:** Creating opportunities for children to become productive members of society
**Reproductive function:** Preserving family presence over time and societal survival
**Economic function:** Providing adequate economic resources
**Health care function:** Providing for physical needs

Family strengths and unique functioning styles (Box 3-4) are significant resources nurses can employ in meeting families' needs. Building on the very things that make a particular family work well and strengthening the family's resources make the family unit even stronger and more capable of negotiating the developmental course of both individual family members and the family unit.

### Vulnerable Families

Certain families lack the supports and security to provide adequately for their children. In some instances social and economic factors have undermined supports for families.

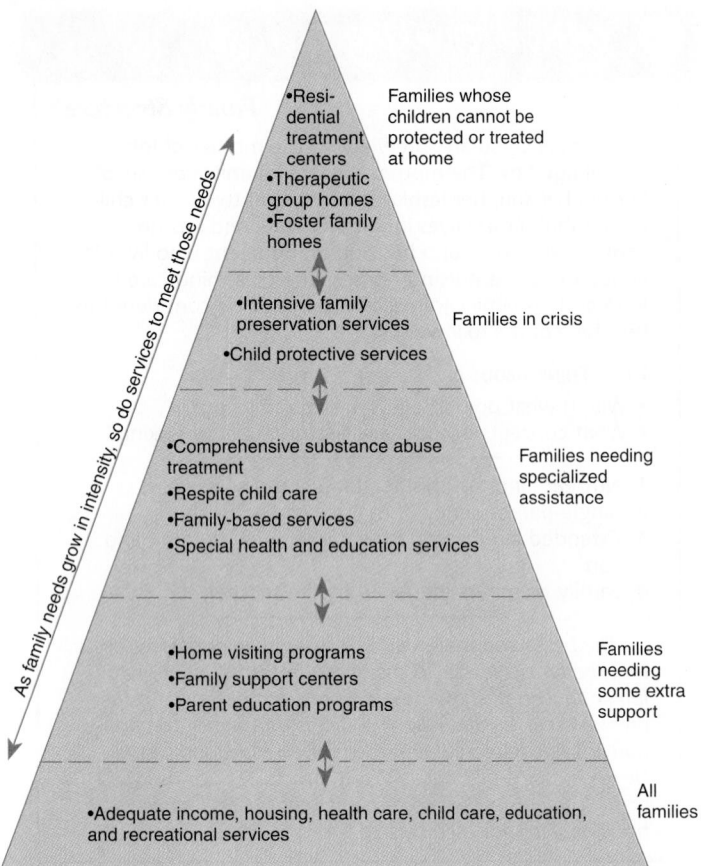

Families whose children cannot be protected or treated at home
•Residential treatment centers
•Therapeutic group homes
•Foster family homes

Families in crisis
•Intensive family preservation services
•Child protective services

Families needing specialized assistance
•Comprehensive substance abuse treatment
•Respite child care
•Family-based services
•Special health and education services

Families needing some extra support
•Home visiting programs
•Family support centers
•Parent education programs

All families
•Adequate income, housing, health care, child care, education, and recreational services

As family needs grow in intensity, so do services to meet those needs

**Fig. 3-3** Building a pyramid of services. When communities are able to offer a pyramid of assistance that matches the pyramid of family needs, problems are likely to be solved or alleviated at earlier stages, when they are easier and less costly to address. (From Children's Defense Fund: *The state of America's children 1998*, Washington, DC, 1998. Used with permission. All rights reserved.)

---

**Box 3-4** ◼ ◼ ◻
**Qualities of Strong Families**

1. A belief and sense of **commitment** toward promoting the well-being and growth of individual family members as well as that of the family unit
2. **Appreciation** for the small and large things that individual family members do well and **encouragement** to do better
3. Concentrated effort to spend **time** and do things together, no matter how formal or informal the activity or event
4. A sense of **purpose** that permeates the reasons and basis for "going on" in both bad and good times
5. A sense of **congruence** among family members regarding the value and importance of assigning time and energy to meet needs
6. The ability to **communicate** with one another in a way that emphasizes positive interactions
7. A clear set of **family rules, values,** and **beliefs** that establishes expectations about acceptable and desired behavior
8. A varied repertoire of **coping strategies** that promote positive functioning in dealing with both normative and non-normative life events
9. The ability to engage in **problem-solving** activities designed to evaluate options for meeting needs and procuring resources
10. The ability to be **positive** and see the positive in almost all aspects of their lives, including the ability to see crisis and problems as an opportunity to learn and grow
11. **Flexibility** and **adaptability** in the roles necessary to procure resources to meet needs
12. A **balance** between the use of internal and external family resources for coping and adapting to life events and planning for the future

From Dunst C, Trivette C, Deal A: *Enabling and empowering families: principles and guidelines for practice,* Cambridge, MA, 1988, Brookline Books.

---

**Box 3-5** ◼ ◼ ◻
**Effective Approaches for Working with Vulnerable Families**

Emphasize the family unit instead of focusing narrowly on an individual child or other family members.
Build on family strengths instead of emphasizing deficits.
Offer preventive services to avert crises instead of merely reacting to emergencies.
Address family needs comprehensively instead of piecemeal.
Treat families with respect and honor cultural differences.
Offer flexible, responsive services instead of rigid, single-purpose services.

From Children's Defense Fund: *The state of America's children 1998,* Washington, DC, 1998. Used with permission. All rights reserved.

---

For example, incomes of young families have sharply declined in recent years, increasing numbers of families are headed by young single mothers, and gaps in health care coverage continue to grow.

Poverty is perhaps the most global and widely used indicator of child well-being (Lerner, Sparks, and McCubbin, 1999). Increased rates of childhood poverty are associated with the following demographic maternal factors: (1) single status, (2) unemployment, (3) lack of high school education, and (4) young age (National Center for Children in Poverty, 1998). Lack of family structure and parenting resources are associated with problems of family life and child development (Lerner, Sparks, and McCubbin, 1999).

A disadvantaged beginning is only part of the problem. Today's families are more isolated from their neighbors and extended families than in the past, leaving them with fewer informal supports in times of crisis. In addition, the neighborhoods in which many of the most vulnerable families live are increasingly plagued by drugs and violence and lack necessary services.

Most families in crisis want to be helped to better protect and nurture their children, and most families can change when offered the right kind of help (Fig. 3-3). Effective approaches for helping vulnerable families tend to share certain characteristics (Box 3-5). Nursing interventions must be therapeutic and not a process that perpetuates the control by some members over others. Should someone disclose that he or she is a victim of domestic violence, guidelines for appropriate responses are listed in the Community Focus box.

In recent years the term **dysfunctional family,** which often refers to a continuum of mildly to highly dysfunctional levels, has become increasingly part of both professional and popular literature, imparting a sense of pathology or sickness about the ways in which certain families function. Families are better served when condescending labels are

## COMMUNITY FOCUS
### Guidelines for Care of Victims of Domestic Violence*

**DO**

Give priority to ensuring the woman's immediate safety.

Recognize her need for a positive response and your support.

Be sensitive to and discuss her fears.

Take her seriously; *believe* her.

Reassure her that the violence is not her fault.

Let her know that she is not alone in being abused.

Remember that her problems may be compounded by racist reactions, language, and cultural barriers; or other reactions to her age, sexuality, or disability.

Remember that her options may be limited by lack of access or resources.

Consult with specialist agencies and individuals.

Check if it is all right to send her letters or to telephone her at home. *Confidentiality is crucial.*

Respect her wishes if she does not want you to make contact at all.

Find out what she wants and see if you can help her achieve it.

Let her know that she does not have to leave home or talk to the women at the local refuge.

Discuss the situation and any options open to her.

Help her explore ways of maximizing her safety, whether she leaves or not.

Find out what other agencies can offer and let her know.

Take personal responsibility when referring her elsewhere.

Keep in contact, if at all possible.

**DON'T**

Ignore your intuition if you suspect a woman is being abused.

Insist on joint sessions with her and the man.

Deceitfully put off a woman if she comes to you for help.

Be flippant or cynical or skeptical.

Ask her what she did to provoke the violence; just ask for the facts.

Just focus on what she alone can do in the situation.

Make choices for her.

Give up on her just because things are taking longer than you think they should.

Give the man the address and telephone number of where she is staying.

Promise to give her a letter or pass on a message to her from him or to facilitate contact in any way.

---

Modified from Cody A: Helping the vulnerable or condoning control within the family: where is nursing? *J Adv Nurs* 23:882-886, 1996.

*The feminine gender and pronoun are used here, but the victim may be of either gender.

avoided. *All* families have strengths as well as vulnerabilities. Nurses who appreciate this will strive to develop assessment skills and use assessment tools that help families identify their strengths, as well as their needs. With this approach, families can not only survive a critical time but learn and grow from the experience.

## FAMILY ROLES AND RELATIONSHIPS

Each individual has a position, or status, in the family structure, and each occupant of a position plays culturally and socially defined roles in interactions within the group.

Within prescribed guidelines for behavior set by the culture, subcultures (including the family group) establish variations in role definition and may specify different requirements for playing the same role. Each family has its own traditions and values and sets its own standards for interaction within and outside the family group. Each determines the experiences the children should have, those they are to be shielded from, and how each of these experiences meets the needs of family members. Conformity to group norms is directly related to the strength and nature of group ties. Where family ties are strong, social control is highly effective, and most members play their roles willingly and with commitment. Conflicts arise when people do not fulfill their roles in ways that meet other family members' expectations, either because they are unaware of the expectations or because they choose not to meet them.

### Parental Roles

In all family groups the socially recognized status of father and mother exists with socially sanctioned roles that prescribe appropriate sexual behavior and childrearing responsibilities. The guides for behavior in these roles serve to control sexual conflict in society and provide for prolonged care of children. The degree to which parents are committed and the way they play their respective roles are influenced by a number of variables. Each individual is affected by a unique socialization experience.

Role definitions are changing as a result of the changing economy and the women's liberation movement. Women are achieving equality with men in education, more of them are entering the labor force, and the number of women who choose to have fewer children or none at all is increasing. During childhood, particularly in the upper and middle classes, the trend is toward deemphasizing the basic male-female characteristics of aggression, dependence, and achievement. As the role of the woman changes, there must necessarily be a change in the complementary role of the man. Fathers are taking a more active role in childrearing and household activities, which is most evident in middle-class families. Marital roles, on the other hand, are most segregated in the lower classes. Redefinition of sex roles in the American family is taking place, but a cultural lag of the persisting traditional role definitions creates role conflicts in many of these families.

### Role Learning

Roles are learned through the socialization process. During all stages of development children learn and practice, through interaction with others and in their play, a set of social roles and something of the characteristics of other roles. They behave in patterned and more or less predictable ways because they learn roles that define mutual expectations in typical and recurring social relationships. Although role definitions are changing, the basic determinants of parenting remain the same. The three determinants of parenting infants and young children are (1) parental personality and psychologic well-being, (2) contextual subsystems of support, and (3) child characteristics

## Box 3-6
### Types of Roles

**Ascribed roles** are those that are strictly defined by the culture, and very little deviation is allowed in modifying them. Ascribed roles apply to general traits such as sex, age, kinship, social class, and ethnic origin. There are culturally determined behaviors that must be adhered to regarding these roles, and they are expected to be learned in the home. For example, a child who attempts to change an ascribed role (such as sex) will be confronted with serious problems.

**Achieved roles** are those acquired through effort, and children must do something to attain them. Achieved roles include educational, occupational, religious, and recreational roles. These are based on performance and are acquired through satisfaction of specified requirements. The direction of these role achievements is strongly influenced by values conveyed to the children by their parents. For example, some parents believe that a college education is essential; others encourage children to seek occupational gratification.

**Adopted roles** are those that are sometimes transient, such as the role of patient or traveler. More often, adopted behavior patterns become fixed into what are known as *character roles* and apply to the unique behaviors that the child displays in a given situation. Such roles as the leader, the follower, the clown, or the show-off are examples of adopted roles. They are frequently adopted when playing the role meets a need or is the response to a complementary role in another.

**Assumed roles** are those related to fantasy and are especially important in childhood. This is one of the dominant means for children's adjustment and socialization. Children continually assume roles of persons they observe in their environment. The environment is a primary resource for learning the conduct that befits their position or status. Assumed roles become a problem only if they persist into the world of reality. For example, a child who persistently plays an infantile role is severely hampered in relationships with peers.

(Foss, 1996). These determinants have been consistent measurements in determining a person's success in fulfilling the parental role.

Role conceptions are transmitted by socializing agents (parents, peers, authority figures) who use positive and negative sanctions to ensure conformity to their norms. Role behaviors positively reinforced by rewards such as love, affection, friendship, and honor are strengthened. Negative reinforcement takes the form of ridicule, withdrawal of love, expressions of disapproval, or banishment. Some types of roles are described in Box 3-6.

In some cultures the role behavior expected of children conflicts with desirable adult behavior. For example, in the United States, children are expected to be submissive in childhood but dominant as adults. This conflict of expectations is known as *role discontinuity*. Other cultures value the same behaviors, such as courage and aggression, both in children and in adults; this provides *role continuity*.

### Role Structuring in Children

One responsibility of the family is to develop culturally appropriate role behavior in the children. Children at a very early age learn to perform in expected ways consistent with their position in the family and culture. The observed behavior of each child is a single manifestation—a combination of social influences as well as individual psychologic processes. In this way the uniting of the child's intrapersonal system (the self) with the interpersonal system (the family) is simultaneously understood as the conduct of the child.

Role structuring initially takes place within the family unit, where the children fulfill a set of roles and respond to

**TABLE 3-3** Family role patterns for siblings

| Job Assignment | Interpersonal Responsibilities |
|---|---|
| **The Firstborn is Responsible for:** | |
| Supporting family rules, values, expectations | The individual family members, rather than for the subsystems or the family as a whole |
| Outcomes, results, products | One parent (often father) and also responsible *to* the same parent |
| A central place in the family in order to be productive | All family members' productivity |
| **The Second-Born is Responsible for:** | |
| Perceiving and supporting the implicit elements in family rules and relationships | Having a unique relationship with everyone in the family |
| Opening clogged channels of communication by making the implicit explicit | One parent (usually mother) and also responsible *to* the same parent |
| Monitoring the quality of performance | The affective state of each family member by supporting his or her emotional needs |
| Acting out discrepancies between the implicit and explicit to force acknowledgment | Working with, or fighting with, if necessary, the first sibling to flush out discrepancies between implicit and explicit rules |
| **The Third-Born is Responsible for:** | |
| The dynamics and quality of the marital relationship | Being connected to both mother and father |
| The balance in all dyadic relationships | Restoring balance in the marital relationship by connecting with each parent |
| Discovering and enforcing rules about the degree and nature of relationship rules, such as closeness, conflict, dependency, intrusiveness, and loyalty | Connecting to all dyadic relationships in the family |
| Identifying family issues | |
| **The Fourth-Born is Responsible for:** | |
| Family unit and harmony | Connecting to each family member to ensure unity and harmony |
| Family purposes and goals | All "garbage" in the family because it disrupts unity and harmony |
| | Acting out the tensions in relationships; can be quite dramatic |

Modified from Hoopes M, Harper J: *Birth order roles and sibling patterns in individual and family therapy,* Rockville, MD, 1987, Aspen.

the complementary roles of their parents and other family members. The roles of the children are shaped primarily by the parents, who apply direct or indirect pressures in an attempt to induce or force children into the desired patterns of behavior or direct their efforts toward modification of the role responses of the child on a mutually acceptable basis. Parents have their own techniques and will determine the course that the process of socialization is to follow. (See Limit-Setting and Discipline, p. 85.)

Research indicates that birth order influences the role each sibling is assigned within the family. When children enter a particular family, they sense the physical, social, and emotional values associated with their own specific role. They then develop characteristic response patterns to fulfill their role. Each sibling position role is created to meet both the family's and the individual's needs. For example, first-born children learn that their job assignment is to produce outcomes that meet with the family's approval and to enforce explicit family rules. Third-born children feel especially responsible for balance in the marital relationship. Four sibling patterns are identified, with the position patterns repeating after the fourth sibling (Table 3-3).

Children respond to life situations according to behaviors learned in reciprocal transactions. As they acquire important role-taking skills, their relationships with others change. For instance, when a teenager is also the mother but lives in a household where the grandmother is a co-resident, the adolescent mother may experience more support for the adolescent role than for the parenting role (Black and Nitz, 1996). Children become proficient at understanding others as they acquire the ability to discriminate their own perspectives from those of others. Children who get along well with others and attain status in the peer group have well-developed role-taking skills.

## Family Size and Configuration

The size and composition of the family directly influence child development. No two children grow in exactly the same environment, although identical twins more nearly approximate this. For example, in a nuclear family with two children—even of the same sex—one will live in a family with an older sibling, whereas the other will be reared in a family with a younger sibling. In a family where there is a 10-year age span between the children, one may be born to a 20-year-old mother and the other to a 30-year-old mother. For the child in each situation, the environment is different.

### Family Size

Parenting practices differ between small and large families. In small families more emphasis is placed on the individual development of the children. Parenting is intensive rather than extensive, and there is constant pressure to measure up to family expectations. Children's development and achievement are measured against that of other children in the neighborhood and social class. In small families there is more democratic participation by the children than in larger families. Adolescents in small families identify more strongly with their parents and rely more on their parents for advice. They have well-developed, autonomous inner

controls as contrasted with adolescents from larger families, who rely more on adult authority.

Children in a large family are able to adjust to a variety of changes and crises. There is more emphasis on the group and less on the individual (Fig. 3-4). Cooperation is essential, often because of economic necessity. The large number of persons sharing a limited amount of space requires a greater degree of organization, administration, and authoritarian control. The control is wielded by a dominant family member—a parent or an older child. The number of children reduces the intimate, one-to-one contact between the parent and any individual child. Consequently, children turn to each other for what they cannot get from their parents. The reduced parent-child contact encourages individual children to adopt specialized roles in an attempt to gain recognition in the family.

Discipline is often administered by older siblings in large families. Siblings are usually better attuned to what constitutes misbehavior, and sibling disapproval or ostracism is frequently a more meaningful disciplinary measure than parental interventions. In situations such as death or illness of a parent, an older sibling assumes responsibility for the family at considerable personal sacrifice. Large families seem to generate a sense of security in the children fostered by sib-

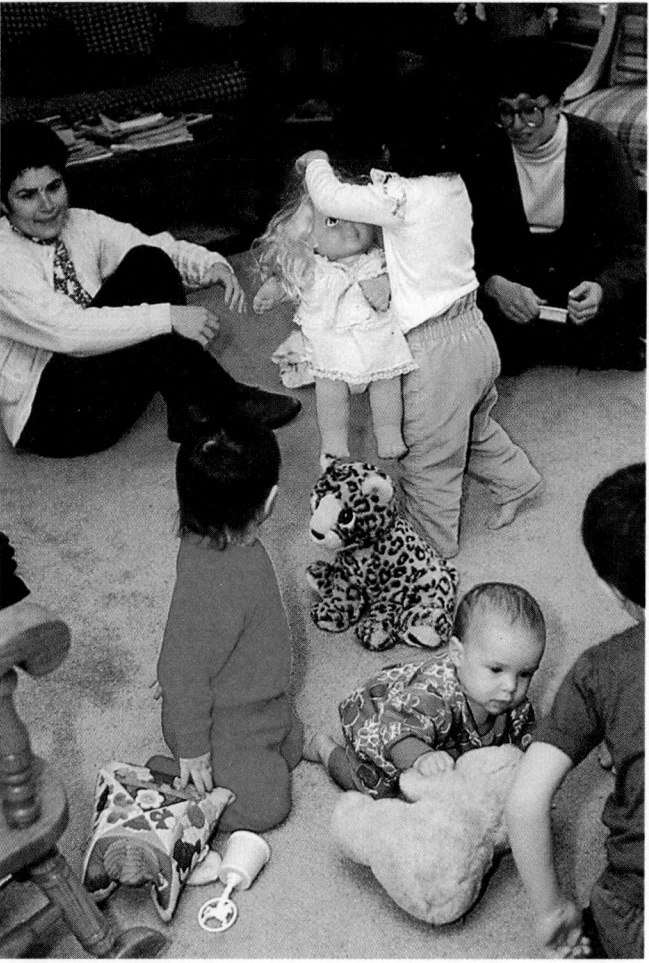

**Fig. 3-4**   Innumerable relationships and activities are possible in a large family.

ling support and cooperation. However, adolescents from a large family are more peer oriented than family oriented.

## Spacing of Children

Age differences between siblings affect the childhood environment but to a lesser extent than does the sex of the siblings. The arrival of a sibling has the greatest impact on the older child, and a 2- to 4-year difference in age appears to be most threatening to the older child. When the older child is very young, the self-image is too immature to be threatened. At an older age the child is better able to understand the situation and therefore is less likely to see the newcomer as a threat, although the child does feel the loss of the only-child status.

In general, the narrower the spacing between siblings, the more the children influence one another, especially in emotional characteristics; the wider the spacing, the greater the influence of the parents. This is not to say that bonds are nonexistent between siblings with large age spans, or that siblings with only a year or two difference in age will always feel a strong bond. However, high accessibility during these developmentally formative years is the almost routine accompaniment of an influential sibling relationship. High-access siblings are generally close in age and the same gender, which promotes access to common life events. They often attend the same school, play with the same friends, date in the same circle, and share a common bedroom and clothing. In essence, it means that just about any spacing can work well if parents handle sibling rivalry sensitively (Silver, 1995).

## Sibling Interaction

Most children have at least one brother or sister. Asked why they chose to have a second child, most parents give as their primary reason the fact that they did not want their firstborn to be an only child. Right or wrong, many persons believe that children develop best within the company of other children.

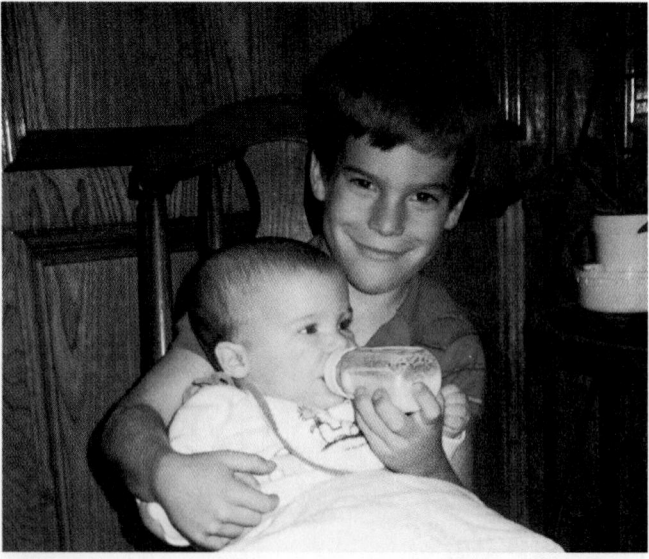

**Fig. 3-5**   Older school-age children often enjoy taking responsibility for the care of a younger sibling.

For a number of years, sibling relationships were viewed from a Freudian perspective that emphasizes the concept of sibling rivalry. However, in recent decades researchers have viewed siblings through developmental or ecologic frameworks and have focused on interactions within family systems (Friedman, 1998). Results of these broader perspectives reveal rich and varied sibling interaction (Fig. 3-5).

Perhaps the sibling relationship's most unique feature is its duration. Likely the longest relationship one will share with another human being, the sibling relationship lasts through a lifetime, often 50 to 80 years, as compared with the child-parent relationship of approximately 30 to 50 years. Siblings spend long periods of time together and come to know each other—at their best and worst—extremely well.

**Sibling Functions.**   Siblings exert power, exchange services, and express feelings in reciprocal ways that are often not revealed explicitly in the presence of parents. They see themselves in their brother or sister, experience life vicariously through their sibling's behavior, and begin to expand on their own possibilities. Siblings can also be touchstones for what the other would *not* like to be, and they tend to use each other as yardsticks for comparison. They are sounding boards for one another; they offer a safe forum for experimenting with new behaviors and roles before using either with parents or nonfamily peers.

Brothers and sisters provide each other with tangible services (e.g., lending money, clothing, toys, sports equipment, teaching a skill), help with childhood problems, provide support in dealing with parents or others outside the family, and may provide an introduction to a new friendship group. Siblings learn to negotiate and bargain, and sometimes to manipulate. Many opportunities arise for conflict and conflict resolution. They learn about sharing, competition, rivalry, and compromise. Siblings can also protect one another from parental-executive abuse of power and can form a coalition to deal with the issues of authority, power, and emotional support. Negotiating with parents is stronger when siblings act together rather than singly.

Siblings interpret the outside world for each other and perform genuine educative functions for the parents. A related function is *pioneering,* wherein one sibling initiates a process, thereby giving permission to the others to follow accordingly. Patterns may include breaking explicit family rules, taking new developmental pathways (such as leaving the family), or adopting different moral or political codes and lifestyles.

Tattling can be an important lever in sibling interactions. On the other hand, there is often a conspiracy of silence among siblings, leaving the parents feeling isolated and excluded. A willingness to make and maintain each other's privacy often serves as a powerful bond of loyalty among the children. It is this loyalty that often distinguishes the relationship between siblings from that between friends.

**More Active Sibling Relationships.**   Sibling relationships vary among cultures. Certain factors, however, may be giving the sibling relationship greater significance in North America than in the past. Shrinking family size, longer life spans, divorce and remarriage, geographic mobility, maternal employment and alternative sources of child care, competitive pressures, stress, and various forms of parental insufficiency may be propelling siblings into greater contact and emotional interdependence than ever before.

For example, siblings often join forces to confront the trauma of divorce. They frequently rely on each other for support when parents remarry. The large number of working mothers means that many young siblings today have large amounts of time when their relationship is not monitored by a personally committed adult. Often an older sibling is required to baby-sit, resulting in children spending more and more time together unsupervised. In a worried, mobile, small-family, high-stress, fast-paced, parent-absent society, children often turn to a brother or sister to meet their needs for contact, constancy, and permanency.

## Ordinal Position

It has been observed for some time that the birth position of children affects their personalities. Parents treat children differently, and sibling interactions are different depending on the children's positions within the family. Also, power is unequally distributed among siblings. Older siblings attempt to dominate younger ones; therefore younger siblings develop interpersonal skills, the ability to negotiate, and an ability to accept unfavorable outcomes to a greater extent than older siblings. Later-born children are obliged to interact with other siblings from birth and seem to be more outgoing and make friends more easily than firstborns. However, children vary tremendously; these generalizations represent averages and do not apply in all situations. General characteristics of children in the various ordinal positions are presented in Box 3-7.

**The Only Child.**   Being the only child in a family has traditionally been considered a disadvantage. Only children have been described as selfish, spoiled, dependent, and lonely. However, a review of 141 research studies indicates that there are no essential personality differences between a child reared alone and one who is reared with one or more siblings (Polit and Falbo, 1987). They display no more evidence of maladjustment or self-centeredness than any other children and tend to strongly resemble firstborn children in such respects as higher educational goals. Only children perform better on cognitive tests, are more mature and cultivated, are more socially sensitive, and demonstrate superiority in language facility.

Only children also enjoy the advantage of having parents who, without the distraction of other children, are able to devote more time to them, talk to them, and stimulate them in intellectual activities. However, parents also exert greater pressure for mature behavior at an early age and for achievement. Relative isolation from peers contributes to intellectual pursuits and encourages a rich fantasy life, independence, and originality.

The effects of being an only child on personality are questionable. Only children do not have the stereotyped concept of sex-appropriate behavior and often exhibit some characteristics associated with both sexes, but the significant influence is the quality of the parent-child relationship. Because of the wide differences among parents, a typical personality cannot be assigned to the only child. An unusually large number of only children live with a single parent, primarily as a result of divorce.

## Multiple Births

A deviation in early development that occurs with variable frequency is multiple births. Twins are not uncommon in the population, but triplets are rare and quadruplets or quintuplets are extremely unusual. In any of these situations the offspring can be of the like or unlike sex (i.e., derived from a single ovum, from multiple ova, or a combination of the two, which can involve one or more cell divisions). The cause of twinning is unknown, but the increase in the number of larger multiples (quintuplets, sextuplets) during recent years has been associated with fertility-enhancing techniques (ovulation-inducing drugs and assisted reproductive techniques such as in vitro fertilization) (Ventura and others, 1997). Since women in their thirties are almost $2\frac{1}{2}$ times as likely as women in their twenties to have higher-order plural births, the rise in the multiple-

---

**Box 3-7** ■ ■ ■
**Influence of Ordinal Position on Children**

**FIRSTBORN CHILDREN**

Are more achievement oriented
Are more dominant
Receive more physical punishment
Are allowed to show more aggression to siblings
Have stronger consciences, are more self-disciplined and inner directed
Are more socially anxious
Are prone to feelings of guilt
Identify more with parents than with peers
Are more conservative
Are subject to greater parental expectations
Begin to speak earlier in life
Demonstrate higher intellectual achievement
Plan better and experience fewer frustrations
Are likely to be most wanted

**MIDDLE CHILDREN**

Have more demands made on them for household help
Are praised less often
Receive less of the parents' time
Learn to compromise and be adaptable
Are less stimulated toward achievement
Are more difficult to characterize because of a variety of positions in family

**YOUNGEST CHILDREN**

Are less dependent than firstborn children
Are less tense, more affectionate, and more good-natured
Tend to identify more with peer group than with parents
Are more flexible in their thinking
Are popular with classmates
Have fewer demands placed on them for household help

**ONLY CHILDREN**

Resemble firstborn children
Are more mature and cultivated
Experience greater parental pressure for mature behavior and achievement
Demonstrate superiority in language facility
Rarely develop into stereotype of spoiled, selfish child
Often enjoy a rich fantasy life as a result of isolation

birth ratio has been associated with increased child-bearing among older women and the expanded use of fertility drugs (Guyer and others, 1999).

Twins are of two distinct types: *identical*, or *monozygotic (MZ)*, and *fraternal*, or *dizygotic (DZ)* (Fig. 3-6 and Box 3-8). In the United States the overall twinning rate is approximately 1 in 80 pregnancies; one third are MZ twins, and two thirds are DZ twins.

A special kind of sibling relationship is observed in twins, although getting along with each other and quarreling are not much different from those behaviors in any other two siblings, especially if they are different-sex fraternal twins. Twins generally tend to work out a relationship that is reasonably satisfactory to both and demonstrate early independence from parental attention. They develop a remarkable capacity for cooperative play and considerable loyalty and generosity toward each other. It is not uncommon for them to evolve a private language between themselves that may interfere with development of the family language.

In a twinship, one member of the pair, to a greater or lesser extent, is more dominant, outgoing, and assertive than the other, often to the consternation of their parents. However, the seemingly more passive twin is able to accomplish as much and get his or her way as frequently as the more assertive twin.

It has also been observed that there is a difference in behavior between identical and fraternal twins. Whereas there is near unison in the actions of identical twins (although they alternate in assuming the leadership), fraternal twins, even of the same sex, do not display this quality. Sibling rivalry can be quite pronounced in fraternal twins, especially in different-sex twins.

Identical twins also differ in their response to the tendency of some parents to treat twins exactly alike. The present philosophy is to determine the degree to which the children demonstrate an inclination toward togetherness. Some twins thrive best when they are constantly in each other's company; others prefer more individuality and separateness. The conservative approach is to allow the children to follow their natural inclinations. Early years of togetherness are often the basis of the children's security. To separate them too early may produce unnecessary stresses. The tendency is to foster individual differences as they are evidenced in order to ease the process of separation when it becomes advisable.

**Parental Adjustment.** The entrance of any new member into a household creates a number of stresses, but with multiple births two or more new members must be incorporated into the family at the same time. The problems are obvious. Two infants must be provided with physical care, including feeding, diapering, and all the purchasing and preparation that accompany the care of any infant. Scheduling becomes crucial, and each advancement in development brings new problems and adjustments (e.g., space and sleeping arrangements, selecting a stroller and other equipment). Care must be observed in selecting toys. As play becomes a serious business, some toys that would be safe and appropriate for a single child become weapons when two infants share a playpen. It is a good idea to select different toys for the children as they grow older and encourage sharing.

It is especially important for parents to maintain relationships with each other and other family members. It is doubly important for parents to arrange time together as often as possible. The **National Organization of Mothers of Twins Clubs, Inc.,*** has local chapters throughout the United States to offer information and support to parents of twins and is highly recommended as a resource for all new

---

*Executive office, PO Box 438, Thompson's Station, TX 37179-0438; www.nomote.org.

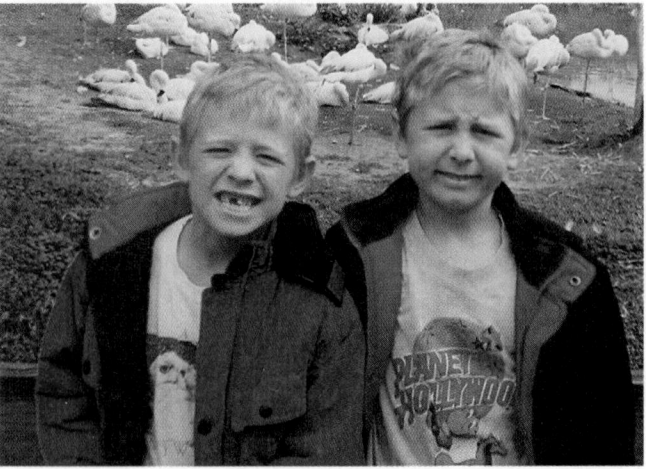

**Fig. 3-6** Fraternal twins.

---

### Box 3-8 ■ ■ ■
### Characteristics of Twins

| MONOZYGOTIC (MZ, IDENTICAL TWINS) | DIZYGOTIC (DZ, FRATERNAL TWINS) |
|---|---|
| Result of one fertilized ovum that became separated early in development | Result of fertilization of two ova |
| Alike physically and genetically | Differ physically and genetically |
| Same sex | May be like or opposite sex |
| Frequency: | Frequency: |
| Occurs uniformly in all populations | Varies among races (highest—African-Americans, lowest—Asians, intermediate—whites) |
| Unaffected by maternal age | More common with advancing maternal age (maximum at age 35-39, then decreases rapidly) |
| Tendency unaffected by heredity | Marked familial tendency Expressed only in the female Fathers appear to transmit disposition toward double ovulation to daughters |
| Similar behavior | Dissimilar behavior; more sibling rivalry |

parents of twins. **TWINS magazine†** is a place to seek and give advice about parenting multiples.

Another problem faced by parents of twins occurs at the time of birth. Not only are the parents faced with double the work and care of newborns, but the process of attachment may also be impeded. The parents first form an attachment to the twins as a unit before they are able to form an attachment to each child individually. (See discussion on multiple births and subsequent children under Promote Parent-Infant Bonding [Attachment], Chapter 8.) Parents are often surprised that this occurs. Other family members, extended family, and even teachers and baby-sitters will experience the same phenomenon to some extent. As they develop, the children, who are facing the task of differentiating themselves from their environment, must learn to differentiate themselves not only from the parent (usually the mother) but from one another as well.

**Promoting Individuation.**   All children proceed through a separation-individuation process as they grow and develop. For twins, the process is complicated in a number of ways. Unlike singletons, twins lack a perception of separateness, and the close physical and emotional attachment between them inhibits development of individuality. In addition, twin children are frequently thought of and treated as a unit, and efforts they make in the direction of individuality are often impeded by others. There are a number of ways in which parents and others can aid twins in achieving individuation (Box 3-9).

---

†twinsmagazine.com.

---

**Box 3-9** ■ ■ □
**Promoting Individuation of Twins**

Select different-sounding names.
Take separate photographs of the children (beginning at birth) so each child will have a picture of "me." Be certain to label each picture.
Avoid dressing children alike.
Use their given names. Avoid referring to them as "the twins."
Take each child on separate short outings occasionally while the other is at home with another family member or a sitter.
Build a one-to-one relationship with each child.
Hold and cuddle each child. Provide frequent body contact with each one.
Play and participate in learning with each child and to the same extent as with a singly born child.
Provide toys according to individual preferences, needs, and interest.
Entertain each as much as feasible. Avoid leaving them to entertain each other for long periods of time.
Provide separate rooms, if possible.
Praise each child individually and, preferably, at different times.
Discipline twins individually.
Provide separate feeding and care schedules according to the needs of the individual child.
Arrange for frequent opportunities for individual contact with other adults.
Encourage play with other children the same age.

---

Modified from Sater J: Appraising and promoting a sense of self in twins, *MCN* 4:218-226, 1979.

# PARENTING
## Motivation for Parenthood

A dominant characteristic in all societies is that adults are expected to become parents and to be gratified by the experience. Pressures of tradition, sentiment regarding the state of parenthood, and religious exhortations to fulfill divine commands of fertility profoundly influence decision making because conformity to social-role expectations is a strong influence in family planning.

In North American society there is a change in the rationale for marriage and parenthood. The modern nuclear family believes that marriage and family are based on romantic love, with maternal love predominant toward children, and that the family is the most important social affiliation. The family members depend on each other for love, support, and nurturance. The postmodern family (dating from about 1960) affirms that marriage, if it occurs and lasts, is based on consensual love. Parenting is seen as shared responsibility, not only with both parents but also with nonparental caregivers. Independence is encouraged for children to pursue their own interests even if that pursuit takes precedence over family events (Elkind, 1995). Although many pregnancies are unplanned, there are numerous reasons why couples decide to initiate a pregnancy. Many consider children a normal part of marriage, others see them as proof of their adulthood, some desire heirs for the family name and fortune, and a few want to fulfill a parent's wish for grandchildren. Having a child in an attempt to save an unstable marriage is a poor reason that usually fails in its goal. However, in most instances the couple sincerely wish to become parents.

Factors that are likely to influence family size are social class, religion, race, financial stability, type of conjugal-role relationships, and the social-psychologic aspects of sexual relations. Of course, how effectively the couple practices contraception may determine whether the family size remains as planned. Also, in the case of divorce and remarriage, an individual may decide to have more children with the new spouse.

## Preparation for Parenthood

The basic goals of parenting are to promote the physical survival and health of the children, to foster the skills and abilities necessary to be a self-sustaining adult, and to foster behavioral capabilities for maximizing cultural values and beliefs. However, new parents approach parenthood with meager experience and scant knowledge, although no other task can compare, in overall consequences, with that of rearing a human being. Parents learn by trial and error, committing the same mistakes that have been committed by countless other parents, but they somehow manage to accomplish the task, becoming more skilled with each additional child. Tradition rather than rational planning furnishes the chief norms for childrearing. Experience in having been nurtured as a child is an essential component of successful parenting.

Their own parents are probably the only persons who parents observe intimately in the parental role; this results in a *generational continuity*—parents rear their own children in much the same way as they themselves were reared. Other essential skills and knowledge parents need in order to feel more comfortable in the parenting role include a basic understanding of childhood growth and development, bathing, feeding, use of play, and interpersonal communication skills. All of this information is integrated throughout this text.

## Goals of Parenting

The family, in order to fulfill one of its primary functions, provides for the caregiving, nurturing, and training of children. In the process of childrearing, parents have at least three basic goals for their children:

1. **Survival:** To promote the physical survival and health of their children, thereby ensuring that the children live long enough to produce children of their own
2. **Economic:** To foster the skills and behavioral capacities that the children will need for economic self-maintenance as adults
3. **Self-actualization:** To foster behavioral capabilities for maximizing cultural values and beliefs

## Transition to Parenthood

Although there is disagreement as to whether or not the birth of a couple's first child should be labeled a crisis, the early weeks of an infant's life call for a couple to make drastic adjustments. Although the parents have anticipated and perhaps prepared for the child's arrival, the birth means the sudden imposition of totally dependent care 24 hours a day for the new member of the family. It may very well be a crisis if the event is perceived as disturbing old habits and relationships and eliciting new responses. It requires role changes, destroys or significantly modifies former relationships, and means adjusting to new role realignments. Whereas previously the roles of a couple were husband and wife, they now become, in addition, father and mother. It is difficult to adjust to being parents, but it is a normal human experience and a tool for personal growth.

The advent of a new family member requires that the family cope with greater financial responsibilities, a possible loss of income, changes in sleeping habits, and less time for the husband and wife to spend with each other (especially if it is a firstborn) and with other children. If the events are perceived as aversive, it could well disrupt the couple's bond. Some investigators find that the birth of a first child results in a reduction of the couple's intimacy and affection, whereas others report that the adjustment to parenthood is only mildly stressful.

### Parental Factors Affecting Transition to Parenthood

The birth of an infant is a highly significant event that alters the behavior of both mothers and fathers. No amount of preparation can truly and fully prepare prospective parents for the constant and immediate needs of an infant. The importance of early parent-infant interactions is addressed in the discussion of the neonate, especially the attachment

process (see Chapter 8). Some of the predominant factors affecting parenting are the age of the parents, the quality of the parental relationship, the amount of previous experience with childrearing, parental support systems, and the effects of stress on parental behavior.

**Parental Age.** The most satisfactory ages for childbearing are established as the years between 18 and 35. During this time parents are considered to be in optimum health, with a predicted life span that allows sufficient time and vigor to raise a family. However, the age at which parents begin their families has changed over the last few decades in the United States, with a substantial increase in the birth rate for women 30 to 44 years of age and a decline for women ages 20 to 29 years (Ventura and others, 1997). Recent statistics report that the number of births for women aged 30 and over has increased since the late 1970s.

Reasons for postponing childbearing are related to more women entering career paths, needs of individuals and couples to achieve educational and occupational goals and attain more financial security, and a sense of commitment in a relationship. Some women who initially decide not to have children change their minds as the "biologic time clock" begins to run out. Although there has been considerable research on the transition to parenthood, the impact of delayed childbearing on the couple, the child, and the family unit has not been fully explored.

**Father Involvement.** Current practices that encourage early father-infant interaction have indicated that fathers appear to be just as intrigued with their newborns as mothers are. (See discussion on paternal engrossment under Promote Parent-Infant Bonding [Attachment], Chapter 8.) Even fathers who have little initial contact with their neonates will become involved with them over the next few months, although the type of interaction will be different from that of the mother (Fig. 3-7). For example, whereas mothers are likely to hold, soothe, care for, or play quietly with their infants, fathers are more boisterous, engaging in more physically stimulating activities that infants seem to enjoy. However, fathers are more than simply playmates. They are often successful at soothing a distressed infant

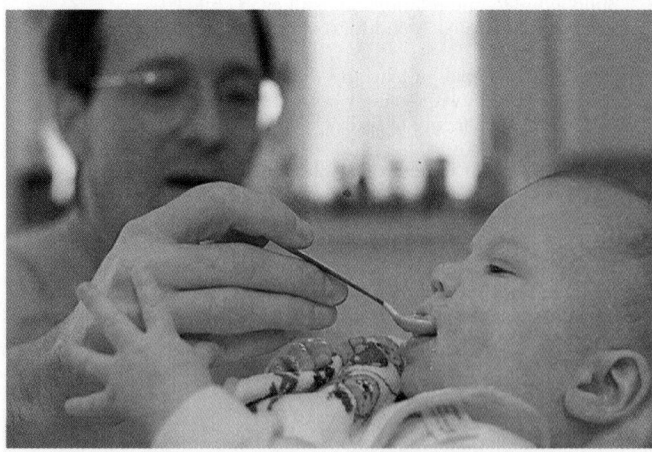

**Fig. 3-7** Fathers who assume care of their children may feel more comfortable and successful in their parenting role.

(Fig. 3-8). Furthermore, a secure attachment to the father can help offset the consequences of an insecure attachment to the mother.

The role of the father is now considered to be essential to a family's health and well-being. The essential role is somewhat diminished because of inadequate role models, a lack of childrearing information and education, and a set of values that may need reevaluation (May, 1996). In fact, one study that covered prebirth to 1 year olds and their fathers showed that the fathers needed education about appropriate expectations of a 3-month-old child and information regarding alternative methods of discipline (Tiller, 1995).

May (1996) suggests a number of ways that a nurse can assist new fathers in relating to their children:

- Have an attitude and willingness to involve the father even when he does not appear to be interested.
- Provide opportunities and places for fathers to learn.
- Ensure that hours are flexible enough to accommodate the father's schedule.
- Promote the strengths that you see in the father and do not make issues of the weaknesses.
- Provide as many opportunities for fathers to hug and embrace their child as possible.
- Encourage new fathers to talk to their father.
- Try to get fathers to talk to other fathers.

**Parenting Education.**    First-time parents who have had more help preparing themselves to be parents experience less stress in the transition than do those who have not. Research suggests that programs designed to take place near the time of or during transition are more helpful in easing transitional stress than are those programs designed to take place earlier in life (e.g., high school programs). (See Influence of the "Experts," p. 88.)

Many parents are looking for ways to be a better parent. Shrifrin (1997) offers a number of suggestions: improving communication by becoming an active listener, being actively involved in the child's education, becoming computer literate, looking at things from the child's point of view, considering his or her temperament, keeping the child healthy with needed checkups and vaccinations, providing the best

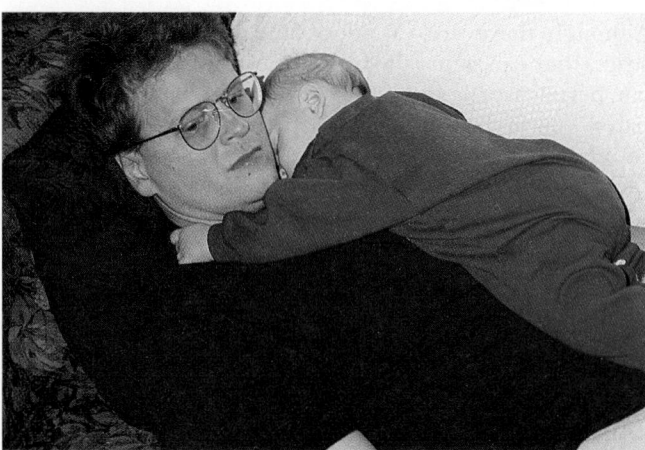

**Fig. 3-8**    The role of the father is essential to a family's health and well-being.

nutritional meals possible, paying attention to safety concerns, spending time with the child, and evaluating the family's overall functioning.

■　■　■

Other factors influencing the transition to the parental role include:

- Parents with previous experience, such as another child, appear to be more relaxed and have less conflict in disciplinary relationships, and they are more aware of normal growth and development expectations.
- The amount of stress experienced by one or both parents may interfere with their ability to exhibit patience and understanding or otherwise cope with their children's behavior.
- Special characteristics of the infant, such as being temperamentally difficult, can cause the parents to lose confidence and doubt their abilities. Also, an infant with special care needs, such as those associated with a disability, can be a significant source of added stress.
- Marital relationships can have a negative effect on parental transition because marital tension or strife can alter caregiving routines and interfere with enjoyment of the infant. Conversely, parents who support and encourage one another serve as a positive influence on establishing a satisfying parental role.

### Support Systems

Successful adaptation to the stress of transition to parenthood involves at least two types of family resources (McCubbin and McCubbin, 1994). First are the *internal resources* of the family, such as adaptability and integration. Changing from an orderly, predictable life to a relatively disordered, unpredictable one is a universal adaptation families must make. Rigid schedules are impossible to maintain, and former activities must be curtailed or abandoned. *Adaptation* is reflected in learning to be patient, becoming better organized, and becoming more flexible. *Integration* involves an attempt of the couple to continue some activities they engaged in before they became parents. In this way couples are able to maintain a sense of continuity and appreciate the importance of the husband-wife relationship.

The second kind of resource for coping with stress is the use of *coping strategies* that strengthen the organization and functioning of the family. These include the use of community resources, the use of social support, and the adoption of a future orientation. Interpersonal supports that provide information, advice, and caretaking are derived from friends, relatives, and neighbors. Relationships with family, friends, and community are essential (Fig. 3-9). For fathers, positive work relationships seem to be especially important; for mothers, activities with friends are important. Arranging for time away from the child or children is also beneficial. Fathers can assume care of the family to allow the mother some time to herself at home or away from the home, even if just for an afternoon or evening. Adoption of a future orientation provides reassurance to parents that things will get better, that they will cope, and that it is realistic to plan for the time when they will be able to engage in self-fulfilling activities.

It is also reassuring to know that others experience ambivalent feelings toward parenthood and share the same difficulties and frustrations. Exchanging ideas and experiences

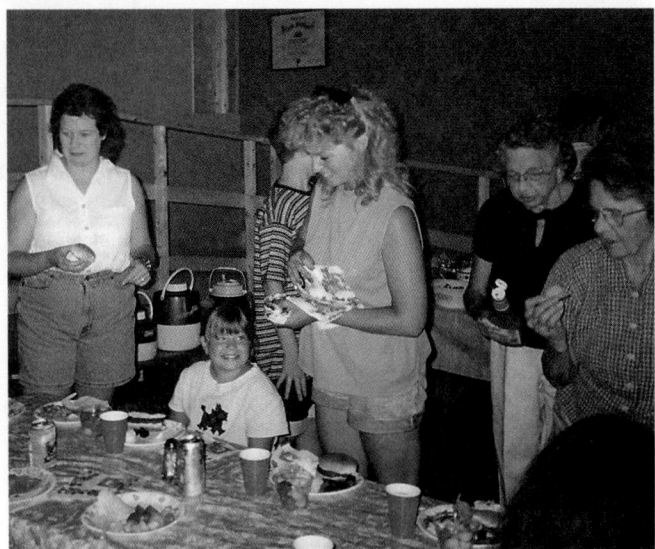

**Fig. 3-9**   Maintaining relationships with the extended family is important.

with other parents provides an opportunity to voice concerns and to learn new ways of coping with the multiple problems of childrearing. Whether it is family, friends, or community resources, parents need persons to whom they can turn for advice, comfort, and assistance—persons with whom they can share the joys and difficulties of childrearing.

## Parenting Behaviors

### Attitudes Toward Childrearing

There are infinite variations in the way parents rear their children. Some are related to cultural influences; others are related to social class and economic resources. The results of numerous studies suggest that parents differ from one another in two major attitudinal continuums.

*Permissiveness-restrictiveness* refers to the degree of autonomy that parents allow their children. Some parents exercise close, restrictive control over much of their children's behavior. They limit their children's freedom of expression by imposing many demands and actively surveying their children's behavior to ensure that they comply with rules and regulations. Permissive parents make few demands and allow their children considerable freedom in exploring their environment, expressing their opinions and emotions, and making decisions about their activities. Many find a balance between the two extremes. It is not uncommon to find that many parents become less restrictive as both they and their children mature.

*Warmth-hostility* refers to how openly or frequently parental affection is expressed and the degree to which affection is mixed with feelings of rejection or hostility. Parents described as warm and nurturant are those who often smile at, praise, and encourage their children while limiting their criticisms, punishments, and signs of disapproval.

Within the wide range of families, the amount of affection that parents show their children may vary considerably and be influenced by cultural factors and individual differ-

ences in the personality and temperament of both the parents and the children. Children who come from homes in which they are loved and accepted display socially acceptable behavior and are generally good-natured, cheerful, friendly, cooperative, and emotionally stable. Because they are loved and accepted themselves, they are able to form satisfactory relationships with others.

Cool, hostile, or rejecting parents are quick to criticize, belittle, punish, or ignore their children while limiting their expressions of affection or approval. It is important to be aware that these measures of parental warmth or coldness reflect parental behavior in a large number of situations. For example, a parent may be cool and rejecting when a child misbehaves but warm and affectionate in other contexts. Such a parent would be considered high in parental warmth. On the other hand, a parent who demonstrates warmth when praising the child but who is critical, punitive, or indifferent in most other situations would be classified as aloof and rejecting. Rejection may be subtle or blatant, and manifestations may be extensive, ranging from neglect and belittling to emotional and physical abuse. Rejecting parents overtly or covertly express feelings of dislike for the child, indicate that the child is unwanted, or state that caring for the child is burdensome.

Children who are rejected develop feelings of insecurity and inferiority; they believe that if they are unworthy of parental love, they must be of no value. Many develop an avoidant relationship with the rejecting parent(s). Others attempt to win parental affection through attention-getting behaviors that frequently serve only to compound the rejecting behavior of the parents. When these tactics fail, the child may become hostile and aggressive or withdrawn and submissive. Sometimes, rejected children find acceptance through identification with peers or gangs. A persistent pattern of rejection can have pervasive and long-range effects on a child's personality. The problems of disturbed parent-child relationships that are severely damaging to children are discussed in relation to some types of the failure-to-thrive syndrome, the abused child, and some of the emotional problems of childhood.

### Parental Styles of Control

Although there are variations and degrees in parenting styles, they can generally be described as either authoritarian, permissive, or authoritative. **Authoritarian,** or **dictatorial,** parents try to control their children's behavior and attitudes through unquestioned mandates. They establish rules and regulations or a standard of conduct that they expect to be followed rigidly and unquestioningly. They value and reward absolute obedience, mute acceptance of their word, and unfailing respect for the family's principles and beliefs. They forcefully punish any behavior that is contrary to parental standards. Parental authority is exercised with little explanation and little involvement of the child in decision making. The message is: "Do it because I say so."

Punishment need not be corporal but may be stern withdrawal of love and approval. The familiar saying—"Children are to be seen, not heard"—typifies this type of childrearing. Careful training often results in rigidly conforming behavior in the children, who tend to be sensitive, shy, self-conscious, retiring, and submissive. They are more apt to be courteous, loyal, honest, and dependable but docile. These behaviors are more typically observed when parental arbitrary power assertion is accompanied by close supervision and a reasonable level of affection. If not, arbitrary power assertion is more likely to be associated with both defiant and antisocial behavior.

*Permissive,* or *laissez-faire,* parents exert little or no control over their children's actions. These well-meaning parents sometimes confuse permissiveness with license. They avoid imposing their own standards of conduct and allow their children to regulate their own activity as much as possible. These parents consider themselves to be resources for the children, not role models. If rules do exist, the parents explain the underlying reason, encourage the children's opinions, and consult them in decision-making processes. They employ lax, inconsistent discipline, do not set sensible limits, and do not prevent the children from upsetting the home routine. The parents rarely punish the children because most behavior is considered acceptable. Consequently, the children, in effect, control the parents. Children of submissive parents are often disobedient, disrespectful, irresponsible, aggressive, and generally defiant of authority.

*Authoritative,* or *democratic,* parents combine some childrearing practices from both of the foregoing extremes. They direct their children's behavior and attitudes by emphasizing the reason for rules and negatively reinforcing deviations. They respect the individuality of each of their children and allow them to voice their objections to family standards or regulations. Parental control is firm and consistent but tempered with encouragement, understanding, and security. Control is focused on the issue, not on withdrawal of love or the fear of punishment. These parents foster "inner-directedness," a conscience that regulates behavior based on feelings of guilt or shame for wrongdoing, not on fear of being caught or punished. Parents' realistic standards and reasonable expectations produce children with high self-esteem who are self-reliant, assertive, inquisitive, content, and highly interactive with other children.

The most successful type of childrearing seems to be the authoritative method. Parents do not set rigid, arbitrary limits but maintain firm control, particularly in areas of parent-child disagreement. Permissiveness is tempered with reasonable and consistent setting of limits. Parental power is shared, and both parents provide leadership but listen to what the children think.

## Limit-Setting and Discipline

In its broadest sense, *discipline* means to teach or refers to a set of rules governing conduct. In a narrower sense, it refers to the action taken to enforce the rules following noncompliance. *Limit-setting* refers to establishing the rules or guidelines for behavior. Generally, the clearer the limits that are set and the more consistently they are enforced, the less need there is for disciplinary action. For

example, it is often suggested that parents should set limits on the amount of time children spend watching television (Bar-on, 2000).

Therefore the initial goal for the family is for the nurse to help parents establish realistic and concrete "rules." Limit-setting and discipline are positive, necessary components of childrearing and serve several useful functions as they help children:

- Test their limits of control
- Achieve in areas appropriate for mastery at their level
- Channel undesirable feelings into constructive activity
- Protect themselves from danger
- Learn socially acceptable behavior

Children want and need limits. Unrestricted freedom is a tremendous threat to their security and safety. Through testing the limits imposed on them, children learn the extent to which they can manipulate their environment, as well as gain reassurance from knowing that others will be there to protect them from potential harm.

### Minimizing Misbehavior

The goals of or reasons for misbehavior may include attention, power, defiance, and a display of inadequacy (the child misses classes because of a fear that he or she is unable to do the work). Children may also misbehave because the rules are not clear or consistently applied. Acting-out behavior, such as a temper tantrum, may represent uncontrolled frustration, anger, depression, or pain.

The best approach is to structure interactions with children so that unacceptable behavior is prevented or minimized. While many parents devise strategies that are most effective for their child, general guidelines include those listed in the Family Home Care box on p. 86.

### General Guidelines for Implementing Discipline

Regardless of the type of discipline used, certain principles are essential in ensuring the efficacy of the approach (See Guidelines box on p. 86.) Many strategies, such as behavior modification, can be implemented effectively only when principles of consistency and timing are followed. A pattern of intermittent or occasional enforcement of limits actually prolongs the undesired behavior because children learn that if they are persistent, the behavior is permitted eventually. Delaying punishment weakens its intent, and practices such as telling the child, "Wait until your father comes home," are not only ineffectual but also convey negative connotations about the other parent.*

### Types of Discipline

To deal with misbehavior, parents need to implement appropriate disciplinary action. Numerous approaches are available, and some have definite advantages over others.

*Reasoning* involves explaining why an act is wrong and is usually appropriate for older children, especially when moral issues are involved. However, young children cannot

---

*For parenting of K-6 children, see childparenting.about.com and kidshealth.org.

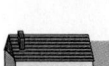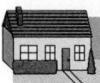

## FAMILY HOME CARE
### Minimizing Misbehavior

Set realistic goals for acceptable behavior and expected achievements.

Structure opportunities for small successes to lessen feelings of inadequacy.

Praise children for desirable behavior with attention and verbal approval.

Structure the environment to prevent unnecessary difficulties (e.g., place fragile objects in inaccessible area).

Set clear and reasonable rules; expect the same behavior regardless of the circumstances, and if exceptions are made, clarify that the change is for one time only.

Teach desirable behavior through own example, such as using a quiet, calm voice rather than screaming.

Review expected behavior before special or unusual events, such as visiting a relative or dinner in a restaurant.

Phrase requests for appropriate behavior positively, such as "Put the book down," rather than "Don't touch the book."

Call attention to unacceptable behavior as soon as it begins; use distraction to change the behavior or offer alternatives to annoying actions, such as a quiet toy for one that is excessively noisy.

Give advance notice or "friendly reminders," such as "When the TV program is over, it is time for dinner" or "I'll give you to the count of three and then we have to go."

Be attentive to situations that increase the likelihood of misbehaving, such as overexcitement or fatigue, or decreased personal tolerance to minor infractions.

Offer sympathetic explanations for not granting a request, such as "I am sorry I can't read you a story now, but I have to finish dinner. Then we can spend time together."

Keep any promises made to children.

Avoid outright conflicts; temper discussions with statements such as "Let's talk about it and see what we can decide together" or "I have to think about it first."

Provide children with opportunities for power and control.

## GUIDELINES
### Implementing Discipline

**Consistency:** Implement disciplinary action exactly as agreed on and for each infraction.

**Timing:** Initiate discipline as soon as child misbehaves; if delays are necessary, such as to avoid embarrassment, verbally disapprove of the behavior and state that disciplinary action will be implemented later.

**Commitment:** Follow through with the details of the discipline, such as timing of minutes; avoid distractions that may interfere with the plan, such as telephone calls.

**Unity:** Make certain that all caregivers agree on the plan and are familiar with the details to prevent confusion and alliances between child and one parent.

**Flexibility:** Choose disciplinary strategies that are appropriate to child's age, temperament, and the severity of the misbehavior.

**Planning:** Plan discipline strategies in advance and prepare child if feasible (e.g., explain use of time-out); for unexpected misbehavior, try to discipline when you are calm.

**Behavior-orientation:** Always disapprove of the behavior, not the child, with such statements as "That was a wrong thing to do. I am unhappy when I see behavior like that."

**Privacy:** Administer discipline in private, especially with older children who may feel ashamed in front of others.

**Termination:** Once the discipline is administered, consider child as having a "clean slate" and avoid bringing up the incident or lecturing.

- Do not rely on explanations or reasoning alone to change behavior.
- Use consistent consequences if the child fails to follow instructions.
- Verbal commands are generally better for initiating a behavior than stopping a behavior.

Unfortunately, reasoning is often combined with *scolding*, which sometimes takes the form of shame or criticism. For example, the parent may state, "You are a bad boy for hitting your brother." Children take such remarks seriously and personally, believing that *they* are bad.

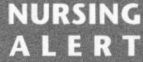

**NURSING ALERT**  When reprimanding children, focus only on the misbehavior, not on the child. Use of "I" messages rather than "you" messages expresses personal feelings without accusation or ridicule. For example, an "I" message attacks the behavior—"I am upset when Johnny is punched; I don't like to see him hurt"—not the child.

be expected to "see the other side" because of their egocentrism. Children in the preoperative stage of cognitive development (toddlers and preschoolers) have a limited ability to distinguish between their point of view and those of others. Sometimes children use "reasoning" as a way of gaining attention. For example, they may misbehave in order for the parents to give them a lengthy explanation of the wrongdoing because negative attention is better than none. When children use this technique, parents may have to end the explanation by stating, "This is the rule, and this is how I expect you to behave. I won't explain it any further."

Blum and others (1995) note that often, verbal reasoning is not effectively used and provide the following suggestions to improve this style of discipline and encourage the development of other modes:

- Warnings or instructions at the time of misbehavior should be brief (about one word per year of age [e.g., "no hitting, time-out" for a 3-year-old]).
- When long explanations are necessary, give them after the punishment, when parent and child are calm.
- Use commands or warnings only when behavior change is very important, and only when the parent is willing to enforce the warning if the child strongly resists.
- If the child does not respond to the first warning, use another discipline strategy.

Positive and negative reinforcement is the basis of *behavior modification* theory—behavior that is rewarded will be repeated; behavior that is not, will be extinguished. Using *rewards* is a positive approach; by encouraging children to behave in specified ways, the tendency to misbehave is lessened. With young children, using paper stars is a very effective method. For older children the "token system" is appropriate, especially if a certain number yields a special reward, such as a trip to the movies or a new book. In planning a reward system, the expected behaviors must be clearly explained to the child and the rewards must be reinforcing. A chart should be used to record the stars or tokens, and every earned reward should be promptly given. Verbal approval should always accompany extrinsic rewards.

**FAMILY HOME CARE**
*Using Consequences*

1. Give the child a choice:
   "Either-or" choices
   "When-then" choices
2. Ask the child to help set the consequences.
3. Make sure consequences are logical.
4. Give only choices you can live with.
5. Keep your tone firm and calm.
6. Give the choice once, then act.
7. Expect testing.
8. Allow the child to try again after experiencing the consequence.

From Popkin M: *Active parenting today*, Atlanta, 1993, Active Parenting Publishers.

**FAMILY HOME CARE**
*Using Time-Out*

Select an area for time-out that is safe, convenient, and unstimulating, but where the child can be monitored, such as the bathroom, hallway, or laundry room.
Determine what behaviors warrant a time-out.
Make sure children understand the "rules" and how they are expected to behave.
Explain to children the process of time-out:
When they misbehave, they will be given *one* warning.
If they do not obey, they will be sent to the place designated for time-out.
They are to sit there for a specified period of time.
If they cry, refuse, or display any disruptive behavior, the time-out period will begin *after* they quiet down.
When they are quiet for the duration of the time, they can then leave the room.
A rule for the length of time-out is *1 minute per year of age;* use a kitchen timer with an audible bell rather than a watch to record the time.
Implement time-out in a public place by selecting a suitable area or explain to children that time-out will be spent immediately on returning home.

(A more formal reward system involving a contract, which is appropriate for older children, is discussed in Chapter 27 under Compliance).

Consistently *ignoring* behavior will eventually extinguish or minimize the act. Although this approach sounds very simple, it is often difficult to implement consistently. Parents frequently "give in" and resort to previous patterns of discipline. Consequently, the behavior is actually reinforced because the child learns that persistence gains parental approval.

For ignoring to be effective, health professionals must devote a fair amount of time toward (1) explaining the approach in detail, (2) recording behavior before the extinction process is instituted to see if a problem exists and to compare results after ignoring is begun, (3) making certain that the parent's attention is the reinforcer, and (4) warning parents of a phenomenon called "response burst," which refers to an *increase* in the child's behavior soon after the process is initiated because the child is "testing" the parents to see if they are serious about the plan.

The strategy of *consequences* involves allowing children to experience the results of their misbehavior and includes three types:

1. **Natural:** Those that occur without any intervention, such as being late and missing dinner
2. **Logical:** Those that are directly related to the rule, such as not being allowed to play with another toy until the used ones are put away
3. **Unrelated:** Those that are imposed deliberately, such as no playing until homework is completed or the use of time-out

Natural or logical consequences are preferred but are effective only when they are meaningful to children. For example, the natural consequence of living in a messy room may do little to encourage cleaning up, but allowing no friends over until the room is neat can be very motivating! Withdrawing privileges is often an unrelated consequence. After the child experiences the consequence, the parent should refrain from any comment, because the usual tendency is for the child to try to place blame for imposing the rule. (See Family Home Care box above.)

*Time-out* is actually a refinement of the common practice of "sending the child to his or her room" and is a type of unrelated consequence. It is also based on the premise of re-

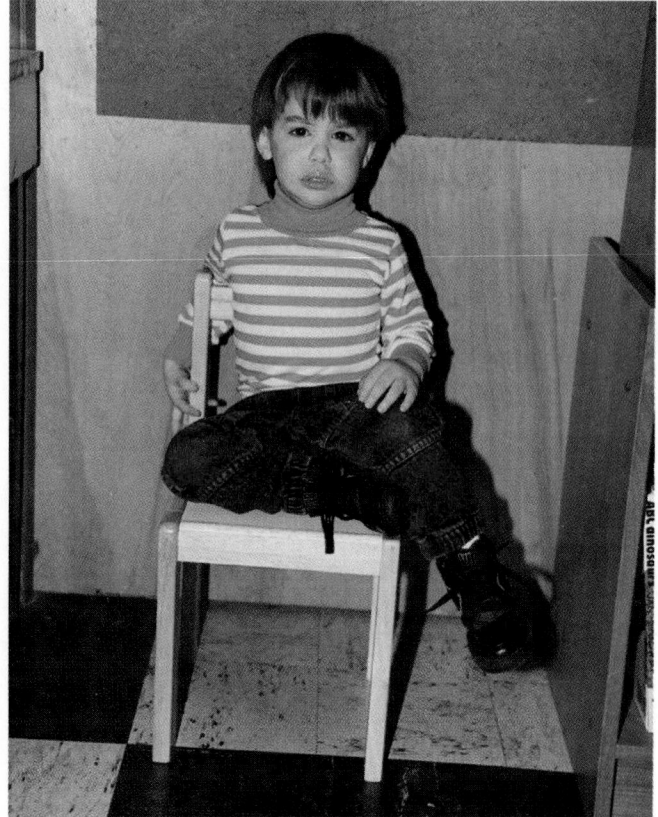

**Fig. 3-10** Time-out is an excellent disciplinary strategy for young children.

moving the reinforcer (i.e., the satisfaction or attention the child is receiving from the activity). (See Family Home Care box above.) When placed in an unstimulating and isolated place, children become bored and consequently agree to behave in order to reenter the family group (Fig. 3-10). Time-out avoids many of the problems of other disciplinary approaches because no physical punishment is involved, no reasoning or scolding is given, and the parent is usually not present for all of the time-out, facilitating his or her ability to consistently apply the punishment. It also offers both the child and the parent a "cooling off" time. To be effective, time-out must be planned in advance.

*Corporal punishment* most often takes the form of spanking. Based on the principles of aversive therapy, inflicting pain through spanking causes a dramatic short-term decrease in the behavior. However, there are some serious flaws in this approach: (1) it teaches children that violence is acceptable; (2) many times the spanking is the result of parental rage and may physically harm the child; and (3) children become "accustomed" to spanking, requiring more severe corporal punishment each time. Consequently, parents may use paddles, whips, or other objects, or they may eliminate a spanking because of their unwillingness to "hit the child harder," a practice that may prolong the behavior.

Spanking can result in severe physical and psychologic injury (Bauman and Friedman, 1998). It can interfere with effective parent-child interaction; children who receive corporal punishment are less likely to learn what they *should* do, because the focus is on what they *should not* do (American Academy of Pediatrics, 1998). In addition, when the parent is not around, the misbehavior is likely to occur, for children have not learned to behave well for their own sake. Parental use of corporal punishment has also been found to interfere with the child's development of moral reasoning.

The use of corporal punishment, a model of violent behavior, is being questioned more in conjunction with concern regarding increasing violence in contemporary society. Unfortunately, the fact remains that many parents practice corporal punishment. Also, the practice continues to play a role in the public education of schoolchildren in many parts of the United States. (See Chapter 17.)

**NURSING ALERT** When nurses encounter parents who use spanking, a basic guide would include that spanking should be used as a last resort and should never be used in public. Parents should use only their hand, apply the hand to the child's bottom only one time, and follow through with a stern message and sometimes additional consequences (Nelms, 1996). Advise parents of the disadvantages of this discipline method and suggest more effective and less dangerous approaches.

## Influence of the "Experts"

Evidence indicates that there have been decided shifts in the overall philosophy of childrearing during the twentieth century. Directions on childrearing, with parental roles and practices defined by the experts, have been transmitted as advice to parents through a steady flow of pamphlets, books, and articles. Recent changes in the opinions of these experts are the result of alterations in the concept of child development and behavior and of research into the effects of parent-child interaction.

The earlier view of child care that advocated rigid scheduling, early weaning and toilet training, and prohibition of devices that provided the child with passive pleasures (such

as pacifiers) has been, for the most part, replaced by an easier, warmer, and more relaxed approach toward coping with child behavior that emphasizes "tender loving care" as the basis for satisfactory physical and emotional well-being. Some believe, however, that this approach generates too much permissiveness and produces some undesirable long-term consequences. The current trend in parenting manuals is to reassure parents that they will not be "perfect" parents, that mistakes are allowed, and that while they should keep trying to do a good job of rearing their children, at the same time they should try to be relaxed and spontaneous, and enjoy their children. These manuals attempt to convey the idea that parents are more capable than they think they are.

Parents turn to guidebooks because of an optimistic belief in progress, a faith in the future, and a typical desire to do better—better than they have been doing, better than their own parents, and better than their relatives and neighbors. Through these popular how-to-parent books, parents can gain some of the accumulated knowledge of significant researchers in child development that they would be unable to acquire by attempting to read and synthesize the original texts. These guidebooks do not attempt to provide all of the answers and are less authoritarian than those of the past. Most are written on the assumption that parents want to raise successful children and need support to view themselves as competent adults whose decisions are valid. Parents must deal with parenting problems on the spot at the same time that they are assimilating helpful advice and new information. They must be made to feel confident in their values and judgment during this process.

In the past, one of the primary deficiencies in how-to books was a disregard for alternate lifestyles, cultural variations, or class differences in the population. For example, the working mother was ignored or discouraged, and daycare was seldom mentioned. Fortunately, recent manuals tend to reflect the realities of our more complex society. Some books have also appeared that offer guidelines for single parents, adoptive parents, parents with a child who is disabled, stepparents, and families in the process of divorce. These are primarily authored by individuals who offer help based on their own experiences or by authorities who have made a study of a special problem. Parents can receive some assistance from these supplemental publications to help them cope with the additional stresses imposed by their special circumstances. Popular parenting manuals vary in their approaches, so it is probably best to suggest that parents review some of those that are available and select at least two for use rather than relying on the advice of a single resource.

## SPECIAL PARENTING SITUATIONS

Parenting is a demanding task under the most ideal circumstances, but when parents and children are faced with situations that deviate from what is considered to be the norm, the potential for family disruption is increased. Some of the issues that are encountered frequently are divorce, single parenthood, blended families, adoption, and dual-career families. The problems associated with children of alcoholic parents, parents with physical disabilities, homeless parents, or incarcerated parents are ones that are not addressed in the following discussions but may be topics that the reader may wish to investigate.

## Parenting the Adopted Child

Adoption establishes the legal relationship of parent and child between persons who are not so related by birth, with the same rights and obligations that exist between children and their biologic parents. In the past the biologic mother alone made the decision to relinquish the rights to her child. In recent years, however, the courts have acknowledged the legal rights of the biologic father regarding this decision. Concerned child advocates have questioned decisions that honor the father's rights when the decision may not be in the best interests of the child. As the rights of the child have become recognized, older children have successfully dissolved their legal bond with their biologic parents to pursue adoption by adults of their choice. Furthermore, there is a growing interest and demand within the gay and lesbian community to adopt. Agencies have developed few specific policies in this regard and face questions about the legal and social ramifications of adopting in a relationship not based on marriage, as well as possible consequences of not developing policies (Sullivan, 1995).

### Motivation for Adoption

People are motivated to adopt a child for different reasons. Most instances involve an adopting couple who find it impossible to have children of their own. However, many people consider adoption for other reasons. Some feel a responsibility to provide a home for a child who needs one; others are able to have more children of their own but are seriously concerned about overpopulation and elect to increase their family through adoption; many families are finding "room for one more" with whom to share their love; families involved in foster care may pursue adopting the child when parental rights are terminated. In addition, single, divorced, and widowed people who believe that they have love and security to offer a child are seeking to adopt. In one longitudinal study of single-parent adoptive homes, it was demonstrated that these homes have the capacity to be successful adoptive placements (Shireman, 1996).

The demand for white infants with no physical or mental problems far exceeds the supply. However, there has been an increase in the number of children with special needs who are finding homes through the adoptive process. These include children with disabilities, older children, children who are of minority or mixed racial ancestry, and children from foreign countries.

The decision to adopt should be a joint one, and various attitudes and feelings must be examined before the couple can assume the responsibility for an adopted child. Most adults assume that they will be able to have children of their own. Discovering that they are unable to do so is often accompanied by feelings of inferiority, doubts about masculinity or femininity, and feelings of guilt or blame in relation to the spouse. These feelings and frustrations, superimposed on the anxious waiting for pregnancy, feelings of loss, endless medical procedures to establish the cause of in-fertility, and failed medical efforts to establish a pregnancy, provide an adoptive couple with their own unique preparation for parenthood.

Whatever motivates a couple to seek adoption as an alternative means of acquiring a family, the decision should be based on emotionally healthy needs. The welfare of the child should be the primary consideration in placement, and such motives as the need to strengthen an unstable marriage, to treat emotional problems (including grief over the death of a child), or to treat psychogenic sterility should be carefully explored. Also, when adoption satisfies the needs of only one of the two parents, the outcome is questionable.

### Sources of Adoptive Children

In the past the major source of adoptable infants was socially unsanctioned pregnancies, primarily of unwed mothers because society accords a very high rating to the married status. Although adoption as a means of creating a family is openly acceptable, having children outside the marriage state is generally met with societal disapproval. However, with the widespread use of contraception, more liberalized abortion laws, and more liberal attitudes toward single parents, the number of these children available for adoption has decreased significantly.

Almost half of the adoptable children in the United States are adopted by relatives, either extended family members or stepparents. Nonrelative adoptions are primarily arranged through licensed social agencies. A small proportion are arranged independently by individuals such as physicians, lawyers, nurses, and members of the clergy. However, the safest and most satisfactory adoptions are those conducted through a licensed social agency, either public or voluntary. Although adoption through an ***authorized agency*** can be time-consuming, with sometimes frustrating and disappointing delays, the decision to pursue an ***independent adoption*** should be made with caution. While independent adoptions are frequently faster than agency adoptions, independent adoptions sometimes result in serious problems. They are generally more costly, and some are arranged by persons seeking a profit. The child's anonymity may not be guaranteed, and the child's health or legal status may be unclear. Also, because independent contractors, unlike adoption agencies, frequently do not investigate the adoptive family, an independent adoption may not always be in the child's best interests.

In recent years the concept of ***open adoption,*** either through an agency or an independent source, has gained greater acceptance. In open adoption, the adoptive parents and the biologic mother (and sometimes father and other family members) meet before the birth of the child and mutually agree to the adoption. Arrangements are often made for the child to have contact with the biologic family throughout the child's lifetime.

In a variant form of open adoption, the biologic mother is invited to write an explanatory letter to the child and the adoptive parents, who usually respond with a letter and pictures. It is a voluntary exchange handled through the agency, which keeps all names and addresses confidential. When these exchanges are eventually read by the adopted children, it helps them realize the circumstances of their adoption.

Risks related to agency adoptions are usually fewer than those encountered in family life. Careful screening of infants can detect all but the more obscure defects, and subsequent development of defects or illnesses is no less predictable than in biologic families. However, inherent emotional difficulties may be intensified in the case of adoption. Common reactions to adoption include anxiety associated with the waiting period until the adoption is legally final, uncertainty regarding whether adoption is the right choice, the parents' concerns about their ability to love and parent the child, and difficulty coping with the reactions and questions of relatives, other children (if any) in the family, and friends. However, bonding can be as strong and immediate for adoptive parents and children as it is for biologic parents—sometimes even stronger.

Adoptive mothers share many of the same initial feelings as birth mothers for their babies and reactions to becoming parents. Both adoptive and birth mothers react to the first moments with their babies with strong and varied emotions ranging from happiness to distress. Adoptive mothers are likely to develop emotional ties to their babies at much the same time that birth mothers do. Bonding is not hindered by the lack of either a biologic relationship or immediate contact with their babies (Fig. 3-11).

## Preparation for Adoption

Unlike biologic parents who prepare for their child's birth with prenatal classes and the support of friends and relatives, adoptive parents have few sources of support and preparation for the new addition to their family. Nurses who offer services to adoptive parents can provide the information, support, and reassurance needed to reduce parental anxiety regarding the adoptive process and refer them to parental support groups that provide guidance for adoptive parents. Such sources can be contacted through a state or county welfare office. Prospective parents seeking information on international adoptions can contact **Families Adopting Children Everywhere, Inc. (FACE).***

---

*PO Box 28058, Northwood Station, Baltimore, MD 21239, (410) 488-2656.

Preadoption counseling should include measures to help parents overcome feelings of inadequacy and make preparations for receiving the child, such as instruction in infant care. Adoptive parents need to prepare for the possibility that the confidentiality or the identity of the biologic parents may not be guaranteed. Some agencies even advise the adoptive parents to maintain an ongoing information store about the natural parents so that they can answer the child's questions and thereby reduce the excessive fantasizing that children may engage in later during identity formation.

## Parenting Adopted Children

Most problems faced by adoptive parents are no different from those encountered by natural parents. All parents want to be good parents, but this desire is often intensified in adoptive parents. Adoptive parents have been portrayed as being more apprehensive and insecure than biologic parents and in need of more assistance. However, adoptive parents may feel the need for less assistance than biologic parents. This feeling is probably due to the adoptive parents' completely voluntary decision to become parents, the relatively long time they had to prepare for parenting, and the maturity associated with adopting.

The sooner infants enter their adoptive homes, the better for purposes of parent-infant attachment; the more caregivers the infant has had before adoption, the more problems are likely to be encountered in attachment. The infant must break the bond with the previous caregiver and form a new bond with the adoptive parents. The difficulties in forming an attachment will depend on the amount of time the infant has spent with earlier caregivers, such as the birth mother, nurse, or adoption agency personnel.

Siblings, adopted or biologic, who are old enough to understand should be included in decisions regarding the commitment to adopt, with reassurance that they are not being replaced (Phillips, 1999). Ways that the siblings can interact with the adopted child should be stressed (Fig. 3-12).

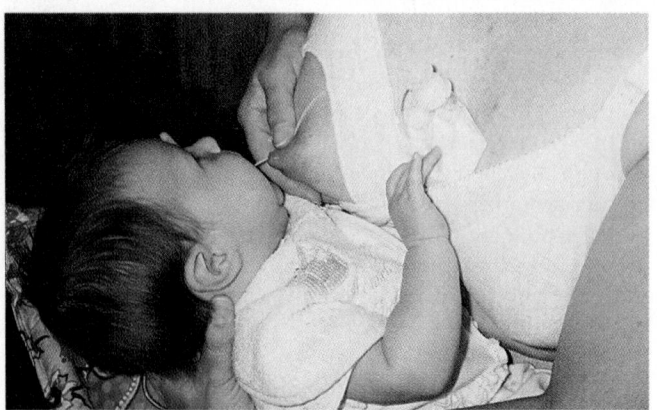

**Fig. 3-11** Mothers of adopted infants can successfully breast-feed. Note the supplemental formula system with the end of the tubing extending 2.5 cm beyond the nipple.

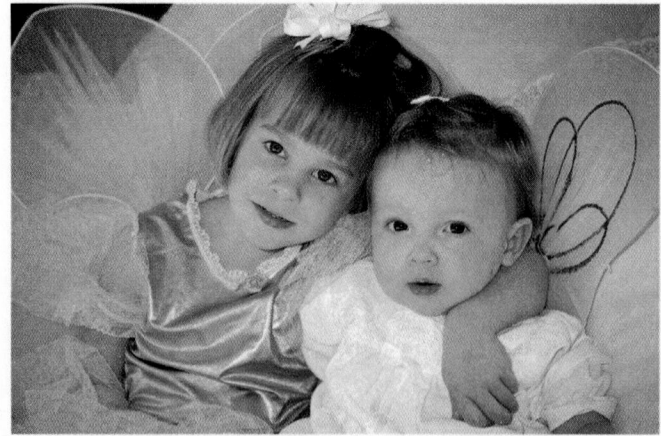

**Fig. 3-12** A big sister lovingly embraces her adopted sister.

Acceptance by extended family members and friends may create additional stresses for the family. Parents are encouraged to discuss the issue of adoption with other members of the family, especially the grandparents, whose feelings and attitudes about adoption may not be compatible with those of the parents. This may be a particularly difficult problem when the adopted children are members of different ethnic groups. It should be made clear to everyone that the child is the parents' child, not their "adopted" child.

**Issues of Origin.** The task of telling children that they are adopted is a cause of deep concern and anxiety. There are no clear-cut guidelines for parents to follow in determining precisely when and at what age children are ready for the information, and parents are naturally reluctant to present the children with such unsettling news. However, it is an important aspect of their parental responsibilities, and although they may be tempted to withhold the fact from the child, it is an essential component of the child's identity. (See Critical Thinking Exercise box.)

## Critical Thinking Exercise

### Parenting the Adopted Child

Twelve-month-old Justin was adopted at birth. His parents tell you that they wonder when they should tell Justin that he is adopted. As the nurse, what nursing actions would you provide for Justin's parents?

FIRST, THINK ABOUT IT . . .

- What precise questions are you trying to answer?
- What would the consequences be if you put your thoughts into action?

1. Reassure them that because Justin was adopted at birth, they do not need to tell him he was adopted.
2. Give Justin's parents some books, pamphlets, and community resources on adoption so that they can decide on their own what to do.
3. Discuss the general understanding that they should tell Justin in a matter-of-fact manner at an early age so that he will always know he was adopted.
4. Recommend that they not tell Justin until he reaches early adolescence and can better understand this information.

*The best response is three. Being adopted can be viewed by the adoptee as part of his unique heritage. Justin's parents chose to have him join the family as a welcomed member. Children join families in many ways, such as biologic heritage or blending of families. Sharing the story of adoption is an important parental responsibility and can be handled much like one shares birth experiences with a biologic child. Most authorities believe that children should be informed at a young enough age that as they grow older they do not remember a time when they did not know they were adopted. Waiting until adolescence is too late. Children have a more difficult adjustment if disclosure occurs when they are older. Giving Justin's parents resources about adoption is appropriate; however, because they have asked you as the nurse for guidance, a more direct approach is best.*

The timing seems to arise naturally as parents become aware of the child's readiness. Most authorities believe that children should be informed at an age young enough so that, as they grow older, they do not remember a time when they did not know that they were adopted. The time must be right for both the parents and the child and is highly individual; it may be when children ask where babies come from, at which time children can also be told the facts of their adoption. If they are told in such a way as to convey the idea that they were active participants in the selection process, they will be less apt to feel that they were abandoned victims in a helpless situation. For example, parents can tell children that their personal qualities drew the parents to them. It is wise for parents who have not previously discussed adoption to tell children that they are adopted before the children enter school to avoid third parties inadvertently telling the children before the parents have had the opportunity to do so. Complete honesty between parents and children usually strengthens the relationship. (See Evidence-Based Practice box on p. 92.)

Earlier advice to adoptive parents stressed the need to treat adopted children exactly the same as any biologic siblings and to make them feel no different. This approach, however, denies the differences that adopted children actually feel. At age 5 or 6, children begin to realize that someone had to give them up for them to be "chosen" by the adoptive family. To deny these feelings may actually hurt the child (Smit, 1996). For both the child and the adoptive parents, it is important to acknowledge the differences in the adoptive situation.

Acknowledging and encouraging discussion of the child's feelings helps the child develop a positive self-image. Once the child has been told about the adoption, the child's feelings about it do not end; rather, adjusting to one's own adoption is a continuous process often characterized by a sense of loss and a search for identity throughout childhood and adolescence and even continuing when adopted children become adults and have their own children. Some will feel a sense of social stigma based on feelings of discrimination because they are unable to provide answers to unknown biologic ties (March, 1995). Adopted children, however, seem to adapt more easily if the family is comfortable with the adoption, talks about the birth circumstances openly, and has acceptance and support from the extended family, friends, and neighbors. When they are emotionally and developmentally ready, adopted children may benefit from learning about their birth parents and may even decide to contact them, although this is usually recommended only after adolescence in closed adoptions because of the identity crises and turmoil surrounding the event.

Children should be encouraged to ask questions. Parents can anticipate many of the questions, although children may hesitate to ask about the birth parents, hoping that the adoptive parents will initiate the discussion. This is probably one of the most difficult tasks facing adoptive parents. However, what is said to the children is less important than the attitudes and feelings that are communicated. Children should be told about their birth parents and the situations

## EVIDENCE-BASED PRACTICE
### Adoption Disclosure

The decision to tell a child about adoption is less of an issue in adoptive families than it was in the past. The argument now concerns when to tell children they are adopted. Some researchers suggest that waiting until the child is 6 to 7 years old allows for better understanding of the factors related to the adoption (Smit, 1996). However children as young as 3 years of age may ask questions about birth and family structure. Common questions asked by young children include: "Where do babies come from?" or "Where do I come from?" These preschool-age children are able to learn the difference between adoption and birth, developing awareness that while everyone is born, some children enter their family through birth while others enter through adoption (Smit, 1999). They are also able to realize that some children live with their birth parents and others live with adoptive parents. Adoptive parents of preschool children should be encouraged to answer their questions because their discussions will help the child prepare to answer questions that will ultimately come from schoolmates and peers. Children as young as 4 years may notice differences in skin, hair, or eye color and may focus on how they look compared with other family members. Parents should be encouraged to emphasize similarities rather than focusing on the differences. Preschool children, because of their vivid imaginations, may exhibit great fear when their adoption is discussed. It is essential to reassure children that their place in the family is permanent and that they will not be taken away (Smit, 1996).

School-age children are able to understand the birth process and are aware of the losses that are associated with adoption (Smit, 1996). Children this age may feel abandoned or blame themselves because their birth parents gave them away. Allowing children to express their feelings and emotions is essential. Some researchers believe that children this age should not be told that the birth mother loved the child so much that she wanted him or her to have a better life. This may cause the child to feel even more abandoned (Donovan, 1990). Simple, concrete explanations such as the following may be most beneficial for school-age children: "Your birth parents had a baby, which was you. They were not able to take care of a baby so they decided to have another family take care of you. We became your family." Parents must understand that children this age will grieve their loss of a birth mother and father.

Adolescents perceive adoption as related to their own sense of identity. When discussions have occurred at a younger age, adolescents usually have dealt with most issues related to adoption. Adolescents want factual information about their adoption. They may fantasize about their birth parents and wish for more details regarding their birth and adoption. Parents should be open and honest with their adopted child and willing to listen to all concerns.

discipline and limit-setting, as any other child (see Critical Thinking Exercise box p. 91). Adoptive parents may experience unwelcome curiosity and even cruel remarks from others about the child's adoption and appearance. Questions about the child's "real" birth parents, jokes that an infertile mother will now get pregnant, or misguided attempts to match physical characteristics of the child with the adoptive parents can be distressing. Nurses in contact with adoptive parents can help counter the effects of these thoughtless remarks by affirming the parental role, asking the parents about the child's arrival, and listening to their reports about the child's development and accomplishments.

**Adolescence.**  Adolescence may be an especially trying time for parents of adopted children. The normal confrontations of adolescents and parents may assume more painful aspects in adoptive families. Adolescents may use their adoption as a tool in defying parental authority or as a justification for aberrant behavior. As they attempt to master the task of identity formation, the feeling of abandonment by their biologic parents may come to awareness or may be intensified. Gender differences in reacting to adoption may surface. It has been shown that girls have more difficulty accepting their sexuality because they may not be able to identify with a nonfertile female parent.

The children fantasize about their parents, and they may feel the need to discover the identity of their biologic parents in order to define themselves and their identity—one of the major tasks of adolescent development. It is important for parents to keep lines of communication open and to reassure youngsters that they understand the need to search for their identities. In some states birth certificates are made legally available to adopted children when they come of age. It is important for parents to be honest with questioning adolescents and to tell them of this possibility (the parents themselves are unable to obtain the birth certificate; it is the children's responsibility if they desire it).

## Special Adoptive Situations

The difficulty in finding infants to adopt has created an increased opportunity for adoptive parents to provide homes for children with special needs. The additional burdens of care for children with physical or emotional disabilities are no different from those of biologic children with similar problems, with the possible exception that adoptive parents are aware of the nature of the disabilities before they receive the children. Such children may be eligible for financial assistance from the Federal 4E Adoption Subsidy Program and additional state programs (Office of Human Development Services, DHHS, 2000). However, adoption of older children or those of a different racial or ethnic origin poses special considerations for both parents and children.

**Older Children.**  Adopting older children constitutes an emotional experience for everyone concerned—children, parents, siblings (if any), and, often, extended family members. It involves a commitment on the part of both the adopting family and the adopted child. Adoptive families should learn as much as possible about the child before they make a final commitment.

Children awaiting adoption are usually from foster homes, group homes, or institutions. Visits between the po-

and circumstances involved to provide as complete a picture as possible.

Parents can anticipate some behavior changes following the disclosure—especially in children who are older. One study found that children who were adopted were two to five times more likely to be referred for psychologic treatment than nonadopted peers (Grotevant and McRoy, 1996). Children may use the fact of their adoption as a weapon to manipulate and threaten parents. There is the inevitable "My real mother would not treat me like this," or "You don't love me as much because I'm adopted." Statements such as these hurt parents and increase their feelings of insecurity so that as parents they may become overpermissive. Adopted children need the same undemanding love, combined with firm

tential adoptive family and the child can take place in the child's present home or on some type of outing during which the individuals involved are able to interact, such as on a picnic or a trip to the zoo or a playground. Visits by the child to the home of the adoptive family begin with short excursions such as an afternoon, then a day, followed by a weekend or a week. The number and frequency of visits depend on the needs of the child and the family. During the visits the child and the family determine whether or not they will be able to make a commitment.

One of the difficulties of rearing adopted older children is helping them to deal with having had another set of parents. In addition to their biologic parents, the children may have lost siblings, grandparents, friends, and personal possessions. Often they have lived in several foster homes in which they formed attachments. They need time and assistance in working through the grief process that is an integral part of any loss. At the same time, they must adjust to a new household and relationships. Children who have experienced many losses and disappointments find adjustment more difficult and take a longer period of time to overcome fear of rejection and to develop affectionate ties to the new family. They grieve for those they left behind and may be afraid to love in case they must again move on.

Children who are adopted after age 2 maintain an image of the previous parenting persons that may cause the adopting parents some insecurity. The parents may not feel as close to these children as they would to children adopted in infancy. It is necessary that children who can remember them maintain an image of the biologic parents. As they grow, children are able to clearly distinguish between the parents who loved and cared for them and those who were merely responsible for their birth. Some of the early difficulties of adaptation are related to the change in surroundings—a change that is difficult for all children.

Early in the process of forming lasting relationships, the families alter routines and activities to accommodate the children and avoid conflicts. The children are excited but somewhat frightened that they will be unable to behave in such a way that will ensure acceptance and prevent their being sent away. Eventually the parents and the children are unable to maintain the host-houseguest roles and behaviors and begin a stormy period of adjustment. The children continually test the families, who must repeatedly reassure the children that they are wanted. The children may withdraw or act angry for months. Many conflicts can arise, particularly in the area of parental expectations and discipline. The children's past experiences, good and bad, are brought to the fore, especially during holidays. Although the children are relieved and happy to be in a new home, they often miss the familiar times and relationships. During this time the families may require considerable support and encouragement from sources outside the immediate family unit.

Eventually, expectations become more realistic, and family members learn to cope more effectively. The children are increasingly able to integrate past with present. They develop trust and confidence in the parents, and all the members develop into a family unit with autonomy, stability, and identification.

**Cross-Racial and International Adoption.**    Adoption of children of racial backgrounds different from that of the family is relatively commonplace. In addition to the problems faced by adopted children of any age, children of a cross-racial adoption must deal with their differentness. It is advised that parents who adopt such children do everything to preserve the adopted children's racial heritage.

> **NURSING ALERT**    As a health care provider, it is important *not* to ask the wrong questions, such as, "Is she yours, or is she adopted?" "What do you know about the 'real' mother?" "Are they really brother and sister?" or "How much did she cost?" (Hostetter and Johnson, 1996).

In international adoptions, adoptive parents are urged to investigate the culture of their children's country, maintain their children's family name as a middle name (in some cultures this is a link to the village of their ancestors), and teach children the history and heroes of their native country. Persons from the children's country can provide information about eating and sleeping patterns that will help the family make the adopted children's adaptation easier. Even music, a few words of the native language, and foods from their native country will appeal to the children's senses.

Although the children are full-fledged members of an adopting family and citizens of the adopted country, if they have a foreign appearance or other decided racial characteristics, problems may be encountered outside the family. Bigotry exists that may appear among relatives and friends. Strangers may make thoughtless comments and talk about the children as though they were not members of the family. It is vital that the family make it clear to others that this is their child and a cherished member of the family.

In international adoptions the medical information the parents receive may be quite complete or very sketchy; weight, height, and head circumference are often the only objective information present in the child's medical record (Miller, 1999; Kronemyer, 2001). Many internationally adopted children were born prematurely, and common health problems such as infant diarrhea and malnutrition may delay growth and development. Some children may have serious or multiple health problems, and this can be very stressful for the parents. Many foreign-born children have not been immunized adequately (Kronemyer, 2001; Miller, 1999; Mitchell and Jenista, 1997). Cultural practices, such as constant holding rather than letting the child explore, may further affect the child's progress. On arrival, regardless of age, some internationally adopted children may experience temporary adjustment problems. Sleep disturbances, malaise without fever, abdominal pain, avoidance of school, and preoccupation with food have all been reported (Hostetter and Johnson, 1996). In addition to giving advice on medical management, nurses should provide these parents with opportunities to discuss their feelings and situations.*

---

*For more information contact the **International Adoption Clinic,** University of Minnesota, Mailcode 211, 420 Delaware St SE, Minneapolis, MN 55455; (614) 624-1164; www.peds.umn.edu

## Parenting and Divorce

Since the mid-1960s there has been a marked change in the stability of families that is reflected in increased rates of divorce, single parenthood, and remarriage. In 1999 the divorce rate for the United States was 4.1 per 1000 total population (Centers for Disease Control and Prevention, 2000). The divorce rate has changed very little since 1987. During the previous decade the rate increased almost yearly, with a peak in 1979. Although almost half of all divorcing couples are childless, over 1 million children experience divorce each year, and most of the children are very young.

The process of divorce begins with a period of marital conflict of varying length and intensity, followed by a separation, the actual legal divorce, and the establishment of different living arrangements (Box 3-10). Because a function of parenthood is to provide for the security and emotional welfare of children, disruption of the family structure often engenders strong feelings of guilt in the parents.

During a divorce, parents' coping abilities may be compromised. The parents may be much too preoccupied with their own feelings, needs, and life changes to be available and supportive to their children. Newly employed parents, usually mothers, are likely to leave children with new caregivers, in strange settings, or alone after school. The parent may also spend more time away from home, searching for or establishing new relationships. Sometimes, however, the adult feels frightened and alone and begins to depend on the child as a substitute for the absent parent. This dependence places an enormous burden on the child.

Common characteristics in the custodial household following separation and divorce include disorder, coercive types of control, inflammable tempers in both parents and children, reduced parental competence, a greater sense of parental helplessness, poorly enforced discipline, and diminished regularity in enforcing household routines. Noncustodial parents also are seldom prepared for the role of visitor, may assume the role of recreational and "fun" parent, and may not have a residence suitable for children's visits. They may be concerned about maintaining the arrangement over the years to follow.

### Impact of Divorce on Children

The results of numerous studies show that divorce has a profound effect on children.

**Family Differences.** The impact of divorce on children depends on a variety of factors, including the age and sex of the children, the outcome of the divorce, and the quality of the parent-child relationship and parental care during the years following the divorce. Family characteristics appear to be more crucial to children's well-being than specific child characteristics such as age or sex. The most important factor is continuing conflict between the divorced parents (Kelly, 2000). Children cope better when parents adopt an attitude of "together for our child while separate for us" (Kelly, 2000; Hetherington and Stanley-Hagan, 1999). High levels of ongoing family conflict are related to problems of social development, emotional stability, and cognitive skills for the child.

Complications sometimes associated with divorce include efforts on the part of one parent to subvert the child's loyalties to the other, abandonment to other caregivers, and adjustment to a stepparent. A major problem occurs when children become the middle persons between the divorced parents. They become the message bearers between the parents, are often quizzed about the activities of the other parent, and have to listen to criticisms from one parent about the other. A nurse may be able to intercede by helping the child get out of the middle by stating "I messages" based on the formula of "I feel . . . (state the feeling) when you . . . (state the source). I would like it if you . . ." This approach may empower the child to feel more in control. For example, the "I message" may be: "I feel uncomfortable when you ask me all those questions about Mom. I would like it if you would talk to her yourself"(Arbuthnot and Gordon, 1995).

Children may feel a sense of shame and embarrassment concerning the family situation. Such feelings cause children to see themselves as different, inferior, or unworthy of love, especially if they feel any responsibility for the family dissolution. Nurses may be in a position to help clarify misconceptions a child may have about the divorce. They can help children to understand that the divorce is not their fault, that they cannot take on the job of getting their parents back together or taking care of the parent (Arbuthnot and Gordon, 1995).

Although the social stigma attached to divorce no longer produces the emotions it did in the past, the stigma may still exist in some small towns and can reinforce children's negative self-image. The lasting effects of divorce depend on the children's and the parents' adjustments to the transition from an intact family to a single-parent family and, often, to a reconstituted family.

**Age- and Sex-Related Responses to Divorce.** Previously it was believed that divorce had a greater impact on younger

---

**Box 3-10** ■ ■ ■
## Stages of the Divorce Process

**ACUTE PHASE**

The married couple make the decision to separate. This phase includes the legal steps of filing for dissolution of the marriage and, usually, the departure of the father from the home. The duration of this phase lasts from several months to over a year and is accompanied by familial stress and a chaotic atmosphere.

**TRANSITIONAL PHASE**

The adults and children assume unfamiliar roles and relationships within a new family structure. This phase is often accompanied by a change of residence, a reduced standard of living and altered lifestyle, a larger share of the economic responsibility being shouldered by the mother, and radically altered parent-child relationships.

**STABILIZING PHASE**

The postdivorce family reestablishes a stable, functioning family unit. Remarriage frequently occurs, with concomitant changes in all areas of family life.

Modified from Wallerstein JS: Children of divorce: stress and developmental tasks. In Garmezy N, Rutter M, editors: *Stress, coping, and development in children,* New York, 1983, McGraw-Hill.

children, but more recent observations indicate that divorce constitutes a major disruption for children in all age-groups. However, the responses (behaviors and feelings) may differ (Box 3-11).

Egocentric preschoolers, who see and understand things only in relation to themselves, assume themselves to be the cause of parental distress and interpret the separation as punishment. They feel sadness and strong feelings of responsibility for the loss of the absent parent. Moreover, they consciously fear that they may be abandoned by the remaining parent. Consequently, it is essential to establish some kind of stability for these children; otherwise they will convert their energies to restabilization efforts rather than to growth and development. They need frequent, repeated, and concrete explanations of what is going to happen to them and how they will be cared for, and assurance that something new will take the place of the old and that they will not be deserted. In order that they do not imagine things, explanations, such as where they will live, who will prepare their meals when the parent is at work, and when they will see the absent parent again, should be specific. They need to focus on reality.

School-age children are able to cope with parental separation better than younger children, even though they feel intense pain, loneliness, and deprivation. Younger children are preoccupied with the departure of one parent, usually the father, and grieve openly and long for his return, fearing replacement. Older children are more likely to perceive one parent as being responsible, become angry with both parents, and express this anger with behavior distressing to one or both parents. School performance may be affected because they are unable to focus on learning; therefore teachers and school counselors should be informed so that they have a better understanding of alterations in the children's behavior and performance. Often children must move to an unfamiliar environment or new neighborhood and form new relationships in addition to coping with the alteration in their family structure. They almost invariably wish for the parents to reunite.

Adolescents may be highly resentful because their lives are already sufficiently difficult and stressful. Although they are able to comprehend the divorce and are less likely to feel responsibility, adolescents find the divorce of their parents extraordinarily painful. Adolescents' sexual identity is affected by disturbed parental relationships, a precipitous deidealization of both parents, and concern about their own future as a marital partner. They are anxious about the availability of money for future needs. However, the separation of the parents may provide some space in which the older adolescent can develop an emotional detachment

---

## Box 3-11 ■ ■ ■
## Feelings and Behaviors of Children Related to Divorce

**INFANCY**

Effects of reduced mothering or lack of mothering
Increased irritability
Disturbance in eating, sleeping, and elimination
Interference with attachment process

**EARLY PRESCHOOL CHILDREN (AGES 2-3 YEARS)**

Frightened and confused
Blame themselves for the divorce
Fear of abandonment
Increased irritability, whining, tantrums
Regressive behaviors (e.g., thumb sucking, loss of elimination control)
Separation anxiety

**LATER PRESCHOOL CHILDREN (AGES 3-5 YEARS)**

Fear of abandonment
Blame themselves for the divorce; decreased self-esteem
Bewilderment regarding all human relationships
Become more aggressive in relationships with others (e.g., siblings, peers)
Engage in fantasy to seek understanding of the divorce

**EARLY SCHOOL-AGE CHILDREN (AGES 5-6 YEARS)**

Depression and immature behavior
Loss of appetite and sleep disorders
May be able to verbalize some feelings and understand some divorce-related changes
Increased anxiety and aggression
Feel abandoned by departing parent

**MIDDLE SCHOOL-AGE CHILDREN (AGES 6-8 YEARS)**

Panic reactions
Feelings of deprivation—loss of parent, attention, money, and secure future
Profound sadness, depression, fear, and insecurity

Feelings of abandonment and rejection
Fear regarding the future
Difficulty expressing anger at parents
Intense desire for reconciliation of parents
Impaired capacity to play and enjoy outside activities
Decline in school performance
Altered peer relationships—become bossy, irritable, demanding, and manipulative
Frequent crying, loss of appetite, sleep disorders
Disturbed routine, forgetfulness

**LATER SCHOOL-AGE CHILDREN (AGES 9-12 YEARS)**

More realistic understanding of divorce
Intense anger directed at one or both parents
Divided loyalties
Able to express feelings of anger
Ashamed of parental behavior
Feel the need for revenge; may wish to punish the parent they hold responsible
Feel lonely, rejected, and abandoned
Altered peer relationships
Decline in school performance
May develop somatic complaints
May engage in aberrant behavior such as lying, stealing
Temper tantrums
Dictatorial attitude

**ADOLESCENTS (AGES 12-18 YEARS)**

Able to disengage themselves from parental conflict
Feel a profound sense of loss—of family, childhood
Feelings of anxiety
Worry about themselves, parents, siblings
Express anger, sadness, shame, embarrassment
May withdraw from family and friends
Disturbed concept of sexuality
May engage in acting-out behaviors

from the family and individualization—normal developmental tasks of adolescence.

Although considerable research has looked at gender differences in children's adjustments to divorce, the findings are not conclusive. In some studies, emotional and behavioral problems in children from divorced families show an increase during adolescence (Hetherington and Stanley-Hagan, 1999). Earlier research on divorce often showed more deleterious effects related to the adjustment of boys. Diminishing gender effects may be attributed to the increased involvement of fathers following divorce. Father involvement may be more important for boys than girls. For some girls, divorce causes them to acquire increased caretaking responsibilities within the family, with the expectation that they will provide parent emotional support as well (Hetherington and Stanley-Hagan, 1999). These responsibilities and expectations may greatly overburden the teenager, who also is in need of support and comfort, and may be the reason that some adolescent girls have demonstrated lowered self-competence and self-worth following divorce.

**Telling the Children.**   Parents are understandably hesitant to tell children about their decision to divorce. A vast majority of parents neglect to discuss with their preschool children either the divorce or the inevitable changes it brings. Without preparation, even children who remain in the family home are confused by the parental separation, and this confusion seems to overpower any soothing effects remaining in the home may have.

Most likely, the children are already experiencing vague, uneasy feelings that are more difficult to cope with than being told truthfully about the situation. If possible, the initial disclosure should include both parents and siblings, followed by later discussions with each child individually. Ample time should be set aside for the discussions, and they should take place during a period of calm, not after an argument. Parents who physically hold or touch their children provide them with a feeling of warmth that is reassuring. The discussions should include the reason for the divorce—minimizing blame—and reassurance that the divorce is not the fault of the children. Children may feel guilty, as though they have somehow failed or are being punished for misbehavior. They wonder what role they played in the divorce or failure to keep the family together.

Parents need not fear crying in front of the children; it gives the children permission to cry also. Children need to ventilate their feelings. They normally feel anger and resentment and should be allowed to communicate these feelings without punishment. They also have feelings of terror and abandonment and long for consistency and order in their lives. One way to support and assure the child is to provide information that the child needs to know. A nurse may have the opportunity to suggest that parents talk over with the children certain issues such as where the child will live and where each parent will be; they should reassure the child that there will be enough money to meet needs and that, although the parents are divorcing, they are not divorcing the children and parental love will not end. Further issues a child may ponder include questions about what will happen on special days like birthdays and holidays, whether both parents will come to school events, and whether the child will still have the same friends (Arbuthnot and Gordon, 1995).

■ ■ ■

Research on the adverse effects of divorce on children should be viewed with some caution and scrutiny. Many of the samples are small, are drawn from one area of the country, or are selected from clinical rather than general populations. The lack of a control group in many studies also limits the conclusions. An area needing further research is the influence of children's temperament and coping abilities on adjustment to divorce.

Although most studies have concentrated on the negative effects of divorce on children, positive outcomes of divorce have been reported. A successful postdivorce family, either as a single-parent or as a reconstituted family, can improve the quality of life for adults and children. Living with conflict is resolved, and a better relationship with one or both parents may result. Children may also have less contact with a disturbed parent. Greater maturity, independence, and commitment to sustaining relationships are also positive outcomes (Kelly, 2000). However, emotional adjustment is closely associated with the child's personal adjustment before the divorce.

### Children's Developmental Tasks Related to Divorce

Most children go through two major phases when adjusting to a divorce: a *crisis phase,* which often lasts for a year or longer and is accompanied by an emotional upheaval that affects the relationship with the custodial parent, and an *adjustment phase,* in which children settle down and begin to adapt to life in a single-parent home.

Psychologic tasks for children following divorce are found in Box 3-12. Successful mastery of the early tasks is linked with maintenance of developmental pace and resumption of schoolwork following an expected period of diminished learning effectiveness and academic performance. Later tasks are associated with a more leisurely pace and extend over the remainder of the growth period.

### Custody and Parenting Partnerships

Traditionally when parents separated, the mother was given custody of the children. Now both parents and the courts are seeking alternatives. The present belief is that neither fathers nor mothers should be awarded custody automatically. Rather, custody should be awarded to the parent who is best able to provide for the children's welfare. In certain situations children experience severe stress when living or spending time with a parent. Some recent court decisions have reflected respect for the rights of children by allowing children to legally sever ties with one or both parents.

In most divorce cases the mother still receives custody of the child with visitation agreements for the father. However, more courts are now awarding custody to fathers. Men usu-

<table>
</table>

## Box 3-12 ■ ■ ■
### Psychologic Tasks for Children After Divorce

**TASK I: UNDERSTANDING THE DIVORCE**

**Young children:** Understand the immediate changes and differentiate fantasy from reality; manage concerns regarding abandonment, placement in foster care, not seeing departed parent again.

**Adolescents/young adults:** Understand what led to marital failure; evaluate parents' actions; draw useful conclusions for their own lives.

**TASK II: STRATEGIC WITHDRAWAL**

Acknowledge concern and provide appropriate help to parents and siblings; remove divorce from being their total focus and get back to their own interests, pleasures, activities, peer relationships, etc.

Parents must help children to remain children to complete this task.

**TASK III: DEALING WITH LOSS**

Deal with loss of intact family and loss of presence of one parent, usually the father.

May be most difficult task.

Deal with feelings of rejection and blame for making one parent leave.

Task is easier if child has good relationship with both parents.

**TASK IV: DEALING WITH ANGER**

Manage anger at parents for deciding to divorce, yet are aware of parents' needs, anxiety, and loneliness.

Diminished anger and forgiveness come about together.

**TASK V: WORKING OUT GUILT**

Deal with sense of guilt for causing marital difficulties and driving wedge between parents.

Need to separate guilty ties and get on with their lives.

**TASK VI: ACCEPTING PERMANENCE OF DIVORCE**

Overcome early denial and fantasies of parents getting back together.

Task may not be completed until parent remarries or child separates from parents and leaves.

**TASK VII: TAKING A CHANCE ON LOVE**

Most important task for growing children—adolescents and young adults.

Remain open to love, commitment, marriage, fidelity.

Able to turn away from parents' model.

Data from Wallerstein J, Blakeslee S: *Second chances: men, women, and children a decade after divorce,* New York, 1989, Ticknor & Fields.

ally make more money and can offer more material benefits than many women are able to provide. The incidence of delinquent support payments to custodial mothers is a matter of universal knowledge and concern. The single-parent family is commonplace, but many divorced mothers with small children move in with parents, other relatives, or friends in some kind of dependent or sharing arrangement.

Often overlooked are the changes that may occur in the children's relationships with other relatives, especially grandparents. Grandparents on the noncustodial side are often kept from their grandchildren; those on the custodial side may be overwhelmed by their adult child's return to the household with the grandchildren.

Two less common custody arrangements are divided custody and joint custody. **Divided,** or **split, custody** means that each parent is awarded custody of one or more of the children, thereby separating siblings. For example, sons might live with the father and daughters might live with the mother. Joint custody takes one of two forms. In **joint physical custody** the parents alternate having the physical care and control of the children on a reasonably equitable basis while maintaining shared parenting responsibilities legally. This type of custody arrangement works well for families who live close to each other and whose occupations allow an active role in the care and rearing of the children. In **joint legal custody** the children reside with one parent, but both parents are the children's legal guardians, and both participate in childrearing (Kelly, 2000).

Co-parenting offers substantial benefits for the family; children can be close to both parents, and life with each parent can be more normal as opposed to the situation of a disciplinarian mother and a recreational father. However, to be successful, the parents must place a high value on the commitment to provide as normal parenting as possible and be able to separate their marital conflicts from the parenting roles. No matter what type of custody arrangement is awarded, the primary consideration is the welfare of the children.

## Single-Parenting

Single-parent status is acquired by means of divorce, separation, or death, or through birth or adoption of a child by a single person. Although divorce rates have stabilized, the number of single-parent households continues to rise. Today, 25% of all children under 18 years of age live in single-parent families, with the majority of single parents being women (U.S. Census Bureau, 2001). It is estimated that at least half of the children born during the 1990s will spend part of their time in a family headed by a divorced, separated, widowed, or never-married mother. Although some women are single parents by choice, most of these women never planned on being single parents, and many feel pressure to marry or remarry.

Managing shortages of money, time, and energy are major concerns of single parents. Studies repeatedly confirm the financial difficulties of single-parent families, particularly in the case of single mothers. Approximately 41% of female-headed families lived in poverty in 1999. Only 31% of mother-headed households receive any child support or alimony (Annie E. Casey Foundation, 2001). In fact, the stigma of poverty may be more keenly felt than the discrimination associated with being a single parent. Nurses are encouraged to avoid seeing single-parent families as a deviant, pathologic, and less functional family system (Campbell and Ford-Gilboe, 1996).

In addition, these families are often forced by their financial status to live in communities where inadequate housing and personal safety are concerns. Moreover, single parents may feel guilty about the time spent away from their children. Divorced mothers from marriages where the father assumed the breadwinning role and the mother the household maintenance and parenting roles have been found to have the most difficulty in adjusting to becoming breadwinners. Many single parents have trouble arranging for adequate child care, and care for sick children is especially difficult to obtain. Single mothers trying to balance work, chores, and child care may frequently give up personal activities, recreation, and even rest.

Literature on the subject of single parents is diverse. Several authors (Elshtain, 1997; Mackey, 1997; Whitehead, 1997) suggest that such large-scale distribution of single parents is harmful to the society as a whole because the children are more likely to be and stay poor, commit crime, and be a source of discipline problems in public education. Zinsmeister (1997) thinks that, because of the absence of the father in most single-parent homes, the mother is overtaxed as both nurturer and disciplinarian and that a lack of a male role model may lead to poor educational performance, truancy, criminal activity, and psychologic problems for children of divorce. However, Skolnick and Rosencranz (1997) state that single-parent families have been unfairly stigmatized, that the harm caused by single or unwed mothers is exaggerated and unfair, and that single motherhood is a legitimate choice (Fig. 3-13).

Supports and resources for single-parent families include health care services that are open evenings and weekends; high-quality child care; respite child care to relieve parental exhaustion and burnout; and parent enhancement centers for advancing education and job skills, providing recreational activities, and offering parenting education. Groups for single-parent fathers and grandparents who are primary caregivers are also important. There is a need on the part of the parent for social contacts and a life separate from the children for the emotional growth of both parent and child. The single parent can find support and encouragement from **Parents Without Partners, Inc.,**\* an organization designed to meet the needs of this increasingly important group.

---

\*International Headquarters, 1650 South Dixie Hwy, Suite 510 Boca Raton, FL 33432; (800) 637-7974; www.parentswithoutpartners.org.

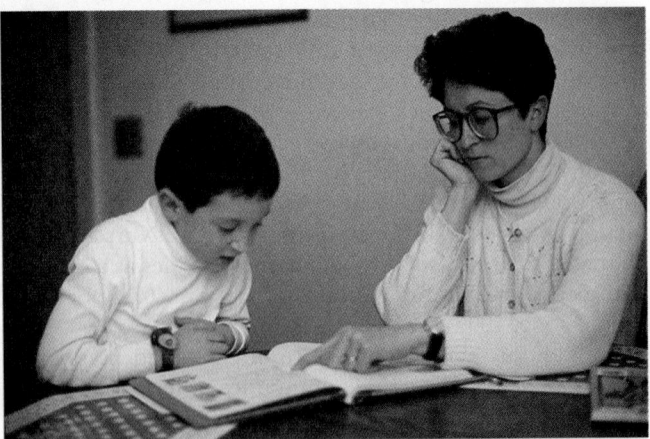

**Fig. 3-13** Working mothers must accomplish numerous tasks as part of their busy day.

### Single Fathers

Fathers who have custody of their children have many of the same problems as divorced mothers. They feel overburdened by the responsibility, depressed, and concerned about their ability to cope with the emotional needs of the children, especially the needs of the girls. The lack of homemaking skills is characteristic of most fathers. They find it difficult at first to coordinate household tasks, school visits, and other activities associated with managing a household alone. Fathers often demand more assistance with household tasks and more independence from their children than custodial mothers do, and they are likely to make use of alternative caregiving and support systems.

## Parenting in Reconstituted Families

In the United States approximately half of all children in homes where parents have divorced will experience yet another major change in their lives—a return to a nuclear family and the sudden acquisition of a stepparent when the custodial parent remarries (Dunn, 1995). The entry of a stepparent into a ready-made family requires adjustments for all of the family members. Some obstacles to the role adjustments and family problem solving include disruption of previous lifestyles and interaction patterns, complexity in the formation of new ones, and lack of social supports. Despite these problems, most children from divorced families want to live in a two-parent home.

### Stepparenting

The term *parenting coalition* has been suggested to describe the situation where there are more than two parents for a child, as in stepfamilies (Visher and Visher, 1995). This term implies the need for cooperation rather than competition between the biologic parents and the stepparents. Cooperative parenting relationships can allow more time for each set of parents to be alone to establish their own relationship. Under ideal circumstances, power conflicts between the two households can be reduced, and tension and anxiety can be lessened for all family members. In addition, the children's self-esteem can be increased, and there is a greater likelihood of continued contact with grandparents.

The development of a parenting coalition requires time and corresponds to the stages of stepfamily development: (1) bonding between the couple, (2) recognition that all parenting adults are important to the children's well-being, (3) definition and clarification of acceptable stepparent roles, and (4) ability to share among adults in both households in terms of childrearing decisions and responsibilities. Flexibility, mutual support, and open communication are critical in successful relationships in stepfamilies and stepparenting situations. Visher and Visher (1995) suggest the following special features of stepfamilies:

- Biologic parents may become angry with each other because of fear of further loss, and their child is caught in the middle, struggling with loyalty conflicts. Helping the parents cooperate helps everyone.
- Children may come and go between their two households. Stresses can be expected during times of transition.

- Discipline is an area of difficulty for most stepfamilies. The stepparent has little power until a stepparent-stepchild relationship has been established. Patience becomes a necessary virtue!
- Children initially may have stronger bonds with their parents than the parent has with the stepparent. One-on-one times help to maintain these relationships and to develop new ones.
- There are differences in family customs and values based on previous family experiences. New family traditions and customs must be negotiated.
- Stepparents are often unfamiliar with the medical history of stepchildren. They also do not have legal rights for authorizing treatments unless written permission is granted by the custodial parent.
- Many of the losses for children in stepfamilies are unrecognized by adults. These losses often can be accepted by adults when they are brought to their attention.
- The parent must require respect of all children and adults in the household to facilitate integration.
- Feelings cannot be forced; it is important to respect the children's wishes regarding their stepparent.
- A "parenting coalition" can do much to relieve tension between a child's two households.
- Stepfamilies can look forward to many rewards. The family must persevere and allow the necessary time for adjustment and integration to take place.

Unfortunately, stepfamilies usually do not seek help to prevent problems from arising. Typically, information and counseling are sought only when problems have surfaced and can no longer be ignored. A preventive rather than remedial approach to stepfamilies and stepparenting is needed (Box 3-13).

### Effects on Children

Although there has been a great deal of research on the impact of divorce on children, there is much less data on the outcomes for children in stepfamilies. Becoming a stepchild is often a stressful transition, especially during initial marital rearrangement (Dunn, 1995). Several transitional factors have been demonstrated to have an effect on children. The relationship with the noncustodial parent usually deteriorates. Divided loyalties between the two sets of parents may be exacerbated. As time goes on, the entry of new children from the remarriage can cause a stepchild from a pre-vious marriage to have less-favored status. In stepfamilies the possibility of a second divorce situation is critical because the children have already experienced significant losses in both relationships, as well as environmental and circumstantial changes. Despite these risks and stresses, studies to date have not demonstrated long-term negative effects on children in remarried families.

## Parenting in Dual-Earner Families

No change in family lifestyle has had more impact than the large numbers of women entering the workplace. As women moved away from the traditional homemaker pattern, the numbers of dual-earner families increased dramatically. Currently, 62% of women with preschool children are employed outside the home (Ulione, 1996). This trend is unlikely to diminish. As a result, the family is subjected to considerable stress as members attempt to meet the challenge of the often competing demands of occupational needs and those regarded as necessary for a rich family life.

Role definitions are frequently altered to arrange an equitable division of time and labor, as well as to resolve conflicts between earlier and later norms, especially those related to the traditional norms of the culture. Overload is a common source of stress in a dual-earner family, and social activities are significantly curtailed. Time demands and scheduling are major problems, and when there are children, the demands can be even more intense; dual-earner couples may increase the strain on themselves in order to avoid creating stress for their children. Although there is no evidence to indicate that the dual-earner lifestyle, as such, is stressful to children, the stress experienced by the parents may affect the children indirectly.

### Working Mothers

Even though working mothers have become the norm in the United States, disapproving attitudes from some health care workers and some child care books, lack of a national policy on child care, and "scripts" from their own childhood of being cared for by an at-home mother contribute to the torn and guilty feelings many working mothers experience (Youngblut and others, 2000).

Child care is critical to the working mother's well-being. The quality of child care is a persistent concern for all working parents. (See Evidence-Based Practice box on p. 100.) Determinants of child care quality are based on health and safety requirements, responsive and warm interaction between staff and children, developmentally appropriate activities, and trained staff, limited group size, age-appropriate caregivers, child ratios, and adequate indoor and outdoor space (Scarr, 1998). In general, the quality of child care is improved by lower ratios, smaller group sizes, and better qualified teachers.

Nurses play an important role in helping families to find suitable sources of child care and to prepare children for this experience. (See Alternate Child Care Arrangements, Chapter 12.) Although families exist in many types, it is more important to know and understand how family process functions (Acock and Demo, 1996).

---

**Box 3-13**

### Tips for "Living in Step"

1. Let relationships develop slowly and naturally. Don't expect too much too soon, from the children, from your spouse, or from yourself.
2. Don't criticize or belittle lost (or new) parents, or try to erase or replace them. Stepparents are additional parents.
3. Expect confused feelings, anxieties, competition for attention, bids for loyalty. Decide on standards of discipline and behavior and stick to them.
4. Communicate. Don't pretend everything is fine if it isn't. Look at problems squarely and deal with them openly.
5. If you need help, admit it and get it. Read a book, get counseling, join a support group, call a family meeting.

From Stein B: Yours, mine, and ours: a look at stepfamilies, *Growing Parent* 12(9):1-5, 1984.

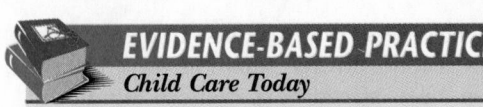

Child care in this country was originally created for three purposes: to support maternal employment opportunities, to promote child development, and to intervene with economically disadvantaged children (Scarr, 1998). There are a variety of child care arrangements in this country including family daycare vs center daycare, licensed vs unlicensed facilities, and nonprofit vs profit daycare. Much discussion has occurred regarding the quality of care provided to children in these settings. There is a consensus that quality daycare includes warm, supportive interactions with adults in a safe, healthy, and stimulating environment where early education and trusting relationships support children's physical, emotional, social, and intellectual development (Scarr, 1998).

Researchers have explored the long-term effects of daycare. Children from low-income families have benefited from quality child care when used as an intervention strategy (Ramey and Ramey, 1992). Children from disadvantaged homes who participated in a child care program showed better school achievement and socialization skills than similar children who did not. For middle- to upper-income families, the long-term effects of child care are less clear. In a large study of 720 young children ages 12 to 60 months, researchers found a small but stastically significant effect of the quality of child care on social adjustment ratings (McCartney and others, 1997). However, in a 4-year follow-up study of 141 of these children, researchers reported no long-term effects of differences in the quality of child care on the children's social, emotional, or behavioral adjustment (Deater-Deckard, Pinkerton, and Scarr, 1996).

Longitudinal studies report that children who attended better quality daycare centers during the preschool period exhibited more social competence, increased empathy for others, and were better liked by their peers than children in poor quality daycare centers (Scarr, 1998). This finding, however, may be masked by the influence of the family.

The effect of daycare on infant development and attachment has been one of the most controversial issues studied since the 1980s. Finally, a study by the National Institute of Child Health and Human Development (NICHD) Early Child Care Research Network demonstrated no relationship among infant age at entry into child care, amount of time spent in infant care, and abnormal attachment behaviors (NICHD Early Child Care Research Network, 1997). Findings did reveal that less sensitive, less well-adjusted mothers were more likely to have insecurely attached infants (Lamb, 2000).

## FOSTER PARENTING

The term *foster care* is defined as placement in an approved living situation away from the family of origin. The living situation may be an approved foster home with other relatives or strangers or a preadoptive home (Carlson, 1996; Hacsi, 1995). Each state provides a standard for the role of foster parent and a process by which to become one. These "parents" are on contract with the state to provide a "home" for children for a limited duration. Most states require about 27 hours of training before being on contract and at least 12 hours of continuing education a year. Foster parents may be required to attend a foster parent support group that is often separate from a state agency. Each state has guidelines regarding the relative health of the prospective foster parents and their families, background checks regarding legal issues for the adults, personal interviews, and a safety inspection of the residence and surroundings.

Foster homes include both kinship and nonrelative placements. Heger and Scannapieco (1995) report that since 1982 the proportion of children in out-of-home care placed with relatives has increased rapidly and substantially, accompanied by a decrease in the number of foster families. Long-term studies indicate that there is relatively little difference in adult functioning between kinship and nonrelative placements (Benedict and others, 1996). As with their nonfoster counterparts, much of the child's adjustment depends on the stability of the family and available resources (Fein, 1995). Even though foster homes are designed to provide short-term care, it is not unusual for children to stay for many years. In these cases, studies indicate that children consider their foster caregivers "family" and express the feeling that the foster family functions like a normal family (Gardner, 1996; Kufeldt, 1995).

Nurses need to be aware that nearly 500,000 children will be in foster care at any given time in the United States (American Academy of Pediatrics, 2000). Carlson (1996) notes that children in foster care tend to have a higher than normal incidence of acute and chronic health problems. These may include developmental, emotional, medical, and dental problems. These children are often at risk because of their previous caretaking environment. Nurses need to implement strategies to provide a better health care system for this vulnerable population of children. Also, assessment skills and case management skills are required to involve other disciplines in meeting the needs of individual foster children and their families (Carlson, 1996).

## ACCOMMODATING CONTEMPORARY PARENTING SITUATIONS

During recent years both the private and government sectors have noted some of the problems contemporary families face. Many of these issues involve working parents. For example, perhaps one of the greatest stressors for the working single parent or for dual-earner families is when a child becomes ill. Frequency of childhood illness, exclusion practices of most licensed child care programs, and employer's limited sick-leave policies are contributing factors. Most agree that a familiar face and familiar place should be goals of sick-child care; therefore many argue that the only place for an ill child is at home with a parent or other relative.

Some employers have become more family focused and give parents time off to be with their sick children. Increasing numbers are also more generous in the amount of time they allow parents—fathers as well as mothers—to remain at home after the birth or adoption of a child. More flexible work schedules and family-oriented legislation can also ease the burden of managing family and work responsibilities. The passage of the **Family and Medical Leave Act (FMLA)** in 1993 set the stage for a greater focus on the issues that contemporary American families face. The FMLA allows eligible employees to take up to 12 weeks of unpaid leave each year to care for newborn or newly adopted children, parents, or spouses who have serious health conditions, or to recover from their own serious health condition.

## KEY POINTS

- Because there is no agreement about the definition of *family*, a family is what an individual considers it to be.
- Three theories that have significant relevance and application to pediatric nursing are family systems theory, family stress theory, and developmental theory.
- Although the traditional family structure has been nuclear or extended, in recent years other forms, such as the single-parent family, have emerged.
- Family size and positioning within the family structure have a strong impact on a child's development.
- Interpersonal skills and a basic understanding of childhood growth and development are two essential areas of focus for parents.
- Parental control tends to be predominantly one of three types: authoritarian, permissive, or authoritative.

- Three areas of special concern to adoptive families include the initial attachment process, the task of telling the children they are adopted, and identity formation during adolescence.
- Marital factors within the home significantly influence a child's development. The impact of divorce on a child depends on the child's age and sex, the outcome, and the quality of the parent-child relationship and parental care following the divorce.
- Single-parenting and stepparenting create adjustment difficulties and stress to the already-demanding parental role. Significant numbers of children will live in a single-parent or reconstituted family at some point.

## REFERENCES

Acock A, Demo D: Family structure, family process, and adolescent well-being, *J Res Adolesc* 6(4):457-488, 1996.

American Academy of Pediatrics, Committee on Early Childhood, Adoption, and Dependent Care: Development issues for young children in foster care (RE0012), *Pediatrics* 106(5):1145-1150, 2000.

American Academy of Pediatrics, Committee on Psychosocial Aspects of Child and Family Health: Guidance for effective discipline, *Pediatrics* 101(4):723-728. 1998.

Annie E. Casey Foundation: *Kids count 2001*, Washington, DC, 2001, Center for the Study of Social Policy.

Arbuthnot J, Gordon D: *Surviving divorce: a student's companion to children in the middle*, Athens, OH, 1995, Center for Divorce Education.

Ariel J, McPherson DW: Therapy with lesbian and gay parents and their children, *J Mar Fam Ther* 26(4):421-432, 2000.

Bar-on ME: The effects of television on child health: implications and recommendations, *Arch Dis Child* 83:289-292, 2000.

Bauman LJ, Friedman SB: Corporal punishment, *Pediatr Clin North Am* 45(2):403-415, 1998.

Benedict M and others: Adult functioning of children who lived in kin versus nonrelative family foster homes, *Child Welfare* 75(5):529-549, 1996.

Black M, Nitz K: Grandmother co-residence, parenting and child development among low income, urban teen mothers, *J Adolesc Health* 18:218-226, 1996.

Blum N and others: Disciplining young children: the role of verbal instruction and reasoning, *Pediatrics* 96(2):336-341, 1995.

Brazelton TB: Working with families: opportunities for early intervention, *Pediatr Clin North Am* 42(1):1-10, 1995.

Campbell J, Ford-Gilboe M: The mother-headed single-parent family: a feminist critique of the nursing literature, *Nurs Outlook* 44(4):173-183, 1996.

Carlson K: Providing health care for children in foster care: a role for advanced practice nurses, *Pediatr Nurs* 22(5):418-421, 1996.

Centers for Disease Control and Prevention: Births, marriages, divorces, and deaths: provisional data for November 1999, *National Vital Statistics Reports*, vol 48, no 17, 2000.

Cody A: Helping the vulnerable or condoning control within the family: where is nursing? *J Adv Nurs* 23:882-886, 1996.

Deater-Deckard A, Pinkerton R, Scarr S: Child care quality and children's behavioral adjustment: a four-year longitudinal study, *J Child Psychol Psychiatry* 37(8):937-948, 1996.

Donovan D: A contrary view on adoption disclosure, *Child Teens Today* 10(10):4-6, 1990.

Dunn J: Step families and children's adjustment, *Arch Dis Child* 73(6):487-489, 1995.

Duvall ER: *Family development*, ed 5, Philadelphia, 1977, JB Lippincott.

Elkind D: The young child in the postmodern world, *Dimens Early Child* 23(3):6-9, 1995.

Elshtain JB: Single-parent families contribute to the breakdown of society. In Swisher KL, editor: *Single-parent families*, San Diego, CA, 1997, Greenhaven Press.

Fein E: Stability and change: initial findings in a study of treatment foster care placements, *Child Youth Serv Rev* 17(3):379-389, 1995.

Foss G: A conceptual model for studying parenting behaviors in immigrant populations, *Adv Nurs Sci* 19(2):74-87, 1996.

Friedman M: *Family nursing: theory and practice*, ed 4, Norwalk, CT, 1998, Appleton-Century-Crofts.

Furukawa S: *The diverse living arrangements of children: summer 1991*, US Bureau of the Census, Current Population Reports, Series P70, No 38, Washington, DC, 1994, US Government Printing Office.

Gardner H: The concept of family: perceptions of children in foster care, *Child Welfare* 75(2):161-182, 1996.

Grotevant H, McRoy R: Emotional disorders in adopted children and youth. In McManus M, editor: Adoption: a lifelong journey for children and families, *Focal Point* 10(1), 1996.

Guyer and others: Annual summary statistics—1998, *Pediatrics* 104(8):1229-1249, 1999.

Hacsi T: From indenture to family foster care: a brief history of child placing, *Child Welfare* 74(1):162-180, 1995.

Heger R, Scannapieco M: From family duty to family policy: the evolution of kinship care, *Child Welfare* 74(1):200-216, 1995.

Hetherington EM, Stanley-Hagan M: The adjustment of children with divorced parents: a risk and resiliency perspective, *J Child Psychol Psychiatry* 40(1):129-140, 1999.

Hostetter M, Johnson D: Medical supervision of internationally adopted children, *Pediatr Basics* 77:10-17, 1996.

Kelly JB: Children's adjustment in conflicted marriage and divorce: a decade review of research, *J Am Acad Child Adolesc Psychiatry* 39(8):963-973, 2000.

Kronemyer B: Providing care for internationally adopted children proves rewarding, *Inf Dis Child* 14(1):15, 2001.

Kufeldt K and others: How children in care view their own and their foster families, *Child Welfare* 74(3):695-715, 1995,

Lamb ME and others: Nonparental child care: context, quality, correlates, and consequences. In Damon W, Sigel IE, Renninger KA, editors: *Handbook of child psychology: child psychology in practice*, ed 5, New York-Toronto, 2000, John Wiley & Sons.

Lerner RM, Sparks EE, McCubbin LD: *Family diversity and family policy: strengthening families for America's children*, Boston, 1999, Kluwer Academic Publishers.

Lynch JM, Murray K: For the love of the children: the coming out process for lesbian and gay parents and stepparents, *J Homosex* 39(1):1-24, 2000.

Mackey WC: Single-parent families contribute to violent crime. In Swisher KL, editor: *Single-parent families*, San Diego, CA, 1997, Greenhaven Press.

March K: Perception of adoption as social stigma: motivation for search and reunion, *J Marriage Fam* 57(3):653-660, 1995.

May J: Fathers: the forgotten parent, *Fam Matters* 22(3):243-246, 1996.

McCartney K and others: Social development in the context of typical center-based child care, *Merrill-Palmer Quarterly* 43(3):426-450, 1997.

McCubbin MA, McCubbin HI: Families coping with illness: the resiliency model of family stress, adjustment, and adaptation. In Danielson CB, Bissel BH, Winstead-Fry P, editors: *Families, health, anl illness*, St Louis, 1994, Mosby.

Miller L: Caring for internationally adopted children, *N Engl J Med* 341(20):1539-1540, 1999.

Mitchell MA, Jenista JA: Health care of the internationally adopted child, part 1. Before and at arrival into the adoptive home, *J Pediatr Health Care* 11(2):51-60, 1997.

National Center for Children in Poverty: Young child poverty in the states—wide variation and significant change. In *Childhood Poverty (Research Brief 1)*, New York, 1998, Columbia University School of Public Health.

National Center for Health Statistics: Advanced report of final natality statistics, 1991, *Monthly Vital Statistics Report*, vol 42, no 2, (suppl: entire issue), 1993.

National Institute of Child Health and Human Development, Early Child Care Research Network: The effects of infant child care on infant-mother attachment security: results of the NICHD Study of Early Child Care, *Child Dev* 68(5):860-879, 1997.

Nelms B: Discipline: we need it now more than ever, *J Pediatr Health Care* 10:193-194, 1996.

Office of Human Development Services, Department of Health and Human Services: Part 1356—requirements applicable to Title IV-E, *Title 45 Public Welfare* CFR Title 50(2), 2000.

Patterson C: Children of lesbian and gay parents, *Child Dev* 63:1025-1042, 1992.

Patterson CJ: Families of the lesbian baby boom: parents' division of labor and children's adjustment, *Dev Psychol* 31:115-123, 1995.

Perrin EC, Kulkin H: Pediatric care for children whose parents are gay or lesbian, *Pediatrics* 97(5):629-635, 1996.

Perrin EC: Technical report: coparent or second-parent adoption by same-sex parents, *Pediatrics* 109(2):341-343, 2002.

Phillips NK: Adoption of a sibling: reactions of biological children at different stages of development, *Am J Orthopsychia* 69(1):122-126, 1999.

Polit D, Falbo T: Only children and personality development, *J Marriage Fam* 49:309-325, 1987.

Ramey C, Ramey S: Early educational interventions with disadvantaged children—to what effect? *Appl Prev Psychol* 1:131-140, 1992.

Rogers RH: *Improvement in the construction and analysis of family life cycle categories*, Kalamazoo, MI, 1962, Western Michigan University.

Scarr S: American child care today, *Am Psychol* 53(2):95-108, 1998.

Shrifin D: Resolved: 10 tips for better parenting in the new year, *AAP News*, Jan 1997.

Shireman J: Single parent adoptive homes, *Child Youth Serv Rev* 18(1):23-36, 1996.

Silver N: The lowdown on spacing children, *Parents* 70(5):86-88, 1995.

Skolnick A, Rosencranz S: The harmful effects of single-parent families are exaggerated. In Swisher KL, editor: *Single-parent families*, San Diego, CA, 1997, Greenhaven Press.

Smit EM: Unique issues of the adopted child: helping parents talk openly and honestly with their child and the community, *J Psychosocial Nurs Ment Health Serv* 34(7):9-36, 1996.

Sullivan A: Policy issues in gay and lesbian adoption, *Adopt Foster* 19(4)21-25, 1995.

Tiller C: Father's parenting attitudes during a child's first year, *J Obstet Gynecol Neonat Nurs* 24(6):508-514, 1995.

US Census Bureau: *Living arrangements of children*, 1996, Washington, DC, 2001, US Government Printing Office, pp 70-74.

Ulione M: Physical and emotional health in dual-earner family members, *Fam Community Health* 19(3):14-20, 1996.

Ventura SJ and others: Report of final natality statistics, 1995, *Monthly Vital Statistics Report*, vol 45, no 11, (suppl), 1997.

Visher E, Visher J: Beyond the nuclear family: resources and implications for pediatricians, *Fam Focused Pediatr* 42(1):31-43, 1995.

Whitehead BD: Single-parent families are harmful. In Swisher KL, editor: *Single-parent families*, San Diego, CA, 1997, Greenhaven Press.

Woodworth R: You're not alone . . . you're one in a million, *Child Welfare League America* 75(5):619-635, 1996.

Youngblut JM and others: Factors influencing single mother's employment status, *Health Care Women International* 21:125-136, 2000, Taylor & Francis.

Zinsmeister K: Divorce harms children. In Swisher KL, editor: *Single-parent families*, San Diego, CA, 1997, Greenhaven Press.

# Chapter 4

# Community-Based Nursing Care of the Child and Family

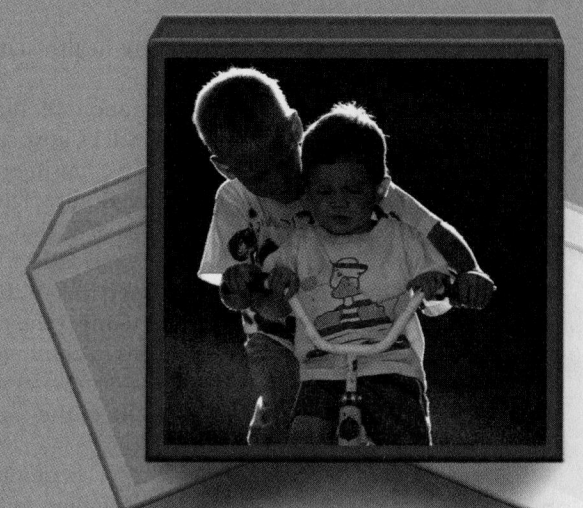

## Chapter Outline

**COMMUNITY HEALTH CONCEPTS, 103**
Community, 103
Demography, 104
Epidemiology, 104

Distribution of Disease, Injury, or
    Illness, 105
Epidemiologic Triangle, 105
Levels of Prevention, 105
**Economics, 106**

**COMMUNITY NURSING PROCESS, 106**
Community Needs Assessment, 107
Community Planning, 107
Community Implementation, 107
Community Evaluation, 107

## Related Topics

*Healthy People 2010:* Perspectives of Pediatric
    Nursing, Ch 1

Measuring the Distribution of Disease, Injury,
    or Illness: Perspectives of Pediatric
    Nursing, Ch 1

Screening: Physical and Developmental
    Assessment of the Child, Ch 7

## COMMUNITY HEALTH CONCEPTS

### Community

Healthy communities provide children not only with quality medical care, but they also provide a nurturing, safe place to live and grow. Healthy communities address concerns through collaboration between and among citizens, businesses, and governmental and private agencies (Flynn and Ivanov, 2000). The health of children and their families is greatly influenced by their community, and nurses can make a significant contribution by working with the community to promote children's health. Nurses working with pediatric populations need to understand the concepts and processes critical to addressing pediatric concerns from a community health perspective.

This chapter focuses on community health nursing as it relates to children. First, it outlines and defines the concepts that serve as the basis of the Community Health Nursing Process. Next it describes the process step by step. It concludes by using the process to address a very real child health concern, childhood obesity.

■ Christine A. Brosnan, PhD, RN, and Sandra Upchurch, PhD, RN, CDE, wrote this chapter.

> **NURSING TIP** Knowing the characteristics of a healthy community will help the nurse develop a plan of care. A healthy community "practices ongoing dialogue, generates leadership, shapes its future, embraces diversity, knows itself, connects people and resources, and creates a sense of community" (*www.healthycommunities.org*).

A *community* can be defined as a group of individuals with shared characteristics or interests who interact with each other (Allender and Spradley, 2001). A community includes children and families, the physical environment, educational facilities, safety and transportation resources, political and governmental agencies, health and social services, communication resources, economic resources, and recreational facilities (Anderson and McFarlane, 2000). Community health initiatives are directed at either the health of the community as a whole or at specific populations within the community who have unique needs. In this context, *populations* can be described as groups of people who live in a community, such as school-age children (American Nurses' Association, 1986). Common values often guide behaviors of populations in relation to health promotion and disease prevention activities. *Target populations* or *subpopulations* are more narrowly defined groups (e.g., obese middle-school children) toward whom nurses direct activities in order to improve the health status of individuals in the group.

*Community care* involves a collaboration of individuals and groups, including health care providers, advocates, governments, managed care organizations, businesses, children, and families within a specific community. The goal of the collaborative effort is to provide services that promote the child health initiatives of *Healthy People 2010.**  Community care is "without walls" in that the services of the health care system are frequently redesigned to meet the changing needs of the community. Those involved in community care partner with the community to identify, plan, intervene, and evaluate activities that improve the health of the community (Anderson and McFarlane, 2000).

*Community health nursing* focuses on promoting and maintaining the health of individuals, families, and groups in the community setting. It is a synthesis of nursing and public health, emphasizing personal responsibility for health and self-care (Allender and Spradley, 2001). At its best, community health nursing empowers communities by enabling members to gain the knowledge and skills needed to fulfill their own needs.

**NURSING TIP** Empowering people with knowledge and skills is not a new idea. Marcus Aurelius reflected this notion many years ago with his well-known quote:

If I give you a fish, you eat for a day.
If I teach you to fish, you eat for a lifetime.

Although community health concepts can be used to address health concerns in any setting, traditional community health settings include the following: home health agencies, schools, doctors' offices, ambulatory health clinics, emergency rooms, triage call centers, insurance agencies, health departments, international relief agencies, health education agencies, juvenile detention facilities, camps, daycare centers, foster care facilities, and rehabilitation agencies. The American Nurses' Association (1986) has established nine standards for community health nursing related to the following categories: theory, data collection, diagnosis, planning, intervention, evaluation, quality assurance and professional development, interdisciplinary collaboration, and research.

The *roles and functions* of the community health nurse continue to evolve. In the future, more pediatric nurses will be working in community settings. The Health Resources and Services Administration (2001) reported that 18.3% of the total registered nurse workforce was employed in a community or public health setting and 9.5% in ambulatory care. Only 59% of registered nurses practiced in hospital settings.

Traditionally, the *roles and functions* of community health nurses included caregiver, advocate, case manager, case finder, counselor, educator, epidemiologist, group process leader, health planner, and manager (Clemen-Stone, McGuire, and Eigsti, 1998). For example, the nurse employed in a pediatric outpatient clinic will function in a number of roles to provide care to a child with Type 2 dia-

betes. The nurse provides case management by coordinating care among the disciplines, counsel by supporting the child and family through developmental crisis, and acts as a case finder by identifying risk factors in the child's siblings.

In recent years, the Institute of Medicine developed a list of *core functions* to guide the work of public health professionals, including nurses. The core functions are directed at providing population-wide services and personal and home services for people at risk (Institute of Medicine, 1988; Allender and Spradley, 2001). The population-wide services are based on assessment of health status monitoring and on disease *surveillance, policy development,* and *assurance* that can be translated into service. A certain skill set has been identified as important for the nurse in a public health setting. Some of the skills needed include the ability to analyze data, measure health status, connect people to organizations, bring about change in organizations, build strength in diversity, build coalitions, develop interdisciplinary teams, and devise approaches to quality improvement (Gebbie and Hwang, 2000). Consequently, the pediatric nurse employed in a managed care environment may be asked to develop a creative approach to teaching children with asthma about peak flow meters during emergency room visits. Included in the request may be a mechanism for evaluating the cost of the approach and the occurrence of repeated emergency room visits.

## Demography

*Demography* is the study of population characteristics. *Demographic characteristics* include age, gender, race and ethnicity, socioeconomic status, and education. Individuals, families, and communities may have demographic characteristics that affect their health risks (Anderson and McFarlane, 2000). *Risk* is the probability of developing a disease, injury, or illness. Age is one of the most important risk factors to consider for disease prevention and the development of certain health conditions. For example, children under age 5 are more likely to have respiratory infections than children ages 5 to 17, and those of the older age group are more likely to suffer fractures and dislocations than children under age 5 (Institute of Medicine, 1998). Gender also plays an important role. Males are at much greater risk of hemophilia A and B than females. Race and ethnicity have long been associated with increased risk for disease and disability, but it is now thought that, aside from genetic predisposition, there is complicated relationship between minority status and socioeconomic status that increases the risk for disease and disability (Smith, 2000). Low socioeconomic status predisposes children to a variety of problems. Poor children are more likely to be hospitalized for pneumonia, asthma, dehydration, and gastroenteritis than children from affluent families (Institute of Medicine, 1998). They are also less likely to be immunized against childhood illnesses (Ortega and others, 2000).

## Epidemiology

*Epidemiology* is the science of population health applied to the detection of morbidity and mortality in a population.

---

*www.health.gov/healthy/people

The epidemiologic process identifies the distribution and causes of disease or injury across a population (Anderson and McFarlane, 2000). It also serves an important component in developing health programs. For example, *Healthy People 2010* incorporated the process to develop a set of health objectives for the United States. Health professionals in community, state, and health care organizations use the objectives as a guide to develop programs that have the greatest impact on the health of children.

## Distribution of Disease, Injury, or Illness

*Morbidity rates* are used to measure disease and injury and, along with *natality and mortality rates,* they present an objective picture of the health status of a community. There are two types of morbidity rates, incidence and prevalence. *Incidence* measures the occurrence of *new* events in a population during a period of time. *Prevalence* measures *existing* events in a population during a period of time (Hennekens and Buring, 1987). For example, the incidence of Type 1 diabetes in a community is estimated by counting the new cases in a population and dividing that figure by the number of people at risk. The prevalence is estimated by counting the existing cases of Type 1 diabetes in a population and dividing that figure by the number of people at risk. Both incidence and prevalence are usually given as rates per 1000, 10,000, or 100,000 population, depending on their frequency. Box 4-1 presents frequently used rates.

## Epidemiologic Triangle

Three factors form the epidemiologic triangle, and their interrelationship alters the risk of acquiring a disease or condition (McKeown and Weinrich, 2000). These factors are agent, host, and environment. An *agent* is responsible for causing a disease and may be an infectious agent such as *Mycobacterium tuberculosis,* a chemical agent such as lead in paint, or a physical agent such as fire. *Host* factors are those that are specific to an individual or group. These may be genetic factors that cannot be controlled or they can be lifestyle factors, for example, food selections or exercise patterns. *Environmental factors* provide a setting and include the climatic conditions in which the host lives as well as factors related to the home, neighborhood, and school.

## Levels of Prevention

Community health programs are based on three classic levels of prevention (Leavell and Clark, 1965). *Primary prevention* focuses on health promotion and prevention of disease or injury. Examples of primary prevention activities include well-child care clinics, immunization programs, safety programs (bike helmets, car seats, seat belts, childproof containers), nutrition programs, environmental efforts (clean air programs), sanitation measures (chlorinated water, garbage removal, sewage treatment), and community parenting classes. *Secondary prevention* focuses on screening and early diagnosis of disease. Examples of secondary interventions include tuberculosis and lead screening programs and mental health counseling for stressful events such as separation, divorce, death, or community natural disasters (e.g., earthquakes, floods, and hurricanes). *Tertiary prevention* focuses on optimizing function for children with disabilities or chronic diseases. Tertiary interventions include rehabilitation and disease management programs for asthma, sickle cell disease, cancer, anorexia, and special education programs for children.

---

### Box 4-1 ■ ■ ■
### Frequently Used Mortality and Morbidity Rates

**CRUDE BIRTH RATE**

$$\frac{\text{Number of births in a population within a time period}}{\text{Total population}} \times 1000$$

**CRUDE DEATH RATE**

$$\frac{\text{Number of deaths in a population within a time period}}{\text{Total population}} \times 1000$$

**CAUSE-SPECIFIC DEATH RATE**

$$\frac{\text{Number of deaths in a population due to a certain disease within a time period}}{\text{Total population}} \times 100,000$$

**AGE-SPECIFIC DEATH RATE**

$$\frac{\text{Number of deaths in a population in a certain age group within a time period}}{\text{Total population in that age group}} \times 100,000$$

**INCIDENCE OF DISEASE**

$$\frac{\text{Number of new events in a population within a time period}}{\text{Total at-risk population}} \times 100,000$$

**PREVALENCE OF DISEASE**

$$\frac{\text{Number of existing events in a population within a time period}}{\text{Total at-risk population}} \times 100,000$$

**Screening.**   Community health nurses are frequently involved in *screening,* a secondary prevention activity. The purpose of screening is to detect and treat disease early in the period of pathogenesis in order to prevent the spread and progression of the disease (Wilson and Jungner, 1968). However, screening is not appropriate for every condition. In a seminal article, Wilson and Jungner described 10 principles for assessing tools that should be used as a reference point when developing screening programs (Box 4-2). Although screening may bring benefit, there is a certain amount of risk associated with any intervention. In the case of screening, there is the psychologic risk associated with false-positive results as well as the danger that a parent may treat a child differently because of early identification of a disease (Clayton, 1999; Kwon and Farrell, 2000). A great deal of planning is required in order to ensure that the benefits of screening exceed the risks and cost.

## Economics

A basic understanding of the *economics* of health care is essential because it enables the nurse to participate in decision making about the worth of children's health programs. Economists theorize that individuals and societies view health as a basic utility, that is, something that is perceived as valuable (Gold and others, 1996). Other basic utilities are food, shelter, and clothing. People are willing to trade resources, such as money and time, for a program or intervention that will improve their health. Economists measure the amount of resources individuals and communities are willing to pay for good health. They also examine how different groups prioritize health care needs and allocate health care dollars. Methods for defining and estimating cost have been well described as has the need for a standardized approach to the measurement of cost and effects (Brosnan and Swint, 2001; Drummond and others, 1997).

Economic evaluation provides objective information to establish the value of a program to the community. An example is an evaluation of a school-based hepatitis B vaccination program by Wilson (2000). He concluded that the percentage of vaccinated sixth-graders increased from 8% without the program to 82% with the program. The higher vaccination rate saves dollars that might eventually be spent to treat these children for hepatitis, cirrhosis, or cancer in the future. Therefore the program resulted in potential cost savings of $24 million when compared to the no-program alternative.

**NURSING TIP**   In today's health care climate of interdisciplinary practice and managed care, nurses are expected to understand basic economic concepts and collaborate with others in applying the methods of cost analysis to their practice. Nurses who are unable to do this risk loss of decision-making responsibilities for themselves and for their patients.

A *cost-effectiveness analysis,* the most common type of economic evaluation, requires a comparison of one program with an alternative. In this type of analysis the costs of nursing interventions are calculated in dollars and end points are calculated in health units (such as lives saved or hospital days avoided). The results are presented in a ratio with costs in the numerator and health units in the denominator. Tengs and others (1995) described the cost effectiveness of 500 health-related interventions in a review of economic studies. The results were presented in cost per life-year saved. As an example, neonatal intensive care for infants weighing 751 to 1000 g costs $5800 per life-year saved compared with that for infants weighing 500 to 750 g, which costs $18,000 per life-year saved.

## COMMUNITY NURSING PROCESS

In community nursing, the focus of the nursing process shifts from the individual child and family to the community or target population. The stages of the process (assessment, diagnosis, planning, intervention, and evaluation) are similar whether the client is one child or a population of children. Only the types of interventions and indicators of wellness and illness differ (Anderson and McFarlane, 2000). *Assessment* is focused on collecting subjective and objective information about the target population in order to *diagnose* problems based on community needs. *Planning* involves the development of community-centered *interventions.* The nurse works with the community to implement a program that enables members to reach their goals and to *evaluate* whether the goals were met. Community nursing is collaborative, and the nurse is one member of a community team that includes other health professionals, educators, politicians, religious leaders, members of public and voluntary organizations, and consumers. The role of the nurse depends on the scope of the project, the target population, and the expertise of team members. For instance, the school nurse may assume a leadership role in planning for the health needs of elementary school children and serve as a panel member on a citywide committee assessing environmental pollution.

# Community Needs Assessment

The assessment phase of the community nursing process is called a *community needs assessment.* Assessment involves the collection of subjective and objective information about a community. Subjective information indicates what community members say are their most important needs and can be determined in a number of ways. One way is to distribute questionnaires to a sample of people living in the community. Another way is to interview community members directly, phoning or meeting with individuals, such as community leaders, who represent the group or who have a special role in the group.

The nurse collects objective information, or data, either by direct observation or through written sources. A windshield tour is one method of direct observation. Nurses drive through a neighborhood and take notes about the environment, including the appearance of houses, the presence of sidewalks and gutters, the number of public areas, etc. Objective information about the health status of the community can also be obtained from such sources as the Chamber of Commerce, census bureaus, libraries, state health departments, and the internet sites of voluntary health organizations and government agencies. Information about service agencies can be found in resource directories compiled by such organizations as the United Way, and population-specific books provided by public and voluntary agencies.

One way to organize an assessment is to use a guide that lists community systems that need to be examined. This process is similar to using a physical assessment guide to examine the different body systems in an individual patient. Anderson and McFarlane (2000) described eight community systems that the nurse should examine: health and social services, communication, recreation, physical environment, education, safety and transportation, politics and government, and economics. During the assessment the nurse studies how well each component in the community functions/interacts to meet the health needs of children. The nurse also identifies the strengths of the community and determines whether any barriers prevent access to care for children and their families.

Once the assessment is completed the community nurse collaborates with team members to analyze the results of surveys and questionnaires, determines if the needs described by community members can be met by existing community agencies, and identifies individuals at highest risk. During the analysis the demographic characteristics and the morbidity and mortality rates in the community are compared to a standard. Comparisons can be made on the basis of time or place. In time comparisons, the nurse contrasts the rates in the current year with the rates during an earlier period. In place comparisons, the nurse contrasts the rates in the community with a standard population. Standard rates may come from another community or from city, state, or national rates. For example, the rate of tuberculosis in a group of preschool children in the *community* in 2002 could be compared to the rate of tuberculosis in preschool children in the *state* in 2002.

A *community health diagnosis* is the reflection of health status, risks, or needs as determined by a causative agent. The format of a community diagnosis is similar to an individual nursing diagnosis in that it identifies a problem (need) and the etiology related to that problem (causative agent). An example of a community nursing diagnosis is "Child abuse related to a violent environment" (Visiting Nurses Association, 1986).

# Community Planning

The nurse collaborates with community members in developing a plan that addresses the needs and problems of the target population. In order to maximize the use of community resources, problems should first be prioritized on the basis of their severity, the felt needs of the community, and the ability of the community nurse to bring about change. Once the problems are prioritized, the nurse works with community members to develop at least one goal for each problem the members will address. *Goals* are outcomes that give direction to interventions and provide a measure of the change the interventions produced. Community interventions frequently take the form of *health programs* for improving the health status of the target population. Community health programs are based on three levels of prevention: primary, secondary, and tertiary. For example, a goal for preventing bicycle injuries is, "Within 1 year all students in the first grade will wear bicycle helmets." The nurse and community members then plan a program that includes a health education program about bicycle safety for students and their parents (primary prevention).

The planning group considers the resources that are already available in the community and those that will be needed for implementing a health program, including personnel, supplies and equipment, office space, phones, and computers. Decisions are made about the timeline of the program, the budget, and strategies that can be used to obtain funding. The nurse may also contact health professionals who have implemented successful programs in other communities; they can provide valuable time-saving tips and suggestions. Program descriptions are found through professional contacts, online resources, and literature reviews. An example of a community assessment and planning project is presented in Box 4-3.

# Community Implementation

During program implementation the nurse and community members carry out the intervention. Whether the program is simple or complex, oversight is needed to ensure that everyone involved is communicating with each other, following the guidelines of the plan, keeping within the timeline, and documenting daily activities and expenses. The documentation will prove invaluable during the evaluation phase of the process.

# Community Evaluation

Evaluation identifies whether the goals and program objectives are met. Various models of program evaluation exist. A structure, process, and outcome method is commonly used by health care organizations. Donabedian (1980) described this approach as:

- *Structure:* Where and by whom is the care delivered in a program?
- *Process:* Was the care delivered using operational standards and within the financial guidelines of the program?
- *Outcome:* What was the impact to health status? Was there an improvement?

Structure focuses on the qualifications of personnel; the adequacy of buildings, offices, supplies, and equipment;

and the characteristics of the target population. Process focuses on the interaction of patients and providers. Process indicators include the number of people who attend a health education program, the number of pamphlets distributed, and the efficiency of the program. Outcome focuses on whether program objectives and community goals were met. Program evaluation should be ongoing so that performance improvement initiatives are monitored and so that an improvement in the way health care is delivered will affect the health status of the target population.

---

## Box 4-3 ■ ■ ■
### Example of Community Assessment and Planning

Sabine is an elementary school with 500 prekindergarten to sixth-grade children. The school nurse has been asked to conduct an assessment of the school community and to develop a plan of care. The school children and their families are the target population.

#### COMMUNITY NEEDS ASSESSMENT

The school nurse formed a team of community members that included parents of students who attend Sabine Elementary School, faculty and staff, health care professionals, local religious leaders, and politicians. The group met at regularly scheduled intervals. Their first task was to complete the community assessment. Team members mailed questionnaires to a random sample of families who had children attending Sabine. They held focus groups with community members to obtain subjective information about the needs of the school community. Team members obtained objective data from the local health department, school records, and the U.S. Census Bureau. The nurse also conducted a windshield tour of the neighborhood surrounding the school. The following information was collected:

*People:* Sabine is located in an ethnically diverse area composed of 30% Hispanics, 30% African-Americans, 30% non-Hispanic whites, and 10% Asians. The ethnicity of students in the school is representative of the surrounding area. Sabine is located in a large southwestern city.

*Safety and Transportation:* School bus service was rated very good to excellent by a majority of those surveyed. Transportation records indicated that the last school bus accident occurred 1 year ago. There were no fatalities, but a number of children were injured. Other accidents occurred 2 years and 10 years prior to the most recent accident.

*Economics:* Although 94% of families had at least one fully employed member, 25% of the families lived below the poverty level. The number below poverty level had not changed in 10 years.

*Education:* Sixty percent of the adult population had a high school diploma, and 10% of this group had completed at least 1 year of college. School attendance at Sabine was higher than overall state attendance rates.

*Communication:* Ninety-five percent of homes had telephones compared with 85% 10 years ago. An estimated 10% of the target population did not speak English, and Spanish was the primary language spoken in this group.

*Recreation:* Few places were available for small children to play. The focus groups recommended more parks and playgrounds.

*Politics and Government:* The school system was strongly centralized and headed by a school superintendent. The city had a mayor and city council.

*Social:* Of those families living below the poverty level, 60% received some type of welfare assistance, including food stamps. The school lunch program served 95% of the children attending the school.

*Health:* The childhood immunization rate for all diseases among children in the community who were 2 years of age was 90%, compared with the national level of 75% (Teitelbaum and Edmunds, 1999). The immunization rate for children attend-

ing Sabine Elementary School was 100%. Vision and hearing screening programs at Sabine resulted in the referral of 5% of the students for vision problems and 2% of the students for hearing problems. Review of student records indicated that all those children referred received diagnostic follow-up and treatment when indicated. Heights and weights were obtained on all students annually and the Body Mass Index (BMI) was determined for each student. BMI is calculated by dividing the weight in kilograms by the square of the height in meters (Flegal and others, 1998). Results indicated that 30% of students were above the 95th percentile for age and sex compared with 11% nationally (Ludwig, Peterson, and Gortmaker, 2001). In focus groups, students and teachers noted that school breakfasts and lunches were high in carbohydrates and fats. They also observed that decreased recess time resulted in decreased student activity during school hours.

Based on the above assessment, the following community diagnoses were made:

1. Increase in injuries related to school bus accidents.
2. Increase in obesity among students compared to the national standard related to high intake of calories and sedentary lifestyle.

#### PLANNING

Team members agreed that the number of school bus accidents should be closely monitored over the next 5 years. However, there was a consensus that increased obesity among students was the priority problem, and the team developed the following *goals:* (1) within 2 years the percentage of students with BMIs above the 95th percentile for age and sex will be 20% and (2) within five years that percentage will be 10%.

Team members reviewed the literature for examples of communities that had experienced similar problems, contacted school and health department officials in other areas of the country, examined the results of successful programs, and planned a health program that addressed the unique needs of the target population. The program was entitled "Sabine Excels in Health." *Program activities* were (1) each September the nurse will address the school's parent association about the program and will discuss the importance of a healthy diet and exercise for all family members, (2) every month teachers will set aside 1 hour to talk with their students about healthy food choices and about the importance of limiting television viewing time, (3) within 6 months school administrators and community members will petition the city to provide a neighborhood park, (4) within 1 year the school dietitian will assess the nutritional value of the current school meals and, if indicated, revise the meal plan to ensure a healthy diet, and (5) within 1 year the school will develop a plan to allow a minimum of 30 minutes of unrestricted play during the school day.

Team members determined the resources needed to implement the program, including personnel, supplies, and equipment. They estimated the total cost of setting up the program and maintaining it for 5 years and applied for funding to the school district and to the city and state health departments. The school nurse and other team members assumed responsibility for the timely implementation and evaluation of the "Sabine Excels in Health" program.

## KEY POINTS

- Caring for children within a community requires a multidisciplinary approach.
- Healthy communities provide children with not only quality medical care but also a nurturing, safe place to live and grow.
- Community health nursing focuses on promoting and maintaining the health of individuals, families, and groups in the community setting.
- Individuals, families, and communities may have demographic characteristics that affect their risk for disease or injury.
- Epidemiology is the science of population health applied to the detection of morbidity and mortality in a population.

- Community health programs are based on three levels of intervention: primary, secondary, and tertiary.
- Economic evaluations provide objective information to establish the value of a program to society.
- A community needs assessment involves collection of subjective and objective information about the community.
- A community health diagnosis is similar to a nursing diagnosis, identified by a problem with defined etiology.
- Program planning and implementation in the community require collaboration between the nurse and community members who are in positions to promote change.
- Evaluation of effective community programs includes consideration of the structure, process, and outcomes of the program.

## REFERENCES

Allender JA, Spradley BW: *Community health nursing: concepts and practice,* Philadelphia, 2001, Lippincott Williams & Wilkins.

American Nurses' Association: *Standards of community health nursing practice,* Kansas City, MO, 1986, The Association.

Anderson ET, McFarlane JM: *Community as partner: theory and practice in nursing,* Philadelphia, 2000, JB Lippincott.

Brosnan CA, Swint JM: Cost analysis: concepts and application, *Public Health Nurs* 18(1):13-18, 2001.

Clayton EW: What should be the role of public health in newborn screening and prenatal diagnosis? *Am J Prev Med* 16(2):111-115, 1999.

Clemon-Stone S, McGuire SL, Eigsti DG: *Comprehensive community health nursing,* St Louis, 1998, Mosby.

Donabedian A: *The definition of quality and approaches to its assessment,* Ann Arbor, MI, 1980, Health Administration Press.

Drummond MF and others: *Methods for the economic evaluation of health care programmes,* ed 2, New York, 1997, Oxford University Press.

Flegal KM and others: Overweight and obesity in the United States: prevalence and trends, *Int J Obes Relat Metab Disord* 22(1):39-47, 1998.

Flynn BC, Ivanov LL: Health promotion through healthy cities. In Stanhope M, Lancaster J: *Community and public health nursing,* St Louis, 2000, Mosby.

Gebbie KM, Hwang I: Preparing currently employed public health nurses for changes in the health system, *Am J Public Health* 90(5):716-721, 2000.

Gold MR and others: Identifying and valuing outcomes. In Gold MR and others, editors: *Cost-effectiveness in health and medicine,* New York, 1996, Oxford University Press.

Health Resources and Services Administration: *The registered nurse population,* Rockville, MD, 2001, US Department of Health and Human Services.

Hennekens CH, Buring JE: *Epidemiology in medicine,* Boston, 1987, Little Brown & Company.

Institute of Medicine: *The future of public health,* Washington, DC, 1988, National Academy Press.

Institute of Medicine: *America's children: health insurance and access to care,* Washington, DC, 1998, National Academy Press.

Kwon C, Farrell PM: The magnitude and challenge of false-positive newborn screening test results, *Arch Pediatr Adoles Med* 154:714-718, 2000.

Leavell HR, Clark EG: *Preventive medicine for the doctor in his community: an epidemiologic approach,* ed 3, New York, 1965, McGraw-Hill.

Ludwig DS, Peterson K, Gortmaker SL: Relation between consumption of sugar-sweetened drinks and childhood obesity: a prospective, observational analysis, *Lancet* 357:505-508, 2001.

McKeown RE, Weinrich SP: Epidemiologic applications. In Stanhope M, Lancaster J: *Community and public health nursing,* St Louis, 2000, Mosby.

Ortega NA and others: The impact of a pediatric medical home on immunization coverage, *Clin Pediatr* 39:89-96, 2000.

Smith GD: Learning to live with complexity: ethnicity, socioeconomic position, and health in Britain and the United States, *Am J Public Health* 90:1694-1698, 2000.

Teitelbaum MA, Edmunds M: Immunization and vaccine-preventable illness, United States, 1992 to 1997, *Stat Bull Metrop Insur Co* 80(2):13-20, 1999.

Tengs TO and others: Five hundred life-saving interventions and their cost-effectiveness, *Risk Anal* 15(3):369-390, 1995.

Visiting Nurse Association of Omaha: *Client management information system for community health nursing agencies,* Rockville, MD, 1986, US Department of Health and Human Services.

Wilson JMG, Jungner G: Principles and practice of screening for disease, *Public Health Papers 34,* Geneva, 1968, World Health Organization.

Wilson T: Economic evaluation of a metropolitan-wide, school-based hepatitis B vaccination program, *Public Health Nurs* 17(3):222-227, 2000.

**Internet Resources**

American Public Health Association: *www.apha.org/*

Children Now, Report Card Guide. *www.childrennow.org/report_guide.html*

Community County Data: *www.communityhealth.hrsa.gov/*

Healthy Communities: *www.healthycommunities.org*

Healthy People 2010: *www.health.gov/healthypeople/*

Kids Count Data, Annie E. Casey Foundation: *www.kidscount.org/*

Medical Matrix, clinical medical resources: *www.medmatrix.org/*

National Safe Kids Web Site: *www.safekids.org*

PubMed, the search service for the National Library of Medicine: *www.ncbi.nlm.nih.gov/PubMed/*

US Census Bureau, national and state census information: *www.census.gov/*

US Department of Education: *www.ed.gov/*

US Department of Health and Human Services: *www.os.dhhs.gov/*

World Health Organization: *www.who.int/*

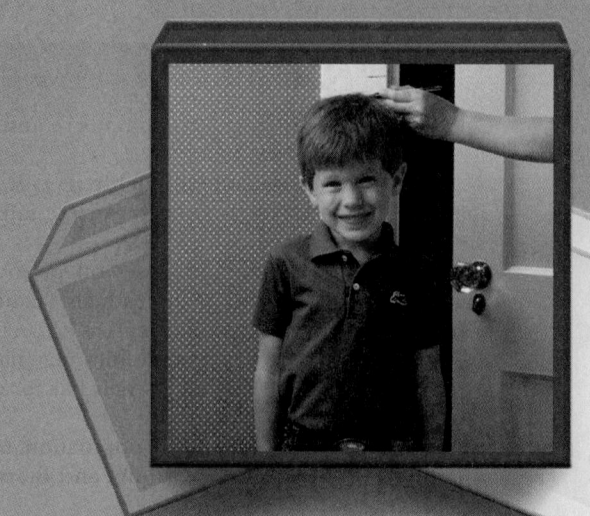

# Chapter 5

# Hereditary Influences on Health Promotion of the Child and Family

## Chapter Outline

**GENETIC INFLUENCES ON HEALTH, 110**
**Heredity in Health Problems, 111**
**Congenital Malformations, 111**
**Chromosome (Cytogenetic) Disorders, 113**
Causes of Chromosome Defects, 113
Errors in Cell Division, 114
Autosomal Chromosome Abnormalities, 116
Sex Chromosome Abnormalities, 116
**Single-Gene (Monogenic) Disorders, 118**
Autosomal Inheritance Patterns, 118
X-Linked Inheritance Patterns, 120
**Gene Variation and Nontraditional Inheritance, 121**
**Mitochondrial Disorders, 122**
**Hereditary Cancer Genes, 122**

**Cytogenetic and Molecular Genetic Diagnosis, 123**
Cytogenetic Diagnostic Techniques, 123
Molecular Diagnostic Techniques, 123
**Multifactorial Disorders, 124**
Disorders of the Intrauterine Environment, 124
**Therapeutic Management of Genetic Disease, 124**
Therapeutic Modalities, 124
Environmental Manipulation, 125
**IMPACT OF HEREDITARY DISORDERS ON THE FAMILY, 125**
**Genetic Screening, 125**
Purposes of Screening, 125

Significance of Screening to Families, 127
**Prenatal Diagnosis, 128**
Indications for Prenatal Testing and Types of Procedures, 128
**Genetic Evaluation and Counseling, 130**
Clients, 130
Counseling Services, 131
Estimation of Risks, 131
Interpretation of Risks, 131
**Role of Nurses in Genetic Counseling and Referral, 132**
Taking a Family History, 133
Follow-Up Care, 134
Supportive Counseling, 135
Burden of Genetic Defect, 136
Barriers to Effective Counseling, 137

## Related Topics

Abnormal Sexual Development, Ch. 11
Birth of a Child with a Physical Defect, Ch. 11
Cleft Lip and/or Cleft Palate, Ch. 11
Communicating with Families, Ch. 6
Cranial Deformities, Ch. 11
Cystic Fibrosis, Ch. 32
Defects in Physical Development, Ch. 11
Down Syndrome, Ch. 24

Family-Centered Care of the Child with Chronic Illness or Disability, Ch. 22
Fetal Alcohol Syndrome, Ch. 11
Fragile X Syndrome, Ch. 24
Guidelines for Communication and Interviewing, Ch. 6
Hypertrophic Pyloric Stenosis, Ch. 33

Malformations of the Central Nervous System, Ch. 11
Multiple Births, Ch. 3
Muscular Dystrophies, Ch. 40
Phenylketonuria, Ch. 9
Retinoblastoma, Ch. 36
Skeletal Defects, Ch. 11

## GENETIC INFLUENCES ON HEALTH

With the beginning of the new millennium we have witnessed the completion of the international Human Genome Project (HGP) to map and sequence the human genome. The information from this project about the 3 billion base pairs of the human genome will open the possibility of changes in every aspect of biology and medicine and have a major impact on health care in the future (International Human Genome Sequencing Consortium, 2001).

■ This chapter was revised by Susan Fernbach RN, BSN.

Much effort is being focused on identifying gene variations. Although as a human species we are 99.9% alike, it may be the 0.1% variation that will help us understand the genetic risk for illnesses. It is hoped that treatment strategies can be devised that are specific to an individual's disease mutation. Another new field of study created by the HGP is the study of how inheritance affects the body's responses to drugs, called *pharmacogenetics*. The hope is that better, safer, and in some cases more powerful drugs can be developed. The information from the HGP may influence more areas than we can currently imagine. Because of this, part of the total budget for the project was allotted to the Ethical, Legal, and Social Implications (ELSI) program to deal with the new genetic information. Research by the ELSI has focused on issues such as genetic discrimination, privacy, and education. It will continue to look at new issues generated by information about our human genome.

Nurses will increasingly be faced with interpreting genetic information in client histories and diagnostic testing, and with assuming responsibility for protecting client privacy (Scanlon and Fibison, 1995). To better counsel families and to anticipate likely problems, the nurse needs a fundamental understanding of the principles of genetics and the importance of heredity and the prenatal environment as etiologic factors in diseases and disorders of childhood. Key terms for understanding genetics are defined in Box 5-1.

## Heredity in Health Problems

Contained within the nucleus of every somatic cell in the human body are approximately 35,000-70,000 *genes,* the genetic material responsible for programming the body's physiologic process and characteristics (International Human Genome Sequencing Consortium, 2001). These genes are composed of segments of DNA (deoxyribonucleic acid) and are organized into structures called *chromosomes,* which are visible only during certain stages of cell division. Alterations of a whole chromosome, a part of a chromosome, or even a single gene can manifest as a genetic disorder. Important to this concept is that this alteration or mutation may have been passed from one or both parents and previous generations, or it may be a new alteration in that individual. It is misleading to regard all genetic disorders as having been "passed through the family."

There is probably a genetic component in all disease processes. In some disorders the genetic defect is known; in others the precise nature of the genetic component is more obscure. In some the disorder is apparent at birth; in others the manifestations do not appear for weeks, months, or years (Table 5-1). Some diseases and disorders are determined by the genetic constitution of the individual, such as muscular dystrophy, Marfan syndrome, and Down syndrome. Other diseases, although genetically determined, do not become clinically apparent until environmental factors precipitate the onset of symptoms. For instance, phenylketonuria is a disorder in which the enzyme to metabolize the protein phenylalanine is lacking. Deleterious effects in the infant are exhibited subsequent to sufficient ingestion of phenylalanine-containing substances, such as milk. Also, the acute symptoms of sickle cell disease are precipitated by certain conditions such as lowered oxygen tension, infection, or dehydration.

Another area in which this interplay of genetic and environmental factors is being investigated is cancer genetics. All cancer is genetic in the sense that cancer cells result from a "sporadic" gene malfunction (acquired mutation). However, only 5% to 10% of all cancers are inherited, which means the gene mutation that predisposes to cancer development was present in the germline. Therefore the individual is prone to cancerous development much earlier in life.

| TABLE 5-1  Characteristic age of onset for manifestations of some genetic diseases | |
| --- | --- |
| **Age of Onset** | **Condition** |
| Lethal during prenatal life | Some chromosome aberrations |
| | Some gross malformations |
| Birth | Congenital malformations |
| | Chromosome aberrations (e.g., Down syndrome) |
| | Some forms of adrenogenital syndrome |
| | Some forms of deafness |
| Soon after birth | Phenylketonuria |
| | Galactosemia |
| | Cystic fibrosis (sometimes) |
| | Maple syrup urine disease |
| Infancy | Sickle cell anemia (sometimes later) |
| | Tay-Sachs disease |
| | Werdnig-Hoffman disease |
| Early childhood | Cystic fibrosis |
| | Duchenne muscular dystrophy |
| | Fragile X syndrome |
| Near puberty | Limb-girdle muscular dystrophy |
| | Some forms of adrenogenital syndrome |
| | Turner syndrome |
| Young adulthood | Acute intermittent porphyria |
| | Hereditary juvenile glaucoma |
| Variable-onset age | Diabetes mellitus (0 to 80 years) |
| | Huntington chorea (15 to 65 years) |
| | Myotonic dystrophy (birth to old age) |

Other disorders result primarily from environmental factors. These include most infectious diseases and trauma. Development of the disease depends on environmental contact with the etiologic agent, but there is strong evidence to indicate a decided genetic element in the susceptibility to most diseases (e.g., tuberculosis, poliomyelitis, and measles in some populations).

Genetic diseases can usually be classified into one of the following broad categories according to the hereditary factors that produce the observed effect: cytogenetic, mitochondrial, monogenetic, or multifactorial. Prenatal environmental influences, such as alcohol exposure and placental abnormalities, are also regarded as being within the realm of genetics because these effects can produce congenital structural, functional, or growth defects. In such cases the chromosomes would be normal although anomalies produced might be indistinguishable phenotypically from a genetically determined anomaly. The important difference is that the defects would not be inheritable because they would not have been caused by a genetic mutation.

## Congenital Malformations

The development of an organism, especially during embryogenesis, is an intricate process in which all parts must be properly integrated to ensure a coordinated whole. The rate must be such that one part is ready when needed by another part; otherwise, either part may cease to grow or may deviate from its normal path. *Congenital anomalies,* or *birth defects,* occur in 2% to 4% of all liveborn children and can

---

**Box 5-1** ■ ■ ■
**Key Genetic Terms**

**Allele**—Alternative forms of a gene occupying same locus on homologous chromosomes

**Association**—Nonrandom cluster of malformations without a specific etiology (e.g., CHARGE or VATER association)

**Autosome**—Chromosome other than a sex (X or Y) chromosome; in normal human cells there are 22 pairs of autosomes and 2 sex chromosomes

**Carrier**—Person who possesses one copy of affected gene and one copy of unaffected gene and is clinically unaffected; however, may have clinically affected offspring because of expansion of mutation, X-linked expression, or recessive pairing with another

**Chromosome aberration**—Addition, loss, or structural abnormality of a chromosome; detectable by cytogenetic analysis

**Congenital**—Condition present at birth, although may not be apparent; causes may be genetic, nongenetic, environmental, or multifactorial

**Cytogenetics**—Study of relationship of microscopic appearance of chromosomes and their behavior during cell division to genotype and phenotype of individual

**Deformation**—Fetal abnormalities due to extrinsic factors (e.g., uterine position); may also show subsequent defects

**Deoxyribonucleic acid (DNA)**—Two-stranded molecule that contains the genes or blueprints responsible for the structure and function of living organisms and allows the transmission of genetic information from one generation to the next
  *Nuclear DNA (nDNA)*—Located in the nucleus of the cell; it contains blueprints for the cells that make up the body
  *Mitochondrial DNA (mtDNA)*—Located in the mitochondria or powerhouse of each cell

**FISH analysis**—Fluorescent in situ hybridization, a process by which chromosomes or portions of chromosomes are painted with fluorescent molecules; technique is useful for identifying chromosomal microdeletions

**Gamete**—One of two cells produced by a gametocyte, male (spermatozoon) and female (ovum), whose union in sexual reproduction initiates development of a new individual

**Genes**—Genetic material (DNA) responsible for programming body's physiologic functions and characteristics

**Genome**—Complete genetic information of an organism, usually described as total number of base pairs; human genome contains 3 billion base pairs

**Genotype**—Genetic constitution that determines the physical and chemical characteristics of an individual

**Germ cell**—Sperm or ovum with DNA complement of 23 unpaired chromosomes

**Human Genome Project**—International research project to map each human gene and sequence the human genome

**Imprinting**—Phenomenon in which an allele at a given locus is altered or inactivated, depending on whether it is inherited from mother or father; implies a functional difference in genes inherited from the two parents and explains some variation in expression

**Inherited (heritable, hereditary)**—Genetic transmission of a particular quality or trait from parent to offspring

**Malformation**—Morphogenic defect of organ, part of organ, or larger region of the body resulting from intrinsically abnormal developmental process
  *Major malformation*—Structural abnormality with serious medical, surgical, or cosmetic consequences
  *Minor malformation*—Has no serious consequences or is normal variation (e.g., extra nipple or umbilical hernia)

**Meiosis**—Cell division that results in reproductive cells (gametes) containing a complement of 23 unpaired chromosomes

**Microdeletion**—Chromosome deletion too small to be detected by standard cytogenetic techniques; can be detected by FISH analysis, which is a molecular cytogenetic technique

**Mitochondrion**—Part of the cell that is responsible for converting nutrients into energy as well as many other specialized tasks; mitochondria are the only part of the body known to have their own separate and unique DNA; mtDNA is inherited exclusively from the mother

**Mitosis**—Cell division resulting in two daughter cells identical to parent cell in chromosome complement (23 pairs) and genetic information

**Monogenetic**—Genetic disease caused by single-gene mutation

**Monosomy**—Chromosome abnormality in which one chromosome of a pair is missing; most monosomies are nonviable

**Mosaicism**—Condition in which an individual harbors two or more genetically distinct cell lines (generally, one cell line is normal and one is abnormal); results from a genetic change after formation of a zygote (i.e., postzygotic event)

**Multifactorial**—Complex interaction of both genetic and environmental factors that produces an effect on individual

**Mutation**—*Structural* or *chemical* alteration in genetic material that when changed remains changed and is transmitted to future generations; usually occurs naturally *(spontaneous)*, or can be *induced* by a variety of external agents, or *mutagens,* including temperature, certain chemicals, and radiation

**Mutation**—*Hereditary* change in genetic material; can be either change in single gene or change in chromosome characteristics; gene mutations can be passed from parent to offspring or can be new mutation in an individual, which is then heritable in offspring

**Nondisjunction**—Failure of two chromatids or two homologous chromosomes to separate during cell division, so that both members of a pair pass to new cell, resulting in trisomy of that chromosome pair, or monosomy in cell that does not receive chromosome

**Pedigree**—Diagram of genetic family tree

**Penetrance**—Frequency with which a heritable trait is manifested in individuals carrying gene

**Phenotype**—Clinically exhibited physical or chemical characteristics of individual; produced by interaction of environment with genotype

**Polygenic**—Inheritance involving many genes at separate loci whose combined, additive effects produce a given phenotype

**Proband (index case)**—Affected individual (regardless of sex) through whom family comes to attention of investigator

**Recessive**—Refers to a gene that produces its effect (is expressed) only when it is present in homozygous state

**Somatic cell**—Body tissue cells with DNA complement of 46 chromosomes

**Sporadic**—Birth defect or disorder occurring as a new case in a family and not inherited

**Syndrome**—Recognized pattern of malformations with a single, specific etiology (e.g., Down syndrome)

**Translocation**—Transfer of all or part of a chromosome to a different chromosome following chromosome breakage; can be balanced, producing no phenotypic effects, or unbalanced, producing severe or lethal effects

**Trisomy**—Condition in which there are three, rather than two, copies of one chromosome in same cell

**X inactivation (Lyon hypothesis)**—In normal female most of genes on one of X chromosomes are inactivated during early embryonic development, such that alleles on active chromosome are allowed full expression

**X-linked**—Refers to gene located on X chromosome and to specific mode of inheritance of such genes

**Zygote**—Conjugation of male and female gametes

arise at any stage of development. There is wide variability in etiologic factors, as well as in type, extent, and frequency of defects. Some defects result when a state present in one phase of development as a normal condition persists into another phase as abnormal. For example, a cleft lip is normal in a young embryo, and a patent ductus arteriosus is essential during fetal life. Any agent that interferes with these complex processes will produce a defect in development ranging in severity from an insignificant local anomaly to complete degeneration.

A few congenital defects are clearly caused by a single gene mutation, some are associated with chromosome abnormalities, and others are produced by known intrauterine environmental factors. However, many of the more common and severe defects (e.g., pyloric stenosis, central nervous system malformations, cataracts, and congenital heart disease) appear to be consistent with multifactorial inheritance.

The types of malformations that can result from genetic and/or prenatal environmental causes can be *major structural abnormalities* with serious medical, surgical, or quality-of-life consequences, or they can be *minor anomalies* or *normal variants* with no serious consequences, such as a sacral dimple, an extra nipple, or an umbilical hernia. Malformations can occur in isolation, such as congenital heart defect, or multiple anomalies may be present. A recognized pattern of malformations due to a single specific cause is called a *syndrome,* such as Down syndrome or fetal alcohol syndrome. A nonrandom pattern of malformations for which an etiology has not been determined is called an *association,* such as *VATER* (vertebral defects, imperforate anus, tracheoesophageal fistula, and radial/renal defects) association. Neural tube defects, cleft lip and/or cleft palate, deafness, congenital heart defects, and mental retardation are examples of anomalies that can occur in isolation or as part of a syndrome or association and can have different etiologies, such as single-gene or chromosome abnormalities, prenatal exposures, or multifactorial causes.

## Chromosome (Cytogenetic) Disorders

*Chromosome* or *cytogenetic disorders* are deviations in either structure or number of a chromosome; the consequences in either situation can be readily observed in the affected individual and are often severe or even lethal. The reason for this is that a numerical or structural chromosome abnormality involves a duplication or loss of at least a few genes, or up to thousands of genes. Although the types of cytogenic disorders are not as varied as those caused by a single gene, the incidence for many of the specific abnormalities is significantly higher than that for any of the single-gene (monogenic) disorders.

A *structural abnormality* involves loss, addition, rearrangement, or exchange of some of the genes of a chromosome. If there is sufficient remaining genetic material to render the organism viable, structural alterations can produce an endless variety of clinical manifestations. These deviations are usually a result of an error in cell division in the sperm or ovum that resulted in that individual, but the parents are chromosomally normal.

Sometimes, however, the chromosome abnormality can be inherited from a parent who is a balanced translocation carrier. Also, fragile, or weak, sites have been identified on both autosomes and on the X chromosome. An X-chromosome fragile site has been associated with physical and mental abnormalities termed *fragile X syndrome.* (See Chapter 24.)

Another relatively rare structural abnormality that can occur is a *ring chromosome.* If a break occurs in the terminal end of both arms of a chromosome, the ends may fuse together, forming a circle. Like any structural alteration of a chromosome, the clinical manifestations depend on which genes are lost.

The normal number of chromosomes in a somatic cell is 23 pairs, or 46 total. Deviations in chromosome number involve the gain or loss of a chromosome and are designated with the suffix *-somy*. A cell that contains one fewer than the total number of chromosomes is called a *monosomy* because of the loss of one member of a chromosome pair; a cell that contains one more than the total number of chromosomes resulting from the addition of an extra member to a normal pair is called a *trisomy*. A number of deviations compatible with life occur in humans, especially those involving the sex chromosomes; the more serious outcomes are related to abnormalities of the autosomes. Trisomies are the chromosome aberrations encountered most commonly by health care workers. Monosomies may occur as often in conceptuses but are usually nonviable. A relatively rare but clinically recognized variation is triploidy, in which there are three chromosomes in every pair, so that the total chromosome number is 69. This condition is lethal in early infancy.

The clinical consequences that attend variations in chromosome number frequently consist of discrete, identifiable syndromes, particularly in regard to the trisomies (see Tables 5-2 and 5-3). The chromosome structural anomalies form a more diverse group of reported physical deviations with few recognized syndromes. Some of the chromosome disorders, such as Down syndrome, can be identified on the basis of physical characteristics but require chromosome analysis to rule out the less common situation of translocation Down syndrome.

### Causes of Chromosome Defects

There is considerable speculation regarding the precise cause of chromosome errors. Ionizing radiation—especially large doses or from occupational exposure—has been found to be a cause of chromosome breaks, rearrangements, and nondisjunction. Autoimmune diseases appear to have a role in the pathogenesis of nondisjunction during cell division. Viruses have also been implicated, especially in relation to chromosome breakage. However, only germ cell chromosome errors or breaks have the potential to cause chromosome abnormalities in offspring. Somatic errors do not have reproductive consequences.

Most of the information regarding factors that cause chromosome errors is related to parental age. The incidence of trisomic births corresponds strongly with increasing maternal age, regardless of the number of pregnancies. For example, the risk for trisomy 21, or Down syndrome, increases dramatically for mothers more than 35 years of age. (See Down Syndrome, Chapter 24.) There is no positive explanation for this observation. However, throughout a lifetime the germ cells are vulnerable to a variety of exogenous influences and to the normal effects of the aging process. Increasing paternal age is not associated with most chromosome abnormalities (Michelena and others, 1993), but it is associated with an increased risk for new mutation cases of autosomal dominant disorders, such as skeletal dysplasias.

## Errors in Cell Division

The process by which chromosomes are distributed to the daughter cells during cell division is very complex and therefore prone to error. These errors can occur during *gamete formation (meiosis)* or in early *postzygotic cell division (mitosis)*. The resulting unequal distribution of genetic material may involve the gain or loss of a whole chromosome or part of a chromosome.

The most common cause of numeric chromosome abnormalities is the process of nondisjunction during cell division. *Nondisjunction* is the failure of separation of homologous chromosomes during meiosis I (Fig. 5-1, *A*) or of sister chromosomes during meiosis II (Fig. 5-1, *B*) or mitosis (Fig. 5-1, *C*). The term *sister chromatid* refers to the pair of strands that constitute a metaphase (a stage of mitosis) chromosome. This failure to separate can result in one or both members of the pair not passing (segregating) to either daughter cell. Nondisjunction can involve either the autosomes or the sex chromosomes. If nondisjunction takes place at meiosis I, the gamete will contain both the maternally and the paternally derived

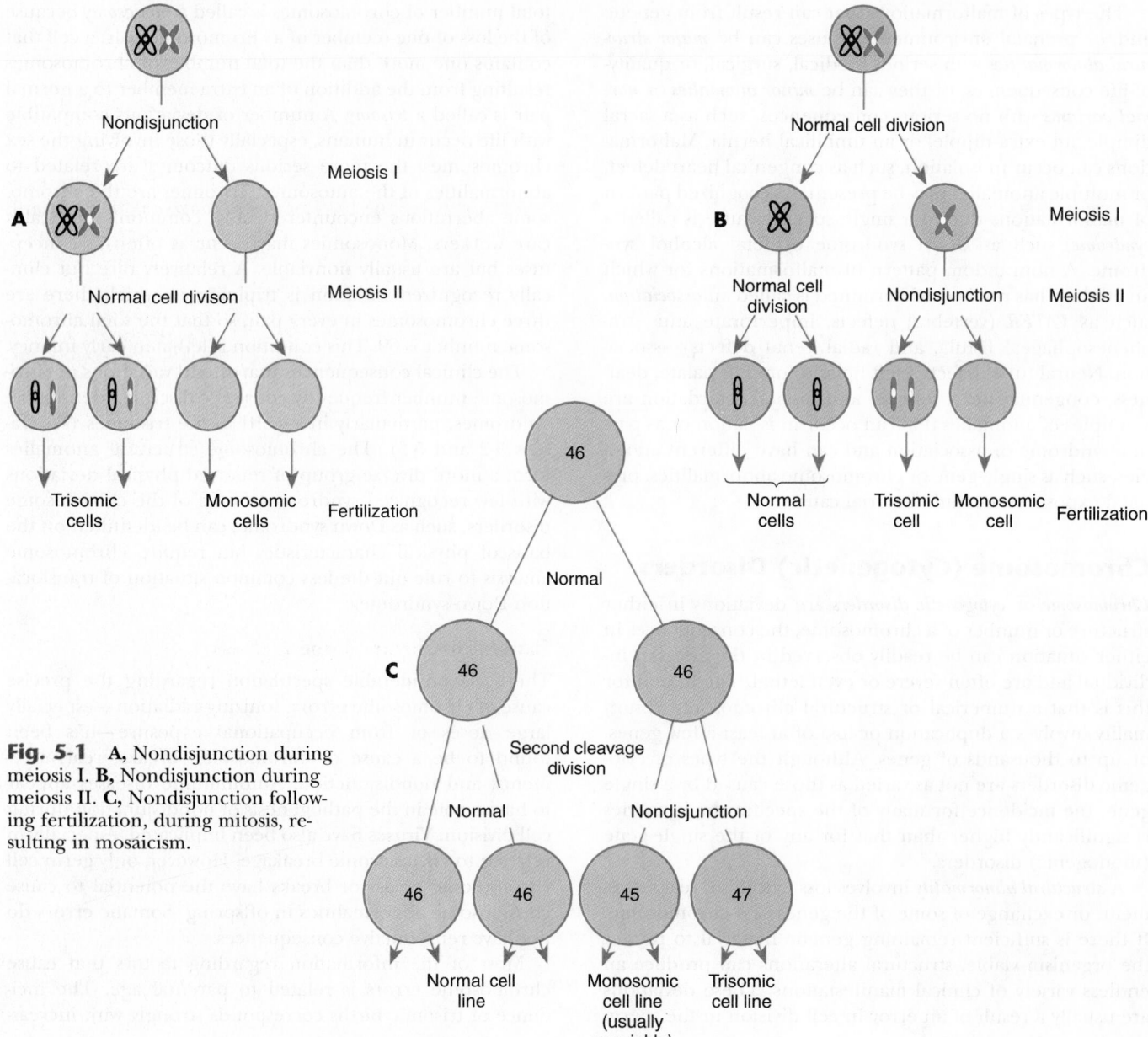

**Fig. 5-1** **A,** Nondisjunction during meiosis I. **B,** Nondisjunction during meiosis II. **C,** Nondisjunction following fertilization, during mitosis, resulting in mosaicism.

chromosomes of the pair involved. If it occurs at meiosis II, the gamete will contain a double complement of either the maternal or the paternal chromosome. In either case the resulting gamete will have too many or too few chromosomes. If this gamete is fertilized with a sperm or ovum with a normal chromosome complement, the resulting fetus will be either trisomic (3) or monosomic (1) for the chromosome pair involved. Monosomies are usually not viable, with the exception of monosomy X (Turner syndrome).

*Mosaicism* is the presence of two or more chromosomally distinct cell lines, usually one normal and one abnormal. This situation occurs when nondisjunction occurs in the later cell divisions (postzygotic) of a chromosomally normal fertilized egg. The abnormality may be either numeric or structural, although numeric mosaicism is the most common type seen clinically. Postzygotic mitotic nondisjunction results in a fetus with two or more cell lines. This early cell division error following fertilization is the most common cause of mosaicism and usually results in a normal and trisomic cell line, although results showing a mosaic Turner syndrome (normal and monosomic X cell line) are seen (see Fig. 5-1, *C*). The percentage, or level, of mosaicism depends on the stage of embryonic development in which the cell division error occurs. If it occurs at the first cell division after fertilization, the level of mosaicism may be as high as 50%. If the cell division error occurs in later development, the abnormal cells may be localized to one cell type, such as the brain tissue or germ cell line (ovaries or testes). The extent of clinical manifestations is determined by the type of tissues that contain cells with abnormal chromosome numbers and the percentage of affected cells, and may vary from near normal to a fully manifested syndrome.

Placental tissue is commonly found to be mosaic and may determine the viability to term of fetuses with chromosome abnormalities. It is now understood that different cells can have different percentages of mosaicism; for example, a parent's germline cells (which produce the sperm and egg) may be mosaic, but other tissues (e.g., skin, blood [somatic cells]) may be normal. Therefore, a phenotypically normal parent could test negative for a mutation from the DNA of the lymphocytes yet carry the gene mutation in his or her germ cell line, with all the attendant risks of transmission. Different percentages of mosaicism in different tissues can also explain variable phenotypic expression.

X inactivation also produces a functional mosaicism. It is also now known that not all of the second X chromosome is inactivated and that inactivation is not random, which further explains variable phenotypic expression in regard to genes on the X chromosome.

A *translocation* is a structural abnormality that involves an exchange of genetic material between two or more chromosomes. A simple translocation results when a break occurs in one arm of each of any two nonhomologous (not paired) chromosomes and the segments below or above the break points change places. A variation of this occurrence, called a *robertsonian translocation,* occurs between acrocentric chromosomes: group D (13, 14, 15) and group G (21, 22). In an *acrocentric chromosome,* the centromere is near one end, so that one arm is much longer than the other. Translocations between those groups involving the No. 21 chromosome can result in an inherited form of Down syndrome, called *translocation Down syndrome,* which accounts for approximately 4.7% to 6.7% of cases (Fig. 5-2).

If there is essentially no loss or gain of genetic material in the exchange, the translocation is **balanced,** or **reciprocal.** Carriers of a balanced translocation are phenotypically normal and occur with a frequency of about 1 in 600 in the general population. These carrier individuals (either male or female) may pass the translocation to their offspring in a balanced or unbalanced form, depending on how the chromosomes segregate to the gametes. If it is passed in the **unbalanced** form, the combination is often lethal, and an early spontaneous abortion occurs. However, the risk of having a liveborn offspring with birth defects associated with the unbalanced translocation is 5% to 20%. Approximately 5% of cases of repeated spontaneous abortion (two or more) can

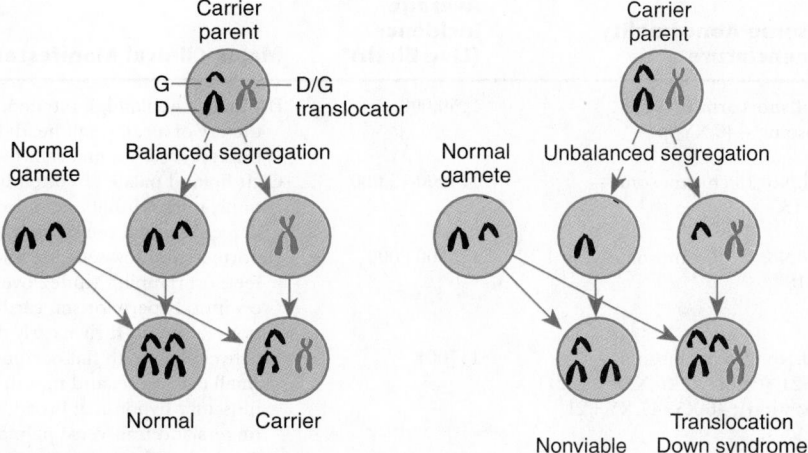

**Fig. 5-2**  Possible offspring from mating of somatically normal carrier of D/G translocation with genetically and somatically normal individual. *D/G,* Translocated chromosomes D and G.

be attributed to a balanced translocation carrier parent. Unlike nondisjunction, translocations are not related to increasing maternal age. Translocations, balanced or unbalanced, can be passed from a carrier parent or be *de novo* (arising as a new change), which subsequently can be passed to future offspring.

## Autosomal Chromosome Abnormalities

Both numeric and structural abnormalities of autosomes account for a variety of syndromes usually characterized by mental deficiencies. A few are associated with a group of characteristics that clearly indicate the precise chromosome anomaly. The first and the most common disorder in which an associated chromosome abnormality was demonstrated is Down syndrome. (See Chapter 24.) The most viable trisomies are trisomy 21 (Down syndrome), trisomy 18 (Edward syndrome), and trisomy 13 (Patau). Nurses often note dysmorphic facial features (Table 5-2), behavioral characteristics such as an unusual cry and poor feeding behavior, and other neurologic manifestations such as hypotonia or abnormal reflex responses, which may alert them to these and other chromosome abnormalities.

*Partial chromosome abnormalities* involve a missing (deletion) or extra (duplication) segment of a chromosome. The features of classic deletion and contiguous gene (microdeletion and microduplication) syndromes are usually less recognizable at birth. Phenotypic effects of these syndromes may include a cluster of known single-gene disorders. The *classic deletion syndromes* can be detected on a routine chromosome analysis and include cri-du-chat (Table 5-2), Wolf-Hirschhorn, and chromosome 18 deletions. *Contiguous gene syndromes* are disorders characterized by a microdeletion or microduplication of smaller chromosome segments, which may require special analysis techniques or molecular testing to detect (Torra and others, 1998). Microdeletion syndromes are more common and may have more clinically obvious phenotypic ef-fects than microduplication syndromes. Examples of these syndromes include Prader-Willi, Angelman (see p. 122), DiGeorge, and Beckwith-Wiedemann.

## Sex Chromosome Abnormalities

The possible mechanisms by which sex chromosome abnormalities may occur are the same as those previously described (i.e., prefertilization nondisjunction during one of the meiotic divisions of gametogenesis in either parent or in the early postfertilization divisions of the zygote). An alteration in the number of sex chromosomes usually does not produce the profound effects that are associated with the autosomal trisomies. Intelligence may be normal or low-normal, or the child may have some learning disabilities, but moderate or severe mental retardation is less common.

*Turner syndrome* (45, X) is essentially the only viable monosomy. It is still extremely lethal prenatally, with 99% of these fetuses being spontaneously aborted. Most girls have one +X chromosome missing from all cells (45, X). Some have mosaic cell lines with some cells 45, X and others 46, XX. The syndrome should be suspected in the newborn period by the presence of lymphedema of the hands and feet and a low posterior hairline, in childhood by a webbed neck and short stature, and at puberty by delayed development and primary amenorrhea (Table 5-3 and Fig. 5-3). The reason for the growth retardation is unknown. The child's growth is usually normal until 3 years of age and then slows, gradually drifting away from the normal growth curve. There is no prepubertal growth spurt, and girls with Turner syndrome are generally infertile. These girls may have difficulty with peer relationships and with understanding social cues. They may exhibit behavioral problems, especially in relation to immature, socially isolated behavior. Most, however, lead productive lives and function as independent adults.

*Klinefelter syndrome*, the most common of all sex chromosome abnormalities, is caused by the presence of one or

---

**TABLE 5-2   Common autosomal aberrations**

| Syndrome | Chromosome Abnormality and Nomenclature | Average Incidence (Live Birth)* | Major Clinical Manifestations |
|---|---|---|---|
| Cri-du-chat | Deletion of short arm of No. 5 chromosome—46,XY,5p− | 1:50,000 | Distinctive weak, high-pitched, mewlike cry resembling the cry of a cat; small head; hypertelorism; failure to thrive; severe mental retardation—profound with age |
| Trisomy 13 (Patau) | Trisomy of No. 13 chromosome—47,XY,+13 | 1:4000-15,000 | Cleft lip and palate (frequently bilateral); ear malformations; microphthalmia; polydactyly; eye defects; cardiac defects; mental retardation; early death |
| Trisomy 18 (Edward) | Trisomy of No. 18 chromosome—47,XY,+18 | 1:3500-8000 | Deformed and low-set ears; micrognathia; rocker-bottom feet; overlapping (index over third) fingers; prominent occiput; hypertelorism; cardiac defects; mental retardation; failure to thrive; early death |
| Trisomy 21 (Down) | Trisomy of No. 21 chromosome—47,XY,+21 (trisomy); 46,XY,+(14;21) (translocation); 46,XY/47,XY,+21 (mosaic) | 1:700† | Brachycephaly with flat occiput; inner epicanthal folds; small ears, nose, and mouth with protruding tongue; muscular hypotonia; broad, short hands with stubby fingers and transverse palmar crease; broad, stubby feet with wide space between big and second toes; cardiac defects; mental retardation; variable life expectancy |

*Data from Nora JJ, Fraser FC: *Medical genetics: principles and practice,* ed 4, Philadelphia, 1994, Lea & Febiger.
†Risk related to maternal age: age 30 years = 1:900; age 35 years = 1:300; age 40 years = 1:100; age 45 years = 1:30.

more additional X chromosomes. The majority of males with this syndrome have a chromosome complement of 47, XXY, but there are numerous variants in the number of extra sex chromosomes. There are no distinctive physical characteristics that are helpful in detecting Klinefelter syndrome before the advent of puberty. Mental impairment of varying degrees is a frequent finding and appears to have a direct relationship to the number of X chromosomes in the cells. The severity of retardation increases with the number of X chromosomes. Characteristic features of the Klinefelter syndrome are listed in Table 5-3 and shown in Fig. 5-4.

The milder physical and mental deficiencies of children with sex chromosome abnormalities compared with children with autosomal abnormalities are due in part to a phenomenon called *X inactivation* or *Lyon hypothesis.* In all body cells one X chromosome is biologically active; if more than one X chromosome is present, most (but not all, as previously thought) of the other(s) (Sack, 1999) are in some way "switched off," or inactivated, during the very early divisions of the zygote and remain so throughout life. Because of the milder effects of sex chromosome abnormalities, many individuals are phenotypically normal and may remain undiagnosed. Sex chromosome mosaicism occurs, which also accounts for some variation in phenotype. The aberrant social behavior described as typical of multiple-Y chromosome abnormalities is thought to have been exaggerated and is more limited to poor impulse control, hyperactivity, and learning disability.

Multiples of the X and Y chromosomes exist, in trisomic or greater numbers (see Table 5-3). Regardless of the number of X chromosomes, the presence of a Y chromosome appears to be a male determining factor. Therapy of sex chromosome disorders consists primarily of hormone treatment to initiate appropriate pubertal sexual development. Growth hormone therapy may be used in girls with Turner

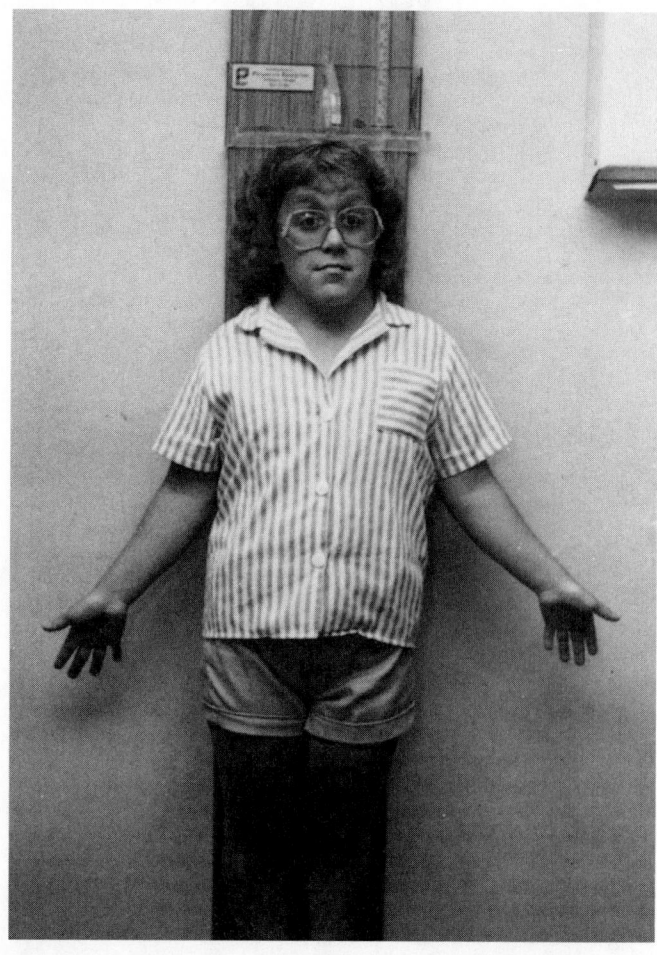

**Fig. 5-3** Turner syndrome in a young girl. Note short stature, webbed neck, increased abduction or carrying angle of forearms, and broad chest with no breast development. (From Hall R, Evered DC: *Color atlas of endocrinology,* ed 2, Chicago, 1990, Year Book Medical Publishers.)

| **TABLE 5-3** | **Common sex chromosome abnormalities** | | | |
|---|---|---|---|---|
| **Syndrome** | **Chromosome Nomenclature** | **Phenotype** | **Occurrence** | **Clinical Manifestations** |
| **Turner** | 45,X | Female | 1:2500 female births* | Short stature; webbed neck; low posterior hairline; shield-shaped chest with widely spaced nipples; usually infertile (see Fig. 5-3) |
| **Triple X** | 47,XXX (can also be 48,XXXX or 49,XXXXX) | Female | 1:850-1250 female births | Normal female characteristics; usually tall; variable mental capacity and behavior; at risk for impaired language, neuromotor problems, learning skills, and psychosocial adaptation; fertile |
| **Klinefelter** | 47,XXY (48,XXYY, 48,XXXY, 49,XXXXY, and so on, mosaics) | Male | 1:850 male births* | Tall with long legs; hypogenitalism; sterile; male secondary sex characteristics may be deficient; gynecomastia (30%); poor psychosocial adjustment (see Fig. 5-4) |
| **XYY male** | 47,XYY (can also be 48,XYYY or mosaic) | Male | 1:900 male births* | Usually normal sex development; tendency to be tall with long head; poor coordination; may demonstrate poor impulse control; at risk for learning disabilities |

*Data from Nora JJ, Fraser FC: *Medical genetics: principles and practice,* ed 4, Philadelphia, 1994, Lea & Febiger.

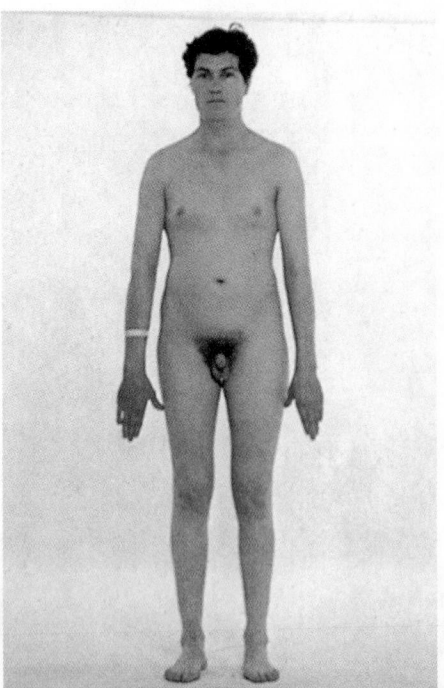

**Fig. 5-4** Klinefelter syndrome. Note these individuals are usually tall with evidence of primary gonadal failure. (From Hall R, Evered DC: *Color atlas of endocrinology,* ed 2, Chicago, 1990, Year Book Medical Publishers.)

syndrome to increase growth velocity and, hopefully, final height (Reiter and others, 2001).

## Single-Gene (Monogenic) Disorders

Disorders that are the result of a defect or mutation of a single gene, rather than a partial or whole chromosome abnormality, are called *single-gene disorders.* These disorders, which generally follow a simple, definite inheritance pattern, are rare individually, but collectively they constitute a significant portion of health problems seen in infants and children. They can involve any system in the body. They can

be of such minor importance that they have little effect on the child or be so severe as to cause serious disability or to be incompatible with life.

The defective or mutated gene cannot be diagnosed by chromosome analysis, because it is at a more basic level of the chromosome, that of the DNA structure. Diagnosis of a single-gene disorder is presented on p. 123. These disease-producing mutant genes are usually distributed or transmitted in families according to basic mendelian principles of dominant or recessive behavior on the autosomes or sex chromosomes (usually the X chromosome). Some generalizations can be applied to dominant and recessive inheritance patterns of the autosomes or sex chromosomes and the resultant diseases and malformations.

Some examples of single-gene disorders, including the inheritance pattern, basic defect, and manifestations, are outlined in Table 5-4.

A number of variables are observed in many disorders that modify the basic inheritance patterns. In addition, there are genetic phenomena that are not explained by traditional mendelian inheritance. These variations and concepts are discussed following presentation of traditional autosomal dominant, recessive, and sex chromosome X-linked patterns.

### Autosomal Inheritance Patterns

**Autosomal Dominant Inheritance.** Children with an autosomal dominant disorder have usually inherited it from an affected parent, although the parent's case may have been mild or undetected. When a first case in a family appears, it is usually as a result of a new mutation. It is being recognized, however, that in rare cases, especially when a second affected child is born, one parent could have germline mosaicism (i.e., the gene mutation for a disorder is only present in the egg or sperm cells). Depending on the degree of disability the condition imposes on the individual and the age of onset, the gene will either die out or continue to be passed on through several generations (Fig. 5-5). For example, Huntington disease, a progressive incapacitating and fatal neuromuscular disease, is usually not manifested until age 40 or later, after the affected person may

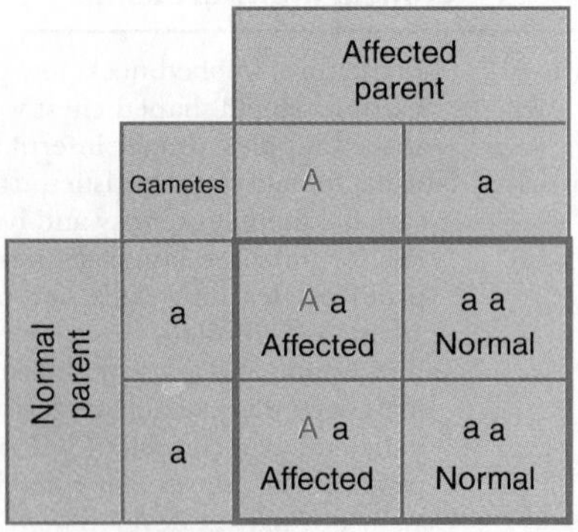

|  |  | Affected parent | |
|---|---|---|---|
|  | Gametes | A | a |
| Normal parent | a | A a Affected | a a Normal |
|  | a | A a Affected | a a Normal |

**Characteristics of autosomal dominant inheritance**

Males and females are affected with equal frequency.
Affected individuals will have an affected parent, although expression may be variable (unless the condition is caused by a new mutation or germline mosaicism).
Children of a heterozygous affected parent have a 50% probability of possessing the defective gene, although it may be nonpenetrant.
Children of affected parents who did not receive the affected gene will have unaffected children.
Traits can be traced vertically through previous generations—a positive family history—unless it is a new mutation, germline mosaicism, or nonpenetrant.
Autosomal dominant disorders are more common than recessive disorders and are usually less severe.

**Fig. 5-5** Possible offspring of mating between normal parents and one heterozygous for an autosomal dominant trait.

**TABLE 5-4**   Partial list of single-gene disorders

| Disease | Inheritance | Basic Defect | Manifestations | Therapy |
|---|---|---|---|---|
| Achondroplasia | Autosomal dominant, new mutation | Defect in ossification at epiphyseal plate (growth portion of bones) | Very short limbs; large head; lordosis | Supportive |
| Albinism (ocular) | Autosomal recessive | Deficiency of tyrosinase: failure to convert tyrosine to dopa, and, hence, lack of melanin synthesis | Lack of pigment in skin, hair, and eyes; eye defects | Symptomatic Avoid exposure to sunlight Ophthalmologic care |
| Cystic fibrosis (Ch. 32) | Autosomal recessive | Defect in pancreatic enzymes | Abnormal secretions; chronic pulmonary disease; malabsorption | Symptomatic, enzyme therapy |
| Fragile X syndrome (Ch. 24) | X-linked dominant | Unknown | Long face; large ears; large testicles; mental retardation | Symptomatic |
| Galactosemia (Ch. 9) | Autosomal recessive | Defect in galactose metabolism | Hypotonia; vomiting; hepatosplenomegaly; cataracts | Galactose-free diet |
| Hemophilia A (Ch. 35) | X-linked recessive | Defect in factor VIII production | Hemorrhage into tissues, joints after injury | Factor VIII replacement therapy |
| Hypothyroidism (familial) | Autosomal recessive | Deficiency of iodotyrosine deiodinase | Lethargy; stunted growth; mental retardation | Early administration of thyroid hormone |
| Maple syrup urine disease | Autosomal recessive | Defective metabolism of branched-chain amino acids | Onset in early infancy; neurologic disorders; odor of urine similar to that of maple syrup | Diet low in branched-chain amino acids |
| Marfan syndrome (arachnodactyly) | Autosomal dominant, new mutation | Defect in elastic fibers of connective tissues | Tall and thin, with long tapering fingers; poorly developed musculature; associated defects include aortic aneurysm, dislocation of optic lens, winged scapula | Supportive Surgical correction of deformities |
| Muscular dystrophy (Duchenne) (Ch. 40) | X-linked recessive, new mutation | Protein dystrophin is absent | Muscular atrophy; progressive deterioration of motor function and mental development | Symptomatic |
| Myotonic dystrophy | Autosomal dominant | Defective calcium metabolism in nerve and muscle cells | Hypotonia; characteristic facial features; respiratory distress; poor feeding; high-arched palate; cataracts; severe neonatal form leads to early death | Symptomatic |
| Neurofibromatosis (von Recklinghausen disease) (Ch. 18) | Autosomal dominant, new mutation | Defect in neural cells— exact mechanism unknown | Café-au-lait spots; multiple fibromas; neurologic and ophthalmologic defects; skeletal anomalies | Symptomatic, surgical removal of tumors |
| Noonan syndrome | Autosomal dominant | Unknown | Small stature; shield-shaped chest; webbed neck; low posterior hairline; narrow maxilla; low-set ears; ptosis; hypertelorism; cardiac anomalies (pulmonic stenosis) | Correct cardiac anomalies Supportive |
| Osteogenesis imperfecta (Ch. 39) | Autosomal dominant, new mutation | Defect in production of type 1 procollagen | Fragile, short, bowed bones; blue sclera; hyperextensible joints; hearing loss | Symptomatic, surgical orthopaedic procedures |
| Phenylketonuria (Ch. 9) | Autosomal recessive | Defect in phenylalanine metabolism | Eczema; poor feeding; seizures; musty smell to urine; mental retardation | Low-phenylalanine diet |
| Tay-Sachs disease (amaurotic familial idiocy) | Autosomal recessive | Deficiency of hexosaminidase; defect in synthesis of gangliosides | Predominantly in Ashkenazi Jews; progressive neurologic deterioration; blindness, cherry red spot in macula; early death | Supportive |
| Thalassemias (Ch. 35) | Autosomal recessive | Defect in synthesis of one or more globin chains of hemoglobin | Anemia; hepatosplenomegaly; thinning of bones | Symptomatic, transfusions |
| Wilson disease | Autosomal recessive | Failure of biliary excretion of copper, leading to copper toxicity | Liver failure; speech abnormalities; tremors; psychiatric and behavior problems | Chelation agents, treatment of liver disease |

have passed on the defective gene to offspring. Incomplete penetrance of autosomal dominant disorders is common, and there is wide variability in expression. Regardless of penetrance or variable expression in the parent, there is a 50% risk of passing on the defective gene to offspring, where it may be fully expressed. Other examples of autosomal dominant disorders include achondroplasia, neurofibromatosis, and Marfan syndrome.

**Autosomal Recessive Inheritance.**   Children who display an autosomal recessive disorder will always be homozygous

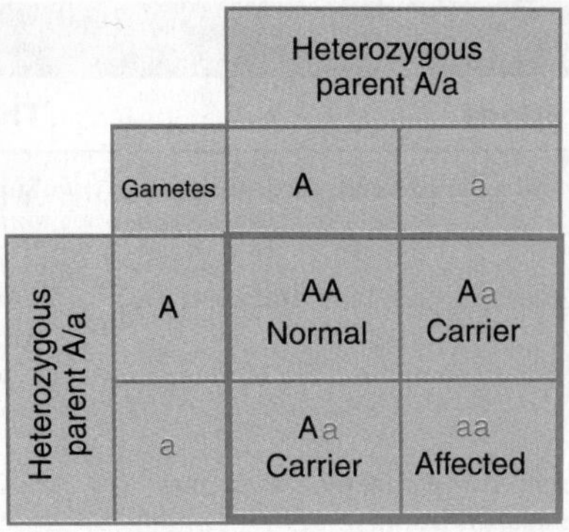

### Characteristics of autosomal recessive inheritance

Males and females are affected with equal frequency.
Affected individuals will have unaffected parents who are heterozygous for the trait.
There is a 1 in 4 (25%) chance that any child of two unaffected heterozygous parents will be affected.
Unaffected siblings of an affected person have a ⅔ risk of being a carrier.
Affected individuals mated to normal individuals will have normal children, all of whom will be carriers.
There is usually no evidence of the trait in previous generations—a negative family history—unless consanguinity is a factor.

**Fig. 5-6** Possible offspring of mating between two parents with a recessive gene on an autosome.

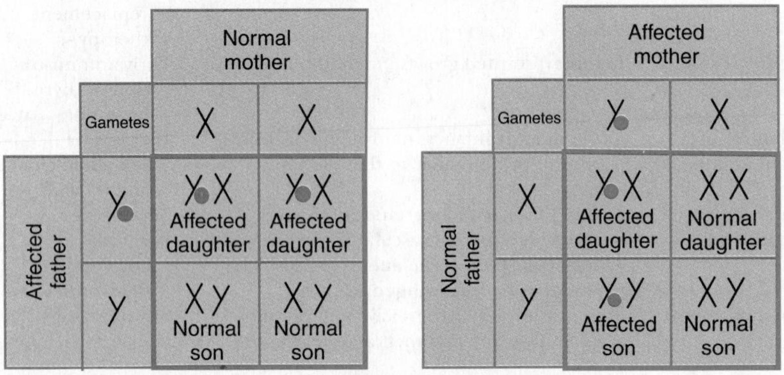

### Characteristics of X-linked dominant inheritance

Affected individuals will have an affected parent.
All the daughters but none of the sons of an affected male have the probability of being affected (although usually more mildly).
Half the sons and half the daughters of an affected female will be affected.
Normal children of an affected parent will have normal offspring.
There are no carriers (although expression may vary).
The inheritance pattern shows a positive family history.

**Fig. 5-7** Sex differences in offspring ratios in X-linked dominant inheritance. *Solid circle,* Dominant allele on X chromosome.

for that trait. The heterozygous person, with only one gene for a rare recessive disorder, remains undetected in the population (Fig. 5-6). It is estimated that each person carries from three to eight genes for a severe genetic disease. For example, 1 in 20 persons in the U.S. and Northern European populations carry the recessive gene for cystic fibrosis. In the African-American population, 1 in 10 persons is a carrier for the sickle cell gene. For phenylketonuria the general population carrier rate is 1 in 50. However, the probability of the mating of two persons who carry the same gene is highly unlikely. The chances are increased if the mating occurs in persons who select a mate because of geographic, ethnic, or religious restrictions or blood relationship *(consanguinity)*. For example, 1 in 30 Ashkenazi Jews is a carrier of the Tay-Sachs disease gene. The age of onset for autosomal recessive disorders is early, and, because they are usually biochemical defects, heterozygote detection and prenatal diagnosis are often possible. Other examples of autosomal recessive disorders include the thalassemias, congenital adrenal hyperplasia, galactosemia, and cystic fibrosis.

### X-Linked Inheritance Patterns

Genes on the X chromosome differ from those on the Y chromosome; therefore the transmission of traits caused by these genes will vary according to the sex of the individual who carries the gene. The two X chromosomes in the female are alike in gene constitution, with two genes for each trait. Genes on the X chromosome have no counterpart on the Y chromosome; therefore a characteristic determined by a gene on the X chromosome is *always* expressed in the male. One of the most significant aspects of X-linked inheritance is the absence of father-to-son transmission. Although it is essential for development of the male phenotype, the Y chromosome carries no known medically significant characteristics.

**X-Linked Dominant Inheritance.** Superficially this pattern resembles an autosomal dominant inheritance pattern (Fig. 5-7). This type of inheritance is relatively uncommon. An example of an X-linked dominant disorder is hypophosphatemic vitamin D–resistant rickets. The inheritance pattern of fragile X syndrome is complex and may not follow the standard X-linked pattern.

**X-Linked Recessive Inheritance.** The abnormal gene behaves as any recessive gene would; that is, its effect is hidden by a normal dominant gene. Therefore, two recessive genes are usually present if manifestations in the female are seen (Fig. 5-8). This rare situation would require the father to be affected and the mother to be a carrier. However, unequal X inactivation can also produce manifestations in a carrier female. New mutations are not uncommon. Examples of X-linked recessive disorders include hemophilia types A and B and Duchenne muscular dystrophy.

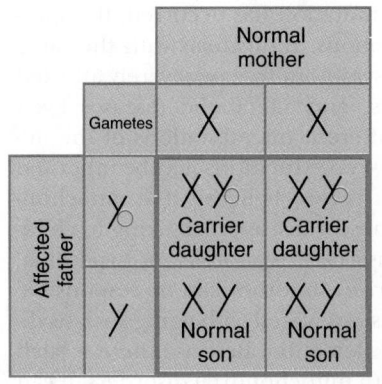

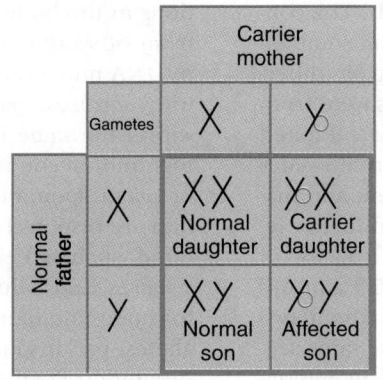

**Characteristics of X-linked recessive inheritance**

Affected individuals are principally males.
Affected individuals will have unaffected parents (except in the rare possibility that the father is affected and the mother is a carrier).
Half the female siblings of an affected male have the probability of being carriers of the trait.
Unaffected male siblings of an affected male cannot transmit the disorder.
Sons of an affected male are unaffected.
Daughters of an affected male are carriers.
The unaffected male children of a carrier female do not transmit the disorder.

**Fig. 5-8**  Sex differences in offspring ratios in X-linked recessive inheritance. *Open circle,* Recessive allele on X chromosome.

## Gene Variation and Nontraditional Inheritance

A number of variables have been observed that explain or modify basic inheritance patterns and the effects of chromosome abnormalities. Some of these variations have been recognized for some time; others are newly discovered phenomena that explain some apparent contradictions in the established patterns of inheritance. Some of the variations involve individual genes, and others involve whole-chromosome behavior but will still affect manifestation of single-gene disorders. Also, some disorders have been reported to follow more than one inheritance pattern in different families (e.g., a classically recessive disorder may occasionally be reported as following a dominant or X-linked pattern in other families).

The most notable of these gene variations is mutation. A *mutation* is any heritable change in the DNA sequence of a gene. Mutations can be a deletion, duplication, or alteration in the base pair sequence (Sack, 1999). A mutation may cause the protein made by that gene to be produced in an altered, less functional form; to be produced in a decreased amount; or to be entirely absent. A gene mutation may have occurred generations ago and be passed down unchanged until it dies out because an individual does not reproduce, or a new gene mutation can occur spontaneously in an individual. Certain disease-producing gene mutations are known to be "old" mutations, such as the mutation that causes fragile X syndrome, and new mutations are seldom if ever identified. Other diseases are known to have a high new mutation rate, such as the 30% to 50% rate for neurofibromatosis and Duchenne muscular dystrophy. This type of definitive determination of a gene mutation is possible only for those single-gene disorders in which the gene site has been located and characterized. Some disorders previously described as exhibiting sporadic occurrence (e.g., Williams syndrome) not attributable to a traditional inheritance pattern may be new mutations with effects such that the individual does not reproduce and the mutation is not passed on to offspring.

*Variable expression* is an important concept that describes differences in the extent and severity of manifestations of genetic diseases. There is a continuum of expression for any affected person from undetectable (mild) to severe clinical manifestation. Therefore a phenotypically normal person may still possess the mutant gene. This situation most often applies to autosomal dominant disorders; for example, a parent of a child with neurofibromatosis may exhibit only a couple of café-au-lait spots. Genomic imprinting and X inactivation, discussed later in this section, may account for some variation in expression and *penetrance,* a term used less often as these new discoveries explain variation in phenotypic manifestation.

The discovery of a new type of mutation in some genetic disorders has helped explain their variation in inheritance patterns and clinical expression (Nelson, 1996). Within genes are sequences of **DNA nucleotide repeats.** A normal gene has a certain number of these repeats; for example, in the fragile X syndrome gene there are about 30 to 50 repeats. Some persons, however, have additional repeats of from 50 to 200, which have been termed **premutations.** These premutations in females are unstable and during meiosis can undergo amplification, expanding to hundreds more repeats, thereby becoming a full mutation and causing the offspring to be affected. Because fragile X is an X-linked disorder, females are less likely to be affected because of the tempering effect of the second X chromosome. These expanding repeats have also been found to occur in myotonic dystrophy, Huntington disease, and spinocerebellar ataxia, which are autosomally transmitted disorders. This expanding-gene discovery exhibits the old concept of **genetic anticipation,** in which certain dominantly inherited disorders to worsen or have an earlier age of onset with succeeding generations (Han and Peschel, 2000). It is believed that additional disorders may be discovered to exhibit this type of mutation. In fact, the first recessively inherited disorder to exhibit an expansion mutation is Friedreich ataxia (Chamberlain, 1996). This disorder usually demonstrates an onset in puberty or early adulthood, depending on the repeat size of the smaller of the two expansion alleles. Recent evidence suggests genetic anticipation may be a factor for the presence of father-son testicular tumors (Han and Peschel, 2000).

Genomic imprinting and uniparental disomy are two genetic phenomena that consider the parental origin of genetic information (i.e., maternally or paternally derived). The concept of *genomic imprinting* refers to modification, in some instances, of genetic material, resulting in phenotypic differences based on whether the genes/chromosomes were from the mother or the father. Genomic imprinting is exhibited during pregnancy, when paternally derived chromosomes seem to positively influence placental development and maternally derived chromosomes seem to positively influence fetal development. It has also been shown to be a factor in some genetic disorders, most classically Prader-Willi and Angelman syndromes. In both of these disorders, about two thirds of affected individuals have a deletion of the same segment of chromosome 15. However, the clinical manifestations of Prader-Willi and Angelman syndromes are markedly different. If the deletion occurs on the paternally derived chromosome 15, the child exhibits Prader-Willi syndrome; if the deletion occurs on the maternally derived chromosome 15, Angelman syndrome is manifested (Jorde, 2002).

*Prader-Willi syndrome* is characterized by central hypotonia, cognitive dysfunction, dysmorphic appearance, behavioral disturbances, hypothalamic hypogonadism, short stature, and obesity, as well as abnormal low body temperature, an increased tolerance to pain, and diminished salivation. In contrast, *Angelman syndrome* (also called happy puppet syndrome) includes severe mental retardation, characteristic facies, abnormal (puppetlike) gait, and paroxysms of inappropriate laughter. Children with Angelman syndrome are usually nonverbal, although they may vocalize (Fridman and others, 2000).

In some cases both copies of a chromosome pair are determined to have come from one parent, either the mother or the father, instead of one from each, a phenomenon called *uniparental disomy* (Fridman and others, 2000). Another example of uniparental disomy has been reported with cystic fibrosis, in which both chromosomes, each with a mutant recessive gene, came from the carrier mother; the father was not a carrier. In cases that appear to be nonpaternity, uniparental disomy may be a factor. One of the several theories about uniparental disomy is that the chromosome pair was originally a trisomy and the father's chromosome was randomly expelled, leaving two copies of the mother's chromosome. Because the chromosomes appear as a normal "pair," diagnosis of this situation is only possible with molecular (DNA) techniques. Uniparental disomy has also been reported with Beckwith-Wiedemann syndrome, which is characterized by overgrowth and hypoglycemia at birth.

## Mitochondrial Disorders

Mitochondrial DNA mutations also account for nontraditional inheritance patterns. Mitochondria are components of the cell cytoplasm involved in energy production.

They perform many different functions in different tissues of the body. They are the only cellular organelles to have their own DNA distinct from nDNA and inheritance is exclusively maternal. A defect in the mtDNA can lead to altered functions of the proteins in some or all of the cells. Because the mitochondria perform so many different functions in the body, when a mutation has occurred, the spectrum of symptoms is enormous. Individuals with the same mtDNA mutation may be symptom free or severely affected with seizures, pancreatitis, and metabolic disease. Even within the same family, different manifestations of the mitochondrial condition are seen. Mutations may be inherited or occur spontaneously. It is now believed that mitochondria are responsible not only for diseases occurring in childhood, such as Leigh disease (with symptoms of hypotonia, seizures, and failure to thrive), but they can be responsible for many common diseases associated with aging such as diabetes, parkinsonism, and dementia. Because there is such variability of expression with mitochondrial disorders, it can be very confusing to determine the diagnosis. However, when a child has an unexplained constellation of symptoms, a mitochondrial disorder should be considered.

Diagnosis of a mitochondrial disorder can be very difficult and therefore genetic counseling may be possible only in a small number of cases. Nuclear DNA mutations can also cause disorders of the mitochondria, and, with the advances in the detection of nDNA mutations, accurate diagnosis and therefore accurate information about recurrence risk and prenatal diagnosis is possible (Thorburn 2001). Currently, treatment for these disorders is symptomatic and some patients show benefits from vitamin and cofactor supplementation. Referral to mitochondrial support groups can be very helpful to parents.

## Hereditary Cancer Genes

As discussed earlier in this chapter, all cancers are "genetic." In DNA, cellular maintenance and repair genes inhibit abnormal cell growth that may become malignant (Williams, 1997). To lose this function, mutations must occur in both alleles of one of these genes. These mutations usually result from exposure to carcinogens, with exposure occurring over a lifetime. Only 5% to 10% of cancer occurs as a single gene abnormality, and in these hereditary cancer syndromes a person is born with a mutation already existing in one of the alleles. For this reason the cancer is much more likely to develop earlier in life. One of the cardinal clues to an inherited cancer syndrome is early onset.

Some of the inherited cancer syndromes for which DNA testing is available and medical surveillance and intervention is indicated in children include retinoblastoma, medullary thyroid carcinoma, familial adenomatous polyposis coli, multiple endocrine neoplasia, and Wilms tumor. Inherited cancer syndromes tend to follow an autosomal dominant inheritance pattern in families.

Testing may help identify family members who could benefit from medical intervention as well as those who do not need the expensive and uncomfortable screening tests. However, the benefits and risks of testing, confidentiality of results, and potential psychologic impact on the child need to be discussed with the parents before testing. Nurses play a key role in identifying and educating families with an increased cancer risk. Available testing can be discussed with these families, and they can be referred for genetic counseling.

# Cytogenetic and Molecular Genetic Diagnosis

## Cytogenetic Diagnostic Techniques

*Chromosome analysis* by *karyotyping,* a pictorial representation of the chromosomes matched by size and banding patterns into pairs from 1 to 22 (the twenty-third pair are the sex chromosomes) is the basis of genetic diagnosis (Fig. 5-9). Numeric and structural abnormalities such as trisomies and translocations are easily seen on chromosome analysis. The most common human cells used to analyze the chromosomes are skin tissue (including fetal skin cells), bone marrow and, most frequently, blood leukocytes obtained by venipuncture. The chromosomes are cultured and examined during mitosis, when they are most visible. Deletions, duplications, and translocations of larger segments of genetic material are visible on routine chromosome analysis. However, microdeletions, microduplications, and fragile sites usually require newer, enhanced resolution techniques that essentially "stretch out" the chromosome, thereby allowing detection of more subtle defects. Another new technique that has enhanced diagnosis of these subtle defects is *fluorescence in situ hybridization (FISH),* which uses radioactive or fluorescent probes in a variety of ways to identify chromosome and DNA abnormalities such as Williams and Prader-Willi syndromes.

## Molecular Diagnostic Techniques

Diagnosis of genetic disorders at the gene level has experienced remarkable advances in technique. Identification of single-gene mutations responsible for some genetic disorders is now possible as more and more genes are being *mapped* (located on a specific chromosome or segment of a chromosome) through efforts as part of the Human Genome Project. In some conditions, such as cystic fibrosis (CF), sickle cell disease, Huntington disease, and fragile

X syndrome, the specific gene/DNA mutations are known and can be detected directly. For other disorders, while the exact gene location is not known, the particular chromosome and specific segment are known. By using "linkage" studies and mapping techniques, the likelihood that an individual has inherited the same chromosome segment as a known affected member of the family can be determined. Use of these techniques allows not only diagnosis of an affected individual but also determination of carrier status and prenatal diagnosis (i.e., whether a fetus is normal, a carrier, or affected). There are over 200 diseases that can be diagnosed by direct or indirect (linkage) DNA testing (Box 5-2). DNA testing "enabling" technologies include Southern blotting and polymerase chain reaction (PCR) as the most common methods. Each method has advantages and disadvantages and is chosen depending on the characteristics of the mutation being tested.

### Box 5-2 ■ ■ ■
### Disorders Detected by DNA-Based Testing

| | |
|---|---|
| Achondroplasia | Huntington disease |
| Apert syndrome | Lesch-Nyhan syndrome |
| Becker muscular dystrophy | Maple syrup urine disease |
| Congenital adrenal hyperplasia | Marfan syndrome |
| Crouzon syndrome | Myotonic dystrophy |
| Cystic fibrosis | Neurofibromatosis type I |
| Duchenne muscular dystrophy | Osteogenesis imperfecta |
| Fragile X syndrome | Phenylketonuria (PKU) |
| Friedreich ataxia | Sickle cell disease |
| Gaucher disease | Spinal muscular atrophy |
| Hemophilia A (factor VIII deficiency) | Spinocerebellar ataxia |
| Hemophilia B (factor IX deficiency) | Tay-Sachs disease |
| | Thalassemia (alpha and beta) |
| | Tuberous sclerosis |

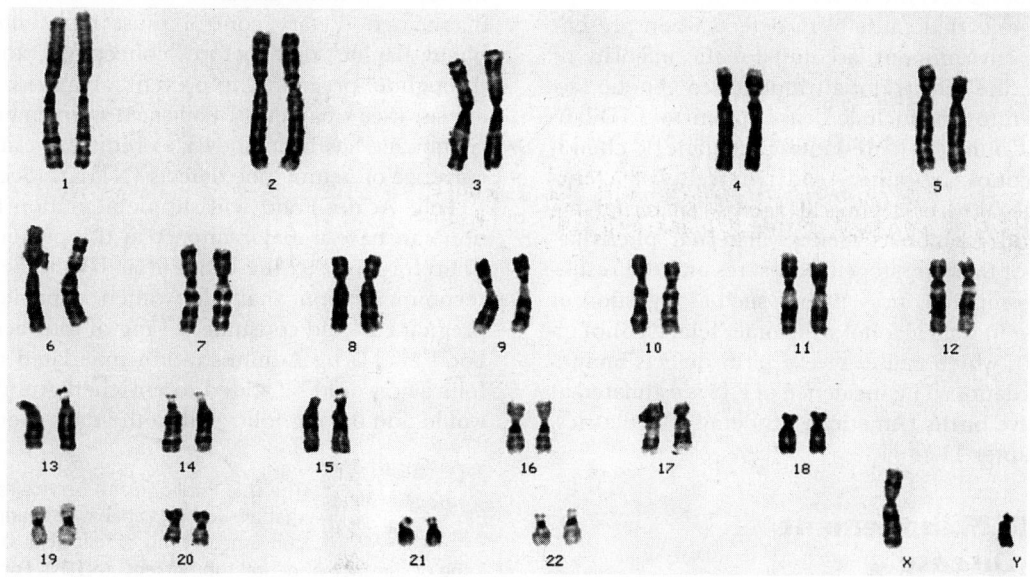

**Fig. 5-9**   Normal male karyotype. (Courtesy HA Chapman Institute of Medical Genetics, Tulsa, Oklahoma.)

## Multifactorial Disorders

A number of diseases and defects that are encountered frequently in the population show an increased incidence in some families but have no clear-cut affected-unaffected classification. Although the incidence is higher than would be expected by chance, no specific mode of inheritance can be identified. In some, environmental factors, including the prenatal environment, appear to play an important role. These conditions are classified as *multifactorial* disorders, in which a genetic susceptibility and appropriate environmental agents interact to produce a disease state. Diseases considered to be multifactorial (at least in isolation) include neural tube defects, cleft lip and cleft palate, many congenital heart defects, congenital hip dislocation, and pyloric stenosis. Determining risks of recurrence is more difficult than for single-gene disorders, but the risk is usually low, less than 10%. For example, anencephaly and/or spina bifida occur in 0.2 to 5 births per 1000 in the general population. The recurrence risk after the first affected child is 3% to 6%. Advances in genetics are enhancing knowledge of multifactorial inheritance to better understand familial risks.

### Disorders of the Intrauterine Environment

The prenatal intrauterine environment can have a profound and permanent effect on a developing fetus, even when chromosome or single-gene abnormalities are not present. Sometimes, however, intrauterine effects occur in tandem with genetic factors. Intrauterine growth retardation (IUGR), for example, can occur with many genetic syndromes, such as Down, Russell-Silver, Prader-Willi, and Turner syndromes (Behrman, Kliegman, and Jenson, 2000), or can occur from nongenetic causes such as maternal alcohol ingestion. Placental abnormalities are increasingly being found to be the etiologic factor in neurodevelopmental disorders (such as cerebral palsy and mental retardation) that were previously attributed to asphyxia during delivery (Bos, Einspieler, and Prechtl, 2001).

*Teratogens,* agents that cause birth defects when present in the prenatal environment, account for the majority of adverse intrauterine effects not attributable to genetic factors. Types of teratogens include drugs (phenytoin [Dilantin], warfarin [Coumadin], tretinoin [Accutane]); chemicals (ethyl alcohol, cocaine, lead); infectious agents (rubella, cytomegalovirus); physical agents (maternal hyperthermia); and metabolic agents (maternal phenylketonuria). Many of these teratogen exposures and the resulting effects are completely preventable, such as ingestion of alcohol resulting in fetal alcohol syndrome/fetal alcohol effects (FAS/FAE), which causes severe birth defects including mental retardation. The incidence of FAS is estimated at 5.2 per 10,000 live births (American Academy of Pediatrics, 2000). (See Chapter 11.)

## Therapeutic Management of Genetic Disease

There is no cure for genetic disease at present, although preventive and corrective therapy is helping to reduce the harmful effects in an increasing number of conditions. Genetic research is making progress in the art of altering the genetic material directly. Meanwhile, the major goal of therapy is modification of the internal or external environment to correct or minimize the effects of the genetic defect.

### Therapeutic Modalities

The therapeutic modalities available for genetic disorders are few when compared with the infinite variety of conditions afflicting the population, but with increased understanding of the basic defects and the technical advances being made, an increasing number of genetic disorders are becoming amenable to treatment.

**Surgical Repair.** Surgical repair of structural defects has made it possible to prolong life in a number of multifactorial disorders, such as congenital heart disease and pyloric stenosis. Numerous facial and limb deformities can be altered by plastic and reconstructive techniques. In cases of familial polyposis coli, surgical removal of the colon eliminates the countless polyps that invariably become cancerous. Splenectomy prevents the trapping of abnormal blood cells in that organ in several hereditary disorders of red blood cells. Early diagnosis and enucleation in retinoblastoma have reduced the mortality from this malignant eye tumor. Fetal surgery may also be performed for some life-threatening anomalies, particularly urinary tract abnormalities.

**Diet Modification.** For disorders in which an enzyme deficiency causes a toxic accumulation of a substance or its by-products, restricting the intake of foods containing the offending substance often prevents irreversible damage from the improper metabolism of these compounds, this dietary control is a life-long recommendation. Examples include the low-phenylalanine diet prescribed for children with phenylketonuria (PKU), elimination of dairy products containing lactose for infants and children with hereditary lactase deficiency, avoidance of foods containing or producing galactose for children with galactosemia, and a diet low in branched-chain amino acids for infants and children with maple syrup urine disease. Women with PKU who have not maintained dietary control must reinstitute a strict low-phenylalanine diet before conception and maintain it throughout pregnancy to prevent a high risk of adverse fetal effects. (See Chapter 9.) Folic acid supplementation preconceptionally has been shown to reduce the incidence or recurrence of neural tube defects (NTDs). (See Chapter 11.)

**Folic Acid.** Folic acid supplementation before conception can have a major impact in the prevention of NTDs. Therefore in 1992 the U.S. Public Health Service made the recommendation that all women capable of becoming pregnant should consume 0.4 mg of folic acid per day. The Food and Drug Administration mandated that as of 1998 folic acid would be added to enriched grain products. This would add 0.1 mg folic acid to the daily diet of the average

> **NURSING ALERT** The U.S. Public Health Service recommends that all women capable of bearing children consume 0.4 mg of folic acid daily to prevent the occurrence of neural tube defects (NTDs). For women who have previously had a pregnancy with an NTD, it is recommended that they consume 4.0 mg folic acid daily to prevent the recurrence of a NTD in a future child.

person. Since that time there has been a 19% reduction in the incidence of NTDs (Honein, 2001).

Women who have previously had a pregnancy affected with an NTD are advised to take 4.0 mg of folic acid per day beginning 1 month before conception and continuing throughout the first trimester of pregnancy. The risk of recurrence in another pregnancy affected by an NTD is reduced by 72% in women following this regimen.

**Product Replacement.** In some deficiency diseases, supplying the missing product that cannot be synthesized prevents undesirable effects. For example, thyroid extract is prescribed to prevent the damaging effects of hypothyroidism and providing the missing blood factors prevents life-threatening and debilitating hemorrhages in persons with hemophilia. Other examples are insulin for diabetes mellitus, growth hormone for growth hormone deficiency, and corticosteroids for adrenogenital syndrome.

**Avoidance of Drugs or Other Substances.** In drug-induced disease, such as glucose-6-phosphate dehydrogenase (G-6-PD) deficiency and the porphyrias, avoidance of the drugs that precipitate a reaction provides a simple preventive measure.

**Removal of Toxic Substances.** Removal of toxic substances that accumulate in vital tissues as a result of a hereditary disease can prevent disabling complications. Some of the deleterious effects of hemochromatosis, a hereditary disorder characterized by an excess accumulation of iron in the liver, heart, and pancreas, can be reduced with the removal of iron by administration of chelating agents or periodic phlebotomies.

**Immunologic Prevention.** The administration of immunoglobulin to Rh-negative mothers following the birth of an Rh-positive infant is effective in preventing Rh-antibody formation that causes hemolytic disease of the newborn in subsequent births.

**Transplantation.** Replacement of nonfunctioning organs with normal organs is increasing the survival of children with defective organs because the problems of tissue incompatibility are better controlled. Examples of organ transplants include the kidneys in hereditary polycystic kidneys, the heart in severe cardiac myopathy, the liver in hepatic atresia, and bone marrow.

**Cofactor Administration.** Diet supplements can be given when the body is unable to synthesize or effectively use some substances needed as cofactors in metabolism, such as vitamin $B_{12}$ in pernicious anemia, in which absorption of this vitamin is absent. Vitamin and cofactor supplementation may be used in the treatment of mitochondrial disease.

**Recombinant DNA.** The transfer of modified genetic material from one organism (a virus) to another causes the viral DNA to become integrated into the cellular DNA of a recipient cell, often a bacteria cell. This recombinant DNA multiplies, producing the missing substance in the host cell. This technology has been applied in growth hormone therapy and factor VIII synthesis.

**Gene Transfer.** Fragments of DNA from a normal gene can be introduced directly into a recipient cell lacking such a gene. This approach has been attempted in humans with the transfer of normal gene copies of β-hemoglobin into bone marrow cells in an effort to treat a form of β-thalassemia and

has been used in sickle cell disease. Gene transfer has also been successfully used in adenosine deaminase deficiency. Gene therapy research has suffered a number of setbacks in clinical research, and the search for safer, more effective ways to transfer genes into human cells continues.

**Other Therapies.** Other methods such as enzyme repression and competitive inhibition are providing effective treatment in some metabolic disorders. Growth hormone therapy is used in Turner and Noonan syndromes. Future therapies include the possibility of replacement or stabilization by injection or oral administration of a substance that the patient lacks.

### Environmental Manipulation

Inherited diseases or defects for which there is no therapeutic modality can be modified to enhance the quality of life for the affected individual. Some examples of environmental manipulation include hearing aids for deaf children, glasses or vision enhancers such as enlarged print and books in braille for the visually impaired, mobilizing devices such as braces and wheelchairs for persons with muscle and bone impairment, prosthetic devices for limb deficiencies, and infant stimulation programs to maximize the potential of children who are mentally retarded.

## IMPACT OF HEREDITARY DISORDERS ON THE FAMILY
### Genetic Screening

Tests to detect the presence of a defective gene are rapidly assuming greater importance in management of genetic disorders as more defects are identified and techniques are developed for easy application. It is probable that with improved technology, mass screening for numerous defects may eventually be a routine procedure. However, to be truly effective, screening programs depend on thorough education of both health professionals and the public regarding these programs and the limitations and implications of testing. The religious, moral, ethical, and legal issues revolving around screening and prenatal diagnosis are extensive and change over time (Farrell, 2001).

### Purposes of Screening

Genetic screening is presumptive identification of an unrecognized genotype in individuals or populations. There are several purposes for this screening: (1) to detect the presence of apparent or nonapparent disease, (2) to provide reproductive information, and (3) to gain information concerning the incidence of a disorder in the population

**Newborn Screening.** Newborn screening began in the 1960s when Dr. Guthrie devised the blood spot test to screen for PKU. Newborn screening for PKU was begun in all states, and currently each state offers screening for a number of additional disorders such as sickle cell anemia, galactosemia, hypothyroidism, congenital adrenal hypoplasia, and others. The disorders selected for newborn screening have been chosen because they meet the following criteria:

- The disease occurs with a significant frequency.
- An inexpensive and reliable method of testing exists.

- There is effective treatment and intervention.
- If untreated, the baby will die or be severely mentally retarded.
- An affected baby may appear normal at birth.

Because many of the conditions tested for are metabolic disorders, it is important that the first newborn screening blood sample be obtained at least 24 hours after the first protein feeding or within the first 72 hours of life. Infants found to be at high risk for a metabolic condition such as PKU or galactosemia are immediately referred to a medical center for testing to confirm the diagnosis and initiate treatment. (See Evidence-Based Practice box.) Mass screening programs have indicated that many disorders are more prevalent than formerly believed. Others that are included in some screening programs are congenital adrenal hyperplasia, maple syrup urine disease, sickle cell disease and other hemoglobinopathies, tyrosinemia, adenosine deaminase deficiency, and various other aminoacidurias and urea cycle disorders.

Newborn screening for CF has been controversial and is offered in only a few states. The Wisconsin Cystic Fibrosis Newborn Screening Project found that identification of affected newborns prevented severe malnutrition and improved long-term growth (Farrell, 2001).

A number of technologies are available for detecting disease—biochemical assays, protein iontophoresis, chromosome analysis, and testing with DNA molecular probes. It is sometimes recommended that the DNA of an affected child be banked and used to identify markers in other family members at a later date, such as in a subsequent pregnancy.

**Screening for Reproductive Information.** Screening for heterozygotes (carriers) can detect unaffected persons with certain genes who, when they mate with an individual who carries a similar gene, are at high risk of producing an affected offspring. These individuals are thus provided with the knowledge they need for use in decisions about family planning. Carriers of a number of diseases can be detected by laboratory tests, but, because of the rarity of these diseases, mass screening is not feasible except in persons or populations known to be at risk. Persons at risk include close relatives of those with an inborn error of metabolism or other detectable disorder, as well as certain ethnic populations known to have a high incidence of a specific disease, such as sickle cell anemia in African-Americans, Tay-Sachs disease in Ashkenazi Jews, and thalassemia in people of Mediterranean ancestry.

This type of screening is sometimes controversial. Screening for carrier status for CF is one such situation that has the potential to create ethical dilemmas. CF is caused by a gene mutation, but there are numerous variations that cause the same phenotypic effect. Only 90% of these mutations are known, meaning that an individual with a CF-causing gene mutation would not be identified as a carrier 10% of the time. Therefore, following screening, a couple may feel safe to proceed with pregnancy yet still have a child with CF. Other possible dilemmas with carrier status screening include marriage partner selection bias based on carrier status and misunderstanding of the implications of carrier status (i.e., that individuals are not affected themselves and that there is only potential risk

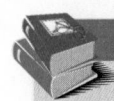

Advances in genetic testing have resulted in the capability of not only diagnosing a genetic disorder in an individual manifesting symptoms, but also determining if an asymptomatic person will manifest the disease in the future or has the potential to transmit disease-producing genetic material to offspring. This capability has tremendous potential to prevent or ameliorate the effects of genetic disease, such as in newborn screening for PKU or sickle cell disease. In some cases, however, it also has the power to cause substantial psychologic distress and anxiety for individuals, and may cause them to make life-altering decisions based on a knowledge of the past or the future that they may wish had remained unknown. As such, the ethical and moral responsibilities of genetic screening and presymptomatic testing can be agonizing for health care professionals, in whom it can elicit uncomfortable feelings of "playing God" or "being a psychic with a crystal ball."

to offspring if the partner is also a carrier). Carrier or presymptomatic testing of children is generally not recommended or performed except in conditions such as familial adenomatous polyposis because the humerous intestinal polyps can become malignant during adolescence. (See Evidence-Based Practice box opposite.)

Careful counseling is necessary with carrier screening to ensure that individuals understand the limitations of testing and the implications of results. Even with careful counseling, there may be significant misunderstanding or misuse of information (Ciske and others, 2001; Farrell and others, 2001).

*Presymptomatic testing* for individuals at risk of an adult-onset disorder, such as Huntington disease, presents different, but equally weighty, dilemmas. Huntington disease is an autosomal dominant inherited disorder characterized by progressive neuromuscular deterioration and dementia, with eventual complete incapacitation and death. The age of onset is approximately 40 ($\pm$12 years) years of age—ironically, after childbearing occurs. Individuals with an affected parent have a theoretic 50% risk of eventually becoming symptomatic. The emotional threat for these individuals as they face an unknown future can be devastating. Now, through DNA testing, it can be determined with 98% accuracy whether they inherited the Huntington gene mutation. For some individuals, the chance that they would find out that they will develop this distressing condition is unbearable, like a delayed death sentence. They would rather not know. Others do want testing in the hope that the news will relieve them of the dread of the unknown and provide direction for their life whether the news is good or bad. Because testing is often of family groups, even those who receive good news may experience survivor guilt if another family member receives bad news. An equally devastating situation has occurred with the discovery of a gene defect that causes inherited breast cancer. Women in these cancer-prone families face an 85% risk of developing breast or ovarian cancer. The dread in some women who have had family members die can be so great that they will undergo a prophylactic mastectomy.

## EVIDENCE-BASED PRACTICE
### Genetic Testing of Children

Many centers offering carrier and presymptomatic testing for adult-onset disorders have struggled with ethical issues surrounding testing of currently healthy children. When a deleterious recessive or dominant gene is identified in a family, parents are often most concerned about future health and reproductive implications for their children. They may request testing for them, unaware of the potential pyschosocial harm in testing asymptomatic children, such as stigmatization, insurance and employment discrimination, disclosure of nonpaternity, potential loss of self-esteem, and disruption of the parent-child bond. Of course, negative results may provide relief, but if other siblings test positive, the child with negative results may feel guilt because he or she was the one to escape.

Most organizations and genetic centers advocate that unless there are clear medical benefits such as early treatment, testing should be postponed until the age of consent (Clark, 1994; Wertz, Fanas, and Reilly, 1994; Williams and Lessick, 1996). At that time, with appropriate counseling regarding the risks and benefits, an informed decision can be made about testing. The issue extends to potential adoption situations as well. Genetic testing of potential adoptees has been likened to "making the child into a commodity undergoing quality control" (Wertz and others, 1994). Testing may also be offered when there is a benefit to another family member and no anticipated harm to the minor (AAP, 2000).

Again, as with any genetic testing, extensive counseling with discussion of benefits and risks is necessary for an informed decision.

The economic consequences of carrier status screening and presymptomatic testing are also foreboding. Technologic advances have outstripped policy making; therefore discrimination in the workplace and in insurance coverage has occurred on the basis of screening and testing results. Many states are enacting legislation to prevent such discrimination, but the complexity has hampered effective statutes, and many issues remain unresolved (Hudson and others, 1995; Williams and Lessick, 1996). Maintaining confidentiality of test results while knowing the possible consequences is an additional sobering burden.

**Screening for Epidemiologic Information.** Public health officials may use screening as a method for monitoring the incidence of diseases or malformations in a population in order to detect environmental or other causes that might significantly influence the incidence of the disorders. For example, geographic and socioeconomic variations in the incidence of NTDs eventually led to research that determined that folic acid supplementation of 0.4 mg per day in women of childbearing age reduces NTD occurrence by as much as 50% (AAP, 1999; Honein and others, 2001).

### Significance of Screening to Families

Mass screening programs have received mixed acceptance from health professionals and the general public. The reasons for controversy include lack of knowledge on the part of health professionals about the testing purposes and implications of results, the public cost of testing (if government funded), and the psychologic implications of learning about carrier status. However, with the success of several well-organized or legislated programs and their significance in the prevention of disease or of the damaging effects of disease, an increasing number of programs are gaining acceptance and support.

Much of family concern regarding screening centers around the issues of informed consent and the use of the screening information. Some states require written consent; some specify the tests to be performed; and some describe the risks, benefits, and the right to be informed of uncertain results, including the implications of an abnormal finding. Institutions may provide classes for families to explain the screening program, provide verbal explanation, or distribute written materials. In some areas exemptions from mandated screening are allowed in certain situations, such as objections on religious grounds if there is a conflict with religious practices and beliefs of an established church.

The nature and purposes of the procedure should be clearly explained to clients in language that they can understand. The issue of divulging unexpected findings is subject to debate. If a genetic trait is detected in a child but not in a parent (such as the sickle cell trait), the question of paternity may be raised. It is also important to help families understand the meaning of *false-positive* test results (indicates a problem exists when it does not) and *false-negative* test results (indicates a problem does not exist when it does).

Release of information to persons other than the family is also subject to debate. At present the reporting of genetic findings is not mandatory as it is for certain contagious diseases, and it is questionable whether this would be desirable. A family may not wish for other family members or even the family practitioner to receive the results of screening. Knowledge of screening results by third parties may lead to insurance or employment discrimination. All of these possibilities should be made clear to families in order to provide them with some selective control.

The social stigma of being the carrier of a defective gene may be a side effect of screening. In some families such knowledge is a source of embarrassment and is damaging to the self-esteem of its members. Teenagers are especially vulnerable to the effects of knowing they carry a specific defective gene at a time when identity formation and peer approval are extremely important. Cultural views regarding this knowledge can have profound effects on the members of some ethnic groups. In some cases, social status within the cultural group can be impaired.

Probably the most important area for nursing practice is teaching. Families need an understanding of why the screening is proposed, what the results mean, and how the family can interpret false-positive and false-negative results (Baroni, Anderson, and Mischler, 1997). Anxiety is greater when families have not received sufficient information about the screening or testing process and its significance for their health. The need for further testing, no matter what the reason, can be extremely stressful to families, and they also have a right to know who assumes the cost of additional testing or retesting—the family or the state. The nurse is a valuable resource in ensuring that families are aware of alternatives and in helping them make the best decision.

## Prenatal Diagnosis

Advances in technology have greatly increased the spectrum and accuracy of prenatal detection of genetic diseases and defects. Prenatal testing provides the means to detect defects that are best corrected soon after delivery, conditions that may require preterm delivery for early correction, conditions that may require cesarean delivery, conditions that may require medical or surgical treatment before birth, and conditions on which a decision may be based to terminate a pregnancy. In addition, a very important benefit is that normal results provide peace of mind for the expectant family. However, even with normal prenatal test results, the birth of a healthy baby cannot be guaranteed.

A variety of techniques are available for diagnosing a number of diseases and defects in the fetus. Some procedures are considered *screening tests,* meaning that the test only indicates a higher risk than expected in the general population or an age-dependent risk. Other methods are *diagnostic tests,* meaning that they determine with a high degree of accuracy the presence or absence of a birth defect or genetic disorder (Table 5-5). Risks of prenatal testing vary, depending on the procedure.

### Indications for Prenatal Testing and Types of Procedures

There is approximately a 2% to 3% risk of a major birth defect or genetic disorder with each pregnancy in the general population regardless of other risk factors such as age or family history. Prenatal diagnostic testing of the general pregnant population is not justified because of the risks, cost, and specificity of diagnostic procedures. Certain general and specific risk factors determine those for whom diagnostic testing, such as amniocentesis, is indicated. Relatively inexpensive and safe screening tests, such as routine ultrasound and maternal serum Trisomy Profile Screen for the remaining population will determine those for whom diagnostic testing is advisable.

**Prenatal Screening Tests.**   The maternal triple marker *Trisomy Profile Screen* blood test is a prenatal screening test offered to all pregnant women under the age of 35 and is

| **TABLE 5-5**   Types of prenatal genetic testing | | | |
| --- | --- | --- | --- |
| **Purpose** | **Advantages** | **Disadvantages** | **Risks** |
| **Triple Marker Screen (Also called Trisomy Profile Screen)** | | | |
| Screening test for NTDs, ventral wall defects, and trisomy pregnancies (e.g., Down syndrome) Detects alpha-fetoprotein (AFP), human chorionic gonadotropin (hCG), and unconjugated estriol (uE3) | Identifies women at higher risk who otherwise would not receive diagnostic testing | Is not diagnostic; only indicates need for further testing False-positive and false-negative results occur | Venipuncture Minimal risk |
| **Ultrasonography** | | | |
| Assesses gestational age, fetal growth, placental sufficiency Detects multiple gestation and structural anomalies Screening and diagnostic test | Detects structural anomalies and effects of intrauterine environment that may not be detected by chromosome analysis | Accuracy depends on skill of ultrasonographer, quality of equipment, and size of defect Does not detect biochemical abnormalities | Noninvasive |
| **Amniocentesis** | | | |
| Chromosome analysis of fetal cells DNA analysis Alpha-fetoprotein (AFP) analysis, other biochemical analyses | Diagnostic for chromosome abnormalities Provides DNA for direct and indirect testing for single-gene disorders High accuracy for detection of NTDs using biochemical analysis | Does not detect structural anomalies not caused by chromosome abnormalities except for neural tube or ventral wall defects (VWDs) Usually not performed until second trimester (14-16 weeks) Results are usually available in 1-3 weeks Relatively expensive | Invasive ½% risk of spontaneous abortion Nongrowth of fetal cells requires repeat procedure |
| **Chorionic Villus Sampling (CVS)** | | | |
| Chromosome analysis of chorionic (fetal) cells DNA analysis | Diagnostic for chromosome abnormalities Provides DNA for direct and indirect testing for single-gene disorders Test is done earlier than amniocentesis (9-12 weeks); therefore results are available earlier | Diagnostic accuracy may be less because of greater risk of maternal cell contamination and false evidence of mosaicism, which may require subsequent amniocentesis Does not detect structural anomalies Relatively expensive Less available than amniocentesis | Invasive Risk of spontaneous abortion 1-2% Controversial evidence of limb-reduction defects |

performed between 15 to 21 weeks of pregnancy. Three chemicals, alpha-fetoprotein (AFP), human chorionic gonadotropin (hCG), and unconjugated estriol (uE3), are synthesized in the fetal liver or yolk sac. By diffusion across the placenta and amnion, these proteins are present in the maternal circulation. The levels can be measured from a blood sample and compared with the norms for that point in gestation.

Neural tube defects (NTDs) such as anencephaly and spina bifida and ventral wall defects (VWDs) such as gastroschisis and omphalocele are associated with exposed fetal membrane and blood vessel surfaces that increase the leakage of AFP into the amniotic fluid and, consequently, the maternal blood. Therefore an elevated AFP level may indicate an increased risk for a neural tube defect (NTD).

The Trisomy Profile Screen can also detect an increased risk for Down syndrome, which may be present when the AFP and uE3 levels are lower and the hCG is elevated.

Certain factors other than NTDs or Down syndrome can cause an abnormal triple marker screening level, such as multiple gestation, incorrectly estimated gestational age, fetal hemorrhage, fetal death, placental abnormalities, or normal variation in the level of protein in the blood. Other factors affecting results that may require correction include maternal diabetes, race, and weight. Further diagnostic testing is indicated for abnormal results that cannot be attributed to any of these factors.

*Ultrasonography* can also be a screening or diagnostic technique, depending on the sophistication of the equipment, the skill of the ultrasonographer, and the type of abnormality seen. Ultrasound screening of all pregnant women can potentially detect major or minor findings that indicate a need for further diagnostic testing. Routine ultrasonography is noninvasive, safe, and a standard screening practice in many countries, yet controversy exists in the United States over its actual benefits vs cost.

High-resolution *ultrasonography* is especially useful for detecting birth defects in which the chromosome analysis is most likely normal, such as with teratogen exposure; in multifactorial conditions, such as isolated congenital heart defect; and in anatomic defects, such as skeletal dysplasias and IUGR. Although equipment and ultrasonographer skill may vary, accuracy can be greater than 90% for detecting major neural tube, cardiac, kidney, and bladder anomalies.

**Prenatal Diagnostic Procedures.** There are general, specific, and ethnic risk factors that may be present in any pregnancy that are indicators for diagnostic testing. The specific testing recommended depends on the identified risk. These may be preexisting risks, personal characteristics, or a newly identified risk for this pregnancy (Box 5-3). General risk factors include age and abnormal triple marker screen results. It is a standard recommendation that women 35 years of age or older be offered amniocentesis, rather than screening, based on an increased risk for Down syndrome, other trisomies, and sex chromosome abnormalities with advancing maternal age (American College of Medical Genetics, 1996). Recent information suggests that amniocentesis should be offered at 31 years of age in twin pregnancies (Meyers and others, 1997). Specific risk factors

are usually identified in the family history, previous pregnancy outcomes, or the mother's medical history. Ethnic risk factors are based on a higher carrier rate frequency for certain genetic diseases in selected populations. Indications for prenatal diagnosis when any of these risk factors are present is based on a greater than general population risk that a genetic defect or disorder will occur in the pregnancy. The specific risk is, of course, different for each situation.

*Amniocentesis* is currently the basis of diagnostic prenatal testing. It is usually performed at 14 to 16 weeks of gestation under ultrasound guidance. Estimated fetal loss following amniocentesis is 0.5%. Amniocentesis provides several types of diagnostic information. First, viable fetal skin cells that have sloughed off and are present in the amniotic fluid are obtained and cultured for chromosome analysis to detect chromosome abnormalities. Chromosome analysis results are obtained in about 7 to 14 days in most facilities and are 99% accurate. Second, DNA may be extracted from the chromosomes for direct DNA and indirect linkage analysis to detect single-gene disorders. Testing for each single-gene disorder is unique; therefore testing of this type is done only when a pregnancy is at high risk for a specific disorder, such as CF. The third type of diagnostic information available from amniocentesis is amniotic fluid AFP levels (AF-AFP). The AFP level in the amniotic fluid is a much more reliable indicator of an NTD or VWD because interfering factors, such as placental diffusion differences, are minimized. Also, an additional test for an enzyme specific to neural tissue acetylcholinesterase (AChE) may be done, which, if positive

---

**Box 5-3** ■ ■ ■
### Indications for Prenatal Diagnosis

**GENERAL RISK FACTORS**

Maternal age ≥35 years at time of delivery or ≥31 years if twin gestation

Elevated or low Trisomy Profile Screen results

**SPECIFIC RISK FACTORS**

Previous child with a structural defect or chromosome abnormality

Previous stillbirth or neonatal death

Structural abnormality in mother or father

Balanced translocation in mother or father

Inherited disorders: cystic fibrosis, metabolic disorders, sex-linked recessive disorders

Medical disease in mother: diabetes mellitus, PKU

Exposure to a teratogen: ionizing radiation, anticonvulsant medicines, lithium, isotretinoin, alcohol

Infection: rubella, toxoplasmosis, cytomegalovirus

Abnormal ultrasound findings

**ETHNIC RISK FACTORS**

| DISORDER | ETHNIC OR RACIAL GROUP |
| --- | --- |
| Tay-Sachs disease | Ashkenazi Jewish, French Canadian |
| Sickle cell anemia | Black African, Mediterranean, Arab, Indian, Pakistani |
| α- and β-thalassemia | Mediterranean, Southern and Southeast Asian, Chinese |

Modified from D'Alton ME, DeCherney AH: Prenatal diagnosis, *N Engl J Med* 328(2):114-120, 1993.

in the presence of an elevated AF-AFP level, is diagnostic of an open NTD.

*Chorionic villus sampling (CVS)* is a less commonly used procedure to obtain cells for chromosome analysis. An advantage of CVS is that it may be performed between 9 and 12 weeks of gestation, either transcervically or transabdominally. The procedure is somewhat controversial because of a slightly higher rate of fetal loss following the procedure. When performed at centers with a large experience the fetal loss rate is approximately the same as for amniocentesis. The accuracy of the chromosome analysis may be slightly less than with amniocentesis because of a greater risk for contamination by maternal cells, and, if mosaicism is detected, a confirmatory amniocentesis at 14 to 16 weeks is recommended.

A few additional diagnostic tests are sometimes used. *Fetal blood sampling* can be performed after 18 weeks of gestation. This procedure is usually done for prenatal evaluation of fetal hematologic abnormalities, inborn errors of metabolism, fetal infection, and rapid chromosome analysis. Fetal blood cells grow rapidly and hematologic and chromosome test results are usually possible in less than 1 week (Sack, 1999). *Fetal biopsy (FB)* is sometimes used to diagnose certain genetic skin disorders and metabolic disorders when DNA studies are unavailable or are uninformative. *Fetal echocardiography* may be performed for further diagnosis when a cardiac defect is noted on ultrasound. Research is underway to improve prenatal diagnostic testing.

A relatively new option for parents at risk of having a child with a genetic disorder is *preimplantation genetic diagnosis.* Through the technique of *in vitro (test tube) fertilization,* the embryo can be tested at the six- to eight-cell stage for the presence of the specific genetic disorder. If found to be normal or a carrier but not affected, the embryo(s) can then be implanted. This technique has been used for Tay-Sachs disease, CF, and some X-linked disorders (Harper, 1996). It was used by a couple who wished not only to avoid the birth of another child affected with Fanconi anemia but also to have a healthy sibling who could provide a human lymphocyte antigen (HLA) match for an affected sibling who needed stem cell transplantation (Verlinsky, 2001).

## Genetic Evaluation and Counseling

In recent years the significance of genetics as an etiologic agent in disease and disability has assumed a more prominent place in the nursing care of infants and children. The expanded recognition of genetic diseases and defects and an increasingly well-informed public is creating a justified demand for genetic evaluation and diagnosis, as well as information regarding risks to present and future generations. Unfortunately, however, persons who need expert genetic counseling often make uninformed decisions on their own or are the victims of well-meaning but equally uninformed relatives, acquaintances, or paraprofessionals. Nurses involved in infant and child care continually encounter families in which there is a risk that a disorder may be transmitted to an offspring, as well as children who may have an undiagnosed genetic disorder that needs expert

evaluation. It is a nurse's responsibility to be alert to situations in which families could benefit from genetic evaluation and counseling, become familiar with facilities in their areas where these services are available, and learn basic genetic principles. In this way, nurses will be able to direct individuals and families to needed services and to be active participants in the genetic evaluation and counseling process. Nurses should be knowledgeable regarding special services that are available to help in the management and support of affected children. Early identification of a genetic disorder allows anticipation of associated conditions and implementation of available preventive measures and therapy to avoid potential complications and to actualize or enhance the child's health potential. It may also prevent the unexpected birth of another affected child in the immediate or extended family.

### Clients

The clients, or persons who seek genetic evaluation and counseling, must first be aware that there is a genetic or potential problem. They may be referred by a family practitioner, a specialist, a nurse, a friend, or a relative, or they may seek counseling as a result of information in the media. Clients who seek counseling expect information, explanation, reassurance, advice, and help in making decisions (Michie, Marteau, and Bobrow, 1997).

Genetic evaluation for diagnostic purposes may occur at any point along the life span. In the newborn period, birth defects are an obvious reason for referral. Beyond the newborn period, indicators for referral include metabolic disorders, developmental delays, growth delays, behavioral problems, cognitive delays, abnormal or delayed sexual development, and medical problems known to be associated with genetic diseases. For example, a preschooler with hyperactivity and autistic-like behaviors may need evaluation for fragile X syndrome, and a 17-year-old girl with primary amenorrhea should be tested for Turner syndrome. In adulthood an asymptomatic individual with a family history of Huntington disease may desire testing to determine his or her risk of becoming symptomatic in the future.

With so many recent advances in genetic testing, it is not at all unusual for a child or adult with long-standing medical problems, including mental retardation, to be referred for reevaluation of his or her condition as a possible genetic disorder that might not have been diagnosable a few years earlier, such as microdeletion disorders or single-gene mutations. If a genetic diagnosis is made, the client will usually be referred back to the primary care physician with recommendations for routine management.

Clients may or may not be affected themselves but may request genetic counseling about the heritability of a trait. Clients might be a young couple contemplating childbearing who are concerned about a disorder in one of their families or who may seek advice because they are related. A couple who are both members of a population at risk for certain diseases may wish to determine whether they carry the harmful gene (e.g., African-Americans and sickle cell anemia, Ashkenazi Jews and Tay-Sachs disease, or persons of Mediterranean ancestry and thalassemia). A couple planning adoption might seek counseling regarding a prospective child. (See Evidence-Based Practice box on p. 127.)

More often, persons who inquire about the possibility of recurrence of a disease or disorder have a child, or had a child who died, with a genetic disease or disorder. They are concerned about their likelihood of having another, similarly affected child and may want to know what reproductive choices are available to them. This advice might be sought before the couple initiates another pregnancy or after the mother is already pregnant. If prenatal diagnostic testing is not done, the history of a condition in an older sibling, such as galactosemia, alerts health personnel to initiate specific and thorough testing for the condition in a newborn. In this way, early therapy can be initiated when indicated, thus minimizing or eliminating the effects of the disease or defect.

Parents need to know the risk in *their particular situation* and how it relates to the random risk for *any* prospective parents. When families understand the risks involved, they can make informed decisions regarding family planning and available prenatal testing. Additional counseling is necessary if abnormal results are obtained so that the couple can decide to continue or terminate the pregnancy. They will need considerable support for either decision (Allen and Mulhauser, 1995). Parents may also have concerns about risks to unaffected siblings and about reproductive implications for their affected and unaffected offspring.

## Counseling Services

The most efficient counseling service consists of a group of specialists, which may include physicians, geneticists, psychologists, biochemists, cytologists, nurses, social workers, and other auxiliary personnel. The services are most often under the leadership of a physician trained in medical genetics, who assumes responsibility for the medical aspects of the problem. The counseling service may serve only as a referral group, or it may conduct a regular clinic service. Most often it is associated with a large medical center, which may have extensive outreach programs with satellite clinics throughout adjacent rural areas. There are also numerous specialty clinics that deal with specific genetic disorders (such as CF, muscular dystrophy, hemophilia, or diabetes) and provide their own genetic counseling services. Unfortunately, these units are concentrated in and around large metropolitan areas. As a result, counseling is not always accessible to the large number of persons who would benefit from the service.

Unlike a medical prognosis, which predicts the outcome of a disease, a genetic prognosis directly involves other persons: the affected child, members of the immediate family, other relatives, and future offspring. For genetic evaluation or follow-up, the geneticist and the counselor usually work together to obtain the family history and pedigree and the medical history of the person being evaluated (including pregnancy, labor, and delivery information), perform a physical examination for dysmorphic features, and order appropriate testing such as biochemical and cytogenetic procedures. A genetic diagnosis may or may not be made initially. Genetic evaluation and counseling is a time-consuming and labor-intensive process. The pediatric nurse can help the

family understand the sometimes lengthy process in arriving at a diagnosis as well as help the family prepare questions for the counseling session.

*Genetic counseling* is a communication process that deals with the human problems associated with the occurrence, or risk of occurrence, of a genetic disorder in a family. This process involves an attempt by one or more appropriately trained persons to help the individual or family:

- Comprehend the medical facts, including the diagnosis, the probable course of the disorder, and the available management
- Appreciate the way heredity contributes to the disorder and the risk of recurrence in specified relatives
- Understand the options for dealing with the risk of recurrence
- Choose the course of action that seems appropriate to them in view of their risk and family goals and act in accordance with that decision
- Make the best possible adjustment to the disorder in an affected family member and to the risk of recurrence of that disorder

## Estimation of Risks

Effective genetic counseling based on a diagnosis or known risk factors requires a thorough evaluation of each situation. The counselor derives risks of occurrence or recurrence from information acquired through a thorough family history, including known genetic information. A careful, detailed family history not only provides a picture of the *proband* (the affected person, or *index case*) in relation to other family members but also may serve to identify others who are similarly affected or who might be presymptomatic or at risk of producing affected children. Analyzing the pattern of affected members of the family can assist in confirming a tentative diagnosis or in determining the level of risk in multifactorial inheritance.

An accurate diagnosis is essential in order to provide specific risk figures. There are over 6000 known inherited disorders, many of which have similar clinical manifestations but different modes of inheritance. For example, symptoms in the early stages of severe X-linked muscular dystrophy appear much like those of the milder autosomal recessive and autosomal dominant varieties, autosomal recessive neurogenic muscular atrophies, and nongenetic poliomyelitis. The significance of the risks related to each type of disorder is readily apparent. For disorders with an unknown or multifactorial cause, recurrence risks are termed *empiric,* meaning they are based on observations of recurrence in similar situations, rather than *theoretic,* meaning they are based on mendelian inheritance patterns.

The mode of inheritance determines the degree of risk in the major categories of genetic disorders (Box 5-4). In general, the more definite and clear-cut the genetics, the greater the risks; as the causative factors become more obscure, the risk of recurrence is less likely.

## Interpretation of Risks

When explaining risk estimates, the counselor does not attempt to make recommendations or decisions for clients. The counselor provides appropriate and accurate information about the nature of the disorder, the extent of the risk involved, the probable consequences, and alternative solutions but remains nondirective, leaving the final decision to

---

**Box 5-4** ▪ ■ ▪
**Estimation of Genetic Risk**

**HIGH-RISK SITUATIONS**

Conditions caused by a factor that segregates during cell division
*Recurrence risk:* 1:10 or greater
Can be predicted with high degree of accuracy
Based on mendelian ratios (theoretic)
*Examples:* Single-gene disorders, translocated chromosome disorders

**MODERATE-RISK SITUATIONS**

Conditions that are multifactorial or sporadic
*Recurrence risk:* Less than 1:10 to 1:100
Based on prior experience and observation of the disorder under similar circumstances (empiric)
*Examples:* Spina bifida, congenital heart defects, most chromosome abnormalities

**RANDOM-RISK SITUATIONS**

Conditions caused by environmental agents and not likely to recur in another pregnancy under normal circumstances unless the agent is still operative
*Recurrence risk:* Approximately 1:30
*Examples:* Rubella syndrome, new mutations, maternal diabetes, fetal alcohol syndrome

---

**Box 5-5** ▪ ■ ▪
**Assessment Clues to Genetic Disorders***

**Major or minor birth defects (anomalies) and dysmorphic features**—Cardiac defect, ear or eye abnormalities, micrognathia, forehead prominence, hairline low-set on forehead or nape of neck, wide-set eyes, epicanthal folds, low-set or unusually shaped ears
**Growth abnormalities**—Short stature, overgrowth, asymmetric growth, IUGR
**Skeletal abnormalities**—Limb abnormalities, asymmetry, scoliosis, hyperextensible joints, hypotonic or hypertonic muscle tone, pectus excavatum, finger or joint abnormalities.
**Vision or hearing problems**—Coloboma, cat's eye, hearing loss, vision loss, congenital or early cataracts
**Metabolic disorders**—Unusual odor of breath, urine, or stool
**Sexual development abnormalities**—Ambiguous genitalia, small penis, delayed onset of puberty, primary amenorrhea, precocious sexual development, large testicles
**Skin disorders**—Unusual pigmentation, café-au-lait spots, dry and scaly skin, skin tumors
**Recurrent infection or immune deficiency**—Ear infections, pneumonia
**Developmental and speech delays or loss of milestones**
**Cognitive delays**—Learning disabilities, mild to severe mental retardation
**Behavioral disorders**—Hyperactivity, attention deficit disorder, autistic-like behavior, aggressive behavior.

*Suggests genetic etiology if two or more findings are present.

---

the persons concerned. In some instances genetic information will increase the family's distress; in others their anxiety will be reduced, depending on their personalities and the meaning that the disorder has for that particular family.

It is helpful to explain risks in different ways and to use examples to aid in understanding the meaning of probabilities. Most people do not have an adequate knowledge of genetics and human biology to fully comprehend these complex concepts. Words and concepts that can be used include "percentages," "chance," "odds," and "likelihood." For example, if a 40-year-old woman has a 1:112 risk of having a child with Down syndrome, other ways to explain it include saying "You have about a 1% chance of having a baby with Down syndrome" or "Out of 112 women your age having a baby, odds are that 1 of them will have a child with Down syndrome." Games of probability can also be used, such as flipping coins, baseball pools, and lotteries.

**NURSING ALERT**
Families may misunderstand probabilities, even when they are fully explained. It is important to impress on them that *each pregnancy is an independent event*. It is not uncommon for parents who are told that a recessive disorder carries a 1:4 risk of recurrence to incorrectly reason that because they already have one affected child the next three will be unaffected. Chance has no memory; the risk is 1:4 for each and every pregnancy.

## Role of Nurses in Genetic Counseling and Referral

Genetic counseling is a professional specialty that requires master's level preparation and board certification because of the crucial nature of the information these professionals provide. However, the number of board-certified genetic counselors is limited; therefore nurses skilled in counseling techniques are in a unique position to help meet the counseling needs of families in which there is a genetic disease or disorder. Public health nurses work with a family in a close, sustained relationship and earn the family's confidence and trust. Genetics nurse specialists,* with advanced preparation in genetic theory, are assuming a prominent position on counseling teams, and practitioners in the specialty areas of maternity and pediatric nursing are often involved with families in which there is a genetic defect. New advances in genetic diagnosis have greatly increased opportunities for, and responsibilities of, nurses in all levels of practice in terms of assessment, referral, education, and counseling (MacDonald, 1997; Greco, 2000).

It is often a nurse who first identifies a need for counseling and referral by identifying the presence of an inherited disorder in a family history or by noting physical, mental, or behavioral abnormalities when performing a nursing assessment (Box 5-5). Guidelines for determining if a genetic referral is indicated are given in the Guidelines box.

A genetic nurse or counselor usually contacts the family before the primary counseling session or diagnostic workup to assess the needs of the family and to attempt to reduce their anxiety. In the interview the nurse takes a family history for pertinent information and explains the clinic procedures carefully. Many families are concerned about such

---

*For additional information contact the **International Society of Nurses in Genetics (ISONG)**, www.nursing.creighton.edu/isong.

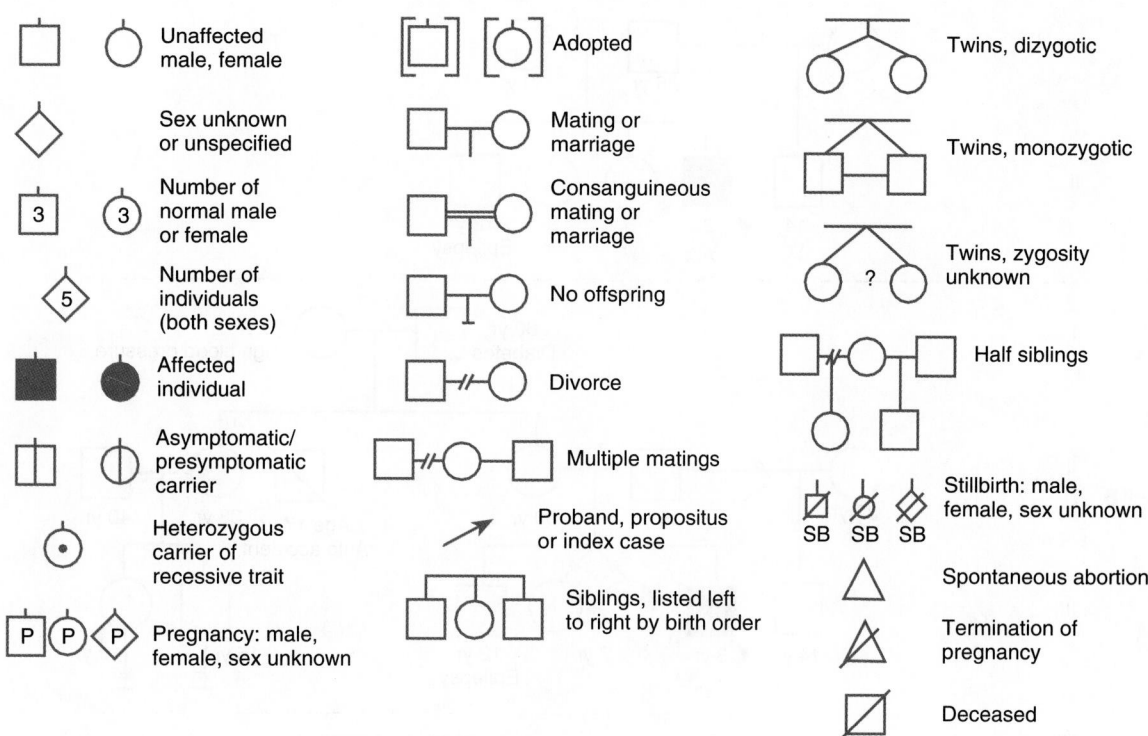

**Fig. 5-10**    Common pedigree symbols.

things as whether they will be required to undress, if blood is to be drawn, if they can accompany the child during the visit, or if they will be told what to do about reproduction. Families who know what to expect are able to gain more from a counseling session.

## Taking a Family History

The person taking a family history during a genetic consultation must allow a liberal amount of time. When possible, it is best to include both parents in the interview in order to elicit information about relatives on both sides of the family. Medical records, birth and death records, family Bibles, and photograph albums are helpful resources, and persons being interviewed should be instructed to bring such items if they are available. It may be necessary to consult other members of the family. The level of education and the degree of understanding vary widely among informants and influence the reliability of the information. There may be reticence on the part of informants, particularly if they view the disorder as something to be ashamed of or in some way threatening. Sometimes true relationships may be concealed, such as illegitimacy or nonpaternity.

Skillful interviewing is necessary in order to obtain essential, but often embarrassing or private, information. Since many parents may not be married, they should be addressed as couples or partners and asked about other unions that may have produced a pregnancy. In eliciting a birth history from the mother and father, the nurse should specifically ask about abortions, miscarriages, and stillbirths as well as live births. To identify all members of the family tree, it is best to

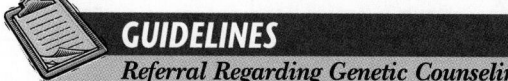

### GUIDELINES
#### Referral Regarding Genetic Counseling

Individuals with a family history of hereditary diseases, birth defects, or developmental problems

Known balanced translocation carriers or parents who have previously had a fetus or child with a chromosome abnormality

Couples with a history of multiple miscarriages, stillbirths, or infertility

Individuals at risk for ethnic-related disorders

Pregnant women exposed to teratogenic agents

Pregnant women of advanced maternal age (≥35 years)

Disorders in which pregnancy could threaten maternal or fetal life or health

ask about pregnancies even of young teenagers. When inquiring about family diseases, it is often necessary to ask the question in different ways. For example, if a client denies any mental retardation in the family, asking other questions, such as about learning problems, being in special education classes, and failing or not completing school, may uncover a family history of cognitive impairment.

The family history is recorded in the form of a *pedigree chart* or *family tree* (in some disciplines the pedigree chart is termed a *genogram*), using standard symbols to indicate persons, relationships, and significant details related to them (Bennett and others, 1995) (Fig. 5-10). Construction of a pedigree begins with the affected child (proband, index case, original patient) and *all* the mother's pregnancies (Fig. 5-11, *A*). Next, the maternal family history is explored

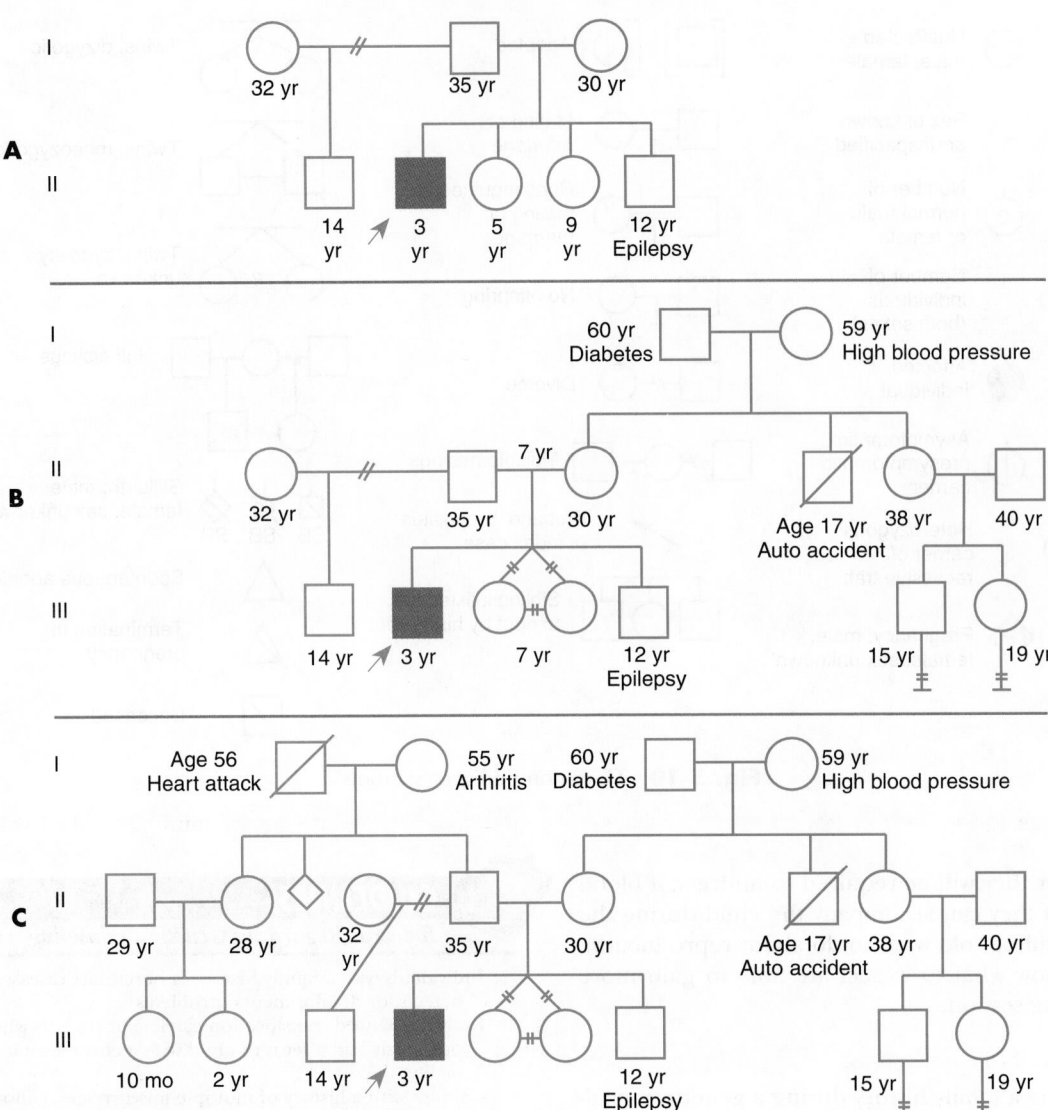

**Fig. 5-11**   Construction of a pedigree. **A,** Proband, siblings, and parents. **B,** Maternal relatives, **C,** Paternal relatives added.

in a similar manner (Fig. 5-11, *B*); then information about relatives on the father's side, as well as any children or pregnancies that may have occurred through the father's previous unions, is gathered in the same manner (Fig. 5-11, *C*). (See Guidelines box.) It is important at this point to determine whether the couple might be related in any way; although contrary to popular belief, this is usually a concern only for first cousins or closer relatives. The first-cousin risk for birth defects is about 5% vs the general population risk of 2% to 3%. The primary risk increase is for autosomal recessive disorders, in which the chance that two individuals carry the same rare, deleterious gene is increased if they are related.

Information to be solicited includes information not only about other affected family members but also about: (1) births (live birth, stillbirths, and abortions [especially spontaneous abortions], including gestational age of pregnancy); (2) infertility problems; (3) matings (legally sanc-

tioned, consanguineous, multiple, unwed, and other complex relationships); (4) health of family members, including any other genetic diseases or disorders or birth defects; and death and causes of death, including early infant deaths. Sometimes the place of birth and ethnic background are significant. For example, the incidence of Tay-Sachs disease is higher in Ashkenazi Jews from eastern Europe than in Jews from other geographic origins. Also, when a pedigree chart is being evaluated, a sister's death in infancy from a congenital heart defect might be genetically significant, whereas a healthy sibling's death from drowning at age 1 year would not. Information concerning first-degree relatives is most important and should be complete.

### Follow-Up Care

The success of counseling is measured by the way in which the family uses the information presented to them. Maintaining contact with the family or referral to an agency that

## GUIDELINES
### Pedigree Construction

1. Begin diagram in the middle of a large sheet of paper.
2. Represent males by a square placed to the left and females by a circle placed to the right.
3. Represent the proband (index case, original patient) with an arrow (if the counselee or patient is different, place a *C* under that person's symbol).
4. Use a horizontal line between a square and a circle for a mating or marriage.
5. Suspend offspring vertically from the mating line and place in order of birth with oldest to the left (regardless of sex).
6. Symbolize generations by Roman numerals, with the earliest generation at the top.
7. Include three generations: grandparents, parents, offspring, siblings, aunts, uncles, and first cousins of proband.
8. Include name of each person, their age, health problems, and date and cause of death. Due to privacy concerns, include only first names of the family you are interviewing.
9. Date the pedigree and update at subsequent visits.

For a detailed description of pedigree construction, see Nelson-Anderson DL, Waters CV: *Genetic connections: a guide to documenting your individual and family health history,* Washington, MO, 1995, Sonters.

### Box 5-6 ■ ■ ■
### Nurse's Role in Genetic Evaluation and Counseling of Families

1. Identify infants and children at risk of a genetic disorder.
2. Obtain family, prenatal, and health history.
3. Assess the family's understanding of the genetic condition.
4. Refer for genetic evaluation and counseling when indicated.
5. Establish a plan of care with the family and coordinate care with other health professionals.
6. Understand the benefits and risks of genetic testing. Educate families about available testing.
7. Maintain privacy and confidentiality of family records and information.
8. Facilitate family access to early child stimulation programs, genetic resources, and support groups.
9. Provide follow-up care and support throughout the lifespan of the child.

can provide a sustained relationship—usually the public health agency in their locality—is one of the most important aspects of the counseling process. Some families choose not to have follow-up visits, but in most instances these visits make the family feel that they have not been abandoned and facilitate the process of adjustment to the problem. A summary letter of the interview or counseling session is helpful to review information presented and reinforce recommendations.

Follow-up visits to the counseling service or in the home provide the family with the opportunity to ask questions that have arisen since previous visits. Often the family members have not really "heard" the information presented to them or have misinterpreted what they have heard, so that it may be necessary to repeat and reinforce counseling. In some disorders a diagnosis in one family member places relatives at risk and is an indication for further testing.

One very important aspect of follow-up care is support and assistance in management of the affected child. For example, a disorder such as PKU requires conscientious diet management; therefore it is important to make certain that the family understands and follows instructions. Genetic and specialty clinics devote a great deal of time and effort to helping families cope with the consequences of genetic disease.

Nurses should be prepared to help families arrive at tentative decisions regarding the future, including family planning, education or institutionalization of a child with a disability, plans for adoption, and any other problems related to the specific situation. Initial and ongoing assessment of the family's coping abilities, resources, and support systems is vital in order to determine their need for additional assistance and support. As with any family who has a child with chronic health care needs, nurses must teach the family to become the child's advocate. Also nurses should be alert for evidence of risk factors that indicate poor adjustment (e.g., child abuse, divorce, or other maladaptive behaviors). Lo-

cating agencies and clinics specializing in a specific disorder or its consequences who can provide services (e.g., equipment, medication, and rehabilitation), educational programs, and parent support groups is part of the nurse's role. Nurses can be instrumental in helping parents start a support group when none is available.

### Supportive Counseling

It requires time and understanding to deal with the emotional tension and anxiety generated in families who are faced with the prospect of a genetic disorder. Knowledge of and the ability to deal with the range of psychologic responses and all their ramifications (e.g., the grief reaction, guilt, anger, and coping mechanisms) are essential components of the nursing role in genetic counseling. Many of these factors determine the degree to which a counselor's message is understood and influence the family's attitudes and the use they make of counseling information.

Timing of the counseling requires careful evaluation. Some families may not be ready to listen immediately after a diagnosis is made or the first time information is presented to them. Families who seek genetic counseling, spontaneously or by referral, are apprehensive and know that decisions made on the basis of the information they receive may alter their lives significantly and may even alter their view of themselves. There may be numerous blocks to getting information across to families. Often they are so angry or frightened that they do not hear what is being said to them; they may feel guilty, embarrassed, or somehow inferior or inadequate. It may take a week or more for the family sufficient time to absorb the initial impact of the situation before they are ready to assimilate any new information.

It is important early in counseling to get a clear understanding of the family's initial concerns, their state of knowledge about the disease, and their attitudes and beliefs concerning the condition, and to determine the kind and amount of information they need or want (Box 5-6). Some are not sure they should be at a counseling service. Whether the persons needing help are parents who have given birth to an affected child, relatives of an affected individual, persons who have been identified as carriers of a deleterious gene, or a couple with a higher-risk pregnancy, their feelings, attitudes, and fears must be addressed.

Careful interviewing and assessment will determine the extent and type of information needed and desired by the clients. Misunderstanding of the counseling information can have many causes. It can be due to cultural differences, the disparity of knowledge between the counselor and the family, and the heightened emotion surrounding genetic counseling. Information often needs to be repeated several times before the family understands the content and its implications.

Guilt and self-blame are natural and universal reactions. Nurses must deal with parents' feelings of guilt about carrying "bad genes" or having "made my child sick." Depending on the type of cytogenetic disorder, the counselor may be able to absolve the parents of guilt by explaining the random nature of segregation during both gamete formation and fertilization and that errors in cell division unique to the pregnancy in question are not likely to happen again and are not inherited. Families often try to "reason" that some unrelated event caused the abnormality (e.g., a fall, a urinary tract infection, or "one glass of wine") before the mother was aware that she was pregnant.

Nurses can provide an opportunity for parents to mourn the loss of the "perfect baby" dreamed of during the pregnancy. Parents may experience emotions of shock and disbelief, denial, guilt, shame, sadness, anger, and hostility at the birth of a baby with a genetic disorder or at the time of diagnosis of an older child's genetic disorder. These reactions are normal responses to information that may permanently change how they view their world.

Parental attachment and adjustment to the baby can be supported and facilitated by nursing interventions. Assessing the parents' understanding of the child's disorder and providing simple and truthful explanations can help them begin to understand their child's health issues. Guiding the parents in recognizing their child's cues, responses, and strengths can be helpful even for experienced parents. A caring attitude conveys the value of their child and, by extension, their value as parents. Help the parents identify their strengths as a family and identify support that is available to them.

If after the genetic evaluation parents do not have an accurate understanding of their child's disorder, follow-up is appropriate. Parents may need to hear the information several times before they begin to understand it. Referral to local and national support groups can be helpful. Contact with a local family that has a child with the same condition can be very helpful for new parents. Privacy and confidentiality are imperative, and both families must give permission before their contact information is given (ANA, 1998).

Sometimes there is comfort in knowing that everyone carries defective genes and that it is mere chance that both members of a couple happen to carry the same abnormal gene. Reactions may be different in situations where one member can pinpoint the "blame" (dominant or X-linked disorders), whereas in recessive disorders there is some reassurance for the couple to know that both of them carry the defective gene. Anxieties generated by superstitions and misconceptions can be dispelled.

Families have a tendency to be more ashamed of a hereditary disorder than of other illnesses. The threat of a hereditary "taint" often creates intrafamilial strife, hostility, and marital or couple disharmony, sometimes to the point of family disintegration. Crisis intervention may be necessary to prevent progressive discord.

A family member may decide not to have children after the diagnosis of a hereditary defect, or the decision to marry may be deferred on the basis of a disorder, even a remote chance of one, in a partner's family. Often these decisions may not be based on accurate information because these individuals may not have been involved in the proband's family's counseling.

Although people may understand the situation intellectually, this may not help them emotionally. A large and vital part of the nurse's role in genetic counseling is that of sympathetic and supportive listener. In addition, ensuring that families have accurate and complete information on which to make an informed decision is a primary goal.

Health information on the Internet is increasingly obtained by families. Nurses can help families evaluate the accuracy of the information. It will be helpful to remind families that frequently information is given about the severely affected child and there may be little available pertaining to the mildly affected child.

## Burden of Genetic Defect

The way in which members of a family respond to the probability of a genetic disorder will depend a great deal on the nature of the condition and the burden, actual or perceived, that it may place on them. A *burden* is considered to be the total amount of distress, economic and emotional, that is placed on persons, their families, and society by the birth of an affected child—the anticipated burden as well as the threat of disability. Various factors that are associated with disorders produce a burden in different ways to determine the total impact on a family. These include severity, chronicity, age of onset, mortality, morbidity, presence or absence of chronic pain, mental retardation, and cosmetic disfigurement. A long-term grieving process, sometimes called *chronic sorrow,* can plague parents of a child with a disability (Olshansky, 1962). It has been described as a normal response to an abnormal situation. Parents may feel acute grief during milestones such as the first day of school or when other children are receiving their drivers' licenses. Parents need support throughout the life span of the child.

In some disorders, such as Down syndrome, the burden of the disease rests primarily on the family rather than on the affected child. In diseases with severe crippling effects, such as muscular dystrophy, the impact of the disease affects both the child and the family. When a genetic disorder is inherited and extended family members are at risk, such as with fragile X syndrome, the parents face the burden of informing the other members. They may be met with disbelief, blame, or hostility, and they may need support in this difficult task (McConkie-Rosell and others, 1995).

All of these matters confront a family when they must make a decision about whether to risk a pregnancy that might result in a child with a disability, and nurses should be prepared to explore these probabilities and the availability of prenatal testing with them. If a pregnancy does result in a fetus or child with a genetic defect or disorder and the family chooses to continue the pregnancy, education about the condition and treatment options helps to provide the best possible outcome for the child.

## Barriers to Effective Counseling

Differences in the ability to comprehend what is said probably interfere most with effective use of counseling information. Clients vary in experiences, education, language, and intellectual level, and even with careful explanation may have difficulty understanding the fundamentals of inheritance. They may be able to repeat information but fail to grasp its significance.

Cultural, religious, and ethnic values determine our responses as well as those of our patients and their families. These values and beliefs influence perceptions of health, disease, sexuality, reproduction, and disability. Whether or not a family finds interventions and genetic testing appropriate is influenced by these beliefs (Weil, 2001).

Sometimes nurses create barriers with their own biases and personal feelings. Some diseases have a special impact on individual nurses, and in such cases it is difficult to be nonjudgmental. For some families, the attempt to be neutral may be viewed as unhelpful rather than noncoercive. By clarifying areas of confusion it is possible to help families make decisions. The basic tenet of genetic counseling is that families should be given all the facts and possible consequences and then be assisted, without coercion, in their problem solving. The decision concerning a course of action must be left to them.

## KEY POINTS

- There is probably a genetic component in all disease processes.
- Genetic diseases are usually classified as those produced by chromosome aberrations, those caused by a single mutant gene, those produced by mitochondrial disorders, or those resulting from interaction of genetic and environmental factors (multifactorial).
- Environmental teratogens and maternal disease may also disrupt fetal development, leading to birth defects.
- Chromosomal disorders are caused by abnormalities in either chromosome structure or number.
- Alterations in chromosome number occur as a result of unequal distribution of genetic material during gamete formation or early cell division of the zygote.
- Disorders caused by a single gene are distributed in families according to predictable mendelian principles of inheritance, although there are exceptions based on nontraditional concepts.
- Mutant genes can be dominant or recessive and can be located on an autosome or an X chromosome.
- Variations in gene action include the regularity with which it is manifested (penetrance), the severity or variability of its expression (expressivity), and the different and seemingly unrelated effects associated with the basic defect (pleiotropy).

- Congenital defects, errors or morphogenic development, may arise at any stage of development and demonstrate wide variability in causative factors.
- Although no cure for genetic disease is presently available, various therapeutic measures are used to modify or correct the basic defect.
- The objectives of genetic screening are to detect the presence of disease in individuals, detect unaffected carriers of a disease, and monitor the incidence of disease or malformations in a population.
- Prenatal testing includes screening through ultrasound and maternal serum alpha-fetoprotein (MS-AFP) testing, and diagnosis by amniocentesis, ultrasound, chorionic villus sampling (CVS), and DNA testing.
- Genetic counseling is directed toward providing individuals and families with information needed to make decisions about a course of action appropriate to them.
- Nurses' roles in genetic counseling include identifying cases, referral for genetic counseling, interviewing families, educating families about their disease and its therapy, and providing follow-up care and support throughout the life span.

## REFERENCES

Allen JF, Mulhauser LC: Genetic counseling after abnormal prenatal diagnosis: facilitating coping in families who continue their pregnancies, *J Genet Counsel* 4:251-265, 1995.

American Academy of Pediatrics, Committee on Genetics: Folic acid for the prevention of neural tube defects (Re 9834), *Pediatrics* 104(2):325-327, 1999.

American Academy of Pediatrics, Committee on Genetics: Molecular genetic testing in

pediatric practice: a subject review, *Pediatrics* 106(6):1494-1497, Review, 2000.

American College of Medical Genetics: *Statement on multiple marker screening in pregnant women,* vol 6, Winter, 1996 (college newsletter).

American Nurses' Association and International Society of Nurses in Genetics: *Statement of the scope and standards of genetics clinical nursing practice,* Washington, DC, 1998, American Nurses' Association.

Baroni MA, Anderson YE, Mischler E: Cystic fibrosis newborn screening: impact of early screening results on parenting stress, *Pediatr Nurs* 23(2):143-151, 1997.

Behrman RE, Kliegman RM, Jenson HA: *Nelson textbook of pediatrics,* ed 16, Philadelphia, 2000, WB Saunders.

Bennett RL and others: Recommendations for standardized human pedigree nomenclature, *Am J Med Genet* 56:745-752, 1995.

Bos AF, Einspieler C, Prechtl HF: Intrauterine growth retardation, general movements, and neurodevelopmental outcome: a review, *Dev Med Child Neurol* 43(1):61–68, 2001.

Chamberlain S: Friedreich's in relief, *Nat Genet* 12(4):344-345, 1996.

Ciske D and others: Genetic counseling and neonatal screening for cystic fibrosis: an assessment of the communication process, *Pediatrics* 107(4):699-705, 2001.

Clark A: The genetic testing of children: report of a working party of the Clinical Genetics Society (UK), *J Med Genet* 31(10):785-797, 1994.

Farrell M, Certain L, Farrell P: Genetic counseling and risk communication services of newborn screening programs, *Arch Pediatr Adolesc Med* 155(2):120-126, 2001.

Farrell P and others: Early diagnosis of cystic fibrosis through neonatal screening prevents severe malnutrition and improves long-term growth, Wisconsin Cystic Fibrosis Neonatal Screening Study Group, *Pediatrics* 107(1):1-13, 2001.

Fridman C and others: Paternal UPD15: further genetic and clinical studies in four Angelman syndrome patients, *Am J Med Genet* 92(5):322-327, 2000.

Greco KE: Cancer genetics nursing: impact of the double helix, *Oncol Nurs Forum* 27(suppl 9):29-36, 2000.

Han S, Peschel RE: Father-son testicular tumors: evidence for genetic anticipation? A case report and review of the literature, *Cancer* 88(10):2319-2325, Review, 2000.

Harper JC: Preimplantation diagnosis of inherited disease by embryo biopsy: an update of the world figures, *J Assist Reprod Genet* 13(2):90-95, 1996.

Honein M and others: Impact of folic acid fortification on the US food supply on the occurrence of neural tube defects, *JAMA* 285(23):2981-2986, 2001.

Hudson KL and others: Genetic discrimination and health insurance: an urgent need for reform, *Science* 270:391-393, 1995.

International Human Genome Sequencing Consortium: Initial sequencing and analysis of the human genome, *Nature* 409:806-921, 2001.

Jorde L: Genes and genetic disease. In McCance KL, Huether, SE: *Pathophysiology,* St Louis, 2002, Mosby.

MacDonald DJ: The oncology nurse's role in cancer risk assessment and counseling, *Semin Oncol Nurs* 3(2):123-128, Review, 1997.

McConkie-Rosell A and others: Dissemination of genetic risk information to relatives in the fragile X syndrome: guidelines for genetic counselors, *Am J Med Genet* 59(4):426-430, 1995.

Meyers C and others: Aneuploidy in twin gestations: when is maternal age advanced? *Obstet Gynecol* 89(2):248–251, 1997.

Michelena MI and others: Paternal age as a risk factor for Down syndrome, *Am J Med Genet* 45(6):679-682, 1993.

Michie S, Marteau TM, Bobrow M: Genetic counseling: the psychological impact of meeting patients' expectations, *J Med Genet* 34(3):237-241, 1997.

Nelson DL: Allelic expansion underlies many genetic diseases, *Growth Genet Horm* 12(1):1-4, 1996.

Olshansky S: Chronic sorrow: a response to having a mentally defective child, *Soc Casework* 43:190-193, 1962.

Reiter EO and others: Early initiation of growth hormone treatment allows age-appropriate estrogen use in Turner's syndrome, *J Clin Endocrinol Metab* 86(5):1936-1941, 2001.

Sack GH: *Medical genetics,* New York, 1999, McGraw-Hill.

Scanlon C, Fibison W: *Managing genetic information: implications for nursing practice,* Washington, DC, 1995, American Nurses' Association Publishing.

Thorburn D, Dahl H: Mitochondrial disorders: genetics counseling, prenatal diagnosis and reproductive options, *Am J Med Genet (Semin Med Genet)* 106(1):102-114, 2001.

Torra R and others: Facilitated diagnosis of the contiguous gene syndrome: tuberous sclerosis and polycystic kidneys by means of haplotype studies, *Am J Kidney Dis* 31(6):1038-1043, 1998.

Verlinsky Y and others: Preimplantation diagnosis for Fanconi anemia combined with HLA matching, *JAMA* 285(24):3130-3133, 2001.

Weil J: Multicultural education and genetic counseling, *Clin Genet* 59(3):143-149, 2001.

Wertz DC, Fanas JH, Reilly PR: Genetic testing for children and adolescents: who decides? *JAMA* 272:875-881, 1994.

Williams JK: Principles of genetics and cancer, *Semin Oncol Nurs* 13(2):68-73, 1997.

Williams JK, Lessick M: Genome research: implications for children, *Pediatr Nurs* 22(1):40-46, 1996.

## Internet Resources

1. Online Mendelian Inheritance in Man
   *www.ncbi.nlm.nih.gov/Omim/*
   Up-to-date online summaries of human genes and genetic disorders

2. Genetic Alliance
   *www.geneticalliance.org/*
   International coalition of individuals, professionals, and genetic support organizations

3. National Human Genome Research Institute
   *www.nhgri.nih.gov/*
   Information on the Human Genome Project: From Maps to Medicine

4. Gene Clinics
   *www.geneclinics.org/*
   A clinical information resource regarding genetic disorders

5. Gene Tests
   *www.genetests.org/*
   A genetic testing resource; a password necessary to enter the site; is easy to obtain

6. Ethical, Legal, and Social Issues (ELSI)
   *www.ornl.gov/hgmis/elsi/elsi.html*
   A program developed to study the issues surrounding the availability of genetic information

7. National Organization of Rare Disorders (NORD)
   *www.rarediseases.org*
   A federation of voluntary health organizations dedicated to helping people with rare "orphan" diseases

8. National Coalition for Health Professional Education in Genetics
   *www.nchpeg.org/*
   Promotes access to information about advances in human genetics

9. National Cancer Institute
   *www.cancernet.nci.nih.gov/index.html*
   Provides accurate and up-to-date cancer information

10. The Health on the Net Code of Conduct Principles
    *www.hon.ch/HONcode/Conduct.html*
    Describes the Health on the Net Foundation code of conduct for medical and health websites, which addresses the reliability and credibility of information

11. United Mitochondrial Disease Foundation
    *www.umdf.org*
    Provides information about mitochondrial defects, including both professional and lay materials

12. Communities of Color and Genetic Policy Project
    *www.sph.umich.edu/genpolicy/*
    Information on two projects designed to provide policy recommendations based on public perceptions and responses to the explosion of genetic technology

13. The Family Village
    *www.familyvillage.wisc.edu/*
    A community that integrates information and resources for families with disabilities

## Chapter 6

# Communication and Health Assessment of the Child and Family

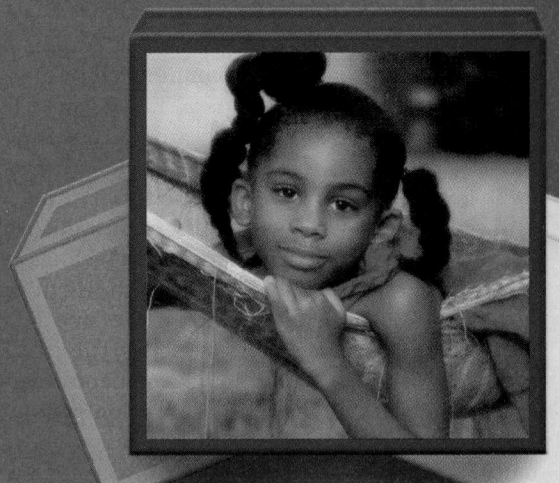

## Chapter Outline

**COMMUNICATION, 139**
**Verbal Communication—The Power of Words, 140**
  Avoidance Language, 140
  Distancing Language, 140
**Nonverbal Communication— Paralanguage, 140**
  Confirming and Disconfirming Behaviors, 140

**GUIDELINES FOR COMMUNICATION AND INTERVIEWING, 141**
**Establishing a Setting for Communication, 141**
  Appropriate Introduction, 141
  Role Clarification and Explanation of the Interview, 141
  Preliminary Acquaintance, 141
  Assurance of Privacy and Confidentiality, 141
**Computer Privacy and Applications in Nursing, 142**
**Telephone Triage and Counseling, 142**

**COMMUNICATING WITH FAMILIES, 143**
**Communicating with Parents, 143**
  Encouraging the Parent to Talk, 143
  Directing the Focus, 144
  Listening, 144
  Using Silence, 145
  Being Empathic, 145
  Defining the Problem, 145
  Solving the Problem, 146
  Providing Anticipatory Guidance, 146
  Avoiding Blocks to Communication, 146
  Communicating with Families Through an Interpreter, 146
**Communicating with Children, 147**
  Communication Related to Development of Thought Processes, 148
**Communication Techniques, 150**

**HISTORY TAKING, 153**
**Performing a Health History, 153**
  Identifying Information, 153
  Chief Complaint, 154
  Present Illness, 154
  Past History, 155
  Pain History, 157
  Family Medical History, 158
  Psychosocial History, 158
  Sexual History, 158
  Review of Systems, 159
**FAMILY ASSESSMENT, 160**
**Assessment of Family Structure, 160**
**Assessment of Family Function, 162**
**NUTRITIONAL ASSESSMENT, 164**
**Dietary Intake, 164**
  Dietary History, 164
**Clinical Examination, 165**
**Evaluation of Nutritional Assessment, 168**

## Related Topics

Developmental Assessment, Ch. 7
Establishing a Support System (Chronic Health Conditions), Ch. 22
Family Structure and Function, Ch. 3
Family Theories, Ch. 3
Growth Measurements, Ch. 7
Immunizations, Ch. 12

Nutritional Disturbances, Ch. 13
Pain Assessment, Ch. 26
Preparation for Procedures, Ch. 27
Sex Education, Chs. 15 and 17
Sexually Transmitted Diseases, Ch. 20
Sleep Problems, Chs. 12 and 15

Social, Cultural, and Religious Influences on Child Health Promotion, Ch. 2
Taking a Family History, Ch. 5
Use of Play in Procedures, Ch. 27
Using Play/Expressive Activities to Minimize Stress, Ch. 26

## COMMUNICATION

Communication is a complex process that includes the perceptions and judgments of all individuals involved. Communication may be verbal, nonverbal, or abstract. *Verbal communication* may involve language and its expression; vocalizations in the form of laughs, moans, and squalls; or the implications of what is not said in light of what has been said. *Nonverbal communication,* often called "body language," includes gestures, movements, facial expressions, postures, and reactions. *Abstract communication* takes such forms as play, artistic expression, symbols, photographs, and choice of clothing. Because it is possible to exert greater conscious control over verbal communication, it is a less reliable indicator of true feelings, especially with children.

**139**

Many factors influence the communication process. To be successful (gratifying), communication must be appropriate to the situation, properly timed, and clearly delivered. This implies that nurses understand and use techniques of effective communication. Verbal and nonverbal messages must be congruous; that is, two or more messages sent via different levels must not be contradictory.

Nurses need to recognize their own feelings and attempt to recognize those of the persons with whom the communicative interchange takes place. Biases and judgments interfere with all aspects of the process. The tendency to approve or disapprove of another's statements inhibits positive reactions. In addition, the transmission and reception of messages may be altered by influences of intimacy or distance, trust or mistrust, security or insecurity, and caring or not caring on the part of the participants. A superficial understanding of communication may generate behaviors that often produce misunderstandings rather than resolutions. The value of effective communication is increased understanding between the nurse, child, and family. Because nursing of infants and children always involves the inclusion of a caregiver, nurses must be able to communicate not only with children of all ages but also with the adults in their lives. The essential issue in communication is to keep lines open and to check perceptions frequently to assess the quality of understanding.

## Verbal Communication— The Power of Words*

Words shape reality, and thus they hold tremendous power. A person can change another's perception of reality by the choice of words that are used. For example, if the diagnosis of cancer is always referred to as a tumor, cyst, malignancy, or carcinoma, patients may never really know that they have cancer. Consequently, they may assume less responsibility for their care than they would if they were aware of the seriousness of the condition. By learning to recognize how patients and health professionals use language to manipulate reality, one can also learn how to change perceptions and communicate more effectively.

### Avoidance Language

Probably the most common way people try to alter reality is by avoiding words that truly describe it. For example, euphemisms such as "passed on" are used instead of the word "death." Avoidance language usually indicates that a person wants to hide something, especially feelings. As a rule, accepting a person's use of euphemisms only serves to perpetuate the fears and never helps the person deal with them. In contrast, use of straightforward, precise, descriptive language lends perspective to the situation and allows the person to discuss the fears. Most often, imagined fears are far worse than the actual reality.

### Distancing Language

Sometimes people use impersonal words, such as "it" or "others," to shield themselves from the painful reality of a situation. For example, parents may state that they know *someone* with a child who is slow and actually be talking about personal fears regarding *their* child. By realizing that parents need to talk about this difficult subject, the nurse can provide sensitive statements that ease them into discussing their situation.

One of the dangers in supporting distancing language is that the parent may effectively deny that a problem exists. To return to the previous example, if the issue of retardation is never approached directly but is allowed to be "someone else's problem," the parents may not seek appropriate care for their child.

Sometimes distancing is desirable because the topic may be too painful to discuss directly. The use of third-person technique (see Box 6-4) may be very therapeutic in allowing an individual the opportunity to indirectly approach a subject and receive feedback but still remain in control.

## Nonverbal Communication— Paralanguage

In addition to the spoken word, messages are relayed through nonverbal means, or *paralanguage*, which involves pitch, pause, intonation, rate, volume, and stress in speech. Young children become very adept at understanding paralanguage; long before they know the meaning of words, they sense anxiety or fear by the rise in pitch or the accelerated rate of the parent's voice. By careful attention to the spoken word, nurses can better understand the meaning of another's verbal message and more accurately control their own paralanguage.

Because most people do not exert conscious control over paralanguage, it is a valuable clue to such things as feelings and concerns. For example, *pausing* may signify a need to formulate thoughts, recall information, or fabricate a story. Frequent pauses, however, often make the speaker sound insecure. Long pauses may mean that the individual needs more information or time to process their thoughts.

*Rate* also sends unspoken messages. Talking too fast usually makes the speaker sound glib and insensitive. Talking slowly with a firm tone and appropriate pauses conveys authority. Therefore a person is much more likely to "hear" instructions if the latter approach is used. Children, in particular, respond attentively to a slow, even, steady voice.

### Confirming and Disconfirming Behaviors

People respond to each other through *confirming behaviors,* such as nodding the head, using direct eye contact, repeating or requesting clarification, and making appropriate comments, or *disconfirming behaviors,* such as tapping fingers or a foot, turning away from the speaker, avoiding eye contact, and interrupting. There is a reciprocal relationship between such behaviors, so nurses need to use confirming behaviors to receive confirmation in return. This "mirroring" effect is particularly evident in children because of their sensitivity to nonverbal cues.

---

*For additional information, please view "Communicating with Children and Families" in *Whaley and Wong's Pediatric Nursing Video Series,* St Louis, 1996, Mosby; (800) 426-4545; www.mosby.com.

# GUIDELINES FOR COMMUNICATION AND INTERVIEWING

The most widely used method of communicating with parents on a professional basis is the interview process. Interviewing, unlike social conversation, is a specific form of goal-directed communication. As nurses converse with children and adults, they focus on individuals to determine the kind of person they are, their usual mode of handling problems, whether help is needed, and the way in which they react to counseling. Developing interviewing skills requires time and practice, but following some guiding principles can facilitate this process. Regardless of whether the interview is formal or informal, an organized approach is most important when using interviewing skills in patient teaching.

## Establishing a Setting for Communication

Part of the success in interviewing depends on the type of physical and psychologic setting the interviewer constructs. Appropriate introduction, role clarification, explanation of the reason for the interview, preliminary acquaintance with the family, and assurance of privacy and confidentiality are prerequisites for establishing a setting that fosters communication.

### Appropriate Introduction

Nurses should introduce themselves to the family, offer a handshake, and ask the name of each family member who is present (Thompson and Wilson, 1996). Address parents or other adults using their appropriate titles, such as "Mr." or "Mrs.," unless they specify a preferred name. Record the preferred name on the medical record. Using formal address or their preferred names, rather than using first names or "mom" or "dad," conveys respect and regard for the parents or other caregivers and the critical role they play in the lives of their children.

At the beginning of the visit, include children in the interaction by asking them their names, ages, and other information. Nurses often direct all questions to adults, even when children are old enough to speak for themselves. This serves to omit one extremely valuable source of information, the patient. When the child is included, follow the general rules for communicating with children given in the Guidelines box on p.147.

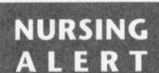 **NURSING ALERT** Nurses must make every effort to sense the world of the child and family as they sense it (Seidel and others, 1999).

### Role Clarification and Explanation of the Interview

During the introduction it is also necessary to clarify the nurse's particular role in the health care delivery system. For example, nurses performing interviews may be pediatric nurse practitioners (PNPs), inpatient staff nurses, clinical nurses, office nurses, visiting nurses, or school nurses. A parent is much more likely to reveal personal information about the child and family if the relevance and importance of the interview are stressed. If this is not done, parents may refuse to elaborate on certain areas because they feel it has no bearing on the "problem." In addition, more than one member of the health team may take a history during the course of a hospital admission. The reason for each interview must be clarified to find out what is at the root of the child's and family's concern to help them deal with the problem (Seidel and others, 1999).

Another reason for role clarification is education of the health consumer. With expanded roles in nursing, it is not unusual for families to think that the examiner is a physician rather than a nurse. Role clarification is especially important because some parents may feel deceived if they later are made aware of the nurse's identity. Because general consumer acceptance of PNPs has been very favorable, it is important to acknowledge their expertise by emphasizing the PNP's role.

### Preliminary Acquaintance

To make the family feel at ease and to develop rapport, begin with some general conversation. Open-ended questions leave the discretion about the extent of the answer to the person responding. Comments such as "How have things been since your last visit?" "Tell me about Johnny," or (to the child) "What do you think is going to happen today?" allow the parent or child to express the main concern in a casual, relaxed atmosphere.

The preliminary acquaintance conversation also reveals how responsive the informant may be to questions. For example, using open-ended statements may lead a person into a lengthy, detailed discussion. In this case direct questions toward specific answers to focus the conversation. At other times a person may respond to open-ended questions with only minimal information; in this case continue to use open-ended questions rather than "yes" or "no" questions.

### Assurance of Privacy and Confidentiality

The place where the interview is conducted is almost as important as the interview itself. The physical environment should allow for as much privacy as possible, with distractions, such as interruptions, noise, or other visible activity, kept to a minimum. At times it is necessary to turn off a television or radio. The environment should also have some play provision for young children to keep them occupied during the parent-nurse interview (Fig. 6-1). Parents who are constantly interrupted by their children are unable to concentrate fully and tend to give short, brief answers to terminate the interview as quickly as possible. (See Critical Thinking Exercise box on p. 142.)

Confidentiality is also an essential component of the initial phase of the interview. Because the interview is usually shared with other members of the health team or the teacher (as in the case of students), be sure to inform the family of the confidential limits of the conversation. If there is concern regarding confidentiality in a situation, such as talking to a parent suspected of child abuse or a teenager contemplating suicide, deal with this directly and inform

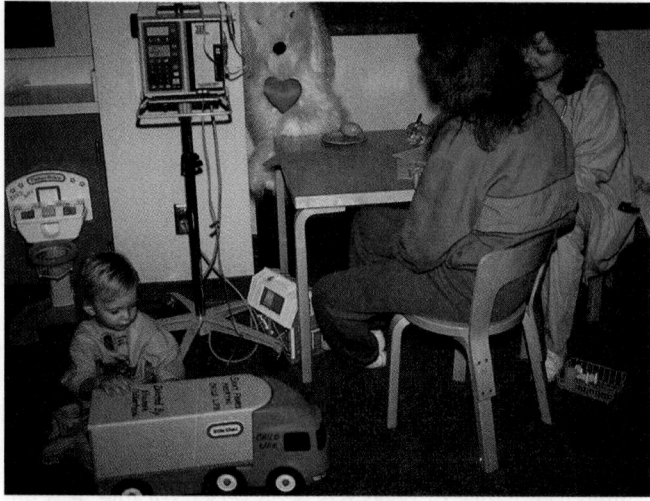

**Fig. 6-1**   Child plays while nurse interviews parent.

 **Critical Thinking Exercise**

*The Interview*

During your interview with Ms. Gaines, 2¹/₂-year-old Jesse continually interrupts the conversation. Although Ms. Gaines has told her several times to be quiet, the interruptions continue. Frustrated, the mother states firmly, "If you don't be good, the nurse will give you a shot." Jesse begins to cry softly and hugs her mother's legs. What would be an appropriate response?

FIRST, THINK ABOUT IT . . .
- Within what point of view are you thinking?
- If you accept your conclusions, what are the implications?

_____

1. State, "Ms. Gaines, don't threaten Jesse that way. Her behavior isn't bothering me."
2. Do nothing, because Jesse has become quiet.
3. State, "Jesse, nurses don't give needles because children are not being quiet. Here are paper and crayons to draw some pictures while your mom and I talk."
4. Hug Jesse and give her crayons and paper to draw.

_____

*The best response is three. The threat of injections or other painful or frightening procedures should never be used to gain a child's cooperation. You want to reassure Jesse about this but at the same time reinforce the need for her to be quiet. The point of view that providing play materials helps keep her occupied is developmentally sound.*

*Although the other responses may seem appropriate, they fail to remove the threat of a "shot" to Jesse and may bear negative implications for your future relationship. In particular, the first response can alienate your relationship with the parent. It also dismisses the issue that the interruptions do bother Ms. Gaines and most likely affect the quality of the interview.*

the person that in such instances confidentiality cannot be ensured. However, the nurse judiciously protects information of a confidential nature (Sullivan, 1997).

**NURSING ALERT**   Nurses must respect patient confidentiality and watch what they say, not only in elevators but also in places where people are waiting, such as cafeteria lines.

## Computer Privacy and Applications in Nursing

The use of computer technology to store and retrieve health information has become widespread. The privacy and security of this health information has generated a growing concern throughout the health care community. Any person accessing health information of a confidential nature is charged with managing safeguards for disclosures because violations might incur civil damages.

In 1994 a committee of the Institute of Medicine recommended a national code of fair health information practices. The suggestion was made that Health Data Organizations (HDOs) should establish data protection units to develop privacy policies and security practices for manual and automated data processing systems. Technologic safeguards and managerial procedures known as *computer security* can be applied to computer hardware and software to ensure that individual privacy is protected (Saba, Pocklington, and Miller, 1997).

Computer and information applications in nursing *(nursing informatics)* are used by 75% of all nurses to record care, access information, and obtain library resources. Two important health care applications are record transmission, including facsimile (fax) and electronic mail (e-mail), and telemedicine. The telemedicine application is capable of two-way video conferencing, transmission of radiographs, and clinical consultation between remote sites and central-

ized resources. Nurses can use these computer applications to make unique interventions that contribute to the health care of families* (Brennan, 1996).

## Telephone Triage and Counseling

Nurses are increasingly becoming responsible for assessment of children's symptoms and clinical judgment for further medical care *(triage)* via telephone report. Most often, health problems are assessed and prioritized according to urgency, and treatment is judiciously provided via telephone services (Kastens, 1998). Successful outcomes are based on the consistency and accuracy of the information provided, and parents are empowered to participate in their child's medical care. Telephone triage care management has increased access to quality health care services, and patient satisfaction has significantly improved. Unnecessary

*Nicoll LH: *Nurses' guide to the Internet*, Philadelphia, 2000, Lippincott; Williams & Wilkins.

---

**Box 6-1** ■ ■ ■
**Telephone Triage Guidelines**

**Date/time**
**Background**
   Name, age, sex
   Chronic illness
   Allergies, current medications, treatments, or recent
   immunizations
**Chief complaint**
**General symptoms**
   Severity
   Duration
   Other symptoms
   Pain
**Systems review**
**Advised to call EMS (911)**
**Advised to see practitioner**
**Advice given for home care**
**Call back if symptoms worsen or fail to improve**

**RESOURCES FOR TELEPHONE TRIAGE PROTOCOLS**

Brown J: *Pediatric telephone medicine: principles, triage and advice,*
   ed 2, Philadelphia, 1994, JB Lippincott.
Murphy KA: *Pediatric triage guidelines,* St Louis, 1997, Mosby.
Schmitt BD: *Pediatric telephone protocols,* Littleton, CO, 1994,
   Decision Press.
Simonsen SM: *Telephone health assessment: guidelines for practice,*
   ed 2, St Louis, 2001, Mosby.

---

emergency room and clinic visits have decreased, saving medical costs and time (less work absence) for families in need of health care. The most common telephone triage call is for a fever. (See Chapter 27.) Approximately 37% of the triage calls related to fever require emergency care, and nearly 50% benefit from home management (Deadrick and Boggess, 1996).

A well-designed telephone triage program is essential for safe, prompt, and consistent-quality health care (Rutenberg, 2000). Telephone triage is more than "just a phone call" because a child's life is a high price to pay for poorly managed or incompetent telephone assessment skills. Typically, general guidelines for telephone triage include screening questions, determining when to immediately refer to Emergency Medicine Services (EMS) (dial 911), and determining when to refer to same-day appointments, appointments in 24 to 72 hours, appointments in 4 days or more, or home care (Box 6-1).

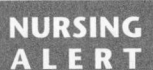 **NURSING ALERT** Legal issues can emerge from errors in telephone triage care management. Always advise that the child should be seen if there is any doubt as to the seriousness of the illness.

## COMMUNICATING WITH FAMILIES

Communicating with the family is a triangular process involving the nurse, parents, and child. Although the following discussion focuses primarily on this triad, in many circumstances significant others, such as siblings, relatives, or other caregivers, may be part of the communication process.

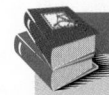 *EVIDENCE-BASED PRACTICE*
*Knowing the patient and family through effective interview skills*

Understanding the patient is highly valued in nursing (Chambers-Evans, Stelling, Godin, 1999). Knowledge goes beyond having objective information about the patient and the disease to include concerns, beliefs, and interpretation of the illness. When the patient is a child, understanding the child's world broadens to include the family. How do nurses come to know families in ways that facilitate care for the child? Unfortunately, meeting the heavy demands of clinical nursing often prevents our empathetic focus on the child in the context of the family (Reynolds, Scott, and Austin, 2000).

Learning to communicate effectively with the child and the family provides important details regarding the unique culture of children and how the world actually appears to them (Docherty and Sandelowski, 1999). Because the interview is an important means of obtaining information from children and families, methods to promote communication should be used. This approach requires listening, understanding, and validating what is being said as well as providing a climate that is sensitive to personal discussion. Exploration of the family's interpretation of the meaning of the experience as well as of the clinical situation provides more in-depth exploration of their needs and concerns.

## Communicating with Parents

Although the parent and child are separate and distinct entities, relationships with the child are frequently mediated via the parent, particularly in the case of younger children. For the most part, information about the child is acquired by direct observation or communicated to the nurse by the parents. Usually it can be assumed that because of the close contact with the child, the parent gives reliable information. Making an assessment of the child requires input from the child (verbal and nonverbal), information from the parent, and the nurse's own observations of the child and interpretation of the relationship between the child and the parent. Counseling and guidance must be directed to the caregiver of infants and small children; when children are old enough to be active participants in their own health maintenance, the parent becomes a collaborator in health care.

### Encouraging the Parent to Talk

Interviewing parents not only offers an opportunity to determine the health and developmental status of the child, but also offers information about all factors that influence the child's life. (See Evidence-Based Practice box.) Whatever the parent sees as a problem should be of concern to the nurse. These problems are not always easy to identify. Be alert for clues and signals a parent uses to communicate worries and anxieties. Careful phrasing with broad, open-ended questions, such as "What is Jimmy eating now?" provides more information than several single-answer questions, such as "Is Jimmy eating what the rest of the family eats?"

Sometimes the parent will take the lead without prompting. At other times it may be necessary to direct another question on the basis of an observation, such as "Connie seems unhappy today," or "How do you feel when David cries?" If the parent appears to be tired or distraught, consider asking, "What do you do to relax?" or "What help do you have with the children?" A comment and question such as "You handle the baby very well; what kinds of experience have you had with babies?" to new parents who appear comfortable with their first child gives positive reinforcement and provides an opening for any questions they might have regarding the care of the infant. Often all that is required to keep parents talking is a nod or saying "yes" or "and then."

When attempting to elicit feelings and covert problem areas, avoid closed-ended questions that begin with "Does . . . ," "Did . . . ," or "Is . . . ," which usually require only a single response. In addition, asking questions such as "Does your son have any problems at school?" subtly implies a lack of parental skills and evokes defensiveness. Instead, say, "What . . . ," "How . . . ," "Tell me about . . . ," and encourage elaboration with "You were saying . . . ," "You say that . . . ," or reflecting back key words or phrases,

## GUIDELINES
### *Culturally Sensitive Interactions*

**NONVERBAL STRATEGIES**

Invite family members to choose where they would like to sit or stand, allowing them to select a comfortable distance.
Observe interactions with others to determine which body gestures (e.g., shaking hands) are acceptable and appropriate. Ask when in doubt.
Avoid appearing rushed.
Be an active listener.
Observe for cues regarding appropriate eye contact.
Learn appropriate use of pauses or interruptions for different cultures.
Ask for clarification if nonverbal meaning is unclear.

**VERBAL STRATEGIES**

Learn proper terms of address.
Use a positive tone of voice to convey interest.
Speak slowly and carefully, not loudly, when families have poor language comprehension.
Encourage questions.
Learn basic words and sentences of family's language, if possible.
Avoid professional terms.
When asking questions, tell family why the questions are being asked, the way in which the information they provide will be used, and how it might benefit their child.
Repeat important information more than once.
Always give the reason or purpose for a treatment or prescription.
Use written information translated into appropriate languages (or dialects). If the family members are illiterate, written translations are useless, and the nurse must consider alternative ways of communicating, such as audio or video recordings.
Offer the services of an interpreter when necessary (see p. 147).
Learn from families and representatives of their culture methods of communicating information without creating discomfort.
Address intergenerational needs (e.g., family's need to consult with others).
Be sincere, open, and honest and, when appropriate, share personal experiences, beliefs, and practices to establish rapport and trust.

such as "He was depressed?" Open-ended questions are nonthreatening and encourage description.

Another useful approach is to elicit information about a topic and compare the answer with the person's perception of what "things" should be. For example, after the parent describes what the child is eating, ask, "What do you think your child should be eating?" If there is a discrepancy between the two answers, ask the parent to comment on how important the difference is. This approach allows the parent to discuss areas of concern that may not be disclosed otherwise.

### Directing the Focus

The ability to direct the focus of the interview while allowing for maximum freedom of expression is one of the most difficult goals in effective communication. One approach is the use of open-ended or broad questions, followed by guiding statements. For example, if the parent proceeds to list the other children by name, say, "Tell me their ages, too." If the parent continues to describe each child in depth, which is not the purpose of the interview, redirect the focus by stating, "Let's talk about the other children later. You were beginning to tell me about Paul's activities at school." This approach conveys interest in the other children but focuses the assessment on the patient.

In the event that the parent has suggested that a problem exists with one of the other children, reintroduce this subject at the end of the interview to assess the need for further family follow-up. Saying to the parent, "Earlier you were mentioning that your older son is having trouble in school. Tell me what you see as the problem," reintroduces this subject, but only in terms of the possible problem.

### Listening

Listening is the most important component of effective communication. When the interviewer engages in active listening, full attention is given to all aspects (verbal, nonverbal, and abstract) of the conversation. Special notation is made of the context, gestures, and subtle changes in voice or expression that may indicate underlying messages. Two of the greatest blocks to listening are environmental distraction and premature judgment.

The attitudes and feelings of the nurse are easily injected into an interview. Often nurses' perceptions of a parent's behavior are influenced by their own perceptions, prejudices, and assumptions, which may include racial, religious, and cultural stereotypes. What may be interpreted as passive hostility or disinterest on the part of a parent may be shyness or an expression of anxiety. For example, in Western cultures eye contact and directness are signs of paying attention. However, in many non-Western cultures, including Native Americans, directness, such as looking someone in the eye, is considered rude. Children are taught to avert their gaze and to look down when being addressed by an adult, especially one with authority (Seidel and others, 1999). Therefore judgments about "listening" need to be made with an appreciation of cultural differences. (See Guidelines box and Chapter 2.)

Although it is necessary to make some preliminary judgments, attempt to listen with as much objectivity as possible by clarifying meanings and attempting to see the situation from the parent's point of view. Effective interviewers use conscious control over their reactions and responses.

Minimal verbal activity with active listening facilitates parent involvement. It is tempting to spend time explaining, describing, and interpreting health information when the opportunity presents itself. However, it is possible to provide effective health education by properly timing the information and presenting only as much as is necessary at the moment.

Careful listening facilitates the use of clues, verbal leads, or signals from the interviewer to move the interview along. Frequent references to an area of concern, repetition of certain key words, and a special emphasis on something or someone serve as cues to the interviewer for the direction of inquiry. Concerns and anxieties are usually mentioned in a casual, offhand manner. Even though they are casual, they are important and deserve more careful scrutiny to identify problem areas. For example, a parent who is concerned about a child's habit of bed-wetting may casually mention that the child's bed was "wet this morning."

Because the interview is almost always triangular—nurse, child, and parent—the parent may wish to convey information in such a way as to prevent the child from hearing it. This requires active listening on the part of the nurse to hear the unspoken message. The following example illustrates this point:

> During a routine health visit the nurse performed a complete history and physical examination on a 4-year-old girl. The child was accompanied by her mother, who appeared to be a reliable, well-informed, and talkative informant. During the child's birth history, the mother gave all the information asked. However, during the family history, the mother stated to the nurse, "I had a hysterectomy 6 years ago." Because the nurse gave no indication of acknowledging the significance of this statement, the mother repeated it, but this time she stressed the "6 years." The nurse, who had not been listening as attentively as she should have been, realized that the mother was telling her something very important. The mother raised her eyebrows and gently shook her head "no," warning the nurse not to explore this area too openly. The nurse correctly read the cues and stated, "Let's return to your health history later."
>
> At the completion of the physical examination, the nurse took the child to the health center's playroom and then took the opportunity to investigate this contradictory information of a "4-year-old child born to a woman with a hysterectomy 6 years ago." The mother revealed that the child was adopted. The mother was greatly concerned because the child was unaware of this and requested the nurse's advice.
>
> Fortunately, the nurse had "listened" carefully enough to realize the significance of this woman's concern and allowed her the opportunity to discuss it in private.

Listening is also helpful in assessing reliability. For example, the answers elicited at the beginning of the interview may differ from those at the end, when the parent feels more confident in revealing problems. It is important to identify any discrepancies and reintroduce those topics for further investigation.

## Using Silence

Silence as a response is often one of the most difficult interviewing techniques to learn. It requires a sense of confidence and comfort on the part of the interviewer to allow the interviewee space in which to think uninterrupted. Silence permits the interviewee to sort out thoughts and feelings and search for responses to questions. It also allows for sharing of feelings in which two or more people absorb the emotion to its depth. Also, silence may be a clue for interviewers to go slower, to reexamine their approach, and not to push too hard (Seidel and others, 1999).

Sometimes it is necessary to break silence and reopen communication. Do this in a way that encourages the person to continue talking about what is considered important. Breaking a silence by introducing a new topic or by prolonged talking essentially terminates the interviewee's opportunity to use the silence. Suggestions for breaking the silence include statements such as "Is there anything else you wish to say?" "I see you find it difficult to continue; how may I help?" or "I don't know what this silence means. Perhaps there is something you would like to put into words but find difficult to say."

## Being Empathic

*Empathy* is the capacity to understand what another person is experiencing from within that person's frame of reference; it is often described as the ability to put oneself in another's shoes. The essence of empathic interaction is accurately understanding another's feelings (Price and Archbold, 1997; White, 1997; Reynolds, Scott, and Jessiman, 1999). Empathy differs from *sympathy,* which is *having* feelings or emotions in common with another person, rather than *understanding* those feelings. Sympathy is not therapeutic in the helping relationship because it leads to feeling emotionally overinvolved and potentially to professional burnout (Yegdich, 1999).

## Defining the Problem

To arrive at a solution to a problem or concern, the nurse and the parent must agree that one exists. Sometimes the parent may believe that there is a problem that the nurse is unable to see. For example, a mother was overly concerned about every small sniffle, sneeze, or cough in her infant, who had been carefully examined and found to be healthy with no evidence of a respiratory problem. On careful questioning, the nurse discovered that a previous child had died of pneumonia in infancy. Consequently, the nurse was able to better understand the mother's concern and could help the mother deal with her anxieties about her infant and teach her how to recognize any need for concern.

Occasionally a problem is identified that the parent denies exists. In this case pursue the situation and either find a way to deal with it or enlist the aid of other health team members. For example, the parents of a child with Down syndrome may refuse to believe that their child is different from any other child of the same age. They may say, "He is just a little slow," or "All the child needs to do is to try harder." A child with an obvious behavior problem may be described by the parents as "just stubborn" or "just behaving that way to spite us." Such statements may be clues that the parents have not progressed past the stage of denial in adjusting to the abnormality of a generalized syndrome.

## Solving the Problem

Once the problem is identified and agreed on by parent and nurse, they can begin to arrive at a solution. A parent who is included in the problem-solving process is more apt to follow through with a course of action. Such questions as "What have you tried so far?" or "What have you thought about doing?" provide leads for exploration and give the parents the feeling that their ideas and solutions are worthwhile. These can be followed by "What prevents you from trying that?" "That sounds like a good plan," or "You seem to be stumped. Have you considered trying this?" Such approaches encourage participation and reinforce rather than belittle parents' efforts to solve problems.

Sometimes a parent arrives at a solution that the nurse does not consider to be the best alternative. If it can be ascertained that it will do no harm and the parents are convinced of its merits, it is usually best to allow them to continue with the plan. A course of action is more likely to be carried out when parents can reach their own conclusions. However, when parental decisions may be hazardous, nurses are obligated to discuss the risks with the family and try to reach a more beneficial solution. Whenever possible, decisions should be theirs, with the nurse serving as a *facilitator* in problem solving.

## Providing Anticipatory Guidance

The ideal way to handle a situation is to deal with it *before* it becomes a problem. The best preventive measure is anticipatory guidance. Traditionally, anticipatory guidance interventions have focused on providing families with information on normal growth and development, and nurturing childrearing practices. For example, one of the most significant areas in pediatrics is injury prevention. Beginning prenatally, parents need specific instructions on home safety. Because of the child's maturing developmental skills, home safety changes must be implemented early to minimize risks to the child.

Many normal developmental changes can disturb unprepared parents, such as a toddler's diminished appetite, negativism, altered sleeping patterns, and anxiety toward strangers. Such topics are discussed in the chapters on health promotion to provide the nurse with knowledge to counsel parents.

However, anticipatory guidance should extend beyond giving information to empowering families to use the information as a means of building competence in their parenting abilities. To achieve this level of anticipatory guidance (Desselle and Pearlmutter, 1997):

- Base interventions on needs identified by the family not by the professional.
- View the family as competent or as having the ability to be competent.
- Provide opportunities for the family to achieve competence.

**NURSING TIP** Often parents need early guidance with their children (Desselle and Pearlmutter, 1997), and anticipatory guidance builds confidence in their parenting skills.

## Avoiding Blocks to Communication

A number of blocks to communication can adversely affect the quality of the helping relationships. Many of these

---

**Box 6-2** ◼ ◼ ◻
**Blocks to Communication**

**COMMUNICATION BARRIERS**

Socializing
Giving unrestricted and sometimes unasked-for advice
Offering premature or inappropriate reassurance
Giving overready encouragement
Defending a situation or opinion
Using stereotyped comments or cliches
Limiting expression of emotion by asking directed, closed-ended questions
Interrupting and finishing the person's sentence
Talking more than the interviewee
Forming prejudged conclusions
Deliberately changing the focus

**SIGNS OF INFORMATION OVERLOAD**

Long periods of silence
Wide eyes and fixed facial expression
Constant fidgeting or attempting to move away
Nervous habits (e.g., tapping, playing with hair)
Sudden disruptions (e.g., asking to go to the bathroom)
Looking around
Yawning, eyes drooping
Frequently looking at a watch or clock
Attempting to change topic of discussion

---

blocks are initiated by the interviewer, such as giving unrestricted advice or forming prejudged conclusions. Another type of block occurs primarily with the interviewees and deals with information overload. When individuals are presented with too much information or information that is overwhelming, they will often demonstrate signals of increasing anxiety or decreasing attention. Such signals should alert the interviewer to give less information or to clarify what has been said. Some of the more common blocks to communication, including signs of information overload, are listed in Box 6-2.

Communication blocks can be corrected by careful analysis of the interview process. One of the best methods for improving interviewing skills is audiotape or videotape feedback. With supervision and guidance, the interviewer can recognize the blocks and consciously avoid them.

## Communicating with Families Through an Interpreter

Sometimes communication is impossible because two people speak different languages. In this case it is necessary to obtain information through a third party, the interpreter. When an interpreter is used, the same guidelines for interviewing are used. Specific guidelines for using an adult interpreter are presented in the Guidelines box.

Communicating with families through an interpreter requires sensitivity to cultural, legal, and ethical considerations. For example, in some cultures using a child as an interpreter is considered an insult to an adult, because children are expected to show respect by not questioning their elders. In some cultures class differences between the interpreter and the family may cause the family to feel intimidated and less inclined to offer information. Therefore choose the interpeter carefully and provide time for the interpreter and family to establish rapport.

## GUIDELINES
### Using an Interpreter

Explain to interpreter the reason for the interview and the type of questions that will be asked.

Clarify whether a detailed or brief answer is required and whether the translated response can be general or literal.

Introduce interpreter to family and allow some time before the actual interview so that they can become acquainted.

Communicate directly with family members when asking questions to reinforce interest in them and to observe nonverbal expressions, but do not ignore interpreter.

Pose questions to elicit only one answer at a time, such as "Do you have pain?" rather than "Do you have any pain, tiredness, or loss of appetite?"

Refrain from interrupting interviewee and interpreter while they are conversing.

Avoid commenting to interpreter about family members because they may understand some English.

Be aware that some medical words, such as "allergy," may have no similar word in another language; avoid medical jargon whenever possible.

Respect cultural differences; it is often best to pose questions about sex, marriage, or pregnancy indirectly—ask about "child's father" rather than "mother's husband."

Allow time following the interview for interpreter to share something that he or she felt could not be said earlier; ask about interpreter's impression of nonverbal clues to communication and family members' reliability or ease in revealing information.

Arrange for family to speak with same interpreter on subsequent visits whenever possible.

Issues of legal and ethical concerns may also arise. For example, in obtaining informed consent through an interpreter, it is important that the family be fully informed of all aspects of the particular procedure that they are consenting to. Issues of confidentiality may arise when someone related to another patient is asked to interpret for the family, thus revealing sensitive information that may be shared with other families on the unit.

When no one else is available to translate, children within the family are often asked to assume this role. In this situation it is important to stress *literal* translation of parent responses. To maximize correct translations, it may be necessary to interrupt the parent and ask the child to translate every few sentences. When using children as interpreters, ask questions directed at specific answers and assess the interpreted translation in terms of nonverbal expressions of communication.*

**NURSING ALERT** When using translated materials, such as a health history form, be sure the informant is literate in the foreign language.

## Communicating with Children

Although the greatest amount of verbal communication may usually be carried out with the parent, do not exclude the child during the interview. Pay attention to infants and younger children through play or by occasionally directing questions or remarks to them. Include older children as active participants.

*Interpreting services are also available through American Telephone and Telegraph (AT&T) by calling (800) 628-8486 or (800) 752-6096.

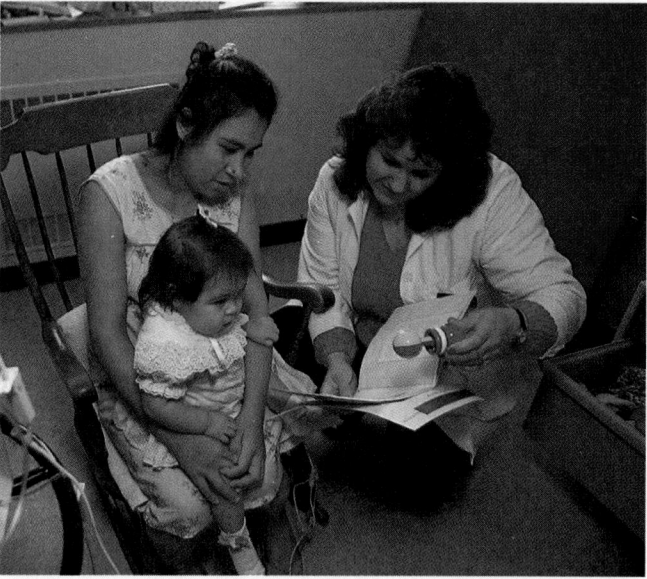

**Fig. 6-2** Nurse assumes position at child's level.

## GUIDELINES
### Communicating with Children

Allow children time to feel comfortable.

Avoid sudden or rapid advances, broad smiles, extended eye contact, or other gestures that may be seen as threatening.

Talk to the parent if child is initially shy.

Communicate through transition objects such as dolls, puppets, or stuffed animals before questioning a young child directly.

Give older children the opportunity to talk without the parents present.

Assume a position that is at eye level with child (Fig. 6-2).

Speak in a quiet, unhurried, and confident voice.

Speak clearly, be specific, and use simple words and short sentences.

State directions and suggestions *positively*.

Offer a choice only when one exists.

Be honest with children.

Allow children to express their concerns and fears.

Use a variety of communication techniques.

In communication with children of all ages, the nonverbal components of the communication process convey the most significant messages. It is difficult to disguise feelings, attitudes, and anxiety when relating to children. They are very alert to surroundings and attach meaning to every gesture and move that is made. This is particularly true with very young children.

Active attempts to make friends with children before they have had an opportunity to evaluate an unfamiliar person tend to increase their anxiety. A helpful tactic is to continue to talk to the child and parent while going about activities that do not involve the child directly, thus allowing the child to observe from a safe position. If the child has a special toy or doll, "talk" to the doll first. Ask simple questions, such as "Does your teddy bear have a special name?" to ease the child into conversation. Other guidelines for communicating with children are presented in the Guidelines box (above). Specific guidelines for preparing children for procedures, a common nursing function, are discussed in Chapter 27.

## Communication Related to Development of Thought Processes

The normal development of language and thought offers a frame of reference in knowing how to communicate with children. Thought processes progress from sensorimotor to perceptual to concrete and finally to abstract, formal operations. The early social communicative development of children has been divided into three stages: (1) *perlocutionary stage*—unintentional communication behavior. (2) *illocutionary stage*—true intent in communication efforts, and (3) *locutionary stage*—intentional communication behaviors and use of symbols (Hoge and Parette, 1995). An understanding of the typical characteristics of these stages provides the nurse with a framework to facilitate social communication (Box 6-3).

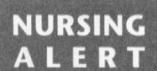 **NURSING ALERT**   Children with special needs may require additional time to process information and formulate a response (Hoge and Parette, 1995).

**Infancy.**   Because they are unable to use words, infants primarily use and understand nonverbal communication. Infants communicate their needs and feelings through nonverbal behaviors and vocalizations that can be interpreted by someone who is around them for a sufficient amount of time. Infants smile and coo when content and cry when distressed. Crying is provoked by unpleasant stimuli from inside or outside, such as hunger, pain, body restraint, or loneliness. Adults interpret this to mean that an infant needs something and consequently try to alleviate the discomfort and reduce tension. Crying (or the desire to cry) persists as a part of everyone's communication repertoire.

---

| **Box 6-3** ■ ■ □ |
| --- |
| **Stages of Communicative Development in Young Children** |

**PERLOCUTIONARY STAGE (0 TO 8-9 MONTHS)**
*Characteristics*
Child is reflexive to stimuli
Increasing purpose in action

**EMERGING ILLOCUTIONARY STAGE (8-9 TO 12-15 MONTHS)**
*Characteristics*
Communicates intentionally with signals and gestures

**CONVENTIONAL ILLOCUTIONARY/EMERGING LOCUTIONARY STAGE (12-15 TO 18-24 MONTHS)**
*Characteristics*
Communicates intentionally with gestures, vocalizations, and
   verbalizations

Modified from Hoge DR, Parette HP: Facilitating communicative development in young children with disabilities, *Transdisciplinary J* 5(2):113-130, 1995.

---

Infants respond to adults' nonverbal behaviors. They become quiet when they are cuddled, patted, or receive other forms of gentle physical contact. They derive comfort from the sound of a voice, even though they do not understand the words that are spoken. Until infants reach the age at which they experience stranger anxiety, they readily respond to any firm, gentle handling and quiet, calm speech. Loud, harsh sounds and sudden movements are frightening.

Older infants' attentions are centered on themselves and their parents; therefore any stranger is a potential threat until proved otherwise. Holding out the hands and asking the child to "come" is seldom successful, especially if the infant is with the parent. If infants must be handled, simply pick them up firmly without gestures. Observe the position in which the parent holds the infant. Most infants have learned to prefer a particular position and manner of handling. In general, infants are more at ease upright than horizontal. Also, hold infants so that they can see their parents. Until they have developed the understanding that an object (in this case the parent) removed from sight can still be present, they have no way of knowing that the object is still there.

**Early Childhood.**   Children under 5 years of age are egocentric. They see things only in relation to themselves and from their point of view. Therefore focus communication on *them*. Tell them what they can do or how they will feel. Experiences of others are of no interest to them. It is futile to use another child's experience as an attempt to gain the cooperation of very small children. Allow them to touch and examine articles that will come in contact with them. A stethoscope bell will feel cold; palpating a neck might tickle. Although they have not yet acquired sufficient language skills to express their feelings and wants, toddlers are able to communicate effectively with their hands to transmit ideas without words. They push an unwanted object away, pull another person to show them something, point, and cover the mouth that is saying something they do not wish to hear.

Everything is direct and concrete to small children. They are unable to work with abstractions and interpret words literally. Analogies escape them because they are unable to separate fact from fantasy. For example, they attach literal meaning to such common phrases as "two-faced," "sticky fingers," or "coughing your head off." Children who are told they will get "a little stick in the arm" may not be able to envision an injection (Fig. 6-3). Therefore avoid using a phrase that might be misinterpreted by a small child. (See Guidelines box under Preparation for Procedures, Chapter 27.)

Use language that is consistent with the child's developmental level. For example, in talking with a toddler, use simple, *short* sentences; repeat words that are *familiar* to the child; and limit descriptions to *concrete* explanations. Be certain that nonverbal messages are consistent with words and actions. For example, do not smile while doing something painful; children may think you enjoy hurting them.

Young children assign human attributes to inanimate objects. Consequently, they fear that objects may jump, bite, cut, or pinch all by themselves. Children do not know that these devices are unable to perform without human direction. To minimize their fear, keep unfamiliar equipment out of view until it is needed.

**School-Age Years.** Younger school-age children rely less on what they see and more on what they know when faced with new problems. They want explanations and reasons for everything but require no verification beyond that. They are interested in the functional aspect of all procedures, objects, and activities. They want to know why an object exists, why it is used, how it works, and the intent and purpose of its user. They need to know what is going to take place and why it is being done to *them* specifically. For example, to explain a procedure such as taking a blood pressure, show the child how squeezing the bulb pushes air into the cuff and makes the "silver" in the tube go up. Let the child operate the bulb. An explanation for the reason might be as simple as "I want to see how far the silver goes up when the cuff squeezes your arm." Consequently, the child becomes an enthusiastic participant.

School-age children have a heightened concern about body integrity. Because of the special importance and value they place on their body, they are overly sensitive to anything that constitutes a threat or suggestion of injury to it. This concern extends to their possessions also, so that they may appear to overreact to loss or threatened loss of treasured objects. Helping children to voice their concerns enables the nurse to provide reassurance and to implement activities that reduce their anxiety. For example, if a shy child dislikes being the center of attention, ignore that particular child by talking and relating to other children in the family or group. When children feel more comfortable, they will usually interject personal ideas, feelings, and interpretations of events.

Older children have an adequate and satisfactory use of language. They still require relatively simple explanations, but their ability to think concretely can facilitate communication and explanation. Commonly they have sufficient experience with health and health workers to understand what is transpiring and generally what is expected of them.

**Adolescence.** As children move into adolescence, they fluctuate between child and adult thinking and behavior. They are riding a current that is moving them rapidly toward a maturity that may be beyond their coping ability. Therefore, when tensions rise, they may seek the security of the more familiar and comfortable expectations of childhood. Anticipating these shifts in identity allows the nurse to adjust the course of interaction to meet the needs of the moment. No single approach can be relied on consistently, and encountering cooperation, hostility, anger, bravado, and a variety of other behaviors and attitudes can be expected. It is as much a mistake to regard the adolescent as an adult with an adult's wisdom and control as it is to confine to the teenager the concerns and expectations of a child.

Frequently adolescents are willing to discuss their concerns with an adult outside the family, and they often welcome the opportunity to interact with a nurse. They are accepting of anyone who displays a genuine interest in them. However, adolescents are quick to reject persons who attempt to impose their values on them, whose interest is feigned, or who appear to have little respect for who they are and what they think or say.

As with all children, adolescents need to express their feelings. Generally, they talk quite freely when given an opportunity. However, what adolescents say cannot always be taken at face value. When emotional factors are involved, the feelings that are interjected into words are as significant as the words that are used. To give support, be attentive, try not to interrupt, and avoid comments or expressions that convey disapproval or surprise. Avoid prying and asking embarrassing questions, and resist any impulse to give advice. Frequently adolescents reveal their feelings or a source of concern or ask a question when they are involved in routine matters such as a physical assessment.

Teenagers characteristically have a language and culture all their own that further sets them apart. To avoid misinterpretation, clarify terms frequently. Occasionally adolescents refuse to answer or answer only in monosyllables. Usually this happens when they are opposed to the contact or do not yet feel safe enough to reveal themselves. In this instance confine discussions to irrelevant topics to reduce the element of threat until such time as they feel more secure. Be alert for signals indicating they are ready to talk. The major sources of concern for adolescents are attitudes and feelings toward sex, substance abuse, relationships with parents, peer-group acceptance, and developing a sense of identity.

**NURSING ALERT**   Recently studies have indicated that family communication patterns significantly influence self-esteem in deaf children. Adolescents whose parents use total communication (speech, finger spelling, and sign language) had higher self-esteem scores than those with parents who used speech only (Desselle and Pearlmutter, 1997).

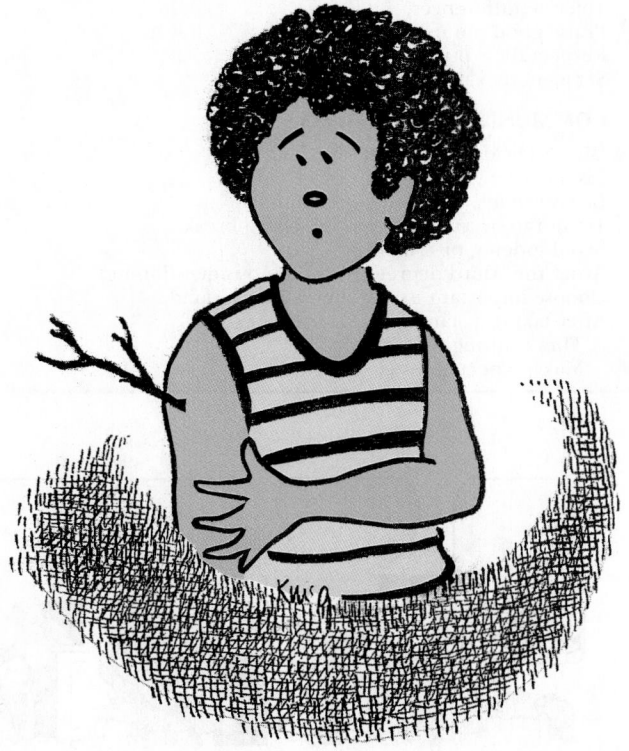

**Fig. 6-3** To a young child the expression "a little stick in the arm" is taken literally.

Interviewing the adolescent presents some special situations. The first may be whether to talk with the adolescent alone, with the adolescent and parents together, or with each individually. Of course, if the adolescent is alone, there is no question, except whether to suggest to the teenager that the parents may be interviewed at another time. If the parents and teenager are together, talking with the adolescent first has the advantage of immediately identifying with the young person, thus fostering the interpersonal relationship. Afterward, the parents can be included in the interview or given an opportunity to talk privately with the nurse. If time constraints are important, such as during history taking, clarify these at the onset to avoid appearing to "take sides" by talking more with one person than with the other.

Confidentiality is of great importance when interviewing adolescents. Explain to parents and teenagers the limits of confidentiality, specifically that young persons' disclosures will not be shared unless they indicate a need for intervention, as in the case of suicidal behavior.

Another dilemma in interviewing adolescents is that two views of a problem frequently exist—the teenager's and the parents'. Clarification of the problem is a major task. However, providing both parties with an opportunity to discuss their perceptions in an open and unbiased atmosphere can, by itself, be therapeutic. Demonstrating positive communication skills can help families communicate more effectively. (See Guidelines box.)

## Communication Techniques

In addition to such conventional interviewing methods as reflection and open-ended questions, there are a number of techniques that encourage family members to express their thoughts and feelings in a less directive and confrontational manner. Several approaches are projective—they present nonspecific material that enables individuals to externalize or project inner aspects of themselves to others.

A variety of verbal techniques can be used to encourage communication. Some of these techniques can be used to pose questions or explore concerns in a less threatening manner. Others can be presented as "word games," which are often well received by children. However, for many children and adults, talking about feelings is difficult and verbal communication may be more stressful than supportive. In such instances several nonverbal techniques can be used to encourage communication.

Both verbal and nonverbal techniques are described in Box 6-4. Because of the importance of play in communicating with children, play is discussed more extensively in the following section. Any of the verbal or nonverbal techniques can give rise to strong feelings that surface unexpectedly. Be prepared to handle them or to recognize when issues go beyond your ability to deal with them. At that point, consider an appropriate referral.

**Play.** Play is a universal language of children. It is one of the most important forms of communication and can be an effective technique in relating to them. Clues about physical, intellectual, and social developmental progress can often be gleaned from the form and complexity of a child's play behaviors. Play requires a minimum of equipment or none at all. Therapeutic play is often used to reduce the trauma of illness and hospitalization (Chapter 26) and to prepare children for therapeutic procedures (Chapter 27).

Because their ability to perceive precedes their ability to transmit, younger infants respond to activities that register on their senses. Patting, stroking, and other skin play con-

---

> ### GUIDELINES
> ### *Communicating with Adolescents*
>
> **BUILD A FOUNDATION**
>
> Spend time together.
> Encourage expression of ideas and feelings.
> Respect their views.
> Tolerate differences.
> Praise good points.
> Respect their privacy.
> Set a good example.
>
> **COMMUNICATE EFFECTIVELY**
>
> Give undivided attention.
> Listen, listen, listen.
> Be courteous, calm, and open-minded.
> Try not to overreact. If you do, take a break.
> Avoid judging or criticizing.
> Avoid the "third degree" of continuous questioning.
> Choose important issues when taking a stand.
> After taking a stand:
>   Think through all options.
>   Make expectations clear.

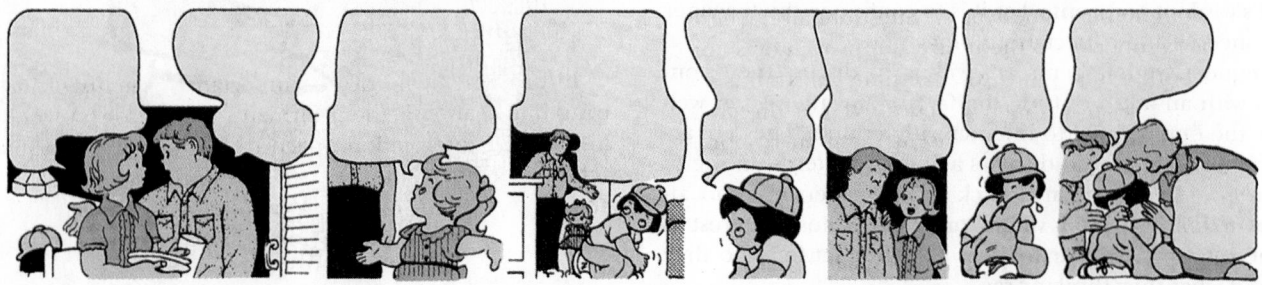

**Fig. 6-4** Filling in the blanks on a comic strip is an effective communication technique with older children.

**Box 6-4** ◼ ◼ ◻
## Creative Communication Techniques with Children

### VERBAL TECHNIQUES

#### "I" Messages

Relate a feeling about a behavior in terms of "I."
Describe effect behavior had on the person.
Avoid use of "you."
 "You" messages are judgmental and provoke defensiveness.
 *Example:* "You" message—"You are being very uncooperative about doing your treatments."
 *Example:* "I" message—"I am concerned about how the treatments are going because I want to see you get better."

#### Third-Person Technique

Involves expressing a feeling in terms of a third person ("he," "she," "they").
Is less threatening than directly asking children how they feel because it gives them an opportunity to agree or disagree without being defensive.
 *Example:* "Sometimes when a person is sick a lot, he feels angry and sad because he cannot do what others can." Either wait silently for a response or encourage a reply with a statement such as "Did you ever feel that way?"
Approach allows children three choices: (1) to agree and, hopefully, express how they feel; (2) to disagree; or (3) to remain silent, in which case they probably have such feelings but are unable to express them at this time.

#### Facilitative Responding

Involves careful listening and reflecting back to patients the feelings and content of their statements.
Responses are empathic and nonjudgmental, and legitimize the person's feelings.
 *Example:* If child states, "I hate coming to the hospital and getting needles," a facilitative response is, "You feel unhappy because of all the things that are done to you."

#### Storytelling

Uses the language of children to probe into areas of their thinking while bypassing conscious inhibitions or fears.
Simplest technique is asking children to relate a story about an event, such as "being in the hospital."
Other approaches:
 Show children a picture of a particular event, such as a child in a hospital with other people in the room, and ask them to describe the scene.
 Cut out comic strips, remove words, and have child add statements for scenes (Fig. 6-4).

#### Mutual Storytelling

Reveals child's thinking and attempts to change child's perceptions or fears by retelling a somewhat different story (more therapeutic approach than storytelling).
Begins by asking child to tell a story about something, followed by another story told by the nurse that is similar to child's tale but with differences that help child in problem areas.
 *Example:* Child's story is about going to the hospital and never seeing his or her parents again. Nurse's story is also about a child (using different names but similar circumstances) in a hospital whose parents visit everyday, but in the evening after work, until the child is better and goes home with them.

#### Bibliotherapy

Uses books in a therapeutic and supportive process.
Provides children with an opportunity to explore an event that is similar to their own but sufficiently different to allow them to distance self from it and remain in control.
General guidelines for using bibliotherapy are:
 Assess child's emotional and cognitive development in terms of readiness to understand the book's message.

Be familiar with the book's content (intended message or purpose) and the age for which it is written.
Read the book to the child if child is unable to read.
Explore the meaning of the book with the child by having child:
 Retell the story
 Read a special section with the nurse or parent
 Draw a picture related to the story and discuss the drawing
 Talk about the characters
 Summarize the moral or meaning of the story

#### Dreams

Often reveal unconscious and repressed thoughts and feelings.
 Ask child to talk about a dream or nightmare.
 Explore with child what meaning dream could have.

#### "What If" Questions

Encourage child to explore potential situations and to consider different problem-solving options.
 *Example:* "What if you got sick and had to go to the hospital?" Children's responses reveal what they know already and what they are curious about; provide opportunity for helping children learn coping skills, especially in potentially dangerous situations.

#### Three Wishes

Involves asking, "If you could have any three things in the world, what would they be?"
If child answers, "That all my wishes come true," ask child for specific wishes.

#### Rating Game

Uses some type of rating scale (numbers, sad to happy faces) to rate an event or feeling.
 *Example:* Instead of asking youngsters how they feel, ask how their day has been "on a scale of 1 to 10, with 10 being the best."

#### Word Association Game

Involves stating key words and asking children to say the first word they think of when they hear the word.
 Start with neutral words and then introduce more anxiety-producing words, such as "illness," "needles," "hospitals," and "operation."
 Select key words that relate to some event in child's life that is relevant.

#### Sentence Completion

Involves presenting a partial statement and having child complete it.
Some sample statements are:
 The thing I like best (least) about school is _____
 _____.
 The best (worst) age to be is _____
 _____.
 The most (least) fun thing I ever did was _____
 _____.
 The thing I like most (least) about my parents is _____
 _____.
 The one thing I would change about my family is _____
 _____.
 If I could be anything I wanted, I would be _____
 _____.
 The thing I like most (least) about myself is _____
 _____.

#### Pros and Cons

Involves selecting a topic, such as "being in the hospital," and having child list "five good things and five bad things" about it.
Is an exceptionally valuable technique when applied to relationships, such as things family members like and dislike about each other.

*Continued*

---

## Box 6-4 ■ ■ ■
## Creative Communication Techniques with Children—cont'd

**NONVERBAL TECHNIQUES**

*Writing*

Is an alternative communication approach for older children and adults.

Specific suggestions include:

Keep a journal or diary.

Write down feelings or thoughts that are difficult to express.

Write "letters" that are never mailed (a variation is making up a "pen pal" to write to).

Keep an account of child's progress from both a physical and an emotional viewpoint.

*Drawing*

Is one of the most valuable forms of communication—both nonverbal (from looking at the drawing) and verbal (from child's story of the picture).

Children's drawings tell a great deal about them because they are projections of their inner selves.

*Spontaneous drawing* involves giving child a variety of art supplies and providing the opportunity to draw.

*Directed drawing* involves a more specific direction, such as "draw a person" or the "three themes" approach (state three things about child and ask child to choose one and draw a picture) (Fig. 6-5).

*Guidelines for evaluating drawings*

Use spontaneous drawings and evaluate more than one drawing whenever possible.

Interpret drawings in light of other available information about child and family.

Interpret drawings as a whole rather than focus on specific details of the drawing.

Consider individual elements of the drawing that may be significant:

*Sex of figure drawn first*—Usually relates to child's perception of own sex role.

*Size of individual figures*—Expresses importance, power, or authority.

*Order in which figures are drawn*—Expresses priority in terms of importance.

*Child's position in relation to other family members*—Expresses feelings of status or alliance.

*Exclusion of a member*—May denote feeling of not belonging or desire to eliminate.

*Accentuated parts*—Usually express concern for areas of special importance (e.g., large hands may be a sign of aggression).

*Absence of or rudimentary arms and hands*—Suggest timidity, passivity, or intellectual immaturity; tiny, unstable feet may be an expression of insecurity, and hidden hands may mean guilt feelings.

*Placement of drawing on the page and type of stroke*—Free use of paper and firm, continuous strokes express security, whereas drawings restricted to a small area and lightly drawn in broken or wavering lines may be a sign of insecurity.

*Erasures, shading, or cross-hatching*—Expresses ambivalence, concern, or anxiety with a particular area.

**Magic**

Uses simple magic tricks to help establish rapport with child, encourage compliance with health interventions, and provide effective distraction during painful procedures.

Although "magician" talks, no verbal response from child is required.

**Play**

Is universal language and "work" of children.

Tells a great deal about children because they project their inner selves through the activity.

*Spontaneous play* involves giving child a variety of play materials and providing the opportunity to play.

*Directed play* involves a more specific direction, such as providing medical equipment or a dollhouse for focused reasons, such as exploring child's fear of injections or exploring family relationships.

---

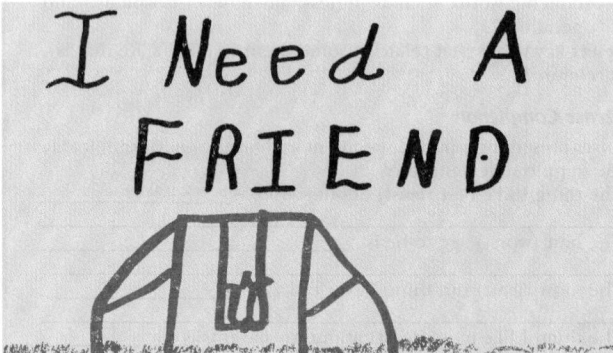

**Fig. 6-5** Using the three themes approach, this child chose the theme, "the first day of school." The drawing and title reveal the child's loneliness and insecurity in a new setting.

vey messages. Repetitive actions, such as stretching infants' arms out to the side while they are lying on their back and then folding them across the chest or raising and revolving the legs in a bicycling motion, will elicit pleasurable sounds. Colorful items to catch the eye or interesting sounds such as a ticking clock, chimes, bells, or singing can be used to attract children's attention.

Older infants respond to simple games. The old game of peekaboo is an excellent means of initiating communication with infants while maintaining a "safe," nonthreatening distance. After this intermittent eye-to-eye contact, the nurse is no longer viewed as a stranger but as someone who is a friend. This can be followed by touch games. Clapping an infant's hands together for pat-a-cake or wiggling the toes for "this little piggy" delights an infant or small child. Much of the nursing assessment can be carried out with the use of games and simple play equipment while the infant remains in the safety of the parent's arms or lap. Talking to a foot or other part of the child's body is an effective tactic.

The nurse can capitalize on the natural curiosity of small children by playing games such as "Which hand do you take?" and "Guess what I have in my hand" or by manipulating items such as a flashlight or stethoscope. Finger games are very useful. More elaborate materials, such as puppets and replicas of familiar or unfamiliar items, serve as excellent means to communicate with small children (see Fig. 6-2). The variety and extent are limited only by the nurse's imagination.

Through play children reveal their perceptions of interpersonal relationships with their family, friends, or hospital personnel. Children may also reveal the wide scope of knowledge they have acquired from listening to others around them. For example, through needle play, children may disclose how carefully they have watched each procedure by precisely duplicating the technical skills. They may also reveal how well they remember those who performed procedures. One child who painstakingly reenacted every detail of a tedious medical procedure also played the role of the physician who had repeatedly shouted at her to be still for the long ordeal. Her anger at him was most evident during the play session and revealed the cause of her abrupt withdrawal and passive hostility toward the medical and nursing staff following the test.

Play sessions serve not only as assessment tools for determining children's awareness and perception of their illness, but also as methods of intervention and evaluation. In the previous example, when the child revealed anger toward the physician, the nurse acted the part of the patient but this time did not accept the physician's harsh commands to stay still. Instead, the nurse said to the physician all the things the child had wished she could say.

Subsequent play sessions can also be used for evaluation of the child's progress. A change in the type of drawing or the theme of the play may indicate progression toward or away from the ability to deal with anxiety.

## HISTORY TAKING

This section deals with interviewing as it relates to the health history. The precise depth and extent of a nursing history vary with its intended purpose. Judgment is used in deciding what data are necessary and relevant for the identification of problems or concerns.

The format used resembles a medical history, but the objective of each assessment area is the identification of nursing diagnoses. The value in following this well-established approach is that it is systematic and familiar to members of the health team. The categories listed in Box 6-5 encompass children's current and past health status and information about their psychosocial environment.

### Performing a Health History

The format used for history taking may be (1) **direct**—the nurse asks for information via direct interview with the informant—or (2) **indirect**—the informant supplies the information by completing some type of questionnaire. The direct method or a combination of both is superior to the indirect approach. However, in view of time constraints, the direct approach is not always practical. If the direct approach cannot be used, review parents' written responses and question them regarding any unusual answers. The categories listed in the box encompass children's current and past health status and information about their psychosocial environment.

#### Identifying Information

Much of the identifying information may already be available from other recorded sources. However, if the parent

---

**Box 6-5 ■ ■ ■**
**Outline of A Pediatric Health History**

**Identifying information**
| | |
|---|---|
| 1. Name | 6. Sex |
| 2. Address | 7. Religion |
| 3. Telephone | 8. Date of interview |
| 4. Birthdate and place | 9. Informant |
| 5. Race/ethnic group | |

**Chief complaint (CC)**—To establish the major *specific* reason for the child's and parents' seeking professional health attention

**Present illness (PI)**—To obtain *all* details related to the chief complaint

**Past history (PH)**—To elicit a profile of the child's previous illnesses, injuries, or operations
| | |
|---|---|
| 1. Birth history (pregnancy, labor, delivery, perinatal history) | 3. Allergies |
| | 4. Current medications |
| | 5. Immunizations |
| 2. Previous illnesses, injuries, or operations | 6. Growth and development |
| | 7. Habits |
| | 8. Pain assessment |

**Family medical history**—To identify the presence of genetic traits or diseases that have familial tendencies and to assess exposure to a communicable disease in a family member and family habits that may affect the child's health, such as smoking and other chemical use

**Psychosocial history**—To elicit information about the child's self-concept

**Sexual history**—To elicit information concerning the child's sexual concerns and activities and any pertinent data regarding adults' sexual activity that influences the child

**Family history**—To develop an understanding of the child as an individual and as a member of a family and a community
1. Family composition
2. Home and community environment
3. Occupation and education of family members
4. Cultural and religious traditions
5. Family function and relationships

**Nutritional assessment**—To elicit information on the adequacy of the child's nutritional intake and need

**Review of systems (ROS)**—To elicit information concerning any potential health problem
| | |
|---|---|
| 1. General | 11. Respiratory |
| 2. Integument | 12. Cardiovascular |
| 3. Head | 13. Gastrointestinal |
| 4. Eyes | 14. Genitourinary |
| 5. Ears | 15. Gynecologic |
| 6. Nose | 16. Musculoskeletal |
| 7. Mouth | 17. Neurologic |
| 8. Throat | 18. Endocrine |
| 9. Neck | 19. Lymphatic |
| 10. Chest | |

---

and youngster seem anxious, use this opportunity to ask about such information to help them feel more comfortable. The school-age child should be able to cooperate fully, whereas the younger child may present the nurse with a challenge.

**Informant.** One of the important elements of identifying information is the informant, the person(s) who furnished the information. Record (1) who the person is (child, parent, or other), (2) an impression of reliability and willingness to communicate, and (3) any special circumstances, such as the use of an interpreter or conflicting answers by more than one person.

Assessing reliability is one of the more important judgments to make. A totally reliable informant will always give

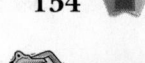

**Type**—Be as specific as possible. With young children, asking the parents how they know the child is in pain may help describe its type, location, and severity. For example, a parent may state, "My child must have a severe earache because she pulls at her ears, rolls her head on the floor, and screams. Nothing seems to help." Help older children describe the "hurt" by asking them if it is sharp, throbbing, dull, aching, or stabbing. Record whatever words they use in quotes.

**Location**—Be specific. "Stomach pains" is too general a description. Children can better localize the pain if they are asked to "point with one finger to where it hurts" or to "point to where Mommy or Daddy would put a Band-Aid." Determine if the pain radiates by asking, "Does the pain stay there or move? Show me with your finger where the pain goes."

**Severity**—Best determined by finding out how it affects the child's usual behavior. Pain that prevents a child from playing, interacting with others, sleeping, and eating is most often severe. Assess pain intensity using a rating scale, such as a numeric scale or faces scale. (See Table 26-2.)

**Duration**—Include the duration, onset, and frequency. Describe this in terms of activity and behavior, such as "pain appeared to last all night, because child refused to sleep and cried intermittently."

**Influencing factors**—Include anything that causes a change in the type, location, severity, or duration of the pain: (1) precipitating events (those that cause or increase the pain), (2) relieving events (those that lessen the pain, such as medications), (3) temporal events (times when the pain is relieved or increased), (4) positional factors (standing, sitting, lying down), and (5) associated events (meals, stress, coughing).

the same correct answers to questions. Be cautious about accepting vague, confused, or contradictory responses to questions. Ask for clarification as needed and make a note in the written record about the informant, such as "Mother, reliability questionable, answers items with hesitation, speaks primarily Spanish, interpreter (Mrs. _____) present for history."

## Chief Complaint

The chief complaint is the specific reason for the child's visit to the clinic, office, or hospital. Six guidelines determine appropriate recording of the chief complaint: it should (1) consist of a brief statement, (2) be restricted to one or two symptoms, (3) refer to a concrete complaint, (4) be recorded in the child's or parent's own words, (5) avoid the use of diagnostic terms or translations, and (6) state the duration of the symptoms.

Elicit the chief complaint by asking open-ended, neutral questions, such as "Tell me what seems to be the matter," "How may I help you?" or "Why did you come here today?" Avoid labeling-type questions, such as "How are you sick?" or "What is the problem?" because the reason for the visit may not be an illness or a problem. For example, the visit may be for a routine health assessment, or the chief complaint may be of a nonphysical nature. If the visit is for a well-child examination, ask, "Before we begin, is there anything of particular concern that you would like to discuss?"

to encourage the parent (or child) to bring up an issue that may not surface during routine interviewing.

Occasionally it is difficult to isolate one symptom or problem as the chief complaint because the parent may identify many. In this situation be as specific as possible when asking questions. For example, ask parents to identify which *one* problem or symptom caused them to seek help *now*.

## Present Illness

The history of the present illness* is a narrative of the chief complaint from its earliest onset through its progression to the present. The four major components are (1) details of *onset*, (2) complete *interval* history (from onset to present), (3) *present* status, and (4) reason for seeking help *now*. The focus of the present illness is on all factors that are relevant to the main problem, even if they have disappeared or changed during the onset, interval, and present status of the complaint.

**Analyzing a Symptom.** Because pain is often the most characteristic symptom denoting the onset of a physical problem, it is used as an example for analysis of a symptom. Assessment includes (1) type, (2) location, (3) severity, (4) duration, and (5) influencing factors. (See Guidelines box; see Pain Assessment, Chapter 26.)

**Determining the Reason for Seeking Help.** The preceding discussion deals primarily with a description of the problem. However, because most chief complaints have a "duration," it follows that something significant must have occurred to motivate the person to seek help at this time. Such factors may be a change in physical status, a change in behavioral reaction, or a result of social pressure. Eliciting such information may alter the possible nursing diagnosis and plan of care. The following example illustrates the potential significance of determining why a person seeks help at a particular time:

> **Chief complaint:** "I can't control my son. It's always been a problem, but for the past year and a half it has become worse."
> **Present history:** Child has had temper tantrums since infancy. He "throws things, hits and kicks people, yells and screams." It occurs whenever he "doesn't get his way." They usually last "a minute or two" and occur almost daily. Mother has responded to them in a variety of ways: hits him, ignores him, takes a special object or privilege away, or insults him. Nothing seems to work. Mother admits that ignoring the behavior is the most difficult approach, and she rarely can do so without eventually hitting or scolding him. Mother is not able to identify why she sought help now.

Physical history revealed nothing unusual. However, the family history disclosed several significant facts, especially that (1) the father had died 2 months earlier, and (2) he had been ill for 1½ years before his death. The nurse focused the history on events that had occurred since the beginning of the father's illness, which coincided with the son's increased behavior problems. The mother revealed that during her husband's illness she had had too little time to concern herself with her son's behavior, other than real-

---

*NOTE: The term *illness* is used in its broadest sense to denote any problem or concern of a physical, emotional, or psychosocial nature. It is actually a history of the chief complaint.

izing that it was a problem. However, after her husband's death she could no longer ignore the severity of her son's behavior or its disruptive effect on the family. As she verbalized these thoughts, she began to identify the specific reason for seeking help now. She stated, "I used to wait for my husband to come home to take the children off my hands. When he was sick, I was too busy worrying about him. But now I am home all alone. When dinnertime comes, there is no one to relieve me."

Although the interventions included several approaches to managing the problem, one of them focused on providing the mother with some freedom from the constant responsibility of parenting. Had the nurse not concentrated on uncovering the mother's reason for seeking help at this particular time, a very important clue in planning care might have been missed.

## Past History

The past history contains information relating to all previous aspects of the child's health status and concentrates on several areas that are ordinarily omitted in the history of an adult, such as the birth history, a detailed feeding history, immunizations, and growth and development. Since a large amount of data is included in this section, use a combination of open-ended and fact-finding questions. For example, begin interviewing for each section with an open-ended statement, such as "Tell me about your child's birth," to provide informants with the opportunity to relate what they think is most important. Ask fact-finding questions related to specific details whenever necessary to focus the interview on certain topics.

**Birth History.**   The birth history includes all data concerning (1) the mother's health during pregnancy, (2) the labor and delivery, and (3) the infant's condition immediately after birth. The extent of the history depends on the child's age—the younger the child, the more detailed the birth history. With older children, parents may question the relevance of inquiry regarding pregnancy and birth. A response that addresses this concern is, "I will be asking you some questions about your pregnancy and _____'s (refer to child by name) birth. Your answers will give me a more complete picture of his (her) overall health."

*Pregnancy, labor, and delivery.*   An obstetric history begins with an overview of the pregnancy, preferably by an open-ended question, such as "How was your pregnancy?" This allows the mother to state what she considered most significant. Most important, ask about the use of medications or other remedies that the mother used to relieve physical symptoms.

Basic information in an obstetric history includes maternal age, number of pregnancies (gravida), outcome of pregnancies (parity), length of gestation, and any complications. (For a more detailed obstetric history refer to maternity texts.) Because emotional factors also affect the outcome of pregnancy and the subsequent parent-child relationship, it is important to investigate (1) concurrent crises during pregnancy and (2) prenatal attitudes toward the fetus.

The topic of parental acceptance of pregnancy is best approached through indirect questioning. Asking parents if the pregnancy was planned is a leading statement because they may respond affirmatively for fear of criticism if the pregnancy was unexpected. Rather, encourage parents to disclose their true reactions by referring to specific facts relating to the pregnancy, such as the spacing between offspring, an extended or short interval between marriage and conception, or the concurrent experience of pregnancy and adolescence. The parent can choose to explore such statements with further explanations or, for the moment, may not be able to reveal such feelings. If the parent remains silent, reintroduce this topic later in the interview.

*Perinatal history.*   The perinatal period is the time from birth to 27 days of life, but the primary focus is on the immediate period after birth and during hospitalization. Specific data include (1) weight and length at birth; (2) loss of weight following delivery; (3) time of regaining birth weight; (4) condition of health immediately after birth, such as quality of cry, level of activity (feeble or vigorous), and color of skin; (5) Apgar score (some parents may be aware of this); and (6) possible problems, such as fever, convulsions, hemorrhage, snuffles (discharge from nasal mucous membranes in infants, generally in congenital syphilis), skin eruptions, desquamation, paralysis, birth injuries, deformities, or congenital anomalies.

**Dietary History.**   Parental concerns related to eating are common. A knowledge of the past history of diet, present dietary intake, and family dietary habits is important to ensure appropriate nursing interventions to ensure optimum nutrition. The detailed dietary history is discussed under Nutritional Assessment (see p. 164.)

**Previous Illnesses, Injuries, and Surgeries.**   When inquiring about past illnesses, begin with a general question, such as "What other illness has your child had?" Parents are most likely to recall serious health problems, so ask specifically about colds, earaches, and common childhood diseases, such as measles, rubella (German measles), chickenpox, mumps, pertussis (whooping cough), diphtheria, scarlet fever, strep throat, tonsillitis, or allergic manifestations. Encourage parents to indicate the onset, symptoms, course, and termination. It is not uncommon for parents to confuse measles with rubella or strep throat with tonsillitis.

In addition to illnesses, ask questions about injuries that required medical intervention, operations, and any other reason for hospitalization, including dates of each incident. It is important to focus on injuries such as falls, poisonings, choking, or burns because these may be potential areas for parental guidance. While obtaining a history of the injury, inquire about events before the injury (who was the child with, where were the parents, had this ever happened before), as well as the parent's immediate action.

Inquiries about the child's emotional reactions to each experience are important. For example, one mother stated that her 4-year-old daughter had recently been admitted to the hospital for respiratory distress and had become very afraid of medical personnel, procedures, and equipment. The nurse realized from this information that the child needed special preparation for the physical examination.

**Allergies.**   Ask about commonly known allergic disorders, such as hay fever and asthma, as well as unusual reac-

tions to drugs, food, latex products (see Spina Bifida, Chapter 11) or other contact agents, such as poisonous plants,
animals, household products, or fabrics. If asked appropriate questions, most people can give reliable information
about drug reactions. (See Guidelines box.)

**NURSING ALERT** Information about allergic reactions to drugs is
essential. Failure to document a serious reaction
places the child at risk if the drug is given; mis-
diagnosing a reaction, such as a serious allergy, may deprive the
child of effective treatment.

**Current Medications.** Inquire about current drug regimens (prescription and nonprescription), including vitamins, antipyretics (especially aspirin), antibiotics, antihistamines, decongestants, or antitussives. List all medications,
including name, dose, schedule, duration, and reason for
administration. Often, parents are unaware of the actual
name of the drug. Whenever possible, ask parents to bring
the containers with them to the next visit, or ask them for
the name of the pharmacy and call for a list of all the child's
recent prescription medications. However, this list will not
include over-the-counter (OTC) medications, which are important to know.

**NURSING ALERT** Inquire about previous administration of any
horse or other foreign serum, recent administration of gamma globulin or blood transfusion,
and anaphylactic reactions to neomycin or chicken eggs.

**Immunizations.** A record of all immunizations is essential. Since many parents are unaware of the exact name and
date of each immunization, the most reliable source of information is a hospital, clinic, or private practitioner's
record. List all immunizations and "boosters," stating (1)
the name of the specific disease; (2) the number of injections; (3) the dosage, if known (sometimes lesser amounts
are given if a reaction is anticipated); (4) the ages when administered; and (5) the occurrence of any reaction following the immunization. (See Immunizations, Chapter 12.)

**Growth and Development.** Questions about growth
and development are an essential part of the child's history.
The American Academy of Pediatrics recommends developmental appraisal at each health visit. (See Recommendations for Health Supervision, Chapter 7.) Asking parents
about their perception of the child's development is important because their concerns are good indicators that a problem exists. Whenever possible, parental responses are compared with existing health records or with current
evaluation of actual growth (height, weight, dentition) and
developmental performance (screening tests, grades in
school, scholastic achievement, play activities, social relationships). (See Development Assessment, Chapter 7.)

The most important previous growth patterns to record
are (1) approximate weight at 6 months, 1 year, 2 years, and
5 years of age; (2) approximate length at 1 and 4 years;
and (3) dentition, including age of onset, number of teeth,
and symptoms during teething. Developmental milestones
include (1) age of holding up head steadily, (2) age of sitting alone without support, (3) age of walking without assistance, and (4) age of saying first words with meaning.

Use specific and detailed questions when inquiring
about developmental milestones. For example, "sitting up"
can mean many different activities, such as sitting propped
up, sitting in one's lap, sitting with support, sitting up alone
but in a hyperflexed position for assisted balance, or sitting
up unsupported with the back slightly rounded. The clue to
misunderstanding of the requested activity is an unusually
early age of achievement.

Probing the area of developmental or intellectual performance can be a delicate one for parents, especially if there is
concern for the child's progress. Therefore, approach such
questioning with broad questions, such as "How is Jimmy doing in school?" rather than with qualifying statements, such
as "Does Jimmy do well in school?" If the parents' response
is vague and general, follow with questions such as "How
does he do in spelling, reading, or math?" Because these
questions are appropriate for older children, address them
directly to the child, as well as to the parent, for comparison
of responses and increased reliability.

**Habits.** Habits are an important area to explore (Box 6-6).
Parents frequently express concerns during this part of the

### GENERAL HISTORY OF CHIEF COMPLAINT

Ask parents/child to describe sleep problems; record in their words.

Inquire about onset, duration, character, frequency, and consistency of sleep problems:

    Circumstances surrounding onset (birth of sibling, start of toilet training, death of significant other, move from crib to bed)

    Circumstances that aggravate problem (i.e., overtiredness, family conflict, or disrupted routine [visitors])

    Remedies used to correct problem and results of interventions

### 24-HOUR SLEEP HISTORY

Time and regularity of meals†

    Family members present

        Activities afterward, especially evening meal

Time of night and day sleep periods

    Hours of sleep and waking

    Hours of being put to bed and taken out of bed

        How bedtime is decided (when child looks tired or at a time decided by parent; do both parents agree on bedtime?)

Prebedtime or nap rituals (bath, bottle- or breast-feeding, snack, television, active or quiet playing, story)

    Mood before nap or bedtime (wide awake, sleepy, happy, cranky)

    Which parent(s) participates in nap or bedtime rituals?

Nap and bedtime rituals

    Where is child allowed to fall asleep? (own bed or crib, couch, parent's bed, someone's lap, other)

    Is child helped to fall asleep? (rocked, walked, patted, given pacifier or bottle, placed in room with light, television, radio, or tape recorder on, other)

    Are patterns consistent each time, or do they vary?

Does child awaken if sleep aids are changed or taken away (placed in own bed, television turned off, other)?

Does child verbally insist that parents stay in room?

Child's behaviors if refuses to go to sleep or stay in room

    If child complains of fears, how convincing are the fears?

Sleep environment

    Number of bedrooms

    Location of bedrooms, especially in relation to parent(s)' room

    Sensory features (light on, door open or closed, noise level, temperature)

Night wakings

    Time, frequency, and duration

    Child's behavior (call out, cry, come out of room, appear frightened, confused, or upset)

    Parent(s)' responses (let child cry, go in immediately, take to own bed, feed, pick up, rock, give pacifier, talk, scold, threaten, other)

    Conditions that reestablish sleep

        Do they always work?

        How long do the interventions take to work?

        Which parent intervenes?

        Do both parents use same or different approach?

Daytime sleepiness

    Occurrence of falling asleep at inappropriate times (circumstances, suddenness and irresistibility of onset, length of sleep, mood on awakening)

    Signs of fatigue (yawning, lying down, as well as overactivity, impulsivity, distractibility, irritability, temper tantrums)

### PAST SLEEP HISTORY

Sleep patterns since infancy, especially age when slept during the night, stopped daytime naps, later bedtime

Response to changes in sleep arrangements (crib to bed, different room or house, other)

Sleep behaviors (restlessness, snoring, sleepwalking, nightmares, partial wakings [young child may wake confused, crying, and thrashing, but does not respond to parent; falls asleep with intervention if not excessively disturbed])

Parent(s)' perception of child's sleep habits (good or poor sleeper, light or deep sleeper, needs little sleep)

Family history of sleep problems (sibling behavior imitated by child; some sleep disorders [e.g., narcolepsy and enuresis] tend to recur in families)

---

Modified from Ferber R: Assessment procedures for diagnosis of sleep disorders in children. In Noshpitz J, editor: *Sleep disorders for the clinician*, London, 1987, Butterworths, pp. 185-193.

*Not all of these areas need to be assessed with every family. For example, if night wakings are not a problem, this section of the interview can be eliminated.

†A convenient point to start the 24-hour history is the evening meal.

---

history. Encourage their input by saying, "Please tell me any concerns you have about your child's habits, activities, or development." Investigate further any concerns that are expressed.

One of the most common concerns relates to sleep. Many children develop a normal sleep pattern, and all that is required during the assessment is a general overview of nighttime sleep and nap schedules. However, a number of children also develop sleep problems. (See Sleep Problems, Chapters 12 and 15.) When sleep problems occur, a more detailed sleep history is required in order to guide appropriate interventions.* (See Guidelines box.)

Habits related to use of chemicals apply primarily to older children and adolescents. If a youngster admits to smoking, drinking, or drug use, ask about the quantity and frequency. Questions such as "Have you ever had a drinking or drug problem?" or "When was the last time you had a drink or took drugs?" may yield more reliable data than questions such as "How much do you drink?" or "How often do you drink or take drugs?" Clarify that "drinking" includes all types of alcohol, such as beer and wine. When quantities such as a "glass" of wine or a "can" of beer are given, ask about the size of the glass or can.

If older children deny use of chemical substances, inquire about past experimentation. Asking, "You mean you never tried to smoke or drink?" implies that the nurse expects some such activity, and the youngster may be more inclined to answer truthfully. Be aware of the confidential nature of such questioning, the adverse effect that the parents' presence may have on the adolescent's willingness to answer, and that self-report may not be an accurate account of chemical abuse.

### Pain History

The Joint Commission on Accreditation of Healthcare Organizations (JCAHO) established pain standards that were

---

*A sleep history and a sleep chart for the family to record the child's daily sleep and wake activities are available in Wong DL, Hess CS: *Wong and Whaley's clinical manual of pediatric nursing*, ed 5, St Louis, 2000, Mosby.

effective for surveys beginning in 2001. The standards require that all patients be assessed for pain. If the patient has acute or chronic pain symptoms, a detailed assessment should be performed and should include a pain intensity measure. (See Chapter 26.) General screening questions such as, "Do you have pain now?" "Have you had pain in the last few months?" can be used.

### Family Medical History

The family medical history is used primarily for the purpose of discovering the potential existence of hereditary or familial diseases in the parents and child, as well as family habits that may affect the child's health, such as smoking and other chemical use. In general, it is confined to first-degree relatives (parents, siblings, and grandparents and their children) and is easily recorded using a pedigree chart or genogram (see Fig. 5-11). Information about each family member includes age, marital status, state of health if living, cause of death if deceased, and any evidence of the following conditions: heart disease, hypertension, hyperlipidemia (see Chapter 34), cancer, diabetes mellitus, obesity, congenital anomalies, allergy, asthma, tuberculosis, sickle cell disease, mental retardation, seizures, mental illness such as depression or psychosis, emotional problems, syphilis, or rheumatic fever. In the case of genetic diseases, inquire about the pattern of family transmission of the disorder. (See Role of Nurses in Genetic Counseling and Referral, Chapter 5.) Confirm the accuracy of the reported disorders by inquiring about the symptoms, course, treatment, and sequelae of each diagnosis.

**Geographic Location.** One of the important areas to explore when assessing the family health history is geographic location, including birthplace and travel to different areas in or outside of the country for identification of possible exposure to communicable diseases. Although the primary interest focuses on the child's temporary residence in various localities, also inquire about close family members' travel, especially during tours of military service or business trips. Children are especially susceptible to parasitic infestation in areas with poor sanitary conditions and to vector-borne diseases, such as those from mosquitoes or ticks in warm and humid or heavily wooded regions.

### Psychosocial History

In the traditional health history a personal and social section is included that concentrates on children's personal status, such as school adjustment and any unusual habits, and on the family and home environment. Because several personal aspects are covered earlier under Growth and Development and under Habits, and the social aspects are discussed in detail under Family Assessment, only those issues related to children's general view of themselves in terms of self-concept are presented here.

Through observation, obtain a general idea of how children handle themselves in terms of confidence in dealing with others and ability to answer questions. Watch the parent-child relationship for the types of messages sent to children about their self-worth. Do the parents treat the child with respect, focusing on strengths, or is the interaction one of constant reprimands, with emphasis on the child's weaknesses and faults? Do the parents help the child learn new coping strategies or support the ones the child uses?

Messages about body image are also conveyed through the parent-child interaction. Does the parent label the child and body parts, such as "bad boy," "skinny legs," or "ugly scar?" Look at how the parent touches the child. Is the child handled gently, with soothing touch used to calm an anxious child, or is the child treated roughly, with slaps or restraint used to force compliance? When the child touches certain parts of the body, such as the genitals, does the parent make comments that suggest a negative connotation?

With older children, many of the communication strategies discussed earlier in the chapter are useful in eliciting more definitive information about their self-concept. Children can write down five things they like and dislike about themselves. Sentence completion statements, such as "The thing I like best (or worst) about myself is _____ ," or "If I could change one thing about myself, it would be _____ ," can be used. Drawing offers numerous possibilities for offering insight. Children can draw a picture of an "ideal person" and then discuss how their characteristics are the same as or different from this portrait. Another activity is to have children make a collage using cutouts from magazines to represent themselves. Through play with puppets, dolls, or stuffed animals, children can reveal how they relate to others, often reflecting their own self-image.

### Sexual History

The sexual history is an essential component of an adolescent health assessment and requires a professional sensitivity when inquiring about personal information (Seidel and others, 1999). The history uncovers areas of concern related to sexual activity, alerts the nurse to circumstances that may indicate screening for sexually transmitted diseases or testing for pregnancy, and provides information related to the need for sexual counseling, such as safe sex practices.

One approach toward initiating a conversation about sexual concerns is to begin with a history of peer interactions. Open-ended statements, such as "Tell me about your social life," or "Who are your closest friends?" generally lead into a discussion of dating and sexual issues. To probe further, include questions about the adolescent's attitudes on such topics as sex education, "going steady," "living together," and premarital sex. Phrase questions to reflect concern and not judgment or criticism of sexual practices.

In any conversation regarding sexual history, be aware of the language that is used in either eliciting or conveying sexual information. Phrases such as "sexually active" have many meanings. "Are you having sex with anyone?" is suggested as the most direct and best understood question. Other questions to ask adolescents include "Are you using any type of contraception? Why not? Have you discussed this relationship with your parents? If you did, what would their reaction be?" If teenagers deny sexual activity, it is just as important to discuss with them their concerns about not being sexually active as it is to discuss concerns with teenagers who are sexually active. Most teenagers tend to

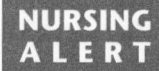

believe "Everyone is doing it but me," and this becomes a major issue for them. Because homosexual experimentation may occur, all sexual contacts should be referred to in nongender terms, such as "anyone" or "partners," rather than "girlfriends" or "boyfriends."

A detailed account of sexual partners is needed if the patient has a history of, displays any of the symptoms of, or asks for treatment of a sexually transmitted disease. A difficult but necessary part of the interview is to determine the sites of possible infection.

The degree of inquiry into the parents' sexual activity depends on many factors. For example, it may be limited to a brief discussion of their plans regarding future children or contraception. In instances in which overt adult sexual activity may be having an adverse effect on the children, a more detailed exploration of this area is warranted. Be sure to

make this decision based on facts learned during the interview, since this line of questioning should never be meaningless prying. If parents ask the relevance of revealing such matters, be prepared to offer a sound and logical explanation. It is every person's right to refuse to disclose personal information, especially if not informed of its significance or value.

## Review of Systems

The review of systems is a specific review of each body system, similar to the order of the physical examination. (See Guidelines box.) Often the history of the present illness provides a complete review of the system involved in the chief complaint. Because asking questions about other body systems may appear unrelated and irrelevant to the parents or child, precede the questioning with an explanation of why the data are needed (similar to the explanation concerning the relevance of the birth history), and reassure the family that the child's main problem has not been forgotten.

> **NURSING ALERT**
> Because sexual diseases can be contracted at any of the body orifices, inform the adolescent that a sexually transmitted disease can be acquired without visible signs of disease at nongenital sites, such as the mouth.

> **NURSING ALERT**
> The database collected during the physical assessment must be organized and documented (Thompson and Wilson, 1996).

## GUIDELINES
### Review of Systems

**General**—Overall state of health, fatigue, recent or unexplained weight gain or loss (period of time for either), contributing factors (change of diet, illness, altered appetite), exercise tolerance, fevers (time of day), chills, night sweats (unrelated to climatic conditions), frequent infections, general ability to carry out activities of daily living

**Integument**—Pruritus, pigment or other color changes, acne, eruptions, rashes (location), tendency toward bruising, petechiae, excessive dryness, general texture, disorders or deformities of nails, hair growth or loss, hair color change (for adolescent, use of hair dyes or other potentially toxic substances, such as hair straighteners)

**Head**—Headaches, dizziness, injury (specific details)

**Eyes**—Visual problems (ask about behaviors indicative of blurred vision, such as bumping into objects, clumsiness, sitting very close to the television, holding a book close to the face, writing with head near desk, squinting, rubbing the eyes, bending the head in an awkward position), cross-eye (strabismus), eye infections, edema of lids, excessive tearing, use of glasses or contact lenses, date of last optic examination

**Nose**—Nosebleeds (epistaxis), constant or frequent running or stuffy nose, nasal obstruction (difficulty in breathing), alteration or loss of sense of smell

**Ears**—Earaches, discharge, evidence of hearing loss (ask about behaviors such as need to repeat requests, loud speech, inattentive behavior), results of any previous auditory testing

**Mouth**—Mouth breathing, gum bleeding, toothaches, toothbrushing, use of fluoride, difficulty with teething (symptoms), last visit to dentist (especially if temporary dentition is complete), response to dentist

**Throat**—Sore throats, difficulty in swallowing, choking (especially when chewing food—may be from poor chewing habits), hoarseness, or other voice irregularities

**Neck**—Pain, limitation of movement, stiffness, difficulty in holding head straight (torticollis), thyroid enlargement, enlarged nodes or other masses

**Chest**—Breast enlargement, discharge, masses, enlarged axillary nodes (for adolescent female, ask about breast self-examination)

**Respiratory**—Chronic cough, frequent colds (number per year), wheezing, shortness of breath at rest or on exertion, difficulty in breathing, sputum production, infections (pneumonia, tuberculosis), date of last chest x-ray examination, and skin reaction from tuberculin testing

**Cardiovascular**—Cyanosis or fatigue on exertion, history of heart murmur or rheumatic fever, anemia, date of last blood count, blood type, recent transfusion

**Gastrointestinal**—(Much of this in regard to appetite, food tolerance, and elimination habits has been asked elsewhere), nausea, vomiting (not associated with eating, may be indicative of brain tumor or increased intracranial pressure), jaundice or yellowing skin or sclera, belching, flatulence, recent change in bowel habits (blood in stools, change in color, diarrhea, and constipation)

**Genitourinary**—Pain on urination, frequency, hesitancy, urgency, hematuria, nocturia, polyuria, unpleasant odor to urine, force of stream, discharge, change in size of scrotum, date of last urinalysis (for adolescent, sexually transmitted disease, type of treatment; for male adolescent, ask about testicular self-examination)

**Gynecologic**—Menarche, date of last menstrual period, regularity or problems with menstruation, vaginal discharge, pruritus, date and result of last Pap smear (include obstetric history as discussed under birth history when applicable); if sexually active, type of contraception

**Musculoskeletal**—Weakness, clumsiness, lack of coordination, unusual movements, back or joint stiffness, muscle pains or cramps, abnormal gait, deformity, fractures, serious sprains, activity level

**Neurologic**—Seizures, tremors, dizziness, loss of memory, general affect, fears, nightmares, speech problems, any unusual habits

**Endocrine**—Intolerance to weather changes, excessive thirst and urination, excessive sweating, salty taste to skin, signs of early puberty

**Lymphatic**—History of frequent infections, enlarged lymph nodes in any region, swelling, tenderness, red streaks

Begin the review of a specific system with a broad statement, such as "How has your child's general health been?" or "Has your child had any problems with his eyes?" If the parent states that there have been past problems with some body function, pursue this with an encouraging statement, such as "Tell me more about that." If the parent denies any problems, ask further about specific symptoms, such as "No headaches, bumping into objects, or squinting?" If the parent reconfirms the absence of such symptoms, record positive statements in the history, such as "Mother denies child is having headaches, bumping into objects, or squinting." In this way, anyone who reviews the health history is aware of exactly what symptoms were investigated.

## FAMILY ASSESSMENT

Assessment of the family, both its structure and function, is one of the most important components of the history. Because the quality of the functional relationship between the patient and family members is a major factor in emotional and physical health, family assessment is discussed separately and in greater detail apart from the more traditional health history.

Family assessment is the collection of data about the composition of the family and the relationships among its members. In its broadest sense, *family* refers to all those individuals who are significant to the nuclear unit, including relatives, friends, and other social groups, such as the school and church. (See Chapter 3.) Although family assessment should not be confused with family therapy, it can and frequently is therapeutic. Involving family members in discussing family characteristics and activities often stimulates productive discussion and insight into family dynamics and relationships.

Because of the time involved in performing an in-depth family assessment as presented here, selectivity is needed in deciding what aspects to explore. During brief contacts with families, a full assessment is not appropriate, and screening with one or two questions from each category may reflect the health of the family system or the potential need for additional assessment. Indications for initiating a comprehensive family assessment are presented in the Guidelines box.

In addition to the discussion of family assessment presented here, assessment issues specific to the family of a child with a chronic illness or disability are included in Chapter 22.

## Assessment of Family Structure

*Family structure* refers to the composition of the family—who lives in the home and those social, cultural, religious, and economic characteristics that influence the child's and family's overall psychobiologic health. (See also Chapters 2 and 3.) Since the information elicited in this part of the history is often the most personal and confidential, include it toward the end of the interview when rapport is established. The most common method of eliciting information on family structure is interviewing family members (Box 6-7). The principal areas of concern are (1) family composition, (2) home and community environment, (3) occupation and education of family members, and (4) cultural and religious traditions.

Family composition is primarily concerned with the immediate members of the household but should also include a review of the family's extended support system. For example, in a single-parent family, the household members may consist of the mother and two children, but the mother's parents may be very significant sources of child care and financial support. Although the interview method can be used to collect information about household members—their relationship, ages, and roles within the family, as well as significant individuals outside the family unit—other efficient methods include those discussed in the following paragraphs. Also inquire about previous marriages, separations, death of spouses, or divorces. Ask about the children's reaction to any of these events, which usually have a tremendous effect on their general physical and emotional health.

Several structural assessment tools are valuable in collecting and recording data about family composition and environment. Like the interview method, these tools also provide information about relationships, although several additional methods should be used to assess family function.

> **NURSING ALERT**  In assessing family composition, it is sometimes difficult to ascertain the status of the adult relationships. If the parent fails to mention the other parent, ask, "Where is the child's father (or mother)?" Avoid saying "husband" or "wife" because this assumes that only marital relationships exist.

Tools that involve drawing have several advantages. They:

- Provide an immediate visual presentation of the family and extended support systems
- Yield extensive information in a short period of time
- Are easily updated
- May stimulate productive and meaningful communication among family members

Additional tools involving drawing are discussed on p. 162 under Assessment of Family Function.

The *genogram* (family tree, family diagram) uses symbols to diagrammatically record data about family structure. It is a modification of the pedigree chart used in genetics to record the family medical history. (See Chapter 5.)

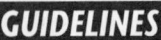

### GUIDELINES
#### Initiating a Comprehensive Family Assessment

Perform a comprehensive assessment on:
    Children receiving comprehensive well-child care
    Children experiencing major stressful life events (e.g., chronic illness, disability, parental divorce, or death of a family member)
    Children requiring extensive home care
    Children with developmental delays
    Children with repeated accidental injuries and those with suspected child abuse
    Children with behavioral or physical problems that suggest family dysfunction as the etiology

## Box 6-7 ▪ ▪ ▪
## Family Assessment Interview

### GENERAL GUIDELINES FOR FAMILY INTERVIEW

Schedule the interview with the family at a time that is most convenient for all parties; include as many family members as possible; clearly state the purpose of the interview

Begin the interview by asking each person's name and their relationship to each other

Restate the purpose of the interview and the objective

Keep the initial conversation general to put members at ease and to learn the "big picture" of the family

Identify major concerns and reflect these back to the family to be certain that all parties perceive the same message

Terminate the interview with a summary of what was discussed and a plan for additional sessions if needed

### STRUCTURAL ASSESSMENT AREAS
#### Family Composition

Immediate members of the household (names, ages, and relationships)

Significant extended family members

Previous marriages, separations, death of spouses, or divorces

#### Home and Community Environment

Type of dwelling/number of rooms/occupants

Sleeping arrangements

Number of floors, accessibility of stairs, elevators

Adequacy of utilities

Safety features (fire escape, smoke detector, guardrails on windows, use of car restraint) and firearms

Environmental hazards (e.g., chipped paint, poor sanitation, pollution, heavy street traffic)

Availability and location of health facilities, schools, play areas

Relationship with neighbors

Recent crises or changes in home

Child's reaction or adjustment to recent stresses

#### Occupation and Education of Family Members

Types of employment

Work schedules

Work satisfaction

Exposure to environmental or industrial hazards

Sources of income and adequacy

Effect of illness on financial status

Highest degree or grade level attained

#### Cultural and Religious Traditions

Religious beliefs and practices

Cultural and ethnic beliefs and practices

Language spoken in home

*Assessment questions include:*

Does the family identify with a particular religious or ethnic group? Are both parents from that group?

How is religious or ethnic background part of family life?

What special religious or cultural traditions are practiced in the home (e.g., food choices and preparation)?

Where were family members born, and how long have they lived in this country?

What language does the family speak most frequently?

Do they speak and understand English?

What do they believe causes health or illness?

What religious or ethnic beliefs influence the family's perception of illness and its treatment?

What methods are used to prevent or treat illness?

How does the family know when a health problem needs medical attention?

Who is the person the family contacts when a member is ill?

Does the family rely on cultural or religious healers or remedies? If so, ask them to describe the type of healer or remedy.

Who does the family go to for support (clergy, medical healer, relatives)?

Does the family experience discrimination because of their race, beliefs, or practices? Ask them to describe.

### FUNCTIONAL ASSESSMENT AREAS
#### Family Interactions and Roles

Interactions refer to ways family members relate to each other

Chief concern is amount of intimacy and closeness among the members, especially spouses

Roles refer to behaviors of people as they assume a different status or position

*Observations include:*

Family members' responses to each other (cordial, hostile, cool, loving, patient, short-tempered)

Obvious roles of leadership vs submission

Support and attention shown to various members

*Assessment questions include:*

What activities do the family perform together?

Whom do family members talk to when something is bothering them?

What are members' household chores?

Who usually oversees what is happening with the children, such as at school or concerning their health?

How easy or difficult is it for the family to change or accept new responsibilities for household tasks?

#### Power, Decision Making, and Problem Solving

Power refers to individual member's control over others in family; manifested through family decision making and problem solving

Chief concern is clarity of boundaries of power between parents and children

One method of assessment involves offering a hypothetical conflict or problem, such as a child failing school, and asking family how they would handle this situation

*Assessment questions include:*

Who usually makes the decisions in the family?

If one parent makes a decision, can the child appeal to the other parent to change it?

What input do children have in making decisions or discussing rules?

Who makes and enforces the rules?

What happens when a rule is broken?

#### Communication

Concerned with clarity and directness of communication patterns

*Observations include:*

Who speaks to whom

If one person speaks for another or interrupts

If members appear disinterested when certain individuals speak

If there is agreement between verbal and nonverbal messages

Further assessment includes periodically asking family members if they understood what was just said and to repeat the message

*Assessment questions include:*

How often do family members wait until others are finished talking before "having their say"?

Do parents or older siblings tend to lecture and preach?

Do parents tend to talk "down" to the children?

#### Expression of Feelings and Individuality

Concerned with personal space and freedom to grow with limits and structure needed for guidance

Observing patterns of communication offers clues to how freely feelings are expressed

*Assessment questions include:*

Is it OK for family members to get angry or sad?

Who gets angry most of the time? What do they do?

If someone is upset, how do other family members try to comfort this person?

Who comforts specific family members?

When someone wants to do something, such as try out for a new sport or get a job, what is the family's response (offer assistance, discouragement, or no advice)?

Although there is a universal list of pedigree symbols, health professionals may not use them. If in doubt regarding which symbol to use, or if one does not exist, write in the word describing the relationship, such as "foster child." Since the genogram is also concerned with the *strength* of family relationships, attachment symbols are often added as additional information on family functioning is obtained. Because a genogram can become complex, it is helpful to circle the nuclear family on the diagram. Instructions for beginning a genogram are similar to those for a pedigree (see Fig. 5-11).

## Assessment of Family Function

Family function is concerned with how the family members behave toward one another and the quality of the relationships. (See Chapter 3.) It is considered the most important component in determining "family health." Assessment of function requires more skill on the part of the interviewer than does assessment of structure and is best approached after structure is assessed. As in assessment of family structure, the more traditional method of eliciting information on family function is interviewing family members. The principal areas of concern are discussed in Box 6-7.

In addition to observing and interviewing the family to assess family function, both questionnaires and drawings can be used as needed to obtain a comprehensive assessment. The following section discusses selected instruments that are reliable and valid but require little formal training and minimal time to administer.

The *Family APGAR (FAPGAR)* is a brief screening questionnaire designed to reflect a family member's satisfaction with the functional state of the family (Smilkstein, Ashworth, and Montano, 1982). (See Appendix A.) The acronym APGAR is for Adaptation, Partnership, Growth, Affection, and Resolve (commitment). The acronym was chosen because it is familiar to health professionals, but it bears no relationship to the Apgar scoring system for newborns.

The questions in Box 6-8 can be used in the interview without the APGAR ratings to elicit similar types of information. It can be completed in about 5 minutes, can be used by families with traditional and alternative lifestyles and from different cultures, and is appropriate for children age 10 years or older. Separate forms have been designed to assess relationships with friends and fellow workers, because these groups represent other significant sources of support.

The responses to the five questions are scored as follows: "Almost always"—2; "Some of the time"—1; and "Hardly ever"—0. Each score is totaled. Scores of 7 to 10 suggest a highly functional family; 4 to 6, a moderately dysfunctional family; and 0 to 3, a severely dysfunctional family. Also, a low score in any single item could signal family dysfunction. The

---

### Box 6-8  ◼ ◼ ◻
### Family APGAR

| DEFINITION | FUNCTION MEASURED BY THE FAMILY APGAR | RELEVANT OPEN-ENDED QUESTIONS |
|---|---|---|
| *Adaptation* is the use of intrafamilial and extrafamilial resources for problem solving when family equilibrium is stressed during a crisis. | How resources are shared, or the degree to which a member is satisfied with the assistance received when family resources are needed. | How have family members aided each other in time of need? |
| *Partnership* is the sharing of decision-making and nurturing responsibilities by family members. | How decisions are shared, or the member's satisfaction with mutuality in family communication and problem solving. | In what way have family members received help or assistance from friends and community agencies? |
| *Growth* is the physical and emotional maturation and self-fulfillment that is achieved by family members through mutual support and guidance. | How nurturing is shared, or the member's satisfaction with the freedom available within the family to change roles and attain physical and emotional growth or maturation. | How do family members communicate with each other about such matters as vacations, finances, medical care, large purchases, and personal problems? |
| | | How have family members changed during the past years? |
| | | How has this change been accepted by family members? |
| | | In what ways have family members aided each other in growing or developing independent lifestyles? |
| | | How have family members reacted to your desires for change? |
| *Affection* is the caring or loving relationship that exists among family members. | How emotional experiences are shared, or the member's satisfaction with the intimacy and emotional interaction that exists in the family. | How have members of your family responded to emotional expressions such as affection, love, sorrow, or anger? |
| *Resolve* is the commitment to devote time to other members of the family for physical and emotional nurturing. It also usually involves a decision to share wealth and space. | How time (and space and money) is shared, or the member's satisfaction with the time commitment that has been made to the family by its members. | How do members of your family share time, space, and money? |

Modified from Smilkstein G: The Family APGAR: a proposal for a family function test and its use by physicians, *J Fam Pract* 6(6):1231-1239, 1978.

family APGAR is not recommended for use with individuals from enmeshed (overly close) or "psychosomatic" families. Persons with health problems, such as asthma, atopic dermatitis, or irritable bowel syndrome, may report falsely high scores (Smilkstein, 1993).

The **Feetham Family Functioning Survey** provides information about family members' *perception* of relationships that contribute to or are affected by family functioning (Feetham, Perkins, and Carroll, 1993).* Although recommended primarily as a research instrument, it can be used clinically without scoring the items to identify areas that may be of concern to the family. The survey consists of 25 ratings of family functioning (household tasks; child care; sexual and marital relationships; interaction with family, children, and friends; community involvement; and sources of emotional support) and two open-ended questions. Each of the questions on family functioning is rated on three 7-point scales of "How much is there now?" "How much should there be?" and "How important is this to me?" (Box 6-9). Discrepancy between the first two ratings, together with the rating of importance, contributes to an assessment of the members' perceptions of family functioning. The survey takes less than 10 minutes to complete and can be used with single-parent and two-parent families (Feetham, Perkins, and Carroll, 1993).

Ideally, a thorough assessment includes observing the child and family in a variety of settings. Undoubtedly, the richest environment for observing a child's development and interactions with family members is the home. Two tools that can be used to assess the child's home environment are the **Home Observation for Management of the Environment (HOME)**† (Caldwell and Bradley, 1984) and the **Home Screening Questionnaire (HSQ)** (Frankenburg and Coons,

---

*The survey is available for a fee from Nursing Systems and Research, Children's National Medical Center, 111 Michigan Ave NW, Washington, DC 20010, (202) 939-4980.
†The forms and an administration manual are available for a fee from the Center for Research on Teaching and Learning, College of Education, University of Arkansas at Little Rock, 2801 S University Ave, Little Rock, AR 72204-1099, (501) 569-3422.

1986).* Both are divided into two age-groups—birth to 3 years of age and 3 to 6 years of age. (See Appendix A.) HOME has an additional inventory for children ages 6 to 10 years; forms are also available for children with moderate to severe disabilities in each of the three age-groups for visual, auditory, orthopaedic, and cognitive impairments.

Some of the HOME items require direct observation, whereas others necessitate questioning of the parents. Each item receives a "yes" or "no" response. The number of "yes" responses correlates with the amount of appropriate environmental stimulation. Any "no" responses indicate possible areas for intervention and counseling. Use of HOME requires about a 1-hour home visit with both the child and the primary caregiver.

The HSQ was developed using HOME as a guide. The 0- to 3-year form consists of 30 items plus a checklist of toys available to the child in the home. The 3- to 6-year form has 34 items and a similar toy checklist. The questions are written at approximately a third- to sixth-grade reading level and, unlike the HOME, can be completed by the parents in any setting in about 15 to 20 minutes. Scoring directions are detailed in the manual and are based on credits for different answers. For each age-group there is a minimum score for determining suspect or nonsuspect results.

The **kinetic family drawing (KFD)** (Burns, 1982; Burns and Kaufman, 1972) involves asking the family member to "Draw your family doing something." In giving directions, offer only a general statement of encouragement to avoid suggesting themes. Drawing the family is appropriate for children over 4 years of age.

The focus of the KFD is not only the family unit but also the activity and interaction of each family member. The drawing describes the person's perspective of family dynamics and his or her place in the family matrix. To evaluate a KFD, either subjective impressions or an objective scoring system may be used (Burns, 1982; Spinetta and others, 1981). Suggestions for evaluating a KFD are listed in the Guidelines box.

---

*The forms and manual are available for a fee from Denver Developmental Materials, Inc, PO Box 6919, Denver, CO 80206-0919, (303) 355-4729.

---

### Box 6-9 ■ ■ ■
#### Sample Questions from the Feetham Family Functioning Survey

The amount of time you spend with your *spouse*.
a. How much is there now?

LITTLE    MUCH
1   2   3   4   5   6   7

b. How much should there be?

LITTLE    MUCH
1   2   3   4   5   6   7

c. How important is this to me?

LITTLE    MUCH
1   2   3   4   5   6   7

---

Reproduced with the permission of Suzanne L. Feetham, PhD, RN, FAAN. Developed from research funded by Division of Nursing, HRA, HHS, NU00632, Wayne State University, Detroit, MI, 1977-1980.

---

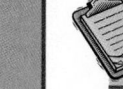

### GUIDELINES
#### *Evaluating Kinetic Family Drawings*

Note omission of family members; if someone is missing, ask child if everyone in the family has been included in the drawing.
Ask child to explain what each family member is doing.
Encourage child to tell as much as possible about the drawing.
Note signs of physical intimacy or distance, such as people close to each other or touching.
Note placement of people in the drawing, such as top or bottom of drawing and proximity to each other.
Note facial expressions, such as happy, sad, blank, or bored.
Note which members are facing each other or turned away from each other and how they are grouped together.

---

Modified from Burns R: *Self-growth in families: kinetic family drawings (KFD)—research and application*, New York, 1982, Brunner/Mazel.

Another useful technique with children and adults is the *conjoint family drawing*. Give the family a large sheet of white paper and a box of colored pencils, pens, or crayons. Ask each member to select a different-color pen and not to exchange colors. Instruct them to work together on a drawing but without talking to each other. After the drawing is completed, ask each member to discuss it. Emphasize the process or "how" the drawing took place, rather than the symbolic meaning of each part. Assess the process by looking at:

- Who initiates the drawing?
- Who uses the most or least space?
- Does anyone infringe on another's "space"?
- Do "subsystems" appear, or is anyone deleted?
- Does someone take the lead in organizing the drawing?
- Who copies another's theme, or who draws something completely different?

The conjoint family drawing is a valuable tool in uncovering family dynamics and relationships. It can be used as a learning experience to help "well" families learn more about themselves. When it is used with dysfunctional families, nurses must have sufficient skill in handling issues and feelings that may arise.

## NUTRITIONAL ASSESSMENT

A nutritional assessment is an essential part of a complete health appraisal. Its purpose is to evaluate the child's nutritional status, the state of balance between nutrient intake and nutrient expenditure or need. A thorough nutritional status assessment includes (1) dietary intake, (2) clinical examination, and (3) biochemical analysis.

## Dietary Intake

Knowledge of the child's dietary intake is a useful and practical component of a nutritional assessment. However, it is also one of the most difficult factors to assess. Individuals' recall of food consumption, especially amounts eaten, is frequently unreliable. In addition, people may be hesitant to reveal their eating patterns if they sense criticism from the nurse. People from different cultures may have difficulty adequately describing the types of food they eat. Despite these obstacles, however, a food intake record is essential. Several methods are available.

### Dietary History

Regardless of the format used in recording food intake, every nutritional assessment should begin with a *dietary history*. The exact questions used to elicit a dietary history vary with the child's age. In general, the younger the child, the more specific and detailed the history should be. Box 6-10 provides a sample dietary history for children. Important additional questions regarding infant feeding are included.

In addition to the broad overview of food intake, the dietary history is concerned with financial and cultural factors that influence food selection and preparation. Because cul-

---

**Box 6-10** ■ ■ ■
**Dietary History**

What are the family's usual mealtimes?
Do family members eat together or at separate times?
Who does the family grocery shopping and meal preparation?
How much money is spent to buy food each week?
How are most foods prepared—baked, broiled, fried, other?
How often does the family or your child eat out?
  What kinds of restaurants do you go to?
  What kinds of food does your child typically eat at restaurants?
Does your child eat breakfast regularly?
Where does your child eat lunch?
What are your child's favorite foods, beverages, and snacks?
  What are the average amounts eaten per day?
  What foods are artificially sweetened?
  What are your child's snacking habits?
  When are sweet foods usually eaten?
  What are your child's toothbrushing habits?
What special cultural practices are followed? What ethnic foods are eaten?
What foods and beverages does your child dislike?
How would you describe your child's usual appetite (hearty eater, picky eater)?
What are your child's feeding habits (breast, bottle, cup, spoon, eats by self, needs assistance, any special devices)?
Does your child take vitamins or other supplements? Do they contain iron or fluoride?
Are there any known or suspected food allergies? Is your child on a special diet?
Has your child lost or gained weight recently?
Are there any feeding problems (excessive fussiness, spitting up, colic, difficulty sucking or swallowing)? Are there any dental problems or appliances, such as braces, that affect eating?

What types of exercise does your child do regularly?
Is there a family history of cancer, diabetes, heart disease, high blood pressure, or obesity?

**ADDITIONAL QUESTIONS FOR INFANTS**

What was the infant's birth weight? When did it double? Triple?
Was the infant premature?
Are you breast-feeding or have you breast-fed your infant?
  For how long?
If you use a formula, what is the brand?
  How long has the infant been taking it?
  How many ounces does the infant drink a day?
Are you giving the infant cow's milk (whole, low-fat, skimmed)?
  When did you start?
  How many ounces does the infant drink a day?
Do you give your infant extra fluids (water, juice)?
If the infant takes a bottle to bed at nap or nighttime, what is in the bottle?
At what age did you start cereal, vegetables, meat or other protein sources, fruit or juice, finger food, table food?
Do you make your own baby food or use commercial foods, such as infant cereal?
Does the infant take a vitamin and mineral supplement? If so, what type?
Has the infant shown an allergic reaction to any food(s)? If so, list the foods and describe the reaction.
Does the infant spit up frequently, have unusually loose stools, or have hard, dry stools? If so, how often?
How often do you feed your infant?
How would you describe your infant's appetite?

tural practices are very prevalent in food preparation, it is important to consider carefully the kinds of questions that are asked and the judgments made in regard to counseling. (See Cultural Awareness box.)

The most common and probably easiest method of assessing daily intake is the *24-hour recall.* The child or parent recalls every item eaten in the past 24 hours and the approximate amounts. The 24-hour recall is most beneficial when it represents a typical day's intake. Some of the difficulties with a daily recall are the family's inability to remember exactly what was eaten and inaccurate estimation of portion size. To increase accuracy of reporting portion sizes, try using food models and asking additional questions. In general, this method is most useful in providing *qualitative* information about the child's diet.

To improve the reliability of the daily recall, have the family complete a *food diary* by recording every food and liquid consumed for a certain number of days. A 3-day record consisting of two weekdays and one weekend day represents most people's eating patterns. To improve compliance, provide specific charts to record intake and ask the family to record items immediately after eating.

A *food frequency questionnaire* or *record* provides information about the number of times in a day, week, or month a child consumes items from the four food groups (Box 6-11). In general, it provides more of a qualitative overview but has

the advantage of avoiding recall based on a "typical" day. It is especially useful when verifying a food history or diary.

## Clinical Examination

A significant amount of information regarding nutritional adequacy is elicited from a clinical examination, especially from assessing the skin, hair, teeth, gums, lips, tongue, and eyes. The hair, skin, and mouth are vulnerable to nutritional deficiency or excess because of the rapid turnover of epithelial and mucosal tissue. Table 6-1 summarizes clinical signs of possible nutritional deficiency or excess. Few are diagnostic for a specific nutrient, and if suspicious signs are

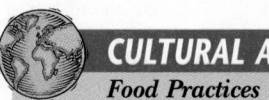

### CULTURAL AWARENESS
#### Food Practices

Because cultural practices are very prevalent in food preparation consider carefully the kinds of questions that are asked and the judgments made in regard to counseling. For example, some cultures, such as Hispanic, African-American, and Native American, include many vegetables, legumes, and starches in their diet that together provide sufficient essential amino acids, even though the actual amount of meat or dairy protein is low. (See Chapter 2 for cultural food practices.)

---

**Box 6-11** ▪ ▪ ▫
**Food Frequency Record***

| Food Group | Number of Servings (day, week) | Serving Size (in cup, tablespoon, or ounce portions) | Food Group | Number of Servings (day, week) | Serving Size (in cup, tablespoon, or ounce portions) |
|---|---|---|---|---|---|
| **BREADS/CEREALS/ RICE/PASTA** | | | **MILK/CHEESE/YOGURT** | | |
| Bread, tortilla | | | Milk | | |
| Cooked pasta, rice, hot cereal | | | Cheese | | |
| Dry cereal (not presweetened) | | | Yogurt | | |
| Crackers | | | Pudding | | |
| Muffins | | | Ice cream | | |
| Other | | | Other | | |
| **VEGETABLES** | | | **OTHER PROTEIN FOODS** | | |
| Yellow or orange | | | Meat | | |
| Green or leafy | | | Fish | | |
| Other | | | Poultry | | |
| | | | Egg | | |
| | | | Peanut butter | | |
| | | | Legumes (dried beans, peas) | | |
| | | | Nuts | | |
| | | | Other | | |
| **FRUITS/JUICE** | | | **FATS/OILS/SWEETS** | | |
| Citrus (orange, grapefruit, tangerine) | | | Butter, oil, margarine, mayonnaise, salad dressing | | |
| Noncitrus | | | Soda, punch | | |
| Other | | | Cake, cookie, etc. | | |
| | | | Candy | | |
| | | | Presweetened cereal | | |

*For comparison of actual intake with recommended intake, see Food Guide Pyramid, Fig. 13-1.

**TABLE 6-1   Clinical assessment of nutritional status**

| Evidence of Adequate Nutrition | Evidence of Deficient or Excess Nutrition | Deficiency/Excess* |
|---|---|---|
| **General Growth** | | |
| Within 5th and 95th percentiles for height, weight, and head circumference | Below 5th or above 95th percentiles for growth | Protein, calories, fats, and other essential nutrients, especially A, pyridoxine, niacin, calcium, iodine, manganese, zinc |
| Steady gain with expected growth spurts during infancy and adolescence | Absence of or delayed growth spurts; poor weight gain | |
| Sexual development appropriate for age | Delayed sexual development | Excess vitamin A, D |
| **Skin** | | |
| Smooth, slightly dry to touch | Hardening and scaling | Vitamin A |
| Elastic and firm | Seborrheic dermatitis | Excess niacin |
| Absence of lesions | Dry, rough, petechiae | Riboflavin |
| Color appropriate to genetic background | Delayed wound healing | Vitamin C |
| | Scaly dermatitis on exposed surfaces | Riboflavin, vitamin C, zinc |
| | Wrinkled, flabby | Niacin |
| | Crusted lesions around orifices, especially nares | Protein and calories |
| | | Zinc |
| | Pruritus | Excess vitamin A, riboflavin, niacin |
| | Poor turgor | Water, sodium |
| | Edema | Protein, thiamin |
| | | Excess sodium |
| | Yellow tinge (jaundice) | Vitamin B$_{12}$ |
| | | Excess vitamin A, niacin |
| | Depigmentation | Protein, calories |
| | Pallor (anemia) | Pyridoxine, folic acid, vitamin B$_{12}$, C, E (in premature infants), iron |
| | | Excess vitamin C, zinc |
| | Paresthesia | Excess riboflavin |
| **Hair** | | |
| Lustrous, silky, strong, elastic | Stringy, friable, dull, dry, thin | Protein, calories |
| | Alopecia | Protein, calories, zinc |
| | Depigmentation | Protein, calories, copper |
| | Raised areas around hair follicles | Vitamin C |
| **Head** | | |
| Even molding, occipital prominence, symmetric facial features | Softening of cranial bones, prominence of frontal bones, skull flat and depressed toward middle | Vitamin D |
| Fused sutures after 18 months | Delayed fusion of sutures | Vitamin D |
| | Hard, tender lumps in occiput | Excess vitamin A |
| | Headache | Excess thiamine |
| **Neck** | | |
| Thyroid not visible, palpable in midline | Thyroid enlarged; may be grossly visible | Iodine |
| **Eyes** | | |
| Clear, bright | Hardening and scaling of cornea and conjunctiva | Vitamin A |
| Good night vision | Night blindness | |
| *Conjunctiva*—Pink, glossy | Burning, itching, photophobia, cataracts, corneal vascularization | Riboflavin |
| **Ears** | | |
| *Tympanic membrane*—Pliable | Calcified bone (hearing loss) | Excess vitamin D |
| **Nose** | | |
| Smooth, intact nasal angle | Irritation and cracks at nasal angle | Riboflavin |
| | | Excess vitamin A |
| **Mouth** | | |
| *Lips*—Smooth, moist, darker color than skin | Fissures/inflammation at corners of mouth | Riboflavin |
| | | Excess vitamin A |
| *Gums*—Firm, coral pink color, stippled | Gums spongy, friable, swollen, bluish red or black color, bleed easily | Vitamin C |

*Nutrients listed are deficient unless specified as excess.

**TABLE 6-1    Clinical assessment of nutritional status—cont'd**

| Evidence of Adequate Nutrition | Evidence of Deficient or Excess Nutrition | Deficiency/Excess |
|---|---|---|
| **Mouth—cont'd** | | |
| *Mucous membranes*—Bright pink, smooth, moist | Stomatitis | Niacin |
| *Tongue*—Rough texture, no lesions, taste sensation | Glossitis | Niacin, riboflavin, folic acid |
| | Diminished taste sensation | Zinc |
| *Teeth*—Uniform white color, smooth, intact | Brown mottling, pits, fissures | Excess fluoride |
| | Defective enamel | Vitamin A, C, D, calcium, phosphorus |
| | Caries | Excess carbohydrates |
| **Chest** | | |
| Infants, shape is almost circular | Depressed lower portion of rib cage | Vitamin D |
| In children, lateral diameter increases in proportion to anteroposterior diameter | Sharp protrusion of sternum | |
| Smooth costochondral junctions | Enlarged costochondral junctions | Vitamin C, D |
| *Breast development*—Normal for age | Delayed development | See General Growth, p. 166, especially zinc |
| **Cardiovascular System** | | |
| Pulse and blood pressure (BP) within normal limits | Palpitations | Thiamine |
| | Rapid pulse | Potassium |
| | | Excess thiamine |
| | Arrhythmias | Magnesium, potassium |
| | | Excess niacin, potassium |
| | Increased BP | Excess sodium |
| | Decreased BP | Thiamine; excess niacin |
| **Abdomen** | | |
| In young children, cylindric and prominent | Distended, flabby, poor musculature | Protein, calories |
| | Prominent, large | Excess calories |
| In older children, flat | Potbelly, constipation | Vitamin D |
| Normal bowel habits | Diarrhea | Niacin |
| | | Excess vitamin C |
| | Constipation | Excess calcium, potassium |
| **Musculoskeletal System** | | |
| *Muscles*—Firm, well-developed, equal strength bilaterally | Flabby, weak, generalized wasting | Protein, calories |
| | Weakness, pain, cramps | Thiamine, sodium, chloride, potassium, phosphorus, magnesium |
| | | Excess thiamine |
| | Muscle twitching, tremors | Magnesium |
| | Muscular paralysis | Excess potassium |
| *Spine*—Cervical and lumbar curves (double S curve) | Kyphosis, lordosis, scoliosis | Vitamin D |
| *Extremities*—Symmetric; legs straight with minimum bowing | Bowing of extremities, knock-knees | Vitamin D, calcium, phosphorus |
| | Epiphyseal enlargement | Vitamin A, D |
| | Bleeding into joints and muscles, joint swelling, pain | Vitamin C |
| *Joints*—Flexible, full range of motion, no pain or stiffness | Thickening of cortex of long bones with pain and fragility, hard tender lumps in extremities | Excess vitamin A |
| | Osteoporosis of long bones | Calcium; excess vitamin D |
| **Neurologic System** | | |
| *Behavior*—Alert, responsive, emotionally stable | Listless, irritable, lethargic, apathetic (sometimes apprehensive, anxious, drowsy, mentally slow, confused) | Thiamine, niacin, pyridoxine, vitamin C, potassium, magnesium, iron, protein, calories |
| | | Excess vitamin A, D, thiamine, folic acid, calcium |
| Absence of tetany, convulsions | Masklike facial expression, blurred speech, involuntary laughing | Excess manganese |
| | Seizures | Thiamine, pyridoxine, vitamin D, calcium, magnesium |
| Intact peripheral nervous system | Peripheral nervous system toxicity (unsteady gait, numb feet and hands, fine motor clumsiness) | Excess phosphorus (in relation to calcium) |
| | | Excess pyridoxine |
| Intact reflexes | Diminished or absent tendon reflexes | Thiamine, vitamin E |

found, they must be confirmed with dietary and biochemical data. Generally, the clinical examination does not reveal children at risk for a deficiency or excess.

An essential parameter of nutritional status is ***anthropometry,*** the measurement of height, weight, head circumference in young children, proportions, skinfold thickness, and arm circumference. Height and head circumference reflect past nutrition, whereas weight, skinfold thickness, and arm circumference reflect present nutritional status, especially of protein and fat reserves. Skinfold thickness measures the body's fat content, since approximately one half of the body's total fat stores are directly beneath the skin. The upper arm muscle circumference correlates with measurements of total muscle mass. Since muscle serves as the body's major protein reserve, this measurement serves as an index of the body's protein stores. Ideally, record growth measurements over a period of time and compare the *velocity* of growth based on previous and present values. Techniques for anthropometric measurement are discussed in Chapter 7 under Growth Measurements.

Numerous ***biochemical tests*** are available for assessing nutritional status and include analysis of plasma, blood cells, urine, or tissues from liver, bone, hair, and fingernails. Many of these tests are complicated and are not performed routinely. Common laboratory procedures for nutritional status include measurement of hemoglobin, hematocrit, transferrin, albumin, creatinine, and nitrogen. Laboratory values

for these tests and more specific nutrient measurements are given in Appendix D.

## Evaluation of Nutritional Assessment

After collecting the data needed for a thorough nutritional assessment, evaluate the findings to plan appropriate counseling. From the data, assess if the child is (1) malnourished, (2) at risk for becoming malnourished, or (3) well nourished with adequate reserves.

Analyze the daily food diary for the variety and amounts of foods suggested in the Food Guide Pyramid. (See Fig. 13-1.) For example, if the list includes no vegetables, inquire about this rather than assume that the child dislikes vegetables, because it could be that none was served on that day. Also, evaluate the information in terms of the family's ethnic practices and financial resources. Encouraging increased protein intake with additional meat may not be feasible for families on a limited budget or may conflict with food practices that use meat sparingly, such as in Asian meal preparation.

Compare findings from clinical examination and anthropometry with the data obtained from the dietary intake. For example, signs of anemia and a dietary record of iron-poor foods suggest laboratory analysis of hemoglobin, hematocrit, and transferrin. Refer any suspicious findings for further evaluation.

## KEY POINTS

- Communication, the most important skill nurses must possess in the care of children, has verbal, nonverbal, and abstract components.
- To effectively establish a setting for communication, nurses must make an appropriate introduction, clarify their role and the purpose of the interview, and ensure privacy and confidentiality.
- When communicating with parents, nurses need to encourage parental involvement, listen carefully, use silence, and be empathic.
- Communication with children must reflect their developmental stage.
- Verbal communication techniques include the third-person technique, use of "I" messages, facilitative responding, storytelling, bibliotherapy, the use of "what if" questions and other word games.

- Nonverbal communication with children may take the form of writing, drawing, magic, and play.
- The objectives of performing a health history are to identify pertinent information, determine the chief complaint, analyze the present illness, secure the past history, and record a family and sexual history.
- Family assessment is the collection of data about family composition and relationships among members; it focuses on home and community environment, occupation and education, and cultural and religious traditions.
- The family function interview examines interaction and roles, power, decision making, problem solving, communication, and expression of feelings and individuality.
- Nutritional assessment is performed by determination of dietary intake, clinical examination, and biochemical analysis.

# REFERENCES

Brennan PF: The future of clinical communication in an electronic environment, *Holistic Nurs Pract* 11(1):97-104, 1996.

Burns R: *Self-growth in families: kinetic family drawings (KFD)—research and application,* New York, 1982, Brunner/Mazel.

Burns RC, Kaufman SH: *Actions, styles, and symbols in kinetic family drawings (KFD): research and applications,* New York, 1972, Brunner/Mazel.

Caldwell B, Bradley R: *Home observation for measurement of the environment,* rev ed, Little Rock, 1984, University of Arkansas.

Chambers-Evans J, Stelling J, Godin M: Learning to listen: serendipitous outcomes of a research teaching experience, *J Adv Nurs* 29(6):1421-1426, 1999.

Deadrick D, Boggess P: *Pediatrics on telephone line.* Paper presented at the First Annual National Conference for Advanced Practice Nurses, Rutgers University, Nov 6-8, 1996.

Desselle DD, Pearlmutter L: Navigating two cultures: deaf children, self-esteem, and parents' communication patterns, *Soc Work Educ* 19(1):23-30, 1997.

Docherty S, Sandelowski M: Interviewing children, *Res Nurs Health* 22(2):177-185, 1999.

Feetham S, Perkins M, Carroll R: Exploratory analysis: a technique for analysis of dyadic data in research of families. In Feetham S and others: *Nursing in families: theory/research/education/practice,* Newport, CA, 1993, Sage Publications.

Frankenburg W, Coons C: Home screening questionnaire: its validity in assessing home environment, *J Pediatr* 108(4):624-626, 1986.

Hoge DR, Parette HP: Facilitating communicative development in young children with disabilities, *Transdisciplinary J* 5(2):113-130, 1995.

Kastens JM: Integrated care management: aligning medical call centers and nurse triage services, *Nurs Econ* 16(6):320-322, 329, 1998.

Price V, Archbold J: What's it all about, empathy? *Nurs Educ Today* 17(2):106-110, 1997.

Reynolds W, Scott PA, Austin W: Nursing, empathy and perception of the moral, *J Adv Nurs* 32(1):235-242, 2000.

Reynolds WJ, Scott B, Jessiman WC: Empathy has not been measured in clients' terms or effectively taught: a review of the literature, *J Adv Nurs* 30(5):1177-1185, 1999.

Rutenberg CD: Telephone triage, *Am J Nurs* 100(3):77-78, 80-81, 2000.

Saba VK, Pocklington DB, Miller, KP: *Nursing and computers,* New York, 1997, Springer.

Seidel HM and others: *Mosby's guide to physical examination,* ed 4, St Louis, 1999, Mosby.

Smilkstein G: Family APGAR analyzed (letter to the editor), *Fam Med* 25(5):293-294, 1993.

Smilkstein G, Ashworth C, Montano D: Validity and reliability of the family APGAR as a test of family function, *J Fam Pract* 15(2):303-311, 1982.

Spinetta J and others: The kinetic family drawing in childhood cancer. In Spinetta J, Deasy-Spinetta P: *Living with childhood cancer,* St Louis, 1981, Mosby.

Sullivan GH: Protecting patients' privacy, *RN* 60(6):55-56, 58-59, 1997.

Thompson JM, Wilson SF: *Health assessment for nursing practice,* St Louis, 1996, Mosby.

White SJ: Empathy: a literature review and concept analysis, *J Clin Nurs* 6(4):253-257, 1997.

Yegdich T: On the phenomenology of empathy in nursing: empathy or sympathy? *J Adv Nurs* 30(1):83-93, 1999.

# Chapter 7

# Physical and Developmental Assessment of the Child

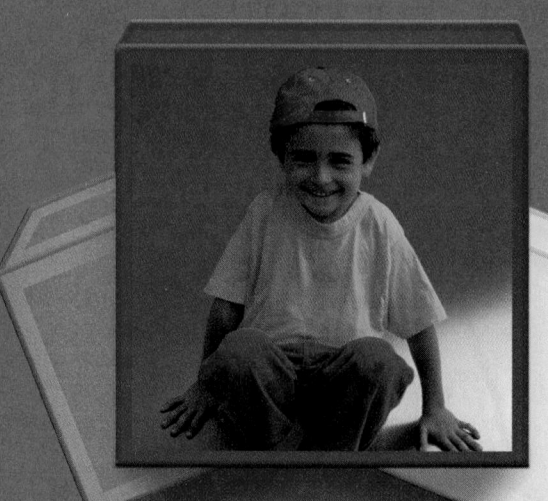

## Chapter Outline

**GENERAL CONCEPTS OF A PEDIATRIC PHYSICAL ASSESSMENT, 171**
**Recommendations for Health Supervision, 171**
**Sequence of the Examination, 171**
**Preparation of the Child, 172**
**PHYSICAL EXAMINATION, 174**
**Growth Measurements, 174**
　Growth Charts, 174
　Length, 175
　Height, 176
　Weight, 177
　Skinfold Thickness and Arm Circumference, 177
　Head Circumference, 177
**Physiologic Measurements, 178**
　Temperature, 178
　Pulse, 179
　Respiration, 179
　Blood Pressure (BP), 182
**General Appearance, 186**
**Skin, 187**
　Factors Influencing Assessment, 187
　Variations in Skin Color, 188
　Texture, 189
　Temperature, 189
　Turgor, 189
　Accessory Structures, 189
**Lymph Nodes, 190**
**Head, 190**
**Neck, 191**
**Eyes, 192**

Inspection of External Structures, 192
Inspection of Internal Structures, 194
Vision Testing, 195
**Ears, 200**
　Inspection of External Structures, 200
　Auditory Testing, 203
　Vestibular Testing, 204
**Nose, 204**
　Inspection of External Structures, 204
　Inspection of Internal Structures, 204
**Mouth and Throat, 206**
　Inspection of Internal Structures, 206
**Chest, 208**
**Lungs, 210**
　Inspection, 210
　Palpation, 211
　Percussion, 212
　Auscultation, 212
**Heart, 213**
　Inspection, 214
　Palpation, 214
　Auscultation, 215
**Abdomen, 217**
　Inspection, 217
　Auscultation, 218
　Percussion, 219
　Palpation, 219
**Genitalia, 220**
　Male Genitalia, 220
　Female Genitalia, 222
**Anus, 223**
**Back and Extremities, 223**

Spine, 223
Extremities, 224
Joints, 225
Muscles, 225
**Neurologic Assessment, 225**
　Behavior, 225
　Cognitive-Perceptual Development, 225
　Motor Functioning, 225
　Sensory Functioning, 225
　Cerebellar Functioning, 226
　Reflexes, 226
　Cranial Nerves, 227
　"Soft" Signs, 228
**GENERAL CONCEPTS OF MENTAL FUNCTION AND PERSONALITY DEVELOPMENT, 230**
**Theoretic Foundations of Personality Development, 230**
　Psychosexual Development (Freud), 230
　Psychosocial Development (Erikson), 231
**Theoretic Foundations of Mental Development, 231**
　Cognitive Development (Piaget), 231
　Moral Development (Kohlberg), 232
　Spiritual Development, 233
**DEVELOPMENTAL ASSESSMENT, 233**
**Denver II, 235**
**Revised Prescreening Developmental Questionnaire (R-PDQ), 237**
**Developmental Screening and Interpretation, 237**

## Related Topics

Altered States of Consciousness, Ch. 37
Assessment of Cardiac Function, Ch. 34
Biologic Development: Adolescent, Ch. 19
Dental Disorders, Ch. 18
Developmental Dysplasia of the Hip, Ch. 11
Disorders Affecting the Skin, Ch. 18

Gynecologic Examination, Ch. 20
Hearing Impairment; Visual Impairment, Ch. 24
History Taking, Ch. 6
Pain Assessment, Ch. 26

Physical Assessment: Newborn, Ch. 8
Preparation for Procedures, Ch. 27
Scoliosis, Ch. 39
Sexually Transmitted Diseases, Ch. 20
Systemic Hypertension, Ch. 34

# GENERAL CONCEPTS OF A PEDIATRIC PHYSICAL ASSESSMENT*

## Recommendations for Health Supervision

The objectives of pediatric health supervision are maintenance of optimum wellness and prevention of illness. The concept of prevention necessitates an orderly and routine schedule of activities—of which physical examination plays an essential role—that are aimed at meeting these two objectives. Box 7-1 provides a recommended schedule for the care of well children who receive competent parenting and who have no serious health problems. Circumstances that may indicate the need for additional visits or procedures include families of diverse socioeconomic and cultural backgrounds, especially those with foreign-born adopted children (Hostetter and Johnson, 1996; Lears, Guth, and Lewandowski, 1998; Mitchell and Jenista, 1997) or foster children (Chernoff and others, 1994; Giorgi:, 2001; Halfon and others, 1994; Horwitz, Simms, and Farrington, 1994; Scahill, 2000), single-parent families, homeless families (Wagner, Menke, and Ciccone, 1995), or those with children who have chronic illnesses or disabilities.

The services required by each child must be individualized by the practitioner. Look for opportunities to review children's previous schedules of health care and to institute specific measures or referrals to update the health record. For example, during hospitalization review children's overall record to ensure that they have had sensory screening, appropriate immunizations, and a yearly dental examination.

## Sequence of the Examination

Ordinarily the examining sequence follows a head-to-toe direction to provide a general guideline for assessing each body area in order to minimize omitting segments of the examination. The typical organization of a physical examination is listed in the chapter outline. In examining children, alter the sequence to accommodate each child's developmental needs, but record the findings according to the tra-

 *For additional information, please view "Pediatric Assessment" in *Whaley and Wong's Pediatric Nursing Video Series,* St Louis, 1996, Mosby; (800) 426-4545; www.mosby.com.

---

### Box 7-1
### Child Preventive Care Timeline

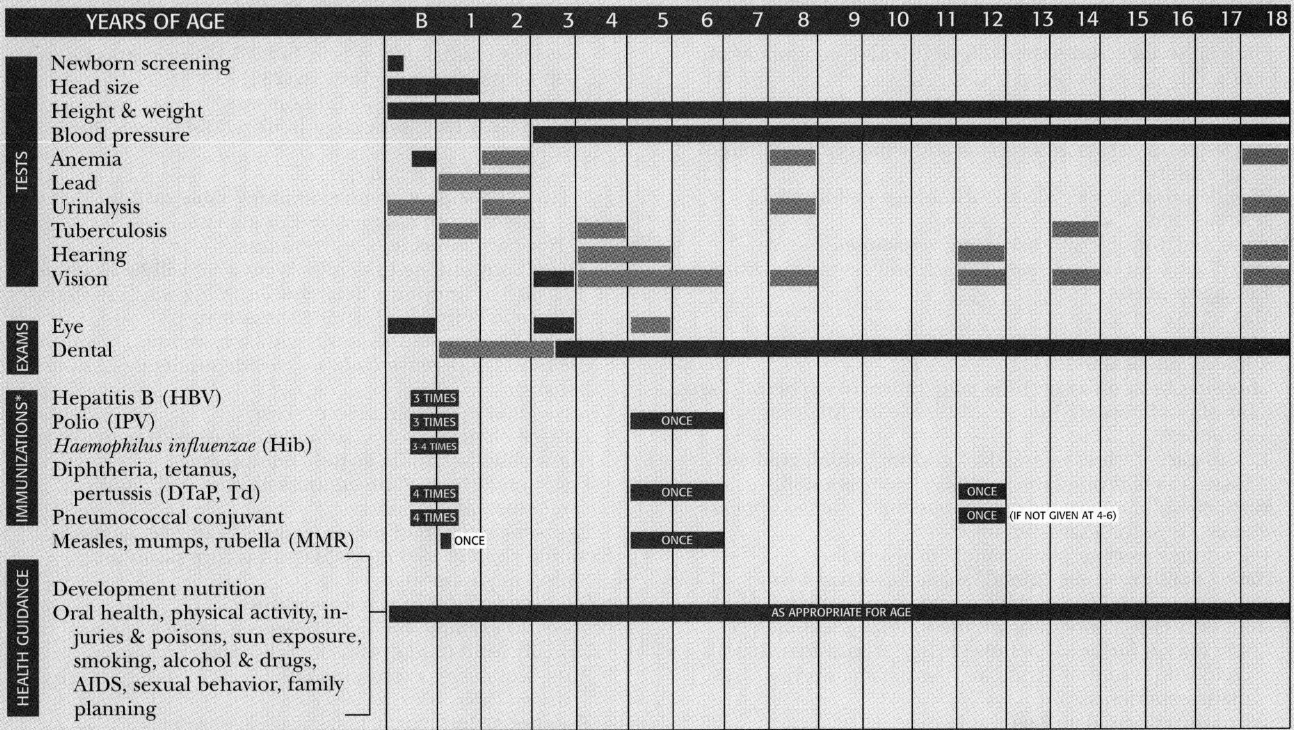

| YEARS OF AGE | B | 1 | 2 | 3 | 4 | 5 | 6 | 7 | 8 | 9 | 10 | 11 | 12 | 13 | 14 | 15 | 16 | 17 | 18 |
|---|---|---|---|---|---|---|---|---|---|---|---|---|---|---|---|---|---|---|---|
| **TESTS** | | | | | | | | | | | | | | | | | | | |
| Newborn screening | ■ | | | | | | | | | | | | | | | | | | |
| Head size | ■■■■ | | | | | | | | | | | | | | | | | | |
| Height & weight | ━━━━━━━━━━━━━━━━━━━━━━━━━━━━━━━━━━━ |
| Blood pressure | | | | ━━━━━━━━━━━━━━━━━━━━━━━━━━ |
| Anemia | ■ | | | | | | | | ■ | | | | | | | | | | ■ |
| Lead | | | ■ | | | | | | | | | | | | | | | | |
| Urinalysis | ■ | | | ■ | | | | | | | | | | | | | | | |
| Tuberculosis | | | | | | | | | | | | | | | | | | | |
| Hearing | | | | | ■ | | | | | | | | ■ | | | | | | |
| Vision | | | | ■ | | | | | | | | | ■ | | | | | | |
| **EXAMS** | | | | | | | | | | | | | | | | | | | |
| Eye | ■ | | | | | ■ | | | | | | | | | | | | | |
| Dental | | | ━━━━━━━━━━━━━━━━━━━━━━━━━━━━━━━━━ |
| **IMMUNIZATIONS*** | | | | | | | | | | | | | | | | | | | |
| Hepatitis B (HBV) | 3 TIMES | | | | | | | | | | | | | | | | | | |
| Polio (IPV) | 3 TIMES | | | | ONCE | | | | | | | | | | | | | | |
| *Haemophilus influenzae* (Hib) | 3-4 TIMES | | | | | | | | | | | | | | | | | | |
| Diphtheria, tetanus, pertussis (DTaP, Td) | 4 TIMES | | | | ONCE | | | | | | | ONCE | | | | | | | |
| Pneumococcal conjuvant | 4 TIMES | | | | | | | | | | | ONCE (IF NOT GIVEN AT 4-6) | | | | | | | |
| Measles, mumps, rubella (MMR) | ■ ONCE | | | | ONCE | | | | | | | | | | | | | | |
| **HEALTH GUIDANCE** | | | | | | | | | | | | | | | | | | | |
| Development nutrition | | | | | | | | | | | | | | | | | | | |
| Oral health, physical activity, injuries & poisons, sun exposure, smoking, alcohol & drugs, AIDS, sexual behavior, family planning | ━━━━━━━━━━━━━━━ AS APPROPRIATE FOR AGE ━━━━━━━━━━━━━━━ |

Key: ■ Recommended by all major authorities.
■ Recommended by some major authorities.

Please note: Children with special risk factors may need more frequent and additional types of preventive care. Some examples:

| RISK FACTOR | PREVENTIVE SERVICES NEEDED |
|---|---|
| Exposure to TB | TB test |
| Sexually active | Pap test (females); syphilis, gonorrhea, chlamydia tests |
| High-risk sexual behavior | AIDS test, hepatitis immunization |
| Drug abuse | AIDS, TB tests, hepatitis immunization |

From *Child health guide: put prevention into practice,* US Department of Health and Human Services, undated, pp. 20-21.
*Author Note: For current immunization information, see Chapter 12.

ditional model. Using developmental and chronologic age as the main criteria for assessing each body system accomplishes several goals:

- Minimizes stress and anxiety associated with assessment of various body parts
- Fosters a trusting nurse-child-parent relationship
- Allows for maximum preparation of the child
- Preserves the essential security of the parent-child relationship, especially with young children
- Maximizes the accuracy and reliability of assessment findings

## Preparation of the Child

Although the physical examination consists of painless procedures, using a tight arm cuff, probing in the ears and mouth, pressing on the abdomen, and listening to the chest with a cold piece of metal can be considerably stressful to a child. Therefore the same considerations discussed in Chapter 27 for preparing children for procedures are followed here. In addition to that discussion, general guidelines related to the examining process are presented in the Guidelines box. The physical examination should be as pleasant as possible as well as educational. (See Atraumatic Care box, p. 178.) With preschool and older children, use a detailed drawing or anatomically correct doll to help them learn about their bodies (Vessey, 1995). The "paper-doll" technique is a useful approach to teaching children about the part of the body being examined (Fig. 7-1). Have the child lie supine on the paper covering, and draw around the body to make an outline. At the conclusion of the visit, the child can take the paper doll home as a memento of the experience.

In most instances children cooperate best when their parents remain with them. However, there are occasions in which older children, particularly adolescents, prefer to be examined alone, such as during the genital examination. The child being examined is commonly accompanied by a sibling, who may be disruptive because of boredom. A helpful tactic is to involve the sibling in the examination by allowing the sibling to hold the stethoscope or a tongue blade; praise the child for the "help" during the assessment.

---

### GUIDELINES
#### *Performing Pediatric Physical Examination*

Perform examination in appropriate, nonthreatening area.
  Have room well-lit and decorated with neutral colors.
  Have room temperature comfortably warm.
  Place all strange and potentially frightening equipment out of sight.
  Have some toys, dolls, stuffed animals, and games available for child.
  If possible, have rooms decorated and equipped for different-age children.
  Provide privacy, especially for school-age children and adolescents.
Provide time for play and becoming acquainted.
Observe behaviors that signal child's readiness to cooperate:
  Talking to nurse
  Making eye contact
  Accepting offered equipment
  Allowing physical touching
  Choosing to sit on examining table rather than parent's lap
If signs of readiness are not observed, use the following techniques:
  Talk to parent while essentially "ignoring" child; gradually focus on child or a favorite object, such as a doll.
  Make complimentary remarks about child, such as appearance, dress, or a favorite object.
  Tell a funny story or play a simple magic trick.
  Have a nonthreatening "friend" available, such as a hand puppet to "talk" to the child for the nurse (see Fig. 7-31, *A*).
If child refuses to cooperate, use the following techniques:
  Assess reason for uncooperative behavior; consider that a child who is unduly afraid may have had a previous traumatic experience.
  Try to involve child and parent in process.
  Avoid prolonged explanations about examining procedure.
  Use a firm, direct approach regarding expected behavior.
  Perform examination as quickly as possible.
  Have attendant gently restrain child.
  Minimize any disruptions or stimulation.
    Limit number of people in room.
    Use isolated room.
    Use quiet, calm, confident voice.

Begin examination in a nonthreatening manner for young children or children who are fearful:
  Use those activities that can be presented as games, such as test for cranial nerves (see Table 7-17) or parts of developmental screening tests (p. 235).
  Use approaches such as "Simon says" to encourage child to make a face, squeeze a hand, stand on one foot, and so on.
  Use "paper-doll" technique.
    Lay child supine on an examining table or floor that is covered with a large sheet of paper.
    Trace around child's body outline.
    Use body outline to demonstrate what will be examined, such as drawing a heart and listening with the stethoscope before performing the activity on child.
If several children in the family will be examined, begin with the most cooperative child to provide modeling of desired behavior.
Involve child in examination process:
  Provide choices, such as sitting on table or in patient's lap.
  Allow child to handle or hold equipment.
  Encourage child to use equipment on a doll, family member, or examiner.
  Explain each step of the procedure in simple language.
Examine child in a comfortable and secure position:
  Sitting in parent's lap
  Sitting upright if in respiratory distress
Proceed to examine the body in an organized sequence (usually head to toe) with the following exceptions:
  Alter sequence to accommodate needs of different-age children (Table 7-1).
  Examine painful areas last.
  In emergency situation, examine vital functions (airway, breathing, and circulation) and injured area first.
Reassure child throughout examination, especially about bodily concerns that arise during puberty.
Discuss findings with family at end of examination.
Praise child for cooperation during examination; give reward such as a small toy or sticker.

**TABLE 7-1**    Age-specific approaches to physical examination during childhood

| Position | Sequence | Preparation |
|---|---|---|
| **Infant** | | |
| Before sits alone: supine or prone, preferably in parent's lap; before 4 to 6 months: can place on examining table<br>After sits alone: use sitting in parent's lap whenever possible<br>If on table, place with parent in full view | If quiet, auscultate heart, lungs, abdomen<br>Record heart and respiratory rates<br>Palpate and percuss same areas<br>Proceed in usual head-to-toe direction<br>Perform traumatic procedures last (eyes, ears, mouth [while crying])<br>Elicit reflexes as body part examined<br>Elicit Moro reflex last | Completely undress if room temperature permits<br>Leave diaper on male<br>Gain cooperation with distraction, bright objects, rattles, talking<br>Have older infants hold a small block in each hand; until voluntary release develops toward end of the first year, infants will be unable to grasp other objects (e.g., stethoscope, otoscope)<br>Smile at infant; use soft, gentle voice<br>Pacify with bottle of sugar water or feeding<br>Enlist parent's aid for restraining to examine ears, mouth<br>Avoid abrupt, jerky movements |
| **Toddler** | | |
| Sitting or standing on or by parent<br>Prone or supine in parent's lap | Inspect body area through play: "count fingers," "tickle toes"<br>Use minimal physical contact initially<br>Introduce equipment slowly<br>Auscultate, percuss, palpate whenever quiet<br>Perform traumatic procedures last (same as for infant) | Have parent remove outer clothing<br>Remove underwear as body part examined<br>Allow to inspect equipment; demonstrating use of equipment is usually ineffective<br>If uncooperative, perform procedures quickly<br>Use restraint when appropriate; request parent's assistance<br>Talk about examination if cooperative; use short phrases<br>Praise for cooperative behavior |
| **Preschool Child** | | |
| Prefer standing or sitting<br>Usually cooperative prone or supine<br>Prefer parent's closeness | If cooperative, proceed in head-to-toe direction<br>If uncooperative, proceed as with toddler | Request self-undressing<br>Allow to wear underpants if shy<br>Offer equipment for inspection; briefly demonstrate use<br>Make up "story" about procedure: "I'm seeing how strong your muscles are" (blood pressure)<br>Use paper-doll technique (see Fig. 7-1)<br>Give choices when possible<br>Expect cooperation; use positive statements: "Open your mouth" |
| **School-Age Child** | | |
| Prefer sitting<br>Cooperative in most positions<br>Younger child prefers parent's presence<br>Older child may prefer privacy | Proceed in head-to-toe direction<br>May examine genitalia last in older child<br>Respect need for privacy | Request self-undressing<br>Allow to wear underpants<br>Give gown to wear<br>Explain purpose of equipment and significance of procedure, such as otoscope to see eardrum, which is necessary for hearing<br>Teach about body functioning and care |
| **Adolescent** | | |
| Same as for school-age child<br>Offer option of parent's presence | Same as for older school-age child | Allow to undress in private<br>Give gown<br>Expose only area to be examined<br>Respect need for privacy<br>Explain findings during examination: "Your muscles are firm and strong"<br>Matter-of-factly comment about sexual development: "Your breasts are developing as they should be"<br>Emphasize normalcy of development<br>Examine genitalia as any other body part; may leave until end |

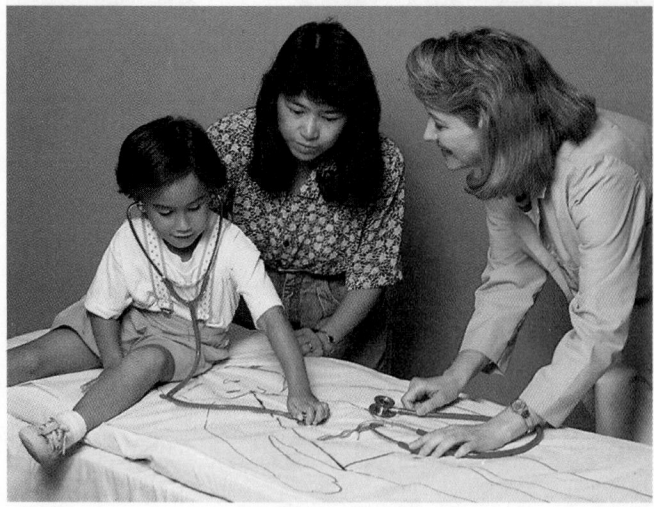

**Fig. 7-1**  Using paper-doll technique to prepare child for physical examination.

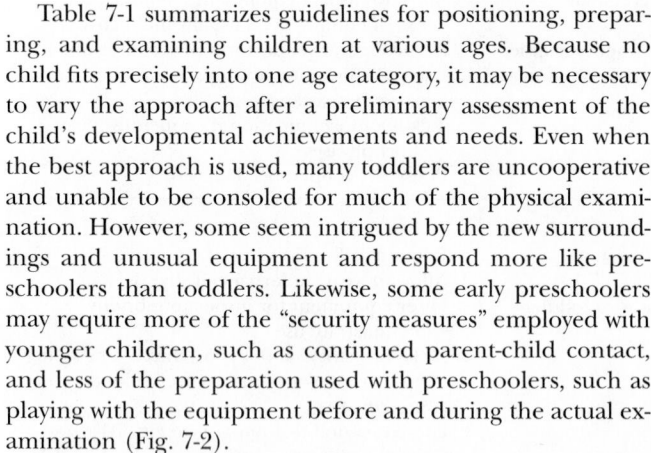

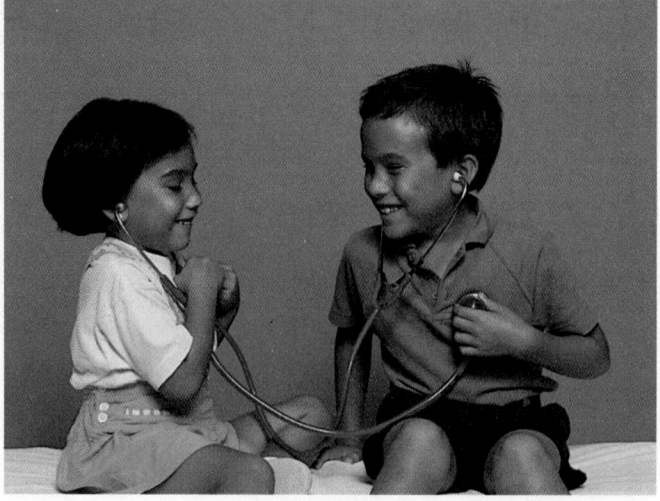

**Fig. 7-2**  Preparing children for physical examination.

Table 7-1 summarizes guidelines for positioning, preparing, and examining children at various ages. Because no child fits precisely into one age category, it may be necessary to vary the approach after a preliminary assessment of the child's developmental achievements and needs. Even when the best approach is used, many toddlers are uncooperative and unable to be consoled for much of the physical examination. However, some seem intrigued by the new surroundings and unusual equipment and respond more like preschoolers than toddlers. Likewise, some early preschoolers may require more of the "security measures" employed with younger children, such as continued parent-child contact, and less of the preparation used with preschoolers, such as playing with the equipment before and during the actual examination (Fig. 7-2).

Although the variations in the general approaches are numerous, some of them are discussed here because they are more common. For example, the suggested sequence may change considerably when the child is in pain or when obvious physical defects are present. In either situation examine the affected area last to minimize distress early in the examination and to focus on normal, healthy, or functioning body parts.

Positioning may also be altered because of physical distress. For example, the child who is having difficulty breathing may not be able to lie down. In this case perform as much of the physical examination as possible with the child in a sitting or slightly reclining position, or complete the examination at another time.

## PHYSICAL EXAMINATION

Although the approach to and sequence of the physical examination differ according to the child's age, the following discussion outlines the traditional model for physical assessment. It emphasizes normal findings, variations from the norm that may cause parents or children concern but that require little or no intervention, and abnormalities that necessitate appropriate referral. The focus here includes all pediatric age-groups; see Chapter 8 for a detailed discussion of a newborn assessment, which describes procedures and findings unique to the neonate.

## Growth Measurements

Measurement of physical growth in children is a key element in evaluating their health status. Physical growth parameters include weight, height (length), skinfold thickness, arm circumference, and head circumference. Values for these growth parameters are plotted on percentile charts, and the child's measurements in percentiles are compared with those of the general population.

### Growth Charts

The most commonly used growth charts in the United States are from the ***National Center for Health Statistics (NCHS).*** The growth charts have been revised to include the body mass index-for-age (BMI-for-age) charts, 3rd and 97th smoothed percentiles for all charts and the 85th percentile for the weight-for-stature and BMI-for-age charts. (See Appendix C.) The data was collected from five national surveys during 1963-1994. The revised charts have eliminated the disjunctions between the curves for infants and other children and have been extended for children and adolescents to 20 years (National Center for Health Statistics, 2000).

The weight-for-age percentile distributions are now continuous between the infant and the older child charts at 24 to 36 months. The length-for-age to stature-for-age and the weight-for-length to weight-for-stature curves are parallel in the overlapping ages of 24 to 36 months. The revised weight-for-stature charts provide a smoother transition from the weight-for-length charts for pre-school–aged children.

The most prominent change to the complement of growth charts for older children and adolescents is the addition of the BMI-for-age growth curves. The BMI-for-age charts were developed with national survey data (1963-1994), excluding data from the 1988-1994 NHANES III survey for children older than 6 years because an increase in body weight and BMI occurred between NHANES III and previous national surveys. Without this exclusion, the 85th and 95th percentile curves would have been higher, and fewer children and adolescents would have been classified as at risk or overweight. Therefore the BMI-for-age growth curves do not represent the current population of children over 6 years of age.

The sex-specific BMI-for-age charts for ages 2 to 20 years replace the 1977 NCHS weight-for-stature charts that were limited to prepubescent boys under 11.5 years of age and statures less than 145 cm, and to prepubescent girls under 19 years of age and statures less than 137 cm. BMI-for-age may be used to identify children and adolescents at the upper end of the distribution who are either overweight (≥95th percentile) or at risk for overweight (≥85th and <95th percentile) (Roche and Guo, 2001). Formulas for determining BMI are available at *www.cdc.gov/nccdphp/dnpa/bmi/bmi-definition.htm* and in Appendix C.

**Breast- and Formula-Fed Infants.** The national survey data better represent the combined size and growth patterns of the general U.S. population (1971 to 1994). Over the past two decades in the United States, approximately one half of all infants were reported ever to have been breast-fed, and approximately one third were breast-fed for 3 months or more. Therefore, compared with the 1977 NCHS growth charts, the nationally representative data on which the revised infant growth charts are based will better represent the combined growth patterns of breast-fed and formula-fed infants in the U.S. population.

With regard to differences in the growth of breast- or formula-fed infants, other research efforts are currently in progress to address this issue. A Working Group of the World Health Organization (WHO) is collecting data at seven international study centers to develop a new set of international growth charts for infants and preschoolers through age 5 years. These charts will be based on the growth of exclusively or predominately breast-fed infants. The basic assumption is that infants from healthy populations, following the current WHO feeding recommendations, are growing optimally. The WHO multicenter growth reference study should be completed in 2002.

**Special Groups.** Although there are differences in size and growth among the major racial and ethnic groups in the United States, these appear to be small and inconsistent. Therefore the revised growth charts include all infants and children whatever their race or ethnicity. Because the growth patterns of preterm, very-low-birth-weight (VLBW) (<1500g) infants are considerably different from those of higher birth-weight term infants and specialized growth charts exist to track the growth of VLBW infants, data for VLBW infants were excluded from the revised charts.

**Versions of the Growth Charts.** Three different versions of the charts are available on *www.cdc.gov/growthcharts*. The first set contains all nine smoothed percentile lines (3rd, 5th, 10th, 25th, 50th, 75th, 90th, 95th, 97th), and the second and third sets contain seven smoothed percentile lines. The sec-

| **TABLE 7-2** Expected growth rates at various ages | |
|---|---|
| **Age** | **Expected Growth Rate (cm/yr)** |
| 1 to 6 months | 18-22 |
| 6 to 12 months | 14-18 |
| 2nd year | 11 |
| 3rd year | 8 |
| 4th year | 7 |
| 5th to 10th years | 5-6 |

From *Human growth and growth disorders: an update,* San Francisco, 1989, Genentech.

ond set contains the 5th and 95th percentile lines, and the third set contains the 3rd and 97th percentile lines at the extremes of the distribution. In addition, the charts for weight-for-stature and BMI-for-age contain the 85th percentile. In all the growth charts, age is truncated to the nearest full month, for example, 1 month (1.0 to 1.9 mo), 11 months (11.0 to 11.9 mo), 23 months (23.0 to 23.9 mo), and so forth.

The three sets of charts are provided to meet the needs of various users. Set 1 shows all of the major percentile curves but may have limitations when the curves are close together, especially at the youngest ages. Most users in the United States may wish to use the format shown in set 2 for the majority of routine clinical applications. (See Appendix C.) Pediatric endocrinologists and others dealing with special populations, such as children with failure to thrive, may wish to use the format in set 3.

Nurses are often responsible for measuring growth in children, so it is essential that they have an understanding of the revised growth charts. Several important differences exist between the 1977 and the revised charts with significant implications for classifying children as underweight or overweight. Nurses need to become familiar with determining BMI, which only requires information about the child's weight and height.* With the increasing number of overweight children in the United States, the BMI charts will become a critical component of children's physical assessment. Children whose growth may be questionable include:

- Children whose height and weight percentiles are widely disparate (e.g., height in the 10th percentile and weight in the 90th percentile, especially with above-average skinfold thickness)
- Children who fail to show the expected growth rates in height and weight, especially during the rapid growth periods of infancy and adolescence (Table 7-2)
- Children who show a sudden increase (except during puberty) or decrease in a previously steady growth pattern

Because growth is a continuous but uneven process, the most reliable evaluation lies in comparing growth measurements over time. It is important to remember that normal growth patterns vary among children the same age (Fig. 7-3).

## Length

Length (or recumbent length) refers to measurements taken when children are supine. Measure recumbent length

---

*BMI = (Weight in pounds ÷ Height in inches ÷ Height in inches) × 703.

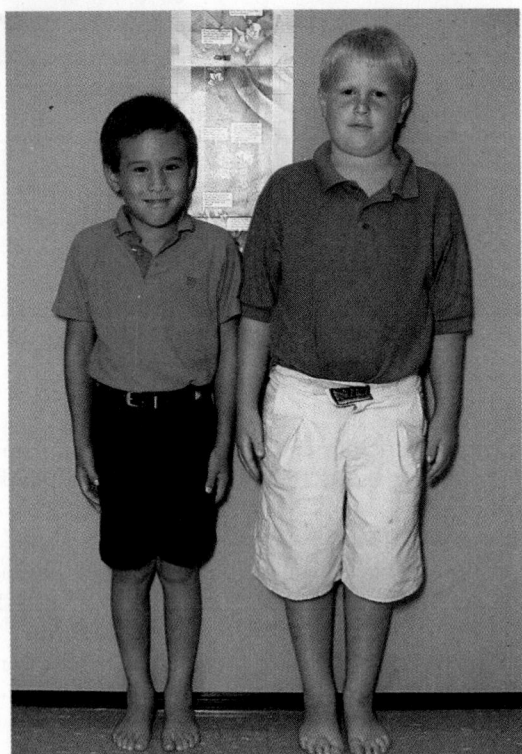

**Fig. 7-3** Children of identical age (8 years) are markedly different in size. The child on the left, of Asian descent, is at the 5th percentile for height and weight. The child on the right is above the 95th percentile for height and weight. However, both children demonstrate normal growth patterns.

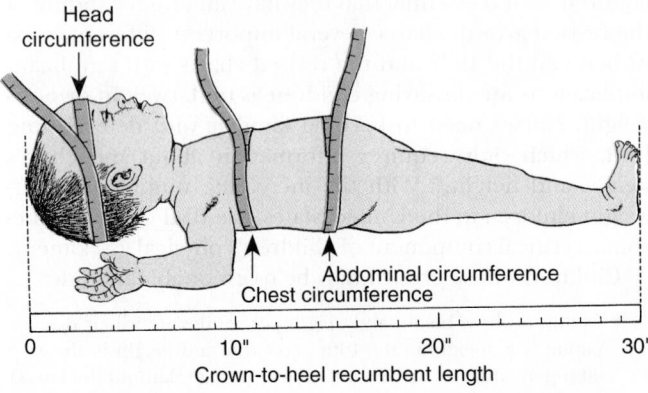

**Fig. 7-4** Measurement of head, chest, and abdominal circumference and crown-to-heel (recumbent) length.

until children are 24 months old (36 months if the birth to 36-month chart is used). Because of the normally flexed position during infancy, fully extend the body by (1) holding the head in midline, (2) grasping the knees together gently, and (3) pushing down on the knees until the legs are fully extended and flat against the table. If using a measuring board, place the head firmly at the top of the board and the heels of the feet firmly against the footboard.

If such a measuring device is not available, measure length by placing the child on a paper-covered surface, marking the end points of the top of the head and the heels of the feet, and measuring between these two points (Fig. 7-4). For

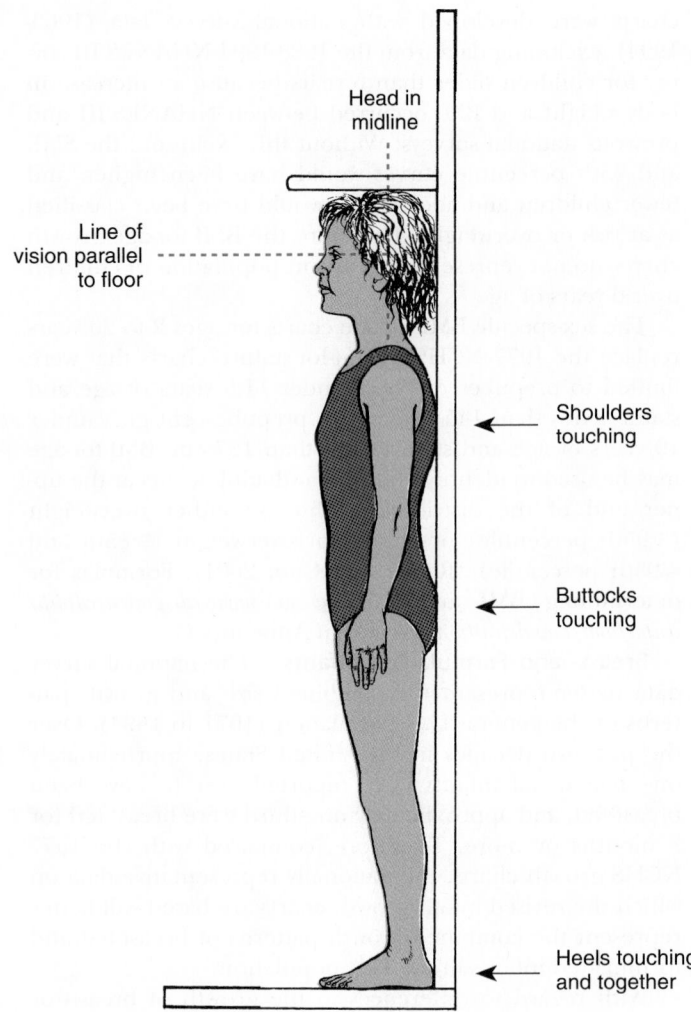

**Fig. 7-5** Measure of height. (Redrawn from *Human growth and growth disorders: an update,* San Francisco, 1989, Genentech.)

accurate measurement hold the writing utensil at a right angle to the table when marking the cephalic point; position the feet with the toes pointing directly to the ceiling when marking the heel point. Regardless of the method used, have someone assist in holding the child's head in midline while you extend the legs and take the measurement.

## Height

Height (or stature) refers to the measurement taken when children are standing upright. Measure height by having the child, with shoes removed, stand as tall and as straight as possible, with the head in midline and the line of vision parallel to the ceiling or floor. Be sure the child's back is to the wall or other vertical flat surface, with the heels, buttocks, and back of the shoulders touching the wall and the medial malleoli touching if possible (Fig. 7-5). Check for and correct any bending of the knees, slumping of the shoulders, or raising of the heels.

**NURSING TIP** Normally height is less if measured in the afternoon rather than in the morning. To minimize this variation, apply modest upward pressure under the jaw or the mastoid processes.

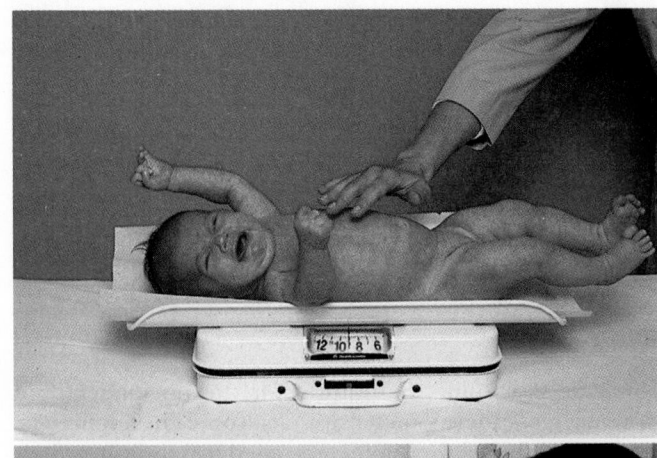

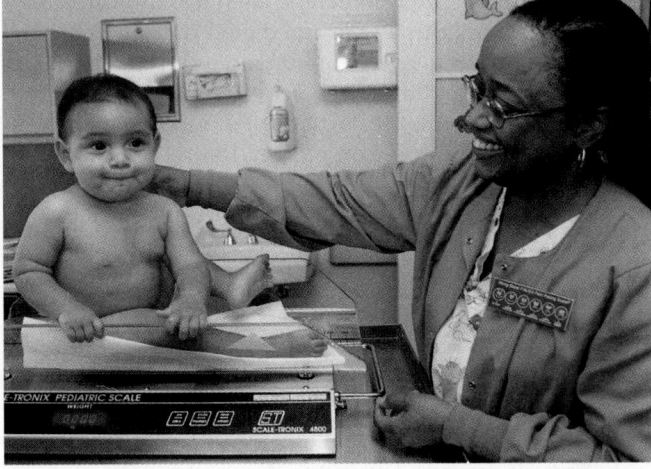

**Fig. 7-6** **A,** Infant on scale. **B,** Child on scale. Note presence of nurse to prevent falls. (**B,** Courtesy Paul Vincent Kuntz, Texas Children's Hospital.)

For the most accurate measurement, use a wall-mounted unit *(stadiometer).* The movable measuring rod of platform scales is accurate only if it maintains a position parallel to the floor and rests securely on the topmost part of the head. To improvise a flat surface for measuring length, attach a paper or metal tape or yardstick to the wall, position the child adjacent to the tape, and place a three-dimensional object, such as a thick book or box, on top of the head. Rest the side of the object firmly against the wall to form a right angle. Measure length or stature to the nearest 1 mm or ⅛ inch.

Occasionally special length measurements are taken, such as *sitting height* or *crown-to-rump length.* (For newborns, see Physical Assessment, Chapter 8.) Normally, sitting height accounts for 70% of total body length at birth, 60% at 2 years, and approximately 52% at age 10 years. In older infants and children determine sitting height by having the child sit against the wall; measure between the vertex of the head and the sitting surface. Although not a usual measurement, this method is used for distinguishing true growth deficiency from genetic small stature.

### Weight

Weight is measured with an appropriately sized beam balance scale, which measures weights to the nearest 10 g or ½ ounce for infants and 100 g or ¼ pound for children, or

with an electronic digital scale. Before weighing the child, balance the scale by setting it at zero and noting if the balance registers exactly in the middle of the mark. If the end of the balance beam rises to the top or bottom of the mark, add more or less weight, respectively. Some scales are designed to allow for self-correction, but others need to be recalibrated by the manufacturer. Scales vary in their accuracy; infant scales tend to be more accurate than adult platform scales, and newer scales are more accurate than older ones, especially at the upper levels of weight measurement. When precise measurements are needed, have a second nurse measure the weight independently.

Measurements are made in a comfortably warm room. When the birth to 36-month growth chart is used, children should be weighed nude. Older children are usually weighed while wearing their underpants or a light gown. Always respect the privacy of all children. If the child must be weighed wearing some article of clothing or some type of special device, such as a prosthesis, note this when recording the weight. Children who are measured for recumbent length are usually weighed on a large platform-type infant scale and placed in a lying-down or sitting position. When weighing infants, place your hand lightly above the body to prevent them from accidentally falling off the scale (Fig. 7-6). For maximum asepsis, cover the scale with a clean sheet of paper between each child's measurement. A study comparing two techniques for weighing young patients revealed no significant differences between the weights of children using an infant scale compared with their indirect weight using an adult scale while being held by a nurse (Vessey and Stueve, 1996). With an indirect weight measurement, the nurse's weight is subtracted from the total weight to determine the child's weight.

### Skinfold Thickness and Arm Circumference

Measures of relative weight and stature cannot distinguish between adiposity and muscularity. One convenient measure of body fat is skinfold thickness. Skinfold thickness is measured with special calipers, such as the *Lange calipers.* The most common sites for measuring skinfold thickness are the triceps (most practical for routine clinical use), subscapula, suprailiac, abdomen, and upper thigh. For greatest reliability, follow the exact procedure for measurement and record the average of at least two measurements of one site. (See Guidelines box on p. 178.)

Arm circumference is an indirect measure of muscle mass. To measure arm circumference, follow the same procedure as for skinfold thickness, except measure the midpoint with a paper or steel tape. Place the tape vertically along the posterior aspect of the upper arm from the acromial process to the olecranon process; half the measured length is the midpoint. Percentiles for triceps skinfold and arm circumference in children are listed in Appendix C and may be used as reference data. However, the percentiles are not standards or norms because all values between the 5th and 95th percentiles are not ranges of normal.

### Head Circumference

Measure head circumference in children up to 36 months of age and in any child whose head size is questionable. Measure the head at its greatest circumference, usually slightly

## GUIDELINES
### Measuring Triceps Skinfold Thickness

With child's right arm flexed 90 degrees at elbow, mark midpoint between acromion and olecranon on posterior aspect of arm.

With arm hanging freely, grasp a fold of skin between thumb and forefinger 1 cm above midpoint.

Gently pull fold away from underlying muscle, and continue to hold until measurement is completed.

Place caliper jaws over skinfold at midpoint mark; if a plastic caliper (e.g., Ross Adipometer) is used, apply pressure with thumb to align lines on caliper; follow directions for using other calipers.

Estimate reading to nearest 1.0 mm, 2 to 3 seconds after applying pressure.

Take measurements until two agree within 1 mm.

## ATRAUMATIC CARE
### Reducing Young Children's Fears

Young children, especially preschoolers, fear intrusive procedures because of their poorly defined body boundaries. Therefore avoid invasive procedures, such as measuring rectal temperature, whenever possible. Also avoid using the word "take" when measuring vital signs because young children interpret words literally and may think that their temperature or other function will be taken away. Say instead, "I want to know how warm you are."

above the eyebrows and pinna of the ears and around the occipital prominence at the back of the skull (see Fig. 7-4). Because head shape can affect location of the maximum circumference, more than one measurement at points above the eyebrows may need to be taken to obtain the most accurate measure. Use a paper or metal tape because a cloth tape can stretch and give a falsely small measurement. For greatest accuracy, use devices with tenths of a centimeter because percentile charts list only 0.5-cm increments.

Plot head size on the appropriate growth chart under head circumference. In general, head and chest circumferences are equal at approximately 1 to 2 years of age. During childhood chest circumference exceeds head size by approximately 5 to 7 cm (2 to 3 inches). (For newborns, see Physical Assessment, Chapter 8.)

## Physiologic Measurements

Physiologic measurements are key elements in evaluating the physical status of vital functions and include temperature, pulse, respiration, and blood pressure. Compare each measurement with normal values for that age-group. (See inside back cover.) In addition, compare present recordings with the values obtained on preceding health visits. For example, a falsely elevated blood pressure reading may not indicate hypertension if previous recent readings have been within normal limits. The isolated recording may indicate some stressful event in the child's life.

As with most procedures carried out with children, older children and adolescents are treated much the same as are adults. However, special consideration must be given to preschool children. (See Atraumatic Care box.)

For best results in obtaining the vital signs of infants, count respirations first (before the infant is disturbed), take the pulse next, and measure temperature last. If vital signs cannot be obtained without disturbing the child, record the child's behavior (e.g., crying) along with the measurement.

### Temperature*

Temperature in healthy or ill children can easily be measured at several body sites via oral, rectal, axillary, ear

canal, or skin route. Substitutes for the no longer used mercury glass thermometer are electronic thermometers, infrared ear-based thermometers, chemical indicator thermometers, skin plastic strips, and digital thermometers, all of which offer advantages (rapid temperature taking, minimal intrusion, and reduced cross contamination) and some disadvantages. (See Evidence-Based Practice box on pp. 180-181 and Table 7-3 on pp. 182-183.) The accuracy of these instruments may differ, and variations in results may occur if the correct technique is not applied (Fig. 7-7), if the child is febrile, or if the child's age is not appropriately considered (Androkites, Werger, and Young, 1998; Erickson, 1999; Loveys and others, 1999; Robinson and others, 1998; Romanovsky and others, 1997).

Currently the most frequently used temperature-measurement devices (Healthcare Product Comparison System, 1996a, 1996b, and 1996c) in children are:

1. *Electronic continuous thermometers.* Measure the patient's temperature during the administration of general anesthesia, treatment of hypothermia or hyperthermia, and other situations that require continuous monitoring.
2. *Electronic intermittent thermometers.* Measure the patient's temperature at oral, rectal, and axillary sites and are used as primary diagnostic indicators.
3. *Infrared thermometers.* Measure the patient's temperature by collecting emitted thermal radiation from a particular site (e.g., ear canal).

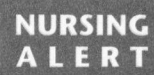

**NURSING ALERT**  Mercury thermometers should not be used because if broken, inhaled vapors can cause significant toxicity (Goldman and Shannon, 2001).

The routine sites for taking temperature are the sublingual pocket, rectum, axilla, and the ear canal. As a general rule in children, temperature is currently taken in the axilla or rectum in infants and young children, and by mouth after the age of 4 to 5 years when the child understands how to hold the thermometer. Ear-based temperature devices may also be a convenient option (Barone and Rowe, 1999).

The time of the device's placement at the measurement site should be noted. No universal agreement exists regarding the length of time mercury thermometers should be kept in place. Recommendations based on research vary from 8 to 10 minutes for an oral reading, 4 minutes for a rectal reading, and 5 minutes for an axillary reading, but there are researchers who recommend longer placements for oral and axillary routes (Barone and Rowe, 1999). These times may also vary widely within practice settings. Elec-

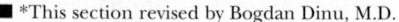

■ *This section revised by Bogdan Dinu, M.D.

tronic devices considerably lower the measurement time to the range of seconds. However, all efforts should be made to obtain an accurate reading, and devices should be kept in place long enough to achieve this.

Based on the classical literature, the normal core-body temperature is 99° to 100° F (actually assessed for research for surgical and intensive care purposes). The peripheral temperature considered normal in the clinical setting registers as 37.0° C (98.6° F) via the oral route. Temperatures taken at different sites may present small variations from the value of a given reference-criterion site (i.e., oral or rectal) (Childs, Harrison, Hodkinson, 1999; Cretel and others, 1999; Irvin, 1999; Wilshaw and others, 1999). Traditionally it has been assumed that rectal temperatures are around 1° C higher (mean) and axillary temperatures around 1° C lower (mean) than oral temperatures. Recent research reinforces that differences among these sites (rectal, axillary, ear, and oral) may show wide and significant variation across studies (Craig and others, 2000).

**NURSING TIP** Because of variations in temperature among rectal, axillary, oral, and ear sites, it is necessary to chart the route along with the recorded temperature reading and to consistently use one route if possible.

Whenever a child feels warm to the touch, the temperature should be immediately measured, even if it was normal only a short time before. The family should be taught the classic signs of increased body temperature such as malaise, low energy level, flushed face and skin, increased respiratory and heart rates, and a "glassy look" to the eyes. The rapid and accurate assessment of a child's temperature can be of great significance to the outcome of a medical condition.

### Pulse

An accurate pulse can be taken radially in children over 2 years of age. However, in infants and young children the apical impulse (heard through a stethoscope held to the chest at the apex of the heart) is more reliable. (See Fig. 7-39 for location of pulses.) Count the pulse for 1 full minute in infants and young children because of possible irregularities in rhythm. However, use shorter counting times (e.g., 15- or 30-second intervals) when frequent apical rates are needed. For greater accuracy, measure the apical rate while the child is asleep; record the child's behavior along with the rate. Pulses may be graded according to the criteria in Table 7-4 on p. 184. Compare radial and femoral pulses at least once during early childhood to detect the presence of circulatory impairment, such as coarctation of the aorta. (See inside back cover for normal rates for pediatric age-groups.)

### Respiration

Count the respiratory rate in the same manner as for the adult patient. Observe abdominal movements in infants because their respirations are primarily diaphragmatic. Because the movements are irregular, count them for 1 full minute for accuracy (see p. 211). (See inside back cover for normal respiratory rates in children.)

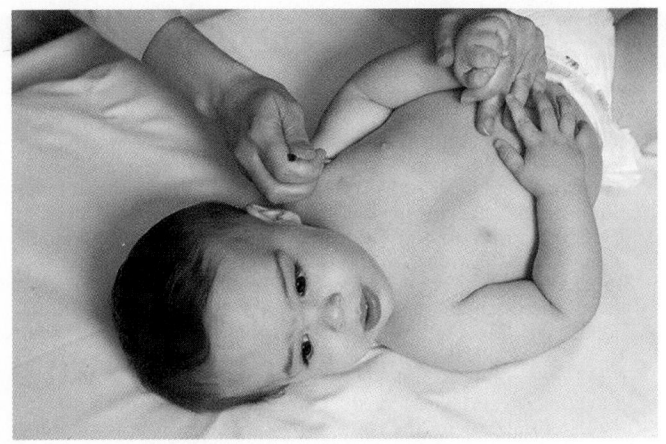

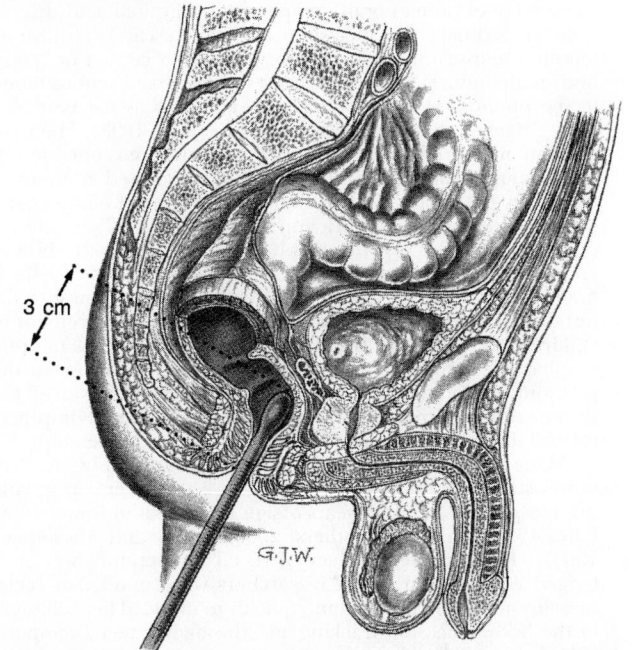

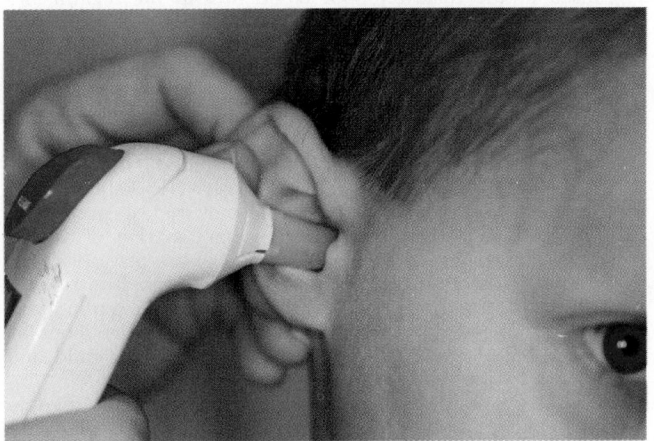

**Fig. 7-7**  **A,** Position for taking axillary temperature. **B,** Cross section of rectum illustrates curve approximately 3 cm from anus, where risk of perforation from thermometer is greatest in infants under 3 months of age. **C,** Position for tympanic temperature measurement. Note ear tug to help straighten the canal for the infrared sensor to focus on the eardrum. (See also Fig. 7-25.)

## EVIDENCE-BASED PRACTICE
### *Route of Temperature Measurement in Children* *

The primary purpose of measuring body temperature is to detect and assess abnormally high or low values. The normal absolute value of the body's temperature is still a challenging issue. The "gold standard" of 37° C (98.6° F) in adults has been questioned; the "new" mean oral temperature, reported as 36.8° C (98.2° F), varies among individuals and can fluctuate by an average of 0.5° C a day (Mackowiack, Wassermann, and Levine, 1992). Body temperature follows a circadian rhythm with a low around 6 AM and a peak about 12 hours later (Lell and others, 2000). The effect of fever on the circadian rhythm is unknown. In healthy adults the core temperature is influenced by exercise, oral intake, and psychologic performance (Aldemir and others, 2000; Latzka and Sawka, 2000; Owens and others, 2000).

In febrile patients the chief concern is the temperature of the brain because very high temperature can cause neural damage. Knowledge of human brain temperature is limited, and this parameter is usually not measured directly. Researchers have attempted to assess the best sites for measuring central or "core" body temperature. The temperature of the mixed venous blood in the pulmonary artery is generally accepted as the best core body ("deep-body") temperature value (Loveys, 1998). The most accurate measurement of core body temperature is obtained by using a pulmonary artery catheter, the method used in intensive care units but which is not completely risk free (Kodavatiganti, Hearn, and Insler, 1999; Prielipp and Morell, 1997). Other acceptable core sites are the esophagus and bladder (Robinson and others, 1998). Jugular vein temperature also closely reflects brain temperature (Ao and others, 2000). In an attempt to determine the most reliable site for temperature measurement in children, researchers found that in anesthetized children, esophageal temperature readings were closest to those in the pulmonary artery (Robinson and others, 1998). However, all the sites mentioned involve invasive thermometry and are impractical and unnecessary for routine temperature measurement.

Many clinicians still consider the rectal route to be the "criterion standard" for routine temperature measurement in children, especially before 5 years of age (Barone and Rowe, 1999; Jaffe, 1995; Jensen and others, 2000; Shann and Mackenzie, 1996). However, the accuracy of rectal temperature was challenged as early as 1954 by researchers who found that rectal measurements did not respond quickly to induced heat changes in the body. This slow tracking and the higher rectal temperature (compared with pulmonary artery temperature) may be caused by the relatively poor blood flow to the rectum and to the insulating property of the stool (Loveys, 1998; Rotello, Crawford, and Terndrup, 1996). Rectal thermometers have been reported to cause perforations and transmission of enteric pathogens, especially in very young children (Barone and Rowe, 1999). To avoid the risk of perforation, the thermometer should be inserted no further than 2.5 cm for toddlers and 1.5 cm for infants. Rectal measurement should be avoided in neutropenic children and after recent anorectal surgery (Hockenberry and Kline, 2001). Although a large number of studies continue to consider rectal temperature an important marker of disease status (Jensen and others, 2000), the rectal site may not be acceptable to parents or children (Craig, 1999). In a British study, 37 of 42 parents interviewed expressed concerns regarding this issue that included fear of hurting the child, anxieties about being accused of sexual abuse, difficulty comforting the child, and concern for the youngster's feelings (Kai, 1993).

Oral temperature assessment, which is currently used in older children and adolescents, may be influenced by many factors, including mouth breathing, crying, eating, drinking, smoking, or location of the thermometer in the mouth. Mastication and smoking both cause significant increases in oral temperature that may persist for over 20 minutes; drinking of hot or cold liquids may cause a significant, but more transient,

change in oral temperature (Rabinowitz and others, 1996). When using an oral mercury thermometer, it must be correctly placed under the tongue, with the mouth closed for 8 to 10 minutes (Barone and Rowe, 1999). Electronic oral thermometers have replaced the traditional mercury glass thermometers. These modern devices substantially reduce the measurement time from 8 minutes to about 20 to 40 seconds. However, the faster the reading, the greater the chance for variability in the results (Erickson, 1999).

Electronic thermometers use an electronic tracking circuity and apply a mathematical/algorithm to calculate the site's temperature. These adjustments may represent a large source of measurement variability. The final displayed temperature value is an estimate of the actual core temperature. Although electronic measurements tend to be accepted today without question, their accuracy may require further validation (Erickson, 1999).

Axillary measurement of temperature has generally been found to underestimate core temperature and to be affected by ambient temperature (Haddock, Merrow, and Swanson, 1996). In several studies the mean axillary temperature was almost always found to be lower than the mean rectal temperature; also, a statistically significant difference was observed when using mercury vs. electronic thermometers for the two sites (Craig and others, 2000). Differences in results can be related to the age of the patient, duration of placement of the device, and the actual medical condition of the child (Craig and others, 2000). The axillary site must be completely dry and the thermometer facing anteriorly with the tip high in the axilla. The optimal axillary measurement time using the traditional mercury thermometer may take up to 11 minutes (Barone and Rowe, 1999). There is a traditional belief that rectal temperature can be estimated by adding 1° C to the temperature taken in the axilla, but studies have shown this to be incorrect (Craig and others, 2000).

Some studies suggest that in children too young to cooperate with oral temperature assessment, the often-preferred method of axillary temperature measurement yields varying and inaccurate results and often does not detect fever (Haddock, Merrow, and Swanson, 1996). Another issue in axillary temperature assessment is that none of the currently available electronic thermometers have offsets for axillary temperature measurement in the rapid "predictive" mode; for accurate axillary temperature measurements the instrument must be kept in place for up to 5 minutes. The convenience of using rapid electronic thermometry, which often requires less than 30 seconds, is diluted by the potential inaccuracy of using sites not intended by the manufacturer. Some manufacturers are developing thermometers with software specific for axillary temperature assessment. Studies have shown that using the more rapid "predictive" mode in electronic thermometers is acceptable for axillary temperatures in newborn infants and premature infants (Bliss-Holtz, 1995).

Thermographs (plastic strip thermometers placed on the skin) have also been found to underestimate core temperature. In comparative studies, liquid crystal forehead devices had the poorest performance with the largest range of error, a 0.5° C to 1° C deviation compared with a rectal control (Kongpanichkul and Bunjongpak, 2000; Loveys, 1998). These strips may also produce false-positive findings: afebrile children diagnosed as having fever (Shann and Mackenzie, 1996). Their performance reportedly can be influenced by such factors as the ambient air temperature (Lewit, Marshall, and Salzer, 1982). Practitioners may find a reason to use plastic strip thermometers when cost, safety and contamination are major issues, such as in community clinics or third world countries (Shann and Mackenzie, 1996; Yotsuyanagi, Yokoi, and Sawada, 1996).

Another site that has rapidly gained favor for temperature measurement is the ear. The ear-based measurement, viewed as one of the easiest and widely used methods, appears to be less reliable than the rectal method (Amoateng-Adjepong, Del-

---

*Revised by Bogdan Dinu, M.D.

Mundo, and Manthous, 1999; ; Cretel and others, 1999; Modell and others, 1998). There is a need for terminology clarification regarding this method (Erickson, 1999). The term *tympanic temperature* (which tends to commonly and inappropriately used for all ear measurements) actually refers to a *direct contact measurement* of the tympanic membrane. Although a good index for core temperature, this method is rather invasive and is mainly recommended for research or surgical and anesthesia purposes (Sato and others, 1996).

Erickson (1999) proposed the term *ear-based temperature* for the routinely taken *auricular temperature,* which is the reading of the *ear-canal temperature* by using a noncontact infrared thermometer, with the probe placed partly into the external ear canal. This thermometer is an optical-electronic detector with an infrared sensor that detects thermal radiation emitted from all of the ear-canal surfaces. When the first clinical infrared ear thermometers were marketed in the 1980s, they were misleadingly termed devices for the tympanic temperature, and this designation has continued. The ear-based temperature depends on many variables: different zones of the tympanum, skin of the canal walls, ear cerumen, size and shape of the ear canal, size and shape of the thermometer, and depth and orientation of the thermometer. Middle ear effusion or foreign bodies (even myringotomy tubes) should not affect the ear-based temperature because they are in thermic equilibrium with the auditory canal and the tympanic membrane (Barone and Rowe, 1999). However, the size of the probe may influence this type of temperature reading because many ear probes are too large to be correctly placed in the canal. Technique is also an important factor. For the sensor to appropriately detect heat, the ear canal must be straightened as is done when using an otoscope.

It was believed that the ear's proximity to the hypothalamus, the body's temperature-regulating center, makes it a good area for reflecting true core temperature, but results of studies conducted both in adults and in children are conflicting and do not entirely support this hypothesis. Henker and Coyne (1995) found that, although mercury and electronic oral, axillary, and rectal temperature readings correlated moderately well (r = .79) with pulmonary artery temperature, the ear-based temperatures had a poor (r<20) correlation. However, in another study, three different brands of ear-based thermometers provided a closer estimate of core temperature than did a rectal measurement (Rotello, Crawford, and Terndrup, 1996). Research studies emphasize that ear-based thermometry is not entirely accurate in infants and toddlers (Lanham and others, 1999).

Overall, ear-based thermometers, although very user friendly, may not appropriately detect and assess fever in children. Researchers have reported a significant difference (5° C) between ear-based and rectal temperatures in febrile patients, suggesting that infrared ear thermometry should not be used in emergency departments for detecting fever in small children (Romanovsky and others, 1997). Similar conclusions were reinforced by Lanham and associates (1999), who found that sensitivity, specificity, and the positive and negative predictive values were unacceptably low for detecting fever in a large group of children younger than 6 years. There was concern that screening with an infrared ear thermometer would miss fever in a large number of children (Lanham and others, 1999).

A large number of studies report that ear-based thermometry (infrared ear-canal thermometer), although time-saving, easy, and simple to use in a great variety of settings, provides significantly less reliability, sensitivity, and accuracy, and may be improper for detecting a serious illness (Amoateng-Adjepong, DelMundo, and Manthous, 1999; Modell and others, 1998; Sievert, Pau, and Weidemann, 1999; Valle, Kildahl-Andersen, and Steinvoll, 2000).

Research studies in children comparing temperatures taken at various sites (rectal, oral, axillary, and ear-based) and using various devices, showed that results vary (Craig and others, 2000). The reason for this variability may be the use of various

"offsets" that mathematically "translate" the collected number into the value displayed on the LCD screen (Erickson, Meyer, and Woo, 1996; Erickson, 1999). Another reason for variation may be the technique used (Weiss and others, 1998) or the condition of the patient (Giuliano and others, 1999). Klein and others (1993) suggest that in order to effectively track temperature in a particular patient, it is important for the site of temperature measurement to remain consistent.

An ideal technique for measuring temperature should be rapid and painless, and it should provide reproducible values that accurately reflect core temperature (Lodha and others, 2000). A review of the literature leads to the conclusion that no single routinely used site for temperature assessment provides unequivocal estimates of core-body temperature. Studies evaluating various devices have yielded contradictory results. What factors might influence these discrepancies? One might be the use of the rectal temperature as the "gold standard" for comparison. The rectal temperature may change slowly and may not always reflect pulmonary artery values. Some authorities caution that "gold standards" are rarely reached because the technology is changing and ever improving. Such may be the case with ear-based sensors, and the ear route may prove to be superior to the rectal site. A poor correlation between the two sites may be a reflection of the ambient temperature on the eardrum (Henker and Coyne, 1995) or may actually indicate more accurate, not less accurate, temperature values from ear thermometry (Rotello, Crawford, and Terndrup, 1996). Because of the inconvenience and patient dissatisfaction with the rectal route, ear-based temperatures may need to be considered the "criterion standard," and, with the continuous technologic improvement of ear-devices, perhaps research findings will support the ear route. Most models of ear sensors use "offsets," or internal calculations (algorithms) that transform the ear temperature into equivalent oral or rectal temperatures. These offsets may be a source of variability that lowers the accuracy of these thermometers because each of these adjustment algorithms is a proprietary secret that differs among thermometer models (Erickson, 1999).

In deciding which route to use for temperature taking, atraumatic care should always be considered. Children are less upset having their temperature taken via the ear route than via the rectal route (Wells and others, 1995). When considering all the findings for and against different sites of temperature measurement, nurses need to think critically about why the information is needed, how clinically significant a small difference in temperature between routes is, and how much the procedure upsets the child and caregiver (Androkites, Werger, and Young, 1998; Irvin, 1999; Smith, 1998; Wilshaw and others, 1999). It is important to remember that although two different methods may correlate well in a number of studies, the accuracy and sensitivity may be questionable.

A thermometer must be sensitive enough to detect fever accurately and in a timely, convenient manner. At the onset of fever and as the temperature rises, it is not enough to know that ear-based temperature rises as rectal temperature rises. The nurse must have an accurate estimate of the actual temperature. A difference in a few tenths of a degree may indicate the need for specific measures such as medication. If children are being assessed as afebrile when they indeed have fever, the proper measures cannot be taken. In one study, parental subjective ability to assess fevers in their children was accurate in approximately 80% of the subjects (Hooker and Houston, 1996). Interestingly, this accuracy is close to the sensitivity reported for some temperature devices (Brennan and others, 1995; Wells and others, 1995), indicating that the parental report of fever without thermometry may be important in temperature assessment, especially when the child is afebrile when seen by the practitioner. There are many factors to consider, and research studies are published frequently as temperature measurement devices improve.

**TABLE 7-3** Comparison of body temperature techniques*

| Description/Procedure | Comments |
|---|---|
| **Mercury Glass Thermometer** | |
| Heat causes mercury to expand and rise in glass tube (No longer recommended for use because of toxicity of mercury if it breaks [Goldman and Shannon, 2001]) | The rectal type has more rounded tip and the oral type a more slender, elongated tip<br>Mercury thermometers should remain in place for an appropriate length of time to accurately measure the temperature |
| **Oral Temperature** | |
| Place device under tongue in right or left posterior sublingual pocket, not in front of tongue<br>Have child keep mouth closed, without biting on thermometer | Oral site indicates rapid changes in core body temperature, but accuracy may be an issue when compared with the rectal site (Jensen and others, 2000)<br>Various factors may affect temperature of mouth, such as mastication, hot or cold beverages, smoking, open-mouth breathing, and ambient temperature (Hooker and Houston, 1996; Rabinowitz and others, 1996) |
| **Axillary Temperature** | |
| Place under arm with tip in center of axilla and kept close to skin, not clothing; hold child's arm firmly against side (Fig. 7-7, A) | Recommended for children who object strongly to rectal temperature but for whom an oral temperature is not feasible<br>Has advantage of avoiding intrusive procedure and eliminating risk of rectal perforation and possible peritonitis<br>May be affected by poor peripheral perfusion (lower value), use of radiant warmers, or brown fat in cold-stressed neonates (higher value) (Bliss-Holtz, 1995; Haddock, Merrow, and Swanson, 1996) |
| **Rectal Temperature** | |
| Place well-lubricated tip not more than 2.5 cm (1 in) into rectum; hold thermometer securely and close to anus<br>May place child in side-lying, supine, or prone position (i.e., supine with knees flexed toward abdomen); cover penis because procedure often stimulates urination<br>A small child may be placed prone across parent's lap | Obtained when no other route or device can be used (e.g., in children whose mental age or temperament prevents cooperation and understanding instructions, and those who have oral or axillary injuries or surgery) (Barone and Rowe, 1999; Jensen and others, 2000)<br>Rectal temperature technique (Fig. 7-7, B)<br>Not recommended in anyone who has had rectal surgery, in children with diarrhea, or in those receiving chemotherapy that affects mucosa or causes neutropenia (Hockenberry and Kline, 2001)<br>Accuracy is affected by stool in rectum (higher value) (Loveys, 1998) |
| **Electronic Thermometer** | |
| Measures temperature with electronic component called **thermistor** mounted at tip of plastic and stainless steel probe, which is connected to electronic recorder; temperature measurement appears on digital display within 60 seconds<br>Probe can be placed in mouth, axilla, or rectum as with mercury thermometer. | Ideally suited for pediatric use because plastic sheath is unbreakable and child's mouth can remain open when oral temperature is taken<br>Accuracy for axillary temperature is supported by some research but not by other studies (Haddock, Merrow, and Swanson, 1996; Wilshaw and others, 1999) |
| **Infrared Thermometry** | |
| Infrared thermometer measures thermal radiation from axilla, ear canal, or tympanic membrane; temperature measurement appears on digital display in approximately 1 sec | Three types of infrared thermometers are available for ear-based use: tympanic, ear-canal, and arterial heat balance via the ear canal (AHBE); often these devices are inappropriately referred to as "tympanic thermometers"; temperatures measured in this way reflect arterial (blood stream) temperature (Pompei and Pompei, 1996; Wilshaw and others, 1999) |

*Revised by Bogdan Dinu, M.D.

## Blood Pressure (BP)

Noninvasive BP measurement is part of a routine vital sign determination. BP should be measured annually in children 3 years of age through adolescence, in children with symptoms of hypertension, in children in emergency rooms and intensive care units, and in high-risk infants. Several authorities also recommend routine measurements in low-risk neonates (Seidel, Rosenstein, and Pathak, 1997).

**Measurement Devices.** The most common method of measuring BP uses *auscultation* and either a *mercury-gravity* or *aneroid sphygmomanometer.* (Goonasekera and Dillon, 2000). Both types are reliable and accurate, but the aneroid type requires recalibration, whereas the mercury-gravity manometer does not.

BP can also be measured using electronic devices that employ oscillometric or Doppler techniques. In *oscillome-*

**TABLE 7-3**   Comparison of body temperature techniques—cont'd

| Description/Procedure | Comments |
|---|---|
| **Infrared Thermometry—cont'd** | |
| *Ear-Based Temperature Sensor* | |
| Insert the covered probe tip gently in ear canal, pointing toward midpoint between opposite eyebrow and sideburns (Childs, Harrison, and Hodkinson, 1999); for most accurate results straighten ear canal for sensor to measure heat appropriate (see Fig. 7-25), take three measurements, and record highest reading<br>Most models use "offsets" for internal calculations that transform ear temperature into approximately equivalent oral or rectal temperatures | Although frequently used in pediatric settings, especially ambulatory clinics, debate continues on accuracy of ear-based thermometry in screening febrile child (Lanham and others, 1999)<br>Because of difficulty with correct placement in young infants' ears, accuracy may be affected at this age group as well (Houlder, 2000; Robinson and others, 1998) |
| *Ear Sensor (Lightouch LTX)†* | |
| Measures infrared heat radiating from canal opening, scans canal for highest temperature reading, and then calculates arterial temperature (correlates highly with core or internal body temperature)<br>Insert hemispheric probe in ear opening; ear tug is not necessary | Available in two sizes; smaller size of LighTouch Ped-Q is for infants and toddlers (Wilshaw and others, 1999)<br>Does not calculate offsets; therefore reading is only for arterial temperature (not equivalent to other sites) |
| *Axillary Sensor (LighTouch LTN)†* | |
| Measures infrared heat energy radiating from axilla<br>Touch covered probe to axilla, depress and release button, remove and read | Can be used on wet skin, in incubators, or under radiant heaters, warming pads, or other heat sources |
| **Digital Thermometer** | |
| Consists of probe that connects to microprocessor chip, which translates signals into degrees and sends temperature measurement to digital display<br>Used like oral mercury thermometer | More accurate and easier to read but somewhat more expensive than mercury or plastic strip thermometer |
| **Liquid Crystal Skin Contact Thermometer (Chemical Dot Thermometer)** | |
| Single-use disposable, flexible thermometer with specific chemical mixture in each circle that changes color to measure temperature increments of two tenths of a degree<br>Two types:<br>　Used like mercury thermometer; kept in mouth (1 min), axilla (3 min), or rectum (3 min); color change is read 10-15 sec after removing thermometer<br>　Wearable, continuous-use thermometer, which is placed under axilla; may be read within 2-3 min after placement and continuously thereafter, discard and replace every 48 hr | May underestimate oral temperature and overestimate axillary temperature (Erickson, Meyer, and Woo, 1996)<br>Easier to read than mercury or plastic strip thermometer<br>Safer than glass thermometer<br>Read thermometer away from heat source (e.g., radiant warmer)<br>For older chemical dot thermometers, if unused thermometer changes color from storage in a warm area (above 35° C [95° F]), place in freezer for 1 hr and then at room temperature for 24 hours before using (Py Ma H Corporation, 1994); newer types do not require special storage (Medical Indicators, Inc., 1999)<br>Wearable, continuous-reading thermometer preferred by parents because it requires minimal disturbance to child (i.e., nurse can just lift child's arm to get a temperature reading) (Rivera and others, 1997) |
| **Plastic Strip Thermometer (Thermograph)** | |
| Changes color in response to temperature changes<br>Place strip on forehead until color change occurs; usually takes less than 15 sec<br>Some strips are used like oral mercury thermometer | Accuracy is variable; may be used for screening (Shann and Mackenzie, 1996)<br>Advantages for home and community use include simple instructions and minimal cost (Valadez, Elmore-Meegan, and Morley, 1995) |

†Manufactured by Exergen Corporation, 51 Water St, Watertown, MA 02472, (800) 422-3006, (617) 923-9911; *www.exergen.com.*

*try,* pressure changes are transmitted through the arterial wall to the pressure cuff, and the oscillations are detected by a pressure-sensitive indicator. Oscillometers have digital readouts for pulse and for systolic, diastolic, and ***mean arterial pressures (MAPs).*** The MAP is not the same as the mean BP, which is the arithmetic average of systolic and diastolic pressures. Rather, MAP is a value somewhat lower than the arithmetic mean. BP readings using oscillometry, such as Dinamap, are generally higher and correlate better with direct radial artery values than with measurements using auscultation (Gillman and Cook, 1995; Ling and others, 1995; Lyew and Jamieson, 1994; Wattigney and others, 1996) (Table 7-5).

Oscillometry also eliminates common problems found with the auscultation method, such as deflating the cuff too rapidly, not hearing the softest sounds, and rounding numbers for the Korotkoff sounds (Goonasekera and Dillon, 2000).

*Doppler ultrasound* translates changes in ultrasound frequency caused by blood movement within the artery to audible sound by means of a transducer in the cuff. Doppler ultrasound is useful for systolic pressure measurement but is unreliable for diastolic pressure measurement. Oscillometric and Doppler instruments are very useful in measuring BP in infants and have largely replaced the flush method (which reflects only the mean BP) and the auscultatory method.

*Selection of cuff.* No matter what type of noninvasive technique is used, the most important factor in accurately measuring BP is the use of an appropriately sized cuff. (*Cuff size* refers only to the inner inflatable bladder, not the cloth covering.) A technique to establish an appropriate cuff size is to choose a cuff having a bladder width that is approximately 40% of the arm circumference midway between the olecranon and the acromion. This will usually be a cuff

bladder that covers 80% to 100% of the circumference of the arm (Fig. 7-8) (NIH, 1996).

Using limb circumference for selecting cuff width more accurately reflects direct arterial BP than using limb length, because this method takes into account the variations in thickness of the arm and the amount of pressure required to compress the artery (Gillman and Cook, 1995) (Table 7-6). For measurements sites other than the upper arms, the limb circumference guidelines can be used, although the shape of the limb (i.e., conical shape of the thigh) may prevent appropriate placement of the cuff and inaccurately reflect intraarterial BP.

Cuffs that are too narrow or too wide affect the accuracy of BP measurements, although wide cuffs tend to affect Bp readings less. If the cuff is too small, the reading on the device is falsely high. If the cuff is too large, the reading is falsely low.

When another site is used, BP measurements using noninvasive techniques may differ. Generally, systolic pressure

| **TABLE 7-4** | Grading of pulses |
|---|---|
| **Grade** | **Description** |
| 0 | Not palpable |
| +1 | Difficult to palpate, thready, weak, easily obliterated with pressure |
| +2 | Difficult to palpate, may be obliterated with pressure |
| +3 | Easy to palpate, not easily obliterated with pressure (normal) |
| +4 | Strong, bounding, not obliterated with pressure |

**TABLE 7-5** Normative oscillometric (Dinamap) BP values (systolic/diastolic, with mean arterial pressure in parentheses)

| Age-Group | Mean | 90th Percentile | 95th Percentile |
|---|---|---|---|
| Newborn (1-3 days) | 65/41 (50) | 75/49 (59) | 78/52 (62) |
| 1 month to 2 years | 95/58 (72) | 106/68 (83) | 110/71 (86) |
| 2-5 years | 101/57 (74) | 112/66 (82) | 115/68 (85) |

From Park M, Menard S: Normative oscillometric blood pressure values in the first 5 years in an office setting, *Am J Dis Child* 143(7):860-864, 1989.

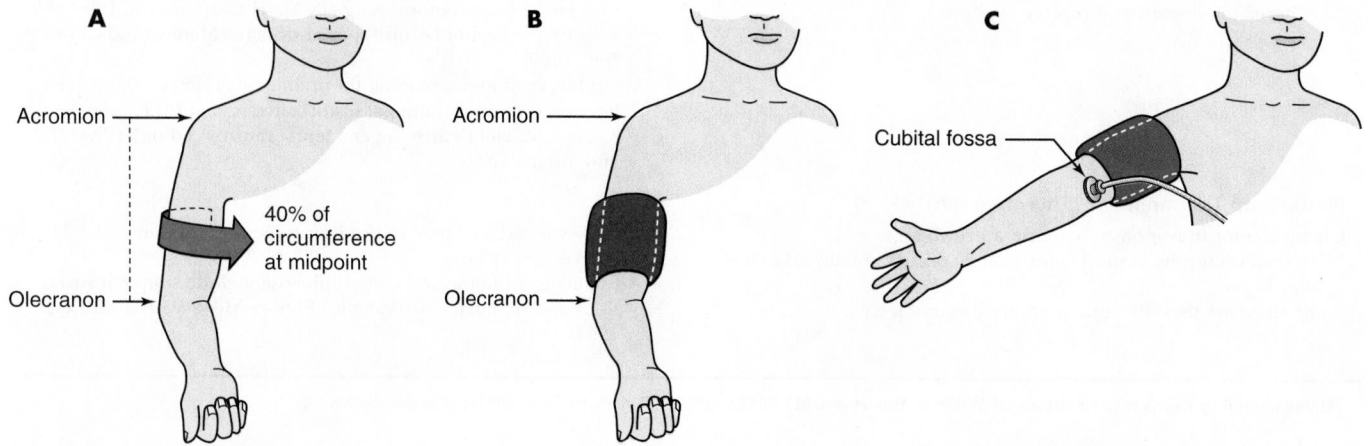

**Fig. 7-8** Determination of proper blood pressure cuff size. **A,** The cuff bladder width should be approximately 40% of the circumference of the arm measured at a point midway between the olecranon and acromion. **B,** Cuff bladder length should cover 80% to 100% of the circumference of the arm. **C,** Blood pressure should be measured with the cubital fossa at heart level. The arm should be supported. The stethoscope bell is placed over the brachial artery pulse, proximal and medial to the cubital fossa, and below the bottom edge of the cuff. (From National Institutes of Health, National Heart, Lung, Blood Institute: *Update on the Task Force Report [1987] on high blood pressure in children and adolescents: a working group report from the National High Blood Pressure Education Program,* NIH Pub No 96-3790, Sept, 1996.)

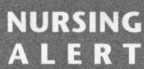

> **NURSING ALERT**
>
> In choosing cuff sizes, use an appropriately sized cuff (Table 7-7). When the correct size is not available, use an oversized cuff rather than an undersized one, or use another site that more appropriately fits the cuff size. Do not choose a cuff based on the name of the cuff (e.g., an "infant" cuff may be too small for some infants).

in the lower extremities (thigh or calf) is greater than pressure in the upper extremities, and systolic BP in the calf is higher than that in the thigh. These differences are listed in Table 7-8 and apply to oscillometric measurements taken on the right extremities with the child supine and the cuff size based on the circumference method (Park, Lee, and Johnson, 1993).

> **NURSING ALERT**
>
> Compare blood pressure in the upper and lower extremities at least once to detect abnormalities, such as coarctation of the aorta, in which the lower extremity pressure is less than the upper extremity pressure.

***Measurement and interpretation.*** Measuring and interpreting BP in infants and children requires additional attention to correct procedure for several reasons: (1) limb sizes vary and cuff selection must accommodate the circumference; (2) excessive pressure on the antecubital fossa affects the Korotkoff sounds; (3) children easily become anxious, which can elevate BP; and (4) BP values change with age and growth.

Age, height, weight, and body mass have been shown to be highly correlated with BP (NIH, 1996). Recent studies indicate that height is a more appropriate index of maturation than weight for use with normative BP data and should be considered when evaluating BP in children. Tables are now available that indicate—when height is taken into account—that more short children (10th percentile for age-sex-specific height) and fewer tall children (90th percentile for age-sex-specific height) are likely to be classified as hypertensive. (See inside back cover for BP tables.)

Although the technique of BP measurement in children is generally the same as that used for adults, certain aspects of the procedure are especially important. (See Guidelines box on p. 186.) Because children are easily upset by unfamiliar procedures, prepare them for BP measurement. For children of preschool age or older, explain each step of the procedure and tell them how the cuff will feel, such as a tight feeling or an arm hug. Use explanations such as "I want to see how strong your muscle is" or "Let's watch the silver rise in the tube."

Because the child should be quiet and relaxed during the procedure, measure BP before performing any anxiety-producing procedures. Infants and small children may be more quiet if the reading is taken while they are sitting in the parent's lap.

Use a pediatric stethoscope and bell for hearing BP sounds in small children and infants. If auscultation is not possible, obtain a systolic reading by palpation; measure the point at which the pulse at the radial or brachial artery reappears as the cuff is deflated. BP should be measured twice,

---

**TABLE 7-6** Recommended bladder dimensions for blood pressure cuffs

| Arm Circumference at Midpoint (cm) | Cuff Name* | Bladder Width (cm) | Bladder Length (cm) |
|---|---|---|---|
| 5-7.5 | Newborn | 3 | 5 |
| 7.5-13 | Infant | 5 | 8 |
| 13-20 | Child | 8 | 13 |
| 24-32 | Adult | 13 | 24 |
| 32-42 | Wide adult | 17 | 32 |
| 42-50 | Thigh | 20 | 42 |

From Frohlich ED and others: Recommendations for human blood pressure determination by sphygmomanometers: report of a special task force appointed by the Steering Committee, American Heart Association, *Circulation* 77:509A, 1988.
*Cuff name does not guarantee that the cuff will be appropriate size for a child within that age range.

---

**TABLE 7-7** Commonly available blood pressure cuffs

| Cuff Name* | Bladder Width (cm) | Bladder Length (cm) |
|---|---|---|
| Newborn | 2.5-4.0 | 5.0-9.0 |
| Infant | 4.0-6.0 | 11.5-18.0 |
| Child | 7.5-9.0 | 17.0-19.0 |
| Adult | 11.5-13.0 | 22.0-26.0 |
| Large arm | 14.0-15.0 | 30.5-33.0 |
| Thigh | 18.0-19.0 | 36.0-38.0 |

From Report of the Second Task Force on Blood Pressure Control in Children—1987, *Pediatrics* 79(1):1-25, 1987.
*Cuff name does not guarantee that the cuff will be appropriate size for a child within that age range.

---

**TABLE 7-8** Differences in oscillometric systolic BP between arm and lower extremity sites in normal children

| Age-Group (Years) | Systolic BP × (Mean ± SD) | |
|---|---|---|
| | Arm-Thigh | Arm-Calf |
| 4-8 | $-7.1 \pm 6.8$ | $-9.3 \pm 7.4$ |
| 9-16 | $-2.4 \pm 7.7$ | $-5.0 \pm 26.9$ |

From Park M, Lee D, Johnson GA: Oscillometric blood pressure in the arm, thigh, and calf in healthy children and those with aortic coarctation, *Pediatrics* 91(4):761-765, 1993.

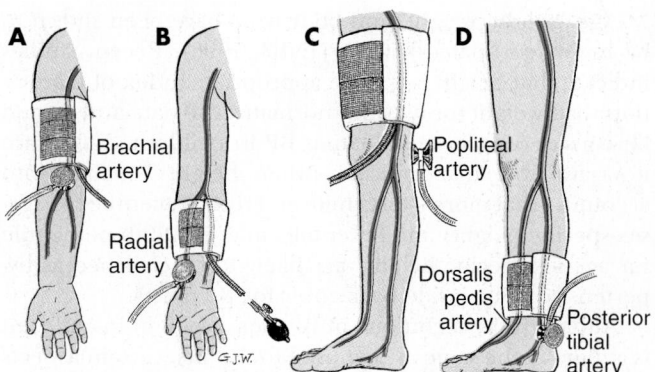

**Fig. 7-9** Sites for measuring blood pressure, **A,** Upper arm. **B,** Lower arm or forearm. **C,** Thigh. **D,** Calf or ankle.

**GUIDELINES**
*Measuring Blood Pressure*

Use an appropriately sized cuff.
Use same position, preferably sitting, and right arm for brachial artery site (Fig. 7-9, *A*).
Use alternate site as needed to accommodate available cuff sizes:
  Use smaller size on forearm: place cuff above wrist and auscultate radial artery (Fig. 7-9, *B*).
  Use larger size on thigh: place cuff above knee and auscultate popliteal artery (Fig. 7-9, *C*).
  Use larger size on calf: place cuff above malleoli or at midcalf and auscultate posterior tibial or dorsal pedal artery (Fig. 7-9, *D*).
Position limb at level of heart.
Rapidly inflate cuff to approximately 20 mm Hg above point at which radial pulse disappears.
Release cuff pressure at a rate of approximately 2 to 3 mm Hg/sec during auscultation of artery.
Read mercury-gravity manometer at eye level.
Record systolic value as onset of a clear tapping sound (first Korotkoff sound).
Record diastolic pressure as:
  Fourth Korotkoff sound (K4) (low-pitched, muffled sound) for children up to age 12 years
  Fifth Korotkoff sound (K5) (disappearance of all sound) for children ages 13 to 18 years
Record also limb, position, cuff size, and method of measurement.
If using electronic monitor, follow manufacturer's instructions and guidelines for correct cuff size.
  With oscillometric device (i.e., Dinamap), can use all four limb sites, but reserve the thigh for last because it is the most uncomfortable.
Stabilize limb during cuff deflation because movement interferes with the device's ability to measure BP accurately.

and the average measurement should be recorded (NIH, 1996).

The average BP readings at various ages throughout childhood using sphygmomanometry are listed on the inside back cover; readings using oscillometry are listed in Table 7-5. A normal BP is defined as a systolic and diastolic BP less than the 90th percentile for age and sex. (See Hypertension, Chapter 25.)

**NURSING ALERT** Published norms for BP, such as those on the inside back cover, are valid only if the same method of measurement (auscultation and limb length for cuff size) is used in clinical practice.

**NURSING TIP** Use the following quick formula for average *systolic BP* using auscultation:

1 to 7 years: Age in years + 90
8 to 18 years: (2 × Age in years) + 83

Use the following quick formula for average *diastolic BP* using auscultation:

1 to 5 years: 56
6 to 18 years: Age in years + 52

## General Appearance

The general appearance of the child is a cumulative, subjective impression of the child's physical appearance, state of nutrition, behavior, personality, interactions with parents and nurse (also siblings if present), posture, development, and speech. Although general appearance is recorded at the beginning of the physical examination, it encompasses all the observations of the child during the interview and physical assessment.

Note the *facies,* the facial expression and appearance of the child. The facies may give clues to children who are in pain; have difficulty breathing; feel frightened, discontent, or happy; are mentally deficient; or are acutely ill.

Observe the *posture, position,* and types of *body movement.* The child with hearing or vision loss may characteristically tilt the head in an awkward position to hear or see better. The child in pain may favor a body part. The child with low self-esteem or a feeling of rejection may assume a slumped, careless, and apathetic pose or posture. Likewise, a child with confidence, a feeling of self-worth, and a sense of security usually demonstrates a tall, straight, well-balanced posture. While observing such "body language," do not interpret too freely but rather record objectively.

Note the child's *hygiene* in terms of cleanliness; any unusual body odor; the condition of the hair, neck, nails, teeth, and feet; and the condition of the clothing. Such observations are excellent clues to possible instances of neglect, inadequate financial resources, housing difficulties (e.g., no running water), or lack of knowledge concerning children's needs.

General appearance includes an overall impression of the child's state of *nutrition.* This impression is more than just a statement describing body weight or stature, such as "slender and tall." It is an estimation of the quality and quantity of nutritional intake. For example, two children can be of the same height and weight, with one appearing overweight because of flabby, loose skin and the other appearing strong, robust, and well-built because of firm, well-defined musculature. Likewise, a small, slender child may be well-nourished with no signs of chronic undernutrition such as bony prominences, protuberant abdomen, flat but-

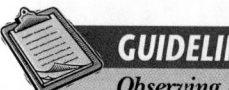

## GUIDELINES
### Observing Behavior

What is the child's overall personality—calm, anxious, tense, content, outgoing, shy, talkative, aggressive, introverted, stable, or moody?

Is the child active, sedentary, fidgety, or restless?

Does the child have a long attention span, or is the child easily distracted?

Does the child sit quietly on the examining table or parent's lap, or does the child climb, run, open doors, and otherwise explore the environment?

How does the child react to commands—with fear or willingness to obey?

How advanced is the child's ability to follow requests? Can the child follow two or three commands in succession without the need for repetition? Is the child attentive to requests, or must they be repeated several times?

Is the child cooperative, belligerent, or argumentative?

What is the child's response to delayed gratification or frustration? Is the child able to withstand momentary discomfort and wait for the requests to be met?

In what tone of voice does the child make requests or talk to the parents?

Does the child seek approval and gain satisfaction from it?

Does the child use eye-to-eye contact during conversation?

Does the child agree with the parent's answers or find reasons to disagree, interrupt, or argue? What is the child's reaction to the nurse—respectful, friendly, reserved, apprehensive, or uninterested?

Is the child interested in the surroundings? Does the child look around the room, ask questions about unfamiliar objects, seem to enjoy exploring them, or attempt to break or destroy them?

Can the child follow directions for using the instruments or imitate their use? Is the child quick or slow to grasp explanations?

tocks, gaunt facies, and poor muscle tone with evidence of wasting.

Compare your impression of the nutritional state with the parents' history of feeding practices. Discrepancies between the two "impressions" may be a valuable area for nutritional counseling. For example, parents who believe that their child is too thin and eats too little—despite evidence of adequate growth and physical signs of proper nutrition—may find it helpful to keep a daily diary in which to calculate the child's cumulative food intake. Many parents are surprised at the quantity of food ingested, even though the amounts at each meal or snack are small.

*Behavior* includes the child's personality; level of activity; reactions to stress, requests, or frustration; interactions with others, primarily the parent and nurse; degree of alertness; and responses to stimuli. It is one of the most important observations to make during a child's health assessment. (See Guidelines box.)

*Development* can be assessed by carefully observing the child, but verify your impressions with screening tests. Various tests for assessing development, speech, vision, and hearing are discussed later in this chapter and in Chapter 24.

Under general appearance, record an overall estimate of the child's speech development, motor skills, degree of coordination, and recent area of achievement. For example, the following statement may apply to an 18-month-old child:

"Motor development advanced for age; climbs, runs, jumps (most recent motor skill); manipulates small objects with ease; excellent coordination and balance; beginning to name many objects; uses two-word phrases; and enjoys 'talking' to self and others."

## Skin

Skin is assessed for color, texture, temperature, moisture, and turgor. Hair is also inspected for color, texture, quality, distribution, and elasticity. Examination of the skin and its accessory structures primarily involves inspection and palpation.

### Factors Influencing Assessment

*Physical factors* related to the examining environment and the child's skin surface can affect accurate assessment. Because colors such as pink, blue, yellow, or orange cast deceiving glows on the skin, conduct the examination in a well-illuminated room with nonglare lighting and neutral color. The room should also be comfortably warm because air-conditioning can cause a cold-induced cyanosis and excessive heat can produce flushing. Poor hygiene and artificial paint on nails or lips also mask a true determination of color. Sometimes it is necessary to clean the skin with soap and water and to remove cosmetics before beginning inspection. Although not a common situation in pediatrics, remember that such factors can hide signs of ecchymoses, petechiae, pallor, or cyanosis.

Texture, temperature, moisture, and turgor can be subjectively inspected, but palpation must be performed for greater accuracy. Clothing always interferes with palpation; thus examine each area of the body nude, either as part of the general overall examination or combined with assessment of each body system. Because texture is affected by climatic exposure, such as cold, sun, and wind, compare the texture of protected areas with that of exposed areas.

*Genetic factors* influence assessment of color. The normal color in light-skinned children varies from a milky white and rosy color to a more deeply hued pink color. In general, cyanosis or bluish discolorations are not normal, except in the newborn (Table 7-9). Dark-skinned children, such as those of Native American, Hispanic, African-American, Latin, Mediterranean, or Asian descent, have inherited various brown, red, yellow, olive green, and bluish tones in their skin, which can falsely alter assessment. For example, some children of Mediterranean origin normally have bluish-tinged lips, which is otherwise suggestive of cyanosis. Asian persons, whose skin is normally of a yellow tone, may appear to be jaundiced. Many African-American individuals often have normal bluish pigmentation of the gums, buccal cavity, borders of the tongue, and nail beds. The visible portion of their sclera may contain speckled deposits of brown melanin that resemble petechiae.

*Physiologic factors* also affect assessment of color. Edema increases the amount of interstitial fluid, thereby increasing the distance between the outermost layers of the epidermis and the pigmented and vascular layers. Consequently, edema decreases the intensity of skin color, sometimes producing a false pallor.

**TABLE 7-9** Differences in color changes of racial groups

| Color Change | Light Skin | Dark Skin |
|---|---|---|
| Cyanosis | Bluish tinge, especially in palpebral conjunctiva (lower eyelid), nail beds, earlobes, lips, oral membranes, soles, and palms | Ashen gray lips and tongue |
| Pallor | Loss of rosy glow in skin, especially face | Ashen gray appearance in black skin. More yellowish brown color in brown skin |
| Erythema | Redness easily seen anywhere on body | Much more difficult to assess; rely on palpation for warmth or edema |
| Ecchymosis | Purplish to yellow-green areas; may be seen anywhere on skin | Very difficult to see unless in mouth or conjunctiva |
| Petechiae | Purplish pinpoints most easily seen on buttocks, abdomen, and inner surfaces of arms or legs | Usually invisible except in oral mucosa, conjunctiva of eyelids, and conjunctiva covering eyeball |
| Jaundice | Yellow staining seen in sclera of eyes, skin, fingernails, soles, palms, and oral mucosa | Most reliably assessed in sclera, hard palate, palms, and soles |

In general, the amount of adipose tissue does not markedly affect skin color, because deposition of fat cells is below the pigmented layers of the skin. Overnutrition may not mean adequate nutrition; pallor that may indicate nutritional iron deficiency is carefully assessed.

Exposure to sunlight stimulates the melanocytes to produce more melanin, thereby increasing skin color. Individuals who are deeply suntanned require as careful observation as those who are genetically dark-skinned.

Assess color changes in areas of the body in which melanin production is least: sclerae, conjunctivae, nail beds, lips, tongue, buccal mucosa, palms, and soles. These areas are rarely affected by edema or the amount of adipose tissue but are sensitive to changes from physical factors, such as the use of cosmetics or poor hygiene.

### Variations in Skin Color

Many of the specific color changes peculiar to the newborn are described in Table 8-3. Differences in assessment of color changes in ethnic groups are presented in Table 7-9.

The skin receives its pigmented color of yellow, brown, or black from melanin and its shades of red or blue from the color of hemoglobin. Oxygenated (saturated) hemoglobin in the superficial capillaries of the dermis gives a rosy, pink glow. Reduced levels of oxygenated hemoglobin reflect a bluish tone through the skin *(cyanosis)*, which is evident when reduced (deoxygenated or desaturated) hemoglobin levels reach at least 5 mg/dl of blood, regardless of the total hemoglobin concentration. In general, with darker skin pigmentation, higher levels of deoxygenated hemoglobin must be present for cyanosis to be evident.

*Pallor,* or paleness, may be a sign of anemia, chronic disease, edema, or shock. However, it may also be a normal complexion characteristic or an indication of indoor living.

Pallor or cyanosis can be compared to the color change normally produced by blanching. For example, in nonpigmented nails, pressing down on the free edge of the nail on the index or middle finger of a child with good skin color produces marked blanching or whitening as compared with the return blood flow. In a child with pallor the difference in color change will be slight. Observe the blanching color change in dark-skinned individuals by gently applying pressure to their lips or gums.

*Erythema,* or redness of the skin, may be the result of increased temperature from climatic conditions, local inflammation, or infection. It may also appear as a sign of skin irritation, allergy, or other dermatoses. The degree of redness reflects the amount of increased blood flow to the area. Note any reddening, and describe the location, size, presence of warmth, itching, type of distribution (e.g., diffuse, clearly circumscribed, parallel to a vein), and presence of characteristic lesions such as macules, papules, or vesicles. (See Chapter 18 for a description of skin lesions.)

*Plethora* is also redness of the skin but is caused by increased numbers of red blood cells as a compensatory response to chronic hypoxia. Intense redness of the lips or cheeks occurs.

Ecchymosis and petechiae are caused by extravasation or hemorrhage of blood into the skin; the only difference between these two conditions is size. *Ecchymoses* are large, diffuse areas, usually black and blue in color, and are typically the result of injuries. Because ecchymotic areas may indicate systemic disorders or child maltreatment, always investigate the reported cause of the bruises, especially when they are located in suspicious areas (e.g., the back or buttocks) rather than on the knees, shins, elbows, or forearms.

*Petechiae* are small, distinct pinpoint hemorrhages 2 mm or less in size and can denote some type of blood disorder, such as decreased platelets in leukemia. Because of their size, ecchymoses are more readily observed than are petechiae, which may be visible only in areas of very light-colored skin. Areas of erythema can be distinguished from ecchymosis or petechiae by blanching the skin. Because erythema is a result of increased blood flow *to* the area, exerting pressure will momentarily empty the engorged vessels and produce blanching. Because the other discolorations are produced by blood leaking *into* tissue spaces, blanching will not occur.

*Jaundice,* a yellow staining of the skin usually caused by bile pigments, is always a significant finding. If a yellow-orange cast is noted in an otherwise healthy child, inquire about the quantity of ingested yellow vegetables, such as carrots. In excess, yellow vegetables produce a yellow-orange color from deposits of carotene in the skin, a condition called *carotenemia.*

## Texture

Palpate the skin for texture, noting moisture and temperature. Note any marks or scars that may indicate healed injuries and inquire about their origin. Normally the skin of young children is smooth, soft, and slightly dry to the touch, not oily or clammy. Note any variations from these findings because they may indicate common problems of childhood such as cradle cap, eczema, diaper rash, or excessive dryness (xeroderma) all over the body from too-frequent bathing, exposure to the weather, or vitamin A deficiency. Excessively moist, clammy skin may indicate serious health problems, particularly heart disease.

## Temperature

Evaluate temperature by symmetrically feeling each part of the body and comparing upper areas with lower ones. Note any distinct difference in temperature. Although not a common anomaly, one of the key signs for coarctation of the aorta is warm upper extremities and cool lower ones. Also observe the skin temperature of the dressed child. Young children produce heat rapidly, and they quickly become overheated if dressed too warmly. Many parents do not realize this and fail to change clothing to accommodate climatic variations.

## Turgor

*Tissue turgor* refers to the amount of elasticity in the skin. To assess turgor, grasp the skin on the abdomen between the thumb and index finger, pull it taut, and quickly release it. Elastic tissue immediately assumes its normal position without residual marks or creases. In children with poor skin turgor, the skin remains suspended or tented for a few seconds before slowly falling back on the abdomen. Skin turgor is one of the best estimates of adequate hydration and nutrition. (See Fig. 28-2.)

While evaluating turgor, inspect for signs of *edema,* which is normally evident as swelling or puffiness. Periorbital edema is a sign of several systemic disorders, such as kidney disease, but it may normally be evident in children who have been crying or sleeping or have allergies. Evaluate for changes in edema according to position, specific location, and response to pressure. For example, in *pitting edema,* pressing a finger into the edematous area causes a temporary indentation.

## Accessory Structures

Inspection of the accessory structures of the skin, namely the hair, nails, and dermatoglyphics, may be performed while the skin is being examined or when the scalp and extremities are being assessed.

Inspect the *hair* for color, texture, quality, distribution, and elasticity. Children's scalp hair is usually lustrous, silky, strong, and elastic. Genetic factors affect the appearance of hair. For example, the hair of black children is usually curlier and coarser than that of white children. Hair that is stringy, dull, brittle, dry, friable, and depigmented may suggest poor nutrition. Note any bald or thinning spots. Although alopecia can be a sign of various skin disorders, such as tinea capitis, loss of hair in infants is often the result of lying in the same position, such as supine for sleeping. A bald-

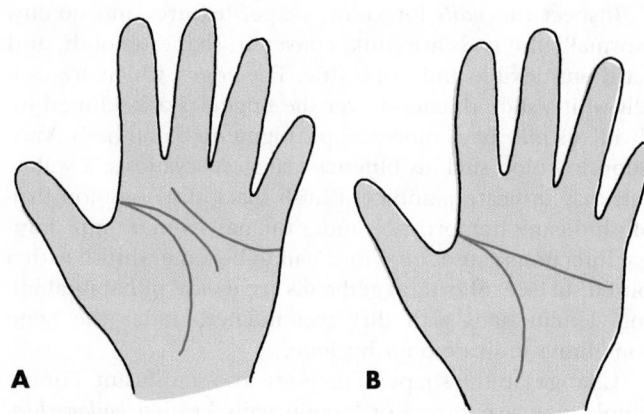

**Fig. 7-10**  Examples of flexion creases on palm. **A,** Normal. **B,** Transpalmar crease.

ing area may be a clue for counseling parents concerning the child's stimulation needs or position changes.

Inspect the hair and scalp for cleanliness. Various ethnic groups condition their hair with oils or lubricants, which will clog the sebaceous glands if not thoroughly washed from the scalp, causing scalp infections. Inspect hair shafts for lice, whose ova appear as grayish translucent flakes. Ova or nits are distinguished from dandruff because the eggs adhere to the hair. If pediculosis capitus (head infested with lice) is suspected, be careful to guard against self-infestation by handwashing and by wearing gloves or using tongue blades to inspect the hair.

Inspect the *scalp* for ticks, which appear as grayish or brown oval bodies. Although they can be found anywhere on the body, the most common sites are exposed parts such as the head. Although not all dog or wood ticks transmit serious disease, always record their presence or removal in case symptoms appear.

Note unusual hairiness anywhere on the body, such on as the arms, legs, trunk, or face. Tufts of hair anywhere along the spine, especially over the sacrum, are significant because they can mark the site of spina bifida occulta.

In older children who are approaching puberty, look for growth of secondary hair as a sign of normally progressing pubertal changes. (See Figs. 19-4 and 19-6.) Note precocious or delayed appearance of hair growth because, although not always suggestive of hormonal dysfunction, it may be of great concern to the early- or late-maturing adolescent.

Inspect the hands. Each individual has a distinct set of handprints and footprints. These patterns, or *dermatoglyphics,* are unique to the individual and vary a great deal in detail and complexity. Flexion creases also appear on the palm of the hand and the sole of the foot. The palm normally shows three flexion creases (Fig. 7-10, *A*). In some situations, such as Down syndrome, the two distal horizontal creases are fused to form a single horizontal crease called a *single palmar crease* or *transpalmar crease* (Fig. 7-10, *B*). If grossly abnormal lines or folds are observed, sketch a picture to describe them and refer the finding to a specialist for further investigation.

Inspect the **nails** for color, shape, texture, and quality. Normally the nails are pink, convex in shape, smooth, and hard but flexible and not brittle. The edges, which are usually white, should extend over the fingers. Dark-skinned individuals may have more deeply pigmented nail beds. Variation in color, such as blueness, suggests cyanosis; a yellow tint may indicate jaundice. Bluish black discoloration usually indicates hemorrhage under the nail from trauma. Fungal infections cause the entire nail to become whitish with a pitted surface. Short, ragged nails are typical of habitual biting. Uncut nails with dirt accumulated under the edge sometimes indicate poor hygiene.

Changes in the shape of nails are also significant. For example, concave curves or "spoon nails," called **koilonychia**, are sometimes seen in iron deficiency anemia. **Clubbing** of the nails is always a significant finding and usually is associated with chronic cyanosis. In clubbing, the base of the nail becomes visibly swollen and feels springy when palpated, rather than firm as in the normal nail. (See Fig. 31-7.)

## Lymph Nodes

Lymph nodes are usually assessed when examining the part of the body where they are located. The usual sites for palpating accessible lymph nodes are shown in Fig. 7-11. The major function of lymph nodes is to collect and filter the lymph of bacteria and other foreign matter as it returns to the circulatory system. Tender, enlarged warm lymph nodes generally indicate infection or inflammation close to their location (Seidel and others, 1999). For example, occipital or postauricular adenopathy is often seen in local scalp in-

fection, such as pediculosis, tick bite, or external otitis. Cervical adenopathy usually accompanies acute infections in or around the mouth or throat. In children, however, small, nontender, movable nodes are frequently normal.

Palpate nodes with the distal portion of the fingers by gently but firmly pressing in a circular motion along the regions where nodes are normally present. During assessment of the nodes in the head and neck, tilt the child's head upward slightly but without tensing the sternocleidomastoid or trapezius muscle. This position facilitates palpation of the **submental, submaxillary, tonsillar,** and **cervical nodes.** Palpate the **axillary nodes** with the child's arms relaxed at the side but slightly abducted. Assess the **inguinal nodes** with the child supine. Note size, mobility, temperature, and tenderness, as well as the parents' reports of any visible change of enlarged nodes.

## Head

Observe the head for general **shape** and **symmetry.** A flattening of one part of the head, such as the occiput, may indicate that the child continually lies in this position. Marked asymmetry is usually abnormal and may indicate premature closure of the sutures (craniosynostosis).

> **NURSING ALERT** Significant head lag after 6 months of age strongly indicates cerebral injury and is referred for further evaluation.

Note **head control** in infants and **head posture** in older children. By 4 months of age, most infants should be able to hold the head erect and in midline when in a vertical position.

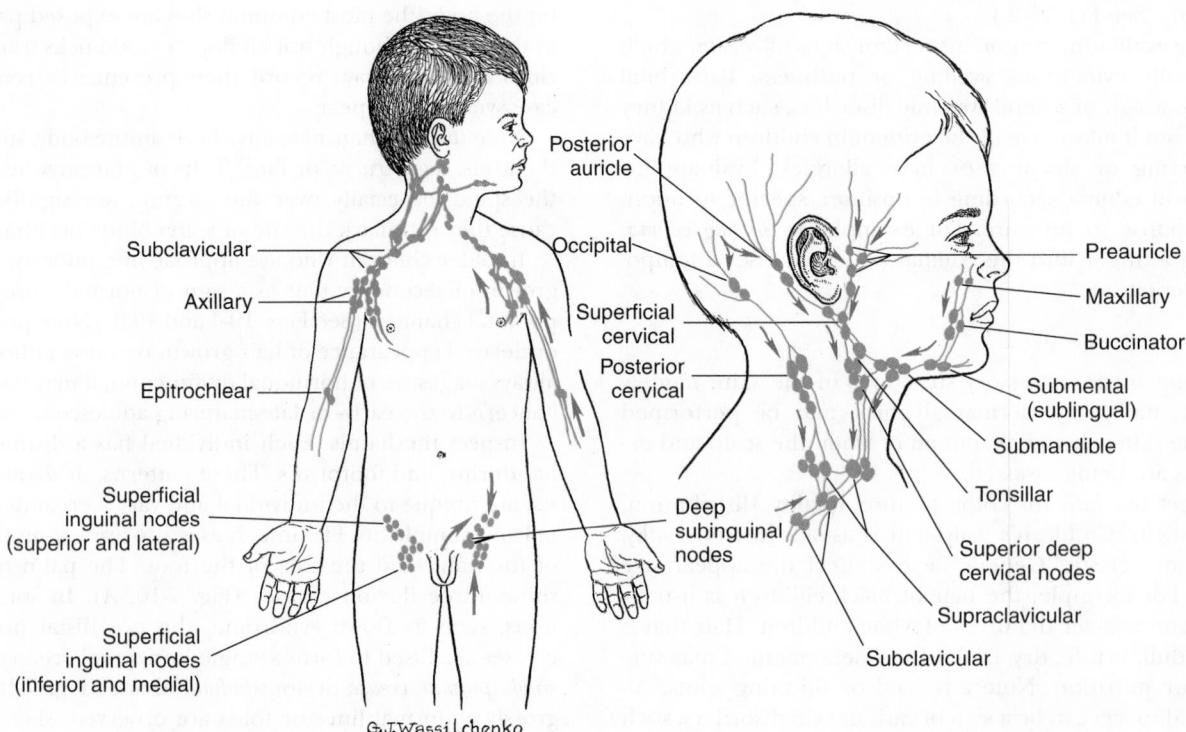

**Fig. 7-11** Location of superficial lymph nodes. *Arrows* indicate directional flow of lymph.

Evaluate range of motion by asking the older child to look in each direction (to either side, up, and down) or by manually putting the younger child through each position. Limited range of motion may indicate *wryneck*, or *torticollis*—a result of injury to the sternocleidomastoid muscle—in which the child holds the head to one side with the chin pointing toward the opposite side.

> **NURSING ALERT**   Hyperextension of the head (opisthotonos) with pain on flexion is a serious indication of meningeal irritation and is referred for immediate medical evaluation. (See Fig. 7-57 for Brudzinski sign.)

Palpate the *skull* for patent sutures, fontanels, fractures, and swellings. Normally the posterior fontanel closes by the second month of life, and the anterior fontanel fuses between 12 and 18 months of age. Early or late closure is noted because either may be a sign of a pathologic condition. (For a more detailed discussion of the cranial bones, see Chapter 8.)

While examining the head, observe the *face* for symmetry, movement, and general appearance. Ask the child to "make a face" to assess symmetric movement and disclose any degree of paralysis. Note any unusual facial proportion, such as an unusually high or low forehead, wide- or close-set eyes, or a small, receding chin.

Also note any unusual swellings or sites of edema that may be associated with specific disorders (e.g., nephrosis or Cushing syndrome) or steroid therapy. Visible and palpable swelling anterior to the earlobe and above the angle of the jaw is characteristic of parotid gland enlargement in mumps, which gives the child a characteristic "chipmunk" appearance.

Generally, the head and face are not auscultated or percussed, with the exception of the *sinuses* (air cavities within certain bones adjacent to the nasal cavity) (Fig. 7-12). The sinuses develop as outpouchings of the nasal airway as the skull bones enlarge throughout infancy and childhood. The maxillary and ethmoid sinuses are present soon after birth (Seidel and others, 1999). The frontal and sphenoid sinuses develop later in childhood. Percuss the sinuses for evidence of pain if there are signs of an infection, such as headache and congestion.

## Neck

Besides assessing motility of the head and neck, inspect the size of the neck and palpate it for associated structures. During infancy the neck is short, with skinfolds between the head and shoulders; it lengthens during the next 3 to 4 years. A short or webbed neck is associated with various anomalies, such as Turner syndrome. Marked edema of the neck may indicate mumps, local throat or mouth infections, or diphtheria. Distended neck veins often indicate difficulty on expiration, such as in asthma or cystic fibrosis.

Palpate the *trachea* by placing the thumb and index finger on each side and sliding them back and forth to note any masses. Normally the trachea is in the midline or slightly to the right of the midline. Note any shift, because it can signify serious lung problems such as a tumor or foreign body in the lung.

Palpate the *thyroid gland*, which is located at the base of the neck. This butterfly-shaped gland straddles the trachea and has two lateral lobes connected by an *isthmus*, or band of glandular tissue. The isthmus is the only portion of the thyroid that is usually palpable, because the lobes that curve posteriorly around the trachea are partially covered by the sternocleidomastoid muscle (Fig. 7-13). Normally the thyroid rises as the child swallows. However, palpating the thyroid takes considerable practice and is especially difficult in an infant, whose neck is short and thick. If any masses are detected in the neck, record and report them for further investigation.

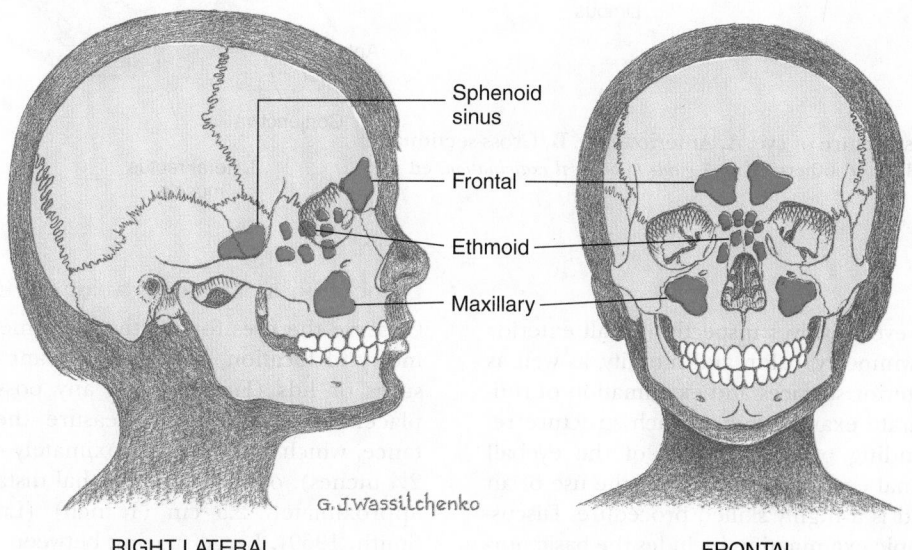

Sphenoid sinus

Frontal

Ethmoid

Maxillary

G.J.Wassilchenko

RIGHT LATERAL                    FRONTAL

**Fig. 7-12**   Location of sinuses.

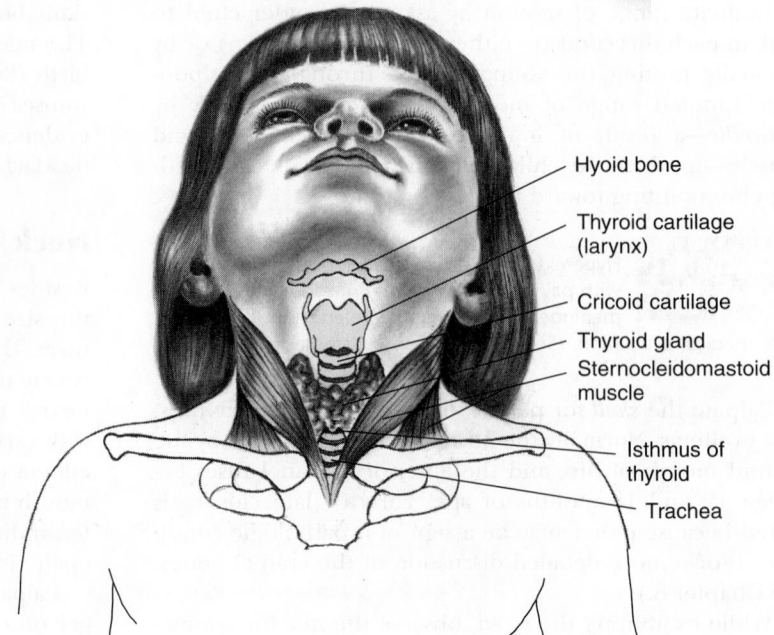

**Fig. 7-13**   Anterior view of structures in neck.

Hyoid bone
Thyroid cartilage (larynx)
Cricoid cartilage
Thyroid gland
Sternocleidomastoid muscle
Isthmus of thyroid
Trachea

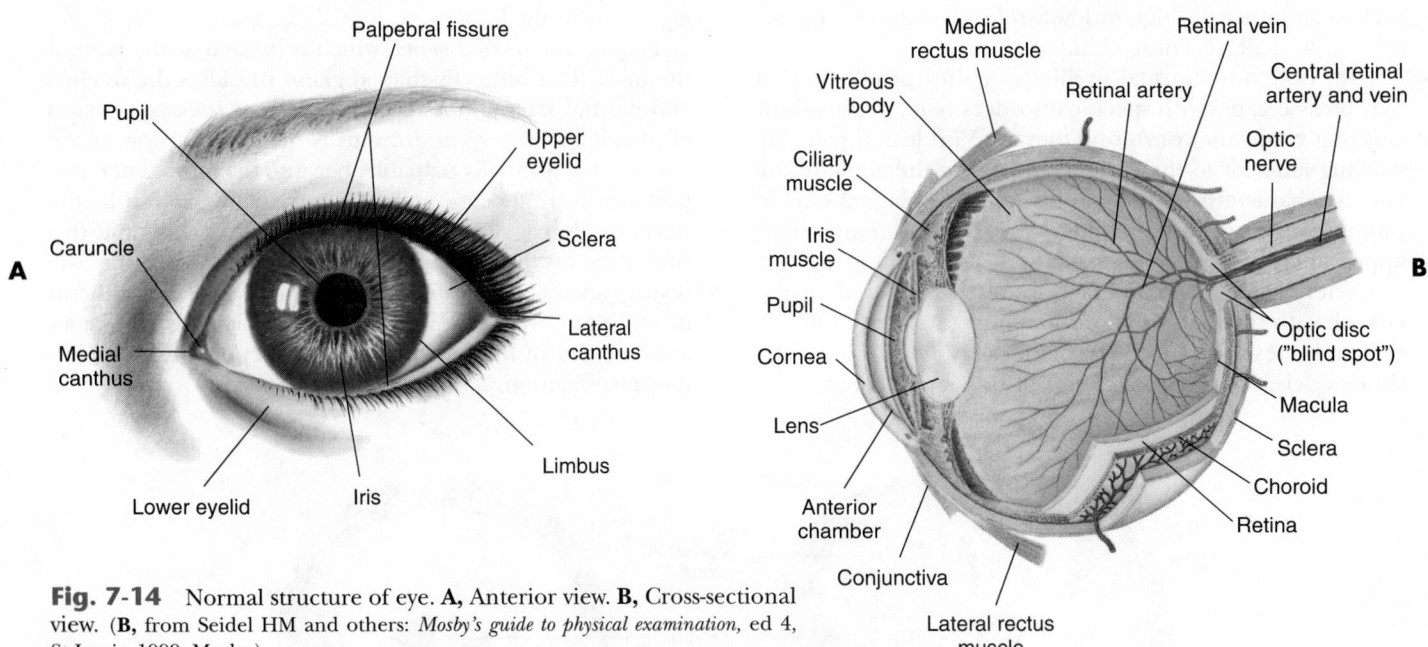

**Fig. 7-14**   Normal structure of eye. **A,** Anterior view. **B,** Cross-sectional view. (**B,** from Seidel HM and others: *Mosby's guide to physical examination*, ed 4, St Louis, 1999, Mosby.)

## Eyes

Examination of the eyes involves inspection of all exterior structures for size, symmetry, color, and motility, as well as inspection of the interior surfaces and examination of retinal structures. Accurate examination of each structure requires an understanding of the anatomy of the eyeball (Fig. 7-14). The retinal examination requires the use of an ophthalmoscope and is a highly skilled procedure. Discussion of the funduscopic examination includes the basic normal findings that the nurse should be able to discern with some practice in using the ophthalmoscope. The third part of the examination involves vision testing.

## Inspection of External Structures

Observe the eyes for relative placement on the face, symmetry of location, and general slant of the palpebral fissures or lids (Fig. 7-15). If any possible abnormality of placement is observed, measure the interpupillary distance, which averages approximately 4.5 to 5.5 cm (1¾ to 2¼ inches), or the inner canthal distance, which averages approximately 2.5 cm (1 inch) (Laestadius, Aase, and Smith, 1969). Large spacing between the eyes is called **hypertelorism.** Although a normal variant in some children, hypertelorism together with other midfacial anomalies may suggest mental retardation.

*Epicanthal folds,* an excess fold of skin extending from the roof of the nose to the inner termination of the eyebrow and partially or completely overlapping the inner canthus of the eye, are commonly found in Asian children (Fig. 7-15, *B*). They may be normally present in non-Asian infants but usually disappear as the child grows older.

Determine the general slant of the *palpebral fissures* or lids by drawing an imaginary line through the two points of the medial canthus and across the outer orbit of the eyes and aligning each eye on the line. Usually the palpebral fissures lie horizontally, but in Asian persons the slant is normally upward (Fig. 7-15, *C*). Because eye abnormalities are common in many chromosomal disorders, be careful to observe and record any deviations from the expected. For example, children with Down syndrome characteristically

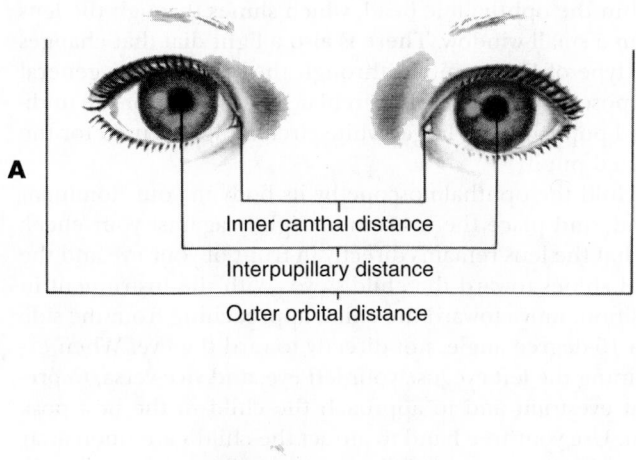

Inner canthal distance
Interpupillary distance
Outer orbital distance

**A**

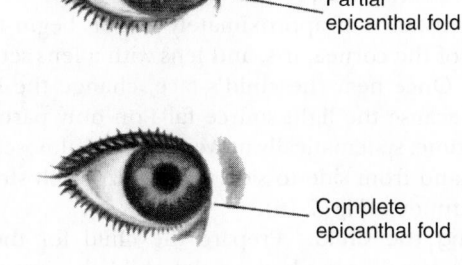

Partial epicanthal fold

**B**

Complete epicanthal fold

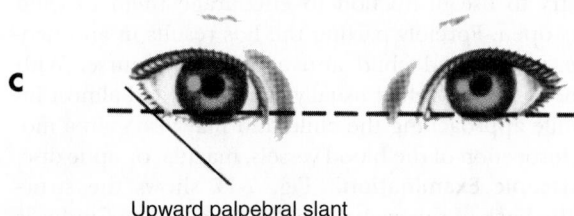

**C**

Upward palpebral slant

**Fig. 7-15  A,** Anatomic landmarks of eye. **B,** Epicanthal folds. **C,** Upward palpebral slant. (Note imaginary line to determine slant.)

demonstrate hypertelorism, epicanthal folds, and upward palpebral slant.

Inspect the *lids* for proper placement on the eye. When the eye is open, the upper lid should fall somewhere between the upper iris and upper rim of the pupil. *Ptosis* refers to a lid that covers part of the pupil or the lower part of the iris. The term *sunset eyes* or the *setting-sun sign* refers to an upper lid that covers no part of the iris, allowing some of the sclera or "white-of-the-eye" to show. Although ptosis and setting-sun sign can be a normal variant of lid placement, either can also be a sign of several disorders.

When the eyes are closed, the lids should completely cover the cornea and sclera. Incomplete closure can result in chronic eye irritation and infection. When the lids are opened or closed, no palpebral conjunctiva should be visible. Malposition of the eyelids includes *ectropion,* a rolling-out of the lids with exposed conjunctiva, and *entropion,* a turning-in of the lid. The latter is normally found in some Asian children. Check to see if the inturned lid causes irritation of the cornea.

The lids are also observed for color (any sign of hemorrhage), size (any evidence of edema), and mobility. Normally the lids contain the same amount of pigmentation as the rest of the skin. Inflammation or erythema along the lid is noted. Some of the more common lid disorders are listed in Box 7-2.

Inspect the lining of the lids, the *palpebral conjunctiva.* Inspect the lower conjunctival sac by pulling the lid down while the child looks up. To evert the upper lid, hold the upper lashes and gently pull *down* and *forward* while the child looks down. If this is not successful, place the stem of a cotton-tipped applicator 1 cm above the edge of the lid margin and gently push down on the lid with the stick and roll the lid upward. As soon as the lid is everted, use the fingers holding the lashes to keep the lid everted.

Normally the conjunctiva appears pink and glossy. Vertical yellow striations along the edge are the *meibomian* or *sebaceous glands* near the hair follicle. Located in the inner or medial canthus and situated on the inner edge of the upper and lower lids is a tiny opening called the *lacrimal punctum.* Note any excessive tearing or inflammation of the lacrimal apparatus.

---

**Box 7-2 ▪ ■ □**

**Inflammations of the Eyelid**

**Hordeolum** or **stye**—Inflammation of sebaceous glands near lashes, usually on lower lid; painful, red, swollen areas

**Internal stye**—Acute inflammation of meibomian (sebaceous) glands of upper lid; if upper lid is everted, stye appears as a yellow line across the tarsus (edge of eyelid)

**Chalazion**—Granulomas or cysts of internal sebaceous glands (meibomian glands); localized, nontender, firm, discrete swellings covered with freely movable skin

**Marginal blepharitis**—Inflammation of edge of lid; red, scaly, crusted lid edges; may include pustules around base of lashes and pus from meibomian glands

**Dacryocystitis**—Inflammation and blockage of lacrimal sac or duct; swelling, redness, and pain, below and to nasal side of inner canthus, with purulent discharge

Observe the lids for blinking movement. Excessive blinking can indicate eyestrain or a nervous habit. Asymmetric or infrequent blinking can be a sign of paralysis or muscle weakness. Test the **blink reflex** by making a quick movement toward the eye.

Inspect the **eyelashes** for distribution, direction of growth, and pigmentation. Normally the upper lashes curl upward and the lower lashes curve downward. Lashes that turn inward toward the eyeball can cause conjunctival irritation.

The **bulbar conjunctiva,** which covers the eye up to the limbus (junction of the cornea and sclera), should be transparent. Dilation of the blood vessels in the conjunctiva makes it appear red. Although this redness is characteristic of many disorders, it can also indicate eyestrain, irritation, or fatigue.

The **sclera,** or white covering of the eyeball, should be clear. Record any yellow staining, because this may indicate jaundice. Tiny black marks in the sclera of heavily pigmented individuals are normal and do not indicate petechiae or the presence of a foreign body. A bluish tone may indicate disorders such as osteogenesis imperfecta or glaucoma.

The **cornea,** or covering of the iris and pupil, should be clear and transparent. Record any opacities, because they can be signs of scarring or ulceration and can interfere with vision. To test for opacities, illuminate the eyeball by shining a light at an angle (obliquely) toward the cornea.

Compare the **pupils** for size, shape, and movement. They should be round, clear, and equal. Test their **reaction to light** by quickly shining a source of light toward the eye and removing it. As the light approaches, the pupils constrict; as the light fades, the pupils dilate. Test **accommodation,** or the focusing ability of the eyes to produce clear vision at different distances, by having the child look at a bright, shiny object at a distance and quickly moving the object toward the face. The pupils constrict as the object is brought near the eye. Normal findings on examination of the pupil may be recorded as **PERRLA,** which means "pupil equal, round, reacts to light and accommodation."

Inspect the **iris** for size, color, and clarity. The iris should be perfectly round; a cleft or notch at its outer edge is called a **coloboma.** Because a visual field defect coincides with the coloboma, report this finding for further ophthalmologic evaluation. Permanent eye color is usually established by 6 to 12 months of age. Lack of usual eye color and a pink glow to the iris are characteristic of **albinism.** The pink color is a reflection of the red reflex of the retina. Black-and-white speckling of the iris, known as **Brushfield spots,** is seen in Down syndrome.

While inspecting the iris and pupil, also look for the **lens.** Normally the lens is not visible while looking into the pupil. White or gray spots usually indicate opacities or cataracts in the lens. Complete opacities prevent funduscopic examination of internal retinal structures.

### Inspection of Internal Structures

**Use of the Ophthalmoscope.** The ophthalmoscope permits visualization of the interior of the eyeball with a system of lenses and a high-intensity light. The "ophthalmic head" contains plus lenses (magnifiers), which are usually indicated by black numbers, and minus lenses (minifiers), which are indicated by red numbers. The lenses are changed by rotating a disk on the outside of the head. These lenses permit clear visualization of eye structures at different distances from the examiner's eye and correct visual acuity differences in the examiner and child.

If the child wears glasses, remove them unless they are worn to correct severe astigmatism, which can cause distortion of the images. The lens of the ophthalmoscope can grossly detect visual acuity problems in the child if the examiner with 20/20 vision (with or without corrective lenses) must use plus or minus lenses to see the retinal structures clearly. With hyperopia, or farsightedness, higher plus or convex lenses are needed; with myopia, or nearsightedness, more minus or concave lenses are used. Use of the ophthalmoscope requires practice to know which lens setting produces the clearest image.

The interior of the eye is illuminated by a light source within the ophthalmic head, which shines through the lens from a small window. There is also a light dial that changes the type of light emitted through the window. For general purposes, the small, white circular light is used for the undilated pupil and the larger white circular light is used for the dilated pupil.

Hold the ophthalmoscope by its body in your dominant hand, and place the instrument lightly against your cheek so that the lens remains directly in front of your eye and the light shines toward the child's eye. With the instrument in position, move toward the child, approaching from the side at a 15-degree angle, not directly toward the eye. When examining the left eye, use your left eye, and vice versa, to prevent eyestrain and to approach the child in the best position. Use your free hand to attract the child's attention away from the instrument's light source and toward a point directly in front of the child to help you move as close as possible to the child. Perform the examination in a dimly lit, but not necessarily dark, room.

From a distance of approximately 1 foot, begin the examination of the cornea, iris, and lens with a lens setting of +8 to +2. Once near the child's face, change the lens to 0 or −2. Because the light source falls on only part of the retina at a time, systematically move the ophthalmoscope up and down and from side to side to visualize each structure within the fundus (Fig. 7-16).

**Preparing the Child.** Prepare the child for the ophthalmic examination by showing the child the instrument, demonstrating the light source and how it shines in the eye, and explaining the reason for darkening the room. For infants and young children who do not respond to such explanations, try to use distraction to encourage them to keep their eyes open. Forcibly parting the lids results in an uncooperative, watery-eyed child and a frustrated nurse. With some practice, a red reflex usually can be elicited almost instantly while approaching the child and may also gain a momentary inspection of the blood vessels, macula, or optic disc.

**Funduscopic Examination.** Fig. 7-17 shows the structures of the back of the eyeball, or the **fundus.** The fundus is immediately apparent as the **red reflex.** The intensity of the color increases in individuals with deeply pigmented skin.

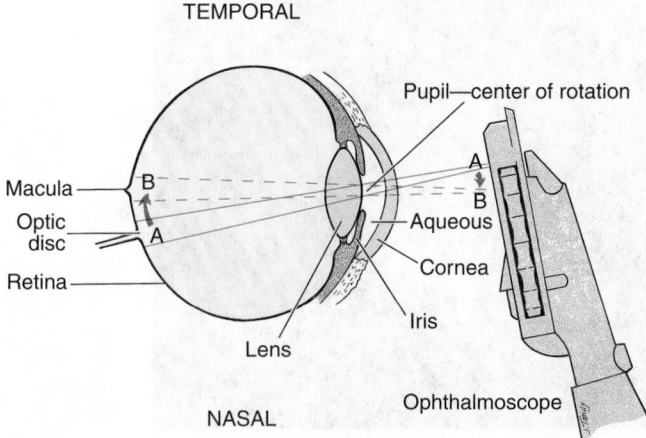

TEMPORAL

Macula
Optic disc
Retina

B
A

Pupil—center of rotation

A
B

Aqueous
Cornea
Iris

Lens

NASAL

Ophthalmoscope

**Fig. 7-16**   Visual axis through ophthalmoscope. **A,** Beam of light and its corresponding visual field is the usual view when approaching child from side at 15-degree angle. **B,** Representation of a direct visualization with child staring at light.

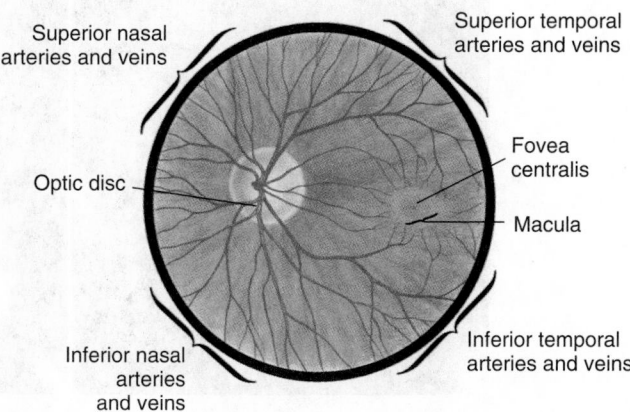

Superior nasal
arteries and veins

Optic disc

Inferior nasal
arteries
and veins

Superior temporal
arteries and veins

Fovea
centralis

Macula

Inferior temporal
arteries and veins

**Fig. 7-17**   Structures of fundus. Interior circle represents approximate size of area seen with ophthalmoscope. (From Seidel HM and others: *Mosby's guide to physical examination,* ed 4, St Louis, 1999, Mosby.)

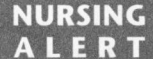 **NURSING ALERT**   A brilliant, uniform red reflex is an important sign because it virtually rules out almost all serious defects of the cornea, aqueous chamber, lens, and vitreous chamber. Record any dark shadows or opacities because they indicate some abnormality in any of these structures.

As the ophthalmoscope is brought closer to the eye, the most conspicuous feature of the fundus is the *optic disc,* the area where the blood vessels and optic nerve fibers enter and exit from the eye. The round or vertically oval disc is creamy pink but lighter than the surrounding fundus and derives its color from the rich capillary network. Its size is important because other structures of the fundus are measured in relationship to the *disc diameter (DD).* Most discs have a small, pale depression in their center, called the *physiologic cup* or *depression,* which represents the blind spot of the retina. It is not always visible but, when large enough to be seen, should not extend to the disc margin. Blurring of the disc margins, loss of the depression, and a bulging disc are important signs of *papilledema,* or swelling of the optic nerve, which clinically indicates increased intracranial pressure.

After the optic disc is located, inspect the area for blood vessels. The *central retinal artery and vein* appear in the depths of the disc and emanate outward with visible branching. The veins are darker in color and approximately one-fourth larger in size than the arteries. A narrow band of light, the *arteriolar light reflex,* is reflected from the center of an artery but does not appear in veins. Normally the branches of the arteries and veins cross each other. Observe the pattern of branching for abnormalities such as notching or indenting at the crossings, tortuosity or dilation of the vessels, or small hemorrhages (dark areas) along the branches. Report any of these findings for further investigation.

Approximately 2 DD temporal to the disc is the *macula,* the area of the fundus with the greatest concentration of visual receptors. It is approximately 1 DD in size and darker in color than the fundus (red reflex) or optic disc. The intensity of the color directly correlates with the individual's skin pigmentation; that is, the darker the skin, the darker the color of the macula. In the center of the macula is a minute glistening spot of reflected light called the *fovea centralis,* the area of most perfect vision.

Although abnormalities of the macula are usually not apparent unless the eye is dilated to permit more detailed inspection, at least note its presence. If locating the macula is difficult, ask the child to look directly at the light. As Fig. 7-16, *B,* shows, a light shone directly into the eye falls on the fovea. However, because this is the most light-sensitive area of the retina, be careful to focus on the macula only momentarily. Record if direct visualization does *not* cause the light to fall on the center of the fovea because strabismus may exist when fixation occurs at a point other than the center of the macula.

### Vision Testing

Several tests are available for assessing vision. The following discussion focuses on four areas: (1) binocularity, (2) visual acuity, (3) peripheral vision, and (4) color vision. Behavioral and physical signs that indicate visual impairment are discussed in Chapter 19.

**Ocular Alignment.**   Normally, by the age of 3 to 4 months children achieve the ability to fixate on one visual field with both eyes simultaneously (binocularity). One of the most important tests for binocularity is alignment of the eyes to detect nonbinocular vision, or strabismus. In *strabismus,* or cross-eye, one eye deviates from the point of fixation. If the malignment is constant, the weak eye becomes "lazy," and the brain eventually suppresses the image produced by that eye. If strabismus is not detected and corrected by age 4 to 6 years, blindness from disuse, known as *amblyopia,* may result.

Tests commonly used to detect malalignment are the corneal light reflex and the cover tests. To perform the *corneal light reflex test,* or *Hirschberg test,* shine a flashlight or the light of the ophthalmoscope directly into the patient's eyes from a distance of about 40.5 cm (16 inches). If the eyes

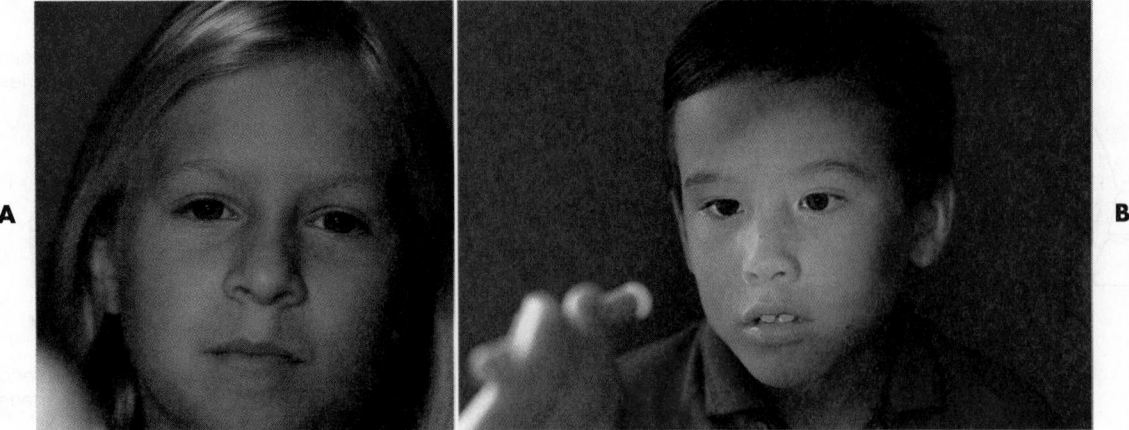

**Fig. 7-18** **A,** Corneal light reflex test demonstrating orthophoric (normal) eyes. **B,** Pseudostrabismus. Inner epicanthal folds cause eyes to appear malaligned; however, corneal light reflexes fall perfectly symmetrically.

## Critical Thinking Exercise

### Vision Screening

Your nursing class will be assisting with EPSDT (Early Periodic Screening, Diagnosis, and Treatment) screens for preschoolers. You are responsible for setting up the area for visual screening. You will need all of the following equipment *except* which?

FIRST, THINK ABOUT IT. . .

• What precise questions are you trying to answer?
• How are you interpreting the information?

1. Snellen acuity charts
2. Pirate patches
3. Penlights
4. A paper or metal tape measure

*The best response is one. Precisely, the question is whether preschoolers know their alphabet. The Snellen chart is inappropriate because it uses letters, and it cannot be assumed that preschoolers know their alphabet. A correct interpretation of the information would lead you to think about all of the appropriate equipment you need for visual screening. The "Lazy E" acuity chart is not ideal, because preschoolers may not have the perceptual abilities needed to determine in which direction the "legs" of the E are pointing. A picture acuity chart or the Blackbird system should be used with this population. Pirate patches serve as eye occluders and are needed for assessing acuity and alignment. Penlights are needed for assessing corneal light reflex and pupil reactivity. A nonstretchable tape measure is used to determine the correct distance for assessing acuity when using an eye chart.*

are *orthophoric,* or normal, the light falls symmetrically within each pupil (Fig. 7-18, *A*). If the light falls off center in one eye, the eyes are malaligned. *Epicanthal folds,* excess folds of skin that extend from the roof of the nose to the inner termination of the eyebrow and that partially or completely overlap the inner canthus of the eye, may give a false impression of malalignment (*pseudostrabismus*) (Fig. 7-18, *B*). Epicanthal folds are often found in Asian children.

Terms for describing the types of strabismus are:

**Esotropia** or **esophoria**—Inward deviation of the eye
**Exotropia** or **exophoria**—Outward deviation of the eye
**Phoria**—Malalignment that is not obvious until fusion is disrupted
**Tropia**—Constant or intermittent malalignment of the eyes; more severe and more likely than phoria to result in amblyopia

In the *cover test,* one eye is covered, and the movement of the *uncovered* eye is observed while the child looks at a near (33 cm, or 13 inches) or distant (3 m, or 10 feet) object. If the uncovered eye does not move, it is aligned. If the uncovered eye moves, a malalignment is present because when the stronger eye is temporarily covered, the misaligned eye attempts to fixate on the object.

In the *alternate cover test,* occlusion is shifted back and forth from one eye to the other, and movement of the eye that was *covered* is observed as soon as the occluder is removed while the child focuses on a point in front of him or her (Nelson, 1998). If normal alignment is present, shifting the cover from one eye to the other will not cause the eye to move. If malalignment is present, eye movement will occur when the cover is moved. Photoscreening uses a camera or video system to examine images of the pupillary reflexes and red reflexes to screen for amblyogenic factors (strabismus), media opacities, and significant refractive errors. The child fixates on a target long enough to obtain the images (Swanson and others, 2002).

**NURSING ALERT** The cover test is usually easier to perform if the examiner uses his or her own hand rather than a card-type occluder (Fig. 7-19). Attractive occluders fashioned like an ice cream cone or happy-face lollipop cut from cardboard are also well received by young children.

In older children the *random-dot-E stereoscopic test* can be used to assess for stereoacuity (depth perception). This test is more likely to detect lesser degrees of eye muscle imbalance. The random-dot-E test cards are held 16 inches from the child's eyes. The child wears stereoscopic glasses while looking straight ahead at the cards. The card set consists of a blank card, a card with a raised E, and a card with a re-

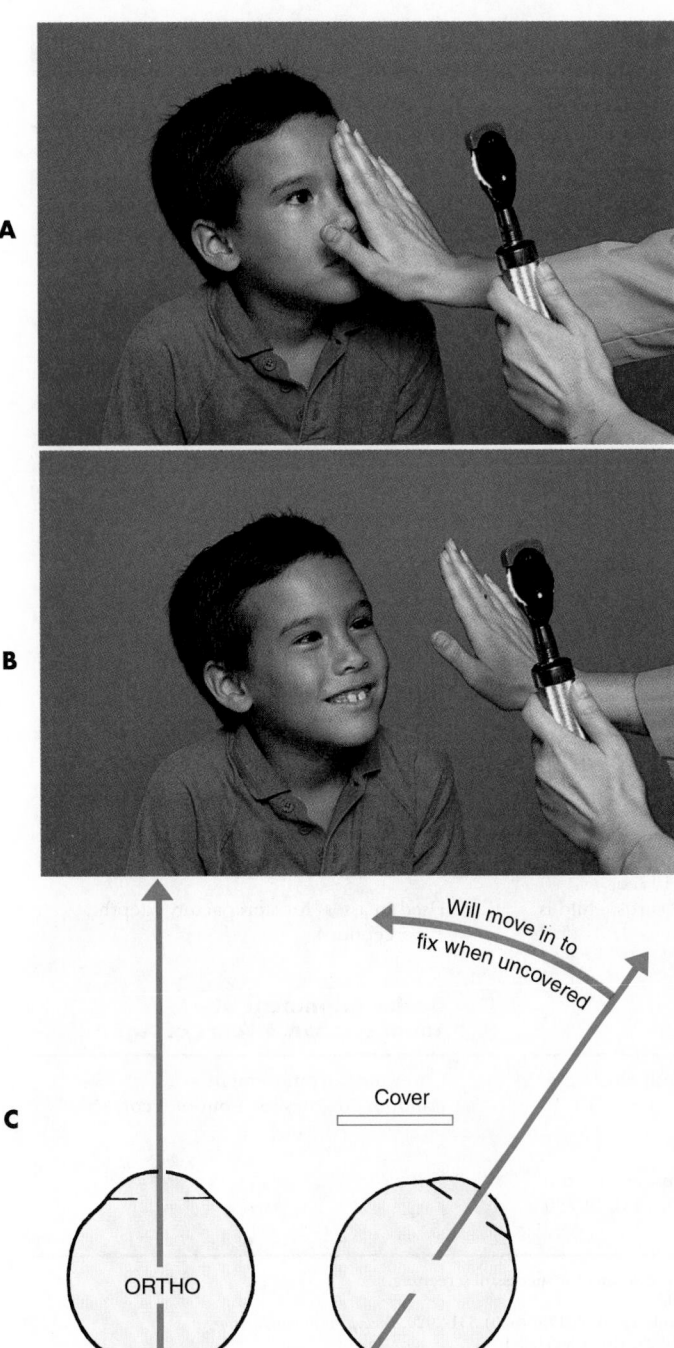

**Fig. 7-19**    Uncover test for strabismus. **A,** Eye is occluded and child is fixated on light source. **B,** If eye does not move when uncovered, eyes are aligned. **C,** Exophoria. As eye is uncovered, it shifts to fixate on object. (**C** from Prior JA, Silverstein JS, Stang JM: *Physical diagnosis: the history and examination of the patient,* ed 6, St Louis, 1981, Mosby.)

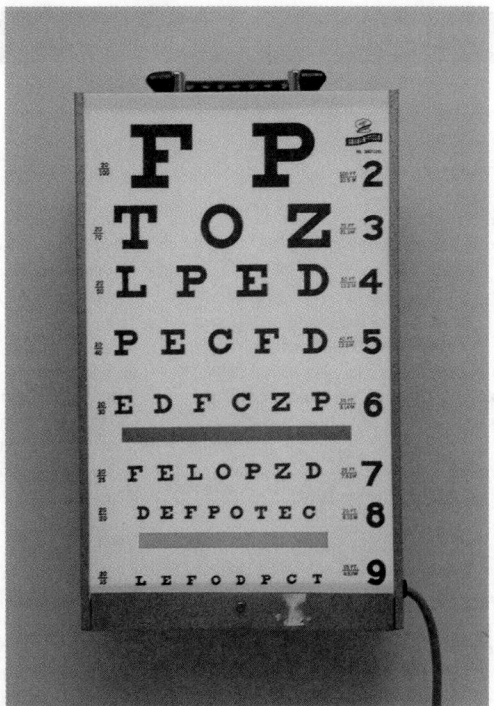

**Fig. 7-20**    Snellen letter chart for testing visual acuity. (Courtesy Paul Vincent Kuntz, Texas Children's Hospital.)

cessed E. The cards are held straight in front of the child, who is asked to identify the E card. The E card should be presented randomly, switching from a right, left, down, right, up, and left presentation of the letter. To pass the test, the child must identify the E correctly in 4 out of 6 attempts.

**Visual Acuity Testing in Children Beyond Infancy.**    The most common test for measuring visual acuity is the *Snellen*

*letter chart,* which consists of lines of letters in decreasing size (Fig. 7-20). (See Appendix B and Critical Thinking Exercise box on p. 196.) During testing, the American Academy of Pediatrics (1996) now recommends that children stand 10 feet from the chart with their heels at the 10-foot line. When screening for visual acuity in children, the child's right eye is tested first by covering the left. Children who wear glasses should be screened wearing the lenses. Tell the child to keep both eyes open during the examination. If the child fails to read the bottom line, move up the chart to the next larger line. Continue up the chart until a line is found that the child can pass. Then begin moving down the chart again until the child fails to read the line. To pass each line, the child must correctly identify 4 out of 6 symbols on the line. Repeat the procedure, covering the right eye. Table 7-10 provides a list of visual screening tests for children and guidelines for referral recommended by the American Academy of Pediatrics (1996).

For children unable to read letters and numbers, the *tumbling E* or *HOTV test* is useful (Coats and Jenkins, 1997). The tumbling E test uses the capital letter E to point in four different directions. The child is then asked to point in the direction the E is facing. The HOTV test consists of a wall chart composed of Hs, Os, Ts, and Vs. The child is given a board containing a large H, O, T, and V. The examiner points to a letter on the wall chart, and the child matches the correct letter on the board held in his or her hand. The tumbling E and HOTV are excellent tests for preschool-age children. When a child is unable to perform the tumbling E or HOTV test, the LH symbol or Allen card test may be used. The Allen card test uses common figures to test the child's

**TABLE 7-10** Visual screening tests for children

| Test | Description | Comments* |
|---|---|---|
| **Tests For Visual Acuity** | | |
| **Snellen Letter†** | Uses letters of English alphabet for testing | For most children above second grade who are familiar with reading the alphabet |
| **Snellen Number†** | Uses numbers for testing | For children who know their numbers |
| **Snellen E (Tumbling E)†** | Uses the capital letter E pointing in four directions; children "read" chart by showing direction of E or using a large duplicate E to match E on chart | For illiterate or non–English-speaking people, preschool children, and grade 1 Preschool children often have difficulty with direction despite adequate vision |
| **Home Eye Test for Preschoolers‡** | Uses a large letter E for demonstration and E chart for testing at 10 feet | For use by parents for children ages 3 to 6 years |
| **Blackbird Preschool Vision Screening System§** | Uses a modified E to resemble a flying bird; children identify which way bird is flying | Designed for children as young as 3 years |
| | Uses flash cards, storytelling, and disposable cardboard eyeglass occluders | |
| **HOTV or Matching Symbol†** | Uses the four letters H, O, T, and V on a chart for testing | For children as young as 3 years Avoids problem with image reversal and eye-hand coordination that can occur with letter E |
| | Child names letters on chart or matches them to a demonstration card | |
| **LH Symbol** | Spiral-bound flash cards of house, apple, circle, and square in different sizes | |
| **Denver Eye Screening Test (DEST)‖** | Uses single cards for letter E, one for demonstration and one for testing | For children 2½ years and older May be reliably used with cooperative children beginning at age 24 months |
| | Also uses **Allen Cards** (picture of a tree, birthday cake, horse and rider, telephone, car, house, and teddy bear) for testing | |
| **Tests for Ocular Alignment** | | |
| **Cover Test** | As child looks at distant object, one eye is occluded to check for movement in uncovered eye; child is tested at 3 m or 10 feet | Can be performed on preschoolers without difficulty |
| **Random-Dot-E Test** | Uses stereoscopic glasses and E cards; child is tested at 40 cm | Used to assess for stereoacuity (depth perception) |

| Referral Criteria¶ | | |
|---|---|---|
| **Visual Acuity at 3–5 Years of Age** | **Visual Acuity at 6 Years and Older** | **Ocular Alignment at Younger Than 3 Years of Age** |
| <4 out of 6 correct at 20 feet; either eye tested at 10 feet monocularly (i.e., <10/20 or 20/40) | <4 out of 6 correct at 15 feet with either eye tested at 10 feet monocularly (i.e., <10/15 or 20/30) | Cover test: any movement Random-dot-E test: <4 out of 6 correct |
| *or* | *or* | |
| Two-line difference between eyes, even within pass range (i.e., 10/12.5 and 10/20 or 20/25 and 20/40) | Two-line difference between eyes, even within pass range (i.e.,10/10 and 10/15 or 20/20 and 20/30) | |

*Ages for testing are based on published reports. Proper instruction of young children is essential for successful screening.
†Available from Good-Lite Co, 1540 Hannah Ave, Forest Park, IL 60130, (708) 366-3860.
‡Available from the National Society to Prevent Blindness, 500 E Remington Rd, Schaumburg, IL 60173, (800) 331-2020, *www.prevent-blindness.org.*
§Available from Blackbird Vision Screening System, PO Box 277424, Sacramento, CA 95827, (916) 363-6884.
‖Available from Denver Developmental Materials, Inc, PO Box 6919, Denver CO 80206-0919, (303) 355-4729.
¶Available from Western Psychological Services, 12031 Wilshire Blvd, Los Angeles, CA 90025-1251, (800) 648-8867.

vision. It is important to assess whether the child is able to identify the pictures before actual vision testing. The examiner walks backward slowly, flipping through the cards and presenting different pictures to the child. The examiner continues to move backward as the child correctly calls out the figures. When the child begins to miss the figure on the cards, the examiner moves forward to confirm that the child is able to identify the figures at that point. All Allen card figures are 20/30 in size. The farthest distance at which the child is able to identify the pictures accurately becomes the numerator, and 30 becomes the denominator. For example, if the child is able to identify the pictures accurately at

15 feet, the visual acuity is recorded as 15/30. This is equivalent to 20/40 or 10/20 visual acuity. The LH symbol test is somewhat different from the Allen card test because it is a spiral-bound set of flash cards. The flash cards contain large pictures of a house, apple, circle, and square. The LH symbol cards contain the symbol size and visual acuity value for a 10-foot testing distance. The visual acuity is determined by the smallest symbols the child is able to identify at 10 feet.

The *Blackbird Preschool Vision Screening System* was developed by a nurse. The screening system uses a modified E that resembles a bird and a story about the Blackbird to help engage children's attention. Testing is done with flash cards or a wall-mounted chart, and the child is instructed to indicate the direction of the bird's flight. The Blackbird System also contains guidelines for vision screening of noncommunicative children, nonreaders, or non-English-speaking children to assist screeners with more difficult-to-test populations, and the *Blackbird Storybook Home Eye Test* is designed for parents to prescreen young children at home.

**Visual Acuity Testing in Infants and Difficult-To-Test Children.**   In newborns vision is tested mainly by checking for *light perception* by shining a light into the eyes and noting responses such as pupillary constriction, blinking, following the light to midline, increased alertness, or refusal to open the eyes after exposure to the light. Although the simple maneuver of checking light perception and eliciting the pupillary light reflex indicates that the anterior half of the visual apparatus is intact, it does not confirm that the infant can see. In other words, this test does not assess whether the barin receives the visual message and interprets the signals.

Another test of visual acuity is the infant's ability to fix on and follow a target at about 2 months of age (Mills, 1999). Although any brightly colored or patterned object can be used, the human face is excellent. Hold the infant upright while moving your face slowly from side to side.

| NURSING ALERT | If visual fixation and following are not present by 3 to 4 months of age, refer for further ophthalmologic evaluation is needed. |
|---|---|

Other signs that may indicate visual loss or other serious eye problems include fixed pupils, strabismus, constant nystagmus, the setting-sun sign, and slow lateral movements. Unfortunately, it is very difficult to test each eye separately; the presence of such signs in one eye could indicate unilateral blindness.

Special tests are available for testing infants and other difficult-to-test children to assess acuity or confirm blindness. Description of normal development of vision and eye movements is found in Table 7-11. For example, in *visually evoked potentials,* the eyes are stimulated with a bright light or pattern, and electrical activity to the visual cortex is recorded through scalp electrodes. Acuity is assessed by using progressively smaller patterns.

**Peripheral Vision.**   In children who are old enough to cooperate, estimate *peripheral vision,* or the visual field of each eye, by having children fixate on a specific point directly in front of them as an object, such as a finger or a pencil, is moved from beyond the field of vision into the range of peripheral vision. Check each eye separately and for each quadrant of vision. Instruct children to say "stop" as soon as they see the object. At that point measure the angle from the anteroposterior axis of the eye (straight line of vision) to the peripheral axis (point at which the object is first seen). Normally children see about 50 degrees upward, 70 degrees downward, 60 degrees nasalward, and 90 degrees temporally. Limitations in peripheral vision may indicate blindness from damage to structures within the eye or to any of the visual pathways.

**TABLE 7-11**   Normal development of vision and eye movements

| Age | Normal Vision and Eye Movements |
|---|---|
| Birth (term) | Fixation<br>Poor following<br>Intermittent strabismus frequently present<br>Visual acuity 20/400 to 20/600 |
| One month | Horizontal following to midline<br>Normal alignment<br>Visual acuity 20/300 |
| Two months | Vertical following begins<br>Normal alignment<br>Visual acuity 20/200 |
| Three months | Good horizontal and vertical following<br>Normal alignment<br>Visual acuity 20/100<br>Accommodation begins<br>Binocularity detectable |
| Six months | Visual acuity 20/20 to 20/30<br>Binocularity well developed |
| Eight to 10 years | End of sensitive period for amblyopia |

From Mills MD: The eye in childhood, *Am Acad Fam Physician* 60:907-918, 1999.

**Color Vision.**   Another important test is for color vision. It is estimated that from 8% to 10% of Caucasian males and less than half that percentage of African-American males have inherited the X-linked disorder known as *color vision deficit* (the less acceptable term is *color blindness*). From 0.5% to 1% of white females are affected. Although the severity of impaired perception of color varies considerably, the two most common types are *protanomaly,* in which the child confuses gray with pink or pale blue with green, and *deuteranomaly,* in which the child confuses gray with pale purple or green. In most of these individuals, the color vision deficit causes no major problems. However, some of the difficulties encountered by individuals with more severe deficits may be an inability to distinguish amber or red traffic lights, failure to see a red brake light on the rear of a car, difficulty in distinguishing green traffic lights from certain types of incandescent street lamps, and a poor sense of color coordination of clothing. For school-age children the greatest difficulty lies in the performance of academic skills that use color as a visual aid. Adolescents may be ineligible for certain vocational opportunities, such as electronics, photography, printing, interior decorating, pharmaceuticals, textiles, police work, and several types of military service.

Tests available for color vision include the *Ishihara test* and the *Hardy-Rand-Rittler (HRR) test.* Each consists of a series of cards (pseudoisochromatic) on which is printed a color field composed of spots of a certain "confusion" color. Against the field is a number or symbol similarly printed in dots and in a color likely to be confused with the field color by a person with a color vision deficit. As a result, the figure or letter is invisible to an affected individual but is clearly seen by a person with color vision. By using the HRR test, which uses symbols rather than numbers, reliable testing can be performed on young children (Nelson, 1998).

Nurses administering the test must be familiar with the testing materials and should be able to inform the parents of the disorder's effects on practical areas of living, its genetic transmission, and its irreversibility.

## Ears

As with the eyes, examination of the ears involves inspection of the external auditory structures, visualization of the internal landmarks using the otoscope, and screening for hearing ability.

### Inspection of External Structures

The entire external earlobe is called the *pinna,* or *auricle,* and is located on each side of the head. Measure the height alignment of the pinna by drawing an imaginary line from the outer orbit of the eye to the occiput or most prominent protuberance of the skull. The top of the pinna should meet or cross this line. Low-set ears are commonly associated with renal anomalies or mental retardation. Measure the angle of the pinna by drawing a perpendicular line from the imaginary horizontal line and aligning the pinna next to this mark. Normally the pinna lies within a 10-degree angle of the vertical line (Fig. 7-21). If it falls outside this area, record the deviation and look closely for other anomalies.

Normally the pinnas extend slightly outward from the skull. Except in newborn infants, ears that are flat against the head or protruding away from the scalp may indicate problems. For example, a mass or swelling makes the pinnas stand forward and may indicate mastoiditis, mumps, or postauricular abscesses. Flattened ears in infants may suggest a frequent side-lying position and may offer a clue to the parents' lack of understanding of the child's stimulation needs.

Fig. 7-22 shows the usual landmarks of the pinna. The *helix* is the prominent outer rim of the pinna. The *antihelix* is a second curved rim that is adjacent and almost parallel to the helix. The *concha* is a deep cavity, within and partly surrounded by the antihelix, that leads into the external auditory canal. Lying anterior to the concha is a prominent protuberance called the *tragus;* opposite to this is the *antitragus,* below which is the *lobule.* In some children the lobule is adherent with the helix in an upward and backward slant. An adherent lobule is considered a normal variation. Each of the major projections of the pinna forms corresponding depressions. There is remarkable similarity among external pinnas; note any deviations because they can be a sign of possible middle ear anomalies and congenital conductive hearing loss.

Inspect the *skin* around the ear for small openings, extra tags of skin, or sinuses. If a sinus is found, note this because it may represent a fistula that drains into some area of the neck or ear. Cutaneous tags represent no pathologic process but may cause parents concern in terms of the child's appearance.

Inspect the ear for general *hygiene.* An otoscope is not necessary to look into the external canal to note the presence of *cerumen,* a waxy substance produced by the ceruminous glands in the outer portion of the canal. If the ear canal appears totally free of cerumen, ask how the ears are cleaned. Occasionally parents insert cotton-tipped swabs or thin objects such as bobby pins into the canal to remove wax. Deep insertion of such objects can damage the drum or walls of the canal and can push the wax against the tympanic membrane to form a plug. It is best to question parents about ear cleaning by remarking how clean the ears are and casually asking how they remove the wax. This approach is more likely to yield an honest answer than is direct questioning about the use of specific instruments.

Advise parents or children to clean the ears with a washcloth and, if they use a swab, to gently wipe only the outermost portion of the canal. Caution them against using any sharp, hard object in the ear. The use of cotton-tipped swabs to clean children's ears has been directly associated with occlusion of the middle ear (Macknin, Talo, and Medendorp, 1994). If the cerumen is hard and dry (appears dark and crusted rather than yellow-brown and soft), it can be softened and removed by instilling 2 or 3 drops of mineral oil into the ear for a few days and then rinsing the canal with an ear syringe. Commercial products (Cerumenex, Murine, Debrox) are also available without prescription to aid in removing dried cerumen. If otitis media is suspected, remove the wax by using lukewarm water and a dental irrigation device, large syringe (without needle), or bulb syringe.

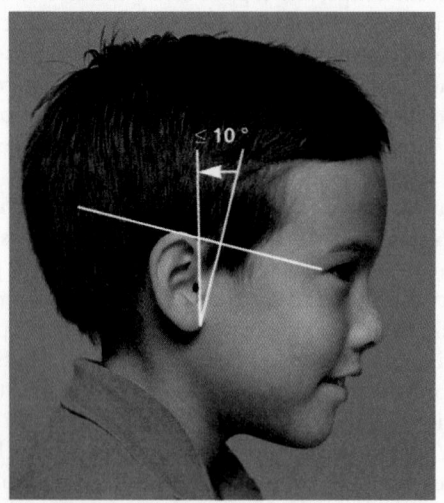

**Fig. 7-21**   Ear alignment.

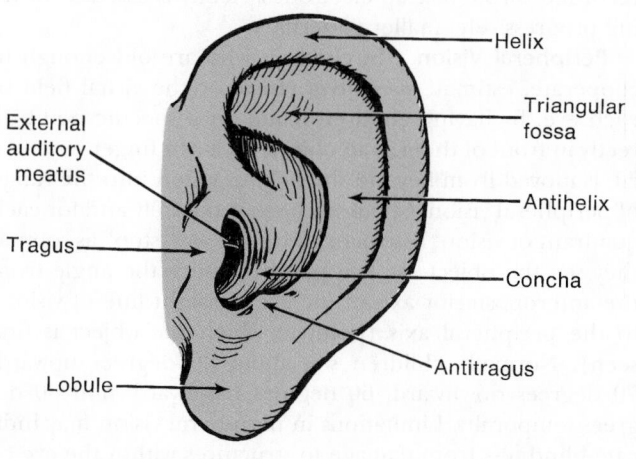

**Fig. 7-22**   Usual landmarks of pinna.

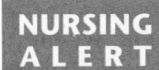

Note the presence, color, and odor of any discharge from the aural canal. If discharge is present in one canal, prevent transmitting potentially infectious material to the other ear or to another child through handwashing and the use of disposable specula or sterilization of reusable specula between each examination.

### Inspection of Internal Structures

**Use of the Otoscope.**   The otic head permits visualization of the tympanic membrane by use of a bright light, a magnifying glass, and a speculum. Some otoscopes have an attachment for a pneumatic device, through which air can be inserted into the canal to determine membrane compliance (movement). The speculum comes in a variety of sizes (2, 3, 4, and 5 mm) to accommodate different canal widths. The largest speculum that fits comfortably into the ear is used to achieve the greatest area of visualization. The lens or magnifying glass is movable, which allows the examiner to insert an object, such as a curette, into the ear canal through the speculum while still viewing the structures through the lens. The handle is the same as for the ophthalmic head and operates similarly.

**Positioning the Child.**   Before beginning the otoscopic examination, position the child properly and restrain if necessary. Older children usually cooperate and do not need to be restrained. However, prepare them for the procedure by allowing them to play with the instrument, demonstrating how it works, and stressing the importance of remaining still. A helpful suggestion is to let them observe you examining the parent's ear. Restraint is needed for younger children because the ear examination upsets them. (See Atraumatic Care box.)

As you insert the speculum into the meatus, move it around the outer rim to accustom the child to the feel of something entering the ear. If examining a painful ear, touch a nonpainful part of the affected ear, then examine the unaffected ear, and finally return to the painful ear. By this time the child is usually less fearful of anything causing discomfort to the ear and will cooperate more.

For their protection and safety, restrain infants and toddlers for the otoscopic examination. There are two general positions of restraint. In one the child sits sideways on the parent's lap with one arm "hugging" the parent and the

### ATRAUMATIC CARE

#### Reducing Distress from Otoscopy in Young Children

Make examining the ear a game by explaining that you are looking for a "big elephant" in the ear. This kind of "fairy tale" is an absorbing distraction and usually elicits cooperation. After the ear has been examined, clarify that "looking for elephants" was only pretending and thank the child for letting you look in his or her ear.

other arm at the side. The ear to be examined is away from the parent. With one arm the parent holds the child's head firmly against his or her chest, and with the other arm "hugs" the child, thereby securing the child's free arm. Examine the ear using the same procedure for holding the otoscope, described later in this section (Fig. 7-23, *A*).

The other position of restraint involves placing the child on the side or abdomen with the arms at the side and the head turned so that the ear to be examined points toward the ceiling. Lean over the child, use the upper part of the body to restrain the arms and upper trunk movements, and use the examining hand to stabilize the head. This position is practical for young infants or for older children who need minimum restraining, but it may not be feasible for other children who protest vigorously. For safety, enlist the parent's help in immobilizing the head by firmly placing one hand above the ear and the other on the child's back or side (Fig. 7-23, *B*).

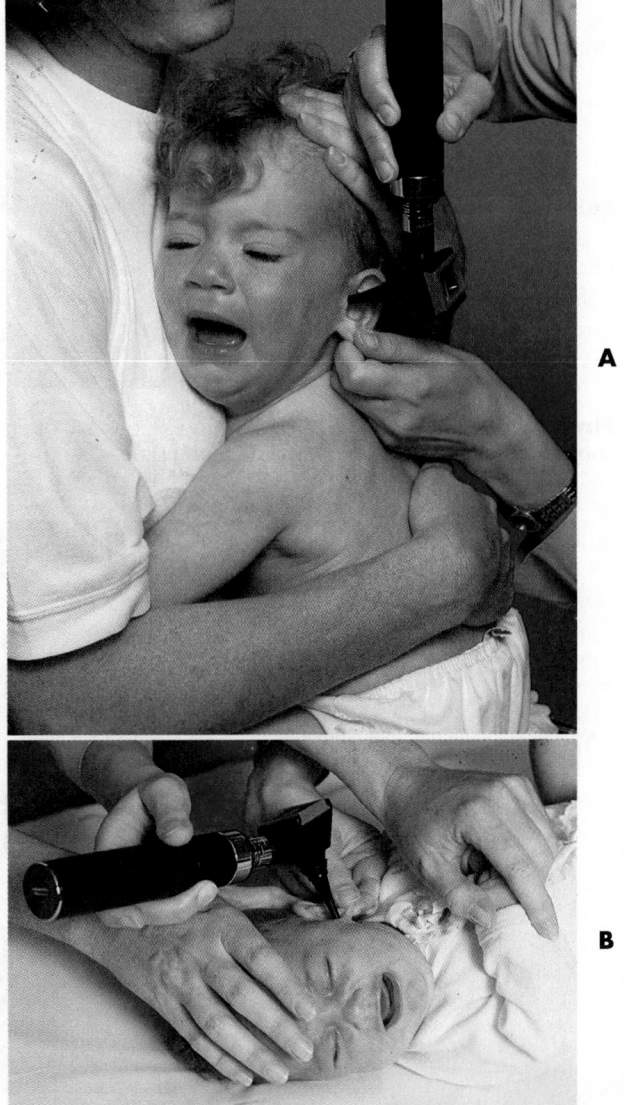

**Fig. 7-23**   Position for restraining child (**A**) and infant (**B**) during otoscopic examination.

If the child is cooperative, examine the ear with the child in a side-lying, sitting, or standing position. One disadvantage to standing is that the child may "walk away" as the otoscope enters the canal. If the child is standing or sitting, tilt the head slightly toward the child's opposite shoulder to achieve a better view of the drum (Fig. 7-24; see Nursing Tip, p. 204).

Grasp the auricle with the thumb and forefinger of the free (usually nondominant) hand. For the two positions of restraint, hold the otoscope upside down at the junction of its head and handle with the thumb and index finger. Place

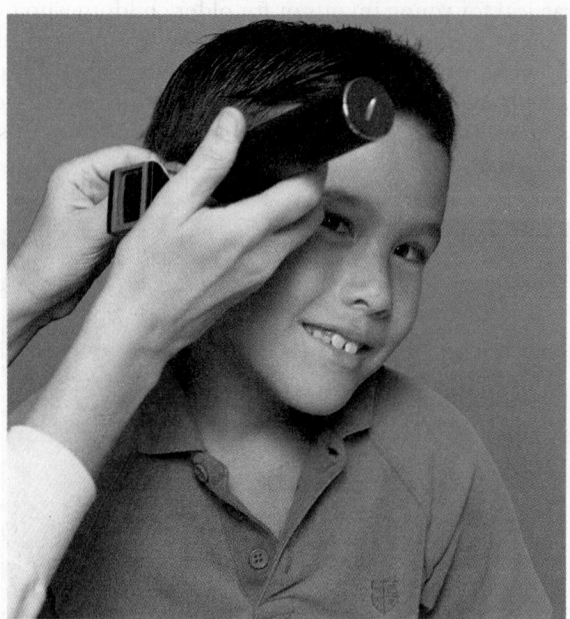

**Fig. 7-24** Positioning head by tilting it toward opposite shoulder for better view of tympanic membrane.

the other fingers against the skull to allow the otoscope to move with the child in case of sudden movement. When examining a cooperative child, hold the handle with the otic head upright or upside down. Use the dominant hand to examine both ears or reverse hands for each ear, whichever is more comfortable.

Before using the otoscope, visualize the external ear and the tympanic membrane as being superimposed on a clock (see Fig. 7-27). The numbers become important geographic landmarks. Introduce the speculum into the meatus between the 3 and 9 o'clock positions in a *downward* and *forward* position. Because the canal is curved, the speculum does not permit a panoramic view of the tympanic membrane unless the canal is straightened. In infants the canal curves upward. To straighten the canal, pull the pinna *down* and *back* to the 6 to 9 o'clock range (Fig. 7-25, *A*).

In older children, usually those over 3 years of age, the canal curves downward and forward. Therefore pull the pinna *up* and *back* toward a 10 o'clock position (Fig. 7-25, *B*). If there is difficulty in visualizing the membrane, try repositioning the head, introducing the speculum at a different angle, and pulling the pinna in a slightly different direction.

In neonates and young infants the walls of the canal are pliable and floppy because of the underdeveloped cartilaginous and bony structures. Therefore the very small 2-mm speculum usually needs to be inserted more deeply into the canal than in older children. Use great care to avoid damaging the walls or drum. Because the small opening of the speculum permits a limited view, systematically inspect each quadrant of the membrane. In older children do not insert the speculum past the cartilaginous (outermost) portion of the canal, usually a distance of 0.60 to 1.25 cm (¼ to ½ inch). The entire canal is approximately 2.5 cm (1 inch) long. Insertion of the speculum into the posterior or bony portion of the canal causes pain (Fig. 7-26).

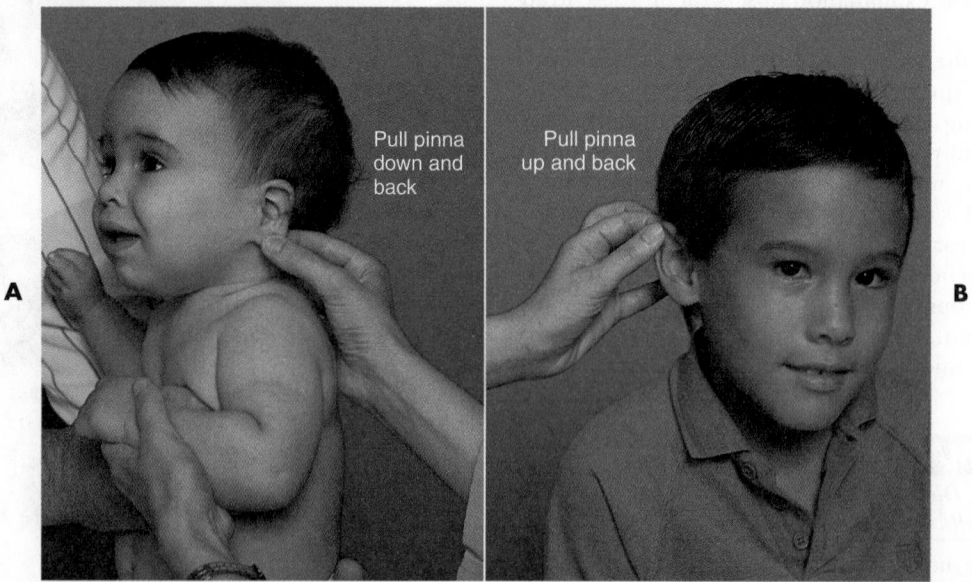

Pull pinna down and back

Pull pinna up and back

**Fig. 7-25** Positioning of eardrum in infant (**A**) and in child over 3 years of age (**B**).

**Otoscopic Examination.** As you introduce the speculum into the external canal, inspect the walls of the canal, the color of the tympanic membrane, the light reflex, and the usual landmarks of the bony prominences of the middle ear (Fig. 7-27).

The **walls** of the external auditory canal are pink, although they are more pigmented in dark-skinned children. Minute hairs are evident in the outermost portion, where cerumen is produced. Note signs of irritation, foreign bodies, or infection.

Foreign bodies in the ear are not uncommon in children and range from erasers to beans. Symptoms may include pain, discharge, and affected hearing. Soft objects, such as paper or insects, can be removed with forceps. Small, hard objects, such as pebbles, can be removed with a suction tip, a hook, or irrigation. However, irrigation is contraindicated if the object is vegetative matter, such as beans or pasta, which swells when in contact with fluid.

| **NURSING ALERT** | If there is any doubt about the type of object in the ear and the appropriate method to remove it, refer the child to the appropriate practitioner. |
|---|---|

The **color** of the **tympanic membrane** is a translucent, light pearly pink or gray. Note marked erythema (which may indicate suppurative otitis media), a dull nontransparent grayish color (sometimes suggestive of serous otitis media), or ashen gray areas (signs of scarring from a previous perforation). A black area usually suggests an unhealed perforation of the membrane; perforations are commonly located at the periphery of the drum. Slight redness is normal in the newborn because of increased vascularity and is often evident in older infants and young children as a result of crying.

The characteristic tenseness and slope of the tympanic membrane cause the light of the otoscope to reflect at approximately the 5 or 7 o'clock position. The **light reflex** is a fairly well-defined cone-shaped reflection, which normally points away from the face.

The **bony landmarks** of the drum are formed by several structures. The **umbo,** or tip of the malleus bone, appears as a small, round, opaque concave spot near the center of the drum. The **manubrium** (long process or handle) of the malleus appears to be a whitish line extending from the umbo upward to the margin of the membrane. At the upper end of the long process near the 1 o'clock position (in the right ear) is a sharp, knoblike protuberance, which represents the **short process** of the malleus. Sometimes a shadow is seen at approximately the 10 or 11 o'clock position. This is the junction of the **incus** and the **stapes** bones.

Note the absence or loss of the light reflex in any of these landmarks because it is probably caused by bulging of the membrane as a result of fluid accumulation in the middle ear. Retraction of the drum with abnormal prominence of the bony landmarks suggests serous otitis media.

## Auditory Testing

Several types of hearing tests are available. Some of them, such as audiometric testing, involve specialized equipment that measures the degree of hearing loss. Others, such as tests for the startle reflex in neonates, are rough estimations of the perception of sound. The nurse must operate under a high index of suspicion for those children who may have conditions associated with hearing loss and who may have developed behaviors that indicate auditory impairment. Types of hearing loss, causes, clinical manifestations, and appropriate treatment are discussed in Chapter 24.

One of the most commonly used tests is **audiometry,** which measures the threshold of hearing for pure-tone frequencies (measured in Hertz [Hz]) at various levels of loudness (measured in decibels [dB]). An audiogram is a record of the audiometric testing.

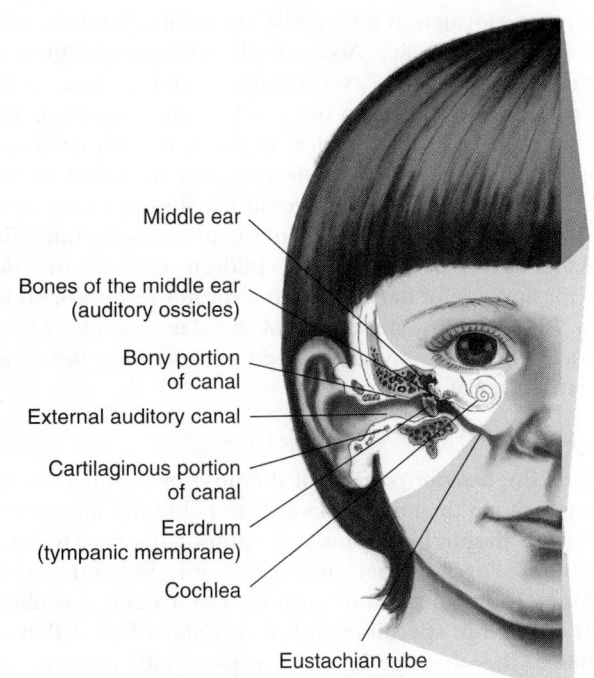

**Fig. 7-26** Cross section of external, middle, and parts of inner ear.

Middle ear
Bones of the middle ear (auditory ossicles)
Bony portion of canal
External auditory canal
Cartilaginous portion of canal
Eardrum (tympanic membrane)
Cochlea
Eustachian tube

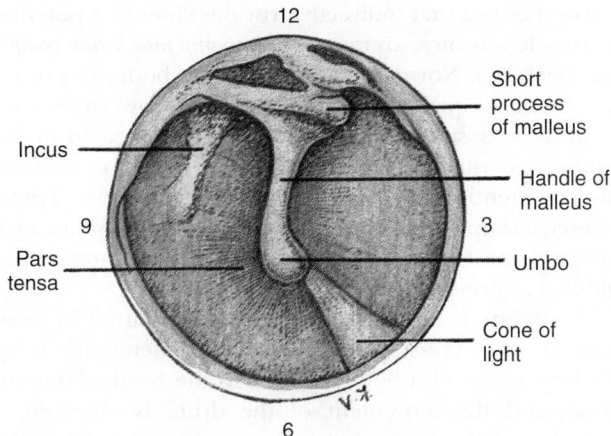

**Fig. 7-27** Landmarks of tympanic membrane with "clock" superimposed. (Modified from Potter PA, Perry AG: *Basic nursing: theory and practice,* ed 2, St Louis, 1991, Mosby.)

12
Incus
Pars tensa
9
Short process of malleus
Handle of malleus
Umbo
3
Cone of light
6

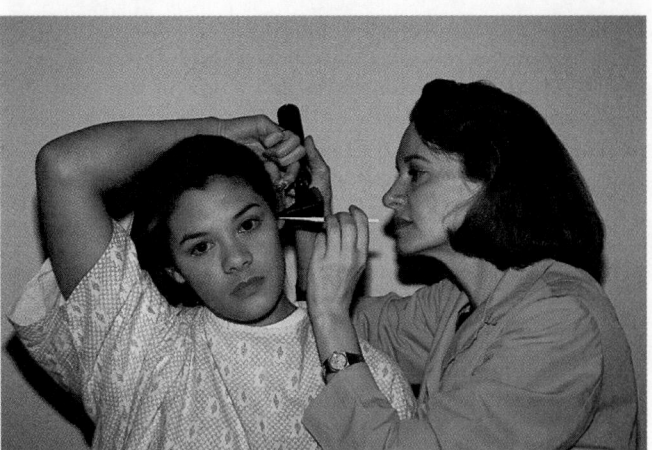

**Fig. 7-28** Having the child tug on the ear to straighten the canal leaves both of the nurse's hands available for the otoscopic examination.

In a **threshold acuity test,** a sound is initially transmitted to the child's ear at a level the child can easily hear; the loudness is then reduced until the child indicates the sound is no longer heard (usually by holding up a hand or pushing a button). This procedure is repeated for frequencies between 500 and 8000 Hz. The sounds are usually delivered through headphones that can be compared to a "space helmet." Because the child will be listening to very soft sounds, audiometry is best performed in a soundproof room.

Audiometry can also be used as a screening test or "sweep check" by presenting several different frequencies at either 20 or 25 dB. The Audioscope incorporates audiometric hearing screening and otoscopy into a single instrument. The Audioscope produces pure tones at 500, 1000, 2000, and 4000 Hz at a fixed hearing level of 25 dB. Failure to respond to any frequency is considered a failure. The instrument is reliable for children 5 years of age and older. Children as young as 3 years of age may be able to respond to the screening if adequately prepared by having a practice session in which they can become acquainted with the directions. Other hearing tests that may be used in infants and children are described in Table 7-12.

Another test that indirectly provides clues to a potential hearing loss is measurement of **tympanic membrane compliance (mobility).** Normally the pressure on both sides of the membrane is equal, allowing the drum to move easily when negative or positive pressure is applied. Decreased or low compliance usually indicates middle ear effusion (otitis media), a potential cause of conductive hearing loss. **Tympanometry,** a simple, reliable, and easily performed procedure, measures the compliance of the tympanic membrane and middle ear pressure.

Membrane compliance can also be measured by **pneumatic otoscopy.** Pressure to the tympanic membrane is applied by means of a bulb attached to the head of the otoscope, and the movement of the drum is observed. A limitation of the test is that the pressures needed to properly assess tympanic membrane mobility and accurately screen for middle ear abnormalities are not known.

**NURSING TIP** Sometimes it takes an extra hand to examine a child's ear—one hand to hold the otoscope, a second hand to straighten the canal, and a third hand to use the bulb (or a curette). The solution is to enlist the child's help (Fig. 7-28). Have the child raise the arm opposite the affected ear up and over the head toward the opposite side. Then ask the child to grasp the upper edge of the earlobe at about the 11 or 1 o'clock position and to pull the lobe gently up and back. With that third "helper" hand, you can use your hands to manipulate the equipment.

## Vestibular Testing

Vestibular testing for inner ear function concerning equilibrium is evaluated in young children by holding them at a 30-degree angle and rotating them in a complete circle in each direction. The normal response is nystagmus (movement of the eyes) in the direction of the rotation while being swung and in the opposite direction when the movement stops. For older children use a swivel chair or have them pivot quickly to one side and then the other.

## Nose

The nose marks the beginning of the passageway through the respiratory tract. It is a sensory organ for olfaction (smell) and is an important organ for filtration, temperature control, and humidification of inspired air. Each of these functions depends on the patency of the passageways and the mucosal lining of the nasal cavity. Inspection is primarily used for assessing the external and internal structures.

### Inspection of External Structures

The nose is located in the middle of the face, just below the eyes and above the lips. Assess its placement and alignment by drawing an imaginary vertical line from the center point between the eyes down to the notch of the upper lip. The nose should lie exactly vertical to this line, with each side exactly symmetric. Note its location, any deviation to one side, and any asymmetry in overall size and in diameter of the nares (nostrils). The **bridge** of the nose is sometimes flat in Asian and African-American children. Observe the **alae nasi** for any sign of flaring, which indicates respiratory difficulty. Always report any flaring of the alae nasi. Fig. 7-29 illustrates the usual landmarks used in describing the external structures of the nose.

### Inspection of Internal Structures

Inspect the **anterior vestibule** of the nose by pushing the tip upward, tilting the head backward, and illuminating the cavity with a flashlight or otoscope without the attached ear speculum. For a deeper view of the inferior and middle turbinates and the middle meatus, use a nasal speculum, such as a 9-mm speculum with a very short barrel that attaches to the otoscope head. Forceps specula are not routinely used in children. Insert the short, wide speculum into the nares, slightly away from the septum, and tilt the otoscope upward to straighten the passageway toward the pos-

**TABLE 7-12**    Selected hearing and tympanic membrane compliance tests*

| Description | Comments |
| --- | --- |
| **Clinical Hearing Tests** | |
| In newborns elicit the startle reflex and observe other neonatal responses to loud noises, such as facial grimaces, blinking, gross motor movement, quiet if crying or crying if quiet, opening the eyes, or ceasing sucking activity. During infancy note child's reaction to a noise. Stand approximately 18 inches away from infant, to the side, and out of child's peripheral field of vision. With the room silent and infant sitting in parent's lap, distracted by some object, make a voice sound such as "ps" or "phth" (high-pitched) or "oo" (low-pitched), ring a bell or a rattle, or rustle tissue paper. | An objective sign of alerting to sound may be an increase in heart rate or respiratory rate. Absence of alerting behaviors suggests hearing loss. Eliciting the startle reflex is used only in infants from birth to 4 months. Test is usually inadequate for children beyond infancy because of their tendency to ignore sounds or be distracted. Compare response of localizing sound to expected age response (see Biologic Development, Chapter 12). |
| **Tympanometry** | |
| Measures tympanic membrane compliance (or mobility) and estimates middle ear air pressure. A soft rubber cuff is pressed over the external canal to produce an airtight seal; an automatic reading of air pressure registers on the machine. | Detects middle ear disease and abnormalities but does not indicate the degree of hearing loss or the interpretation of sound. Difficult to perform in young children because of inability to maintain an adequate seal or excessive movement by the child. |
| **Conduction Tests** | |
| **Rinne test**—Stem of tuning fork is placed against the mastoid bone until the sound ceases to be audible. Tuning fork is then moved so that the prongs are held near, but not touching, the auditory meatus. Child should again hear the sound **(Rinne positive)**. If sound is not again audible **(Rinne negative)**, some abnormality is interfering with the conduction of air through the external and middle chambers. | Requires the cooperation and ability of the child to signal when the sound is no longer audible and when it is again heard. Not useful for most children before preschool age. |
| **Weber test**—Stem of tuning fork is held in the midline of the head. Child should hear the sound equally in both ears **(Weber positive)**. With air conductive loss, child will hear the sound better in the affected ear **(Weber negative)**. | Often not suitable for young children because of their difficulty in discriminating between "better, more, or less." |
| **Audiometry** | |
| Electrical audiometer measures the threshold of hearing for pure-tone frequencies and loudness. A sound is transmitted to the child's ear and reduced until child indicates the sound is no longer heard; this procedure is repeated for several sounds covering the range found in conversation. In an air conduction audiogram the sounds are transmitted through earphones. In a bone conduction audiogram the sounds are passed through a plaque placed over the mastoid bone. | Provides valuable information regarding the severity of the hearing loss, the sound cycles involved, and the possible location of the defect. Requires specialized training of personnel, expensive equipment, and cooperation from the child in terms of confirming the perception of sound. For children ages 24 months to approximately 5 years, play audiometry can be used; it is based on behavior modification and involves reinforcement for correct response. |
| **Otoacoustic Emissions (OAEs)** | |
| Special OAE analyzer delivers a rapid series of clicks to the ear through a probe fitted with a tympanometry tip that is inserted closely in the external auditory canal. The presence of OAEs, defined as sound energy emitted by the cochlea that is believed to be generated by movement of the outer hairs of the organ of Corti, is usually associated with normal or near-normal cochlear sensitivity; with hearing losses of 40dB or more, it is unlikely that the emissions are present (Callison, 1999). | Preferred method of screening neonates for sensorineural hearing loss (ototoxicity and noise-induced hearing loss). Requires specialized equipment. Minimal training is required. Infants must be in a quiet sleep for testing. Results do not indicate severity of cochlear damage; should be followed by ABR (see below). |
| **Auditory Brainstem Response (ABR)** | |
| Through electrode wires attached to the infant's or child's scalp, electrical or brain wave potentials generated within the auditory system are transmitted to a computer for analysis (Silverman, 1998). Following repetitive acoustic stimulation, the waveforms from a normal sleeping or quiet infant consist of several peaks and valleys that reflect activations of neural structures of the brain. | Requires expensive equipment and specialized training of personnel. |

*Any child who is suspected of a hearing loss because of poor performance using screening tests is referred for special audiometric or ABR testing.

terior wall of the cavity. Avoid pushing against the septum, because doing so causes pain. In general, inspection is adequate without the speculum unless a closer examination of the nasal membranes is warranted. If using the nasal speculum, explain the process to the child in a way similar to the preparation given for using the otoscope.

Note the *color* of the *mucosal lining,* which is normally redder than the oral membranes, and any swelling, discharge, dryness, or bleeding. Nasal membranes that are abnormally pale, grayish pink, and swollen suggest nasal allergies. Red, swollen membranes are usually characteristic of the common cold. These differences in appearance are important diagnostic clues to distinguishing between allergy and cold symptoms.

Normally there should be no discharge from the nose. However, a watery discharge is normal if the child has been crying. A thin, clear exudate at other times may indicate allergies, chronic rhinitis, or sinusitis. Purulent discharge is caused by infection and can indicate upper respiratory tract infections resulting from either a viral or a bacterial agent. A foul odor and discharge from one nostril may be caused by a foreign body. If possible, remove the object with forceps (tweezers). If it is deep in the cavity, refer the child to a more experienced practitioner.

Looking deeper into the nose, inspect the *turbinates,* or *concha,* which are plates of bone enveloped by mucous membrane that jut into the nasal cavity. The turbinates greatly increase the surface area of the nasal cavity as air is inhaled. The spaces or channels between the turbinates are called the *meatus* and correspond to each of the three turbinates. Normally the front end of the inferior and middle turbinates and the middle meatus can be seen. The turbinates should be the same color as the lining of the vestibule. Note enlarged, boggy, pale, grayish mucosa. Swollen turbinates greatly occlude the passageways for entry of air.

Also inspect the *septum,* which should equally divide the vestibules. Note any deviation, especially if it causes an occlusion of one side of the nose. A perforation may be evident within the septum. If this is suspected, shine the light of the otoscope into one naris and look for light coming through the perforation to the other nostril.

Because olfaction is an important function of the nose, testing for smell may be done at this point or as part of cranial nerve assessment (see Table 7-17).

## Mouth and Throat

The mouth is the beginning of the passageway to the digestive tract, but it also functions in the entry or exit of air. The major structure of the exterior of the mouth is the *lips.* Inspection of the lips for color is discussed in the section on skin (p. 187). Note any deviations, such as *cheilitis,* which is the presence of painful, inflamed, and dried cracks or fissures of the lips. Cheilitis may be caused by exposure to harsh climatic conditions, habitual licking or biting of the lips, mouth breathing from respiratory distress, or dehydration, particularly with fever. *Cheilosis,* or angular stomatitis, is fissuring at the angles or corners of the lips and may indicate deficiencies of riboflavin or niacin.

Observe for lesions on the lips. The herpes simplex virus produces singular or clusters of vesicular eruptions, often called "cold sores." The lip may also be the site of a primary syphilitic chancre, which appears as a firm nodule that ulcerates and crusts.

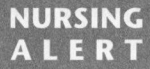

**NURSING ALERT** Whenever potentially infectious lesions are examined, be sure to wear gloves and to wash hands after removing gloves.

### Inspection of Internal Structures

The mouth and throat are divided into three areas: (1) the *oral cavity,* which extends from the lips to the palatopharyngeal arches; (2) the *oropharynx,* which extends from the epiglottis to the lower edge of the adenoids; and (3) the *nasopharynx,* which extends from above the lower edge of the adenoids to the nasal cavity. The major structures that are visible on examination within the oral cavity and oropharynx are the mucosal lining of the lips, cheeks, gums (gingiva), teeth, tongue, palate, uvula, tonsils, and posterior oropharynx (Fig. 7-30). Other pharyngeal structures that are not visible on examination are the epiglottis, lingual tonsils, and pharyngeal tonsils or adenoids.

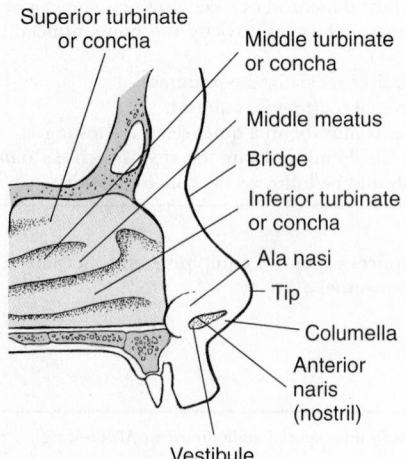

Superior turbinate or concha
Middle turbinate or concha
Middle meatus
Bridge
Inferior turbinate or concha
Ala nasi
Tip
Columella
Anterior naris (nostril)
Vestibule

**Fig. 7-29** External landmarks and internal structures of the nose.

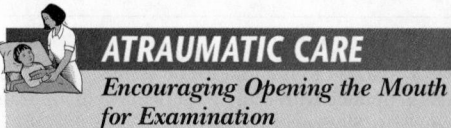

**ATRAUMATIC CARE**
*Encouraging Opening the Mouth for Examination*

Perform the examination in front of a mirror.
Let child first examine someone else's mouth, such as the parent, the nurse, or a puppet (Fig. 7-31, *A*), and then examine child's mouth.
Instruct child to tilt the head back slightly, breathe deeply through the mouth, and hold the breath; this action lowers the tongue to the floor of the mouth without using a tongue blade.

With a cooperative child, almost the entire examination can be performed without the use of a tongue blade. Ask the child to open the mouth wide, to move the tongue in different directions for full visualization, and to say "ahh," which depresses the tongue for a full view of the back of the mouth (tonsils, uvula, oropharynx). For a closer look at the buccal mucosa or lining of the cheeks, ask children to use their fingers to move the outer lip and cheek to one side. (See Atraumatic Care box.)

Infants and toddlers usually resist attempts to keep the mouth open. Because inspecting the mouth is an upsetting part of the examination, reserve this inspection until last (with examination of the ears) or perform it during episodes of crying. If the child resists opening the mouth, pinch the nostrils closed; this forces the child to open the mouth to breathe. Use a tongue blade to depress the tongue. Place it along the *side* of the tongue, not the center-back area, where the gag reflex is elicited. Fig. 7-31, *B*, illustrates proper positioning of the child for oral examination.

Inspect all areas lined with **mucous membranes** (inside the lips and cheeks, gingiva, underside of tongue, palate, back of pharynx). The membranes should be bright pink, smooth, glistening, uniform, and moist. Note any deviations, such as color, white patches or ulcerations, bleeding, and sensitivity. Reddened areas with white ulcerated centers may be canker sores (aphthae), which may be caused by trauma to the gums during toothbrushing or chewing. White curdy plaques or patches anywhere on the oral mucosa—but particularly on the surface of the tongue and hard palate—that bleed when scraped are signs of moniliasis (candidiasis).

While observing the lining of the mouth, note any odor (halitosis). Mouth odors are characteristic of a number of important health problems such as poor dental hygiene, gingival disease, chronic constipation, dehydration, malnutrition, or systemic illness. A sudden, foul odor in the mouth may indicate a foreign body in the nose, particularly a bean or pea.

Inspect the **teeth** for number in each dental arch, hygiene, and occlusion or bite. (See Teething, Chapter 12.) Discoloration of tooth enamel with obvious plaque (whitish coating on the surface of the teeth) is a sign of poor dental hygiene and indicates a need for dental counseling. Brown spots in the crevices of the crown of the tooth or between the teeth may be caries (cavities). Chalky white to yellow or brown areas on the enamel may indicate fluorosis (excessive fluoride ingestion). Teeth that appear greenish black may be stained temporarily from ingestion of supplemental iron.

Evaluate malocclusion or the poor biting relationship of the teeth in terms of (1) how the jaws relate to each other in vertical, transverse, and anteroposterior directions (e.g., the "bucktoothed" appearance that results when the maxilla is forward in relation to the mandible); (2) how the teeth are aligned; and (3) how the teeth interdigitate when in occlusion. (See Thumb Sucking, Chapter 12.)

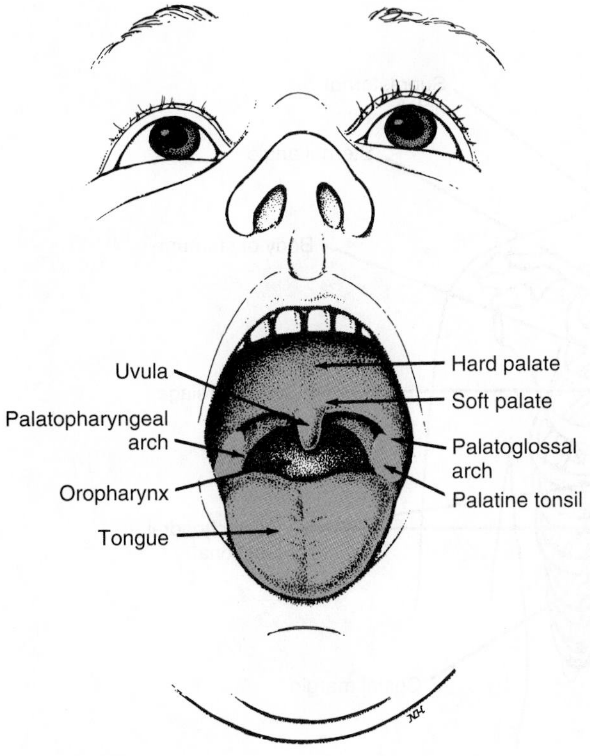

Uvula

Palatopharyngeal arch

Oropharynx

Tongue

Hard palate

Soft palate

Palatoglossal arch

Palatine tonsil

**Fig. 7-30**   Interior structures of mouth.

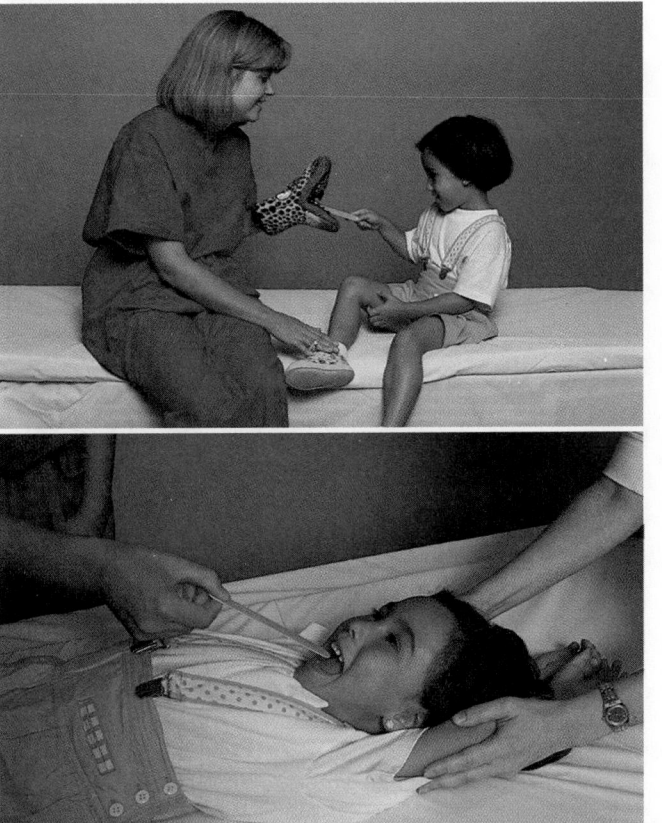

A

B

**Fig. 7-31**   **A,** Encouraging child to cooperate. **B,** Positioning child for examination of mouth.

Examine the *gums* surrounding the teeth. The color is normally coral pink and the surface texture is stippled, similar to the appearance of orange peel. In dark-skinned children the gums are more deeply colored, and a brownish area is often observed along the gum line. Note if the gums are inflamed; redness, puffiness along the gum line, and a tendency to bleed are signs of gingivitis. Counsel the child and family about good dental hygiene, especially flossing.

Inspect the *tongue* for the presence of papillae, small projections that contain several taste buds each and give the tongue its characteristic rough appearance. Note changes in the surface texture, such as (1) "geographic tongue," unusual patterns of papillae formation and denuded areas; (2) coated tongue, such as in candidiasis; or (3) an exceptionally beefy red and swollen tongue, which is a sign of various systemic diseases.

Note the size and mobility of the tongue, especially protrusion, which is often seen in children with mental retardation. Normally the tip of the tongue extends to the lips. If the child is unable to move the tongue forward to this point, the frenulum—the central band of mucous membrane that attaches the tongue to the floor of the mouth—may be too short. "Tongue-tie" can result in speech problems.

The roof of the mouth consists of the *hard palate,* near the front of the cavity, and the *soft palate,* toward the back of the pharynx, which has a small midline protrusion called the *uvula.* Inspect both carefully to be sure they are intact. Sometimes there is a pinpoint cleft in the soft palate that may go undetected unless carefully inspected. Such a cleft is especially important if the uvula is bifid, or separated into two appendages. A submucosal cleft may result in speech problems later on because air is not effectively trapped for vocalization. The arch of the palate should be dome-shaped. A narrow, flat roof or highly arched palate affects the placement of the tongue and can cause feeding and speech problems. Test the movement of the uvula by eliciting a gag reflex, which moves the uvula upward.

While inspecting the recesses of the oropharynx, note the size and color of the *palatine tonsils.* They are normally the same color as the surrounding mucosa, glandular rather than smooth in appearance, and barely visible over the edge of the palatoglossal arches. Enlargement, redness, and white patches on the tonsils and surrounding area may indicate suppurative tonsillitis or pharyngitis. Report these findings for further evaluation.

## Chest

Although the thoracic cavity houses two vital organs, the heart and the lungs, the anatomic structures of the chest wall are important sources of information concerning cardiac and pulmonary function, skeletal formation, and secondary sexual development. Inspect the chest for size, shape, symmetry, movement, breast development, and the presence of the bony landmarks formed by the ribs and sternum.

The *rib cage* consists of 12 ribs and the sternum, or breast bone, located in the midline of the trunk (Fig. 7-32). The first seven ribs, often called *true ribs,* attach directly to the

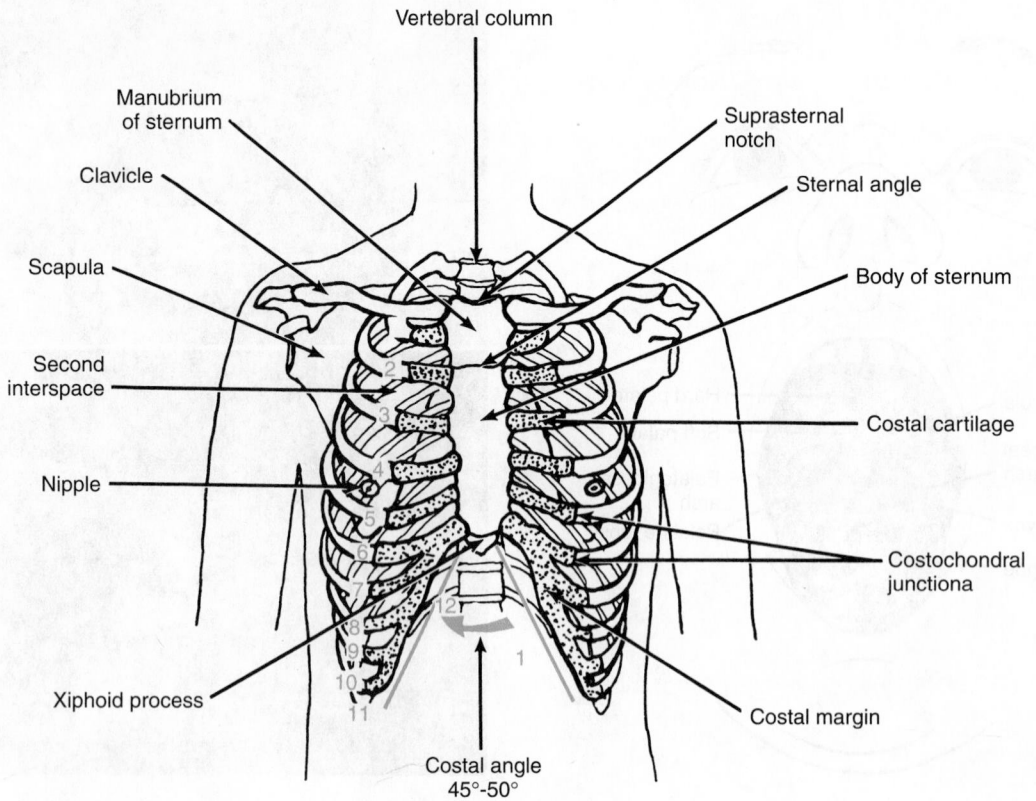

**Fig. 7-32** Rib cage.

costal cartilages of the sternum at the costochondral junction. The next five ribs are called *false ribs* because they do not attach directly to the costal cartilages of the sternum. The eighth, ninth, and tenth ribs attach to the costal cartilages below the seventh rib; the last two ribs, often called *floaters,* have no direct attachment to the sternum or anterior ribs other than their posterior attachment to the vertebral column.

The *sternum* is composed of three main parts. The *manubrium,* the uppermost portion, can be felt at the base of the neck at the *suprasternal notch.* The largest segment of the sternum is the body, which forms the *sternal angle (angle of Louis)* as it articulates with the manubrium. At the end of the body is a small, movable process called the *xiphoid.* The angle of the costal margin as it attaches to the sternum is called the *costal angle* and is normally about 45 to 50 degrees. These bony structures are important landmarks in the location of ribs and intercostal spaces. The first rib attaches directly to the manubrium. The second rib attaches directly to the body of the sternum below the sternal angle. The sternal angle is felt as a ridge a few centimeters below the suprasternal notch. The space immediately below a rib is its corresponding *intercostal space (ICS).*

Become familiar with locating and properly numbering each rib, because ribs are geographic landmarks for palpating, percussing, and auscultating underlying organs. Normally all the ribs can be counted by palpating inferiorly from the second rib. The tip of the eleventh rib can be felt laterally, and the tip of the twelfth rib can be felt posteriorly. Other helpful landmarks include the nipples, which are usually located between the fourth and fifth ribs or at the fourth interspace and, posteriorly, the tip of the scapula, which is located at the level of the eighth rib or interspace. In children with thin chest walls, correctly locating the ribs presents little difficulty.

The *thoracic cavity* is also divided into segments by drawing imaginary lines on the chest and back. Fig. 7-33 illustrates the anterior, lateral, and posterior divisions.

Measure the *size* of the chest by placing the tape around the rib cage at the nipple line (see Fig. 7-4). For greatest accuracy take at least two measurements—one during inspiration and the other during expiration—and record the average. Chest size is important mainly in comparison with its relationship to head circumference (see p. 178). Always report marked disproportions because most are caused by abnormal head growth, although some may be a result of altered chest shape, such as barrel chest or pigeon chest.

During infancy the *shape* of the chest is almost circular (barrel-shaped), with the anteroposterior (front-to-back) diameter equaling the transverse or lateral (side-to-side) diameter. As the child grows, the chest normally increases in the transverse direction, causing the anteroposterior diameter to be less than the lateral diameter. A barrel-shaped chest in an older child is a significant sign of chronic obstructive lung disease, such as asthma or cystic fibrosis. Other variations of the normal configuration are *pigeon breast,* or *pectus carinatum,* in which the sternum protrudes outward and increases the anteroposterior diameter; and *funnel chest,* or *pectus excavatum,* in which the lower portion

of the sternum is depressed. A severe depression may impair cardiorespiratory function and may indicate the presence of an underlying heritable connective tissue disorder, such as Marfan syndrome (Kalangos and others, 1995). In general, neither condition causes pathologic dysfunction but often causes parents and children concern regarding acceptable physical appearance.

Ordinarily the *costal angle* made by the lower costal margin and the sternum is approximately 45 degrees. A larger angle is characteristic of the lung diseases that also cause a barrel-shaped chest. A smaller angle may be a sign of malnutrition. While inspecting the rib cage, note the junction of the ribs to the costal cartilage (costochondral junction) and sternum. Normally the points of attachment are fairly smooth. Swellings or blunt knobs along either side of the sternum, known as the *rachitic rosary,* may indicate vitamin D deficiency. Another variation in shape that may either be normal or suggest rickets (vitamin D deficiency) is *Harrison groove,* a depression or horizontal groove in which the diaphragm leaves the chest wall. Marked flaring of the rib cage below the groove is usually an abnormal finding.

Body *symmetry* is always an important notation during inspection. Asymmetry in the chest may indicate serious un-

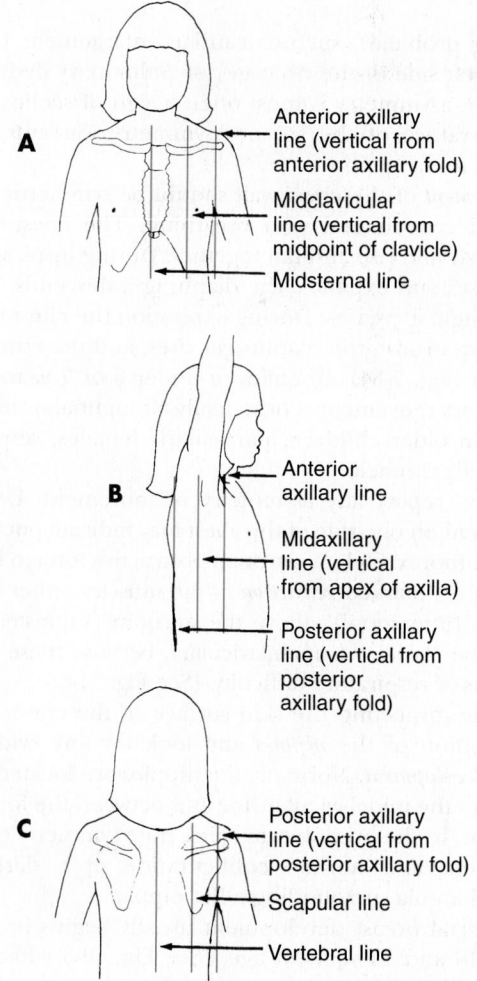

**Fig. 7-33** Landmarks of chest. **A,** Anterior. **B,** Right lateral. **C,** Posterior.

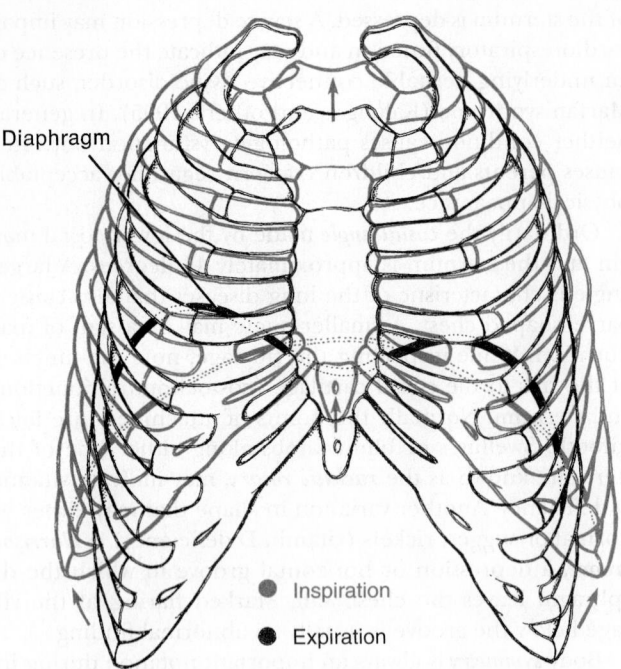

Diaphragm

● Inspiration

● Expiration

**Fig. 7-34**  Movement of chest during respiration.

derlying problems, such as cardiac enlargement (bulging on the left side of the rib cage) or pulmonary dysfunction. However, asymmetry is most often a sign of scoliosis, a lateral curvature of the spine. Asymmetry warrants further medical investigation.

*Movement* of the chest wall should be symmetric bilaterally and coordinated with breathing. The chest and abdomen should rise and fall together. During inspiration the chest rises and expands, the diaphragm descends, and the costal angle increases. During expiration the chest falls and decreases in size, the diaphragm rises, and the costal angle narrows (Fig. 7-34). In children under 6 or 7 years of age, respiratory movement is principally abdominal or diaphragmatic. In older children, particularly females, respirations are chiefly thoracic.

Always report any asymmetry of movement. Decreased movement on one side of the chest may indicate pneumonia, pneumothorax, atelectasis, or an obstructive foreign body. Always report marked *retraction* of the muscles either between the ribs (intercostal), above the sternum (suprasternal), or above the clavicles (supraclavicular), because these findings are signs of respiratory difficulty. (See Fig. 31-6.)

While inspecting the skin surface of the chest, observe the position of the *nipples* and look for any evidence of *breast development.* Normally the nipples are located slightly lateral to the midclavicular line and between the fourth and fifth ribs. In the prepubertal child, note symmetry of nipple placement and normal configuration of a darker pigmented areola surrounding a flat nipple.

Pubertal breast development usually begins in girls between 10 and 14 years of age. (See Fig. 19-3.) Record any precocious or delayed breast development, as well as evidence of any other secondary sexual characteristics. In males gynecomastia may be caused by hormonal or systemic

disorders, but more commonly it is a result of adipose tissue from obesity or a transitory body change during early puberty. In either situation investigate the child's feelings regarding breast enlargement.

In adolescent females who have achieved sexual maturity, palpate the breasts for evidence of any masses or hard nodules. Use this opportunity to discuss the importance of routine breast self-examination. Although carcinoma of the breast is rare in women under 20 years of age, stress the value of routine breast self-examination so that it becomes a practiced habit during later years. The vast majority of palpable masses are benign (West and others, 1995). Many clinically diagnosed breast masses do not require surgery and may resolve over a 6-month period. An ultrasound of the breast is useful in distinguishing a solid lesion from a cystic lesion (Boothroyd and Carty, 1994). Emphasize this fact to decrease any fear or concern that results when a mass is felt.

## Lungs

The lungs are situated inside the thoracic cavity, with one lung on each side of the sternum. Each lung is divided into an *apex,* which is slightly pointed and rises above the first rib; a *base,* which is wide and concave and rides on the dome-shaped diaphragm; and a body, which is divided into *lobes.* The right lung has three lobes—the upper, middle, and lower. The left lobe has only two lobes, the upper and lower, because of the space occupied by the heart. The two surfaces of the lung are the *costal surface,* which faces the chest wall and backs up to the vertebral column, and the *mediastinal surface,* which faces the space lying between the lungs, the mediastinum. The center of the mediastinal surface is called the *hilus,* where the bronchus and blood vessels enter the lung (Fig. 7-35, *A*).

Examination of the lungs requires knowledge of their location and their relationship to the rib cage. The trachea bifurcates slightly below the level of the sternal angle. The apex of each lung rises approximately 2 to 4 cm above the inner third of the clavicles. The lower costal margin crosses the sixth rib at the midclavicular line and the eighth rib at the midaxillary line. The posterior base of the lungs crosses the eleventh rib at the vertebral line. The upper border of the right middle lobe parallels the inferior surface of the fourth rib. Fig. 7-35 illustrates the position of the lobes within the thoracic cavity during relaxation. Respiration causes displacement of the lobes upward (expiration) or downward (inspiration).

### Inspection

Inspection of the lungs primarily involves observation of respiratory movements, which are discussed below. Evaluate respirations for (1) rate (number per minute), (2) rhythm (regular, irregular, or periodic), (3) depth (deep or shallow), and (4) quality (effortless, automatic, difficult, or labored). Also note the character of breath sounds, such as noisy, grunting, snoring, or heavy. Usual terms for describing various patterns of respiration are listed in Box 7-3.

Always evaluate respiratory rate in relation to general physical status. For example, tachypnea is expected with

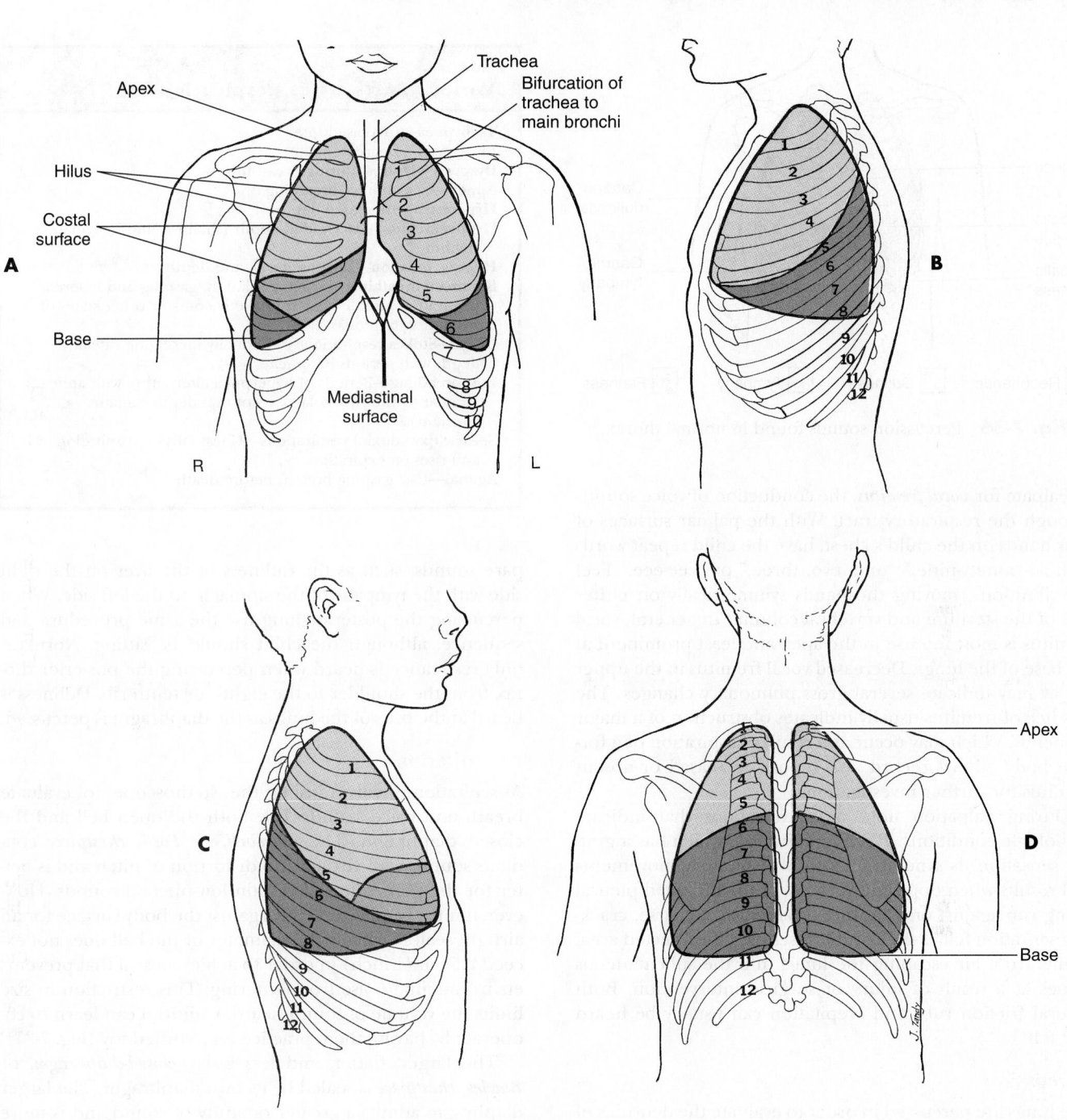

**Fig. 7-35**    Location of lobes of lungs within thoracic cavity. **A,** Anterior view. **B,** Left lateral view. **C,** Right lateral view. **D,** Posterior view.

fever because the respiratory rate increases four breaths per minute for every degree of Fahrenheit elevation in temperature. The usual ratio of breaths to heartbeats is 1:4. (See inside back cover for normal respiratory rates at various ages.)

## Palpation

Evaluate *respiratory movements* by placing each hand flat against the child's back or chest with the thumbs in midline along the lower costal margin of the lungs. The child should be sitting during this procedure and, if cooperative, should take several deep breaths. During respiration the hands will move with the chest wall. Assess the amount of respiratory excursion and note any asymmetry of movement. Normally in older children the posterior base of the lungs descends 5 to 6 cm (approximately 2 inches) during a deep inspiration.

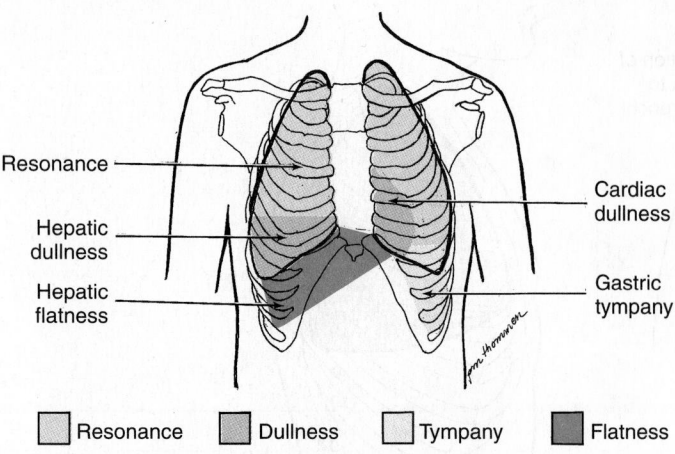

**Fig. 7-36** Percussion sounds found in normal thorax.

Palpate for *vocal fremitus,* the conduction of voice sounds through the respiratory tract. With the palmar surfaces of your hands on the child's chest, have the child repeat words such as "ninety-nine," "one, two, three," or "eee-eee." Feel the vibrations, moving the hands symmetrically on either side of the sternum and vertebral column. In general, vocal fremitus is most intense in the apex and least prominent at the base of the lungs. Decreased vocal fremitus in the upper airway may indicate several gross pulmonary changes. The absence of fremitus usually indicates obstruction of a major bronchus, which may occur as a result of aspiration of a foreign body. Always record and report decreased or absent fremitus for further investigation.

During palpation note other vibrations that indicate pathologic conditions. *Pleural friction rub,* which has a grating sensation, is synchronous with respiratory movements and results when opposing surfaces of the inflamed pleural lining rub against one another. *Crepitation,* a coarse, crackling sensation felt as the hand presses over the affected area, results from air escaping the lungs into the subcutaneous tissues as a result of injury or surgical intervention. Both pleural friction rubs and crepitation can usually be heard and felt.

## Percussion

The lungs are percussed in order to evaluate the densities of the underlying organs. Fig. 7-36 illustrates the expected percussion sounds within the anterior thorax. *Resonance* is heard over all the lobes that are not adjacent to other organs. *Dullness* is heard beginning at the fifth interspace in the right midclavicular line. Percussing downward to the end of the liver, a *flat sound* is heard because the liver no longer overlies the air-filled lung. *Cardiac dullness* is felt over the left sternal border from the second to the fifth interspace and medially to the midclavicular line. Below the fifth interspace on the left side, *tympany* results from the air-filled stomach. Always record and report deviations from these expected sounds.

In percussing the chest, begin over the anterior lung from apex to base, usually with the child supine or sitting. Percuss each side of the chest in sequence in order to compare sounds, such as the dullness of the liver on the right side with the tympany of the stomach on the left side. When percussing the posterior lung use the same procedure and sequence, although the child should be sitting. Normally only resonance is heard when percussing the posterior thorax from the shoulder to the eighth or tenth rib. Dullness is heard at the base of the lungs as the diaphragm is percussed.

## Auscultation

Auscultation involves using the stethoscope to evaluate breath and voice sounds. Use both the open bell and the closed diaphragm. The *open-bell,* or *Ford, chestpiece* conducts sounds with virtually no distortion of pitch and is better for the perception of certain low-pitched sounds. However, it must be placed firmly against the body surface for an airtight seal. Normally the diameter of the bell does not exceed 2.5 cm (1 inch) in order to achieve a seal that prevents environmental noise from entering. This restriction in size limits the volume of sound heard. Children can learn to cooperate by having them practice on a stuffed toy (Fig. 7-37).

The larger, flatter, and less bulky *closed-diaphragm,* or *Bowles, chestpiece* is sealed by its own diaphragm. The larger diaphragm admits a greater quantity of sound and is more sensitive to high-pitched sounds. The diaphragm filters out low-frequency vibrations so that sounds appear to be of higher pitch than when heard through the bell. The self-sealing diaphragm can be placed on a bony or small chest, although a close-fitting seal is still recommended in order to decrease the admittance of environmental sounds. In infants and small children, especially premature infants, use a specially sized pediatric diaphragm to achieve sufficient skin contact and to localize sounds in segmented areas of the chest. Listen for breath sounds as the child inspires deeply. (See Guidelines and Atraumatic Care boxes.)

Breath sounds in the lungs are classified as vesicular, bronchovesicular, or bronchial (Box 7-4). *Absent or diminished breath sounds* are always an abnormal finding and warrant investigation. Fluid, air, or solid masses in the pleural

## GUIDELINES
### Effective Auscultation

Try to make sure child is relaxed and not crying, talking, or laughing. Record if child is crying.
Check that room is comfortable and quiet.
Warm stethoscope before placing it against skin.
Apply firm pressure on chestpiece but not enough to prevent vibrations and transmission of sound.
Avoid placing stethoscope over hair or clothing, moving it against skin, breathing on tubing, or sliding fingers over chestpiece, which may cause sounds that falsely resemble pathologic findings.
Use a symmetric and orderly approach to compare sounds.

## ATRAUMATIC CARE
### Encouraging Deep Breaths

Ask child to "blow out" the light on an otoscope or pocket flashlight; discreetly turn off the light on the last try so the child feels successful.
Place a cotton ball in child's palm; ask child to blow the ball into the air and have parent catch it.
Place a small tissue on the top of a pencil and ask child to blow the tissue off.
Have child blow a pinwheel, a party horn, or bubbles.

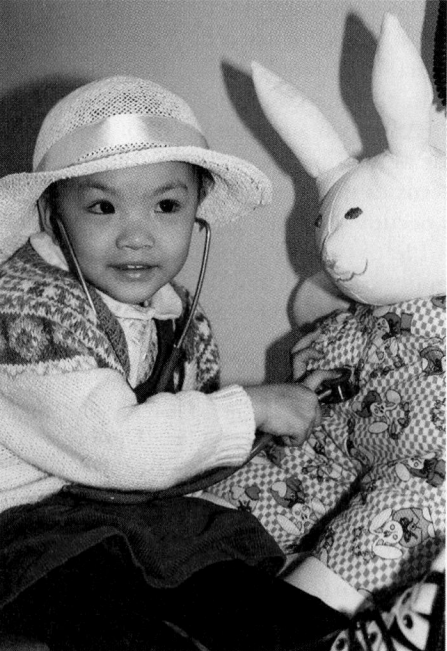

**Fig. 7-37** Child practicing on a stuffed toy to learn how nurses listen to the lungs.

space interfere with the conduction of breath sounds; in young children breath sounds are easily transmitted through the thin chest wall, and unilateral breath sounds may not be heard. Diminished breath sounds in certain segments of the lung suggest pulmonary areas that may benefit from postural drainage and percussion. Increased breath sounds following pulmonary therapy indicate improved passage of air through the respiratory tract.

*Voice sounds* are also part of auscultation of the lung. Vocal resonance or voice sounds are normally heard, but the syllables are indistinct. Elicit them in the same manner as for vocal fremitus, except listen with the stethoscope. Consolidation of lung tissue produces three types of abnormal voice sounds: (1) *whispered pectoriloquy* (words are whispered, and syllables are heard); (2) *bronchophony* (spoken words are not distinguishable, but the vocal resonance is increased in intensity and clarity); and (3) *egophony* ("ee" is heard as the nasal sound "ay" through the stethoscope). Decreased or absent vocal resonance is caused by the same conditions that affect vocal fremitus.

Various pulmonary abnormalities produce **adventitious sounds** that are not normally heard over the chest. They are not alterations of normal breath sounds but are additional abnormal sounds (Table 7-13). Considerable practice with an experienced tutor is necessary to differentiate the various types of adventitious sounds.* Often it is best to describe the type of sound heard in the lungs rather than to try to label it correctly.

*A suggested resource for becoming familiar with normal and abnormal lung sounds is *Lung Sounds: A Practical Guide* (second edition) by R. Wilkins, J. Hodgkin, and B. Lopez (1996, Mosby) (book and audiotape).

### Box 7-4
### Classification of Normal Breath Sounds

**VESICULAR BREATH SOUNDS**
Heard over entire surface of lungs, with exception of upper intrascapular area and area beneath manubrium.
Inspiration is louder, longer, and higher pitched than expiration.
Sound is soft, swishing noise.

**BRONCHOVESICULAR BREATH SOUNDS**
Heard over manubrium and in upper intrascapular regions where trachea and bronchi bifurcate.
Inspiration is louder and higher in pitch than in vesicular breathing.

**BRONCHIAL BREATH SOUNDS**
Heard only over trachea near suprasternal notch.
Inspiratory phase is short, and expiratory phase is long.

The other important adventitious sound is the pleural friction rub. Its sound can be simulated by cupping one hand to the ear and rubbing a finger of the other hand across the cupped hand. The most common site for a friction rub to be heard is the lower anterolateral chest wall (between the midaxillary and midclavicular lines), the area of greatest thoracic mobility.

## Heart

Knowledge of the anatomy and physiology of the normal heart is essential in order to properly evaluate the findings. In addition to the following discussion, the normal circulation of the blood through the heart chambers, major blood vessels, and valves is discussed in Chapter 34.

The heart is situated in the thoracic cavity between the lungs in the mediastinum and above the diaphragm (Fig. 7-38). Approximately two thirds of the heart lies within the left side of the rib cage, with the other third on the right side as it crosses the sternum. Most of the anterior cardiac surface is occupied by the right ventricle. Part of the right atrium and left ventricle also faces anteriorly, whereas the left atrium lies primarily in a posterior position.

The heart is positioned in the thorax like a trapezoid:

- **Vertically** along the right sternal border (RSB) from the second to the fifth rib
- **Horizontally (long side)** from the lower right sternum to the fifth rib at the left midclavicular line (LMCL)
- **Diagonally** from the left sternal border (LSB) at the second rib to the LMCL at the fifth rib
- **Horizontally (short side)** from the RSB and LSB at the second intercostal space (ICS)—base of the heart

The most important skill in examining the heart is auscultation, performed when the child is quiet. Inspection and palpation also yield important information. However, percussion is of little value in assessing cardiac size or function.

## Inspection

When examining the chest, note any obvious bulging, especially on the left side, which may indicate cardiac enlargement. Observe the child sitting in a semi-Fowler position, and look at the anterior chest wall from an angle, comparing both sides of the rib cage with each other. Normally they are symmetric. In children with thin chest walls, a pulsation may be visible.

Because comprehensive evaluation of cardiac function is not limited to the heart, also consider other findings, such as the presence of all pulses (especially the femoral pulses) (Fig. 7-39), distended neck veins, clubbing of the fingers, peripheral cyanosis, edema, blood pressure, and respiratory status.

## Palpation

Use palpation to determine the location of the **apical impulse (AI)**, the most lateral cardiac impulse that may correspond to the apex. The AI is found:

- Just lateral to the LMCL and fourth ICS in children <7 years of age
- At the LMCL and fifth ICS in children >7 years of age

Although the AI gives a general idea of the size of the heart (with enlargement, the apex is lower and more lat-

**TABLE 7-13    Description of abnormal lung sounds**

| Term | Characteristics | Similar Sound | Cause |
|---|---|---|---|
| Coarse crackle | Discontinuous, interrupted explosive sounds<br>Loud, low in pitch | Agitating a container of moderately heated salt | Air passing through larger airways containing fluid |
| Fine crackle | Discontinuous, interrupted explosive sounds<br>Less loud than above and of shorter duration; higher in pitch than coarse crackles | Strands of hair rolled between fingers; separating self-adhering fasteners | Air passing through smaller airways containing fluid |
| Wheeze | Continuous sounds<br>High-pitched; a hissing sound | Two marble plates coated with oil are suddenly separated | Airway narrowed by asthma or partially obstructed by tumor or foreign body |
| Rhonchus | Continuous sounds<br>Low-pitched; a snoring sound | Cooing of a wood pigeon, croaking of a frog, or snoring | Large upper airway partially obstructed by thick secretions |

Data from Ward J: Lung sounds: easy to hear, hard to describe, *Respir Care* 34(1):763-770, 1989; and Murphy R, Holford S: Lung sounds, *Respir Care* 25(7):763-770, 1980.

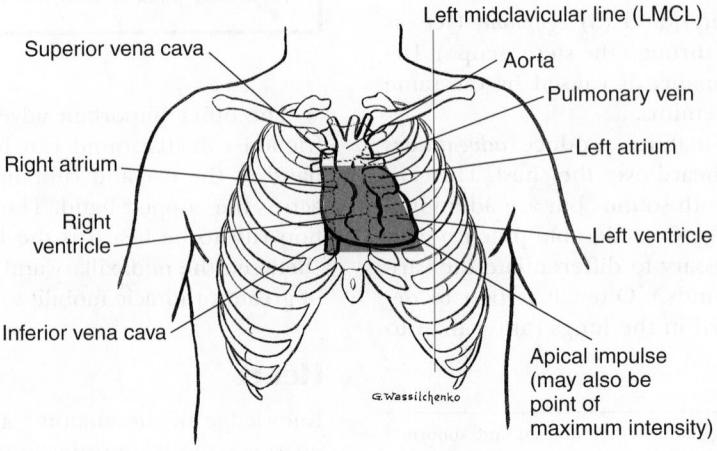

**Fig. 7-38**   Position of heart within thorax.

eral), its normal location is quite variable, making it a rather unreliable indicator of heart size.

The *point of maximum intensity (PMI)*, as the name implies, is the area of most intense pulsation. Usually the PMI is located at the same site as the AI, but it can occur elsewhere. For this reason, these two terms should not be used interchangeably.

*Thrills* are palpable vibrations most commonly produced by the flow of blood from one chamber of the heart to another through a narrowed or abnormal opening, such as a stenotic valve or a septal defect. Thrills are best felt with the ball of the hand (palmar surface at the base of the fingers) and during expiration. They feel similar to the placing of one's hand on a purring cat.

*Pericardial friction rubs* are scratchy, high-pitched grating sounds; they are similar to pleural friction rubs except that they are not affected by changes in respiration. This is a useful clue in differentiating the two rubs—pleural rubs cease if the child holds the breath, whereas pericardial rubs do not. Both thrills and rubs are abnormal; report them for further evaluation.

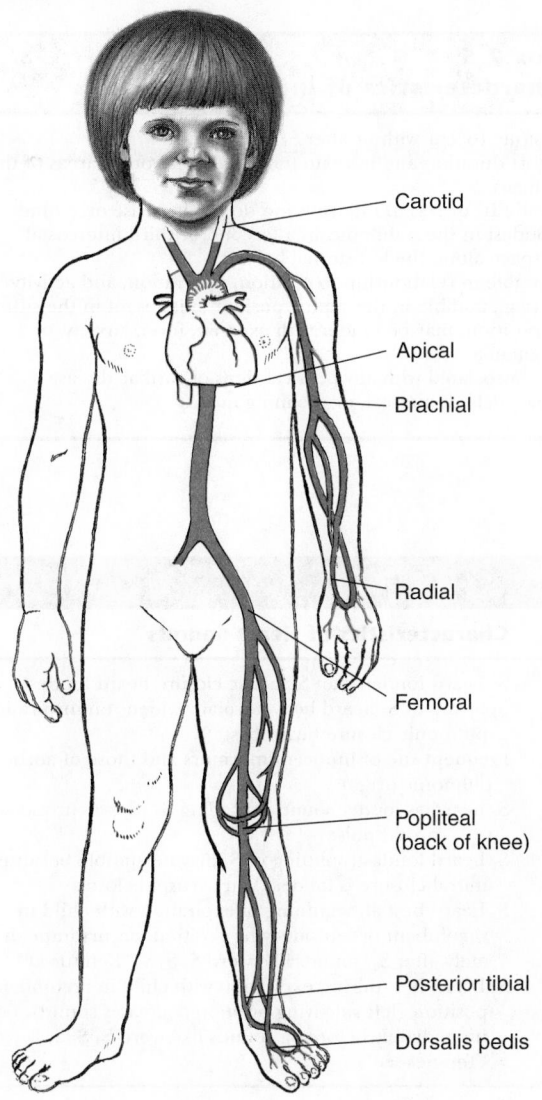

**Fig. 7-39**  Location of pulses.

During palpation assess *capillary refill time*—an important test of peripheral circulation. Blanch the nail bed with sustained pressure for a few seconds and then release the pressure. The time it takes for the nail to return to its original color is the capillary refill time.

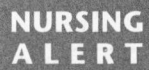

**NURSING ALERT**  Capillary refill should be brisk—less than 2 seconds; prolonged refill may be associated with poor systemic perfusion.

### Auscultation

**Origin of Heart Sounds.**  The heart sounds are produced by the opening and closing of the valves and the vibration of blood against the walls of the heart and vessels. Normally two sounds—$S_1$ and $S_2$—are heard and correspond respectively to the familiar "lub-dub" often used to describe the sounds. $S_1$ is caused by closure of the *tricuspid* and *mitral valves* (sometimes called the *atrioventricular valves*). $S_2$ is the result of closure of the *pulmonic* and *aortic valves* (sometimes called *semilunar valves*). Normally the split of the two sounds in $S_2$ is distinguishable and widens during inspiration. *Physiologic splitting* is a significant normal finding.

**NURSING ALERT**  "Fixed splitting," in which the split in $S_2$ does not change during inspiration, is an important diagnostic sign of atrial septal defect.

Two other heart sounds—$S_3$ and $S_4$—may be produced. $S_3$ is the result of vibrations produced during ventricular filling. It is normally heard in some children and young adults but is considered abnormal in older individuals. $S_4$ is caused by the recoil of vibrations between the atria and ventricles following atrial contraction at the end of diastole. It is rarely heard as a normal heart sound and indicates the need for further cardiac evaluation.

Another important category of heart sounds is *murmurs,* which are produced by vibrations within the heart chambers or in the major arteries from the back-and-forth flow of blood. (For a more detailed discussion, see Assessment of Cardiac Function, Chapter 34.) Murmurs are classified as:

**Innocent**. No anatomic or physiologic abnormality exists.
**Functional**. No anatomic cardiac defect exists, but a physiologic abnormality such as anemia is present.
**Organic**. A cardiac defect with or without a physiologic abnormality exists.

The description and classification of murmurs are skills that require considerable practice and training. In general, recognize murmurs as distinct swishing sounds that occur in addition to the normal heart sounds and record the (1) *location* of the area of the heart in which the murmur is heard best, (2) *time* of the occurrence of the murmur within the $S_1S_2$ cycle, (3) *intensity* (evaluation in relationship to the child's position), and (4) *loudness*. The usual subjective method of grading the loudness or intensity of a murmur is listed in Table 7-14. Characteristics of innocent murmurs as opposed to organic murmurs are described in Box 7-5.

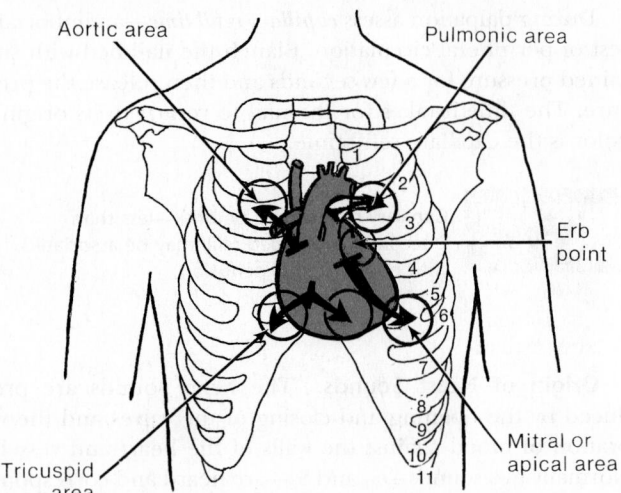

**Fig. 7-40** Direction of heart sounds for anatomic valve sites and areas used *(circled)* for auscultation.

Other abnormal sounds, such as ejection clicks, snaps, gallops, and hums, are beyond the scope of this discussion. The best approach is to become familiar with normal heart sounds and to refer any questionable heart sound for further evaluation.*

**Differentiating Normal Heart Sounds.** Fig. 7-40 illustrates the approximate anatomic position of the valves within the heart chambers. Note that the anatomic location of the valves does not correspond to the area where the sounds are heard best. The auscultatory sites are located in the direction of the blood flow through the valves.

Normally $S_1$ is louder at the apex of the heart in the mitral and tricuspid area, and $S_2$ is louder near the base of the heart in the pulmonic and aortic area. Listen to each sound by inching down the chest (Table 7-15). Also auscultate the fol-

---

*A suggested resource for becoming familiar with normal and abnormal heart sounds is *Heart Sounds and Murmurs: A Practical Guide* (third edition), by B.B. Erickson (1997, Mosby) (book and audiotape).

**TABLE 7-14** Grading of the intensity of heart murmurs

| Grade | Description |
|-------|-------------|
| I | Very faint; often not heard if child sits up |
| II | Usually readily heard; slightly louder than grade I; audible in all positions |
| III | Loud, but not accompanied by a thrill |
| IV | Loud, accompanied by a thrill |
| V | Loud enough to be heard with the stethoscope barely touching the chest; accompanied by a thrill |
| VI | Loud enough to be heard with the stethoscope not touching the chest; often heard with the human ear close to the chest; accompanied by a thrill |

**Box 7-5** ■ ■ □
**Characteristics of Innocent Murmurs**

Systolic (occur with or after $S_1$)
Short duration and have no transmission to other areas of the heart
Grade III or less in intensity and do not increase over time
Loudest in the pulmonic area (second or third intercostal space along the left sternal border)
Variable in relationship to position, respiration, and activity (e.g., audible in the supine position but absent in the sitting position; may be louder with exercise, fever, anxiety, or anemia)
Not associated with any physical signs of cardiac disease
Low-pitched, musical, or groaning quality

**TABLE 7-15** Sequence of auscultating heart sounds*

| Auscultatory Site | Chest Location | Characteristics of Heart Sounds |
|-------------------|----------------|--------------------------------|
| Aortic area | Second right intercostal space close to sternum | $S_2$ heard louder than $S_1$; aortic closure heard loudest |
| Pulmonic area | Second left intercostal space close to sternum | Splitting of $S_2$ heard best, normally widens on inspiration; pulmonic closure heard best |
| Erb point | Second and third left intercostal space close to sternum | Frequent site of innocent murmurs and those of aortic or pulmonic origin |
| Tricuspid area | Fifth right and left intercostal space close to sternum | $S_1$ heard as louder sound preceding $S_2$ ($S_1$ synchronous with carotid pulse) |
| Mitral or apical area | Fifth intercostal space, left midclavicular line (third to fourth intercostal space and lateral to left midclavicular line in infants) | $S_1$ heard loudest; splitting of $S_1$ may be audible because mitral closure is louder than tricuspid closure<br>$S_3$ heard best at beginning of expiration with child in recumbent or left side-lying position, occurs immediately after $S_2$, sounds like word $S_1 S_2 S_3$ "Ken-tuc-ky"<br>$S_4$ heard best during expiration with child in recumbent position (left side-lying position decreases sound), occurs immediately before $S_1$, sounds like word $S_4 S_1 S_2$ "Ten-nes-see" |

*Use both diaphragm and bell chestpieces when auscultating heart sounds. Bell chestpiece is necessary for low-pitched sounds of murmurs, $S_3$, and $S_4$.

lowing areas for sounds, such as murmurs, which may radiate to these sites: the sternoclavicular area above the clavicles and manubrium, the area along the sternal border, the area along the left midaxillary line, and the area below the scapulae.

**NURSING TIP**   To distinguish between $S_1$ or $S_2$ heart sounds, simultaneously palpate the carotid pulse with the index and middle finger and listen to the heart sounds; $S_1$ is synchronous with the carotid pulse.

Auscultate the heart with the child in at least two positions: sitting and reclining. If adventitious sounds are detected, further evaluate them with the child standing, sitting and learning forward, and lying on the left side. For example, atrial sounds such as $S_4$ are heard best with the child in a recumbent position and usually fade if the child sits or stands.

Evaluate heart sounds for the following: (1) *quality* (should be clear and distinct, not muffled, diffuse, or distant); (2) *intensity,* especially in relation to the location or auscultatory site (should not be weak or pounding); (3) *rate* (should be the same as the radial pulse); and (4) *rhythm* (should be regular and even).

A particular arrhythmia that occurs normally in many children is *sinus arrhythmia,* in which the heart rate increases with inspiration and decreases with expiration. Differentiate this rhythm from a truly abnormal arrhythmia by having children hold their breath. In sinus arrhythmia, cessation of breathing causes the heart rate to remain steady. Variations in patterns of heart rate or pulse are listed in Box 7-6.

As with respiratory rate, always evaluate heart rate in relation to general physical status. For example, the pulse rate is usually increased by 8 to 10 beats per minute for each degree of Fahrenheit elevation in temperature. Athletic children occasionally have lower heart rates, which represent a highly developed and efficient heart muscle. (See inside back cover for normal heart rates at various ages.)

## Abdomen

Examination of the abdomen involves the usual four skills, except that the order is altered. Start with inspection and follow with auscultation, percussion, and palpation because the latter three maneuvers may distort the normal abdominal sounds. The sequence of examination changes according to the age and cooperativeness of the child. All four types of assessment are commonly performed at different times. For example, auscultate for bowel sounds following evaluation of heart and lung sounds at the beginning of the examination when the child is quiet. Use inspection at any time during the examination. Percuss after lung percussion, and palpate toward the end of the examination, when the child is relaxed and more trusting.

Knowledge of the anatomic placement of the abdominal organs is essential in differentiating normal, expected findings from abnormal ones (Fig. 7-41). The *abdominal cavity* is the portion of the trunk from directly beneath the diaphragm and thoracic cavity to the region of the pelvic cavity. For descriptive purposes the abdominal cavity is divided into four quadrants by drawing a vertical line midway from the sternum to the pubic symphysis and a horizontal line across the abdomen through the umbilicus (Fig. 7-41). This method of division actually includes the pelvic cavity. Each section is designated as follows:

- Right upper quadrant (RUQ)
- Right lower quadrant (RLQ)
- Left upper quadrant (LUQ)
- Left lower quadrant (LLQ)

The abdominal cavity contains the major organs of digestion, and the pelvic cavity houses the internal reproductive organs, the lower parts of the digestive tract, and the urinary bladder. In infancy the bladder is an abdominal organ.

### Inspection

Inspect the *contour* of the abdomen with the child in the erect position and supine position. Normally the abdomen of infants and young children is quite cylindric and, in the erect position, fairly prominent because of the physiologic lordosis of the spine. In the supine position the abdomen appears flat. During adolescence the usual male and female contours of the pelvic cavity change the shape of the ab-

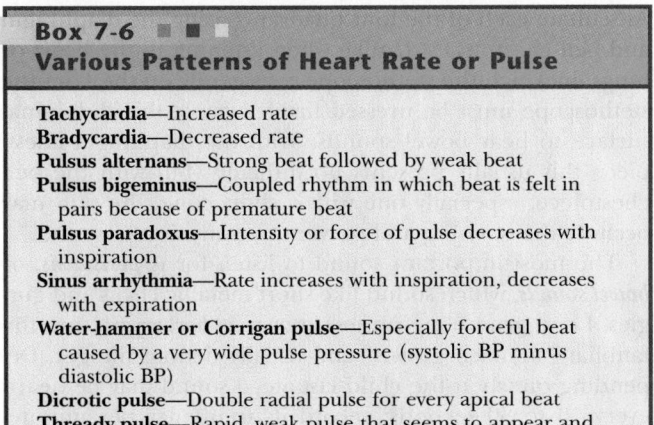

**Box 7-6**
### Various Patterns of Heart Rate or Pulse

**Tachycardia**—Increased rate
**Bradycardia**—Decreased rate
**Pulsus alternans**—Strong beat followed by weak beat
**Pulsus bigeminus**—Coupled rhythm in which beat is felt in pairs because of premature beat
**Pulsus paradoxus**—Intensity or force of pulse decreases with inspiration
**Sinus arrhythmia**—Rate increases with inspiration, decreases with expiration
**Water-hammer or Corrigan pulse**—Especially forceful beat caused by a very wide pulse pressure (systolic BP minus diastolic BP)
**Dicrotic pulse**—Double radial pulse for every apical beat
**Thready pulse**—Rapid, weak pulse that seems to appear and disappear

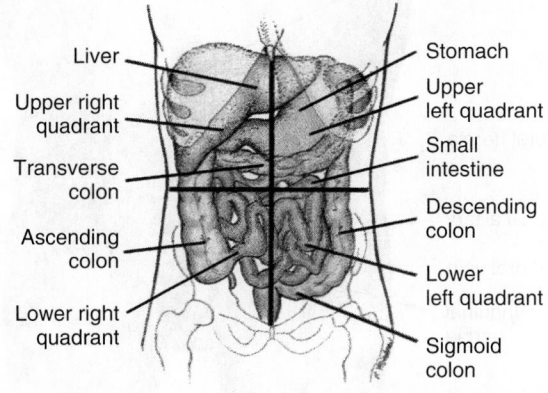

**Fig. 7-41**   Location of structures in abdomen. Cross rules divide cavity into quadrants. (From Potter PA, Perry AG: *Basic nursing: theory and practice,* ed 4, St Louis, 1999, Mosby.)

domen to form characteristic adult curves, especially in the female.

The *size* and *tone* of the abdomen also give some indication of general nutritional status and muscular development. A large, prominent, flabby abdomen is often seen in obese children, whereas a concave abdomen suggests undernutrition. Carefully note a protruding abdomen, which may indicate pathologic states such as abdominal distention, ascites, tumors, or organomegaly. A protuberant abdomen with spindly extremities and flat, wasted buttocks suggests severe malnutrition that may occur from inadequate protein-energy intake or from diseases such as cystic fibrosis. A midline protrusion from the xiphoid to the umbilicus or pubic symphysis usually indicates *diastasis recti,* or failure of the rectus abdominis muscles to join in utero. In a healthy child a midline protrusion is usually a variation of normal muscular development.

> **NURSING ALERT**  A tense, boardlike abdomen is a serious sign of paralytic ileus and intestinal obstruction.

The *skin* covering the abdomen should be uniformly taut, without wrinkles or creases. Sometimes silvery, whitish striae are seen, especially if the skin has been stretched as in obesity or with distention resulting from ascites. Note any scars, ecchymotic areas, excessive hair distribution, or distended veins. Superficial veins may be visible in thin, light-skinned children, but distended veins are an abnormal finding and suggest vascular or abdominal obstruction or abdominal distention.

Observe *movement* of the abdomen. In infants and thin children *peristaltic waves* may be visible through the abdominal wall. They are best observed by standing at eye level to and across from the abdomen. Always report this finding because visible peristaltic waves most often indicate pathologic states, particularly intestinal obstruction such as pyloric stenosis. Abdominal movement in relation to respiration is discussed on p. 210.

Inspect the *umbilicus* for herniation, discharge, hygiene, and fistulas, such as a patent *urachus* (an abnormal connection between the umbilicus and bladder). If a herniation is present, palpate the sac for abdominal contents and estimate the approximate size of the opening. *Umbilical hernias* are common in infants, especially in African-American children. Because "home remedies" for treatment, such as taping coins over the umbilicus or using "belly binders," may be harmful to the skin and actually delay natural closure, ask parents whether such procedures have been used and advise against continuing their use. Umbilical hernias normally protrude and expand when the child coughs, cries, or strains.

Hernias may exist elsewhere on the abdominal wall, such as in the inguinal or femoral region (Fig. 7-42). An *inguinal hernia* is a protrusion of peritoneum through the abdominal wall in the inguinal canal. It occurs mostly in males, is often bilateral, and may be visible as a mass in the scrotum. To locate a hernia, slide the little finger into the external inguinal ring at the base of the scrotum and ask the child to cough. If a hernia is present, it will hit the tip of the finger.

**NURSING TIP**  If the child is too young to cough, have the child blow up a balloon or laugh to raise the intraabdominal pressure sufficiently to demonstrate the presence of an inguinal hernia.

A *femoral hernia,* which occurs more commonly in girls, is felt or seen as a small mass on the anterior surface of the thigh just below the inguinal ligament in the femoral canal (a potential space medial to the femoral artery). Feel for a hernia by placing the index finger of your right hand on the child's right femoral pulse (left hand for left pulse) and the middle ring finger flat against the skin toward the midline. The ring finger lies over the femoral canal, where the herniation occurs. Palpation of hernias in the pelvic region, particularly inguinal ones, is often part of the examination of genitalia.

## Auscultation

Auscultate each of the four quadrants using the diaphragm and bell chestpieces. Unlike when listening to the heart or lungs, in which the stethoscope rests gently on the skin, the stethoscope must be pressed firmly against the abdominal surface to hear bowel sounds. With the diaphragm chestpiece this usually presents no difficulty, but with the bell chestpiece, especially one with a short cone, the skin may occlude the opening and prevent transmission of sound.

The most important sound to listen for is *peristalsis,* or *bowel sounds,* which sound like short metallic clicks and gurgles. Loud grumbling noises, known as *borborygmi,* are the familiar "stomach growls" and usually denote hunger. Depending on when the child last ate, a sound may be heard every 10 to 30 seconds; record its frequency per minute. Bowel sounds may be stimulated by stroking the abdominal surface with a fingernail. Always report hyperperistalsis or

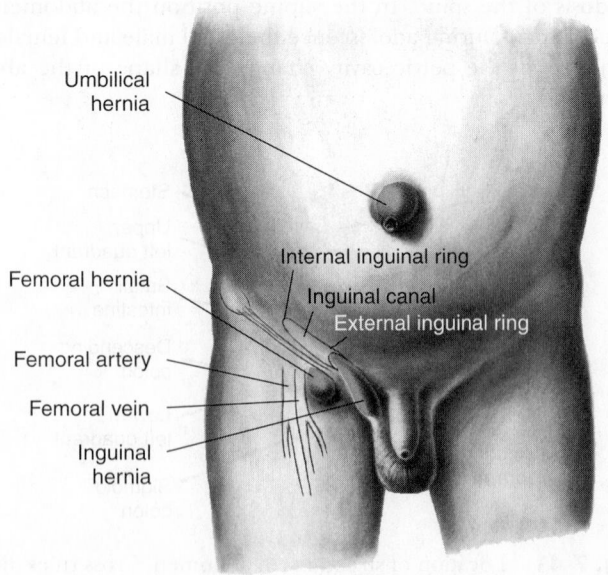

Umbilical hernia

Femoral hernia

Femoral artery

Femoral vein

Inguinal hernia

Internal inguinal ring

Inguinal canal

External inguinal ring

**Fig. 7-42**   Location of hernias.

an absence of bowel sounds because either usually denotes an abdominal disorder.

Various other sounds may be heard in the abdominal cavity. Normally the pulsation of the aorta is heard in the epigastrium. Always refer sounds that resemble murmurs (called *bruits*), hums, or rubs for further evaluation.

## Percussion

Percuss the abdomen in the same manner as with percussion of the lungs (see Fig. 7-36). Normally dullness or flatness is heard on the right side at the lower costal margin because of the location of the liver. Tympany is typically heard over the stomach on the left side and in the rest of the abdomen. An unusually tympanitic sound, like the beating of a tight drum, denotes air in the stomach, which is commonly caused by mouth breathing. However, this sound can also indicate a pathologic condition such as low intestinal obstruction or paralytic ileus. Lack of tympany may occur normally when the stomach is full after a meal, but in other situations it may signal the presence of fluid or solid masses. Refer for further investigation any variations in percussion tones not explained by normal physiologic processes.

## Palpation

Two types of palpation are performed: superficial and deep. For *superficial palpation* place the hand lightly against the skin and feel each quadrant, noting any areas of tenderness, muscle tone, and superficial lesions such as cysts. Also test skin turgor, which is discussed on p. 189.

Because superficial palpation is often perceived as tickling, use techniques to minimize this sensation. (See Atraumatic Care box.) Telling the child to stop laughing only draws attention to the sensation and decreases cooperation. Always note tenderness or pain anywhere in the abdomen

during superficial palpation. There are two types of abdominal pain:

1. **Visceral,** which arises from the viscera or internal organs, such as the intestines, and is usually dull, poorly localized, and difficult for the patient to describe
2. **Somatic,** which arises from the walls or linings of the abdominal cavity, such as the peritoneum, and is generally sharp, well-localized, and more easily described

When assessing abdominal pain, remember that children often respond with an "all-or-none" reaction—either there is no pain or there is great pain. Using a pain measurement scale helps children more specifically rate pain intensity and distinguish pain from fear. (See Pain Assessment, Chapter 26.) One approach is to ask children "how thin" and "how fat" they can make themselves. If this produces discomfort, some degree of peritoneal irritation is probably present.

**NURSING TIP** When a child complains of abdominal pain, observe whether the child's eyes are opened or closed during palpation of the abdomen. The natural reaction of patients with genuine abdominal tenderness is to watch the palpating hand carefully.

Elicit *rebound tenderness,* or *Blumberg sign,* if the child complains of abdominal pain. Press firmly over part of the abdomen distal to the area of tenderness and release the pressure suddenly. Rebound tenderness is present if the child feels pain in the original area of tenderness. This response is found only when the peritoneum overlying a diseased organ is inflamed, such as in appendicitis.

Use *deep palpation* for palpating organs and large blood vessels and for detecting masses and tenderness not discovered during superficial palpation. If the child complains of abdominal pain, palpate that area of the abdomen *last.* Normally palpation of the midepigastrium causes pain as pressure is exerted over the aorta, but this should not be confused with visceral or somatic tenderness.

Palpate the abdominal organs by pressing them against your free hand, which is placed on the child's side (Fig. 7-43). Begin palpation in the lower quadrants and proceed upward

## ATRAUMATIC CARE

### Promoting Relaxation During Abdominal Palpation

Position child comfortably, such as in a semireclining position in the parent's lap, with knees flexed.

Warm the hands before touching the skin.

Use distraction, such as telling stories or talking to child.

Teach child to use deep breathing and to concentrate on an object.

Give infant a bottle or pacifier.

Begin with light, superficial palpation and gradually progress to deeper palpation.

Palpate any tender or painful areas last.

Have child hold the parent's hand and squeeze it if palpation is uncomfortable.

Use the nonpalpating hand to comfort child, such as placing the free hand on child's shoulder while palpating the abdomen.

To minimize sensation of tickling during palpation:

Have children "help" with palpation by placing their hand over the palpating hand.

Have them place their hand on the abdomen with the fingers spread wide apart and palpate between their fingers.

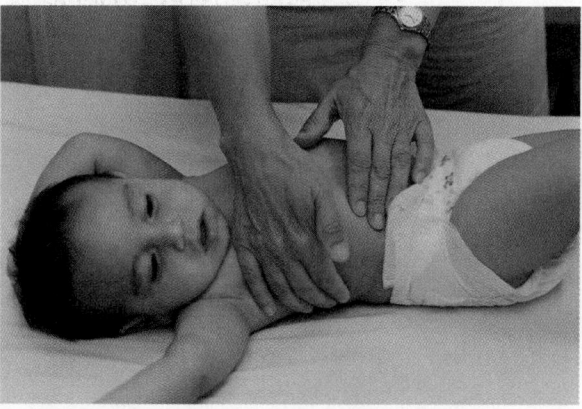

**Fig. 7-43** Palpation of abdominal organs. (Courtesy Paul Vincent Kuntz, Texas Children's Hospital.)

to avoid missing the edge of an enlarged liver or spleen. Except for palpating the liver, successful identification of other organs, such as the spleen, kidney, and part of the colon, requires considerable practice with tutored supervision.

The lower edge of the *liver* is sometimes palpable in infants and young children as a superficial mass 1 to 2 cm (⅜ to ¾ inch) below the right costal margin (the distance is sometimes measured in fingerbreadths). Normally the liver descends during inspiration as the diaphragm moves downward. This downward displacement should not be mistaken for a sign of hepatomegaly. In older children the liver often is not palpable.

Palpate the *spleen* by feeling it between the hand placed against the back and the one palpating the left upper quadrant. The spleen is much smaller than the liver and is positioned behind the fundus of the stomach. The tip of the spleen may be felt during inspiration as it descends within the abdominal cavity. It is sometimes palpable 1 to 2 cm below the left costal margin in infants and young children.

> **NURSING ALERT**
> If the liver is palpable 3 cm below the right costal margin or the spleen is palpable more than 2 cm below the left costal margin, these organs are enlarged—a finding that is always reported for further medical investigation.

Other anatomic structures that are sometimes palpable in children include the kidney, bladder, cecum, and sigmoid colon. Palpation of the *kidney,* which is discussed in Chapter 8 under assessment of the neonate, is quite difficult because of its deep position within the abdominal cavity. Normally only the tip of the right kidney is palpable because of its lower placement within the cavity, and it is best felt during inspiration. The *bladder* may be palpated slightly above the pubic symphysis in infants and young children. It descends deeper into the pelvic cavity during adolescence, when it is not palpable except if distended. Occasionally parts of the colon are palpable. The *cecum* is a soft, gas-filled mass in the right lower quadrant. The *sigmoid colon* is felt as a sausage-shaped mass that is freely movable over the pelvic brim in the left lower quadrant; it is normally tender.

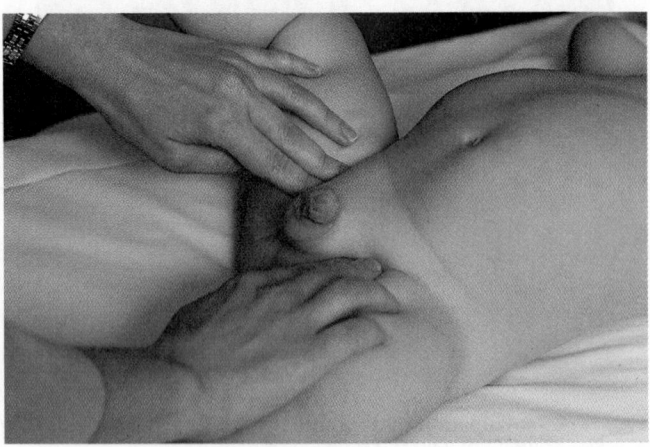

**Fig. 7-44** Palpating for femoral pulses.

Although most of these structures are not routinely felt, be aware of their relative location and characteristics to avoid mistaking them for abnormal masses that require additional investigation. The most common palpable mass in children is feces, which may be associated with pain in the right lower quadrant from a distended cecum. In sexually active pubescent females a palpable mass in the lower abdomen may be a pregnant uterus.

During palpation of the abdomen locate the *femoral pulses* by placing the tips of two or three fingers (index, middle, and/or ring) along the inguinal ligament about midway between the iliac crest and pubic symphysis. Feel both pulses simultaneously to make certain they are equal and strong (Fig. 7-44).

> **NURSING ALERT**
> Absence of femoral pulses is a significant sign of coarctation of the aorta and is referred for medical evaluation.

When examining the abdomen, test the *abdominal reflexes* by scratching the skin toward the umbilicus. The normal response is for the umbilicus to move toward the stimulus or quadrant that was stroked. Normally the response may be absent in children under 1 year of age. Although there is great variability in correctly eliciting a response, note and report asymmetry or absence of response.

## Genitalia

Examination of the genitalia conveniently follows assessment of the abdomen, while the child is still supine. In adolescents, inspection of the genitalia may be left to the end of the examination. This part of the physical appraisal is usually uneventful for infants or toddlers but begins to be anxiety-producing for older preschoolers, school-age children, and adolescents, mainly because of their concern for modesty and privacy. (See Atraumatic Care box.)

In examining the genitalia, wear gloves whenever touching body substances. It might be helpful for the adolescent to know that wearing gloves also prevents skin-to-skin contact.

The genital examination is an excellent time for eliciting questions of concern about body functioning or sexual activity. Also use this opportunity to increase or reinforce the child's knowledge of reproductive anatomy by naming each body part and explaining its function. For example, many females are unaware of the existence of two openings within the vulva. They assume that the passage of urine occurs from the vagina. For males, this part of the health assessment is an opportune time to teach testicular self-examination.

### Male Genitalia

Note the external appearance of the glans and shaft of the penis, the prepuce, the urethral meatus, and the scrotum (Fig. 7-45). The size of the *penis* is generally small in infants and young boys until puberty, when it begins to increase in both length and width. A very small penis may actually be an enlarged clitoris in a genetically female child. In an obese child the penis often looks abnormally small because of the folds of skin partially covering it at the base. An enlarged penis in a young child may denote precocious puberty. Be familiar with normal pubertal growth of the external male genitalia in order to compare the findings with the expected sequence of maturation. (See Fig. 19-6.)

Examine the *glans* (head of the penis) and *shaft* (portion between the perineum and prepuce) for signs of swelling, skin lesions, inflammation, or other irregularities. Any of these signs may indicate underlying disorders, especially sexually transmitted diseases. Consider the possibility of sexual abuse, especially in young children, if sexually transmitted disease is present.

If the child is uncircumcised, inspect the *prepuce*, or *foreskin*, covering the glans. In infants the prepuce is normally tight and is not retracted for examination because accidental tearing of the thin membrane may cause later scarring and adhesion formation. In children *gently* retract the foreskin to examine the glans and the meatus and then *replace it*. A tight foreskin that cannot be retracted in older boys is called *phimosis*.

Carefully inspect the *urethral meatus* for location and evidence of discharge. Normally the urethral meatus is centered at the tip of the shaft. An opening on the ventral, or underneath, side of the glans or shaft is called *hypospadias*. An opening on the dorsal, or top, part of the penis is termed *epispadias*. If the urethral meatus opens into the perineum at the junction of the scrotum, look for signs suggesting ambiguous genitalia. If feasible during inspection, note the strength and direction of the urinary stream during micturition.

### ATRAUMATIC CARE
**Examination of Genitalia**

Offer older children and adolescents the choice of whether or not they wish to be accompanied by a family member. Whenever possible, the sex of the examiner should also be an option for the teenager. Studies show that some young people feel more comfortable with an examiner of the same sex, although males and females report feeling comfortable with a female examiner (Neinstein and others, 1989). For females, the semisitting position is less stressful than the supine position for the pelvic examination.

Examine the genitalia matter-of-factly, placing no more emphasis on this part of the assessment than on any other segment. Explain each step of the examination before it is performed, such as checking the scrotum for an inguinal hernia. If male adolescents have an erection during the examination, reassure them that this is a normal involuntary reflex to touch, not a sexual response, and complete the rest of the examination. It helps to relieve children's and parents' anxiety by stating the findings (e.g., "Everything looks fine here").

If it is necessary to ask questions about deviations, such as about discharge or difficulty in urinating, respect the child's privacy by covering the lower abdomen with the gown or underpants. To prevent embarrassing interruptions, keep the door or curtain closed and post a "do not disturb" sign. Have a drape ready to cover the genitalia if someone enters the room.

One of the most important factors in successfully performing an atraumatic examination is to recognize any personal fears or anxieties and deal with them. Transfer of anxiety, especially in the beginning practitioner, can increase the child's concern or fear.

Observe the size of the *scrotum.* In infants the scrota appear large in relation to the rest of the genitalia. Normally the left scrotum hangs lower than the right, and both hang freely from the perineum behind the penis. Note scrota that are small or close to the perineum or that have any midline separation, which could be enlarged labia. An abnormally large scrotal sac may indicate an inguinal hernia, a hydrocele, or inflammation of the internal reproductive structures, particularly the epididymis.

The skin of the scrotum is usually loose and highly rugated (wrinkled). During early adolescence the skin normally becomes redder and coarser. In dark-skinned children the scrota are more deeply pigmented. Report a smooth, shiny surface with pigmentation that varies markedly from the surrounding skin.

Also note *hair distribution.* Normally no pubic hair is present before puberty. Soft downy hair at the base of the penis is an early sign of pubertal maturation. In older adolescent males hair distribution is diamond-shaped and extends from the anus to the umbilicus.

While palpating the scrotum, feel for the testes, epididymis, spermatic cords and, if present, inguinal hernias. The two *testes* are felt as small ovoid bodies, approximately 1.5 to 2 cm (½ to ¾ inch) long—one in each scrotal sac. They do not enlarge until puberty, when they approximately double in size. Normally the testes descend during the last trimester of uterine development, usually by the eighth month of gestation. Therefore undescended testes *(cryptorchidism)* is a common finding in premature infants.

Palpating for the presence of the testes requires an understanding of the normal anatomy and physiology of the coverings of the testes and scrotal sac. The scrotum and testes are surrounded by cremasteric fascia, which extends to the cremaster muscle. This muscle attaches to a point in the abdomen and extends downward along the inner surface of the thigh. The muscle or *cremasteric reflex* is stimulated by cold, touch, emotional excitement, or exercise. When contracted, this muscle causes the skin of the scrotum to shrink and pulls the testes higher into the pelvic cavity.

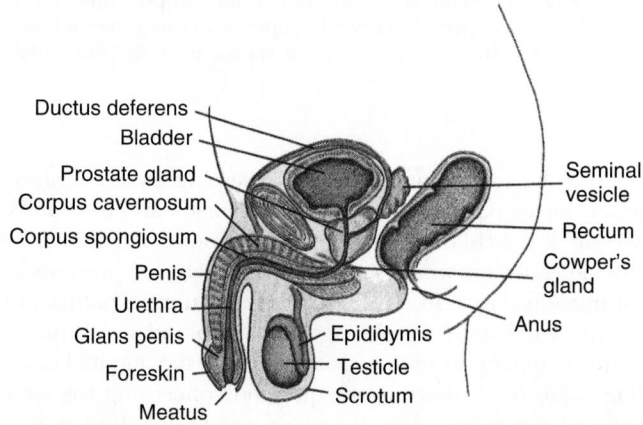

**Fig. 7-45** Major structures of genitalia in uncircumcised postpubertal male. (From Potter PA, Perry AG: *Basic nursing: theory and practice*, ed 4, St Louis, 1999, Mosby.)

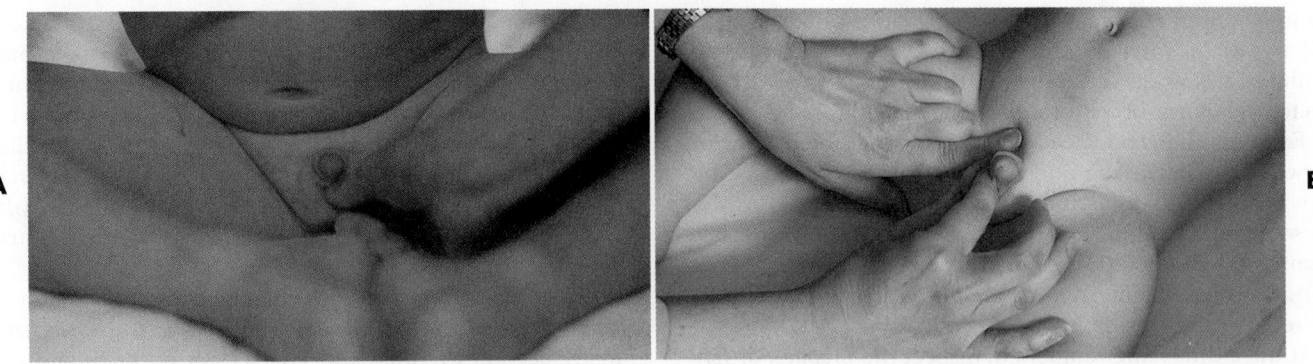

**Fig. 7-46** **A,** Preventing cremasteric reflex by having child sit in " tailor" position. **B,** Blocking inguinal canal during palpation of scrotum for descended testes.

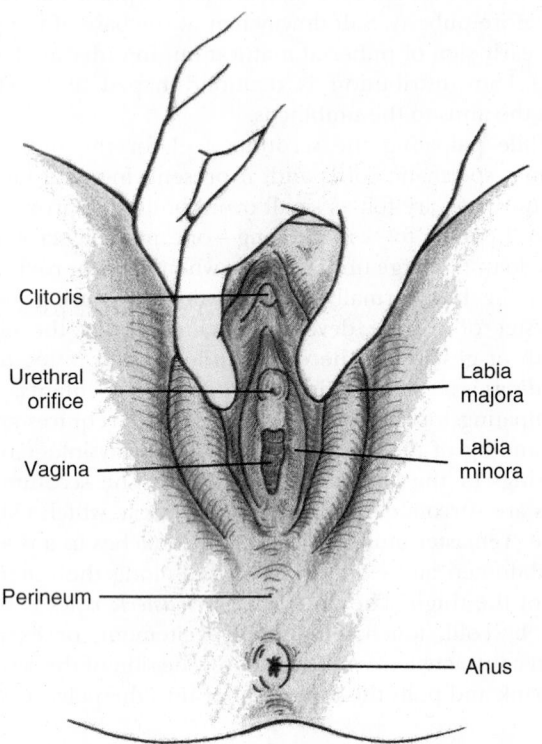

Clitoris

Urethral orifice

Vagina

Labia majora

Labia minora

Perineum

Anus

**Fig. 7-47** External structures of genitalia in postpubertal female. Labia are spread to reveal deeper structures. (From Potter PA, Perry AG: *Basic nursing: theory and practice*, ed 4, St Louis, 1999, Mosby.)

Several measures are useful in preventing the cremasteric reflex during palpation of the scrotum. First, warm the hands. Second, if the child is old enough, examine him in a tailor or "Indian" position, which stretches the muscle and prevents its contraction (Fig. 7-46, *A*). Third, block the normal pathway of ascent of the testes by placing the thumb and index finger over the upper part of the scrotal sac along the inguinal canal (Fig. 7-46, *B*). If there is any question concerning the existence of two testes, place the index and middle fingers in a scissors fashion to separate the right and left scrota. If after using these techniques the testes have not been palpated, feel along the inguinal canal and perineum to locate masses that

may be undescended testes. Although undescended testes may descend at any time during childhood and are checked at each visit, report the failure to palpate testes.

The *epididymis* is a vertical ridge of soft nodular tissue behind the testes. The *spermatic cord* consists of the blood vessels, nerves, lymphatic glands, and the ductus deferens of the testes. Note and report any masses, swelling, or tenderness.

### Female Genitalia

The examination of female genitalia is limited to the inspection and palpation of external structures. If a vaginal examination is required, an appropriate referral is made unless the nurse is qualified to perform the procedure. A convenient position for examination of the genitalia involves placing the young child supine on the examining table or in a semireclining position on the parent's lap, with the feet supported on your knees as you sit facing the child. Divert the child's attention from the examination by instructing her to try to keep the soles of her feet pressed against each other. Separate the labia majora with the thumb and index finger to expose the labia minora, urethral meatus, and vaginal orifice. Have the child use her hands "to help."

Inspect the genitalia for size and location of the structures of the *vulva* or *pudendum* (area of the external genital organs) (Fig. 7-47). The *mons pubis* is a pad of adipose tissue over the symphysis pubis. At puberty the mons is covered with hair, which extends along the labia. The usual pattern of female *hair distribution* is an inverted triangle. The appearance of soft downy hair along the labia majora is an early sign of sexual maturation.

The *clitoris,* an erectile organ located at the anterior end of the labia minora, is covered by a small flap of skin, the *prepuce.* Note its size because, although variable, a large protruding clitoris may represent an underdeveloped phallus.

The *labia majora* are two thick folds of skin running posteriorly from the mons to the posterior commissure of the vagina. Internal to the labia majora are two folds of skin, the *labia minora.* Although the labia are prominent in the newborn, they gradually atrophy and are almost invisible until their enlargement during puberty.

The inner surface of the labia should be pink and moist. Note any skin lesions such as chancres, blisters, or warts (condylomata acuminata) because they may be sexually transmitted. Observe the size of the labia and any evidence of fusion, which may suggest male scrota. Normally no masses are palpable within the labia. However, in genitalia of an ambiguous nature, palpable masses may represent descended testes.

The urethral meatus and vaginal orifice are located in the space between the labia, the *vestibule.* The **urethral meatus** is located posterior to the clitoris and is surrounded by Skene glands and ducts. Although not a prominent structure, the meatus appears as a small V-shaped slit. Note its location, especially if it opens from the clitoris or inside the vagina. Gently palpate the glands, which are common sites of cysts.

The *vaginal orifice* is located posterior to the urethral meatus. Its appearance is variable depending on individual anatomy and sexual activity. Ordinarily examination of the vagina is limited to inspection. However, in the presence of signs suggesting ambiguous genitalia, refer or perform a manual examination to determine if a vaginal vault exists.

In virgins a thin, crescent-shaped or circular membrane called the *hymen* may cover part of the vaginal opening. In some instances, it completely occludes the orifice. After rupture, small rounded pieces of tissue called *caruncles* remain. Although an imperforate hymen denotes lack of penile intercourse, a perforate one does not necessarily indicate sexual activity. (See Sexual Abuse, Chapter 16.)

> **NURSING ALERT**
> In females who have been circumcised, the genitalia will appear different. Do not show surprise or disgust, but note the appearance and discuss the procedure with the young woman. (See Cultural Awareness box on p. 272.)

Surrounding the vaginal opening are *Bartholin glands,* which secrete a clear, mucoid fluid into the vagina for lubrication during intercourse. Palpate the ducts for cysts and note the discharge from the vagina, which is usually clear or whitish. Variations in appearance (e.g., white and cheesy or yellow-green) and odor may indicate infection. Sudden, foul-smelling, and profuse discharge may suggest a foreign body inside the vaginal vault. The presence of feces or urine from the vagina indicates a fistula from the rectum or urethra. Note any swelling, inflammation, or prolapsed area around the vagina and refer for further gynecologic evaluation.

## Anus

Following examination of the genitalia, observe the anal area, preferably by placing the child on the abdomen. Note the general firmness of the buttocks and symmetry of the gluteal folds. Assess the tone of the anal sphincter by eliciting the *anal reflex.* Scratching or gently pricking the anal area results in an obvious quick contraction of the external anal sphincter.

Inspect the sphincter area for *fissures,* small cuts or tears in the mucosa that are painful and often lead to constipation because the child refrains from defecating; *prolapse* of the rectum, which is evident as a tubelike protrusion that can be retracted manually; *polyps,* cherry-red protrusions that often cause bleeding; and *hemorrhoids,* dark protrusions of blood vessels. Report any of these findings for further medical investigation. Note any *mucosal tabs,* benign protrusions of skin attached to the anal sphincter.

Inspect the skin around the anal area for lesions, the most common of which are caused by diaper rash. If the child complains of perianal itching, testing for pinworms is recommended.

## Back and Extremities

### Spine

Observe the general *curvature* of the spine. Normally the back of a newborn is rounded or C-shaped from the thoracic and pelvic curves. The development of the cervical and lumbar curves approximates development of various motor skills, such as cervical curvature with head control, and gives the older child the typical double-S curve.

Marked curvatures in posture are abnormal. (See Fig. 39-34.) *Scoliosis,* lateral curvature of the spine, is an important childhood problem, especially in females. Although scoliosis may be palpated by feeling along the spine and noting a sideways displacement, more objective tests include the following:

- With the child standing erect, clothed only in underpants (and bra if older girl), observe from behind, noting asymmetry of the shoulders and hips.
- With the child bending forward so that the back is parallel to the floor, observe from the side, noting asymmetry or prominence of the rib cage.

A slight limp, a crooked hemline, or complaints of a sore back are other signs and symptoms of scoliosis.

Inspect the *back,* especially along the spine, for any tufts of hair, dimples, or discoloration. A small dimple (usually with a tuft of hair), called a *pilonidal cyst,* may indicate an underlying spina bifida occulta. Palpate the spine to identify the presence or absence of each spiny process of the vertebrae.

*Mobility* of the vertebral column is easily assessed in most children because of their propensity for constant motion during the examination. To specifically test mobility, ask the child to sit up from a prone position or to do a modified sit-up exercise. Maintaining a rigid straightness when performing these maneuvers is considered abnormal and may indicate central nervous system infection or irritation. However, some individuals who are unable to relax, despite normal skeletal function, may also retain a rigid posture.

Movement of the cervical spine is an important diagnostic sign for neurologic problems, such as meningitis. Normally movement of the head in all directions is effortless.

> **NURSING ALERT**
> Hyperextension of the neck and spine, called *opisthotonos,* which is accompanied by pain when the head is flexed, is always referred for immediate medical evaluation.

## Extremities

Inspect each extremity for symmetry of length and size; refer any deviation for orthopaedic evaluation. Count the fingers and toes to be certain of the normal number. This normalcy is so often taken for granted that an extra digit (*polydactyly*) or fusion of digits (*syndactyly*) may go unnoticed. Also inspect the fingers and toes for any evidence of clubbing, cyanosis, disorders of the nails (including habitual nail biting), and general hygiene. These are discussed in more detail under assessment of the skin (p. 187). If there is any doubt regarding symmetry of leg length, measure the legs from the anterior iliac spine (felt as the point of the pelvis) to the medial malleolus (ankle bone).

Inspect the arms and legs for *temperature, color, tenderness,* and *masses.* The temperature in each extremity should be equal, although the feet may normally be colder than the hands. Coolness denotes decreased circulation, such as from occlusion of a blood vessel, whereas heat indicates increased blood flow, such as from an infection or inflammation. Enlargement of bone, such as from swelling, with redness, heat, and tenderness needs further evaluation. It may signify trauma, infection, or an underlying disease process (e.g., sickle cell disease). A solid mass palpable along a bone with or without pain may be a tumor. Although not all masses are malignant, they must be evaluated further.

Because accidental fractures are common in children, be familiar with assessing orthopaedic injuries. The five main criteria are (1) pain, (2) pulse, (3) paresthesia (abnormal sensation, such as numbness), (4) pallor, and (5) paralysis. Palpation over a possible fractured bone may elicit *crepitation,* a grating sound produced by movement of the broken ends of the bone.

Assess the *shape* of bones. Several variations of bone shape may be observed in children. Although many of them cause parents concern, most are benign and require no treatment. *Bowleg,* or *genu varum,* is lateral bowing of the tibia. It is clinically present when the child stands with the medial malleoli

(rounded prominence on either side of the ankle) in apposition and the space between the knees is greater than approximately 5 cm (2 inches) (Fig. 7-48). Toddlers are usually bowlegged after they begin to walk until all of their lower back and leg muscles develop. Unilateral or asymmetric bowleggedness present beyond the age of 2 to 3 years, particularly in African-American children, may represent a pathologic condition that requires further investigation.

*Knock-knee,* or *genu valgum,* is the opposite of bowleg; the knees are close together but the feet are spread apart. Use the same method of assessment as for genu varum, but measure the distance between the malleoli, which should be less than 7.5 cm (3 inches) (Fig. 7-49). Knock-knee is normally present in children from approximately 2 to 7 years of age. Knock-knee that is excessive (as measured roentgenographically by the tibiofemoral angle), asymmetric, accompanied by shortened stature, or evident in a child nearing puberty requires further evaluation.

Observe the *feet* for arch development and correct gait. Infants' and toddlers' feet appear flat because the foot is normally wide and the arch is covered by a fat pad. Development of the arch occurs naturally from the action of walking. Normally at birth the feet are held in a valgus (outward) or varus (inward) position. To determine whether a foot deformity at birth is the result of intrauterine position or development, scratch the outer, then inner, side of the sole. If the foot position is self-correctable, it will assume a right angle to the leg.

Assess *gait* by having the child walk; estimate the angle of gait, which is the angle between the axis of the foot (imaginary line drawn through center of foot) and the line of progression (Fig. 7-50). Normally the feet turn outward less than 30 degrees and inward less than 10 degrees. Variations in foot positions are described in Chapter 11.

Toddlers have a "toddling" or broad-based gait, which facilitates walking by lowering the center of gravity. As the child reaches preschool age, the legs are brought closer to-

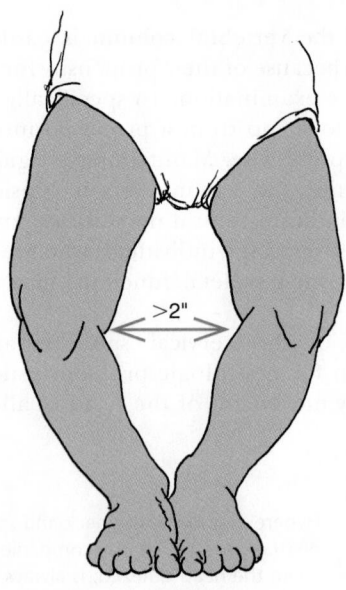

**Fig. 7-48** Bowleg.

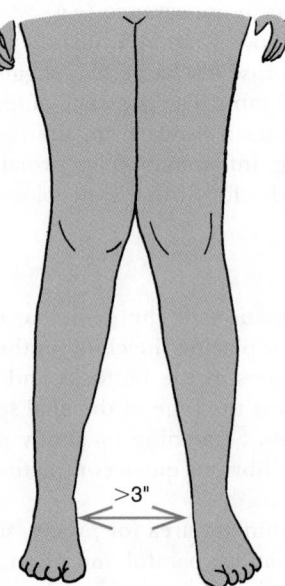

**Fig. 7-49** Knock-knee.

gether. By school age the walking posture is much more graceful and balanced.

The most common gait problem in young children is *pigeon toe,* or *toeing in,* which usually results from torsional deformities such as internal tibial torsion (abnormal rotation or bowing of the tibia). Tests for tibial torsion include measuring the thigh-foot angle, which requires considerable practice for accuracy.

Observe for walking on the toes. Toe walking, in the absence of neuromuscular disorders, is normal in infants. If it persists longer than 3 months, refer the child for an orthopaedic evaluation.

Test the *plantar* or *grasp reflex* while examining the feet. Exert firm but gentle pressure, with the tip of the thumb against the lateral sole of the foot from the heel upward to the little toe and then across to the big toe. The normal response in children who are walking is flexion of the toes. *Babinski sign,* the dorsiflexion of the big toe and fanning of the other toes, is normal during infancy but abnormal after about 1 year or when locomotion begins. (See Fig. 8-9.) A positive Babinski sign after age 1 year indicates spinal cord lesions and requires further neurologic examination.

### Joints

Evaluate the joints for *range of motion.* Normally this requires no specific testing other than observing the child's movements during the examination. However, check the hips for signs of congenital dislocation. (See Developmental Dysplasia of the Hip, Chapter 11.) Report any evidence of joint immobility or hyperflexibility.

Palpate the joints for *heat, tenderness,* and *swelling.* These signs, as well as redness over the joint, may indicate infection or any of the collagen diseases and warrant further investigation.

### Muscles

Note symmetry and quality of muscle development, tone, and strength. Observe *development* by looking at the shape and contour of the body in both a relaxed and a tensed state. Estimate *tone* by grasping the muscle and feeling its firmness when it is relaxed and contracted. A common site for testing tone is the biceps muscle of the arm. Children are usually willing to "make a muscle" by clenching their fist.

Estimate *strength* by having the child use an extremity to push or pull against resistance, as in the following examples:

**Arm strength.** Child holds the arms outstretched in front of the body and tries to raise the arms while downward pressure is applied.
**Hand strength.** Child shakes hands with nurse and squeezes one or two fingers of the nurse's hand.
**Leg strength.** Child sits on a table or chair with the legs dangling and tries to raise the legs while downward pressure is applied.

Note symmetry of strength in the extremities, hands, and fingers and report any evidence of paresis or weakness.

## Neurologic Assessment

The assessment of the nervous system is the broadest and most diverse because every human function—physical and emotional—is controlled by neurologic impulses. This discussion focuses primarily on a general appraisal of behavior, cognitive-perceptual development, sensory and cerebellar functioning, deep tendon reflexes, the cranial nerves, and "soft" signs.

### Behavior

There is no special testing for behavior. It is instead an overall impression of the child's personality, affect, level of activity, social interaction, and attention span. Some aspects of assessing behavior are discussed elsewhere (see p. 187). Difficulties at home, at school, and in social situations suggest the need for additional psychologic assessment.

*State of consciousness* is a specific area for behavior under neurologic assessment. Hyperirritability, hyporeactivity, lethargy, delirium, stupor, or coma requires immediate referral. Levels of consciousness are described in Chapter 37. Always question parents' perceptions of changes in behavior, which usually precede an altered level of consciousness.

### Cognitive-Perceptual Development

Cognitive-perceptual development is best assessed using a standard screening test. Adaptive and speech-comprehension development are significant indicators of intellectual functioning. If intellectual or perceptual impairment is suspected or if learning difficulties exist, refer the child to an appropriate developmental specialist for further evaluation. "Soft" signs that should suggest minimum or borderline brain dysfunction are discussed at the conclusion of this section (p. 228).

### Motor Functioning

Motor ability primarily involves assessment of voluntary muscle contraction and acquisition of age-specific developmental milestones for gross and fine motor skills (see Developmental Assessment, p. 233). One of the most important milestones in motor development is *head control.* Because development proceeds in the cephalocaudal direction, head lag suggests early brain damage. Head control is usually acquired by 4 months of age although, as discussed in Chapter 8, even the newborn demonstrates some head control.

Also observe *handedness.* Infants and toddlers may show preference for one hand, but they usually do not display marked preference until the preschool years. The sole use of one hand may indicate paresis on the opposite side. A school-age child's failure to demonstrate handedness suggests failure of the brain to develop dominance, but its diagnostic significance is controversial.

### Sensory Functioning

Sensory functioning is assessed mainly in terms of the sensory cranial nerves (in particular, vision and hearing) and

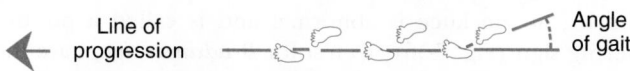

**Fig. 7-50**  Measurement of angle of gait.

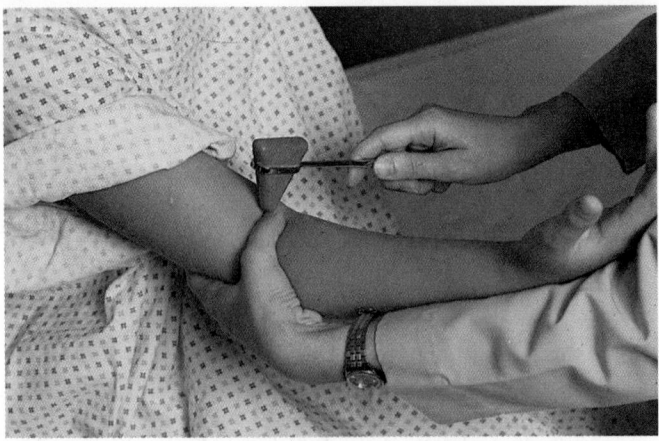

**Fig. 7-51** Testing for biceps reflex. Hold child's partially flexed elbow in palm of hand with your thumb over antecubital space. Strike thumbnail with hammer. Normal response is partial flexion of forearm.

peripheral sensation. This discussion is devoted to the testing of peripheral sensation. Testing of the cranial nerves is discussed on p. 227, and vision and auditory testing are discussed on pp. 195 and 203, respectively.

**Peripheral Sensation.** With children old enough to cooperate, assess *sensory discrimination* by performing the activities in Box 7-7 with the child's eyes closed. Because these tests are similar to playing a game, consider introducing them at the beginning of the examination to decrease the child's anxiety and foster trust.

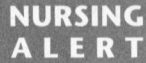 **NURSING ALERT** Decreased sensation and hyperesthesia (excessive sensation) are abnormal and must be referred for further neurologic evaluation.

## Cerebellar Functioning

The cerebellum mainly controls balance and coordination. Much of the assessment of cerebellar functioning involves observing the child's posture, body movements, gait, and development of fine and gross motor skills. Tests such as balancing on one foot and the heel-to-toe walk in the Denver II also assess balance. Test *coordination* by asking the child to reach for a toy, button clothes, tie shoes, or draw a straight line on a piece of paper, provided the child is old enough to accomplish these activities.

Several tests for cerebellar function are described in Box 7-8 and can be performed as games. When the Romberg test is performed, stay beside the child if there is a possibility that the child may fall.

School-age children should be able to perform these tests, although preschoolers normally can bring the finger only within 5 to 7.5 cm (2 to 3 inches) of their nose. Difficulty in performing these exercises indicates a poor sense of position (especially with the eyes closed) and incoordination (especially with the eyes open). Coordination can also be

tested by any sequence of rapid successive movements, such as quickly touching each finger with the thumb of the same hand. Cerebellar testing is particularly significant in children with symptoms of hyperactivity or learning difficulty.

## Reflexes

Testing reflexes is an important part of the neurologic examination. Persistence of primitive reflexes, loss of reflexes, or hyperactivity of deep tendon reflexes is usually the result of a cerebral insult. The following discussion is primarily concerned with reflexes found in children past infancy. The primitive reflexes of the newborn are discussed in Chapter 8.

Elicit reflexes by using the rubber head of the reflex hammer, flat part of the finger, or side of the hand. Use your hand or finger if the child is easily frightened by equipment. Although testing reflexes is a simple procedure to perform, the child may inhibit the reflex by unconsciously tensing the muscle. To avoid tensing, distract younger children with toys or by talking to them. Have older children grasp their two hands in front of them and try to pull them apart.

Several *superficial reflexes,* such as the abdominal, cremasteric, anal, and plantar, are present. These have been discussed throughout the chapter. *Deep tendon reflexes* are stretch reflexes of a muscle. The most common deep tendon reflex is the knee jerk, or patellar reflex (sometimes called quadriceps reflex). The reflexes normally elicited are described in Figs. 7-51 to 7-55. Use the grading system in Table 7-16 to evaluate reflexes. Report absent or hyperactive reflexes for further evaluation.

Several other reflexes are normally present or absent but are not elicited unless specific indications exist. For example, the Kernig sign and the Brudzinski sign are elicited in the presence of symptoms that suggest meningeal irritation. To test for *Kernig sign,* have the child lie supine with the leg flexed at the hip and knee. Resistance or pain on extending the leg at the knee is abnormal and is called a positive Kernig sign (Fig. 7-56). To test for *Brudzinski sign,* have the child lie supine, and flex the child's head. If this causes pain or causes the knees and hips to flex involuntarily, the Brudzinski sign is positive (Fig. 7-57).

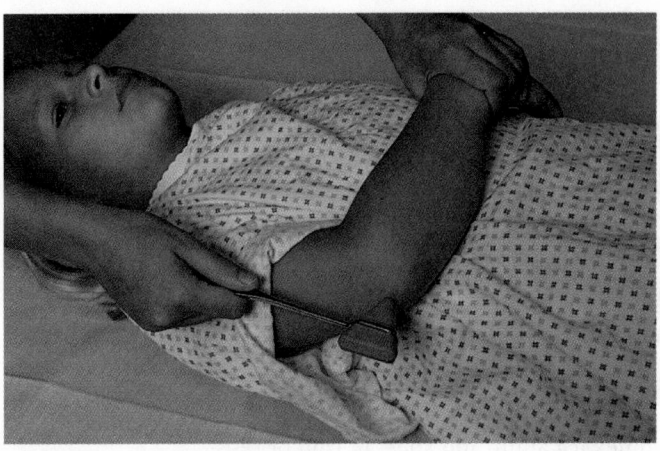

**Fig. 7-52**   Testing for triceps reflex. Child is placed supine, with forearm resting over chest, and triceps tendon is struck. *Alternate procedure:* child's arm is abducted, with upper arm supported and forearm allowed to hang freely. Triceps tendon is struck. Normal response is partial extension of forearm.

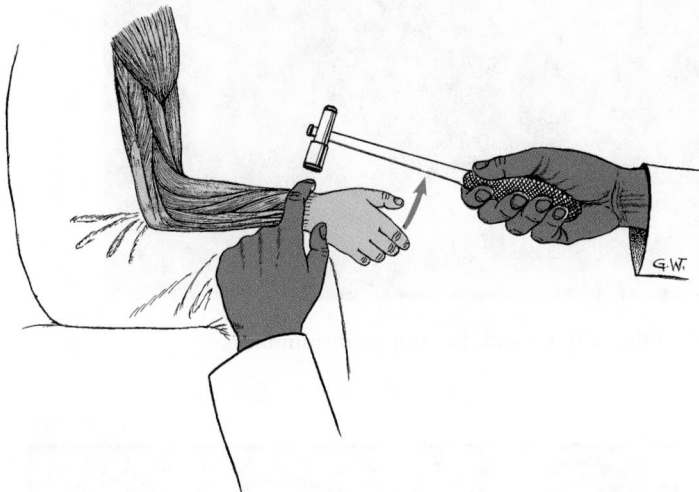

**Fig. 7-53**   Testing for brachioradialis reflex. Place child's forearm on child's lap (if sitting) or abdomen (if supine) with arm flexed at elbow and palm down. Strike radius approximately 1 inch (depending on child's size) above wrist. Normal response is flexion of forearm and supination (turning upward) of palm.

| TABLE 7-16 | Grading of reflexes |
|---|---|
| **Grade** | **Description** |
| 4+ | Extremely brisk, hyperactive |
| 3+ | Brisker than normal |
| 2+ | Average, normal |
| 1+ | Diminished |
| 0+ | Absent |

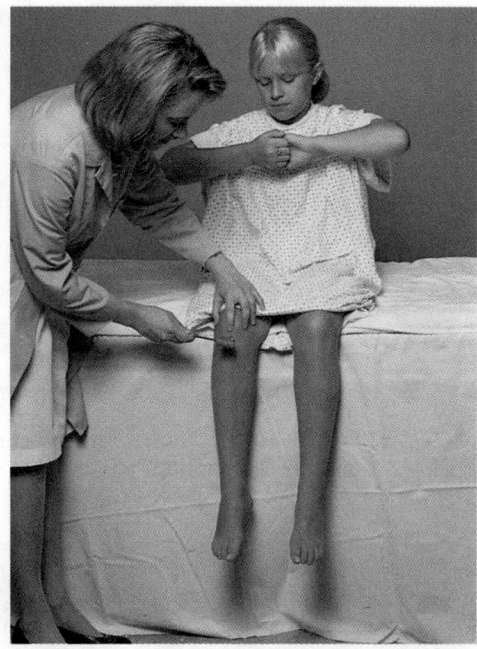

**Fig. 7-54**   Testing for patellar, or knee jerk, reflex using distraction. Child sits on edge of examining table (or on parent's lap) with lower legs flexed at knee and dangling freely. Patellar tendon is tapped just below kneecap. Normal response is partial extension of lower leg.

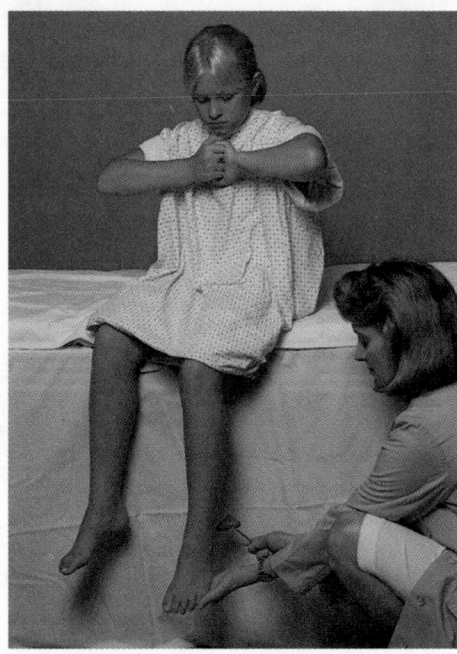

**Fig. 7-55**   Testing for Achilles reflex. Use same position for eliciting knee jerk reflex. Support foot lightly in your hand and strike Achilles tendon. Normal response is plantar flexion of foot (foot pointing downward, or "planting" toward floor).

## Cranial Nerves

Assessment of the cranial nerves is an important area of neurologic assessment (Table 7-17). With young children, present the tests as games at the beginning of the examination to encourage trust and security. The cranial nerve test could also be included when each "system" is examined, such as tongue movement and strength, gag reflex, swallowing, cardinal positions of gaze (Fig. 7-58), and position of the uvula during examination of the mouth.

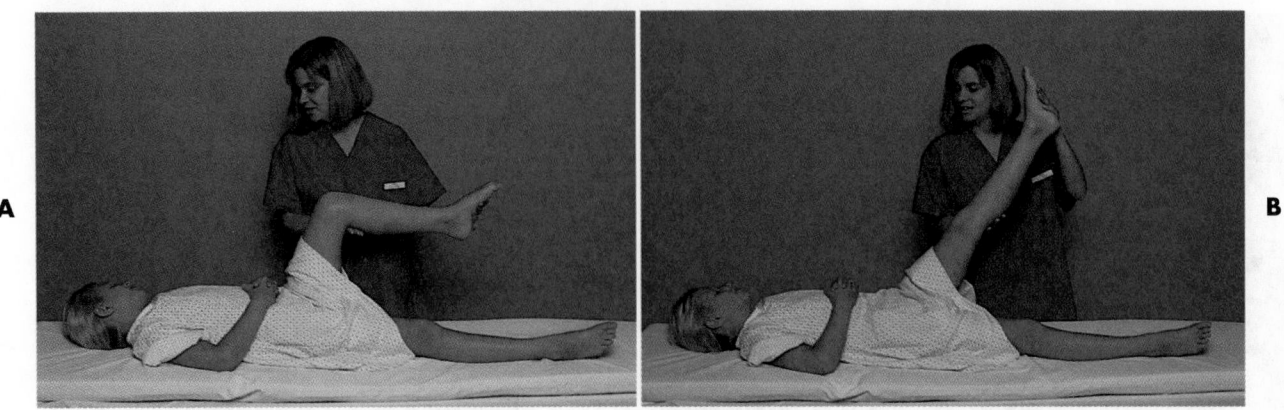

**Fig. 7-56** **A,** Testing for Kernig sign. Have child flex leg at hip and knee. **B,** Pain or resistance on extension is abnormal.

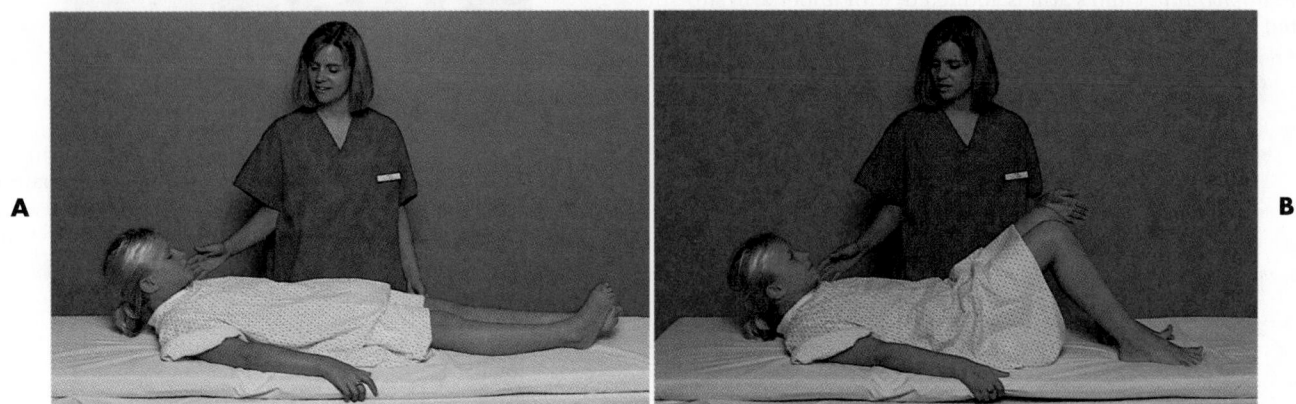

**Fig. 7-57** **A,** Testing for Brudzinski sign. Ask child to flex head. **B,** Pain or involuntary flexion of knees and hips is abnormal.

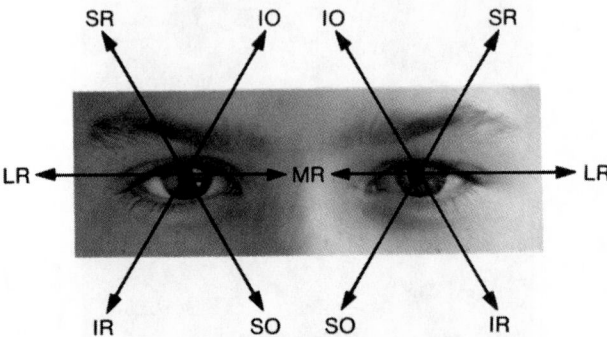

**Fig. 7-58** Testing cardinal positions of gaze.

---

**Box 7-9** ■ ■ ■
**Neurologic "Soft" Signs**

Short attention span
Unusual body movement, such as mirroring
Poor coordination and sense of position
Excessive, sustained, and purposeless movement (hyperactivity)
Hypoactivity
Impulsiveness
Labile emotions
Distractibility
No established handedness
Language and articulation problems
Perceptual deficits (space, form, movement, time)
Problems with learning, especially reading, writing, and arithmetic

---

### "Soft" Signs

One of the difficulties in assessing the nervous system is differentiating clearly between normal and abnormal findings (sometimes referred to as "hard" signs). There is a gray area called "soft" signs—findings that are normal in a young child but disappear in the normal course of maturation.

Soft signs represent the persistence of a more primitive form of behavior or response and a failure to perform the age-specific activity. Although the list of soft signs is long and the controversy concerning their significance far from resolved, some of the classic signs are listed in Box 7-9.

## TABLE 7-17   Assessment of cranial nerves

**Distribution/Function Test**

### I—Olfactory Nerve

Olfactory mucosa of nasal cavity
Smell

With eyes closed, have child identify odors such as coffee, alcohol from a swab, or other smells; test each nostril separately

### II—Optic Nerve

Rods and cones of retina, optic nerve
Vision

Check for perception of light, visual acuity, peripheral vision, color vision, and normal optic disc

### III—Oculomotor Nerve

Extraocular muscles (EOM) of eye:
   Superior rectus (SR)—moves eyeball up and in
   Inferior rectus (IR)—moves eyeball down and in
   Medial rectus (MR)—moves eyeball nasally
   Inferior oblique (IO)—moves eyeball up and out
Pupil constriction and accommodation
Eyelid closing

Have child follow an object (toy) or light in the six cardinal positions of gaze (see Fig. 7-58)
Check pupils for reaction to light
Check for proper placement of lid

### IV—Trochlear Nerve

Superior oblique (SO) muscle—moves eye down and out

Have child look down and in (see Fig. 7-58)

### V-Trigeminal Nerve

Muscles of mastication
Sensory: face, scalp, nasal and buccal mucosa

Have child bite down hard and open jaw; test symmetry and strength
With child's eyes closed, see if child can detect light touch in the mandibular and maxillary regions
Test corneal and blink reflex by touching cornea lightly (approach from the side so that child does not blink before cornea is touched)

### VI—Abducens Nerve

Lateral rectus (LR) muscle—moves eye temporally

Have child look toward temporal side (see Fig. 7-58)

### VII—Facial Nerve

Muscles for facial expression
Anterior two thirds of tongue (sensory)

Have child smile, make a funny face, or show teeth to see symmetry of expression
Have child identify a sweet or salty solution; place each taste on anterior section and sides of protruding tongue; if child retracts tongue, solution will dissolve toward posterior part of tongue

### VIII—Auditory, Acoustic, or Vestibulocochlear Nerve

Internal ear
Hearing and balance

Test hearing; note any loss of equilibrium or presence of vertigo

### IX—Glossopharyngeal Nerve

Pharynx, tongue
Posterior one third of tongue (sensory)

Stimulate posterior pharynx with a tongue blade; child should gag
Test sense of sour or bitter taste on posterior segment of tongue

### X—Vagus Nerve

Muscles of larynx, pharynx, some organs of gastrointestinal system; sensory fibers of root of tongue, heart, lung, and some organs of gastrointestinal system

Note hoarseness of voice, gag reflex, and ability to swallow
Check that uvula is in midline; when stimulated with a tongue blade, should deviate upward and to stimulated side

### XI—Accessory Nerve

Sternocleidomastoid and trapezius muscles of shoulder

Have child shrug shoulders while applying mild pressure; with examiner's hands placed on shoulders, have child turn head against opposing pressure on either side; note symmetry and strength

### XII—Hypoglossal Nerve

Muscles of tongue

Have child move tongue in all directions; have child protrude tongue as far as possible; note any midline deviation
Test strength by placing tongue blade on one side of tongue and having child move it away

## GENERAL CONCEPTS OF MENTAL FUNCTION AND PERSONALITY DEVELOPMENT

Personality and cognitive skills develop in much the same manner as biologic growth—new accomplishments build on previously mastered skills. Many aspects depend on physical growth and maturation. This section does not provide a comprehensive account of the multiple facets of personality and behavior development. Many aspects are integrated with the child's emotional and social development and are discussed in later chapters with various age-groups. Table 7-18 summarizes some of the developmental theories.

## Theoretic Foundations of Personality Development

According to Freud, all human behavior is energized by psychodynamic forces, with this psychic energy being divided among three components of personality: the id, the ego, and the superego. The *id,* the *unconscious mind,* is the inborn component that is driven by instincts. The id obeys the pleasure principle of immediate gratification of needs regardless of whether the object or action can actually do so. The *ego,* the *conscious mind,* serves the reality principle. It functions as the conscious or controlling self that is able to find a realistic means for gratifying instincts while blocking the irrational thinking of the id. The *superego,* the *conscience,* functions as the moral arbitrator and represents the ideal. It is the mechanism that prevents individuals from expressing undesirable instincts that might threaten the social order.

### Psychosexual Development (Freud)

Freud considered the sexual instincts to be significant in personality development. However, he used the term *psychosexual* to describe any **sensual pleasure.** During childhood certain regions of the body assume a prominent psychologic significance as the source of new pleasures and new conflicts gradually shifts from one part of the body to another at particular stages of development:

**Oral stage (birth to 1 year).** During infancy the major source of pleasure seeking is centered on oral activities such as sucking, biting, chewing, and vocalizing. Children may prefer one of these over the others, and the preferred method of oral gratification can provide some indication of the personality they develop.

**Anal stage (1 to 3 years).** Interest during the second year of life centers in the anal region as sphincter muscles develop and children are able to withhold or expel fecal material at will. At this stage the climate surrounding toilet training can have lasting effects on children's personalities.

**Phallic stage (3 to 6 years).** During the phallic stage the genitals become an interesting and sensitive area of the body. Children recognize differences between the sexes and become curious about the dissimilarities. This is the period around which the controversial issues of the Oedipus and Electra complexes, penis envy, and castration anxiety are centered.

**Latency period (6 to 12 years).** During the latency period children elaborate on previously acquired traits and skills. Physical and psychic energy are channeled into the acquisition of knowledge and vigorous play.

**Genital stage (age 12 and over).** The last significant stage begins at puberty with maturation of the reproductive system and production of sex hormones. The genitals become the major source of sexual tension and pleasure, but energies are also invested in forming friendships and preparing for marriage.

**TABLE 7-18**   Summary of personality, cognitive, and moral development theories

| Stage/Age | Psychosexual Stages (Freud) | Psychosocial Stages (Erikson) | Cognitive Stages (Piaget) | Moral Judgment Stages (Kohlberg) |
|---|---|---|---|---|
| **I Infancy** Birth to 1 year | Oral sensory | Trust vs mistrust | Sensorimotor (birth to 2 years) | |
| **II Toddlerhood** 1-3 years | Anal-urethral | Autonomy vs shame and doubt | Preoperational thought, preconceptual phase (transductive reasoning, e.g., specific to specific) (2-4 years) | Preconventional (premoral) level    Punishment and obedience orientation |
| **III Early childhood** 3-6 years | Phallic-locomotion | Initiative vs guilt | Preoperational thought, intuitive phase (transducive reasoning) (4-7 years) | Preconventional (premoral) level    Naive instrumental orientation |
| **IV Middle childhood** 6-12 years | Latency | Industry vs inferiority | Concrete operations (inductive reasoning and beginning logic) (7-11 years) | Conventional level    Good-boy, nice-girl orientation    Law-and-order orientation |
| **V Adolescence** 12-19 years | Genitality | Identity and repudiation vs identity confusion | Formal operations (deductive and abstract reasoning) (11-15 years) | Postconventional or principled level    Social-contract orientation    Universal ethical principle orientation (no longer included in revised theory) |
| **VI Early adulthood** | | Intimacy and solidarity vs isolation | | |
| **VII Young and middle adulthood** | | Generativity vs self-absorption | | |
| **VIII Later adulthood** | | Ego integrity vs despair | | |

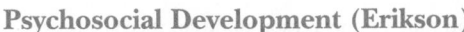

## Psychosocial Development (Erikson)

The most widely accepted theory of personality development is that advanced by Erikson (1963). Although built on Freudian theory, it is known as the theory of *psychosocial* development and emphasizes a healthy personality as opposed to a pathologic approach. Erikson also uses the biologic concepts of critical periods and epigenesis, describing key conflicts or core problems that the individual strives to master during critical periods in personality development. Successful completion or mastery of each of these core conflicts is built on the satisfactory completion or mastery of the previous core.

Each psychosocial stage has two components—the favorable and the unfavorable aspects of the core conflict—and progression to the next stage depends on resolution of this conflict. No core conflict is ever mastered completely but remains a recurrent problem throughout life. No life situation is ever secure. Each new situation presents the conflict in a new form. For example, when children who have satisfactorily achieved a sense of trust encounter a new experience (e.g., hospitalization), they must again develop a sense of trust in those responsible for their care in order to master the situation. Erikson's life span approach to personality development consists of eight stages; however, only the first five relating to childhood are included here:

1. **Trust vs mistrust (birth to 1 year).** The first and most important attribute to develop for a healthy personality is a basic *trust*. Establishment of basic trust dominates the first year of life and describes all of a child's satisfying experiences at this age. Corresponding to Freud's oral stage, it is a time of "getting" and "taking in" through all the senses. Trust exists only in relation to something or someone; therefore consistent, loving care by a mothering person is essential to its development. *Mistrust* develops when trust-promoting experiences are deficient or lacking or when basic needs are inconsistently or inadequately met. Although shreds of mistrust are sprinkled throughout the personality, from a basic trust in parents stems trust in the world, other people, and oneself. The result is *faith* and *optimism.*
2. **Autonomy vs shame and doubt (1 to 3 years).** Corresponding to Freud's anal stage, the problem of *autonomy* can be symbolized by the holding onto and letting go of the sphincter muscles. The development of autonomy during the toddler period is centered around children's increasing ability to control their bodies, themselves, and their environment. They want to do things for themselves by using their newly acquired motor skills of walking, climbing, and manipulating and their mental powers of selection and decision making. Much of their learning is acquired through imitating the activities and behavior of others. Negative feelings of *doubt* and *shame* arise when children are made to feel small and self-conscious, when their choices are disastrous, when others shame them, or when they are forced to be dependent in areas in which they are capable of assuming control. The favorable outcomes are *self-control* and *willpower.*
3. **Initiative vs guilt (3 to 6 years).** The stage of *initiative* corresponds to Freud's phallic stage and is characterized by vigorous and intrusive behavior, enterprise, and a strong imagination. Children explore the physical world with all of their senses and powers. They develop a conscience. No longer guided only by outsiders, there is an inner voice that warns and threatens. Children sometimes undertake goals or activities that are in conflict with those of parents or others, and being made to feel that their activities or imaginings are bad produces a sense of *guilt.* Children must learn to retain a sense of initiative without impinging on the rights and privileges of others. The lasting outcomes are *direction* and *purpose.*
4. **Industry vs inferiority (6 to 12 years).** The stage of *industry* is the latency period of Freud. Having achieved the more crucial stages in personality development, children are ready to be workers and producers. They want to engage in tasks and activities that they can carry through to completion; they need and want real achievement. Children learn to compete and cooperate with others, and they learn the rules. It is a decisive period in their social relationships with others. Feelings of *inadequacy* and *inferiority* may develop if too much is expected of them or if they believe they cannot measure up to the standards set for them by others. The ego quality developed from a sense of industry is *competence.*
5. **Identity vs role confusion (12 to 18 years).** Corresponding to Freud's genital period, the development of *identity* is characterized by rapid and marked physical changes. Previous trust in their bodies is shaken, and children become overly preoccupied with the way they appear in the eyes of others as compared with their own self-concept. Adolescents struggle to fit the roles they have played and hope to play with the current roles and fashions adopted by their peers, to integrate their concepts and values with those of society, and to come to a decision regarding an occupation. Inability to solve the core conflict results in *role confusion.* The outcome of successful mastery is *devotion* and *fidelity* to others and to values and ideologies.

# Theoretic Foundations of Mental Development

The term *cognition* refers to the process by which developing individuals become acquainted with the world and the objects it contains. Children are born with inherited potentialities for intellectual growth, but they must develop into that potential through interactions with the environment. By assimilating information through the senses, processing it, and acting on it, they come to understand relationships between objects and between themselves and their world. With cognitive development, children acquire the ability to reason abstractly, to think in a logical manner, and to organize intellectual functions or performances into higher-order structures. Language, morals, and spiritual development emerge as cognitive abilities advance.

## Cognitive Development (Piaget)

Cognitive development consists of age-related changes that occur in mental activities. The best-known theory regarding children's thinking, and a more comprehensive developmental theory than those already described, has been developed by the Swiss psychologist Jean Piaget (1969). According to Piaget, intelligence enables individuals to make adaptations to the environment that increase the probability of survival; through their behavior individuals establish and maintain equilibrium with the environment.

Piaget proposes three stages of reasoning: (1) *intuitive,* (2) *concrete operational,* and (3) *formal operational.* When children enter the stage of concrete logical thought at approximately 7 years of age, they are able to make logical inferences, classify, and deal with quantitative relationships about concrete things. Not until adolescence are they able to reason abstractly with any degree of competence.

According to Piaget, children proceed through the stages of mental activity in an orderly and sequential manner. The mechanisms that enable them to adapt to new situations and to move from one stage to the next are assimilation and accommodation. By *assimilation* children incorporate new knowledge, skills, ideas, and insights into cognitive schemes (Piaget uses the term *schema\**) already familiar to them. For new situations that do not fit into an established schema, children *accommodate.* They change and organize existing schemas to solve more difficult tasks and form new schemas. Children's understanding of a new experience is based on all relevant previous experiences. They achieve equilibrium over and over again by applying schemas already available to them. Thus children achieve an accurate understanding of reality and come to deal with increasingly complex problems in an increasingly effective manner.

One of the most prominent criticisms of Piaget's theory is that it ignores the important concept of unconscious motivation and its impact on behavior. Nor does it account for individual differences and unevenness in cognitive development—children may demonstrate more advanced behavior in one area than in another. Although it emphasizes biologic factors in human development, Piaget's theory provides one of the dominant frameworks for understanding children's thinking. Piaget was very conservative in his descriptions of children's abilities. Recent studies indicate that children, especially preschool children, are capable of more advanced thought than Piaget acknowledged.

**Development of Logical Thinking.** Piaget believed there are four major stages in the development of logical thinking. Each stage is derived from and builds on the accomplishments of the previous stage in a continuous, orderly process. The course of intellectual development is both maturational and invariant and is divided into the following periods, subperiods, and stages (ages are approximate):

**Sensorimotor (birth to 2 years).** The sensorimotor stage of intellectual development consists of six substages that are governed by sensations in which simple learning takes place (See Chapters 12 and 14.) Children progress from reflex activity through simple, repetitive behaviors to imitative behavior. They develop a sense of "cause and effect" as they direct behavior toward objects. Problem solving is primarily trial and error. They display a high level of curiosity, experimentation, and enjoyment of novelty and begin to develop a sense of self as they are able to differentiate themselves from their environment. They become aware that objects have *permanence*—the objects exist even when no longer visible. Toward the end of the sensorimotor period, children begin to use language and representational thought.

**Preoperational (2 to 7 years).** The predominant characteristic of the preoperational stage of intellectual development is *egocentrism,* which in this sense does not mean selfishness or self-centeredness but rather the inability to put oneself in the place of another. Children interpret objects and events not in terms of general properties but in terms of their relationships or their use to them. They are unable to see things from any perspective other than their own; they cannot see another's point

of view, nor can they see any reason to do so. (See Cognitive Development [Piaget], Chapter 14.)

Preoperational thinking is concrete and tangible. Children cannot reason beyond the observable, and they lack the ability to make deductions or generalizations. Thought is dominated by what they see, hear, or otherwise experience. However, they are increasingly able to use language and symbols to represent objects in their environment. Through imaginative play, questioning, and other interactions, they begin to elaborate concepts and to make simple associations between ideas. In the latter stage of this period their reasoning is *intuitive* (e.g., the stars need to go to bed just as they do) and they are only beginning to deal with problems of weight, length, size, and time. Reasoning is also *transductive*—because two events occur together, they cause each other, or knowledge of one characteristic is transferred to another (e.g., all women with big bellies have babies).

**Concrete operations (7 to 11 years).** At this age thought becomes increasingly logical and coherent. Children are able to classify, sort, order, and otherwise organize facts about the world to use in problem solving. They develop a new concept of permanence—*conservation.* (See Cognitive Development [Piaget], Chapter 17.) That is, they realize that physical factors such as volume, weight, and number remain the same even though outward appearances are changed. They are able to deal simultaneously with a number of different aspects of a situation. They do not have the capacity to deal in abstraction; they solve problems in a concrete, systematic fashion based on what they can perceive. Reasoning is *inductive.* Through progressive changes in thought processes and relationships with others, thought becomes less self-centered. Children can consider points of view other than their own. Thinking has become socialized.

**Formal operations (11 to 15 years).** Formal operational thought is characterized by adaptability and flexibility. Adolescents can think in abstract terms, use abstract symbols, and draw logical conclusions from a set of observations. For example, they can solve the following question: If *A* is larger than *B*, and *B* is larger than *C*, which symbol is the largest? (The answer is *A*.) They can make hypotheses and test them; they can consider abstract, theoretic, and philosophic matters. Although they may confuse the ideal with the practical, most contradictions in the world can be dealt with and resolved.

## Moral Development (Kohlberg)

It is theorized that children develop moral reasoning in an invariant developmental sequence. To understand the stages in the development of moral judgment, it is important to be aware of the stages of logical thought and its relationship to cognitive development and moral behavior. Moral development is based on cognitive developmental theory and consists of three major levels, each with two stages (Kohlberg, 1968).

Kohlberg's theory allows for prediction of behavior but pays little attention to individual differences. Questions arise relative to observed sex differences in attainment of the various sequences of moral development (Holstein, 1976). It has been argued that the theory was derived from interviews with male adults and may not reflect feminine moral reasoning (Gilligan, 1977).

The *preconventional level* of morality parallels the preconceptual level of cognitive development and intuitive thought. At this level morality is external because children conform to rules imposed by authority figures. Culturally

---

*A schema is a pattern of action or thought.

oriented to the labels of good/bad and right/wrong, children integrate these labels in terms of the physical or pleasurable consequences of their actions. The two stages of this level are:

**Stage 1: The punishment-and-obedience orientation.** Children determine the goodness or badness of an action in terms of its consequences. They avoid punishment and obey unquestioningly those who have the power to determine and enforce the rules and labels. They have no concept of the underlying moral order that supports these consequences.

**Stage 2: The instrumental-relativist orientation.** The right behavior consists of that which satisfies the child's own needs (and sometimes the needs of others). Although elements of fairness, reciprocity, and equal sharing are evident, they are interpreted in a very practical, concrete manner without the elements of loyalty, gratitude, or justice.

At the *conventional level* children are concerned with conformity and loyalty; actively maintaining, supporting, and justifying the social order; and personal expectations of those significant in their lives. They value the maintenance of family, group, or national expectations regardless of consequences. This level correlates with the concrete operational stage in cognitive development and consists of two stages:

**Stage 3: The interpersonal concordance or "good boy-nice girl" orientation.** Behavior that meets with approval and pleases or helps others is viewed as good. Conformity to the norm is the "natural" behavior, and one earns approval by being "nice."

**Stage 4: The "law and order" orientation.** Obeying the rules, doing one's duty, showing respect for authority, and maintaining the social order is the correct behavior. The rules and authority can be social or religious, depending on which is most valued.

At the *postconventional, autonomous,* or *principled level* children have reached the cognitive formal operational stage, and they endeavor to define moral values and principles that are valid and applicable beyond the authority of the groups and persons holding these principles. This level is not associated with the individual's identification with these groups. This third level has two stages, but stage 6 has been eliminated because Kohlberg determined that it is so rarely attained that it serves no useful purpose in a discussion such as this:

**Stage 5: The social-contract, legalistic orientation.** Correct behavior tends to be defined in terms of general individual rights and standards that have been examined and agreed on by the entire society. Although procedural rules for reaching consensus become important, with emphasis on the legal point of view, there is also emphasis on the possibility of changing law in terms of societal needs and rational considerations. Agreement and contract outside the legal realm are binding elements of obligation.

The most advanced level of moral development is one in which self-chosen ethical principles guide decisions of conscience. These are abstract, ethical, and universal principles of justice and human rights with respect for the dignity of persons as individuals. It is believed that few persons reach this stage of moral reasoning.

## Spiritual Development

Spiritual beliefs are closely related to the moral and ethical portion of children's self-concepts and as such must be considered as part of their basic needs assessment. Children need to have meaning, purpose, and hope in their lives, and the need for confession and forgiveness is present even in very young children. The research in spiritual development is both limited and subject to criticism, particularly in relation to age-stage theories. However, the stage theories provide a useful means for the reader to assess the approximate level of development for any given child. Extending beyond religion (an organized set of beliefs and practices), spiritually affects the whole person: mind, body, and spirit.

Fowler (1974) has identified seven stages in the development of faith, five of which parallel and are closely associated with cognitive and psychosocial development in childhood:

**Stage 0: Undifferentiated.** This stage of development encompasses the period of infancy, in which there is no concept of right or wrong, no beliefs, and no convictions to guide behavior. However, the beginnings of a faith are established with the development of basic trust through relationships with the primary caregiver.

**Stage 1: Intuitive-projective.** Toddlerhood is primarily a time of imitating the behavior of others. Children imitate the religious gestures and behaviors of others without comprehending the meaning or significance of the activities. During the preschool years children assimilate some of the values and beliefs of their parents. Parental attitudes toward moral codes and religious beliefs convey to children what they consider good and bad. Children follow parental beliefs as part of their daily lives rather than through an understanding of their basic concepts.

**Stage 2: Mythical-literal.** Through the school-age years spiritual development parallels cognitive development and is closely related to children's experiences and social interactions. Most children have a strong interest in religion during the school-age years. The existence of a deity is accepted, and petitions to an omnipotent being are important and expected to be answered; good behavior is rewarded, and bad behavior is punished. Children's developing conscience bothers them when they disobey. They have a reverence for many thoughts and matters and are able to articulate their faith. They may even begin to question its validity.

**Stage 3: Synthetic-convention.** As children approach adolescence, they become increasingly aware of spiritual disappointments. They recognize that prayers are not always answered (at least on their own terms). They begin to reason, to question some of the established parental religious standards, and to drop or modify some religious practices.

**Stage 4: Individuating-reflexive.** Adolescents become more skeptical and begin to compare the religious standards of their parents with the standards of others. They attempt to determine which to adopt and incorporate into their own set of values. They also begin to compare religious standards with the scientific viewpoint. It is a time of searching rather than reaching. Adolescents are uncertain about many religious ideas but will not achieve profound insights until late adolescence or early adulthood.

## DEVELOPMENTAL ASSESSMENT

One of the most essential components of a complete health appraisal is assessment of developmental functioning (Johnson, 2000). *Screening procedures* are designed to identify quickly and reliably those children whose developmental level is below normal for their age and who therefore may require further investigation. They also provide a

**TABLE 7-19** Biologic risk factors warranting systematic and regular developmental screening

| Prenatal or Perinatal | Postnatal |
|---|---|
| Birth weight less than 1000 g | Meningitis |
| Chronic lung disease of prematurity | Brain or spinal cord trauma |
| Apgar score of 0–3 at 5 minutes | Lead poisoning |
| ECMO therapy* | Chronic serous otitis media |
| Hyperbilirubinemia requiring exchange transfusion | Seizure disorder |
| Grade III or IV intraperiventricular hemorrhage | Severe chronic illness (cystic fibrosis, cancer) |
| Periventricular leukomalacia | Child abuse or neglect |
| Neonatal seizures | |
| Documented systemic infection, congenital or acquired | |
| Intrauterine growth retardation | |
| Maternal phenylketonuria | |
| Materanl human immunodeficiency virus infection | |
| Maternal use of anticonvulsants | |
| Family history of childhood deafness or blindness | |

From Levine MD, Carey WB, Crocker AC: *Developmental-behavioral pediatrics,* Philadelphia, 1999, WB Saunders.
*ECMO, extracorporeal membrane oxygenation.

**TABLE 7-20** Selected infant and preschool screening tests and parent questionnaires

| Name | Age Range | Time (min) | Source |
|---|---|---|---|
| Bayley Infant Neurodevelopmental Screener (BINS) | 3–24 months | 10–15 | The Psychological Corporation P.O. Box 839954 San Antonio, TX 78238-3954 (800) 228-0752 |
| Denver II | 0–6 years | 30–45 | Denver Developmental Materials P.O. Box 371075 Denver, CO 80237-5075 (303) 355-4729*; (800) 419-4729 |
| Batelle Developmental Inventory | 0–8 years | 30 | Riverside Publishing Company 425 Spring Lake Drive Itasca, IL 60143-2079 (800) 323-9540 |
| Parents' Evaluation of Developmental Status (PEDS) | 0–8 years | 5 | Ellsworth & Vandermeer Press 4405 Scenic Drive Nashville, TN 37204 (615) 386-0061 *www.pedstest.com* |
| Ages and Stages Questionnaire (ASQ) | 4–48 months | 10–15 | Paul H. Brookes Publishing Co., Inc. P.O. Box 10624 Baltimore, MD 21285-0624 (800) 638-3775 |
| Brigance Screens | 0–7 years | 10–15 | Curriculum Associates P.O. Box 2001 N. Billerica, MA 01862-0901 (800) 225-0248 |
| Early Screening Inventory-Revised | 3–6 years | 10–15 | Rebus Inc. P.O. Box 4479 718 N. University Avenue Ann Arbor, MI 48106 (800) 435-3085 |
| Early Language Milestone Scale (ELM) | 0–3 years | 1–3 | PRO-ED 8700 Shoal Creek Boulevard Austin, TX 78758 (800) 897-3202 |
| Clinical Adaptive Text—Clinical Linguistic and Auditory Milestone Scale (CAT—CLAMS) | 0–3 years | 10–20 | |

From Levine MD, Carey WB, Crocker AC: *Developmental-behavioral pediatrics,* Philadelphia, 1999, WB Saunders.
*Denver Prescreening Developmental Questionnaire and Home Screening Questionnnaire are also available from this source.

**TABLE 7-21** Standardized tests that may be used in pediatric developmental assessment of the school-age child

| Test | Age Range (Years) | Domains of Function |
|------|-------------------|---------------------|
| Peabody Picture Vocabulary Test | 3–adult | Receptive vocabulary |
| Goodenough Draw-A-Person | 3–15 | Visual-motor integration |
| Gesell Figures | 3–12 | Visual-motor integration |
| Stanford-Binet Memory Test | 2–adult | Auditory memory |
| Wide Range Achievement Test | 5–adult | Reading, spelling, arithmetic |
| Durrell Test of Reading Comprehension | 5–adult | Reading comprehension |
| Boder Word Recognition Inventory | 5–adult | Decoding and spelling |
| Word Attack (Woodcock-Johnson) | 6–adult | Phonology |
| Rapid Automatized Naming Test | 5–adult | Fluency/automaticity |
| Block Design (WISC-III) | 6–16 | Nonverbal reasoning |
| Vocabulary (WISC-III) | 6–16 | Verbal reasoning |
| Kaufman Brief Intelligence Test | 4–adult | Intelligence quotient |

From Levine MD, Carey WB, Crocker AC: *Developmental-behavioral pediatrics,* Philadelphia, 1999, WB Saunders.

means for recording objective measurements of present developmental functioning for future reference. Since the passage of P.L. 99-457, the Education of the Handicapped Act Amendments of 1986, much greater emphasis has been placed on developmental assessment of children with disabilities; nurses can play a vital role in providing this service. Situations placing children at increased risk for developmental delays are found in Table 7-19 (Romeo, 2002).

In selecting a screening test, be aware of the instrument's *validity*—the extent to which it measures what it purports to measure. When screening for a single disease that is diagnosed by a single test, such as anemia, one can use criteria such as sensitivity, specificity, and predictive value of a positive finding. Although these criteria may not be appropriate for developmental tests, such as the Denver II, they are commonly used.

*Sensitivity* is the percentage of children with true problems who are correctly detected; approximately 80% is preferable. The other 20% of children have problems that are not detected *(false-negatives)* (Glascoe, 2000). *Specificity* is the percentage of children without problems who are correctly detected. Because there are many more children without problems, 90% is preferable. The other 10% of children without problems are identified as having problems *(false-positives)*.

Validity may also be based on the accuracy with which the *standard norms* have been established (e.g., the accuracy of the growth norms used to establish the growth curve). Such norms are most appropriate when screening the child's status

(e.g., growth and development) and are determined by a host of factors such as genetics, nutritional intake, and opportunities to learn. As a result, deviant global measures of growth or development may reflect a variety of conditions, some of which may be pathologic. For instance, a child's language development may be delayed in comparison with that of other children because of a hearing impairment, neglect, mental retardation, or an emotional disorder. Therefore, it is not appropriate to compare the child's development with any one test because few, if any, currently available diagnostic tests are equally accurate in detecting developmental delays in speech, language, fine and gross motor activities, and emotional and intellectual development (Frankenburg, 1994a).

There are several types of screening tests available which include parent screening tools, examiner check lists, and direct examination instruments. Table 7-20 describes selected infant and preschool screening tests, and Table 7-21 lists tools that can be used with the school-age child. These screening tests can be administered in a variety of settings—home, school, daycare center, hospital, or clinic.

## Denver II

The most widely used developmental screening tests for young children have been the series of tests developed by Dr. William Frankenburg and his colleagues in Denver, Colorado. The oldest and best known, the *Denver Developmental Screening Test (DDST)* and its revision, the *DDST-R,* have been revised, restandardized, and renamed the *Denver II.* Before administering the Denver II, the examiner should be trained by and receive a certificate from a master instructor who has been trained by the Denver faculty.* The Denver II differs from the DDST in number of items, test form, interpretation, and referral. (See Appendix B.) The previous total of 105 items has been increased to 125, including an increase from 21 DDST to 39 Denver II language items. Items that had been difficult to administer or interpret have been modified or eliminated. Many items that were previously tested by parental reports now require observation by the examiner.

Each item was evaluated to determine if significant differences exist on the basis of sex, ethnic group, maternal education, and place of residence. Items for which clinically significant differences exist were replaced, or if retained, are discussed in the Technical Manual. When evaluating children who are delayed on one of these items, the examiner can look up norms for the subpopulations to consider if the delay may be caused by sociocultural or environmental differences.

The items on the test form are arranged in the same format as the DDST-R. The norms for the distribution bars have been updated with the new standardization data but retain the 25th, 50th, 75th, and 90th percentile divisions. The test form contains a place to rate the child's behavioral

---

*Forms and complete instructions are available from Denver Developmental Materials, Inc, PO Box 371075, Denver, CO 80237-5075, (303) 355-4729, (800) 419-4729.

characteristics (compliance, interest in surroundings, fearfulness, and attention span).

To determine relative areas of advancement and areas of delay, sufficient items should be administered to establish the basal and ceiling levels in each sector. By scoring appropriate items as "pass," "fail," "refusal," or "no opportunity" and by relating such scores to the age of the child, each item can be interpreted as described in Box 7-10. To identify cautions, all items intersected by the age line are administered. To screen solely for developmental delays, only the items located totally to the *left* of the child's age line are administered. Criteria for referral are based on the availability of resources in the community (see Box 7-10).

Research on the Denver II's validity and accuracy is in the beginning stages. One study found that most children with even subtle developmental problems were identified. However, almost half of the children without developmental problems received suspect scores, resulting in a high rate of overreferrals (Glascoe and others, 1992). To minimize overreferrals, a decision for referral depends not only on the results of the Denver II but also on the availability of local resources for diagnosis and treatment and on the practitioner's clinical judgment after considering the child's developmental history, general health status, and social, cultural, and emotional environment (Frankenburg, 1994a).

Although it is not the purpose of this discussion to detail the instruction manual, some points concerning preparation, administration, and interpretation of the Denver II are important to stress. Before beginning the screen, ask if the child was born prematurely and correctly calculate the adjusted age. Up to 24 months of age, allowances are made for infants born prematurely by subtracting the number of

weeks of missed gestation from their present age and testing them at the adjusted age. For example, a 16-week-old infant who was born 4 weeks early is tested at a 12-week adjusted age level. Explain to the parents and child, if appropriate, that the screenings are *not* intelligence tests but a method of showing what the child can do at a particular age. Emphasize that the child is *not* expected to perform each item on the test.

Tell the parent before the screening begins that the results of the child's performance will be explained after all the items have been concluded. It is the nurse's responsibility to properly inform parents about any testing or screening procedure before its administration so that they are fully aware of its purpose and intent.

Prepare toddlers and preschoolers for the procedure by presenting it as a game. The Denver II often is an excellent way to begin a health appraisal because it is nonthreatening, requires no painful or unfamiliar procedures, and capitalizes on the child's natural activity of play. Because children are easily distracted, perform each item quickly and present only one toy from the kit at a time. After that toy's purpose is concluded, such as building a tower of blocks or identifying its color, replace the toy in the bag and take out another one. Temporary factors that may interfere with the child's performance include fatigue, illness, fear, hospitalization, separation from the parent, or general unwillingness to perform the activities. In addition, undiagnosed mental retardation, hearing loss, vision loss, neurologic impairment, or a familial pattern of slow development greatly influences the child's performance.

Following completion of the Denver II, ask the parent if the child's performance was typical of behavior at other times. If the parent replies affirmatively and the child's cooperation was satisfactory, explain the results. Emphasize all successful items first, then those items the child failed but was not expected to pass, and finally those items that were delays. If the parent replies that the child's performance was not typical of usual behavior, it is best to defer any scoring or discussion of results, especially if the refusals yield a suspect score. In this situation reschedule testing for a time when the child is more likely to cooperate.

In explaining a normal score, focus on how well the child performed and reinforce the parents' efforts in satisfactorily stimulating their child. In addition to assessing the child's present developmental level, the Denver II can be used to guide parents toward those activities that are appropriate, although not necessarily expected, for the child's age. By testing for items to the right of the age line (ones the child is not expected to perform), children with advanced development and who may be gifted can be identified.

In explaining delays, carefully note the parent's response, especially indications of casual acceptance, such as "He'll catch up," or questions such as, "Does this mean my child is retarded?" Be aware of personal anxieties during these situations and refrain from giving reassurances such as, "I'm sure he will do better the next time." Rather, respond to parents' questions honestly yet with appropriate flexibility and concern and stress the need for further developmental testing.

---

## Box 7-10 ■ ■ □
## Denver II Scoring

### INTERPRETATION OF DENVER II SCORES

**Advanced:** Passed an item completely to the *right* of the age line (passed by fewer than 25% of children at an age older than the child)

**OK:** Passed, failed, or refused an item intersected by the age line between the 25th and 75th percentiles

**Caution:** Failed or refused items intersected by the age line on or between the 75th and 90th percentiles

**Delay:** Failed an item completely to the *left* of the age line; refusals to the left of the age line may also be considered delays, because the reason for the refusal may be inability to perform the task

### INTERPRETATION OF TEST

**Normal:** No delays and a maximum of one caution

**Suspect:** One or more delays and/or two or more cautions

**Untestable:** Refusals on one or more items completely to the left of the age line or on more than one item intersected by the age line in the 75th to 90th percentile area

### RECOMMENDATIONS FOR REFERRAL FOR SUSPECT AND UNTESTABLE TESTS

Rescreen in 1 to 2 weeks to rule out temporary factors.

If rescreen is suspect or untestable, use clinical judgment based on the following: number of cautions and delays, which items are cautions and delays, rate of past development, clinical examination and history, availability of referral resources.

## Revised Prescreening Developmental Questionnaire (R-PDQ)

The R-PDQ is a revision of the original PDQ (Frankenburg, Fandal, and Thorton, 1987). Advantages of the R-PDQ include the addition and arrangement of items to be more age-appropriate, simplified parent scoring, and easier comparison with Denver II norms for professionals. The R-PDQ is a parent-answered prescreen consisting of 150 questions from the Denver II, although only a subset of questions are asked for each age-group. The form may need to be read to less-educated caregivers.

Four different forms are available and are selected on the basis of age: orange (0 to 9 months), purple (9 to 24 months), gold (2 to 4 years), and white (4 to 6 years). (See Appendix B.) The caregiver answers the questions until (1) three "NOs" are circled (they do not need to be consecutive) or (2) all of the questions on both sides of the form have been answered. Scoring is based on the number of delays. Children who have no delays are considered to be developing normally. If a child has one delay, the caregiver is provided with age-appropriate developmental activities to pursue with the child; a rescreen with the R-PDQ is performed 1 month later. If on rescreening a child has one or more delays, the Denver II is administered as soon as possible. If a child has two or more delays on the first screening with the R-PDQ, the Denver II is administered as soon as possible.

## Developmental Screening and Interpretation

Although screening tests are an effective method of applying the knowledge of children's expected rate of development to a large segment of the population, they are only as successful as the individual's expertise in administering them. Because many of the screening tests are devised to be used by paraprofessionals, there are inherent risks in screening if such individuals are not properly trained or supervised. For example, false-positives can label the child as developmentally delayed and cause problems that otherwise might not have existed. False-negatives can prevent children with problems from receiving the help they need.

Screening tests should not be used for diagnosis but to determine whether further assessment is needed. Screening tests should be used only for their specific purpose and should be culturally sensitive (Levine, Carey, and Crocker, 1999).

Nurses administering developmental screening or supervising paraprofessionals' testing need to assess the child's "whole picture" and not rely solely on any screening procedure. Development, like growth and health, is a dynamic process. Tests such as the Denver II should be used as part of *developmental surveillance,* a continuous comprehensive primary health care approach that includes the parents as partners with professionals (Frankenburg, 1994b). Evaluation of the child's total well-being is the result of evaluating data from a comprehensive health and family history, physical examination, and developmental screening.

## KEY POINTS

- The most common approach to examining children follows a head-to-toe sequence.
- Growth measurements during the physical examination focus on length, height, weight, skinfold thickness, and arms and head circumference. Assessment of growth is measured against standard growth charts to determine a child's status in comparison with other children of the same age.
- Measurements of temperature, pulse, respiration, and blood pressure require accurate assessment techniques to provide useful data.
- The general appearance of a child is a cumulative and subjective impression of physical appearance, state of nutrition, behavior, personality, interactions with parents and nurse, posture, development, and speech.
- Assessment of the skin, which primarily involves inspection and palpation, focuses on color, texture, temperature, moisture, and turgor. The nurse needs to be aware of both physiologic and ethnic factors that may affect these areas.
- In assessment of the lymph nodes, the nurse examines by palpation the part of the body in which the glands are located.
- The head is inspected for shape, symmetry, mobility, and head control.

- Assessment of the neck includes palpation of the trachea and thyroid gland.
- Examination of the eyes includes placement and alignment, inspection of external and internal structures, and vision testing.
- Ears are examined for placement and alignment, inspection of external and internal structures, and auditory testing.
- The lungs are examined by methods of inspection, palpation, percussion, and auscultation.
- Auscultation is the most important procedure for examining the heart.
- Heart murmurs are classified as innocent, functional, or organic and should be evaluated for location, timing, intensity, and loudness.
- Abdominal assessment follows an orderly sequence of inspection, auscultation, percussion, and palpation, because palpation may distort normal abdominal sounds.
- Examination of the genitalia may be anxiety-provoking in the child, and the nurse must avoid transferring personal anxiety.
- Neurologic assessment addresses behavior, cognitive-perceptual development, motor functioning, sensory and cerebellar functioning, reflexes, cranial nerves, and soft signs.

- The Denver II, a major revision and a restandardization of the DDST, differs from the DDST in items included in the test, the test form, the interpretation of scoring, and referral criteria. Both tests are composed of four categories: personal-social, fine motor-adaptive, language, and gross motor.
- According to Freud's psychosexual theory, during childhood certain regions of the body assume a prominent psychologic significance as the source of new pleasures.
- Erikson's psychosocial theory emphasizes the concept of critical periods in personality development, when children strive to master core conflicts. Each successive stage is built on the successful completion of early stages.
- Piaget's theory of cognitive development describes children's progress through stages of mental activity in an orderly and sequential manner that enables them to adapt to the environment.
- Moral and spiritual development are accomplished in conjunction with cognitive development.

# REFERENCES

Aldemir H and others: A comparison of the immediate effects of moderate exercise in the late morning and late afternoon on core temperature and cutaneous thermoregulatory mechanisms, *Chronobiol Int* 17(2):197-207, 2000.

American Academy of Pediatrics, Committee on Practice and Ambulatory Medicine, Section on Ophthalmology: Eye examination and vision screening in infants, children, and young adults, *Pediatrics* 98(1):153-157, 1996.

Amoateng-Adjepong Y, Del Mundo J, Manthous CA: Accuracy of an infrared tympanic thermometer, *Chest* 115(4):1002-1005, 1999.

Androkites AL, Werger AM, Young ML: Comparison of axillary and infrared tympanic membrane thermometry in a pediatric oncology outpatient setting, *J Pediatr Oncol Nurs* 15(4):216-222, 1998.

Ao H and others: Jugular vein temperature reflects brain temperature during hypothermia, *Resuscitation* 45(2):111-118, 2000.

Barone MA, Rowe PC: Pediatric procedures. In McMillan JA, DeAngelis CD, Feigin RD, editors: *Oski's pediatrics—principles and practice*, ed 3, Philadelphia, 1999, Lippincott Williams & Wilkins.

Bliss-Holtz J: Methods of newborn infant temperature monitoring: a research review, *Issues Compr Pediatr Nurs* 18(4):287-298, 1995.

Boothroyd A, Carty H: Breast masses in childhood and adolescence, *Pediatr Radiol* 24(2):81-84, 1994.

Brennan DF and others: Reliability of infrared tympanic thermometry in the detection of rectal fever in children, *Ann Emerg Med* 25(1):21-30, 1995.

Callison DM: Early identification and intervention of hearing-impaired infants, *J Otolaryngol Clin North Am* 32(6):1009-1018, 1999.

Chernoff R and others: Assessing the health status of children entering foster care, *Pediatrics* 93(4):594-601, 1994.

Childs C, Harrison R, Hodkinson C: Tympanic membrane temperature as a measure of core temperature, *Arch Dis Child* 80(3):262-266, 1999.

Coats DK, Jenkins RH: Vision assessment of the pediatric patient: refinements, *Am Acad Opthalmol* 1(1):1-12, 1997.

Craig J: Recording tympanic temperature, *Paediatr Nurs* 11(6):10, 1999.

Craig JV and others: Temperature measured at the axilla compared with rectum in children and young people: systematic review, *BMJ* 320(7243):1174-1178, 2000.

Cretel E and others: A comparative study of body temperature using rectal and tympanic measurement, *Rev Med Intern* 20(11):981-984, 1999.

Erickson EH: *Childhood and society*, ed 2, New York, 1963, WW Norton.

Erickson RS: The continuing question of how best to measure body temperature, *Crit Care Med* 27(10):2307-2310, 1999.

Erickson RS, Meyer LT, Woo TM: Accuracy of chemical dot thermometers in critically ill adults and young children, *Image J Nurs Sch* 28(1):23-28, 1996.

Fowler JW: Toward a developmental perspective on faith, *Relig Educ* 68:207-219, 1974.

Frankenburg WK: Preventing developmental delays: is developmental screening sufficient: I. Developmental screening and the Denver II, *Pediatrics* 93(4):586-589, 1994a.

Frankenburg WK: Preventing developmental delays: is developmental screening sufficient? II. Partners in health care, *Pediatrics* 93(4):589-593, 1994b.

Frankenburg WK, Fandal LA, Thornton S: Revision of Denver Prescreening Developmental Questionnaire, *J Pediatr* 110(4):653-657, 1987.

Gilligan C: In a different voice: woman's conception of self and morality, *Harvard Educ Rev* 47:481-517, 1977.

Gillman MW, Cook NR: Blood pressure measurement in childhood epidemiological studies, *Circulation* 92(4):1049-1057, 1995.

Giorgi AZ: AAP says international adoptees need careful vaccination screening, *Inf Dis Child* 14(1);12-14, 2001.

Giuliano KK and others: Temperature measurement in critically ill orally intubated adults: a comparison of pulmonary artery core, tympanic, and oral methods, *Crit Care Med* 27(10):2188-2193, 1999.

Glascoe, FP: Early detection of developmental and behavioral problems, *Pediatr Rev* 21(8):272-280, 2000.

Glascoe FP and others: Accuracy of the Denver-II in developmental screening, *Pediatrics* 89(6 Pt 2):1221-1225, 1992.

Goldman LR, Shannon MW: Technical report: mercury in the environment: implications for pediatricians, *Pediatrics* 108(1):197-205, 2001.

Goonasekera CDA, Dillon MJ: Measurement and interpretation of blood pressure, *Arch Dis Child* 82(3):261-265, 2000.

Haddock BJ, Merrow DL, Swanson MS: The falling grace of axillary temperatures, *Pediatr Nurs* 22(2):121-125, 1996.

Halfon N and others: National health care reform, Medicaid and children in foster care, *Child Welfare* 73(2):99-115, 1994.

Healthcare Product Comparison System: *Thermometers, electronic, continuous*, Plymouth Meeting, PA, 1996a, ECRI.

Healthcare Product Comparison System: *Thermometers, electronic, intermittent*, Plymouth Meeting, Pa, 1996b, ECRI.

Healthcare Product Comparison System: *Thermometers, infrared, ear*, Plymouth Meeting, Pa, 1996c, ECRI.

Henker R, Coyne C: Comparison of peripheral temperature measurements with core temperature, *AACN Clin Issues* 6(1):21-30, 1995.

Hockenberry M, Kline NE: Nursing support of the child with cancer. In Pizzo PA, Poplack DP, editors: *Principles and practices of pediatric oncology*, ed 4, Philadelphia, 2001, JB Lippincott.

Holstein C: Irreversible, stepwise sequence in the development of moral judgement: a longitudinal study of males and females. *Child Dev* 47:51-61, 1976.

Hooker EA, Houston H: Screening for fever in an adult emergency department: oral vs tympanic thermometry, *South Med J* 89(2):230-234, 1996.

Horwitz SM, Simms MD, Farrington R: Impact of developmental problems on young children's exits from foster care, *J Dev Behav Pediatr* 15(2):105-110, 1994.

Hostetter MK, Johnson D: Medical examination of the internationally adopted child: screening for infectious diseases and developmental delay, *Postgrad Med* 99(4):70-72, 75-77, 81-82, 1996.

Houlder LC: The accuracy and reliability of tympanic thermometry compared to rectal and axillary sites in young children, *Pediatr Nurs* 26(3):311-314, 2000.

Irvin SM: Comparison of the oral thermometer versus the tympanic thermometer, *Clin Nurs Spec* 13(2):85-89, 1999.

Jaffe DM: What's hot and what's not: the gold standard for thermometry in emergency medicine, *Ann Emerg Med* 25(1):97-99, 1995.

Jensen BN and others: Accuracy of digital tympanic, oral, axillary, and rectal thermometers compared with standard rectal mercury thermometers, *Eur J Surg* 166(11):848-851, 2000.

Johnson CP: Using developmental and behavioral screening tests, *Pediatr Rev* 21(8):255-256, 2000.

Kai J: Parents' perceptions of taking babies' rectal temperature, *BMJ* 307(6905):660-662, 1993.

Kalangos A and others: Correction of pectus excavatum combined with open heart surgery in a patient with Marfan's syndrome, *Thorac Cardiovasc Surg* 43(4):220-222, 1995.

Klein DG and others: A comparison of pulmonary artery, rectal, and tympanic membrane temperature measurement in the ICU, *Heart Lung* 22(5):435-441, 1993.

Kodavatiganti R, Hearn CJ, Insler SR: Bleeding from a pulmonary artery catheter temperature connection port, *J Cardiothorac Vasc Anesth* 13(1):75-77, 1999.

Kohlberg L: Moral development. In Sills DL, editor: *International encyclopedia of the social sciences,* New York, 1968, MacMillan.

Kongpanichkul A, Bunjongpak S: A comparative study on accuracy of liquid crystal forehead, digital electronic axillary, infrared tympanic with glass-mercury rectal thermometer in infants and young children, *J Med Assoc Thai* 83(9):1068-1076, 2000.

Laestadius N, Aase J, Smith D: Normal inner canthal and outer orbital dimensions, *J Pediatr* 74(3):465-468, 1969.

Lanham DM and others: Accuracy of tympanic temperature readings in children under 6 years of age, *Pediatr Nurs* 25(1):39-42, 1999.

Latzka WA, Sawka MN: Hyperhydration and glycerol: thermoregulatory effects during exercise in hot climates, *Can J Appl Physiol* 25(6):536-545, 2000.

Lears MK, Guth KJ, Lewandowski L: International adoption: a primer for pediatric nurses, *Pediatr Nurs* 24(6):578-586, 1998.

Lell B and others: The circadian rhythm of body temperature is preserved during malarial fever, *Wien Klin Wochenschr* 112(23):1014-1015, 2000.

Levine MD, Carey WB, Crocker AC: *Developmental-behavioral pediatrics,* Philadelphia, 1999, WB Saunders.

Lewit EM, Marshall CL, Salzer JE: An evaluation of a plastic strip thermometer, *JAMA* 247(3):321-325, 1982.

Ling J and others: Clinical evaluation of the oscillometric blood pressure monitor in adults and children based on the 1992 AAMI SP-10 standards, *J Clin Monit* 11(2):123-130, 1995.

Lodha R and others: Is axillary temperature an appropriate surrogate for core temperature? *Indian J Pediatr* 67(8):571-574, 2000.

Loveys AA: Measuring temperatures, *Pediatr Infect Dis J* 17(10):920-921, 1998.

Loveys AA and others: Comparison of ear to rectal temperature measurements in infants and toddlers, *Clin Pediatr (Phila)* 38(8):463-466, 1999.

Lyew MA, Jamieson JW: Blood pressure measurement using oscillometric finger cuffs in children and young adults: a comparison with arm cuffs during general anaesthesia, *Anaesthesia* 49(10):895-899, 1994.

Macknin ML, Talo H, Medendorp SV: Effect of cotton tipped swab use on earwax occlusion, *Clin Pediatr* 33(1):14-18, 1994.

Mackowiak MD, Wasserman SS, Levine M: A critical appraisal of 98.6° F, the upper limit of the normal body temperature, and other legacies of Carl Reinhold August Wunderlich, *JAMA* 268(12):1578-1580, 1992.

Medical Indicators, Inc: Nex Temp™ single-use clinical thermometers: the quick, accurate, "no-hassle" way to take a temp, *NCFI* Jan 1999.

Mills MD: The eye in childhood, *Am Fam Physician* 60(3):907-918, 1999.

Mitchell MAS, Jenista JA: Health care of the internationally adopted child, *J Pediatr Health Care* 11(2):51-60, 1997.

Modell JG and others: Unreliability of the infrared tympanic thermometer in clinical practice: a comparative study with oral mercury and oral electronic thermometers, *South Med J* 91(7):649-654, 1998.

National Center for Health Statistics: CDC growth charts: United States, *Advance Data* 314:entire issue, 2000.

National Institutes of Health, National Heart, Lung, and Blood Institute: *Update on the Task Force Report (1987) on high blood pressure in children and adolescents: a working group report from the National High Blood Pressure Education Program,* NIH Pub No 96-3790, Sept, 1996, NIH.

Neinstein L and others: Comfort of male adolescents during general and genital examination, *J Pediatr* 115(3):494-497, 1989.

Nelson LB: *Harley's pediatric ophthalmology,* ed 4, Philadelphia, 1998, WB Saunders.

Owens DS and others: Diurnal variations in the mood and performance of highly practiced young women living under strictly controlled conditions, *Br J Psychol* 91(pt 1):41-60, 2000.

Park M, Lee D, Johnson CA: Oscillometric blood pressure in the arm, thigh and calf in healthy children and those with aortic coarctation, *Pediatrics* 92(4):761-765, 1993.

Piaget J: *The theory of stages in cognitive development,* New York, 1969, McGraw-Hill.

Pompei F, Pompei M: *Physicians reference handbook on temperature,* Watertown, MA, 1996, Exergen Corporation.

Prielipp RC, Morell R: Debate: The pulmonary artery catheter, is it safe to use or not to use. Con: Swan song for the Swan-Ganz? *J Clin Monit* 13(5):339-340, 1997.

Py Ma H Corporation: *Tempa Dot single use thermometer: technical information,* Flemington, NJ, 1994, The Corporation.

Rabinowitz RP and others: Effects of anatomic site, oral stimulation, and body position on estimates of body temperature, *Arch Intern Med* 156(7):777-780, 1996.

Rivera AY and others: Evaluation of a liquid crystal contact thermometer in children with fever, *J Investig Med* 45(1), 1997.

Robinson JL and others: Comparison of esophageal, rectal, axillary, bladder, tympanic, and pulmonary artery temperatures in children, *J Pediatr* 133(4):553-556, 1998.

Roche AF, Guo S: The new growth charts, *Pediatr Basics* 94:2-13, 2001.

Romanovsky AA and others: A difference of 5 degrees C between ear and rectal temperatures in a febrile patient, *Am J Emerg Med* 15(4):383-385, 1997.

Romeo, S: Developmental screening in children, *Advan Nurs Pract* 55-58, 2002.

Rotello LC, Crawford L, Terndrup TE: Comparison of infrared ear thermometer derived and equilibrated rectal temperatures in estimating pulmonary artery temperatures, *Crit Care Med* 24(9):1501-1506, 1996.

Sato KT and others: Reexamination of tympanic membrane temperature as a core temperature, *J Appl Physiol* 80(4):1233-1239, 1996.

Scahill M: The healthcare needs of children in foster care, *J Soc Pediatr Nurs* 5(4):183-184, 2000.

Seidel HM, Rosenstein BJ, Pathak A: *Primary care of the newborn,* ed 2, St Louis, 1997, Mosby.

Seidel HM and others: *Mosby's guide to physical examination,* ed 4, St Louis, 1999, Mosby.

Shann F, Mackenzie A: Comparison of rectal, axillary, and forehead temperatures, *Arch Pediatr Adolesc Med* 150(1):74-78, 1996.

Sievert U, Pau HW, Weidemann T: The "ear fever thermometer"—studies of ear thermography, *Laryngorhinootologie* 78(7):397-400, 1999.

Silverman CA: Ear, nose and throat disorders, *J Prim Care* 25(3):545-581, 1998.

Smith J: Are electronic thermometry techniques suitable alternatives to traditional mercury in glass thermometry techniques in the paediatric setting? *J Adv Nurs* 28(5):1030-1039, 1998.

Swanson JT and others: Use of photoscreening for children's vision screening, *Pediatrics* 109(3):524-525, 2002.

Valadez JJ, Elmore-Meegan M, Morley D: Comparing liquid crystal thermometer readings and mercury thermometer readings of infants and children in a traditional African setting. Implications for community-based health, *Trop Geogr Med* 47(3):130-133, 1995.

Valle PC, Kildahl-Andersen O, Steinvoll K: Infrared tympanic thermometry compared to mercury thermometers, *Tidsskr Nor Laegeforen* 120(1):15-17, 2000.

Vessey JA: Developmental approaches to examining young children, *Pediatr Nurs* 21(1):53-56, 1995.

Vessey JA, Stueve DL: A comparison of two techniques for weighing young children, *Pediatr Nurs* 22(4):327-330, 1996.

Wagner JD, Menke EM, Ciccone JK: What is known about the health of rural homeless families? *Public Health Nurs* 12(6):400-408, 1995.

Wattigney WA and others: Utility of an automatic instrument for blood pressure measurement in children: the Bogalusa Heart Study, *Am J Hypertens* 9(3):256-262, 1996.

Weiss ME and others: A comparison of temperature measurements using three ear thermometers, *Appl Nurs Res* 11(4):158-166, 1998.

Wells N and others: Does tympanic temperature measure up? *MCN* 20(2):95-100, 1995.

West KW and others: Diagnosis and treatment of symptomatic breast masses in the pediatric population, *J Pediatr Surg* 30(2):182-187, 1995.

Wilshaw R and others: A comparison of the use of tympanic, axillary, and rectal thermometers in infants, *J Pediatr Nurs* 14(2):88-93, 1999.

Yotsuyanagi T, Yokoi K, Sawada Y: Facial injury by mercury from a broken thermometer, *J Trauma* 40(5):847-849, 1996.

# Chapter **8**

# Health Promotion of the Newborn and Family

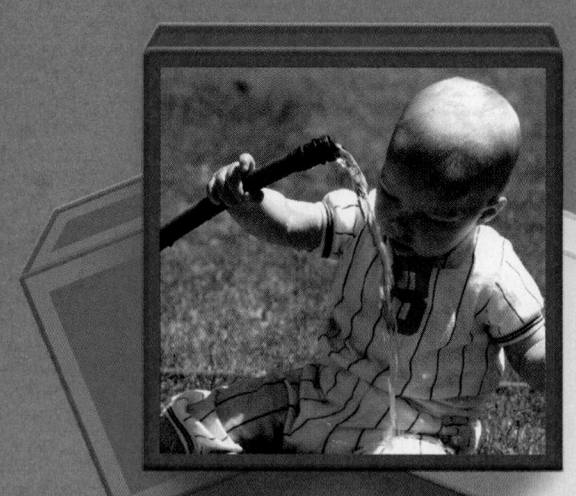

## Chapter Outline

**ADJUSTMENT TO EXTRAUTERINE LIFE, 240**
**Immediate Adjustments, 240**
    Respiratory System, 240
    Circulatory System, 241
**Physiologic Status of Other Systems, 241**
    Thermoregulation, 241
    Hemopoietic System, 241
    Fluid and Electrolyte Balance, 242
    Gastrointestinal System, 242
    Renal System, 242
    Integumentary System, 242
    Musculoskeletal System, 243
    Defenses Against Infection, 243

Endocrine System, 243
Neurologic System, 243
Sensory Functions, 243
**NURSING CARE OF THE NEWBORN AND FAMILY, 244**
**Assessment, 244**
    Initial Assessment: Apgar Scoring, 244
    Transitional Assessment: Periods of Reactivity, 245
    Behavioral Assessment, 245
    Assessment of Attachment Behaviors, 247
    Clinical Assessment of Gestational Age, 247
    Physical Assessment, 250

**Nursing Diagnoses, 263**
**Planning, 263**
**Implementation, 264**
    Maintain a Patent Airway, 265
    Maintain a Stable Body Temperature, 265
    Protect from Infection and Injury, 265
    Provide Optimum Nutrition, 273
    Promote Parent-Infant Bonding (Attachment), 282
    Prepare for Discharge and Home Care, 286
**Evaluation, 288**
*Nursing Care Plan: The Normal Newborn and Family, 289*

## Related Topics

Administration of Medication, Ch. 27
Ambiguous Genitalia, Ch. 11
Birth Injuries, Ch. 9
Blood Specimens, Ch. 27
Cardiac Development and Function: Embryologic Development, Ch. 34
Changes in Fluid Volume Related to Growth, Ch. 28

Congenital Heart Disease, Ch. 34
Dermatologic Problems in the Newborn, Ch. 9
Diaper Dermatitis, Ch. 13
Fluoride, Ch. 14
The High-Risk Newborn and Family, Ch. 10
Motor Vehicle Injuries, Chs. 12 and 14
Multiple Births, Ch. 3

Neonatal Pain, Ch. 10
Nutrition, Ch. 12
Physical Examination, Ch. 7
Sibling Rivalry, Ch. 14
The Skin, Ch. 18

## ADJUSTMENT TO EXTRAUTERINE LIFE

The most profound physiologic change required of the newborn is transition from fetal or placental circulation to independent respiration. The loss of the placental connection means the loss of complete metabolic support, especially the supply of oxygen and the removal of carbon dioxide. The normal stresses of labor and delivery produce alterations of placental gas exchange patterns, acid-base balance in the blood, and cardiovascular activity in the neonate. Factors that interfere with this normal transition or increase fetal *asphyxia* (a condition of hypoxemia, hypercapnia, and acidosis) will affect the fetus's adjustment to extrauterine life.

## Immediate Adjustments

### Respiratory System

The most critical and immediate physiologic change required of the newborn is the onset of breathing. The stimuli that help initiate respiration are primarily chemical and

---

■ David Wilson, MS, RNC, revised this chapter.

thermal. *Chemical factors* in the blood (low oxygen, high carbon dioxide, and low pH) initiate impulses that excite the respiratory center in the medulla. The primary *thermal stimulus* is the sudden chilling of the infant, who leaves a warm environment and enters a relatively cooler atmosphere. This abrupt change in temperature excites sensory impulses in the skin that are transmitted to the respiratory center.

The significance of *tactile stimulation* is questionable. Descent through the birth canal and normal handling during delivery, such as drying the skin, probably have some effect on initiation of respiration. Slapping the newborn's heel or buttocks has no beneficial effect. Moreover, it can waste precious time in the event of respiratory difficulty and can cause additional damage if cerebral trauma has occurred.

The initial entry of air into the lungs is opposed by the surface tension of the fluid that filled the fetal lungs and alveoli. However, fetal lung fluid is removed by the pulmonary capillaries and lymphatic vessels. Some fluid is also removed during the normal forces of labor and delivery. As the chest emerges from the birth canal, fluid is squeezed from the lungs through the nose and mouth. Following complete emergence of the neonate's chest, a brisk recoil of the thorax occurs. Air enters the upper airway to replace the lost fluid. In cesarean birth the chest is not compressed, and the newborn may need additional respiratory support.

In the alveoli the surface tension of the fluid is reduced by *surfactant,* a substance produced by the alveolar epithelium that coats the alveolar surface. The effect of surfactant in facilitating breathing is discussed in relation to respiratory distress syndrome. (See Chapter 10.)

## Circulatory System

Equally important as the initiation of respiration are the circulatory changes that allow blood to flow through the lungs. These changes occur more gradually and are the result of pressure changes in the lungs, heart, and major vessels. The transition from fetal circulation to postnatal circulation involves the functional closure of the fetal shunts: the foramen ovale, the ductus arteriosus, and eventually the ductus venosus. (For a brief review of fetal circulation, see Chapter 34.)

Once the lungs are expanded, the inspired oxygen dilates the pulmonary vessels, which decreases pulmonary vascular resistance and consequently increases pulmonary blood flow. As the lungs receive blood, the pressure in the right atrium, right ventricle, and pulmonary arteries decreases. At the same time, there is a progressive rise in systemic vascular resistance and an increased volume of blood as a result of cord clamping. This increases the pressure in the left side of the heart. Because blood flows from an area of high pressure to one of low pressure, the circulation of blood through the fetal shunts is reversed. (See Fig. 34-2.)

The most important factor controlling ductal closure is the increased oxygen concentration of the blood. Secondary factors are the fall in endogenous prostaglandins and acidosis. The foramen ovale closes functionally at or soon after birth from compression of the two portions of the atrial septum. The ductus arteriosus is closed functionally by the fourth day. Anatomic closure from deposition of

fibrin and cell products takes considerably longer. Because of the reversible flow of blood through the ductus arteriosus during the early neonatal period, functional murmurs are occasionally heard.

## Physiologic Status of Other Systems

### Thermoregulation

Next to establishing respiration, heat regulation is most critical to the newborn's survival. Although the newborn's capacity for heat production is adequate, several factors predispose the newborn to excessive heat loss. First, the newborn's large surface area facilitates heat loss to the environment. The normal metabolic rate per unit weight of the newborn is about twice that of the adult, but the neonate's surface area per unit weight is about three times that of the adult. Consequently, the infant produces only two thirds as much heat as an adult but loses twice as much heat per unit area. However, the large body surface is partially compensated for by the newborn's usual position of flexion, which decreases the amount of surface area exposed to the environment.

The second factor that retards the conservation of body heat is the newborn's thin layer of subcutaneous fat. Since core body temperature is approximately 1° F higher than surface body temperature, this temperature gradient (difference) causes a heat transfer from a higher to lower temperature.

A third factor is the newborn's mechanism for producing heat. Unlike the child or adult, who can increase heat production through shivering, the chilled neonate cannot shiver but produces heat through *nonshivering thermogenesis (NST).* NST is produced by stimulating cellular respiration; the resulting oxygen consumption can be three times the amount of any other body tissue (Bliss-Holtz, 1993). (See Thermoregulation, Chapter 10.) A thermogenic source unique to the full-term newborn is *brown adipose tissue (BAT),* or *brown fat,* which owes its name to its larger content of mitochondrial cytochromes. BAT has a greater capacity for heat production through intensified metabolic activity than does ordinary adipose tissue. Heat generated in the brown fat is distributed to other parts of the body by the blood, which is warmed as it flows through the layers of this tissue. Superficial deposits of brown fat are located between the scapulae, around the neck, in the axillae, and behind the sternum. Deeper layers surround the kidneys, trachea, esophagus, some major arteries, and adrenals. The location of the brown fat may explain why the nape of the neck often feels warmer than the rest of the body, and brown fat can affect the accuracy of axillary temperature measurement (see p. 256).

Although concern is usually for newborns' ability to conserve heat, they also can have difficulty dissipating heat in an overheated environment. This increases the risk of hyperthermia.

### Hemopoietic System

The *blood volume* of the newborn depends on the amount of placental transfer of blood. The blood volume of the full-term infant is about 80 to 85 ml/kg of body weight. Immediately after birth the total blood volume averages 300 ml, but, depending on how long the infant is attached to the placenta, as much as 100 ml can be added to the blood volume. The blood values for the newborn are listed in Appendix D.

## Fluid and Electrolyte Balance

Changes occur in the **total body water volume,** extracellular fluid volume, and intracellular fluid volume during the transition from fetal to postnatal life. Early in gestation the fetus is composed almost entirely of water and at term is 73% fluid, as compared with 58% in the adult. There is more extracellular fluid than intracellular fluid in the fetus, but this shifts progressively throughout postnatal life, probably because of the growth of cells at the expense of extracellular fluid. The infant has a proportionately higher ratio of extracellular fluid than the adult and consequently has a higher level of total body sodium and chloride and a lower level of potassium, magnesium, and phosphate. (See Chapter 28.)

A very important aspect of fluid balance is its relationship to other systems. The rate of fluid exchange is seven times greater in the infant than in the adult, and the infant's **rate of metabolism** is twice as great in relation to body weight. As a result, twice as much acid is formed, leading to more rapid development of acidosis. In addition, the immature kidneys cannot sufficiently concentrate urine to conserve body water. These three factors make the infant more prone to problems of dehydration, acidosis, and overhydration.

## Gastrointestinal System

The ability of the newborn to digest, absorb, and metabolize foodstuff is adequate but limited in certain functions. **Enzymes** are available to catalyze proteins and simple carbohydrates (monosaccharides and disaccharides), but deficient production of pancreatic amylase impairs utilization of complex carbohydrates (polysaccharides). A deficiency of

pancreatic lipase limits the absorption of fats, especially with ingestion of foods that have a high saturated fatty acid content, such as cow's milk.

The **liver** is the most immature of the gastrointestinal organs. The activity of the enzyme **glucuronyl transferase** is reduced, affecting the conjugation of bilirubin with glucuronic acid, which contributes to the physiologic jaundice of the newborn. The liver is also deficient in forming plasma proteins. The decreased plasma protein concentration probably plays a role in the edema usually seen at birth. Prothrombin and other coagulation factors are also low. The liver stores less glycogen at birth than later in life. Consequently, the newborn is prone to hypoglycemia, which may be prevented by early and effective feeding, especially breast-feeding.

Some **salivary glands** are functioning at birth, but the majority do not begin to secrete saliva until about age 2 to 3 months, when drooling is common. The stomach capacity is limited to about 90 ml; thus the infant requires frequent small feedings. Newborns who breast-feed usually have more frequent feedings and more frequent stools than infants who receive formula.

The infant's **intestine** is longer in relation to body size than that in the adult. Therefore there are a larger number of secretory glands and a larger surface area for absorption as compared with the adult's intestine. There are rapid peristaltic waves and simultaneous nonperistaltic waves along the entire esophagus. These waves, called the **migrating motor complex (MMC),** propel nutrients forward. The relative immaturity of the MMC, combined with decreased lower esophageal sphincter (LES) pressure, inappropriate relaxation of the LES, and delayed gastric emptying, make regurgitation a common occurrence. Progressive changes in the stooling pattern indicate a properly functioning gastrointestinal tract (Box 8-1).

## Renal System

All structural components are present in the renal system, but there is a functional deficiency in the kidney's ability to concentrate urine and to cope with conditions of fluid and electrolyte fluctuations, such as dehydration or a concentrated solute load.

Total volume of urinary output per 24 hours is about 200 to 300 ml by the end of the first week. However, the bladder involuntarily empties when stretched by a volume of 15 ml, resulting in as many as 20 voidings per day. The first voiding should occur within 24 hours. The urine is colorless and odorless and has a specific gravity of approximately 1.020.

## Integumentary System

At birth all of the structures within the skin are present, but many of the functions of the integument are immature. The two layers of the skin, the **epidermis** and **dermis,** are loosely bound to each other and are very thin. **Rete pegs,** which later in life anchor the epidermis to the dermis, are not developed. Slight friction across the epidermis, such as from rapid removal of tape, can cause separation of these layers and blister formation or loss of the epidermis. In term infants the transitional zone between the cornified and living layers of the epidermis is effective in preventing fluid from reaching the skin surface.

The *sebaceous glands* are very active late in fetal life and in early infancy because of high levels of maternal androgens. They are most densely located on the scalp, face, and genitalia and produce the grayish white, greasy vernix caseosa that covers the infant at birth. Plugging of the sebaceous glands causes *milia.*

The *eccrine glands,* which produce sweat in response to heat or emotional stimuli, are functional at birth, and palmar sweating on crying reaches levels equivalent to those of anxious adults by 3 weeks of age. Observing palmar sweating is helpful in assessing pain. The eccrine glands produce sweat in response to higher temperatures than those required in adults, and the retention of sweat may result in *miliaria.* The *apocrine glands,* sweat glands that develop as attachments to hair follicles, remain small and nonfunctional until puberty.

The growth phases of *hair follicles* usually occur simultaneously at birth. During the first few months the synchrony between hair loss and regrowth is disrupted, and there may be overgrowth of hair or temporary alopecia. Boys' hair grows faster than girls' hair, and in both sexes scalp hair growth is slower at the crown.

Because the amount of *melanin* is low at birth, newborns are lighter skinned than they will be as children. Consequently, infants are more susceptible to the harmful effects of the sun.

## Musculoskeletal System

At birth the *skeletal system* contains larger amounts of cartilage than ossified bone, although the process of ossification is fairly rapid during the first year. The nose, for example, is predominantly cartilage at birth and is frequently flattened by the force of delivery. The six skull bones are relatively soft and not yet joined. The sinuses are incompletely formed as well.

Unlike the skeletal system, the *muscular system* is almost completely formed at birth. Growth in the size of muscular tissue is caused by hypertrophy, rather than hyperplasia, of cells.

## Defenses Against Infection

The infant is born with several defenses against infection. The first line of defense is the *skin* and *mucous membranes,* which protect the body from invading organisms. The second line of defense is the *cellular elements* of the immunologic system, which produces several types of cells capable of attacking a pathogen. The *neutrophils* and *monocytes* are phagocytes, cells that engulf, ingest, and destroy foreign agents. *Eosinophils* also probably have a phagocytic property because in the presence of foreign protein they increase in number. The *lymphocytes* (T- and B-cells) are capable of being converted to other cell types, such as monocytes and antibodies. Although the phagocytic properties of the blood are present in the infant, the inflammatory response of the tissues to localize an infection is immature.

The third line of defense is the formation of specific *antibodies* to an antigen. This process requires exposure to various foreign agents for antibody production to occur. Infants are generally not capable of producing their own immunoglobulins (Ig) until the beginning of the second month of life, but they receive considerable passive immunity in the form of IgG from the maternal circulation and from human milk (see p. 274). They are protected against most major childhood diseases, including diphtheria, measles, poliomyelitis, and rubella, for about 3 months, provided that the mother has developed antibodies to these illnesses.

## Endocrine System

Ordinarily, the endocrine system of the newborn is adequately developed, but its functions are immature. For example, the posterior lobe of the pituitary gland produces limited quantities of *antidiuretic hormone (ADH),* or *vasopressin,* which inhibits diuresis. This renders the newborn highly susceptible to dehydration.

The effect of maternal *sex hormones* is particularly evident in the newborn. The labia are hypertrophied, and the breasts in both sexes may be engorged and secrete milk (witch's milk) during the first few days of life to as long as 2 months of age. Female newborns may have *pseudomenstruation* (more often seen as a milky secretion rather than actual blood) from a sudden drop in progesterone and estrogen levels.

## Neurologic System

At birth the nervous system is incompletely integrated but sufficiently developed to sustain extrauterine life. Most neurologic functions are *primitive reflexes.* The *autonomic nervous system* is crucial during transition because it stimulates initial respirations, helps maintain acid-base balance, and partially regulates temperature control.

*Myelination* of the nervous system follows the cephalocaudal-proximodistal (head-to-toe—center-to-periphery) laws of development and is closely related to the observed mastery of fine and gross motor skills. *Myelin* is necessary for rapid and efficient transmission of some, but not all, nerve impulses along the neural pathway. Tracts that develop myelin earliest are the sensory, cerebellar, and extrapyramidal. This accounts for the acute senses of taste, smell, and hearing, as well as the perception of pain, in the newborn. All *cranial nerves* are myelinated except the optic and olfactory nerves.

## Sensory Functions

The newborn's sensory functions are remarkably well developed and have a significant effect on growth and development, including the attachment process.

**Vision.**   At birth the eye is structurally incomplete. The *fovea centralis* is not yet completely differentiated from the macula. The *ciliary muscles* are also immature, limiting the ability of the eyes to accommodate and fixate on an object for any length of time. The *pupils* react to light, the blink reflex is responsive to a minimal stimulus, and the corneal reflex is activated by a light touch. *Tear glands* usually do not begin to function until 2 to 4 weeks of age.

The newborn has the ability to momentarily fixate on a bright or moving object that is within 20 cm (8 inches) and in the midline of the visual field. In fact, the infant's ability to fix-ate or coordinate movement is greater during the first hour of life than during the succeeding several days. *Visual acuity* is reported to be between 20/100 and 20/400, depending on the vision measurement techniques. (See Table 7-12.)

The infant also demonstrates visual preferences: medium colors (yellow, green, pink) over dim or bright colors (red, orange, blue); black-and-white contrasting patterns, especially geometric shapes and checkerboards; large objects with medium complexity rather than small, complex objects; and reflecting objects over dull ones.

**Hearing.**  Once the amniotic fluid has drained from the ears, the infant probably has *auditory acuity* similar to that of an adult. The newborn is able to detect a loud sound of about 90 decibels and reacts with a startle reflex. The new-born's response to sounds of low frequency and high frequency differs; the former, such as a heartbeat, metronome, or lullaby, tends to decrease an infant's motor activity and crying, whereas the latter elicits an alerting reaction.

There is an early sensitivity to the sound of human voices and to specific speech sounds. For example, infants younger than 3 days of age can distinguish the mother's voice from that of other females. As early as 5 days, new-borns can differentiate between stories read by the mother's voice (in utero) vs stories read by another woman's voice after birth.

The internal and middle *ear* structures are large at birth, but the external canal is small. The mastoid process and the bony part of the external canal have not yet developed. Consequently, the tympanic membrane and facial nerve are very close to the surface and can be easily damaged.

**Smell.**  Newborns react to strong odors such as alcohol or vinegar by turning their heads away. Breast-fed infants are able to smell breast milk and will cry for their mothers when the breasts are engorged and leaking. Infants are also able to differentiate the breast milk of their mother from the breast milk of other women by smell. Maternal odors are believed to influence the attachment process and successful breast-feeding. Unnecessary routine washing of the breasts may interfere with establishment of early breast-feeding.

**Taste.**  The newborn can distinguish between tastes, and various types of solutions elicit differing facial reflexes. A tasteless solution elicits no facial expression; a sweet solution elicits an eager suck and a look of satisfaction; a sour solution causes the usual puckering of the lips; and a bitter liquid produces an angry, upset expression. Newborns prefer glucose and water to sterile water.

**Touch.**  The newborn perceives tactile sensation in any part of the body, although the face (especially the mouth), hands, and soles of the feet seem to be most sensitive. There is increasing documentation that touch and motion are essential to normal growth and development. Gentle patting of the back or rubbing of the abdomen usually elicits a calming response from the infant. However, painful stimuli, such as a pinprick, elicit an upset response.

# NURSING CARE OF THE NEWBORN AND FAMILY

## ■ Assessment*

The newborn requires thorough, skilled observation to ensure a satisfactory adjustment to extrauterine life. Physical assessment following delivery can be divided into four phases: (1) the initial assessment using the Apgar scoring system, (2) transitional assessment during the periods of re-activity, (3) assessment of gestational age, and (4) systematic physical examination. In addition, the nurse must be aware of those behaviors that signal successful attachment between the infant and parents. Awareness of the expected normal findings during each assessment process helps the nurse recognize any deviation that may prevent the infant from progressing uneventfully through the early postnatal period. With increasingly shorter hospitalizations, accomplishing a thorough newborn assessment and parent teaching has become a challenge (see p. 287).

### Initial Assessment: Apgar Scoring

The most frequently used method to assess the newborn's immediate adjustment to extrauterine life is the *Apgar scoring system* (Papile, 2001). The score is based on observation of heart rate, respiratory effort, muscle tone, reflex irritability, and color (Table 8-1). Each item is given a score of 0, 1, or 2. Evaluations of all five categories are made 1 and 5 minutes after birth and are repeated until the infant's condition stabilizes. Total scores of 0 to 3 represent severe distress, scores of 4 to 6 signify moderate difficulty, and scores of 7 to 10 indicate absence of difficulty in adjusting to extrauterine life. Many healthy newborns do not achieve a score of 10 because the body is not completely pink. The Apgar score is affected by the degree of physiologic imma-

---

*For additional information, please view "Pediatric Assessment" in *Whaley and Wong's Pediatric Nursing Video Series*, St Louis, 1996, Mosby; (800) 426-4545; www.mosby.com.

| TABLE 8-1 | Infant evaluation at birth—Apgar scoring system | | |
|---|---|---|---|
| **Sign** | **0** | **1** | **2** |
| Heart rate | Absent | Slow, <100 | >100 |
| Respiratory effort | Absent | Irregular, slow, weak cry | Good, strong cry |
| Muscle tone | Limp | Some flexion of extremities | Well-flexed |
| Reflex irritability | No response | Grimace | Cry, sneeze |
| Color | Blue, pale | Body pink, extremities blue | Completely pink |

turity, infection, congenital malformations, maternal sedation or analgesia, and neuromuscular disorders (American Academy of Pediatrics and American College of Obstetricians and Gynecologists, 1996; Hegyi and others, 1998).

The Apgar score reflects the general condition of the infant at 1 and 5 minutes based on the five parameters described above. The Apgar score is not a tool, however, that stands on its own to either interpret past events or predict future events linked to the infant's eventual neurologic or physical status. There has been a considerable amount of discussion and controversy in the past about Apgar scoring because of its misuse as an indicator for the presence or absence of perinatal asphyxia in the medicolegal field (American Academy of Pediatrics and American College of Obstetricians and Gynecologists, 1996). In addition, the Apgar score is not used to determine the newborn's need for resuscitation at birth.

## Transitional Assessment: Periods of Reactivity

The newborn exhibits behavioral and physiologic characteristics that can at first appear to be signs of stress. However, during the initial 24 hours changes in heart rate, respiration, motor activity, color, mucus production, and bowel activity occur in an orderly, predictable sequence, which is normal and indicates lack of stress. Distressed infants also progress through these stages but at a slower rate.

For 6 to 8 hours after birth the newborn is in the *first period of reactivity.* During the first 30 minutes the infant is very alert, cries vigorously, may suck a fist greedily, and appears very interested in the environment. At this time the neonate's eyes are usually open, suggesting that this is an excellent opportunity for mother, father, and child to see each other. Because the newborn has a vigorous suck reflex, this is an opportune time to begin breast-feeding. The newborn usually grasps the nipple quickly, satisfying both mother and child. This is particularly important to remember, because it is likely that after this initially highly active state the infant may be quite sleepy and uninterested in sucking. Physiologically the respiratory rate can be as high as 80 breaths/min, crackles may be heard, heart rate may reach 180 beats/min, bowel sounds are active, mucus secretions are increased, and temperature may decrease slightly.

After this initial stage of alertness and activity, the infant enters the *second stage* of the first reactive period, which generally lasts 2 to 4 hours. Heart and respiratory rates decrease, temperature continues to fall, mucus production decreases, and urine or stool is usually not passed. The infant is in a state of sleep and relative calm. Any attempt at stimulation usually elicits a minimal response. Because of the decrease in body temperature, avoid undressing or bathing the infant during this time.

The *second period of reactivity* begins when the infant wakes from this deep sleep; it lasts about 2 to 5 hours and provides another excellent opportunity for child and parents to interact. The infant is again alert and responsive, heart and respiratory rates increase, the gag reflex is active, gastric and respiratory secretions are increased, and passage of meconium commonly occurs. This period is usually over when the amount of respiratory mucus has decreased. Following this stage is a period of stabilization of physiologic systems and a vacillating pattern of sleep and activity.

### Behavioral Assessment

Another important area of assessment is observation of behavior. Infants' behavior helps shape their environment, and their ability to react to various stimuli affects how others relate to them. The principal areas of behavior for newborns are sleep, wakefulness, and activity, such as crying.

One method of systematically assessing the infant's behavior is use of the *Brazelton Neonatal Behavioral Assessment Scale (BNBAS)* (Brazelton and Nugent, 1996). The BNBAS is an interactive examination that assesses the infant's response to 28 items organized according to the clusters in Box 8-2. It is generally used as a research or diagnostic tool and requires special training.

In addition to its use as an initial and ongoing tool to assess neurologic and behavioral responses, the scale can be used as an assessor of initial parent-child relationships, as a preventive instrument that identifies the caregiver as one who may benefit from a role model, and as a guide for parents to help them focus on their infant's individuality and to develop a deeper attachment to their child. Studies have demonstrated that by showing parents the unique characteristics of their infant, a more positive perception of the infant develops, with increased interaction between infant and parent.

**Patterns of Sleep and Activity.**  Newborns begin life with a systematic schedule of sleep and activity that is initially evident during the periods of reactivity. For the next 2 to 3 days it is not unusual for infants to sleep almost constantly in order to recover from the exhausting birth process.

Infants have six distinct sleep-wake states, which represent a particular form of neural control (Table 8-2). As gestational and postconceptional maturity increases, each state becomes more precisely defined according to the behaviors observed. State is defined as a "group of characteristics that regularly occur together" (Blackburn and Loper, 1992) and are comprised of body activity, eye and facial movements, respiratory pattern, and response to internal and external stimuli. The six sleep-wake states are: quiet (deep) sleep, ac-

---

**Box 8-2  ■ ■ ■**
### Clusters of Neonatal Behaviors in Brazelton Neonatal Behavioral Assessment Scale

*Habituation*—Ability to respond to and then inhibit responding to discrete stimulus (light, rattle, bell, pin-prick) while asleep
*Orientation*—Quality of alert states and ability to attend to visual and auditory stimuli while alert
*Motor performance*—Quality of movement and tone
*Range of state*—Measure of general arousal level or arousability of infant
*Regulation of state*—How infant responds when aroused
*Autonomic stability*—Signs of stress (tremors, startles, skin color) related to homeostatic (self-regulating) adjustment of the nervous system
*Reflexes*—Assessment of several neonatal reflexes

| **TABLE 8-2** States of sleep and activity* | |
|---|---|
| **State/Behavior** | **Implications for Parenting** |
| **Deep Sleep (Quiet)**<br>Closed eyes<br>Regular breathing<br>No movement except for occasional sudden bodily twitch<br>No eye movement | Continue usual house noises because external stimuli do not arouse infant<br>Leave infant alone if sudden loud noise awakens infant and child cries<br>Do not attempt to feed |
| **Light Sleep (Active)**<br>Closed eyes<br>Irregular breathing<br>Slight muscular twitching of body<br>Rapid eye movements (REM) under closed eyelids<br>May smile | External stimuli that did not arouse infant during regular sleep may minimally arouse child<br>Periodic groaning or crying is usual; do not interpret as an indication of pain or discomfort |
| **Drowsy**<br>Eyes may be open<br>Irregular breathing<br>Active body movement variable, with occasional mild startles | Most stimuli arouse infant but may return to sleep state<br>Pick infant up during this time rather than leaving in crib<br>Provide mild stimulus to awaken<br>May enjoy nonnutritive sucking |
| **Quiet Alert**<br>Eyes wide open and bright<br>Responds to environment by active body movement and staring at close-range objects<br>Minimal body activity<br>Regular breathing<br>Focuses attention on stimuli | Satisfy infant's needs such as hunger or nonnutritive sucking<br>Place infant in area of home where activity is continuous<br>Place toys in crib or playpen<br>Place objects within 17.5-20 cm (7-8 inches) of infant's view<br>Intervene to console |
| **Active Alert**<br>May begin with whimpering and slight body movement<br>Eyes open<br>Irregular breathing | Remove intense internal or external stimuli because infant has increased sensitivity to stimuli |
| **Crying**<br>Progresses to strong, angry crying and uncoordinated thrashing of extremities<br>Eyes open or tightly closed<br>Grimaces<br>Irregular breathing | Comforting measures that were effective during alert state are usually ineffective<br>Rock and swaddle to decrease crying<br>Intervene to reduce fatigue, hunger, or discomfort |

*Portions adapted from Blackburn S, Loper DL: *Maternal, fetal, and neonatal physiology: a clinical perspective*, Philadelphia, 1992, WB Saunders.

tive (light) sleep, drowsy, awake (quiet), active alert, and crying. Infants respond to internal and external environmental factors by controlling sensory input and regulating the sleep-wake states; the ability to make smooth transitions between states is called **state modulation.** The ability to regulate sleep-wake states is essential in the neurobehavioral development of the infant. The more immature the infant, the less able he or she is able to cope with factors, external or internal, that affect the sleep-wake patterns.

Recognition and knowledge of sleep-wake states is important in the planning of nursing care. It is also important for nurses to help parents and caregivers understand the significance of the infant's behavioral responses to daily caregiving and how these states can be altered. A classic example is the newborn who feeds vigorously in the active alert state rather than the deep sleep state. The neurologic assessment of a newborn in the active alert state will differ significantly from that of the deep sleep state. Newborns typically spend as much as 16 to 18 hours sleeping and do not necessarily follow a pattern of light-dark diurnal rhythm; with increasing age sleep-wake states will change, with increasing amounts of time spent in awake alert states and decreasing amounts of sleep time. Approximately 50% of total sleep time is spent in irregular or rapid eye movement sleep.

**Cry.** The newborn should begin extrauterine life with a strong, lusty cry. The sounds produced by crying can be described as hunger, anger, pain, and "bid for attention" cries. Discomfort (pain) sounds initially consist of gasps and cries in which the consonant *H* is clearly distinguishable. The duration of crying is as highly variable in each infant as is the duration of sleep patterns. Some newborns may cry for as little as 5 minutes or as much as 2 hours or more per day.

Variations in the initial cry can indicate abnormalities. A weak, groaning cry or grunting during expiration usually indicates a possible respiratory disturbance. Absent, weak, or constant crying may suggest a pathologic state such as tension pneumothorax or perinatal asphyxia. A high-pitched, shrill cry may be a sign of increased intracranial pressure. Crying status alone, however, is not a diagnostic tool.

## Assessment of Attachment Behaviors

One of the most important areas of assessment is careful observation of those behaviors thought to indicate the formation of emotional bonds between the newborn and family, especially the mother. Although the terms *bonding* and *attachment* are sometimes referred to as separate phenomena, with **bonding** representing the development of emotional ties from parent to infant and **attachment** representing the emotional ties from infant to parent, in this discussion and in the one on p. 284, the terms are used interchangeably to denote both processes.

Unlike physical assessment of the neonate, which has concrete guidelines to follow, assessment of parent-child attachment requires much more skill in terms of observation and interviewing. The assessment process is even more challenging with the trend toward shortened hospital stays for mothers and their newborn infants. However, rooming-in of mother and infant and open invitations for father, siblings, and grandparents facilitate recognition of behaviors that demonstrate positive or negative attachment. Guidelines for assessment of bonding behaviors are presented in the Guidelines box.

Talking to the parents uncovers many variables that can affect the development of attachment and parenting. (See also Child Maltreatment, Chapter 16.) What expectations do they have for this child? In other words, how similar are their predictions of the fantasy child and their realizations about the real child? Encourage them to talk about their relationship with their own parents because the type of parenting that parents received as children influences their childrearing practices. Is this a planned birth? How do they see the addition of a dependent family member affecting their lifestyle? What arrangements have they made for such changes in lifestyle? What "support system" or significant others are available for assistance? What are their views regarding childrearing?

The labor process also significantly affects the immediate attachment of mothers to their newborn children. Factors such as a long labor, feeling tired or "drugged" after delivery, and problems with breast-feeding can delay the development of initial positive feelings toward the newborn.

During pregnancy, and often even before conception occurs, parents develop an image of the "ideal or fantasy infant." The unborn child has an imagined appearance, pattern of behavior, expected accomplishments, and predetermined effect on the lifestyle of the family. At birth the fantasy infant becomes the real infant. How closely the dream child resembles the real child influences the bonding process. Assessing such expectations during pregnancy and at the time of the infant's birth allows identification of discrepancies in the parents' view of the fantasy child vs the real child.

The **Neonatal Perception Inventory (NPI)** (Broussard, 1979) assesses the mother's perception of her real infant compared with her image of an "average" infant. It has been hypothesized that for optimum mothering to occur, the mother needs to see her infant as better than an "average" baby. Mothers who do not rate their infants as better than average may be at risk for developing parenting abilities that fail to meet the infant's needs. The NPI II (completed

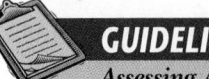

### GUIDELINES
#### Assessing Attachment Behavior

When the infant is brought to the parents, do they reach out for the child and call the child by name?

Do the parents speak about the child in terms of identification—whom the infant looks like; what appears special about their child over other infants?

When parents are holding the infant, what kind of body contact is there—do parents feel at ease in changing the infant's position; are fingertips or whole hands used; are there parts of the body they avoid touching or parts of the body they investigate and scrutinize?

When the infant is awake, what kinds of stimulation do the parents provide—do they talk to the infant, to each other, or to no one? How do they look at the infant—direct visual contact, avoidance of eye contact, or looking at other people or objects?

How comfortable do the parents appear in terms of caring for the infant? Do they express any concern regarding their ability or disgust for certain activities, such as changing diapers?

What type of affection do they demonstrate to the newborn, such as smiling, stroking, kissing, or rocking?

If the infant is fussy, what kinds of comforting techniques do the parents use, such as rocking, swaddling, talking, or stroking?

---

4 weeks after delivery) accurately predicted later childhood adjustment problems, whereas the NPI I (completed 1 to 2 days after the infant's birth) did not (Broussard, 1976). In follow-up studies over a 19-year period (Broussard, 1984), infants who were negatively perceived had the greatest risk for developing behavioral and emotional disorders.

Because attachment involves a mutually reciprocal interchange, observing the interaction between parent and infant is very important. An excellent opportunity exists during feeding. A useful instrument for systematically describing the parent's and infant's behaviors is the **Feeding Scale** developed by the **National Child Assessment Satellite Training (NCAST) program** (Barnard, 1994). It consists of 76 behavioral items; 50 items describe the parent's behavior regarding (1) sensitivity to cues, (2) response to child's distress, (3) social-emotional growth fostering, and (4) cognitive growth fostering. Twenty-six items focus on the child's behavior in terms of (1) clarity of cues and (2) responsiveness to parent. The results can be shared with the parent to encourage discussion of feelings about the infant and to highlight behaviors of the dyad that foster successful interaction. The Feeding Scale is appropriate for use with infants during the first year. Training to become a certified tester is available through the **NCAST** program.*

### Clinical Assessment of Gestational Age

Assessment of gestational age is an important criterion because perinatal morbidity and mortality are related to gestational age and birth weight. A frequently used method of determining gestational age is the **Simplified Assessment of Gestational Age** by Ballard, Novack, and Driver (1979)

---

*For information contact Jean F. Kelly, PhD, Director, NCAST, University of Washington, Box 357920, Seattle, WA 98195, (206) 543-8528, fax (206) 685-3284; e-mail: ncast@u.washington.edu.

(Fig. 8-1, *A*). The Ballard scale, an abbreviated version of the *Dubowitz scale,* can be used to measure gestational ages of infants between 35 and 42 weeks (Dubowitz and Dubowitz, 1977). It assesses six external physical and six neuromuscular signs. Each sign has a number score, and the cumulative score correlates with a maturity rating of from 26 to 44 weeks of gestation.

The "new" *Ballard Scale,* a revision of the original scale, can be used with newborns as young as 20 weeks of gestation. The tool has the same physical and neuromuscular sections but includes −1 and −2 scores that reflect signs of extremely premature infants, such as fused eyelids; imperceptible breast tissue; sticky, friable, transparent skin; no lanugo; and square-window (flexion of wrist) angle of greater than 90 degrees (see Fig. 8-1, *A,* and the description of the tests in Box 8-3). The examination of infants with a gestational age of 26 weeks or less should be performed at a postnatal age of less than 12 hours. For infants with a gestational age of at least 26 weeks, the examination can be performed up to 96 hours after birth. To ensure accuracy, it is recommended that the initial examination be performed within the first 48 hours of life. Neuromuscular adjustments following birth in extremely immature neonates require that a follow-up examination be performed to further validate neuromuscular criteria (Trotter, 1996). The scale overestimates gestational age by 2 to 4 days in infants younger than 37 weeks of gestation, especially at gestational ages of 32 to 37 weeks (Ballard and others, 1991). In a recent study,

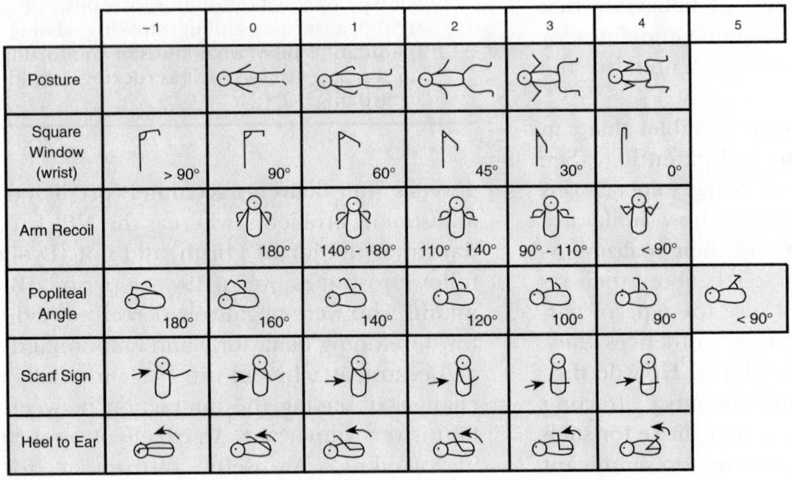

## ESTIMATION OF GESTATIONAL AGE BY MATURITY RATING

**Fig. 8-1** **A,** Ballard Scale for newborn maturity rating. Expanded scale includes extremely premature infants and has been refined to improve accuracy in more mature infants. (**A** from Ballard JL and others: New Ballard Score expanded to include extremely premature infants, *J Pediatr* 119:417, 1991.)

the Ballard scale was shown to overestimate gestational age of infants less than 28 weeks by as much as 1.3 to 3.3 weeks (Donovan and others, 1999), so other indices of gestational age must also be used in this age-group.

**Weight Related to Gestational Age.** The weight of the infant at birth also correlates with the incidence of perinatal morbidity and mortality. Birth weight alone, however, is a poor indicator of gestational age and fetal maturity. Maturity implies functional capacity—the degree to which the neonate's organ systems are able to adapt to the requirements of extrauterine life. Therefore gestational age is more closely related to fetal maturity than is birth weight.

Because heredity influences size at birth, it is important to note the sizes of other family members as part of the assessment process.

Classification of infants at birth by both weight and gestational age provides a more satisfactory method for predicting mortality risks and providing guidelines for management of the neonate. The infant's birth weight, length, and head circumference are plotted on standardized graphs that identify normal values for gestational age (Fig. 8-1, *B*). The infant whose weight is ***appropriate for gestational age (AGA)*** (between the 10th and 90th percentiles) can be presumed to have grown at a normal rate regardless of the

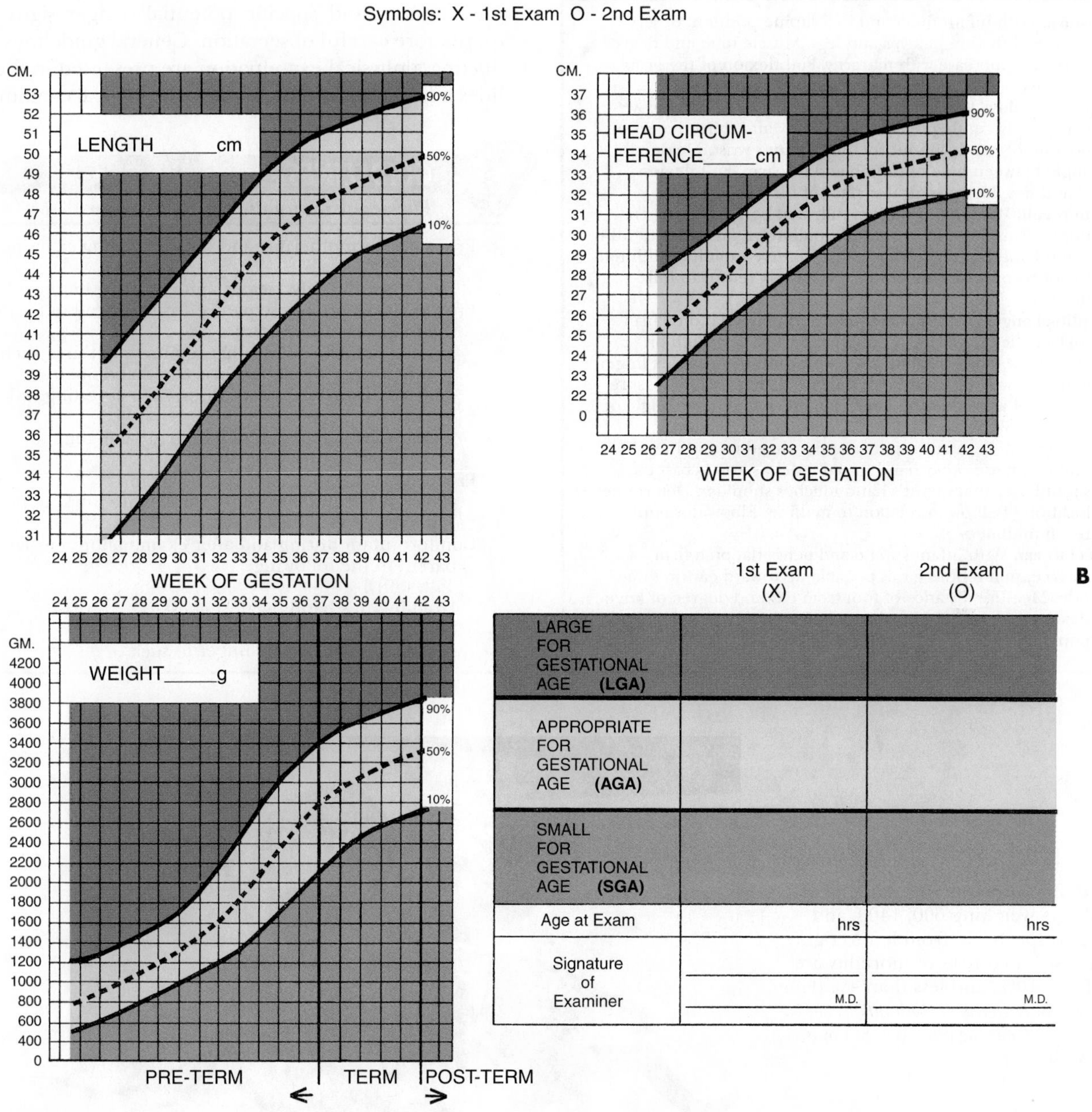

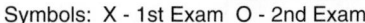

**Fig. 8-1—cont'd    B,** Newborn classification based on maturity and intrauterine growth. (**B** modified from Lubchenko LC, Hansman C, Boyd E: *J Pediatr* 37:403, 1966 and Battaglia FC, Lubchenko LC: *J Pediatr* 71:159, 1967.)

length of gestation—preterm, term, or postterm. The infant who is *large for gestational age (LGA)* (above the 90th percentile) can be presumed to have grown at an accelerated rate during fetal life; the *small-for-gestational-age (SGA)* infant (below the 10th percentile) can be presumed to have grown at a retarded rate during intrauterine life. When gestational age is determined according to the Ballard scale, the newborn will fall into one of the following nine possible categories for birth weight and gestational age: AGA—term,

preterm, postterm; SGA—term, preterm, postterm; LGA—term, preterm, postterm. Fig. 8-2 illustrates the disparity between birth weights of three preterm infants of the same gestational age of 32 weeks. Infants with birth weights of 600 g have over a 50% mortality rate, those weighing 1400 g have a 25% to 50% mortality rate, and infants weighing 2750 g have less than a 4% mortality rate. Therefore birth weight influences mortality—the lower the birth weight, the higher the mortality. The same is true for gestational age—the lower the gestational age, the higher the mortality.

## Physical Assessment

The discussion of physical examination focuses on normal findings, variations from the norm that require little or no intervention, and specific potential danger signs that require more careful observation. General guidelines for conducting a physical examination are presented in the Guidelines box. Table 8-3 summarizes the physical examination of

---

**Box 8-3** ▪ ■ □
### Tests Used in Assessing Gestational Age

**Posture.** With infant quiet and in a supine position, observe degree of flexion in arms and legs. Muscle tone and degree of flexion increase with maturity. Full flexion of the arms and legs = 4.

**Square window.** With thumb supporting back of arm below wrist, apply gentle pressure with index and third fingers on dorsum of hand without rotating infant's wrist. Measure angle between base of thumb and forearm. Full flexion (hand lies flat on ventral surface of forearm) = 4.

**Arm recoil.** With infant supine, fully flex both forearms on upper arms, hold for 5 seconds; pull down on hands to fully extend and rapidly release arms. Observe rapidity and intensity of recoil to a state of flexion. A brisk return to full flexion = 4.

**Popliteal angle.** With infant supine and pelvis flat on a firm surface, flex lower leg on thigh and then flex thigh on abdomen. While holding knee with thumb and index finger, extend lower leg with index finger of other hand. Measure degree of angle behind knee (popliteal angle). An angle of less than 90 degrees = 5.

**Scarf sign.** With infant supine, support head in midline with one hand; use other hand to pull infant's arm across the shoulder so that infant's hand touches shoulder. Determine location of elbow in relation to midline. Elbow does not reach midline = 4.

**Heel to ear.** With infant supine and pelvis flat on a firm surface, pull foot as far as possible up toward ear on same side. Measure distance of foot from ear and degree of knee flexion (same as popliteal angle). Knees flexed with a popliteal angle of less than 10 degrees = 4.

---

## GUIDELINES
### *Physical Examination of the Newborn*

Provide a normothermic and nonstimulating examination area.
   Undress only body area examined to prevent heat loss.
Proceed in an orderly sequence (usually head to toe) with the following exceptions:
   Perform all procedures that require quiet first, such as auscultating the lungs, heart, and abdomen.
   Perform disturbing procedures, such as testing reflexes, last.
   Measure head, chest, and length at same time to compare results.
Proceed quickly to avoid stressing infant.
   Check that equipment and supplies are working properly and are accessible.
Comfort infant during and after examination; involve parent in the following:
   Talk softly.
   Hold infant's hands against chest.
   Swaddle and hold.
   Give pacifier or gloved finger to suck.

---

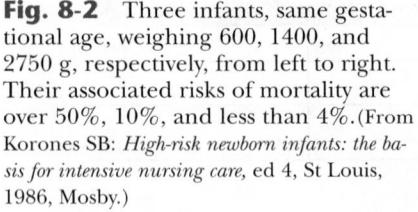

**Fig. 8-2** Three infants, same gestational age, weighing 600, 1400, and 2750 g, respectively, from left to right. Their associated risks of mortality are over 50%, 10%, and less than 4%. (From Korones SB: *High-risk newborn infants: the basis for intensive nursing care*, ed 4, St Louis, 1986, Mosby.)

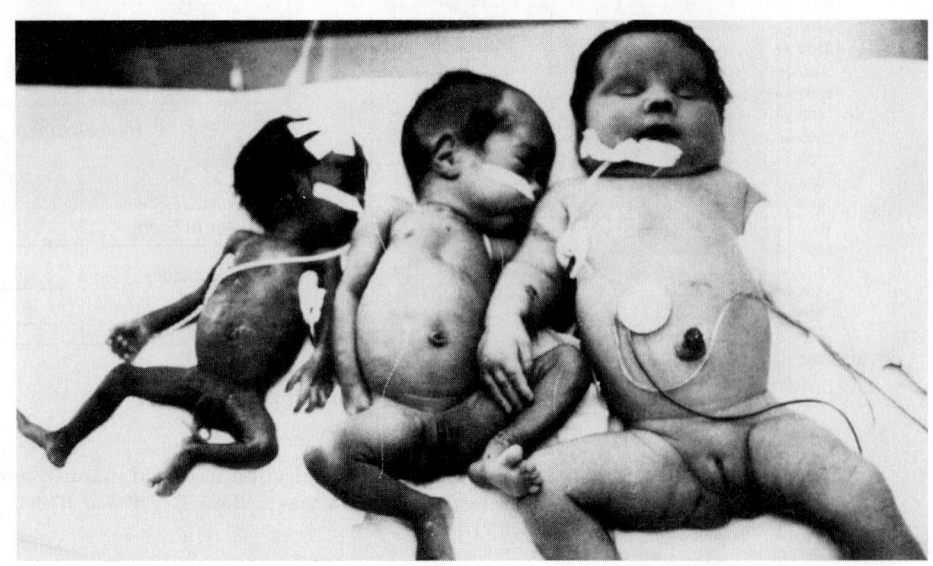

**TABLE 8-3**    Summary of physical assessment of the newborn

| Usual Findings | Common Variations/ Minor Abnormalities | Potential Signs of Distress/ Major Abnormalities |
|---|---|---|
| **General Measurements** | | |
| *Head circumference*—33-35 cm (13-14 inches); about 2-3 cm (1 inch) larger than chest circumference | Molding after birth may decrease head circumference | Head circumference <10th or >90th percentile |
| *Chest circumference*—30.5-33 cm (12-13 inches) | Head and chest circumference may be equal for first 1-2 days after birth | |
| *Crown-to-rump length*—31-35 cm (12.5-14 inches); approximately equal to head circumference | | |
| *Head-to-heel length*—48-53 cm (19-21 inches) | | |
| *Birth weight*—2700-4000 g (6-9 pounds) | Loss of 10% of birth weight in first week; regained in 10-14 days | Birth weight <10th or >90th percentile |
| **Vital Signs** | | |
| **Temperature** | | |
| Axillary—36.5°-37° C (97.9°-98° F) | Crying may increase body temperature slightly | Hypothermia |
| | Radiant warmer will falsely increase axillary temperature | Hyperthermia |
| **Heart Rate** | | |
| Apical—120-140 beats/min | Crying will increase heart rate; sleep will decrease heart rate | Bradycardia—Resting rate below 80-100 beats/min |
| | During first period of reactivity (6 to 8 hours), rate can reach 180 beats/min | Tachycardia—Rate above 160-180 beats/min |
| | | Irregular rhythm |
| **Respirations** | | |
| 30-60 breaths/min | Crying will increase respiratory rate; sleep will decrease respiratory rate | Tachypnea—Rate above 60 breaths/min |
| | During first period of reactivity (6 to 8 hours), rate can reach 80 breaths/min | Apnea—20 seconds or more |
| **Blood Pressure (BP)** | | |
| Oscillometric—65/41 mm Hg in arm and calf | Crying and activity will increase BP | Oscillometric systolic pressure in calf 6-9 mm Hg less than in upper extremity (sign of coarctation of aorta) |
| | Placing cuff on thigh may agitate infant; thigh BP may be higher than arm or calf BP by 4-8 mm Hg | |
| **General Appearance** | | |
| *Posture*—Flexion of head and extremities, which rest on chest and abdomen | *Frank breech*—Extended legs, abducted and fully rotated thighs, flattened occiput, extended neck | Limp posture, extension of extremities |
| **Skin** | | |
| At birth, bright red, puffy, smooth | Neonatal jaundice after first 24 hours | Progressive jaundice, especially in first 24 hours |
| Second to third day, pink, flaky, dry | Ecchymoses or petechiae caused by birth trauma | Cracked or peeling skin |
| Vernix caseosa | *Milia*—Distended sebaceous glands that appear as tiny white papules on cheeks, chin, and nose | Generalized cyanosis |
| Lanugo | | Pallor |
| Edema around eyes, face, legs, dorsa of hands, feet, and scrotum or labia | *Miliaria* or *sudamina*—Distended sweat (eccrine) glands that appear as minute vesicles, especially on face | Mottling |
| *Acrocyanosis*—Cyanosis of hands and feet | | Grayness |
| *Cutis marmorata*—Transient mottling when infant is exposed to decreased temperature, stress, or overstimulation | *Erythema toxicum*—Pink papular rash with vesicles superimposed on thorax, back, buttocks, and abdomen; may appear in 24 to 48 hours and resolve after several days | Plethora |
| See Critical Thinking Exercise box, p. 255 | | Hemorrhage, ecchymoses, or petechiae that persist |
| | | *Sclerema neonatorum*—Hard and stiff skin |
| | | Poor skin turgor |
| | *Harlequin color change*—Clearly outlined color change as infant lies on side; lower half of body becomes pink or red, and upper half is pale | Rashes, pustules, or blisters |
| | | *Café-au-lait spots*—Light brown spots |
| | | *Nevus flammeus*—Port-wine stain |

*Continued*

**TABLE 8-3** Summary of physical assessment of the newborn—cont'd

| Usual Findings | Common Variations/ Minor Abnormalities | Potential Signs of Distress/ Major Abnormalities |
|---|---|---|
| **Skin—cont'd** | *Mongolian spots*—Irregular areas of deep blue pigmentation, usually in sacral, lumbar, and gluteal regions; seen predominantly in newborns of African, Native American, Asian, or Hispanic descent (see figure at right) <br> *Telangiectatic nevi ("stork bites")*—Flat, deep pink, localized areas usually seen on back of neck | 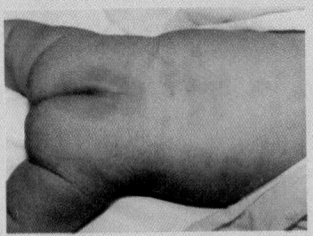 |
| **Head** <br> *Anterior fontanel*—Diamond shaped, 2.5-4.0 cm (1-1.75 inches) (see Fig. 8-6) <br> *Posterior fontanel*—Triangular, 0.5-1 cm (0.2-0.4 inch) <br> Fontanels should be flat, soft, and firm <br> Widest part of fontanel measured from bone to bone, not suture to suture | Molding following vaginal delivery <br> Third sagittal (parietal) fontanel <br> Bulging fontanel when crying <br> *Caput succedaneum*—Edema of soft scalp tissue <br> *Cephalhematoma (uncomplicated)*— Hematoma between periosteum and skull bone | Fused sutures <br> Bulging or depressed fontanels when quiet <br> Widened sutures and fontanels <br> *Craniotabes*—Snapping sensation along lambdoid suture that resembles indentation of Ping-Pong ball |
| **Eyes** <br> Lids usually edematous <br> Color—Slate gray, dark blue, brown <br> Absence of tears <br> Presence of red reflex <br> Corneal reflex in response to touch <br> Pupillary reflex in response to light <br> Blink reflex in response to light or touch <br> Rudimentary fixation on objects and ability to follow to midline | Epicanthal folds in Asian infants <br> Searching nystagmus or strabismus <br> *Subconjunctival (scleral) hemorrhages*— Ruptured capillaries, usually at limbus | Pink color of iris <br> Purulent discharge <br> Upward slant in non-Asians <br> Hypertelorism (3 cm or greater) <br> Hypotelorism <br> Congenital cataracts <br> Constricted or dilated fixed pupil <br> Absence of red reflex <br> Absence of pupillary or corneal reflex <br> Inability to follow object or bright light to midline <br> Yellow sclera |
| **Ears** <br> Position—Top of pinna on horizontal line with outer canthus of eye <br> Startle reflex elicited by a loud, sudden noise <br> Pinna flexible, cartilage present | Filled aural canals prevent visualization of tympanic membranes <br> Pinna flat against head <br> Irregular shape or size <br> Pits or skin tags | Low ear placement <br> Absence of startle reflex in response to loud noise (see text) <br> Minor abnormalities may be signs of various syndromes, especially renal |
| **Nose** <br> Nasal patency <br> Nasal discharge—Thin white mucus <br> Sneezing | Flattened, bruised, or slightly deviated | Nonpatent canals <br> Thick, bloody nasal discharge <br> Flaring of nares (alae nasi) <br> Copious nasal secretions or stuffiness (may be minor) |
| **Mouth and Throat** <br> Intact, high-arched palate <br> Uvula in midline <br> Frenulum of tongue <br> Frenum of upper lip <br> Sucking reflex—Strong and coordinated <br> Rooting reflex <br> Gag reflex <br> Extrusion reflex <br> Absent or minimal salivation <br> Vigorous cry | *Natal teeth*—Teeth present at birth; benign but may be associated with congenital defects <br> *Epstein pearls*—Small, white epithelial cysts along midline of hard palate | Cleft lip <br> Cleft palate <br> Large, protruding tongue or posterior displacement of tongue <br> Profuse salivation or drooling <br> *Candidiasis (thrush)*—White, adherent patches on tongue, palate, and buccal surfaces <br> Nasogastric tube placement impossible <br> Hoarse, high-pitched, weak, absent, or other abnormal cry |

**TABLE 8-3**  Summary of physical assessment of the newborn—cont'd

| Usual Findings | Common Variations/<br>Minor Abnormalities | Potential Signs of Distress/<br>Major Abnormalities |
|---|---|---|
| **Neck** | | |
| Short, thick, usually surrounded by skinfolds<br>Tonic neck reflex | *Torticollis* (wry neck)—Head held to one side with chin pointing to opposite side | Excessive skinfolds<br>Resistance to flexion<br>Absence of tonic neck reflex<br>Fractured clavicle |
| **Chest** | | |
| Anteroposterior and lateral diameters equal<br>Slight sternal retractions evident during inspiration<br>Xiphoid process evident<br>Breast enlargement | Funnel chest (pectus excavatum)<br>Pigeon chest (pectus carinatum)<br>Supernumerary nipples<br>Secretion of milky substance from breasts ("witch's milk") | Depressed sternum<br>Marked retractions of chest and intercostal spaces during respiration<br>Asymmetric chest expansion<br>Redness and firmness around nipples<br>Wide-spaced nipples |
| **Lungs** | | |
| Respirations chiefly abdominal<br>Cough reflex absent at birth, present by 1-2 days in term infants<br>Bilateral equal bronchial breath sounds | Rate and depth of respirations may be irregular, periodic breathing<br>Crackles shortly after birth | Inspiratory stridor<br>Expiratory grunting<br>Retractions<br>Persistent irregular breathing<br>Periodic breathing with repeated apneic spells<br>Seesaw respirations (paradoxical)<br>Unequal breath sounds<br>Persistent fine crackles<br>Wheezing<br>Diminished breath sounds<br>Peristaltic sounds on one side, with diminished breath sounds on same side |
| **Heart** | | |
| Apex—Fourth to fifth intercostal space, lateral to left sternal border<br>$S_2$ slightly sharper and higher in pitch than $S_1$ | *Sinus arrhythmia*—Heart rate increases with inspiration and decreases with expiration<br>Transient cyanosis on crying or straining | *Dextrocardia*—Heart on right side<br>Displacement of apex, muffled<br>Cardiomegaly<br>Murmurs<br>Thrills<br>Persistent cyanosis<br>Hyperactive precordium |
| **Abdomen** | | |
| Cylindric in shape<br>*Liver*—Palpable 1-3 cm below right costal margin<br>*Spleen*—Tip palpable at end of first week of age<br>*Kidneys*—Palpable 1-2 cm above umbilicus<br>*Umbilical cord*—Bluish white at birth with two arteries and one vein<br>*Femoral pulses*—Equal bilaterally | Umbilical hernia<br>*Diastasis recti*—Midline gap between recti muscles<br>*Wharton's jelly*—Unusually thick umbilical cord content | Abdominal distention<br>Localized bulging<br>Distended veins<br>Absent bowel sounds<br>Enlarged liver and spleen<br>Ascites<br>Visible peristaltic waves<br>Scaphoid or concave abdomen<br>Green umbilical cord<br>Presence of only one artery in cord<br>Urine or stool leaking from cord<br>Palpable bladder distention following scanty voiding<br>Absent femoral pulses<br>Cord bleeding or hematoma |
| **Female Genitalia** | | |
| Labia and clitoris usually edematous<br>Urethral meatus behind clitoris<br>Vernix caseosa between labia<br>Urination within 24 hours | *Pseudomenstruation*—Blood-tinged or mucoid discharge<br>Hymenal tag | Enlarged clitoris with urethral meatus at tip<br>Fused labia<br>Absence of vaginal opening<br>Meconium from vaginal opening<br>No urination within 24 hours<br>Masses in labia<br>Ambiguous genitalia |

*Continued*

**TABLE 8-3** Summary of physical assessment of the newborn—cont'd

| Usual Findings | Common Variations/ Minor Abnormalities | Potential Signs of Distress/ Major Abnormalities |
|---|---|---|
| **Male Genitalia** | | |
| Urethral opening at tip of glans penis<br>Testes palpable in scrotum<br>Scrotum usually large, edematous, pendulous, and covered with rugae; usually deeply pigmented in dark-skinned ethnic groups<br>Smegma<br>Urination within 24 hours | Urethral opening covered by prepuce<br>Foreskin not retractable<br>*Epithelial pearls*—Small, firm, white lesions at tip of prepuce<br>Erection or priapism<br>Testes palpable in inguinal canal<br>Scrotum small | *Hypospadias*—Urethral opening on ventral surface of penis<br>*Epispadias*—Urethral opening on dorsal surface of penis<br>*Chordee*—Ventral curvature of penis<br>Testes not palpable in scrotum or inguinal canal<br>No urination within 24 hours<br>Inguinal hernia<br>Hypoplastic scrotum<br>*Hydrocele*—Fluid in scrotum<br>Masses in scrotum<br>Meconium from scrotum<br>Discoloration of testes (blue or purple)<br>Ambiguous genitalia |
| **Back and Rectum** | | |
| Spine intact, no openings, masses, or prominent curves<br>Trunk incurvation reflex<br>Anal reflex<br>Patent anal opening<br>Passage of meconium within 48 hours of birth | Green liquid stools in infant under phototherapy<br>Delayed passage of meconium in very-low-birth-weight neonates | Anal fissures or fistulas<br>Imperforate anus<br>Absence of anal reflex<br>No meconium within 36-48 hours<br>Pilonidal cyst or sinus<br>Tuft of hair along spine<br>Spina bifida (any degree) |
| **Extremities** | | |
| Ten fingers and toes<br>Full range of motion (ROM)<br>Nail beds pink, with transient cyanosis immediately after birth<br>Creases on anterior two thirds of sole<br>Sole usually flat<br>Symmetry of extremities<br>Equal muscle tone bilaterally, especially resistance to opposing flexion<br>Equal bilateral brachial pulses | Partial syndactyly between second and third toes<br>Second toe overlapping into third toe<br>Wide gap between first (hallux) and second toes<br>Deep crease on plantar surface of foot between first and second toes<br>Asymmetric length of toes<br>Dorsiflexion and shortness of hallux | *Polydactyly*—Extra digits<br>*Syndactyly*—Fused or webbed digits<br>*Phocomelia*—Hands or feet attached close to trunk<br>*Hemimelia*—Absence of distal part of extremity<br>Hyperflexibility of joints<br>Persistent cyanosis of nail beds<br>Yellowing of nail beds<br>Sole covered with creases<br>Transverse palmar (simian) crease<br>Fractures<br>Decreased or absent ROM<br>*Dislocated or subluxated hip*<br>   Limitation in hip abduction<br>   Unequal gluteal or leg folds<br>   Unequal knee height (Allis or Galeazzi sign)<br>   Audible clunk on abduction (Ortolani sign)<br>Asymmetry of extremities<br>Unequal muscle tone or range of motion |
| **Neuromuscular System** | | |
| Extremities usually maintain some degree of flexion<br>Extension of an extremity followed by previous position of flexion<br>Head lag while sitting, but momentary ability to hold head erect<br>Able to turn head from side to side when prone<br>Able to hold head in horizontal line with back when held prone | Quivering or momentary tremors | *Hypotonia*—Floppy, poor head control, extremities limp<br>*Hypertonia*—Jittery, arms and hands tightly flexed, legs stiffly extended, startles easily<br>Asymmetric posturing (except tonic neck reflex)<br>*Opisthotonic posturing*—Arched back<br>Signs of paralysis<br>Tremors, twitches, and myoclonic jerks<br>Marked head lag in all positions |

the newborn. (See Chapter 7 for further discussion of examination techniques.)

**General Measurements.** Several important measurements of the newborn are significant when compared with each other, as well as when recorded over time on a graph. For the full-term infant, average *head circumference* is between 33 and 35 cm (13 to 14 inches). Head circumference may be somewhat less immediately after birth because of the molding process that occurs during vaginal delivery. Usually by the second or third day the normal size and contour of the skull have replaced the molded one.

*Chest circumference* is 30.5 to 33 cm (12 to 13 inches). Head circumference is usually about 2 to 3 cm (about 1 inch) greater than chest circumference. Because of the molding of the head during delivery, these measurements may initially appear equal. However, if the head is significantly smaller than the chest, microcephaly or premature closure of the sutures (craniostenosis) is suspected. If the head is more than 4 cm (1¾ inches) larger than the chest in circumference and this relationship remains constant or increases over several days, then hydrocephalus must be considered. Other causes of increased head circumference are caput succedaneum, cephalhematoma, and subdural hematoma. Prematurity and intrauterine malnutrition also can cause the head measurement to be significantly larger than the chest circumference, but this is because of decreased chest size, not increased head circumference.

## Critical Thinking Exercise

### Newborn Physical Assessment

A young, first-time, single mother is examining her newborn daughter, who is only 2 hours old. She seems to be preoccupied with her daughter's face and makes the following statement: "She looks OK, but these white pimples on her face really bother me." Which of the following would provide the mother with the most accurate information?

FIRST, THINK ABOUT IT . . .

• What precise question are you trying to answer?
• Within what point of view are you thinking?

1. "Those pimples will go away in a few days if you apply skin moisturizer."
2. "You should discuss those with your pediatrician when she comes in later."
3. "Those 'pimples' are just immature sweat glands that all newborns have until they are a few weeks old."
4. "Just don't touch those, or they will get infected!"

*The best response is three. The "pimples" are milia, immature sweat glands that are common in newborns. The other answers do not adequately address the mother's concerns that her newborn is somehow different from others or that her newborn's appearance has been altered by birth. The mother's point of view may be very different from the nurse's, and she requires precise, accurate information to cope with her concern.*

Head circumference may also be compared with *crown-to-rump* length, or sitting height. Crown-to-rump measurements are usually 31 to 35 cm (12.5 to 14 inches) and are approximately equal to head circumference. The relationship of the head and crown-to-rump measurements is more reliable than that of the head and chest. Severn (1994) noted that neonatal head circumference and crown-to-rump length provide a more accurate means for identifying infants at risk; head circumference was shown to be equal to or up to 1 cm more than crown-to-rump length in 62% of the infants examined and determined to be normocephalic.

*Head-to-heel* length is also measured. Because of the usual flexed position of the infant, extend the leg completely when measuring total body length. The average length of the newborn is 48 to 53 cm (19 to 21 inches) (Fig. 8-3).

*Abdominal circumference* in the newborn may be measured just above the level of the umbilicus. Because the umbilical cord is still attached, making measurements across the umbilicus (see Fig. 7-4) is too variable in newborns. Measuring the abdominal circumference below the umbilical region is also unsuitable because bladder status may affect the reading. In the event of abdominal distention, serial measurements are taken to determine changes in girth (Conner, 1996).

Measure *body weight* soon after birth because weight loss occurs fairly rapidly. Normally the newborn loses up to 10% of the birth weight by 3 to 4 days of age because of loss of excessive extracellular fluid and meconium, as well as limited food intake, especially in breast-fed infants. The birth weight is regained by the tenth day of life. Most newborns weigh 2700 to 4000 g (6 to 9 pounds), the average weight being about 3400 g (7½ pounds). Accurate birth weights and lengths are important because they provide a baseline for assessment of risk status and future growth.

Another category of measurements is vital signs. *Axillary temperatures* are taken because insertion of a thermometer into the rectum can cause perforation of the mucosa. (See Fig. 7-7, *B*.) Core (internal) body temperature varies according to the period of reactivity but should be 36.5° to 37.6° C (97.7° to 99.7° F). Skin temperature is slightly lower than core body temperature. Therefore, axillary tempera-

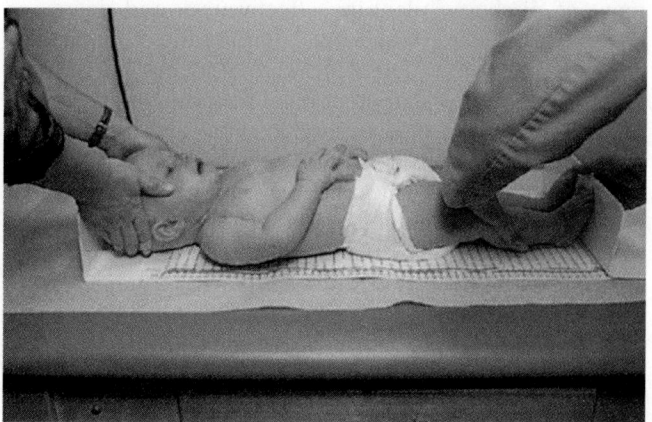

**Fig. 8-3** Measurement of infant length.

ture may be less than rectal or tympanic membrane temperature, although the difference is small (as little as 0.2° F) between axillary and rectal sites (Yetman and others, 1993). Because brown adipose tissue is located in the axillary pocket, axillary readings may be elevated whenever nonshivering thermogenesis (NST) occurs (see p. 241). However, axillary readings may be normal in cold-stressed infants when NST is not triggered or is overwhelmed (Bliss-Holtz, 1993). There is also controversy regarding the accuracy of tympanic membrane sensors for measuring temperature in infants and children.

The single best method for determining the newborn infant's temperature in any given situation remains elusive when considering the available studies. There is controversy regarding the accuracy of tympanic membrane sensors. Bliss-Holtz (1993) compared axillary and tympanic membrane temperatures in neonates and found that tympanic membrane temperature measurements were helpful in determining the infant's thermal state. However, other studies have found tympanic membrane temperatures to have high variability according to neonatal environment (bassinet or open crib, radiant warmer, and incubator) (Hicks, 1996; Leick-Rude and Bloom, 1998) and limited usefulness for use in critically ill neonates (Weiss, Poeltler, and Gocka, 1993; Wilshaw and others, 1999). One study concluded that tympanic membrane temperatures were unacceptable for detecting fever in children under 6 years of age (Lanham and others, 1999). Bliss-Holtz (1995) and Yetman and others (1993) concluded that infrared tympanic membrane technology has yet to meet current clinical needs for use in newborn infants. Infrared axillary and digital thermometers are used in many neonatal units because they give rapid readings and are easy to clean; studies demonstrate their usefulness in well term newborns (Sganga and others, 2000), whereas accuracy with critically ill neonates is less predictable (Seguin and Terry, 1999; Wilshaw and others, 1999). Skin temperature readings have also been found to vary with probe site placement, bed type, environmental temperature, and the use of blankets, clothing, and nesting devices (Leick-Rude and Bloom, 1998). Advantages of digital thermometers in neonatal care include relatively easy readibility by parents and caretakers in the home, improvement of discharge planning effectiveness, and decreased risk of breakage and associated complications compared to glass thermometers. The American Academy of Pediatrics (2001) has issued a statement recommending that mercury thermometers no longer be used in clinics and homes to decrease mercury exposure hazard.

In most studies regarding newborn temperature, the glass mercury thermometer is the gold standard against which other methods are compared. There is no universal agreement on placement times for glass thermometers, although 3 minutes for rectal temperature and 5 minutes for axillary temperature are considered to be adequate.

Nurses must be cognizant of the many variables involved (site—axillary, rectal, tympanic, skin; environment—radiant warmer, open crib, incubator, clothing, or nesting; purpose—fever, possible sepsis [in which case the temperature may be lower than normal in newborns], and thermoregulation in

the transition phase; instrument—electronic, digital, infrared) and be able to make clear clinical decisions based on accurate and objective data. Cost effectiveness (nursing care time and instrument operation cost) and potential cross-contamination risks must also be considered when evaluating neonatal temperature measurement (Sganga and others, 2000). Further research is needed to perfect thermometers that accurately reflect the infant's core temperature in order to effectively plan nursing care and maintain a stable temperature.

*Pulse* and *respirations* vary according to the periods of reactivity and to the infant's behavior but are usually in the range of 120 to 140 beats/min and 30 to 60 breaths/min, respectively. Both are counted for a full 60 seconds to detect irregularities in rate, rhythm, and quality. The heart rate is taken apically with a stethoscope, and the femoral arteries are palpated for equality of strength or fullness.

Measurement of **blood pressure (BP)** provides useful baseline data and may indicate cardiovascular problems. However, routine BP measurement on healthy full-term neonates is not recommended because it is a poor predictor for hypertension later in life (American Academy of Pediatrics, 1993). BP is most easily and accurately assessed using oscillometry (Dinamap) although the device is less reliable when the mean arterial BP is below 35 mm Hg (Fig. 8-4). Oscillometric blood pressures are more accurate when the newborn is in quiet or sleep state and an appropriate cuff width–to–arm or calf ratio of 0.45 to 0.70 (approximately ½ to ¾) is used (Nutnarumit, Yang, and Bada-Ellzey, 1999). It is also recommended that an average of two to three BP measurements be taken in sick infants and that the mean BP be used because there is less error than when using systolic and diastolic readings. The average oscillometric systolic/diastolic BP is 65/41 mm Hg at 1 to 3 days of age (Park and Menard, 1989). Compare BP in the upper and lower extremities, which should be equal.

Calf BP measurements are comparable to brachial pressures in newborns and infants less than 1 year of age and are often more accessible. For consistency, it is recommended that baseline calf and brachial pressures be taken initially and the site documented (Axton and others, 1995).

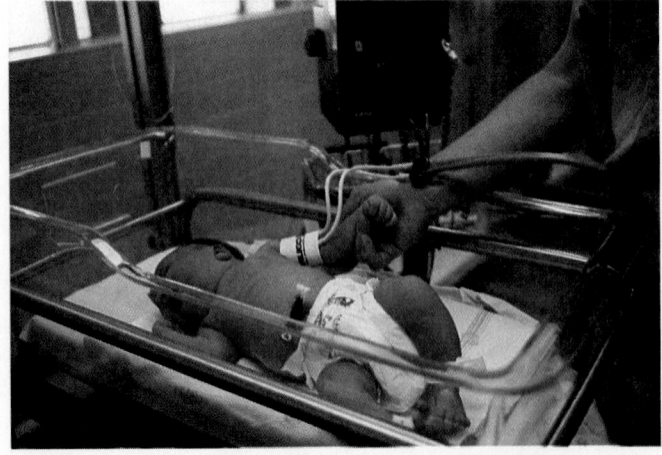

**Fig. 8-4** Measurement of blood pressure using oscillometry.

> **NURSING ALERT** Systolic oscillometric BP in the calf that is 6 to 9 mm Hg less than systolic BP in the upper arm is a sign of possible coarctation of the aorta and should be reported for further evaluation (Park and Lee, 1989).

A suggested schedule for monitoring heart and respiratory rates and temperature is on admission to the nursery and then once every 8 hours until discharge. However, this schedule may vary according to institutional policy. Any change in the infant, such as in color, breathing, muscle tone, or behavior, necessitates more frequent monitoring.

**General Appearance.**   In the full-term newborn the *posture* is one of flexion, a result of in utero position (Fig. 8-5). Most infants are born in a vertex (head first) presentation and keep the head flexed, with the chin resting on the upper chest. The arms are flexed at the elbows and rest, folded, on the chest with hands clenched or fisted. The legs are flexed at the knees, the hips are flexed with thighs resting on the abdomen, and the feet are dorsiflexed against the anterior aspect of the legs. The vertebral column is also flexed.

Note any deviation from this very characteristic fetal position. For example, preterm, as well as hypoxic, infants do not assume an attitude of total flexion but rather one of limp or hypotonic extension. Nonvertex presentations also result in variations in posture. In breech presentations the posture will depend on the presenting part; a frank breech presentation results in extended legs, abducted and fully rotated thighs, a flattened head on top, and a neck that appears elongated.

Observe the infant's *behavior,* especially the degree of alertness, drowsiness, and irritability, which are common signs of neurologic problems. Mentally ask the following questions when assessing behavior:

- Is the infant awakened easily by a loud noise?
- Is the infant comforted by rocking, sucking, or cuddling?
- Do there seem to be periods of deep and light sleep?
- When awake, does the infant seem satisfied after a feeding?
- What stimuli elicit responses from the infant?

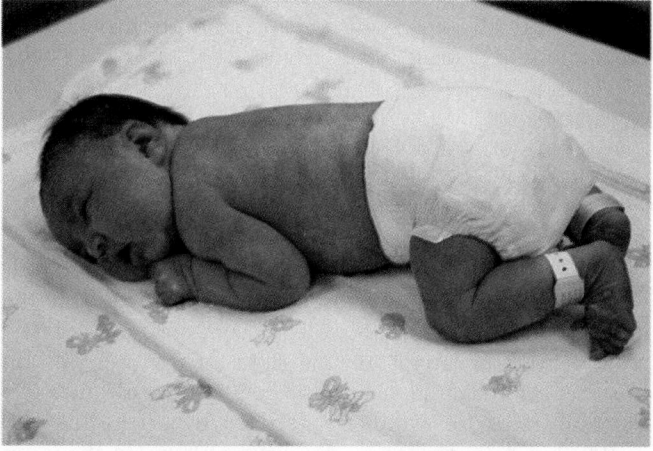

**Fig. 8-5**   Flexion position of neonate.

**Skin.**   The *texture* of the newborn's skin is velvety smooth and puffy, especially about the eyes, the legs, the dorsal aspect of the hands and feet, and the scrotum or labia.

Skin *color* depends on racial and familial background and varies greatly among newborns. In general, the Caucasian infant is usually pink to red; the African-American newborn may appear a pinkish or yellowish brown. Infants of Hispanic descent may have an olive tint or a slight yellow cast to the skin. Infants of Asian descent may be a rosy or yellowish tan. The color of Native American newborns depends on the tribe and can vary from a light pink to a dark reddish brown. By the second or third day the skin turns to its more natural tone and is drier and flakier.

Observe the color of the skin in relation to activity, position, and temperature changes. In general, the infant becomes redder when crying and may demonstrate transient periods of cyanosis during the first few hours of life (not associated with apnea or bradycardia). Several other color changes and minor skin blemishes that may be noted on the skin are described in Table 8-3.

At birth the skin is covered with a grayish white, cheese-like substance called *vernix caseosa,* a mixture of sebum and desquamating cells. If it is not removed during the bath, it will dry and disappear by about 24 to 48 hours. A fine, downy hair called *lanugo* is present on the skin, especially on the forehead, cheeks, shoulders, and back.

**Head.**   General observation of the *contour* of the head is important because molding occurs in almost all vaginal deliveries. In a vertex delivery the head is usually flattened at the forehead, with the apex rising and forming a point at the end of the parietal bones and the posterior skull or occiput dropping abruptly. The usual, more oval contour of the head is apparent by 1 to 2 days after birth. The change in shape occurs because the bones of the cranium are not fused, allowing for overlapping of the edges of these bones to accommodate to the size of the birth canal during delivery. Such molding does not occur in infants born by cesarean section unless there has been prolonged labor or the head has been engaged in the pelvis.

Six bones—the frontal, occipital, two parietals, and two temporals—constitute the cranium. Between the junctions of these bones are bands of connective tissue called *sutures.* At the junction of the suture are wider spaces of unossified membranous tissue called *fontanels.* The two most prominent fontanels are the *anterior fontanel,* formed by the junction of the sagittal, coronal, and frontal sutures, and the *posterior fontanel,* formed by the junction of the sagittal and lambdoid sutures (Fig. 8-6, *A*).

> **NURSING TIP**   The location of the sutures is easily remembered because the coronal suture "crowns" the head, and the sagittal suture "separates" the head.

Two other fontanels—the *sphenoidal* and *mastoid*—are normally present but are not usually palpable. An additional third fontanel located between the anterior and posterior fontanels along the sagittal suture is found in some neonates but is also found in some infants with Down syndrome. Always record the presence of this sagittal or parietal fontanel.

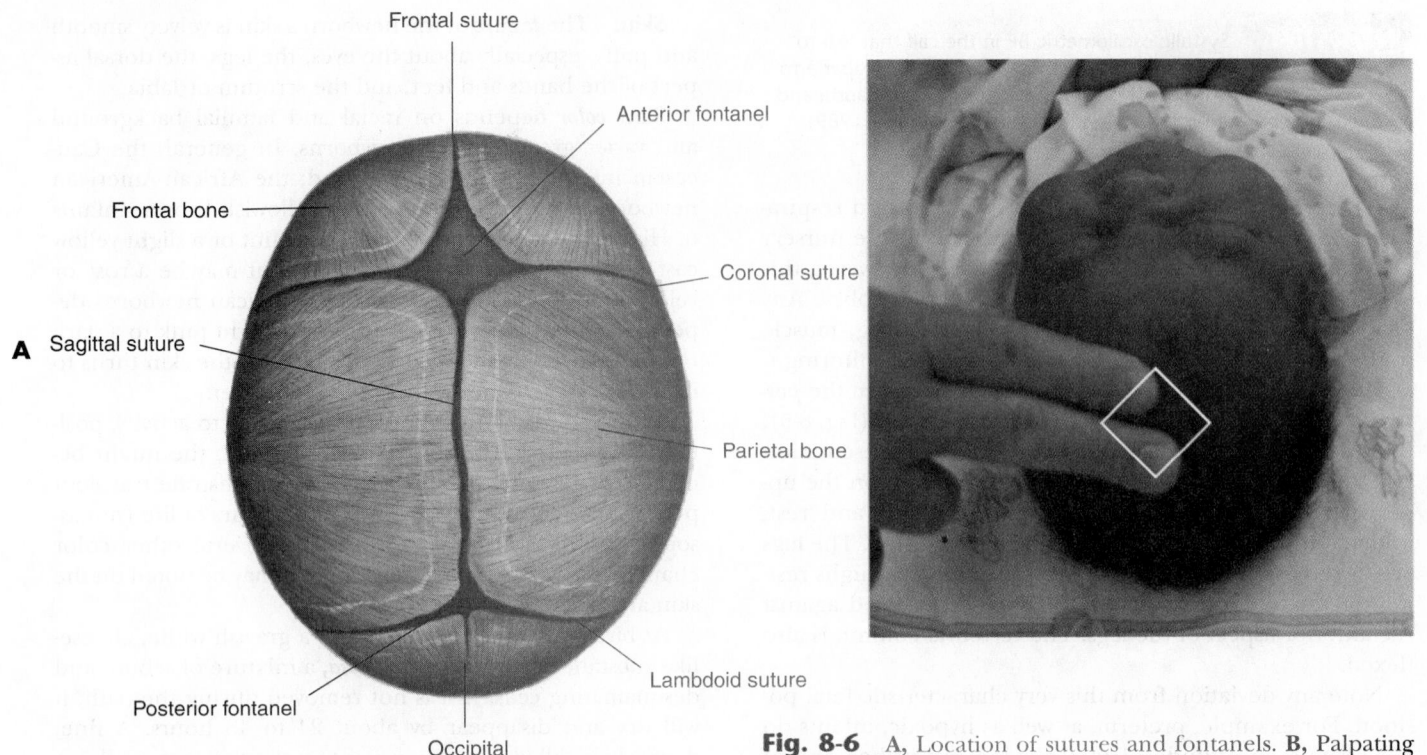

**Fig. 8-6** **A,** Location of sutures and fontanels. **B,** Palpating anterior fontanel.

Palpate the skull for all sutures and fontanels by using the tip of the index finger and running it along the ends of the bones (Fig. 8-6, *B*). Sutures feel like cracks between the skull bones; fontanels feel like wider "soft spots" at the junction of sutures. Note their size, shape, molding, and any abnormal closure.

The anterior fontanel is diamond shaped and measures 4 to 5 cm (about 2 inches) at its widest point (from bone to bone, rather than from suture to suture). The posterior fontanel is triangular, measuring between 0.5 and 1 cm (less than ½ inch) at its widest part. It is easily located by following the sagittal suture toward the occiput. The posterior fontanel may not be palpable after birth because of edema (caput) or other cranial molding.

The fontanels should feel flat, firm, and well demarcated against the bony edges of the skull. Frequently pulsations are visible at the anterior fontanel. Coughing, crying, or lying down may temporarily cause the fontanels to bulge and become more taut.

**NURSING ALERT** Always record and report a widened, tense, bulging fontanel (sign of increased intracranial pressure) and a markedly sunken, depressed fontanel (sign of dehydration or malformation).

Palpate the skull for any unusual masses or prominences, particularly those resulting from birth trauma, such as caput succedaneum or cephalhematoma. (See Chapter 9.) Because of the pliability of the skull, exerting pressure at the margin of the parietal and occipital bones along the lambdoid suture may produce a snapping sensation similar to the indentation of a Ping-Pong ball. This phenomenon, known as *physiologic craniotabes,* may be found normally, especially in newborns of breech birth, but also may indicate hydrocephalus, congenital syphilis, or rickets.

Assess the degree of *head control.* Although *head lag* is normal, the newborn has some ability to control the head in certain positions. If the supine infant is pulled from the arms into a semi-Fowler position, head lag and hyperextension occur (Fig. 8-7, *A*). However, as infants are brought forward into a sitting position, they attempt to control their heads in an upright position. As the head falls forward onto the chest, many infants attempt to right it into the erect position. If they are held in ventral suspension (i.e., held prone above and parallel to the examining surface), the head is held in a straight line with the spinal column (Fig. 8-7, *B*). When lying on the abdomen, newborns have the ability to lift the head slightly, turning it from side to side. Marked head lag is seen in neonates with Down syndrome, prematurity, hypoxia, and metabolic and neurologic disorders.

**NURSING ALERT** Report evidence of excessive head lag and observe for other signs of neurologic deficit.

**Eyes.** Because newborns tend to keep their eyes tightly closed, begin the examination of the eyes by observing the lids for edema, which is normally present for the first 2 days after delivery. A lateral upward slope of the eyes with an inner epicanthal fold may indicate Down syndrome. Observe the eyes for symmetry and for hypertelorism (see p. 193) but do not measure the distance between the inner canthi unless there is cause for further investigation. *Tears*

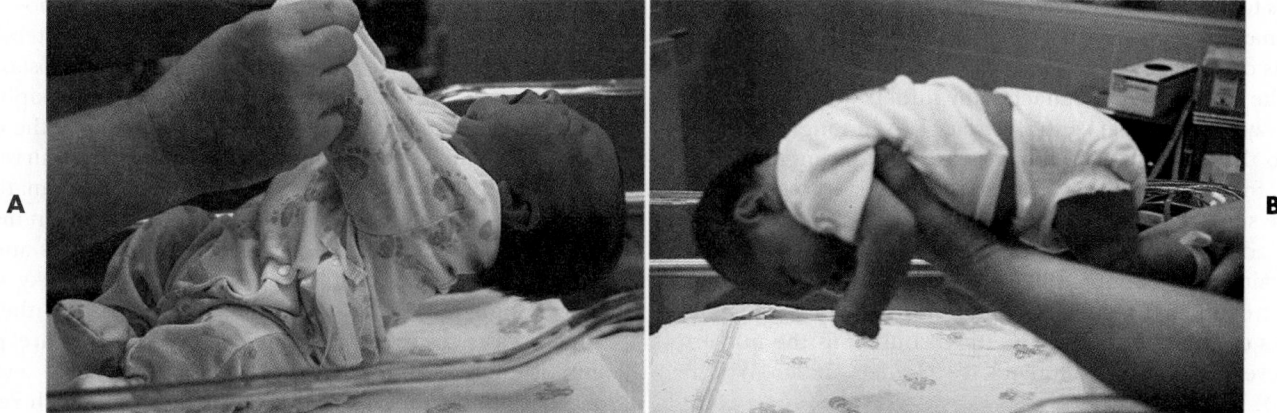

**Fig. 8-7**   Head control in infant. **A,** Inability to hold head erect when pulled to sitting position. **B,** Ability to hold head erect when placed in ventral suspension.

may be present at birth, but purulent discharge from the eyes shortly after birth is abnormal.

> **NURSING ALERT**   Report purulent discharge, which may signify *ophthalmia neonatorum* (infectious conjunctivitis of the newborn).

To visualize the surface structures of the eye, hold the infant supine and gently lower the head. The eyes will usually open, similar to the mechanism of a doll's eyes. The *sclera* should be white and clear.

Examine the cornea for the presence of any opacities or haziness. The *corneal reflex* is present at birth but is generally not elicited unless brain or eye damage is suspected. The pupil usually responds to light by constricting. Absence of the *pupillary reflex,* particularly by 3 weeks of age, suggests blindness. A fixed, dilated, or constricted pupil may indicate anoxia or brain damage. A searching *nystagmus* is common after birth. *Strabismus* is a normal finding because of the lack of binocularity.

Note the color of the *iris.* Most light-skinned newborns have slate gray or dark blue eyes, whereas dark-skinned infants have brown eyes. Absence of color is characteristic of albinism.

Although it is difficult to perform a complete funduscopic examination of the retina, always try to elicit a *red reflex* (see p. 194).

> **NURSING ALERT**   Always record and report absence of the red reflex. It may indicate the presence of retinal hemorrhages or congenital cataracts.

**Ears.**   Examine the ears for position, structure, and auditory function. The *pinna* is often flattened against the side of the head from pressure in utero. An otoscopic examination is ordinarily not performed, because the canals are filled with vernix caseosa and amniotic fluid, making visualization of the tympanic membrane difficult. Periauricular skin tags, sinuses, misshapen or low-set ears may be familial or associated with other congenital defects such as trisomy 18 and renal defects.

Assess *auditory ability* by making a sharp, loud noise close to the infant's head and noting the presence of the *startle reflex* (see Table 8-4) or twitching of the eyelids. Note, however, that the absence of a response to a loud noise in the newborn is not diagnostic for hearing deficit. Full-term newborns have the ability to habituate to noxious stimuli such as noise and may not react every time to a loud noise. Also, be aware of newborns considered at risk for hearing loss so that early testing can be performed (see Universal Newborn Hearing Screening, p. 268). (See Auditory Testing, Chapter 7; Hearing Impairment, Chapter 24.)

> **NURSING ALERT**   Always report the consistent absence of any behavioral response to a sudden noise, an indication of possible hearing deficit.

**Nose.**   Assess patency of the *nasal canals* by holding your hand over the infant's mouth and one canal and noting the passage of air through the unobstructed opening. If nasal patency is questionable, report it, because most newborns are obligatory nose breathers and are unable to breathe orally in response to nasal occlusion.

The *shape* of the nose is usually flattened after birth, and bruises are common, especially if forceps were used. Thin, white mucus is very common in the newborn, but a thick, bloody nasal discharge should be evaluated. *Sneezing* is very common.

> **NURSING ALERT**   Always report flaring of the nares because it is a serious sign of air hunger from respiratory distress.

**Mouth and Throat.**   The mouth is inspected for its existing structures. The *palate* is normally high arched and somewhat narrow. Inspect the hard and soft palates for any clefts, which warrant further investigation. A common finding is *Epstein pearls*—small, white, epithelial cysts along both sides of the midline of the hard palate. They are insignificant and disappear in several weeks.

The *frenulum* of the upper lip is a band of thick, pink tissue that lies under the inner surface of the upper lip and extends to the maxillary alveolar ridge. It usually disappears as the maxilla grows. It is particularly evident when the infant yawns or smiles.

The *lingual frenulum* attaches the underside of the tongue midway between the ventral surface of the tongue and the tip to the lower palate. In some cases a tight lingual frenulum, formerly referred to as tongue-tie, may restrict adequate sucking. Further evaluation may be required to ascertain adequate sucking, particularly in breast-fed infants (Masaitis and Kaempf, 1996; Wiessinger and Miller, 1995). The treatment for a tight lingual frenulum in infancy remains controversial; snipping the frenulum in the nursery, however, is not recommended (Godley, 1994; Wright, 1995).

Elicit the *sucking reflex* by placing a nipple or gloved finger in the infant's mouth. The infant should exhibit a strong, vigorous suck. To stimulate the *rooting reflex,* stroke the cheek and note the infant's response of turning toward the stimulated side and sucking (Fig. 8-8). Assess the *gag reflex* when using a tongue blade to visualize the oropharynx.

Inspect the *uvula* while the infant is crying and the chin is depressed. However, it may be retracted upward and backward during crying. Tonsillar tissue is generally not seen in the newborn. *Natal teeth* (teeth present at birth as opposed to *neonatal teeth*—teeth that erupt during the first month of life) are seen infrequently and erupt chiefly at the position of the lower central incisors. They are reported because they are frequently found with developmental abnormalities and syndromes, including cleft lip and palate. Most natal teeth are loosely attached. However, current thinking suggests preserving them until they exfoliate naturally (McDonald and Avery, 1999), unless breast-feeding is impaired by the neonate biting the breast or the teeth are very loose (Wright, 2000).

**Neck.** Because the newborn's neck is short and covered with folds of tissue, for adequate assessment allow the head to fall gently backward in slight hyperextension while supporting the back in a slightly raised position. Observe for range of motion, shape, and any abnormal masses, and palpate each clavicle for possible fractures. (See Fractures, Chapter 9.)

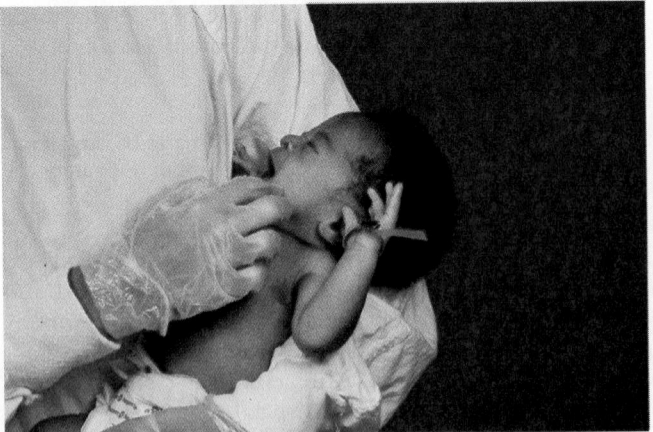

**Fig. 8-8** Eliciting rooting reflex. (From Seidel HM and others: *Mosby's guide to physical examination,* ed 3, St Louis, 1995, Mosby.)

**Chest.** The *shape* of the newborn's chest is almost circular because the anteroposterior and lateral diameters are equal. The ribs are very flexible, and slight intercostal retractions are normally seen on inspiration. The xiphoid process is commonly visible as a small protrusion at the end of the sternum. The sternum is raised and slightly curved.

Inspect the *breasts* for size, shape, and nipple formation, location, and number. Breast enlargement appears in many newborns of either sex by the second or third day and is caused by maternal hormones. Occasionally a milky substance (sometimes called *witch's milk*) is secreted by the infant's breasts. Infrequently, *supernumerary nipples* are present; if these are found, the kidneys should be evaluated because of the association of extra nipples with renal anomalies.

**Lungs.** The normal *respirations* of the newborn are irregular and abdominal, and the rate is between 30 and 60 breaths/min. Periods of *apnea* lasting more than 20 seconds are abnormal and may be accompanied by bradycardia. After the first forceful breaths required to initiate respiration, subsequent breaths should be easy and fairly regular in rhythm. Occasional irregularities occur in relation to crying, sleeping, and feeding. *Periodic breathing* is commonly seen in term newborns and consists of rapid nonlabored respirations followed by pauses of less than 20 seconds; periodic breathing may be more prominent during sleep and is not accompanied by status changes such as cyanosis or bradycardia.

Perform auscultation when the infant is quiet. Bronchial breath sounds should be equal bilaterally. Report any differences in auscultatory findings between symmetric sites. *Crackles* soon after birth indicate areas of atelectasis, which represent the normal transition of the lungs to extrauterine life. However, wheezes, persistence of crackles, and stridor should be reported.

**Heart.** *Heart rate* may range from 100 to 180 beats/min shortly after birth and, when the infant's condition has stabilized, from 120 to 140 beats/min. Palpate to find the *point of maximum intensity (PMI),* which is usually in the fourth to fifth intercostal space, medial to the left midclavicular line. The PMI gives some indication of the location of the heart, which may be displaced in conditions such as diaphragmatic hernia or pneumothorax. *Dextrocardia,* an anomaly wherein the heart is on the right side of the body, should be reported (the abdominal organs may also be reversed) along with associated circulatory abnormalities.

**NURSING TIP** Because auscultation of neonatal breath sounds and heart tones is often difficult for the untrained ear, practice auscultating one parameter at a time. Close your eyes and mentally block out the extraneous sounds heard, such as room noise or neonatal movement; offer the newborn a pacifier. Auscultation of a murmur and decreased air movement in specific lung fields requires patience and practice; it may require auscultating the heart tones or breath sounds for 1 to 3 minutes each.

Auscultation of the specific components of the *heart sounds* is difficult because of the rapid rate and effective transmission of respiratory sounds. However, the *first (S₁)* and *sec-*

ond (S₂) sounds should be clear and well-defined; the second sound is somewhat higher in pitch and sharper than the first. *Murmurs* are very frequently heard in the newborn, especially over the base of the heart or at the left sternal border in the third or fourth interspace. Ordinarily they are not associated with specific cardiac defects (Fuloria and Kreiter, 2002) because they frequently represent the incomplete functional closure of fetal shunts. (Grading of heart murmurs is discussed in Chapter 7.) However, always record and report any murmur or other unusual sounds.

**Abdomen.**   The normal *contour* of the abdomen is cylindric and prominent with visible veins. Bowel sounds are heard within the first 15 to 20 minutes after birth. Visible peristaltic waves may be observed in thin newborns but should not be seen in well-nourished infants.

Inspect the **umbilical cord** to determine the presence of two arteries, which look like papular structures, and one vein, which has a larger lumen than the arteries and a thinner vessel wall. At birth the cord appears bluish white and moist. After clamping, it begins to dry and appears a dull, yellowish brown. It progressively shrivels in size and turns greenish black.

If the umbilical cord appears unusually large in diameter at the base, inspect for the presence of a hematoma or small omphalocele. If the cord is clamped over an existing omphalocele, part of the intestine will be clamped, causing tissue necrosis. One practical rule of thumb is to cut the cord distally 4 to 5 inches from a questionable enlargement until further examination is carried out by a practitioner. The extra length can later be cut once normal anatomy has been identified.

Palpate after inspecting the abdomen. The **liver** is normally palpable 1 to 3 cm (about ½ to 1 inch) below the right costal margin. The tip of the **spleen** can sometimes be felt, but a palpable spleen more than 1 cm below the left costal margin suggests enlargement and warrants further investigation. Although both **kidneys** should be palpated, this maneuver requires considerable practice. When felt, the lower half of the right kidney and the tip of the left kidney are 1 to 2 cm above the umbilicus. During examination of the lower abdomen, palpate for **femoral pulses**, which should be strong and equal bilaterally.

> **NURSING ALERT**   Always report absent or weak femoral pulses for further evaluation.

**Female Genitalia.**   Normally the *labia majora* and *minora* (the minora may be more prominent) and *clitoris* are edematous, especially following a breech delivery. However, carefully inspect the labia and clitoris to identify any evidence of ambiguous genitalia or other abnormalities. Normally in a female the urethral opening is located behind the clitoris. Any deviation from this may mistakenly suggest that the clitoris is a small penis, which can occur in conditions such as adrenal hyperplasia.

Virtually all female newborns have hymens, and this fact should be noted on the chart for future reference in case of suspected sexual abuse. A **hymenal tag** is occasionally visible from the posterior opening of the vagina. It is composed of tissue from the hymen and the labia minora and usually disappears in several weeks. Generally, the vaginal vault is not inspected.

*Vaginal discharge* may be noted during the first week of life. This pseudomenstruation is a manifestation of the abrupt decrease in maternal hormones and usually disappears by 2 to 4 weeks of age. *Fecal discharge* from the vaginal opening indicates a rectovaginal fistula and is always reported. Vernix caseosa may be present in large amounts between the labia. Vigorous attempts to remove all the vernix through bathing is avoided to prevent tissue damage. With routine bathing and care, vernix will disappear after several days.

**Male Genitalia.**   Inspect the penis for the **urethral opening,** which is located at the tip. However, the opening may be totally covered by the **prepuce,** or **foreskin,** which covers the **glans penis.** A tight prepuce is a very common finding in newborns and does not indicate phimosis. It should not be forcefully retracted; locating the urinary meatus is usually possible without retracting the foreskin (Fletcher, 1994). *Smegma,* a white cheesy substance, is commonly found around the glans penis, under the foreskin. An erection is common in the newborn. Small, white, firm lesions called **epithelial pearls** may be seen at the tip of the prepuce.

The *scrotum* may be large, edematous, and pendulous in the full-term neonate, especially in the infant born in breech position. It is more deeply pigmented in dark-skinned infants. A noncommunicating **hydrocele** commonly occurs unilaterally and disappears within a few months. Always palpate the scrotum for the presence of *testes.* (See Chapter 7.) A discolored or dusky scrotum, scrotal edema, or palpation of a small mass should be reported to the practitioner because these may be a sign of testicular torsion (Juretschke, 2000). In small newborns, particularly premature infants, the undescended testes may be palpable within the inguinal canal. Absence of the testes may also be a sign of ambiguous genitalia, especially when accompanied by a small scrotum and penis. *Inguinal hernias* may or may not be manifested immediately after birth. A hernia is more easily detected when the infant is crying. Palpable **lymph nodes** are most commonly found in the inguinal area.

**Back and Anus.**   Inspect the *spine* with the infant prone. The shape of the spine is gently rounded, with none of the characteristic S-shaped curves seen later in life. Any abnormal openings, masses, dimples, or soft areas are noted. A protruding sac anywhere along the spine, but most commonly in the sacral area, indicates some type of *spina bifida.* A small sinus, which may or may not be communicating with the spine, is a *pilonidal sinus.* It is frequently covered with a tuft of hair. Although it may have no pathologic significance, a pilonidal cyst may indicate the existence of spina bifida occulta or be a portal of entry into the spinal column. With the infant still prone, note symmetry of the gluteal folds. Report any evidence of asymmetry; tests for developmental dysplasia of the hip are performed by skilled examiners. (See Chapter 11.)

The presence of an anal orifice and passage of meconium during the first 24 to 48 hours of life indicates *anal pa-*

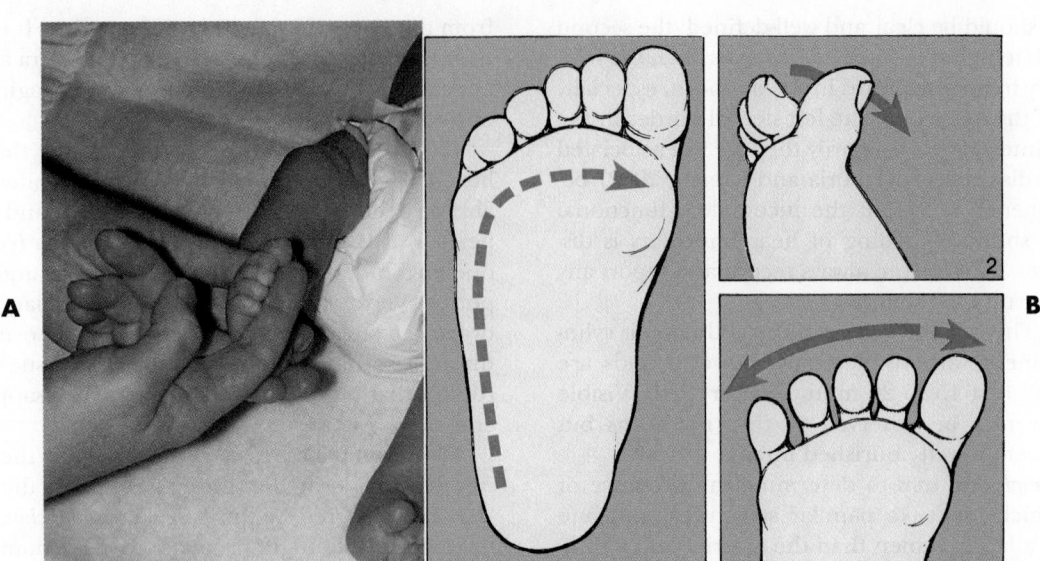

**Fig. 8-9** **A,** Plantar or grasp reflex. **B,** Babinski reflex. *1,* Direction of stroke. *2,* Dorsiflexion of big toe. *3,* Fanning of toes. (**A** from Zitelli BJ, Davis HW: *Atlas of pediatric physical diagnosis,* ed 3, St Louis, 1997, Mosby.)

*tency.* If an imperforate anus is suspected and not readily visible, insert a small catheter into the anal opening.

| **NURSING ALERT** | Do not use a gloved finger or rectal thermometer to test for anal patency because of the risk of mucosal perforation; also, the smaller diameter of the thermometer may pass through even a severely stenotic anus. Always report failure to pass meconium by 48 hours. |
|---|---|

With the infant still prone, gently separate the buttocks to inspect the anal area for the presence of *fissures,* or small cracks, in the mucosa. Anal fissures are a common cause of constipation and blood in the stool because the infant refuses to strain during defecation in order to avoid pain. Asymmetry of the mucosal folds around the sphincter also suggests fissures.

**Extremities.** Examine the extremities for symmetry, range of motion, and signs of malformation or trauma. Count the *fingers* and *toes,* and note supernumerary digits *(polydactyly)* or fusion of digits *(syndactyly).* A partial syndactyly between the second and third toes is a common variation seen in otherwise normal infants. More extensive fusion is abnormal and reported.

Observe *range of motion* of the extremities throughout the entire examination. The newborn will demonstrate full range of motion in the elbow, hip, shoulder, and knee joints. Movements should be symmetric, smooth, and unrestricted. The absence of arm movement signals a potential birth injury paralysis such as Klumpke or Erb-Duchenne palsy (Alexander and Kuo, 1997). (See Birth Injuries, Chapter 9.) An asymmetric or partial Moro reflex should alert the practitioner to further evaluate upper extremity mobility. Examine the lower extremities for limb length, symmetry, and hip abduction and flexion (Alexander and Kuo, 1997).

Examine the *nails;* the nail beds should be pink, although slight blueness is evident in acrocyanosis. Persistent *cyanosis* of the nail beds may indicate anoxia or vasoconstriction. *Yellowing* of the nail beds may indicate intrauterine distress, postmaturity, or hemolytic disease. *Short* or *absent nails* are seen in premature infants, whereas *long nails,* extending over the ends of the fingers, are characteristic of postmature newborns.

The *palms* of the hands should have the usual creases. (See Fig. 7-10.) A *transverse palmar crease (simian crease)* suggests Down syndrome but may also be a normal finding. The full-term newborn usually has creases covering the entire sole of the foot. In postmature infants the sole is covered with deep creases, and in premature infants the creases may partially cover the upper two thirds of the sole or may be absent. The *soles* are flat with prominent fat pads. Any foot abnormalities are noted.

Two reflexes are elicited. The first is the *grasp reflex.* Touching the palms of the hands or soles of the feet near the base of the digits causes flexion or grasping (Fig. 8-9, *A*). The other is the *Babinski reflex.* Stroking the outer sole of the foot upward from the heel across the ball of the foot causes the big toe to dorsiflex and the other toes to hyperextend (Fig. 8-9, *B,* and Table 8-4).

Inspect the extremities for evidence of fractures from birth trauma. The clavicle, humerus, and femur are most commonly involved. Limitation of movement, crepitus, visible deformity, asymmetry of reflexes, and malposition of the site suggest a fracture.

Also assess *muscle tone.* By attempting to extend a flexed extremity, determine if tone is equal bilaterally. Extension of any extremity is usually met with resistance, and when released, the extremity returns to its previous flexed position. *Hypotonia* suggests some degree of hypoxia, neurologic disorder, or Down syndrome. *Asymmetry* of muscle tone may indicate a degree of paralysis from damage to the brain or

**TABLE 8-4** Assessment of reflexes in the newborn

| Reflexes | Expected Behavioral Responses |
|---|---|
| **Localized** | |
| *Eyes* | |
| Blinking or corneal reflex | Infant blinks at sudden appearance of a bright light or at approach of an object toward cornea; persists throughout life |
| Pupillary | Pupil constricts when a bright light shines toward it; persists throughout life |
| Doll's eyes | As head is moved slowly to right or left, eyes lag behind and do not immediately adjust to new position of head; disappears as fixation develops; if persists, indicates neurologic damage |
| *Nose* | |
| Sneeze | Spontaneous response of nasal passages to irritation or obstruction; persists throughout life |
| Glabellar | Tapping briskly on glabella (bridge of nose) causes eyes to close tightly |
| *Mouth and Throat* | |
| Sucking | Infant begins strong sucking movements in response to stimulation; persists throughout infancy, even without stimulation, such as during sleep |
| Gag | Stimulation of posterior pharynx by food, suction, or passage of a tube causes infant to gag; persists throughout life |
| Rooting | Touching or stroking the cheek along side of mouth causes infant to turn head toward that side and begin to suck; should disappear at about age 3-4 months but may persist for up to 12 months (see Fig. 8-8) |
| Extrusion | When tongue is touched or depressed, infant responds by forcing it outward; disappears by age 4 months |
| *Extremities* | |
| Grasp | Touching palms of hands or soles of feet near base of digits causes flexion of hands and toes (see Fig. 8-9, *A*): palmar grasp lessens after age 3 months, to be replaced by voluntary movement; plantar grasp lessens by 8 months of age |
| Babinski | Stroking outer sole of foot upward from heel and across ball of foot causes toes to hyperextend and hallux to dorsiflex (see Fig. 8-9, *B*); disappears after age 1 year |
| Ankle clonus | Briskly dorsiflexing foot while supporting knee in partially flexed position results in one to two oscillating movements ("beats"); eventually no beats should be felt |
| **Mass** | |
| Moro (startle) | Sudden jarring, noise, or change in equilibrium causes sudden extension and abduction of extremities and fanning of fingers, with index finger and thumb forming a C shape, followed by flexion and adduction of extremities; then arms abduct and elbows flex, hands remain clenched, and legs may weakly flex; infant may cry (Fig. 8-10); disappears after age 3-4 months, usually strongest during first 2 months |
| Perez | While infant is prone on a firm surface, thumb is pressed along spine from sacrum to neck; infant responds by crying, flexing extremities, and elevating pelvis and head; lordosis of the spine, as well as defecation and urination, may occur; disappears by age 4-6 months |
| Asymmetric tonic neck | When infant's head is turned to one side, arm and leg extend on that side, and opposite arm and leg flex (Fig. 8-11); disappears by age 3-4 months, to be replaced by symmetric positioning of both sides of body |
| Trunk incurvation (Galant) reflex | Stroking infant's back alongside spine causes hips to move toward stimulated side; disappears by age 4 weeks |
| Dance or step | If infant is held so that sole of foot touches a hard surface, there is a reciprocal flexion and extension of the leg, simulating walking (Fig. 8-12); disappears after age 3-4 weeks, to be replaced by deliberate movement |
| Crawl | When placed on abdomen, infant makes crawling movements with arms and legs; disappears at about age 6 weeks (Fig. 8-13) |
| Placing | When infant is held upright under arms and dorsal side of foot is briskly placed against hard object, such as table, leg lifts as if foot is stepping on table; age of disappearance varies |
| Landau | When suspended prone on examiner's hand, the infant will demonstrate a reflex extension of the trunk, causing an upward curvature of the spine with lifting of the head |

CNS. Failure to move the lower limbs suggests a spinal cord lesion or injury. Sustained rhythmic *tremors, twitches,* and *myoclonic jerks* characterize neonatal seizures or may indicate neonatal abstinence syndrome. (See Neonatal Seizures and Drug Exposed Infants, Chapter 10.) Sudden jerking movements, quivering, or momentary tremors are usually normal.

**Neurologic System.** Assessing neurologic status is a critical part of the physical examination of the newborn. Much of the neurologic testing takes place during evaluation of body systems, such as eliciting localized reflexes and observing posture, muscle tone, head control, and movement. However, several important mass (total body) reflexes also need to be elicited. Test these at the end of the examination, because they may disturb the infant and interfere with auscultation. These reflexes, as well as several local reflexes,

are described in Table 8-4. Record and report the absence, asymmetry, persistence, or weakness of a reflex.

## ✳ Nursing Diagnoses

A number of nursing diagnoses are prominent in the nursing care of the newborn and family, and others specific to individual cases become evident. The most common nursing diagnoses are outlined in the Nursing Care Plan on pp. 289-291.

## ✳ Planning

The goals for the newborn and family are as follows:

1. Infant will maintain a patent airway.
2. Infant will maintain a stable body temperature.
3. Infant will experience no infections or injuries.

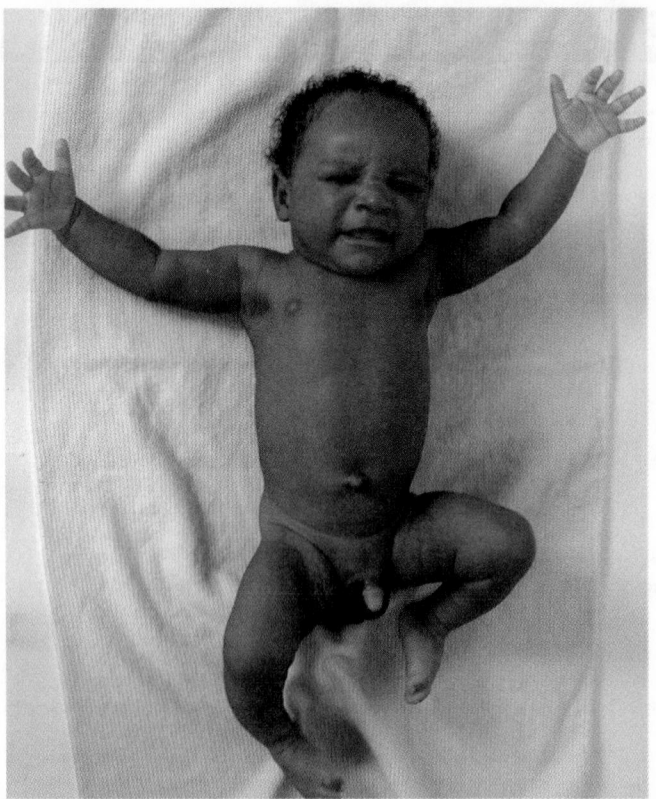

**Fig. 8-10** Moro reflex. (Courtesy Paul Vincent Kuntz, Texas Children's Hospital.)

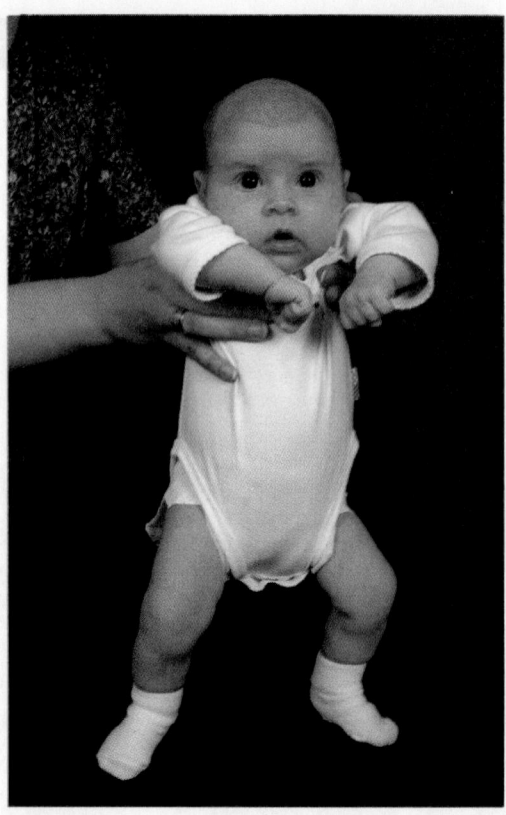

**Fig. 8-12** Dance reflex. (Courtesy Paul Vincent Kuntz, Texas Children's Hospital.)

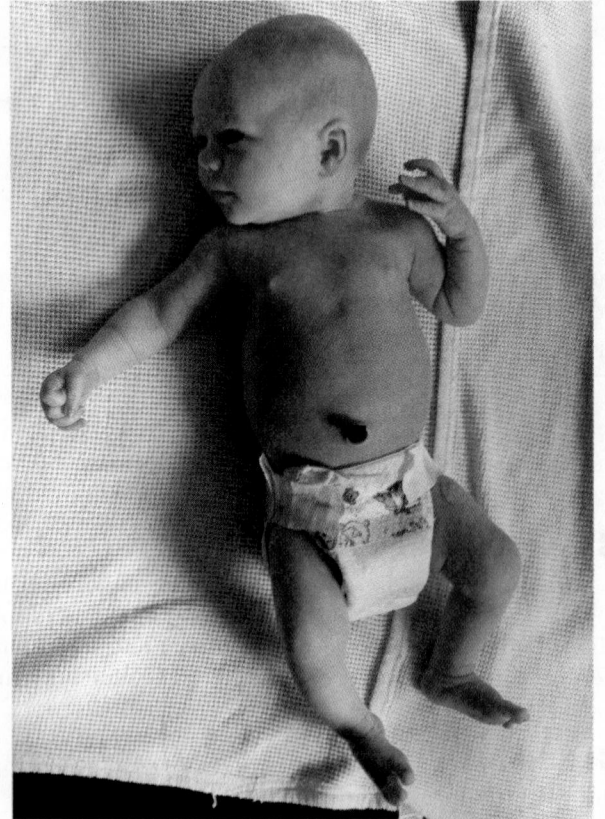

**Fig. 8-11** Tonic neck reflex. (Courtesy Paul Vincent Kuntz, Texas Children's Hospital.)

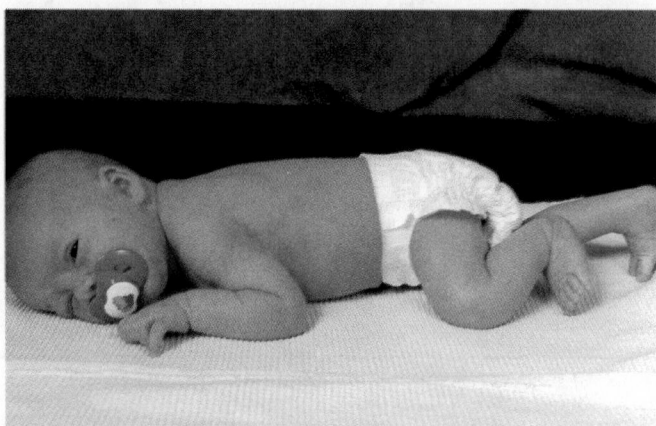

**Fig. 8-13** Crawl reflex. (Courtesy Paul Vincent Kuntz, Texas Children's Hospital.)

4. Infant will receive optimum nutrition.
5. Family will exhibit attachment behavior.
6. Family will be prepared for discharge and home care.

## ✖ Implementation

The following discussion focuses on nursing care after the infant has been delivered. A more detailed discussion of the birth and immediate care of the neonate can be found in any of the many excellent maternity texts.

## Maintain a Patent Airway

Establishing a patent airway, the primary objective in the delivery room, is the responsibility of the attending physicians and nurses. However, maintaining a patent airway continues to be a priority, with attention to proper positioning of the infant to facilitate drainage of secretions, especially after feeding (see Fig. 8-18).

The American Academy of Pediatrics (2000a) recommends the supine position during sleep for all newborns. This recommendation is based on the association between sleeping prone and sudden infant death syndrome. (See Chapter 13.) Since the initial recommendation in 1992 that all infants be placed in the supine sleep position, there has not been an evidenced increase in the number of complications, such as choking or vomiting (Malloy, 2002).

A bulb syringe is kept near the infant and is used if suctioning is required. Used bulb syringes should be replaced every 24 hours in the hospital and boiled for 10 minutes after use in the home to prevent bacterial contamination.*

> **NURSING ALERT**
> To avoid aspiration of amniotic fluid or mucus, clear the pharynx first, then the nasal passages. Compress the bulb *before* insertion to prevent forcing secretions into the bronchi.

If more forceful removal of secretions is required, mechanical suction is used. Use of the proper-size catheter and correct suctioning technique is essential in order to prevent mucosal damage and edema. Gentle suctioning is necessary to prevent laryngospasm, reflex bradycardia, and other cardiac arrhythmias from vagal stimulation. Oropharyngeal suctioning is performed for 5 seconds with sufficient time between each attempt to allow the infant to reoxygenate.

The stomach may be emptied (aspirated) to remove amniotic fluid that may cause abdominal distention and interfere with the establishment of respiration. Passing a catheter to the stomach also rules out esophageal atresia. Vital signs are closely monitored, and any indication of respiratory distress is immediately reported.

> **NURSING ALERT**
> Signs of respiratory distress include tachypnea, grunting, flaring alae nasi, intercostal retractions, stridor, abnormal breath sounds, cyanosis, or pallor.

## Maintain a Stable Body Temperature

Conserving the newborn's body heat is an essential nursing goal. At birth a major cause of heat loss is *evaporation,* the loss of heat through moisture. The amniotic fluid that bathes the infant's skin favors evaporation, especially when combined with the cool atmosphere of the delivery room. Heat loss through evaporation is minimized by rapidly drying the skin and hair with a warmed towel and placing the infant in a heated environment.

Another source of heat loss is *radiation,* the loss of heat to cooler solid objects in the environment that are not in direct contact with the infant. Loss of heat through radiation increases as these solid objects become colder and closer to the infant. The temperature of ambient (surrounding) air in the incubator essentially has no effect on loss of heat through radiation. This is a critical point to remember when attempting to maintain a constant temperature for the infant, because even when the temperature of the ambient air is optimum, the infant can become hypothermic. The use of radiant heating devices, such as heat lamps or phototherapy lights, with an incubator may cause overheating of the infant, because the neonate cannot effectively dissipate radiant heat through the Plexiglas wall of the incubator. For this same reason, an incubator should not be exposed to direct sunlight.

An example of radiant heat loss is the placement of the incubator close to a cold window or air conditioning unit. The cold from either source will cool the walls of the incubator and subsequently the body of the neonate. To prevent this, the incubator is placed as far away as possible from walls, windows, or ventilating units. If heat loss continues to be a problem, a radiant warmer may be placed over the infant or the infant and mother.

Heat loss can also occur through conduction and convection. *Conduction* involves loss of heat from the body from direct contact of skin with a cooler solid object; it is minimized by placing the infant on a padded, covered surface rather than directly on a hard table and by providing insulation with clothes and blankets. Placing the newborn very close to the mother, such as in her arms or on her abdomen immediately after delivery, is physically beneficial in terms of conserving heat, as well as fostering maternal attachment.

*Convection* is similar to conduction, except that heat loss is aided by surrounding air currents. For example, placing the infant in the direct flow of air from a fan or air conditioner vent causes rapid heat loss through convection. Transporting the neonate in a crib with solid sides reduces airflow around the infant.

## Protect from Infection and Injury

The most important practice for preventing cross-infection is thorough handwashing of all individuals involved in the infant's care. A common ritual in many newborn nurseries is the use of cover gowns and "scrub" clothes to prevent infection. Several studies have shown that this practice is ineffective and costly. Benefits to discontinuing the practice of gowning may include saving staff time in procedures and the cost of laundering and stocking gowns (Pelke and others, 1994). Several other procedures to prevent infection include eye care, umbilical care, bathing, and care of the circumcision. Artificial and long fingernails are discouraged in neonatal care because the former have been implicated in the transmission of *Pseudomonas* (Moolenaar and others, 2000; Foca and others, 2000); contaminated hand lotions have also been suspected in one outbreak of *Pseudomonas* (Becks and Lorenzoni, 1995). Vitamin K is administered to protect against hemorrhage. In addition, several safety measures are practiced, particularly in terms of proper identification, and screening tests are used to detect various disorders.

---

*Home care instructions for using a bulb syringe are available in Wong DL, Hess CS: *Wong and Whaley's clinical manual of pediatric nursing,* ed 5, St Louis, 2000, Mosby.

**Identification.**   Proper identification of the newborn is absolutely essential. The nurse must verify that identifying bands are securely fastened, usually on the ankles, and verify the information (name, sex, mother's admission number, date, and time of birth) against the birth records and the child's actual sex. Some institutions use methods of infant identification such as a color photograph kept in the medical record, storage of blood for DNA genotyping, and electronic surveillance systems for infant security. Footprinting or fingerprinting is *not* currently recommended for newborn identification (American Academy of Pediatrics and American College of Obstetricians and Gynecologists, 1997); however, footprinting continues to be practiced in many institutions. Electronic tags that give off a radio frequency are also being used to prevent newborn abductions (Quayle, 1997). Another measure to decrease infant abduction is to discontinue the publication of birth announcements in the local newspaper. Mother-newborn units are encouraged to develop a proactive infant abduction plan (Geller, 2000).

The nurse needs to discuss safety issues with the mother the first time the infant is brought to her. It has been recently reported by the **National Center for Missing and Exploited Children (NCMEC)*** that 56% of infant abductions occur in the mother's room (Carroll, 2000). A written copy of the safety instructions should also be given to the parent. Parents are instructed to look at identification badges of nurses and hospital personnel who come to take infants and not to relinquish their infants to anyone without proper identification. Some hospital employees in newborn and maternity areas wear color-coded badges or symbols that are changed frequently to decrease the likelihood of infant abduction. Mothers are also advised not to leave the infant alone in the crib while they shower or use the bathroom; rather, they should ask to have the infant returned to the nursery if a family member is not present in the room. Parents and staff are encouraged to use a password system when the newborn is taken from the room as a routine security measure (Carroll, 2000). The nurse should document in the chart that these instructions were given and that appropriate identification band checks are routinely made throughout each shift. Nursing staff are also educated re-

---

*(800) THE-LOST or (800) 843-5678; www.missingkids.org. Another resource is *Creating a Secure Workplace: Effective Policies and Practices in Health Care,* available from American Hospital Publishing, (800) 621-6902; www.amphi.com.

garding the "typical" abductor profile and to be constantly aware of visitors with unusual behavior.

The typical profile of an abductor is a female between the ages of 15 and 44 who often has a large build and low self-esteem; she may be emotionally disturbed because of the loss of her own child or inability to conceive and may have a strained relationship with her husband or partner. The typical abductor may also be seen visiting the newborn nursery or neonatal intensive care unit (NICU) area before the abduction and may ask questions about the care of or the health of a specific newborn. The abductor may familiarize herself with the hospital routine and may also impersonate a health care worker. Parents are made aware of the fact that infant safety measures must be implemented in the home as well, because home abductions are also a potential threat (Carroll, 2000).

**Eye Care.**   Prophylactic eye treatment against **ophthalmia neonatorum,** infectious conjunctivitis of the newborn, includes the use of (1) silver nitrate (1%) solution, (2) erythromycin (0.5%) ophthalmic ointment or drops, or (3) tetracycline (1%) ophthalmic ointment or drops (preferably in single-dose ampules or tubes) (Guidelines box). *Chlamydia trachomatis* is the major cause of ophthalmia neonatorum in the United States. Silver nitrate is effective against gonococcal conjunctivitis.

Topical antibiotics (tetracycline and erythromycin), and silver nitrate, have not proved to be effective in the prevention and treatment of chlamydial conjunctivitis. A 14-day course of oral erythromycin or an oral sulfonamide may be given for chlamydial conjunctivitis (American Academy of Pediatrics 2000b). The administration of oral erythromycin to infants less than 6 weeks old has been associated with the development of infantile hypertrophic pyloric stenosis; therefore parents should be informed of the potential risks and signs of the illness (American Academy of Pediatrics, 2000b).

Although eye prophylaxis is mandatory in the United States, health care facilities are free to choose specific drugs. Effective prophylaxis may be better directed at treating maternal chlamydial infection.

Because studies on maternal attachment emphasize that in the first hour of life a newborn has a greater ability to focus on coordinated movement than at any other time during the next several days and because eye contact is very important in the development of maternal-infant bonding, the routine administration of silver nitrate or antibiotics can be postponed for up to 1 hour. However, there must be some kind of checklist to ensure that the drug is given.

**Vitamin K Administration.**   Shortly after birth, vitamin K is administered as a single intramuscular dose of 0.5 to 1 mg to prevent hemorrhagic disease of the newborn. (See Chapter 9.) Normally, vitamin K is synthesized by the intestinal flora. However, because the infant's intestine is sterile at birth and because breast milk contains low levels of vitamin K, the supply is inadequate for at least the first 3 to 4 days. The major function of vitamin K is to catalyze the synthesis of prothrombin in the liver, which is needed for blood clotting and coagulation. The vastus lateralis muscle is the traditionally recommended injection site, but the ventrogluteal (not dorsogluteal) muscle can be used.

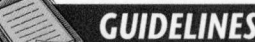

## GUIDELINES
### Ophthalmia Neonatorum Prophylaxis

Clean the eyelids with sterile cotton and sterile water if needed.
Separate lids and apply 2 drops or a 1 to 2 cm (½ inch) ribbon of ointment in each conjunctival sac.
Massage lids to ensure spread of the medication.
Wipe excess medication from eye with sterile cotton 1 minute after application.
Do not rinse eyes with sterile normal saline.

A single dose of oral vitamin K was not as effective as a single intramuscular dose in preventing hemorrhagic disease of the newborn; however, a 3-dose oral regimen was proven to be effective (Puckett and Offringa, 2000).

The oral form should be given at birth (2.0 mg) and again at 1 to 2 weeks, with a third dose at 4 weeks usually only to breast-fed infants. If diarrhea occurs in an exclusively breast-fed infant, the dose should be repeated (American Academy of Pediatrics, 1993).

**Hepatitis B (HBV) Vaccine Administration.**   To decrease the incidence of HBV in children and its serious consequences, cirrhosis and liver cancer, in adulthood, the first of three doses of HBV vaccine is recommended between birth and 2 months of age for all newborns born to hepatitis B surface antigen (HBsAg)-negative mothers. The injection is given in the vastus lateralis muscle. This muscle is used because this site is associated with a better immune response than the dorsogluteal area (although this muscle typically is not used in infants in the United States) (American Academy of Pediatrics, 2000b). (See Immunizations, Chapter 12.) Giving the infant concentrated oral sucrose can reduce the pain of the injection (Allen, White, and Walburn, 1996).

Premature infants born to HBsAg-negative mothers should be vaccinated just before hospital discharge, provided that the infant weighs 2000 g or more; the vaccination should be delayed until 2 months of age if the infant weighs less than 2000 g. Infants born to HBsAg-positive mothers should be immunized within 12 hours after birth with HBV vaccine and hepatitis B immune globulin (HBIG) at separate sites, regardless of gestational age or birth weight (American Academy of Pediatrics, 2002d).

**Newborn Screening for Disease.**   A number of congenital disorders can be detected in the newborn period by blood sampling so that early intervention may take place to decrease the long-term effects and cost of such illnesses. There is currently no national policy regulating newborn screening; therefore, the extent of newborn screening has been largely determined by state laws and individual practice. All states now mandate screening tests for PKU and congenital hypothyroidism (see Chapters 9 and 35); many states also have programs that include screening for sickle cell disease and galactosemia. However, concern has recently been voiced regarding the inconsistency among states in screening for such conditions based on cost, population demographics, resource availability, and political environment. To address these issues, a national Task Force on Newborn Screening was formed by the American Academy of Pediatrics and other federal health agencies, and from this group a number of resolutions and policies have emerged to better address the issue of newborn screening (American Academy of Pediatrics, 2000d). It is not within the scope of this text to discuss the resolutions of the Task Force and the reader is referred to the AAP 2000d reference, which includes a full summary of those resolutions and recommendations.

The nurse's responsibility is to educate parents regarding the importance of screening and to collect appropriate specimens at the recommended time (after 24 hours of age). With early newborn discharge before 24 hours, adequate screening for PKU requires a follow-up test within 2 weeks (American Academy of Pediatrics and American College of Obstetricians and Gynecologist, 1997). Accurate screening depends on good-quality blood spots on approved filter paper forms. The blood should completely saturate the filter paper spot on one side only. The paper should not be handled, placed on wet surfaces, or contaminated with any substance, such as coffee or tea. (See Atraumatic Care box.)

The American Academy of Pediatrics and American College of Obstetricians and Gynecologists (1997) also recommends routine prenatal and perinatal human immunodeficiency virus (HIV) counseling and testing for all pregnant women. Benefits of early identification of HIV-infected infants are early antiretroviral therapy and aggressive nutritional supplementation; appropriate changes in their immunization schedule; monitoring and evaluating of immunologic, neurologic, and neuropsychologic functions for possible changes caused by antiretroviral

---

### ATRAUMATIC CARE
#### Heel Punctures

Repeated heel lancing may be needed to obtain sufficient blood for the filter paper spot test. The use of automated lancet devices such as Tenderfoot* have been found to cause less pain and require fewer punctures than using manual lance blades (Blain-Lewis, 1992; Paes and others, 1993). The benefit of applying the topical anesthetic EMLA (eutectic mixture of local anesthetic) to reduce pain has been inconclusive (Fitzgerald, Millard, and McIntosh, 1989; Taddio and others, 1998). Newborns given 2 ml of oral sucrose solution (25% or 50%) demonstrated a significant reduction in crying time and heart rate after 3 minutes in comparison with controls (given sterile water) during heelstick sampling for serum bilirubin concentrations (Haouari and others, 1995). In a similar study of healthy preterm infants exposed to heelsticks for blood work, crying was significantly decreased in those infants receiving intraoral sucrose solution compared with a control group receiving only intraoral sterile water (Ramenghi and others, 1996). Healthy term newborns who were cuddled and then given 2 ml of a 50% oral sucrose solution during heelstick PKU testing showed decreased pain responses on the Neonatal Infant Pain Scale (NIPS) (Overgaard and Knudsen, 1999). Sucrose is typically administered by giving 2 ml of the oral solution 2 minutes before the procedure or by using a pacifier that is coated several times with the solution both before and during the procedure. The pacifier method appears to produce greater analgesia both from the sucrose and the sucking (Blass and Watt, 1999). The mother's holding the infant in skin-to-skin contact has also been shown to significantly reduce the child's distress during the procedure (Gray, Watt, and Blass, 2000).

Amethocaine, a 4% topical anethetic gel, has been shown to be as effective as EMLA in decreasing some sources of pain (Bishai and others, 1999; McCafferty and others, 1997) but was not found to be effective in significantly decreasing the pain of heelsticks in newborns (Jain, Rutter, and Ratnayaka, 2001); this gel, however, is currently licensed for use in infants 1 month or older. Amethocaine gel has the purported advantages of becoming effective 30 minutes after application and lasting up to 3 to 4 hours for surface pain (McCafferty, Woolfson, and Boston, 1989).

An approximate 25% sucrose solution is made by mixing 1 teaspoon of granulated (table) sugar with 4 teaspoons of sterile water (see p. 272).

---

*Manufactured by International Technidyne, Inc, Edison, NJ.

therapy; initiation of special educational needs; evaluation for the need of other therapies, such as immunoglobulin for the prevention of bacterial infections; tuberculosis screening and treatment; and management of communicable disease exposures. As a result of virologic diagnostic techniques such as HIV culture, polymerase chain reaction, and immune complex–dissociated p24 antigen, diagnosis of HIV infection can be made in almost 50% of infants at birth and in 95% or more of infants by 1 to 3 months of age.*

**Universal Newborn Hearing Screening.** It has been estimated that screening children for hearing loss by risk factors alone fails to identify approximately 50% of all newborns with a congenital hearing loss. Furthermore, infants who are hard of hearing and deaf yet receive intervention before the age of 6 months maintain appropriate language development matching their cognitive abilities through the age of 5 years (Yoshinaga-Itano and others, 1998). For these reasons the Joint Committee on Infant Hearing, American Academy of Pediatrics (2000e), now recommends universal hearing screening of all newborns before discharge from the birthing hospital. Infants may be screened for hearing loss by auditory brainstem response or evoked otoacoustic emissions. Newborns who fail the initial screening require referral for outpatient retesting and intervention by 1 month of age; newborns who do not receive initial screening before discharge should also be tested by 1 month (American Academy of Pediatrics, 2000d).

**Bathing.** Bath time is an opportunity for the nurse to accomplish much more than general hygiene. It is an ex-

---

*For information on several diseases that may be included in newborn screening, see Table 1, p. 393, in American Academy of Pediatrics: Newborn screening: a blueprint for the future, *Pediatrics* 106(2):393, 2000.

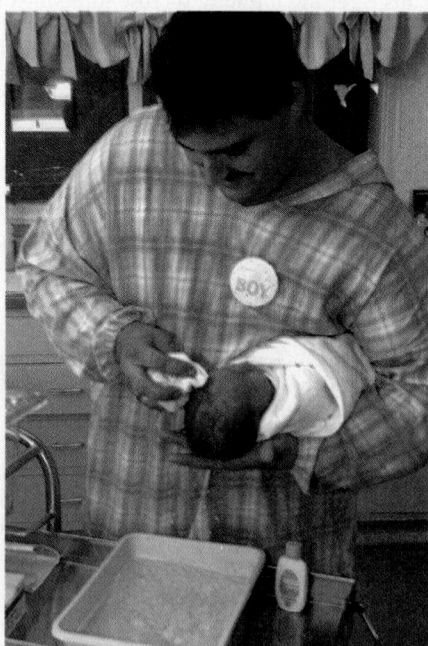

**Fig. 8-14** Bath time is an excellent opportunity for parents to learn about their newborn.

cellent time for observations of the infant's behavior, state of arousal, alertness, and muscular activity. Bathing is usually performed after the vital signs have stabilized, especially the temperature.

With the possibility of transmission of HBV and HIV via maternal blood and blood-stained amniotic fluid, the traditional timing of the newborn's bath has been questioned. Studies indicate that healthy term newborns with a stable body temperature can be bathed as early as 1 hour of age without experiencing problems, provided that effective thermoregulation measures are taken after the bath (Penny-MacGillivray, 1996; Varda and Behnke, 2000). The newborn must be considered a potential contamination source until proved otherwise. As part of *standard precautions,* nurses should wear gloves when handling the newborn until blood and amniotic fluid are removed by bathing.

The bath time provides an opportunity for the nurse to involve the parents in the care of their child, to teach correct hygiene procedures, and for parents to learn about their infant's individual characteristics (Fig. 8-14). The bath may also be used to help parents learn and better understand their newborn's behavioral characteristics using the BNBAS (Karl, 1999). The appropriate types of bathing supplies and the need for safety in terms of water temperature and supervision of the infant at all times during the bath are stressed.

Parents are encouraged to examine every finger and toe of their infant during bathing. Frequently normal variations such as milia, erythema toxicum (rash), or "stork bites" cause parents much worry because they are unaware of the insignificance of such findings. Minor birth injuries may appear as major defects to them. Explaining how these occurred and when they will disappear reassures parents of their infant's normalcy. Common variations are discussed further in Chapter 9.

One of the most important considerations in skin cleansing is preservation of the skin's "acid mantle," which is formed from the uppermost horny layer of the epidermis, sweat, superficial fat, metabolic products, and external substances such as amniotic fluid, microorganisms, and chemicals. The infant's skin surface has a pH of about 5 soon after birth, and the bacteriostatic effects of this pH are significant. Consequently, only plain warm water should be used for routine bathing. If a cleanser is needed, Dove (Fragrance-Free) has a neutral pH and is mild (Darmstadt and Dinulos, 2000). Alkaline soaps, oils, powder, and lotions are not used because they alter the acid mantle, thus providing a medium for bacterial growth. Talcum powder has the added risk of aspiration if it is applied close to the infant's face. Corn starch powder may also cause respiratory problems and aspiration (Silver, Sagy, and Rubi, 1996). (See Diaper Dermatitis, Chapter 13.)

Parents should be involved in a discussion regarding the newborn's bath at home. It is recommended that for the first 2 to 4 weeks the infant be bathed no more than two or three times per week with a plain warm sponge bath. This practice will help maintain the integrity of the newborn's skin and allow time for the umbilical cord to dry completely.

Routine daily bathing for newborns is no longer recommended because it washes away the skin's protective coating (Darmstadt and Dinulos, 2000; Marbut and Loan, 1996).

Cleansing proceeds in the cephalocaudal (head-to-toe) direction. A washcloth is used and turned so that a clean part touches the skin with each stroke. The eyes are carefully wiped from the inner to the outer aspect of the lid. The face is cleansed next. The scalp is usually wiped, although it is sometimes necessary to shampoo the hair. Shampooing is best accomplished by positioning the infant's head over a small basin, lathering the scalp with a mild soap, and rinsing by pouring water from a small vessel over the head into the basin. The rest of the body is kept covered during this procedure. The head is dried quickly to prevent heat loss from evaporation.

The rest of the body is washed in a similar manner. Vigorous rubbing to remove vernix is unnecessary and may cause more harm than good (Darmstadt and Dinulos, 2000).

The genitalia of both sexes require careful cleansing. Cleansing of the vulva is done in a front-to-back direction. The bath is a perfect opportunity to stress this part of hygiene to the mother, for both the infant's and her protection against urinary tract infection.

Cleansing the male genitalia involves washing the penis and scrotum. Sometimes smegma needs to be removed by wiping around the glans. The foreskin is not retracted because it is normally tight in newborns. It remains adhered to the glans for approximately 3 to 14 years.

**NURSING ALERT** If an infant is not to be circumcised, the parents are taught how to cleanse under and around the foreskin by *moving it gently only as far as it will go* and returning it to its normal position. Leaving the prepuce in a retracted position constricts the blood vessels supplying the glans penis, causing edema.

Once the foreskin can be easily retracted, the boy should be taught to gently wash the glans with soap, rinsing well afterward. During the act of urination, retraction of the foreskin will help avoid irritation of the glans with urine. Parents are also instructed to be aware of the signs of urinary tract infections, which may be more common in uncircumcised infant males. Symptoms include irritability or fussiness on urination (from discomfort), voiding in small amounts and frequently, and unusual voiding urgency (Westbrooks, 1996).

The buttocks and anal area are thoroughly cleansed of any fecal material.

A diaper is applied after the bath. It should fit snugly around the thighs and abdomen to prevent urine from leaking. Diapers are fastened with the back side overlapping the front side to allow full flexion of the hips.

The nurse should discuss the choice of cloth or disposable diapers with parents.* In the United States the most commonly used diapers are disposable paper diapers. Other choices are home-laundered or commercially laundered cloth diapers. A number of factors—cost, convenience, skin care benefits, infection control, and environmental concerns—influence the relative merits of these three diaper types. In general, home-laundered diapers are the least expensive when human labor cost is not included. Once human labor cost is included, the price difference between disposable diapers, diaper service reusable diapers, and home-laundered diapers is quite small, although paper diapers tend to cost the most. Disposable diapers are the most convenient, although a diaper service eliminates the need to shop for replacement diapers.

Disposable diapers with absorbent gelling material have benefits related to preserving healthy skin, preventing diaper dermatitis, especially beyond the neonatal period (see Chapter 13), and controlling contamination of the environment because of their better containment of urine and feces. (See Community Focus box.)

**Care of the Umbilicus.** Because the umbilical stump is an excellent medium for bacterial growth, various methods of cord care are practiced. None has proved to be superior, with regard to minimizing bacterial growth. Regardless of the type of treatment, the diaper is placed below the cord to avoid irritation and wetness on the site. Parents are instructed regarding stump deterioration and proper umbilical care. The stump deteriorates through the process of dry gangrene. Cord separation time is influenced by a number of factors, including type of cord care, type of delivery, and other perinatal events. The average cord separation time is 10 to 14 days; however, this may vary depending on the type of cord care used.

Studies addressing the issue have led many to question the effectiveness of routine cord care with antiseptics such as triple dye, hexachlorophene, chlorhexidine, and alcohol (Dore and others, 1998; Krebs, 1998). Other studies have shown that although antiseptic and antibiotic cord treatments minimize bacterial growth, the time to cord drying and separation was increased (Zupan and Garner, 2000). Because the incidence of omphalitis has diminished significantly over the last 30 years in developing countries, the ev-

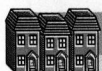

**COMMUNITY FOCUS**
*Environmental Impact of Diapers*

The most controversial issue surrounding the discussion of disposable vs cloth diapers has been their effect on the environment. Disposable diapers are discarded as solid waste in landfills, whereas waste from laundered diapers is disposed of as treated sewage. The main differences between solid waste and treated sewage are cost and possibly sanitation, with solid waste being more expensive. The manufacture and disposal of cloth and paper diapers affect energy resources and the environment differently. Paper diapers consume more raw materials and generate more solid waste. Cloth diapers, especially home-laundered ones, use more water and energy and create more water and air pollution. When health professionals are asked about the effect of diapers on the environment, they must answer with a balanced view based on the health advantages of paper diapers and the different uses of resources for paper or cloth diapers.

---

*A resource for families is *Parent Pages: A Guide to Skin Care,* available from Procter & Gamble, 1 Procter & Gamble Plaza, Cincinnati, OH 45202, (800) 543-0480; www.pampers.com.

idence appears to support simply keeping the cord clean and dry as being as safe as using antibiotics (Zupan and Garner, 2000). Nurses working in neonatal care must evaluate the available studies and compare the risks and benefits regarding the method of cord care within their own population of patients. Regardless of the method used, nurses must include cord care teaching in discharge planning because it has been demonstrated to be a big concern of parents once the newborn is discharged (Ford and Ritchie, 1999).

It takes a few more weeks for the cord base to heal completely following cord separation. During this time care consists of keeping the base clean and dry and may include wiping it with alcohol.

> **NURSING ALERT**
>
> Instruct parents to report any signs of cord infection, such as presence of erythema and malodorous, purulent discharge, to their health care professional.

> **NURSING ALERT**
>
> With early hospital discharge newborns may be discharged before it is safe to remove the cord clamp. Teach the parent how to safely remove the clamp once the newborn is at least 24 hours old and no oozing from the cord is noted.

**Circumcision.** Circumcision, the surgical removal of the foreskin on the glans penis, is usually done in the hospital, although it is not a common practice in most countries. Despite the frequency of the procedure in the United States, there is still much controversy regarding the benefits and risks. One study that has received considerable criticism since its publication, demonstrated a ninefold increase in urinary tract infections in uncircumcised boys during the first year of life (Bartman, 2001, letter; Schoen, Colby, and Ray, 2000) (Box 8-4). The American Academy of Pediatrics (1999) issued a new circumcision policy statement that states that the medical benefits of male newborn circumcision are not sufficiently significant to recommend it as a routine procedure. This policy statement reverses its earlier 1989 policy statement that concluded that, although the circumcision procedure had associated risks, newborn male circumcision did provide certain potential medical benefits, including reduction of urinary tract infections and sexually transmitted diseases, particularly acquired HIV infection. The new statement emphasizes parental autonomy to determine what is in the best interest of their male newborn infant. The policy advises the physician to ensure that parents have been given accurate and unbiased information about the risks, benefits, and alternatives before making an informed choice and that they understand that circumcision is an elective procedure. In addition to examining the medical benefits of male newborn circumcision, the Academy for the first time in their circumcision policy history recommended that if parents decide to have their male infant circumcised, procedural analgesia should be provided.

This policy statement has direct implications for nurses caring for newborns and their families. First, because nurses are in a unique position to help educate parents regarding the care of their newborns, they must take responsibility for ensuring that each parent has accurate and unbiased information by which to make an informed decision. Parents need to know the options for pain control, especially the choice of topical or injected anesthesia, and their option of observing the procedure.* Second, in the event that anesthesia is not used, the nurse should use every nonpharmacologic intervention that can reduce the pain of this operative procedure. (See Atraumatic Care box.) Despite adequate scientific evidence that newborns feel and respond to pain, circumcisions are still being performed in the United States with either insufficient analgesia or no analgesia at all. Nurses can use the Academy's policy statement to advocate more effectively for the use of optimal pain relief during circumcision.

Four types of anesthesia and analgesia are used in newborns undergoing circumcision: ring block, dorsal penile nerve block (DPNB), topical anesthetic such as EMLA (prilocaine-lidocaine), and oral sucrose. Oral acetaminophen and comfort measures such as music, sucking on a pacifier, and soothing voices have not proved to be solely effective in reducing the pain of circumcision (Williamson, 1997).

Studies demonstrate that DPNB is more effective at reducing the effects of circumcision pain than EMLA, EMLA is more effective than placebo cream, and ring block is the most effective method (Lander and others, 1997; Taddio and others, 1997; Williamson, 1997).

The topical application of 2 g of EMLA to the penis before circumcision has also been effective in reducing the pain of circumcision. An occlusive dressing must be placed over the cream, which must be applied approximately 1 hour before the procedure. Although this preparation may be perceived as complicated and requiring too much advance notice, it is equally important to remember that most

---

### Box 8-4
### Risks and Benefits of Neonatal Circumcision

| RISKS | BENEFITS |
|---|---|
| Complications: | Prevention of penile cancer |
|   Hemorrhage |   and posthitis (inflamma- |
|   Infection |   tion of prepuce) |
|   Dehiscence (separation of | Decreased incidence of bal- |
|     approximated edges of skin) |   anitis (inflammation of |
|   Meatitis (from loss of |   glans) and, possibly, |
|     protective foreskin) |   urinary tract infection in |
|   Adhesions |   infant males as well as |
|   Concealed penis |   some sexually transmitted |
|   Urethral fistula |   diseases later in life |
|   Meatal stenosis | Prevention of complications |
| Pain in unanesthetized infants |   associated with later |
|   (long-term consequences |   circumcision |
|   unknown, but short-term | Preservation of male's body |
|   stresses include increased |   image that is consistent |
|   heart rate, behavior changes, |   with peers (in countries |
|   prolonged crying, increased |   where procedure is |
|   cortisol levels, and decreased |   common) |
|   blood oxygenation) | |

---

*Circumcision: Information for Parents* is available from the American Academy of Pediatrics, 141 Northwest Point Blvd, Elk Grove Village, IL 60009-1098, (888) 227-1770, fax: (847) 228-1281; www.aap.org.

newborns are kept NPO for 1 to 2 hours before the procedure to prevent aspiration. The use of EMLA cream was not associated with methemoglobinemia, the only serious but very rare complication from the prilocaine. However, localized rash has been associated with EMLA when used for circumcision. Benini and others (1993) reported effective pain amelioration during circumcision with the use of EMLA. Further evaluations of circumcision analgesia reveal that EMLA remains an effective agent in reducing neonatal pain (Taddio, Ohlsson, and Ohlsson, 2000).

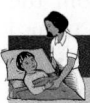

## ATRAUMATIC CARE
*Guidelines for Pain Management During Neonatal Circumcision*

### PHARMACOLOGIC INTERVENTIONS

#### Use of Topical Anesthetic Only

One hour before the procedure, administer acetaminophen (e.g., Tylenol, 15 mg/kg) as ordered by the practitioner.

Place a thick layer (1 g) of EMLA* cream around the penis where the prepuce (foreskin) attaches to the glans. Avoid placing cream on the tip of the penis where EMLA may come in contact with urethral opening.

Cover the penis with a "finger cot" that is cut from a vinyl or latex glove, or a piece of plastic wrap, and secure bottom of covering with tape. Avoid using Tegaderm or large amounts of tape on the skin because removing the adhesive causes pain and can irritate the fragile skin.

If the infant urinates during the time EMLA is applied (1 hour) and a significant amount of EMLA is removed, reapply the cream and covering. The total application of EMLA should not exceed a surface area of 10 cm² (1.25 × 1.25 inches).

Remove cream with clean cloth or tissue. Blanching of skin is an expected reaction to EMLA's application under an occlusive dressing; erythema and some edema may occur also.

During procedure, give the infant a sucrose solution. To make an approximate 24% sucrose solution, add 1 teaspoon of table sugar to 4 teaspoons of sterile water. Use this solution to coat the pacifier (recoat several times before and during the procedure) or administer 2 ml to the tongue 2 minutes before the procedure.

Following procedure, apply petrolatum or A&D ointment on a 2 × 2 dressing before diapering infant to prevent the wound from adhering to the dressing or diaper.

Administer acetaminophen as ordered by the practitioner 4 hours after the initial dose; give additional doses as needed but not to exceed 5 doses in 24 hours or a maximum dose of 75 mg/kg/day.

#### Use of Dorsal Penile Nerve Block (DPNB) or Ring Block

One hour before the procedure administer acetaminophen as ordered by the practitioner.

One hour before procedure, apply EMLA. For the DPNB apply EMLA to the prepuce as described previously and at the penile base. For the ring block apply EMLA to the prepuce as described previously and to the shaft of the penis. A topical anesthetic should be used in conjunction with the dorsal penile nerve block or ring block to avoid the pain of injecting the anesthetic.

Use a 30-gauge needle to administer the lidocaine.† For the DPNB, 0.4 ml of the lidocaine is infiltrated at the 10:30 o'clock and 1:30 o'clock positions in Buck's fascia at the penile base. For the ring block, 0.4 ml of lidocaine is infiltrated subcutaneously on each side of the shaft of the penis below the prepuce.

For maximum anesthesia, wait 5 minutes following the injection of lidocaine. An alternative anesthetic agent is chloroprocaine, which is as effective as lidocaine after 3 minutes.

During the circumcision, administer sucrose as described previously.

Apply A&D ointment or petrolatum as described previously.

Administer acetaminophen as described previously.

### NONPHARMACOLOGIC INTERVENTIONS (TO ACCOMPANY PRECEDING PHARMACOLOGIC INTERVENTIONS)

If Circumstraint board is used, pad with blankets or other thick, soft material such as "lamb's wool." A more comfortable, padded, and physiologic restraint that places the infant semi-reclining can also decrease distress (Stang and others, 1997).‡

Provide the parents, caregiver, or another staff member with the option to hold the infant during the procedure or to be present during the circumcision.

Swaddle the upper body and legs to provide warmth and containment and to reduce movement.

If the patient is not swaddled and is unclothed, use a radiant warmer to prevent hypothermia. Shield infant's eyes from overhead lights.

Prewarm any topical solutions to be used in sterile preparation of the surgical site by placing in a warm blanket or towel.

Play infant relaxation music§ before, during, and after procedure; allow parents or other caregiver the option to provide the music of choice.

Following the procedure, remove restraints and swaddle. Immediately have the parent, other caregiver, or nursing staff hold the infant. Continue to have the infant suck on pacifier or offer feeding.

Data from Broadman LM and others: Post-circumcision analgesia: a prospective evaluation of subcutaneous ring block of the penis, *Anesthesiology* 67:339-402, 1987; Howard CR, Howard FM, Weitzman ML: Acetaminophen analgesia in neonatal circumcision: the effect on pain, *Pediatrics* 93(4):641-646, 1994; Lander J and others: Comparison of ring block, dorsal penile nerve block, and topical anesthesia for neonatal circumcision, *JAMA* 278:2157-2162, 1997; Mintz MR, Grillo R: Dorsal penile nerve block for circumcision, *Clin Pediatr* 28:590-591, 1989; Serour F, Mandelberg A, Mori J: Slow injection of local anesthetic will decrease pain during dorsal penile nerve block, *Acta Anesthesiol Scand* 42:926-928, 1998; Spencer DM and others: Dorsal penile nerve block in neonatal circumcision: chloroprocaine versus lidocaine, *Am J Perinatol* 9(3):214-218, 1992; Stang H and others: Beyond dorsal penile nerve block: a more humane circumcision, *Pediatrics* 100(2):E3, 1997 (*www.pediatrics.org/cgi/content/full/100/2/e3*); Stevens B and others: The efficacy of sucrose for relieving procedural pain in neonates—a systematic review and meta-analysis, *Acta Pediatr* 86:837-842, 1997; Taddio A and others: Efficacy and safety of lidocaine-prilocaine cream (EMLA) for pain during circumcision, *N Engl J Med* 336(17):1197-1201, 1997.

*NOTE: On March 11, 1999, the FDA approved the use of EMLA in infants age 37 weeks of gestation. Although the package insert lists under "Warnings" that patients taking drugs associated with drug-induced methemoglobinemia, such as acetaminophen, are at greater risk for developing methomoglobinemia, there have been no reported cases of this complication occurring in children taking acetaminophen and using EMLA. In fact, there is no evidence that acetaminophen is a methemoglobin-inducing drug in humans (Prescott LF: *Paracetamol (acetaminophen): a critical bibliographic review*, Bristol, 1996, Taylor & Francis). The only reported cases of methemoglobinemia from acetaminophen have been in cats and dogs (Hjelle JJ, Grauer GF: Acetaminophen-induced toxicosis in dogs and cats, *J Am Vet Med Assoc* 188(7):742-749, 1986).

†NOTE: In one study, the use of buffered lidocaine, which normally reduces the stinging sensation of lidocaine, did not provide effective anesthesia for DPNB (Stang and others, 1997). The study on slow injection of the anesthetics lidocaine and bupivacaine compared 40 vs 80 seconds in patients ages 15-53 years (Serour, Mandelberg, and Mori, 1998).

‡For information on the Stang Circ Chair, contact Pedicraft, 4134 Augustine Rd, Jacksonville, FL 32207, (800) 223-7649; e-mail: info@pedicraft.com; *www.pedicraft.com*.

§Suggested infant relaxation music: *Heartbeat Lullabies* by Terry Woodford. Available from Baby-Go-To-Sleep Center, Audio Therapy Innovations, Inc, PO Box 550, Colorado Springs, CO 80901, (800) 537-7748.

An interesting concept of combination analgesia with a Mogen clamp was shown to significantly reduce newborn pain (Taddio and others, 2000). In this study one group of newborns was given acetaminophen before the procedure, and EMLA was applied to the foreskin and abdomen 1 hour before the procedure; a DPNB was administered and the newborn was given a concentrated sucrose solution during the procedure. When compared with the group circumcised with the Gomco clamp and EMLA alone, the group receiving a combination of analgesics received significantly better scores on the Neonatal Facial Coding System and infant cry duration measurements.

A seemingly unconventional method for providing pain relief for circumcision is the use of intraoral sucrose. In studies on neonatal heelsticks and circumcision, crying during the procedure was reduced with the intake of 2 ml of a 12% sucrose solution in comparison with sterile water intake, which had no perceived effects on decreasing pain (Stevens and others, 1997). This has led investigators to question whether sucrose has an antinociceptive effect in infants (Blass and Hoffmeyer, 1991). Other researchers have investigated stronger sucrose solutions (25% and 50%) for heelsticks in full-term and preterm infants with positive results (Haouari and others, 1995; Ramenghi and others, 1996). The administration of a concentrated dose of oral sucrose and nonnutritive sucking have proved to be effective in decreasing procedural pain (venipuncture, heelstick, circumcision) in term and preterm infants in comparison to no treatment (Herschel and others, 1998; Stevens and others, 1997; Stevens and others, 1999; Stevens, Yamada, and Ohlsson, 2001). Therefore it is imperative that nurses use this nonpharmacologic pain treatment for procedures such as circumcision, venipuncture, and heelstick in their own practice.

Circumcision is usually performed in the nursery. It should not be performed immediately after delivery because of the neonate's unstabilized physiologic status and increased susceptibility to stress. Preoperative nursing care includes allowing the infant nothing by mouth before the procedure to prevent aspiration of vomitus (about 1-2 hours), checking for a signed consent form, and adequately restraining the infant, usually on a special board (Fig. 8-15) or physiologic circumcision restraint chair. The circumcision chair is padded and allows free movement of the newborn's extremities without compromising the surgical field. In addition, the chair allows the infant to sit at a 30- to 45-degree angle, and it is adjustable to accomodate smaller newborns (Stang and others, 1997). All of the equipment used for the procedure, such as gloves, instruments, dressings, and draping towels, must be sterile.

The procedure involves freeing the foreskin from the glans penis by using a scalpel, Gomco or Mogen (Cultural Awareness box) clamp, or Plastibell. In the *Gomco technique* the foreskin is clamped, cut with a scalpel, and removed; the clamp crushes the nerve endings and blood vessels, promoting hemostasis. In the *Plastibell procedure* the foreskin is removed using a plastic ring and a string tied around the foreskin like a tourniquet. The excess foreskin is trimmed. In about 5 to 8 days the plastic ring separates and falls off.

Once the procedure is completed, the infant is released from the restraints and comforted. If the parents were not present during the procedure, they are informed of the infant's status and reunited with their son.

Care of the circumcision depends on the type of procedure. If a clamp (Gomco or Mogen) was used, a petrolatum gauze dressing may be applied loosely to prevent adherence to the diaper. If the Plastibell was applied, no special dressing is required. Because the area is tender, the diaper is applied loosely to prevent friction against the penis. The circumcision is evaluated for excessive bleeding in the first few hours following the procedure, and the first void is recorded. A recommended standard is to evaluate the site every 30 minutes for at least 2 hours and then at least every 2 hours thereafter (Williamson, 1997).

**NURSING TIP** To check for the first void in disposable diapers made of absorbent gelling material, pinch the crotch of the diaper for a "clumpy, doughy" feeling because these diapers will feel dry despite voiding.

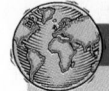

## CULTURAL AWARENESS
### Circumcision

In the Jewish culture circumcision is performed during a ceremony called a *berith*, or *brit*, which takes place on the eighth day of life. A specially trained professional known as a *mohel* stretches the prepuce over the glans, pulling it through a slit in a shield (usually a Mogen clamp) and cutting it with a knife. The traditional technique is not sterile, and bleeding is controlled by tight bandaging around the penis (Cohen and others, 1992). The infant may be given some sweet wine before the procedure. Blankets instead of straps are usually used to restrain the infant to a board, and the parents are present (Trochtenberg, 1990).

Female circumcision (mutilation) is also practiced, particularly in Africa, the Middle East, and Southeast Asia—and in immigrants from these countries to the United States, Australia, Canada, and Europe. In the most extensive operation (excision or infibulation) the clitoris, labia minora, and medial aspects of the labia majora are removed. The remaining labia majora are sewn closed, except for a small opening for urine and menses (American Academy of Pediatrics, 1998; McCleary, 1994). Anesthesia is used very rarely. In African and Asian cultures, female circumcision is used to prove virginity and to reduce sexual pleasure, thus promoting fidelity. The World Health Organization condemns all forms of female genital mutilation (Female Genital Mutilation, 1994).

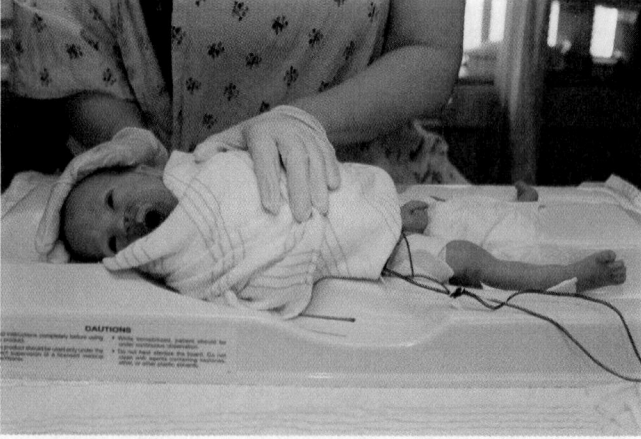

**Fig. 8-15** Proper positioning of infant in Circumstraint. (Courtesy Paul Vincent Kuntz, Texas Children's Hospital.)

Normally, on the second day a yellowish white exudate forms as part of the granulation process. This is not a sign of infection and is not forcibly removed. As healing progresses, the exudate disappears. Parents are educated to report any evidence of bleeding, unusual swelling, or absence of voiding to the practitioner. (See Critical Thinking Exercise box.)

## Provide Optimum Nutrition

Selection of a feeding method is one of the major decisions faced by parents. The options for infant feeding must be explored during the antepartum period when parents are better able to understand the importance of infant nutrition and the choices available. Nurses should be at the forefront in providing the parent(s) with accurate and unbiased information needed to make a conscientious informed decision regarding feeding method. In general, there are two primary choices: human milk and commercially prepared cow's milk–based formula. There are significant nutritional, economic, and psychologic advantages and differences between these two methods (Box 8-5).

**Human Milk.** Human milk is the best option for infant nutrition up to 1 year of age. Breast milk consists of a number of micronutrients that are termed *bioavailable,* meaning these nutrients are available in quantities and qualities that make them easily digestible by the newborn's intestine and

absorbed for energy and growth. Breast milk offers a variety of immunologic properties that are found exclusively in human milk. In general human milk has been shown to be effective in protecting the newborn against respiratory infections, gastrointestinal infections caused by enterococci, otitis media, numerous allergies, and atopy (Beaudry, Dufour, and Marcoux, 1995; Dewey, Heinig, and Nommsen-Rivers, 1995; Scariati, Grummer-Strawn, and Fein, 1997). The fat content of human milk is composed of lipids, triglycerides, and cholesterol; cholesterol is an essential element for brain growth. The function of these lipids is to allow optimal intestinal absorption of fatty acids and provide essential fatty acids (EFAs) and polyunsaturated fatty acids (PUFAs). Furthermore lipids contribute approximately 50% of the total calories in human milk (Lawrence and Lawrence, 1999). Although the overall fat content in human milk is higher than cow's milk–based formula, it is used more efficiently by the infant.

The primary source of carbohydrate in human milk is lactose, which is present in higher concentrations (6.8 g/dl) than cow's milk–based formula (4.9 g/dl). Other carbohydrates found in human milk include glucose, galactose, and glucosamine. The carbohydrates serve not only as a large percentage of the total calories in human milk but they also have a protective function; the oligosaccharides in human milk stimulate the growth of *Lactobacilus bifidus* and prevent bacteria from adhering to epithelial surfaces (Lawrence and Lawrence, 1999).

Human milk also contains the two proteins, whey (lactalbumin) and casein (curd), in a ratio of approximately 60:40

---

## Critical Thinking Exercise

### Newborn Home Circumcision Care

You visit the Andersons, who went home after a 24-hour stay following the birth of their son, Jason, who is now 3½ days old. The father asks you about Jason's circumcision care; he is concerned about a yellow crusted exudate that has formed on the glans of the penis. Jason had a Gomco circumcision. Your assessment reveals that Jason is voiding without any problems, there is no bleeding from the site, and the urinary meatus is intact. What should you tell the Andersons in order to continue caring for the circumcision site?

FIRST, THINK ABOUT IT . . .

• What concepts or ideas are central to your thinking?
• What are you taking for granted; what assumptions are you making?

1. The circumcision has become infected, and antibiotics will be necessary.
2. The exudate is a part of the normal healing process; the penis should be cleansed gently with water at least once a day.
3. The Andersons have not been properly caring for the circumcision site and should be taught proper care.
4. The newborn will need to be referred to the practitioner for further inspection of the circumcision site.

*The best response is two. A yellow crusted exudate is commonly seen on the glans penis and is a normal aspect of healing that is often observed during the healing stages. A correct assumption is that the newborn does not need antibiotics or a subsequent visit to the practitioner. Reinforce that the care the Andersons have been giving is appropriate and praise their efforts.*

---

**Box 8-5** ■ ■ ■
### Advantages of Human Milk

**HUMAN MILK**

Contains adequate (not excessive) protein; has greater quantities of certain amino acids, including cystine and taurine

Contains more lactalbumin (produces easily digested curds) than casein (produces large, hard curds)

Contains more lactose, which in the gut stimulates growth of microorganisms, which synthesize some B vitamins and produce organic acids that may retard growth of harmful bacteria

Contains more monounsaturated fatty acids, which enhance absorption of fat and calcium

Contains adequate (not excessive) minerals with exception of fluoride (low)

Amounts of iron and zinc are low but more readily absorbed

Contains less calcium and phosphorus but a more favorable ratio of the minerals, which prevents excessive calcium excretion

Contains adequate amounts of vitamins A, B complex, and E; vitamin C content depends on maternal intake; vitamin D is low but more readily absorbed (vitamins C, D, and E are low in cow's milk, but K is higher)

Contains growth modulators that modify growth or maturation

Offers several immunologic benefits: contains various immunoglobulins (Ig), especially IgA; macrophages, granulocytes, T- and B-cell lymphocytes; and other factors that inhibit bacterial growth

Has laxative effect

Is economical, readily available, and sanitary

Has psychologic benefits of a close bond between infant and mother during feeding

(80:20 in most cow-milk–based formula). This ratio in human milk makes it more digestible and produces the soft stools seen in infants who breast-feed. Thus human milk has a laxative effect and constipation is rare. The whey protein, lactoferrin, in human milk has iron-binding characteristics with bacteriostatic capabilities, particularly against gram-positive and gram-negative aerobes, anaerobes, and yeasts (Lawrence and Lawrence, 1999).

Lysozyme is found in large quantities in human milk with bacteriostatic functions against gram-positive bacteria and enterobacteriacae. Human milk also contains numerous other host defense factors such as macrophages, granulocytes, and T- and B-lymphocytes. Casein in human milk greatly enhances the absorption of iron, thus preventing iron-dependent bacteria from proliferating in the gastrointestinal tract (Biancuzzo, 1999). Secretory immunoglobulin A (IgA) is found in high levels in colostrum, but levels gradually decrease over the first 14 days of life. Secretory IgA is an immunoglobulin that prevents viruses and bacteria from invading the intestinal mucosa in breast-fed newborns, thus protecting them from infections. This whey protein is also believed to play an important role in preventing the development of allergies (Biancuzzo, 1999).

Several digestive enzymes also present in human milk include amylases, lipases, proteases, and ribonucleases, which enhance digestion and absorption of various nutrients (Lawrence and Lawrence, 1999).

The amounts of lipid and water-soluble vitamins as well as electrolytes, minerals, and trace elements in human milk are sufficient for infant growth, development, and energy needs during the first 6 months of life. Several studies have shown that feeding infants human milk produces children with higher intelligence than their cow's milk–based formula-fed counterparts (Anderson, Johnstone, and Remley, 1999; Lanting and others, 1994).

Additional beneficial components of human milk include prostaglandins, epidermal growth factor, desoxyhexanoic acid (DHA), arachidonic acid (AA), taurine, carnitine, cytokine, interleukins, and natural hormones such as thyroid-releasing hormone, gonadotrophin-releasing hormone, and prolactin.

There are also variations in human milk related to the timing of the lactation cycle. Colostrum, for example, is rich in immunoglobulins and vitamin K and has a higher protein content than mature milk; however, it has a lower fat content. Transitional milk replaces colostrum when the mother's milk supply starts increasing, and eventually mature milk becomes the primary milk source. There is also diurnal variation in the biochemistry of mature human milk. Human milk also varies with respect to gestational age; preterm human milk differs from mature milk in its biochemical composition (Lawrence and Lawrence, 1999). Nonphysiologic advantages of human milk are discussed under Breast-Feeding.

**Breast-Feeding.** *Human milk* is the preferred form of nutrition for the full-term infant. *Healthy People 2010* has a goal to increase breast-feeding rates in the United States to 75% in early postpartum and to 50% for mothers who continue to breast-feed for at least 6 months (*Healthy People 2010*, 1999). A survey by Ross (Ross Mothers Survey, 2000) indicates that 68.4% of women breast-fed in early postpartum and 31.4% still breast-fed at 6 months. The incidence of breast-feeding in the United States declined in the 1980s, but other data show an overall increase of more than 14% in the number of mothers initiating breast-feeding in the hospital. In addition, there was an increase (19.3%) in the number of mothers breast-feeding at 6 months. Breast-feeding incidence increased across all socioeconomic groups but was greater among groups who historically have been less likely to breast-feed: African-American women; mothers less than 20 years old; primiparas; women with grade school education only; residents of the South Atlantic region; participants in the Women, Infants, and Children (WIC) program; and mothers employed full time outside the home. Breast-feeding rates were highest among older, multiparous college-educated women in western states, not enrolled in WIC, not employed outside the home but with a higher disposable income, and whose infants were of normal birth weight (Ryan, 1997). There is also concern that the increasingly early discharge of new mothers from hospitals, more aggressive marketing of infant formulas to the public, and more employed mothers have contributed to the decline of breast-feeding in the previous decade.

There is evidence that hospital practices intended to provide optimum maternal-newborn health may instead undermine breast-feeding. Early separation of mother and newborn, delays in initiating breast-feeding, conflicting information by health care workers, provision of formula in the hospital and in discharge packs, and formula coupons given at discharge have been implicated in the decline of breast-feeding following discharge. Rooming-in correlated positively with successful breast-feeding, whereas the use of a pacifier was associated with earlier weaning from breast to bottle. Changing hospital practices that were perceived as detrimental to breast-feeding significantly improved the overall duration of breast-feeding in one study (Wright, Rice, and Wells, 1996). Although some studies have shown that the availability of commercial formula from hospital discharge packs may influence mothers to bottle-feed (Wright, Rice, and Wells, 1996), other studies have found no such effect (Dungy and others, 1997; Donnelly and others, 2000).

In a recent survey breast-feeding mothers indicated that the determining factors for changing to bottle-feeding included the mother's perception of the father's attitude toward breast-feeding and the mother's uncertainty regarding the amount of milk the infant would receive (Arora and others, 2000). These findings have important implications for involving fathers in education and discussion regarding breast-feeding before and during the pregnancy.

The American Academy of Pediatrics (1998b) has reaffirmed its position on recommending exclusive breast-feeding until at least 1 year of age as the best form of infant nutrition. The Academy also supports programs that enable women to continue breast-feeding after returning to work. In its support of breast-feeding practices, the Academy further discourages the advertisement of infant formula to breast-feeding mothers and distribution of formula discharge packs without the advice of a health care provider.

The *Baby-Friendly Hospital Initiative (BFHI)* is a joint effort of the World Health Organization and the United Nations Children's Fund to encourage, promote, and support breast-feeding as the model for optimum infant nutrition. Ten research-supported practices were developed by BFHI as a guideline for maternity facilities worldwide to promote breast-feeding (Kyenkya-Isabirye, 1992; Wright, Rice, and Wells, 1996) (Box 8-6).

In addition to the physiologic qualities of human milk, the most outstanding psychologic benefit of breast-feeding is the close maternal-child relationship. The infant is nestled very close to the mother's skin, can hear the rhythm of her heartbeat, can feel the warmth of her body, and has a sense of peaceful security. The mother has a very close feeling of union with her child and feels a sense of accomplishment and satisfaction as the infant suckles milk from her.

Human milk is the most economical form of feeding. It is always available, ready to serve at room temperature, and free of contamination. The projected monetary savings for a population of breast-feeding infants in relation to preventive medicine have been estimated and are considered to be significant (Ball and Wright, 1999; Montgomery and Splett, 1997). Although human milk is not sterile, healthy full-term infants can tolerate varying amounts of nonpathogenic and pathogenic organisms. The protection against infection can provide additional cost savings in terms of fewer medical visits and less time lost from work for the employed mother.

Breast-feeding may also offer protection against obesity, allergy, diabetes, and atherosclerosis although the evidence is inconclusive. Breast-fed infants, especially beyond 2 to 3 months of age, tend to grow at a satisfactory but slower rate than bottle-fed infants (Dewey and others, 1991). In-fants who are exclusively breast-fed have decreased amount of free fat, thus the tendency for breast-fed infants to appear leaner than their counterparts fed formula (Butte and others, 2000; Dewey and others, 1993). Only recently have National Center for Health Statistics' (NCHS) growth charts* been adjusted to reflect exclusively breast-fed infants who have a slower growth rate during the first several months of life. By the age of 12 to 15 months breast-fed infants weigh approximately the same as their bottle-fed counterparts.

Contraindications to breast-feeding include (Lawrence and Lawrence, 1999):

- Maternal cancer therapy
- Hepatitis C virus (HCV) in mother
- Active tuberculosis not under treatment in mother
- HIV in mother
- Galactosemia in infant
- Cytomegalovirus (CMV)—primary risk is to premature infants receiving CMV-infected donor milk, not to infected mother's infant, who already has CMV
- Maternal substance abuse (e.g., cocaine and marijuana)
- Human T-cell leukemia virus type 1 (HTLV-1)

Mastitis is usually not a contraindication if the discomfort is tolerable.

Breast-feeding can also be done with twin births (and other multiples). If the infants are full term, they can begin feedings immediately after birth (Fig. 8-16). Simultaneous feeding promotes the rapid production of milk needed for both infants and makes the milk that would normally be lost in the letdown reflex available to one of the twins. When only one infant is hungry, the mother should feed singly. She should also alternate breasts when feeding each infant and avoid favoring one breast for one infant. The sucking patterns of infants vary, and each infant needs the visual stimulation and exercise that alternating breasts provides.

A disadvantage of breast-feeding to many mothers is the perceived inconvenience of loss of freedom and indepen-

---

*In order to access the NCHS growth charts go to the National Health and Nutrition Examination Survey (NHANES) home page www.cdc.gov/nchs/nhanes.htm and then go to the growth chart site.

---

> **Box 8-6** ■ ■ ■
> **Ten Steps to Successful Breast-Feeding**
>
> Every facility providing maternity services and care for newborn infants should:
> 1. Have a written breast-feeding policy that is routinely communicated to all health care staff.
> 2. Train all health care staff in skills necessary to implement this policy.
> 3. Inform all pregnant women about the benefits and management of breast-feeding.
> 4. Help mothers initiate breast-feeding within a half-hour of birth.
> 5. Show mothers how to breast-feed, and how to maintain lactation even if they should be separated from their infants.
> 6. Give newborn infants no food or drink other than breast milk, unless medically indicated.
> 7. Practice rooming-in—allow mothers and infants to remain together—24 hours a day.
> 8. Encourage breast-feeding on demand.
> 9. Give no artificial teats or pacifiers (also called dummies or soothers) to breast-feeding infants.
> 10. Foster the establishment of breast-feeding support groups and refer mothers to them on discharge from the hospital or clinic.
>
> From Kyenkya-Isabirye M: UNICEF launches the Baby-Friendly Hospital Initiative, *MCN* 17(4):177-179, 1992; and Wright A, Rice S, Wells S: Changing hospital practices to increase the duration of breastfeeding, *Pediatrics* 97(5):669-676, 1996.

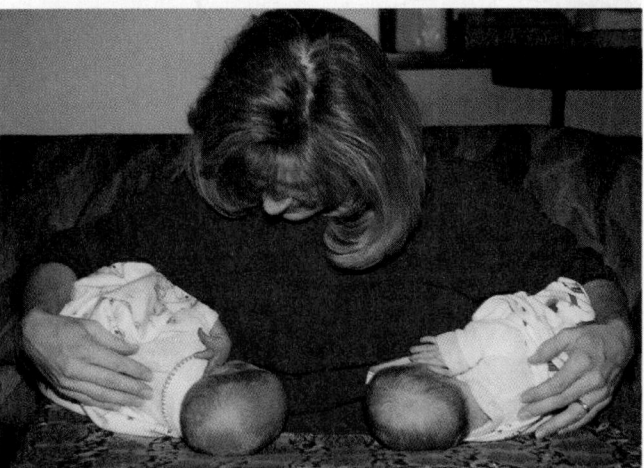

**Fig. 8-16**   Simultaneous breast-feeding of twins.

dence. Being committed to feeding the infant every 2 to 3 hours can be overwhelming, especially to women with multiple responsibilities. Many women resume their careers shortly after their pregnancy and prefer to use bottle-feeding. However, breast-feeding and employment are possible, and suggestions for the mother are discussed in Chapter 12. Although breast-feeding is the preferred form of infant feeding, mothers' decisions regarding their preferences must be supported and respected. (See Critical Thinking Exercise box.)

Successful breast-feeding probably depends more on the mother's desire to breast-feed, satisfaction with breast-feeding, and available support systems than on any other factors. Contrary to popular belief, breast-feeding is not instinctive. Mothers need support, encouragement, and assistance during their postpartum hospital stay and at home to enhance their opportunities for success and satisfaction.

Three main criteria have been proposed as essential in promoting breast-feeding: correct sucking technique, absence of a rigid feeding time schedule, and correct positioning of the infant at the breast to achieve latch-on. Correct sucking for breast-feeding is defined as a wide-open mouth, tongue under the areola, and expression of milk by slow, deep sucking (Fig. 8-17).

The following interventions promote breast-feeding:

- Frequent and early breast-feeding, especially during the first hour of life; immediate skin-to-skin contact; rooming-in; feeding on demand; and careful control of drugs
- Direct modeling of the importance of breast-feeding by health care providers, such as implementing demand nursing with no formula supplementation and decreased emphasis on infant formula products
- Increased information and support to mothers following discharge, especially phone follow-up
- Early breast pumping every 2 to 3 hours for 20 minutes bilaterally if the newborn is unable to nurse immediately (increases oxytocin production and thus milk production)

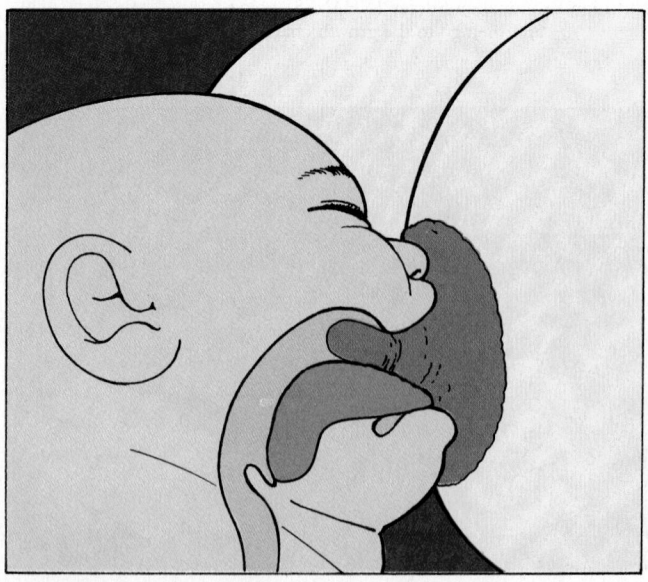

**Fig. 8-17** The tongue is under the areola, with the tip of the nipple at the back of the wide-open mouth.

Nurses play a very significant role in the breast-feeding decision and must make themselves available to families for guidance and support. Several excellent books and organizations, such as **La Leche League International,** * are available as resources for professionals and breast-feeding mothers.

***Breast-Feeding Problems.*** Many mothers have concerns regarding breast-feeding, and, with earlier discharge from postpartum units, common problems, such as engorgement and painful nipples, may occur after the mother is at home. New mothers are often concerned about their milk supply, and excessive anxiety can affect successful lactation. (See Family Focus box).

---

*1400 N Meacham, Schaumburg, IL 60173, (800) LA-LECHE, (800) 525-3243; www.lalecheleague.org. In Canada: Box 29, 18C Industrial Dr, Chesterville, Ontario, KOC 1HO, (613) 448-1842.

 **Critical Thinking Exercise**

### Breast-Feeding and Returning to Work

Amy S. has delivered a 4.1 kg baby girl and wishes to breast-feed in the delivery room. Following successful feeding, Amy comments to her husband about wishing she could continue breast-feeding at home. Your further assessment reveals that Amy must return to work within 6 to 8 weeks to maintain their financial status and believes she will have to stop breast-feeding. Amy is considering switching to bottle-feeding after going home. What is the best solution that you might suggest to meet Amy's needs and those of her family?

FIRST, THINK ABOUT IT . . .

- What information are you using?
- How are you interpreting that information?

---

1. Discontinue breast-feeding now to begin decreasing milk production and to prevent becoming too disappointed.
2. Continue breast-feeding in the hospital, then stop when she goes home.
3. Continue breast-feeding, and, when the time nears for her return to work, consult with a professional about available options to continue breast-feeding while returning to work.
4. Discuss with her husband the possibility of not returning to work.

---

*The best response is three. Amy may continue to breast-feed after discharge. Discussing options later will give her and her husband time to think about the options available that will meet their family's, as well as Amy's, needs. It is important to discuss with families that returning to work and continuing breast-feeding is a very viable option; mothers may pump during breaks at work, store the milk, and have the breast milk fed by bottle while they are away. Often mothers may not be aware of this information. Infants adapt to taking milk by bottle and continue breast-feeding after a successful period of effective breast-feeding. To discontinue breast-feeding now is a poor option because Amy may decide once she gets home to resume breast-feeding; the milk supply may then be limited by interrupting breast-feeding at this time.*

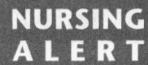 **NURSING ALERT**  Encourage frequent feedings to increase milk production rather than use of supplemental formula or solid foods.

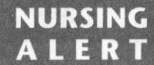 **NURSING ALERT**  The use of pacifiers in the early period of breast-feeding has been associated with earlier interruption of breast-feeding and weaning to bottle.

The more common breast-feeding problems and the interventions to correct them are summarized in Table 8-5. Most of these problems can be easily remedied, provided that the mother receives the attention needed to identify the concern. Assessment should include a detailed history of the complaint, examination of the breasts, and observation of the breast-feeding. (See Guidelines box.)

Many breast-feeding problems respond rapidly to simple interventions, such as correcting the infant's feeding position. However, the mother needs continual reassurance of success and the support that allows her the needed rest and relaxation to nurse her infant. Referral to supportive agencies, such as local groups of **La Leche League International,** or to a lactation specialist may be beneficial.

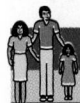 ## FAMILY FOCUS
### Breast-Feeding and Infant Weight Gain

Mothers whose breast-fed infants fail to gain weight according to the standard growth curves may be told that their milk, although nutritionally good for the baby from an immunologic standpoint, lacks fat for adequate growth. In addition there are numerous anecdotal reports of mothers who are told by relatives to stop breast-feeding the infant because he/she does not weigh as much as the same-age infant who is being bottle fed. There is evidence, however, which indicates that the 1977 standard growth charts may not reflect normal growth patterns of infants who are breast-fed. Infants who are breast-fed grow more rapidly during the first 2 months of life, but growth is slower from 3 to 12 months when compared with the previous NCHS growth reference data charts. In the second year of life, breast-fed infants gain weight faster than is reflected by reference charts, and by 24 months their average weight approximates current growth charts (Dewey and others, 1995).

It has been suggested that perhaps breast-fed infants grow slower in the first few months of life as a result of protein deficiency; however, in a study of breast-fed infants receiving an additional 20% higher protein intake, the growth rate remained the same as for infants who were exclusively breast-fed (Dewey and others, 1996). Breast-fed infants are leaner and have less body fat than formula-fed infants, but growth in head circumference is greater in the breast-fed group. Even with the introduction of solid foods at 5 to 6 months, breast-fed infants demonstrate self-regulation in regard to energy intake. The conclusions from the studies are that infants who are breast-fed during the first year of life, even with the introduction of solids at 4 to 6 months, are at risk for being labeled as "growth deficient" when compared with 1977 NCHS growth charts (Dewey and others, 1995). In 2000 NHANES revised the growth charts to reflect differences in growth in infants who are breast- and bottle-fed. The new growth charts may be downloaded from the CDC website: *www.cdc.gov/ growthcharts/.*

Nurses can share these findings with parents to allay fears of an inadequate milk supply, which can discourage mothers from continuing to breast-feed. Also, an evaluation of growth, especially if weight falls below the 5th percentile, must be viewed carefully to avoid the diagnosis of failure to thrive in infants with no other evidence of inadequate nutrition. (See Chapter 12.)

**Bottle-Feeding.**  Bottle-feeding generally refers to the use of bottles for feeding commercial or evaporated milk formula rather than using the breast, although in some instances human milk may be expressed and fed with a bottle. Bottle-feeding is an acceptable method of feeding. However, nurses should not assume that new parents automatically know how to bottle-feed their infant. Parents who choose bottle-feeding also need support and assistance in meeting their infant's needs.

Providing newborns with nutrition is only one aspect of the feeding. Holding them close to the body while rocking or cuddling them helps to ensure the emotional component of feeding. Like breast-fed infants, bottle-fed infants need to be held on alternate sides of the lap to expose them to different stimuli. The feeding should not be hurried. Even though they may suck vigorously for the first 5 minutes and seem to be satisfied, they should be allowed to continue sucking. Infants need at least 2 hours of sucking a day. If there are six feedings per day, then about 20 minutes of sucking at each feeding provides for oral gratification.

**NURSING TIP**  An angled bottle is preferable to a straight bottle because it encourages more physiologic positioning of the infant, improves the infant's comfort level, and decreases the need for burping (Farber, Van Fossen, and Koontz, 1995).

After feedings, infants are positioned on the right side to permit the feeding to flow toward the lower end of the stomach and to allow any swallowed air to rise above fluid and through the esophagus (Fig. 8-18). This position prevents regurgitation and distention. To maintain the side-lying position, a small blanket roll can be placed snugly behind the back. During sleep, only the supine position is used.

 ## GUIDELINES
### Observing the Breast-Feeding Pair

Position of mother, her body language, and any possible tension
Position of infant: child's ventral (front) surface should be next to mother's ventral surface with the face directly in front of the breast ("tummy to tummy"); the infant cannot swallow if the head has to turn to the breast
Position of mother's hand on the breast: using the thumb and index finger to compress the areola (the C-hold) and support the breast facilitates infant's ability to grasp the areola properly
Flanged position of infant's lips on the areola: the lips should gently grasp most of the areola, with the lower lip covering more of the areola than the upper lip
Baby's chin, not the nose, is touching mother's breast (Newman and Pitman, 2000)
Use of alternate breasts and feeding time on each breast
Technique to break suction: should release suction using fingers between the areola and lips; should not pull infant from the breast abruptly

**TABLE 8-5** Common breast-feeding problems

| Problem | Comments/Interventions |
|---|---|
| **Engorgement** | Best intervention is *prevention* with proper deep areolar latch on and frequent nursing on both breasts for complete emptying of ducts<br>If engorgement occurs, infant is unable to properly grasp distended areola<br>Interventions:<br>  Express manually small amount of milk; electric pump may be beneficial for some<br>  Use warm compresses or a warm shower *before feeding*; for severely engorged breasts, cold compresses may be helpful to reduce vascularity *after feeding*<br>  Compress areola with fingers to facilitate infant's grasp (C-hold)<br>  Use well-fitting nursing brassiere and wear 24 hours a day<br>  For excessive discomfort, take aspirin, ibuprofen or acetaminophen 30 minutes before feeding<br>  Massage breasts; vary position of infant's mouth on nipple and areola |
| **Painful nipples** | Most common causes are poor feeding technique, improper care of breasts, and/or poor hygiene with bacterial or fungal infection<br>If left untreated, discomfort may cause mother to terminate breast-feeding<br>Interventions for care of breasts:<br>  Avoid soaps, oils, or self-prescribed treatments<br>  Apply small amount of breast milk to areola after feeding and let dry<br>  Air nipples as much as possible; use heat (60-watt bulb placed 18 inches away or hair dryer on low setting)<br>  Change breast pads frequently; avoid plastic-backed pads (may trap moisture)<br>Interventions related to feeding:<br>  Start let-down reflex by manual expression before putting infant to breast<br>  Begin nursing with less affected breast, then nurse on affected side<br>  Position infant properly at breast to achieve deep areolar grasp<br>  Change infant's position<br>  For excessive discomfort, take analgesics 30 minutes before feeding; apply ice to nipples after feeding |
| **Delayed let-down reflex** | Reflex essential to delivery of milk from alveoli and smaller milk ducts into larger lactiferous ducts and sinuses<br>Controlled primarily by release of prolactin and oxytocin<br>Pain, stress, and anxiety can interfere with reflex<br>Interventions:<br>  Provide quiet, relaxing atmosphere for nursing (e.g., soothing music, privacy, pillows for positioning, decreased distractions)<br>  Stroke breast gently<br>  Apply warmth to breast<br>  May need to use oxytocin nasal spray to induce reflex (used only in newborn period) |
| **Inadequate milk supply** | Production of milk depends on supply and demand<br>Rarely is related to organic causes, such as decreased glandular tissue but may occur after breast augmentation surgery<br>Interventions:<br>  **Avoid use of supplemental formula feedings before breast-feeding is well established** to prevent nipple preference and satiation (infant will not be hungry enough to breast-feed)<br>  Reassure mother that her milk supply will be adequate and depends on frequent nursing<br>  Encourage more frequent nursing (at least six to eight times daily, initially at both breasts)<br>  Encourage adequate rest, nutrition, and fluids (increased fluids, however, have not been shown to increase milk production)<br>  Monitor infant's growth; in some cases formula supplementation may be indicated; an alternative to bottle-feeding is use of a supplemental feeding device consisting of a plastic bag or syringe for formula and a thin feeding tube that is placed next to mother's nipple during nursing |
| **Plugged ducts** | May occur at any time, especially during first 6 weeks<br>Continue breast-feeding every 2-3 hours<br>Massage breasts before feedings<br>Apply ice compresses to breasts between feedings for 10-15 minutes and apply warm compresses before pumping or feeding<br>Alternate feeding positions, positioning infant's chin toward obstructed area |
| **Mastitis** | Inflammation or infection in mammary gland or tissue by *Staphylococcus aureus*; results from inadequate emptying of ducts or from cracks in nipple skin; may be associated with fever and flu-like symptoms<br>Prevention: see Plugged ducts, above, if mastitis occurs, current treatment is 10 days of antibiotics (usually amoxicillin or cephalexin, started 24 hours after onset of symptoms)<br>Continue breast-feeding during this time to keep breast well drained (unless contraindicated for medical reasons such as systemic illness) |
| **Unsuccessful latch-on** | Improper positioning of infant at breast, inability to achieve deep areolar grasp, sleepiness, or improper suckling technique may be the cause of this common problem; flat, large, or inverted nipples may also be a factor<br>Mother and newborn must be anatomically positioned so that infant's mouth is in full contact with breast; mother should use C-hold; newborn's mouth is opened wide, and most of areola is grasped (see Fig. 8-17), especially with lower lip; frequent audible swallowing should be heard as evidence of spontaneous and successful suckling<br>Anatomic problems such as flat or inverted nipples are managed by mother wearing shells to elongate or make nipples more accessible |

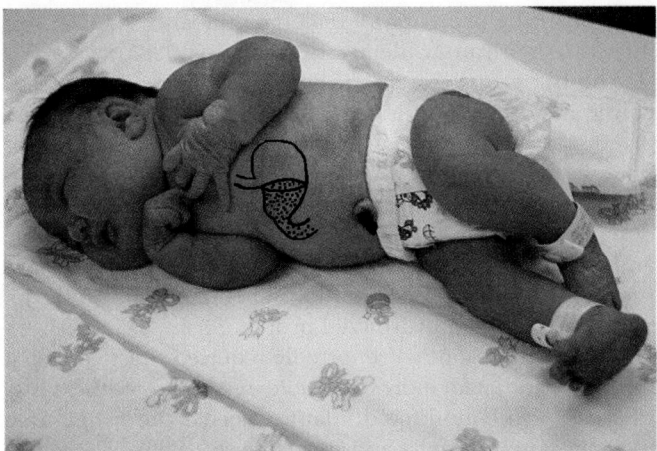

**Fig. 8-18** Right-side lying position after feeding while awake. Supine positioning is recommended during sleep.

Propping the bottle is discouraged for the following reasons:

- It denies the infant the important component of close human contact.
- The infant may aspirate formula while sleeping.
- It may facilitate the development of middle ear infections. As the infant lies flat and sucks, milk that has pooled in the pharynx becomes a suitable medium for bacterial growth. Bacteria then enters the eustachian tube, which leads to the middle ear, causing acute otitis media.
- It encourages continuous pooling of formula in the mouth, which can lead to caries when the teeth erupt. (See Chapter 14.)

*Preparation of Formula.* The two traditional ways of preparing formula are the terminal heat method (all of the utensils and formula are boiled together for 25 minutes) and the aseptic method (the equipment is boiled separately, after which the formula is poured into the bottles). Because of improved sanitary conditions in developed countries, neither of these methods is essential. The clean technique is satisfactory, including using a dishwasher. Persons preparing the formula wash their hands well and then wash all of the equipment used to prepare the formula, including the cans of formula or evaporated milk. The formula is prepared and bottled immediately before each feeding. Warming the formula is optional. Any milk remaining in the bottle after the feeding is discarded because it is an excellent medium for bacterial growth. Opened cans of formula are covered and refrigerated until the next feeding.

**NURSING ALERT** Warming bottles in the microwave oven is not recommended because of the risk of burns from bottles exploding or the hot temperature of the fluid.

Recommendations for labeling infant formulas require that the directions for preparation and use of the formula include pictures and symbols for nonreading individuals. In addition, manufacturers are translating the directions into foreign languages, such as Spanish and Vietnamese, to prevent misunderstanding and errors in formula preparation.

**NURSING ALERT** Impress on families that the proportions *must not be altered*—neither diluted to extend the amount of formula nor concentrated to provide more calories.

**Feeding Schedules.** Ideally, feeding schedules should be determined by the infant's hunger. *Demand feedings* are given when the infant signals readiness. *Scheduled feedings* are arranged at predetermined intervals. Some hospitals routinely feed infants every 3 to 4 hours. Although this may be satisfactory for bottle-fed infants, it hinders the breast-feeding process. Since breast-fed infants tend to be hungry every 2 to 3 hours because of the easy digestibility of the milk, they should be fed on demand.

Supplemental feedings should *not* be offered to breast-fed infants before lactation is well established because they may satiate the infant and may cause nipple preference. Supplemental water is not needed in breast-fed infants, even in hot climates (Sachdev and others, 1991). Satiated infants suck less vigorously at the breast, and milk production depends on the breast being emptied at each feeding. If milk is allowed to accumulate in the ducts, causing breast engorgement, ischemia results, suppressing the activity of the acini or milk-secreting cells. Consequently, milk production is reduced. In addition, the process of sucking from a bottle is different from breast nipple compression. The relatively inflexible rubber nipple prevents the tongue from its usual rhythmic action. Infants learn to put the tongue against the nipple holes to slow down the more rapid flow of fluid. When infants use these same tongue movements during breast-feeding, they may push the human nipple out of the mouth and may not grasp the areola properly.

Usually by 3 weeks of age, lactation and a feeding schedule are well established. Bottle-fed infants retain about 2 to 3 ounces of formula at each feeding and are fed approximately six times a day. The quantity of formula consumed is based on the caloric need of 108 kcal/kg/day; therefore a newborn who weighs 3 kg requires 324 kcal/day. Because commercial formula for term infants has 20 kcal/oz, about 16 ounces (480 ml) will provide the daily caloric requirement. Breast-fed infants may feed as frequently as 10 to 12 times a day. Larger infants are able to retain increased amounts because of greater stomach capacity; as a result, they generally sleep through the night sooner than smaller infants or breast-fed infants.

**Feeding Behavior.** Five behavioral stages occur during successful feeding. Recognizing these steps can assist nurses in identifying potential feeding problems caused by improper feeding techniques (see discussion of NCAST Feeding Scale, p. 247). *Prefeeding behavior,* such as crying or fussing, demonstrates the infant's level of arousal and degree of hunger. To encourage the infant to grasp the breast properly, it is preferable to begin feeding during the quiet alert state, before the infant becomes upset. *Approach behavior* is indicated by sucking movements or the rooting reflex. *Attachment behavior* includes those activities that occur from the time the infant receives the nipple and sucks (sometimes more pronounced during initial attempts at breast-feeding). *Consummatory behavior* consists of coordinated sucking and swallowing. Persistent gagging might indicate unsuccessful consummatory behavior. *Satiety behavior* is observed when infants let the parent know that they are satisfied, usually by falling asleep.

> **NURSING ALERT** Do not use microwaving to defrost frozen human milk. High-temperature microwaving (72° C to 98° C [162° to 208° F]) destroys the antiinfective factors. The safety of low-temperature microwaving (20° to 53° C [68° to 127° F]) is questionable (Quan and others, 1992). It is best to thaw human milk in the refrigerator for a day. To thaw frozen milk quickly, place frozen milk container under cool or lukewarm running tap water or place in a bowl of lukewarm water (Biancuzzo, 1999).

**Commercially Prepared Formulas.** The analysis of human and whole cow's milk indicates that the latter is unsuitable for infant nutrition. Whole cow's milk has a high protein content, low fat and lipid content, and there has been evidence that it may cause intestinal bleeding and lead to iron-deficiency anemia in infants. There has also been some question regarding the unmodified protein content of whole cow's milk, which may trigger an undesired immune response and thus increase the incidence of allergies in children at an early age.

Commercially prepared formulas are cow's milk–based formulas that have been modified to closely resemble the nutritional content of human milk. These formulas are altered from cow's milk by removing butterfat, decreasing the protein content, and adding vegetable oil and carbohydrate. Some cow's milk–based formulas have demineralized whey added to yield a whey:casein ratio of 60:40. The standard cow's milk–based formulas, regardless of the commercial brand, have essentially the same compositions of vitamins, minerals, protein, carbohydrates, and essential amino acids, with minor variations such as the source of carbohydrate (Akers and Groh-Wargo, 1999; Tigges, 1997). Standard cow's milk–based formulas are also sold as low-iron and iron-fortified; however, only the iron-fortified formulas meet the iron requirements of infants (Akers and Groh-Wargo, 1999).

There are three main categories of infant formulas: (1) *cow's milk–based formulas,* available commercially in 20 kcal/fl oz as liquid (ready to feed), as powder (requires dilution with water), or as concentrated liquid (requires dilution with water); (2) *soy-based formulas,* available commercially in ready-to-feed 20 kcal/fl oz powder and concentrated liquid forms, commonly used for children who are lactose- or cow's milk protein–intolerant; and (3) *casein- or whey-hydrolysate formulas,* commercially available in ready-to-feed and powder forms and used primarily for children who cannot tolerate or digest cow's milk or soy-based formulas (Wilson and Bowman, 2000).

The American Academy of Pediatrics (1998a) recommends the use of soy protein–based formulas for infants with galactosemia, hereditary lactase deficiency, documented IgE allergies caused by cow's milk, and documented evidence of lactose intolerance. Soy protein–based formulas, however, have not been proved to be effective against colic or in the prevention of allergy in healthy or high-risk infants (American Academy of Pediatrics, 1998a).

The last group, casein- or whey-hydrolysate formulas, is considered to be less antigenic than either cow's milk–based or soy-based formulas. The protein hydrolysate formulas (casein and whey) are derived from cow's milk–based formula by a process of heat, filtration, and enzyme treatment designed to break the peptide chains into more digestible and nonallergic proteins. The hydrolysate formulas have the reported disadvantage of tasting bad. In one study, infants who were fed hydrolyzed protein formulas in early infancy (at 1 to 2 months) reportedly acquired a taste for such formulas and had more favorable reactions to the taste, whereas 7- to 8-month-old infants rejected the hydrolysate formula taste (Menella and Beauchamp, 1996). Those formulas can be made more palatable by adding a hypoallergenic flavoring additive such as Vari-Flavor (Christie, 1999).

> **NURSING ALERT** It is unsafe and unnecessary to warm formula in the microwave because the heat is not equally distributed. The bottle may remain at a cooler temperature than the liquid inside, which may burn the infant. Warming a bottle under a warm water flow is sufficient. There is no evidence that infants prefer warm formula to that kept at room temperature (Akers and Groh-Wargo, 1999).

Neocate is an extensively hydrolyzed amino acid formula, designed for infants who are sensitive to cow's milk–based, soy-based, and partially hydrolyzed casein- and whey-based formulas. This formula is available in powder form and is relatively expensive. Additionally, a wide variety of formulas are manufactured for infants and children with special needs; it is not within the scope of this text to discuss each one, and many are found in Table 8-6.

*Follow-up formulas* are marketed as a transitional formula for infants older than 6 months who are also eating solid foods. These generally contain a higher percentage of calories from protein and carbohydrate sources, a higher amount of iron and vitamins, and a lower amount of fat than standard cow's milk–based formulas. Many nutrition experts and the American Academy of Pediatrics (1998b), however, discount the necessity of follow-up formulas if the infant is receiving an adequate amount of solid food containing sufficient iron, vitamins, and minerals.

**Alternate Milk Products.** In the United States few infants are fed *evaporated milk formula,* and its use is not recommended by the American Academy of Pediatrics. However, it has many advantages over whole milk. It is readily available in cans, needs no refrigeration if unopened, is less expensive than commercial formula, provides a softer, more digestible curd, and contains more lactalbumin and a higher calcium/phosphorus ratio. Disadvantages of evaporated milk for infant nutrition include low iron and vitamin C concentrations, excessive sodium and phosphorus, decreased vitamin A and D (except in fortified forms), and poorly digested fat (Akers and Groh-Wargo, 1999).

A common rule for preparing evaporated milk formula is diluting the 13-ounce can of milk with 19½ ounces of water

**TABLE 8-6**   Normal and special infant formulas*

| Formula (Manufacturer) | Protein Source | Carbohydrate Source | Fat Sources | Indications for Use | Comments (Nutritional Considerations) |
|---|---|---|---|---|---|
| **Human and Cow's Milk Formulas** | | | | | |
| **Human breast milk** | Mature human milk; whey/casein ratio—60;40 | Lactose | Mature human milk | For all full-term infants except those with galactosemia; may also be used with low-birth-weight infants | Recommended sole form of feeding for first 12 months; nutritionally complete |
| **Evaporated cow's milk formulas** | Milk protein; whey/casein ratio—18;82 | Lactose, sucrose | Butterfat | For full-term infants with no special nutritional requirements | Supplement with iron and vitamin C; A and D if not fortified; fluoride if fluoridated water is not used for formula preparation (after 6 mo) |
| **Commercial Infant Formulas** | | | | | |
| **Enfamil** (Mead Johnson) | Nonfat cow's milk, demineralized whey; whey/casein ratio—60:40 | Lactose | Palm olein, soy, coconut, HOSun oils† | For full-term and premature infants with no special nutritional requirements | Available fortified with iron, 12 mg/L Also available in 22 and 24 cal/oz |
| **Similac** (Ross) | Nonfat cow's milk; whey/casein ratio—48:52 | Lactose | Soy, coconut oils, and high-oleic safflower oil | For full-term and premature infants with no special nutritional requirements | Available fortified with iron, 1.8 mg/100 cal, nucleotides, 72 mg/L Also available in 22 and 24 cal/oz with iron |
| **Good Start** (Carnation) | Hydrolyzed whey | Lactose, maltodextrin | Palm olein, soy, safflower, coconut oils | For full-term infants | Lower osmolality; lower protein, calcium, sodium, vitamin E; less expensive in comparison to other brand-name formulas |
| **Similac Neosure** (with iron) | Nonfat cow's milk, whey/casein ratio—50:50 | Corn syrup and lactose | MCT oils‡ | Preterm infants, 22 cal/oz | Protein, 2.6 g/100 cal Phosphorus, 62 mg/100 cal Calcium, 105 mg/100 cal |
| **Enfamil AR** (Mead Johnson) | Nonfat milk; demineralized whey | Lactose, rice starch, maltodextrin | Palm olein, soy, coconut, HOSun oils | Mild gastroesophageal reflux | Iron fortified |
| **Enfamil Lipil** (Mead Johnson) | Whey, nonfat cow's milk | Lactose | Palm olein, soy, coconut, HOSun oils, mortierella alpina oil, crypthecodinum cohnii oil | For full-term infants | Iron fortified; contains docosahexaenoic acid (DHA) and arachidonic acid (ARA), which are important in development of brain and eyes |
| **For Milk Protein—Sensitive Infants ("Milk Allergy"), Lactose Intolerance** | | | | | |
| **Prosobee** (Mead Johnson) | Soy protein isolate | Corn syrup solids | Palm, soy, coconut, HOSun oils | With milk protein allergy, lactose intolerance, lactase deficiency, galactosemia | Hypoallergenic, zero band antigen; lactose- and sucrose-free |
| **Isomil** (Ross) | Soy protein isolate | Corn syrup, sucrose | Soy, coconut oils | With milk protein allergy, lactose intolerance, lactase deficiency, galactosemia | Hypoallergenic; lactose-free |
| **Isomil DF** (Ross) | Soy protein isolate | Hydrolyzed corn starch | Soy, coconut oils | For use during diarrhea in infants >6 mo and toddlers | Lessens amount and duration of watery stools; contains fiber |
| **Lactofree** (Mead Johnson) | Milk protein isolate | Corn syrup solids | Palm olein, soy, HOSun oils | With lactose intolerance, lactase deficiency, galactosemia | Lactose-free |
| **Similac Lactose Free** (Ross) | Milk isolate | Sucrose, glucose oligomers | Soy, coconut oil | With lactose malabsorption | Iron fortified |

*All formulas provide 20 kcal/oz except as noted in product information from the formula manufacturers. For the most current information, consult product labels or package enclosures.
†HOSun, high-oleic sunflower.
‡MCT, medium-chain triglycerides.
Each of the major formula companies (Ross and Mead Johnson) have a variety of formulas in 22 and 24 cal/oz, with high or low iron concentrations intended for use in preterm infants. In addition, major retail companies manufacture their own brands of term infant formulas that comply with the Food and Drug Administration guidelines for infant formula composition.

*Continued*

**TABLE 8-6**　Normal and special infant formulas—cont'd

| Formula (Manufacturer) | Protein Source | Carbohydrate Source | Fat Sources | Indications for Use | Comments (Nutritional Considerations) |
|---|---|---|---|---|---|
| **For Infants with Malabsorption Syndromes, Milk Allergy (Hydrolysate Formulas)** | | | | | |
| **RCF** (Ross Carbohydrate Free) (Ross) | Soy protein isolate | | Soy, coconut oils | With carbohydrate intolerance | Carbohydrate is added according to amount infant will tolerate |
| **Portagen** (Mead Johnson) | Sodium caseinate | Corn syrup solids, sucrose, lactose | MCT (coconut source), corn oil | For impaired fat absorption secondary to pancreatic insufficiency, bile acid deficiency, intestinal resection, lymphatic anomalies | Nutritionally complete |
| **Nutramigen** (Mead Johnson) | Casein hydrolysate, L-amino acids§ | Corn syrup solids, modified corn starch | Corn, soy oils | For infants and children sensitive to food proteins; use in galactosemic patients | Nutritionally complete; hypoallergenic formula; lactose- and sucrose-free |
| **Pregestimil** (Mead Johnson) | Casein hydrolysate, L-amino acids | Corn syrup solids, modified corn starch, dextrose | MCT, soy, HOSun oils | Disaccharidase deficiencies, malabsorption syndromes, cystic fibrosis, intestinal resection | Nutritionally complete; easily digestible protein, carbohydrate, and fat; lactose- and sucrose-free |
| **Alimentum** (Ross) | Casein hydrolysate, L-amino acids | Sucrose, modified tapioca starch | MCT, oleic, soy oils | For infants and children sensitive to food proteins or with cystic fibrosis | Nutritionally complete; hypoallergenic formula; lactose-free |
| **Specialty Formulas** | | | | | |
| **Neocate**‖ | Free amino acids | Corn syrup solids | MCT, safflower oils | For infants sensitive to cow's milk, soy, and hydrolyzed protein formulas | Nutritionally complete; lactose free; high osmolality; low fat |
| **Similac PM 60/40** (Ross) | Whey protein concentrate, sodium caseinate (60:40 ratio) | Lactose | Coconut, corn oils | For newborns predisposed to hypocalcemia and infants with impaired renal, digestive, and cardiovascular functions | Low calcium, potassium, and phosphorus; relatively low solute load; Na = 7 mEq/L; available in powder only |
| **Diet Modifiers** | | | | | |
| **Polycose** (Ross) | | Glucose polymers (corn syrup solids) | | Used to increase calorie intake, as in failure-to-thrive infants | Carbohydrate only; a powdered or liquid calorie supplement; powder, 23 kcal/tbsp |
| **Moducal** (Mead Johnson) | | Hydrolyzed corn starch | | Used to increase carbohydrate intake | Carbohydrate only; a powdered calorie supplement: 30 kcal/tbsp |
| **Casec** (Mead Johnson) | Calcium caseinate | | | Used to increase protein intake | Protein only; negligible fat and no carbohydrate |
| **MCT Oil** (Mead Johnson) | | | 90% MCT (coconut source) | Supplement in fat malabsorption conditions | Fat only; 8.3 kcal/g; 115 kcal/tbsp |

§L-Amino acids include L-cystine, L-tyrosine, and L-tryptophan, which are reduced in hydrolyzed, charcoal-treated casein.
‖Scientific Hospital Supplies, Gaithersburg, MD.

and adding 3 tablespoons of sugar or commercially processed corn syrup.

Evaporated milk must not be confused with condensed milk, which is a form of evaporated milk with 45% more sugar. Because of its high carbohydrate concentration and disproportionately low fat and protein content, condensed milk is not used for infant feeding. Likewise, skim milk and low-fat milk must not be used because they are deficient in caloric concentration, significantly increase the renal solute load and water demands, and deprive the body of essential fatty acids.

Goat's milk is a poor source of iron and folic acid. It has an excessively high renal solute load as a result of its high protein content, making it unsuitable for infant nutrition.

Some parents believe that goat's milk is less allergenic than other available milk sources and may feed it to their infants to reduce allergic milk reactions. However, infants who indeed have a reaction to foreign proteins in cow's milk will likewise react to the foreign proteins in goat's milk (Fomon, 1993). Raw, unpasteurized milk from any animal source is unacceptable for infant nutrition.

### Promote Parent-Infant Bonding (Attachment)

The process of parenting is based on a mutual relationship between parent and infant. As more is learned of the complexity of neonates and of their potential for influencing and shaping their environments, particularly their interaction with significant others, it is apparent that promoting

**TABLE 8-6**   Normal and special infant formulas—cont'd

| Formula (Manufacturer) | Protein Source | Carbohydrate Source | Fat Sources | Indications for Use | Comments (Nutritional Considerations) |
|---|---|---|---|---|---|
| **Diet Modifiers** | | | | | |
| **Similac Natural Care Human Milk Fortifier** (Ross) | Nonfat cow's milk; whey protein concentrate | Hydrolyzed corn starch, lactose | MCT, coconut, soy oils | For low-birth-weight infants; fed mixed with human milk or fed alternately with human milk; improves vitamin/mineral content of human milk | Protein 2.7 g/100 cal osmolality—300 mOsm/kg water, 24 cal/oz; low iron; liquid not intended as sole source of nutrients |
| **Similac Human Milk Fortifier** (Ross) | Whey protein, nonfat dry milk | Corn syrup solids | MCT oil | For breast milk fortification in preterm infants | Fortification in excess of 1 package per 25 ml human milk is not recommended |
| **Enfamil Human Milk Fortifier** (Mead Johnson) | Whey protein concentrate, casein | Corn syrup solids, lactose | Trace | For low-birth-weight infants; fed mixed with human milk; increases protein, calories, calcium, phosphorus, and other nutrients | Used only as human milk fortifier, not as separate formula |
| **For Infants with Phenylketonuria¶** | | | | | |
| **Lofenalac** (Mead Johnson) | Casein hydrolysate, L-amino acids | Corn syrup solids, modified tapioca starch | Corn oil | For infants and children | 111 mg phenylalanine per quart of formula (20 cal/oz); must be supplemented with other foods to provide minimal phenylalanine |
| **Phenyl-free** (Mead Johnson) | L-Amino acids | Sucrose, corn syrup solids, modified tapioca starch | Corn, coconut oils | For children over 1 year of age | Phenylalanine-free; permits increased supplementation with normal foods |
| **Phenex-1** (Ross) | L-Amino acids | Hydrolyzed corn starch | Soy, coconut, palm oils | For infants | Phenylalanine-free; fortified with L-tyrosine, L-glutamine, L-carnitine, taurine; contains vitamins, minerals, trace elements |
| **Phenex-2** (Ross) | L-Amino acids | Hydrolyzed corn starch | Soy, coconut, palm oils | For children and adults | Phenylalanine-free; fortified with L-tyrosine, L-glutamine, L-carnitine, taurine; contains vitamins, minerals, trace elements |
| **Pro-Phree** (Ross) | None | Hydrolyzed corn starch | Soy, coconut, palm oils | For infants and toddlers requiring reduced protein intake | Must be supplemented with protein; has vitamins, minerals, trace elements; fortified with L-carnitine and taurine |

¶Ross Laboratories and Mead Johnson manufacture several specialty formulas for metabolic disorders for infants. For a comprehensive list of metabolic disease formulas the reader should contact either Ross Laboratories or Mead Johnson.

positive parent-child relationships necessitates an understanding of factors involved in identifying behavioral steps in attachment, variables that enhance or hinder this process, and methods of teaching parents ways to develop a stronger relationship with their children, especially by recognizing potential problems (see Assessment of Attachment Behaviors, p. 247).

**Infant Behavior.**   Nurses must appreciate the individuality and uniqueness of each infant. According to the individual temperament, the infant will change and shape the environment, which will undoubtedly influence future development. Obviously, an infant who sleeps 20 hours a day will be exposed to fewer stimuli than one who sleeps 16 hours a day. In turn, each infant will likely elicit a different

response from parents. The infant who is quiet, undemanding, and passive may receive much less attention than the infant who is responsive, alert, and active. Behavioral characteristics such as irritability and consolability can influence the ease of transition to parenthood and the parent's perception of the infant.

Nurses can positively influence the attachment of parent and child. The first step is recognizing individual differences and explaining to parents that such characteristics are normal. For example, some people believe that infants sleep throughout the day, except for feedings. For some newborns this may be true, but for many it is not. Understanding that the infant's wakefulness is part of biologic rhythm and not a reflection of inadequate parenting can be crucial in promoting healthy parent-child relationships. Another aspect of helping parents concerns supplying guidelines on how to enhance the infant's development during awake periods. Placing the child in a crib to stare at the same mobile every day is not exciting, but carrying the infant into each room as one does daily chores can be fascinating. A few suggestions can make life more stimulating for the infant and gratifying for the parents (Box 8-7).

**Maternal Attachment.** Research has suggested that there is a *maternal sensitive period* immediately and for a short time after birth when parents have a unique ability to attach to their infants (Klaus, Kennell, and Klaus, 1995). Mothers demonstrate a predictable and orderly pattern of behavior during the development of the attachment process. When mothers are presented with their nude infants, they begin to examine the infant with their fingertips, concentrating on touching the extremities, and then proceed to massage and encompass the trunk with their entire hands. Assuming the *en face position,* in which the mother's and infant's eyes meet in visual contact in the same vertical plane, is significant in the formation of affectional ties (Fig. 8-19). Although similar patterns of touching have been observed, additional studies demonstrate different patterns for mothers, as well as the same pattern for nonmaternal persons, such as male and female nurses. Consequently, nurses must exercise caution in interpreting behaviors such as touching.

Several studies have attempted to substantiate the long-term benefits of providing parents with opportunities to optimally bond with their infant during the initial postpartum period. Although there has been some evidence that increased parent-child contact encourages prolonged breastfeeding and may minimize the risks of parenting disorders, conclusions about the long-term effects of such early intervention on parenting and child development must be viewed cautiously. In addition, some authorities claim that the emphasis on bonding has been unjustified and may lead to guilt and fear in parents who did not have early contact with their infant. There is also concern over the literal interpretation of "sensitive" or "critical" to imply that without early contact, optimum bonding cannot occur or, conversely, that early contact alone is sufficient to ensure competent parenting.

Certainly, it should be stressed to parents that, although early bonding may be valuable, it does not represent an "all or none" phenomenon. Throughout the child's life there will be multiple opportunities for the development of parent-child attachment. Bonding is a complex process that develops gradually and is influenced by numerous factors, only one of which is the type of initial contact between the newborn and parent.

Another component of successful maternal attachment is the concept of *reciprocity* (Brazelton, 1974). As the mother responds to the infant, the infant must respond to the mother by some signal, such as sucking, cooing, eye contact, grasping, or molding (conforming to other's body during close physical contact). The first step is *initiation,* in which interaction between infant and parent begins. Next is *orientation,* which establishes the partners' expectations of each other during the interaction. Following orientation is *acceleration* of the attention cycle to a peak of excitement. The infant reaches out and coos, both arms jerk forward, the head moves backward, the eyes dilate, and the face brightens. After a short time, *deceleration* of the excitement and *turning away* occur, in which the infant's eyes shift away from mother's and the child grasps his or her own shirt. During this cycle of nonattention, repeated verbal or visual attempts to reinitiate the infant's attention are ineffective. This deceleration and turning away probably prevent the infant from being overwhelmed by excessive stimuli. In a good interaction both partners have synchronized their attention-nonattention cycles. Parents or other caregivers who do not allow the infant to turn away and who continually attempt to maintain visual contact may encourage the infant to turn off the attention cycle and thus prolong the nonattention phase.

Although this description of reciprocal interacting behavior is usually observed in the infant by 2 to 3 weeks of age, nurses can use this information to teach parents how to interact with their infant. Recognizing the attention vs

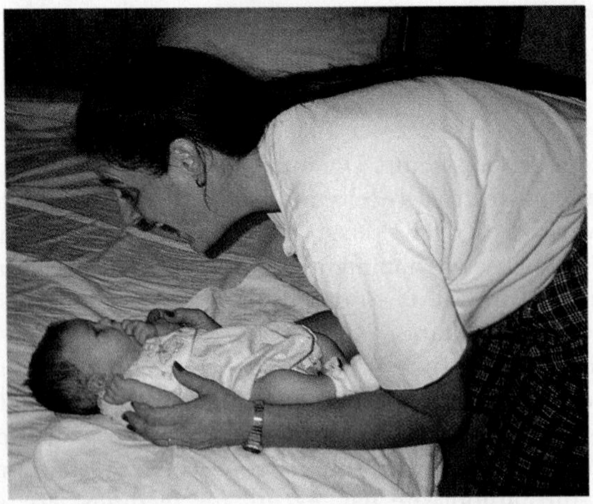

**Fig. 8-19**   En face position between parent and infant can be significant in attachment process.

**Box 8-7**

**How to Make the Infant's World More Exciting***

Infant prefers animated and auditory objects.
Infant enjoys novelty, quickly tires of seeing same objects; mobile should be changed frequently.
Infant prefers to look at medium-intensity colors and contrasting colors, such as black and white.
Infant likes geometric shapes and checkerboards; prefers patterns over straight lines.
Contrasting lights and reflective surfaces such as mirrors are especially interesting.
But most of all, nothing is as fascinating as the human face and voice!

*Objects should be placed about 20 cm (8 inches) away from infant.

nonattention cycles and understanding that the latter is not a rejection of the parent helps parents develop competence in parenting.

**Paternal Engrossment.** Fathers also show specific attachment behaviors to the newborn. This process of *paternal engrossment,* forming a sense of absorption, preoccupation, and interest in the infant, includes (1) visual awareness of the newborn, especially focusing on the beauty of the child; (2) tactile awareness, often expressed in a desire to hold the infant; (3) awareness of distinct characteristics with emphasis on those features of the infant that resemble the father; (4) perception of the infant as perfect; (5) development of a strong feeling of attraction to the child that leads to intense focusing of attention on the infant; (6) experiencing a feeling of extreme elation; and (7) feeling a sense of deep self-esteem and satisfaction. These responses are greatest during the early contacts with the infant and are intensified by the neonate's normal reflex activity, especially the grasp reflex and visual alertness. In addition to behavioral reactions, fathers also demonstrate physiologic responses such as increased heart rate and blood pressure during interactions with their newborns. In one study the attachment scores of inexperienced or first-time fathers were not significantly different from the attachment scores of experienced fathers. The researchers found support for the concept that the love relationship a father develops for a second or subsequent child is as strong and unique as for the first child (Ferketich and Mercer, 1995).

The process of engrossment has significant implications for nurses. It is imperative to recognize the importance of early father-infant contact in performing these behaviors. Fathers need to be encouraged to express their positive feelings, especially if such emotions are contrary to any popular belief that fathers should remain stoic. If this is not clarified, fathers may feel confused and attempt to suppress the natural sensations of absorption, preoccupation, and interest in order to conform with societal expectations.

Mothers also need to be aware of the responses of the father toward the newborn, especially because one of the consequences of paternal preoccupation with the infant is less overt attention toward the mother. If both parents are able to share their feelings, each can appreciate the process of attachment toward their child and will avoid the unfortunate conflict of being insensitive and unaware of the other's needs. In addition, a father who is encouraged to form a relationship with his newborn is less likely to feel excluded and abandoned once the family returns home and the mother directs her attention toward caring for the infant.

Ideally, the process of engrossment should be discussed with parents before the delivery, such as in prenatal classes, to reinforce the father's awareness of his natural feelings toward the expected child. Focusing on the future experience of seeing, touching, and holding one's newborn may also help expectant fathers become more comfortable in accepting their paternal feelings. This in turn can assist them in being more supportive toward the mother, especially as labor and delivery draw near.

At the infant's birth the nurse can play a vital role in helping the father express engrossment by assessing the neonate in front of the couple; pointing out normal characteristics; encouraging identification through consistent referral to the child by name; encouraging the father to cuddle, hold, talk to, or feed the infant; and demonstrating whenever necessary the soothing powers of caressing, stroking, and rocking the child (Fig. 8-20). Fathers are encouraged to be with the mother during labor and delivery, to spend time alone with the mother and newborn after delivery, and to "room in" with the mother and infant.

The nurse watches for the same indications of affection from the father as those expected in the mother, such as visual contact in the en face position and embracing the infant close to the body. When present, such behaviors are reinforced. If such responses are not obvious, the nurse needs to assess the father's feelings regarding this birth, cultural beliefs that may prevent his expression of emotions, and other factors in order to help him facilitate a positive attachment during this critical period.

**Siblings.** Although the attachment process has been discussed almost exclusively in terms of the parents and infants, it is essential that nurses be aware of other family members, such as siblings; grandparents, and members of the extended family, who need preparation for the acceptance of this new child. Young children in particular need sensitive preparation for the birth to minimize sibling jealousy.

In support of *family-centered care,* there is an increasing trend to allow siblings to visit the mother on the postpartum unit and to hold the newborn (Fig. 8-21). Another trend has been the presence of siblings at childbirth. Unlike sibling visitation, the evidence supporting this practice has been controversial, yet the nature of truly providing family-centered care encompasses siblings, grandparents, and other significant persons form the extended family unit (Tomlinson, Bryan, and Esau, 1996). The American Academy of Pediatrics (2000b) supports the presence of siblings at childbirth and visitation of the newborn and mother; basic guidelines for infection control and adult supervision are also recommended.

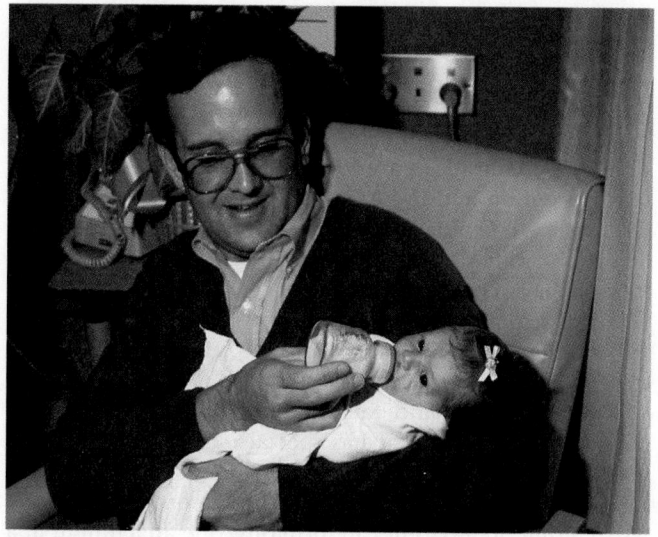

**Fig. 8-20**  Desire to hold the infant and participate in caregiving activities is an indication of paternal engrossment.

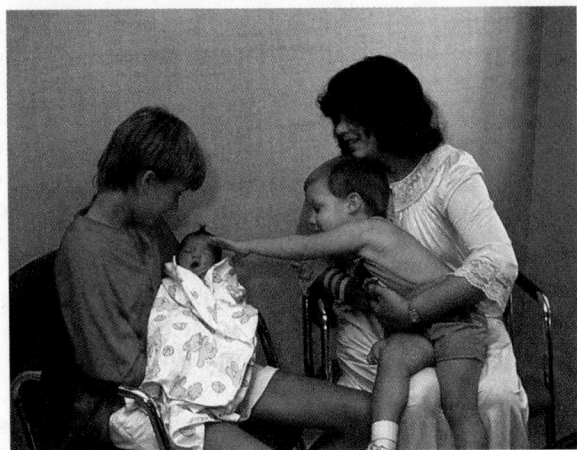

**Fig. 8-21** Sibling visitation shortly after birth can be significant in the attachment process.

Children exhibit different degrees of involvement in the birth process. Young children often fall asleep toward the end of delivery. Some reported benefits include children's increased knowledge of the birth process, less regressive behavior following the birth, and more mothering and caregiving behavior toward the infant. Some practitioners add facilitated family bonding and assimilation of the newborn into the family as positive outcomes. Parents whose children attended the birth have echoed these same benefits and have expressed their desire to repeat the experience should another pregnancy occur. Despite these positive findings, opponents believe that allowing children to observe a delivery could lead to emotional difficulties, although there is no research to support this contention. As research mounts, birthing centers that allow siblings at the birth are developing more definitive guidelines, such as an age requirement of at least 4 to 5 years, the presence of a supportive person for the sibling only, and an adequate sequence of preparation in which parents explore all options for preparing their other children.

From observations during sibling visitation, there is evidence that sibling attachment occurs. However, the en face position is assumed much less often among the newborn and siblings than between mother and newborn, and when this position is used, it is brief. Siblings focus more on the head or face than on touching or talking to the infant. The siblings' verbalizations are focused less on attracting the infant's attention and more on addressing the mother about the newborn. Children who have established a prenatal relationship with the fetus have demonstrated more attachment behaviors, supporting the suggestion of encouraging prenatal acquaintance. Additional research is needed to establish theories on sibling bonding as have been constructed for parental bonding.

**Multiple Births and Subsequent Children.** A component of attachment that has special meaning for families with multiple births, *monotropy* refers to the principle that a person can become optimally attached to only one individual at a time. If a parent can form only one attachment at a time, how can all the siblings of a multiple birth receive optimum emotional care?

There is very little research on bonding and multiple births, and even less is known about paternal engrossment and sibling attachment. In regard to maternal-twin bonding, the conclusions of different authors vary. Some report that mothers bond equally to each twin at the time of birth, even if one twin is ill. Others suggest that mothers of twins may take months or even years to form individual attachments and even longer if the twins are identical.

Nurses can be instrumental in promoting bonding at multiple births. The most important principle is to assist the parents in recognizing the individuality of the children, especially in monozygotic (identical) twins. The mother should visit with each newborn, including a sick infant, as much as possible after birth. Rooming-in and breast-feeding are encouraged. Any characteristics that are unique to each child are emphasized, and each infant is called by name, rather than calling them "the twins." Asking the family questions such as "How do you tell Sally and Amy apart?" and "In what ways are Sally and Amy different and similar?" helps point out their individual characteristics. Behaviors on the BNBAS can be used to illustrate these differences and to stress effective strategies for dealing with multiple personalities at the same time. Co-bedding of twins or other multiples may also be encouraged in the hospital and home to maintain the bond between siblings that was formed in utero (Della Porta, Aforismo, and Butler-O'Hara, 1998). (Other strategies for promoting individualism are discussed under Multiple Births in Chapter 3.)

Another area of attachment that has received minimal attention is maternal bonding of multiparous mothers. Research suggests that there are several additional tasks to "taking on" a second child. These include:

- Promoting acceptance and approval of the second child
- Grieving and resolving the loss of an exclusive dyadic relationship with the first child
- Planning and coordinating family life to include a second child
- Reformulating a relationship with the first child
- Identifying with the second child by comparing this child with the first child in terms of physical and psychologic characteristics
- Assessing one's affective capabilities in providing sufficient emotional support and nurturance simultaneously to two children

Employed mothers who have a second child report fewer concerns regarding general aspects of separation from their child and the effect of separation on the child, but they have similar concerns regarding separation because of employment as they had with the first child. It appears that although experience may decrease some concerns, it may not minimize others.

## Prepare for Discharge and Home Care

With increasingly shorter postpartum stays, as well as a trend toward *mother-infant care,* also called *dyad* or *couplet care,* discharge planning, referral, and home visiting have become important components of comprehensive newborn care. First-time, as well as "experienced," parents benefit from guidance and assistance with the infant's care, such as breast- or bottle-feeding, and with the family's integration of a new member, particularly sibling adjustment.

To assess and meet these needs, teaching must begin early, ideally *before the birth.* Not only is the postpartum stay

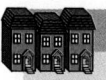

**COMMUNITY FOCUS**
*Early Newborn Discharge Checklist*

Feeding—Adequate latch-on demonstrated for breast-feeding newborn; successfully feeding 2 to 3 ounces of formula every 3 to 4 hours with minimal spitting up and absence of vomiting; wet diapers indicate adequate hydration and intake

Elimination—Voiding every 4 to 6 hours or more often; stool—one stool passed in first 24-28 hours

Circumcision—Evidence of voiding; nonbleeding circumcision (does not require pressure)

Color—Pink centrally and buccal mucosa moist; no evidence of jaundice in first 24 hours

Cord—Triple dye or other antibacterial, drying agent applied per institution protocol (see Care of the Umbilicus, p. 269)

Newborn screening—Completed PKU and others per state law

Vital signs—Stable heart rate, respiratory rate, and temperature for at least 8 to 12 hours; no apnea

Activity—Wakeful periods before feedings; moves all extremities

Home visit or primary practitioner visit—Appointment made within 2 to 3 days after discharge

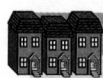

**COMMUNITY FOCUS**
*Newborn Home Care Following Early Discharge**

Wet diapers—3 to 4 per day in first 10-14 days, then 6 to 10 per day

Breast-feeding—Successful latch-on and feeding every 1½ to 3 hours daily

Formula feeding—Successfully, voiding as above, taking 2 to 3 ounces every 3 to 4 hours

Circumcision—Wash with warm water only; yellow exudate forming, nonbleeding, Plastibell intact 48 hours

Stools—At least one soft stool every 48-72 hours (bottle-feeding), or two to three per day (breast-feeding)

Color—Pink to ruddy when crying; pink centrally when at rest or asleep

Activity—Has four to five wakeful periods per day and alerts to environmental sounds and voices

Jaundice—Physiologic jaundice (not appearing in first 24 hours), feeding, voiding, and stooling as noted above *or* practitioner notification for suspicion of pathologic jaundice (appears within 24 hours of birth, ABO/Rh problem suspected), decreased activity, poor feeding, dark orange skin color persisting > fifth day in light-skinned newborn

Cord—Kept above diaper line; nonodorous; drying

Vital signs—Heart rate 120 to 140 beats/min at rest; respiratory rate 30 to 55 at rest without evidence of sternal retractions, grunting, or nasal flaring; temperature 36.3° to 37° C (97.3° to 98.6° F) axillary

Position of sleep—Back

———
*Any deviation from the above or suspicion of poor newborn adaptation should be reported to the practitioner at once.

short (12 to 24 hours) but mothers are also in the *taking-in phase*, where they demonstrate passive and dependent behaviors. Therefore, on the first postpartum day, women may not be able to absorb large amounts of information. This time may need to be spent highlighting essential aspects of care, such as infant safety and feeding. Parents may also be given a list of mother and infant care topics as part of the nursing admission history to choose issues they wish to review. Concerns before discharge should focus on newborn feeding patterns, stool cycles, jaundice, and excessive crying.

Since the institution of early postpartum discharge for the mother and infant in 1992, there has been concern among health care workers that this group of patients is not receiving adequate care, and that infant morbidities will increase significantly. Although legislation has been enacted guaranteeing most mothers a minimum of 48 hours' hospitalization, studies indicate that many mothers are leaving the hospital as early as 8 to 12 hours after vaginal delivery. The American Academy of Pediatrics (1995) has established guidelines for early postpartum discharge; these include minimum discharge criteria such as single birth, uncomplicated vaginal delivery, no evidence of jaundice within the first 24 hours, and maintenance of adequate thermoregulation without external heat source. The Academy emphasizes that the primary care physician rather than an insurance company should make the determination of appropriate discharge time. Because it is obvious that the trend for early postpartum discharge will not be reversed, health care workers must continue to work within the confines of available resources and time to maintain adequate quality of care for mothers and infants.

Many concerns have been expressed regarding early discharge and newborn rehospitalizations for dehydration, jaundice, breast-feeding failure, congenital heart disease, and certain congenital metabolic diseases such as PKU. Studies in various parts of the United States continue to show, however, that rehospitalizations, emergency room visits, and

infant morbidities have not significantly increased in the last several years (Kotagal and others, 1999; Gries, Phyall, and Barfield, 2000; Danielson and others, 2000). One study (Malkin and others, 2000) indicated that infants discharged early (less than 30 hours) were more likely to die of infections and heart problems than infants discharged later, yet this has not been well substantiated in larger studies.

To better meet the needs of mothers being discharged soon after delivery, many institutions have implemented programs to provide early follow-up postpartum care at no additional cost to the mother (Brown and Johnson, 1998; Lieu and others, 2000; Locklin and Jansson, 1999). (See Community Focus boxes.)

Although many mothers and newborns may be safely discharged within 12 to 24 hours without detriment to their health, others may require a longer stay (Weekly and Neumann, 1997). Follow-up home care within days (or even hours after discharge when minor problems are anticipated) appears to be the emerging trend in an effort to curtail hospital costs and provide adequate maternal-newborn care with minimal complications. Despite the changing spectrum of well-newborn health care, the nurse's role continues to be that of providing ongoing assessments of each mother-newborn dyad to ensure a safe transition to home and a successful adaptation into the family unit (Weekly and Neumann, 1997). (See Evidence-Based Practice box on p. 311.)

With family structures changing, it is essential that nurses identify the primary caregiver, which may not always be the mother but may be a father, grandparent, or baby-sitter. Depending on the family composition, the mother's primary support system in the care of the newborn may not always be the traditional husband or male companion.

Nurses should not assume that terminology associated with mother-infant care is understood. Words relating to the anatomy (e.g., "meconium," "labia," "edema," and "genitalia") and to breast-feeding (e.g., "areola," "colostrum," and "let-down reflex") may be unfamiliar to mothers. Mothers with other children do not necessarily understand more words, and young age and less education decrease comprehension.

An essential area of discharge counseling is the safe transport of the newborn home from the hospital. Ideally this information should be provided *before* delivery to allow parents an opportunity to purchase a suitable infant car safety seat restraint. An emerging trend is to hold the birthing center or hospital liable for any harm incurred as result of discharging a newborn without ensuring that the child is safely secured in an appropriate car safety seat restraint.

When purchasing a car safety seat restraint, parents should consider cost and convenience. The convertible-type seats are more expensive initially but cost less than two separate systems. Convenience is a major factor, because a cumbersome restraint may be used less and improperly. Before buying a car safety seat restraint, it is best to try out different models. For example, some types are too large for subcompact cars. Asking friends about the advantages and disadvantages of their restraints is helpful, but borrowing their car seat or purchasing a used one can be dangerous. Parents should use only a restraint that has directions for use and a certification label stating that it complies with federal motor vehicle safety standards (both should be on the seat). They should not use a restraint that has been involved in a crash. Some service clubs and hospitals have loan programs for restraints. Information about approved models and other aspects of car safety seat restrains is available from several organizations and sources.*

Parents are cautioned against placing an infant in the front seat of a car with a passenger-side air bag. Infants weighing less than 9.07 kg (20 pounds) or younger than 1 year should always be placed in a rear-facing child safety seat in the back seat of the car (Centers for Disease Control and Prevention, 1997).

In the United States and Canada, all states and provinces have mandated the use of child restraints. Therefore hospitals and birthing centers should have policies regarding the safe discharge of a newborn in a car safety seat and provisions for parents to learn to use the device correctly. Parents are more likely to use a restraint correctly and consistently if the proper use of one is demonstrated and its necessity is stressed.

Although federal safety standards do not specify the *minimum* weight of an infant and the appropriate type of restraint, newborns weighing 2 kg (4 pounds 8 ounces) receive relatively good support in convertible seats with a seat back-to-crotch strap height of 14 cm (5½ inches) or less. Rolled blankets and towels may be needed between the crotch and legs to prevent slouching and can be placed along the sides to minimize lateral movements. Seats with shields (large padded surfaces in front of the child) and armrests (found on some other models) are unacceptable because of their proximity to the infant's face and neck. (For a discussion of appropriate car restraints for preterm infants, see p. 369, and for infants, see Motor Vehicle Injuries in Chapters 12 and 14.)

> **NURSING ALERT**
> Padding is **never** placed underneath or behind the infant because it creates slack in the harness, leading to the possibility of the child's ejection from the seat in the event of a crash. In vehicles with front passenger-side air bags, the rear-facing safety seat must be placed in the back seat to avoid injury to the infant from the released air bag forcing the safety seat against the vehicle seat or passenger door.

The use of an appropriate car safety seat restraint is also encouraged to prevent injuries to children riding in airplanes. The Federal Aviation Administration recommends that children less than 4 years old ride in an approved safety restraint seat to prevent harm during turbulent weather, landing, and takeoff (American Academy of Pediatrics, 2002b).

## ❖ Evaluation

The effectiveness of nursing interventions is determined by continual reassessment and evaluation of care based on the following observational guidelines:

1. Observe infant's color and respiratory patterns.
2. Monitor axillary temperature regularly; observe for signs of temperature instability such as respiratory distress.
3. Observe for any evidence of infection, especially at the umbilicus or site of circumcision; check identification bands; check medical record for documentation of prophylactic eye treatment, vitamin K injection, HBV vaccine, and metabolic screening tests.
4. Monitor daily weight.
5. Observe interactions between infant and family members; interview family regarding their feelings about the newborn.
6. Observe parents' ability to provide care for infant; interview parents regarding any concerns about infant's care at home.
7. Observe parents' correct use of car safety seat restraint on discharge.

The *expected outcomes* are described in the Nursing Care Plan on pp. 289-291.

---

*__American Academy of Pediarics,__ 141 Northwest Point Blvd, Elk Grove Village, IL 60007, (888) 227-1770, fax: (847) 228-1281; www.aap.org/family/carseatguide.htm; and local division of traffic safety or __National Highway Traffic Safety Administration Auto Safety Hotline,__ (800) 424-9393. For children with special needs, contact the National Easter Seal Society, (800) 221-6827, and ask about Special KARS (Kids Are Riding Safe). Guidelines for car seat safety are available in Wong DL, Hess CS: *Wong and Whaley's clinical manual of pediatric nursing,* ed 5, St Louis, 2000, Mosby.

# Nursing Care Plan
## The Normal Newborn and Family

---

**NURSING DIAGNOSIS:** Ineffective airway clearance related to excess mucus, improper positioning

**PATIENT GOAL 1:** Will maintain a patent airway
- **Nursing Interventions/Rationales**

Suction mouth and nasopharynx with bulb syringe as needed
    Compress bulb before insertion and aspirate pharynx, then nose, *to prevent aspiration of fluid*
With mechanical suction, limit each suctioning attempt to 5 seconds, with sufficient time between attempts *to allow reoxygenation*
Position infant on right side after feeding *to prevent aspiration*
Position infant on back during sleep *to decrease risk of sudden infant death syndrome*
Perform as few procedures as possible on infant during first hour and have oxygen ready for use if respiratory distress should develop
Take vital signs according to institutional policy and more frequently if necessary
    Observe for signs of respiratory distress and report any of the following immediately:
    Apnea
    Tachypnea
    Grunting, stridor
    Abnormal breath sounds
    Flaring alae nasi
    Cyanosis or pallor
    Retractions
Keep diapers, clothing, and blankets loose enough *to allow maximum lung (abdominal) expansion and to avoid overheating*
Clean nares of any secretions during bath or when necessary
Check for patent nares

- **EXPECTED OUTCOMES**

Airway remains patent
Breathing is regular and unlabored
Respiratory rate is within normal limits (see inside back cover for normal limits)

---

**NURSING DIAGNOSIS:** Risk for imbalanced body temperature related to immature temperature control, change in environmental temperature

---

**PATIENT GOAL 1:** Will maintain stable body temperature
- **NURSING INTERVENTIONS/RATIONALES**

Dry thoroughly and remove wet linen immediately following birth
Wrap infant snugly in a warmed blanket
Place infant in a preheated environment (under radiant warmer or next to mother, skin-to-skin contact)
Place infant on a padded, covered surface
Take infant's temperature on arrival at nursery or mother's room; proceed according to hospital policy regarding method and frequency of monitoring
Maintain room temperature between 24° and 25.5° C (75° to 78° F) and humidity about 40% to 50%
Give initial bath according to hospital policy
    Prevent chilling of infant during bath

Postpone bath if there is any question regarding stabilization of body temperature
Dress infant in a shirt and diaper and swaddle in a blanket or cover with blanket
Provide infant with a head covering if heat loss is a problem, *because large surface area of head favors heat loss*
Keep infant away from drafts, air conditioning vents, or fans
Place infant in a recessed cubicle with walls high enough to *shield from cross-ventilation*
Warm all objects used to examine or cover infant (e.g., place them under radiant warmer)
Uncover only one area of body for examination or procedures
Postpone circumcision until after temperature stabilizes, or use radiant warmer during procedure
Be alert to signs of hypothermia or hyperthermia

- **EXPECTED OUTCOME**

Infant's temperature remains at optimum level (36.5° to 37.5° C [97.7° to 99.5° F])

---

**NURSING DIAGNOSIS:** Risk for infection or inflammation related to deficient immunologic defenses, environmental factors, maternal disease

---

**PATIENT GOAL 1:** Will exhibit no evidence of infection

- **NURSING INTERVENTIONS/RATIONALES**

Wash hands before and after caring for each infant
Wear gloves when in contact with body secretions
Use of cover gowns is controversial *because studies show they do not decrease infection rates but do increase costs*
Make certain appropriate eye prophylaxis has been carried out
Check eyes daily for evidence of inflammation or discharge
Keep infant from potential sources of infection (e.g., persons with respiratory or skin infections, improperly prepared food sources, other unclean items)
Clean vulva in posterior direction *to prevent fecal contamination of vagina or urethra;* stress this to parents
While cleaning penis, do not retract foreskin; gently wipe away smegma
Maintain asepsis during circumcision
*If infant has been circumcised, cover area with a petrolatum jelly gauze dressing (except when Plastibell is used) *to prevent adherence to diaper*
Check for voiding and bleeding after circumcision; disposable diaper may feel dry when wet, but crotch area will feel "clumpy" or "doughy" and heavy
Keep umbilical stump clean and dry
Place diapers below umbilical stump
Assess cord daily for odor, color, and drainage
*Apply antibacterial agent and/or alcohol to cord as appropriate
*Administer hepatitis B vaccine (HBV) in vastus lateralis muscle as status warrants
Avoid artificial fingernails, nail covers

- **EXPECTED OUTCOMES**

Infant exhibits no evidence of infection or inflammation
Eyes remain clear with no evidence of irritation
Genital area is free of irritation
Cord appears dry, surrounding area free of infection
Infant receives HBV vaccine

---

*Dependent nursing action.

*Continued*

# Nursing Care Plan
## The Normal Newborn and Family—cont'd

**NURSING DIAGNOSIS:** Risk for trauma related to physical helplessness

**PATIENT GOAL 1:** Will be clearly and correctly identified

- **NURSING INTERVENTIONS/***RATIONALES*

Make certain infant is properly identified *for placement with correct mother*

    Ensure that identification (ID) band(s) are properly and securely placed

    Check infant's ID band often *to ensure correct infant identity*

Discuss safety issues with parents, especially mother, *to prevent possible abduction*

Observe staff's ID badge and give infant only to properly identified personnel

Never leave infant alone

- **EXPECTED OUTCOMES**

Infant is clearly and correctly identified at all times

Parents observe safety practices

ID bands remain in place

**PATIENT GOAL 2:** Will have no physical injury

- **NURSING INTERVENTIONS/***RATIONALES*

Avoid using rectal thermometer *because of risk of rectal perforation*

Never leave infant unsupervised on a raised surface without sides *to prevent falls*

Always close diaper pins (if used) and place them away from infant's body

Keep pointed or sharp objects away from infant

Keep own fingernails short and trimmed; avoid jewelry that can scratch infant

Use appropriate methods of handling and transporting infant

- **EXPECTED OUTCOME**

Infant remains free of physical injury

**PATIENT GOAL 3:** Will exhibit no evidence of bleeding

- **NURSING INTERVENTIONS/***RATIONALES*

*Administer vitamin K intramuscularly, in vastus lateralis muscle

Check circumcision site; assess for any oozing *that may indicate bleeding tendencies*

- **EXPECTED OUTCOME**

Infant exhibits no evidence of bleeding

**NURSING DIAGNOSIS:** Imbalanced nutrition: less than body requirements (risk) related to immaturity, parental knowledge deficit

**PATIENT GOAL 1:** Will receive optimum nutrition

- **NURSING INTERVENTIONS/***RATIONALES*

Assess strength of suck and coordination with swallowing *to identify possible problem affecting feeding*

Offer initial intake according to parent's preference, hospital policy, and practitioner's protocol

Prepare for demand feeding of breast-fed infants; night feedings determined by condition and preferences of mother

Offer bottle-fed infants 1 to 2 ounces of formula every 3 to 4 hours or on demand (intake will vary with age)

Support and assist breast-feeding mothers during initial feedings and more frequently if necessary

Avoid routine water or supplemental feedings for breast-feeding infants because they may *decrease the desire to suck and cause nipple preference*

Encourage father or other support person to remain with mother to help her and infant with positioning, relaxation, and reinforcement

Encourage father or other support person to participate in bottle-feeding

Place infant on right side after feeding *to prevent aspiration* (place infant supine for sleep)

Observe stool pattern

- **EXPECTED OUTCOMES**

Infant demonstrates strong suck

Infant retains feedings

Infant receives an adequate amount of nutrients (specify amount and frequency of feedings)

Infant loses less than 10% of birth weight; regains birth-weight by 10 to 14 days of age

**NURSING DIAGNOSIS:** Interrupted family processes related to maturational crisis, birth of term infant, change in family unit

**PATIENT (FAMILY) GOAL 1:** Will exhibit parent-infant attachment behaviors

- **NURSING INTERVENTIONS/***RATIONALES*

As soon after delivery as possible, encourage parents to see and hold infant; place newborn close to face of parents *to establish visual contact*

Ideally, perform eye care after initial meeting of infant and parents, within 1 hour after birth *when infant is alert and most likely to visually relate to parent*

Identify for parents specific behaviors manifested by infant (e.g., alertness, ability to see, vigorous suck, rooting behavior, and attention to human voice)

Discuss with parents their expectations of fantasy child vs real child if indicated

Encourage parents to "talk out" their labor and delivery experience; identify any events that signify loss of control to either parent, especially mother

Identify behavioral steps in attachment process, and evaluate those aspects that could be considered positive and those that may represent inadequate or delayed parenting

Encourage family to room-in or to call for infant frequently if not rooming-in

Observe and assess reciprocity of cues between infant and parent *to identify behaviors that may need strengthening*

Assist parents in recognizing attention-nonattention cycles and in understanding their significance

*Dependent nursing action.

# Nursing Care Plan
## The Normal Newborn and Family—cont'd

### PATIENT (FAMILY) GOAL 1:—cont'd

• **NURSING INTERVENTIONS/***RATIONALES***—cont'd**

Assess variables affecting development of attachment through observing infant and parent and interviewing each parent or other significant caregiver

• **EXPECTED OUTCOMES**

Parents establish contact with infant immediately or soon after birth

Parents demonstrate attachment behaviors, such as touch, eye contact, naming and calling infant by name, talking to infant, participating in caregiving activities

Parents recognize attention-nonattention cycles

### PATIENT (SIBLING) GOAL 2: Will demonstrate adjustment and attachment behaviors toward newborn

• **NURSING INTERVENTIONS/***RATIONALES***

Allow to visit and touch newborn when feasible

Explain physical features of newborn, such as bald head, umbilical stump and clamp, circumcision, *to lessen any fear siblings might have*

Explain to siblings realistic expectations regarding newborn's abilities and needs
  Requires complete care
  Is not a playmate

Encourage siblings to participate in care at home *to make them feel part of the experience*

Encourage parents to spend individual time with other children at home *to reduce feelings of jealousy toward new sibling*

• **EXPECTED OUTCOME**

Siblings express interest in newborn and realistic expectations for their age

### PATIENT (FAMILY) GOAL 3: Will be prepared for discharge and home care

• **NURSING INTERVENTIONS/***RATIONALES***

Discuss with parents correct preparation of formula
  Stress that proportions must not be altered to dilute or concentrate the formula
  Discourage microwaving of bottles *to avoid burns*

Encourage use of support persons, such as lactation specialist or members of La Leche League, for assistance with breast-feeding

Instruct in other aspects of newborn care
  Bathing
  Umbilical cord and circumcision care
  Recognize states of activity for optimum interaction (see Table 8-3)

Encourage participation in parenting classes, if offered

Discuss importance and proper use of federally approved car seat restraints
  If infant is small, advise parents to use rolled blankets and towels in crotch area to *prevent slouch and along sides to minimize lateral movement*, but never use padding underneath or behind infant *because it creates slack in harness, leading to possible ejection from seat in a crash*
  Refer to organizations that may rent car seat restraints

If parent-infant attachment is at risk, refer to appropriate agencies (social services, family and child services, at-risk programs)

• **EXPECTED OUTCOMES**

Family demonstrates ability to provide care for infant

Family keeps appointments for follow-up care

Infant rides home in federally approved car seat restraint

Family members avail themselves of needed services

---

# KEY POINTS

- Transition from fetal or placental circulation to independent respiration is the most important physiologic change required of the newborn.

- Chemical and thermal factors help initiate the neonate's first breaths.

- Circulatory changes in the neonate result from shifts in pressure in the heart and major vessels and from functional closures of the fetal shunts.

- The newborn's large surface area, thin layer of subcutaneous fat, and unique mechanism for producing heat predispose the newborn to excessive heat loss.

- The infant's high rate of metabolism is closely correlated with the rate of fluid exchange, which is seven times greater in the infant than in the adult.

- The skin and mucous membranes, the reticuloendothelial system, and antibodies are the first, second, and third lines of defense against infection.

- Apgar scoring, the initial assessment of the newborn, focuses on heart rate, respiratory effort, muscle tone, reflex irritability, and color.

- Physical assessment of the newborn includes clinical assessment of gestational age, general measurements, general appearance, head-to-toe assessment, and parent-infant attachment or bonding.

- Neurologic assessment focuses on reflexes and posture, muscle tone, head control, and movement and is best accomplished during the general physical examination.

- Behavioral assessment of newborns with the Brazelton Neonatal Behavioral Assessment Scale examines responses to seven categories: habituation, orientation, motor performance, range of state, regulation of state, autonomic regulation, and reflexes.

- An instrument for assessing the reciprocal interchange between parent and infant is the NCAST Feeding Scale.

- Physical care for the newborn includes maintaining a patent airway, maintaining a stable body temperature, protecting from infection and injury, and providing optimal nutrition.
- Although the attachment, or bonding, process primarily affects infants and parents, siblings and other family members also play an important role.

- With short postpartum stays teaching should begin before birth and continue after discharge with telephone and/or home follow-up.
- An essential aspect of discharge teaching is ensuring the newborn's safe transportation home in a federally approved, backward-facing car safety seat restraint.

# REFERENCES

Akers SM, Groh-Wargo SL: Normal nutrition during infancy. In Samour PQ, Helm KK, Lang CE, editors: *Family handbook of pediatric nutrition*, ed 2, Gaithersburg, MD, 1999, Aspen.

Alexander M, Kuo KN: Musculoskeletal assessment of the newborn, *Orthop Nurs* 16(1):21-31, 1997.

Allen KD, White DD, Walburn JN: Sucrose as an analgesic agent for infants during immunization injections, *Arch Pediatr Adolesc Med* 150(3):270-274, 1996.

American Academy of Pediatrics: Car safety seats: a guide for families—2002, *www.aap.org/family/carseatguide.htm,* 2002b.

American Academy of Pediatrics: Changing concepts of sudden infant death syndrome: implications for infant sleeping environment and sleep position, *Pediatrics* 105(3):650-656, 2000a.

American Academy of Pediatrics, Committee on Bioethics: Female genital mutilation, *Pediatrics* 102(1):153-156, 1998.

American Academy of Pediatrics, Committee on Environmental Health: Technical report: mercury in the environment: implications for pediatricians, *Pediatrics* 108(1):197-205, 2001.

American Academy of Pediatrics, Committee on Fetus and Newborn: Hospital stay for healthy term newborns, *Pediatrics* 96(4):788-790, 1995.

American Academy of Pediatrics, Committee on Fetus and Newborn: Routine evaluation of blood pressure, hematocrit, and glucose in newborns, *Pediatrics* 92(3):474-476, 1993.

American Academy of Pediatrics, Committee on Fetus and Newborn, and American College of Obstetricians and Gynecologists, Committee on Obstetric Practice: Use and abuse of the Apgar Score, *Pediatrics* 98(1):141-142, 1996.

American Academy of Pediatrics, Committee on Infectious Diseases: Recommended childhood immunization schedule—United States, 2002, *Pediatrics* 109(1):162-163, 2002a.

American Academy of Pediatrics, Committee on Infectious Diseases, Pickering L, editor: *2000 Red book report of the Committee on Infectious Diseases*, ed 25, Elk Grove Village, IL, 2000b, The Academy.

American Academy of Pediatrics, Committee on Nutrition: *Pediatric nutrition handbook*, Elk Grove Village, IL, 1998b, The Academy.

American Academy of Pediatrics, Committee on Nutrition: Soy-protein–based formulas: recommendations for infant feedings, *Pediatrics* 101(1):148-153, 1998a.

American Academy of Pediatrics and American College of Obstetricians and Gynecologists: *Guidelines for perinatal care*, ed 4, Elk Grove Village, IL, 1997, The Academy.

American Academy of Pediatrics: Serving the family from birth to the medical home: newborn screening: a blueprint for the future, *Pediatrics* 106(2 pt. 2):389-427, suppl, 2000c.

American Academy of Pediatrics, Task Force on Circumcision: Circumcision policy statement, *Pediatrics* 103(3):686-693, 1999.

American Academy of Pediatrics: Year 2000 position statement: principles and guidelines for early hearing detection and intervention programs, *Pediatrics* 106(4):798-824, 2000d.

American Academy of Pediatrics, Vitamin K Ad Hoc Task Force: Controversies concerning vitamin K and the newborn, *Pediatrics* 91(5):1001-1003, 1993.

Anderson JW, Johnstone BM, Remley DT: Breastfeeding and cognitive development: a meta-analysis, *Am J Clin Nutr* 70(4):525-535, 1999.

Arora S and others: Major factors influencing breastfeeding rates: mother's perception of father's attitude and milk supply, *Pediatrics* 106(5):e67, 2000.

Axton SE and others: Comparison of brachial and calf blood pressures in infants, *Pediatr Nurs* 21(4):323-326, 1995.

Ball TM, Wright AL: Health care costs of formula-feeding in the first year of life, *Pediatrics* 103(suppl 4):S870-S876, 1999.

Ballard JL, Novak KK, Driver M: A simplified score for assessment of fetal maturation of newly born infants. *J Pediatr* 95(5):769-774, 1979.

Ballard JL and others: New Ballard Score expanded to include extremely premature infants, *J Pediatr* 119:417-423, 1991.

Barnard K: *NCAST feeding manual*, Seattle, WA, 1994, University of Washington.

Bartman T: Newborn circumcision and urinary tract infections (letter), *Pediatrics* 107(1):210-214, 2001.

Beaudry M, Dufour R, Marcoux S: Relation between infant feeding and infections during the first six months of life, *J Pediatr* 126(2):191-197, 1995.

Becks VE, Lorenzoni NM: *Pseudomonas aeruginosa* outbreak in a neonatal intensive care unit: a possible link to contaminated hand lotion, *Am J Infect Control* 23(6):396-398, 1995.

Benini F and others: Topical anesthesia during circumcision in newborn infants, *JAMA* 270(7):850-853, 1993.

Biancuzzo M: *Breastfeeding the newborn: clinical strategies for nurses*, St Louis, 1999, Mosby.

Bishai R and others: Relative efficacy of amethocaine gel and lidocaine-prilocaine cream for port-a-cath puncture in children, *Pediatrics* 104(3):e31, 1999.

Blackburn ST, Loper DL: *Maternal, fetal, and neonatal physiology: a clinical perspective*, Philadelphia, 1992, WB Saunders.

Blain-Lewis N: Comparative studies of bruising and healing after heelstick, *Neonat Intensive Care* 5(5):18-21, 1992.

Blass EM, Hoffmeyer LB: Sucrose as an analgesic for newborn infants, *Pediatrics* 87(2):215-218, 1991.

Blass EM, Watt LB: Suckling- and sucrose-induced analgesia in human newborns, *Pain* 83(3):611-623, 1999.

Bliss-Holtz J: Determination of thermoregulatory state in full-term infants, *Nurs Res* 42(1):204-207, 1993.

Bliss-Holtz J: Methods of newborn infant temperature monitoring: a research review, *Issues Compr Pediatr Nurs* 18(4):287-298, 1995.

Brazelton TB: Mother-infant reciprocity. In Klaus M and others, editors: *Maternal attachment and mothering disorders*, New Brunswick, NJ, 1974, Johnson & Johnson Baby Products.

Brazelton TB, Nugent JK: *Neonatal behavioral assessment scale*, London, 1996, MacKeith Press.

Broussard ER: Neonatal prediction and outcome at 10/11 years, *Child Psychiatr Hum Dev* 7(2):85-93, 1976.

Broussard ER: Assessment of the adaptive potential of the mother-infant system: the Neonatal Perception Inventories, *Semin Perinatol* 3(1):91-100, 1979.

Broussard ER: The Pittsburgh firstborns at age nineteen years. In Call J, Calerson E, Tyson R, editors: *Frontiers of infant psychiatry*, vol 2, New York, 1984, Basic Books.

Brown SG, Johnson BT: Enhancing early discharge with home follow-up: a pilot project, *J Obstet Gynecol Neonat Nurs* 27(1):33-38, 1998.

Butte NF and others: Infant feeding mode affects early growth and body composition, *Pediatrics* 106(6):1355-1366, 2000.

Carroll V: Infant abduction: lowering the risk, *AWHONN Lifelines* 3(6):25-27, 2000.

Centers for Disease Control and Prevention: Update: fatal air bag-related injuries to children—United States, 1993-1996, *JAMA* 277(1):11-12, 1997.

Christie L: Food hypersensitivities. In Samour PQ, Helm KK, Lang CE, editors: *Handbook of pediatric nutrition,* ed 2, Gaithersburg, MD, 1999, Aspen.

Cohen HA and others: Postcircumcision urinary tract infection, *Clin Pediatr* 31(6):322-324, 1992.

Conner GK: Abdomen assessment. In Tappero EP, Honeyfield ME: *Physical assessment of the newborn: a comprehensive approach to the art of physical examination,* ed 2, Petaluma, CA, 1996, NICU Ink.

Danielson B and others: Newborn discharge timing and readmissions: California, 1992-1995, *Pediatrics* 106(1):31-39, 2000.

Darmstadt GL, Dinulos JG: Neonatal skin care, *Pediatr Clin North Am* 47(4):757-782, 2000.

Della Porta K, Aforismo D, Butler-O'Hara M: Co-bedding of twins in the neonatal intensive care, *Pediatr Nurs* 24(6):529-531, 1998.

Dewey KG, Heinig MJ, Nommsen-Rivers LA: Differences in morbidity between breast-fed and formula-fed infants, *J Pediatr* 126(5 part 1):696-702, 1995.

Dewey KG and others: Do exclusively breast-fed infants require extra protein? *Pediatr Res* 39(2):303-307, 1996.

Dewey KG and others: Breastfed infants are leaner than formula-fed infants at 1 year of age: the DARLING study, *Am J Clin Nutr* 57(2):140-145, 1993.

Dewey K and others: Adequacy of energy intake among breast-fed infants in the DARLING study: relationships to growth velocity, morbidity, and activity levels, *J Pediatr* 119(4):538-547, 1991.

Donnelly A and others: Commercial hospital discharge packs for breastfeeding women, *Cochrane Database Syst Rev* 2000(2):CD002075, 2000.

Donovan EF and others: Inaccuracy of Ballard scores before 28 weeks' gestation, *J Pediatr* 135(2 pt 1):147-152, 1999.

Dore S and others: Alcohol versus natural drying for newborn cord care, *J Obstet Gynecol Neonat Nurs* 27(6):621-627, 1998.

Dubowitz LMS, Dubowitz V: *Gestational age of the newborn,* Menlo Park, CA, 1977, Addison-Wesley.

Dungy CI and others: Hospital infant formula discharge packages: do they affect the duration of breast-feeding? *Arch Pediatr Adolesc Med* 151(7):724-729, 1997.

Farber SD, Van Fossen RL, Koontz SW: Quantitative and qualitative video analysis of infants feeding: angled- and straight-bottle feeding systems, *J Pediatr* 126(6):S118-S124, 1995.

*Female genital mutilation, AAP News* 10(2):3, 1994.

Ferber R, Kryger M: *Principles and practice of sleep medicine in the child,* Philadelphia, 1995, WB Saunders.

Ferketich SL, Mercer RT: Paternal-infant attachment of experienced and inexperienced fathers during infancy, *Nur Res* 44(1):31-37, 1995.

Fitzgerald M, Millard C, McIntosh N: Cutaneous hypersensitivity following peripheral tissue damage in newborn infants and its reversal with topical anesthesia, *Pain* 39:31-36, 1989.

Fletcher MA: Physical assessment and classification. In Avery GB, Fletcher MA, MacDonald MG, editors: *Neonatalogy: pathophysiology and management of the newborn,* ed 4, Philadelphia, 1994, JB Lippincott.

Foca M and others: Endemic *Pseudomonas aeruginosa* infection in a neonatal intensive care unit, *N Engl J Med* 343(10):695-700, 2000.

Fomon SJ: *Infant nutrition,* St Louis, 1993, Mosby.

Ford LA, Ritchie JA: Maternal perceptions of newborn umbilical cord treatments and healing, *J Obstet Gynecol Neonat Nurs* 28(5):501-506, 1999.

Fuloria M, Kreiter S: The newborn examination. Part 1. Emergencies and common abnormalities involving the skin, head, neck, chest, and respiratory and cardiovascular systems, *Am Fam Physician* 65(1):61-68, 2002.

Geller M: Infant abduction in the hospital setting, *QRC Advisor* 16(5):1-4, 2000.

Godley FA: Frenuloplasty with a buccal mucosal graft, *Laryngoscope* 104(3):378-381, 1994.

Gray L, Watt L, Blass EM: Skin-to-skin contact is analgesic in healthy newborns, *Pediatrics* 105(1):110-111, 2000, *www.pediatrics.org/cgi/content/full/105/1/e14.*

Gries DM, Phyall G, Barfield WD: Evaluation of early discharge program for infants after childbirth in a military population, *Mil Med* 165(8):616-621, 2000.

Haouari N and others: The analgesic effect of sucrose in full-term infants: a randomised controlled trial, *BMJ* (6993):310:1498-1500, 1995.

*Healthy People 2010: Healthy People 2010 www.health.gov/healthypeople.*

Hegyi T and others: The Apgar score and its components in the preterm infant, *Pediatrics* 101(1):77-81, 1998.

Herschel M and others: Neonatal circumcision. Randomized trial of a sucrose pacifier for pain control, *Arch Pediatr Adolesc Med* 152(3):279-284, 1998.

Hicks MA: A comparison of the tympanic and axillary temperatures of the preterm and term infant, *J Perinatol* 16(4):261-267, 1996.

Jain A, Rutter N: Does topical amethocaine gel reduce the pain of venipuncture in newborn infants? A randomised double blind controlled trial, *Arch Dis Child Fetal Neonatal Ed* 83(3):F207-210, 2000.

Jain A, Rutter N, Ratnayaka M: Topical amethocaine gel for pain relief of heel prick blood sampling: a randomised double blind controlled trial, *Arch Dis Child Fetal Neonatal Ed* 84(1):F56-F59, 2001.

Juretschke LJ: Unilateral neonatal testicular torsion, *J Obstet Gynecol Neonat Nurs* 29(5):451-456, 2000.

Karl DJ: The interactive newborn bath using infant neurobehavior to connect parents and newborns, *MCN* 24(6):280-286, 1999.

Klaus MH, Kennell JH, Klaus PH: *Bonding: building the foundations of secure attachment and independence,* Menlo Park, CA, 1995, Addison-Wesley.

Kotagul UR and others: Safety of early discharge of Medicaid newborns, *JAMA* 282(12):1150-1156, 1999.

Krebs TL: Is cord care necessary? *Mother Baby J* 3(2):5-12, 1998.

Kumar SL, Dhanireddy R: Time of first stool in premature infants: effect of gestational age and illness severity, *J Pediatr* 127(6):971-974, 1995.

Kyenkya-Isabirye M: UNICEF launches the Baby-Friendly Hospital Initiative, *MCN* 17(4):177-179, 1992.

Lander J and others: Comparison of ring block, dorsal penile nerve block, and topical anesthesia for neonatal circumcision: a randomized controlled trial, *JAMA* 278(24):2157-2162, 1997.

Lanham DM and others: Accuracy of tympanic temperature readings in children under 6 years of age, *Pediatr Nurs* 25(1):39-42, 1999.

Lanting CI and others: Neurological differences between 9-year-old children fed breast-milk or formula-milk as babies, *Lancet* 344(8933):1319-1322, 1994.

Lawrence RA, Lawrence RM: *Breastfeeding: a guide for the medical profession,* ed 5, St Louis, 1999, Mosby.

Leick-Rude MK, Bloom LF: A comparison of temperature-taking methods in neonates, *Neonatal Network* 17(5):21-37, 1998.

Lieu TA and others: A randomized comparison of home and clinic follow-up visits after early postpartum hospital discharge, *Pediatrics* 105(5):1058-1065, 2000.

Locklin MP, Jansson MJ: Home visits: strategies to protect the breast-feeding newborn at risk, *J Obstet Gynecol Neonatal Nurs* 28(1):33-40, 1999.

Malkin JD and others: Infant mortality and early postpartum discharge, *Obstet Gynecol* 96(2):183-188, 2000.

Malloy MH: Trends in postneonatal aspiration deaths and reclassification of sudden infant death syndrome: impact of the "Back to Sleep" program, *Pediatrics* 109(4):661-665, 2002.

Marbut KK, Loan LA: Newborn hygiene: to bathe or not to bathe, *Mother Baby J* 1(6):25-30, 1996.

Masaitis NS, Kaempf JW: Developing a frenotomy policy at one medical center: a case study approach, *J Hum Lactation* 12(3):229-232, 1996.

McCafferty DF and others: Effect of percutaneous local anaesthetics on pain reduction during pulse dye laser treatment of portwine stains, *Br J Anaesth* 78(3):286-289, 1997.

McCafferty DF, Woolfson AD, Boston V: In vivo assessment of percutaneous local anaesthetic preparations, *Br J Anaesth* 62(1):17-21, 1989.

McCleary PH: Female genital mutilation and childbirth: a case report, *Birth* 21(4):221-223, 1994.

McDonald RE, Avery DR: *Dentistry for the child and adolescent,* ed 7, St Louis, 1999, Mosby.

Menella JA, Beauchamp GK: Developmental changes in the infant's acceptance of protein-hydrolysate formulas and its relation to mothers' eating habits, *J Dev Behav Pediatr* 17(6):386-391, 1996.

Montgomery DL, Splett PL: Economic benefit of breast-feeding infants enrolled in WIC, *J Am Diet Assoc* 97(4):379-385, 1997.

Moolenaar RL and others: A prolonged outbreak of *Pseudomonas aeruginosa* in a neonatal intensive care unit: did staff fingernails play a role in disease transmission? *Infect Control Hosp Epidemiol* 21(2):80-85, 2000.

Newman J, Pitman T: *The ultimate breastfeeding book of answers,* Roseville, CA, 2000, Prima Publishing.

Nuntnarumit P, Yang W, Bada-Ellzey HS: Blood pressure measurements in the newborn, *Clin Perinatol* 26(4):981-996, 1999.

Overgaard C, Knudsen A: Pain-relieving effect of sucrose in newborns during heel prick, *Biol Neonat* 75(2):279-284, 1999.

Paes B and others: A comparative study of heel-stick devices for infant blood collection, *Am J Dis Child* 147(3):346-348, 1993.

Papile LA: The Apgar score in the 21st century, *N Engl J Med* 344(7):519-520, 2001.

Park M, Lee D: Normative arm and calf blood pressure values in the newborn, *Pediatrics* 83(2):240-243, 1989.

Park M, Menard S: Normative oscillometric blood pressure values in the first 5 years in an office setting, *Am J Dis Child* 143(7):860-864, 1989.

Pelke S and others: Gowning does not affect colonization or infection rates in a neonatal intensive care unit, *Arch Pediatr Adolesc Med* 148(1):1016-1020, 1994.

Penny-MacGillivray T: A newborn's first bath: when? *J Obstet Gynecol Neonat Nurs* 25(6):481-487, 1996.

Puckett RM, Offringa M: Prophylactic vitamin K for vitamin K deficiency bleeding in neonates (Cochrane Review), *Cochrane Database Syst Rev* 2000(4):CD002776, 2000.

Quan R and others: Effects of microwave radiation on antiinfective factors in human milk, *Pediatrics* 89(4):667-669, 1992.

Quayle C: Robbing the cradle: hospitals have learned the hard way that one baby stolen is one too many, *Health Facilities Manag* 10(8):20-27, 1997.

Ramenghi LA and others: Reduction of pain response in premature infants using intraoral sucrose, *Arch Dis Child* 74:F126-F128, 1996.

Ryan AS: The resurgence of breastfeeding in the United States, *Pediatrics* 99(4):596(E12), 1997.

Ross Products Division, Abbott Laboratories: *Mother's survey*, Columbus OH, 2000, The Company, *www.ross.com/aboutRoss/survey.pdf.*

Sachdev H and others: Water supplementation in exclusively breastfed infants during summer in the tropics, *Lancet* 337(8747):929-933, 1991.

Scariati PD, Grummer-Strawn LM, Fein SB: A longitudinal analysis of infant morbidity and the extent of breastfeeding in the United States, *Pediatrics* 99(6):e5, 1997.

Schoen EJ, Colby CJ, Ray GT: Newborn circumcision decreases incidence and costs of urinary tract infections during first year of life, *Pediatrics* 105(4):789-793, 2000.

Seguin J, Terry K: Neonatal infrared axillary thermometry, *Clin Pediatr* 38(1):35-40, 1999.

Serour F, Mandelberg A, Mori J: Slow injection of local anesthetic will decrease pain during dorsal penile nerve block, *Acta Anaesthesiol Scand* 42(8):926-928, 1998.

Severn CB: Head circumference–crown-rump length: practical measurements for neonatal screening, *Neonat Intensive Care* 7(4):52-57, 1994.

Sganga A and others: A comparison of four methods of normal newborn temperature measurement, *MCN* 25(2):76-79, 2000.

Silver P, Sagy M, Rubin L: Respiratory failure from corn starch aspiration: a hazard of diaper changing, *Pediatr Emerg Care* 12(2):108-110, 1996.

Stang HJ and others: Beyond dorsal penile nerve block: a more humane circumcision, *Pediatrics* 100(2):e3, 1997, *www.pediatrics.org/cgi/content/full/100/2/e3.*

Stevens B and others: The efficacy of sucrose for relieving procedural pain in neonates—a systematic review and meta-analysis, *Acta Paediatr* 86(8):837-842, 1997.

Stevens B and others: The efficacy of developmentally sensitive interventions and sucrose for relieving procedural pain in very low birth weight infants, *Nurs Res* 48(1):35-43, 1999.

Stevens B, Yamada J, Ohlsson A: Sucrose for analgesia in newborn infants undergoing procedures, (Cochrane Review), *Cochrane Database Syst Rev* 2001(4):CD001069, 2001.

Taddio A and others: Efficacy and safety of lidocaine-prilocaine cream for pain during circumcision, *N Engl J Med* 336(17):1197-1201, 1997.

Taddio A and others: A systematic review of lidocaine-prilocaine cream (EMLA) in the treatment of acute pain in neonates, *Pediatrics* 101(2):e1, 1998, *www.pediatrics.org/cgi/content/full/101/2/e1.*

Taddio A and others: Combined analgesia and local anesthesia to minimize pain during circumcision, *Arch Pediatr Adolesc Med* 154(5):620-623, 2000.

Taddio A, Ohlsson K, Ohlsson A: Lidocaine-prilocaine cream for analgesia during circumcision in newborn boys, *Cochrane Database Syst Rev* 2000(2):CD000494, 2000.

Tigges BB: Infant formulas: practical answers for common questions: *Nurse Pract* 22(8):70, 73, 77-80, 1997.

Tomlinson PS, Bryan AA, Esau AL: Family centered intrapartum care: revisiting an old concept, *J Obstet Gynecol Neonat Nurs* 25(4):331-337, 1996.

Trochtenberg DS: Neonatal circumcision, *N Engl J Med* 323(17):1206, 1990 (letter to the editor).

Trotter CW: Gestational age assessment. In Tappero EP, Honeyfield ME, editors: *Physical assessment of the newborn: a comprehensive approach to the art of physical examination*, Petaluma, CA, 1996, NICU Ink.

Varda KE, Behnke RS: The effect of timing the initial bath on newborn's temperature, *J Obstet Gynecol Neonat Nurs* 29(1):27-32, 2000.

Weekly SJ, Neumann ML: Speaking up for baby: the case for individualized neonatal discharge plans, *AWHONN Lifelines* 1(1):24-29, 1997.

Weinberg S: An alternative to meet the needs of early discharge: the tender beginnings postpartum visit, *MCN* 19:339-342, 1994.

Weiss ME, Poeltler D, Gocka I: Infrared tympanic thermometry for neonatal temperature assessment, *J Obstetric Gynecol Neonat Nurs* 23(9):798-803, 1993.

Westbrooks C: Ask the experts: what should be taught to new parents about care of their son's uncircumcised penis? *AWHONN Voice* 4(1):7, 1996.

Wiessinger D, Miller M: Breastfeeding difficulties as a result of tight lingual and labial frena: a case report, *J Hum Lactation* 11(4):313-316, 1995.

Williamson ML: Circumcision anesthesia: a study of nursing implications for dorsal penile nerve block, *Pediatr Nurs* 23(10):59-63, 1997.

Wilshaw R and others: A comparison of the use tympanic, axillary, and rectal thermometers in infants, *J Pediatr Nurs* 14(2):88-93, 1999.

Wilson D, Bowman C: Infant nutrition: building blocks for the future, *Mother Baby J* 5(4):17-22, 2000.

Wright A, Rice S, Wells S: Changing hospital practices to increase the duration of breastfeeding, *Pediatrics* 97(5):669-676, 1996.

Wright JE: Tongue-tie, *J Paediatr Child Health* 31(4):276-278, 1995.

Wright JT: Normal formation and development defects of human dentition, *Pediatr Clin North Am* 47(5):975-1000, 2000.

Yetman RJ and others: Comparison of temperature measurements by an aural infrared thermometer with measurements by traditional rectal and axillary techniques, *J Pediatr* 122(5):769-773, 1993.

Yoshinaga-Itano C and others: Language of early- and late-identified children with hearing loss, *Pediatrics* 102(5):1161-1171, 1998.

Zupan J, Garner P: Topical umbilical cord care at birth, *Cochrane Database Syst Rev* 2000(2):CD001057, 2000.

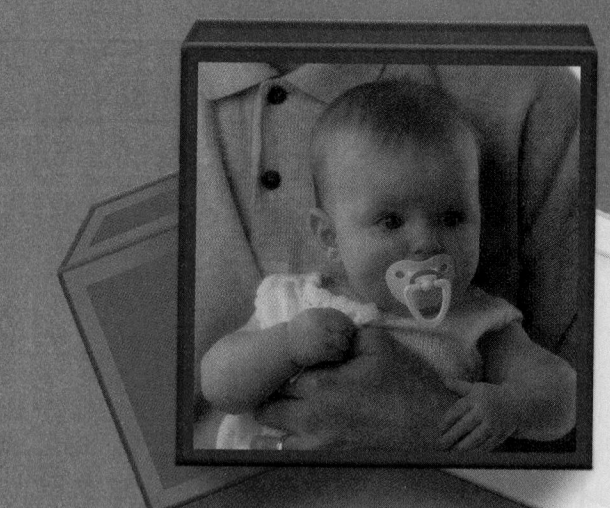

# Chapter 9

# Health Problems of the Newborn

## Chapter Outline

**BIRTH INJURIES, 295**
**Soft Tissue Injury, 295**
**Head Trauma, 296**
    Caput Succedaneum, 296
    Subgaleal Hemorrhage, 296
    Cephalhematoma, 297
**Fractures, 298**
**Paralyses, 298**
    Facial Paralysis, 298
    Brachial Palsy, 299
    Phrenic Nerve Paralysis, 299
**DERMATOLOGIC PROBLEMS IN THE NEWBORN, 300**
**Erythema Toxicum Neonatorum, 300**

**Candidiasis, 300**
**Bullous Impetigo, 301**
**"Birthmarks," 301**
**PROBLEMS RELATED TO PHYSIOLOGIC FACTORS, 303**
**Hyperbilirubinemia, 303**
    Pathophysiology, 304
    Physiologic Jaundice, 304
    *Nursing Care Plan: The Newborn with Hyperbilirubinemia, 313*
**Hemolytic Disease of the Newborn (HDN), 310**
    Blood Incompatibility, 310
**Hypoglycemia, 316**

**Hyperglycemia, 317**
**Hypocalcemia, 318**
**Hemorrhagic Disease of the Newborn, 319**
**INBORN ERRORS OF METABOLISM (IEMs), 319**
**Congenital Hypothyroidism (CH), 320**
**Phenylketonuria (PKU), 322**
**Galactosemia, 324**
**PROBLEMS CAUSED BY PERINATAL ENVIRONMENTAL FACTORS, 325**
**Infectious Agents, 325**
**Chemical Agents, 326**
**Fetal Alcohol Syndrome, 326**
**Radiation, 330**

## Related Topics

Birth of a Child with a Physical Defect, Ch. 11
Blood Specimens, Ch. 27
The Child with Cognitive, Sensory, or Communication Impairment, Ch. 24
Congenital Adrenogenital Hyperplasia, Ch. 38
Diaper Dermatitis, Ch. 13
Family-Centered Care of the Child with Chronic Illness or Disability, Ch. 22
Genetic Evaluation and Counseling, Ch. 5
Genetic Screening, Ch. 5
Health Promotion of the Newborn and Family, Ch. 8
The High-Risk Newborn and Family, Ch. 10
Infants of Diabetic Mothers, Ch. 10

## BIRTH INJURIES

Birth injuries occur during the birth process. They are most likely to occur when the infant is large, the presentation is breech, the delivery is precipitous, forceful extraction is used, or inexperienced practitioners manage the delivery.

Many injuries are minor and resolve spontaneously in a few days; others, although minor, require some degree of intervention. Still others can be serious and even fatal. Part of the nurse's responsibility is to identify such injuries so that appropriate interventions can be initiated as soon as possible. Birth injuries can be classified according to the type of body structure involved (Box 9-1).

■ David Wilson, MS, RNC, revised this chapter.

## Soft Tissue Injury

Various types of soft tissue injury may be sustained during the process of birth, primarily in the form of bruises and abrasions secondary to dystocia. Soft tissue injury usually occurs when there is some degree of disproportion between the presenting part and the maternal pelvis (cephalopelvic disproportion). Common types of soft tissue injury are listed in Box 9-2. The use of forceps to facilitate a difficult vertex delivery may produce discoloration or abrasions of the same configuration as the forceps on the sides of the neonate's face. Petechiae or ecchymoses may be observed on the presenting part after a breech or brow delivery. After a difficult or precipitous delivery, the sudden release of pressure on the head can produce scleral hemorrhages or generalized pe-

---

**Box 9-1 ■ ■ □**
**Types of Physical Injuries at Birth**

**SOFT TISSUE INJURY**
Erythema
Abrasion
Petechiae
Ecchymoses
Subcutaneous fat necrosis
Subconjunctival (scleral) hemorrhage
Retinal hemorrhage
Hemorrhage into abdominal organ(s)

**HEAD INJURY**
Caput succedaneum
Subgaleal hemorrhage
Cephalhematoma
Fracture (depressed or linear)
Intracranial hemorrhage

**NEUROLOGIC INJURY**
Subdural or epidural hematoma
Facial paralysis
Brachial palsy (Erb-Duchenne paralysis, Klumpke palsy)
Phrenic nerve palsy (diaphragmatic paralysis)
Spinal cord injury

---

**Box 9-2 ■ ■ □**
**Common Types of Soft Tissue Injury**

**Erythema and abrasions**—Usually the result of the application of forceps; discoloration is the same configuration as the instrument
**Petechiae**—Nonraised, pinpoint hemorrhages caused by a sudden increase and then release of pressure during passage through the birth canal; may be seen on the chest, face, and head
**Ecchymoses**—Small hemorrhagic areas (larger than petechiae) that may occur after traumatic, precipitous, or breech delivery
**Subcutaneous fat necrosis**—Clearly outlined masses located in the subcutaneous tissues that are firm to the overlying skin but movable over the underlying tissue; most likely caused by traumatic manipulation during delivery
**Subconjunctival (scleral) hemorrhages**—The result of rupture of capillaries in the sclera from pressure on the fetal head during delivery; most common location is the limbus of the iris
**Retinal hemorrhages**—Flame-shaped, irregular, or round areas of bleeding in the retina from excessive pressure on the fetal head during delivery; extensive areas may indicate subdural hematoma or brain trauma

---

techiae over the face and head. Petechiae and ecchymoses may also appear on the head, neck, and face of an infant born with a nuchal cord, giving the infant's face a cyanotic appearance. A well-defined circle of petechiae and ecchymoses may also be seen on the occipital region of the newborn's head when a vacuum suction cup is applied during delivery. Rarely, lacerations occur during cesarean section.

These traumatic lesions generally fade spontaneously and without treatment within a few days. However, petechiae may be a manifestation of an underlying bleeding disorder and is evaluated.

### Nursing Considerations

Nursing care is directed primarily toward assessing the injury, maintaining asepsis of the area to prevent breakdown and infection, and providing an explanation and reassurance to the parents. An accurate description of the injury is recorded to facilitate subsequent comparative nursing evaluations (e.g., extent of petechiae).

Regardless of how benign the injury, parents are concerned and mourn the loss of the expected "perfect" infant. Explanations of the cause and treatment, if any, need to be thorough and repeated frequently. If the injury is temporarily disfiguring, such as extensive facial bruising, nurses can demonstrate acceptance of the child through their example of sensitive, personal care of the infant.

## Head Trauma

Head trauma that occurs during the birth process is usually benign but occasionally results in more serious injury. The injuries that produce serious trauma, such as intracranial hemorrhage and subdural hematoma, are discussed in relation to neurologic disorders in the newborn. (See Chapters 10

and 37.) Skull fractures are discussed with other fractures sustained during the birth process. The three most common types of extracranial hemorrhagic injury are caput succedaneum, subgaleal hemorrhage, and cephalhematoma.

### Caput Succedaneum

The most commonly observed scalp lesion is caput succedaneum, a vaguely outlined area of edematous tissue situated over the portion of the scalp that presents in a vertex delivery (Fig. 9-1, *A*). The swelling consists of serum and/or blood that has accumulated in the tissues above the bone. Typically the swelling extends beyond the bone margins and may be associated with overlying petechiae or ecchymosis. It is present at or shortly after birth. No specific treatment is needed, and the swelling subsides within a few days.

### Subgaleal Hemorrhage

Subgaleal hemorrhage is bleeding into the subgaleal compartment (Fig. 9-1, *B*). The *subgaleal compartment* is a potential space that contains loosely arranged connective tissue; it is located beneath the galea aponeurosis, the tendinous sheath that connects the frontal and occipital muscles and forms the inner surface of the scalp. The injury occurs as a result of forces that compress and then drag the head through the pelvic outlet (Moe and Page, 1998). There have been reports of concern regarding the increased use of the vacuum extractor at birth and an association with cases of subgaleal hemorrhage, neonatal morbidity, and deaths (Garas and others, 2001; Ross, Fresquez, and El-Haddad, 2001; Towner and others, 1999); however, the rates are reportedly declining (Putta and Spencer, 2000). The bleeding extends beyond bone, often posterior into the neck, and continues after birth, with the potential for serious complications.

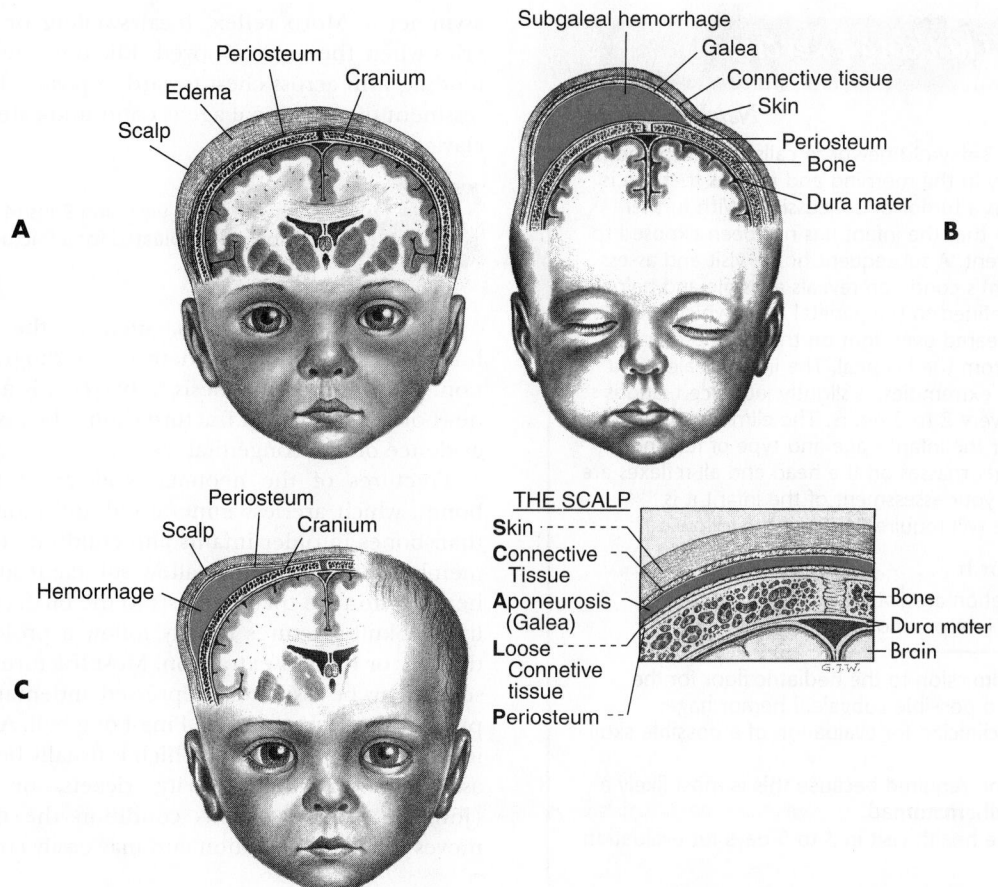

**Fig. 9-1**  **A,** Caput succedaneum. **B,** Subgaleal hemorrhage. **C,** Cephalhematoma. (A and C from Seidel HM and others: *Mosby's guide to physical examination,* ed 4, St Louis, 1999, Mosby.)

Early detection of the hemorrhage is vital; serial head circumference measurements and inspection of the back of the neck for increasing edema and a firm mass are essential. A boggy scalp, pallor, tachycardia, and increasing head circumference may also be early signs of a subgaleal hemorrhage (Putta and Spencer, 2000). Computed tomography (CT) or magnetic resonance imaging (MRI) are useful in confirming the diagnosis. Replacement of lost blood and clotting factors are required in acute cases of hemorrhage. An early sign of subgaleal hemorrhage is a forward and lateral positioning of the newborn's ears as the hematoma extends posteriorly. Monitoring the infant for changes in level of consciousness and a decrease in the hematocrit are also key to early recognition and management. An increase in serum bilirubin levels may be seen as a result of the degrading blood cells within the hematoma.

## Cephalhematoma

A cephalhematoma is formed when blood vessels rupture during labor or delivery to produce bleeding into the area between the bone and its periosteum. The injury occurs most often with primiparous women and is often associated with forceps delivery and vacuum extraction. Unlike caput succedaneum, the boundaries of the cephalhematoma are sharply demarcated and do not extend beyond the limits of

the bone (Fig. 9-1, *C*). The cephalhematoma may involve one or both parietal bones. The occipital bones are less commonly affected, and the frontal bones are rarely affected. The swelling is usually minimal or absent at birth and increases in size on the second or third day. Blood loss is usually not significant.

No treatment is indicated for uncomplicated cephalhematoma. Most lesions are absorbed within 2 weeks to 3 months. Lesions that result in severe blood loss to the area or that involve an underlying fracture require further evaluation. Hyperbilirubinemia may result during resolution of the hematoma. A local infection can develop and is suspected when a sudden increase in swelling occurs.

## Nursing Considerations*

Nursing care is directed toward assessment and observation of the common scalp injuries and vigilance in observing for possible associated complications such as skin breakdown, infection, or, rarely, acute blood loss and hypovolemia. Because these visible injuries resolve spontaneously, parents need reassurance of their usual benign nature. (See Critical

*For additional information, please view "Pediatric Nursing: Newborn Assessment" in *Whaley and Wong's Pediatric Nursing Video Series,* St Louis, 1996, Mosby; (800) 426-4545; www.mosby.com.

*Critical Thinking Exercise*

### Newborn Head

The mother of a 3-day-old newborn calls you at the home health office early in the morning and reports that she is afraid her son has a tumor or concussion. With further inquiry you learn that the infant has not been exposed to any traumatic event. A subsequent home visit and assessment of the infant's condition reveals a visible and palpable soft mass confined to the parietal area, which the mother says appeared overnight on the second day after their discharge from the hospital. The infant is alert and active, moves all extremities, is slightly jaundiced, and is breast-feeding every 2 to 3 hours. The elimination pattern is appropriate for the infant's age and type of feeding. There are no other masses on the head and all reflexes are intact. Based on your assessment of the infant it is expected that he will require which of the following?

FIRST, THINK ABOUT IT . . .
- What information are you using?
- How are you interpreting that information?

1. Immediate admission to the pediatric floor for the evaluation of a possible subgaleal hemorrhage.
2. A visit to the clinician for evaluation of a possible skull fracture.
3. No intervention required because this is most likely a benign cephalhematoma.
4. A return home health visit in 3 to 5 days for evaluation of jaundice.

*The best response is three. Interpreting the information correctly, you realize that a cephalhematoma does not cross scalp suture lines and may appear unilaterally or bilaterally within hours after delivery. The infant's activity level and other evaluative data exclude a subgaleal hemorrhage. A skull fracture in the newborn period is rare and may or may not involve edema. If neurologic signs are normal, no treatment is necessary unless it is a depressed fracture. The fourth answer would apply if the infant had moderate jaundice at this time because breast-feeding combined with a hematoma may exacerbate jaundice.*

Thinking Exercise box and earlier discussion under Soft Tissue Injury.)

## Fractures

Fracture of the *clavicle,* or collarbone, is the most common birth injury. It is often associated with difficult vertex or breech deliveries of infants of greater-than-average size. *Crepitus* (the coarse, crackling sensation produced by the rubbing together of fractured bone fragments) is often felt or heard on further examination, and radiographs usually reveal a complete fracture with overriding of the fragments. A palpable spongy mass, representing localized edema and hematoma, may also be a sign of a fractured clavicle (Reiners and others, 2000).

The newborn with a fractured clavicle may have no symptoms, but a fracture should be suspected if an infant has limited use of the affected arm, malposition of the arm, an asymmetric Moro reflex, focal swelling or tenderness, or cries when the arm is moved. Eliciting the scarf sign (extending arm across chest toward opposite shoulder) for assessment of gestational age is contraindicated if a fractured clavicle is suspected.

**NURSING ALERT** Any newborn weighing 9 lbs (4.5 kg) or more should be evaluated for a fractured clavicle.

Fractures of *long bones,* such as the femur or the humerus, are difficult to detect by radiographic examination. Although osteogenesis imperfecta is a rare finding, a newborn infant with a fracture should be assessed for other evidence of this congenital disorder.

Fractures of the neonatal *skull* are uncommon. The bones, which are less mineralized and more compressible than bones in older infants and children, are separated by membranous seams that allow sufficient alteration in the head contour so that it adjusts to the birth canal during delivery. Skull fractures usually follow a prolonged, difficult delivery or forceps extraction. Most fractures are linear, but some may be visible as depressed indentations that compress or decompress like a Ping-Pong ball. A similar finding in neonates is *craniotabes,* which is usually benign or may be associated with prematurity, rickets, or hydrocephalus (Johnson, 1996). In this condition the cranial bone(s) moves freely on palpation and may easily compress.

### Nursing Considerations

Often no intervention may be prescribed other than proper body alignment, careful dressing and undressing of the infant, and handling and carrying techniques that support the affected bone. For example, if the infant has a fractured clavicle, it is important to support the upper and lower back rather than pull the infant up from under the arms. Occasionally, for immobilization and relief of pain, the arm on the side of the fractured clavicle may be secured against the body by pinning the sleeve to the shirt or by applying a triangular sling or figure-8 bandage.

Linear skull fractures usually require no treatment. A Ping-Pong type fracture may require decompression by surgical intervention. Decompression of a depressed skull fracture may be accomplished with the use of a vacuum extractor suction device (Pollak and others, 1999). The infant is carefully observed for signs of neurologic complications. The parents of an infant with a fracture of any bone should be involved in caring for the infant during hospitalization as part of discharge planning for care at home.

## Paralyses

### Facial Paralysis

Pressure on the facial nerve during delivery may result in injury to cranial nerve VII. The primary clinical manifestations are loss of movement on the affected side, such as an inability to completely close the eye, drooping of the corner of the mouth, and absence of wrinkling of the forehead and nasolabial fold (Fig. 9-2). The paralysis is most noticeable

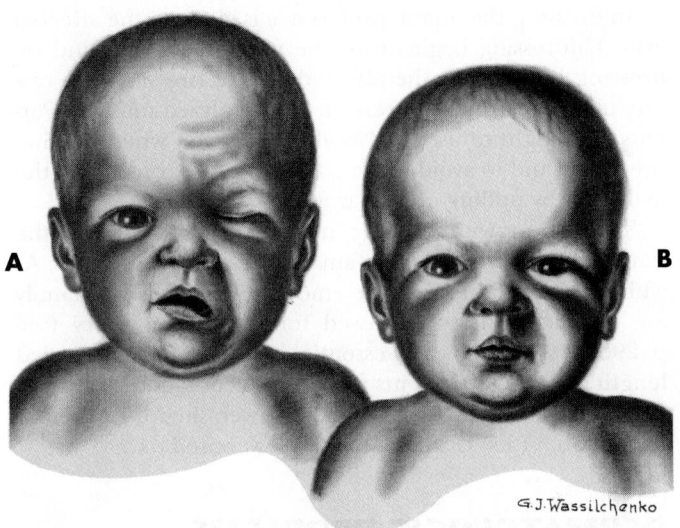

**Fig. 9-2  A,** Paralysis of right side of face 15 minutes after forceps delivery. Absence of movement on affected side is especially noticeable when infant cries. **B,** Same infant 24 hours later.

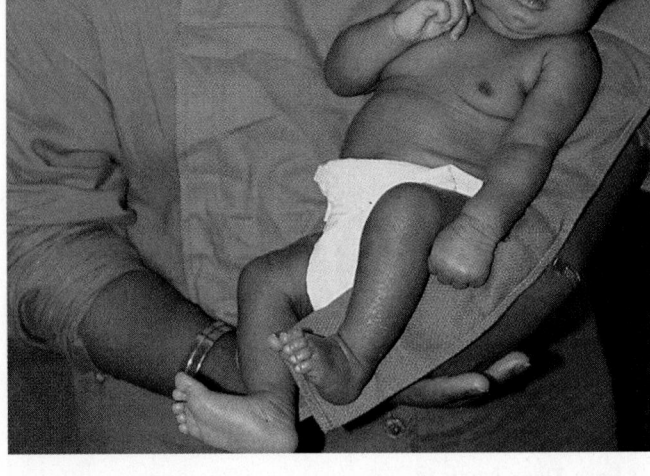

**Fig. 9-3** Left-sided brachial plexus (Erb) palsy. Note extended, internally rotated arm and pronated wrist on affected side.

when the infant cries. The mouth is drawn to the unaffected side, the wrinkles are deeper on the normal side, and the eye on the involved side remains open.

No medical intervention is necessary. The paralysis usually disappears spontaneously in a few days but may take as long as several months.

## Brachial Palsy

Brachial plexus injury results from forces that alter the normal position and relationship of the arm, shoulder, and neck. *Erb palsy (Erb-Duchenne paralysis)* is caused by damage to the upper plexus and usually results from a stretching or pulling away of the shoulder from the head. The less common lower plexus palsy, or *Klumpke palsy,* results from severe stretching of the upper extremity while the trunk is relatively less mobile.

The clinical manifestations of Erb palsy are related to the paralysis of the affected extremity and muscles. The arm hangs limp alongside the body. The shoulder and arm are adducted and internally rotated. The elbow is extended, and the forearm is pronated, with the wrist and fingers flexed; a grasp reflex may be present because finger and wrist movement remain normal (Alexander and Kuo, 1997) (Fig. 9-3). In lower plexus palsy the muscles of the hand are paralyzed, with consequent wrist drop and relaxed fingers. In a third and more severe form of brachial palsy, the entire arm is paralyzed and hangs limp and motionless at the side. The Moro reflex is absent on the affected side for all forms of brachial palsy.

Treatment of an affected arm is aimed at preventing contractures of the paralyzed muscles and maintaining correct placement of the humeral head within the glenoid fossa of the scapula. Complete recovery from stretched nerves usually takes 3 to 6 months. However, avulsion of the nerves (complete disconnection of the ganglia from the spinal cord that involves both anterior and posterior roots) results in permanent damage. For those injuries that do not improve spontaneously by 3 months, surgical intervention may be needed to relieve pressure on the nerves or to repair the nerves with grafting (Volpe, 2001). Repeated injections of botulinum toxin type A into the triceps muscles of some children has been effective in reducing muscle contractures after birth-related brachial plexus injuries (Rollnik and others, 2000).

## Phrenic Nerve Paralysis

Phrenic nerve paralysis results in diaphragmatic paralysis as demonstrated by ultrasonography, which shows paradoxical chest movement and an elevated diaphragm. Initially, chest radiography may not demonstrate an elevated diaphragm in the acute period. The injury sometimes occurs in conjunction with brachial palsy. Respiratory distress is the most common and important sign of injury. Because injury to the phrenic nerve is usually unilateral, the lung on the affected side does not expand and respiratory efforts are ineffectual. The infant is positioned on the affected side to facilitate maximum expansion of the uninvolved lung. Breathing is primarily thoracic, and cyanosis, tachypnea, or complete respiratory failure may be seen. Pneumonia and atelectasis on the affected side may also occur.

## Nursing Considerations

Nursing care of the infant with facial nerve paralysis involves aiding the infant in sucking and helping the mother with feeding techniques. A comprehensive evaluation of the infant's oral motor skills by an infant feeding specialist is recommended in order to develop an effective multidisciplinary feeding regimen. Because part of the mouth cannot close tightly around the nipple, the use of a soft rubber nipple with a large hole may be helpful but should be used carefully to

### Incomplete Moro Reflex

During a particularly busy evening in a mother-newborn care unit, you are asked by a curious new father why his newborn daughter startles so easily when the crib is accidentally bumped. While you are explaining the Moro reflex and eliciting the reflex as a demonstration to the father, you note that the newborn (weight 9 pounds, 10 ounces) does *not* exhibit a complete Moro reflex. Her left arm does not rise from the mattress surface when the Moro is elicited. Further examination indicates that both clavicles are intact with palpation, the right arm flexes appropriately when the Moro is elicited, and the newborn's left hand and fingers open and close spontaneously. Based on this information and a history of a difficult delivery, you suspect that this newborn will likely require which of the following interventions?

FIRST, THINK ABOUT IT . . .
• What conclusions are you reaching?
• If you accept the conclusions, what are the implications?

1. A full arm cast because she has a fractured arm as a result of trauma.
2. Immobilization of the affected arm on the upper abdomen.
3. Placing the arm in a splint with elbow flexion at a 90-degree angle.
4. Gentle passive range-of-motion exercises for the arm, elbow, and wrist q.i.d.

*The best response is two. Brachial plexus (Erb) palsy is the most likely diagnosis. The infant with a fracture of a long bone such as the humerus will also display edema of the affected extremity. Splinting the arm is no longer recommended with a brachial plexus injury. Passive range-of-motion exercises are recommended once it has been ascertained that there is no fracture involved.*

prevent choking. The infant may require partial gavage feeding and supplemental oral stimulation with a minimal amount of formula to prevent aspiration. Breast-feeding is not contraindicated, but the mother will need additional assistance in helping the infant grasp and compress the areolar area.

If the lid of the eye on the affected side does not close completely, artificial tears can be instilled as needed to prevent drying of the conjunctiva, sclera, and cornea. The lid may be taped shut to prevent accidental injury. If eye care is needed at home, the parents are taught the procedure for administering eye drops before the infant is discharged from the nursery. (See Chapter 27.)

Nursing care of the newborn with brachial palsy is concerned primarily with proper positioning of the affected arm. The affected arm should be gently immobilized on the upper abdomen; passive range-of-motion exercises of the shoulder, wrist, elbow, and fingers are initiated following careful evaluation. Wrist flexion contractures may be prevented with the use of supportive splints.

In dressing the infant, preference is given to the affected arm. Undressing begins with the unaffected arm, and redressing begins with the affected arm to prevent unnecessary manipulation and stress on the paralyzed muscles. Parents are taught to use the "football" position when holding the infant and to avoid picking the child up from under the axillae or by pulling on the arms.

The infant with phrenic nerve paralysis requires the same nursing care as any infant with respiratory distress. As with other birth injuries, the emotional needs of the family are similar to those discussed for soft tissue injury (see p. 296). Follow-up is also essential because of the extended length of recovery. Parents may wish to contact the **Brachial Plexus Palsy Foundation** and visit the web site for further information.* (See Critical Thinking Exercise box.)

## DERMATOLOGIC PROBLEMS IN THE NEWBORN
### Erythema Toxicum Neonatorum

*Erythema toxicum neonatorum,* also known as *"flea bite dermatitis"* or *"newborn rash,"* is a benign, self-limiting eruption that usually appears within the first 2 or 3 days of life. The 1- to 3-mm lesions are firm, pale yellow or white papules or pustules on an erythematous base, which resemble flea bites. Erythema toxicum may appear as one or two isolated "flea bites" or as multiple lesions; the rash commonly disappears from one location and reappears elsewhere hours later. The rash appears most commonly on the face, proximal extremities, trunk, and buttocks, but it may be located anywhere on the body except the palms and soles. The rash may be more obvious during crying episodes. There are no systemic manifestations, and successive crops of lesions heal without pigmentation changes. The rash usually lasts approximately 5 to 7 days.

The etiology is unknown. However, a smear of the pustule shows numerous eosinophils and a relative absence of neutrophils. Bacterial, fungal, or viral cultures should be obtained when the diagnosis is questionable. Although no treatment is necessary, parents are usually concerned about the rash and need to be reassured of its benign and transient nature.

### Candidiasis

*Candidiasis,* also known as *moniliasis,* is not uncommon in the newborn. *Candida albicans,* the organism usually responsible, may cause disease in any organ system. It is a yeastlike fungus (produces yeast cells and spores) that can be acquired from a maternal vaginal infection during delivery, by person-to-person transmission (especially from poor handwashing technique), or from contaminated hands, bottles, nipples, or other articles. Mucocutaneous, cutaneous, and disseminated candidiasis are observed in this age-

*210 Spring Haven Circle, Royersford, PA 19468, www.membrane.com/bpp/index.html

group. It is usually a benign disorder in the neonate and is often confined to the oral and diaper regions. (See Diaper Dermatitis, Chapter 13.)

*Oral candidiasis (thrush)* is characterized by white adherent patches on the tongue, palate, and inner aspects of the cheeks. It is often difficult to distinguish from milk. The infant may refuse to suck because of pain in the mouth.

> **NURSING ALERT** Candidiasis can be distinguished from coagulated milk when attempts to remove the patches with a tongue blade are unsuccessful, usually resulting in bleeding from the scraped surfaces.

This condition tends to be acute in the newborn (rarely appears in first week of life) and chronic in older infants and young children. Thrush appears when the oral flora are altered as a result of antibiotic therapy or poor handwashing by the infant's caregiver. Although the disorder is usually self-limiting, spontaneous resolution may take as long as 2 months, during which time lesions may spread to the larynx, trachea, bronchi, and lungs and along the gastrointestinal tract. The disease is treated with good hygiene, application of a fungicide, and correction of any underlying disturbance. The source of infection, usually the mother, should be treated to prevent reinfection.

Topical application of 1 ml of nystatin (Mycostatin) over the surfaces of the oral cavity four times a day or every 6 hours is usually sufficient to prevent spread of the disease or prolongation of its course. Several other drugs may be used, including amphotericin B (Fungizone), clotrimazole (Lotrimin, Mycelex), fluconazole (Diflucan), or miconazole (Monistat, Micatin) given intravenously, orally, or topically. Gentian violet solution may be used in addition to one of the antifungal drugs in chronic cases of oral thrush; however, the former does not treat gastrointestinal candida and may be irritating to the oral mucosa. To prevent relapse, therapy should be continued for at least 3 days after the lesions disappear. Nystatin in combination with an oral systemic antifungal drug may be more effective in treating oral thrush (Hoppe, 1997).

### Nursing Considerations

Nursing care is directed toward preventing spread of the infection and correct application of the prescribed topical medication. For candidiasis in the diaper area, the caregiver is taught to keep the diaper area clean and to apply the medication to affected areas as prescribed. (See Diaper Dermatitis, Chapter 13.)

Oral nystatin is administered after feedings. The medication is distributed over the surface of the oral mucosa and tongue with an applicator or syringe; the remainder of the dose is deposited in the mouth to be swallowed by the infant to treat any gastrointestinal lesions. The intravenous administration of amphotericin B must be closely monitored to prevent tissue damage and phlebitis.

In addition to good hygienic care, other measures to control thrush include rinsing the infant's mouth with plain water after each feeding before applying the medication and boiling reusable nipples and bottles for at least 20 minutes after a thorough washing (spores are heat-resistant). Pacifiers should be boiled for at least 20 minutes once daily, and the nipples of breast-feeding mothers should be treated to prevent reinfection. Older infants can introduce *Candida* into their mouths with hands contaminated by contact with diaper dermatitis. Placing clothes over the diaper can prevent this cycle of self-infection.

## Bullous Impetigo

*Bullous impetigo (impetigo neonatorum)* is an infectious superficial skin condition most often caused by various strains of *Staphylococcus aureus*. It is characterized by the eruption of bullous vesicular lesions on previously untraumatized or intact skin. The lesions may appear on any body surface and sometimes become widespread, but the usual distribution involves the buttocks, perineum, trunk, face, and extremities. They vary in size from a few millimeters to several centimeters, contain turbid fluid, and are easily ruptured. The bullae rupture in 1 to 2 days, leaving a superficial red, moist, denuded area with very little crusting. In extreme cases the condition may be mistaken for thermal injury (Scales, Fleischer, and Krowchuk, 1997).

Treatment usually involves the administration of oral antibiotics and topical application of mupirocin (Bactroban). Recovery is usually rapid and uneventful.

### Nursing Considerations

Once the diagnosis is suspected, the infant is isolated until therapy is instituted to prevent spread of the infection to other infants. Persons who have come in contact with the infant are investigated to determine a possible source of the infecting organism. Other infants in the nursery should be scrutinized for early detection of any evidence of infection. Parents and other visitors are instructed regarding precautions for the prevention of infection, especially through handwashing and standard precautions. (See Infection Control, Chapter 27.)

In older infants the arms may need to be confined to prevent scratching the lesions by using elbow restraints, by pulling the undershirt sleeves over the hands and securing the openings with tape, or by applying mittens. If restraints of any kind are used, the infant is allowed freedom of movement at supervised times. Rocking, cuddling, and holding during feeding are essential components of care.

## "Birthmarks"

Discolorations of the skin are common findings in the newborn infant. (See discussion on skin assessment under Physical Assessment, Chapter 8.) Most, such as mongolian spots or telangiectatic nevi, involve no therapy other than reassuring parents of the benign nature of these discolorations. However, some can be the manifestation of a disease that suggests further examination of the child and other family members (e.g., multiple flat, light brown *café-au-lait spots* often characterize the autosomal-dominant hereditary disorder neurofibromatosis and are common findings in Albright syndrome).

Darker or more extensive lesions demand further scrutiny; excision of the lesion is recommended when feasible or when excisional biopsy is performed. Such lesions include the reddish brown solitary nodule that appears on the face or upper arm and usually represents a spindle and epithelioid cell nevus *(juvenile melanoma)*; a *giant pigmented nevus (bathing trunk nevus)*, a dark brown to black irregular plaque that is at risk of transformation to malignant melanoma; and the dark brown or black macules that become more numerous with age *(junctional* or *compound nevi)*.

Vascular birthmarks may be divided into the following categories: vascular malformations and vascular tumors (hemangiomas). *Vascular stains (malformations)* are permanent lesions that are present at birth and are initially flat and erythematous. Any vascular structure, capillary, vein, artery, or lymphatic, may be involved. The two most common vascular stains are the *port-wine stain* and *nevus flameus*. The port-wine lesions are pink, red, or, rarely, purple stains of the skin that thicken, darken, and proportionately enlarge as the child grows (Fig. 9-4, *A*). The nevus flameus ("stork bite" or "salmon patch") is usually located on the glabella or nape of the neck (Dohil, Baugh, and Eichenfield, 2000).

Port-wine stains may also be associated with structural malformations, such as glaucoma or leptomeningeal angiomatosis (tumor of blood or lymph vessels in the pia-arach-noid, or *Sturge-Weber syndrome)* or bony and/or muscular overgrowth *(Klippel-Trénaunay-Weber syndrome)*. Children with port-wine stains on the eyelids, forehead, cheeks, or on extremities should be monitored for these syndromes with periodic ophthalmologic examination, neurologic imaging, and measurement of extremities (see Fig. 9-4, *A*).

The treatment of choice for port-wine stains is the use of the flashlamp pulsed dye laser. A series of treatments are usually needed. (See Atraumatic Care box.) The treatments can significantly lighten or completely clear the lesions with almost no scarring or pigment change (Marcus and Goldberg, 1996).

*Capillary hemangiomas,* also sometimes referred to as *strawberry hemangiomas,* are benign cutaneous tumors that involve only capillaries. These are often not apparent at birth but may appear within a few weeks, enlarge considerably during the first year of life, and tend to resolve spontaneously by 2 to 3 years of age. These hemangiomas are bright red, rubbery nodules with a rough surface and a well-defined margin (Fig. 9-4, *B*).

*Cavernous venous hemangiomas* involve deeper vessels in the dermis and have a bluish red color and poorly defined margins. These latter forms may be associated with the trapping of platelets *(Kasabach-Merritz syndrome)* and subsequent thrombocytopenia (Szlachetka, 1998).

Although most hemangiomas usually require no treatment because of their high rate of spontaneous involution, some vision and airway obstruction may necessitate therapy. The pulsed dye laser can effectively reduce some hemangiomas; systemic prednisone administered for 2 to 3 weeks or longer may also deter further growth. Subcutaneous injections of interferon alpha-2A or interferon alpha-2B may be required if prednisone therapy and the pulsed dye laser fail to control a problematic hemangioma (Soumekh, Adams, and Shapiro, 1996); however, associated side effects may outweigh the benefits of therapy in some cases (Dohil, Baugh, and Eichenfield, 2000).

### ATRAUMATIC CARE
#### Laser Therapy

The laser pulse feels like the sharp snap of a rubber band on the skin, and each treatment may involve from 15 to 100 pulses. Therefore children should be given a general anesthetic, sedation, and/or a topical anesthetic, such as EMLA (eutectic mixture of local anesthetics [prilocaine 2.5% and lidocaine 2.5%]) or amethocaine gel 4%* (McCafferty and others, 1997).

---

*Not available in the United States.

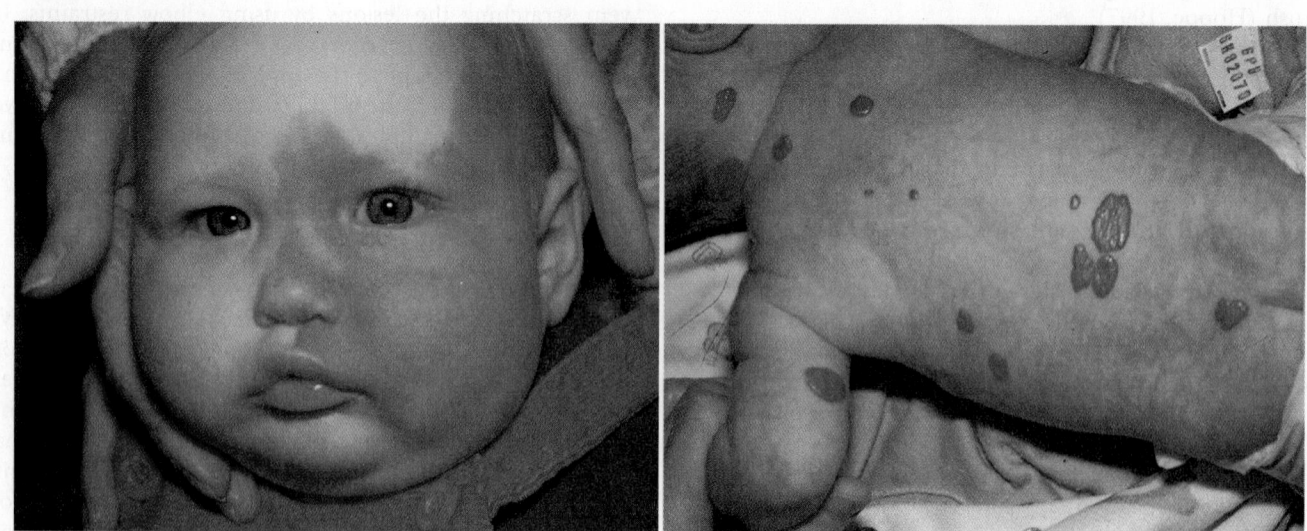

**Fig. 9-4**  **A,** Port-wine stain. **B,** Strawberry hemangioma. (From Zitelli BJ, Davis HW: *Atlas of pediatric physical diagnosis,* ed 3, St Louis, 1997, Mosby.)

## Nursing Considerations

Birthmarks, especially those on the face, are upsetting to parents. Families need an explanation of the type of lesion, its significance, and possible treatment.* They can benefit from seeing photographs of other infants before and after treatment for port-wine stains or after the passage of time for hemangiomas. Pictures taken to follow the involution process may further help parents gain confidence that progress is taking place.

If laser therapy is performed, the lesion will have a purplish black appearance for 7 to 10 days, after which the blackness will fade and give way to redness with an eventual lightening of the treated area. During the treatment phase parents are cautioned to avoid any trauma to the lesion or picking at the scab. The infant's fingernails are trimmed as an added precaution. Washing the area gently with water and dabbing it dry is adequate, although in some cases a topical antibiotic ointment may be used. No salicylates should be given during the treatment phase because they

---

*Information is available from **Hemangioma HOPE** (814) 898-1054; www.hemangiomahope.org and **Vascular Birthmarks Foundation,** (877) VBF-LOOK days, (877) VBF-4646 evenings and weekends; www.birthmark.org/.

decrease the effects of the therapy. The infant should be kept out of the sun for several weeks and then protected with a sunscreen of at least SPF 15. Complications associated with laser treatment include possible secondary infection, keloid or pyogenic granuloma formation, localized dermatitis, and hyperpigmentation or hypopigmentation (Vanderhoof, Doidge, and Maughan, 1998).

# PROBLEMS RELATED TO PHYSIOLOGIC FACTORS

## Hyperbilirubinemia

The term *hyperbilirubinemia* refers to an excessive level of accumulated bilirubin in the blood and is characterized by *jaundice*, or *icterus*, a yellowish discoloration of the skin and other organs. Hyperbilirubinemia is a common finding in the newborn and in most instances is relatively benign. However, in extreme cases, it can indicate a pathologic state.

Hyperbilirubinemia may result from increased unconjugated or conjugated bilirubin. The unconjugated form (Table 9-1) is the type most commonly seen in newborns. The following discussion of hyperbilirubinemia is limited to unconjugated hyperbilirubinemia.

---

**TABLE 9-1**  Comparison of major types of unconjugated hyperbilirubinemia*

| Physiologic Jaundice | Breast-Feeding–Associated Jaundice (Early Onset) | Breast Milk Jaundice (Late Onset) | Hemolytic Disease |
|---|---|---|---|
| **Cause** | | | |
| Immature hepatic function plus increased bilirubin load from red blood cell (RBC) hemolysis | Decreased milk intake related to fewer calories consumed by infant before mother's milk is well-established; enterohepatic shunting | Possible factors in breast milk that prevent bilirubin conjugation<br>Less frequent stooling | Blood antigen incompatibility causes hemolysis of large numbers of RBCs<br>Liver unable to conjugate and excrete excess bilirubin from hemolysis |
| **Onset** | | | |
| After 24 hours (preterm infants, prolonged) | Second to fourth day | Fifth to seventh day | During first 24 hours (levels increase faster than 5 mg/dl/day) |
| **Peak** | | | |
| 72-90 hours | Third to fifth day | Tenth to fifteenth day | Variable |
| **Duration** | | | |
| Declines on fifth to seventh day | Variable | May remain jaundiced for 3-12 weeks or more | Dependent on severity and treatment |
| **Therapy** | | | |
| Phototherapy if bilirubin levels increase significantly (rise in bilirubin greater than 5 mg/dl/day) | Frequent (10-12 times/day) breast-feeding<br>Phototherapy for bilirubin 17-22 mg/dl in healthy term infants (Maisels, 1994) and continue breast-feeding; possibly alternate formula feedings; avoid glucose water and water supplementation | Increase frequency of breast-feeding; use no supplementation such as glucose water; cessation of breast-feeding no longer recommended<br>If bilirubin levels reach 16 mg/dl, may discontinue breast-feeding for 12 hours; if bilirubin levels decrease, breast-feeding can resume<br>May include home phototherapy without discontinuing breast-feeding | *Postnatal*—Phototherapy; if severe, exchange transfusion<br>*Prenatal*—Transfusion (fetus)<br>Prevent sensitization (Rh incompatibility) of Rh-negative mother with RhIG (RhoGAM) |

*Table depicts patterns of jaundice in term infants; patterns in preterm infants will vary according to factors such as gestational age, birth weight, and illness.

## Pathophysiology

*Bilirubin* is one of the breakdown products of hemoglobin that results from red blood cell (RBC) destruction. When RBCs are destroyed, the breakdown products are released into the circulation, where the hemoglobin splits into two fractions: heme and globin. The globin (protein) portion is used by the body, and the heme portion is converted to *unconjugated bilirubin,* an insoluble substance bound to albumin.

In the liver the bilirubin is detached from the albumin molecule and, in the presence of the enzyme *glucuronyl transferase,* is conjugated with glucuronic acid to produce a highly soluble substance, *conjugated bilirubin glucuronide,* which is then excreted into the bile. In the intestine, bacterial action reduces the conjugated bilirubin to urobilinogen, the pigment that gives stool its characteristic color. Most of the reduced bilirubin is excreted through the feces; a small amount is eliminated in the urine (Fig. 9-5).

Normally the body is able to maintain a balance between the destruction of RBCs and the use or excretion of byproducts. However, when developmental limitations or a pathologic process interferes with this balance, bilirubin accumulates in the tissues to produce jaundice. Possible causes of hyperbilirubinemia in the newborn are:

- Physiologic (developmental) factors (prematurity)
- An association with breast-feeding or breast milk
- Excess production of bilirubin (e.g., hemolytic disease, biochemical defects, bruises)
- Disturbed capacity of the liver to secrete conjugated bilirubin (e.g., enzyme deficiency, bile duct obstruction)

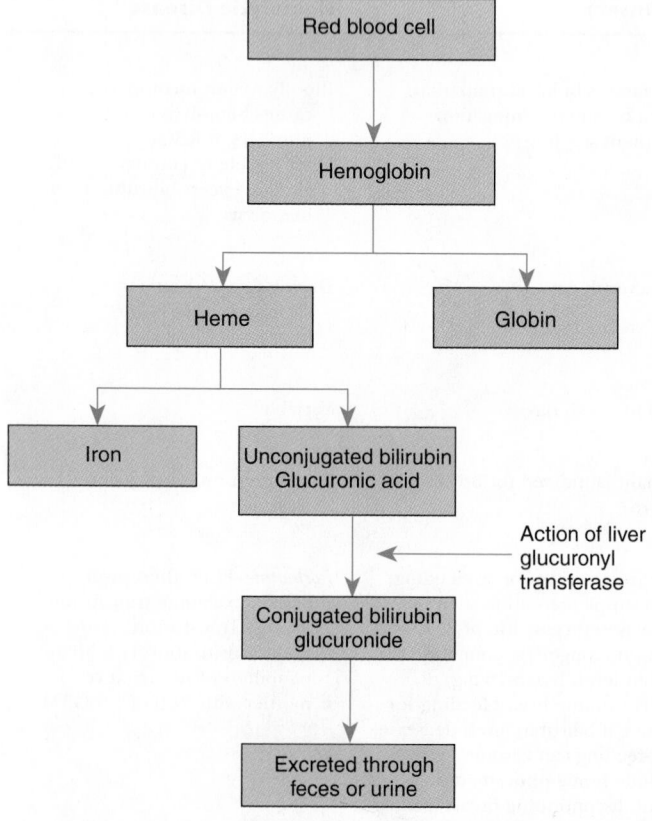

**Fig. 9-5** Formation and excretion of bilirubin.

- Combined overproduction and underexcretion (increased hemolytic process)
- Some disease states (e.g., hypothyroidism, galactosemia, infant of a diabetic mother)
- Genetic predisposition to increased production (Native Americans, Asians)

The first two causes, physiologic factors and an association with breast-feeding, are discussed in the following sections; the third major cause (hemolytic disease) is presented on p. 310.

**Complications.** Unconjugated bilirubin is highly toxic to neurons; therefore an infant with severe jaundice is at risk of developing *bilirubin encephalopathy* (also referred to as kernicterus), a syndrome of severe brain damage resulting from the deposition of unconjugated bilirubin in brain cells. *Kernicterus* describes the yellow staining of the brain cells that may result in bilirubin encephalopathy (Maisels, 1994). The damage occurs when the serum concentration reaches toxic levels, regardless of cause. There is evidence that a fraction of unconjugated bilirubin crosses the blood-brain barrier in neonates with physiologic hyperbilirubinemia. When certain pathologic conditions exist in addition to elevated bilirubin levels, there is an increase in the permeability of the blood-brain barrier to unconjugated bilirubin and, thus, potential irreversible damage. The exact level of serum bilirubin required to cause damage is not yet known.

Multiple factors contribute to bilirubin neurotoxicity; therefore, *serum bilirubin levels alone do not predict the risk of brain injury.* Factors that enhance the development of bilirubin encephalopathy include respiratory acidosis, lowered serum albumin levels, intracranial infections such as meningitis, and abrupt fluctuations in blood pressure. In addition, any condition that increases the metabolic demands for oxygen or glucose (e.g., fetal distress, hypoxia, hypothermia, or hypoglycemia) also increases the risk of brain damage despite lower serum levels of bilirubin. The administration of hypertonic solutions such as glucose and sodium bicarbonate in acutely ill infants, which causes a sudden rise in serum osmolality, has also been implicated as a contributing factor in the development of bilirubin encephalopathy.

The signs of bilirubin encephalopathy are those of central nervous system depression or excitation. Generally, the clinical symptoms appear after the peak plasma bilirubin level has been established for several hours. Prodromal symptoms consist of decreased activity, lethargy, irritability, and a loss of interest in feeding. Within several days these subtle findings are followed by rigid extension of all four extremities, opisthotonos, fever, irritable cry, and seizures. Those who survive may eventually show evidence of neurologic damage, such as mental retardation, attention deficit hyperactivity disorder, delayed or abnormal motor movement (especially ataxia or athetosis), behavior disorders, perceptual problems, or sensorineural hearing loss.

## Physiologic Jaundice

The most common cause of hyperbilirubinemia is the relatively mild and self-limited *physiologic jaundice,* or *icterus neonatorum.* Unlike hemolytic disease of the newborn (see p. 310), physiologic jaundice is not associated with any pathologic process. Although almost all newborns experience elevated bilirubin levels, only about half demonstrate observable signs of jaundice.

Two phases of physiologic jaundice have been identified in term infants. In the first phase bilirubin levels gradually increase to approximately 6 mg/dl on the third day of life, then decrease to a plateau of 2 to 3 mg/dl by the fifth day. Bilirubin levels maintain a steady plateau state in the second phase without increasing or decreasing until approximately 12 to 14 days, at which time levels decrease to the normal value of <1 mg/dl (Maisels, 1994; Volpe, 2001). This pattern varies according to racial group, method of feeding (breast vs bottle), and gestational age (Maisels, 1994). In preterm infants, serum bilirubin levels may peak as high as 10 to 12 mg/dl at 4 to 5 days and decrease slowly over a period of 2 to 4 weeks (Blackburn, 1995; Gartner, 1994).

Infants of Asian descent (as well as Native Americans) have mean bilirubin levels almost twice those seen in Caucasians or African-Americans. An increased incidence of hyperbilirubinemia is seen in newborns from certain geographic areas, particularly areas around Greece. These populations may have glucose-6-phosphate dehydrogenase (G6PD) deficiency, which can cause acute hemolytic anemia. Hyperbilirubinemia also develops in a small number of newborns with Crigler-Najjar syndrome, an inherited disorder in which there is an absence of glucuronyl transferase. Infants with metabolic disorders such as galactosemia or hypothyroidism may also develop hyperbilirubinemia.

**Mechanisms Involved in Physiologic Jaundice.** On average, newborns produce twice as much bilirubin as do adults because of higher concentrations of circulating erythrocytes and a shorter life span of RBCs (only 70 to 90 days, in contrast to 120 days in older children and adults). In addition, the ability of the liver to conjugate bilirubin is reduced because of limited production of glucuronyl transferase. Newborns also have a lower plasma-binding capacity for bilirubin because of lower albumin concentrations than older children. Normal changes in hepatic circulation following birth may contribute to excessive demands on liver function.

Normally, conjugated bilirubin is reduced to *urobilinogen* by the intestinal flora and excreted in feces. However, the sterile and less motile newborn bowel is initially less effective in excreting urobilinogen. In the newborn intestine the enzyme β-glucuronidase is able to convert conjugated bilirubin into the unconjugated form, which is subsequently reabsorbed by the intestinal mucosa and transported to the liver. This process, known as *enterohepatic circulation*, or *shunting*, is accentuated in the newborn and is thought to be a primary mechanism in physiologic jaundice (Blackburn, 1995). Feeding (1) stimulates peristalsis and produces more rapid passage of meconium, thus diminishing the amount of reabsorption of unconjugated bilirubin; and (2) introduces bacteria to aid in the reduction of bilirubin to urobilinogen. Colostrum, a natural cathartic, facilitates meconium evacuation.

**Jaundice in Breast-Feeding Infants.** Breast-feeding is associated with an increased incidence of jaundice. Two types have been identified. *Breast-feeding–associated jaundice (early-onset jaundice)* begins at 2 to 4 days of age and occurs in approximately 10% to 25% of breast-fed newborns. The jaundice is related to the process of breast-feeding and probably results from decreased caloric and fluid intake by breast-fed infants before the milk supply is well established, because fasting is associated with decreased hepatic clearance of bilirubin (Porter and Dennis, 2002).

*Breast milk jaundice (late-onset jaundice)* begins at age 5 to 7 days and occurs in 2% to 3% of breast-fed infants. Rising levels of bilirubin peak during the second week and gradually diminish. Despite high levels of bilirubin that may persist for 3 to 12 weeks, these infants are well. The jaundice may be caused by factors in the breast milk (pregnanediol, fatty acids, and β-glucuronidase) that either inhibit the conjugation or decrease the excretion of bilirubin. Less frequent stooling by breast-fed infants may allow for extended time for reabsorption of bilirubin from stools.

**Clinical Manifestations.** The most obvious sign of hyperbilirubinemia is jaundice, the yellowish discoloration primarily of the sclera, nails, or skin. As a rule, jaundice that appears within the first 24 hours is caused by hemolytic disease of the newborn, sepsis, or one of the maternally derived diseases such as diabetes mellitus or infections. Jaundice that appears on the second or third day, peaks on the third to fourth day, and declines on the fifth to seventh day is usually the result of physiologic jaundice. The intensity of the jaundice is not always related to the degree of hyperbilirubinemia.

**Diagnostic Evaluation.** The degree of jaundice is determined by serum bilirubin measurements. Normal values of unconjugated bilirubin are 0.2 to 1.4 mg/dl. In the newborn, levels must exceed 5 mg/dl before jaundice (icterus) is observable (see Table 9-1). It is important to note, however, that the evaluation of jaundice is not based solely on serum bilirubin levels, but also on the timing of the appearance of clinical jaundice, gestational age at birth, age in days since birth, family history including maternal Rh factor, evidence of hemolysis, feeding method, infant's physiologic status, and progression of serial serum bilirubin levels. The following critera are indicators of pathologic jaundice that, when present, warrant further investigation as to the cause. It is not an all-inclusive list; other factors are also evaluated:

- Appearance of jaundice within 24 hours of birth
- Persistent jaundice after 1 (term neonate) or 2 (preterm) weeks
- Total serum bilirubin levels >12 to 13 mg/dl
- Increase in serum bilirubin >5 mg/dl/day
- Direct bilirubin >1.5 to 2 mg/dl

Noninvasive monitoring of bilirubin via cutaneous reflectance measurements (*transcutaneous bilirubinometry*) allows for repetitive estimations of bilirubin. These devices work well on dark- and light-skinned infants and correlate fairly well with serum determinations of bilirubin levels in full-term infants. With shorter maternity stays, the value of transcutaneous bilirubin measurements as an assessment tool in follow-up home care has been demonstrated in a homogenous population (Ruchala, Seibold, and Stemsterfer, 1996). However, because transcutaneous bilirubin measurements are affected by race, gestational age, and birth weight, their use in heterogenous populations remains limited. Once phototherapy has been initiated, transcutaneous bilirubinometry is no longer useful as a screening tool.

Some studies describe the use of hour-specific serum bilirubin levels to predict newborns at risk for rapidly rising levels, which may not occur until after discharge. Using a nomogram with three levels (high, intermediate, or low risk) of rising values would assist in the determination of which newborns might need further evaluation after discharge. This would require universal bilirubin screening, possibly at the same time as the routine newborn profile (phenylketonuria, galactosemia, and others) (Bhutani, Johnson, and Sivieri, 1999; Johnson and Bhutani, 1998). Newer technologies that may soon be available for monitoring neonatal serum bilirubin values include carbon monoxide indices in exhaled breath (carbon monoxide is produced when RBCs are broken down) (Wheeler, 2000) and the use of a transcutaneous bilirubin meter (BiliCheck) that measures the total serum bilirubin and provides a prediction of risk for hyperbilirubinemia in newborns before discharge (Bhutani and others, 2000).

**Therapeutic Management.** The primary goals in the treatment of hyperbilirubinemia are to prevent bilirubin encephalopathy and, as in any blood group incompatibility, to reverse the hemolytic process (see p. 310). The main form of treatment involves the use of phototherapy. Exchange transfusion is generally used for reducing dangerously high bilirubin levels that occur with hemolytic disease.

The pharmacologic management of hyperbilirubinemia with phenobarbital has centered primarily on the infant with hemolytic disease and is most effective when given to the mother several days before delivery. Phenobarbital promotes (1) hepatic glucuronyl transferase synthesis, which increases bilirubin conjugation and hepatic clearance of the pigment in bile, and (2) protein synthesis, which may increase albumin for more bilirubin binding sites. However, the use of phenobarbital in either the antenatal or the postnatal period has not proved to be as effective as other treatments in reducing bilirubin. Bilirubin production in the newborn can be decreased by inhibiting heme oxygenase—an enzyme needed for heme breakdown (to biliverdin)—with *metalloporphyrins,* especially tin-protoporphyrin and tin-mesoporphyrin. The use of heme-oxygenase inhibitors provides a preventive approach to hyperbilirubinemia (Martinez and others, 1999).

Full-term infants with jaundice may also benefit from early initiation of feedings and frequent breast-feeding. These preventive measures are aimed at promoting increased intestinal motility, decreasing enterohepatic shunting, and establishing normal bacterial flora in the bowel to effectively enhance the excretion of unconjugated bilirubin.

**Phototherapy.** Phototherapy consists of the application of fluorescent light to the infant's exposed skin. Light promotes bilirubin excretion by *photoisomerization,* which alters the structure of bilirubin to a soluble form *(lumirubin)* for easier excretion.

Studies indicate that blue fluorescent light is most effective in reducing bilirubin. However, because blue light alters the coloration of the infant, the normal light of fluorescent bulbs in the spectrum of 420 to 460 nm is often preferred so that the infant's skin can be better observed for color (jaundice, pallor, cyanosis) or other conditions. For phototherapy to be effective, the infant's skin must be fully exposed to an adequate amount of light. When serum bilirubin levels are rapidly increasing or approximating critical levels, double or intensive phototherapy is recommended; this technique involves the application of conventional overhead lamps while the infant is lying on a fiberoptic blanket. The color of the infant's skin does not influence the efficacy of phototherapy. Best results occur within the first 24 to 48 hours of treatment. Phototherapy alone is not effective in the management of hyperbilirubinemia where levels are at a critical level or are rising rapidly; it is designed primarily for the treatment of mild to moderate hyperbilirubinemia.

An alternative to traditional phototherapy "bililights" is the *fiberoptic blanket* or *panel* (Wallaby,* Biliblanket†), which consists of a light-generating illuminator, a bundle of plastic fibers affixed to a panel that distributes the energy, and a soft, disposable, light-permeable cover to protect the infant. The blanket delivers therapeutic light consistently and continuously to the infant and achieves the same photoisomerization as conventional phototherapy. The fiberoptic blanket is especially suited for home phototherapy. The portable blanket permits more infant-parent interaction, as well as better temperature control because the infant can be covered. It also eliminates the need for using eye patches (*if the infant's eyes are not exposed to a direct light source*) and placing the lights at the correct distance. However, special caution should be taken to prevent exposing the fragile skin of extremely immature or compromised infants to the fiberoptic blanket because dermal injury has been reported (Woo, 1998).

The American Academy of Pediatrics (1994) practice parameter provides suggestions for initiating phototherapy in healthy term infants (Table 9-2). The authors emphasize that the initiation of phototherapy should always be based on individual clinical judgment rather than serum bilirubin levels alone.

Preterm infants have a higher risk of developing pathologic jaundice at lower serum bilirubin levels than healthy term infants because of associated illness factors that may alter the blood-brain barrier's susceptibility to bilirubin (Gartner, 1994). Therefore the recommendation for starting phototherapy in infants weighing 1500 g is at levels of 5 to 8 mg/dl; for those weighing <1500 to 1999 g, levels of 8 to 12 mg/dl; and for those weighing 2000 to 2499 g, levels of 11 to 14 mg/dl (Maisels, 1994). However, each infant should be carefully evaluated with other illness and risk factors in mind, rather than depending on absolute values for all infants in a specific group.

Phototherapy has not been found to cause long-term adverse effects. The effectiveness of treatment is determined by a decrease in serum bilirubin. Concurrently, the infant's

---

*Fiberoptic Medical Products, Inc, Allentown, PA.
†Ohmeda, Columbia, MO.

**TABLE 9-2** Management of hyperbilirubinemia in the healthy term newborn

| Age (Hours) | TSB Level mg/dl (μmol/L)* | | | |
|---|---|---|---|---|
| | Consider Phototherapy | Phototherapy | Exchange Transfusion if Intensive Phototherapy Fails | Exchange Transfusion and Intensive Phototherapy |
| ≤24† | — | — | — | — |
| 25-48 | ≥12 (170) | ≥15 (260) | ≥20 (340) | ≥25 (430) |
| 49-72 | ≥15 (260) | ≥18 (310) | ≥25 (430) | ≥30 (510) |
| >72 | ≥17 (290) | ≥20 (340) | ≥25 (430) | ≥30 (510) |

From American Academy of Pediatrics, Provisional Committee for Quality Improvement and Subcommittee on Hyperbilirubinemia: Practice parameter: management of hyperbilirubinemia in the healthy newborn, *Pediatrics* 94(4):558-562, 1994.
*TSB indicates total serum bilirubin.
†Term infants who are clinically jaundiced at ≤24 hours old are not considered healthy and require further evaluation.

total physical status is assessed continually because the suppression of jaundice by phototherapy may mask signs of sepsis, hemolytic disease, or hepatitis.

**Management of Breast-Feeding Jaundice.** Recommendations for prevention and management of early-onset jaundice in breast-fed infants are to monitor for early stooling, initiate early and frequent breast-feeding, and discourage the use of dextrose water, formula, or water. The infant's weight, voiding, and stooling along should be evaluated along with the breast-feeding pattern (Lawrence and Lawrence, 1999).

Bilirubin levels are monitored in late-onset jaundice and treatment options vary. If the serum bilirubin levels remain above 16 mg/dl for more than 24 hours, breast-feeding may be interrupted for 12 hours and repeat levels drawn; with a serum bilirubin level decrease of 2 mg/dl or more, the infant may resume breast-feeding if levels are below 15 mg/dl. In the event that levels do not drop significantly, further evaluation is necessary (Lawrence and Lawrence, 1999). It is not within the scope of this text to discuss the full spectrum of treatment possibilities; therefore, other sources should be consulted. Whenever possible, parents should be offered the option of continuing breast-feeding, provided that the jaundiced infant is being closely monitored for additional contributing factors. Home phototherapy and continued breast-feeding is an option for the family with a jaundiced newborn.

**Prognosis.** Early recognition and treatment of neonatal hyperbilirubinemia prevents unnecessary medical therapies, parent-infant separation, breast-feeding disruption and possibly failure, and the potential for bilirubin encephalopathy. The characteristic features of bilirubin encephalopathy include sensorineural hearing loss, dental enamel hypoplasia, gaze paralysis, athetosis (involuntary writhing movements), and delayed motor skills; intellectual impairment is reported to be mild.

## Nursing Considerations

### Assessment

Part of the routine physical assessment includes observing for evidence of jaundice at regular intervals. Jaundice is most reliably assessed by observing the infant's skin color from head to toe and the color of the sclerae and mucous membranes. Applying direct pressure to the skin, especially over bony prominences such as the tip of the nose or the sternum, causes blanching and allows the yellow stain to be more pronounced. Also, bilirubin (especially at high levels) is not uniformly distributed in skin. The nurse observes the infant in natural daylight for a true assessment of color.

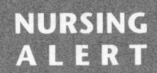

**NURSING ALERT** Evidence of jaundice that appears before the infant is 24 hours of age is an indication for assessing bilirubin levels.

The transcutaneous bilirubin meter is a useful screening device and is used to detect neonatal jaundice in full-term infants. Because phototherapy reduces the accuracy of the instrument, its value is limited to assessments made before the initiation of phototherapy. Institutions in which the device is used set up their own criteria based on their experience with their particular instrument. Blood samples are also taken for the measurement of bilirubin in the laboratory.

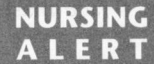

**NURSING ALERT** While blood is drawn, phototherapy lights are turned off, and the blood is transported in a covered tube to avoid a false reading as a result of bilirubin destruction in the test tube.

With short hospital stays, jaundice may appear after discharge. A careful history from the parents may reveal significant familial patterns of hyperbilirubinemia (older siblings of the infant). Other considerations in assessment include the ethnic origin of the family (e.g., higher incidence in Asian infants), type of delivery (e.g., induction of labor), and infant characteristics such as weight loss after birth, gestational age, sex, and presence of any bruising. The method and frequency of feeding are assessed.

### Nursing Diagnoses

After the nursing assessment, a number of nursing diagnoses become evident. The most likely diagnoses are outlined and discussed in the Nursing Care Plan on pp. 313-314. Others may be apparent in individual cases.

### Planning

The goals for the infant with hyperbilirubinemia and the family are as follows:

1. Infant will receive appropriate therapy as needed to reduce serum bilirubin levels.

2. Infant will experience no complications from therapy.
3. Family will receive emotional support.
4. Family will be prepared for home phototherapy (if prescribed).

## Implementation

Basic nursing care of the child with hyperbilirubinemia differs from that of any newborn infant only in management of specific therapy. (See Nursing Care of the Newborn and Family, Chapter 8, and Nursing Care of High-Risk Newborns, Chapter 10.)

Prevention of physiologic and breast-feeding jaundice may be possible with early introduction of feedings and frequent nursing without water supplementation. Every effort is made to provide an optimum thermal environment to reduce metabolic needs.

**Phototherapy.** The infant who receives phototherapy is placed nude under the light source and repositioned frequently to expose all body surface areas to the light. Once phototherapy has been initiated, frequent (every 6 to 12 hours) serum bilirubin levels are necessary because visual assessment of jaundice is no longer considered valid.

Several precautions are instituted to protect the infant during phototherapy. The infant's eyes are shielded by an opaque mask to prevent exposure to the light (Fig. 9-6). The eye shield should be properly sized and correctly positioned to cover the eyes completely but prevent any occlusion of the nares. The infant's eyelids are closed before the mask is applied because the corneas may become excoriated if they come in contact with the dressing. The newborn's eyes are checked at least every 4 to 6 hours for evidence of discharge, excessive pressure on the lids, or corneal irritation. Eye shields are removed during feedings, which provide the opportunity for visual and sensory stimulation. A special light-permeable phototherapy diaper, Bilibottoms,* or bikini diaper fashioned with a face mask may be used to cover the genitalia and buttocks.

---

*Available from Bilibottoms, Inc, 10 Laurel Dr, Hershey, PA 17033, (717) 533-0995; www.bilibottoms.com

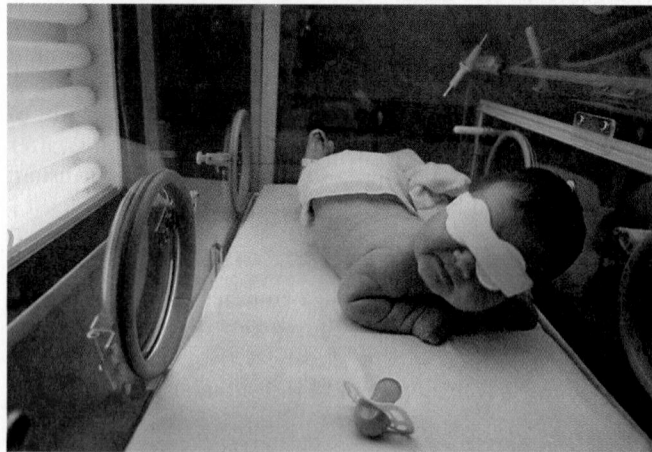

**Fig. 9-6** Infant under phototherapy unit. Note that the eyes are shielded and a diaper is used to contain the diarrheal stools.

The phototherapy unit may be combined with a radiant heat warmer or servocontrolled incubator to provide an optimum thermal environment. The thermistor should be attached to the infant or covered with a reflector patch so that it is not exposed to direct radiation. This may require changing the sensor from the abdomen to the back according to the infant's position. Placing the sensor on the infant's side reduces the need for frequent changes. Vital signs are taken at least every 4 hours to ensure that the infant's body temperature is normothermic.

Infants who are in an open crib must have a protective Plexiglas shield between them and the fluorescent lights to minimize the amount of undesirable ultraviolet light reaching their skin and to protect them from accidental bulb breakage. Their temperature is closely monitored to prevent hyperthermia or hypothermia. Maintaining the infant in a flexed position with rolled blankets along the sides of the body helps maintain heat and provides comfort.

Accurate charting is another important nursing responsibility and includes (1) times that phototherapy is started and stopped, (2) proper shielding of the eyes, (3) type of fluorescent lamp (by manufacturer), (4) number of lamps, (5) distance between surface of lamps and infant (should be no less than 18 inches), (6) use of phototherapy in combination with an incubator or open bassinet, (7) photometer measurement of light intensity, and (8) occurrence of side effects.

**Side Effects of Phototherapy.** Minor side effects for which the nurse should be alert include loose, greenish stools; transient skin rashes; hyperthermia; increased metabolic rate; dehydration; electrolyte disturbances, such as hypocalcemia; and priapism. To prevent or minimize these effects, the temperature is monitored to detect early signs of hypothermia or hyperthermia, and the skin is observed for evidence of dehydration and drying, which can lead to excoriation and breakdown. Oily lubricants or lotions are not used on the skin in order to prevent increased tanning, or a "frying" effect. Full-term infants receiving phototherapy may require additional fluid volume to compensate for insensible and intestinal fluid loss. Because phototherapy enhances the excretion of unconjugated bilirubin through the bowel, loose stools may indicate accelerated bilirubin excretion. Frequent stooling can cause perianal irritation; therefore meticulous skin care, especially keeping the skin clean and dry, is essential.

Once phototherapy is permanently discontinued, there is often a subsequent increase in the serum bilirubin level, often called the "rebound effect"; this is usually transient and resolves without resuming therapy.

Another reaction to phototherapy is the **bronze-baby syndrome,** in which the serum, urine, and skin turn grayish brown several hours after the infant is placed under the light. This reaction is probably caused by retention of a bilirubin breakdown product of phototherapy, possibly copper porphyrin. The syndrome almost always occurs in infants who have elevated *conjugated* hyperbilirubinemia and some degree of cholestasis. The browning generally resolves following discontinuation of phototherapy.

**Family Support.** Parents need reassurance concerning their infant's progress. All of the procedures are explained to familiarize them with the benefits and risks. Parents need to be reassured that the naked infant under the bilirubin light is warm and comfortable. Parents may be concerned about the eye shields because "blindness" is a frightening experience. Eye shields are removed when the parents are visiting to facilitate the attachment process. The parents can be reassured that the neonate is accustomed to darkness after months of intrauterine existence and benefits a great deal from auditory and tactile stimulation. (See Family Focus box.)

The initiation of any treatment requires *informed consent* by the parents for the therapy prescribed; however, in the case of phototherapy considerable anxiety may rightfully occur when such words as "kernicterus" and "brain damage" are used to describe possible effects of nontreatment. It is imperative that nurses remain sensitive to parents' feelings and information needs during this process; an important nursing intervention is the assessment of the parents' understanding of the treatment involved and clarification of the nature of the therapy. One of the most important nursing interventions is recognition of breast-feeding jaundice. Lack of familiarity among health professionals has caused many newborns prolonged hospitalization, termination of breast-feeding, and unnecessary phototherapy. Care of the new mother may include supporting successful and frequent breast-feeding. Parents also need reassurance of the benign nature of the jaundice and encouragement to resume breast-feeding if temporary cessation is prescribed. Unfortunately, jaundice increases the risk of breast-feeding being discontinued and development of the vulnerable child syndrome—the belief of parents that their child has suffered a "close call" and is vulnerable to serious injury. (See Critical Thinking Exercise box.)

**Discharge Planning and Home Care.**  With short hospital stays, mothers and infants may be discharged before evidence of jaundice is present. It is imperative that the nurse discuss signs of jaundice with the mother because any clinical symptoms will probably appear at home. Parents are taught to evaluate the number of voids and evidence of adequate breast-feeding once the infant is at home and are encouraged to bring the newborn to the hospital, clinic, or primary care practitioner if there are indications of hyperbilirubinemia (Wheeler, 2000). Home visits within 2 to 3 days following discharge to evaluate feeding and elimination patterns and jaundice are becoming routine for some health care organizations. (See Evidence-Based Practice box on p. 311.)

If home phototherapy is instituted, the hospital or home health care nurse is usually responsible for teaching family members and assessing their abilities to implement the treatment safely and in a timely manner. General guidelines for home care preparation and education are discussed in

---

**FAMILY FOCUS**

*Phototherapy and Parent-Infant Interaction*

The traditional use of phototherapy has evoked concerns regarding a number of psychobehavioral issues, including parent-infant separation, potential social isolation, decreased sensorineural stimulation, altered biologic rhythms, altered feeding patterns, and activity changes. Parental anxiety is greatly increased, particularly at the sight of the newborn blindfolded and under special lights. The interruption of breast-feeding for phototherapy is a potential deterrent to successful maternal-infant attachment and interaction. Because research has demonstrated that bilirubin catabolism occurs primarily within the first few hours of the initiation of phototherapy, there is increased support for the removal of the infant from treatment for feeding and holding. Intermittent phototherapy may be just as effective as continuous therapy when used correctly. The benefits of stopping phototherapy for parental feeding and holding outweigh concerns related to the clearance of bilirubin in the healthy term newborn with mild-to-moderate hyperbilirubinemia. Home phototherapy offers an additional opportunity to foster parent-infant attachment.

---

### Critical Thinking Exercise

*Jaundice*

A 10-day-old full-term newborn is brought to the hospital laboratory for a follow-up serum bilirubin measurement. While waiting for laboratory results, the mother becomes tearful and expresses concern that the baby may have a serious illness because of her breast milk and a high bilirubin level. The baby, although quite jaundiced, is well-hydrated and alert. The mother says the baby has been breast-feeding every 3 to 4 hours and empties both breasts. In addition, the baby has a normal elimination pattern. The physician has recommended that she interrupt breast-feeding for 24 hours. The total bilirubin level is 18 mg/dl. Given these facts and the mother's concern, what is the best intervention?

FIRST, THINK ABOUT IT . . .

- What information are you using?
- If you accept the conclusion, what are the implications?

1. Encourage the mother to further verbalize her concerns about having a child with possible brain damage.
2. Encourage the mother to use an automatic breast pump to maintain her milk supply.
3. Prepare for an exchange transfusion to decrease the infant's bilirubin level.
4. Suggest that the mother consider stopping breast-feeding to prevent further jaundice.

*The best response is two. The age of the baby, health status, and feeding pattern support the concept of hyperbilirubinemia caused in part by breast-feeding. If you accept the conclusion that breast milk jaundice is a normal physiologic occurrence, the implications may be that the mother needs further reassurance that she may resume breast-feeding once the bilirubin level starts decreasing (usually within 24 hours of interrupting breast-feeding).*

*The first intervention is not correct because of the infant's healthy, well-nourished status and the fact that kernicterus is not a likely occurrence given the clinical findings. An exchange transfusion is not appropriate therapy in this particular situation, and discontinuing breast-feeding is almost always unnecessary.*

Chapters 8 (Early Newborn Discharge Checklist), 25, and 26. Written instructions and supervision of care—especially the application of eye shields, if needed—are essential. The minor side effects of phototherapy are reviewed, and parents may need instruction in taking axillary temperatures and recording times and amounts of feedings and the number of wet diapers and stools. Regardless of how benign the disorder or the therapy, parents need support and understanding. Siblings also benefit from an explanation of the therapy to allay fears or misconceptions.

In jaundice associated with breast-feeding, follow-up blood studies are usually required to assess the progress of the jaundice. If temporary cessation of breast-feeding is prescribed, mothers should be taught to pump the breasts every 3 to 4 hours to maintain lactation; the expressed milk is frozen for use after breast-feeding is resumed.

## ✷ Evaluation

The effectiveness of nursing interventions is determined by continual reassessment and evaluation of care based on the following observational guidelines:

1. Observe skin color; review bilirubinometric and/or laboratory findings.
2. Evaluate feeding and elimination pattern.
3. Check placement of eye shields; observe skin for signs of dehydration; monitor infant's temperature.
4. Interview family members and observe parent-infant interactions.

The *expected outcomes* are described in the Nursing Care Plan on pp. 313-314.

## Hemolytic Disease of the Newborn (HDN)

Hyperbilirubinemia in the first 24 hours of life is most often the result of HDN (erythroblastosis fetalis), an abnormally rapid rate of RBC destruction. Anemia caused by this destruction stimulates the production of RBCs, which in turn provides increasing numbers of cells for hemolysis. Major causes of increased erythrocyte destruction are isoimmunization (primarily Rh) and ABO incompatibility.

### Blood Incompatibility

The membranes of human blood cells contain a variety of *antigens,* also known as *agglutinogens,* substances capable of producing an immune response if recognized by the body as foreign. The reciprocal relationship between antigens on RBCs and antibodies in the plasma causes *agglutination* (clumping). In other words, antibodies in the plasma of one blood group (except the AB group, which contains no antibodies) produce agglutination when mixed with antigens of a different blood group. In the *ABO blood group system* the antibodies occur naturally. In the *Rh system* the person must be exposed to the Rh antigen before significant antibody formation takes place and causes a sensitivity response known as *alloimmunization.*

**Rh Incompatibility (Alloimmunization).** The Rh blood group consists of several antigens (with D being the most prevalent). For simplicity, only the terms *Rh-positive* (presence of antigen) and *Rh-negative* (absence of antigen) are used in this discussion. (See Autosomal Inheritance Patterns, Chapter 5.) The presence or absence of the naturally occurring Rh factor determines the blood type.

Ordinarily, no problems are anticipated when the Rh blood types are the same in both mother and fetus or if the mother is Rh-positive and the infant is Rh-negative. Difficulty may arise when the mother is Rh-negative and the infant is Rh-positive. Although the maternal and fetal circulations are separate, fetal RBCs (with antigens foreign to the mother) sometimes gain access to the maternal circulation through minute breaks in the placental vessels. The mother's natural defense mechanism responds to these alien cells by producing anti-Rh antibodies.

Under normal circumstances, this process of alloimmunization has no effect on the fetus during the first pregnancy with an Rh-positive fetus, because the initial sensitization to Rh antigens rarely occurs before the onset of labor. However, with the increased risk of fetal blood being transferred to the maternal circulation during placental separation, maternal antibody production is stimulated. During a subsequent pregnancy with an Rh-positive fetus, these previously formed maternal antibodies to Rh-positive blood cells enter the fetal circulation, where they attach to and destroy fetal erythrocytes (Fig. 9-7). Multiple gestation, abruptio placenta, placenta previa, manual removal of the placenta, and cesarean delivery increase the incidence of transplacental hemorrhage and subsequent alloimmunization.

Because the condition begins in utero, the fetus attempts to compensate for the progressive hemolysis by accelerating the rate of erythropoiesis. As a result, immature RBCs *(erythroblasts)* appear in the fetal circulation, hence the term *erythroblastosis fetalis.*

There is wide variability in the development of maternal sensitization to Rh-positive antigens. Sensitization may occur during the first pregnancy if the woman previously received an Rh-positive blood transfusion. No sensitization may occur in situations in which a strong placental barrier prevents transfer of fetal blood into the maternal circulation. In approximately 10% to 15% of sensitized mothers, there is no hemolytic reaction in the newborn. In addition, some Rh-negative women, even though exposed to Rh-positive fetal blood, are immunologically unable to produce antibodies to the foreign antigen (Neal, 2001).

In the most severe form of erythroblastosis fetalis *(hydrops fetalis),* the progressive hemolysis causes fetal hypoxia, cardiac failure, generalized edema (anasarca), hydrops, and effusions into the pericardial, pleural, and peritoneal spaces. The fetus may be delivered stillborn or in severe respiratory distress. Maternal RhIG administration, early intrauterine detection of alloimmunization by ultrasonography, and chorionic villus sampling and subsequent treatment by fetal blood transfusions have dramatically improved the outcome of affected fetuses (Gruslin-Giroux and Moore, 1997; Schumacher and Moise, 1996).

**ABO Incompatibility.** Hemolytic disease can also occur when the major blood group antigens of the fetus are different from those of the mother. The major blood groups are A, B, AB, and O. The incidence of these blood groups

## EVIDENCE-BASED PRACTICE
### Newborn Jaundice, Early Discharge, and Breast-Feeding

The demand for cost containment in the United States continues to change current models of health care delivery. This is evident in perinatal care because delivery of a healthy-appearing newborn by a healthy mother essentially represents a "wellness" event. There is concern, however, for mothers and newborns who do not fit into the wellness model yet are discharged home as early as 6 to 12 hours after delivery. These mother-infant pairs may not be considered "high risk" during hospitalization because of the seemingly healthy course of their short hospital stays, but the infant may become high risk at home.

Nurses are the primary educators for mother-infant pairs. However, mothers in the early postpartum period are not able to absorb large amounts of information (Rubin, 1961). There is evidence that maternal cognitive deficits in the first postpartum day may impair the mother's inability to adequately retain infant care information (Eidelman and Kaitz, 1996).

Many factors require the nurse's expertise in the postpartum period when caring for the mother-newborn pair. It is essential to assess the newborn during the hospital stay for subtle cues that may impair future healthy outcomes and adaptation. The newborn must first make a successful transition to extrauterine existence to survive at home. Cardiopulmonary, digestive, eliminatory, and thermoregulatory functions must be well-established. Many newborns do not successfully accomplish an effective latch-on with a regular breast-feeding pattern until after discharge. It may take as long as 3 to 4 days to establish adequate production of maternal milk. Therefore in-hospital assessments of feeding adaptation are often inadequate—a newborn effectively sucking on a pacifier or bottle nipple does not automatically indicate breast-feeding will be successful.

Another factor to consider is that most newborns do not become visibly jaundiced until rather late in the second or third day of life, often before the mother's milk supply has been adequately established. Breast-fed newborns tend to have more clinical jaundice than those who are bottle-fed (Maisels and Newman, 1998). If the mother is either unsuccessful in establishing breast-feeding or lacks confidence in her infant caregiving skills, there is potential for compounding the problem—increasing jaundice and the inability to successfully nourish the infant. Yet if early discharge has occurred, this mother-newborn pair is often no longer considered to be within the health care system, where guidance and help can be given. Pascale and others (1996) identified a strong relationship between short hospital stays, jaundice, dehydration, and unsuccessful breast-feeding in a sample of healthy term newborns. These researchers stress the importance of ensuring that breast-feeding is proceeding well and that adequate teaching regarding complications occurs before discharge.

It has been previously hypothesized that kernicterus, or bilirubin encephalopathy, does not occur in the healthy breast-fed infant. There have been reports of kernicterus occurring in seemingly healthy breast-fed term infants without hemolytic disease or sepsis (Maisels and Newman, 1995). Others have reported increased readmission rates for hyperbilirubinemia following early discharge in term breast-fed infants (Seidman and others, 1995). Grupp-Phelan and colleagues (1999) found that newborns sent home early (<30 hours) were more likely to be readmitted within 2 weeks for jaundice than newborns with longer stays (>2 days). Furthermore, newborns readmitted were more likely to have been born to primiparas, teenagers younger than 18, and women on Medicaid. Newborns discharged early before a weekend (Thursday through Saturday) were more likely to be readmitted than those discharged Sunday through Wednesday, suggesting that the inability to access the primary care provider over the weekend had an impact on newborn readmission rates. These researchers concluded, however, that ending early discharge practices will probably not prevent newborn readmissions. JCAHO (Joint Commission on Accreditation of Healthcare Organizations) recently issued an alert to hospitals urging them to monitor newborns being discharged home for jaundice and educate parents about jaundice in an attempt to decrease the incidence of neonatal kernicterus (Joint Commission, 2001).

What then is the solution to the complexity of early discharge, newborn jaundice, and the effective establishment of breast-feeding? Home visits by a perinatal nurse for each mother-newborn pair within 2 to 3 days after discharge may be an effective solution. Some health care providers have implemented this model, often with variations such as phone consults after discharge in addition to home visits (Brown, Towne, and York, 1996). A home visit program also works well with breast-feeding education and support for new mothers discharged early (Johnson, Brennan, and Flynn-Tymkow, 1999). In a study of inner-city infants discharged early, more visits were made to the primary health care clinic in the first month of life than those who were not discharged early (Cooper and others, 1996). In yet another study, hospital readmission of infants showed a strong association with breast-feeding (81%); 94% of the infants readmitted with jaundice or dehydration were breast-fed in comparison to the control group (67%), who were neither jaundiced nor breast-fed. The researchers proposed that discharge before the successful establishment of breast-feeding was a major factor in readmission rates (Soskolne and others, 1996). One final question was posed by the researchers: If hospital costs are decreased by shorter postpartum stays, could not some of the costs of readmission be prevented through adequate follow-up? The establishment of community health centers where maternal-newborn follow-up care may occur is a viable option.

A number of health care organizations have established clinics where mothers may return for a postpartum visit within 2 to 3 days of discharge to receive counseling regarding newborn jaundice, elimination patterns, and feeding (breast or bottle). There were reports of a decrease in the incidence of newborn readmissions and an increase in breast-feeding rates when such services are available to mothers and newborns (Keppler and Roudebush, 1999; Nelson, 1999). One program instituted a practical discharge information sheet for parents, and physicians were encouraged to use the hyperbilirubinemia risk nomogram (Bhutani and others, 2000) in order to decrease the number of potential newborn problems and readmissions related to early postpartum discharge (LaReau, 2000). Home visits or clinic facilities where patients may return shortly after discharge for assistance are no doubt helpful in many areas, yet there exists a large percentage of persons in the United States who do not have insurance coverage for a pediatrician or clinic visit. A large indigent population with transportation, economic, and social problems presents logistic challenges for health care planners in regard to follow-up care after early discharge so that newborn problems that occur after discharge may be effectively managed (Jackson and others, 2000).

One might question whether a new model of perinatal health care delivery is emerging or is a rebirth of the days when public health nurses visited new mothers in the home to assist with delivery and subsequent maternal-newborn care. Are early home visits a tenable solution to early discharge, breast-feeding success, and assessment of newborn well-being, including resolution of jaundice without negative outcomes? What about the increasing mobility of the population today? Are there maternal-newborn pairs who *do not wish to have* home visits? Clearly there are situations wherein every model of care, regardless of its seeming practicality and decreased cost, will not meet the needs of every mother-newborn pair. Just as there are deficits in seeking prenatal care despite widespread availability, there will be those infants whose health care needs remain unmet unless creative nurses are active in the development and implementation of new models of care.

The perinatal nurse is faced with the challenge of ensuring that the newborn makes an effective transition to extrauterine life, assessing for evidence of associated problems such as jaundice, and assisting the mother in establishing effective breast-feeding. As health care delivery models change, nurses will be found in nontraditional settings and in the home providing the care formerly provided in acute care institutions. (See Prepare for Discharge and Home Care, Chapter 8).

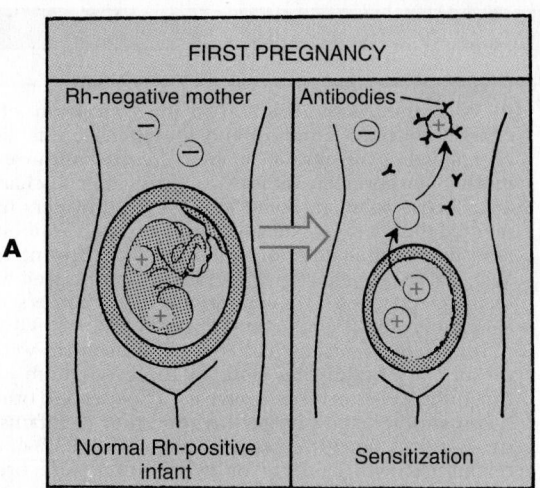
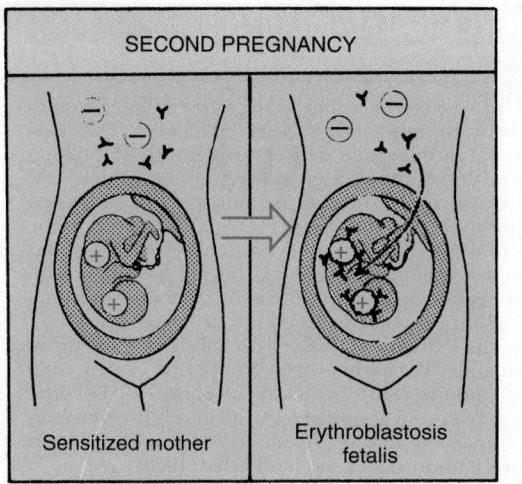

**Fig. 9-7** Development of maternal sensitization to Rh antigens. **A,** Fetal Rh-positive erythrocytes enter maternal system. Maternal anti-Rh antibodies are formed. **B,** Anti-Rh antibodies cross placental barrier and attach to fetal erythrocytes.

**TABLE 9-3** ABO relationships of antigens/antibodies and donor-recipient compatibility

| Blood Group (Phenotype) | Genotype | RBC Antigens | Plasma Antibodies | RBC Compatibility | |
|---|---|---|---|---|---|
| | | | | As Donor to Type | As Recipient From Type |
| A | AA,AO | A | B | AB,A | O,A |
| B | BB,BO | B | A | AB,B | O,B |
| AB | AB | A and B | None | AB | O,A,B,AB |
| O | OO | None | A and B | AB,A,B,O | O |

**TABLE 9-4** Potential maternal-fetal ABO incompatibilities

| Maternal Blood Group | Incompatible Fetal Blood Group |
|---|---|
| O | A or B |
| B | A or AB |
| A | B or AB |

varies according to race and geographic location. In the North American white population, 46% have type O blood, 42% have type A blood, 9% have type B blood, and 3% have type AB blood.

The presence or absence of antibodies and antigens determines whether agglutination will occur (Table 9-3). Antibodies in the plasma of one blood group (except the AB group, which contains no antibodies) will produce agglutination (clumping) when mixed with antigens of a different blood group. Naturally occurring antibodies in the recipient's blood cause agglutination of a donor's RBCs. The agglutinated donor cells become trapped in peripheral blood vessels, where they hemolyze, releasing large amounts of bilirubin into the circulation.

The most common blood group incompatibility in the neonate is between a mother with O blood group and an infant with A or B blood group. (See Table 9-4 for possible ABO incompatibilities.) Naturally occurring anti-A or anti-B antibodies already present in the maternal circulation cross the placenta and attach to fetal RBCs, causing hemolysis. Usually the hemolytic reaction is less severe than in Rh incompatibility. Unlike the Rh reaction, ABO incompatibility may occur in the first pregnancy. The risk of significant hemolysis in subsequent pregnancies is thought to be unchanged from the first (Luchtman-Jones, Schwartz, and Wilson, 1997).

**Clinical Manifestations**

Jaundice appears shortly after birth (during the first 24 hours), and serum levels of unconjugated bilirubin rise rapidly. Anemia results from the hemolysis of large numbers of erythrocytes, and hyperbilirubinemia and jaundice result from the liver's inability to conjugate and excrete the excess bilirubin. Most newborns with HDN are not jaundiced at birth. However, hepatosplenomegaly and varying degrees of hydrops may be evident. If the infant is severely affected, hydrops, anemia and hypovolemic shock are apparent. Hypoglycemia may occur as a result of pancreatic cell hyperplasia.

**Diagnostic Evaluation**

The diagnosis of alloimmunization can be made early in the pregnancy by chorionic villus sampling to determine fetal blood group and type; drawbacks to the procedure include

# Nursing Care Plan
## The Newborn with Hyperbilirubinemia

**NURSING DIAGNOSIS:** Risk for injury from breakdown products of red blood cells in greater numbers than normal and functional immaturity of liver

**PATIENT GOAL 1:** Will receive appropriate therapy if needed to accelerate bilirubin excretion

- **NURSING INTERVENTIONS/*RATIONALES***

Initiate early feedings *to enhance excretion of bilirubin in the stool*

Assess skin for evidence of jaundice, *which indicates rising bilirubin levels*

Check bilirubin levels with blood levels and/or transcutaneous bilirubinometry *to determine rising levels*

Note time of initial jaundice *to distinguish physiologic jaundice (appears after 24 hours) from jaundice due to hemolytic disease or other causes (appears before 24 hours)*

Assess infant's overall status, especially factors (e.g., hypoxia, hypothermia, hypoglycemia, and respiratory acidosis) *that increase the risk of altering the blood-brain barrier*

Initiate phototherapy as prescribed

- **EXPECTED OUTCOMES**

Newborn begins feeding soon after birth

Newborn is exposed to prescribed light source

**PATIENT GOAL 2:** Will experience no complications from phototherapy

- **NURSING INTERVENTIONS/*RATIONALES***

Shield infant's eyes*

Make certain that lids are closed before applying shield *to prevent corneal irritation*

Check eyes every 4-6 hours for drainage or irritation

Place infant nude under light *for maximum skin exposure*

Change position frequently, especially during the first several hours of treatment, *to increase body surface exposure*

Monitor body temperature *to detect hypothermia or hyperthermia*

Check axillary temperature

Chart duration of therapy, type of lights, distance of lights from infant, use of open or closed bassinet, and shielding of infant's eyes *to document correct use of phototherapy*

With increased stooling, cleanse skin frequently *to prevent perianal irritation*

Avoid use of oily applications on skin *to prevent burning*

Ensure adequate fluid intake *to prevent dehydration*

- **EXPECTED OUTCOME**

Infant displays no evidence of eye irritation, dehydration, temperature instability, or skin breakdown

**PATIENT GOAL 3:** Will experience no complications from exchange transfusion (if therapy required)

- **NURSING INTERVENTIONS/*RATIONALES***

Give infant nothing by mouth before procedure (usually for 2 to 4 hours) *to prevent aspiration*

Check donor blood for correct blood group and Rh type *to*

---

*May not be required for fiberoptic blanket.

*prevent transfusion reaction*

Assist practitioner during procedure; ensure asepsis *to prevent infection*

Keep accurate records of amounts of blood infused and withdrawn *to maintain proper blood volume*

Maintain optimum body temperature of infant during procedure *to prevent hypothermia and cold stress or hyperthermia*

Observe for signs of exchange transfusion reaction (tachycardia or bradycardia, respiratory distress, dramatic change in blood pressure, temperature instability, and rash) *to initiate therapy promptly*

Have resuscitation equipment (supplemental oxygen, airway, manual resuscitation bag, endotracheal tube, and laryngoscope) at bedside *to be prepared for an emergency*

Check umbilical site for bleeding or infection

Monitor vital signs during and following transfusion *to detect complications such as cardiac arrhythmias*

- **EXPECTED OUTCOMES**

Infant exhibits no signs of adverse effects from exchange transfusion

Vital signs remain within normal limits (see inside back cover for normal variations)

There is no evidence of infection or bleeding at infusion site

**NURSING DIAGNOSIS:** Interrupted family processes related to infant with potentially adverse physiologic response

**PATIENT (FAMILY) GOAL 1:** Will receive emotional support

- **NURSING INTERVENTIONS/*RATIONALES***

Discontinue phototherapy during family visiting; remove infant's eye shields *to promote family interaction*

Emphasize benign nature of physiologic jaundice *to prevent undue parental concern and potential overprotection of child*

Assure family that skin will regain normal pigmentation

Advise breast-feeding mothers of possibility of prolonged jaundice

Emphasize benign nature of jaundice and benefits of human milk *to prevent early termination of breast-feeding*

Evaluate breast-feeding latch-on and mother's comfort level with feeding process before discharge

Encourage frequent breast-feeding

- **EXPECTED OUTCOME**

Family demonstrates an understanding of therapy and prognosis

**PATIENT (FAMILY) GOAL 2:** Will be prepared for home phototherapy (if prescribed)

- **NURSING INTERVENTIONS/*RATIONALES***

Assess family's understanding of jaundice and proposed therapy *to ensure optimum results and safety*

*Continued*

## Nursing Care Plan

## The Newborn with Hyperbilirubinemia—cont'd

Instruct family regarding:

Placement and care of phototherapy device or fiberoptic unit

Proper eye care*

Apply eye patches

Close lids before applying patches

Be certain patches fit snugly with no possibility of light leaks

Remove patches when light is discontinued—during feeding, bathing, and other caregiving activities, at least once every 4 to 6 hours

Proper positioning while under phototherapy device*

Rotate to expose all areas of skin

―――――――――
*May not be required for fiberoptic blanket.

Keep infant nude or dressed in mini-diaper

Providing increased fluid intake

Measuring axillary temperature

Keeping log of time spent under light, infant's color, feeding patterns, amount of feedings, number of voids and stools

Observing for signs of lethargy, change in sleeping pattern, any difficulty arousing infant, changes in stooling or voiding

Keeping diaper area clean and dry

Importance of bilirubin tests as prescribed

• EXPECTED OUTCOME

Family demonstrates ability to provide home phototherapy for infant (specify learning and methods of demonstration)

―――――――――

possible early spontaneous abortion and the risk of fetomaternal hemorrhage and alloimmunization. Another diagnostic method to determine alloimmunization is an amniocentesis using polymerase chain reaction (PCR) to determine the fetal blood type, hemoglobin, hematocrit, and presence of maternal antibodies (Schumacher and Moise, 1996). Percutaneous umbilical fetal blood sampling (PUBS) is considered to be the most accurate means for assessing the severity of fetal hemolytic disease in the absence of fetal hydrops (Bowman, 1999). With either method the determination of an Rh-negative fetus requires no further treatment. Ultrasonography is considered an important adjunct in the detection of alloimmunization; alterations in the placenta, umbilical cord, and amniotic fluid volume, as well as the presence of fetal hydrops, can be detected with high-resolution ultrasonography and allow early noninvasive treatment before the development of erythroblastosis (Gruslin-Giroux and Moore, 1997; Whitecar and Moise, 2000). Erythroblastosis fetalis caused by Rh incompatibility can also be assessed by evaluating rising anti-Rh antibody titers in the maternal circulation (*indirect Coombs test*) or by testing the optical density of amniotic fluid (delta $OD_{450}$ test), because bilirubin discolors the fluid. Ultrasonography may also be used to detect fetal anemia in the non-hydroptic fetus (Mari, 2000).

The disease in the newborn is suspected on the basis of the timing and appearance of jaundice (see Table 9-1) and can be confirmed postnatally by detecting antibodies attached to the circulating erythrocytes of affected infants (*direct Coombs test* or *direct antiglobulin test* [*DAT*]). The Coombs test is routinely performed on cord blood samples from infants born to Rh-negative mothers.

### Therapeutic Management

The primary aim of therapeutic management of alloimmunization is prevention. Postnatal therapy usually entails phototherapy for mild cases and exchange transfusion for more severe forms. In severe cases of hydrops aggressive interven-

tions such as pericardial and pleural fluid aspiration, mechanical ventilatory support, and inotrope therapy may be required for stabilization. Although phototherapy may control bilirubin levels in mild cases, the hemolytic process may continue, causing severe anemia between 7 and 21 days of life.

**Prevention of Rh Alloimmunization.** The administration of Rho immune globulin (RhIG), a human gamma globulin concentrate of anti-D, to all *unsensitized* Rh-negative mothers after delivery or abortion of an Rh-positive infant or fetus prevents the development of maternal sensitization to the Rh factor. The injected anti-Rh antibodies are thought to destroy (by subsequent phagocytosis and agglutination) fetal RBCs passing into the maternal circulation before they can be recognized by the mother's immune system. Because the immune response is blocked, anti-D antibodies and memory cells (which produce the primary and secondary immune responses, respectively) are not formed. The inhibition of memory cell formation is especially important because memory cells provide long-term immunity by initiating a rapid immune response once the antigen is reintroduced (McCance and Heuther, 1998).

To be effective, RhIG (such as RhoGAM) must be administered to unsensitized mothers within 72 hours (but possibly as long as 3 to 4 weeks) after the first delivery, miscarriage, or abortion, and repeated after subsequent pregnancies. The administration of RhIG at 26 to 28 weeks gestation further reduces the risk of Rh alloimmunization. RhIG is not effective against existing Rh-positive antibodies in the maternal circulation. The use of a heme-oxygenase inhibitor, such as tin-mesoprophyrin (given IM to the newborn), has proved effective in the preventive treatment of hyperbilirubinemia (Martinez and others, 1999).

**NURSING ALERT**   RhIG is administered intramuscularly, not intravenously, and only to Rh-negative women with a negative Coombs test—**never** to the infant or father.

**Intrauterine Transfusion.**   Infants of mothers already sensitized may be treated by intrauterine transfusion, which consists of infusing blood into the umbilical vein of the fetus. The need for therapy is based on the antenatal diagnosis of alloimmunization by determining the optical density of amniotic fluid (by amniocentesis) as an index of fetal hemolysis, or by serial ultrasonography, which may detect the presence of fetal hydrops as early as 16 weeks of gestation (Bowman, 1999; Schumacher and Moise, 1996). With ultrasound technology fetal transfusion may be accomplished directly via the umbilical vein, infusing Rh O-negative packed RBCs to raise the fetal hematocrit to 40%; fetal movement and transfusion risks are minimized by administering a muscle paralyzing drug for temporary fetal paralyzation. The frequency of intrauterine transfusions may vary according to institution yet may be as often as every 2 weeks until the fetus reaches pulmonary maturity at approximately 37 to 38 weeks of gestation (Gruslin-Giroux and Moore, 1997; Schumacher and Moise, 1996). Long-term follow-up studies of children who had severe hemolytic anemia and intrauterine transfusions demonstrate appropriate intellectual growth and development (Hudon and others, 1998). The use of intraperitoneal blood transfusions is employed less commonly for alloimmunization because of higher associated fetal risks; however, it may be used for cases in which intravascular access is impossible.

**Exchange Transfusion.**   Exchange transfusion, in which the infant's blood is removed in small amounts (usually 5 to 10 ml at a time) and replaced with compatible blood (Rh-negative blood), is a standard mode of therapy for treatment of severe hyperbilirubinemia that is unresponsive to phototherapy and is the treatment of choice for severe hyperbilirubinemia and hydrops caused by Rh incompatibility. Exchange transfusion removes the sensitized erythrocytes, lowers the serum bilirubin level to prevent bilirubin encephalopathy, corrects the anemia, and prevents cardiac failure. Indications for exchange transfusion include rapidly increasing serum bilirubin levels and hemolysis despite aggressive phototherapy (see Table 9-2). The criteria for exchange transfusion in preterm infants vary according to associated illness factors. An infant born with hydrops fetalis or signs of cardiac failure is a candidate for immediate exchange transfusion with fresh whole blood.

For exchange transfusion, fresh whole blood is typed and cross-matched to the mother's serum. The amount of donor blood used is usually double the blood volume of the infant, which is approximately 85 ml/kg body weight. The two-volume exchange transfusion replaces approximately 85% of the neonate's blood.

An exchange transfusion is a sterile surgical procedure. A catheter is inserted into the umbilical vein and threaded into the inferior vena cava. Depending on the infant's weight, 5 to 10 ml of blood is withdrawn within 15 to 20 seconds, and the same volume of donor blood is infused over 60 to 90 seconds. If the blood has been citrated (addition of citrate phosphate dextrose adenine to prevent coagulation), calcium gluconate may be given after the infusion of each 100 ml of donor's blood to prevent hypocalcemia.

**ABO Incompatibility.**   The treatment for ABO hemolytic disease is early detection and implementation of phototherapy for the reduction of hyperbilirubinemia. The initial diagnosis is often more difficult because the direct Coombs test may be negative or weakly reactive. The presence of jaundice within the first 24 hours, elevated serum bilirubin levels, RBC spherocytosis, and increased erythrocyte production are diagnostic of ABO incompatibility. In some centers intravenous immune globulin transfusions are used in combination with phototherapy to treat ABO incompatibility (Hammerman and others, 1996). Exchange transfusion is not commonly required for ABO incompatibility except when phototherapy fails to decrease bilirubin concentrations.

**Prognosis.**   The severe anemia of alloimmunization may result in stillbirth, shock, congestive heart failure, poor feeding, or poor weight gain. Complications from exchange transfusion are uncommon.

### Nursing Considerations

The initial nursing responsibility is recognizing jaundice. The possibility of hemolytic disease can be anticipated from the prenatal and perinatal history. Prenatal evidence of incompatibility, maternal blood type O, and a positive Coombs test are cause for increased vigilance for early signs of jaundice in an infant.

If an exchange transfusion is required, the nurse prepares the infant and the family and assists the practitioner with the procedure. Documentation of blood volumes exchanged, including the amount of blood withdrawn and infused, the time of each procedure, and the cumulative record of the total volume exchanged, are kept. Vital signs, monitored electronically, are evaluated frequently and correlated with the removal and infusion of blood. If signs of cardiac or respiratory problems occur, the procedure is stopped temporarily and resumed once the infant's cardiorespiratory function stabilizes. The nurse also observes for signs of transfusion reaction.

**NURSING ALERT**   Signs of blood exchange transfusion reaction include:
Tachycardia or bradycardia
Respiratory distress
Dramatic change in blood pressure
Temperature instability
Rash

Throughout the procedure attention must be given to the infant's thermoregulation. Hypothermia increases oxygen and glucose consumption, causing metabolic acidosis. Not only do these consequences hinder the infant's overall physical ability to withstand the long procedure, but they also inhibit the binding capacity of albumin and bilirubin and the hepatic enzymatic reactions, thus increasing the risk of kernicterus. Conversely, hyperthermia damages the donor erythrocytes, elevating the free potassium content and predisposing the infant to cardiac arrest.

The exchange transfusion is performed under a radiant warmer. However, the infant is usually covered with sterile drapes that may prevent the radiant heat from sufficiently warming the skin; a temperature-controlled warming pad under the infant may prevent hypothermia during the procedure. The blood is also warmed (using specially designed devices, never microwave ovens) before infusion.

After the procedure is completed, the nurse inspects the umbilical site for evidence of bleeding. Usually the catheter remains in place in case repeated exchanges are required.

**Family Support.**   Parents often feel guilty because they think they have caused the blood incompatibility. Parents should never be made to feel responsible or negligent. They are encouraged to verbalize and express their thoughts. Actions that were taken to prevent any problems, such as frequent antepartum examinations and blood tests, should be referred to and praised.

## Hypoglycemia

Hypoglycemia is present when the newborn's blood glucose concentration is lower than the body's requirement for cellular energy and metabolism. However, the precise definition of hypoglycemia for every newborn in regard to gestational age, birth weight, metabolic needs, and illness- or wellness-state remains quite controversial. Cornblath and others (2000) have suggested an operational threshold at which interventions to increase serum glucose levels should be instituted to prevent serious effects. For the healthy term infant, born after an uneventful pregnancy and delivery, recommendations are to monitor glucose levels only if risk factors are present (see following) or there are clinical manifestations of hypoglycemia; in these infants a plasma glucose less than 45 mg/dl (2.5 mmol/L) requires intervention. Healthy term, breast-fed newborns may not fit into this category because human milk appears to provide adequate substrate (Cornblath and others, 2000). Hoseth and others (2000) evaluated blood glucose levels in healthy term, breast-fed infants and found that there was no significant hypoglycemia in all but 2 of the 223 infants during the first 4 days of life. Maternal tobacco use, method of delivery, and anesthetic were found not to have affected the infants' glucose levels.

In infants who are at risk for altered metabolism as a result of maternal illness factors (diabetes, pregnancy-induced hypertension, terbutaline administration) or newborn factors (perinatal hypoxia, infection, hypothermia, polycythemia, congenital malformations, hyperinsulinism, small for gestational age, fetal hydrops), it is recommended that close observation and blood glucose levels be monitored within 2 to 3 hours of birth. If the newborn has a blood glucose below 36 mg/dl (2.0 mmol/L), intervention such as breast or bottle feeding should be instituted; if levels remain low despite feeding, intravenous dextrose is warranted. In such infants the treatment should be aimed at maintaining the blood glucose levels above 45 mg/dl (2.5 mmol/L) (Cornblath and others, 2000). Blood glucose levels for infants with severe hyperinsulinism may need to be higher (60 mg/dl; 3.3 mmol/L) to prevent serious effects. Hypoglycemia in preterm infants requires further studies, but it has been suggested that values be maintained above 47 mg/dl (2.6 mmol/L) (Cornblath and others, 2000).

Studies have shown that infants with blood glucose values below 47 mg/dl had decreased cognitive and motor abilities later in life (Lucas, Morley, and Cole, 1988). There is additional evidence that fetal glucose concentrations should optimally be above 50 mg/dl for appropriate brain development to occur (Marconi and others, 1993).

Other normal glucose values for neonatal hypoglycemia are often cited by different authors; the decision regarding when to treat the hypoglycemic newborn is not based on a single plasma glucose value but on a number of clinical factors (Cowett, 1999; Schwartz, 1997; Stanley and Baker, 1999).

### Pathophysiology

After birth the infant must supply nutrients to meet energy requirements for maintaining body temperature, respiration, muscular activity, and regulation of blood glucose. Glucose is derived primarily from glycogen stores deposited in the liver, heart, and skeletal muscles during the last trimester of pregnancy.

The brain is especially dependent on adequate glucose supply for appropriate function. There is evidence of a major shift in energy metabolism from glucose to carbohydrate in newborns during the first several hours of life, thus the importance for provision of adequate energy substrate. Although newborns demonstrate the ability to use ketones and amino acids as energy substrate, there are certain limitations; infants with severe hyperinsulinism are unable to compensate metabolically and require more glucose than normal. Conditions that decrease the availability of substrate or prevent appropriate metabolism of available substrate, place the infant at risk for hypoglycemia. These include but are not limited to intrauterine growth failure, prematurity, maternal diabetes, maternal use of hypoglycemic drugs, maternal administration of tocolytics such as terbutaline and ritodrine, intrapartum administration of glucose, perinatal hypoxia, infection, hypothermia, polycythemia, fetal hydrops, inborn errors of metabolism such as galactosemia, certain congenital malformations, endocrine disorders, abnormal extrauterine transition, and failure to receive adequate perinatal nutrition. The different types of neonatal hypoglycemia may be categorized and include:

**Early transitional neonatal**—Large-for-gestational-age or normal-size infants who appear to suffer from transient hyperinsulinism
**Classic transient neonatal**—Infants who suffered intrauterine malnutrition that depleted glycogen and fat stores (small-for-gestational-age [SGA] and polycythemic infants)
**Secondary-associated**—A response to perinatal stresses that increase the infant's metabolic needs relative to glycogen stores (associated with birth asphyxia, intracranial hemorrhage, and congenital anomalies)
**Recurrent, severe**—Caused by an enzymatic or metabolic-endocrine defect such as chronic hyperinsulinism

### Clinical Manifestations

The signs of hypoglycemia are usually vague and often indistinguishable from those observed in other newborn conditions, such as hypocalcemia, septicemia, central nervous system disorders, or cardiorespiratory problems. Because the brain depends on glucose for energy, cerebral signs such as jitteriness, tremors, twitching, weak or high-pitched cry, lethargy, hypotonia, limpness, seizures, and coma are prominent. Other clinical manifestations are cyanosis, apnea, rapid and irregular respirations, sweating, eye rolling, and refusal to feed. The symptoms often are transient but recurrent.

### Diagnostic Evaluation

Diagnosis is confirmed by direct analysis of blood glucose concentration. Two consecutive specimens of blood should be analyzed because of the many factors that can affect correct readings.

> **NURSING ALERT** Proper handling of the specimen is essential because storage at room temperature increases glycolysis. Accurate readings can be facilitated by storing the blood sample on ice to slow cellular metabolism or by removing the red blood cells through centrifugation.

Blood glucose levels may be determined with a reagent strip such as Dextrostix or Chemstrip-BG, which may be read manually or with a glucose reflectance meter. Although simple procedures, the tests are very sensitive and must be performed correctly to prevent a false reading. The accuracy of reagent strips at low levels (<40 mg/dL) is unreliable for clinical screening of hypoglycemia (Cornblath and Ichord, 2000).

A number of bedside blood glucose meters (glucometers) are used to screen newborns for hypoglycemia. The reliability of such meters in the neonate (term and preterm) has been adequately established. However, strict quality monitoring, regular calibration, and adherence to strict protocols are necessary to ensure accuracy (Brooks, 1997; Innanen and others, 1997; Martin and others, 1997). The most accurate method is the laboratory analysis of serum glucose. Blood specimens may be obtained from heel, arterial, or venous punctures. (See Atraumatic Care box.) The American Academy of Pediatrics (1993) does not recommend universal screening for hypoglycemia in full-term neonates.

### Therapeutic Management

Intravenous infusion of glucose is one method of treating hypoglycemia. In full-term infants who are borderline hypoglycemic and clinically asymptomatic, the early institution of bottle-feeding or breast-feeding may reestablish normoglycemia, thus avoiding the need for intravenous glucose. Infants who are at increased risk for developing hypoglycemia should have their blood glucose measured within 1 hour after birth. The procedure should be repeated every 1 to 2 hours for the first 6 to 8 hours, then every 4 to 6 hours for 2 days.

Oral glucose feedings are often used as a treatment for hypoglycemia in healthy newborns; however, formula and breast milk are just as effective. Hypoglycemia can be prevented in most instances by the initiation of early feeding in normoglycemic newborns. Breast-fed infants should be put

**ATRAUMATIC CARE**
*Blood Glucose Testing*

To obtain an optimal amount of blood with minimal bruising and squeezing, prewarm the heel with a warm cloth for 10 minutes and use a spring-loaded automatic puncture device such as Tenderfoot. An optical bedside glucose monitor calibrated to neonatal hematocrit is more reliable than reagent strips (Cornblath and others, 2000). Heel bruising in preterm infants was decreased when an automatic incision device was used instead of a manual lancet (Vertanen and others, 2001).

to breast as soon as possible after delivery. (See Infants of Diabetic Mothers, Chapter 10, for management of hypoglycemia related to hyperinsulinemia.)

### Nursing Considerations

Much of the nursing responsibility for the infant with hypoglycemia involves identification of the problem through careful observation of physical status. Another concern is to reduce environmental factors, such as cold stress and respiratory difficulty, that predispose the infant to the development of a decreased blood glucose level. The use of proper feeding techniques promotes adequate ingestion of nutrients, particularly carbohydrates.

Major nursing objectives also include preventing, anticipating, and recognizing potential dangers of concentrated dextrose infusion. Too-rapid infusion of the hypertonic solution can cause circulatory overload, hyperglycemia, and intracellular dehydration. Maintaining the ordered flow rate with an intravenous pump and checking and charting hourly intake decreases the chance of such hazards. If the intravenous infusion has been temporarily discontinued, the rate is not increased to make up for the fluid lost during the interruption.

The infusion is administered through a peripheral vein to increase hemodilution of the concentrated solution and to prevent irritation of the vessel walls. Extravasation of the fluid into the surrounding area can cause tissue sloughing. Termination of the glucose solution must be gradual to prevent hypoglycemia caused by hyperinsulinism.

Because hypoglycemia may be a symptom of some other underlying pathophysiologic process, parents are usually very concerned about their infant's progress, particularly because these infants do not feed well or behave responsively. Nurses need to be aware of parents' thoughts, allow them to express their feelings, and keep them aware of the infant's progress.

## Hyperglycemia

Hyperglycemia in the newborn is usually defined as a blood glucose concentration greater than 125 mg/dl in the full-term infant or greater than 150 mg/dl in the preterm infant. Affected infants are usually low-birth-weight infants who are unable to tolerate intravenous glucose infusions at the usual rate. The glucose intolerance is probably related to general immaturity of the usual regulatory mechanisms. Increased blood glucose levels may also occur in infants with sepsis or decreased insulin sensitivity (such as infants with transient diabetes mellitus), infants receiving methylxanthines, and infants who are stressed (infants with respiratory distress syndrome, infants undergoing surgical procedures).

Hyperglycemia is usually asymptomatic but detected on routine screening. Most often, hyperglycemia is treated by reducing the infant's glucose intake. Insulin infusion is sometimes administered to very-low-birth-weight infants who require but are unable to tolerate IV dextrose solutions with concentrations greater than 5 g/dl.

### Nursing Considerations

Blood glucose is monitored frequently, especially in the infant receiving insulin. This requires numerous heelsticks, and sites should be rotated to minimize tissue damage. (See Blood Specimens, Chapter 27.) Urinary output is carefully measured to detect any evidence of glycosuria and possible osmotic diuresis.

As in the care of all infants, parents are given a careful explanation of the therapy, provided with frequent progress reports, and given support to reduce anxiety. (See Nursing Care of High-Risk Newborns, Chapter 10.)

## Hypocalcemia

As with many conditions in the neonate, hypocalcemia is difficult to differentiate from other disorders (sepsis, meningitis, narcotic withdrawal, hypoglycemia), and the etiology is ill-defined. There are two times during the neonatal period when the incidence is highest. *Early-onset hypocalcemia,* which appears within the first 24 to 48 hours, is the more common form and typically affects the preterm or small-for-gestational-age infant who has experienced perinatal hypoxia. An infant born to a diabetic mother may also experience early hypocalcemia. Symptoms include jitteriness, prolonged QT interval, apnea, cyanotic episodes, a high-pitched cry, and abdominal distention.

*Late-onset hypocalcemia,* which is not apparent until after the first 3 to 4 days of life, is commonly referred to as *cow's milk-induced hypocalcemia* or *neonatal tetany.* It is observed in well-nourished infants who are fed modified cow's milk, such as evaporated milk formula. Cow's milk, which has a high phosphorus content, produces hyperphosphatemia and a resultant hypocalcemia by either increasing calcium deposition in the bone and soft tissues, enhancing the hypocalcemic effect of calcitonin, or inhibiting the calcemic response to parathyroid hormone (Demarini, Mimouni, and Tsang, 1997). Late hypocalcemia may also be seen in infants with intestinal malabsorption, hyperinsulinemia hypoparathyroidism, or hypomagnesemia. Hypocalcemia may also occur as a result of the administration of phosphate enemas (Walton and others, 2000).

The manifestations of neonatal tetany reflect neuromuscular irritation—twitching, tremors, and focal or generalized convulsive seizures that can be triggered by even minor stimuli and vary in duration from a few seconds to several minutes. Neonatal tetany is rarely seen in industrialized countries because of the prevalent use of commercial formula or human milk as the newborn's primary source of nutrition.

### Diagnostic Evaluation

Diagnosis of hypocalcemia is confirmed with serum electrolyte determinations. Normal neonatal serum calcium values are usually in the range of 7.0 to 8.5 mg/dl (1.75 to 2.12 mmol/L).

In full-term infants hypocalcemia is indicated at total serum calcium levels below 7.8 to 8 mg/dl (1.95 to 2.0 mmol/L) or ionized calcium levels (the biologically important fraction of calcium) below 4.4 mg/dl (1.1 mmol/L) (Demarini, Mimouni, and Tsang, 1997). Most clinicians consider the serum ionized calcium to be the best standard for monitoring blood calcium activity.

### Therapeutic Management

In most instances early-onset hypocalcemia is temporary and resolves in 1 to 3 days. Restoration of a normal calcium level is facilitated by early feedings, physiologic correction of hypoparathyroidism and, sometimes, administration of calcium supplements.

Treatment of hypocalcemia involves intravenous administration of 10% calcium gluconate. The drug is administered slowly over 10 to 30 minutes or as a continuous infusion. Rapid intravenous calcium administration may cause cardiac dysrhythmias and circulatory collapse. The heart rate and blood pressure should be electronically monitored. Care must be taken to ascertain that the infusion device is positioned within the vein because extravasation into surrounding tissue causes local necrosis, calcification, and sloughing. Intramuscular administration of calcium gluconate is contraindicated because it precipitates in the tissue, causing necrosis. If the infant can tolerate oral fluids, oral doses of calcium are given. Caution must be exercised in the use of oral calcium salts because of their hypertonicity and subsequent effects on the bowel of at-risk infants.

### Nursing Considerations

Nursing care of the infant with hypocalcemia is directed toward identifying the cause of the manifestations observed and administering calcium. The infant is monitored continuously during intravenous infusions. Calcium gluconate can cause tissue necrosis and scar formation; therefore it is recommended that the scalp veins be avoided. Calcium gluconate is also incompatible with a number of drugs, most notably sodium bicarbonate ($NaHCO_3$), which is often given for metabolic acidosis. To prevent tissue necrosis, the infusion site is observed carefully and changed as needed.

The nurse also observes for signs of acute hypercalcemia (vomiting, bradycardia). If such symptoms occur, the injection or infusion is discontinued and the practitioner is notified. Seizure precautions are instituted because seizures are common. Minor stimuli (e.g., picking the infant up for a feeding or a sudden jarring of the crib) can provoke tremors or seizures. During the acute phase, the environment around the infant is manipulated to allow for maximal rest and minimal activity.

The restlessness, irritability, and seizure activity of the hypocalcemic infant are of much concern to the parents. The nurse supports the parents during the hospitalization and emphasizes that the condition will subside rapidly with no subsequent ill effects. During the acute phase, parents are advised to disturb the infant as little as possible. However, as soon as the calcium level rises they are encouraged to hold and feed the infant in order to reestablish parent-child attachment.

If the infant is discharged on formula feedings supplemented with calcium salts, the parents are taught the correct procedure for diluting the mineral in the formula and are advised to use only the prescribed formula.

## Hemorrhagic Disease of the Newborn

Hemorrhagic disease of the newborn is a bleeding disorder that occurs as a result of a vitamin K deficiency. Hemorrhagic disease of the newborn may be classified according to appearance as early, classic, or late onset. Newborn vitamin K stores are virtually absent, and there is a moderate deficiency of prothrombin activity, which decreases until approximately 72 hours after birth and then begins to increase. Consequently, vitamin K–dependent coagulation factors (II, VII, IX, X) are significantly reduced. In addition, the newborn's sterile intestinal tract is unable to synthesize the vitamin until feedings have begun.

Signs and symptoms of hemorrhagic disease typically appear early within hours of birth and can include oozing from the umbilicus or circumcision site, bloody or black stools, hematuria, ecchymoses on the skin and scalp, epistaxis, or bleeding from punctures. *Classic* hemorrhagic disease usually occurs 1 to 7 days after birth; signs and symptoms are the same as those seen with early-onset disease. Diagnosis can be confirmed in the presence of prolonged prothrombin time (PT) and partial thromboplastin time (PTT) accompanied by normal platelet count and fibrinogen level.

A late form of hemorrhagic disease *(late-onset)* appears at approximately 2 to 12 weeks of age. This form occurs in totally or predominantly breast-fed infants who did not receive adequate vitamin K prophylaxis at birth. Although vitamin K levels in breast milk appear to be lower than in cow's milk–based formulas, the results of previous studies indicate that hemorrhagic disease occurred in infants who were exclusively breast-fed and who did not receive the standard prophylaxis at birth or were given a single dose of oral vitamin K (Lawrence and Lawrence, 1999). Manifestations of late-onset disease include evidence of intracranial hemorrhage, deep ecchymoses, bleeding from the gastrointestinal tract, and/or bleeding from mucous membranes, skin punctures, or surgical incisions.

### Therapeutic Management

The goal of management is prevention of hemorrhagic disease of the newborn with prophylactic administration of vitamin K. In the United States, intramuscular administration of vitamin K (AquaMEPHYTON and Mephyton) in a dose of 0.5 to 1 mg once during the first 24 hours of life is a standard practice. The current recommendation to prevent hemorrhagic disease in infants who are breast-fed is to provide intramuscular vitamin K at birth and for the mother to have a well-balanced diet (Lawrence and Lawrence, 1999). Oral vitamin K preparations are unavailable in the United States but may be given in other countries. A single oral dose of vitamin K may be inadequate to raise serum vitamin K levels; therefore, it is recommended that oral doses of vitamin K be given shortly after birth, at 1 to 2 weeks, and a third dose at one month to prevent hemorrhagic disease (Lawrence and Lawrence, 1999; Puckett and Offringa, 2000). The use of prophylactic vitamin K is not routinely practiced in all countries. Despite the recent controversy surrounding the use of vitamin K in newborns and a possible link to childhood cancer, its use continues to be strongly recommended for the prevention of hemorrhage (American Academy of Pediatrics and American College of Obstetricians and Gynecologists, 1997; Buck, 2001).

In newborns with hemorrhagic disease, treatment is the same as the preventive measures except that the vitamin may be given intravenously to prevent a hematoma at an intramuscular site. Bleeding usually ceases within 2 to 4 hours of vitamin K administration.

### Nursing Considerations

Nursing care is directed primarily toward prevention and involves careful administration of the vitamin into the vastus lateralis muscle or ventrogluteal (not dorsogluteal) muscle. In instances in which this procedure is not routinely carried out (e.g., home births or emergency deliveries), the nurse observes for signs of the disorder and notifies the practitioner for appropriate diagnosis and treatment. Breast-feeding mothers are encouraged to increase their intake of foods containing vitamin K, primarily vegetables. The best sources are green vegetables, especially broccoli.

According to one study, even at the recommended daily dietary intake of 1 $\mu$g/kg/day, breast-feeding mothers had suboptimal levels of vitamin K in their milk. Maternal oral vitamin K supplements of 5 mg/day increased the human milk concentration of the vitamin to acceptable levels (Greer and others, 1997).

## INBORN ERRORS OF METABOLISM (IEMs)

IEMs include a large number of inherited diseases caused by the absence or deficiency of a substance essential to cellular metabolism, usually an enzyme. When the normal metabolic process is interrupted as a result of a missing enzyme, an accumulation of substances precedes the interruption, the end product of the process is absent, or the process takes an alternate metabolic pathway. The consequence is manifested as an illness. Most IEMs are characterized by abnormal protein, carbohydrate, or fat metabolism.

All biochemical processes are under genetic control, and each consists of a complex sequence of reactions. Fig. 9-8, *A,* schematically represents a portion of a normal metabolic pathway. A *substrate* (the substance on which an enzyme acts) is converted to a product through the action of a specific enzyme. A *metabolic pathway* consists of many such reactions, or steps; each step depends on the previous reaction, and each is catalyzed by a specific enzyme.

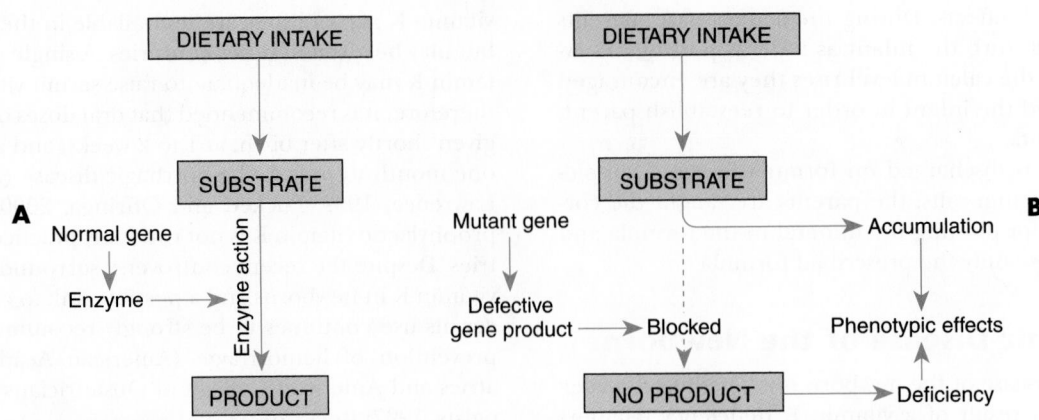

**Fig. 9-8**  Metabolic pathway. **A,** Normal metabolic pathway. **B,** Effect of defective gene action.

A specific gene is responsible for the production of a specific enzyme in the metabolic pathway. Fig. 9-8, *B*, illustrates the interruption of this process by a change in a gene that interferes with the synthesis of an essential enzyme. A block in the normal pathway can produce the following:

- Accumulation of the substances preceding the block, such as galactose in galactosemia or phenylalanine in phenylketonuria
- A deficiency in the product, such as thyroxine in familial hypothyroidism
- An increase in the products of alternate metabolic pathways when these pathways are used, such as the production of phenylketones in phenylketonuria

These effects of defective gene action are observable in the individual as diseases.

The mode of inheritance in IEMs is almost always autosomal recessive. The heterozygote has one gene with a normal effect and is still able to produce the enzyme in sufficient amounts to carry out the metabolic function under normal circumstances. Therefore the heterozygote does not exhibit symptoms of the disorder. The homozygote, who inherits a defective gene from both parents, has no functioning enzyme and thus is clinically affected.

Individually, different IEMs are rare; collectively they account for a significant proportion of health problems in children. It is becoming possible to detect and screen for an increasing number of IEMs—to detect the presence of the disease in the heterozygote, the newborn, and the fetus. With most IEMs, early diagnosis and prompt treatment are essential to prevent a relentless course of physical and mental deterioration. Prenatal diagnosis provides for special care of the infant immediately after birth. Neonatal screening is useful in detecting many disorders after a few days of life, but it is less helpful in detecting symptoms early in the neonatal period. Nurses caring for neonates must be certain that screening is performed, especially in infants who are discharged early, born at home, or in neonatal intensive care units. (See Genetic Screening, Chapter 5.) Most screening tests require a heel puncture to obtain sufficient blood to completely cover circles on special blotting paper. (See Atraumatic Care box on p. 317 for measures to reduce the pain of lancing and squeezing the heel and see Newborn Screening, Chapter 8.)

Some nonspecific manifestations—including lethargy, poor feeding, vomiting, diarrhea, hypoglycemia, metabolic acidosis, respiratory distress, apnea, hypothermia, coma, and seizures—are observed in a wide variety of genetic and acquired disorders. The time of onset may be important. Most IEMs produce no symptoms during the first 24 hours of life. Other manifestations that may indicate an IEM include jaundice, hepatomegaly, unusual odor (sweat, urine), abnormal eating patterns (food aversions, vomiting after eating certain foods), coarse facial features, macroglossia, abnormal hair, dysmorphic features, and abnormal eye findings (e.g., cataracts, retinal changes). A family history of neonatal deaths (within the same sibling group, in males, or among family members) alerts the observer to the possibility of an IEM. The initial recognition of signs that might indicate an IEM is the responsibility of health professionals, including nurses.

Although there are many IEMs, only three are selected for discussion because they can be identified in the neonatal period and because reasonable success has been achieved with treatment. (Other IEMs are outlined in Table 5-4.)

## Congenital Hypothyroidism (CH)

CH (sometimes called by the undesirable term "cretinism") is a deficiency of thyroid hormones believed to be present at birth. Results of screening tests in the United States indicate that CH occurs in approximately 1 of every 3600 to 5000 newborns (American Academy of Pediatrics, 1996). Infants with Down syndrome have a much higher rate of either permanent or transient forms of the disorder. Also, a higher incidence of other congenital abnormalities has been observed in infants with CH.

A number of etiologic factors are implicated in hypothyroidism, and the condition may be permanent or transient. *Permanent CH* can result from defective thyroid gland development, an enzymatic defect in thyroxine synthesis, or (rarely) pituitary dysfunction. *Transient hypothyroidism* results from intrauterine transfer of goiter-inducing substances (such as the antithyroid drugs and expectorants given for asthma), which inhibit thyroid secretion. Although self-limiting, this type is potentially fatal because the infant's thyroid is unable to produce its own hormones once the maternal supply is terminated. In addition, regardless of etiology, a large goiter in a neonate may cause total obstruction of the airway. Many preterm infants have hypothyroidism (hypothyroxinemia) at birth as a result of hypothalamic and pituitary immaturity. However, this type is transient and requires no treatment.

## Clinical Manifestations

The severity of the disorder depends on the amount of thyroid tissue present. Usually the newborn does not exhibit obvious signs of hypothyroidism, probably because of the exogenous source of prenatal thyroid hormone supplied by the maternal circulation. However, subtle signs such as poor feeding, lethargy, prolonged jaundice, respiratory difficulty, cyanosis, constipation, hoarse cry, large fontanels, and bradycardia may be seen shortly after birth. In addition, infants with CH may be born postterm (>40 weeks) and/or have a birth weight over 4 kg (8 lbs 8 oz) (Kirsten, 2000). Clinical manifestations may be delayed in infants with a functional remnant of thyroid gland, infants with some types of familial hypothyroidism, and breast-fed infants, who may not display symptoms until weaned.

Classic features of untreated CH usually appear after approximately 6 weeks of life and include typical facial features (depressed nasal bridge, short forehead, puffy eyelids, and large tongue); thick, dry, mottled skin that feels cold to the touch; coarse, dry, lusterless hair; abdominal distention; umbilical hernia; hyporeflexia; bradycardia; hypothermia; hypotension with narrow pulse pressure; anemia; and widely patent cranial sutures. Bone age is greatly retarded from birth. The most serious consequence is delayed development of the nervous system, which leads to severe mental retardation. The severity of the intellectual deficit is related to the degree of hypothyroidism and the duration of the condition before treatment. Other nervous system manifestations include slow, awkward movements and abnormal deep tendon reflexes (often referred to as "hung-up" because the relaxation phase after the contraction is slow).

## Diagnostic Evaluation

Diagnosis is aimed at early identification of the disorder to prevent the serious effects on mental development as a result of delayed treatment. Neonatal screening consists of an initial filter-paper blood-spot thyroxine ($T_4$) measurement followed by measurement of thyroid-stimulating hormone (TSH) in infants with low $T_4$ values. Tests are mandatory in all 50 U.S. states. Although a heelstick blood sample for the spot test is best obtained between 2 and 6 days of age, specimens are usually taken within the first 24 to 48 hours or before discharge as part of a concurrent screen for other metabolic defects. Early screening can result in overdiagnosis (false-positives) but is preferable to missing the diagnosis.

Screening results that show a low level of $T_4$ (<6 mg/dL) and a high level of TSH (>50 $\mu$IU/ml) indicate CH and the need for further tests to determine the cause of the disease (reference values for infants >7 days old per Polk and Fisher, 1998). Additional tests include serum measurement of $T_4$, $T_3$ resin uptake, free $T_4$, and thyroid-bound globulin

(TBG). Tests of thyroid gland function (thyroid scan and uptake) usually involve oral administration of a radioactive isotope of iodine ($^{131}I$) and measurement of iodine uptake by the thyroid, usually within 24 hours. In CH, $T_4$ $T_3$ and free $T_4$ levels are low and thyroid uptake of $^{131}I$ is decreased. Skeletal radiography is employed to assess bone age.

In the newborn, thyroid function studies are elevated in comparison with values in older children; thus it is important to document the timing of the tests. In preterm and sick full-term infants, thyroid function tests are usually lower than in the healthy full-term infant; a repeat $T_4$ and TSH may be evaluated after 30 weeks (corrected age) in newborns born before that time and after resolution of the acute illness in the sick full-term infant.

## Therapeutic Management

Treatment involves lifelong thyroid hormone replacement therapy that begins as soon as possible after diagnosis to abolish all signs of hypothyroidism and to reestablish normal physical and mental development. The drug of choice is synthetic levothyroxine sodium (Synthroid or Levothroid). Regular measurement of thyroxine levels is important in ensuring optimum treatment. Bone age surveys are also performed to ensure optimum growth.

**Prognosis.** If treatment is started shortly after birth, normal physical growth and intelligence are possible. The most significant factor adversely affecting eventual intelligence appears to be inadequate treatment, which may be related to noncompliance.

## Nursing Considerations

The most important nursing objective is early identification of the disorder. Nurses caring for neonates must be certain that screening is performed, especially in infants who are preterm, discharged early, or born at home. Although the screening test is very specific, some children may not be identified, and nurses in community health need to be aware of the earliest signs of the disorder. Parental remarks about an unusually "quiet and good" baby together with any of the early physical manifestations should lead to a suspicion of hypothyroidism, which requires a referral for specific tests. Unfortunately, some parents harbor guilt about their impressions of the infant before the diagnosis because the child's inactivity may not have alerted them to a problem, with the result that treatment is delayed.

Once the diagnosis is confirmed, parents need an explanation of the disorder and the necessity of lifelong treatment. The importance of compliance with the drug regimen in order for the child to achieve normal growth and development must be stressed (Harrell and Murray, 1998). Because the drug is tasteless it can be crushed and added to formula, water, or food. If a dose is missed, twice the dose should be given the next day. Unless there are maternal contraindicative factors, breast-feeding is acceptable in infants with hypothyroidism (Lawrence and Lawrence, 1999). Parents also need to be aware of signs indicating overdose, such as rapid pulse, dyspnea, irritability, insomnia, fever, sweating, and weight loss. Ideally they should know how to count the pulse and be instructed to withhold a dose and consult their practitioner if the pulse rate is above a certain value. Signs of inadequate treatment are fatigue, sleepiness, decreased appetite, and constipation.

If the diagnosis was delayed past early infancy, the chance of permanent mental retardation is great. Parents need the same guidance in caring for their child as do others who have an offspring with cognitive impairment. (See Chapter 24.) They need an opportunity to discuss their feelings regarding late recognition of the disorder. Although treatment will not reverse the intellectual deficit, it may prevent further damage. Genetic counseling is important, especially if the disorder is caused by an inborn error of thyroid hormone synthesis, which is autosomal recessive. (See Chapter 5 for a discussion of genetic counseling.)

## Phenylketonuria (PKU)

PKU, a genetic disease inherited as an autosomal-recessive trait, is caused by an absence of the enzyme needed to metabolize the essential amino acid *phenylalanine.* The disorder is detected in 1 in 10,000 to 12,000 live births and primarily affects Caucasian children, with the incidence highest in those living in the United States or Northern Europe; frequency of PKU also varies among states in the United States (Koch, 1999). It is very rare in the African, Jewish, and Japanese populations.

Classic PKU is at one end of a spectrum of conditions known as *hyperphenylalaninemia.* Because rarer forms are the result of a deficiency of other enzymes and are diagnosed and treated differently, the following discussion of PKU is limited to the severe, classic form.

### Pathophysiology

In PKU the hepatic enzyme *phenylalanine hydroxylase,* which normally controls the conversion of phenylalanine to tyrosine, is absent. This results in the accumulation of phenylalanine in the bloodstream and urinary excretion of abnormal amounts of its metabolites, the phenyl acids (Fig. 9-9). One of these phenyl ketones, *phenylpyruvic acid,* gives urine the characteristic musty odor associated with this disease and is responsible for the term *phenylketonuria.*

Amino acids produced by the metabolism of phenylalanine are absent in PKU. One of these, *tyrosine,* is needed to form the pigment melanin and the hormones epinephrine and thyroxine. Decreased melanin production results in similar phenotypes of most children with PKU—blond hair, blue eyes, and fair skin that is particularly susceptible to eczema and other dermatologic problems. Children with a genetically darker skin color may be red haired or brunette.

Accumulation of phenylalanine and, presumably, the decreased levels of the neurotransmitters dopamine and tryptophan affect the normal development of the brain and central nervous system, resulting in defective myelinization, cystic degeneration of the gray and white matter, and disturbances in cortical lamination. Mental retardation occurs

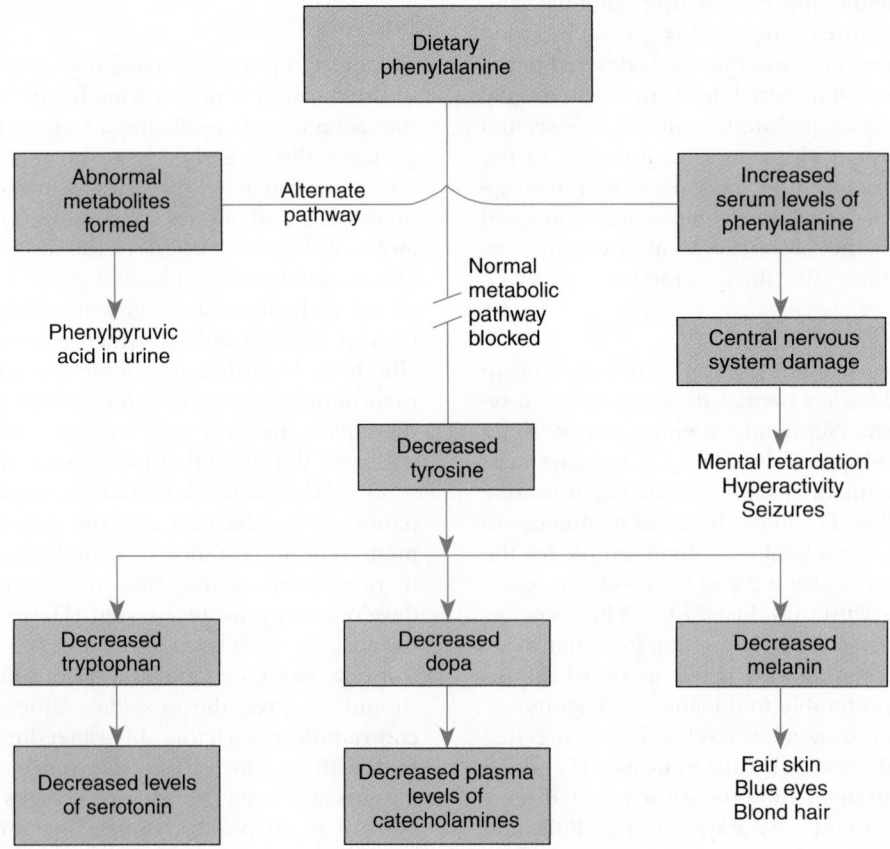

**Fig. 9-9** Metabolic errors and consequences in PKU.

*before* the metabolites are detected in the urine and will progress if ingested phenylalanine levels are not lowered.

## Clinical Manifestations

Clinical manifestations of PKU include failure to thrive, frequent vomiting, irritability, hyperactivity, and unpredictable, erratic behavior. Older children commonly display bizarre or schizoid behavior patterns such as fright reactions, screaming episodes, head banging, arm biting, disorientation, failure to respond to strong stimuli, and catatonia-like positions. Many of the severely retarded children have seizures, and approximately 80% of untreated persons with PKU demonstrate abnormal electroencephalographs, regardless of whether overt seizures occur. Fortunately, this manifestation is rarely seen because of early detection and treatment.

## Diagnostic Evaluation

The objective in diagnosing or treating the disorder is to prevent mental retardation. The most commonly used test for screening newborns is the *Guthrie blood test,* a bacterial inhibition assay for phenylalanine in the blood. *Bacillus subtilis,* present in the culture medium, grows if the blood contains an excessive amount of phenylalanine. The normal range of blood phenylalanine concentration in newborns is 0.5-1 mg/dl (Koch, 1999). If performed properly, this test detects serum phenylalanine levels greater than 4 mg/dl (normal value is 1.6 mg/dl). Only fresh heel blood, not cord blood, can be used for the test.

> **NURSING ALERT**
>
> Avoid "layering" the blood specimen on the special Guthrie paper. Layering is placing one drop of blood on top of the other or overlapping the specimen. This practice results in a falsely high reading, which will restrict the amount of protein intake and thus decrease the amount of food that the child with PKU may receive. Best results are obtained by collecting the specimen with a pipette from the heelstick and spreading the blood uniformly over the blot paper.

The screening test is most reliable if the blood sample is taken after the infant has ingested a source of protein. Because of early discharge of newborns, recommendations for screening include (1) collecting the initial specimen as close as possible to discharge and no later than 7 days, (2) obtaining a subsequent sample by 2 weeks of age if the initial specimen is collected before the newborn is 24 hours old, and (3) designating a primary care provider to all newborns before discharge for adequate newborn screening follow-up (American Academy of Pediatrics, 1996). A second screening test, the McCamon-Robins fluoromatic assay test, is reported to be useful in the detection of PKU in samples drawn when the infant is 12 to 24 hours old (Koch, 1999).

A major concern is that a significantly large number of infants are *not* rescreened for PKU after early discharge and are at risk for a missed or delayed diagnosis. Special consideration must be given to screening infants born at home who have no hospital contact.

Because of the possibility of variant forms of hyperphenylalaninemia, a natural protein challenge test is recommended after approximately 3 months of dietary treatment to confirm the diagnosis of classic PKU.

## Therapeutic Management

Treatment of PKU involves the restriction of dietary protein. Because the genetic enzyme is intracellular, systemic administration of phenylalanine hydroxylase is of no value. Phenylalanine cannot be eliminated because it is an essential amino acid in tissue growth. Therefore dietary management must meet two criteria: (1) meet the child's nutritional need for optimum growth, and (2) maintain phenylalanine levels within a safe range.

The diet is calculated to allow 20 to 30 mg of phenylalanine per kilogram of body weight per day, which should maintain serum phenylalanine levels between 2 and 8 mg/dl. Significant brain damage is likely to occur when levels are greater than 11 to 15 mg/dl. In the United States, a level of 2-10 mg/dl is recommended for children and 2-12 mg/dl for adults (Koch, 1999). At levels less than 2 mg/dl the body begins to catabolize its protein stores, resulting in growth retardation. The daily amounts are individualized for each child and require frequent changes on the basis of appetite, growth and development, and blood phenylalanine and tyrosine levels. For optimal growth to occur, the diet is initiated no later than 3 weeks of age.

Because all natural food proteins contain approximately 15% phenylalanine, specially prepared milk substitutes, such as Lofenalac or Phenex-1, are prescribed for the infant. These products are made from specially treated enzymatic casein hydrolysate, which provides only 0.4% phenylalanine (28.5 mg/8 ounces). They also contain minerals and vitamins to provide a balanced nutritional formula. Medium chain triglyceride (MCT) and vegetable oils and glucose polymers (Polycose) may be added to infant formulas to provide adequate calories. Tyrosine and several other amino acids are supplied in the formula. Because of the low phenylalanine content of breast milk, total or partial breastfeeding may be possible with close monitoring of phenylalanine levels (Lawrence and Lawrence, 1999). In one study, early breast-feeding in infants with PKU before diagnosis was shown to be a positive factor in the neurodevelopmental performance of the same children during the school-age years (Riva and others, 1996). Diet substitutes for older children, such as Phenyl-Free2 (Mead Johnson) and Phenex-2 (Ross), contain no phenylalanine and allow for greater exchanges with natural low-phenylalanine foods in the diet, leading to a more normal diet.

A low-phenylalanine diet is begun as soon as possible after birth and maintained through adulthood. To evaluate the effectiveness of dietary treatment, frequent monitoring of blood phenylalanine and tyrosine levels is necessary. Achievement of optimal outcomes should also include periodic monitoring of intellectual, neurologic, behavioral, and neuropsychologic parameters (NIH Consensus Statement, 2001). Because phenylalanine levels greater than or equal to 20 mg/dl in mothers with PKU affect the normal embryologic development of the fetus, women with PKU must resume a low-phenylalanine diet *before* pregnancy. These women should also be counseled about the risk that their child might have PKU (approximately 1/120), and reproductive options should be discussed.

**Prognosis.** Early recognition and treatment of infants with PKU greatly improves their chances for achieving normal cognitive development; however, the outcomes vary. Even with adequate dietary control, a high percentage of children and adults exhibit some degree of intellectual impairment. However, there is evidence that different clinical outcomes in dietary-treated PKU individuals may occur as a result of varying blood-brain barrier phenylalanine transport characteristics, which may require specific diet management (Weglage and others, 2001). In one study neurologic examinations of adults who had early dietary restrictions (<3 months of age) revealed subtle symptoms of brain damage (Pietz and others, 1998). Other studies reveal mixed results in adult outcomes in patients with early-treated PKU and neurobehavior (Griffiths and others, 2000; Pietz and others, 1998; Ris and others, 1997). There is evidence of severe emotional disturbance in adolescents and adults with PKU not on a restricted diet. However, large populations of adults with early-treated PKU have not been studied in relation to motor, intellectual, and cognitive skills. Koch (1999) suggests that early-treated patients have excellent outcomes. It is clear however that maintaining dietary restrictions in later childhood and early adulthood have an important role in reducing the effects of the disease (Poustie and Rutherford, 2000).

### Nursing Considerations

The principal nursing considerations involve teaching the family regarding the dietary restrictions. Although the treatment may sound simple, the task of maintaining such a strict dietary regimen is very demanding, especially for older children and adolescents. Foods with low phenylalanine levels (e.g., some vegetables [except legumes], fruits, juices, and some cereals, breads, and starches) must be measured to provide the prescribed amount of phenylalanine. Most high-protein foods, such as meat and dairy products, are either eliminated or restricted to small amounts.

Maintaining the diet during infancy presents few problems. Solid foods such as cereal, fruits, and vegetables are introduced as usual to the infant. Difficulties arise as the child gets older. A decreased appetite and refusal to eat may reduce intake of the calculated phenylalanine requirement. The child's increasing independence may inhibit absolute control of what he or she eats. Either factor can result in decreased or increased phenylalanine levels. During the school years, peer pressure becomes a major force in deterring the child from eating the prescribed foods or abstaining from high-protein foods such as milkshakes or ice cream. Limitations of this diet are best illustrated by an example: a quarter-pound hamburger may provide a 2-day phenylalanine allowance for a school-age child. Illness and growth spurts will increase the body's need for this essential amino acid. Adolescence is a particularly difficult period, and limiting foods containing phenylalanine in adolescents with PKU is challenging. Special camps to educate adolescent girls with PKU regarding appropriate food intake demonstrated short-term effects in decreasing blood phenylalanine levels (Singh and others, 2000).

The assistance of a registered nutritionist is essential. Parents need a basic understanding of the disorder and practical suggestions regarding food selection and preparation. A number of support groups for parents of children with PKU are available nationwide. Many Internet resources are also available that contain valuable information regarding dietary counseling and food options. Meal planning is based on an exchange list. As soon as children are old enough, usually by early preschool, they should be involved in the daily calculation, menu planning, and formula preparation. A computer, voice-activated calculator, cards, or colored beads can help children keep track of the daily allowance of phenylalanine foods. A system of goal setting, self-monitoring, contracts, and rewards can promote compliance in adolescents.

Preparation of the formula can present some challenges. The formula tends to be lumpy and has a distinctive odor and taste that has been described as similar to potato but more bitter. A blender or mixer dissolves the powder more easily; a rechargeable hand mixer can be used when traveling. Although the taste is virtually impossible to camouflage, adding orange Tang, fruit-flavored powdered punch, or strawberry or chocolate Quik helps vary the flavor somewhat without greatly altering the phenylalanine content. The chocolate-flavored formula can be heated and served as hot cocoa or frozen into popsicles.

**Family Support.** In addition to the problem related to a child with a chronic disorder (see Chapter 22), the parents have the burden of knowing that they are carriers of the defect and must make serious decisions regarding future children. Prenatal testing is now available to detect the presence of the defective gene in heterozygotes. Genetic counseling is especially important for an affected child, who theoretically has a 50% chance of bearing an affected offspring. (See Genetic Counseling, Chapter 5, and Family Focus box.)

### Galactosemia

Galactosemia is a rare autosomal-recessive disorder that affects approximately 1 out of 50,000 births. It involves an in-

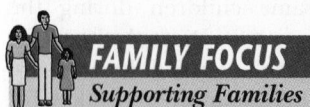

**FAMILY FOCUS**
*Supporting Families*

I am a registered nurse and the mother of a child diagnosed with PKU; I also have three siblings with PKU. As a parent I was devastated when I received a phone call informing me that my son's blood level was high and that he has PKU. The nurse attempted to comfort me by saying that she understood how I felt and what I was going through. I wanted to scream "No, you don't know how I feel and what I am going through!" but didn't because I realized she thought she was helping me. For this reason it is so important for nurses to be aware of what we say when parent(s) face a crisis such as the diagnosis of chronic disease in their child. It is often best to say nothing at all. A sincere "I'm sorry" can mean a lot.

L.E., RN

born error of carbohydrate metabolism in which the hepatic enzyme *galactose 1-phosphate uridine transferase (UDP-galactose transferase)* is absent. This enzyme is one of three needed for the conversion of galactose to glucose (Fig. 9-10). There is considerable genetic variability in enzyme deficiency, with some children having partial transferase activity.

As galactose accumulates in the blood, several organs are affected. Hepatic dysfunction leads to cirrhosis, resulting in jaundice in the infant by the second week of life. The spleen subsequently becomes enlarged as a result of portal hypertension. Cataracts are usually recognizable by 1 or 2 months of age; cerebral damage, manifested by the symptoms of lethargy and hypotonia, is evident soon afterward. Infants with galactosemia appear normal at birth, but within a few days of ingesting milk (which has a high lactose content) they begin to vomit and lose weight. *Escherichia coli* sepsis is also a common initial clinical sign (American Academy of Pediatrics, 1996). Death during the first month of life is not infrequent in untreated infants.

### Diagnostic Evaluation

Diagnosis is made on the basis of the infant's history, physical examination, galactosuria, increased levels of galactose in the blood, or decreased levels of UDP-galactose transferase activity in erythrocytes. The infant may display characteristics of malnutrition; signs of dehydration, decreased muscle mass, and body fat may be evident (Chung, 1997). Newborn screening for this disease is required in most states. Heterozygotes can also be identified, because heterozygotic individuals have significantly lower levels of the essential enzyme. Although asymptomatic, such individuals have been noted to spontaneously dislike and therefore limit the ingestion of galactose-containing foods.

### Therapeutic Management

Treatment of galactosemia consists of eliminating all milk and lactose-containing foods, including breast milk. During infancy, lactose-free formulas are used, with soy-protein formula being the feeding of choice (American Academy of Pediatrics, 1998). Typically baby cereals are added to the infant's diet at 4 to 6 months; baby fruit juices and baby-food fruits and vegetables are gradually introduced at 5 to 8 months. Commercially prepared baby foods should be carefully evaluated because some have been found to contain large amounts of free galactose (Gropper and others, 2000).

If galactosemia is suspected, supportive treatment and care are implemented, including monitoring for hypoglycemia, liver failure, bleeding disorders, and *E. coli* sepsis (American Academy of Pediatrics, 1996).

**Prognosis.**  Follow-up studies of children treated from birth or within the first 2 months of life after symptoms appear have found long-term complications, such as ovarian dysfunction, cataracts, abnormal speech, cognitive impairment, growth retardation, and motor delay (Widhalm, da Cruz, and Koch, 1997). Studies have revealed that eliminating sources of galactose does not significantly improve the outcome. New therapeutic strategies, such as enhancing residual transferase activity, replacing depleted metabolites, or using gene replacement therapy, are needed to improve the prognosis for these children.

### Nursing Considerations

Nursing interventions are similar to those for PKU, except that dietary restrictions are easier to maintain because many more foods are allowed. However, reading food labels very carefully for the presence of any form of lactose, especially dairy products, is mandatory. Many drugs, such as penicillin, contain lactose as filler and must also be avoided. Unfortunately, lactose is an unlabeled ingredient in pharmaceuticals (see Family Support [for PKU], p. 324).

## PROBLEMS CAUSED BY PERINATAL ENVIRONMENTAL FACTORS
### Infectious Agents

The range of pathologic conditions produced by infectious agents is large, and the difference between the maternal and fetal effects caused by any one agent is also great. Some maternal infections, especially viral infections during early gestation, can result in fetal loss or malformations because of viral effects on organogenesis, and the fetal immunologic system is unable to prevent the dissemination of infectious agents to the various tissues.

Not all prenatal infections produce teratogenic effects. Furthermore, the clinical picture of disorders caused by transplacental transfer of infectious agents is not always well defined. One group of viral agents can cause remarkably similar manifestations, and it is not uncommon to test for all

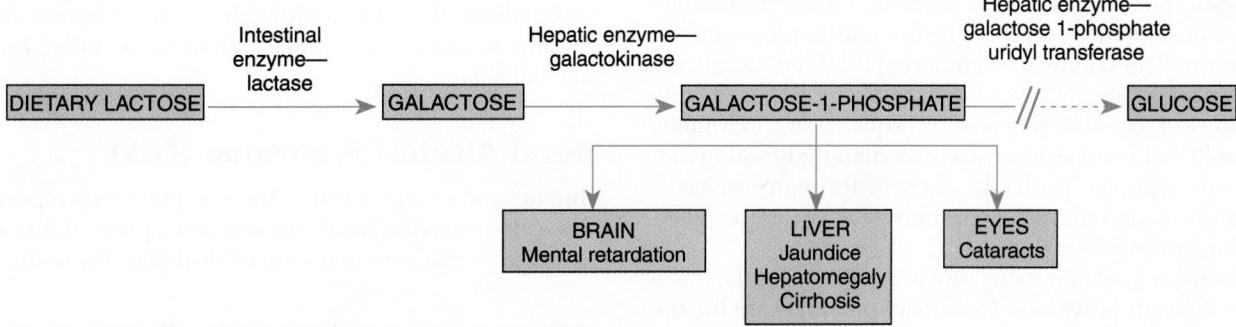

**Fig. 9-10**  Metabolic errors and consequences in galactosemia.

when a prenatal infection is suspected. This is the so-called *TORCH* complex, an acronym for:

**T** Toxoplasmosis
**O** Other (e.g., hepatitis, parvovirus)
**R** Rubella
**C** Cytomegalovirus infection
**H** Herpes simplex virus

To determine the causative agent in a symptomatic infant, tests are performed to rule out each of these infections. The "O" category may involve testing for several viral infections (e.g., hepatitis, varicella zoster, measles, mumps, parvovirus, and listeriosis). Since the TORCH acronym was first developed, other agents have been identified that cause similar neonatal illnesses that were not included in the original set. Therefore, it is recommended that all possible causative agents be investigated. Bacterial infections are not included in the TORCH workup because they are usually identified by clinical manifestations and readily available laboratory tests. The incidence of gonococcal conjunctivitis (ophthalmia neonatorum) and chlamydial conjunctivitis has been significantly reduced by prophylactic measures at birth. (See Chapter 8.) Human immunodeficiency virus (HIV) infection, a growing prenatal and postnatal concern, is discussed in Chapter 35. The major maternal infections, their possible teratogenic effects, and specific nursing considerations are outlined in Table 9-5.

### Nursing Considerations

One of the major goals in care of infants suspected of having an infectious disease is identification of the causative organism. Until the diagnosis is established, standard precautions are implemented according to institutional policy. In suspected cytomegalovirus and rubella infections, pregnant personnel are cautioned to avoid contact with the infant. Herpes simplex virus (HSV) is easily transmitted from one infant to another; therefore the risk of cross-contamination is reduced or eliminated by wearing gloves for patient contact. The hospital infection control department provides guidelines for the type and duration of precautions. Careful handwashing is the most important nursing intervention in reducing the spread of any infection.

Special feeding techniques may need to be implemented for infants with feeding difficulties, and infants subject to seizures are protected from adverse environmental stimuli. Specimens need to be obtained for laboratory examinations, and the infant and parents need to be prepared for diagnostic procedures. When possible, long-term disabilities are prevented by early evaluation and implementation of therapy. The family is taught any special handling techniques needed for the care of their infant and signs of complications or possible sequelae. If sequelae are inevitable, the family will need assistance in determining how they can best cope with the problems, such as through assistance with home care, referral to appropriate agencies, or placement in an institution for care.

The major goal of nursing care is prevention of these disorders through provision of adequate prenatal care for the expectant mother and precautions regarding exposure to potentially harmful infections.

## Chemical Agents

The relationship of the fetal and maternal circulations allows for the interchange of chemical substances across the placental membrane. The limited metabolic capabilities of the fetal liver and its immature enzyme and transport systems render the unborn child ill equipped for maintaining homeostasis when chemical disturbances are imposed by the mother or the environment. This includes both substances produced by the mother in response to a disease state (such as diabetes) and exogenous substances ingested or inhaled by the mother.

The teratogenic effect of drugs is not believed to have an effect on developing tissue until day 15 of gestation, when tissue differentiation begins to take place. Before that time, drugs usually have little effect, because they are believed to have an insignificant affinity for undifferentiated tissue. Also, until implantation takes place, at approximately 7 days after conception, the embryo is not exposed to maternal blood that contains the drug. However, some drugs may affect the uterine lining, making it unsuitable for implantation. Drugs administered between days 15 and 90 may produce an effect if the tissue for which the drug has an affinity is in the process of differentiation at that time. After 90 days, when differentiation is complete, most fetal tissues are believed to be relatively resistant to teratogenic effects of drugs. However, the impact on ongoing neurologic development is not known.

One drug recognized for its carcinogenic effect is *diethylstilbestrol (DES)*. Large doses of this hormone given to pregnant women to prevent abortion cause adenocarcinoma of the vagina in a significant proportion of the female offspring when they reach adolescence and early adulthood. There are recent reports that male offspring of women who received DES are at higher risk for testicular cancer.

### Nursing Considerations

Expectant mothers are cautioned against ingesting any medication without first consulting a practitioner. To help ensure that fewer women will inadvertently take some chemical that might be harmful to the fetus, medications labels are now required to include information regarding the possible teratogenic effects of the drug. Excessive use of some very commonplace drugs, such as alcohol (see following discussion), valproic acid, and isotretinoin (Accutane), has been shown to produce characteristic malformations in the fetus.

Nurses should be aware of **Birth Defect Research for Children, Inc. (BDRC),** * which offers help and information to families with children with defects caused by maternal exposure to drugs, chemicals, radiation, or other environmental agents.

## Fetal Alcohol Syndrome (FAS)

Infants and children with FAS were previously reported to have characteristic facial and associated physical features attributed to excessive ingestion of alcohol by the mother dur-

---

*Birth Defect Research for Children Inc (BDRC), 930 Woodcock Rd, Suite 225, Orlando, FL 32803, (800) 313-2232 or (407) 895-0802; www.birthdefects.org

ing pregnancy. It has since been shown that infants may not initially display the dysmorphic facial features; these are believed to be more well-defined with increasing age during childhood.

The three categories for diagnosis of FAS are (1) growth retardation, both prenatal and postnatal, including microcephaly; (2) dysmorphic facial features (midfacial); and (3) central nervous system involvement (cognitive impair-

| **TABLE 9-5**   Infections acquired from mother before, during, or after birth* | |
|---|---|
| **Fetal or Newborn Effect** | **Comments and Nursing Considerations†** |
| **Human Immunodeficiency Virus (HIV)** | |
| No significant difference between infected and uninfected infants at birth in some instances<br>Embryopathy reported by some observers:<br>  Depressed nasal bridge<br>  Mild upward or downward obliquity of eyes<br>  Long palpebral fissures with blue sclerae<br>  Patulous lips<br>  Ocular hypertelorism<br>  Prominent upper vermilion border | Transmitted: transplacentally; during vaginal delivery; potentially in breast milk<br>Recommended treatment: administer zidovudine (AZT) alone or zidovudine and lamivudine until delivery to HIV-positive mother; untreated mother may be treated at delivery with a 2-dose regimen of nevirapine, administer nevirapine to newborn after delivery; in newborn whose mother is on AZT, same may be given after birth<br>Cesarean section in HIV-positive mother is recommended to reduce transmission<br>Chemoprophylaxis against *Pneumocystis carinii* pneumonia (PCP) in HIV-exposed infants: drug of choice is s.o. trimethoprimsulfamethoxazole (Bactrim, Septra)<br>Documented routine HIV education and routine testing with consent for all pregnant women in the United States is recommended |
| **Chickenpox (Varicella-zoster virus [VZV])** | |
| Intrauterine exposure—congenital varicella syndrome: limb dysplasia, microcephaly, cortical atrophy, chorioretinitis, cataracts, cutaneous scars, other anomalies, auditory nerve palsy, mental retardation<br>Severe symptoms (rash, fever) and higher mortality in infant whose mother develops varicella 5 days before to 2 days after delivery | Transmitted: first trimester (fetal varicella syndrome); perinatal period (infection)<br>Treatment: exposed infants—varicella-zoster immune globulin (VZIG) to infants born to mothers with onset of disease within 5 days before or 2 days after delivery (7 days before and 7 days after in United Kingdom)<br>Isolation precautions 21 days after birth (if hospitalized)<br>Prevention: universal immunization of all children with varicella (Var) vaccine |
| ***Chlamydia* Infection *(Chlamydia Trachomatis)*** | |
| Conjunctivitis, pneumonia | Transmitted: last trimester or perinatal period<br>Standard ophthalmic prophylaxis for gonococcal ophthalmia neonatorum (topical antibiotics, silver nitrate, or povidone-iodine) is not effective in treatment or prevention of chlamydia ophthalmia.<br>Treatment: oral erythromycin 14 days |
| **Coxsackievirus (Group B enterovirus-nonpolio)** | |
| Poor feeding, vomiting, diarrhea, fever; cardiac enlargement, arrhythmias, congestive heart failure; lethargy, seizures, meningeal involvement<br>Mimics bacterial sepsis | Transmitted: peripartum<br>Treatment: supportive; IVIG in neonatal infections |
| **Cytomegalovirus (CMV)** | |
| Variable manifestation from asymptomatic to severe<br>Microcephaly, cerebral calcifications, chorioretinitis<br>Jaundice, hepatosplenomegaly<br>Petechial or purpuric rash<br>Neurologic sequelae: seizure disorders, sensorimotor deafness, mental retardation | Infection acquired at birth, shortly thereafter, or via human milk is not associated with clinical illness<br>Transmitted: throughout pregnancy<br>Affected individuals excrete virus<br>Virus detected in urine or tissue by electron microscopy<br>Avoid kissing affected child<br>Pregnant women should avoid close contact with known cases<br>Treatment: antimetabolites, antiviral agent |
| **Erythema Infectiosum (Parvovirus B19)** | |
| Fetal hydrops and death from anemia and heart failure, early exposure<br>Anemia from later exposure<br>No teratogenic effects established<br>Ordinarily, low risk of ill effect to fetus | Transmitted: transplacentally<br>First trimester infection most serious effects<br>Pregnant health care workers should not care for patients who might be highly contagious (e.g., child with sickle cell anemia, aplastic crisis)<br>Routine exclusion of pregnant women from workplace where disease is occurring is not recommended |

*This table is not an exhaustive representation of all perinatally transmitted infections. For further information regarding specific diseases or treatment not listed here, the reader is referred to American Academy of Pediatrics, Committee on Infectious Diseases: *2000 Red book report of the Committee on Infectious Diseases*, ed 25, Elk Grove Village, IL, The Academy.

†Isolation precautions depend on institutional policy (see Infection Control, Chapter 27).

*Continued*

**TABLE 9-5** Infections acquired from mother before, during, or after birth—cont'd

| Fetal or Newborn Effect | Comments and Nursing Considerations |
|---|---|
| **Gonococcal Disease (Neisseria gonorrhoeae)** | |
| Ophthalmitis | Transmitted: last trimester or perinatal period |
| Neonatal gonococcal arthritis, septicemia, meningitis | Apply prophylactic medication to eyes at time of birth |
| | Obtain smears for culture |
| | Treatment: penicillin |
| **Hepatitis B Virus (HBV)** | |
| May be asymptomatic at birth | Transmitted: transplacentally; contaminated maternal fluids or secretions during delivery |
| Acute hepatitis, changes in liver function | Treatment: hepatitis B immune globulin (HBIG) to all infants of HB₂AG-positive mothers within 12 hours of birth |
| | Prevention: universal immunization of all infants with Hep B vaccine (see Immunizations, Chapter 12) |
| **Herpes, Neonatal (Herpes simplex virus)** | |
| Cutaneous lesions: vesicles at 6 to 10 days of age; may be no lesions | History of genital infection in mother or partner in 50% of cases |
| Disseminated disease resembles sepsis; encephalitis in 60%-70% | Transmitted: intrapartum either ascending or direct contact, especially primary infection |
| Visceral involvement: granulomas | Cesarean sections sometimes a preventive measure for mothers with active lesions |
| Early nonspecific signs: fever, lethargy, poor feeding, irritability, vomiting | Vaginal delivery of infants of mothers with recurrent infection thought to be at lower risk |
| May include hyperbilirubinemia, seizures, flaccid or spastic paralysis, apneic episodes, respiratory distress, lethargy, or coma | Suggest infants room-in with mother in private room |
| | Treatment: acyclovir (intravenous) to newborn |
| **Listeriosis (Listeria monocytogenes)** | |
| Acquired in late pregnancy: stillborn or acutely ill; may die within an hour after birth | Transmitted: transplacentally or by aspiration of secretions at birth |
| Late onset: septicemia; meningitis | Segregate infants until cultures are negative |
| **Rubella, Congenital (rubella virus)** | |
| Eye defects: cataracts (unilateral or bilateral), microphthalmia, retinitis, glaucoma | Transmitted: first trimester; early second trimester |
| CNS signs: microcephaly, seizures, severe mental retardation | Pregnant women should avoid contact with all affected persons, including infants with rubella syndrome |
| Congenital heart defects: patent ductus arteriosus | Emphasize vaccination of all unimmunized prepubertal children, susceptible adolescents, and women of childbearing age (nonpregnant) |
| Auditory: high incidence of delayed hearing loss | Caution women against pregnancy for at least 3 months after vaccination |
| Intrauterine growth retardation | |
| Hyperbilirubinemia, meningitis, thrombocytopenia, hepatomegaly | |
| **Syphilis, Congenital (Treponema pallidum)** | |
| Stillbirth, prematurity, hydrops fetalis | Transmitted: transplacentally; can be anytime during pregnancy or at birth |
| May be asymptomatic at birth and in first few weeks of life or may have multisystem manifestations: hepatosplenomegaly, lymphadenopathy, hemolytic anemia, and thrombocytopenia | Most severe form of syphilis |
| Copper-colored maculopapular cutaneous lesions (usually after first few weeks of life), mucous membrane patches, hair loss, nail exfoliation, snuffles (syphilitic rhinitis), profound anemia, poor feeding, pseudoparalysis of one or more limbs, dysmorphic teeth (older child) | Strict isolation of infant |
| | Treatment: IV penicillin |
| | Evaluate cerebrospinal for neurosyphilis |
| **Toxoplasmosis (Toxoplasma gondii)** | |
| May be asymptomatic at birth (70%-90% of cases) or maculopapular rash, lymphadenopathy, hepatosplenomegaly, jaundice, thrombocytopenia | Transmitted: throughout pregnancy |
| Hydrocephaly, cerebral calcifications, chorioretinitis (classic triad) | Predominant host for organism is cats |
| Microcephaly, seizures, mental retardation, deafness | May be transmitted through cat feces, poorly cooked or raw infected meats |
| Encephalitis, myocarditis, hepatosplenomegaly, anemia, jaundice, diarrhea, vomiting, purpura | Caution pregnant women to avoid contact with cat feces (e.g., emptying cat litter boxes) |
| | Treatment: sulfonamides (Septra, Bactrim), pyrimethamine (Daraprim) |

ment, irritability, hyperactivity, behavioral problems, and hypotonia). Any single or multiple combination of these may be present in addition to a history of maternal alcohol consumption. The diagnosis of FAS is complicated by the absence of a specific single biologic marker and manifesta-

tions that are often seen in other childhood conditions (Stoler and Holmes, 1999).

A number of children and adults who demonstrate cognitive, behavioral, and psychosocial problems without the facial dysmorphia and growth retardation are referred to as having

**Box 9-3 ■ ■ □**
**Major Features of Fetal Alcohol Syndrome***

**FACIAL FEATURES**

　　Short palpebral fissures
　　Hypoplastic philtrum (vertical ridge in upper lip)
　　Thinned upper lip
　　Short, upturned nose
　　Hypoplastic maxilla
　　Micrognathia or prognathia in adolescence
　　Retrognathia in infancy

**NEUROLOGIC**

　　Mental retardation
　　Motor retardation
　　Microcephaly
　　Poor coordination
　　Hypotonia
　　Hearing disorders

**BEHAVIOR**

　　Irritability (infancy)
　　Hyperactivity (child)

**GROWTH**

　　Disproportionately low weight to height
　　Prenatal growth retardation
　　Persistent postnatal growth lag

---

*For a comprehensive list of FAS birth defects, see Fig. 1, in *Pediatrics* 106(2):359, 2000.

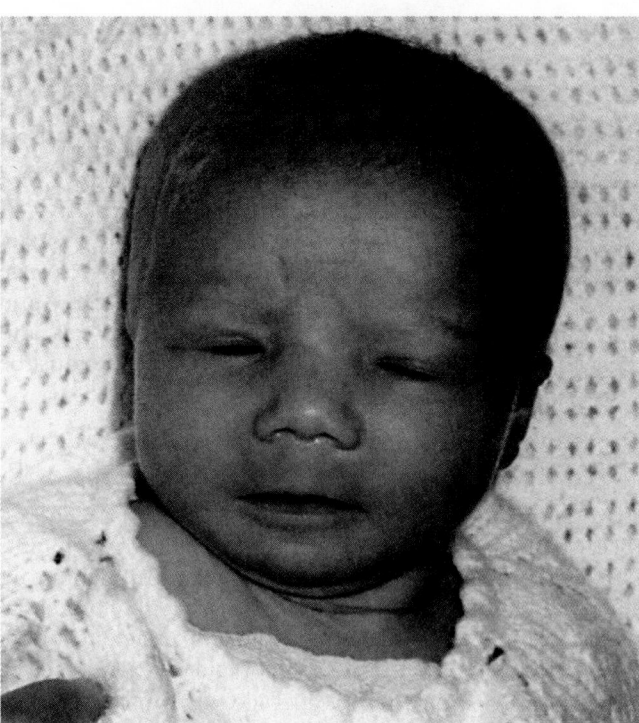

**Fig. 9-11**   Fetal alcohol syndrome. (From Markiewicz M, Abrahamson E: *Diagnosis in color: neonatology,* St Louis, 1999, Mosby.)

*fetal alcohol effects (FAEs);* however, some have suggested that this term be abandoned because it lacks specificity in the diagnosis of FAS and may include children who do not in fact have the syndrome itself (Aase, Jones, and Clarren, 1995).

The Institute of Medicine has recently proposed a nomenclature, including the terms *alcohol-related neurodevelopmental disorder (ARND)* and *alcohol-related birth defects (ARBD)* to replace FAE and FAS in describing conditions in which there is a history of maternal alcohol exposure and an outcome that confirms the effects of such exposure (American Academy of Pediatrics, 2000).

FAS is recognized as the leading cause of mental retardation (American Academy of Pediatrics, 2000). The incidence of FAS is on the rise in the United States despite public warnings, including the U.S. Surgeon General's warning that consumption of alcohol during pregnancy may cause mental retardation and other defects. At the time of this writing, the reported incidence of FAS was 5.2 per 10,000 live births in the United States, with higher rates being reported in certain subgroups (30 per 10,000 live births in Native Americans) (Centers for Disease Control, 1997; American Academy of Pediatrics, 2000). The reported incidence of maternal alcohol consumption during pregnancy has also risen dramatically during the 1991 to 1995 period despite widespread education and information regarding periconceptual and gestational effects of drinking (Alcohol consumption, 1997).

Alcohol (ethanol and ethyl alcohol) interferes with normal fetal development; the effects on the fetal brain are per-

manent, and even moderate use of alcohol during pregnancy may cause long-term postnatal difficulties, including impaired maternal-infant attachment. Because there is no known safe level of alcohol consumption in pregnancy, women who plan to become pregnant should stop consuming alcohol at least 3 months before they plan to conceive.

It is not the degree of alcohol intake in the mother that is related to the presence of abnormalities in the fetus; rather, it is the amount consumed in excess of the liver's ability to detoxify it that places the fetus at risk. The liver's capacity to detoxify alcohol is limited and inflexible—when the liver receives more alcohol than it is able to handle, the excess is continually recirculated until the organ is able to reduce it to carbon dioxide and water. This circulating alcohol has a special affinity for brain tissue. Other factors that contribute to the teratogenic effects include toxic acetyl aldehyde (a degradation by-product of ethanol) and other substances that may be added to the alcohol. Poor nutritional state, smoking, polydrug intake, and poor prenatal care may further compound the problem when alcohol abuse is observed.

The effects on the fetal brain are reflected in central nervous system manifestations of FAS (Box 9-3). Mental retardation, hearing disorders, and a variety of defects in craniofacial development are prominent features (Fig. 9-11). MRI studies of children with diagnosed FAS revealed a high incidence of midbrain anomalies, particularly micrencephaly (Swayze and others, 1997). Some affected infants display physical features of the syndrome; behaviors, however, are nonspecific in newborns and may therefore pass undetected. These include difficulty in establishing respirations, irritability, lethargy, seizure activity, tremulousness, poor suck reflex, and abdominal distention. Affected infants frequently develop metabolic problems and have other birth defects, such as cardiac anomalies, hemangioma, eye and ear anomalies, and neural tube defects (spina bifida).

The initial difficulties in the newborn period are managed by preventing stimulation that might precipitate seizures, providing sedation and antiseizure therapy, and providing general supportive measures. The defects and their effects are irreversible, so the major emphasis must be aimed at prevention in the prenatal period.

### Nursing Considerations

Nursing care of affected infants involves the same assessment and observations that are employed for any high-risk infant. (See Chapter 10.) Poor feeding is characteristic of infants with FAS and can be a significant problem throughout infancy. Strategies to provide individualized developmental care are aimed at reducing noxious environmental stimuli and helping the infant achieve self-regulation. (See Developmental Care, Chapter 10.) Special emphasis is placed on monitoring weight gain, analyzing feeding behaviors, and devising strategies to promote nutritional intake.

The effects of FAS have been identified in adolescents and young adults, primarily in relation to growth deficiencies, delayed motor development, and cognitive impairment. In one study children who were exposed to only small amounts of alcohol prenatally showed more aggressiveness, delinquent behavior, and attention problems at 6 to 7 years of age compared to nonexposed controls (Sood and others, 2001). Facial characteristics tend to be more subtle than in infants and children. Early diagnosis and intervention are reported to be beneficial for reducing the effects of alcohol exposure on the growing child (Stoler and Holmes, 1999); therefore nurses should be actively involved in identifying and referring children exposed to alcohol prenatally.

The dangers of heavy drinking are known, and women with a history of excessive alcohol ingestion should be counseled regarding the risks to the fetus. It should be emphasized to all women that there is no known "safe" amount of alcohol intake during pregnancy that will preclude either FAS or FAE. Furthermore, FAS/FAE is a *totally preventable*

birth defect. A change in drinking habits even as late as the third trimester (when brain growth in the fetus is greatest) is associated with improved fetal outcome.*

## Radiation

Ionizing radiation in large doses has been shown to be both mutagenic and teratogenic in humans. Pelvic irradiation of pregnant women—from natural background radiation that is present everywhere in varying degrees, from occupational exposure, or from diagnostic or therapeutic procedures—is believed to be hazardous to the embryo, although the extent of teratogenicity and the exact dosage required to induce somatic change are still under investigation. Radiation may damage the conceptus at any time during its prenatal existence, and it is known that rapidly dividing and differentiating cells, such as those of the embryo, have increased radiosensitivity. As with other teratogens, the type of effect produced is closely correlated with the stage of development at which the radiation exposure occurs.

Although data are incomplete, there are indications that a larger number of chromosome abnormalities occur in children born to parents who have been exposed to increased preconception radiation. This finding is consistent with the observation that chromosome abnormalities are highest in infants of older mothers, and there is an increased frequency of chromosomally abnormal fetuses born to parents with occupational exposure to radiation. To help prevent the possibility of radiation damage, it is advisable (1) to avoid unnecessary radiation exposure, such as elective radiographs, in women of childbearing age except during the 2 weeks immediately following menstruation; (2) to ask if pregnancy is a possibility; and (3) to advise both men and women who have lower abdominal or pelvic radiographs to avoid conception for several months. Also, the harmful effects of maternal radioactive iodine (RAI) therapy on the fetal thyroid gland have led to the conclusion that termination of pregnancies that occur during RAI therapy should be considered.

---

*Further information is available from **National Organization on Fetal Alcohol Syndrome (NOFAS),** 216 G Street, North East, Washington, DC 20002, (202) 785-4585; www.nofas.org, and **Fetal Alcohol Syndrome Branch,** Division of Birth Defects, Child Development, and Disability and Health, Centers for Disease Control and Prevention, Atlanta, GA, www.cdc.gov/ncbddd/fas.

---

## KEY POINTS

- Problems of the newborn may be attributed to birth injuries, transient metabolic illnesses, and inborn errors of metabolism.
- The forces of labor and delivery may cause soft tissue injury, head trauma, fractures, and paralysis.
- The most common forms of paralysis in the newborn are facial nerve, brachial plexus, and phrenic nerve palsies.
- Common skin problems of the newborn include erythema toxicum, candidiasis, bullous impetigo, and "birthmarks," especially port-wine stains and hemangiomas.

- Because of their immature physiologic status, infants may be predisposed to hyperbilirubinemia, hypoglycemia, hyperglycemia, and hypocalcemia.
- Hyperbilirubinemia is classified according to the two types of bilirubin: unconjugated and conjugated. In the newborn, it may result from excess production of bilirubin, decreased capacity of the liver to conjugate bilirubin, and/or deconjugation of bilirubin in the neonatal intestine (enterohepatic shunting).
- The primary treatment of unconjugated hyperbilirubinemia is phototherapy.

- Hemolytic disease of the newborn is characterized by abnormally rapid destruction of RBCs as a result of blood incompatibility between mother and fetus.
- Hypoglycemia can often be prevented with the initiation of early feedings.
- Hemorrhagic disease of the newborn is characterized by oozing from the umbilicus or circumcision site, bloody or black stools, hematuria, ecchymoses, and epistaxis.
- The most significant IEMs are congenital hypothyroidism, PKU, and galactosemia.
- Thyroid replacement medication is required to treat congenital hypothyroidism.

- Dietary control is the treatment of choice for PKU and galactosemia.
- Prenatal environmental conditions are responsible for high-risk problems in some newborns, especially selected maternal viral and bacterial infections and maternal alcohol ingestion.
- Risk of perinatal HIV transmission may be greatly reduced with maternal HIV testing and subsequent administration of antiviral medications, if indicated. The risk of transmission may be further reduced by cesarean delivery and administering antiviral medications to the newborn.

# REFERENCES

Aase JM, Jones KL, Clarren SK. Do we need the term "FAE"? *Pediatrics* 95(3):428-430, 1995 (commentary).

Alcohol consumption among pregnant and childbearing-aged women—United States, 1991 and 1995, *MMWR* 46(16):346-350, 1997.

Alexander M, Kuo KN: Musculoskeletal assessment of the newborn, *Orthop Nurs* 16(10):21-31, 1997.

American Academy of Pediatrics, Committee on Fetus and Newborn: Routine evaluation of blood pressure, hematocrit, and glucose in newborns, *Pediatrics* 92(3):474-476, 1993.

American Academy of Pediatrics, Committee on Genetics: Newborn screening facts, *Pediatrics* 98(3):473-481, 1996.

American Academy of Pediatrics, Committee on Nutrition: Soy protein-based formulas: recommendations for use in input feeding, *Pediatrics* 101(1):148-153, 1998.

American Academy of Pediatrics, Committee on Substance Abuse and Committee on Children with Disabilities: Fetal alcohol syndrome and alcohol-related neurodevelopmental disorders, *Pediatrics* 106(2):358-361, 2000.

American Academy of Pediatrics, Provisional Committee for Quality Improvement and Subcommittee on Hyperbilirubinemia: Practice parameter: management of hyperbilirubinemia in the healthy term newborn, *Pediatrics* 94(4):558-562, 1994.

American Academy of Pediatrics and American College of Obstetricians and Gynecologists: *Guidelines for perinatal care*, ed 4, Elk Grove Village, IL, 1997.

Bhutani VK and others: Noninvasive measurement of total serum bilirubin in a multiracial predischarge newborn population to assess the risk of severe hyperbilirubinemia, *Pediatrics* 106(2):e17, 2000.

Bhutani VK, Johnson L, Sivieri EM: Predictive ability of a predischarge hour-specific serum bilirubin for subsequent significant hyperbilirubinemia in healthy term and near-term newborns, *Pediatrics* 103(1):6-14, 1999.

Blackburn S: Hyperbilirubinemia and neonatal jaundice, *Neonatal Network* 14(7):15-25, 1995.

Bowman JD: Hemolytic disease (erythroblastosis fetalis). In Creasy RD, Resnik R, editors: *Maternal-fetal medicine*, ed 4, Philadelphia, 1999, WB Saunders.

Brooks C: Neonatal hypoglycemia, *Neonatal Network* 16(2):15-21, 1997.

Brown LP, Towne SA, York R: Controversial issues surrounding early postpartum discharge, *Nurs Clin Am* 31(2):333-339, 1996.

Buck ML: Vitamin K for the prevention of bleeding in newborns, *Pediatr Pharmacotherapy* 7(10):7-10, 2001.

Centers for Disease Control and Prevention: Surveillance for fetal alcohol syndrome using multiple sources, Atlanta, GA, 1981-1989, *MMWR* 46(47):1118-1120, 1997.

Chung M: Galactosemia in infancy: diagnosis, management, and prognosis, *Pediatr Nurs* 23(6):563-569, 1997.

Cooper WO and others: Use of health care services by inner-city infants in an early discharge program, *Pediatrics* 98(4):686-691, 1996.

Cornblath M and others: Controversies regarding definition of neonatal hypoglycemia: suggested operational thresholds, *Pediatrics* 105(5):1141-1145, 2000.

Cornblath M, Ichord R: Hypoglycemia in the neonate, *Semin Perinatol* 24(2):136-149, 2000.

Cowett RM: Neonatal hypoglycemia: a little goes a long way, *J Pediatr* 134(4):389-391, 1999.

Demarini S, Mimouni FB, Tsang RC: Disorders of calcium, phosphorous, and magnesium metabolism. In Fanaroff AA, Martin RJ, editors: *Neonatal-perinatal medicine: diseases of the fetus and infant,* ed 6, St Louis, 1997, Mosby.

Dohil MA, Baugh WP, Eichenfield LF: Vascular and pigmented birthmarks, *Pediatr Clin North Am* 47(4):783-812, 2000.

Eidelman AI, Kaitz M: Maternal postpartum cognitive deficits and early discharge of infants, *Pediatrics* 98(3):516, 1996 (letter to the editor).

Garas T and others: Perinatal morbidity: a comparison of vacuum delivery and spontaneous delivery, *Obstet Gynecol* 97(4 Suppl 1):S64, 2001.

Gartner LM: Neonatal jaundice, *Pediatr Rev* 15(11):422-432, 1994.

Greer FR and others: Improving the vitamin K status of breastfeeding infants with maternal vitamin K supplements, *Pediatrics* 99(1):88-92, 1997.

Griffiths PV and others: Wechsler subscale IQ and subtest profile in early treated phenylketonuria, *Arch Dis Child* 82(3):209-215, 2000.

Gropper SS and others: Free galactose content of fresh fruits and strained fruit and vegetable baby foods: more foods to consider for the galactose-restricted diet, *J Am Diet Assoc* 100(5):573-575, 2000.

Grupp-Phelan J and others: Early newborn hospital discharge and readmission for mild and severe jaundice, *Arch Pediatr Adolesc Med* 153(12):1283-1288, 1999.

Gruslin-Giroux A, Moore TR: Erythroblastosis fetalis. In Fanaroff AA, Martin RJ, editors: *Neonatal-perinatal medicine: diseases of the fetus and infant,* ed 6, St Louis, 1997, Mosby.

Hammerman C and others: Intravenous immune globulin in neonatal ABO isoimmunization: factors associated with clinical efficacy, *Biol Neonate* 70(2):69-74, 1996.

Harrell G, Murray PD: Diagnosis and management of congenital hypothyroidism, *J Perinat Neonat Nurs* 11(4):75-83, 1997.

Hoppe JE: Treatment of oropharyngeal candidiasis and candidal diaper dermatitis in neonates and infants: review and reappraisal, *Pediatr Infect Dis J* 16(9):885-894, 1997.

Hoseth E and others: Blood glucose levels in a population of healthy, breast fed, term infants of appropriate size for gestational age, *Arch Dis Child Fetal Neonatal Ed* 83(2):F117-F119, 2000.

Hudon L and others: Long-term neurodevelopmental outcome after intrauterine transfusion for the treatment of fetal hemolytic disease, *Am J Obstet Gynecol* 179(4):858-863, 1998.

Innamen VT and others: Point-of-care glucose testing in the neonatal intensive care unit is facilitated by the use of the Ames Glucometer Elite electrochemical glucose meter, *Pediatrics* 130(1):151-155, 1997.

JCAHO: Sentinel event alert: kernicterus threatens healthy newborns, Issue 18, April, 2001, *http://www.jcaho.org/edu_pub/sealert/sea18.html.*

Jackson GL and others: Problem identification in apparently well neonates: implications for early discharge, *Clin Pediatr* 39(10):581-590, 2000.

Johnson CB: Head, eyes, ears, nose, mouth and neck assessment. In Tappero EP, Honeyfield ME, editors: *Physical assessment of the newborn: a comprehensive approach to the art of physical assessment,* ed 2, Petaluma, CA, 1996, NICU Ink.

Johnson TS, Brennan RA, Flynn-Tymkow CD: A home visit program for breastfeeding education and support, *J Obstet Gynecol Neonat Nurs* 28(5):480-485, 1999.

Johnson L, Bhutani VK: Guidelines for management of the jaundiced term and near-term infant, *Clin Perinatol* 25(3):555-574, 1998.

Keppler AB, Roudebush JL: Postpartum follow-up care in a hospital-based clinic: an update on an expanded program, *J Perinat Neonat Nurs* 13(1):1-14, 1999.

Kirsten D: The thyroid gland: physiology and pathophysiology, *Neonatal Network* 19(8):11-26, 2000.

Koch RK: Issues in newborn screening for phenylketonuria, *Am Fam Physician* 60(5): 1462-1466, 1999.

LaReau AR: A new approach to early discharge, *Contemp Pediatr* 17(10):73-80, 2000.

Lawrence RA, Lawrence RM: *Breastfeeding: a guide for the medical profession,* ed 5, St Louis, 1999, Mosby.

Lucas A, Morley R, Cole TJ: Adverse neurodevelopmental outcome of moderate neonatal hypoglycemia, *BMJ* 297(6659): 1304-1308, 1988.

Luchtman-Jones L, Schwartz AL, Wilson DB: The blood and hematopoietic system. In Fanaroff AA, Martin RJ: *Neonatal-perinatal medicine: diseases of the fetus and infant,* ed 6, St Louis, 1997, Mosby.

Maisels MJ: Jaundice. In Avery GB, Fletcher MA, MacDonald MG, editors: *Neonatology: pathophysiology and management of the newborn,* ed 4, Philadelphia, 1994, JB Lippincott.

Maisels MJ, Newman TB: Kernicterus in otherwise healthy, breast-fed term newborns, *Pediatrics* 96(4):730-733, 1995.

Maisels MJ, Newman TB: Jaundice in full-term and near-term babies who leave the hospital within 36 hours: a pediatrician's nemesis, *Clin Perinatol* 25(2):295-302,1998.

Marconi A and others: An evaluation of fetal glucogenesis in intrauterine growth retarded pregnancies: steady state fetal and maternal enrichments of plasma glucose at cordocentesis, *Metabolism* 42(7):860-864, 1993.

Mari G: Noninvasive diagnosis by doppler ultrasonography of fetal anemia due to maternal red-cell alloimmunization, *N Engl J Med* 342(1):9-14, 2000.

Marcus J, Goldberg DJ: Lasers in dermatology: a nursing perspective, *Dermatol Nurs* 8(3):181-193, 1996.

Martin S and others: Comparison of two methods of bedside blood glucose screening in the NICU: evaluation of accuracy and reliability, *Neonatal Network* 16(2): 39-43, 1997.

Martinez J and others: Control of severe hyperbilirubinemia in full-term newborns with the inhibitor of bilirubin production Sn-mesoporphyrin, *Pediatrics* 103(1):1-5, 1999.

McCafferty DF and others: Effect of percutaneous local anaesthesia on pain reduction during pulse dye laser treatment of

portwine stains, *Br J Anaesth* 78(3):286-289, 1997.

McCance K, Huether S: *Pathophysiology: the biological basis for disease in infants and children,* ed 3, St Louis, 1998, Mosby.

Moe P, Paige PL: Neurologic disorders. In Merenstein GB, Gardner SL: *Handbook of neonatal intensive care,* ed 4, St Louis, 1998, Mosby.

Neal JL: RhD isoimmunization and current management modalities, *JOGNN* 30(6):589-607, 2001.

Nelson VR: The effect of newborn early discharge follow-up program on pediatric urgent care utilization, *J Pediatr Health Care* 13(2):58-61, 1999.

NIH Consensus Development Conference Statement: Phenylketonuria: screening and management, October 16-18, 2000, *Pediatrics* 108(4):972-982, 2001.

Pascale JA and others: Breastfeeding, dehydration, and shorter maternity stays, *Neonatal Network* 15(7):37-43, 1996.

Pietz J and others: Neurological outcome in adult patients with early-treated phenylketonuria, *Eur J Pediatr* 157(10):824-830, 1998.

Polk DH, Fisher DA: Disorders of the thyroid gland. In Taeusch HW, Ballard RA, editors: *Avery's diseases of the newborn,* ed 7, Philadelphia, 1998, WB Saunders.

Pollak L and others: Revival of non-surgical management of neonatal depressed skull fractures, *J Paediatr Child Health* 35(1): 96-97, 1999.

Porter ML, Dennis BL: Hyperbilirubinemia in the term newborn, *Am Fam Physician* 65(4):599-606, 613-614, 2002.

Poustie VJ, Rutherford P: Dietary interventions for phenylketonuria, *Cochrane Database Syst Rev* (2):CD001304, 2000.

Puckett RM, Offringa M: Prophylactic vitamin K for vitamin K deficiency bleeding in neonates, *Cochrane Database Syst Rev* 4:CD002776, 2000.

Putta LV, Spencer JP: Assisted vaginal delivery using the vacuum extractor, *Am Fam Physician* 62(6):1316-1320, 2000.

Reiners CH and others: Palpable spongy mass over the clavicle, an underutilized sign of clavicular fracture in the newborn, *Clin Pediatr* 39(12):695-698, 2000.

Ris MD and others: Adult psychosocial outcome in early-treated phenylketonuria, *J Inherit Metab Dis* 20(4):499-508, 1997.

Riva E and others: Early breastfeeding is linked to higher intelligence quotient scores in dietary treated phenylketonuric children, *Acta Paediatr* 85(1):56-58, 1996.

Rollnik JD and others: Botulinum toxin treatment of cocontractions after birth-related brachial plexus lesions, *Neurology* 55(1):112-114, 2000.

Ross MG, Fresquez M, El-Haddad MA: Impact of FDA advisory on reported vacuum-assisted delivery and morbidity, *J Fetal Matern Med* 9(6):321-326, 2001.

Rubin R: Puerperal change, *Nurs Outlook* 9(12):753-755, 1961.

Ruchala PL, Seibold L, Stemsterfer K: Validating assessment of neonatal jaundice with transcutaneous bilirubin measurement, *Neonatal Network* 15(4):33-37, 1996.

Scales J, Fleischer AB, Krowchuk DP: Bullous impetigo, *Arch Pediatr Adolesc Med* 151(11): 1168-1169, 1997.

Schumacher B, Moise KJ: Fetal transfusion for red blood cell alloimmunization in pregnancy, *Obstet Gynecol* 88(1):137-148, 1996.

Schwartz RP: Neonatal hypoglycemia: how low is too low? *J Pediatr* 31(2):171-173, 1997.

Seidman DS and others: Hospital readmission due to neonatal hyperbilirubinemia, *Pediatrics* 96(4):727-729, 1995.

Singh RH and others: Impact of a camp experience on phenylalanine levels, knowledge, attitudes, and health beliefs relevant to nutrition management of phenylketonuria in adolescent girls, *J Am Diet Assoc* 100(7):797-803, 2000.

Sood B and others: Prenatal alcohol exposure and childhood behavior at age 6 to 7 years: dose-response effect, *Pediatrics* 108(2):E34, 2001.

Soskolne EI and others: The effect of early discharge and other factors on readmission rates of newborns, *Arch Pediatr Adolesc Med* 150(3):373-379, 1996.

Soumekh B, Adams GL, Shapiro RS: Treatment of head and neck hemangiomas with recombinant interferon alpha 2B, *Ann Otol Rhinol Laryngol* 105(3):201-205, 1996.

Stanley CA, Baker L: The causes of neonatal hypoglycemia, *N Engl J Med* 340(15): 1200-1201, 1999.

Stoler JM, Holmes LB: Under-recognition of prenatal alcohol effects in infants of known alcohol abusing women, *J Pediatr* 135(4):430-436, 1999.

Swayze VW and others: Magnetic resonance imaging of brain anomalies in fetal alcohol syndrome, *Pediatrics* 99(2):232-240, 1997.

Szlachetka DM: Kasabach-Merritt syndrome: a case review, *Neonatal Network* 17(1):7-15, 1998.

Towner D and others: Effect of mode of delivery in nulliparous women on neonatal intracranial injury, *N Engl J Med* 341(23): 1709-1714, 1999.

Vanderhoof SL, Doidge WW, Maughan T: Flashlamp-pumped pulsed dye laser treatment of vascular birthmarks, *AORN J* 67(6):1214-1223, 1998.

Vertanen H and others: An automatic incision device for obtaining blood samples from the heel of preterm infants causes less damage than a conventional manual lancet, *Arch Dis Child Fetal Neonatal Ed* 84(1):F53-F55, 2001.

Volpe JJ: *Neurology of the newborn,* ed 4, Philadelphia, 2001, WB Saunders.

Walton DM and others: Morbid hypocalcemia associated with phosphate enema in a six-week-old infant, *Pediatrics* 106(3): e37, 2000.

Weglage J and others: Individual blood-brain barrier phenylalanine transport determines clinical outcome in phenylketonuria, *Ann Neurol* 50(4):463-467, 2001.

Wheeler BJ: Kernicterus: ancient history or ongoing threat? *Mother Baby J* 5(2):21-30, 2000.

Whitecar PW, Moise KJ: Sonographic methods to detect fetal anemia in red blood cell alloimmunization, *Obstet Gynecol Surv* 55(4):240-250, 2000.

Widhalm K, da Cruz M, Koch M: Diet does not ensure normal development in galatosemia, *J Am Coll Nutr* 16(3):204-208, 1997.

Woo EK: Device errors: biliblanket phototherapy light, *Nursing* 28(8):79, 1998.

# Chapter 10

# The High-Risk Newborn and Family

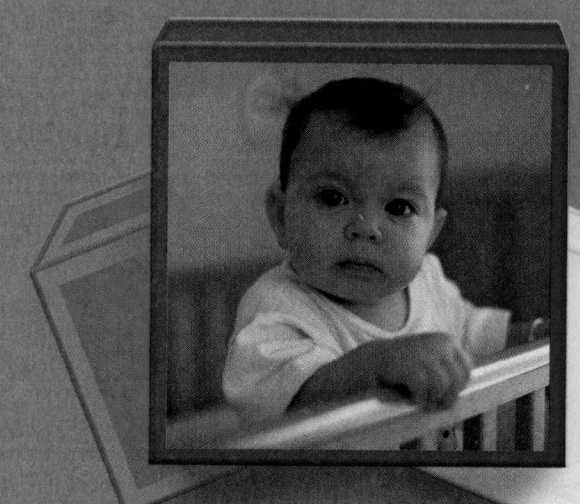

## Chapter Outline

**GENERAL MANAGEMENT OF HIGH-RISK NEWBORNS, 334**
**Identification of High-Risk Newborns, 334**
  Classification of High-Risk Newborns, 334
**Intensive Care Facilities, 334**
  Organization of Services, 335
  Transporting High-Risk Newborns, 335

**NURSING CARE OF HIGH-RISK NEWBORNS, 335**
**Assessment, 335**
  Systematic Assessment, 336
  Monitoring Physiologic Data, 337
**Nursing Diagnoses, 338**
**Planning, 338**
**Implementation, 338**
  Respiratory Support, 338
  Thermoregulation, 338
  Protection from Infection, 341
  Hydration, 341
  Nutrition, 342
  Feeding Resistance, 348
  Skin Care, 349
  Administration of Medications, 350

Neonatal Pain, 351
Developmental Outcome, 357
Facilitating Parent-Infant Relationships, 366
Discharge Planning and Home Care, 368
Neonatal Loss, 369
**Evaluation, 371**
*Nursing Care Plan: The High-Risk Infant, 371*

**HIGH-RISK CONDITIONS RELATED TO DYSMATURITY, 374**
**Preterm Infants, 374**
**Postmature Infants, 376**

**HIGH RISK RELATED TO DISTURBED RESPIRATORY FUNCTION, 376**
**Apnea of Prematurity (AOP), 376**
**Respiratory Distress Syndrome (RDS), 379**
**Meconium Aspiration Syndrome (MAS), 388**
**Extraneous Air Syndromes (Air Leaks), 389**
**Bronchopulmonary Dysplasia (BPD), 390**

**HIGH RISK RELATED TO INFECTIOUS PROCESSES, 393**
**Sepsis, 393**
  Sources of Infection, 393
**Necrotizing Enterocolitis (NEC), 395**

**HIGH RISK RELATED TO CARDIOVASCULAR/HEMATOLOGIC COMPLICATIONS, 397**
**Patent Ductus Arteriosus (PDA), 397**
**Persistent Pulmonary Hypertension of the Newborn (PPHN), 397**
**Anemia, 398**
**Polycythemia, 399**
**Retinopathy of Prematurity (ROP), 399**

**HIGH RISK RELATED TO NEUROLOGIC DISTURBANCE, 400**
**Perinatal Hypoxic-Ischemic Brain Injury, 400**
**Germinal Matrix–Intraventricular Hemorrhage (GM/IVH), 401**
**Intracranial Hemorrhage (ICH), 403**
  Subdural Hemorrhage, 403
  Subarachnoid Hemorrhage, 403
  Intracerebellar Hemorrhage, 403
**Neonatal Seizures, 403**

**HIGH RISK RELATED TO MATERNAL CONDITIONS, 404**
**Infants of Diabetic Mothers (IDMs), 404**
**Drug-Exposed Infants, 406**
  Opiate Exposure, 406
**Cocaine Exposure, 407**
**Infants of Mothers Who Smoke, 408**

## Related Topics

Administration of Medication, Ch. 27
Assessment (Newborn), Ch. 8
Birth of a Child with a Physical Defect, Ch. 11
Birth Injuries, Ch. 9
Bodily Injury and Pain, Ch. 26
Clinical Assessment of Gestational Age, Ch. 8
Congenital Diaphragmatic Hernia, Ch. 11
Discharge Planning and Home Care, Ch. 26
Esophageal Atresia with Tracheoesophageal Fistula, Ch. 11

Family-Centered Home Care, Ch. 25
Fetal Alcohol Syndrome, Ch. 9
Gastroschisis, Ch. 11
Hyperbilirubinemia, Ch. 9
Hypocalcemia, Ch. 9
Hypoglycemia, Ch. 9
Immunizations, Ch. 12
Infant Mortality, Ch. 1
Infectious Agents, Ch. 9
Latex Allergy, Ch. 11

Maintaining Healthy Skin, Ch. 27
Malformations of the Central Nervous System, Ch. 11
Nursing Care of the Surgical Neonate, Ch. 11
Omphalocele, Ch. 11
Pain Assessment; Pain Management, Ch. 26
Problems Caused by Perinatal Environmental Factors, Ch. 9
Promotion of Parent-Infant Bonding (Attachment), Ch. 8

# GENERAL MANAGEMENT OF HIGH-RISK NEWBORNS

## Identification of High-Risk Newborns

The *high-risk neonate* can be defined as a newborn, regardless of gestational age or birth weight, who has a greater-than-average chance of morbidity or mortality because of conditions or circumstances superimposed on the normal course of events associated with birth and the adjustment to extrauterine existence. The high-risk period encompasses human growth and development from the time of *viability* (the gestational age at which survival outside the uterus is believed to be possible, or as early as 23 weeks of gestation) up to 28 days following birth and includes threats to life and health that occur during the prenatal, perinatal, and postnatal periods.

---

■ Carol Turnage, MSN, RN, CNS; Marlene Walden, PhD; and David Wilson, MS, RNC, revised this chapter.

---

Assessment and prompt intervention in life-threatening perinatal emergencies often make the difference between a favorable outcome and a lifetime of disability. The nurse in the newborn nursery is familiar with the characteristics of neonates and recognizes the significance of serious deviations from expected observations. When the need for specialized care can be anticipated and planned for, the probability of successful outcome is increased.

### Classification of High-Risk Newborns

High-risk infants are most often classified according to birth weight, gestational age, and predominant pathophysiologic problems. The more common problems related to physiologic status are closely associated with the state of maturity of the infant and usually involve chemical disturbances (e.g., hypoglycemia, hypocalcemia) and consequences of immature organs and systems (e.g., hyperbilirubinemia, respiratory distress, hypothermia). Because high-risk factors are common to several specialty areas, particularly obstetrics, pediatrics, and neonatology, specific terminology is needed to describe the developmental status of the newborn (Box 10-1).

Formerly, weight at birth was considered to reflect a reasonably accurate estimation of gestational age. That is, if an infant's birth weight exceeded 2500 g (5½ pounds), the infant was considered to be mature. However, accumulated data have shown that intrauterine growth rates are not the same for all infants and that other factors (e.g., heredity, placental insufficiency, and maternal disease) influence intrauterine growth and the birth weight of the infant. From these data a more definitive and meaningful classification system that encompasses birth weight, gestational age, and neonatal outcome has been developed. It has also been determined that the lowest perinatal mortality is found in the infant who weighs between 3000 and 4000 g and whose gestational age is more than 36 weeks (Behrman and Shiono, 1997). (See Fig. 8-2 for size comparison of newborn infants.)

Many perinatal problems can be anticipated before delivery. Prenatal testing and labor monitoring have reduced the incidence of perinatal mortality, and specialized care of the distressed newborn is improving the survival rate. If the infant is likely to require special therapy at or soon after birth, plans can be made for the delivery to take place at a hospital with the facilities to provide such care. In this way there is no delay in initiating needed care, and some of the hazards associated with transporting the sick newborn are averted. Prenatal evaluation of fetal well-being and advanced surgical and anesthetic techniques have made intrauterine treatment of certain pathologic conditions possible, thus enhancing the neonate's chances for survival (Reed and Blumer, 1997).

## Intensive Care Facilities

Awareness of the unique characteristics of perinatal disorders has generated the provision of neonatal intensive care units (NICUs) in major medical facilities. Rapid advances in the understanding of the pathophysiology of the neonate and the increased capacity to apply this knowledge have emphasized the need for appropriate settings in which to care for the seriously ill infant. Advancements in electronics and biochemistry, new methods for monitoring cardiorespiratory function, microtechniques for biochemical determination from minute quantities of blood, noninvasive monitoring, and new methods for assisted ventilation and conservation of body heat have made it possible to effectively manage the newborn with serious illness.

Intensive care of the ill and immature newborn requires specialized knowledge and skill in a number of areas of expertise. Much of the equipment long used in the care of the critically ill adult is unsuited to the singular needs of the very small infant; therefore commonplace apparatus have been modified to meet these needs. Examples of modifications include ventilators that deliver small volumes of oxygen in the proper concentration and pressure, infusion pumps that deliver very small amounts accurately, and radiant heat warmers that provide a constant source of warmth and allow maximum access to the infant. Most important, intensive care has created a need for highly skilled personnel trained in the art of neonatal intensive care.

The diversity of special care needs requires that the unit be arranged for graduated care of the infant population. There should be adequate facilities and skilled personnel to provide one-to-one nursing care for each seriously ill infant, as well as a means for graduation to one-to-three or one-to-four nursing care in a convalescent area where infants require less intensive care until they are ready to leave the unit.

## Organization of Services

The most efficient organization of services is a regionalized system consisting of facilities within a designated geographic area. Neonatal intensive care facilities may provide three prescribed levels of care with special equipment, skilled personnel, and ancillary services concentrated in a centralized institution:

Level I facility—Provides management of normal maternal and newborn care but can identify high-risk pregnancies and high-risk neonates early and implement emergency care in the event of complications

Level II facility—Provides a full range of maternity and newborn care and is equipped to manage the majority of maternal and neonatal complications, depending on the resources available

Level III facility—Offers the full range of maternal and newborn services of a level II facility and has the capacity to provide care for the most complex neonatal complications; at least one full-time neonatologist is on the staff

## Transporting High-Risk Newborns

When the infant at risk is identified or anticipated, arrangements are made for care in the intensive care facility. There is no question that the uterus is the ideal transport unit for the infant with anticipated difficulties; therefore whenever possible the mother is taken where special care is available for her delivery.

Some infants develop difficulties after a seemingly normal pregnancy and uncomplicated labor. Because it is impossible to always predict when infants will require intensive care, a coordinated system is needed to ensure them an optimum opportunity for survival. Each hospital that delivers infants should be able to provide for appropriate neonatal stabilization and arrange for transport to a tertiary care facility. The infant must be kept warm, be adequately oxygenated (including intubation if indicated), have vital signs and oxygen saturation monitored and, when indicated, receive an IV infusion. The infant is transported in a specially designed incubator unit that contains a complete life-support system and other emergency equipment that can be carried by ambulance, van, plane, or helicopter.

The transport team may consist of one or more of the highly trained persons from the NICU: a neonatologist (or a fellow in neonatology), a respiratory therapist, and one or more nurses. The professional assigned to accompany the infant must be constantly alert to every change in the infant's condition and able to intervene appropriately. The neonate who must be moved from one place to another within the hospital (e.g., to surgery, from delivery room to nursery) is transported in an incubator or radiant warmer and accompanied by the necessary personnel and equipment.

# NURSING CARE OF HIGH-RISK NEWBORNS

Because the majority of infants admitted to intensive care facilities are born before the estimated date of delivery, the major discussion of problems related to the high-risk neonate are directed toward the preterm infant. (See p. 376 for a description of the characteristics of preterm infants.) The incidence of neonatal complications (e.g., respiratory distress and hypoglycemia) is highest in this group, and often other high-risk factors (e.g., sepsis and congenital malformations) are found in association with prematurity. Nursing problems encountered in the intensive care nursery are discussed, followed by a consideration of common complications. Nursing care of high-risk infants with more serious disorders is examined in relation to specific high-risk conditions.

## ⁘ Assessment

At birth the newborn is given a cursory, yet thorough, assessment to determine any apparent problems and identify those that demand immediate attention. This examination is primarily concerned with the evaluation of cardiopulmonary and neurologic functions. The assessment includes the assignment of an Apgar score (see Chapter 8) and an evaluation for any obvious congenital anomalies or evidence of neonatal distress. Delivery rooms are equipped with a special resuscitation area where infants with evidence of distress are stabilized and evaluated before being transported to the NICU for therapy and more extensive assessment. (See Clinical Assessment of Gestational Age, Chapter 8.)

Maintaining detailed, ongoing records of all activities and observations is an important responsibility of nurses in the intensive care setting. Knowledge about and operation of complex pieces of equipment and mechanical devices are inherent in the care of the ill neonate. However, sophisticated monitoring and life-support systems cannot replace the vigilance and constant scrutiny of the infant by experienced personnel.

## Systematic Assessment

A thorough systematic physical assessment is an essential component in the care of the high-risk infant. (See Guidelines box.) Subtle changes in feeding behavior, activity, color, oxygen saturation ($SaO_2$), or vital signs often indicate an underlying problem. The preterm infant, especially the extremely-low-birth-weight (ELBW) infant, is ill equipped to withstand prolonged physiologic stress and may die within minutes of exhibiting abnormal symptoms if the underlying pathologic process is not corrected. The alert nurse is aware of subtle changes and reacts promptly to implement interventions that promote optimum functioning in the high-risk neonate. Changes in the infant's status are noted through ongoing observations of the infant's adaptation to the extrauterine environment.

Observational assessments of the high-risk infant are made according to the infant's acuity; the critically ill infant requires close observation and assessment of respiratory function, including continuous pulse oximetry, electrolytes, and evaluation of blood gases. Accurate documentation of the infant's status is an integral component of nursing care. With the aid of continuous, sophisticated cardiopulmonary monitoring, nursing assessments and daily care may be coordinated to allow for minimal handling of the infant (especially the VLBW or ELBW infant) to decrease the effects of environmental stress.

# GUIDELINES
## Physical Assessment

### GENERAL ASSESSMENT

Using electronic scale, weigh daily or more often if necessary.
Measure length and head circumference periodically.
Describe general body shape and size, posture at rest, ease of breathing, presence and location of edema.
Describe any apparent deformities.
Describe any signs of distress: poor color, mottling, hypotonia.

### RESPIRATORY ASSESSMENT

Describe shape of chest (barrel, concave), symmetry, presence of incisions, chest tubes, or other deviations.
Describe use of accessory muscles: nasal flaring or substernal, intercostal, or subclavicular retractions.
Determine respiratory rate and regularity.
Auscultate and describe breath sounds: stridor, crackles, wheezing, diminished sounds, areas of absence of sound, grunting, diminished air entry, equality of breath sounds.
Determine whether suctioning is needed.
Describe cry if not intubated.
Describe ambient oxygen and method of delivery; if intubated, describe size of tube, type of ventilator and settings, and method of securing tube.
Determine oxygen saturation by pulse oximetry and partial pressure of oxygen and carbon dioxide by transcutaneous oxygen ($tcPO_2$) and transcutaneous carbon dioxide ($tcPCO_2$).

### CARDIOVASCULAR ASSESSMENT

Determine heart rate and rhythm.
Describe heart sounds, including any murmurs.
Determine the point of maximum intensity (PMI), the point at which the heartbeat sounds and palpates loudest (a change in the PMI may indicate a mediastinal shift).
Describe infant's color (may be of cardiac, respiratory, or hematopoietic origin): cyanosis, pallor, plethora, jaundice, mottling.
Assess color of mucous membranes and lips.
Determine blood pressure. Indicate extremity used and cuff size; check each extremity at least once.
Describe peripheral pulses, capillary refill (<2 to 3 seconds), peripheral perfusion (mottling).
Describe monitors, their parameters, and whether alarms are in "on" position.

### GASTROINTESTINAL ASSESSMENT

Determine presence of abdominal distention: increase in circumference, shiny skin, evidence of abdominal wall erythema, visible peristalsis, visible loops of bowel, status of umbilicus.
Determine any signs of regurgitation, and time related to feeding; character and amount of residual if gavage fed; if nasogastric tube in place, describe type of suction, drainage (color, consistency, pH, guaiac).
Describe amount, color, consistency, and odor of any emesis.
Palpate liver margin.
Describe amount, color, and consistency of stools; check for occult blood and/or reducing substances if ordered or indicated by appearance of stool.
Describe bowel sounds: presence or absence (must be present if feeding).

### GENITOURINARY ASSESSMENT

Describe any abnormalities of genitalia.
Describe amount (as determined by weight), color, pH, labstick findings, and specific gravity of urine (to screen for adequacy of hydration).
Check weight (the most accurate measure for assessment of hydration).

### NEUROLOGIC-MUSCULOSKELETAL ASSESSMENT

Describe infant's movements: random, purposeful, jittery, twitching, spontaneous, elicited; level of activity with stimulation; evaluate based on gestational age.
Describe infant's position or attitude: flexed, extended.
Describe reflexes observed: Moro, sucking, Babinski, plantar reflex, and other age-appropriate reflexes.
Determine level of response and consolability.
Determine changes in head circumference (if indicated); size and tension of fontanels, suture lines.
Determine pupillary responses in infant >32 weeks of gestation.

### TEMPERATURE

Determine skin and axillary temperature.
Determine relationship to environmental temperature.

### SKIN ASSESSMENT

Describe any discoloration, reddened area, signs of irritation, blisters, abrasions, or denuded areas, especially where monitoring equipment, infusions, or other apparatus come in contact with skin; also check and note *any* skin preparation used (e.g., povidone-iodine, tape).
Determine texture and turgor of skin: dry, smooth, flaky, peeling, etc.
Describe any rash, skin lesion, or birthmarks.
Determine whether intravenous infusion catheter or needle is in place, and observe for signs of infiltration.
Describe parenteral infusion lines: location, type (arterial, venous, peripheral, umbilical, central, peripheral central venous); type of infusion (medication, saline, dextrose, electrolyte, lipids, total parenteral nutrition); type of infusion pump and rate of flow; type of catheter or needle; and appearance of insertion site.

## Monitoring Physiologic Data

Most neonates under intensive observation are placed in a controlled thermal environment and monitored for heart rate, respiratory activity, and temperature. The monitoring devices are equipped with an alarm system that indicates when the vital signs are above or below preset limits. However, it is essential to check the apical heart rate and compare it with the monitor reading.

The placement of electrodes is a continual nursing problem because of the lack of flat areas on the neonate's chest, the limited space for alternating sites, the size of the electrodes, and irritation from the adhesive. Electrodes for cardiac monitors can often be applied to the back or the upper arms to provide relief for chest areas; nonadhesive limb electrodes eliminate possible skin irritation from tape. Hydrogel electrodes are gentler to the skin and are easily removed by lifting an edge from the skin and moistening with plain water to release the adhesive (Lund and others, 1997). If the same electrode is reapplied to the skin, the hydrogel should be rinsed with plain water to remove accumulated sodium from perspiration, which can eventually irritate the skin. It is important to follow the manufacturer's directions for care and handling of electrodes to avoid malfunction or burns to sensitive skin.

Blood pressure (BP) is monitored routinely in the sick neonate by either internal or external means. Direct recording with arterial catheters is often used but carries the risks inherent in any procedure in which a catheter is introduced into an artery. An umbilical venous catheter may also be used to monitor the neonate's central venous pressure. Oscillometry (Dinamap) or Doppler transcutaneous apparatus are simple, effective means for detecting alterations in systemic BP (hypotension or hypertension). Normal BP ranges for healthy premature infants are listed in Table 10-1. Infants who have birth asphyxia, have low Apgar scores, or are mechanically ventilated have lower systolic and diastolic pressures. Infants whose mothers are hypertensive have higher BPs (Hegyi and others, 1996).

In the NICU frequent laboratory examinations and their interpretation are integral parts of the ongoing assessment of infants' progress. Accurate intake and output records are kept on all infants. An accurate output can be obtained by collecting urine in a plastic urine collection bag specifically made for premature infants (see Urine Specimens, Chapter 27) or by weighing the diapers, which is the simplest and least traumatic means of measuring urinary output. The preweighed wet diaper is weighed on a gram scale, and the gram weight of the urine is converted directly to milliliters (e.g., 25 g = 25 ml).

One study showed that urine obtained from cloth diapers and disposable diapers containing absorbent gelling material (AGM) yielded inaccurate results for urine specific gravity, pH, and protein. Urine samples obtained from 100%-cotton cottonballs strategically placed in the diaper proved to be the most accurate (Kirkpatrick, Alexander, and Cain, 1997).

**NURSING TIP** When small volumes of urine are measured, superabsorbent disposable diapers, especially when kept closed, give more accurate volume measurements than cloth diapers because they are less affected by evaporative losses (Wong and others, 1992).

Plastic collecting devices can be used when it is necessary to collect urine for laboratory examination. Because volume normally voided is insufficient to float the standard urometer, a refractometer requiring only a single drop of urine may be used. A drop of urine can be aspirated with a syringe from the wet diaper or from cotton balls in the diaper.

Blood examinations are a necessary part of the ongoing assessment and monitoring of the sick newborn's progress. The tests most often performed are blood glucose, bilirubin, electrolytes, calcium, hematocrit, and blood gases. Samples may be obtained by heelstick, by venipuncture, by arterial puncture, or by an indwelling catheter in an umbilical vein, umbilical artery, or peripheral artery. (See Atraumatic Care box.) In one study, heel warming before lancing with an automated device (Tenderfoot, International Technidyne

### ATRAUMATIC CARE
#### Heel punctures

Wrapping the foot in a warm, damp washcloth or disposable diaper is a simple way to create adequate vasodilation for a heel puncture. The use of an automated lancing device may not require heel warming, however, and may decrease the physiologic stress and tissue trauma. Commercial warm packs are also available that protect the infant from thermal injury by providing a specific temperature range. Some studies found that blood sampling in newborns by venipuncture vs. heel lance was less painful when measured by neonatal pain scales, and the researchers recommend venipuncture for blood sampling (Shah and Ohlsson, 2001). An eutectic mixture of local anesthetics (EMLA) and topical amethocaine gel, although safe, did not appear to offer advantages in newborns when used to avoid the pain of heel lances (Jain, Rutter, and Ratnayaka, 2001; Stevens and others, 1999a). Nonpharmacologic interventions such as swaddling, nonnutritive sucking, facilitated tucking, skin-to-skin contact, and oral sucrose appear to be effective in decreasing or negating the pain experience in some neonates, yet further studies are needed to confirm these findings and make further recommendations (Stevens and Ohlsson, 2000; Gibbins and Stevens, 2001). Oral sucrose and nonnutritive sucking appear to be very effective in decreasing neonatal procedural pain (Noerr, 2001; Stevens and others, 1999b).

**TABLE 10-1**  Blood pressure ranges in different weight groups of healthy premature infants*

| Birth Weight (g) | Systolic (mm Hg) | Diastolic (mm Hg) |
|---|---|---|
| 501-750 | 50-62 | 26-36 |
| 751-1000 | 48-59 | 23-36 |
| 1001-1250 | 49-61 | 26-35 |
| 1251-1500 | 46-56 | 23-33 |
| 1501-1750 | 46-58 | 23-33 |
| 1751-2000 | 48-61 | 24-35 |

Modified from Hegyi T and others: Blood pressure ranges in premature infants. I. The first hours of life, *J Pediatr* 124(4):630, 1994.
*Defined as infants without a history of maternal hypertension, Apgar scores of less than 3 at 1 minute and less than 6 at 5 minutes, pneumothorax, hematocrit <0.32, serum pH <7.1, use of dopamine, infusion of erythrocytes or colloid, mechanical ventilation, or cardiopulmonary resuscitation.

Corporation, Edison, NJ) offered no particular advantage in relation to the amount of blood flow obtained and amount of heel squeezing required when compared with an unwarmed heel. Phlebotomists noted infants cried less and appeared less distressed when the automated device was used; also the heel incision was perceived to heal more readily with the automated device (Johnson and others, 2000).

When numerous blood samples must be drawn, it is important to maintain an accurate record of the amount of blood being removed, especially in ELBW and VLBW infants, who can ill afford to have their blood supply depleted during the acute phase of their illness. Although not widely available in most units, the development of laser beam technology for drawing capillary blood samples may reduce the risk of accidental injuries and infections in neonates. These precision devices break the skin with a tiny laser beam, causing less trauma than sharp lancets (Meehan, 1998). When infants require close monitoring of oxygenation, pulse oximetry, a noninvasive measurement of the saturation or percent of oxygen in the hemoglobin, is typically used. Although used less frequently than pulse oximetry, some situations warrant the monitoring of transcutaneous oxygen ($tcPO_2$) and carbon dioxide ($tcPCO_2$). The nurse notes changes in oxygenation (or other aspects being monitored) associated with handling and adjusts the infant's care accordingly. The frequency of vital signs is determined by the infant's acuity level (seriousness of condition) and response to handling.

**Safety Measures.** The proliferation of equipment technology over the past few years has increased the dangers associated with its use, especially performance malfunction and electrical hazards. Malfunction includes things such as inaccurate monitor function, erratic delivery rates in infusion devices, and low or high suction in pumps. Electrical hazards are related to improper use of equipment or defective equipment, wiring, or grounding.

Parents need to be instructed regarding safety precautions and observations. They are usually uncomfortable around the equipment and atmosphere of an intensive care unit and therefore appreciate an explanation of the purposes and functions of the devices and pertinent safety aspects. Visiting siblings, especially toddlers, must be supervised closely to avoid their "playing" with the equipment and inadvertently causing harm to the neonate. Although most NICUs are closed units, parents must also be educated and informed about specific safety measures designed to prevent neonatal abduction. Most institutions have their own protocols for preventing such an occurrence. (See Protect from Infection and Injury, Chapter 8.)

## Nursing Diagnoses

Many nursing diagnoses may be evident after a careful assessment of the infant at risk. Some apply to all infants; others vary according to the needs and characteristics of individual infants and their families. The nursing diagnoses that represent general guides for nursing intervention are found in the Nursing Care Plan on pp. 371-375. Because a number of health problems accompany the high-risk infant, the nurse is also alert to other conditions and complications discussed later in this chapter and elsewhere in the book.

## Planning

The nursing care plan for the high-risk infant depends to a large extent on the diagnosis of the health problem that places the infant at risk. However, the following are basic goals for all high-risk infants and their families:

1. Infant will exhibit adequate oxygenation.
2. Infant will maintain stable body temperature.
3. Infant will exhibit no evidence of nosocomial infection.
4. Infant will receive adequate hydration and nutrition.
5. Infant will maintain skin integrity.
6. Infant will exhibit normal intracranial pressure and no evidence of intraventricular hemorrhage (unless preexisting condition).
7. Infant will experience no pain or a reduction of pain.
8. Infant receives appropriate developmental support and care.
9. Family receives appropriate support, including preparation for home care or for infant's death.

## Implementation

### Respiratory Support

The primary objective in the care of high-risk infants is to establish and maintain respiration. Many infants require supplemental oxygen and assisted ventilation. All infants require appropriate positioning in order to ensure an open airway and to maximize oxygenation and ventilation. Oxygen therapy is provided on the basis of the infant's requirements and illness (see Respiratory Distress Syndrome, p. 379, and Oxygen Therapy, p. 383).

### Thermoregulation

Concurrent with the establishment of respiration, the most crucial need of the LBW infant is application of external warmth. Prevention of heat loss in the distressed infant is absolutely essential for survival, and maintaining a neutral thermal environment is a challenging aspect of neonatal intensive nursing care. Heat production is a complicated process that involves the cardiovascular, neurologic, and metabolic systems, and the immature neonate has all the problems related to heat production that are faced by the full-term infant. (See Thermoregulation, Chapter 8.) However, LBW infants are placed at further disadvantage by a number of additional problems. They have an even smaller muscle mass and fewer deposits of brown fat for producing heat, lack insulating subcutaneous fat, and have poor reflex control of skin capillaries.

**Pathophysiology.** The immature neonate, unable to increase activity and lacking a shivering response, produces heat primarily through increased metabolic processes. Some heat continues to be generated by liver, heart, brain, and skeletal muscles, but the major source of increased heat production during cold stress is *nonshivering thermogenesis.* Norepinephrine, secreted by the sympathetic nerve endings in response to chilling, stimulates fat metabolism in the richly vascularized brown adipose tissue to produce internal heat, which is then conducted through the blood to surface tissues. A significant increase in metabolism requires increased oxygen consumption.

The consequences of cold stress that produce additional hazards to the neonate are (1) hypoxia, (2) metabolic acidosis, and (3) hypoglycemia. Increased metabolism in response to chilling creates a compensatory increase in oxygen and calorie consumption.

Norepinephrine, released in response to cold stress, causes pulmonary vasoconstriction, which further reduces the effectiveness of pulmonary ventilation. This decrease in oxygen intake diminishes the supply available for glucose metabolism. As a result, glucose is broken down by an alternate, hypoxic pathway (anaerobic glycolysis) that generates increased lactic acid formation. This, together with acid end products of brown fat metabolism, contributes to the acidotic state. Anaerobic metabolism dissipates glycogen at a greatly increased rate over aerobic metabolism, thus precipitating hypoglycemia. This condition is especially marked when glycogen stores are diminished at birth and when there is inadequate caloric intake after birth.

**Maintaining Thermoneutrality.**   To delay or prevent the effects of cold stress, at-risk newborns are placed in a heated environment immediately following birth, where they remain until they are able to independently maintain *thermal stability*—the capacity to balance heat production and conservation and heat dissipation. Because overheating produces an increase in oxygen and calorie consumption, the infant is also jeopardized in a hyperthermic environment. A *neutral thermal environment* is one that permits the infant to maintain a normal core temperature with minimum oxygen consumption and calorie expenditure. Studies indicate that optimum thermoneutrality cannot be predicted for every high-risk infant's needs.

Thermal regulation in both VLBW and ELBW infants may require air temperature ranges higher than body core temperature. VLBW and ELBW infants, with thin skin and almost no subcutaneous fat, can control body heat loss or gain only within a very limited range of environmental temperatures. In these infants heat loss from radiation, evaporation, and transepidermal water loss is three to five times greater than in larger infants, and a decrease in body temperature is associated with an increase in mortality.

The three primary methods for maintaining a neutral thermal environment are the use of an incubator, a radiant warming panel and an open bassinet with cotton blankets (Fig. 10-1). The healthy, term infant dressed and under blankets can maintain a certain temperature within a wider range of environmental temperatures; however, the close observations required with a high-risk infant are best accomplished if the infant remains partially unclothed. The incubator should always be prewarmed before placing an infant in it. The use of *double-walled incubators* significantly improves the infant's ability to maintain a desirable temperature and reduces energy expenditure related to heat regulation. The infant is clothed and warmly wrapped in blankets when removed from the warm environment of the incubator for feeding or cuddling. Inside or outside the incubator, head coverings are effective in preventing heat loss. A fabric-insulated cap is more effective than one fashioned from stockinette (Blackburn and Loper, 1992).

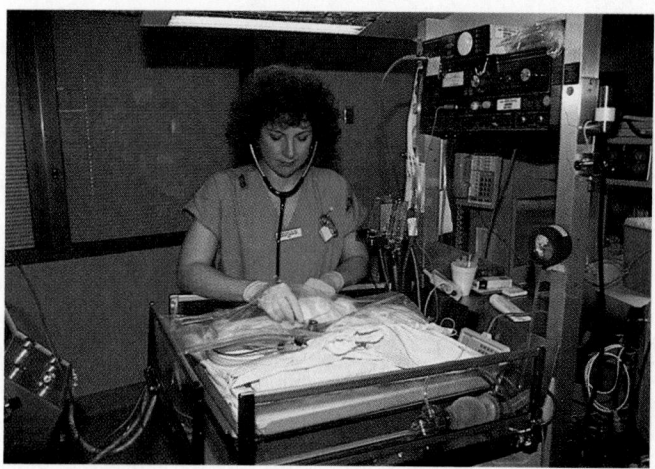

**Fig. 10-1**   Infant under overhead warming unit.

An effective means for maintaining the desired range of temperature in the infant is the use of an *automatically controlled (servocontrolled) incubator.* The mechanism, when set at the upper and lower limits of the desired circulating air temperature range, adjusts automatically in response to signals from a thermal sensor attached to the abdominal skin. If the infant's temperature drops, the warming device is triggered to increase heat output. The servocontrol is usually set to a desired skin temperature between 36° and 36.5°C (96.8° to 97.7°F) (Blake and Murray, 1998). In some cases, an incubator may be inadequate to maintain thermal stability in the ELBW infant during the immediate postnatal period, thus requiring the use of a radiant warmer.

Disadvantages are always inherent in any mechanical device; therefore an important part of nursing assessment is to compare the infant's temperature with the temperature in the incubator. For example, if the infant's temperature fluctuates in response to sepsis, the servocontrolled mechanism would respond by decreasing or increasing the ambient air temperature. However, if the skin probe becomes detached from the infant's skin, the incubator may falsely register a low skin temperature, causing the incubator temperature to rise and overheat the infant.

*Convective heat loss* occurs when infants are exposed to increased air flow velocity and turbulence (e.g., drafts from doors, ventilation system, opening and closing incubator portholes and side panels). The infant being cared for in a radiant warmer will also experience convective heat losses in response to ventilation drafts and traffic flow around the bed; these losses may be partially countered with plastic wrap placed directly on the infant's body or stretched over the side guards of the warmer unit (Fig. 10-2). Oxygen or any source of air, such as an oxygen mask or tube, should not blow directly on the infant's face. Oxygen concentrated around the head, such as that supplied to a hood, must be warmed and humidified.

*Radiant heat loss* is one of the greatest threats to temperature regulation in the incubator, because the temperature of circulating air within has no influence on heat loss to cooler surfaces without, such as windows, walls, or a lower nursery temperature. Such losses can be effectively reduced

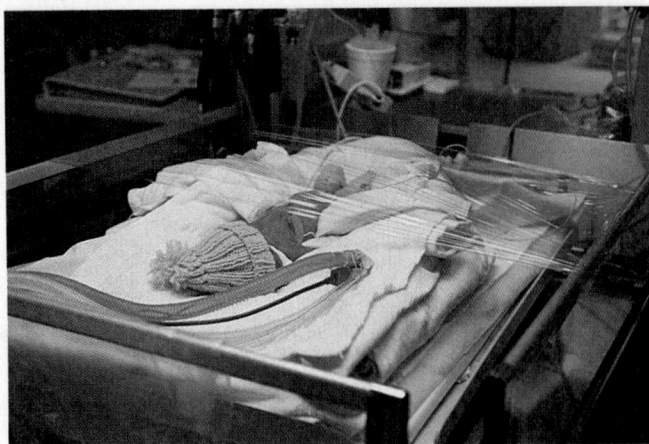

**Fig. 10-2** Infant under plastic wrap, which produces a draft-free environment.

with the use of double-walled incubators; the infant will radiate heat to the inner wall, which is surrounded by the warmed incubator air. The use of a dark cloth incubator cover further reduces radiant heat loss and provides some protection from exterior light sources. Appropriate physiologic monitoring (cardiorespiratory and pulse oximetry) will alert the nurse to any problems the infant may be experiencing while in the darkened environment, which would, of course, warrant visual assessment of the infant's status. (See Critical Thinking Exercise box.)

A high-humidity atmosphere contributes to body temperature maintenance by reducing *evaporative heat loss.* Humidity is provided in some incubators by circulating air over a heated water reservoir, which has the additional advantage of decreasing heat loss by convection as the air flows over the infant. Because stagnant, warm water provides an excellent breeding medium for microorganisms, the reservoir is emptied every 8 to 24 hours and replaced with sterile distilled water. The recommended humidity is 50% to 65%; higher humidity and a warmer environment are recommended for VLBW infants.

A number of "microenvironments" may be used with the VLBW and ELBW infant to minimize evaporative and insensible water losses. These include items such as bubble wrap blankets, humidified reservoirs for incubators, humidified tents, humidified Plexiglas boxes with plastic wrap coverings, and plastic wrap blankets (Horns and Cusson, 1994). The use of emollient cream to prevent transepidermal water loss has varying results (Lambe, 2001). Because of the ever-present danger of infection, many nurseries no longer use water in incubators.

*Conductive heat loss* can be reduced by warming all items that come in direct contact with the infant, such as scales, radiographic film, blankets, and the hands of caregivers. Warming the items before use can reduce this source of heat loss (e.g., storing blankets in a warming unit ready for use and placing a freestanding warming unit or a heat lamp over a scale before weighing an infant).

Although the open radiant warmer unit allows easier access to the infant, there is an inherent increase in evaporative water loss (and evaporative heat loss) from the skin, especially in ELBW and VLBW infants. Transepidermal water

losses (also called insensible water loss [IWL]) may be increased by as much as 50% to 200%, thus predisposing the infant to dehydration; daily fluid requirements are generally increased to compensate for such losses. The use of plastic wrap over the ELBW or VLBW infant in a radiant warmer will help reduce IWL and convective losses. Plexiglas heat shields are not recommended for use in radiant warmers because they block radiant heat waves.

The infant being cared for in a radiant warmer is kept warm using the servocontrol method. Air temperature manual control should not be used because of the danger of overheating the infant. A reflective aluminum temperature probe cover is used to allow proper function of the servocontrol heating unit. Traditionally, the temperature probe is placed over a nonbony, well-perfused tissue area such as the abdomen, flank, or back. In general, the probe site is changed when the infant's position is changed to avoid the probe coming in contact with the bed surface and potentially trapping heat at the probe site, causing an abnormal ambient temperature. However, frequent probe changes may result in epidermal stripping and disruption of skin integrity; two probes may be used to avoid frequent changing, yet this is less cost effective. Blackburn and others (2001) found that abdominal and back skin temperatures varied considerably based on the infant's position and the probe position; when infants were positioned prone and the probe was on the abdomen the skin temperature rose. The researchers concluded that changing probe sites with repositioning may result in unstable body temperatures, that a consistent method of probe placement is needed, and that placement of the probe on the lateral abdomen may allow for frequent position changes (supine and prone) without the difficulties that occur when the infant lies on the probe.

As with incubators used in servocontrol, a dislodged probe or placement of the infant prone over the skin probe will cause inaccurate skin temperature readings and subsequent hypothermia or hyperthermia—with either being undesirable. The use of sterile cloth or disposable drapes will also block radiant heat waves in a radiant warmer; during such procedures the use of a warmed blanket under the infant is appropriate. Clothing an infant on servocontrol in an incubator or radiant warmer is not recommended; head covering and foot covering (socks or booties) may be used with discretion.

Prolonged exposure to cold stress in the sick or preterm infant may have disastrous results from which recovery may not be possible, particularly in the ELBW or VLBW infant. In one study, 45% of VLBW infants delivered in a tertiary center were hypothermic (body temperature less than 36.3°C [97.6°F]); the lower the birth weight and gestational age, the greater the degree of hypothermia. The hypothermic infants were also acidemic, and some required pharmacologic intervention (Loughead, Loughead, and Reinhart, 1997). This study further emphasizes the need for thermoregulation measures to be taken in the labor and delivery area and during transport to the NICU. The use of plastic wrap; careful drying; a cloth head cap; the prewarming of equipment such as scales, stethoscopes, and incubators; and prompt placement of the VLBW or ELBW newborn in a proper heat source is essential for the prevention of further morbidity.

Hyperthermia may cause equally untoward effects because high-risk infants typically have a limited ability to perspire, thus heat dissipation is decreased. In high-risk neonates hyperthermia is usually a result of overheating rather than hypermetabolism. Therefore adequate knowledge of proper care and use of external heating devices, such as radiant warmers or incubators, is as important as knowing the conditions for which they are being used.

## Protection from Infection

Protection from infection is an integral part of all newborn care, but preterm and sick neonates are particularly susceptible. Thorough, meticulous, and frequent handwashing is the foundation of a preventive program. This includes *all* persons who come in contact with infants and their equipment. After handling another infant or equipment, no one should ever touch an infant without first washing hands.

Personnel with infectious disorders are either barred from the unit until they are no longer infectious or are required to wear suitable shields, such as masks or gloves, to reduce the likelihood of contamination. In some areas an annual influenza vaccination is recommended for NICU personnel. Standard precautions as a method of infection control are instituted in all nursery areas to protect the infants and staff. (See Chapter 27.) In some areas special clothing furnished by the institution is worn by everyone working in the unit. Fresh scrub dresses or suits are put on before entering the unit and are changed any time they become contaminated. When personnel leave the unit, the scrub clothing is protected by a cover gown that is removed and then discarded in the laundry hamper before the wearer reenters the unit. The benefit of "gowning" by visitors and hospital staff to control infection is not supported by research (Altimier, Lott, and McCain, 1996). Because of the monetary savings hospitals are reaping from decreasing the availability of hospital-laundered "scrubs" and the lack of conclusive data showing that home-laundered scrubs are ineffective in infection control (Kiehl, Wallace, and Warren, 1997), many neonatal units no longer require staff to wear hospital-laundered scrubs. The practice of wearing home-laundered scrub clothes varies according to unit and institutional policy.

Periodic epidemiologic studies (at least quarterly or monthly is recommended) are carried out in the NICU to evaluate the incidence and types of nosocomial infections and the number and types of bacteria colonized from indwelling lines (catheters) and blood, endotracheal (ET) tube secretions, and cerebrospinal fluid cultures. Specific trends are monitored and reported to the proper institutional authorities. Readmission of infants from home or admission of infants delivered in unsterile conditions or infants suspected of having communicable illnesses is handled per institutional protocol. Such infants should be at least physically isolated from other highly susceptible high-risk infants initially. (See American Academy of Pediatrics and American College of Obstetricians and Gynecologists [1997] for further infection control recommendations, including nursery care of infants with specific communicable diseases.)

## Hydration

High-risk infants often receive supplemental parenteral fluids to supply additional calories, electrolytes, and/or water. Adequate hydration is particularly important in preterm infants because their extracellular water content is higher (70% in full-term infants and up to 90% in preterm infants), their body surface area is larger, and the capacity for osmotic diuresis is limited in preterm infants' underdeveloped kidneys. Therefore these infants are highly vulnerable to fluid depletion.

Parenteral fluids may be given to the high-risk neonate via several routes depending on the nature of the illness, the duration and type of fluid therapy, and unit preference. Common routes of fluid infusion include peripheral, peripherally inserted central venous (or percutaneous central venous), surgically inserted central venous or arterial and, at times, umbilical venous or umbilical arterial catheterization. The preferred sites for peripheral intravenous infusions in neonates are the peripheral veins on the dorsal surfaces of the hands or feet. Alternative sites are scalp veins and antecubital veins. Special precautions and frequent observations (at least once every hour) must accompany the use of peripheral lines with hypertonic solutions (dextrose 10% to 15%) and hyperalimentation. In many neonatal centers the percutaneous central venous catheter (PCVC), also commonly called the peripherally inserted central venous catheter (PICC), is used for intravenous hydration therapy and medication administration because of less expense and decreased neonatal trauma, and because the procedure may be performed by specially trained nurses (Trotter, 1996).

If peripheral sites are exhausted by long-term therapy, percutaneous central venous lines or a venous cutdown (usually inserted in the saphenous or antecubital vein) may be used. The increased use of small-gauge percutaneous catheters has reduced the need for an incision or "cutdown" option.

In most facilities NICU nurses insert peripheral intravenous catheters and maintain the infusions. Intravenous fluids must always be delivered by continuous infusion pumps that deliver minute volumes at a preset flow rate. The catheter is secured to the skin with transparent tape, with care taken not to cause undue pressure from the needle hub and tubing. Because ELBW and VLBW infants are highly vulnerable to any fluid shifts, infusion rates are very carefully regulated and are checked hourly to prevent tissue damage from extravasation, fluid overload, or dehydration (Wilson, 2001). Pulmonary edema, congestive heart failure, patent ductus arteriosus, and intraventricular hemorrhage may occur with fluid overload. Dehydration may cause electrolyte disturbances (particularly $Na^+$), with potentially serious central nervous system (CNS) effects.

Small, fragile peripheral blood vessels are subject to rupture and subsequent infiltration. This situation is compounded by the use of infusion pumps that continue to infuse fluid into surrounding tissues. Observations are especially important when using hypertonic solutions (calcium, sodium bicarbonate, albumin 25%) and intravenous drugs (antibiotics and vasoactive drugs such as dopamine and dobutamine), which can cause severe tissue damage. With the increased use of flexible catheters and small intravenous catheter shields, the use of arm boards and limb restraints is usually unnecessary. If used, restraints are checked frequently to ensure that no harm to the patient's extremity occurs and that peripheral circulation is adequate.

Infants who are ELBW, tachypneic, receiving phototherapy, or in a radiant warmer have increased insensible water

**NURSING ALERT** Nurses should be constantly alert for signs of infiltration (e.g., redness, edema, or color change of tissue; blanching at site) and for signs of overhydration (weight gain over 30 g/24 hr, periorbital edema, tachypnea, tachycardia, and crackles on lung auscultation).

losses that require appropriate fluid adjustments. Nurses must monitor fluid status by daily (or more frequent) weights; accurate intake and output of all fluids, including medications and blood products; specific gravity; dipstick measurements of urine; and evaluation of serum electrolyte levels. ELBW infants often require more frequent monitoring of these parameters because of their inordinate transepidermal fluid loss, immature renal function, and propensity to dehydration or overhydration. Intolerance of even dextrose 5% is not uncommon in the ELBW infant, with subsequent glycosuria and osmotic diuresis. Alterations in behavior, alertness, or activity level in these infants receiving intravenous fluids may signal an electrolyte imbalance, hypoglycemia, or hyperglycemia. The nurse is also observant for tremors or seizures in the VLBW or ELBW infant, because these may be a sign of hyponatremia or hypernatremia.

A common problem observed in infants who have an umbilical catheter in place is vasoconstriction of peripheral vessels, which can seriously impair circulation. The response is triggered by arterial vasospasm caused by the presence of the catheter, the infusion of fluids, or injection of medication. Blanching of the buttocks, genitalia, or legs or feet is an indication of vasospasm. The problem is recognized promptly and reported to the practitioner. The nurse must also observe for signs of thrombi in infants with umbilical venous or arterial lines. The precipitation of microthrombi in the vascular bed with the use of such catheters is commonly manifested by a sudden bluish discoloration seen in the toes, called "cath toes." The problem is promptly reported to the practitioner because failure to alleviate the existing pathology may result in the loss of toes or even a foot or leg.

**NURSING ALERT** Circulatory effects are observed first in the toes but may extend to include the legs and buttocks. The toes first flush and then turn a mulberry color, and if the condition is not corrected, there may be serious complications involving the loss of a limb. The infant with an umbilical venous or arterial catheter should also be observed closely for catheter dislodging and subsequent bleeding or hemorrhage; urinary output, renal function, and gastrointestinal (GI) function are also evaluated in these infants. Although the intent of such catheters is to effectively deliver intravenous fluids (and sometimes medications) and to obtain arterial blood gas samples, they are not without inherent complications.

## Nutrition

Optimal nutrition is critical in the management of ELBW, VLBW, and LBW preterm infants, but there are difficulties in providing for their nutritional needs. The various mechanisms for ingestion and digestion of foods are not fully developed; the more immature the infant, the greater the problem. In addition, the nutritional requirements for this group of infants are not known with certainty. It is known that all preterm infants are at risk because of poor nutritional stores and several physical and developmental characteristics.

**Physiologic Characteristics.**   An infant's need for rapid growth and daily maintenance must be met in the presence of several anatomic and physiologic disabilities. Although some sucking and swallowing activities are demonstrated before birth and in premature infants, coordination of these mechanisms does not occur until approximately 32 to 34 weeks of gestation, and they are not fully synchronized until 36 to 37 weeks. Initial sucking is not accompanied by swallowing, and esophageal contractions are uncoordinated. The gag reflex may not be developed until 36 weeks of gestation. Consequently, infants are highly prone to aspiration and its attendant dangers. As infants mature, the suck-swallow pattern develops but is slow and ineffectual, and these reflexes may also become easily exhausted.

As with most full-term infants, preterm infants have poor muscle tone in the area of the lower esophageal (cardiac) sphincter. This causes milk in the stomach to be easily regurgitated into the esophagus, where it can trigger the chemoreceptors and cause apnea (vagal stimulation) and bradycardia and increase the risk of aspiration. The stomach has a very limited capacity in preterm infants and is easily overdistended, further compromising respiration.

Physiologically, preterm infants (LBW, not ELBW or VLBW) have approximately the same capacity to digest and absorb protein as full-term infants. However, carbohydrates and fats are less well tolerated. The secretion of lactase, a late-developing enzyme, is low in infants born before 34 weeks of gestation; therefore formulas containing lactose may not be well tolerated. Although amylase is deficient in preterm infants, an alternative enzyme (glucoamylase) is able to compensate in most neonates so that they are able to tolerate moderate amounts of starch. Preterm infants are inefficient in digesting and absorbing lipids, especially the saturated triglycerides of cow's milk, because they have low levels of pancreatic lipase and low bile acid.

**Nutritional Needs.**   The demand for nutrients in LBW infants is much higher than that in larger infants, and individual infants vary in activity level, ease of achieving basal energy expenditure, thermoneutrality, physical condition, and efficacy of nutrient absorption. The American Academy of Pediatrics, Committee on Nutrition (1998), recommends an energy intake of 105 to 130 kcal/kg/day (taken enterally) for most preterm infants to achieve a satisfactory growth rate. Increased calories may be provided if growth is not satisfactory using these parameters.

The caloric requirements of preterm infants are shown in Table 10-2. Because most of the nutritional stores are accumulated in the final months of gestation, preterm infants are also hampered by low stores of calcium, iron, phosphorus, proteins, and vitamins A and C.

The amount and method of feeding are determined by the size and condition of the infant. Nutrition can be provided by either the parenteral or enteral route or by a com-

**TABLE 10-2**   Estimated energy requirement in low-birth-weight infant

| Energy Expenditure | kcal/kg/day |
| --- | --- |
| Total energy used | 40-60 |
| Resting metabolic rate | 40-50 |
| Activity | 0-5 |
| Thermoregulation | 0-5 |
| Energy synthesis | 15 |
| Stored energy | 20-30 |
| Stool loss (energy) | 15 |
| Energy intake | 90-120 |

Modified from American Academy of Pediatrics, Committee on Nutrition: *Pediatric nutrition handbook*, ed 4, Evanston, IL, 1998, The Academy; and European Society of Pediatric Gastroenterology and Nutrition (ESPGAN): *Nutrition and feeding of preterm infants*, Oxford, England, 1987, Blackwell Scientific Publications.

bination of the two. Infants who are ELBW, VLBW, or critically ill have often been fed exclusively by the parenteral route because of their inability to digest and absorb enteral nutrition. Illness factors resulting in hypoxia and major organ immaturity further preclude the use of enteral feeding until the infant's condition has stabilized; necrotizing enterocolitis (NEC) has previously been associated with enteral feedings in acutely ill or distressed infants. (See section on NEC in this chapter.)

Total parenteral nutritional support of acutely ill infants may be accomplished with commercially available intravenous solutions specifically designed to meet the infant's nutritional needs, including protein, amino acids, trace minerals, vitamins, carbohydrates (dextrose), and fat (lipid emulsion). Daily monitoring of weight, electrolytes, renal function, calcium, triglycerides (or lipoprotein), and hydration status is carried out to ensure adequate therapy. Equally important as nutrition is the necessity to maintain adequate serum glucose homeostasis in sick preterm infants who may be dependent on exogenous glucose sources for several days or weeks. Cornblath and Ichord (2000) recommend that in sick preterm infants an operational threshold blood glucose value of 45 to 50 mg/dl (2.6 to 2.8 mmol/L) be maintained; healthy, feeding preterm infants may tolerate lower levels (30 to 35 mg/dl; 1.7 to 2.0 mmol/L) the first day of life without adverse neurologic effects.

Recent studies have shown that there are benefits to the early introduction of small amounts of enteral feedings in metabolically stable preterm infants (Evans and Thureen, 2001). These *minimal enteral feedings* (trophic feedings, GI priming) have been shown to simulate the infant's GI tract, preventing mucosal atrophy and subsequent enteral feeding difficulties. Minimal enteral feedings with as little as 0.1 to 4 ml/kg formula or breast milk may be given by gavage as early as the third or seventh postnatal day. An increased incidence of NEC in those VLBW infants fed enterally was not substantiated (Berseth, 1995; Schanler and others, 1999).

Schanler and others (1999) studied 171 premature infants (26 to 30 weeks) randomly assigned by diet (human milk or preterm formula), presence or absence of GI priming, and tube feeding method (continuous or intermittent bolus). There was no difference in the time to full oral feeding regardless of the method used. GI priming was not associated with any adverse outcomes and was related to improved calcium and phosphorus retention, higher calcium levels and alkaline phosphatase activity, and decreased intestinal transit times. Infants receiving intermittent bolus feedings showed significantly less feeding intolerance and demonstrated better weight gain than continuously fed infants. Morbidity was lower for infants who received the greater number of human milk feedings.

There is still some controversy regarding the type of enteral feeding that best meets the nutritional needs of LBW infants. The predominant view supports the use of milk from an infant's own mother or modified premature infant formulas. Commercial formulas have been designed specifically to meet the needs of small preterm infants and provide for adequate growth and metabolic stability. (See Table 8-6.) Prepared formulas have the added advantage of allowing more concentrated feedings.

Milk produced by mothers whose infants are born before term contains higher concentrations of protein, sodium, chloride, and immunoglobulin A (IgA). Thus mothers appear to be the preferred source of milk for their preterm infants. Growth factors, hormones, prolactin, calcitonin, thyroxine, steroids, and taurine (an essential amino acid) are also found in human milk. The milk produced by mothers for their infants changes in content over the first 30 days postnatally, at which time it is similar to full-term human milk. Infants fed with their own mother's milk display a more rapid rate of growth in all parameters and require a shorter length of time to regain birth weight. Premature infants who received unfortified human milk during their hospitalization demonstrated better intellectual performance scores at 7½ to 8 years of age compared to children who received formula (Schanler, 2001). Improved psychomotor development at 18 months has also been observed in preterm infants fed donor human milk compared with formula-fed preterm infants. It has been reported that once the mother's milk "matures" (around 3 to 4 weeks postnatally), it is not adequate for optimal growth to occur in the LBW infant.

LBW infants (<1500 g) who are exclusively fed unfortified human milk demonstrate decreased growth rates and nutritional deficiencies even beyond the hospitalization period. Inadequacies of calcium, phosphorus, protein, sodium, vitamins, and energy are seen in these infants (Schanler, 2001). Although fortified human milk (FHM) is associated with a slower rate of growth, studies show it supplies adequate nutrition. Preterm infants fed FHM have shorter hospital stays and less infection and NEC than infants given preterm formulas. Fortifiers are commercially available usually as a liquid or powder containing protein, carbohydrate, calcium, phosphorus, magnesium, sodium, and varied amounts of zinc, copper, and vitamins. Because fortifiers do not contain sufficient iron, an exogenous source must be administered after enteral feeding. FHM should be mixed daily and stored in a refrigerator to be used within 24 hours (Schanler, 2001).

The antiinfective attributes of human milk provide additional advantages for preterm infants. Secretory IgA concentration is higher in the milk from mothers of preterm infants than in the milk from mothers of full-term infants. IgA is important in the control of bacteria in the intestinal tract, where it inhibits adherence and proliferation of bacteria on epithelial surfaces. Additional protection from infection is provided by leukocytes, lactoferrin, and lysozyme, all of which are in human milk.

In a retrospective medical record review, the incidence and severity of retinopathy of prematurity was less in human milk–fed preterm infants than those given formula. Fewer developed advanced retinopathy, and none of them required retinal surgery.

NEC has been shown in several studies to be higher in formula-fed infants than in preterm infants fed human milk. Another report suggests that severity of NEC is lessened and the prevalence of intestinal perforation lowered when human milk constitutes the feeding for preterm infants (Schanler, 2001).

Preterm infants exclusively fed FHM have demonstrated significantly decreased NEC, fewer positive blood cultures, and decreased need for antibiotics. In one study infants fed FHM also received more skin-to-skin (STS) contact with their mothers and shorter hospital stays. Schanler (2001) suggests that STS contact might potentially stimulate the enteromammary immune system to produce specific antibodies against nosocomial pathogens in the nursery. Gastric emptying is improved with human milk feedings for preterm infants, primarily because of increased intestinal lactase and possibly decreased intestinal permeability. Finally, the psychologic advantages the mother gets from using her own milk cannot be overlooked.

The use of donor human milk must be carefully evaluated in reference to transmission of infections such as cytomegalovirus and human immunodeficiency virus (HIV). Pasteurization of donor human milk appears to kill HIV but is also harmful to leukocytes, milk lipids, and lactoferrin.

Although the timing of the first feeding has been a matter of controversy, most authorities now believe that early feeding (provided that the infant is medically stable) reduces the incidence of complicating factors such as hypoglycemia, dehydration, and the degree of hyperbilirubinemia. The feeding regimen used varies in different units. The initial enteral feeding is usually not attempted until infants have adapted to extrauterine existence as evidenced by adequate oxygenation, evidence of GI motility, including passage of meconium, and stable cardiopulmonary status (see p. 369 for discharge nutrition).

**Nipple Feeding.** Vigorous infants can be fed from a nipple with little difficulty, whereas compromised preterm infants will require alternative methods. The amount to be fed is determined largely by the infant's weight gain and tolerance of previous feeding and is increased by small increments until a satisfactory caloric intake is ensured.

The rate of increase that is well tolerated varies from one infant to another, and determining this rate is often a nursing responsibility. Preterm infants require more time and patience to feed than full-term infants, and the oral-pharyngeal mechanism may be stressed by an attempt to feed too rapidly. It is important not to tire the infants or overtax their

## Critical Thinking Exercise

### Infant Feeding

The mother of a 4-pound, 36-week preterm infant who has only recently started nipple feeding expresses concern that the feeding takes 25 to 30 minutes and that the infant has one or two apneic episodes during feedings. The infant is gaining approximately 20 to 30 g per day, and axillary temperature has been 36.6°C (97.9°F) throughout the day. To assist the mother in understanding aspects of feeding a preterm infant, what should be your best response?

FIRST, THINK ABOUT IT . . .

• Within what point of view are you thinking?
• What conclusions are you reaching?

1. Suggest that the mother let the experienced nurse feed the infant until the mother learns to feed correctly.
2. Recommend that the mother use a softer, pliable nipple to allow the infant to feed faster.
3. Encourage the mother to continue feeding the infant, with frequent rest periods or pauses.
4. Explain to the mother that the infant will require all feedings to be given by gavage, because the infant is so small and has apnea.

*The best response is three. It is not uncommon for preterm infants to experience apnea with nipple feedings. Frequent short breaks in feeding allow for swallowing and breathing to occur.*

*Option two is incorrect. The common belief that a soft nipple is more desirable is incorrect. Expediency in feeding is not always the major goal. Because the infant is demonstrating adequate weight gain, there is no reason to gavage feed or suspect pathologic apnea as suggested in option four. Option one is incorrect because it discounts the mother's involvement in the care of her infant.*

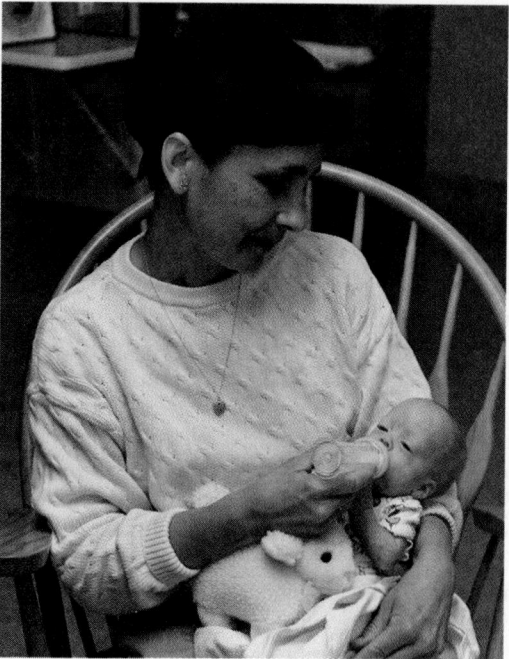

**Fig. 10-3**   Position for nipple-feeding premature infant.

mittent feedings by gavage are instituted until they gain enough strength and coordination to use the nipple.

> **NURSING ALERT**   Poor feeding behaviors such as apnea, bradycardia, cyanosis, pallor, and decreased oxygen saturation in any infant who has previously fed well may indicate an underlying illness.

Although the nurse's role in relation to feeding depends on the institution, the following are suggested nursing responsibilities: (1) recognize feeding readiness cues; (2) identify feeding behaviors typical of preterm infants; (3) understand the infant's history and current medical condition; (4) consider environment, behavioral state, time of day, nipple type, and positioning; (5) understand rationale for different facilitation techniques and use appropriately; (6) evaluate feeding ability and tolerance; and (7) identify infants with poor progress, structural defects, or abnormal feeding patterns who would benefit from specific therapy.

A developmental approach to feeding considers the individual infant's readiness rather than initiating feedings based on weight and age. Feeding readiness is determined by each infant's medical status, energy level, ability to sustain a brief quiet alert state, gag reflex (demonstrated with gavage tube insertion), spontaneous rooting and sucking behaviors, and functional sucking reflex (Hunter, 2001).

Nipple feeding within a developmental framework involves three steps (Ancona and others, 1998):

1. Assessing individual physiologic, motor, and state behaviors during feeding
2. Individualizing the feeding plan based on specific infant cues
3. Fostering parental skill and confidence with feeding

capacity to retain the feedings (Fig. 10-3). When infants require a prolonged time (more than 30 minutes) to complete a feeding, gavage feeding may be considered for the next time. (See Critical Thinking Exercise box.)

The decision regarding when to start nipple feeding is somewhat controversial. In many cases the decision is based on an evaluation of the infant's postnatal age (>34 weeks), weight, activity level, respiratory status (absence of apnea and adequate oxygen saturation levels), and strong sucking capabilities. Pickler, Mauck, and Geldmaker (1997) emphasize that there is no universally accepted criteria for the initiation and advancement of bottle-feedings in preterm infants. This study found that a slower rate of progression to full bottle-feeding and discharge positively correlated with a lower gestational age at birth and prolonged assisted ventilation.

Infant behavioral organizational skills, such as the ability to maintain a quiet alert state and display engagement cues and the absence of uncontrolled apnea, have also been shown to influence the preterm infant's successful transition to oral feedings (Mandich, Ritchie, and Mullett, 1996). When infants are unable to tolerate bottle-feedings, inter-

Preterm infants at 32 to 34 weeks postconception who were fed based on individual feeding readiness cues progressed to full oral feedings sooner and gained more weight on a lower volume of intake compared to control infants fed on a schedule (Hubler and others, 1997).

The goal of feeding must be well understood. A key concept is recognizing the difference between a successful feeding (volume and time) and a successful feeder (infant ability and enjoyment); this is the difference between task and developmental feeding techniques. Planning the progression and nature of feedings requires close monitoring and careful documentation. Baseline assessment data is collected before each feeding and observed during and after the feeding to make a comparative evaluation of feeding success. Assessment is ongoing throughout the feeding, and facilitation techniques are chosen based on the individual infant's responses to improve the chance for feeding success and tolerance. Feeding stress and performance (Box 10-2) are evaluated and documented. Planning is done in collaboration with the health care team and family before the next feeding to determine appropriate strategies for the infant. Examples of ways to facilitate feeding are found in Box 10-3. A key ingredient for success is choosing an appropriate nipple.

The nipple used should be relatively firm and stable. Although a high-flow, pliable nipple requires less energy to use, it may provide a flow rate that is too rapid for some preterm infants to manage without risk of aspiration. A firmer nipple facilitates a more "cupped" tongue configuration and allows for a more controlled, manageable flow rate.

Twenty preterm infants around 34 weeks gestation (±1.6 weeks) who were fed through a nipple that allowed milk flow only during active sucking demonstrated enhanced proficiency (volume taken during the first 5 minutes compared to total ordered volume), efficiency of feeding, and more total volume ingested than control infants fed using traditional nipples (Lau and others, 1997).

Prodding techniques to encourage sucking can increase the risk of aspiration, especially if adequate breathing opportunities are not provided. The preterm infant has difficulty managing rapid or continuous milk flow with suck, swallow, and breathing coordination when the nipple is manipulated frequently by twisting or turning; the bottle is moved up and down or in and out of the mouth; or by moving the infant's jaw up and down (not the same as cheek and jaw support). The infant will try to continue to suck or swallow at the risk of physiologic and behavioral consequences.

The infant is positioned in the feeder's arms or placed semiupright in the lap (see Fig. 10-3) and is held with the back curved slightly to simulate the position assumed naturally by most full-term newborns. Stroking the infant's lips, cheeks, and tongue before feeding helps promote oral sensitivity.

Hill and colleagues (2000) used cheek and jaw support for preterm infants between 32 and 34 weeks to facilitate feeding. Supported infants had fewer and shorter pauses during feeding and had higher postfeeding oxygen saturations than infants not receiving oral support. There was no

---

**Box 10-2** ■ ■ ■
**Feeding Stress Cues**

**STATE ORGANIZATION AND ENDURANCE**
- ☐ Decreased arousal
- ☐ Awake but no energy
- ☐ Irritable
- ☐ Fatigues quickly within first 5 minutes

**PHYSIOLOGIC**
- ☐ Tachypnea
- ☐ Nasal flaring, retractions (increased work of breathing)
- ☐ Decreased oxygen saturation
- ☐ Apnea, bradycardia
- ☐ Color change to dusky or pale

**ORAL MOTOR**
- ☐ Unable to control fluid bolus (leaking milk out of mouth)
- ☐ High-pitched sounds
- ☐ Gulping
- ☐ Coughing, choking
- ☐ Multiple swallows without pausing for breath

Modified from Ancona J and others: Improving outcomes through a developmental approach to nipple feeding, *J Nurs Care Qual* 12(5):1-4, 1998.

---

**Box 10-3** ■ ■ ■
**Feeding Facilitation Techniques for Preterm Infants**

**ENVIRONMENT**
- ☐ Prepare calm, quiet area with dim lighting and no distractions
- ☐ Ensure restful environment between feedings

**DIRECT CARE**
- ☐ Avoid trial oral feedings after stressful procedures
- ☐ Choose slightly firm nipple with slower flow
- ☐ Gently arouse to alert state
- ☐ Swaddle in gentle flexion with infant's hands midline and toward face
- ☐ Support positioning with infant cradled close to body in semi-upright or upright position, with neck in neutral to slightly flexed position
- ☐ Continuously observe physiologic, behavioral, and oral-motor functioning
- ☐ Provide adequate breathing and rest periods for infants who cannot pace themselves by gently removing nipple or, if that is too stressful, tip bottle gently downward to drain milk from nipple
- ☐ Provide firm but gentle jaw and cheek support for problems with latching onto nipple (weak seal, loss of milk bolus)
- ☐ Institute "developmental burping" on shoulder with postural support and gentle back rubbing in an upward motion to stimulate burp
- ☐ Recognize infant's limits and when to stop feeding
- ☐ Gavage the rest of the feeding as needed
- ☐ Schedule plenty of undisturbed rest between feedings

**FAMILY SUPPORT AND EDUCATION**
- ☐ Model appropriate feeding techniques
- ☐ Provide opportunity for feeding
- ☐ Educate on infant cues and measuring feeding success

Modified from Hunter J: The neonatal intensive care unit. In Case-Smith J, editor: *Occupational therapy for children*, ed 4, St Louis, 2001, Mosby.

difference between groups in oxygen saturation, heart rate, and respiratory rate during feeding, indicating the technique is as safe as traditional feeding techniques. This technique uses the thumb and index finger to provide gentle pressure (inward and forward) on the cheeks and the third finger to lift and stabilize the jaw under the mandible where the base of the tongue resides.

Bottle-feedings are continued if infants are able to tolerate the feedings and take the required amount. The infant is best fed when fully alert. Drowsy infants feed more slowly, and liquid is more likely to fill the relaxed pharynx before the infant swallows, causing choking. It is believed that many digestive powers require signal stimulation to respond. Some premature infants respond more slowly than full-term infants; therefore the feeding interval, as well as the amount of the feeding, is individualized. Preterm infants are often slow feeders and require patience, frequent rest periods, and burping (or bubbling).

> **NURSING ALERT**  An increase in gastric residuals, abdominal distention, bilious vomiting, temperature instability, apneic episodes, and bradycardia may indicate early NEC and should be called to the attention of the practitioner.

Feeding tolerance and feeding success are not entirely the same concept. Feeding tolerance is evaluated by the following: (1) soft abdomen; (2) absence of abdominal distention or visible bowel loops on the skin surface; (3) minimal or no aspirated gastric residual; (4) presence of bowel sounds; (5) usual frequency, color, and consistency of stools; (6) minimal to no spitting or vomiting; (8) infant's continued interest in feeding; and (9) consistent behavior pattern. Successful oral feeding should be safe, functional, and pleasurable (Biber and others, 1995). Success can be measured by an infant's ability to (1) participate in feeding with energy, (2) coordinate sucking and swallowing with adequate pauses for breathing, (3) maintain vital signs and oxygenation within normal limits, (4) maintain normal muscle tone in face and body, (5) complete feeding in about 20 to 25 minutes, (6) manage liquid bolus with minimal or no loss of liquid from mouth, (7) sustain alertness for feeding, (8) maintain strength and endurance for entire feeding, and (9) measure appropriate-for-age on standard growth curve. A preterm infant's success with feeding is first measured in terms of safety and functionality. Nurturing by holding close, but not socializing, during a feeding creates a warm and pleasurable experience. Later, after the infant is a competent feeder, socialization will enrich both parents' and infant's mealtime enjoyment.

**Breast-feeding.**  The American Academy of Pediatrics (1997) recommends human milk as the preferred food for all infants, including sick newborns and preterm infants (with rare exceptions). The Academy recognizes that the choice of what to feed is the parents' prerogative but advise that the parents should be provided with complete and accurate information on the benefits and methods of breast-feeding so they can make an informed decision. Barriers to initiation and continuation of breast-feeding include physi-

cian indifference, misinformation, lack of prenatal education about breast-feeding, distracting hospital policies, lack of follow-up, working mother, unsupportive work environment, lack of support from family or society, hospital discharge packs or coupons for formula, and media portrayal of bottle-feeding.

Studies indicate that even small preterm infants are able to breast-feed if they have adequate sucking and swallowing reflexes and there are no other contraindications, such as respiratory complications, or concurrent illness (Bier and others, 1993; Meier and Brown, 1996). Mothers who wish to breast-feed their preterm infants are encouraged to pump their breasts until their infants are sufficiently stable to tolerate breast-feeding.

The use of a bilateral breast pump at least four times daily by mothers of preterm infants may decrease the time spent in pumping, thus allowing more time to be spent with the infant. Bilateral pumping did not increase milk production significantly over alternate-breast pumping (Groh-Wargo and others, 1995).

Appropriate guidelines for the storage of *expressed mother's milk (EMM)* should be followed to decrease the risk of milk contamination and destruction of its beneficial properties.

Preterm infants may be able to successfully breast-feed earlier than previously believed (28 to 36 weeks); in addition, preterm infants who are breast-fed rather than bottle-fed demonstrate fewer oxygen desaturation episodes, absence of bradycardia, warmer skin temperature, and better coordination of breathing, sucking, and swallowing (Gardner, Snell, and Lawrence, 1998). The preterm infant should be carefully evaluated for readiness to breast-feed, including assessment of behavioral state, ability to maintain body temperature outside an artificial heat source, respiratory status, and readiness to suckle at the mother's breast. The latter may be accomplished with nonnutritive sucking at the breast during STS (kangaroo) contact so the mother and newborn may become accustomed to each other (Gardner, Snell, and Lawrence, 1998). Nasal cannula oxygen may also be provided during breast-feeding on the basis of the infant's assessed requirements.

Time, patience, and dedication on the part of the mother and the nursing staff are needed to help infants with breast-feeding. The process is begun slowly—beginning with one oral feeding daily and gradually increasing the feedings as the infant tolerates them. Supplementary bottle-feeding is inefficient because the infant expends energy and calories to feed twice. Feeding more often, supplementing with gavage feeding, or using a training nipple is more energy and calorie efficient. Breast-feeding the preterm infant often requires additional guidance by a lactation consultant as well as continued support and encouragement by the nursing staff. In addition, postdischarge breast-feeding often requires further guidance, counseling, and support.

Social support for the mother is a major influence on the decision to breast-feed. To be effective advocates for mothers of all ethnicities, nurses must understand the cultural aspects related to sources of support, whether positive or negative, on breast-feeding choices (Riordan and Gill-Hopple, 2001). African-American women, for example, identify pre-

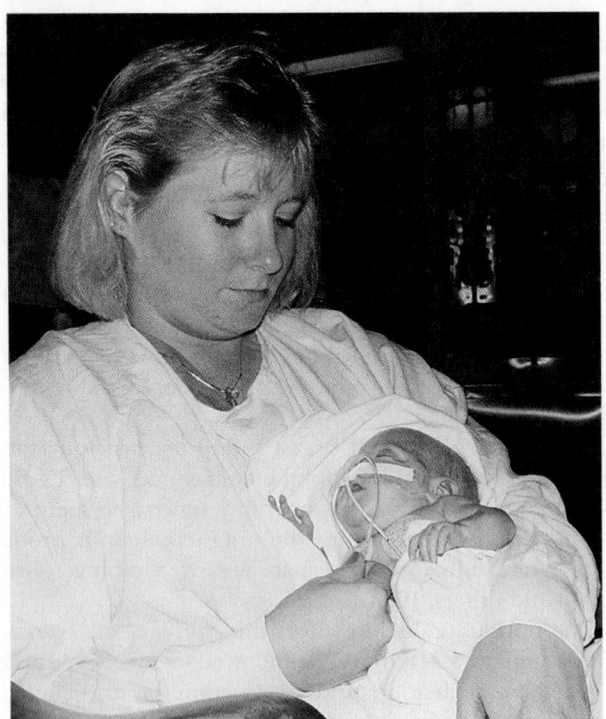

**Fig. 10-4**   Infant held during gavage feeding. Note oxygen source held in the vicinity of the face.

natal health care providers and friends as influential in decisions regarding breast-feeding. They tend to breast-feed less than women from other cultures and should be provided with appropriate information on breast-feeding by health care providers.

Breast-feeding materials are available from organizations such as Best Start Social Marketing* and La Leche League International.†

**Gavage Feeding.**   Gavage feeding is a safe means of meeting the nutritional requirements of infants who are less than 32 weeks of gestation or weigh less than 1500 g. These infants are usually too weak to suck effectively, are unable to coordinate swallowing, and lack a gag reflex. Gavage feedings may be provided by continuous drip regulated by infusion pump or by intermittent bolus feedings. Studies have demonstrated an overall decrease in total milk fat concentration delivery when continuous gavage infusions are administered, which suggests that intermittent gavage of EMM be administered when possible (Schanler, 1995). Intermittent gavage feeding is used as an energy-conserving technique for infants learning to nipple feed who become excessively tired, listless, or cyanotic.

A size 5 or 8 French feeding tube is usually used to instill the formula, and the usual methods for determining correct placement are used. (See Chapter 27 for technique.) Although the more relaxed cardiac sphincter makes passage

of the tube easier, there may be changes in heart rate and blood pressure in response to vagal stimulation. The procedure is best accomplished when an infant is in a prone or a right side-lying position with the head slightly elevated. It is preferable to insert the tube through the mouth rather than the nares. Nasal insertion obstructs nose breathing and may irritate the delicate nasal mucosa. Passage through the mouth also provides an opportunity to observe the sucking response. However, because of less stimulation of the gag reflex, nasal tube gavage may be used in certain situations, such as in older preterm infants who need supplementation after nipple feeding but who fight, gag, and vomit with oral tube management.

The stomach is aspirated, the contents measured, and the aspirate returned as part of the feeding. However, this practice may vary, depending on circumstances and individual unit protocol. The amount of aspirate depends on the length of time since the previous feeding or concurrent illness. Whether or not the amount of the aspirate is deducted from the total feeding varies among units. Some advocate deducting to avoid overdistending the stomach. For example, if a feeding is 25 ml and the aspirate is 5 ml, the aspirate is returned plus 20 ml of feeding for a total of 25 ml. In other units the amount is determined on an individual basis.

The formula is allowed to flow by gravity, and the length of time varies. This procedure is not used as a timesaving method for the nurse. Complications of indwelling tubes include the obstructed nares, mucous plugs, purulent rhinitis, epistaxis, infection, and possible stomach perforation.

The infant may be held during gavage feedings by the caregiver or parent (Fig. 10-4). Oxygen may be supplied via nasal cannula to facilitate handling. It is not recommended that the infant be removed from a primary source of oxygen (e.g., a hood or tent) for feedings because doing so decreases oxygen availability. Flow-by oxygen may be given for brief episodes of desaturation, but this is inadequate for the duration of feedings, either by gavage or nipple. Also, nonnutritive sucking on a pacifier helps infants associate the sucking with the feeling of satiety. When compared with other LBW infants, those who are allowed *nonnutritive sucking* are ready for bottle-feeding earlier, require fewer tube feedings, demonstrate better weight gain, are discharged earlier, and have fewer complications. Nonnutritive sucking also increases oxygenation during tube feeding.

### Feeding Resistance

Any feeding technique that bypasses the mouth precludes the opportunity for the affected child to "practice sucking and swallowing, or the opportunity to experience normal hunger and satiation cycles." Infants may demonstrate aversion to oral feedings by such behaviors as averting the head to the presentation of the nipple, extruding the nipple by tongue thrust, gagging, or even vomiting.

Developmental delays have been noted in perceptual-motor performance as measured by standard tests, although intellectual function remains within normal limits. Other observations include disinterest in or active resistance to oral play, diminished spontaneity and motivation, and shal-

---

*Best Start Social Marketing, 3500 E Fletcher Ave, #519, Tampa, FL 33613-4708, (800)277-4975; www.hmhb.org/pub_breast.html.
†La Leche League, International, PO Box 4079, Schaumburg, IL 60618, (847) 519-9585 (order department); www.lalecheleague.org/.

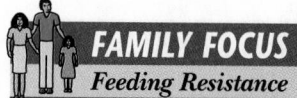

## FAMILY FOCUS
### Feeding Resistance

Our son was in the NICU for several months. Now at 6 years of age he is normal in every way except one—he refuses almost all food. He lives on a diet of mashed bananas, mashed potatoes, fruit juice, milk, and a daily multivitamin/mineral pill. Getting him to eat has been a 6-year battle that we have lost. Now I know that simple oral stimulation techniques could have prevented this problem. Please tell nurses the importance of these interventions when any infant is NPO for a prolonged time.

A mother and a nurse

---

low interpersonal relationships, probably related to the absence of some early incorporative patterns of normal oral experiences. The longer the period of nonoral feeding, the more severe the feeding problems, especially if this period occurs during a time when the infant progresses from reflexive to learned and voluntary feeding actions. During infancy the mouth is the primary instrument for reception of stimulation and pleasure.

Infants identified as being at risk for feeding resistance should be provided with regular oral stimulation based on the child's developmental level. Those who exhibit feeding aversion should begin a stimulation program to overcome resistance and acquire the ability to take nourishment by the oral route. Because management requires long-term commitment, successful implementation of a plan for oral stimulation depends on maximal parental involvement and promotion of primary nursing. (See Family Focus box.) Key components and interventions are listed in Box 10-4.

### Skin Care

The skin of premature infants is characteristically immature. Because of its increased sensitivity and fragility, no alkaline-based soap that might destroy the "acid mantle" of the skin is used. The increased permeability of the skin facilitates absorption of ingredients. All skin products (e.g., alcohol or povidone-iodine) are used with caution; the skin is rinsed with water afterward because these substances may cause severe irritation and chemical burns in LBW infants.

The skin is easily excoriated and denuded; therefore, care must be taken to avoid damage to the delicate structure. The total skin is thinner than that of full-term infants and lacks "rete pegs," appendages that anchor the epidermis to the dermis. Therefore there is less cohesion between the thinner skin layers. Adhesives used after heelsticks or to secure monitoring equipment or intravenous infusions may excoriate the skin or adhere to the skin surface so well that the epidermis can be separated from the dermis and pulled away with the tape. The use of a zinc oxide base HyTape* (pink tape) is encouraged to minimize epidermal stripping; the tape is flexible, waterproof, and washable. The use of skin barriers protects healthy skin and helps excoriated skin heal.

It is unsafe to use scissors to remove dressings or tape from the extremities of very small and immature infants because it is easy to snip off tiny extremities or nick loosely attached skin. Solvents used to remove tape are avoided because they tend to dry and burn the delicate skin. Guidelines for skin care are listed in the Guidelines box on p. 350.

During skin assessment of preterm infants, nurses are alert to the subtle signs that indicate zinc deficiency, a common problem in these infants. Breakdown usually occurs in the areas around the mouth, buttocks, fingers, and toes. In VLBW infants it may also occur in the creases of the neck, wrists, ankles, and around wounds. Zinc deficiency is most likely to appear in infants with sepsis, those experiencing nasogastric losses, or those who have had surgery. Suspicious lesions are reported to the practitioner so that zinc supplements can be prescribed. In most preterm infants the skin barrier properties resemble those of the term infant by 2 to 3 weeks postnatal age, regardless of gestational age at birth.

Although no studies comparing the effectiveness of different commercially available neonatal bedding has been done, a number of products are useful in minimizing skin problems. General information about bedding is described in the Guidelines box on p. 364. Particularly vulnerable areas of the skin such as the ears, occiput, scapula, and hips can be protected with products (Kuller, 2001) such as Spenco Gel Pads.* Children's Medical Ventures Inc. makes

---

### Box 10-4
### Components of a Care Plan to Prevent or Overcome Feeding Resistance

Stimulate normal feeding interactions.
  Hold and cuddle infant in en face feeding position.
  Engage in eye contact with infant.
  Engage in verbal interaction with infant as tolerated.
Overcome oral hypersensitivity (sensitivity to intraoral stimulation).
  Provide oral stimulation.
  When external oral stimulation is tolerated, attempt gentle massage of gums and tongue (use finger or soft rubber item).
  Massage gums from center and move toward molar region, and move gradually from anterior to posterior.
  Withdraw stimulus and close child's mouth if child gags.
Encourage oral exploration.
  Assist child in mouthing hands, fingers, toes, or soft rubber toys.
  Play oral games (e.g., blowing a kiss, kissing an object [toy animal]).
Provide oral feedings.
  Introduce small volumes (even 3 to 5 ml) as early as possible.
  Offer feedings consistently (formula).
  Avoid force feeding.
Provide feeding stimulation during tube feedings.
  Hold child in feeding position.
  Provide nonnutritive sucking during bolus feedings.
  Give oral feedings before tube feedings.
  Give bolus feedings in response to hunger when possible rather than on predetermined schedule.
Provide nonnutritive sucking to encourage use of oral musculature.

Data from Orr MJ, Allen SS: Optimal oral experiences for infants on long-term total parenteral nutrition, *Nutr Clin Pract* 9:288-295, 1986.

---

*HyTape Corporation, PO Box 540, Patterson, NY 12563, (800) 248-0101.

*Spenco Medical Corp, Waco, TX.

# GUIDELINES
*Neonatal Skin Care*

## GENERAL SKIN CARE

### Assessment

☐ Assess skin every day or once a shift for redness, dryness, flaking, scaling, rashes, lesions, excoriation, or breakdown.
☐ Evaluate and report abnormal skin findings and analyze for possible causation.
☐ Intervene according to interpretation of findings or physician order.

### Bathing

*Initial bath*

☐ Assess for stable temperature a minimum of 2 to 4 hours before first bath.
☐ Use cleansing agents with neutral pH or minimal dyes or perfume, in water
☐ Do not completely remove vernix.
☐ Bathe preterm infant <32 weeks in sterile water alone.

### Routine

☐ Decrease frequency of baths to every second or third day by daily cleansing of eye, oral, and diaper areas and pressure points.
☐ Use cleanser or soaps no more than 2-3 times a week.
☐ Avoid rubbing skin during bathing or drying.
☐ Immerse stable infants fully (except head) in an appropriate-sized tub.
☐ Use swaddled immersion bathing technique: slow unwrapping after gently lowering into water for sensitive, but stable, infants needing assistance with motor system reactivity.

### Emollients

Follow hospital protocol or consider the following:
☐ Apply petroleum-based ointment without preservative sparingly to body (avoid face, head) every 6 to 12 hours during the first 2 to 4 weeks for infants <32 weeks (except when neonate is in radiant heat source).

Modified from Kuller JM: Skin breakdown: risk factors, prevention, and treatment, *NINR* 1(1):33-42, 2001; Johnson FE, Maikler VE: Nurses' adoption of the AWHONN/NANN Neonatal Skin Care Project, *NINR* 1(1):59-67, 2001; Lund CH, Kuller J, Lott JW: Neonatal skin care: clinical outcomes of the AWHONN/NANN evidence-based clinical practice guideline, *J Obstet Gynecol Neonat Nurs* 30(1):41-51, 2001; Taquino LT: Promoting wound healing in the neonatal setting: process versus protocol, *J Perinat Neonat Nurs* 14(1):108-118, 2000; Lund C, Lane A, Raines DA: Neonatal skin care: the scientific basis for practice, *J Obstet Gynecol Neonat Nurs* 28(3):241-254, 1999; Malloy MB, Perez-Woods R: Neonatal skin care: prevention of skin breakdown, *Pediatr Nurs* 17(1):41-48, 1991.

☐ Apply emollient as needed to infants >32 weeks for dry, flaking skin.

### Adhesives

☐ Decrease use as much as possible.
☐ Use transparent adhesive dressings to secure IVs, catheters, and central lines.
☐ Use hydrogel or limb electrodes.
☐ Consider pectin barriers (Hollihesive,* Duoderm†) beneath adhesives to protect skin.
☐ Secure pulse oximeter probe or electrodes with elasticized dressing material (carefully avoid restricting blood flow).
☐ Do not use adhesive remover, solvents, and bonding agents.
☐ Avoid removing adhesives for at least 24 hours after application.
☐ Adhesive removal can be facilitated using water, mineral oil, or petrolatum.
☐ Remove adhesives or skin barriers slowly, supporting the skin underneath with one hand and gently peeling away the product from the skin with the other hand.‡

### Antiseptic Agents

☐ Apply before invasive procedures.
☐ Apply povidone-iodine two times, air dry for 30 seconds; remove completely with sterile water or sterile saline solution following procedure.
☐ Avoid use of alcohol.

### Transepidermal Water Loss (TEWL)

Minimize TEWL and heat loss in small premature infants <30 weeks by:
☐ Measuring ambient humidity during first weeks of life.
☐ Considering an increase in humidity to >70% by using one or more of the following options or hospital guidelines:
  Transparent dressings.
  Emollient application every 6 to 8 hours or according to hospital protocol.
  Servocontrolled humidifying incubator.

*Houister, Libertyville, IL.
†ConvaTec/Bristol-Myers Squibb Co, Princeton, NJ.
‡*Caution:* Scissors are not to be used for tape or dressing removal because of hazard of cutting skin or amputating tiny digits.

a Gel Support* for preventing skin breakdown in patients with decreased mobility. Other developmentally supportive products by Children's Medical Ventures include positioning aids like the gel-filled wedgie and gel pillows and mattresses. The gel mattress is suggested for use with oscillating ventilators and during extracorporeal membrane oxygenation (ECMO) to minimize vibration and reduce pressure.

Skin injuries have been reported during use of phototherapy blankets. Caution is warranted in using these products with extremely premature infants or infants with birth trauma, poorly perfused skin, hypotension, or bacterial contamination of the bed or humidified incubator. Manufacturers of phototherapy blankets recommend the following during therapy: monitor color of skin, observe for rashes or excoriation, keep skin clean with warm water, promptly clean perineum after stooling, reposition every 2

hours, carefully monitor cleanliness and skin integrity, and avoid direct contact of blanket with infant's skin.

Sun protection and use of sunscreen should be discussed with parents before discharge. Older infants with chronic conditions who are allowed to go outside for a brief outing will also need sun protection. While the use of sunscreen in infants less than 6 months old remains controversial, the American Academy of Pediatrics (1999a) recommends using it on small areas such as the face and extremities when clothing, hats, and shade do not offer adequate protection. Sun exposure should be avoided between 10 AM and 4 PM and on cloudy days because clouds do not protect against ultraviolet radiation.

## Administration of Medications

Administration of therapeutic agents, such as drugs, ointments, intravenous infusions, and oxygen, requires judicious handling and meticulous attention to detail. The com-

*Children's Medical Ventures Inc, Norwell, MA.

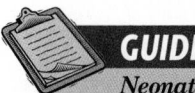

## GUIDELINES
*Neonatal Skin Care—cont'd*

### SKIN BREAKDOWN

#### Prevention

- Decrease pressure from externally applied forces using water, air, or gel mattresses, sheepskin, or cotton bedding.
- Provide adequate nutrition, including protein, fat, and zinc.
- Apply transparent adhesive dressings to protect arms, elbows, and knees from friction injury.
- Use tracheostomy and gastrostomy dressings for drainage and relief of pressure from trach or G tube (Hydrasorb or Lyofoam).†
- Use emollient in the diaper area (groin and thighs) to reduce urine irritation.

#### Treating Skin Breakdown

- Irrigate wound every 4 to 8 hours with warm half-strength normal saline (NS) using a 30 ml or larger syringe and 20-gauge teflon cathether.
- Culture wound and treat if signs of infection are present (excessive redness, swelling, pain on touch, heat, or resistance to healing).
- Use transparent adhesive dressing for uninfected wounds.
- Apply hydrogel with or without antibacterial or antifungal ointments (as ordered) for infected wounds (may need to moisten before removal).
- Use hydrocolloid for deep, uninfected wounds (leave in place for 5 to 7 days) or as an ostomy barrier and to improve appliance adhesion; warm barrier in hand for several minutes to soften before applying to skin.
- Avoid use of antiseptic solutions for wound cleansing (used for intact skin only).

#### Treating Diaper Dermatitis

- Maintain clean, dry skin; use absorbent diapers and change often.
- If mild irritation occurs, use petrolatum barrier.
- For developing dermatitis, apply a generous quantity of zinc-oxide barrier.
- For severe dermatitis, identify cause and treat (frequent stooling from spina bifida, severe opiate withdrawal, or malabsorption syndrome).
- Treat *Candida albicans* with antifungal ointment or cream.

†ConvaTec/Bristol-Myers Squibb Co, Princeton, NJ.

- Avoid powders and antibiotic ointments (not recommended). (See Cord and Circumcision Care, Chapter 8.)

### OTHER SKIN CARE CONCERNS

#### Use of Substances on Skin

- Evaluate all substances that come in contact with infant's skin.
- Before using any topical agent, analyze components of preparation and:
  Use sparingly and only when necessary.
  Confine use to smallest possible area.
  Whenever possible and appropriate, wash off with water.
  Monitor infant carefully for signs of toxicity and systemic effects.

#### Use of Thermal Devices

- Avoid heat lamps because of increased potential for burns. If needed, measure actual temperature of exposed skin every 15 minutes.
- When using heating pads (Aqua-K pads):
  Change infant's position every 15 minutes initially and then every 1 to 2 hours.
  Preset temperature of heating pads <40°C (104°F).
- When using preheated transcutaneous electrodes:
  Avoid use on infants <1000 g.
  Set at lowest possible temperature (<44°C [111.2°F]) and secure with plastic wrap.
  Use pulse oximetry rather than transcutaneous monitoring whenever possible.
- When prewarming heels before phlebotomy, avoid temperatures >40°C.
- Warm ambient humidity, direct away from infant; use aerosolized sterile water and maintain ambient temperature so as not to exceed 40°C.
- Document use of all heating devices.

#### Use of Fluid Therapy/Hemodynamic Monitoring

- Be certain fingers or toes are visible whenever extremity is used for IV or arterial line.
- Secure catheter or needle with transparent dressing/tape to promote easy visualization of site.
- Assess site hourly for signs of ischemia, infiltration, and inadequate perfusion (check capillary refill).
- Avoid use of restraints (e.g., armboards); if used, check that they are secured safely and not restricting circulation or movement (check for pressure areas).
- Use commercial IV protector (i.e., I.V. House) with minimal tape.

putation, preparation, and administration of drugs in minute amounts often require collaboration between nurses, physicians, and pharmacists to reduce the chance for error. In addition, the immaturity of an infant's detoxification mechanisms and inability to demonstrate symptoms of toxicity (e.g., signs of auditory nerve involvement from ototoxic drugs such as gentamycin) complicate drug therapy and require that nurses be particularly alert for signs of adverse reaction. (See Administration of Medication, Chapter 27.)

Nurses should be aware of the hazards of administering bacteriostatic and hyperosmolar solutions to infants. Benzyl alcohol, a common preservative in bacteriostatic water and saline, has been shown to be toxic to newborns and should not be used to flush intravenous catheters or to dilute or reconstitute medications. It is recommended that medications with preservatives such as benzyl alcohol be avoided whenever possible. Nurses must read labels carefully to detect the

presence of preservatives in any medication to be administered to an infant.

Hyperosmolar solutions present a potential danger to preterm infants. Hyperosmolar solutions given orally to infants can produce clinical, physiologic, and morphologic alterations, the most serious of which is NEC. Oral or parenteral medications should be sufficiently diluted to prevent complications related to hyperosmolality.

## Neonatal Pain

It has long been believed that the nerve pathways of newborn infants are not sufficiently myelinated to transmit painful stimuli, that the infant does not possess sufficiently integrated cortical function to interpret or recall pain experiences, and that the risk of anesthesia is too great to justify any possible benefit of pain relief (Anand and Hickey, 1987; McLaughlin and others, 1993; Hadjistavropoulos and others, 1997; Shapiro, 1989). Nurses have been found to hold similar beliefs and to give significantly higher pain intensity ratings to full-term as opposed to preterm neonates (Shapiro, 1993). Consequently, invasive procedures are performed on preterm infants without an anesthetic.

This traditional view has been refuted by a number of research studies that indicate that both preterm and full-term infants perceive and react to pain in much the same manner as children and adults. Evidence indicates that pain pathways, cortical and subcortical centers needed for pain perception, and neurochemical systems associated with pain transmission and modulation are intact and functional in the neonate. Pain perception has both physiologic and psychologic components, and it is accepted that newborns recognize and respond to painful stimuli. However, pain is a sensation with strong emotional associations, and the consciousness of the newborn to the perception of pain has not been agreed on by researchers (Anand and others, 1999). Therefore, the term *nociception* (the perception by the *nerves* of injurious influences or painful stimuli) is often used to discuss pain in the neonate.

**Pain Physiology.** Five physiologic components are required for successful transmission of painful stimuli and for perception of pain. These components include sensory receptors (A-delta and C-polymodal fibers) that receive painful stimuli, tracts to the brain that transmit painful stimuli, centers in the brain that interpret stimuli as painful, chemical neuromediators that are responsible for the transmission of stimuli throughout the entire process, and descending control systems that modulate or alter pain transmission and at times suppress the perception of pain. A-delta neurons are generally thinly myelinated, whereas C-polymodal neurons are unmyelinated (Anand and Hickey, 1987; Anand and Carr, 1989).

Researchers have discovered that the physiologic components required to perceive pain begin to develop early in fetal life. Pain receptors begin to appear in the fetus around the seventh week. These receptors spread to all cutaneous and mucous surfaces by the twentieth week. The tracts to the brain that develop in the anterior horn cells of the spinal cord are present and undergo myelination during the second and third trimesters. The tracts are completely myelinated by 30 weeks. Limited myelination has been argued in the past to be the reason there is a lack of pain perception in the neonate. Myelination, however, is not required for pain transmission (C-fibers) and is responsible only for increasing the speed of transmission. Slower transmission in the neonate due to incomplete myelination is offset by the shorter distance an impulse must travel in the neonate vs the adult (Anand and Hickey, 1987).

By 20 weeks of gestation each cortex of the brain has a full complement of neurons. This suggests the functional ability of the centers in the brain that are responsible for interpreting painful stimuli. Chemical neuromediators and their receptors appear in the dorsal horn of the spinal cord at 12 and 16 weeks of gestation. The descending control systems that modulate and alter the perception of pain are the only physiologic component not available to the neonate. These control systems do not develop until after birth, which suggests that newborns are potentially more sensitive

---

**Box 10-5 ■ ■ ■**
**Manifestations of Acute Pain in the Neonate**

**PHYSIOLOGIC RESPONSES**
Vital signs: observe for variations
   Increased heart rate
   Increased blood pressure
   Rapid, shallow respirations
Oxygenation
   Decreased transcutaneous $O_2$ saturation (tcPO$_2$)
   Decreased arterial $O_2$ saturation (SaO$_2$)
Skin: observe color and character
   Pallor or flushing
   Diaphoresis
   Palmar sweating
Other observations
   Increased muscle tone
   Dilated pupils
   Decreased vagal nerve tone
   Increased intracranial pressure
   Laboratory evidence of metabolic or endocrine changes
      Hyperglycemia
      Lowered pH
      Elevated corticosteroids

**BEHAVIORAL RESPONSES**
Vocalizations: observe quality, timing, and duration
   Crying
   Whimpering
   Groaning
Facial expression: observe characteristics, timing, orientation of eyes and mouth (see Figs. 10-5 and 10-6)
   Grimaces
   Brow furrowed
   Chin quivering
   Eyes tightly closed
   Mouth open and squarish
Body movements and posture: observe type, quality, and amount of movement or lack of movement; relationship to other factors
   Limb withdrawal
   Thrashing
   Rigidity
   Flaccidity
   Fist clenching
Changes in state: observe sleep, appetite, activity level
   Changes in sleep/wake cycles
   Changes in feeding behavior
   Changes in activity level
   Fussiness, irritability
   Listlessness

---

to pain than adults (Anand and Hickey, 1987; Fitzgerald, 1995).

**Pain Assessment.** Assessment of pain in the preverbal child is difficult, especially in the neonate, because the most reliable indicator of pain, self-report, is not possible. Evaluation must be based on physiologic changes and behavioral observations (Box 10-5). Although behaviors such as vocalizations, facial expressions, body movements, and general state are common to all infants, they vary with different situations. Crying associated with pain is more intense and sustained (Fig. 10-5). Facial expression is the most consistent and specific characteristic; scales are available to systematically evaluate facial features, such as eye squeeze, brow bulge, and open mouth and taut tongue (Fig. 10-6) (Grunau and Craig, 1987; Grunau, Johnston, and Craig, 1990; Hadjistavropoulos and others, 1997). Most infants re-

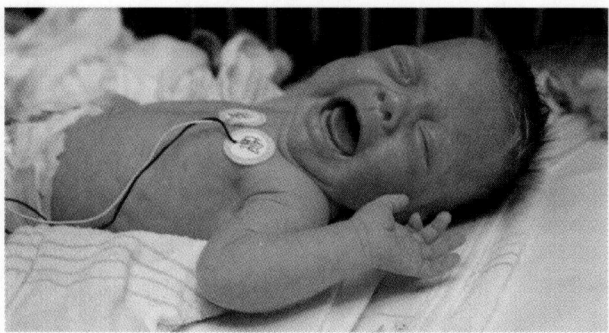

**Fig. 10-5** Full, robust crying of preterm infant following heelstick. (Courtesy Halbouty Premature Nursery, Texas Children's Hospital, Houston, Texas; photo by Paul Vincent Kuntz.)

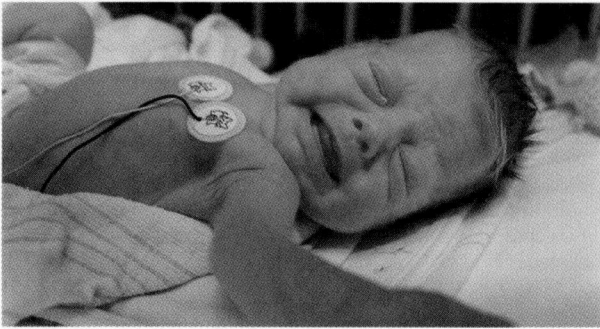

**Fig. 10-6** The face of pain after heelstick. Note eye squeeze, brow bulge, nasolabial furrow, and wide-spread mouth. (Courtesy Halbouty Premature Nursery, Texas Children's Hospital, Houston, Texas; photo by Paul Vincent Kuntz.)

spond with increased body movements, but the infant may be experiencing pain even when lying quietly with eyes closed. The preterm infant's response to pain may be behaviorally blunted or absent. In addition, infants in awake or alert states demonstrate a more robust reaction to painful stimuli than infants in sleep states (Grunau and Craig, 1987; Johnston and others, 1999; Stevens, Johnston, and Horton, 1994; Stevens and others, 1996). Also an infant receiving a muscle-paralyzing agent (vecuronium) will be incapable of a behavioral or visible pain response.

Although regular use of pain assessment tools can better assist caregivers in determining if the infant is in pain, caregivers must consider the infant's maturity, behavioral state, energy resources available to respond, and whether risk factors for pain are present. In infants with diminished ability to respond robustly to pain, it is imperative to presume that pain exists in all situations that are usually considered painful for adults and children, even in the absence of behavioral or physiologic signs.

> **NURSING ALERT**  When in doubt about pain in infants, base your decision on the following rule: Whatever is painful to an adult or child is painful to an infant regardless of gestational age unless proved otherwise.

Several pain assessment tools have been developed for the assessment of pain in the neonate (Table 10-3). One pain assessment tool used by nurses in the neonatal intensive care setting is called the ***CRIES.*** This tool has been developed for use by nurses who work with premature and full-term infants. The CRIES is an acronym for the physiologic and behavioral indicators of pain used in the tool. The indicators include crying, requiring increased oxygen, increased vital signs, expression, and sleeplessness. Each indicator is scored from 0 to 2—similar to the Apgar score for neonates. The total possible pain score, which represents the worst pain, is 10. A pain score greater than 4 should be considered significant. This tool has been tested for reliability and validity for postoperative pain in infants between the ages of 32 weeks of gestation and 20 weeks postterm (Bildner and Krechel, 1996; Krechel and Bildner, 1995).

The ***Premature Infant Pain Profile (PIPP)*** is unique because it has been developed specifically for preterm infants

(Stevens and others, 1996). The category "gestational age at time of observation" gives a higher pain score to infants with lower gestational age. Infants who are asleep 15 seconds before the painful procedure also receive additional points for their blunted behavioral responses to painful stimuli. The other observational categories are listed in Table 10-3.

The ***Neonatal Pain and Sedation Scale (NPASS)*** was originally developed to measure pain/sedation in preterm infants following surgery. It measures five criteria (see Table 10-3) in two dimensions (pain and sedation) and may be used in neonates as young as 23 weeks gestation up to infants 100 days old. Extra points are added in the pain scale dimension for preterm infants based on gestational age.

**Memory of Pain.**   Premature infants are subjected to a variety of repeated noxious stimuli, including multiple heel sticks, venipuncture, endotracheal intubation and suctioning, arterial sticks, chest tube placement, and lumbar puncture. Research has found that infants born between 27 and 31 weeks gestation are submitted to an average of 134 painful procedures in the first 2 weeks of life alone (Stevens and others, 1999a; 1999b). The effects of pain caused by such procedures are not fully known, but researchers have begun to investigate the potential consequences. Fitzgerald, Millard, and McIntosh (1989) recorded evidence of hypersensitivity to repeated heel lance procedures in premature infants born at 27 to 32 weeks gestational age.

The memory of pain has been a well-investigated phenomenon. Neither adults nor infants have the capacity to remember the sensation of pain. Only the experiences associated with pain can be remembered (Anand and Hickey, 1987). Grunau and others (1994) demonstrated the phenomenon of memory in toddlers with a history of ELBW and long stays in the NICU. These toddlers had significantly higher somatic complaints of unknown origin than children who had been full-term healthy infants.

Barba and others (1991) hypothesized that a repeated painful experience may cause the newborn to eventually recognize the activities of the event and demonstrate early memory capacities. They analyzed the behavioral and physiologic responses of 20 full-term newborns to repeated heel lancing. With another 20 full-term newborns as a control group, they repeated the exact same steps of the heel lance

**TABLE 10-3**    Summary of pain assessment scales for infants

| Tools and Authors/Ages of Use | Reliability and Validity | Variables and Scoring Range | |
|---|---|---|---|
| **Postoperative Pain Score (POPS)** | | | |
| Attia J and others: Measurement of postoperative pain and narcotic administration in infants using a new clinical scoring system, *Anesthesiology* 67(3A):A532, 1987.<br>*Ages of use:* 1-7 months | Not tested by original authors<br>Later tested by Joyce BA and others (1994); high interrater agreement (reliability); discriminant validity ($p < 0.0001$); reliability with high Cronbach alpha ranging from .79-.88 | Sleep (0-2)<br>Facial expression (0-2)<br>Quality of cry (0-2)<br>Spontaneous motor activity (0-2)<br>Spontaneous excitability (0-2)<br>*Scoring range:* 0 = worst pain, 20 = no pain | Flexion fingers/toes (0-2)<br>Sucking (0-2)<br>Tone (0-2)<br>Consolability (0-2)<br>Sociability (0-2) |
| **Neonatal Infant Pain Scale (NIPS)** | | | |
| Lawrence J and others: The development of a tool to assess neonatal pain, *Neonatal Network* 12(6):59-66, 1993.<br>*Ages of use:* average gestational age 33.5 weeks | Interrater reliability = .92 and .97<br>Construct validity using ANOVA between before, during, and after procedure scores: F = 18.97, df = 2.42, $p < .001$<br>Concurrent validity between NIPS and VAS using Pearson correlations = .53-.84<br>Internal consistency using Cronbach alpha = .95, .87, and .88 for before, during, and after procedure scores | Facial expression (0-1)<br>Cry (0-2)<br>Breathing patterns (0-1)<br>*Scoring range:* 0 = no pain; 7 = worst pain | Arms (0-1)<br>Legs (0-1)<br>State of arousal (0-1) |
| **Pain Assessment Tool (PAT)** | | | |
| Hodgkinson K and others: Measuring pain in neonates: evaluating an instrument and developing a common language, *Aust J Adv Nurs* 12(1):17-22, 1994.<br>*Ages of use:* 27 weeks gestational age–full term | No reliability or validity discussed by original authors | Posture/tone (1-2)<br>Sleep pattern (0-2)<br>Expression (1-2)<br>Color (0-2)<br>Cry (0-2)<br>*Scoring range:* 4 = no pain; 20 = worst pain | Respirations (1-2)<br>Heart rate (1-2)<br>Saturations (0-2)<br>Blood pressure (0-2)<br>Nurse's perception (0-2) |
| **Pain Rating Scale (PRS)** | | | |
| Joyce BA and others: Reliability and validity of preverbal pain assessment tools, *Issues Comp Pediatr Nurs* 17:121-135, 1994.<br>*Ages of use:* 1-36 months | Interrater agreement: $r = .65-.84$, $p < 0.0001$<br>Discriminant validity: statistically significant $t$ tests ($p < .0001$) | 0—smiling, sleeping, no change when moved/touched<br>1—takes small amount orally, restless, moving, cries<br>2—not drinking/eating, short periods of cries, distracted with rocking or pacifier<br>3—change in behavior, irritable, arms/legs shake/jerk, facial grimace<br>4—flailing, high-pitched wailing, parents request pain medication, unable to distract<br>5—sleeping prolonged periods interrupted by jerking, continuous crying, rapid and shallow respirations<br>*Scoring range:* 0 = no pain; 5 = worst pain | |
| **CRIES** | | | |
| Krechel SW, Bildner J: CRIES: a new neonatal postoperative pain measurement score: initial testing of validity and reliability, *Pediatr Anaesth* 5:53-61, 1995. | Concurrent validity between CRIES and POPS = 0.73 ($p < 0.0001$, $n = 1382$); Spearman correlation between subjective report and POPS and CRIES = 0.49 ($p < 0.0001$, $n > 1300$) | Crying (0-2)<br>Requires increased oxygen (0-2)<br>Increased vital signs (0-2)<br>Expression (0-2)<br>Sleepless (0-2)<br>*Scoring range:* 0 = no pain; 10 = worst pain | |

procedure, but without puncturing the skin. As hypothesized, the experimental group demonstrated responses indicating awareness of the forthcoming painful event, whereas the control group did not. These findings seem to indicate infants' memory of events and their ability to perceptually categorize information.

A study by Wong (1992) specifically investigated the effect of prior pain experiences on the physiologic and behavioral responses of infants to an injection. The findings of this study revealed that infants with high pain history scores had significantly more physical distress or anger expressions than infants with low pain history scores. An implication of this study is the preliminary evidence that past pain influences present pain responses.

Another study found that there were increasing pain scores in unanesthetized circumcised infants ages 4 to

## TABLE 10-3   Summary of pain assessment scales for infants—cont'd

| Tools and Authors/Ages of Use | Reliability and Validity | Variables and Scoring Range | |
|---|---|---|---|
| **CRIES—cont'd** | | | |
| *Ages of use:* 32-60 weeks gestational age | Discriminant validity using before and after analgesia scores: Wilcoxon Sign Rank Test = mean decline of 3.0 units ($p < 0.0001$, $n = 74$) Interrater reliability using Spearman correlation coefficient: $r = 0.72$ ($p < 0.0001$, $n = 680$) | | |
| **Premature Infant Pain Profile (PIPP)** | | | |
| Stevens B and others: Premature Infant Pain Profile: development and initial validation, *Clin J Pain* 12:13-22, 1996. See also Ballantyne and others, 1999. *Ages of use:* 28-40 weeks gestational age | Internal consistency using Cronbach alpha = 0.75-0.59; standardized item alpha for 6 items = 0.71 Construct validity using handling vs painful situations: statistically significant differences (paired $t = 12.24$, two-tailed $p < 0.0001$, and Mann-Whitney U = 765.5, $p < 0.00001$) and using real vs sham heelstick procedures with infants aged 28-30 weeks gestational age ($t = 2.4$, two-tailed $p < 0.02$, and Mann-Whitney U = 132 $p < 0.016$) and with full-term males undergoing circumcision with topical anesthetic vs placebo ($t = 2.6$, two-tailed $p < 0.02$, or nonparametric equivalent Mann-Whitney U test, U = 145.7, two-tailed $p < 0.02$) | Gestational age (0-3) Behavioral state (0-3) Heart rate (0-3) Oxygen saturation (0-3) Brow bulge (0-3) *Scoring range:* 0 = no pain; 21 = worst pain | Eye squeeze (0-3) Nasolabial furrow (0-3) |
| **Scale for Use in Newborns (SUN)** | | | |
| Blauer T, Gerstmann D: A simultaneous comparison of three neonatal pain scales during common NICU procedures, *Clin J Pain* 14(1):39-47, 1998. *Ages of use:* 0-28 days | No reliability; face validity, content validity, construct validity using extreme groups | CNS state (0-4) Breathing (0-4) Heart rate (0-4) Mean BP (0-4) *Scoring range:* 0 = no pain; 28 = worst pain; average baseline score 10-14; a 2 represents normal or baseline value | Movement (0-4) Tone (0-4) Face (0-4) |
| **Neonatal Pain, Agitation, and Sedation Scale (NPASS)** | | | |
| Puchalski M, Hummel P: Loyola University Chicago, Loyola University Medical Center. *Ages of use:* Birth (23 weeks gestational age) and term newborns up to 100 days | Interrater reliability using ICC: .95 CI for pre- and post-intervention pain scale; .95 CI for pre- and post-intervention sedation scale Internal consistency (Cronbach alpha): Pre-intervention pain scale, 0.75 and 0.71 raters 1 and 2 Post-intervention pain scale, 0.25 and 0.27 raters 1 and 2 Pre-intervention sedation scale, 0.88 and 0.81 raters 1 and 2 Post-intervention sedation scale, 0.86 and 0.89 raters 1 and 2 | Cry/irritability (0-2) Behavior/state (0-2) Facial expression (0-2) Extremities/tone (0-2) Vital signs—HR, RR, BP, $SaO_2$ (0-2) *Scoring range:* Pain score: 0-10 (0 = no pain; 10 = intense pain) Sedation score: 0-10 (0 = no sedation; 10 = deep sedation) | |

6 months as compared to those circumcised with EMLA or with a placebo analgesic. Among the infants, the circumcised group with EMLA showed less pain response to vaccination. The study postulates that unanesthetized circumcision may induce long-lasting changes in infant pain behavior because of alterations in the infant's central neural processing of painful stimuli (Taddio and others, 1997).

**Consequences of Untreated Pain in Infants.** Despite current research on the neonate's experience of pain, infant pain often remains inadequately managed. The mismanagement of infant pain is partially the result of misconceptions regarding the effects of pain on the neonate as well as a lack of knowledge of immediate and long-term consequences of untreated pain. Infants respond to noxious stimuli through physiologic indicators (increased heart rate and blood pressure, variability in heart rate and intracranial pressure [ICP], and decreases in $SaO_2$ and skin blood flow) and behavioral indicators (muscle rigidity, facial expression, crying, withdrawal, and sleeplessness) (Anand, Grunau, and Oberlander, 1997; Bildner and Krechel, 1996). The physiologic and behavioral indicators, as well as a variety of neurophysiologic responses to noxious stimulation, are responsible for acute and long-term consequences of pain (Box 10-6).

Two studies have investigated the effects of blood pressure and transcutaneous oxygen changes and crying on premature infants in the NICU. Perry and others (1990) found significant increases in arterial blood pressure values and a significant decrease in $tcPO_2$ saturation in response to han-

dling procedures in the NICU. The greatest changes were in response to arterial puncture procedures, echocardiogram, chest vibration, and endotracheal suctioning. Arterial puncture, chest vibration, and suctioning have been reported as painful procedures (Anand and Hickey, 1987). Peak blood pressure changes were plotted according to infant weight. A safe peak blood pressure value for each weight group was noted, above which the majority of infants subsequently developed periventricular-intraventricular hemorrhage (Perry and others, 1990).

Brazy (1988) also observed infants in the NICU to determine the effects of crying on cerebral oxygen delivery and blood volume fluctuations in the brain. Significant oscillatory changes in blood volume and oxygen supply were noted in response to crying. Brazy reported that similar changes have been associated with movement and blood pressure peaks, resulting in a high risk for intraventricular hemorrhage (IVH).

Anand and Hickey (1987) described additional responses of infants to painful stimuli from their own unpublished and other scientific studies. Chemical and hormonal responses were observed following noxious stimuli without the use of an anesthetic or analgesic. Such responses included increased $\beta$-endorphin secretion (an endogenous opioid), increased plasma renin activity, increased plasma epinephrine and norepinephrine, increased catecholamines, growth hormone, glucagon, aldosterone, and other corticosteroids. The result of these chemical and hormonal increases include the breakdown of fat and carbohydrate stores, prolonged hyperglycemia, and increased serum lactate, pyruvate, total ketone bodies, and nonesterified fatty acids. Such consequences can be attributed to a greater morbidity for neonates in the NICU. Several experimental studies revealed a significant decrease in these responses when adequate analgesia was used before the painful procedure. One study showed that with the standardization of postoperative pain management strategies for infants in the NICU, the following improvements were noted: (1) decreased length of time to extubation, (2) decreased length of stay, (3) better fluid management, and (4) reduced side effects of opioids. The authors also noted improved pain management documentation, decreased cost, and decreased nursing time (Furdon and others, 1998). (See Atraumatic Care box.)

An experience known as the "windup" phenomenon has been attributed to a decreased pain threshold and chronic pain. Central and peripheral mechanisms that occur in re-

---

**Box 10-6** ■ ■ ■
## Consequences of Untreated Pain in Infants

**ACUTE CONSEQUENCES**
Periventricular-intraventricular hemorrhage
Increased chemical and hormone release
Breakdown of fat and carbohydrate stores
Prolonged hyperglycemia
Higher morbidity for NICU patients
Memory of painful events
Hypersensitivity to pain
Prolonged response to pain
Inappropriate innervation of the spinal cord
Inappropriate response to nonnoxious stimuli
Lower pain threshold

**POTENTIAL LONG-TERM CONSEQUENCES**
Higher somatic complaints of unknown origin
Greater physiologic and behavioral responses to pain
Increased prevalence of neurologic deficits
Psychosocial problems
Neurobehavioral disorders
Cognitive deficits
Learning disorders
Poor motor performance
Behavioral problems
Attention deficits
Poor adaptive behavior
Inability to cope with novel situations
Problems with impulsivity and social control
Learning deficits
Emotional temperament changes in infancy or childhood
Accentuated hormonal stress responses in adult life

Data from Anand KJ, Hickey P: Pain and its effects in the human neonate and fetus, *N Engl J Med* 317:1321-1329, 1987; Anand KS, Grunau RE, Oberlander TF: Developmental character and long-term consequences of pain in infants and children, *Child Adolesc Psychiatr Clin North Am* 6(4):703-724, 1997; Barba B and others: Pain memory in full-term newborn, *J Pain Symptom Manage* 6:206, 1991; Fitzgerald M: Pain in infancy: some unanswered questions, *Pain Reviews* 2:77-91, 1995; Fitzgerald M, Millard C, McIntosh N: Cutaneous hypersensitivity following peripheral tissue damage in newborn infants and its reversal with topical anaesthesia, *Pain* 39:31-36, 1989; Grunau RVE and others: Early pain experience, child and family factors as precursors of somatization: a prospective study of extremely premature and full-term children, *Pain* 56:353-359, 1994; Langland J, Langland P: Pain in the neonate and fetus (letter to the editor), *N Engl J Med* 318:1398, 1988; Penticuff J: Neonatal nursing ethics: toward a consensus, *Neonatal Network* 5:7-16, 1987; Perry E and others: Blood pressure increases, birth weight–dependent stability boundary, and intraventricular hemorrhage, *Pediatrics* 85:727-732, 1990; Sexson W and others: Auditory conditioning in the critically ill neonate to enhance interpersonal relationships, *J Perinatol VI,* 20-23, 1986; Wong DL: *Physiological responses, facial expressions, and cry of infants during immunization in relation to their pain history,* Ann Arbor, MI, 1992, University Microfilm (order number 9321617).

---

## ATRAUMATIC CARE
### Use of Opioids and Extubation Practice

Traditional belief holds that the continued use of opioids for neonates in the postoperative period results in prolonged intubation. Consequently, traditional practice is to discontinue all opioids several hours before and after extubation, preventing pain relief. Furdon and others (1998) found that continuous opioid infusion in infants without an underlying pulmonary or neurologic pathologic condition actually shortened the time to extubation and caused no problems of respiratory depression that required reintubation.

sponse to noxious tissue injury have been studied in an attempt to explain a prolonged neonatal response to pain characteristic of the "windup" phenomenon. Following exposure to noxious stimuli, multiple levels of the spinal cord experience an altered excitability. This altered excitability may cause nonnoxious stimuli, such as routine nursing care and handling, to be perceived as noxious stimuli. The nonnoxious stimuli produce the same physiologic response to stress that noxious stimuli would produce, leading to chronic pain. Long-term exposure to chronic pain may be responsible for more biologic and clinical consequences in critically ill premature infants than acute pain (Anand, Grunau, and Oberlander, 1997).

Researchers have found that nerve damage resulting from tissue injury stimulates collateral nerve growth by surrounding undamaged nerves. This collateral growth is responsible for inappropriate innervation in the spinal cord, which processes information from the surrounding undamaged nerves (Anand, Grunau, and Oberlander, 1997). Based on evidence from the study of human infants and adult rats exposed to neonatal pain, additional long-term consequences of neonatal pain include potential emotional temperament changes in infancy or childhood, accentuated hormonal stress responses in adult life, a documented preference for alcohol, and decreased exploratory behaviors (Anand, Grunau, and Oberlander, 1997).

Consequences of a history of ELBW and early pain exposure that may be attributed to pain and environmental stress include increased prevalence of neurologic deficits, psychosocial problems, and neurobehavioral disorders. Additional sequelae include cognitive deficits, learning disorders, poor motor performance, behavioral problems, attention deficits, poor adaptive behavior, inability to cope with novel situations, problems with impulsivity and social control, and learning deficits (Anand, Grunau, and Oberlander, 1997).

The limited available knowledge with respect to the consequences of infant pain suggests serious potential deleterious effects of untreated pain (Box 10-6). Prevention of acute pain and treatment of chronic pain have been documented as beneficial in reducing the morbidity and mortality associated with frequent exposure to pain in premature infants (Anand and Carr, 1989; Anand and Hickey, 1987; Anand and Hickey, 1992). Nurses who care for infants and children should consider the potential acute and long-term effects of pain on their young patients and be active advocates in treating and preventing pain.

**Pain Management.** Morphine and fentanyl are the most widely used opioid analgesics for pharmacologic management of neonatal pain. Continuous or bolus epidural or intravenous infusion of opioids provides effective and safe pain control (Farrington and others, 1993; Haberkern and others, 1996). Other methods of relieving pain are epidural/intrathecal infusion, local and regional nerve blocks, and topical anesthetics (Choonara, 1992; Ochsenreither, 1997; Taddio and others, 1998; Yaster and others, 1994). (See Pain Management, Chapter 26, for more information on pharmacologic management of pain in the infant.)

Parents are universally concerned that their infants are suffering pain during procedures (Franck, Scurr, and Couture, 2001). Nurses need to address these concerns and encourage the parents to speak with the health care professionals involved. Parents have the right to withhold consent for invasive procedures and are entitled to honest answers from those responsible for the infant's care. When permissible, they can also help provide comfort measures for the infant.

## Developmental Outcome

Neonatal intensive care, along with rapid improvements in technology, is associated with improved survival of critically ill newborn and preterm infants. Survival rates have increased to 93% for VLBW infants (1001 to 1500 g), 85% for ELBW infants (751 to 1000 g), and about 50% for infants weighing 501 to 750 g (Msall and Tremont, 2000). With decreasing mortality, morbidity rates have remained stable. At highest risk for unfavorable outcomes are preterm infants compromised during the neonatal period by respiratory distress syndrome (RDS), bronchopulmonary dysplasia (BPD), NEC, sepsis, anemia, IVH, hydrocephalus, meningitis, or seizures (McGrath, Sullivan, and Lester, 2000; Vohr and others, 2000). These serious sequelae of prematurity correlate with the degree of immaturity, demonstrating the relationship of increasing morbidity with decreasing gestational age. A greater incidence of cerebral palsy (CP), attention deficit hyperactivity disorder (ADHD), visual-motor deficits, mild to severe cognitive disabilities, hearing loss, speech and language impairment, and neuromotor problems have been reported in outcome studies of preterm infants (Cherkes-Julkowski, 1998; Hack and others, 2000; Msall and Tremont, 2000; McGrath, Sullivan, and Lester, 2000). Delayed expressive and receptive language has been reported in former LBW infants at 24 months of age (Byrne and others, 1993).

These deficits may contribute to later academic difficulties, with increased need for special education classes, additional learning resources, and diagnosis of learning disabilities. Twenty percent to 65% of former VLBW or LBW infants with no major disabling conditions reportedly require special education or additional school services (McGrath, Sullivan and Lester, 2000). A recent study comparing VLBW and infants of normal birth weight found that the VLBW group had significantly poorer mathematical skills, more frequent grade retention, and required 2.8 times more special academic assistance (Schraeder and others, 1997).

The presence of neurodevelopmental impairment also occurs in preterm infants who have been spared the complications of IVH, sepsis, and hypoxemia, moving through the NICU with seemingly few problems. Conversely, there are preterm infants who do very well and function at age level without evidence of neurobehavioral limitations. Improved developmental outcomes are more likely for these survivors of early gestation and LBW when emphasis is placed on providing the finest medical and nursing care within a developmentally supportive framework. This philosophy requires caregivers to evaluate their own knowledge, skills, and attitudes and expand their thinking beyond the traditional medical and nursing models of care.

**Developmental Assessment.** Individualized developmental care has been reported to have numerous positive effects on medical and neurobehavioral outcomes in high-risk newborn infants. These benefits include fewer days on the ventilator or with oxygen supplementation, lower postconception age at oxygen weaning, less time to complete oral feeding, fewer incidences of IVH, shorter hospital stay, lower hospital charges, less severe BPD, higher scores on the Assessment of Preterm Infant Behavior (APIB) at 42 to 44 weeks, less need for sedation when critically ill, and better scores on Bayley Scales of Infant Development at 9, 18, and 36 months (Als, 1982; Als, 1986; Als and others, 1986; Als and others, 1994; Fleischer and others, 1995; Heller and others, 1997; Westrup and others, 2000).

One approach to NICU care is based on Als (1982) Synactive Theory of Infant Development that provides the framework for understanding the preterm infant's development. The model proposes a systematic method for observing NICU infants to collect information concerning each infant's competencies, vulnerabilities, and thresholds. This information forms the basis for planning individualized care appropriate for a particular infant (Table 10-4). The major assumption of this model states that infants, even ELBW infants, can communicate through physical and behavioral responses that provide us with the best information for planning their care. Communication by the infant is seen through three subsystems of functioning (autonomic, motor, and state) that can be readily observed in the clinical setting during rest, care, or procedures, and while recovering from care or procedures. Responses by an infant's autonomic (physiologic), motor, and state systems to the environment, physical care, or procedures help the nurse to make necessary adjustments in technique to optimize the infant's stability and functioning.

Because each infant is unique, supportive developmental care requires ongoing data collection of moment-by-moment responses and flexible care to address the infant's cues. For example, an infant who demonstrates altered vital signs and even apnea after being weighed might benefit from swaddled weighing to support the infant's competence and organization during a stressful procedure. (See Critical Thinking Exercise box.)

Knowledge of behavioral assessment and infant development assist the nurse in providing care that supports each infant's ongoing functioning in a manner consistent with current evidence. Nurses have the greatest impact on the daily routine experienced by their tiny patients. It is important to understand the different stages of infant development in order to provide the most effective nursing care.

The CNS is undergoing rapid and significant change during the preterm infant's stay in the NICU. This vulnerable period of brain growth, differentiation, and organization is combined with the challenge of developing in environmental conditions that are not typical for the fetus and newborn (Blackburn and VandenBerg, 1998). Brain organization peaks from about 20 weeks gestation to several years after birth. The product of this complex process is establishment of an elaborate circuitry unique to the human brain.

**Behavioral State Organization.** Traditional nursing placed emphasis on interpreting physiologic data as the basis of caregiving. Developmentally supportive care uses both physiologic and behavioral information to better understand the needs of infants in the NICU setting. Behavioral states are highly individualized and formed by experience, maturation, circadian rhythms, and genetic inheritance (Mayes, 2000). The emerging availability and regulation of arousal states mark a balancing of CNS inhibitory and excitatory processes that impact attention states and also mark executive functions (prefrontal cortex) that influence information processing and learning as well as socialization. State organization has been described as a gating mechanism that protects the cortex from overstimulation and promotes coordination between attentional, executive, and sensory cortical systems.

Infant responsiveness to environmental stimuli depends on the quality, amount, and availability of particular states of arousal. States can be organized into five levels of arousal (Table 10-5). Transitional states such as drowsiness are not considered true states but are in-between levels of arousal in which the infant either moves toward wakefulness or back into sleep.

Distinct sleep and awake states are observable by 28 weeks gestation (Holditch-Davis, 1998; Glass, 1994). Young preterm infants spend 70% or more of their time in active sleep. Developmental maturation for the young preterm infant is seen by a decrease in the amount of active sleep with an increase in quiet sleep, awake periods, and crying. Around 30 to 32 weeks, quiet alert states with some focused attention can be observed. Before 28 weeks, attempts to attend to stimuli may have physiologic consequences for the immature infant

## Critical Thinking Exercise

### Developmental Care

You are getting ready to feed a 4-week-old infant born at 28 weeks of gestation. While taking vital signs, you notice that the infant's color is pink but slightly mottled; he is yawning, extending his arms and legs, and splaying his fingers. Oxygen saturation by pulse oximetry indicates a reading within the lower range of normal for this infant. You recognize these behaviors as manifestations of what neonatal event?

FIRST, THINK ABOUT IT . . .

• What precise questions are you trying to answer?
• How are you interpreting the information?

1. Preterm behavior
2. Subtle seizures
3. Stress
4. Onset of infection

*The best response is three. Precisely, recall that preterm neonates may exhibit these signs and others (see Box 10-3) when they are not able to habituate to external stimuli, including routine handling. Interpreting this information alone does not indicate subtle seizure activity or infection. They are normal preterm behaviors but signal the infant's need for "time-out."*

**TABLE 10-4**  Synactive theory of development: neurobehavioral subsystems

| Subsystem | Signs of Stress | Signs of Stability |
|---|---|---|
| **Autonomic** | **Physiologic instability** | **Physiologic stability** |
| Respiratory | Tachypnea, pauses, gasping, sighing | Smooth, stable respirations, regular rate and pattern |
| Color | Mottled, flushed, dusky, pale or gray | Pink, stable color |
| Visceral | Hiccups, gagging, choking, spitting up, grunting and straining as if having a bowel movement; coughing, sneezing, yawning | Absence of hiccups, gagging, spitting up, etc. |
| Autonomic | Tremors, startles, twitches | Absence of tremors, startles, twitches |
| **Motor** | **Fluctuating tone, lack of control over movement, activity and posture** | **Consistent tone, controlled or improved movement, activity, and posture** |
| Flaccidity | Low tone in trunk; limp, floppy upper and lower extremities; limp, drooping jaw (gape face) | Tone consistent and appropriate for postconception age |
| Hypertonicity | Arm or leg extensions, arm(s) outstretched with fingers splayed in salute gesture, fingers stiffly outstretched, trunk arching, neck hyperextended | Well-maintained posture<br>Smooth, controlled movements |
| Hyperflexion | Trunk, extremities, fisting | Successful motor strategies for self-regulation (see self-regulation below) |
| Activity | Squirming; frantic diffuse activity or little or no activity or responsiveness | |
| **State** | **Disorganized quality to state behaviors, including range of available states, maintenance of state control, and transition from one state to another** | **Easy-to-read state behaviors that are maintained; calm, focused alertness, well-modulated sleep** |
| Sleep | Whimpering sounds, facial twitching, irregular respirations, fussing, grimacing, restless appearance | Clear, well-defined sleep states, periods of quiet, restful sleep |
| Awake | Glazed, unfocused look, staring, worried or pained expression, hyperalert or panicked appearance, eye roving, crying, cry-face, actively averting gaze or closing eyes, irritability, prolonged awake periods, inconsolability, frenzy | Alert with bright, shiny eyes, focused attention on object or person, animated expression (e.g., cheek softening, frowning, "ooh face," cooing, smiling)<br>Robust crying<br>Good calming, consolability |
| | Abrupt or rapid state changes | Smooth changes between states, full range of sleep/wake states |
| **Other State-Related Behaviors and Attention-Interaction** | **Efforts to attend to and interact with environmental stimulation elicits signs of stress and disorganized subsystem functioning** | **Responsive to auditory, visual, and social stimuli** |
| Autonomic | Physiologic instability of varying degrees with autonomic, respiratory, color, and visceral responses | Responsiveness to stimuli well-maintained and prolonged |
| Motor | Fluctuating tone, increased motor activity, progressively frantic diffuse activity if stimulation continues | Actively seeking auditory stimulus, minimal motor activity |
| State | Roving eyes, gaze averting, glazed-unfocused look or worried, panicked expression, weak cry, cry-face, irritability | Bright, shiny-eyed, alert, and attentive expression |
| | Closed eyes and sleep-like withdrawal | |
| | Abrupt state changes | Sustained awake and alert state |
| | Signs of stress when presented with more than one type of stimulus at a time | Shifting attention smoothly to more than one type of stimulation |

**Self-Regulation: Infant's efforts to achieve, maintain, or regain a balanced, stable, and relaxed state of subsystem functioning and integration; success of these efforts will vary among infants depending on maturity, available self-regulatory skills, and overall subsystem organization**

Examples of self-regulatory strategies include:
  Motor—Foot bracing against a boundary or blanket nest, hand holding, grasping hands together, hand to mouth or face, grasping blanket, tubing, tucking trunk, sucking, position changes
  State—Lowering state from high arousal to quiet alert or sleep state; releasing energy by rhythmic, robust crying; focused attention and orientation

**Facilitation by caregivers through environmental modifications or developmental care techniques can aid the infant's own self-regulatory abilities when environmental challenges exceed the infant's capabilities**

Modified from Als H: Toward a synactive theory of development: promise for the assessment and support of infant individuality, *Inf Mental Health J* 3(4):229-243, 1982; Als H: A synactive model of neonatal behavior organization: framework for the assessment of neurobehavioral development in the premature infant and for support of infants and parents in the neonatal intensive care environment, *Phys Occup Ther Pediatr* 6:3-55, 1986; Hunter JG: The neonatal intensive care unit. In Case-Smith J, Allen AS, Pratt PN, editors: *Occupational therapy for children*, ed 4, St Louis, 2001, Mosby.

**TABLE 10-5** Arousal states

| State | Description |
|---|---|
| Deep sleep | Regular breathing, eyes closed with no movement of eyes under lid, relaxed face, little or no movement or activity except for possible startle response |
| Active sleep | Sometimes called light sleep, may see rapid eye movements (REM) under closed lids, low activity level, breathing regular or irregular, occasional sighing or smiling |
| Drowsy | Eyes open or closed, unfocused expression, activity level varied |
| Quiet awake | Different qualities of alerting: |
| Robust | Bright, shiny appearance to eyes, focused attention, minimal motor activity |
| Low level | Dull or unfocused eyes, little energy, appears to look through an object or caregiver |
| Hyperalert | Wide eyes, panicked expression, may fixate on an object or caregiver very intensely and have trouble breaking away |
| Active awake | Active, eyes open or closed, fussy but not crying robustly |
| Crying | Highest level of arousal, agitated, rhythmic, and robust crying |

*Modified from Als H: *Manual for the naturalistic observation of newborn behavior, Newborn Individualized Developmental Care and Assessment Program (NIDCAP)*, Boston, 1995, Harvard Medical School.

(Blackburn, 1998). Responsiveness to sound and touch is greater during active or light (rapid eye movement [REM]) sleep, resulting in longer periods of vulnerability to sleep disturbance (Holditch-Davis, 1998). Maturation continues throughout the first year of life. By 6 months, the amount of quiet sleep is greater than that of active sleep. By 1 year, infants usually sleep 10 to 12 hours at night and take one to two naps during the day. Preterm infants generally demonstrate shorter night sleep and awaken more frequently than term infants. Other maturational changes include organization of the standard sleep cycle and electroencephalogram (EEG) sleep patterns comparable to adults. Neurologic insults, severity of illness, hyperbilirubinemia, and prenatal exposure to drugs can alter behavioral state patterns (Holditch-Davis, 1998; Prechtl, 1992).

Physiologic parameters vary depending on level of arousal (Holditch-Davis, 1998). Heart rate is higher during waking periods but more variable during active sleep. Blood pressure is higher during wakefulness. Cerebral blood flow is greater during active sleep (greater during quiet sleep in term infants). Respiratory rates fluctuate more and are higher in active sleep. Arterial oxygen and carbon dioxide levels are decreased in active sleep when compared to quiet sleep or awake states. Hypoventilation and poorly coordinated chest wall and abdominal movements are reported for active sleep. Apneic pauses of less than 20 seconds are more frequent in active than quiet sleep in term and preterm infants.

Nursing care should be timed to the responsiveness of the infant as much as possible to optimize developing sleep organization and enhancement of alerting as it emerges. Sensory stimulation can influence behavioral state as seen by either increased or decreased infant arousal when presented with a stimulus, its removal, and the type of stimulus (e.g. loud bell or soft lullaby). The quality of each state, its duration, and the movement between states provides information concerning how well organized the state is and how much state control the infant has. Protection of sleep is an important goal for both the preterm and term infant. Environmental modifications and timing of care to provide longer episodes of undisturbed sleep should be planned into care. Preterm infants <34 weeks who received four 1½-hour naps (two at night and one during the evening and one during the day) demonstrated a significantly faster decline in apneic episodes than control infants (Torres, and others, 1997); these infants also gained more weight per day than controls.

Nurses can also support transitions between states. Gentle arousal to wakefulness by soft speech or gentle touch before caregiving is preferable to the traditional model in which care is begun without warning and with abrupt disruption of sleep. Slow movements and gentle handling support quiet alerting or return to sleep without periods of arousal after care is over. Nurses should facilitate return to sleep or interact with a quietly alert infant after care events.

An infant's state of arousal allows for communication of responses that are valuable for individualized caregiving. Observing state patterns and individual responses of infants, nurses can better know their patients and support behavioral state organization. This knowledge can also be shared with parents to foster intimacy between parent and child.

**Sensory System.** Research with animal fetuses and infants has shown that atypical sensory experiences, whether overstimulating or depriving, can modify the developing brain (Glass, 1994; Lickliter, 2000a). In fact, much of the cerebral cortex is associated with the sensory system. Most sensory systems develop prenatally and are capable of functioning before birth. Onset of function of each sensory system proceeds in the same order for each individual (e.g., tactile, vestibular, gustatory-olfactory, auditory, and visual). The visual system becomes functional after birth. Sensory input provided before the stimulation would typically occur has been shown to interfere with perceptual and behavioral development (Lickliter, 2000b).

The normal experience for the preterm infant is within the womb and for the term infant is the home environment with a few primary caregivers. These environments are vastly different from the NICU. The NICU experience for the high-risk infant is made up of external conditions and interactions with caregivers. Often that experience is overstimulating to later-developing sensory systems (i.e., auditory and visual) and understimulating to earlier ones (i.e., tactile, vestibular, gustatory-olfactory). Alterations in the sensory environment may have developmental consequences. It is important for the nurse to consider the following while caring for high-risk infants: (1) timing of stimulation in relation to the expected experience of an infant's current developmental stage, (2) amount of stimulation provided or denied, (3) type of stimulation, and (4) the infant's response to the stimulation (Lickliter, 2000b).

Tactile sensation begins around the mouth of the fetus at approximately the seventh week of gestation. By the fifteenth week, cutaneous sensitivity has spread to the rest of the face, palms of hands, soles of feet, trunk, arms, legs, tongue, and mucous membranes. By the age of viability, infants in the NICU have sophisticated perioral sensation and perceive pressure, pain, and temperature (Als, 1999). Touch in the NICU frequently involves routine, sometimes impersonal, caregiving and procedures that are either intrusive or painful. Even nonpainful care has been associated with adverse responses in premature infants.

Preterm infants demonstrate cry expression, grimacing, and knee and leg flexion during major reposition changes (Evans and others, 1997). Hypoxemia, associated with nonpainful or routine caregiving activities such as suctioning, repositioning, taking vital signs, changing diapers, and removing electrodes, has been reported (Evans, 1991). Other physiologic changes include blood pressure changes, heart rate changes, and respiratory rhythm and rate alterations (Browne, 2000; Evans, 1991; Peters, 1992). Nursing activities that are painful or especially intrusive, such as needle puncture, suctioning, and chest physiotherapy, have resulted in acute decreases in $SaO_2$ and behavioral state changes in preterm infants ranging from 23 to 37 weeks gestation (Zahr and Balian, 1995). Increased motor activity, agitation, crying, and startle reflex have also been described as negative behavioral responses to touch (Browne, 2000).

Rest is often disrupted by frequent handling with periods of undisturbed rest reportedly no longer than 2 to 59 minutes (Appleton, 1997). Pohlman and Beardslee (1987) found that 56% of those disruptions are from moderately to highly intrusive care by nurses. They observed only 8.2% of nursing contacts as comforting. "Clustering" care to provide adequate rest periods without handling has been advocated; however, if the cluster is overwhelming and prolonged the immature or ill infant is at risk for physiologic and behavioral compromise (Peters, 1999).

Touch is the first sensory system to develop and forms the basis for early communication between infants and caregivers. In particular, touch is a powerful means of emotional exchange for parents and infants. Positioning and handling techniques are used to promote comfort and minimize stress, while creating a balance between nurturing care and necessary interventions.

**Therapeutic Handling.** Using the developmental model of supportive care, the nurse closely monitors physiologic and behavioral signs to promote organization and well-being of high-risk infants during handling (Box 10-7). The type, timing, and amount of handling are carefully considered using the infant's current age, condition, vulnerabilities, thresholds for stress, and capabilities as reference. Because touch can be disruptive to maturing sleep/wake states, attempts should be made to avoid waking an infant for care or nurturing. Sleep deprivation may affect secretion of growth hormone and interfere with growth and development (Hunter, 1996).

Respectful approach before touching an infant allows more time for transition and adaptation from being alone to being handled. Softly calling an infant by name and then gently placing a hand on the body signals care is beginning

---

**Box 10-7 ■ ■ ■**
**Considerations for Tactile Interventions in the NICU**

1. Modify all handling and touch so that it is supportive and calming
2. Consider sleep/wake states and behavioral cues to determine optimal times for handling and touch
3. Adjust handling and touch based on continual observation of infant autonomic and behavioral responses
4. Ensure appropriate touch opportunities for parents aside from routine caregiving
5. Encourage parents to be primary providers of social touch
6. Avoid using massage with vulnerable high-risk infants (e.g., medically unstable, LBW infants <32 weeks; easily disorganized, low threshold infants; chronically ill infants with BPD or cardiac disorders known to display physiologic and behavioral disorganization, etc.)
7. Assist parents in identifying the most appropriate type of touch and handling for their infant
8. Teach infant cues to parents for monitoring responses to handling and touch
9. Weigh the risk/benefit for any tactile intervention

---

and alleviates the abrupt interruption that frequently precedes caregiving. The infant's own cues can be used by the nurse to determine optimal times for caregiving rather than adhering to a rigid schedule. The best time for care is when an infant is awake. If the care or procedure cannot be postponed, then gentle arousal prepares the infant without the sudden, unexpected rushed caregiving characteristic of traditional care. Abrupt transitions can disrupt even organized functioning of an infant's autonomic, motor, and state subsystems.

Infants who are unable to maintain a gently flexed position during repositioning or care procedures may benefit from containment. Gently holding the infant's arms and legs in a tucked, flexed position close to the body can be accomplished using hands or blanket swaddling. "Facilitated tucking" before a heelstick procedure was shown to decrease physiologic and behavioral distress in preterm infants as young as 25 weeks gestational age (Corff and others, 1995). Blanket swaddling and nesting or containment has been shown to decrease physiologic and behavioral stress during routine care procedures such as bathing, weighing, and heel lance (Fearon and others, 1997; Neu and Browne, 1997; Peters, 1992, 1998).

Because repositioning has been associated with significant physiologic distress in immature infants, sudden postural changes should be avoided. Slow turning while containing the infant's extremities in a gently tucked, midline position may reduce the impact of this procedure.

Stroking preterm infants who are not physiologically stable has been reported to result in behavioral signs of distress such as gasping, grunting, gaze aversion, and decreased $tcPO_2$ levels (Harrison and others, 1996; Oehler, 1985). Increased periods of oxygen desaturation in preterm infants between 27 and 33 weeks were reported to occur during usual parent-infant interactions that varied in type and amount of handling (Harrison, Leeper, and Yoon, 1990). Some infants experience apnea and bradycardia during massage or tactile/kinesthetic stimulation (Glass, 1994). Individual infants show varied responses to tactile intervention, further supporting the need for close monitoring of behavioral and physiologic parameters (Harrison, Leeper, and Yoon, 1990; Harrison and Woods, 1991).

Other investigators have reported positive benefits of massage on stable, growing preterm infants. Infants around 31 weeks gestation weighing between 1000 and 2000 g demonstrated significant weight gain; had more active, alert periods during sleep/wake observations; exhibited more mature orientation, motor, habituation, and range of state behaviors on Brazelton's Newborn Behavior Assessment Scale (BNBAS); and spent fewer days in the hospital than those provided only routine care (Field and others, 1986; Scafidi and others, 1990). Wheeden and others (1993) studied 30 preterm infants (mean gestational age 30 weeks) prenatally exposed to cocaine. The massaged infants averaged 28% more weight gain, and had fewer postnatal complications, decreased stress behaviors, and more mature motor behaviors on the Brazelton scales.

Vickers and others (2000) evaluated literature relevant to infant massage, gentle touch, and *gentle human touch (GHT).* The researchers concluded that available studies, although demonstrating advantages to massage for preterm infants, lack sound methodologic bases on which firm recommendations can be made to advocate widescale use of this intervention.

*Kangaroo care (KC),* or *STS holding,* has been advocated for fostering neurobehavioral development and supporting parent-infant intimacy and attachment. STS contact is maintained with the diaper-clad infant resting prone and semi-upright on the bared chest of either parent, who encloses the infant in their own clothing to facilitate temperature stability. KC is reported to reduce incidence of severe illness and nosocomial infection, support breast-feeding duration until discharge, and improve maternal satisfaction (Conde-Agudelo, 2000). Hurst and others (1997) reported a significant increase in milk volume in mothers providing KC to stable, ventilated LBW infants (mean 27.7 weeks gestation) compared to a non-KC control group. Others have reported advantages that include maintenance of skin temperature, reduction of apnea and bradycardia, stable tcPO₂ level, increased frequency and duration of quiet sleep, less time crying, and lower activity levels during KC (Roberts, Paynter, and McEwan, 2000). KC has been successfully initiated in stable preterm infants who weigh less than 1000 g (Neu, Browne, and Vojir, 2000).

However, in a recent study of preterm infants (mean gestational age 29 weeks), KC was associated with a significant increase in bradycardia, less regular breathing, and hypoxemia. Temperatures were increased (measured rectally) every 2 hours (Bohnhorst and others, 2001). Although adverse effects are not usually associated with KC, monitoring is important to avoid potential harmful effects and should include cardiorespiratory parameters, body temperature, and oxygenation.

Infants appear to be most vulnerable during the transfer from bed to parent and back to bed when KC is provided. A study was done of fifteen ventilated preterm infants (mean

weight 1094 g) who were randomly assigned to one of two transfer techniques, either parent or nurse-to-parent, alternating methods for 2 consecutive days of KC holding (Neu Browne, and Vojir, 2000). Regardless of the transfer method, SaO₂ decreased and heart rate increased during transfer but returned to baseline during KC. Duskiness, decreased muscle tone, decreased self-regulatory behaviors, and more caregiver facilitation were observed during transfer. Physiologic and behavioral stability was observed in all infants during and after KC. Heart rate and SaO₂ were less variable during KC than during the pre-KC period, and muscle tone and self-regulatory behaviors improved during the post-KC period. Both techniques required a brief period of disconnection from the ventilator during the transfer that may have influenced oxygenation. Handling and repositioning necessary to prepare and move an infant into the KC position may result in similar disorganizing responses as previously described with routine nursing care.

Some parents may be uncomfortable with KC. Thirty mother-infant pairs were randomly assigned (Roberts, Paynter, and McEwan, 2000) to provide either KC or *conventional cuddling (CC)* to their preterm infants (mean gestational age 31 weeks). The only difference between treatments was that CC infants wore clothes when held by their mothers. There was no significant difference in weight gain, temperature maintenance, duration of breast-feeding, or length of hospital stay between the two groups. The data suggested equal benefits of KC and CC. CC affords parents another option for social touch in the NICU.

**Co-Bedding Multiples.**   Co-bedding is the practice of bedding twins or other multiples in the same crib or incubator (Fig. 10-7). It is based on the idea that extrauterine adaptation is facilitated by continued physical contact with the intrauterine partner (Walden, 1999; Nyqvist and Lutes, 1998). There is little evidence supporting or refuting the use of co-bedding in the NICU; however, bed sharing after discharge, whether with parents or siblings and regardless of infant sleep position, reportedly increases the incidence of unexplained death (sudden infant death syndrome [SIDS]) in infants (Thogmartin, Siebert, and Pellan, 2001).

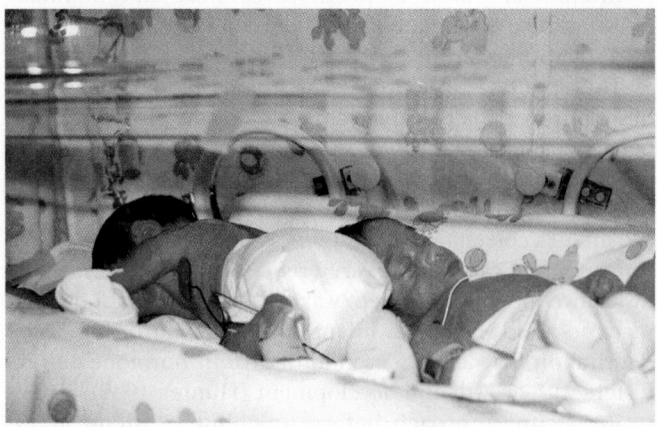

**Fig. 10-7**   Co-bedding. Twins are placed next to each other in one incubator. (Courtesy Kathy Conner, RN, Hillcrest Medical Center, Tulsa, Oklahoma)

The American Academy of Pediatrics (2000) recommends that bed sharing with infants be avoided by adults and other children or siblings in the home. Nursing staff must be sure that parents are aware of the hazards of this practice at home, especially if co-bedding is practiced in the NICU.

Co-bedding is approved in some institutions around the country. A care protocol is usually defined with inclusion or exclusion criteria to identify infants who might benefit (Nyqvist and Lutes, 1998). Special attention must be paid to identification of the paired infants and their personal medications and equipment. It is recommended that body temperature be closely monitored, particularly on initiation, interruption, or termination of co-bedding, to avoid thermal stress.

**Therapeutic Positioning.**   The American Academy of Pediatrics (2000) recommends the supine sleeping position for healthy infants in the first year of life as a preventive measure for SIDS. Prone sleeping has decreased from over 70% to about 20% in the United States since the guidelines were published. Although SIDS remains the highest cause of infant death after the neonatal period (28 days), the rate has decreased by over 40% with the advent of supine sleeping. (See Sudden Infant Death Syndrome, Chapter 12.)

Parents of infants in the NICU should be educated on the safe sleeping position at home as part of discharge instructions. Supportive positioning in the NICU for acutely ill or recovering infants may look very different from the Academy's recommendations, depending on each infant's changing clinical condition, maturation, and readiness for the supine sleeping position and minimal bedding (Lockridge and others, 1999). It is important for staff to realize that routine care practices in the NICU may serve as a model for parents and, without proper instruction, they may reproduce at home the environment and care techniques they have observed in the NICU. Position and bedding choices in the unit, such as prone positioning, nests, and sheepskin, may be lethal for infants who have been discharged home.

Infants in the NICU are at increased risk for acquiring position-related deformities for a variety of reasons. Illness, weakness, low tone, immature motor control, the effects of gravity, and treatments such as ECMO or sedation are a few of the factors associated with prolonged immobility or decreased spontaneous movement (Hunter, 2001). Common position-related deformities include:

- Shoulder retraction and scapular adduction causing upper extremity external rotation, resulting in a persistent "W" positioning of the arms; can interfere with later midline skills that form the foundation for feeding, crawling, reaching, and midline play with objects (Georgieff and Bernbaum, 1986).
- Lower extremity external rotation deformities occurring when the trunk and pelvis are flat on the mattress, causing extreme hip abduction and outward rotation of the lower limbs or the frog-leg appearance (Downs and others, 1991).
- Neck extension and arching posture often observed in infants pulling away from endotracheal tubes or nasal prongs during mechanical ventilation or nasal continuous positive airway pressure (NCPAP).
- Motor asymmetries reported in premature infants who are <32 weeks or SGA, occurring more often than in full-term infants even after 4 months corrected age (de Groot, Hopkins, and Touwen, 1997).

Therapeutic positioning is used to reduce the potential for acquired positional deformities that can affect motor development, play skills, attractiveness, and social attachment (Hunter, 1996). Positioning can affect stability and comfort, and each infant must be observed for the effects of any position and after repositioning. A position may also need to be adapted to accommodate necessary medical equipment or particular conditions, such as myelomeningocele where the supine position is contraindicated. Deciding on which position and supportive aids are to be used requires the caregiver consider the medical and developmental risks and benefits unique to a specific infant and situation. (See Guidelines boxes.)

The goal of therapeutic positioning for preterm and high-risk infants is to provide adequate support and containment as indicated to sustain flexed and midline postures, in an attempt to minimize positional deformities and assist infants in remaining calm and organized (Hunter, 2001).

The supine position requires support for the weak or immature infant. Because this position can create the most disorganization, attention must be paid to sustaining this position comfortably using positioning aids or blanket boundaries that support the head, trunk, and extremities according to the general positioning principles.

Although the prone position may appear to be the easiest to maintain, mistakes are often made with babies who are unable to sustain rounded shoulders, trunk, and pelvis without assistance. Use of a prone roll or positioner has been shown to prevent scapular-humeral tightness and shoulder retraction commonly seen as a result of this position (Figs. 10-8 and 10-9) (Monfort and Case-Smith, 1997).

**Auditory Environment.**   The auditory system of the human fetus is mature enough for sound to produce physiologic effects as early as 23 weeks gestation (Graven, 2000). Physical and behavioral responses to sudden, loud NICU noise have been observed in premature and term infants (Anderssen, Nicolaisen, and Gabrielsen, 1993; Gadeke and others, 1969; Jurkovica and Aghova, 1989; Long, Lucey, and Philip, 1980; Wharrad and Davis, 1997; Zahr and Balian, 1995). Some studies suggest that continuous noise exposure at 60 decibels (dB) or louder may potentiate the ef-

---

## GUIDELINES
### *General Considerations for Positioning*

- ☐ Neutral or slightly flexed neck
- ☐ Gently rounded shoulders (no flattened posture against bed as in supine or prone positions)
- ☐ Elbows flexed
- ☐ Hands to face or midline as position allows
- ☐ Trunk slightly rounded with pelvic tilt
- ☐ Hips partially flexed and adducted to near midline (not medial or neutral alignment) and knee flexion (no frog leg or externally rotated hips flat against bed)
- ☐ Secure lower boundary for foot-bracing

Modified from Biber P and others: When to seek consultation. In Creger PJ, Browne JV: *Developmental interventions for preterm and high-risk infants: self-study modules for professionals,* Tucson, 1995, Therapy Skill Builders.

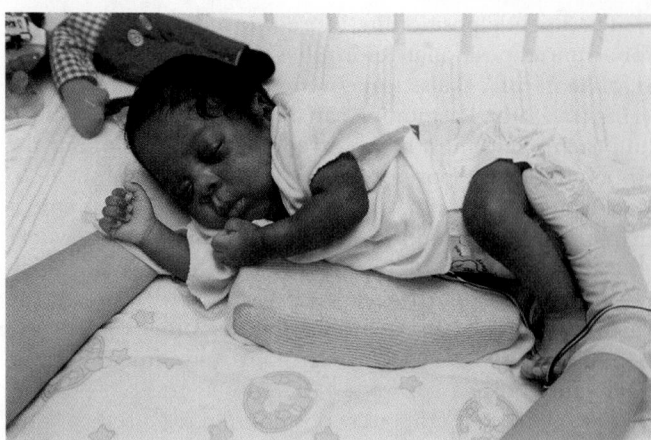

**Fig. 10-8** Preterm infant slowly and gently transitioned to prone position on prone roll designed with stockingnette-covered foam cut to individual specifications to prevent flattening of shoulders and pelvis against the mattress and to support a stable breathing base for the infant. (Courtesy Halbouty Premature Nursery, Texas Children's Hospital, Houston, Texas; photo by Paul Vincent Kuntz.)

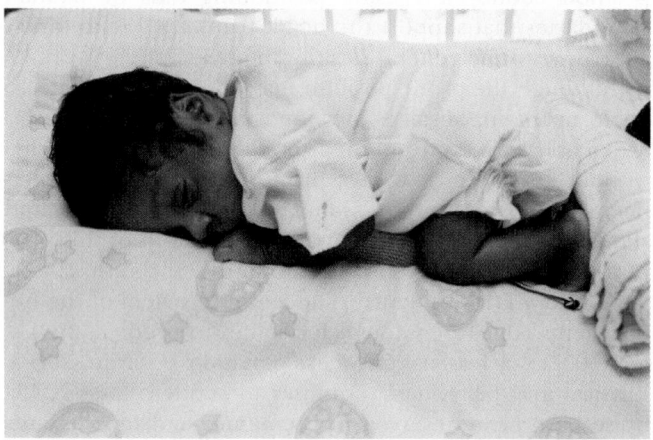

**Fig. 10-9** Preterm infant positioned on prone roll. (Courtesy Halbouty Premature Nursery, Texas Children's Hospital, Houston, Texas; photo by Paul Vincent Kuntz.)

fects of ototoxic medications (Jauhiainen, Kohonen, and Jauhiainen, 1972; Dayal, Kokshanian, and Mitchell, 1971).

These data demonstrate that infants in the NICU are capable of perceiving and responding to sounds around them. The primary auditory environment in fetal life is made up of the maternal voice, respirations, heartbeat, and intestinal sounds. Soon after birth, newborn infants demonstrate preference for their own mother's voice and the language heard in utero (Gerhardt and Abrams, 2000). The acoustic environment of most NICUs is vastly different from the uterine and home milieu. Currently there are no data on the effects of long-term exposure to NICU noise levels. Of serious concern is the increased risk of sensorineural hearing loss (Blackburn, 1998; Veen and others, 1993) and language delays in infants born prematurely (Byrne and others, 1993). Cochlear dysfunction is responsible for most of the permanent hearing loss discovered in children (Hall, 2000). NICU

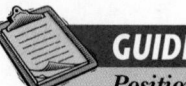

## GUIDELINES
### Positioning

1. Bedding and positioning aids must be individually determined to meet the needs of the infant. Soft bedding, such as sheepskin, secure nesting, and boundaries or swaddling, is used for those infants requiring such devices to maintain comfortable positioning and to prevent skin problems. Waterbeds (Fowler and others, 1997), or gel or water pillows (Marsden, 1980) are recommended to avoid abnormal head molding.
2. Calm, organized behavior may be improved by use of the following strategies:
   a. Prone position to facilitate improved oxygenation and ventilation.
   b. Side-lying position, well supported with swaddling, commercial containment devices, or a heavy blanket roll surrounding the infant's flexed back, to promote midline hands-together or hands-to-face movements.
   c. Swaddling to provide the most secure containment and to be used in combination with other positioning devices as needed.
3. Repositioning is usually indicated every 2 to 3 hours or when care must be provided. An infant may demonstrate behavioral cues that suggest discomfort and the need for positional change.
4. Oversized diapers may result in hips maintained in the externally rotated and abducted "frog-leg" posture. Appropriately sized commercial diapers are available and should be used to preserve normal hip alignment.
5. Tension from lines or tubing such as endotracheal tubes, naso- or orogastric tubes, cardiac leads, or intravenous lines may result in deforming pressures or postures and should be avoided.
6. Repositioning is often stressful for sick or preterm infants. Caregivers can reduce the stress of this necessary procedure with containment of the extremities and/or a pacifier for a brief time after moving the infant.
7. Once repositioned, the infant's breathing pattern, color, oxygen saturation, heart rate, respiratory rate and pattern, behavioral cues, stability of position should be monitored and whether positioning principles have been followed.
8. Finally, a very important consideration is that caregivers continually observe each infant's emerging capabilities to determine appropriate positioning and bedding options. Infants who begin to fight containment or boundaries or those who have matured beyond the need for positioning devices and can maintain a flexed posture unassisted should be allowed to do so.
9. Daily physical activity has been shown to enhance bone growth and development in LBW preterm infants (Moyer-Mileur and others, 2000). It is important to avoid restrictive swaddling or nesting that inhibits infants from all movement or pushing against their boundaries. Such practice could prove detrimental to motor development.
10. Supine positioning at least 2 weeks before discharge should be initiated so that infants can adjust to the home sleeping position.

Modified from Hunter J: The neonatal intensive care unit. In Case-Smith J, editor: *Occupational therapy for children*, ed 4, St Louis, 2001, Mosby.

noise may interfere with developing auditory pathways and mask socially relevant sounds of the human voice necessary for language development.

The timing, amount, and type of sound must be considered to create an environment supportive for each infant at varying stages of development. Recommendations for the sound environment of the term and premature newborn have been developed by the Physical and Developmental Environment of the High-Risk Infant Center, Study Group on NICU Sound, and the Expert Review Panel (Graven, 2000). Nurses can make a significant impact on the sound environment. Personal attention to one's own contribution includes lowering the voice during conversation or laughter, gently closing incubator doors and cabinet drawers, responding quickly to suspend alarms, giving report some distance away from the bedside, eliminating radios for personal use, and keeping access doors closed. Achieving an appropriate sound environment may even require renovation using improved design and material with respect to acoustic impact. When the sound environment is softened, it becomes possible to provide infants with the natural voices of their parents, an important stimulus during early development. Although earmuffs have been shown to reduce noise levels by 7 to 12 dB (Zahr and de Traversay, 1995), caution is warranted in using them for more than short-term attenuation of sound, such as during a loud procedure like magnetic resonance imaging (MRI). A more enriched sound environment can be provided for older infants who are medically stable. Sleep is facilitated when environmental noise is not disruptive, promoting the maturation of more organized sleep state behavior. Finally, maintaining recommended sound levels in the NICU may prove beneficial and include some or all of the following: (1) increased physiologic stability, (2) improved growth, (3) more natural and consistent neurosensory maturation, (4) enhanced parent-infant interaction and subsequent attachment, and (5) fewer speech and language difficulties (Graven, 2000).

**Visual Environment.**   Vision is the least mature of the newborn's senses. The preterm infant's eyes undergo significant maturation and differentiation of the retina and its connections to the visual cortex that typically occur in utero during the last trimester of pregnancy (Glass, 1994; Hunter, 2001). The fetus resides in a dark womb, although very small amounts of red or long-wavelength light can penetrate. Development of the visual system in utero is genetically coded and requires no light (Graven, 2001). The infant's other sensory systems are developing in a protected environment where visual stimulation is not provided. A current concern is that early, intense visual stimulation for preterm infants could adversely affect visual pathways and alter the developmental course for other sensory systems. This is called "sensory interference" (Lickliter, 1999b).

Visual functioning in preterm infants is more limited than that in term infants who, although limited in ability to focus (accommodation to near and far distances) and discriminate (acuity), will actively explore the environment. Preterm infants are less responsive to visual stimulation and have even less acuity and accommodation than term infants. The ability to visually attend occurs around 30 to 32 weeks, and the infant may become stressed if the visual stimulus is intense and prolonged. Glass (1994) questions the need for patterned stimulation, suggesting that just because an infant is able to respond to a stimulus does not necessarily mean that level of stimulation is beneficial for the infant. Strong visual stimulation such as high-contrast black and white patterns can evoke an obligatory staring response by the immature infant who is unable to break away from it. This behavior is neither appropriate nor desired.

A variety of lighting conditions exist for NICUs from continuous 24-hour illumination, continuous dim lighting, day/night cycled lighting, or unpredictable periods of light/dark depending on staff or situations. Ambient lighting in some NICUs is reported to range from 40 to 150 footcandles (ftc) during the day with levels over 1500 ftc if sunlight is added (Glass, 1994; Blackburn, 1998). These levels drop dramatically at night if light is cycled to reported levels of 5 to 9 ftc (Fielder and Merrick, 2000).

The Committee to Establish Recommended Standards for Newborn ICU Design (1999) recommends that ambient lighting be adjustable at each bedside through a range of 1 and 60 ftc (approximately 10 to 600 lux, another measure of illumination). The American Academy of Pediatrics (1999a) recommends separate procedure lighting of no more than 100 to 150 ftc (1080 to 1620 lux). Both groups warn that UV radiation from fluorescent fixtures should be reduced using plastic or glass shields because it is potentially damaging to the retina. Continuous exposure to intense, white fluorescent light has been associated with chromosome damage, alterations in circadian rhythms and the sleep/wake cycle, changes in endocrine and gonad function, changes in vitamin D synthesis, and suppression of melatonin (Hunter, 2001; Shanahan and Czeisler, 2000)

Factors influencing the light exposure of an infant include: (1) location in the unit, (2) position in bed, (3) light source, (4) treatments, and (5) certain examinations (Fielder and Merrick, 2000). When natural lighting from windows is present, the seasons and climate will affect light exposure. Bed location and infant position can result in different light exposure, depending on room arrangement and direction of light sources. Supine positioning with lights on overhead can be particularly disturbing with full exposure to both eyes. Side-lying or prone positioning usually results in more intense exposure to the upper eye. The intensity of the light source must also be considered and whether it is adjustable to lower levels. Phototherapy for neonatal jaundice is a common treatment for preterm infants with light exposures between about 200 to 280 ftc (2400 to 3000 lux) and small amounts of UV from 330 to 400 nanometers (nm). This treatment usually lasts for several days and infants receive protection with the use of eye patches. Ninety percent of the light from a phototherapy device can be blocked with securely attached eye patches. Photokeratitis from UV exposure and retinal injury associated with the blue-light photochemical mechanism mandate careful and continuous protection of the eyes of infants during phototherapy (Fielder and Merrick, 2000).

Staff need to carefully consider the impact of visual stimuli on the NICU infant. For preterm infants whose visual system is undergoing maturation, it is probably more prudent to provide stimulation to the earlier-developing senses first and minimize the impact of the NICU visual milieu on the infant. As attention and alerting emerge, the most appropriate visual stimulus is most likely to be the human face, especially that of the parent. Box 10-8 (Glass, 1994; White,

## Box 10-8 ■ ■ □
### Visual Stimulation: Considerations for Infants

1. Lower ambient light levels by dimming lights or using incubator covers for lower birth weight and gestational age infants
2. Facilitate eye opening and visual attention in older preterm and term infants by dimming overhead lights
3. Direct procedure lights toward the necessary visual field and away from infants' eyes when performing tasks that require visual acuity such as intravenous catheter insertion
4. Shield infants' eyes from bright procedure lights or full ambient lighting as needed during exams, treatments, or procedures
5. Avoid placing a cloth over the face or using eye patches that provide tactile irritation unless necessary for phototherapy or special circumstances
6. Ensure eye patches are securely in place during phototherapy
7. Introduce day/night cycling of lighting in the NICU and intermediate nursery before discharge
8. Avoid bright lights directed in infants' eyes
9. Consider the human face the most appropriate visual stimulation in early infancy
10. Avoid leaving visual stimuli in the beds of infants who cannot escape from it
11. Provide appropriate visual stimuli or toys for recovering term or older infants

## Box 10-9 ■ ■ □
### Psychologic Tasks of Parents of a High-Risk Infant

Work through the events surrounding labor and delivery.
Acknowledge that the infant's life is endangered and begin anticipatory grieving process.
Confront and recognize feelings of inadequacy and guilt in not delivering a healthy child.
Adapt to the neonatal intensive care environment.
Resume parental relationships with the sick infant and initiate the caregiving role.
Prepare to take the infant home.

Modified from Siegel R, Gardner SL, Merenstein GB: Families in crisis: theoretical and practical considerations. In Merenstein GB, Gardner SL: *Handbook of neonatal intensive care*, ed 4, St Louis, 1998, Mosby.

1999; Hunter, 2001; Mirmiran and Ariagno, 2000) provides some suggested approaches to visual stimulation in the NICU.

## Facilitating Parent-Infant Relationships

Because of their physiologic instability, preterm infants are immediately separated from their mothers and surrounded by a complex, impenetrable barrier of glass windows, mechanical equipment, and special caregivers. There is increasing evidence to indicate that the emotional separation that accompanies the physical separation of mothers and infants interferes with the normal maternal-infant attachment process discussed in Chapter 8. Maternal attachment is a cumulative process that begins before conception, strengthens by significant events during pregnancy, and matures through maternal-infant contact during the neonatal period.

When an infant is sick, the necessary physical separation appears to be accompanied by an emotional estrangement in the parents, which may seriously damage the capacity for parenting their infant. This detachment is further hampered by the tenuous nature of the infant's condition. When survival is in doubt, parents may be reluctant to establish a relationship with their infant. They prepare themselves for the death of the infant while continuing to hope for recovery. This anticipatory grief (see Chapter 23) and hesitancy to embark on a relationship are evidenced by behaviors such as delay in giving the infant a name, reluctance in visiting the nursery (or when they do visit, focusing on equipment and treatments rather than on their infant), and hesitancy to touch or handle the infant when given the opportunity.

Comprehensive management of high-risk newborns includes encouraging and facilitating parental involvement rather than isolating parents from their infant and associated care (Box 10-9). This is particularly important in relation to mothers; to reduce the effects of physical separation, mothers are united with their newborns at the earliest opportunity. Preparing the parents to see their infant for the first time is a nursing responsibility.

Before the first visit, the parents are prepared for their infant's appearance, the equipment attached to the child, and some indication of the general atmosphere of the unit. The initial encounter with the intensive care unit is a stressful experience, and the frightening array of people, equipment, and activity is likely to be overwhelming. A book of photographs or pamphlets describing the NICU environment (infants in incubators or under radiant warmers, monitors, mechanical ventilators, and intravenous equipment) provides a useful and nonthreatening introduction to the NICU.

Parents are encouraged to visit their infant as soon as possible. Even if they saw the infant at the time of transport or shortly after birth, the infant may have changed considerably, especially if there are a number of medical and equipment requirements associated with the infant's hospitalization. At the bedside the nurse should explain the function of each piece of equipment and the role it plays in facilitating recovery. Explanations may often need to be patiently repeated because parents' anxiety over the infant's condition and the surroundings may prevent them from really "hearing" what is being said. When possible, some items related to therapy can be removed; for example, phototherapy can be temporarily discontinued and eye patches removed to permit eye-to-eye contact.

Parents appreciate the support of a nurse during the initial visit with their infant, but they may also appreciate some time alone with the infant. It is important during the early visits to emphasize the positive aspects of their infant's behavior and development so that parents can focus on their infant as an individual rather than on the equipment that surrounds the child. For example, the nurse may describe the infant's spontaneous behaviors during care, such as grasp, sucking, and movement, or make comments about the infant's biologic functions. Most institutions have open visiting policies so that parents and siblings may visit as often as they wish.

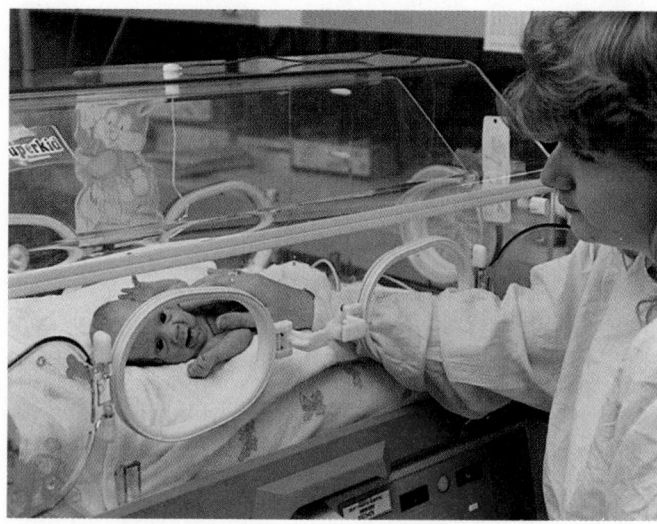

**Fig. 10-10** Encouraging interaction of mother and her premature infant in intensive care unit facilitates mother-infant attachment process.

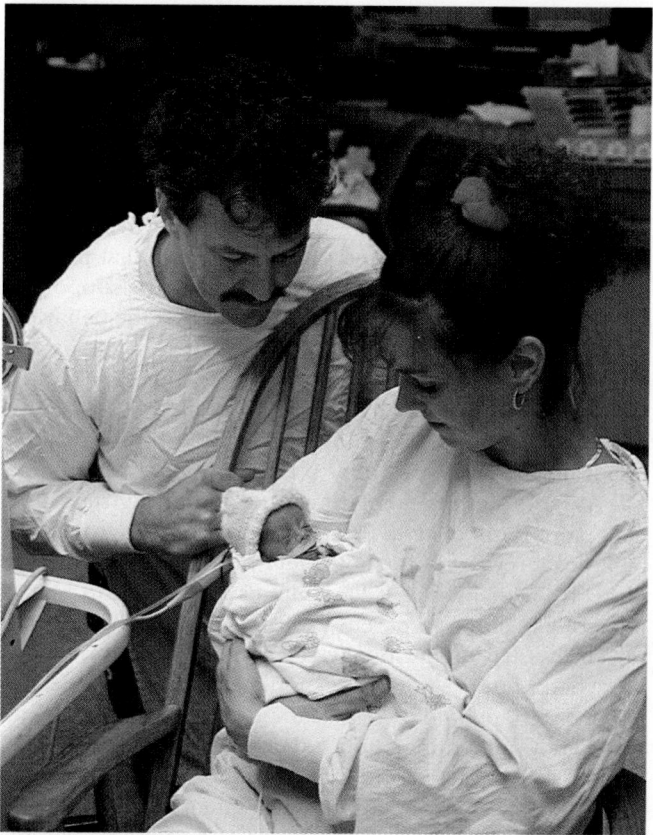

**Fig. 10-11** Mother and father visit their newborn infant.

Parents vary greatly in the degree to which they are able to interact with their infant. Some may wish to touch or hold their infant during the first visit, whereas others may not feel comfortable enough even to enter the nursery. These reactions depend on a variety of prenatal and postnatal factors, such as the parity of the mother and her preparation before birth; the size, condition, and physical appearance of the infant; and the type of treatment the infant is receiving. It is essential to recognize that the individualized pacing and quality of the interactions are more important than an early onset of these interactions. Parents may not be receptive to early and extended infant contact because they need time to adjust to the impact of an infant with birth problems and must be helped to grieve before acceptance of their infant can occur.

The parents' inability to focus on their infant is a clue for the nurse to assist the parents in expressing feelings of guilt, anxiety, helplessness, inadequacy, anger, and ambivalence. Nurses can help parents deal with these distressing feelings and recognize that they are normal responses shared by other parents. It is important to point out and reinforce the positive aspects of parents' behavior and interactions with their infant.

Most parents feel shaky and insecure about initiating interaction with their infant. Nurses can sense parents' level of readiness and offer encouragement in these initial efforts. Parents of premature infants follow the same acquaintance process as do parents of term infants. They may quickly proceed through the process or may require several days, or even weeks, to complete the process. Parents begin by touching their infant's extremities with their fingertips and poking the infant tenderly, and then proceed to caresses and fondling (Fig. 10-10). Touching is the first act of communication between parents and child. Parents need to be prepared for their infant's exaggerated and generalized startle responses to touch so that they will not interpret these as negative reactions to their overtures. It may be necessary to limit tactile stimuli when the infant is critically ill and labile, but the nurse can offer other options, such as speaking softly or sitting at the bedside.

Parents of acutely ill preterm infants may express feelings of helplessness and lack of control. Involving the parent in some type of caregiving activity, no matter how minor it may seem to the nurse, enables the parent to "take on" a more active role. Examples of such caregiving for the acutely ill infant who cannot be held and is seemingly not responding positively include moistening the infant's lips with a small amount of sterile water on a cotton-tipped swab or slipping the diaper from under the infant when it is wet or soiled.

Eventually parents begin to endow their infant with an identity—as part of the family. When an infant no longer appears as a foreign object and begins to take on aspects of family members, such as the father's chin or the sister's nose, nurses can facilitate this incorporation. Parents are encouraged to bring in clothes, a toy, a stuffed animal, or a family snapshot for their infant, and the nurse can help parents set goals for themselves and for the infant. Parents may become involved by reading a children's storybook or nursery rhymes in a soft, soothing voice. Some families tape record the parents' voices telling or reading stories and play the tapes when the infant is able to cope with such stimuli. Feeding schedules are discussed, and parents are encouraged to visit at times when they can become involved in the care of their infant (Fig. 10-11).

Throughout the parent-infant acquaintance process, the nurse listens carefully to what the parents say in order to assess their concerns and their progress toward incorporating their infant into their lives. The manner in which parents refer to their infant and the questions they ask reveal their worries and feelings and can serve as valuable clues to future relationships with the infant. The alert nurse is attuned to these subtle indications of parents' needs, which provide guidelines for nursing intervention. Often all that the parents need is reassurance that they will have the support of the nurse during caregiving activities and that the behaviors about which they are concerned are normal reactions and will disappear as the infant matures (e.g., an exaggerated Moro reflex or inability to coordinate swallowing).

Parents need guidance in their relationships with their infant and assistance in their efforts to meet their infant's physical and developmental needs. The nursing staff must help parents understand that their preterm infant offers few behavioral rewards and show them how to accept small rewards from their infant. The infant's reactions and behaviors are explained to parents, who take their infant's jerky, rejective behavior personally. They need reassurance that these behaviors are not a reflection on their parenting skills. Parents are taught to recognize their infant's cues regarding stimulation, handling, and other interaction, especially aversive behaviors that indicate a need for rest. Nurses need to include parents in planning their infant's care.

Above all, nurses must encourage and reinforce parents during their caregiving activities and interactions with their infant in order to promote healthy parent-child relationships. It is also helpful for the parents to have contact and communication with the infant's primary nurse and associate primary nurse. This decreases the amount of different information given to parents and often instills confidence that while the parents cannot be at their infant's bedside 24 hours a day, there are competent and caring nurses whom they may call to inquire about the infant's status. Periodic parent conferences involving the primary practitioner, primary nurse, and associate primary nurse serve to clarify misunderstandings or problems related to the infant's condition. Other members of the NICU team, such as the perinatal social worker or surgeon, may become involved as necessary.

**Siblings.** In the past, concerns about sibling visitation in the NICU focused on fears of infection and disruption of nursing routines. These fears have not been substantiated, and sibling visits should be a part of the normal operation of NICUs.

The birth of a preterm infant is a difficult time for siblings, who rely on the support of understanding parents. When the happy anticipation is changed to sadness, worry, and altered routines, siblings are bewildered and deprived of their parents' attention. They know something is wrong, but they have only a dim understanding of what it is. Concern about the negative effects on visiting siblings of seeing the ill newborn has not been confirmed. Children have not hesitated to approach or touch the infant, and children less than 5 years of age have been less reluctant than older children; in addition, there have been no measurable differences between previsit and postvisit behaviors.

The potential benefits of sibling visits must be weighed against exposure of the child to the environment of the NICU. Children must be prepared for the unfamiliar NICU atmosphere, but contact with the infant appears to have a positive effect on siblings by helping them to deal with the reality rather than the bizarre fantasies that are characteristic of young children. Such visits also help to bond the family as a unit.

**Support Groups.** Parents need to feel they are not alone. Parent support groups have been of immeasurable value to families of infants in the NICU. Some groups consist of parents who have infants in the hospital and share the same anxieties and concerns. Other groups include parents who have had infants in the NICU and who have dealt with the crisis effectively. The groups are usually under the leadership of a staff person and involve physicians, nurses, and social workers, but it is the parents who can offer other parents something that no one else can provide.

The **Family Support America** (formerly **Family Resource Coalition**)* is a North American network of family support programs designed to help families of preterm infants. An excellent resource for parents of preterm infants is the book by J. Zaichkin, *Newborn Intensive Care: What Every Parent Needs to Know* (1996).† This resource has technical and anecdotal information regarding different problems facing preterm infants, common treatments and therapies, preparation for home discharge, and home care for the preterm infant. Another resource for parents wanting more information about kangaroo care is by S.M. Ludington-Hoe, *Kangaroo Care: The Best You Can Do to Help Your Preterm Infant* (1993).‡

## Discharge Planning and Home Care

Parents become very apprehensive and excited as the time for discharge approaches. They have many concerns and insecurities regarding the care of their infant. They fear the child may still be in danger, that they will be unable to recognize signs of distress or illness in their infant, and that the infant may not yet be ready for discharge. Nurses need to begin early to assist parents in acquiring or increasing their skills in the care of their infant. Appropriate instruction must be provided and sufficient time allowed for the family to assimilate the information and learn the continuing special care requirements. Where rooming-in or other live-in arrangements are available, parents can stay for a few days and nights and assume the care of their infant under the supervision and support of the nursery staff.

There should be appropriate medical and nursing follow-up and referrals to services that can benefit the family, including developmental follow-up. Parents of preterm infants should also be given adequate information about immunizations with other discharge planning information. Home health agencies provide nursing supervision, counseling, and referrals for nursing visits. With the trend toward

---

*20 N Wacker Dr, Suite 1100, Chicago, IL 60606, (312) 338-0900; www.familysupportamerica.org.
†Available from NICU Ink, Petaluma, CA, (707) 762-2646 or (888) 642-8465; www.neonatalnetwork.com/nicuink/.
‡Available from Bantam/Random House, New York; www.randomhouse.com.

early discharge, many hospital-based home health care agencies become involved in the follow-up and care of the NICU "graduate" in the home. For the parents of an infant being discharged with equipment such as an oxygen tank, apnea monitor, or even a ventilator, discharge planning requires multidisciplinary collaborative practice to ensure that the family has not only the appropriate resources but also the available assistance for dealing with the infant's needs. Organized support groups are a part of many communities, including those discussed previously, those designed for parents of infants who require special care because of specific defects or disabilities, and those for parents of multiple births. (See Chapter 3.) Some manufacturers provide for the special needs of such infants. For example, premature size disposable diapers are available from the manufacturers of Pampers.*

Car seat safety is an essential aspect of discharge planning, and infants less than 37 weeks of gestation should have a period of observation in an appropriate car seat to monitor for possible apnea, bradycardia, and decreased $SaO_2$. Several models can be adapted for small infants with the placement of blanket rolls on each side of the infant to support the head and trunk. For adequate support without slumping, the seat back-to-crotch strap distance must be 14 cm (5½ inches) or less; a small rolled blanket may be placed between the crotch strap and the infant to reduce slouching. The distance from the lower harness strap to the seat bottom should be 10 inches or less to decrease the potential for the harness straps to cross the infant's ears (American Academy of Pediatrics, 1996). A car seat restraint without a shield is recommended and if the infant needs to be supine a crash-tested car bed may be used (American Academy of Pediatrics, 2002). The Centers for Disease Control and Prevention also recommends that infants less than 1 year old and weighing less than 20 pounds not be placed in rear-facing child-safety seats on the passenger side of cars with air bags because of the increased risk of injury when the air bag is inflated. Additional guidelines are available from the American Academy of Pediatrics (1996; 2002), including a video tape for the safe transportation of premature and LBW infants. (See Chapter 12 for a discussion of infant car restraints and AAP website: *www.aap.org* for a list of appropriate car seats for infants.)

An important part of discharge planning and care of the preterm infant is nutrition for continued growth, thus choice of feeding must be carefully addressed. Human milk should be fortified according to the infant's corrected age and physiologic needs. An enriched postdischarge formula (usually 22 cal/oz) is required for preterm infants born at less than 36 weeks to meet appropriate growth standards (Lucas and others, 2001; Carver and others, 2001). Term infant formulas are not considered adequate for proper growth in preterm infants. (See Table 8-6.)

The term *vulnerable child syndrome* is applied to physically healthy children who are perceived by their parents to be at high risk for medical or developmental problems. The syndrome has been observed in parents of children who have had an earlier illness or injury from which they had not been expected to recover. The family continues to perceive the child as fragile, vulnerable, "different," and as having needs that warrant special status in the family, which adversely affects the child's and family's behavior. The parents may lack confidence in their parenting ability that persists beyond the illness. The parents may also become overly indulgent and have difficulty setting limits, resulting in interference with normal development. Consequently, the child becomes dependent, demanding, and out of control. Overprotection and frequent visits to the health care provider are characteristic.

Problems that may arise in the high-risk newborn include overfeeding, underfeeding, feeding resistance, aversion to human touch or interaction, and difficulty separating the child from the parent. To help parents deal with the stress of home care for the infant, nurses can help families to discuss their fears and anxieties, which are exaggerated in parents of preterm infants, and encourage the family to create a normal routine in caring for the infant. Parents need to learn the normal developmental delays expected of premature infants and the importance of setting disciplinary limits and schedules. Continued explanations and clarification of the infant's true health status and ongoing support of the parents' efforts are important aspects of follow-up care.

## Neonatal Loss

The precarious nature of many high-risk infants makes death a very real and ever-present possibility. Although infant mortality has been reduced sharply with improved technology, the mortality rate is still greatest during the neonatal period. Nurses in the NICU are the persons who must prepare the parents for an inevitable death and facilitate a family's grieving process after an expected or unexpected death.

The loss of an infant has special meaning for the grieving parents. It represents a loss of a part of themselves (especially for mothers), a loss of the potential for immortality that offspring represent, and the loss of the dream child that has been fantasized throughout the pregnancy. There is a sense of emptiness and failure. In addition, when an infant has lived for such a short time, there may be few, if any, pleasant memories to serve as a basis for the identification and idealization that are part of the resolution of a loss.

To help parents understand that the death is a reality, it is important that they be encouraged to hold their infant before death and, if possible, be present at the time of death so that their infant can die in their arms if they choose. Many who deny the need to hold the infant later regret the decision.

Parents are given the opportunity to actually "parent" the infant in any manner they wish or are able to do before and after the death. This may include seeing, touching, holding, caressing, and talking to their infant privately; the parents may also wish to bathe and dress the infant. If parents are hesitant about seeing their dead infant, it is advisable to keep the body in the unit for a few hours, because many parents change their minds after the initial shock of the death.

---

*Procter & Gamble; to place order, phone toll-free (800) 543-4932; in Ohio: (800) 582-2623.

Parents may need to see and hold the infant more than once—the first time to say "hello" and the last time to say "good-bye." If parents wish to see the infant after the body has been taken to the morgue, the infant should be retrieved, wrapped in a blanket, rewarmed in a radiant warmer, and taken to the mother's room or other private place. The nurse should stay with the parents and provide them an opportunity for private time alone with their dead infant. Individual grief responses of the mother and father should be recognized and handled appropriately; gender differences and cultural and religious beliefs will affect the parents' grief responses (Wallerstedt and Higgins, 1996).

Some units have implemented a hospice approach for families with infants for whom the decision has been made not to prolong life and who are receiving only palliative care. A special "family" room is set aside and contains all supportive equipment needed for the care of the infant. It also provides a homelike atmosphere for the family. All hospice services are available to the family, and the infant remains under the care and supervision of a primary nurse on the NICU staff. (See Chapter 23 for further discussion of hospice care.)

A photograph of the infant taken before or after death is highly desirable. Parents may wish to have a special family portrait taken with the infant and other family members; this often helps personalize and make the experience more tangible. The parents may not wish to see the photograph at the time of death, but the chance to refer to it later will help to make their infant seem more real, which is a part of the normal grief process. A photograph of their infant being held by the hand or touched by an adult offers a more positive image than a morgue type of photograph. Many NICUs have a bereavement or memory packet made up for the grieving parents, which may include the infant's handprints and footprints, a lock of hair, the bedside name card and, as appropriate to the family's religious beliefs, a certificate of baptism. The photographs and other personal effects of the deceased infant were perceived as critically important in the grieving process by one group of parents in a recent survey. Parents often indicated that the photographs were helpful in the remembrance of the infant's actual appearance during this stressful period (Anderson, 2001). In some units special knitted clothing is made by hospital volunteer groups and donated for dressing the infant postmortem. Other tangible remembrances of the child can be provided, such as name tags, armbands, and locks of hair. Naming the deceased infant is an important step in the grieving process. Some parents may hesitate to give the newborn a name that had been chosen during the pregnancy for their special "baby." However, having a tangible person for whom to grieve is an important component of the grieving process.

A primary nurse who is familiar to the family should be present during the discussion about the dead or dying infant. An *RTS (Resolve Through Sharing)* or bereavement counselor is often involved in helping the family through this difficult period. The nurse should talk with parents openly and honestly about funeral arrangements because few of them have had experience with this aspect of death.

Many funeral homes now offer inexpensive arrangements for these special cases. Someone from the NICU should take the responsibility for acquiring this type of information. It is often helpful to parents for the NICU to have a list of local funeral homes, services offered, and a price for the service offered. Families need to be informed of the options available, but it is preferable to encourage a funeral because the ritual provides an opportunity for parents to feel the support of friends and relatives. A clergyman of the appropriate faith may be notified if the parents wish. Issues regarding an autopsy or organ donation (when appropriate) are approached in a multidisciplinary fashion (primary practitioner and primary nurse) with respect, tact, and consideration of the family's wishes. (See also Grief and Perinatal Loss in Merenstein and Gardner, 1998.)

Before the parents leave the hospital, they are given the telephone number of the unit (if they do not have it) and invited to call any time they have any further questions. Many intensive care units make it a point to contact the parents following a neonatal death to assess the parents' coping mechanisms, evaluate the grieving process, and provide support as needed. Several organizations are available to offer support and understanding to families who have lost a newborn, including **The Compassionate Friends**\* and **Aiding Mothers and Fathers Experiencing Neo-Natal Death (AMEND).**† (See Chapter 23 for further discussion of the family and the grief process.)

Nurses who care for critically ill infants also experience grief; NICU nurses may feel helpless and sorrowful. It is important that such grief be allowed and that nurses attend the funeral or memorial service as a part of working through the grief process. Nurses may fear that showing emotion is unprofessional and that the expression of grief is a "loss of control" issue; these fears are unfounded. Studies have demonstrated that to continue to be effective managers and providers of care, nurses must be allowed to grieve and support each other through the process (Downey and others, 1995).

**Baptism.** Many Christian parents wish to have their child baptized if death is anticipated or is a decided possibility. Whenever possible, it is most desirable that a representative of the parents' faith (e.g., a Roman Catholic priest or a Protestant minister) perform such a ritual. When death is imminent, a nurse or a physician can perform the baptism by simply pouring water on the infant's forehead (a medicine dropper is a convenient means) while repeating the words, "I baptize you in the name of the Father and of the Son and of the Holy Spirit." This includes a birth of any gestational age, particularly when the parents are of the Roman Catholic faith.

When the faith of the parents is uncertain, a conditional baptism can be carried out by saying, "If you are capable of receiving baptism, I baptize you in the name of the Father and of the Son and of the Holy Spirit." The fact of the baptism is recorded in the infant's chart, and a notice is placed

---

\*PO Box 3696, Oak Brook, IL 60522-3696, (630) 990-0010, (877) 969-0010; www.compassionatefriends.org.
†Contact Maureen Connelly, 4324 Berrywick Terrace, St Louis, MO 63128, (314) 487-7582.

on the crib or incubator. Parents are informed at the first opportunity.

## ✚ Evaluation

The effectiveness of nursing interventions is determined by continual reassessment and evaluation of care based on the following observational guidelines:

1. Take vital signs and perform respiratory assessments at time intervals based on infant's condition and needs; observe infant's respiratory efforts and response to therapy; check functioning of equipment; review laboratory test results.
2. Measure abdominal skin and axillary temperatures at specified intervals.
3. Observe infant's behavior and appearance for evidence of sepsis.

4. Assess for hydration; assess and measure fluid intake; observe infant during feeding; measure amount of formula or parenteral intake; weigh daily.
5. Observe infant's skin for signs of irritation and breakdown.
6. Observe infant for evidence of increased intracranial pressure or signs of IVH.
7. Observe infant's physiologic and behavioral response to pain and pain-relief interventions.
8. Observe infant's response to developmental care.
9. Observe parental interaction with infant; interview family regarding their feelings, concerns, and readiness for home care.
10. Assess family and observe their behaviors during and after the death of their infant.

The *expected outcomes* are listed in the Nursing Care Plan following on pp. 371-375.

# Nursing Care Plan
## The High-Risk Infant*

**NURSING DIAGNOSIS:** Ineffective breathing pattern related to pulmonary and neuromuscular immaturity, decreased energy, and fatigue

**PATIENT GOAL 1:** Will exhibit adequate oxygenation parameters (specify)

- **NURSING INTERVENTIONS/RATIONALES**

Position for optimum air exchange
　Place prone when feasible *because this position results in improved oxygenation, better-tolerated feedings, and more organized sleep-rest patterns*
　Place supine with neck slightly extended and nose pointing to ceiling in "sniffing" position *to prevent any narrowing of airway*
Avoid neck hyperextension *because it reduces diameter of trachea*
Observe for deviations from desired functioning; recognize signs of distress—grunting, cyanosis, nasal flaring, apnea
Suction *to remove accumulated mucus from nasopharynx, trachea, and endotracheal tube*
Suction only as necessary based on assessment (e.g., auscultation of chest, evidence of decreased oxygenation, increased infant irritability)
Never suction routinely *because it may cause bronchospasm, bradycardia caused by vagal nerve stimulation, hypoxia, and increased intracranial pressure (ICP), predisposing infant to intraventricular hemorrhage (IVH)*
Use proper suctioning technique *because improper suctioning can cause infection, airway damage, pneumothoraces, and IVH*
Use two-person suction technique *because assistant can provide immediate hyperoxygenation before and after catheter insertion*
†Carry out percussion, vibration, and postural drainage only as prescribed *to facilitate drainage of secretions*
Avoid using Trendelenburg position *because it can contribute to increased ICP and reduced lung capacity from gravity pushing organs against diaphragm*
During diaper changes, raise infant slightly under hips and not by raising feet and legs *to avoid elevation of intracranial pressure*
Use semiprone or side-lying position *to prevent aspiration in infant with excessive mucus or who is being fed*

Observe for signs of respiratory distress—nasal flaring, retractions, tachypnea, apnea, grunting, cyanosis, low oxygenation saturation ($SaO_2$)
Carry out regimen prescribed for supplemental oxygen therapy (maintain ambient $O_2$ concentration at minimum $FiO_2$ level based on arterial blood gases, $SaO_2$, and transcutaneous oxygen [$tcPO_2$])
Maintain neutral thermal environment *to conserve utilization of $O_2$*
Closely monitor blood gas measurements, $tcPO_2$ and $SaO_2$ readings *to prevent hypoxemia and acidemia*
Apply and manage monitoring equipment correctly (i.e., cardiac or oxygen)
Demonstrate understanding of function of respiratory support apparatus:
　Mechanical ventilation apparatus
　Insufflation bags with masks and endotracheal tube adaptor
　Oxygen hoods and tents
　Humidifier warmers
Observe and assess infant's response to ventilation and oxygenation therapy

- **EXPECTED OUTCOMES**

Airway remains patent
Breathing provides adequate oxygenation and $CO_2$ removal
Respiratory rate and pattern is within appropriate limits for age and weight (specify)
Arterial blood gases and acid-base balance are within normal limits for gestational age
Tissue oxygenation is adequate

**NURSING DIAGNOSIS:** Ineffective thermoregulation related to immature temperature control and decreased subcutaneous body fat

**PATIENT GOAL 1:** Will maintain stable body temperature

- **NURSING INTERVENTIONS/RATIONALES**

Place infant in incubator, radiant warmer, or warmly clothed in open crib *to maintain stable body temperature*
Monitor axillary temperature in unstable infants (use skin probe or air temperature control; check function of servocontrolled mechanism when used)

---

*Relates primarily to LBW infant with weight of 1500 to 2500 g.
†Dependent nursing action.

# Nursing Care Plan
## The High-Risk Infant—cont'd

**PATIENT GOAL 1—cont'd**

- **NURSING INTERVENTIONS/*RATIONALES*—cont'd**

Regulate servocontrolled unit or air temperature control as needed *to maintain skin temperature within accepted thermal range*

Use plastic heat shield as appropriate *to decrease heat and water losses*

Monitor for signs of hyperthermia—redness, flushing, diaphoresis (rarely)

Check temperature of infant in relation to ambient temperature and temperature of heating unit *to decrease radiant heat loss*

Avoid situations that might predispose infant to heat loss, such as exposure to cool air, drafts, bathing, cold scales, or cold mattress

Monitor serum glucose values *to ensure euglycemia*

- **EXPECTED OUTCOME**

Infant's body temperature remains within normal range for postconception age (specify)

> **NURSING DIAGNOSIS:** Risk for infection related to deficient immunologic defenses

**PATIENT GOAL 1:** Will exhibit no evidence of nosocomial infection

- **NURSING INTERVENTIONS/*RATIONALES***

Ensure that all caregivers wash hands before and after handling infant *to minimize exposure to infective organisms*

Ensure that all equipment in contact with infant is clean or sterile

Prevent personnel with upper respiratory tract or communicable infections from coming into direct contact with infant

Isolate other infants who have infections according to institutional policy

Instruct health care workers and parents in infection control procedures

†Administer antibiotics as ordered

Ensure strict asepsis with invasive procedures and equipment such as peripheral IV therapy, lumbar punctures, and arterial/venous catheter insertion

- **EXPECTED OUTCOME**

Infant exhibits no evidence of nosocomial infection

> **NURSING DIAGNOSIS:** Imbalanced nutrition: less than body requirements (risk) related to inability to ingest nutrients because of immaturity and/or illness

**PATIENT GOAL 1:** Will receive adequate nourishment, with caloric intake to maintain positive nitrogen balance and exhibit appropriate weight gain

- **NURSING INTERVENTIONS/*RATIONALES***

†Maintain parenteral fluid or total parenteral nutrition therapy as ordered

Monitor for signs of intolerance to total parenteral therapy, especially protein and glucose

Assess readiness to nipple feed, especially ability to coordinate swallowing and breathing

Nipple feed infant if strong sucking, swallowing, and gag reflexes are present (usually at gestational age of 34 to 35 weeks) *to minimize risk of aspiration*

Follow unit protocol for advancing volume and concentration of formula *to avoid feeding intolerance*

Use orogastric feeding if infant tires easily or has weak sucking, gag, or swallowing reflexes *because nipple feeding may result in weight loss*

Assist mother with expressing breast milk *to establish and maintain lactation until infant can breast-feed*

Assist mother with breast-feeding when feasible and desirable

- **EXPECTED OUTCOMES**

Infant receives an adequate amount of calories and essential nutrients

Infant demonstrates a steady weight gain (approximately 20 to 30 g/day) once past acute phase of illness

> **NURSING DIAGNOSIS:** Risk for fluid volume deficit or excess related to immature physiologic characteristics of preterm infant and/or illness

**PATIENT GOAL 1:** Will exhibit adequate hydration status

- **NURSING INTERVENTIONS/*RATIONALES***

Monitor fluid and electrolytes closely with therapies that increase insensible water loss (IWL) (e.g., phototherapy, radiant warmer)

Implement strategies to minimize IWL such as plastic covering, increased ambient humidity, emollient application

Ensure adequate parenteral/oral fluid intake

Assess state of hydration (e.g., skin turgor, blood pressure, edema, weight, mucous membranes, urine specific gravity, electrolytes, fontanel)

Regulate parenteral fluids closely *to avoid dehydration, overhydration, or extravasation*

Avoid administering hypertonic fluids (e.g., undiluted medications, concentrated glucose infusions) in peripheral veins *to prevent excess solute load on immature kidneys and fragile veins*

Monitor urinary output and laboratory values *for evidence of dehydration or overhydration* (adequate urinary output 1-2 ml/kg/hr)

Minimize use of adhesives and antiseptic agents *to preserve intact skin barrier*

- **EXPECTED OUTCOME**

Infant exhibits evidence of fluid homeostasis

> **NURSING DIAGNOSIS:** Risk for impaired skin integrity related to immature skin structure, immobility, decreased nutritional state, invasive procedures

**PATIENT GOAL 1:** Will maintain skin integrity

- **NURSING INTERVENTIONS/*RATIONALES***

See Guidelines box on neonatal skin care, p. 350-351

---

†Dependent nursing action.

# Nursing Care Plan
## The High-Risk Infant—cont'd

- **EXPECTED OUTCOME**

Skin remains clean and intact with no evidence of irritation or injury

> **NURSING DIAGNOSIS:** Risk for injury from variable cerebral blood flow, systemic hypertension or hypotension, and decreased cellular nutrients (glucose and oxygen) related to immature central nervous system and physiologic stress response

**PATIENT GOAL 1:** Will receive care to prevent injury and maintain appropriate systemic and cerebral blood flow, as well as adequate cerebral glucose and oxygen; will not exhibit evidence of IVH (unless preexisting condition)

- **NURSING INTERVENTIONS/**_RATIONALES_

Decrease environmental stimulation *because stress responses, especially increased blood pressure, increase risk of elevated ICP*

Establish a routine that provides for undisturbed sleep/rest periods *to eliminate or minimize times of stress*

Use minimal handling and handle or disturb infant only when absolutely necessary (see Therapeutic Handling, p. 361)

Keep extra diapers under buttocks to facilitate changing soiled diapers; raise infant's hips, not feet and legs

Organize (cluster) care during normal waking hours as much as possible *to minimize sleep disruption and frequent intermittent noise*

Close and open drapes and dim lights *to allow for day/night schedule*

Cover incubator with cloth and place "do not disturb" sign nearby *to decrease light and alert others to infant's rest period*

Refrain from loud talking or laughing

Limit number of visitors and staff near infant at one time

Explain meaning of unfamiliar sounds to family

Keep equipment noise to minimum:

    Turn alarms as low as safely possible

    Attend to alarms and telephones immediately

    Place bedside equipment, such as ventilator or IV pump, away from head of bed

    Turn outflow valve from ventilator away from infant's ear

    Perform treatments requiring equipment at one time

    Turn off bedside equipment that is not in use, such as suction and oxygen

    Avoid loud, abrupt noises, such as discarding items in trash can, dropping items, placing items on top of incubator, closing doors and drawers, heavy traffic

    Turn off any radios or televisions

    May place soft earmuffs on infant for loud procedures (see Auditory Environment, p. 363)

Assess and manage pain using pharmacologic and nonpharmacologic methods *because pain increases blood pressure*

Recognize signs of physical stress and overstimulation *to institute appropriate interventions promptly*

Avoid hypertonic medications and solutions *because they increase cerebral blood flow*

Elevate head of bed or mattress between 15 and 20 degrees *to decrease ICP*

Maintain adequate oxygenation *because hypoxia increases cerebral blood flow and ICP* (see interventions under nursing diagnosis of ineffective breathing pattern on p. 371)

Avoid any sudden turning of head to side, *which restricts carotid artery blood flow and adequate oxygenation to brain*

- **EXPECTED OUTCOME**

Infant exhibits no evidence of increased ICP or IVH

> **NURSING DIAGNOSIS:** Pain related to procedures, diagnosis, treatment, handling

**PATIENT GOAL 1:** Will experience no pain or a reduction of pain

- **NURSING INTERVENTIONS/**_RATIONALES_

Recognize that infants, regardless of gestational age, feel pain

Assess for pain using a clinically appropriate neonatal pain assessment tool (see Table 10-3)

†Administer analgesics as prescribed, advocate for effective pain control

Use nonpharmacologic pain measures appropriate to infant's age and condition: repositioning, swaddling, containment, cuddling, rocking, music, reducing environmental stimulation, tactile comfort measures (stroking, patting), oral sucrose, and nonnutritive sucking

Assess effectiveness of nonpharmacologic pain measures *because some measures (e.g., stroking) may increase premature infant's distress*

Encourage parents to provide comfort measures when possible

Convey an attitude of sensitivity and compassion for infant's discomfort

Discuss with family their concerns about infant's pain

Encourage family to speak with health practitioner about their concerns

- **EXPECTED OUTCOME**

Infant exhibits no or minimal signs of pain

> **NURSING DIAGNOSIS:** Delayed growth and development related to preterm birth, unnatural NICU environment, separation from parents

**PATIENT GOAL 1:** Will attain normal growth and development potential

- **NURSING INTERVENTIONS/**_RATIONALES_

Provide optimum nutrition *to ensure steady weight gain and brain growth*

Provide regular periods of undisturbed rest *to decrease unnecessary $O_2$ use and caloric expenditure*

Provide age-appropriate developmental intervention, including positioning

Recognize signs of overstimulation (flaccidity, yawning, staring, active averting, irritability, crying) *so that infant is allowed to rest* (see Table 10-4)

---

†Dependent nursing action.

*Continued*

## *Nursing Care Plan*
## The High-Risk Infant—cont'd

**PATIENT GOAL 1—cont'd**

• **NURSING INTERVENTIONS**/*RATIONALES*—cont'd

Promote parent-infant interaction *because it is essential for normal growth and development*

Promote self-regulating behaviors (e.g., midline, flexed extremities, hands to mouth, and "nesting") (see Table 10-4)

• **EXPECTED OUTCOMES**

Infant exhibits a steady weight gain once past the acute phase of illness

Infant is exposed only to appropriate stimuli

Infant demonstrates quiet alert state interspersed with uninterrupted sleep periods

> **NURSING DIAGNOSIS:** Interrupted family processes related to situational/maturational crisis, knowledge deficit (birth of a preterm and/or ill infant), interruption of parental attachment process

**PATIENT (FAMILY) GOAL 1:** Will be informed of infant's progress

• **NURSING INTERVENTIONS**/*RATIONALES*

Prioritize information *to help parents understand most important aspects of care, signs of improvement, or deterioration in infant's condition*

Encourage parents to ask questions about child's status

Answer questions, facilitate expression of concern regarding care and prognosis

Be honest; respond to questions with correct answers *to establish trust*

Encourage mother and father to visit and/or call unit often *so they are informed of infant's progress*

Emphasize positive aspects of infant's status *to encourage sense of hope*

• **EXPECTED OUTCOME**

Parents express feelings and concerns regarding infant and prognosis and demonstrate understanding and involvement in care

**PATIENT (FAMILY) GOAL 2:** Will exhibit positive attachment behaviors

• **NURSING INTERVENTIONS**/*RATIONALES*

Encourage parents to visit as soon as possible *so that attachment process is initiated*

Encourage parents to:
Visit infant frequently
Touch, hold, and caress infant as appropriate for infant's physical condition
Become actively involved in infant's care
Bring clothing to dress infant as soon as condition permits

Reinforce parents' endeavors *to increase their self-confidence*

Be alert to signs of tension and stress in parents

Enable parents to spend time alone with infant

Help parents interpret infant's responses; comment regarding any positive response and signs of overstimulation or fatigue

Help parents by demonstrating infant care techniques and offering support

Identify resources (e.g., transportation, child care) *to enable parents to visit*

• **EXPECTED OUTCOMES**

Parents visit infant soon after birth and at frequent intervals

Parents relate positively with infant (e.g., call infant by name, look at and touch infant)

Parents provide care for infant and demonstrate an attitude of comfort in relationships with infant

Parents identify signs of stress or fatigue in infant

**PATIENT (SIBLINGS) GOAL 3:** Will exhibit positive attachment behaviors

• **NURSING INTERVENTIONS**/*RATIONALES*

Encourage siblings to visit infants when feasible

Explain environment, events, appearance of infant, and why infant cannot come home *to prepare them for visiting*

Provide photos of infant or other items if siblings are unable to visit

Encourage siblings to make pictures or bring other small items, such as a letter or drawing, for infant and place in incubator or crib

• **EXPECTED OUTCOMES**

Siblings visit infant in NICU or nursery

Siblings exhibit an understanding of explanations (specify)

Siblings receive infant-related items (specify)

---

# HIGH-RISK CONDITIONS RELATED TO DYSMATURITY

## Preterm Infants

Prematurity accounts for the largest number of admissions to an NICU. The immaturity places infants at risk for not only neonatal complications (e.g., hyperbilirubinemia and respiratory distress syndrome, which is highest in the preterm infant) but also for other high-risk factors (e.g., congenital anomalies in association with prematurity).

### Etiology

Most of the aspects concerning high-risk neonates are related to prematurity; however, the actual cause of prematurity is not known in most instances. The incidence of prematurity is lowest in the middle to high socioeconomic classes, in which pregnant women are generally in good health, are well nourished, and receive prompt and comprehensive prenatal care. The incidence is highest in the lower socioeconomic classes, in which a combination of deleterious circumstances is present. Other factors, such

## Nursing Care Plan
### The High-Risk Infant—cont'd

**PATIENT (FAMILY) GOAL 4:** Will be prepared for home care

- **NURSING INTERVENTIONS/*RATIONALES***

Assess readiness of family (especially mother or other primary caregiver) to care for infant in home setting *to facilitate parents' transition to home with infant*

Teach necessary infant care techniques and observations

Encourage parent(s), when possible, to spend one or two nights in a hospital predischarge room before discharge with infant *to foster confidence in caring for infant at home*

Reinforce follow-up medical care

Refer to appropriate agencies or services *so that needed assistance is provided*

Encourage and facilitate involvement with parent support group or refer to appropriate support group(s) *for ongoing support*

Offer family opportunity to learn infant cardiopulmonary resuscitation and response to choking incident

- **EXPECTED OUTCOMES**

Family demonstrates ability to provide care for infant

Family members state how and when to contact available services

Family members recognize importance of follow-up medical care

---

**NURSING DIAGNOSIS:** Anticipatory grieving related to unexpected birth of high-risk infant, grave prognosis, and/or death of infant

---

**PATIENT (FAMILY) GOAL 1:** Will acknowledge possibility of child's death and demonstrate healthy grieving behaviors

- **NURSING INTERVENTIONS/*RATIONALES***

Provide family with the opportunity to hold their infant before death and, if possible, to be present at the time of death

Support family's decision for terminating life support

Arrange for or perform appropriate baptism rite for infant

Provide family with the opportunity to see, touch, hold, bathe, caress, examine, and talk to their infant privately before and after death

Keep infant's body available for a few hours *to give family members who are hesitant an opportunity to see deceased infant if they change their minds;* rewarm as necessary

Provide photographs taken before and after infant's death for family *to refer to at a later time to make infant real*

Take photograph of infant being held or touched by an adult; avoid morgue-type photograph *because it depersonalizes child*

Dress infant in an appropriate dress or suit *to personalize child*

Provide other tangible remembrances of the child (e.g., name tags, identification band, lock of hair, footprints, blanket)

Encourage family to name infant if they have not done so

Identify resources to assist with funeral arrangements *to facilitate parental grieving*

- **EXPECTED OUTCOME**

Family discusses the reality of the death and conveys an attitude of realization

**PATIENT (FAMILY) GOAL 2:** Will receive adequate emotional and physical support

- **NURSING INTERVENTIONS/*RATIONALES***

Be available to family *to provide support*

Provide appropriate religious spiritual support (e.g., clergy)

Discuss infant's illness and death with family

Talk with family openly and honestly about funeral arrangements

Have information available regarding inexpensive services in the community

Inform family of all options available *so that they can make informed decisions*

Provide opportunity for family to call the unit if they have any questions regarding infant's illness and death

May contact family after the death *to assess coping and status of grieving process*

Refer family to appropriate support group(s) *for ongoing support*

- **EXPECTED OUTCOMES**

Family grieves for infant's death appropriately

Family demonstrates appropriate (influenced by cultural, religious, and social factors) grieving behaviors over infant's death

---

as multiple pregnancies, pregnancy-induced hypertension, and placental problems that interrupt the normal course of gestation before completion of fetal development, are responsible for a large number of preterm births.

The outlook for preterm infants is largely, but not entirely, related to the state of physiologic and anatomic immaturity of the various organs and systems at the time of birth. Infants at term have advanced to a state of maturity sufficient to allow a successful transition to the extrauterine

environment. Infants born prematurely must make the same adjustments but with functional immaturity proportional to the stage of development reached at the time of birth. The degree to which infants are prepared for extrauterine life can be predicted to some extent by estimated gestational age. (See Clinical Assessment of Gestational Age, Chapter 8.) An understanding of prenatal development provides some concept of the status of the systems, at various stages of development, that must cope with functional changes that occur with birth.

## Characteristics

Preterm infants have a number of distinct characteristics at various stages of development. Identification of these characteristics provides valuable clues to the gestational age and hence to the physiologic capabilities of infants. The general, outward physical appearance changes as the fetus progresses to maturity. Characteristics of skin, general attitude (or posture) when supine, appearance of hair, and amount of subcutaneous fat provide cues to a newborn's physical development. Observation of spontaneous, active movements and response to stimulation and passive movement contribute to the assessment of neurologic status. The appraisal is made as soon as possible after admission to the nursery because much of the observation and management of infants depends on this information.

On inspection, preterm infants are very small and appear scrawny because they lack or have only minimal subcutaneous fat deposits and have a proportionately large head in relation to the body, which reflects the cephalocaudal direction of growth. The skin is bright pink (often translucent, depending on the degree of immaturity), smooth, and shiny (may be edematous), with small blood vessels clearly visible underneath the thin epidermis. The fine lanugo hair is abundant over the body (depending on gestational age) but is sparse, fine, and fuzzy on the head. The ear cartilage is soft and pliable, and the soles and palms have minimal creases, resulting in a smooth appearance. The bones of the skull and the ribs feel soft, and the eyes may be closed. Male infants have few scrotal rugae, and the testes are undescended; the labia and clitoris are prominent in females. Fig. 10-12 compares the features of full-term and preterm infants.

In contrast to full-term infants' overall attitude of flexion and continuous activity, preterm infants are inactive and listless. The extremities maintain an attitude of extension and remain in any position in which they are placed. Reflex activity is only partially developed—sucking is absent, weak, or ineffectual; swallow, gag, and cough reflexes are absent or weak; and other neurologic signs are absent or diminished. Physiologically immature, many preterm infants are unable to maintain body temperature, have limited ability to excrete solutes in the urine, and have increased susceptibility to infection. A pliable thorax, immature lung tissue, and an immature regulatory center lead to periodic breathing, hypoventilation, and frequent periods of apnea. They are more susceptible to biochemical alterations such as hyperbilirubinemia and hypoglycemia (see Chapter 9), and they have a higher extracellular water content that renders them more vulnerable to fluid and electrolyte derangements. Preterm infants exchange fully half of their extracellular fluid volume every 24 hours compared with one seventh of the volume in adults.

The soft cranium is subject to characteristic unintentional deformation, or "preemie head," caused by positioning from one side to the other on a mattress. The head looks disproportionately longer from front to back, is flattened on both sides, and lacks the usual convexity seen at the temporal and parietal areas. This positional molding is often a concern to parents and may influence the parents' perception of the infant's attractiveness and their responsiveness to the infant. Frequent repositioning of the infant and positioning on a waterbed or gel mattress can reduce or minimize cranial molding.

## Therapeutic Management

When delivery of a preterm infant is anticipated, the intensive care nursery is alerted and a team approach implemented. Ideally, a neonatologist, an advanced practice nurse, a staff nurse, and a respiratory therapist are present for the delivery. Infants who do not require resuscitation are immediately transferred in a heated incubator to the NICU, where they are weighed and where intravenous lines, oxygen therapy, and other therapeutic interventions are initiated as needed. Resuscitation is conducted in the delivery area until infants can be safely transported to the NICU. Ongoing care is described elsewhere in the chapter and is not repeated in this section.

## Nursing Considerations

As with therapeutic management, nursing care is individualized for each infant. See appropriate discussions under Nursing Care of High-Risk Newborns for details of care.

# Postmature Infants

Infants born of a gestation that extends beyond 42 weeks as calculated from the mother's last menstrual period (or by gestational age assessment) are considered to be postmature, or postterm, regardless of birth weight. This constitutes 3.5% to 15% of all pregnancies. The cause of delayed birth is unknown. Some infants are appropriate for gestational age but show the characteristics of progressive placental dysfunction. These infants, often called postmature infants, display the characteristics of infants who are 1 to 3 weeks of age, such as absence of lanugo, little if any vernix caseosa, abundant scalp hair, and long fingernails. The skin is often cracked, parchmentlike, and desquamating. A common finding in postmature infants is a wasted physical appearance that reflects intrauterine deprivation. Depletion of subcutaneous fat gives them a thin, elongated appearance. The little vernix caseosa that remains in the skin-folds may be stained a deep yellow or green, which is usually an indication of meconium in the amniotic fluid.

There is a significant increase in fetal and neonatal mortality in postterm infants as compared with those born at term. They are especially prone to fetal distress associated with the decreasing efficiency of the placenta, macrosomia, congenital anomalies, and meconium aspiration syndrome. The greatest risk occurs during the stresses of labor and delivery, particularly in infants of *primigravidas,* or women delivering their first child. Cesarean section or induction of labor is usually recommended when infants are significantly overdue.

# HIGH RISK RELATED TO DISTURBED RESPIRATORY FUNCTION

## Apnea of Prematurity (AOP)

AOP is a common phenomenon in the preterm infant. Rarely observed in full-term infants, the prevalence of apneic spells increases the younger the gestational age. Ap-

**CLINICAL EVALUATION**

|  PRETERM | TERM |

**Posture**—The preterm infant lies in a "relaxed attitude," limbs more extended; the body size is small, and the head may appear somewhat larger in proportion to the body size. The term infant has more subcutaneous fat tissue and rests in a more flexed attitude.

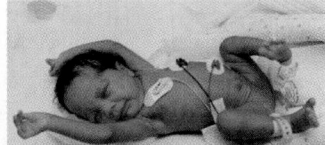 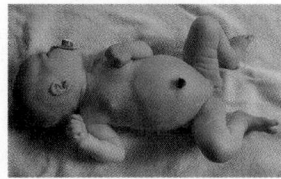

**Ear**—The preterm infant's ear cartilages are poorly developed, and the ear may fold easily; the hair is fine and feathery, and lanugo may cover the back and face. The mature infant's ear cartilages are well formed, and the hair is more likely to form firm, separate strands.

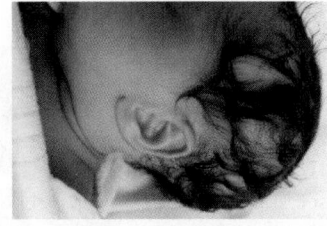 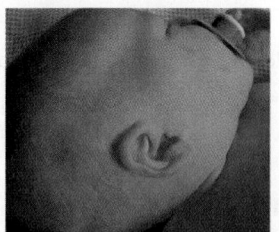

**Sole**—The sole of the foot of the preterm infant appears more turgid and may have only fine wrinkles. The mature infant's sole (foot) is well and deeply creased.

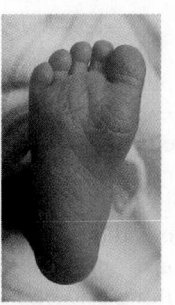 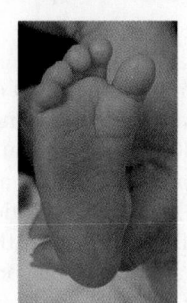

**Female genitalia**—The preterm female infant's clitoris is prominent, and labia majora are poorly developed and gaping. The mature female infant's labia majora are fully developed, and the clitoris is not as prominent.

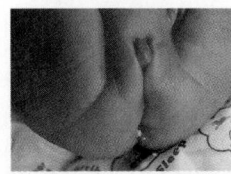 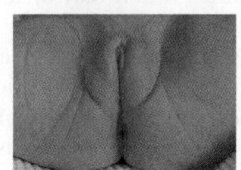

**Male genitalia**—The preterm male infant's scrotum is undeveloped and not pendulous; minimal rugae are present, and the testes may be in the inguinal canals or in the abdominal cavity. The term male infant's scrotum is well developed, pendulous, and rugated, and the testes are well down in the scrotal sac.

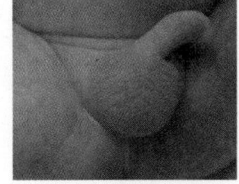 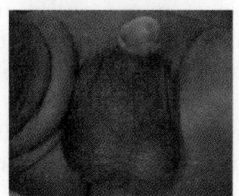

**Scarf sign**—The preterm infant's elbow may be easily brought across the chest with little or no resistance. The mature infant's elbow may be brought to the midline of the chest, resisting attempts to bring the elbow past the midline.

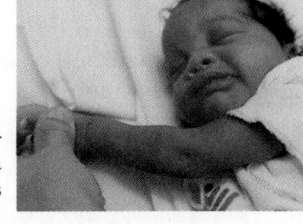 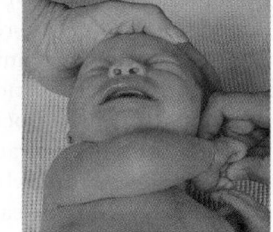

**Fig. 10-12**  Clinical and neurologic examinations comparing preterm and full-term infants. (Data from Pierog SH, Ferrara A: *Medical care of the sick newborn,* ed 2, St Louis, 1976, Mosby; photos courtesy Paul Vincent Kuntz, Texas Children's Hospital.)

*Continued*

**NEUROLOGIC EVALUATION**

PRETERM                                                    TERM

Grasp reflex—The preterm infant's grasp is weak; the term infant's grasp is strong, allowing the infant to be lifted up from the mattress.

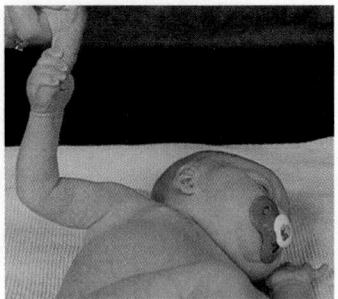

Heel-to-ear maneuver—The preterm infant's heel is easily brought to the ear, meeting with no resistance. This maneuver is not possible in the term infant, since there is considerable resistance at the knee.

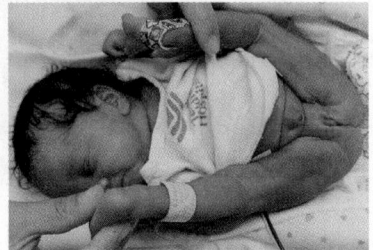
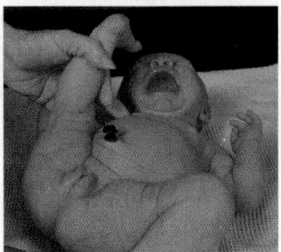

**Fig. 10-12—cont'd** For legend, see p. 377. (Data from Pierog SH, Ferrara A: *Medical care of the sick newborn,* ed 2, St Louis, 1976, Mosby; photos courtesy Paul Vincent Kuntz, Texas Children's Hospital.)

proximately one third of infants less than 32 weeks of gestation and more than one half apparently healthy infants less than 30 weeks of gestation have apneic spells. Characteristically, preterm infants are periodic breathers; they have periods of rapid respiration separated by periods of very slow breathing, and often there are short periods during which there are no visible or audible respirations. Apnea is primarily an extension of this periodic breathing and can be defined as a lapse of spontaneous breathing for 20 or more seconds, which may or may not be followed by bradycardia and color change.

AOP may be further classified according to origin. The three recognized classifications are as follows: (1) *central apnea*—absence of diaphragmatic and other respiratory muscle function that causes a lack of respiratory effort and occurs when the CNS does not transmit signals to the respiratory muscles; (2) *obstructive apnea*—air flow ceases because of upper airway onstruction, yet chest and/or abdominal wall movement is present; (3) *mixed apnea*—a combination of central and obstructive apnea, representing the most common form of apnea seen in preterm infants (Theobald and others, 2000). AOP should not be confused with apnea of infancy. (See Chapter 13.)

### Pathophysiology

Although the cause of AOP is unknown, it probably reflects the immature and poorly refined neurologic and chemical respiratory control mechanisms. These infants are not as responsive to hypercarbia and hypoxemia, and their neurons have fewer dendritic associations than those of the more mature infant. The respiratory reflexes of these infants are significantly less mature, which may be a contributing factor in the etiology. Overall weakness of the muscles of the tho-

rax, diaphragm, and upper airway may also contribute to apneic episodes in the preterm infant. In addition, apnea is characteristically observed during periods of REM sleep.

### Clinical Manifestations

A number of factors that appear to promote the incidence of apnea in preterm neonates can be treated. Apnea can be anticipated in infants with any of a variety of circumstances (Box 10-10); conversely, one of these disorders may be suspected in infants with persistent apneic spells. Although apnea is an expected event in preterm neonates, it should not be designated as such until all other causes have been ruled out. The observation of apnea is a reason to screen for any of the causes listed in Box 10-10.

### Therapeutic Management

It has been found that administration of methylxanthines (aminophylline, theophylline, or caffeine) is often effective in reducing the frequency of primary apnea-bradycardia spells in newborns. Theophylline and caffeine act as CNS stimulants to breathing. Neonates who receive these drugs have their serum drug levels measured regularly and must be closely observed for symptoms of toxicity. Serum drug levels are determined by the infant's weight, gestational age, and postnatal age and are maintained within a therapeutic range such as 6 to 13 $\mu$g/ml (Bhatt-Mehta and others, 1996). Caffeine has come to the forefront of pharmacologic therapy for AOP because it has fewer side effects than theophylline, requires dosing once daily, has more predictable plasma concentrations, has slower elimination, and has a wider therapeutic range (trough, 5-20 $\mu$g/ml). Cafcit (caffeine citrate) (Roxane Laboratories, Columbus, OH) has been approved for use in preterm infants with AOP; it is

## Box 10-10 ■ ■ ■
### Possible Causes of Apnea of Prematurity

Prematurity
Airway obstruction with mucus or milk, or poor positioning
Anemia, polycythemia
Dehydration
Cooling or overheating
Hypoxemia
Hypercapnia or hypocapnia
Hypoglycemia
Hypocalcemia
Hyponatremia
Sepsis, meningitis
Seizures
Increased vagal tone (in response to suctioning nasopharynx, gavage tube insertion, reflux of gastric contents, endotracheal intubation)
CNS depression from pharmacologic agents
Intraventricular hemorrhage (IVH)
Patent ductus arteriosus, congestive heart failure
Depression following maternal obstetric sedation
Infants with respiratory distress, pneumonia, inborn errors of metabolism such as hyperammonemia, congenital defects of the upper airways

available in injectable and oral form. Because theophylline is metabolized into caffeine, serum levels of both drugs should be routinely monitored to prevent toxicity. Urine intake and output should be closely monitored because both caffeine and theophylline act as mild diuretics.

> **NURSING ALERT**
> Signs of theophylline or caffeine toxicity are tachycardia (rate greater than 180 to 190 beats/min) at rest, vomiting, irritability, restlessness, diuresis, dysrhythmias, jitteriness, and gastritis (hemorrhagic).

### Nursing Considerations

Management of apnea consists of monitoring respiration and heart rate routinely in all preterm infants and preventing contributing conditions. Mechanical apnea monitors provide a means of alerting the staff to cessation of respiration according to a preset delay time—usually 15 to 20 seconds. Effective monitoring devices do not make alert nursing observation unnecessary. Any mechanical device is subject to malfunction. Without close observation, even of monitored infants, many unidentified episodes of prolonged apnea and severe bradycardia may occur. Nursing observation combined with monitoring is the most effective means of identifying neonatal apnea.

> **NURSING ALERT**
> When the alarm sounds, infants are first assessed for color and for presence of respiration. If they display the usual color and respirations, the nurse should investigate possible causes of a false alarm, such as faulty lead placement, detached or disconnected leads, improper alarm setting, or mechanical failure.

If begun early, gentle tactile stimulation (e.g., rubbing the back or chest gently, turning the infant to a supine position) will stop most apneic spells. If tactile stimulation fails to reinstitute respiration, the nose and oropharynx are suctioned and flow-by 100% oxygen is administered; if breathing does not begin, the chin is raised gently to open the airway, and sufficient pressure is applied with a resuscitation mask and bag to lift the rib cage. The infant is never shaken. After breathing is restored, the infant is assessed for possible precipitating factors, such as temperature, abdominal distention (if not observed earlier), and oxygen content (if any) being delivered before the episode. The use of pulse oximetry has helped in the detection of the onset of an apneic episode. It is important that nurses document episodes of apnea. A careful record is maintained regarding the number of apneic spells, the appearance of the infant during and after attacks, and whether the infant self-recovers or whether tactile stimulation or other measures are needed to restore breathing. Persistent and repeated periods of apnea may be treated by mechanical ventilation or CPAP.

Subsequent investigation into the possible cause of the apneic episode is vital to the care of the preterm infant because it may be a signal of an underlying condition such as sepsis or IVH. Bradycardia may occur with apnea because there is decreased delivery of oxygen to the myocardium.

Various methods devised to provide an intermittent stimulus for breathing, such as oscillating beds and water beds, have achieved variable success in the treatment of AOP.

## Respiratory Distress Syndrome (RDS)

Respiratory distress is a name applied to respiratory dysfunction in neonates and is primarily a disease related to developmental delay in lung maturation. The terms *respiratory distress syndrome* and *hyaline membrane disease (HMD)* are most often applied to this severe lung disorder, which is not only responsible for more infant deaths than any other disease but also carries the highest risk in terms of long-term respiratory and neurologic complications. (See Chapter 32 for a discussion of adult RDS.) It is seen almost exclusively in preterm infants. The disorder is rare in drug-exposed infants or infants who have been subjected to chronic intrauterine stress (e.g., maternal preeclampsia or hypertension). Respiratory distress of a nonpulmonary origin in neonates may also be caused by sepsis, cardiac defects (structural or functional), exposure to cold, airway obstruction (atresia), IVH, hypoglycemia, metabolic acidosis, acute blood loss, and drugs. Pneumonia in the neonatal period is respiratory distress caused by bacterial or viral agents and may occur alone or as a complication of RDS.

### Pathophysiology

Preterm infants are born before the lungs are fully prepared to serve as efficient organs for gas exchange. This appears to be a critical factor in the development of RDS. Although the precise cause is still undetermined, several features in the development of the disorder have been established, and there are a number of interdependent relationships that complicate the situation.

There is evidence of fetal respiratory activity before birth. The lungs make respiratory movements, and fluid is excreted through the alveoli. Because the final unfolding of

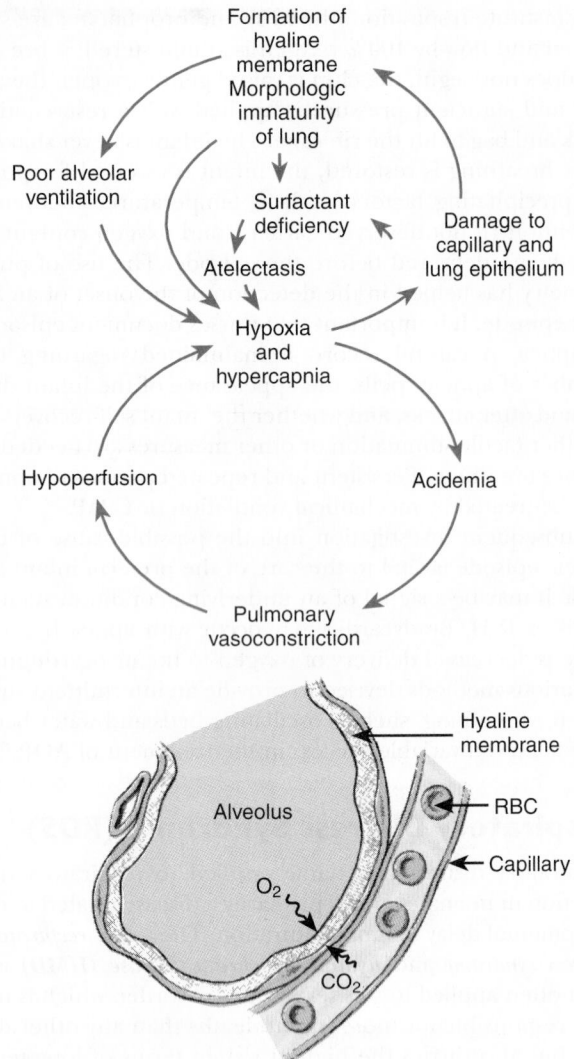

**Fig. 10-13** Interdependent relationship of factors involved in pathology of respiratory distress syndrome. (From Pierog SH, Ferrara A: *Medical care of the sick newborn*, ed 2, St Louis, 1976, Mosby.)

the alveolar septa, which increases the surface area of the lungs, occurs during the last trimester of pregnancy, premature infants are born with numerous underdeveloped and many uninflatable alveoli. There is limited pulmonary blood flow, which results from the collapsed state of the fetal lungs—from poor vascular development in general and an immature capillary network in particular. Because of increased pulmonary vascular resistance, the major portion of fetal blood is shunted from the lungs by way of the ductus arteriosus and foramen ovale. (See Cardiac Development and Function, Chapter 34.)

At birth, infants must initiate breathing and keep the previously fluid-filled lungs inflated with air. At the same time, the pulmonary capillary blood flow must be increased approximately tenfold to provide for adequate lung perfusion and to alter the intracardiac pressure that closes the fetal cardiac structures. Most full-term infants successfully accomplish these adjustments, but preterm infants with respiratory distress are unable to do so. Although numerous factors are involved, most authorities believe that the central factor responsible for this adaptation is normal development of the surfactant system.

*Surfactant* is a surface-active phospholipid secreted by the alveolar epithelium. Acting much like a detergent, this substance reduces the surface tension of fluids that line the alveoli and respiratory passages, resulting in uniform expansion and maintenance of lung expansion at low intraalveolar pressure. Immature development of these functions produces consequences that seriously compromise respiratory efficiency. Deficient surfactant production causes unequal inflation of alveoli on inspiration and the collapse of alveoli on end expiration. Without surfactant, infants are unable to keep their lungs inflated and therefore exert a great deal of effort to reexpand the alveoli with each breath. It has been estimated that each breath requires as much negative pressure (60 to 75 cm $H_2O$) as the initial lung expansion at birth. To expend this amount of energy, infants use more oxygen than they take in, which rapidly leads to exhaustion. With increasing exhaustion they are able to open fewer and fewer alveoli. This inability to maintain lung expansion produces widespread atelectasis.

In the absence of alveolar stability (normal functional residual capacity) and with progressive atelectasis, pulmonary vascular resistance (PVR) increases, whereas with normal lung expansion it would decrease. Consequently, there is hypoperfusion to the lung tissue, with a decrease in effective pulmonary blood flow. The increase in PVR causes partial reversion to the fetal circulation, with a right-to-left shunting of blood through the persisting fetal communications—the ductus arteriosus and foramen ovale.

Inadequate pulmonary perfusion and ventilation produce hypoxemia and hypercapnia. Pulmonary arterioles, with their thick muscular layer, are markedly reactive to diminished oxygen concentration. Thus a decrease in oxygen tension causes vasospasm in the pulmonary arterioles that is further enhanced by a decrease in blood pH. This vasoconstriction contributes to a marked increase in PVR. In normal ventilation with increased oxygen concentration, the ductus arteriosus constricts and the pulmonary vessels dilate to decrease PVR (Fig. 10-13).

Prolonged hypoxemia activates anaerobic glycolysis, which produces increased amounts of lactic acid. An increase in lactic acid causes metabolic acidosis; inability of the atelectic lungs to blow off excess carbon dioxide produces respiratory acidosis. Lowered pH causes further vasoconstriction. With deficient pulmonary circulation and alveolar perfusion, $PaO_2$ continues to fall, pH falls, and the materials needed for surfactant production are not circulated to the alveoli.

Pulmonary edema observed in the early stages of RDS also contributes to impaired gas exchange. Factors believed to facilitate this fluid accumulation in the lungs include renal immaturity or insufficiency resulting from hypoxemia, high fluid intake and patent ductus arteriosus, left ventricular dysfunction associated with papillary muscle necrosis, low serum protein concentration and low colloid osmotic pressure, increased alveolar surface tension that enhances the shift of interstitial fluid to alveolar spaces, oxygen toxicity, and high plasma vasopressin.

*Pulmonary interstitial emphysema* develops in preterm infants with RDS and immature lungs as a result of overdistention of distal airways; this condition further complicates adequate oxygenation in the immature airways (see Extraneous Air Syndromes, p. 389).

Deficiencies in other systems contribute to respiratory distress. For example, a high threshold of the respiratory center to afferent stimuli and weak or absent gag and cough reflexes reflect the immaturity of the nervous system. In addition, the persistence of fetal hemoglobin, so beneficial in prenatal existence, may place the infant at a disadvantage during respiratory distress. Although the binding power of fetal hemoglobin for oxygen is much greater than in adult hemoglobin, this increased affinity also causes less oxygen to be released to the tissues at normal oxygen tension. In the newborn the arterial oxygen concentration must fall to a lower level for bound oxygen to be released from fetal hemoglobin.

A hyaline membrane is formed as hypoxemia and the increased pulmonary vascular pressure cause transudation of fluid into the alveoli. Necrotic cells from damaged alveoli plus the fibrin in the transudate form a membranous layer that lines the alveoli and inhibits gas exchange. The presence of the hyaline membrane contributes to respiratory difficulties by greatly diminishing lung distensibility, or *compliance,* the elastic quality of lung tissue that permits expansion in response to a given amount of applied pressure during inspiration. Affected lungs are stiffer and require far more pressure than do normal lungs to achieve an equal amount of expansion. The major factors that produce respiratory distress syndrome in immature infants are summarized in Table 10-6.

RDS is a self-limiting disease. Following a period of deterioration (approximately 48 hours) and in the absence of complications, affected infants begin to improve by 72 hours. Often heralded by the onset of diuresis, this improvement has been attributed primarily to increased production and greater availability of surface-active material.

## Clinical Manifestations

Infants with RDS can develop respiratory distress either acutely or over a period of hours, depending on the acuity of pulmonary immaturity, associated illness factors, and gestational maturity. The observable signs produced by the pulmonary changes usually begin to appear in infants who apparently achieve normal breathing and color soon after birth. In a matter of a few hours, breathing gradually becomes more rapid (greater than 60 breaths/min). Infants may display retractions—suprasternal or substernal, and supracostal, subcostal, or intercostal—which result from a compliant chest wall. Weak chest wall muscles and the highly cartilaginous nature of the rib structure produce an abnormally elastic rib cage. Thus considerable negative pressure is wasted as the infant attempts to produce higher intrathoracic pressure changes. During this early period the infant's color may remain satisfactory, and auscultation reveals air entry. Some of the criteria for evaluating respiratory distress in infants are illustrated in Fig. 10-14.

**TABLE 10-6   Major factors in respiratory distress syndrome**

| Cause | Effect |
| --- | --- |
| Increased surface tension of alveoli (surfactant deficiency) | Alveolar collapse; atelectasis; increased difficulty of breathing |
| Impaired gas exchange | Hypoxemia and hypercapnia with respiratory acidosis |
| Increased pulmonary vascular resistance | Hypoperfusion of pulmonary circulation |
| Hypoperfusion (with hypoxemia) | Tissue hypoxia and metabolic acidosis |
| Increased transudation of fluid into lungs | Hyaline membrane formation; impaired gas exchange |

Within a few hours, respiratory distress becomes more obvious. The respiratory rate continues to increase (to 80 to 120 breaths/min), and breathing becomes more labored. It is significant to note that infants will increase the *rate* rather than the *depth* of respiration when in distress. Substernal retractions become more pronounced as the diaphragm works hard in an attempt to fill collapsed air sacs. Fine inspiratory rales can be heard over both lungs, and there is an audible expiratory grunt. This grunting, a useful mechanism observed in the earlier stages of RDS, serves to increase end-expiratory pressure in the lungs, thus maintaining alveolar expansion and allowing gas exchange for an additional brief period. Flaring of the nares is also a sign that accompanies tachypnea, grunting, and retractions in respiratory distress. Central cyanosis (a bluish discoloration of oral mucous membranes and generalized body cyanosis) is a late and serious sign of respiratory distress. Initially cyanosis may be abolished by supplemental oxygen. The use of pulse oximetry and arterial blood gas sampling obviates the necessity for dependence on color to determine oxygen requirements.

At this point the respiratory distress may gradually decrease over 12 to 24 hours with eventual recovery, or it may increase in severity. In distressed infants cyanosis becomes more marked despite increases in ambient oxygen concentration. Often there is pallor caused by peripheral vasoconstriction, but it is often masked by cyanosis. The infants become flaccid and unresponsive and begin to display frequent apneic episodes. Chest auscultation reveals diminished breath sounds. The chances of recovery without assisted ventilation are then very small. Severe RDS is often associated with a shocklike state, as manifested by diminished cardiac inflow and low arterial blood pressure. As a result of extreme pulmonary immaturity, decreased glycogen stores, and lack of accessory muscles, the ELBW and VLBW infant may have severe RDS at birth, therefore bypassing the aforementioned steps in the development of RDS.

Infants with RDS who survive the first 96 hours have a reasonable chance for recovery. Complications of RDS include those described as complications of positive pressure ventilation (see p. 385). Associated complications (of prematurity and RDS) include patent ductus arteriosus and congestive heart failure, IVH, BPD, NEC, and neurologic sequelae.

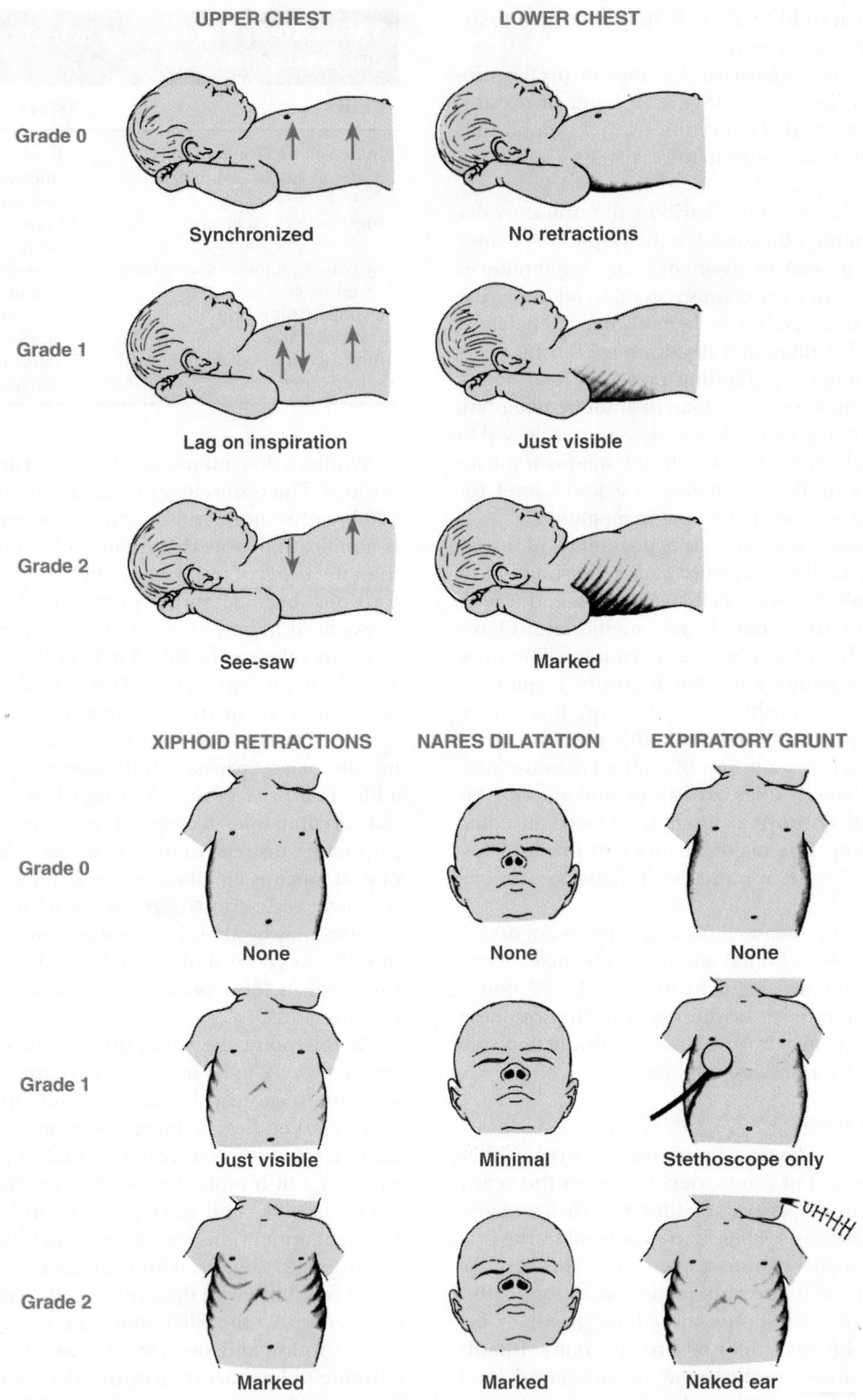

**Fig. 10-14** Criteria for evaluating respiratory distress. (Modified from Silvermann WA, Anderson DH: A controlled clinical trial of effects of water mist on obstructive respiratory signs, death rate, and necropsy findings among premature infants, *Pediatrics* 17:1, 1956.)

## Diagnostic Evaluation

Laboratory data are nonspecific, and the abnormalities observed are identical to those observed in numerous biochemical abnormalities of the newborn (i.e., the findings of hypoxemia, hypercapnia, and acidosis). Specific tests are used to determine complicating factors, such as blood glucose (to test for hypoglycemia), serum calcium (to test for hypocalcemia), blood gas measurements for serum pH (to test for acidosis), and Pao$_2$ (to test for hypoxia). Pulse oximetry is an important component for determining hypoxia. Other special examinations may be used to diagnose or rule out complications.

Radiographic findings characteristic of RDS include (1) a diffuse granular pattern over both lung fields that closely resembles ground glass and represents alveolar atelectasis, and (2) dark streaks, or bronchograms, within the ground glass areas that represent dilated, air-filled bronchioles. It is important to distinguish between RDS and pneumonia in infants with respiratory distress.

**Prenatal Diagnosis.**   Fetal lung maturity depends on gestational age, except in some specific instances that may not be known until the time of labor or delivery. Functional maturity of the fetal lung can be determined by using surfactant phospholipids in amniotic fluid as indicators of maturity. The most commonly tested is the *lecithin/sphingomyelin (L/S) ratio,* which measures the relationship between these two lipids during gestation. Phospholipids are synthesized by fetal alveolar cells, and the concentrations in amniotic fluid change during gestation. Initially there is more sphingomyelin, but at approximately 32 to 33 weeks the concentrations become equal; sphingomyelin then diminishes and lecithin increases significantly until the fetus has developed sufficient surfactant to maintain alveolar stability at approximately 35 weeks. An L/S ratio of 2:1 in nondiabetic mothers indicates relative assurance of the absence of risk of RDS.

Other key surfactant compounds (also phospholipids) that are needed to stabilize surfactant are phosphatidylcholine (PC) and phosphatidylglycerol (PG). Without these compounds lecithin is not functional as a surfactant. Concentrations of PC parallel those of lecithin, peaking at 35 weeks and then gradually decreasing. At 36 weeks PG appears in amniotic fluid and increases until term. By measuring these phospholipids—L/S ratio, PC, and PG—the maturity of the lungs can be estimated with a high degree of accuracy. Pregnancies complicated by maternal illnesses such as diabetes and hypertension may be associated with acceleration (before 33 weeks) or delay (later than 37 weeks) in fetal lung maturation.

Other, but less commonly used, methods have been devised to provide rapid, inexpensive, and accurate measures of lung maturity. These include the "shake" or "bubble" test, in which stable foam or bubbles form when amniotic fluid is shaken in the presence of ethanol, and the tap test, in which abundant bubbles appear in a test tube of amniotic fluid with 6N hydrochloric acid and diethyl ether. Tests designed to evaluate amniotic fluid turbidity for fetal lung maturity include visual inspection for the presence of vernix, the optical density test, and lamellar body number density test.

Increasing evidence has shown that certain *antioxidant enzymes,* which develop late in gestation, have an important role in protecting alveoli and airway cells from damage by oxygen radicals that appear in hyperoxic states (as in the infant attempting to adapt to an extrauterine existence). The antioxidant system (AOS) has no effect on fetal lung maturity, but when it is deficient there is more damage to the already compromised alveoli and airway cells.

Another test currently being used to evaluate fetal lung maturity is the *TDx Fetal Lung Maturity (FLM) assay,* which determines PG levels in amniotic fluid or neonatal tracheal aspirates. The FLM test is faster than L/S ratio determination (<1 hour vs 4 to 5 hours) and is reported to predict the absence of RDS with greater accuracy; a level of 50 or more is predictive of fetal lung maturity (Steinfeld and others, 1992). Recent evidence suggests that African-American fetuses have lower TDx FLM predictive values for fetal lung maturity than were previously demonstrated in a mixed population (Berman and others, 1996). TDx FLM may also be used in the postnatal period to determine the presence of RDS as a result of surfactant deficiency by collecting tracheal aspirate samples (Giacoia and others, 1995).

Lamellar bodies, representing the storage form of surfactant, are found in amniotic fluid in increasing quantities with the advancement of gestational age and lung maturity. A quantitative count of lamellar bodies has been reported to be as accurate as the L/S ratio in the determination of fetal lung maturity. The count can be obtained faster than the L/S ratio, thus making it clinically appealing (Neerhof and others, 2001; Wijnberger and others, 2001).

## Therapeutic Management

The treatment of RDS is largely supportive and includes all the general measures required for any premature infant as well as those instituted to correct imbalances. The supportive measures most crucial to a favorable outcome are (1) maintain adequate ventilation and oxygenation with either an oxygen hood or mechanical ventilation, (2) maintain acid-base balance, (3) maintain a neutral thermal environment, (4) maintain adequate tissue perfusion and oxygenation, (5) prevent hypotension, and (6) maintain adequate hydration and electrolyte status. Nipple and gavage feedings are contraindicated in any situation that creates a marked increase in respiratory rate because of the greater hazards of aspiration. In addition, administering substrate to the infant with transient hypoxia places the infant at risk for NEC. Nutrition is provided by parenteral therapy during the acute stage of the disease.

**Oxygen Therapy.**   The goals of oxygen therapy are to provide adequate oxygen to the tissues, prevent lactic acid accumulation resulting from hypoxia, and, at the same time, avoid the potentially negative effects of oxygen volutrauma. Numerous methods have been devised to improve oxygenation (Table 10-7). All require that the gas be warmed and humidified before entering the respiratory tract. If the infant does not require ventilatory assistance, oxygen can be given via a plastic hood placed over the infant's head to supply variable concentrations of humidified oxygen. (See Oxygen Therapy, Chapter 31.) If oxygen saturation of blood cannot be maintained at a satisfactory level and the carbon dioxide level (Paco$_2$) rises, infants will require ventilatory assistance.

Continuous positive airway pressure (CPAP) or continuous distending pressure (CDP), the application of 3 to 8 cm of water (positive) pressure to the airway, uses the infant's spontaneous respiration to improve oxygenation by helping prevent alveolar collapse and increasing diffusion time. CPAP may be delivered via nasal prongs or an endotracheal tube. Ventilation with CPAP is done entirely by the infant. If

**TABLE 10-7** Common methods for assisted ventilation in neonatal respiratory distress*

| Method | Description | How Provided |
|---|---|---|
| **Conventional Methods** | | |
| Continuous positive airway pressure (CPAP) or continuous distending pressure (CDP) | Provides constant distending pressure to airway in spontaneously breathing infant | Nasal prongs Endotracheal tube |
| Positive end-expiratory pressure (PEEP)† | Provides increased end-expiratory pressure during expiration and between mandatory breaths, which prevents alveolar collapse; maintains residual airway pressure | Endotracheal intubation and either volume-limited or pressure-limited ventilator |
| Intermittent mandatory ventilation (IMV)† | Allows infant to breathe spontaneously at own rate but provides mechanical cycled respirations and pressure at regular preset intervals | Endotracheal intubation and ventilator |
| **Alternative Methods** | | |
| **High-frequency ventilation (HFV)** | | |
| High-frequency positive-pressure ventilation (HFPPV) | Low-compliant circuit provides high gas flow through circuit: operates at rates between 60 and 150 breaths/min | Conventional infant ventilators; endotracheal tube |
| High-frequency oscillation (HFO) | Applies high-frequency, low-volume, sine-wave flow oscillations to airway at rates between 480 and 1200 breaths/min | Variable-speed piston pump (or loud-speaker, fluidic oscillator); endotracheal tube |
| High-frequency jet ventilation (HFJV) | Uses a separate, parallel, low-compliant circuit and injector port to deliver small pulses or jets of fresh gas deep into airway at rates between 250 and 900 breaths/min | May be used alone or with low-rate IMV; endotracheal tube |
| Synchronized intermittent mandatory ventilation (SIMV) | Synchronizes mechanically delivered breaths to the onset of spontaneous patient breaths; assist/control mode facilitates full inspiratory synchrony; involves signal detection of onset of spontaneous respiration from abdominal movement, thoracic impedance, and airway pressure or flow changes | Patient-triggered infant ventilator with signal detector and assist/control mode; endotracheal tube |

*For a more detailed review of assisted ventilation, see Askin DF: *Acute respiratory care of the neonate,* ed 2, Petaluma, CA, 1997, NICU Ink.
†Also referred to as conventional ventilation (vs HFV).

oxygenation is not improved and the infant requires assisted ventilation, intermittent mandatory ventilation (IMV) or continuous positive-pressure ventilation (CPPV) is used with positive end-expiratory pressure (PEEP). This allows infants to breathe at their own rate but provides positive pressure at regular preset intervals, with end-expiratory pressure to prevent alveolar collapse and overcome airway resistance. Additional components involved in IMV are peak inspiratory pressure (PIP) and rate (number of breaths per minute). The PIP is the maximum amount of positive pressure applied to the infant on inspiration. The total amount of pressure transmitted to the airway throughout an entire respiratory cycle is called the mean airway pressure (MAP). Increasing MAP in infants with severe RDS correlates positively with improved oxygenation by maintaining functional residual capacity and overcoming the resistive forces of the atelectatic lung. The MAP is affected by changes in the PEEP, PIP, and inspiratory/expiratory (I/E) ratio. Although MAP is now recognized as the major determinant of oxygenation, this does not imply that simply increasing MAP alone will automatically improve oxygenation (Harris and Wood, 1996).

If adequate oxygenation cannot be maintained and hypercarbia persists, infants may benefit from one of the three high-frequency ventilation (HFV) modalities. HFV delivers gas at very rapid rates to provide adequate minute volumes using lower proximal airway pressures by way of high-frequency positive-pressure ventilation (HFPPV), high-frequency oscillation (HFO), or high-frequency jet ventilation (HFJV). HFJV and HFO are believed to benefit the preterm infant with RDS by enhancing the distribution and diffusion of respiratory gases; efficient $CO_2$ elimination independent of mean lung volumes is but one of the advantages of these modalities (Mammel and Boros, 1996). HFV is recommended for intractable respiratory failure, especially for infants with pulmonary air leaks and pulmonary interstitial emphysema. It is primarily a short-term therapy and is believed to reduce the incidence of volutrauma, which often complicates oxygen therapy in preterm infants. Volutrauma is believed to be a key factor in the development of BPD/CLD. However, there is an increased incidence of necrotizing tracheitis, pneumopericardium, and hypotension reported with HFJV. Additional potential advantages of HFV over conventional ventilation are active elimination of carbon dioxide and the ability to ventilate infants with persistent pulmonary hypertension.

Improved technologic advances have made available to preterm or sick neonates a form of mechanical ventilatory assistance used primarily in adults—synchronized intermittent mandatory ventilation (SIMV). With this method mechanically delivered breaths are synchronized to the onset of spontaneous infant breaths. The net effect is to produce full respiratory synchrony rather than asynchronous respiratory efforts (commonly called "fighting the ventilator")

## Critical Thinking Exercise

### Respiratory Distress Syndrome

A 32-week preterm infant requires mechanical ventilation for the treatment of respiratory distress syndrome as a result of surfactant deficiency. The nurse is aware of problems associated with prematurity and RDS, such as hypoglycemia. Problems for which you are particularly vigilant in light of the use of positive pressure ventilation with this infant and the knowledge of pathology include what?

FIRST, THINK ABOUT IT . . .
- What precise question are you trying to answer?
- What conclusions are you reaching?

1. Meconium aspiration
2. Transient tachypnea
3. Air leaks
4. Persistent pulmonary hypertension

*The best response is three. The precise question is focused on the fact that infants who are preterm and lack adequate surfactant have immature alveoli and increased surface tension that predispose them to the development of air leaks during positive pressure ventilation. It is correct to conclude that the other three options are neonatal respiratory conditions usually unrelated to RDS of the type in which surfactant deficiency is the major pathology.*

that are believed to significantly impede the ability to adequately oxygenate infants without sedation or muscle paralysis. With SIMV the patient may breathe spontaneously between mechanical breaths. In the "assist-control" mode a mechanical breath is delivered each time a spontaneous respiration is detected; the "control" mode includes the delivery of a mechanical breath at a regular rate if the patient fails to initiate a spontaneous respiration. Additional benefits of SIMV are improved oxygenation, decreased incidence of pulmonary air leaks (pneumothorax), decreased use of sedation, and decreased time on mechanical ventilation.

**Complications of Positive Pressure Ventilation.** Although lifesaving, oxygen therapy is not without hazards. Positive pressure introduced by mechanical apparatus has caused an increased incidence of air leaks that produce complications, such as pulmonary interstitial emphysema, pneumothorax, and pneumomediastinum (see p. 389). Other complications directly related to positive pressure include BPD/CLD and various problems associated with intubation, such as nasal, tracheal, or pharyngeal perforation; stenosis; inflammation; palatal grooves; subglottic stenosis; tube obstruction; and infection. (See Critical Thinking Exercise box.)

**Nitric Oxide.** Inhaled nitric oxide (NO) has emerged as a significant treatment modality for neonates with conditions that cause persistent pulmonary hypertension, pulmonary vasoconstriction, and subsequent acidosis and severe hypoxia. Infants with conditions such as meconium aspiration syndrome, pneumonia, sepsis, and congenital diaphragmatic hernia with pulmonary hypoplasia have often required ECMO in an attempt to reverse pulmonary

hypertension. NO is a colorless, highly diffusible gas that has been shown to cause smooth muscle relaxation and reduce pulmonary vasoconstriction and subsequent pulmonary hypertension when inhaled into the lungs. NO may be administered through the ventilator circuit and blended with oxygen. It attaches readily to hemoglobin and is thus deactivated so that systemic vasculature is not affected. NO is toxic in large quantities, but the amount required to induce pulmonary vasculature relaxation (6 to 20 ppm) is well below toxic levels.

Studies of term and near-term infants being treated with NO for respiratory failure have demonstrated optimal success rates (Finer and Barrington, 2001). In most cases reversal of persistent pulmonary hypertension of the newborn (PPHN) without ECMO was achieved in infants with MAS, RDS, and in perioperative congenital heart disease and sepsis (Davidson and others, 1998; Kinsella and Abman, 2000). One exception is the study of newborns with congenital diaphragmatic hernia who required ECMO after NO and whose morbidity/mortality was not significantly improved with inhaled NO (Neonatal Inhaled Nitric Oxide Study Group, 1997; Finer and Barrington, 2001). Surfactant replacement therapy may be performed in combination with inhaled NO therapy in infants with inadequate pulmonary maturity. Nursing care of the infant receiving inhaled NO is the same as for the newborn with RDS; continual assessment of respiratory status and response to treatment is essential.

**Liquid Ventilation.** Infants who may not be candidates for NO or ECMO may benefit from the administration of liquid ventilation. Although seemingly an unusual concept, liquid ventilation appears to have two main benefits over other technologies such as surfactant replacement because the fluid-filled lung, even when surfactant-deficient, demonstrates increased compliance. Uniformly filling the lung with fluid diminishes surface tension, reducing required inflation pressures and subsequent barotrauma in preterm and sick term neonates. Additional advantages of using liquid ventilation with perfluorocarbons are the increased removal of pulmonary debris such as meconium, distention of lung parenchyma, and its use as a medium or transporter of drugs such as antibiotics and surfactant directly into the smaller capillaries of the lung, which are usually unreachable (or at least uniformly so) in neonatal pulmonary disorders such as meconium aspiration.

*Perfluorocarbons (PFCs)* are inert liquids derived by replacing all the carbon-bound hydrogen atoms on organic compounds with fluorine. PFCs are clear, odorless, inert, and require no metabolism by the kidneys or liver. Oxygen and carbon dioxide are highly soluble in PFCs, which are removed from the body by evaporation. No adverse histologic, biochemical, or toxic effects have been identified in these substances, making them highly attractive as a medium for liquid ventilation (Cox, Wolfson, and Shaffer, 1996).

The two main techniques for liquid ventilation delivery are *total (or tidal) liquid ventilation (TLV)* and *partial liquid ventilation (PLV)*, sometimes called *perfluorocarbon-assisted gas exchange (PAGE)*. With PLV the lungs are filled with perfluorocarbons during the inspiratory phase (which is somewhat slower than regular gas ventilation), with a filling volume equal to functional residual capacity through the ET tube. Gas ventilation is interspersed with PFC insertion until the desired effects are achieved. In TLV, oxygenated PFC is continuously instilled into the lungs with special equipment. Once gas exchange and lung mechanics improve, the neonate is weaned from ventilatory support, often within a matter of hours. In both systems PFCs lost to evaporation are replaced through the mechanical ventilation system to achieve the desired results. Liquid ventilation may be used in conjunction with ECMO and NO. PFC fluids are radiopaque and may be used to assess the lungs for ventilation-perfusion function and to view anatomic lung structures.

The nursing care of the infant on liquid ventilation is similar to the care of any infant on conventional gas ventilation. Special attention to lung sounds and adequacy of therapy by assessment of arterial blood gases is imperative; with TLV actual breath sounds will not be auscultated; fine rales and coarse rhonchi may be auscultated with PLV. Attention is given to the positioning of the neonate, suctioning only when indicated and assessing for complications related to the infant's status or the equipment being used for gas and liquid delivery. Heart tones will be much more distinct with liquid ventilation because sound wave transmission is increased with fluids. The infant is evaluated for signs of a pneumothorax and signs of deteriorating pulmonary status. Vital signs are assessed according to the severity of the infant's condition. Liquid ventilation has also been shown to be effective in the treatment of persistent pulmonary hypertension, congenital diaphragmatic hernia, meconium aspiration, and pneumonia. Perhaps the most attractive feature of liquid ventilation with the use of PFCs is the relative safety of its use in neonates, even critical preterm neonates, with practically no reported adverse physiologic sequelae such as IVH or sepsis. Clinical trials have thus far demonstrated the efficacy of partial liquid ventilation for respiratory illnesses in the sick term and preterm neonate; however, it is a complex and costly procedure (Valls-I-Soler, Alvarez, and Gastiasoro, 2001). Liquid ventilation is used in a few centers nationwide. Further randomized neonatal clinical trials need to be completed for the procedure to be fully accepted (Greenspan, Woolfson, and Shaffer, 2001). Liquid ventilation may be useful in older children with pulmonary insufficiency and in adults with respiratory distress syndrome (ARDS).

**Medical Therapies.** The treatment of the infant with RDS requires the establishment of one or more intravenous lines to maintain hydration and nutrition, monitor arterial blood gases, and administer medications.

Systemic antibiotics may be administered during the acute phase for sepsis (see Sepsis, p. 393). The administration of a neuromuscular blocking agent (for muscle paralysis) and phenobarbitol, fentanyl, or sodium pentobarbital (Nembutal) (for sedation) is individualized according to the infant's response to illness. Methylxanthines (theophylline or caffeine) are administered to treat apnea and to prepare for weaning VLBW and ELBW infants from mechanical ventilation. Inotropes such as dopamine and dobutamine may be required to support the infant's systemic blood pressure and maintain effective cardiac output during the acute phase of illness.

It is not uncommon for high-risk neonates, including those with RDS, to receive a blood transfusion (often packed red blood cells) to replace the blood volume lost from frequent sampling during the acute phase of illness. In addition, preterm infants experience anemia of prematurity as a result of inadequate responses to erythropoietin. Therapy (administered subcutaneously three times a week) with recombinant erythropoietin has proved to be effective in reducing the number of blood transfusions required for anemia of prematurity (Luchtman-Jones, Schwartz, and Wilson, 1997). In some studies, however, a significant overall reduction has not been observed (Strauss, 2001; Vamvakas and Strauss, 2001) (see Anemia, p. 398).

**Surfactant.** The administration of exogenous surfactant to preterm neonates with RDS has become an accepted and common therapy in most neonatal centers worldwide. Numerous clinical trials involving the administration of exogenous surfactant to infants with or at high risk for RDS demonstrate improvements in blood gas values and ventilator settings, decreased incidence of pulmonary air leaks, decreased deaths from RDS, and an overall decreased infant mortality rate (American Academy of Pediatrics, 1999b). Exogenous surfactant is derived from a natural source (e.g., human [obtained from donor's amniotic fluid], porcine, or bovine) or from the production of artificial surfactant. Commercially available surfactant products include Exosurf Neonatal, a synthetic colfosceril surfactant*; beractant (Survanta), a bovine surfactant†; and Curosurf, a porcine surfactant.‡

Studies have shown mixed results in comparing one surfactant product with another. In one study there were fewer complications and earlier improvement with natural (vs. synthetic) surfactant use (Soll and Blanco, 2001). Additional benefits of surfactant replacement therapy include decreased oxygen requirements and MAP within hours of administration and an overall decrease in the incidence of pulmonary air leaks. To date, long-term improvement in the decrease of BPD/CLD and IVH has not been evidenced in all clinical trials.

Complications seen with surfactant administration include pulmonary hemorrhage and mucus plugging. Additional studies are under investigation for the potential benefits of surfactant in infants with meconium aspiration, infectious pneumonia, and lung hypoplasia concomitant with congenital diaphragmatic hernia (Wiswell, 2001). ARDS may also respond favorably to surfactant administration. Surfactant may be administered at birth as a prophylactic treatment of RDS or later in the course of RDS as a rescue treatment. Studies found improved clinical outcomes and fewer adverse effects when surfactant is administered prophylactically to infants at risk for developing RDS (Soll and Morley, 2001). Surfactant is administered via the ET tube directly into the infant's trachea; the exact number of doses (single vs multiple) that is most effective has yet to be determined. Nursing responsibilities with surfactant ad-

*Burroughs Wellcome Company, Research Triangle Park, NC.
†Ross Laboratories, Columbus, OH.
‡Ghiesi Company, Parma, Italy.

ministration include assistance in the delivery of the product, collection and monitoring of arterial blood gases, scrupulous monitoring of oxygenation with pulse oximetry or tcPO$_2$, and assessment of the infant's tolerance of the procedure. Once surfactant is absorbed, there is usually an increase in respiratory compliance that requires adjustment of ventilator settings to decrease MAP and prevent overinflation or hyperoxemia. Suctioning is usually delayed for an hour or so (depending on the type of surfactant, delivery system, and unit protocol) to allow maximum effects to occur. Current research is in progress to investigate the possibility of delivering an aerosolized surfactant. This method would decrease the problems associated with current delivery systems (contamination of the airway, interruption of mechanical ventilation, and loss of the drug in the endotracheal tubing from reflux).

**Prevention.**  The most successful approach to prevention of RDS is prevention of premature delivery, especially in elective early delivery and cesarean section. Improved methods for assessing the maturity of the fetal lung by amniocentesis, although not a routine procedure, allow a reasonable prediction of adequate surfactant formation (see Diagnostic Evaluation, p. 382). Because estimation of a delivery date can be miscalculated by as much as 1 month, such tests are particularly valuable when scheduling an elective cesarean section. Studies indicate that the combination of maternal glucocorticoid administration before delivery and surfactant administration postnatally has a synergistic effect on neonatal lungs, with the net result being a decrease in infant mortality, decreased incidence of IVH, fewer pulmonary air leaks, and fewer problems with pulmonary interstitial emphysema and RDS (Andrews and others, 1995; Volpe, 2001).

## Nursing Considerations

Care of infants with RDS involves all the observations and interventions previously described for high-risk infants. In addition, the nurse is concerned with the complex problems related to respiratory therapy and the constant threat of hypoxemia and acidosis that complicates the care of patients in respiratory difficulty.

The respiratory therapist, an important member of the neonatal intensive care team, is often responsible for the maintenance of respiratory equipment. Although it may be the responsibility of the respiratory therapist to regulate the apparatus, nurses should understand the equipment and be able to recognize when it is not functioning correctly. The most essential nursing function is to observe and assess the infant's response to therapy. Continuous monitoring and close observation are mandatory because an infant's status can change rapidly and because oxygen concentration and ventilation parameters are prescribed according to the infant's blood gas measurements, tcPO$_2$ readings, and pulse oximetry readings.

Changes in oxygen concentration are based on these observations. The amount of oxygen administered, expressed as the fraction of inspired air (FIO$_2$), is determined on an individual basis according to pulse oximetry and/or direct or indirect measurement of arterial oxygen concentration.

Capillary samples collected from the heel (see Chapter 27 for procedure) are useful for pH and PacO$_2$ determinations but *not* for oxygenation status. Continuous transcutaneous or pulse oximetry readings are recorded at least hourly. Blood sampling is performed after ventilator changes for the acutely ill infant and thereafter when clinically indicated.

In infants with RDS who are acutely ill and/or extremely preterm, an umbilical arterial catheter (UAC) may be used to draw arterial blood for monitoring oxygenation. This method, although initially invasive and therefore performed by the practitioner with sterile precautions, allows for blood sampling without repeated peripheral arterial punctures. The catheter is inserted via one of the umbilical arteries to the premeasured desired position (either at the level of the diaphragm, T6-T8, or between L3-L4) and rests in the descending aorta. Continuous arterial pressure monitoring may be carried out with an "in-line" transducer. Practices vary regarding medication administration via a UAC. The nurse is aware of the potential hazards associated with these catheters (infection, hemorrhage, thrombus formation and subsequent vessel occlusion, arterial vasospasm) and implements monitoring and observation strategies to promptly intervene should complications occur (see Hydration, p. 341). An umbilical venous catheter (UVC) may be used separately or in conjunction with the UAC, depending on the severity of the infant's illness, the fluid requirements, and practice. UVCs have historically been associated with more complications than UACs, including hepatic necrosis, intestinal ischemia, and hypertension. When monitored properly, both types of catheters can be used to administer hyperalimentation to the critically ill neonate with RDS.

Mucus may collect in the respiratory tract as a result of the infant's pulmonary condition. Secretions interfere with gas flow and predispose the infant to obstruction of the passages, including the ET tube. Suctioning should be performed only when necessary and should be based on individual infant assessment, which includes auscultation of the chest, evidence of decreased oxygenation, excess moisture in the ET tube, or increased infant irritability. Before suctioning, hyperventilation and/or hyperoxygenation may be used to prevent hypoxemia; however, the efficacy of these procedures has not been well established (Swartz, Noonan, and Edwards-Beckett, 1996). Instillation of 0.25 to 0.5 ml of sterile normal saline in the ET tube before insertion of the suction catheter may aid in removing secretions, but its value is unproven.

> **NURSING ALERT**  Suctioning is not an innocuous procedure (may cause bronchospasm, bradycardia because of vagal nerve stimulation, hypoxia, and increased ICP, predisposing the infant to IVH) and should *never* be carried out on a routine basis. Improper suctioning technique can also cause infection, airway damage, or even pneumothoraces.

When nasopharyngeal passages, the trachea, or the ET tube is being suctioned, the catheter should be inserted gently but quickly; intermittent suction is applied as the catheter is withdrawn. It is imperative that the time the airway is obstructed by the catheter be limited to no more than 5 seconds, because continuous suction removes air from the lungs along with the mucus. It is recommended that the "two-person" suctioning procedure be used on infants who are acutely ill and who do not tolerate any procedure without profound decreases in oxygen saturation, BP, and heart rate. However, this procedure may not be necessary with an in-line suction device. The object of suctioning an artificial airway is to maintain patency of that airway, not the bronchi. Suction applied beyond the ET tube can cause traumatic lesions of the trachea. The $FIO_2$ should be increased by 10% before suctioning to compensate for a decrease in $FIO_2$ during the procedure. (See Chapter 31.) The use of in-line suction catheters may decrease airway contamination and hypoxia.

> **NURSING ALERT**
>
> The pulse oximeter is observed before, during, and after suctioning to provide an ongoing assessment of oxygenation status and to prevent hypoxemia.

Research indicates that suctioning to a point where the catheter meets resistance and is then withdrawn causes trauma to the tracheobronchial wall. In order to remove secretions without damage to the tracheobronchial mucosa, the suction catheter is premeasured and inserted to a predetermined depth to avoid extension beyond the ET tube. The practice of suctioning patients on mechanical ventilation has undergone close scrutiny in recent years; further studies are needed to validate this practice and to determine the best methods for maintaining a patent airway without compromising the patient's well-being (Copnell and Fergusson, 1995; Swartz, Noonan, and Edwards-Beckett, 1996).

Removal of secretions can be further facilitated by positioning and application of percussion and vibration to the thoracic wall. The technique and positioning for postural drainage, percussion, and vibration are outlined in Chapter 31. However, the Trendelenburg position should not be used with preterm infants because it can contribute to increased ICP. Percussion and vibration are poorly tolerated in most ELBW and VLBW infants, often resulting in hypoxia, rib fractures, bruising, and further atelectasis. Chest physiotherapy should be carefully evaluated according to the infant's condition and with consideration of benefit risk factors. Chest percussion and vibration for the removal of secretions may benefit infants with meconium aspiration (except in the acute phase) and BPD more than preterm infants with RDS.

The most advantageous positions for facilitating an infant's open airway are on the side with the head supported in alignment by a small folded blanket or, when on the back, positioned to keep the neck slightly extended. With the head in the "sniffing" position, the trachea is opened to its maximum; hyperextension reduces the tracheal diameter in neonates. The supported side-lying position can also be used effectively (see Therapeutic Positioning, p. 363).

Inspection of the skin is part of routine infant assessment. Position changes and the use of water pillows are helpful in guarding against skin breakdown.

Mouth care is especially important when infants are receiving nothing by mouth, and the problem is often aggravated by the drying effect of oxygen therapy. Drying and cracking can be prevented by good oral hygiene using sterile water. Irritation to the nares or mouth that occurs from appliances used to administer oxygen may be reduced by the use of a water-soluble ointment (see Skin Care, p. 350). (See Nursing Care Plan: The Infant with Respiratory Distress Syndrome.*)

The nursing care of an infant with RDS is a demanding role; meticulous attention must be given to subtle changes in the infant's oxygenation status. The importance of attention to detail cannot be overemphasized, particularly in regard to medication administration.

## Meconium Aspiration Syndrome (MAS)

Meconium aspiration is a serious condition that accounts for a substantial number of neonatal fatalities. It occurs when a fetus has been subjected to fetal asphyxia or other intrauterine stress that causes relaxing of the anal sphincter and passage of meconium into the amniotic fluid. The majority of meconium aspiration occurs with the first breath. However, a severely compromised fetus may aspirate in utero. At delivery of the chest and initiation of the first breath, infants inhale fluid and meconium into the nasooropharynx.

### Pathophysiology

MAS involves the passage of meconium in utero as a result of hypoxic stress. It occurs primarily in full-term and postterm infants but has been reported in infants less than 37 weeks of gestation. Once the meconium is swallowed or inhaled by the fetus, any gasping activity occurring as a result of intrauterine stress may cause the rather sticky and tenacious product to become aspirated into the lower airways. The net results are partial airway obstruction, air trapping, hyperinflation distal to the obstruction, and atelectasis caused by surfactant displacement. A "ball-valve" situation exists wherein gas flows into the lungs on inspiration but is trapped there on exhalation as a result of the small airway diameter. As the infant struggles to take in more air (air hunger), even more meconium may be aspirated. Hyperinflation, hypoxemia, and acidemia result in increased pulmonary vascular resistance.

In turn, shunting of blood through the ductus arteriosus (right-to-left) occurs because of increased resistance to blood flow through the pulmonary arteries (and to the lungs), leading to further hypoxemia and acidosis. Ductal shunting increases with hypoxia; some blood may enter the left atrium (LA) from the right atrium (RA) via the foramen ovale because there is a net decrease in blood returning to the LA via the pulmonary venous system, thus preventing closure of the foramen ovale. This pathologic process is essentially persistence of the fetal circulation; it is commonly referred to as persistent pulmonary hypertension of the newborn and is discussed later in this chapter. The air trapping of MAS causes overdistention of the alveoli and often

---

*In Wong DL, Hess C: *Wong and Whaley's clinical manual of pediatric nursing*, ed 5, St Louis, 2000, Mosby.

air leaks. There is evidence that meconium contributes to the destruction of surfactant, thus increasing surface tension and further predisposing the alveoli to decreased functional capacity.

### Clinical Manifestations

Infants who have released meconium in utero for some time before birth are stained from green meconium stools (those with more recent meconium passage may not be stained), tachypneic, hypoxic, and often depressed at birth. They develop expiratory grunting, nasal flaring, and retractions similar to those experienced by infants with RDS. They may initially be cyanotic or pale as well as tachypneic, and they may demonstrate the classic barrel chest from hyperinflation. The infants are often stressed, hypothermic, hypoglycemic, and hypocalcemic. Severe meconium aspiration progresses very rapidly to respiratory failure. These infants exhibit profound respiratory distress with gasping, ineffective ventilations, marked cyanosis and pallor, and hypotonia.

### Diagnostic Evaluation

At birth, meconium can often be visualized via laryngoscopy in the respiratory passages and vocal cords. Chest radiographs show uneven distribution of patchy infiltrates, air trapping, hyperexpansion, and atelectasis. Air leaks may be seen as the illness progresses; oxygenation will be poor, as evidenced by pulse oximetry and arterial blood gases. These infants may quickly develop metabolic and respiratory acidosis. Echocardiography assists in the diagnosis of right-to-left shunting of blood away from the pulmonary system.

### Therapeutic Management

Prevention of meconium aspiration begins with suctioning the mouth, nose, and posterior pharynx just after the head is delivered and the chest is still compressed in the birth canal. Following delivery, the need for tracheal suctioning is based on infant assessment. Infants who are vigorous with strong, stable respiratory effort, good muscle tone, and heart rate greater than 100 beats/min should not undergo tracheal suctioning but should be closely monitored (Kattwinkel, 2000). On the other hand, infants who demonstrate poor respiratory effort, low heart rate, and poor tone should be rapidly intubated, suctioned appropriately, and resuscitated according to clinical status postsuctioning.

Infants with respiratory distress are admitted to the NICU. Management of MAS consists of ventilatory support, exogenous surfactant administration, intravenous fluids, and systemic antibiotics. Because these infants are prone to develop persistent pulmonary hypertension, they are maintained somewhat hyperoxic and alkalotic as a precautionary measure and may be candidates for ECMO therapy, HFV, or NO (see Nitric Oxide, p. 385). Management of severe MAS may require neuromuscular blocking with agents such as pancuronium or vecuronium to effectively mechanically ventilate the hypoxic infant who is struggling (called "fighting the vent") (see Persistent Pulmonary Hypertension of the Newborn, p. 397). Complications are managed symptomatically or as described under the specific disorder.

### Nursing Considerations

Nursing considerations are the same as for any high-risk neonate. See nursing care in oxygen therapy, persistent pulmonary hypertension, and other complications.

## Extraneous Air Syndromes (Air Leaks)

Extraneous air syndromes, extraalveolar air accumulation, and air leaks are names applied to various clinically recognized disorders produced as a result of alveolar rupture and subsequent escape of air to tissues in which air is not normally present. Extraneous air collection (1) may occur spontaneously in normal neonates, (2) can result from congenital renal/pulmonary malformations, and (3) often complicates underlying respiratory disease and its therapy (e.g., positive pressure ventilation, especially when high distending pressures are required).

Following alveolar rupture, air often vents directly into the pleural space to create a *pneumothorax.* Air may vent into the perivascular interstitium, a condition called *pulmonary interstitial emphysema (PIE).* PIE may be seen on radiographs as early as 2 to 3 hours after birth in ELBW and VLBW infants with severe RDS. Localized PIE may resolve by itself or may be a precursor to pneumothorax. High-frequency ventilation has been reported to improve the outcome in infants with PIE (Korones, 1996). Air can dissect along the perivascular sheaths to eventually enter the mediastinum and cause *pneumomediastinum.* More extensive leaks involve the pericardium (manifested as *pneumopericardium*) or emphysema in the cervical, subcutaneous, or retroperitoneal soft tissues.

### Clinical Manifestations

Spontaneous pneumothorax usually occurs during the first few breaths after birth, primarily in full-term or postterm infants, and is evident by the gradual onset of symptoms of respiratory distress after arrival in the nursery. Improper use of positive-pressure ventilation in resuscitation may cause air leaks; mechanical positive pressure ventilation may contribute to an increase in the incidence of air leaks; however, there are cases, such as in extreme prematurity and meconium aspiration, in which air leaks may not be altogether preventable. It can be suspected on the basis of respiratory manifestations and a shift in location of maximum intensity of heart sounds and absent or diminished breath sounds (although breath sounds may not be altered because of the small diameter of the chest and auscultation of referred breath sounds). In preterm infants being mechanically ventilated, an air leak may demonstrate hypotension, bradycardia, decreased or absent breath sounds unilaterally, decreased oxygenation (by pulse oximetry), and cyanosis, none of which respond to efforts for oxygenation (a resuscitation bag connected to the ET tube and provision of manual ventilations). An air leak may contribute to an increased incidence of IVH in preterm infants. A tension pneumothorax occurs more frequently in infants requiring ventilatory assistance. There may also be chest asymmetry, altered cardiac sounds (diminished, shifted, or muffled), a palpable liver and spleen, and subcutaneous emphysema.

Infants on HFV may demonstrate an air leak by a sudden decrease in systemic pressure or an absence of chest movement (because of difficulty in auscultation of the chest with such modalities). The otherwise healthy full-term infant may exhibit only mild to moderate signs of respiratory distress.

> **NURSING ALERT**
> Early manifestations of pneumothorax include tachypnea, restlessness and irritability, lethargy, grunting, nasal flaring, and retractions. Pneumothorax during ventilatory assistance is evident from abrupt and profound duskiness or cyanosis; significant declines in heart rate, arterial blood pressure, and pulse pressure; and poor peripheral perfusion.

## Therapeutic Management

Diagnosis is confirmed by transillumination of the chest with a fiberoptic light and/or radiographic examination. Treatment is urgent. Evacuation of trapped air is accomplished by chest tube insertion into the pleural space through a small chest incision. The chest tube is then attached to continuous water-seal drainage. A dry suction control drainage system not requiring water is also available. Needle aspiration serves as an emergency measure until a chest tube can be inserted. Pneumomediastinum seldom requires treatment, but pneumopericardium is managed by needle aspiration or pericardial tube drainage. The full-term newborn with a small tension pneumothorax may require only oxygen therapy and intravenous nutrition for a brief period if respiratory distress is not severe. One treatment modality that may be used for these infants is a *nitrogen washout*. The infant is placed in a hood or tent with 100% oxygen, and a gradient is created in the lungs wherein enhanced absorption of the trapped pleural air is accomplished.

## Nursing Considerations

The most important nursing function, which is most effective for early detection, is close vigilance for the possibility of an air leak in susceptible infants. Nurses maintain a high level of suspicion in (1) infants with RDS with or without positive-pressure ventilation, (2) infants with meconium-stained amniotic fluid or MAS, (3) infants with radiographic evidence of interstitial or lobar emphysema, (4) infants who required resuscitation at birth, or (5) infants receiving continuous positive airway pressure or positive-pressure ventilation. For infants at risk, needle aspiration equipment (30-ml syringe, three-way stopcock, and 23- to 25-gauge butterfly needles) should be at the bedside for emergency use.

The general nursing care of the infant with an extraneous air syndrome is the same as that for all high-risk neonates. Respiratory management is similar to that for infants with RDS. Assessing breath sounds frequently, monitoring the efficacy of gas exchange, and regulating oxygen therapy according to the needs of the infants are vital nursing functions. Care of chest tubes is an additional responsibility and is similar to, but not always the same as, that with older children (Merenstein and Gardner, 1998). Attention to pain management with the procedure is vital in these preverbal and significantly stressed infants.

## Bronchopulmonary Dysplasia (BPD)

**BPD,** also known as *chronic lung disease (CLD),* is a pathologic process that may develop in primarily ELBW and VLBW infants with RDS. BPD may also develop in infants with MAS, persistent pulmonary hypertension, pneumonia, and cyanotic heart disease. Infants who survive are at risk for frequent hospitalization because of their borderline respiratory reserve, hyperactive airway, and increased susceptibility to respiratory infection.

BPD/CLD is operationally defined in clinical trials as (1) history of mechanical ventilation, oxygen dependency, and abnormal pulmonary radiographic findings at 28 days of age or (2) the same characteristic findings at 36 weeks postmenstrual age (Cole and Fiascone, 2000). An inverse relationship to the incidence of BPD/CLD and birthweight is emphasized in the Vermont-Oxford Network report where a 60% incidence was reported for ELBW (501 to 750 g) vs 21% for infants weighing 1001 to 1250 g. Risk factors for BPD/CLD include surfactant use (increased survival of ELBW and LBW infants), prenatal and postnatal (nosocomial) infections, patent ductus arteriosus (PDA), and fluid balance (Marshall and others, 1999; Cole and Fiascone, 2000; Bancalari, 2001).

The more severe form of BPD/CLD usually begins with severe respiratory failure secondary to RDS or with pneumonia requiring mechanical ventilation with high airway pressure and oxygen supplementation during the first few days of life (Bancalari, 2001). Since the advent of antenatal glucocorticoid therapy, surfactant replacement, and new ventilator strategies, a "new" BPD/CLD is emerging as well (Bancalari, 2001; Cole and Fiascone, 2000). These infants experience a milder initial respiratory course but continue to require ventilatory support or oxygen supplementation and show radiographic pulmonary changes characteristic with BPD/CLD.

### Pathophysiology

The pathogenesis of BPD/CLD is complex and multifactorial. BPD/CLD begins with the immature lung that undergoes an initial injury leading to a chronic inflammatory process that results in recurrent injury and abnormal healing (Cole and Fiascone, 2000; Bancalari, 2001). A variety of mechanisms have been related to the initial injury: (1) prenatal infection (inflammatory process before birth), (2) mechanical ventilation (volutrauma, intubation), (3) supplemental oxygen (oxygen-derived free radicals), (4) increased pulmonary blood flow from PDA, or (5) postnatal infection.

The pulmonary changes are characterized by interstitial edema and epithelial swelling followed by thickening and fibrotic proliferation of the alveolar walls and squamous metaplasia of the bronchiolar epithelium. Areas of atelectasis and cystlike foci of hyperaeration are visible on radiographs between 10 and 20 days of life and persist for weeks; however, some infants may not demonstrate cystic foci. In addition, ciliary activity is paralyzed by high oxygen concentrations that interfere with the ability to clear the lung of mucus, thus aggravating airway obstruction and atelectasis. As the infant's lungs begin healing, the process is altered, possibly by continuous high oxygenation, inadequate nutrition, or vitamin E deficiency, resulting in decreased surface for $O_2$ and $CO_2$ exchange. The overall results of this process are hypercarbia, hypoxemia, and subsequent inability to wean successfully from mechanical ventilation.

As survival of immature preterm infants (less than 28 weeks gestation) increases, the occurrence of BPD/CLD also increases. Despite the fact that management of $O_2$ therapy, volutrauma, fluids, and PDA has improved, BPD/CLD is still on the rise in ELBW and VLBW infants.

The marked similarity between BPD/CLD and *Wilson-Mikity syndrome,* in which the lungs of premature infants exhibit alveolar thickening and cystlike patterns of hyperventilation, has led some investigators to theorize that the two disorders may be part of a continuous spectrum of the same lung disease. Other diseases associated with similar radiographic findings include congenital heart disease and viral pneumonia caused by cytomegalovirus. There are no laboratory alterations that confirm a diagnosis; diagnosis is made on the basis of radiographic findings, oxygen or positive-pressure ventilation >28 days, signs of respiratory distress, and a history of requiring mechanical ventilation in the first week of life for more than 3 days.

## Therapeutic Management

The first approach to management is prevention of the disorder in susceptible infants. Despite previous theorization that surfactant administration to preterm infants would eradicate BPD/CLD, studies so far have failed to show a significant decrease of BPD/CLD in infants receiving surfactant for prophylaxis or rescue. To reduce the risk of volutrauma when positive pressure ventilation is being used, the lowest peak inspiratory pressure necessary to obtain adequate ventilation is maintained, and the lowest level of inspired oxygen is used to maintain adequate oxygenation. Fluid administration is carefully controlled and restricted. Drug or surgical intervention is indicated when there is significant shunting of blood through the PDA.

There is no specific treatment for BPD/CLD except to maintain adequate arterial blood gases with the administration of oxygen and to avoid progression of the disease. Corticosteroid (dexamethasone) therapy has been shown to benefit infants with BPD/CLD by decreasing the pulmonary inflammatory response and improving oxygenation and gas exchange, resulting in earlier weaning from mechanical assistance. However, complications such as sepsis, hypertension, hyperglycemia, glycosuria, and occult positive stools and an overall lack of decreased mortality in such infants has caused this therapy to remain controversial. In light of recent studies that show an increased incidence of periventricular leukomalacia, neuromotor abnormalities, cerebral palsy, decreased cerebral cortical gray matter volume, and adverse long-term neurologic outcome, the risk may not outweigh the benefits of this treatment (American Academy of Pediatrics and Canadian Paediatric Society, 2002; Murphy, 2001; Thebaud and others, 2001). Other adverse effects of this long-acting, potent glucocorticoid have been reported: growth retardation, hyperglycemia, hypertension, infection, GI hemorrhage, and cardiomyopathy. Weaning infants from the ventilator is difficult and must be accomplished gradually.

These infants do not tolerate excessive or even normal amounts of fluid well and have a tendency to accumulate interstitial fluid in the lungs, which aggravates the condition.

Oral diuretics are used to control interstitial fluid. Nebulized or metered dose inhaler (MDI) bronchodilators (albuterol) and inhaled steroids may be effective and promote improvement in infants with chronic lung disease. Theophylline improves lung compliance and reduces expiratory resistance in ventilated infants with BPD/CLD. Oral electrolyte supplements are given to replace those lost with concurrent oral diuretics and renal water losses.

Growth and development are often delayed in infants with BPD/CLD, which is related in part to the difficulties in providing adequate nutrition and in part to the lack of normal sensory stimulation because of prolonged hospitalization. Children with BPD/CLD have metabolic needs far greater than those of the average infant. This can create a problem for the caregiver, who must meet the goals of adequate nutrition while avoiding overhydration, especially if the child is ill, eats poorly, or has cardiopulmonary instability. The infant may be further compromised by gastroesophageal reflux, a frequent complication in premature infants. (See Chapter 33.)

Osteopenia commonly occurs in infants with BPD/CLD and in preterm infants, with higher incidence among the infants with BPD/CLD, presumably because of low calcium and vitamin D intake secondary to the calciuric effects of diuretic therapy.

*RSV immune globulin* (RSV-IGIV, RespiGam) and *palivizumab* (Synagis) have been shown to be effective agents in diminishing the complications of respiratory syncitial virus (RSV). RSV is a common cause for hospitalization and mortality in growing preterm neonates, including those with BPD/CLD. RespiGam is given intravenously over several hours, preferably before the beginning of RSV season and repeated once a month during the peak season. Palivizumab is preferred over RespiGam because it can be given intramuscularly to high-risk infants, does not interfere with other immunizations, and has few side effects (American Academy of Pediatrics, 1998). Palivizumab is administered in a dose of 15 mg/kg once a month, usually beginning in October and ending in May. In the first full season in which palivizumab was used as a preventive measure for RSV, hospitalization rates among preterm infants and infants with BPD/CLD were significantly reduced (Sorrentino and Powers, 2000). (See Respiratory Syncitial Virus, Chapter 32.)

**Prognosis.**   Reports vary regarding the mortality rate for BPD/CLD. The hospital stay is often long because of the infant's need for supplemental oxygen, although home oxygen therapy provides selected infants the opportunity for discharge. However, a significant proportion of deaths occur after discharge from the hospital. A nasal cannula provides an acceptable way to administer oxygen for the dependent infant to promote development of motor and social skills. Long-term problems seen in older children who had BPD/CLD as infants include growth failure, airway hyperreactivity, hyperexpansion, increased incidence of respiratory infections, and airway obstruction.

A study of school-age children compared pulmonary function, nutritional status, anthropometric measurements, body composition, intelligence, and resting energy expenditure in three distinct groups: BPD/CLD, term control, and preterm control. The researchers found that the BPD/CLD group had decreased pulmonary function, lower bone mineral density, and lower intelligence scores than their counterpart term and preterm controls. Both BPD/CLD and preterm children were of shorter stature and had significantly lower intelligence scores than the term group (Giacoia and others, 1997).

### Nursing Considerations

Infants with BPD/CLD expend considerable energy in their efforts to breathe; therefore it is important that they receive plenty of opportunities for rest and additional calories. Growth records provide clues to the need for change in their diets, and some infants require nutritional supplements. Because these infants tire easily and because large quantities of formula might compromise respiration, small, frequent feedings are better tolerated. Reducing environmental stimuli and subsequent hypoxia is an important aspect in the care of these infants. Close attention to the infant's behavioral cues is important in the older infant with BPD/CLD because these cues may signal $CO_2$ retention.

Adequate hydration is extremely important because greater amounts of fluid are lost through respiration, and secretions must be thinned sufficiently to facilitate removal by suctioning. However, because BPD/CLD increases lung permeability, many infants are subject to pulmonary edema and require fluid restriction.

Because the growing infant with BPD/CLD has a restricted fluid intake, has higher than average caloric requirements, and often requires many oral medications, the nurse is challenged by the complexity of care involved. Infants with BPD/CLD may become difficult or maladaptive feeders if they are aware of hunger yet compromised by not being able to eat fast enough to satiate that hunger because of the increased labor of breathing. Individualized nursing care aimed at increasing oxygenation needs during feedings, decreasing environmental stimuli, fortifying feedings, and providing more contact with a primary caregiver may facilitate the infant's care. Feeding schedules should be individualized as much as possible. Oral medications that taste bad to the infant may be given at times separate from feedings to enhance feeding time as a pleasant experience rather than one associated with forced oral administration of medications. Adjustments to overall fluid administration requirements are made, taking into account that the oral medications are also fluids. Regurgitated medications and feedings need to be dealt with in regard to fluid and caloric needs and the amount of absorption of medication that occurs before emesis.

Parents are extremely anxious regarding the prognosis when their infant has BPD/CLD. In addition, the lengthy hospitalization interferes with parent-child relationships and deprives the infant of parental stimulation. Nurses should encourage the parents to visit the infant and become involved in the routine care. The parents need to be informed regarding medical care, equipment, and procedures related to their infant and taught procedures such as suctioning and chest physiotherapy.

The older infant with BPD/CLD should be provided with normal nurturing and developmental opportunities appropriate to the infant's condition and abilities. Careful monitoring of physiologic and behavioral systems during any activity is necessary so that activity can be stopped before the infant becomes irritable or tired. Opportunities out of bed in an infant seat or on a floor mat with a nurse or therapist provides one-on-one interaction that can enhance the infant's experience of the world and people. Irritability has been associated with infants who have BPD/CLD, making their care often challenging and sometimes frustrating (see Developmental Outcome, p. 357). Some strategies to facilitate infant coping during prolonged hospitalization include (1) decreased number of unfamiliar caregivers, (2) increased access to their parents, (3) predictability in schedule and caregivers, (4) consistency of care routines and practices, (5) pleasurable opportunities for play and socialization within physical tolerance, (6) adequate nutrition, and (7) uninterrupted rest cycles with diurnal variation to facilitate biologic rhythms. Parental involvement is critical because they are the one constant for the infant.

**Home Care.** Because the availability of home cardiac and apnea monitors and home oxygen therapy has increased, many infants with BPD/CLD can be discharged when they are gaining weight and their oxygen need is low. Home care is desirable to promote parent-infant bonding, minimize health care costs, and prevent nosocomial infections. Preparation for home care requires education and considerable reassurance. (See Chapter 26.) Management of home monitoring equipment and home oxygen therapy is stress provoking, but most families become comfortable with the machinery while their infant is still in the hospital. Families must be reminded about their infant's increased risk of infection and cautioned regarding contact with persons who have respiratory infections. Because of their minimum respiratory reserve, these infants can be threatened by even a minor illness.

Some infants are discharged with tracheostomies on oxygen supplementation or home ventilators. Discharge teaching and home care nursing (minimum of 2 weeks to several months) is crucial to the safe and successful transition of these infants into the community and home setting. Parents are taught how to advocate for appropriate home care and supplies in anticipation of future needs.

Because of the high mortality rate in the first year, parents are taught cardiopulmonary resuscitation* and how to manage any other emergency that might be anticipated for their infant. Helping families cope with their anxieties and reas-

---

**NURSING ALERT**
Nurses must be alert to signs of both overhydration and underhydration, such as weight changes, electrolytes, output measurements, urine specific gravity, and signs of edema.

---

*Home care instructions are available in Wong DL, Hess CS: *Wong and Whaley's clinical manual of pediatric nursing* ed 5, St Louis, 2000, Mosby.

suring them of their ability to manage the care of their infant are important nursing functions. Parents need follow-up in the home and the comfort of knowing that help is only a telephone call away.

# HIGH RISK RELATED TO INFECTIOUS PROCESSES

## Sepsis

Sepsis, or septicemia, refers to a generalized bacterial infection in the bloodstream. Neonates are highly susceptible to infection as a result of diminished nonspecific (inflammatory) and specific (humoral) immunity, such as impaired phagocytosis, delayed chemotactic response, minimal or absent immunoglobulin A and immunoglobulin M (IgA and IgM), and decreased complement levels. Because of the infant's poor response to pathogenic agents, there is usually no local inflammatory reaction at the portal of entry to signal an infection, and the resulting symptoms tend to be vague and nonspecific. Consequently, diagnosis and treatment may be delayed.

Although the mortality from sepsis has diminished, the incidence of septicemia has not. Nursery epidemics are not infrequent, and the high-risk infant has a four times greater chance of developing septicemia than does the normal neonate. The frequency of infection is almost twice as great in male infants as in females and also carries a higher mortality for males. Other factors increasing the risk of infection are prematurity, invasive procedures such as peripheral IV therapy and ET tubes, steroid use for chronic lung disease, and nosocomial exposure to a number of pathogens in the NICU. Proper handling of formula and supplies such as syringes and gavage tubes is vital to the prevention of infection.

Breast-feeding has a protective benefit against infection. Colostrum contains agglutinins that are effective against gram-negative bacteria. Human milk contains large quantities of IgA and iron-binding protein that exert a bacteriostatic effect on *Escherichia coli.* Human milk also contains macrophages and lymphocytes that promote a local inflammatory reaction.

## Pathophysiology

The premature withdrawal of the placental barrier leaves infants vulnerable to most common viral, bacterial, fungal, and parasitic infections. Immune substances, primarily immunoglobulin G (IgG), are normally acquired from the maternal system and stored in fetal tissues during the final weeks of gestation to provide newborns with passive immunity to a variety of infectious agents. Early birth interrupts this transplacental transmission; thus preterm infants have a low level of circulating IgG; the concentrations of immune substances directly relate to the length of gestation. IgA, which plays a role in defense against viral infections, and IgM, with properties that are most efficient in dealing with gram-negative organisms, are not transferred to the fetus, which leaves infants highly vulnerable to invasion by these organisms.

Defense mechanisms of neonates are further hampered by a low level of complement, diminished opsonization ability, monocyte dysfunction, and a reduced number and inefficient functioning of circulating leukocytes. Furthermore, these leukocytes with diminished motility and phagocytic capacity are unable to concentrate their limited numbers selectively at the site of infection. In addition, a hypofunctioning adrenal gland contributes only a meager antiinflammatory response. Consequently, these deficiencies permit rapid invasion, spread, and multiplication of organisms.

### Sources of Infection

Sepsis in the neonatal period can be acquired prenatally across the placenta from the maternal bloodstream or during labor from ingestion or aspiration of infected amniotic fluid. Prolonged rupture of the membranes always presents a risk for maternal-fetal transfer of pathogenic organisms. In utero transplacental transfer can occur with organisms and viruses such as cytomegalovirus, toxoplasmosis, and *Treponema pallidum* (syphilis), which cross the placental barrier during the latter half of pregnancy.

Early sepsis (less than 3 days) is acquired in the perinatal period; infection can occur from direct contact with organisms from the maternal gastrointestinal and genitourinary tracts. The most common infecting organisms are group B streptococcus (GBS) and *E. coli,* which may be present in the vagina. *E. coli* accounts for approximately two thirds of all cases of sepsis caused by gram-negative organisms. GBS has emerged as an extremely virulent organism in neonates, with a high (50%) death rate in affected infants. In a multicenter study of early onset sepsis in VLBW infants, *Haemophilus influenzae* was the third most common causative organism; coagulase-negative staphylococci also emerged in early-onset sepsis in VLBW neonates (Stoll and others, 1996). Other pathogens that are harbored in the vagina and may infect the infant include gonococci, *Candida albicans,* herpes simplex virus (type II), *Listeria* organisms, and chlamydia.

Late sepsis (1 to 3 weeks following birth) is primarily nosocomial, and the offending organisms are usually staphylococci, *Klebsiella,* enterococci, and *Pseudomonas.* Coagulase-negative staphylococcus, considered to be primarily a contaminant in older children and adults, is commonly found to be the cause of septicemia in ELBW and VLBW infants. Bacterial invasion can occur through sites such as the umbilical stump; the skin; mucous membranes of the eye, nose, pharynx, and ear; and internal systems such as the respiratory, nervous, urinary, and GI systems.

Postnatal infection is acquired by cross-contamination from other infants, personnel, or objects in the environment. Bacteria that are commonly called "water bugs" (because they are able to grow in water) are found in water supplies, humidifying apparatus, sink drains, suction machines, most respiratory equipment, and indwelling venous and arterial catheters used for infusions, blood sampling, and monitoring vital signs. Neonatal sepsis is most common in the infant at risk, particularly the preterm infant or the infant born following a difficult or traumatic labor and delivery, who is least capable of resisting such bacterial invasion. These organisms are often transmitted by the personnel from person to person or object to person by poor handwashing and inadequate housecleaning.

## Clinical Manifestations

A few neonatal infections (e.g., pyoderma, conjunctivitis, omphalitis, and mastitis) are easily recognized. However, systemic infections are characterized by subtle, vague, nonspecific, and almost imperceptible physical signs. Often the only complaint concerning an infant's progress is "failure to do well," not looking "right," or nonspecific respiratory distress. Rarely is there any indication of a local inflammatory response, which would suggest the portal of entry into the bloodstream. The presence of bacteria is indicated by a specific characteristic. For example, *Pseudomonas* organisms produce necrotic purplish skin lesions, and group B β-hemolytic streptococci usually result in severe respiratory distress, periods of apnea, and a chest radiograph similar to that of RDS.

All body systems tend to show some indication of sepsis, although often there is little correlation between the manifestations and the etiologic factors involved. For example, seizures and fever, a universal feature of infection in older children, may be absent in neonates. It is usually the nursing observation of subtle changes in the appearance and behavior of infants that leads to the detection of infection. The nonspecific, early signs are hypothermia and changes in color, tone, activity, and feeding behavior; in addition,

sudden episodes of apnea and unexplained desaturations may signal an infection. Significantly, similar signs may be manifestations of a number of clinical conditions unrelated to sepsis, such as hypoglycemia, hypocalcemia, heroin withdrawal, or CNS disorders.

Preterm infants, particularly ELBW and VLBW infants, are highly suspect for early sepsis and pneumonia occurring concurrently with RDS because preterm delivery has been increasingly shown to be associated with a maternal bacterial pathogen. ELBW and VLBW infants are also highly susceptible to fungal and viral infections; investigation for such agents should be implemented when sepsis is suspected in this population. Because meningitis is a common sequela of sepsis, the neonate is evaluated for bacterial growth in cerebrospinal fluid (CSF); clinical signs of neonatal meningitis, particularly in VLBW infants, may not demonstrate typical features of older infants. Clinical signs that may indicate possible neonatal sepsis are listed in Box 10-11.

## Diagnostic Evaluation

Because sepsis is so easily confused with other neonatal disorders, the definitive diagnosis is established by laboratory and radiographic examination. Isolation of the specific organism is always attempted through cultures of blood, urine, and CSF. Blood studies may show signs of anemia, leukocytosis, or leukopenia. Leukopenia is usually an ominous sign because of its frequent association with high mortality. An elevated number of immature neutrophils, decreased or increased total neutrophils, and changes in neutrophil morphology also suggest an infectious process in the neonate. Other diagnostic data that are helpful in the determination of neonatal sepsis include C-reactive protein and interleukins, specifically interleukin-6 (Kuster and others, 1998; Bomela and others, 2000; Kallman and others, 1999; Horns, 2000).

## Therapeutic Management

In addition to the institution of vigorous therapeutic measures, early recognition and diagnosis are essential to increase the infant's chance for survival and reduce the likelihood of permanent neurologic damage. Diagnosis of sepsis is often based on suspicion of initial clinical signs and symptoms, and antibiotic therapy is initiated before laboratory results are available for confirmation and identification of the exact organism. Treatment consists of circulatory support, respiratory support, aggressive administration of antibiotics, and immunotherapy.

Supportive therapy usually involves administration of oxygen (if respiratory distress or hypoxia is evident), careful regulation of fluids, correction of electrolyte or acid-base imbalance, and temporary discontinuation of oral feedings. Blood transfusion may be needed to correct anemia and shock, and electronic monitoring of vital signs and regulation of the thermal environment are mandatory.

Antibiotic therapy is continued for 7 to 10 days if cultures are positive, discontinued in 3 days if cultures are negative and the infant is asymptomatic, and most often administered via IV infusion. Antifungal and/or antiviral therapies are implemented as appropriate, depending on causative

---

**Box 10-11** ■ ■ ■
### Manifestations Observed in Neonatal Sepsis

**GENERAL SIGNS**
Infant generally "not doing well"
Poor temperature control—hypothermia, hyperthermia (rare)

**CIRCULATORY SYSTEM**
Pallor, cyanosis, or mottling
Cold, clammy skin
Hypotension
Edema
Irregular heartbeat—bradycardia, tachycardia

**RESPIRATORY SYSTEM**
Irregular respirations, apnea, or tachypnea
Cyanosis
Grunting
Dyspnea
Retractions

**CENTRAL NERVOUS SYSTEM**
Diminished activity—lethargy, hyporeflexia, coma
Increased activity—irritability, tremors, seizures
Full fontanel
Increased or decreased tone
Abnormal eye movements

**GASTROINTESTINAL SYSTEM**
Poor feeding
Vomiting
Diarrhea or decreased stooling
Abdominal distention
Hepatomegaly
Hemoccult-positive stools

**HEMATOPOIETIC SYSTEM**
Jaundice
Pallor
Petechiae, ecchymosis
Splenomegaly

agents. Transfusions with fresh, irradiated granulocytes or polymorphonuclear leukocytes obtained from adult donors by continuous-flow centrifugation leukapheresis have been introduced as therapy for bacterial sepsis. The results have proved to be highly effective in lowering mortality from this disease. Intravenous immunoglobulin therapy has also proved effective as a prophylactic measure against infection and for the treatment of documented infections.

**Prognosis.** The prognosis for neonatal sepsis is variable. Severe neurologic and respiratory sequelae may occur in ELBW and VLBW infants as a result of early-onset sepsis. Late-onset sepsis and meningitis may also result in poor outcomes for immunocompromised neonates. The trend in antenatal screening, diagnosis, and treatment of maternal group B streptococcus has positively affected infection rates in some centers among full-term infants, although not all studies report enthusiastic results, perhaps because of the existence of a number of screening and treatment protocols (Gilson and others, 2000; Locksmith, Clark, and Duff, 1999; Gervasio and others, 2001).

The introduction of new markers (interleukins) for neonatal sepsis may prove to be particularly helpful in differentiating true sepsis from RDS early on and guiding antibiotic therapy (Horns, 2000; Kallman and others, 1999). Future experimental methods being explored to combat infection in neonates include monoclonal antibody therapy, fibronectin infusion, and lymphokine enhancement.

### Nursing Considerations

Nursing care of the infant with sepsis involves observation and assessment as outlined for any high-risk infant. Recognition of the existing problem is of paramount importance; it is usually the nurse who observes and assesses infants and identifies that "something is wrong" with them. Awareness of the potential modes of infection transmission also helps the nurse identify those at risk for developing sepsis. Much of the care of infants with sepsis involves the medical treatment of the illness. Knowledge of the side effects of the specific antibiotic and proper regulation and administration of the drug are vital. Because the volume of fluid required to administer antibiotics via Soluset or Buretrol would seriously compromise a small infant, antibiotics are usually administered via a special injection port near the infusion site. The medication is administered slowly by mechanical pump.

Prolonged antibiotic therapy poses additional hazards for affected infants. Oral antibiotics, if administered, destroy intestinal flora responsible for the synthesis of vitamin K, which can reduce blood coagulability. In addition, antibiotics predispose the infant to growth of resistant organisms and superinfection from fungal or mycotic agents, such as *C. albicans.* Nurses must be alert for evidence of such complications. Nystatin oral suspension may be administered for prophylaxis against oral candidiasis.

A number of specimens may be needed to help identify the cause and source of the infection. It is recommended that the fully flexed position be avoided for obtaining spinal fluid and that the side-lying position (modified with neck extension) or sitting position be used for obtaining spinal fluid specimens. Continual cardiorespiratory and pulse

oximetry monitoring provides an ongoing assessment of the infant's condition during the procedure.

Part of the total care of infants with sepsis is to decrease any additional physiologic or environmental stress. This includes providing an optimum thermoregulated environment and anticipating potential problems such as dehydration or hypoxia. Precautions are implemented to prevent the spread of infection to other newborns, but to be effective, activities must be carried out by all caregivers. Proper handwashing, the use of disposable equipment (e.g., linens, catheters, feeding supplies, and IV equipment), disposing of excretions (e.g., vomitus and stool), and adequate housekeeping of the environment and equipment are essential. Because nurses are the most consistent caregivers involved with sick infants, it is usually their responsibility to oversee that all phases of isolation are maintained by everyone.

Another aspect of caring for infants with sepsis involves observation for signs of complications, including meningitis and septic shock, a severe complication caused by toxins in the bloodstream.

A number of viral agents, namely cytomegalovirus, herpes, hepatitis, and HIV, may also be transmitted to the fetus from the mother. When acquired prenatally (congenital), these viruses represent a serious threat to the infant's life. (See Table 9-5 for viral infections.)

## Necrotizing Enterocolitis (NEC)

NEC is an acute inflammatory disease of the bowel with increased incidence in preterm and other high-risk infants; it is most common in infants who are preterm. Three factors appear to play an important role in the development of NEC: intestinal ischemia, colonization by pathogenic bacteria, and substrate (formula feeding) in the intestinal lumen.

### Pathophysiology

The precise cause of NEC is still uncertain, but it appears to occur in infants whose GI tract has suffered vascular compromise. Intestinal ischemia of unknown etiology, immature GI host defenses, bacterial proliferation, and feeding substrate are now believed to have a multifactorial role in the etiology of NEC. Prematurity remains the most prominent risk factor in the development of NEC (McElhinney and others, 2000).

The damage to mucosal cells lining the bowel wall is great. Diminished blood supply to these cells causes their death in large numbers; they stop secreting protective, lubricating mucus; and the thin, unprotected bowel wall is attacked by proteolytic enzymes. Thus the bowel wall continues to swell and break down; it is unable to synthesize protective IgM, and the mucosa is permeable to macromolecules (e.g., exotoxins), which further hampers intestinal defenses. Gas-forming bacteria invade the damaged areas to produce ***pneumatosis intestinalis,*** the presence of air in the submucosal or subserosal surfaces of the bowel.

### Clinical Manifestations

The prominent clinical signs of NEC are a distended (often shining) abdomen, gastric retention, and blood in the stools.

Because NEC closely mimics or resembles septicemia, the infant may have that "not looking well" appearance. Nonspecific signs include lethargy, poor feeding, hypotension, apnea, vomiting (often bile-stained), decreased urine output, and hypothermia. The onset is usually between 4 and 10 days after the initiation of feedings, but signs may be evident as early as 4 hours of age and as late as 30 days. NEC in full-term infants almost always occurs in the first 10 days of life; late-onset NEC is confined primarily to preterm infants and coincides with the onset of feedings after passing through the acute phase of an illness such as RDS.

## Diagnostic Evaluation

Radiographic studies show a sausage-shaped dilation of the intestine that progresses to marked distention and the characteristic pneumatosis intestinalis—"soapsuds," or the bubbly appearance of thickened bowel wall and ultralumina. There may be air in the portal circulation or free air observed in the abdomen, indicating perforation. Laboratory findings may include anemia, leukopenia, leukocytosis, metabolic acidosis, and electrolyte imbalance. In severe cases coagulopathy (disseminated intravascular coagulation [DIC]) and/or thrombocytopenia may be evident. Organisms are often cultured from blood, although bacteremia or septicemia may not be prominent early in the course of the disease.

## Therapeutic Management

Treatment of NEC begins with prevention. Oral feedings may be withheld for at least 24 to 48 hours from infants who are believed to have suffered birth asphyxia and as long as deemed necessary from ELBW and VLBW infants. Breast milk is the preferred enteral nutrient because it confers some passive immunity (IgA), macrophages, and lysozymes.

*Minimal enteral feedings* (trophic feeding, GI priming) have gained acceptance with no increased incidence of NEC. Early experience shows that such feedings may in fact be protective against NEC in nonasphyxiated preterm infants (Schanler and others, 1999; Newell, 2000). Some researchers, however, dispute the advantages of such feedings in prevention of NEC (Tyson and Kennedy, 2000). Others have demonstrated a reduction of risk of NEC by 84% following the implementation of a standardized feeding protocol in infants weighing 1250 to 2500 g and who are less than 35 weeks gestation (Kamitsuka, Horton, and Williams, 2000).

Medical treatment of confirmed NEC consists of discontinuation of all oral feedings, institution of abdominal decompression via nasogastric suction, administration of IV antibiotics, and correction of extravascular volume depletion, electrolyte abnormalities, acid-base imbalances, and hypoxia. Replacing oral feedings with parenteral fluids decreases the need for oxygen and circulation to the bowel. Serial abdominal radiograph films (every 4 to 6 hours in the acute phase) are taken to monitor for possible progression of the disease to intestinal perforation.

**Prognosis.** With early recognition and treatment, medical management is increasingly successful. If there is progressive deterioration under medical management or evidence of perforation, surgical resection and anastomosis are performed. Extensive involvement may necessitate establishment of an ileostomy, jejunostomy, or colostomy. Sequelae in surviving infants include short-bowel syndrome or short-gut-syndrome (SGS) (see Chapter 33), colonic stricture with obstruction, fat malabsorption, and failure to thrive secondary to intestinal dysfunction. Intestinal transplantation has been successful in some former preterm patients with NEC-associated SGS who had already developed life-threatening TPN-related complications. Over 50% of these patients survived with improved quality of life. Transplantation may be a life-saving option for infants who previously faced high morbidity and mortality (Vennarecci, 2000).

## Nursing Considerations

Nursing responsibilities begin with early recognition. The nurse is a key factor in the prompt recognition of the early warning signs of NEC. Because the signs are similar to those observed in many other disorders of the newborn, nurses must constantly be aware of the possibility of this disease.

> **NURSING ALERT** Observe for indications of early development of NEC by checking the abdomen frequently for distention (measuring abdominal girth, measuring residual gastric contents before feedings, and listening for the presence of bowel sounds) and performing all routine assessments for high-risk neonates.

When the disease is suspected, the nurse assists with diagnostic procedures and implements the therapeutic regimen. Vital signs, including blood pressure, are monitored for changes that might indicate bowel perforation, septicemia, or cardiovascular shock, and measures are instituted to prevent possible transmission to other infants. It is especially important to avoid rectal temperatures because of the increased danger of perforation. To avoid pressure on the distended abdomen and to facilitate continuous observation, infants are often left undiapered and positioned supine or on the side.

Conscientious attention to nutritional and hydration needs is essential, and antibiotics are administered as prescribed. The time at which oral feedings are reinstituted varies considerably but is usually at least 7 to 10 days following diagnosis and treatment. Sterile water or electrolyte solution may be given initially and followed by dilute human milk (if available) or elemental formula such as Pregestimil. The concentration is gradually increased as tolerated until the infant is again taking full-strength feedings.

Because NEC is an infectious disease, one of the most important nursing functions is control of infection. Strict handwashing is the primary barrier to spread, and confirmed multiple cases are isolated. Persons with symptoms of a GI should not care for these or any other infants.

The infant who requires surgery requires the same careful attention and observation as any infant with abdominal surgery, including ostomy care (as applicable). This disorder is one of the most common reasons for performing ileostomies on newborns. Throughout the medical and surgical management of infants with NEC, the nurse is continually alert to signs of complications, such as septicemia, DIC, hypoglycemia, and other metabolic derangements.

# HIGH RISK RELATED TO CARDIOVASCULAR/ HEMATOLOGIC COMPLICATIONS

## Patent Ductus Arteriosus (PDA)

A common complication of severe respiratory disease in preterm infants is PDA. It occurs in the majority of preterm infants under 1200 g, and the incidence diminishes in direct relationship to increasing birth weight. During fetal life the ductus remains patent through the vasodilatory action of prostaglandins within its tissues. Postnatally the increase in oxygen tension has a constricting effect on the ductus, but it may reopen in preterm infants in response to the lowered oxygen tension associated with respiratory impairment.

Lack of ductal smooth muscle in premature infants also prolongs patency of the ductus arteriosus. Functional closure occurs usually within 3 to 4 days, but complete anatomic closure with fibrosis and permanent sealing of the lumen may take up to 2 to 3 weeks.

### Clinical Manifestations

Signs of PDA may appear within the first week of life. Early signs are increased $PaCO_2$, decreased $PaO_2$, increased $FIO_2$, and recurrent apnea. Other signs include bounding peripheral pulses, wide pulse pressure with decreased diastolic blood pressure, pericardial hyperactivity, cardiomegaly, and a systolic or continuous murmur usually referred to as a "machinery-type" murmur heard loudest in systole. If the PDA is wide open, a murmur may not be heard. Spontaneous closure usually occurs (usually within 12 weeks), but in infants with severe lung involvement the left-to-right shunting of blood leads to life-threatening pulmonary insufficiency. Confirmation of the diagnosis is by echocardiography.

### Therapeutic Management

Therapy consists of careful fluid regulation, respiratory support, diuretic therapy, and administration of indomethacin, a prostaglandin synthetase inhibitor that has been successful in constricting the ductus in critically ill preterm infants. However, because the drug has been found to inhibit platelet function and affect renal function in neonates, close monitoring for bleeding and renal dysfunction is necessary. If a ductus reopens following cessation of therapy, readministration of the medication may produce a favorable response; as many as four doses may be used to accomplish ductal closure. Surgical ligation may be necessary if medical therapy is unsuccessful because ductal shunting is perceived as an important contribution to respiratory distress.

### Nursing Considerations

Nursing observations are important in the recognition and management of PDA. Assisting in early detection, assessing cardiovascular status carefully, and monitoring for complications following implementation of therapy are nursing responsibilities. The focus of activities related to therapy includes collection of specimens for laboratory examination, continued assessment of renal function (adequate urinary output, any abnormal laboratory findings such as blood urea nitrogen [BUN] and creatinine levels), and observation for any bleeding tendencies (Hematest-positive stools or gastric aspirate, oozing from heelsticks or venipuncture sites, and laboratory evidence of clotting abnormalities).

Postoperative care includes monitoring for pneumothorax or atelectasis on the affected side, assessment for bleeding and signs or symptoms of infection, supportive respiratory care, and pain management. Other nursing observations and management are the same as for the high-risk infant and the infant with PDA. (See Chapter 34.)

## Persistent Pulmonary Hypertension of the Newborn (PPHN)

PPHN, formerly known as *persistent fetal circulation (PFC)*, is a condition in which affected infants display severe pulmonary hypertension, with pulmonary artery pressure levels equal to or greater than systemic pressure, and large right-to-left shunts through both the foramen ovale and the ductus arteriosus. PPHN is a group of disorders having varied causes yet common presenting features and may be classified according to causative etiology (Walsh and Stork, 2001). Because full development of pulmonary arterial musculature occurs late in gestation, PPHN is primarily a condition of near-term, full-term, or postterm infants, many of whom were products of complicated pregnancies or deliveries. The condition is often associated with aspiration (especially meconium aspiration), congenital diaphragmatic hernia with severe respiratory distress, cold stress, respiratory distress (e.g., RDS or pneumonia), and septicemia (group B streptococcus). PPHN is believed to be precipitated by perinatal factors, such as perinatal asphyxia, that cause or contribute to vasoconstriction of the pulmonary vasculature.

PPHN can also be either primary or secondary. Primary PPHN occurs when the pulmonary vascular system fails to open with the initial respiration at birth; secondary PPHN results from hypoxic stress that increases pulmonary vascular resistance and causes a return to fetal cardiopulmonary circulation. PPHN is most commonly observed in infants at 35 to 44 weeks of gestation who have a history of perinatal asphyxia, metabolic acidosis, or sepsis and respiratory distress within the first 24 hours. The infants become hypoxic and display marked cyanosis, tachypnea with grunting and retractions, and decreased peripheral perfusion. A loud pulmonary component of the second heart sound and, sometimes, a systolic ejection murmur are present. Diagnosis is established from clinical signs and diagnostic tests, including chest radiography, ECG, and echocardiography.

### Therapeutic Management

Early recognition and management of conditions that contribute to or cause hypoxia and pulmonary vascular vasoconstriction is the primary goal in the prevention of PPHN. Additional treatment includes careful fluid regulation and evaluation of intravascular fluid volume. Supplemental oxygen is administered to reduce hypoxia and decrease pulmonary vasoconstriction. Assisted ventilation, often by HFV, is required if hypoxia is severe; this ventilation is accompanied by paralysis with a neuromuscular blocking agent to minimize opposition to the respirator. Vasodilators, such as tolazoline, are sometimes prescribed to decrease pulmonary vascular resistance, thereby decreasing right-to-left shunting and increasing cardiac output. Additional drug therapy used in the management of PPHN includes sodium bicarbonate or tromethamine (THAM) to maintain appropriate acid-base balance, volume expanders such as albumin or plasma, and the vasopressors dopamine, dobutamine, and nitroprusside to increase systemic vascular resistance (DeBoer and Stephens, 1997). The use of inhaled NO has been successfully used to reverse pulmonary vascular vasoconstriction and is often attempted before other therapies such as ECMO (see Nitric Oxide, p. 385). Liquid ventilation may also be advantageous for the treatment of PPHN, but clinical trials in neonates with this condition have yet to be completed (see Liquid Ventilation, p. 385).

Another approach to management of infants with pulmonary complications is the use of *extracorporeal membrane oxygenation (ECMO)* with a modified heart-lung machine. Blood is shunted from a catheter in the right atrium or right internal jugular vein by gravity to a servoregulated roller pump, pumped through a membrane lung and a small heat exchanger, and returned to the systemic circulation via a major artery, such as the carotid artery, to the aortic arch. A venovenous approach (femoral vein) may be used, thus avoiding the need to ligate the carotid artery. ECMO provides oxygen to the circulation and allows the lungs to rest. The goal of ECMO is to "buy time" for the severely injured lung to heal while effectively oxygenating major organ systems, including the brain, heart, kidneys, and lungs (Fig. 10-15). ECMO is very labor intensive and thus expensive. Technical malfunctions may occur, requiring frequent monitoring of the equipment and the patient's response to treatment. Typically, two nurses, or a nurse and a perfusionist, are required as minimum staffing for the ECMO patient; more staff, including a respiratory therapist, are required in the acute phase. ECMO requires heparinization of the blood and blood circuit; for this reason it is not used in infants less than 35 weeks of ges-

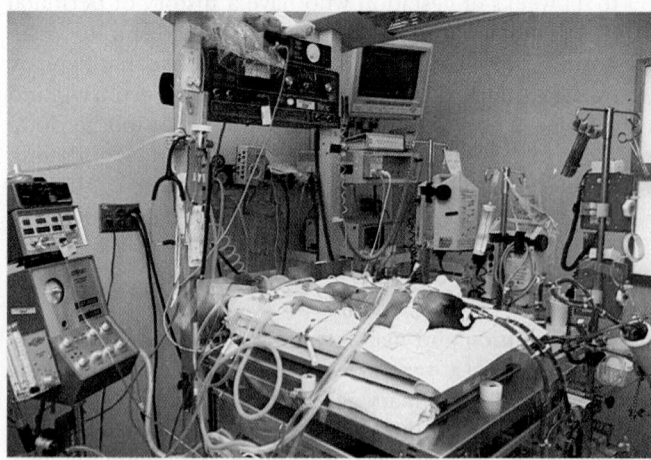

**Fig. 10-15** Infant on extracorporeal membrane oxygenation (ECMO).

tation who are prone to IVH. Bleeding is one of the major complications associated with ECMO. Some neonatal units have experienced a decrease in the need for ECMO with increased use of exogenous surfactant, inhaled NO, and high-frequency oscillatory ventilation (HFOV) for neonatal hypoxemic respiratory failure (Hintz and others, 2000).

### Nursing Considerations

The nursing care for PPHN is the same as for infants with severe respiratory difficulties and infants supported by mechanical ventilation and cardiovascular support. The infant with PPHN is often the sickest on the unit, depending on the causative factors and reaction to treatment. Because handling for any reason causes a decrease in arterial oxygen concentration, the stresses imposed by routine care must be weighed against the risk of iatrogenic hypoxia. It is important to decrease noxious stimuli that cause hypoxia and to use clustered nursing interventions that keep nonsedated infants calm. Continuous monitoring of oxygenation, temperature, central venous pressure, vital signs, blood pressure, and acid-base balance decreases the need for physical manipulation and disturbance. Infants are further assessed for response to treatments, including intravenous therapy, fluids and electrolytes, and the provision of exogenous glucose.

## Anemia

Preterm infants tend to develop anemia that is more severe and that appears earlier than in more mature infants. It may be a result of hemorrhage occurring during pregnancy and/or labor and delivery (loss of placental integrity, anomalies of the umbilical cord, fetomaternal hemorrhage), hemorrhage occurring during the neonatal period (intracranial hemorrhage, visceral trauma), or blood disorders (hemolytic disease, thrombocytopenia). Anemia may also be iatrogenic from blood withdrawn in the NICU for laboratory tests. Physiologic characteristics of prematurity tend to contribute to the development of anemia (i.e., a decreased red blood cell mass at birth and a drop in the production of hemoglobin and shortened survival time of the red blood cells). This lag in hematopoiesis during continued growth results in physiologic anemia, probably as a consequence of diminished erythropoietin values.

Fortunately, even VLBW infants are able to accommodate the GI absorption of iron required for their high needs. Iron is supplied in iron-fortified formulas or iron supplements as both a preventive and therapeutic measure. Transfusions with packed red blood cells are often required for severe anemia, usually for replacement of blood loss resulting from iatrogenic measures. At 4 to 12 weeks of age "physiologic anemia" reaches a peak, at which time infants sometimes display signs that suggest true anemia.

### Nursing Considerations

One of the most common causes of anemia in acutely ill preterm infants is blood loss associated with frequent sampling for blood gas and metabolic analyses. Therefore an important nursing responsibility is careful monitoring and recording of all blood drawn for tests. It is surprising how easily and rapidly the small total blood volume of preterm infants is depleted by repeated withdrawals. Replacement in light of hepatitis and HIV transmission is less frequent than previously. Investigations into the effectiveness of *recombinant human erythropoietin (r-HuEPO)* administration to increase erythrocyte production and decrease the need for blood transfusion in high-risk neonates have yielded mixed results. Recent studies found only a modest decrease in the overall volume of blood transfused to preterm infants weighing 1000 g or less who received r-HuEPO therapy (Vamvakas and Strauss, 2001). Ringer and others (1998) proposed that some critically ill infants may require and receive transfusion before r-HuEPO has time to stimulate erythropoiesis and that r-HuEPO therapy may be more effective in moderately ill infants who develop anemia of prematurity later and who have not sustained large phlebotomy losses within the first few weeks of life. Factors that are reported to significantly contribute to anemia of prematurity are large phlebotomy losses and the lack of standardized transfusion criteria (Ohls, 2000; Lin and others, 2000). Ohls (2000) contends that attention to blood amounts lost to phlebotomy and transfusion guidelines, in addition to standard r-HuEPO therapy, will likely decrease the necessity for frequent transfusions. Therapy with r-HuEPO may be administered weekly via either the intravenous or subcutaneous route.

Observation for signs of anemia is a vital nursing function. The signs of anemia in the preterm infant are poor feeding, decreased oxygen saturation, systolic murmur, dyspnea, tachycardia, tachypnea, diminished activity, and pallor. However, some infants may not display all of these signs. Poor weight gain may be an indication of a lowered hemoglobin level. (Nursing precautions and observations during blood transfusion are discussed in Chapter 35.)

## Polycythemia

The current definition of polycythemia is a venous hematocrit of 65% or more (Armentrout and Huseby, 2002). With a hematocrit above 65%, blood flow becomes increasingly sluggish and hyperviscous, resulting in hypoperfusion of organs. Polycythemia may result from in utero twin-to-twin transfusion and maternal-fetal transfusion, delayed cord clamping or stripping of the umbilical cord, or intrapartum asphyxia. The small-for-gestational-age infant is the most at risk for polycythemia; increased red blood cell consumption of glucose further predisposes the infant to hypoglycemia. Among infants with polycythemia there is a high incidence of cardiopulmonary distress symptoms (PPHN, cyanosis, and apnea), seizures, hyperbilirubinemia, and GI abnormalities.

Appropriate therapy for correcting metabolic disturbances (e.g., hypoxia, hypoglycemia, and hyperbilirubinemia) is implemented, and lowering blood viscosity by partial plasma exchange transfusion may be considered in symptomatic cases.

### Nursing Considerations

Nursing care involves watching for signs of polycythemia (e.g., plethora, peripheral cyanosis, respiratory distress, lethargy, jitteriness or seizure activity, hypoglycemia, hyperbilirubinemia) and assisting with diagnostic tests and therapeutic procedures. (Care of the infant with hyperbilirubinemia is discussed in Chapter 9.)

## Retinopathy of Prematurity (ROP)

Although often discussed in relation to respiratory dysfunction, ROP is a disorder involving blood vessels. ROP is a term used to describe all phases of retinal changes observed in preterm infants. The older term, *retrolental fibroplasia (RLF),* describes the cicatricial changes that characterize the later stages in the most severely affected infants. ROP is primarily, but not exclusively, a disease of premature infants. The incidence and severity of the disease correlates with the degree of the infant's maturity—the younger the gestational age, the greater the likelihood of the development of ROP, with extremely preterm infants being the group most at risk. There have been documented cases of ROP in term infants who received no oxygen therapy (Korones, 1996).

In addition to immaturity, numerous factors have been implicated in the cause of ROP, including hyperoxemia and hypoxemia, hypercarbia and hypocarbia, PDA, prostaglandin synthetase inhibitors, apnea, intralipid administration, IVH, infection, vitamin E and A deficiency, lactic acidosis, maternal diabetes, prenatal complications, exposure to light, and genetic factors. Previously considered to be an iatrogenic disease related to hyperoxia, ROP is now believed to be a complex disease of prematurity with multiple causes and therefore difficult to completely prevent.

The LIGHT-ROP study (Reynolds and others, 1998; Phelps and Watts, 2001) supports the conclusion that light reduction is not the solution for preventing ROP and resulting vision loss in preterm infants. There is still the question whether light affects the developing visual system through cerebral visual impairment (Fielder and Merrick, 2000). The effects of light exposure when such stimuli would not normally be present may result in aberrant cortical pathways for the visual system.

### Pathophysiology

ROP is characterized by severe vascular constriction in the immature retinal vasculature, followed by hypoxia in those areas. This appears to stimulate vascular proliferation of retinal capillaries into the hypoxic areas, where veins become numerous and dilate. As new vessels proliferate toward the lens, the aqueous humor and vitreous humor become turbid. The retina becomes edematous, and hemorrhages separate the retina from its attachment. Advanced scarring occurs from the retina to the lens, destroying the normal architecture of the eye. This extensive retinal detachment and scarring result in irreversible blindness.

### Diagnostic Evaluation

A system of classification (International Classification of Retinopathy of Prematurity [ICROP]) has been established to describe the location and extent of the developing vasculature involved. Normal vascular growth proceeds in an orderly fashion from the disc toward the *ora serrata,* the irregular anterior margin of the retina. The stages of ROP are outlined in Box 10-12. ROP is further classified by location

**Box 10-12** ■ ■ ■
**Stages of Retinopathy of Prematurity**

1. A demarcation line (separates the avascular retina anteriorly from the vascularized retina posteriorly)
2. A ridge (formed from the demarcation line with the height and width, occupies volume, and extends beyond the plane of the retina)
3. A ridge with extraretinal fibrovascular proliferation
4. Retinal detachment

"Plus" disease—increased dilation and tortuosity of peripheral retinal vessels (e.g., Stage 2 plus ROP)

Data from an International Classification of Retinopathy of Prematurity, *Pediatrics* 74:127-133, 1984; Merenstein GB, Gardner SL: *Handbook of neonatal intensive care,* ed 4, St Louis, 1998, Mosby; and Phelps DL: Retinopathy of prematurity, *Pediatr Clin North Am* 40(4):705-714, 1993.

of damage in the retina and by the extent of abnormally developing vascularization.

### Therapeutic Management

The management and treatment of ROP is primarily aimed at preventing fluctuations in arterial concentrations of oxygen in preterm neonates. It has been previously believed and taught that high oxygen concentrations in preterm infants contributed to the development of ROP. Initial studies indicate, however, that ROP is a multifactorial disease, primarily of preterm neonates, and oxygen saturation do not appear to be the causative factor. In some studies it has been reported that increased oxygen saturations (96% to 99%) may decrease the progression of ROP (The STOP-ROP Multicenter Study Group, 2000). Studies indicate also that decreasing ambient light exposure in preterm infants did not decrease the incidence of ROP (Phelps and Watts, 2001). The early recognition of ROP, treatment, and follow-up are essential components of disease management. The American Academy of Pediatrics, American Academy of Pediatric Ophthalmology and Strabismus, and the American Academy of Ophthalmology (1997) have issued a joint statement for appropriate screening guidelines in an effort to prevent and reduce the effects of the disease in preterm infants. An initial screening examination is recommended in infants <1500 g and/or a gestational age of <28 weeks at 4 to 6 weeks of age, or between 31 and 33 weeks postconception age, with additional follow-up. These guidelines may soon be revised because some studies have shown that intervention earlier than 31 to 33 weeks postconception age is needed to detect early ROP in ELBW infants (Subhani and others, 2001). With increased survival of extremely preterm infants, most authorities agree that the incidence of ROP is not likely to decrease until definitive causative factors are identified.

Although prevention is the primary goal of therapeutic management, treatment of retinal pathology is directed toward arresting the proliferation process. Cryotherapy and laser therapy are the most effective treatments when performed by a pediatric ophthalmologist.

### Nursing Considerations

The nursing care of extremely preterm infants and those at risk for development of ROP should focus on decreasing constant bright environmental light and stimuli and decreasing or avoiding events known to cause fluctuations in systemic blood pressure and oxygenation. Individualized care of the preterm infant is essential to aid in further decreasing the incidence of ROP.

Intraoperative nursing care for the infant undergoing either cryotherapy or laser surgery involves proper infant identification, stabilization and monitoring of vital signs as required, monitoring of IV therapy, and administration of the necessary medications. Postoperative nursing care also includes monitoring the infant for signs of pain and appropriate pain management as needed. After surgery the infant's eyelids will be edematous and closed; parents are informed of this preoperatively. Eye medications are administered as needed, and the infant's tolerance of these medications is monitored closely. Most infants are able to nipple feed once awake and alert in the postoperative period, depending on the feeding situation before surgery; breast-feeding infants should also be allowed to feed. When the infant suffers partial or complete visual impairment, the parents need a considerable amount of support and assistance in meeting the special developmental needs of the infant. (See Chapter 25.)

## HIGH RISK RELATED TO NEUROLOGIC DISTURBANCE

Neurologic complications are observed with increased frequency in preterm infants and in infants born following a difficult labor and delivery. A disproportionately high incidence of perinatal encephalopathy and psychomotor retardation is found in the high-risk infant population, especially ELBW and VLBW infants. Preterm infants are also more vulnerable to cerebral insults (e.g., hypoxia) and chemical alterations (e.g., decreased blood glucose). In addition, fragility and increased permeability of capillaries and prolonged prothrombin time predispose the preterm infant's brain to trauma when delicate structures are subjected to increased pressure, such as the forces of labor, high ventilatory pressures, fluid and electrolyte imbalances, sepsis, acidosis, and seizure activity. All of these factors contribute to intracranial insults, including traumatic bleeding in the newborn, which consists of four major types: intraventricular, subdural, primary subarachnoid, and intracerebellar.

### Perinatal Hypoxic-Ischemic Brain Injury

Hypoxic-ischemic brain injury, or hypoxic-ischemic reperfusion injury, is the most common cause of neurologic impairment observed in term and preterm infants. The brain damage usually results from asphyxia before, during, or after delivery. Ischemia and hypoxemia may occur simultaneously, or one may precede the other. The fetal brain is somewhat protected against mild hypoxic events but may be damaged when there is a decrease in cerebral blood flow, oxygen and nutrients such as glucose, and systemic blood pressure. Subsequent reperfusion following the event may further result in bleeding of the fragile capillaries, as well as tissue ischemia. ***Hypoxic-ischemic encephalopathy (HIE)*** is the resultant cellular damage from hypoxic-ischemic injury that causes the clinical manifestations observed in each case. Such clinical manifestations are variable and may be either mild, moderate, or severe. In some infants there may be little or no residual damage observed. In general, hypoxia that is severe enough to cause HIE will also cause damage to other organs such as the liver, kidneys, myocardium, and GI tract (Fenichel, 1997). In the preterm infant HIE may occur in conjunction with intraventricular hemorrhage. As a consequence of prematurity and general organ and system immaturity, the preterm infant may also suffer hypoxic-ischemic brain damage in the neonatal period as a result of altered cerebral blood flow, systemic hypotension, and decreased cellular nutrients (blood glucose and oxygen).

The site of the hypoxic-ischemic injury will vary according to the infant's gestational age. In the term infant the primary ischemic damage is parasagittal cerebral injury with cortical necrosis (deeper region of the brain). In the preterm infant, the primary ischemic lesion is in the white matter near the ventricles or periventricular with resultant ***periventricular leukomalacia (PVL)*** (Volpe, 2001).

### Clinical Manifestations

The neurologic signs that indicate encephalopathy appear within the first hours after the hypoxic episode, with manifestations of bilateral cerebral dysfunction. The infant may be stuporous or comatose. Seizures begin after 6 to 12 hours in approximately 50% of the infants, and they become more frequent and severe by 12 to 24 hours. Between 24 and 72 hours there may be deterioration in the level of consciousness, and after 72 hours there may be persistent stupor, abnormal tone (usually hypotonia), and evidence of disturbances of sucking and swallowing. Muscular weakness of the hips and shoulders is observed in full-term infants, and lower limb weakness occurs in premature infants. Apneic episodes are seen in approximately 50% of the affected infants.

Improvement in the neurologic deficiencies is highly variable and difficult to predict. Infants who demonstrate the most rapid initial improvement appear to have the best prognosis. Myocardial failure and acute tubular necrosis are frequent complications. The major long-term sequelae of hypoxic-ischemic injury are mental retardation, seizures, and CP.

### Therapeutic Management

Treatment involves aggressive resuscitation at birth, supportive care to provide adequate ventilation and prevent aggravating the existing hypoxia, and measures to maintain cerebral perfusion and prevent cerebral edema. Seizures are managed as described in the discussion on p. 403. However, prevention is the most important therapy, and every effort should be made to recognize high-risk pregnancies, monitor the fetus, and initiate appropriate therapy early.

### Nursing Considerations

Nursing care is primarily the same as for any high-risk infant: careful assessment and observation for signs that might indicate cerebral hypoxia or ischemia, monitoring of ventilatory and IV therapy, observation and management of seizures, and general supportive care to infants and parents, including guidelines for management in the event of cognitive impairment. (See Chapter 24.)

## Germinal Matrix–Intraventricular Hemorrhage (GM/IVH)

GM/IVH is known by a variety of terms according to the locus of bleeding: ***intraventricular hemorrhage (IVH), periventricular hemorrhage (PVH),*** and ***subependymal-intraventricular hemorrhage (SE/IVH).*** Most authorities use the term IVH to describe this disorder, which is responsible for a significant percentage of seriously ill infants and neonatal mortality. The incidence of IVH ranges from 15% to 39%. IVH is extremely common in preterm infants, especially ELBW and VLBW infants less than 32 weeks of gestation; the degree of neonatal immaturity correlates with the incidence of hemorrhage, and subsequent neurologic handicap is not uncommon (Volpe, 2001).

### Pathophysiology

During the early months of prenatal development there is an extensive but fragile vascular network in the region of the ventricles that receives a disproportionately large amount of cerebral blood flow. Toward term, more blood is directed to the germinal matrix located in the periventricular region near the caudate nuclei of the cerebrum. Therefore preterm infants are subject to bleeding in this heavily vascularized region, especially during events that are likely to cause fluctuations in cerebral blood flow, such as hypoxic episodes and the associated increased venous pressure. In IVH the bleeding originates in these capillaries. The blood may rupture through the ependymal lining of the ventricles and fill all or part of the ventricular system. Under pressure the ventricular system can dilate and cause acute hydrocephalus. Eventually, obliterative arachnoiditis may develop and obstruct the flow of CSF. In severe cases the hemorrhage extends into the cerebral parenchyma. Table 10-8 lists the classification of degrees of IVH.

Several clinical features are associated with IVH, such as birth asphyxia, early gestational age, low birth weight, respiratory distress, dysynchronous breathing on ventilatory therapy, pneumothorax, low blood glucose, noxious stimulation, hypercarbia, coagulation and platelet disorders, and hypotension. Posthemorrhagic hydrocephalus and damage to the periventricular white matter of the brain (such as in grade 4) are major determinants in relation to associated chronic problems and prognosis.

### Clinical Manifestations

Volpe (2001) classifies clinical manifestations of IVH into the following three categories:

1. **Catastrophic deterioration**—Begins within minutes to hours of the insult with a coma or deep stupor, respiratory abnormalities such as apnea and hypoventilation, fixed pupils, decerebrate posturing, generalized tonic seizures, flaccid quadriparesis, and cardiac arrhythmias.

**TABLE 10-8** Severity of germinal matrix intraventricular hemorrhage

| Grade | Extent of Hemorrhage | Percentage of Infants Affected |
|-------|----------------------|-------------------------------|
| Grade I | Germinal matrix hemorrhage with minimal to no IVH | 35 |
| Grade II | IVH in roughly 10% to 50% of ventricle | 40 |
| Grade III | IVH with lateral ventricular distention | 25 |
| Grade III+ | IVH and a periventricular hemorrhagic infarction* | 15 |

Data modified from Volpe JJ: *Neurology of the newborn,* ed 4, Philadelphia, 2001, WB Saunders.
*Periventricular hemorrhage is a separate category.

2. **Saltatory deterioration**—More subtle; signs appear over several hours, may stop altogether, then reappear; signs consist of altered level of consciousness, hypotonia, subtle abnormal eye position and movements, decreased spontaneous or abnormal movements and an abnormally tight popliteal angle; respiratory abnormalities are observed in some cases.
3. **Clinically silent deterioration**—Often overlooked clinically, but a sudden unexplained decrease in hematocrit may be the only clinical sign of IVH.

Approximately 50% of all IVHs occur on the first postnatal day of life, 25% on the second, 15% on the third, and 10% on or after the fourth day of life (Volpe, 2001).

### Diagnostic Evaluation

When IVH is suspected or the infant is at risk, studies of intracranial structures are performed by ultrasonography, computed tomography (CT), or magnetic resonance imaging (MRI). In many NICUs screening with cranial ultrasonography is performed at the bedside (via the anterior fontanel) within hours of birth if there is suspicion of IVH or within 4 to 7 days for high-risk infants <32 weeks of gestation. Lumbar puncture (LP) may be helpful in the diagnosis of IVH. A PET (positron emission tomography) scan may also be helpful in identifying cerebral blood flow in and around the site of the hemorrhage.

### Therapeutic Management

The treatment of IVH is aimed at prevention; prevention of prematurity and any events that may lead to IVH is foremost. The maintenance of adequate oxygenation by decreasing iatrogenic events is the key to keeping ELBW and VLBW infants neurologically intact. A number of factors associated with prematurity and RDS may predispose the preterm infant to IVH, including acidosis, electrolyte imbalances and rapid fluid shifts (extracellular to intracellular), administration of hyperosmolar solutions (such as NaHCO₃), and hypotension followed by rapid volume expansion. Medical treatment aimed at preventing IVH with vitamin E, maternal vitamin K, pancuronium (to decrease BP fluctuations), ibuprofen, phenobarbitol, ethamsylate, magnesium sulfate, indomethacin, and surfactant (for RDS) has met with varying degrees of success. Antenatal be-

tamethasone administration has played a significant role in the reduction of IVH in preterm infants (Volpe, 2001).

Treatment is both preventive and supportive in the event of IVH; prompt detection by clinical signs and/or periodic ultrasonography are key elements in implementing strategies to prevent further damage. Posthemorrhagic hydrocephalus is a common occurrence within 1 month of the event. Serial LPs may be used to decrease the amount of CSF and thus decrease ventricular size. A closed reservoir may be attached to an intraventricular shunt, with the reservoir tapped or drained intermittently to relieve pressure on the ventricles. Ventricular dilation (grade III to grade III+) may be managed with shunting (ventriculoperitoneal) or a temporary external ventricular drainage (EVD). Drugs such as acetazolamide may be administered to decrease CSF production.

The long-term outcome of IVH is variable and unpredictable and is influenced by the size of the hemorrhage and the extent of parenchymal involvement. Infants with small lesions have an excellent prognosis for neurologic outcome (Hill and Volpe, 1994).

### Nursing Considerations

In addition to routine observations and management, nursing care is directed toward prevention of fluctuations in cerebral blood flow. It has been observed that some nursing procedures increase ICP. For example, there is a marked increase in BP during endotracheal suctioning in preterm infants, and head positioning produces measurable changes in ICP. It has been found that ICP is highest when infants are in the dependent position and decreases when the head is in a midline position and elevated 30 degrees.

Cerebral pressure is lower when infants are in a midline position as opposed to a right side-lying position. When the head is turned to the right without body alignment, the resulting venous congestion creates hydrostatic pressure fluctuations that increase ICP. Infants encumbered with tubes and monitoring equipment are more difficult to turn while maintaining head-body alignment.

Other interventions that may reduce the risk of increased ICP include avoiding interventions that cause crying (such as painful procedures). Crying (which essentially creates a Valsalva effect) can impede venous return, increase cerebral blood volume, and compromise cerebral oxygenation in LBW infants. Rapid volume expansion following hypotension (primarily in preterms) and administration of hyperosmolar solutions such as NaHCO₃ should be avoided. Because air leaks such as pneumothorax produce variable cerebral blood flow, rapid detection and intervention is a key component of nursing care of the high-risk infant. Monitoring serum blood glucose levels and preventing hypoglycemia is also an important factor in keeping the infant neurologically intact. An attitude of minimum handling of infants at high risk is used in many units because routine nursing care has been shown to cause fluctuations in cerebral blood flow. In addition, research has implicated noxious external stimuli (e.g., pain and noise) as having a potential role in stimulation that may lead to IVH. Care includes evaluating manipulations and handling and administering analgesics to reduce discomfort.

# Intracranial Hemorrhage (ICH)

ICH in neonates, although manifested in the same ways as those described in older children, occurs with different frequencies and different degrees of severity.

## Subdural Hemorrhage

A subdural hematoma is a life-threatening collection of blood in the subdural space. It is most often produced by the stretching and tearing of the large veins in the *tentorium cerebelli,* the dural membrane that separates the cerebrum from the cerebellum. With improved obstetric care this condition has become relatively uncommon; however, it is especially serious because of the inaccessibility of the hematoma to aspiration by subdural tap. Less commonly, hemorrhage occurs when veins in the subdural space over the surface of the brain are torn. (See Head Injury, Chapter 37.)

## Subarachnoid Hemorrhage

Subarachnoid hemorrhage, the most common type of intracranial hemorrhage, occurs in term infants as a result of trauma and in preterm infants as a result of the same types of events that cause IVH. Small hemorrhages are the most common. Bleeding is of venous origin, and underlying contusion may also occur.

## Intracerebellar Hemorrhage

Intracerebellar hemorrhage is a common finding on postmortem examination of the premature infant and can be a primary hemorrhage in the cerebellum associated with skull compression during abrupt, precipitous delivery, or it may occur secondary to extravasation of blood into the cerebellum from a ventricular hemorrhage. In the full-term infant the bleeding may follow a difficult delivery.

## Nursing Considerations

Nursing care is the same as care of the infant with IVH or with perinatal hypoxic-ischemic brain injury.

# Neonatal Seizures

Seizures in the neonatal period are usually the clinical manifestation of a serious underlying disease. The most common cause of seizures in the neonatal period (for term and preterm) is hypoxic ischemic encephalopathy secondary to perinatal asphyxia (Volpe, 2001). Although not life threatening as an isolated entity, seizures constitute a medical emergency because they signal a disease process that may produce irreversible brain damage. Consequently, it is imperative to recognize a seizure and its significance so that the cause, as well as the seizure, can be treated (Box 10-13).

## Pathophysiology

The features of neonatal seizures are different from those observed in the older infant or child. For example, the well-organized, generalized tonic-clonic seizures seen in older children are rare in infants, especially preterm infants. The newborn brain, with its immature anatomic and physiologic status and less cortical organization, is insufficient to allow ready development and maintenance of a generalized seizure. The advanced degree of development of limbic structures with connections to the diencephalon and brainstem probably accounts for the higher frequency of seizure manifestations that originate in these structures, such as oral movements, oculomotor deviations, and apnea.

## Clinical Manifestations

Seizures in newborns may be subtle and barely discernible or grossly apparent. Because most neonatal seizures are subcortical, they do not have the etiologic and prognostic significance of seizures in children. The type of seizure is seldom important because one may produce any of a variety of manifestations. Neonatal seizures can be divided into four major types. These classifications are outlined in order of frequency in Table 10-9 and consist of clonic, tonic, myoclonic, and subtle seizures (Volpe, 2001). Clonic, multifocal clonic, and migratory clonic seizures are more common in term infants.

---

**Box 10-13**
## Causes of Neonatal Seizures

**METABOLIC**
Hypoglycemia; hyperglycemia
Hypernatremia, hyponatremia
Hypocalcemia
Hypomagnesemia
Pyridoxine deficiency
Aminoacidurias (e.g., phenylketonuria, maple syrup urine disease)
Hyperammonemia

**TOXIC**
Uremia
Bilirubin encephalopathy (kernicterus)

**PRENATAL INFECTIONS**
Toxoplasmosis
Syphilis
Cytomegalovirus
Herpes simplex
Hepatitis

**POSTNATAL INFECTIONS**
Bacterial meningitis
Viral meningoencephalitis
Sepsis
Brain abscess

**TRAUMA AT BIRTH**
Hypoxic brain injury
Intracranial hemorrhage
Subarachnoid, subdural hemorrhage
IVH

**MALFORMATIONS**
CNS agenesis
Hydroencephalopathy
Parencephalopathy
Tuberous sclerosis

**MISCELLANEOUS**
Degenerative disease
Benign familial neonatal seizures
Narcotic withdrawal

**TABLE 10-9** Classification of neonatal seizures

| Type | Characteristics |
|------|-----------------|
| **Clonic** | Slow rhythmic jerking movements |
| | Approximately 1 to 3 per second |
| *Focal* | Involves face, upper or lower extremities on one side of body |
| | May involve neck or trunk |
| | Infant is conscious during event |
| *Multifocal* | May migrate randomly from one part of the body to another |
| | Movements may start at different times |
| **Tonic** | Extension/stiffening movements |
| *Generalized* | Extensions of all four limbs (similar to decerebrate rigidity) |
| | Upper limbs are maintained in a stiffly flexed position (resembles decorticate rigidity) |
| *Focal* | Sustained posturing of a limb |
| | Asymmetric posturing of trunk or neck |
| **Subtle** | May develop in either full-term or preterm infants but are more common in preterm |
| | Often overlooked by inexperienced observers |
| | Signs: |
| |    Horizontal eye deviation |
| |    Repetitive blinking or fluttering of the eyelids, staring |
| |    Sucking or other oral-buccal-lingual movements |
| |    Arm movements that resemble rowing or swimming |
| |    Leg movements described as pedaling or bicycling |
| |    Apnea (common) |
| | Signs may appear alone or in combination |
| **Myoclonic** | Rapid jerks that involve flexor muscle groups |
| *Focal* | Involves upper extremity flexor muscle group |
| *Multifocal* | No EEG discharges observed |
| | Asynchronous twitching of several parts of the body |
| *Generalized* | No associated EEG discharges observed |
| | Bilateral jerks of upper and lower limbs |
| | Associated with EEG discharges |

*Adapted from Volpe J: Neonatal seizures. In Volpe J: *Neurology of the newborn,* ed 4, Philadelphia, 2001, WB Saunders.

*Jitteriness* or tremulousness in the newborn is a repetitive shaking of an extremity or extremities that may be observed with crying, may occur with changes in sleeping state, or may be elicited with stimulation. Jitteriness is relatively common in newborns, and in a mild degree may be considered normal during the first 4 days of life. Jitteriness can be distinguished from seizures by several characteristics: jitteriness is not accompanied by ocular movement as are seizures; the dominant movement in jitteriness is tremor, whereas seizure movement is clonic jerking that cannot be stopped by flexion of the affected limb; and jitteriness is highly sensitive to stimulation, whereas seizures are not. Further evaluation is indicated if jittery movements persist beyond the fourth day, if the movements are persistent and prolonged after a stimulus, or if they are easily elicited with minimal stimulus.

A *tremor* is defined as repetitive movements of both hands (with or without movement of legs or jaws) at a frequency of 2 to 5 per second and lasting more than 10 min-utes. It is common in newborn infants and has a variety of causes, including neurologic damage, hypoglycemia, and hypocalcemia. In most instances tremors are of no pathologic significance.

### Diagnostic Evaluation

Early evaluation and diagnosis of seizures is urgent. In addition to a careful physical examination, the pregnancy and family histories are investigated for familial and prenatal causes. Blood is drawn for glucose and electrolyte examination, and CSF is obtained for examination for gross blood, cell count, protein, glucose, and culture. Electroencephalography (EEG) may help identify subtle seizures but is less helpful in establishing a diagnosis. Other diagnostic procedures, such as CT and echoencephalography, may be indicated.

### Therapeutic Management

Treatment is directed toward prevention of cerebral damage and involves correction of metabolic derangements, respiratory and cardiovascular support, and suppression of the seizure activity. The underlying cause is treated (e.g., glucose infusion for hypoglycemia, calcium for hypocalcemia, and antibiotics for infection). If needed, respiratory support is provided for hypoxia, and anticonvulsants may be administered, especially when the other measures fail to control the seizures. Phenobarbital has been the drug of choice given intravenously or orally and is used if seizures are severe and persistent. Other drugs that may be used are fosphenytoin sodium, phenytoin (Dilantin), lorazepam, and diazepam (Valium).

### Nursing Considerations

The major nursing responsibilities in the care of infants with seizures are to recognize when the infant is having a seizure so that therapy can be instituted, to carry out the therapeutic regimen, and to observe the response to the therapy and any further evidence of seizures or other symptomatology. Assessment and other aspects of care are the same as for all high-risk infants. Parents need to be informed of their infant's status, and the nurse should reinforce and clarify the explanations of the practitioner. The infant's behaviors need to be interpreted for the parents, and the infant's responses to the treatment must be anticipated and their significance explained. Parents are encouraged to visit their infant and perform the parenting activities consistent with the plan of care. Seizures are a frightening phenomenon and generate a great deal of anxiety and fear, which is easily compounded by the justifiable concern of the staff. Providing support and guidance is an important nursing function.

# HIGH RISK RELATED TO MATERNAL CONDITIONS

## Infants of Diabetic Mothers (IDMs)

Before insulin therapy, few women with diabetes were able to conceive; for those who did, the mortality rate for both mother and infant was high. The morbidity and mortality of IDMs have been significantly reduced as a result of effective control of maternal diabetes and an increased understanding of fetal disorders. Because infants born to women with gestational diabetes mellitus (GDM) are at risk for the same complications as IDMs, the following discussion of IDMs includes infants born to those with GDM.

The severity of the maternal diabetes affects infant survival. Severity of maternal diabetes is determined by the duration of the disease before pregnancy, age of onset, extent of vascular complications, and abnormalities of the current pregnancy such as pyelonephritis, diabetic ketoacidosis, pregnancy-induced hypertension, and noncompliance. The single most important factor influencing fetal well-being is the euglycemic status of the mother. It has been found that reasonable metabolic control that begins before conception and continues during the first weeks of pregnancy can prevent malformation in an IDM. Elevated levels of hemoglobin $A_{1C}$ during the first trimester appear to be associated with a higher incidence of congenital malformations.

## Effects of Diabetes on the Fetus

Hypoglycemia may appear a short time after birth and in IDMs is associated with increased insulin activity in the blood. A standardized definition for neonatal hypoglycemia remains elusive and quite controversial. At best, authorities agree that reliance on a single numeric value for every clinical situation is inadequate (see Therapeutic Management section). Hypoglycemia in the IDM is related to hypertrophy and hyperplasia of the pancreatic islet cells, thus a resultant transient state of hyperinsulinism.

High maternal blood sugar levels during fetal life provide a continual stimulus to the fetal islet cells for insulin production. This sustained state of hyperglycemia promotes fetal insulin secretion that ultimately leads to excessive growth and deposition of fat, which probably accounts for the infants who are LGA, or macrosomic. When the neonate's glucose supply is removed abruptly at the time of birth, the continued production of insulin soon depletes the blood of circulating glucose, creating a state of hyperinsulinism and hypoglycemia within 1½ to 4 hours, especially in infants of mothers with class C diabetes or beyond (classes D through R). Precipitous drops in blood glucose levels can cause serious neurologic damage or death.

Tests of fetal well-being are performed routinely on the expectant mother with diabetes. Screening for neural tube defects by evaluating maternal serum alpha fetoprotein levels is recommended at 16 weeks of gestation; ultrasonography (US) is performed at 18 to 20 weeks to determine fetal size and to rule out the presence of fetal anomalies. US may be repeated periodically during the course of fetal development. After 30 weeks of gestation a nonstress test (NST) for assessment of fetal and placental function should be performed weekly (Suevo, 1997). If the NST is nonreactive, further studies such as a contraction stress test or Biophysical Profile should be performed. Before delivery, fetal lung maturation tests via amniocentesis are carried out, including lecithin/sphingomyelin ratio, phosphatidylglycerol, and disaturated phosphatidylcholine measurements. In the IDM, the presence of phosphatidylglycerol in the amniotic fluid is the best predictor of normal neonatal respiratory function.

## Clinical Manifestations

Infants of diabetic mothers have a characteristic appearance. They are usually macrosomic for their gestational age, very plump and full-faced, liberally coated with vernix caseosa, and plethoric. The placenta and umbilical cord are also larger than average. However, infants of mothers with advanced diabetes may be SGA, may have IUGR, or may be AGA because of the maternal vascular (placental) involvement. There is an increase in congenital anomalies in IDMs in addition to a high susceptibility to hypoglycemia, hypocalcemia, hyperbilirubinemia, hypomagnesemia, and RDS. Hyperinsulinemia and hyperglycemia in the diabetic mother may be a factor in reducing fetal surfactant synthesis, thus contributing to the development of RDS. Morbidities in IDMs are the result of exposure to elevated glucose and ketone levels, placental insufficiency, and prematurity. Although large, these infants may be delivered before term due to maternal complications or increased fetal size.

## Therapeutic Management

The most effective management of IDMs is careful monitoring of serum glucose levels and observation for accompanying complications such as RDS. The infants are examined for the presence of any anomalies or birth injuries, and blood studies for initial determinations of glucose, calcium, hematocrit, and bilirubin are obtained on a regular basis. Cornblath and others (2000) suggest the use of operational thresholds at which hypoglycemia should be closely monitored and treated; the researchers recommend close observation in infants with known risk factors such as maternal diabetes, with close observation if plasma glucose values are below 36 mg/dl (2.0 mmol/L). If a feeding fails to increase the glucose levels in such cases or if abnormal signs develop, intravenous glucose should be administered to maintain glucose levels above 45 mg/dl (2.5 mmol/L). A newborn with levels at or below 25 mg/dl should receive intravenous glucose. Cornblath and others (2000) further recommend that therapeutic glucose levels be kept at or above 60 mg/dl (3.3 mmol/L) in neonates with profound, recurrent, or persistent hyperinsulinemic hypoglycemia.

Because the hypertrophied pancreas is so sensitive to blood glucose concentrations, the administration of oral glucose may trigger a massive insulin release, resulting in rebound hypoglycemia. Therefore feedings of breast milk or formula begin within the first hour after birth provided that the infant's cardiorespiratory condition is stable (would not feed infant with RDS). Some practitioners prefer early feedings of nonglucose carbohydrates, such as inert sugar or galactose, because they are less insulinogenic. Approximately half of IDMs do very well and adjust without complications. Infants born to mothers with uncontrolled diabetes may require IV infusion of dextrose. Oral and IV intake may be titrated to maintain adequate blood sugar levels. Frequent blood glucose determinations are needed for the first 2 days of life to assess the degree of hypoglycemia present at any given time. Testing blood taken from the heel with reagent strips and portable reflectance meters (glucometer) is a simple and effective screening evaluation that can then be confirmed by laboratory examination.

## Nursing Considerations

The nursing care of IDMs involves early examination for congenital anomalies, signs of possible respiratory or cardiac problems, maintenance of adequate thermoregulation, early introduction of carbohydrate feedings as appropriate, and monitoring serum blood glucose levels. The latter is of particular importance because many hypoglycemic infants may remain asymptomatic. IV glucose infusion requires careful monitoring of the site and the neonate's reaction to therapy; high glucose concentrations (>12.5%) should be infused via a central line instead of a peripheral site. Because macrosomic infants are at risk for problems associated with a difficult delivery, they are monitored for birth injuries such as brachial plexus injury and palsy, fractured clavicle, and phrenic nerve palsy. Additional monitoring of the infant for associated problems (RDS, polycythemia, hypocalcemia, poor feeding, and hyperbilirubinemia) with this condition is also a vital nursing function.

## Drug-Exposed Infants*

### Opiate Exposure

Narcotics, which have a low molecular weight, readily cross the placental membrane and enter the fetal system. When the mother is a habitual user of narcotics, especially heroin or methadone, the unborn child may also become passively physiologically addicted to the drug, which places such infants at risk during the early neonatal period. *Neonatal abstinence syndrome (NAS)* is the term used by many to describe the set of behaviors exhibited by the infant exposed to chemical substances in utero.

### Clinical Manifestations

Most infants of drug-dependent mothers appear normal at birth but may begin to exhibit signs of drug withdrawal within 12 to 24 hours if the mother has been taking heroin by itself. If mothers have been taking methadone, the signs appear somewhat later—anywhere from 1 or 2 days to 2 to 3 weeks or more after birth. The clinical manifestations of withdrawal may fall into one or all of the following categories: CNS, GI, respiratory, and autonomic nervous signs (Kandall, 1999). The manifestations become most pronounced between 48 and 72 hours of age and may last from 6 days to 8 weeks, depending on the severity of the withdrawal (Box 10-14).

In a study of polydrug use during pregnancy the most prominent signs of withdrawal were increased tone, increased respiratory rate, disturbed sleep, fever, excessive sucking, and loose watery stools. Others signs observed in this study included projectile vomiting, mottling, crying, nasal stuffiness, hyperactive Moro reflex, and tremors (D'Apolito and Hepworth, 2001). Although these infants

---

*It is important to note that the term *addiction* is often associated with behaviors whereby the person seeks the drug(s) in order to experience a high, euphoria, escape from reality, or satisfy a personal need. Newborns are not addicted in a behavioral sense, yet they may experience mild to strong physiologic signs as a result of the mother's drug use. Therefore, to say that an infant born to a mother who uses substances is addicted is incorrect; *drug-exposed newborn* is a better term, which implies intrauterine drug exposure.

---

> ### Box 10-14 ■ ■ ⬜
> ### Signs of Withdrawal in the Neonate
>
> | | |
> |---|---|
> | Irritability | Tachypnea (>60/min) |
> | Tremors | Excoriations (knees, face) |
> | Shrill cry | Mottling (skin) |
> | Hypertonicity of muscles | Sneezing |
> | Frantic sucking of hands | Yawning |
> | Poor feeding | Vomiting, often projectile |
> | Hyperactivity | Temperature instability |
> | Perspiring | Loose diarrheal stools |
> | Fever | Seizures |
> | Nasal stuffiness | Sleep disturbances |

suck avidly on fists and display an exaggerated rooting reflex, they are poor feeders with uncoordinated and ineffectual sucking and swallowing reflexes.

One observation in a large percentage of these infants is generalized perspiring, which is unusual in newborn infants. It is significant that although drug-exposed infants have some tachypnea, cyanosis, and/or apnea, they rarely develop RDS when born near term. Apparently, heroin or stress factors in the intrauterine environment cause accelerated lung maturation even with a high incidence of prematurity.

Not all infants of heroin-addicted mothers will show signs of withdrawal. Because of irregular and varying degrees of drug use, quality of drug, and mixed drug usage by the mother, some infants display mild or variable manifestations. Most manifestations are the vague, nonspecific signs characteristic of infants in general; therefore it is important to differentiate between drug withdrawal and other disorders before specific therapy is instituted. Other states (e.g., hypocalcemia, hypoglycemia, or sepsis) often coexist with the drug withdrawal.

Infants who do not display the signs of fetal alcohol syndrome (see p. 326) but are born to mothers who are also heavy alcohol drinkers have significantly more tremors, hypertonia, restlessness, excessive mouthing movements, crying, and inconsolability than infants of addicted mothers who do not consume alcohol during pregnancy. A concern regarding substance abuse is that many of the mothers often use several drugs, such as tranquilizers, sedatives, narcotics, amphetamines, phencyclidine (PCP), marijuana, and other psychotropic agents. Of increasing concern in the United States is the number of newborns who are exposed to methamphetamines in utero.

### Therapeutic Management

The treatment of the drug-exposed infant initially consists of modulating the environment to decrease external stimuli. Drug therapies to decrease withdrawal side effects include administration of phenobarbital, morphine, chlorpromazine, diazepam, or methadone.

### Nursing Considerations

When possible, the nursery personnel are alerted to the likelihood of drug-exposed infants. If the mother has had good prenatal care, the practitioner is aware of the problem and therapy may have been instituted before delivery. However, a number of mothers deliver their infants without the benefit of adequate care, and the addiction is unknown to health care personnel at the time of delivery. The degree of narcosis or withdrawal is closely related to the amount of drug the mother has habitually taken, the length of time she has been taking the drug, and her drug level at the time of delivery. The most severe symptoms are observed in the infants of mothers who have taken large amounts of drugs over a long period. In addition, the nearer to the time of delivery that the mother takes the drug, the longer it takes the child to develop withdrawal, and the more severe the manifestations. The infant may not exhibit withdrawal symptoms until 7 to 10 days after delivery.

Once the presence of NAS is identified in an infant, nursing care is directed toward reducing the external stimuli that might trigger hyperactivity and irritability (e.g., dimming the lights and decreasing noise levels), providing adequate nutrition and hydration, and promoting maternal-infant relationships. Providing care on demand rather than a fixed or set schedule may help reduce irritability for infants who promptly have their needs met. Appropriate individualized developmental care may be implemented, such as care with preterm infants to facilitate self-consoling and self-regulating behaviors (see Table 10-4). Irritable and hyperactive infants have been found to respond to comforting, movement, containment, and close contact. Wrapping snugly (swaddling), pacifier, and gentle holding or rocking are used to calm and nurture a disorganized infant (Jorgensen, 1999). Arranging nursing activities to reduce the amount of disturbance helps to decrease exogenous stimulation.

The Neonatal Abstinence Scoring System has been developed to monitor infants in an objective manner and evaluate the infant's response to clinical and pharmacologic interventions (Finnegan, 1985). This system is also designed to assist nurses and other health care workers in evaluating the severity of the infant's withdrawal symptoms.

Loose stools and poor intake and regurgitation following feeding predispose the infants to malnutrition, dehydration, and electrolyte imbalance. An oral opioid such as morphine may be administered to control loose watery stools (D'Apolito and Hepworth, 2001). It takes considerable time and patience to ensure that these infants receive a sufficient caloric and fluid intake.

Hyperactive infants must be protected from skin abrasions on the knees, toes, and cheeks that are caused by rubbing on bed linens while lying on their abdomens. Monitoring and recording the activity level and its relationship to other activities, such as feeding and preventing complications, are important nursing functions.

A valuable aid to anticipating problems in the newborn is recognizing drug abuse in the mother. Unless the mother is enrolled in a methadone rehabilitation program, she seldom risks calling attention to her habit by seeking prenatal care. Consequently, infants and mothers are exposed to the additional hazards of obstetric and medical complications. Moreover, the nature of heroin addiction makes the user susceptible to disorders such as infection (hepatitis B, HIV), foreign body reaction, and the hazards of inadequate nutrition and preterm birth. Methadone treatment does not pre-

vent withdrawal reaction in neonates, but the clinical course may be modified. Also, intensive psychologic support of mothers is a factor in the treatment and reduction of perinatal mortality. Experience has indicated that mothers are usually anxious and depressed, lack confidence, have poor self-image, and have difficulty with interpersonal relationships. They may have a psychologic need for the pregnancy and an infant.

Initial symptoms or the recurrence of withdrawal symptoms may develop after discharge from the hospital; therefore it is important to establish rapport and maintain contact with the family so that they return for treatment if this occurs. The demands of the drug-exposed infant on the caregiver are enormous and nonrewarding in terms of positive feedback. The infants are difficult to comfort, and they cry for long periods, which can be especially trying for the caregiver after the infant's discharge from the hospital. Long-term follow-up to evaluate the status of the infant and family is very important. Sudden infant death syndrome (SIDS) and HIV are observed more commonly in infants born to users of methadone and heroin.

An important aspect of nursing care is the identification of an infant who was exposed to drugs in utero; observation of signs mentioned previously may warrant further investigation so prompt treatment may be implemented. Meconium sampling for intrauterine drug exposure is reported to provide more screening accuracy than urine because drug metabolites accumulate in meconium (Kandall, 1999; Ostrea, 2001).

There are many problems relating to the disposition of infants of drug-dependent mothers. Those who advocate separation of mothers and children argue that the mothers are not capable of assuming responsibility for their infant's care, that child care is frustrating to them, and that their existence is too disorganized and chaotic. Others encourage the maternal-infant bond and recommended a protected environment such as a therapeutic community, a halfway house, or continuous ongoing, supportive services in the home after discharge. Careful evaluation and the cooperative efforts of a variety of health professionals are required whether the choice is foster home placement or supportive follow-up care of mothers who keep their infants.

## Cocaine Exposure

Cocaine, the number one illicit drug in the United States, has multiple modes of use. However, use of the relatively inexpensive and easily administered "crack" form is increasing at an alarming rate, especially among pregnant women and women of childbearing age (Askin and Diehl-Jones, 2001; Eyler, Behnke, and Conlon, 1998). Because crack vaporizes at relatively low temperatures, it is smoked and absorbed in large quantities through pulmonary vasculature. The drug readily enters the placenta, placing the fetus at risk (Malanga and Kosofsy, 1999).

Cocaine is a CNS stimulant and peripheral sympathomimetic, and the effects on the fetus may be direct or indirect. Indirect effects include fetal hypoxemia secondary to impaired uterine blood flow. Cocaine also appears to affect fetal cardiac function and suppress the fetal immune system. The difficulties encountered by cocaine-exposed infants are compounded when the mother takes the drug in conjunction with other illicit drugs (Askin and Diehl-Jones, 2001). Studies have found that women who use cocaine in pregnancy are less likely to have adequate prenatal care, are more likely to smoke tobacco and consume alcohol, are more likely to be malnourished, and are more likely to have sexually transmitted diseases than nonusers (Tronick and Beeghly, 1999). These variables compound the problem of drug exposure and effects on the fetus.

### Clinical Manifestations

Infants who are exposed to cocaine in utero may demonstrate no immediate untoward effects. Previous reports of catastrophic neurologic effects have been published, yet there is considerable variability in findings because of poor maternal history reliability, maternal polydrug use, prematurity, poor social environment, and poor specificity in detecting cocaine exposure. Researchers point out, however, that there are negative effects of habitual cocaine use in pregnancy, many of which may be too subtle to notice in the newborn and infancy period (Askin and Diehl-Jones, 2001). Clinical manifestations of intrauterine cocaine exposure include IUGR; decreased head circumference; association with preterm delivery; NEC, cerebral infarcts; respiratory disturbances such as apnea, cardiac arrhythmias, transient EEG abnormalities; and IVH (Askin and Diehl-Jones, 2001; Chiriboga and others, 1999). Other findings related to neurobehavioral effects include sleep disturbances, increased tone, jitteriness, delayed language acquisition, behavioral problems in school, poor impulse control, hypertonia, abnormal reflexes, poor BNBAS scores, significant cognitive delays the first 2 years, and poor responses to auditory, arousal, and visual stimuli (Chiriboga and others, 1999; Delaney-Black and others, 1998; Eyler, Behnke, and Conlon, 1998; Schuler and Nair, 1999; Singer and others, 2002). Environmental as well as sociodemographic factors likely play an important role in the outcome of children exposed to cocaine in utero.

### Therapeutic Management

Infants exposed to cocaine alone are less likely to demonstrate signs of withdrawal. Regardless of the type of drug or substance to which the newborn was exposed, treatment begins with prompt identification of a potential problem by obtaining a comprehensive maternal history, identifying potential risks associated with exposure, and maintaining a safe environment. Newborn urine, hair, or meconium sampling may be required to identify drug exposure and implement appropriate early interventional therapies aimed at minimizing the consequences of intrauterine drug exposure.

### Nursing Considerations

Nursing care of cocaine-exposed infants is similar to that of infants exposed to other drugs. Individualized assessment should be carried out to determine appropriate intervention strategies. If hypertonicity and sleep disturbance is identified, the environment should be modified accordingly to decrease noxious stimuli. The use of swaddling, containment, gentle rocking, nonnutritive sucking and undisturbed periods of rest may help promote self-containment and state regulation. As previously noted, tissue samples may be required for identification of drug exposure. Because cocaine is easily passed in breast milk (Chasnoff, Lewis, and Squires, 1987), mothers should be counseled accordingly regarding avoidance of breast-feeding. A fussy newborn may be interpreted by caretakers to be consistently hungry and thus overfeeding and vomiting may be problematic. Provision of a safe environment in which the mother and newborn may interact is imperative. Opportunities for appropriate family bonding and attachment should be provided as with any other newborn. Because a large percentage of women who use cocaine during pregnancy have sexually transmitted diseases, viral titers and hepatitis screening for the newborn should be considered (Askin and Diehl-Jones, 2001).

Referral to early intervention programs, including child health care, parental drug treatment, individualized developmental care, and parenting education, is essential in promoting optimum outcomes for these children. Children exposed to maternal cocaine use often live in impoverished conditions, putting them at high risk for cognitive delays, poor child health care, and inadequate nutrition; they would benefit from an early intervention program (Tronick and Beeghly, 1999). Comprehensive health care services for both mother and child may be provided at one location "one stop–shopping model" (Tanney and Lowenstein, 1997). It is essential that nurses caring for these infants and their mothers do the following: understand the depth of the problem of prenatal drug exposure; have a positive attitude toward cocaine-using mothers and their children; be aware of community resources; encourage positive parenting (Pokorni and Stanga, 1996); and be proactive in the legislative arena (Maier, 1995).

## Infants of Mothers Who Smoke

Cigarette smoking during pregnancy is clearly associated with significant birth weight deficits—up to 440 g in full-term newborns—and there is a definitive dose-response relationship between the number of cigarettes smoked by the mother and these deficits. This dose-related response also affects the Apgar scores. The number of infants with low Apgar scores is nearly four times higher for infants whose mothers smoked three packs per day than for infants whose mothers smoked none or only one pack per day. Large studies indicate that 21% to 39% of the incidence of low birth weight is attributable to maternal cigarette smoking.

The rate of preterm births is increased in mothers who smoke, but the infants are smaller at *all* stages of gestation. They show fetal growth retardation in length, weight, and chest and head circumference; these deficits are not related to maternal appetite or weight gain. The concentrations of two pharmacologically active substances found in tobacco—nicotine and cotinine—have been found to be higher in newborns of mothers who smoke than in the mothers themselves. In addition, these substances are secreted in breast milk and have a half-life of 70 to 80 minutes. It has also been shown that cigarette smoking has detrimental effects beyond the neonatal period, with deficits in growth, intellectual and emotional development, and behavior. Maternal smoking and passive smoking by household members has been correlated with an increased incidence of SIDS (Leach and others, 1999), respiratory tract illnesses (Jorgensen, 1999), spontaneous abortion, premature rupture of membranes, preterm delivery, and deficits in learning and behavior (Bennett, 1999). (See Passive Smoking, Chapter 32.)

## Nursing Considerations

Nurses are prime candidates for disseminating information to expectant mothers regarding smoking-related risks. Mothers who stop or substantially reduce smoking during pregnancy improve the quality of life for their unborn infants. Infants of expectant mothers who were given information, support, encouragement, practical guidance, and behavior modification during pregnancy delivered infants with significantly higher birth weights than did controls. If mothers continue to smoke while breast-feeding, they should be encouraged to do so *immediately after* breast-feeding to reduce the amount of nicotine and cotinine in the breast milk. Smoking has been shown to decrease milk production in the breast-feeding mother (Lawrence and Lawrence, 1999). All efforts should be made to avoid second-hand smoke in infants born with respiratory or cardiac problems and those born prematurely.

## KEY POINTS

- High-risk neonates may be defined as newborns, regardless of gestational age or birth weight, who have a greater than average chance of morbidity or mortality because of conditions or circumstances superimposed on the normal course of events associated with birth and adjustment to extrauterine existence.
- Identification of high-risk newborns may occur during any one of the following stages: preconceptual, prenatal, natal, or postnatal.
- High-risk infants may be classified according to birthweight, gestational age, and morbidity factors.
- Newborn intensive care units are categorized according to the population served and the degree of treatment.
- General management of the newborn entails immediate care, protection from infection, monitoring of physiologic data (including heart rate, respiratory activity, temperature, and blood pressure), laboratory data, and systematic assessment of the high-risk infant.
- Assessment of the newborn includes a general assessment, respiratory assessment, cardiovascular assessment, GI assessment, genitourinary assessment, neurologic-musculoskeletal assessment, skin assessment, and temperature.
- Because many of their metabolic processes are immature, high-risk newborns are placed in a heated environment to help maintain thermoneutrality.

- Because of the immature, fragile skin of preterm infants, the nurse should use caution when applying topical preparations and, when possible, avoid adhesives.
- Meeting the high-risk infant's nutritional needs requires specific knowledge of physiologic characteristics, the infant's particular needs, and methods of feeding.
- Delayed development in high-risk neonates is a concern; developmental interventions are individualized to ameliorate the effects and increase infant well-being.
- Parental involvement in the care of high-risk infants is important, and nurses should encourage parent-infant relationships from birth to discharge.
- Prematurity accounts for the largest number of admissions to an NICU.
- Several severe respiratory conditions place the infant at high risk: AOP, RDS, MAS, extraneous air syndromes, and BPD. Therapeutic management of respiratory distress syndrome includes oxygen therapy and assisted ventilation.
- Newborns are highly susceptible to infection, particularly septicemia.
- Cardiovascular complications in the high-risk infant may include PDA and PPHN.
- Neurologic disturbances in the high-risk newborn may include perinatal hypoxic-ischemic brain injury, IVH, intracranial hemorrhage, and neonatal seizures.
- Maternal conditions that pose a threat to the newborn include diabetes and substance abuse.

## REFERENCES

Als H: A synactive model of neonatal behavioral organization: framework for the assessment of neurobehavioral development in the premature infant and for support of infants and parents in the neonatal intensive care environment, *Phys Occup Ther Pediatr* 6(1):3-55, 1986.

Als H: Reading the premature infant. In Goldson E, editor: *Nurturing the premature infant: developmental interventions in the neonatal intensive care nursery*, New York, 1999, Oxford University Press.

Als H: Toward a synactive theory of development: promise for the assessment and support of infant individuality, *Inf Mental Health J* 3(4):229-243, 1982.

Als H and others: Individualized behavioral and environmental care for the very low birth weight preterm infant at high risk for bronchopulmonary dysplasia: neonatal intensive care unit and developmental outcome, *Pediatrics* 78(6):1123-1132, 1986.

Als H and others: Individualized developmental care for the very low birth weight preterm infant: medical and neurofunctional effects, *JAMA* 272(11):853-858, 1994.

Altimier LB, Lott JW, McCain G: Research utilization: evaluating the use of hospital cover gowns in a neonatal intensive care unit, *Neonat Intensive Care* 9(7):52-56, 58, 1996.

American Academy of Pediatrics: Car safety seats: a guide for families, 2002, *www.aap.org/family/carseatguide.htm.*

American Academy of Pediatrics: Changing concepts of sudden infant death syndrome: implications for infant sleeping environment and sleep position, *Pediatrics* 105(3):650-656, 2000.

American Academy of Pediatrics, Committee on Environmental Health: Ultraviolet light: a hazard to children, *Pediatrics* 104(2):328-333, 1999a.

American Academy of Pediatrics, Committee on Fetus and Newborn: Surfactant replacement therapy for respiratory distress syndrome, *Pediatrics* 103(3):684-686, 1999b.

American Academy of Pediatrics, Committee on Infectious Diseases and Committee on Fetus and Newborn: Prevention of respiratory syncitial virus infections: indications for the use of palivizumab and update on the use of RSV-IVIG, *Pediatrics* 102(5):1211-1214, 1998.

American Academy of Pediatrics, Committee on Injury and Poison Prevention and Committee on Fetus and Newborn: Safe transportation of premature and low birth weight infants, *Pediatrics* 97(5):758-762, 1996.

American Academy of Pediatrics, Committee on Nutrition: *Pediatric nutrition handbook*, ed 4, Evanston, IL, 1998, The Academy.

American Academy of Pediatrics, Section on Ophthalmology, Retinopathy of Prematurity Subcommittee: Screening examination of premature infants for retinopathy of prematurity, *Pediatrics* 100(2):273, 1997.

American Academy of Pediatrics, Work Group on Breastfeeding: Breastfeeding and the use of human milk, *Pediatrics* 100(6):1036-1039, 1997.

American Academy of Pediatrics and American College of Obstetricians and Gynecologists: *Guidelines for perinatal care*, ed 4, Elk Grove Village, IL, 1997, The Academy and College.

American Academy of Pediatrics and Canadian Paediatric Society: Postnatal corticosteroids to treat or prevent chronic lung disease in preterm infants, *Pediatrics* 109(2): 330-338, 2002.

Anand KJ, Carr DB: The neuroanatomy, neurophysiology, and neurochemistry of pain, stress, and analgesia in newborns and children, *Pediatr Clin North Am* 36(4):795-822, 1989.

Anand KJ, Hickey P: Pain and its effects in the human neonate and fetus, *N Engl J Med* 317(21):1321-1329, 1987.

Anand K, Hickey P: Halothane-morphine compared with high-dose sufentanil for anesthesia and postoperative analgesia in neonatal cardiac surgery, *N Engl J Med* 326(1):1-9, 1992.

Anand KS, Grunau RE, Oberlander TF: Developmental character and long-term consequences of pain in infants and children, *Child Adolesc Psychiatr Clin North Am* 6(4):703-724, 1997.

Anand KJS and others: Consciousness, behavior, and clinical impact of the definition of pain, *Pain Forum* 8(2):64-73, 1999.

Ancona J and others: Improving outcomes through a developmental approach to nipple feeding, *J Nurs Care Qual* 12(5): 1-4, 1998.

Anderson KV: The one thing you can never take away: perinatal bereavement photographs, *MCN* 26(1):123-128, 2001.

Anderssen SH, Nicolaisen RB, Gabrielsen GW: Autonomic response to auditory stimulation, *Acta Paediatr* 82(11):913-918, 1993.

Andrews EB and others: Antenatal steroids and neonatal outcomes in controlled trials of synthetic surfactant replacement, *Am J Obstet Gynecol* 173(1):290-295, 1995.

Appleton SM: "Handle with care": an investigation of the handling received by preterm infants in intensive care, *J Neonat Nurs* 3(1):23-27, 1997.

Armentrout DC, Huseby V: Practice guidelines: neonatal polycythemia, *J Pediatr Healthcare* 16(1):40-42, 2002.

Askin DF, Diehl-Jones B: Cocaine: effects of in utero exposure on the fetus and neonate, *J Perinat Neonat Nurs* 14(4):83-102, 2001.

Ballantyne M and others: Validation of the premature infant pain profile in the clinical setting, *Clin J Pain* 15(4):297-303, 1999.

Bancalari E: Changes in the pathogenesis and prevention of chronic lung disease of prematurity, *Am J Perinatol* 18(1):1-5, 2001.

Barba B and others: Pain memory in full-term newborn, *J Pain Symptom Manage* 6(1):206, 1991.

Behrman RE, Shiono PH: Neonatal risk factors. In Fanaroff AA, Martin RJ, editors: *Neonatal-perinatal medicine: diseases of the fetus and infant*, ed 6, St Louis, 1997, Mosby.

Bennett AD: Perinatal substance abuse and the drug-exposed neonate, *Adv Nurs Pract* 7(5):32-36, 1999.

Berman S and others: Racial differences in the predictive value of the TDx fetal lung maturity assay, *Am J Obstet Gynecol* 175(1): 73-77, 1996.

Berseth CL: Minimal enteral feedings, *Clin Perinatol* 22(1):195-205, 1995.

Bhatt-Mehta V and others: Prospective evaluation of two dosing equations for theophylline in premature infants, *Pharmacotherapy* 16(5): 769-776, 1996.

Biber P and others: When to seek consultation. In Creger PJ, Browne JV: *Developmental interventions for preterm and high-risk infants: self-study modules for professionals*, Tucson, 1995, Therapy Skill Builders.

Bier JAB and others: Breast-feeding of very low birth weight infants, *J Pediatr* 123(5): 773-778, 1993.

Bildner J, Krechel SW: Increasing staff nurse awareness of postoperative pain management in the NICU, *Neonatal Network* 15(1):11-16, 1996.

Blackburn ST, VandenBerg KA: Assessment and management of neonatal neurobehavioral development. In Kenner C, Lott JW, Flandermeyer AA, editors: *Comprehensive neonatal nursing: a physiologic perspective*, ed 2, Philadelphia, 1998, WB Saunders.

Blackburn ST, Loper DL: *Maternal, fetal, and neonatal physiology: a clinical perspective*, Philadelphia, 1992, WB Saunders.

Blackburn S: Environmental impact of the NICU on developmental outcomes, *J Pediatr Nurs* 13(5):279-289, 1998.

Blackburn S and others: Neonatal thermal care, part III: the effect of infant position and temperature probe placement, *Neonatal Network* 20(3):25-30, 2001.

Blake WW, Murray JA: Heat balance. In Merenstein GB, Gardner SL, editors: *Handbook of neonatal intensive care*, ed 4, St Louis, 1998, Mosby.

Bohnhorst B and others: Skin-to-skin (kangaroo) care, respiratory control, and thermoregulation, *J Pediatr* 138(2):193-197, 2001.

Bomela HN and others: Use of C-reactive protein to guide duration of empiric antibiotic therapy in suspected early neonatal sepsis, *Pediatr Infect Dis J* 19(6):531-535, 2000.

Brazy JE: Effects of crying on cerebral blood volume and cytochrome aa3, *J Pediatr* 112(3):457-461, 1988.

Browne JV: Considerations for touch and massage in the neonatal intensive care unit, *Neonatal Network* 19(1):61-64, 2000.

Byrne J and others: Language development in low birth weight infants: the first two years of life, *J Dev Behav Pediatr* 14(1):21-27, 1993.

Carver JD and others: Growth of preterm infants fed nutrient-enriched or term formula after hospital discharge, *Pediatrics* 107(4):683-689, 2001.

Chasnoff IJ, Lewis DE, Squires L: Cocaine intoxication in breast fed infant, *Pediatrics* 80(6):836-838, 1987.

Cherkes-Julkowski M: Learning disability, attention-deficit disorder, and language impairment as outcomes of prematurity: a longitudinal descriptive study, *J Learning Disabilities* 31(3):294-306, 1998.

Chiriboga CA and others: Drug-response effect on fetal cocaine exposure on newborn neurologic function, *Pediatrics* 103(1):79-85, 1999.

Choonara I: Management of pain in newborn infants, *Semin Perinatol* 16(1):32-40, 1992.

Cole CH, Fiascone JM: Strategies for prevention of neonatal chronic lung disease, *Semin Perinatol* 24(6):445-462, 2000.

Committee to Establish Recommended Standards for Newborn ICU Design: Recommended standards for newborn ICU design, 1999, http://www.nd.edu/~kkolberg/frmain.htm.

Conde-Agudelo A, Diaz-Rossello JL, Belizan JM: Cochrane Neonatal Review: Kangaroo mother care to reduce morbidity and mortality in low birthweight infants, http://www.nichd.nih.gov/cochraneneonatal/Vickers/Vickers.htm, 2000.

Copnell B, Fergusson D: Endotracheal suctioning: time-worn ritual or timely intervention? *Am J Crit Care* 4(2):100-105, 1995.

Cornblath M, Ichord R: Hypoglycemia in the neonate, *Semin Perinatol* 24(2):136-149, 2000.

Cornblath M and others: Controversies regarding definition of neonatal hypoglycemia: suggested operational thresholds, *Pediatrics* 105(5):1141-1145, 2000.

Corff KE and others: Facilitated tucking: a nonpharmacologic comfort measure for pain in preterm neonates, *J Obstet Gynecol Neonat Nurs* 24(2):144-147, 1995.

Cox CA, Wolfson MR, Shaffer TH: Liquid ventilation: a comprehensive review, *Neonatal Network* 15(3):31-43, 1996.

D'Apolito K, Hepworth JT: Prominence of withdrawal symptoms in polydrug-exposed infants, *J Perinat Neonat Nurs* 14(4):46-60, 2001.

Davidson D and others: Inhaled nitric oxide for the treatment of persistent pulmonary hypertension of the term newborn: a randomized, double-masked, placebo-controlled, dose-response, multicenter study, *Pediatrics* 101(3):325-334, 1998.

Dayal VS, Kokshanian A, Mitchell DP: Combined effects of noise and kanamycin, *Ann Otol Rhinol Laryngol* 80(6):897-902, 1971.

DeBoer S, Stephens, D: Persistent pulmonary hypertension of the newborn: case study and pathophysiology review, *Neonatal Network* 16(1):7-13, 1997.

de Groot L, Hopkins B, Touwen B: Motor asymmetries in preterm infants at 18 weeks corrected age and outcomes at 1 year, *Early Hum Dev* 48(1-2):35-46, 1997.

Delaney-Black V and others: Prenatal cocaine exposure and child behavior, *Pediatrics* 102(4):945-950, 1998.

Downey V and others: Dying babies and associated stress in NICU nurses, *Neonatal Network* 14(1):41-45, 1995.

Downs JA and others: Effect of intervention on the development of hip posture in very preterm babies, *Arch Dis Child* 66(7):197-201, 1991.

Evans JC and others: Pain behaviors in LBW infants accompany some "nonpainful caregiving procedures," *Neonatal Network* 16(3):33-40, 1997.

Evans JC: Incidence of hypoxemia associated with caregiving in premature infants, *Neonatal Network* 10(2):17-23, 1991.

Evans RA, Thureen PJ: Early feeding strategies in preterm and critically ill neonates, *Neonat Network* 20(7):7-18, 2001.

Eyler FD, Behnke M, Conlon M: Birth outcome from a prospective, matched study of prenatal/crack use. II. Interactive and dose effects on neurochemical assessment, *Pediatrics* 101(2):237-241, 1998.

Farrington EA and others: Continuous intravenous morphine infusion in postoperative newborn infants, *Am J Perinatol* 10(1):84-87, 1993.

Fearon I and others: Swaddling after heel lance: age-specific effects on behavioral recovery in preterm infants, *J Dev Behav Pediatr* 18(4):222-232, 1997.

Fenichel GM: *Clinical pediatric neurology: a signs and symptoms approach*, Philadelphia, 1997, WB Saunders.

Field TM and others: Tactile/kinesthetic stimulation effects on preterm neonates, *Pediatrics* 77(5):654-658, 1986.

Fielder AR, Merrick JM: Environmental light and the preterm infant, *Semin Perinatol* 24(4):291-298, 2000.

Finer NN, Barrington KJ: Nitric oxide for respiratory failure in infants born at or near term, *Cochrane Database Syst Rev* (2):CD000399, 2001.

Finnegan LP: Neonatal abstinence. In Nelson N, editor: *Current therapy in neonatal perinatal medicine 1985-1986*, Toronto, 1985, BC Decker.

Fitzgerald M: Pain in infancy: some unanswered questions, *Pain Rev* 2:77-91, 1995.

Fitzgerald M, Millard CM, McIntosh N: Cutaneous hypersensitivity following peripheral tissue damage in newborn infants and its reversal with topical anaesthesia, *Pain* 39(1):31-36, 1989.

Fleisher BE and others: Individualized developmental care for very low birthweight premature infants improves medical and neurodevelopmental outcome in the neonatal intensive care unit, *Clin Pediatr* 34(10):523-529, 1995.

Fowler K and others: Water beds may be useful in preventing scaphocephaly in preterm very low birth weight neonates, *J Perinatol* 17(5):397, 1997.

Franck LS, Scurr K, Couture S: Parent views of infant pain and pain management in the neonatal intensive care unit, *Newborn Inf Nurs Rev* 1(2):106-113, 2001.

Furdon S and others: Outcome measures after standardized pain management strategies in postoperative patients in the NICU, *J Perinat Neonat Nurs* 12(1):58-69, 1998.

Gädeke R and others: The noise level in a children's hospital and the wake-up threshold in infants, *Acta Paediatr Scand* 58(2):164-170, 1969.

Gardner SL, Snell BJ, Lawrence RA: Breastfeeding the neonate with special needs. In Merenstein GB, Gardner SL, editors: *Handbook of neonatal intensive care*, ed 4, St Louis, 1998, Mosby.

Georgieff M, Bernbaum J: Abnormal shoulder girdle muscle tone in premature infants during their first 18 months of life, *Pediatrics* 77(5):664-669, 1986.

Gerhardt KJ, Abrams RM: Fetal exposures to sound and vibroacoustic stimulation, *J Perinatol* 20(8 Pt 2):S21-S30, 2000.

Gervasio CT and others: Early-onset neonatal group B streptococcal sepsis: intrapartum antibiotic prophylaxis in the clinical setting, *J Perinatol* 21(1):9-14, 2001.

Giacoia GP and others: Tracheal TDx fetal lung maturity test for assessing lung maturity in newborns with respiratory distress, *Am J Perinatol* 12(6):420-424, 1995.

Giacoia GP and others: Follow-up of school-age children with bronchopulmonary dysplasia, *J Pediatr* 130(3):400-408, 1997.

Gibbins S, Stevens B: State of the art: pain assessment and management in high-risk infants, *Newborn Inf Nurs Rev* 1(2):85-96, 2001.

Gilson GJ and others: Prevention of group B streptococcus early-onset neonatal sepsis: comparison of the Center for Diseases Control and Prevention screening-based protocol to a risk-based protocol in infants at greater than 37 weeks' gestation, *J Perinatol* 29(8 pt 1):491-495, 2000.

Glass P: The vulnerable neonate and the neonatal intensive care environment. In Avery GB, Fletcher MA, MacDonald MG, editors: *Neonatology: pathophysiology and management of the newborn*, ed 4, Philadelphia, 1994, JB Lippincott.

Graven SN: *Light and early visual development*. Presented at the Annual Conference on The Physical and Developmental Environment of the High-Risk Infant, St Petersburg Beach, FL, 2001.

Graven SN: Sound and the developing infant in the NICU: conclusions and recommendations for care, *J Perinatol* 20(8 Pt 2):S88-S93, 2000.

Greenspan JS, Woolfson MR, Shaffer TH: Liquid ventilation, *Semin Perinatol* 24(6):396-405, 2001.

Groh-Wargo S and others: The utility of a bilateral breast pumping system for mothers of premature infants, *Neonatal Network* 14(8):31-36, 1995.

Grunau RV, Craig, KD: Pain expression in neonates: facial action and cry, *Pain* 28(3):395-410, 1987.

Grunau RV, Johnston CC, Craig KD: Neonatal facial and cry responses to invasive and noninvasive procedures, *Pain* 42(3):295-305, 1990.

Grunau RV and others: Early pain experience, child and family factors as precursors of somatization: a prospective study of extremely premature and full-term children, *Pain* 56(3):353-359, 1994.

Haberkern CM and others: Epidural and intravenous bolus morphine for postoperative analgesia in infants, *Can J Anaesth* 43(12):1203-1210, 1996.

Hack M and others: Neurodevelopment and predictors of outcomes of children with birth weights of less than 1000 g, *Arch Pediatr Adolesc Med* 154(7):725-731, 2000.

Hadjistavropoulos HD and others: Judging pain in infants: behavioural, contextual, and developmental determinants, *Pain* 73(3):319-324, 1997.

Hall JW: Development of the ear and hearing, *J Perinatol* 20(8 Pt 2):S12-S20, 2000.

Harris TR, Wood BR: Physiologic principles. In Goldsmith JP, Karotkin EH, editors: *Assisted ventilation of the neonate*, ed 3, Philadelphia, 1996, WB Saunders.

Harrison L and others: Effects of gentle human touch on preterm infants: pilot study results, *Neonatal Network* 15(2):35-41, 1996.

Harrison LL, Leeper JD, Yoon M: Effects of early parent touch on preterm infants' heart rates and arterial oxygen saturation levels, *J Adv Nurs* 15(8):877-885, 1990.

Harrison LL, Woods S: Early parental touch and preterm infants, *J Obstet Gynecol Neonat Nurs* 20(4):299-306, 1991.

Hegyi T and others: Blood pressure ranges in premature infants. II. The first week of life, *Pediatrics* 97(3):336-342, 1996.

Heller C and others: Sedation administered to very low birth weight premature infants, *J Perinatol* 17(2):107-112, 1997.

Hill A, Volpe JJ: Neurologic disorders. In Avery GB, Fletcher MA, MacDonald MG, editors: *Neonatology: pathophysiology and management of the newborn*, ed 4, Philadelphia, 1994, JB Lippincott.

Hill AS, Kurkowski TB, Garcia J: Oral support measures used in feeding the preterm infant, *Nurs Res* 49(1):2-10, 2000.

Hintz SR and others: Decreased use of neonatal extracorporeal membrane oxygenation (ECMO): how new treatment modalities have affected ECMO utilization, *Pediatrics* 106(6):1339-1343, 2000.

Holditch-Davis D: Neonatal sleep-wake states. In Kenner C, Lott JW, Flandermeyer AA, editors: *Comprehensive neonatal nursing: a physiologic perspective*, ed 2, Philadelphia, 1998, WB Saunders.

Horns KM, Cusson RM: Physiologic and methodologic issues: neonatal insensible water loss, *Neonatal Network* 13(5):83-86, 1994.

Horns KM: Neoteric physiologic and immunologic methods for assessing early-onset neonatal sepsis, *J Perinat Neonat Nurs* 13(4):50-66, 2000.

Hubler E and others: Infant regulation of nipple feeding progression, *Pediatrics* 100(3):S508-S509, 1997.

Hunter J: The neonatal intensive care unit. In Case-Smith J, editor: *Occupational therapy for children*, ed 4, St Louis, 2001, Mosby.

Hunter J: The neonatal intensive care unit. In Case-Smith J, Allen AS, Pratt PN, editors: *Occupational therapy for children*, ed 3, St Louis, 1996, Mosby.

Hurst NM and others: Skin-to-skin holding in the neonatal intensive care unit influences maternal milk volume, *J Perinatol* 17(3): 213-217, 1997.

Jain A, Rutter N, Ratnayaka M: Topical amethocaine gel for pain relief of heel prick blood sampling: a randomized double blind controlled trial, *Arch Dis Child Fetal Neonatal Ed* 84(1):F56-F69, 2001.

Jauhiainen T, Kohonen A, Jauhiainen M: Combined effect of noise and enomycin on the cochlea, *Acta Otolaryngol* 73(5):387-390, 1972.

Johnson KJ and others: Neonatal laboratory blood sampling: comparison of results from arterial catheters with those from an automated capillary device, *Neonatal Network* 19(1):27-34, 2000.

Johnston C and others: Factors explaining lack of response to heel stick in preterm newborns, *J Obstet Gynecol Neonat Nurs* 28(6):587-594, 1999.

Jorgensen KM: The drug-exposed infant: physiology, signs and symptoms, *NANN Central Lines* 15(2):1-2, 8-9, 11, 1999.

Jurkovicova J, Aghova L: Evaluation of the effects of noise exposure on various body functions in low birth weight newborns, *Act Nerv Super* 31(3):228-229, 1989.

Kallman J and others: Contribution of interleukin-6 in distinguishing between mild respiratory disease and neonatal sepsis in the newborn infant, *Acta Paediatr* 88(8): 880-884, 1999.

Kamitsuka MD, Horton MK, Williams MA: The incidence of necrotizing enterocolitis after introducing standardized feeding schedules for infants between 1250 and 2500 grams and less than 35 weeks gestation, *Pediatrics* 105(2):379-384, 2000.

Kandall SR: Treatment strategies for drug-exposed neonates, *Clin Perinatol* 26(1):231-243, 1999.

Kattwinkel J, editor: *Textbook of neonatal resuscitation*, ed 4, Elk Grove Village, IL, 2000, American Academy of Pediatrics and American Heart Association.

Kiehl E, Wallace R, Warren C: Tracking perinatal infection: is it safe to launder your scrubs at home? *MCN* 22(2):195-197, 1997.

Kinsella JP, Abman SH: Inhaled nitric oxide: current and future uses in neonates, *Semin Perinatol* 24(6):387-395, 2000.

Kirkpatrick JM, Alexander J, Cain RM: Recovering urine from diapers: are test results accurate? *MCN* 22(2):96-102, 1997.

Korones SB: Complications: bronchopulmonary dysplasia, air leak syndromes, and retinopathy of prematurity. In Goldsmith JP, Karotkin EH, editors: *Assisted ventilation of the neonate*, ed 3, Philadelphia, 1996, WB Saunders.

Krechel SW, Bildner J: CRIES: a new neonatal postoperative pain measurement score: initial testing of validity and reliability, *Pediatr Anaesth* 5(1):53-61, 1995.

Kuller JM: Skin breakdown: risk factors, prevention, and treatment, *NINR* 1(1):33-42, 2001.

Kuster H and others: Interleukin-1 receptor antagonist and interleukin-6 for early diagnosis of neonatal sepsis 2 days before clinical manifestations, *Lancet* 352(9136):1271-1277, 1998.

Lambe MB: Topical agents in infants, *Newborn Infant Nurs Rev* 1(1):25-34, 2001.

Lau C and others: Oral feeding in low birth weight infants, *J Pediatr* 130(4):561-569, 1997.

Lawrence RA, Lawrence RM: *Breastfeeding: a guide for the medical profession*, ed 5, St Louis, 1999, Mosby.

Leach CEA and others: Epidemiology of SIDS and explained sudden infant deaths, *Pediatrics* 104(4):e43, 953-954, 1999.

Lickliter R: The role of sensory stimulation in perinatal development: insights from comparative research for care of the high-risk infant, *J Dev Behav Pediatr* 21(6):437-447, 2000b.

Lickliter R: Atypical perinatal sensory stimulation and early perceptual development: insights from developmental psychobiology, *J Perinatol* 20(8 Pt 2):S45-S54, 2000a.

Lickliter R: *Sensory interference: practical issues*. Presented at the Annual Conference on The Physical and Developmental Environment of the High-Risk Infant, Clearwater Beach, FL, 1999.

Lin JC and others: Phlebotomy overdraw in the neonatal intensive care nursery, *Pediatrics* 106(2):e19, 2000.

Lockridge T and others: Back to sleep: is there room in that crib for both AAP recommendations and developmentally supportive care? *Neonatal Network* 18(5):29-33, 1999.

Locksmith GJ, Clark P, Duff P: Maternal and neonatal infection rates with three different protocols for prevention of group B streptococcal disease, *Am J Obstetr Gynecol* 180(2 pt 1):416-422, 1999.

Long JG, Lucey JF, Philip AGS: Noise and hypoxemia in the intensive care nursery, *Pediatrics* 65(1):143-145, 1980.

Loughead MK, Loughead JL, Reinhart MJ: Incidence and physiologic characteristics of hypothermia in the very low birth weight infant, *Pediatr Nurs* 23(1):11-15, 1997.

Lucas A and others: Randomized trial of nutrient-enriched formula versus standard formula for postdischarge preterm infants, *Pediatrics* 108(3):703-711, 2001.

Luchtman-Jones L, Schwartz AL, Wilson DB: The blood and hematopoietic system. In Fanaroff AA, Martin RJ, editors: *Neonatal-perinatal medicine: diseases of the fetus and infant*, ed 6, St Louis, 1997, Mosby.

Lund CH and others: Disruption of barrier function in neonatal skin associated with adhesive removal, *J Pediatr* 131(3):367-372, 1997.

Maier NP: Examining the feasibility of hospital-based intervention for mothers and their drug-exposed neonates, *Pediatr Nurs* 21(2):169-172, 1995.

Malanga CJ, Kosofsky BE: Mechanism of action of drugs of abuse on the developing fetal brain, *Clin Perinatol* 26(1):17-37, 1999.

Mammel MC, Boros SJ: High-frequency ventilation. In Goldsmith JP, Karotkin EH, editors: *Assisted ventilation of the neonate*, ed 3, Philadelphia, 1996, WB Saunders.

Mandich MB, Ritchie SK, Mullett M: Transition times to oral feeding in premature infants with and without apnea, *J Obstet Gynecol Neonat Nurs* 25(9):771-776, 1996.

Marsden DJ: Reduction of head flattening in preterm infants, *Dev Med Child Neurol* 22(4):507-509, 1980.

Marshall DD and others: Risk factors for chronic lung disease in the surfactant era: a North Carolina population-based study of very low birth weight infants, *Pediatrics* 104(6):1345-1450, 1999.

Mayes LC: A developmental perspective on the regulation of arousal states, *Semin Perinatol* 24(4):267-279, 2000.

McElhinney DB and others: Necrotizing enterocolitis in neonates with congenital heart disease: risk factors and outcomes, *Pediatrics* 106(5):1080-1087, 2000.

McGrath MM, Sullivan MC, Lester MC: Longitudinal neurologic follow-up in neonatal intensive care unit survivors with various neonatal morbidities, *Pediatrics* 106(6):1397-1405, 2000.

McLaughlin CR and others: Neonatal pain: a comprehensive survey of attitudes and practices, *J Pain Symptom Manage* 8(1):7-16, 1993.

Meehan RM: Heelsticks in neonates for capillary blood sampling, *Neonatal Network* 17(1):17-24, 1998.

Meier PP, Brown LP: Breastfeeding for mothers and low birth weight infants, *Nurs Clin North Am* 31(2):351-365, 1996.

Merenstein GB, Gardner SL: *Handbook of neonatal intensive care*, ed 4, St Louis, 1998, Mosby.

Mirmiran M, Ariagno RL: Influence of light in the NICU on the development of circadian rhythms in preterm infants, *Semin Perinatol* 24(4):247-257, 2000.

Monfort K, Case-Smith J: The effects of a neonatal positioner on scapular rotation, *Am J Occup Therapy* 51(5):378-384, 1997.

Moyer-Mileur LJ and others: Daily physical activity program increases bone mineralization and growth in preterm very low birth weight infants, *Pediatrics* 106(5):1088-1092, 2000.

Msall ME, Tremont MR: Functional outcomes in self-care, mobility, communication, and learning in extremely low-birth weight infants, *Clin Perinatol* 27(2):381-401, 2000.

Murphy BP and others: Impaired cerebral cortical matter growth after treatment with dexaethasone for neonatal chronic lung disease, *Pediatrics* 107(2):217-221, 2001.

Neerhof DO and others: Lamellar body counts: a concensus on protocol, *Obstet Gynecol* 97(2):318-320, 2001.

Neonatal Inhaled Nitric Oxide Study Group (NINOS): Inhaled nitric oxide and hypoxic respiratory failure in infants with congenital diaphragmatic hernia, *Pediatrics* 99(6):838-845, 1997.

Neu M, Browne JV: Infant physiologic and behavioral organization during swaddled versus unswaddled weighing, *J Perinatol* 17(3):193-198, 1997.

Neu M, Browne JV, Vojir C: The impact of two transfer techniques used during skin-to-skin care on the physiologic and behavioral responses of preterm infants, *Nurs Res* 49(4):215-223, 2000.

Newell SJ: Enteral feeding the micropremie, *Clin Perinatol* 27(1):221-234, 2000.

Noerr B: Sucrose for neonatal procedural pain, *Neonatal Network* 20(7):63-67, 2001.

Nyqvist KH, Lutes LM: Co-bedding twins: a developmentally supportive care strategy, *J Obstet Gynecol Neonat Nurs* 27(4):450-456, 1998.

Ochsenreither J: Epidural analgesia in infants, *Neonatal Network* 16(6):79-84, 1997.

Oehler JM: Examining the issue of tactile stimulation for preterm infants, *Neonatal Network* 4(3):25-33, 1985.

Ohls RK: The use of erythropoeitin in neonates, *Clin Perinatol* 27(3):681-696, 2000.

Ostrea E: Understanding drug testing in the neonate and the role of meconium analysis, *J Perinat Neonat Nurs* 14(4):61-82, 2001.

Perry E and others: Blood pressure increases, birth weight-dependent stability boundary, and intraventricular hemorrhage, *Pediatrics* 85(5):727-732, 1990.

Peters KL: Does routine nursing care complicate the physiologic status of the premature neonate with respiratory distress syndrome? *J Perinat Neonat Nurs* 6(2):67-84, 1992.

Peters KL: Infant handling in the NICU: does developmental care make a difference? An evaluative review of the literature, *J Perinat Neonat Nurs* 13(3):83-109, 1999.

Phelps DL, Watts JL: Early light reduction for preventing retinopathy of prematurity in very low birth weight infants, *Cochrane Neonatal Review: http://www.nichd.nih.gov/cochraneneonatal/Phelps/Phelps.htm*, 2001.

Pickler RH, Mauck HG, Geldmaker B: Bottle-feeding histories of preterm infants, *J Obstet Gynecol Neonat Nurs* 26(4):414-420, 1997.

Pohlman S, Beardslee C: Contacts experienced by neonates in intensive care environments, *MCN* 16:207-226, 1987.

Pokorni JL, Stanga J: Serving infants and families affected by maternal cocaine abuse. I, *Pediatr Nurs* 22(5):439-442, 1996.

Prechtl HFR: The organization of behavioral states and their dysfunction, *Semin Perinatol* 16(4):258-263, 1992.

Reed MD, Blumer JL: Pharmacologic treatment of the fetus. In Fanaroff AA, Martin RJ, editors: *Neonatal-perinatal medicine: diseases of the fetus and infant*, ed 6, St Louis, 1997, Mosby.

Reynolds JD and others: Lack of efficacy of light reduction in preventing retinopathy of prematurity. Light Reduction in Retinopathy of Prematurity (LIGHT-ROP) Cooperative Group, *New Engl J Med* 338(22):1572-1576, 1998.

Ringer SA and others: Variations in transfusion practice in neonatal intensive care, *Pediatrics* 101(2):194-200, 1998.

Riordan J, Gill-Hopple K: Breastfeeding care in multicultural populations, *J Obstet Gynecol Neonat Nurs* 30(2):216-223, 2001.

Roberts KL, Paynter C, McEwan B: A comparison of kangaroo mother care and conventional cuddling care, *Neonatal Network* 19(4):31-35, 2000.

Scafidi FA and others: Massage stimulates growth in preterm infants: a replication, *Inf Behav Dev* 13:167-188, 1990.

Schanler RJ: The evidence for breastfeeding, *Pediatr Clin North Am* 48(1):207-219, 2001.

Schanler RJ: Suitability of human milk for the low-birthweight infant, *Clin Perinatol* 22(1):207-222, 1995.

Schanler RJ and others: Feeding strategies for premature infants: randomized trial of gastrointestinal primimg and tube-feeding method, *Pediatrics* 103(2):434-439, 1999.

Schraeder BD and others: Academic achievement and educational resource use of very low birth weight (VLBW) survivors, *Pediatr Nurs* 23(1):21-25, 1997.

Schuler ME, Nair P: Brief report: frequency of maternal cocaine use during pregnancy and infant neurobehavioral outcome, *J Pediatr Psychol* 24(6):511-514, 1999.

Shah V, Ohlsson A: Venepuncture versus heel lance for blood sampling in term neonates, *Cochrane Database Syst Rev* (2):CD001452, 2001.

Shanahan TL, Czeisler CA: Physiological effects of light on the human circadian pacemaker, *Semin Perinatol* 24(4):299-320, 2000.

Shapiro CR: Nurses' judgments of pain in term and preterm newborns, *J Obstet Gynecol Neonat Nurs* 22(1):41-47, 1993.

Shapiro CR: Pain in the neonate: assessment and intervention, *Neonatal Network* 8(1):7-21, 1989.

Singer LT and others: Cognitive and motor outcomes of cocaine-exposed infants, *JAMA* 287(15):1952-1960, 2002.

Soll RF, Blanco F: Natural surfactant extract versus synthetic surfactant for neonatal respiratory distress syndrome, *Cochrane Database Syst Rev* (2):CD000144, 2001.

Soll RF, Morley CJ: Prophylactic selective use of surfactant in preventing morbidity and mortality in preterm infants, *Cochrane Database Syst Rev* (2):CD000510, 2001.

Sorrentino M, Powers T: Effectiveness of palivizumab: evaluation of outcomes from the 1998 to 1999 respiratory syncitial virus season. The Palivizumab Outcomes Study Group, *Pediatr Infect Dis* 19(11):1068-1071, 2000.

Steinfeld JD and others: The utility of the TDx test in the assessment of fetal lung maturity, *Obstet Gynecol* 79:460-464, 1992.

Stevens B, Johnston C, Horton L: Factors that influence the behavioral pain responses of premature infants, *Pain* 59(1):101-109, 1994.

Stevens B, Ohlsson A: Sucrose for analgesia in newborn infants undergoing painful procedures, *Cochrane Database Syst Rev* (2):CD001069, 2000.

Stevens B and others: Management of pain from heel lance with lidocaine-prilocaine (EMLA): is it safe and efficacious in preterm infants? *J Dev Behav Pediatr* 20(14):216-221, 1999a.

Stevens B and others: Premature Infant Pain Profile: development and initial validation, *Clin J Pain* 12(1):13-22, 1996.

Stevens B and others: The efficacy of developmentally sensitive interventions and sucrose for relieving procedural pain in very low birth weight neonates, *Nurs Res* 48(1):35-42, 1999b.

Stoll BJ and others: Early-onset sepsis in very low birth weight neonates: a report from the National Institute of Child Health and Human Developmental Neonatal Research Network, *J Pediatr* 129(1):72-80, 1996.

Strauss RG: Managing the anemia of prematurity: red blood cell transfusions versus recombinant erythropoietin, *Transfus Med Rev* 15(3):213-223, 2001.

Subhani M and others: Screening guidelines for retinopathy of prematurity: the need for revision in extremely low birth weight infants, *Pediatrics* 107(4):656-659, 2001.

Suevo D: The infant of the diabetic mother, *Neonatal Network* 16(5):25-33, 1997.

Swartz K, Noonan DM, Edwards-Beckett J: A national survey of endotracheal suctioning techniques in the pediatric population, *Heart Lung* 25(1):52-60, 1996.

Taddio A and others: Effect of neonatal circumcision on pain response during subsequent routine vaccination, *Lancet* 349(9052):599-603, 1997.

Taddio A and others: A systematic review of lidocaine-prilocaine cream (EMLA) in the treatment of acute pain in neonates, *Pediatrics* 101(7):299, 1998.

Tanney MR, Lowenstein V: One-stop shopping: description of a model program to provide primary care to substance-abusing women and their children, *J Pediatr Health Care* 11(1):20-25, 1997.

The STOP-ROP Multicenter Study Group: Supplemental therapeutic oxygen for prethreshold retinopathy of prematurity (STOP-ROP), a randomized, controlled trial. I: primary outcomes, *Pediatrics* 105(2):295-310, 2000.

Thebaud B, Lacaze-Masmonteil T, Watterberg K: Commentaries: postnatal glucocorticoids in very preterm infants: "The good, the bad, and the ugly?" *Pediatrics* 107(2):413-415, 2001.

Theobald K and others: Apnea of prematurity: diagnosis, implications for care, and pharmacologic management, *Neonatal Network* 19(6):17-24, 2000.

Thogmartin JR, Siebert Jr CF, Pellan WA: Sleep position and bed-sharing in sudden infant deaths: an examination of autopsy findings, *J Pediatr* 138(2):212-217, 2001.

Torres C and others: Effect of standard rest periods on apnea and weight gain in preterm infants, *Neonatal Network* 16(8):35-43, 1997.

Tronick EZ, Beeghly M: Prenatal cocaine exposure, child development, and the compromising effects of cumulative risk, *Clin Perinatol* 26(1):151-171, 1999.

Trotter CW: Percutaneous central venous catheter-related sepsis in the neonate: an analysis of the literature from 1990 to 1994, *Neonatal Network* 15(3):15-28, 1996.

Tyson JE, Kennedy KA: Minimal enteral nutrition for promoting feeding tolerance and preventing morbidity in parenterally fed infants, *Cochrane Database Syst Rev* (2):CD000504, 2000.

Valls-I-Soler A, Alvarez FJ, Gastiasoro E: Liquid ventilation: from experimental use to clinical application, *Biol Neonate* 80(suppl 1):29-33, 2001.

Vamvakas EC, Strauss RG: Meta-analysis of controlled clinical trials: studying the efficacy of rHuEPO in reducing blood transfusions in the anemia of prematurity, *Transfusion* 41(3):406-415, 2001.

Veen S and others: Hearing loss in very preterm and very low birthweight infants at the age of 5 years in a nationwide cohort, *Int J Pediatr Otorhinolaryngol* 26(1):11-28, 1993.

Vennarecci G and others: Intestinal transplantation for short gut syndrome attributable to necrotizing enterocolitis, *Pediatrics* 105(2):1-5, 2000.

Vickers A and others: Cochrane Neonatal Review: Massage for promoting growth and development of preterm and/or low birth-weight infants, *http://www.nichd.nih.gov/cochraneneonatal/Vickers/Vickers.htm*, 2000.

Vohr BR and others: Neurodevelopmental and functional outcomes of extremely low birth weight infants in the National Institute of Child Health and Human Development Neonatal Research Network, 1993-1994, *Pediatrics* 105(6):1216-1226, 2000.

Volpe JJ: *Neurology of the newborn*, ed 4, Philadelphia, 2001, WB Saunders.

Walden M: *Co-bedding twins/multiples: is togetherness a good thing?* Presented at Annual Perinatal Symposium, Houston, 1999, Baylor College of Medicine.

Wallerstedt C, Higgins P: Facilitating perinatal grieving between the mother and father, *J Obstet Gynecol Neonat Nurs* 25(5):389-394, 1996.

Walsh MC, Stork EK: Persistent pulmonary hypertension of the newborn: rational therapy based on pathophysiology, *Clin Perinatol* 28(3):609-628, 2001.

Westrup B and others: A randomized, controlled trial to evaluate the effects of the Newborn Individualized Developmental Care and Assessment Program in a Swedish setting, *Pediatrics* 105(1 Pt 1):66-72, 2000.

Wharrad HJ, Davis AC: Behavioral and autonomic responses to sound in pre-term and full-term babies, *Br J Audiol* 31(5):315-329, 1997.

Wheeden A and others: Massage effects on cocaine-exposed preterm neonates, *J Dev Behav Pediatr* 14(5):318-322, 1993.

White R: *Lighting strategies that address the needs of babies and staff.* Presented at the Annual Conference on The Physical and Developmental Environment of the High-Risk Infant, Clearwater Beach, Fla, 1999.

Wijnberger LD and others: The accuracy of lamellar body count and lecithin/sphyngomyelin ratio in the prediction of neonatal respiratory distress syndrome: a meta-analysis, *Br J Obstetr Gynecol* 108(6):583-588, 2001.

Wilson D: Starting neonatal IVs: practical tips, *Mother Baby J* 5(1):11-18, 2000.

Wiswell TE: Expanded uses of surfactant therapy, *Clin Perinatol* 28(3):695-711, 2001.

Wong DL: *Physiological responses, facial expressions, and cry of infants during immunization in relation to their pain history*, Ann Arbor, MI, 1992, University Microfilm (order number 9321617).

Wong DL and others: Diapering choices: a critical review of the issues, *Pediatric Nurs* 18(1):41-54, 1992.

Yaster M and others: Local anesthetics in the management of acute pain in children, *J Pediatr* 124(2):165-176, 1994.

Zahr LK, Balian S: Responses of premature infants to routine nursing interventions and noise in the NICU, *Nurs Res* 44(3):179-185, 1995.

Zahr LK, de Traversay J: Premature infant responses to noise reduction by earmuffs: effects on behavioral and physiologic measures, *J Perinatol* 15(6):448-455, 1995.

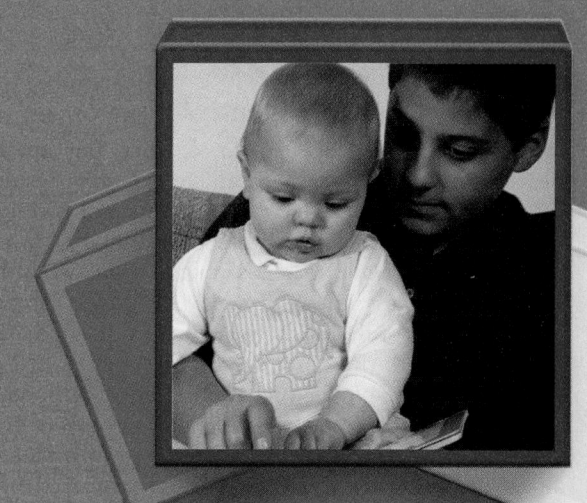

# Chapter 11

# Conditions Caused by Defects in Physical Development

## Chapter Outline

**DEFECTS IN PHYSICAL DEVELOPMENT, 415**
**Prenatal Development, 416**
Fetal Growth and Differentiation, 416
Sensitive Periods in Prenatal Development, 416
**Birth of a Child with a Physical Defect, 416**
**Nursing Care of the Surgical Neonate, 419**

**MALFORMATIONS OF THE CENTRAL NERVOUS SYSTEM (CNS), 423**
**Defects of Neural Tube Closure, 423**
**Anencephaly, 425**
**Spina Bifida (SB)/Myelodysplasia, 425**
**Myelomeningocele (Meningomyelocele), 425**
**Latex Allergy, 433**
*Nursing Care Plan: The Infant with Myelomeningocele, 434*
**Hydrocephalus, 436**

**CRANIAL DEFORMITIES, 443**
**Microcephaly, 444**
**Craniosynostosis, 444**
**Craniofacial Abnormalities, 445**
**Plagiocephaly, 446**
**SKELETAL DEFECTS, 446**
**Developmental Dysplasia of the Hip (DDH), 446**
**Congenital Clubfoot, 451**
**Metatarsus Adductus (Varus), 453**
**Skeletal Limb Deficiency, 453**
**DISORDERS OF THE GASTROINTESTINAL (GI) TRACT, 454**
**Cleft Lip (CL) and/or Cleft Palate (CP), 454**
*Nursing Care Plan: The Child with Cleft Lip and/or Cleft Palate, 461*
**Esophageal Atresia (EA) and Tracheoesophageal Fistula (TEF), 463**
*Nursing Care Plan: The Infant with Esophageal Atresia and Tracheoesophageal Fistula, 467*

**Anorectal Malformations, 466**
**Biliary Atresia, 470**
**Abdominal Wall Defects, 472**
Omphalocele, 472
Gastroschisis, 473
**HERNIAS, 474**
**Umbilical Hernia, 474**
**Congenital Diaphragmatic Hernia (CDH), 475**
**Inguinal Hernia, 477**
**Femoral Hernia, 478**
**DEFECTS OF THE GENITOURINARY (GU) TRACT, 478**
**Phimosis, 479**
**Hydrocele, 479**
**Cryptorchidism (Cryptorchism), 480**
**Hypospadias, 481**
**Epispadias/Exstrophy Complex, 482**
**Obstructive Uropathy, 484**
**Ambiguous genitalia, 487**

## Related Topics

Alternative Feeding Techniques, Ch. 27
Anaphylaxis, Ch. 29
Assessment (Newborn), Ch. 8
Autosomal Inheritance Patterns, Ch. 5
Birth Injuries, Ch. 9
"Birthmarks," Ch. 9
Cerebral Palsy, Ch. 40

Family-Centered Home Care, Ch. 25
Health Promotion of the Newborn and Family, Ch. 8
The High-Risk Newborn and Family, Ch. 10
Hypertrophic Pyloric Stenosis, Ch. 33
Multifactorial Disorders, Ch. 5
Neonatal Pain, Ch. 10

Osteogenesis Imperfecta, Ch. 39
Pain Assessment; Pain Management, Ch. 26
Preparation for Procedures; Surgical Procedures, Ch. 27
Promotion of Parent-Infant Bonding (Attachment), Ch. 8

## DEFECTS IN PHYSICAL DEVELOPMENT

*Congenital malformations,* also called *congenital anomalies* or *birth defects,* may be caused by genetic or environmental factors, but not all congenital defects are malformations

---

■ David Wilson, MS, RNC, edited and revised sections of this chapter.

(e.g., inborn errors of metabolism and mental retardation). However, this chapter is primarily concerned with structural abnormalities and with the impact on the family of the birth of a child with a physical defect. The genetic basis of physical defects is discussed in Chapter 5, and other specific disorders are presented as appropriate throughout the book.

## Prenatal Development

### Fetal Growth and Differentiation

Development consists of two distinct but interrelated processes: growth and differentiation. *Growth* results when cells divide and synthesize new proteins and is reflected in increased size and weight. It is accomplished by two mechanisms: (1) *hyperplasia* (increase in cell number) and (2) *hypertrophy* (increase in cell size). Hyperplasia is the predominant form of growth during the embryonic period. Although the rate slows during later stages of gestation, cell division continues in variable degrees throughout childhood. Hypertrophy is more prominent during later periods of growth.

Each organ and tissue has a typical growth pattern, and all organs progress from a stage characterized by an increase in cell number to one of growth by increase in cell size. Any interference with this pattern of growth results in a reduction in the size and weight of that organ. However, the consequences of the inhibiting factor depend on whether the insult is inflicted during a period of hyperplasia or during a period of hypertrophy. Interference with growth during a period of cell proliferation is likely to cause irreversible growth retardation of that organ with a permanent deficit in overall cell numbers. Interruption of growth during cell enlargement is usually only temporary and can be overcome with proper intervention.

*Differentiation* is the process by which early cells are systematically modified and specialized to form all of the tissues necessary to ensure an organized, coordinated individual. Each step in this process depends on successful completion of a previous step. Anything that interferes with one of these steps, such as a mutant gene or environmental agent, will cause an arrest in the development of that particular tissue or organ. Divergence from the normal course of development will result in maldevelopment of a part or, if it occurs at an early age, a sequence of distortions causing more severe or multiple malformations.

There appears to be a relationship between the incidence of one congenital anomaly and the presence of additional anomalies in an affected child. For example, there is an association between malformed ears and kidney abnormalities that reflects a common developmental stage. The knowledge of the stage of development for a variety of organs and systems provides a valuable clue for the examiner. When one defect is observed, closer scrutiny may reveal defects in another organ or system related to the same stage of development.

Extremely rapid development and change take place during the first 8 to 12 weeks of fetal life, and the beginnings of all major organ systems *(organogenesis)* are formed. The embryo begins to acquire the specific functions needed to integrate these organs and organ systems into an organized, coordinated whole. It is also the period during which the organism is most vulnerable to structural disturbance from environmental hazards.

### Sensitive Periods in Prenatal Development

Every organ, system, and body part goes through a period during which it experiences the most rapid cell division and differentiation. During this time the organism displays a marked susceptibility to injurious influences. These specific stages of crucial developmental advancement are termed *sensitive,* or *critical periods,* and the major impact of environmental factors on development always coincides with these periods. The origin or method by which prenatal growth processes are disturbed to produce a structural or functional defect is termed *teratogenesis* (from the Greek *teratos,* "monster," and *genesis,* "production"). An agent capable of producing such an effect is a *teratogen.* (See Congenital Defects Caused by Prenatal Environmental Factors, Chapter 9.)

The sensitive periods for all organs or parts do not occur simultaneously. A part that is susceptible to adverse influences at one particular time may be resistant to the same influences at other periods of development. At the same time, another part may be highly sensitive at that moment. Susceptibility to environmental influences decreases as organ formation advances—the younger the organism and the fewer the cells, the greater is the extent of involvement when an adverse influence is applied.

During the period of intensive differentiation, most teratogenic agents are highly effective and may produce a variety of deformities. The type of defect that is produced depends on which organ is most susceptible at the time of application. The susceptibility of most tissues to teratogenic influences decreases rapidly in the later periods of development, which are characterized by growth and elaboration of established organs. However, some tissues, particularly those of the central nervous system (CNS), are sensitive to varying degrees throughout fetal life and even beyond. Fig. 11-1 illustrates the approximate times of critical differentiation for some of the major organs and systems.

## Birth of a Child with a Physical Defect

### Parental Responses

Part of the preparation for childbirth involves fantasies and images of the expected infant. Normally, parents hope for a perfect child, but at the same time, they fear that the infant will be abnormal. This fear is often expressed by the expectant parents when they state that their concern is not whether the child is a girl or a boy, but just that the infant is healthy. One of the first things the mother wants confirmed at the time of birth is: "Is my baby all right?" In many instances there is some discrepancy between the parents' idealized child and the infant the mother delivers, as, for example, the birth of a boy when they had hoped for a girl. Resolution of this discrepancy is a developmental task of parenthood and is essential to the establishment of a healthy parent-child relationship. If this discrepancy is major, as with the birth of an infant with a birth defect or when the wishes of the parents are unrealistic, the resulting emotional stress may be overwhelming.

The more severe the defect, the greater the impact of the experience, especially for the mother. The birth of a child with a physical imperfection abruptly ends the psychologic attachment the mother has formed during pregnancy with the idealized child. She and the father must now deal with loss of the anticipated healthy child while they face meeting the demands of the affected child for care and affection. The birth of an infant with a defect evokes the same psychologic reaction as the death of a child. The need for the

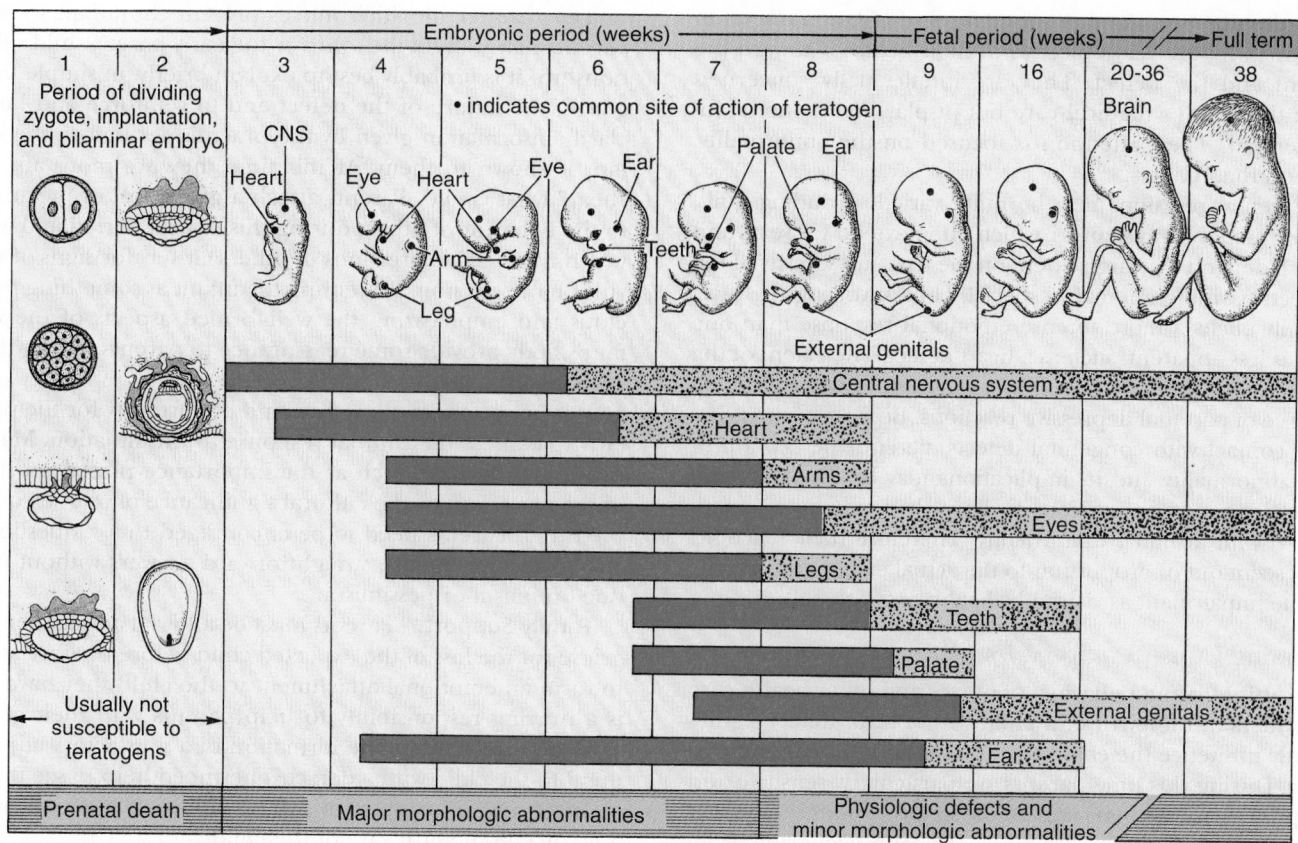

**Fig. 11-1**   Sensitive, or critical, periods in human development. Solid color denotes highly sensitive periods; stippled color indicates stages when embryo is less sensitive to teratogens. (From Moore KL: *The developing human: clinically oriented embryology,* ed 4, Philadelphia, 1988, WB Saunders.)

parents to grieve for the loss of the expected child while adapting to the care of the child with a disability places overwhelming demands on them at a time when their own psychologic and physiologic resources have been depleted by the birth experience. The impact of this new and unexpected burden inhibits the accomplishment of the grief work that normally follows a loss.

The grief reaction experienced by parents at the birth of a child with a physical disability is the same as the response that follows the loss of any valued or significant object. The parents experience shock, frustration, and anger at what has happened to them, and they ask themselves, "Why? Why me?" Parents may feel shame and embarrassment, often with feelings of personal failure and guilt. Frequently the mother believes that she might have caused harm to the unborn child, and she may associate the condition with wrongdoing or evil thoughts, especially if the pregnancy was unwanted initially. She may believe the defect to be a result of passive or active attempts to terminate the pregnancy, such as deliberate attempts to induce abortion or failure to obtain prenatal care or comply with the practitioner's instructions. The father may react to the situation by becoming withdrawn from the newborn and the mother; anger is not uncommon and may be directed at health care workers involved in the child's care. Inwardly the father may blame himself for the child's "imperfection" yet project that blame to others. The mother may not understand the father's withdrawal, and this may further compound her emotional feelings.

There is a phase of overwhelming **shock,** accompanied by weeping and feelings of helplessness. To deal with stress and anxiety, parents use defense mechanisms that have provided protection in the past. A very common response is ***disbelief*** and ***denial,*** which may be short-lived or may last for many months. They do not appear to "hear" what is told to them about their child, and they behave as though nothing is wrong with the child. However, denial during the shock phase of the grief process can serve as a constructive means for parents to deal with the sudden and profound impact of the initial stress until they are better able to cope with the situation.

When parents are unable to face the reality of the infant's condition, they may ***withdraw*** from the situation either physically or emotionally. They frequently become incapacitated and unable to function in their usual manner. They may avoid interpersonal contacts. Unable to face relatives and friends for fear of the reactions they may encounter, parents choose the protection of isolation. They feel as though they are alone in a world all their own. Avoidance behaviors on the part of others, including health workers, contribute to this withdrawal and compound the feelings of loneliness that are so common in parents of an affected infant.

Parents may extend this avoidance behavior to include each other or the infant. They seem to be unable to face the infant, and visiting patterns may become sporadic or nonexistent. Sometimes it takes time for the parents to master their own feelings before they are able to deal constructively with the situation. A more subtle form of isolation is seen in parents who are very objective in their behavior toward the infant and the defect. They are intellectually concerned with the infant's medical care but display no emotional involvement. Their attention is focused on the abnormality, not on the infant.

Parental reactions may be quite varied, including guilt, anger, anxiety, and sadness, which often extend for years and which depend to a large extent on the type and severity of the defect. A visible anomaly, especially one involving the face, usually elicits a more intense emotional response than one that is less apparent, such as a heart defect. The extent of the impairment cannot be used as a criterion to determine the degree of parental depressive reactions. Because of their limited contact with congenital defects, parents' perception of the abnormality and its implications may be distorted, and much depends on previous feelings they may have experienced with a similar abnormality. Therefore their reactions may seem out of proportion to the actual extent and severity of the impairment as viewed by health professionals.

## Nursing Considerations

The attitudes and behaviors of nurses and other health care providers at the birth of a child with a birth defect significantly influence the effect that the situation has on the parents. During this time parents are particularly sensitive and responsive to the behaviors of those with whom they are in contact. Therefore the reactions of health professionals toward the infant and the parents provide cues to the parents that can affect their feelings toward the infant and themselves. Parents are the persons who exert the greatest influence on the growth and development of the child, and the initial relationship with the child significantly affects the subsequent course of interaction.

**Initial Contact.** The first indication that all is not well often occurs at the time of delivery. The atmosphere of happy anticipation suddenly changes to one laden with anxiety. Even when the mother is unable to see the infant, she may sense with terrifying awareness the heightened and prolonged tension in the room, which conveys to her that something is seriously wrong. Health professionals, unprepared for this disturbing experience, find it difficult to cope with their own feelings and react with frustration and resentment toward a situation that they are powerless to change. As a result, they may forget about or retreat from the parents, who at this moment are suffering the most.

Most physicians and nurse midwives believe that it is their responsibility to inform the parents of a congenital anomaly. At the time of delivery, unless a pediatrician or nurse practitioner is in attendance, there is a delay while the practitioner is involved with the mother's care. During this period the mother, unable to see her child and feeling the tense atmosphere, will believe either that the child is normal but that others do not share her enthusiasm or that the child has a defect that is so terrible that the professional people in the room are unable to talk about it. A nurse, the person who is most likely to be free to support the mother and who is familiar with most common congenital anomalies, can make truthful statements about the defect.

The manner in which nurses present the infant to the parents may well set the tone for the early parent-child relationship. It is probably best to explain briefly, in simple language, the nature of the defect and to reinforce and help clarify information given by the practitioner before the infant is shown to them. At this time they are more apt to "hear" what is said. Parents attach a great deal of meaning to the behavior of others during this critical period and will watch the facial expressions of others closely for signs of revulsion or rejection. Presenting the infant as something precious and emphasizing the well-formed aspects of the infant's body provide some reassurance to parents during this crisis period.

It is important to allow time and opportunity for the parents to express their initial response to the situation. Many issues may surface, such as the importance placed on this particular infant or the cultural significance of one sex over the other. Parents need to be encouraged to ask questions and to receive honest, straightforward answers without undue optimism or pessimism.

**Family Support.** Parents must be allowed ample time to grieve for the loss of the expected child before they are able to form an emotional attachment to the child they have. It is a nursing responsibility to help parents with their grief work and to facilitate the formation of a satisfactory adjustment to the child with a defect. They need help to see their infant as a *person*, support in coping with their situation, and guidance in physical care of the child.

Nurses who understand the grief response will be prepared to support the parents through this necessary process. This is particularly important with the birth of a child with a defect, because the parents may not begin to invest any feeling for the child until they are able to talk about and work through their feelings of disappointment, resentment, guilt, and helplessness. Parents need to talk, and the supportive nurse is one who creates and maintains an atmosphere that encourages expression of feelings. Open expression is difficult for many people, and the parent(s) may hesitate to display intense feelings. Containing those feelings expends considerable energy that would be better used later on to develop a relationship with the infant. Nurses therefore need to listen closely for cues that indicate areas of discomfort or readiness to talk.

Parents may not be ready to talk about their feelings during the first few days following the birth. Their dream has vanished, and when others avoid them, it is often interpreted as another abandonment. Staying near and available tells them that they are not alone and that someone cares about them and their feelings. What is said to them is also important. Cliches such as "You will be able to have more children" or "It could be a lot worse" are not a comfort to the parents. Such behavior implies that this infant is not important, and this behavior may destroy the parents' trust.

Initiating a discussion about matters that were of concern to others in a similar situation may help the parents to know that their feelings are natural. Parents need to be allowed silence and solitude if this is their wish. The parents are likely to be angry and will often direct this anger at anyone at hand—physicians, nurses, friends, and families who have normal children. Directing their frustrations at a nonjudgmental target helps parents to relieve some of their distress. Nurses must be prepared to accept any or all of the parental reactions and defenses—anger, hostility, rejection, dependency—without anger and without withdrawing from the situation. If nurses make themselves available to the parents for support, they can often find nonthreatening ways to help, comfort, and support. Most important, nurses need to promote communication and understanding within the family and help strengthen family interpersonal relationships.

**Care of the Infant.**   Many parents are very uneasy about handling their infant and require support and encouragement in their caregiving tasks. A longer period of dependency is needed by these parents to regroup their resources for coping. Although they should not feel forced to care for the infant until they are ready for the responsibility, they should be given opportunities to assume care of the infant as soon as possible to help them deal with the reality of the infant's condition. Parents' responses are highly individual and must be evaluated on this premise. However, all parents need sympathetic, patient, and understanding help to gain feelings of adequacy in the care of their child and to facilitate development of a positive relationship with the infant later on. As anxiety and the intensity of emotional responses abate, parents begin to feel more comfortable with the infant and more confident in their ability to provide needed care.

**Supplying Information.**   Parents need to have accurate, up-to-date information given to them early and in language they can understand. Because they do not hear all that is said the first time it is told to them, they want careful, repeated explanations about the child's defect, the treatments outlined, and what will be expected of them. Parents often misinterpret information, another reason for repeated explanations. Often the nurse's responsibility is to explain, interpret, and clarify information that has been given by the practitioner and to answer questions. Following the basic concepts of informational needs assessment, the nurse determines what the parents know and proceeds from that point. One cannot assume that the parents' failure to ask questions means they understand. Most parents have little or no knowledge of basic anatomy or physiology; therefore pictures and other visual aids can be used effectively to explain both normal and deviant structures.

Teaching the parents to provide the special care that is frequently required for an infant with a physical defect is an important nursing responsibility. Special feeding, holding, and positioning techniques need to be explained and demonstrated. Anticipatory guidance regarding problems that are unique to each abnormality reduces apprehension and stimulates the parents to institute preventive measures and to make alert observations.

Numerous agencies and organizations offer services to families of children with congenital defects. Some provide services for a variety of conditions; others are devoted to specific disorders. They help families with ongoing problems and with anticipating problems they will encounter in raising a child with a defect, including financial burdens. Many have local support groups. All have unique and specialized services designed to help support the family and aid parents in their problem solving. Among those that include most types of defects and diseases are the **National Easter Seal Society for Crippled Children and Adults,**\* the **March of Dimes-Birth Defects Foundation,**† and the **Birth Defect Research for Children, Inc.,**‡ most of which have branches in all major cities and communities. The state **Program for Children with Special Health Needs** (formerly Crippled Children's Services) is also a prime source of assistance. (See Nursing Care Plan: The Child with Chronic Illness or Disability, Chapter 22.)

# Nursing Care of the Surgical Neonate

Advances in early detection of defects (including prenatal diagnosis), surgical techniques, and anesthesia have made it possible for correction or amelioration of many physical defects in the newborn period. In some centers fetal surgery for the correction of life-threatening anomalies has improved the outcome for the newborn without compromising the mother's health. Some newborns have anomalies that require surgery during the neonatal period, often as emergencies. Fortunately, most malformations are correctable with a high degree of success, even those that are dramatic in their presentation.

## Preoperative Care

Most of the problems encountered with the infant undergoing surgery have been discussed in relation to the high-risk infant (e.g., airway maintenance, cardiovascular support, thermoregulation, fluid and electrolyte balance, and nutritional needs). Electronic monitoring of cardiovascular and respiratory status is implemented and maintained, as well as regular comprehensive assessments. (See Systematic Assessment, Chapter 10.) Monitoring and assessments are continued in the postoperative period. Some congenital defects are often associated with other anomalies; therefore assessment should include careful observation for evidence of complications related to these.

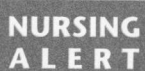 **NURSING ALERT**   A preoperative assessment of the infant's behavior is essential because postoperative deviations may be a manifestation of pain or unstable condition.

Before surgery the infant will usually require a peripheral intravenous (IV) line for fluids and glucose; any electrolyte problems, as well as anemia, are corrected. In some instances a blood product such as packed red blood cells or whole blood is placed on reserve in case blood loss is anticipated. Prophylactic antibiotic administration may begin before surgery, and the infant is observed for any evidence of infection. In addition to routine care, special attention is di-

---

\*230 W Monroe St, Suite 1800, Chicago, IL 60606-4802, (312) 726-6200, 800-221-6827; www.easter-seals.org.
†1275 Mamaroneck Ave, White Plains, NY 10605, (914) 428-7100, (888) MODIMES; www.modimes.org.
‡930 Woodcock Rd, Suite 225, Orlando, FL 32803, (407) 895-0802 or (800) 313-2232; www.birthdefects.org.

rected to specific defects, such as abdominal decompression, protection and management of open lesions, and specific measurements (e.g., abdominal girth, head dimensions). (See also discussion of specific defects.)

Compounding the initial shock of having an infant born with a physical defect, the parents are often further traumatized by the prospect of surgery, sometimes shortly after birth. The parents are provided with accurate information regarding the type of surgical procedure anticipated, method of anesthesia, and, most important, what to expect postoperatively. (Parents are sometimes mentally unprepared for the infant's appearance postoperatively; likewise, some may have false hopes or expectations that the infant will be perfect following surgery.) The parents are also assured that the infant's pain management needs will be evaluated and met postoperatively.

When an infant is transported to a tertiary center for surgery shortly after birth, it is helpful for the nurse to stay in contact with the parents, especially the mother, regarding the infant's condition. Snapshots and even videos, when possible, are helpful tools to allay the mother's anxiety; without seeing her infant and without adequate communication, the mother's anxiety and fears about her infant's condition may be far worse than the reality. During this time the father may serve as the vital link of information between the mother, siblings, and the tertiary center where the infant is undergoing surgery.

### Postoperative Care

Surgery imposes significant stresses on the neonate, especially the preterm or ill infant. The assessment and observations remain much the same as for preoperative care, with the additional problems related to surgery, such as anesthesia and pain. It is essential to maintain physiologic stability to avoid undesirable consequences. Because the neonate is subject to many adverse effects of stress in all physiologic parameters, continual vigilance is mandatory.

Many of the physiologic problems to which the neonate is vulnerable have been discussed in relation to assessment and nursing care of the normal newborn (Chapter 8) and the high-risk infant (Chapter 10). Optimum ventilation, cardiac function, thermoregulation, fluid regulation, care of the operative site, and pain management are primary concerns (Table 11-1). Some of the possible reactions, their probable cause, and the nursing responsibilities are further outlined in Table 11-2.

**TABLE 11-1** Critical guidelines for neonatal postoperative care

| Nursing Responsibilities | Rationale |
| --- | --- |
| **Airway Maintenance*** Monitor respirations, especially if extubated Monitor oxygenation with pulse oximetry and arterial blood gases as necessary Monitor and observe color | Effects of anesthetics, surgery, and pain may decrease respiratory effort; alteration in acid-base balance may reflect early respiratory or metabolic response to surgical interventions |
| **Circulation*** Monitor heart rate Monitor peripheral perfusion—note color and temperature of extremities; capillary refill should be 2 to 3 seconds Monitor blood pressure | A decrease in cardiac output may be seen peripherally before a decrease in blood pressure because of compensatory mechanisms |
| **Fluids, Electrolytes, and Glucose** Evaluate hydration status (overhydration vs dehydration) by weighing neonate postoperatively Monitor electrolytes Perform bedside glucose monitoring using glucometer | An increase or decrease in fluids given intraoperatively is reflected in weight before external signs of hydration are evident A change in electrolyte status often indicates hydration status Stress response to surgery may be evidenced by elevated serum glucose; bedside monitoring is faster than laboratory analysis; physician's order may not be necessary |
| **Thermoregulation*** Maintain a neutral thermal environment Monitor axillary temperature | Effects of anesthetics, exposure to cold, and metabolic response to surgery may decrease body temperature |
| **Operative Site** Observe surgical site and skin status Observe dressings for drainage, bleeding, and amount of output from drainage tubes | Loss of blood may require transfusion; chest tubes, catheters, gastrostomies not draining properly may impair operative site and status |
| **Pain Management** Assess need for analgesics with a neonatal pain scale (see Neonatal Pain, Chapter 10) Implement comfort measures Administer analgesics as needed to prevent pain (see Pain Management, Chapter 26) | Neonate may not be capable of demonstrating pain response but is capable of perceiving pain Major surgery without adequate anesthetics and analgesics can increase postoperative mortality and morbidity |

*Suggested interval for monitoring vital signs postoperatively in neonate: every 15 minutes × 4, every 30 minutes × 2, every 1 hour × 6, then every 2 hours for 24 hours. More frequent monitoring may be needed based on nurse's judgment of infant's status.

**TABLE 11-2**   Possible effects of surgery on selected systems

| Physiologic Response | Nursing Responsibilities |
|---|---|
| **Cardiovascular System** | |
| Hypotension related to:<br>  Large doses of anesthetic<br>  Vasodilation (narcotics)<br>  Myocardial depression (anesthetic agents)<br>  Impaired venous return<br>Hypertension related to:<br>  Hypervolemia, pain, hypercarbia<br>  Increased intracranial pressure (ICP),<br>    vasoconstrictor drugs<br>Tachycardia related to:<br>  Compensation for hypovolemia<br>  Pain<br>  Certain drugs<br>Bradycardia related to:<br>  Hypoxemia (most commonly)<br>  Vagal stimulation<br>  Increased ICP (certain drugs)<br>Vasoconstriction related to:<br>  Hypothermia | Observe for signs of low cardiac output: tachycardia, poor perfusion (prolonged capillary filling; normal is 2-3 seconds in newborn), weak or absent peripheral pulses, decreased intensity of heart sounds, decreased urine specific gravity<br>Observe for signs of congestive heart failure: tachycardia, increased peripheral vasoconstriction (skin changes such as mottling), pulmonary venous engorgement (respiratory distress)<br>Monitor laboratory data (glucose, electrolytes, acid-base balance, hemoglobin, and hematocrit)<br>Administer blood products, vasoactive drugs, cardiotonics as prescribed<br>Monitor and maintain fluid balance, including blood loss<br>Provide ventilatory support as needed |
| **Respiratory System** | |
| Increased respiratory rate related to physiologic characteristics<br>Airway obstruction related to:<br>  Bronchospasm<br>  Laryngeal edema<br>  Mucous plugs<br>Compressed lung tissue related to:<br>  Air, fluid, or blood in pleural cavities<br>  Anatomic defects of diaphragm<br>  Intrinsic pulmonary lesions<br>Ventilation/perfusion imbalance related to:<br>  Atelectasis<br>  Inadequate respiratory effort<br>  Pulmonary edema<br>  Pneumothorax<br>Hypoventilation related to:<br>  Termination of anesthesia<br>  Administration of narcotics, hypocarbia, cold stress, lack of surgical stimulus<br>  Extubation | Observe respiratory rate and symmetry, breath sounds (pitch, intensity, quality, duration, location), color, use of accessory muscles, signs of airway obstruction (decreased breath sounds, decreased $Po_2$, respiratory distress, improper head alignment), signs of respiratory distress (marked retractions, nasal flaring, grunting, tachypnea, cyanosis), signs of impaired diaphragmatic movement (distended abdomen, constrictive dressings)<br>Monitor oxygenation/ventilation, laboratory data<br>Administer oxygen in amount and manner prescribed<br>Position for optimum ventilation<br>Alleviate any impediment to diaphragmatic expansion |
| **Immune System** | |
| Subject to infection related to:<br>  Inability to generate rapid and effective immune defenses<br>  Effects of anesthetics and surgery may mask assessment data | Observe for evidence of sepsis (bradycardia, temperature instability, poor feeding, change in activity level, irregular respiration or apnea), GI disturbances, evidence of abnormal clotting (bleeding from punctures, surgical sites)<br>Monitor for signs of pulmonary or cardiovascular compromise<br>Monitor fluid administration to maintain vascular volume<br>Administer antibiotics as ordered |
| **Endocrine System** | |
| Hypoglycemia related to:<br>  Surgical stress<br>  Rapid depletion of glycogen stores<br>  Decreased gluconeogenesis with stress<br>Hyperglycemia related to:<br>  Surgical stress<br>  Decreased insulin activity<br>Hypothermia<br>Hypocalcemia related to:<br>  Immaturity<br>  Stress<br>  Decreased parathyroid hormone secretion<br>Hypomagnesemia related to:<br>  Hypocalcemia | Observe for apnea, tachypnea, lethargy, pallor, tremors, or seizures<br>Monitor serum glucose levels (bedside glucometer); verify abnormal values with laboratory sample<br>Administer supplemental glucose as prescribed<br>Monitor urinary output (1 to 2 ml/kg/hr)<br>Maintain neutral thermal environment<br>Monitor serum calcium levels<br>Observe for lethargy, vital sign instability, apnea, irritability, jitteriness, seizures<br>Administer supplemental calcium if prescribed<br>Observe for neuromuscular excitability (tetany, seizures)<br>Monitor serum magnesium levels in infants with above signs |

Data from Rushton CH: The surgical neonate: principles of nursing management, *Pediatr Nurs* 14:141-151, 1988.

*Continued*

**TABLE 11-2** Possible effects of surgery on selected systems—cont'd

| Physiologic Response | Nursing Responsibilities |
| --- | --- |
| **Renal System** | |
| Inability to concentrate urine and excrete waste related to:<br>　Immature renal function<br>　Decreased cardiac output<br>　Hypovolemia | Observe for amount and characteristics of urinary output<br>Monitor renal function, drug levels, intravascular volume |
| **Gastrointestinal (GI) System** | |
| Abdominal distention related to:<br>　Hypoactive bowel<br>　Obstruction<br>Hypoactivity related to:<br>　Bowel surgery<br>　Peritonitis<br>　Perforation<br>Hyperactivity related to:<br>　Obstruction<br>Feeding modification related to:<br>　GI surgery (see specific GI surgeries) | Monitor bowel sounds (hyperactivity or hypoactivity)<br>Observe for skin color and integrity (erythema of abdominal wall, prominent veins), abdominal distention (e.g., serial abdominal girth measurements)<br>Palpate abdomen for tenderness<br>Palpate abdomen for organomegaly, evidence of masses<br>Observe frequency, volume, and characteristics of vomiting and vomitus; frequency, volume, and characteristics of stools<br>Delay enteral feedings if prescribed<br>Monitor parenteral feedings and fluid therapy<br>Provide alternative enteral feedings as prescribed (gavage, gastrostomy)<br>Begin and monitor oral feedings as prescribed<br>Provide ostomy care if indicated |
| **Neurologic System** | |
| Hypothermia related to:<br>　See Thermoregulation, below<br>Seizures related to:<br>　Hypoxemia<br>　Hypoglycemia<br>　Hypocalcemia<br>Unresponsiveness<br>Stress related to:<br>　Surgical procedure<br>Pain (see discussion on p. 423) | See Thermoregulation, below<br>Monitor serum calcium, glucose<br>Observe for any seizure activity, unresponsiveness, evidence of pain, signs of hypoglycemia or hypocalcemia (see Chapter 10)<br>Administer sedatives, analgesics, antiepileptic drugs, glucose, calcium as prescribed |
| **Hemopoietic System** | |
| Anemia related to:<br>　Blood loss<br>Hyperviscosity related to:<br>　Polycythemia<br>　Decreased RBC deformability<br>　Plasma protein abnormalities due to third spacing<br>Polycythemia related to:<br>　Chronic hypoxia<br>Coagulation defects related to:<br>　Inherited coagulation defects<br>　Physiologic coagulation factor defects<br>　Transitory coagulation disturbances<br>　Platelet abnormalities | Monitor any blood loss<br>Monitor laboratory data<br>Administer blood or blood products as ordered<br>Observe for complications related to hemopoietic dysfunction and blood administration |
| **Fluid and Electrolyte Disturbances** | |
| Abnormal fluid losses related to:<br>　Blood loss<br>　Fluid shifts (e.g., losses to interstitial tissues [third space])<br>　Transudated fluid<br>　GI, renal, wounds, drains<br>　Membrane injury from sepsis or injury<br>　Insensible fluid losses from open wounds, exposed viscera, immature skin (prematurity) | Observe for evidence of dehydration or overhydration (see Chapter 28)<br>Monitor laboratory data<br>Monitor blood pressure, central venous pressure<br>Weigh daily or more frequently as needed<br>Monitor vital signs<br>Monitor fluid and electrolyte administration<br>Administer albumin, electrolytes |

**TABLE 11-2**   Possible effects of surgery on selected systems—cont'd

| Physiologic Response | Nursing Responsibilities |
|---|---|
| **Acid-Base Balance** | |
| Acid-base disturbance related to: | Monitor acid-base status |
|   Cold stress | Monitor respirations (see above) |
|   Respiratory embarrassment | Administer bicarbonate or other buffer as prescribed |
|   GI disturbances | Maintain neutral thermal environment (see Thermoregulation, below) |
|   Infectious processes | |
|   Surgery | |
|   Immature buffering mechanisms | |
| Acidosis related to: | |
|   Ventilatory insufficiency (respiratory acidosis) | |
|   Ischemic tissue damage | |
|   Cold stress | |
| **Thermoregulation** | |
| Hypothermia related to: | Monitor environmental and infant's core and skin temperatures |
|   Unstable regulatory mechanisms | Maintain optimum thermal environment |
|   Heat loss from large surface area, open wounds, defects | Observe for evidence of hypothermia: peripheral vasoconstriction, apnea, cyanosis, decreased body temperature, respiratory distress, tachycardia |
|   Depletion of glycogen stores and metabolism of brown fat | Minimize heat loss; conserve heat and provide external warmth as needed, including coverings for head and extremities |
|   Immaturity of thermoregulation (see Thermoregulation, Chapter 10) | Warm any blood and irrigating solutions |
| | Observe for seizure activity |

Data from Rushton CH: The surgical neonate: principles of nursing management, *Pediatr Nurs* 14:141-151, 1988.

Because of the respiratory characteristics of newborns, some compromising responses may be anticipated. The newborn's poor chest wall stability, smaller and more reactive airways, fewer and smaller alveoli, and poorly developed accessory muscles contribute to respiratory dysfunction. Compression by intrapleural fluid, air, blood, or a distended abdomen can further compromise pulmonary efforts. Respiratory distress is a common problem in preterm infants. Many postoperative neonates require mechanical ventilation, which may be further influenced by the type, duration, and urgency of the surgery. Mechanical ventilation may be continued in extensive surgical cases to allow for pain management postoperatively. Neonates are highly subject to acidosis and hypoxia and require continuous monitoring of oxygen and acid-base status. Preterm infants will require close monitoring for respiratory complications from general anesthesia.

Cardiovascular support is of particular importance because the immature sympathetic innervation of the myocardium makes the neonate particularly sensitive to vagal stimulation induced by many postoperative procedures, such as nasogastric (NG) tubes, endotracheal (ET) tubes, and suctioning. Any evidence of early compensation for diminished cardiac output is noted, and interventions are implemented before decompensation occurs.

Careful management of fluid and electrolyte status is vital to neonatal surgical care. The natural tendency for rapid fluid shifts related to characteristics of the neonate (see Chapter 28) may be aggravated by stress and any abnormal losses associated with some surgical procedures. (See Hydration, Chapter 10.)

**Pain Management.**   During the postoperative period it is essential to assess and manage neonatal pain. This task is somewhat complicated by the variability with which neonates respond to painful stimuli and the lack of physiologic responses that may occur as a result of anesthesia. The use of muscle-paralyzing agents may further obviate physiologic manifestations of pain in the postoperative period. It is often noted that the more preterm or physiologically immature the infant, the more difficult it becomes to measure pain responses, particularly when major surgery is involved. Because infants of any gestational age are capable of experiencing pain and likewise are capable of being adversely affected by pain during and after operative procedures, it is important to advocate for appropriate pharmacologic therapy to ameliorate neonatal pain. Both pharmacologic and nonpharmacologic pain management therapies may be used in the postoperative period to effectively reduce neonatal pain. (See Neonatal Pain, Chapter 10.)

# MALFORMATIONS OF THE CENTRAL NERVOUS SYSTEM (CNS)*
## Defects of Neural Tube Closure

Abnormalities that are derived from the embryonic neural tube *(neural tube defects [NTDs])* constitute the largest group of congenital anomalies consistent with multifactorial inheritance. Normally the spinal cord and cauda equina are encased in a protective sheath of bone and meninges (Fig. 11-2, *A*). Failure of neural tube closure produces defects of varying degrees (Box 11-1). They may involve the entire length of the neural tube or may be restricted to a small area.

■ *\*Amy Nadel Romanczuk, MSN, RN, CNS, revised this section.*

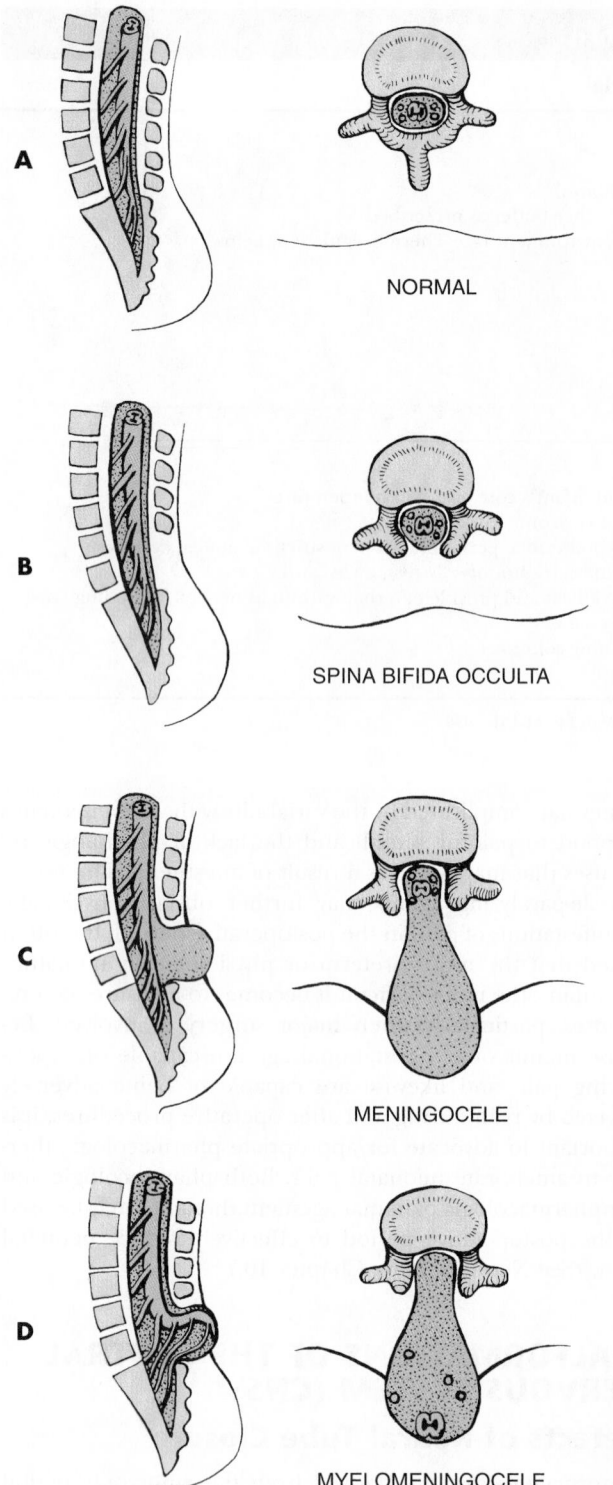

**Fig. 11-2** Midline defects of osseous spine with varying degrees of neural herniations. **A,** Normal. **B,** Spina bifida occulta. **C,** Meningocele. **D,** Myelomeningocele.

---

## Etiology

Two of the defects, *anencephaly* and *spina bifida (SB)*, occur in association with one another more often than would be expected by chance, suggesting a common origin. The CNS defects may alternate in siblings, which also tends to support the theory of a common origin. The incidence of SB is higher in girls than in boys, and it is three times more likely to occur in whites than in African-Americans. It is now known that 50% or more (American Academy of Pediatrics, 1999) of the cases of SB occur as a result of nutritional deficiency (i.e., folic acid deficiency); the remaining causes are multifactorial (Sarwark, 1996).

Studies have shown that women at high risk for having a child with an NTD because they had previously delivered an infant or fetus with SB, anencephaly, or encephalocele significantly reduced the recurrence rate by taking supplements of the *B vitamin folic acid* before conception (American Academy of Pediatrics, 1999). *Folate* is a generic term for food compounds that have the biologic activity of folic acid, although folates in food are generally not as well absorbed as is folic acid. Other factors possibly involved in the etiology of NTDs include maternal heat exposure (i.e., hot tubs, saunas), valproic acid (an antiepileptic drug), and familial tendency.

The American Academy of Pediatrics (1999) recommends daily intake of folic acid for all women of childbearing age. The recommended 0.4-mg daily dose is supplied safely in many multivitamin preparations. Because the greatest risk factor is a previous pregnancy affected by NTDs, women in this category should increase their daily folic acid dose to 4 mg, under a practitioner's supervision, beginning at least 1 month before they plan a pregnancy and through the first trimester because the neural tube closes about 1 month after conception. A 50% to 70% reduction in NTDs is anticipated with folic acid supplementation. As of January 1998, the Food and Drug Administration (FDA) authorized the fortification of cereal grains (including corn meal, grits, and wheat flour) with folic acid. It remains important for all women of childbearing age to take a multivitamin with 0.4 mg folic acid daily (American Academy of Pediatrics, 1999; Centers for Disease Control and Prevention, 1999).

**NURSING ALERT**   Supplementation of 4.0 mg of folate should not be met through the use of multivitamin preparations alone because of the risk of excessive ingestion of other vitamins. Excess folate can mask symptoms of vitamin $B_{12}$ deficiency, and excess vitamin A may cause birth defects.

The following discussion of NTDs is limited to the two most common types: anencephaly, a defect incompatible with life, and SB, in particular, myelomeningocele, an abnormality that causes significant disability.

## Anencephaly

Anencephaly, the most serious NTD, is a congenital malformation in which both cerebral hemispheres are absent. The condition is incompatible with life, and many affected infants are stillborn. For those who survive, no specific treatment is available. The infants have an intact brainstem and are able to maintain vital functions (such as temperature regulation and cardiac and respiratory function) for a few hours to several weeks but eventually die of respiratory failure.

Traditionally these infants have been provided comfort measures, but with no effort at resuscitation. Ethical and moral questions are encountered regarding treatment and withdrawal of support systems (e.g., feedings) if the newborn survives the first few days of life, as well as use of the organs for donor transplants. During this time the family requires emotional support and counseling to cope with the birth of an infant with a fatal defect.

## Spina Bifida (SB)/Myelodysplasia

*Myelodysplasia* refers broadly to any malformation of the spinal canal and cord. Midline defects involving failure of the osseous (bony) spine to close are called *spina bifida,* the most common defect of the CNS. SB is categorized into two types: spina bifida occulta and spina bifida cystica.

*Spina bifida occulta* refers to a defect that is not visible externally. It occurs most commonly in the lumbosacral area (L5 and S1) (Fig. 11-2, *B*). Routine radiographic examinations indicate that the disorder may be seen in as many as 10% to 30% of the general population (Lutkenhoff, 1999). However, it may not be apparent unless there are associated cutaneous manifestations or neuromuscular disturbances.

Superficial cutaneous indications include a skin depression or dimple (which may also mark the outlet of a dermal sinus tract that extends to the subarachnoid space), portwine angiomatous nevi, dark tufts of hair, and soft, subcutaneous lipomas. These signs may be absent, appear singly, or be present in combination.

If associated neurologic involvement is present, the defect is known as *occult spinal dysraphism.* The spinal cord or roots can be distorted by fibrous bands and adhesions, an intraspinal lipoma (fatty tumor) or subcutaneous lipoma (lipomyelomeningocele), a dermoid or epidermoid cyst, diastematomyelia (spinal cord split in two), or a tethered cord (Dias and Li, 1998). The usual cause is abnormal adhesion, or *tethering,* to a bony or fixed structure, resulting in trac-

tion on the spinal cord and cauda equina. (See Figs. 40-6 and 40-8 for areas innervated by specific spinal nerves.)

Neuromuscular disturbances usually consist of progressive or static changes in gait with foot weakness, foot deformity, and/or bowel and bladder sphincter disturbances. Manifestations may not be evident until the child walks or is toilet trained.

Plain radiography is employed to disclose the precise bony defect in the symptomatic lesion and to establish the diagnosis in the suspected, nonsymptomatic occult variety. Magnetic resonance imaging (MRI) is the most sensitive tool for evaluating the defect. Computed tomography (CT), ultrasonography, and myelography are also used to differentiate between SB occulta and other spinal disorders.

*Spina bifida cystica* refers to a visible defect with an external saclike protrusion. The two major forms of SB cystica are *meningocele,* which encases meninges and spinal fluid, but no neural elements (Fig. 11-2, *C*), and *myelomeningocele* (or *meningomyelocele*), which contains meninges, spinal fluid, and nerves (Fig. 11-2, *D*). Meningocele is not associated with neurologic deficit, which occurs in varying, often serious, degrees in myelomeningocele. Clinically the term *spina bifida* is used to refer to myelomeningocele.

## Myelomeningocele (Meningomyelocele)

Myelomeningocele develops during the first 28 days of pregnancy when the neural tube fails to close and fuse at some point along its length. It may be detected prenatally or at birth, accounts for 90% of spinal cord lesions, and may be located at any point along the spinal column. Usually the sac is encased in a fine membrane that is prone to tears through which cerebrospinal fluid (CSF) leaks. In other instances the sac may be covered by dura, meninges, or skin, in which instances there is rapid and spontaneous epithelialization. The largest number of myelomeningoceles are found in the lumbar or lumbosacral area (Fig. 11-3). The location and magnitude of the defect determine the nature and extent of neurologic impairment. When the defect is located below the second lumbar vertebra, the nerves of the cauda equina are involved, giving rise to symptoms such as flaccid, areflexic partial paralysis of the lower extremities and varying degrees of sensory deficit. Unlike a spinal cord injury, the degree of deficit is not necessarily uniform on both sides but may vary between extremities, depending on the compromise to specific nerves from malformation or tethering.

The anomaly most frequently associated with myelomeningocele is *hydrocephalus;* 80% to 85% of children with SB will develop hydrocephalus (Rintoul and others, 2002). Although present at birth, hydrocephalus may not be apparent until shortly thereafter, or after the primary closure of the opening on the back. Careful monitoring of head circumference, fontanel tension, and ventricular size by head ultrasonography can indicate its presence. Hydrocephalus can occur because the NTD itself disrupts the flow of cerebrospinal fluid. In many cases a *Chiari malformation* (type 2) is responsible (see p. 437). Chiari malformation is present,

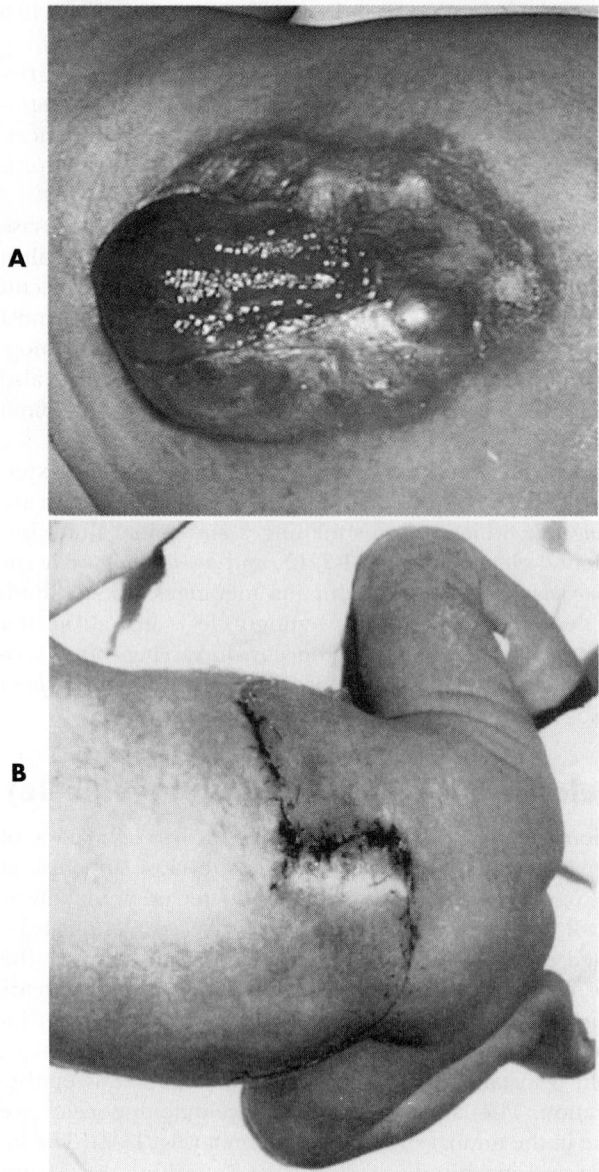

**Fig. 11-3 A,** Meningomyelocele before surgery. (An antibacterial dressing was used.) **B,** Repair of meningomyelocele. (**A** from Zitelli BJ, Davis HW: *Atlas of pediatric physical diagnosis,* ed 3, St Louis, 1997, Mosby; **B** courtesy MC Gleason, MD, San Diego. From Novak JC, Broom BL: *Ingalls and Salerno's maternal and child health nursing,* ed 8, St Louis, 1995, Mosby.)

though asymptomatic, in most children with SB. It can, however, adversely affect respiratory function, causing episodic apnea. Other clinical symptoms of problematic Chiari malformation include stridor, hoarse cry from vocal cord paralysis, feeding difficulties, and, in older children, a worsening of upper extremity function.

## Pathophysiology

The pathophysiology of SB is best understood when related to the normal formative stages of the nervous system. At approximately 20 days of gestation a decided depression, the neural groove, appears in the dorsal ectoderm of the embryo. During the fourth week of gestation the groove deep-

ens rapidly, and its elevated margins develop laterally and fuse dorsally to form the neural tube. Neural tube formation begins in the cervical region near the center of the embryo and advances in both directions—caudally and cephalically—until by the end of the fourth week of gestation the ends of the neural tube, the anterior and posterior neuropores, are closed.

The primary defect in neural tube malformations is believed by most authorities to be a failure of neural tube closure. However, there is evidence to indicate that the defects are a result of splitting of the already-closed neural tube as a result of an abnormal increase in CSF pressure during the first trimester.

## Clinical Manifestations

The manifestations of SB vary widely according to the degree of the spinal defect. The defect is readily apparent on inspection. The degree of neurologic dysfunction is directly related to the anatomic level of the defect and thus the nerves involved. Sensory disturbances usually parallel motor dysfunction. The upper level of sensory and motor impairment can be determined by observation of the infant's response to a pinprick over the legs and trunk. The infant will respond to the sensory stimulus with limb movement, arousal, and crying. When withdrawal activity is used to determine the lowest level of spinal cord function, the response to pinprick should begin above the lesion.

Defective nerve supply to the bladder affects both sphincter and detrusor tone, which often causes constant dribbling of urine or produces overflow incontinence. This can often be mistaken for normal voiding patterns in the newborn. Some infants with SB, however, are able to void in a stream and achieve complete bladder emptying with each void.

Frequently there is poor anal sphincter tone and poor anal skin reflex, which result in lack of bowel control and sometimes rectal prolapse. Rectal temperatures are avoided in affected infants. If the defect is located below the third sacral vertebra, there is no motor impairment, but there may be saddle anesthesia with bladder and anal sphincter paralysis.

Sometimes the denervation to the muscles of the lower extremities will produce joint deformities in utero. These are primarily flexion or extension contractures, talipes valgus or varus contractures, kyphosis, lumbosacral scoliosis, and hip dislocations. The extent and severity of these associated orthopaedic deformities again depend on the degree of nerve involvement. Most flexion deformities result from the pull of stronger, fully innervated muscles acting without the counterpull of their nonfunctioning paralyzed antagonists. See Box 11-2 for summary of clinical manifestations of SB cystica and occulta.

## Diagnostic Evaluation

The diagnosis is made on the basis of clinical manifestations and examination of the meningeal sac. Diagnostic measures used to evaluate the brain and spinal cord include MRI, ultrasonography, CT, and myelography.

Laboratory examinations are used primarily to determine causative organisms in the major complications of my-

### Box 11-2
## Clinical Manifestations of Spina Bifida

**SPINA BIFIDA CYSTICA**

Sensory disturbances usually parallel motor dysfunction
  Below second lumbar vertebra:
    Flaccid, partial paralysis of lower extremities
    Varying degrees of sensory deficit
    Overflow incontinence with constant dribbling of urine
    Lack of bowel control
    Rectal prolapse (sometimes)
  Below third sacral vertebra:
    No motor impairment
    Bladder and anal sphincter paralysis
Joint deformities (sometimes produced in utero):
  Talipes valgus or varus (foot) contractures
  Kyphosis
  Lumbosacral scoliosis
  Hip dislocation

**SPINA BIFIDA OCCULTA**

Frequently no observable manifestations
May be associated with one or more cutaneous manifestations:
  Skin depression or dimple
  Port-wine angiomatous nevi
  Dark tufts of hair
  Soft, subcutaneous lipomas
May be neuromuscular disturbances:
  Progressive disturbance of gait with foot weakness
  Bowel and bladder sphincter disturbances

elomeningocele—meningitis and urinary tract infections. Infants with urinary incontinence require urinalysis, culture, and evaluation of blood urea nitrogen (BUN) and creatinine clearance.

**Prenatal Detection.**   It is possible to determine the presence of some major open NTDs prenatally. Ultrasonographic scanning of the uterus and elevated maternal concentrations of alpha-fetoprotein (AFP or MS-AFP), a fetal-specific gamma-1 globulin, in amniotic fluid may indicate the presence of anencephaly or myelomeningocele. (See Chapter 5.) The optimum time for performing these diagnostic tests is between 16 and 18 weeks of gestation, before AFP concentrations normally diminish and in sufficient time to permit a therapeutic abortion. It is recommended that such diagnostic procedures be considered for all mothers who have borne an affected child, and testing is offered to all pregnant women. In addition, elective prelabor cesarean birth may result in less motor dysfunction. Early closure of the myelomeningocele sac through fetal surgery is also being evaluated to see if such an intervention might prevent injury to the exposed spinal cord tissue and possibly improve neurologic outcomes in the affected infant (Tulipan and Bruner, 1998; Olutoye and Adzick, 1999).

## Therapeutic Management

Management of the child who has a myelomeningocele requires a multidisciplinary approach involving the specialties of neurology, neurosurgery, pediatrics, urology, orthopaedics, rehabilitation, physical therapy, occupational therapy, and social service, as well as intensive nursing care in a variety of specialty areas. The collaborative efforts of these specialists are focused on (1) the myelomeningo-

cele and the problems associated with the defect—hydrocephalus, paralysis, orthopaedic deformities, and genitourinary abnormalities; (2) possible acquired problems that may or may not be associated, such as meningitis, hypoxia, and hemorrhage; and (3) other abnormalities, such as cardiac or gastrointestinal malformations. Many hospitals have implemented routine outpatient care by multidisciplinary teams to provide the complex follow-up needed for children with myelodysplasia (Chambers and others, 1996; Rauen, 1995).

**Initial Care.**   Care of the newborn involves prevention of infection; neurologic assessment, including observation for associated anomalies; and dealing with the impact of the anomaly on the family. Most authorities believe that early closure, within the first 24 to 72 hours, offers the most favorable outcome, especially in regard to morbidity and mortality from serious infection. Early closure, preferably in the first 12 to 18 hours, not only prevents local infection and trauma to the exposed tissues, but also avoids stretching of other nerve roots, which may occur as the meningeal sac expands during the first 24 hours after birth, thus preventing further motor impairment.

A variety of neurosurgical and plastic surgical procedures are employed for skin closure without disturbing the neural elements or removing any portion of the sac. The objective is satisfactory skin coverage of the lesion and meticulous closure. Wide excision of the large membranous covering may damage functioning neural tissue.

Associated problems are assessed and managed by appropriate surgical and supportive measures. Shunt procedures provide relief from imminent or progressive hydrocephalus (see p. 436). Meningitis, urinary tract infection, and pneumonia are treated with vigorous antibiotic therapy and supportive measures. Surgical intervention for Chiari malformation (a downward herniation of the brain into the brainstem) is indicated only when the child is symptomatic (i.e., high-pitched crowing cry, respiratory difficulties, oral/motor difficulties).

Improved surgical techniques do not alter the major physical disability and deformity or chronic urinary tract and pulmonary infections that affect the quality of life for these children. Superimposed on these physical problems are the effects that the disorder has on family life and finances and on school and hospital services.

**Orthopaedic Considerations.**   According to most orthopaedists, musculoskeletal problems that will affect later locomotion should be evaluated early, and treatment, where indicated, should be instituted without delay. Neurologic assessment will determine the neurosegmental level of the lesion, recognition of spasticity and progressive paralysis, the potential for deformity, and functional expectations. Orthopaedic management includes prevention of joint contractures, correction of the deformity, prevention of skin breakdown, and obtaining the best possible ambulatory function. The status of the neurologic deficit remains the most important factor in determining the child's ultimate functional abilities.

Great diversity is observed in patterns of musculoskeletal involvement. The hip flexors and adductors are innervated by L1 to L3, whereas extensors and abductors are innervated by L5 to S1. Consequently, there is often an imbalance in muscle pull around a joint. Children with lesions at L2 or above have some hip flexion and are usually confined to a wheelchair for mobility. Children with lesions at L2 to L5 have strong hip flexors and are candidates for crutches and braces, although the majority use a wheelchair most of the time. At levels L3 and L4 there is usually an imbalance between sensory and motor nerve involvement, and hip dislocation is often a problem. Children with sacral lesions are able to walk, but some may require ankle bracing.

Physical therapy and orthopaedic management of children with myelomeningocele is a continuous process to achieve optimum function and ambulation when possible. Problems such as Arnold-Chiari malformation, hydrocephalus, and a tethered spinal cord can complicate expectations. Controversies exist over the orthopaedic management of dislocated hips, scoliosis, and kyphosis.

A variety of devices are available to provide mobility to children with spinal cord lesions, including lightweight braces, special "walking" devices, and custom-built wheelchairs. (See Chapter 39.) Corrective procedures, when indicated, are best initiated at an early age so that the child will not lag significantly behind age-mates in developmental progress. Where there is little hope for lower extremity functioning, surgery is seldom recommended.

**Management of Genitourinary Function.\*** Myelomeningocele is one of the most common causes of neuropathic (neurogenic) bladder dysfunction among children. Myelomeningocele affects approximately 1 in 1000 infants born in the United States, and as many as 90% will experience subsequent voiding dysfunction. In infants the goal of treatment is to preserve renal function. In older children the goal is to preserve renal function *and* achieve optimum urinary continence (Bellinger, 1996; Fernandes and others, 1994). Urinary incontinence is a chronic, often debilitating problem for the child. In addition, the neuropathic bladder may produce **urinary system distress,** characterized by symptomatic urinary tract infections, ureterohydronephrosis, vesicoureteral reflux, or renal insufficiency. The characteristics of bladder dysfunction in children vary according to the level of the neurologic lesion and the influence of bony growth and development of the spine. In addition, the presence of an Arnold-Chiari defect and subsequent hydrocephalus has the potential to affect bladder function, although spinal influences are predominant (Kelalis, King, and Belman, 1992).

During infancy, urinary incontinence is normally physiologic, but urinary system distress may occur. Ongoing urologic monitoring is essential, and there is growing evidence that early intervention, based on evaluation during the neonatal period and *before* complications occur has the following benefits: (1) improves bladder function, (2) reduces the subsequent risk of urinary system distress, and (3) reduces the need for reconstructive surgery of the lower urinary tract (Holzbierlein and others, 2000; Kaefer and oth-

ers, 1999). Ultrasonography of the bladder and ureters as well as routine urinalysis (and urine cultures when indicated) are used to detect urinary system distress before renal function is compromised. In addition, urodynamic testing is used to identify bladder dysfunction that predisposes the child to urinary system distress. These conditions include high pressure detrusor hyperreflexia (reflex contractions of the detrusor muscle) with vesicosphincter dyssynergia (incoordination of detrusor and sphincter muscles), low bladder wall compliance (poor distensibility of the bladder wall causing increased intravesical pressures during urine filling and storage), or detrusor areflexia (absence of detrusor contractions caused by the spinal defect).

Infants may have one of several predominant neuropathic bladder disorders. Detrusor contractions associated with vesicosphincter dyssynergia are particularly common. Some infants are able to empty the bladder efficiently despite incoordination between the sphincter mechanism and detrusor, but the majority experience chronic residual urine, urinary tract infections, or more serious types of urinary system distress. A minority of infants have poor detrusor contraction strength or detrusor areflexia (absence of contractions). This condition is particularly damaging to the urinary system when it coexists with low bladder wall compliance and an elevated detrusor leak point pressure. Low bladder wall compliance occurs when collagen or fibrosis causes stiffening of the bladder wall. This stiffened bladder wall raises intravesical pressures, obstructing the bladder, ureters, and, ultimately, the nephron. The impact of low bladder wall compliance is directly related to the influence of the bladder outlet. Among children with myelodysplasia, the urethral muscles are typically weakened, and much of the muscle tissue is replaced by collagen. As a result, the sphincter is fixed, so that it neither closes efficiently to prevent urinary leakage nor opens well to allow urinary flow with a detrusor contraction. When the magnitude of the pressure required to drive urine across the abnormal sphincter is greater than 40 cm $H_2O$ (the detrusor leak point pressure) and the compliance of the bladder wall is low (<10 cm $H_2O$), the risk of urinary system distress is high (Gray, 1993).

In contrast, a small number of infants experience effective detrusor contractions without vesicosphincteric dyssynergia. Effective bladder evacuation is likely among this group, and the incidence of urinary system distress during the first year of life is low (Kelalis, King, and Belman, 1992).

As the child grows, detrusor hyperreflexia is often replaced by deficient detrusor contraction strength and **stress urinary incontinence (SUI)** (leakage produced by physical exertion). The bladder wall is often poorly compliant (producing chronically elevated intravesical pressures), and the bladder outlet, while incompetent, obstructs the outflow of urine. When the detrusor leak point pressure exceeds 40 cm $H_2O$, the child is predisposed to chronic urinary leakage and urinary distress symptoms, including recurrent urinary tract infections and reflux. When the detrusor leak point pressure is lower than 40 cm $H_2O$, urinary leakage is more severe, although the risk of urinary system distress is lessened. Thus the child with more severe urinary inconti-

---

■ \*Mikel Gray, PhD, CUNP, CCCN, FAAN, wrote this section.

nence is less predisposed than the "drier" child to serious urinary infections.

Infants with myelomeningocele and a neurogenic bladder who are not at risk for urinary system distress are managed by diaper containment and watchful waiting. The infant empties the bladder into a diaper, the urine is routinely monitored for infection, and the upper urinary tracts are monitored for evidence of urinary system distress (dilation of the ureters, renal pelves, or collecting systems) via serial ultrasonography.

In contrast, children with evidence of urinary system distress, or those considered at risk based on early urodynamic testing, are placed on *clean intermittent catheterization (CIC),* typically in combination with an antispasmodic medication such as oxybutynin or propantheline (Holzbierlein and others, 2000; Kaefer and others, 1999; Wu, Baskin, and Kogan, 1997). Anticholinergic medications are prescribed because they reduce detrusor muscle tone and reduce bladder pressures during both urine filling and storage and during micturition. CIC is not intended to prevent spontaneous voiding; instead, it ensures routine, regular bladder evacuation, further preventing deleterious elevation of intravesical pressures. Usually, the parents are taught to catheterize the infant every 3 hours during the day and once each night. Follow-up evaluation, consisting of serial ultrasonography and urinalysis, is completed every 3 to 6 months as indicated.

Infants with significant urinary system distress and hostile neuropathic bladder dysfunction at birth sometimes require temporary urinary diversion to ensure adequate urine outflow and prevent further damage to the upper urinary tracts. A *vesicostomy* is a relatively simple procedure wherein the anterior bladder wall is brought to the abdominal wall, creating a small stoma for urinary drainage. Urine is contained via a diaper, but double diapering or use of a larger diaper that can be placed higher on the abdomen is necessary for adequate urine containment. Meticulous skin care is needed because the perineal skin is exposed to continuous urinary leakage.

Among older children the quest for continence typically begins with a CIC program. The parents are taught the procedure, and the child is taught to self-catheterize as soon as possible, usually by the sixth year of life. The child with detrusor hyperreflexia and dyssynergia often responds well to antispasmodic medications and CIC. In contrast, the child with poor bladder wall compliance and SUI often requires a combination of antispasmodic medications to reduce intravesical filling pressures and an $\alpha$-sympathetic agonist (such as imipramine, pseudoephedrine, or phenylpropanolamine) to enhance sphincter competence. Unfortunately, the combination of medications and CIC is typically only partly effective, and more aggressive interventions are often required to render the neuropathic bladder both continent and free from its predisposition toward producing urinary system distress.

When continence cannot be attained by conservative measures, surgery is considered. *Augmentation enterocystoplasty* is a surgical procedure that increases bladder capacity, reverses or halts the deleterious effects of the poorly compliant bladder wall, and reduces harmfully high bladder pressures caused by detrusor hyperreflexia with vesi-

cosphincter dyssynergia (Gray, 1993). A detubularized segment of large or small bowel, as well as a wedge of the fundus of the stomach, has been used to successfully augment bladder capacity. The choice of segment varies according to the surgeon's preference and the status of the patient's urinary and gastrointestinal systems. Large and small bowel segments produce significant volumes of mucus that may clog catheters used for CIC. Augmentation with the stomach produces less mucus, and its acidic secretions may reduce the urinary system's predisposition to infection.

Even though augmentation of the bladder may improve or resolve urinary leakage related to detrusor hyperreflexia or urinary system distress caused by low bladder wall compliance, the SUI produced by the abnormal sphincter mechanism typically persists. Several surgical procedures may be used to correct this intrinsic sphincter deficiency. The *Mitrofanoff procedure* uses the appendix to provide an alternative route for intermittent catheterization (Kaefer and others, 1997). The appendix is removed from the colon and used to create a continent conduit between the abdominal wall and the bladder. The resulting stoma is relatively small and produces minimal mucus. The ureter may be used as an alternative to the appendix for some children. When intrinsic sphincter deficiency produces only mild stress urinary leakage, the construction of a Mitrofanoff route alone may be sufficient to achieve continence between catheterization episodes. However, when SUI is more severe, a suburethral sling or suburethral collagen injection is used to alleviate intrinsic sphincter deficiency.

The *suburethral sling* is a slip of fascia or synthetic material that is placed below the proximal third of the urethra. The sling may be placed in a fashion that uses only very slight tension to obstruct the urethra and prevent SUI. The sling may be used for both boys and girls, and the procedure can be completed at the same time the augmentation enterocystoplasty is constructed. The surgeon carefully avoids excessive tension when placing the sling to avoid ischemia or other complications. Following augmentation enterocystoplasty and placement of a suburethral sling, the patient can expect to evacuate the bladder by CIC of the appendicial Mitrofanoff route or the urethra if a Mitrofanoff route has not been constructed.

Suburethral injection of *glutaraldehyde cross-linked (GAX) collagen* also may be used to alleviate or prevent SUI caused by intrinsic sphincter deficiency (Bennett and others, 1995). Collagen is used to bulk or expand the urethral tissue, promoting coaptation (approximation) of the mucosa. The collagen implant complements the urethra's ability to form a watertight seal, rather than obstructing the urethral lumen. Collagen may be injected using different approaches. *Transurethral collagen* is injected through the working channel of a cystoscope. *Transperineal collagen* is directed underneath the urethra using a needle inserted through the perineal skin. In this case, the location of the urethra is confirmed by simultaneous cystoscopic visualization of the urethra. The *antegrade approach* requires creation of a suprapubic cystostomy tract. A flexible cystoscope is then inserted through the cystostomy tract, and collagen is injected into the proximal urethra. Multiple injections may be required to achieve optimum continence. Subsequent injections may be required when the collagen is dissipated or reabsorbed by the body over a period of years.

The *artificial urinary sphincter* provides another alternative for the management of intrinsic sphincter deficiency in the child with myelomeningocele. The device consists of a urethral cuff, abdominal reservoir, and control pump. In the activated position, the cuff is filled, and the pressure of this cuff closes the urethral lumen. During micturition, the control pump is used to baffle fluid from the urethral cuff to the abdominal reservoir, opening the urethra for micturition or catheterization. However, because of the significant risk for infection, need for revision with growth, and mechanical failure, the popularity of the artificial urinary sphincter has declined.

Uncommonly, children with myelodysplasia who have urinary system distress or incontinence that is intractable to other treatments may undergo urinary diversion (Kelalis, King, and Belman, 1992). Whenever possible, a continent urinary diversion is constructed using large or small bowel or a portion of the stomach. An *enterocystoplasty* is constructed by removing a segment of bowel from the intestinal stream (see p. 429). The bladder is then evacuated using CIC. Rarely, when intermittent catheterization is deemed unfeasible because of psychosocial or physiologic factors, an incontinence diversion is constructed.

Because of advances in neurogenic bladder management, adolescents and young adults with myelomeningocele and neurogenic bladders have been followed for up to 30 years without evidence of deterioration in renal function (Peeker and others, 1997). Nevertheless, urinary and fecal incontinence are common, and these conditions lead to significant, and sometimes devastating, problems with growth and developmental tasks, including establishing independence, as well as social and intimate relationships. This observation underscores the need to aggressively manage both continence and the threat of urinary system distress from an early age and to establish an expectation of social continence critical to providing these patients with the skills they need to thrive as adolescents and adults. Newborns with SB and normal urodynamics require close follow-up during the first several years of life to prevent deterioration in urodynamic status as a result of neurologic deterioration (Tarcan and others, 2001).

**Bowel Control.** Some degree of fecal continence can usually be achieved in most children with myelomeningocele with diet modification, regular toilet habits, and prevention of constipation and impaction. However, it is frequently a lengthy process. Fiber supplements, laxatives, suppositories, and enemas aid in producing a pattern of regular evacuation.

*Prognosis.* The early prognosis for the child with myelomeningocele depends on the neurologic deficit present at birth, including motor ability and bladder innervation and the presence of associated cerebral anomalies. Early surgical repair of the spinal defect, antibiotic therapy to reduce the incidence of meningitis and ventriculitis, prevention of urinary system dysfunction, and early detection and correction of hydrocephalus have significantly increased the survival rate of such children. Based on current medical knowledge and ethical considerations, aggressive management is favored for the child with myelomeningocele.

*Prevention.* The widespread use of folic acid among women of childbearing age is expected to significantly decrease the incidence of SB. It has been estimated that a daily intake of 0.4 mg of folic acid in women of childbearing age will prevent 50% to 70% of all cases of NTDs (Centers for Disease Control and Prevention [CDC], 1999). In fact, studies indicate there is a coincident decrease in NTDs since periconceptual folic acid public awareness campaigns were instituted (Stevenson and others, 2000; Evans and others, 2001). For women who have had a previous pregnancy affected by NTDs, this intake is increased to 4 mg under supervision of a practitioner beginning 1 month before a planned pregnancy and continuing during the first trimester. Supplementation of 4 mg of folate should not be given solely in multivitamin preparations because of the risk of overdose of other vitamins. However, despite the recommendations of several health care and public agencies for the daily intake of 0.4 folic acid in the periconceptual period, a recent survey revealed that only 42% of women of childbearing age actually follow these guidelines (CDC, 2001). Awareness of the benefits of folic acid for the prevention of birth defects was highest in women ages 25 to 29 years, college educated, married, Caucasian, and not considered overweight. These results indicate that nurses and other health care workers have an important task in disseminating information that may decrease the incidence of birth defects in children by promoting maternal consumption of folic acid.* To ensure adequate daily intake of the recommended amount of folic acid, women must take a folic acid supplement, eat a fortified breakfast cereal containing 100% of the Recommended Dietary Allowance (RDA) of folic acid (Kellogg's Product 19, General Mills Total, Multigrain Cheerios Plus), or increase their consumption of fortified foods (cereal, bread, rice, grits, pasta) and foods naturally rich in folate (green leafy vegetables and citrus fruits).

> **NURSING ALERT** Because approximately one half of all pregnancies in the United States are unplanned (Henshaw, 1998), adolescent girls and women of child-bearing age need to be educated about the necessity of folic acid to prevent NTDs. The daily dose of 0.4 mg (400 $\mu$g) is most easily obtained from a multivitamin supplement.

## Nursing Considerations

### ■ Assessment

At the time of delivery an examination is performed to assess the intactness of the membranous cyst. During transport to the nursery every effort is made to prevent trauma to this protective covering. In addition to the routine assessment of the newborn (see Chapter 8), the infant is assessed for the level of neurologic involvement. Movement of

---

*Information is available from the Centers for Disease Control and Prevention. "Flo" CDC, NCEH, BDPG, MS F-45 4770 Buford Highway NE, Atlanta, GA 30341, (888) 232-6789; e-mail: Floacdc.gov; www.cdc.gov/ncbddd/folicacid; March of Dimes Resource Center, 1275 Mamaroneck Ave, White Plains, NY 10605; (888) MODIMES; www.modimes.org.

extremities or skin response, especially an anal reflex, that might provide clues to the degree of motor or sensory impairment is noted. It is important to observe the infant's behavior in conjunction with the stimulus because limb movements can be induced in response to spinal cord reflex activity that has no connection with the higher centers. Observation of urinary output, especially if a diaper remains dry, may indicate urinary retention. The head circumference is measured daily (see Chapter 7), and the fontanels are examined for signs of tension or bulging.

> **NURSING ALERT** Avoid measuring rectal temperatures in infants with SB. Because bowel sphincter function is frequently affected, the thermometer can cause irritation and rectal prolapse.

## ▓ Nursing Diagnoses

Following the nursing assessment a number of nursing diagnoses become evident. The most likely diagnoses are outlined and discussed in the Nursing Care Plan on pp. 434-435. Others may be apparent in individual cases.

## ▓ Planning

The goals for the infant with myelomeningocele and the family include the following:

1. Infant will not experience damage to the myelomeningocele sac.
2. Infant will not experience complications.
3. Family will receive support and education.

## ▓ Implementation

The basic needs of the infant with a myelomeningocele are essentially the same as for any newborn infant. (See Chapter 8.) Special needs related to the defect and potential complications are discussed in the following section. As the child matures, the problems increase and involve all aspects of daily living; therefore care is directly related to the child's habilitation at each stage of development.

**Care of the Myelomeningocele Sac.** The infant is usually placed in an incubator or radiant warmer so that temperature can be maintained without clothing or covers that might irritate the delicate lesion. When an overhead warmer is used, the dressings over the defect require more frequent moistening because of the dehydrating effect of the radiant heat. Before surgical closure the myelomeningocele is prevented from drying by the application of a sterile, moist, nonadherent dressing over the defect. The moistening solution is usually sterile normal saline. Dressings are changed frequently (every 2 to 4 hours), and the sac is closely inspected for leaks, abrasions, irritation, or any signs of infection. The sac must be carefully cleansed if it becomes soiled or contaminated. Sometimes the sac ruptures during delivery or transport, and any opening in the sac greatly increases the risk of infection to the CNS.

> **NURSING ALERT** Observe for early signs of infection, such as elevated temperature (axillary), irritability, lethargy, and nuchal rigidity, and for signs of increased intracranial pressure (ICP), which might indicate developing hydrocephalus.

> **NURSING TIP** To prevent preoperative stool contamination of the SB defect, obtain a surgical drape (such as Steri Drape*). Cut a portion of the drape to fit the infant's sacrum, using nonlatex tape to secure the drape to the sacrum. The rest of the drape is placed loosely over the dressing covering the defect, thus preventing exposure to stool.

**Positioning.** One of the most important and challenging aspects of the early care of the infant with myelomeningocele is positioning. Before surgery the infant is kept in the prone position to minimize tension on the sac and the risk of trauma. The prone position allows for optimum positioning of the legs, especially in cases of associated hip dysplasia. A variety of aids, including diaper rolls, pads, small sandbags, or specially designed frames and appliances, can be used to maintain the desired position.

The prone position affects other aspects of the infant's care. For example, in this position the infant is more difficult to keep clean, pressure areas are a constant threat, and feeding becomes a problem. The infant's head is turned to one side for feeding. Fortunately, most defects are repaired early, and the infant can be held for feeding soon after surgery. Physical therapy consultation may be sought for difficult positioning problems. Occupational therapy consultation may be needed for difficulty with oral-motor skills that may indicate complications due to Chiari malformation.

**General Care.** Diapering the infant may be contraindicated until the defect has been repaired and healing is well advanced or epithelialization has taken place. The padding beneath the diaper area is changed as needed to keep the skin dry and free of irritation. When urinary retention is detected (the bladder is still an abdominal organ in early infancy), CIC is employed.† Because the bowel sphincter is frequently affected, there may be continual passage of stool, often misinterpreted as diarrhea, which is a constant irritant to the skin and a source of infection to the spinal lesion.

Areas of sensory and motor impairment are subject to skin breakdown and therefore require meticulous care. Placing the infant on a pressure-reducing mattress or mattress overlay may be needed to prevent pressure on the knees and ankles. (See Skin Care, Chapter 10, and Maintaining Healthy Skin, Chapter 27.)

Gentle range-of-motion exercises are sometimes carried out to prevent contractures, and stretching of contractures is performed when indicated. However, these exercises may be restricted to the foot, ankle, and knee joint. When the hip joints are unstable, stretching against tight hip flexors or adductor muscles, which act much like bowstrings, may aggravate a tendency toward subluxation. A physical therapy consultation is usually obtained.

Some infants with unrepaired myelomeningocele are unable to be held in the arms and cuddled as unaffected infants are, so their need for tactile stimulation is met by caressing, stroking, and other comfort measures. To facilitate handling and reduce parental anxiety, the infant can recline on a pillow placed in the parent's lap. Black-and-white

---

*3M, St Paul, MN.

†Home care instructions for performing CIC are available in Wong DL, Hess CS: *Wong and Whaley's clinical manual of pediatric nursing*, ed 5, St Louis, 2000, Mosby.

drawings or geometric shapes can be placed within the infant's view, and other stimulation usually provided for infants is appropriate. All infants respond to pleasant sounds. (See Developmental Outcome, Chapter 10.)

Ophthalmic complications occur frequently in children with SB and hydrocephalus. The sudden appearance of a squint, other ocular motility, or papilledema usually denotes hydrocephalus and is reported. Shunt surgery is the first priority but may not restore normal ocular motility and visual function. Ophthalmologic follow-up, particularly in those children with shunts, is generally included in the multidisciplinary plan of care.

**Postoperative Care.** Postoperative care of the infant with myelomeningocele involves the same basic care as that of any postsurgical infant—monitoring vital signs, weight, and intake and output; maintaining body temperature; assessing and relieving pain; providing nourishment; and observing for signs of infection. The wound is managed according to the directions of the surgeon, and general care is continued as preoperatively.

The prone position is maintained after operative closure, although many neurosurgeons allow a side-lying or partial side-lying position unless it aggravates a coexisting hip dysplasia or permits undesirable hip flexion. This offers an opportunity for position changes, which reduces the risk of pressure sores and facilitates feeding. Once the effects of anesthesia have subsided and the infant is alert, feedings may be resumed unless there are other anomalies or associated complications.

Nursing assessments are carried out for implementation of comfort measures in the postoperative period. The infant can be held upright against the body, with care taken to avoid pressure on the operative site. In the case of an unusually large defect, skin grafting may be required for wound closure; the infant must then be kept prone postoperatively with as little movement as possible to prevent tension on the skin graft.

The nurse can assist in determining the extent of neuromuscular involvement. Movement of the extremities or skin response, especially an anal reflex, that might provide clues to the degree of motor or sensory status is noted. The head circumference is measured daily (see Chapter 7), and the fontanels are examined for signs of tension or bulging. The nurse is also alert to early signs of infection, such as elevated or decreased temperature (axillary), irritability, lethargy, and nuchal rigidity, and to signs of increased ICP. Catheterization may be needed for urine retention. Although it may not have been a problem preoperatively, swelling around the operative site may cause transient urine retention, which resolves in 2 to 5 days.

**Family Support and Home Care.** As soon as the parents are able to cope with the infant's condition, they are encouraged to become involved in care. They need to learn how to continue at home the care that has been initiated in the hospital—positioning, feeding, skin care, and range-of-motion exercises when appropriate. Parents are taught clean catheterization technique when prescribed. The family needs to know the signs of complications and how to reach assistance when needed.

As the child grows and develops, parents need guidance to encourage and stimulate the infant to accomplish age-appropriate developmental tasks within the limits imposed by the disabilities. Upper limb movement can be stimulated early by placing the infant on the floor in a prone position with toys within reach. Activities that encourage body consciousness, such as rolling over and pulling to a sitting position, are encouraged at the appropriate times. Creeping and crawling, even in a limited way, help the child to explore the environment. The parents may need help to modify appliances and activities normally expected of a growing child. For example, the child who is paraplegic is encouraged to use the arms and shoulders as much as possible. When the infant is sitting in an infant seat, stroller, high chair, or feeding table, the hips can be supported, a footrest provided, and hard-soled shoes worn to maintain the feet in correct alignment and to protect the insensitive feet from trauma. A standing table, frame, or parapodium is helpful for a variety of activities, and it is best for the child to begin supported weight bearing and standing as close as possible to the expected time for standing to occur.

It is important for the family to understand the nature of sensory deficit in a child with a spinal defect. The child will be insensitive to pressure or other sources of tissue injury. Therefore the family must be alert to hot or cold items that could cause thermal injury to tissues and remember to inspect the skin regularly for signs of pressure, especially over bony prominences. Because of sensory impairment, the child is unaware of bladder discomfort; therefore signs of urinary tract infections may be easily overlooked. Urinary tract infection is often considered when the child becomes ill.

The long-range planning with and support of the parents and newborn begin in the hospital and extend throughout childhood. Nurses assume an important role as a central member of the health team. As a coordinator the nurse reviews information with the family, takes responsibility for family teaching, and acts as a liaison between inpatient and outpatient services. The child will need numerous hospitalizations over the years, and each one will be a source of stress to which the younger child is especially vulnerable.

Changes in functional ability, particularly those in the lower extremities, bowel, or bladder, may indicate the presence of a tethered cord, one that is bound down or restricted in an abnormal position by scar tissue. These symptoms usually occur after a growth spurt and can best be detected with MRI. Tethering can be repaired surgically but, unfortunately, may recur.

Habilitation involves solving not only problems of self-help and locomotion but also the most distressing problem of incontinence, which threatens the child's social acceptability. Assistance with preparing the child and the school regarding the special needs of children with disabilities helps provide a better initial adjustment to broader social experiences. Numerous organizations and agencies are able to offer assistance and support to children and families. (See Family Focus box.) The **Spina Bifida Association of America**\* provides

---

\*4590 McArthur Blvd NW, Suite 250, Washington, DC 20007, (202) 944-3285 or (800) 621-3141, fax: (202) 944-3295, e-mail: spinabifida@aol.com.

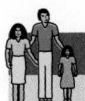

**FAMILY FOCUS:**
*Additional references for families
and professionals on spina bifida*

Kriegsman K, Zaslow E, D'Zmura-Rechsteiner: *Taking
charge: teenagers talk about life and physical disabilities,*
Bethesda, MD, 1992, Woodbine House.
Lutkenhoff M, editor: *Children with spina bifida: a parent's
guide,* Bethesda, MD, 1999, Woodbine House.
Lutkenhoff M, Oppenheimer S, editors: *Spinabilities: a
young person's guide to spina bifida,* Bethesda, MD, 1997,
Woodbine House.
Rowley-Kelly F, Reigel D: *Teaching the student with spina
bifida,* Baltimore, MD, 1993, Paul H Brooks.
Sandler A: *Living with spina bifida: a guide for families and
professionals,* Chapel Hill, NC, 1997, University of North
Carolina Press.

**Box 11-3** ■ ■ ■
**Medical Conditions Associated
with Risk of Latex Allergy**

Spina bifida
Urogenital anomalies
Imperforate anus
Tracheoesophageal fistula
VATER association (*v*ertebral defects, imperforate *a*nus, *tra*-
cheo*e*sophageal fistula, and *r*adial and *r*enal dysplasia)
Preterm infants
Ventriculoperitoneal shunt
Mental retardation
Cerebral palsy
Quadriplegia
Multiple surgeries
Atopy

Data from Slater JE: *J Allergy Clin Immunol* 94:139-149, 1994; Alenius H
and others: *Int Arch Allergy Immunol* 102:61-66, 1993; Centers for Disease
Control: *MMWR* 38:9-10, 1989; and Landwehr LP, Lane G, Leung DYM:
*Am J Asthma Allergy Pediatr* 4:205-210, 1994.

services and support for families of children with spinal
lesions.

The multiple aspects of care of the child with a disability
are discussed in Chapter 22. Complex problems associated
with partial or complete lower extremity paralysis are discussed in Chapters 39 and 40 and include bowel and bladder control, orthopaedic appliances, and the observation
and management of complications, especially urinary tract
infections (see Chapter 30) and pressure necrosis (see
Wounds, Chapter 18).

## ▓ Evaluation

The effectiveness of nursing interventions is determined by
continual reassessment and evaluation of care based on the
following observational guidelines:

1. Inspect the spinal lesion, take appropriate measurements
   (weight, vital signs, head circumference), observe the child's
   general health status, and check completed care against the
   preoperative checklist.
2. Take vital signs, inspect the operative site (or preoperative
   lesion), inspect the skin (especially dependent and pressure
   areas), measure the head circumference, and assess the range
   of motion of the lower extremities.
3. Observe parent-infant interactions, as well as behaviors of
   family members, and interview family members regarding their
   feelings and concerns.

The *expected outcomes* are described in the Nursing Care
Plan on pp. 434-435.

## Latex Allergy

Latex allergy was identified as being a serious health hazard
when a report linked intraoperative anaphylaxis with latex
in children with SB. One study suggests that the allergy is
disease related in that SB patients have a disease-associated
propensity for latex sensitization (Zsolt and others, 1999).
These children are at high risk for developing latex allergy
because of repeated exposure to latex products during
surgery and from numerous procedures (Mazon and others, 2000). Allergic reactions range from urticaria, wheezing, watery eyes, and rashes to anaphylactic shock. More severe reactions tend to occur when latex comes in contact

**GUIDELINES**
*Identifying Latex Allergy*

Does your child have any symptoms, such as sneezing,
coughing, rashes, or wheezing, when handling rubber
products (balloons, tennis or Koosh balls, adhesive
bandage strips) or when in contact with rubber hospital
products, such as gloves or catheters?
Has your child ever had an allergic reaction during
surgery?
Does your child have a history of rashes, asthma, or allergic
reactions to medication or foods, especially milk, kiwi,
bananas, or chestnuts?
How would you identify or recognize an allergic reaction in
your child?
What would you do if an allergic reaction occurred?
Has anyone ever discussed latex or rubber allergy or sensitivity with you?
Has the child had any allergy testing?
When did the child last come in contact with any type of
rubber product? Were you present?

Modified from Romanczuk A: Latex use with infants and children: it
can cause problems, *MCN* 18(4):208-212, 1993.

with mucous membranes, wet skin, the bloodstream, or an
airway. There also can be cross-reactions to a number of
foods (e.g., banana, avocado, kiwi, chestnut) (Kellet, 1997;
Landwehr and Boguniewicz, 1996; Sussman and Beezhold,
1997). In addition to patients with SB, high-risk populations
include patients with urogenital anomalies or multiple surgeries as well as health care workers (Poley and Slater, 2000).
See Box 11-3 for medical conditions associated with SB. The
incidence of latex allergy in children with SB ranges from
an estimated 18% to 67% (Kellett, 1997).

The most important goals are prevention of latex allergy
and identification of children with a known hypersensitivity.
(See Guidelines box.) High-risk and latex-allergic individuals must be managed in a *latex-safe* environment. Care must
be taken so that they do not come in direct or secondary
contact with products or equipment containing latex at any

## Nursing Care Plan
## The Infant with Myelomeningocele

---

**NURSING DIAGNOSIS:** Risk for infection related to presence of infective organisms, nonepithelialized meningeal sac, paralysis

**PATIENT GOAL 1:** Will experience minimized risk of central nervous system infection

- **NURSING INTERVENTIONS/RATIONALES**

Position infant *to prevent contamination from urine and stool*

Cleanse myelomeningocele carefully with sterile normal saline if it becomes soiled or contaminated

*Apply sterile dressings and moisten with sterile solution as ordered (normal saline, antibiotic) *to prevent drying of sac*

*Administer antibiotics as prescribed

Monitor closely for signs of infection (elevated temperature, irritability, lethargy, nuchal rigidity) *to prevent delay in treatment*

Administer similar care to operative site postoperatively

- **EXPECTED OUTCOME**

Meningeal sac remains clean, intact, and exhibits no evidence of infection

**PATIENT GOAL 2:** Will experience minimized risk of urinary tract infection

- **NURSING INTERVENTIONS/RATIONALES**

Avoid urethral contamination with stool *to prevent introduction of infective organisms into urinary tract*

Carry out meticulous perineal hygiene *to remove infective organisms*

Monitor urinary output for retention *to minimize risk of infection due to stasis of urine*

*Administer antibiotics as prescribed

*Administer urinary tract antiseptics if prescribed

Ensure adequate fluid intake *to increase urination and prevent bacterial growth*

- **EXPECTED OUTCOME**

Infant exhibits no evidence of urinary tract infection

---

*Dependent nursing action.

---

**NURSING DIAGNOSIS:** Risk for trauma related to delicate spinal lesion

**PATIENT GOAL 1:** Will not experience trauma to spinal lesion or surgical site

- **NURSING INTERVENTIONS/RATIONALES**

Handle infant carefully *to prevent damage to meningeal sac or surgical site*

Place infant in prone position, or side-lying position if permitted, *to minimize tension on the meningeal sac or surgical site*

Apply protective devices around sac (e.g., a surgical plastic drape, cut to fit and taped below the sac by the sacrum and loosely draped over the sac) *to provide a protective shield*

Modify routine nursing activities (e.g., feeding, making bed, comforting activities) *to prevent trauma*

- **EXPECTED OUTCOMES**

Meningeal sac remains intact

Surgical site heals without trauma

---

**NURSING DIAGNOSIS:** Risk for impaired skin integrity related to paralysis, continual dribbling of urine, and feces

**PATIENT GOAL 1:** Will not experience skin irritation

- **NURSING INTERVENTIONS/RATIONALES**

Change diapers as soon as soiled, if diapered, *to keep skin clean, dry, and free of irritation*

Keep perianal area clean and dry

Place infant on pressure-reducing surface *to reduce pressure on knees and ankles during prone positioning*

Gently massage healthy skin during cleansing and application of lotion *to increase circulation*

- **EXPECTED OUTCOME**

Skin remains clean and dry with no evidence of irritation

---

time during medical treatment. Allergy testing has been used to identify latex allergy with varying success. Skin prick testing and provocation testing carry the risk of allergic reaction or anaphylaxis. Several commercially available assays can be very useful in confirming latex allergy. To date, none of these tests demonstrates complete diagnostic reliability and should not be the sole determinent of the presence or absence of an allergic response to latex.

The radioallergosorbent test (RAST) has been used to measure the serum level of latex-specific immunoglobulin E (IgE). The RAST has been shown to be 90% to 95% sensitive (Kellett, 1997). Pretreatment with antihistamines and steroids (dexamethasone) before and after surgery to reduce the possibility of a serious reaction remains controversial because it may interfere with healing.

Because children who have SB are prone to develop an allergy to latex, reducing exposure, from birth on, hopefully will decrease the chance of allergy development. Latex, a natural product derived from the rubber tree, is used in combination with other chemicals to give elasticity, strength, and durability to many products.

Avoiding contact with latex is the most important intervention. The establishment of a latex-safe environment is being accomplished in many health care facilities where patients and health care workers are at risk. In addition, there are published lists of products, such as vinyl gloves, that may be substituted for latex (see footnote to Box 11-4). In the health care arena it is important to use products with the lowest potential risk of sensitizing patients and staff members. User labeling for latex-containing devices that come

## *Nursing Care Plan*
## The Infant with Myelomeningocele—cont'd

**NURSING DIAGNOSIS:** Risk for trauma related to impaired cerebrospinal fluid circulation

**PATIENT GOAL 1:** Will not experience adverse effects of increased intracranial pressure (ICP)

• **NURSING INTERVENTIONS/***RATIONALES*

Measure occipitofrontal circumference daily *to detect increased ICP and developing hydrocephalus*

Observe for signs of increased ICP, *which might indicate developing hydrocephalus:*
　Irritability
　Lethargy
　Infant
　　Cries when picked up or handled; quiets when lies still
　　Increased occipitofrontal circumference
　　Separated sutures
　　Change in level of consciousness
　Child
　　Headache (especially in morning)
　　Apathy
　　Confusion

Minimize stressful events (e.g., pain) *because stress increases blood pressure, a main determinant of ICP* (see Pain Assessment and Pain Management, Chapter 26)

• **EXPECTED OUTCOME**

Evidence of increased ICP and hydrocephalus is detected early, and appropriate interventions are implemented

**NURSING DIAGNOSIS:** Risk for injury related to repeated exposure to latex products and development of latex allergy

**PATIENT GOAL 1:** Will experience minimal exposure to latex

• **NURSING INTERVENTIONS/***RATIONALES*

Identify children with latex allergy (see Guidelines box on p. 433)

Maintain a latex-free environment *to reduce exposure*

Educate family members and other caregivers (i.e., daycare workers, teachers) about:
　Risk of latex allergy and items to avoid *to reduce exposure*
　Signs of allergy (from hives, rash, and wheezing to anaphylaxis) *to detect a reaction quickly*
　Emergency treatment, including use of anaphylaxis kit and summoning emergency medical services, *to prevent delay in treatment*

• **EXPECTED OUTCOME**

Child does not develop allergic reactions to latex

**NURSING DIAGNOSIS:** Risk for injury related to neuromuscular impairment

**PATIENT GOAL 1:** Will experience no or minimized risk of hip and lower extremity deformity

• **NURSING INTERVENTIONS/***RATIONALES*

Carry out passive range-of-motion exercises *to prevent contractures;* do not push past point of resistance *to prevent trauma*

Carry out muscle stretching when indicated *to prevent contractures*

Maintain hips in slight to moderate abduction *to prevent dislocation;* maintain feet in neutral position *to prevent contractures*

Use diaper rolls, pads, stuffed animals, or specially designed appliances *to maintain desired position*

• **EXPECTED OUTCOMES**

Lower extremities maintain flexibility

Hips and lower extremities are maintained in correct articulation and alignment

See also:

Nursing Care Plan: The Child with Chronic Illness or Disability, Chapter 22

Nursing Care Plan: The Child in the Hospital, Chapter 26

Nursing Care Plan: The Family of the Child Who Is Ill or Hospitalized, Chapter 26

---

into contact directly or indirectly with live human tissue has been proposed by the FDA (1996).*

The American Nurses' Association (ANA) (1997) has issued a position statement on latex allergies emphasizing that all health care institutions abandon the unnecessary use of latex gloves and provide low-allergen, powder-free latex gloves in other settings. Procedures for the identification and treatment of latex-sensitive patients, provision of latex-free medical products, and reporting of allergic events related to latex medical devices to the Food and Drug Administration MedWatch Program are also strongly advocated by the ANA. In addition, the ANA recommends that each health care facility have a multidisciplinary task force to develop occupational health guidelines to ensure a safe environment for health care workers to minimize latex exposure, identify those at risk for reaction to latex, and accommodate the needs of latex-sensitive employees.

**NURSING ALERT** Ask *all* patients about allergic reactions to latex, not only those at risk, during the health interview with the parent and/or child. Be sure this is a routine part of all preoperative and preprocedural histories. Stress the importance of the allergy history to *all* personnel (e.g., phlebotomists).

---

*Additional information regarding latex allergy may be found at the following web sites: www.latexallergyhelp.com, www.latex-allergy.org, latexallergylinks.tripod.com, and www.sbaa.org. See additional sites in Mitchell NA: Innovative informations: latex allergy: accessing information on the Internet, *J Emerg Nurs* 32(1):51-52, 1997.

---

**Box 11-4** ■ ■ □
**Selected Items Possibly Containing Latex***

**MEDICAL ITEMS**

Adhesive bandage strips
Airways, masks (oxygen)
Anesthesia vent circuits, bags
Blood pressure cuffs and tubing
Bulb syringe
Catheters (indwelling, condom)
Cardiopulmonary resuscitation (CPR) manikins
Chux (washable rubber)
Crutches (axillary, hand pads)
Dressings and wraps (various)
Elastic bandages
Electrode pads, bulbs
Endotracheal tubes
Finger cots
Gloves (sterile and examining, surgical and medical)
Heparin lock adapter
Intravenous tubing, injection ports, bags, burets
Medication vials
Nasogastric tubes
Penrose drains
Pulse oximeters
Spacer (metered dose inhaler)
Stethoscope tubing
Suction tubing
Syringes (disposable)
Tape (cloth adhesive, paper)

Tourniquet
Urodynamics rectal pressure catheters
Wheelchair cushions, tires

**HOME AND COMMUNITY ITEMS†**

Art supplies (paint, markers, glue)
Balloons (not Mylar)
Balls (Koosh, tennis, bowling)
Chewing gum
Cleaning/kitchen gloves
Condoms, contraceptive sponges, diaphragms
Dental dams and equipment
Rubber pants
Diaphragms
Elastic exercisers
Elastic on legs, waist of clothing, some disposable diapers
Feeding nipples
Foam rubber lining on splints, braces
Infant toothbrush-massager
Pacifier
Racquet handles
Rubberbands
Water toys, swim and scuba equipment
Wheelchair cushions, tires
Zippered plastic storage bags

---

Modified from Meeropol E, Romanczuk A, editors: *Latex in the hospital environment*, Washington, DC, 1997, Spina Bifida Association.
*It is very difficult to obtain full and accurate information on the latex content of certain products, which may vary among companies and product series. Double-checking with suppliers before use with latex-allergic individuals is strongly recommended. For an updated list of latex-free items (medical and community) and alternative products call (800) 621-3141 or to download a list access *www.sbaa.org*, Spina Bifida Association of America, 4590 MacArthur Blvd NW, Suite 250, Washington, DC 20007-4226.
†Latex-free products for home and community may be ordered from: Alternative Resource Catalog (Latex-free products for daily living) (800) 618-3129 or (630) 587-2705, and Cetra Latex-Free Supplies (888) LATEX-NO.

---

The identification of those sensitive to latex is best accomplished through careful screening of *all* patients. (See Guidelines box, p. 433, for questions related to latex allergy.)

Children with latex allergy should carry some form of allergy identification, such as a Medic-Alert bracelet. Education programs regarding latex allergy are aimed at those who care for high-risk groups, such as children with SB, and may include relatives, school nurses, teachers, child care workers, and baby-sitters. In addition to educating caregivers about the child's exposure to medical products that contain latex, nurses need to inform them of common nonmedical latex objects (Box 11-4). Items brought to the hospital, such as floral bouquets, are also screened for latex toys or balloons. Parents should also be given literature explaining signs and symptoms of latex hypersensitivity and appropriate emergency treatment. (See Anaphylaxis, Chapter 29.)

## Hydrocephalus

Hydrocephalus is a syndrome, or sign, resulting from disturbances in the dynamics of CSF, which may be caused by various diseases. The advent of MRI and CT scanning has provided valuable information about the pathophysiology of hydrocephalus. Although prenatal diagnosis is having an impact on the current prevalence of neural defects at birth, congenital hydrocephalus occurs in 3 of every 1000 live births

(McGee and Burkett, 2000). The causes are diverse, from either congenital or acquired conditions. Congenital hydrocephalus is usually a result of a maldevelopment or, less commonly, an intrauterine infection. Acquired hydrocephalus can be caused by infection, neoplasm, or hemorrhage.

### Pathophysiology

To appreciate the condition, an understanding of the dynamics of CSF and the relationship between the various structures that make up the ventricular and subarachnoid spaces is necessary (Fig. 11-4). The two mechanisms by which CSF is formed include secretion by the choroid plexuses and lymphatic-like drainage by the extracellular fluid of the brain. CSF circulates throughout the ventricular system and is then absorbed within the subarachnoid spaces by a mechanism that is not entirely clear.

**Ventricular Circulation.** The fluid flows from the lateral ventricles through the *foramen of Monro* to the third ventricle, where it combines with fluid secreted into the third ventricle. From there CSF flows through the *aqueduct of Sylvius* into the fourth ventricle, where more fluid is formed; it then leaves the fourth ventricle by way of the lateral *foramen of Luschka* and the midline *foramen of Magendie* and flows into the *cisterna magna*. From there CSF flows to the cerebral and cerebellar subarachnoid spaces, where it is absorbed. A large portion is absorbed through the arachnoid

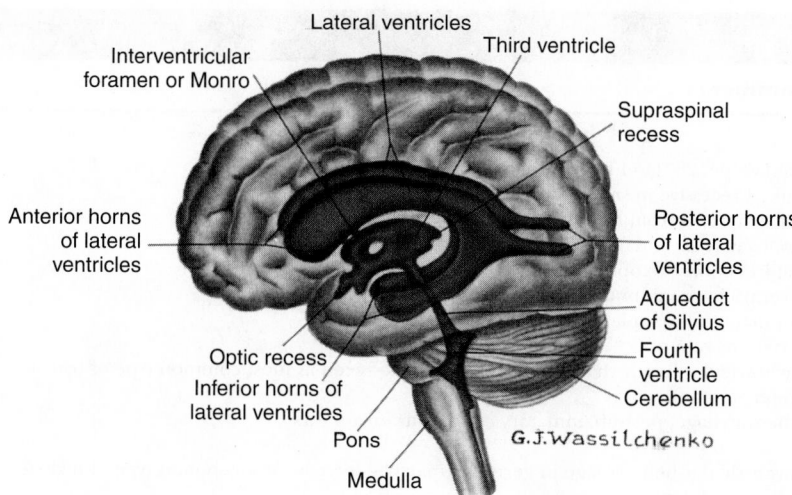

**Fig. 11-4** Cerebral ventricular system. (From Thompson JM and others: *Mosby's clinical nursing,* ed 4, St Louis, 1997, Mosby.)

villi, but the sinuses, veins, brain substance, and dura also participate in absorption.

**Mechanisms of Fluid Imbalance.** The causes of hydrocephalus are varied, but the result is either (1) impaired absorption of CSF fluid within the subarachnoid space *(communicating hydrocephalus)* or (2) obstruction to the flow of CSF through the ventricular system *(noncommunicating hydrocephalus).* Rarely, a tumor of the choroid plexus causes increased CSF secretion. Any imbalance of secretion and absorption causes an increased accumulation of CSF in the ventricles, which become dilated and compress the brain substance against the surrounding rigid bony cranium. When this occurs before fusion of the cranial sutures, it provides enlargement of the skull, as well as dilation of the ventricles. In children under 10 to 12 years of age, previously closed suture lines, especially the sagittal suture, may become diastatic or opened.

Most cases of noncommunicating hydrocephalus are a result of developmental malformations. Although the defect usually is apparent in early infancy, it may become evident at any time from the prenatal period to late childhood or early adulthood. Other causes include neoplasms, intrauterine infections, and trauma. An obstruction to the normal flow can occur at any point in the CSF pathway to produce increased pressure and dilation of the pathways proximal to the site of obstruction. Table 11-3 describes the most frequent sites of obstruction and the consequences.

Developmental defects (e.g., Arnold-Chiari malformations [see following discussion], aqueduct stenosis, aqueduct gliosis, and atresia of the foramina of Luschka and Magendie [Dandy-Walker syndrome]) account for most cases of hydrocephalus from birth to 2 years of age. *Dandy-Walker malformation* represents a disorder of the midline CNS indicative of marked genetic and etiologic factors. A female predominance of 3:1 is noted. Hydrocephalus is so often associated with myelomeningocele that all such infants should be observed for its development. In the remainder of cases there is a history of intrauterine infection (toxoplasmosis, cytomegalovirus), perinatal hemorrhage (anoxic or traumatic), and neonatal meningoencephalitis (bacterial or viral). In older children hydrocephalus is most often a result of intracranial masses (vascular anomalies, cysts, tumors), preexisting developmental defects, intracranial infections, trauma, or hemorrhage.

**Arnold-Chiari Malformations (ACMs).** ACM is a brain defect involving posterior fossa contents; the major types are described in Table 11-3. The type 2 malformation, seen almost exclusively with myelomeningocele, is characterized by herniation of a small cerebellum, medulla, pons, and fourth ventricle into the cervical spinal canal through an enlarged foramen magnum. The resulting obstruction of CSF flow causes the hydrocephalus.

## Clinical Manifestations

The three factors that influence the clinical picture in hydrocephalus are the acuity of onset, timing of onset, and the presence of associated structural malformations. In infancy before closure of the cranial sutures, head enlargement is the predominant sign, whereas in older infants and children the lesions responsible for hydrocephalus produce other neurologic signs through pressure on adjacent structures.

**Infancy.** In infants with hydrocephalus, the head grows at an abnormal rate, although the first signs may be bulging fontanels with or without head enlargement (Fig. 11-5). The anterior fontanel is tense, often bulging, and nonpulsatile. Scalp veins are dilated and markedly so when the infant cries. With the increase in intracranial volume, the bones of the skull become thin and the sutures become palpably separated to produce the *cracked-pot sound (Macewen sign)* on percussion of the skull. There may be frontal protrusion, or *frontal bossing,* with depressed eyes, and the eyes may be rotated downward, producing a *setting-sun sign,* in which the sclera may be visible above the iris. Pupils are sluggish, with unequal response to light.

The infant is irritable and lethargic, feeds poorly, and may display changes in level of consciousness, opisthotonos (often extreme), and lower extremity spasticity. The infant cries when picked up or rocked and quiets when allowed to lie still. Early infantile reflexes may persist, and normally expected responses may not appear, indicating failure in the development of normal cortical inhibition.

**TABLE 11-3** Sites and types of hydrocephalus

| Site and Type | Causes and Comments |
| --- | --- |
| **Noncommunicating Hydrocephalus** | |
| *Site:* Aqueduct of Sylvius | Accounts for 33% (Volpe, 2001) of hydrocephalus |
| *Type:* Stenosis or atresia | Congenital (X-linked recessive in small number) |
| | Insidious onset of symptoms from birth to adulthood |
| Gliosis | Postinflammatory, usually secondary to perinatal infection or hemorrhage |
| | Prenatal maternal infection (toxoplasmosis) |
| Obstructive | Tumors of third ventricle or midbrain |
| | Ependymitis from maternal toxoplasmosis |
| | Congenital aneurysm of vein of Galen |
| *Type:* Posthemorrhagic | Blood from intraventricular hemorrhage in germinal matrix—seen as most common type of hydrocephalus in preterm infants |
| *Site:* Fourth ventricle or subarachnoid pathway | Intraventricular hemorrhage, postinflammatory conditions, or tumors |
| *Type:* Posthemorrhagic | Blood from intraventricular hemorrhage in germinal matrix—seen as most common type of hydrocephalus in preterm infants |
| *Site:* Fourth ventricle and foramen magnum | Accounts for 50% of all hydrocephalus |
| *Type:* Chiari malformations | Accounts for 28% to 40% of fourth ventricle obstructions |
| Type 1 | A neural tube defect with herniation of medulla through foramen magnum; may be asymptomatic in childhood; similar to type 2, but more mild |
| Type 2 (Arnold-Chiari malformation) | A more severe defect; downward displacement of brainstem, fourth ventricle, and lower parts of cerebellum through foramen magnum with fixed attachment of spinal cord at site of a myelomeningocele |
| Type 3 (Absence or occlusion of ventricles) | High cervical or occipitocervical myelomeningocele with cervical herniation through body defect |
| | Congenital (Dandy-Walker syndrome) caused by obstruction of foramina of Luschka and Magendie |
| | Tumors of posterior fossa (e.g., medulloblastoma) cause pressure on surrounding tissues to produce obstruction |
| | Less often: subdural hematoma, bacterial or granulomatous meningitis |
| **Communicating Hydrocephalus** | |
| *Site:* Arachnoid villi and cisterna magna | Obstruction by thick arachnoid membrane or meninges |
| *Type:* Meningitis | Bacterial or granulomatous |
| | Acute phase: clumping of purulent fluid in drainage channels |
| | Chronic phase: organization of blood and exudate that results in fibrosis of subarachnoid spaces |
| Prenatal maternal infections | Toxoplasmosis, cytomegalic inclusion disease, mumps |
| Meningeal malignancy | Secondary to leukemia or lymphoma |
| Arachnoid cyst | Located in basal cistern or (uncommon) over cerebral cortex |
| Tuberculosis, fungal, or parasitic infection | More common in children ages 2 to 10 years |

Infants with ACM may exhibit behaviors that reflect cranial nerve dysfunction as a result of brainstem compression, including swallowing difficulties, stridor, apnea, aspiration, respiratory difficulties, and arm weakness.

The preterm infant with posthemorrhagic hydrocephalus may not exhibit any clinical signs and symptoms other than a gradual increase in head circumference. Ventricular dilation is assessed by ultrasonography or CT scanning in preterm infants at high risk for intraventricular hemorrhage.

If hydrocephalus is allowed to progress, development of lower brainstem functions is disrupted, as manifested by difficulty in sucking and feeding and a shrill, brief, high-pitched cry. Eventually the skull becomes enlarged, and the cortex is destroyed. If the hydrocephalus is rapidly progressive, the infant may display emesis, somnolence, seizures, and cardiopulmonary distress.

**Childhood.** The signs and symptoms in early to late childhood are caused by increased ICP, and specific manifestations are related to the focal lesion. Most commonly resulting from posterior fossa neoplasms and aqueduct stenosis, the clinical manifestations are primarily those associated with space-occupying lesions, (i.e., headache on awakening with improvement following emesis or upright posture, papilledema, strabismus, and extrapyramidal tract signs such as ataxia [see Chapter 36]). As with infants, the child will be irritable, lethargic, apathetic, confused, and often incoherent. In one of the congenital defects with later onset (by age 3 months), the Dandy-Walker syndrome, characteristic manifestations are a bulging occiput, nystagmus, ataxia, and cranial nerve palsies.

Manifestations of ACM in children over 3 years of age are related to spinal cord dysfunction rather than brainstem compression as observed in infants. Commonly seen are scoliosis proximal to the level of the myelomeningocele (usually associated with ACM) and development of upper extremity spasticity, which may progress to weakness and atrophy. Cranial nerve deficits are rare.

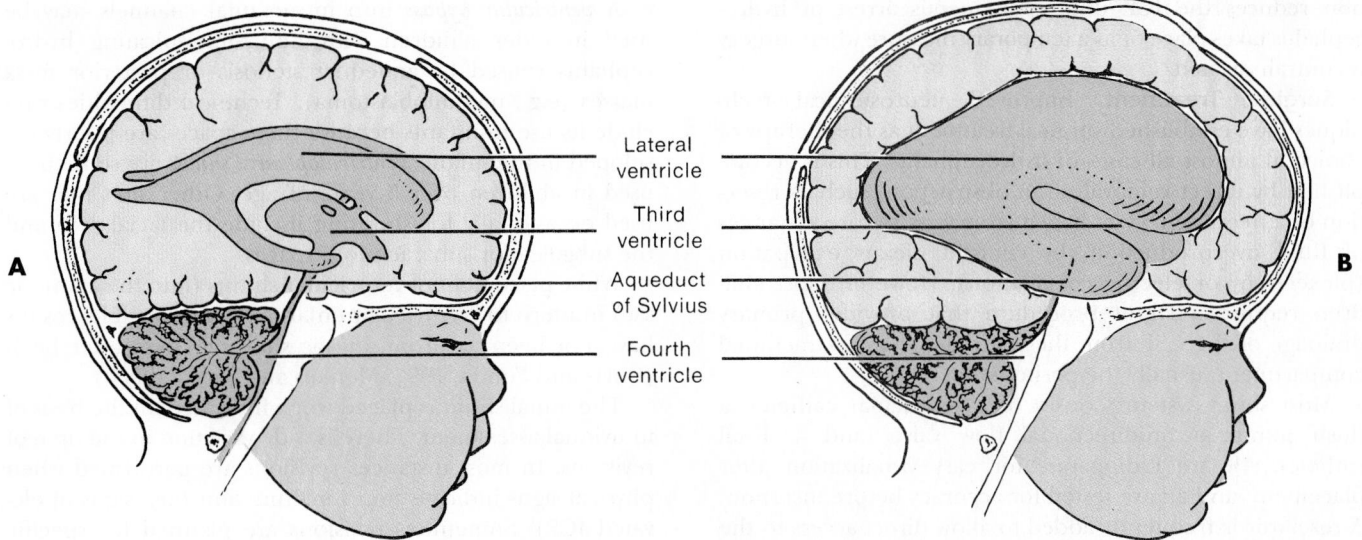

**Fig. 11-5**    Hydrocephalus: a block in flow of cerebrospinal fluid. **A,** Patent cerebrospinal fluid circulation. **B,** Enlarged lateral and third ventricles caused by obstruction of circulation—stenosis of aqueduct of Sylvius.

## Diagnostic Evaluation

Antenatal diagnosis of hydrocephalus is possible with fetal ultrasonography as early as 14 weeks of gestation (Bulas and Fonda, 1997). Delivery is not currently recommended until fetal lung maturity has been achieved.

In infancy the diagnosis of hydrocephalus is based on head circumference that crosses one or more grid lines on the measurement chart within a period of 2 to 4 weeks and on associated neurologic signs that are present and progressive. However, other diagnostic studies are needed to localize the site of CSF obstruction. Routine daily head circumference measurements are carried out in infants with myelomeningocele, hemorrhage, or intracranial infections. In evaluation of a premature infant, specially adapted head circumference charts are consulted to distinguish abnormal head growth from rapid head growth that takes place normally.

The primary diagnostic tools for detecting hydrocephalus are CT and MRI (Fig. 11-6). Some sedation is usually required because the child must remain absolutely still for an accurate picture. Diagnostic evaluation of children who have symptoms of hydrocephalus after infancy is similar to that employed in those with a suspected intracranial tumor. In the neonate, echoencephalography is useful in comparing the ratio of lateral ventricle to cortex. Sometimes isotope ventriculograms are used to assess the flow and patency of existing shunts and to check the size of the ventricles.

Problems in differential diagnosis are related to the child whose head circumference is greater than the 95th percentile but whose head growth parallels the normal growth curve. It is sometimes valuable to measure the parental occipitofrontal circumference (OFC) to detect a possible normal familial characteristic (benign familial megalencephaly). (See Table 37-2 for diagnostic tests for neurologic evaluation.)

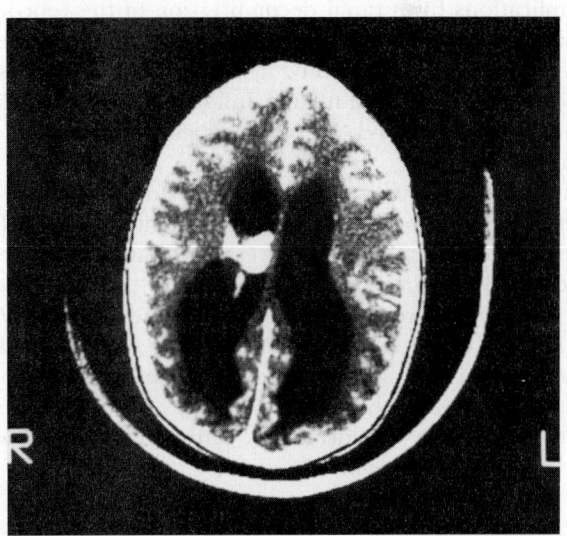

**Fig. 11-6**    CT scan reveals enlarged ventricles of child with hydrocephalus.

## Therapeutic Management

The treatment of hydrocephalus is directed toward (1) relief of the hydrocephalus, (2) treatment of complications, and (3) management of problems related to the effect of the disorder on psychomotor development. The treatment is, with few exceptions, surgical.

Medical therapy has been largely disappointing. Many newborn infants with progressive cranial enlargement secondary to intracranial hemorrhage demonstrate spontaneous stabilization and resolution. Serial lumbar punctures and medications have been used with varying success. The administration of acetazolamide and isosorbide or furosemide is somewhat beneficial in decreasing the production of CSF in selected cases of slowly progressive disease. The medication reduces the ICP until spontaneous arrest of hydrocephalus takes place or as a temporary measure when surgery is contraindicated.

**Surgical Treatment.** Improved neurosurgical techniques have established surgical treatment as the therapy of choice in almost all cases of hydrocephalus. This is accomplished by direct removal of an obstruction, such as resection of a neoplasm, cyst, or hematoma, or, in rare instances of fluid overproduction, by choroid plexus extirpation (plexectomy or electric coagulation). However, most children require a shunt procedure that provides primary drainage of the CSF from the ventricles to an extracranial compartment, usually the peritoneum.

Most shunt systems consist of a ventricular catheter, a flush pump, a unidirectional flow valve, and a distal catheter. All are radiopaque for easy visualization after placement, and all are tested for accuracy before insertion. A reservoir is frequently added to allow direct access to the ventricular system for administration of medications and removal of fluid. In all models the valves are designed to open at a predetermined intraventricular pressure and close when the pressure falls below that level, thus preventing backflow of fluid. High-pressure valves are used to prevent complications from rapid decompression of the ventricles. Medium-pressure valves are used in most children, especially those with long-standing hydrocephalus. Low-pressure valves are used in small infants. Infants should not be held in a prolonged head-down position because this interferes with flow of CSF.

The preferred procedure is the *ventriculoperitoneal (VP) shunt,* especially in neonates and young infants (Fig. 11-7). There is greater allowance for excess tubing, which minimizes the number of revisions needed as the child grows. Since it requires repeated lengthening, the *ventriculoatrial (VA) shunt* (ventricle to right atrium) is reserved for older children who have attained most of their somatic growth and children with abdominal pathology. The VA shunt is contraindicated in children with cardiopulmonary disease or elevated CSF protein.

A *ventricular bypass* into intracranial channels may be used in older children with noncommunicating hydrocephalus caused by aqueduct stenosis or posterior fossa masses (e.g., medulloblastoma). Technical difficulties preclude its use in infants because these spaces are poorly developed in the infant. *Ventriculopleural shunts* are sometimes used in children over 5 years of age. Other sites that are used occasionally for shunting include the facial vein and the subgaleal or subarachnoid spaces.

While placement of ventricular shunts (into the amniotic sac) in utero for ventricular enlargement is possible, results have not been as promising as shunting soon after birth (Bulas and Fonda, 1997; Menkes and Sarnat, 2000).

The initial shunt is placed when indicated on the basis of individual assessment. There is wide variation in the time of revisions. In most instances revisions are performed when physical signs indicate shunt malfunction (i.e., signs of elevated ICP). Sometimes revisions are planned for specific times during development. The initial success rate is relatively high; however, shunts are associated with complications that interfere with continued shunt function or that threaten the life of the child.

*Endoscopic third ventriculostomy* is a procedure that has potential for greater independence from VA or VP shunting in children with noncommunicating hydrocephalus. In this procedure a small opening is made in the floor of the third ventricle, allowing CSF to flow freely through the previously blocked ventricle, thus bypassing the aqueduct of Sylvius. Children with SB and anatomic ventricular malformations are reportedly poor candidates for this procedure, as are children with bleeding disorders and those who have had previous radiotherapy (Walker and Meijer, 1995). Reports of the success of endoscopic third ventriculostomy in children vary; however, as surgical techniques and advances continue, it is expected that neonates and small children will be successfully treated with this procedure rather than with conventional shunting (Grant and McLone, 1997; Lawton, Meyers, and Donahue, 1997; Murshid, 2000).

**Complications.** The major complications of VP shunts are infection and malfunction. All shunts are subject to mechanical difficulties, such as kinking, plugging, or separation and migration of tubing. Malfunction is most often caused by mechanical obstruction either within the ventricles from particulate matter (tissue or exudate) or at the distal end from thrombosis or displacement as a result of growth. Functional obstruction of a shunt's antisiphon device remains a common complication. The probability of shunt malfunction within 6 months was 8% in one study (Williams, Hayes, and McCool, 1996). The child with a shunt obstruction often presents as an emergency with clinical manifestations of increased ICP, frequently accompanied by worsening neurologic status.

The most serious complication, shunt infection, can occur at any time, but the period of greatest risk is 1 to 2 months following placement. The infection may be a result of intercurrent infections at the time of shunt placement. Infections include sepsis, bacterial endocarditis, wound infection, shunt nephritis, meningitis, and ventriculitis. In a survey of shunt infections, gram-positive organisms (*Staphy-*

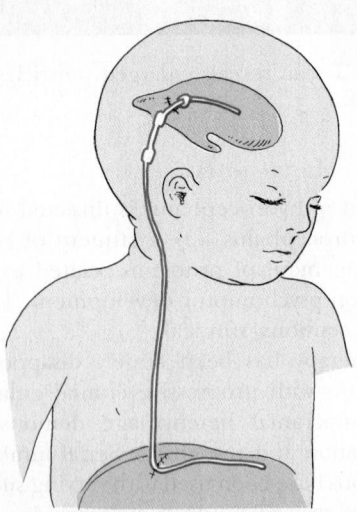

**Fig. 11-7** Ventriculoperitoneal shunt. Catheter is threaded beneath the skin.

*lococcus epidermidis, Staphylococcus aureus*) were most commonly isolated; *Propionibacterium acnes* was predominant in adolescents. Shunt malfunction (33%), fever (26%), wound or shunt tract inflammation (22%), and abdominal pain were the most common presenting symptoms of shunt infection in the study (Williams, Hayes, and McCool, 1996). Brain abscess associated with colonic perforation and infection with a gram-negative enteric organism suggests an ascending shunt infection in a child who has a VP shunt. Meningitis and ventriculitis are of greatest concern because any complicating CNS infection is a significant predictor of intellectual outcome. Infection is treated with antibiotics administered intravenously or intrathecally for a minimum of 7 to 10 days. A persistent infection requires removal of the shunt until the infection is controlled. *External ventricular drainage (EVD),* or external ventriculostomy, is used until CSF is sterile. EVD allows removal of CSF from a tube placed in the child's ventricle that flows by gravity into a collection device.

The primary reasons for inserting an EVD include unstable child status, increased ICP which is difficult to stabilize, or infection of an existing VP shunt; the EVD may drain CSF intermittently or continuously according to need, but drainage and ICP monitoring is not an option unless a fiberoptic monitor is used (Pope, 1998). The EVD is a closed system comprised of transparent pliable tubing, a collection bag and, at times, a drip chamber between the tubing and the collection bag. The EVD is placed at the level of the child's external auditory meatus with the head at a 20- to 30-degree elevation, depending on physician preference. Elevating the EVD above this level decreases the flow of CSF, and placing the device below the level of the external meatus increases the flow. Ambulation or sitting up in bed or chair usually requires that the tubing be clamped to prevent imbalance in CSF drainage. In addition, the EVD is a closed sterile system and should be handled as such in relation to emptying the device or changing the scalp dressing. Accurate and frequent documentation of the incision site, amount, color, and consistency of drainage into the device, and the child's vital and neurologic signs are an important part of the nursing care. Complications related to an EVD include infection, meningitis, and tentorial herniation as a result of imbalance in CSF drainage (Pope, 1998). In preterm infants with intraventricular hemorrhage requiring CSF drainage, a *ventricular access drain (VAD)* may be temporarily inserted (Hudgins, Boydston, and Gilbreath, 1998); this system is similar to the EVD but has an access port for frequent taps and can be used to administer antibiotics and thrombolytic agents such as urokinase.

Another serious shunt-related complication is subdural hematoma caused by too rapid reduction of ICP and size. This usually can be averted by careful assessment of ICP before insertion of the shunt and use of correct valvular pressure. Other complications that may occur include peritonitis, abdominal abscesses, perforation of abdominal organs by catheter or trochar (at the time of insertion), fistulas, hernias, and ileus. Children who require shunts because of noncommunicating hydrocephalus often need shunt lengthening as body growth occurs. This procedure usually involves replacing the distal catheter below the valve during the toddler period and again before the growth acceleration of puberty.

**Prognosis.**   The prognosis of children with treated hydrocephalus depends largely on the size of the cerebral mantle before shunt placement, the amount of irreversible brain damage before shunting, and the cause of the hydrocephalus. For example, malignant tumors may have a high mortality regardless of other complicating factors.

Untreated, hydrocephalus has a 50% to 60% mortality rate caused by the disorder or intercurrent illnesses. In the survivors there is a high incidence of subnormal intellectual capacity, and a large majority have major physical and disabling neurologic handicaps such as ataxia, spastic diplegia, poor fine motor coordination, and perceptual deficits. Spontaneous arrest of head growth occurs occasionally in approximately 40% of those with near-normal intelligence.

Surgically treated hydrocephalus in patients with little or no evidence of irreversible brain damage has a survival rate of about 90%, with the highest incidence of mortality occurring within the first year of treatment. Of the surviving children, approximately two thirds are intellectually normal. Inattentiveness and hyperactivity are significant behavioral problems in children with both hydrocephalus and mental retardation. The presence of additional medical problems in infancy, including ocular defects, is the most significant variable associated with a high likelihood of mental retardation.

Children with communicating hydrocephalus and myelomeningocele are thought to have a better prognosis than children with permanent atrophy as a result of meningitis, aqueductal stenosis, or Dandy-Walker malformation (Volpe, 2001).

### Nursing Considerations

Preoperatively the infant with suspected hydrocephalus is observed carefully for signs of increasing ventricular size and increasing ICP. In infants the head is measured daily at the point of largest measurement—the occipitofrontal circumference (OFC). (See Chapter 7 for technique.) To avoid the likelihood of wide discrepancies, the point at which the measurements are taken is indicated on the head with a marking pen. Fontanels and suture lines are gently palpated for size, signs of bulging, tenseness, and separation. An infant with hydrocephalus and normal ICP will display bulging under certain circumstances such as straining or crying; therefore such accompanying behavior is noted. Irritability, lethargy, or seizure activity, as well as altered vital signs and feeding behavior, may indicate advancing pathology.

**NURSING ALERT**   In the toddler a headache and lack of appetite are two of the earliest common signs of shunt malfunction.

In older children, who are usually admitted to the hospital for elective or emergency shunt revision, the most valuable indicator of increasing ICP is an alteration in the child's level of consciousness and interaction with the environment. Changes are identified by observing and comparing present behavior with customary behavior, sleep patterns, developmental capabilities, and habits obtained through a detailed history and a baseline assessment. This baseline information serves as a guide for postoperative assessment and evaluation of shunt function.

General nursing care of the infant with hydrocephalus may present special problems. Maintaining adequate nutrition often requires flexible feeding schedules to accommodate diagnostic procedures, because feeding before or after handling can precipitate vomiting. Small feedings at more frequent intervals are often better tolerated than larger ones spaced farther apart. These infants are often difficult to feed and require extra time and innovation.

The nurse is responsible for preparing the child for diagnostic tests such as MRI or a CT scan and for assisting with procedures such as a ventricular tap, which is often performed to relieve excessive pressure and to obtain CSF during the preoperative period. Sedation is required because the child must remain absolutely still during diagnostic testing. A variety of drugs are available for sedation. (See Chapter 27 for preparing children for procedures.) If surgery is anticipated, IV infusions should not be placed in a scalp vein.

**NURSING TIP** Oral administration of chloral hydrate, a bitter-tasting liquid, may be given to an infant by the "nipple method." Place the nipple without the bottle in the mouth, add 5 ml of dextrose water to initiate sucking, then add the sedative, and finish with another 5 ml of dextrose water.

Fortunately, almost all children with hydrocephalus are recognized, and treatment is begun early. For those children with significant head enlargement, care must be exercised to see that the head is well supported when the infant is fed or moved to prevent extra strain on the infant's neck, and measures must be taken to prevent development of pressure areas. Not infrequently, infants with irreversible brain damage or with severe developmental defects such as hydranencephaly, in which both cerebral hemispheres fail to develop and are replaced with a membranous sac filled with CSF, are placed in long-term care facilities specially designed for care of these infants.

**Postoperative Care.**   In addition to routine postoperative care and observation, the infant or child is positioned carefully on the unoperated side to prevent pressure on the shunt valve. The child is kept flat to help avert complications resulting from too rapid reduction of intracranial fluid. When the ventricular size is reduced too rapidly, the cerebral cortex may pull away from the dura and tear the small interlacing veins, producing a subdural hematoma. This is not a problem in children with elective shunt revision because their intraventricular size and pressure have been normal. The surgeon indicates the position to be maintained and the extent of activity allowed. If there is increased ICP, the surgeon will prescribe the head of the bed to be elevated or allow the child to sit up to enhance gravity flow through the shunt. Different types of shunt mechanisms exist, so pumping the shunt to check function in the immediate postoperative period is performed at the surgeon's discretion and according to the manufacturer's recommendation.

Observation for signs of increased ICP, which indicate obstruction of the shunt, is continued. Neurologic assessment includes pupil dilation (pressure causes compression or stretching of the oculomotor nerve, producing dilation on the same side as the pressure) and blood pressure (hypoxia to the brainstem causes variability in these vital signs). The child is also observed for abdominal distention because CSF may cause peritonitis or a postoperative ileus as a complication of distal catheter placement.

Intake and output are carefully monitored. Children are often placed on fluid restriction with nothing by mouth (NPO) for 24 to 48 hours. The IV infusion is closely monitored to prevent fluid overload. Routine feeding is resumed after the prescribed NPO period, but the presence of bowel sounds is determined before feeding children with VP shunts.

Because infection is the greatest hazard of the postoperative period, nurses are continually on the alert for the usual manifestations of CSF infection, which may include elevated temperature, poor feeding, vomiting, decreased responsiveness, and seizure activity. There may be signs of local inflammation at the operative sites and along the shunt tract. Antibiotics are administered by the IV route as ordered, and the nurse may also need to assist with intraventricular instillation. The incision site is inspected for leakage, and any suspected drainage is tested for glucose, an indication of CSF. (See Critical Thinking Exercise box.)

Meticulous skin care is continued postoperatively, with extra care taken to prevent tissue damage from pressure. Pressure-reducing beds or mattresses may be needed to prevent pressure on prominent areas. The skin is inspected regularly for any signs of pressure, irritation, or infection.

**Family Support.**   Specific needs and concerns of parents during periods of hospitalization are related to the reason for the child's hospitalization (shunt revision, infection, diagnosis) and the diagnostic and surgical procedures to which the child must be subjected. Parents may have very little understanding of anatomy; therefore, they need further exploration and reinforcement of information that was given to them by the physician and neurosurgeon, as well as information about what they can expect. They are especially frightened of any procedure that involves the brain, and the fear of retardation or brain damage is very real and pervasive. Nurses can allay their anxiety with explanations of the rationale underlying the various nursing and medical activities such as positioning or testing and by simply being available and willing to listen to their concerns.

To prepare for the child's discharge and home care, the parents are instructed on how to recognize signs that indicate shunt malfunction or infection. Active children may have injuries, such as a fall, that can damage the shunt, and the tubing may pull out of the distal insertion site or become disconnected during normal growth. It is also important for the nurse to encourage families to enroll infants and toddlers with hydrocephalus into an early childhood development program. Depending on the degree of initial damage and the underlying cause, many children may have normal intellectual development.

The management of hydrocephalus in a child is a demanding task for both the family and health professionals,

## Critical Thinking Exercise

### Hydrocephalus

A 3-week-old infant is 8 days postoperative for shunt placement for hydrocephalus that developed following a primary repair of a meningomyelocele. The infant weighs 7.5 pounds and has been taking 90 to 120 ml of formula every 4 hours without problems. Within the last few hours the infant has become agitated and fussy and took only 15 ml of formula. Given the history and the fact that the infant has a VP shunt, what is the best intervention?

FIRST, THINK ABOUT IT . . .
- What conclusions are you reaching?
- If you accept the conclusions, what are the implications?

1. Request sedation for the infant.
2. Gavage the rest of the feeding to make up the calories and fluids required.
3. Pump the shunt reservoir with the infant in Trendelenburg position.
4. Measure the OFC; observe the shunt site for redness, edema, and drainage; take an axillary temperature; and call the neurosurgeon.

*The best response is four. The most common cause of such behavior in infants with shunts is shunt failure, which is an important conclusion. Infection may be a cause of failure; therefore monitoring the temperature and evaluating the shunt site is also important.*

*Arbitrary pumping of the shunt may cause more problems and should be performed only when indicated by the neurosurgeon. Sedation is not indicated in this instance, or at least not until the infant's neurologic status has been evaluated. Gavage feeding may replenish the infant's caloric and fluid requirements but is not the priority; poor feeding often indicates shunt failure and subsequent increased ICP. Vomiting, setting-sun sign, and greatly increased OFC may not be seen in newborns with increased ICP.*

and helping the family cope with the child's difficulties is an important nursing responsibility. Children with hydrocephalus have lifelong special health care needs. The nurse can provide optimum primary health care, including advice on immunizations, treatments for common infectious conditions, or child care and school precautions. The overall aim is to establish realistic goals and an appropriate educational program that will assist the child in achieving the optimum potential. Families can be referred to community agencies for support and guidance. The **National Hydrocephalus Foundation (NHF)*** and the **Hydrocephalus Association**† provide information on the condition for families, and the NHF assists interested groups in establishing local organizations.

Anticipatory guidance will prepare parents for possible problems and help them to avoid being overprotective of

*12413 Centialia Rd, Lakewood, CA 90715-1623, (562) 402-3523; www. nhfonline.org.
†870 Market St, Suite 955, San Francisco, CA 94102, (415) 732-7040; www.hydroassoc.org. A booklet entitled *About Hydrocephalus—A Book for Parents* is available in English or Spanish.

the child. There need be few restrictions placed on the child's activities (mainly contact sports), and the child is encouraged to live as would any other youngster of the same age and abilities. Parents need support and encouragement in coping with the child and problems the child may encounter in relationships with peers and others. Reactions of other children when the child has a noticeably enlarged head or requires shaving at times of revision are stressful situations for both the child and the parents. (See Chapter 22 for problems and coping with the child with a disability. See Nursing Care Plan: The Infant with Hydrocephalus.*)

## CRANIAL DEFORMITIES

In the normal newborn the cranial sutures are separated by membranous seams several millimeters wide. For the first few hours to 1 to 2 days after birth, the cranial bones are highly mobile, which allows the cranial bones to mold and slide over one another, adjusting the circumference of the head to accommodate to the changing shape and character of the birth canal. The principal sutures in the infant's skull are the sagittal, coronal, and lambdoidal sutures, and the major soft areas at the juncture of these sutures are the anterior and posterior fontanels. (See Fig. 8-6.)

Following birth, growth of the skull bones occurs in a direction *perpendicular* (at right angles) to the line of the suture, and normal closure occurs in a regular and predictable order. Although there are wide variations in the age at which closure takes place in individual children, solid union of all sutures is not completed until very late childhood. Normally, sutures and fontanels are ossified by the following ages:

**8 weeks**—Posterior fontanel closed
**6 months**—Fibrous union of suture lines and interlocking of serrated edges
**18 months**—Anterior fontanel closed
**10 to 12 years**—Sutures cannot be separated by ICP

Closure of a suture before the expected time inhibits the perpendicular growth. Since normal increase in brain volume requires expansion, the skull is forced to grow in a direction *parallel* to the fused suture. This alteration in skull growth always produces a distortion of the head shape when the underlying brain growth is normal. The small head with closed sutures and a normal shape is a result of deficient brain growth; the suture closure is secondary to this brain growth failure. Failure of brain growth is not secondary to suture closure.

Various types of cranial deformities are encountered in early infancy. These include the enlarged head with frontal protrusion, or bossing (characteristic of hydrocephalus), the parietal bossing that is seen in chronic subdural hematoma, the small head, and a variety of skull deformities (Fig. 11-8). Some occur during prenatal development; in others, head circumference is usually within normal limits at birth, and the deviation from normal development becomes apparent with advancing age.

*In Wong DL, Hess CS: *Wong and Whaley's clinical manual of pediatric nursing*, ed 5, St Louis, 2000, Mosby.

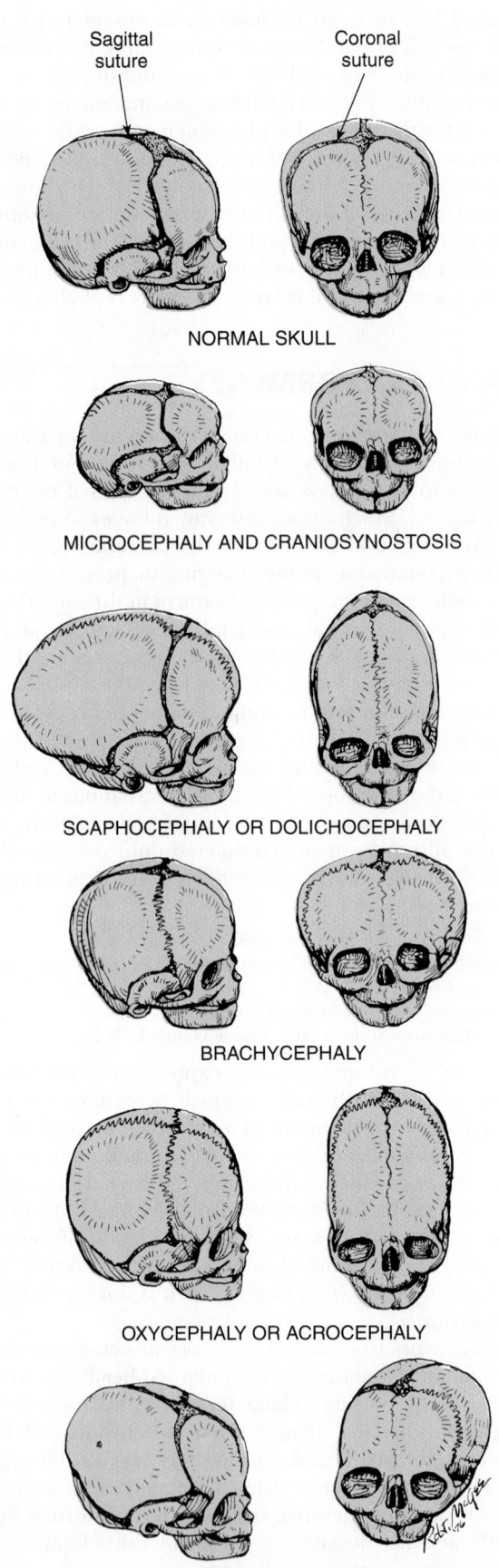

**Fig. 11-8** Craniostenosis. Abnormal head configuration resulting from premature closing of cranial sutures.

## Microcephaly

*Primary microcephaly* reflects a small brain and may be caused by an autosomal-recessive disorder, a chromosome abnormality, or application of a toxic stimulus during the period of induction and major cell migration in prenatal development. These stimuli may be irradiation (especially between 4 and 20 weeks of gestation), maternal infection (notably toxoplasmosis, rubella, or cytomegalovirus), or chemical agents. *Secondary microcephaly* can result from a variety of insults that occur during the third trimester of pregnancy, the perinatal period, or early infancy. Infection, trauma, metabolic disorders, and anoxia are all capable of causing decreased brain growth and early closure of cranial sutures. Microcephaly is defined as an OFC greater than 3 standard deviations below the mean for age and sex (Haslam, 2000).

In both types the neurologic manifestations range from decerebration, complete unresponsiveness, and/or autistic behavior to mild motor impairment, educable mental retardation, and/or mild hyperkinesis. There appears to be a decided relationship between microcephaly and mental retardation of varying degrees; however, not all children with microcephaly are mentally retarded (Haslam, 2000).

### Nursing Considerations

There is no treatment. Nursing care is supportive and may be directed toward helping parents adjust to rearing a child with cognitive impairment. (See Chapter 24.)

## Craniosynostosis

Craniosynostosis is defined as the premature closure at birth of one or more cranial sutures (Menkes and Sarnat, 2000). In craniosynostosis the clinical picture depends on which sutures close, the duration of the closure process, and the success or failure of the other sutures to compensate by expansion (see Fig. 11-8). Focal hydrodynamic mechanisms are involved in the compensatory skull changes seen in craniosynostosis. Brain atrophy and an underlying motor delay account for the position-induced skull changes. Craniosynostosis is also a common feature of children with Crouzon, Apert (Box 11-5), Pfeiffer, and Jackson-Weiss syndromes. Prenatal maternal smoking has been implicated as a cause of this condition; however, conclusive evidence has yet to be confirmed (Alderman and others, 1997; McIntyre, 1997). Diagnosis is established with CT scan, and MRI is useful in identifying accompanying brain abnormalitites. Increased ICP is more frequent in children with more than one prematurely fused suture.

The most common form of craniosynostosis is premature closure of the sagittal suture with resulting elongation of the skull in the anteroposterior direction. A similar head shape is seen as a result of postnatal position maintenance in some premature infants; however, in this case there is no premature closure of sutures. Craniosynostosis causes some increase in ICP, which may or may not cause mental retardation but can result in progressive papilledema, optic atrophy, and eventual blindness.

Trigonocephaly, or metopic craniosynostosis, represents a premature closure of the metopic suture in utero, a congenital problem that is familial and may not require surgical treatment. The metopic suture occurs where the right and left frontal bones meet on the forehead. Craniosynostosis of the metopic suture may be an autosomal dominantly inherited disorder not associated with functional brain or other abnormalities.

### Therapeutic Management

Treatment, if any, involves surgical excision of long bars of bone along or parallel to the fused suture. Various surgical procedures are employed in an effort to release the fused suture and direct growth. Lining the bony margins of the suture with silicone to delay closure is infrequently used. Surgery is performed to achieve the best possible cosmetic effect and, in severe cases, to relieve cerebral pressure symptoms and complications. The advised timing of suture release is before 6 months of age for best cosmetic and neurodevelopmental results.

Evidence suggests that early surgical intervention results in more positive outcomes with this condition, particularly in trigonocephaly. Mortality and morbidity was significantly higher in children with kleeblattschädel (cloverleaf skull) deformity and in children with multiple fused sutures (Sloan and others, 1997).

### Nursing Considerations

Nursing care primarily involves the early identification of persistent cranial molding weeks after regular birth molding would have resolved and referral for follow-up. In the postoperative period, nursing care includes observation for changes in neurologic status, hemorrhage, or infection. Following cranial surgery, pressure bandages may be applied to reduce swelling.

Because of the type of bone surgery involved with craniosynostosis, blood loss can be large. Therefore the hematocrit and hemoglobin are carefully monitored. Parents may also wish to provide a compatible blood donor for their infant. Nurses need to inform and guide parents through this blood bank procedure.

Most children will have substantial swelling of the eyelids postoperatively; careful handling and talking to the child may help allay fears when the eyelids are swollen shut. Eye care should be limited to gentle cleansing with a moist cloth. Pain management measures should be instituted in infants experiencing postoperative pain as they would for older children or adults. Fluids and adequate hydration are essential; oral feedings are resumed as soon as possible for hydration and for the nutritive sucking needs of the infant.

Early surgical management of craniosynostosis allows proper expansion of the brain and the creation of an acceptable appearance. Parents require special support and education during this time, especially from other parents whose infants have undergone similar operations. The nurse can serve as a liaison for this type of parental support.

## Craniofacial Abnormalities

Craniofacial abnormalities are those deformities involving the skull and facial bones. They have a low incidence rate in the population, but their effects can be psychologically devastating to affected children and their families. Deformities caused by abnormal growth of cranial bone(s) are listed in Box 11-5.

Most craniofacial anomalies are compatible with life, and all efforts are made to help the child and family live as normal a life as any other child. Advances in microscopic, orthopedic, neurologic, and plastic reconstructive surgery techniques have made it possible for children with craniofacial anomalies not only to survive beyond childhood, but also live a fulfilling life without the social stigmas of past decades. These children, however, may continue to face erroneous assumptions of mental handicap or retardation because of their appearance. Many hospitals in the United States now have craniofacial multidisciplinary teams dedicated to the purpose of helping the child and family achieve optimum potential for intellectual growth, physical competence, and social acceptance. Web sites are provided by many of these institutions and may be accessed for updated information on the condition, new treatments, and support groups.

### Therapeutic Management

Craniofacial surgical correction involves peeling the patient's face away from the skull and remolding the understructures. Parts can be brought together, the skull reshaped, and bone fragments removed or reshaped. The procedures are performed at various ages, depending on the anomaly, in craniofacial centers specializing in this pediatric problem. The timing of surgery is before school entry and is determined on an individual basis to ensure normal growth and development. Depending on the abnormality, other surgeries are performed, such as mandibular and digit correction. Following surgery, continued growth conforming to the inborn abnormality is unlikely.

### Nursing Considerations

Nursing efforts are directed toward preparation for surgery (there may be several surgical procedures over a period of time), postoperative care similar to care of any child with cranial surgery, and support of the child and family. There

---

**Box 11-5**

**Cranial Abnormalities Associated with Abnormal Bone Growth**

**Crouzon syndrome**—Craniofacial dysostosis (abnormal ossification of fetal cartilages) with shallow orbits and underdevelopment of the middle third of the face

**Apert syndrome**—Craniosynostosis resulting in a prominent forehead; may be extracranial abnormalities, such as syndactyly (webbing) of fingers and toes and cardiac defects

**Treacher Collins syndrome**—Asymmetric facial deformity including absent cheekbones, underslung jaw, and small chin; there is also downward slant of the eyes and other minor defects

**Pierre Robin syndrome**—Displacement of the chin as a result of micrognathia (mandibular hypoplasia) or retrognathia (normal-sized mandible positioned posteriorly); there is also glossoptosis with obstruction of the airway, and a cleft palate may be present

is frequently adjustment to the unfamiliar body image, which may be as traumatic as the previous deformity. A helmet may be worn to protect the operative site and bone grafts for varying lengths of time ranging from 6 months to 2 years. Follow-up care is very important.

## Plagiocephaly

Plagiocephaly is a rhomboid-shaped deformity that occurs in at least 1 of 300 live births and is rarely caused by brain malformation or unilateral suture stenosis. The rapidly growing infant head is easily molded by continued pressure against a surface, such as the uterine wall or a mattress. As a result, the skull is progressively flattened. There has been an increase in the number of children with plagiocephaly in recent years, primarily believed to be a result of the increased prevalence of supine sleeping in infants to prevent sudden infant death syndrome (SIDS). It is important to note that this *positional plagiocephaly* does not involve cranial suture stenosis and may be resolved by rotating the side of the head on which the infant sleeps and by placing the infant prone while awake and being observed (American Academy of Pediatrics, 2000a). Sometimes a helmet is used (see following discussion). **Congenital torticollis** (wry neck) is also a prevalent cause of positional plagiocephaly; torticollis occurs as a result of sustained contraction of the sternocleidomastoid muscle in utero (Raco and others, 1999).

### Therapeutic Management

Therapies available for the treatment of positional plagiocephaly include rotating the infant's head position each week (when asleep on the back), allowing the infant tummy time when awake and being observed, and in severe cases helmet or band therapy. Helmet therapy involves the use of a polypropylene device, which is large enough to fit the largest diameter of the head. The helmet is worn 23 hours a day for a prescribed period (usually 3 months); this therapy is most effective up to 9 months of age (McGee and Burkett, 2000). A dynamic orthotic cranioplasty (DOC) band also may be used as a corrective device to dynamically mold prominent areas of the skull and allow flattened areas to grow (Dias and Veetai, 1998). However, most believe that the head shape will change in most cases of mild to moderate plagiocephaly (without craniosynostosis) and do not advocate the use of these devices. Surgical treatment of plagiocephaly is primarily reserved for severe cases of true lambdoid synostosis (Dias and Veetai, 1998). When plagiocephaly is caused by torticollis, exercises for rotation and lateral bending of the neck are prescribed—often as much as five times daily—to correct the head shape (McGee and Burkett, 2000).

### Nursing Considerations

An important nursing function is helping to identify infants with significant plagiocephaly and refer them for further evaluation. It is also important to help parents understand the importance of placing the infant to sleep on the back to prevent SIDS and to alternate head positions during sleep to prevent occipital molding. Parents need encouragement and reinforcement to implement stretching exercises for

plagiocephaly associated with torticollis. Another important nursing function is to provide counseling and reassurance to parents that positional plagiocephaly does not affect brain growth or function. Nursing care of the surgical patient is the same as that for other children undergoing similar surgery. Care of the child receiving helmet therapy involves teaching parents the importance of making certain that the child wears the device as prescribed.

## SKELETAL DEFECTS*

This discussion is limited to those defects in development that are most common, that are amenable to therapy, and that involve nurses to a considerable extent. Less common defects and disorders are listed in Table 11-4.

### Developmental Dysplasia of the Hip (DDH)

The broad term *developmental dysplasia of the hip* describes a spectrum of disorders related to abnormal development of the hip that may develop at any time during fetal life, infancy, or childhood. A change in terminology from congenital hip dysplasia (CHD) and congenital dislocation of the hip (CDH) to DDH more properly reflects the varying onset and types of hip abnormalities in which there is a shallow acetabulum, subluxation, or dislocation (Box 11-6). The incidence of hip instability of some kind is approximately 10 per 1000 live births. The incidence of frank dislocation or dislocatable hip is 1 per 1000 live births (Wall, 2000). The left hip is involved in 60% of the cases, the right hip in 20%, and both hips in 20%. Eighty percent of the patients are female. Caucasian children have a higher incidence of devel-

---

■ *Jean Brown, MS, RNC, revised this section.

---

| Box 11-6 ■ ■ ⬜ |
| :--- |
| **Degrees of Developmental Dysplasia of the Hip** |

**Acetabular dysplasia** (or **preluxation**)—The mildest form, in which there is neither subluxation nor dislocation. The dysplasia reflects an apparent delay in acetabular development evidenced by osseous hypoplasia of the acetabular roof, which is oblique and shallow, although the cartilaginous roof is comparatively intact. The femoral head remains in the acetabulum.

**Subluxation**—Accounts for the largest percentage of congenital hip dysplasias. Subluxation implies incomplete dislocation or disclosable hip and is sometimes regarded as an intermediate state in the development from primary dysplasia to complete dislocation. The femoral head remains in contact with the acetabulum, but a stretched capsule and ligamentum teres cause the head of the femur to be partially displaced. Pressure on the cartilaginous roof inhibits ossification and produces a flattening of the socket.

**Dislocation**—The femoral head loses contact with the acetabulum and is displaced posteriorly and superiorly over the fibrocartilaginous rim. The ligamentum teres is elongated and taut.

opmental dysplasia than other groups (Maher, Salmond, and Pellino, 1998).

## Etiology and Pathophysiology

The cause of DDH is unknown, but certain factors such as gender, birth order, family history, intrauterine position, delivery type, joint laxity, and postnatal positioning are believed to affect the risk of DDH. Predisposing factors associated with DDH may be divided into three broad categories: (1) physiologic, (2) mechanical, and (3) genetic.

*Physiologic factors* that may influence development of hip abnormalities are maternal hormone secretion and mechanical factors of intrauterine posture. Toward the end of pregnancy there is increased maternal pelvic laxity mediated by maternal hormone secretion (principally estrogen), which affects the fetal joints as well. All joints are more lax in the newborn period, and the greater incidence of hip dislocation in females may be explained by their greater reactivity to the maternal hormones.

*Mechanical factors* that affect the hip and leg position indicate an association between a higher incidence of developmental hip deformities with breech presentations and cesarean section (often necessitated by abnormal intrauterine position). The position of the legs in frank breech position (i.e., with the hips acutely flexed and knees extended) is an important factor in the etiology of hip dislocation. The larger number of firstborn children (about one half of all children with DDH are firstborn) may be related to this factor, because the breech position in first deliveries is nearly always a frank breech. Other prenatal factors that contribute to hip dysplasia include oligohydramnios, twinning, and large infant size. (See Cultural Awareness box.)

*Genetic factors* include a positive family history. If one child has DDH, there is a 6% chance that each sibling will also have it. If one parent and one child have DDH, the risk to subsequent children is 36%.

Three degrees of DDH are illustrated in Fig. 11-9 and outlined in Box 11-6. Also, mounting evidence lends sup-

| **TABLE 11-4** Congenital defects involving the skeleton | | |
|---|---|---|
| **Disorder** | **Description and Anatomic Variation** | **Therapy** |
| Achondroplasia | Inherited (autosomal dominant)<br>Defect in ossification at the epiphyseal plate, resulting in very short limbs, large head, and lordosis | None |
| Osteogenesis imperfecta | Inherited (autosomal dominant, autosomal recessive)<br>Characterized by brittle, fragile, and easily fractured bones<br>Intrauterine fractures may produce congenital deformities | Reduction of fractures<br>Careful handling of extremities<br>See Chapter 39 |
| Pes planus (flatfoot) | Normal finding in infancy<br>May be result of muscular weakness in older child | Rarely indicated<br>Wedge on inner side of heel and sole for persistent or severe cases |
| Pes valgus | Eversion of entire foot, but sole rests on ground | Exercises |
| Pes varus | Inversion of entire foot, but sole rests on ground | Exercises |
| Metatarsus valgus | Eversion of forefoot while heel remains straight<br>Also called toeing out or duck walk | Passive exercises |
| Talipes deformities | See p. 451 | See p. 452 |
| Supernumerary digits (polydactyly) | Excessive number of fingers, toes, or both; usually inherited (autosomal dominant) | No treatment, or amputation of extra digits to improve function or for cosmetic reasons |
| Genu varum (bowleg) | May be congenital, result of rickets, or caused by osteochondrosis of proximal tibial epiphysis | Corrective splinting<br>Osteostomy in severe or neglected cases |
| Genu recurvatum (back knee) | Congenital, result of prenatal developmental defect or abnormal intrauterine position<br>Developmental, result of postnatal trauma or infection | Repeated corrective casting<br>Exercises |
| Klippel-Feil syndrome | Absence of one or more cervical vertebrae and two or more fused together<br>Neck short and limited in motion<br>Sometimes kyphosis and scoliosis | Rarely indicated<br>Scapula brought down and fixed if marked deformity or loss of function<br>Bracing of spinal deformities |
| Arachnodactyly (Marfan syndrome) | Inherited (autosomal dominant)<br>Abnormal length of fingers, toes, and extremities; hypermobility of joints; defects of spine and chest (pigeon breast); other associated abnormalities | Supportive measures |
| Congenital spine deformities | Kyphosis, scoliosis, lordosis, hemivertebrae, or a combination of these | Prevention of progression of defect with growth<br>Casting, bracing<br>Operative stabilization of affected vertebrae |
| Arthrogryposis multiplex congenita | Incomplete fibrous ankylosis of many or all joints (except spine and jaw) associated with hypoplasia of attached muscles<br>Contracture deformities—some extension, others flexion | Bracing, splinting, corrective surgery, and rehabilitation efforts |

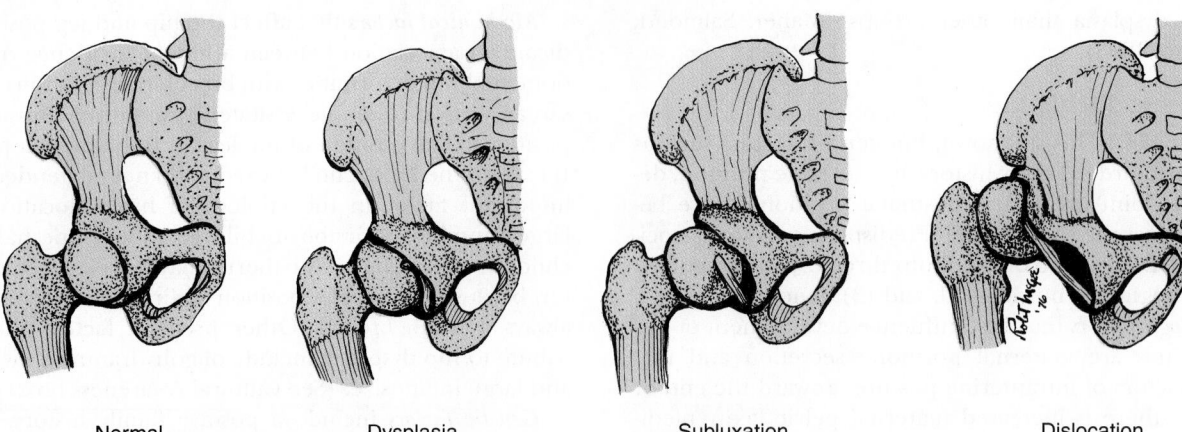

| Normal | Dysplasia | Subluxation | Dislocation |

**Fig. 11-9** Configuration and relationship of structures in developmental dysplasia of the hip.

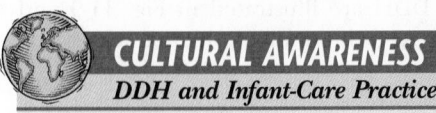

### CULTURAL AWARENESS
#### DDH and Infant-Care Practices

A striking relationship exists between the development of dislocation and methods of handling infants. Among the cultures with the highest incidence of dislocation (Navajo Indians and Canadian Eskimos), newly born infants are tightly wrapped in blankets or other swaddling material or are strapped to cradle boards. In cultures where mothers carry infants on their backs or hips in the widely abducted straddle position, such as in the Far East and Africa, the disorder is virtually unknown.

port to the suggestion that there are two types of DDH: the common type due to laxity of the supporting capsule and another type as a result of an abnormality of the acetabulum. The excessive laxity of the joint may prevent detection in early infancy. The femoral head remains in contact with the acetabulum until additional stress (such as standing) moves it away.

### Clinical Manifestations

The diagnosis of DDH should be made in the **newborn period** if possible, since treatment initiated before 2 months of age achieves the highest rate of success. In the newborn period dysplasia usually appears as hip joint laxity rather than as outright dislocation. Subluxation and the tendency to dislocate can be demonstrated by the Ortolani or Barlow tests. With the infant quiet and relaxed in the supine position on a firm surface and the legs facing the examiner, the hips are flexed (not forced) at right angles and the knees are flexed. The examiner places the middle finger of each hand over the greater trochanter and the thumbs on the inner side of the thigh at a point opposite the lesser trochanter. The knees are carried to midabduction, and each hip joint is submitted, one at a time, first to forward pressure exerted behind the trochanter and then to backward pressure exerted from the thumbs in front as the opposite joint is held steady. If the femoral head can be felt to slip forward into the acetabulum on pressure from behind, it is dislocated **(Ortolani test)** (Fig. 11-10, *D*). Sometimes an audible "clunk"

can be heard on exit or entry of the femur out of or into the acetabulum. If, on pressure from the front, the femoral head is felt to slip out over the posterior lip of the acetabulum and immediately slips back in place when pressure is released, the hip is said to be dislocatable or "unstable" **(Barlow test).**

**NURSING ALERT** These tests must be performed by an experienced clinician to prevent fracture or other damage to the hip. If these tests are performed too vigorously in the first 2 days of life, when the hip subluxates freely, persistent dislocation may occur.

The Ortolani and Barlow tests are most reliable from birth to 2 or 3 months of age. Adduction contractures develop at about 6 to 10 weeks, and the Ortolani sign disappears. After this time the most sensitive test is limited hip abduction (Fig. 11-10, *B*). Other signs are shortening of the limb on the affected side **(Galleazzi sign, Allis sign)** (Fig. 11-10, *C*), **asymmetric thigh and gluteal folds** (Fig. 11-10, *A*), and **broadening of the perineum** (in bilateral dislocation). Weight bearing may precipitate a transition from subluxation to dislocation in unrecognized cases.

A common cause of decreased hip abduction in the newborn is pelvic obliquity in which one side of the pelvis is higher than the other. This is thought to be caused by intrauterine positioning and will resolve on its own (Alexander and Kuo, 1997).

In the **older infant** and **child** the affected leg will be shorter than the other, with telescoping or piston mobility; that is, the head of the femur can be felt to move up and down in the buttock when the extended thigh is first pushed toward the child's head and then pulled distally. Instability of the hip on weight bearing delays walking and produces a characteristic **limp** and **toe walking.** When the child stands first on one foot and then on the other (holding onto a chair, rail, or someone's hands), bearing weight on the affected hip, the pelvis tilts downward on the normal side instead of upward as it would with normal stability **(Trendelenburg sign)** (Fig. 11-10, *E*). The practitioner should test the child for at least 30 seconds. In both unilateral and

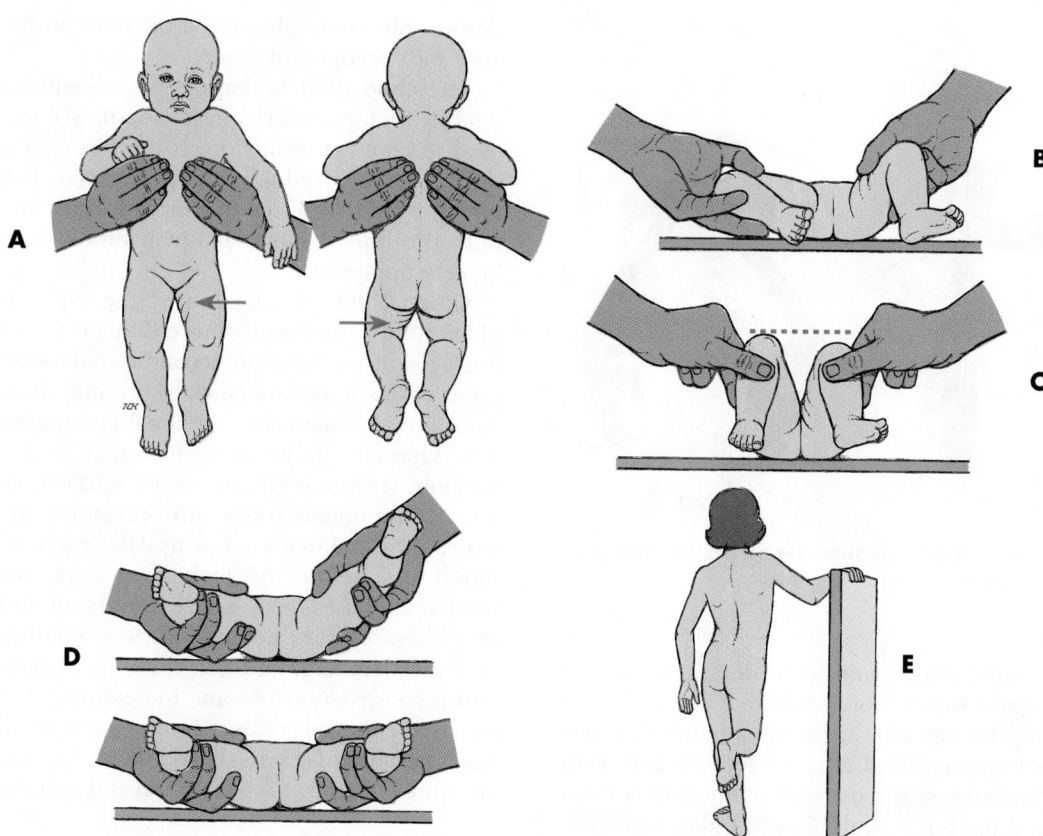

**Fig. 11-10** Signs of developmental dysplasia of the hip. **A,** Asymmetry of gluteal and thigh folds. **B,** Limited hip abduction, as seen in flexion. **C,** Apparent shortening of the femur, as indicated by the level of the knees in flexion. **D,** Ortolani click (if infant is under 4 weeks of age). **E,** Positive Trendelenburg sign or gait (if child is weight bearing).

bilateral dislocations the greater trochanter is prominent and appears above a line from the anterosuperior iliac spine to the tuberosity of the ischium. The child with bilateral dislocations has marked *lordosis* and a peculiar *waddling gait.*

### Diagnostic Evaluation

The primary diagnostic tools in the newborn period are the assessment techniques just described. DDH is often not detected at the initial examination after birth; thus all infants should be carefully monitored for hip dysplasia at follow-up visits throughout the first year of life.

Radiographic examination in early infancy is not reliable because ossification of the femoral head does not normally take place until the third to sixth month of life. However, the cartilaginous head can be visualized directly with real-time high-resolution ultrasonography. The use of ultrasonography as a screening tool for all infants to detect DDH has been proposed. However, it has been associated with a high incidence of false-positive results and overtreatment. Ultrasound technology has been reported to be effective as an adjunct to abnormal physical findings in some cases of DDH and as a tool to evaluate proper hip positioning in the Pavlik harness. The ultrasonographic examination can detect slight subluxations and dislocations as well as monitor progress over time.

In older infants and children, radiographic examination is useful in confirming the diagnosis. An upward slope in the roof of the acetabulum (the acetabular angle) greater than 40 degrees with upward and outward displacement of the femoral head is a frequent finding in older children.

A CT scan may be useful to assess the position of the femoral head relative to the acetabulum following closed reduction and casting. Arthrography can confirm stability and is useful in obtaining and evaluating closed reduction.

### Therapeutic Management

Treatment is begun as soon as the condition is recognized because early intervention is more favorable to the restoration of normal bony architecture and function. The longer treatment is delayed, the more severe the deformity, the more difficult the treatment, and the less favorable the prognosis. The treatment varies with the age of the child and the extent of the dysplasia. The goal of treatment is to obtain and maintain a safe, congruent position of the hip joint in order to promote normal hip joint development.

**Newborn to Six Months.** The hip joint is maintained by dynamic splinting in a safe position with the proximal femur centered in the acetabulum in an attitude of flexion. A variety of abduction devices are available for maintaining the femur in the acetabulum. Of these, the *Pavlik harness* is

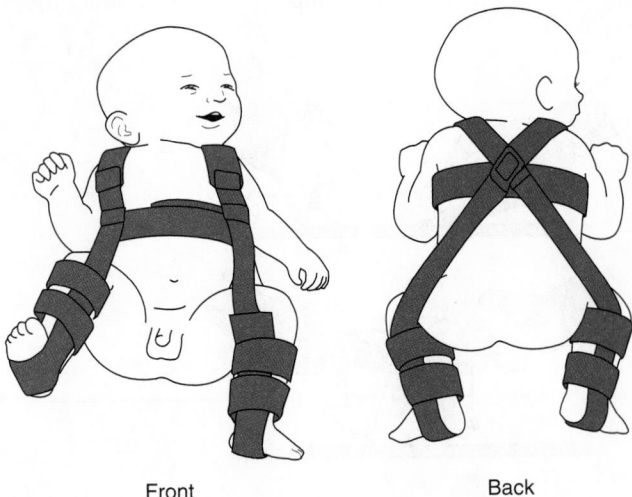

Front          Back

**Fig. 11-11** Child in Pavlik harness. (From Ball JW: *Mosby's pediatric patient teaching guides,* St Louis, 1998, Mosby.)

the most widely used device, and with time, motion, and gravity the hip works into a more abducted, reduced position (Fig. 11-11). The rate of reduction is about 95% effective with early treatment and if hips are reducible at birth (Wall, 2000). The harness is a dynamic splint that is worn continuously until the hip is clinically and radiographically stable, usually about 3 to 5 months. It is highly effective when the device is well constructed, follow-up care is adequate, and the parents follow instructions in its use. The Pavlik harness does not rigidly immobilize the hip but acts to prevent hip extension or adduction. Because of the infant's rapid growth rate, the straps should be checked every 1 to 2 weeks for possible adjustments (Novacheck, 1996); improper positioning may cause vascular or nerve damage.

When adduction contracture is present, other devices (such as skin traction) are employed to slowly and gently stretch the hip to full abduction, after which wide abduction is maintained until stability is attained. When there is difficulty in maintaining stable reduction, a hip spica cast is applied and changed periodically to accommodate the child's growth. After 3 to 6 months, sufficient stability is acquired to allow transfer to a removable protective abduction brace. The duration of treatment depends on development of the acetabulum but is usually accomplished within the first year.

**NURSING ALERT** The former practice of double- or triple-diapering for DDH is not recommended because it promotes hip extension, thus worsening proper hip development.

**Six to Eighteen Months.** In this age-group the dislocation is not recognized until the child begins to stand and walk, when attendant shortening of the limb and contractures of hip adductor and flexor muscles become apparent. Gradual reduction by traction is used for approximately 3 weeks. An individualized home traction program may be developed for the child preoperatively to decrease the length of hospitalization and maintain the home environment.

Written directions should be provided to increase compliance with preoperative care.

The child then undergoes an attempted closed reduction of the hip under general anesthesia; an arthrogram is used to confirm reduction. If the hip is not reducible, an open operative reduction is performed. Following reduction, the child is placed in a hip spica cast for 2 to 4 months until the hip is stable, at which time a flexion-abduction brace is applied.

**Older Child.** Correction of the hip deformity in the older child is inherently more difficult than in the preceding age-groups because secondary adaptive changes and other etiologic factors (such as juvenile rheumatoid arthritis or nonambulatory cerebral palsy) complicate the condition. Operative reduction, which may involve preoperative traction, tenotomy of contracted muscles, and any one of several innominate osteotomy procedures designed to construct an acetabular roof, is usually required. After cast removal and before weight bearing is permitted, range-of-motion exercises help restore movement. Other rehabilitative measures may include muscle strengthening, a period of crutch walking, and gait training. Successful reduction and reconstruction become increasingly difficult after the age of 4 years and are usually impossible or inadvisable after age 6 because of severe shortening and contracture of muscles and deformity of the femoral and acetabular structures.

### Nursing Considerations

Nurses are in a unique position to detect DDH in the newborn. During the infant assessment process and routine nurturing activities, the hips and extremities are inspected for any deviations from normal. Observation for unequal gluteal and thigh folds is routine, and nurses who have been educated to perform the Ortolani and Barlow tests should refer the infant with a positive test result to the practitioner. The ambulatory child who displays a limp or an unusual gait is referred for evaluation. This may indicate an orthopaedic or neurologic problem. Nonambulatory children with cerebral palsy are also assessed for evidence of dislocation.

**NURSING ALERT** Observations during routine care, such as diapering, provide an opportunity to observe the infant for limited movement and a wide perineum, which is an indication to assess for leg shortening, unequal gluteal and thigh folds, and limited abduction.

**Care of the Child in a Reduction Device.** The major nursing problems in the care of an infant or child in a cast or other device are related to maintenance of the device and adapting nurturing activities to meet the needs of the infant or child. Generally, treatment, as well as follow-up care, of these children is carried out in a clinic, practitioner's office, or outpatient unit. Hospitalization may be necessary for cast application or brace fitting but seldom exceeds 24 to 48 hours. Longer hospitalization is required for open reduction.

**Family Support and Home Care.** The primary nursing goal is teaching parents to apply and maintain the reduction device. The Pavlik harness allows for easy handling of the infant and usually produces less apprehension in the parent than heavy braces and casts. It is important that parents understand the correct use of the appliance, which may or may not allow for its removal during bathing. When the infant has a harness that is not removed, a sponge bath is recommended.

The following instructions for preventing skin breakdown are stressed:

- Always put an undershirt (or a shirt with extensions that close at the crotch) under the chest straps and put knee socks under the foot and leg pieces to prevent the straps from rubbing the skin.
- Check frequently (at least two or three times a day) for red areas under the straps and the clothing.
- Gently massage healthy skin under the straps once a day to stimulate circulation. In general, avoid lotions and powders, because they can cake and irritate the skin.
- Always place the diaper *under* the straps.

The parents are permitted to pad shoulder straps at pressure points if desired, but unbuckling or removal is determined on the basis of the family's level of understanding and the degree of deformity in the hip. In general, parents are not encouraged to adjust the harness without supervision. The child should be examined by the practitioner before any adjustment is attempted to ascertain that the hips are in correct placement before the harness is resecured.

Casts and braces offer more challenging nursing problems, since they cannot be removed for routine care, although sometimes the practitioner allows a brace to be removed for bathing. Care of an infant or small child with a cast requires nursing innovation to reduce irritation and to maintain cleanliness of both the child and the cast, particularly in the diaper area. The importance of spica cast care should be emphasized when providing instructions. The life of the cast should be prolonged so as to hold the legs and hips in proper position postoperatively and prevent an unnecessary cast change.

Cast care and observation are discussed in Chapter 39 and therefore are not elaborated on here. However, inasmuch as DDH is almost the exclusive reason for application of casts in early infancy, some of the problems specific to that age-group are mentioned.

Parents are taught the proper care of the cast (or brace) and are helped to devise means for maintaining cleanliness. A disposable superabsorbent (newborn-size) diaper is tucked beneath the entire perineal opening of the cast. A larger (toddler-size) diaper can be applied and fastened over the small diaper and cast.

For tightly fitting casts, transparent film dressing can be cut into strips as for petalling (see Chapter 39), and one edge can be applied to the cast edge and the other directly to the perineum; this forms a continuous waterproof bridge between the perineum and the cast to prevent leakage. An additional advantage to the use of this dressing material is that it keeps both the skin and the cast dry while allowing for observation of the skin beneath the dressing.

Older infants and small children may stuff bits of food, small toys, or other items under the cast; parents are alerted to this possibility so that suitable preventive measures, such as placing clothing over the cast, can be initiated.

Feeding the infant in a hip spica cast or brace offers problems of positioning. Very young infants can be fed in the supine position with the head elevated, and, with the infant's hips and legs supported on a pillow at the side, the parent can cuddle the infant during feeding. A somewhat similar position can be used for breast-feeding (i.e., with the infant supported on pillows or held in a "football" hold facing the mother with the legs behind her). An alternate position is to hold the infant upright on the mother's lap with the legs of the infant astride the mother's legs.

Infants who are able to sit up can be fed in a feeding table or modified high chair. Parents may be able to fashion a tilt board with a padded seat or an adjustable chair. The table or chair provides an excellent place for the child to play in an upright position. The child's car seat is also a vital consideration. Some hospitals have a child passenger safety program. A loan program for the appropriate automotive safety restraint may be offered to the parents, or referral to an agency that provides for this service may be made by the nurse or social worker.*

It is important for nurses, parents, and other caregivers to understand that these children need to be involved in all of the activities of any child in the same age-group. Toys are chosen that can be used in a prone position on the floor or in the seats devised for feeding and other activities. Confinement in a cast or appliance should not exclude children from family (or unit) activities. They can be held astride a lap for comfort and transported to areas of activity. The child may be allowed to walk in a cast or brace. An adapted wheelchair or stroller can offer mobility to the older infant or child. (See Chapter 39 for further discussion of care of a child in a spica cast.†)

## Congenital Clubfoot

Congenital clubfoot is a complex deformity of the ankle and foot that includes forefoot adduction, midfoot supination, hindfoot varus, and ankle equinus. Also referred to as *talipes equinovarus (TEV)*, congenital clubfoot involves bone deformity and malposition with soft tissue contracture (Fig. 11-12). This condition requires early evaluation and treatment for optimum correction. TEV is the most frequently occurring type of clubfoot (approximately 95%), although other variations may be seen and are generally described according to the position of the ankle and foot (Box 11-7).

The incidence of clubfoot is 1 to 2 per 1000 live births. Males are affected twice as often as females. Bilateral clubfeet occur in 50% of the cases. A positive family history is associated with increased incidence. Incidence varies with geographical location with the lowest incidence in China and the highest in Polynesia.

---

*For additional information contact the **Automotive Safety for Children Program,** James Whitcomb Riley Hospital for Children, Indiana University School of Medicine, 575 West Dr, Room 004, Indianapolis, IN 46202, (317) 274-7722 (in Indianapolis) (800) 543-6227, *www.preventinjury.org*.
†Home care instructions for caring for the child in a cast are available in Wong DL, Hess CS: *Wong and Whaley's clinical manual of pediatric nursing,* ed 5, St Louis, 2000, Mosby.

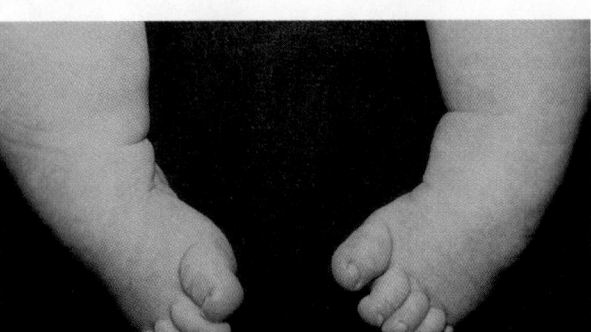

**Fig. 11-12** Bilateral congenital talipes equinovarus (congenital clubfoot) in 2-month-old infant. (From Zitelli BJ, Davis HW: *Atlas of pediatric physical diagnosis*, ed 3, St Louis, 1997, Mosby.)

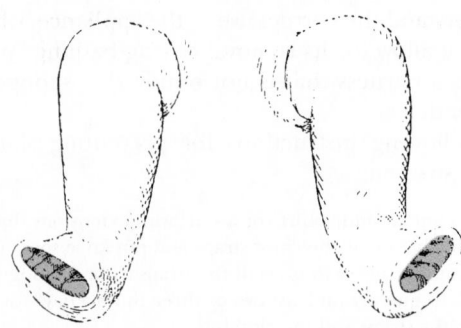

**Fig. 11-13** Feet casted for correction of bilateral congenital talipes equinovarus. (From Brashear HR Jr, Raney RB: *Handbook of orthopaedic surgery*, ed 10, St Louis, 1986, Mosby.)

> **Box 11-7** ■ ■ ■
> ## Common Foot Malformations
>
> **Talipes varus**—An inversion or a bending inward
> **Talipes valgus**—An eversion or a bending outward
> **Talipes equinus**—Plantar flexion, in which the toes are lower than the heel
> **Talipes calcaneus**—Dorsiflexion, in which the toes are higher than the heel

Clubfoot may be further divided into three categories: (1) *positional clubfoot* (also called *transitional, mild,* or *postural clubfoot*), which is believed to occur primarily from intrauterine crowding and responds to simple stretching and casting; (2) *syndromic* (or *tetralogic*) *clubfoot,* which is associated with other congenital abnormalities such as myelomeningocele (myelodysplasia) or arthrogryposis and is a more severe form of clubfoot that is often resistant to treatment; and (3) *congenital clubfoot,* also referred to as *idiopathic* or *true clubfoot,* which may occur in an otherwise normal child and has a wide range of rigidity and prognosis. The third category may be detected in utero by ultrasonography and is the most common type of TEV seen.

### Pathophysiology

The exact cause of clubfoot remains unknown. However, there is a strong familial tendency, with a 1 in 10 chance that a parent with clubfoot will have an affected offspring (Kyzer and Stark, 1995). Other possible theories as to the cause of clubfoot include arrested fetal developmental of skeletal and soft tissue during gestational weeks 9 to 10, when foot development occurs; abnormal neuromuscular dysfunction or muscle abnormalities; and possibly a defect in the primary germ plasma, resulting in ankle dysplasia. Cases of clubfoot have been observed as a possible result of distal limb *amniotic banding,* a condition in which the amnion forms constrictive bands around a limb in utero, cutting off the circulation to the limb and resulting in further abnormal or arrested development.

### Diagnostic Evaluation

Clubfoot is readily apparent at birth if it has not been previously detected antenatally. A careful yet comprehensive physical assessment of the affected foot (or feet) should be carried out once detection has occurred for appropriate decisions to be made regarding treatment and discussion of possible treatment plans and prognosis with the parents. The affected foot (or feet) is usually smaller and shorter, with an empty heel pad and a transverse plantar crease. When the defect is unilateral, the affected limb is usually shorter and some calf atrophy may be present. Anteroposterior and lateral (maximal dorsiflexion) radiographs are useful in the determination of the type and severity of clubfoot; ultrasonography may also be used. A thorough hip examination should be done on all infants with a clubfoot. An increased risk of hip dysplasia is associated with clubfoot deformities.

### Therapeutic Management

The goal of treatment for clubfoot is to achieve a painless, plantigrade, and stable foot. Once the diagnosis is established, treatment is ideally initiated in the newborn period and involves three stages: (1) correction of the deformity, (2) maintenance of the correction until normal muscle balance is regained, and (3) follow-up observation to avert possible recurrence of the deformity.

Serial casting is begun immediately or shortly after birth. Successive casts allow for gradual stretching of skin and tight structures on the medial side of the foot (Fig. 11-13). Manipulation and casting are repeated frequently (every few days for 1 to 2 weeks, then at 1- to 2-week intervals) to accommodate the rapid growth of early infancy. The affected extremity, or extremities, are casted until maximum correction is achieved, usually within 8 to 12 weeks. During this period, it is important to avoid overcorrection wherein a "rocker bottom" foot is created. A radiograph is then taken to evaluate the relationship of the bones to each other. Failure to achieve normal alignment indicates the need for surgical intervention. The typical age for surgery is generally between 6 months and 1 year of age (Thompson and Scoles, 2000).

Surgical intervention for clubfoot involves pin fixation and the releasing of tight joints and tendons. Casting of the affected foot and leg is performed, and after 2 or 3 months, a varus-prevention brace is used to maintain correction. With severe deformities, repeated surgical tendon or joint releases may be necessary.

**Prognosis.** Some feet respond to treatment readily; some respond only to prolonged, vigorous, and sustained efforts; and the improvement in others remains disappointing even with maximum effort. Parents should realize that outcomes are not always predictable and depend on the severity of the deformity, age of the child at initial intervention, compliance with treatment protocols, and development of bones, muscles, and nerves. Surgical intervention does not restore the ankle to an entirely normal state, with the affected foot and leg remaining smaller and thinner than the unaffected side. Ankle range of motion following surgery may be even less than it was preoperatively. Many children with surgically corrected clubfoot, however, are able to walk without a limp and run and play (Hoffinger, 1996).

### Nursing Considerations

Nursing care of the child with nonsurgical correction of clubfoot is the same as it is for any child who has a cast. (See Chapter 39.) The child will spend a considerable time in a corrective device; therefore nursing care plans include both long-term and short-term goals. Conscientious observation of skin and circulation is particularly important in young infants because of their normally rapid growth rate. Since treatment and follow-up care are handled in the orthopaedist's office, clinic, or outpatient department, parent education and support are important in nursing care of these children.

Parents need to understand the diagnosis, the overall treatment program, the importance of regular cast changes, and the role they play in the long-term effectiveness of the therapy. Reinforcing and clarifying the orthopaedic surgeon's explanations and instructions, providing emotional support, teaching parents about care of the cast or appliance (including vigilant observation for potential problems; see discussion of cast care on p. 451 and in Chapter 39), and encouraging parents to facilitate normal development within the limitations imposed by the deformity or therapy are all part of nursing responsibilities.

## Metatarsus Adductus (Varus)

Metatarsus adductus, or metatarsus varus, is probably the most common congenital foot deformity. In most instances it is a result of abnormal intrauterine positioning and is usually detected at birth. It may occur bilaterally in 50% of newborns, and 10% of affected children will have developmental dysplasia of the hip (Cooperman and Thompson, 1997). The deformity is characterized by medial adduction of the toes and forefoot, frequently associated with inversion, and convexity of the lateral border of the (kidney-shaped) foot. Unlike TEV, with which it is often confused, the angulation occurs at the tarsometatarsal joint while the heel and ankle

remain in a neutral position. This deformity often causes a pigeon-toed gait in the child.

Management depends on the rigidity of the deformity. Most children under the age of 18 months with mild valgus or varus deformities do not require treatment because the defect corrects itself in time. When treatment is needed, correction can usually be accomplished by gentle manipulation and passive stretching of the foot, which the parent is taught to perform. Repeated and consistent stretching is continued for the first 6 weeks, after which the treatment is based on the flexibility of the foot. If the child is able to actively overcorrect the deformity voluntarily on stimulation, continued stretching is generally sufficient. If the foot cannot be actively or passively overcorrected, the feet are stretched and manipulated and held with casts or orthoses.

### Nursing Considerations

The nursing role primarily involves identifying the defect so that early therapy and instruction of the parents can be instigated. The nurse teaches the parents how to hold the heel firmly and to stretch the forefoot. If casting is needed, the nurse instructs the parents in cast care and observation. (See Chapter 39.)

## Skeletal Limb Deficiency

Congenital limb deficiencies, or reduction malformations, are manifested by loss of functional capacity of varying degrees. They are characterized by underdevelopment of skeletal elements of the extremities. The range of malformation can extend from minor defects of the digits to serious abnormalities such as *amelia,* absence of an entire extremity, or *meromelia,* partial absence of an extremity, which includes *phocomelia* (seal limbs), an interposed deficiency of long bones with relatively good development of hands and feet attached at or near the shoulder or the hips. In some instances prenatal destruction of limbs may occur, but most reduction deformities are believed to be primarily defects of development (*agenesis, aplasia*).

### Pathophysiology

Limb deficiencies can be attributed to both heredity and environment, and they can originate at any stage of limb development. Formation of limbs may be suppressed at the time of limb bud formation, or there may be interference in later stages of differentiation and growth. Heredity appears to play a prominent role, and prenatal environmental insults have been implicated in a number of cases, such as the well-publicized *thalidomide* tragedy in the late 1950s and early 1960s, which demonstrated a clear relationship between the time of exposure of the pregnant woman to the antiemetic drug and the presence and type of limb deformity in the newborn. A number of reports suggest that absence or shortening of the digits is associated with *chorionic villus sampling,* especially if the procedure is performed before 10 to 12 weeks of gestation; however, the incidence and relationship remain uncertain. The Centers for Disease Control and Prevention (1995) recommends that parents be counseled regarding the risks and benefits of chorionic villus sampling.

> **NURSING ALERT**  Parents of children with limb deficiencies should be referred for genetic counseling.

## Therapeutic Management

Children with congenital limb deficiencies should be fitted with prosthetic devices whenever possible, and a functional replacement should be applied at the earliest possible stage of development in an attempt to match the motor readiness of the infant. This favors natural progression of prosthetic use. For example, an infant with an upper extremity deficiency is fitted with a simple passive device such as a mitten prosthesis between 3 and 6 months of age, when limb exploration is active, sitting is beginning (with the extremities needed for support), and bilateral hand activities are to be encouraged. Lower limb prostheses are applied when the infant is ready to pull to a standing position.

In preparation for prosthetic devices, surgical modification is often necessary to ensure the most favorable use of the device because severe deformity can interfere with its effective use. Phocomelic digits are preserved for controlling switches of externally powered appliances in the upper extremities. Digits (in both the upper and lower extremities) provide the child with surfaces for tactile exploration and stimulation. Prostheses are replaced to accommodate growth and increasing capabilities of the child.

### Nursing Considerations

Prosthetic application training and habilitation are most successfully carried out in a center that specializes in meeting the special needs of these children, especially very young children and those with multiple amputations. Specialized limb deficiency clinics are most helpful to parents and provide an introduction to support groups for both parents and affected children. Parents must encourage the child in making age-commensurate adjustments to the environment. Although these children need assistance, overprotection may produce overdependency with later maladjustment to school and other situations.

## DISORDERS OF THE GASTROINTESTINAL (GI) TRACT

Congenital defects of the GI tract can involve any portion from the mouth to the anus. Most are apparent at birth or shortly thereafter and are anomalies in which normal growth ceased at a crucial stage of embryonic development, leaving the structure in an embryonic form or only partially completed. The result may be atresia, malposition, nonclosure, or any number of variations.

*Atresia* is absence of a normal opening or normally patent lumen. Atresia at any point along the length of the GI tract creates an obstruction to the normal progress of nutrients and secretions. The most common anomalies requiring surgical intervention are atresias of the esophagus, intestine, and anus. The congenital defects considered in this chapter include abnormalities of the lip and palate, esophagus, and anus. Some malformations of the GI tract are considered here rather than in Chapter 33 because they are identified at birth and are cause for considerable parental concern.

## Cleft Lip (CL) and/or Cleft Palate (CP)

CL with or without CP is the most common craniofacial malformation and occurs with a frequency of 1 in 700 live births. Isolated CP has an incidence of approximately 1 in 2000 live births. CL with or without CP is more common in males, and CP alone is more common in females. CL appears more often in Native Americans and Asians and less frequently in African-Americans. See Table 11-5 for a comparison of the two defects.

CL results from incomplete fusion of the embryonic structures surrounding the primitive oral cavity. The cleft may be unilateral or bilateral and is often associated with abnormal development of the external nose, nasal cartilages, nasal septum, and maxillary alveolar ridges. It may or may not be associated with CP. The extent of the cleft varies greatly from an indentation in the lip to a deep and wide fissure extending to the nostril. In severe clefts the nostril on the affected side is low and the nose is deviated to that side. With bilateral CL the midportion of the upper lip is unattached on both sides and may be displaced forward. Dental anomalies, such as missing, malpositioned, or deformed teeth, are common on the side of the cleft.

CP occurs when the primary and secondary palatine plates fail to fuse during embryonic development. CPs vary greatly in degree and may involve only the soft palate or may extend into the hard palate. The cleft may occur only in the midline of the posterior palate but may extend to the nostril on one or both sides. Wide central palatal clefts may be accompanied by partial or complete absence of nasal septal development, resulting in communication between the nasal and oral cavities. Occasionally, small clefts of the soft palate may be difficult to identify. A *submucous cleft palate* may be present; this form of CP may be difficult to identify initially because the palatal cleft is covered by the mucous membrane of the roof of the mouth. The submucous cleft palate may be associated with a cleft or bifid uvula and may lead to subsequent speech problems in some cases.

### Etiology

Many factors appear to be involved in the etiology of CL and CP, and evidence indicates that CL with or without CP is developmentally and genetically different from isolated CP. The majority of cases appear to be consistent with the concept of multifactorial inheritance as evidenced by an increased incidence in relatives and a higher concordance in monozygotic twins than in dizygotic twins. Siblings of children with CL with or without CP have an increased risk of the same anomaly but not of CP alone, and vice versa.

There are many recognized syndromes that include CL and CP as a feature. Some of these syndromes are a result of

**TABLE 11-5** Comparison of cleft lip and cleft palate

| | Cleft Lip | Cleft Palate |
|---|---|---|
| Incidence | 1:7800 | 1:2000 |
| Inheritance | Multifactorial inheritance, environmental factors, familial occurrence<br>Male predominance | Associated with syndromes (chromosomal), familial occurrence, environmental factors such as maternal alcohol ingestion, or smoking or teratogens<br>Female predominance |
| Anatomy | Unilateral or bilateral<br>May involve external nose, nasal cartilages, nasal septum, maxillary alveolar ridges, and dental anomalies | Soft palate and/or hard palate<br>Midline of posterior palate<br>May involve nostril and absence of nasal septal development (communication with oral and nasal cavity) |
| Management | Surgical—Z-plasty<br>First few weeks of life if no respiratory, oral, or systemic infections occur | First few weeks of life if stable before development of speech |
| Short-term problems (before repair) | Feeding, possibly | Feeding—aspiration; growth failure |
| Special postoperative care | Suture line protection and care<br>Position—right side or upright in infant seat; avoid prone positioning to protect suture line<br>Special feeding—Breast-feeding, slow-flow nipple, plastic squeezable bottle, Haberman feeder, Breck feeder—until suture line heals | May be prone, supine, or side-lying<br>Breast-feeding, feeding cup, Haberman feeder, slow-flow nipple, Breck feeder; avoid spoon, fork (also tongue blade and other objects that could damage suture line) |
| Long-term problems | Social acceptance (depends on success of repair), orthodontic if associated with CP | Speech, otitis media, possible hearing loss, upper respiratory tract infections<br>Orthodontic<br>Feeding<br>Social acceptance (voice changes, facial appearance if with CL) |

chromosome abnormalities, and environmental factors or teratogens may be responsible for clefts at a critical point in embryonic development. Drugs such as phenytoin, valproic acid, thalidomide, and the pesticide dioxin are known to cause CL/CP. Maternal nutrition, especially folic acid deficiency, has been linked to clefting in humans as have maternal alcohol ingestion and smoking during pregnancy (Bender, 2000). There is evidence that maternal smoking early in pregnancy is associated with a 1.5- to 2-fold increase in the risk for orofacial clefts, especially isolated clefts, with the risk increasing proportionately with the number of cigarettes smoked (Shaw and others, 1996).

## Pathophysiology

Development of the primary and secondary palates takes place at different times and involves different developmental processes. CL with or without CP results from failure of the maxillary processes to fuse with the nasal elevations on the frontal prominence, which normally occurs during the sixth week of gestation (Fig. 11-14, *A*). Merging of the upper lip at the midline is completed between the seventh and eighth weeks of gestation. There is evidence, however, that in some cases separation may be a result of rupture subsequent to fusion.

Fusion of the secondary palate (hard and soft palates) takes place later in development, between the seventh and twelfth weeks of gestation (Fig. 11-14, *B* to *D*). At the time the primary palate is completed, the two lateral palatine processes are situated in a vertical position at the side of the tongue. In the process of migrating to a horizontal position, they are, for a short time, separated by the tongue. With de-

velopment of the neck and jaws, the tongue moves downward, allowing the palatine processes to fuse with each other and with the primary palate to form the roof of the mouth. If there is delay in this movement, or if the tongue fails to descend soon enough, the remainder of development proceeds but the palate never fuses.

## Diagnostic Evaluation

A cleft that involves the lip with or without CP is readily apparent at birth and is one of the defects that elicits the most severe emotional reactions in parents. CL can be diagnosed in utero by ultrasonography as early as 14 to 16 weeks gestation (Mitchell and Wood, 2000); fetal surgical repair of CL, however, is considered to have too many associated risks, and neonatal repair may be accomplished with minimal complications (Bender, 2000). Prenatal diagnosis of CL and CP is becoming more common. An important initial assessment in the diagnostic evaluation is to determine if the defect is isolated or one feature of a broader syndrome. Palpation of the hard and soft palate and uvula with a gloved finger, as well as inspection of the oral cavity and its structures, are an important part of the newborn physical examination. (See Chapter 8.) The degree of malformation of the CL or CP can then be evaluated (Figs. 11-15 and 11-16). Clefts of the lip may be unilateral or bilateral, and the extent of the cleft and degree of nasal deformity are variable. CP can occur with CL or as an isolated deformity. As with CL, the degree of deformity varies and may involve only the uvula or may extend through both the soft and hard palates. The severity of the CP has an impact on feeding problems; the infant is unable to generate negative pressure and create suction in the oral cavity. This impairs feeding even though in most cases the infant's ability to swallow is normal.

### Therapeutic Management

Treatment of the child with CL is surgical and usually involves no long-term interventions other than possible scar revision. However, management of CP involves the cooperative efforts of a multidisciplinary health care team—including pediatrics, plastic surgery, orthodontics, otolaryngology, speech and language pathology, audiology, nursing, and social work—to provide optimum results. Treatment continues over a long

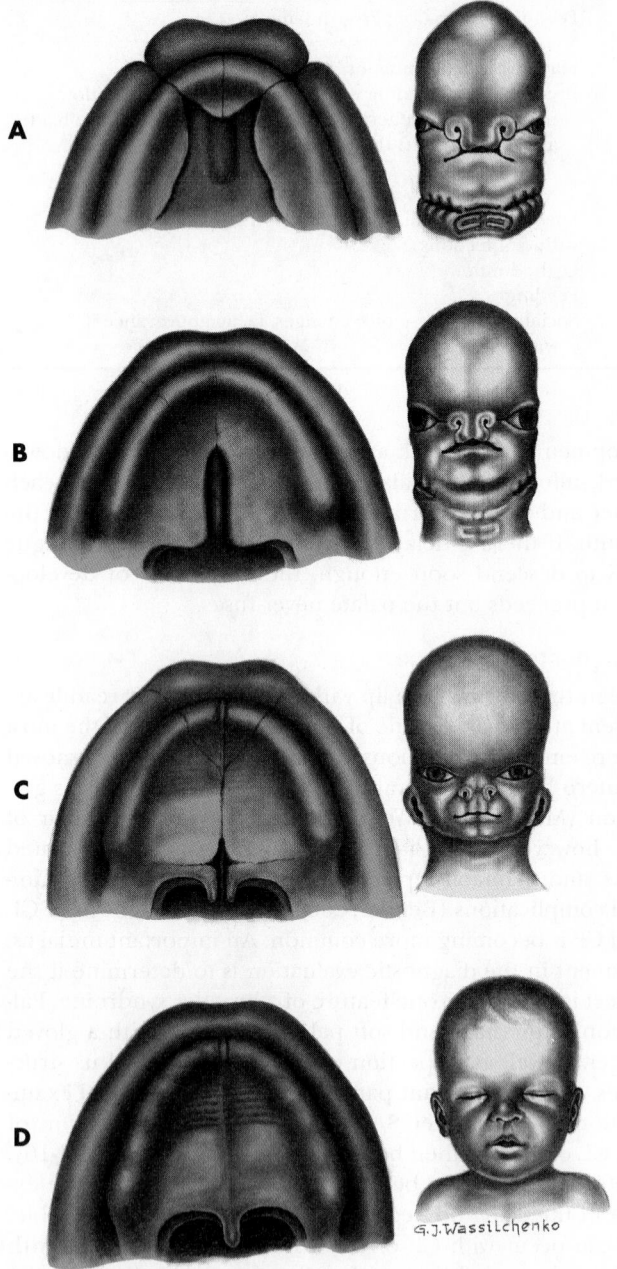

**Fig. 11-14** **A** to **D,** Stages in palatine development. See text for discussion.

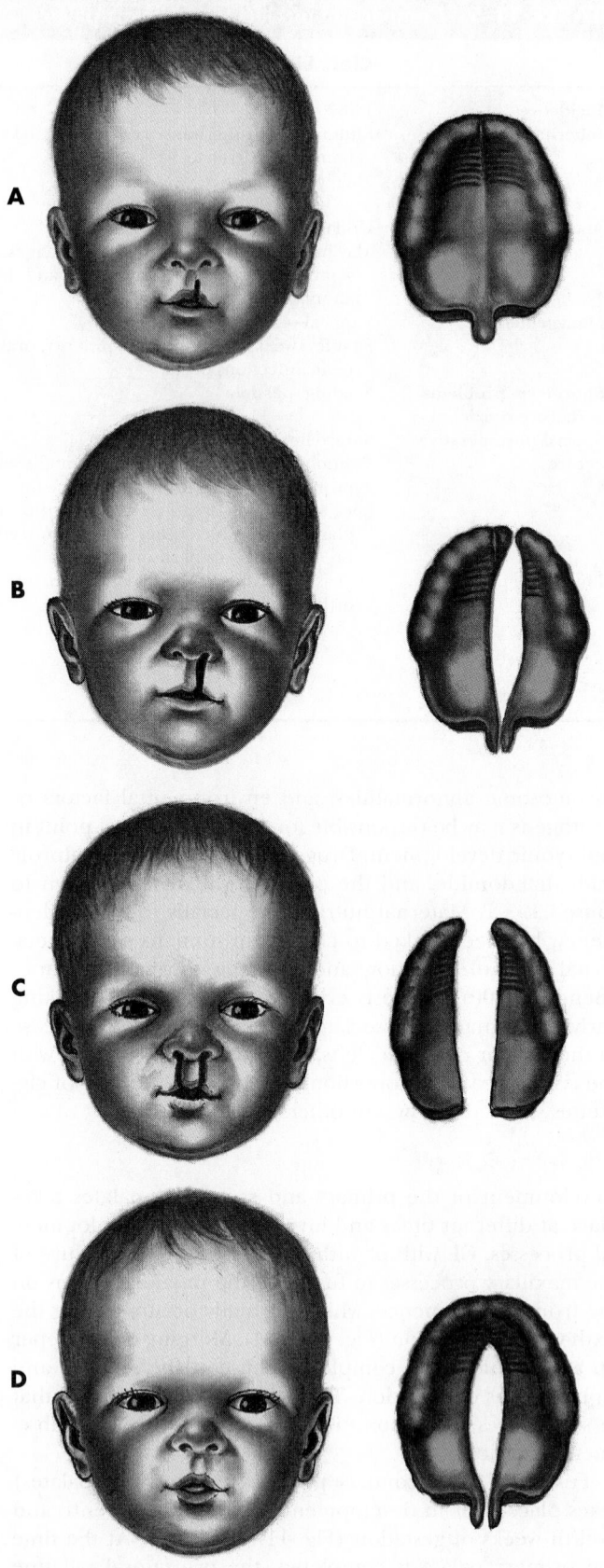

**Fig. 11-15** Variations in clefts of lip and palate at birth. **A,** Notch in vermilion border. **B,** Unilateral cleft lip and cleft palate. **C,** Bilateral cleft lip and cleft palate. **D,** Cleft palate.

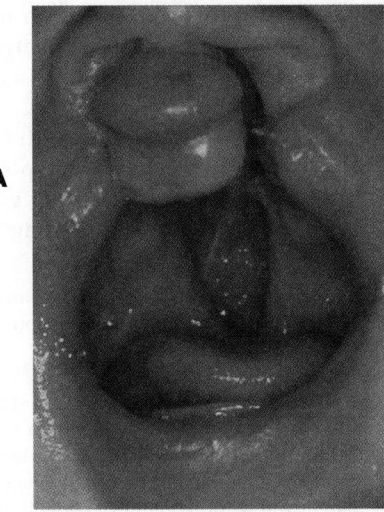
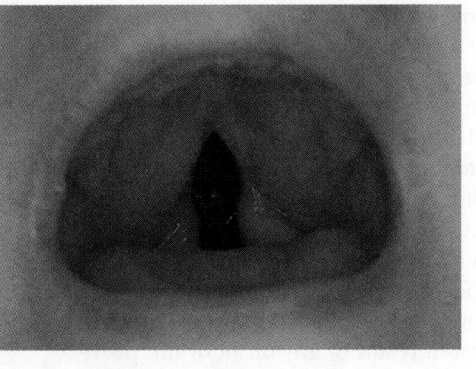

**Fig. 11-16  A,** Bilateral cleft lip with complete cleft palate. Cleft extends from the soft to the hard palate, exposing the nasal cavity. **B,** Midline cleft of the soft palate. (From Zitelli BJ, Davis HW: *Atlas of pediatric physical diagnosis,* ed 3, St Louis, 1997, Mosby; **B** courtesy Barbara Elster, Cleft Palate Center, Pittsburgh.)

time, but, even after completion of a program of health care, the child will probably retain defects of speech, facial appearance, and other problems related to the cleft. Management of both defects is directed toward surgical closure of the cleft, prevention of complications, and facilitation of normal growth and development of the child.

**Surgical Correction: CL.**  Closure of the lip defect precedes that of the palate, usually during the first weeks of life. Surgical correction is performed when the infant is free of any oral, respiratory, or systemic infection. The method of repair of the CL involves one of several staggered suture lines (Z-plasty) to minimize notching of the lip from retraction of scar tissue and to lengthen the lip.

Improved surgical techniques have minimized deformity related to scar retraction, but optimum cosmetic results are difficult to obtain in severe defects. In the absence of infection or trauma, healing takes place with little scar formation. Remaining physical characteristics in the older child are residual nasal deformity, a mildly protruding lower lip, and a somewhat flattened lower third of the upper lip, usually with an abnormally shaped red lip margin. Not infrequently, revisions may be required at a later age. Animal studies in which intrauterine repair of a CL took place demonstrate better healing of the lip than is typically seen with conventional repair.

**Surgical Correction: CP.**  CP repair was previously postponed until a later age than repair of the CL in order to take advantage of palatal changes that occur with normal growth.

With advanced surgical and anesthetic techniques, many surgeons are performing palatal repairs in the neonatal period (Sandberg, Magee, and Denk, 2002). However, the timing of repairs remains controversial. Most surgeons prefer to close the cleft before the child develops faulty speech habits. Persistent velopharyngeal insufficiency, manifested by nasal regurgitation and nasal speech, may require a posterior pharyngeal flap procedure or palate bone grafting at a later time.

**Long-Term Problems.**  The care of children with CL and CP often involves a group of specialists who meet

periodically to examine the child and consult with each other and with the parents. Even with adequate anatomic closure, the majority of children with CL and CP have some degree of speech impairment that requires speech therapy. The physical problems are a result of inefficient functioning of the muscles of the soft palate and nasopharynx, improper tooth alignment, and varying degrees of hearing loss.

Improper drainage of the middle ear, as a result of inefficient function of the eustachian tube, causes increased pressure in the middle ear and contributes to recurrent otitis media, which leads to hearing impairment in some children with CP. The insertion of pressure-equalizing (PE) tubes has become standard procedure in the child with CL/CP and is performed at the same time as other surgical procedures (such as cleft lip repair) to facilitate fluid drainage from the middle ear and prevent recurrent otitis media.

Extensive orthodontics and prosthodontics are usually needed to correct problems of malposition of the teeth and maxillary arches. There may be missing teeth, or the teeth may be malformed or malpositioned, which can interfere with feeding. In addition, a significant number of these children have an inadequate nasal airway that forces them to breathe through the mouth, which also contributes to oral deformity. Children with both CL and CP often require several stages of orthodontic therapy. The *first stage* (at birth to 18 months) is concerned with aligning the maxillary segments into a near-normal relationship. This is frequently done before lip closure in severely expanded segments to facilitate a primary lip closure. The *second stage* (at 2 to 5 years) consists of repositioning maxillary segments and/or correcting a dental crossbite (a condition in which the upper teeth close inside the lower teeth) in an attempt to allow the primary teeth to develop in a normal relationship. The *third stage* of therapy (at 10 to 11 years) takes place during the mixed-dentition stage and involves correction of faulty occlusion. In the *fourth stage* (at 12 to 18 years) treatment of the permanent teeth is accomplished in much the same manner as for any adolescent except for alignment and spacing in the cleft area.

Often, temporary or permanent dental prostheses are necessary to replace missing teeth; these assist in chewing and produce a more pleasing cosmetic effect. Special dental plates, called *obturators,* are sometimes used to mechanically close clefts in the palate to facilitate feeding and speech until permanent closure is attempted. However, any appliance must be checked periodically to ensure a proper fit and to see that it is performing its intended function.

A major problem for a child with CP may be defective speech. This can occur as a result of any or all of the previously discussed complications: insufficient palate function, faulty dentition, and hearing loss. CP interferes with speech sounds in the mouth that are normally made through interaction of the throat and palatine muscles. Improper tooth alignment can pose a mechanical hazard to development of clear speech, and hearing loss from middle ear infection is an additional impediment because of difficulty in interpreting sounds. With isolated CL, no speech problems should be anticipated. The child with CP usually requires the services of a speech therapist.

Some of the more difficult long-term problems are related to social adjustment of the child. In one study infants with CL or CP had significant cognitive and motor delays at 5 months when compared with a control group; at 13 months, only infants with CP showed delays in motor development. At 36 months all of the toddlers with CL or CP showed significantly lower performance in fine motor, gross motor, and expressive language in comparison with the 25-month-old toddlers with CL or CP (Neiman and Savage, 1997). One study found that children with CL/CP were at greater risk for developmental problems during the second year of life than previously expected (Kapp-Simon and Krueckeberg, 2000). The better the physical care, the better the chance for emotional and social adjustment, although the presence of the defect and the degree of residual disability are not always directly related to a satisfactory adjustment. Physical defects are a threat to the self-image, and abnormal speech quality is an impediment to social expression.

## Nursing Considerations

## Assessment

Since CL is readily visible at birth, assessment consists of describing the location and extent of the defect and looking for an accompanying palatine cleft during crying. CP without CL is detected by palpating the palate with the gloved finger during the newborn assessment.

The birth of an infant with a cosmetic, as well as a functional, disability is especially traumatic to the family. Consequently, the nursing assessment is also concerned with the emotional reaction of the family to the infant and the defect.

## Nursing Diagnosis

Following a thorough nursing assessment, a number of nursing diagnoses become evident. The most likely diagnoses are outlined and discussed in the Nursing Care Plan on pp. 461-462. Others may be apparent in individual cases.

## Planning

The goals of care for the infant with CL and CP are related to preoperative care, short-term postoperative care, and long-term management. The major goals of care for the infant and family include the following:

**Preoperative care:**
1. Family will cope with the impact of an infant with a defect.
2. Infant will receive optimum nutrition.
3. Infant will be prepared for surgery.

**Postoperative care:**
1. Infant will experience no trauma and minimal or no pain.
2. Infant will receive optimal nutrition.
3. Infant will experience no complications.
4. Infant and family will receive adequate support.
5. Family will be prepared for care at home and the long-term needs of a child with CP.

## Implementation

The immediate nursing problems in the care of an infant with CL and CP deformities are related to feeding the infant and dealing with the parental reaction to the defect. Facial deformities are particularly disturbing to parents; CL, especially, is a disfiguring, visible defect that may generate a strong negative response in parents. During the initial phase following the birth of an infant with CL and/or CP, it is important for the nurse to place emphasis not only on the infant's physical needs but also on the parents' emotional needs. The concept that infants with CL and/or CP are at increased risk for failure of maternal attachment has recently been challenged. In a few studies, maternal-infant attachment was not negatively affected when measured at 1 year of age (Speltz and others, 1997) and at 24 months (Maris and others, 2000).

The nurse should encourage expression of parental grief and fears, which may promote attachment in the preoperative period. It is especially important to emphasize the positive aspects of the infant's physical appearance and to express optimism regarding surgical correction while acknowledging the parents' concern. The manner of handling the infant should convey to the parents that the infant is indeed a precious human being. (See Birth of a Child with a Physical Defect, p. 416.)

**Feeding.** Feeding the newborn with CL/CP can be difficult, and teaching the parent to successfully feed the child is perhaps one of the most significant and challenging roles the nurse will encounter. Growth failure in infants with CL and/or CP has been attributed to preoperative feeding difficulties. Following surgical repair most infants with isolated CL or CP and no associated syndrome gain weight successfully or achieve adequate weight and height for age (Lee, Nunn, and Wright, 1997).

Clefts of the lip or palate reduce the infant's ability to suck, which interferes with compression of the areola and renders breast-feeding and bottle-feeding difficult. Liquid taken into the mouth tends to escape via the CP through the nose. Feeding is best accomplished with the infant's head in an upright position, either held in the caregiver's

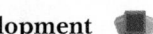

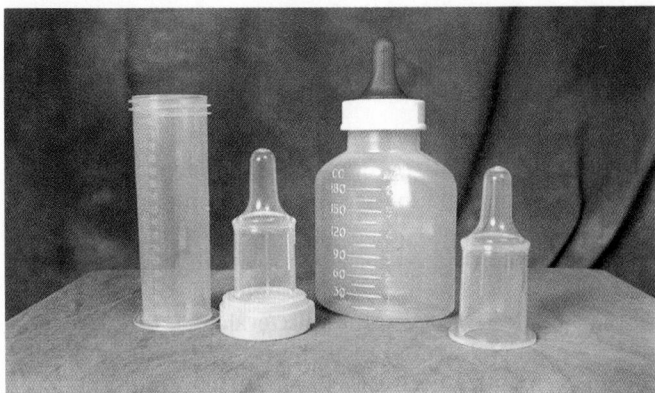

**Fig. 11-17**  Some devices used to feed an infant with a cleft lip and palate. (Courtesy Paul Vincent Kuntz, Texas Children's Hospital.)

hand or cradled in the arm. Standard bottle nipples may be unsuitable for these infants, who are unable to generate the suction required; therefore special nipples or other feeding devices are needed. A number of special feeding devices are available for feeding the infant with CL/CP, and some are more successful than others, depending on a number of factors (Fig. 11-17). One device is the Cleft Lip/Cleft Palate Nurser* which consists of a squeezable plastic bottle and a cross-cut nipple. The Haberman Feeder† may also be used successfully in infants with a poor or disorganized suck. The Haberman Feeder has a specially designed valve and nipple to adjust the flow of milk to the infant and avoid choking or gagging. A gravity flow nipple‡ attached to a squeezable plastic bottle allows formula to be deposited into the mouth of the infant with CL/CP.

Using these various types of nipples for feeding also has the advantage of helping to meet the infant's sucking needs. Muscle development is especially important for later development of speech. The nipple is positioned in such a way that it is compressed by the infant's tongue and existing palate. If a single-slit nipple is used, the slit is placed vertically so that the infant will be able to produce and stop the flow of milk by alternately opening and closing the opening. No matter which type of nipple is used, gentle, steady pressure on the base of the bottle reduces the chance of choking or coughing, and the person doing the feeding should resist the temptation to remove the nipple because of the noise the infant makes or for fear that the infant will choke. An indication that the infant needs to stop feeding momentarily is the *facial signal,* which involves elevated eyebrows and a wrinkled forehead; the nipple may be gently removed to allow swallowing of formula in the mouth without upsetting the infant (Richard, 1991). These infants need frequent burping because they have a tendency to swallow excessive amounts of air.

When the infant has trouble with nipple feeding, a rubber-tipped medicine dropper, Asepto syringe, or Breck feeder (a

---

*Mead Johnson & Company, Evansville, IN.
†Medela Inc, McHenry, IL 60051.
‡Ross Laboratories, Columbus, OH.

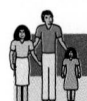

## FAMILY FOCUS
*Breast-Feeding the Infant with Cleft Lip and/or Cleft Palate*

Many health professionals and parents assume that successful breast-feeding is impossible because of the CL/CP. On the contrary, breast-feeding is not only possible, it has several benefits, including the normal integration of the infant into the family, fewer problems with otitis media, and passive immunity to upper respiratory tract infections. In addition, breast-feeding enhances normal muscular movements of the mouth and face, and benefits normal speech development. Breast-fed infants are also better able to regulate the flow of milk into the oral cavity during sucking, thus decreasing the chance of choking and/or aspirating. In several studies infants with CL/CP were breast-fed shortly after surgical repair; there were no complications observed in this group, and they gained weight more quickly and were discharged sooner than infants with CL/CP repair who were fed by cup (Jackson and Beal, 1997; Darzi, Chowdri, and Bhat, 1996; Cohen, 1997). A modified Hotz-type plate may be used to help infants with CL/CP breast-feed successfully (Kogo and others, 1997). There are varied results in anecdotal reports of breast-feeding the infant with CL/CP (Conversations, 1997; Beckler, 1997).

If the mother intended to breast-feed before delivery, she is encouraged and helped to do so as soon as possible after birth. If available, the services of a lactation expert or of a local La Leche League leader (Chapters 8 and 9) should be used. Breast-feeding the infant with CL/CP requires a team approach. Because CL/CP presents a variety of different physiologic differences, one particular position for feeding may be more successful than another (Lawrence and Lawrence, 1999). Breastfeeding the infant with CL/CP requires time and patience on part of the mother, infant, and nurse; the nurse should encourage the mother in this endeavor yet recognize that some infants may not be able to entirely breast-feed. In such cases the infant may be fed expressed breast milk, which has many benefits and the mother is encouraged to use kangaroo care (skin-to-skin contact) and nonnutritive suckling at the breast. (See Chapter 10.)

---

large syringe with soft rubber tubing) may provide an efficient, safe feeding device. The rubber extension should be sufficiently long to extend well back into the mouth to reduce the likelihood of regurgitation through the nose. The formula is deposited on the back of the tongue, and the flow is controlled by bulb or syringe compression that is adjusted to the infant's needs. With some infants, spoon feeding works best, especially if the formula is slightly thickened with cereal.

Breast-feeding is also an option. The nipple is positioned and stabilized well back in the oral cavity so that tongue action facilitates milk expression. However, the suction required to stimulate milk may be absent initially; therefore a breast pump may be useful before nursing to stimulate the let-down reflex. (See Family Focus box.)

Regardless of the feeding method used, the mother should begin to feed the infant as soon as possible. In this way she is able to help determine the method best suited to her and the infant and to become adept in the technique before discharge.

**Preoperative Care.**  In preparation for the surgical repair, the parents are frequently instructed to accustom the infant to some of the needs of the early postoperative period. In some cases it is important for the infant who has a

CL repair to avoid the prone position postoperatively, even when awake; therefore, it is helpful to accustom the infant to lying on the back or side to reduce the irritability and resistance associated with any change in routine. If elbow restraints are to be used, it may be helpful to place the infant in restraints periodically before admission and to feed the infant in the manner to be used postoperatively. Some craniofacial surgery teams encourage the transition to cup-feeding before CP surgery, and this feeding method is used postoperatively as well. Preoperative preparation, including medication, is determined by the surgeon and anesthesiologist.

**Postoperative Care: CL.** The major efforts in the postoperative period are directed toward protecting the operative site. Following CL repair *(cheiloplasty)*, a lip protective device may be used to prevent trauma to the suture line. Elbow restraints may be applied immediately following surgery to prevent the infant from rubbing the suture line, although this practice has been abandoned by many surgeons (Sandberg, Denk, and Magee, 2002; Woods and Jurkiewicz, 1999). It is advisable to pin the cuffs of the restraints to the infant's clothing to keep the restraints in place.

An older infant who is able to roll over may require a jacket restraint in addition to arm restraints, to prevent rolling onto the abdomen and rubbing the face on the bed. It is important to remove the restraints at regular intervals, such as every 2 hours, to allow for exercising the arms, to provide relief from restrictions, and to observe the skin for signs of irritation. Removing restraints also offers an opportunity for cuddling and body contact. Adequate analgesia is recommended to relieve postoperative pain; sedation is sometimes needed for a very restless, anxious infant.

Clear liquids are offered when the infant has fully recovered from the anesthesia, and breast or bottle feeding is usually resumed as tolerated. The suture line is carefully cleansed of formula or serosanguineous drainage as needed. A thin layer of antibiotic ointment may be prescribed for application to the suture line after cleansing. Meticulous care of the suture line is a nursing responsibility because inflammation or infection will interfere with optimum healing and the ultimate cosmetic effect of the surgical repair.

The infant should be positioned to prevent airway obstruction by secretions, blood, or the tongue. Gentle aspiration of mouth and nasopharyngeal secretions may be necessary to prevent aspiration and respiratory complications. Because of vascularity of the lip and palate, postoperative care involves monitoring operative sites for bleeding; excessive swallowing may be a sign of bleeding and swallowing blood (Sandberg, Magee, and Denk, 2002).

**Postoperative Care: CP.** The child with a CP repair *(palatoplasty)* is allowed to lie on the abdomen, especially immediately postoperatively. The child may resume feedings by bottle, breast, or cup shortly after surgery. Many plastic surgeons will not permit a small spoon to be used, although a wide spoon may be acceptable if the caregiver does not insert the spoon into the mouth, where it might damage the suture line.

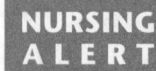 **NURSING ALERT** Avoid the use of suction or objects in the mouth such as tongue depressors, thermometers, spoons, or straws.

Following surgery, parents can assist palatal function by stimulating the child to use simple words that require coordination of the speech apparatus, encouraging chewing and frequent swallowing to exercise throat and palatine muscles, and engaging in blowing games to help close off the posterior palate. The speech therapist evaluates the individual needs of the child and directs the parents in specific activities to facilitate speech development. The more children are encouraged to use speech, the sooner they will gain self-confidence and assurance in social situations.

Throughout the child's therapy, the ultimate goal should be the development of a healthy personality and self-esteem. Several agencies provide services and information for children with CL/CP and their families. These include the **American Cleft Palate Craniofacial Association,** the **Cleft Palate Foundation,*** the **Birth Defect Research for Children (BDRC),†** the **March of Dimes-Birth Defects Foundation,‡** and **International Institute for Birth Defects.§**

## ■ Evaluation

The effectiveness of nursing interventions is determined by continual reassessment and evaluation of care based on the following guidelines:

**Preoperative care:**
1. Discuss infant's condition with parents relative to their understanding, feelings, and concerns regarding the defect.
2. Observe parental interactions with infant and encourage active involvement in infant's care.
3. Assist parents (primary caretakers) with feedings and maintain clear airway.
4. Discuss anticipated surgical plans with parents relative to realistic expectations of surgical results and infant's appearance and extent of parental involvement in postoperative care.

**Postoperative care:**
1. Inspect operative site and keep clean.
2. Prevent damage to operative site by restraining infant (elbow restraints) as necessary, and position infant for optimal comfort and clear airway.
3. Observe infant for pain cues and administer analgesics as needed.
4. Assist parents with feedings and encourage involvement in infant's care.
5. Observe operative site for signs of infection or tissue compromise.
6. Assist parents and family with plans for home discharge, anticipated follow up, and long-term care needs.

The *expected outcomes* are described in the Nursing Care Plan on pp. 461-462.

---

*1218 Grandview Ave, Pittsburgh, PA 15211-1239 (800) 242-5338; www.cleft.com
†930 Woodcock Rd, St 225, Orlando, FL 32803, (407) 895-0802 or (800) 313-2232; www.birthdefects.org
‡1275 Mamaroneck Ave, White Plains, NY 10605, (914) 428-7100; www.modimes.org In Canada: Aboutface, 99 Crowns Lane, 4th Floor, Toronto, Ontario, Canada M5R3P4, (416) 944-3223 or (800) 665-3223; www.interlog.com/~abtface
§PO Box 1304, West Babylon, NY 11704; www.cleft.net

# Nursing Care Plan
## The Child with Cleft Lip and/or Cleft Palate

### PREOPERATIVE CARE

**NURSING DIAGNOSIS:** Imbalanced nutrition: less than body requirements related to physical defect

**PATIENT GOAL 1:** Will consume adequate nourishment

- **NURSING INTERVENTIONS/**_RATIONALES_

Administer diet appropriate for age (specify)

Assist mother with breast-feeding if this is mother's preference, because the newborn with either defect can breast-feed

Position and stabilize nipple well back in oral cavity _so that tongue action facilitates milk expression_

Stimulate let-down reflex manually or with breast pump before nursing _because suction required to stimulate milk may be absent initially_

Modify feeding techniques to adjust to defect _because infant's ability to suck is reduced_

Hold child in upright (sitting) position _to minimize risk of aspiration_

Use special feeding appliances as needed _that compensate for infant's feeding difficulty_

Try to nipple-feed infant _to meet infant's need for sucking and to promote muscle development for speech_

Position nipple between infant's tongue and existing palate _to facilitate compression of nipple_

When using devices without nipples (e.g., Breck feeder, Asepto syringe), deposit formula on back of tongue _to facilitate swallowing_ and adjust flow according to infant's swallowing _to prevent aspiration_

Bubble (burp) frequently _because of tendency to swallow excessive amounts of air_

Encourage parents to begin feeding infant as soon as possible _so that they become adept in feeding technique before discharge_

Monitor weight _to assess adequacy of nutritional intake_

- **EXPECTED OUTCOMES**

Infant consumes an adequate amount of nutrients (specify amount)

Infant exhibits appropriate weight gain

**NURSING DIAGNOSIS:** Risk for impaired parenting related to infant with a highly visible physical defect

**PATIENT (FAMILY) GOAL 1:** Will demonstrate acceptance of infant

- **NURSING INTERVENTIONS/**_RATIONALES_

Allow expression of feelings _to encourage family's coping_

Convey attitude of acceptance of infant and family _because parents are sensitive to affective attitudes of others_

Indicate by behavior that child is a valuable human being _to encourage acceptance of infant_

Describe results of surgical correction of defect

Use photographs of satisfactory results _to encourage feeling of hope_

Arrange meeting with other parents who have experienced a similar situation and coped successfully

- **EXPECTED OUTCOMES**

Family discusses feelings and concerns regarding child's defect, its repair, and future prospects

Family exhibits an attitude of acceptance of infant

See also Nursing Care Plan: The Child Undergoing Surgery, Preoperative Care, Chapter 27

### POSTOPERATIVE CARE

**NURSING DIAGNOSIS:** Risk for trauma of the surgical site related to surgical procedure, dysfunctional swallowing

**PATIENT GOAL 1:** Will experience no trauma to operative site

- **NURSING INTERVENTIONS/**_RATIONALES_

Position on back or side or in infant seat (CL) _to prevent trauma to operative site and to maintain open airway_

Use nontraumatic feeding techniques _to minimize risk of trauma_

Restrain elbows only as necessary _to prevent access to operative site_

Avoid placing objects in the mouth following CP repair (suction catheter, tongue depressor, straw, pacifier, small spoon) _to prevent trauma to operative site_

Prevent vigorous and sustained crying _that can cause tension on sutures_

Cleanse suture line gently after feeding and as necessary in manner ordered by surgeon (CL) _because inflammation or infection will interfere with healing and the cosmetic effect of surgical repair_

Teach cleansing and restraining procedures, especially when infant will be discharged before suture removal _to minimize complications after discharge_

Observe for bleeding at operative site and excessive swallowing _to promote healing and prevent potential aspiration_

- **EXPECTED OUTCOME**

Operative site remains undamaged

**PATIENT GOAL 2:** Will exhibit no evidence of aspiration

- **NURSING INTERVENTIONS/**_RATIONALES_

Position _to allow for drainage of mucus_ (partial side-lying position, semi-Fowler position) and _to prevent aspiration of formula_

- **EXPECTED OUTCOME**

Child manages secretions and formula without aspiration

_Continued_

## Nursing Care Plan
### The Child with Cleft Lip and/or Cleft Palate—cont'd

---

**NURSING DIAGNOSIS:** Imbalanced nutrition: less than body requirements related to difficulty eating following surgical procedure

---

**PATIENT GOAL 1:** Will consume adequate nourishment

• **NURSING INTERVENTIONS/*RATIONALES***

Monitor IV fluids (if prescribed)

Administer diet appropriate for age and as prescribed for postoperative period (specify)

Involve family in determining best feeding methods *because family assumes feeding responsibility at home*

Modify feeding technique *to adjust to defect and surgical repair*

Feed in sitting position *to minimize risk of aspiration*

Use special appliances *that compensate for feeding difficulties without causing trauma to operative site*

Bubble frequently *because of tendency to swallow large amounts of air*

Assist with breast-feeding if method of choice

Teach feeding and suctioning techniques to family *to ensure optimum home care*

• **EXPECTED OUTCOMES**

Infant consumes an adequate amount of nutrients (specify amounts)

Family demonstrates ability to carry out postoperative care

Infant exhibits appropriate weight gain

---

*Dependent nursing action.

---

**NURSING DIAGNOSIS:** Acute pain related to surgical procedure

---

**PATIENT GOAL 1:** Will experience optimum comfort level

• **NURSING INTERVENTIONS/*RATIONALES***

Assess behavior and vital signs for evidence of pain

*Administer analgesics and/or sedatives as ordered

Remove restraints periodically while supervised *to exercise arms, provide relief from restrictions, and observe skin for signs of irritation*

Provide cuddling and tactile stimulation and other nonpharmacologic interventions *as needed for optimum comfort*

Involve parents in infant's care *to provide comfort and sense of security*

• **EXPECTED OUTCOME**

Infant appears comfortable and rests quietly

---

**NURSING DIAGNOSIS:** Interrupted family processes related to child with a physical defect, hospitalization

---

**PATIENT (FAMILY) GOAL 1:** Will receive adequate support

• **INTERVENTIONS AND EXPECTED OUTCOMES**

Refer family to appropriate agencies and support groups

See also:

Nursing Care Plan: The Family of the Child Who Is Ill or Hospitalized, Chapter 26

Nursing Care Plan: The Child with Chronic Illness or Disability, Chapter 22

---

Sometimes the infant will have difficulty breathing following surgery because it is often necessary to alter an established pattern of breathing and adjust to breathing through the nose. This is frustrating but seldom requires more than positioning and support.

The elbows may be restrained to keep the hands away from the mouth, and the parents are instructed to maintain this precaution at home until the palate is healed. They should be instructed to remove the restraints at frequent intervals to allow the child to exercise the arms. The infant should be assessed for pain postoperatively. Opiates may be prescribed for the first 24 to 48 hours postoperatively, or longer if needed, and acetaminophen may be given thereafter.

The older infant is usually discharged on a blenderized or soft diet, which parents are instructed to continue until the surgeon directs them to do otherwise. They should be cautioned against allowing the child to eat hard items such as toast, hard cookies, or potato chips, which could damage the newly repaired palate.

**Preparation for Discharge and Home Care.** Parents are encouraged to participate in the care of the infant as soon as possible following surgery. They should be taught the proper feeding method. Parents should also be taught

to cleanse the suture line to free any crust that might form and to replace elbow restraints (if used). Car seat restraint appropriate to the infant's condition should be carefully evaluated and discussed with the parents before discharge. Infant sleep position should also be discussed based on the infant's condition and the AAP recommendation for supine sleeping in infants. (See Chapter 12.)

**Long-Term Family Guidance.** The problems of parents in the care of an infant with CP may extend well beyond the initial acceptance and adjustment to the defect and surgical correction. These families need support and encouragement by health care professionals and guidance in activities that facilitate the most normal life for the child. Financial stressors are often cited by parents as being the most difficult issue to deal with when the child has a craniofacial anomaly. However, with the combined efforts of the family and the health care team, the majority of these infants achieve a satisfactory long-term outcome. Parents need to understand the therapy and the purpose of any appliance. They should be taught proper care and placement of the device and that establishing good mouth care and proper brushing habits is especially important for these children.

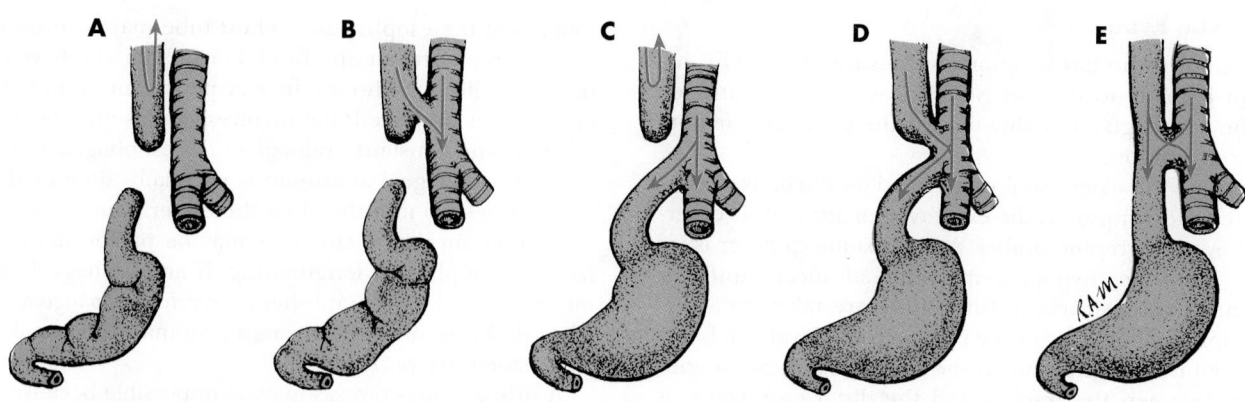

**Fig. 11-18**   Five most common types of esophageal atresia (EA) and tracheoesophageal fistula (TEF). (See text for discussion.)

Because of the increased risk of middle ear infection, the ears are examined regularly, and hearing tests are scheduled early and repeated periodically throughout childhood. It is particularly important to emphasize the need for an ear examination when the child has symptoms of an upper respiratory tract infection. When treatment can be implemented early, the chances are greater that permanent damage to the ear can be avoided. Parents should be alerted to signs of any hearing impairment in the child in order to obtain needed help and prevent progression of any deficit. (See Chapter 24.)

The parents are also provided with guidance in helping the child to develop normal speech. They should encourage the child's early attempts to make sounds. Some parents erroneously believe that the child may form poor speech habits if he or she tries to speak before the palate is repaired. However, attempting to delay speech further hampers this development.

## Esophageal Atresia (EA) and Tracheoesophageal Fistula (TEF)

Congenital EA and TEF are rare malformations that represent a failure of the esophagus to develop as a continuous passage and a failure of the trachea and esophagus to separate into distinct structures. These defects may occur as separate entities or in combination, and without early diagnosis and treatment they pose a serious threat to the infant's well-being.

The incidence is estimated to be from 1 in 3000 to 4500 live births. There appears to be an equal sex incidence, but the birth weight of most affected infants is significantly lower than average, and there is an unusually high incidence of prematurity in infants with EA. A history of maternal polyhydramnios is common.

Associated anomalies include cardiovascular, vertebral, renal, anorectal, limb, and radius deformities. EA/TEF is a component of **VATER** or **VACTERL association,** an acronym describing associated anomalies. Cardiac anomalies occur most frequently in EA/TEF; therefore, all patients should undergo a workup for associated anomalies.

### Pathophysiology

The esophagus develops from the first segment of the embryonic gut. During the fourth and fifth weeks of gestation, the foregut normally lengthens and separates longitudinally; each longitudinal portion fuses to form two parallel channels (the esophagus and the trachea) that are joined only at the larynx. Anomalies involving the trachea and esophagus are caused by defective separation, incomplete fusion of the tracheal folds following this separation, or altered cellular growth during embryonic development.

The most commonly encountered form of EA and TEF (80% to 95% of cases) is one in which the proximal esophageal segment terminates in a blind pouch and the distal segment is connected to the trachea or primary bronchus by a short fistula at or near the tracheal bifurcation (Fig. 11-18, *C*). The second most common type, (5% to 8%), consists of a blind pouch at each end, widely separated and with no communication to the trachea; this is known as "pure EA" (Fig. 11-18, *A*). Less frequently, an otherwise normal trachea and esophagus are connected by a fistula; this is commonly referred to as "H type" (Fig. 11-18, *E*). Extremely rare anomalies involve a fistula from the trachea to the upper esophageal segment (Fig. 11-18, *B*) or to both the upper and lower segments (Fig. 11-18, *D*).

### Clinical Manifestations

The presence of EA is suspected in a newborn with frothy saliva in the mouth and nose, drooling, choking, and coughing. If fed, the infant may swallow normally but suddenly cough and gag, with return of fluid through the nose and mouth. The infant may become cyanotic and apneic because of aspiration of formula or saliva.

In the infant who has EA with a distal TEF (type C), the stomach becomes distended with air, and thoracic and abdominal compression (especially during crying) cause the gastric contents to be regurgitated through the fistula and into the trachea, producing a chemical pneumonitis. When the upper segment of the esophagus opens directly into the trachea (types B and D), the infant is in danger of aspirating any swallowed material. Cyanosis or choking during feeding may be the only symptom of type E fistula.

## Diagnostic Evaluation

In a newborn who has symptoms suggestive of EA/TEF, an attempt is made to pass an NG/orogastric (OG) catheter into the esophagus. Inability to pass the catheter warrants further evaluation.

Although the diagnosis is established on the basis of clinical signs and symptoms, the exact type of anomaly is determined by radiographic studies. A radiopaque catheter is inserted into the hypopharynx and advanced until it encounters an obstruction. Chest films are taken to ascertain esophageal patency or the presence and level of a blind pouch. Films that show air in the stomach indicate a connection between the trachea and the distal esophagus in types C, D, and E. Complete absence of air in the stomach is seen in both types A and B. Occasionally, fistulas are not patent, which makes their presence more difficult to diagnose. A careful bronchoscopic examination may be performed to visualize the fistula.

The presence of *polyhydramnios* (accumulation of more than 2000 ml of amniotic fluid) prenatally is a clue to the possibility of EA in the unborn infant, especially if the defect is type A, B, or C. With these types of EA/TEF, amniotic fluid normally swallowed by the fetus is unable to reach the GI tract to be absorbed and excreted by the kidneys. The result is an abnormal accumulation of amniotic fluid or polyhydramnios.

## Therapeutic Management

The treatment of EA and TEF includes maintenance of a patent airway, prevention of pneumonia, gastric or blind pouch decompression, supportive therapy, and surgical repair of the anomaly. Since type C is the most common, the discussion is directed primarily toward that defect.

When EA with a TEF is suspected, the infant is immediately deprived of oral intake, IV fluids are initiated, and the infant is positioned to facilitate drainage of secretions and decrease the likelihood of aspiration. Accumulated secretions are suctioned frequently from the mouth and pharynx. A double-lumen catheter should be placed into the upper esophageal pouch and attached to intermittent or continuous low suction. The infant's head is kept in an upright position so that fluid collected in the pouch is easily removed and to prevent aspiration of gastric contents. Since aspiration pneumonia is almost inevitable and appears early, broad-spectrum antibiotic therapy is often instituted.

**Surgical Correction.** Most malformations can be corrected surgically in one operation or staged with two or more procedures. The success depends on early diagnosis before complications occur and on the presence and severity of other associated anomalies and illness factors, including prematurity. With measures instituted to prevent aspiration pneumonia and to ensure adequate hydration and nutrition, surgery may be postponed to allow for more effective treatment of pneumonia and physiologic stabilization so that the infant can better withstand the complex surgery. The delay also offers an opportunity for further evaluation and assessment to rule out any associated anomalies and to optimize respiratory support.

The surgery consists of a thoracotomy with division and ligation of the TEF and an end-to-end or end-to-side anastomosis of the esophagus. A chest tube may be inserted to drain intrapleural air and fluid. For infants who have multiple anomalies, or who are in very poor condition, a staged operation is preferred that involves gastrostomy, ligation of the TEF, and constant drainage of the esophageal pouch. A delayed esophageal anastomosis is usually attempted after several weeks to months when the upper pouch elongates.

Further surgical techniques may be performed later to facilitate esophageal lengthening. If an esophageal anastomosis cannot be accomplished, a *cervical esophagostomy* (to allow drainage of saliva through a stoma in the neck) and gastrostomy are performed.

A primary anastomosis may be impossible because of insufficient length of the two segments of esophagus. In these cases an esophageal replacement procedure using a part of the colon or gastric tube interposition may be necessary to bridge the missing esophageal segment.

Endotracheal intubation may be required because many of these infants have *tracheomalacia.* Tracheomalacia may occur as a result of weakness in the tracheal wall that exists when a dilated proximal pouch compresses the trachea early in fetal life.

This condition may also occur as a result of inadequate intratracheal pressure causing abnormal tracheal development. Tracheomalacia occurs in 10% to 20% of infants with EA/TEF, in varying degrees and may require surgical intervention in severe cases.

**Prognosis.** The survival rate is nearly 100% in otherwise healthy children. Most deaths are the result of extreme prematurity or other lethal associated anomalies.

Potential complications following the surgical repair of EA and TEF depend on the type of defect and surgical correction. Complications of an EA and TEF repair include an anastomotic leak, strictures due to tension or ischemia, esophageal motility disorders causing dysphagia, respiratory compromise, and gastroesophageal reflux. Anastomotic esophageal strictures may cause dysphagia, choking, and respiratory distress. The strictures are often treated with routine esophageal dilation. Feeding difficulties are often present for months or years postoperatively, and the infant must be followed closely to ensure adequate weight gain, growth, and development. At times the infant must be fed via gastrostomy or jejunostomy in order to receive adequate caloric intake.

## Nursing Considerations

### ■■ Assessment

Nursing responsibility for detection of this serious malformation begins immediately after birth. The defect is suspected in any infant who has an excessive amount of frothy saliva in the mouth and unexplained episodes of cyanosis. Cyanosis is usually a result of laryngeal spasm caused by overflow of saliva into the larynx from the proximal esophageal pouch or aspiration, and normally resolves after removal of the secretions from the oral pharynx by suctioning. In addition, a history of maternal polyhydramnios and a small-for-gestational-age infant should alert the nurse to investigate further. The passage of a small-gauge orogastric feeding tube via the mouth into the stomach during the initial nursing physical assessment is helpful to rule out a TEF or other obstructive defects.

Ideally, the condition is diagnosed before the initial feeding. As mentioned previously, if fed, the infant may swallow normally but suddenly coughs and gags, and the fluid is aspirated or returns through the nose and mouth. For this reason, it has been customary for the nurse to give the infant plain water for the first feeding or to be present when a parent feeds the child in order to observe the infant's response. This practice, however, should not preclude the infant from early breast-feeding unless there is a strong suspicion of EA.

> **NURSING ALERT**   Any infant who has an excessive amount of frothy saliva in the mouth or difficulty with secretions and unexplained episodes of cyanosis should be suspected of having an EA/TEF and referred immediately for medical evaluation.

## Nursing Diagnoses

Following the initial assessment, a number of nursing diagnoses become evident. The most likely diagnoses are outlined and discussed in the Nursing Care Plan on pp. 467-468. Others may be apparent in individual cases.

## Planning

The broad goals for an infant with EA and a TEF and the family are as follows:

1. Infant will experience no respiratory distress.
2. Infant will receive adequate nutrition.
3. Infant will experience no complications related to airway management.
4. Infant and family will receive adequate support.

## Implementation

The infant is placed in an incubator or a radiant warmer, and humidified oxygen is administered in the event of respiratory distress. Intubation and assisted mechanical ventilation may be necessary if the infant is in respiratory distress.

**Preoperative Care.**  The mouth and nasopharynx are carefully suctioned, and the infant is placed in an optimum position to facilitate drainage and avoid aspiration. The most desirable position for a newborn who is suspected of having the typical EA with a TEF (e.g., type C) is supine (or sometimes prone) with the head elevated on an inclined plane of at least 30 degrees. This positioning serves to minimize the reflux of gastric secretions at the distal esophagus into the trachea and bronchi, especially when intraabdominal pressure is elevated.

It is imperative that any secretions that can be a source of aspiration be removed at once. Until surgery the blind pouch is kept empty by intermittent or continuous suction through an indwelling double-lumen or Replogle catheter passed orally or nasally to the end of the pouch. Because the catheter has a tendency to become clogged with secretions, it is irrigated frequently with normal saline and replaced as needed. Sometimes a gastrostomy tube is inserted and left

open so that any air entering the stomach through the fistula can escape, thus minimizing the danger of gastric contents being regurgitated into the trachea. The gastrostomy tube is emptied by gravity drainage.

Feedings through the gastrostomy tube and irrigations with fluid are contraindicated before surgery in the infant with a distal TEF. Nursing interventions include respiratory assessment, airway management, thermoregulation, fluid and electrolyte management, and parenteral nutritional support.

Often the infant must be transferred to a hospital with specialized care units. Care is exercised to maintain the desired position and continue suctioning during transport. Parents are advised of the infant's condition and provided with necessary support and information.

**Postoperative Care.**  Postoperative care for these infants is the same as for any high-risk newborn. The infant is returned to a radiant warmer, the double-lumen NG/OG catheter is attached to low suction or gravity drainage, parenteral nutrition is provided, and the gastrostomy tube (if a gastrostomy is performed) is returned to gravity drainage until the infant can tolerate feedings. Tracheal suction should only be done using a premeasured catheter and with extreme caution to avoid injury to the suture line.

If tolerated, gastrostomy feedings may be initiated and continued until the esophageal anastomosis is healed. Before oral feedings are initiated and the chest tube is removed a contrast study or esophogram is performed to verify the integrity of the esophageal anastomosis.

The initial attempt at oral feeding must be carefully observed to make certain that the infant is able to swallow without choking. Oral feedings are begun with sterile water, followed by frequent small feedings of breast milk or formula. Until the infant is able to take a sufficient amount by mouth, oral intake may need to be supplemented by bolus or continuous gastrostomy feedings. Ordinarily the infant is not discharged until oral fluids are taken well. The gastrostomy tube may be removed before discharge or maintained for supplemental feedings at home.

**Special Problems.**  Upper respiratory tract complications are a threat to life in both the preoperative and postoperative periods. In addition to pneumonia, there is a constant danger of respiratory distress resulting from atelectasis, pneumothorax, and laryngeal edema. Any persistent respiratory difficulty after removal of secretions is reported to the surgeon immediately. The infant is monitored for anastomotic leaks and signs of infection such as purulent chest tube drainage, an increased white blood cell count, and temperature instability.

In the infant awaiting esophageal replacement surgery, the upper esophageal segment may be drained by means of a cervical esophagostomy. An esophagostomy is difficult to care for because the skin may become irritated by moisture from the continued discharge of saliva. Frequent removal of drainage followed by application of a layer of protective ointment, barrier dressing, and/or a collection device is usually sufficient treatment. An enterostomal nurse may provide helpful guidance in the prevention and treatment of skin breakdown.

For the infant who requires esophageal replacement, nonnutritive sucking is provided by a pacifier. Sometimes small amounts of water or formula are given orally; the liquid drains from the esophagostomy but allows the infant to develop mature sucking patterns and with other appropriate oral stimulation can prevent feeding resistance. (See Chapter 10.) Infants who remain NPO for an extended period and have not received oral stimulation frequently have difficulty eating by mouth after corrective surgery and may develop oral hypersensitivity and food aversion. They require patient, firm guidance in learning the techniques of taking food into the mouth and swallowing after repair. A referral to a multidisciplinary feeding behavior program may be necessary.

**Family Support, Discharge Planning, and Home Care.** One of the difficulties in TEF is the immediate transfer of the sick infant to the intensive care unit and sometimes lengthy hospitalization. The attachment process is facilitated by encouraging parents to visit the infant, participate in his or her care where appropriate, and express their feelings regarding the infant's condition. The nurse in the intensive care unit should assume responsibility for ensuring that the parents are kept fully informed of the infant's progress.

Preparing parents for discharge of their infant involves teaching the techniques that will be continued at home, such as careful suctioning, oral or gastrostomy feeding, and skin care. The parents are taught child or infant behaviors that might be expected after corrective surgery, such as those that indicate that the infant needs to be suctioned, signs of respiratory difficulty, and signs that indicate constriction of the esophagus (poor feeding, dysphagia, drooling, or regurgitating undigested food).

Parents are reminded that it is particularly important to guard against the infant swallowing foreign objects. They are instructed to cut solid food into small pieces, teach the child to chew thoroughly, give frequent sips of liquid to help swallow food, and avoid foods such as whole hot dogs or large pieces of meat that may become lodged in the esophagus.

Many infants will have some degree of tracheomalacia; therefore parents should be educated regarding the signs and symptoms. Parents are instructed to be alert for signs of respiratory distress, and discharge planning should include teaching parents and other caretakers infant cardiopulmonary resuscitaction (CPR). Because many infants with EA and a TEF will develop gastroesophageal reflux, precautions should be initiated. (See Gastroesophageal Reflux, Chapter 33.)

Discharge planning should include attainment of needed equipment and home nursing services to assist with ongoing assessment of the child and continuity of care. (See Home Care, Chapter 25.)

### ■ Evaluation

The effectiveness of nursing interventions is determined by continual reassessment and evaluation of care based on the following observational guidelines:

1. Monitor infant's respiratory status.
2. Monitor weight daily; observe infant's eating behavior.
3. Inspect surgical site; observe infant's behavior; monitor vital signs.
4. Observe and interview family members regarding their understanding, feelings, and concerns regarding infant's condition or treatment.

The *expected outcomes* are described in the Nursing Care Plan on pp. 467-468.

## Anorectal Malformations

Anorectal malformations are among the more common congenital malformations caused by abnormal development with an incidence of approximately 1 in 4000 to 5000 births. These malformations may range from simple imperforate anus to include other associated complex anomalies of genitourinary and pelvic organs, which may require extensive treatment for fecal, urinary, and sexual function. Anorectal malformations may occur in isolation or as a part of VACTERL association (see p. 463). These anomalies are classified according to the newborn's gender and abnormal anatomic features, including genitourinary defects (Box 11-8). The classifications of high, intermediate, and low do not accurately describe the specific anomaly.

*Rectal atresia and stenosis* occurs when the anal opening appears normal and there is a midline intergluteal groove, but the infant experiences difficulty in passing meconium stool; there is usually no fistula between the rectum and urinary tract. This defect may not become apparent until later in infancy when the infant has a history of difficult stooling, abdominal distention, and ribbon-like stools.

A *persistent cloaca* is a complex anorectal malformation in which the rectum, vagina, and urethra drain into a common channel opening into the perineum. The single channel opens to the exterior via the urethral site (Fig. 11-19, *A*).

*Imperforate anus* includes several forms of malformation without an obvious opening (Fig. 11-20) and there is frequently a fistula from the distal rectum to the perineum or genitourinary system. A *fistula* is an abnormal communication between the rectum and genitourinary system or perineum (Fig. 11-19, *B* and *C*). The fistula may be evidenced when meconium is evacuated through the vaginal opening,

---

**Box 11-8** ■ ■ ■
**Classification of Anorectal Malformations**

**MALE DEFECTS**
Perineal fistula
Rectourethral bulbar fistula (Fig. 11-19, *C*)
Rectourethral prostatic fistula
Rectovesicular (bladder neck) fistula
Imperforate anus without fistula
Rectal atresia and stenosis

**FEMALE DEFECTS**
Perineal fistula
Vestibular fistula
Imperforate anus without fistula
Rectal atresia and stenosis
Cloaca (Fig. 11-19, *A*)

From Peña A, Hong A: Advances in the management of anorectal malformations, *Am J Surg* 180(5):370-376, 2000.

# Nursing Care Plan
## The Infant with Esophageal Atresia and Tracheoesophageal Fistula

**NURSING DIAGNOSIS:** Ineffective airway clearance related to abnormal opening between esophagus and trachea or obstruction to swallowing

**PATIENT GOAL 1:** Will maintain patent airway

- **NURSING INTERVENTIONS/*RATIONALES***

Suction as necessary *to remove accumulated secretions from oropharynx*

Position supine with head elevated on an inclined plane (at least 30 degrees) *to decrease pressure against thoracic cavity and to minimize reflux of gastric secretions up distal esophagus and into trachea and bronchi*

Administer oxygen per unit guidelines (pulse oximetry, blood gases) *to help relieve respiratory distress*

Avoid use of resuscitation bag/mask *because it may introduce air into stomach and intestines, creating additional pressure in the thoracic cavity*

Administer nothing by mouth *to prevent aspiration*

Maintain intermittent or continuous suction of esophageal segment, if ordered preoperatively, *to keep blind pouch empty of secretions*

Leave gastrostomy tube, if present, open to gravity drainage *so that air can escape, minimizing risk of regurgitation of gastric contents into trachea*

- **EXPECTED OUTCOMES**

Airway remains patent
Infant does not aspirate secretions
Respirations remain within normal limits

**NURSING DIAGNOSIS:** Impaired (difficulty) swallowing related to mechanical obstruction

**PATIENT GOAL 1:** Will receive adequate nourishment

- **NURSING INTERVENTIONS/*RATIONALES***

Administer gastrostomy feedings as prescribed *to provide nourishment until oral feedings are possible*

Progress to oral feedings as prescribed according to infant's condition and surgical correction

Observe closely *to make certain infant is able to swallow without choking*

Monitor intake, output, and weight *to assess adequacy of nutritional intake*

Give infant pacifier *to provide for nonnutritive sucking*

Teach family appropriate feeding techniques *to prepare for discharge*

- **EXPECTED OUTCOME**

Infant receives sufficient nourishment and exhibits a satisfactory weight gain

**PATIENT GOAL 2:** Patient will learn to take oral feedings (following complete repair)

- **NURSING INTERVENTIONS/*RATIONALES***

Introduce foods one at a time *to evaluate tolerance of food item*

Provide age-appropriate foods with various textures and flavors *to stimulate interest in eating*

Begin with pureed foods and progress to more solid food as child shows readiness

Cut food in small, noncylindrical pieces *to prevent choking*

Avoid foods such as whole hot dogs, raw vegetables, or large pieces of meat *to decrease risk of choking*

Teach child to chew foods well *to decrease risk of choking*

Refer to speech or occupational therapist, if appropriate, *to facilitate learning*

- **EXPECTED OUTCOME**

Child takes an adequate amount of nourishment and displays no evidence of feeding resistance, malnutrition, or dysphagia

**NURSING DIAGNOSIS:** Risk for injury related to surgical procedure

**PATIENT GOAL 1:** Will not experience trauma to surgical site

- **NURSING INTERVENTIONS/*RATIONALE***

Suction only with catheter premeasured to a distance that does not reach to surgical site *to prevent trauma to mucosa*

- **EXPECTED OUTCOME**

Child does not exhibit evidence of injury to surgical site

**NURSING DIAGNOSIS:** Anxiety related to difficulty swallowing, discomfort from surgery

**PATIENT GOAL 1:** Will experience a sense of security without discomfort

- **NURSING INTERVENTIONS/*RATIONALES***

Provide tactile stimulation (e.g., cuddling, rocking) *to facilitate optimum development and promote comfort*

Administer mouth care *to keep mouth clean and mucous membranes moist*

Offer pacifier frequently *to provide nonnutritive sucking*

*Administer analgesics as prescribed

Encourage parents to participate in child's care *to provide comfort and security*

- **EXPECTED OUTCOMES**

Infant rests calmly, is alert when awake, and engages in nonnutritive sucking
Mouth remains clean and moist
Child experiences no or minimal pain

---

*Dependent nursing action.

*Continued*

## Nursing Care Plan
### The Infant with Esophageal Atresia and Tracheoesophageal Fistula—cont'd

**NURSING DIAGNOSIS:** Interrupted family processes related to child with a physical defect

**PATIENT (FAMILY) GOAL 1:** Will be prepared for home care of child

- **NURSING INTERVENTIONS/*RATIONALES***

Teach family skills and observations needed for home care:
  Positioning *to prevent aspiration*
  Signs of respiratory distress *to prevent delay in treatment*
  Signs of complications—refusal to eat, dysphagia, increased coughing—*so practitioner can be notified*
  Acquiring needed equipment and services

Infant CPR
Care of gastrostomy and esophagostomy when infant has staged surgery, including techniques such as suctioning, feeding, care of operative site and/or ostomies, dressing changes, *to ensure appropriate care after discharge*

- **EXPECTED OUTCOME**

Family demonstrates ability to provide care to infant, an understanding of signs of complications, and appropriate actions
See also:
Nursing Care Plan: The Family of the Child Who Is Ill or Hospitalized, Chapter 26
Nursing Care Plan: The High-Risk Infant, Chapter 10

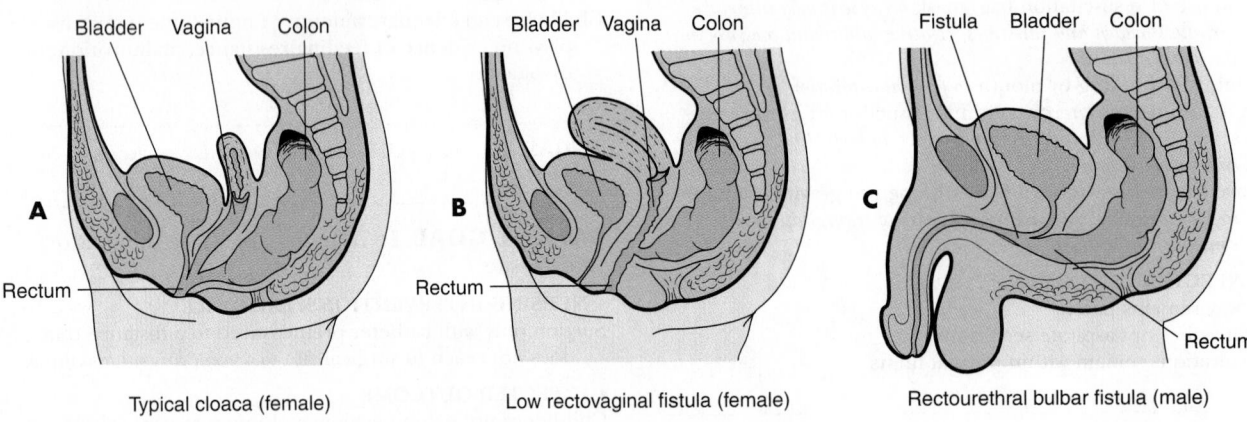

Typical cloaca (female)          Low rectovaginal fistula (female)          Rectourethral bulbar fistula (male)

**Fig. 11-19** Anorectal malformations. **A,** Typical cloaca (female). **B,** Low rectovaginal fistula (female). **C,** Rectourethral bulbar fistula (male).

the perineum below the vagina, the male urethra, or the perineum under the scrotum. The presence of meconium on the perineum does not indicate anal patency. A fistula may not be apparent at birth, but, as peristalsis increases, meconium is forced through the fistula into the urethra or onto the newborn's perineum.

### Pathophysiology

During embryonic development the *cloaca* becomes the common channel for the developing urinary, genital, and rectal systems. The cloaca is divided at the sixth week of gestation into an anterior urogenital sinus and a posterior intestinal channel by the urorectal septum. After the lateral folds join the urorectal septum, separation of the urinary and rectal segments takes place. Further differentiation results in the anterior genitourinary system and the posterior anorectal channel. An interruption of this development will lead to incomplete migration of the rectum to its normal perineal position.

### Diagnostic Evaluation

The diagnosis of an anorectal malformation is based on the physical finding of an absent anal opening. Other symptoms

may include abdominal distention, vomiting, absence of meconium, or presence of meconium in the urine. Additional physical findings with an anorectal malformation are a flat perineum and the absence of a midline intergluteal groove. The appearance of the perineum alone does not accurately predict the extent of the defect and associated anomalies; genitourinary and spinal/vertebral anomalies associated with anorectal malformations should be considered when an anomaly is noted. EA with or without TEF, cardiac defects, and spinal or vertebral anomalies may occur in association with anorectal malformations, and the infant should be carefully evaluated for the presence of these and other anomalies. A perineal fistula (see Box 11-8) may be diagnosed by clinical observation. The presence of a prominent anal dimple and a band of skin tissue commonly known as a *bucket handle* is indicative of a perineal fistula (Peña and Hong, 2000). Abdominal and pelvic ultrasonography is performed to further evaluate the infant's anatomic malformation. An IV pyelogram (IVP) and a voiding cystourethrogram are performed to evaluate associated anomalies involving the urinary tract. Other diagnostic examinations that may be performed include a pelvic MRI, radiography, and fluoroscopic examination of pelvic anatomic contents.

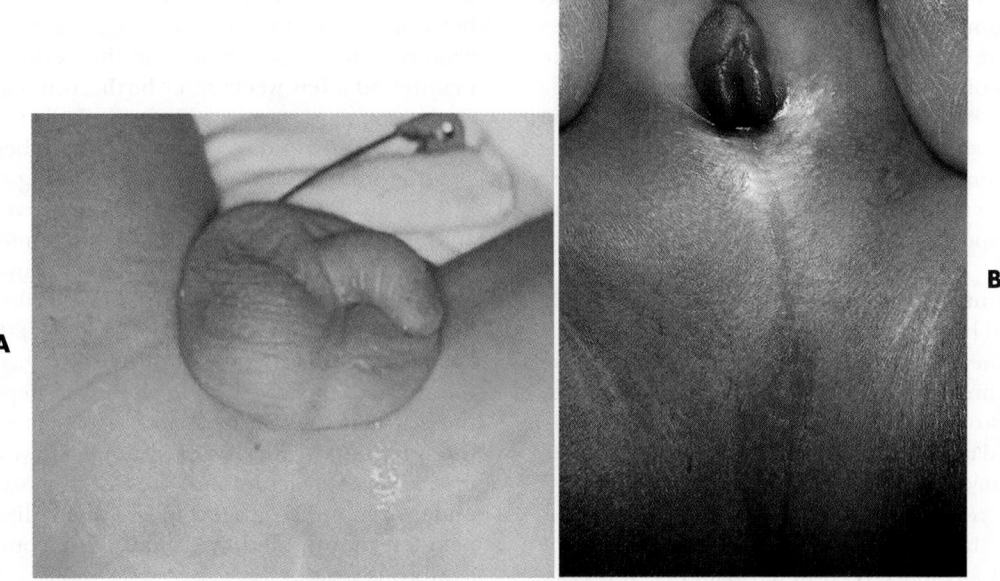

**Fig. 11-20   A,** No visible external opening is consistent with high imperforate anus defect; absence of intergluteal cleft is also common. **B,** Imperforate anus in the female, commonly associated with cloacal anomaly, which manifests as a single perineal opening on perineum. (From Zitelli BJ, Davis HW: *Atlas of pediatric physical diagnosis,* ed 3, St Louis, 1997, Mosby.)

## Therapeutic Management

The primary management of anorectal malformations is surgical. Once the defect is identified steps are taken to rule out associated life-threatening defects, which need immediate surgical intervention. Provided there are no immediate life-threatening problems, the newborn is stabilized and made NPO for further evaluation. IV fluids are provided to maintain glucose and fluid balance. Current recommendation is that surgery be delayed at least 24 hours to properly evaluate for the presence of a fistula and possibly other anomalies (Peña and Hong, 2000).

For the newborn with a perineal fistula an *anoplasty* is performed, which involves moving the fistula opening to the center of the sphincter and enlarging the rectal opening. A program of anal dilations is usually initiated when the child returns for the 2-week check-up (Guardino, 2000). Feedings are started soon after surgical repair and breastfeeding is encouraged because it causes less constipation (Guardino, 2000). In neonates with anomalies such as cloaca (female), rectourethral prostatic fistula (male), and vestibular fistula (female), a descending *colostomy* is performed to avoid fecal contamination of the distal imperforate section and subsequent urinary tract infection in infants with urorectal fistulas.

The *posterior sagittal anorectoplasty (PSRAP)* is a common surgical procedure for the repair of anorectal malformations in infants approximately 1 month after the initial colostomy. In this procedure the repair is made via a posterior midline sacral approach in order to dissect the different muscle groups involved without damaging strategic innervation of pelvic structures, so that optimal postoperative bowel continence is achieved (Peña, 1992). A laparotomy may be required if the rectum is unidentifiable by the posterior approach. Additional management following successful repair involves a program of anal dilations, colostomy closure, and a bowel management program.

**Prognosis.**   The long-term prognosis depends on such factors as the type of defect, anatomy of the sacrum and vertebra, quality of muscles, and the success of the surgery.

Parents are instructed in perineal and wound care or care of the colostomy as needed. Anal dilations may be necessary for some infants. Parents are advised to observe stooling patterns and to observe for signs of anal stricture or complications. Information on dietary modifications and administration of medications is included in counseling. Nurses have a vital role in assisting families of children with anorectal malformations to provide optimal care for the child so that bowel management is successful and quality of life enhanced for the child and family. (See Nursing Care Plan: The Infant with Anorectal Malformation.*)

The presence of a flat or "rocker" bottom and no midline groove will usually have a poor prognosis for bowel continence because of associated neurologic, muscular, and anatomic problems (Flake and Ryckman, 1997). When the internal anal sphincter is absent, incontinence is a common long-term problem. These children may achieve socially acceptable continence over time with the aid of a bowel management program. Other potential complications following surgical treatment of anorectal anomalies include strictures, recurrent rectourinary fistula, mucosal prolapse, and constipation.

## Nursing Considerations

The first nursing responsibility is assisting in identification of anorectal malformations. A newborn who does not pass

---

*In Wong DL, Hess CS: *Wong and Whaley's clinical manual of pediatric nursing,* ed 5, St Louis, 2000, Mosby.

stool within 24 hours following birth or has meconium that appears at a location other than the anal opening requires further assessment. Preoperative care includes diagnostic evaluation, GI decompression, and IV fluids.

Preoperative PSRAP care often involves irrigation of the distal stoma to prevent fecal contamination of the operative site. During this time parents must be given accurate yet simple information regarding the infant's appearance post-operatively and expectations as to their level of involvement in the child's care.

Postoperative nursing care following anoplasty is primarily directed toward healing of the surgical site without other complications. When a colostomy is needed, postoperative nursing care is directed toward maintaining appropriate skin care at the stoma site, management of postoperative pain, IV fluids, and administration of antibiotics. (See Chapter 27 for colostomy care.)

Parents need reassurance when a colostomy is performed regarding the child's appearance and their ability to care for the child at home. With much patience and reassurance, parents learn how to provide optimal care of the skin and the appliance, while maintaining an appropriate bond with the child. It is imperative that nursing care focus on empowering parents to love and care for the child and be sensitive to cues that there is a disruption in the parent's ability to care for the child. Postoperative NG decompression may be required with laparostomy, and nursing care should focus on maintenance of appropriate drainage.

**Family Support, Discharge Planning, and Home Care.** Long-term follow-up is essential for children with complex malformations. Following the definitive pull-through procedure, toilet training may be delayed. Complete continence is seldom achieved at the usual age of 2 to 3 years. Prevention of constipation is important; therefore breast-feeding is encouraged. If cow's milk–based formula is used, a mild laxative may be prescribed. Bowel habit training, diet modification, and administration of stool softeners or fiber help children slowly improve bowel management, but optimum results may not be achieved until later childhood or adolescence. Support and reassurance during the slow progression to normal function are essential.

## Biliary Atresia

Biliary atresia, or *extrahepatic biliary atresia (EHBA)*, is a progressive inflammatory process that causes both intrahepatic and extrahepatic bile duct fibrosis, resulting in eventual ductal obstruction. The incidence of biliary atresia is between 1 in 10,000 to 25,000 live births. There does not seem to be a racial or genetic predilection, although there is a female predominance of 1.4:1 (Whitington, 1996). Associated malformations include polysplenia, intestinal atresia, and malrotation of the intestine. Biliary atresia, if untreated, usually leads to cirrhosis, liver failure, and death in the first 2 years of life.

### Pathophysiology

The exact cause of biliary atresia is unknown, although immune mechanisms or viral injury may be responsible for the progressive process that results in complete obliteration of the bile ducts. Biliary atresia is not seen in the fetus or stillborn or newborn infant. This suggests that biliary atresia is acquired late in gestation or in the perinatal period and is manifested a few weeks after birth. Although congenital infections such as cytomegalovirus, rubella virus, Epstein-Barr virus, rotavirus, and reovirus type 3 have been implicated as a cause of hepatocellular damage leading to biliary atresia, no specific agent has been identified in every case (McEvoy and Suchy, 1996; Sokol, 2001). Immune-mediated bile duct injury from viral exposure and immaturity of the neonatal immune system may play a role in the destruction of bile ducts and development of EHBA (Sokol, 2001). Early in the course of the disease, the intrahepatic ducts are patent from the intralobular ductules to the porta hepatis. The size of these structures is variable and is correlated with the age of the infant and with bile excretion following surgical treatment. These structures are present in most affected infants under 2 months of age but gradually disappear over the next few months and by 4 months are completely replaced by fibrous tissue.

The degree of involvement of the extrahepatic biliary ducts is also variable. Most commonly the entire extrahepatic system is involved in the obliterative process, but some infants have a patent proximal portion of the extrahepatic duct or patency of the gallbladder, cystic duct, and common bile duct. Microscopic examination of the liver tissue reveals cholestasis with absent or diminished bile duct proliferation and fibrosis.

### Clinical Manifestations

Many infants with biliary atresia are full term and appear healthy at birth. If jaundice persists beyond 2 weeks of age, especially if the direct (conjugated) bilirubin is elevated, biliary atresia should be suspected. The urine may be dark, and the stools often become progressively more *acholic* or gray, indicating absence of bile pigment. Hepatomegaly is present early in the course of the disease, and the liver is firm on palpation. The serum aminotransferase, alkaline phosphatase, and gamma glutamyl transpeptidase (GGTP) levels are usually elevated.

*Orthotopic liver transplantation (OLT)* is now considered to be the definitive therapy for biliary atresia. The portoenterostomy offers increased survivability for children with EHBA up to as much as 5 years, but fibrosis and cirrhosis may occur despite adequate bile drainage as the child ages. Furthermore, portoenterostomy increases the chances of finding a suitable donor organ before the patient reaches end-stage liver disease. Complications following liver transplantation include obstruction and bile leaks at the biliary anastomosis, portal hypertension, hemorrhage, infection, and rejection. Immunosuppressive drugs are required following transplantation, including corticosteroids and cyclosporine. Immunosuppressive drugs FK-506 (Prograf) and OKT3 are currently being used following liver transplantation to enhance survival rates.

Medical management of biliary atresia is primarily supportive. It includes nutritional support with infant formulas that contain medium-chain triglycerides and essential fatty acids. Supplementation with fat-soluble vitamins (A, D, E, K), a multivitamin, and minerals, including iron, zinc, and selenium, is usually required. Aggressive nutritional support in the form of continuous tube feedings or total parenteral nutrition may be indicated for moderate to severe failure to thrive; the enteral solution should be low in sodium. Phenobarbital may be prescribed following hepatic portoenterostomy to stimulate bile flow, and ursodeoxycholic acid may be used to decrease cholestasis and the intense pruritus (itching) from jaundice. In cases of advanced liver dysfunction, management is the same as in infants with cirrhosis. (See Chapter 33.)

**Prognosis.** Untreated biliary atresia results in progressive cirrhosis and death in most children by 2 years of age. The Kasai portoenterostomy does improve the prognosis, but it is not a cure. Biliary drainage can often be achieved if the surgery is performed before the intrahepatic bile ducts are destroyed, usually by 8 weeks of age; otherwise the prognosis is poor. Long-term survival has been reported in children who underwent portoenterostomy (Carceller and others, 2000). However, even with successful bile drainage, many children ultimately develop liver failure and require liver transplantation.

The advances in surgical techniques for liver transplantation and the development of immunosuppressive and antifungal drugs have significantly improved the success of transplantation. Surgical techniques such as reduced-size and split-liver transplantation and retransplantation have contributed to a projected 10-year patient survival rate of more than 75% for children (Van der Werf and others, 1998). The major obstacle remains the shortage of suitable infant donors.

In infants with delayed diagnosis, or in children in whom surgery has failed to provide adequate bile drainage, there is progression of liver disease. Cirrhosis and splenomegaly occur with hypoalbuminemia, ascites, and coagulopathy. Fat malabsorption and malnutrition result in severe failure to thrive. Severe pruritus may also be present as the disease progresses. The severity of pruritis intensifies as the jaundice progresses as the result of disease advancement.

## Diagnostic Evaluation

Early diagnosis is key to the survival of the child with EHBA; the outcome in children surgically treated before 2 months of age is much better than in patients with delayed treatment. The diagnosis of biliary atresia is suspected on the basis of the history, physical findings, and laboratory studies. Laboratory tests include a complete blood count, serum bilirubin levels, and liver function studies. Additional laboratory analyses, including alpha$_1$-antitrypsin level, TORCH titers (see p. 326), hepatitis serology, alpha-fetoprotein, and urine cytomegalovirus, may be indicated to rule out other conditions that cause cholestasis and jaundice. An abdominal sonogram is usually performed to identify potential causes of extrahepatic obstruction, such as a choledochal cyst. The patency of the extrahepatic biliary system will be demonstrated by a nuclear scintiscan using technetium 99m iminodiacetic acid ($^{99m}$Tc-IDA) (**HIDA**). If there is no evidence of radioactive material excreted into the duodenum, biliary atresia is the most probable diagnosis. A liver biopsy may also be useful in the diagnosis in many cases of biliary atresia. The definitive diagnosis of biliary atresia is further

established during an exploratory laparotomy and an intraoperative cholangiogram that demonstrates complete obstruction at some level of the biliary tree. Laparoscopy and laparoscopic-guided cholangiography has also been successfully performed to avoid the invasive effects of exploratory laparotomy (Hay and others, 2000).

### Therapeutic Management

The primary treatment of biliary atresia is *hepatic portoenterostomy (Kasai procedure)*. This surgical procedure involves dissection of the porta hepatis to expose an area through which bile may drain (Fig. 11-21). A *roux-en-Y* jejunal limb is then anastomosed to the porta hepatis (a Y-shaped anastomosis performed to provide bile drainage without reflux). There are several variations of this procedure. In approximately 80% to 90% of infants with biliary atresia who are operated on when younger than 10 weeks of age, bile drainage is achieved (Halamek and Stevenson, 1997; Ryckman and others, 1993). However, progressive cirrhosis still occurs in many children, and up to 80% to 90% will eventually require liver transplantation (Andres, 1996). Complications following the portoenterostomy procedure include ascending cholangitis, cirrhosis, portal hypertension, and GI bleeding. Prophylactic antibiotics are given following the Kasai procedure to minimize the risk of ascending cholangitis.

### Nursing Considerations

There are many important nursing interventions for the child with biliary atresia. Education regarding all aspects of the treatment plan and the rationale for therapy should be provided to the family members. In the immediate postoperative period following a hepatic portoenterostomy, nursing

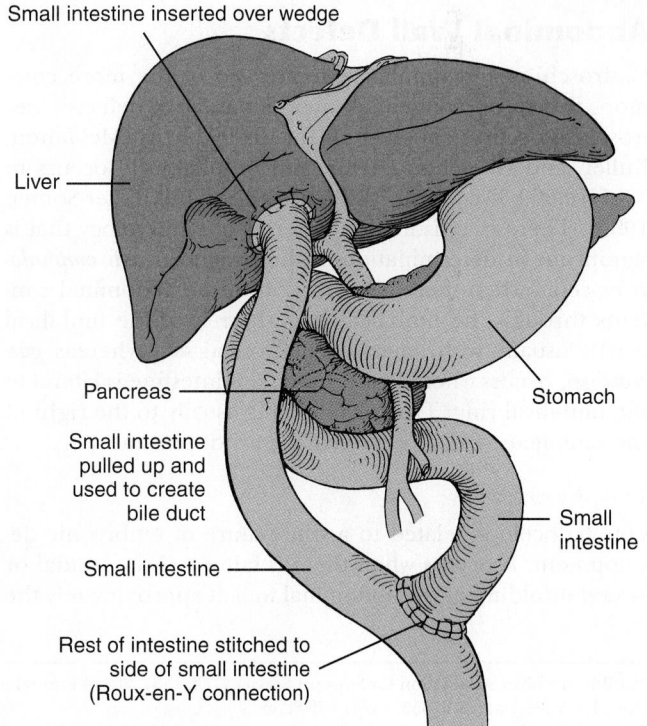

**Fig. 11-21** Biliary atresia—Kasai procedure.

care is similar to that following any major abdominal surgery. If an interrupted jejunal conduit has been performed, the family will need to be taught how to care for the two stomas and how to refeed the bile following feedings. Teaching includes the proper administration of medications. Administration of nutritional therapy, including special formulas, vitamin and mineral supplements, tube feedings, or parenteral nutrition, is an essential nursing responsibility. Growth failure in such infants is common, and increased metabolic needs combined with ascites, pruritus, and nutritional anorexia constitute a challenge for care. The caregivers are taught how to monitor and administer nutritional therapy in the home. Pruritus may be a significant problem that can be relieved by drug therapy or comfort measures such as baths in colloidal oatmeal compounds and trimming of fingernails. The risk of complications of biliary atresia, such as cholangitis, portal hypertension, GI bleeding, and ascites, should be explained to the caregivers.

These children and their families require special psychosocial support. The uncertain prognosis, discomfort, and waiting for transplantation can produce considerable stress. (See Cirrhosis, Chapter 33.) In addition, extended hospitalizations, as well as pharmacologic and nutritional therapy, can impose significant financial burdens on the family, as with any chronic condition. The expertise of a multidisciplinary health care team including physicians, nurses, nutritionists, pharmacists, and social workers is often needed. Parent support groups can be very beneficial. The **Children's Liver Association for Support Services (CLASS)*** and the **Biliary Atresia and Liver Transplant Network, Inc. (BALT)†** provide educational materials, programs, and support systems for parents of children with liver disease.

## Abdominal Wall Defects

Gastroschisis and omphalocele are two of the more common forms of congenital abdominal wall defects; gastroschisis occurs in about 1 to 3 in 10,000 births (McMahon, Kuller, and Chescheir, 1996), and omphalocele occurs in 3 of 10,000 live births (Kilby, Lander, and Usher-Somer, 1999). There is a distinction in terms of embryology that is significant in determination of the prognosis. An *omphalocele* occurs when there is herniation of the abdominal contents through the umbilical ring (hernia of the umbilical cord), usually with an intact peritoneal sac, whereas *gastroschisis* occurs when the herniation of intestine is lateral to the umbilical ring. This herniation is usually to the right of the umbilicus, and a peritoneal sac is not present.

### Omphalocele

Omphalocele is related to a true failure of embryonic development. It occurs when there is failure of the caudal or lateral infolding of the abdominal wall at approximately the third week of gestation. With the deficiency in the abdominal wall, the bowel is unable to complete its return to the abdomen between the tenth and twelfth weeks of gestation.

The omphalocele is usually covered only by a translucent peritoneal sac (Fig. 11-22). The sac may contain only a small portion of the bowel or most of the bowel and other abdominal viscera, such as the liver. If the sac ruptures, the abdominal contents become exposed. Omphalocele often is associated with other anomalies, including cardiac, neurologic, skeletal, and genitourinary anomalies; imperforate anus; ileal atresia; and bladder exstrophy. Omphalocele is also associated with trisomies 13, 18, and 21 (Down syndrome).

A small omphalocele may go undetected at first glance and appeal as a bulge in the umbilical cord; it is, therefore, imperative that an unusually large umbilical cord be inspected for omphalocele before clamping to prevent possible damage to bowel tissue (Donlon, Furdon, and Clark, 2002). (See Umbilical Cord Care, Chapter 8.)

With the increasing frequency of and improvements in prenatal ultrasonography, prenatal diagnosis of some abdominal wall defects is being accomplished. The benefits of prenatal ultrasonographic diagnosis include the ability to transfer the mother to a tertiary care center, where pediatric surgeons and a neonatal intensive care unit are available to assist with care following delivery. Delivery at a regional center has had better outcomes with shorter hospitalization and fewer hospital charges.

Initial management after delivery includes loosely covering the exposed abdominal contents and membranes with a bowel bag or saline-soaked pads and a plastic drape to prevent excessive fluid loss, drying, and temperature instability. IV fluids and antibiotics are administered, and a further evaluation for other associated anomalies is completed. Bowel decompression with a Silastic double-lumen catheter is also performed.

Following initial medical management and stabilization, surgical closure of the omphalocele is performed. The sac is resected, contents are reduced into the abdominal cavity, and an attempt is made to close the abdominal fascia with sutures. The abdominal wall may need to be stretched. If there is an intestinal atresia, a bowel resection may be performed, possibly involving a diverting stoma.

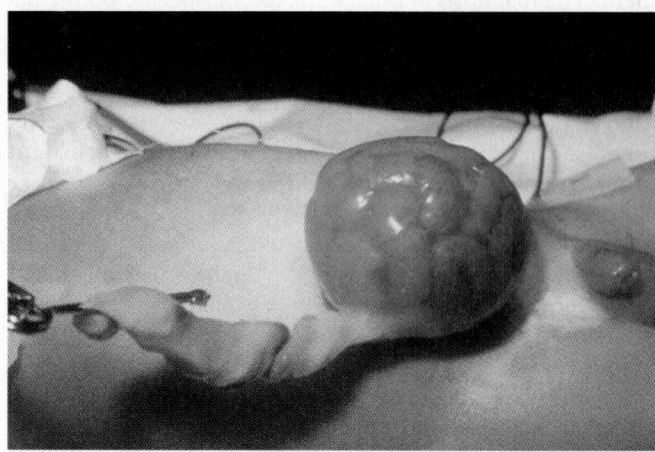

**Fig. 11-22** Omphalocele in membraneous sac.

*Children's Liver Association for Support Services (CLASS), 26444 Emerald Dove Dr, Valencia, CA 91355, (877) 679-8256; www.classkids.org.
†Biliary Atresia and Liver Transplant Network, Inc (BALT), 3835 Richmond Ave, Box 190, Staten Island, New York 10312-3828, (718) 987-6200; www.transweb.org

When a primary closure of the defect is not possible because of the small size of the abdominal cavity or an extremely large omphalocele, staged reduction is accomplished and a silo is created with a sheet of Silastic material that is sutured to the edges of the skin following removal of the sac. The abdominal contents are placed in the abdomen, and the abdominal wall is stretched before the silo is placed. Following surgery, the silo may be suspended using mild tension from the top of the incubator or radiant warmer. An antibacterial ointment is applied to the silo and suture lines to prevent local infection. Usually the silo is compressed on a daily basis. At the end of approximately 7 to 10 days, the infant is returned to the operating room and the silo is removed. The abdominal fascia and skin are then closed with sutures.

Postoperatively these infants often require mechanical ventilation and parenteral nutrition for several days. Postoperative complications include infection, evisceration, intestinal volvulus, obstruction, and development of a ventral hernia.

## Gastroschisis

Gastroschisis occurs when the bowel herniates through a defect in the abdominal wall to the right of the umbilical cord and through the rectus muscle (Fig. 11-23). There is no membrane covering the exposed bowel. Controversy exists regarding the etiology of gastroschisis. It has been suggested that at some point between the bowel's stay in the umbilical cord and the completion of fixation, a tear occurs at the base of the umbilical cord, allowing the intestine to herniate. The gap between the cord and the tear is filled in by skin, giving the appearance of a defect in the abdominal wall to the right of the umbilical cord. The base of the defect is narrow, and the lack of membranes results in thickening and foreshortening of the bowel. Gastroschisis is rarely associated with other major congenital anomalies; however, jejunoileal atresia, ischemic enteritis, and malrotation may occur as a result of the defect itself.

Initial management is similar to that for omphalocele. The exposed bowel is loosely covered in saline-soaked pads, and the abdomen wrapped in a plastic drape or bowel bag. IV fluids and antibiotics are administered, and a double-lumen NG tube is inserted for bowel decompression.

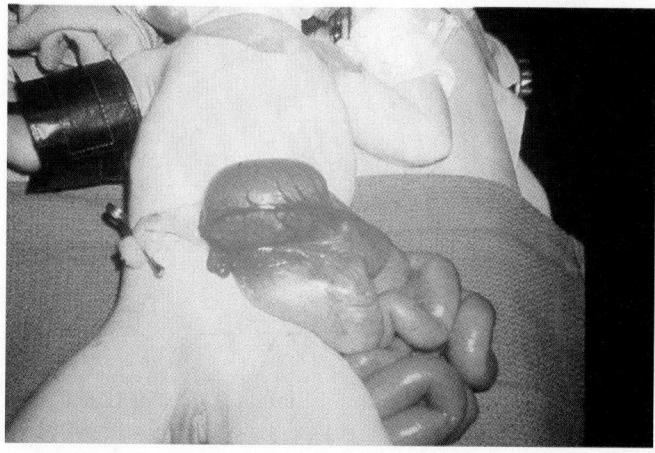

**Fig. 11-23** Gastroschisis with nonmatted bowel.

Adequate thermoregulation and fluid management are extremely important for both omphalocele and gastroschisis. During surgery the abdominal wall is stretched and the mass of bowel is replaced in the abdomen. If primary closure is not possible, a silo is performed similar to that in an omphalocele. The silo is reduced over a period of several days, at which time it is removed surgically and the defect is closed.

Infants with gastroschisis have traditionally been operated on within 24 hours of birth because of temperature instability, risk of infection in the unprotected bowel, and fluid loss. In some centers, for infants with gastroschisis, silo placement over the unprotected bowel is performed in the neonatal intensive care unit, followed by elective repair at a later date. The reported advantages to this approach (vs. immediate surgical repair) are a gradual reduction of abdominal contents, fewer intraoperative complications, and shorter length of stay (Minkes and others, 2000).

Postoperatively most infants require mechanical ventilation and parenteral nutrition because many infants have a prolonged ileus. Respiratory distress may occur postoperatively because of increased abdominal pressure. Other complications include infection, intestinal obstruction, vena cava compression, and a subsequent decrease in blood flow to the lower extremities.

### Prognosis

Advanced surgical techniques, improved parenteral nutrition delivery systems, and better medical management have improved the prognosis for the newborn with an abdominal wall defect. Survival estimates for infants with gastroschisis differ from 88.5% (Forrester and Merz, 1999) to 100% for low-risk (simple) and 91% for high-risk (complex) cases (Molik and others, 2001). Survival rates for omphalocele are reported to be 71% (Forrester and Merz, 1999; Kitchanan and others, 2000). Because 67% of newborns with omphalocele often have serious associated congenital anomalies, such as cardiac and chromosome anomalies, the prognosis for survival of such infants is not as predictable or as positive as it is for those with gastroschisis.

### Nursing Considerations

Nursing care is similar to that for any high-risk infant. In addition, infection is a constant threat before surgery, and careful positioning and handling are needed to prevent rupture of the omphalocele sac, herniated bowel, or disturbance of the Silastic material used for gradual reduction. Viscera should be protected with saline-soaked pads and plastic drape placed over the defect. Heat and fluid loss from the exposed viscera are major concerns in the preoperative period; therefore thermoregulation is critical. Fluid replacement is vital and must compensate for losses. The GI tract is decompressed via an NG tube before surgery to aid in bowel reduction. Postoperative care includes monitoring for signs of complications and assessment of bowel function. Parenteral nutritional support may be necessary when ileus persists. It may require several days or weeks for normal bowel function to return before enteral feeding can be initiated.

**Family Support, Discharge Planning, and Home Care.** Because these abdominal defects are visible and may be shocking to parents, immediate emotional support at the time of birth is essential. The family needs a brief explanation of the defect and reassurance that their child is in no immediate danger (unless circumstances are different). After the parents have had time to interact with their newborn, they should be informed about the surgical treatment and postoperative care. (See Critical Thinking Exercise box.) At the time of discharge from the hospital, many of these infants are receiving oral feedings, but extended parenteral nutrition may be required if malabsorption and prolonged ileus occur. Oral stimulation during the period of receiving nothing by mouth is essential to prevent oral aversion, which often requires the involvement of a speech therapist to retrain the infant to suck and swallow. (See Feeding Resistance, Chapter 10.) Continuity of care may be ensured by a referral to a home health care agency, especially if long-term nutritional support is required.

## HERNIAS

A *hernia* is a protrusion of a portion of an organ or organs through an abnormal opening. The danger from herniation arises when the protrusion is constricted, impairing circulation, or when the protrusion interferes with the function or development of other structures. The herniations of concern in this section are those that protrude through the diaphragm, the abdominal wall, or the inguinal canal.

### Umbilical Hernia

The umbilical hernia is the most common hernia in infants. It occurs when fusion of the umbilical ring is incomplete at the point where the umbilical vessels exit the abdominal wall. It affects African-Americans more often than Caucasians and low-birth-weight infants and premature infants more often than full-term infants. An umbilical hernia usually is an isolated defect, but it may be present in association with other congenital anomalies, such as Down syndrome (trisomy 21) and trisomies 13 and 18. The size of the defect is variable, and the protrusion is more prominent when the infant is crying (Fig. 11-24). *Incarceration,* in which the hernia is constricted and cannot be reduced manually, is rare; usually the defect resolves spontaneously by 3 to 5 years of age. If the hernia persists beyond this age, it is usually surgically corrected on an elective basis.

#### Nursing Considerations

The appearance of an umbilical hernia may be disconcerting to parents; therefore, they need reassurance that the defect usually is not harmful. Taping or strapping the abdomen to flatten the protrusion does not aid in resolution and can produce skin irritation.

---

### Critical Thinking Exercise

#### Abdominal Wall Defect

A 2800-g newborn is noted to have a large mass of intestinal contents covering the exterior abdomen and protruding from around the umbilical cord; this event was not anticipated. The mother is 23 years old and single; the father is not involved. The maternal grandmother is present at the delivery and notices the defect. She is visibly shocked. The newborn is not in any respiratory distress. Given these facts, what is the best intervention at this time?

FIRST, THINK ABOUT IT . . .

• What information are you using?
• What would the consequences be if you put your thoughts into action?

---

1. Cover the defect with a blanket, show the newborn to the mother, and make no mention of the defect until the pediatrician arrives.
2. Prepare for immediate endotracheal intubation because this is a life-threatening defect.
3. Allow the mother to hold the newborn briefly while protecting the defect with moist saline gauze.
4. Discuss with the mother surgical options for correction of the defect.

---

*The best response is three. The mother and newborn are not at immediate risk for any health complications that would preclude a short but meaningful time for interaction.*

*The mother and grandmother need to be reassured that the infant will be completely evaluated on arrival in the nursery (or neonatal intensive care unit) by other health care professionals and that surgical correction is the most probable treatment. Discussing the surgical options immediately after birth is not the best intervention and may bear negative consequences; this discussion may be better received after the mother has had some time to examine the newborn and react to others in the immediate surroundings. The other health care workers' reactions will play an important part in the mother's perception of her newborn in relation to acceptance of the newborn. The action of covering the baby with a blanket and hiding the defect will only enhance the mother's anxiety and may interfere with her attachment to the infant. There is no need to prepare for intubation at this time, because no respiratory distress is noted.*

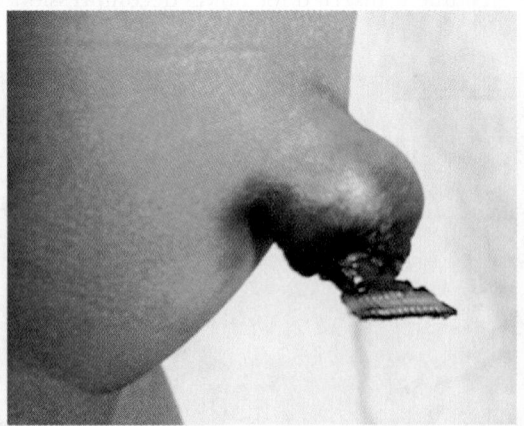

**Fig. 11-24**  Newborn with an umbilical hernia. (From Zitelli BJ, Davis HW: *Atlas of pediatric physical diagnosis,* ed 3, St Louis, 1997, Mosby.)

Nursing care of the child with an umbilical hernia repair is essentially the same as that of other minor GI surgery. The procedure may be performed on an outpatient basis, and a pressure dressing is maintained for approximately 48 hours postoperatively. The child is observed for complications related to a hematoma or respiratory compromise as a result of general anesthesia. Oral fluids are generally well tolerated postoperatively, and strenuous activity or play is restricted for 2 to 3 weeks.

# Congenital Diaphragmatic Hernia (CDH)

CDH results when there is failure of the transverse septum and the pleuroperitoneal folds to completely develop and form the diaphragm. The most common type of CDH (90%) is a left posterolateral defect, also known as a Bochdalek hernia, because the herniation occurs through the foramen of Bochdalek. If the diaphragm does not form completely, the intestines and other abdominal structures, such as the liver, can enter the thoracic cavity, compressing the lung. Lung growth may be arrested on the affected side and to a lesser degree on the contralateral side. Respiration is further compromised by hypoplasia and compression of the lung, including the airways and blood vessels. Pulmonary hypoplasia and pulmonary hypertension have also been recently recognized as components in the pathology of CDH in addition to the anatomic defect. This serious defect requires prompt recognition and aggressive treatment to reduce its high mortality. The incidence of CDH is approximately 0.3 in 3300 live births (Katz, Wiswell, and Baumgart, 1998).

## Clinical Manifestations

The most common manifestation of CDH is acute respiratory distress in the newborn. Entrance of air into the intestines following birth further compromises respiration. Infants with a CDH may be dyspneic and cyanotic and have a scaphoid abdomen (because of abdominal contents in the chest); cardiac output is impaired, and the infant will exhibit signs and symptoms of shock.

## Diagnostic Evaluation

Prenatal diagnosis of CDH as early as the twenty-fifth week of gestation is possible. The three main features detected by ultrasonography that confirm the diagnosis are polyhydramnios, mediastinal shift, and the presence of loops of bowel in the chest cavity. In severe cases fetal hydrops is evident. Low maternal serum alpha-fetoprotein (MS-AFP) levels are seen in cases of CDH; however, the finding is not specific for this anomaly.

Antenatal diagnosis of CDH is reported to have the following advantages: (1) counseling the family regarding pregnancy alternatives and potential problems of the neonatal period; (2) continuation of the pregnancy and further management, including possible antenatal treatment; and (3) transport of the fetus with a CDH in utero to a tertiary center for management. A multidisciplinary team of neonatologists, neonatal nurses, and pediatric surgeons can intervene early in the acute phase to improve the infant's chances for survival and a positive outcome.

After birth, the diagnosis of CDH may depend on the type of hernia present. In the majority of cases the diagnosis is suspected on the basis of the clinical manifestations and is confirmed by a chest radiograph. The chest radiograph shows fluid and air-filled loops of intestine in the affected side of the chest. The mediastinum may be shifted to the unaffected side, and auscultation may reveal decreased breath sounds on the affected side.

## Therapeutic Management

**Fetal Surgery.**   Advances in fetal diagnostic and surgical techniques have led to intrauterine repair of CDH in certain cases. Previously, attempts to repair CDH in utero were often unsuccessful, possibly because of associated anomalies restricting fetal lung growth and preterm delivery. Recent fetal surgical repair of CDH is done when it occurs as an isolated anomaly with liver herniation into the chest, at gestational age less than 26 weeks, and with an adequate LH (lung/head) ratio (Howell, Von Nessen, and Burns, 2000).

Tracheal obstruction has been shown to expand the lungs and push the abdominal contents back into the abdomen, thus producing larger, functional lungs. This technique, **PLUG (plug the lung until it grows),** has been used in human fetuses to increase fetal lung growth. At the time of delivery the fetal chest is delivered by cesarean section, but the lower body remains in utero with functional placental circulation until the fetal trachea has been cleared and an effective airway established; this is called the **EXIT (ex utero intrapartum treatment)** procedure. Preliminary results with these methods have not yielded favorable outcomes; mortality resulting from pulmonary causes and prematurity is high (Flake and others, 2000; Harrison, 2000). Intrauterine diaphragmatic repair has been associated with the onset of premature labor, but fetal endoscopic repair of CDH has prevented preterm delivery in some cases (Katz, Wiswell, and Baumgart, 1998). Only a few major medical centers in the United States are involved in fetal surgical repair of CDH.

**Post-Birth.**   Many infants with a CDH require immediate respiratory assistance, which includes endotracheal intubation and GI decompression with a double-lumen catheter to prevent further respiratory compromise. At birth, bag and mask ventilation is contraindicated to prevent air from entering the stomach and especially the intestines, further compromising pulmonary function. Positioning the infant with the head and chest elevated higher than the abdomen will facilitate downward displacement of the abdominal organs. In infants with mild respiratory distress, oxygen may be given by hood; however, close attention to the infant's acid-base status is imperative in the management and prevention of pulmonary hypertension. Low ventilatory positive pressure and the lowest mean airway pressure possible combined with rapid ventilatory rates (80 to 120 breaths/min) may serve to reduce the incidence of pulmonary leaks from over-inflation of the unaffected lung. Another strategy that has demonstrated considerable success in the management of

CDH is the use of *permissive hypercapnia* wherein hyperventilation is not employed in order to reduce iatrogenic lung injury and barotrauma; preductal $SpO_2$ is maintained at 90, $pCO_2$ is ignored, and metabolic acidosis is corrected with buffers instead of hyperventilation (Juretschke, 2001). There is considerable controversy regarding the respiratory management of persistent pulmonary hypertension and CDH (Katz, Wiswell, and Baumgart, 1998; Muratore and Wilson, 2000).

IV fluids are initiated during the stabilization period. An umbilical arterial catheter may be placed for monitoring arterial blood gases and for provision of adequate glucose. A transcutaneous oxygen pressure monitor or pulse oximeter may be placed preductally (right hand) and postductally (left hand, arm, or either foot) to monitor the amount of ductal shunting through the patent ductus arteriosus. An umbilical arterial catheter will help monitor postductal arterial oxygen tension ($Pao_2$). Ductal shunting of deoxygenated blood occurs when pressure in the pulmonary artery is equal to or less than peripheral blood pressure. If pulmonary hypertension is severe, with decreased pulmonary venous return, right atrial pressure will be greater than left atrial pressure, resulting in shunting of blood through the foramen ovale. The net results of these events cause further hypoxia, hypercarbia, and acidosis.

Further preoperative stabilization may include the use of opioids, such as fentanyl, and a paralyzing agent, such as pancuronium, in infants who are agitated and resisting ventilation. An inotropic drug such as dopamine may be used to support systemic blood pressure and improve cardiac output. Tolazoline may be used to promote pulmonary vascular vasodilation and decrease the amount of pulmonary hypertension. (See Persistent Pulmonary Hypertension of the Newborn, Chapter 10.)

Because acidosis increases pulmonary hypertension and consequently shunting of unoxygenated blood away from the lungs, it is imperative to monitor acid-base status closely. Prevention of acidosis may be accomplished with sodium bicarbonate continuous infusion and hyperventilation; tromethamine (THAM) may also be used in place of sodium bicarbonate. Close attention to the infant's thermoregulation status (maintain neutral thermal environment) and glucose requirements during the acute phase are also a priority of care. The use of high-frequency jet ventilation and/or high-frequency oscillation to manage the infant with a CDH is used in many tertiary centers with varying results; ventilatory management is individualized on the basis of the infant's response and requirements. Surfactant replacement therapy may also be used to stabilize neonates with CDH (Juretschke, 2001). The use of inhaled nitric oxide to relieve pulmonary hypertension of CDH has also been used in some cases with mixed results (Muratore and Wilson, 2000). (See Nitric Oxide, Surfactant Replacement Therapy, and ECMO, Chapter 10.)

Traditional management has been early surgical repair of the defect. However, increased survival rates have been reported with surgery following a period of preoperative stabilization that may include placing the infant on extracorporeal membrane oxygenation (ECMO) or high-frequency ventilation. Operative treatment involves returning the abdominal organs to the abdomen and repairing the diaphragmatic defect. Postoperative management involves continuation of ventilatory therapy, monitoring of acid-base balance, and even maintaining the infant in a slightly alkalotic state to prevent or decrease the effects of pulmonary hypertension. In addition, gastric decompression, thermoregulation, sedation, and maintenance of adequate cardiac output and peripheral perfusion are continued. Following surgery for CDH, the infant may at first show marked improvement in ventilatory status; the infant may then gradually deteriorate with the combined effects of hypoxemia and pulmonary hypertension. For this reason, close attention to acid-base balance and ventilatory requirements during the postoperative period will help prevent a potentially irreversible poor outcome. If paralysis is continued in the postoperative period, appropriate pain management should not be overlooked. The infant may return from surgery with one or two chest tubes, which require close monitoring.

**Prognosis.** CDH is a complex problem of pulmonary hypoplasia, immature lungs, and other associated problems. The overall mortality rates for CDH are decreasing as the pathophysiology is better understood in relation to current treatment modalities. Current data suggests overall survival rates of 80% to 90% (Muratore and Wilson, 2000). Surgical repair of the defect alone, whether in utero or postbirth, does not resolve the infant's problems related to organ immaturity. Long-term complications of CDH include chronic lung disease, gastroesophageal reflux, feeding problems, recurrent diaphragmatic herniation, pneumonia, growth failure, and impaired motor and cognitive function. In one study 75% of infants with CDH required rehospitalization for complications within the first year of life (Katz, Wiswell, and Baumgart, 1998).

## Nursing Considerations

Assessment of the infant at birth is an integral component of nursing care. This is accentuated in life-threatening cases such as CDH, where prompt recognition of neonatal respiratory distress, cyanosis, a scaphoid abdomen, and a possible mediastinal shift would alert the nurse to investigate further. Any one or a combination of these signs may signal the presence of CDH. A newborn in respiratory distress at birth who does not initially respond to resuscitation is further evaluated for CDH; endotracheal intubation is an option for providing adequate oxygenation until CDH is ruled out as a cause of the distress. If CDH is diagnosed prenatally and the infant is in distress, endotracheal intubation is required to prevent further accumulation of air in the stomach and intestines and subsequent respiratory compromise. (See Critical Thinking Exercise box.)

**NURSING ALERT** Any newborn infant with a scaphoid abdomen, moderate to severe respiratory distress, decreased breath sounds unilaterally, and a history of polyhydramnios should be suspected of having a CDH. Ventilation should not be given with bag and mask to prevent further intestinal air and subsequent respiratory compromise.

Preoperative care involves prompt recognition, resuscitation, and stabilization of the infant, including ventilatory support, blood gas monitoring, and administration of IV fluids. The stomach is decompressed with a double-lumen tube, and the infant is observed for signs of impaired cardiac output, acidosis, and hypoxemia.

The infant may be positioned on the affected side to take advantage of gravity, which facilitates expansion of the unaffected lung and reduces the likelihood of overexpansion into the unaffected side. Postoperative care includes the routine observations discussed in the care of the high-risk infant. Close observation to detect signs of respiratory distress or fluid and electrolyte imbalances is an important nursing function. The infant is closely monitored for signs of mediastinal shift, pulmonary air leak, and infection. Hypovolemia as a result of third-spacing of intravascular fluids may occur; correction with salt-free albumin is one option for treatment of hypovolemia.

Nursing care of the infant with a CDH is also aimed at reducing stimulation either from care activities such as routine suctioning or from environmental factors such as noise and light. Measures that further reduce infant stress, such as management of pain, should be a routine aspect of care for the infant with a CDH. It is not uncommon for the infant with a CDH to be the sickest patient and thus the most demanding of nursing care.

## Critical Thinking Exercise

### Congenital Diaphragmatic Hernia

A prenatal ultrasonographic examination has revealed the presence of a congenital diaphragmatic hernia in the fetus of a 31-year-old woman who has had two previous cesarean sections. A repeat C-section is carried out, and the newborn is placed under a radiant warmer for stabilization; the weight is approximately 3.5 kg. The newborn is cyanotic, has copious oral secretions, and demonstrates gasping respiratory effort. What is the most important initial intervention?

FIRST, THINK ABOUT IT . . .

• What precise question are you trying to answer?
• What information are you using?

1. Place the infant in Trendelenburg position to facilitate drainage of secretions.
2. Begin bag and mask ventilation with 100% oxygen and a proper-size face mask.
3. Prepare moist, warm saline gauze pads to place over the congenital defect.
4. Suction the oropharynx and prepare a 4-mm endotracheal tube and stylet for immediate intubation.

*The best response is four. In most cases the infant with a CDH and respiratory distress will benefit the most from intubation for airway maintenance.*

*Air from the manual resuscitation bag will enter the stomach and intestines in the chest cavity, further compromising respiratory status. There is no outward defect to cover, and the Trendelenburg position is contraindicated because it increases pressure of organs against lungs.*

Because of the serious nature of the condition and the urgency of treatment, the parents are in great need of ongoing support and education regarding postoperative care. The infant with a CDH may require long-term hospitalization and care; this further places the infant at risk for delayed acceptance and integration into the family unit. As soon as medically possible, the parents should be involved in the daily care of their child.

## Inguinal Hernia

Inguinal hernias account for approximately 80% of all childhood hernias and occur more frequently in boys (roughly 5:1) than in girls. These hernias have an incidence of approximately 10 to 20 per 1000 live births, with 30% occurring in preterm infants (Kapur, Caty, and Glick, 1998; Pelosi, 2000).

### Pathophysiology

Inguinal hernia is derived from persistence of all or part of the processus vaginalis, the tube of peritoneum that precedes the testicle through the inguinal canal into the scrotum during the eighth month of gestation. Following descent of the testicle, the proximal portion of the processus vaginalis normally atrophies and closes, whereas the distal portion forms the tunica vaginalis, which envelops the testicle in the scrotum. When the upper portion fails to atrophy, the abdominal fluid or an abdominal structure can be forced into it, creating a palpable bulge or mass. The persistent sac may end at any point along the inguinal canal; it may stop at the inguinal ring or extend all the way into the scrotum (Fig. 11-25). The hernial sac is present at birth but does not usually become apparent until the infant is able to build up sufficient intraabdominal pressure to open the sac, usually at 2 to 3 months of age.

### Clinical Manifestations

This very common defect is asymptomatic unless the abdominal contents are forced into the patent sac. Most often it appears as a painless inguinal swelling that varies in size. It disappears during periods of rest or is reducible by gentle compression; it appears when the infant cries or strains or when the older child strains, coughs, or stands for a long period. The defect can be palpated as a thickening of the cord in the groin, and the *silk glove sign* can be elicited by rubbing together the sides of the empty hernial sac.

Sometimes the herniated loop of intestine becomes partially obstructed, producing variable symptoms that may include fretfulness and irritability, tenderness, anorexia, abdominal distention, and difficulty defecating. Occasionally the loop of bowel becomes incarcerated (irreducible), with symptoms of complete intestinal obstruction that, left untreated, will progress to strangulation and gangrene. Incarceration occurs more often in infants under 10 months of age.

### Therapeutic Management

The treatment for hernias is prompt, elective surgical repair in the healthy child as soon as the defect is diagnosed. Because there is a significant incidence of bilateral involvement, many surgeons advocate exploration of both sides.

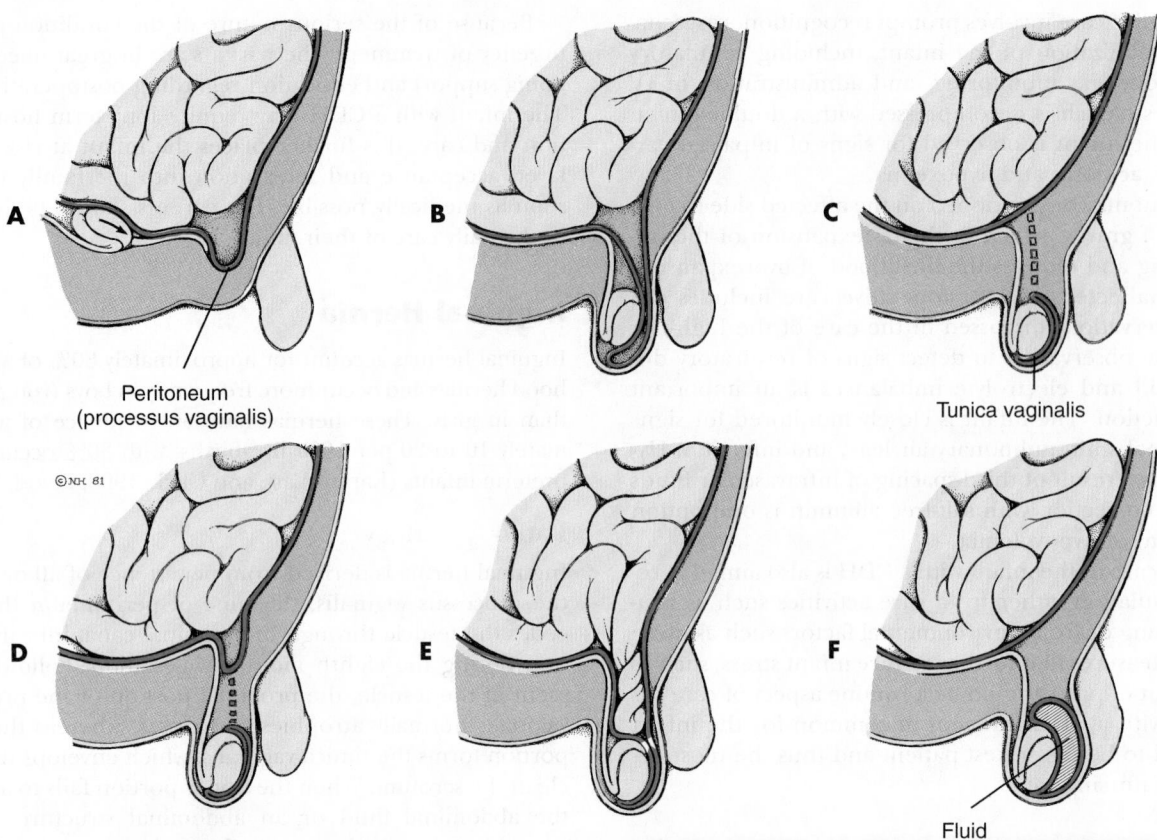

**Fig. 11-25** Development of inguinal hernias. **A** and **B,** Prenatal migration of processus vaginalis. **C,** Normal. **D,** Partially obliterated processus vaginalis. **E,** Hernia. **F,** Hydrocele.

## Nursing Considerations

Prompt recognition of an inguinal hernia is imperative. The hernia may first be noticed when the infant is crying or straining (Valsalva maneuver) to stool. An inguinal hernia is brought to the attention of the practitioner for a definitive diagnosis (vs. hydrocele). Nursing care of the infant or child with an inguinal hernia involves preoperative preparation of the infant and appropriate explanation to the parents of the child's expected postoperative status. Most hernia repairs can be managed on an outpatient basis. The preterm infant usually will have hernia repair several days before discharge from the neonatal intensive care unit (provided one is present and diagnosed). The former preterm infant diagnosed after discharge is admitted the day of surgery and, after repair, is observed for 12 to 24 hours for occurrence of apnea and bradycardia (Kapur, Caty, and Glick, 1998).

Postoperatively the wound is kept clean and dry, and infant's pain is managed appropriately. In infants and small children who are not yet toilet trained, the wound may be covered with an occlusive dressing or left without a dressing. Changing diapers as soon as they become damp helps reduce the chance of irritation or infection of the incision.

Parents are instructed to give the child sponge baths for 2 to 5 days and to change diapers frequently. There are no restrictions placed on the infant's or toddler's activity, but older children are cautioned against lifting, pushing, wrestling or fighting, bicycle riding, and athletics for about 3 weeks.

If surgery is postponed, parents need to be taught the signs of incarcerated hernia, simple measures to reduce it (a warm bath, avoidance of upright positioning, and comfort measures to reduce crying), and where to call for assistance if relief is not obtained in a reasonably short time.

## Femoral Hernia

Femoral hernias are rare in children, with a reported incidence of less than 0.5% (Kapur, Caty, and Glick, 1998). When they occur, there is a higher incidence in girls than in boys. Initial symptoms are a swelling in the groin area associated with severe abdominal pain and cramping. Treatment and management are the same as for inguinal hernia. Incarceration and strangulation are frequent complications.

## DEFECTS OF THE GENITOURINARY (GU) TRACT*

External defects of the GU tract are usually obvious at birth. The anatomic location of these defects frequently causes more psychologic concern to parents than does the actual

---

◼ *Mikel Gray, PhD, CUNP, CCCN, FAAN, revised this section.

**TABLE 11-6**  Renal anomalies

| Anomaly | Description and Nursing Implications |
| --- | --- |
| **Anomalies of the Kidneys** | |
| *Anomalies of Number* | |
| Bilateral agenesis | Fatal anomaly associated with Potter facies and multisystem congenital defects |
| Unilateral agenesis | Occurs in approximately 1:1500 live births; may be discovered on routine examination; parents and child may be counseled regarding advisability of avoiding contact sports |
| Supernumerary kidneys | Rare anomaly; intervention indicated if obstruction or infection of anomalous kidney occurs |
| *Anomalies of Rotation* | Rotation of kidney from its usual relationship to spine; malrotation is not by itself significant, but it is often associated with clinically significant defects, including renal ectopia or fusion |
| *Anomalies of Ascent* | Incomplete ascent of kidney caused by abnormal ureteral bud development; ectopic kidneys are usually located in pelvis; obstruction and infection occasionally occur; abnormally high ascent (intrathoracic kidney) is particularly rare; associated obstruction is rare; crossed renal ectopia occurs when both kidneys ascend on single side of retroperitoneum; renal fusion is possible when crossed ectopia occurs |
| *Anomalies of Fusion* | Fusion of kidneys occurs when renal masses meet during embryonic development; horseshoe kidney is union of inferior portions of two kidneys crossing midline; fusion also may occur with crossed renal ectopia |
| **Anomalies of the Renal Pelvis and Ureters** | |
| Bifid renal pelvis | Duplication of renal pelvis; may slightly increase risk of urinary tract infections |
| Incomplete ureteral duplication | Partial duplication of ureter that opens into single orifice in bladder; peristalsis and evacuation of upper urinary tract may be adversely affected |
| Complete ureteral duplication | Complete duplication of ureters with separate orifices noted in bladder; reflux of lower ureteral segment is common; upper ureteral segment may be obstructed |
| Ureteral ectopia | Ureteral orifice opens into a structure other than bladder base; urethra and vagina are common sites of ectopia; obstruction or continuous urinary incontinence occurs depending on site of ectopic ureteral orifice; defects of associated kidney are common |
| Ureterocele | Bulging dilation of intravesical ureteral segment; ureterocele may obstruct bladder outlet and is often associated with ureteral duplication |

condition or treatment. The timing of medical and surgical procedures for correction of these defects has important implications for children. Surgery involving sexual organs can be particularly disruptive to preschoolers, who fear punishment, retaliation, body mutilation, or castration. Therefore the trend is toward early correction of visible genital defects, preferably without multiple-stage repairs. Renal anomalies, which are typically not obvious at birth, are described in Table 11-6.

# Phimosis

Phimosis is a narrowing or stenosis of the preputial opening of the foreskin that prevents retraction of the foreskin over the glans penis. It is a normal finding in infants and young boys and usually disappears as the child grows and the distal prepuce dilates. Occasionally the narrowing obstructs the flow of urine, resulting in a dribbling stream or even ballooning of the foreskin with accumulated urine during voiding.

*Balanitis* is an inflammation or infection of the phimotic foreskin, which occurs occasionally and is managed as any other inflammation or infection. Severe phimosis is treated surgically by circumcision.

## Nursing Considerations

Proper hygiene of the phimotic foreskin in infants and young boys consists of external cleansing during routine bathing. The foreskin should not be forcibly retracted, because it may create scarring, which can prevent future retraction. Furthermore, retraction of the tight foreskin can result in *paraphimosis,* a condition in which the retracted foreskin cannot be replaced in its normal position over the glans. This causes edema and venous congestion created by constriction by the tight band of foreskin—a urologic emergency that requires immediate evaluation.

# Hydrocele

Hydrocele is the presence of fluid in the processus vaginalis and is a result of the same developmental process as inguinal hernia (Fig. 11-25, *F*). A hydrocele in which the upper segment of the processus vaginalis has been obliterated but the tunica vaginalis still contains peritoneal fluid is called a *noncommunicating hydrocele.* This type of hydrocele is common in newborns and often subsides spontaneously as fluid is gradually absorbed (Gill, 1998).

A *communicating hydrocele* is one in which the processus vaginalis remains open and into which peritoneal fluid may be forced by intraabdominal pressure and gravity. The length of the hydrocele depends on the length of the processus vaginalis and may extend into the tunica vaginalis within the scrotum. The hydrocele is asymptomatic except for a palpable bulge in the inguinal or scrotal area. Unlike a hernia, the hydrocele may not be reducible and may not be produced by a sudden increase in intraabdominal pressure (such as straining). The scrotum appears to be larger after an active day and smaller in the morning. Because a communicating hydrocele represents a patent processus vaginalis, it can predispose the child to herniation; therefore, surgical repair is indicated if spontaneous resolution does not take place by 1 year of age.

### Nursing Considerations

The nursing care of the infant with a hydrocele is essentially the same as that for inguinal hernia. Parents are advised that there is often temporary swelling and discoloration of the scrotum that resolves spontaneously.

## Cryptorchidism (Cryptorchism)

Cryptorchidism is failure of one or both testes to descend normally through the inguinal canal into the scrotum. Absence of testes within the scrotum can be a result of (1) *undescended (cryptorchid) testes,* (2) *retractile testes,* or (3) *anorchia* (absence of testes). Undescended testes can be categorized further according to location:

**Abdominal**—Proximal to the internal inguinal ring
**Canalicular**—Between the internal and external inguinal rings
**Ectopic**—Outside the normal pathways of descent between the abdominal cavity and the scrotum

The incidence of cryptorchidism is approximately 33% in preterm males and 3% to 4% in full-term males; by the age of 1 year the incidence decreases to less than 1% and does not change thereafter.

### Pathophysiology

Testicular development is influenced by a number of genes, but the dominant one is located on the Y chromosome (Thomas, 1999). This gene stimulates the medullary sex cords of the embryonic gonad to differentiate into secretory Sertoli cells. Beginning around week 7, these cells secrete a glycoprotein, müllerian inhibiting substance, that leads to development of a male genital system. Testicular descent is a critical element of the development of the male genital system. This descent occurs in two phases; the first is dominated by müllerian inhibiting substance and the second phase by testosterone. Between weeks 8 and 15 a cord-like structure, the gubernaculum, extends from the developing testis (located in the lower abdomen) to the labioscrotal swelling. The fetus grows, but the length of this gubernaculum remains relatively fixed, anchoring the testis to the developing inguinal canal (transabdominal migration) in preparation for the second phase of descent. This second phase begins around weeks 25 to 30 and is characterized by shrinkage of the gubernaculum under the influence of testosterone, causing the testis to migrate down the inguinal canal and into a scrotal position (transinguinal migration). Descent is also characterized by protrusion of peritoneum, the processus vaginalis, that closes before birth.

*Cryptorchidism* occurs when one or both testes fail to descend through the inguinal canal and into the scrotum. Several processes may slow or arrest testicular descent, including endocrinologic abnormalities affecting the hypothalamic-pituitary-testicular axis, denervation of the genitofemoral nerve, traction of the gubernaculum, abnormal development of the epididymis, or premature birth. Cryptorchid testes are often accompanied by congenital hernias and abnormal testes, and they are at risk for subsequent torsion.

An *ectopic testis* emerges outside the inguinal ring into the perineum, femoral area, or lies in a transverse scrotal or prepenile location. The most common site is the superficial inguinal pouch. Ectopia is postulated to occur because of obstruction of the scrotal inlet, scarring (fibrosis) of the gubernaculum, or other mechanical anomalies.

*Anorchia* is the complete absence of a testis. Anorchia is suspected whenever one or both testes cannot be palpated in the patient with cryptorchidism. In some cases, bilateral anorchidism is associated with genotypic and phenotypic abnormalities, but it is commonly associated with a normal karyotype (46XY) and normal genital development. This observation supports the hypothesis that, in most cases, anorchidism represents degeneration rather than agenesis of the testes (vanishing testes or testicular regression syndrome).

The cryptorchid or ectopic testis must be differentiated from anorchia because of the risk for malignant degeneration and subfertility when the testis is left in an extrascrotal location. This differentiation may be resolved by an imaging study, such as a ultrasonography, or it may require surgical exploration.

*Retractile testes* can be found at any level within the path of testicular descent, but they are most commonly identified in the groin. Fortunately, they are not truly cryptorchid; instead, they are introverted to an inguinal or abdominal position because of an overactive *cremasteric reflex.* The cremasteric reflex, observed as withdrawal of the testis above the scrotum and into the inguinal canal in response to various stimuli including exposure to cool temperatures, is active during infancy and peaks around age 4 to 5 years. Unlike the cryptorchid testis, the retractile testis can be gently moved into the scrotum without residual tension and does not require treatment.

### Clinical Manifestations

A nonpalpable testis is typically observed by the parent or detected during routine physical examination by a nurse practitioner or physician. If one testis is not palpable, the affected hemiscrotum will appear smaller than the other, while both hemiscrota appear small with bilateral nonpalpable testes. In the case of retractile testes, the parents may report intermittently observing the testis in the scrotum, interspersed with periods when it cannot be visualized or palpated. Frequently, the retractile testis will be observed in the scrotum when child is being bathed in warm water.

### Diagnostic Evaluation

It is important to differentiate the true undescended testis from the more common retractile testis. Retractile testes can be "milked" or pushed back into the scrotum, but truly undescended ones cannot. For examination, the cremasteric reflex can be obviated by placing the child in a squatting position or by applying firm finger pressure on the external ring before palpating the abdomen or genitalia. (See Fig. 7-46.)

Undescended testes may be felt along the inguinal canal, but those in the abdominal cavity usually cannot. Ultrasonography, computed tomography, MRI, and abdominal laparoscopy are sometimes employed to verify cryptorchidism in children undergoing orchiopexy; laparoscopy has been shown to be the most accurate means for locating non-palpable testes (Pillai and Besner, 1998). Suggestions to employ in diagnostic examination include:

- An undescended testis is usually smaller and softer than its descended mate.
- A well-developed rugous scrotum usually indicates normal testicular descent (may be confused by the presence of a hydrocele or inguinal hernia).
- A retractile testis is usually bilateral (the cremasteric reflex is equally brisk on both sides).
- A testis can usually be distinguished from a lymph node by its elastic nature. A testis is mobile and can be massaged down into the scrotum, although it will spring back into the canal.
- Application of soap, cornstarch, or talcum powder to the tip of the examiner's fingers facilitates massaging the inguinal canal.

***Acquired undescended testes*** in children who have had normally descended testes are relatively uncommon. Therefore evaluation of the testes should continue to be a part of the routine physical assessment.

### Therapeutic Management

A retractile testis that can be manipulated into the scrotum will eventually assume a satisfactory scrotal position without medical or surgical intervention. The diagnosis is not made at a single examination, and parents are asked if they have observed the testes in the scrotum at some time. If so, the anomaly probably represents the retractile variety and the parents can be reassured. By 1 year of age, cryptorchid testes will descend spontaneously in approximately 75% of cases in both full-term and preterm infants. In contrast, true undescended testes rarely descend spontaneously after 1 year of age.

A trial of hormone therapy with luteinizing hormone-releasing hormone (nasal spray) and human chorionic gonadotropin (injection) may be attempted; however, surgical treatment is the preferred management (Pillai and Besner, 1998). If the testes do not descend spontaneously, *orchiopexy* is performed before the child's second birthday, preferably between 1 and 2 years of age. Surgical repair is done to (1) prevent damage to the undescended testicle by exposure to the higher degree of body heat in the undescended location, thus maintaining future fertility; (2) decrease the incidence of tumor formation, which is higher in undescended testicles; (3) avoid trauma and torsion; (4) close the processus vaginalis; and (5) prevent the cosmetic and psychologic handicap of an empty scrotum. Because of the increased propensity toward neoplastic changes (even after orchiopexy), cryptorchid testes are better observed in the scrotal position, where they can be routinely palpated.

The timing of the surgery is important, as it is in any genital surgery. Orchiopexy is usually performed between 6 and 24 months of age. Fewer psychologic effects and a higher rate of fertility may be achieved when repair takes place at an early age. Having both testes in the scrotum by school age prevents psychologic problems related to body image and peer-group embarrassment, since the empty scrotum is smaller in size and altered in shape.

In the routine surgical procedure for undescended testes, the testes are brought down into the scrotum and secured in that position without tension or torsion. A simple orchiopexy for a palpable testis can usually be performed in an outpatient surgical unit. Intraabdominal testes require considerable surgical skill because of technical problems resulting from variations in the length of the spermatic cord, and overnight hospitalization may be necessary. In most cases the family can be reassured of normal function in adulthood.

### Nursing Considerations

The postoperative nursing care is directed toward prevention of infection and instructing parents in home care of the child, including pain control. Infection is prevented by carefully cleansing the operative site of stool and urine. Observation of the wound for complications and activity restrictions are discussed. Parents are concerned about the future fertility of the child, and the family is counseled regarding the prognosis and the optimum time for discussing it with the child—ideally as a part of sex education.

## Hypospadias

Hypospadias refers to a condition in which the urethral opening is located below the glans penis or anywhere along the ventral surface (underside) of the penile shaft (Fig. 11-26). The incidence of hypospadias is reported to be 1 out of 300 live births with 10% to 15% of affected newborns having a first-degree male relative (sibling or father) with the same condition (Bukowski and Zeman, 2001). In very mild cases the meatus is just below the tip of the penis. In the most severe malformations the meatus is located on the perineum between the halves of the scrotum (bifid scrotum). ***Chordee,*** or ventral curvature of the penis, results from the replacement of normal skin with a fibrous band of tissue and usually accompanies more severe forms of hypospadias. In addition,

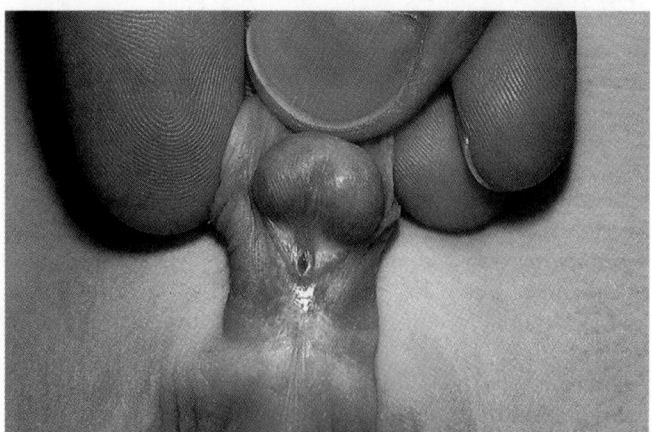

**Fig. 11-26**  Hypospadias. (Courtesy H. Gil Rushton, MD, Children's National Medical Center, Washington, DC.)

the foreskin is usually absent ventrally and, when combined with chordee, gives the organ a hooded and crooked appearance. In severe cases the altered appearance may leave the infant's gender in doubt at birth because the perineal position of the meatus may be mistaken for a female urethra. Because undescended testes may also be present, the small penis may appear to be an enlarged clitoris. In any case of ambiguous genitalia, further study, such as chromosome analysis, is essential. (See Ambiguous Genitalia, p. 487.)

### Surgical Correction

The principal objectives of surgical correction are (1) to enhance the child's ability to void in the standing position with a straight stream, (2) to improve the physical appearance of the genitalia for psychologic reasons, and (3) to preserve a sexually adequate organ. Many procedures have been described that accomplish one or more of these goals. The choice of surgical procedure is affected primarily by the severity of the defect and the presence of associated anomalies. *Glandular hypospadias* (defect noted at the glans penis) may be corrected by a *glans approximation procedure (GAP)* or a *meatal advancement glanuloplasty (MAGPI)* procedure. The GAP requires approximation of the nonjoined urethral opening with lengthening of the urethra and de-epithelialization of skin at the lateral edges of the defect. While the procedure is relatively simple, the potential for urethrocutaneous fistula is significant. The MAGPI requires a dorsal meatotomy with incision of the tissue between the urethral meatus and the glanular groove. The dorsal epithelium is then advanced distally, and care is taken to avoid disrupting the urethra. The ventral skin is then approximated, redundant tissue is carefully excised, and the defect is closed.

More *distal hypospadias* defects typically require alternative approaches. The *Mathieu procedure* may be used for distal hypospadias defects when sufficient ventral skin is present. A skin flap is mobilized that is large enough to reach the tip of the penis. The flap is freed with as much subcutaneous tissue attached as is feasible. Urethral reconstruction is accomplished by reversing the meatal-based flap distally to the glans penis. Specific strategies are used to provide adequate vascular supply to the mobilized skin grafts and to prevent fistula formation. When ventral skin volume is deficient, an *island flap repair* may be used. This procedure requires more extensive use of skin grafts to create the new urethra and close the defect.

Commonly, the chordee that often coexists with a hypospadias defect is repaired by release of the ventral skin described previously. When the chordee persists, additional procedures, such as a *flip-flap procedure, transverse island flap urethroplasty,* or *Mustarde procedure,* may be indicated. Again, more extensive skin flap mobilization is required, and additional reconstruction is used to ensure penile straightening.

Increased surgical experience and improvements in technique have reduced the number of staged procedures needed for hypospadias defects. However, a staged procedure is indicated in particularly severe defects with marked deficits of available skin for mobilization of flaps and in rare cases when scrotal transposition occurs.

The preferred time for surgical repair is 6 to 18 months of age, before the child has developed body image and castration anxiety. Surgical repair of hypospadias as early as 3 months of age has been successful with no higher incidence of complications. Occasionally a short course of testosterone is administered preoperatively to achieve additional penile size to facilitate the surgery.

### Nursing Considerations

Every male newborn should be examined carefully for signs of hypospadias. If the nurse suspects even mild hypospadias, this is reported to the practitioner because circumcision may be delayed to save the foreskin for material to be used in the repair.

Preparation of parents for the type of procedure to be done and the expected cosmetic result helps avert later problems. Frequently parents are informed of what is to be surgically corrected but are not advised of what to expect as a reasonable consequence. As a result, they are greatly disappointed to see a physically imperfect penis. If children are old enough to understand what is occurring, they are also prepared for the operation and the expected outcome.

Hypospadias repair may require some type of urinary diversion with a silicone stent or feeding tube to promote optimum healing and to maintain the position and patency of the newly formed urethra. Sedation may be required for the excessively irritable or restless child, and pain is controlled with analgesics. Epidural anesthesia using a local anesthetic and/or analgesic may be used for the repair and postoperative pain management.

Parents are taught to care for the indwelling catheter or stent and irrigation technique if indicated. They need to know how to empty the urine bag and how to avoid kinking, twisting, or blockage of the catheter or stent. Often the child is discharged with a catheter or stent emptying directly into the diaper. To prevent infection, a tub bath should be avoided until the stent has been removed. An antibacterial ointment may be applied to the penis daily for infection control. In older children a urine collection device can be used. Parents are taught how to tape the drainage bag to the leg to allow the child to be mobile and *never* to clamp off a catheter. An extra bag is sent home with the family in case of tears or leakage. The family is advised to encourage the child to increase fluid intake. Straddle toys, sandboxes, swimming, and rough activities are avoided until allowed by the surgeon.

## Epispadias/Exstrophy Complex

Bladder exstrophy is a severe defect of the GU system characterized by externalization of the bladder, splaying of the urethra with failure of tubular formation, and diastasis (separation) of the pelvic bone (Figs. 11-27 and 11-28). Epispadias is a defect of the urinary system characterized by failure of urethral canalization similar to that seen in exstrophy. Both of these defects are part of a complex of congenital

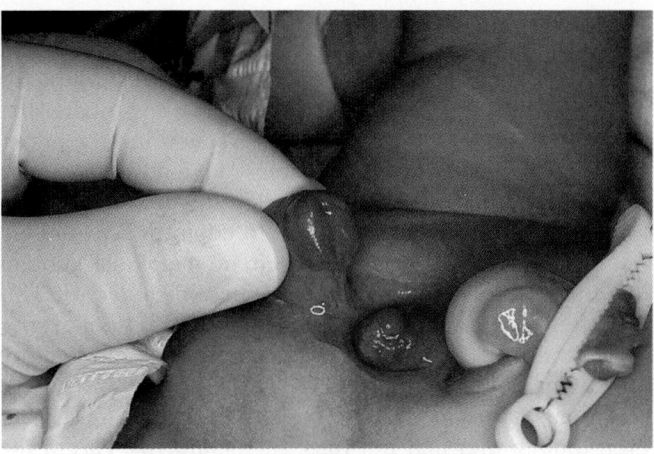

**Fig. 11-27** Newborn with bladder extrophy and epispadias. (Courtesy Tim Yancy, St. Francis Hospital, Tulsa, OK.)

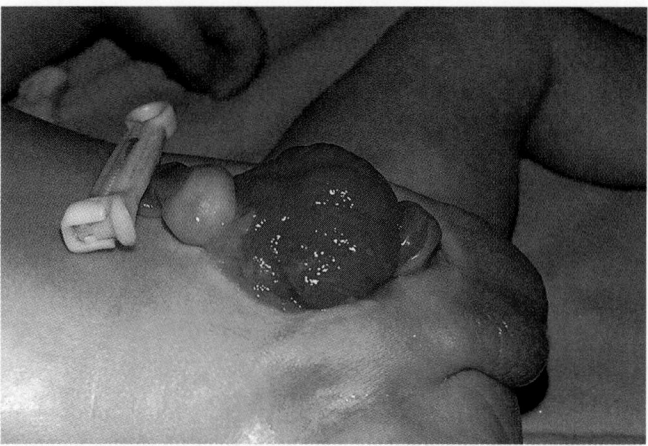

**Fig. 11-28** Exstrophy of bladder. (Courtesy H. Gil Rushton, MD, Children's National Medical Center, Washington, DC.)

anomalies of GU development that range from relatively mild defects (such as glandular epispadias, or a defect on the dorsal surface [topside] of the penile shaft) to severe defects involving multiple organ systems (such as cloacal exstrophy). Fortunately, the incidence of exstrophy/epispadias complex anomalies is small. Exstrophy is estimated to occur in 1 of 10,000 to 50,000 live births; the defect is reportedly more common in males (3:1 ratio to 6:1 ratio) than females (Grady, Carr, and Mitchell, 1999).

## Pathophysiology

Exstrophy results from failure of the abdominal wall and underlying structures, including the ventral wall of the bladder, to fuse in utero. As a result, the lower urinary tract is exposed and the everted bladder appears bright red through the abdominal opening. This is accompanied by a constant seepage of urine from the exposed ureteral orifices, making the area malodorous and susceptible to infection. The constant accumulation of urine on the surrounding skin produces tissue ulceration and further infection. Progressive renal damage from infection and obstruction may cause renal failure if left untreated.

In males the defect is almost always associated with epispadias and may include other problems, such as undescended testes, a short penis, or inguinal hernia. The sexual handicap in males may be severe because the penis protrudes inadequately. In females the genitalia may be affected, with a cleft or bifid clitoris, completely separated labia, and absent vagina. In either sex, separation of the pubic bones causes difficulty in walking, such as a waddling gait.

## Therapeutic Management

The objectives of treatment are (1) preservation of renal function, (2) attainment of urinary control, (3) adequate reconstructive repair for psychologic benefit, and (4) prevention of urinary tract infections, and (5) preservation of optimum external genitalia with continence and sexual function. The correction of an epispadias or bladder exstrophy defect is complex and typically requires multiple surgi-

cal procedures, as well as ongoing management of the urinary system (Canning, Koo, and Duckett, 1996; Grady, Carr, and Mitchell, 1999). For the child with exstrophy, the bladder is closed during the neonatal period, preferably within the first 1 to 2 days of life. Before closure, the bladder is covered with clear plastic wrap or a thin film dressing *without* adhesive. Petroleum jelly is avoided because it tends to damage the bladder mucosa. Following bladder closure, the neonate is monitored for urinary output and for signs of urinary tract or wound infection. At the time of closure, the pelvic diastasis is corrected to prevent the abnormal, waddling gait that occurs when pelvic bone defects are not addressed. Umbilical and inguinal herniorrhaphies may be completed with initial closure in order to reduce the risk of subsequent incarceration, particularly for boys.

During the next 3 to 5 years, urine drains freely from the urethra, which has no sphincter mechanism. This period should allow the bladder to gain capacity while the child grows and matures before subsequent surgical repair. The parents are taught to recognize the signs of urinary tract infection, and the urinary system is regularly monitored via urinalysis and ultrasonographic imaging.

The second phase of exstrophy management is repair of the epispadias and creation of a urethral sphincter mechanism. Epispadias repair should lengthen and straighten the penis to a dependent position and provide a distal urethra adequate for urination and ejaculation. Creation of a urethral sphincter mechanism requires closure of the bladder neck and tubulization of the proximal urethra. Several surgical procedures may be used to accomplish these goals.

Additional procedures may be required for the child with exstrophy. Creation of a urethral sphincter may provide insufficient continence. In this case, suburethral collagen injections or implantation of an artificial urinary sphincter may be performed. Occasionally the bladder fails to achieve an adequate functional capacity and augmentation enterocystoplasty is required. This procedure is typically combined with the creation of a Mitrofanoff appendicial stoma because catheterization is particularly difficult after reconstruction of the proximal urethra (see p. 429).

Sexual function of the child with bladder exstrophy also requires surgical reconstruction. In boys, the testes are typically cryptorchid, and bilateral orchiopexy procedures are combined with reconstruction of the bifid scrotum. In girls, surgical enlargement of the vaginal introitus may be needed to permit intercourse. In both genders, plastic surgery to reduce scarring of the genital area or to create an umbilicus may significantly improve the child's body image and emerging sexual identity.

### Nursing Considerations

Physical care of the unrepaired defect includes meticulous hygiene of the bladder area to prevent infection and excoriation of the surrounding tissue. A sterile nonadherent dressing is placed over the exposed bladder area to prevent infection and to keep the diaper from adhering to the mucosa. An ointment may be prescribed for the surrounding skin to protect it from the constantly draining urine. If external compression is used, the skin is inspected periodically for evidence of pressure necrosis.

Other aspects of preoperative care are similar to those for any major abdominal surgery. If a urine specimen is needed, it can be obtained by allowing urine to drip into a container while holding the child prone over a basin or by aspirating some urine directly from the bladder area into a medicine dropper or syringe. If a sterile specimen is needed for evaluation of existing infection, the former procedure is preferable, but a sterile container must be used. A mechanical and/or bowel preparation may be required.

Postoperative nursing care following bladder neck reconstruction and antireflux surgery (ureteral reimplantation) includes routine wound care and careful monitoring of urinary output from the bladder and/or ureteral drainage tubes. Care following a penile lengthening, chordee release, and urethral reconstruction is similar to care following hypospadias repair.

In addition to routine postsurgical care, nursing following a continent diversion includes wound care, observation of nasogastric suction (surgery requires bowel resection), and measurement and observation of urinary output. In most cases a continent urinary diversion can be surgically created. Clean intermittent catheterization* is used to regularly empty the urinary reservoir.

**Family Support and Home Care.** One of the most devastating aspects of exstrophy of the bladder is its appearance. Although the actual physical care is not difficult, it is not easy for parents to assume responsibility for what to them seems an enormous task because of the emotional impact of the defect.

Parents should be instructed regarding a realistic outcome of surgery because unrealistic expectations of the cosmetic and functional result may leave them very disappointed and discouraged. When possible, continuous care

---

*Home care instructions for clean intermittent catheterization are available in Wong DL, Hess CS: *Clinical manual of pediatric nursing,* ed 5, St Louis, 2000, Mosby.

by one nurse helps the family adjust to all aspects of recovery. As difficult as it was for parents to adjust to the defect at the time of the child's birth, it may be equally disturbing for them to accept the fact that surgical closure does not ensure normal urination and that urinary diversion may be necessary. It is helpful to discuss the long-range advantages of a permanent urinary diversion. A well-fitting ileostomy bag allows the child almost unrestricted freedom in activities enjoyed by other children and results in no major alteration in toileting, except emptying the bag at periodic intervals. This is extremely important to older children and adolescents, who want to be accepted as one of the group and deplore any stigma of being different.

Parents often worry about the child's sexual adjustment, even though they may not voice such concerns. Part of the nursing admission history is directed toward evaluating the parents' (and child's if appropriate) expectation of the surgical repair, knowledge of the possibility of eventual urinary diversion, and feelings concerning this permanent change in body function.

When the infant is discharged with an unrepaired defect, diapers are placed over the defect and are changed frequently to prevent infection, ulceration, and odor. Parents are taught to recognize the signs of urinary tract infection (see Chapter 30) and to report a suspected infection to the practitioner. General infant care remains unchanged except for sponge baths rather than immersion in water.

Even with improved reconstructive surgery for these patients, substantial psychologic support and guidance are needed to help them adjust to their fears of inadequate penile size, appearance of the genitalia, potential inability to procreate, and rejection by peers, especially the opposite sex. Ongoing discussion groups for parents and children are particularly useful in promoting resolution of these fears and allowing for optimum psychologic adjustment, particularly during adolescence.

## Obstructive Uropathy

Structural or functional abnormalities of the urinary system can obstruct the normal flow of urine and compromise function. The area proximal to the site of obstruction is exposed to increased intraluminal pressure, dilation, and urinary stasis. For example, when the bladder outlet is obstructed, the renal pelves and both ureters may become distended, a condition called *ureterohydronephrosis.* However, if one ureterovesical junction is obstructed, the entire ureter and renal pelvis of that side will be affected and the contralateral system will remain normal in appearance and function. Similarly, if the ureteropelvic junction becomes obstructed, the renal pelvis and calyces will become dilated, a condition called *hydronephrosis.*

Obstruction may be congenital or acquired, unilateral or bilateral, complete or incomplete, and chronic or acute (Fig. 11-29). Boys are affected more commonly than girls, but an obstructive uropathy is suspected whenever a child experiences a congenital urinary system defect. Table 11-7 provides a summary of common obstructive sites in children and their nursing implications.

**TABLE 11-7** Common causes of obstructive uropathy in children

| Obstructive Site | Description and Nursing Implications |
| --- | --- |
| Calyx | Congenital infundibular stenosis, intrinsic blockage from a stone, inflammation, or tumor causes calyceal dilation or a diverticulum; the obstructed calyx is typically asymptomatic but it is clinically significant when it serves as a reservoir for infection |
| Ureteropelvic junction | Intrinsic stenosis or extrinsic blockage caused by an anomalous blood vessel, kink, or fibrous band; often detected on prenatal ultrasonography or when diuresis causes acute onset flank pain; a radionuclide scan is used to determine the severity of obstruction and subsequent treatment |
| Ureterovesical junction | Congenital megaureter (congenital obstruction due to unknown cause), acquired intrinsic blockage from stone, tumor, or inflammation, or extrinsic obstruction from tumor; the megaureter may be asymptomatic or may cause urinary tract infection, hematuria, or an abdominal mass |
| Bladder and urethra | Low bladder wall compliance or blockage of the bladder outlet caused by bladder neck contracture or hypertrophy, urethral valves, urethral polyp; congenital urethral obstruction is detected by observing the infant's initial urination; straining or failure to urinate within the first 12-24 hours of life indicates potentially serious urinary system obstruction |
| Functional obstruction | Vesicosphincteric dyssynergia due to spinal anomalies (such as myelodysplasia or spinal injury) or functional causes (Hinman syndrome) often leads to ureterohydronephrosis, vesicoureteral reflux, and chronic voiding dysfunction |

## Pathophysiology

The pathophysiologic changes produced by obstruction are influenced by the location and severity of the blockage and by the presence of complicating factors, such as infection. When the kidney is obstructed, the papilla is flattened, the distal nephron is dilated, and, if the obstruction persists, glomerular filtration is greatly diminished or arrested. Unless the obstruction is relieved, these changes become irreversible, leading to renal insufficiency and atrophy of the affected kidney.

Several factors may magnify the destructive changes associated with obstruction. During the neonatal period the immature kidneys have a higher vascular resistance than do the kidneys of the older child or adult. This condition, combined with the immaturity of the parenchyma, accelerates the occurrence of irreversible renal damage in response to obstruction. Infection also magnifies the destructive changes associated with urinary obstruction. In contrast to the adult, pyelonephritis in the developing kidney of the infant or child leads to renal scarring that reduces the potential for further growth.

Fortunately, when obstruction is restricted to one kidney, compensatory growth occurs in the contralateral kidney. In the infant and child, compensatory growth includes both hypertrophy (enlargement of existing nephrons) and hyperplasia (replication of new cells). Unfortunately, this cannot completely compensate for the loss of renal function created by obstruction of one kidney. Research has identified the presence of a humorally mediated renotrophic factor that modulates this compensation (Chevalier, 1996; Gillenwater and others, 1996).

Obstruction also affects the smooth muscle of the renal pelvis, ureter, and bladder. Obstruction of the ureter and renal pelvis causes dilation in an attempt to overcome the obstruction by stronger peristaltic contractions. Unfortunately, the process of dilation ultimately leads to urinary stasis and loss of smooth muscle tone unless the obstruction is relieved. The detrusor smooth muscle is also affected by obstruction of the bladder outlet. Like the ureter, the bladder initially responds by increasing the force and duration of its

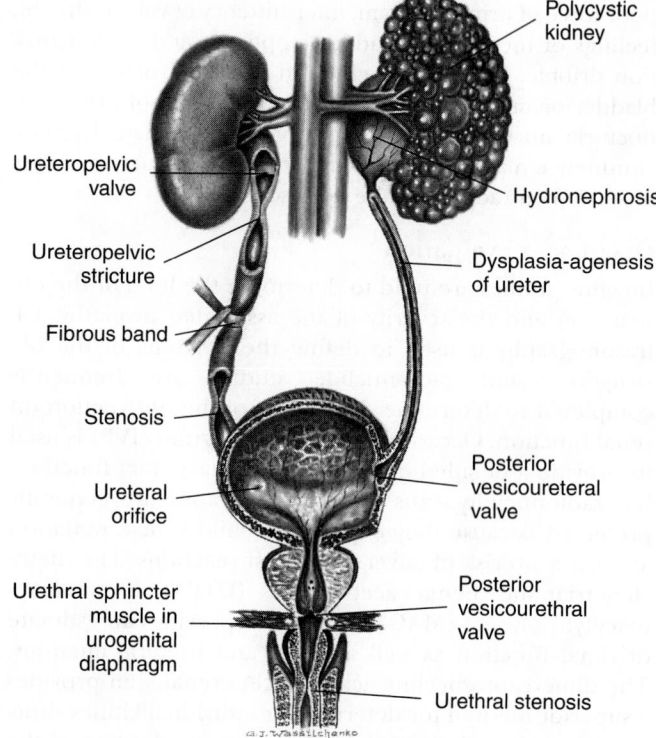

**Fig. 11-29** Major sites of urinary tract obstruction.

contractions. However, when the obstruction persists, the bladder wall becomes trabeculated and the effectiveness of the detrusor contractions is compromised. In addition to these changes, obstruction of the bladder causes neurologic changes that predispose the bladder to unstable (hyperactive) contractions and subsequent urge incontinence.

## Clinical Manifestations

The clinical manifestations of obstructive uropathy depend on the location of the obstructing lesion, its severity, and the underlying cause. Occasionally, ureteropelvic junction (UPJ) obstruction is diagnosed when a child experiences flank pain during an episode of diuresis. However, these conditions are more frequently diagnosed on routine prenatal ultrasonographic examination or when a mass is observed during routine newborn examination. Congenital ureteral obstruction also may be asymptomatic, or the obstruction may cause urinary infections or an abdominal mass. In contrast, obstruction of the renal pelvis, ureter, or ureteropelvic junction due to a urinary calculus produces a characteristic pain called **renal colic.** This pain is characterized by discomfort in the flank, lower back, or lower abdomen. The discomfort is typically intense, and it is not relieved by changes in position. Renal colic typically occurs in the early morning hours and persists until the stone passes or is removed. Narcotic analgesia is frequently required to manage the pain produced by an obstructing stone.

Obstruction of the bladder produces lower urinary tract symptoms. These symptoms are closely related to those produced by other dysfunctional voiding conditions, including detrusor instability and urinary retention. Symptoms include poor force of urinary stream, intermittency of voided stream, feelings of incomplete bladder emptying, and postmicturition dribble. In addition, children with obstruction of the bladder or urethra may experience frequency of urination, nocturia, nocturnal enuresis, or urgency to urinate. Urge incontinence may occur, particularly when obstruction causes unstable contractions of the detrusor muscle.

## Diagnostic Evaluation

Imaging studies are used to determine the level of the obstruction and the severity of the associated uropathy. Ultrasonography is used to define the anatomy of the obstruction, and radionuclide studies are frequently completed to determine the impact of the obstruction on renal function. Occasionally an IV pyelogram (IVP) is used to provide a detailed evaluation of urinary tract function, but radionuclide scans or ultrasonography are generally preferred because they expose the child to less radiation and carry no risk of adverse contrast reactions. The diethylenetriamine penta acetic acid (DTPA) or mercaptoacetyltriglycine (MAG3) renal scan provides an estimate of renal function as well as renal and ureteral anatomy. The dimercaptosuccinic acid (DMSA) renal scan provides a superior method for determining individual kidney function, but this technique does not allow visualization of the renal pelves, ureters, or bladder.

## Therapeutic Management

The management of obstructive uropathy depends on the magnitude of the obstruction and the likelihood that renal function will be compromised unless aggressive intervention is undertaken (Chevalier and Howards, 1998). For example, UPJ obstruction causing hydronephrosis in the neonate may or may not require surgical intervention. In contrast, posterior urethral valve obstruction requires aggressive intervention to prevent progressive, severe, obstructive uropathy affecting the entire urinary system. Whenever feasible, obstruction is treated by a surgical procedure that directly ablates the obstructive lesion. For example, UPJ obstruction is ideally treated by pyelotomy, ure-

thral valves by endoscopic ablation, or obstructing calculi by extracorporeal or endoscopic shock-wave lithotripsy. Urinary flow is temporarily diverted during the postoperative period via a urethral catheter, ureteral stent, or pyelostomy tube (tube inserted directed into the renal pelvis) until postoperative edema subsides and adequate urinary outflow is achieved.

In contrast, transient or permanent urinary diversion may be required for the child with severe obstructive uropathy causing renal insufficiency who is not able to undergo surgery or who has irreversible damage to the lower urinary tract causing an ongoing threat to renal function. Transient diversion can be created at the level of the renal pelvis (pyelostomy), the ureters (ureterostomy), or the bladder (vesicostomy), depending on the level of the obstruction. The stomas created from these procedures are not typically pouched in the neonate; instead, the infant's diaper may be placed higher on the abdomen or a two-diaper system may be used to ensure urinary containment. Permanent urinary diversion may involve an incontinent stoma (the Bricker conduit) or a continent urinary diversion incorporating the bowel, stomach, or a ureter. In contrast to transient diversions, these procedures are reserved for older children and require ongoing pouching or intermittent catheterization.

**Prognosis.** The prognosis depends on the type of obstruction, the degree of irreversible renal damage, whether renal dysplasia is present, the age at which the diagnosis was established, and the severity of complications. Despite the improvements in corrective surgery, some patients develop renal failure, which may evolve over a highly variable period of time that can extend into adulthood. Renal failure can result from hypoplasia-dysplasia, pyelonephritic scarring, and other proposed mechanisms that cause progressive nephron loss. Careful follow-up of children should extend throughout childhood and adolescence, especially when any degree of renal insufficiency is present.

## Nursing Considerations

Nursing goals in urinary tract obstruction include helping to identify cases, assisting with diagnostic procedures, and caring for children with complications. (See Chapter 30.) Preparing parents and children for procedures, especially urinary diversion procedures, is a major nursing responsibility. (See Preparation for Procedures, Chapter 27.)

Parents and children need emotional support and counseling during the lengthy management of these disorders. Parents are the primary target during infancy and very early childhood, when most reparative surgery is performed. They will need assistance in managing the apparatus that accompanies many temporary and permanent repair procedures. Many children are discharged with ureteral drainage systems in place that must be protected from damage, and the danger of infection is a constant concern. Parents are taught to care for the equipment and recognize the signs of possible obstruction or infection within the system. (See Discharge Planning and Home Care, Chapter 26.)

Children with external diversional systems will need psychologic support and guidance, especially as they reach adolescence and body image concerns assume more prominence. Those with progressive renal deterioration may face the prospect of dialysis and/or transplantation and the emotional aspects that accompany these procedures.

## Ambiguous Genitalia

The birth of a child with ambiguous genitalia is a situation that constitutes a crisis quite different from that of many other congenital anomalies. Uncertain gender is a potential lifetime social tragedy for the child and family. Furthermore, the electrolyte disturbances that accompany conditions such as congenital adrenal hyperplasia can be life-threatening. The identification of appropriate gender must be done with precision and accuracy. The assignment of gender is a complex process; the newborn should be examined by a multidisciplinary team that includes a geneticist, a pediatric urologist, an endocrinologist, a pediatrician, and a pediatric surgeon. Although a rapid assignment of gender will help allay some of the parents' anxiety, an erroneous gender determination requiring a later change is even more stressful for the family. The parents may be advised to tell relatives and friends that the newborn has a congenital malformation of the external genitalia that will require some time for doctors to determine the child's sex.

### Etiology

Genetic sex is determined at the time of conception and depends on whether the ovum is fertilized by a sperm bearing an X chromosome or one bearing a Y chromosome. The phenotypic evidence of gender depends on whether subsequent processes proceed normally: differentiation of primitive gonads, differentiation and development of internal duct systems, and differentiation and development of external genitalia. The normal order of events can be altered by abnormalities of the chromosomal complement, defects of embryogenesis, or biochemical (hormonal) abnormalities. Disturbances in any of these processes will lead to abnormal development evidenced by the presence of ambiguous genitalia at birth.

**Normal Genitalia and Reproductive Organ Development.**   For the first 6 weeks of life, the developing embryo is morphologically asexual, neither male nor female. The primitive, bipotential (able to form either a testicle or an ovary) gonad consists of an outer layer (the cortex) and an inner medulla. Differentiation into testes or ovaries takes place during the seventh and eighth weeks of gestation. At this time, in the male the medullary portion develops and the cortical zone regresses; in the female the cortex is preserved while the medulla regresses. Active factors from the male testes cause the müllerian duct system to regress. Without these factors the primitive gonad has an inherent tendency to feminize. The embryonic ovary develops in the absence of male hormone stimulation.

The final stage of genitalia and reproductive organ development is differentiation of the external genitalia, which in the early embryo consists of a urogenital sinus, two lateral labioscrotal swellings, and an anteriorly situated genital tubercle. Depending on the presence or absence of male hormones, the genital tubercle differentiates into a penis or a cli-

toris. In response to testicular androgens, the labiosacral folds fuse to form a scrotum and the ventral skin of the penis; the urethral folds form the perineal and penile urethra. Without the influence of masculinizing secretions, the urethral folds do not fuse and instead become the labia minora, the labiosacral folds remain unfused to separate into the labia majora, and the urogenital sinus differentiates into a lower vagina and the vaginal and urethral openings (Fig. 11-30).

**Abnormal Genitalia and Reproductive Organ Development.**   Disturbances in the normal order of events in gender determination will produce abnormal genitalia and reproductive organ development with the presence of ambiguous or indeterminate external genitalia at birth. Ambiguous genitalia can be variable and may often closely conform to one gender or the other. In some forms, the external sexual structures represent those of a normal male or female, whereas the karyotype is the direct opposite. A situation in which the phenotypic gender differs from the chromosomal gender is often termed *intersex.*

A failure or abnormality in any of the four steps of genitalia and reproductive organ development can lead to abnormal development in subsequent stages. The mechanisms and sites of defective development include:

**Abnormal gender determination**—Chromosome abnormalities result in disturbance of secondary sexual characteristics and reproductive organ development. (See Chapter 5.)

**Abnormal differentiation of gonads**—When induction of the bipotential gonad fails, gender differentiation proceeds in the direction of the female phenotype, regardless of karyotype.

**Abnormal differentiation of ductal systems**—Biologic inactivity of androgenic male organizer substances or insensitivity of ductal tissue to the action of these substances results in a persistent female duct system, which leads to the presence of a uterus and uterine tubes.

**Abnormal secretion of or tissue insensitivity to testicular androgen**—Complete failure of male hormone secretion produces female external genitalia in a genetic male. Partial or incomplete failure results in incomplete masculinization with ambiguity of the external genitalia. The genetic female fetus exposed to large amounts of androgenic hormone may exhibit varying degrees of masculinization of the external genitalia (congenital adrenal hyperplasia).

### Types of Abnormalities

Some disorders with abnormal genitalia development are not characterized by ambiguous genitalia in the newborn period. For example, the most common sex chromosome disorders do not become apparent until later childhood, adolescence, or even young adulthood, when the individual seeks medical attention because of problems of delayed development or infertility. The four conditions producing ambiguous genitalia in the newborn that require prompt and accurate evaluation are the masculinized female, the incompletely masculinized male, the presence of both male and female sexual organs, and mixed gonadal dysgenesis.

Ambiguous genitalia in the newborn is often a result of virilization in the female by adrenal androgens after the time of early gonadal differentiation. The most common type, *congenital adrenogenital hyperplasia (CAH),* is an inherited deficiency of adrenal corticoid hormones. (See Chapter 38.) The resulting decrease in cortisol stimulates pitu-

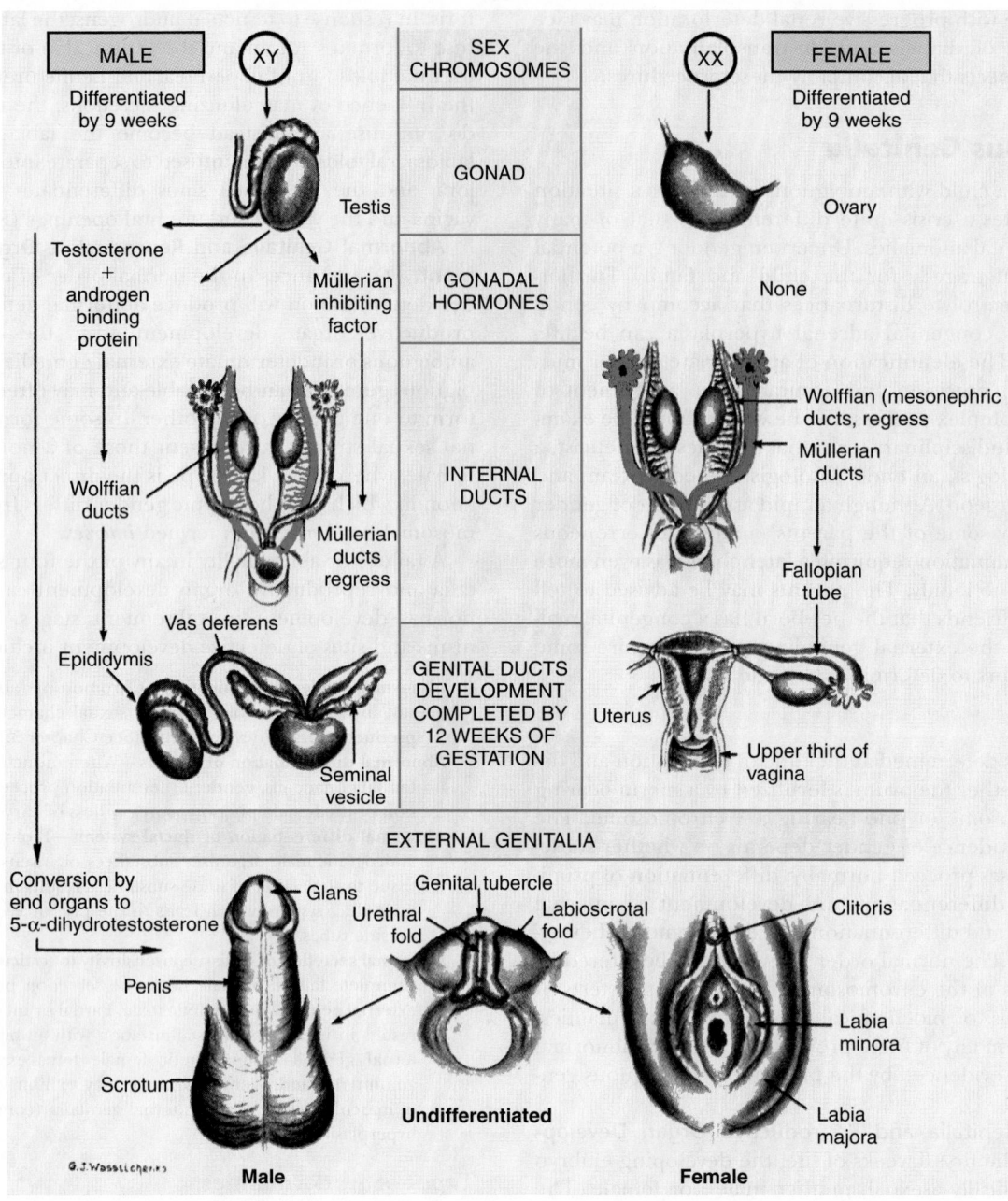

**Fig. 11-30** Sex organ differentiation in male and female. (From Thompson JM and others: *Mosby's manual of clinical nursing*, ed 2, St Louis, 1989, Mosby.)

itary secretion of adrenocorticotropic hormone (ACTH), which causes the adrenal cortex to increase production of adrenal hormones, including the androgens. Because the adrenal gland differentiates later than the gonadal duct system but before differentiation of the external genitalia, masculinization of the external genitalia is the predominant feature. The internal female anatomy is normal. CAH is the only intersex problem that is life-threatening and should be considered in any situation where the child's gender is doubtful.

The external genitalia in the incompletely masculinized male may be incompletely male, ambiguous, or completely female. The complex nature of virilization offers numerous opportunities for disturbance in the process. Defects may be a result of deficient production of fetal androgen, deficiency in any of the enzymes needed for testosterone biosynthesis, or unresponsiveness or subresponsiveness of genital structures to testosterone. Individuals who may be either genetic males or females with *both* ovarian and testicular tissues, with an ovary on one side and a testis on the other, or a combination of ovotestis are rare. The external genitalia may be male (possibly cryptorchid with a micropenis) or normal female, but are ambiguous in the majority of cases.

*Mixed gonadal dysgenesis,* in which affected infants are sex chromosome mosaics, is the second most common disorder.

## TABLE 11-8   Ambiguous genitalia

| Normal Findings | Ambiguous Findings |
| --- | --- |
| **Male** | |
| Penile shaft protrudes from perineum and hangs freely | Micropenis (less than 2.5 to 3 cm [0.8 to 1.0 inches] in newborn) may be enlarged clitoris |
| Urethral meatus centered at tip of glans penis | Urethral meatus anywhere along dorsal or ventral surface of penis, especially on perineum |
| Two scrotal sacs hang freely, covered with loose, wrinkled skin | Small scrotum with smooth, tight skin and any degree of separation in midline may be enlarged labia |
| Palpable testes in each scrotum | Absent testes may be undescended; if combined with small scrotum, may be evidence of enlarged labia |
| **Female** | |
| Small clitoris at anterior end of labia | Enlarged clitoris that protrudes from labia may be small penis |
| Urethral meatus located between clitoris and vagina | Urethal meatus located in clitoris may suggest small penis |
| Labia minora prominent in newborn but atrophied and almost absent in prepubertal female; completely separated from clitoris to posterior vault of vagina; on palpation, no masses in labia | Prominent labia, partially or completely fused with palpable masses on each side, may be small scrotum with testes |

### Box 11-9 ■ ■ ■
### Assessment to Determine a Gender Assignment

**History**—Previous miscarriages (may help identify chromosome aberrations); maternal ingestion of steroids; relatives with ambiguous genitalia or who had an unexplained death in the first weeks of life; maternal ovarian tumor in pregnancy

**Physical examination**—Presence of palpable gonads strongly suggests a male genotype; uterus may be palpable by rectal exam; stretch length of penis to measure location of urethral orifice; location of vaginal orifice

**Chromosome analysis**—Detects chromosome abnormalities and precise genetic karyotype; results are available in 2 to 3 days

**Endoscopy, ultrasonography, and radiographic contrast studies**—Reveal presence, absence, or nature of internal genital and urinary structures

**Biochemical tests**—Include 17-ketosteroids, 17-hydroxycorticoids, and urinary pregnanediol; urinary steroid excretion patterns help detect several of the adrenal cortical syndromes (CAH)

**Laparotomy or gonad biopsy**—In some instances is the only way to arrive at a definitive diagnosis.

(See Errors in Cell Division, Chapter 5.) Genitalia vary greatly, but in those who appear predominantly female, the dysplastic testis may cause masculinization at puberty. The external appearance of the genitalia is described in Table 11-8.

### Diagnostic Evaluation

Diagnostic tools and the significant findings that help determine sex and assist in making a gender assignment are outlined in Box 11-9.

### Therapeutic Management

The assignment of a gender to the infant in whom it is doubtful constitutes a psychosocial emergency. The long-term implications are such that a hasty decision based on appearance alone may be disastrous, and the optimum gender of rearing may not be the same as the genetic or gonadal gender.

The overall goal of management is to enable the affected child to grow into a well-adjusted, psychosocially stable person who is able to identify with the assigned gender and is content with same (Lerman, McAleer, and Kaplan, 2000). Current recommendations for gender assignment involve a number of factors, including.

1. Age at presentation; gender identity is believed to be established by 2½ years of age; therefore changing the child's gender beyond this age is not recommended.

2. Male sexual orientation may be in part determined by the amount of androgen exposure in utero; therefore extent of brain virilization should be evaluated.

3. Females with CAH, or overvirilization, are often successfully managed with steroids and surgical reconstruction of female genitalia.

4. Males with severe hypsopadias and cryptorchidism (undervirilization) may be successfully reared as males, and surgical repair of both defects has been reported to be successful.

5. The child with mixed gonadal dysgenesis may be assigned a gender on the basis of anatomy present and potential for surgical reconstruction; however long-term studies are lacking as to the success of such management (Lerman, McAleer, and Kaplan, 2000).

6. Male infants with micropenis may respond to testosterone and be successfully reared as boys with the possible exception of those with cloacal exstrophy and penile agenesis (Lerman, McAleer, and Kaplan, 2000).

Clearly the decision for gender assignment in cases of ambiguous genitalia is a difficult one and the approach of "one size fits all" is not applicable. In some cases children may reach puberty and request gender reassignment (Phornphutkul, Fausto-Sterling, and Gruppuso, 2000). Each child must be considered individually with adequate input from family and extensive diagnostic evaluation. Families often require long-term counseling and follow-up to ensure the welfare of the child and security in the assigned gender. The American Academy of Pediatrics (2000) has recently recommended guidelines for the diagnosis and management of such children in an effort to minimize trauma to the child and family.

### Nursing Considerations

Families need a great deal of support and encouragement from nurses and other members of the health team to cope with this emotionally charged situation. Parents are confused, anxious, and overwhelmed by feelings of guilt and shame. They may pressure the health care team for immediate gender assignment because they are concerned about the child and the child's future and because they must face questioning relatives and friends. The best approach is honesty. The disorder should be treated as any other disorder, and no attempt should be made to camouflage the problem. The sequence of embryologic events leading to the defect can be explained using correct terminology to describe abnormalities of genitalia and reproductive organs. An understanding of the anomaly assists parents in explaining the defect to others, just as with any other physical defect. It requires sympathy and understanding to deal with parental anxiety during this trying period and to guide them throughout the long-term management. (See Chapter 22.)

## KEY POINTS

- Congenital malformations or anomalies, or "birth defects," are present at birth and are a result of genetic or nongenetic influences.
- Typical reactions of parents to an infant with a physical defect include grief over "loss" of a perfect child, shock, and withdrawal.
- The nurse's primary roles in care of an infant with a physical defect are caregiver, provider of family support, and supplier of information.
- Surgery initiates a number of physiologic responses, including cardiovascular, respiratory, endocrine, renal, gastrointestinal, immune, neurologic, and fluid and electrolyte.
- One of the largest groups of congenital anomalies includes those associated with the embryonic neural tube, the most common of which are spina bifida and myelomeningocele.
- Folic acid supplementation in women before and during pregnancy prevents as many as 50% to 70% of the cases of neural tube defects, anencephaly, and spina bifida.
- Care of the infant and child with myelomeningocele requires both immediate and long-term professional supervision. Associated problems include infection, neurologic damage, impaired renal function, musculoskeletal impairment, and latex allergy.
- Hydrocephalus is a symptom of an underlying brain pathology, demonstrated by impaired absorption of CSF or obstruction to the flow of CSF within the ventricles.
- Therapy for hydrocephalus involves relief of the hydrocephalus, treatment of the underlying brain pathology if possible, prevention and/or treatment of complications, and management of problems related to psychomotor development.
- Treatment of DDH involves maintaining the head of the femur correctly positioned in the acetabulum by means of an external device, usually the Pavlik harness.

- Treatment of clubfoot involves manual overcorrection of the deformity, maintenance of the correction until normal muscle balance is gained, and follow-up observation to detect possible recurrence of the deformity.
- CL deformities are repaired at the earliest opportunity; CP repair may be delayed to take advantage of growth changes.
- Management of CP involves a multidisciplinary approach to care involving professionals from surgery, medicine, nursing, social work, dentistry, speech therapy, and audiology.
- Major nursing challenges with infants born with either cleft involve feeding. Breast-feeding is possible and is encouraged if this is the mother's choice.
- TEF is an abnormal connection between the esophagus and the trachea, placing the untreated infant at risk for life-threatening pulmonary aspiration.
- Anorectal defects are often associated with other congenital anomalies, such as those involving the GI tract and kidneys.
- Congenital diaphragmatic hernia may be diagnosed in the first trimester of pregnancy and usually causes moderate to severe respiratory distress at birth.
- Umbilical and inguinal hernias are common in children and require minor surgical intervention with excellent postoperative recovery.
- Abdominal wall defects, omphalocele and gastroschisis, require careful nursing care involving thermoregulation, fluid management, and prevention of infection pre- and postoperatively.
- GU tract defects are repaired early to promote normal function and psychosocial adjustment.
- In cases of ambiguous genitalia, gender assignment is established following careful evaluation of prenatal and postnatal influences, karyotype, anatomic features, surgical possibilities, future fertility, and potential sexual function.

## REFERENCES

Alderman BW and others: Diagnostic practice and the estimated prevalence of craniosynostosis in Colorado, *Arch Pediatr Adolesc Med* 151(2):159-164, 1997.

Alexander M, Kuo KN: Musculoskeletal assessment of the newborn, *Orthop Nurs* 16(1):21-31, 1997.

American Academy of Pediatrics, Committee on Genetics: Folic acid for the prevention of neural tube defects, *Pediatrics* 104(2 pt 1): 325-327, 1999.

American Academy of Pediatrics, Committee on Genetics: Evaluation of the newborn with developmental anomalies of the external genitalia, *Pediatrics* 106(1):138-142, 2000.

American Academy of Pediatrics, Task Force on Infant Sleep Position and Sudden Infant Death Syndrome: Changing concepts of sudden infant death syndrome: implications for infant sleeping environment and sleep position, *Pediatrics* 105(3):650-656, 2000a.

American Nurses' Association: Position statement on latex allergy, *Okla Nurse* 42(4):32-33, 1997.

Andres JM: Neonatal hepatobiliary disorders, *Clin Perinatol* 23(2):321-352, 1996.

Beckler L: Cleft palates, *AWHONN Lifelines* 1(6):11, 1997 (letter).

Bellinger MF: Myelomeningocele and neuropathic bladder. In Gillenwater JY and others, editors: *Adult and pediatric urology,* ed 3, St Louis, 1996, Mosby.

Bender PL: Genetics of cleft lip and palate, *J Pediatr Nurs* 15(4):242-249, 2000.

Bennett JK and others: Collagen injections for intrinsic sphincter deficiency in the neuropathic urethra, *Paraplegia* 33(12):697-700, 1995.

Bukowski TP, Zeman PA: Hypospadias: of concern but correctable, *Contemp Pediatr* 18(2):89-109, 2001.

Bulas DI, Fonda JS: Prenatal evaluation of fetal anomalies, *Pediatr Clin North Am* 44(3):537-553, 1997.

Canning DA, Koo HP, Duckett JW: Anomalies of the bladder and cloacae. In Gillenwater JY and others, editors: *Adult and pediatric urology*, ed 3, St Louis, 1996, Mosby.

Carceller A and others: Past and future of biliary atresia, *J Pediatr Surg* 35(5):717-720, 2000.

Centers for Disease Control and Prevention: Chorionic villus sampling and amniocentesis: recommendations for prenatal counseling, *MMWR* 44(RR-9):1, 1995.

Centers for Disease Control and Prevention: Knowledge and use of folic acid by women in childbearing age—United States, 1995 and 1998, *MMWR* 48(16):325-327, 1999.

Centers for Disease Control and Prevention: Knowledge and use of folic acid among women of reproductive age—Michigan, 1998, *MMWR* 50(10):185-189, 2001.

Chambers GK and others: Assessment of the appropriateness of services provided by a multidisciplinary myelomeningocele clinic, *Pediatr Neurosurg* 24(1):92-97, 1996.

Chevalier RL: Growth factors and apoptosis in neonatal ureteral obstruction, *J Am Soc Nephrol* 7(8):1098-1105, 1996.

Chevalier RL, Howards SS: Renal function in the fetus, neonate and child. In Walsh PC and others, editors: *Campbell's urology*, ed 7, Philadelphia, 1998, WB Saunders, Harcourt.

Cohen M: Immediate unrestricted feeding of infants following cleft lip and palate repair, *Br J Plast Surg* 50(2):143, 1997 (letter to editor).

Conversations with colleagues: Breastfeeding and cleft palates, *AWHONN Lifelines* 1(4):23, 1997.

Cooperman DR, Thompson GH: Congenital abnormalities of the upper and lower extremities and spine. In Fanaroff AA, Martin RJ, editors: *Neonatal-perinatal medicine: diseases of the fetus and infant*, ed 6, St Louis, 1997, Mosby.

Darzi MA, Chowdri NA, Bhat AN: Breast feeding or spoon feeding after cleft lip repair: a prospective, randomised study, *Br J Plast Surg* 49(1):24-26, 1996.

Dias MS, Li V: Pediatric neurosurgical disease, *Pediatr Clin North Am* 45(6):1539-1578, 1998.

Dias MS, Veetai L: Pediatric neurosurgical disease, *Pediatr Clin North Am* 45(6):1539-1578, 1998.

Donlon CR, Furdon SA, Clark DA: Look before you clamp: delivery room examination of the umbilical cord, *Advan Neonatal Care* 2(1):19-26, 2002.

Evans MI and others: Impact of folic acid supplementation in the United States: markedly diminished high maternal serum AFPs, *Obstet Gynecol* 97(suppl 1):S42, 2001.

Fernandes ET and others: Neurogenic bladder dysfunction in children: review of pathophysiology and current management, *J Pediatr* 124(1):1-7, 1994.

Flake AW, Ryckman FC: Selected anomalies and intestinal obstruction. In Fanaroff AA, Martin RJ, editors: *Neonatal-perinatal medicine: diseases of the fetus and infant*, ed 6, St Louis, 1997, Mosby.

Flake AW and others: Treatment of severe congenital diaphragmatic hernia by fetal tracheal occlusion: clinical experience with fifteen cases, *Am J Obstet Gynecol* 183(5):1059-1066, 2000.

Forrester MB, Merz RD: Epidemiology of abdominal wall defects, Hawaii, 1986-1997, *Teratology* 60(3):117-123, 1999.

Gill FT: Umbilical hernia, inguinal hernias, and hydroceles in children: diagnostic clues for optimal patient management, *J Pediatr Health Care* 12(5):231-235, 1998.

Gillenwater JY and others: *Adult and pediatric urology*, ed 3, St Louis, 1996, Mosby.

Grady RW, Carr MC, Mitchell ME: Complete primary closure of bladder exstrophy. Epispadias and bladder exstrophy repair, *Urol Clin North Am* 26(1):95-109, 1999.

Grant JA, McLone DG: Third ventriculostomy: a review, *Surg Neurol* 47(3):210-212, 1997.

Gray ML: Anatomy related to urinary function. In Broadwell DB, Parrish RS, Saunders RC, editors: *Child health nursing*, Philadelphia, 1993, JB Lippincott.

Gross SM and others: Inadequate folic acid intakes are prevalent among young women with neural tube defects, *J Am Diet Assoc* 101(3):342-345, 2001.

Guardino KO: Anorectal malformations in children. In Wise BV and others, editors: *Nursing care of the general pediatric surgical patient*, Gaithersburg, MD, 2000, Aspen.

Halamek LP, Stevenson DK: Neonatal jaundice and liver disease. In Fanaroff AA, Martin RJ, editors: *Neonatal-perinatal medicine: diseases of the fetus and infant*, ed 6, St Louis, 1997, Mosby.

Harrison MR: Surgically correctable fetal disease, *Am J Surg* 180(5):335-342, 2000.

Haslam RHA: The nervous system. In Behrman RE, Kliegman RM, Jenson HB, editors: *Nelson textbook of pediatrics*, ed 16, Philadelphia, 2000, WB Saunders.

Hay SA and others: Neonatal jaundice: the role of laparoscopy, *J Pediatr Surg* 35(12):1706-1709, 2000.

Henshaw SK: Unintended pregnancy in the United States, *Fam Plann Perspect* 30(1):24-29, 46, 1998.

Hoffinger SA: Evaluation and management of pediatric foot deformities, *Pediatr Clin North Am* 43(5):1091-1111, 1996.

Holzbeierlein J and others: The urodynamic profile of myelodysplasia childhood with spinal closure during gestation, *J Urol* 164(4):1336-1339, 2000.

Howell LJ, SK Von Nessen, Burns KM: Fetal surgery. In Wise BV and others, editors: *Nursing care of the general pediatric surgical patient*, Gaithersburg, MD, 2000, Aspen.

Hudgins RJ, Boydston WR, Gilbreath CL: Treatment of posthemorrhagic hydrocephalus in the preterm infant with a ventricular access device, *Pediatr Neurosurg* 29(6):309-313, 1998.

Jackson IT, Beal B: Early feeding after cleft repair, *Br J Plast Surg* 50(2):217, 1997 (letter to editor).

Juretschke LJ: Congenital diaphragmatic hernia: update and review, *JOGNN* 30(3):259-268, 2001.

Kaefer M and others: Continent urinary diversion: the Children's Hospital experience, *J Urol* 157(4):1394-1399, 1997.

Kaefer M and others: Improved bladder function after prophylactic treatment of the high risk neurogenic bladder in newborns with myelomeningocele, *J Urol* 162(3 pt 2):1068-1071, 1999.

Kapp-Simon KA, Krueckeberg S: Mental development in infants with cleft lip and/or palate, *Cleft Palate Craniofac J* 37(1):65-70, 2000.

Kapur P, Caty MG, Glick PL: Pediatric hernias and hydroceles, *Pediatr Clin North Am* 45(4):773-789, 1998.

Katz AL, Wiswell TE, Baumgart S: Contemporary controversies in the management of congenital diaphragmatic hernia, *Clin Perinatol* 25(1):219-248, 1998.

Kelalis PP, King LR, Belman AB, editors: *Clinical pediatric urology*, Philadelphia, 1992, WB Saunders.

Kellett PB: Latex allergy: a review, *J Emerg Nurs* 23(1):27-36, 1997.

Kilby MD, Lander A, Usher-Somers M: Exomphalos (omphalocele), *Prenat Diagn* 18(12):1283-1288, 1998.

Kitchanan S and others: Neonatal outcome of gastroschisis and exomphahalos: a 10-year review, *J Paediatr Child Health* 36(5):428-430, 2000.

Kogo M and others: Breast feeding for cleft lip and palate patients, using the Hotz-type plate, *Cleft Palate Craniofac J* 34(4):351-353, 1997.

Kyzer SP, Stark SL: Congenital idiopathic clubfoot deformities, *AORN J* 61(3):492-505, 1995.

Landwehr LP, Boguniewicz M: Current perspectives on latex allergy, *J Pediatr* 128(3):305-312, 1996.

Lawrence RA, Lawrence RM: *Breastfeeding: a guide for the medical profession*, ed 5, St Louis, 1999, Mosby.

Lawton KH, Meyers M, Donahue EM: Current practices and advances in pediatric neurosurgery, *Nurs Clin North Am* 32(1):73-96, 1997.

Lee J, Nunn J, Wright C: Height and weight achievement in cleft lip and palate, *Arch Dis Child* 76(1):70-72, 1997.

Lerman SE, McAleer IM, Kaplan GW: Sex assignment in cases of ambiguous genitalia and its outcome, *Urology* 55(1):8-11, 2000.

Lutkenhoff M, editor: *Children with spina bifida: a parent's guide*, Bethesda, MD, 1999, Woodbine House.

Maher AB, Salmond SW, Pellino TA, editors: *Orthopaedic nursing*, ed 2, Philadelphia, 1998, WB Saunders.

Maris CL and others: Are infants with orofacial clefts at risk for insecure mother-child attachments? *Cleft Palate Craniofac J* 37(3):257-265, 2000.

Mazon A and others: Latex sensitization in children with spina bifida: follow-up comparative study after two years, *Ann Allergy Asthma Immunol* 84:207-210, 2000.

McEvoy CF, Suchy FJ: Biliary tract disease in children, *Pediatr Clin North Am* 43(1):75-98, 1996.

McGee S, Burkett KW: Identifying common pediatric neurosurgical conditions in the primary care setting, *Nurs Clin North Am* 35(1):61-85, 2000.

McIntyre F: Craniosynostosis, *Am Fam Physician* 55(4):1173-1178, 1997.

McMahon MJ, Kuller JA, Chescheir NC: Prenatal ultrasonographic findings associated with short bowel syndrome in two fetuses with gastroschisis, *Obstet Gynecol* 4(pt 2):676-678, 1996.

Menkes JH, Sarnat HB: Malformations of the central nervous system. In Menkes JH, Sarnat HB, editors: *Child neurology*, ed 6, Philadelphia, 2000, Lippincott Williams & Wilkins.

Minkes RK and others: Routine insertion of a Silastic spring-loaded silo for infants with gastroschisis, *J Pediatr Surg* 35(6):843-846, 2000.

Mitchell JC, Wood RJ: Management of the cleft lip and palate in primary care, *J Pediatr Health Care* 14(1):13-19, 2000.

Molik KA and others: Gastroschisis: a plea for risk categorization, *J Pediatr Surg* 36(1): 51-55, 2001.

Muratore CS, Wilson JM: Congenital diaphragmatic hernia: where are we and where do we go from here? *Semin Perinatol* 24(6):418-428, 2000.

Muratore CS and others: Pulmonary morbidity in 100 survivors of congenital diaphragmatic hernia monitored in a multidisciplinary clinic, *J Pediatr Surg* 36(1):133-140, 2001.

Murshid WR: Endoscopic third ventriculostomy: towards more indications for the treatment of non-communicating hydrocephalus, *Minim Invasive Neurosurg* 43(2):75-82, 2000.

Neiman GS, Savage H: Development of infants and toddlers with clefts from birth to three years of age, *Cleft Palate Craniofac J* 34(3):218-225, 1997.

Novacheck TF: Developmental dysplasia of the hip, *Pediatr Clin North Am* 43(4):829-848, 1996.

Olutoye OO, Adzick NS: Fetal surery for myelomeningocele, *Semin Perinatol* 23(6):462-473, 1999.

Peeker R and others: The urological fate of young adults with myelomeningocele: a three decade follow-up study, *Eur Urol* 32(2):213-217, 1997.

Pelosi L: The role of the advanced practice nurse in pediatric general surgery, *Nurs Clin North Am* 35(1):159-170, 2000.

Penã A: Current management of anorectal anomalies, *Surg Clin North Am* 72(6):1393-1416, 1992.

Penã A, Hong A: Advances in the management of anorectal malformations, *Am J Surg* 180(5):370-376, 2000.

Phornphutkul C, Fausto-Sterling A, Grupposo PA: Gender self-reassignment in an XY adolescent female born with ambiguous genitalia, *Pediatrics* 106(1):135-137, 2000.

Pillai SB, Besner GE: Pediatric testicular problems, *Pediatr Clin North Am* 45(4):813-830, 1998.

Poley GE, Slater JE: Latex allergy, *J Allergy Clin Immunol* 105(6 pt 1):1054-1062, 2000.

Pope W: External ventriculostomy: a practical application for the acute care nurse, *J Neurosci Nurs* 30(3):185-190, 1998.

Raco A and others: Congenital torticollis in association with craniosynostosis, *Childs Nerv Syst* 15(4):163-168, 1999.

Rauen K, editor: *Guidelines for spina bifida health care services throughout life*, Washington, DC, 1995, Spina Bifida Association of America.

Richard M: Feeding the newborn with cleft lip and/or palate: the enlargement, stimulate, swallow rest (ESSR) method, *J Pediatr Nurs* 6(5):317-321, 1991.

Rintoul NE and others: A new look at myelomenigoceles: functional level, vertebral level, shunting, and the implications for fetal intervention, *Pediatrics* 109(3):409-413, 2002.

Ryckman FC and others: Improved survival in biliary atresia patients in the present era of liver transplantation, *J Pediatr Surg* 28(3):382-386, 1993.

Sandburg DJ, Magee WP, Denk MJ: Neonatal cleft lip and cleft palate repair, *AORN J* 75(3):490-499, 2002.

Sarwark JF: Spina bifida, *Pediatr Clin North Am* 43(5):1151-1159, 1996.

Shaw GM and others: Orofacial clefts, parental cigarette smoking, and transforming growth factor-alpha gene variants, *Am J Human Genetics* 58(3):551-561, 1996.

Sloan GM and others: Surgical treatment of craniosynostosis: outcome analysis of 250 consecutive patients, *Pediatrics* 100(1):124, 1997.

Sokol RJ: Etiopathogenesis of biliary artresia, *Sem Liver Disease* 21(4):517-524, 2001.

Speltz ML and others: Early predictors of attachment in infants with cleft lip and/or palate, *Child Dev* 68(1):12-25, 1997.

Stevenson R and others: Decline in prevalence of neural tube defects in a high-risk region of the United States, *Pediatrics* 106(4):677-683, 2000.

Sussman GL, Beezhold DH: Latex allergy: a clinical perspective, *Surg Serv Manage* 4(2):25-28, 1997.

Tarcan T and others: Long-term followup of newborns with myelodysplasia and normal urodynamic findings: is followup necessary? *J Urol* 165(2):564-567, 2001.

Thomas DFM: Embryology. In: Mundy AR and others, editors: *The scientific basis of urology*, Oxford, GB, 1999, Isis Medical.

Thompson GH, Scoles PV: Bone and joints disorders: orthopedic problems. In Behrman RE, Kliegman RM, Jenson HB, editors: *Nelson textbook of pediatrics*, ed 16, Philadelphia, 2000, WB Saunders.

Tulipan N, Bruner JP: Myelomeningocele repair in utero: a report of three cases, *Pediatr Neurosurg* 28(4):177-180, 1998.

Van der Werf WJ and others: Infant pediatric liver transplantation results equal those for older pediatric patients, *J Pediatr Surg* 33(1):20-23, 1998.

Volpe JJ: *Neurology of the newborn*, ed 4, Philadelphia, 2001, WB Saunders.

Walker J, Meijer JG: Neuroendoscopic third ventriculostomy: a nursing perspective, *J Neurosci Nurs* 27(2):78-82, 1995.

Wall EJ: Practical primary pediatric orthopedics, *Nurs Clin North Am* 35(1):95-113, 2000.

Walsh DS, Adzick NS: Fetal surgical intervention, *Am J Perinatol* 17(6):277-283, 2000.

Whitington PF: Chronic cholestasis of infancy, *Pediatr Clin North Am* 43(1):1-77, 1996.

Woods RJ, Jurkiewicz MJ: Plastic and reconstructive surgery. In Schwartz S, editor: *Principles of surgery*, ed 7, Philadelphia, 1999, McGraw-Hill.

Williams DG, Hayes J, McCool S: Shunt infections in children: presentation and management, *J Neurosci Nurs* 28(3):155-162, 1996.

Wu HY, Baskin LS, Kogan BA: Neurogenic bladder dysfunction due to myelomeningocele: neonatal versus childhhod treatment, *J Urol* 157(6):2295-2297, 1997.

Zsolt S, and others: Latex sensitization in spina bifida appears disease-associated, *J Pediatr* 134(3):344-348, 1999.

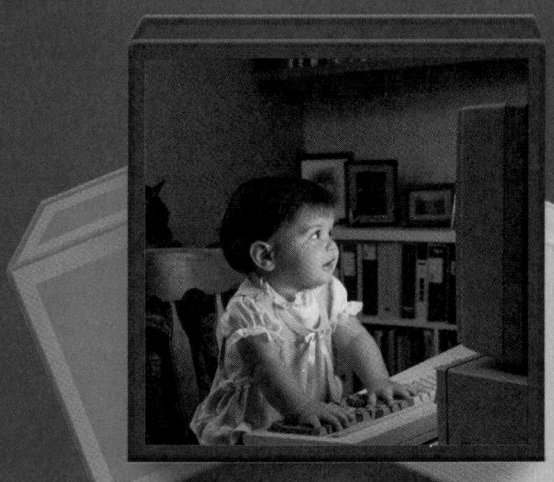

Chapter **12**

# Health Promotion of the Infant and Family

## Chapter Outline

**PROMOTING OPTIMUM GROWTH AND DEVELOPMENT, 494**
**Biologic Development, 494**
    Proportional Changes, 494
    Sensory Changes, 495
    Maturation of Systems, 496
    Fine Motor Development, 498
    Gross Motor Development, 498
**Psychosocial Development, 501**
    Developing a Sense of Trust
        (Erikson), 501
**Cognitive Development, 502**
    Sensorimotor Phase (Piaget), 502
**Development of Body Image, 504**
**Development of Sexual Identity, 504**
**Social Development, 504**
    Attachment, 504
    Language Development, 506
    Personal-Social Behavior, 506
    Play, 507
**Temperament, 507**
    Childrearing Practices Related to
        Temperament, 509

**Coping with Concerns Related to Normal
    Growth and Development, 514**
    Separation Anxiety and Stranger Fear, 514
    Spoiled Child Syndrome, 515
    Limit-Setting and Discipline, 516
    Alternate Child Care
        Arrangements, 516
    Thumb Sucking and Use of
        Pacifier, 518
    Teething, 519
    Infant Shoes, 519
**PROMOTING OPTIMUM HEALTH
DURING INFANCY, 520**
**Nutrition, 520**
    The First 6 Months, 520
    The Second 6 Months, 521
    Selection and Preparation of Solid
        Foods, 522
    Food Storage, 523
    Method of Introduction, 523
    Weaning, 524
**Sleep and Activity, 525**
    Sleep Problems, 525

**Dental Health, 527**
**Immunizations, 527**
    Schedule for Immunizations, 528
    Recommendations for Routine
        Immunizations, 530
    Recommendations for Selected
        Immunizations, 535
    Reactions, 535
    Contraindications/Precautions, 535
    Administration, 538
**Injury Prevention, 541**
    Aspiration of Foreign Objects, 541
    Suffocation, 544
    Motor Vehicle Injuries, 545
    Falls, 546
    Poisoning, 547
    Burns, 547
    Drowning, 548
    Bodily Damage, 548
    Nurse's Role in Injury
        Prevention, 548
**Anticipatory Guidance—
    Care of Families, 550**

## Related Topics

Animal Bites, Ch. 18
Communicable Diseases, Ch. 16
Dental Health, Ch. 14
Health Problems During Infancy, Ch. 13
Infant Mortality, Ch. 1
Ingestion of Injurious Agents, Ch. 16
Injuries—The Leading Killer, Ch. 1

Injury Prevention, Ch. 14
Intramuscular Administration (of
    Medication), Ch. 27
Limit-Setting and Discipline, Ch. 3
Paroxysmal Abdominal Pain (Colic), Ch. 13
Preschool and Kindergarten Experience, Ch. 15

Promotion of Parent-Infant Bonding
    (Attachment), Ch. 8
Provision of Optimum Nutrition, Ch. 8
Separation Anxiety, Ch. 26
Sudden Infant Death Syndrome (SIDS), Ch. 13
Sunburn, Ch. 18
Temperament, Ch. 14

# PROMOTING OPTIMUM GROWTH AND DEVELOPMENT

## Biologic Development

At no other time in life are physical changes and developmental achievements so dramatic as during infancy. All body systems undergo progressive maturation. Concurrent development of skills increasingly allows infants to respond to the environment. Acquisition of these fine and gross motor skills occurs in an orderly head-to-toe and center-to-periphery (cephalocaudal-proximodistal) sequence.

### Proportional Changes

Growth is very rapid during the first year, especially during the initial 6 months. Infants gain 680 g (1½ pounds) per month until age 5 months, when the birth weight has at least doubled. An average weight for a 6-month-old child is 7.26 kg (16 pounds). Weight gain decreases by half that amount during the second 6 months. By 1 year of age the infant's birth weight has tripled, to an average weight of 9.75 kg (21½ pounds). Infants who are breast-fed beyond 4 to 6 months of age typically gain less weight than those who are bottle-fed, yet head circumference is more than adequate (Lawrence and Lawrence, 1999). (See Family Focus Box, p. 277.)

Height increases by 2.5 cm (1 inch) per month during the first 6 months and by half that amount per month during the second 6 months. Increases in length occur in sudden spurts rather than in a slow, gradual pattern. Average height is 65 cm (25½ inches) at 6 months and 74 cm (29

---

■ David Wilson, MS, RNC, revised this chapter.

inches) at 12 months. By 1 year birth length has increased by almost 50%. This increase occurs mainly in the trunk rather than the legs and contributes to the characteristic physique of the older infant (see Fig. 12-9, *A*).

Head growth is also rapid and an important determinant of brain growth. During the first 6 months head circumference increases approximately 2 cm (3/4 inch) per month from birth to 3 months, 1 cm per month from 4 to 6 months, and decreases to 0.5 cm (1/4 inch) per month during the second 6 months (Johnson and Blasco, 1997). The average size is 43 cm (17 inches) at 6 months and 46 cm (18 inches) at 12 months. By 1 year of age head size has increased by almost 33%. Closure of the cranial sutures occurs, with the posterior fontanel fusing by 6 to 8 weeks of age and the anterior fontanel closing by 12 to 18 months of age (the average age being 14 months). It is important to note that infant growth is strongly influenced by genetic, metabolic, environmental, and nutritional factors; thus, the previous statements are general guidelines only. Appropriate growth charts reflecting weight for length and head circumference should be used in each case to determine appropriate growth parameters.

Expanding head size reflects the growth and differentiation of the nervous system. By the end of the first year the brain has increased in weight approximately two and one half times. Maturation of the brain is exhibited in the dramatic developmental achievements of infancy (see Table 12-3). The primitive reflexes (see Table 8-4) are replaced by voluntary, purposeful movement, and new reflexes that influence motor development appear (Box 12-1).

The chest assumes a more adult contour, with the lateral diameter becoming larger than the anteroposterior diameter. The chest circumference approximately equals head circumference by the end of the first year. The heart grows less rapidly than does the rest of the body. Its weight is usually doubled by 1 year of age in comparison with body weight, which triples during the same period. The size of the heart is still large in relation to the chest cavity; its width is approximately 55% of the chest width.

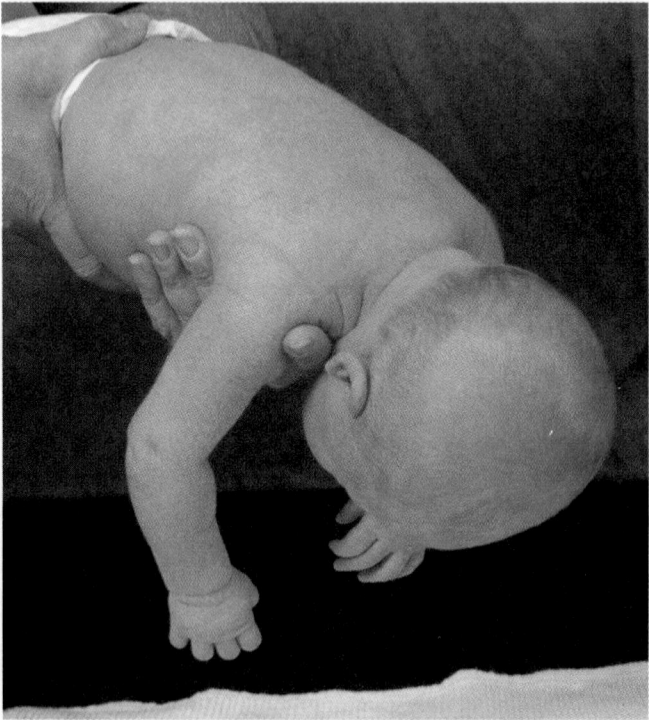

**Fig. 12-1**  Parachute reflex. (Courtesy Paul Vincent Kuntz, Texas Children's Hospital.)

---

> **Box 12-1** ■ ■ ☐
> ## Neurologic Reflexes That Appear During Infancy
>
> **Labyrinth-righting**—Infant in prone or supine position is able to raise head; appears at 2 months, strongest at 10 months
> **Neck-righting**—While infant is supine, head is turned to one side; shoulder, trunk, and finally pelvis will turn toward that side; appears at 3 months, until 24-36 months
> **Body-righting**—A modification of the neck-righting reflex in which turning hips and shoulders to one side causes all other body parts to follow; appears at 6 months, until 24-36 months
> **Otolith-righting**—When body of an erect infant is tilted, head is returned to upright, erect position; appears at 7-12 months, persists indefinitely
> **Landau**—When infant is suspended in a horizontal prone position, the head is raised and legs and spine are extended; appears at 6-8 months, until 12-24 months
> **Parachute**—When infant is suspended in a horizontal prone position and suddenly thrust downward, hands and fingers extend forward as if to protect against falling (Fig. 12-1); appears at 7-9 months, persists indefinitely

## Sensory Changes

During infancy, visual acuity gradually improves and binocular fixation is established. The major developmental characteristics of vision during infancy are listed in Box 12-2.

*Binocularity,* or the fixation of two ocular images into one cerebral picture (fusion), begins to develop by 6 weeks of age and should be well established by age 4 months (Fig. 12-2). Lack of binocular vision results in strabismus and must be detected early to prevent permanent blindness.

*Depth perception (stereopsis)* begins to develop by age 7 to 9 months but may exist earlier as an innate safety mechanism. Studies have demonstrated that even 2- to 3-month-old infants distinguish depth. At approximately 7 months the parachute reflex appears and may be a protective response during a fall (see Fig. 12-1 and Box 12-1).

Infants have a *visual preference* for looking at the human face; this preference also has a developmental sequence. At age 6 weeks infants show more interest in a picture of a face with eyes than in one without eyes. By 10 weeks of age a picture with both eyes and eyebrows elicits more response,

and by 20 weeks of age the mouth is also necessary. By age 6 months infants respond to facial expressions and can distinguish between familiar and strange faces. This is about the time that separation anxiety is manifested (see p. 505).

With progressive myelination of the auditory pathway, the specific responses of locating sound replace the generalized response of the neonate. The major developmental characteristics of hearing are listed in Box 12-3. (For further discussion of hearing and the senses of smell, taste, and touch, see Chapter 8.)

---

### Box 12-2 ■ ■ □
### Major Developmental Characteristics of Vision

| AGE (WEEKS) | DEVELOPMENT |
|---|---|
| Birth | Visual acuity 20/100-20/400* |
| | Pupillary and corneal (blink) reflexes present |
| | Able to fixate on moving object in range of 45 degrees when held 20-25 cm (8-10 inches) away |
| | Cannot integrate head and eye movements well (doll's eye reflex—eyes lag behind if head is rotated to one side) |
| 4 | Can follow in range of 90 degrees |
| | Can watch parent intently as he or she speaks to infant |
| | Tear glands begin to function |
| | Visual acuity is hyperoptic because of less spheric eyeball than in adult |
| 6-12 | Has peripheral vision to 180 degrees |
| | Binocular vision begins at age 6 weeks, is well established by age 4 months |
| | Convergence on near objects begins by age 6 weeks, is well developed by age 3 months |
| | Doll's eye reflex disappears |
| 12-20 | Recognizes feeding bottle |
| | Able to fixate a 1.25 cm (½ inch) block |
| | Looks at hand while sitting or lying on back |
| | Able to accommodate to near objects |
| 20-28 | Adjusts posture to see an object |
| | Able to rescue a dropped toy |
| | Develops color preference for yellow and red |
| | Able to discriminate between simple geometric forms |
| | Prefers more complex visual stimuli |
| | Develops hand-eye coordination |
| 28-44 | Can fixate on very small objects |
| | Depth perception begins to develop |
| | Lack of binocular vision indicates strabismus |
| 44-52 | Visual acuity, 20/40-20/60 |
| | Visual loss may develop if strabismus is present |
| | Can follow rapidly moving objects |

*Measurement of visual acuity differs according to testing procedures. (See Chapter 7.)

---

### Box 12-3 ■ ■ □
### Major Developmental Characteristics of Hearing

| AGE (WEEKS) | DEVELOPMENT |
|---|---|
| Birth | Responds to loud noise by startle or Moro reflex |
| | Responds to sound of human voice more readily than to any other sound |
| | Low-pitched sounds, such as lullaby, metronome, or heartbeat, have quieting effect |
| 8-12 | Turns head to side when sound is made at level of ear |
| 12-16 | Locates sound by turning head to side and looking in same direction (see Fig. 12-2) |
| 16-24 | Locates sound by turning head to side and then looking up or down |
| 24-32 | Locates sounds by turning head in a curving arc |
| | Responds to own name |
| 32-40 | Localizes sounds by turning head diagonally and directly toward sound |
| 40-52 | Knows several words and their meaning, such as "no," and names of members of the family |
| | Learns to control and adjust own response to sound, such as listening for the sound to occur again |

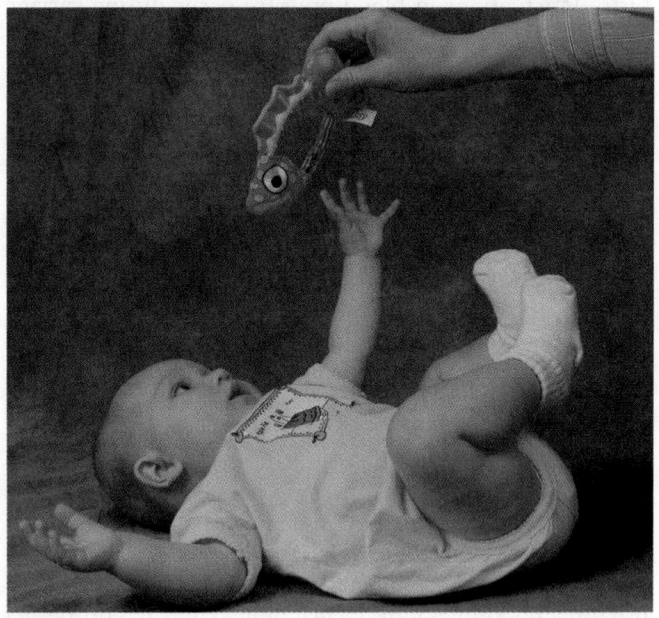

**Fig. 12-2** Three-month-old infant focuses on visual object and reaches toward it. (Courtesy Paul Vincent Kuntz, Texas Children's Hospital.)

## Maturation of Systems

Other organ systems also change and grow during infancy. The *respiratory* rate slows somewhat (see inside back cover) and is relatively stable. Respiratory movements continue to be abdominal. Several factors predispose the infant to more severe and acute respiratory problems. The close proximity of the trachea to the bronchi and its branching structures rapidly transmits an infectious agent from one anatomic location to another. The short, straight eustachian tube closely communicates with the ear, allowing infection to ascend from the pharynx to the middle ear. In addition, the inability of the immune system to produce immunoglobulin A (IgA) in the mucosal lining provides less protection against infection in infancy than during later childhood. The ability of the entire respiratory tract to produce mucus is diminished, decreasing the humidification of the large volume of inspired air.

Although the lumen of the trachea and bronchi enlarges during infancy, it remains small in comparison with the total size of the lung, maintaining high resistance to the volume of air inspired. The small airways are easily blocked by edema, mucus, or a foreign body. The pliant (flexible) rib cage has less elastic recoil, and during respiratory distress the work of breathing is increased. In addition, the volume of dead space (that amount of air needed to fill the respiratory passages with each breath) is large, requiring the infant to breathe approximately twice as fast as the adult to provide the body with the needed amount of oxygen.

The *heart rate* slows (see inside back cover), and the rhythm is often *sinus arrhythmia* (rate increases with inspiration and decreases with expiration). Blood pressure also changes during infancy (see inside back cover). Systolic pressure rises during the first 2 months as a result of the increasing ability of the left ventricle to pump blood into the systemic circulation. Diastolic pressure decreases during the first 3 months then gradually rises to values close to those at birth. Fluctuations in blood pressure occur during varying states of activity and emotion.

Significant *hemopoietic changes* occur during the first year. (See Appendix D.) Fetal hemoglobin (HgbF) is present up to the first 5 months, with adult hemoglobin steadily increasing through the first half of infancy. Fetal hemoglobin results in a shortened survival of red blood cells (RBCs) and thus a decreased number of RBCs. A common result at 2 to 3 months of age is *physiologic anemia.* High levels of HgbF are thought to depress the production of erythropoietin, a hormone released by the kidney that stimulates RBC production.

Maternally derived iron stores are present for the first 5 to 6 months and gradually diminish, which also accounts for lowered hemoglobin levels toward the end of the first 6 months. The occurrence of physiologic anemia is not affected by an adequate supply of iron. However, when erythropoiesis is stimulated, iron stores are necessary for the formation of adequate amounts of hemoglobin.

The *digestive processes* are relatively immature at birth. Although term newborn infants have some limitations in digestive function, studies indicate that human milk has properties that partially compensate for decreased digestive enzymatic activity, thus enabling the infant to receive optimal nutrition during the first several months of life (Blackburn and Loper, 1992). The enzyme *ptyalin* (also called *amylase*) is present in small amounts but usually has little effect on the foodstuffs because of the small amount of time the food stays in the mouth. Gastric digestion in the stomach consists primarily of the action of hydrochloric acid and rennin, an enzyme that acts specifically on the casein in milk to cause the formation of curds—coagulated semisolid particles of milk. The curds cause the milk to be retained in the stomach long enough for digestion to occur.

Digestion also takes place in the duodenum, where pancreatic enzymes and bile begin to break down protein and fat. Secretion of the pancreatic enzyme *amylase,* which is needed for digestion of complex carbohydrates, is limited until about the fourth to sixth month of life. *Lipase* is also limited, and infants do not achieve adult levels of fat absorption until 4 to 5 months of age. *Trypsin* is secreted in sufficient quantities to catabolize protein into polypeptides and some amino acids.

The immaturity of the digestive processes is evident in the appearance of stools. During infancy, solid foods (e.g., peas, carrots, corn, and raisins) are passed incompletely broken down in the feces. An excessive quantity of fiber easily disposes the child to loose, bulky stools.

During infancy the stomach enlarges to accommodate a greater volume of food. By the end of the first year the infant is able to tolerate three meals a day and an evening bottle and may have one or two bowel movements daily. However, with any type of gastric irritation the infant is vulnerable to diarrhea, vomiting, and dehydration. (See Chapters 28 and 29.)

The liver is the most immature of all the gastrointestinal organs throughout infancy. The ability to conjugate bilirubin and secrete bile is achieved after the first couple of weeks of life. However, the capacities for gluconeogenesis, formation of plasma protein and ketones, storage of vitamins, and deaminization of amino acids remain relatively immature for the first year of life.

Maturation of the sucking, swallowing and breathing reflexes and the later eruption of teeth parallel the changes in the gastrointestinal tract and prepare the infant for the introduction of solid foods.

*Sucking* activity is observed in utero as early as 15 to 18 weeks gestation. Weak, disorganized mouthing movements may be noted at 27 to 28 weeks gestation, yet complete maturation of sucking, swallowing, and breathing patterns are not reported to be present until 35 to 36 weeks (Wolf and Glass, 1992). Sucking is further divided into *nutritive* and *nonnutritive;* the latter is observed in infants of all ages and is reported to be primarily for the purpose of satisfying the basic sucking urge. On the other hand, nutritive sucking has as its primary purpose the intake of food. *Suckling* is a term often used in denoting breast-feeding (Lawrence and Lawrence, 1999), yet use of the term often varies among different sources.

*Swallowing (deglutition)* is the ability to collect the food (bolus) and propel it into the esophagus. During the *infantile (visceral) swallow reflex* (Fig. 12-3, *A*) food lies in a shallow groove on the top (dorsum) of the tongue. As the

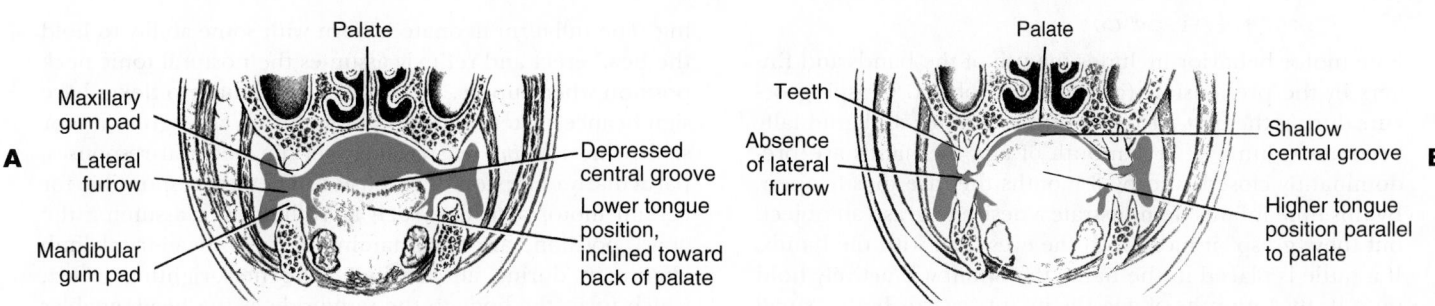

**Fig. 12-3**  Comparison of (**A**) infantile (visceral) swallow reflex and (**B**) mature (somatic) swallow reflex.

tongue is pressed upward toward the palate, the milk flows by gravity down the sloping tongue and along the sides of the mouth in lateral furrows between the tongue, cheek, and gum pads. As the bolus moves downward, the posterior wall of the pharynx comes forward to displace the soft palate. This swallowing process is efficient for fluids but not for solids.

As the infant grows, the tongue becomes smaller in proportion to the oral cavity and attains greater motility, the orofacial muscles develop, and teeth erupt. Consequently, the *mature (somatic) swallow reflex* (Fig. 12-3, *B*) is significantly different. The tongue remains behind the central incisors, and the mandible no longer thrusts forward. The dorsum of the tongue is less concave and remains higher and parallel, not inclined, against the palate; the lateral furrows are absent because of tooth eruption. Tongue pressure and movement against the hard palate pushes the bolus back into the pharynx.

Infants also exhibit a special reflex called the *Santmyer swallow.* When a puff of air is directed at the face, the infant will exhibit a reflex swallow.

The *immunologic system* undergoes numerous changes during the first year. The term newborn receives significant amounts of maternal immunoglobulin G (IgG), which for approximately 3 months confers immunity against many antigens to which the mother was exposed. During this time the infant begins to synthesize IgG; approximately 40% of adult levels are reached by 1 year of age. Significant amounts of IgM are produced at birth yet specificity is decreased, thus limiting recognition of certain pathogens. Adult levels of IgM are reached by 9 to 12 months of age. The production of IgA, IgD, and IgE is much more gradual, and maximum levels are not attained until early childhood.

Secretory IgA is not present at birth but is found in saliva and tears by 2 to 5 weeks. IgA is present in large amounts in human colostrum; this is believed to have a protective role in the gastrointestinal tract against many bacteria such as *Escherichia coli* and viruses such as poliovirus. The function and quantity of T-lymphocytes, lymphokines, and complement is reduced in early infancy, thus preventing optimal response to certain bacteria and viruses.

During infancy *thermoregulation* becomes more efficient; the ability of the skin to contract and of muscles to shiver in response to cold increases. The peripheral capillaries respond to changes in ambient temperature to regulate heat loss. The capillaries constrict in response to cold, conserving core body temperature and decreasing potential evaporative heat loss from the skin surface. The capillaries dilate in response to heat, decreasing internal body temperature through evaporation, conduction, and convection. Shivering (*thermogenesis*) causes the muscles and muscle fibers to contract, generating metabolic heat, which is distributed throughout the body. Increased adipose tissue during the first 6 months insulates the body against heat loss.

A shift in *total body fluid* occurs. At birth 75% of the infant's body weight is water, and there is an excess of extracellular fluid (ECF). As the percentage of body water decreases, so does the amount of ECF—from 40% at term to 20% in adulthood. The high proportion of ECF, which is composed of blood plasma, interstitial fluid, and lymph, predisposes the infant to a more rapid loss of total body fluid and, consequently, dehydration.

The immaturity of the *renal structures* also predisposes the infant to dehydration. Complete maturity of the kidney occurs during the latter half of the second year, when the cuboidal epithelium of the glomeruli becomes flattened. Before this time the filtration capacity of the glomeruli is reduced. Urine is voided frequently and has a low specific gravity (1.000 to 1.010).

The *endocrine system* is adequately developed at birth, but its functions are immature. The interrelatedness of all the endocrine organs has a major effect on the function of any one gland. The lack of homeostatic control because of various functional deficiencies renders the infant especially vulnerable to imbalances in fluid and electrolytes, glucose concentration, and amino acid metabolism.

For example, corticotropin (ACTH) is produced in limited quantities during infancy. ACTH acts on the adrenal cortices to produce their hormones, particularly the glucocorticoids and aldosterone. Because the feedback mechanism between ACTH and the adrenal cortex is immature during infancy, there is much less tolerance for stressful conditions, which affect fluid and electrolytes and the metabolism of fats, proteins, and carbohydrates. In addition, although the islets of Langerhans produce insulin and glucagon during fetal life and early infancy, blood sugar levels tend to remain labile, particularly under conditions of stress.

## Fine Motor Development

Fine motor behavior includes the use of the hands and fingers in the prehension (grasp) of an object. Grasping occurs during the first 2 to 3 months as a reflex and gradually becomes voluntary. At 1 month of age the hands are predominantly closed, and by 3 months they are mostly open. By this time infants demonstrate a desire to grasp an object, but they "grasp" it more with the eyes than with the hands. If a rattle is placed in the hand, the infant will actively hold onto it. By 4 months of age the infant regards both a small pellet and the hands and then looks from the object to the hands and back again. By 5 months the infant is able to voluntarily grasp an object.

Gradually the palmar grasp (using the whole hand) is replaced with a pincer grasp (using the thumb and index finger). By 8 to 9 months of age the infant uses a crude pincer grasp (Fig. 12-4) and by 10 months of age the pincer grasp is sufficiently established to enable infants to pick up a raisin and other finger foods. By 11 months the infant has progressed to a neat pincer grasp (Fig. 12-5).

By 6 months of age infants have increased manipulative skill. They hold their bottle, grasp their feet and pull them to their mouth, and feed themselves a cracker. By 7 months they transfer objects from one hand to the other, use one hand for grasping, and hold a cube in each hand simultaneously. They enjoy banging objects and will explore the movable parts of a toy.

By 10 months of age infants can deliberately let go of an object and will offer it to someone. By 11 months they put objects into a container and like to remove them. By age 1 year infants try to build a tower of two blocks but fail.

## Gross Motor Development

Gross motor behavior includes developmental maturation in posture, head balance, sitting, creeping, standing, and walking. The full-term neonate is born with some ability to hold the head erect and reflexly assumes the postural tonic neck position when supine. Several of the primitive reflexes have significance in terms of development of later gross motor skills. The *righting reflexes* elicit certain postural responses, particularly of flexion or extension. They are responsible for certain motor activities, such as rolling over, assuming the crawl position, and maintaining normal head-trunk-limb alignment during all activities. The neck-righting reflex, which turns the body to the same side as the head, enables the child to roll over from supine to prone. Other reflexes, such as the otolith-righting and labyrinth-righting reflexes, enable the infant to raise the head (see Box 12-1).

The asymmetric tonic neck reflex, which persists from birth to 3 months, prevents the infant from rolling over. The symmetric tonic neck reflex, which is evoked by flexing or extending the neck, helps the infant to assume the crawl position. When the head and neck are extended, the extensor tone of the upper extremities and the flexor tone of the lower extremities increase. The child extends the arms and bends the knees. Because of the strong flexor tone of the lower extremities, the infant may initially crawl backward before crawling forward. This reflex disappears when neurologic maturity allows actual crawling to occur because independent limb movement is required.

**Head Control.**   The full-term newborn can momentarily hold the head in midline and parallel when the body is suspended ventrally and can lift and turn the head from side to side when prone. (See Fig. 8-7.) This is not the case when the infant is lying prone on a pillow or soft surface; infants do not have the head control to lift their head out of the depression of the object and therefore risk suffocation. Marked head lag is evident when the infant is pulled from a lying to a sitting position. By 3 months of age infants can hold their head well beyond the plane of the body. By 4 months of age infants can

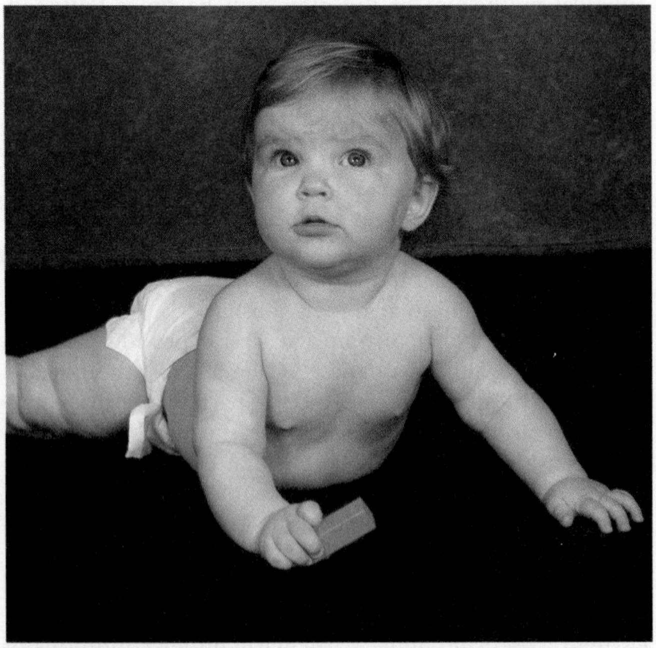

**Fig. 12-4**   Crude pincer grasp at 8 to 10 months of age. (Courtesy Paul Vincent Kuntz, Texas Children's Hospital.)

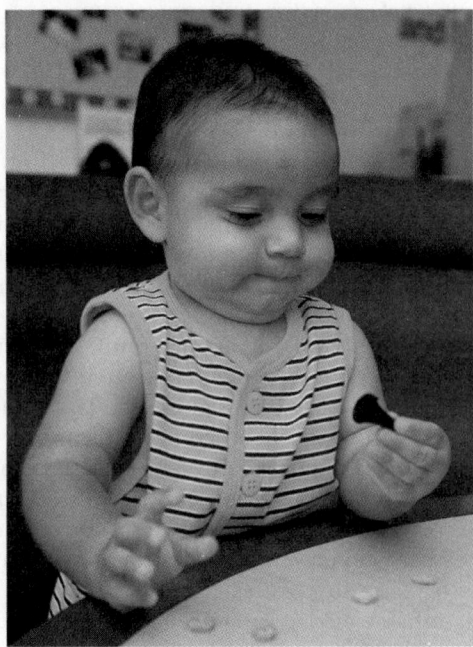

**Fig. 12-5**   Neat pincer grasp at 11 months of age. (Courtesy Paul Vincent Kuntz, Texas Children's Hospital.)

lift the head and front portion of the chest approximately 90 degrees above the table, bearing their weight on the forearms. Only slight head lag is evident when the infant is pulled from a lying to a sitting position, and by 4 to 6 months head control is well established (Figs. 12-6 and 12-7).

**Rolling Over.** Newborns may roll over accidentally because of their rounded back. The ability to willfully turn from the abdomen to the back occurs at 5 months, and the ability to turn from the back to the abdomen occurs at 6 months. It is noteworthy that the parachute reflex (see Fig. 12-1), which elicits a protective response to falling, appears at 7 months.

**Sitting.** The ability to sit follows progressive head control and straightening of the back (Fig. 12-8). For the first

2 to 3 months the back is uniformly rounded. The convex cervical curve forms at approximately 3 to 4 months of age, when head control is established. The convex lumbar curve appears when the child begins to sit, at about age 4 months. As the spinal column straightens, the infant can be propped in a sitting position. By age 7 months infants can sit alone, leaning forward on their hands for support. By age 8 months they can sit well while unsupported and begin to explore their surroundings in this position rather than in a lying position. By 10 months they can maneuver from a prone to a sitting position.

**Locomotion.** Locomotion involves acquiring the ability to bear weight, propel forward on all four extremities, stand

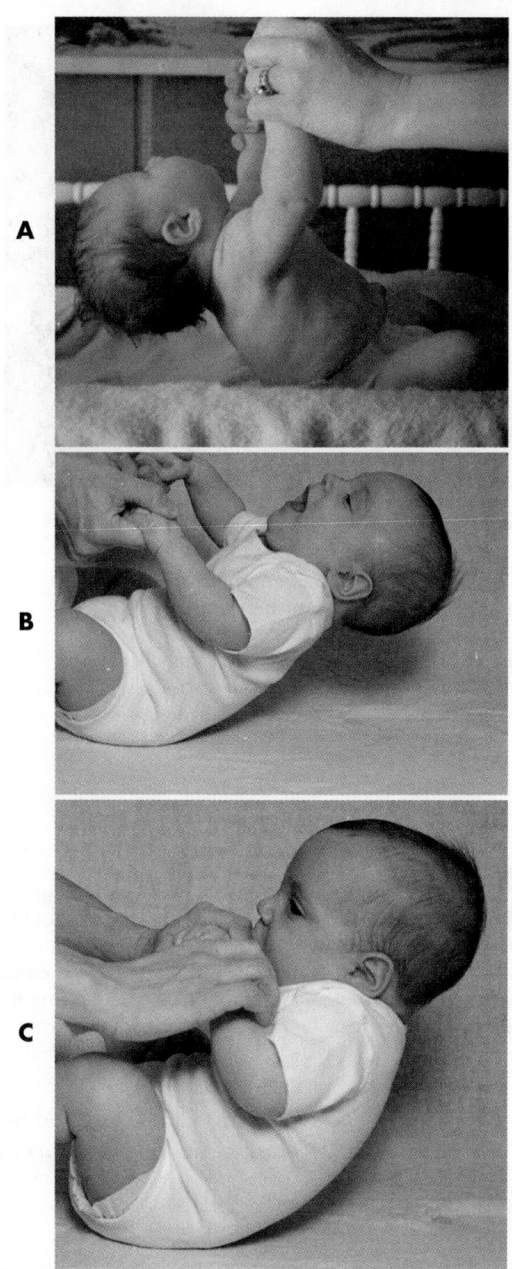

**Fig. 12-6** Head control while pulled to sitting position. **A,** Complete head lag at 1 month. **B,** Partial head lag at 2 months. **C,** Almost no head lag at 4 months.

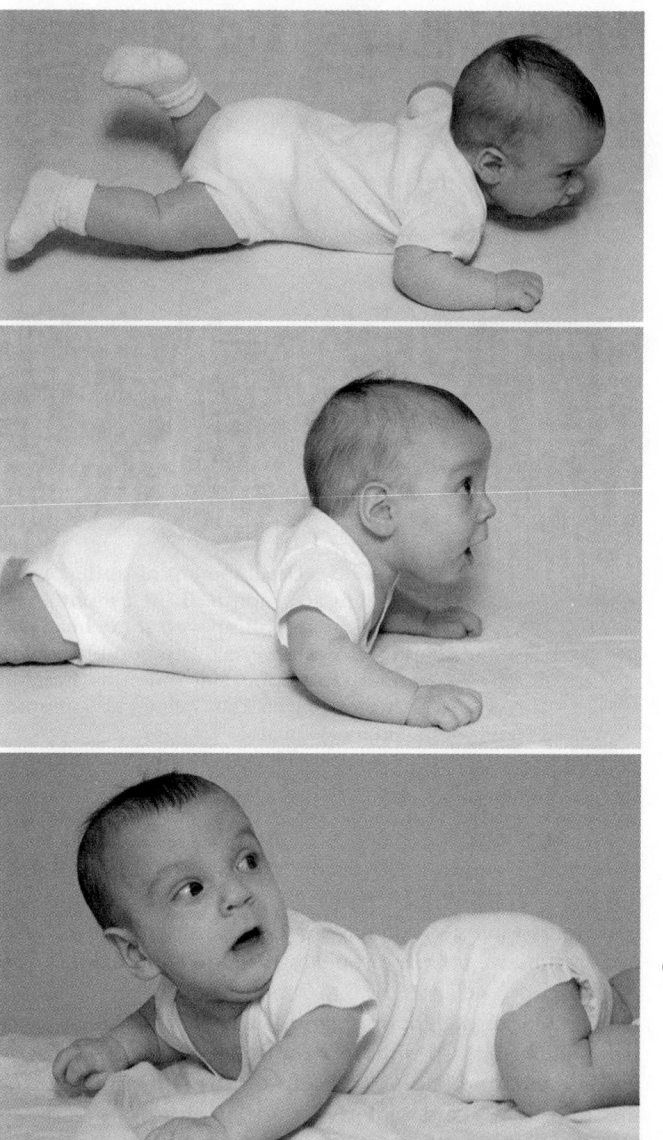

**Fig. 12-7** Head control while prone. **A,** Infant momentarily lifts head at 1 month. **B,** Infant lifts head and chest 90 degrees and bears weight on forearms at 4 months. **C,** Infant lifts head, chest, and upper abdomen and can bear weight on hands at 6 months. Note how this position facilitates turning from abdomen to back.

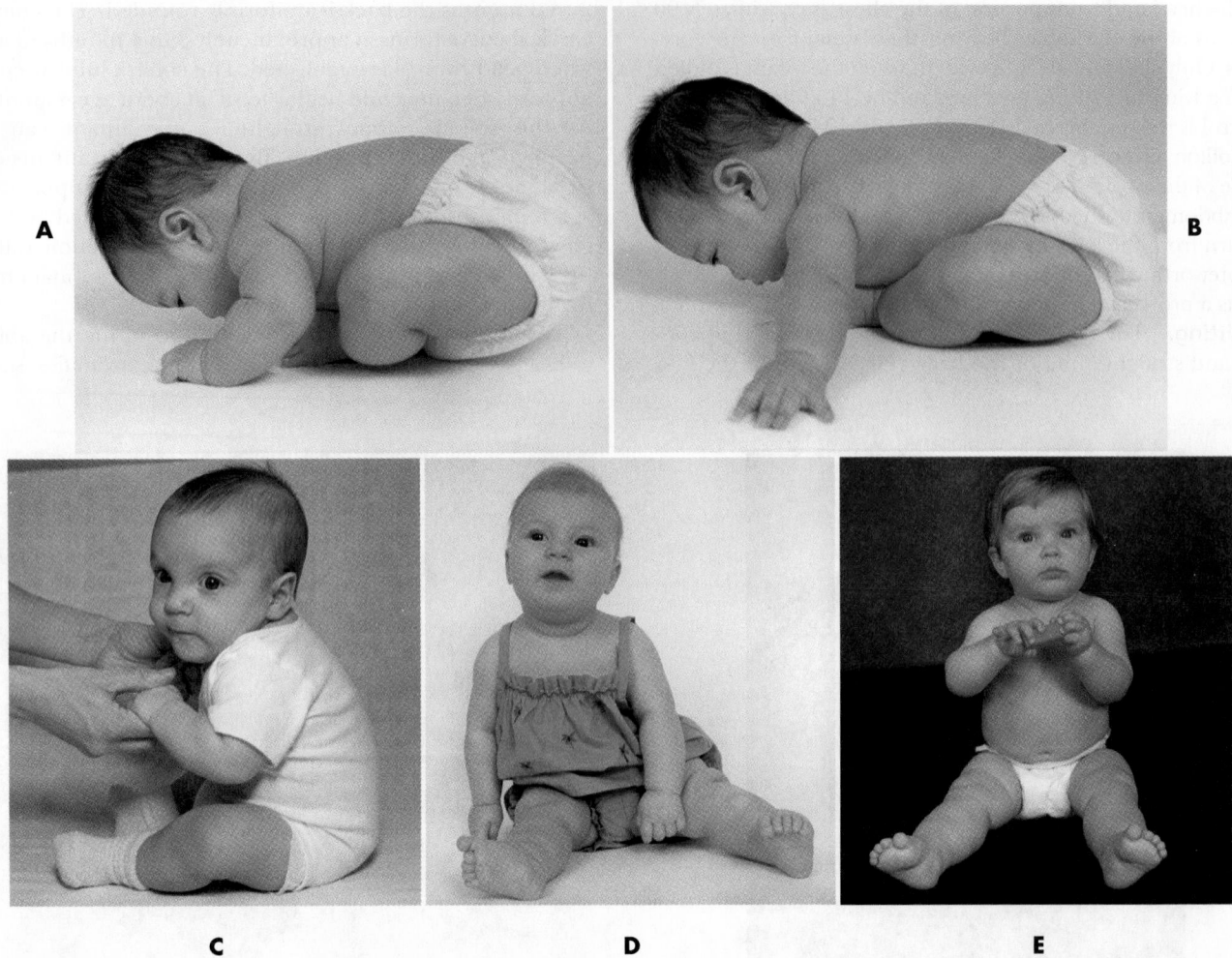

**Fig. 12-8** Development of sitting. **A,** Back is completely rounded; infant has no ability to sit upright at 1 month. **B,** At 2 months, exhibits more control; back is still rounded, but infant can try to pull up with some head control. **C,** Back is rounded only in lumbar area; infant is able to sit erect with good head control at 4 months. **D,** Infant can sit alone, leaning on hands for support, at 7 months. **E,** Infant sits without support at 8 months. Note the transferring of objects that occurs at 7 months. (*A, B, D,* and *E* courtesy Paul Vincent Kuntz, Texas Children's Hospital.)

upright with support and, finally, walk alone (Fig. 12-9). Following a cephalocaudal pattern, infants 4 to 6 months old have increasing coordination in their arms. Initial locomotion results in infants propelling themselves backward by pushing with the arms. By 6 to 7 months of age they are able to bear all their weight on their legs with assistance. *Crawling* (propelling forward with belly on floor) progresses to *creeping* on hands and knees (with belly off floor) by 9 months. At this time they stand while holding onto furniture and can pull themselves to the standing position, but they are unable to maneuver back down except by falling. By 11 months they walk while holding onto furniture or with both hands held, and by age 1 year they may be able to walk with one hand held. A number of infants attempt their first independent steps by their first birthday.

**NURSING ALERT** An infant who does not pull to a standing position by 11 to 12 months of age should be further evaluated for possible developmental dysplasia of the hip (see Chapter 11). Although there is considerable variation among infants in regard to the achievement of these milestones, they provide guidelines for early intervention.

Infants' motor age (development) can be assessed by calculating a *motor quotient (MQ)* using the following formula:

$$MQ = \frac{\text{Motor age (MA)}}{\text{Chronologic age (CA)}} \times 100$$

For example, if a 12-month-old infant begins to creep, the motor quotient is 9 (MA for this skill) ÷ 12 (CA) × 100,

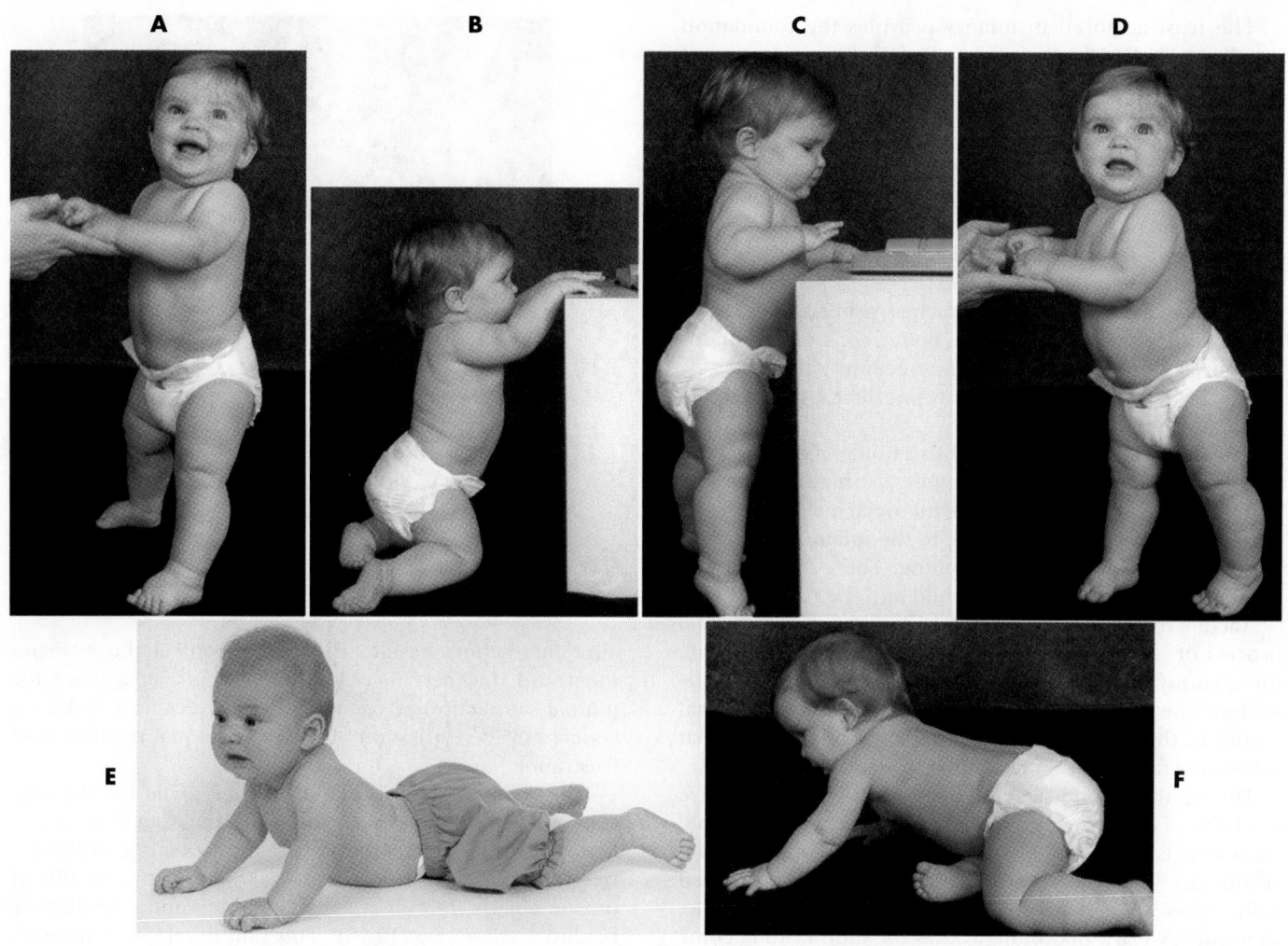

**Fig. 12-9**  Development of locomotion. **A,** Infant bears full weight on feet by 7 months. **B,** Infant can maneuver from sitting to kneeling position by 8 months. **C,** Infant can stand holding onto furniture at 8-9 months. **D,** While standing, infant takes deliberate step at 9-10 months. **E,** Infant crawls with abdomen on floor and pulls self forward and then **F,** creeps on hands and knees at 9 months. (Courtesy Paul Vincent Kuntz, Texas Children's Hospital.)

or 75. Values above 85 are considered within normal limits, values below 70 are abnormal, and values between 70 and 85 are borderline (Johnson and Blasco, 1997).

## Psychosocial Development

### Developing a Sense of Trust (Erikson)

Erikson's phase I (birth to 1 year) is concerned with *acquiring a sense of trust* while *overcoming a sense of mistrust.* Erikson was a neo-Freudian who incorporated much of Freud's theory. (See Chapter 7.) The trust that develops is a trust of self, of others, and of the world. Infants "trust" that their feeding, comfort, stimulation, and caring needs will be met. The crucial element for the achievement of this task is the quality of both the parent (caregiver)-child relationship and the care the infant receives. The provi-

sion of food, warmth, and shelter by itself is inadequate for the development of a strong sense of self. The infant and parent must jointly learn to satisfactorily meet their needs in order for mutual regulation of frustration to occur. When this synchrony fails to develop, mistrust is the eventual outcome. Frustration is heightened in situations in which the parent(s) is an adolescent who does not understand the infant's behavioral cues due to his/her own self-centered phase of development.

Failure to learn "delayed gratification" leads to mistrust. Mistrust can result either from too much or too little frustration. If parents always meet their children's needs before the children signal their readiness, infants will never learn to test their ability to control the environment. If the delay is prolonged, infants will experience constant frustration and eventually mistrust others in their efforts to satisfy them. Therefore consistency of care is essential.

The trust acquired in infancy provides the foundation for all succeeding phases. Trust allows infants a feeling of physical comfort and security, which assists them in experiencing unfamiliar, unknown situations with a minimum of fear. Erikson has divided the first year of life into two oral/social stages. During the first 3 to 4 months, food intake is the most important social activity in which the infant engages. The newborn can tolerate little frustration or delay of gratification. Primary *narcissism* (total concern for oneself) is at its height.

However, as bodily processes such as vision, motor movements, and vocalization become better controlled, infants use more advanced behaviors to interact with others. For example, rather than cry, infants may put their arms up to signify a desire to be held.

The next social modality involves a mode of reaching out to others through *grasping.* Grasping is initially reflexive, but even as a reflex it has a powerful social meaning for the parents. The reciprocal response to the infant's grasping is the parents' holding on and touching. There is pleasurable tactile stimulation for both the child and the parents.

Tactile stimulation is extremely important in the total process of acquiring trust. The degree of mothering skill, the quantity of food, or the length of sucking does not determine the quality of the experience. Rather, it is the total nature of the quality of the interpersonal relationship that influences the infant's formulation of trust.

During the second stage, the more active and aggressive modality of *biting* occurs. Infants learn that they can hold onto what is their own and can more fully control their environment. During this stage infants may be confronted with one of their first conflicts. If they are breast-feeding, they quickly learn that biting causes the mother to become upset and withdraw the breast. Yet biting also brings internal relief from teething discomfort and a sense of power or control.

This conflict may be solved in a variety of ways. The mother may wean the infant from the breast and begin bottle-feeding, or the infant may learn to bite substitute "nipples," such as a pacifier, and retain pleasurable breast-feeding. The successful resolution of this conflict strengthens the mother-child relationship because it occurs at a time when infants are recognizing the mother as the most significant person in their life.

## Cognitive Development

### Sensorimotor Phase (Piaget)

The theory most commonly used to explain *cognition,* or the ability to know, is that of Piaget. The period from birth to 24 months is termed the *sensorimotor phase* and is composed of six stages; however, because this discussion is concerned with ages birth to 12 months, only the first four stages are discussed (Table 12-1; see Table 14-1 for the stages from 13 to 24 months).

During the sensorimotor phase infants progress from reflex behaviors to simple repetitive acts to imitative activity. Three crucial events take place during this phase. The first event involves *separation,* in which infants learn to separate themselves from other objects in the environment. They re-

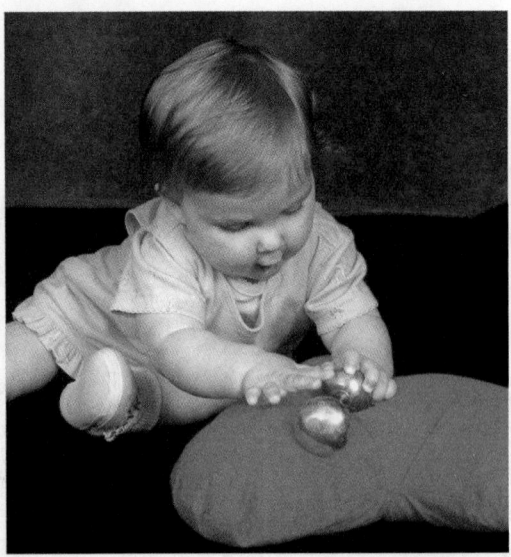

**Fig. 12-10**   Nine-month old is able to find hidden object under pillow. (Courtesy Paul Vincent Kuntz, Texas Children's Hospital.)

alize that others besides themselves control the environment and that certain readjustments must take place for mutual satisfaction to occur. This coincides with Erikson's concept of the formation of trust and mutual regulation of frustration.

The second major accomplishment is achieving the concept of *object permanence,* or the realization that objects that leave the visual field still exist. A typical example of the development of object permanence is when infants are able to pursue objects they observe being hidden under a pillow or behind a chair (Fig. 12-10). This skill develops at approximately 9 to 10 months of age, which corresponds to the time of increased locomotion skills.

The last major intellectual achievement of this period is the ability to use *symbols,* or *mental representation.* The use of symbols allows the infant to think of an object or situation without actually experiencing it. The recognition of symbols is the beginning of the understanding of time and space.

The first stage, from birth to 1 month, is identified by the infant's *use of reflexes.* At birth the infant's individuality and temperament are expressed through the physiologic reflexes of sucking, rooting, grasping, and crying. The repetitious nature of the reflexes is the beginning of associations between an act and a sequential response. When infants cry because they are hungry, a nipple is put in the mouth, and they suck, feel satisfaction, and sleep. They are assimilating this experience while perceiving auditory, tactile, and visual cues. This experience of perceiving certain patterns, or "ordering," provides a foundation for the subsequent stages.

The second stage, *primary circular reactions,* marks the beginning of the replacement of reflexive behavior with voluntary acts. During the period from 1 to 4 months, activities such as sucking or grasping become deliberate acts that elicit certain responses. The beginning of accommodation is evident. Infants incorporate and adapt their reactions to the environment and recognize the stimulus that produced a response. Previously they would cry until the nipple was

**TABLE 12-1**   Sensorimotor phase during infancy*

| Stage/Age | Cognitive Development | Behavior |
|---|---|---|
| **I. Use of reflexes**<br>**Birth–1 month** | Repetitious use of reflexes establishes a pattern of experiences<br>Totally narcissistic (self-centered) being | Mostly reflexive (sucking, swallowing, rooting, grasping, crying)<br>Little or no tolerance for frustration of delayed gratification |
| **II. Primary circular reactions**<br>**1-4 months** | Use of reflexes is gradually replaced by voluntary activity<br>Recognition of causality occurs when repetition of events causes one stimulus to produce a consistent response<br>Beginning notion of temporal space of time occurs as infant realizes the progression of an orderly sequence of events<br>Beginning separation of self from others<br>Learns from type of interaction between object or individual rather than from object itself<br>Engages in an activity for the pleasure of the activity more than for its result | Recognizes familiar faces and objects (e.g., bottle)<br>Shows anticipation before feeding<br>Awareness of strange surroundings indicates memory<br>Discovers parts of own body—plays with hands, fingers, feet<br>Becomes bored when left alone<br>Shows no separation anxiety unless caregiver's skill differs from usual routine |
| **III. Secondary circular reactions**<br>**4-8 months** | Intentional activity replaces repetitious activity that did not produce a desired result<br>Beginning of object permanence when object is beyond perceptual range<br>Progressive idea of time; awareness of before and after in a sequence of events<br>Able to imitate selective activity from several events<br>Further separation of self from environment<br>Idea of quality and quantity<br>Beginning recognition of symbols as type of communication | Secures objects by pulling on a string<br>Searches for objects that have fallen<br>Shows separation anxiety<br>Able to tolerate some frustration and delayed gratification<br>Imitates sounds and simple gestures<br>Great interest in mirror image (see Fig. 12-11)<br>Beginning independence in self-feeding<br>Shows displeasure if activity is inhibited<br>Language development; attracts attention by methods other than crying<br>Realizes that parents are present even if not in visual field |
| **IV. Coordination of secondary schemas and their application to new situations**<br>**9-12 months** | Concept of object permanence advances; beginning of intellectual reasoning<br>Associates symbols with events, but classification is based on own experience<br>Distinguishes objects from the related activity and perceives them as objects<br>Distinguishes end products from their means; attempts to remove barriers to achieve the end | Actively searches for a hidden object (see Fig. 12-10)<br>Comprehends meanings of words and simple commands<br>Knows that gestures (bye-bye, kiss) have certain meanings<br>Is able to put objects in a container<br>Works to get toy that is out of reach<br>Ventures away from parent to explore surroundings |

*For phases during toddlerhood, see Table 14-1.

brought to the mouth. Now they associate the nipple with the sound of the parent's voice. They accommodate this new piece of information and adapt by ceasing to cry when they hear the voice—before receiving the nipple. What is taking place is a realization of causality and a recognition of an orderly sequence of events. The environment is taken in with all the senses and with whatever motor ability is present.

The *secondary circular reactions* stage is a continuation of primary circular reactions and lasts until 8 months of age. In this stage the primary circular reactions are repeated and prolonged for the response that results. Grasping and holding now become shaking, banging, and pulling. Shaking is performed to hear a noise, not solely for the pleasure of shaking. Quality and quantity of an act become evident. "More" or "less" shaking produces different responses. Causality, time, deliberate intention, and separateness from the environment begin to develop.

Three new processes of human behavior occur. *Imitation* requires the differentiation of selected acts from several events. By the second half of the first year infants can imitate sounds and simple gestures. *Play* becomes evident as they take pleasure in performing an act after they have mastered it. Much of infants' waking hours are absorbed in sensorimotor play. *Affect* (outward manifestation of emotion and feeling) is seen as infants begin to develop a sense of permanency. During the first 6 months infants believe that an object exists only for as long as they can visually perceive it. In other words, out of sight—out of mind. Affect to external objects is evident when the object continues to be present or remembered even though it is beyond the range of perception. Object permanence is a critical component of parent-child attachment and is seen in the development of separation anxiety at 6 to 8 months of age (p. 505).

During the fourth sensorimotor stage, *coordination of secondary schemas and their application to new situations,* infants use previous behavioral achievements primarily as the foundation for adding new intellectual skills to their expanding repertoire. This stage is largely transitional. Increasing motor skills allow for greater exploration of the environment. They begin to discover that hiding an object does not mean that it is gone but that removing an obstacle will reveal the object. This marks the beginning of intellectual reasoning. Furthermore, they can experience an event by observing it, and they begin to associate symbols with events (e.g., "bye-bye" with "Daddy goes to work"), but the classification is purely their own. In this stage they learn from the object itself; this is in contrast to the second stage, in which infants learn from the type of interaction between objects or individuals. Intentionality is further developed in that infants now actively attempt to remove a barrier to the desired (or undesired) action (see Fig. 12-10). If something is in their way, they attempt to climb over it or push it away. Previously an obstacle would cause them to give up any further attempt to achieve the desired goal.

## Development of Body Image

The development of body image parallels sensorimotor development. Infants' kinesthetic and tactile experiences are the first perceptions of their body, and the mouth is the principal area of pleasurable sensations. Other parts of the body are primarily objects of pleasure—the hands and fingers to suck and the feet to play with. As physical needs are met, they feel comfort and satisfaction with their body. Messages conveyed by the caregivers reinforce these feelings. For example, when infants smile, they receive emotional satisfaction from others who smile back.

Achieving the concept of object permanence is basic to the development of self-image. By the end of the first year

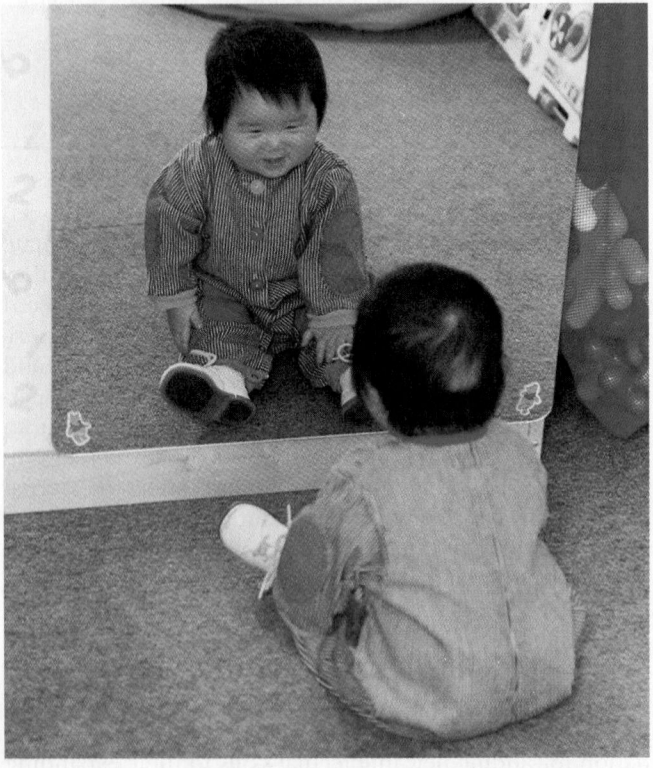

**Fig. 12-11** Nine-month-old infant enjoying own image in mirror.

infants recognize that they are distinct from their parents. At the same time there is increasing interest in their image, especially in the mirror (Fig. 12-11). As motor skills develop, they learn that parts of the body are useful; for example, the hands bring objects to the mouth, and the legs help them move to different locations. All of these achievements transmit messages to them about themselves. Therefore it is important to transmit positive messages to infants about their bodies.

## Development of Sexual Identity

Sexual identity is reported to begin in utero because hormonal influences, which are not entirely understood. At birth the child is named and significant others, especially the parents, act certain ways toward the infant because of its gender. Touch is crucial to infant development and plays a primary role in sexual development. Infants have a great oral sensitivity, which is manifested through sucking and mouthing. They enjoy skin-to-skin contact and explore their own body for pleasure. Infants are capable of genital self-stimulation to orgasm; erections in male infants are common. Parents' responses to these early manifestations of sexuality influence children's evolving attitudes; therefore a healthy, accepting response by parents is important.

## Social Development

Infants' social development is initially influenced by their reflexive behavior, such as the grasp, and eventually depends primarily on the interaction between them and the principal caregivers. Attachment to the parent is increasingly evident during the second half of the first year. In addition, tremendous strides are made in communication and personal-social behavior. Play is a major socializing agent and provides the stimulation needed to learn from interactions with the environment.

### Attachment

The importance of human physical contact cannot be overemphasized. Parenting is not an instinctual ability but a learned, acquired process. The attachment of parent and child, which begins before birth and assumes even more importance at birth (see Chapter 8), continues during the first year. In the following discussion of attachment, the word "mother" is used in the broad context of the consistent caregiver with whom the child relates more than anyone else. However, in society's changing social climate and sex-role stereotypes, this person may very well be the father. Studies on father-child attachment demonstrate that stages similar to maternal attachment occur and that fathers are more involved in child care when mothers are employed (although mothers continue to do the majority of infant care) (Jones and Heermann, 1992). Additional research has shown that inexperienced, first-time fathers are as capable as experienced fathers of developing a close attachment with their infants (Ferketich and Mercer, 1995).

Children who had insecure attachment to their teenage mothers were found to have a strong attachment to the grandmother who was also a primary caretaker (Patterson,

1997). With many single-parent families in existence, a grandmother (or other significant caretaker) may become the primary caretaker. It is important for nurses to recognize that infant-parent attachments may be present or absent in situations wherein caretaker roles are less well-defined by those involved.

Attachment progresses during infancy, with the child assuming an increasingly significant role. Two components of cognitive development are required for attachment: (1) the ability to discriminate the mother from other individuals and (2) the achievement of object permanence. Both of these processes prepare the infant for an equally important aspect of attachment—separation from the parent. Separation-individuation should occur as a harmonious, parallel process with emotional attachment.

During the formation of attachment to the parent, the infant progresses through four distinct but overlapping stages. For the first few weeks infants respond indiscriminately to anyone. Beginning at approximately 8 to 12 weeks of age, they cry, smile, and vocalize more to the mother than to anyone else but continue to respond to others, whether familiar or not. At approximately 6 months of age, infants show a distinct preference for the mother. They follow her more, cry when she leaves, enjoy playing with her more, and feel most secure in her arms. About 1 month after showing attachment to the mother, many infants begin attaching to other members of the family, most often the father.

Infants acquire other developmental behaviors that influence the attachment process. These include (1) differential crying, smiling, and vocalization (more to mother than to anyone else), (2) visual-motor orientation (looking more at mother, even if she is not close), (3) crying when mother leaves the room, (4) approaching through locomotion (crawling, creeping, or walking), (5) clinging (especially in presence of a stranger), and (6) exploring away from mother while using her as a secure base.

There is increasing evidence that childhood behavior disorders such as attention-deficit hyperactivity disorder (ADHD) and oppositional defiant disorder/conduct disorder have origins in an altered infant-parent attachment or the caregiving environment during infancy (Shaw and others, 2001).

**Effects of Prolonged Separation.** Attachment is considered so critical to optimum child development that many researchers have documented the effects of prolonged and early separation on infants in the absence of quality parent substitutes. Some of the most famous research on emotional deprivation has been done by John Bowlby, John Robertson, and René Spitz. Bowlby (1969) studied the effects of the infant's separation from the mother and noted severe mental and physical retardation, particularly if emotional deprivation occurred during the first 3 years of life. He observed that progressive retardation could be arrested or reversed if no further emotional deprivation occurred after the first 2 years, whereas prolonged, severe deprivation beginning early in the first year and lasting for 3 years led to severe permanent effects. Among these were the inability to form trusting, intimate interpersonal relationships, language impairment, and deficiency in abstract thinking. Robertson (1953) and Bowlby (1969) found typical behavioral reactions of infants who were

hospitalized and separated from their mothers. (See Separation Anxiety, Chapter 26.)

Spitz (1945) studied the effects of emotional deprivation on children raised in foundling homes or institutions. The infants were cared for by one nurse who had responsibility for eight children. Although the caregiver might be a loving, motherly person, she lacked the time necessary to devote individual attention and stimulation to each child. As a result, the children were delayed in physical growth, were more susceptible to disease, and demonstrated decreasing developmental quotients over a 2-year period. Spitz found that children developed normally if given one-to-one attention by a mother substitute.

Although these studies represent extreme examples of young children reared in environments essentially devoid of quality mothering, rather than temporary separation such as daycare, the question remains regarding the long-term effects of separation and other stresses on children.

*Reactive attachment disorder (RAD)* is a psychologic and developmental problem that stems from maladaptive or absent attachment between the infant and parent and may persist into childhood and even adulthood. Signs of RAD are usually seen before the age of 5 in infants who had insecure attachments to the mother or other primary caretaker (American Psychiatric Association, 2000). The child may manifest behaviors such as not being cuddly with parents, failing to make eye contact with significant others, having poor impulse control, and being destructive to self and others (Reber, 1996). Maltreated and orphaned children often are diagnosed with this complex disorder. Without early intervention, some of these children fail to develop a conscience and suffer from an antisocial personality disorder that may lead to criminal acts.

Based on such findings, nurses need to assess each family with the understanding that stress may or may not be necessarily harmful and that children can adapt even under adverse conditions. Individual risk factors that influence a child's coping ability are evaluated, and tools such as the Revised Infant Temperament Questionnaire (see p. 507) are used to assess "goodness of fit." When parental separation occurs, every effort is made to help the family provide suitable caregiver substitutes for the child. Individuals who are warm, responsive, and interactive with the infant during separation can significantly minimize the physiologic and behavioral effects. The child's plasticity and resiliency in coping are stressed to the family to minimize their feelings of responsibility and guilt.

**Separation Anxiety.** Between the ages of 4 and 8 months the infant progresses through the first stage of separation-individuation and begins to have some awareness of self and mother as separate beings. At the same time, object permanence is developing, and the infant is aware that the parent can be absent. Therefore separation anxiety develops and is manifested through a predictable sequence of behaviors.

During the early second half of the first year infants protest when placed in their crib, and a short time later they object when the mother leaves the room. Infants may not notice the mother's absence if they are absorbed in an activity. However, when they realize her absence, they protest. From this point on they become very alert to her activities and whereabouts. By 11 to 12 months they are able to anticipate her imminent departure by watching her behaviors, and they begin to protest *before* she leaves. At this point many parents learn to postpone alerting the child to their departure until just before leaving.

**Stranger Fear.** As infants demonstrate attachment to one person, they correspondingly exhibit less friendliness to others. Between ages 6 and 8 months fear of strangers and stranger anxiety become prominent and are related to infants' ability to discriminate between familiar and nonfamiliar people. Behaviors such as clinging to the parent, crying, and turning away from the stranger are common (Fig. 12-12). Suggestions for coping with stranger fear and separation anxiety are discussed on p. 514.

## Language Development

The infant's first means of verbal communication is crying. Crying as a biologic sign conveys a message of urgency and signals displeasure, such as hunger. However, crying is also a social event that affects the development of the parent-infant relationship—either by its absence, which usually has a positive effect on parents, or its presence, which may evoke a negative response or persuade parents to minister to the child's physical or emotional needs.

In the first few weeks of life, crying has a reflexive quality and is mostly related to physiologic needs. Infants cry for 1 to 1½ hours a day up to 3 weeks of age and then build up to 2, and even 4, hours by 6 weeks. Crying tends to decrease by 12 weeks. It is thought that the increase in crying for no apparent reason during the first few months may be related to the discharge of energy and the maturational changes in the central nervous system. During the end of the first year infants cry for attention, from fear (especially stranger fear), and from frustration, usually in response to their developing but inadequate motor skills.

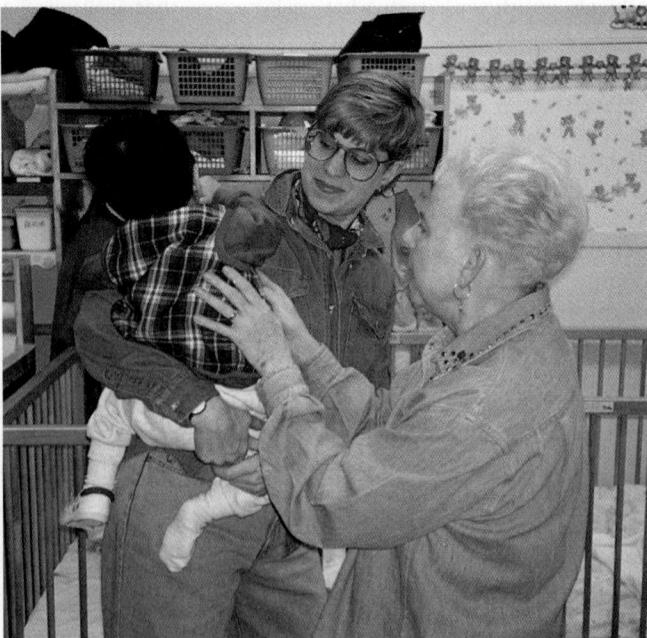

**Fig. 12-12** Stranger fear behaviors include clinging to the parent and turning away from a stranger.

Many parents state that they can distinguish between different types of cry and from these messages are able to interpret the infant's needs. However, crying can be a source of acute distress for parents, especially the inconsolable crying of colic. (See Chapter 13.) Parents benefit from an explanation of the variability of crying among infants and an assurance that periods of "unexplained fussiness" are normal. Some parents may need guidance in consoling techniques, such as holding, swaddling, massaging, caressing, rocking, walking, or stimulating sucking.

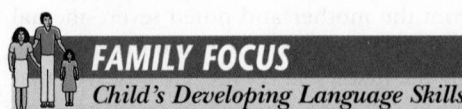

**NURSING ALERT** Be alert to parents' reports about maternal postpartum depression and infant crying because these concerns may indicate a stressed mother-infant relationship.

Vocalizations heard during crying eventually become syllables and words (e.g., the "mama" heard during vigorous crying). Infants vocalize as early as 5 to 6 weeks of age by making small throaty sounds. By 2 months they make single vowel sounds such as *ah*, *eh*, and *uh*. By 3 to 4 months the consonants *n*, *k*, *g*, *p*, and *b* are added, and the infants coo, gurgle, and laugh aloud. By 6 months they imitate sounds, add the consonants *t*, *d*, and *w* and combine syllables (e.g., "dada"), but they do not ascribe meaning to the word until 10 to 11 months of age. (See Family Focus box.) By 9 to 10 months they comprehend the meaning of the word "no" and obey simple commands accompanied by gestures. By age 1 year they can say three to five words with meaning and may understand as many as 100 words (Johnson and Blasco, 1997). Because language development is based on expressive (ability to make thoughts, ideas, and desires known to others) and receptive skills (ability to understand the words being spoken), it is important that infants are exposed to expressive speech (Johnson and Blasco, 1997) and that delays in achieving milestones are carefully evaluated for potential hearing loss. (See Universal Newborn Hearing Screening, Chapter 8.)

## Personal-Social Behavior

Personal-social behavior includes the child's personal responses to the environment. It is the area most influenced by external stimuli but, as in the other fields of behavior, it follows certain developmental laws. Personal-social behavior implies communication with one's self and with others. It provides the foundation for the successful mastery of skills such as feeding, control of bodily functions, independence, and cooperativeness in play.

**FAMILY FOCUS**
*Child's Developing Language Skills*

During the acquisition of new language skills the child temporarily may stop using other recently learned sounds or words. This is often distressing for parents, who have waited in anticipation for the words "dada" or "mama." Because these sounds are commonly replaced by other vocalizations, they may not be repeated for several weeks. Nurses can reassure parents that the child will again say these special words and with increased meaning.

Infants have the ability to shape their environment and to elicit certain responses. Newborns show visual preference for the human face and, as early as 1 week of age, begin to watch the parent intently as he or she speaks to them. As they regard the parent's face, activity diminishes, their head bobs up and down, and their mouth moves, almost as if they were trying to say something.

By 6 to 8 weeks a social smile in response to pleasurable stimuli is present. This has a profound effect on family members and is a tremendous stimulus for evoking continued responses from others. By 3 months infants show considerable interest in the environment—excitement when a toy is presented, refusal to be left alone, recognition of parent, and demonstration of pleasure by squealing. By 4 months they laugh aloud and enjoy strange, novel stimuli.

By 6 months infants are very personable. They play games such as peekaboo when their head is hidden in a towel, signal their desire to be picked up by extending their arms, and show displeasure when a toy is removed or their face is washed. There is increasing demonstration of their ability to control the environment. The acquisition of fine and gross motor skills allows much more independence in movement.

By the second half of the first year infants understand simple discipline, such as the meaning of the word "no" or a scolding remark. They comprehend different facial expressions and are sensitive to emotional changes in others. Imitation is developing during this time. They imitate actions and noises by 7 months, sounds by 8 months, and games such as pat-a-cake and peekaboo by 10 months.

From 11 months onward they are increasingly independent. They are learning to feed themselves; are using their fingers, spoon, and cup (with much spilling); and can help with dressing by putting the foot out for a shoe or pushing the arm through the sleeve. They not only comprehend the meaning of "no," but they shake their head to indicate "no." They can follow simple directions and gladly perform for others to attract and prolong attention.

### Play

Play during infancy represents the various social modalities observed during cognitive development. The activity of infants is primarily narcissistic and revolves around their own body. As discussed under Development of Body Image, body parts are primarily objects of play and pleasure.

During the first year, play becomes more sophisticated and interdependent. From birth to 3 months infants' responses to the environment are global and largely undifferentiated. Play is dependent; pleasure is demonstrated by a quieting attitude (1 month), a smile (2 months), and a squeal (3 months). From 3 to 6 months infants show more discriminate interest in stimuli and begin to play alone with a rattle or a soft stuffed toy or with someone else. There is much more interaction during play. By 4 months of age they laugh aloud, show preference for certain toys, and become excited when food or a favorite object is brought to them. They recognize an image in a mirror, smile at it, and vocalize to it.

By 6 months to 1 year play involves sensorimotor skills. Actual games such as peekaboo and pat-a-cake are played. Verbal repetition and imitation of simple gestures occurs in response to demonstration. Play is much more selective, not only in terms of specific toys but also in terms of "playmates." Although play is solitary or one-sided, infants choose with whom they will interact. At 6 to 8 months they usually refuse to play with strangers. Parents are definite favorites, and infants know how to attract their attention. At 6 months they extend the arms to be picked up, at 7 months cough to make their presence known, at 10 months pull the parent's clothing, and at 12 months call them by name. This represents a tremendous advance from the newborn who signaled biologic needs by crying to express displeasure.

Stimulation is as important for psychosocial growth as food is for physical growth. Knowledge of developmental milestones allows nurses to guide parents regarding proper play for infants. It is not sufficient to place a mobile over a crib and toys in a playpen for a child's optimum social, emotional, and intellectual development. Play must provide interpersonal contact and recreational and educational stimulation. Infants need to be *played with,* not merely be *allowed to play.* Although the type of play infants engage in is called **solitary,** this is only a figurative, not literal, term to denote one-sided play. The types of toys given to the child is much less important than the quality of personal interaction that occurs.

Table 12-2 lists play activities appropriate for the developmental level of the infant in terms of motor, language, and personal-social achievements. Although the activities are grouped according to the major mode of stimulation provided, there is overlap in many instances. In addition, play activities suggested for one age-group may be appropriate for older infants but inappropriate for younger ones.

## Temperament

The infant's temperament or behavioral style influences the type of interaction that occurs between the child and parents and other family members. In assessing a child's temperament, it is the parents' perception of the child and the degree of fit between their expectations and the child's actual temperament that are important. The more dissonance or lack of harmony between the child's temperament and the parent's ability to accept and deal with the behavior, the more risk for subsequent parent-child conflicts. (See Evidence-Based Practice box on p. 509.)

The *Revised Infant Temperament Questionnaire (RITQ)* (Carey and McDevitt, 1978) can be used as a screening tool with parents. The questionnaire focuses on nine temperament variables, but the 95 questions relate specifically to activities such as sleep, feeding, play, diapering, and dressing. The scores from the RITQ help identify the child's temperamental style. Use of the RITQ is well accepted by parents and should be accompanied by an adequate explanation of the results. In discussing the results, it is best to avoid descriptors such as "difficult" by describing such infants in terms of characteristics such as "intense" or "less predictable." The Early Infancy Temperament Questionnaire (EITQ) is a 76-item parent questionnaire that was adapted from the RITQ to evaluate temperament characteristics of infants 1 to 4 months old, whereas the RITQ is best suited

**TABLE 12-2**   Play during infancy

| Age (months) | Visual Stimulation | Auditory Stimulation | Tactile Stimulation | Kinetic Stimulation |
|---|---|---|---|---|
| **Suggested Activities** | | | | |
| **Birth-1** | Look at infant at close range<br>Hang bright, shiny object within 20-25 cm (8-10 inches) of infant's face and in midline<br>Hang mobiles with black-and-white designs | Talk to infant; sing in soft voice<br>Play music box, tape, or CD | Hold, caress, cuddle<br>Keep infant warm<br>May like to be swaddled | Rock infant; place in cradle<br>Use carriage for walks |
| **2-3** | Provide bright objects<br>Make room bright with pictures or mirrors<br>Take infant to various rooms while doing chores<br>Place infant in infant seat for vertical view of environment | Talk or sing to infant<br>Include in family gatherings<br>Expose to various environmental noises other than those of home<br>Use rattles, wind chimes | Caress infant while bathing, at diaper change<br>Comb hair with a soft brush<br>Massage with lotion | Use infant swing<br>Take in car for rides<br>Exercise body by moving extremities in swimming motion<br>Use cradle gym |
| **4-6** | Place infant in front of unbreakable mirror<br>Give brightly colored toys to hold (small enough to grasp) | Talk to infant; repeat sounds infant makes<br>Laugh when infant laughs<br>Call infant by name<br>Crinkle different papers by infant's ear<br>Place rattle or bell in hand | Give infant soft squeeze toys of various textures<br>Allow to splash in bath<br>Place nude on soft, furry rug and move extremities | Use swing or stroller<br>Bounce infant in lap while holding in standing position<br>Support infant in sitting position; let infant lean forward to balance self<br>Place infant on floor to crawl, roll over, sit |
| **6-9** | Give infant large toys with bright colors, movable parts, and noisemakers<br>Place unbreakable mirror where infant can see self<br>Play peekaboo, especially hiding face in a towel<br>Make funny faces to encourage imitation<br>Give ball of yarn or string to pull apart | Call infant by name<br>Repeat simple words such as "dada," "mama," "bye-bye"<br>Speak clearly<br>Name parts of body, people, and foods<br>Tell infant what you are doing<br>Use "no" only when necessary<br>Give simple commands<br>Show how to clap hands, bang a drum | Let infant play with fabrics of various textures<br>Have bowl with foods of different sizes and textures to feel<br>Let infant "catch" running water<br>Encourage "swimming" in large bathtub or shallow pool<br>Give wad of sticky tape to manipulate | Hold upright to bear weight and bounce<br>Pick up, say "up"<br>Put down, say "down"<br>Place toys out of reach; encourage infant to get them<br>Play pat-a-cake |
| **9-12** | Show infant large pictures in books<br>Take infant to places where there are animals, many people, different objects (shopping center)<br>Play ball by rolling it to child, demonstrate "throwing" it back<br>Demonstrate building a two-block tower | Read infant simple nursery rhymes<br>Point to body parts and name each one<br>Imitate sounds of animals | Give infant finger foods of different textures<br>Let infant mess and squash food<br>Let infant feel cold (ice cube) or warm objects, say what temperature each is<br>Let infant feel a breeze (fan blowing) | Give large push-pull toys<br>Place furniture in a circle to encourage cruising<br>Turn in different positions |
| **Suggested Toys** | | | | |
| **Birth-6** | Nursery mobiles<br>Unbreakable mirrors<br>See-through crib bumpers<br>Contrasting colored sheets | Music boxes<br>Musical mobiles<br>Crib dangle bells<br>Small-handled clear rattle | Small stuffed animals<br>Soft clothes*<br>Soft or furry quilt*<br>Soft mobiles | Rocking crib/cradle<br>Weighted or suction toy<br>Infant swing |
| **6-12** | Various colored blocks<br>Nested boxes or cups<br>Books with rhymes and bright pictures<br>Strings of big beads<br>Simple take-apart toys<br>Large ball<br>Cup and spoon<br>Large puzzles<br>Jack-in-the box | Rattles of different sizes, shapes, tones, and bright colors<br>Squeaky animals and dolls<br>Records with light, rhythmic music | Soft, different-texture animals and dolls<br>Sponge toys, floating toys<br>Squeeze toys<br>Teething toys<br>Books with textures/objects, such as fur and zipper | Activity box for crib<br>Push-pull toys<br>Wind-up swing |

*Remove from crib when put to sleep to avoid possible suffocation (see p. 583).

## EVIDENCE-BASED PRACTICE
### Effect of Infant Temperament on Parenting

Although the importance of temperament is generally acknowledged, its influence on parenting is less clear, and studies often report conflicting findings. However, there is evidence that infant temperament does affect parenting, at least in terms of parents' perception of their parenting role.

An "easy" child is apt to make parents feel more thankful and content in their parenting role, whereas a less adaptable and predictable, more fussy infant may cause parents, especially mothers, to be depressed (Mayberry and Alfonso, 1993). Infants who are labeled easy (approximately two thirds) are reported to fall into three subcategories: (1) social, playful, happy, attention-seeking; (2) gentle, tender, affectionate, and sensitive; and (3) variable, changeable, and adaptable (Johnson and Blasco, 1997). Infants who are less predictable in their behavior, such as sleeping, feeding, and general satisfaction, cause parents to feel less competent and to experience less ease in transition to parenthood. Mothers, especially of first-born children, report having major concerns regarding the behavior of "difficult" infants and of having to make large family adjustments because of their infants.

Infants with "difficult" temperaments also tend to have more colic, injuries, and night waking. About one third of infants may be categorized as difficult or slow to warm up (Johnson and Blasco, 1997). These children sleep approximately 2 hours less at night and 1 hour less during the day than the "easy" child. Children's sleep behavior probably influences parental perceptions of their temperament, but exactly what effect these variables have on parenting is unclear (Scher and others, 1992). There is evidence that having a "difficult" child mobilizes parents to provide a more responsive home environment (Houdlin, 1987). One study found that among the various temperament types, the "difficult" group had higher intelligence quotients if the family was of higher socioeconomic status. It might be that in order to deal with the child's negative behaviors, the parents pay more attention to the child (Maziade and others, 1987). Such findings emphasize the tremendous challenge, as well as the opportunity, that exists in rearing these children.

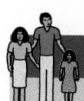

## FAMILY FOCUS
### Difficult Temperament and Preterm Infants

Parents typically rate preterm, low-birth-weight infants as being more difficult than full-term infants (Langkamp, Kim, and Pascoe, 1998). Parents are often concerned that the difficult temperament is permanent and results from the many negative and painful hospital experiences. The family can be reassured that although these infants may be difficult to parent for the first 6 months of corrected age (chronologic age minus amount of prematurity), over time the infants tend to become less difficult (Medoff-Cooper, 1995). Most of the studies indicating that preterm infants are more difficult to console were performed before wide-scale implementation of individualized developmental care for such infants; kangaroo care and assisting the infant in self-regulation behaviors may in fact change current thought. By enabling the preterm infant to experience more positive caretaking and less stressful stimuli, such infants may be found in the future to be less temperamental.

Parents may find the following book helpful: *The Fussy Baby* by W. Sears (Franklin Park, Ill, 1989, La Leche League International).

---

for infants 4 months old and older (Medoff-Cooper, Carey, and McDevitt, 1993).

With knowledge of the infant's temperament, nurses are better able to (1) provide parents with background information that will help them see their child in a better perspective, (2) offer a more organized picture of their child's behavior and possibly reveal distortions in their perceptions of the behavior, and (3) guide parents regarding appropriate childrearing techniques.

### Childrearing Practices Related to Temperament

Most parents realize that their infant is born with unique characteristics, and few parents of difficult infants need to be told of the challenge of caring for them. However, very few parents are aware of the significance of the temperamental characteristics and of constructive approaches to dealing with them. The following are examples of interventions that promote more positive parenting of infants with different temperament styles.*

---

*Recommended resources for parents are *The Difficult Child* by S.K. Turecki and L. Tonner (2000, Bantam Books) www.randomhouse.com, and *Know Your Child: An Authoritative Guide for Today's Parents* by S. Chess and A. Thomas (1996, Jason Aronson, Inc); www.aronson.com.

"Difficult" children may respond better to scheduled feedings and structured caregiving routines than demand feedings and frequent changes in daily routines. These children sleep less and may need more structured approaches to bedtime to prevent bedtime problems. "Highly distractible children" may require additional soothing measures such as swinging, rocking, or being carried in a pack that the parent wears across the chest or back. Children with "high activity" levels require vigilant watching, and parents need to take extra precautions in safeguarding the home. These children benefit from increased opportunities for gross motor activity to constructively channel their energy.

The child who is "slow to warm up" may demonstrate more stranger fear than other children and may require gradual and frequent preparation for new situations, such as substitute child care. Even the "easy child" can present problems in that the parents may need reminders to feed the child who sleeps for prolonged intervals and rarely cries. They may need to "retrain" the child because of the ease of developing habits such as keeping the child up late or sleeping with the youngster, which may later become troublesome.

Appropriate counseling based on awareness of the child's temperament can greatly enhance the quality of interaction between parents and infant. Even just letting parents know that "difficult" traits are innate can relieve feelings of guilt and incompetence. (See Family Focus box.)

■   ■   ■

Knowledge of the developmental sequence allows the nurse to assess normal growth and minor or abnormal deviations, helps parents gain realistic expectations of their child's ability, and provides guidelines for suitable play and stimulation. Parents who lack knowledge of child growth and development may set inappropriate behavioral expectations for their children. Emphasizing the child's developmental rather than chronologic age strengthens the parent-child relationship by fostering trust and lessening frustration. Therefore the importance of a thorough understanding and appreciation of the growth and development of children cannot be overemphasized.

Because of the complexity of the developmental process during the first 12 months, Table 12-3 is presented to help or-

**TABLE 12-3**   Growth and development during infancy

| Age (months) | Physical | Gross Motor | Fine Motor |
|---|---|---|---|
| 1 | Weight gain of 150 to 210 g (5 to 7 ounces) weekly for first 6 months<br>Height gain of 2.5 cm (1 inch) monthly for first 6 months<br>Head circumference increases by 2 cm (¾ inch) monthly for first 3 months<br>Primitive reflexes present and strong<br>Doll's eye reflexes and dance reflex fading<br>Obligatory nose breathing (most infants) | • Assumes flexed position with pelvis high but knees not under abdomen when prone (at birth, knees flexed under abdomen)<br>• Can turn head from side to side when prone; lifts head momentarily from bed (see Fig. 12-7, *A*)<br>Has marked head lag, especially when pulled from lying to sitting position (see Fig. 12-6, *A*)<br>Holds head momentarily parallel and in midline when suspended in prone position<br>Assumes asymmetric tonic neck reflex position when supine<br>When held in standing position, body limp at knees and hips<br>In sitting position back is uniformly rounded, absence of head control (see Fig. 12-8, *A*) | Hands predominantly closed<br>Grasp reflex strong<br>Hand clenches on contact with rattle |
| 2 | Posterior fontanel closed<br>Crawling reflex disappears | • Assumes less flexed position when prone—hips flat, legs extended, arms flexed, head to side<br>Less head lag when pulled to sitting position (see Fig. 12-6, *B*)<br>Can maintain head in same plane as rest of body when held in ventral suspension<br>When prone, can lift head almost 45 degrees off table<br>When held in sitting position, head is held up but bobs forward (see Fig. 12-8, *B*)<br>Assumes asymmetric tonic neck reflex position intermittently | Hands often open<br>Grasp reflex fading |
| 3 | Primitive reflexes fading | Able to hold head more erect when sitting, but still bobs forward<br>Has only slight head lag when pulled to sitting position<br>Assumes symmetric body positioning<br>Able to raise head and shoulders from prone position to a 45- to 90-degree angle from table; bears weight on forearms<br>When held in standing position, able to bear slight fraction of weight on legs<br>Regards own hand | • Actively holds rattle but will not reach for it<br>Grasp reflex absent<br>Hands kept loosely open<br>Clutches own hand; pulls at blankets and clothes |
| 4 | Head circumference increases by 1 cm<br>Drooling begins<br>• Moro, tonic neck, and rooting reflexes have disappeared | • Has almost no head lag when pulled to sitting position (see Fig. 12-6, *C*)<br>• Balances head well in sitting position (see Fig. 12-8, *C*)<br>Back less rounded, curved only in lumbar area<br>Able to sit erect if propped up<br>Able to raise head and chest off surface to angle of 90 degrees (see Fig. 12-7, *B*)<br>Assumes predominant symmetric position<br>• Rolls from back to side | • Inspects and plays with hands; pulls clothing or blanket over face in play<br>Tries to reach objects with hand but overshoots<br>Grasps object with both hands<br>Plays with rattle placed in hand, shakes it, but cannot pick it up if dropped<br>Can carry objects to mouth |

• Milestones representing essential integrative aspects of development that lay the foundation for the achievement of more advanced skills.

ganize and clarify the data already discussed. Although all milestones are important, some represent essential integrative aspects of development that lay the foundation for achievement of more advanced skills. These essential milestones are designated by a square (■) in the table. The table represents the average monthly age at which various skills are attained. It must be remembered that, although the sequence is the same, the rate will vary among children.

| Sensory | Vocalization | Socialization/Cognition |
|---|---|---|
| ■ Able to fixate on moving object in range of 45 degrees when held at a distance of 20-25 cm (8-10 inches)<br>Visual acuity approaches 20/100*<br>Follows light to midline<br>Quiets when hears a voice | Cries to express displeasure<br>Makes small, throaty sounds<br>Makes comfort sounds during feeding | Is in sensorimotor phase—stage I, use of reflexes (birth–1 month), and stage II, primary circular reactions (1-4 months)<br>Watches parent's face intently as she or he talks to infant |
| Binocular fixation and convergence to near objects beginning<br>When supine, follows dangling toy from side to point beyond midline<br>Visually searches to locate sounds<br>Turns head to side when sound is made at level of ear | ■ Vocalizes, distinct from crying<br>Crying becomes differentiated<br>Coos<br>Vocalizes to familiar voice | ■ Demonstrates social smile in response to various stimuli |
| ■ Follows object to periphery (180 degrees)<br>■ Locates sound by turning head to side and looking in same direction<br>Begins to have ability to coordinate stimuli from various sense organs | ■ Squeals aloud to show pleasure<br>Coos, babbles, chuckles<br>Vocalizes when smiling<br>"Talks" a great deal when spoken to<br>Less crying during periods of wakefulness | Displays considerable interest in surroundings<br>Ceases crying when parent enters room<br>Can recognize familiar faces and objects, such as feeding bottle<br>Shows awareness of strange situations |
| Able to accommodate to near objects<br>Binocular vision fairly well established<br>Can focus on a 1.25-cm (½-inch) block<br>Beginning eye-hand coordination | Makes consonant sounds *n, k, g, p, b*<br>■ Laughs aloud<br>Vocalization changes according to mood | Is in stage III, secondary circular reactions<br>Demands attention by fussing; becomes bored if left alone<br>Enjoys social interaction with people<br>Anticipates feeding when sees bottle or mother if breast-feeding<br>Shows excitement with whole body, squeals, breathes heavily<br>Shows interest in strange stimuli<br>Begins to show memory |

*Degree of visual acuity varies according to vision measurement procedure used.

*Continued*

**TABLE 12-3**  Growth and development during infancy—cont'd

| Age (months) | Physical | Gross Motor | Fine Motor |
|---|---|---|---|
| 5 | Beginning signs of tooth eruption<br>Birth weight doubled | No head lag when pulled to sitting position<br>When sitting, able to hold head erect and steady<br>Able to sit for longer periods when back is well supported<br>Back straight<br>When prone, assumes symmetric positioning with arms extended<br>▪ Can turn over from abdomen to back<br>When supine, puts feet to mouth | ▪ Able to grasp objects voluntarily<br>Uses palmar grasp, bidextrous approach<br>Plays with toes<br>Takes objects directly to mouth<br>Holds one cube while regarding a second one |
| 6 | Growth rate may begin to decline<br>Weight gain of 90 to 150 g (3 to 5 ounces) weekly for next 6 months<br>Height gain of 1.25 cm (½ inch) monthly for next 6 months<br>▪ Teething may begin with eruption of two lower central incisors<br>▪ Chewing and biting occur | When prone, can lift chest and upper abdomen off table bearing weight on hands (see Fig. 12-7, C)<br>When about to be pulled to a sitting position, lifts head<br>Sits in high chair with back straight<br>Rolls from back to abdomen<br>When held in standing position, bears almost all of weight<br>Hand regard absent | Resecures a dropped object<br>Drops one cube when another is given<br>Grasps and manipulates small objects<br>Holds bottle<br>Grasps feet and pulls to mouth |
| 7 | Eruption of upper central incisors<br>Parachute reflex appears (see Fig. 12-1) | When supine, spontaneously lifts head off table<br>▪ Sits, leaning forward on hands (see Fig. 12-8, D)<br>When prone, bears weight on one hand<br>Sits erect momentarily<br>Bears full weight on feet (see Fig. 12-9, A)<br>When held in standing position, bounces actively | ▪ Transfers objects from one hand to the other (see Fig. 12-8, E)<br>Has unidextrous approach and grasp<br>Holds two cubes more than momentarily<br>Bangs cube on table<br>Rakes at a small object |
| 8 | Begins to show regular patterns in bladder and bowel elimination | ▪ Sits steadily unsupported (see Fig. 12-8, E)<br>Readily bears weight on legs when supported; can maneuver from sitting to kneeling position (see Fig. 12-9, B)<br>Adjusts posture to reach an object | Has beginning pincer grasp using index, fourth, and fifth fingers against lower part of thumb<br>Releases objects at will<br>Rings bell purposely<br>Retains two cubes while regarding third cube<br>Secures an object by pulling on a string<br>Reaches persistently for toys out of reach |
| 9 | Eruption of upper lateral incisor may begin | Creeps on hands and knees<br>Sits steadily on floor for prolonged time (10 minutes)<br>Recovers balance when leans forward but cannot do so when leaning sideways<br>▪ Pulls self to standing position and stands holding onto furniture (see Fig. 12-9, B-D) | ▪ Uses thumb and index finger in crude pincer grasp (see Fig. 12-4)<br>Preference for use of dominant hand now evident<br>Grasps third cube<br>Compares two cubes by bringing them together |

▪ Milestones representing essential integrative aspects of development that lay the foundation for the achievement of more advanced skills.

| Sensory | Vocalization | Socialization/Cognition |
|---|---|---|
| Visually pursues a dropped object<br>Is able to sustain visual inspection of an object<br>Can localize sounds made below the ear | Squeals<br>Makes vowel cooing sounds interspersed with consonant sounds (e.g., *ah-goo*) | Smiles at mirror image<br>Pats bottle or breast with both hands<br>More enthusiastically playful, but may have rapid mood swings<br>Is able to discriminate strangers from family<br>Vocalizes displeasure when object is taken away<br>Discovers parts of body |
| Adjusts posture to see an object<br>Prefers more complex visual stimuli<br>Can localize sounds made above the ear<br>Will turn head to the side, then look up or down | ▪ Begins to imitate sounds<br>▪ Babbling resembles one-syllable utterances—*ma, mu, da, di, hi*<br>Vocalizes to toys, mirror image<br>Takes pleasure in hearing own sounds (self-reinforcement) | Recognizes parents; begins to fear strangers<br>Holds arms out to be picked up<br>Has definite likes and dislikes<br>Begins to imitate (cough, protrusion of tongue)<br>Excites on hearing footsteps<br>Laughs when head is hidden in a towel<br>▪ Briefly searches for a dropped object (object permanence beginning)<br>Frequent mood swings—from crying to laughing with little or no provocation |
| ▪ Can fixate on very small objects<br>Responds to own name<br>Localizes sound by turning head in a curving arch<br>Beginning awareness of depth and space<br>Has taste preferences | ▪ Produces vowel sounds and chained syllables—*baba, dada, kaka*<br>Vocalizes four distinct vowel sounds<br>"Talks" when others are talking | ▪ Increasing fear of strangers; shows signs of fretfulness when parent disappears<br>Imitates simple acts and noises<br>Tries to attract attention by coughing or snorting<br>Plays peekaboo<br>Demonstrates dislike of food by keeping lips closed<br>Exhibits oral aggressiveness in biting and mouthing<br>Demonstrates expectation in response to repetition of stimuli |
|  | Makes consonant sounds *t, d,* and *w*<br>Listens selectively to familiar words<br>Utterances signal emphasis and emotion<br>Combines syllables, such as *dada*, but does not ascribe meaning to them | Increasing anxiety over loss of parent, particularly mother, and fear of strangers<br>Responds to word "no"<br>Dislikes dressing, diaper change |
| Localizes sounds by turning head diagonally and directly toward sound<br>Depth perception increasing | Responds to simple verbal commands<br>Comprehends "no-no" | Parent (mother) is increasingly important for own sake<br>Shows increasing interest in pleasing parent<br>Begins to show fears of going to bed and being left alone<br>Puts arms in front of face to avoid having it washed |

*Continued*

**TABLE 12-3**  Growth and development during infancy—cont'd

| Age (months) | Physical | Gross Motor | Fine Motor |
|---|---|---|---|
| 10 | Labyrinth-righting reflex is strongest—when infant is in prone or supine position, is able to raise head | Can change from prone to sitting position<br>Stands while holding onto furniture, sits by falling down<br>Recovers balance easily while sitting<br>While standing, lifts one foot to take a step (see Fig. 12-9, *D*) | Crude release of an object beginning<br>Grasps bell by handle |
| 11 | Eruption of lower lateral incisors may begin | When sitting, pivots to reach toward back to pick up an object<br>▪ Cruises or walks holding onto furniture or with both hands held | Explores objects more thoroughly (e.g., clapper inside bell)<br>Has neat pincer grasp (see Fig. 12-5)<br>Drops object deliberately for it to be picked up<br>Puts one object after another into a container (sequential play)<br>Able to manipulate an object to remove it from tight-fitting enclosure |
| 12 | ▪ Birth weight tripled<br>▪ Birth length increased by 50%<br>Head and chest circumference equal (head circumference 46 cm [18 inches])<br>Has total of six to eight deciduous teeth<br>Anterior fontanel almost closed<br>Landau reflex fading<br>Babinski reflex disappears<br>Lumbar curve develops: lordosis evident during walking | ▪ Walks with one hand held<br>Cruises well<br>▪ May attempt to stand alone momentarily; may attempt first step alone<br>Can sit down from standing position without help | Releases cube in cup<br>Attempts to build two-block tower but fails<br>Tries to insert a pellet into a narrow-necked bottle but fails<br>Can turn pages in a book, many at a time |

▪ Milestones representing essential integrative aspects of development that lay the foundation for the achievement of more advanced skills.

## Coping with Concerns Related to Normal Growth and Development

### Separation Anxiety and Stranger Fear

A number of fears can appear during infancy. However, the fear that causes many parents concern is fear related to strangers and separation. Although erroneously interpreted by some as a sign of undesirable, antisocial behavior, stranger fear and separation anxiety are important components of a strong, healthy parent-child attachment. Nevertheless, this period can present difficulties for the parent and child. Parents may be more confined to the home because baby-sitters are violently protested by the infant. To accustom the infant to new people, parents are encouraged to have close friends or relatives visit often. This provides for other persons with whom the child is comfortable and who can give parents time for themselves.

Infants also need opportunities to safely experience strangers. Usually toward the end of the first year infants begin to venture away from the parent and demonstrate curiosity about strangers. If allowed to explore at their own rate, many infants eventually "warm up." If parents hold the child away from their face, the infant can observe while maintaining close physical contact.

A number of factors influence the intensity of a child's stranger fears:

▪ Sex, age, and size of the stranger—female, younger age, and smaller size (including kneeling or sitting rather than standing) being less stressful
▪ Approach—loud, sudden, intrusive approach causing more distress
▪ Child's proximity to parent—closer to parent (on parent's lap rather than in infant seat) being less stressful

| Sensory | Vocalization | Socialization/Cognition |
|---|---|---|
| | • Says "dada," "mama" with meaning<br>Comprehends "bye-bye"<br>May say one word (e.g., "hi," "bye," "no") | Inhibits behavior to verbal command of "no-no" or own name<br>Imitates facial expressions; waves bye-bye<br>Extends toy to another person but will not release it<br>• Develops object permanence<br>Repeats actions that attract attention and cause laughter<br>Pulls clothes of another to attract attention<br>Plays interactive games such as pat-a-cake<br>Reacts to adult anger; cries when scolded<br>Demonstrates independence in dressing, feeding, locomotive skills, and testing of parents<br>Looks at and follows pictures in a book |
| | Imitates definite speech sounds | Experiences joy and satisfaction when a task is mastered<br>Reacts to restrictions with frustration<br>Rolls ball to another on request<br>Anticipates body gestures when a familiar nursery rhyme or story is being told (e.g., hold toes and feet in response to "This little piggy went to market")<br>Plays game up-down, "so big," or peekaboo<br>Shakes head for "no" |
| Discriminates simple geometric forms (e.g., circle)<br>Amblyopia may develop with lack of binocularity<br>Can follow rapidly moving object<br>Controls and adjusts response to sound; listens for sound to recur | • Says three to five words besides "dada," "mama"<br>Comprehends meaning of several words (comprehension always precedes verbalization)<br>Recognizes objects by name<br>Imitates animal sounds<br>Understands simple verbal commands (e.g., "Give it to me," "Show me your eyes") | Shows emotions such as jealousy, affection (may give hug or kiss on request), anger, fear<br>Enjoys familiar surroundings and explores away from parent<br>Is fearful in strange situation; clings to parent<br>May develop habit of "security blanket" or favorite toy<br>Has increasing determination to practice locomotor skills<br>• Searches for an object even if it has not been hidden, but searches only where object was last seen |

Consequently, the best approach for the stranger (who may be the nurse) is to talk softly, meet the child at eye level (to appear smaller), maintain a safe distance from the infant, and avoid sudden, intrusive gestures, such as holding the arms out and smiling broadly.

Parents also may wonder whether they should encourage the child's clinging, dependent behavior, especially if there is pressure from others who view this as "spoiling" (see following discussion). Parents need to be reassured that such behavior is healthy, desirable, and necessary for the child's optimum emotional development. If parents can reassure the infant of their presence, the infant will learn to realize that they are still there even if not physically present. Talking to infants when leaving the room, allowing them to hear one's voice on the telephone, and using transitional objects (e.g., a favorite blanket or toy) reassures them of the parent's continued presence.

This is a no less trying but necessary time for infants, because parents cannot always be with the child. An excellent example of necessary separation is bedtime. Fear of going to bed or being left alone in the dark commonly occurs during the second half of the first year. Fear at bedtime is only one of the many bedtime problems that can occur in young children and is discussed on p. 525 and in Chapter 15.

## Spoiled Child Syndrome

A common concern of parents is that too much attention can "spoil" a child. Many of the recommendations for promoting attachment, such as attending to the infant's needs to establish trust, accepting fear of strangers and separation from parent, and holding and rocking the crying child, are described by parents as methods of spoiling. However, research on parents' response to crying during early infancy does not support the contention that "picking up a crying baby" leads to spoiling. Ainsworth (1982) found that the amount an infant cried during the first 3 months had no correlation with the frequency of crying during the rest of the first year. However, the degree of maternal responsiveness to crying did. Parents who were less responsive, such as not picking up the infant immediately on crying, had infants who cried *more* than those of parents who responded promptly to crying. Parents of colicky infants less than 3 months old who responded to the crying with increased attention successfully decreased the overall crying time.

If "too much attention" does not cause spoiling in early infancy, parents need to understand what "spoiling" really is and how it differs from normal behavior that may mimic aspects of spoiling. The *spoiled child syndrome* has been defined as "excessive self-centered and immature behavior, resulting from the failure of parents to enforce consistent, age-appropriate limits" (McIntosh, 1989). Spoiled children demand to have their own way, are inconsiderate of others, and have intrusive, obstructive, and manipulative behavior. Indulging children, when combined with clear expectations and limits, does not cause spoiling. However, indulgence with failure to provide guidelines for acceptable behavior can result in a "spoiled brat."

Several age-related normal behaviors and child characteristics can be mistaken for evidence of spoiling:

- Crying during early infancy that may or may not be associated with colic
- Toddler behaviors such as negativism, persistent exploration, and temper tantrums
- Children with difficult temperaments or ADHD
- Children experiencing extreme stress from marital discord, abuse, substance abuse, or mental illness in a parent

With anticipatory guidance regarding expected but challenging behaviors and situations that may produce extreme stress in children, parents should feel comfortable in loving their infant without fear of spoiling. However, as the infant gets older, parents need assistance in providing limits that prevent normal, disruptive behaviors, such as temper tantrums, from becoming problems.

## Limit-Setting and Discipline

As infants' motor skills advance and mobility increases, parents are faced with the need to set safe limits (see discussion of nurse's role in injury prevention on p. 548). Although there are numerous disciplinary techniques, some are more appropriate for this age than others. Parents can begin discipline using a negative voice and stern eye-to-eye contact. When more definitive measures must be used, one of the most effective approaches is time-out. The basic principles are the same as those discussed in Chapter 3, except that the place for time-out needs to be commensurate with the child's abilities. For example, the playpen is better for most infants than a chair. Although parents may be concerned with instituting discipline during infancy, it is important to stress that the earlier effective disciplinary methods are employed, the easier it is to continue these approaches.

## Alternate Child Care Arrangements

For many parents, especially working mothers, the need for locating safe and competent child care facilities for the infant is an increasingly difficult problem—one that is compounded by the number of mothers working outside the home. Over the past 30 years there has been a marked shift in child-care arrangements, with fewer children cared for at home and more children cared for in group centers or other settings.

**Types of Child Care.** The basic types of care are inhome care, either in the parents' or caregivers' home (family daycare), and center-based care, usually in a daycare center. *Inhome care* may consist of a full-time baby-sitter or nanny who lives in the home, a full-time baby-sitter who comes to the home, cooperative arrangements such as exchange baby-sitting, and family daycare. A licensed *family daycare home* typically provides care and protection for up to five children for part of a 24-hour day and does not include informal arrangements such as exchange baby-sitting or caregivers in the child's own home. The five children include the family daycare provider's own children younger than 5 years of age living in the home. Many family daycare homes operate without a license and may care for large numbers of infants without adequate staff and facilities.

*Center-based care* usually refers to a licensed daycare facility that provides care for six or more children, for 6 or more hours in a 24-hour day. *Work-based group care* is another option that is becoming increasingly popular as employers recognize the benefit of providing quality and convenient child care to their employees. *Sick-child care* may also be available for times when the youngster is ill. Such programs are often located in community hospitals and some corporations.

**Guiding Parents in Selecting Child Care.** A major nursing responsibility is guiding parents in locating suitable facilities that have a well-qualified staff. State licensing agencies can help parents identify daycare centers that accept children of specific age-groups and are convenient to home and work. Their records are available to the public and provide reports from the health, safety, and fire departments; periodic evaluations from the licensing agency; complaints filed against the center; and qualification of the center's employees. State-licensed programs are supposed to abide by established standards, which represent the *minimum* requirements and safeguards. However, enforcement of the standards is sometimes inadequate. Early childhood programs may also belong to a voluntary accreditation system, the National Academy of Early Childhood Programs, which serves as a model for *optimum* care.* References from other

---

*Information about the accreditation criteria and procedures of the National Academy of Early Childhood Programs is available from the **National Association for the Education of Young Children,** 1509 16th St NW, Washington, DC 20036, (800) 424-2460 or (202) 232-8777; fax: (202) 328-1846; www.naeyc.org. These criteria are excellent guidelines for evaluating child care facilities. Other resources are *Child Care: What's Best for Your Family* and a number of other child care pamphlets available from the **American Academy of Pediatrics,** 141 Northwest Point Blvd, Elk Grove Village, IL 60007, (888) 227-1770; www.medem.com, then enter "Medical Library" for pamphlet titles, and *Parent's Guide to Day Care,* available from the **National Association of Pediatric Nurse Associates and Practitioners (NAPNAP),** 1101 Kings Highway North, Suite 206, Cherry Hill, NJ 08034-1912, (877) 662-7627 or (856) 667-1773, fax: (856) 667-7187; www.napnap.org.

parents are also helpful, provided they have investigated the center carefully and have remained involved with the agency's activities.

Other areas for parents to evaluate are the center's daily program, teacher qualifications, nurturing qualities of caregivers, student-to-staff ratio, discipline policy, environmental safety precautions, provision of meals, sanitary conditions, adequate indoor/outdoor space per child, and fee schedule. Although fees vary considerably, a program that charges a minimum fee may also be providing minimum services. In terms of an overall evaluation, *there is no substitute for a personal observation of the facility.* Parents should arrange to meet the director and some of the employees, especially those who would be caring for the child. Resources to familiarize parents with characteristics of quality child care and checklists to systematically evaluate the center and make comparisons with other facilities can help parents make successful choices.

The same conscientious attention is applied to locating competent baby-sitters. References from other employers are essential, and there is no substitute for observing the interaction between the individual and the child. Although very young infants need little if any preparation for the introduction of a new caregiver, older infants may benefit from a gradual placement to reduce stranger fear. (See Preschool and Kindergarten Experience, Chapter 15.) At all times the parent should have the right to visit the child, and regular conferences should be established to review the child's progress.

One of the areas that is increasingly important in selecting child care is the center's health practices, however, parents often do not check the center for health and safety features. Substantial evidence shows that children, especially those under age 3 years in daycare centers, have more illnesses—especially diarrhea, otitis media, respiratory tract infections (especially if the caregiver smokes), hepatitis A, meningitis, and cytomegalovirus—than children cared for in their home (Alho and others, 1993). The strongest predictor of risk of illness is the number of unrelated children in the room. Proactive infection control measures and education of staff have been effective in reducing the incidence of upper respiratory infections, diarrhea, and rotavirus (Uhari and Mottonen, 1999; Denehy, 2000; Roberts and others, 2000a; Roberts and others, 2000b). Parents should inquire about the center's policy regarding the attendance and care of sick children.

Another concern is the frequency of injuries in daycare centers and daycare homes. Reports on daycare homes found a high rate of safety hazards, even higher than in daycare centers. Other reports indicate that injuries, especially falls on playgrounds, commonly occur in daycare centers. Studies indicate that boys are more likely to sustain daycare center playground injuries than girls; these injuries primarily occurred late in the morning (Ulione and Dooling, 1997; Alkon and others, 1999). What is less clear is whether these risks are greater than those in the child's own home; preliminary data suggest that the risk is not greater (Briss and others, 1994; Rivara and others, 1989). State regulations regarding playground safety, choking, and firearms safety are often poorly monitored (Runyan and others, 1991; Ulione, 1997).

Nurses play an important role in infection control and injury prevention. Not only can they advise parents regarding the evaluation of a center's sanitary and safety practices, but they can also take an active part in educating staff in measures to minimize the transmission of infection and injury. For example, in centers caring for children who are not toilet trained, reducing environmental contamination with urine and feces is an important infection control issue. Some studies have shown that disposable superabsorbent diapers contain urine and feces better and result in less environmental contamination than cloth diapers (Kubiak and others, 1993). In one study, diaper type (cloth vs disposable) made no significant difference in frequency or intensity of fecal contamination in four separate child daycare centers (Holaday and others, 1995). Nurses can discuss the advantages of disposable vs cloth diapers with staff (Wong and others, 1992). Guidelines for diapering and toileting recommended by the **American Public Health Association** and the **American Academy of Pediatrics** (1992) include (Fig. 12-13):*

- Handwashing by children and personnel after diaper changing and toileting
- Using disposable paper diapers, single-unit reusable cloth diapers with an inner cotton lining attached to an outer water-

*Child care guidelines can be ordered from American Academy of Pediatrics, 141 Northwest Point Blvd, PO Box 747, Elk Grove Village, IL 60009, (888) 227-1770, fax: (847) 228-1281; www.aap.org. Use ISBN: 0875532055 when ordering guidelines.

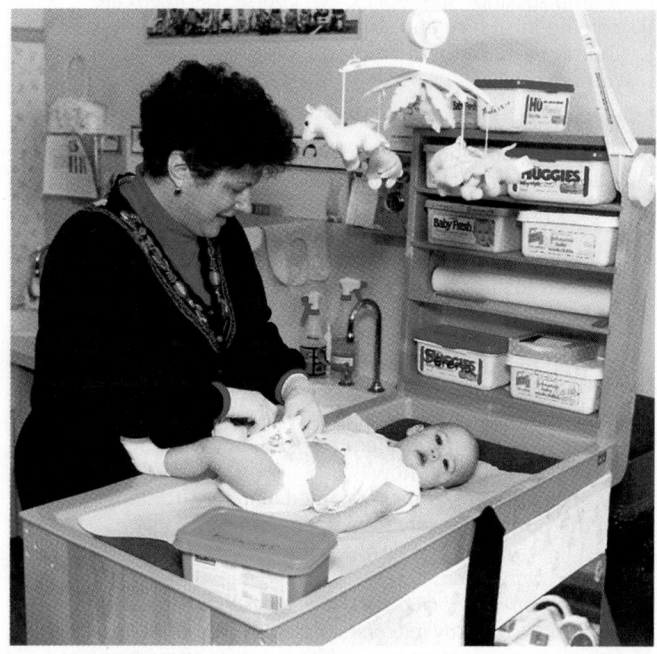

**Fig. 12-13**  Prevention of urine- and fecal-borne infections requires sanitary practices during diaper changes, such as discarding paper diapers in a covered receptacle, changing paper covers on the diaper-changing surface, and having facilities for handwashing nearby. Soiled cloth diapers and clothing are stored in a plastic bag for transport home.

proof cover, or cloth diapers with a separate overwrap if removed as one unit and not reused until cleaned and disinfected

■ Changing diapers as soon as they are soiled

■ Never rinsing cloth diapers, although fecal contents can be flushed down the toilet

■ Sending soiled cloth diapers and clothing home in a sealed plastic bag

■ Cleaning the diaper-changing surface properly and using it only for this purpose

The nurse should also encourage parents to discuss their feelings regarding the child's separation from home, particularly guilt about leaving the child in someone else's care when the parent returns to work. Practical ways of alleviating anxiety and improving the quality of time spent with the child include planning a household schedule that divides major chores into smaller ones, combining household duties with a childcare activity, such as cleaning the bathroom while the child is bathing, and providing time for relaxation and activity with the child.

### Thumb Sucking and Use of Pacifier

Sucking is the infant's chief pleasure and may not be satisfied by breast- or bottle-feeding. It is such a strong need that

## Critical Thinking Exercise

### Thumb Sucking

During a well-child visit you observe that Mrs. Lopez persistently takes the thumb out of her 10-month-old daughter, Maria's, mouth. You ask if she has concerns about the thumb sucking. She replies, "Of course. Her teeth are coming in so nice and straight and I don't want the thumb to make them crooked." What is an appropriate response?

FIRST, THINK ABOUT IT . . .

• What information are you using?

• How are you interpreting that information?

1. "Sucking on a thumb or pacifier is very common in young children, especially in infants. It satisfies their need to suck and helps them to comfort themselves. Sometimes, making an issue of the sucking can cause it to last longer."

2. "Thumb sucking is perfectly normal and children stop when they are ready. So don't worry about it."

3. "If thumb sucking continues when most of her teeth are in, it will make them crooked. But we don't need to worry about it now."

4. "You are right to be concerned. Let her suck longer on the bottle to satisfy her sucking needs."

*The best response is one. The response provides factual information in a nonjudgmental manner that invites further discussion. You may interpret options two and three as partly correct in regard to thumb sucking, but they offer premature reassurance. Option four is incorrect and at 10 months of age, infants should be relying less, not more, on bottle-feeding, which can lead to excessive intake of milk, juice, or other sweetened beverages in place of solid foods and to dental caries. (See Weaning, p. 524, and Dental Health, p. 527.)*

infants who are deprived of sucking, such as those with a cleft lip repair, will suck on their tongues. Some newborns are born with sucking blisters on their hands from in utero sucking activity. The benefits of nonnutritive sucking have been documented, such as increased weight gain in premature infants and decreased crying (Pickler and Frankel, 1995).

Problems arise when parents are overly concerned about the sucking of the fingers, thumb, or pacifier and attempt to restrain this natural tendency. Before giving advice, nurses should investigate the parents' feelings and base guidance on this information. (See Critical Thinking Exercise box.)

During infancy and early childhood there appears to be no need to restrain nonnutritive sucking of the fingers unless the habit extends into the late preschool years. Malocclusion may occur if thumb sucking persists past 4 years of age or 6 years as indicated by some authorities (Johns, Miller, and Hochstetler, 1998; Van Norman, 2001), or when the permanent teeth erupt. A number of studies have shown that pacifier use in infancy is associated with a higher incidence of malocclusion, regardless of the pacifier type (orthodontic vs. standard nipple) (Nowak and Warren, 2000).

Thumb sucking in one study of breast-feeding infants was not associated with a decrease in the incidence of breast-feeding (Aarts and others, 1999).

There are studies linking the early introduction of a pacifier with less frequent breast-feeding, (Aarts and others, 1999; Howard and others, 1999; Vogel, Hutchison, and Mitchell, 2001), early termination of breast-feeding, and early weaning from the breast. Biancuzzo (1999) suggests that health care workers must maintain a commonsense approach to pacifier usage and breast-feeding. Parents should be informed of the relationship between pacifier use and early termination of breast-feeding so that an informed decision can be made. Furthermore, pacifier use should not replace actual feeding or suckling; prohibiting pacifier use will not ensure an increase in the length of breast-feeding, and there should be an emphasis on allowing the infant to control the pace, frequency, and termination of feeding rather than allowing the pacifier (or anything else) to become the focus of the interaction.

The use of a pacifier in infants has also been suggested as a causative factor in the increase in episodes of acute otitis media (Niemela, Uhari, and Mottonen, 1995). However, a 29% decrease in the incidence of acute otitis media was reported in clinics when parents were encouraged to use a pacifier for infants less than 18 months old when the child was going to sleep rather than on a continuous basis (Niemela and others, 2000). The effect of continual pacifier use on early speech and language development is unknown, but the pacifier may decrease the child's desire to imitate sounds and affect intelligibility. Parents need to be alerted that continual dependency on a pacifier may influence social and speech development.

If the child uses a pacifier, safety considerations in purchasing one must be stressed. Parents should be cautioned against altering a pacifier, thus making it more dangerous. (See Aspiration of Foreign Objects, p. 541.) To decrease dependence on nonnutritive sucking in young infants, sucking pleasure can be increased by prolonging feeding time. A small-holed, firm nipple causes stronger sucking and slower feeding. Also, the parent's excessive use of the pacifier to calm the child should be explored. It is not unusual for parents to place a pacifier in the infant's mouth as soon as crying begins, thus reinforcing a pattern of distress-relief.

At the time of this writing, there is no evidence that pacifier use and nonnutritive sucking in preterm infants has any effect on the initiation and length of breast-feeding. Nonnutritive sucking should not be withheld from preterm infants, especially when performed in conjunction with the use of concentrated sucrose for pain management.

Thumb sucking reaches its peak at age 18 to 20 months and is most prevalent when the child is hungry, sick, or tired. Persistent thumb sucking in a listless, apathetic child always warrants investigation. It may be a sign of an emotional problem between parent and child or of boredom, isolation, and lack of stimulation.

## Teething

One of the more difficult periods in the infant's (and parents') life is the eruption of the deciduous (primary) teeth, often referred to as teething. The age of tooth eruption shows considerable variation among children, but the order of their appearance is fairly regular and predictable (Fig. 12-14). The first primary teeth to erupt are the lower central incisors, which appear at approximately 6 to 8 months of age. These are followed closely by the upper central incisors.

**NURSING TIP** A quick guide to assessment of deciduous teeth during the first 2 years is: *age of the child in months − 6 = number of teeth.* For example: 8 months of age − 6 = 2 teeth at this time.

The exact mechanisms responsible for the eruption of teeth are not fully understood. The growth of the root, dentin, and pulp of the tooth; the pressure exerted against the periodontal tissue; and hormonal control of pituitary growth hormone and thyroid hormone are some of the theories under investigation.

Teething is a physiologic process; some discomfort is common as the crown of the tooth breaks through the periodontal membrane. Some children show minimum evidence of teething, such as drooling, increased finger-sucking, or biting on hard objects. Others are very irritable, have difficulty sleeping, mild temperature elevation, ear-rubbing, and decreased appetite for solid foods. Generally, signs of illness such as fever (over 102° F), vomiting, or diarrhea are not symptoms of teething but of illness and may warrant further investigation (Macknin and others, 2000).

Because teething pain is a result of inflammation, cold is soothing. Giving the child a frozen teething ring or an ice cube wrapped in a washcloth helps relieve the inflammation. Several nonprescription topical anesthetic ointments are available, such as Baby Ora-Jel. The active ingredient in most of them is benzocaine. If such products are used, parents are advised to apply them correctly. In the event of persistent irritability that affects sleeping and feeding, systemic analgesics such as acetaminophen or ibuprofen can (if age appropriate) be given; however, parents should know that this is a temporary measure.

**NURSING ALERT** The use of teething powders or procedures such as cutting or rubbing the gums with aspirin are discouraged because ingestion of the powder, infection or irritation of the tissue, or aspiration of the aspirin can occur. Hard candy may cause accidental choking or aspiration and should be avoided at this age.

## Infant Shoes

Many parents are unaware of the type of shoes that are appropriate for the older infant and buy expensive infant shoes because of misleading advertising claims. Inflexible shoes that have hard soles can be detrimental by delaying walking, aggravating intoeing and outtoeing, and impeding the development of supportive foot muscles. Therefore counseling parents regarding footwear should begin when infants are 6 months old—well before they are walking.

It is helpful to begin by explaining to parents that changes in the feet occur during infancy and early childhood as locomotion and weight bearing progress. At birth the feet are flat because the arches are protected by fat pads on the soles of the feet. As the bones in the arches develop, the pads disappear and the feet begin to assume a mature shape. A normal arch is determined by proper alignment of all the bones and development of the surrounding musculature, not by the height of the arch.

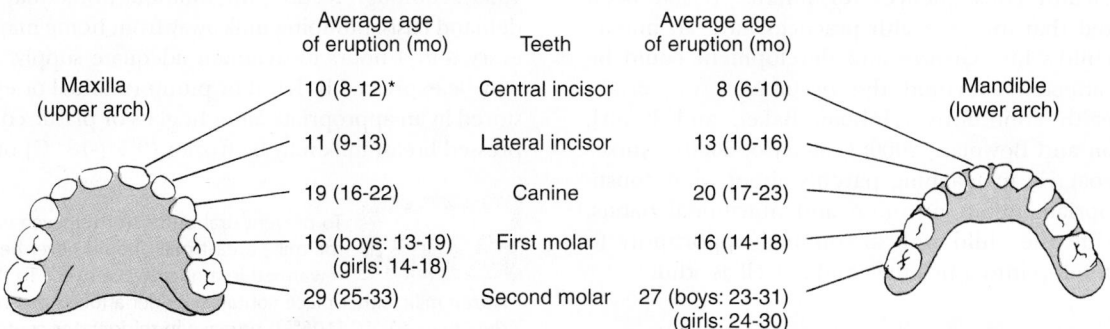

| Maxilla (upper arch) | Average age of eruption (mo) | Teeth | Average age of eruption (mo) | Mandible (lower arch) |
|---|---|---|---|---|
| | 10 (8-12)* | Central incisor | 8 (6-10) | |
| | 11 (9-13) | Lateral incisor | 13 (10-16) | |
| | 19 (16-22) | Canine | 20 (17-23) | |
| | 16 (boys: 13-19) (girls: 14-18) | First molar | 16 (14-18) | |
| | 29 (25-33) | Second molar | 27 (boys: 23-31) (girls: 24-30) | |

**Fig. 12-14** Sequence of eruption of primary teeth. *Range represents ±1 standard deviation or 67% of subjects studied. (Data from McDonald RE, Avery DR: *Dentistry for the child and adolescent,* ed 6, St Louis, 1994, Mosby.)

When children begin walking, the main reason for shoes is *protection*. To provide protection, the shoe should retain its fit, be made of durable material with a smooth interior and few construction seams to irritate the skin, and be soft and flexible, especially in the toe area. A high-top shoe is not necessary for support but may be helpful in keeping the foot in the shoe. A good infant/toddler shoe is one that can easily be bent in half by squeezing the heel and toe with the thumb and index finger (Wall, 2000).

A good shoe conforms to the anatomic shape of the foot, with a rounded toe and sufficient toe room. During weight bearing there should be at least the space of half the width of the thumbnail, or 1.25 cm (½ inch), between the end of the longest toe and the shoe. Roomy and square-toed socks allow for proper growth and alignment. Inexpensive but well-constructed sneakers or soft-leather moccasin-type shoes are suggested as adequate footgear for walking infants.

Even if the shoes are fitted properly, frequent changes are needed to accommodate the infant's rapidly growing feet. Shoe size changes at approximately 3-month intervals between 12 to 36 months; during this time the child's foot should be measured every 3 months. Curled toes when shoes are removed and redness and irritation of the skin on the bottom of the toes indicate the need for a larger size.

## PROMOTING OPTIMUM HEALTH DURING INFANCY

### Nutrition

Ideally, discussion of optimum nutrition should begin prenatally with the decision to breast- or bottle-feed the newborn. The choice for either is highly individual and is discussed in Chapter 8. This section is primarily concerned with infant nutrition during the next 12 months, when growth needs and developmental milestones ready the child for the introduction of solid foods. The relatively simple feeding plan for infants, especially during the first 6 months, allows the nurse ample opportunity to educate parents regarding the nutritional needs of their child and to prepare them for the addition of solid foods.

There is concern however that despite adequate availability of optimum nutrient sources, parents are not feeding infants appropriately. These practices may have far reaching long-term health consequences for infants. It has been demonstrated that infant health practices have an impact upon the child's life. Growth and development could be negatively affected as could the occurrence of certain chronic health conditions (Hobbie, Baker, and Bayerl, 2000; Wilson and Bowman, 2000; Calamaro, 2000). Nurses must be proactive in teaching parents about what constitutes appropriate infant nutrition and nutritional habits, which provide the child with an optimal opportunity to grow and develop into a healthy child as well as adult.

### The First 6 Months

Human milk is the most desirable complete diet for the infant during the first 6 months. In most cases, healthy term infants being breast-fed by a mother with a well-balanced diet may not need any vitamin or mineral supplementation with the exception of iron by 4 to 6 months of age (when fetal stores are depleted). Although breast milk is relatively low in iron, it is more readily absorbed than iron-fortified formula. Supplements of vitamin D (400 IU daily) may be indicated if the mother's vitamin D intake is inadequate. Recent cases of nutritional rickets in children who were exclusively breast-fed beyond 6 months and received little exposure to ultraviolet light or had dark skin and were not supplemented with vitamin D has focused concern on supplementation with vitamin D (Kreiter and others, 2000; Centers for Disease Control and Prevention, 2001). Fluoride supplementation in exclusively breast-fed children is not required for the first 6 months because of the risk of fluorosis; however, fluoride supplementation may be necessary if the breast-feeding mother's water supply does not contain the required amount of fluoridation (see p. 527). Infants who are breast- or bottle-fed do not require additional fluids, especially water or juice, during the first 4 months of life. Excessive feeding of water may result in water intoxication, failure to thrive, and hyponatremia (Ruth-Sanchez and Greene, 1997). Even in hot climates additional water or fluids are not recommended for breast-fed infants.

Cultural beliefs and values often influence infant feeding practices. Health care professionals may benefit from understanding the multicultural feeding practices that parents choose for their infant. Traditional feeding practices include offering a variety of liquids or foods, such as sugared wine, water, or honey, during the first few days of life and thereafter. Honey should be avoided in the first 12 months because of the risk of botulism. Socializing the infant to food flavors of the family's culture is common in addition to continuing breast-feeding for periods of 2 to 4 years (Coletta, Bartholmey, Menella, 1996).

Employed mothers can continue breast-feeding with guidance and encouragement. Mothers are encouraged to set realistic goals for employment and breast-feeding, with accurate information regarding the costs, risks, and benefits of available feeding options. Many mothers may find that a program of breast-pumping when away from home and bottle-feeding the infant the expressed milk with or without formula supplementation is successful. Expressed breast milk may be stored in the refrigerator (4° C or 39° F) without danger of bacterial contamination for up to 5 days (Lawrence and Lawrence, 1999). Although feeding the infant at home may occur on a demand basis, pumping milk away from home may be needed every 3 to 4 hours to maintain adequate supply. Breast milk may be expressed by hand or pump (manual or electric) and stored in an appropriate air-tight glass or plastic container. Expressed breast milk may be frozen (0°F [-18° C] or lower) for

> **NURSING ALERT**
>
> To prevent oral burns from uneven warming of the milk, breast milk should never be thawed or rewarmed in a microwave oven. To thaw the frozen milk, either place container under a lukewarm water bath (less than 40.5°C [105°F]) or place in refrigerator overnight. (*Note:* Warming expressed milk in a microwave decreases the availability of antiinfective properties and vitamin C and causes a separation of milk layers, which affects fat content.)

up to 12 months, but care should be taken to prevent freezer burn. Health care workers and new mothers may find the booklet "Working and Breastfeeding—Can You Do It? Yes, You Can!" by Johnson & Johnson helpful.*

In addition to efficient breast pumping, mothers also need child care by a trusted individual or agency and support and assistance from significant others. Like all breastfeeding mothers, these women must have proper nutrition and rest for adequate lactation. Maternal fatigue is considered the biggest threat to successful breast-feeding in employed mothers (Corbett-Dick and Bezek, 1997). With a schedule of work and child care, careful planning is required to successfully manage the demands of both responsibilities. (See Family Focus box on p. 525.)

An acceptable alternative to breast-feeding is commercial iron-fortified formula. Like human milk, it supplies all the nutrients needed by the infant for the first 6 months.

> **NURSING ALERT**
>
> If infants are being fed powdered or concentrated formula, they may receive a substantial amount of lead from tap water, placing them at risk for lead poisoning. Bottled water is a relatively safe alternative to tap water.

Unmodified whole cow's milk, low-fat cow's milk, skim milk, other animal milks, and imitation milks are not acceptable as a major source of nutrition for infants because of poor digestability, an increased risk of contamination, and a lack of components needed for appropriate growth. Whole milk can cause iron deficiency anemia in infants, presumably from occult gastrointestinal blood loss, but not all research supports this etiology (Fuchs and others, 1993). Pasteurized whole cow's milk is deficient in iron, zinc, and vitamin C and has a high renal solute load, which makes it undesirable for infants less than 12 months of age (American Academy of Pediatrics, 1998).

> **NURSING ALERT**
>
> Whole milk should not be introduced to infants until after 1 year of age (American Academy of Pediatrics, 1998).

The amount of formula per feeding and the number of feedings per day vary among infants, but general guidelines are given in Table 12-4. Infants on demand feeding usually determine their own feeding schedule, but some infants, especially those with "easy" temperaments, may need a more planned schedule based on average feeding patterns to ensure sufficient nutrients.

The addition of solid foods before 4 to 6 months of age is not recommended. Solid foods during the early months are not yet compatible with the ability of the gastrointestinal tract and nutritional needs of the infant. Furthermore feeding solids exposes infants to food antigens that may produce food protein allergy. Despite these recommendations, and lacking scientific evidence to support such practices, many parents

*Developed by **National Healthy Mothers, Healthy Babies Coalition,** 121 N Washington St, Suite 300, Alexandria, VA 22314, (703) 836-6110; www.hmhb.org.

**TABLE 12-4**   Volume of formula per feeding and number of feedings per day*

| Age in Months (Midpoint) | Formula Consumed per Feeding | | Feedings per Day |
|---|---|---|---|
| | (ml)† | (oz) | |
| 1 | 94.6 | 3.2 | 6.6 |
| 2 | 124.2 | 4.2 | 6.4 |
| 3 | 162.7 | 5.5 | 5.4 |
| 4 | 162.7 | 5.5 | 5.5 |
| 5 | 162.7 | 5.5 | 4.8 |
| 6 | 177.4 | 6.0 | 4.7 |
| 7 | 171.5 | 5.8 | 4.4 |
| 8 | 180.4 | 6.1 | 4.5 |
| 9 | 168.6 | 5.7 | 4.0 |
| 10 | 183.4 | 6.2 | 4.0 |
| 11 | 201.1 | 6.8 | 4.0 |
| 12 | 174.5 | 5.9 | 3.9 |

From Ross Laboratories, 1989.
*Infants fed human milk or a combination of cow's milk, human milk, and formula are excluded.
†1 fluid ounce = 29.573 ml.

introduce solids as early as 2 weeks of age. In such cases rice cereal is often added to the formula so the infant will sleep better at night or to enhance weight gain (Calamaro, 2000; Wilson and Bowman, 2000; Assisting new mothers, 2001).

Developmentally, infants are not ready for solid food. The extrusion (protrusion) reflex is strong and often causes food to be pushed out of the mouth. Infants instinctively suck when given food. Because of their limited motor abilities, infants are unable to deliberately push food away or avoid feeding. Therefore early introduction of solids is a type of forced feeding that may lead to excessive weight gain and increased predisposition to allergies and iron deficiency anemia. Fruit juices are not required in the first 6 months; there are no studies demonstrating benefits of giving fruit juice to infants, yet many parents perceive this practice as beneficial.

> **NURSING ALERT**
>
> Dietary fat should not be restricted in infancy. Substituting skim or low-fat milk is unacceptable because the essential fatty acids are inadequate and the solute concentration of protein and electrolytes, such as sodium, is too high.

## The Second 6 Months

During the second half of the first year human milk or formula continues to be the primary source of nutrition. Fluoride supplementation begins depending on the infant's intake of fluoridated tap water (see p. 527). If breast-feeding is discontinued, a commercial iron-fortified formula should be substituted. Formulas specially marketed for older infants or follow-up formulas offer no advantages over other infant formulas and provide excessive protein (American Academy of Pediatrics, 1998).

The major change in feeding habits is the addition of solid foods to the infant's diet. Physiologically and develop-

## Box 12-4 ■ ■ ■
### Developmental Milestones Associated with Feeding

| AGE (MONTHS) | BEHAVIOR |
|---|---|
| Birth | Sucking, rooting, and swallowing reflexes |
| | Feels hunger and indicates desire for food by crying; expresses satiety by falling asleep |
| | Extrusion reflex is strong |
| 3-4 | Extrusion reflex is fading |
| | Beginning eye-hand coordination |
| 4-5 | Can approximate lips to the rim of a cup |
| 5-6 | Can use fingers to feed self a cracker |
| 6-7 | Chews and bites |
| | May hold own bottle, but may not drink from it (prefers for it to be held) |
| 7-9 | Refuses food by keeping lips closed; has preferences |
| | Holds a spoon and plays with it during feeding |
| | May drink from a straw |
| | Drinks from a cup with assistance |
| 9-12 | Picks up small morsels of food (finger foods) and feeds self |
| | Holds own bottle and drinks from it |
| | Drinks from a cup but spills some of the contents |
| | Uses a spoon with much spilling |

mentally, the infant 4 to 6 months of age is in a transition period. By this time the gastrointestinal tract has matured sufficiently to handle more complex nutrients and is less sensitive to potentially allergenic foods. Tooth eruption is beginning and facilitates biting and chewing. The extrusion reflex has disappeared, and swallowing is more coordinated to allow the infant to accept solids easily. Head control is well developed, which permits infants to sit with support and purposely turn the head away to communicate disinterest in food. Voluntary grasping and improved eye-hand coordination gradually allow infants to pick up finger foods and feed themselves. Their increasing sense of independence is evident in their desire to hold the bottle and try to "help" during feeding. The major developmental milestones associated with feeding are listed in Box 12-4.

### Selection and Preparation of Solid Foods

The choice of solid foods to introduce first is variable but should meet the reasons for feeding solids, such as supplying nutrients not found in formula or breast milk. Iron-fortified infant cereal is generally introduced first because of its high iron content (7 mg/3 tablespoons of prepared dry cereal). Commercially prepared ready-to-serve dry cereals for infants include rice, barley, oatmeal, and high-protein cereals; rice is usually suggested as an initial food because of its easy digestibility and low allergenic potential. Cereals such as Cream of Farina are not used because infant commercial cereals are a better source of iron. Some of the commercial baby cereals are combined with fruit. There is little nutritional benefit from these preparations, and they are more expensive. New foods should be added one at a time, and therefore parents should avoid cereal combinations when beginning a new grain.

Infant cereal may be mixed with formula in a bowl until whole milk is given. If the infant is breast-fed, the cereal is mixed with expressed breast milk or water. After 6 months of age, fruit juices can be mixed with the dry cereal; the vitamin C content of the juice enhances the absorption of iron in the cereal. Because of their benefit as a source of iron, infant cereals should be continued until the child is 18 months of age.

Fruit juice can be offered from a cup for its rich source of vitamin C and as a substitute for milk for one feeding a day. Certain juices (e.g., apple, pear, prune, sweet cherry, peach, and grape) are avoided because they contain high amounts of fructose and sorbitol and may cause abdominal pain, diarrhea, or bloating in some children. White grape juice is reported to be better absorbed and safe for infants this age (no more than 5 oz/day) without causing GI distress (Calamaro, 2000). Studies have shown that excessive fruit juice consumption (12 or more oz/day) in young children increases the likelihood of short stature and childhood obesity (Dennison, Rockwell, and Baker, 1997) and nonorganic failure to thrive (Smith and Lifshitz, 1994). Because vitamin C is naturally destroyed by heat, juice is not warmed. Juice containers are always kept covered and refrigerated to prevent further vitamin loss.

**NURSING ALERT** Offer fruit juice from a cup, rather than a bottle, to prevent the development of dental caries. (See Low-Cariogenic Diet, Chapter 14.)

The addition of other foods is arbitrary. A common sequence is strained fruits followed by vegetables and, finally, meats. Some clinicians prefer to add vegetables before fruit. Only one solid is introduced every 5 to 7 days so that a reaction to a particular food will be distinguished. If foods are introduced early, citrus fruits, meats, and eggs are still delayed until after 6 months of age because of their potential cause allergy. At 6 months foods such as a cracker or zwieback can be offered as a type of finger and teething food. By 8 to 9 months junior foods and nutritious finger foods such as a firmly cooked vegetable, raw pieces of fruit (except grapes), or cheese can be given. By 1 year well-cooked table foods are served.

The introduction of solid foods into the infant's diet at this age is primarily for taste and chewing experience. The majority of the infant's caloric needs are derived from the primary milk source (human or formula); therefore, solids should not be perceived as a substitute for milk until the child is older than 12 months. Studies have shown that the addition of solids to the diet of exclusively breast-fed infants does not significantly increase overall caloric intake or weight gain (Heinig and others, 1993; Dewey, 2001).

Commercially prepared baby foods are the most commonly used types of food served to infants in the United States. They are convenient and contain no added salt or sugar, but they are relatively expensive. An alternative is preparing baby foods at home, which is a simple and inexpensive process. Fruits and vegetables can be steamed in a small amount of water and pureed in a blender or food processor. Many of them, such as ripe banana, can be mashed fine with a fork. Fruits such as apples or pears require little or no water in the cooking process. Vegetables such as carrots, potatoes, or string beans require additional water in the cooking and blending process.

Preferably, home-prepared infant foods should be fresh or frozen, because canned foods, other than those prepared for infants, may contain excessive sodium or sugar or be a source of lead from the container. If sweetening is needed, refined sugar can be used, but honey and corn syrup are avoided because of the risk of infant botulism. There is no evidence that the addition of salt to foods, such as peas, increases the infant's acceptance of the new food (Sullivan and Birch, 1994).

## Food Storage

Storage of commercial baby food requires a few simple rules. Unopened jars can remain on the shelf until the manufacturer's expiration date, which is on the container. Opened jars are refrigerated and can be used for a couple of days. If the infant does not finish a jar of food at one time, a portion of the food is removed from the jar using a clean spoon. If a clean spoon is not used, bacteria are introduced and the salivary enzymes on the feeding spoon begin to digest unused portions of the food. Dried baby foods are prepared in individual portions, thus eliminating storage problems and waste of unused food.

For convenience, home-prepared baby foods can be made in advance and frozen in small jars or in special plastic bags that are sealed by heat and reheated by placing them in boiling water. If microwave heating is used, the food is mixed thoroughly and checked to ensure a safe temperature before feeding. The temperature of the container may not indicate the heat intensity of the food, which can result in an oral burn. Individual portions of food can be frozen in ice cube trays, transferred to a large container, and individually defrosted as needed. With reasonable care in the preparation and storing of foods, there is little need to worry about bacterial contamination.

> **NURSING ALERT** Although microwaving of bottles and baby food is not recommended, it remains a common practice. Guidelines have been developed for microwave heating of refrigerated formula, and these should be given to the family. (See Family Home Care box.)

## Method of Introduction

When the spoon is first introduced, infants often push it away and appear dissatisfied. Some patience and skill are required to overcome this initial response. A small-bowled, straight, long-handled spoon, similar to a demitasse spoon, allows a small portion of food to be placed toward the back of the tongue. Food that is placed on the front of the tongue and pushed out is simply scooped up and refed. As infants become accustomed to the spoon, they will more eagerly accept the food and eventually open the mouth in anticipation (or keep it closed in dislike). Because the introduction of food is a new experience, spoon feeding should be attempted after ingestion of some breast milk or formula

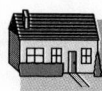

### FAMILY HOME CARE
#### Microwave Heating of Refrigerated Infant Formula

Before heating
    Heat only 4 oz or more
    Heat only *refrigerated* formula
    Always *stand* the bottle up
    Always leave bottle top *uncovered* to allow heat to escape
Heating instructions (full power)
    4-oz bottles
        Heat for no more than 30 seconds
    8-oz bottles
        Heat for no more than 45 seconds
Serving instructions
    Always replace nipple assembly; *invert* 10 times (vigorous shaking is unnecessary)
    Formula should be cool to the touch; formula warm to the touch may be too hot to serve
    Always *test* formula; place several drops on your tongue or on top of the hand (not the inside wrist)

From Sigman-Grant M, Bush G, Anantheswaran R: Microwave heating of infant formula: a dilemma resolved, *Pediatrics* 90(3):414, 1992.

to associate this activity with a pleasurable and satisfying experience. Trying to introduce a food *after* the entire milk feeding is usually useless because the infant is satiated and has no inclination to try something new.

After several spoon feedings, food can be introduced at the beginning of a meal. It is best to introduce many foods during the first year, when the infant is more likely to eat them because of a hearty appetite resulting from a rapid growth rate. During the toddler years eating becomes less of an adventure, and strong food preferences become evident.

Each new food item is introduced at an interval of 5 to 7 days to allow for identification of food allergies. New foods are fed in small amounts, from 1 teaspoon to a few tablespoons. As the amount of solid food increases the child will decrease the intake of breast milk or formula to approximately 1 L per day.

Because feeding is a learning process as well as a means of nutrition, new foods are given alone to allow the child to learn new tastes and textures. Sometimes it is necessary to camouflage a new food by mixing it with another favorite food to encourage the child to try it, but this should not become a routine. Food should not be mixed in the bottle and fed through a nipple with a large hole in healthy infants. This deprives the child of the pleasure of learning new tastes and developing a discriminating palate. It can also cause problems with poor chewing of food later in life because of lack of experience. Guidelines for the introduction of new foods are given in the Family Home Care box on p. 524.*

Introducing solid foods can be an exciting time for parent and child. Most infants are good eaters and enjoy eating from a spoon and later feeding themselves. However, the transition from "parent doing it" to "baby doing it" can be a

---

*A recommended resource is *Starting Solids: A Guide for Parents and Child Care Providers*, available from the **National Association of Pediatric Nurse Associates and Practitioners (NAPNAP)**, 1101 Kings Highway North, Suite 206, Cherry Hill, NJ 08034-1931, (609) 667-1773, fax: (609) 667-7187; www.napnap.org.

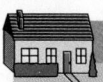

## FAMILY HOME CARE
### Feeding During the First Year

### BIRTH TO 6 MONTHS (BREAST- OR BOTTLE-FEEDING)

#### Breast-Feeding

Most desirable complete diet for first half of year.*
Requires supplements of vitamin D (400 units) if mother's diet is inadequate or if child has minimal ultraviolet light exposure.

#### Formula

Iron-fortified commercial formula is a complete food for the first half of the year.*
Requires fluoride supplements (0.25 mg) when the concentration of fluoride in the drinking water is below 0.3 parts per million (ppm) after 6 months of age.
Evaporated milk formula requires supplements of vitamin C, iron, and fluoride (in accordance with the fluoride content of the local water supply after 6 months of age).

### 6 TO 12 MONTHS (SOLID FOODS)

May begin to add solids by 5 to 6 months of age.
First foods are strained, pureed, or finely mashed.
Finger foods such as teething crackers, raw fruit, or vegetables can be introduced by 6 to 7 months.
Chopped table food or commercially prepared junior foods can be started by 9 to 12 months.
With the exception of cereal, the order of introducing foods is *variable;* a recommended sequence is weekly introduction of other foods, beginning with fruit, then vegetables, and then meat. (Some clinicians prefer to introduce vegetables first.)
Avoid foods that have potential for choking: hot dogs, nuts, grapes, raw carrots, popcorn, and hard candies.

#### Method of Introduction

Introduce solids when infant is hungry.
Begin spoon feeding by pushing food to back of tongue because of infant's natural tendency to thrust tongue forward.

Use small spoon with straight handle; begin with 1 or 2 teaspoons of food; gradually increase to about 1 tablespoon per year of age.
Introduce one food at a time, usually at intervals of 5 to 7 days, to identify food allergies.
Never introduce foods by mixing them with the formula in the bottle.

#### Cereal

Introduce commercially prepared iron-fortified infant cereals and administer daily until 18 months.
Rice cereal is usually introduced first because of its low allergenic potential.
Can discontinue supplemental iron once cereal is given.

#### Fruits and Vegetables

Applesauce, bananas, and pears are usually well tolerated.
Avoid fruits and vegetables marketed in cans that are not specifically designed for infants because of variable and sometimes high lead content and addition of salt, sugar, and/or preservatives.
Offer dilute fruit juice only from a cup, not a bottle, to reduce the development of bottle caries (limit to no more than 4 oz daily).

#### Meat, Fish, and Poultry

Avoid fatty meats (sausage, wieners).
Prepare by baking, broiling, steaming, or poaching.
Include organ meats such as liver, which has a high iron, vitamin A, and vitamin B complex content.
If soup is given, be sure all ingredients are familiar to child's diet.
Avoid commercial meat/vegetable combinations because protein is low.

#### Eggs and Cheese

Serve egg yolk hard boiled and mashed, soft cooked, or poached.
Introduce egg white in small quantities (1 tsp) toward end of first year to detect an allergy.
Use cheese as a substitute for meat and as finger food.

---

*Breast-feeding or commercial formula feeding for up to 12 months of age is recommended. After 1 year, whole cow's milk can be given if there is no history of atopy.

---

trying experience, particularly for those who value a clean house or who view cleaning up the mess as a waste of time. The infant's first, second, and often twentieth try at self-feeding or cup feeding is a sloppy experience. Finger foods such as soft fruits or vegetables are just as good playthings as food; they can be squeezed, smeared, squashed, and thoroughly painted on oneself, others, and the surrounding environment. However, all of this is part of learning, and mastery follows many accidents.

If parents find this experience distressing, a few suggestions may prove helpful. The feeding area should have a floor that can be easily wiped and is relatively far from walls, upholstered furniture, or drapes. A hand-held portable vacuum is helpful in cleaning up crumbs. Messes are confined to one area if the child is seated in a high chair rather than allowed to crawl or walk around while drinking or eating. Infants should be expected to get themselves covered with food; therefore a large bib (plastic can be wiped easily but needs to be removed after feeding) should be used, as well as washable clothes that are easily removed. In a carpeted eating area a bed sheet or washable drop cloth can be

spread under the high chair to save on clean up time and avoid frustration; one can expect the infant to drop food at this stage. High chairs can be thoroughly cleaned in a shower. Outdoor dining provides an excellent opportunity for practicing with a cup, spoon, or fingers because accidents are simple to hose or sweep away. Children cannot be pressured into eating neatly or developing table manners before manipulative skill is acquired.

If older infants suddenly refuse to eat, the feeding process should be investigated. It is not unusual for an 11-month-old infant to become stubborn, push the spoon away, and refuse to open the mouth. The child may not be content with having a spoon to play with while someone else does the feeding. Helping parents understand the child's growing need for independence may prevent many temper tantrums and power struggles later on.

### Weaning

Defined as the process of giving up one method of feeding for another, *weaning* usually refers to relinquishing the breast or bottle for a cup. In Western societies this is generally regarded as a major task for infants and is often seen as a potentially traumatic experience. It is psychologically significant because the infant is required to give up a major source of oral pleasure and gratification.

Other cultural groups define weaning in relation to significant life events (e.g., teething) or reaching a specific age. A culturally sensitive approach may consider the weaning process as beginning in utero, with the transmission of food flavors via amniotic fluid, and extending through childhood as the infant becomes accustomed to culturally indigenous foods introduced by the parents (Coletta, Bartholmey, and Menella, 1996).

There is no one time for weaning that is best for every child, but generally most infants show signs of readiness during the second half of the first year. They have learned that good things come from a spoon. Their increasing desire for freedom of movement may lessen their desire to be held close for feedings. They are acquiring more control over their actions and can easily manipulate a cup to their lips (even if it is held upside down!). Imitation becomes a powerful motivator by age 8 or 9 months, and they enjoy using a cup or glass like others do.

Weaning should be gradual by replacing one bottle- or breast-feeding at a time. The nighttime feeding is usually the last feeding to be discontinued. It is advisable never to begin allowing a child to take a bottle of milk to bed—this is a major cause of baby bottle caries in deciduous teeth. If breast-feeding is terminated before 5 or 6 months of age, weaning should be to a bottle to provide for the infant's continued sucking needs. If discontinued later, weaning can be directly to a cup, especially by age 12 to 14 months. Any sweet liquid, such as fruit juice, should be given in a cup.

## Sleep and Activity

Sleep patterns vary among infants, with active infants typically sleeping less than placid children. Generally, by 3 to 4 months of age most infants have developed a nocturnal pattern of sleep that lasts from 9 to 11 hours. The total daily sleep is approximately 15 hours. The number of naps per day varies, but infants may take one or two naps by the end of the first year. Breast-fed infants usually sleep for shorter periods, with more frequent waking, especially during the night, than do bottle-fed infants. Because of the trend toward breast-feeding, sleep norms such as those previously described, which were based primarily on bottle-fed infants, may not be relevant. (See Family Focus box.) (For a discussion of sleep position, see Sudden Infant Death Syndrome, Chapter 13.)

Most infants are naturally active and need no encouragement to be mobile. However, problems can arise when devices such as playpens, strollers, commercial swings, and walkers are used excessively. These items restrict movement and prevent infants from exploring and developing gross motor skills. Contrary to popular belief, walkers do not enhance coordination and are dangerous if tipped over or placed near stairs. The American Academy of Pediatrics, Committee on Injury and Poison Prevention (1995) recommends a ban on the sale of infant walkers due to the large number of injuries.

### FAMILY FOCUS
#### Breast-Feeding and Infant Sleep Patterns

Sleep patterns vary greatly among infants, with temperament and type of feeding considered important factors. Typically, bottle-fed infants sleep through the night sooner than breast-fed infants. However, parents should be encouraged to make feeding choices that promote optimum nutrition and meet the needs of the infant, as well as themselves (Walker, 1993). A study by Pinilla and Birch (1993) demonstrated that the sleep pattern of breast-fed infants could be modified to encourage longer nighttime sleep intervals—a possible benefit for the working mother and an incentive to continue breast-feeding. A two-step procedure of behavioral training was used.

The first phase began soon after birth. The parents were instructed to try not to hold, rock, or nurse their infants to sleep; to accentuate differences in environmental cues for day and nighttime hours (e.g., high levels of stimulation during the day but low levels during the night); to feed the infant at a focal feeding time each night (between 10:00 PM and midnight); and to make sure the infant was really complaining before picking him or her up.

When the infant was 3 weeks old, the second phase began. The goal was to "stretch" nighttime feeding intervals by breaking the association between awakening at night (between midnight and 5:00 AM) and being fed. Parents were instructed not to leave the infant alone crying; rather, alternative interventions were encouraged: reswaddling, patting, diapering, or walking the infant in lieu of feeding. If the infant continued to cry after these interventions, a feeding was offered.

The results: by 8 weeks all of the "trained" breast-fed infants slept from midnight to 5:00 AM, compared with 23% of the untrained (control) group. Both groups had similar milk intakes and weight gain. This research indicates that frequent night waking and feeding is not an essential element of breast-feeding. Nurses can offer suggestions to parents to prolong nighttime sleep for the infant and themselves. In fact many of the steps in the training plan help prevent the development of problems associated with nighttime feeding and night crying—regardless of the feeding method.

**NURSING ALERT**   Formal infant exercise programs do not provide any long-term benefit to normal infants, and the possibility for damage to the infant's skeletal system exists. For these reasons, such programs are not recommended (American Academy of Pediatrics, 1988).

### Sleep Problems

Concerns regarding sleep are common during infancy. Sometimes these concerns are as basic as parents' questioning if the infant needs additional sleep. In this case it is best to investigate the reason for their concern, stressing the individual needs of each child. Infants who are active during wakeful periods and growing normally are sleeping a sufficient amount of time.

However, a number of more serious concerns require intervention. Sleep disturbances of physiologic origin are rare with the exception of colic, which is discussed in Chapter 13. The more common sleep disturbances are a learned pattern or developmental characteristic of some infants (Table 12-5). Although many families may report sleep problems typical of

**TABLE 12-5** Selected sleep disturbances during infancy and early childhood

| Disorder/Description | Management |
|---|---|
| **Nighttime Feeding\*** | |
| Child has a prolonged need for middle-of-night bottle- or breast-feeding | Increase daytime feeding intervals to 4 hours or more (may need to be done gradually) |
| Child goes to sleep at the breast or with a bottle | Offer last feeding as late as possible at night; may need to gradually reduce amount of formula or length of breast-feeding |
| Awakenings are frequent (may be hourly) | Offer no bottles in bed |
| Child returns to sleep after feeding; other comfort measures (e.g., rocking or holding) are usually ineffective | Put to bed *awake* |
| | When child is crying, check at progressively longer intervals each night; reassure child but do not hold, rock, take to parent's bed, or give bottle or pacifier |
| **Developmental Night Crying** | |
| Child age 6-12 months with undisturbed nighttime sleep now awakes abruptly; may be accompanied by nightmares | Reassure parents that this phase is temporary |
| | Enter room immediately to check on child but keep reassurances *brief* |
| | Avoid feeding, rocking, taking to parent's bed, or any other routine that may initiate trained night crying |
| **Trained Night Crying\* (Inappropriate Sleep Associations)** | |
| Child typically falls asleep in place other than own bed (e.g., rocking chair or parent's bed) and is brought to own bed while asleep; on awakening, cries until usual routine is instituted (e.g., rocking) | Put child in own bed when *awake* |
| | If possible, arrange sleeping area separate from other family members |
| | When child is crying, check at progressively longer intervals each night; reassure child but do not resume usual routine |
| **Refusal to Go to Sleep\*** | |
| Child resists bedtime and comes out of room repeatedly | Evaluate if hour of sleep is too early (child may resist sleep if not tired) |
| Nighttime sleep may be continuous, but frequent awakenings and refusal to return to sleep may occur and become a problem if parent allows child to deviate from usual sleep pattern | Assist parents in establishing consistent before-bedtime routine and enforcing consistent limits regarding child's bedtime behavior |
| | If child persists in leaving bedroom, close door for progressively longer periods |
| | Use reward system with child to provide motivation |
| **Nighttime Fears** | |
| Child resists going to bed or wakes during the night because of fears | Evaluate if hour of sleep is too early (child may fantasize when nothing to do but think in dark room) |
| Child seeks parent's physical presence and falls asleep easily with parent nearby, unless fear is overwhelming | Calmly reassure the frightened child; keeping a night-light on may be helpful |
| | Use reward system with child to provide motivation to deal with fears |
| | Avoid patterns that can lead to additional problems (e.g., sleeping with child or taking child to parent's room) |
| | If child's fear is overwhelming, consider desensitization (e.g., progressively spending longer periods of time alone; consult professional help for protracted fears) |
| | Distinguish between nightmares and sleep terrors (confused partial arousals) (see Table 15-3) |

Modified from Ferber R: Behavioral "insomnia" in the child, *Psychiatr Clin North Am* 10(4):641-653, 1987.
\*Guidelines for parents in dealing with these sleep problems are in Wong DL, Hess CS: *Wong and Whaley's clinical manual of pediatric nursing*, ed 5, St Louis, 2000, Mosby.

these patterns, interventions are offered *only* when the pattern is disruptive to the family. (See Cultural Awareness box.)

When a sleeping problem is presented, a careful assessment is essential. (See Guidelines box on p. 157.) Charting sleep habits both before and after interventions is also an important strategy.\* Questions regarding the frequency and duration of waking, the usual bedtime routine, the number of nighttime feedings, the perceived problem (e.g., how much disruption the behavior generates), and the attempted interventions are important in planning effective approaches designed for the specific sleep problem. A common suggestion given for any type of sleep problem—"let

the child cry until falling asleep"—is very difficult to implement and is inappropriate for certain conditions. Once the parents relent and console the child, they have only reinforced the crying.

An equally effective and more atraumatic approach to night crying, known as *graduated extinction,* is to let the child cry for progressively longer times between *brief* parental interventions that consist only of reassurance—not rocking, holding, or using the bottle or pacifier. For example, the parents may check on the child every 5 minutes during the first night and progressively extend this interval by 5 minutes on successive nights (Ferber and Kryger, 1995).

Families who cannot tolerate unexpected crying spells while everyone else is asleep can try the two-step approach. Graduated extinction is used during naps and at bedtime

\*A 2-week sleep record for families is available in Wong DL, Hess CS: *Wong and Whaley's clinical manual of pediatric nursing*, ed 5, St Louis, 2000, Mosby.

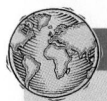

## CULTURAL AWARENESS
### The Family Bed

Co-sleeping, or the "family bed," in which parents allow the children to sleep with them, is a relatively common and accepted practice, especially among African-American, Hispanic, and Asian families, such as the Japanese (Schachter and others, 1989). Other groups that are adopting co-sleeping include (1) single parents, whose need for company may encourage this practice; (2) working parents, who desire the closeness at night that was lost during the day; and (3) parents who have had an issue about sleep or separation in their own past (Brazelton, 1990). Recent studies, however, have demonstrated that co-sleeping is associated with a higher incidence of SIDS-like deaths in infants, most likely as a result of suffocation (Drago and Dannenburg, 1999). One particular study found that a shared sleep surface was the site of death in 47% of cases whereas only 8.4% of deaths involved infants who were found nonprone and sleeping alone (Kemp and others, 2000). Suffocation by a co-sleeper was also found to be a factor in another study of SIDS-like deaths (Carroll-Pankhurst and Mortimer, 2001). The clinical implication for nurses is that parents should be given complete information regarding bedsharing and its risks; there appear to be no advantages to bedsharing in relation to decreasing SIDS deaths, and there may be disadvantages if co-sleepers are not cautious.

until the parents retire. If the child cries during the night, the parents use comforting measures. However, once the child is partially trained, step 2 is initiated—the use of graduated extinction at all times.

The best way to prevent sleep problems is to encourage parents to establish bedtime rituals that do not foster problematic patterns. One of the most constructive is placing infants *awake* in their own crib. When infants are accustomed to falling asleep somewhere else, such as in their parent's arms, and then being transferred to their crib, they awaken in unfamiliar surroundings and are unable to fall asleep until the routine is repeated. Also, the bed should be used for sleeping only—not as a playpen. It is advisable not to hang playthings over or on the bed; in this way the child associates the bed with sleep, not with activity. Although the interventions described previously and in Table 12-5 are usually successful, it is much easier to prevent the problem with appropriate counseling during the early months of the infant's life.*

## Dental Health

Good dental hygiene begins as soon as the primary teeth erupt. The teeth and gums are initially cleaned by wiping with a damp cloth; toothbrushing is too harsh for the tender gingiva. The caregiver can stabilize the infant by cradling the child with one arm and using the free hand to cleanse the teeth. Oral hygiene can be made pleasant by singing or talking to the infant. There are no clear guidelines regarding when toothbrushing should begin; however, it is recommended that the first dental visit occur at or

---

*An excellent resource for parents is *Solve Your Child's Sleep Problems* by Richard Ferber (1986, Simon & Schuster Trade, [800] 223-2336; www.simonsays.com). Also available in Spanish.

around 1 year of age (Nowak and Warren, 2000). It is generally recommended that a small, soft-bristled toothbrush be used as more teeth erupt and the infant adjusts to the routine of cleaning. Water is preferred to toothpaste, which the infant will swallow (and if the toothpaste is fluoridated, the infant may ingest excessive amounts of fluoride).

*Fluoride,* an essential mineral for building caries-resistant teeth, is needed beginning at 6 months of age if the infant does not receive water with an adequate fluoride content. The American Academy of Pediatrics, Committee on Nutrition (1998) no longer recommends fluoride supplementation from birth to 6 months. The fluoride dosage has been decreased from earlier recommendations because of an increased occurrence of dental fluorosis from excessive fluoride ingestion. The latest recommendation is to give children 6 months to 3 years of age 0.25 mg fluoride daily if water fluoride content is less than 0.3 ppm (parts per million) (American Academy of Pediatrics, 1998).

Dietary considerations are also important because habits begun during infancy tend to continue into later years. Foods with concentrated sugar are used sparingly (if at all) in the infant's diet. The practice of coating pacifiers with honey or using commercially available hard-candy pacifiers is discouraged. Besides being cariogenic, honey also may cause infant botulism, and parts of the candy pacifier can be aspirated (see p. 543). Parents need to be counseled regarding the detrimental effects of frequent and prolonged bottle- or breast-feeding during sleep, when the sweet milk or other fluid, such as juice, bathes the teeth, producing *nursing caries.* (See Chapter 14 for a more extensive discussion of dental care, including bottle caries.)

## Immunizations

One of the most dramatic advances in pediatrics has been the decline of infectious diseases during the twentieth century because of the widespread use of immunization for preventable diseases. Although many of the immunizations can be given to individuals of any age, the recommended primary schedule begins during infancy and, with the exception of boosters, is completed during early childhood. Therefore the discussion of childhood immunizations for diphtheria, tetanus, pertussis (DTaP using acellular pertussis); polio; measles, mumps, rubella (MMR); *Haemophilus influenzae* type b (Hib); hepatitis B virus (HBV); pneumococcal conjugate vaccine (PCV); and chickenpox (Var) is included under health promotion during infancy. Selected vaccines generally reserved for children considered at high risk for the disease are discussed here and as appropriate throughout the text. (See Communicable Diseases, Chapter 16, for a discussion of several of the diseases for which vaccines are available.) All vaccines currently licensed for use in the United States are listed in Box 12-5.

To facilitate an understanding of immunizations, key terms are defined in Box 12-6. Although in this discussion the terms *vaccination* and *immunization* are used interchangeably in reference to active immunization, they are not synonymous because the administration of an immunobiologic such as a vaccine cannot automatically be equated with the development of adequate immunity.

## Box 12-5

### Licensed Vaccines and Toxoids Available in the United States and Recommended Routes of Administration

**VACCINE/ROUTE**

Adenovirus*/oral
Anthrax/subcutaneous
Bacillus of Calmette and Guérin (BCG)/intradermal or subcutaneous
Cholera/subcutaneous, intramuscular, or intradermal†
Diphtheria-tetanus-pertussis (DTP)/intramuscular
DTP-*Haemophilus influenzae* type b conjugate (DTP-Hib)‡/intramuscular
DTaP-Hib conjugate‡/intramuscular
Diphtheria-tetanus-acellular pertussis (DTaP)/intramuscular
Hepatitis A/intramuscular
Hepatitis B/intramuscular§
*Haemophilus influenzae* type b conjugate (Hib)‡/intramuscular
Hib conjugate—Hepatitis B/intramuscular
Influenza/intramuscular
Japanese encephalitis/subcutaneous
Lyme disease/intramuscular
Measles/subcutaneous
Measles-rubella/subcutaneous
Measles-mumps-rubella (MMR)/subcutaneous
Meningococcal/subcutaneous
Mumps/subcutaneous
Pertussis/intramuscular
Plague/intramuscular
Pneumococcal/intramuscular or subcutaneous
Poliovirus vaccine, inactivated (IPV)/subcutaneous
Poliovirus vaccine, oral (OPV)
Rabies/intramuscular or intradermal‖
Rubella/subcutaneous
Tetanus/intramuscular
Tetanus-diphtheria (Td or DT)/intramuscular
Typhoid (parenteral)/subcutaneous¶
Typhoid (Ty21a)/oral
Varicella/subcutaneous
Yellow fever/subcutaneous

Modified from American Academy of Pediatrics: Active and Passive Immunization. In Pickering LK, editor: *2000 Red book: report of the Committee on infectious Diseases,* ed 25, Elk Grove Village, IL, 2000, American Academy of Pediatrics.
*Available only to the U.S. Armed Forces.
†The intradermal dose is lower than the subcutaneous dose.
‡May be administered in combination products or as reconstituted products with DTP or DTaP if approved by the FDA for the child's age and if administration of other vaccine is justified.
§Not administered in dorsogluteal muscle (buttock) because of possible reduced immunologic response.
‖The intradermal dose of rabies vaccine, human diploid cell (HDCV), is lower than the intramuscular dose and is used only for preexposure vaccination. **Rabies vaccine, adsorbed (RVA) should not be used intradermally.** Another rabies vaccine PCEC (purified chicken embryo cell culture), RabAvert, may be given by intramuscular route only for preexposure or postexposure prophylactic use in persons who are sensitive to the other rabies vaccines.
¶Booster doses may be administered intradermally unless vaccine that is acetone-killed and dried is used.

## Box 12-6

### Key Immunization Terms

**Immunization**—Inclusive term denoting the process of inducing or providing active or passive immunity *artificially* by administering an immunobiologic
**Immunity**—An inherited or acquired state in which an individual is resistant to the occurrence or the effects of a specific disease, particularly an infectious agent
**Natural immunity**—Innate immunity or resistance to infection or toxicity
**Acquired immunity**—Immunity from exposure to the invading agent, either bacteria, virus, or toxin
**Active immunity**—Immune bodies are actively formed against specific antigens, either *naturally* by having had the disease clinically or subclinically or *artificially* by introducing the antigen into the individual
**Passive immunity**—Temporary immunity by transfusing immune globulins or antitoxins either *artificially* from another human or from an animal that has been actively immunized against an antigen or *naturally* from the mother to the fetus via the placenta
**Antibody**—A protein, found mostly in serum, that is formed in response to exposure to a specific antigen
**Antigen**—A variety of foreign substances, including bacteria, viruses, toxins, and foreign proteins that stimulate the formation of antibodies
**Attenuate**—Reduce the virulence (infectiousness) of a pathogenic microorganism by such measures as treating it with heat or chemicals or cultivating it on a certain medium
**Immunobiologic**—Antigenic substances (e.g., vaccines and toxoids) or antibody-containing preparations (e.g., globulins and antitoxins) from human or animal donors, used for active or passive immunization or therapy
*Vaccine*—A suspension of live (usually attenuated) or inactivated microorganisms (e.g., bacteria, viruses, or rickettsiae) or fractions of the microorganism administered to induce immunity and prevent infectious disease or its sequelae
*Toxoid*—A modified bacterial toxin that has been made nontoxic but retains the ability to stimulate the formation of antitoxin
*Antitoxin*—A solution of antibodies (e.g., diphtheria antitoxin and botulinum antitoxin) derived from the serum of animals immunized with specific antigens and used to confer passive immunity and for treatment
*Immune globulin (IG)* or *intravenous immune globulin (IVIG)*—A sterile solution containing antibodies from large pools of human blood plasma; primarily indicated for routine maintenance of immunity of certain immunodeficient persons and for passive immunization against measles and hepatitis A
*Specific immune globulins*—Special preparations obtained from blood plasma from donor pools preselected for a high antibody content against a specific antigen (e.g., hepatitis B immune globulin, varicella zoster immune globulin, rabies immune globulin, tetanus immune globulin, vaccinia immune globulin, and cytomegalovirus immune globulin); as with IG and IVIG, do not transmit hepatitis B virus, human immunodeficiency virus (HIV), or other infectious diseases
**Vaccination**—Originally meant inoculation with vaccinia smallpox virus to make a person immune to smallpox; currently denotes physical act of administering any vaccine or toxoid

## Schedule for Immunizations

In the United States two organizations—the **Advisory Committee on Immunization Practices (ACIP)** of the **U.S. Public Health Service Centers for Disease Control and Prevention (CDC)** and the **Committee on Infectious Diseases** of the **American Academy of Pediatrics (AAP)**—govern the recommendations for immunization policies and procedures. In Canada, recommendations are from the **National Advisory Committee on Immunization** under the authority of the Minister of National Health and Welfare. Because ACIP is concerned primarily with national health issues and the Committee on Infectious Diseases formulates its recommendations for infants and children who receive regular health care, there are occasionally different perspectives in each group's recommendations. The policies of each committee are *recommendations,* not rules, and they change as a result of advances in the

**TABLE 12-6**   Recommended childhood immunization schedule—United States, 2002

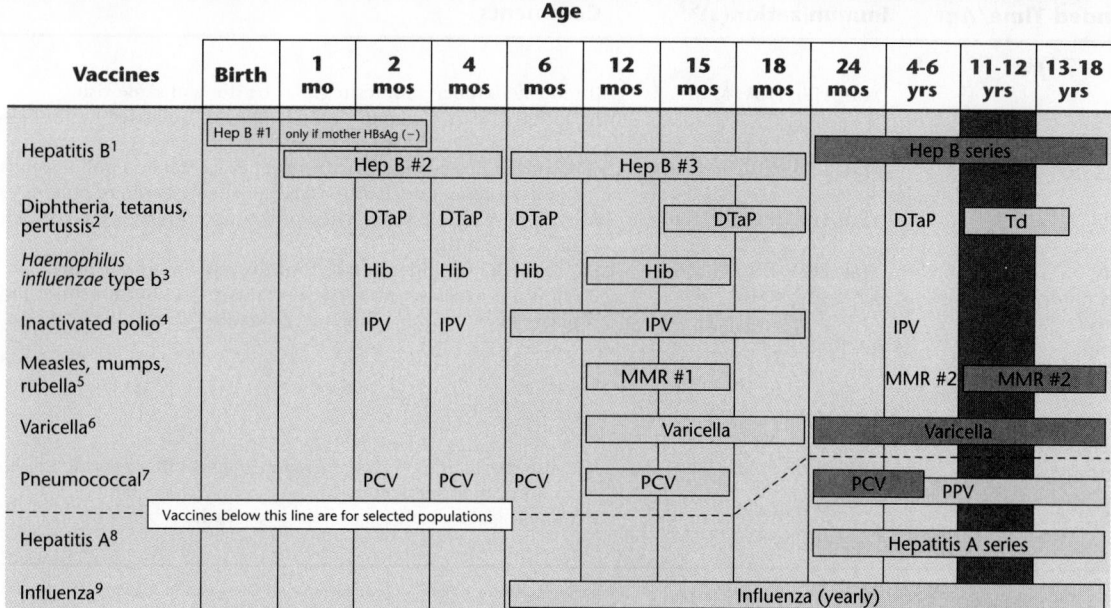

| Vaccines | Birth | 1 mo | 2 mos | 4 mos | 6 mos | 12 mos | 15 mos | 18 mos | 24 mos | 4-6 yrs | 11-12 yrs | 13-18 yrs |
|---|---|---|---|---|---|---|---|---|---|---|---|---|
| Hepatitis B[1] | Hep B #1 | only if mother HBsAg (−) | | | | | | | | | Hep B series | |
| | | Hep B #2 | | | | Hep B #3 | | | | | | |
| Diphtheria, tetanus, pertussis[2] | | DTaP | DTaP | DTaP | | DTaP | | | DTaP | | Td | |
| Haemophilus influenzae type b[3] | | Hib | Hib | Hib | | Hib | | | | | | |
| Inactivated polio[4] | | IPV | IPV | | IPV | | | | IPV | | | |
| Measles, mumps, rubella[5] | | | | | | MMR #1 | | | | MMR #2 | MMR #2 | |
| Varicella[6] | | | | | | Varicella | | | | Varicella | | |
| Pneumococcal[7] | | PCV | PCV | PCV | PCV | | | | PCV | PPV | | |
| Hepatitis A[8] | | | | | | | | | Hepatitis A series | | | |
| Influenza[9] | | | | | Influenza (yearly) | | | | | | | |

Vaccines below this line are for selected populations

| Range of Recommended Ages | Catch-Up Vaccination | Preadolescent Assessment |

**From American Academy of Pediatrics, Committee on Infectious Diseases: Recommended childhood immunization schedule, United States, 2002, *Pediatrics* 109 (1):162-164, 2002.**

This schedule indicates the recommended ages for routine administration of currently licensed childhood vaccines, as of December 1, 2001, for children through age 18 years. Any dose not given at the recommended age should be given at any subsequent visit when indicated and feasible. ▇ Indicates age groups that warrant special effort to administer those vaccines not previously given. Additional vaccines may be licensed and recommended during the year. Licensed combination vaccines may be used whenever any components of the combination are indicated and the vaccine's other components are not contraindicated. Providers should consult the manufacturers' package inserts for detailed recommendation.

1. **Hepatitis B vaccine (Hep B).** All infants should receive the first dose of hepatitis B vaccine soon after birth and before hospital discharge; the first dose may also be given by age 2 months if the infant's mother is HBsAg-negative. Only monovalent hepatitis B vaccine can be used for the birth dose. Monovalent or combination vaccine containing Hep B may be used to complete the series; four doses of vaccine may be administered if combination vaccine is used. The second dose should be given at least 4 weeks after the first dose, except for Hib-containing vaccine which cannot be administered before age 6 weeks. The third dose should be given at least 16 weeks after the first dose and at least 8 weeks after the second dose. The last dose in the vaccination series (third or fourth dose) should not be administered before age 6 months. *Infants born to HBsAg-positive mothers* should receive hepatitis B vaccine and 0.5 mL hepatitis B immune globulin (HBIG) within 12 hours of birth at separate sites. The second dose is recommended at age 1-2 months and the vaccination series should be completed (third or fourth dose) at age 6 months.
*Infants born to mothers whose HBsAg status is unknown* should receive the first dose of the hepatitis B vaccine series within 12 hours of birth. Maternal blood should be drawn at the time of delivery to determine the mother's HBsAg status; if the HBsAg test is positive, the infant should receive HBIG as soon as possible (no later than age 1 week).
2. **Diphtheria and tetanus toxoids and acellular pertussis vaccine (DTaP).** The fourth dose of DTaP may be administered as early as age 12 months, provided 6 months have elapsed since the third dose and the child is unlikely to return at age 15-18 months. **Tetanus and diphtheria toxoids (TD)** is recommended at age 11-12 years if at least 5 years have elapsed since the last dose of tetanus and diphtheria toxoid-containing vaccine. Subsequent routine Td boosters are recommended every 10 years.
3. *Haemophilus influenzae* type b (Hib) conjugate vaccine. Three Hib conjugate vaccines are licensed for infant use. If PRP-OMP (PedvaxHib® or ComVax® [Merck]) is administered at ages 2 and 4 months, a dose at age 6 months is not required. DTaP/Hib combination products should not be used for primary immunization in infants at ages 2, 4 or 6 months, but can be used as boosters following any Hib vaccine.
4. **Inactivated polio vaccine (IPV).** An all-IPV schedule is recommended for routine childhood polio vaccination in the United States. All children should receive four doses of IPV at ages 2 months, 4 months, 6-18 months, and 4-6 years.
5. **Measles, mumps, and rubella vaccine (MMR).** The second dose of MMR is recommended routinely at age 4-6 years but may be administered during any visit, provided at least 4 weeks have elapsed since the first dose and that both doses are administered beginning at or after age 12 months. Those who have not previously received the second dose should complete the schedule by the 11-12 year old visit.
6. **Varicella vaccine.** Varicella vaccine is recommended at any visit at or after age 12 months for susceptible children, i.e. those who lack a reliable history of chickenpox. Susceptible persons aged ≥13 years should receive two doses, given at least 4 weeks apart.
7. **Pneumococcal vaccine.** The heptavalent **pneumococcal conjugate vaccine (PCV)** is recommended for all children age 2-23 months. It is also recommended for certain children age 24-59 months. **Pneumococcal polysaccharide vaccine (PPV)** is recommended in addition to PCV for certain high-risk groups. See *MMWR* 2000;49(RR-9);1-35.
8. **Hepatitis A vaccine.** Hepatitis A vaccine is recommended for use in selected states and regions, and for certain high-risk groups; consult your local public health authority. See *MMWR* 1999;48(RR-12);1-37.
9. **Influenza vaccine.** Influenza vaccine is recommended annually for children age ≥6 months with *certain risk factors* (including but not limited to asthma, cardiac disease, sickle cell disease, HIV, diabetes; see *MMWR* 2001;50(RR-4);1-44), and can be administered to all others wishing to obtain immunity. Children aged ≤12 years should receive vaccine in a dosage appropriate for their age (0.25 mL if age 6-35 months or 0.5 mL if aged ≥3 years). Children aged ≤8 years who are receiving influenza vaccine for the first time should receive two doses separated by at least 4 weeks.

**For additional information about vaccines, vaccine supply, and contraindications for immunization, please visit the National Immunization Program Website at *www.cdc.gov/nip* or call the National Immunization Hotline at 800-232-2522 (English) or 800-232-0233 (Spanish).**

**Approved by the Advisory Committee on Immunization Practices (*www.cdc.gov/nip/acip*), the American Academy of Pediatrics (*www.aap.org*), and the American Academy of Family Physicians (*www.aafp.org*).**

field of immunology. Nurses need to realize the purpose of each organization, view immunization practices in light of the needs of an individual child and the community, and keep informed of the latest advances and changes in policy.

The recommended age for beginning primary immunizations of infants is within 2 weeks of birth, or in special circumstances, at birth (Table 12-6). Children born prematurely should receive the *full dose* of each vaccine at the ap-

**TABLE 12-7** Recommended immunization schedules for children not immunized in the first year of life[a]

| Recommended Time/Age | Immunization(s)[b,c] | Comments |
|---|---|---|
| **Younger Than 7 Years** | | |
| First visit | DTaP, Hib, HBV, MMR | If indicated, tuberculin testing may be done at same visit. |
| | | If child is 5 years of age or older, Hib is not indicated in most circumstances. |
| Interval after first visit | | |
| 1 month (4 weeks) | DTaP, IPV, HBV, Var[d] | The second dose of IPV may be given if accelerated poliomyelitis immunization is necessary, such as for travelers to areas where polio is endemic. |
| 2 months | DTaP, Hib, IPV | Second dose of Hib is indicated only if first dose was received when younger than 15 months. |
| ≥8 months | DTaP, HBV, IPV | IPV and HBV are not given if third doses were given earlier. |
| Age 4-6 years (at or before school entry) | DTaP, IPV, MMR[e] | DTaP is not necessary if fourth dose was given after fourth birthday; IPV is not necessary if third dose was given after fourth birthday. |
| Age 11-12 years | See Table 12-6 | |
| **7-12 Years** | | |
| First visit | HBV, MMR, Td, IPV | |
| Interval after first visit | | |
| 2 months (8 weeks) | HBV, MMR,[e] Var,[d] Td, IPV | IPV also may be given 1 month after first visit if accelerated poliomyelitis immunization is necessary. |
| 8-14 months | HBV,[f] Td, IPV | IPV is not given if third dose was given earlier. |
| Age 11-12 years | See Table 12-6 | |

From American Academy of Pediatrics, Committee on Infectious Diseases, Pickering L, editor: *2000 Red book: report of the Committee on Infectious Diseases,* ed 25, Elk Grove Village, IL, 2000, The Academy.

*HBV,* Hepatitis B virus vaccine; *Var,* varicella vaccine; *DTaP,* diphtheria and tetanus toxoids and acellular pertussis vaccine; *Hib, Haemophilus influenzae* type b conjugate; *IPV,* inactivated poliovirus; *MMR,* live measles, mumps, rubella; *Td,* adult tetanus toxoid (full dose) and diphtheria toxoid (reduced dose), for children ≥7 years and adults.

[a]Table is not completely consistent with all package inserts. For products used, also consult manufacturer's package insert for instructions on storage, handling, dosage, and administration. Biologics prepared by different manufacturers may vary, and package inserts of the same manufacturer may change. Therefore the physician should be aware of the contents of the current package insert.

[b]If all needed vaccines cannot be administered simultaneously, priority should be given to protecting the child against those diseases that pose the greatest immediate risk. In the United States, these diseases for children younger than 2 years usually are measles and *H. influenzae* type b infection; for children older than 7 years, they are measles, mumps, and rubella. Before 13 years of age, immunity against hepatitis B and varicella should be ensured.

[c]DTaP, HBV, Hib, MMR, and Var can be given simultaneously at separate sites if failure of the patient to return for future immunizations is a concern.

[d]Varicella vaccine can be administered to susceptible children any time after 12 months of age. Unvaccinated children who lack a reliable history of chickenpox should be vaccinated before their thirteenth birthday.

[e]Minimal interval between doses of MMR is 1 month (4 weeks).

[f]HBV may be given earlier in a 0-, 2-, and 4-month schedule.

propriate chronologic age. Recommended schedules for children not immunized during infancy are included in Table 12-7.

Table 12-8 describes immunization schedules for Canadian children. Children who began primary immunization at the recommended age but fail to receive all the doses do not need to begin the series again but instead receive only the missed doses. For situations in which there is doubt that the child will return for immunization according to the optimum schedule, HBV, DTaP, IPV (poliovirus vaccine), MMR, varicella, and Hib vaccines can be administered simultaneously. Parenteral vaccines are given in separate syringes in different injection sites (American Academy of Pediatrics, 2001).

## Recommendations for Routine Immunizations

**Hepatitis B Virus (HBV).** HBV is an important pediatric disease because HBV infections that occur during childhood and adolescence can lead to fatal consequences from cirrhosis or liver cancer during adulthood. Up to 90% of infants infected perinatally and 25% to 50% of children infected before age 5 years become HBV carriers. In addition, the incidence of HBV infection increases rapidly during adolescence (American Academy of Pediatrics, 2001). Past immunization strategies targeted several high-risk groups, including health care workers and others in contact with blood and body fluids, recipients of certain blood products (such as those with hemophilia), heterosexuals with multiple partners, sexually active homosexual and bisexual males, intravenous drug abusers, immigrants from countries in which HBV is widespread, and children born to mothers who are HBV surface antigen (HBsAg)–positive. To improve immunization rates, current recommendations include immunizations for all newborns. Both term and preterm infants born to mothers whose HBsAg status is positive or unknown should receive hepatitis B vaccine and hepatitis B immune globulin (HBIG) 0.5 ml within 12 hours of birth at two different injection sites. In the late 1990s, HBV contained small amounts of mercury (thimerosal) as a preservative, which generated concern regarding possible mercury poisoning in infants and led to a subsequent decrease in HBV immunization rates in newborns. There is, however, a new preservative-free HBV (Recombivax HB, Pediatrics*) and the Centers for Disease Control and Prevention (2001) strongly recommends that HBV immunization occur in newborns before discharge from the birth hospital. The American Academy of Pediatrics (2001a) also encourages immunization of all children by age 11 years.

*Merck and Company, West Point, PA.

**TABLE 12-8**   Routine immunization for infants and children—Provincial and territorial schedules, Canada, 1998

| Province or Territory | DTaP (Months) | Polio-IPV (Months) | Hib (Months) | Td/ Td-IPV (Years) | First Dose MMR (Months) | Year Second Dose MMR/MR Introduced | | Measles Catch-up Campaigns |
|---|---|---|---|---|---|---|---|---|
| | | | | | | 18 Months | 4 to 6 Years | |
| Alberta | 2, 4, 6, 18 and 4 to 6 years | 2, 4, 6, 18 and 4 to 6 years | 2, 4, 6, 18 | 14 to 16: Td | 12 | | 1996 MMR | 1997 monovalent measles vaccine grades 1-12* |
| British Columbia | 2, 4, 6, 18 and 4 to 6 years† | 2, 4, 6, 18 and 4 to 6 years† | 2, 4, 6, 18 | 14 to 16: Td | 12 | 1996 MMR | | 1996 MR vaccine 18 months to grade 12 |
| Manitoba | 2, 4, 6, 18 and 5 years | 2, 4, 6, 18 and 5 years | 2, 4, 6, 18 | 15: Td | 12 | | 1996 MMR | 1996 MR vaccine kindergarten to grade 6 |
| New Brunswick | 2, 4, 6, 18 and 4 to 6 years‡ | 2, 4, 6, 18 and 4 to 6 years | 2, 4, 6, 18 | 14 to 16: Td-IPV§ | 12 | 1997 MMR | | No program |
| Newfoundland | 2, 4, 6, 18 and 4 to 6 years | 2, 4, 6, 18 and 4 to 6 years | 2, 4, 6, 18 | 14 to 16: Td-IPV | 12 | 1996 MMR | | No program |
| Nova Scotia | 2, 4, 6, 18 and 4 to 6 years | 2, 4, 6, 18 and 4 to 6 years | 2, 4, 6, 18 | 14 to 16: Td-IPV | 12 | | 1996 MMR | No program |
| Northwest Territories | 2, 4, 6, 18 and 4 to 6 years¶ | 2, 4, 6, 18 and 4 to 6 years¶ | 2, 4, 6, 18 | 14 to 16: Td-IPV** | 12 | 1996 MMR | | 1996 MR vaccine kindergarten to grade 12 |
| Ontario | 2, 4, 6, 18 and 4 to 6 years†† | 2, 4, 6, 18 and 4 to 6 years†† | 2, 4, 6, 18 | 14 to16: Td-IPV‡‡ | 12 | | 1996 MMR | 1996 monovalent measles vaccine; junior kindergarten to grade 13 |
| Prince Edward Island | 2, 4, 6, 18 and 4 to 6 years | 2, 4, 6, 18 and 4 to 6 years | 2, 4, 6, 18 | 14 to 16: Td-IPV | 15 | 1997 MMR§§ | 1996 MMR§§ | 1996 monovalent measles vaccine; grades 1 to 12 |
| Quebec | 2, 4, 6, 18 and 4 to 6 years | 2, 4, 6, 18 and 4 to 6 years¶¶ | 2, 4, 6, 18 | 14 to 16: Td-IPV¶¶ | 12 | 1996 MMR | | 1996 monovalent measles vaccine; 18 months to grade 12 |
| Saskatchewan | 2, 4, 6, 18 and 4 to 6 years*** | 2, 4, 6, 18 and 4 to 6 years*** | 2, 4, 6, 18 | 14 to 16: TD††† | 12 | 1996 MR vaccine | | 1996 MR vaccine; preschool, grades 6, 8, 9, 12 |
| Yukon Territory | 2, 4, 6, 18 and 4 to 6 years‡‡‡ | 2, 4, 6, 18 and 4 to 6 years‡‡‡ | 2, 4, 6, 18 | 14-16: Td-IPV | 12 | 1996 MMR | | 1996 MMR; 18 months to kindergarten; grades 1 to 12 monovalent measles vaccine |

*The Alberta catch-up campaign in 1997 primarily used monovalent measles. A small amount of measles, mumps, and rubella (MMR) and measles and rubella (MR) was initially used in school outbreaks pending availability of multidose monovalent measles vaccine. †In British Columbia, the fifth dose of diphtheria, pertussis, tetanus, and acellular polio (DTaP) and inactive polio virus (IPV) vaccines at four to six years of age is not necessary if the fourth dose was given after the fourth birthday. ‡In New Brunswick, whole cell pertussis vaccine used through 1997. §In New Brunswick, polio vaccine at 14 to 16 years of age is not required if the child has completed the primary series and received one or more doses of oral polio vaccine (OPV) in the past. ¶In Northwest Territories, the fifth dose of DTaP and IPV at four to six years of age is not necessary if the fourth dose was given after the fourth birthday. **In Northwest Territories, polio vaccine at 14 to 16 years of age is not required if the child has completed the primary series and received one or more doses of OPV in the past. ††In Ontario, the fifth dose of DTaP and IPV at four to six years of age is not necessary if the fourth dose was given after the fourth birthday. ‡‡In Ontario, polio vaccine at 14 to 16 years of age is not required if the child has completed the primary series and received one or more doses of OPV in the past. OPV was used routinely from January 1990 through March 1993. §§In Prince Edward Island, the four- to six-year booster program began in April 1996 and a second dose program for 18-month olds began April 1997. As of April 2000, the four- to six-year program will be discontinued. ¶¶In Quebec, polio vaccine doses at four to six years of age and at 14 to 16 years of age are omitted if OPV was used for earlier doses. ***In Saskatchewan, the fifth dose of DTaP and IPV at four to six years of age is not necessary if the fourth dose was given after the fourth birthday. †††In Saskatchewan, polio vaccine at 14 to 16 years of age is given only if one dose of OPV was not received in the past. ‡‡‡In the Yukon Territory, the fifth dose of DTaP and IPV at four to six years of age is not necessary if the fourth dose was given after the fourth birthday. Td Tetanus-diphtheria toxoid (adult type).
From Paediatrics & Child Health: Canadian National Report on Immunization, 1998, *J Canadian Paediatr Soc*, vol 4, supp C, July/August 1999; *www.hc-sc.gc.ca/main/lcdc/web/publicat/paediatr/vol4supc/pch_j_e.html.*
*Note:* one dose of varicella vaccine (Varivax) is recommended for children under 12 years of age who are at risk for varicella; no booster is recommended at this time. Children over 12 years of age who are at risk of contracting varicella should have 2 doses of Varivax, at least 28 days apart. Statement on recommended use of varicella virus vaccine—CCDR, vol 25 ACS1, May 1999.
Pneumococcal vaccine is recommended for all children age 2 and over who are in a high-risk group except in Prince Edward Island and Quebec provinces.
Influenza vaccine is recommended for children in a high-risk group for influenza except in Prince Edward Island province.
Other vaccines such as BCG and meningococcal may be required within certain populations in Canada. See Canadian Paediatric Society immunization Web site for more information: *www.hc_sc.gc.ca/main/lcdc/web/publicat/paediatr/vol4supc/pch_j_e.html.*

**TABLE 12-9** Recommended dosages of hepatitis B vaccines*

| | Vaccine† | |
|---|---|---|
| | **Recombivax HB‡** Dose, $\mu$g (mL) | **Engerix-B§ Dose,** $\mu$g (mL) |
| Infants of HBsAg-negative mothers, children and adolescents younger than 20 years of age | 5 (0.5) | 10 (0.5) |
| Infants of HBsAg-positive mothers (HBIG [0.5 ml] also is recommended) | 5 (0.5) | 10 (0.5) |
| Adults 20 years of age or older | 10 (1.0) | 20 (1.0) |
| Patients undergoing dialysis and other immunosuppressed adults | 40 (1.0)‖ | 40 (2.0)¶ |

From American Academy of Pediatrics, Committee on Infectious Diseases, Pickering LK, editor: *2000 Red book: report of the Committee on Infectious Diseases,* ed 25, Elk Grove Village, IL, 2000, The Academy.

*HBsAg indicates hepatitis B surface antigen; HBIG, Hepatitis B Immune Globulin.
†Vaccines should be stored at 2°C to 8°C (36°F to 46°F). Freezing destroys effectiveness. Both vaccines are administered in a 3-dose schedule. A 2-dose schedule, administered at 0 and 4 to 6 months later, is available for adolescents 11–15 years of age using the adult dose of Recombivax HB (10 $\mu$g).
‡Available from Merck and Co, West Point, PA. A combination of hepatitis B (Recombivax, 5 $\mu$g) and *Haemophilus influenzae b* (PRP-OMP) vaccine is licensed for use at 2, 4, and 12 to 15 months of age (Comvax).
§Available from SmithKline Beecham Pharmaceuticals, Philadelphia, Pa. The US Food and Drug Administration has approved this vaccine for use in an optional 4-dose schedule at 0, 1, 2, and 12 months.
‖Special formulation for dialysis patients.
¶Two 1.0-ml doses given in 1 site in a 4-dose schedule at 0, 1, 2, and 6 to 12 months.

The vaccine is given intramuscularly in the vastus lateralis in newborns or in the deltoid for older infants and children. Regardless of age, the dorsogluteal site is avoided because it has been associated with low antibody seroconversion rates, indicating a reduced immune response (Zuckerman, Cockcroft, and Zuckerman, 1992). No data exist regarding the seroconversion when the ventrogluteal site is used. The vaccine can be safely administered simultaneously at a separate site with DTaP, MMR, and Hib vaccines. Dosage depends on the child's age and the type of vaccine used (Table 12-9).

**Hepatitis A.** Hepatitis A virus (HAV) has recently been recognized as a significant child health problem, particularly in communities with unusually high infection rates. HAV is spread by the fecal-oral route and from person-to-person contact, by ingestion of contaminated food or water, but rarely by blood transfusion. The illness has an abrupt onset with fever, malaise, anorexia, nausea, abdominal discomfort, dark urine, and jaundice being the most common clinical signs of infection. In children under 6 years of age, who represent approximately one third of all cases of HAV, the disease may be asymptomatic, and jaundice is rarely evident. Children living in communities with high infection rates should be immunized with either HAVRIX or VAQTA vaccine, given by the intramuscular route in the deltoid. These vaccines are recommended for children 2 years of age and older, in two doses administered at least 6 months apart. States in which hepatitis A is mandatory are Arizona, Oklahoma, Alaska, New Mexico, South Dakota, Idaho, Nevada, Oregon, Utah, California, and Washington. (Prevention of hepatitis A, 1999). For further information see footnote "8" in Table 12-6.

**Diphtheria.** Diphtheria vaccine is commonly administered (1) in combination with tetanus and pertussis vaccines (DTaP) or DTaP and Hib vaccines for children younger than 7 years of age, (2) in combination with a conjugate *H. in-* *fluenzae* type B vaccine (see Table 12-6), (3) in a combined vaccine with tetanus (DT) for children younger than 7 years of age who have some contraindication to receiving pertussis vaccine, (4) in smaller doses (15% to 20% of that in DTaP or DT) with tetanus vaccine (Td) for use in children age 7 years and older, or (5) as a single antigen when combined antigen preparations are not indicated. Although the diphtheria vaccine does not produce absolute immunity, protective antitoxin persists for 10 years or more when given according to the recommended schedule, and boosters are given every 10 years for life.

**Tetanus.** Three forms of tetanus vaccine—tetanus toxoid, tetanus immune globulin (TIG) (human), and tetanus antitoxin (usually horse serum)—are available. Tetanus toxoid is used for routine primary immunization, usually in one of the combinations listed for diphtheria, and provides protective antitoxin levels for 10 years or more.

For wound management, passive immunity is available with TIG. In persons with a history of two previous doses of tetanus toxoid, a booster dose of the toxoid can be given. Separate syringes and different sites are used when tetanus toxoid and TIG are given concurrently. Table 12-10 presents a summary of the recommended procedure for tetanus prophylaxis in wound management.

**Pertussis.** Pertussis vaccine is recommended for all children 6 weeks through 6 years of age (up to the seventh birthday) who have no neurologic contraindications to its use. It is not given to children 7 years or older because the risk of receiving the vaccine increases as the incidence, severity, and fatality of the disease decrease.

Currently, two forms of pertussis vaccine are available in the United States. The *whole-cell pertussis vaccine* is prepared from inactivated cells of *Bordetella pertussis* and contains multiple antigens. In contrast, the *acellular pertussis vaccine* contains one or more immunogens derived from the *B. pertussis* organism. The highly purified acellular vaccine is associated

**TABLE 12-10**   Guide to tetanus prophylaxis in routine wound management, 1997

| History of Adsorbed Tetanus Toxoid (Doses) | Clean, Minor Wounds | | All Other Wounds* | |
|---|---|---|---|---|
| | Td† | TIG | Td† | TIG |
| Unknown or <three | Yes | No | Yes | Yes |
| ≥Three‡ | No§ | No | No|| | No |

Data from American Academy of Pediatrics, Committee on Infectious Diseases, Pickering L, editor: *2000 Red book: report of the Committee on Infectious Diseases,* ed 25, Elk Grove Village, Ill, 2000, The Academy.
*Such as, but not limited to, wounds contaminated with dirt, feces, soil, and saliva, puncture wounds, avulsions, and wounds resulting from missiles, crushing, burns, and frostbite.
†For children <7 years old: DTaP (DT, if pertussis vaccine is contraindicated) is preferred to tetanus toxoid alone. For persons ≥7 years of age, Td is preferred to tetanus toxoid alone.
‡If only three doses of *fluid* toxoid have been received, then a fourth dose of toxoid, preferably an adsorbed toxoid, should be given.
§Yes, if >10 years since last dose.
||Yes, if >5 years since last dose. (More frequent boosters are not needed and can accentuate side effects.)

with fewer local and systemic reactions than those occurring with the whole-cell vaccine in children of similar age. The acellular pertussis vaccine is recommended by the American Academy of Pediatrics (2001) for the first three immunizations and is usually given at 2, 4, and 6 months of age with diphtheria and tetanus (DTaP). Four forms of acellular pertussis vaccine are currently licensed for use in infants: Acel-Imune, Tripedia, Certiva, and Infanrix (diphtheria, tetanus toxoid, and acellular pertussis conjugate). Either the acellular or whole-cell vaccine may be given for the fourth and fifth doses, but the acellular is preferred. It is also recommended that the first three DTaP vaccinations be from the same manufacturer; the fourth dose may be from a different manufacturer. The child who has received one or more whole-cell vaccines may complete the series of five with the acellular vaccine.

**Polio.**   In July 1999 the ACIP recommended an all-IPV schedule for routine childhood polio vaccination. All children should receive four doses of IPV at 2 months, 4 months, 6 to 18 months, and 4 to 6 years of age (American Academy of Pediatrics, 2001).

The change from the exclusive use of OPV to the exclusive use of IPV is related to the rare risk of *vaccine-associated polio paralysis (VAPP)* from OPV. The exclusive use of IPV eliminates the risk of VAPP but is associated with an increased number of injections and increased cost. Taylor and others (2001) found that the switch from OPV to IPV has not had a negative impact on the immunization status of young children.

**Measles.**   The measles (rubeola) vaccine is given at 12 to 15 months of age. During the course of measles outbreaks, the vaccine can be given any time after 6 months of age, followed by a second inoculation after age 12 months.

Because of continued outbreaks of measles among unvaccinated preschool-age children and among vaccinated school-age children and college students, a second measles immunization is recommended at 4 to 6 years of age (at school entry) or revaccination by 11 to 12 years of age if only the measles vaccine has been administered (American Academy of Pediatrics, 2001). Revaccination should include all individuals born after 1956 who have not received two doses of measles vaccine after 12 months of age. Individuals born before this date are thought to be immune from exposure to natural measles virus.

**Mumps.**   Mumps virus vaccine is recommended for children at 12 to 15 months of age and is typically given in combination with measles and rubella. It should not be administered to infants younger than 12 months because persisting maternal antibodies can interfere with the immune response.

Because of recent outbreaks of the disease, especially in children 10 to 19 years of age, mumps immunization is recommended for all individuals born after 1957 who may be susceptible to mumps (i.e., those who have no history of having had the disease or vaccine and when there is no laboratory evidence of immunity).

**Rubella.**   Rubella is a relatively mild infection in children, but in a pregnant woman the actual infection presents serious risks to the developing fetus. Therefore the aim of rubella immunization is actually protection of the unborn child rather than the recipient of the immunization.

Rubella immunization is recommended for all children at 12 to 15 months of age and is administered in a combined form with measles and mumps vaccine. Increased emphasis should also be placed on vaccinating all unimmunized prepubertal children and susceptible adolescents and adult women in the childbearing age-group.

Because the live attenuated virus may cross the placenta and theoretically present a risk to the developing fetus, rubella vaccine is currently not given to any pregnant woman. Although this is standard practice, current evidence from women who received the vaccine while pregnant and delivered unaffected offspring indicates that the risk to the fetus is negligible. In addition, there is no reported danger of administering rubella vaccine to a child if the mother is pregnant.

***Haemophilus influenzae* type b (Hib).**   Hib conjugate vaccines provide protection against a number of serious infections caused by Hib, especially bacterial meningitis, epiglottitis, bacterial pneumonia, septic arthritis, and sepsis (Hib is not associated with the viruses that cause influenza, or "flu"). Several Hib vaccines are available; some are combination vaccines, such as *Comvax* (Hib and HBV) (see Table 12-14). These conjugate vaccines connect Hib to a nontoxic form of another organism, such as meningococcal protein or diphtheria protein. There is *no* antibody response to these nontoxic proteins, but they significantly improve the antibody response to Hib, especially in infants.

The use of combination vaccines provides equivalent immunogenicity and decreases the number of injections an infant receives; however, it is important that they be given to the appropriate-age child.

When possible, the Hib conjugate vaccine used at the first vaccination should be used for all subsequent vaccinations in the primary series. All Hib vaccines are administered by intramuscular injection using a separate syringe and at a site separate from any concurrent vaccinations.

**Varicella.**   Administration of the cell-free live-attenuated varicella vaccine *(Varivax)* is recommended for healthy children 12 to 18 months of age. A single dose of 0.5 ml should be given by subcutaneous injection. From the age of 19 months to the thirteenth birthday, a single dose of varicella vaccine may be given at any time to children who may be susceptible, either by lack of proof of varicella vaccination, serologic testing, or a reliable history of having never had varicella infection (American Academy of Pediatrics, 2000a). The vaccine should be kept frozen in the lyophilized form (stable particles that readily go into solution) and used within 30 minutes of being reconstituted to ensure viral potency (American Academy of Pediatrics, 2000a).

Varicella vaccine may be administered simultaneously with MMR. However, separate syringes and injection sites should be used. If they are not administered simultaneously, the interval between administration of varicella vaccine and MMR should be at least 1 month. Varicella vaccine may also be given simultaneously with DTaP, IPV, HBV, and/or Hib (American Academy of Pediatrics, 2001; Infectious Diseases in Children, 2002).

**Pneumococcal (Prevnar).**   A seven-valent *Streptococcus pneumoniae* conjugate vaccine (PCV7)* has been approved for use in children under 2 years of age. Streptococcal pneumococci are responsible for a number of bacterial infections in children under 2, which may cause serious morbidity and mortality. Among these are generalized infections such as septicemia and meningitis, or localized infections such as otitis media, sinusitis, and pneumonia. These illnesses are particularly problematic in children who attend daycare facilities and in those who are immune compromised. PCV7 is expected to prevent pneumococcal illnesses that have become resistant to penicillin and to significantly decrease the incidence of otitis media and pneumonia (Murray, 2001). The vaccine is administered at 2, 4, and 6 months, with a fourth dose at 12 to 15 months of age; children 7 to 11 months old may receive three doses as long as they are 6 to 8 weeks apart and a fourth dose at 12 to 15 months; children 12 to 23 months who have not been immunized with the pneumococcal vaccine may be given two doses, 6 to 8 weeks apart. PCV7 is also recommended for all children under 24 months and older children (24 to 59 months) with the following: sickle cell disease; functional or anatomic asplenia; nephrotic syndrome or chronic renal failure; conditions associated with immunosuppression, such as solid organ transplantation, drug therapy, or cytoreduction therapy (including long-term systemic corticosteroid therapy); congenital immune deficiency; HIV infection; cere-

---

**ATRAUMATIC CARE**
*Immunizations*

To minimize local reactions from vaccines:
Select a needle of adequate length (1 inch [2.5 cm] in infants) to deposit the antigen deep in the muscle mass.
Needle length is an important factor and must be considered for each individual child; fewer reactions to immunizations are observed when the vaccine is given deep into the muscle rather than into subcutaneous tissue; contrary to previous thought, deep intramuscular tissue has a better blood supply and fewer pain receptors than adipose tissue, thus providing an optimal site for immunizations with fewer side effects (Zuckerman, 2000).
Inject into the vastus lateralis or ventrogluteal muscle; the deltoid may be used in children 18 months of age or older or in infants receiving HBV vaccine.
Use an air bubble to clear the needle after injecting the vaccine (theoretically beneficial but unproved).
To minimize pain:
Apply the topical anesthetic EMLA to the injection site and cover with an occlusive dressing for at least 1 hour.
Apply a vapocoolant spray (i.e., ethyl chloride or FluoriMethane) directly to the skin or to a cotton ball, which is placed on the skin for 15 seconds immediately before the injection (Reis and Holubkov, 1997).
In preschool children use distraction, such as telling the child to "take a deep breath and blow and blow and blow until I tell you to stop."
*Note:* Changing the needle on the syringe after drawing up the vaccine and before injecting it has not been shown to decrease local reactions. In children 4 to 6 years of age, the administration of sequential injections or simultaneous injections of vaccines did not alter their perceptions of distress, but parents preferred the simultaneous method (Horn and McCarthy, 1999).

---

brospinal fluid leaks; chronic cardiovascular disease (e.g., congestive heart failure or cardiomyopathy); chronic pulmonary disease (e.g., emphysema or cystic fibrosis, but not asthma); chronic liver disease (e.g., cirrhosis); or living in special environments or social settings in which the risk of invasive pneumococcal disease or its complications is very high (e.g., Alaska Native, African-American, and certain American Indian populations) (American Academy of Pediatrics, 2000b).

The 23PS (pneumococcal polysaccharide 23) is not recommended for children younger than 24 months who do not have one of the high-risk conditions described previously. One dose of 23PS is recommended in children older than 23 months who have one of the high-risk conditions after primary immunization with PCV7. (See American Academy of Pediatrics, 2000b, Table 3 for PCV7 and 23PS schedule.)

**Influenza.**   The influenza vaccine is now recommended for children 6 months and older with risk factors including but not limited to the following: asthma, cardiac disease, HIV, diabetes, and sickle cell disease. Influenza vaccine may also be given to other children of appropriate age whose parents wish them to be immunized against the flu. Children who have a reported anaphylactic hypersensitivity to eggs should not receive the vaccine.

The vaccine is administered in early fall before the flu season begins and is repeated yearly for ongoing protection. The intramuscular vaccine is administered as two separate doses

---

*Prevnar, Wyeth-Lederle, Philadelphia, PA.

**TABLE 12-11   Recommendations for selected nonmandated vaccines**

| Description | Administration/Precautions |
|---|---|
| **Meningococcal Polysaccharide Vaccine (Menomune)**<br><br>Affords protection against *Neisseria meningitidis;* serogroups A, C, Y, and W-135.<br>Recommended for children 2 years and older with terminal complement deficiencies and anatomic or functional asplenia.<br>Meningococcal vaccine has also been recommended by ACIP for college freshmen living in dormitories because of higher rates of meningococcal disease.<br>Meningococcal vaccine is expected to be licensed for universal administration to infants within the next 2 to 4 years (Baltimore and Jenson, 2001). | Subcutaneous injection.<br>Duration of protection unknown.<br>Safety during pregnancy not established. |
| **Lyme Disease Vaccine (LYMErix)**<br><br>Affords protection against infection with the spirochete *Borrelia burgdorferi,* which causes Lyme disease (LD).<br>Recommended for individuals 15 to 70 years of age who are at high risk for LD from significant exposure to tick habitats in endemic areas (northeast and north-central United States) and for those who have been infected with LD.<br>Although the vaccine is not currently recommended for children under 15 because of safety issues, its use might be considered in situations where LD poses a significantly high risk (Lutwick and Abramson, 2000). | Intramuscular injection in deltoid muscle.<br>Administered on 0-, 1-, and 12-month schedule. Doses 2 and 3 should be given several weeks before *B. burgdorferi* season, which usually begins in April (i.e., first dose should be given in mid-February). |

Data from American Academy of Pediatrics, Committee on Infectious Diseases, Pickering L, editor: *2000 Red book: report of the Committee on Infectious Diseases,* ed 25, Elk Grove Village, IL, 2000, The Academy.

2 weeks apart in first-time recipients under the age of 8 years. The dose is 0.25 ml for children aged 3 to 35 months and 0.5 ml for children 3 years and above. The vaccine may be given simultaneously with other vaccines but at a separate site (American Academy of Pediatrics, 2002). The vaccine is administered yearly because different strains of influenza are used each year in the manufacture of the vaccine.

## Recommendations for Selected Immunizations

Several additional vaccines are recommended for children at high risk for particular diseases. Most of these children have chronic disorders or impaired immune systems that make them more susceptible to certain infections than the general population. Selected immunizations are presented in Table 12-11. Others, such as the rabies vaccine, are discussed elsewhere in this text.

## Reactions

Vaccines for routine immunizations are among the safest and most reliable drugs available. However, minor side effects do occur following many of the immunizations and, rarely, a serious reaction may result from the vaccine (Table 12-12).

With inactivated antigens, such as DTaP, side effects are most likely to occur within a few hours or days of administration and are usually limited to local tenderness, erythema, and swelling at the injection site; low-grade fever; and behavioral changes (drowsiness, fretfulness, eating less, prolonged or unusual cry). Local reactions tend to be less severe when a needle of sufficient length to deposit the vaccine in the muscle is used. (See Atraumatic Care box.) Rarely, more severe reactions may occur, especially with pertussis and varicella. Reactions to DTaP tend to be more severe if they occurred with a previous immunization.

Hib vaccine is one of the safest vaccines available but may be associated with low-grade fever and mild local reactions at the site of injection, which resolve rapidly.

Unlike the inactivated antigens, live attenuated virus vaccines such as MMR multiply for days or weeks, and unfavorable reactions and "vaccine-associated" disorders can occur up to 30 to 60 days. These reactions are usually mild, although reactions to rubella tend to be more troublesome in older children and adults.

## Contraindications/Precautions

Nurses need to be aware of the reasons for withholding immunizations—both for the child's safety in terms of avoiding reactions and for the child's maximum benefit from receiving the vaccine. Unfounded fears and lack of knowledge regarding contraindications can needlessly prevent a child from having protection from life-threatening diseases.

The contraindications to the usual childhood vaccines are presented in Table 12-13. A general discussion of specific concerns follows.

There is growing concern that public awareness via the Internet and television may have a negative affect on the current rates of immunization. Parental objections to childhood immunizations for philosophic or religious reasons are said to account for less than 1% of the nonvaccinated pediatric population, yet clusters of such groups may contribute to outbreaks of vaccine-preventable disease (Lutwick, 2000). It is not uncommon for a seemingly vaccine-associated catastrophic illness in one child to receive much attention in the media, possibly prompting parents to question the safety of vaccination. Recent attention has been given to the possible association between increased rates of childhood autism and the MMR vaccine, yet studies show the lack of data to support

**TABLE 12-12** Possible side effects of recommended childhood immunizations and nursing responsibilities

| Immunization | Reaction | Nursing Responsibilities |
|---|---|---|
| Hepatitis B virus | Well tolerated, few side effects | Explain to parents reason for this immunization<br>Consider that cost for 3 injections may be a factor |
| Diphtheria | Fever usually within 24-48 hours<br>Soreness, redness, and swelling at injection site<br>Behavioral changes: drowsiness, fretfulness, anorexia, prolonged or unusual crying | Nursing responsibilities for DTP apply to immunizations for diphtheria, tetanus, and pertussis<br>Instruction for DTP: advise parents of possible side effects |
| Tetanus | Same as for diphtheria but may include urticaria and malaise<br>All may have delayed onset and last several days<br>Lump at injection site may last for weeks, even months, but gradually disappears | Recommend prophylactic use of acetaminophen at time of DTP immunization and every 4-6 hours for a total of 3 doses<br>Advise parents to notify practitioner *immediately* of any unusual side effects, such as those listed under pertussis in Table 12-13 |
| Pertussis | Same as for tetanus but may include loss of consciousness, convulsions, persistent inconsolable crying episodes, generalized or focal neurologic signs, fever (temperature at or above 40.5° C [105° F]), systemic allergic reaction | Before administering next dose of DTP, inquire about reactions, especially those listed under pertussis in Table 12-13 |
| *Haemophilus influenzae* type b | Mild local reactions (erythema, pain) at injection site<br>Low-grade fever | Advise parents of possible mild side effects |
| Poliovirus (IPV) | No serious adverse effects have been associated with the currently available product; rare adverse reactions, however, cannot be excluded. Trace amounts of neomycin, streptomycin, and polymyxin B may be present in IPV (American Academy of Pediatrics, 2000a). | Advise parents of safety of IPV, (i.e., no vaccine-associated polio paralysis with inactivated virus) |
| Measles | Anorexia, malaise, rash, and fever may occur 7 to 10 days after immunization<br>Rarely (estimated risk 1:1 million doses) encephalitis may occur | Advise parents of more common side effects and use of antipyretics for fever<br>If a persistent fever with other obvious signs of illness occurs, have parents notify physician immediately |
| Mumps | Essentially no side effects other than a brief, mild fever | See general comment to parents* |
| Rubella | Fever, lymphadenopathy, or mild rash that lasts 1 or 2 days within a few days after immunization<br>Arthralgia, arthritis, or paresthesia of the hands and fingers may occur approximately 2 weeks after vaccination and is more common in older children and adults | Advise parents of side effects, especially of time delay before joint swelling and pain; assure them that these symptoms will disappear<br>May recommend use of acetaminophen for pain |
| Varicella | Pain, tenderness, or redness at the injection site<br>Mild, vaccine-associated maculopapular or varicelliform rash at the vaccine site or elsewhere | Advise parents of possible side effects<br>May recommend use of acetaminophen for pain |
| Hepatitis A | No severe reactions have been reported<br>Local erythema may occur in some cases | Explain to parents and teens rationale for immunization<br>Encourage parents in high-risk areas to immunize children, especially teens and preteens |
| Pneumococcal (PCV7) | Fever, fussiness, decreased appetite, drowsiness, local erythema, interrupted sleep, diarrhea, vomiting, and hives<br>*Note:* These reported reactions occurred in a small sample population; the combined reactions were equal to or less than the number of reactions experienced in children receiving DtaP and MMR, yet are reported here because of the relative newness of the vaccine | Explain to parents benefits and rationale for vaccination in children younger than 2 years and older than 2 years if in high-risk category (see p. 534) |

*General comment to parents regarding each immunization: benefit of being protected by immunization is believed to greatly outweigh risk from the disease.

such a conclusion (Dales, Hammer, and Smith 2001). Nurses should be at the forefront in providing parents with appropriate information regarding childhood immunization benefits, contraindications, side effects, and effects of nonvaccination on the child's health. For several decades pertussis vaccine was considered a rare cause of serious, permanent brain damage or death. After reviewing recent studies, experts have concluded that whole-cell pertussis vaccine has not been proved to cause neurologic damage (American Academy of Pediatrics, 2000a). Previous contraindications to whole-cell pertussis vaccination are now considered precautions.

The general contraindication for all immunizations is a severe febrile illness. This precaution avoids adding the risk of adverse side effects from the vaccine to an already ill child or mistakenly identifying a symptom of the disease as having been caused by the vaccine. The presence of minor illnesses

## TABLE 12-13   Contraindications and precautions to vaccinations*

| True Contraindications and Precautions | Not Contraindications (Vaccines May Be Administered) |
|---|---|
| **General for All Vaccines (DTP/DTaP, IPV, MMR, Hib, Hepatitis B, Hepatitis A, Var, PCV)** | |
| *Contraindications* | *Not Contraindications* |
| Anaphylactic reaction to a vaccine contraindicates further doses of that vaccine | Mild to moderate local reaction (soreness, redness, swelling) following a dose of an injectable antigen |
| Anaphylactic reaction to a vaccine constituent contraindicates the use of vaccines containing that substance | Mild acute illness with or without low-grade fever |
| Moderate or severe illnesses with or without a fever | Current antimicrobial therapy |
| | Convalescent phase of illnesses |
| | Prematurity (same dosage and indications as for normal, full-term infants) |
| | Recent exposure to an infectious disease |
| | History of penicillin or other nonspecific allergies or family history of such allergies |
| **Diphtheria, Tetanus, Pertussis or Acellular Pertussis (DTP/DTaP)** | |
| *Contraindication* | *Not Contraindications* |
| Encephalopathy within 7 days of administration of previous dose of DTP | Temperature of <40.5° C (104.8° F) following a previous dose of DTP |
| *Precautions†* | Family history of seizures‡ |
| Fever of ≥40.5° C (104.8° F) within 48 hours after vaccination with a prior dose of DTP | Family history of sudden infant death syndrome |
| Collapse or shocklike state (hypotonic-hyporesponsive episode) within 48 hours of receiving a prior dose of DTP | Family history of an adverse event following DTP administration |
| Seizures within 3 days of receiving a prior dose of DTP‡ | |
| Persistent, inconsolable crying lasting ≥3 hours within 48 hours of receiving a prior dose of DTP | |
| **Inactivated Polio (IPV)** | |
| *Contraindication* | *Not Contraindications* |
| Anaphylactic reaction to neomycin, streptomycin, or polymyxin B | Breast-feeding |
| *Precaution†* | Mild diarrhea |
| Pregnancy | |
| **Measles, Mumps, Rubella (MMR)** | |
| *Contraindications* | *Not Contraindications* |
| Pregnancy | Tuberculosis or positive PPD skin test |
| Known altered immunodeficiency (hematologic and solid tumors, congenital immunodeficiency, and long-term immunosuppressive therapy) | Simultaneous TB skin testing§ |
| | Breast-feeding |
| | Pregnancy of mother of recipient |
| *Precautions†* | Immunodeficient family member or household contact |
| Recent immune globulin (IG) administration | Infection with HIV |
| IG products and MMR should not be given simultaneously; if unavoidable, give at different sites and revaccinate or test for seroconversion in 3 months; if IG is given first, MMR should not be given for at least 3-6 months, depending on the dose; if MMR is given first, IG should not be given for 2 weeks | Nonanaphylactic reactions to eggs or neomycin |
| Thrombocytopenia/thrombocytopenia purpura | |
| ***Haemophilus Influenzae* Type b (Hib)** | |
| *Contraindication* | *Not a Contraindication* |
| None identified | History of Hib disease |

From American Academy of Pediatrics, Committee on Infectious Diseases, Pickering LK, editor: *2000 Red book: report of the Committee on Infectious Diseases,* ed 25, Elk Grove Village, IL, 2000, The Academy.

*This information is based on the recommendations of the Advisory Committee on Immunization Practices (ACIP) and those of the Committee on Infectious Diseases (Red Book Committee) of the American Academy of Pediatrics (AAP). Sometimes these recommendations vary from those contained in the manufacturer's package inserts. For more detailed information, providers should consult the published recommendations of the ACIP, AAP, and the manufacturer's package inserts.

†The events or conditions listed as precautions, although not contraindications, should be carefully reviewed. The benefits and risks of administering a specific vaccine to an individual under the circumstances should be considered. If the risks are believed to outweigh the benefits, the vaccination should be withheld; if the benefits are believed to outweigh the risks (e.g., during an outbreak or foreign travel), the vaccination should be administered. Whether and when to administer DTP to children with proven or suspected underlying neurologic disorders should be decided on an individual basis. It is prudent on theoretic grounds to avoid vaccinating pregnant women.

‡Acetaminophen given before administering DTP and thereafter every 4 hours for 24 hours should be considered for children with a personal or family history of seizures in siblings or parents.

§Measles vaccination may temporarily suppress tuberculin reactivity. If testing cannot be done the day of MMR vaccination, the test should be postponed for 4 to 6 weeks.   *Continued*

**TABLE 12-13   Contraindications and precautions to vaccinations—cont'd**

| True Contraindications and Precautions | Not Contraindications (Vaccines May Be Administered) |
| --- | --- |
| **Hepatitis B Virus (HBV)** | |
| *Contraindication* | *Not a Contraindication* |
| Anaphylactic reaction to common baker's yeast | Pregnancy |
| **Varicella** | |
| *Contraindications* | *Not a Contraindication* |
| Immunocompromised individuals (e.g., HIV, acute lymphocytic leukemia) | Breast-feeding |
| Pregnancy | |
| Children receiving corticosteroids | |
| **Hepatitis A** | |
| *Contraindication* | *Not a Contraindication* |
| Sensitivity to alum (component) or phenoxyethanol (in Havrix) | Pregnancy |
| **Pneumococcal (PCV7)** | |
| *Contraindications* | *Not Contraindications* |
| Pregnancy | Concurrent administration with DTaP, MMR, Var, IPV, Hib, HbOC, |
| Children >24 months unless in high-risk category (see p. 534) | hepatitis B, hepatitis A (unknown) |
| Previous sensitivity | |

From American Academy of Pediatrics, Committee on Infectious Diseases, Pickering LK, editor: *2000 Red book: report of the Committee on Infectious Diseases*, ed, 25, Elk Grove Village, IL, 2000, The Academy.

such as the common cold is *not* a contraindication. Live virus vaccines are generally not administered to anyone with an altered immune system, because multiplication of the virus may be enhanced, causing a severe vaccine-induced illness.

Another contraindication to live virus vaccines (MMR and varicella) is the presence of recently acquired passive immunity through blood transfusions, immunoglobulin, or maternal antibodies. Administration of MMR and varicella should be postponed for a *minimum* of 3 months after passive immunization with immunoglobulins and blood transfusions (except washed red blood cells, which do not interfere with the immune response). Suggested intervals between administration of immune globulin preparations and MMR and varicella depend on the type of immune product and dosage. If the vaccine and immunoglobulin are given simultaneously because of imminent exposure to disease, the two preparations are injected at sites far from each other. Vaccination should be repeated after the suggested intervals unless there is serologic evidence of antibody production.

Pregnancy is a contraindication to mumps, measles, and rubella vaccines, although the risk of fetal damage is primarily theoretic. Breast-feeding is not a contraindication for any vaccine.

A final contraindication is a known allergic response to a previously administered vaccine or a substance in the vaccine. (See DTP in Table 12-13.) Measles, mumps, and rubella virus vaccines contain minute amounts of neomycin; measles and mumps vaccines, which are grown on chick embryo tissue cultures, are not believed to contain significant amounts of egg cross-reacting proteins. Therefore only a history of anaphylactoid reaction to neomycin or to the vaccine itself is considered a contraindication to their use. To identify the rare child who may not be able to receive the vac-

cines, a careful allergy history is taken. (See Guidelines box, "Taking a Drug Allergy History," Chapter 6.) If the child has a history of anaphylaxis, it is reported to the practitioner before administering the vaccine. Contact dermatitis to neomycin is not considered to be a contraindication to immunization. Evidence indicates that children who are egg-sensitive are not at increased risk for untoward reactions to MMR vaccine. Furthermore, skin testing of egg-allergic children with vaccine has failed to predict immediate hypersensitivity reactions (American Academy of Pediatrics, 2000a).

### Administration

The principal precautions in administering immunizations include proper storage of the vaccine to protect its potency and institution of recommended procedures for injection. The nurse must be familiar with the manufacturer's directions for storage and reconstitution of the vaccine. For example, if the vaccine is to be refrigerated, it should be stored on a center shelf, not on the door, where frequent temperature increases from opening the refrigerator can alter the vaccine's potency. For protection against light the vial can be wrapped in aluminum foil. Periodic checks are established to ensure that no vaccine is used after its expiration date.

The DTP (or DTaP) vaccines contain the adjuvant alum to retain the antigen at the injection site and prolong the stimulatory effect. Because subcutaneous or intracutaneous injection of the adjuvant can cause local irritation, inflammation, or abscess formation, excellent intramuscular injection technique must be used. (See Evidence-Based Practice box.) (See Atraumatic Care box on p. 534.)

The total series requires several injections, and every attempt is made to rotate the sites and administer the injections as painlessly as possible. (See discussion on intramus-

## EVIDENCE-BASED PRACTICE

### Appropriate Site for Intramuscular Injection* in Infants and Toddlers

Infants and toddlers receive more immunizations than any other age child. Although a number of vaccines are available in conjugate form, infants may receive as many as four to five injections per clinic visit. It is well known that this age group also has a smaller muscle mass for injectable medications than any other age group, thus placing them at risk for more pain and potential side effects from injected medications. Many immunizations require intramuscular (IM) administration for maximal effectiveness (Table 12-14). It is imperative that nurses administering vaccines and other medications to infants and toddlers use an appropriate site, needle size, and amount of medication for the child's size, in addition to the five rights of drug administration, to minimize adverse effects. Common complications of IM injection include abscess, gangrene, fibrosis and muscle contractures, nerve injury, and local and systemic reactions (erythema, pain, limited mobility) (Beecroft and Kongelbeck, 1994). A number of local systemic reactions have been recently witnessed in clinical settings by the author wherein either an inappropriate site, needle size, or amount of medication administered caused a localized reaction of erythema, pain, and limited limb mobility. Most of these local reactions may be avoided by injecting the drug deep into the muscle at an appropriate site for the child's age and size.

Length of needle and size of muscle mass is an important consideration when administering IM injections such as immunizations and antibiotics. There is a paucity of research regarding IM medication administration in children, particularly infants and toddlers. Studies in adults indicate that injection pain can be minimized by deep IM administration because muscle tissue has fewer nerve endings and medications are absorbed faster than those administered subcutaneously (Zuckerman, 2000). Immunizations such as DTaP and hepatitis A and B contain an aluminum adjuvant which, if injected into subcutaneous tissue, increases the incidence of local reactions. Inadvertent injection into subcutaneous tissue may be caused by use of a needle too short to reach IM tissue (Zuckerman, 2000). One study found that 4-month-old infants experienced fewer local side effects (redness, tenderness, and swelling) when immunizations were administered into the anterior aspect of the thigh with a 25-mm (1-inch) needle as opposed to the shorter 16-mm (5/8-inch) needle (Diggle and Deeks, 2000). In another study, needle length was compared to injection method, that is, a longer needle (25 mm or 1 inch) was preferred for injection when bunching the skin and injecting, whereas a shorter needle (5/8 inch or 16 mm) was perceived as causing fewer localized reactions when the injection was administered with the skin being held taut (Grosswasser and others, 1997). However, conclusions of the study fail to address whether needle lengths were applicable to both the deltoid and vastus lateralis. Beecroft and Redick (1990) cited numerous differences of opinion regarding IM injection technique among pediatric nurses, highlighting how little agreement there is among nursing texts evaluated in regards to injection site and technique. This concern was further expressed in a nursing journal column when a nurse noted that there were discrepancies in IM administration technique when injections were given to her child (Winslow and Jacobson, 1997). In a study of DTP immunizations administered to infants 7 months and younger, only 84.6% of injections were administered at the correct site (anterior thigh); an alarming number were given in the dorsogluteal and deltoid muscles (Daly, Johnston, and Chung, 1992). Beecroft and Kongelbeck (1994) evaluated pediatric IM injections and concluded that the ventrogluteal site is the site of choice in children of all ages and that there were no reports in the literature of complications at this site. The ventrogluteal site is relatively free of important nerves and vascular

structures, the site is easily identified by landmarks, and the subcutaneous tissue is thinner in that area (Beecroft and Kongelbeck, 1994). To date, no reports can be found in the literature to refute the claims made by these researchers.

The American Academy of Pediatrics (2000a) recommends that vaccines containing adjuvants such as aluminum (DTaP, hepatitis A and B, DT, Td) be given deep into the muscle to prevent local reactions. In addition, a 5/8-inch needle may be adequate for injections in small infants, and a 7/8-to 1-inch needle be used in infants 4 months and older. The deltoid muscle may be used for immunizations in toddlers, older children, and adolescents. When multiple vaccines are given, two may be given in the thigh (anterior and lateral) because of its larger size. The dorsogluteal muscle should be avoided in infants and toddlers, and perhaps even in smaller preschoolers with smaller muscle mass, because of the possibility of damaging the sciatic nerve. No research or supportive data was found regarding the amount of medication to be given at the different sites in infants and toddlers, although a table from one text has suggested amounts; the basis for these recommendations is unknown. In general, 1 ml of medication is recommended for infants less than 12 months; however, no data can be found to refute or support such a recommendation. Furthermore, small and preterm infants may only tolerate up to ½ ml in each muscle to prevent local complications. In summary, it is evident that there remains some discrepancy in actual clinical practice regarding IM injection sites, amount of drug injected, and needle size in infants and toddlers. Further research is needed to address the following issues:

☐ What is the appropriate muscle in which an IM injection can be administered with fewest adverse effects in infants and toddlers?

☐ What is the appropriate needle size based on the infant or toddler's age and weight?

☐ What is the largest safe amount of medication that can be given to infants and toddlers based on weight and muscle size?

A number of simple nursing measures can be carried out to minimize the pain of multiple IM injections in infants and toddlers. One important factor is to change the needle after a medication is drawn from a rubber top vial before injecting into the muscle to prevent injection of latex particles into the muscle. The use of EMLA or a topical vapocoolant spray may also decrease pain at the injection site.

Until further research is available to refute or support these recommendations, the anterior aspect of the thigh (ventrogluteal) is considered the best site for IM injection in infants and toddlers. In newborns the vastus lateralis is also an acceptable site. The dorsogluteal and deltoid sites should be avoided in infants because muscle mass is small and sciatic nerve damage may occur with dorsogluteal injection. Needle length should be chosen carefully according to the infant's muscle mass, and, until further research is available to refute or support these recommendations the following may be considered acceptable:

☐ Preterm or small infants and newborns—5/8 to 7/8 inches (16 to 22 mm).

☐ Infants 4 months old and older—consider at least 1-inch (25-mm) needle, unless muscle mass is decreased as a result of illness or weight.

☐ Toddlers—1- to 1½ inch (25-mm) needle, depending on muscle size.

Further research is needed to provide optimal care to infants and children receiving IM injections such as immunizations and antibiotics.

---

*See also Chapter 27, Intramuscular Administration.

**TABLE 12-14**  Product brand names, manufacturers/distributors, and route of administration for principal childhood vaccine types

| Product | Brand Name/Manufacturer/Distributor | Type |
|---|---|---|
| **DTaP**—Diphtheria and tetanus toxoids and acellular pertussis vaccine | Acel-Imune (WLV)<br>Certiva (NAV, distributed by ALI)<br>Infanrix (SBB, distributed by SB)<br>Tripedia (CON, distributed by PMC) | IM |
| **DTaP-Hib**—Diphtheria and tetanus toxoids and acellular pertussis and *Haemophilus influenzae* type b vaccine | TriHIBit* (ActHIB Hib reconstituted with Tripedia DTaP; distributed by PMC) | IM |
| **DTwP**—Diphtheria and tetanus toxoids and whole-cell pertussis vaccine | Tri-Immunol† (WLV) | IM |
| **DTwP-Hib**—Diphtheria and tetanus toxoids and whole-cell pertussis and *Haemophilus influenzae* type b vaccine | ActHIB Hib reconstituted with DTwP (CON; distributed by PMC)<br>Tetramune (WLV) | IM |
| **HepA**—Hepatitis A vaccine | Havrix (SBB, distributed by SB) Vaqta (MRK) | IM |
| **HepB**—Hepatitis B vaccine | Engerix-B (SBB, distributed by SB)<br>Recombivax HB (MRK) | IM |
| **Hib**—*Haemophilus influenzae* type b conjugate vaccine<br>　**HbOC**—Oligosaccharides conjugated to diphtheria $CRM_{197}$ toxin protein | HibTITER (WLV) | IM |
| 　**PRP-OMP**—Polyribosylribitol phosphate polysaccharide conjugated to a meningococcal outer membrane protein | PedvaxHIB (MRK) | |
| 　**PRP-T**—Polyribosylribitol phosphate polysaccharide conjugated to tetanus toxoid | ActHIB (PMSV, distributed by CON, PMC)<br>OmniHIB (PMSV, distributed by SB) | |
| 　**PRP-D**—Polyribosylribitol phosphate polysaccharide conjugated to diphtheria toxoid | ProHIBiT (CON, distributed by PMC) | |
| **Hib-HepB**—*Haemophilus influenzae* type b and hepatitis B vaccine | Comvax (Hib component = PRP-OMP) (MRK) | IM |
| **IPV**—Trivalent inactivated polio vaccine (killed Salk type) | IPOL (PMSV, distributed by CON, PMC) | IM or SQ |
| **MMR**—Measles, mumps, rubella vaccine | M-M-R II (MRK) | SQ |
| **Pneumococcal (PCV7)** | Prevnar (WLV) | IM |
| **Var**—Varicella (chickenpox) vaccine | Varivax (MRK) | SQ |

Modified from American Academy of Pediatrics: Combination vaccines for childhood immunization: recommendations of the Advisory Committee on Immunization Practices (ACIP), the American Academy of Pediatrics (AAP), and the American Academy of Family Physicians (AAFP), *Pediatrics* 103(5):1072, 1999.
*ALI,* Ross Products Division, Abbott Laboratories, Inc; *CON,* Connaught Laboratories, Inc; *MRK,* Merck & Co, Inc; *NAV,* North American Vaccine, Inc; *PMC,* Pasteur Mérieux Connaught; *PMSV,* Pasteur Mérieux Sérums & Vaccins, SA; *SBB,* SmithKline Beecham Biologicals; *SB,* SmithKline Beecham Pharmaceuticals; *WLV,* Wyeth-Lederle vaccines; *IM,* intramuscular injection; *SQ,* subcutaneous injection.
*As of April 10, 1999, TriHIBit was licensed only for the fourth dose, recommended at age 15 to 18 months in the vaccination series.
†Manufacture discontinued.

cular injections in Chapter 27.) When two or more injections are given at separate sites, the order of injections is arbitrary. Some practitioners suggest injecting the less painful one first. Some believe this is DTP (or DTaP), whereas others suggest the MMR or Hib vaccine. Still others advocate injecting at two sites simultaneously (requires two operators).

A recent study found that children between the ages of 4 and 6 years rated sequential injections for immunizations vs. simultaneous injections as being equally stressful (Horn and McCarthy, 1999). Parents in the study preferred simultaneous immunization injections.

Because allergic reactions can occur after injection of vaccines, appropriate precautions are taken. (See Nursing Alert about anaphylactic reation in Chapter 36.)

One of the most important features of injecting vaccines is adequate penetration of the muscle for deposition of the drug intramuscularly and not subcutaneously. Two injection techniques have been studied to determine the best needle length for the deltoid and vastus lateralis sites. If the muscle is grasped or bunched, a needle length of 25 mm (1 inch) is recommended. If the muscle is stretched or flattened, a needle length of 16 mm (⅝ inch) is adequate (Groswasser and others, 1997). Unfortunately, the conclusions of the study fail to address if these lengths apply to both muscles. From the data, it appears more likely that the recommendations apply to the thigh muscle only. Research

regarding the safest site—the ventrogluteal muscle—is not available.

Practitioners are required to fully inform families of the risks and benefits of the vaccines. The U.S. Public Health Service has developed a series of vaccine information pamphlets. Health professionals need to provide parents with sufficient time to read the information, discuss the vaccines to determine caregivers' understanding, address parents' concerns, and correct any misinformation. Because nurses often administer vaccines, they may have the responsibility for adequately informing parents of the nature, prevalence, and risks of the disease; the type of immunization product to be used; the expected benefits and the risk of side effects of the vaccine; and the need for accurate immunization records. Referring to immunizations as "baby shots" and limiting the discussion to vague statements about the vaccines are unacceptable practices.

Another important nursing responsibility is accurate documentation. Each child should have an immunization record for parents to keep, especially for families who move frequently. Although immunization rates have increased significantly, health care professionals should use every opportunity to encourage complete immunization of all children. (See Community Focus boxes.)

The following information is documented on the medical record: day, month, and year of administration; manu-

*Improving Immunization Rates Among Children and Adolescents*

Strategies that may increase compliance include giving parents vaccine information at the time of the newborn's discharge, mailing reminder cards, making immunization services readily available, removing barriers to vaccination (such as long waiting times and appointment-only systems), and taking every opportunity to immunize children when they enter a health care facility (such as emergency departments, clinics, private offices, and hospitals).

Despite improving vaccination rates among infants and young children, *adolescents* are often incompletely immunized. An immunization update is an important part of adolescent preventive care, especially at 11 to 12 years of age. With the exception of pregnant teenagers, all adolescents should receive a second dose of the *measles, mumps,* and *rubella (MMR) vaccine* unless they have documentation of two MMR vaccinations following the first 12 months of life. All adolescents who have not previously completed the three-dose series of the *hepatitis B (HBV) vaccine* should initiate or complete the series at age 11 to 12 years.

Adolescents ages 11 to 12 years and no later than 16 years should receive a booster dose of *diphtheria-tetanus (Td) vaccine* if they have received the primary series of vaccinations and if no dose has been received during the previous 5 years. Unvaccinated adolescents who lack a reliable history of chickenpox should receive the *varicella virus vaccine* at age 11 to 12 years.

*Hepatitis A vaccine* should be given to adolescents who are traveling or living in countries where the hepatitis A virus is endemic or in communities where there are high rates of hepatitis A, chronic liver disease, intravenous drug users, or males who have sex with other males. Adolescents who have chronic disorders or underlying medical conditions that place them at high risk for complications associated with the disease, such as influenza, should receive the appropriate vaccines (see p. 529).

**Meningococcal** vaccine should be considered for adolescents before or when entering college, especially if planning to live in a college dormitory.

*Keeping Current on Vaccine Recommendations*

It is much easier to keep current if you know where to look for the official recommendations of the **American Academy of Pediatrics (AAP)** and the **Centers for Disease Control and Prevention's (CDC) Advisory Committee on Immunization Practices (ACIP)**. The primary sources are publications and the Internet. You can also contact each organization to request information:

> **American Academy of Pediatrics**
> 141 Northwest Point Blvd.
> PO Box 747
> Elk Grove Village, IL 60009
> (888) 227-1770
> Fax: (847) 228-1281
> Web site: *www.aap.org*

> **Centers for Disease Control and Prevention**
> 1600 Clifton Rd. NE
> Atlanta, GA 30333
> (404) 639-3311
> Information Hotline: (800) 232-2522 or (800) 232-7468
> International Travel Hotline: (877) 394-8747
> Spanish Hotline: (800) 232-0233
> Web site: *www.cdc.gov;* National Immunization Program at CDC: *www.cdc.gov/nip*

The American Academy of Pediatrics' **Report of the Committee on Infectious Diseases,** known as the **Red Book,** is an authoritative source of information on vaccines and other important pediatric infectious diseases. However, it lacks an in-depth review and reference list of controversial issues. The recommendations in the *Red Book* first appear in the journal **Pediatrics** and/or the **AAP News.** Typically, the most recent immunization schedule appears in the January issue of the journal.

A publication of the CDC, **Morbidity and Mortality Weekly Report (MMWR),** contains comprehensive reviews of the literature, as well as important background data regarding vaccine efficacy and side effects. To receive an electronic copy, send an e-mail message to *listserv@listserv.cdc.gov.* The body content should read: *SUBscribe mmwr-toc.* Electronic copy also is available from the CDC's web site at *www.cdc.gov/* or from the CDC's file transfer protocol server at *ftp.cdc.gov.* To subscribe for a paper copy, contact:

**Superintendent of Documents**
U.S. Government Printing Office
Washington, DC 20402
(202) 512-1800

**Immunization Gateway: Your Vaccine Fact-Finder** at *www.immunofacts.com* provides direct links to all of the best vaccine resources on the Internet.

*Vaccine information statements (VISs)* are available by calling your state or local health department. They can also be downloaded from the **Immunization Action Coalition's** web site at *www.immunize.org/vis/* or CDC's web site at *www.cdc.gov/nip/publications/vis/.* Some translations are available.

*Note:* The Wong Update series on the Internet at *www.mosby.com/WOW* routinely includes information on changes in immunization information.

---

facturer, expiration date, and lot number of vaccine; and the name, address, and title of the person administering the vaccine. Additional data to record are the site and route of administration and evidence that the parent or legal guardian gave informed consent before the immunization was administered. Any adverse reactions after the administration of any vaccine are reported to the **Vaccine Adverse Event Reporting System (VAERS).***

In response to the concerns of manufacturers, practitioners, and parents of children with serious vaccine-associated injuries, the *National Childhood Vaccine Injury Act (NCVIA)* of 1986 and the *Vaccine Compensation Amendments* of 1987 were passed. Basically, these laws are designed to provide fair compensation for children who are inadvertently injured and provide greater protection from liability for vaccine manufacturers and providers.

## Injury Prevention

Injuries are a major cause of death during infancy, especially for children 6 to 12 months old. Constant vigilance, awareness, and supervision are essential as the child gains

increased locomotor and manipulative skills that are coupled with an insatiable curiosity about the environment. Table 12-15 lists the major developmental achievements of each period during infancy and the appropriate injury prevention plan.

### Aspiration of Foreign Objects

Asphyxiation by foreign material in the respiratory tract, combined with mechanical suffocation, is one of the leading

---

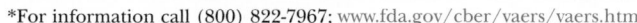

*For information call (800) 822-7967; www.fda.gov/cber/vaers/vaers.htm

**TABLE 12-15** Injury prevention during infancy

| Major Developmental Accomplishments | | Injury Prevention |
|---|---|---|

**Age: Birth-4 Months**

Involuntary reflexes, such as the crawling reflex, may propel infant forward or backward, and the startle reflex may cause the body to jerk

May roll over

Increasing eye-hand coordination and voluntary grasp reflex

**Aspiration**

Not as great a danger to this age-group, but should begin practicing safeguarding early (see under Age: 4-7 Months)

Never shake baby powder directly on infant; place powder in hand and then on infant's skin; store container closed and out of infant's reach

Hold infant for feeding; do not prop bottle

Know emergency procedures for choking*

Use pacifier with one-piece construction and loop handle

**Suffocation/drowning**

Keep all plastic bags stored out of infant's reach; discard large plastic garment bags after tying in a knot

Do not cover mattress with plastic

Use a firm mattress and loose blankets; no pillows

Make sure crib design follows federal regulations and mattress fits snugly—crib slats <2⅜ inches (6 cm) apart

Position crib away from other furniture and away from heaters

Do not tie pacifier on a string around infant's neck

Remove bibs after meal

Never leave infant alone in bath of any kind

Do not leave infant under 12 months alone on adult or youth mattress or "beanbag" type pillows

**Falls**

Always raise crib rails

Never leave infant on a raised, unguarded surface

When in doubt as to where to place child, use floor

Restrain child in infant seat and never leave child unattended while the seat is resting on a raised surface

Avoid using a high chair until child can sit well with support

**Poisoning**

Not as great a danger to this age-group, but should begin practicing safeguards early (see under Age: 4-7 Months)

**Burns**

Install smoke detectors in home

Use caution when warming formula in microwave oven; shake bottle and check temperature of liquid before feeding

Check bathwater temperature before placing child in same

Do not pour hot liquids when infant is close by, such as sitting on lap

Beware of cigarette ashes that may fall on infant

Do not leave infant in sun for more than a few minutes; keep exposed areas covered or use an appropriate sun screen

Wash flame-retardant clothes according to label directions

Use cool-mist vaporizers

Check surface heat of car restraint before placing child in seat

**Motor vehicles**

Transport infant in federally approved, rear-facing car seat,* preferably in back seat

Do not place infant on seat (of care) or in lap

Do not place child in a carriage or stroller behind a parked car

Do not place infant or child in front passenger seat with an air bag

Do not leave child unattended in car

**Bodily damage**

Avoid sharp, jagged objects such as scissors

Keep diaper pins closed and away from infant

**Age: 4-7 Months**

Rolls over

Sits momentarily

Grasps and manipulates small objects

Resecures a dropped object

Has well-developed eye-hand coordination

Can focus on and locate very small objects

**Aspiration**

Keep buttons, beads, syringe caps, bottle caps, and other small objects out of infant's reach

Keep floor free of any small objects

Do not feed infant hard candy, nuts, food with pits or seeds, or whole or circular pieces of hot dog

Exercise caution when giving teething biscuits, because large chunks may be broken off and aspirated

Do not feed infant while child is lying down

Inspect toys for removable parts

Keep baby powder, if used, out of reach—use sparingly

Discard used button-sized batteries; store new batteries in safe area

Keep telephone number of local poison control center (usually listed in front of telephone directory) by main telephone

Keep address of residence written next to primary telephone for sitters, friends, or relatives—in emergency address may not be easily remembered

*Community and home care instructions for care of the choking infant and for use of child safety seats are available in Wong DL, Hess CS: *Wong and Whaley's clinical manual of pediatric nursing,* ed 5, St Louis, 2000, Mosby.

causes of fatal injury in children younger than 1 year. In one survey, choking was the fourth leading cause of death in infants (Brenner and others, 1999). The size, shape, and consistency of foods or objects are important determinants of fatal obstruction. For example, small spheric or cylindric and pliable objects (less than 3.2 cm, or 1¼ inches) are more likely to completely obstruct the airway. Unfortunately, common household items can be deadly to infants.

As soon as infants have the ability to find their mouth, they are vulnerable to aspiration of small objects, such as those left within reach or removable parts of objects that may on initial inspection appear safe. All toys must be carefully inspected for potential danger. Many toys that make noise or rattle, for example, have small beads inside. A broken or cracked toy can be dangerous because the beads can easily be aspirated while the infant has the toy in the mouth. Stuffed animals are another potentially dangerous toy if any of the parts, such as the eyes or nose, are removable buttons or plastic pieces. An active infant can grab a low-hanging mobile and quickly chew off a small piece. As soon as the infant crawls or plays on the

**TABLE 12-15**    Injury prevention during infancy—cont'd

| Major Developmental Accomplishments | Injury Prevention | |
| --- | --- | --- |

**Age: 4-7 Months—cont'd**

Mouthing is very prominent

Can push up on hands and knees

Crawls backward

**Suffocation**

Keep all latex balloons out of reach

Remove all crib toys that are strung across crib or playpen when child begins to push up on hands or knees or is 5 months old

Avoid storing large quantities of cleaning fluid, paints, pesticides, and other toxic substances

Discard used containers of poisonous substances

Do not store toxic substances in food containers

**Burns**

Keep faucets out of reach

Place hot objects (cigarettes, candles, incense) on high surface and away from curtains or blinds

Limit exposure to sun; apply sunscreen

**Motor vehicles**

See under Age: Birth-4 Months

**Falls**

Restrain in a high chair

Keep crib rails raised to full height

**Poisoning**

Make sure that paint for furniture or toys does not contain lead

Place toxic substances on a high shelf or in locked cabinet

Hang plants or place on high surface rather than on floor

**Bodily damage**

Give toys that are smooth and rounded, preferably made of wood or plastic

Avoid long, pointed objects as toys

Avoid toys that are excessively loud

Keep sharp objects out of infant's reach

**Age: 8-12 Months**

Crawls/creeps

Stands, holding onto furniture

Stands alone

Cruises around furniture

Walks

Climbs

Pulls on objects

Throws objects

Is able to pick up small objects; has pincer grasp

Explores by putting objects in mouth

Dislikes being restrained

Explores away from parent

Increasing understanding of simple commands and phrases

**Aspiration**

Keep small objects off floor, furniture, and out of reach of children

Take care in feeding solid table food to ensure that very small pieces are given

Do not use beanbag toys or allow child to play with dried beans

See under Age: 4-7 Months

**Suffocation/drowning**

Keep doors of ovens, dishwashers, refrigerators, coolers, and front-loading clothes washers and dryers closed at all times

If storing an unused appliance, such as a refrigerator, remove the door

Supervise contact with inflated balloons; immediately discard popped balloons, and keep uninflated balloons out of reach

Fence swimming pools

Always supervise when near any source of water, such as cleaning buckets, drainage areas, toilets

Keep bathroom doors closed

Eliminate unnecessary pools of water

Keep one hand on child at all times when in tub

Do not leave a full tub of water within child's access

**Falls**

Fence stairways at top and bottom if child has access to either end†

Dress infant in safe shoes and clothing (soles that do not "catch" on floor, tied shoelaces, pant legs that do not touch floor)

Avoid walkers, especially near stairs

Ensure that furniture is sturdy enough for child to pull self to standing position and cruise

Pad objects such as table corners at the child's head level

Also suggest temporarily pad brick fireplace hearths because many children fall and hit head on these

Keep sharp metal fireplace implements out of child's reach

**Poisoning**

Administer medications as a drug, not as a candy

Do not administer medications unless so prescribed by a practitioner

Replace medications and poisons immediately after use; replace caps properly if a child-protector cap is used

Have syrup of ipecac in home; use only if advised

**Burns**

Place guards in front of or around any heating appliance, fireplace, or furnace

Keep electrical wires hidden or out of reach

Place large, unremovable plastic guards over electrical outlets; place furniture in front of outlets

Keep hanging tablecloths out of reach (child may pull down hot liquids or heavy or sharp objects)

†Information on many items such as cribs or walkers available from US Consumer Product Safety Commission; (800) 638-CPSC; *www.cpsc.gov/*.

floor, the floor must be kept free of any small articles that can be picked up and swallowed, such as coins and buttons.

When infant *clothes* are purchased, the type of closure is important. A front button can easily be pulled off and swallowed.

*Food items* are the second most common cause of aspiration, and the most common offenders are hot dogs, candy, nuts, and grapes. When new foods are given to the child, nuts, hard candies, marshmallows, large amounts of peanut butter, or fruits with pits or seeds are avoided. When traveling (especially in airplanes) or entertaining, snack foods such as peanuts and popcorn are kept away from young children. If given to young children, hot dogs must be cut into small, irregular pieces rather than served whole or sliced into sections because their size (diameter), round shape, and consistency allow for complete occlusion of the airway. Perhaps the most dangerous foods are dried beans, which, if aspirated, enlarge when they come in contact with the wet mucosa and block the airway.

*Pacifiers* can also be dangerous because the entire object may be aspirated if it is small, or the nipple and shield may become detached from the handle and become lodged in the pharynx. Improvised pacifiers, such as those made from a padded nipple, also present dangers. The nipple may separate from the plastic collar and be aspirated. To prevent the hazards of improvised pacifiers, only safe commercial types should be used, if at all. Candy pacifiers pose dangers because the candy portion can dislodge from the circular base and be aspirated. To be safe, pacifiers should have the following:

- Sturdy, one-piece construction with material that is nontoxic, flexible, and firm but not brittle
- An easily grasped handle
- A mouthguard that cannot be separated from the nipple, has two ventilating holes, and is too large to be aspirated
- No detachable ribbon or string
- A label warning against tying the pacifier around the infant's neck

Using a syringe to accurately measure and dispense oral liquid medications to young children has become common practice. However, the *syringe cap* is a potential aspiration hazard. As a precaution, keep parts of medication devices out of the reach of children and be certain the cap is removed before dispensing medication. Other items that may easily be aspirated include soda and fruit juice bottle tops or caps, aluminum soda can pop-top rings that tear off easily, and small key rings (less than 1½ inch in diameter).

Even safety devices can be dangerous. To prevent tampering, items (such as baby food jars) may be covered with a plastic oversleeve. The *tear-down strip* can be aspirated and is very difficult to locate because it is clear.

Another hazardous substance if aspirated is *baby powder,* which is usually a mixture of talc (hydrous magnesium silicate) and other silicates. Although the use of talc has been discouraged, it is a common baby care product that can cause severe and often fatal aspiration pneumonia. Improperly using powder by sprinkling it directly on the skin creates a cloud of talc dust that is easily inhaled. Parents are advised of the danger of baby powder and are discouraged from using it. If they prefer to use a powder, a cornstarch preparation can be substituted. (See Diaper Dermatitis, Chapter 13.) Whenever a powder is used, it is placed in the hand and then applied to the skin, never shaken directly from the container to the skin.

## Suffocation

Mechanical suffocation includes suffocation by covering of the airway (i.e., mouth and nose), by pressure on the throat and chest, and by exclusion of air, such as by refrigerator entrapment. Suffocation was second only to homicide as the leading cause of death in infants, according to a recent survey (Brenner and others, 1999). Nonfood items cause the majority of deaths in young children. *Latex balloons,* whether partially inflated, uninflated, or popped, are the leading cause of pediatric choking deaths from children's products. They should be kept away from infants and young children. Even the practice of inflating latex gloves to amuse children in health care settings may pose a danger, especially if the child is latex-sensitive. Future deaths may be avoided by changing balloon design and materials and substituting mylar or paper balloons.

**NURSING ALERT**  Encourage adults to: Blow up balloons for children, supervise children's balloon play, pick up and dispose of broken balloon pieces, warn older children of dangers of chewing or sucking on balloons, and substitute Mylar or paper balloons for latex balloons.

The *bed* or *crib* poses a number of hazards. An infant who is placed in a bed under tucked-in blankets and sheets can be caught under them and unable to wriggle free. (See Sudden Infant Death, Chapter 13.) Baby pillows filled with plastic foam beads that make them resemble small bean bags are dangerous; very young infants are suffocated when the pillow contours to the face and blocks the airway. There are potential dangers in adults sleeping with a small infant because of the possibility of their rolling over and smothering the child. The incidence of infant suffocation by an adult when bed sharing increased during the period from 1980 to 1997 (Drago and Dannenberg, 1999). The most common causes of infant suffocation were wedging between a bed or mattress and a wall and oronasal obstruction by a plastic bag.

Infant strangulation may occur if the infant's head becomes caught between the crib slats and mattress or objects close to the crib. Suffocation deaths are not confined to cribs; ill-fitting mattresses in adult or youth beds, bunk beds, and waterbeds have also been reported. According to U.S. federal regulation the distance between crib slats should not be more than 2⅜ inches (approximately 6 cm), roughly the width of three adult fingers. Mattresses and bumper pads should fit snugly against the slats. A general rule is that the mattress is too small if two adult fingers can be placed between the mattress and crib or bed side. A temporary solution is to place large, rolled towels in the space to create a snug fit.

Corner post extensions on cribs are another source of strangulation. Children have died when their clothing caught on raised corner posts as they climbed out of the crib. Voluntary manufacturing standards state that corner post extensions not exceed 1/16 inch. However, the safety of *any* extension is questionable. Decorative extensions need to be removed from cribs. Ideally, information regarding correct crib design should be given prenatally, before parents have purchased or borrowed a crib.*

Mesh-sided playpens and cribs can result in death if the sides are left in the lowered position. Infants have suffocated when they fell off the edge of the mattress and the head or chest was compressed between the floorboard and mesh side. Parents should be advised of this danger and encouraged to *always* keep the sides locked securely in the up position whenever the child is in the playpen or crib.

The crib should be positioned away from large furniture, because children who crawl out of the crib may become caught between the two objects. Cribs should also be located away from windows, where drape or blind cords can become wrapped around the infant's neck.

---

*A number of parent education pamphlets—*Crib Safety Tips* and *Is Your Used Crib Safe?*—are available from the **US Consumer Product Safety Commission,** Publication Request, Washington, DC 20207, (800) 638-2772; www.cpsc.gov. Additional free information is available from the **Danny Foundation,** 3158 Danville Blvd, PO Box 680, Alamo, CA 94507, (800) 83-DANNY; www.dannyfoundation.org

Another cause of suffocation is *plastic bags.* Large plastic bags used over garments are very lightweight and can easily and quickly be wrapped around the head of an active infant or pressed against the face. For this reason, pillows and mattresses should not be covered with plastic. Older infants may play with a plastic bag and accidentally pull it over their heads. Because plastic is nonporous, suffocation occurs in a matter of minutes.

*Cords* located near the infant or tied around the infant's neck can potentially cause strangulation. Bibs are removed after meals, and objects such as pacifiers are never hung on a string around the infant's neck. This is a common practice in some cultures that can be remedied by tying a *short* string to a pacifier and pinning the string to the child's shirt.

Toys that have strings attached, such as a telephone, or toys that are tied to cribs or playpens can be hazards because the string can become wrapped around the child's neck or the child can become entrapped in the toy. As a precaution, all cords should be less than 30 cm (12 inches) long. Crib toys should be hung high enough that the infant cannot become entangled in them and should no longer be used once the child is able to reach them.

If applied too loosely or left unfastened, restraining straps can be a hazard. For example, a child may slide off a high chair beneath the tray and become strangled on the loose strap. All straps should be fastened securely.

## Motor Vehicle Injuries

Automobile injuries are the leading cause of accidental death in children older than 1 year of age (MMWR, 2001). However, a significant number of infants are injured or die from improper restraint within the vehicle, most often from riding on the lap of another occupant. All infants must be secured in a U.S. federally approved restraint rather than held or placed on the seat of the car. There is no safe alternative. Recent reports indicate that child restraint use decreases with increasing age of children and increasing number of occupants. Lack of proper child restraint continues to be a major factor in fatal accidents involving children (Murphy, 1999). A Task Force on Community Preventive Services from the Department of Health and Human Services recommends community-wide information and enforcement campaigns for use of child safety seats, incentive and education programs for use of child safety seats, and a lower legal blood alcohol concentration for young drivers (MMWR, 2001).

Infant restraints are designed either as an infant-only model (Fig. 12-15) or as a convertible infant-toddler model. Either restraint is a semireclined seat that faces the *rear* of the car. A rear-facing car seat provides the best protection for the disproportionately heavy head and weak neck of a young child. This position minimizes the stress on the neck by spreading the forces of a frontal crash over the entire back, neck, and head; the spine is supported by the back of the car seat. If the seat were faced forward, the head would whip forward because of the force of the crash, creating enormous stress on the neck.

The restraint is anchored to the vehicle with the vehicle's seat belt, and the restraint has a harness system for securing the infant. Some harness systems require a clip to keep the

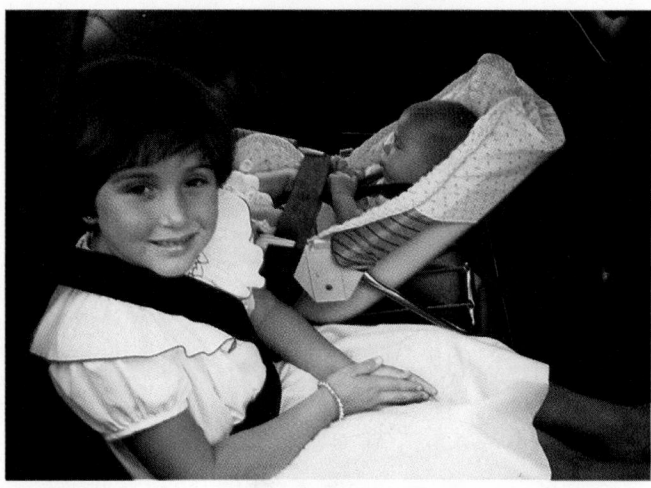

**Fig. 12-15**  Federally approved infant car restraint. Note placement in middle of backseat and use of car lap/shoulder belt for older child.

**NURSING ALERT**  Infants should face the rear from birth to 20 pounds and as close to 1 year of age as possible.

shoulder straps correctly positioned. Although many infant restraints can be recliners, they are used in the car only in the position specified by the manufacturer.

The backseat is the safest area of the car. Severe injuries and deaths in children have occurred from air bags deploying on impact in the front passenger seat (Grisoni and others, 2000; McKay and Jolly, 1999). If the backseat is not an option, an infant restraint may be positioned in the front seat provided that the seat belt can be locked into position and there is *no* passenger-side air bag. If there is a passenger-side air bag and the child has special health care needs or constant observation is recommended by the practitioner and no other adult is available to ride in the back seat with the child, an on/off switch may be installed to prevent the air bag from deploying and injuring the child riding in the front seat. Another condition that may arise is the use of vehicles without a back seat; in such cases it is best that the front passenger seat be placed as far back as possible and appropriate child safety restraint employed.

**NURSING ALERT**  Rear-facing infant safety seats must not be placed in the front seats of cars equipped with an air bag on the passenger side. If an infant safety seat is placed in the passenger seat with an air bag, the child could be seriously injured if the air bag is released because rear-facing infant seats extend closer to the dashboard (Fig. 12-16).*

---

*An air bag safety fact sheet is available from the **American Academy of Pediatrics,** 141 Northwest Point Blvd, Elk Grove Village, IL 60009, (888) 227-1770, fax: (847) 228-1281; www.aap.org; for carseats, www.aap.org and the **Insurance Institute for Highway Safety,** 1005 N Glebe Rd, Arlington, VA 22201, (703) 247-1500, fax: (703) 247-1678; www.highwaysafety.org

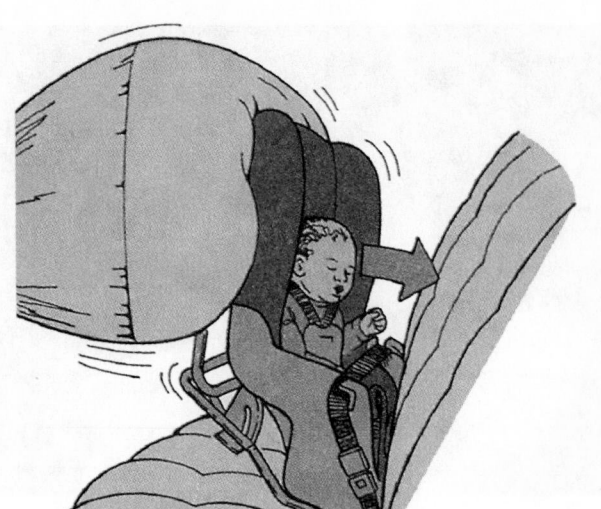

**Fig. 12-16** An air bag could strike a child safety seat, seriously injuring the infant. (Redrawn from AAP News: *Health Alert,* 10(4):22, 1994.)

Despite widespread education and publicity regarding seat belt safety restraint and the danger of front seat air bags for children, surveys indicate that children are still placed in potentially lethal situations of either improper seat restraint or in a front seat with an air bag (Ferguson, Wells, and Williams, 2000; Wittenberg, Nelson, and Graham, 1999).

For restraints to be effective, they must be used properly. Dressing the infant in an outfit with sleeves and legs allows the harness to hold the child securely in the seat. A small blanket or towel rolled tightly can be placed on either side of the head to minimize movement and keep the infant's hips against the back of the seat. Padding between the infant's legs and crotch is added to prevent slouching. Thick, soft padding is not placed under the infant or behind the back because during the impact the padding will compress, leaving the harness straps loose. (For further discussion of restraints, see Chapter 14.)

### Falls

Falls are most common after 4 months of age when the infant has learned to roll over, but they can occur at any age. The best advice is never to place a child of any age unattended on a raised surface that has no type of guardrails. When in doubt, the safest place is the floor. Even though young infants cannot climb over a partially raised crib rail, it is best to form a habit of raising the rail all the way, because someday that infant will be able to climb out. Crib sides should have a latching device that cannot be easily released. The welds attaching the crib corner locks to the corner posts should not be cracked or broken. If the welds are damaged, the bedspring could fall to the floor. Ideally, cribs should be placed on carpeted, not hard, floors.

Another danger area for falling is the *changing table,* which is usually high and narrow. Although these tables have a restraining belt, children are never left unattended, even when restrained. The best way to avoid needing to leave is to arrange the area with all necessary articles within easy reach so that the child is always in full sight of the caregiver. It takes only a fraction of a second for an infant to fall off. During the latter half of the first year, infants usually resist dressing and diapering and may be difficult to manage. If there is danger that the child is strong enough to resist restraining, the infant should be changed on a safer surface, such as a clean floor.

*Infant seats, high chairs, walkers,* and *swings* present additional opportunities for falls. If the *infant seat* is placed on a table or bed, the child should never be left unrestrained or unattended. The same rule is essential for other baby equipment, particularly when the child has learned to crawl and to stand up. Small infants can slip through a high chair if a protective harness is not used. The danger of falls from being unrestrained also applies to shopping carts. *High chairs* are designed for older infants who can sit well and who are tall enough to have the tray at the level of their chest or abdomen. *Infant walkers* are responsible for a number of different types of injuries that occur because the walker tipped over or fell down stairs. Parents need to be warned of these dangers and encouraged to keep a constant vigil on their child's activities; the use of walkers should be discouraged. The American Academy of Pediatrics Committee on Injury and Poison Prevention (1995) does not recommend the use of walkers. In response to the large number of accidents and deaths associated with infant walkers, several manufacturers made modifications on these products to prevent falls down stairs. The new models should have a label or sign indicating "meets new safety standard." Infant walkers may still pose a risk for climbing up to reach dangerous objects and should be carefully supervised. One alternative is to use a stationary play station with a seat similar to a walker. There is no evidence that infant walkers help infants walk sooner.

Once infants are mobile, they should not be allowed to crawl unsupervised on any raised surface, near stairs, or near any water reservoir. Gates should be used at the *bottom* and *top* of *stairs,* because both present dangers to the crawling and climbing infant. However, certain types of gates can present hazards. Freestanding enclosures constructed of criss-crossed wood slats that expand and contract can trap the head or neck when children attempt to climb over them. If these types of gates are used, they must be securely fastened to prevent mobility of the slats.

As children begin to pull themselves to a standing position, *heavy objects,* such as unsturdy furniture, televisions, CD players, or any free-standing item (e.g., wrought iron fish tank stands or concrete birdbath), can be extremely dangerous if pulled down on top of the child. To prevent injury from furniture tipping over, televisions should be placed on lower furniture and as far back as possible. Angle braces or anchors can secure furniture to walls.

Even when the environment is made safe, infants may sometimes literally trip over their own feet from *clothing.* Slippery socks; hard, slick soles on shoes or rubber soles that can catch, especially on a carpet; and long pants or pajama bottoms can easily upset a child's balance. Such dangers need to be pointed out to parents, especially when infants are taking their first steps.

## Poisoning

Poisoning is one of the major causes of death in children younger than 5 years of age. The highest incidence occurs in the 2-year-old group, with the second highest incidence occurring in 1-year-old children. Infants who do not crawl are relatively free from the danger of poisonous agents by virtue of immobility. However, once locomotion begins, danger from poisoning is present almost everywhere. There are more than 500 toxic substances in the average home, with approximately one third of all poisonings occurring in the kitchen.

The major reason for ingestion of poisons is *improper storage.* To protect the infant, toxic agents should not be placed on a low shelf, table, or floor. Drugs that are kept in a purse pose additional dangers; if the handbag is given to infants to play with, they may open it and ingest the drug.

*Plants* are another source of poisoning for infants. Plants are commonly placed on the floor, and the leaves or flowers are attractive and easy to pull off. More than 700 species of plants are known to cause illness or death.

Another danger is ingestion of the *button-sized batteries* used in devices such as hearing aids, calculators, watches, and cameras. Because they are bright and shiny, they are attractive to children. However, they can cause severe morbidity, even death, if lodged in the esophagus. The strong alkali in a battery can leak and cause a severe caustic burn. As a precaution, small batteries must be safely stored and discarded where young children cannot easily retrieve them.

Not all poisonings result from ingestion—*inhalation* is another possible route, such as inhaling chlorine vapors from household cleaning or pool supplies. Passive cocaine toxicity has occurred in young children exposed to freebase cocaine ("crack") smoking by adults. Children should be protected from environments in which inhaled toxins exist. (For a discussion of passive or second-hand tobacco smoke, see Chapter 32.)

The only sure way to prevent poisoning is to remove toxic agents, which means placing containers out of the infant's reach or contact. Because crawling infants soon become climbing toddlers, it is best to keep all toxic agents, especially drugs, in a locked cabinet. Special plastic hooks can be attached to the inside of cabinet doors to keep them securely closed (Fig. 12-17). Firm thumb pressure is required to unlatch the hook, and small children are usually unable to manipulate them. Locks are best, but for frequently used cleaning agents, such as those often kept under a kitchen sink, hooks are a practical alternative.

With several hundred toxic substances in each house, locking them all up can present a problem; however, careful planning can help. A large surplus of cleaning agents, furniture polishes, laundry additives, paints, insecticides, and solvents should be avoided. Used poison containers should be promptly discarded and not used to store another poison without adequately marking the package. Potentially hazardous substances should not be stored in any type of food container. A popular container used to store toxic liquids is a soda or pop bottle. A child who is unaware of the dangerous contents is vulnerable to poisoning. Parents should know the location of local poison control centers and call in

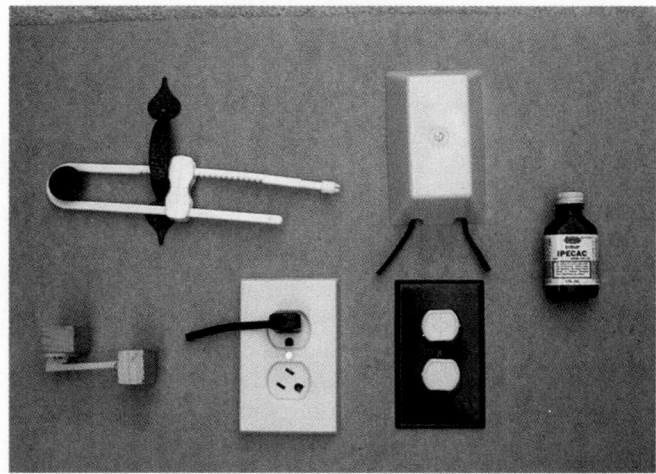

**Fig. 12-17**   Safety demonstration board. *Clockwise from lower left:* Cabinet latches, shock guard for electrical outlet, syrup of ipecac, and two types of outlet covers (white cover is passive device that automatically covers outlet when plug is removed).

the event of a suspected poisoning. Emergency measures for poisoning are discussed in Chapter 16.

## Burns

Scalding from water that is too hot, excessive sunburn, and burns from house fires, electrical wires, sockets, and heating elements such as radiators, registers, and floor furnaces cause a significant number of deaths and many more injuries in infants. The infant's skin is particularly sensitive to irritation, and the mechanisms for temperature perception are not completely developed. As a general precaution, all homes should have smoke alarms installed near the bedroom areas and on each level of the building.

Scald burns from *hot tap water* can be prevented by lowering the hot water heater to a safe temperature of 49°C (120°F). In addition, the bathwater should be checked before the infant is placed in the water. Scalds can also occur from bathing infants in the kitchen sink when the garbage disposal, occluded with debris, causes the draining dishwasher effluent to back up into the sink. The temperature of the effluent from a dishwasher is typically that of the maximum water temperature of the household water heater, but many dishwashers are equipped with heating elements that heat water to an even higher temperature. As a precaution, instruct caregivers to avoid bathing small children in the kitchen sink while the dishwasher is running.

If formula or food is warmed in a *microwave oven,* it must be checked before feeding because the container may remain cool while the contents are hot. Oropharyngel burns from the contents of baby bottles heated in a microwave have been reported (Weiner and O'Connell, 1995). Another danger is explosion of the bottle from the buildup of steam. Because of these dangers, microwaving infant formula or food should be avoided or done using the guidelines in the Family Home Care box on p. 523. The handles of cooking utensils should be turned toward the back of the stove. When the infant is underfoot, pouring hot liquids and cooking with hot oil are avoided. Hanging tablecloths are also placed out of the infant's reach to prevent pulling hot items off the table.

*Sunburn* can be a source of a first- or second-degree burn. Exposure to direct sunlight should be avoided for the first 6 months. When infants are in the sun, the body, especially the face and head, should be covered. Sunscreen can be used on older infants but should be used on small areas of the body and sparingly in infants under 6 months (American Academy of Pediatrics, 1999). (See Sunburn, Chapter 18.) Although dark-skinned infants burn less readily, their thin skin can become sunburned and needs protection.

*Electrical outlets* should be covered with protective plastic caps that prevent the child from sucking on the outlet or putting objects such as hairpins into it (see Fig. 12-17). Live wires are placed out of reach so that curious infants cannot chew on them and break the rubber coating. Infants should not be allowed to play near television sets, stereo units, or other appliances, whether these units are turned on or off, because infants cannot determine when the appliance is safe.

Any *heat-producing element* should have a guard placed in front of it. Fireplaces should be well screened because they are very appealing and within easy access. Small portable heaters should be placed on a high surface. Floor furnaces should have barrier gates to prevent children from crawling or walking over them. Burning cigarettes, candles, and incense should be kept out of reach, and infants should not be held by a smoking adult because falling ashes are a hazard, especially to the eyes. Heated-mist vaporizers are a source of burns and should not be used. If humidity is needed, only cool mist vaporizers are safe.

By law, all infant sleepwear must be flame retardant. Unfortunately, this does not apply to all *infant clothing*. Flame-retardant fabric must never be viewed as the ultimate protection against burns. Repeated washing reduces the flame-retardant properties, and the use of soap or bleach destroys the protection. If sleepwear is home sewn, parents are advised to look for specially treated, flame-retardant fabric.

Another type of thermal injury occurs when children are exposed to excessive heat during confinement in poorly ventilated *vehicles*. The practice of leaving the windows open a couple of inches is not protective. The nurse should caution parents never to leave children in parked cars, especially when the automobile is in direct sunlight.

Children can also be burned by overheated metal hardware and vinyl seats in cars parked in the sun. As a precaution, the surface heat of car restraints should be determined before placing children in them. Covering the restraints and hardware (such as metal latches on seat belts) may be necessary to prevent skin burns. An additional safeguard is buying a light-colored restraint, which absorbs less heat.

## Drowning

Drowning in this age-group can occur in only inches of water. Consequently, infants should **always** be supervised in a bathtub, hot tub, or near a source of water such as a swimming pool, lake, toilet, or bucket. Organized swimming instruction is not recommended for children under 4 years of age because it may lead to a false sense of security. No infant can be expected to learn the elements of water safety or to react appropriately in an emergency. Therefore all young children need to be considered at risk when near water (American Academy of Pediatrics, 1993). Infants and toddlers are also at increased risk of infection and convulsions from swallowing large amounts of water.

## Bodily Damage

Injuries can occur in numerous ways. Sharp, jagged-edged objects can cause wounds in the skin. Long-pointed articles, such as the common toothpick or fork, can be poked into the eye or ear, causing serious damage. Such articles should be safely stored away from the infant's reach; forks are best avoided for self-feeding until the child has mastered the spoon, usually by age 18 months.

In addition to hazards such as aspiration, small articles can be placed in the ear or nose, and excessive noise from toys can result in sensorineural hearing loss. Although toys with the highest noise levels are model airplanes, air guns, and toy cap guns, even common squeaking toys used by young children may be harmful if placed close to the ear.

A disturbing trend exists in that there is an overall increase in the number of infant deaths attributed to *homicide*. Over a 9-year study period, 6.4% of 10,370 infant injury deaths occurred as a result of homicide (Brenner and others, 1999). Specific interventions must be set in place to protect infants from harm, especially in entirely preventable situations.

Another commonly unrecognized danger to infants is animal attacks. As newcomers to the home, helpless infants can provoke jealousy in animals, especially dogs and cats. Parents must be constantly vigilant to protect the child from household pets and farm animals. (See Animal Bites, Chapter 18.)

## Nurse's Role in Injury Prevention

The task of injury prevention begins to be appreciated only when the potential environmental dangers to which infants are vulnerable are considered. Nurses must be aware of the possible causes of injury in each age-group in order for *anticipatory* preventive teaching to occur. For example, the guidelines for injury prevention during infancy presented in Table 12-15 should be discussed *before* the child reaches the susceptible age-group. Preventive teaching ideally occurs during pregnancy. Two thirds of all injuries to children occur in the home, and therefore the importance of safety cannot be overemphasized. A home safety checklist can be presented to parents to increase their awareness of danger areas in the home and assist them in implementing safety devices and practices *before* their absence can inflict injury on infants. (See Family Home Care box.) In addition, displays such as a safety demonstration board (see Fig. 12-17) can be helpful in familiarizing parents with inexpensive, commercial devices that can be used in the home to prevent injuries.

**NURSING TIP** To help parents appreciate the dangers present in their home to young children, suggest that they get eye level with the floor to survey the environment from a child's view.

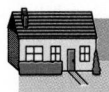

## FAMILY HOME CARE
### Child Safety Home Checklist

### SAFETY: FIRE, ELECTRICAL, BURNS

☐ Guards in front of or around any heating appliance, fireplace, or furnace (including floor furnace)*
☐ Electrical wires hidden or out of reach*
☐ No frayed or broken wires; no overloaded sockets
☐ Plastic guards or caps over electrical outlets, furniture in front of outlets*
☐ Hanging tablecloths out of reach, away from open fires*
☐ Smoke detectors tested and operating properly
☐ Kitchen matches stored out of child's reach*
☐ Large, deep ashtrays throughout house (if used)
☐ Small stoves, heaters, and other hot objects (cigarettes, candles, coffee pots, slow cookers) placed where they cannot be tipped over or reached by children
☐ Hot water heater set at 49°C (120°F) or lower
☐ Pot handles turned toward back of stove, center of table
☐ No loose clothing worn near stove
☐ No cooking or eating hot foods or liquids with child standing nearby or sitting in lap
☐ All small appliances, such as iron, turned off, disconnected, and placed out of reach when not in use
☐ Cool, not hot, mist vaporizer used
☐ Fire extinguisher available on each floor and checked periodically
☐ Electrical fuse box and gas shutoff accessible
☐ Family escape plan in case of a fire practiced periodically; fire escape ladder available on upper-level floors
☐ Telephone number of fire or rescue squad and address of home with nearest cross street posted near phone

### SAFETY: SUFFOCATION AND ASPIRATION

☐ Small objects stored out of reach*
☐ Toys inspected for small removable parts or long strings*
☐ Hanging crib toys and mobiles placed out of reach
☐ Plastic bags stored away from young child's reach, large plastic garment bags discarded after typing in knots*
☐ Mattress or pillow not covered with plastic or in manner accessible to child*
☐ Crib design according to federal regulations (crib slats less than 2⅜ inches [6 cm] apart) with snug-fitting mattress*†
☐ Crib positioned away from other furniture or windows*
☐ Portable playpen gates up at all times while in use*
☐ Accordion-style gates not used*
☐ Bathroom doors kept closed and toilet seats down*
☐ Faucets turned off firmly*
☐ Pool fenced with locked gate
☐ Proper safety equipment at poolside
☐ Electric garage door openers stored safely and garage door adjusted to rise when door strikes object
☐ Doors of ovens, trunks, dishwashers, refrigerators, and front-loading clothes washers and dryers kept closed*

---

*Safety measures are specific for homes with young children. All safety measures should be implemented in homes where children reside and visit frequently, such as those of grandparents or baby-sitters.
†Federal regulations are available from US Consumer Product Safety Commission, (800) 638-CPSC; *www.cpsc.gov.*
‡Community and home care instructions for infant cardiopulmonary resuscitation and infant/child choking are available in Wong DL, Hess CS: *Wong and Whaley's clinical manual of pediatric nursing,* ed 5, St Louis, 2000, Mosby.

☐ Unused appliance, such as a refrigerator, securely closed with lock or doors removed*
☐ Food served in small, noncylindric pieces*
☐ Toy chests without lids or with lids that securely lock in open position*
☐ Buckets and wading pools kept empty when not in use*
☐ Clothesline above head level
☐ At least one member of household trained in basic life support (CPR) including first aid for choking‡

### SAFETY: POISONING

☐ Toxic substances, including batteries, placed on a high shelf, preferably in locked cabinet
☐ Toxic plants hung or placed out of reach*
☐ Excess quantities of cleaning fluid, paints, pesticides, drugs, and other toxic substances not stored in home
☐ Used containers of poisonous substances discarded where child cannot obtain access
☐ Telephone number of local poison control center and address of home with nearest cross street posted near phone
☐ Syrup of ipecac in home containing two doses per child
☐ Medicines clearly labeled in childproof containers and stored out of reach
☐ Household cleaners, disinfectants, and insecticides kept in their original containers, separate from food and out of reach
☐ Smoking in areas away from children

### SAFETY: FALLS

☐ Nonskid mats, strips, or surfaces in tubs and showers
☐ Exits, halls, and passageways in rooms kept clear of toys, furniture, boxes, or other items that could be obstructive
☐ Stairs and halls well lighted, with switches at both top and bottom
☐ Sturdy handrails for all steps and stairways
☐ Nothing stored on stairways
☐ Treads, risers, and carpeting in good repair
☐ Glass doors and walls marked with decals
☐ Safety glass used in doors, windows, and walls
☐ Gates on top and bottom of staircases and elevated areas, such as porch, fire escape*
☐ Guardrails on upstairs windows with locks that limit height of window opening and access to areas such as fire escape*
☐ Crib side rails raised to full height; mattress lowered as child grows*
☐ Restraints used in high chairs, walkers, or other baby furniture; preferably walkers not used*
☐ Scatter rugs secured in place or used with nonskid backing
☐ Walks, patios, and driveways in good repair

### SAFETY: BODILY INJURY

☐ Knives, power tools, and unloaded firearms stored safely or placed in locked cabinet
☐ Garden tools returned to storage racks after use
☐ Pets properly restrained and immunized for rabies
☐ Swings, slides, and other outdoor play equipment kept in safe condition
☐ Yard free of broken glass, nail-studded boards, other litter
☐ Cement birdbaths placed where young child cannot tip them over*

---

Injury prevention requires protection of the child and education of the caregiver. Nurses in ambulatory care settings, health maintenance centers, or visiting nurse agencies are in a most favorable position for injury education. This does not exclude nurses in inpatient facilities, who could use visiting times as an excellent opportunity for discussing this topic. Although early postpartum discharge may be restrictive, this is an excellent opportunity to introduce the family to infant safety and safety for other children in the household as well. Pamphlets, safety checklists, and brief information sessions describing potential dangers and remedies aimed at preventing injury can be an effective way to help the new family get off to a good beginning with the new infant.

One approach to teaching injury prevention is to relate why children in various age-groups are prone to specific types of injuries. Stressing prevention is just as important as emphasizing the *why* of the injury. However, injury prevention must also be practical. Asking parents for their ideas leads to realistic suggestions that can be followed. For instance, bathroom cleaning agents, cosmetics, and personal care items can be placed on a top shelf in the linen closet, and towels or sheets can be stored on the lower shelves and floor.

If an injury has occurred, the nurse should not be too quick to admonish the parent. Injuries do not always indicate neglect. It is a difficult task to watch children carefully without overprotecting or unnecessarily confining them. Small falls help older children learn the dangers of heights. Touching a hot object once can emphasize to the child the pain of a burn. Allowing children to explore while maintaining consistent, age-appropriate limits is sound advice.

Parents need to remember that infants and young children cannot anticipate danger or understand when it is or is not present. A dead electrical wire may present no actual harm, but if the child is allowed to play with it, a poor behavior is enforced and will be practiced when the child encounters a live wire. Although it is always wise to explain why something is dangerous, it must be remembered that small children need to be physically removed from the situation.

It is not easy to teach safety, supervise closely, and refrain from saying "no" a hundred times a day. Parents become acutely aware of this dilemma as soon as the infant learns to crawl. Preventing injuries to children is usually the first reason for limit-setting and discipline, but limits are also set to prevent damage to valuable household objects. When small children are in the home, dangerous objects must be removed or guarded and valuable articles placed out of reach.

When children are taught the meaning of "no," they should also be taught what "yes" means. Children should be praised for playing with suitable toys, their efforts at behaving or listening should be reinforced, and innovative and creative recreational toys should be provided for them. Infants love to tear paper and avidly pursue books, magazines, or newspapers left on the floor. Instead of always scolding them for destroying a valued book, child-safe books (such as those constructed of fabric) can be kept available for them to play with. If they enjoy pots and pans, a cabinet can be arranged with safe utensils for them to explore.

One additional factor must be stressed concerning injury prevention and education. Children are imitators; they copy what they see and hear: *practicing safety teaches safety,* which applies to parents and their children and to nurses and their clients. Saying one thing but doing another confuses children and can lead to difficulties as the child grows older.

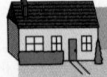

## FAMILY HOME CARE
### *Guidance During Infant's First Year*

**FIRST 6 MONTHS**

Teach car safety with use of federally approved restraint, facing rearward, in the middle of the back seat—not in a seat with an air bag.

Understand each parent's adjustment to newborn, especially mother's postpartal emotional needs.

Teach care of infant and help parents to understand his or her individual needs and temperament and that the infant expresses wants through crying.

Reassure parents that infant cannot be spoiled by too much attention during the first 4 to 6 months.

Encourage parents to establish a schedule that meets needs of child and themselves.

Help parents understand infant's need for stimulation in environment.

Support parents' pleasure in seeing child's growing friendliness and social response, especially smiling.

Plan anticipatory guidance for safety.

Stress need for immunization.

Prepare for introduction of solid foods.

**SECOND 6 MONTHS**

Prepare parents for child's "stranger anxiety."

Encourage parents to allow child to cling to them and avoid long separation from either.

Guide parents concerning discipline because of infant's increasing mobility.

Encourage use of negative voice and eye contact rather than physical punishment as a means of discipline.

Encourage showing most attention when infant is behaving well, rather than when infant is crying.

Teach injury prevention because of child's advancing motor skills and curiosity.

Encourage parents to leave child with suitable caregiver to allow some free time.

Discuss readiness for weaning.

Explore parents' feelings regarding infant's sleep patterns.

## Anticipatory Guidance— Care of Families

Childrearing is no easy task; it presents challenges to both new parents and "seasoned" parents. With society's changing roles and mores, combined with a highly mobile population, there is little stability for traditional role models and time-honored methods of raising children. As a result, parents look to professionals for guidance. Nurses are in an advantageous position to render assistance and suggestions. Every phase of a child's life has its particular traumas—toilet training for toddlers, unexplained fears for preschoolers, and identity crises for adolescents. For parents of an infant some challenges center around dependency, discipline, increased mobility, and safety. Major areas for parental guidance during the first year are listed in the Family Home Care box.

## KEY POINTS

- Biologic development of the child encompasses proportional changes; sensory changes, including binocularity, depth perception, and visual preference; maturation of biologic systems; fine motor development; and gross motor development.
- Erikson's theory of psychosocial development (birth to 1 year) is concerned with acquiring a sense of trust while overcoming a sense of mistrust.
- Piaget's theory of cognitive development, as it applies to the infant, focuses on the sensorimotor phase, which includes the use of reflexes, primary circular reactions, secondary circular reactions, and coordination or secondary schemata and their application to new situations.
- Development of body image begins in infancy; by 1 year of age infants recognize that they are distinct from their parents.
- Social development of the infant is guided by attachment, language development, personal-social behavior, and participation in play.
- Temperament influences the type of interaction that occurs between the child and parents and siblings.
- Parents are faced with many concerns, including infant fears, daycare, limit-setting and discipline, thumb sucking and pacifier use, teething, and choice of infant shoes.
- Breast milk is the most desirable food for the infant for the first 6 to 12 months. Commercial formula is an acceptable choice for infant nutrition when breast-feeding is not an option, followed by gradual introduction of solid food during the second 6 months. Whole milk is not recommended until after 12 months.
- Common sleep problems that develop during infancy—and that are easily prevented—are associated with night crying and feeding. Nurses should instruct the parents, after careful assessment, in strategies to deal with the specific problem.
- Cleaning the teeth regularly and appropriate dietary intake promote good dental health.
- Because injuries are a major cause of death during infancy, parents should be alerted to aspiration of foreign objects, suffocation, falls, poisoning, burns, motor vehicle injuries, and bodily damage, as well as preventive actions needed to make the environment safe for infants.
- Recommended routine immunizations include those for hepatitis B virus, hepatitis A (in some states), diphtheria, tetanus, pertussis, polio, measles, mumps, rubella, pneumococcal, chickenpox, influenza, and *Haemophilus influenzae* type b.
- Recommended immunizations for selected groups of children are Lyme, hepatitis A, and meningococcal vaccines.

## REFERENCES

Aarts C and others: Breastfeeding patterns in relation to thumb sucking and pacifier use, *Pediatrics* 104(4):e50, 1999.

Ainsworth M: Early caregiving and later patterns of attachment. In Klaus M, Robertson M, editors: *Birth, interaction, and attachment*, Skillman, NJ, 1982, Johnson & Johnson Baby Products.

Alho OP and others: Control of the temporal aspect when considering risk factors for acute otitis media, *Arch Otolaryngol Head Neck Surg* 119(4):444-449, 1993.

Alkon A and others: The epidemiology of injuries in 4 child care centers, *Arch Pediatr Adolesc Med* 153(12):1248-1254, 1999.

American Academy of Pediatrics, Committee on Environmental Health: Ultraviolet light: a hazard to children, *Pediatrics* 104(2): 328-333, 1999.

American Academy of Pediatrics, Committee on Infectious Diseases, Pickering L, editor: *2000 Red book: report of the Committee on Infectious Diseases,* ed 25, Elk Grove Village, IL, 2000a, The Academy.

American Academy of Pediatrics, Committee on Infectious Diseases: Policy statement: recommendations for the prevention of pneumococcal infections, including the use of pneumococcal conjugate vaccine (Prevnar), pneumococcal polycaccharide vaccine, and antibiotic prophylaxis, *Pediatrics* 106(2):362-367, 2000b.

American Academy of Pediatrics, Committee on Infectious Diseases: Recommended childhood immunization schedule, United States, January-December, 2001, *Pediatrics* 107(1):202-204, 2001.

American Academy of Pediatrics, Committee on Infectious Diseases: Recommended childhood immunization schedule—United States, 2002, *Pediatrics* 109(1):162-164, 2002.

American Academy of Pediatrics, Committee on Injury and Poison Prevention: Drowning in infants, children and adolescents, *Pediatrics* 92(2):292-294, 1993.

American Academy of Pediatrics, Committee on Injury and Poison Prevention: Injuries associated with infant walkers, *Pediatrics* 95(5):778-780, 1995.

American Academy of Pediatrics, Committee on Sports Medicine: Infant exercise programs, *Pediatrics* 82(5):800, 1988.

American Academy of Pediatrics, Committee on Nutrition: *Pediatric nutrition handbook,* ed 4, Elk Grove Village, IL, 1998, The Academy.

American Public Health Association and American Academy of Pediatrics: *Caring for our children: national health and safety performance standards: guidelines for out-of-home child care programs,* Washington, DC, 1992, The Association.

American Psychiatric Association: *Diagnostic and statistical manual of mental disorders,* ed 4, Washington, DC, 2000, the Association.

Assisting new mothers with infant feeding when breastfeeding is not an option: PBM educational symposium, *Pediatr Nurs* 27(1):47-60, 2001.

Baltimore RS, Jenson HB: Editorial commentary: meningococcal vaccine: new recommendations for immunization of college freshmen, *Curr Opin Pediatr* 3(1):47-50, 2001.

Beecroft PC, Redick SA: Intramuscular injection practices of pediatric nurses: site selection, *Nurs Educ* 15(4):23-28, 1990.

Beecroft PC, Kongelbeck SR: How safe are intramuscular injections? *AACN Clin Issues* 5(2):207-215, 1994.

Biancuzzo M: *Breastfeeding the newborn: clinical strategies for nurses,* St Louis, 1999, Mosby.

Blackburn ST, Loper DL: *Maternal, fetal, and neonatal physiology: a clinical perspective,* Philadelphia, 1992, WB Saunders.

Bowlby J: *Attachment and loss,* vol 1, New York, 1969, Basic Books.

Brazelton T: Parent-infant cosleeping revisited, *Ab Initio* 2(1):1-7, 1990.

Brenner RA and others: Deaths attributable to injuries in infants, United States, 1983-1991, *Pediatrics* 103(5):968-974, 1999.

Briss PA and others: A nationwide study of the risk of injury associated with day care center attendance, *Pediatrics* 93(3):364-368, 1994.

Calamaro CJ: Infant nutrition in the first year of life: tradition or science? *Pediatr Nurs* 26(2):211-215, 2000.

Carey WB, McDevitt SC: Revision of the infant temperament questionnaire, *Pediatrics* 61(5):735-739, 1978.

Carroll-Pankhurst C, Mortimer EA: Sudden infant death syndrome, bedsharing, parental weight, and age at death, *Pediatrics* 107(3):530-536, 2001.

Centers for Disease Control and Prevention: Impact of the 1999 AAP/USPHS joint statement on thimerosal in vaccines on hepatitis B vaccination practices, *MMWR* 50(6):94-97, 2001.

Centers for Disease Control and Prevention: Severe malnutrition among young children-Georgia, January 1997-June 1999, *MMWR* 50(12):224-227, 2001.

Coletta F, Bartholmey S, Menella JA: Flavor bridges: a critical link in ethnic feeding recommendation, *Pediatr Basic* 77(summer):1-8, 1996.

Committe on Infectious Diseases in Children: Give varicella vaccine at same time as MMR vaccine or wait 30 days, *Infect Dis Child* 15(1):22, 2002.

Corbett-Dick P, Bezek SK: Breastfeeding promotion for the employed mother, *J Pediatr Health Care* 11(1):12-19, 1997.

Dales L, Hammer SJ, Smith NJ: Time trends in autism and in MMR immunization coverage in California, *JAMA* 285(9):1183-1185, 2001.

Daly JM, Johnston W, Chung Y: Injection sites utilized for DPT immunizations in infants, *J Community Health Nurs* 9(2):87-94, 1992.

Dennehy PH: Transmission of rotavirus and other pathogens in the home, *Pediatr Infect Dis J* 19(10):S103-S105, 2000.

Dennison BA, Rockwell HL, Baker SL: Excess fruit juice consumption by preschool-aged children is associated with short stature and obesity, *Pediatrics* 99(1):15-22, 1997.

Dewey KG: Nutrition, growth, and complementary feeding of the breastfed infant, *Pediatr Clin North Am* 48(1):87-105, 2001.

Diggle L, Deeks J: Effect of needle length on incidence of local reactions to routine immunisation in infants aged 4 months: randomised controlled trial, *BMJ* 321(7266):931-933, 2000.

Drago DA, Dannenberg AL: Infant mechanical suffocating deaths in the United States, 1980-1997, *Pediatrics* 103(5):e59, 1999.

Ferber R, Kryger M: *Principles and practice of sleep medicine in the child,* Philadelphia, 1995, WB Saunders.

Ferguson SA, Wells JK, Williams AF: Child seating position and restraint use in three states, *Inj Prev* 6(1):24-28, 2000.

Ferketich SL, Mercer RT: Paternal-infant attachment of experienced and inexperienced fathers during pregnancy, *Nurs Res* 44(1):31-37, 1995.

Fuchs G and others: Gastrointestinal blood loss in older infants: impact of cow milk versus formula, *J Pediatr Gastroenterol Nutr* 16(1):4-9, 1993.

Grisoni ER and others: Pediatric airbag injuries: the Ohio experience, *J Pediatr Surg* 35(2):160-162, 2000.

Groswasser J and others: Needle length and injection technique for efficient intramuscular vaccine delivery in infants and children evaluated through an ultrasonographic determination of subcutaneous and muscle layer thickness, *Pediatrics* 100(3 pt 1):400-403, 1997.

Heinig MJ and others: Intake and growth of breast-fed and formula-fed infants in relation to the timing of introduction of complementary foods: the DARLING study, *Acta Paediatr* 82(12):999-1006, 1993.

Hobbie C, Baker S, Bayerl C: Parental misunderstanding of basic infant nutrition: misinformed feeding choices, *J Pediatr Health Care* 14(1):26-31, 2000.

Holaday B and others: Diaper type and fecal contamination in child day care, *J Pediatr Health Care* 9(2):67-74, 1995.

Horn MI, McCarthy AM: Children's responses to sequential versus simultaneous immunization injections, *J Pediatr Health Care* 13(1):18-23, 1999.

Houldin A: Infant temperament and the quality of the childbearing environment, *Matern Child Nurs J* 16(2):131-143, 1987.

Howard CR and others: The effects of early pacifier use on breastfeeding duration, *Pediatrics* 103(3):e33, 1999.

Johns RM, Miller L, Hochstetler J: Mother and baby dental care, *Mother Baby J* 3(3):15-22, 1998.

Johnson CP, Blasco PA: Infant growth and development, *Pediatr Rev* 18(7):224-242, 1997.

Jones L, Heermann J: Parental division of infant care: contextual influences and infant characteristics, *Nurs Res* 41(4):228-234, 1992.

Kemp JS and others: Unsafe sleep practices and an analysis of bedsharing among infants dying suddenly and unexpectedly: results of a four-year, population-based, death-scene investigation study of sudden infant death syndrome and related deaths, *Pediatrics* 106(3):e41, 2000.

Kreiter SR and others: Nutritional rickets in African American breast-fed infants, *J Pediatr* 137(2):153-157, 2000.

Kubiak M and others: Comparison of stool containment in cloth and single-use diapers using a simulated infant feces, *Pediatrics* 91(3):632-636, 1993.

Langkamp DL, Kim Y, Pascoe JM: Temperament of preterm infants at 4 months of age: maternal ratings and perceptions, *J Dev Behav Pediatr* 19(6):391-396, 1998.

Lawrence RA, Lawrence RM: *Breastfeeding: a guide for the medical profession,* ed 5, St Louis, 1999, Mosby.

Lutwick LI, Abramson JM: Pediatric immunization for the future: Lyme disease vaccine and beyond, *Pediatr Clin North Am* 47(2):465-479, 2000.

Lutwick SM: Pediatric vaccine compliance, *Pediatr Clin North Am* 47(2):427-434, 2000.

Macknin ML and others: Symptoms associated with infant teething: a prospective study, *Pediatrics* 105(4):747-752, 2000.

Mayberry LJ, Affonso DD: Infant temperament and postpartum depression: a review, *Health Care Women Int* 14(2):201-211, 1993.

Maziade M and others: Temperament and intellectual development: a longitudinal study from infancy to four years, *Am J Psychiatry* 144(2):144-150, 1987.

McIntosh B: Spoiled child syndrome, *Pediatrics* 83(1):108-114, 1989.

McKay MP, Jolly BT: A retrospective review of air bag deaths, *Acad Emerg Med* 6(7):708-714, 1999.

Medoff-Cooper B: Infant temperament: implications for parenting from birth through 1 year, *J Pediatr Nurs* 10(3):141-145, 1995.

Medoff-Cooper B, Carey WB, McDevitt SC: The Early Infancy Temperament Questionnaire, *J Dev Behav Pediatr* 14(4):230-231, 1993.

Motor-vehicle occupant injury: strategies for increasing use of child safety seats, increasing use of safety belts, and reducing alcohol-impaired driving, *MMWR* 50(RR7):1-13, 2001.

Murphy JM: Pediatric occupant car safety: clinical implications based on recent literature, *Pediatr Nurs* 25(2):137-148, 1999.

Murray DL: Preventing and managing pneumococcal disease, *Contemp Pediatr* 18(3 suppl):10-17, 2001.

Niemela M and others: Pacifier as a risk factor for acute otitis media: a randomized, controlled trial of parental counseling, *Pediatrics* 106(3):483-488, 2000.

Niemela M, Uhari M, Mottonen M: A pacifier increases the risk of recurrent acute otitis media in children in day care centers, *Pediatrics* 96(5 pt 1):884-888, 1995.

Nowak AJ, Warren JJ: Infant oral health and oral habits, *Pediatr Clin North Am* 47(5):1043-1066, 2000.

Patterson DL: Adolescent-mothering: child-grandmother attachment, *J Pediatr Nurs* 12(4):228-237, 1997.

Pickler R, Frankel H: The effect of non-nutritive sucking on preterm infants' behavioral organization and feeding performance, *Neonatal Network* 14(2):83, 1995.

Pinilla T, Birch LL: Help me make it through the night: behavioral entrainment of breast-fed infant's sleep patterns, *Pediatrics* 91(2):436-444, 1993.

Prevention of hepatitis A through active or passive immunization: recommendations of the Advisory Committee on Immunization Practices (ACIP), *MMWR* 48(RR12):1-37, Oct. 1, 1999.

Reber K: Children at risk for reactive attachment disorder: assessment, diagnosis, and treatment. *Progress: Fam Sys Res Ther* 5:83-98, 1996, Encino, CA, Phillips Graduate Institute.

Reis EC, Holubkov R: Vapocoolant spray is equally effective as EMLA cream in reducing immunization pain in school-aged children, *Pediatrics* 100(6):1025, 1997.

Reider M, Schwartz C, Newman J: Patterns of walker use and walker injury, *Pediatrics* 78(3):488-493, 1986.

Rivara FP and others: Risk of injury to children less than 5 years of age in day care versus home care settings, *Pediatrics* 84(6):1011-1016, 1989.

Roberts L and others: Effect of infection control measures on the frequency of upper respiratory infection in child care: a randomized, controlled trial, *Pediatrics* 105(4 pt 1):738-742, 2000a.

Roberts L and others: Effect of infection control measures on the frequency of diarrheal episodes in child care: a randomized, controlled trial, *Pediatrics* 105(4 pt 1): 743-746, 2000b.

Robertson J: Some responses of young children to the loss of maternal care, *Nurs Times* 49:382-386, 1953.

Runyan CW and others: Analysis of US child care safety regulations, *Am J Public Health* 81(8):981-985, 1991.

Ruth-Sanchez V, Greene CV: Water intoxication in a three day old: a case presentation, *Mother Baby J* 2(4):5-11, 1997.

Schachter F and others: Cosleeping and sleep problems in Hispanic-American urban young children, *Pediatrics* 84(3):522-530, 1989.

Scher A and others: Toddlers' sleep and temperament: reporting bias or a valid link?

A research note, *J Child Psychol Psychiatry* 33(7):1249-1254, 1992.

Shaw DS and others: Infant and toddler pathways leading to early externalizing disorders, *J Am Acad Child Adolesc Psychiatry* 40(1):36-43, 2001.

Smith MM, Lifshitz F: Excess fruit juice consumption as a contributing factor in nonorganic failure to thrive, *Pediatrics* 93(3):438-443, 1994.

Spitz RA: Hospitalism: an inquiry into the genesis of psychiatric conditioning in early childhood. In Fenechel D and others, editors: *Psychoanalytic studies of the child*, vol 1, New York, 1945, International University Press.

Sullivan SA, Birch LL: Infant dietary experience and acceptance of solid foods, *Pediatrics* 93(2):271-277, 1994.

Taylor JA and others: Impact of the change to inactivated poliovirus vaccine on the immunization status of young children in the United States: a study from pediatric research in office settings and the National Medical Association, *Pediatrics* 107(6):e90, 2001.

Uhari M, Mottonen M: An open randomized controlled trial of infection in child daycare centers, *Pediatr Infect Dis J* 18(8):672-677, 1999.

Uhari M: A eutectic mixture of lidocaine and prilocaine for alleviating vaccination pain in infants, *Pediatrics* 92(5):719-721, 1993.

Ulione MS: Health promotion and injury prevention in a child developmental center, *J Pediatr Nurs* 12(3):148-154, 1997.

Ulione MS, Dooling M: Preschool injuries in child care centers: Nursing strategies for prevention, *J Pediatr Health Care* 11(3): 111-116, 1997.

Van Norman RA: Why we can't afford to ignore prolonged digit-sucking, *Contemp Pediatr* 18(6):61-81, 2001.

Vogel A, Hutchison B, Mitchell E: The impact of pacifier use on breastfeeding: a prospective cohort study, *J Paediatr Child Health* 37(1):58-63, 2001.

Walker M: To the editor: sleep, feeding and opinions, *Pediatrics* 9(6):883-884, 1993.

Wall EJ: Practical primary pediatric orthopedics, *Nurs Clin North Am* 35(1):95-113, 2000.

Weiner GM, O'Connell JE: Oropharyngeal burns from microwave ovens: case report and review of the literature, *J Otolaryngol* 24(6):368-369, 1995.

Wilson D, Bowman C: Infant nutrition: building blocks for the future, *Mother Baby J* 5(4):17-21, 2000.

Winslow EH, Jacobson AF: Research for practice: pediatric IM injections: one size does not fit all, *Am J Nurs* 97(11):20, 1997.

Wittenberg E, Nelson TF, Graham JD: The effect of passenger airbags on child seating behavior in motor vehicles, *Pediatrics* 104(6):1247-1250, 1999.

Wolf L, Glass RP: *Feeding and swallowing disorders in infancy: assessment and management*, San Antonio, TX, 1992, Therapy Skill Builders.

Wong DL and others: Diapering choices: a critical review of the issues, *Pediatr Nurs* 18(1):41-54, 1992.

Zuckerman J: The importance of injecting vaccines into muscle, *BMJ* 321(7271): 1237-1238, 2000.

Zuckerman JN, Cockcroft A, Zuckerman AJ: Site of injection for vaccination, *BMJ* 305(6862):1158, 1992.

# Chapter 13

# Health Problems During Infancy

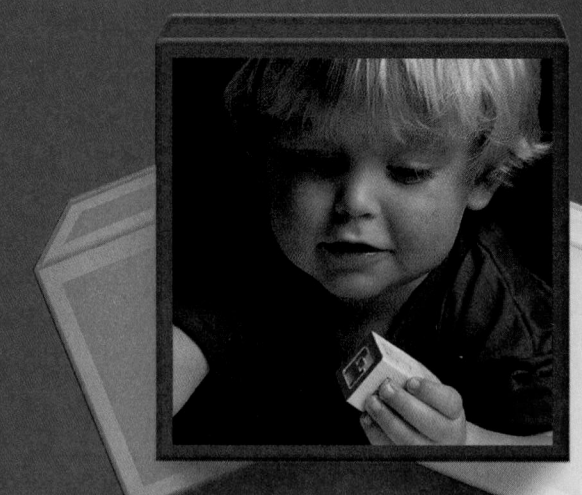

## Chapter Outline

**NUTRITIONAL DISTURBANCES, 554**
**Vitamin Disturbances, 554**
**Mineral Disturbances, 555**
**Vegetarian Diets, 560**
**Nursing Considerations, 560**
**Protein and Energy Malnutrition (PEM), 566**
    Kwashiorkor, 566
    Marasmus, 567
**Food Sensitivity, 568**

Cow's Milk Allergy, 569
    Lactose Intolerance, 570
**FEEDING DIFFICULTIES, 571**
**Improper Feeding Technique, 571**
**Regurgitation and "Spitting Up," 571**
**Paroxysmal Abdominal Pain (Colic), 571**
**Rumination, 574**
**Failure to Thrive (FTT), 574**

**SKIN DISORDERS, 578**
**Diaper Dermatitis, 578**
**Seborrheic Dermatitis, 580**
**Atopic Dermatitis (AD) (Eczema), 580**
**DISORDERS OF UNKNOWN ETIOLOGY, 582**
**Sudden Infant Death Syndrome (SIDS), 582**
    Infants at Risk for SIDS, 584
**Apnea of Infancy (AOI), 585**

## Related Topics

Anaphylaxis, Ch. 29
Apnea of Prematurity, Ch. 10
Asthma, Ch. 32
Autism, Ch. 24
Breast-Feeding Problems, Ch. 8
Candidiasis, Ch. 9
Cardiopulmonary Resuscitation, Ch. 31

The Child with Cognitive, Sensory, or
    Communication Impairment, Ch. 24
Dental Health, Chs. 12 and 14
Diarrhea, Ch. 29
Disorders Affecting the Skin, Ch. 18
Family-Centered Care of the Child with
    Chronic Illness or Disability, Ch. 22

Family-Centered Care of the Child with Life-
    Threatening Illness, Ch. 23
Feeding Resistance, Ch. 10
Gastroesophageal Reflux, Ch. 33
Iron Deficiency Anemia, Ch. 35
Nutritional Assessment, Ch. 6

# NUTRITIONAL DISTURBANCES

## Vitamin Disturbances

Vitamins are an essential food element and function in small quantities by regulating specific metabolic activity, usually by acting as *coenzymes.* When vitamin coenzymes enter the body, they are combined with a protein *apoenzyme* that has been synthesized within the cell to form a *holoenzyme.* The quantity of apoenzymes any cell can produce limits the body's ability to make use of excessive vitamins. A deficiency of the vitamin directly affects the metabolic activity it regulates. However, regular ingestion of excessive amounts of vitamins may produce a toxic effect.

True vitamin deficiencies are relatively uncommon in the United States, although subclinical deficiencies are seen in population subgroups where dietary intake is imbalanced. A

study revealed that only 1 in 5 children ages 2 to 18 years regularly consumed five or more servings of fruit and vegetables per day. In the same group approximately 50% of the children surveyed consumed less than one serving of fruit per day, with boys eating more fruit than girls. The most common vegetable consumed by children and adolescents were potatoes in the form of French fries (Krebs-Smith and others, 1996).

The fat-soluble vitamins, A, D, E, and K are commonly found in food sources and are stored in the liver and adipose tissues. Vitamin K is also synthesized by intestinal bacteria, and vitamin D is synthesized in the skin with exposure to ultraviolet light. Vitamin K is essential for proper blood clotting, and deficiency is seen primarily in the newly born infant. (See Chapter 8.)

Vitamin A deficiency correlates with increased morbidity and mortality in children with measles. Complications from

■ David Wilson, MS, RNC, revised this chapter.

diarrhea and infections are often increased in infants and children with vitamin A deficiency.

Because widespread screening for vitamin A deficiency is not feasible or practical in the United States, children within certain population groups perceived to be at high risk for the deficiency should be carefully evaluated. These groups include: (1) toddler and preschool children who typically have a low intake of fruits and vegetables; (2) children living at or below the poverty level; (3) children who have inadequate health care and/or immunizations; (4) children who have other nutritional deficiencies, such as iron deficiency anemia; (5) children who have recently immigrated from other countries where measles mortality is high and/or vitamin A deficiency is prevalent; (6) children with inadequate absorptive and digestive function as a result of an underlying medical condition such as celiac disease or short bowel syndrome; and (7) children with immunodeficiency (American Academy of Pediatrics, 2000a; Stephens, Jackson, and Gutierrez, 1996). The American Academy of Pediatrics recommends that vitamin A supplementation be considered in children hospitalized with measles and associated complications (diarrhea, croup, pneumonia), especially children between the ages of 6 months and 2 years (American Academy of Pediatrics, 2000a).

Vitamin D–deficiency rickets, once rarely seen because of vitamin D–fortified milk, has increased (Hartman, 2000; Centers for Disease Control and Prevention, 2001). Populations at risk include (1) children breast-fed by vitamin D-deficient mothers or breast-fed longer than 6 months without vitamin D supplementation by a mother with inadequate vitamin D intake; (2) individuals who are exposed to minimal sunlight because of their particular clothing, religious or cultural beliefs, housing in areas of high pollution, or dark skin pigmentation; (3) children with diets that are low in sources of vitamin D and calcium; and (4) individuals who use milk products not supplemented with vitamin D (e.g., yogurt* or raw cow's milk) as the primary source of milk. Children may also be at risk secondary to disorders or their treatment. For example, vitamin deficiencies of the fat-soluble vitamins A and D may occur in malabsorptive disorders. Preterm infants may develop rickets in the second month of life as a result of inadequate intake of vitamin D, calcium, and phosphorus.

Of equal, if not greater, concern is the overuse of vitamins, especially as a part of alternative therapies (McGuire and others, 2000). Parents should be cautioned not to exceed the upper limits of vitamin intake according to the new RDAs (see Dietary Reference Intakes, p. 564). An excessive dose of a vitamin is generally defined as 10 or more times the recommended dietary allowance, although the fat-soluble vitamins, especially A and D, tend to cause adverse reactions at lower doses. With the addition of vitamins to commercially prepared foods, the potential for *hypervitaminosis* has increased, especially when combined with the excessive use of vitamin supplements. Hypervitaminosis of A and D presents the greatest problems, because these fat-soluble vitamins are stored in the body. Vitamin D is the most likely of all vitamins

to cause adverse reactions in relatively small overdoses. However, there appears to be variance in the tolerance to different vitamin intakes. For example, two children ingesting excessive amounts of vitamin A may not both demonstrate clinical features of intoxication.

The water-soluble vitamins C, B complex, biotin, and pantothenic acid are also found in various food sources when a well-balanced diet is consumed. These vitamins are absorbed with water in the intestine and are excreted in the urine. It has been reported that in children ages 7 to 18 years, approximately one third of the children and two thirds of adolescent girls consume less than the recommended amount of vitamin $B_6$ (pyridoxine).

Folate (vitamin $B_9$, folic acid) deficiency has been linked to a number of congenital birth defects, primarily neural tube defects. Folic acid taken before conception and during early pregnancy can reduce the risk of neural tube defects such as spina bifida by as much as 70%. It is now recommended that all women of childbearing age take folic acid supplementation of 0.4 mg if dietary intake of folic acid is inadequate or unknown. Drugs such as oral contraceptives and antidepressants may decrease folic acid absorption; thus women on such drugs should consider supplementation. (See Spina Bifida, Chapter 11.)

The water-soluble vitamins, niacin, $B_6$, and C, can also cause adverse reactions by the following mechanisms:

- May have direct adverse effects, especially niacin and $B_6$
- May lead to dependency states with development of deficiency symptoms when the vitamin is abruptly discontinued, such as ascorbic acid
- May mask signs of a disease, such as vitamin C and interference with Clinitest results (common dipstick test used to detect glucose or acetone in urine) in diabetes
- May interact with drugs or other vitamins, such as folic acid's effect on reducing serum phenytoin levels
- May be combined with high doses of fat-soluble vitamins, such as high-dose multisupplement preparation

**NURSING ALERT**   Educate childbearing adolescent females about the need for folic acid to prevent neural tube birth defects. It is most easily obtained from a daily multivitamin supplement.

Deficiencies and excesses of vitamins A, B complex, C, D, E, and K are summarized in Table 13-1. General nursing considerations are discussed on p. 560, and specific interventions are presented in Table 13-1.

## Mineral Disturbances

A number of minerals are essential nutrients. The *macrominerals* refer to those with daily requirements greater than 100 mg and include calcium, phosphorus, magnesium, sodium, potassium, chloride, and sulfur. *Microminerals,* or *trace elements,* have daily requirements of less than 100 mg and include several essential minerals and those whose exact role in nutrition is still unclear. The greatest concern with minerals is deficiency, especially iron deficiency anemia. (See Chapter 35.) However, other minerals that may be inadequate in children's diets, even with supplementation,

---

*Yogurt does not contain adequate amounts of vitamins A and D yet is an acceptable source of calcium and phosphorous.

*Text continued on p. 560*

## TABLE 13-1 Vitamins and their nutritional significance

| Physiologic Functions/Sources | Results of Deficiency or Excess | Nursing Considerations |
|---|---|---|
| **Vitamin A (Retinol)*** <br><br> *Functions* <br> Necessary component in formation of pigment rhodopsin (visual purple) <br> Formation and maintenance of epithelial tissue <br> Normal bone growth and tooth development <br> Needed for growth and spermatogenesis <br> Involved in thyroxine formation <br> Antioxidant <br><br> *Sources* <br> *Natural form*—Liver, kidney, fish oils, milk and nonskimmed milk products, egg yolk <br> *Provitamin A (carotene)*—Carrots, sweet potatoes, squash, apricots, spinach, collards, broccoli, cabbage, artichokes | *Deficiency* <br> Night blindness <br> Keratinization (hardening and scaling) of epithelium <br>   Xerophthalmia (hardening and scaling of cornea and conjunctiva) <br>   Phrynoderma (toad skin) <br>   Drying of respiratory, gastrointestinal, and genitourinary tracts <br> Defective tooth enamel <br> Retarded growth <br> Impaired bone formation <br> Decreased thyroxine formation <br><br> *Excess* <br> *Early signs*—Irritability, anorexia, pruritus, fissures at corners of nose and lips <br> *Later signs*—Hepatomegaly, jaundice, retarded growth, poor weight gain, thickening of the cortex of long bones with pain and fragility, hard tender lumps in extremities and occiput of the skull <br> May cause birth defects from excessive maternal intake <br> NOTE: Overdose results from ingestion of large quantities of the vitamin only, not the provitamin; large amounts of carotene (carotenemia) cause yellow or orange discoloration of the skin (not the sclera, urine, or feces as in jaundice) but none of the above symptoms | Encourage foods rich in vitamin A, such as whole cow's milk (after 12 months) <br> As milk consumption decreases, encourage foods rich in vitamin A <br> Ensure adequate intake in preterm infants (formula or human milk) <br> Advise parents of safe use of supplements in child with measles <br><br><br> Emphasize correct use of vitamin supplements and potential hazards of excess <br> Investigate child's dietary habits to calculate approximate intake; if excessive, remove supplemental source (e.g., daily feeding of liver) <br> Advise parents of the benign nature of carotenemia; treatment is avoidance of excess pigmented fruits or vegetables, especially carrots; skin color returns to normal in 2 to 6 weeks |
| **Vitamin B₁ (Thiamine)†** <br><br> *Functions* <br> Coenzyme (with phosphorus) in carbohydrate metabolism <br> Needed for healthy nervous system <br><br> *Sources* <br> Pork, beef, liver, legumes, nuts, whole or enriched grains and cereals, green vegetables, fruits, milk, brown rice | *Deficiency* <br> *Gastrointestinal*—Anorexia, constipation, indigestion <br> *Neurologic*—Apathy, fatigue, emotional instability, polyneuritis, tenderness of calf muscles, partial anesthesia, muscle weakness, paresthesia, hyperesthesia, decreased or absent tendon reflexes, convulsions, and coma (in infants) <br> *Cardiovascular*—Palpitations, cardiac failure, peripheral vasodilation, edema <br> **Beriberi** (wet and dry forms) <br>   *Wet*—may be confused with congestive heart failure <br>   *Dry*—high-marching gait <br><br> *Excess* <br> Headache <br> Irritability <br> Insomnia <br> Rapid pulse <br> Weakness | Vitamin B complex <br> Encourage foods rich in B vitamins <br> Stress proper cooking and storage techniques to preserve potency, such as minimum cooking of vegetables in small amount of liquid; storage of milk in opaque container <br> Advise against fad diets that severely restrict groups of food, such as vegetarianism (vegans or macrobiotics) <br> Explore need for vitamin supplements when dieting or when using goat milk (which is not recommended) exclusively for infant feeding (deficient in folic acid) or when the breast-feeding mother is a strict vegetarian (vitamin B₁₂) <br> Emphasize correct use of vitamin supplements and potential hazards of excesses |
| **Vitamin B₂ (Riboflavin)†** <br><br> *Functions* <br> Coenzyme (with phosphorus) in carbohydrate, protein, and fat metabolism <br> Maintains healthy skin, especially around mouth, nose, and eyes <br><br> *Sources* <br> Milk and its products, eggs, organ meat (liver, kidney, and heart), enriched cereals, some green leafy vegetables,‡ legumes | *Deficiency* <br> Ariboflavinosis <br> *Lips*—Cheilosis (fissures at corners of lips), perlèche (inflammation at corners of lips) <br> *Tongue*—Glossitis <br> *Nose*—Irritation and cracks at nasal angle <br> *Eyes*—Burning, itching, tearing, photophobia, corneal vascularization, cataracts <br> *Skin*—Seborrheic dermatitis, delayed wound healing and tissue repair <br><br> *Excess* <br> Paresthesia, pruritus | Same as vitamin B complex |

*Fat soluble.
†Water soluble.
‡Green leafy vegetables include spinach, broccoli, kale, turnip greens, mustard greens, collards, dandelion greens, and beet greens.

**TABLE 13-1** Vitamins and their nutritional significance—cont'd

| Physiologic Functions/Sources | Results of Deficiency or Excess | Nursing Considerations |
|---|---|---|
| **Niacin (Nicotinic Acid, Nicotinamide)†** | | |
| *Functions* | *Deficiency* | Same as vitamin B complex |
| Coenzyme (with riboflavin) in protein and fat metabolism | Pellagra | If used as hypolipidemic agent, stress safe dosage to prevent child's accidental ingestion |
| Needed for healthy nervous system, skin, and normal digestion | *Oral*—Stomatitis, glossitis | |
| May lower cholesterol | *Cutaneous*—Scaly dermatitis on exposed areas | |
| | *Gastrointestinal*—Anorexia, weight loss, diarrhea, fatigue | |
| *Sources* | *Neurologic*—Apathy, anxiety, confusion, depression, dementia | |
| Meat, poultry, fish, peanuts, beans, peas, whole or enriched grains except corn and rice | Death | |
| | *Excess* | |
| Milk and its products are sources of tryptophan (60 mg of tryptophan = 1 mg of niacin) | Release of vasodilator, histamine (flushing, decreased blood pressure, increased cerebral blood flow; aggravates asthma) | |
| | Dermatologic problems (pruritus, rash, hyperkeratosis, acanthosis nigricans) | |
| | Increased gastric acidity (aggravates peptic ulcer disease) | |
| | Hepatotoxicity | |
| | Increased serum uric acid levels | |
| | Elevated plasma glucose levels | |
| | Certain cardiac arrhythmias | |
| **Vitamin B$_6$ (Pyridoxine)†** | | |
| *Functions* | *Deficiency* | Same as vitamin B complex |
| Coenzyme in protein and fat metabolism | Scaly dermatitis, weight loss, anemia, retarded growth, irritability, convulsions, peripheral neuritis | Stress proper cooking and storing techniques to preserve potency |
| Needed for formation of antibodies, hemoglobin | | Cook food covered in small amount of water |
| Needed for utilization of copper and iron | *Excess* | Store in light-resistant container |
| Aids in conversion of tryptophan to niacin | Peripheral nervous system toxicity (unsteady gait, numb feet and hands, clumsiness of hands, sometimes perioral numbness) | |
| *Sources* | May cause peptic ulcer disease or seizures | |
| Meats, especially liver and kidney, cereal grains (wheat and corn), yeast, soybeans, peanuts, tuna, chicken, salmon | | |
| **Folic Acid (Folacin); Reduced Form is Called Folinic Acid or Citrovorum Factor†** | | |
| *Functions* | *Deficiency* | Same as vitamin B complex |
| Coenzyme for single-carbon transfer (purines, thiamin, hemoglobin) | Macrocytic anemia, bone marrow depression, glossitis, intestinal malabsorption | Stress proper cooking and storing techniques to preserve potency |
| Necessary for formation of red blood cells | | Cook food covered in small amount of water |
| Prevents neural tube defects (i.e., myelomeningocele) | *Excess* | Do not soak food in water |
| | Rare because megadoses not available over the counter | Store in light-resistant container |
| *Sources* | May cause insomnia and irritability | Women of childbearing age should receive RDA (0.4 mg/day) to prevent neural tube defects |
| Green leafy vegetables,‡ cabbage, asparagus, liver, kidney, nuts, eggs, whole grain cereals, legumes, bananas | | |
| **Vitamin B$_{12}$ (Cobalamin)†** | | |
| *Functions* | *Deficiency* | Same as vitamin B complex |
| Coenzyme in protein synthesis; indirect effect on formation of red blood cells (particularly on formation of nucleic acids and folic acid metabolism) | Pernicious anemia | Consider supplementation in case of strict vegetarian mother who is breastfeeding |
| | (One form of deficiency from absence of intrinsic factor in gastric secretions) | |
| Needed for normal functioning of nervous tissue | General signs of severe anemia | |
| | Lemon-yellow tinge to skin | |
| | Spinal cord degeneration | |
| | Delayed brain growth | |

*Fat soluble.
†Water soluble.
‡Green leafy vegetables include spinach, broccoli, kale, turnip greens, mustard greens, collards, dandelion greens, and beet greens.

*Continued*

## TABLE 13-1 Vitamins and their nutritional significance—cont'd

| Physiologic Functions/Sources | Results of Deficiency or Excess | Nursing Considerations |
|---|---|---|
| **Vitamin B$_{12}$ (Cobalamin)—cont'd**<br>*Sources*<br>Meat, liver, kidney, fish, shellfish, poultry, milk, eggs, cheese, nutritional yeast, sea vegetables | *Excess*<br>Excess is rare | |
| **Biotin†**<br>*Functions*<br>Coenzyme in carbohydrate, protein, and fat metabolism<br>Interrelated with functions of other B vitamins<br><br>*Sources*<br>Liver, kidney, egg yolk, tomatoes, legumes, nuts | *Deficiency*<br>Deficiency is uncommon because synthesized by bacterial flora<br><br>*Excess*<br>Unknown | Same as vitamin B complex |
| **Pantothenic Acid†**<br>*Functions*<br>Coenzyme in carbohydrate, protein, and fat metabolism<br>Synthesis of amino acids, fatty acids, and steroids<br><br>*Sources*<br>Liver, kidney, heart, salmon, eggs, vegetables, legumes, whole grains | *Deficiency*<br>Deficiency is uncommon because of its multiple food sources and synthesis by bacterial flora<br><br>*Excess*<br>Minimum toxicity (occasional diarrhea and water retention) | Same as vitamin B complex |
| **Vitamin C (Ascorbic Acid)†**<br>*Functions*<br>Essential for collagen formation<br>Increases absorption of iron for hemoglobin formation<br>Enhances conversion of folic acid to folinic acid<br>Affects cholesterol synthesis and conversion of proline to hydroxyproline<br>Probably a coenzyme in metabolism of tyrosine and phenylalanine<br>May play role in hydroxylation of adrenal steroids<br>May have stimulating effect on phagocytic activity of leukocytes and formation of antibodies<br>Antioxidant agent (spares other vitamins from oxidation)<br><br>*Sources*<br>Citrus fruits, strawberries, tomatoes, potatoes, cabbage, broccoli, cauliflower, green peppers, spinach, papaya, mango, cantaloupe, watermelon, enriched fruit juice | *Deficiency*<br>**Scurvy**<br>*Skin*—Dry, rough, petechiae, perifollicular hyperkeratotic papules (raised areas around hair follicles)<br>*Musculoskeletal*—Bleeding muscles and joints, pseudoparalysis from pain, swelling of joints, costochondral beading (scorbutic rosary)<br>*Gums*—Spongy, friable, swollen, bleed easily, bluish red or black color, teeth loosen and fall out<br>*General disposition*—Irritable, anorexic, apprehensive, in pain, refuses to move, assumes semifroglike position when supine (scorbutic pose)<br>Signs of anemia<br>Decreased wound healing<br>Increased susceptibility to infection<br><br>*Excess*<br>Diarrhea<br>Increased excretion of uric acid and acidification of urine (may cause urate precipitation and formation of oxalate stones)<br>Hemolysis<br>Impaired leukocytosis activity<br>Damage to beta cells of pancreas and decreased insulin production<br>Reproductive failure<br>"Rebound scurvy" from withdrawal of large amounts | Encourage foods rich in vitamin C<br>Investigate infant's diet for sources of vitamin, especially when cow's milk (after 12 months) is principal source of nutrition<br>Stress proper cooking and storing techniques to preserve potency<br>  Wash vegetables quickly; do not soak in water<br>  Cook vegetables in covered pot with minimum water and for short time; avoid copper or cast iron cookware<br>  Do not add baking soda to cooking water<br>  Use fresh fruits and vegetables as soon as possible; store in refrigerator<br>  Store juice in airtight, opaque container<br>  Wrap cut fruit or eat soon after exposing to air<br>In caring for child with scurvy:<br>  Position for comfort and rest<br>  Handle very gently and minimally<br>  Administer analgesics as needed<br>  Prevent infection<br>  Provide good oral care<br>  Provide soft, bland diet<br>  Emphasize rapid recovery when vitamin is replaced<br>Emphasize correct use of vitamin supplement and potential hazards of excess |

*Fat soluble.
†Water soluble.
‡Green leafy vegetables include spinach, broccoli, kale, turnip greens, mustard greens, collards, dandelion greens, and beet greens.

**TABLE 13-1**   Vitamins and their nutritional significance—cont'd

| Physiologic Functions/Sources | Results of Deficiency or Excess | Nursing Considerations |
|---|---|---|
| **Vitamin D₂ (Ergocalciferol) and D₃ (Cholecalciferol)*** | | |
| *Functions*<br>Absorption of calcium and phosphorus and decreased renal excretion of phosphorus<br><br>*Sources*<br>Direct sunlight<br>Cod liver oil, herring, mackerel, salmon, tuna, sardines<br>*Enriched food sources*—Milk, milk products, enriched cereals, margarine, breads, many breakfast drinks | *Deficiency*<br>**Rickets**<br>*Head*—Craniotabes (softening of cranial bones, prominence of frontal bones), deformed shape (skull flat and depressed toward middle), delayed closure of fontanels<br>*Chest*—Rachitic rosary (enlargement of costochondral junction of ribs), Harrison groove (horizontal depression in lower portion of rib cage), pigeon chest (sharp protrusion of sternum)<br>*Spine*—Kyphosis, scoliosis, lordosis<br>*Abdomen*—Potbelly, constipation<br>*Extremities*—Bowing of arms/legs, knock-knee, saber shins, instability of hip joints, pelvic deformity, enlargement of epiphysis at ends of long bones<br>*Teeth*—Delayed calcification, especially of permanent teeth<br>*Rachitic tetany*—Seizures | Encourage foods rich in vitamin D, especially fortified cow's milk (after 12 months)<br>In breast-fed infants encourage use of vitamin D supplements if maternal diet inadequate or infant exposed to minimal sunlight<br>Any child who is 12-13 months old and healthy but does not or cannot pull to a standing position should be evaluated for rickets<br>Prevent infection<br>Observe for possibility of overdose from supplements<br>If prescribed, supervise proper use of orthopaedic splints or braces |
| | *Excess*<br>*Acute*—Vomiting, dehydration, fever, abdominal cramps, bone pain, convulsions, and coma<br>*Chronic*—Lassitude, mental slowness, anorexia, failure to thrive, thirst, urinary urgency, polyuria, vomiting, diarrhea, abdominal cramps, bone pain, pathologic fractures<br>*Calcification of soft tissue*—Kidneys, lungs, adrenal glands, vessels (hypertension), heart, gastric lining, tympanic membrane (deafness)<br>Osteoporosis of long bones<br>Elevated serum levels of calcium and phosphorus | Same as vitamin A; may include low-calcium diet during initial therapy |
| **Vitamin E (Tocopherol)*** | | |
| *Functions*<br>Production of red blood cells and protection from hemolysis<br>Muscle and liver integrity<br>Coenzyme factor in tissue respiration<br>Minimizes oxidation of polyunsaturated fatty acids and vitamins A and C in intestinal tract and tissues<br>Possible role in treatment and prevention of bronchopulmonary dysplasia and retinopathy of prematurity is under investigation<br><br>*Sources*<br>Vegetable oils, wheat germ oil, milk, egg yolk, muscle meats, fish, whole grains, nuts, legumes, spinach, broccoli | *Deficiency*<br>Hemolytic anemia from hemolysis caused by shortened life of red blood cells, especially in preterm infants, and focal necrosis of tissues<br>Causes infertility in rats, but not in humans (does *not* increase human male virility or potency)<br><br>*Excess*<br>Little is known: less toxic than other fat-soluble vitamins | Initiate early feeding in preterm infants; may need supplementation |
| **Vitamin K*** | | |
| *Functions*<br>Catalyst for production of prothrombin and blood-clotting factors II, VII, IX, and X by the liver<br><br>*Sources*<br>Pork, liver, green leafy vegetables‡ (spinach, kale, cabbage), tomatoes, egg yolk, cheese | *Deficiency*<br>Hemorrhage<br><br>*Excess*<br>Hemolytic anemia in individuals who are deficient in glucose-6-phosphate dehydrogenase | Administer prophylactically to all newborns (see Chapter 9)<br>Other indications include intestinal disease, lack of bile, prolonged antibiotic therapy; may be used in management of blood-clotting time when anticoagulants such as warfarin (Coumadin) and dicumarol (bishydroxycoumarin), which are vitamin K antagonists, are used |

*Fat soluble.
†Water soluble.
‡Green leafy vegetables include spinach, broccoli, kale, turnip greens, mustard greens, collards, dandelion greens, and beet greens.

include calcium, phosphorus, magnesium, and zinc. Low levels of zinc can cause nutritional failure to thrive.

The regulation of mineral balance in the body is a complex process. Dietary extremes of mineral intake can cause a number of mineral-mineral interactions that could result in unexpected deficiencies or excesses. For example, excessive amounts of one mineral, such as zinc, can result in a deficiency of another mineral, such as copper, even if sufficient amounts of copper are ingested. This is thought to be a result of competition in the process of absorption because of (1) displacement of one mineral by another on the molecule necessary for their uptake from the lumen in the intestinal cell or (2) competition for pathways through the intestinal wall or into the bloodstream. Therefore megadose therapy with one mineral may not cause adverse effects from an excess but rather from a deficiency in a competing mineral.

Deficiencies can also occur when various substances in the diet interact with minerals. For example, iron, zinc, and calcium can form insoluble complexes with phytates and/or oxalates (substances found in plant proteins), which impairs the bioavailability of the mineral. This type of interaction is important in vegetarian diets because plant foods, such as soy, are high in phytates. Contrary to popular opinion, spinach is not a rich source of iron or calcium because of its high oxalate content.

Deficiencies and excesses of the essential macrominerals and microminerals are summarized in Table 13-2. General nursing considerations are discussed following, and specific interventions are discussed in the table.

## Vegetarian Diets

The importance of vegetarian diets and their relationship to potential nutritional deficiencies in children cannot be overemphasized. The stricter the vegetarian diet, the more difficult it becomes to ensure adequate nutrition for infants and children. The major types of vegetarianism are:

**Lacto-ovovegetarians,** who exclude meat from their diet but eat milk and eggs and rarely fish

**Lactovegetarians,** who exclude meat and eggs but drink milk

**Pure vegetarians (vegans),** who eliminate any food of animal origin, including milk and eggs

**Zen macrobiotics,** who are even more restrictive than pure vegetarians; small amounts of fruits, vegetables, and legumes are allowed

**Semi-vegetarians,** who consume a lacto-ovovegetarian diet with some fish and poultry; this is an increasingly popular form of vegetarianism and poses little or no nutritional risk to infants unless dietary fat and cholesterol intake is severely restricted

Many individuals who are concerned about healthful diets subscribe to vegetarian diets that are not typified by the above categories. Therefore, during nutritional assessment it is necessary to clearly list exactly what the diet includes and excludes.*

---

*Further information regarding vegetarian diets may be found at the **Vegetarian Resource Group (VRG),** PO Box 1463, Baltimore, MD 21203, (410) 366-VEGE; www.vrg.org.

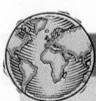

## CULTURAL AWARENESS
### Vegetarian Diets

In the United States strict vegetarian diets are common among members of Black Muslim or Seventh-Day Adventist faiths. Achieving a nutritionally adequate vegetarian diet is not difficult, but it requires careful planning and knowledge of nutrient sources. For children the lacto-ovovegetarian diet is nutritionally adequate; however, the vegan diet requires supplementation with vitamins D and $B_{12}$, particularly for children ages 2 to 12 years. There have been reported cases of severe neurologic impairment in infants with vitamin $B_{12}$ deficiency whose mothers were on a vegan diet (Graham, Arvela, and Wise, 1992). Infants on a vegan diet should be breast-fed for the first 6 months and preferably for 1 year, fed solid foods after about 4 months, and receive iron-fortified cereal for at least 18 months. The use of juices containing vitamin C with foods high in iron will further improve iron absorption. If cow's or human milk is not given, fortified soy milk is recommended. Other approaches toward increasing vitamin D and calcium intake in the diet that may be accepted are inclusion of fatty fish (herring, salmon, sardines, trout, tuna) and less fiber, because high fiber intake limits mineral absorption by decreasing intestinal transit time and binding calcium, iron, and other minerals.

The lacto-ovovegetarian diet is associated with the fewest deficiencies, although protein intake needs to be monitored. The lactovegetarian diet may also be low in protein as well as iron. The major deficiencies in the stricter vegetarian diets are inadequate protein for growth, inadequate calories for energy and growth, poor digestibility of many of the natural, unprocessed foods, especially for infants, and deficiencies of vitamin $B_6$, niacin, thiamine, riboflavin, vitamin D, iron, calcium, and zinc. Because vegetarian diets eliminate the major sources of complete proteins (those proteins with all the essential amino acids in amounts needed to support physiologic functions), protein deficiency can occur. (See Cultural Awareness box.) Strict vegetarian diets also require supplements of vitamin $B_{12}$ and vitamin D. Vitamin D is essential if exposure to sunlight is inadequate (<5 to 15 minutes per day on the hands, arms and face) or in persons who are dark-skinned or who live in northern latitudes or cloudy or smoky areas (American Dietetic Association, 1997).

Iron deficiency anemia and rickets may also be seen in children on strict vegetarian diets as a result of consuming plant foods such as unrefined cereals, which impairs the absorption of iron, calcium, and zinc.

## Nursing Considerations

Identification of nutrient imbalance is the initial nursing goal and requires assessment based on a dietary history and physical examination for signs of deficiency or excess. (See Nutritional Assessment, Chapter 6.) Once assessment data are collected, this information is evaluated against standard intakes to identify areas of concern. The most widely used standard is the *Recommended Dietary Allowances (RDAs)*, developed by the *National Academy of Sciences, Food and Nutrition Board.* The RDAs are not average requirements but recommendations intended to meet the physiologic needs of

*Text continued on p. 564*

**TABLE 13-2**   Minerals and their nutritional significance

| Physiologic Functions/Sources | Results of Deficiency or Excess | Nursing Considerations |
|---|---|---|
| **Calcium***<br>*Functions*<br>Bone and tooth development and mainte-<br>nance (in combination with phosphorus)<br>Muscle contractions, especially the heart<br>Blood clotting<br>Absorption of vitamin $B_{12}$<br>Enzyme activation<br>Nerve conduction<br>Integrity of intracellular cement substances<br>and various membranes<br><br>*Sources*<br>Dairy products, egg yolk, sardines, canned<br>salmon with bones, dark green leafy vege-<br>tables (except spinach), soybeans, dried<br>beans, and peas | *Deficiency*<br>Rickets<br>Impaired growth, especially of bones and<br>teeth<br><br>*Excess*<br>Drowsiness, extreme lethargy<br>Impaired absorption of other minerals<br>(iron, zinc, manganese)<br>Calcium deposits in tissues (renal failure) | Encourage foods rich in calcium, especially<br>dairy products<br>Caution that oxalates in leafy vegetables<br>(spinach), oxalates in chocolates, and a<br>high phosphorus intake (especially from<br>carbonated beverages) can decrease<br>calcium absorption<br>Discourage use of whole cow's milk in new-<br>borns because the phosphorus-to-calcium<br>ratio favors excretion of calcium<br>Advise against fad diets, especially those that<br>restrict dairy products<br>Emphasize correct use of calcium supplement,<br>especially adequate intake of vitamin D for<br>calcium absorption, and the possible interac-<br>tion between megadoses of calcium and<br>resulting deficiency states of other minerals |
| **Chloride***<br>*Functions*<br>Acid-base and fluid balance<br>Enzyme activation in saliva<br>Component of hydrochloric acid in stomach<br><br>*Sources*<br>Salt, meat, eggs, dairy products, many<br>prepared and preserved foods | *Deficiency*<br>Acid-base disturbances (hypochloremic<br>alkalosis, dehydration); occurs mostly<br>in combination with sodium loss<br><br>*Excess*<br>Acid-base disturbance | Deficiency and excess are unusual; most diets<br>supply adequate chloride (usually in combi-<br>nation with sodium)<br>Disease states such as excessive vomiting can<br>necessitate chloride replacement |
| **Chromium†**<br>*Functions*<br>Involved in glucose metabolism and energy<br>production<br><br>*Sources*<br>Meat, cheese, whole-grain breads and cereals, le-<br>gumes, peanuts, brewer's yeast, vegetable oils | *Deficiency*<br>Possible abnormal glucose metabolism<br><br>*Excess*<br>Unknown | No specific recommendations are needed |
| **Copper†**<br>*Functions*<br>Production of hemoglobin<br>Essential component of several enzyme systems<br><br>*Sources*<br>Organ meats, oysters, nuts, seeds, legumes,<br>corn-oil margarine | *Deficiency*<br>Anemia, leukopenia, neutropenia<br><br>*Excess*<br>Severe vomiting and diarrhea<br>Hemolytic anemia | Deficiency from inadequate food sources is<br>less likely than from excess intake of other<br>minerals, especially zinc and possibly iron;<br>therefore emphasize the correct use of any<br>vitamin supplement<br>Caution against cooking acidic foods in<br>unlined copper pots, which can lead to<br>chronic and toxic accumulation of copper |
| **Fluoride†**<br>*Functions*<br>Formation of caries-resistant teeth<br>Strong bone development<br><br>*Sources*<br>Fluoridated water and foods or beverages pre-<br>pared with fluoridated water; fish, tea, com-<br>mercially prepared chicken for infants | *Deficiency*<br>Increased susceptibility to tooth decay<br><br>*Excess*<br>**Fluorosis** (mottling and/or pitting of<br>enamel)<br>Severe bone deformities | In areas with optimally fluoridated water,<br>encourage sufficient intake to supply recom-<br>mended amount of fluoride<br>In areas of unfluoridated water or when ready-<br>to-use formula, bottled water, or breast milk<br>is used, stress the importance of fluoride<br>supplements in infants ≥6 mos (see Chap-<br>ters 12 and 14)<br>In areas with excess fluoride in the water, con-<br>sider the use of bottled water for drinking<br>and possibly cooking to reduce the fluoride<br>intake to safe levels<br>Fluoride has the narrowest range of safe and<br>adequate intake; therefore stress the impor-<br>tance of storing supplements in a safe area |

*Macrominerals—required intake >100 mg/day.
†Microminerals or trace elements—required intake <100 mg/day.

*Continued*

## TABLE 13-2 Minerals and their nutritional significance—cont'd

| Physiologic Functions/Sources | Results of Deficiency or Excess | Nursing Considerations |
| --- | --- | --- |
| **Iodine†**<br><br>*Functions*<br>Production of thyroid hormone<br>Normal reproduction<br><br>*Sources*<br>Seafood, kelp, iodized salt, sea salt, enriched bread, milk (from dairy processing) | *Deficiency*<br>**Goiter** (enlarged thyroid from decreased thyroxine formation)<br><br>*Excess*<br>Unknown from food sources; may occur from ingestion of iodine preparations such as saturated solutions of potassium iodide (SSKI) | Encourage use of iodized salt for individuals living far from the sea<br>If iodine preparations are in the home, stress the importance of safe storage |
| **Iron†**<br><br>*Functions*<br>Formation of hemoglobin and myoglobin<br>Essential part of several enzymes and proteins<br><br>*Sources*<br>Liver, especially pork, followed by calf, beef, and chicken; liverwurst, red meat, poultry, clams, oysters, beans, ham, whole grains, iron-enriched infant formula and cereal, enriched cereals and bread, legumes, nuts, seeds, green leafy vegetables (except spinach), dried fruits, potatoes, molasses, tofu, prune juice | *Deficiency*<br>**Anemia** (see Chapter 35)<br><br>*Excess*<br>Hemosiderosis (excess iron storage in various tissues of the body, especially the spleen, liver, lymph glands, heart, and pancreas)<br>Hemochromatosis (excess iron storage with cellular damage) | Encourage foods rich in iron<br>Discourage excessive milk consumption, especially more than 1 L per day (milk is a very poor source of iron)<br>If iron supplements are prescribed, teach parents factors that affect absorption (Box 13-1)<br>Stress the importance of storing iron supplements in a safe area<br>To increase consumption of iron:<br>  Make meatloaf by adding up to ½ pound ground liver to 1 pound ground beef; when the seasonings and other ingredients have been added, it is impossible to tell the meat loaf contains liver<br>  Make a trail mix snack with nuts, pumpkin and sunflower seeds, raisins, and dried apricots; serve as a snack with a high–vitamin C juice to improve iron absorption; give to children who can safely eat nuts and seeds |
| **Magnesium\***<br><br>*Functions*<br>Bone and tooth formation<br>Protein production<br>Nerve conduction to muscles<br>Activation of enzymes needed for carbohydrate and protein metabolism<br><br>*Sources*<br>Whole grains, nuts, soybeans, meat, green leafy vegetables (uncooked), tea, cocoa, raisins | *Deficiency*<br>Tremors, spasm<br>Irregular heartbeat<br>Muscular weakness<br>Lower extremity cramps<br>Convulsions, delirium<br><br>*Excess*<br>Nervous system disturbances due to imbalance in calcium-to-magnesium ratio | Deficiency and excess are unusual, except in disease states such as prolonged vomiting or diarrhea or kidney dysfunction, where replacement may be needed |
| **Manganese†**<br><br>*Functions*<br>Activation of enzymes involved in reproduction, growth, and fat metabolism<br>Normal bone structure<br>Nervous system functioning<br><br>*Sources*<br>Nuts, whole grains, legumes, green vegetables, fruit | *Deficiency*<br>Unknown<br><br>*Excess*<br>Unknown | No specific recommendations are needed |
| **Molybdenum†**<br><br>*Functions*<br>Essential component of several oxidative enzymes<br><br>*Sources*<br>Legumes, whole grains, organ meats, some dark green vegetables | *Deficiency*<br>Very rare; diagnosed in patients on total parenteral nutrition<br><br>*Excess*<br>Produces secondary copper deficiency (growth failure, anemia, and disturbed bone development) | No specific recommendations are needed |

\*Macrominerals—required intake >100 mg/day.
†Microminerals or trace elements—required intake <100 mg/day.

**TABLE 13-2**   Minerals and their nutritional significance—cont'd

| Physiologic Functions/Sources | Results of Deficiency or Excess | Nursing Considerations |
|---|---|---|
| **Phosphorus\*** | | |
| *Functions* | *Deficiency* | Dietary deficiency is uncommon, although prolonged use of antacids can produce deficiency, in which case supplementation is recommended |
| Bone and tooth development (in combination with calcium) | Weakness, anorexia, malaise, bone pain | |
| Involved in numerous chemical reactions, including protein, carbohydrate, and fat metabolism | *Excess* | To preserve calcium-to-phosphorus ratio in newborns, discourage use of whole cow's milk until 12 months old |
| Acid-base balance | Produces secondary calcium deficiency from disturbed calcium-to-phosphorus ratio | |
| *Sources* | | |
| Dairy products, eggs, meat, poultry, legumes, carbonated beverages | | |
| **Potassium\*** | | |
| *Functions* | *Deficiency* | Dietary deficiency and excess are unlikely, although disease states such as prolonged nausea and vomiting or the use of diuretics can result in hypokalemia; in such instances encourage replacement with oral potassium supplements |
| Acid-base and fluid balance (major extracellular fluid areas) | Cardiac arrhythmias | |
| Nerve conduction | Muscular weakness | |
| Muscular contraction, especially the heart | Lethargy | |
| Release of energy | Kidney and respiratory failure | |
| | Heart failure | |
| *Sources* | *Excess* | |
| Bananas, citrus fruit, dried fruits, meat, fish, bran, legumes, peanut butter, potatoes, coffee, tea, cocoa | Cardiac arrhythmias | |
| | Respiratory failure | |
| | Mental confusion | |
| | Numbness of extremities | |
| **Selenium†** | | |
| *Functions* | *Deficiency* | Deficiency and excess are uncommon in North America, although selenium deficiency can occur in patients on prolonged total parenteral nutrition; in these instances supplementation is required |
| Antioxidant, especially protective of vitamin E | Keshan disease (cardiomyopathy in children; found in China) | |
| Protects against toxicity of heavy metals | Kashin-Beck disease—a degenerative osteoarticular disease endemic to Tibet; iodine deficiency is a risk factor for disease | |
| Associated with fat metabolism | | |
| *Sources* | *Excess* | |
| Seafood, organ meats, egg yolk, whole grain, chicken, meat, tomatoes, cabbage, garlic, mushrooms, milk | Eye, nose, and throat irritation | |
| | Increased dental caries | |
| | Liver and kidney degeneration | |
| **Sodium\*** | | |
| *Functions* | *Deficiency* | Deficiency intake is very rare, although losses secondary to nausea, vomiting, excessive sweating, and use of diuretics can occur and require replacement |
| Acid-base and fluid balance (major extracellular fluid cation) | Dehydration | |
| Cell permeability; absorption of glucose | Hypotension | Encourage parents to limit excessive use of salt in preparing foods and limit commercial foods with high sodium content (smoked meats) |
| Muscle contraction | Seizures | |
| | Muscle cramps | |
| *Sources* | *Excess* | Avoid electrolyte-free water intake in infants and supplementation with water; may cause hyponatremia and seizures (see Chapter 8) |
| Table salt, seafood, meat, poultry, numerous prepared foods | Edema | |
| | Hypertension | |
| | Intracranial hemorrhage | |
| **Sulfur\*** | | |
| *Functions* | *Deficiency* | No specific recommendations are needed |
| Essential component of cell protein, especially of hair and skin | Unknown | |
| Enzyme activation | *Excess* | |
| Associated with energy metabolism | Unknown | |
| Detoxification of certain chemical reactions | | |
| *Sources* | | |
| Dairy products, eggs, meat, fish, nuts, legumes | | |

\*Macrominerals—required intake >100 mg/day.
†Microminerals or trace elements—required intake <100 mg/day.

*Continued*

**TABLE 13-2**   Minerals and their nutritional significance—cont'd

| Physiologic Functions/Sources | Results of Deficiency or Excess | Nursing Considerations |
|---|---|---|
| **Zinc†** | **Deficiency** | Encourage food sources rich in zinc, especially protein |
| **Functions** | Loss of appetite | Caution that fiber, phytates, oxalates, tannins (in tea or coffee), iron, and calcium adversely affect zinc absorption |
| Component of about 100 enzymes | Diminished taste sensation | |
| Synthesis of nucleic acids and protein in immune system and coagulation | Delayed healing | |
| Release of vitamin A from liver | *Skin lesions*—Erythematous, crusted lesions around body orifices | Recognize groups at risk for zinc deficiency, such as vegetarians, whose diets may have restricted or low meat content and high fiber, phytate content; and patients with malabsorption syndromes |
| Improved wound healing with vitamin C | Alopecia | |
| | Diarrhea | |
| **Sources** | Growth failure | |
| Seafood (especially oysters), meat, poultry, eggs, wheat, legumes | Retarded sexual maturity | Emphasize correct use of zinc supplements and the possible interaction with other minerals |
| | **Excess** | |
| | Vomiting and diarrhea | |
| | Malaise, dizziness | |
| | Anemia, gastric bleeding | |
| | Impaired absorption of calcium/copper | |

*Macrominerals—required intake >100 mg/day.
†Microminerals or trace elements—required intake <100 mg/day.

---

**Box 13-1** ■ ■ ■
**Factors That Affect Iron Absorption**

| INCREASE ABSORPTION | DECREASE ABSORPTION |
|---|---|
| *Acidity (low pH)*—Administer iron between meals (gastric hydrochloric acid) | *Alkalinity (high pH)*—Avoid any antacid preparation |
| *Ascorbic acid (vitamin C)*—Administer iron with juice, fruit, or multivitamin preparation | *Phosphates*—Milk is unfavorable vehicle for iron administration |
| Vitamin A | *Phytates*—Found in cereals |
| Calcium | *Oxalates*—Found in many fruits and vegetables (plums, currants, green beans, spinach, sweet potatoes, tomatoes) |
| Tissue need | |
| Meat, fish, poultry | *Tannins*—Found in tea, coffee |
| Cooking in cast iron pots | Tissue saturation |
| | Malabsorptive disorders |
| | Disturbances that cause diarrhea or steatorrhea |
| | Infection |

---

almost every healthy person. To meet the needs of those with the highest requirements, the RDAs will exceed most people's requirements. Therefore children consuming less than the RDAs are not necessarily consuming an inadequate diet, but they are more likely at risk for deficiency than those who are consuming nutrients in amounts equal to the RDAs.

The *Institute of Medicine (IOM)* has developed guidelines for nutritional intake that encompass the RDAs yet extend their scope to include additional parameters related to nutritional intake. The *Dietary Reference Intakes (DRIs)* are comprised of four categories. These include *estimated average requirements (EARs)* for age and gender categories, *tolerable upper-limit (UL)* nutrient intakes that are associated with a low risk of adverse effects, *adequate intakes (AIs)* of nutrients, and *new standard RDAs.* The new guidelines present information about lifestyle factors that may affect nutrient function, such as caffeine intake and exercise, and about how the nutrient may be related to chronic disease. The first DRIs published included calcium, magnesium, phosphorus, vitamin D, and fluoride. Additional groups of nutrients being evaluated by communities developing DRIs include folate and other B vitamins, dietary antioxidants, micronutrients, macronutrients, trace elements, electrolytes, and food components such as dietary fiber. The comprehensive set of guidelines covers nutrient effects across the life span, including pregnancy and lactation. With the increased interest in nutrition, illness, and health, this reference will serve to better educate the general population and health care workers for improved nutrition and health.*

Several organizations have published dietary advice for the public. The *Dietary Guidelines for Americans* encourage eating a variety of foods, maintaining ideal body weight, consuming adequate starch and fiber, and limiting intake of fat, cholesterol, sugar, salt, and alcohol. The *Food Guide Pyramid (FGP)*, which replaces the basic four food groups, is used to convey nutrition information to the public and applies to children as young as 2 years of age (Fig. 13-1).

The new FGP includes pictures aimed at younger children. The different food groups and servings are the same, yet the foods are made to appear more realistic. Names of the groups have also been reduced for children to better understand. The tip of the pyramid emphasizes a decrease in the consumption of fats and sweets (Box 13-2).

Because one of the best assurances of nutritional adequacy is eating a variety of foods, families need guidelines for selecting foods that provide essential nutrients without exceeding energy requirements. With a varied diet most children do not need vitamin or mineral supplements. There are no restrictions on the availability of toxic doses of

---

*For information on the DRIs go to IOM web site: www.iom.edu. At this site either use the site's search engine for DRIs or go to the IOM site map: Ongoing Studies—Dietary Reference Intakes, or call (202) 334-1732.

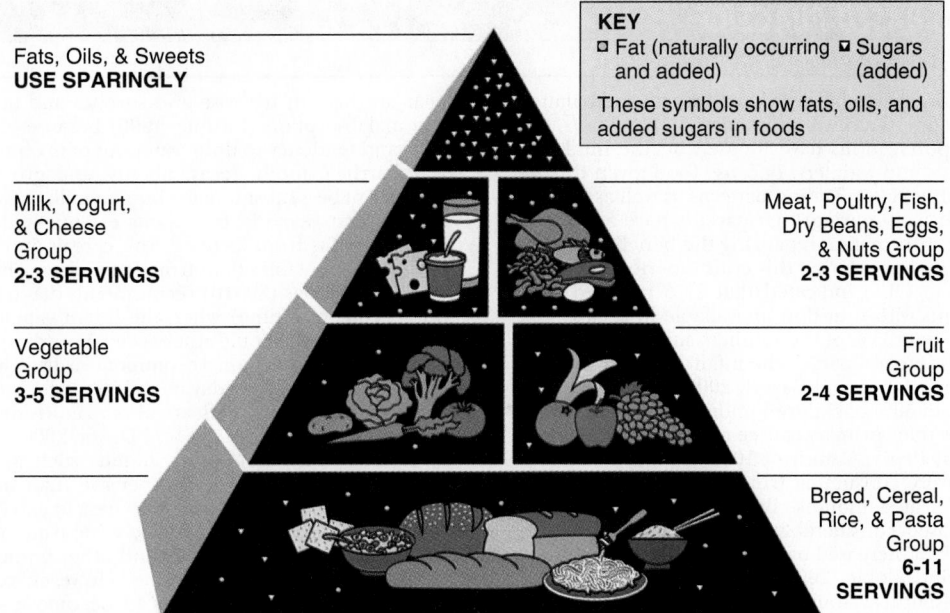

**Fig. 13-1** Food Guide Pyramid: a guide to daily food choices. (Courtesy US Department of Agriculture, 1996.)

vitamins or minerals. Nurses need to inquire about alternative therapies that include vitamin or mineral supplements and inform families of the potential dangers from excess vitamins or minerals. The idea that "more is better" is probably best dispelled by a simple explanation of the body's inability to use more than the needed requirement.

Achieving a nutritionally adequate vegetarian diet (with the exception of the strictest diets) is not difficult, but it requires careful planning and knowledge of nutrient sources. For children the lacto-ovovegetarian diet is nutritionally adequate; however, the vegan diet requires supplementation with vitamins D and B$_{12}$ for children ages 2 to 12 years. Infants should be breast-fed for the first 6 months and preferably for 1 year, be introduced to some solid foods after about 4 months, and receive iron-fortified cereal for at least 18 months. The American Dietetic Association (1997) recommends iron supplementation in infants exclusively breast-fed after 4 to 6 months by vegetarian mothers and no dietary fat restrictions in vegetarian children younger than 2 years. The use of vitamin C juices (in moderate amounts, not as a milk substitute) with foods high in iron will further improve iron absorption. (See Evidence-Based Practice box on p. 566.) Breast milk from vegetarian mothers can be deficient in vitamin B$_{12}$; supplementation of both mother and child is advisable. If cow's or human milk or commercial infant formula is not given, fortified soy milk is recommended. A variety of foods should be introduced during the early years to ensure a well-balanced intake.

**NURSING ALERT** When solid foods are introduced, the safety and digestibility of the selections must be considered. Raw fruits with seeds, vegetables, and nuts are hazardous for infants and young children because of the danger of aspiration. Beans, grain cereals, and vegetables should be served well-cooked and mashed during infancy.

---

**Box 13-2 ■ ■ ■**
**Food Guide Pyramid: Sample Serving Sizes**

**BREAD, CEREAL, RICE, AND PASTA GROUP**
1 slice of bread
1 ounce of ready-to-eat cereal
½ cup of cooked cereal, rice, or pasta

**VEGETABLE GROUP**
1 cup of raw leafy vegetable
½ cup of another vegetable, cooked or chopped raw
¾ cup of vegetable juice

**FRUIT GROUP**
1 medium apple, banana, or orange
½ cup of chopped, cooked, or canned fruit
¾ cup of fruit juice

**MILK, YOGURT, AND CHEESE GROUP**
1 cup of milk or yogurt
1½ ounces of natural cheese
2 ounces of processed cheese

**MEAT, POULTRY, FISH, DRY BEANS, EGGS, AND NUTS GROUP**
2-3 ounces of cooked lean meat, poultry, or fish
½ cup of cooked dry beans, 1 egg, or 2 tablespoons of peanut butter count as 1 ounce of lean meat

---

To ensure sufficient protein in the diet, foods with incomplete proteins (those that do not have all of the essential amino acids) must be eaten at the same meal with other foods that supply the missing amino acids. The three basic combinations of foods consumed by vegetarians that generally provide the appropriate amounts of essential amino acids are:

1. **Grains** (cereal, rice, pasta) and **legumes** (beans, peas, lentils, peanuts)

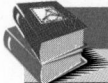

## EVIDENCE-BASED PRACTICE
### Infants and Juice Intake

Do infants need fruit juice to bolster vitamin stores and balance their diet in the second 6 months of infancy?

Several recent publications have focused on the intake of fruit juices in infants and toddlers. Because food given during the first year may affect later feeding patterns as well as growth and development, it is important that parents have adequate, unbiased, scientific information regarding the benefits and adverse effects of taking juice during this critical period. A recent survey of mothers in Ohio indicated that 17% believed fruit juice provides infants with nutrition unavailable in breast milk or formula. In addition 35% of the mothers surveyed believed that fruit juice is an integral part of the infant's diet in the first year of life (Hobbie, Baker, and Bayerl, 2000). Another study found that more than 50% of children under 1 year of age were given apple juice as their primary source of daily-required fruit servings (Dennison, 1996). A study of 1000 infants in England showed that 25% were consuming fruit juice and 14.6% were given herbal drinks at 4 months. By 8 months the volume of milk had decreased considerably, and the intakes of juice and herbal drinks had increased by 55% and 14%, respectively (Emmett, North, and Noble, 2000). A survey of low-income rural mothers in Kentucky found that fruit juice was being given to infants as early as 1 to 2 months of age (Barton, 2001). Some studies have correlated an increased amount of juice intake in toddlers and preschoolers with short stature, obesity, and growth failure (Dennison, Rockwell, and Baker, 1997); however, others have refuted these claims (Skinner and others, 1999; Skinner and Carruth, 2001).

Are fruit juices bad for infants? Essentially the answer is "no" provided that (1) juices, as well as other milk substitutes, are not given in amounts that negate the benefits of human milk or infant formula; (2) juices do not cause gastrointestinal malabsorption problems and diarrhea; and (3) juices are not given in a manner that would cause tooth decay. Juices such as apple and pear are high in fructose and sorbitol and may cause diarrhea and malabsorption (Lifshitz, 1996) because of their high osmolality and tendency to draw water out of the intestine. The results are diarrhea, tooth decay, obesity, and growth failure. Juices should not be a substitute for human milk or formula intake during the first year of life. Infants essentially derive more nutritional benefits from fortified iron cereals and small amounts of semi-solid vegetables than from fruit juices. The American Academy of Pediatrics (2001b) recommends that fruit juices be introduced (one at a time) when the infant is able to drink from a cup; the amount should not exceed 5 oz/day (Calamaro, 2000). Authorities in nutrition recommend a fruit juice intake of no more than 10 to 12 oz/day in children 2 to 6 years old as long as adequate amounts of milk are also taken (American Academy of Pediatrics, 1998a; Doucette and Dwyer, 2000).

Infants like sweet-tasting liquids such as juice. Juice and juice drinks are often less expensive than milk and formula. Juice and juice products are also easy to carry around in a bottle without refrigeration. At face value fruit juice appears to be a good alternative when soda and other nonmilk beverages are compared for nutritional value. However, parents should be cautioned not to allow juices to become a substitute for the daily milk products infants need to grow healthy bodies. Only pasteurized and 100% fruit juices should be given to infants and toddlers because fresh-squeezed may be contaminated with *Salmonella* (Peregrin, 2001). Dental decay can be minimized by giving juice in a cup, rather than in a bottle. Unfortified juices do not provide adequate amounts of vitamin C. Fruit juice drinks are often sold as fruit juice when in fact they are flavored sugar products and may contain minimal amounts of vitamins and minerals. Finally, any excessive use of fruit juice or drink in infants may cause multiple health problems because they are essentially empty calories that do not support proper growth and development.

---

2. **Grains** and **milk products** (milk, cheese, yogurt)
3. **Seeds** (sesame, sunflower) and **legumes**

## Protein and Energy Malnutrition (PEM)

Malnutrition continues to be a major health problem in the world today, particularly in children under 5 years of age. Lack of food, however, is not always the primary cause for malnutrition. In many developing and underdeveloped nations, *diarrhea* is a major factor in malnutrition. Additional factors are bottle-feeding (in poor sanitary conditions), inadequate knowledge of proper child care practices, parental illiteracy, economic and political factors, and simply the lack of food. The most extreme forms of malnutrition, or protein energy malnutrition (PEM), are kwashiorkor and marasmus.

In the United States milder forms of PEM are seen, although the classic cases of marasmus and kwashiorkor may also occur. Unlike developing countries, where the main reason for PEM is inadequate food, in the United States PEM occurs despite ample dietary supplies (see Failure to Thrive, p. 574).

### Kwashiorkor

Kwashiorkor has been defined in the past as primarily a deficiency of protein with an adequate supply of calories. A diet consisting mainly of starch grains or tubers provides adequate calories in the form of carbohydrates but an inadequate amount of high-quality proteins. There is evidence, however, supporting a multifactorial etiology, including cultural, psychologic, and infective factors that may interact to place the child at risk for kwashiorkor. A mycotoxin mold, *aflatoxin,* has been implicated in the etiology of this disease; the mold has been found to grow on stored grains and to be present in large numbers in the intestines of children with kwashiorkor. Taken from the Ga language (Ghana), the word *kwashiorkor* means "the sickness the older child gets when the next baby is born" and aptly describes the syndrome that develops in the first child, usually between 1 and 4 years of age, when weaned from the breast once the second child is born.

**Pathophysiology and Clinical Manifestations.** The pathophysiology of kwashiorkor results in part from protein deficiency, both in quantity and quality. Because protein is essential for tissue growth and cell repair, all body systems are affected, but rapidly growing cells, such as those of the epithelium and mucosa, are most severely damaged. The skin is scaly and dry and has areas of depigmentation. Several dermatoses may be evident, partly resulting from the vitamin deficiencies. Permanent blindness results from the severe lack of vitamin A. Immunity is severely affected and is of considerable importance in the development of infections.

Mineral deficiencies are common, especially iron, calcium, and zinc. Acute zinc deficiency is a common complication of severe PEM and results in skin rashes, loss of hair,

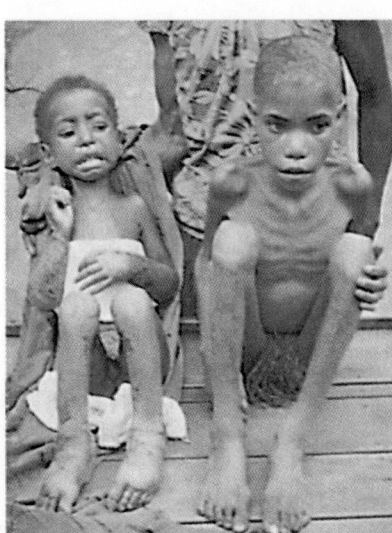

**Fig. 13-2** Children suffering from kwashiokor (*left*) and marasmus (*right*) as a result of inadequate energy intake. (From Grodner MG, Anderson SL, DeYoung SL: *Foundations and clinical applications of nutrition: a nursing approach,* St Louis, 1996, Mosby.)

impaired immune response and susceptibility to infections, digestive problems, night blindness, changes in affective behavior, defective wound healing, and impaired growth. Its depressant effect on appetite further limits food intake. There is evidence that doubling the amount of oral zinc supplementation in children under 5 years who have acute persistent diarrhea decreases the length and severity of diarrhea episodes (Bhutta and others, 2000).

With kwashiorkor the hair is thin, dry, coarse, and dull. Depigmentation is common, and patchy alopecia may occur. There is loss of weight in conjunction with generalized edema from the hypoalbuminemia. The edema often masks the severe muscular atrophy, making the children appear less debilitated than they actually are (Fig. 13-2). Total body water increases, but total body potassium decreases with retention of sodium, causing signs of hypokalemia and hypernatremia.

Diarrhea commonly occurs from a lowered resistance to infection and further complicates the electrolyte imbalance. A large number of fatalities in children with kwashiorkor occurred in those who developed human immunodeficiency virus (HIV) infection, many of whom were breast-fed (Brewster, Manary, and Graham, 1997). Gastrointestinal disturbances occur, such as fatty infiltration of the liver and atrophy of the acini cells of the pancreas. Protein deficiency increases the child's susceptibility to infection, which eventually results in death. Behavioral changes are evident as the child grows progressively more irritable, lethargic, withdrawn, and apathetic. Fatal deterioration may be caused by diarrhea and infection or as the result of circulatory failure.

## Marasmus

Marasmus results from general malnutrition of both calories and protein. It is a common occurrence in underdeveloped countries during times of drought, especially in cul-

tures where adults eat first; the remaining food is often insufficient in quality and quantity for the children.

Marasmus is usually a syndrome of physical and emotional deprivation and is not confined to geographic areas where food supplies are inadequate. It may be seen in children with failure to thrive, where the cause is not solely nutritional but primarily emotional. Marasmus may be seen in infants as young as 3 months of age if breast-feeding is not successful and there are no suitable alternatives.

***Marasmic-kwashiorkor*** is a form of PEM in which clinical findings of both kwashiorkor and marasmus are evident; the child has edema, severe wasting, and stunted growth. In marasmic-kwashiorkor the child suffers from inadequate nutrient intake and superimposed infection. Fluid and electrolyte disturbances, as well as hypothermia and hypoglycemia, are associated with a poor prognosis.

**Pathophysiology and Clinical Manifestations.**   Marasmus is characterized by gradual wasting and atrophy of body tissues, especially subcutaneous fat (see Fig. 13-2). Children with the condition appear to be very old; their skin is flabby and wrinkled, unlike children with kwashiorkor, who appear more rounded from the edema. Fat metabolism is less impaired than in kwashiorkor, so that vitamin A deficiency is usually minimal or absent.

In general, the clinical manifestations of marasmus are similar to those seen in kwashiorkor with the following exceptions: with marasmus there is no edema from hypoalbuminemia or sodium retention, which contributes to a severely emaciated appearance; no dermatoses caused by vitamin deficiencies; little or no depigmentation of hair or skin; moderately normal fat metabolism and lipid absorption; and smaller head size and slower recovery following treatment.

As in kwashiorkor, body metabolism is minimal, and maintaining body temperature is complicated by lack of subcutaneous fat. The child is fretful, apathetic, withdrawn, and so lethargic that prostration often occurs. Intercurrent infection with debilitating diseases such as tuberculosis, parasitosis, and dysentery is common. Severe, chronic malnutrition in infancy results in decreased brain growth and has implications for the child's future mental capacity.

## Therapeutic Management

The treatment of PEM includes providing a diet with quality proteins, carbohydrates, vitamins, and minerals. When PEM occurs as a result of diarrhea (see also Diarrhea, Chapter 29), three management goals are identified: (1) rehydration with an oral rehydration solution (ORS) that also replaces electrolytes, (2) administration of medications such as antibiotics and antidiarrheals, and (3) provision of adequate nutrition either by breast-feeding or a proper weaning diet. When the child is too ill to tolerate oral fluids, intravenous administration of fluids and electrolytes will be required to prevent death.

## Nursing Considerations

Provision of essential physiologic needs, such as rest, individually tailored activity, and protection from infection, is paramount. Because children are usually weak and withdrawn, they depend on others for feeding. Hygiene may be distressing because of the poor integrity of the skin, and decubiti are a constant threat. Appropriate developmental stimulation should be provided also.

A larger problem is the prevention of these conditions through education concerning the importance of proper nutrition, whether breast-feeding or bottle-feeding, when being weaned to semisolid foods. Because children with marasmus may suffer from emotional starvation as well, care should be consistent with care of the child with failure to thrive (see p. 574).

## Food Sensitivity

Food sensitivity is a general term that includes any type of adverse reaction to food or food additives. Food sensitivities can be divided into two broad categories:

1. **Food allergy** or **hypersensitivity,** which refers to those reactions involving immunologic mechanisms, usually immunoglobulin E (IgE); the reactions may be immediate or delayed and mild or severe, such as an anaphylactic reaction.
2. **Food intolerance,** which refers to those reactions involving known or unknown nonimmunologic mechanisms; lactose intolerance is an example of a reaction that looks like allergy but is due to deficiency of the enzyme lactase.

However, this classification is not universally accepted; therefore the terms *food sensitivity, hypersensitivity, allergy,* and *intolerance* are often used interchangeably. The American Academy of Allergy and Immunology further suggests defining food-induced reactions according to the following: *adverse food reactions, food hypersensitivity (allergy), food anaphylaxis, food intolerance, food idiosyncrasy, food toxicity or poisoning, anaphylactoid reaction to food, pharmacologic food reaction,* and *metabolic food reaction* (American Academy of Pediatrics, 1998a).

Food allergy is caused by exposure to *allergens,* usually proteins (but not the smaller amino acids) that are capable of inducing IgE antibody formation ("sensitization") when ingested. *Sensitization* refers to the initial exposure of an individual to an allergen, resulting in an immune response; subsequent exposure induces a much stronger response that is clinically apparent. Consequently, food hypersensitivity typically occurs after the food has been ingested one or more times. In infants an allergic response can occur with the first ingestion because of transplacental sensitization in utero or because of sensitization to the substance passed through breast milk. Allergens can also produce an allergic response when inhaled or injected, but these routes rarely apply to food allergens. (See also discussion of asthma in Chapter 32.) The most common food allergens are eggs, cow's milk, peanuts, soy, wheat, corn, nuts from trees, shell fish, and fish (Sicherer, 2001) (Box 13-3).

Food allergies can occur at any time but are common during infancy, because the immature intestinal tract is more permeable to proteins than the mature intestinal tract, thus increasing the likelihood of an immune response. Allergies in general demonstrate a genetic component: children who have one parent with allergy have a 50% or greater risk of developing allergy; children who have

both parents with allergy have up to a 100% risk of developing allergy. Allergy with a hereditary tendency is referred to as *atopy.* Some infants with atopy can be identified at birth from elevated levels of IgE in cord blood.

Deaths have been reported in children who suffered an anaphylactic reaction to food. Onset of the reactions occurred shortly after ingestion (5 to 30 minutes). In most of the children the reactions did not begin with skin signs, such as hives, red rash, and flushing, but rather as an acute asthma attack. Parents, teachers, and daycare workers should be educated regarding signs and symptoms of food hypersensitivity reactions. Those with food sensitivity should avoid unfamiliar foods, as well as restaurants that do not disclose food ingredients. Hidden ingredients in prepared foods have been implicated as a potential source.

> **NURSING ALERT** Patients with extremely sensitive food allergies should wear a medical identification bracelet and have an injectible epinephrine cartridge (Epipen) readily available. (See Anaphylaxis, Chapter 29.)

Although the reason is unknown, many children "outgrow" their food allergies. Children who are allergic to more than one food may develop tolerance to each food at a different time. The most common allergens, such as soy, are outgrown less readily than other food allergens. Because of the tendency to lose the hypersensitivity, allergenic foods should be reintroduced into the diet after a period of abstinence (usually a year or more) to evaluate if the food can be

---

**Box 13-3** ■ ■ ■
**Hyperallergenic Foods/Sources**

**Milk\***: Ice cream, butter, margarine (if it contains dairy products), yogurt, cheese, pudding, baked goods, wieners, bologna, canned creamed soups, instant breakfast drinks, powdered milk drinks, milk chocolate

**Eggs\***: Mayonnaise, creamy salad dressing, baked goods, egg noodles, some cake icing, meringue, custard, pancakes, French toast, root beer

**Wheat\***: Almost all baked goods, wieners, bologna, pressed or chopped cold cuts, gravy, pasta, some canned soups

**Legumes:** Peanuts,\* peanut butter or oil, beans, peas, lentils

**Nuts\***: Some chocolates, candy, baked goods, cherry soda (may be flavored with a nut extract), walnut oil

**Fish or shellfish\***: Cod liver oil, pizza with anchovies, Caesar salad dressing, any food fried in same oil as fish

**Soy\***: Soy sauce, teriyaki or worcestershire sauce, tofu, baked goods using soy flour or oil, soy nuts, soy infant formulas or milk, soybean paste, tuna packed in vegetable oil, many margarines

**Chocolate:** Cola beverages, cocoa, chocolate-flavored drinks

**Buckwheat:** Some cereals, pancakes

**Pork, chicken:** Bacon, wieners, sausage, pork fat, chicken broth

**Strawberries, melon, pineapple:** Gelatin, syrups

**Corn:** Popcorn, cereal, muffins, cornstarch, corn meal, corn bread, corn tortilla

**Citrus fruits:** Orange, lemon, lime, grapefruit; any of these in drinks, gelatin, juice, or medicines

**Tomatoes:** Juice, some vegetable soups, spaghetti, pizza sauce, catsup

**Spices:** Chili, pepper, vinegar, cinnamon

---

\*Most common allergens.

safely added to the diet. Foods that are associated with severe anaphylactic reactions, however, will continue to present a lifelong risk and must be avoided (Anderson, 1997).

Breast-feeding is now considered to be a primary consideration for avoiding atopy in families with known food sensitivities; however, there is evidence that cow's milk protein is transferred via human milk, causing some infants to have hypersensitivity reactions (Jarvinen, Makinen-Kiljunen, and Suomalainen, 1999). The breast-feeding mother is encouraged to avoid allergenic foods such as peanuts, tree nuts, soy, and fish during the first 6 to 8 months of breast-feeding. In addition, supplementation, if required, is best with hydrolysated, *not soy* formulas (American Academy of Pediatrics, 1998b). The strategies listed in the Guidelines box are those recommended by most authorities for infants with a family history of atopy.*

## Cow's Milk Allergy

Cow's milk allergy is a multifaceted disorder representing adverse systemic and local gastrointestinal reactions to cow's

---

*Further information for parents of infants with food allergies is available from the **American Academy of Allergy, Asthma, and Immunology,** 611 E Wells St, Milwaukee, WI 52202, (800) 822-2762; www.aaai.org. Information is also available from the **Food Allergy Network,** (800) 929-4040; www.foodallergy.org, on school food allergy program and food allergy resources.

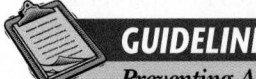

## GUIDELINES
### *Preventing Atopy in Children*

**IDENTIFY CHILDREN AT RISK**

Family history of allergy
Increased IgE in cord blood and postnatal serum
Dry, flaky skin

**PRENATAL PRECAUTIONS (LAST TRIMESTER)**

Avoid any known food allergens
Avoid milk and other dairy products, peanuts, and eggs
Minimize ingestion of other hyperallergenic foods (see Box 13-3)

**POSTNATAL PRECAUTIONS**

Breast milk or casein/whey hydrolysate formula (e.g., Nutramigen, Pregestimil, Alimentum) or amino acid-based formula (Neocate) exclusively for at least 6 months
No solid food for first 6 months
No cow's milk or soy formula for 12 months
No egg, fish, corn, citrus, peanuts, nuts, or chocolate for 12 to 18 months
One new food added at 5 to 7-day intervals to identify possible reaction

**ENVIRONMENTAL CONTROL**

Limited exposure to dust mites, molds, furry animals, and cigarette smoke

---

Data from Johnstone D: Strategy for intervention of food allergy in infants, *Int Pediatr* 4(4):319-325, 1989; Zeiger R and others: Effectiveness of dietary manipulation in the prevention of food allergy in infants, part 2, *J Allergy Clin Immunol* 78 (1 pt 2):224-238, 1986; and Wood RA: Prospects for the prevention of allergy in children, *Curr Opin Pediatr* 8(6):601-605, 1995.

---

milk protein. (This discussion is centered on cow's milk protein found in commercial infant formulas; *whole milk* is not recommended for infants under 12 months of age.) The hypersensitivity may be manifested within the first 4 months of life through a variety of signs and symptoms (Box 13-4) that may appear within 45 minutes of milk ingestion or after a period of several days. The diagnosis may initially be made from the history, although the history alone is not diagnostic; the timing and diversity of clinical manifestations vary greatly. For example, cow's milk allergy may be manifested as colic (see p. 571), gastroesophageal reflux, chronic constipation, or sleeplessness in an otherwise healthy infant.

**Diagnostic Evaluation.** A number of diagnostic tests may be performed, including stool analysis for blood, eosinophils, and leukocytes (both frank and occult bleeding can occur from the colitis), serum IgE levels, skin-prick or scratch testing, and radioallergosorbent test (RAST) (measures IgE antibodies to specific allergens in serum by radioimmunoassay). Both skin testing and RAST may help identity the offending food, but the results are not always conclusive. No single diagnostic test is considered to be definitive for the diagnosis (Wylie, 1996; Baron, 2000).

The most definitive diagnostic strategy is elimination of cow's milk, followed by challenge testing after improvement of symptoms. Challenge testing involves reintroducing small quantities of cow's milk to the diet to detect resurgence of symptoms; at times challenge testing involves the use of a placebo so that the parent is unaware of or "blind" to the timing of allergen ingestion. A double-blind placebo-controlled food challenge (DBPCFC) is the gold standard for diagnosing food allergies, yet is not used very often for cow's milk allergy in infants (Baron, 2000).

> **NURSING ALERT**   Careful observation of the child is required during a challenge test because of the possibility of anaphylactic reaction.

**Therapeutic Management.** Treatment of cow's milk allergy is elimination of cow's milk–based formula and all other dairy products. For infants fed cow's milk formula, this primarily involves changing the formula to a casein hydrolysate milk formula (Pregestimil, Nutramigen, or Alimentum), in which the protein has been broken down (or "predigested") into its amino acids through enzymatic hy-

---

**Box 13-4**
### Common Clinical Manifestations of Cow's Milk Sensitivity

| GASTROINTESTINAL | RESPIRATORY | OTHER SIGNS AND SYMPTOMS |
|---|---|---|
| Diarrhea | Rhinitis | Eczema |
| Vomiting | Bronchitis | Excessive crying |
| Colic | Asthma | Pallor (from |
| Wheezing | Sneezing | anemia secondary |
| Gastroesophageal reflux | Coughing | to chronic blood |
| | Chronic nasal discharge | loss in GI |
| Bloody stools | | tract) |
| Rectal bleeding | | Fussiness/irritability |

drolysis. Although the American Academy of Pediatrics (1998b) recommend the use of hydrolyzed formulas for cow's milk–protein allergy, many practitioners may start a soy formula instead. Approximately 50% of infants who are sensitive to cow's milk protein will also demonstrate sensitivity to soy, yet soy is less expensive than protein hydrolysate formula. Another choice is the amino acid–based formula, Neocate. Goat's milk is not an acceptable substitute because it cross-reacts with cow's milk protein, is deficient in folic acid, and is unsuitable as the only source of calories. Infants who are breast-fed but have symptoms of cow's milk hypersensitivity are treated by eliminating all peanuts and tree nuts from the lactating mother's diet, and possibly eggs and milk, depending on the mother's motivation for compliance (American Academy of Pediatrics, 1998a). If maternal dairy intake is restricted, vitamin D and calcium supplementation should be considered to prevent deficiency. Infants are maintained on the milk-free diet for 1 or 2 years, after which time very small quantities of milk are reintroduced; eggs and fish may be introduced at 2 to 3 years of age.

**Nursing Considerations.** The principal nursing objectives are identification of potential milk allergy and appropriate counseling of parents regarding substitute formulas. Parents will often interpret gastrointestinal symptoms such as spitting up and a loose stool or fussiness as an indication that the infant is allergic to cow's milk and switch the infant to a variety of formulas in an attempt to resolve the problem. In fact, 28% of parents reported their infants as being allergic to cow's milk–based formula, yet extensive testing revealed that only 8% were truly sensitive to cow's milk protein (Sicherer, 2001). Parents need much reassurance regarding the needs of nonverbal infants when such an array of symptoms are evidenced. Endless nights of lost sleep and a crying infant may promote feelings of parenting inadequacy and role conflict, thus aggravating the situation. Nurses can reassure parents that many of these symptoms are common and the reasons are often never found yet the child does achieve appropriate growth and development; acute symptoms are reported to the practitioner for further evaluation. The protein hydrolysate formulas tend to be less palatable and more expensive than milk-based formulas. Consequently, the child's reluctance to accept the new formula may be a problem. This can be overcome by adding

## FAMILY HOME CARE
### Controlling Symptoms of Lactose Intolerance

In infants substitute soy-based formula for cow's milk formula or human milk.

Limit milk consumption to one glass at a time.

Drink milk with other foods rather than alone.

Eat hard cheese, cottage cheese, or yogurt instead of drinking milk.

Use enzyme tablets (Lactaid, Lactrase, Dairy Ease) to predigest the lactose in milk or supplement the body's own lactase (add tablets to milk or sprinkle on dairy products such as ice cream).

Eat small amounts of dairy foods daily to help colonic bacteria adapt to ingested lactose.

nonnutritive, hypoallergenic flavor packets (Christie, 1999) or by introducing the formula gradually over a few days using 1 ounce of new formula to 7 ounces of old formula, then 2 to 6 ounces, 3 to 5, and as needed. Parents also need to be reassured that the infant will receive complete nutrition from the new formula and will suffer no ill effects from the absence of cow's milk.

Once solid foods are started, parents need guidance in avoiding milk products, although many children reportedly outgrow cow's milk protein sensitivity by 3 to 4 years of age (Sicherer, 2001) (see Box 13-3). Carefully reading all food labels helps avoid exposure to prepared foods containing milk products.

### Lactose Intolerance

Lactose intolerance refers to at least three different entities that involve a deficiency of the enzyme **lactase,** which is needed for the hydrolysis or digestion of lactose in the small intestine (lactose is hydrolyzed into glucose and galactose). *Congenital lactase deficiency* occurs soon after birth once the newborn has consumed lactose-containing milk (human milk or commercial formula). This inborn error of metabolism involves the complete absence or severely reduced presence of lactase, is extremely rare, and requires lifelong lactose-free or extremely reduced lactose diet (McBean and Miller, 1998).

*Late-onset lactase deficiency,* sometimes referred to as *primary lactase deficiency,* is the most common type of lactose intolerance and is manifested usually around 3 to 7 years of age, although the time of onset is variable. This decrease in intestinal lactase is not a disease but is considered a normal physiologic process (McBean and Miller, 1998). Ethnic groups with a high incidence of lactase deficiency include Asians, southern Europeans, Arabs, Israelis, and African-Americans.

Lactose intolerance or *secondary lactase deficiency* may also occur secondary to damage of the intestinal lumen, which decreases or destroys the enzyme lactase. Cystic fibrosis, sprue, kwashiorkor, or infections such as giardiasis, HIV, or rotavirus may cause a temporary or permanent lactose intolerance.

The primary symptoms of lactose intolerance include abdominal pain, bloating, flatulence, and diarrhea. The onset of symptoms occurs within 30 minutes to several hours of lactose consumption. Infants with congenital lactase deficiency may have severe watery diarrhea and stools positive for reducing substances (Baron, 2000).

Lactose intolerance may be diagnosed on the basis of the history and improvement with a lactose-reduced diet. The breath hydrogen test is used to positively diagnose the condition. Breath samples in lactose-deficient individuals will yield a higher percentage of hydrogen (20 ppm or more above baseline). The breath hydrogen test is difficult to perform in infants and small toddlers. Direct endoscopic visualization of the gastric mucosa and digestive fluid sampling is one alternative diagnostic method for lactase deficiency (Baron, 2000).

Treatment of lactose intolerance is elimination of offending dairy products or the use of enzyme replacement. (See Family Home Care box.) In infants, soy-based formula can be substituted for cow's milk formula or human milk

(American Academy of Pediatrics, 1998b). Most people are able to tolerate small amounts of lactose (Srinivasan and Minocha, 1998). Milk taken at meals may be better tolerated than when taken alone. Pretreated milk (with microbial-derived lactase) is reported to be effective in improving lactose absorption. Because dairy products are a major source of calcium and vitamin D, supplementation of these nutrients is needed to prevent deficiency. Yogurt contains inactive lactase enzyme, which is activated by the temperature and pH of the duodenum; this lactase activity substitutes for the lack of endogenous lactase. Fresh yogurt may be tolerated better than frozen yogurt.

**Nursing Considerations.**   Nursing care is similar to the interventions discussed for cow's milk allergy: assisting in establishing a definitive diagnosis before switching formula in infant or eliminating dairy products in older child; explaining the dietary restrictions to the family; identifying alternative sources of calcium such as yogurt; explaining the importance of supplementation; and discussing sources of lactose, especially hidden sources such as its use as a bulk agent in certain medications, and ways of controlling the symptoms. (See Family Home Care box.) Parents are advised to check with the pharmacist regarding the avoidance of lactose-containing medications when obtaining medication.*

# FEEDING DIFFICULTIES

## Improper Feeding Technique

A common cause of feeding problems is improper feeding technique. A satisfactory feeding requires a number of mechanical skills, such as placing the infant to the breast properly (see Chapter 8, Breast-feeding); holding the bottle at an angle that allows fluid, not air, to flow into the nipple; "reading" the infant's cues for burping or satiation; and holding the infant during feeding, rather than propping the bottle. A number of other problems can also occur singly or in combination, such as feeding too much or too little food; feeding too often, especially during the night, or too infrequently; selecting inappropriate foods for the infant's physiologic and motor development; and incorrectly preparing formula. While such feeding problems are more common in first-time inexperienced parents, they can also occur with seasoned parents who are unprepared for an infant with different needs or less clear cues of hunger or satiation.

Most of these feeding problems are easily corrected with reassurance, guidance and demonstration. Early assessment is essential to prevent complex problems from developing between parent and child at mealtime.

## Regurgitation and "Spitting Up"

The return of small amounts of food after a feeding is a common occurrence during infancy. It should not be confused with actual vomiting, which can be associated with a number of disturbances that may be insignificant or serious.

It is usually benign, although persistent regurgitation necessitates medical evaluation to rule out gastroesophageal reflux. For clarification the following terms are defined:

**Regurgitation**—Return of undigested food from the stomach, usually accompanied by burping

**Spitting up**—Dribbling of unswallowed formula from the infant's mouth immediately after a feeding

The normal occurrence of regurgitation or spitting up should be explained to parents, especially to those who are unduly concerned about it. Regurgitation can be reduced by some simple measures, such as frequent burping during and after feeding, minimum handling during and after feeding, and positioning the child on the right side with the head slightly elevated after feeding. The inconvenience of spitting up can be managed with the use of absorbent bibs on the infant and protective cloths on the parent.

Sometimes frequent dribbling of formula causes excoriation of the corners of the mouth, chin, and neck. Keeping the area dry promotes healing but can be difficult to maintain. Helpful suggestions include applying a thin film of petrolatum or A and D Ointment to the affected areas after cleansing and using absorbent nonplastic-lined terry-cloth bibs, which are changed frequently.

## Paroxysmal Abdominal Pain (Colic)

Colic is generally described as paroxysmal abdominal pain or cramping that is manifested by loud crying and drawing the legs up to the abdomen. Other definitions include variables such as duration of cry greater than 3 hours a day, occurring more than 3 days per week, and parental dissatisfaction with the child's behavior. Some studies report an increase in symptoms (fussiness and crying) in the late afternoon or evening; however, in some infants the onset of symptoms occurs at another time. Colic is more common in young infants under the age of 3 months than in older infants, and infants with "difficult" temperaments are more likely to be colicky. Despite the obvious behavioral indications of pain, the infant with colic gains weight and usually thrives.

### Etiology

Among the theories that have been investigated as potential causes are too rapid feeding, overeating, swallowing excessive air, improper feeding technique (especially in positioning and burping), and emotional stress or tension between parent and child. Although all of these may occur, there is no evidence that one factor is consistently present. In some infants colic may be a sign of cow's milk allergy or intolerance, and eliminating cow's milk products from the infant's diet and the diet of lactating mothers can reduce the symptoms. Parental smoking has also been associated with colic.

Some investigators discount the biologic causes of colic and attribute the problem to parents' ineffective responses to the infant's crying or too little carrying of the infant. The incidence of colic differs markedly among social classes—with more parents with a higher socioeconomic status reporting colic. A possible explanation may be greater acceptance of an infant's crying behavior among lower social groups.

*Parents may find updated resources on lactose intolerance at www. lactose.net.

Carbohydrate malabsorption is a commonly accepted cause of colic because of the infant's clinical signs during the crying episodes (Balon, 1997). However, excessive air swallowing and colonic fermentation leading to intestinal gas as a cause of colic has been discounted (Sferra and Heitlinger, 1996). Infant temperament has also been postulated as a cause of colic (Jacobson and Melvin, 1995). One theory suggests that there is a dysregulation of the brain-gut neural pathways, primarily in the right hemisphere, resulting in a disruption of neurochemical balance of dopamine and subsequent manifestations of crying and fussiness (Friedman, 1996).

## Therapeutic Management

Management of colic should begin with an investigation of diagnosable causes, such as cow's milk allergy. If a sensitivity to cow's milk is strongly suspected, a trial substitution of another formula, such as a casein hydrolysate (Nutramigen, Alimentum, Pregestimil), is warranted. Soy formulas are usually avoided because of the possibility of sensitivity to soy protein as well. When no specific inciting agent can be found, the supportive measures discussed under Nursing Considerations are employed. (See Cultural Awareness box.)

The use of drugs, including sedatives, antispasmodics, antihistamines, and antiflatulents, is sometimes recommended. The most commonly used sedatives are phenobarbitol, hydroxyzine hydrochloride (Atarax), and chloral hydrate. Simethicone (Mylicon) may also help allay the symptoms of colic. It is important to note that in most controlled studies none of these drugs completely reduce the symptoms of colic (Balon, 1997; Treem, 1994).

Two European studies found a significant decrease in the amount of crying time of colicky infants who were fed whey hydrolyzed formula (Lucassen and others, 2000) or a casein hydrolyzed formula (Jakobsson and others, 2000); in the latter study infants were known to be sensitive to cow's milk protein at entry to the study. In an extensive review of reported treatments for colic, Garrison and Christakis (2000) noted that the most promising results occurred with dietary changes such as feeding hypoallergenic formulas, treating with herbal tea, and decreasing the infant's environmental

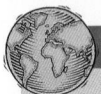

## CULTURAL AWARENESS
### Colic

Herbal teas (chamomile, vervain, licorice, fennel, and balm mint) containing natural antispasmodic properties are used as a remedy for colic in Israel. According to one study, infants given herbal tea (vs a placebo) showed significant improvement in irritability and crying associated with colic (Weizman and others, 1993).

## FAMILY HOME CARE
### Relieving Colic

Place infant prone over a covered hot-water bottle, heated towel, or covered heating pad.
Massage infant's abdomen.
Respond immediately to the crying.
Change infant's position frequently; walk with child's face down and with body across parent's arm, with parent's hand under infant's abdomen, applying gentle pressure (Fig. 13-3).
Use a front carrier for transporting infant.
Swaddle infant tightly with a soft, stretchy blanket.
Place infant in a wind-up swing.
Take infant for car rides or outside for a change in environment.
Use bottles that minimize air swallowing (curved bottle and/or inner collapsible bag).
Use a commercial device* in the crib that stimulates the vibration and sound of a car ride or plays soothing "noise," in utero sounds, or music.†
Provide smaller, frequent feedings; burp infant during and after feedings using the shoulder position or sitting upright, and place infant in an upright seat after feedings.
Introduce a pacifier for added sucking.
In breast-fed infants, mother should avoid all milk products for a trial period.
If household members smoke, avoid smoking near infant; preferably confine smoking activity to outside of home.
Give appropriate dose of acetaminophen elixir or suppository if suggested by health professional; not recommended for daily use.
If nothing reduces the crying, place infant in crib and allow to cry; periodically hold and comfort child and put down again.

*Sweet Dreems, Inc, Sleep Tight Order Department, 4710 E Walnut St, Westerville, OH 43081; (800) NO COLIC, (800) 662-6542; www.colic.com.
†Suggested infant relaxation music: "Heartbeat Lullabies" by Terry Woodford. Available from Baby-Go-To-Sleep Center, Audio Therapy Innovations, Inc, PO Box 550, Colorado Springs, CO 80901; (800) 537-7748; www.babygotosleep.com.
Helpful information may also be found at www.colichelp.com.

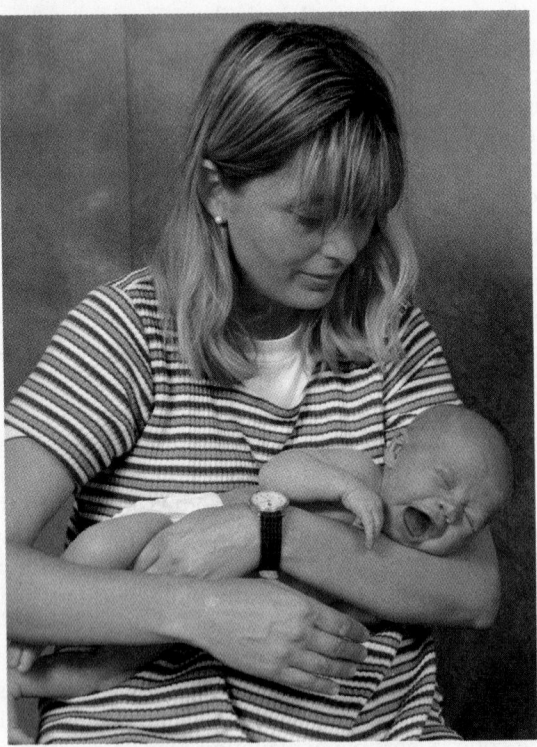

**Fig. 13-3** The "colic carry" may be comforting to an infant with colic. (Courtesy Paul Vincent Kuntz, Texas Children's Hospital.)

stimuli. Additional findings suggest that breast-feeding mothers' avoidance of exposure to foods such as peanuts, nuts, and cow's milk may play a small role in the amelioration of colicky symptoms. Infants who were treated with lactase in two of the studies evaluated did not have a significant change in crying and fussiness (Garrison and Christakis, 2000). Herbal tea (chamomile), offered at the onset of colic episodes, as much as 3 times a day with a maximum dose of 150 ml, was effective in reducing symptoms of colic in 57% of the infants studied (Weizman and others, 1993).

## Nursing Considerations

The initial step in managing colic is to take a thorough, detailed history of the usual daily events. Areas that should be stressed include (1) the infant's diet; (2) the diet of the breast-feeding mother; (3) the time of day when crying occurs; (4) the relationship of the crying to feeding time; (5) the presence of specific family members during the crying and habits of family members, such as smoking; (6) activity of the mother or usual caregiver before, during, and after the crying; (7) characteristics of the cry (duration, intensity); (8) measures used to relieve the crying and their effectiveness; and (9) the infant's stooling, voiding, and sleeping patterns. Of special emphasis is a careful assessment of the feeding process via demonstration by the parent.

If cow's milk sensitivity is suspected, breast-feeding mothers should follow a milk-free diet (see Box 13-3) for a minimum of 3 to 5 days in an attempt to reduce symptoms in the infant. Mothers need to be cautioned that some nondairy creamers may contain calcium caseinate, a cow's milk protein. If a milk-free diet is helpful, lactating mothers may need calcium supplements to meet the body's requirement. Bottle-fed infants may improve with the same dietary modifications as for the child with cow's milk allergy (see p. 569).

When no cause can be identified, it is preferable to determine the time of the onset of crying and attempt to manipulate the circumstances associated with it. For example, some infants have episodes of colic around the family's dinner time, when all household members are home and often tired and busy. The overstimulating, more tense atmosphere may upset the infant. Changing the evening routine, such as encouraging someone else to prepare dinner, preparing dinner earlier in the day, and feeding the infant in a quieter area of the house, may help. Other approaches for relieving colic are listed in the Family Home Care box. Parents are encouraged to try as many of these approaches as possible because not all are effective for every infant. (See Family Focus and Critical Thinking Exercise boxes.) One study confirmed that children with colic (as infants) were

---

### FAMILY FOCUS
#### Colic

Although colic is considered a minor ailment, the presence of a colicky, crying, irritable infant can have an intense emotional impact on parent-child attachment and family relationships. Parents, especially mothers, often relate histories of a daily routine that is laden with feelings of frustration, anger, despair, and helplessness. A vicious cycle ensues in which the parent's own anxiety may be transferred to the infant, further increasing the tension, irritability, and crying.

One of the most important areas of nursing concern is the support of parents during the colic period. It should be stressed that despite the crying and obvious pain, the infant is doing well. Colic disappears spontaneously, usually by 3 to 4 months of age, although guarantees should never be given, because it may continue for much longer. The parent, especially the mother, may be encouraged to leave the house and arrange for some free time. Most important, it should be emphasized that colic does not indicate poor or inadequate parenting. Parents' negative feelings toward the infant and insecurities regarding their parenting abilities are normal. Parents are encouraged to talk about such feelings, because active listening may do more to relieve the colic syndrome than offering stereotyped advice, remedies, and glib statements such as "Don't worry about it; your child will eventually outgrow the colicky spells."

Parents may find the following books supportive and informative: *Crying Baby, Sleepless Nights: Why Your Baby Is Crying and What You Can Do About It* by Sandy Jones, Linda Ziedrich, and Mariah Thompson, 1992, Harvard Common Press; and *The Fussy Baby Book: Parenting Your High-Need Child from Birth to Five* by William Sears and Martha Sears., 1996, Little Brown & Co.

---

### Critical Thinking Exercise
#### Colic

During a routine clinic visit you notice that the mother of a 2-month-old infant appears very tired, gets easily confused answering simple questions, and mentions that the infant cries much more than her first child did and for no apparent reason. You direct the focus of the interview on the infant's behavior preceding the crying spells; feeding habits, including dietary history; and patterns of sleep. The mother suspects that the infant has colic. What would be the best response to this mother?

FIRST, THINK ABOUT IT . . .

- What is the purpose of your thinking?
- What would the consequences be if you put your thoughts into actions?

1. "Are you concerned that maybe you have done something wrong with this child?"
2. "You must feel a little frustrated about this situation; can you tell me more about your concerns and how you are managing?"
3. "Colic is a complex problem for which there are few solutions other than giving the child medications and tolerating the crying the best way possible."
4. "We have some pamphlets on colic in the lobby; after you see the doctor, be sure to pick one up and read it at home."

*The best response is two. The purpose is to allow the mother time to express her feelings about the colicky infant, as well as her own fears, and open the door for a discussion of some solutions to the problem. Options three and four end the discussion and are inappropriate nursing actions. Option one is too direct a question at this point in the interview and may suggest a concern the mother never had or may intensify any guilt.*

more emotional than most children at age 4, yet there were no serious side effects or complications of the problem in those in the study. At 4 years of age the children evaluated were developing appropriately physically and mentally (Canivet, Jakobsson, and Hagander, 2000).

## Rumination

Rumination is the active, voluntary return of swallowed food into the mouth. The food is then rechewed, partially or completely reswallowed, or expelled. Technically, this is not a feeding problem, because infant ruminators usually have fairly good appetites. However, in some instances rumination may lead to progressive malnutrition, marasmus (Thame, Burton and Forrester, 2000), and even death, because considerable food and fluid loss can occur.

Rumination differs from regurgitation, which is involuntary. The ruminating infant makes purposeful movements of the mouth, tongue, and stomach in an attempt to force food back into the oropharynx. On successful rumination the infant is obviously satisfied with the activity.

Organic causes for rumination are rarely found, although the possibility of gastroesophageal reflux should be investigated in the differential diagnosis. It may also be seen in mentally handicapped children. However, it is most often considered a result of a disturbed parent-child relationship. The factors culminating in the disorder may be similar to those described in nonorganic failure to thrive. Some authorities believe rumination is a conditioned behavioral response to an increased need for self-stimulation or parental attention.

Treatment typically involves psychotherapy to provide improved parenting ability or behavior-modification techniques to modify eating patterns. Behavioral approaches vary but may include increased attention, such as holding before, during, and after meals.

### Nursing Considerations

The primary objective is to terminate the ruminating behavior and restore a nurturing environment. A structured feeding plan, similar to those used to feed the child with nonorganic failure to thrive (see p. 577), may be required in addition to behavior modification. Parents need to learn how to feed the child, and follow-up after discharge is essential to prevent a recurrence of the behavior.

## Failure to Thrive (FTT)

FTT is a sign of inadequate growth resulting from inability to obtain and/or use calories required for growth. FTT has no universal definition, although one of the more common parameters is a weight (and sometimes height) that falls below the 5th percentile for the child's age. Some authorities prefer the 3rd percentile as a criterion, but the widely used National Center for Health Statistics growth charts include only the 5th, not the 3rd, percentile in their measurements. Growth measurements alone are not used to diagnose FTT. Rather, the finding of a persistent deviation from an established growth curve is cause for concern.

Three general categories of FTT are the following:

1. **Organic failure to thrive (OFTT)**—Result of a physical cause, such as congenital heart defects, neurologic lesions, microcephaly, chronic renal failure, gastroesophageal reflux, malabsorption syndrome, endocrine dysfunction, cystic fibrosis, or acquired immunodeficiency syndrome (AIDS).
2. **Nonorganic failure to thrive (NFTT)**—Has a definable cause that is unrelated to disease. NFTT is most often the result of psychosocial factors, such as inadequate parental knowledge of nutrition; deficiency in maternal care or a disturbance in maternal-child attachment; or a disturbance in the child's ability to separate from the parent, leading to food refusal to maintain attention.
3. **Idiopathic failure to thrive**—Unexplained by the usual organic and environmental etiologies but may also be classified as NFTT. Both categories of NFTT account for the majority of cases of FTT.

Traditionally the category of NFTT has implied a disturbance in the parent-child interaction. However, this is not always the case. Many other factors can lead to inadequate feeding of the infant, such as the following:

**Poverty**—Lack of funds to buy sufficient food; may dilute formula to extend available supply; uninsured, no primary care practitioner, or homeless

**Health beliefs**—Use of fad diets; excessive concern with preventing conditions such as obesity or hypercholesterolemia

**Inadequate nutrition knowledge**—Cultural confusion of newly arrived immigrants who are unaware of appropriate food selections in American markets; parents with cognitive impairment and parents who are teens or who had inadequate parenting from broken or distressed families

**Family stress**—Overwhelming involvement with another chronically ill child; any number of other stresses (financial, marital, excessive parenting and employment responsibilities, single parent employed full-time, depression, substance abuse, acute grief)

**Feeding resistance**—Result of nonoral nutritional therapy early in life (e.g., severe prematurity, extracorporeal membrane oxygenation [ECMO], severe cleft lip/palate repaired late, congenital diaphragmatic hernia)

**Insufficient breast milk**—Result of a number of different causes (fatigue, illness, poor release of milk, breast surgery augmentation, lack of maternal confidence or support)

In these instances parent education and provision of necessary supports (financial or psychosocial) are successful in correcting the reason for the malnutrition. Dealing with families in which a child has NFTT because of a parent-child disturbance is much more difficult and is the focus of the nursing care discussion.

### Diagnostic Evaluation

Diagnosis is initially made from evidence of growth failure. If FTT is recent, the weight, but not the height, is below accepted standards (usually the 5th percentile); if FTT is long-standing, both weight and height are low, indicating chronic malnutrition. Additional diagnostic procedures include a complete health and dietary history (including perinatal history), physical examination for evidence of organic causes, developmental assessment, and a family assessment. Other tests (lead toxicity, anemia, stool reducing substances, occult blood, ova and parasites, alkaline phosphatase, and zinc levels) are selected *only* as indicated to rule out organic problems. To prevent the overuse of diagnostic procedures,

NFTT should be considered *early* in the differential diagnosis. To avoid the social stigma of NFTT during the early investigative phase, many health care workers use the term *growth delay (or failure)* until the actual cause is established.

## Therapeutic Management

Regardless of the cause of FTT, the treatment is directed at reversing the malnutrition. The goal is to provide sufficient calories to support "catch-up" growth—a rate of growth greater than the expected rate for age. Any coexisting medical problems are treated.

In most cases of NFTT a multidisciplinary team of physician, nurse, dietitian, child-life specialist, occupational therapist, pediatric feeding specialist, and social worker or mental health professional is needed to deal with the multiple problems. Efforts are made to relieve any additional stresses on the family by offering referrals to welfare agencies or supplemental food programs.

## Prognosis

The prognosis for NFTT is related to the cause. If the parents have simply been ignorant of the infant's needs, teaching may remedy the child's limited caloric intake and permanently reverse the growth failure. Inadequate or infrequent feeding periods by the infant's primary caretaker are often observed to be the cause of NFTT in conjunction with family disorganization. Factors related to poor prognosis are severe feeding resistance, lack of awareness in and cooperation from the parent(s), low family income, low maternal educational level, adolescent mother, and early age of onset of NFTT. Many of these children are below normal in intellectual development, have poorer language development and less well-developed reading skills, attain lower social maturity, and have a higher incidence of behavioral disturbances. Such findings indicate that a long-term plan is needed for the optimal development of these children.

## Nursing Considerations

Caring for the child with NFTT presents many nursing challenges, whether treatment takes place in the hospital, clinic, or home. Providing a positive feeding environment, teaching the parent successful feeding strategies, and supporting the child and family are essential components of care.

Nurses play a critical role in the diagnosis of NFTT through their assessment of the child, parents, and family interactions. (See Evidence-Based Practice box.) Knowl-

## EVIDENCE-BASED PRACTICE
### Failure to Thrive

A 4-month-old boy, Derek, is under your care on the pediatric unit with an initial diagnosis of FTT secondary to inadequate maternal care. Derek's birth weight was 9 pounds 6 ounces, and he now weighs 10 pounds 8 ounces. His mother, Rhonda, is $18\frac{1}{2}$ years old, and Derek is her first baby. She lives at home with her parents, and the biologic father is not involved. She is in the room with Derek when you go in to do your morning assessment. Derek has an intravenous intermittent infusion device in his left hand, his color is pink, and he is actively playing with a squeeze toy; he turns toward your voice and holds eye contact with you before looking at his mom and then starting to cry. Rhonda picks him up and consoles him with a soothing voice. Once you complete Derek's physical assessment, what would be the next step in assessing the cause of the growth failure?

Talk to Rhonda and obtain some data from her regarding Derek's feeding patterns, and at the same time, observe some of her physical caretaking capabilities. (*NOTE:* You spoke with the physician earlier this morning, and she indicated that Rhonda's poor parenting skills are the cause of Derek's growth failure.) Rhonda interacts appropriately with Derek, and it is approaching feeding time, so you watch as she prepares his formula. He has had three to four formula changes in the first few months as a result of suspicion of cow's milk–based formula intolerance. Derek is now taking Nutramigen with 2 tablespoons of fortified rice cereal per ounce of formula. While Rhonda feeds her son, you inquire about his feeding habits at home—feeding times, amounts fed, social context surrounding feedings, and stooling patterns. Rhonda points out that Derek "spits up a lot after his feeding." Further inquiry reveals that Derek becomes very fussy during feedings, with a taut abdomen, arching of his back, and excessive flatus. During this particular feeding you observe this occurring, yet Rhonda's interactions during feeding appear totally appropriate. She makes eye contact with Derek, talks to him, holds the bottle in an upright position, and burps him after about every ounce of formula taken. Her parents are present, and they do not give cues or indications that this behavior is any different; in fact, they report that when they take turns feeding Derek, he demonstrates the same behaviors. You note that Derek has hyperactive bowel sounds,

and he spits up roughly 1 to $1\frac{1}{2}$ ounces of undigested formula 30 minutes after the feeding.

What is your next step in this process? Derek is being appropriately hydrated with intravenous fluids and appears comfortable after spitting up. Derek's behavior patterns also fit with colic, except for the spitting up. While it is not a nursing function to establish a diagnosis, it is appropriate to assess and plan interventions to meet the child's needs. You might conclude that Derek does not appear to have FTT as a result of poor parenting and continue providing care for him and his mother to meet their needs. At the same time, you continue to support and encourage Rhonda in her parenting abilities and her parents for their help and support.

Derek eventually gains weight and is sent home 2 days later with plans for a follow-up visit by a home health nurse to see if he is continuing to gain weight. The home health care team reports that Rhonda's parenting behaviors at home are more than adequate and that he is doing better but continues to spit up and have fussy spells during feedings. The next day Derek is admitted with severe vomiting and occult blood in stools (guaiac-positive stools) to the emergency department of another local hospital. The pediatric surgeon diagnoses hypertrophic pyloric stenosis. Derek has surgery that evening and goes home 2 days later.

Lessons learned from this actual scenario are as follows:

☐ The report of FTT should be carefully followed with extensive evaluation of the multiple social and biologic factors involved.
☐ Switching formulas is common in infants when spitting up, diarrhea, and/or gastrointestinal distress are noted—on average, infants may have 3 to 3.5 formula changes during the early investigative phase (Treem, 1994).
☐ Parents (mothers) know their child's behavior better than nurses and other health care workers, often even despite their seeming lack of parenting skills. Believe them and substantiate with appropriate assessments.
☐ Colic, gastroesophageal reflux, cow's milk protein intolerance, and hypertrophic pyloric stenosis are common causes of infant feeding problems.

edge of the characteristics of children with NFTT and their families is essential in helping identify these children and hastening the confirmation of a correct diagnosis. Accurate assessment of initial weight and height and daily weight, as well as recording of all food intake, is mandatory. The feeding behavior of the child is documented, as well as the parent-child interaction during feeding, other caregiving activities, and play. An excellent feeding observation instrument is the *Nursing Child Assessment Satellite Training (NCAST) Feeding Scale,* which is designed to assess the feeding interaction of infants up to 12 months of age (Barnard and others, 1993).* (See Nutritional Assessment, Chapter 6.)

A 25-item observational scale, the *Feeding Checklist,* was developed specifically for the purpose of observing mother-infant dyads with NFTT. The checklist has helped nurses and other health care professionals in the objective assessment of key aspects of infant and toddler feeding situations related to NFTT (MacPhee and Schneider, 1996).

The approximate developmental age should be assessed on admission by administering an appropriate developmental test. Only after objective measurements are available is a plan of care for stimulation outlined. The nursing admission history and ongoing assessment should also focus on the following characteristics that have been identified in many of these children and their parents.

**The Child.** Besides showing obvious signs of malnutrition and delayed development, children with NFTT may interact differently from children with OFTT. They may display intense interest in inanimate objects, such as a toy, but much less interest in social interactions. They are often vigilant of people at a distance but become increasingly distressed as they come closer. They may dislike being touched or held and avoid face-to-face contact. However, when held, they protest briefly on being put down and are apathetic when left alone.

Often there is a history of difficult feeding, vomiting, sleep disturbance, and excessive irritability. Patterns such as crying during feedings, vomiting, hoarding food in the mouth, ruminating after feeding, refusal to switch from liquids to solids, and aversion behavior, such as turning from food or spitting food, become attention-seeking mechanisms to prolong the attention received at mealtime. In addition, chronic reduction in calories can lead to appetite depression, which compounds the problem.

A feature of many children with NFTT is their irregularity (low rhythmicity) in activities of daily living. Some of these children typify the "difficult" temperament pattern. However, another type is the passive, sleepy, lethargic infant who does not wake up for feedings. Parents who have been advised of "demand feeding schedules" may be unsure of whether to wake the child or let the child sleep. Because of their inexperience and lack of guidance, parents may develop a pattern of infrequent feeding that is inadequate to meet the infant's nutritional needs. Such characteristics in a

child do not necessarily result in NFTT. Rather, a complex set of variables is significant, such as the degree of *fit* between the child's temperament and that of the parents. Because the personalities of infants can have definite effects on the parent-child attachment process, identifying such situations of disharmony may be one approach toward prevention and anticipatory guidance.

**The Parents.** Some parents are at increased risk for attachment problems because of (1) isolation and social crisis, (2) inadequate support systems, such as teenage and single mothers, and (3) poor parenting role models when they were children. Other factors that should be considered are lack of education; physical and mental health problems, such as physical and sexual abuse, depression, or drug dependence; immaturity, especially in adolescent parents; and lack of commitment to parenting, such as giving priority to other ventures such as entertainment or employment. Often these parents and their families are under stress and in multiple chronic emotional, social, and financial crises.

■ ■ ■

Planning needs to begin as soon as the problem is identified, whether care is on an outpatient basis or hospitalization is required. The priority nursing goal is providing the infant with sufficient nutrients for growth. More specific nursing care depends on the identified cause of FTT. If an organic cause is confirmed, care is related primarily to management of the disorder. If the problem is one of inadequate knowledge regarding child feeding, parental education is required. When serious psychosocial factors are involved, hospitalization may be needed, and additional interventions are required to meet the needs of both the child and the family.

Because part of the difficulty between parent and child is dissatisfaction and frustration, the child should have a primary core of nurses when hospitalized (Fig. 13-4). Depend-

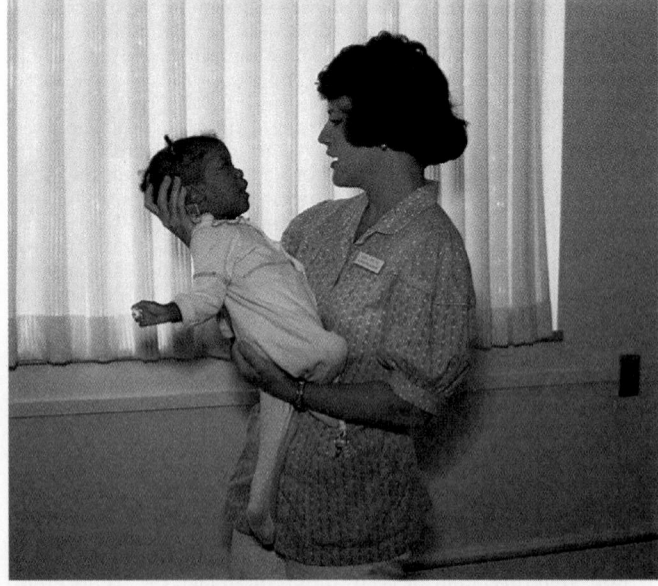

**Fig. 13-4** A consistent nurse is important in developing trust with infants who have nonorganic failure to thrive.

---

*Training is required to use the Feeding Scale, and information on the training program is available from Jean F. Kelly, PhD, Director, NCAST, WJ-10, University of Washington, Seattle, WA 98195, (206) 543-8528; e-mail: ncast@u.washington.edu.

ing on the cause of NFTT, most children are treated on an outpatient basis.

Because many of these children are responding to stimuli that have led to the negative feeding patterns, the first goal is to structure the feeding environment to encourage eating. Initially staff members may need to feed these children to assess thoroughly the difficulties encountered during the feeding process and to devise strategies that eliminate or minimize such problems. General guidelines for the feeding process are outlined in the Guidelines box.

## Nutritional Management

Four primary goals in the nutritional management of FTT are to (1) correct nutritional deficiencies and achieve appropriate weight for height, (2) allow for catch-up growth, (3) restore optimal body composition, and (4) educate the parents or primary caregivers regarding the child's nutritional requirements and appropriate feeding methods (Maggioni and Lifshitz, 1995; Corrales and Utter, 1999).

Age-appropriate foods are selected. To increase caloric intake in formula-fed infants, supplements such as carbohy-

drate additives (8 kcal/tsp) or medium-chain triglycerides (MCTs), may be added slowly, in 2 kcal/oz increments every 2 to 3 days to yield up to 28 or 30 kcal/oz. In young infants, the final caloric density of the formula should not exceed 24 kcal/oz because of the higher osmolality and renal solute load, which may be poorly tolerated (Peterson, 1993). Other carbohydrate additives include rice cereal and vegetable oil. Because vitamin and mineral deficiencies may occur, multivitamin supplementation, including zinc and iron, is recommended. For toddlers, the addition of nonfat dry milk to 24 kcal/oz formula or whole cow's milk and some foods is recommended to increase caloric density. Signs of intolerance to the formula should be carefully monitored. Breast-fed infants with NFTT may require caloric supplementation. One suggested method is to add 1 teaspoon of 24 kcal/oz formula to 3 ounces of breast milk (Corrales and Utter, 1999).

Because maladaptive feeding practices often contribute to growth failure, parents are given specific step-by-step directions for formula preparation, as well as a written schedule of feeding times. The excessive consumption of sweetened juices (Smith and Lifshitz, 1994) and sweets such as candy, which are empty calorie sources, have been implicated in the development of NFTT. Juices should be avoided in children with growth failure until adequate weight gain has been achieved with appropriate milk sources, then given in amounts not to exceed 4 oz/day.

The use of behavior-modification techniques in older infants and toddlers may be required to interrupt poor feeding patterns. Feeding times may actually involve "struggles of will" in cases of maladaptive feedings that result in NFTT. These behaviors are quite different from the occasional toddler behavior of food refusal, which is primarily developmental, not pathologic. The association of appropriate food with good or bad behaviors and consequent rewards may be part of the complex problem. Usually only in extreme cases of malnourishment are tube feedings or intravenous therapy required.

Besides attending to the physical needs of the child, the interdisciplinary team must plan care for appropriate developmental care. Once an approximate developmental age is established, a planned program of play is begun. A child-life specialist may be involved to implement and supervise the developmental care program. Every effort is made to teach the parent how to play and interact with the child.

Nursing care of these children involves a "family systems" approach. In other words, for the entire family to become healthy, each member must be helped to change. Care of the parents is aimed at helping them improve their feelings of self-esteem through positive, successful parenting skills. Initially this necessitates providing an environment in which they feel welcomed and accepted.

Teaching infant care techniques to the parents is begun through *example* and *demonstration,* not by lecturing. As the nurse perceives the infant's cues, these are emphasized to the parents. For example, during a feeding the nurse might comment that the infant is still hungry because the child sucks vigorously. When the infant is satisfied, the nurse points out that the infant is signaling this by releasing the

---

## GUIDELINES

### Feeding Children with Nonorganic Failure to Thrive

**Provide a primary core of staff to feed the child.** The same nurses are able to learn the child's cues and respond consistently.

**Provide a quiet, unstimulating atmosphere.** A number of these children are very distractible, and their attention is diverted with minimal stimuli. Older children do well at a feeding table; younger children should be held.

**Maintain a calm, even temperament throughout the meal.** Negative outbursts may be commonplace in this child's habit formation. Limits on eating behavior definitely need to be provided, but they should be stated in a firm, calm tone. If the nurse is hurried or anxious, the feeding process will not be optimized.

**Talk to the child by giving directions about eating.** "Take a bite, Lisa" is appropriate and directive. The more distractible the child, the more directive the nurse should be to refocus attention on feeding. Positive comments about feeding are actively given.

**Be persistent.** This is perhaps one of the most important guidelines. Parents often give up when the child begins negative feeding behavior. Calm perseverance through 10 to 15 minutes of food refusal will eventually diminish negative behavior. Although forced feeding is avoided, "strictly encouraged" feeding is essential.

**Maintain a face-to-face posture with the child when possible.** Encourage eye contact and remain with the child throughout the meal.

**Introduce new foods slowly.** Often these children have been exclusively bottle-fed or fed inappropriate foods for age and development. If acceptance of solids is a problem, begin with pureed food and, once accepted, advance to junior and regular solid foods.

**Follow the child's rhythm of feeding.** The child will set a rhythm when the previous conditions are met.

**Develop a structured routine.** Disruption in their other activities of daily living has great impact on feeding responses, so bathing, sleeping, dressing, and playing, as well as feeding, are structured. The nurse or parent should feed the child in the same way and place as often as possible. The length of the feeding should also be established (usually 30 minutes).

strong suck, closing the eyes, and breathing deeply and more slowly.

At the same time, the parents are offered an opportunity to care for the infant without having demands made on them. Whenever the parents participate, they are praised and encouraged to continue caring for the child.

Social agencies that can provide financial or housing assistance to lessen the stress of everyday life are also contacted. (See Nursing Care Plan: The Child with Nonorganic Failure to Thrive.*)

# SKIN DISORDERS

## Diaper Dermatitis

Dermatitis in the diaper area is encountered frequently by nurses in all pediatric settings. Approximately 35% of young children demonstrate some degree of diaper dermatitis, and about 5% have severe rash (intense erythema, scaling, papules, and ulcerations). The peak age for diaper dermatitis is 9 to 12 months and may be associated with decreased frequency of diaper changes and modifications in diet, such as the change from breast milk to formula and the introduction of solids. The incidence is greater in bottle-fed infants than in breast-fed infants.

### Pathophysiology and Clinical Manifestations

Diaper dermatitis is caused by prolonged and repetitive contact with an irritant, principally urine, feces, soaps, detergents, ointments, and friction. Although the obvious irritant in the majority of incidences is urine and feces, the specific components that contribute to irritation include a combination of factors (Fig. 13-5).

Prolonged contact of the skin with diaper wetness affects several skin properties. It produces higher friction, greater abrasion damage, increased transepidermal permeability, and increased microbial counts. Therefore, healthy skin becomes less resistant to potential irritants.

---

*In Wong DL, Hess CS: *Wong and Whaley's clinical manual of pediatric nursing,* ed 5, St Louis, 2000, Mosby.

Although ammonia was once thought to cause diaper rash because of the association between the strong odor on diapers and dermatitis, ammonia alone is not sufficient. The irritant quality of urine is related to an increase in pH from the breakdown of urea in the presence of fecal urease. The increased pH promotes the activity of fecal enzymes, principally proteases and lipases, which act as irritants. Fecal enzymes also increase the permeability of skin to bile salts, another potential irritant in feces. The decreased incidence of diaper dermatitis in breast-fed infants is believed to be related to this interaction between pH and fecal enzymes, because feces from breast-fed infants have lower fecal enzyme activity and lower pH.

The eruption of diaper dermatitis can be manifested primarily on convex surfaces or in the folds (intertriginous areas), and the lesions can represent a variety of types and configurations. Eruptions involving the skin in most intimate contact with the diaper (e.g., the convex surfaces of buttocks, inner thighs, mons pubis, and scrotum) but sparing the folds are likely to be caused by chemical irritants, especially from urine and feces (Fig. 13-6). Other causes are detergents or soaps from inadequately rinsed cloth diapers or the chemicals (alcohol) in disposable wipes.

Perianal involvement is usually the result of chemical irritation from feces, especially diarrheal stools. *Candida albicans* infection produces bright red, confluent lesions with raised borders and often with satellite lesions (Fig. 13-7). The infected area usually includes the folds and is painful. Risk factors for development of *Candida* infection are an altered immune status and antibiotic therapy.

### Therapeutic Management

Treatment is primarily related to the measures discussed under Nursing Considerations. For inflammations that do not respond to these interventions, topical glucocorticoid preparations are sometimes required. If steroids are prescribed, their use is limited to low-potency preparations, such as 1% hydrocortisone cream. Combined antifungals with potent halogenated topical steroids, such as clotrimazole/betamethasone disproprionate (Lotrisone) and nystatin/triamcinolone (Mycolog), are avoided because their

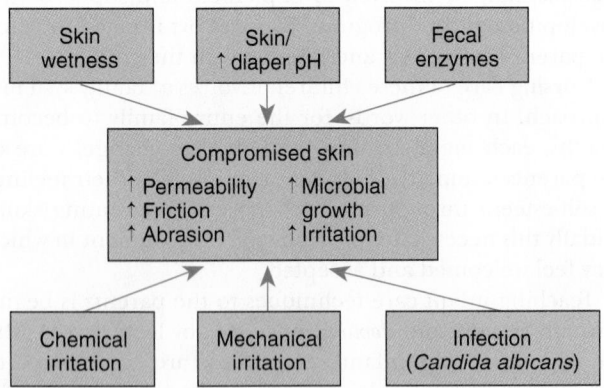

**Fig. 13-5** Principal factors involved in development of diaper dermatitis.

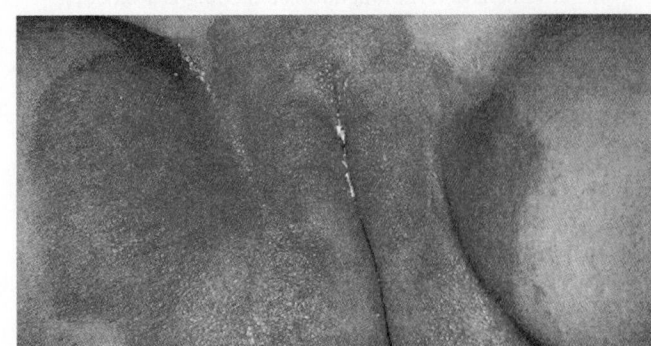

**Fig. 13-6** Irritant diaper dermatitis. Note sharply demarcated edges. (From Habif TP: *Clinical dermatology: a color guide to diagnosis and therapy,* ed 3, St Louis, 1996, Mosby.)

use on compromised thin skin increases systemic absorption (Ward and others, 2000). Potential side effects include striae, epidermal atrophy, suppression of the pituitary-adrenal axis, cessation of longitudinal growth, and Cushing syndrome from chronic use. Topical antifungals are used to treat *Candida* infections and include clotrimazole, miconazole, ketoconazole, and nystatin ointment (Boiko, 1997; Lund, 1999). When *Candida* is present elsewhere, oral administration of a fungicide is advised because the gastrointestinal tract is usually the source of infection. (See Candidiasis, Chapter 9.)

### Nursing Considerations

Nursing interventions are aimed at altering the three factors considered to produce dermatitis—wetness (hydration), pH, and fecal irritants. The most significant factor amenable to intervention is the moist environment created in the diaper area. Changing the diaper as soon as it becomes wet eliminates a large part of the problem, and removing the diaper to expose intact skin to air facilitates drying as long as fecal contamination of the skin does not occur, in which case the skin is again exposed to possible injury (Lund, 1999). The use of a hair dryer or heat lamp is not recommended because they can cause burns. Also, on denuded skin, dry heat delays healing. Instead, occlusive ointments or dressings are applied to provide a moist healing environment for open wounds and to protect the skin from further irritation. (See Ostomies, Chapter 27.) A protective barrier such as zinc oxide prevents skin injury and allows the skin to heal (Lund, 1999; Ward and others, 2000). In the event of diaper dermatitis caused by fungal and contact irritants, a layer of antifungal powder or cream under a zinc oxide–based skin barrier ointment may be used, but care must be taken to avoid mixing the two preparations together (Lund, 1999). A hydrogel barrier cream was shown to be more effective than petrolatum-based cream in the treatment of contact dermatitis in a recent comparative study involving children and adults (Draelos, 2000).

Diaper construction has a significant impact on the incidence and severity of diaper dermatitis. Superabsorbent disposable diapers reduce diaper dermatitis. They contain an absorbent gelling material that binds water tightly to decrease skin wetness, maintains pH control by providing a buffering capacity, and decreases skin irritation by preventing mixing of urine and feces in the diaper (Wong and others, 1992). The improved containment of urine and feces is also a very important factor in decreasing contamination of the environment, such as in daycare centers, and spread of disease.

Another advance is the addition of an inner layer or topsheet that is impregnated with petrolatum (Ultra Pampers with Tender Touch Liner*). The liner transfers the petrolatum to the skin, where it acts as a barrier to moisture and irritants. Studies show that this formulation reduces skin erythema and excess hydration (Baldwin and others, 1998; Odio and others, 2000).

Guidelines for controlling diaper rash are presented in the Family Home Care box. Some caregivers may choose to apply a powder that may contain either talc or cornstarch. A common misconception about using cornstarch on skin is that it promotes the growth of *C. albicans*. Both cornstarch and talc do not support growth of the fungi under conditions normally found in the diaper area. Cornstarch is also more effective in reducing friction and tends to cake less than talc when the skin is wet. On the basis of these properties and its safety in terms of inhalation injury, cornstarch is the preferred product. Talc should not be used.

Special care must be taken to avoid cuts from diaper tape fasteners, which may occur if the child has outgrown the diaper. Also, if the diaper fastener is removed to check for dryness and replaced, the adhesive may come loose and cause skin cuts.

---

*Manufactured by Procter & Gamble Company, Cincinnati, OH 45224, (800) 285-6064; www.pampers.com.

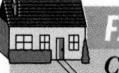

## FAMILY HOME CARE
### Controlling Diaper Rash

Keep skin dry*.
   Use superabsorbent disposable diapers to reduce skin wetness.
   If using cloth diapers, use only overwraps that allow air to circulate; avoid rubber pants.
   Change diapers as soon as soiled, especially with stool, whenever possible, preferably once during the night.
   Expose healthy or only slightly irritated skin to air, not heat, to dry completely.
   Apply ointment, such as zinc oxide or petrolatum, in thick layer to protect skin, especially if skin is very red or has moist, open areas.
      Avoid removing skin barrier cream with each diaper change; remove waste material and reapply skin barrier cream.
      To completely remove ointment, especially zinc oxide, use mineral oil; do not wash vigorously.
Avoid overwashing the skin, especially with perfumed soaps or commercial wipes that may be irritating.
   May use a moisturizer or nonsoap cleanser, such as cold cream or Cetaphil, to wipe urine from skin.
   Gently wipe stool from skin using water and mild cleanser, such as Dove.

---

*Powder helps keep the skin dry, but talc is very dangerous if breathed into the lungs. Plain cornstarch or cornstarch-based powder is safer. When using any powder product, shake it first into your hand, then apply it to the diaper area. Store the container away from the infant's reach; keep container closed when not in use.

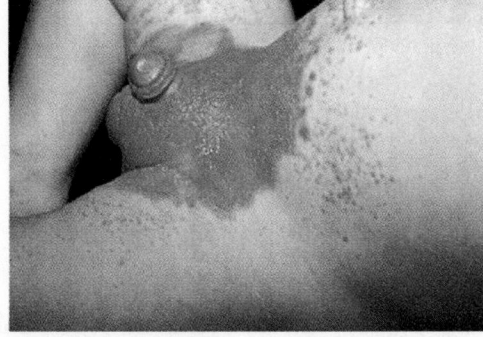

**Fig. 13-7** Candidiasis of diaper area. Note beefy red central erythema with satellite pustules. (From Weston WL, Lane AT, Morelli JG: *Color textbook of pediatric dermatology*, ed 2, St Louis, 1996, Mosby.)

## Seborrheic Dermatitis

Seborrheic dermatitis is a chronic, recurrent, inflammatory reaction of the skin that occurs most commonly on the scalp (cradle cap) but may involve the eyelids (blepharitis), external ear canal (otitis externa), nasolabial folds, and inguinal region. The cause is unknown, although it is more common in early infancy when sebum production is increased and is thought to be linked to the overgrowth of *Pityrosporum yeast*. The lesions are characteristically thick, adherent, yellowish, scaly, oily patches that may or may not be mildly pruritic. If pruritus is present, the infant may be irritable. Unlike atopic dermatitis, seborrheic dermatitis is not associated with a positive family history for allergy and is very common in infants shortly after birth and is also common after puberty. Diagnosis is made primarily by the appearance and location of the crusts or scales.

### Nursing Considerations

Cradle cap may be prevented with adequate scalp hygiene. Not infrequently, parents omit shampooing the infant's hair from fear of damaging the "soft spots" or fontanels. The nurse should discuss how to shampoo the infant's hair and emphasize that the fontanel is like skin anywhere else on the body—it does not puncture or tear with mild pressure.

When seborrheic lesions are present, the treatment is mainly directed at removing the crusts. Parents are taught the appropriate procedure to clean the scalp, which may necessitate a demonstration. Shampooing should be done daily with a mild soap or commercial baby shampoo; medicated shampoos are usually not needed, but an antiseborrheic shampoo containing sulfur and salicylic acid may be used. The shampoo is applied to the scalp and allowed to remain on until the crusts are softened, and then the scalp is thoroughly rinsed. Using a fine-tooth comb or a soft facial brush after shampooing helps remove the loosened crusts from the strands of hair.

## Atopic Dermatitis (AD) (Eczema)

Eczema or eczematous inflammation of the skin refers to a descriptive category of dermatologic diseases and not to a specific etiology. AD is a type of pruritic eczema that usually begins during infancy and is associated with allergy with a

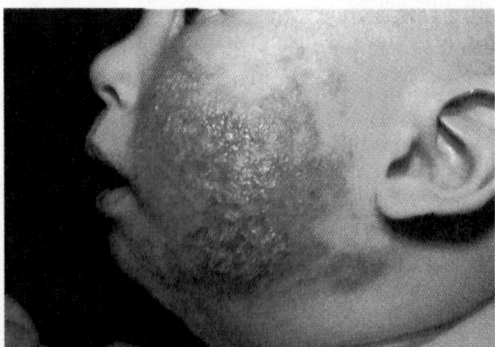

**Fig. 13-8** Infantile atopic dermatitis with oozing and crusting of lesions. (From Weston WL, Lane AT, Morelli JG: *Color textbook of pediatric dermatology*, ed 2, St Louis, 1996, Mosby.)

hereditary tendency *(atopy)*. AD presents in three forms based on the age of the child and the distribution of lesions:

1. **Infantile (infantile eczema)**—Usually begins at 2 to 6 months of age and generally undergoes spontaneous remission by 3 years of age.
2. **Childhood**—May follow the infantile form; it occurs at 2 to 3 years of age, and 90% of the children will manifest the disease by age 5 years.
3. **Preadolescent and adolescent**—Begins at about 12 years of age and may continue into the early adult years or indefinitely.

Because the disease often begins within the first 6 months of life (Raimer, 2000), this discussion is restricted to the infantile form of atopic dermatitis.

The diagnosis of AD is based on a combination of history and morphologic findings (Box 13-5). Children with the disease have a lower threshold for cutaneous itching, and many authorities believe the dermatologic manifestations appear subsequent to scratching from the intense pruritus. For example, infants will rub their faces against bed linen,

---

**Box 13-5** ■ ■ ■
**Clinical Manifestations of Atopic Dermatitis**

**DISTRIBUTION OF LESIONS**
**Infantile form**—Generalized, especially cheeks, scalp, trunk, and extensor surfaces of extremities (Fig. 13-8)
**Childhood form**—Flexural areas (antecubital and popliteal fossae, neck), wrists, ankles, and feet
**Preadolescent and adolescent form**—Face, sides of neck, hands, feet, and antecubital and popliteal fossae (to a lesser extent)

**APPEARANCE OF LESIONS**
Infantile form
Erythema
Vesicles
Papules
Weeping
Oozing
Crusting
Scaling
Often symmetric
Childhood form
Symmetric involvement
Clusters of small erythematous or flesh-colored papules or minimally scaling patches
Dry and may be hyperpigmented
Lichenification (thickened skin with accentuation of creases)
Keratosis pilaris (follicular hyperkeratosis) common
Adolescent/adult form
Same as childhood manifestations
Dry, thick lesions (lichenified plaques) common
Confluent papules

**OTHER MANIFESTATIONS**
Intense itching
Unaffected skin dry and rough
African-American children likely to exhibit more papular and/or follicular lesions than Caucasian children
May exhibit one or more of the following:
Lymphadenopathy, especially near affected sites
Increased palmar creases (many cases)
Atopic pleats (extra line or groove of lower eyelid)
Prone to cold hands
Pityriasis alba (small, poorly defined areas of hypopigmentation)
Facial pallor (especially around nose, mouth, and ears)
Bluish discoloration beneath eyes ("allergic shiners")
Increased susceptibility to unusual cutaneous infections (especially viral)

and crawling (a form of scratching) results in irritation of knees and elbows. Lesions will disappear if the scratching is stopped.

The majority of children with infantile AD have a family history of eczema, asthma, food allergies, or allergic rhinitis, which strongly supports a genetic predisposition. The cause is unknown but may be related to abnormal function of the skin, including alterations in perspiration, peripheral vascular function, and heat tolerance. The chronic disease is better in humid climates and worse in fall and winter, when homes are heated and environmental humidity is lower. The disorder can be controlled but not cured. House dust mites, certain foods, mold, and animal hair may play a role in the etiology of AD. Some research points to an immunologic basis. Many children (80%) with AD have elevated IgE levels, and a T-cell dysfunction has been proposed (Romeo, 1995). IgE food sensitization has been found to be a major risk factor for atopic dermatitis in infancy (Hill and others, 2000). It has also been suggested that children with AD have a blunted immune response to endogenous cortisol, thus the possible explanation for children who do not respond well to steroid therapy (Schneider and Lester, 1996).

## Therapeutic Management

The major goals of management are to (1) hydrate the skin, (2) relieve pruritus, (3) reduce flare-ups or inflammation, and (4) prevent and control secondary infection. Most of the general measures for managing AD serve to reduce pruritus, as well as other aspects of the disease. General management includes avoiding exposure to skin irritants or allergens, avoiding overheating, avoiding skin moisture loss, improving skin hydration, and administering medications such as antihistamines, topical steroids, and (sometimes) mild sedatives as indicated.

Enhancing skin hydration and preventing dry, flaky skin can be accomplished in a number of ways, depending on the child's skin characteristics and individual needs. A tepid bath with a mild soap (Dove or Neutrogena), no soap or an emulsifying oil, followed immediately by application of an emollient (within 3 minutes) assists in trapping moisture and preventing moisture loss. Bubble baths and harsh soaps should be avoided. The bath may need to be repeated once or twice daily, depending on the child's status; excessive bathing without emollient application only dries out the skin. Some lotions are not effective and emollients should be chosen carefully to prevent excessive skin drying. Aquaphor, Cetaphil, and Eucerin are acceptable lotions for skin hydration. A nighttime bath, followed by emollient application and dressing in soft cotton pajamas, may help alleviate much of the nighttime pruritus.

Sometimes colloid baths, such as the addition of 2 cups of cornstarch to a tub of warm water, provide temporary relief of itching and may help the child sleep if given before bedtime. Cool, wet compresses are soothing to the skin and provide antiseptic protection.

Moderate or severe pruritus is usually relieved by administration of oral antihistamine drugs (hydroxyzine [Atarax] or diphenhydramine [Benadryl]), the amount tailored to the individual child. Nonsedating antihistamines such as loratidine (Claritin) or fexofenadine (Allegra) may be pre-ferred for daytime pruritis relief. Because pruritus increases at night, a mildly sedating antihistamine may be needed.

Occasional flare-ups require the use of topical steroids to diminish inflammation. Low-, moderate-, or high-potency topical corticosteroids are prescribed, depending on the degree of involvement, the area of the body to be treated, the age of the child, potential for local side effects (striae, skin atrophy, and pigment changes), and the type of vehicle to be used (e.g., cream, lotion, ointment). Medical management of secondary skin infections with systemic antibiotics is an important part of the treatment of AD. Coal tar preparations may also be used to hydrate the skin yet are considered cumbersome because of staining of clothing.

Acute flare-ups may require the use of wet wraps. One method is to apply a light coat of topical corticosteroid, then wrap the child in cool wet towels for 10 minutes (warm towels slightly in the winter to prevent heat loss). Once the towels are removed, the steroid ointment is reapplied, followed by a moisturizer (Raimer, 2000). Care must be taken, however, not to use excessive wet wraps as these may cause skin maceration and secondary infections (Leung, Tharp, and Boguniewicz, 1999).

There is controversy regarding prevention of atopic dermatitis by limiting the exposure of infants at risk to allergens both prenatally and postnatally. Studies have shown a decrease in atopic eczema in breast-fed infants at risk for atopy whose mothers avoided known allergens while lactating; however, further evidence is needed to substantiate the findings (Kramer, 2001). Although conclusive evidence for preventive strategies is lacking, the precautions in the Guidelines box on p. 569 may be recommended. Chinese herbal tea and phototherapy with ultraviolet light, such as psoralen plus ultraviolet A (PUVA), may also be used for the treatment of AD (Schneider and Lester, 1996; Raimer, 2000). Additional therapies that have been used with some success in adults and children with AD include immunosuppressant therapy with cyclosporine, topical immunosuppressants such as tacrolimus (Protopic), interferons (alpha and gamma), and essential fatty acids (Raimer, 2000). In children 2 years and older, 1% topical pimecrolimus (Elidel) has proved effective in the treatment of AD (Eichenfield and others, 2002).

## Nursing Considerations

The child with AD presents a nursing challenge. Controlling the intense pruritus is imperative if the disorder is to be successfully managed, because scratching leads to the formation of new lesions and may cause secondary infection. In addition to the medical regimen, other measures can be taken to prevent or minimize the scratching. Fingernails and toenails are cut short, kept clean, and filed frequently to prevent sharp edges. Gloves or cotton socks may need to be placed over the hands and pinned to shirtsleeves. One-piece cotton outfits with long sleeves and long pants also decrease direct contact with the skin. If gloves or socks are used, the child needs time to be free from such restrictions. An excellent time to remove any protective devices is during the bath or after receiving sedative or antipruritic medication.

Conditions that increase itching are eliminated when possible. Woolen clothes or blankets, rough fabrics, and furry stuffed animals are removed. Because heat and humidity cause perspiration, which intensifies the itching, proper dress for climatic conditions is essential. Pruritus is often precipitated by exposure to the irritant effects of certain components of common products such as soaps, detergents, fabric softeners, perfumes, diaper wipes, and powders. Most children experience less itching when soft cotton fabrics are worn next to the skin. During cold months, synthetic fabrics (not wool) should be used for overcoats, hats, gloves, and snowsuits. Exposure to latex products, such as gloves and balloons, should also be avoided.

Clothes and sheets are laundered in a mild detergent and rinsed thoroughly in clear water (without fabric softeners or antistatic chemicals). Putting the clothes through a second complete wash cycle without using detergent minimizes the amount of residue remaining in the fabric.

Preventing infection is usually accomplished by preventing scratching. Personal hygiene is maintained as described previously. Baths are given as prescribed, the water is kept tepid, and soaps (except as indicated) and bubble baths are avoided, as well as the use of oils and powders. Skinfolds and diaper areas need frequent cleansing with plain water. A room humidifier or vaporizer may benefit children with extremely dry skin. The lesions are examined for signs of infection—usually the presence of honey-colored crusts with surrounding erythema. Any signs of infection are reported to the practitioner.

> **NURSING ALERT** If the child is being treated with baths for hydration, it is imperative that the emollient preparation be applied immediately following bathing (while the skin is still slightly moist) to prevent drying.

Wet soaks or compresses are applied, and medications for pruritus or infection are administered as directed. The family is given explicit written instructions on the preparation and use of soaks, special baths, and topical medications, including the order of application if more than one is prescribed. Directions are worded in language the family understands. It is important to emphasize that one thick application of a topical medication is *not* equivalent to several thin applications and that excessive use of an agent, particularly steroids, can be hazardous. If children have difficulty remaining still for a 10- or 15-minute soak, bath, or dressing application, these can be carried out at nap time or when the child is engrossed in television, a story, or playing with tub toys.

Because adequate rest is also important for these children, who are usually fretful and irritable, planning meals, baths, medications, and treatments during awake periods is paramount. During periods of irritability, these children tend to have a poor appetite, which is worsened by restriction of their usual foods.

Diet modification is another source of frustration to parents. When a hypoallergenic diet is prescribed, parents need help in understanding the reason for the diet and guidelines for avoiding hyperallergenic foods (see Box 13-3).

Because hypoallergenic diets take time before visible effects are apparent, parents need reassurance that results may not be seen immediately. If airborne allergens also worsen the eczema, the family is counseled regarding measures to "allergy proof" the home. (See Asthma, Chapter 32.)

**Family Support.\*** Parents can be assured that the lesions will not produce scarring (unless secondarily infected) and that the disease is not contagious. However, the child will be subject to repeated exacerbations and remissions. Spontaneous and permanent remission takes place at approximately 2 to 3 years of age in most children with the infantile disorder.

Perhaps it is because the physical problems seem insurmountable during periods of acute exacerbation that the emotional stress becomes so intense for the family members. They need time to discuss negative feelings and to be reassured that these feelings are expected, normal, acceptable, and healthy, provided there is an emotional outlet to dissipate pent-up energy. During acute phases, efforts aimed at relieving as much anxiety as possible in both parents and child have a beneficial emotional and physical effect because stress tends to aggravate the severity of the condition. (See Nursing Care Plan: The Child with Atopic Dermatitis [Eczema].†)

# DISORDERS OF UNKNOWN ETIOLOGY
## Sudden Infant Death Syndrome (SIDS)

SIDS is defined as the sudden death of an infant under 1 year of age that remains unexplained after a complete postmortem examination, including an investigation of the death scene and a review of the case history. In the United States mortality from SIDS has declined more than 40% since 1992 (American Academy of Pediatrics, 2000b). The dramatic decrease is attributed to the "Back to Sleep" campaign‡ (see following section) (Malloy, 2002). SIDS is the third leading cause of death in children between the ages of 1 month and 1 year and claimed the lives of almost 2500 infants in 1998 (Guyer and others, 1999). Table 13-3 summarizes the major epidemiologic characteristics of SIDS.

### Etiology

Numerous theories have been proposed regarding the etiology of SIDS; however, the cause is unknown. The most compelling hypothesis is that SIDS is related to a brainstem abnormality in the neurologic regulation of cardiorespiratory control. Abnormalities include prolonged sleep apnea, increased frequency of brief inspiratory pauses, excessive periodic breathing, and impaired arousal responsiveness to increased carbon dioxide or decreased oxygen. However, sleep apnea is not the cause of SIDS. The vast majority of infants with apnea do not die, and only a minority of SIDS victims have documented **apparent life-threatening events (ALTEs).** (See Apnea of Infancy, p. 585.) A theory that has been disproved associated SIDS with diphtheria, tetanus, and pertussis vaccines.

---

\*Parents may also find helpful information at the Eczema Connection, PO Box 1101, Windsor, CT 06095; www.eczema.cc/.
†In Wong DL, Hess CS: *Wong and Whaley's clinical manual of pediatric nursing*, ed 5, St Louis, 2000, Mosby.
‡"Back to Sleep" materials may be ordered by calling (800) 505-CRIB; faxing requests to (301) 496-7101; or writing to NICHD/Back to Sleep, 31 Center Drive, Room 2A32, Bethesda, MD 20892-2425.

| **TABLE 13-3** | Epidemiology of SIDS |
|---|---|
| **Factors** | **Occurrence** |
| Incidence | 0.7:1000 live births |
| Peak age | 2 to 4 months; 95% occur by 6 months |
| Sex | Higher percentage of males affected |
| Time of death | During sleep |
| Time of year | Increased incidence in winter |
| Racial | Greater incidence in Native Americans, African-Americans, and Hispanics |
| Socioeconomic | Increased incidence in lower socioeconomic class |
| Birth | Higher incidence in: Premature infants, especially LBW infants Multiple births* Neonates with low Apgar scores Infants with central nervous system disturbances and respiratory disorders such as bronchopulmonary dysplasia Increasing birth order (subsequent siblings as opposed to firstborn child) Infants with a recent history of illness |
| Sleep habits | Prone position; use of soft bedding; overheating (thermal stress); cosleeping with adult, especially on soft bedding |
| Feeding habits | Lower incidence in breast-fed infants |
| Siblings | May have greater incidence |
| Maternal | Young age; cigarette smoking, especially during pregnancy; poor prenatal care; substance abuse (heroin, methadone, cocaine) |

*Although a rare event, simultaneous death of twins from SIDS can occur.

Maternal smoking, both prenatally and postnatally, has been proposed as a possible cause of SIDS, as has poor prenatal care and low maternal age (Leach and others, 1999). In fact, maternal smoking during pregnancy has emerged in numerous epidemiologic studies as a major factor in SIDS, and smoke in the infant's environment after birth has also been shown to have a possible relationship with the incidence of SIDS (American Academy of Pediatrics, 2000b). It has been postulated that 12% of all SIDS deaths could be prevented with prenatal maternal smoking cessation (Pollack, 2001). One mechanism that has been proposed as a link between maternal smoking and SIDS is a decrease in the infant's ability to arouse to auditory stimuli in mothers who smoked prenatally (Franco and others, 1999). Increased nicotine concentrations in lung tissue were found in children who died from SIDs compared to a group of conrol children (McMartin and others, 2002).

Co-sleeping, or bed sharing, has been reported to have a positive association with SIDS. Recent evidence implicates a shared sleep surface in 47.1% of SIDS cases in St. Louis between 1994 and 1997; additional findings in the study included infants found prone (61%), infants sleeping on a surface not intended for infant sleep (75.9%), and the head or face covered by bedding (29.4%). SIDS deaths of infants found nonprone and alone on an appropriate sleep surface accounted for only 8.4% of the SIDS cases examined (Kemp and others, 2000). The American Academy of Pediatrics (2000b) recognizes that co-sleeping may be hazardous under certain conditions and recommends that adults follow the same safeguards in the bed as in the crib. The bed sharer should not smoke or use substances, such as alcohol

or drugs, which may impair arousal. Parents may consider placing the infant's crib next to their own as an alternative to co-sleeping. Co-sleeping with infants at risk for SIDS has not been shown to be preventive.

Studies from countries other than the United States link sleep habits with an increased risk of SIDS. Prone sleeping may cause oropharyngeal obstruction or affect thermal balance or arousal state. A recent study found that healthy term infants had significantly impaired arousal from active and quiet sleep states when sleeping prone (Horne and others, 2001). Rebreathing of carbon dioxide by infants in the prone position is also a possible cause for SIDS. Infants sleeping prone and on soft bedding may not be able to move their heads to the side, thus increasing the risk of suffocation and lethal rebreathing. Evidence from other countries and the United States shows an increased incidence of SIDS in infants placed in a side-lying position, thus the side-lying position is no longer recommended for infants sleeping at home, daycare, or hospitals (unless medically indicated). A recent study revealed that 20.4% of SIDS cases occurred in child care settings; thus parents must discuss nonprone sleeping with daycare workers (Moon, Patel, and Shaefer, 2000).

Soft bedding such as waterbeds, sheepskins, beanbags, pillows, or quilts should be avoided for infant sleeping surfaces. Bedding items such as stuffed animals or toys should be removed from the crib while the infant is asleep. Most preterm infants being discharged from the hospital should be placed in a supine sleeping position unless there are special factors that predispose to airway obstruction. One postulated cause of SIDS has been suggested to be a prolonged Q-T interval; however, at the time of this writing there seems to be no strong evidence to support universal testing of newborns for prolonged Q-T interval or to support this as a cause of SIDS (American Academy of Pediatrics, 2000b).

Since the Back to Sleep campaign in 1992 advocating nonprone sleeping for infants, an increase in the incidence of positional *plagiocephaly* has been observed. (See Chapter 11.) It is recommended that an infant's head position be alternated during sleep time to prevent plagiocephaly. Infants may be placed prone during awake periods to prevent positional plagiocephaly and to encourage development of upper shoulder girdle strength (American Academy of Pediatrics, 2000b). (See Evidence-Based Practice box on p. 584.) One recent study indicated breast-feeding during the first 16 weeks of life decreased the likelihood of SIDS (Alm and others, 2002).

**NURSING ALERT**    Research findings have important implications for practices that may reduce the risk of SIDS, such as avoiding smoking during pregnancy and near the infant, encouraging supine sleeping positions, avoiding soft, moldable mattresses and pillows, and avoiding overheating during sleep.

Although the etiology is unknown, autopsies reveal consistent pathologic findings, such as pulmonary edema and intrathoracic hemorrhages, that confirm the diagnosis of SIDS. Consequently, autopsies should be performed on all infants suspected of dying of SIDS, and findings should be shared with the parents as soon as possible after the death.

For decades nurses have been taught to place newborns and infants on their tummies or sides to sleep in order to prevent aspiration and subsequent asphyxia. Nurses instructed parents to do the same. In the early 1990s, however, research data from New Zealand suggested that infants placed prone to sleep were more likely to die of SIDS than those who were placed in a nonprone (supine) position. "Nonsense, that cannot be!" those of us who worked with newborns and infants said. In 1992 the Back to Sleep campaign was initiated to encourage physicians, nurses, and other health professionals to inform parents about placing newborns and infants in a side lying or nonprone position to sleep in order to decrease the risk of SIDS. This recommendation was later amended to propose that infants be placed only in a supine sleep position because infants placed in the side-lying position might role over to a prone position and be at greater risk for SIDS. Since 1992, the incidence of SIDS in the United States has decreased by more than 40% to an all-time low of 0.7 per 1000 live births (American Academy of Pediatrics, 2000b). In 1992 SIDS was the leading cause of death in infants less than 1 year old; SIDS is now the third leading cause of death, preceded by congenital anomalies and prematurity (Moon, 2001). Yet research indicates that approximately 20% of all infants under the age of 6 months are still being placed in a side-lying or prone position to sleep despite findings in New Zealand, Great Britain, Australia, and the United States that the supine sleeping position has not been associated with an increase in the number of asphyxiation events or deaths in this age group (American Academy of Pediatrics, 2000b). Additional research from Australia supports the theory that supine sleeping does not increase the incidence of mortality as a result of gastric contents being aspirated into the trachea (Byard and Beal, 2000).

Recent research from 94 Iowa hospitals indicates that a large number of newborns are still being placed in side-lying sleep positions; 51.4% of those surveyed indicated that the rationale for placing the newborn on the side was out of fear of asphyxiation (Hein and Pettit, 2001). Parents who hear physicians and nurses encourage them to place the infant supine at home may be confused by witnessing hospital workers placing infants prone or in side-lying positions in the nursery or mother-infant care unit. It is imperative that research be evaluated carefully, and, while it is true that old habits die hard, it is time for nurses to be the front-line proponents for saving the lives of thousands of infants yearly by helping parents and caregivers understand the importance of preventing SIDS by putting infants to sleep on their back—at home, in the hospital nurseries, and in daycare facilities.

Postmortem findings in SIDS and accidental suffocation or intentional suffocation such as in Munchausen syndrome by proxy (see Child Maltreatment, Chapter 16) are practically the same. Individuals with less experience and training in performing autopsies, such as coroners instead of medical examiners, may or may not correctly identify some deaths as SIDS. Therefore mortality statistics can vary in different regions.

### Infants at Risk for SIDS

Certain groups of children are at increased risk for SIDS:

- Infants with one or more severe ALTEs requiring cardiopulmonary resuscitation or vigorous stimulation (see p. 585)
- Preterm infants who continue to have apnea at the time of hospital discharge
- Siblings of two or more SIDS victims
- Infants with certain types of diseases or conditions, such as central hypoventilation

Home monitoring and/or the use of respiratory stimulant drugs is recommended for these groups of children. No diagnostic tests exist to predict which infants, including those in the above groups, will survive, and home monitoring is no guarantee of survival. There is no evidence that home monitoring decreases the incidence of SIDS (American Academy of Pediatrics, 2000b).

Whether subsequent siblings of one SIDS infant are at increased risk for SIDS is unclear. Even if the increased risk is correct, families have a 99% chance that their subsequent child will *not* die of SIDS. Home monitoring is not recommended for this group of children, but it is often used by practitioners and may even be requested by parents.

### Nursing Considerations

Nurses have a vital role in preventing SIDS by educating families about the risk of prone sleeping position in infants from birth to 6 months of age, using appropriate bedding surfaces, and the dangers of co-sleeping. It is reported that 20% of all infants in the United States are still placed in a prone or side-lying sleep position (American Academy of Pediatrics, 2000b; Willinger and others, 2000). *Nurses **must** be proactive in further decreasing the incidence of SIDS;* postpartum discharge planning, newborn discharges, follow-up home visits, well-baby clinic visits, and immunization visits provide an excellent opportunity to educate parents in these matters.

Loss of a child from SIDS presents several crises with which the parents must cope. In addition to grief and mourning for the death of their child, the parents must face a tragedy that was sudden, unexpected, and unexplained. The psychologic intervention for the family must deal with these additional variables. This discussion focuses primarily on the objectives of care for families experiencing SIDS, rather than on the process of grief and mourning, which is explored in Chapter 23.

One approach toward delineating the nursing care plan for these families is to base it on the usual sequence of events that occurs after the infant is found. This approach encompasses the different areas in which nurses may be involved with the family.

**Finding the Infant.** Usually it is the mother who finds the child dead in the crib. Typically, the child is in a disheveled bed, with blankets over the head, and huddled into a corner. Frothy, blood-tinged fluid fills the mouth and nostrils, and the infant may be lying face down in the secretions, suggesting that he or she bled to death. The diaper is wet and full of stool, which is consistent with a cataclysmic type of death. The hands may be clutching the sheets, as if the child were in distress before death. The initial appearance of the child combined with the shock of such an unexpected event adds to the horror that the parents must face.

Often the mother is alone and must deal with her initial shock, panic, grief, questions of the other siblings, and the decision of where to find help. The first persons to arrive may be the police and ambulance attendants. They should handle the situation by asking few questions; giving *no* indication of wrongdoing, abuse, or neglect; making sensitive judgments concerning any resuscitation efforts for the child; and comforting the members of the family as much as possible. These individuals should be properly informed about SIDS in order to recognize its characteristic signs and should tell parents that their child probably died of a condition called sudden infant death syndrome, which cannot be predicted or prevented. A compassionate, sensitive approach to the family during the very first few minutes can help spare them some of the overwhelming guilt and anguish that commonly follow this type of death.

**Arriving at the Emergency Department.** The first contact that nurses typically have with these families is in the emergency department, when the infant is seen by a physician in order to be pronounced dead. Usually there is no attempt at resuscitation. During the time in the emergency department several aspects warrant special consideration. Parents are asked only factual questions, such as when they found the infant, how he or she looked, and whom they called for help. Any remarks that may suggest responsibility, such as why didn't they go in earlier, didn't they hear the infant cry out, was the head buried in a blanket, or were the other siblings jealous of this child, are avoided.

The events that took place when help arrived are discussed. If resuscitation was attempted, the infant may have fractured ribs, internal bleeding, and traumatic bruising, which can simulate physical abuse. Also, if statements were made that were misguided, such as "This looks like suffocation," they can be corrected before parents harbor them in their minds as indications of their guilt. The discussion of an autopsy should be presented at this time, emphasizing that a diagnosis cannot be confirmed until the postmortem examination is completed. Instructions about the autopsy and funeral arrangements may need to be repeated or put in writing. If the mother was breast-feeding, she needs information about abrupt discontinuation of lactation.

Another important aspect of compassionate care for these parents is allowing them to say good-bye to their child. Before they go into the examining room, any blood, emesis, or excreta is removed from the child, the body is covered partially with a sheet or blanket, and the room is put in order, especially if instruments and equipment were used. These are the parents' last moments with their child, and they should be as quiet, meaningful, peaceful, and undisturbed as possible. Parents are encouraged to hold their infant before leaving the emergency department (McClain and Shaefer, 1996). The child's belongings are packaged for the parents to take home if they wish. Because the parents leave the hospital without their infant, it is helpful to accompany them to the car or arrange for someone else to take them home. A debriefing session may help health care workers who dealt with the family and deceased infant to deal with feelings that are often engendered when a SIDS victim is brought into the acute care facility (O'Donnell and Gaedeke, 1995). Comprehensive guidelines have been recently published for health professionals involved in SIDS investigations to assist the family and at the same time to determine that the infant's death was not the result of other factors such as child maltreatment (American Academy of Pediatrics, 2001a).

**Returning Home.** When the parents return home, they should be visited by a competent, qualified professional as soon after the death as possible. Printed material that contains excellent information about SIDS (available from the national organizations*) should be provided.

During the initial visit the parents are helped to gain an intellectual understanding of the syndrome. The nursing objectives are to assess what the parents have been told, what they think happened, and how they have explained this to the other siblings, other family members, and friends.

Some parents are able to discuss their feelings openly, and the nurse supports this coping skill. However, others may be reluctant to express their grief, and the nurse may help these parents bring their feelings out into the open. When the unexpected death of a child occurs, it is not uncommon for one parent to place blame on the other for the child's death. Parents may also experience feelings of guilt over the child's death; if they had checked earlier, the child might still be alive. It is important that the nurse assist parents in working through these feelings to prevent marital disruption in addition to the loss of the loved child.

The nurse can encourage the expression of emotions by asking about crying and feeling sad, angry, or guilty. It is an attempt to provoke a display of emotion, not just an admission of a feeling. During this session the parents should be helped to explore their usual coping mechanisms and, if these are ineffectual, to investigate new approaches. For example, one parent may refrain from discussing the death for fear of upsetting the other parent, but each may need to hear how the other feels.

Ideally, the number of visits and plans for subsequent intervention need to be flexible. For example, the siblings may initially appear accepting of the explanation and well-adjusted but may later refuse to go to sleep or ask questions about graves or funerals, indicating their need for further help in dealing with the death. Parents facing the question of a subsequent child will need support. Both the birth of a subsequent child and the survival of that child, especially past the age of death of the previous child, are important transitional stages for parents.

Because the mourning process continues for *at least* a year and because most health plans do not cover periodic visits to the family to evaluate their progress, referrals to other parents who have lost a child to SIDS should be considered.

## Apnea of Infancy (AOI)

AOI generally refers to pathologic apnea in infants of more than 37 weeks gestation. The clinical presentation of AOI is an *apparent life-threatening event (ALTE)* (previously referred

---

*American Sudden Infant Death Syndrome (SIDS) Institute, 2480 Windy Hill Rd, Suite 380, Marietta, GA 30067, (800) 232-SIDS (in Georgia, [800] 847-SIDS); www.sids.org. The Sudden Infant Death Syndrome Alliance, 1314 Bedford Ave, Suite 210, Baltimore, MD 21208, (800) 221-SIDS. National SIDS Resource Center, 2070 Chain Bridge Rd, Suite 450, Vienna, VA 22182, (703) 821-8955; www.sidscenter.org

to by the inaccurate and misleading expression, "near-miss SIDS") that is described as:

- Frightening to the observer, who fears the child died or would have died without vigorous intervention
- Some combination of:
  Apnea—Cessation of breathing for 20 seconds or more
  Color change—Cyanosis or pallor but sometimes plethora
  Marked change in muscle tone—Usually extreme limpness
  Choking or gagging

AOI can be a symptom of many disorders, including sepsis, seizures, upper airway abnormalities, gastroesophageal reflux, hypoglycemia or other metabolic problems, impaired regulation of breathing during sleep or feeding, or a result of intentional poisoning by a caregiver. Abnormal physical properties of pulmonary surfactant have been identified in some children with recurrent ALTE (Silvestri and Weese-Mayer, 1996). However, in about half the cases no cause is identified. Infants with a history of ALTEs are at increased risk for SIDS, but these children constitute less than 7% of all SIDS victims. A diagnosis of AOI is made when no identifiable cause for the ALTE is found.

A recent multicenter consortium study (Collaborative Home Infant Monitoring Evaluation or CHIME) of infants on home apnea monitoring suggests that apnea, bradycardia, and desaturation events are more common in healthy term, preterm, and siblings of SIDS victims than previously theorized (Jobe, 2001; Ramanathan and others, 2001). Findings of the CHIME study further suggest that such cardiorespiratory events are not precursors to SIDS, and that current home apnea monitors may miss critical incidences of apnea or bradycardia in some infants. The postconception age at which critical cardiorespiratory events occurred in preterm infants monitored was <43 weeks, whereas most cases of SIDS are known to occur at 44 postconception weeks or older (Ramanathan and others, 2001). These findings do not, however, justify wide-scale termination of home monitoring for infants who have documented evidence of apnea, bradycardia, or oxygen desaturation events that may be life-threatening (Jobe, 2001).

## Diagnostic Evaluation

The most widely used diagnostic test is continuous recording of cardiorespiratory patterns (cardiopneumogram or pneumocardiogram). Four-channel (or multichannel pneumogram) pneumocardiograms monitor heart rate, respirations (chest impedance), nasal airflow, and oxygen saturation. A more sophisticated test, polysomnography ("sleep study"), also records brain waves, eye and body movements, esophageal manometry, and end-tidal carbon dioxide measurements. However, none of these tests can predict risk. Some children with normal results may still have subsequent apneic episodes.

## Therapeutic Management

Treatment usually involves continuous home monitoring of cardiorespiratory rhythms and/or the use of methylxanthines (respiratory stimulant drugs, such as theophylline or caffeine). Therapeutic levels are typically 6 to 10 or 13 μg/ml of theophylline and 10 to 20 μg/ml of caffeine. The criteria

for discontinuing the monitoring is based on the infant's clinical condition. A general guideline for discontinuation is when infants with ALTEs have gone 2 or 3 months without significant numbers of episodes requiring intervention.

## Nursing Considerations

The diagnosis of AOI engenders great anxiety and concern in parents, and the institution of home monitoring presents additional physical and emotional burdens. Parents of infants on home apnea monitors report experiencing emotional distress, especially depression and hostility, during the first few weeks following hospital discharge (Abendroth and others, 1999). For parents of a SIDS victim who have a new infant on home apnea monitoring, the anxiety is compounded by the uncertainty of the future of the living child and grief for the lost child. Home apnea monitoring may offer some predictability and control over the current child's survival through the period of uncertainty (Maclean, 1999). If monitoring is required, the nurse can be a major source of support to the family in terms of education about the equipment, observation of the infant's status, and immediate intervention during apneic episodes, including cardiorespiratory resuscitation (CPR). (See Critical Thinking Exercise box.) To help the family cope with the numer-

 *Critical Thinking Exercise*

### Home Apnea Monitoring

A family has just brought their newborn home on an apnea monitor. The diagnosis is apnea of prematurity. You are the nurse making the first home visit. Which of the following should you *not* expect to find?

FIRST, THINK ABOUT IT . . .

- What is the purpose of your thinking?
- How are you interpreting the information?

1. The parent appears knowledgeable about monitor use, responses to alarms, and CPR.
2. The infant's respiratory status is stable and color is good.
3. The monitor is plugged into an extension cord.
4. The family appears anxious.

*The best response is three. The purpose of your thinking may focus on safety, and medical equipment should not be plugged into extension cords. If necessary, furniture and equipment should be rearranged so that an appropriate outlet can be used. Regarding the other answers, parents should be well-trained in caring for the child on an apnea monitor before being sent home. You may interpret the information to indicate that the nurse usually only needs to review procedures. However, if parents do not have the necessary information and skills, training should be a priority on the first home visit. Anxiety is common for the first 4 to 8 weeks of home apnea monitoring. An infant with a diagnosis of apnea of prematurity should appear healthy and should not evidence respiratory distress. Signs to the contrary necessitate immediate contact with the family's practitioner.*

ous procedures they must learn, adequate preparation before discharge and written instructions are essential. In the first few weeks following discharge, parents may benefit by having a practitioner readily available to answer questions regarding false alarms and for other technical assistance* (Abendroth, 1999).

Several types of home monitors are available (see Family Home Care box), and most hospitals select the model that the infant will use at home. Nurses, especially those involved in the care at home, must become familiar with the equipment, including its advantages and disadvantages. Safety is a major concern, because monitors can cause electrical burns and electrocution. The following precautions are recommended:

- Remove leads from infant when not attached to monitor.
- Unplug power cord from electrical outlet when cord is not plugged into monitor.
- Use safety covers on electrical outlets to discourage children from inserting objects into a socket.

---

*Community and home care instructions for apnea monitoring and CPR are available in Wong DL, Hess CS: *Wong and Whaley's clinical manual of pediatric nursing,* ed 5, St Louis, 2000, Mosby. Educational materials may also be obtained from the **American SIDS Institute,** 2480 Windy Hill Rd, Suite 380, Marietta, GA 30067.

## FAMILY HOME CARE
### Using Apnea Monitors

Use the monitor as instructed by the practitioner.
Do not adjust the monitor to eliminate false alarms. Adjustments could compromise the monitor's effectiveness.
Place the monitor on a firm surface away from the crib and drapes; plug power cord directly into a wall socket with a three-pronged outlet.
Do not sleep in the same bed as a monitored infant.
Keep pets and children away from the monitor and infant.
Keep the monitor away from possible electrical interferences such as appliances (e.g., electric blankets, televisions, air conditioners, remote telephones).
Check the monitor several times a day to be sure the alarm is working and that it can be heard from room to room. Be sure the caregiver can reach the monitor quickly (in less than 30 seconds).
Periodically check the monitor's breath detection indicator and battery or charger connections.
Be aware that strong signals from nearby radio and television stations, airports, ham radios, cellular phones, or police stations could interfere with the monitor. Check for interference if the monitor is to be operated in these areas.
Read the monitor's user manual carefully; report problems promptly.
Inform community utility and rescue squads of home monitoring as appropriate.
Keep emergency numbers near phones in the home.
Practice safety precautions:
Remove leads when infant is not attached to the monitor.
Unplug the power cord from the electrical outlet when the cord is not plugged into the monitor.
Use safety covers on electrical outlets to prevent children from inserting objects into a socket.

---

Data primarily from *FDA Safety Alert: Important Tips for Apnea Monitor Users,* Department of Health and Human Services, Rockville, MD, 1990.

Siblings should be supervised when near the infant and taught that the monitor is not a toy. Other safety practices include informing local utility and rescue squads of the home monitoring in case of an emergency. Telephone numbers for these services should be posted near all telephones in the home.

**NURSING ALERT** Parents are encouraged to focus on the infant when an alarm sounds, not the machine. Is the infant pink in color centrally and breathing? Help parents attend to the infant's needs rather than to the monitor.

Caregivers need detailed information regarding proper attachment of the electrodes to the infant's chest with impedance monitors that detect chest movement. The electrodes are placed in the midaxillary line, at a space one or two fingerbreadths below the nipple (Fig. 13-9). Adhesive electrodes are attached directly to the skin. For home use, electrodes attached to a belt that is placed around the child's trunk are preferred. The belt is positioned so that the electrodes contact the skin in the same area as shown in Fig. 13-9. Monitors may have memory chips that allow for event recording, which can be an effective tool in evaluating the use of the monitor and reported frequency of alarms.

Monitors are effective only if they are used. They do not prevent death but alert the caregiver to the ALTE in time to intervene. The need to use the monitor and to respond appropriately to alarms must be stressed. Noncompliance can result in the infant's death.

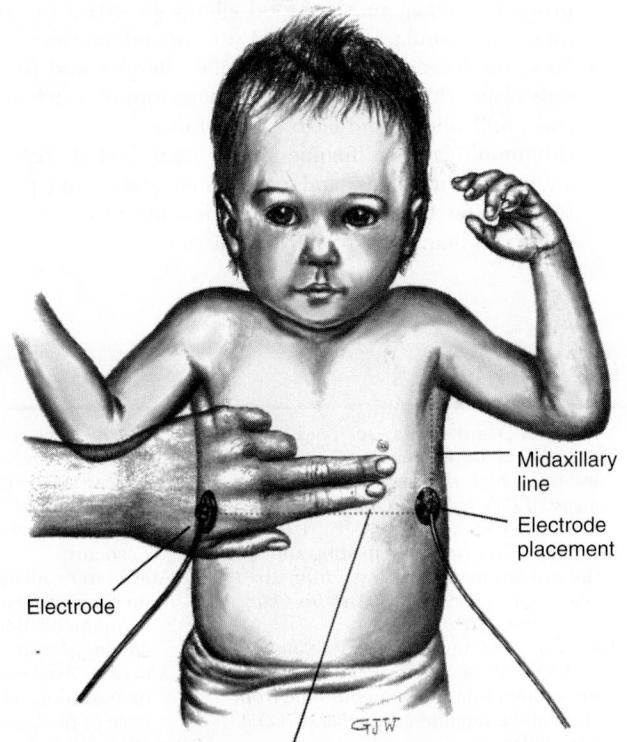

Midaxillary line

Electrode placement

Electrode

Two fingerbreadths below nipple

**Fig. 13-9**   Electrode placement for apnea monitoring. In small infants, one fingerbreadth may be used.

> **NURSING ALERT**
>
> If the infant is apneic, gently stimulate the trunk by patting or rubbing it. If the infant is prone, turn to the back and flick the feet. If there is still no response, begin CPR and activate the EMS—"Call 911!" Never vigorously shake the child. No more than 10 to 15 seconds are spent on stimulation before implementing CPR.

**Family Support.** Although AOI is not a chronic illness, many of the stresses observed during the monitoring period are characteristic of those of families with chronically ill children. Parents report increased stress, including concern for the child's survival, fear of incompetency in assuming home responsibility, inadequate respite care, social isolation, constant work, and fatigue. Siblings are affected, as well as the affected child, who may be characterized as "spoiled" and have developmental delays. To deal with these potential effects, nurses need to employ the same interventions as those discussed for children with chronic illness (see Chapter 22) and be aware of the need for referral when difficulties are suspected.

To lessen the continuous responsibility of monitoring, other family members, such as grandparents, should be taught how to manipulate the equipment, read and interpret the signals, and administer CPR. They are encouraged to stay with the infant for regular periods to allow parents respite. Support groups of other families who have successfully completed monitoring can also be of benefit. Because baby-sitters are difficult to locate, support group members or nursing students may be potential sources of qualified caregivers.

## KEY POINTS

- Common nutritional disturbances of infancy include vitamin and mineral disturbances, some types of vegetarian diets, protein and calorie malnutrition, and food intolerance.
- Mineral disturbances may be caused by mineral-mineral interactions and mineral-diet interactions.
- Food consumption varies among vegetarians; therefore, a detailed dietary assessment is essential for planning adequate intakes, particularly in children and pregnant and lactating women.
- Protein and energy malnutrition may occur as a complication of underlying disease or as a result of fad diets, lack of parental education about infant nutrition, inappropriate management of food allergy, incorrect preparation of formula, or poor food storage and handling.
- Food intolerance encompasses food allergies and food sensitivities during infancy, the most serious of which are cow's milk allergy and lactose intolerance.
- Common feeding difficulties in the infant include regurgitation, spitting up, and paroxysmal abdominal pain (colic). Less frequent but serious feeding problems include rumination and failure to thrive.

- Treatment of colic may involve change in feeding practices, correction of a stressful environment, and support of the parent.
- Failure to thrive may be classified as organic, resulting from some physical cause, or nonorganic, resulting from psychosocial factors involving the child and caregiver (e.g., maternal deprivation), environmental causes (e.g., inadequate parental knowledge of child feeding), or unexplained causes.
- Common skin disorders of infancy are diaper dermatitis, seborrheic dermatitis, and atopic dermatitis.
- Sudden infant death syndrome (SIDS) is the third leading cause of death in children between the ages of 1 month and 1 year.
- Evidence linking SIDS to the prone sleeping position has led to the recommendation that infants sleep supine.
- The primary nursing responsibility in care associated with SIDS and other conditions of unknown etiology is emotional support of the family.
- Children with apnea of infancy receive home monitoring to alert the family to an apparent life-threatening event.

## REFERENCES

Abendroth D and others: Do apnea monitors decrease emotional distress in parents of infants at high risk for cardiopulmonary arrest? *J Pediatr Health Care* 13(2):50-57, 1999.

Alm B and others: Breast-feeding and the sudden infant death syndrome in Scandinavia, 1992-1995, *Arch Dis Child* 86(6):400-402, 2002.

American Academy of Pediatrics, Committee on Child Abuse and Neglect: Distinguishing sudden infant death syndrome from child abuse fatalities, *Pediatrics* 107(2):437-441, 2001a.

American Academy of Pediatrics, Committee on Infectious Diseases, Pickering L, editor: 2000 *Red book: report of the Committee on Infectious Diseases*, ed 25, Elk Grove Village, IL, 2000a, The Academy.

American Academy of Pediatrics, Committee on Nutrition: *Pediatric nutrition handbook*, ed 4, Elk Grove Village, IL, 1998a, The Academy.

American Academy of Pediatrics, Committee on Nutrition: Soy protein–based formulas: recommendations for its use in infant feeding, *Pediatrics* 101(1):148-153, 1998b.

American Academy of Pediatrics, Committee on Nutrition: The use and misuse of fruit juice in pediatrics, *Pediatrics* 107(5):1210-1213, 2001b.

American Academy of Pediatrics, Task Force on Infant Sleep Position and Sudden Infant Death Syndrome: Changing concepts of sudden infant death syndrome: implications for infant sleeping environment and sleep position, *Pediatrics* 105(3):650-656, 2000b.

American Dietetic Association: ADA Reports: Position of the American Dietetic Association: vegetarian diets, *J Am Diet Assoc* 97(11):1317-1321, 1997.

Anderson JA: Milk, eggs and peanuts: food allergies in children, *Am Fam Physician* 56(5):1365-1373, 1997.

Baldwin S and others: *New directions in infant diaper design: beneficial effects of a petrolatum based formulation transferred from the diaper to the skin during use*, Cincinnati, OH, 1998, Procter & Gamble.

Balon AJ: Management of infantile colic, *Am Fam Physician* 55(1):235-242, 1997.

Barnard K and others: Measurement and meaning of parent-child interaction. In Morrison F, Lord C, Keating D, editors: *Applied developmental psychology*, vol 3, New York, 1993, Academic Press.

Baron ML: Assisting families in making appropriate feeding choices: cow's milk protein allergy versus lactose intolerance, *Pediatr Nurs* 26(5):516-520, 2000.

Barton SJ: Infant feeding practices of low-income rural mothers, *MCN* 26(2):93-97, 2001.

Bhutta ZA and others: Therapeutic effects of oral zinc in acute and persistent diarrhea in children in developing countries: pooled analysis of randomized controlled trials, *Am J Clin Nutr* 72(6):1516-1522, 2000.

Boiko S: Diapers and diaper rashes, *Dermatol Nurs* 9(1):33-39, 43, 46, 66, 70, 1997.

Brewster DR, Manary MJ, Graham SM: Case management of kwashiorkor: an intervention project at seven nutrition rehabilitation centres in Malawi, *Eur J Clin Nutr* 51(3):139-147, 1997.

Byard RW, Beal SM: Gastric aspiration and sleeping position in infancy and early childhood, *J Paediatr Child Health* 36(4):403-405, 2000.

Calamaro CK: Infant nutrition in the first year of life: tradition or science? *Pediatric Nurs* 26(2):211-215, 2000.

Canivet C, Jakobsson I, Hagander B: Infantile colic. Follow-up at four years of age: still more emotional, *Acta Paediatr* 89(1):3-7, 2000.

Centers for Disease Control and Prevention: Severe malnutrition among young children-Georgia, January 1997–June 1999, *MMWR* 50(12):224-227, 2001.

Christie L: Food hypersensitivities. In Samour PQ, Helm KK, Lang CE, editors: *Handbook of pediatric nutrition*, ed 2, Gaithersburg, MD, 1999, Aspen.

Corrales KM, Utter SL: Failure to thrive. In Samour PQ, Helm KK, Lang CE, editors: *Handbook of pediatric nutrition*, ed 2, Gaithersburg, MD, 1999, Aspen.

Dennison BA: Fruit juice consumption by infants and children: a review, *J Am Coll Nutr* 15(5 Suppl):4S-11S, 1996.

Dennison BA, Rockwell HL, Baker SL: Excess fruit juice consumption by preschool-aged children is associated with short stature and obesity, *Pediatrics* 99(1):15-22, 1997.

Doucette RE, Dwyer JT: Is fruit juice a "no-no" in children's diets? *Nutr Rev* 58(6):180-183, 2000.

Draelos ZD: Hydrogel barrier/repair creams and contact dermatitis, *Am J Contact Dermatol* 11(4):222-225, 2000.

Eichenfield LF and others: Safety and efficacy of pimecrolimus (ASM 981) cream 1% in the treatment of mild and moderate atopic dermatitis in children and adolescents, *J Am Acad Dermatol* 46(4):495-504, 2002.

Emmett P, North K, Noble S: Types of drinks consumed by infants at 4 and 8 months of age: a descriptive study. The ALSPAC Study Team, *Public Health Nutr* 3(2):211-217, 2000.

Franco P and others: Prenatal exposure to cigarette smoking is associated with a decrease in arousal in infants, *J Pediatr* 135(1):34-38, 1999.

Friedman EH: Infantile colic, *Arch Pediatr Adolesc Med* 150(6):770-771, 1996.

Garrison MM, Christakis DA: Early childhood: colic, child development, and poisoning prevention: a systematic review of treatments for childhood colic, *Pediatrics* 106(1 pt 2 suppl):184-190, 2000.

Graham SM, Arvela OM, Wise GA: Long-term neurologic consequences of nutritional vitamin B$_{12}$ deficiency in infants, *J Pediatr* 121(5):710-714, 1992.

Guyer B and others: Annual summary of vital statistics—1998, *Pediatrics* 104(6):1229-1246, 1999.

Hartman JJ: Vitamin D deficiency rickets in children: prevalence and need for community education, *Orthop Nurs* 19(1):63-69, 2000.

Hein HA, Pettit SF: Back to sleep: good advice for parents but not for hospitals? *Pediatrics* 107(3):537-539, 2001.

Hill DJ and others: The association of atopic dermatitis in infancy with immunoglobulin E food sensitization, *J Pediatr* 134(7):475-479, 2000.

Hobbie C, Baker S, Bayerl C: Parental understanding of basic infant nutrition: misinformed feeding choices, *J Pediatr Health Care* 14(1):26-31, 2000.

Horne RS and others: The prone sleeping position impairs arousability in term infants, *J Pediatr* 138(6):793-795, 2001.

Jacobson D, Melvin N: A comparison of temperament and maternal bother in infants with and without colic, *J Pediatr Nurs* 10(3):181-188, 1995.

Jakobsson I and others: Effectiveness of casein hydrolysate feedings in infants with colic, *Acta Paediatr* 89(1):18-21, 2000.

Jarvinen KM, Makinen-Kiljunen S, Suomalainen H: Cow's milk challenge through human milk evokes immune responses in infants with cow's milk allergy, *J Pediatr* 135(4):506-512, 1999.

Jobe AH: Editorial: what do home monitors contribute to the SIDS problem? *JAMA* 285(17):2244-2245, 2001.

Kemp JS and others: Unsafe sleep practices and an analysis of bedsharing among infants dying suddenly and unexpectedly: results of a four-year, population-based, death-scene investigation study of sudden infant death syndrome and related deaths, *Pediatrics* 106(3):e41, 2000.

Kramer MS: Maternal antigen avoidance during lactation for preventing atopic diseases in infants of women at high risk, *Cochrane Library* 1(4p):2001.

Krebs-Smith SM and others: Fruit and vegetable intakes of children and adolescents in the United States, *Arch Pediatr Adolesc Med* 150(1):81-86, 1996.

Leach CEA and others: Epidemiology of SIDS and explained sudden infant deaths, *Pediatrics* 104(4):e43, 1999.

Leung DYM, Tharp M, Boguniewicz M: Atopic dermatitis (atopic eczema). In Freedberg IM and others, editors: *Fitzpatrick's dermatology in general medicine*, ed 5, New York, 1999, McGraw-Hill.

Lifshitz F: Weaning foods. The role of fruit juice in the diets of infants and children, *J Am Coll Nutr* 15(suppl):s1-s3, 1996.

Lucassen PLBJ and others: Infantile colic: crying time reduction with a whey hydrolysate: a double-blind, randomized, placebo-controlled trial, *Pediatrics* 106(6):1349-1354, 2000.

Lund C: Prevention and management of infant skin breakdown, *Nurs Clin North Am* 34(4):907-920, 1999.

Maclean B: Parenting at-risk infants in the face of uncertainty: home apnea monitoring of subsibs, *J Pediatr Nurs* 14(3):201-209, 1999.

MacPhee M, Schneider J: A clinical tool for nonorganic failure-to-thrive feeding interactions, *J Pediatr Nurs* 11(1):29-39, 1996.

Maggioni A, Lifshitz F: Nutritional management of failure to thrive, *Pediatr Clin North Am* 42(4):791-809, 1995.

Malloy, MH: Trends in postneonatal aspiration deaths and reclassification of sudden infant death syndrome: impact of the "Back to Sleep" program, *Pediatrics* 109(4):661-665, 2002.

McBean LD, Miller GD: Allaying fears and fallacies about lactose intolerance, *J Am Diet Assoc* 98(6):671-676, 1998.

McClain ME, Shaefer SJM: Supporting families after sudden infant death, *J Psychosoc Nurs* 34(4):30-34, 1996.

McGuire JK and others: Fatal hypermagnesemia in a child treated with megavitamin/megamineral therapy, *Pediatrics* 105(2):414, 2000.

McMartin KI and others: Lung tissue concentrations of nicotine in sudden infant death syndrome, *J Pediatr* 140(2):205-209, 2002.

Mitchell EA: Co-sleeping and sudden infant death syndrome, *Lancet* 348(9040):1466, 1996.

Moon RY, Patel KM, Shaefer SJM: Sudden infant death syndrome in child care settings, *Pediatrics* 106(2):295-300, 2000.

Moon RY: Are you talking to parents about SIDS? *Contemporary Pediatr* 18(3):122-129, 2001.

Odio MR and others: Continuous topical administration of a petrolatum formulation by disposable diaper. 2. Effects on skin condition, *Dermatology* 299(3):238-243, 2000.

O'Donnell JK, Gaedeke MK: Sudden infant death syndrome, *Crit Care Nurs Clin North Am* 7(3):473-481, 1995.

Peregrin T: Practice points. Getting back to basics: tips for squeezing the juice controversy, *J Am Diet Assoc* 101(4):437, 2001.

Peterson KE: Failure to thrive. In Queen PM, Lang CE, editors: *Handbook of pediatric nutrition*, Gaithersburg, MD, 1993, Aspen.

Pollack HA: Sudden infant death syndrome, maternal smoking during pregnancy and effectiveness of smoking cessation intervention, *Am J Public Health* 91(3):432-436, 2001.

Raimer SS: Managing pediatric atopic dermatitis, *Clin Pediatr* 39(1):1-14, 2000.

Ramanathan R and others: Cardiorespiratory events recorded on home monitors: comparison of healthy infants with those at increased risk for SIDS, *JAMA* 285(17):2199-2243, 2001.

Romeo SP: Atopic dermatitis: the itch that rashes, *Pediatr Nurs* 221(2):157-162, 1995.

Schneider LC, Lester MR: Office pediatrics: atopic disease, rhinitis and conjunctivitis, and upper respiratory infections, *Curr Opin Pediatr* 8(6): 531-540, 1996.

Sferra TJ, Heitlinger LA: Gastrointestinal gas formation and infantile colic, *Pediatr Clin North Am* 43(2):489-507, 1996.

Sicherer SH: Diagnosis and management of childhood food allergy, *Curr Probl Pediatr* 31(2):39-57, 2001.

Silvestri JM, Weese-Mayer DE: Respiratory control disorders in infancy and childhood, *Curr Opin Pediatr* 8(3):216-220, 1996.

Singhal A and others: Clinical safety of iron-fortified formulas, *Pediatrics* 105(3):e38, 2000.

Skinner JD and others: Fruit juice intake is not related to children's growth, *Pediatrics* 103(1):58-63, 1999.

Skinner JD, Carruth BR: A longitudinal study of children's juice intake and growth: the juice controversy revisited, *J Am Diet Assoc* 101(4):432-437, 2001.

Smith MM, Lifshitz F: Excess fruit juice consumption as a contributing factor in nonorganic failure to thrive, *Pediatrics* 93(3):438, 1994.

Srinivasan R, Minocha A: When to suspect lactose intolerance: symptomatic, ethnic, and laboratory clues, *Postgrad Med* 104(3): 109-123, 1998.

Stephens D, Jackson PL, Gutierrez Y: Subclinical vitamin A deficiency: a potentially unrecognized problem in the United States, *Pediatr Nurs* 22(5):377-389, 1996.

Thame MM, Burton KA, Forrester TE: The human ruminant, *West Indian Med J* 49(2): 172-174, 2000.

Treem WR: Infant colic: a pediatric gastroenterologist's perspective, *Pediatr Clin North Am* 41(5):1121-1137, 1994.

Ward DB and others: Characterization of diaper dermatitis in the United States, *Arch Pediatr Adolesc Med* 154(9):943-945, 2000.

Weizman Z and others: Efficacy of herbal tea preparation in infantile colic, *J Pediatr* 122(4):650-652, 1993.

Willinger M and others: Factors associated with caregiver's choice of infant sleep position, 1994-1998: The National Infant Sleep Position Study, *JAMA* 283(16):2135-2142, 2000.

Wong DL and others: Diapering choices: a critical review of the issues, *Pediatr Nurs* 18(1):41-54, 1992.

Wylie R: Cow's milk protein allergy and hypoallergenic formulas, *Clin Pediatr* 35(10):497-500, 1996.

# Chapter 14

# Health Promotion of the Toddler and Family

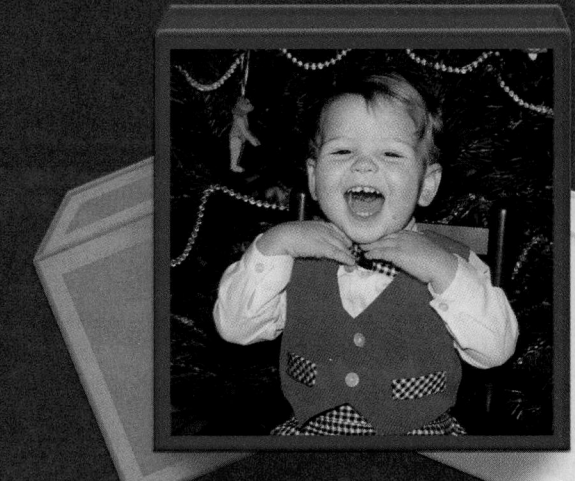

## Chapter Outline

**PROMOTING OPTIMUM GROWTH AND DEVELOPMENT, 591**
**Biologic Development, 592**
    Proportional Changes, 592
    Sensory Changes, 592
    Maturation of Systems, 592
    Gross and Fine Motor
        Development, 593
**Psychosocial Development, 594**
    Developing a Sense of Autonomy
        (Erikson), 594
**Cognitive Development, 594**
    Sensorimotor Phase (Piaget), 594
    Preconceptual Phase (Piaget), 596
**Moral Development, 597**
    Preconventional or Premoral Level
        (Kohlberg), 597
**Spiritual Development, 598**
**Development of Body Image, 598**

**Development of Sexuality, 598**
**Social Development, 598**
    Individuation-Separation, 598
    Language Development, 599
    Personal-Social Behavior, 599
    Play, 600
**Toys, 601**
    Selecting Toys, 601
    Toy Safety, 601
**Temperament, 601**
**Coping with Concerns Related
    to Normal Growth and
    Development, 603**
    Toilet Training, 603
    Sibling Rivalry, 605
    Temper Tantrums, 607
    Negativism, 608
    Coping with Stress, 608

**PROMOTING OPTIMUM HEALTH DURING TODDLERHOOD, 609**
**Nutrition, 609**
    Nutritional Counseling, 610
**Sleep and Activity, 611**
**Dental Health, 611**
    Regular Dental Examinations, 611
    Removal of Plaque, 611
    Fluoride, 613
    Low-Cariogenic Diet, 613
**Injury Prevention, 616**
    Motor Vehicle Injuries, 616
    Drowning, 620
    Burns, 620
    Poisoning, 622
    Falls, 622
    Aspiration and Suffocation, 623
    Bodily Damage, 623
**Anticipatory Guidance—Care of Families, 624**

## Related Topics

Animal Bites, Ch. 18
Attachment, Ch. 12
Dental Disorders, Ch. 18
Enuresis, Ch. 18
Family Influences on Child Health
    Promotion, Ch. 3

Fears, Ch. 15
Ingestion of Injurious Agents, Ch. 16
Injuries—The Leading Killer, Ch. 1
Injury Prevention: Infant, Ch. 12; Preschooler,
    Ch. 15

Limit-Setting and Discipline, Ch. 3
Sleep Problems, Ch. 12
Social, Cultural, and Religious Influences on
    Child Health Promotion, Ch. 2
Spiritual Development, Ch. 15

## PROMOTING OPTIMUM GROWTH AND DEVELOPMENT

The term *terrible twos* has often been used to describe the toddler years, the period from 12 to 36 months of age. It is a time of intense exploration of the environment as children attempt to find out how things work, what the word "no" means, and the power of temper tantrums, negativism,

and obstinacy. "Getting into things" is their way of learning about their world, especially relationships. Successful mastery of the tasks of this age requires a strong foundation of trust during infancy and frequently necessitates guidance from others when parent and toddler face the struggles of toilet training, limit-setting, and sibling rivalry. Nurses who understand the dynamics of growth and development of the toddler can help families deal effectively with the tasks of this age.

■ Patricia Schwartz, PhD, RNC, revised this chapter.

# Biologic Development

## Proportional Changes

Growth slows considerably during toddlerhood. The average *weight* at 2 years is 12 kg (27 pounds). The average weight gain is 1.8 to 2.7 kg (4 to 6 pounds) per year. The birth weight is quadrupled by 2½ years of age. The rate of increase in height also slows. The usual increment is an addition of 7.5 cm (3 inches) per year and occurs mainly in elongation of the legs rather than the trunk. The average *height* of a 2-year-old is 86.6 cm (34 inches). In general, adult height is about twice the child's height at 2 years of age. Accurate measurement of height and weight during the toddler years should reveal a steady growth curve that is steplike in nature rather than linear (straight), which is characteristic of the growth spurts during the early childhood years.

The rate of increase in *head circumference* slows somewhat by the end of infancy, and head circumference is usually equal to chest circumference by 1 to 2 years of age. The usual total increase in head circumference during the second year is 2.5 cm (1 inch). Then the rate of increase slows until age 5 years, when the increase is less than 1.25 cm (½ inch) per year. The anterior fontanel closes between 12 and 18 months of age.

*Chest circumference* continues to increase in size and exceeds head circumference during the toddler years. Its shape also changes as the transverse or lateral diameter exceeds the anteroposterior diameter. After the second year the chest circumference exceeds the abdominal measurement, which, in addition to the growth of the lower extremities, gives the child a taller, leaner appearance. However, the toddler retains a squat, "pot-bellied" appearance because of the less well-developed abdominal musculature and short legs (Fig. 14-1). The legs retain a slightly bowed or curved appearance during the second year from the weight of the relatively large trunk.

## Sensory Changes

*Visual acuity* of 20/40 is considered acceptable during the toddler years. Full binocular vision is well developed, and any evidence of persistent strabismus should receive professional attention as early as possible to prevent amblyopia. Depth perception continues to develop but, because of the child's lack of motor coordination, falls from heights remain a persistent danger.

The senses of *hearing, smell, taste,* and *touch* become increasingly well developed, coordinated with each other, and associated with other experiences. All of the senses are used to explore the environment. Toddlers will visually inspect an object by turning it over; they may taste it, smell it, and touch it several times before they are satisfied with their investigation. They will shake it to see if it makes noise and vigorously test its durability.

Another example of the integrated function of the senses is the toddler's development of specific *taste preferences*. The child is much less likely than infants to try a new food because of its appearance or smell, not just its taste. Nonsensory associations with objects also take on significance. For example, if parents refuse a particular food because of their dislike, they will transfer this negative connotation to the child before the child has had an opportunity to taste it. Awareness of these factors is important in several areas of childrearing, such as feeding, teaching socially acceptable habits, and reinforcing appropriate behavioral responses to various situations.

*Touch* continues to be very important to the toddler. Descending development of the spinal tract is evidenced by increased sensation in the lower extremities, such as tickling the feet. Pleasant tactile sensations soothe and comfort the toddler, especially in times of stress or fatigue.

## Maturation of Systems

Most of the physiologic systems are relatively mature by the end of toddlerhood. By the end of the first year, all of the *brain* cells are present but continue to increase in size. Myelination of the spinal cord is almost complete by 2 years of age, which parallels the completion of most of the gross motor skills associated with locomotion. Brain growth is 75% completed by the end of 2 years.

Development of various areas of the brain seems to correspond with the progressive intellectual capacity of the child. Various areas of the cerebral cortex undergo specific changes as developmental progress occurs, such as the Broca area for speech and cortical areas for control of the legs, hands, feet, and sphincters. Because this neuromotor organization is so inclusive, complex, and intricate, the child is limited in the ability to attend to any one aspect of behavior for more than a few minutes.

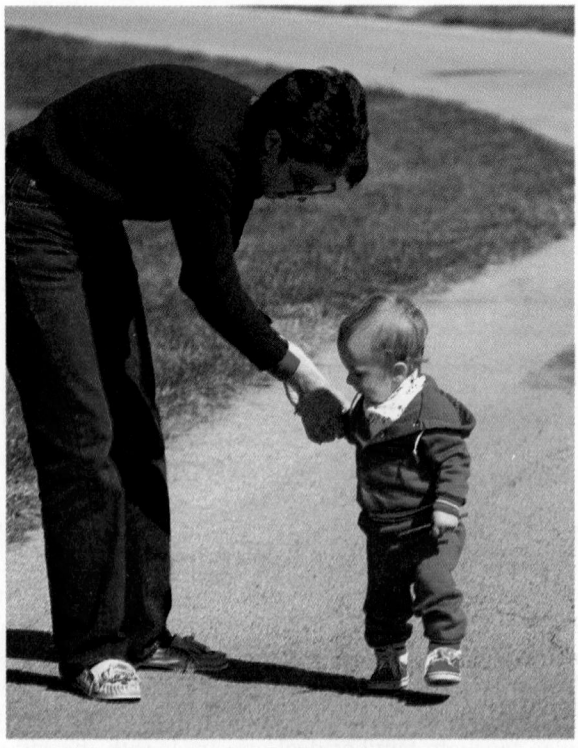

**Fig. 14-1** Typical toddling gait.

Between 2 and 3 years of age, coordination and consolidation of these voluntary functions allow the toddler to listen better, look longer, and have an extended attention span. Although postural control is increasingly developed as myelination of the spinal cord advances, the immaturity of this control, combined with the child's limited experiences and the lack of visual perception, makes simple acts such as seating oneself in a chair or climbing down stairs difficult tasks.

Volume of the *respiratory tract* and growth of associated structures continue to increase during early childhood, lessening some of the factors that predisposed the child to frequent and serious infections during infancy. However, the internal structures of the ear and throat continue to be short and straight, and the lymphoid tissue of the tonsils and adenoids continues to be large. As a result, otitis media, tonsillitis, and upper respiratory tract infections are common. The respiratory and heart rates slow, and the blood pressure increases (see inside back cover). Respirations continue to be abdominal.

The *digestive processes* are fairly complete by the beginning of toddlerhood. The acidity of the gastric contents continues to increase and has a protective function because it is capable of destroying many types of bacteria. Stomach capacity increases to allow for the usual schedule of three small meals a day.

One of the more prominent changes of the gastrointestinal system is the voluntary control of elimination. With complete myelination of the spinal cord, control of anal and urethral sphincters is gradually achieved. The physiologic ability to control the sphincters occurs somewhere between ages 18 and 24 months. Bladder capacity also increases considerably. By 14 to 18 months of age the child is able to retain urine for up to 2 hours or longer.

The *skin* functionally matures during early childhood. The epidermis and dermis are more tightly bound together, increasing their resistance to infection and irritation and creating a more effective barrier against fluid loss. Production of sebum is minimal, which contributes to the development of dry skin. The eccrine glands are functional during early childhood and react to changes in temperature, but they produce very minimal amounts of sweat. Hair grows thicker and coarser and usually darkens and loses some curliness. Fine hair is evident on the lower arms and legs. Production of adipose tissue declines as hyperplasia of muscle cells increases. With the concurrent growth of the lower extremities, the child assumes more adultlike proportions.

Under conditions of moderate variation in temperature, the toddler rarely has the difficulties of the young infant in maintaining *body temperature.* The capillaries are able to conserve core body temperature by constricting in response to cold and dilating in response to heat. Shivering, an involuntary act that results in rhythmic muscle contraction, which increases cellular metabolism, producing heat, is much more effective as a source of thermogenesis. The child also learns mechanisms to control body temperature—putting on clothing when cold or removing it when warm.

The *defense mechanisms* of the tissues and blood, particularly phagocytosis, are much more efficient in the toddler than in the infant. The production of antibodies is well established. Immunoglobulin G (IgG), which neutralizes microbial toxins, reaches adult levels by the end of the second year of life. Passive immunity from maternal transfer during fetal life disappears by the beginning of toddlerhood. Immunoglobulin M (IgM), which responds to artificial immunizing techniques and combats serious infection, attains adult levels during late infancy. Immunoglobulins A, D, and E increase gradually, not reaching eventual adult levels until later childhood. Many young children demonstrate a sudden increase in colds and minor infections when entering daycare or preschool because of the exposure to new antigens.

## Gross and Fine Motor Development

The major *gross motor skill* during the toddler years is the development of locomotion. By 12 to 13 months of age toddlers walk alone, using a wide stance for extra balance; by age 18 months they try to run but fall easily. Between 2 and 3 years of age, refinement of the upright, biped position is evident in improved coordination and equilibrium. By age 2 years toddlers can walk up and down stairs, and by age 2½ years they jump, using both feet, stand on one foot for a second or two, and manage a few steps on tiptoe. By the end of the second year they stand on one foot, walk on tiptoe, and climb stairs with alternate footing.

*Fine motor development* is demonstrated in increasingly skillful manual dexterity. Once the pincer grasp is achieved, usually at 9 to 10 months of age, toddlers combine this skill with other developing sensory and cognitive abilities. For example, by age 12 months they are able to grasp a very small object. At age 15 months they can drop a pellet into a narrow-necked bottle. Casting or throwing objects and retrieving them becomes an almost obsessive activity at about 15 months. By 18 months of age they can throw a ball overhand without losing their balance.

Visual perception of geometric shapes is also evident at this time. At age 12 months children selectively look at a round hole in a special form board but are unable to insert a round object. By age 15 months they promptly place the round object in the hole, even if the board is revised or turned upside down. Spatial relations also are evident in their ability to build a tower with blocks: by age 18 months, a tower of three to four blocks; by age 24 months, a tower of six to seven blocks; and by age 30 months, a tower of eight blocks or more.

Fine motor skill and visual ability are demonstrated in toddlers' progressive adeptness in manipulating a pencil or crayon. By age 15 months they will scribble spontaneously and by age 24 months will imitate a circular stroke and a vertical line. By the end of the toddler period, copying a circle and imitating a cross are possible.

Mastery of gross and fine motor skills is evident in all phases of the child's activity, such as play, dressing, language comprehension, response to discipline, social interaction, and propensity for injuries. Activities occur less in isolation and more in conjunction with other physical and mental abilities to produce a purposeful result. For example, the toddler walks to reach a new location, releases a toy to pick it up or to choose a new one, and scribbles to look at the image produced. The possibilities of the exploration, investigation, and manipulation mastery of the environment—and its hazards—are endless.

## Psychosocial Development

Toddlers are faced with the mastery of several important tasks. If the need for basic trust has been satisfied, they are ready to give up dependence for control, independence, and autonomy. Some of the specific tasks include:

- Differentiation of self from others, particularly the mother
- Toleration of separation from parents
- Ability to withstand delayed gratification
- Control over bodily functions
- Acquisition of socially acceptable behavior
- Verbal means of communication
- Ability to interact with others in a less egocentric manner

Mastery of these goals is only begun during late infancy and the toddler years, and such tasks as developing interpersonal relationships with others may not be completed until adolescence. However, crucial foundations for successful completion of such developmental tasks are laid during these early formative years.

### Developing a Sense of Autonomy (Erikson)

According to Erikson, the developmental task of toddlerhood is acquiring a sense of **autonomy** while overcoming a sense of **doubt** and **shame.** As infants gain trust in the predictability and reliability of their parents, environment, and interaction with others, they begin to discover that their behavior is their own and that it has a predictable, reliable effect on others. However, although they are aware of their will and control over others, they are confronted with the conflict of exerting autonomy and relinquishing the much enjoyed dependence on others. Exerting their will has definite negative consequences, whereas retaining dependent, submissive behavior is generally rewarded with affection and approval. However, continued dependency creates a sense of doubt regarding their potential capacity to control their actions. This doubt is compounded by a sense of shame for feeling this urge to revolt against others' will and a fear that they will exceed their own capacity for manipulating the environment. The latter fear is a basis for instituting limit-setting and consistent discipline at this age. Without appropriate limits on what is acceptable vs nonacceptable behavior, children have no guidelines for establishing the end points of their ability to control.

Just as the infant has the social modalities of grasping and biting, the toddler has the newly gained modality of holding on and letting go. To hold on and let go is evident with the use of the hands, mouth, eyes, and, eventually, the sphincters when toilet training is begun. These social modalities are expressed constantly in the child's play activities, such as casting or throwing objects; taking objects out of boxes, drawers, or cabinets; holding on tighter when someone says, "No, don't touch"; and spitting out food as taste preferences become very strong.

Several characteristics, especially negativism and ritualism, are typical of toddlers in their quest for autonomy. As toddlers attempt to express their will, they often act with **negativism,** the persistent negative response to requests. The words "no" or "me do" can be the sole vocabulary. Emotions become very strongly expressed, usually in rapid mood swings. One minute toddlers can be engrossed in an activity, and the next minute they might be violently angry because they were unable to manipulate a toy or open a door. If scolded for doing something wrong, they can have a temper tantrum and almost instantaneously pull at the parent's legs to be picked up and comforted. Understanding and coping with these swift changes is often difficult for parents. Many parents find the negativism exasperating and, instead of dealing constructively with it, give in to it, which further threatens children in their search for learning acceptable methods of interacting with others (see p. 608).

In contrast to negativism, which frequently disrupts the environment, **ritualism,** the need to maintain sameness and reliability, provides a sense of comfort. Toddlers can venture out with security when they know that familiar people, places, and routines still exist. One can easily understand why change, such as hospitalization, represents such a threat to these children. Without the comfortable rituals, there is little opportunity to exert autonomy. Consequently, dependency and regression occur (see p. 609).

Erikson focuses on the development of the **ego,** which may be thought of as reason or common sense, during this phase of psychosocial development. There is a struggle as the child deals with the impulses of the **id** and attempts to tolerate frustration and learn socially acceptable ways of interacting with the environment. The ego becomes evident as the child is able to tolerate delayed gratification.

There is also a rudimentary beginning of the **superego,** or conscience, which is the incorporation of the morals of society and the process of acculturation. With the development of the ego, children further differentiate themselves from others and expand their sense of trust within themselves. But as they begin to develop awareness of their own will and capacity to achieve, they also become aware of their ability to fail. This ever-present awareness of potential failure creates doubt and shame. Successful mastery of the task of autonomy necessitates opportunities for self-mastery while withstanding the frustration of necessary limit-setting and delayed gratification. Opportunities for self-mastery are present in appropriate play activities, toilet training, the crisis of sibling rivalry, and successful interactions with significant others.

## Cognitive Development

### Sensorimotor Phase (Piaget)

The period from 12 to 24 months of age is a continuation of the final two stages of the sensorimotor phase (Table 14-1). During this time the cognitive processes develop rapidly and at times seem similar to mature thinking. However, reasoning skills are still quite primitive and need to be understood to effectively deal with the typical behaviors of this-age child. The main cognitive achievement of early childhood is the acquisition of language, which represents mental symbolism.

## TABLE 14-1    Sensorimotor and preconceptual phases during toddlerhood*

| Stage/Age | Cognitive Development | Behavior |
|---|---|---|
| **Sensorimotor** | | |
| V. Tertiary circular reactions 13-18 months | Active experimentation to achieve previously unattainable goals<br>Increased concept of object permanence<br>Differentiation of oneself from objects<br>Early traces of memory<br>Beginning awareness of spatial, causal, and temporal relationships<br>Able to enter into an action at any point without reproducing the entire sequence | Insatiable curiosity about the environment<br>Uses all sensory cues for exploration<br>Ventures away from parent for longer periods<br>Uses physical skills to achieve a particular goal<br>Can find hidden objects, but only in first location<br>Able to insert a round object into a hole<br>Fits smaller objects into each other (nesting)<br>Gestures "up" and "down"<br>Puts objects into a container and takes them out<br>Realizes that "out of sight" is not out of reach; opens doors and drawers to find objects<br>Gains comfort from parent's voice even if the parent is not visually present |
| VI. Invention of new means through mental combinations 19-24 months | Awareness of object permanence regardless of the number of invisible displacements<br>Can infer a cause while only experiencing the effect<br>Imitation is increasingly symbolic<br>Beginning sense of time in terms of anticipation, memory, and ability to wait<br>Egocentricism in thought and behavior<br>Global organization of thought | Searches for an object through several hiding places<br>Will infer a cause by associating two or more experiences (such as candy missing, sister smiling)<br>Imitates words and sounds of animals<br>Imitates adult behavior (domestic mimicry)<br>Follows directions and understands requests<br>Uses words "up," "down," "come," and "go" with meaning<br>May sit and wait for meals at the table for short period of time<br>Has some sense of time; waits in response to "just a minute"; may use word "now"<br>Refers to self by name<br>Engages in parallel play; demonstrates awareness of ownership<br>Very concerned with ritualistic, routinized schedule |
| **Preconceptual** | | |
| 2-4 years† | Increased use of language as mental symbolization<br>Egocentricism still present in thought, play, and behavior<br>Increased sense of time, space, causality<br>See Box 14-1 | Uses two- to three-word phrases<br>Increased vocabulary<br>Refers to self by pronoun<br>Possessive of own toys, uses word "mine"<br>Begins to use past tense of verbs<br>Uses phrases "going to," "in a minute," "today," "all done"<br>Uses many future-oriented words, such as "tomorrow," "next day," "afternoon," but poor conception of passage of time<br>Follows directions using prepositions, such as "up," "behind," "under," "in back of," and so on |

*For the previous four stages during early infancy see Table 12-1.
†Cognitive development and behavior apply primarily to ages 24 to 36 months.

In the fifth stage, *tertiary circular reactions* (from 13 to 18 months of age), the child uses active experimentation to achieve previously unattainable goals. Newly acquired physical skills are increasingly important for the function they serve rather than for the acts themselves. The child incorporates the old learning of secondary circular reactions and applies the combined knowledge to new situations, with emphasis on the results of the experimentation. In this way there is the beginning of rational judgment and intellectual reasoning. During this stage there is further differentiation of oneself from objects. This is evident in the child's increasing ability to venture away from the parent and to tolerate longer periods of separation.

Awareness of a causal relationship between two events is apparent. After flipping a light switch, toddlers are aware that a reciprocal response occurs. However, they are not able to transfer that knowledge to new situations. Therefore, every time they see what appears to be a light switch, they must reinvestigate its function. Such behavior demonstrates the beginning of categorizing data into distinct classes, subclasses, and so on. There are innumerable examples of this type of behavior as toddlers repeatedly explore the same object each time it appears in a new place. A classic example is their curiosity about electrical outlets. Even if they receive a shock from one of them, they will adamantly poke, taste, and inspect every other outlet. This inability to transfer information leaves toddlers particularly vulnerable to injuries. However, traces of memory are evident because they will usually avoid the outlet where the shock occurred.

Because classification of objects is still rudimentary, the appearance of an object denotes its function. For example, if the child's toys are stored in a paper bag or large container, there is no difference between that toy receptacle and the garbage pail or laundry basket. If allowed to turn over the toy receptacle, the child will just as quickly do the same to other similar objects because, in the child's mind, there is no difference. Expecting toddlers to judge which receptacles are permissible to explore and which are not is inappropriate for this age-group. Instead, the forbidden object, such as the garbage pail, should be placed out of reach.

The discovery of objects as objects leads to an awareness of their spatial relationships. Children are able to recognize different shapes and their relationship to each other. For example, they can fit slightly smaller boxes into each other (nesting) and can place a round object into a hole, even if the board is turned around, upside down, or reversed. However, they cannot do the same thing with a square until 2 years of age. Children are also aware of space and the relationship of their body to dimensions such as height. They will stretch, stand on a low stair or stool, and pull a string to reach an object.

Object permanence has also advanced. Although they still cannot find an object that has been displaced and is no longer visible or has been moved from under one pillow to another without their seeing the change, toddlers are increasingly aware of the existence of objects behind closed doors, in drawers, and under tables. Parents are usually acutely aware of this developmental achievement, because they find high places and locked cabinets to be the only areas inaccessible to toddlers. Parents also experience toddlers' protest behaviors when the parents leave because toddlers are aware that their parents are absent when they cannot see them.

During ages 19 to 24 months the child is in the final sensorimotor stage, *invention of new means through mental combinations.* This stage completes the more primitive, autistic thought processes of infancy and prepares the way for more complex mental operations during the phase of preoperational thought. One of the most dramatic achievements of this stage is in the area of object permanence. Children will now actively search for an object in several potential hiding places. In addition, they can infer a cause when only experiencing the effect. They can infer that an object was hidden in any number of places even if they only saw the original hiding place.

Imitation displays deeper meaning and understanding. Earlier, imitation was very concrete and action oriented. For example, "bye-bye" was a behavioral response more than a conceptual gesture of departure. Now it has a broader meaning, such as Daddy is going to work, it is time for a walk, or something is no longer present. There is greater symbolization to imitation.

One type of symbolic imitation is *domestic mimicry*, the imitation of household activity. Toddlers are acutely aware of others' actions and attempt to copy them in gestures and in words. They can imitate the parents' performance of a household task both physically and verbally (Fig. 14-2). Parents often remark how accurately they see themselves in their child when the child engages in domestic mimicry. Such activity is part of the child's learning sex-role behavior. Identification with the parent of the same sex becomes apparent by the second year and represents the child's intellectual ability to differentiate models of behavior and to imitate them appropriately.

The conception of time is still embryonic, but children have some sense of timing in terms of anticipation, memory,

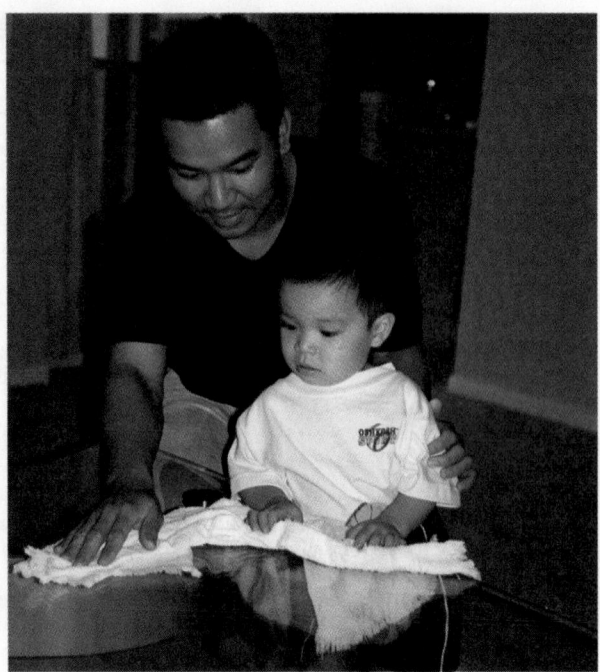

**Fig. 14-2** Domestic mimicry is common during toddlerhood.

and the limited ability to wait. They may listen to the command, "Just a minute," and behave appropriately. However, their sense of timing is exaggerated—1 minute can last an hour. Toddlers' limited attention spans also indicate their sense of immediacy and concern for the present.

*Egocentrism,* or the inability to envision situations from perspectives other than one's own, is evident in all aspects of toddlers' behavior. They see, experience, and live every event in reference to themselves. A common example of egocentric behavior is the toddler who takes a toy away from another child. The child is concerned only with playing with the toy and is unable to conceptualize that taking the toy away will make the other child unhappy.

### Preconceptual Phase (Piaget)

At approximately 2 years of age the child enters the preconceptual phase of cognitive development, which lasts until about age 4 years. The preconceptual phase is a subdivision of the *preoperational phase,* which spans ages 2 to 7 years. The preconceptual phase is primarily one of transition that bridges the purely self-satisfying behavior of infancy and the rudimentary socialized behavior of latency. The principal characteristics of this stage are egocentric use of language and dependence on perception in problem solving (Thomas, 1996a).

During ages 2 to 4 years children learn a variety of words and there is an increasing use of language. In fact, toddlers talk a lot. Speech is primarily of two types—egocentric or socialized. *Egocentric speech* consists of repeating words and sounds for the pleasure of hearing oneself and is not intended to communicate. This *collective monologue* reflects the child's lingering self-centeredness.

*Socialized speech* is for communication; however, it is still egocentric in that children communicate about themselves to

## Box 14-1 ■ ■ ■
## Characteristics of Preoperational Thought

**Egocentrism**—Unable to envision situations from perspectives other than one's own.
  *Example:* If a person is positioned between the toddler and another child, the toddler, who is facing the person, will explain that both children can see the middle person's face. The young child is unable to realize that the other person views the middle person from a different perspective, the back.
  *Implication:* Avoid moralizing about "why" something is wrong if it requires an understanding of someone else's feelings or opinion. Telling a child to stop hitting because hitting hurts the other person is often ineffective because, to the aggressor, it may not hurt to hit someone else. Instead, emphasize that hitting is not allowed.

**Transductive**—Reasons from the particular to the particular.
  *Example:* Child refuses to eat a food because something previously eaten did not taste good.
  *Implication:* Accept child's reasoning; offer refused food at different time.

**Global organization**—Changes in any one part of the whole changes the entire whole.
  *Example:* Child refuses to sleep in room because location of bed is changed.
  *Implication:* Accept child's reasoning; use same bed position or introduce change slowly.

**Centration**—Focuses on one aspect rather than considering all possible alternatives.
  *Example:* Child refuses to eat a food because of its color, even though its taste and smell are acceptable.
  *Implication:* Accept child's reasoning.

**Animism**—Attributes lifelike qualities to inanimate objects.
  *Example:* Child scolds stairs for making child fall down.
  *Implication:* Join child in the "scolding." Keep frightening objects out of view.

**Irreversibility**—Unable to undo or reverse the actions initiated physically.
  *Example:* When told to stop doing something, such as talking, child is unable to think of opposite activity.
  *Implication:* State requests or instructions *positively* (e.g., "Be quiet").

**Magical**—Believes that thoughts are all-powerful and can cause events.
  *Example:* Child wishes someone dead; then if the person dies; child feels at fault because of the "bad" thought that made the death happen.
  Calling children "bad" because they did something wrong makes children feel as if they are bad.
  *Implication:* Clarify that thoughts do not make things happen and that child is not responsible.
  Use "I" messages rather than "you" messages to communicate thoughts, feelings, expectations, or beliefs without imposing blame or criticism. Emphasize that the act is bad, not the child.

**Inability to conserve**—Unable to understand the idea that a mass can be changed in size, shape, volume, or length without losing or adding to the original mass (instead, children judge what they see by the immediate perceptual clues given to them).
  *Example:* If two lines of equal length are presented in such a way that one appears longer than the other, child will state that one line is longer even if child measures both lines with a ruler or yardstick and finds that each has the same length.
  *Implication:* Change the most obvious perceptual clue to reorient child's view of what is seen. For example, give medicine in a small medicine cup, rather than a large cup because child will imagine that the large vessel contains more liquid. If child refuses the medicine in the small cup, pour it into a large cup, because the liquid will appear to be less in a tall, wide container. Give a large flat cookie rather than a thick small one, or do the reverse with meat or cheese; child will usually eat larger size of favorite food and smaller size of less favorite food.

---

others. Before age 3 most speech is directed at self-fulfillment or self-reference, such as, "Want drink," or "I do," and is directed mostly toward adults. Because children think that everyone else's world is the same as theirs, they expect others to understand their verbal messages even when limited information is conveyed.

*Preoperational thinking* implies that children cannot think in terms of *operations*—the ability to manipulate objects in relation to each other in a logical fashion. Rather, toddlers think primarily based on their perception of an event. Problem solving is based on what they see or hear directly rather than on what they recall about objects and events (Box 14-1).

Within the second year the child increasingly uses language symbolically and is concerned with the "why" and "how" of things. For example, a pencil is "something to write with" and food is "something to eat." However, such mental symbolization is closely associated with prelogical reasoning. For instance, a needle is "something that hurts." Such painful experiences take on new significance because memory is associated with the specific event and fears are likely to develop, such as resistance to people who wear white uniforms or rooms that look like the practitioner's office. Sometimes the child's ability to recall events is underestimated, and little thought is given to the preparation for visits to a hospital or other health facility, resulting in fears that can

last a lifetime. Because of the vulnerability of these early years, it is essential to prepare children for new experiences, whether it is a new baby-sitter or a visit to the dentist.

## Moral Development

### Preconventional or Premoral Level (Kohlberg)

Toddlers' development of moral judgment is at the most basic level. There is little, if any, concern for why something is wrong. Young children behave because of the freedom or restriction that is placed on actions. In the *punishment and obedience orientation,* whether an action is good or bad depends on whether it results in reward or punishment. If children are punished for it, the action is bad. If they are not punished, the action is good, regardless of the meaning of the act. For example, if parents allow hitting, the child will perceive that hitting is good because it is not associated with punishment (Thomas, 1996a). By the age of 36 months, developmental aspects of conscience have been reported (Kochanska, 1997).

The type of discipline also affects children's moral development. When parents use power to control behavior, such as physical punishment or withholding privileges, children receive a negative view of morals, especially toward authority figures, such as law enforcement agencies. When parents withdraw love or attention, children behave primarily because of guilt, rather than from an internalization of morals. However, when parents give explanations for the misbehavior and try to help children change through positive approaches, such as consequences or rewards, children feel less hostility and are more likely to base their actions on an analysis of why an act may be wrong. Of course, the effect of discipline is not limited to the toddler years, and the sole use of explanation is inappropriate. Because parents usually establish disciplinary techniques at this time, the use of constructive approaches should begin early. (See Limit-Setting and Discipline, Chapter 3.)

## Spiritual Development

Because of their immature cognitive processes, toddlers have only a vague idea of God and religious teachings. However, routines such as saying prayers before meals or at bedtime can be very important and comforting. Toward the end of toddlerhood, when children are in preoperational thought, there is some advancement of their understanding of God. Religious teachings, such as concerning reward or fear of punishment (heaven or hell), may influence their behavior and moral development (Barnes and others, 2000). (See Chapter 15.)

## Development of Body Image

As in infancy, the development of body image closely parallels cognitive development. With increasing motor ability, toddlers recognize the usefulness of body parts and gradually learn their respective names. They also learn that certain parts of the body have various meanings; for example, during toilet training, the genitalia become significant and cleanliness is emphasized. By 2 years of age there is recognition of sexual differences and reference to self by name and then by pronoun.

Once they begin preoperational thought, toddlers can use symbols to represent objects, but their thinking may lead to inaccuracies. For example, if someone who is pregnant is called "fat," they will describe all "fat" ladies (sometimes even men!) as having babies. There is a beginning recognition of words used to describe physical appearance, such as "pretty," "handsome," or "big boy." Such expressions eventually influence how children view their own bodies, and such labeling (negative or positive) becomes part of their body image.

Although there has been little research done on body image development in young children, it is evident that body integrity is poorly understood and that intrusive experiences are threatening because they fear their blood and insides will leak out (Colson and Dworkin, 1997). For example, during a physical assessment toddlers forcefully resist procedures such as examining the ear or mouth and taking a rectal temperature. Toddlers also have unclear body boundaries and may associate nonviable parts, such as feces, with essential body parts. This can be seen in the toddler who is upset by flushing the toilet and watching the stool disappear.

Nurses can assist parents in fostering a positive body image in their child by encouraging them to avoid negative labels, such as "skinny arms" or "chubby legs"—self-perceptions that can last a lifetime. Body parts, especially those related to elimination and reproduction, should be called by their correct names. Respect for the body should be practiced.

## Development of Sexuality

Just as toddlers explore their environment, they also explore their bodies and find that touching certain body parts is pleasurable. Genital fondling (masturbation) can occur and involves manual stimulation, as well as posturing movements (especially in young girls) such as tightening of the thighs or mechanical pressure applied to the pubic or suprapubic area (Lidster and Horsburgh, 1994). Other demonstrations of sensual activities include rocking, swinging, and hugging people and toys. Parental reactions to toddlers' sexual behavior will influence the children's own attitudes and should be accepting rather than critical (Finan, 1997).

Children in this age-group are learning vocabulary associated with anatomy, elimination, and reproduction. Certain associations between words and functions become significant and can influence future sexual attitudes. For example, if parents refer to the genitalia as dirty, especially in the context of elimination, the child may transfer this association between genitalia and "dirty" to sexual functions.

Sex-role differences become obvious to children and are evident in much of their imitative play. Early attitudes are formed about affectional behaviors between adults from observing parental and other adult sexual/sensual activities. (See Sex Education, Chapter 15.)

## Social Development

### Individuation-Separation

A major task of the toddler period is differentiation of self from significant others, usually the mother. The differentiation process consists of two phases: *separation,* the children's emergence from a symbiotic fusion with the mother, and *individuation,* those achievements that mark children's assumption of their individual characteristics in the environment (Mahler, Pine, and Bergman, 2000). Although the process begins during the latter half of infancy, the major achievements occur during the toddler years.

Toddlers have an increased understanding and awareness of object permanence and some ability to withstand delayed gratification and tolerate moderate frustration. They begin to lose some of their previous resistance to separation yet appear to become even more concerned about the parent's whereabouts. They have learned from experience that parents exist when physically absent. Repetition of events such as going to bed without the parents but waking to find them again reinforces the reliability of such brief separations. Consequently, toddlers are able to venture away from their parents for brief periods because of the security of knowing that the parent will be there when they return. Verbal and visual reassurance from the parent gradually replaces some of the previous need to be physically close for comfort.

Toddlers also show less fear of strangers, but only when their parents are present. When left alone with a stranger, they are very fearful and acutely anxious; manifest depressive behavior, such as crying and withdrawal; and may become restless, hyperactive, or passive, reverting to regressive behaviors. Such reactions may be evident when a child is left with a baby-sitter, during the initial days of preschool or daycare, or if the child is hospitalized. (See Chapter 26.)

These behaviors are not pathologic or harmful if parents realize how desperately their children need them. In fact, indiscriminate friendliness toward strangers and lack of anxiety during separation from parents may be reasons for concern. Sensitive, perceptive parents will be aware of the child's need for increased love, affection, and attention when they are together. An attitude such as "They will get used to the baby-sitter" will not help young children positively tolerate separation.

Parents often need help in realizing the necessity of preparing children for an inevitable separation. Particularly with the firstborn, parents tend to overprotect children, shield them from any anxiety-producing experience, and insulate them from less than immediate gratification. Although this is not necessarily harmful, especially if opportunities for independence are allowed later, it does not prepare children for unexpected events. A typical example is the birth of a sibling. The child is faced with the crisis of sibling rivalry, as well as separation from the parent. No wonder the child will not welcome the infant—the intruder caused the mother to leave! Allowing children to experience brief periods of separation early during infancy prepares them for such experiences later. Indeed, they may still manifest the typical behaviors of protest, but they will also have learned that their mother or father always returns. Therefore it is easy to appreciate the tremendous loss that the death of a parent represents for young children; unlike their other experiences with separation, this time the parent will not return.

Transitional objects, such as a favorite blanket or toy, provide security for young children, especially when they are separated from parents, are dealing with a new stress, or are just fatigued (Fig. 14-3). Security objects often become so important to toddlers that they refuse to have them taken away. Such behavior is normal; there is no need to discourage this tendency. During separations, such as daycare, hospitalization, or even staying overnight with a relative, transitional objects should be provided to minimize any feelings of fear or loneliness.

Learning to tolerate and master brief periods of separation is an important developmental task of children in this age-group. In addition, it is a necessary component of parenting because brief periods of separation from their children allow parents to recoup their energy and patience and to minimize directing their irritations and frustrations at the children.

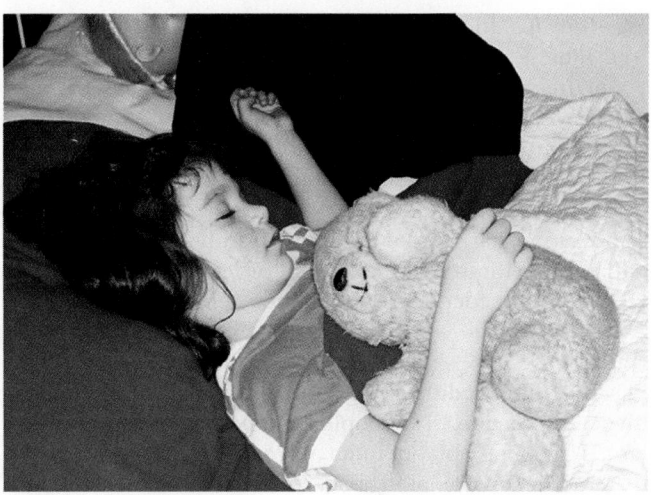

**Fig. 14-3** Transitional objects, such as a warm and fuzzy stuffed animal, are sources of security to a toddler.

## Language Development

The most striking characteristic of language development during early childhood is the increasing level of comprehension. Although the number of words acquired—from about 4 at 1 year of age to approximately 300 at age 2 years—is notable, *the ability to understand speech is much greater than the number of words the child can say.* This is particularly evident in bilingual families where the vocabulary may be delayed, but comprehension in either language is appropriate (Chiocca, 1998).

At age 1 year the child uses one-word sentences or holophrases. The word "up" can mean "pick me up" or "look up there." For the child the one word conveys the meaning of a sentence, but to others it may mean many things or nothing. During this age about 25% of the vocalizations are intelligible. By the age of 2 years the child uses multiword sentences by stringing together two or three words, such as the phrases, "mama go bye-bye" or "all gone," and approximately 65% of the speech is understandable.

## Personal-Social Behavior

One of the most dramatic aspects of development in the toddler is personal-social interaction. Parents frequently wonder why their manageable, docile, lovable infant has turned into a determined, strong-willed, volatile-tempered little "tyrant." In addition, the tyrant can swiftly and unpredictably revert back to the adorable infant. All of this is part of "growing up" and is evident in such areas as dressing, feeding, playing, and establishing self-control.

Toddlers are developing skills of independence, which are evident in all areas of behavior. By age 15 months children feed themselves, drink well from a covered cup, and manage a spoon, with considerable spilling. By age 24 months they use a spoon well and by age 36 months may be using a fork. Between ages 2 and 3 years they eat with the family and like to help with chores such as setting the table or removing dishes from the dishwasher, but they lack table manners and may find it difficult to sit through the family's entire meal (see Table 14-4).

In dressing, toddlers also demonstrate strides in independence. The 15-month-old child helps by putting the arm or foot out for dressing and pulls shoes and socks off. The 18-month-old child removes gloves, helps with pullover shirts, and may be able to unzip. By age 2 years the toddler removes most articles of clothing and puts on socks, shoes, and pants without regard for right or left and back or front. Help is still needed to fasten clothes.

### Play

Play magnifies toddlers' physical and psychosocial development. Interaction with people becomes increasingly important. The solitary play of infancy progresses to *parallel play*—the toddler plays alongside, not with, other children. Although sensorimotor play is still prominent, there is

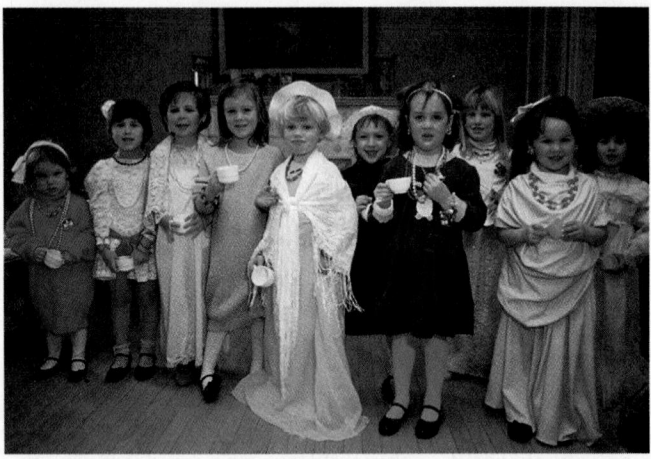

**Fig. 14-4** Young children enjoy dressing up.

much less emphasis on the exclusive use of one sensory modality. The toddler inspects the toy, talks to the toy, tests its strength and durability, and invents several uses for it.

Play assumes many forms and serves several functions (Table 14-2). These youngsters benefit from a wide variety of play interactions (alone, with other children, with adults), environments (own home, other children's homes, park), and activities (active, quiet, organized, unstructured).

Imitation is one of the most distinguishing characteristics of play and enriches children's opportunity to engage in fantasy. With less emphasis on sex-stereotyped toys, play objects such as dolls, carriages, dollhouses, dishes, cooking utensils, child-sized furniture, trucks, and dress-up clothes are used by both sexes, although boys will often display more gender-specific preferences than girls (Martin, Eisenbud, and Rose, 1995) (Fig. 14-4).

Increased locomotive skills make push-pull toys, stick horses, straddle trucks or cycles, a small, low gym and slide, variously sized balls, and rocking horses appropriate for the energetic toddler. Finger paints, thick crayons, chalk, chalkboard, paper, and puzzles with large, simple pieces use the child's developing fine motor skills. Interlocking blocks in varied sizes (but large enough to avoid aspiration) and shapes provide hours of fun and, during later years, are useful objects for creative and imaginative play.

Talking is a form of play for the toddler, who enjoys musical toys such as age-appropriate cassette tape players and recorders, "talking" dolls and animals, and toy telephones. Appropriate children's television programs are excellent for children in this age-group, who learn to associate words with visual images. Toddlers also enjoy "reading" stories from a picture book and imitating the sounds of animals.

Tactile play is also important for the exploring toddler. Water toys, a sandbox with pail and shovel, finger paints, soap bubbles, and clay provide excellent opportunities for

| **TABLE 14-2**   Play during toddlerhood | | |
|---|---|---|
| **Physical Development** | **Social Development** | **Mental Development and Creativity** |
| **Suggested Activities** | | |
| Provide space in which to encourage physical activity | Provide replicas of adult tools and equipment for imitative play | Provide for water play |
| Provide sandbox, swing, and other scaled-down playground equipment | Permit child to "help" with adult tasks | Encourage building, drawing, and coloring |
| | Encourage imitative play | Provide various textures in objects for play |
| | Provide toys and activities that allow for expression of feelings | Provide large boxes and other safe containers for imaginative play |
| | Allow child to play with some actual items used in the adult world; for example, let child help wash dishes or play with pots and pans and other utensils (check for safety) | Read stories appropriate to age |
| | | Monitor television viewing |
| **Suggested Toys** | | |
| Push-pull toys | Music and a record player or tape recorder | Wooden puzzles |
| Rocking horse, stick horse | Purse | Cloth picture books |
| Riding toy | Housekeeping toys (broom, dishes) | Paper, finger paint, thick crayons |
| Balls | Toy telephone | Blocks |
| Blocks (unpainted) | Dishes, stove, table and chairs | Large beads to string |
| Pounding board | Mirror | Wooden shoe for lacing |
| Low gym and slide | Puppets, dolls, stuffed animals (check for safety [e.g., no button eyes]) | Appropriate TV programs |
| Pail and shovel | | |
| Containers | | |
| Play dough | | |

creative and manipulative recreation. Parents sometimes forget the fascination of feeling slippery cream, catching airy bubbles, squeezing and reshaping clay, or smearing paints. These types of unstructured activities are as important as educational play to allow children freedom of expression.

## Toys

Toys are the inanimate objects with which children interact, and cognitive development appears to be related to the variety and accessibility of objects for children to explore, experiment with, and come to know. Access to playthings, particularly during the earlier years, correlates with the accessibility of caregivers who make objects available, react to children's responses to the objects, encourage further exploration, and talk about what is happening. Consequently, although they can be significant in themselves, playthings assume an especially important aspect as a medium of social interchange.

### Selecting Toys

The type of toys chosen by and provided for children can facilitate learning and development in the areas just described. Toys that are small replicas of the culture and its tools help children assimilate their culture and learn sex and occupational roles. Toys that require pushing, pulling, rolling, and manipulating teach children about the physical properties of the items and help to develop muscles and coordination. Rules and the basic elements of cooperation and organization are learned through board games.

Because they can be employed in a variety of ways, raw materials or multidimensional toys are best for enhancing skills and stimulating the imagination. Through manipula-

tion, playthings such as boxes, clay, and blocks can assume a multitude of symbolic objects and inspire creative impulses. For example, building blocks can be used to construct a variety of things, to count, and to learn shapes and sizes. "Educational" toys are less flexible. There are several ways in which families can encourage children's toy play. (See Family Home Care box.)

Play materials need not be expensive or elaborate. Infants and small children derive enjoyment from simple kitchen utensils such as wooden spoons and small plastic plates to bang, pot lids to clang together, and a nest of measuring spoons to rattle. Empty cartons, especially oversized ones used to pack furniture for shipping, can assume the function of clubrooms, hideaways, and other private places. For small children, a large mound of dirt (3 to 4 feet high) can become a place for rolling toy cars and balls and digging holes during summer and a place for sliding in winter. Paper is a fascinating and versatile raw material for children of any age, and most books on toy materials include recipes for play dough and finger paint.

### Toy Safety

The selection of toys and play equipment is a joint effort between parents and children, but evaluating their safety is the responsibility of the adult. Government agencies do not inspect and police all toys on the market. Therefore adults who purchase play equipment, supervise purchases, or allow children to use play equipment need to evaluate such equipment for its safety, including toys that are gifts or those that are purchased by the children themselves. (See Family Home Care box on p. 602.) They should also be alert to notices of toys determined to be defective and recalled by the manufacturers. Parents and health care workers can obtain information on a variety of recalled products and can report potentially dangerous toys and child products to the **U.S. Consumer Product Safety Commission (CPSC)\*** or, in Canada, the **Canadian Toy Testing Council.†**

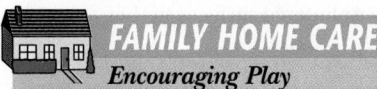

## FAMILY HOME CARE
### Encouraging Play

Realize that play teaches skills and abilities that are the center of intelligence.
Play with your child.
Help your child select a play activity.
Be flexible, creative, and willing to do the unconventional.
Remain available, giving your child the opportunity to indicate the desired level of adult involvement.
Offer encouragement by expressing interest and genuine praise in your child's activity.
Do not turn every play activity into an educational lesson.
Challenge your child from time to time when new skills are learned.
Present new levels of difficulty.
Have available a balanced variety of toys encompassing numerous areas of development.
Respect your child's likes and dislikes; remember that learning is best acquired in an enjoyable situation.
Observe your child at play to learn favorite types of toys and activities.
Enroll your child in a play group that meets several times a week, or hire a baby-sitter who can act as a playmate.

From Lewis M, Block JR: Toy play: IQ building, *Mother's Manual*, pp 31-32, Sept/Oct 1982; and Rollins J: Meeting the child's developmental needs through play. In Smith DP and others, editors: *Comprehensive child and family nursing skills*, St Louis, 1991, Mosby.

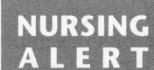 **NURSING ALERT**   Remind parents to request toddler toys when purchasing children's meals at fast-food restaurants.

## Temperament

Temperamental characteristics of children during infancy tend to predominate during toddlerhood. Most difficult infants remain difficult during early childhood, but the easy infants also become less easy (Belsky, Woodworth, and Crnic, 1996). In addition, mothers are more likely to rate children as difficult at ages 1 to 3 years than earlier (Gross and Conrad, 1995; O'Brien, 1996). It is not surprising for parents to see toddlers as more challenging, especially considering the typical negativistic traits of this age-group. Parents of easy infants may be particularly distressed by the behavior change, whereas parents of difficult children may be more prepared,

*CPSC hotline: (800) 638-CPSC.
†22 Hamilton Ave North, Ottowa, Ontario, Canada K1Y 1V6, (613) 729-7101.

## FAMILY HOME CARE
### Toy Safety*

### SELECTION

Select toys that suit the skills, abilities, and interests of children.

Select toys that are safe for the specific child; look for a label that indicates the intended age-group. Toys that are safe for one age may not be safe for another.

For infants, toddlers, and all children who still mouth objects, avoid toys with small parts that may pose a fatal choking hazard or aspiration hazard. Toys in this category are usually labeled as "Not recommended for children under 3 years."

For infants, avoid toys with strings or cords that are 7 inches or longer, because they may cause strangulation.

For all children under 8 years, avoid electric toys with heating elements.

For children under 5 years, avoid arrows or darts.

Check for safety labels such as "flame retardant" or "flame resistant."

Select toys durable enough to survive rough play; look for sturdy construction such as tightly secured eyes, nose, or any small parts.

Select toys light enough that they will not cause harm if one falls on a child.

Look for toys with smooth, rounded edges. Avoid toys with sharp edges that can cut or that have sharp points. Points on the inside of the toy can puncture if the toy is broken.

Avoid toys with any shooting or throwing objects that can injure eyes.

This includes toys with which other missiles, such as sticks or pebbles, might be used as substitutes for the intended projectiles.

Arrows and darts used by children should have blunt tips and be manufactured from resilient materials; make certain the tips are securely attached.

Make certain that materials in toys are nontoxic.

Avoid toys that make loud noises that might be damaging to a child's hearing.

Even some squeaking toys are too loud when held close to the ear.

If selecting caps for cap guns, look for the label required by federal law to be on boxes or packages of caps, which states: "Warning—Do not fire closer than 1 foot to the ear. Do not use indoors."

Make certain that arrows or darts have soft tips, rubber suction cups, or other protective tips. Check to be certain that tips are secure.

If selecting a toy gun, be certain that the barrel or the entire gun is brightly colored to avoid being mistaken for a real gun.

Check toy instructions for clarity. They should be clear to an adult and, when appropriate, to the child.

### SUPERVISION

Maintain a safe play environment.

Remove and discard plastic wrappings on toys immediately; they could suffocate a child.

Remove large toys, bumper pads, and boxes from playpens; an adventuresome child can use such items as a means of climbing or falling out.

Set "ground rules" for play.

Supervise young children closely during play.

Teach children how to use toys properly and safely.

Instruct older children to keep their toys away from younger brothers, sisters, and friends.

Keep children who are playing with riding toys away from stairs, hills, traffic, and swimming pools.

Establish and enforce rules regarding protective gear.

Insist that children wear helmets when using bicycles, skateboards, or in-line skates.

Insist that children wear gloves and wrist, elbow, and knee pads when using skateboards or in-line skates.

Instruct children on electrical safety.

Teach children the proper way to unplug an electric toy—pull on the plug, not the cord.

Teach children to beware of electrical appliances and even electrically operated playthings; often children are unfamiliar with the hazards of electricity in association with water.

Teach children the safe use of utensils that under certain circumstances can cause injury—scissors, knives, needles, heating elements, or loops, long string, or cord.

### MAINTENANCE

Inspect old and new toys regularly for breakage, loose parts, and other potential hazards.

Look for jagged or sharp edges or broken parts that might constitute a choking hazard.

Check movable parts to make certain they are attached securely to the toys; sometimes pieces that are safe when attached to the toy become a danger when detached.

Examine all outdoor toys regularly for rust and weak or sharp parts that could become a danger to a child.

Check electrical cords and plugs for cracked or fraying parts.

Maintain toys in good repair, without signs of possible hazards such as sharp edges, splinters, weak seams, or rust.

Make repairs immediately, or discard out of reach of children.

Sand sharp wooden toys or splintered surfaces so they are smooth.

Use only paint labeled "nontoxic" to repaint toys, toy boxes, or children's furniture.

### STORAGE

Provide a safe place for children to store toys.

Select a toy chest or toy box that is ventilated, is free of self-locking devices that could trap a child inside, and has a lid designed not to pinch a child's fingers or fall on a child's head.

To avoid entrapment and suffocation, containers other than toy chests used for storage purposes should be fitted with spring-loaded support devices if they have a hinged lid.

Teach children to store toys safely in order to prevent accidental injury from stepping, tripping, or falling on a toy.

Playthings meant for older children and adults should be safely stowed away on high shelves, in locked closets, or in other areas unavailable to younger children.

*Another helpful resource is *Toy Safety: Guidelines for Parents* from **American Academy of Pediatrics,** Division of Publications, 141 Northwest Point Blvd, PO Box 927, Elk Grove Village, IL 60009-0927, (800) 433-9016.

---

because of a previously troublesome year, or be overwhelmed by the additional behaviors. The use of the **Toddler Temperament Scale** can assist in identifying temperamental characteristics that benefit from individualized approaches to childrearing (Fullard, McDevitt, and Carey, 1984). The **Toddler Behavior Assessment Questionnaire (TBAQ)** has also proved to be a reliable assessment of toddler temperament, as well as behaviors (Goldsmith, 1996). For practitioners in a busy setting, asking parents about their impression of the child's temperament yields information that can help professionals gain a greater understanding of the parent-child interactional process (Brayden and Poole, 1995).

Although temper tantrums are common in toddlers, certain temperament characteristics make some children more prone to such outbursts. Active, intensely responding children are apt to demonstrate yelling, screaming, and flinging behavior during tantrums. Parents benefit from being forewarned about extreme outbursts and the knowledge that the intensely negative behavior is not abnormal and is tempered by the child's intensely happy moods (Brayden and Poole, 1995; Pavuluri and Luk, 1996; Porrata, 1998; Zuckerman and Frank, 1999).

Discipline is also influenced by temperament. Easy children generally respond well to mild forms of discipline, including a stern voice and sustained eye contact. However, difficult children often need more structured types of discipline, such as time-out or rewards, and the effectiveness of one approach may be short-lived. Efforts at preventing misbehavior are especially important with children who have persistent natures. (See Limit-Setting and Discipline, Chapter 3.) Without "friendly warnings" such children often have difficulty terminating an activity. These children may be punished for behavior that is merely typical of their temperament, and, if the unwarranted punishment continues, the pattern can develop into a behavior problem (Brayden and Poole, 1995). Slow-to-warm-up children may also present challenges, especially when this characteristic is combined with the toddler's usual fear of strangers. These children require gradual introduction to new situations, such as daycare and baby-sitters.

■ ■ ■

Table 14-3 presents a summary of the major features of growth and development for the age-groups of 15, 18, 24, and 30 months. The key developmental ages are 18 and 24 months, although the chronologic ages of 15 and 30 months are also significant. Fifteen months of age is a particularly integrative period of developmental achievement because it represents the completion or fruition of many skills that were unperfected at 1 year of age.

## Coping with Concerns Related to Normal Growth and Development

### Toilet Training

One of the major tasks of toddlerhood is toilet training. The physical ability to control the anal and urethral sphincters is achieved sometime after the child is walking, probably between ages 18 and 24 months. However, complex psychophysiologic factors are also required for readiness. The child must be able to recognize the urge to let go and hold on and be able to communicate this sensation to the parent. In addition, there is probably some necessary motivation in the desire to please the parent by holding on, rather than pleasing oneself by letting go.

Usually physiologic and psychologic readiness is not complete until ages 18 to 24 months. By this time the child has mastered the majority of essential gross motor skills, can communicate intelligibly, is less in conflict with self-assertion and negativism, and is aware of the ability to control the body and please the parent. A child-oriented approach to toilet train-

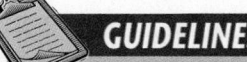

## GUIDELINES
### Assessing Toilet Training Readiness

**PHYSICAL READINESS**

Voluntary control of anal and urethral sphincters, usually by ages 18 to 24 months
Ability to stay dry for 2 hours; decreased number of wet diapers; waking dry from nap
Regular bowel movements
Gross motor skills of sitting, walking, and squatting
Fine motor skills to remove clothing

**MENTAL READINESS**

Recognizes urge to defecate or urinate
Verbal or nonverbal communicative skills to indicate when wet or has urge to defecate or urinate
Cognitive skills to imitate appropriate behavior and follow directions

**PSYCHOLOGIC READINESS**

Expresses willingness to please parent
Able to sit on toilet for 5 to 10 minutes without fussing or getting off
Curiosity about adults' or older sibling's toilet habits
Impatience with soiled or wet diapers; desire to be changed immediately

**PARENTAL READINESS**

Recognizes child's level of readiness
Willing to invest the time required for toilet training
Absence of family stress or change, such as a divorce, moving, new sibling, or imminent vacation

ing is recommended (Stadtler, Gorski, and Brazelton, 1999). One of the most important responsibilities of nurses is to help parents identify the readiness signs in their child. (See Guidelines box.)*

Most children demonstrate readiness for toilet training at approximately 18 months of age. The training process can usually be initiated between the ages of 18 and 24 months. The majority of children achieve daytime continence of urine by the age of 30 to 36 months and nighttime continence of urine by 37 to 48 months (Stadtler, Gorski, and Brazelton, 1999). Girls often exhibit readiness for toilet training and achieve complete training at an earlier age than boys (Largo and others, 1999).

A number of techniques can be helpful when initiating training, and cultural differences should be considered. (See Cultural Awareness box on p. 604.) One is the selection of a potty chair and/or use of the toilet. A freestanding potty chair allows children a feeling of security (Fig. 14-5). Planting the feet firmly on the floor also facilitates defecation (Doughty, 1996). Another option is a portable seat attached to the regular toilet, which may ease the transition from potty chair to regular toilet. Placing a small bench under the feet helps to stabilize the child's position. It is probably best to keep the potty in the bathroom and to let the child observe the excreta being flushed down the toilet to

---

*A helpful brochure is *Toilet Training: A Parent's Guide,* available from the **American Academy of Pediatrics,** 141 Northwest Point Blvd, PO Box 927, Elk Grove Village, IL 60009-0927, (888) 227-1770; fax: (847) 228-1281; www.aap.org

**TABLE 14-3** Growth and development during toddler years

| Age (months) | Physical | Gross Motor | Fine Motor |
|---|---|---|---|
| 15 | Steady growth in height and weight<br>Head circumference 48 cm (19 inches)<br>Weight 11 kg (24 pounds)<br>Height 78.7 cm (31 inches) | Walks without help (usually since age 13 months)<br>Creeps up stairs<br>Kneels without support<br>Cannot walk around corners or stop suddenly without losing balance<br>Assumes standing position without support<br>Cannot throw ball without falling | Constantly casting objects to floor<br>Builds tower of two cubes<br>Holds two cubes in one hand<br>Releases a pellet into a narrow-necked bottle<br>Scribbles spontaneously<br>Uses cup well but rotates spoon |
| 18 | Physiologic anorexia from decreased growth needs<br>Anterior fontanel closed<br>Physiologically able to control sphincters | Runs clumsily, falls often<br>Walks up stairs with one hand held<br>Pulls and pushes toys<br>Jumps in place with both feet<br>Seats self on chair<br>Throws ball overhand without falling | Builds tower of three to four cubes<br>Release, prehension, and reach well-developed<br>Turns pages in a book two or three at a time<br>In drawing, makes stroke imitatively<br>Manages spoon without rotation |
| 24 | Head circumference 49 to 50 cm (19.5 to 20 inches)<br>Chest circumference exceeds head circumference<br>Lateral diameter of chest exceeds anteroposterior diameter<br>Usual weight gain of 1.8 to 2.7 kg (4 to 6 pounds)<br>Usual gain in height of 10 to 12.5 cm (4 to 5 inches)<br>Adult height approximately double height at 2 years<br>May have achieved readiness for beginning daytime control of bowel and bladder<br>Primary dentition of 16 teeth | Goes up and down stairs alone with two feet on each step<br>Runs fairly well, with wide stance<br>Picks up object without falling<br>Kicks ball forward without overbalancing | Builds tower of six to seven cubes<br>Aligns two or more cubes like a train<br>Turns pages of book one at a time<br>In drawing, imitates vertical and circular strokes<br>Turns doorknob, unscrews lid |
| 30 | Birth weight quadrupled<br>Primary dentition (20 teeth) completed<br>May have daytime bowel and bladder control | Jumps with both feet<br>Jumps from chair or step<br>Stands on one foot momentarily<br>Takes a few steps on tiptoe | Builds tower of eight cubes<br>Adds chimney to train of cubes<br>Good hand-finger coordination; holds crayon with fingers rather than fist<br>Moves fingers independently<br>In drawing, imitates vertical and horizontal strokes, makes two or more strokes for cross |

## CULTURAL AWARENESS
### Toilet Training

The timing, method, and significance of toilet training are influenced by cultural practices. For many families in China, the timing is liberal, the method is unique, and the significance is low. Children are diapered during infancy. Once they are walking, they wear loose pants with a long slit between the legs, and they eliminate on the ground. This practice may continue until the child is 5 years of age. In cold weather, a piece of cloth, like a "curtain," may be inserted. However, the Chinese have a concept that the buttocks are not susceptible to cold, so this is not a common practice.

associate these activities with usual practices. If a potty chair is not available, having the child sit *facing* the toilet tank provides added support (Fig. 14-6). Practice sessions should be limited to 5 or 10 minutes, and a parent should stay with the child, practicing sanitary habits after every session. Children should be praised for cooperative behavior and/or successful evacuation. Dressing children in easily removed clothing; using training pants, "pull-on" diapers, or panties; and encouraging imitation by watching others are other helpful suggestions. Forcing children to sit on the potty for long periods, spanking them for having accidents, and other methods of negative control are avoided (Taubman, 1997).

Parents need to give clear instructions to toddlers to encourage elimination. For example, the parent can explain the steps for "going potty" by demonstration, by using a "potty-training" video, or by using a doll. It may also be helpful to stress to children that when they feel the urge to eliminate, they have time to get to the toilet and then urinate or defecate. The entire process of elimination is new to toddlers, and relationships between bodily functions and habits that adults take for granted may not be clear to children.

| Sensory | Vocalization | Socialization |
|---|---|---|
| Able to identify geometric forms; places round object into appropriate hole<br>Binocular vision well-developed<br>Displays an intense and prolonged interest in pictures | Uses expressive jargon<br>Says four to six words, including names<br>"Asks" for objects by pointing<br>Understands simple commands<br>May use head-shaking gesture to denote "no"<br>Uses "no" even while agreeing to the request | Tolerates some separation from parent<br>Less likely to fear strangers<br>Beginning to imitate parents, such as cleaning house (sweeping, dusting), folding clothes, mowing lawn<br>Feeds self using covered cup with little spilling<br>May discard bottle<br>Manages spoon but rotates it near mouth<br>Kisses and hugs parents, may kiss pictures in a book<br>Expressive of emotions, has temper tantrums |
| | Says 10 or more words<br>Points to a common object, such as shoe or ball, and to two or three body parts | Great imitator ("domestic mimicry")<br>Manages spoon well<br>Takes off gloves, socks, and shoes and unzips<br>Temper tantrums may be more evident<br>Beginning awareness of ownership ("my toy")<br>May develop dependency on transitional objects, such as "security blanket" |
| Accommodation well-developed<br>In geometric discrimination, able to insert square block into oblong space | Has vocabulary of approximately 300 words<br>Uses two- to three-word phrases<br>Uses pronouns "I," "me," "you"<br>Understands directional commands<br>Gives first name; refers to self by name<br>Verbalizes need for toileting, food, or drink<br>Talks incessantly | Stage of parallel play<br>Has sustained attention span<br>Temper tantrums decreasing<br>Pulls people to show them something<br>Increased independence from mother<br>Dresses self in simple clothing |
| | Gives first and last name<br>Refers to self by appropriate pronoun<br>Uses plurals<br>Names one color | Separates more easily from mother<br>In play, helps put things away, can carry breakable objects, pushes with good steering<br>Begins to notice sex differences; knows own sex<br>May attend to toilet needs without help except for wiping |

(See Fears, Chapter 15.) It is also wise to use the same words each time for urination and defecation (e.g., "pee-pee" and "poo-poo").

Bowel training is usually accomplished before bladder training because of its greater regularity and predictability; however, training may also begin with voiding (Issenman, Filmer, and Gorski, 1999). There is a stronger sensation for defecation than for urination, and the sensation of defecation can be brought to the child's attention. In fact, nighttime bladder training may not be completed until 4 or 5 years of age, and even later training is normal (Luxem and others, 1997). Limiting fluid intake before the children's hour of sleep and waking them once around midnight may help decrease the incidence of bed-wetting but do not teach voluntary control. Boys may begin toilet training in the stand-up position or by sitting on a potty chair or toilet. Imitating other males is a powerful motivating force.

Daytime accidents are also common, particularly during periods of intense activity. Young children become so engrossed in play activity that if they are not reminded, they will wait until it is too late to reach the bathroom. Therefore, frequent reminders and trips to the toilet are necessary.

### Sibling Rivalry

The term *sibling rivalry* refers to the natural jealousy and resentment of children to a new child in the family. It typically involves the arrival of a new infant but may be associated with anyone who joins the family. A common example is the merging of stepfamilies. However, the following discussion focuses on the response to a newborn.

Toddlers do not hate or resent the infant but do resent the changes that this additional sibling brings, especially the separation from the mother during the birth. Studies suggest that no matter the culture, older siblings experience

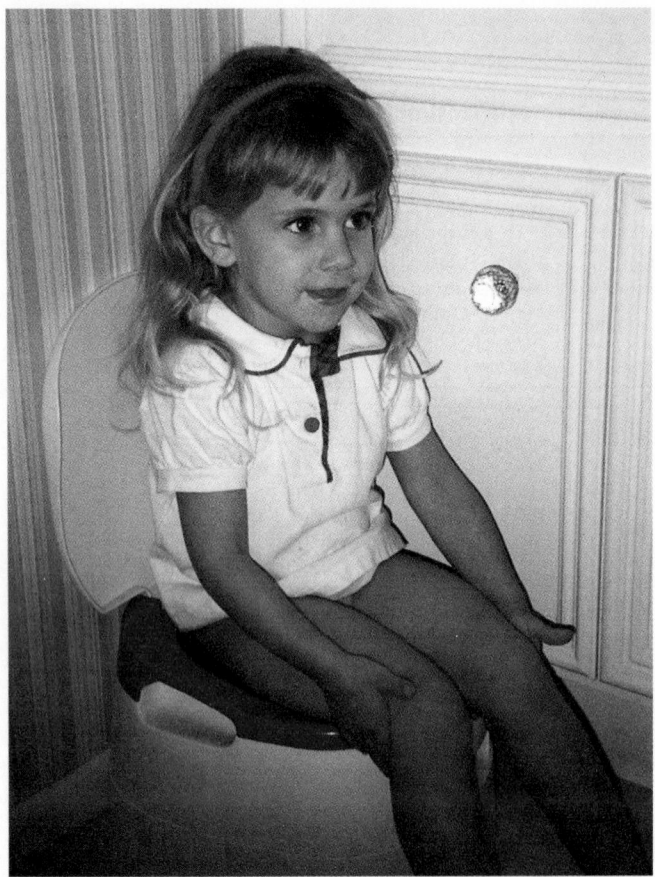

**Fig. 14-5** Children may begin toilet training sitting on a small toilet.

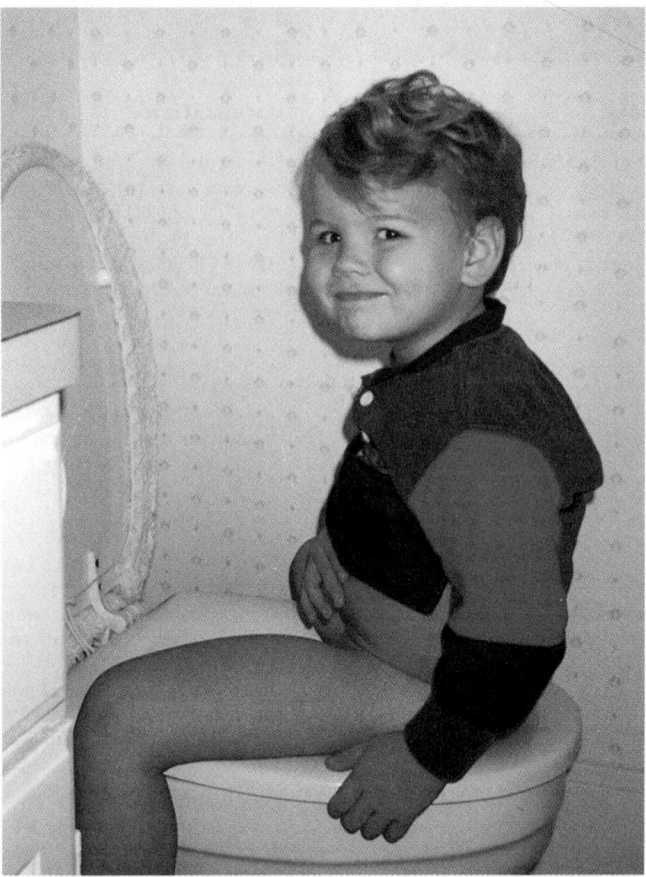

**Fig. 14-6** Sitting in reverse fashion on a regular toilet provides additional security to a young child.

stress with the birth of a new baby (Yamamoto and others, 1996). The parents now share their love and attention with someone else, the usual routine is disrupted, and toddlers may lose their crib and/or room—all at a time when they thought they were in control of their world. Sibling rivalry tends to be most pronounced in the firstborn, who experiences "dethronement" (loss of sole parental attention). It also seems to be most difficult for young children, particularly in terms of mother-child interaction.

Preparation of children for the birth of a sibling is quite individual, but age dictates some important considerations. Time is a vague concept for toddlers. Preparing children too soon for the birth may lessen their interest by the time the event occurs. A good time to start talking about the new baby is when toddlers become aware of the pregnancy and the changes occurring in the home in anticipation of the new member. Jealousy can develop from feeling left out; because fantasy dictates reality, fear of the unknown can lead to fear of abandonment, separation anxiety, and insecurity. To avoid additional stresses when the newborn arrives, anticipated changes, such as moving the toddler to a different room or bed, should be done well in advance of the birth.

Toddlers need to have a realistic idea of what the newborn will be like. Telling them that a new playmate will come home soon sets up unrealistic expectations. Rather, parents should stress the activities that will take place when the baby arrives home, such as diapering, bottle- or breastfeeding, bathing, and dressing. At the same time, parents should emphasize which routines will stay the same, such as reading stories or going to the park. If toddlers have had no contact with an infant, it is a good idea to introduce them to one, if feasible. Providing a doll on which toddlers can imitate parental behaviors is another excellent strategy. They can tend to the doll's needs (diapering, feeding) at the same time the parent is performing similar activities for the infant, then progress to helping with the sibling (Fig. 14-7).

Pregnancy is an abstraction for toddlers. They need concrete illustrations of how the baby is growing inside the mother. It is an excellent opportunity for introducing aspects of reproduction and sexuality. Seeing simple pictures of the uterus and fetus and feeling the fetus move help the child feel involved in the experience. Children also benefit from "siblings" classes that may be part of prenatal sessions. They learn about the characteristics of infants and are taught simple tasks of caring for the new baby (Kramer, 1996). There is some evidence that participation in a sibling preparation class can decrease sibling rivalry behaviors and help mothers cope better with their children's behaviors (Sawicki, 1997; Storr and Robinson, 1998). Books can also help children prepare for birth and cope with sibling rivalry.

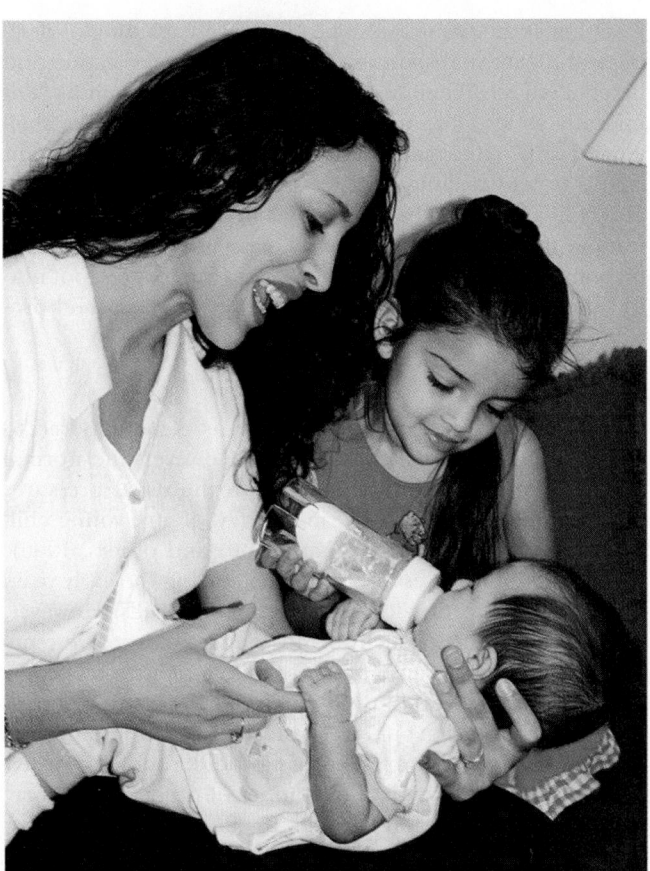

**Fig. 14-7** To minimize sibling rivalry, parents should include the toddler during caregiving activities.

When the new baby arrives, toddlers sense the changed focus of attention. Visitors may initiate problems when they inadvertently favor the infant with attention and presents while neglecting the older child. Parents can minimize this by alerting visitors to the toddler's needs, having small presents on hand for the toddler, and including the child in the visit as much as possible. The toddler can also help with the care of the newborn by getting diapers and doing other small tasks. It is important to involve toddlers in their new sibling's care, because even young infants learn to respond to the sounds of their siblings' voices.

How children exhibit jealousy is complex. Some will overtly hit the infant, push the child off the parent's lap, or pull the bottle or breast from the infant's mouth. More often the expressions of hostility and resentment are much more subtle and covert.

Firstborn children are especially sensitive to a newborn's arrival (Gottlieb and Baillies, 1995; Teti and others, 1996). Toddlers may verbally express a wish that the infant "go back inside Mommy," or they will revert to more infantile forms of behavior, such as demanding a bottle, soiling their diaper, clinging for attention, using baby talk, or aggressively acting out toward others. The latter is particularly common in preschoolers, who may seem accepting of the new sibling at home but behave poorly in daycare or preschool. This is a form of displacement that says, "I can't let my parents know how I feel, so I will tell you." Encouraging parents to explore how their older child is acting with other caregivers is an important aspect of intervention.

Regardless of how well-adjusted and accepting toddlers or preschoolers appear, infants must be protected by supervising the interaction between siblings. Other safety considerations are "baby proofing" the house and instructing children regarding the dangers to infants of small, sharp, or pointed objects. Crib rails should be kept fully raised and the mattress lowered to discourage toddlers from picking up the infant. Infant seats or bassinets should be placed on the floor so that young children cannot pull them off a raised surface to see or play with the baby.

The first few weeks at home with a newborn and toddler can be challenging for parents. Assuring them that this period will pass, that the toddler will learn to accept the changes in lifestyle, and that the newborn will sleep through the night is part of the intervention. Allowing parents to talk about their feelings of ambivalence and frustration and suggesting ways of dealing with the sibling jealousy help all members of the family with this experience. Indeed, sibling rivalry is so common regardless of the children's ages that it is a part of family life. Suggestions such as spending time with each child, letting children settle their arguments, and accepting angry feelings while teaching children appropriate ways to express hostility are general guidelines for dealing with the eventual conflicts between brothers and sisters.

## Temper Tantrums

As toddlers strive for autonomy, they are confronted with many obstacles, such as the physical inability to complete a task (e.g., attempting to build a tower of blocks) or imposed rules or demands that interfere with their activity (e.g., time to go to sleep after listening to one story). Fatigue may simply lower a child's tolerance to frustration.

As the frustration builds, children may "explode" with activity to release their tension (Brayden and Poole, 1995). Typically they may lie down on the floor, kick their feet, and scream. Head banging, head rolling, and breath holding are other behaviors some children use. Although these actions are very disturbing to observe, they usually do not become behavior problems or indicate behaviorally difficult children (Brayden and Poole, 1995; DiMario, 2001). Parents should be told that breath holding and fainting from lack of oxygen cause no physical harm because the accumulation of carbon dioxide stimulates the respiratory control center to initiate breathing. However, head banging may cause injury, and the child requires protection, such as being held or being placed in a protected environment.

The best approach toward extinguishing attention-seeking behavior is to ignore it (no verbal or eye contact with the child), provided that the behavior is not inflicting injury. The parent should remain close by and after the tantrum has subsided offer a toy or a favorite activity to substitute for the ungranted request and to reward the posttantrum behavior. When tantrums occur because the child refuses to comply, the parent can ignore it for a few minutes but may have to physically carry the child if the request must be met, such as getting in the car or going to bed (Grover, 1996).

When tantrums do occur, it is important for parents to intervene *immediately* to prevent their own buildup of angry feelings and the inability to calmly ignore the behavior. Frequently temper tantrums can be avoided by using an approach for minimizing misbehavior, such as time-out. (See Limit-Setting and Discipline, Chapter 3.)*

Temper tantrums are common during the toddler years and essentially represent normal developmental behaviors. However, temper tantrums can be signs of serious problems. Nurses should be alert to situations that require further evaluation. (See Guidelines box.)

## Negativism

One of the more difficult aspects of rearing toddlers is related to their persistent negative "no" response to every request. The negativism is not an expression of being stubborn or disrespectful, but a necessary assertion of control. One method of dealing with the negativism is by reducing the opportunities for a "no" answer. Asking the child, "Do you want to go to sleep now?" is almost certain to be met with an emphatic "no." A more appropriate approach is to tell the child when it will be time to go to sleep (preferably within a specific time frame, such as "after reading a story") and proceed accordingly.

In their attempt to exert control, children like to make choices. When confronted with appropriate choices, such as "You can have a peanut butter-and-jelly sandwich or chicken noodle soup for lunch," they are more likely to choose one than automatically say no. However, if their response is negative, parents should make the choice for the child. This behavior is frustrating for both the child and the parent. Parents need to respond in a calm, reassuring manner. Anger and yelling reinforce the negative behavior (Brayden and Poole, 1995). Many of the suggestions for preventing misbehavior in Chapter 3 also help minimize negativism.

---

*A helpful brochure is *Temper Tantrums: A Normal Part of Growing Up,* available from the **American Academy of Pediatrics,** 141 Northwest Point Blvd, PO Box 927, Elk Grove Village, IL, 60009-0927, (888) 227-1770; fax: (847) 228-1281; www.aap.org.

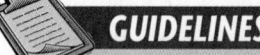

## GUIDELINES
### *Identifying Children with Problem Tantrums*

Parents express concern; feel angry, sad, and helpless; and/or report nothing positive about the child.
Child is younger than 1 year or older than 4 years.
Tantrums occur regularly in school.
Tantrums are associated with aggressive, violent behavior (e.g., injures self or others).
There is a history of other concerns, such as sleep disorders, food refusal, or extreme difficulty with separation.
Child holds breath and faints during tantrums.
Child displays unusual flirtatiousness or extreme modesty (suggests possible sexual abuse).

---

Modified from Needlman R, Howard B, Zuckerman B: Temper tantrums: when to worry, *Contemp Pediatr* 6(8):12-14, 1989.

Other strategies may also be effective in avoiding or dealing with negative responses. Toddlers like to play games and be challenged. When asked to do something, such as "Put on your shoes," the toddler may quickly respond if challenged with "I bet I can put my shoes on first." An important rule is to let the child win. Another approach is to use humor, which can get the task done and defuse anger or frustration. If the child refuses to put on the shoes, a humorous response is for the adult to try to squeeze his or her foot into the shoe. Hopefully, the game will end with the child proclaiming, "No, my shoes," and putting them on.

## Coping with Stress

Adults rarely think of young children as being exposed to stress or suffering its consequences. However, the normal demands of growing up coupled with the usual pressures most families experience mean that few, if any, young children are reared stress-free (Yamamoto and others, 1996). Small amounts of stress are beneficial during the early years to help children develop effective coping skills. However, excessive stress is destructive, and young children are especially vulnerable because of their limited ability to cope.

To deal with stress in their children's lives, parents must be aware of the signs of stress and be able to identify the source. The normal stresses during toddlerhood are listed in Box 14-2. In addition, any number of other stresses may be imposed on children, such as alternative caregiving arrangements, birth of a sibling, marital discord, relocation, or illness (Yamamoto and others, 1996). Watching children at play can identify stressors. For example, one child was

---

### Box 14-2 ■ ■ ■
### Sources of Stress in Toddlers

**Negativism**—Does not like to take orders; may be contrary
**Regression**—Fears losing newly learned skills; may feel helpless
**Rigidity**—Wants own way; is upset when rituals are disrupted; dislikes interference; difficulty coping with disrupted family routines (e.g., divorce, daycare, maternal employment)
**Lack of sociability**—Engages in solitary or parallel play but is generally disinterested in socializing
**Self-centeredness**—Believes the world revolves around her or him; does not want to share; seen with arrival of sibling
**Separation anxiety**—Fears being separated from parent
**Stranger anxiety**—Fears strangers; is shy
**Toilet training**—Especially if begun before the child is ready
**Bedtime**—Dislikes being ordered to bed; may fear bedwetting or separation from parents; may have terrifying dreams
**Tantrums**—May revert to temper tantrums or destructive behavior; may hit or bite
**Security object**—May have a security object that if lost or misplaced leads to great emotional upset
**Overdoing**—May become overstimulated or overtired
**Fears**—In particular, may include animals or anything that makes a loud noise
**Illness and hospitalization**—Source of many stressors: separation, pain, regression, rigidity, fears, and so on
**Violence**—Exposure to family or community violence or excess exposure to media violence

---

Modified from Kuczen B: *Childhood stress: don't let your child be a victim,* New York, 1987, Dell Publishing.

seen pounding on a doll, yelling "Go away! Go away!" The parent was quick to observe that the child's recent irritability was probably caused by the stress of a new sibling. Other signs of increased stress in a toddler's life may include increased thumb sucking, aggressive behavior, and biting (Berkowitz, 1996; Brayden and Poole, 1995).

The best approach to dealing with stress is prevention—monitoring the amount of stress in children's lives so that levels exceeding their coping ability do not occur. In many instances this is as simple as increasing the child's rest periods to allow for quiet recovery time. Often it involves adequately preparing the child for change, such as daycare or a new sibling. It also requires helping the child cope with stress. Play is an excellent vehicle for releasing anger or frustration, and toys such as drums, play nails and hammer, clay, and play dough provide alternative methods of dissipating anxiety. They also begin to teach socially acceptable ways of dealing with such feelings. Another approach is the use of relaxation and imagery. Even young children can learn to "let their bodies go limp like a rag doll" or "imagine floating on a cloud."

*Regression* is a retreat from a present pattern of functioning to past levels of behavior. It usually occurs in instances of stress, when one attempts to cope by reverting to patterns of behavior that were successful in earlier stages of development. Regression is common in toddlers because almost any additional stress lessens their ability to master present developmental tasks. Any threat to their autonomy, such as illness, hospitalization, separation, or adjustment to a sibling, represents a need to revert to earlier forms of behavior, such as increased dependency; refusal to use the potty chair; temper tantrums; demand for the bottle, stroller, or crib; and loss of newly learned motor, language, social, and cognitive skills.

At first, such regression appears acceptable and comfortable for children, but on closer inspection it becomes evident that the loss of newly acquired achievements is frightening and threatening, because children are aware of their total helplessness in the recent past. Parents, too, become concerned about regressive behavior and frequently in their efforts to deal with it force the child to cope with an additional source of stress—the pressure to live up to expected standards. Brazelton (1994; 1995) suggests that these predictable times of regression, or *touchpoints,* are an opportunity to prepare parents for the next step in their child's development.

When regression does occur, the best approach is to ignore it while praising existing patterns of appropriate behavior. The child is saying, "I can't cope with this present stress and accomplish this new skill as well, but I will eventually if given patience and understanding." For this reason, it is advisable not to introduce new areas of learning when an additional crisis is present or expected, such as beginning toilet training shortly before a sibling is born or during a brief period of hospitalization.

*Fears* are very common during this age and include fear of annihilation, going to sleep, animals, and engines, with the greatest fear continuing to be fear of strangers and separa-

tion from parents or other usual caregivers. Because fear of strangers and separation begins in infancy, it is discussed in Chapter 12. The other fears often escalate in the preschool period and consequently are discussed in Chapter 15.

## PROMOTING OPTIMUM HEALTH DURING TODDLERHOOD
### Nutrition

During the period from 12 to 18 months of age, the growth rate slows, resulting in a slight adjustment from the previous caloric requirement of 108 kcal/kg (50 kcal/lb) of body weight during early infancy to 102 kcal/kg (46 kcal/lb) during the next 2 years (American Academy of Pediatrics, 1998; Lucas, 1999). Protein requirements also decrease slightly, from 2.2 to 1.5 g/kg for infants to 1.2 g/kg for toddlers, but are still higher than at succeeding ages to meet the demands of muscle tissue growth and high activity level (Forgac, 1995). Fluid needs drop from the infant requirement of approximately 140 ml/kg to the toddler requirement of 115 ml/kg. The reduced fluid requirement represents a decrease in the relative total body water and an increase in fluid within the cells (intracellular fluid).

The requirements for most vitamins and minerals increase slightly during toddlerhood. The need for minerals such as iron, calcium, and phosphorus may be difficult to meet, considering the characteristic food habits of children in this age-group. Milk intake, the chief source of calcium and phosphorus, should average 2 to 3 cups a day. More than a quart of milk consumption daily considerably limits the intake of solid foods, resulting in a deficiency of dietary iron, as well as other nutrients. After 2 years of age children can be given skim or low-fat milk to reduce daily total fat to less than 30% of calories, saturated fatty acids to less than 10% of calories, and cholesterol to less than 300 mg (Stewart and others, 1999). Other measures to reduce dietary fat include using lean meats, fat-modified products (such as low-fat cheese), and low-fat cooking. Because less fat in children's diet can also mean fewer calories and nutrients, caregivers must know what kinds of food to choose (Dennison, Jenkins, and Rockwell, 2000).

At approximately 18 months of age most toddlers manifest this decreased nutritional need and decreased appetite in a phenomenon known as *physiologic anorexia.* They become picky, fussy eaters with strong taste preferences (Carruth and others, 1998). They may eat voraciously one day and almost nothing the next. They are increasingly aware of the nonnutritive function of food: the pleasure of eating, the social aspect of mealtime, and the control of refusing food. They are influenced by factors other than taste when choosing food. If a family member refuses to eat something, children are likely to imitate that response. If the plate is overfilled, they are likely to push it away, overwhelmed by its size. If food does not appear or smell appetizing, they will probably not try it. Conversely, if food is served attractively and referred to in appealing ways, such as calling an apple slice an "apple cookie" or half a hard-boiled egg a "canoe," children will often try new foods. In essence, mealtime is more closely associated with psychologic components than with nutritional ones, and nutritional counseling must address the characteristics of this age-group.

## Nutritional Counseling

Eating habits established in the first 2 or 3 years of life tend to have lasting effects on subsequent years. If food is used as a regard or sign of approval, a child may overeat for non-nutritive reasons. If food is forced and mealtime is consistently unpleasant, the usual pleasure associated with eating may not develop. Mealtimes should be enjoyable rather than times for discipline or family arguments. The social aspect of mealtime may be distracting for young children; therefore an earlier feeding hour may be appropriate. Young children are unable to sit through a long meal and become restless and disruptive. This is particularly common when children are brought to the table just after active play. Calling them in 15 minutes before mealtime allows them ample opportunity to get ready for eating while settling down their active minds and bodies.

For some young children, sitting at the table may be more disruptive than functional. Frequent nutritious snacks can replace a meal. "Grazing"—nibbling and snacking—is a good way to ensure proper nutrition, provided that appropriate foods are offered. Between-meal snacks can provide significant nutrition, especially calories, protein, carbohydrate, calcium, and vitamin C.

The method of serving food also takes on more importance during this period. Toddlers need to feel in control and to have a sense of achievement. Giving them large, adult-size portions contributes to their feeling overwhelmed. In general, what is eaten is much more significant than how much is consumed. Serving sizes need to be appropriate for age.

**NURSING TIP** A general guide to the serving size of food is 1 tablespoon of solid food per year of age or one fourth to one third the adult portion size. Use the tablespoon guide for easily measured foods such as vegetables or rice. Use the fraction guide for milk, bread, or fruit (Dietz and Stern, 1999).

It is often a good idea to offer less than toddlers may eat and let the child ask for more. Young children tend to like less spicy, bland foods, although this is a culturally determined preference. Substitutions should be provided for foods that they do not enjoy, but this practice should be used sparingly to avoid catering to all toddlers' eating requests.

The ritualism of this age also dictates certain principles in feeding practices. Toddlers like to have the same dish, cup, or spoon every time they eat. They may reject a favorite food simply because it is served in a different utensil. If one food touches another, they often refuse to eat it. Mixed foods, such as stews or casseroles, are also rarely favorites. Because toddlers are unpredictable in their table manners, it is best to use plastic dishes and cups, for both economic and safety reasons. For some children a regular mealtime schedule also contributes to their desire and need for predictability and ritualism.

Appetite and food preferences are sporadic during these years. A child may enjoy one food for 3 days in a row and then suddenly refuse to eat it again for days. Such food fads or "jags" do not ensure a well-balanced diet, but attempts to alter them are met with bitter resentment and unwavering obstinacy. It is preferable to accept such extremes and offer other foods in small portions. Generally, the child will choose another "favorite food" that may compensate for the nutritional inadequacy. Introducing at least three items from the groups in the Food Guide Pyramid at each meal helps develop a variety of taste preferences and well-balanced habits. For snacks, several small pieces of food (carrot sticks, cheese blocks, raisins, crackers, sliced cold meat, apple slices) can be placed in an ice cube tray for a pick-and-choose menu. Fruit juices should not be offered as a replacement for fruit snacks. Juices should be limited to less than 12 ounces per day. In one study, children drinking more than that had an increased incidence of obesity and short stature (Dennison, Rockwell, and Baker, 1997). A sample menu for toddlers is given in Box 14-3.

Developmentally, most children by 12 months of age are eating the same food prepared for the rest of the family. Some may have mastered using a cup with occasional spilling, although most cannot adeptly use a spoon until 18 months of age or later (Table 14-4) and generally prefer using their fingers. Some children find weaning easy and voluntarily relinquish the bottle by the first birthday. Others are unable to give up that pleasure and require a bottle before bedtime or occasionally during the day (Fig. 14-8). Allowing children to

---

**Box 14-3** ■ ■ □

### Sample Menu for Toddlers Based on Food Guide Pyramid*

| | |
|---|---|
| **Breakfast** | ½ cup dry, unsweetened cereal |
| | ½ cup orange juice |
| | 4 oz low-fat milk† |
| **Snack** | ½-1 whole banana |
| **Lunch** | 1 tbsp peanut butter |
| | 2 tsp all-fruit preserves |
| | 1 slice whole-wheat bread |
| | 2 tbsp peas |
| | 4 oz low-fat milk† |
| **Snack** | 2 graham crackers |
| | 4 oz low-fat milk |
| **Dinner** | 1 chicken leg, roasted, without skin |
| | ¼-½ cup macaroni and cheese |
| | 2 tbsp green beans, cooked |
| | 2 tbsp carrots, cooked |
| | 4-6 oz low-fat milk† |
| **Snack** | ½ cup frozen yogurt |

**TOTAL SERVINGS**

| | |
|---|---|
| Bread, cereal, rice, pasta | 6-7 |
| Vegetable | 3 |
| Fruit | 3-4 |
| Milk, yogurt, cheese | 2-3 |
| Meat, poultry, fish, dried beans, eggs, nuts | 2 |

*Use fats, oils, and sweets sparingly. Increase fluids with servings of water. Serving sizes are minimums for nutritional adequacy. Many children eat more.
†Substitute whole milk if child is younger than 24 months.

give up the bottle when they are ready is preferable to forcing the issue.

Some toddlers reject all solid food in preference for the bottle, a practice that can be discouraged by gradually diluting the milk with water to make it less satisfying and introducing foods at times when the child is most likely to be hungry, such as on awakening. Occasionally it may be necessary to withhold bottle-feedings, as well as other between-meal foods and fluids other than water, until the child is hungry enough to eat solid foods. Forcing the child to eat solid foods usually results in conflicts and does little to establish healthy eating habits.

## Sleep and Activity

Total sleep time decreases only slightly during the second year and averages about 12 hours. Most children take one nap a day, and by the end of the second or third year many relinquish this habit. The activity level is high, and there is rarely a problem with too little physical exercise, provided that inappropriate restrictions are not instituted. With increasing numbers of young children being cared for outside the home, attention to the kinds of activity provided is important. For example, children with high activity levels may benefit from an environment in which outdoor play is encouraged.

Sleep problems, especially going to bed and falling asleep, are common and are probably related to fears of separation. Bedtime rituals (same hour of sleep, snack, quiet activity) are helpful, and transitional objects, such as a favorite stuffed animal or blanket, can ease the insecurity at bedtime. For problems that persist, the interventions outlined in Table 12-5 should be employed.

## Dental Health

### Regular Dental Examinations

Ideally, the child should see a dentist (or *pedodontist,* a pediatric dentist) soon after the first teeth erupt, usually around 1 year of age (American Academy of Pediatric Dentistry, 1996). During these visits the dentist can begin to develop a relationship with the child (see Atraumatic Care box); assess oral health, including the use of a pacifier or thumb sucking; teach parents correct methods of dental hygiene; and provide nutritional counseling, especially in relation to preventing nursing caries (see p. 615).

### Removal of Plaque

The objective of oral hygiene is removal of *plaque,* soft bacterial deposits that adhere to the teeth and cause dental *caries* (decay) and *periodontal* (gum) *disease.* The most effective methods for plaque removal are brushing and flossing. Several brushing techniques exist, although there is no universal agreement regarding the best method. One that is suitable for cleaning the primary teeth is the *scrub method.* The tips of the bristles are placed firmly at a 45-degree angle against the teeth and gums, and are moved back and forth in a vibratory motion. The ends of the bristles should be moving gently to avoid damaging the gums and enamel. All of the surfaces of the teeth are cleaned in this manner except the lingual (inner or tongue side) surfaces of the

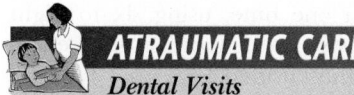

**ATRAUMATIC CARE**
*Dental Visits*

Initial visits to the dentist should be nontraumatizing. Because toddlers react negatively to new and potentially frightening experiences, the initial visit can center around meeting the dentist, seeing the equipment, and sitting in the chair. Avoid statements such as "It won't hurt," because they suggest possible discomfort. If the child is uncooperative, the dentist may just look at the teeth and reserve a more thorough examination for another visit. Modeling can also be effective—the child can observe procedures performed on the parent or a cooperative sibling. This type of conditioning is very important in preparing the child for future experiences.*

---

*A book to help prepare the child is *When Your Child Goes to the Dentist* by Fred Rogers, available from Family Communications, 4802 Fifth Ave., Pittsburgh, PA 15213, (412) 687-2990.

| TABLE 14-4   Developmental milestones associated with feeding | |
|---|---|
| **Age (months)** | **Development** |
| 12-18 | Drools less |
| | Drinks well from cup with lid but may drop it when finished |
| | Holds cup with both hands |
| | Begins to use a spoon but turns it before reaching mouth |
| 24 | Can use a straw and a cup |
| | Chews food with mouth closed and shifts food in mouth |
| | Distinguishes between finger and spoon foods |
| | Uses spoon correctly but with some spilling |
| 36 | Spills small amount from spoon |
| | Begins to use fork; holds it in fist |
| | Uses adult pattern of chewing, which involves rotary action of jaw |

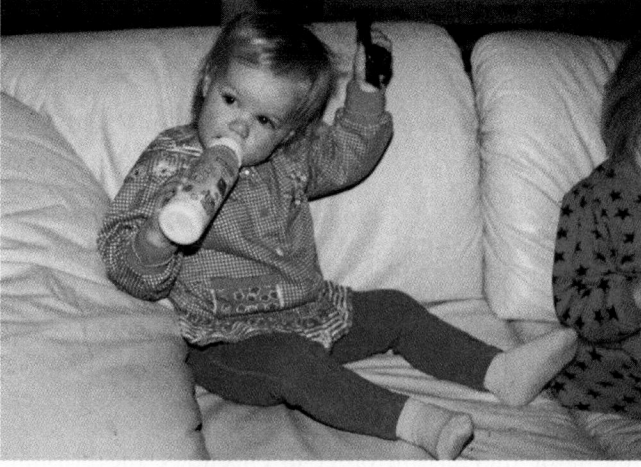

**Fig. 14-8**   Some children find relinquishing the bottle difficult. Prolonged and frequent bottle-feeding can lead to iron deficiency anemia and nursing caries.

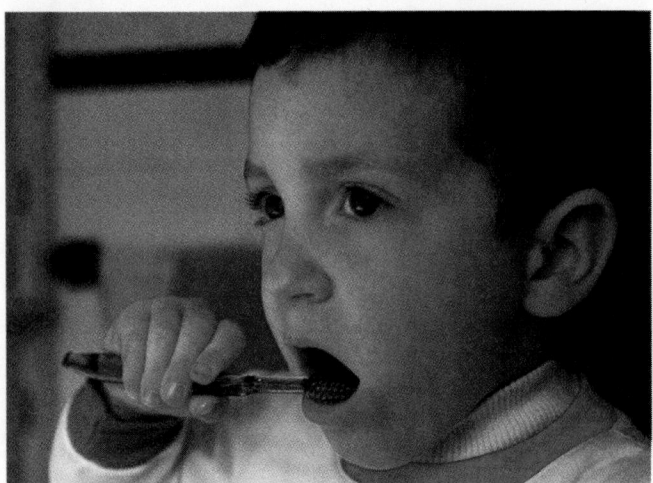

**Fig. 14-9**   Young children can participate in toothbrushing.

front teeth. To clean these surfaces, the toothbrush is placed vertical to the teeth and moved up and down. Only a few teeth are brushed at one time, using six to eight strokes for each section. A systematic approach is used so that all surfaces are thoroughly cleaned.

Young children are only able to brush the mandibular occlusive surface (lower arch, top surface) and the front labial surface (outer or lip side) (Osgasawara, Watanabe, and Kasahara, 1992) (Fig. 14-9). Therefore the most effective cleaning is done by parents (Fig. 14-10). Several positions facilitate access to the mouth and help stabilize the head for comfort:

- Stand with child's back toward adult. (When done in front of a bathroom mirror, both child and adult can see what is being done in the mirror.)
- Sit on a couch or bed with child's head resting in adult's lap.
- Sit on the floor or a stool with child's head resting between adult's thighs.

**NURSING TIP** To encourage children to open their mouths, ask them to "tweet like a bird" to brush the front teeth and to "roar like a lion" to brush the back teeth. Sing, tell stories, or talk to children during teeth cleaning to prevent boredom.

For effective cleaning, a small toothbrush with soft, rounded, multitufted nylon bristles that are short and uniform in length is recommended. Nylon bristles dry more rapidly after use and retain their shape better than natural bristles. Toothbrushes are replaced as soon as the bristles are frayed or bent. With young children, brushing may be more easily accompanied using only water because many children dislike the foam from toothpaste and the foam interferes with visibility. There is also the danger of swallowing fluoridated toothpaste. (See following discussion under Fluoride.) When using toothpaste, children should select the flavor they like in order to encourage the brushing habit.

After the teeth have been cleaned, flossing removes plaque and debris from between the teeth and below the

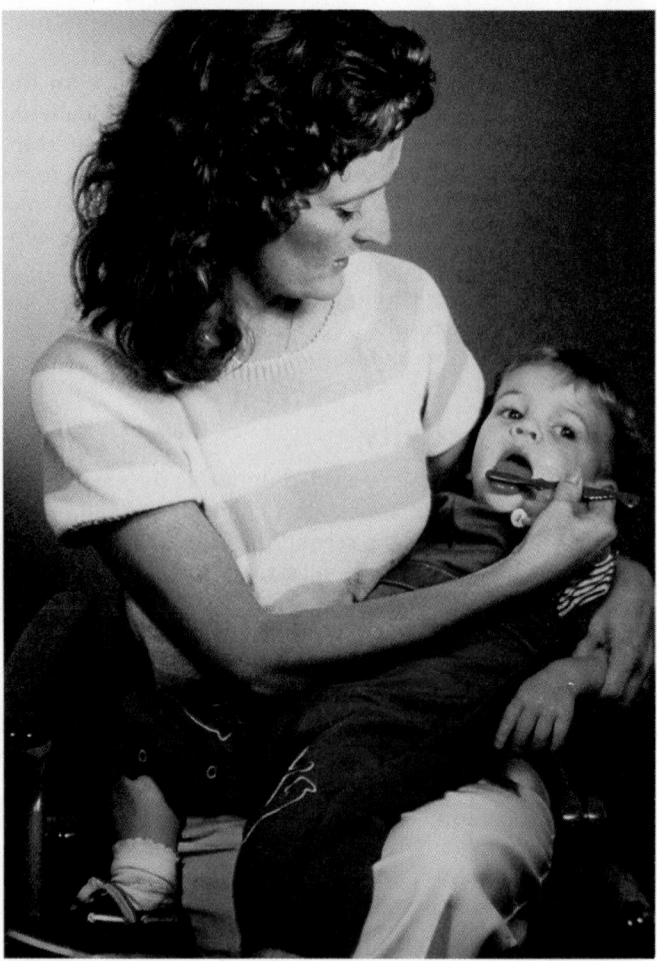

**Fig. 14-10**   The most effective cleaning of the teeth is done by parents.

gum margin where brushing cannot reach. Even if the teeth are widely spaced, flossing is necessary to remove debris below the gum line to prevent *gingivitis* (inflammation of the gums). Because young children do not have the dexterity to manipulate the floss, parents are taught the procedure. The type of floss (waxed or unwaxed, fine, and so on) that easily slides between the teeth is chosen. A length of dental floss about 45 cm (18 inches) long can either be tied in a circle or wrapped around the fingers. The circle method may be easier for children to learn. Floss holders are also available and offer the advantage of only one hand being needed for flossing, freeing the other hand to stabilize the child's head.

With about 2.25 cm (1 inch) of floss held tautly against the thumbs, the floss is gently inserted between two teeth, wrapped around the base of the tooth in a C shape, and directed *below* the gingival margin to remove plaque. The floss is then moved toward the occlusal (biting) surface of the tooth to remove plaque between the teeth as well. This sweeping motion is repeated a few times on every tooth surface, using a clean segment of floss.

A disclosing agent used before brushing is helpful in identifying plaque. It also helps motivate children to clean their teeth, because plaque is invisible. After cleaning, the mouth is inspected to ensure that all traces of plaque have been removed. Where plaque remains, the teeth are re-brushed until the red color is gone.

Although it is generally recognized that thorough plaque removal once a day is sufficient, cleaning the teeth more frequently increases the probability of effective cleaning (McDonald and Avery, 1999; Nomak and Warren, 2000). Ideally, the teeth should be cleaned as soon as possible after each meal and especially before bedtime, and the child should be given nothing to eat or drink except water after the night brushing. At those times when brushing is impractical, the *swish-and-swallow method* will remove some debris. With a mouthful of water, the child rinses the mouth and swallows, repeating the procedure three or four times.

## Fluoride

When adequate amounts of fluoride are ingested before eruption of the teeth and to a lesser extent afterward, the enamel is more resistant to caries. Fluoride replaces the hydroxyl ion in the calcium hydroxyapatite molecule to form calcium fluorapatite, which alters the crystal of the tooth, making it more resistant to acid solubility. The changes in crystalline structure also affect the anatomy of the tooth—the cusps are shorter and the crevices smaller—thus facilitating plaque removal.

Fluoridation of water is the most cost-effective method of ensuring sufficient intake of the mineral. Before the widespread use of fluoride in beverages, food, dental products, and dietary supplements, children in fluoridated communities experienced about a 60% reduction in caries as compared with youngsters in nonfluoridated communities (fluoride concentration generally below 0.3 ppm [parts per million]) (American Academy of Pediatric Dentistry, 1996; Reeves, 1996).

It is now recommended that fluoride supplementation be withheld from birth to 6 months. Supplements are not needed when the level of fluoride in water is greater than 0.6 ppm (Table 14-5) (American Academy of Pediatric Dentistry, 1996).

A major disadvantage of supplementation is compliance, cost, and the potential for excessive intake. Supplements are considerably more expensive than community water fluoridation, and adhering to a daily administration schedule for 16 years (when the third-molar crowns, or "wisdom teeth," are completely calcified) is difficult for many families.

A fluoride dentifrice reduces caries even further when the water supply is fluoridated, because it imparts a topical benefit to the teeth (Featherstone, 1999). However, a concern with fluoride toothpaste used in conjunction with other sources of fluoride is excessive fluoride ingestion by young children and the possibility of *fluorosis*, a condition characterized by an increase in the degree and extent of the enamel's porosity. It can cause staining of the teeth (chalky white to yellow or brown) and, in more severe forms, pitting of the enamel. The prevalence of the moderate to severe form is increasing (Warren and Levy, 1999). Fluorosis is not a health concern but may be a cosmetic concern for af-

| | Water Fluoride Content (in PPM)† | | |
|---|---|---|---|
| **TABLE 14-5**   Fluoride supplementation* | | | |
| Age | <0.3 | 0.3-0.6 | >0.6 |
| Birth-6 months | 0 | 0 | 0 |
| 6 months-3 years | 0.25 | 0 | 0 |
| 3-6 years | 0.50 | 0.25 | 0 |
| 6-16 years | 1.00 | 0.50 | 0 |

From American Academy of Pediatrics, Committee on Nutrition: Fluoride supplementation for children, *Pediatrics* 95(5):777, 1995.
*Fluoride daily doses are given in milligrams. 2.2 mg sodium fluoride contains 1 mg fluoride.
†Parts per million (ppm).

fected children. Fluorosis is directly related to the fluoride dosage and occurs in areas with high levels of natural fluoridation, as well as in nonfluoridated areas as a result of ingesting excessive fluoride from additional sources, such as beverages (including bottled water), processed foods, dental products, and supplements. Ingesting excessive fluoride after age 5 or 6 years does not result in fluorosis, because the permanent teeth, except for the third-year molars, are completely calcified.

As a safeguard, the child's use of toothpaste should be supervised to prevent swallowing of excessive amounts. Only a "pea-sized" amount of toothpaste should be placed on the young child's toothbrush (DenBesten and Ko, 1996). Fluoride rinses, which also offer topical benefits, are not recommended for children under 6 years of age because of the likelihood of their swallowing the liquid (American Academy of Pediatric Dentistry, 1996). As with any drug, acute toxicity (over 5 mg/kg) can occur from ingestion of large quantities of fluoride (Mallatt and Smith, 1996). A lethal dose for children is estimated to be 32 to 64 mg/kg (Heifetz and Horowitz, 1986). (See Community Focus and Evidence-Based Practice boxes on p. 614.)

Nurses have a responsibility to ensure an optimum fluoride regimen for children and to counsel families regarding correct use of supplements. The nurse should have knowledge of the fluoride content of the community water supply and provide instruction to parents regarding correct administration of fluoride drops or tablets. Supplements should remain in the mouth for 30 seconds before swallowing and be taken on an empty stomach. Afterward, the child should not drink or eat for 30 minutes. All fluoride products (toothpaste, supplements, and rinse) need to be stored away from young children to prevent poisoning. If the water supply is fluoridated, parents are encouraged to use water to prepare drinks and foods.

## Low-Cariogenic Diet

Diet is critical to developing good teeth because the carious process depends primarily on fermentable sugars, especially sucrose. Refined table sugar is not the only concentrated sweet food that is cariogenic. Natural foods, including honey, molasses, corn syrup, and dried fruits, such as raisins, are highly cariogenic (O'Sullivan and Curzon, 2000). Com-

## COMMUNITY FOCUS
### An Optimum Fluoride Regimen in Young Children

Base recommendations on the fluoride concentration in child's drinking water, including bottled water, filtered and well water, and processed food.

If the water is fluoridated, encourage use of tap water for drinking and for preparation of formula (except soy formula, which has twice the fluoride of regular formula), frozen-concentrated juices, powdered mixes, soups, ice, and gelatin.

If the water is nonfluoridated or contains less than 0.6 ppm fluoride, or if child refuses to drink tap water or refuses drinks/foods made with tap water, consider fluoride supplements.

If the water, such as water from some wells or springs, has concentration of fluoride above recommended level, encourage use of bottled nonfluoridated water for drinking.

Encourage supervision of toddler when brushing teeth or using a fluoridated mouthrinse to prevent overingestion of fluoridated topical supplement.

Use fluoridated toothpaste.

Consider other sources of fluoride from diet, such as tea.

If fluoride supplements are needed, give special instructions to family, including:
- ☐ Supplements should be given on an empty stomach without calcium-rich products, such as milk or cheese.
- ☐ No food or drink should be given for at least 30 minutes.
- ☐ Drops should be placed on tongue, mixed with saliva, and swished around in the mouth so that fluoride will come in contact with the teeth.
- ☐ Chewable tablets should be chewed and then mixed with saliva and swished in mouth for 30 seconds so that fluoride will come in contact with the teeth.
- ☐ Store fluoride products away from toddlers to avoid overingestion.
- ☐ Keep only a 4-month supply.
- ☐ Administer supplement at same time daily; post reminders if necessary.

Stress that dental appointments should be scheduled every 6 months for professional topical fluoride treatment.

Fluoride rinses are usually only suggested for children at high cariogenic risk or over the age of 6 years.

Modified from Hess C and others: Fluoride too little or too late, *Pediatr Nurs* 10(6):397-403, 1984; and American Academy of Pediatric Dentistry: Reference manual 1996-1997, *Pediatr Dent* 18(6):24-28, 37, 1996.

## EVIDENCE-BASED PRACTICE
### Fluoride

Pediatric dental caries remains a major health care issue. In an effort to decrease the rising numbers of dental caries in childhood, the U.S. Public Health Service included two fluoride-related objectives in the Healthy People 2000 Initiative (*Healthy People 2000*, 1991). Using a baseline of 62% in 1989, the Healthy People 2000 fluoridation objective proposed to raise the proportion of people served by optimally fluoridated community water systems to 75% and to increase the proportion of children receiving dietary fluoride supplements but not optimally fluoridated water to 85%. Over 20 states and the District of Columbia have met these standards (Hinman, Sterritt, and Reeves, 1996).

An important reduction in caries has been noted as a result of optimum fluoride exposure and improved dental care despite an apparent increase in sugar consumption by children (Kandelman, 1997; Reeves, 1996). But with the decrease in pediatric dental caries, the incidence of mild to moderate fluorosis may be increasing (Pendrys, Katz, and Morse, 1996).

All sources of fluoride, including drinking water, dentifrices, fluoride supplements, and other foods and beverages, should be investigated (Warren and Levy, 1999), and parents should be asked about dental hygiene habits at home (Levy and others, 2000; Villena, 2000). For areas where community water sources are not optimally fluoridated (such as well water in rural areas) or where fluoridated tap water is not used by choice, the current recommendations for supplementation should be maintained (Moss, 1999). Even in communities with community fluoridation water supplies, most of the fluoride exposure in children is from fluoridated dentifrices, not from the water (Rojas-Sanchez and others, 1999).

All health care professionals, including nurses, must take an active role in educating the public on proper use of supplements, especially dentifrices like toothpaste (Bentley, Ellwood, and Davies, 1999; Levy and Guha-Chowdhury, 1999). Considering all the sources of fluoride can help the health care provider and parent in the prevention of both dental caries and fluorosis (Levy and others, 1995; Guha-Chowdury, Drummond, and Smillie, 1996).

How knowledgeable are you? Do you know the fluoride content of your local water supply, including well water? Do you know how to obtain this information? In many areas water analysis results can be obtained from dental schools or the public health or water departments. Are dosages of dietary supplements of fluoride increased at 2 to 3 years of age and continued until 16 years of age? Do you know what other sources of fluoride are being used? Do you know how much toothpaste is being applied to the toddler's toothbrush? Are there school fluoridation programs and educational programs on proper dental hygiene? What strategies could be used in your community to improve the dental care of children?

plex carbohydrates, such as breads, potatoes, and pasta, also contribute to caries because they lower the plaque pH. (See Dental Disorders, Chapter 18.)

Ideally, concentrated sugars and high-carbohydrate snacks should be eliminated. However, since this is impractical, some suggestions can be helpful. The first is that *the frequency with which sugar is consumed is more important than the total amount eaten*. Therefore, when sweets are eaten, they are less damaging if consumed immediately after a meal rather than as a snack between meals. When sweets are served as the dessert, the teeth can be cleaned afterward, decreasing the amount of time the sugar is in the mouth.

The form of sugar is also important. The more cariogenic foods are those that are sticky or hard because they remain in the mouth longer. Consequently, sucking on lollipops is more cariogenic than eating a chocolate bar.

These suggestions can help parents plan "treats" in a way that is less damaging to the teeth. In addition, parents

should be aware of foods that are good snacks and that contribute less to tooth decay (Table 14-6). Some snacks do not contribute to tooth decay and may actually protect against it. Aged cheeses, such as cheddar, may alter the pH and retard bacterial growth. Sugarless gum chewed for about 20 minutes after eating may also protect against cavities by stimulating saliva that neutralizes acid (Durward and Thou, 1997), and saliva itself may have caries-protective factors (Featherstone, 1999). The artificial sweeteners saccharin and aspartame are noncariogenic, and sorbitol has low cariogenic potential (Kandelman, 1997).

Likewise, parents should know about hidden sources of sugar, such as numerous prescription and nonprescription drugs, and many popular cereals, including the "all natural"

**TABLE 14-6**   Lower cariogenic snack foods

| Good Snacks Eaten Alone | Snacks Better Served with Meals |
|---|---|
| **Breads and Cereals** | |
| Popcorn and other seeds | Breads and cereals, pasta, crackers, potato products, pretzels, all sweet baked goods |
| **Fruit and Vegetables** | |
| All raw, fresh, frozen, or water-packed fruits or vegetables or their juices prepared without addition of sugars* | All items prepared or used with the addition of sugars,* dried fruits such as raisins, catsup, gelatin |
| **Meats** | |
| Meat of all kinds, including luncheon meats, leftovers, and smoked meat; nuts, peanuts, peanut butter*; bean dips* | Meats prepared with sugars,* candy-coated nuts |
| **Dairy Products** | |
| Milk—whole, low-fat, skim, or buttermilk; cheese, especially cheddar; plain yogurt; dips and spreads*; flavored drinks*; hard-boiled eggs | Chocolate milk, malts, shakes, cocoa, ice cream, ice milk, sherbet, other dairy desserts, flavored yogurt |

*Check labels for added sugars. Look for (cane, maple, brown) sugar (sucrose), molasses, invert sugar, honey, dextrose (glucose), (modified) corn (sugar, syrup, sweetener, solids), lactose, levulose (fructose), and carob.

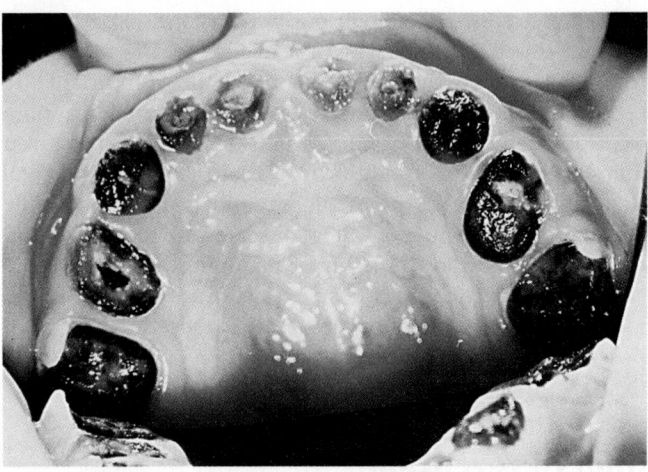

**Fig. 14-11**   Nursing caries. Note extensive carious involvement of maxillary primary incisors. (Courtesy Bruce Carter, DDS, Texas Children's Hospital, Houston, Texas.)

**TABLE 14-7**   Sucrose content of selected cereals

| Cereal (1-ounce serving) | Sucrose (grams/1-ounce serving) |
|---|---|
| Shredded Wheat | 0 |
| Cheerios | 1 |
| Cornflakes | 2 |
| Total | 3 |
| Rice Krispies | 3 |
| Raisin Bran (Post) | 7 |
| Kellogg's Low-Fat Granola | 8 |
| Quaker 100% Natural Cereal | 9 |
| Honey Nut Cheerios | 10 |
| Frosted Rice | 11 |
| Frosted Flakes | 12 |
| Froot Loops | 13 |
| Apple Jacks | 14 |
| Honey Smacks | 15 |
| Raisin Bran (Kellogg) | 19 |

variety (Table 14-7). Reading food labels is *essential* in eliminating sources of sucrose.

A special form of tooth decay in children between 18 months and 3 years of age is *early childhood caries (ECC)* or *baby bottle tooth decay (BBTD),* which occurs when the child is placed in the crib or bed with a bottle of milk, juice, soda pop, or sweetened water at nap or bedtime, or uses the bottle as a pacifier while awake (Reisine and Douglass, 1998). Frequent nocturnal breast-feeding for prolonged periods also leads to extensive destruction of the teeth (American Academy of Pediatric Dentistry, 1996). The practice of coating pacifiers in honey can also contribute to caries and may be a potential source of botulism poisoning. Other factors that may contribute to nursing caries include sleep difficulties, a strong-tempered child, single parenting, and less fluoride supplementation or professional counseling (van Everdingen and others, 1996). As the sweet liquid pools in the mouth, the teeth are bathed for several hours in this cariogenic environment. The maxillary (upper) incisors and sometimes molars are affected most because the mandibular (lower) teeth are thought to be protected by the lower lip, tongue, and saliva (Fig. 14-11). Severely de-

cayed teeth may require the application of stainless steel crowns, with or without white fronts, to preserve the spacing until the permanent teeth erupt.

Prevention involves eliminating the bedtime bottle completely, feeding the last bottle before bedtime, substituting a bottle of water for sweet liquids (Petter, Hourihane, and Rolles, 1995), not using the bottle as a pacifier, and never coating pacifiers in sweet substances. Juice in bottles, especially commercially available ready-to-use bottles, is discouraged, since the beverage is especially damaging because the sugar is more readily converted to acid (Siener, Rothman, and Farrar, 1997). Juice should always be offered in a cup in order to avoid prolonging the bottle-feeding habit.

**NURSING ALERT**   Primary teeth are important to maintain spacing and placement for permanent teeth. The response to an accidental dislodgment of a primary tooth in a toddler is to place the tooth in milk or saliva and notify the child's dentist. The dentist may be able to replace the tooth in the socket.

**NURSING ALERT**   The incidence of nursing caries is especially prevalent in Native American (Indian and Alaskan) children (>50%). Research has shown that education programs are effective in decreasing the incidence for these children (Bruerd and Jones, 1996; Weinstein and others, 1999).

Nurses are in an excellent position to counsel parents regarding this habit, especially if it occurs during a hospitalization. Although the child may need the comfort of the bottle at this stressful time, parents can be shown photographs depicting the typical tooth destruction and given literature about the condition.* Over an extended hospital stay, children can be gradually weaned from the bedtime bottle or given a bottle of water. Health professionals should never contribute to the habit by propping bottles for convenience during feedings. Nurses in clinics or offices should look for children with bottles used for nonnutritive purposes, because these youngsters tend to sleep with their bottles (Von Berg, Sanders, and Weddell, 1995).

## Injury Prevention

Injuries cause more deaths in the age-group 4 years and younger than in any other childhood period except adolescence. In addition, the injury death rate has remained relatively unchanged during the past decade, whereas the corresponding rates from all other causes of death combined have declined significantly. The prominence of injury as the leading cause of death among toddlers and preschoolers underscores the need to emphasize safety awareness among parents and other caregivers, such as personnel in alternative care settings, such as daycare facilities (Kopjar and Wickizer, 1996). Child protection and adult education are key determinants in injury prevention.

---

*Sources of information about nursing caries and other aspects of child dental health include the **National Institute of Dental Research,** Building 31, 31 Center Dr, MFC-2290, Bethesda, MD 20892-2290, (301) 496-4261; www.nidr.nih.gov; **Academy of Pediatric Dentistry,** 211 E Chicago Ave, Suite 700, Chicago, IL 60611, (312) 337-2169 or (800) 544-2174 (outside Illinois); www.aapd.org; **American Dental Association,** 211 E Chicago Ave, Chicago, IL 60611, (312) 440-2593 or (800) 621-8099 (outside Illinois); www.ada.org; and **Canadian Dental Association,** 1815 Alta Vista Dr, Ottawa, Ontario K1G 3Y6, (613) 523-1770. Guidelines for children's dental care are available in Wong DL, Hess CS: *Wong and Whaley's clinical manual of pediatric nursing,* ed 5, St Louis, 2000, Mosby.

A major factor in the increase of injuries during early childhood is the unrestricted freedom achieved through locomotion combined with an unawareness of danger within the environment. Specific categories of injuries and appropriate prevention are best understood by associating them with the major developmental achievements of young children (Table 14-8). The discussions of injuries in Chapters 1 and 12 are also relevant to safety concerns at this age.

### Motor Vehicle Injuries

Motor vehicle injuries cause more accidental deaths in all pediatric age-groups after age 1 year than any other type of injury or disease and are responsible for almost one half of all accidental deaths among children ages 1 to 4 years. Many of the deaths are caused by injuries within the car when restraints have not been used or have been used improperly (Halopka, 1999). Approved restraints properly installed and applied can reduce the majority of fatalities and injuries (American Academy of Pediatrics, 1996).

Nurses have a responsibility for educating parents regarding the importance of car restraints and their proper use. Five types of restraints are available: (1) infant-only devices, (2) convertible models for both infants and toddlers, (3) boosters, (4) safety belts, and (5) devices for children with special needs. (See Chapter 22.) Some cars come equipped with seats that convert to car restraints. The infant-type restraints are discussed in Chapter 12; the convertible restraints and boosters are included here.

The *convertible restraint* is suitable for infants in the rear-facing position and for toddlers in the forward-facing position (Fig. 14-12). The transition point for switching to the forward-facing position is defined by the manufacturer but is generally at a body weight of 9 kg (20 pounds) (American Academy of Pediatrics, 1996). Convertible safety seats should be used until the child weighs at least 40 pounds regardless of age and as long as the child fits properly into the seat (American Academy of Pediatrics, 2002). The restraint consists of a molded hard plastic or metal frame with en-

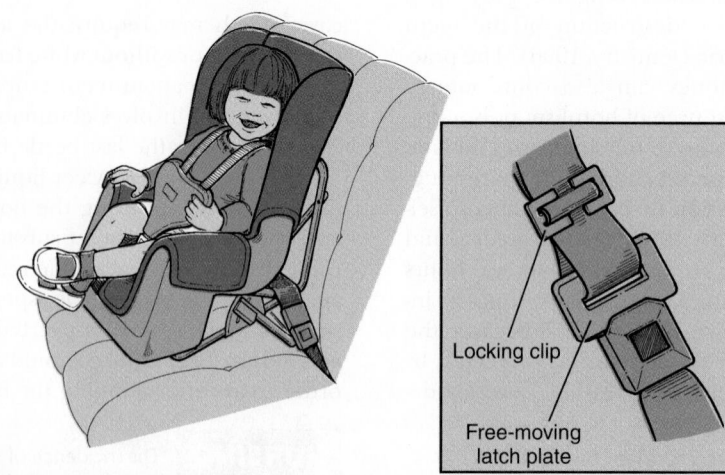

Locking clip

Free-moving
latch plate

**Fig. 14-12** Convertible seat in forward-facing position for older infants and children. *Inset:* Use of locking clip.

**TABLE 14-8   Injury prevention during early childhood**

| Developmental Abilities Related To Risk of Injury | Injury Prevention |
|---|---|
| Walks, runs, and climbs<br>Able to open doors and gates<br>Can ride tricycle<br>Can throw ball and other objects | **Motor vehicles**<br>Use federally approved car restraint; if restraint is not available, use lap belt<br>Supervise child while playing outside<br>Do not allow child to play on curb or behind a parked car<br>Do not permit child to play in pile of leaves, snow, or large cardboard container in trafficked area<br>Supervise tricycle riding<br>Lock fences and doors if not directly supervising children<br>Teach child to obey pedestrian safety rules<br>    Obey traffic regulations; walk only at crosswalks and when traffic signal indicates it is safe to cross<br>    Stand back a step from curb until it is time to cross<br>    Look left, right, and left again and check for turning cars before crossing street<br>    Use sidewalks; when there is no sidewalk, walk on left, facing traffic<br>    Wear light colors at night and attach fluorescent material to clothing |
| Able to explore if left unsupervised<br>Has great curiosity<br>Helpless in water, unaware of its danger; depth of water has no significance | **Drowning**<br>Supervise closely when near any source of water, including buckets<br>Keep bathroom doors and lid on toilet closed<br>Have fence around swimming pool and lock gate<br>Teach swimming and water safety (not a substitute for protection) |
| Able to reach heights by climbing, stretching, standing on toes, and using objects as a ladder<br>Pulls objects<br>Explores any holes or opening<br>Can open drawers and closets<br>Unaware of potential sources of heat or fire<br>Plays with mechanical objects | **Burns**<br>Turn pot handles toward back of stove<br>Place electric appliances, such as coffee maker, frying pan, and popcorn popper, toward back of counter<br>Place guardrails in front of radiators, fireplaces, or other heating elements<br>Store matches and cigarette lighters in locked or inaccessible area; discard carefully<br>Place burning candles, incense, hot foods, ashes, embers, and cigarettes out of reach<br>Do not let tablecloth hang within child's reach<br>Do not let electrical cord from iron or other appliance hang within child's reach<br>Cover electrical outlets with protective devices<br>Keep electrical wires hidden or out of reach<br>Do not allow child to play with electrical appliance, wires, or lighters<br>Stress danger of open flames; teach what "hot" means<br>Always check bathwater temperature; adjust hot-water heater temperature to 48.9° C (120° F) or lower; do not allow children to play with faucets<br>Apply a sunscreen with SPF 15 or higher when child is exposed to sunlight |
| Explores by putting objects in mouth<br>Can open drawers, closets, and most containers<br>Climbs<br>Cannot read warning labels<br>Does not know safe dose or amount | **Poisoning**<br>Place all potentially toxic agents (including plants) in a locked cabinet or out of reach<br>Replace medications and poisons immediately; replace child-resistant caps properly<br>Refer to medications as drugs, not as candy<br>Do not store large surplus of toxic agents<br>Promptly discard empty poison containers; never reuse to store a food item or other poison<br>Teach child not to play in trash containers<br>Never remove labels from containers of toxic substances<br>Have syrup of ipecac in home; use only if advised<br>Know number and location of nearest poison control center (usually listed in front of telephone directory) |
| Able to open doors and some windows<br>Goes up and down stairs<br>Depth perception unrefined | **Falls**<br>Keep screen in window, nail securely, and use guardrail<br>Place gates at top and bottom of stairs<br>Keep doors locked or use child-resistant doorknob covers at entry to stairs, high porch, or other elevated area, such as laundry chute<br>Remove unsecured or scatter rugs<br>Apply nonskid mat in bathtub or shower<br>Keep crib rails fully raised and mattress at lowest level<br>Place carpeting under crib and in bathroom<br>Keep large toys and bumper pads out of crib or playpen (child can use these as "stairs" to climb out), then move to youth bed when child is able to crawl out of crib<br>Avoid using walkers, especially near stairs<br>Dress in safe clothing (soles that do not "catch" on floor, tied shoelaces, pant legs that do not hang on floor)<br>Keep child restrained in vehicles; never leave unattended in shopping cart or stroller<br>Supervise at playgrounds; select play areas with soft ground cover and safe equipment (see Guidelines box, p. 618) |

*Continued*

**TABLE 14-8**   Injury prevention during early childhood—cont'd

| Developmental Abilities Related To Risk of Injury | Injury Prevention |
| --- | --- |
| Puts things in mouth<br>May swallow hard or nonedible pieces of food | **Choking and suffocation**<br>Avoid large, round chunks of meat, such as whole hot dogs (slice lengthwise into short pieces)<br>Avoid fruit with pits, fish with bones, dried beans, hard candy, chewing gum, nuts, popcorn, grapes, marshmallows<br>Choose large, sturdy toys without sharp edges or small removable parts<br>Discard old refrigerators, ovens, and so on; if storing old appliance, remove doors<br>Keep automatic garage door transmitter in inaccessible place<br>Select safe toy boxes or chests without heavy, hinged lids<br>Keep venetian blind strings out of child's reach<br>Remove drawstrings from clothing |
| Still clumsy in many skills<br>Easily distracted from tasks<br>Unaware of potential danger from strangers or other people | **Bodily damage**<br>Avoid giving sharp or pointed objects—such as knives, scissors, or toothpicks—especially when walking or running<br>Do not allow lollipops or similar objects in mouth when walking or running<br>Teach safety precautions (e.g., to carry fork or scissors with pointed end away from face)<br>Store all dangerous tools, garden equipment, and firearms in locked cabinet<br>Be alert to danger of animals, including household pets<br>Use safety glass and decals on large glassed areas, such as sliding glass doors<br>Teach personal safety<br>  Teach name, address, and phone number and to ask for help from appropriate people (cashier, security guard, policeman) if lost; have identification on child (sewn in clothes, inside shoe)<br>  Avoid personalized clothing in public places<br>  Teach child never to go with a stranger<br>  Teach child to tell parents if anyone makes child feel uncomfortable in any way<br>  Always listen to child's concerns regarding others' behavior<br>  Teach child to say "no" when confronted with uncomfortable situations |

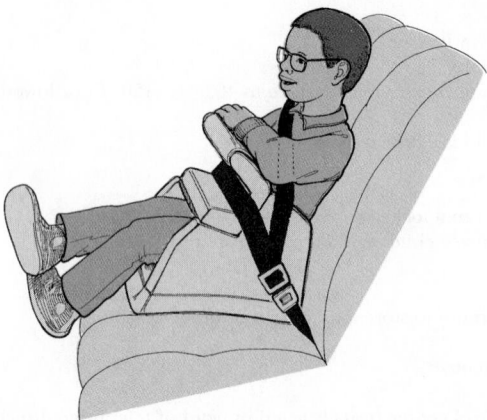

**Fig. 14-13**   Automobile booster seat. Note placement of shoulder strap (away from neck and face).

**GUIDELINES**
*Playground Safety*

Be certain play equipment has no sharp edges, corners, or projections.
Make sure that concrete footings are not exposed.
Examine area for a safe, resilient surface under equipment, such as sand or wood chips, to reduce the impact from a fall.
Be certain that size of equipment matches child.
Make sure there are no holes or other places where fingers, arms, legs, and necks could get caught.
  The incline of a slide should not exceed 30 degrees and should have evenly spaced rungs for climbing and protective "tunnels."
  S-hooks on swings must be closed.
Check for litter, broken glass, exposed wires, electrical outlets, or animal excreta.

ergy-absorbing padding and a special harness system designed to hold the child firmly in the seat and distribute the forces to body areas that can withstand the impact.

Convertible restraints use different types of harness systems: a *five-point harness* that consists of a strap over each shoulder, one on each side of the pelvis, and one between the legs (all five come together at a common buckle); a *padded shield* that uses shoulder straps attached to a shield that is held in place by a crotch strap; and a *T-shield* that has retracting shoulder straps attached to a flat chest shield with a rigid stalk that attaches to a restraint between the legs (see Fig. 14-12).

*Boosters* are not restraint systems like the convertible devices because they depend on the vehicle belts to hold the child and booster in place. Boosters are of two types: a *low-shield model* that primarily uses a lap belt (Fig. 14-13) and a *belt-positioning model* that uses a lap/shoulder belt. The combination lap/shoulder belt is preferred to the low-shield model (American Academy of Pediatrics, 1996).

Some older model restraints require the use of a top anchor (tether) strap to prevent the child from pitching forward in a crash. If the tether strap is not used, up to 90% of the restraint's protection is lost. Instructions for proper installation of the tether strap and permanent bracket are in-

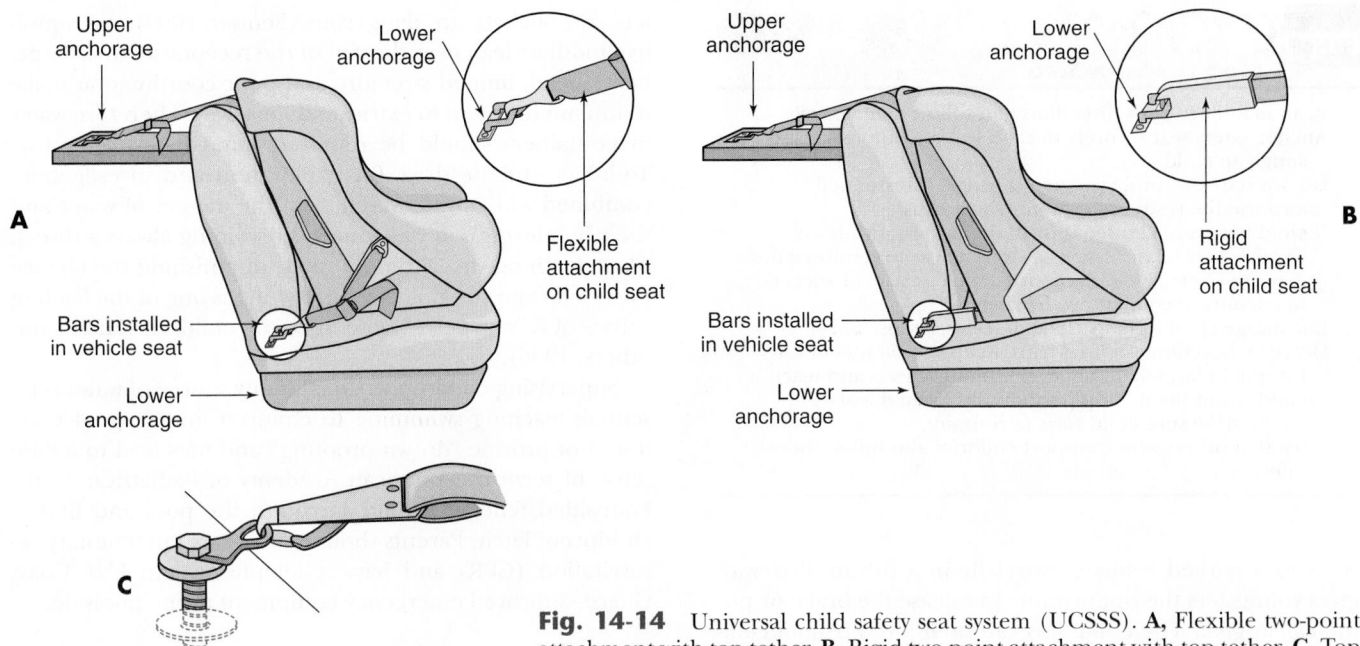

**Fig. 14-14**   Universal child safety seat system (UCSSS). **A,** Flexible two-point attachment with top tether. **B,** Rigid two-point attachment with top tether. **C,** Top tether. (Courtesy US Department of Transportation, National Highway Traffic Safety Administration.)

cluded with the car restraint. Cars with free-sliding latch plates on the lap/shoulder belt require the use of a metal locking clip to keep the belt in a tight-holding position. The locking clip is threaded onto the belt above the latch plate (see inset, Fig. 14-12). If parents have cars with automatic lap/shoulder belts, they need to have additional lap belts installed to properly secure the restraint.

Children should use specially designed car restraints until they weigh at least 60 pounds or are 8 years old (American Academy of Pediatrics, 1996). Children who outgrow the convertible restraint may still be able to ride safely in a booster seat until the midpoint of the head is higher than the vehicle seat back. If a car safety seat is not available, the lap belt provides more protection than no restraint (except for infants, for whom there is no safe alternative to approved restraint devices). Shoulder-only automatic belts are designed to protect adults. Children should use the manual shoulder belts in the rear seat. Air bags do not take the place of child safety seats or seat belts and can be lethal to young children (American Academy of Pediatrics, 1996).

A universal child safety seat system (UCSSS) was implemented as a requirement starting in the fall of 1999 for all new automobiles and child safety seats. This system provides a uniform anchorage consisting of two lower anchorages and one upper anchorage in the rear seat of the vehicle. New child safety seats will have a hook, buckle, strap, or other connector that attaches to the anchorage (Fig. 14-14). Seat belts will no longer be used to anchor child safety seats in newer vehicles. The first phase requires all new cars to have an upper anchorage. By fall of 2002, all new cars must have the entire UCSSS.*

The safest area of the car for children of any age is the middle of the back seat. Children should not ride in the front seat of any air bag–equipped car, except in emergencies, and then the vehicle seat must be as far back as possible (American Academy of Pediatrics, 1996).

> **NURSING ALERT**   Safety belts should be worn low on the hips, snug, and not on the abdominal area. Children should be taught to sit up straight to allow for proper fit. The shoulder belt is used *only* if it does not cross the child's neck or face.

For any restraint to be effective, it must be used consistently and properly (Martinez, 1996). Examples of misuse include misrouting of the vehicle seat belt through the restraint, failing to use the vehicle seat belt through the restraint, failing to use a tether strap, failing to use the restraint's harness system, and incorrectly positioning the child, especially facing infants forward instead of rearward. To address these issues, nurses must stress correct use of car restraints and rules that ensure compliance and can emphasize to parents that children riding in car safety seats are generally better behaved than children left unrestrained. (See Family Home Care box on p. 620.)*

Injuries may also occur during sudden stops when objects are left unrestrained. On sudden impact, a loose ball becomes a projectile. Therefore all items should be secured or stored in the trunk.

Children should never ride in the open back of a truck; the danger of falls can be compounded by another vehicle striking the child. In addition, leaving children unsuper-

---

*U.S. Department of Transportation, National Highway Traffic Safety Administration, 400 Seventh St SW, Washington, DC 20590, (800) 424-9393; www.nhtsa.dot.gov.

*More detailed guidelines for car seat safety are available in Wong DL, Hess CS: *Wong and Whaley's clinical manual of pediatric nursing,* ed 5, St Louis, 2000, Mosby.

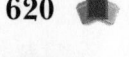

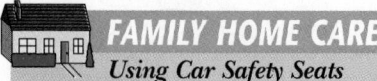

**FAMILY HOME CARE**
*Using Car Safety Seats*

Read manufacturer's directions and follow them exactly.
Anchor safety seat securely to car's seat and apply harness snugly to child.
Do not start car until everyone is properly restrained.
*Always* use the restraint, even for short trips.
If child begins to climb out or undo harness, firmly say, "No." It may be necessary to stop the car to reinforce the expected behavior. Use rewards, such as stars or stickers, to encourage cooperative behavior.
Encourage child to help attach buckles, straps, and shields.
Decrease boredom on long trips. Keep special toys in car for quiet play; talk to child; point out objects and teach child about them. Stop periodically. If child wishes to sleep, make sure child stays in restraint.
Insist that others who transport children also follow these safety rules.

vised in a parked vehicle, especially in a private driveway, gives youngsters the opportunity to release the brake or put the car in gear. The child also can be injured from a collision to or a fall from a bicycle-towed trailer or bicycle-mounted child seat (Powell and Tanz, 2000).

Children over 3 years of age are often involved in pedestrian traffic injuries (Wills and others, 1997). Because of their gross motor skills of walking, running, and climbing and their fine motor skills of opening doors and fence gates, they are likely to be in hazardous areas when unsupervised. Unaware of danger and unable to approximate the speed of a car, they are hit by moving vehicles. Running after a ball, playing in a pile of leaves or snow or inside a cardboard box, riding a tricycle, and playing behind a parked car or near the curb are common activities that may result in a vehicular tragedy. A precaution when children are playing in driveways is to attach to the tricycle a pole with a bright flag that is high enough to be visible through an automobile's back window. Another safeguard is a device that beeps when the vehicle is driven in reverse to alert children to the oncoming car, van, or truck.

Preventing vehicular injuries involves protecting and educating children about the dangers presented by moving or parked vehicles. Although preschool children are too young to be trusted to always obey, the parent should emphasize looking for moving vehicles before crossing the street, teach the color of traffic lights for stop and go, and stress the need for following traffic officers' signals. Most important, what is preached must be practiced. Children learn through imitation, and consistency reinforces learning.

## Drowning

Drowning, not including drowning from water transportation, ranks second among boys and third among girls ages 1 to 4 years as a cause of accidental death. Drowning rates in toddlers have changed little despite attempts at prevention strategies (Fenner, 2000). With well-developed skills of locomotion, toddlers are able to reach potentially dangerous areas, such as bathtubs (Schmidt and Madea, 1995), swimming pools, wading pools, irrigation ditches, post holes, hot tubs, and lakes. Even unlikely sources of water, such as toi-

lets and buckets, are dangerous (Fenner, 2000). As inquisitive toddlers lean over the rim of the receptacle, their large, heavy head, limited strength, and poor coordination make it difficult for them to extricate themselves. Therefore water in containers should be removed immediately after use. Toddlers' intense drive for exploration and investigation, combined with an unawareness of the danger of water and their helplessness in water, makes drowning always a threat. Also, death occurs within minutes, diminishing the chance for rescue and survival. Near-drowning is one of the leading causes of a "vegetative" state in young children (Habib and others, 1996).

Supervising children when near any source of water is essential; teaching swimming to children under age 4 years does not provide "drown proofing" and may lead to a false sense of security (American Academy of Pediatrics, 2000). Four-sided fencing should surround the pool and have a childproof latch. Parents should know cardiopulmonary resuscitation (CPR) and have a telephone and U.S. Coast Guard–approved emergency equipment at the poolside.

## Burns

Burns rank second to motor vehicle injuries among girls and third among boys in this age-group as a cause of accidental death. Toddlers' ability to climb, stretch, and reach objects above their heads makes any hot surface a potential source of danger. Scalds from children pulling pots with hot liquids, especially oil and grease, on top of themselves are a major source of burns. As a precaution, pot handles should be turned toward the back of the stove, and electric pots (e.g., coffee maker, frying pan, slow cooker, popcorn maker), including cords, should be placed out of reach. Ideally, the knobs for controlling the range burners should be out of reach, not on the front panel where nimble fingers can turn them on and accidentally touch the hot burner. Oven doors should be closed whenever the oven is turned on or when it is cooling. The outside of doors of automatic self-cleaning ovens may become hot and, if touched, could cause a burn (Yen and others, 2001). Microwave ovens present much less of a burn hazard to toddlers because the outside remains cool, and they are often inaccessible, although foods heated in microwaves can scald children (Dixon, Burd, and Roberts, 1997).

Other sources of heat, such as radiators, fireplaces, accessible furnaces, kerosene heaters, or wood-burning stoves, should have guards placed in front of them (Becker and Cartotto, 1999). The tops of some of these heaters are designed to become hot enough to boil water to provide humidity. They are hazardous if touched or if the pan of water is spilled. Portable electric heaters must be placed in a high area, well out of reach of climbing young children.

Hot objects such as candles, incense, hot embers and ashes, cigarettes, pots of tea or coffee, or irons must be placed away from children. The flame of a candle and the smoke of a cigarette invite investigation. Ashtrays with a center well are preferred to prevent the cigarette from falling off the rim, and adults should try not to smoke, cook, or drink hot liquids when children are nearby. If tablecloths are used, the edges should be placed out of reach to prevent

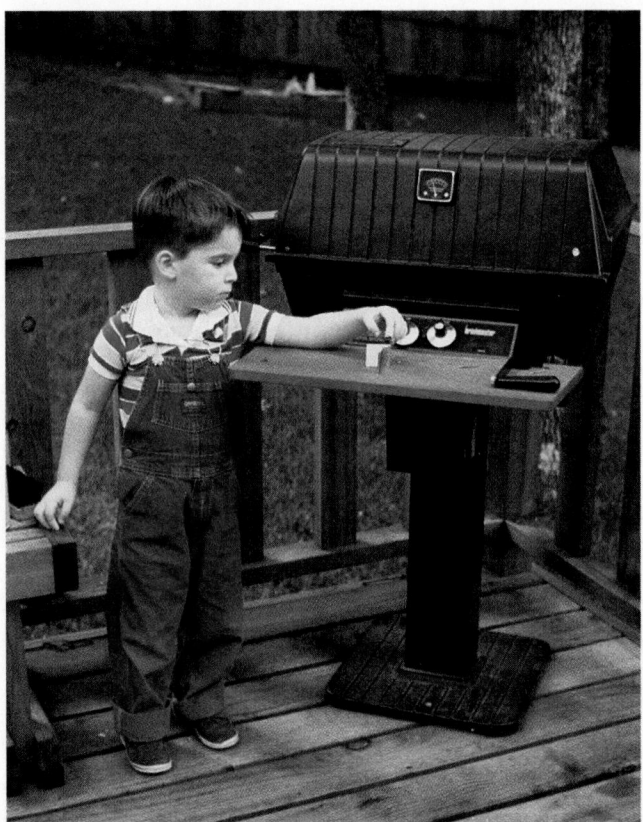

**Fig. 14-15** Matches are a potentially deadly hazard for young children.

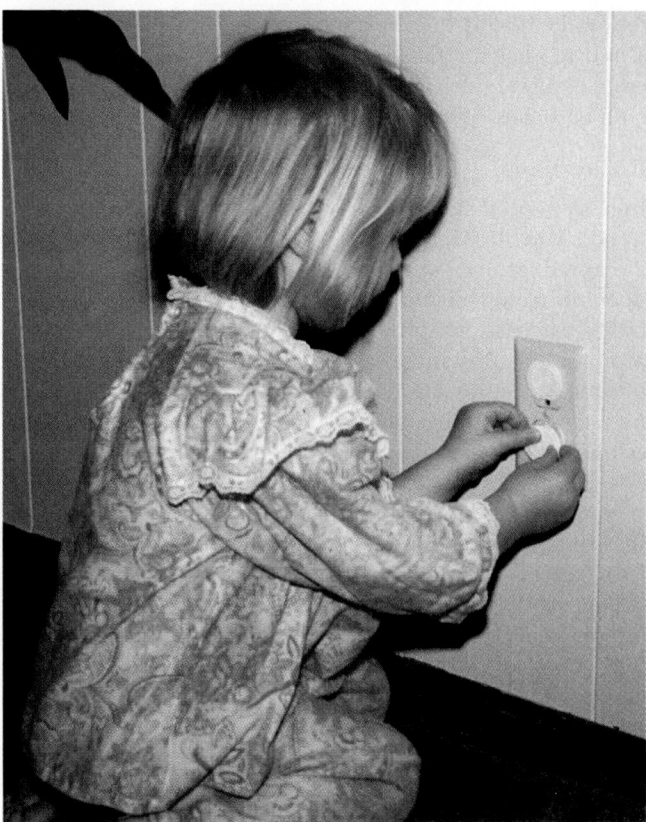

**Fig. 14-16** Special plastic caps in electrical sockets prevent young fingers from exploring dangerous areas.

injuries from both burns and falling objects. When children are near smoldering fires (campfires, brush fires, fires buried on the beach), wearing shoes can help protect the feet from burns.

Flame burns represent one of the most fatal types of burns and commonly occur when children play with matches and accidentally set themselves (and the home) on fire (Fig. 14-15). All matches must be stored safely away from children, and parents need to teach children the dangers of playing with matches (Ying and Ho, 2001). In addition, all homes should have smoke detectors installed to alert the occupants of a fire. A safety plan for immediate escape is also essential.

Electrical burns represent an immediate danger to children. With the ability to manipulate small, thin objects, they are able to insert hairpins or other conductive articles into electrical sockets. Young toddlers may explore outlets and wires by mouthing them. Because saliva is an excellent conductor, the chance for a severe circumoral electrical burn is great (Thomas, 1996b; Milano, 1999). Electrical outlets should have protective guards plugged into them when not in use or be made inaccessible by placing furniture in front of them when feasible (Fig. 14-16). Children should not be allowed to play with electrical cords, appliances, or batteries, which should be kept out of reach as much as possible (Rabban and others, 1997).

An example of an appliance that interests children and can present a hazard is an electric popcorn popper. Chil-

dren can become so excited by the popping that they may inadvertently pull the electrical cord and popper off the table, resulting in a burn from contact with the hot oil, corn, or appliance. Steam from a microwaved bag of popcorn (or other foods) can also cause burns.

Scald burns are the most common type of thermal injury in children. A scalding burn is often caused by high-temperature tap water, which children come in contact with either as a result of turning on the hot-water faucet, falling into a bathtub of hot water, or deliberate abuse (Harre, Field, and Polzer-Debruyne, 1998; Huyer and Corkum, 1997). Besides the obvious prevention of always supervising youngsters when they are near tap water and checking bath-water temperatures, a recommended passive prevention is to limit household water temperatures to less than 49° C (120° F). At this temperature it takes 10 minutes for exposure to the water to cause a full-thickness burn. Conversely, water temperatures of 54° C (130° F), the usual setting of most water heaters, expose household members to the risk of full-thickness burns within 30 seconds. Nurses can help prevent such burns by advising parents of this common household danger and recommending that they readjust the water heater to a safe temperature. A meat or candy thermometer is a convenient way to measure water temperature. An easy-to-read hot-water gauge that changes color to show water temperatures between 120° and 150° F is available; it shows "hot," "cool," or "OK" water temperature. A special device can also be added to the faucet that reduces the water flow if the set temperature is reached. Scalding also often occurs when the curious child tries to sip a parent's coffee or tea and spills the boiling liquid down the chin and chest (Eadie, Williams, and Dickson, 1995).

## Poisoning

Ingestion of toxic agents is common during early childhood. The highest incidence occurs in children in the 2-year-old group. Although in many instances poisoning does not result in mortality, it may cause significant morbidity, such as esophageal stricture from lye ingestion. Mouthing activity increases toddlers' risk of poisoning; exploring objects by tasting them is part of children's curious investigation. Young children's taste is not refined or discriminating. Because of their curious nature, children under 6 years of age are more likely to eat unusual, distasteful substances. Although young children may be able to identify some items as poisonous, they do not understand the toxic effects of ingesting excessive amounts of a familiar drug, such as vitamins or iron (Anderson and others, 2000; Morris, 2000). Almost every nonfood substance is potentially harmful, including many house plants (Lamminpaa

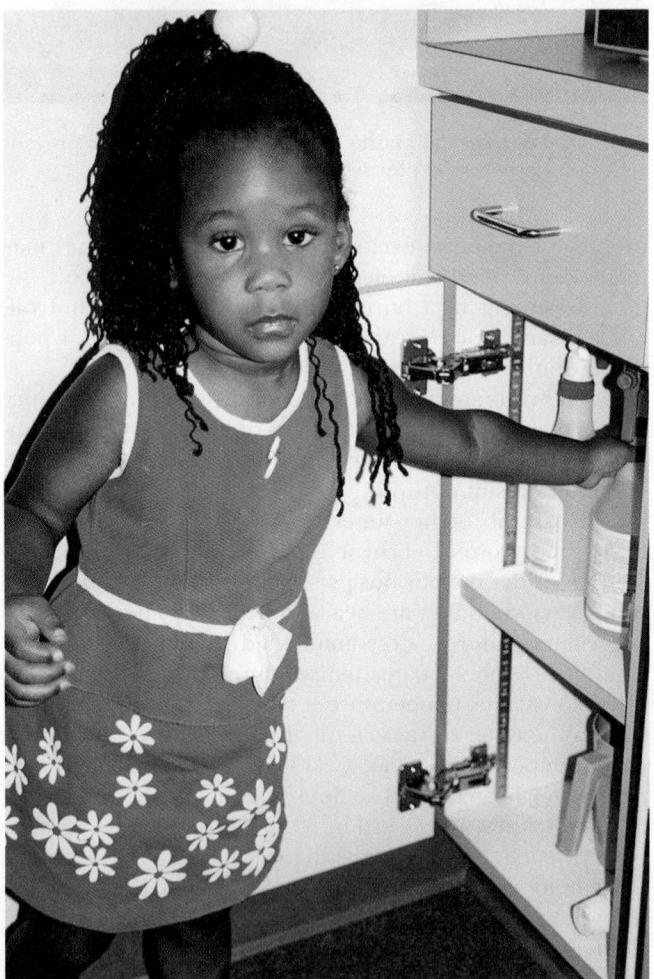

**Fig. 14-17**   Children are most likely to ingest substances that are on their level, such as cleaning agents stored under sinks, rat poison, plants, or diaper pail deodorants.

and Kinos, 1996), and by 2 years of age toddlers are able to climb most heights, open most drawers or closets, and unscrew most lids. By trial and error, they also manage to undo tops of bottles, plastic containers, aerosol cans, and jars.

However, they are most likely to ingest substances that are on their level, such as plants, cleaning agents stored under sinks, rat poison (Parson and others, 1996), or diaper pail deodorants, especially when stored in the kitchen, bathroom, laundry, or garage. Child-resistant tops are required on some substances, such as prescription drugs, but many young children have opened such "safe" caps. In addition, pharmacists often transfer drugs to regular containers for the elderly, who may have difficulty with child-resistant closures. Newer forms of drugs, such as transdermal patches (nicotine or fentanyl) (Woolf and others, 1996; Woolf and others, 1997) and cough-suppressant lozenges, have created additional dangers because they are not packaged with safety caps and in the case of lozenges look like candy.

Many potentially toxic substances are not protected with safety caps and must be stored properly. Even common household items, such as mouthwash that contains ethanol (alcohol), can be toxic to young children.

The major reason for poisoning is improper storage (Fig. 14-17). The guidelines suggested in Chapter 12 apply to children in this age-group as well. However, unlike infants, who are unable to reach certain heights or unlatch inventive locks, young children manage to find access to many high-level, tight-security places. For this age-group, only a locked cabinet is safe.

Parents should have two doses of ipecac syrup for each child in the home, know its proper use and administration, and have the phone number and location of the nearest poison control center (Burda and Burda, 1997). Emergency and preventive measures for accidental poisoning are discussed in Chapter 16.

## Falls

Falls are still a hazard to children in this age-group, although by the later part of early childhood, gross and fine motor skills are well developed, decreasing the incidence of falls down stairs or from chairs. However, playground injuries are common (Mayr and others, 1995; Playground Safety, 1999). Children need to be taught safety at play areas, such as no horseplay on high slides or jungle gyms, *sitting* on swings, and staying away from moving swings (Mayr and others; 1995; McEvoy, Montana, and Panettieri, 1996). Other guidelines for playground safety are listed in the Guidelines box on p. 618.

The climbing and running activity of the typical toddler is complicated by total neglect for and lack of appreciation of danger, immature coordination, and a high center of gravity. Falling from stairs is a major cause of injury, with more children in this age-group sustaining head injuries than older children (Chiaviello, Christoph, and Bond, 1994). Gates must be placed at both ends of stairs. Accessible windows that are left open during warm weather must be screened or guarded with a rail. Falling from open windows is a major cause of accidental death in urban lower socioeconomic groups. Doors leading to stairwells or porches must be locked. A convenient type of lock is a sliding bar or hook that can be attached to the door and frame at a level higher than the child can reach, provided that inventive youngsters do not pull a chair over to unlatch the device.

Another source of falls is from cribs and vehicles. In addition to crib rails being fully raised, the mattress should be kept at the lowest position, and toys or bumper pads that may be used as steps to climb out should be removed. Ideally, the floor should be carpeted. Once children reach a height of 89 cm (35 inches), they should sleep in a bed rather than a crib. If a bunk bed is selected, parents should be aware of possible dangers: falls and head entrapment between the mattress and guardrail or between the supporting mattress slats. If the beds are constructed of tubular metal or if the brackets holding the mattress are metal, parents should check for breaks or cracks in the metal and welds, which may lead to collapse and injury. Children who sleep on the top bunk should be 6 years or older.

Unrestrained children can fall from high chairs, shopping carts, carriages, and car seats (Smith and others, 1996; Harrell, 1997). Therefore proper restraint and adequate supervision are essential.

Clothing can also increase the chance of falling. Slippery shoes or socks, rubber-soled shoes that "catch" on the floor and rug, and loose or cuffed pants can easily make a child fall. Simple safety measures, such as checking clothing and shoes, keeping shoelaces tied with double knots, or using self-adhering closures, can prevent such needless injuries.

### Aspiration and Suffocation

Usually by 1 year of age children chew well, but they may have difficulty with large pieces of food, such as meat or whole hot dogs, and with hard foods, such as nuts or dried beans. Young children cannot discard pits from fruit or bones from fish like older children. It takes practice to learn how to chew gum without swallowing it. Therefore the same precautions as discussed for infants regarding food selection must be implemented. (See Chapter 12.)

Play objects for toddlers must still be chosen with an awareness of the danger of small parts. Large, sturdy toys without sharp edges or removable parts are safest. Coins, paper clips, pull tabs on cans, thumbtacks, nails, screws, jewelry (especially pierced earrings), and all types of pins are common household objects that can cause significant harm if swallowed or aspirated. Because of the danger of aspiration, parents should be taught emergency procedures for choking.* (See Airway Obstruction, Chapter 31.)

One cause of death by traumatic asphyxiation is from electrically operated garage doors. Young children playing in the garage may become trapped under the door. Although the automatic doors should reverse when striking an object, they may not do so when hitting a flexible object or one that is very close to the ground. Precautions include placing controls where they are inaccessible to children, such as high on a wall and in a locked car, and instructing

children that the transmitter is not a toy. Periodically the door should be checked to be certain it reverses when striking an object. Another cause of traumatic asphyxiation and strangulation is the drawstring on jackets or hoods. These drawstrings, especially when near the head, can get caught in playground equipment and cause strangulation (Pless, 1996).

Suffocation is less frequent from causes seen during infancy (Drago and Dannenberg, 1999) but is an ever-present threat from old refrigerators, ovens, and other large appliances. Toddlers can climb inside these appliances, and if they close the door behind them, they will be trapped inside. Discarding old appliances or removing all doors during storage prevents such tragic injuries. Toddlers may also suffocate when toy boxes with heavy, hinged lids accidentally close on their head or neck. Parents should be advised of this danger and encouraged to buy storage chests with lightweight, removable covers.

### Bodily Damage

Toddlers are still clumsy in many of their skills and can seriously harm themselves when walking while holding a sharp or pointed object or having food or objects such as spoons in their mouths. Preventing such occurrences is the best approach with toddlers. With preschoolers, teaching safety is most important. The child should be taught that when walking with a pointed object, such as a fork, knife, or scissors, the pointed end is held away from the face. Dangerous garden or workshop equipment and *all firearms* should be stored in a locked cabinet (Denno and others, 1996; Azrael, Miller, and Hemenway, 2000). Power lawn mowers are especially dangerous, and young children should not be allowed in an area where a mower is being used, nor should they be taken for a ride on a mower or allowed to operate the device (Alonso and Sanchez 1995; Vosburgh and others, 1995; Mayer and others, 1998). The American Academy of Pediatrics (2001) recommends that children under the age of 6 remain indoors during mowing and that children be at least 12 years of age before operating a power mower (16 years for a ride-on mower). Safety education should include respect for firearms and their proper and appropriate use, including nonpowder guns, such as air guns and rifles, which cause serious penetrating injuries (Milroy and others, 1998). In addition, the child should be warned of and protected against potential danger from animals. (See Bodily Damage, Chapter 12, and Animal Bites, Chapter 18.)

Toys can be a source of danger, and safety must be a prime consideration when selecting toys. (See Family Home Care box on p. 602.) Most toys have age ranges written on them to designate their safety, but this must be tempered with knowledge of the specific child's readiness.

Household safety should be practiced and includes the usual precautions recommended for any age-group. (See Family Home Care box on p. 549.) An additional safeguard for young children is the use of safety glass in doors, windows, and tabletops and the application of decals on glassed areas to lessen the likelihood of running through glass. Also, children should not be allowed to run, jump, wrestle,

---

*Home care instructions on caring for the choking child are available in Wong DL, Hess CS: *Wong and Whaley's clinical manual of pediatric nursing,* ed 5, St Louis, 2000, Mosby.

## FAMILY HOME CARE
### Guidance During Toddler Years

### AGES 12 TO 18 MONTHS

Prepare parents for expected behavioral changes of toddler, especially negativism and ritualism.

Assess present feeding habits and encourage gradual weaning from bottle and increased intake of solid foods.

Stress expected feeding changes of physiologic anorexia, presence of food fads and strong taste preferences, need for scheduled routine at mealtimes, inability to sit through an entire meal, and lack of table manners.

Assess sleep patterns at night, particularly habit of a bedtime bottle, which is a major cause of dental caries, and procrastination behaviors that delay hour of sleep.

Prepare parents for potential dangers of the home, particularly motor vehicle, poisoning, and falling injuries; give appropriate suggestions for childproofing the home.

Discuss need for firm but gentle discipline and ways in which to deal with negativism and temper tantrums; stress positive benefits of appropriate discipline.

Emphasize importance for both child and parents of brief, periodic separations.

Discuss new toys that use developing gross and fine motor, language, cognitive, and social skills.

Emphasize need for dental supervision, types of basic dental hygiene at home, and food habits that predispose to caries; stress importance of supplemental fluoride.

### AGES 18 TO 24 MONTHS

Stress importance of peer companionship in play.

Explore need for preparation for additional sibling; stress importance of preparing child for new experiences.

Discuss present discipline methods, their effectiveness, and parents' feelings about child's negativism; stress that nega-tivism is important aspect of developing self-assertion and independence and is not a sign of spoiling.

Discuss signs of readiness for toilet training; emphasize importance of waiting for physical and psychologic readiness.

Discuss development of fears, such as darkness or loud noises, and of habits, such as security blanket or thumb sucking; stress normalcy of these transient behaviors.

Prepare parents for signs of regression in time of stress.

Assess child's ability to separate easily from parents for brief periods under familiar circumstances.

Allow parents opportunity to express their feelings of weariness, frustration, and exasperation; be aware that it is often difficult to love toddlers at times when they are not asleep!

Point out some of the expected changes of the next year, such as longer attention span, somewhat less negativism, and increased concern for pleasing others.

### AGES 24 TO 36 MONTHS

Discuss importance of imitation and domestic mimicry and need to include child in activities.

Discuss approaches toward toilet training, particularly realistic expectations and attitude toward accidents.

Stress uniqueness of toddlers' thought processes, especially through their use of language, poor understanding of time, causal relationships in terms of proximity of events, and inability to see events from another's perspective.

Stress that discipline still must be quite structured and concrete and that relying solely on verbal reasoning and explanation leads to confusion, misunderstanding, and even injuries.

Discuss investigation of preschool or daycare center toward completion of second year.

---

or play ball in areas where glass litter may be a hazard (Makary, 1998).

## Anticipatory Guidance— Care of Families

Understanding toddlers is fundamental to successful child-rearing. Nurses, particularly those in ambulatory or child health centers, are in a most favorable position to assist parents in meeting the tasks and needs of children in this age-group. Anticipatory guidance in each of the areas presented in the Family Home Care box can prevent future problems.

Advice is sometimes not the sole answer. Actual assistance, such as being available for home visiting or telephone consulting, should be a part of the nurse's flexible repertoire of interventions. Whether parents are experiencing the challenges of rearing a first or a subsequent child, they benefit from sharing their feelings, frustrations, and satisfactions. They need adult companionship, shared childrearing responsibilities, and periodic separations from their children. For single parents such goals can be especially difficult to achieve. Part of a nurse's responsibility is to provide opportunities for parents to express their feelings and meet their emotional and physical needs.

## KEY POINTS

- The toddler stage, extending over ages 12 to 36 months, is a period of intense exploration of the environment.
- Biologic development during the toddler years is characterized by the acquisition of fine and gross motor skills that allow children to master a wide variety of activities.
- Although most of the physiologic systems are mature by the end of toddlerhood, development of certain areas of the brain is still occurring, allowing for greater intellectual capacity.

- Locomotion is the major gross motor skill acquired during toddlerhood, followed by increased eye-hand coordination.
- Specific tasks in the psychosocial development of a toddler include differentiating self from others, tolerating separation from parent, coping with delayed gratification, controlling bodily functions, acquiring socially acceptable behavior, communicating verbally, and interacting with others in a less egocentric manner.

- According to Erikson, the major developmental task of toddlerhood is acquiring a sense of autonomy while overcoming a sense of doubt and shame.
- In Piaget's sensorimotor and preconceptual phases of development, the toddler experiments by incorporating the old learning of secondary circular reactions with new skills and applies this knowledge to new situations. There is the beginning of rational judgment, an understanding of causal relationships, and discovery of objects as objects.
- Preconceptual thought is characterized by centration, global organization of thought processes, animism, and irreversibility.
- Language is the major cognitive achievement in toddlerhood.
- The most striking characteristic of language development during early childhood is the increasing level of comprehension.
- Discipline, or a punishment-obedience orientation, aids in children's moral development.

- Development of body image occurs with increasing motor ability, at which point toddlers recognize the importance and capacity of body parts.
- The two phases of differentiation of self from significant others are separation and individuation.
- Parental concerns during the toddler years include toilet training, coping with sibling rivalry, dealing with temper tantrums and negativism, and coping with stress.
- Nutrition is important at this stage because eating habits established in toddlerhood tend to have lasting effects in subsequent years.
- Regular dental examinations, fluoride supplementation, removal of plaque, and provision of a low-cariogenic diet promote optimum dental health.
- Because of increased locomotion, toddlers are at high risk for sustaining injuries. Fatal injuries are primarily the result of motor vehicle accidents, drownings, and burns.

## REFERENCES

Alonso JE, Sanchez FL: Lawn mower injuries in children: a preventable impairment, *J Pediatr Orthop* 15(1):83-89, 1995.

American Academy of Pediatric Dentistry: Reference manual 1996-97, *Pediatr Dent* 18(6):24-77, 1996.

American Academy of Pediatrics, Committee on Injury and Poison Prevention: Selecting and using the most appropriate car safety seats for growing children: guidelines for counseling parents, *Pediatrics* 97(5):761-763, 1996.

American Academy of Pediatrics, Committee on Injury and Poison Prevention: Selecting and using the most appropriate car safety seats for growing children: guidelines for counseling parents, *Pediatrics* 109(3):550-553, 2002.

American Academy of Pediatrics, Committee on Nutrition: *Pediatric nutrition handbook*, ed 4, Elk Grove Village, IL, 1998, American Academy of Pediatrics.

American Academy of Pediatrics, Committee on Sports Medicine and Committee on Injury and Poison Prevention: Swimming programs for infants and toddlers, *Pediatrics* 105(4):868-870, 2000.

American Academy of Pediatrics: Lawn mower–related injuries to children, *Pediatrics* 107(6):1480-81, 2001.

Anderson BD and others: Retrospective analysis of ingestions of iron containing products in the United States: are there differences between chewable vitamins and adult preparations, *J Emerg Med* 19(3):255-258, 2000.

Azrael D, Miller M, Hemenway D: Are household firearms stored safely? It depends on whom you ask, *Pediatrics* 106(3):31, 2000.

Barnes and others: Spirituality, religion, and pediatrics: intersecting worlds of healing, *Pediatrics* 106(4 suppl):899-908, 2000.

Becker L, Cartotto R: The gas fireplace: a new burn hazard in the home, *J Burn Care Rehabil* 20(1 pt 1):86-89, 1999.

Belsky J, Woodworth S, Crnic K: Trouble in the second year: three questions about family interaction, *Child Dev* 67(2):556-578, 1996.

Bentley EM, Ellwood RP, Davies RM: Fluoride ingestion from toothpaste by young children, *Br Dent J* 186(9):460-462, 1999.

Berkowitz C: Thumbsucking and other habits. In Berkowitz C, editor: *Pediatrics: a primary care approach*, Philadelphia, 1996, WB Saunders.

Brayden RM, Poole SR: Common behavioral problems in infants and children, *Prim Care* 22(1):81-97, 1995.

Brazelton TB: *Touchpoints*, Cambridge, MA, 1994, Perseus Publishing.

Brazelton TB: Working with families. Opportunities for early intervention, *Pediatr Clin North Am* 42(1):1-9, 1995.

Bruerd B, Jones C: Preventing baby bottle tooth decay: eight-year results, *Public Health Rep* 111(1):63-65, 1996.

Burda AM, Burda NM: The nation's first poison control center: taking a stand against accidental childhood poisoning in Chicago, *Vet Hum Toxicol* 39(2):115-119, 1997.

Carruth BR and others: The phenomenon of "picky eater": a behavioral marker in eating patterns of toddlers, *J Am Coll Nutr* 17(2):180-186, 1998.

Chiaviello CT, Christoph RA, Bond GR: Stairway-related injuries in children, *Pediatrics* 94(5):679-681, 1994.

Chiocca EM: Language development in bilingual children, *Pediatr Nurs* 24(1):43-47, 1998.

Colson ER, Dworkin, PH: Toddler development, *Pediatr Rev* 18(8):255-257, 1997.

DenBesten P, Ko HS: Fluoride levels in whole saliva of preschool children after brushing with 0.25 g (pea-sized) as compared to 1.0 g (full-brush) of a fluoride dentifrice, *Pediatr Dent* 18(4):277-280, 1996.

Dennison BA, Jenkins PL, Rockwell HL: Development and validation of an instru-

ment to assess child dietary fat intake, *Prev Med* 31(3):214-224, 2000.

Dennison BA, Rockwell HS, Baker SL: Excess fruit juice consumption by preschool-aged children is associated with short stature and obesity, *Pediatrics* 99(1):15-22, 1997.

Denno DM and others: Safe storage of handguns, *Arch Pediatr Adolesc Med* 150(9):927-931, 1996.

Dietz W, Stern L: *American Academy of Pediatrics guide to your child's nutrition*, New York, 1999, Villard.

DiMario FJ: Prospective study of children with cyanotic and pallid breath-holding spells, *Pediatrics* 107(2):265-269, 2001.

Dixon JJ, Burd DA, Roberts DG: Severe burns resulting from an exploding teat on a bottle of infant formula milk heated in a microwave oven, *Burns* 23(3):268-269, 1997.

Doughty D: A physiologic approach to bowel training, *J Wound Ostomy Continence Nurs* 23(1):46-56, 1996.

Drago DA, Dannenberg AL: Infant mechanical suffocation deaths in the United States, 1980-1997, *Pediatrics* 103(5):e59, 1999.

Durward C, Thou T: Dental caries and sugar-containing liquid medicines for children in New Zealand, *NZ Dent J* 93(414):124-129, 1997.

Eadie PA, Williams R, Dickson A: Thirty-five years of pediatric scalds: are lessons being learned? *Br J Plast Surg* 48(2):103-105, 1995.

Featherstone JD: Prevention and reversal of dental caries: role of low level fluoride, *Community Dent Oral Epidemiol* 27(1):31-40, 1999.

Fenner P: Drowning awareness, prevention and treatment, *Aust Fam Physician* 29(11):1045-1049, 2000.

Finan SL: Promoting healthy sexuality: guidelines for infancy through preschool, *Nurs Pract* 22(10):79-80, 83-86, 88, 1997.

Forgac MT: Timely statement of the American Dietetic Association: dietary guidance for healthy children, *J Am Diet Assoc* 95(3):370, 1995.

Fullard W, McDevitt S, Carey W: Assessing temperament in one to three year old children, *J Pediatr Psychol* 9(2):205-217, 1984.

Goldsmith HH: Studying temperament via construction of the Toddler Behavior Assessment Questionnaire, *Child Dev* 67(12):218-235, 1996.

Gottlieb LN, Baillies J: Firstborns' behaviors during a mother's second pregnancy, *Nurs Res* 44(6):356-362, 1995.

Gross D, Conrad B: Temperament in toddlerhood, *J Pediatr Nurs* 10(3):146-151, 1995.

Grover G: Temper tantrums. In Berkowitz C, editor: *Pediatrics: a primary care approach*, Philadelphia, 1996, WB Saunders.

Guha-Chowdhury N, Drummond BK, Smillie AC: Total fluoride intake in children aged 3-4 years—a longitudinal study, *J Dent Res* 75(7):1451-1457, 1996.

Habib DM and others: Prediction of childhood drowning and near-drowning morbidity and mortality, *Pediatr Emerg Care* 12(4):255-258, 1996.

Halopka D: Every ride a safe ride, *J Pediatr Health Care* 13(6):308-310, 1999.

Harre N, Field J, Polzer-Debruyne A: New Zealand children's involvement in home activities that carry a burn or scald risk, *Inj Prev* 4(4):266-271, 1998.

Harrell WA: Epidemiology of shopping cart-related injuries to children, *Arch Pediatr Adolesc Med* 151(1):105-106, 1997.

*Healthy people 2000: national health promotion and disease prevention objectives*, Washington, DC, 1991, US Public Health Service.

Heifetz SB, Horowitz HS: Amounts of fluoride in self-administered dental products: safety considerations for children, *Pediatrics* 77(6):876-882, 1986.

Hinman AR, Sterritt GR, Reeves TG: The US experience with fluoridation, *Community Dent Health* 13(suppl 2):5-9, 1996.

Huyer DW, Corkum SH: Reducing the incidence of tap-water scalds: strategies for physicians, *CMAJ* 156(6):841-844, 1997.

Issenman RM, Filmer RB, Gorski PA: A review of bowel and bladder control development in children: how gastrointestinal and urologic conditions related to problems in toilet training, *Pediatrics* 103(6):1346-1354, 1999.

Kandelman D: Sugar, alternative sweeteners and meal frequency in relation to caries prevention: new perspectives, *Br J Nutr* 77(suppl 1):121-128, 1997.

Kochanska G: Multiple pathways to conscience for children with different temperaments: from toddlerhood to age 5, *Dev Psychol* 33(2):228-240, 1997.

Kopjar B, Wickizer T: How safe are day care centers: day care versus home injuries among children in Norway, *Pediatrics* 97(1):43-47, 1996.

Kramer L: What's real in children's fantasy play? Fantasy play across the transition to becoming a sibling, *J Child Psychol Psychiatry* 37(3):329-337, 1996.

Lamminpaaa A, Kinos M: Plant poisonings in children, *Hum Exp Toxicol* 15(3):245-249, 1996.

Largo RH and others: Development of bladder and bowel control: significance of prematurity, perinatal risk factors,

psychomotor development and gender, *Eur J Pediatr* 158(2):115-122, 1999.

Levy SM, Guha-Chowdhury N: Total fluoride intake and implications for dietary fluoride supplmentation, *J Public Health Dent* 59(4):211-223, 1999.

Levy SM and others: Infants' fluoride ingestion from water, supplements and dentifrices, *J Am Dent Assoc* 126(12):1625-1632, 1995.

Levy SM and others: Factors affecting dentifrice use and ingestion among a sample of U.S. preschoolers, *Pediatr Dent* 22(5):389-394, 2000.

Lidster CA, Horsburg ME: Masturbation—beyond myth and taboo, *Nurs Forum* 29(3):18-27, 1994.

Lucas B: Nutrition in childhood. In Mahan LLK, Escott-Stupp S: *Krause's food, nutrition, and diet therapy*, ed 10, Philadelphia, 1999, WB Saunders.

Luxem MC and others: Behavioral medical treatment of pediatric toilet refusal, *Dev Behav Pediatr* 18(1):34-41, 1997.

Mahler MS, Pine F, Bergman A: *The psychological belief of the human infant: symbiosis and individuation*, New York, 2000, Basic Books.

Makary MA: Reported incidence of injuries caused by street glass among urban children in Philadelphia, *Inj Prev* 4(2):148-149, 1998.

Mallatt ME, Smith CE: Acute fluoride ingestion: recognition and management, *J Indiana Dent Assoc* 75(3):23-24, 26, 1996.

Martin CL, Eisenbud L, Rose H: Children's gender-based reasoning about toys, *Child Dev* 66(5):1453-1471, 1995.

Martinez R: Improving air bags, *Ann Emerg Med* 28(6):709-710, 1996.

Mayer JP and others: A randomized trial of an intervention to prevent lawnmower injuries in children, *Pat Educ Couns* 34(3):239-246, 1998.

Mayr J and others: Playground accidents, *Acta Paediatr* 84(5):573-576, 1995.

McDonald RE, Avery DR: *Dentistry for the child and adolescent*, ed 6, St Louis, 1999, Mosby.

McEvoy M, Montana B, Panettieri M: A nursing intervention to ensure a safe playground environment, *J Pediatr Health Care* 10(5):209-216, 1996.

Milano M: Oral electrical and thermal burns in children: review and report of case, *ASDC J Dent Child* 66(2):116-119, 85, 1999.

Milroy CM and others: Air weapon fatalities, *J Clin Pathol* 51(7):525-529, 1998.

Morris CC: Pediatric iron poisonings in the United States, *South Med J* 93(4):352-358, 2000.

Moss SJ: The case for retaining the current supplementation schedule, *J Public Health Dent* 59(4):259-262, 1999.

Nomak AJ, Warren JJ: Infant oral health and oral habits, *Pediatr Clin North Am* 47(5):1043-1066, 2000.

O'Brien M: Child-rearing difficulties reported by parents of infants and toddlers, *J Pediatr Psychol* 21(3):433-446, 1996.

Osgasawara T, Watanabe T, Kasahara H: Readiness for tooth brushing of young children, *ASDC J Dent Child* 59(5):353-359, 1992.

O'Sullivan EA, Curzon ME: A comparison of acidic dietary factors in children with and without dental erosion, *ASDC J Dent Child* 67(3):186-192, 2000.

Parson BJ and others: Rodenticide poisoning among children, *Aust NZ J Public Health* 20(5):488-492, 1996.

Pavuluri MN, Luk SL: Pattern of preschool behavior problems in New Zealand, using the Behavior Checklist, *J Paediatr Child Health* 32(2):132-137, 1996.

Pendrys DG, Katz RV, Morse DE: Risk factors for enamel fluorosis in a nonfluoridated population, *Am J Epidemiol* 143(8):808-815, 1996.

Petter LP, Hourihane JO, Rolles CJ: Is water out of vogue? A survey of the drinking habits of 2-7 year olds, *Arch Dis Child* 72(2):137-140, 1995.

Playground safety—United States, 1998-1999, *MMWR* 48(16):329-332, 1999.

Pless IB: Childhood injury prevention: time for tougher measures, *CMAJ* 155(10):1417-1419, 1996.

Porrata JL: Eliminating temper tantrums in a four-year old by parent eliciting incompatible behavior, *Percept Mot Skills* 86(1):42, 1998.

Powell EC Tanz RR: Tykes and bikes: injuries associated with bicycle-towed child trailers and bicycle-mounted child seats, *Arch Pediatr Adolesc Med* 154(4):351-353, 2000.

Rabban and others: Mechanisms of pediatric electrical injury. New implications for product safety and injury prevention, *Arch Pediatr Adolesc Med* 151(7):696-700, 1997.

Reeves TG: Status and strategic plans for fluoridation: Centers for Disease Control and Prevention perspective, *J Public Health Dent* 56(5):242-245, 1996.

Reisine S, Douglass JM: Psychosocial and behavioral issues in early childhood caries, *Community Dent Oral Epidemiol* 26(suppl 1):32-44, 1998.

Rojas-Sanchez F and others: Fluoride intake from foods, beverages and dentifrice by young children in communities with negligibly and optimally fluoridated water: a pilot study, *Community Dent Oral Epidemiol* 27(4):288-297, 1999.

Sawicki JA: Sibling rivalry and the new baby: anticipatory guidance and management strategies, *Pediatr Nurs* 23(3):298-302, 1997.

Schmidt P, Madea B: Death in the bathtub involving children, *Forensic Sci Int* 72(2):147-155, 1995.

Siener K, Rothman D, Farrar J: Soft drink logos on baby bottles: do they influence what is fed to children? *ASDC J Dent Child* 64(1):55-60, 1997.

Smith GA and others: Injuries to children related to shopping carts, *Pediatrics* 97(2):161-165, 1996.

Stadtler AC, Gorski PA, Brazelton TB: Toilet training methods, clinical interventions, and recommendations, *Pediatrics* 103(6):1359-1362, 1999.

Stewart KJ and others: Dietary fat and cholesterol intake in young children compared with recommended levels, *J Cardiopulm Rehabil* 19(2):112-117, 1999.

Storr GB, Robinson P: Preparing kids for the new baby, *Can Nurs* 94(3):33-35, 1998.

Taubman B: Toilet training and toileting refusal for stool only: a prospective study, *Pediatrics* 99(1):54-58, 1997.

Teti DM and others: And baby makes four: predictors of attachment security among preschool-age firstborns during the transition to siblinghood, *Child Dev* 67(2): 579-596, 1996.

Thomas RM: *Comparing theories of child development,* ed 4, Belmont, CA, 1996a, Wadsworth.

Thomas SS: Electrical burns of the mouth: still searching for an answer, *Burns* 22(2): 137-140, 1996b.

van Everdingen T and others: Parents and nursing-bottle caries, *ASDC J Dent Child* 63(4):271-274, 1996.

Villena RS: An investigation of the transverse technique of dentifrice application to reduce the amount of fluoride dentifrice for young children, *Pediatr Dent* 22(4): 312-317, 2000.

Von Berg MM, Sanders BJ, Weddell JA: Baby bottle tooth decay: a concern for all mothers, *Pediatr Nurs* 21(6):515-519, 1995.

Vosburg CL and others: Lawn mower injuries of the pediatric foot and ankle: observations on prevetion and management, *J Pediatr Orthop* 15(4):504-510, 1995.

Warren JJ, Levy SM: Systemic fluoride: sources, amounts, and effects of ingestion, *Dent Clin North Am* 43(4):695-711, 1999.

Weinstein P and others: Dental experiences and parenting practices of Native American mothers and caretakers: what we can learn for the prevention of baby bottle tooth decay, *ASDC J Dent Child* 66(2):120-126, 1999.

Wills KE and others: Patterns and correlates of supervision in child pedestrian injury. The Kids 'N' Cars research team, *J Pediatr Psychol* 22(1):89-104, 1997.

Woolf A and others: Self-poisoning among adults using multiple transdermal nicotine patches, *J Toxicol Clin Toxicol* 34(6):691-698, 1996.

Woolf A and others: Childhood poisoning involving transdermal nicotine patches, *Pediatrics* 99(5):e4, 1997.

Yamamoto K and others: Across six nations: stressful events in the lives of children, *Child Psychiatry Hum Dev* 26(3):139-150, 1996.

Yen KL and others: Household oven doors: a burn hazard in children, *Arch Pediatr Adolesc Med* 155(1):84-86, 2001.

Ying SY, Ho WS: Playing with fire—a significant cause of burn injury in children, *Burns* 27(1):39-41, 2001.

Zuckerman BS, Frank DA: Infancy and toddler years. In Levine MD and others, editors: *Developmental-behavioral pediatrics,* ed 3, Philadelphia, 1999, WB Saunders.

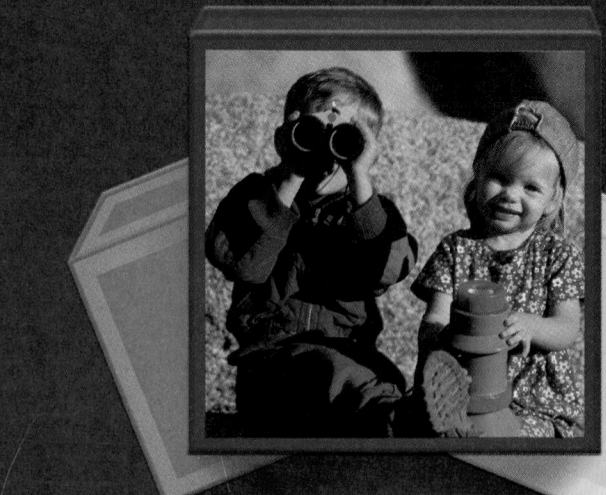

# Chapter 15

# Health Promotion of the Preschooler and Family

## Chapter Outline

**PROMOTING OPTIMUM GROWTH AND DEVELOPMENT, 628**
**Biologic Development, 628**
　Gross and Fine Motor Behavior, 629
**Psychosocial Development, 630**
　Developing a Sense of Initiative
　　(Erikson), 630
　Oedipal Stage (Freud), 630
**Cognitive Development, 631**
　Preoperational Phase (Piaget), 631
**Moral Development, 631**
　Preconventional or Premoral Level
　　(Kohlberg), 631

**Spiritual Development, 632**
**Development of Body Image, 632**
**Development of Sexuality, 632**
**Social Development, 632**
　Language, 633
　Personal-Social Behavior, 633
　Play, 633
**Temperament, 636**
**Coping with Concerns Related to Normal
　Growth and Development, 636**
　Preschool and Kindergarten
　　Experience, 636
　Sex Education, 637

Gifted Children, 640
Aggression, 641
Speech Problems, 642
Stress, 642
Fears, 642
**PROMOTING OPTIMUM HEALTH
DURING THE PRESCHOOL YEARS, 644**
**Nutrition, 644**
**Sleep and Activity, 645**
　Sleep Problems, 645
**Dental Health, 646**
**Injury Prevention, 646**
**Anticipatory Guidance—Care of Families, 647**

## Related Topics

Alternate Child Care Arrangements, Ch. 12
Cognitive Development, Ch. 14
Dental Health, Ch. 14
Draw-A-Person Test, Ch. 7

Habits (Sleep), Ch. 6
Injury Prevention, Ch. 14
Limit-Setting and Discipline, Ch. 3
School Phobia, Ch. 18

Sibling Rivalry, Ch. 14
Speech Impairment, Ch. 24
Temper Tantrums, Ch. 14
Working Mothers, Ch. 3

## PROMOTING OPTIMUM GROWTH AND DEVELOPMENT

The combined biologic, psychosocial, cognitive, spiritual, and social achievements during the *preschool period* (3 to 5 years of age) prepare preschoolers for their most significant change in lifestyle—entrance into school. Their control of bodily systems, experience of brief and prolonged periods of separation, ability to interact cooperatively with other children and adults, use of language for mental symbolization, and increased attention span and memory ready them for the next major period—the school years. Successful achievement of previous levels of growth and development is essential for

preschoolers to refine many of the tasks that were mastered during the toddler years.

### Biologic Development

The rate of physical growth slows and stabilizes during the preschool years. The average *weight* is 14.6 kg (32 pounds) at 3 years, 16.7 kg (36.75 pounds) at 4 years, and 18.7 kg (41.25 pounds) at 5 years. The average weight gain remains approximately 2.3 kg (5 pounds) per year.

Growth in *height* also remains steady at a yearly increase of 6.75 to 7.5 cm (2.5 to 3 inches) and generally occurs by elongation of the legs rather than the trunk. The average height is 95 cm (37.25 inches) at 3 years, 103 cm (40.5 inches) at 4 years, and 110 cm (43.25 inches) at 5 years.

■ Christine Chordas, MSN, RN, CPNP, revised this chapter.

*Physical proportions* no longer resemble those of the squat, potbellied toddler. The preschooler is slender but sturdy, graceful, agile, and posturally erect. There is little difference in physical characteristics according to sex, except as dictated by factors such as dress and hairstyle.

Most organ systems can adjust to moderate stress and change. During this period most children are toilet trained. For the most part, motor development consists of increases in strength and refinement of previously learned skills, such as walking, running, and jumping. However, muscle development and bone growth are still far from mature. Excessive activity and overexertion can injure delicate tissues. Good posture, appropriate exercise, and adequate nutrition and rest are essential for optimal development of the musculoskeletal system.

### Gross and Fine Motor Behavior

Walking, running, climbing, and jumping are well established by 36 months. Refinement in eye-hand and muscle coordination is evident in several areas. At age 3 the preschooler rides a tricycle, walks on tiptoe, balances on one foot for a few seconds, and broad jumps. By age 4 the child skips and hops proficiently on one foot (Fig. 15-1) and catches a ball reliably. By age 5, the child skips on alternate feet, jumps rope, and begins to skate and swim.

Achievement in fine motor development is evident in the child's increasingly skillful manipulation. Drawing shows several advancements in the perception of shape and the development of fine muscle coordination. The 3-year-old child copies a circle and imitates a cross and vertical and horizontal lines. The writing instrument is held with the fingers rather than in the fist. The child scribbles or scrawls drawings but can name what has been drawn. The 3-year-old is not able to draw a complete stick figure but draws a round circle, later adds facial features, and by age 5 or 6 years can draw several parts (head, arms, legs, body, and facial features). Between 4 and 5 years of age the child can trace a cross and copy a square. The triangle and diamond are usually the last geometric figures to be mastered, sometime between ages 5 and 6.

As children progress from scribbling to picture making, they advance through four distinguishable stages (Kellogg,

1969). In the *placement stage* 15-month-old children place their very earliest spontaneous scribblings on the paper in a specific placement pattern, such as in the center, all over, across the lower half, or across the page in a diagonal direction (Fig. 15-2). Approximately 17 different placement patterns appear by age 2 years and, once developed, are never lost.

By 3 years of age children are in the *shape stage.* They draw single-line outline forms such as rectangles, circles, ovals, crosses, and other odd shapes. As soon as they draw diagrams, they almost immediately progress to the *design stage,* in which simple forms are drawn together to make structured designs. When two diagrams are united, the resulting design is called a *combine.* Three or more united di-

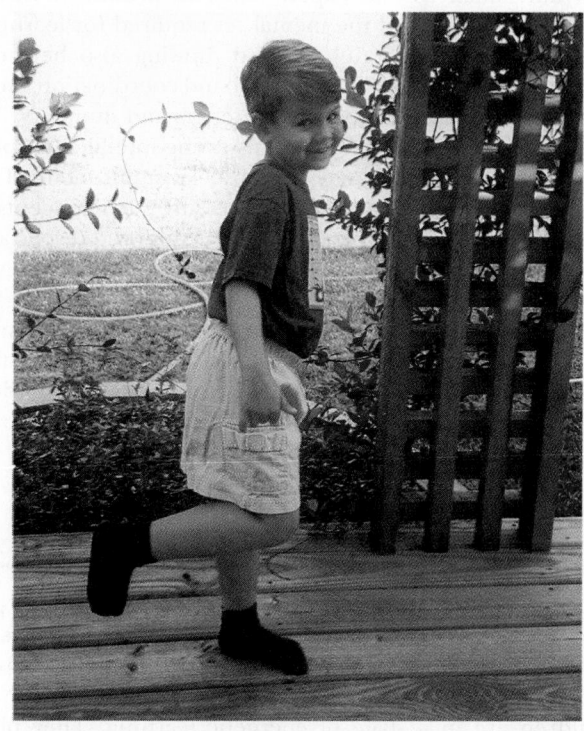

**Fig. 15-1**  A 4-year-old child has sufficient balance to hop on one foot.

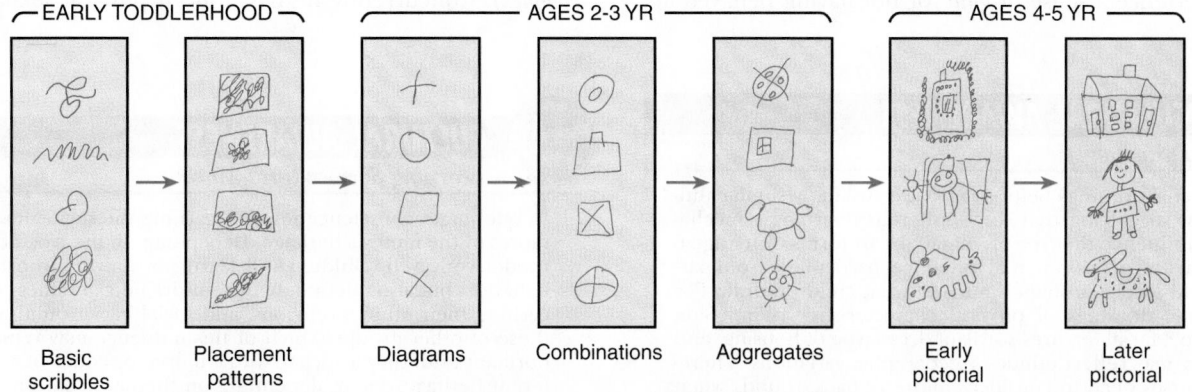

**Fig. 15-2**  Sequential development in self-taught art. (From Kellogg R: Understanding children's art. In *Readings in psychology today,* Del Mar, Calif, 1969, Communications/Research/Machine.)

agrams produce an *aggregate.* Between the ages of 4 and 5 most children enter the *pictorial stage,* in which their designs are recognizable as familiar objects. Early pictorial drawings are suggestive of human figures, houses, animals, and trees. Later pictorial drawings are more clearly defined and recognizable; they are not representations of the actual object but esthetically satisfying structures that *resemble* familiar objects. For example, the initial human figure drawing is a circle with arms attached to the head. It is more an aggregate drawing than any attempt to copy a human figure. Drawings of animals follow the human figure drawing but are only a slight modification, such as attaching ears to the top of the head.

Kellogg suggests that uninhibited scribbling and drawing are necessary for children to learn to read and that children who have been free to experiment and produce abstract forms have developed the mental set required for learning symbolic language. Scribbling and drawing also help develop the fine muscle skills and eye-hand coordination eventually required for making precise letters and numbers.

Drawing is also a tool used for assessing intelligence, personality development, and psychosocial adjustment. The precise value of using drawing to measure such concepts is still an inexact science. However, children (especially school-age children) do reveal thoughts about themselves in their drawings. It is generally not necessary to have indepth knowledge of children's drawings to make assumptions about their significance. Being receptive to all the clues, both verbal and nonverbal, is essential to understanding how and what children are communicating to others. (See Cultural Awareness box.)

## Psychosocial Development

### Developing a Sense of Initiative (Erikson)

If preschoolers have mastered the tasks of the toddler period, they are ready to face the developmental endeavors of the preschool period. Erikson maintains that the chief psychosocial task of this period is acquiring a sense of *initiative.* Children are in a stage of energetic learning. They play, work, and live to the fullest and feel a real sense of accomplishment and satisfaction in their activities. Conflict arises when children overstep the limits of their ability and inquiry and experience a sense of *guilt* for not having behaved ap-

propriately. Feelings of guilt, anxiety, and fear may also result from thoughts that differ from expected behavior.

A particularly stressful thought is wishing one's parent dead. As a sense of rivalry or competition develops between the child and the same-sex parent, the child may think of ways to get rid of the interfering parent. In most situations this contest is resolved when the child strongly identifies with the same-sex parent and peers during the school years. However, if that parent dies before the identification process is completed, the preschooler can be overwhelmed with feelings of guilt for having wished and therefore "caused" the death. Clarifying for children that wishes cannot make events occur is essential in helping them overcome their guilt and anxiety.

Development of the *superego,* or *conscience,* starts toward the end of the toddler years and is a major task for preschoolers. Learning right from wrong and good from bad is the beginning of morality. (See Cultural Awareness box.) Children in this age-group are generally unable to understand the reasons why something is acceptable or unacceptable. They are aware of appropriate behavior primarily through punishment or reward and rely almost completely on parental principles for developing their own moral judgment. Verbal enforcement of limits is much more effective. For example, to prevent injuries, parents need to supervise young children and tell them not to run into the street. The preschooler is much more aware of danger and can be relied on to listen and obey in most instances. If allowed to disagree and question, they will develop socially acceptable behavior and independence in thought and action.

### Oedipal Stage (Freud)

As soon as children comprehend their separateness as persons, they begin to realize that there are categories of objects, such as things, people, males, females, children, and adults. One of the principal goals in further differentiation of oneself from others is learning sex differences and sexually appropriate behavior.

Freud described this goal in psychosexual terms and labeled the period the *oedipal,* or *phallic,* stage. Conflict arises when the male child realizes that his father is much stronger and more powerful than he. Subconsciously he wishes that his father were dead so he could marry his mother *(Oedipus complex).* Concurrently he has noticed physical sexual dif-

### CULTURAL AWARENESS
*Drawings*

Children's drawings before age 6 are strikingly similar universally, suggesting that some inherent neurologic mechanisms influence the type of self-taught art forms. After age 6 cultural and environmental influence, particularly from parents and teachers, shapes much of what children draw. For example, drawings of physical characteristics (skin color, hair type, facial features), style of dress, type of housing, and scenery may reflect ethnic or geographic variations. Therefore nurses need to consider children's backgrounds when interpreting drawings.

### CULTURAL AWARENESS
*Learning Sociocultural Mores*

Developing a conscience implies learning the sociocultural mores of the family's heritage. Depending on the type of attitudes conveyed, children will learn not only appropriate behaviors but also tolerant, biased, or prejudicial values concerning their ethnic, religious, and social background and those of other groups. Much of this influence may remain dormant until they associate with children or adults of a different heritage. Then, depending on the particular group, they may be accepted or ostracized for their attitudes.

ferences, specifically that boys have a penis and girls do not. In his mind he surmises that girls have lost their penis for some wrongdoing. His guilt regarding his feelings toward his father makes him fear the same punishment of mutilation, resulting in the **castration complex.** Girls have similar wishes to marry their father and kill their mother (the **Electra complex**). However, girls do not fear castration; rather they experience **penis envy** (desire to have a penis). The resolution of the Oedipus or Electra complex is identification with the same-sex parent.

## Cognitive Development

One of the tasks related to the preschool period is readiness for school and scholastic learning. Many of the thought processes of this period are crucial for achieving such readiness, and it is intentional that the child begins school between ages 5 and 6 rather than earlier.

### Preoperational Phase (Piaget)

Piaget's cognitive theory does not include a period specifically for children 3 to 5 years old. The **preoperational phase** comprises the age span from 2 to 7 years and is divided into two stages: the **preconceptual phase,** ages 2 to 4, and the phase of **intuitive thought,** ages 4 to 7.

One of the main transitions during these two phases is the shift from totally egocentric thought to social awareness and the ability to consider other viewpoints (Fig. 15-3). Egocentricity, however, is still evident. Children are able to think and verbalize their mental processes without having to act out their thinking. They can think of only one idea at a time and are unable to think of all parts in terms of the whole.

Language continues to develop during the preschool period. Speech remains primarily a vehicle of egocentric communication. Preschoolers assume that everyone thinks as they do and that a brief explanation of their thinking makes them understood by others. Because of this self-referenced,

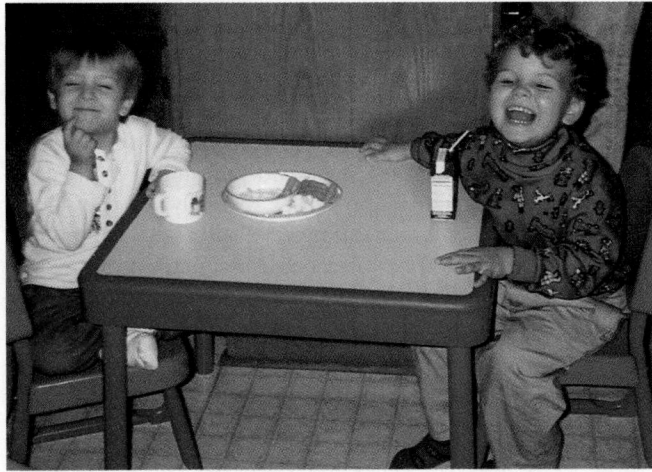

**Fig. 15-3**  Preschool children enjoy friends and often use nonverbal messages to communicate.

egocentric verbal communication, it is often necessary to explore and understand young children's thinking through other, nonverbal approaches. For children in this age-group, the most enlightening and effective method is **play,** which becomes the child's way of understanding, adjusting to, and working out life's experiences. Because of a child's rich imagination and unlimited ability to invent and imitate, all types of play hold therapeutic and communicative value.

Preschoolers increasingly use language without comprehending the meaning of words, particularly concepts of right and left, causality, and time. Children may use the concepts correctly but only in the circumstances in which they have learned them. For example, they may know how to put on shoes by remembering that the buckle is always on the outside of the foot. However, if different shoes have no buckles, they cannot reason which shoe fits which foot. They do not understand the concept of **right and left.**

Superficially, **causality** resembles logical thought. Preschoolers explain a concept as they have heard it described by others, but their understanding is limited. An example is the concept of time. Because **time** is still incompletely understood, the child interprets it according to his or her own frame of reference, such as "A long time means until Christmas." Consequently, time is best explained in relation to an event, such as "Your mother will visit you after you finish your lunch." Avoiding words such as "yesterday," "tomorrow," "next week," or "Tuesday" to express when an event is expected to occur and associating time with usual expected daily occurrences help children learn about temporal relationships while increasing their trust in others' predictions.

Preschoolers' thinking is often described as **magical thinking.** Because of their egocentrism and transductive reasoning, they believe that thoughts are all-powerful. Such thinking places them in the vulnerable position of feeling guilty and responsible for bad thoughts that may coincide with the occurrence of a wished event. A typical example is wishing a new sibling dead. If that sibling does die, young children think their wish caused the death. Their inability to reason the cause and effect of illness or injury makes it especially difficult for them to understand such events.

Preschoolers believe in the power of words and accept their meaning literally. A significant example of this type of thinking is calling children "bad" because they did something wrong. In their minds telling children that they are bad means that they are bad. For this reason it is better to relate such words to the act by saying, for example, "That was a bad thing to do."

## Moral Development

### Preconventional or Premoral Level (Kohlberg)

Young children's development of moral judgment is at the most basic level. There is little, if any, concern for why something is wrong. They behave because of the freedoms or restrictions placed on actions. In the **punishment and obedience orientation,** children (approximately ages 2 to 4 years) judge whether an action is good or bad according to whether it results in reward or punishment. If children are punished for it, the action is bad. If they are not punished, the action is good, regardless of the meaning of the act. For example, if parents allow hitting, the child will perceive that hitting is good because it is not associated with punishment.

From approximately 4 to 7 years of age children are in the stage of *naive instrumental orientation*, in which actions are directed toward satisfying their needs and, less commonly, the needs of others. There is a very concrete sense of justice. Reciprocity or fairness involves the philosophy of "You scratch my back and I'll scratch yours," with no thought of loyalty or gratitude (Thomas, 1996).

## Spiritual Development

Children's knowledge of faith and religion is learned from significant others in their environment, usually from parents and their religious practices (Kenny, 1999). However, young children's understanding of spirituality is influenced by their cognitive level. Preschoolers have a concrete conception of a God with physical characteristics often like an imaginary friend. They understand simple stories and memorize short prayers, but their understanding of the meaning of these rituals is limited. They benefit from concrete representations of religious practices, such as picture books and small statues.

Development of the conscience is strongly linked to spiritual development. At this age children are learning right from wrong and behave correctly to avoid punishment. Wrongdoing provokes feelings of guilt, and preschoolers often misinterpret illness as punishment for real or imagined transgressions. It is important that children view God as one who bestows unconditional love, rather than as a judge of good or bad behavior. Praying to God and observing religious traditions can help children through stressful periods, such as hospitalization (Hart and Schneider, 1997).

## Development of Body Image

The preschool years play a significant role in the development of body image. With increasing comprehension of language, preschoolers recognize that individuals have undesirable and desirable appearances. They recognize differences in skin color and racial identity and are vulnerable to learning prejudices and biases. They are aware of the meaning of words such as "pretty" or "ugly," and they reflect the opinions of others regarding their own appearance. By 5 years of age children compare their size with their peers' and can become conscious of being large or short, especially if others refer to them as "so big" or "so little" for their age. One study reported that negative associations between weight status and self-concept are present in girls as young as 5 years of age (Davison and Birch, 2001).

Despite the advances in body image development, preschoolers have poorly defined body boundaries and little knowledge of their internal anatomy. Intrusive experiences are frightening, especially those that disrupt the integrity of the skin (e.g., injections and surgery). There is a fear that all of their blood and "insides" can leak out if the skin is "broken." Therefore the use of bandages is critical when caring for a preschooler.

## Development of Sexuality

Sexual development during the preschool years is a very important phase to a person's overall sexual identity and beliefs. Preschoolers are forming strong attachments to the opposite-sex parent while identifying with the same-sex parent. *Sex typing*, or the process by which an individual develops the behavior, personality, attitudes, and beliefs appropriate for his or her culture and sex, occurs through several mechanisms during this period. Probably the most powerful mechanisms are childrearing practices and imitation. The ways in which parents dress, hold, cuddle, caress, discipline, and talk to their child express some aspect of sexually oriented behavior. Studies increasingly demonstrate that gender identification is not solely biologic or genetic but primarily a result of complex postnatal psychologic factors and that most children are aware of their sex and the expected set of related behaviors by $1\frac{1}{2}$ to $2\frac{1}{2}$ years of age. Although toddlers might be aware of their particular sex, they do not possess the language and cognitive skills to investigate sexual identity as fully as preschoolers.

As sexual identity develops beyond gender recognition, modesty and fears of mutilation may become a concern. There is sex-role imitation, and "dressing up" like Mommy or Daddy is an important activity. Attitudes and responses of others to role-playing can condition the child to views of self or others. For example, comments such as "Boys shouldn't play with dolls" can influence a boy's masculine self-concept.

Sexual exploration may be more pronounced now than ever before, particularly in terms of exploring and manipulating the genitals. Questions about sexual reproduction may come to the forefront in the preschooler's search for understanding. (See Sex Education, p. 637, and also Chapters 17 and 19).

## Social Development

During the preschool period the *individuation-separation* process is completed. Preschoolers have overcome much of their anxiety associated with strangers and the fear of separation of earlier years. They relate to unfamiliar people easily and tolerate brief separations from parents with little or no protest. However, they still need parental security, reassurance, guidance, and approval, especially when entering preschool or elementary school. Prolonged separation, such as that imposed by illness and hospitalization, is difficult; however, preschoolers respond very well to anticipatory preparation and concrete explanation. They can cope with changes in daily routine much better than toddlers but may develop more imaginary fears. They gain security and comfort from familiar objects such as toys, dolls, or photographs of family members. They are able to work through many of their unresolved fears, fantasies, and anxieties through play, especially if guided with appropriate play objects (e.g., dolls or puppets) that represent family members, health professionals, and other children.

## Language

Language during the preschool years becomes more sophisticated and complex. Both cognitive ability and environment, particularly consistent role models, influence vocabulary, speech, and comprehension (Huttenlocher, 1998). Language becomes a major mode of communication and social interaction. Vocabulary increases dramatically, from 300 words at age 2 to more than 2100 words at the end of 5 years. Sentence structure, grammatical usage, and intelligibility also advance to a more adult level. Preschool children may be bilingual. (See Cultural Awareness box.)

Children between the ages of 3 and 4 form sentences of approximately three to four words and include only the words most essential to convey a meaning. Such speech is often termed *telegraphic* because of its brevity. Three-year-old children ask many questions and use plurals, correct pronouns, and the past tense of verbs. They name familiar objects, such as animals, parts of the body, relatives, and friends. They can give and follow simple commands. They talk incessantly, regardless of whether anyone is listening to or answering them. They enjoy musical or talking toys or dolls and imitate new words proficiently.

From ages 4 to 5 preschoolers use longer sentences of four to five words and use more words to convey a message, such as prepositions, adjectives, and a variety of verbs. They follow simple directional commands, such as "Put the ball on the chair," but can carry out only one request at a time. They answer questions such as "What do you do when you are hungry?" by describing the appropriate action. The pattern of asking questions is at its peak, and children usually repeat the question until they receive an answer.

By age 6, children can use all parts of speech correctly, except for deviations from the rule. They can define simple objects and actions by describing their use, shape, or general category of classification, rather than simply describing their outward appearance. For example, they define a ball as "round, something you bounce, or a toy," rather than describe its color. They can give some opposites, such as "If Mommy is a woman, Daddy is a man." They also can describe an object according to its composition, such as "A spoon is made of metal."

## Personal-Social Behavior

The pervasive ritualism and negativism of toddlerhood gradually diminish during the preschool years. Although self-assertion is still a major theme, preschoolers demonstrate their sense of autonomy differently. They are able to verbalize their request for independence and perform independently because of their much-refined physical and cognitive

development. By 4 or 5 years of age they need little if any assistance with dressing, eating, or toileting (Fig. 15-4). They can also be trusted to obey warnings of danger, although 3- or 4-year-old children may exceed their boundaries at times.

Preschoolers are much more sociable and willing to please. They have internalized many of the standards and values of the family and culture. However, by the end of early childhood they begin to question parental values and compare them with those of their peer group and other authority figures. As a result, they may be less willing to abide by the family's code of conduct. Preschoolers become increasingly aware of their position and role within the family. Although this is a more secure age for experiencing the addition of another sibling, relinquishing the position of first or youngest is still difficult and requires appropriate preparation (Sawicki, 1997). (See Sibling Rivalry, Chapter 14.)

## Play

Various types of play are typical of this period, but preschoolers especially enjoy *associative play*, group play in similar or identical activities but without rigid organization or rules. Play should provide for physical, social, and mental development (Table 15-1).

Play activities for physical growth and the refinement of motor skills include jumping, running, and climbing. Tricycles, wagons, gym and sports equipment, sandboxes, wading

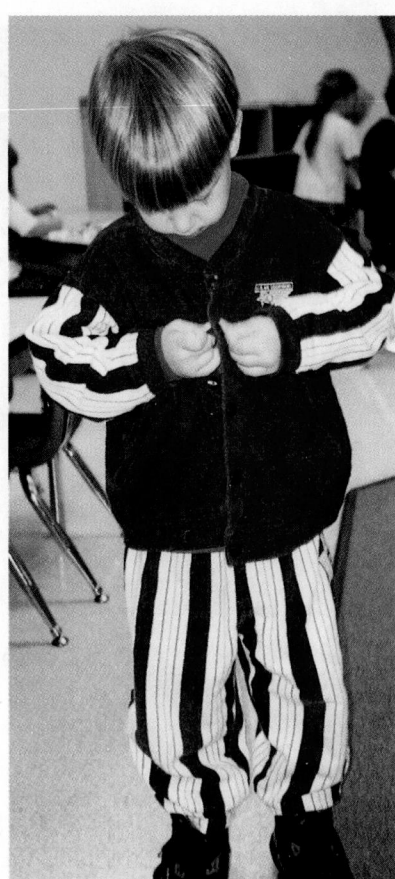

**Fig. 15-4** Most preschoolers are able to dress themselves but need help with more difficult items of clothing.

---

### CULTURAL AWARENESS
#### *Bilingual Children*

Many children in the United States are bilingual. One study reported that learning a second language does not adversely affect language development and proficiency of the primary language (Winsler and others, 1999). Nurses need to be aware of what language the child speaks at home and whether or not the child is bilingual.

| **TABLE 15-1** Play during preschool years | | |
| --- | --- | --- |
| **Physical Development** | **Social Development** | **Mental Development and Creativity** |
| **Suggested Activities** | | |
| Provide space for the child to run, jump, and climb | Encourage interaction with neighborhood children | Encourage creative efforts with raw materials |
| Teach child to swim | Intervene when children become destructive | Read stories |
| Teach simple sports and activities | Enroll child in preschool | Monitor television viewing |
| | | Attend theater and other cultural events appropriate to child's age |
| | | Take short excursions to park, seashore, museums, zoo |
| **Suggested Toys** | | |
| Medium-height slide | Child-size playhouse | Books |
| Adjustable swing | Dolls, stuffed toys | Jigsaw puzzles |
| Vehicles to ride | Dishes, table | Musical and rhythmic toys (xylophone, toy piano, drum, horns) |
| Tricycle | Ironing board and iron | Picture games |
| Wading pool | Cash register, toy typewriter | Blunt scissors, paper, glue |
| Wheelbarrow | Trucks, cars, trains, airplanes | Newsprint, crayons, poster paint, large brushes, easel, finger paint |
| Sled | Play clothes for dress-up | Flannel board and pieces of felt in colors and shapes |
| Wagon | Doll carriage, bed, high chair | Records, tapes |
| Skates, speed graded to skill | Medical kits | Blackboard and chalk (colored and white) |
| Sandbox | Nails, hammer, saw | Wooden and plastic construction sets |
| | Grooming aids, play makeup or shaving kits | Magnifying glass, magnet |
| | | Educational computer programs |
| | | Markers, paint, crayons |

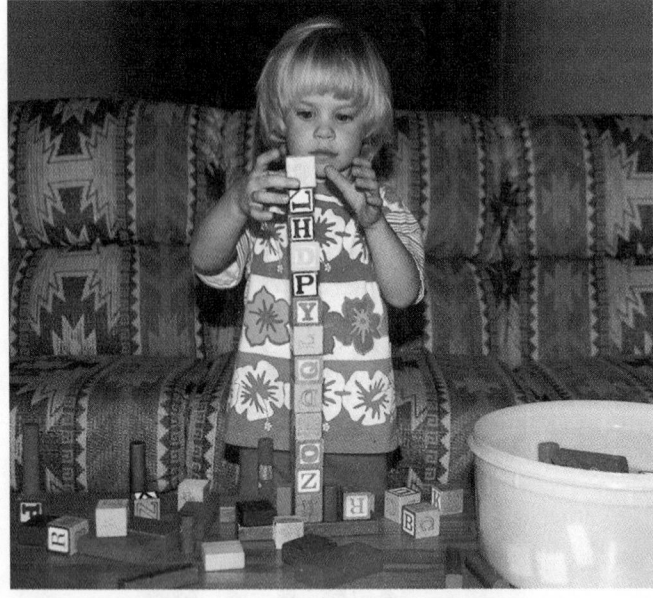

**Fig. 15-5** Preschoolers enjoy a sense of accomplishment from activities such as building blocks.

pools, and winter sleds can help develop muscles and coordination. Activities such as swimming, skating, and skiing teach safety and help develop muscles and coordination.

Manipulative, constructive, creative, and educational toys provide for quiet activities, fine motor development, and self-expression. Easy construction sets, large blocks of various sizes and shapes, a counting frame, alphabet or number flash cards, paints, crayons, simple carpentry tools, musical toys, illustrated books, simple sewing or handicraft sets, large puzzles, and clay are suitable toys (Fig. 15-5). Electronic games and computer programs are especially valuable in helping children learn basic skills, such as letters and simple words. Although their attention span is still short, preschoolers are beginning to enjoy crafts, especially with the guidance and assistance of adults. A helpful rule in planning creative activities is one simple project per year of age. For example, a 3-year-old child usually has the patience to decorate three eggs but will become bored and restless with more.

Probably the most characteristic and pervasive preschooler activity is *imitative, imaginative,* and *dramatic play.* Dress-up clothes, dolls, housekeeping toys, dollhouses, telephones, farm animals and equipment, village sets, trains, trucks, cars, planes, hand puppets, and medical kits provide hours of self-expression (Fig. 15-6). Probably at no other time is the reproduction of the behavior of significant adults so absorbing as in 4- and 5-year-old children. (See Critical Thinking Exercise box.) Toward the end of the preschool period, children are less satisfied with make-believe or pretend objects and enjoy actually doing the activity, such as cooking and carpentry.

Television and videotapes also have their places in children's play, although each should be only one part of their total repertoire of social and recreational activities. Parents and other caregivers should supervise the selection of programs, preview programs for appropriateness, and schedule limited hours for television viewing (Vessey, Yim-Chiplis, and MacKenzie, 1998). Children enjoy and learn from edu-

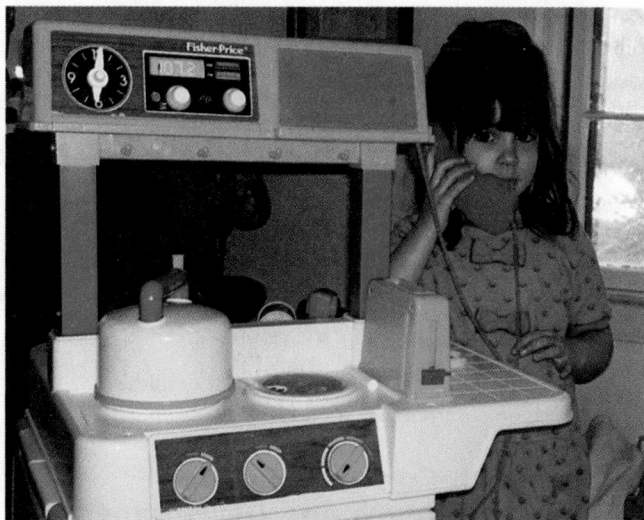

**Fig. 15-6** Imaginative and imitative play is typical of preschoolers.

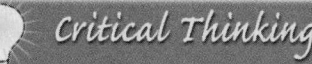

### Critical Thinking Exercise

#### Imitative Play

In her bedroom 4-year-old Juanita is playing with her dolls. She pretends one doll is "Mommy" and is talking on the telephone: "Be quiet! Can't you see that I am busy? This is an important call. Go away." She hangs up the phone and chooses another doll, pokes it, and cries, "You're bad. Mommy doesn't like you."

Juanita's mother, Mrs. Ortiz, hears this play conversation and realizes she says similar things to Juanita when she is on the telephone. What advice would you give Mrs. Ortiz?

FIRST, THINK ABOUT IT . . .

- What concepts or ideas are central to your thinking?
- How are you interpreting the information?

1. Reassure her that imitation is a normal and healthy activity in 4-year-olds.
2. Suggest that she use a telephone recorder to return calls at more convenient times.
3. Inquire about her reactions to the play conversation and discuss possible ways to avoid the situation.
4. Refer the child to a psychologist for further assessment of the apparent child-mother conflict.

*The best response is three. You want to capitalize on the mother's awareness of the possible messages the child's play has revealed. Your goal is also to empower the parent to find reasonable options that accommodate her lifestyle, which is an important concept in parenting.*

*Although a telephone recorder is one option, it may not be the best one. Also, you may interpret this play behavior as typical of preschoolers, and premature reassurance will not address the issue or solutions. More assessment is needed before suggesting a referral.*

cational programs. Television can become an interactive activity when adults view programs with children and discuss program content.

Play is so much a part of the young child's life that reality and fantasy become blurred. The make-believe is reality during play and becomes fantasy only when toys are put away or dress-up clothes are removed. It is no wonder that *imaginary playmates* are so much a part of this age period.

The appearance of imaginary companions usually occurs between the ages of 2½ and 3 years, and for the most part such playmates are relinquished when the child enters school. There seems to be a relationship between the level of intelligence and the presence of the imaginary companion. One study reported that birth order, combined with characteristics of imaginativeness and a predisposition to engage in fantasy, characterized children with imaginary companions (Bouldin and Pratt, 1999).

Imaginary companions serve many purposes; they become friends in times of loneliness, they accomplish what the child is still attempting, and they experience what the child wants to forget or remember. It is not unusual for the "friend" to have a myriad of vices and be blamed for wrongdoing. Sometimes the child hopes to escape punishment by saying, "My friend Brian broke the glass." At other times the preschooler may fantasize that the "companion" misbehaved and play the role of parent. This becomes a way of assuming control and authority in a safe situation.

Parents often worry about their child having imaginary playmates, not realizing how normal and useful they are. They need to be reassured that the child's fantasy is a sign of health that helps to differentiate between make-believe and reality. Parents can acknowledge the presence of the imaginary companion by calling him or her by name and even agreeing to simple requests such as setting an extra place at the table, but they should not allow the child to use the playmate to avoid punishment or responsibility. For ex-

ample, if the child blames the companion for messing up a room, the parents need to state clearly that the child is the only person they see and therefore the child is responsible for cleaning up. (See Critical Thinking Exercise box on p. 636.)

Children also benefit from play that occurs between them and a parent. *Mutual play* fosters development from birth through the school years and provides enriched opportunities for learning. Through mutual play, parents can provide tactile and kinesthetic experiences, can maximize verbal and language abilities, and can offer praise and encouragement for exploration of the world. Additionally, mutual play encourages positive interactions between the parent and the child, strengthening their relationship. Recommendations for mutual play should reflect the child's developmental level and can incorporate readily available items found in the home or community (musical tapes, CDs, puppets) (Gottesman, 1999).*

*Recommended books for suggestions on mutual play include *Quick and Fun Learning Activities*, books by Teacher Created Material, Inc, 6421 Industry Way, Westminster, CA 92683, (714) 891-7895.

### Imaginary Playmates

Mrs. Petner tells you, the nurse, that her 2½-year-old daughter, Kimberly, has an imaginary playmate named Alison. She was not very concerned about this until Kimberly started putting a plate on the table for Alison at mealtimes. What is the best reply?

FIRST, THINK ABOUT IT . . .

• What is the purpose of your thinking?
• What are you taking for granted, and what assumptions are you making?

1. "This is highly unusual behavior for children this age and indicates giftedness."
2. "This is normal for children this age, and it is fine to allow her to set a place for her imaginary playmate."
3. "It is best not to allow Kimberly to include her imaginary playmate in activities such as mealtimes."
4. "It is important that Kimberly separate reality from fantasy, and a referral to a mental health professional is indicated."

*The best response is two. Imaginary playmates are normal at this age and serve many purposes. Educate parents that they can acknowledge the presence of an imaginary companion as long as the child does not use the playmate to avoid punishment or responsibility. A referral is not necessary. Although the assumption may be that the child is gifted, this one behavior does not indicate that this is true.*

## Temperament

Temperament influences children's social development and interactions. The importance of temperament during early childhood is discussed in Chapters 12 and 14. Because temperamental characteristics tend to remain stable, the same considerations in terms of childrearing apply during the preschool years.

One major concern in the preschool age-group is the effect of temperament on adjustment in group situations, especially school, and the long-term consequences of temperamental characteristics. In particular, the degree of adaptability to new situations, intensity of response, distractibility, amount of persistence, mood, and activity level may influence a child's chances for success in school. Consequently, parents can benefit from suggestions that can promote preschoolers' adjustment. For example, children who are slow to warm up need gradual introduction to new situations and may benefit from the parent's presence until they have settled in. Children with high activity levels tend to adjust better to environments that allow freedom of movement, rather than a structured or regimented classroom. The more awareness parents have of their children's unique behaviors, the better able they are to inform teachers or other caregivers of the children's needs and successful approaches to handling the youngsters.

The *Behavioral Style Questionnaire* can be used to identify temperamental characteristics in children who are in the age range of 3 to 7 years (McDevitt and Carey, 1978). Simply asking mothers to rate their child as being either much easier than, easier than, as easy as, more difficult than, or much more difficult than the average child may also be a valuable screening method. The Parents' Evaluation of Developmental Status (PEDS) (Glascoe, 2001) elicits parents' concerns about their child's developmental and behavioral status. This form helps health care providers to determine the need to refer and when to provide advice about childrearing, developmental issues, and other psychosocial concerns.

■　■　■

The major developmental achievements for children 3, 4, and 5 years old are summarized in Table 15-2 on pp. 638-639.

## Coping with Concerns Related to Normal Growth and Development

### Preschool and Kindergarten Experience

Some children are home-schooled, but many children attend some type of early childhood program, usually preschool or a daycare center. Group care has become commonplace with the large number of mothers presently employed outside the home. The effects of early education and stimulation on children have increasingly gained recognition and importance. Because social development widens to include age-mates and other significant adults, preschool provides an excellent vehicle for expanding children's experiences with others. It is also excellent preparation for entrance into elementary school.

In preschool or daycare centers children are exposed to opportunities for learning group cooperation, adjusting to various sociocultural differences, and coping with frustration, dissatisfaction, and anger. If activities are tailored to provide mastery and achievement, children increasingly feel success, self-confidence, and personal competence. Whether or not structured learning is imposed is less important than the social climate, type of guidance, and attitude toward the children that is fostered by the teacher or leader. With a teacher who is aware of preschoolers' developmental abilities and needs, children will learn from the activity provided. Most programs incorporate a daily schedule of quiet play, active outdoor activity, group activities such as games and projects, creative or free play, and snack and rest periods.

Preschool is particularly beneficial for children who lack a peer-group experience, such as an only child, and for children from impoverished homes. It provides extensive stimulation for language, physical, and social development. It also is excellent preparation for kindergarten. For a child from a poor home, elementary school can be so overwhelming that all learning is impeded by the sensory overload. Regular school places many more demands on children for prolonged attention, self-disciplined behavior, and demonstrated progress in performance and achievement than does the less-structured atmosphere of preschool.

One of the issues that parents face is the child's readiness for preschool or kindergarten. There are no absolute indicators for school readiness, but the child's social maturation, especially attention span, is as important as academic readiness.

Using a developmental screening tool that addresses cognitive (especially language), social, and physical milestones can identify children who may benefit from further diagnostic testing. Developmental screening focuses on the potential to learn and differs from readiness testing, which stresses the specific skills the child has acquired (e.g., counts to 10, prints letters of the alphabet, knows days of week) (Glascoe, 2001).

School readiness is influenced by a child's life experiences, development, learning ability, and the degree to which school expectations of children entering are reasonable, appropriate, and supportive of individual differences. Schools must be able to respond to a diverse range of abilities and must provide meaningful contexts for children's learning rather than focusing primarily on isolated skill acquisition (National Association for the Education of Young Children [NAEYC], 1995). Programs should provide comprehensive services to ensure that a wide range of individual needs are met, support parents' roles in supporting their child's development and learning, and provide a variety of firsthand experiences and learning activities either directly to children or through parent participation (NAEYC, 1995).

Health care providers can be helpful in guiding parents in selecting enriched social and educational early intervention programs and schools. Careful selection of early childhood education is intrinsic to future learning and development. Licensed and regulated programs are mandated to abide by established standards, which represent minimum requirements and safeguards. The importance of regulation is to protect children from harm and to promote the conditions essential for a child's healty development and learning. NAEYC supports early childhood regulation on all levels.*

Other areas to evaluate are the facility's daily program, teacher qualifications, staff-to-student ratio, discipline policy, environmental safety precautions, provision of meals, sanitary conditions, adequate indoor and outdoor space per child, and fee schedule. References from other parents help to evaluate a facility, but personal observation of the facility is recommended. Encourage parents to meet the director and some of the employees at a few facilities to make an informed choice.

Important in selecting child care centers is evaluating the facility's health practices. Children in daycare centers, especially those under 3 years of age, have more illnesses, especially diarrhea, hepatitis A, meningitis, otitis media, respiratory tract infections, and cytomegalovirus, than children not in daycare centers (Rovers and others, 1999). Health care providers can advise parents regarding the evaluation of a facility's sanitary practices and can actively participate in educating staff in measures to minimize infection (Lafontaine and Bedard, 1997).

**Preparing the Child.**   Children need preparation for the preschool or kindergarten experience.* For young children these programs represent a change from their usual home environment and prolonged separation from their parents. Even if children have been cared for by a baby-sitter or in a group setting, preschool and kindergarten differ because the individualized attention may be less, the program may be more structured, and learning may be expected.

The nurse helps parents assess children's readiness in terms of age, physical ability, and cognitive and social development (see Table 15-2). For example, a group experience may be difficult for young children with short attention spans. These children may require a different type of experience that provides for more individualized attention.

Before children begin the school experience, the parents should present the idea as exciting and pleasurable. Talking to them about activities such as painting, building with blocks, or enjoying swings and other outdoor equipment allows children to fantasize about the forthcoming event in a positive manner. When the first day of school arrives, the parents should behave confidently. Such behavior requires parents to have resolved their own feelings regarding the experience.

Parents should introduce their child to the teacher and the facility. In some instances it is helpful if the parents remain for at least some part of the first day until the child is comfortable and at ease. If parents stay, they should be available to the child but inconspicuous. A full-day routine is often too overwhelming for a child and needs to be shortened to a morning or afternoon session. Another action that can decrease separation anxiety is providing the school with detailed information about the child's home environment, such as familiar routines, favorite activities, food preferences, names of siblings or pets, and personal habits. Such information helps the child feel familiar in the strange surroundings. A school that automatically requests this information demonstrates the staff's awareness of each child's needs, and the parent has a valuable clue to evaluating the quality of the program. Transitional objects, such as a favorite toy, may also help the child bridge the gap from home to school.

### Sex Education

Preschoolers have experienced a tremendous amount of information during their short lifetimes. Although their thinking may not be mature, they search constantly for explanations and reasons that are logical and reasonable to them. The word "why" seems to supplant the word "no," which was common in toddlerhood. It is only natural that as they learn about "me," they will also want to know "why me," and "how me." Questions such as "Where do babies come from?" are as casual as "Why is the sky blue?" "What makes it rain?" or

---

*Information about the accreditation criteria and procedures of the National Academy of Early Childhood Programs is available from the National Association for the Education of Young Children, 1834 Connecticut Ave NW, Washington, DC 20009, (202) 232-8777 or (800) 424-2460, www.naeyc.org

---

*Recommended books for preparing young children for daycare or school include *Going to School* by Anne Civardi and Stephen Cartwright (EDC Publishing), *Little Bear Goes to Kindergarten* by Jutta Langreuter and Vera Sobat (Millbrook Press), *My First Day of School* by PK Hallinan (Ideals Children's Books), and *Going to Daycare* and *When Your Child Goes to School* by Fred Rogers (GP Putnam's Sons).

**TABLE 15-2** Growth and development during preschool years

| Age (years) | Physical | Gross Motor | Fine Motor | Language |
|---|---|---|---|---|
| 3 | Usual weight gain of 1.8 to 2.7 kg (4 to 6 pounds)<br>Average weight of 14.6 kg (32 pounds)<br>Usual gain in height of 6.75-7.5 cm (2.5-3 inches)<br>Average height of 95 cm (37.25 inches)<br>May have achieved nighttime control of bowel and bladder | Rides tricycle<br>Jumps off bottom step<br>Stands on one foot for a few seconds<br>Goes up stairs using alternate feet, but may still come down using both feet on step<br>Broad jumps<br>May try to dance, but balance may not be adequate | Builds tower of nine or ten cubes<br>Builds bridge with three cubes<br>Adeptly places small pellets in narrow-necked bottle<br>In drawing, copies a circle, imitates a cross, names what has been drawn, cannot draw stick figure but may make circle with facial features | Has vocabulary of approximately 900 words<br>Uses primarily "telegraphic" speech<br>Uses complete sentences of three to four words<br>Talks incessantly regardless of whether anyone is paying attention<br>Repeats sentence of six syllables<br>Asks many questions<br>Begins to sing songs |
| 4 | Average weight of 16.7 kg (36.75 pounds)<br>Average height of 103 cm (40.5 inches)<br>Birth length is doubled<br>Maximum potential for development of amblyopia | Skips and hops on one foot<br>Catches ball reliably<br>Throws ball overhand<br>Walks down stairs using alternate feet | Uses scissors successfully to cut out picture following outline<br>Can lace shoes, but may not be able to tie bow<br>In drawing, copies a square, traces a cross and diamond, adds three parts to stick figure | Has vocabulary of 1500 words or more<br>Uses sentences of four to five words<br>Questioning is at peak<br>Tells exaggerated stories<br>Knows simple songs<br>Obeys four prepositional phrases, such as "under," "on top of," "beside," "in back of," or "in front of"<br>Names one or more colors<br>Comprehends analogies, such as, "If ice is cold, fire is _____" |
| 5 | Average weight of 18.7 kg (41.25 pounds)<br>Average height of 110 cm (43.25 inches)<br>Eruption of permanent dentition may begin<br>Handedness is established (approximately 90% are righthanded) | Skips and hops on alternate feet<br>Throws and catches ball well<br>Jumps rope<br>Skates with good balance<br>Walks backward with heel to toe<br>Balances on alternate feet with eyes closed | Ties shoelaces<br>Uses scissors, simple tools, and pencil very well<br>In drawing, copies a diamond and triangle; adds seven to nine parts to stick figure; prints a few letters, numbers, or words, such as first name | Has vocabulary of approximately 2100 words<br>Uses sentences of six to eight words, with all parts of speech<br>Names coins (e.g., nickel, dime)<br>Names four or more colors<br>Describes drawing or pictures with much comment<br>Knows names of days of week, months, and other time-associated words<br>Knows composition of articles, such as "A shoe is made of _____"<br>Can follow three commands in succession |

"Who is that?" It is the *way* in which questions about procreation are answered that conditions children, even the youngest, to separate these questions from others about their world. If these questions are answered honestly and as matter-of-factly as any other inquiry, children will continue to search for answers. If they are answered with a "tall tale" or an anxious "You are too young to know about that," children will learn to keep such questions to themselves. Unfortunately, as they harbor these silent mysteries, they formulate their own theories to explain birth. Because magical thinking need not be based on logic or fact, any fantastic and often terrifying explanation can substitute for the truth.

Two rules govern answering sensitive questions about topics such as sex. The first is to *find out what children know and think*. By investigating the theories children have produced as a reasonable explanation, parents can not only give correct information but also help children understand why their explanation is inaccurate. Another reason for ascertaining what the child thinks before offering any information is that the "unasked for" answer may be given. For example, 4-year-old Lauren asked her father, "Where did I come from?" Both parents quickly took this inquiry as a clue for offering sex education. After the explanation, Lauren exclaimed, "I don't know about all that! All I know

| Socialization | Cognition | Family Relationships |
|---|---|---|
| Dresses self almost completely if helped with back buttons and told which shoe is right or left<br>Has increased attention span<br>Feeds self completely<br>Can prepare simple meals, such as cold cereal and milk<br>Can help to set table; can dry dishes without breaking any<br>May have fears, especially of dark and of going to bed<br>Knows own sex and sex of others<br>Play is parallel and associative; begins to learn simple games but often follows own rules; begins to share | Is in preconceptual phase<br>Is egocentric in thought and behavior<br>Has beginning understanding of time; uses many time-oriented expressions; talks about past and future as much as about present; pretends to tell time<br>Has improved concept of space as demonstrated in understanding of prepositions and ability to follow directional command<br>Has beginning ability to view concepts from another perspective | Attempts to please parents and conform to their expectations<br>Is less jealous of younger sibling; may be opportune time for birth of additional sibling<br>Is aware of family relationships and sex-role functions<br>Boys tend to identify more with father or other male figure<br>Has increased ability to separate easily and comfortably from parents for short periods |
| Very independent<br>Tends to be selfish and impatient<br>Aggressive physically as well as verbally<br>Takes pride in accomplishments<br>Has mood swings<br>Shows off dramatically, enjoys entertaining others<br>Tells family tales to others with no restraint<br>Still has many fears<br>Play is associative<br>    Imaginary playmates are common<br>    Uses dramatic, imaginative, and imitative devices<br>    Sexual exploration and curiosity demonstrated through play, such as being "doctor" or "nurse" | Is in phase of intuitive thought<br>Causality is still related to proximity of events<br>Understands time better, especially in terms of sequence of daily events<br>Judges everything according to one dimension, such as height, width, or order<br>Immediate perceptual clues dominate judgment<br>Is beginning to develop less egocentrism and more social awareness<br>May count correctly but has poor mathematic concept of numbers<br>Obeys because parents have set limits, not because of understanding of right and wrong | Rebels if parents expect too much, such as impeccable table manners<br>Takes aggression and frustration out on parents or siblings<br>"Do's" and "don'ts" become important<br>May have rivalry with older or younger siblings; may resent older sibling's privileges and younger sibling's invasion of privacy and possessions<br>May "run away" from home<br>Identifies strongly with parent of opposite sex<br>Is able to run simple errands outside the home |
| Less rebellious and quarrelsome than at age 4 years<br>More settled and eager to get down to business<br>Not as open and accessible in thoughts and behavior as in earlier years<br>Independent but trustworthy; not foolhardy; more responsible<br>Has fewer fears; relies on outer authority to control world<br>Eager to do things right and to please; tries to "live by the rules"<br>Has better manners<br>Cares for self totally, occasionally needing supervision in dress or hygiene, especially teeth<br>Not ready for concentrated close work or small print because of slight farsightedness and still-unrefined eye-hand coordination<br>Play is associative; tries to follow rules but may cheat to avoid losing | Begins to question what parents think by comparing them with age-mates and other adults<br>May notice prejudice and bias in outside world<br>Is more able to view other's perspective, but tolerates differences rather than understanding them<br>May begin to show understanding of conservation of numbers through counting objects, regardless of arrangement<br>Uses time-oriented words with increased understanding<br>Very curious about factual information regarding world | Gets along well with parents<br>May seek out parent more often than at age 4 years for reassurance and security, especially when entering school<br>Begins to question parents' thinking and principles<br>Strongly identifies with parent of same sex, especially boys with their fathers<br>Enjoys activities such as sports, cooking, shopping with parent of same sex |

is Mary came from New York and I want to know where I was born."

Regardless of whether children are given sex education, they will engage in games of sexual curiosity and exploration. At approximately 3 years of age children are aware of the anatomic differences between the sexes and are very concerned with how the other "works." This is not really "sexual" curiosity because many children are still unaware of the reproductive function of the genitals. Their curiosity is for the eliminative function of the anatomy. Little boys wonder how girls can urinate without a penis, so they watch girls go to the bathroom. Because they cannot see anything but the stream of urine coming out, they want to observe further. "Doctor play" is often a game invented for just such investigation. Little girls are no less curious about boys' anatomy. It is very intriguing to have a closer inspection of this "thing" that girls do not have.

One question that parents often have is how to handle such sexual curiosity. A positive approach is to neither condone nor condemn the behavior but to express that if children have questions they should ask the parents; the parents should then encourage the children to engage in some other activity. In this way children can be helped to understand that there are ways in which their sexual curiosity can be satisfied other than through playing investigative games. This in no way condemns the act but stresses alternative methods by which to seek solutions and answers. Allowing children unrestricted permissiveness only intensifies their anxiety and concern, because exploring and searching usually yield little evidence to satisfy their curiosity.

Occasionally parents are faced with special dilemmas (e.g., when a child accidentally witnesses sexual intercourse). When such an event occurs, parents must remember that sex education is much more than textbook facts. It is part of a broader concept called *sexuality;* two people unite intimately because of the special relationship they have together (Wright, 1997). Intercourse is not a physical act apart from feeling or emotion but a private act that two people share to express caring and for pleasure. Such an explanation does not deny the child's right to be curious; nor does it deny the request because the wish is bad or dangerous. On the contrary, it teaches appropriate social behavior and, in particular, stresses the meaningful, intimate relationship between two adults. When children witness sexual acts, parents should use the opportunity immediately to communicate that sex is healthy and natural. However, to prevent subsequent interruptions, children are cautioned to always knock first; if they are too young to understand or comply, a lock on the door is appropriate.

The second rule for giving information is to *be honest.* It is true that much of the correct information will be forgotten or misunderstood by the preschooler, but what is more important is that the correct information can be restated until the child absorbs and comprehends the facts. Even though the correct anatomic words may be hard to pronounce or even more difficult to remember, they become important for explaining other concepts later on. Nurses have the opportunity to contribute to early sex education by conveying accurate information regarding genital terms during physical examinations.

Honesty does not imply imparting every fact of life or allowing excessive permissiveness in sexual curiosity. A child who asks one question is looking for one answer. When they are ready, children will ask about the other "unfinished" parts of the story. Sooner or later they will wonder how the "sperm meets the egg" and "how the baby gets out," but it is best to wait until they ask.

If parents offer too much information, the child will simply become bored or end the conversation with an irrelevant question. Parents worry a great deal about whether they can "harm" their children with "too much" information or tell them things they will not understand. In general, knowledge is not harmful. In fact, experts advise parents to tell their children a bit more than they think their children can understand (Finan, 1997). It does not matter if they do not understand everything parents say. What matters is that parents are approachable.

When the child does not ask questions, parents and health professionals should take advantage of natural opportunities to discuss reproduction, such as talking about someone who is pregnant or discussing a television program or movie about biologic aspects. Many excellent books on sex education are available for preschool children at public

libraries, and the **Sexuality Information and Education Council of the United States (SIECUS),*** local chapters of **Planned Parenthood Federation of America,†** and the **American Academy of Pediatrics‡** have bibliographies of suggested reading material. Parents should read the book *before* giving or reading it to a child.

Another concern for some parents is *masturbation,* or self-stimulation of the genitals. This occurs at any age for a variety of reasons and, if not excessive, is normal and healthy. In one study describing the development of sexual behavior in children, preschoolers exhibited developmentally appropriate behavior including touching genital areas in public or at home (Schoentjes, Deboutte, and Friedrich, 1999). For preschoolers it is a part of sexual curiosity and exploration. If parents are concerned about masturbation in their children, it is essential for nurses to investigate the circumstances associated with the activity because it may be an expression of anxiety, boredom, or unresolved conflicts. For example, a boy who repeatedly touches his penis is not masturbating for pleasure but may be reassuring himself that it is intact. Children who openly and publicly masturbate are inviting a reaction, such as discipline, punishment, or criticism. They may be overwhelmed by their sexual feelings and are asking others to help them channel these feelings into more constructive outlets. Masturbation, like other forms of sex play, is a private act, and parents should emphasize this to children when teaching them socially acceptable behavior.

## Gifted Children

The importance of identifying gifted children and their needs is increasingly being recognized. Although the definition of *gifted* varies, a broad view, reflected in the term *gifted/talented,* considers signs of giftedness to be specific academic aptitude, creative or productive thinking, leadership ability, ability in the visual or performing arts, and psychomotor ability, either singly or in combination. Giftedness can exist in children who have learning disorders or attention deficit–hyperactivity disorder (ADHD) or who are underachievers (Robinson and Olszewski-Kubilius, 1996). Most children are identified as gifted when they enter school or are referred by parents or teachers and receive IQ tests. However, not all gifted children are identified, which may result in the tragic loss of the opportunity to develop their potential (Feiring and others, 1997). Consequently, nurses who are aware of the behavioral and developmental characteristics of giftedness can assess children's mental and physical capabilities and assist in early identification (Box 15-1).

Gifted children can present unique challenges to parents. They often demand increased stimulation as infants and continue to seek a great deal of attention from their parents. Their high energy level and persistence can lead to discipline problems similar to those seen in children with

---

*130 W 42nd St, Suite 350, New York, NY 10036, (212) 819-9770; www.siecus.org.

†National office: 810 7th Ave, New York, NY 10019, (212) 541-7800, (800) 829-7732; www.plannedparenthood.org.

‡AAP Publications, 141 Northwest Point Blvd, PO Box 747, Elk Grove Village, IL 60009-0747, (800) 433-9016, fax: (847) 228-1281, www.aap.org.

## Box 15-1 ■ ■ ■
### Characteristics of Gifted Children

Asynchrony across developmental domains
Advanced language and reasoning skills
Conversation and interests like older children and adults
Insatiable curiosity; perceptive questions
Rapid and intuitive understanding of concepts
Impressive long-term memory
Ability to hold problems in mind that are not yet figured out
Ability to make connections between one concept and another
Interest in patterns and relationships
Advanced sense of humor (for age)
Courage in trying new pathways of thinking
Pleasure in solving and posing new problems
Capacity for independent, self-directed activities
Talent in a specific area: drawing, music, games, math, reading
Sensitivity and perfectionism
Intensity of feeling and emotion

From Robinson NM, Olszewski-Kubilius PM: Gifted and talented children: issues for pediatricians, *Pediatr Rev* 17(12):428, 1996. Used with permission. American Academy of Pediatrics.

difficult temperaments. Parents may be intimidated by having a child smarter than themselves and be hesitant to set limits. However, gifted children are children first and have the same needs for love, security, and consistent controls as other youngsters. Sometimes children's above-average skills in one area cause adults to exaggerate their abilities in all areas and thus expect excessively mature behavior. Parents may mislabel slower achievement in a particular skill as lack of trying, when really it represents children's natural progression of abilities. These children benefit from academic settings that provide enrichment and accelerated learning commensurate with their capabilities. Consequently, early identification of gifted/talented children and appropriate parental guidance can be critical to the optimal development and emotional adjustment of children (Jaffe, 2000).

Informational materials on parenting gifted and talented children can be obtained from **The National Association for Gifted Children*** and **The Council for Exceptional Children,†** as well as local associations.

## Aggression

The term *aggression* refers to behavior that attempts to hurt a person or destroy property. Aggression differs from anger, which is a temporary emotional state, but anger may be expressed through aggression. Hyperaggressive behavior in preschoolers is characterized by unprovoked physical attacks on other children and adults, destruction of others' property, frequent intense temper tantrums, extreme impulsivity, disrespect, and noncompliance.

Aggression is influenced by a complex set of biologic, sociocultural, and familial variables. There is evidence that gender differences exist and that males are more aggressive than females (Stormshak and others, 2000). Parenting practices,

specifically those that include punitive interactions, low levels of warmth, and physically aggressive parenting, may contribute to oppositional and aggressive behavior problems. In many cases coercive parent-child interactions contribute to the development of aggression. Recognizing parents and children at risk for negative interactions and behavior is the first step. Programs that train caregivers to implement behavioral change strategies have been shown to be effective, while talking alone with parents has been ineffective (Vanderheyden and Witt, 2000). Other factors that tend to increase aggressive behavior are frustration, modeling, and reinforcement.

*Frustration,* or the continual thwarting of self-satisfaction by parental disapproval, humiliation, punishment, and insults, can lead children to act out against others as a means of release. Especially if they fear their parents, these children will displace their anger on others, particularly peers and other authority figures. This type of aggression often applies to the child who is "well behaved" at home but a discipline problem at school or a "bully" among playmates.

*Modeling,* or imitating the behavior of significant others, is a powerful influencing force in preschoolers. Children who see their parents as physically or verbally abusive are observing behavior that they come to know as acceptable (Hart and others, 1998). Also, early harsh discipline may lead to aggressive behavior (Brenner and Fox, 1998). Another aspect of modeling is establishing a double standard for acceptable conduct. For example, in some families aggression is synonymous with masculinity, and boys are encouraged to defend themselves. Although defending one's rights is to be encouraged for both sexes, at times the principle of "toughness" or "standing up for yourself" is not tempered with judgment, fairness, or equality but becomes an excuse for ruling and dominating others. Such permissive aggression can produce extreme anxiety in children because it makes them feel out of control, even though outwardly they may appear to be the "boss" or "bully."

Another significant source for modeling is television. Numerous studies have found a positive correlation between viewing violent programs and immediate aggression. Consequently, parents need encouragement to supervise programming, especially for those children with aggressive tendencies (Villani, 2001). The American Academy of Pediatrics (2001a) offers a list of recommendations for healthy television viewing.

*Reinforcement* can also shape aggressive behavior and is closely associated with modeling "masculine" behavior. Sometimes the reward for aggressive behavior is negative (e.g., punishment or disapproval) yet reinforcing because it brings attention. For example, children who are ignored by their parents until they hit a sibling learn that this act attracts attention. Parents who permit aggressive behavior by not interfering communicate silent, implicit approval of such acts.

One of the tasks of preschoolers is learning socially acceptable behavior and the ability to control and redirect aggression toward the appropriate source. Parents can help children by modeling the appropriate behavior and encouraging children to express themselves verbally. For example, rather than condoning the hitting of another child for taking a toy, parents can suggest that the child state how he or she feels, such as "I am angry when you take my ball. Give it back."

Children should not be made to feel guilty or ashamed for being angry or frustrated. When children recognize these feelings, they are better able to channel them into constructive, not destructive, outlets. One of the earliest demonstrations of aggression is temper tantrums. (See Chapter 14.) Parents can handle them constructively by not attending to or reinforcing them and by helping children find control through appropriate play situations. In this way, young children learn to acknowledge such feelings and express them in alternate ways, such as pounding on clay or hitting a punching bag. When children are out of control, they may need to be physically restrained or removed from the scene to prevent them from hurting themselves or others.

Sometimes the type of discipline used to extinguish other forms of unacceptable behavior actually promotes aggressive behavior. For example, if the child is spanked for the act, aggression is being used to "teach" a lesson against aggression. Parental permissiveness and lack of discipline, often alternating with extreme punishment, may also foster aggressiveness (Stormshak and others, 2000). The combined use of time-out and reinforcement for solitary play is an effective intervention for aggression. In addition, minimizing anger and frustration can lead to fewer opportunities for acting-out behavior.

When extreme behaviors, such as aggression, are present in a child, parents are often concerned about the need for professional help. Generally, the difference between "normal" and "problematic" behavior is not the behavior itself but its *quantity* (number of occurrences), *severity* (interference with social or cognitive functioning), *distribution* (different manifestations), *onset* (when the behavior started), and *duration* (at least 4 weeks). When aggressive tendencies are evaluated, these factors are assessed to distinguish between behaviors typically seen at various ages and those that may represent an underlying problem. Extreme aggression requires professional treatment and is often difficult to change.*

## Speech Problems

The most critical period for speech development occurs between 2 and 4 years of age. During this period children are using their rapidly growing vocabulary faster than they can produce the words. This failure to master sensorimotor integrations results in *stuttering* or *stammering* as children try to say the word they are already thinking about. This dysfluency in speech pattern is a *normal* characteristic of language development (Ambrose and Yairi, 1999) and usually passes, provided caregivers speak clearly and do not complete the child's sentences and overcorrect mistakes. However, when parents or other significant caregivers place undue emphasis or stress on it, an abnormal speech pattern may develop.

The best therapy for speech problems is prevention and early detection. Common causes of speech problems are hearing loss, developmental delay, and lack of verbal stimulation (American Academy of Pediatrics, 2001c). Referral for further evaluation and treatment may be necessary to prevent a problem from interfering with learning. Anticipatory preparation of parents for expected developmental norms may allay caregiver concerns.

Children pressured into producing sounds ahead of their developmental level may develop *dyslalia* (articulation problems) or revert to using infantile speech. Prevention involves discussing with parents the usual achievement of speech production during childhood. The *Denver Articulation Screening Examination (DASE)* is an excellent tool for assessing articulation skills in the child and for explaining to parents the expected progression of sounds. (See Appendix B.)

## Stress

Although for parents the preschool years generally are less troublesome than toddlerhood, this period presents children with many unique stresses. Some are innate and stem from preschoolers' unique understanding of the world, such as fears. Others are imposed, such as beginning school. Although minimal amounts of stress are beneficial during the early years to help children develop effective coping skills, excessive stress is harmful. Young children are especially vulnerable because of their limited capacity to cope.

To help parents deal with stress in their child's life, they must be aware of signs of stress and be helped to identify the source (Box 15-2). In addition, any number of other stresses may be present, such as the birth of a sibling, marital discord, relocation, or illness. The best approach to dealing with stress is prevention. It is important to monitor the amount of stress in the child's life so that levels exceeding coping ability do not occur. In many instances structuring the child's schedule to allow rest and preparing the child for change, such as entering school, are sufficient measures.

Because stress is a constant aspect of daily living, it is not too early to help preschool children learn to cope with it. They can learn the meaning of the word "stress" and recognize physical signs of a stress reaction, such as a rapid pulse, a pounding heart, or fatigue. Teaching children relaxation and imagery is very effective. Young children can learn to "let their bodies go limp like a rag doll." Parents can use stories to help their child imagine pleasurable events. As language skills improve, preschoolers are encouraged to talk about their feelings and explore other ways of expressing emotions. Play is an excellent vehicle for venting anger or frustration, and toys such as drums, clay, and punching bags provide alternative methods of dissipating anxiety. Toys also begin to teach socially acceptable ways of dealing with such feelings.

## Fears

The greatest number and variety of real and imagined fears are present during the preschool years and include fear of the dark, being left alone (especially at bedtime), animals (particularly large dogs and snakes), ghosts, sexual matters

---

*Information on temperament and child development can be found at www.dbpeds.org.

## Box 15-2
### Sources of Stress in Preschoolers

**THREE YEAR OLD**

**Stubbornness**—Although is developing an interest in social relationships and a concept of "we," may lapse into uncooperative behavior

**Belongings**—Guards possessions

**Jealousy**—Particularly when it comes to parents' love

**Separation anxiety**—Difficulty leaving the parent

**Stranger anxiety**—Expresses fear being around someone unknown

**Confusion**—Cannot always discriminate between fantasy and reality

**Fears**—May be precipitated by imagination; may also fear dogs or other animals

**Speech**—May stutter or stumble over words

**Activity level**—Seems to be in perpetual motion; may exhaust himself or herself

**Mealtime**—May forget to eat or lose interest in food

**Nap or bedtime**—May fear bad dreams, the dark, or missing out on some fun while asleep

**Destructiveness**—May damage or destroy objects

**Questions**—Continually asks "why," and is upset if trusted adults do not respond or do not know the answer

**FOUR YEAR OLD**

**Insecurity**—May develop nervous habits such as nail biting, facial tics, thumb sucking, genital manipulation, eye blinking, or nose picking; may insist on bringing a familiar item from house to preschool

**Companionship**—Enjoys interacting with friends, although there may be many quarrels

**Belongings**—Protects possessions

**Sex**—Interested in the human body; may engage in exhibitionism

**Activity level**—Enjoys running, jumping, and slamming doors; may be punished for disruptive behavior

**Fears**—Picks up fears from adults; may fear dark room or anything perceived as "creepy"

**Attention**—Likes to talk and is frustrated if ignored or put off

**FIVE YEAR OLD**

**Approval**—Parents' love and acceptance are vital; seeks praise

**School**—May have difficulty adjusting to kindergarten

**Separation anxiety**—Particularly fears loss of mother

**Worrying**—May develop irrational fears, take information out of context, or fret over a misinterpreted, overheard conversation

**Belongings**—Protects possessions

**Procrastination**—Delays completing chores or activities

**Name-calling**—Insults others to boost self-image but is upset when he or she is the victim of mockery

Modified from Kuczen B: *Childhood stress: don't let your child be a victim,* New York, 1982, Delacorte Press, pp 15-17.

---

(castration), and objects or persons associated with pain (Muris, Merckelbach, and Prins, 2000). The exact cause of children's fears is unknown. Freudians believe that the upsurge of fears during the preschool years results from the anxiety of being injured and mutilated (castration complex). Piaget views fears as a product of the type of thinking in this age-group. Preschoolers are caught between the egocentric thinking of infants, which protects them from imagined fears, and the more logical thought processes of school-age children, which help explain and dispel potential fears. Children in the preconceptual stage still engage in egocentric thought but are now able to imagine an event without actually experiencing it. For example, seeing someone hurt is sufficient for realizing what the hurt must be like and for consequently fearing that hurt. This is commonly observed in medical practice. When watching another child getting an injection, the preschooler may become very upset, almost as if he or she received the injection.

The concept of *animism* (ascribing lifelike qualities to inanimate objects) helps explain why children fear objects. For example, one child refused to use the toilet after watching a television commercial in which the toilet bowl was portrayed as turning into a monster.

One fear peculiar to this age is fear of annihilation. Because of poorly defined body boundaries and improved cognitive abilities, young children develop concerns related to loss of body parts, such as their body going down the drain. Because preschool children cannot understand concepts of size, they cannot understand that their body is too large to disappear down the drain.

Preschoolers are also likely to develop parent-induced fears. When parents demonstrate their fears, these concerns are communicated to the children. Such fears tend to be long-lasting and difficult to dispel.

The best way to help children overcome their fears is by actively involving them in finding practical methods to deal with frightening experiences. This may be as simple as keeping a dim night-light in the child's bedroom for assurance or letting the child bathe a doll so that the child can observe that large objects cannot go down the drain. In this way, the experience that created the fear in the child can be reconstructed without involving the child directly as the victim. The child is allowed alternative methods by which to feel in control while overcoming fear.

Exposing children to the feared object in a safe situation provides a type of conditioning, or *desensitization.* For instance, children who are afraid of dogs should never be forced to approach or touch one, but they may be gradually introduced to the experience by watching other children play with the animal. This type of modeling, demonstrating fearlessness in others, can be very effective if children are allowed to progress at their own rate.

Usually by 5 or 6 years of age children relinquish these fears. Explaining the developmental sequence of fears and their gradual disappearance may help parents feel more secure in handling preschoolers' fears.

Sometimes fears do not subside with simple measures or developmental maturation. When children experience severe fears that disrupt family life, professional help is required. Successful training programs may include (1) muscle relaxation, (2) guided imagery, (3) positive self-talk or reciting brave statements, or (4) thought stopping or repeating reassuring statements that block fearful thoughts. Rewards or "tokens" may be given for "bravery" and not being afraid.

Such interventions can be applied in clinical settings to reduce fears (e.g., of being alone or of painful procedures).

## PROMOTING OPTIMUM HEALTH DURING THE PRESCHOOL YEARS

### Nutrition

Nutritional requirements for preschoolers are fairly similar to those for toddlers (U.S. Department of Agriculture, 1999). The requirement for calories per unit of body weight continues to decrease slightly to 90 kcal/kg, for an average daily intake of 1800 calories. Fluid requirements may also decrease slightly (to approximately 100 ml/kg daily) but depend on activity level, climatic conditions, and state of health. Protein requirements are 1.2 g/kg for an average daily consumption of 24 g (Food and Nutrition Board, 1989).

The American Academy of Pediatrics Committee on Nutrition (1998) recommends that by 5 years of age saturated fatty acid consumption should be less than 10% of total caloric intake; total fat over several days should be no more than 30% and no less than 20% of total caloric intake. Evidence supports the efficacy of limiting fat intake, and negative health effects have not been reported (Johnson, 2000). However, it is important that the diet contain adequate nutrients. The recommendation for daily calcium intake for children 4 to 8 years old is 800 mg (Food and Nutrition Board, 1997). Milk and dairy products provide the most important source of calcium. Eating less fat does not require drinking less milk but perhaps replacing higher fat milk with lower or non-fat milk. In children over 2 years of age, intake of fiber, fruits, and vegetables should equal the child's age plus 5 in grams/day. This translates into five servings of fruits and vegetables each day (Johnson, 2000).

There is some concern that excessive consumption of fruit juices has adverse health effects such as dental caries and gastrointestinal symptoms (Johnson, 2000). The relationship between fruit juice, growth effects, and obesity is unclear. It is advisable to counsel moderation in fruit juice consumption and at the same time provide suggestions for more appropriate sources of nutrients such as ascorbic acid, folate, and potassium. The American Academy of Pediatrics (2001b) recommends the intake of fruit juice to be limited to 4 to 6 ounces per day for children ages 1 to 6 years.

The U.S. Department of Agriculture (1999) adapted the Food Guide Pyramid for young children aged 2 to 6 years. The foods depicted are those commonly eaten by children in this age-group, and the illustrations emphasize the importance of physical activity. Parents and caregivers can provide opportunities for children to learn to like a variety of nutritious foods by exposing them to these foods.

Some preschoolers still have food habits typical of toddlers, such as food fads and strong taste preferences. When children reach 4 years of age, they seem to enter another period of finicky eating, which is generally characteristic of the more rebellious behavior of children in this age-group. By age 5 years children are more agreeable to trying new foods, especially if encouraged by an adult who allows the child to help with food preparation or experiments with a new taste or different dish (Fig. 15-7). Mealtime can become a battle if parents expect excellent table manners. A 5-year-old child is usually ready for the "social" side of eating, but the younger child still has difficulty sitting quietly through a long family meal.

The amount and variety of foods consumed by young children vary greatly from day to day (Dennison, Rockwell, and Baker, 1998). Consequently, parents sometimes worry about the quantity of food consumed by preschoolers. In general, the quality is much more important than the quantity, which should be stressed during nutritional counseling. There is some evidence that children self-regulate their caloric intake. If they eat less at one meal, they compensate at another meal or snack.

One approach toward lessening parental concern is advising parents to keep a weekly record of everything the child eats. In particular, the need for measuring the amount of food, such as setting aside ½ cup of vegetables and serving the child from this premeasured amount, is stressed to provide a more accurate estimate of food intake at each meal. When parents look at the food chart at the end of the week, they are usually amazed at how much the child has consumed. In general, preschoolers consume only slightly more than toddlers, or approximately half of an adult's portion. Resources are available for the health care provider and the caregiver to help build healthy eating habits for children.*

---

*Nutritional resources for the health care provider include: American Academy of Pediatrics, Committee on Nutrition: *Pediatric nutrition handbook*, Elk Grove, IL, 1998, The Academy. Nutritional resources for parents and caregivers include: *Guide to Your Child's Nutrition* and *Fit for a King: The Smart Kid's Guide to Food and Fun*. To order contact the American Academy of Pediatrics at (888) 227-1770 or visit www.aap.org.

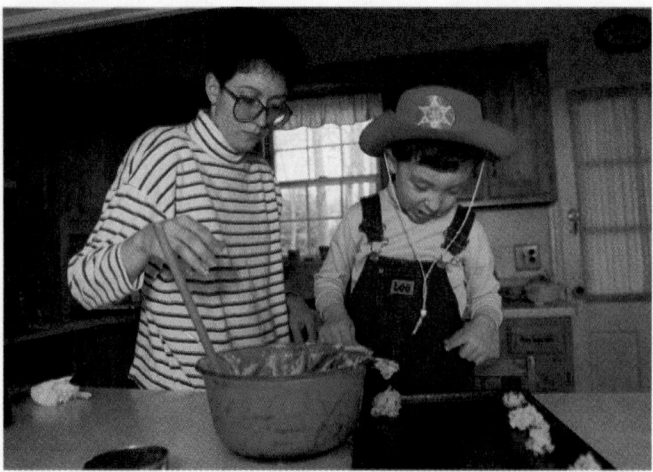

**Fig. 15-7** Preschool children enjoy helping adults and are more likely to try new foods if they are included in the preparation.

> **NURSING ALERT** Obesity has increased over the last two decades in young children. Efforts to provide a healthy diet and to encourage physical activity should begin early to help children achieve optimal health (Johnson, 2000).

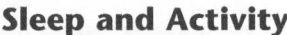

## Sleep and Activity

Sleep patterns vary widely, but the average preschooler sleeps approximately 12 hours a night and infrequently takes daytime naps. Waking during the night is common throughout early childhood and may be related to social rather than developmental factors (Thiedke, 2001).

Motor activity levels continue to be high and allow preschoolers to explore their environment, begin learning physical games and sports, and interact with others. Motor activity is therefore encouraged. Quiet activities, such as television, are increasingly appealing and can become an unhealthy substitute for active play.

Preschoolers' increased gross motor abilities and coordination provide them the opportunity to engage in many physical activities, if only at a novice level. Whether young children should begin formalized training in an activity at this early age is controversial. Training programs must consider the child's physical and psychological immaturity (Maffulli, 2001). Readiness must be determined individually. The American Academy of Pediatrics encourages free play, a variety of physical activities, a noncompetitive atmosphere, and an emphasis on fun and safety.

### Sleep Problems

The preschool years are a prime time for sleep disturbances. As toddlers and preschoolers cope with autonomy, separation, and object permanence, they begin to have more sleep problems (Thiedke, 2001). Some have trouble going to sleep, especially after so much activity and stimulation during the day. Others may develop bedtime fears, wake during the night, or have nightmares or sleep terrors. Still others may prolong the inevitable bedtime through elaborate rituals.

Recommendations for handling a sleep disturbance are offered only after a thorough assessment has been completed. (See Guidelines box on p. 157.) Cultural traditions may dictate sleep practices contrary to certain well-accepted professional recommendations. Therefore parents' perceptions of a sleep habit may not consider it to be a problem. (See Cultural Awareness box on p. 646.)

Interventions differ greatly; for example, nightmares and sleep terrors require very different approaches (Table 15-3). For children who delay going to bed, a recommended approach involves counseling parents about the importance of a consistent bedtime ritual and emphasizing the normalcy of this type of behavior in young children. Attention-seeking behavior is ignored, and the child is not taken into the parents' bed or allowed to stay up past a reasonable hour. Other measures that may be helpful include keeping a light on in the room, providing transitional objects, such as a favorite toy, or leaving a drink of water by the bed.

Helping children slow down before bedtime also contributes to less resistance to going to bed. One approach is

| **TABLE 15-3**   Comparison of nightmares to sleep terrors | |
| --- | --- |
| **Nightmares** | **Sleep Terrors** |
| **Description** | |
| A scary dream; takes place during REM sleep and is followed by full waking | A partial arousal from very deep (stage IV, non-REM) sleep |
| **Time of Distress** | |
| After the dream is over child wakes and cries or calls, not during the nightmare itself | During the terror itself, as child screams and thrashes; afterward is calm |
| **Time of Occurrence** | |
| In the second half of the night, when dreams are most intense | Usually 1 to 4 hours after falling asleep, when non-REM sleep is deepest |
| **Child's Behavior** | |
| Crying in younger children, fright in all; these behaviors persist even though the child is awake | Initially child may sit up, thrash, or run in a bizarre manner, with eyes bulging, heart racing, and profuse perspiring; may cry, scream, talk, or moan; there is apparent fright, anger, and/or obvious confusion, which disappears when child is fully awake |
| **Responsiveness to Others** | |
| Child is aware of and reassured by another's presence | Child is not very aware of another's presence, is not comforted, and may push person away and scream and thrash more if held or restrained |
| **Return to Sleep** | |
| May be considerably delayed because of persistent fear | Usually rapid; often difficult to keep child awake |
| **Description of Dream** | |
| Yes (if old enough) | No memory of a dream or of yelling or thrashing |
| **Interventions** | |
| Accept dream as real fear | Observe child for a few minutes, *without interfering,* until child becomes calm or wakes fully |
| Sit with child; offer comfort, assurance, and sense of protection | Intervene only if necessary to protect child from injury |
| Avoid taking child to own bed | Guide child back to bed if needed |
| Consider professional counseling for recurrent nightmares unresponsive to above approaches | Stress to parents that sleep terrors are a normal, common phenomenon in preschoolers that requires relatively little intervention |

Modified from Ferber R: *Solve your child's sleep problems,* New York, 1985, Simon & Schuster.

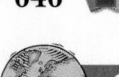

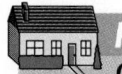

## FAMILY HOME CARE
### Guidance During Preschool Years

**AGE 3 YEARS**

Prepare parents for child's increasing interest in widening personal relationships.
Encourage enrollment in preschool.
Emphasize importance of setting limits.
Prepare parents to expect exaggerated tension-reduction behaviors, such as need for "security blanket."
Encourage parents to offer child choices.
Prepare parents to expect marked changes at 3½ years, when child becomes insecure and exhibits emotional extremes.
Prepare parents for normal dysfluency in speech and advise them to avoid focusing on the pattern.
Prepare parents to expect extra demands on their attention as a reflection of child's emotional insecurity and fear of loss of love.
Warn parents that equilibrium of 3 year old will change to the aggressive, out-of-bounds behavior of 4 year old.
Inform parents to anticipate a more stable appetite with more food selections.
Stress need for protection and education of child to prevent injury. (See Injury Prevention, Chapter 14.)

**AGE 4 YEARS**

Prepare parents for more aggressive behavior, including motor activity and offensive language.
Prepare parents to expect resistance to parental authority.
Explore parental feelings regarding child's behavior.
Suggest some type of respite for primary caregivers, such as placing child in preschool for part of the day.
Prepare parents for child's increasing sexual curiosity.
Emphasize importance of realistic limit-setting on behavior and appropriate disciplinary techniques.
Prepare parents for highly imaginative 4 year old who indulges in "tall tales" (to be differentiated from lies) and for child's imaginary playmates.
Prepare parents to expect nightmares or an increase in them.
Provide reassurance that a period of calm begins at 5 years of age.

**AGE 5 YEARS**

Inform parents to expect tranquil period at 5 years.
Help parents to prepare child for entrance into school environment.
Make sure immunizations are up to date before entering school.
Suggest that nonemployed mothers (or fathers if appropriate) consider own activities when child begins school.
Suggest swimming lessons for child.

---

to establish limited rituals that signal readiness for bed, such as a bath or story. Parents can reinforce the pattern by stating, "After this story it is bedtime," and consistently carrying through the routine. If anticipated extra stimulation (e.g., having visitors arrive at the children's bedtime) disrupts this routine, it is advisable to settle children in bed beforehand.

Television viewing just before bedtime can cause bedtime resistance and delay sleep onset. One study reported that viewing habits associated most significantly with sleep disturbance were increased amounts of television viewing and increased television viewing at bedtime, especially with a television in the child's room (Owens and others, 1999). Assessing sleep patterns and educating families about the development of healthy sleep behaviors should be incorporated into every well-child visit.

## Dental Health

By the beginning of the preschool period, the eruption of the deciduous (primary) teeth is complete. Dental care is essential to preserve these temporary teeth and to teach good dental habits. (See Chapter 14.) Although preschoolers' fine motor control is improved, they still require assistance and supervision with brushing, and flossing should be performed by parents. Professional care and routine prophylaxis, especially fluoride supplements, should be continued. Routine dental care is recommended at a 6-month or a 12-month interval depending on the family history, the child's dental development, and the presence or absence of dental disease (Martof, 2001).

Trauma to teeth during this period is not uncommon, and prompt evaluation by a dentist is warranted if oral trauma occurs. Preservation of the space previously occupied by an evulsed tooth is necessary for proper eruption of the secondary tooth.

## Injury Prevention

Because of improved gross and fine motor skills, coordination, and balance, preschoolers are less prone to falls than

toddlers. They tend to be less reckless, listen more to parental rules, and are aware of potential dangers, such as hot objects, sharp instruments, and dangerous heights. Putting objects in the mouth as part of exploration has all but ceased, but poisoning is still a danger. Children as young as 4½ years old have been shown to engage in risk-taking behaviors. Cognitive ability may play a role in injury avoidance especially in girls, who are less daring and risk taking. Intervention strategies targeted at risk populations need to be part of safety education (Kennedy and Lipsitt, 1998). Pedestrian motor vehicle injuries increase because of activities such as playing in the street, riding tricycles, running after balls, or forgetting safety regulations when crossing streets. In general, the guidelines suggested for injury prevention in Tables 12-15 and 14-8 may apply to children in this age-group as well. However, emphasis is now on protection and education for safety and potential hazards. Because preschoolers are great imitators, it is essential that parents set a good example by "practicing what they preach." Children quickly observe discrepancies between what they are told to do and what they observe. Establishing habits at this time, such as wearing bicycle helmets, can create long-term safety behaviors.

## Anticipatory Guidance— Care of Families

The preschool years present fewer childrearing difficulties than the earlier years, and this stage of development is facilitated by appropriate anticipatory guidance in the areas already discussed. (See Family Home Care box.) There is also a shift in injury prevention from protection to educa-tion. For example, at this age the use of electrical outlet caps may be removed with verbal explanations given of why danger exists and how to avoid it.

During this period an emotional transition between parent and child occurs. Although children are still attached to their parents and accept all their values and beliefs, they are nearing the period of life when they will question previous teachings and prefer the companionship of peers. Entry into school marks a separation for both parents and children. Parents may need help in adjusting to this change, particularly if the mother has focused her daily activities on home responsibilities. As a child begins preschool or elementary school, the mother may need to seek activities outside the home, such as community involvement or a career. In this way all family members are adjusting to change, which is part of the process of growth and development.

## KEY POINTS

- The preschool years comprise the period from 3 to 5 years of age—a time considered critical for emotional and psychologic development.
- Biologic development in the preschool period is characterized by mature organ systems and refinement in gross and fine motor behavior, as evidenced by participation in activities such as running, riding a tricycle, and drawing.
- According to Erikson, acquiring a sense of initiative is the chief psychosocial task of the preschooler. Development of the superego occurs during this period, and the conscience begins to emerge.
- According to Freudian theory, preschoolers are in the oedipal stage. Resolution of this stage occurs when children strongly identify with the parent of the same sex.
- According to Piaget, the preschool age is characterized by intuitive or prelogical thinking and a move toward logical thought processes through advanced and complex-learning, language, and understanding of causality.
- The seeds of moral development are planted during the preschool period. According to Kohlberg, children are in the stage of naive instrumental orientation, in which they are concerned with satisfying their own needs and, less frequently, the needs of others.

- Social development includes further individuation-separation, more sophisticated language, greater independence, and more complex, imaginative forms of play.
- Areas of special concern to parents during the preschool period are the preschool and kindergarten experience, sex education, speech problems, stress, and fears.
- In selecting a school, parents should inquire about daily programs, teacher qualifications, accreditation, student-staff ratio, safety, meals, fees, and health practices. Licensing, regulation, and accreditation are intrinsic factors to look for when selecting early education programs.
- Two rules that govern answering questions about sex and other sensitive issues are finding out what the child thinks and being honest.
- Preschool aggression may result from frustration, modeling behavior, and reinforcement.
- Fears constitute a great part of the preschool period; objects, potential annihilation, and parent-induced fears are common sources.
- Health promotion includes proper nutrition, adequate sleep, proper dental care, and injury prevention.

## REFERENCES

Ambrose NG, Yairi, E: Normative disfluency data for early childhood stuttering, *J Speech Lang Hear Res* 42:895-909, 1999.

American Academy of Pediatrics: Committee on Nutrition: *Pediatric nutrition handbook,* Elk Grove, IL, 1998, The Academy.

American Academy of Pediatrics: Committee on Public Education: Children, adolescents, and television, *Pediatrics* 107(2): 423-426, 2001a.

American Academy of Pediatrics: Committee on Sports Medicine and Fitness and Committee on School Health: Physical fitness

and activity in school, *Pediatrics* 105(5): 1156-1157, 2000.

American Academy of Pediatrics: Guide to your child's symptoms [online] available: *www.aap.org,* 2001c.

American Academy of Pediatrics: Press Release: AAP warns parents and pediatricians that fruit juice is not always the healthiest choice [online] available: *www.aap.org,* 2001b.

Anderson JE: Co-sleeping: can we ever put the issue to rest? *Contemp Pediatr* 107(6): 98-120, 2000.

Bouldin P, Pratt C: Characteristics of preschool and school-age children with imaginary companions, *J Genet Psychol* 160(4): 397-410, 1999.

Brenner V, Fox RA: Parental discipline and behavior problems in young children, *J Genet Psychol* 159(2):251-256, 1998.

Davison KK, Birch LL: Weight status and self-concept in young girls, *Pediatrics* 107(1):46-53, 2001.

Dennison BA, Rockwell HL, Baker SL: Fruit and vegetable intake in young children, *J Am Coll Nutr* 17(4):371-378, 1998.

Feiring C and others: Early identification of gifted minority kindergarten students in Newark, NJ, *Gifted Child Q* 41(3):76-82, 1997.

Finan SL: Promoting healthy sexuality: guidelines for infancy through preschool, *Nurs Pract* 22(10):79-80, 83-86, 88, 1997.

Food and Nutrition Board, National Research Council: *Recommended dietary allowances,* ed 10, Washington, DC, 1989, National Academy Press.

Food and Nutrition Board: *Dietary reference intakes for calcium, phosphorous, magnesium, vitamin D, and fluoride,* Washington, DC, 1997, National Academy Press.

Glascoe FP. Are overreferrals on developmental screening tests really a problem? *Arch Pediatr Adolesc Med* 155(1):54-59, 2001.

Gottesman, MM: Playing to learn: the work of children and their parents, *J Pediatr Health Care* 13(5):259-262, 1999.

Hart CH and others: Overt and relational aggression in Russian nursery school–aged children: parenting style and marital linkages, *Dev Psychol* 34(4):687-697, 1998.

Hart D, Schnieder, D: Spiritual care for children with cancer, *Semin Oncol Nurs* 13(4):263-270, 1997.

Huttenlocher J: Language input and language growth, *Prev Med* 27(2):195-199, 1998.

Jaffe AC: The gifted child, *Pediatr Rev* 21(7):240-242, 2000.

Johnson RK: Changing eating and physical activity patterns of US children, *Proc Nutr Soc* 59(2):295-301, 2000.

Kellogg R: Understanding children's art. In *Readings in psychology today,* Del Mar, CA, 1969, Communications/Research/Machines.

Kennedy CM, Lipsitt LP: Risk-taking in preschool children, *J Pediatr Nurs* 13(2):77-84, 1998.

Kenny G: Assessing children's spirituality: what is the way forward? *Br J Nurs* 8(1):28, 30-32, 1999.

LaFontaine G, Bedard L: The prevention of infections in child daycare centers: potential influential factors, *Can J Public Health* 88(4):250-254, 1997.

Latz S, Wolf AW, Lozoff B: Cosleeping in context: sleep practices and problems in young children in Japan and the United States, *Arch Pediatr Adolesc Med* 153(4):339-346, 1999.

Maffulli N: Conference report: sports injuries in children, *Orthop Sports Med* 5(2):e1-3, 2001.

Martof A: Consultation with the specialist: dental care, *Pediatr Rev* 22(1):13-15, 2001.

McDevitt S, Carey W: The measurement of temperament in 3-7 year old children, *J Child Psychol Psychiatry* 19(3):245-253, 1978.

Muris P, Merckelbach H; Prins E: How serious are common childhood fears? II. The parent's point of view, *Behav Res Ther* 38(3):813-818, 2000.

National Association for the Education of Young Children, Position statement on school readiness [online] available: *www.naeyc.org,* 1995.

Owens J and others: Television-viewing habits and sleep disturbance in school children, *Pediatrics* 104(3):e27-40, 1999.

Robinson NM, Olszewski-Kubilius PM: Gifted and talented children: issues for pediatricians, *Pediatr Rev* 17(12):427-434, 1996.

Rovers MM and others: Day-care and otitis media in young children: a critical review, *Eur J Pediatr* 158(1):1-6, 1999.

Sawicki JA: Sibling rivalry and the new baby: anticipatory guidance and management strategies, *Pediatr Nurs* 23(3):298-309, 1997.

Schoentjes E, Deboutte D, Friedrich W: Child sexual behavior inventory: a Dutch-speaking normative sample, *Pediatrics* 104(4):885-893, 1999.

Stormshak and others: Parenting practices and child disruptive behavior problems in early elementary school, *J Clin Child Psychol* 29(1):17-29, 2000.

Thiedke CC: Sleep disorders and sleep problems in childhood, *Am Fam Physician* 63(2):277-284, 2001.

Thomas RM: *Comparing theories of child development,* ed 4, Belmont, Calif, 1996, Brooks-Cole.

US Department of Agriculture, Center for Nutrition Policy and Promotion: Tips for using the Food Guide Pyramid for young children 2 to 6 years old, *Program Aid 1647,* March 1999, *www.usda.gov/cnpp.*

Vanderheyden A, Witt JC: Proven practices for reducing aggression and noncompliant behaviors exhibited by young children at home and at school, *J La State Med Soc* 152(10):485-496, 2000.

Vessey JA, Yim-Chiplis PK, MacKenzie NR: Effects of television viewing on children's development, *Pediatr Nurs* 23(5):483-485, 1998.

Villani S: Impact of media on children and adolescents: a 10-year review research, *J Am Acad Child Adolesc Psychiatry* 40(4):392-401, 2001.

Winsler A and others: When learning a second language does not mean losing the first: bilingual language development in low-income, Spanish-speaking children attending bilingual preschool, *Child Dev* 70(2):349-362, 1999.

Wright K: Anticipatory guidance: developing a healthy sexuality, *Pediatr Ann Suppl* 26(2):142-145, 1997.

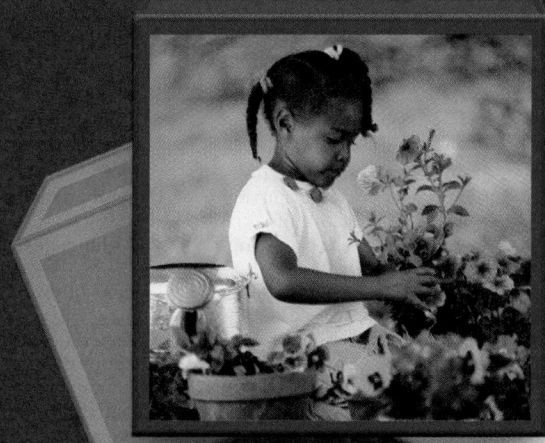

# Chapter 16

# Health Problems of Early Childhood

## Chapter Outline

**INFECTIOUS DISORDERS, 649**
**Communicable Diseases, 649**
*Nursing Care Plan: The Child with
a Communicable Disease, 662*
**Conjunctivitis, 662**
**Stomatitis, 664**
**INTESTINAL PARASITIC DISEASES, 665**
**General Nursing Considerations, 665**
**Giardiasis, 666**
**Enterobiasis (Pinworms), 667**
**INGESTION OF INJURIOUS AGENTS, 668**
**Principles of Emergency Treatment, 669**

Assessment, 669
Gastric Decontamination, 670
Prevention of Recurrence, 673
**Heavy Metal Poisoning, 675**
**Lead Poisoning, 675**
Children and Lead, 676
Causes of Lead Poisoning, 676
Anticipatory Guidance, 679
Screening for Lead Poisoning, 679
**CHILD MALTREATMENT, 683**
**Child Neglect, 683**
Types of Neglect, 683

**Physical Abuse, 684**
Munchausen Syndrome by Proxy
(MSBP), 684
Factors Predisposing to Physical
Abuse, 684
**Sexual Abuse, 685**
Characteristics of Abusers and Victims, 686
Initiation and Perpetuation
of Sexual Abuse, 686
**Nursing Care of the Maltreated Child, 687**
*Nursing Care Plan: The Child Who
Is Maltreated, 694*

## Related Topics

Collection of Specimens, Ch. 27
Compliance, Ch. 27
Controlling Elevated Temperatures, Ch. 27
Disorders Affecting the Skin, Ch. 18
Failure to Thrive, Ch. 13
Gynecologic Examination, Ch. 20
Health Practices, Ch. 2

Immunizations, Ch. 12
Infection Control, Ch. 27
Maintaining Healthy Skin, Ch. 27
Mechanisms Involved in Immunity, Ch. 35
Pain Assessment; Pain Management, Ch. 26
Pertussis (Whooping Cough), Ch. 32

Poisoning, Ch. 14
Posttraumatic Stress Disorder, Ch. 18
Rape, Ch. 20
Seizure Disorders, Ch. 37
Skin Lesions, Ch. 18
Stool Specimens, Ch. 27

# INFECTIOUS DISORDERS

## Communicable Diseases

The incidence of common childhood communicable diseases has declined greatly since the advent of immunizations. Serious complications resulting from such infections have been further reduced through the use of antibiotics and antitoxins. However, infectious diseases do occur, and nurses must be familiar with the infectious agent in order to recognize the disease and institute appropriate preventive and supportive interventions. To facilitate understanding of communicable diseases, several terms are defined in Box 16-1.

---

■ Nicole Sevier, MSN, RN, CPNP, revised this chapter.

### Nursing Considerations

The more common communicable diseases of childhood, their therapeutic management, and specific nursing care are described in Table 16-1. The following is a general discussion of nursing considerations for communicable diseases. The reader is also referred to Chapter 18 for a discussion of nursing care for dermatologic conditions.

### ▪▪ Assessment

Identification of the infectious agent is of primary importance to prevent exposure to susceptible individuals. Nurses in ambulatory clinics, emergency departments, preschools or regular schools, child care centers, and practitioners' offices are often the first persons to see signs of a communi-

---

**Box 16-1** ■ ■ ■
### Key Communicable Disease Terms

**Communicable disease**—An illness caused by a specific infectious agent or its toxic products through a direct or indirect mode of transmission of that agent from a reservoir

**Epidemic**—A disease occurring in a greater-than-expected number of cases in a community

**Endemic**—A disease occurring regularly within a geographic location

**Pandemic**—A disease affecting large portions of the population throughout the world

**Infectious agent**—An organism, such as bacteria or virus, that is capable of producing infection or infectious disease

**Reservoir**—Environment in which an infectious agent lives and multiplies and on which it depends for survival; humans are the most common reservoir of infections that are capable of producing disease in other humans

**Host**—A person, or other living animal, that affords subsistence to an infectious agent under natural conditions

**Source of infection**—The person, object, or substance from which an infectious agent passes immediately to the host; may be the reservoir (e.g., humans) or any one of the several modes of transmission (e.g., contaminated water)

**Carrier**—A person or animal that harbors an infectious agent without apparent clinical disease and serves as a potential source of infection

**Contact**—A person or animal that has been in association with an infected person, animal, or a contaminated environment that might provide an infective agent

**Mode of transmission**—Mechanism by which an infectious agent is transported from the reservoir to a susceptible human host. Types of transmission include the following:

   *Direct*—Direct and immediate transfer of infectious agents either by direct contact (touching, biting, kissing, or sexual intercourse) or droplet spread usually limited to a distance of about 1 meter or less (sneezing, coughing, spitting, singing, or talking)

   *Indirect*—Contact with contaminated objects or another infected source

   **Vehicle**—Any object serving as an intermediate means by which an infectious agent is transported from the reservoir to the host (usually fomites, water, soil, food, or biologic products such as plasma)

   **Vector**—Arthropods or other invertebrates that transmit infection by inoculation or deposition of infectious agents on skin, food, or other objects

   **Airborne**—Dissemination of microbial aerosols usually into the respiratory tract; may be droplet nuclei or dust (e.g., fungus spores separated from dry soil by wind)

**Incubation period**—Time interval between infection or exposure to disease and appearance of initial symptoms

**Period of communicability**—Time or times during which an infectious agent may be transferred directly or indirectly from an infected person to another person

**Prodromal period**—Interval between the time when early manifestations of disease appear to the time when overt clinical syndrome is evident

**Control measures**—Methods used to prevent spread of the organism; most common methods are immunizations, health education, medical treatment of infected person, and isolation or quarantine

**Isolation**—Separation of infected persons from noninfected persons for the period of communicability under conditions that will prevent transmission of the etiologic agent

**Quarantine**—Restriction of activities of persons who have been exposed to a communicable disease until the incubation period has expired

---

cable disease, such as a rash or sore throat. The nurse must operate under a high index of suspicion for common childhood diseases in order to identify potentially infectious cases and to recognize diseases that require medical intervention. An example is the common complaint of a sore throat. Although most often a symptom of a minor viral infection, a sore throat can signal diphtheria or a streptococcal infection such as scarlet fever. Each of these bacterial conditions requires appropriate medical treatment to prevent serious sequelae.

Assessment of the following is helpful in identifying potentially communicable diseases: (1) recent exposure to a known case, (2) *prodromal symptoms* (symptoms that occur between early manifestations of the disease and its overt clinical syndrome) or evidence of constitutional symptoms, such as a fever or rash (see Table 16-1), (3) immunization history, and (4) history of having the disease. Immunizations are available for many diseases, and infection usually confers lifelong immunity; therefore the possibility of many infectious agents can be eliminated on the basis of these two criteria.

### ❖ Nursing Diagnoses

A number of nursing diagnoses are prominent in the care of the child with a communicable disease, and others specific to individual cases become evident. The most common

nursing diagnoses are presented in the Nursing Care Plan on pp. 662-663.

### ❖ Planning

In addition to identification of the communicable disease (see Assessment), the principal goals for the child and family are as follows:

1. Child will not spread the infection to others.
2. Child will not experience complications.
3. Child will have minimal discomfort.
4. Child and family will receive adequate emotional support.

### ❖ Implementation

Many of the diseases require only supportive measures until the illness runs its course. Children are usually cared for at home until the disease is no longer communicable and until they feel well enough to resume normal activity.

**Prevent Spread.** Prevention consists of two components: prevention of the disease and control of its spread to others. Primary prevention rests almost exclusively on immunization. (See Immunizations, Chapter 12.)

Control measures to prevent spread of the disease include appropriate techniques to reduce the risk of cross-transmission of infectious organisms between patients and to protect health care workers from organisms harbored by patients. If the child is hospitalized, the facility's policies for

---

**Box 16-2** ■ ■ ▪
**Antiviral Medications Used to Treat Varicella and Zoster**

*Acyclovir (Zovirax):* Oral or intravenous; used in otherwise healthy children and adults
*Valcyclovir (Valtrex):* Oral; available for adults
*Famciclovir (Famvir):* Oral; available for adults
*Foscarnet (Foscavir):* Intravenous; effective against resistant strains of VZV

---

infection control are followed. (See Infection Control, Chapter 27.) The most important procedure to stress is handwashing. Persons directly caring for the child or handling contaminated articles must wash their hands before beginning care of another patient. The child is instructed to practice good handwashing technique after toileting and before eating. For diseases spread by droplets, the nurse instructs the family in measures aimed at reducing airborne transmission. The child who is old enough should use a tissue to cover the face during coughing or sneezing; otherwise the parent should cover the child's mouth with a tissue and then discard the tissue. The usual hygiene measures of not sharing eating and drinking utensils should be stressed to the family (American Academy of Pediatrics, 2000).

**NURSING ALERT** If a child is admitted to the hospital with an undiagnosed exanthema, strict isolation is instituted until a diagnosis is confirmed. Childhood communicable diseases requiring airborne precautions are diphtheria, measles, varicella zoster, and chickenpox (American Academy of Pediatrics, 2000).

**Prevent Complications.** Although most youngsters recover without any difficulty, certain groups of children are at risk for serious, even fatal, complications from communicable diseases, especially the viral diseases of chickenpox and erythema infectiosum (EI). Children with an immunodeficiency—those receiving steroid or other immunosuppressive therapy, those with a generalized malignancy, or lymphoma, or those with an immunologic disorder—are at risk for viremia from replication of the *varicella-zoster virus (VZV)** in the blood.

VZV causes two distinct diseases: *varicella (chickenpox)* and *zoster (herpes zoster or shingles).* Varicella occurs primarily in children under 15 years of age. However, it remains in latent form in the nerve roots and may be reactivated causing herpes zoster, an intensely painful condition that is localized to one or more dermatomes (body area innervated by a particular segment of the spinal cord) (Kakourou and others, 1998). Patients who are immunocompromised and healthy infants under 1 year of age (who also have reduced

---

*Educational materials for health care providers and families may be obtained from the **Varicella Zoster Virus Research Foundation,** 40 East 72nd St, New York, NY 10021; or Glaxo Wellcome, Inc, 3030 Cornwallis Rd, Research Triangle Park, NC 27709, (919) 248-3000 or (888) 825-5249; www.glaxowellcome.com.

---

**FAMILY FOCUS**
*Use of Acyclovir for Chickenpox*

Acyclovir decreases the number of varicella lesions, speeds healing of lesions, and shortens the duration of fever, itching, lethargy, and anorexia. The drug has little toxicity, and side effects are rare. Despite these benefits, however, the American Academy of Pediatrics (2000) does not recommend its use in otherwise healthy children with varicella. This group's main argument rests on the cost-benefit ratio.

Families, however, may view the cost-benefit issue differently. For many parents a sick child at home means loss of more than half a day from work. Caring for an irritable child is also exhausting. Because the main advantage is in lessening the severity of the illness, both the child and the parents benefit. With this in mind, nurses should be aware of the issues regarding treatment of chickenpox and discuss the options with the family.* The cost of therapy may be considerably less than the loss of income. Hopefully, with universal varicella vaccination, the incidence of this very common childhood disease will decrease dramatically, making the treatment decision for the family a moot point. (See Immunizations, Chapter 12.)

---

*For more information and a parent brochure on the drug, contact Glaxo Wellcome, PO Box 13398, Research Triangle Park, NC, 27709 1 (888) 825-5249, *www.glaxowellcome.com.*

immunity) are at a higher risk for reactivation of VZV, causing herpes zoster, probably as a result of a deficiency in cellular immunity (Bilgrami and others, 1999).

*Varicella-zoster immune globulin (VZIG)* may be given to high-risk children after exposure to chickenpox to prevent the development of varicella. Antiviral agents (Box 16-2) may also be used to treat varicella infections in children who are at increased risk for severe varicella or its complications. Other risk groups include otherwise healthy, nonpregnant individuals 12 years of age or older; children older than 12 months with a chronic cutaneous or pulmonary disorder; those receiving long-term salicylate therapy (because of the possible risk of Reye syndrome); and possibly children receiving short, intermittent, or aerosolized courses of corticosteroids. VZIG should be given to newborns as soon as possible after delivery if the mother has had an onset of VZV from 5 days before to 2 days after delivery (American Academy of Pediatrics, 2000). Because the long-term effects of antiviral agents on the fetus are unknown, they are not recommended for pregnant women with uncomplicated varicella. (See Family Focus box.) Maternal varicella infection before 20 weeks of gestation is associated with only a small risk of malformations in the fetus (Chapman, 1998).

Children with hemolytic disease, such as sickle cell disease, are at risk for aplastic anemia from EI. The *human parvovirus (HPV)* infects and lyses red blood cell precursors, thus interrupting the production of red blood cells. Therefore the virus may precipitate a severe aplastic crisis in patients who need increased red blood cell production to maintain normal cell volumes. Because the fetus depends on a high rate of red blood cell production and has an immature immune system, the fetus may develop severe anemia as a result of HPV infection in the mother.

*Text continued on p. 660*

**TABLE 16-1** Communicable diseases of childhood

**Disease**

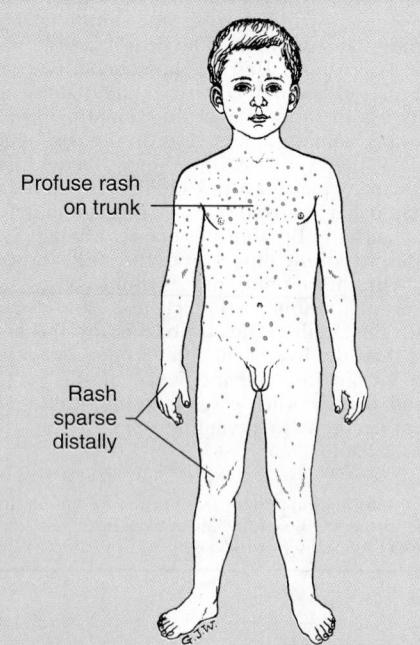

Profuse rash on trunk

Rash sparse distally

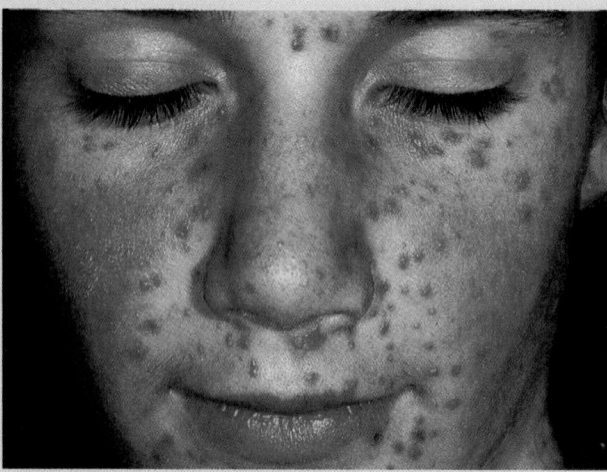

**Fig. 16-1** Chickenpox (varicella). (From Habif TP: *Clinical dermatology: a color guide to diagnosis and therapy*, ed 3, St Louis, 1996, Mosby.)

**Chickenpox (Varicella)** (Fig. 16-1)

*Etiology:* Varicella zoster virus (VZV)

*Source:* Respiratory secretions; to a lesser degree vesicular skin lesions (scabs not infectious)

*Transmission:* Direct contact, droplet (airborne) spread, and contaminated objects

*Incubation period:* 2 to 3 weeks, usually 13 to 17 days

*Period of communicability:* 1 day before eruption of lesions (prodromal period) to the time when all lesions have crusted

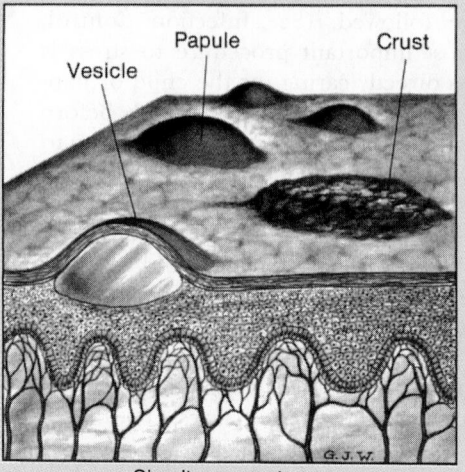

Papule    Crust

Vesicle

Simultaneous stages of lesions in chickenpox

**Diphtheria**

*Etiology: Corynebacterium diphtheriae*

*Source:* Respiratory secretions, skin, and other lesions

*Transmission:* Direct contact with infected person, a carrier, or contaminated articles

*Incubation period:* Usually 2 to 5 days, possibly longer

*Period of communicability:* Variable; until virulent bacilli are no longer present (identified by three negative cultures); usually 2 weeks but as long as 4 weeks

| Clinical Manifestations | Therapeutic Management/Complications | Nursing Considerations |
|---|---|---|
| *Prodromal stage:* Slight fever, malaise, and anorexia for first 24 hours; rash highly pruritic; begins as macule, rapidly progresses to papule and then vesicle (surrounded by erythematous base, breaks easily and forms crusts); all three stages (papule, vesicle, crust) present in varying degrees at one time<br>*Distribution:* Centripetal, spreading to face and proximal extremities but sparse on distal limbs and less on areas not exposed to heat (i.e., from clothing or sun)<br>*Constitutional signs and symptoms:* Fever, irritability from pruritus | *Treatment and supportive care:* Antiviral agent acyclovir (Zovirax), varicella-zoster immune globulin (VZIG) after exposure in high-risk children<br>*Supportive:* Diphenhydramine hydrochloride or antihistamines to relieve itching; skin care to prevent secondary bacterial infection<br>*Complications:*<br>   Secondary bacterial infections (abscesses, cellulitis, pneumonia, sepsis)<br>   Encephalitis<br>   Varicella pneumonia<br>   Hemorrhagic varicella (tiny hemorrhages in vesicles and numerous petechiae in skin)<br>   Chronic or transient thrombocytopenia | Maintain strict isolation in hospital<br>Isolate child in home until vesicles have all dried, and isolate immunosuppressed children from infected children<br>Administer skin care: give bath and change clothes and linens daily; administer topical calamine lotion; keep child's fingernails short and clean; apply mittens if child scratches<br>Administer antihistamines and antiviral agents<br>If older child, reason with child regarding danger of scar formation from scratching<br>Avoid use of aspirin; use acetaminophen for fever control |
| Vary according to anatomic location of pseudomembrane<br>*Nasal:* Resembles common cold, serosanguineous mucopurulent nasal discharge without constitutional symptoms; may be frank epistaxis<br>*Tonsillar/pharyngeal:* Malaise; anorexia; sore throat; low-grade fever; smooth, adherent, white or gray membrane; lymphadenitis<br>*Laryngeal:* Fever, hoarseness, cough, potential airway obstruction, apprehension, dyspneic retractions, cyanosis | *Treatment and supportive care:* Antitoxin (usually intravenously); preceded by skin or conjunctival test to rule out sensitivity to horse serum<br>Antibiotics (penicillin or erythromycin)<br>Complete bed rest (prevention of myocarditis)<br>Tracheostomy for airway obstruction<br>Treatment of infected contacts and carriers<br>*Complications:*<br>   Myocarditis<br>   Neuritis<br>   Toxemia<br>   Septic shock<br>   Death | Maintain strict isolation in hospital<br>Participate in sensitivity testing; have epinephrine available<br>Administer antibiotics; observe for signs of sensitivity to penicillin<br>Administer complete care to maintain bed rest<br>Use suctioning as needed to maintain patent airway<br>Observe respirations for signs of obstruction<br>Administer humidified oxygen if prescribed |

*Continued*

**TABLE 16-1** Communicable diseases of childhood—cont'd

**Disease**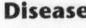

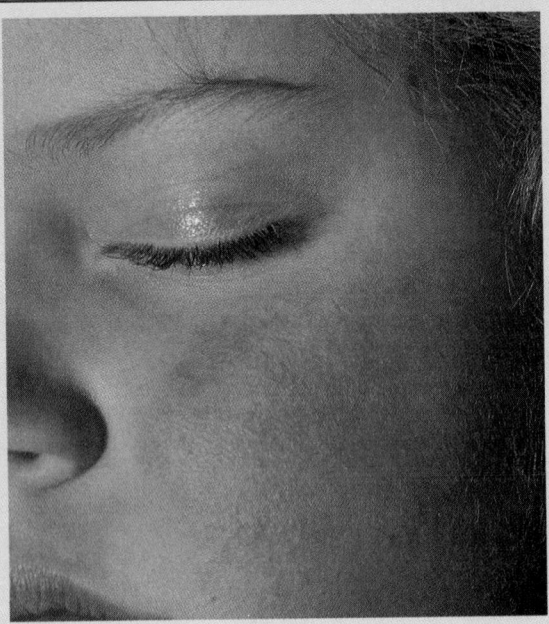

**Fig. 16-2** Erythema infectiosum. (From Habif TP: *Clinical dermatology: a color guide to diagnosis and therapy*, ed 3, St Louis, 1996, Mosby.)

**Erythema Infectiosum (Fifth Disease)** (Fig. 16-2)

*Etiology:* Human parvovirus B19 (HPV)
*Source:* Infected persons
*Transmission:* Unknown; possibly respiratory secretions and blood
*Incubation period:* 4 to 14 days, may be as long as 20 days
*Period of communicability:* Uncertain but before onset of symptoms in most children; also for approximately 1 week after onset of symptoms in children with aplastic crisis

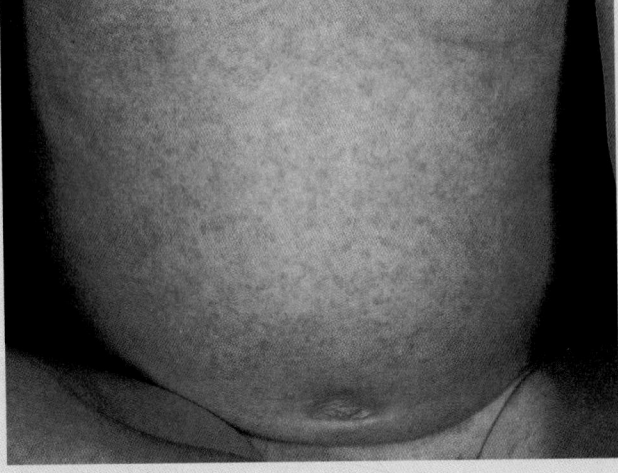

**Fig. 16-3** Roseola infantum. (From Habif TP: *Clinical dermatology: a color guide to diagnosis and therapy*, ed 3, St Louis, 1996, Mosby.)

**Exanthema Subitum (Roseola)** (Fig. 16-3)

*Etiology:* Human herpes virus type 6 (HHV-6)
*Source:* Unknown
*Transmission:* Unknown (occurs between 6 months and 3 years of age)
*Incubation period:* Usually 5-15 days
*Period of communicability:* Unknown

| Clinical Manifestations | Therapeutic Management/Complications | Nursing Considerations |
| --- | --- | --- |
| Rash appears in three stages:<br>I—Erythema on face, chiefly on cheeks, "slapped cheek" appearance; disappears by 1 to 4 days<br>II—Approximately 1 day after rash appears on face, maculopapular red spots appear, symmetrically distributed on upper and lower extremities; rash progresses from proximal to distal surfaces and may last a week or more<br>III—Rash subsides but reappears if skin is irritated or traumatized (sun, heat, cold, friction)<br>In children with aplastic crisis, rash is usually absent and prodromal illness includes fever, myalgia, lethargy, nausea, vomiting, and abdominal pain | ***Treatment and supportive care:*** Antipyretics, analgesics, antiinflammatory drugs. Blood transfusion for transient aplastic anemia as needed<br>***Complications:***<br>Self-limited or chronic arthritis; arthralgia (Moore, 2000)<br>May result in fetal death if mother infected during pregnancy but no evidence of congenital anomalies<br>Aplastic crisis in children with hemolytic disease or immune deficiency<br>Myocarditis (rare)<br>Encephalitis (rare) | Isolation of child not necessary, except hospitalized child (immunosuppressed or with aplastic crises) suspected of HPV infection is placed on respiratory isolation<br>Pregnant women: need not be excluded from workplace where HPV infection is present; explain low risk of fetal death to those in contact with affected children |
| Persistent high fever, greater than 102° F, for 3 to 4 days in child who appears well<br>Precipitous drop in fever to normal with appearance of rash; atypical exanthem subitum can occur without rash<br>***Rash:*** Discrete rose-pink macules or maculopapules appearing first on trunk, then spreading to neck, face, and extremities; nonpruritic, fades on pressure, appears 2 to 3 days after onset of fever, and lasts 1 to 2 days<br>***Associated signs and symptoms:***<br>Cervical/postauricular lymphadenopathy, injected pharynx, cough, coryza | ***Treatment and supportive care:*** Nonspecific<br>Antipyretics to control fever<br>***Complications:***<br>Recurrent febrile seizures (possibly from latent infection of central nervous system that is reactivated by fever)<br>Encephalitis (rare)<br>Hepatitis<br>Meningitis | Administer antipyretics as needed<br>If child is prone to seizures, discuss appropriate precautions, possibility of recurrent febrile seizures (Stoeckle, 2000) |

*Continued*

**TABLE 16-1**    Communicable diseases of childhood—cont'd

**Disease**

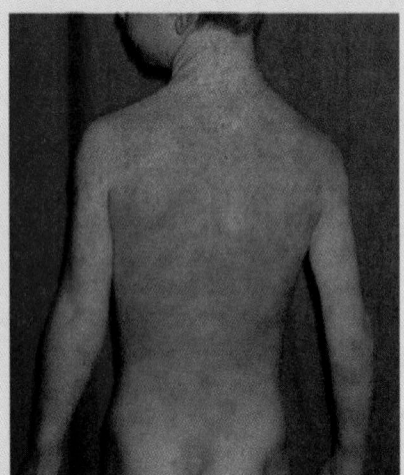

**First day of rash**    **Third day of rash**

Koplik spots on buccal mucosa (see inset)

Confluent maculopapules

Rash discrete

Discrete maculopapules

**Fig. 16-4**    Measles (rubeola). (Clinical view from Seidel HM and others: *Mosby's guide to physical examination,* ed 4, St Louis, 1999, Mosby; Koplik spots from Zitelli BJ, Davis HW: *Atlas of pediatric physical diagnosis,* ed 3, St Louis, 1997, Mosby.)

**Measles (Rubeola)** (Fig. 16-4)

*Etiology:* Virus
*Source:* Respiratory secretions, blood, and urine
*Transmission:* Usually by direct contact with droplets of infected person
*Incubation period:* 10 to 20 days
*Period of communicability:* From 4 days before to 5 days after rash appears but mainly during prodromal (catarrhal) stage

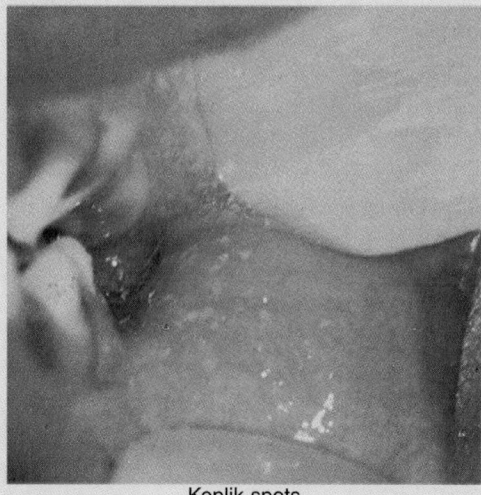

Koplik spots

**Mumps**

*Etiology:* Paramyxovirus
*Source:* Saliva
*Transmission:* Direct contact with or droplet spread from an infected person
*Incubation period:* 14 to 21 days
*Period of communicability:* Most communicable immediately before and after swelling begins

**Pertussis (Whooping Cough)**

*Etiology:* Bordetella pertussis
*Source:* Respiratory secretions
*Transmission:* Direct contact or droplet spread from infected person; indirect contact with freshly contaminated articles
*Incubation period:* 5 to 21 days, usually 10
*Period of communicability:* Greatest during catarrhal stage before onset of paroxysms and may extend to fourth week after onset of paroxysms

| Clinical Manifestations | Therapeutic Management/Complications | Nursing Considerations |
|---|---|---|
| *Prodromal (catarrhal) stage:* Fever and malaise, followed in 24 hours by coryza, cough, conjunctivitis, Koplik spots (small, irregular red spots with a minute, bluish white center first seen on buccal mucosa opposite molars 2 days before rash); symptoms gradually increase in severity until second day after rash appears, when they begin to subside<br>*Rash:* Appears 3 to 4 days after onset of prodromal stage; begins as erythematous maculopapular eruption on face and gradually spreads downward; more severe in earlier sites (appears confluent) and less intense in later sites (appears discrete); after 3 to 4 days assumes brownish appearance, and fine desquamation occurs over areas of extensive involvement<br>*Constitutional signs and symptoms:* Anorexia, malaise, generalized lymphadenopathy | *Treatment and supportive care:* Vitamin A supplementation (see text p. 660) Bed rest during febrile period; antipyretics Antibiotics to prevent secondary bacterial infection in high-risk children<br>*Complications:*<br>  Otitis media<br>  Pneumonia<br>  Bronchiolitis<br>  Obstructive laryngitis and laryngotracheitis<br>  Encephalitis | Isolation until fifth day of rash; if hospitalized, institute respiratory precautions<br>Maintain bed rest during prodromal stage; provide quiet activity<br>*Fever:* Instruct parents to administer antipyretics; avoid chilling; if child is prone to seizures, institute appropriate precautions (fever spikes to 40° C [104° F] between fourth and fifth days)<br>*Eye care:* Dim lights if photophobia present; clean eyelids with warm saline solution to remove secretions or crusts; keep child from rubbing eyes; examine cornea for signs of ulceration<br>*Coryza/cough:* Use cool mist vaporizer; protect skin around nares with layer of petrolatum; encourage fluids and soft, bland foods<br>*Skin care:* Keep skin clean; use tepid baths as necessary |
| *Prodromal stage:* Fever, headache, malaise, and anorexia for 24 hours, followed by jaw or ear pain that is aggravated by chewing<br>*Parotitis:* By third day, parotid gland(s) (either unilateral or bilateral) enlarge(s) and reach(es) maximum size in 1 to 3 days; accompanied by pain and tenderness | *Treatment and supportive care:* Analgesics for pain and antipyretics for fever Intravenous fluid may be necessary for child who refuses to drink or vomits because of meningoencephalitis<br>*Complications:*<br>  Sensorineural deafness<br>  Postinfectious encephalitis<br>  Myocarditis<br>  Arthritis<br>  Hepatitis<br>  Epididymo-orchitis<br>  Sterility<br>  Meningitis<br>  Encephalitis | Isolation during period of communicability; institute respiratory precautions during hospitalization<br>Maintain bed rest during prodromal phase until swelling subsides<br>Give analgesics for pain<br>Encourage fluids and soft, bland foods; avoid foods that require chewing<br>Apply hot or cold compresses to neck, whichever is more comforting<br>To relieve orchitis, provide warmth and local support with tight-fitting underpants (stretch bathing suit works well) |
| *Catarrhal stage:* Begins with symptoms of upper respiratory tract infection, such as coryza, sneezing, lacrimation, cough, and low-grade fever; symptoms continue for 1 to 2 weeks, when dry, hacking cough becomes more severe<br>*Paroxysmal stage:* Cough most often occurs at night and consists of short, rapid coughs followed by sudden inspiration associated with a high-pitched crowing sound or "whoop"; during paroxysms cheeks become flushed or cyanotic; vomiting often follows attack; stage generally lasts 4 to 6 weeks, followed by convalescent stage | *Treatment and supportive care:* Hospitalization required for infants, children who are dehydrated, or those who have complications<br>Bed rest<br>Administration of pertussis-immune globulin<br>Humidified oxygen<br>Antimicrobial therapy (e.g., erythromycin)<br>Adequate hydration<br>*Complications:*<br>  Pneumonia<br>  Atelectasis<br>  Otitis media<br>  Seizure<br>  Hemorrhage (subarachnoid, subconjunctival, epistaxis)<br>  Dehydration<br>  Hernia<br>  Prolapsed rectum | Isolation during catarrhal stage; if hospitalized, institute respiratory precautions<br>Maintain bed rest as long as fever present<br>Provide restful environment and reduce factors that promote paroxysms (dust, smoke, sudden change in temperature, chilling, activity, excitement); keep room well ventilated<br>Encourage fluids; offer small amount of fluids frequently; refeed child after vomiting<br>Provide high humidity (humidifier or tent); suction as needed<br>Observe for signs of airway obstruction (restlessness, apprehension, retractions, cyanosis) |

*Continued*

**TABLE 16-1** Communicable diseases of childhood—cont'd

**Disease**

**Poliomyelitis**

*Etiology:* Enteroviruses, three types: type 1—most frequent cause of paralysis, both epidemic and endemic; type 2—least frequently associated with paralysis; type 3—second most frequently associated with paralysis

*Source:* Feces and oropharyngeal secretions

*Transmission:* Direct contact with persons with apparent or inapparent active infection; spread via fecal-oral and pharyngeal-oropharyngeal routes

*Incubation period:* Usually 7 to 14 days, with range of 5 to 35 days

*Period of communicability:* Not exactly known; virus is present in throat and feces shortly after infection and persists for approximately 1 week in throat and 4 to 6 weeks in feces

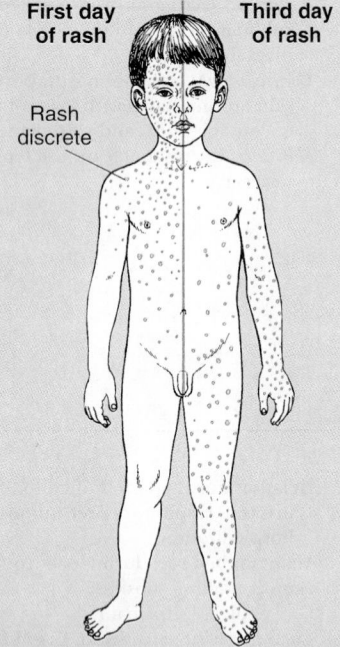

First day of rash

Third day of rash

Rash discrete

**Rubella (German Measles)** (Fig. 16-5)

*Etiology:* Rubella virus

*Source:* Respiratory secretions; virus also present in blood, stool, and urine

*Transmission:* Direct contact and spread via infected person; indirectly via articles freshly contaminated with nasopharyngeal secretions, feces, or urine

*Incubation period:* 14 to 21 days

*Period of communicability:* 7 days before to approximately 5 days after appearance of rash

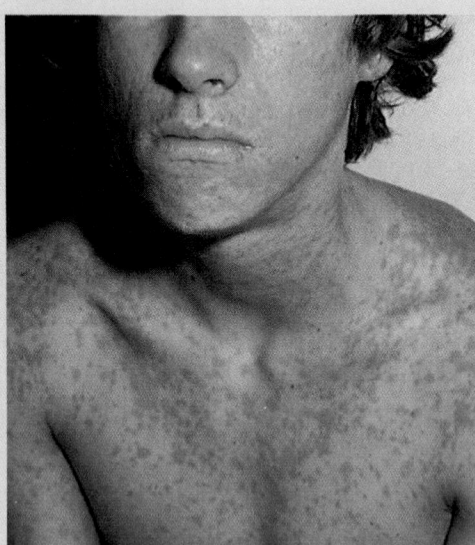

**Fig. 16-5** Rubella (German measles). (Clinical view from Zitelli BJ, Davis HW: *Atlas of pediatric physical diagnosis,* ed 3, St Louis, 1997, Mosby; courtesy Dr. Michael Sherlock.)

| Clinical Manifestations | Therapeutic Management/Complications | Nursing Considerations |
|---|---|---|
| May be manifested in three different forms:<br>*Abortive or inapparent*—Fever, uneasiness, sore throat, headache, anorexia, vomiting, abdominal pain; lasts a few hours to a few days<br>*Nonparalytic*—Same manifestations as abortive but more severe, with pain and stiffness in neck, back, and legs<br>*Paralytic*—Initial course similar to nonparalytic type, followed by recovery and then signs of central nervous system paralysis | *Treatment and Supportive Care:* No specific treatment, including antimicrobials or gamma globulin<br>Analgesics<br>Complete bed rest during acute phase<br>Assisted respiratory ventilation in case of respiratory paralysis<br>Physical therapy for muscles following acute stage<br>*Complications:*<br>  Permanent paralysis<br>  Respiratory arrest<br>  Hypertension<br>  Kidney stones from demineralization of bone during prolonged immobility | Maintain complete bed rest<br>Administer mild sedatives as necessary to relieve anxiety and promote rest<br>Participate in physiotherapy procedures (use of moist hot packs and range-of-motion exercises)<br>Position child to maintain body alignment and prevent contractures or decubiti; use foot board<br>Encourage child to move; administer analgesics for maximum comfort during physical activity<br>Observe for respiratory paralysis (difficulty in talking, ineffective cough, inability to hold breath, shallow and rapid respirations); have tracheostomy tray at bedside |
| *Prodromal stage:* Absent in children, present in adults and adolescents; consists of low-grade fever, headache, malaise, anorexia, mild conjunctivitis, coryza, sore throat, cough, and lymphadenopathy; lasts for 1 to 5 days, subsides 1 day after appearance of rash<br>*Rash:* First appears on face and rapidly spreads downward to neck, arms, trunk, and legs; by end of first day, body is covered with a discrete, pinkish red maculopapular exanthema; disappears in same order as it began and is usually gone by third day<br>*Constitutional signs and symptoms:* Occasionally low-grade fever, headache, malaise, and lymphadenopathy | *Treatment and Supportive Care:* No treatment necessary other than antipyretics for low-grade fever and analgesics for discomfort<br>*Complications:*<br>  Rare (arthritis, encephalitis, or purpura); most benign of all childhood communicable diseases; greatest danger is teratogenic effect on fetus | Reassure parents of benign nature of illness in affected child<br>Use comfort measures as necessary<br>Isolate child from pregnant women |

*Continued*

**TABLE 16-1 Communicable diseases of childhood—cont'd**

**Disease**

**Scarlet Fever** (Fig. 16-6)

*Etiology:* Group A β-hemolytic streptococci
*Source:* Respiratory secretions
*Transmission:* Direct contact with infected person or droplet spread; indirectly by contact with contaminated articles, ingestion of contaminated milk or other food
*Incubation period:* 2 to 4 days, with range of 1 to 7 days
*Period of communicability:* During incubation period and clinical illness approximately 10 days; during first 2 weeks of carrier phase, although may persist for months

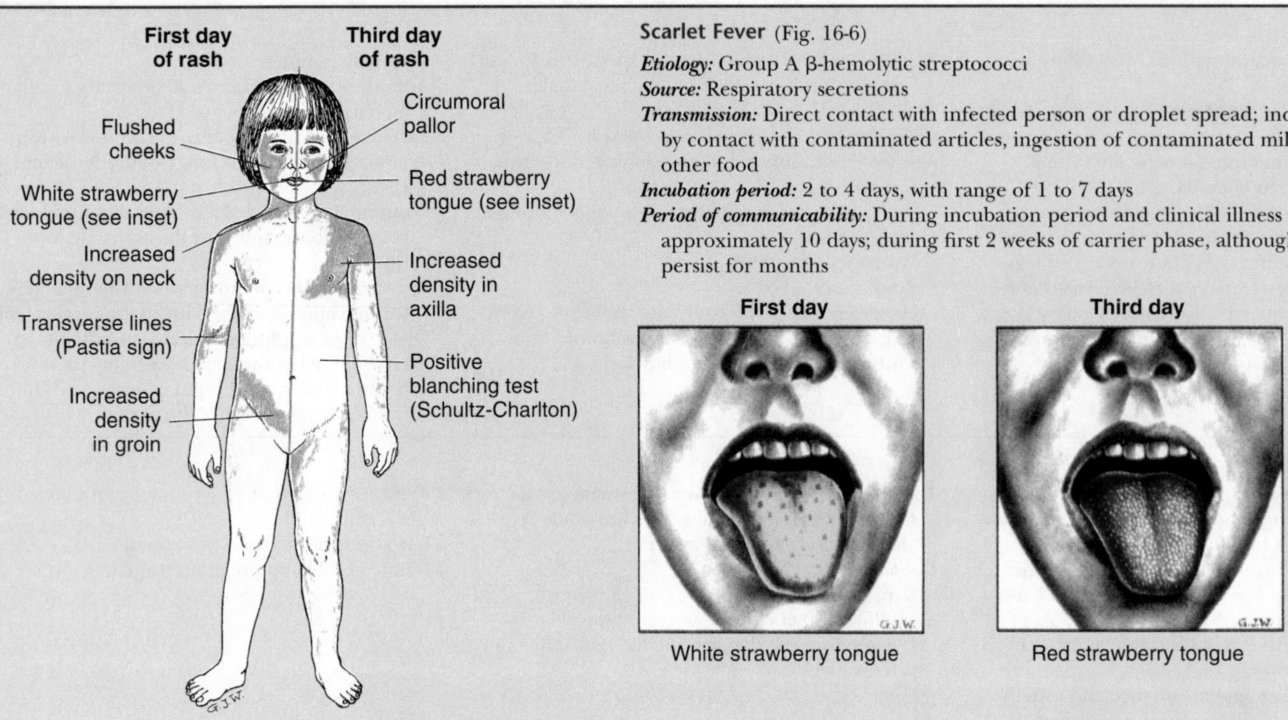

First day of rash
Third day of rash
Flushed cheeks
Circumoral pallor
White strawberry tongue (see inset)
Red strawberry tongue (see inset)
Increased density on neck
Increased density in axilla
Transverse lines (Pastia sign)
Positive blanching test (Schultz-Charlton)
Increased density in groin
First day
Third day
White strawberry tongue
Red strawberry tongue

**Fig. 16-6** Scarlet fever.

> **NURSING ALERT** High-risk children who have signs of communicable diseases are referred to the practitioner immediately. School nurses are responsible for warning the parents about recent outbreaks of communicable diseases to prevent the children's exposure to known cases.

Prevention of complications from diseases such as diphtheria and scarlet fever necessitates compliance with antibiotic therapy. With oral preparations the need to complete the entire course of therapy is stressed. (See Compliance, Chapter 27.)

Recent evidence suggests that vitamin A supplementation reduces both morbidity and mortality in measles and that all children with severe measles should be given vitamin A supplements (Semba, 1999). The American Academy of Pediatrics (2000), based on available data, recommends vitamin A supplementation in the following selected circumstances:

- Patients 6 months to 2 years of age hospitalized with measles and its complications (e.g., croup, pneumonia, diarrhea)
- Patients over 6 months of age who have measles and any of the following risk factors (and who are not already receiving vitamin A): immunodeficiency, clinical evidence of vitamin A deficiency, impaired intestinal absorption, moderate to severe malnutrition (including that associated with eating disorders), and recent immigrants from areas with high mortality rates from measles

A single oral dose of 200,000 IU for children at least 1 year old (half that dose for children 6 to 12 months of age) is recommended. The higher dose may be associated with vomiting and headache for a few hours. The dose should be repeated the next day and at 4 weeks for children with ophthalmologic evidence of vitamin A deficiency (American Academy of Pediatrics, 2000).

> **NURSING ALERT** Although the risk of vitamin A toxicity from these doses (they are 100 to 200 times the recommended dietary allowance) is very low, nurses should instruct parents on safe storage of the drug to avoid accidental ingestion. Ideally, vitamin A should be dispensed in the age-appropriate unit dose to prevent excessive administration and possible toxicity.

**Provide Comfort.** Many of the communicable diseases cause skin manifestations that are annoying or uncomfortable. The chief discomfort from most of the rashes is itching, and measures such as cool baths (usually without soap or with oatmeal preparations) and lotions (e.g., calamine) are helpful.

> **NURSING ALERT** When lotions with active ingredients such as diphenhydramine are used, they are applied sparingly, especially over open lesions, where excessive absorption can lead to drug toxicity. These lotions should be avoided in children simultaneously receiving oral diphenhydramine.

To avoid overheating, which increases itching, children should wear lightweight, loose, nonirritating clothing and

| Clinical Manifestations | Therapeutic Management/Complications | Nursing Considerations |
| --- | --- | --- |
| *Prodromal stage:* High fever, vomiting, headache, chills, malaise, abdominal pain<br><br>*Enanthema:* Tonsils enlarged, edematous, reddened, and covered with patches of exudate; in severe cases appearance resembles membrane seen in diphtheria; pharynx is edematous and beefy red; during first 1 to 2 days tongue is coated and papillae become red and swollen (white strawberry tongue); by fourth or fifth day white coat sloughs off, leaving prominent papillae (red strawberry tongue); palate is covered with erythematous punctate lesions<br><br>*Exanthema:* Rash appears within 12 hours after prodromal stage; red pinhead-sized punctate lesions rapidly become generalized but are absent on face, which becomes flushed with striking circumoral pallor; rash is more intense in folds of joints; by end of first week desquamation begins (fine, sandpaper-like on torso; sheet-like sloughing on palms and soles), which may be complete by 3 weeks or longer | *Treatment and supportive care:* Penicillin (or erythromycin in penicillin-sensitive children); fever should subside 24 hours after beginning therapy<br>Antibiotic therapy for newly diagnosed carriers (nose or throat cultures positive for streptococci)<br>Bed rest during febrile phase, analgesics for sore throat<br>*Complications:*<br>  Otitis media<br>  Peritonsillar abscess<br>  Sinusitis<br>  Glomerulonephritis<br>  Carditis, polyarthritis (uncommon) | Institute respiratory precautions until 24 hours after initiation of treatment<br>Ensure compliance with oral antibiotic therapy (intramuscular benzathine penicillin G [Bicillin] may be given if compliance is questionable)<br>Maintain bed rest during febrile phase; provide quiet activity during convalescent period<br>Relieve discomfort of sore throat with analgesics, gargles, lozenges, antiseptic throat sprays, and inhalation of cool mist<br>Encourage fluids during febrile phase; avoid irritating liquids (citrus juices) or rough foods; when child is able to eat, begin with soft diet<br>Advise parents to consult practitioner if fever persists after beginning therapy |

keep out of the sun. If the child persists in scratching, the nails are kept short and smooth; mittens and clothes with long sleeves or legs may be needed. For severe itching, an antipruritic medication such as diphenhydramine (Benadryl) or hydroxyzine (Atarax) may be required, especially when the child desires to sleep.

An elevated temperature is common, and both antipyretic medicine (acetaminophen [Tylenol] or ibuprofen [Children's Motrin or Children's Advil]) and environmental manipulation are implemented. (See Controlling Elevated Temperatures, Chapter 27.) The use of aspirin for fever control is avoided because of the associated risk of Reye syndrome.

A sore throat, another common symptom, is managed with lozenges, saline rinses (if the child is old enough to cooperate), and analgesics. Because most children have a poor appetite during an illness, bland foods and increased liquids (such as broth, juice, gelatin, and flavored ice pops) are usually preferred. During the early stages of the disease children voluntarily curtail their activity. Although bed rest is beneficial, it should not be imposed unless specifically indicated (e.g., with pertussis). During periods of irritability, quiet activity (e.g., reading, music, television, puzzles, coloring) helps distract children from the discomfort.

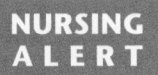

**NURSING ALERT**

The occurrence of a communicable disease provides the opportunity to ask parents about the child's immunization status and reinforce the benefits of vaccines for children.

**Support Child and Family.** Most communicable diseases are benign, but they produce considerable concern and anxiety for some parents. Often the occurrence of a disease such as chickenpox is the first time the child is acutely uncomfortable. Parents need assistance to cope effectively with manifestations of the illness, such as intense itching. Sometimes a visiting nurse may be beneficial to help the family develop a plan of care and encourage compliance with any treatments.

The family and child need reassurance that recovery from the disease is generally rapid. However, visible signs of the dermatosis may be present for some time after the child is well enough to resume the usual activities. For example, children with chickenpox may return to school 5 days after onset of the rash, or sooner if all lesions are crusted (American Academy of Pediatrics, 2000). (See Atraumatic Care box.)

**ATRAUMATIC CARE**

*Returning to School with Visible Skin Lesions*

When the disease involves noticeable signs, such as the crusts of chickenpox, the child benefits from preparation before returning to school. For example, the parent can discuss the child's physical appearance with the teacher and/or school nurse and request that they explain the child's condition to classmates.

## ✖ Evaluation

The effectiveness of nursing interventions is determined by continual reassessment and evaluation of care based on the following observational guidelines:

1. Observe or inquire about family members' use of control measures; observe for signs of disease in household contacts.
2. Monitor vital signs, especially temperature; inquire about the identification of high-risk contacts and appropriate isolation of the contact; observe or inquire about compliance with antibiotic or antiviral therapy.
3. Inquire about effectiveness of comfort measures.
4. Interview family and child regarding their feelings and concerns, especially when child returns to school.

The *expected outcomes* are described in the Nursing Care Plan on pp. 662-663.

## Conjunctivitis

Acute conjunctivitis, inflammation of the conjunctiva, occurs from a variety of causes that are typically age related. In newborns conjunctivitis can occur from infection during birth, most often from *Chlamydia trachomatis* (inclusion conjunctivitis) or *Neisseria gonorrhoeae*. These organisms, as well as herpes simplex virus (HSV), cause serious ocular damage. In infants recurrent conjunctivitis may be a sign of nasolacrimal (tear) duct obstruction. In children the usual causes are viral, bacterial, allergic, or related to a foreign body. Bacterial infection accounts for most instances of acute conjunctivitis in children. Diagnosis is made primarily from the clinical manifestations (Box 16-3), although cultures of purulent drainage may be needed to identify the specific cause.

# Nursing Care Plan
## The Child with a Communicable Disease

> **NURSING DIAGNOSIS:** Risk for infection related to susceptible host and infectious agents

### PATIENT GOAL 1: Will not become infected

- **NURSING INTERVENTIONS/RATIONALES**

Be highly suspicious of infectious diseases, especially in susceptible children

Identify high-risk children (e.g., those with an immunodeficiency or hemolytic disease) to whom communicable disease may be fatal; in case of an outbreak, advise parents to confine child to the home *to avoid exposure*

Participate in public education and service programs regarding prophylactic immunizations, method of spread of communicable diseases, proper preparation and handling of food and water supplies, control of animal vectors in regard to reservoirs of disease (not a factor in childhood communicable disease but in other infectious illness such as malaria), or screening programs to identify streptococcal infections

- **EXPECTED OUTCOME**

Susceptible children do not contract the disease

### PATIENT GOAL 2: Will not spread disease

- **NURSING INTERVENTIONS/RATIONALES**

Institute appropriate infection control practices (see Chapter 27)

Make referral to public health nurse when necessary *to ensure appropriate procedures in the home*

Work with families *to ensure compliance with therapeutic regimens*

Identify close contacts who may require prophylactic treatment (e.g., specific immune globulin or antibiotics)

Report disease to local health department if appropriate

- **EXPECTED OUTCOME**

Infection remains confined to original source

### PATIENT GOAL 3: Will exhibit no evidence of complications

- **NURSING INTERVENTIONS/RATIONALES**

Ensure compliance with therapeutic regimen (e.g., bed rest, antiviral therapy, antibiotics, adequate hydration)

Avoid giving aspirin to children with viral illness *because of the possible risk of Reye syndrome*

Institute seizure precautions if febrile convulsions are a possibility

Monitor temperature; *unexpected elevations may signal an infection*

Maintain good body hygiene *to reduce risk of secondary infection of lesions*

Offer small, frequent sips of water or favorite drinks *to ensure adequate hydration* and soft, bland foods (gelatin, pudding, ice cream, soups) *because many children are anorectic during an illness;* feed again after vomiting; observe for signs of dehydration

- **EXPECTED OUTCOME**

Child exhibits no evidence of complications such as infection or dehydration

> **NURSING DIAGNOSIS:** Pain related to skin lesions, malaise

### PATIENT GOAL 1: Will experience minimal discomfort

- **NURSING INTERVENTIONS/RATIONALES**

Use cool-mist vaporizer, gargles, and lozenges *to keep mucous membranes moist*

Cleanse eyes with physiologic saline solution *to remove secretions or crusts*

Keep skin clean; change bedclothes and linens at least daily

Maintain meticulous oral hygiene

Keep child cool *because overheating increases itching*

Give cool baths and apply lotion such as calamine *to decrease itching*

## Therapeutic Management

Treatment of conjunctivitis depends on the cause. Viral conjunctivitis is self-limiting, and treatment is removal of the accumulated secretions. Bacterial conjunctivitis is usually treated with topical antibacterial agents such as polymyxin and bacitracin (Polysporin), sodium sulfacetamide (Sulamyd), or trimethoprim and polymyxin (Polytrim) (Yetman and Coody, 1997). Drops may be used during the day, with an ointment at bedtime because the ointment preparation remains in the eye longer. Ointments are usually not used in the daytime because they blur vision. Corticosteroids are avoided because they reduce ocular resistance to bacteria. Supportive treatment includes removal of the accumulated secretions. (Prevention of neonatal conjunctivitis, or ophthalmia neonatorum, is discussed in Chapter 8.)

## Nursing Considerations

Nursing goals include keeping the eye clean and properly administering ophthalmic medication. Accumulated secretions are always removed by wiping from the inner canthus downward and outward, away from the opposite eye. Warm, moist compresses, such as a clean washcloth wrung out with hot tap water, are helpful in removing the crusts. Older children can loosen the crusts during a warm shower. Compresses are *not* kept on the eye, because an occlusive covering promotes bacterial growth. Medication is instilled immediately after the eyes have been cleaned and according to correct procedure. (See Chapter 27.)

Prevention of infection in other family members is an important consideration with bacterial conjunctivitis. The child's washcloth and towel are kept separate from those

# Nursing Care Plan
## The Child with a Communicable Disease—cont'd

Assess need for pain medication (see Chapter 26)
Employ nonpharmacologic pain reduction techniques (see Chapter 26)
*Administer analgesics, antipyretics, and antipruritics as needed

- **EXPECTED OUTCOMES**

Skin and mucous membranes are clean and free of irritants
Child exhibits minimal evidence of discomfort (specify)

> **NURSING DIAGNOSIS:** Impaired social interaction related to isolation from peers

**PATIENT GOAL 1:** Will have some understanding of reason for isolation

- **NURSING INTERVENTIONS/***RATIONALES*

Explain reason for confinement and use of any special precautions *to increase child's understanding of restrictions*
Allow child to play with gloves, mask, and gown (if used) *to facilitate positive coping*

- **EXPECTED OUTCOME**

Child demonstrates understanding of restrictions

**PATIENT GOAL 2:** Will have opportunity to participate in suitable activities

- **NURSING INTERVENTIONS/***RATIONALES*

Always introduce self to child; allow child to see face before donning isolation masks, if required
Provide diversionary activity
Encourage parents to remain with child during hospitalization *to decrease separation and provide companionship*
Encourage contact with friends via telephone
Prepare child's peers for altered physical appearance, such as with chickenpox, *to encourage peer acceptance*

- **EXPECTED OUTCOMES**

Child engages in suitable activities and interactions
Peers accept child

> **NURSING DIAGNOSIS:** Risk for impaired skin integrity related to scratching from pruritus

**PATIENT GOAL 1:** Will maintain skin integrity

- **NURSING INTERVENTIONS/***RATIONALES*

Keep nails short and clean *to minimize trauma and secondary infection*
Apply mittens or elbow restraints *to prevent scratching*
Dress in lightweight, loose, and nonirritating clothing *because overheating increases itching*
Cover affected areas (long sleeves, pants, one-piece outfit) *to prevent scratching*
Bathe in cool water with colloidal oatmeal
Avoid use of soap, *which causes drying of skin*
Apply soothing lotions (sparingly on open lesions *because absorption of drug is increased*) to decrease pruritus
Avoid exposure to heat or sun, *which can aggravate rash* (e.g., chickenpox)

- **EXPECTED OUTCOME**

Skin remains intact

> **NURSING DIAGNOSIS:** Interrupted family processes related to child with an acute illness

**PATIENT GOAL 1:** Will receive adequate emotional support

- **NURSING INTERVENTIONS/***RATIONALES*

Inform parents of treatment options, especially antiviral agents for varicella
Reinforce family's effort to carry out plan of care
Provide assistance when necessary, such as visiting nurse *to help with home care*
Keep family aware of child's progress *to encourage optimistic attitude*
Stress rapidity of recovery in most cases *to decrease anxiety*

- **EXPECTED OUTCOMES**

Family continues to comply with expectations
Family seeks needed support

*Dependent nursing action.

## Box 16-3 ■ ■ ■
## Clinical Manifestations of Conjunctivitis

**BACTERIAL CONJUNCTIVITIS**

   Purulent drainage
   Crusting of eyelids, especially on awakening
   Inflamed conjunctiva
   Swollen lids

**VIRAL CONJUNCTIVITIS**
*General*

   Usually occurs with upper respiratory tract infection
   Serous (watery) drainage
   Inflamed conjunctiva
   Swollen lids

*Hemorrhagic*

   Caused by specific virus, enterovirus 70
   Severe inflammation
   Subconjunctival hemorrhage
   Photophobia (sensitivity to light)

**ALLERGIC CONJUNCTIVITIS**

   Itching
   Watery to viscous stringy discharge
   Inflamed conjunctiva
   Swollen lids

**CONJUNCTIVITIS CAUSED BY FOREIGN BODY**

   Tearing
   Pain
   Inflamed conjunctiva

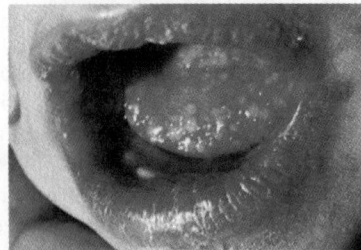

**Fig. 16-7**  Primary gingivostomatitis. (From Thompson JM and others: *Clinical nursing*, St Louis, 1986, Mosby.)

**NURSING ALERT**  Signs of serious conjunctivitis include reduction or loss of vision, ocular pain, photophobia, exophthalmos (bulging eyeball), decreased ocular mobility, corneal ulceration, and unusual patterns of inflammation (e.g., the perilimbal flush associated with iritis or localized inflammation associated with scleritis). If a patient has any of these signs, refer immediately to an ophthalmologist (Ruppert, 1996).

used by others. Tissues used to clean the eye are disposed of properly. The child should not rub the eyes and should be instructed in good handwashing technique.

## Stomatitis

Stomatitis is inflammation of the oral mucosa, which may include the cheek, lip, tongue, gingiva, palate, and floor of the mouth. It may be infectious or noninfectious and may be caused by local or systemic factors. Aphthous stomatitis and herpetic stomatitis are typically seen in children. Children with immunosuppression and those receiving chemotherapy or head and neck radiotherapy are at high risk for developing mucosal ulceration and herpetic stomatitis. (See Managing Side Effects of Treatment, Chapter 36.)

*Aphthous stomatitis (aphthous ulcer, canker sore)* is a benign but painful condition; the cause is unknown. Its onset is usually associated with mild traumatic injury (biting the cheek, hitting the mucosa with a toothbrush, or a mouth appliance rubbing on the mucosa), allergy, and emotional stress. Typ-

ically these lesions are painful, small, whitish ulcerations surrounded by a red border. They are distinguished from other types of stomatitis by healthy adjacent tissues, absence of vesicles, and no systemic illness. The ulcers persist for 4 to 12 days and heal uneventfully. Over the past decade a syndrome of periodic fever, aphthous stomatitis, pharyngitis, and cervical adenitis (or PFAPA) has been described, the cause of which is unknown (Feder, 2000). Children with PFAPA grow normally and exhibit no long-term sequelae.

*Herpetic gingivostomatitis (HGS)* is caused by the herpes simplex virus, most often type 1, and may occur as a primary infection or recur in a less severe form known as recurrent herpes labialis (commonly called "cold sores" or "fever blisters"). The primary infection usually begins with a fever; the pharynx becomes edematous and erythematous, and vesicles erupt on the mucosa, causing severe pain (Fig. 16-7). Cervical lymphadenitis often occurs, and the breath has a distinctly foul odor. The disease can last 5 to 14 days, with varying degrees of severity.

In the recurrent form the vesicles appear on the lips, usually singly or in groups. The precipitating factors for the cold sores include emotional stress, trauma (often related to dental procedures), immunosuppression, or exposure to excessive sunlight.

### Therapeutic Management

Treatment for both types of stomatitis is aimed at relief of symptoms, primarily pain. Acetaminophen is usually sufficient for mild cases, but stronger analgesics such as codeine may be needed for more severe HGS. Topical anesthetics are helpful and include over-the-counter preparations such as Orabase, Anbesol, and Kank-a. Lidocaine (Xylocaine Viscous) can be prescribed for the child who can keep 1 teaspoon of the solution in the mouth for 2 to 3 minutes and then expectorate the drug. A mixture of equal parts of diphenhydramine (Benadryl) elixir and Maalox provides mild analgesia, antiinflammatory properties, and a protective coating for the lesions. Specific treatment for children with severe cases of HGS is the use of antiviral agents (Olin and others, 2000).

### Nursing Considerations

The chief nursing goals for children with stomatitis are relief of pain and prevention of spread of the herpes virus. Analgesics and topical anesthetics are used as needed to

**TABLE 16-2**   Selected intestinal parasites

| Clinical Manifestations | Comments |
| --- | --- |
| **Ascariasis—*Ascaris lumbricoides* (Common Roundworm)** | |
| Light infections: asymptomatic<br>Heavy infections: anorexia, irritability, nervousness, enlarged abdomen, weight loss, fever, intestinal colic<br>Severe infections: intestinal obstruction, appendicitis, perforation of intestine with peritonitis, obstructive jaundice, pneumonitis | Transferred to mouth by way of contaminated food, fingers, or toys<br>Largest of the intestinal helminths<br>Affects principally young children 1-4 years of age<br>Prevalent in warm climates |
| **Hookworm Disease—*Necator americanus*** | |
| Light infections in well-nourished individuals: no problems<br>Heavier infections: mild to severe anemia, malnutrition<br>May be itching and burning followed by erythema and a papular eruption in areas to which the organism migrates | Transmitted by discharging eggs on the soil and in turn picking up infection from direct skin contact with contaminated soil<br>Wearing shoes is recommended, although children playing in contaminated soil expose many skin surfaces |
| **Strongyloidiasis—*Strongyloides stercoralis* (Threadworm)** | |
| Light infection: asymptomatic<br>Heavy infection: respiratory signs and symptoms; abdominal pain, distention; nausea and vomiting; diarrhea—large, pale stools, often with mucus<br>Threat to life in children with weakened immunologic defenses | Transmission is same as for hookworm, except autoinfection common<br>Older children and adults affected more often than young children<br>Severe infections may lead to severe nutritional deficiency |
| **Visceral Larva Migrans—*Toxocara canis* (Dogs); Intestinal Toxocariasis—*Toxocara cati* (Cats)** | |
| Depends on reactivity of infected individual<br>May be asymptomatic except for eosinophilia<br>Specific diagnosis difficult | Transmitted by direct contamination of hands from contact with dog, cat, or objects; or ingestion of soil<br>Dogs and cats should be kept away from areas where children play; sandboxes are especially important transmission areas<br>Periodic deworming of diagnosed dogs and cats |
| **Trichuriasis—*Trichuris trichiura* (Whipworm)** | |
| Light infections: asymptomatic<br>Heavy infections: abdominal pain and distention, diarrhea | Transmitted from contaminated soil, vegetables, toys, and other objects<br>Most common in warm, moist climates<br>Occurs most often in undernourished children living in unsanitary conditions |

provide relief, especially before meals to encourage food and fluid intake. Drinking fluids through a straw is helpful in avoiding the painful lesions. Mouth care is encouraged; the use of a very soft-bristled toothbrush or disposable foam-tipped toothbrush provides gentle cleaning near ulcerated areas.

Careful handwashing is essential when caring for children with HGS. Because the infection is autoinoculable, children should keep their fingers out of the mouth; contaminated hands also can infect other body parts. Very young children may need elbow restraints to ensure compliance. All articles placed in the mouth are cleaned thoroughly. Newborns and individuals with immunosuppression should not be exposed to infected children.

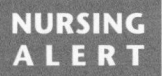 **NURSING ALERT**   When examining herpetic lesions, wear gloves. The virus easily enters breaks in the skin and can cause herpetic whitlow of the fingers.

Because herpes infection is often associated with sexual transmission, the nurse should explain to parents and older children that HGS is usually caused by type 1 HSV, the type not associated with sexual activity.

## INTESTINAL PARASITIC DISEASES

Intestinal parasitic diseases, including helminths (parasitic worms) and protozoa, constitute the most common infections in the world. In the United States the incidence of intestinal parasitic disease, especially giardiasis, has increased among young children who attend daycare centers. Young children are especially at risk because of typical hand-mouth activity and uncontrolled fecal habits.

Intestinal parasitic infections in humans are caused by various infecting organisms. This discussion is limited to the two most common parasitic infections among children in the United States—giardiasis and pinworms. Table 16-2 describes the outstanding features of other helminths that belong to the family of nematodes. Most nematodes (any organism belonging to the class of tapered cylindric helminths), with the exception of threadworm and *Toxocara*, are effectively treated with mebendazole, or albendazole (Table 16-3).

### General Nursing Considerations

Nursing responsibilities related to intestinal parasitic infections involve assisting with identification of the parasite,

**TABLE 16-3** Drugs used to treat intestinal parasitic infections

| Drug | Indication | Side Effects | Comments |
|---|---|---|---|
| Albendazole (Albenza) | Giardiasis<br>Mixed helminthic infections | Headache<br>Nausea/vomiting<br>Abdominal pain<br>Increased LFTs | May be used in children >2 years old.<br>To be taken with high-fat foods<br>Monitor liver functions.<br>Monitor CBC after 1 month and then every 2 weeks. |
| Furazolidone (Furoxone) | Giardiasis | Nausea<br>Vomiting<br>Headache | Contraindicated during pregnancy<br>Hemolysis possible in glucose-6-phosphate dehydrogenase (G6PD) deficiency |
| Mebendazole (Vermox) | Enterobiasis | Occasional, transient abdominal pain<br>Diarrhea in massive infection with expulsion of worms | Also used for hookworm, roundworm, and whipworm<br>Tablets may be chewed, crushed, or mixed with food<br>Not recommended during pregnancy<br>Recommended for children over 2 years |
| Metronidazole (Flagyl) | Giardiasis | Nausea<br>Diarrhea<br>Vomiting<br>Metallic taste<br>Abdominal cramps<br>Headache | May be ineffective in children receiving phenobarbital<br>Not recommended during pregnancy, but may be used if initial treatment with paromomycin fails |
| Piperazine citrate (Antepar) | Enterobiasis | Nausea<br>Vomiting<br>Diarrhea<br>Abdominal cramps<br>Urticaria | Side effects are rare with recommended dose<br>May exacerbate seizures in children with seizure disorders |
| Pyrantel pamoate (Antiminth) | Enterobiasis | Nausea<br>Vomiting<br>Diarrhea<br>Abdominal cramps<br>Tenesmus | Side effects are rare with recommended dose<br>Little published data on safety in pregnant women and children under 2 years of age<br>Protect drug from light |
| Pyrvinium pamoate (Povan) | Enterobiasis | Nausea<br>Vomiting<br>Diarrhea<br>Abdominal cramps | Warn parents that drug stains stool and vomitus bright red, as well as clothing or skin if in contact with drug<br>Swallow tablets whole to avoid staining teeth |
| Thiabendazole (Mintezol) | *Toxacara*<br>Mixed helminthic infections | Dry mucous membranes<br>Drowsiness<br>Dizziness<br>Headache<br>Impaired alertness and coordination<br>Nausea/vomiting | Use with caution in patients with renal or hepatic dysfunction<br>Warn parents of drowsiness and dizziness in child<br>Administer after meals |

treating the infection, and preventing initial infection or reinfection. Identification of the organism is accomplished by laboratory examination of substances containing the worm, its larvae, or ova. Most are identified by examining fecal smears from the stools of persons suspected of harboring the parasite. Fresh specimens are best for revealing parasites or larvae; therefore collected specimens should be taken directly to the laboratory for examination. If this is not feasible, the specimen is placed in a container with a preservative. Parents need clear instructions on obtaining an adequate sample and the number of samples required. (See Collection of Specimens, Chapter 27.)

In most parasitic infections examination of other family members, especially children, may be carried out to identify those who are similarly affected. Nurses often assume the responsibility for directing and instructing the families in the collection and disposition of specimens. The treatment regimen may need further explanation and reinforcement, particularly when it involves other household members and the care of clothing and bed linen. When other members are treated, the family needs to understand the nature of transmission and that in some cases the medication must be repeated in 2 weeks to 1 month to kill the organisms that have hatched since initial treatment.

The nurse's most important function in relation to these parasites is preventive education of children and families regarding good hygiene and health habits. Careful handwashing before eating or handling food and after using the toilet is the most important precautionary method. Other preventive practices are listed in the Community Focus box.

## Giardiasis

Giardiasis is caused by the protozoan, *Giardia lamblia* (also called *G. intestinalis*, *G. duodenalis*, and *Lamblia intestinalis*). It is the most common intestinal parasitic pathogen in the United States; its prevalence among children in daycare centers may range from 17% to over 50% during outbreaks (Cody, Sottnek, and O'Leary, 1994). Risk factors for children

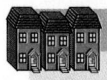

## COMMUNITY FOCUS
### *Preventing Intestinal Parasitic Disease*

Always wash hands and fingernails with soap and water before eating and handling food and after toileting.

Avoid placing fingers in mouth and biting nails.

Discourage children from scratching bare anal area.

Use superabsorbent disposable diapers to prevent leakage.

Change diapers as soon as soiled and dispose of diapers in closed receptacle out of children's reach.

Do not rinse diapers in toilet.

Disinfect toilet seats and diaper-changing areas; use dilute household bleach (10% solution) or Lysol and wipe clean with paper towels.

Drink water that is specially treated, especially if camping.

Wash all raw fruits and vegetables or any food that has fallen on the floor or ground.

Avoid growing foods in soil fertilized with human excreta.

Teach children to defecate only in a toilet not on the ground.

Keep dogs and cats away from playgrounds or sandboxes.

Avoid swimming in pools frequented by diapered children.

Wear shoes outside.

---

attending daycare centers include longer duration of total attendance, increased weekly attendance, low family income, and large family size (four or more members) (Furness, Beach, and Roberts, 2000).

### Life Cycle, Pathogenesis, and Transmission

Infection begins with ingestion of the cysts, the nonmotile stage of the protozoa. Activated by stomach acid, the cysts pass into the duodenum. Following excystation, trophozoites (parasites in their active feeding stage) emerge and colonize the distal duodenum and proximal jejunum. As the cycle continues, the cysts are passed in feces; they are not infective initially but must complete a process of maturation that requires hours to days. Cysts can survive in the environment for months. The mechanism of pathogenesis is not known.

Chief modes of transmission are fecal-oral route, water (especially pools frequented by diapered infants, mountain lakes, and streams), food, and animals, especially puppies. In children, fecal-oral transmission is the most likely cause.

### Clinical Manifestations

Although individuals infected with giardiasis may be asymptomatic, young children (especially infants) usually manifest symptoms at an early stage, such as diarrhea, vomiting, anorexia, and failure to thrive. Children over 5 years of age most often complain of abdominal cramps with intermittent loose stools and constipation. The stools may be malodorous, watery, pale, greasy, and may float. Most infections resolve spontaneously in 4 to 6 weeks, except in rare instances in which the infection becomes chronic and may last for months or years. The chronic form is usually associated with intermittent loose, foul-smelling stools with or without abdominal bloating, flatulence, sulfur-tasting belches, epigastric pain, vomiting, arthropathy, headache, or weight loss because of malabsorption.

### Diagnostic Evaluation

Unlike most other intestinal parasites, *G. lamblia* is not easily diagnosed from stool specimens. Because *Giardia* organisms are excreted in a highly variable pattern, three or more stool specimens collected over several weeks may be necessary to identify the trophozoites or cysts. Other tests that detect *Giardia* antigen in the stool, such as counterimmunoelectrophoresis (CIE) and enzyme-linked immunosorbent assay (ELISA), are available.

### Therapeutic Management

Metronidazole (Flagyl) is the drug of choice for treatment of giardiais. Other drugs available for treatment of giardiasis are furazolidone (Furoxone) and albendazole (Albenza) (see Table 16-3). For pregnant women who need treatment, paromomycin may be used first, followed by metronidazole if the initial treatment is unsuccessful (Furness, Beach, and Roberts, 2000).

### Nursing Considerations

The most important nursing consideration is prevention of giardiasis, especially among the children and staff at daycare centers. Attention to meticulous sanitary practices, especially during diaper changes, is essential. (See Community Focus box.) Nurses can play an important role in educating daycare staff regarding appropriate sanitation. (See Alternate Child Care Arrangements, Chapter 12.)

Once children are infected, family education regarding administration of the drug is essential. If other household members are infected, the nurse should inquire about their understanding and management of the disease.

## Enterobiasis (Pinworms)

Enterobiasis, or pinworm infection is caused by the nematode *Enterobius vermicularis*. It is universally present in temperate climatic zones. Transmission is favored in crowded conditions, such as classrooms and daycare centers.

### Life Cycle, Pathogenesis, and Transmission

Infection begins when the eggs are ingested or inhaled (the eggs float in the air). The eggs hatch in the upper intestine, mature in 2 to 8 weeks, and migrate to the cecal area. The females then mate, migrate out the anus, and lay up to 17,000 eggs (American Academy of Pediatrics, 2000). The movement of the worms on skin and mucous membrane surfaces causes intense itching. Because the surface of the eggs is durable and adhesive, they easily adhere to almost any surface. As the child scratches, eggs are deposited on the hands and under the fingernails. The typical hand-to-mouth activity of youngsters makes them especially prone to continual reinfection. Pinworm eggs also persist in the environment for 2 to 3 weeks, contaminating anything they contact, such as toilet seats, doorknobs, bed linen, underwear, shared toys and baths, and food.

### Clinical Manifestations

The principal symptom of pinworms is intense perianal itching. However, in young children who have difficulty verbalizing this discomfort, general irritability, restlessness, poor sleep, bed-wetting, distractibility, and short attention span should arouse suspicion that the disorder is present. In females the worms may migrate to the vagina and urethra to cause infection.

### Diagnostic Evaluation

The most common test for diagnosing pinworms is the tape test (see Nursing Considerations below). The worms may also be identified by using a flashlight to inspect the anal area 2 to 3 hours after the child is asleep. It is best not to have placed underpants on the child to avoid disturbing the child as much as possible. Finding worms can be very upsetting to parents, and this fact should be considered before recommending this procedure.

### Therapeutic Management

The drugs available for treatment of pinworms include mebendazole (Vermox), pyrantel pamoate (Antiminth), piperazine phosphate, and pyranted pamote (Anthelmintic). The drug of choice is mebendazole, which is safe, effective, and convenient and has few side effects. However, mebendazole is not recommended for children under 2 years of age. Because pinworms are easily transmitted, all household members are treated. The drugs should be repeated in 2 weeks to prevent reinfection. Frequent changing of underclothes and bedsheets may reduce continued transmission. Because of the high frequency of reinfection, families should be informed that recurrence is common. Repeated infections should be treated in the same manner as the first one.

### Nursing Considerations

Nursing care is directed at identifying the parasite, eradicating the organism, and preventing reinfection. Parents need clear, detailed instructions for the *tape test*. A loop of

transparent (not "frosted," or "magic") tape, sticky side out, is placed around the end of a tongue depressor, which is then firmly pressed against the child's perianal area. A convenient commercially prepared tape is also available. Pinworm specimens are collected in the morning as soon as the child awakens and *before* the child has a bowel movement or bathes. The procedure may need to be repeated more than once before eggs are collected. Parents are instructed to place the tongue blade or commercial tape in a glass jar or loosely in a plastic bag so that it can be brought in for microscopic examination. For specimens collected in the hospital, practitioner's office, or clinic, the tape is placed smoothly on a glass slide, sticky side down, for examination.

Compliance with the drug regimen is usually excellent because the duration of treatment is typically one dose. However, the family is reminded of the need to take a second dose in 2 weeks. Posting a reminder on the refrigerator door or bathroom mirror is helpful.

To prevent reinfection, washing all clothes and bed linen in hot water and vacuuming the house may be recommended. However, there is little documentation of the effectiveness of these measures because pinworms survive on so many surfaces. Helpful suggestions include handwashing after toileting and before eating, disposing of diapers in a closed receptacle as soon as they are soiled, keeping the child's fingernails short to minimize the chance of ova collecting under the nails, dressing children in one-piece pant outfits, and daily showering rather than tub bathing.

## INGESTION OF INJURIOUS AGENTS

Since the passage of the Poison Prevention Packaging Act of 1970, which provides that certain potentially hazardous drugs and household products be sold in child-resistant

---

**TABLE 16-4** Most commonly reported poisoning in children less than 6 years of age

| Substance | Total Number | % |
|---|---|---|
| **Nonpharmaceuticals** | | |
| Cosmetics/personal care products (perfume, Cologne, aftershave)* | 153,057 | 13.3 |
| Cleaning products (hypochlorite ["household"] bleach, pine oil disinfectant) | 123,575 | 10.7 |
| Plants (nontoxic gastrointestinal irritants, oxalates) | 79,287 | 6.9 |
| Foreign bodies/toys/miscellaneous (dessicants, thermometer, bubble-blowing solutions) | 76,268 | 6.6 |
| Insecticides, pesticides | 43,107 | 3.7 |
| Arts, crafts, and office supplies (pens, ink) | 29,225 | 2.5 |
| Hydrocarbons (gasoline) | 24,468 | 2.1 |
| **Pharmaceuticals** | | |
| Analgesics (pediatric acetaminophen, nonsteroidal antiinflammatory drugs [NSAIDs, excludes aspirin], especially ibuprofen) | 87,471 | 7.6 |
| Topicals (diaper care products) | 65,561 | 5.7 |
| Cough and cold preparations | 63,951 | 5.5 |
| Vitamins (pediatric and adult multiple vitamins with iron, no fluoride) | 38,651 | 3.3 |
| Gastrointestinal preparations (antacids, laxatives) | 36,133 | 3.1 |
| Antimicrobials (antibiotics) | 34,940 | 3.0 |
| Antihistamines (diphenhydramine) | 24,981 | 2.2 |
| Hormones and hormone antagonists (oral contraceptives, corticosteroids) | 23,661 | 2.0 |

Data from Litovitz T and others: 1996 Annual Report of the American Association of Poison Control Centers Toxic Exposure Surveillance System, *Am J Emerg Med* 18(5):517-574, 2000.
*Most common substances in each category are in parenthesis. Substances ingested are not necessarily most toxic but often represent ready availability.

containers, the incidence of poisonings in children has decreased dramatically. Nevertheless, poisoning remains a significant health concern despite these advances, with most cases occurring in children under 6 years of age. Children are poisoned by a variety of substances (Table 16-4), although not all common household items are likely to produce serious problems. Many poisonings reflect the ready accessibility of the product in the home, where 90% of poisonings occur. A number of poisonings occur elsewhere, especially in a grandparent's or friend's home as well as at unlikely sites such as health care facilities and schools. Although the reported incidence of ingested substances varies, the most commonly ingested poisons are the following (Box 16-4) (Litovitz and others, 2000; Powers, 2000).

- Cosmetics and personal care products (perfume, cologne, aftershave)
- Cleaning products (hypochlorite ["household"] bleach, pine oil disinfectants)
- Analgesics (Tylenol, ibuprofen)
- Plants (nontoxic gastrointestinal irritants, oxalates) (Boxes 16-5 and 16-6)
- Foreign bodies, toys, and miscellaneous substances (desiccants, thermometers, bubble-blowing solutions)

**NURSING ALERT** The following five commonly used and easily available drugs (first four are over-the-counter) can cause serious or fatal consequences if as little as ¼ teaspoon or ½ tablet is ingested: methyl salicylate, camphor, topical imidazolines (sympathomimetics such as those contained in Visine, Afrin, Otrivin, and Clear Eyes), benzocaine, and diphenoxylate/atropine (Lomotil and others). Stress to parents the importance of keeping such drugs away from children. If these agents are ingested, advise parents to seek medical treatment immediately. Emesis is not induced for camphor, topical imidazolines, or Lomotil ingestions (Powers, 2000).

The developmental characteristics of young children predispose them to poisoning by ingestion. Infants and toddlers explore their environment through oral experimentation. Because the sense of taste is less discriminatory at this age, many unpalatable substances are ingested. In addition, toddlers and preschoolers are developing autonomy and initiative, which increase their curiosity and noncompliant behavior. Imitation is also a powerful motivator, especially when combined with a lack of awareness of danger.

This section is primarily concerned with the immediate emergency treatment of ingestion of injurious agents. Specific management of corrosive, hydrocarbon, acetaminophen, salicylate, plant, and iron poisoning is summarized in Box 16-4. Because of the importance of lead poisoning among young children, ingestion of lead is discussed separately. Appropriate suggestions for poison prevention are discussed on p. 673 and in Chapter 14.

## Principles of Emergency Treatment

A poisoning may or may not require emergency intervention, but in every instance medical evaluation is necessary to initiate appropriate action. Parents are advised to call the regional **poison control center (PCC)** *before* initiating any intervention. The regional PCC telephone number (usually listed in the front of the telephone directory) should be posted near each phone in the house.* (See Critical Thinking Exercise box.)

Based on the initial telephone assessment, the PCC counsels the parents to begin treatment at home and/or to bring the child to an emergency facility. When a call is taken, the caller's name and telephone number are recorded so that contact can be reestablished if the connection is interrupted. Because most poisonings are managed outside health care facilities, usually at the patient's home, expert advice is essential in minimizing adverse effects. When the exact quantity or type of ingested toxin is not known, admission to a hospital for laboratory evaluation and surveillance for signs of poisoning (Box 16-7 on p. 672) is critical during the postingestion period.

General guidelines for emergency treatment of poisoning are listed in the Emergency Treatment box on p. 673. Selected interventions, especially those that require professional intervention, are discussed next.

### Assessment

The first and most important principle in dealing with a poisoning is to treat the child first, not the poison. This necessitates an immediate concern for life support; vital signs are taken and respiratory and/or circulatory support instituted as needed. The victim's condition is routinely reevaluated. The increased recovery rate from acute poisonings is largely attributable to vigorous use of supportive measures after symptoms appear.

*Also available by calling (800) 555-1212 from any state in the United States or contacting the **American Association of Poison Control Centers**, 3201 New Mexico Ave, Suite 310, Washington, DC, 20016, (202) 362-7217; www.aapcc.org.

### Critical Thinking Exercise

#### Poisoning

Mrs. Berry, a neighbor, calls you. She is very upset because her 2-year-old son has eaten several chewable multivitamins with iron. She asks you if she should give syrup of ipecac. What should you advise her to do first?

FIRST, THINK ABOUT IT . . .

- What are you taking for granted, and what assumptions are you making?
- How are you interpreting the information?

1. Call the poison control center.
2. Give an antiemetic.
3. Dilute the poison with several glasses of water.
4. Wait to see if the child develops symptoms.

*The best response is one. The poison control center will advise her of home treatment, such as using ipecac. The goal is to remove the poison, not dilute it, which makes option three inappropriate. The most toxic ingredient in the multivitamin is iron, which produces symptoms after several hours. Treatment, if needed, should begin long before symptoms appear.*

---

### Box 16-4 ■ ■ ☐
### Selected Poisonings in Children

#### CORROSIVES (STRONG ACIDS OR ALKALI)

Drain, toilet, or oven cleaners
Electric dishwasher detergent (liquid, because of higher pH, is more hazardous than granular)
Mildew remover
Batteries
Clinitest tablets
Denture cleaners
Bleach

#### Clinical Manifestations

Severe burning pain in mouth, throat, and stomach
White, swollen mucous membranes, edema of lips, tongue, and pharynx (respiratory obstruction); oral ulcerations
Violent vomiting (hemoptysis)
Drooling and inability to clear secretions
Signs of shock
Anxiety and agitation

#### Comments

Household bleach is a commonly ingested corrosive but rarely causes serious damage
Liquid corrosives cause more damage than granular preparations

#### Treatment

Inducing emesis is contraindicated (vomiting redamages the mucosa)
Dilute corrosive with water or milk (usually no more than 120 ml [4 oz])
*Do not neutralize.* Neutralization can cause an exothermic reaction (which produces heat and causes increased symptoms or produces a thermal burn in addition to a chemical burn)
Maintain patent airway
Administer analgesics
Do not allow oral intake
Esophageal stricture may require repeated dilations and/or surgery

#### HYDROCARBONS

Gasoline
Kerosene
Lamp oil
Mineral seal oil (found in furniture polish)
Lighter fluid
Turpentine
Paint thinner and remover

#### Clinical Manifestations

Gagging, choking, and coughing
Nausea
Vomiting
Alterations in sensorium, such as lethargy
Weakness
Respiratory symptoms of pulmonary involvement
 Tachypnea
 Cyanosis
 Retractions
 Grunting

#### Comments

Immediate danger is aspiration (even small amounts can cause bronchitis and chemical pneumonia)
Gasoline, kerosene, lighter fluid, mineral seal oil, and turpentine cause severe pneumonia

#### Treatment

Inducing emesis is generally contraindicated
Gastric decontamination and gastric emptying are questionable, even when the hydrocarbon contains a heavy metal or pesticide; if gastric lavage must be performed, a cuffed ET tube should be in place before lavage because of a high risk of aspiration
Symptomatic treatment of chemical pneumonia includes high humidity, oxygen, hydration, and antibiotics for secondary infection

#### ACETAMINOPHEN
#### Clinical Manifestations

Occurs in four stages
1. Initial period (2 to 4 hours after ingestion): nausea, vomiting, sweating, pallor
2. Latent period (24 to 36 hours): patient improves
3. Hepatic involvement (may last up to 7 days and be permanent): pain in right upper quadrant, jaundice, confusion, stupor, coagulation abnormalities
4. Patients who do not die during hepatic stage gradually recover

#### Comments

Most common drug poisoning in children
Occurs primarily from acute ingestion
Toxic dose is 150 mg/kg or greater in children
Toxicity from chronic therapeutic use is rare but may occur with ingestion of approximately 150 mg/kg/day, or about double the recommended maximum therapeutic dose (90 mg/kg/day) of acetaminophen, for several days (Douidar, Al-Khalil, and Habersang, 1994); toxicity is more likely in children with hepatic dysfunction (McDonough, 1998)

#### Treatment

Antidote N-acetylcysteine (NAC) (Mucomyst) can usually be given orally but is first diluted in fruit juice or soda because of the antidote's offensive odor
Given as one loading dose and usually 17 maintenance doses in different dosages
May be given intravenously, but use is investigational

---

Shock may occur following ingestion of several types of household poisons, particularly corrosives. Therefore measures to reduce the effects of shock, such as provision of warmth and rest and elevation of legs and head to the level of the heart to promote venous drainage, are important. Maintenance of respiratory function may require insertion of an airway and/or mechanical ventilation.

The emergency department nurse's responsibility is to be prepared for immediate intervention with any of the necessary equipment. Because time and speed are critical factors in recovery from serious poisonings, anticipation of potential problems and complications may mean the difference between life and death.

### Gastric Decontamination

In general, the immediate treatment is to remove the ingested poison by inducing vomiting, adsorbing the toxin with activated charcoal, performing gastric lavage, or increasing bowel motility (catharsis). An antidote is usually administered after gastric decontamination and does not negate the need for gastric decontamination. Because of continuing controversy regarding the use of these measures

## Box 16-4 ■ ■ ■
## Selected Poisonings in Children—cont'd

### ASPIRIN (ASA)
#### Clinical Manifestations

Acute poisoning
  Nausea
  Disorientation
  Vomiting
  Dehydration
  Diaphoresis
  Hyperpnea
  Hyperpyrexia
  Oliguria
  Tinnitus
  Coma
  Convulsions
Chronic poisoning
  Same as above but subtle onset (often mistaken for viral illness)
Dehydration, coma, and seizures may be more severe
Bleeding tendencies

#### Comments

May be caused by acute ingestion (severe toxicity occurs with 300 to 500 mg/kg)
May be caused by chronic ingestion (i.e., more than 100 mg/kg/day for 2 or more days); can be more serious than acute ingestion
Time to peak serum salicylate can vary with enteric aspirin or the presence of concretions (bezoars)

#### Treatment

Home use of ipecac for moderate toxicity
Hospitalization for severe toxicity
Emesis, lavage, activated charcoal, and/or cathartic
Lavage will not remove concretions of ASA
Activated charcoal is important early in ASA toxicity
Sodium bicarbonate transfusions to correct metabolic acidosis, and urinary alkalinization may be effective in enhancing elimination. Urinary alkalinization is very difficult to achieve. Be aware of the risk for fluid overload and pulmonary edema
External cooling for hyperpyrexia
Anticonvulsants
Oxygen and ventilation for respiratory depression
Vitamin K for bleeding
In severe cases, hemodialysis (not peritoneal dialysis) may be used

### IRON

Mineral supplement or vitamin containing iron

#### Clinical Manifestations

Occurs in five stages
1. Initial period ($\frac{1}{2}$ to 6 hours after ingestion) (if child does not develop gastrointestinal symptoms in 6 hours, toxicity is unlikely): vomiting, hematemesis, diarrhea, hematochezia (bloody stools), gastric pain
2. Latency (2 to 12 hours): patient improves
3. Systemic toxicity (4 to 24 hours after ingestion): metabolic acidosis, fever, hyperglycemia, bleeding, shock, death (may occur)
4. Hepatic injury (48 to 96 hours): seizures, coma
5. Rarely, pyloric stenosis develops at 2 to 5 weeks

#### Comments

Factors related to frequency of iron poisoning include:
  Widespread availability
  Packaging of large quantities in individual containers
  Lack of parental awareness of iron toxicity
  Resemblance of iron tablets to candy (e.g., M & Ms)
  Toxic dose is based on the amount of elemental iron in various salts (sulfate, gluconate, fumarate), which ranges from 20% to 33%; ingestions of 60 mg/kg are considered dangerous

#### Treatment

#### Emesis or lavage

For toxic doses lavage may be necessary for all chewable tablets or liquids if spontaneous vomiting has not occurred
Chelation therapy with deferoxamine in severe intoxication (may turn urine a red to orange color)
If intravenous deferoxamine is given too rapidly, hypotension, facial flushing, rash, urticaria, tachycardia, and shock may occur; stop the infusion, maintain the intravenous line with normal saline, and notify the practitioner immediately

### PLANTS

Plants listed in Boxes 16-5 and 16-6, p. 672

#### Clinical Manifestations

Depends on type of plant ingested
May cause local irritation of oropharynx and entire gastrointestinal tract
May cause respiratory, renal, and central nervous system symptoms
Topical contact with plants can cause dermatitis

#### Comments

Some of the most commonly ingested substances
Rarely cause serious problems, although some plant ingestions can be fatal
Can also cause choking and allergic reactions

#### Treatment

Induce emesis
Wash from skin or eyes
  Supportive care as needed

---

(except antidotes), each toxic ingestion should be treated individually (Perry and Shannon, 1996; Powers, 2000). The

**NURSING ALERT** The use of an emetic is generally contraindicated in conditions that increase the risk of aspiration and when regurgitation of the poison, such as a corrosive, redamages the mucosa of the esophagus and pharynx. Emesis is also contraindicated in cases in which there is existing or potential for rapid onset of central nervous system depression, dystonias (unusual muscle tone or movements), or seizures.

preferred method for use in the home is to administer *ipecac syrup,* an emetic that exerts its action by directly stimulating the vomiting center and by having an irritant effect on the gastric mucosa.

Proper administration of ipecac is essential. (See Emergency Treatment box on p. 673.) Ipecac is available in 1-ounce (30-ml) vials. However, the label information does not include directions for a second dose if the child fails to vomit after the first dose. Therefore parents need clear instructions for proper use and dose. As a precaution, parents are advised to have full doses of ipecac for *each child* in the home, carry the

## Box 16-5 ■ ■ □
### Poisonous Plants

| PLANT | TOXIC PARTS |
|---|---|
| Apple | Leaves, seeds |
| Apricot | Leaves, stem, seed pits |
| Azalea | All parts |
| Buttercup | All parts |
| Cherry (wild or cultivated) | Twigs, seeds, foliage |
| Daffodil | Bulbs |
| Dumb cane, dieffenbachia | All parts |
| Elephant ear | All parts |
| English ivy | All parts |
| Foxglove | Leaves, seeds, flowers |
| Holly | Berries and leaves |
| Hyacinth | Bulbs |
| Ivy | Leaves |
| Mistletoe* | Berries, leaves |
| Oak tree | Acorn, foliage |
| Philodendron | All parts |
| Plum | Pit |
| Poinsettia† | Leaves |
| Poison ivy, poison oak | Leaves, fruit, stems, smoke from burning plants |
| Pothos | All parts |
| Rhubarb | Leaves |
| Tulip | Bulbs |
| Water hemlock | All parts |
| Wisteria | Seeds, pods |
| Yew | All parts |

*Eating one or two berries or leaves is probably nontoxic.
†Toxic if ingested in massive quantities.

## Box 16-6 ■ ■ □
### Nonpoisonous Plants

| | |
|---|---|
| African violet | Piggyback begonia |
| Aluminum plant | Piggyback plant |
| Asparagus fern | Prayer plant |
| Begonia | Rubber tree |
| Boston fern | Snake plant |
| Christmas cactus | Spider plant |
| Coleus | Swedish ivy |
| Gardenia | Wax plant |
| Grape ivy | Weeping fig |
| Jade plant | Zebra plant |

## Box 16-7 ■ ■ □
### Common Signs of Poisoning

**GENERAL SIGNS**
*Gastrointestinal System*
Abdominal pain
Vomiting
Diarrhea
Anorexia

*Respiratory/Circulatory System*
Depressed respirations
Labored respirations
Unexplained cyanosis
Signs of shock
Delayed capillary refill;
Increased, weak pulse
Decreased blood pressure
Increased, shallow respiration
Pallor
Cool, clammy skin

*Central Nervous System*
Seizures
Overstimulation
Loss of consciousness
Dizziness
Stupor, lethargy
Coma

**SPECIFIC SIGNS**
*Corrosives*
Severe burning pain in mouth, throat, stomach
White, swollen, and/or ulcerated mucous membranes; edema of lips, tongue, pharynx (respiratory obstruction)
Violent vomiting, hemoptysis
Drooling and inability to clear secretions
Signs of shock
Anxiety and agitation

*Hydrocarbons*
Gagging, choking, coughing
Nausea
Vomiting
Alterations in sensorium (e.g., lethargy)
Weakness
Respiratory symptoms of pulmonary involvement; tachypnea, cyanosis, retractions, grunting

*Salicylates*
Nausea
Disorientation
Vomiting
Dehydration
Diaphoresis
Hyperpnea
Hyperpyrexia
Oliguria
Tinnitus
Coma
Seizures

emetic when traveling, and be certain that other caregivers (baby-sitters or relatives) have the emetic available. Because children share activities, it is not uncommon for more than one child to ingest the toxic substance. In an emergency ipecac can be obtained from an all-night pharmacy, convenience store, emergency squad, or emergency department and is inexpensive. Ipecac should only be used when recommended by the Poison Control Center or a physician.

If oral fluids are given following administration of ipecac, clear liquids are preferred to provide better visualization of pill fragments. For maximum benefit in removing the poison, ipecac should be administered within 1 hour of a toxic ingestion.

The safety of ipecac has been questioned. One reason is the increased number of drug ingestions for which induced emesis is contraindicated. Medications such as calcium channel blockers and benzodiazepines either produce a rapid onset of adverse symptoms (e.g., sedation, seizures, coma) or exaggerate the vagal response induced by gagging, which can lead to significant bradycardia. Under either circumstance, uncontrolled vomiting becomes an undesirable and unsafe event (Perry and Shannon, 1996). Concern also exists regarding ipecac's ready availability, specifically its abuse by individuals with anorexia nervosa and bulimia and by parents who intentionally poison their children with ipecac (Munchausen syndrome by proxy) (Hughes and Corbo-Richert, 1999).

If the child is admitted to an emergency facility, *gastric lavage* may also be performed to empty the stomach of the toxic agent. Lavage is indicated for young infants for whom ipecac is contraindicated, for patients who are comatose or seizing or require a protected airway, or if the ingested poison is rapidly absorbed (strychnine or cyanide). The use of lavage in petroleum distillate poisoning remains controversial because of the danger of aspiration. When lavage is performed, the largest-diameter tube that can be inserted is used to facilitate passage of gastric contents.

Another method of decontaminating the stomach is the use of *activated charcoal,* an odorless, tasteless, fine black powder that adsorbs many compounds, creating a stable complex. It is mixed with water, saline cathartic, or sorbitol to form a slurry. Slurries are neither gritty nor distasteful but resemble black mud. Sorbitol, an artificial sweetener, is added to a commercial preparation (Actidose) as a flavoring and a cathartic. If the child refuses to take the charcoal, it is given by nasogastric tube.

Activated charcoal (without sorbitol) is also used in multiple doses to reduce systemic absorption of many toxic agents, even overdoses of some intravenous drugs. After absorption, some toxic substances will reenter the lumen of the gastrointestinal tract by passive diffusion when the concentration of the substance in the gut is lower than that in the blood. Adsorption of the toxin by charcoal keeps the concentration gradient high so that diffusion continues. Ice cream, milk, or chocolate milk are not used because these substances can decrease the adsorptive power of activated charcoal (Soud and Rogers, 1998). The best additive to use is diet soda.

**NURSING TIP**   To increase the child's acceptance of activated charcoal, mix it with diet soda and serve through a straw and in an opaque glass with a cover, such as a disposable coffee cup and lid or an ordinary cup covered with aluminum foil or placed inside a paper bag. Many flavorings and sweeteners, such as those found in ice cream and sherbet, have been found to take up binding sites on the activated charcoal and decrease its effectiveness.

Some authorities suggest that activated charcoal should replace ipecac as the home remedy. Although activated charcoal is safe and highly effective in preventing adsorption of many poisons, arguments against its home use include (1) availability—not a stock item in all stores; (2) dosage—1 g/kg, which is a much larger volume than ipecac and more difficult for parents to administer; and (3) compliance—children often refuse to drink the black liquid.

Three types of complications can occur with the use of activated charcoal: aspiration (usually in patients with impaired gag reflexes), constipation or intestinal obstruction, and electrolyte imbalances caused by activated charcoal or cathartics (most commonly magnesium compounds) (Diamant and others, 1994).

*Cathartics,* such as sorbitol, magnesium citrate, or magnesium sulfate, may be administered to stimulate evacuation of the bowel, thus decreasing systemic absorption of the poison and aiding in removal of the charcoal. However, the beneficial effects of cathartics are not well established. In addition, excessive amounts of a cathartic, such as sorbitol, can cause severe dehydration in infants from fluid loss in the stool. The use of cathartics remains controversial.

In a minority of poisonings, specific *antidotes* are available to counteract the poison. These are highly effective and should be available in all emergency facilities. The supply of antidotes should be checked routinely and replaced as used or according to expiration dates. Among the more commonly employed antidotes are *N*-acetylcysteine (Mucomyst) for acetaminophen poisoning, oxygen for carbon monoxide

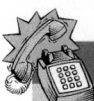

# EMERGENCY TREATMENT
## Poisoning

1. Assess the victim
   Take vital signs; reevaluate regularly.
   Initiate cardiorespiratory support if needed.
   Treat other symptoms, such as seizures.
2. Terminate exposure:
   Empty mouth of pills, plant parts, or other material.
   Flush eyes continuously with normal saline (room-temperature tap water at home) for 15 to 20 minutes.
   Flush skin and wash with soap and a soft cloth; remove contaminated clothes, especially if a pesticide, acid, alkali, or hydrocarbon is involved.
   Bring victim of an inhalation poisoning into fresh air.
   Give one sip of water to dilute ingested poison.
3. Identify the poison
   Question the victim and witnesses.
   Look for environmental cues (empty container, nearby spill, odor on breath) and save all evidence of poison (container, vomitus, urine).
   Be alert to signs and symptoms of potential poisoning in absence of other evidence, including symptoms of ocular or dermal exposure.
   Call poison control center for immediate advice regarding treatment.
4. Remove poison and prevent absorption
   Induce vomiting; administer ipecac if ordered:
   ☐ 6 to 12 months: 5 to 10 ml; do not repeat.*
   ☐ 1 to 12 years: 15 ml; repeat dosage *once* if vomiting has not occurred within 20 minutes.
   ☐ Over 12 years: 30 ml; repeat dosage *once* if vomiting has not occurred within 20 minutes.
   Do not induce vomiting if:
   ☐ Victim is comatose, in severe shock, or having seizures, or has lost the gag reflex.
   ☐ Poison is a low-viscosity hydrocarbon (unless it contains a more toxic substance [e.g., pesticide or heavy metal]) or a strong acid or alkali.
   Place child in side-lying, sitting, or kneeling position with head below chest to prevent aspiration.
   Administer activated charcoal (with a cathartic if necessary); usual dose 1 g/kg.
   If a child needs activated charcoal, *do not* give ipecac first.

---

*Inducing emesis in infants less than 6 months of age is contraindicated. Ipecac can be administered safely only in a health care facility because of the high risk of aspiration.

inhalation, naloxone for opioid overdose, flumazenil (Romazicon) for benzodiazepine (Valium, Versed) overdose, Digibind for digoxin toxicity, and antivenin for certain poisonous bites. The use of an antidote does not negate the need for gastric decontamination.

## Prevention of Recurrence

The ultimate objective is to prevent poisonings from occurring or recurring. One effective counseling method is first to discuss the difficulties of constantly watching and safeguarding young children. (See Family Focus box on p. 674). In this way the challenging task of raising children can lead to a discussion of injury prevention as one part of the parental role. This approach also incorporates other contributory causes for the incident, such as inadequate support systems, marital discord, discipline techniques (especially use of physical punishment), maternal distress, or

## FAMILY FOCUS
### Poisoning

A poisoning is more than a physical emergency for the child. It usually represents an emotional crisis for the parents, particularly in terms of guilt, self-reproach, and insecurity in the parenting role. The emergency department is no place to admonish the family for negligence, lack of appropriate supervision, or failure to safe-proof the home. Rather, it is a time to calm and support the child and parents while unaccusingly exploring the circumstances of the injury. If the nurse prematurely attempts to discuss ways of preventing such an incident from recurring, the parents' anxiety will block out any suggestions or offered guidance. Therefore it is preferable for the nurse to delay the discussion until the child's condition is stabilized or, if the child is discharged immediately after emergency treatment, to make a public health referral or send a packet of information.

### Box 16-8 ■ ■ □
### Questionnaire for Poison Prevention

1. Where do I store cleaning products, medicines, laundry aids, and garden supplies?
2. What do I keep under the sink in the kitchen and bathroom?
3. Do I have any medicines (e.g., pain relievers, tranquilizers, birth control pills, antacids) in my purse?
4. Are all the medicines and household products clearly labeled and in their original container?
5. Do I refer to medicine as candy to encourage my child to take it?
6. Are any medications left on the table or kitchen counter or kept in a purse or diaper bag for handy use?
7. Do I keep drugs prescribed for previous illnesses?
8. Is my child out of sight when I take medicine?
9. When using any medicine or household product, do I keep my eye on it at all times, put it away immediately after use, or put it down where my child cannot get it?
10. Are any of my garden plants or houseplants poisonous?
11. Do all cabinets that store toxic products have a lock on them?
12. What is stored in the garage or basement?
13. Are paints, gasoline, solvents, insecticides, poisons, and fertilizers either on a high shelf or locked in a cabinet?
14. Do I teach my child never to touch any nonfood item without asking me first?

### TABLE 16-5 Teaching strategy for parent education and preparation for accidental poisoning

| Question | Intervention |
|---|---|
| If you suspected that your child had ingested (eaten) a poison, what would you do first? | If answer is to call the poison control center, ask for more specifics, such as how to find the phone number |
| | If answer does not include knowledge of local poison control center, supply information |
| | Stress necessity of not wasting time and of saving all evidence of poisoning |
| Do you have ipecac syrup in your home? | If answer is yes, make sure parent(s) know to **call the poison center first** before giving ipecac |
| | If answer is no, supply correct information |
| Should you always make the child vomit? | If answer is no, acknowledge the correct answer and determine that the parent knows to call the regional PCC before administering ipecac |
| | If answer is yes, supply correct information regarding the need to call the PCC before administering ipecac |
| | Emphasize that instructions on container of household products are minimal and sometimes inaccurate for emergency treatment; the regional poison control center should always be contacted before giving emetic agents |
| If you suspected that your child had taken a poison, but there were no signs of illness and the child denied doing so, what would you do? | Emphasize need to always contact the regional poison control center immediately rather than waiting for signs or believing the child |

any disruption in the family or family activities, such as vacations, moves, visitors, illnesses, or births. A visit to the home, especially after a repeat poisoning situation, is recommended as part of the follow-up care to assess hazards, including family factors, and to evaluate appropriate safe-proofing measures. One method of identifying risk areas is to ask specific questions or to have the parent complete a questionnaire designed to isolate factors that predispose children to poisoning.

**NURSING TIP** Encourage parents to bend down to the child's eye level and survey the home environment for potential hazards. Have the parents try to open cabinets and reach shelves from this height to access poisons.

Box 16-8 is a sample questionnaire of items that may determine what environmental manipulation is needed to

"poison-proof" homes. A teaching plan designed to assess parents' preparedness in case of an accidental poisoning and to supply appropriate strategy and instruction where necessary is presented in Table 16-5. Such tools enable nurses to counsel families systematically and efficiently in the area of injury prevention.

*Passive measures* (those that do not require active participation) have been the most successful in preventing poisoning and include using child-resistant closures and limiting the number of tablets in one container. Other preventive methods include the use of warning labels, such as stickers or a skull and crossbones, to alert children to potential dangers. Also, some products (e.g., nail polish remover, furniture polish) are now available with a bittering agent to discourage large ingestions. However, the effectiveness of such measures is questionable (Rodgers and Tenenbein, 1994). One study found that children actually preferred to touch labeled containers after undergoing education incorporating stickers (Vernberg, Culver-Dickinson, and Spyker, 1984). Also, skull and crossbones labels may make products look like pirate toys and make them attractive to children.

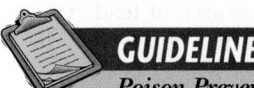

## GUIDELINES
### Poison Prevention

Assess possible contributing factors in occurrence of injury, such as discipline, parent-child relationship, developmental ability, environmental factors, and behavior problems.

Institute anticipatory guidance for possible future injuries based on child's age and maturational level.

Refer to visiting nurse agency to evaluate home environment and need for safe-proofing measures.

Provide assistance with environmental manipulation when necessary, such as lead removal.

Educate parents regarding safe storage of toxic substances. (See Family Home Care box on p. 549.)

Advise parents to take drugs out of sight of children.

Advise parents to make sure that all toxic substances are stored safely.

Teach children the hazards of ingesting nonfood items.

Advise parents against using plants for teas or medicine.

Discuss problems of discipline and children's noncompliance, and offer strategies for effective discipline.

Instruct parents regarding correct administration of drugs for therapeutic purposes and to discontinue drug if there is evidence of mild toxicity.

Advise parents to have syrup of ipecac available—two doses for each child in the family—but to use only if advised to do so by poison control center or practitioner.

Encourage grandparents or other frequent caregivers to keep syrup of ipecac in home.

Post number of regional poison control center with emergency phone list by telephone.

Include by the telephone the home address with nearest cross street in case an ambulance is needed. (In an emergency family members may not remember the house address, and baby-sitters may not know the information.)

However, these measures alone are not sufficient to prevent poisoning; *active measures* (those that require participation) are essential. Guidelines for preventing the occurrence or recurrence of a poisoning, with emphasis on proper storage of poisonous agents, are listed in the Guidelines box.

Even in the busiest health care facilities, poison prevention can be effective. Reminding parents of the telephone number of the local PCC, encouraging them to have ipecac in the home for emergency use, and counseling them on correct use of the emetic can increase their readiness in the event of a poisoning. (See Nursing Care Plan: The Child with Poisoning.*)

## Heavy Metal Poisoning

Heavy metal poisoning can occur from the ingestion of a variety of substances, the most common being lead. Other sources that are important in terms of children are iron (see Box 16-4) and mercury. *Mercury toxicity*, a rare form of heavy metal poisoning, has occurred in children from a variety of sources, such as broken thermometers or thermostats, bro-

*In Wong DL: *Wong and Whaley's clinical manual of pediatric nursing*, ed 5, St Louis, 2000, Mosby.

ken fluorescent lights, and the use of old interior latex house paint (Etzel, 2000). Elemental mercury (also called metallic mercury or quicksilver) is nontoxic if ingested and the gastrointestinal tract is healthy (e.g., has no fistulas or ulcers). However, mercury is volatile at room temperature and enters the bloodstream after it is inhaled, causing toxicity (tremors, memory loss, insomnia, gingivitis, diarrhea, anorexia, weight loss). The classic form of mercury poisoning is called *acrodynia* (or "painful extremities").

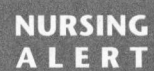 Mercury thermometers are no longer recommended for use because, if broken, inhaled vapors can cause significant toxicity.

Heavy metals have an affinity for certain essential tissue chemicals, which must remain free for adequate cell functioning. When metals are bound to these substances, cellular enzyme systems are inactivated. Treatment involves *chelation*—the use of a chemical compound that combines with the metal for rapid and safe excretion.

## Lead Poisoning

Poisoning from lead in the environment has been a problem throughout history and throughout the world. In the United States, the problem facing young children today began in the early 1900s when white lead, in concentrations as great as 50%, was added to paints and when tetra-ethyl lead was added to gasoline as an antiknock compound (American Academy of Pediatrics, 1998).

Fortunately, the use of lead in paint and leaded gasoline has been banned in the United States. Following this change in policy, the average blood lead level in the United States for people ages 1 to 74 years dropped from 12.8 $\mu$g/dl in 1980 to 2.3 $\mu$g/dl in 1994 (American Academy of Pediatrics, 1998). Yet the nature of lead as a basic chemical element still is part of the heritage of leaded paint and gasoline use. Because it does not decompose or break down into smaller particles, lead deposited in the past is still present in the soil near heavily trafficked areas. Coupled with deteriorating lead-based paint falling from the exterior of nearby houses, soil becomes a significant pathway by which lead poisoning can occur. Bare soil used as a play area contributes to the lead exposure of young children because lead-contaminated dust from these areas is tracked into the home.

The greatest problem remains the presence of many older homes with deteriorating lead-based paint. These homes were usually built before 1950, especially in the case of interior leaded paint. In 1978 the use of lead in household paint was banned. Consequently, homes built between 1900 and 1950 are most likely to contain lead-based paint. Those built from 1950 through 1978 may contain lead-based paint, especially on exterior surfaces; the older the home, the more likely it is that lead-based paint was used. A few homes built in the 2 years after 1978 may even contain this paint, because products remaining on store shelves were sold and used. Chipping, flaking, and chalking lead-based paint contributes to the environmental dust found in households. Although there may be new layers of paint over old lead-based ones, all layers are involved when deterioration occurs (Fisher and Vessey, 1998; Porter and Severtson, 2000).

## Children and Lead

In the United States, much research has been done on lead and its effects.* During the first half of the 1900s, health advocates designed studies to prove that lead is absorbed by the body, is not fully eliminated, and has toxic effect. In the early 1970s the Surgeon General issued a formal statement regarding lead poisoning and its potential toxicity. In 1971 the passage of the Lead Paint Poisoning Prevention Act provided the early funds to screen children for lead poisoning. Young children absorb approximately 50% of the lead to which they are exposed, whereas adults absorb approximately 10%. Children's bodies are much more receptive to lead, thus creating a more efficient and thorough process of absorption. A child does not need to eat loose paint chips to be exposed to the toxin; normal hand-to-mouth behavior, coupled with the presence of lead dust in the environment, is the usual method of poisoning (Jacob and others, 2000).

Children 6 years of age and younger are most vulnerable to the effects of lead. In addition, a disproportionate number of minority children have elevated lead levels. Any child, however, is at risk for becoming lead poisoned if lead-hazardous conditions are present in the environment (American Academy of Pediatrics, 1998; Binder and others, 1996; Lanphear and others, 2002).

## Causes of Lead Poisoning

Although there are numerous sources of lead that can result in exposure in children (Box 16-9), the major cause of lead poisoning of children in the United States is almost always deteriorating lead-based paint. The pathway for the exposure may be in food, air, or water; in most instances of acute childhood lead poisoning, the exposure is household dust and bare soil from yards contaminated with lead (Centers for Disease Control, 2000; American Academy of Pediatrics, 1998).

Lead enters a child's body through ingestion, inhalation or, in the case of an unborn child, through placental transfer when the mother is exposed. The most common route is ingestion either from hand-to-mouth behavior via contaminated hands, fingers, toys, or pacifiers or, less often, from eating sweet-tasting loose paint chips found in the home or play area. Inhalation becomes the route when exposure occurs during the deleading (abatement) process of house renovation or remodeling activities, which generate lead dust in the air (American Academy of Pediatrics, 1998). A pregnant woman who is exposed to lead is inadvertently exposing her unborn child. When measured, a mother's lead level is nearly the same as that of her unborn child. A level of lead not harmful to an adult woman can be quite harmful to the fetus (Gulson and others, 1997).

Because of family, cultural, or ethnic traditions, a source of lead may be a routine part of life for a child. Nurses must educate themselves about the practices of their patients and

identify when such products may be a source of lead. The use of pottery or dishes containing lead may be an issue, as well as the use of folk remedies for stomachaches or the use of cosmetics. (See Cultural Awareness box.) Some hobbies and occupations of adult family members may contribute to lead hazards carried into the household on clothes, shoes, or skin (American Academy of Pediatrics, 1998). Nurses are often in a position to observe or elicit information about these practices and educate families about their potential harm.

## Pathophysiology and Clinical Manifestations

When lead enters the body, it disperses to different areas or compartments. Through an equilibration process, it moves between the blood, tissues, organs, bones, and teeth. Most of the lead found in circulating blood is in the erythrocytes. This portion of the body burden is only about 5%. Lead ultimately settles in the bones and teeth, where it remains inert and in storage. This makes up the largest portion of the body burden, approximately 75% to 90%. The remaining lead is found in organs and tissues, including the brain and nervous system. Lead can affect any part of the body, but the renal, neurologic, and heme systems are seriously affected (Fig. 16-8) (Morrissey-Ross, 2000).

The *hematologic system* is one of the first to show the effects of lead poisoning. When a child's blood lead level

---

### Box 16-9 ■ ■ ■
### Sources of Lead*

Lead-based paint in deteriorating condition
Lead solder
Lead crystal
Battery casings
Lead fishing sinkers
Lead curtain weights
Lead bullets
Some of these may contain lead
   Ceramics ware
   Water
   Pottery
   Pewter
   Dyes
   Industrial factories
   Vinyl miniblinds
   Playground equipment
   Collectible toys
   Artists' paints
   Pool cue chalk
Occupations and hobbies involving lead
   Battery and aircraft manufacturing
   Lead smelting
   Brass foundry work
   Radiator repair
   Construction work
   Bridge repair work
   Painting contracting
   Mining
   Ceramics work
   Stained glass making
   Jewelry making

*The US Consumer Product Safety Commission issues alerts and recalls for products that contain lead and may unexpectedly pose a hazard to young children.

---

*Additional information may be obtained from the **Alliance to End Childhood Lead Poisoning,** www.aeclp.org.

rises, the hematologic system reacts, demonstrating the effects from lead (see Diagnostic Evaluation). There is a relationship between anemia and lead poisoning. Children who are iron deficient absorb lead more readily than those with sufficient iron stores. It may be that lead attaches to the site where iron ordinarily binds within a red blood cell. Many children who have lead poisoning also have iron deficiency anemia. However, many children with lead poisoning have signs of anemia, such as low hemoglobin, but are not deficient in iron (Jacob and others, 2000).

In general, the blood serves as a useful site with which to monitor the lead poisoning status of a particular child. Important measurements include the blood lead and the indicators of anemia, such as hemoglobin or hematocrit and mean corpuscular volume (MCV). In addition, laboratory studies of iron status, such as serum ferritin, serum iron, and total iron-binding capacity, are useful in determining the health management needs of a child with lead poisoning. Serum ferritin is considered the most sensitive indicator of iron status, but it may be altered by an acute illness, such as a viral infection (American Academy of Pediatrics, 1998).

Other changes in the blood are related to lead poisoning. Basophilic stippling (alteration in microscopic appearance) occurs less often in children with mild lead poisoning. Delta-

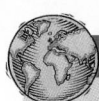

## CULTURAL AWARENESS
### Sources of Lead

In some cultures the use of traditional ethnic remedies or foods that contain lead may increase children's risk of lead poisoning. These remedies include:

**Azarcon** (Mexico)—For digestive problems; a bright orange powder; usual dose is ¼-1 teaspoon, often mixed with oil, milk, or sugar or sometimes given as a tea; sometimes a pinch is added to a baby bottle or tortilla dough for preventive purposes

**Greta** (Mexico)—A yellow-orange powder, used in the same way as azarcon

**Paylooah** (Southeast Asia)—Used for rash or fever; an orange-red powder given as ½ teaspoon straight or in a tea

**Surma** (India)—Black powder applied to the inner lower eyelid that is used as a cosmetic to improve eyesight

**Unknown ayurvedic** (Tibet)—Small, gray-brown balls used to improve slow development; two balls are given orally three times a day.

**Tamarindo jellied, fruit candy** (Mexico)—Fruit candy packaged in ceramic jars (which are lead contaminated).

**Lozeena** (Iraq)—A bright orange powder used by Iraqis to color meat and rice.

---

Modified from Lead poisoning associated with use of traditional ethnic remedies—California, 1991-1992, *MMWR* 42(27):521-524, 1993 and from Lead poisoning associated with imported candy and powdered food coloring—California and Michigan, *MMWR* 47(48):1041-1043, 1998.

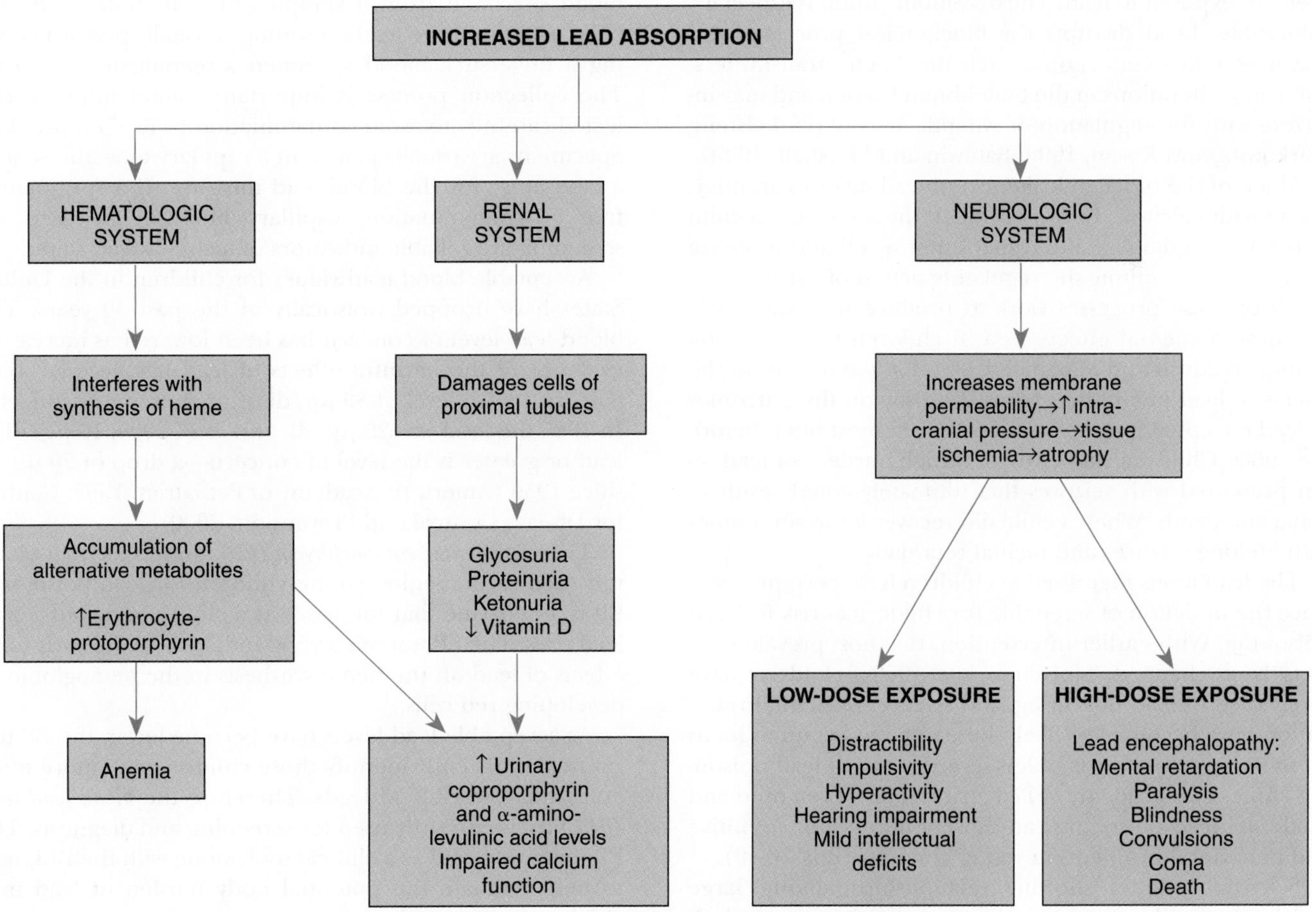

---

```
                    ┌─────────────────────────────┐
                    │  INCREASED LEAD ABSORPTION  │
                    └─────────────────────────────┘
          ┌──────────────────┬─────────────────────────┐
┌──────────────────┐  ┌──────────────┐        ┌──────────────────┐
│   HEMATOLOGIC    │  │    RENAL     │        │    NEUROLOGIC    │
│     SYSTEM       │  │   SYSTEM     │        │     SYSTEM       │
└──────────────────┘  └──────────────┘        └──────────────────┘
```

| HEMATOLOGIC SYSTEM | RENAL SYSTEM | NEUROLOGIC SYSTEM |
| --- | --- | --- |
| Interferes with synthesis of heme | Damages cells of proximal tubules | Increases membrane permeability→↑ intracranial pressure→tissue ischemia→atrophy |
| Accumulation of alternative metabolites ↑Erythrocyte-protoporphyrin | Glycosuria Proteinuria Ketonuria ↓ Vitamin D | |
| Anemia | ↑ Urinary coproporphyrin and α-amino-levulinic acid levels Impaired calcium function | |

**LOW-DOSE EXPOSURE**

Distractibility
Impulsivity
Hyperactivity
Hearing impairment
Mild intellectual deficits

**HIGH-DOSE EXPOSURE**

Lead encephalopathy:
Mental retardation
Paralysis
Blindness
Convulsions
Coma
Death

**Fig. 16-8**   Main effects of lead on body systems.

aminolevulinic acid, an enzyme altered by lead poisoning, is not an indicator that is used clinically (Babcock, 2000).

As a child recovers from lead poisoning, the blood reflects the resolution process through laboratory test values. Children whose laboratory values reflect severe anemia eventually develop normal values when given the proper nutrition and treatment for iron deficiency (Baldwin and Marshall, 1999). In cases of extreme elevations of lead, it may take many months for the values to return to normal, even when the child has been chelated numerous times.

Although adults have been shown to suffer adverse renal effects from occupational lead exposure, few studies document *renal effects* in children at other than extremely high lead levels. Logically, it can be hypothesized that lead can affect the renal integrity of children as well as adults. One study found a relationship between blood lead concentrations and elevation of N-acetyl-beta-D-glucosaminidase (NAG), which is a sensitive indicator of renal effects in adults from lead poisoning and from diabetes and nephrotoxic medicines in children (Verberk and others, 1996). Therefore the renal system of a child is still a potential target for the harmful effects of lead (Baldwin and Marshall, 1999). Because chelating agents are excreted through the kidneys, nurses caring for children undergoing this treatment must be aware of the need for monitoring the renal system.

The *neurologic system* is of most concern when young children are exposed to lead. The developing brain is especially vulnerable. Lead disrupts the biochemical processes and may have a direct effect on the release of neurotransmitters, may cause alterations in the blood-brain barrier, and may interfere with the regulation of synaptic activity (Finkelstein, Markowitz, and Rosen, 1998; Baldwin and Marshall, 1999).

Much of the biochemical effect of lead involves an interaction with calcium. Lead may block the ability of calcium to reach a regulatory site. It may enter a cell and mobilize calcium or may mimic the regulating action of calcium.

All of these processes work to produce the neurologic and developmental effects seen in children with lead poisoning (Baldwin and Marshall, 1999). Early research on the effects of lead in children focused mostly on the outcomes of lead encephalopathy, a condition seen most often before the 1960s. Children with extremely high burdens of lead often presented with seizures that ultimately could result in coma and death. When a child did recover it was sometimes with lifelong seizures and mental retardation.

The lead levels identified in children have become lower since the initiation of screening for children at risk for lead poisoning. With earlier intervention, the most prevalent effects have changed. Since the late 1960s, children have rarely died of lead poisoning, and seizures or mental retardation have become less likely. Research has begun to focus on the long-term effects of less severe forms of lead poisoning (American Academy of Pediatrics, 1998). Even mild and moderate lead poisoning can cause a number of cognitive and behavioral problems in young children (Box 16-10).

Scientific studies showing relationships among large numbers of children do not demonstrate the potential ef-

---

**Box 16-10** ◼ ◼ ◻
## Long-Term Effects of Lead Poisoning

| NEUROCOGNITIVE EFFECTS | BEHAVIORAL EFFECTS |
| --- | --- |
| Developmental delays | Aggression |
| Lowered IQ scores | Hyperactivity |
| Speech and language problems | Impulsivity |
| Reading skill deficits | Delinquency |
| Visual-spatial problems | Disinterest |
| Visual-motor problems | Withdrawal |
| Learning disabilities | |
| Lowered academic success | |

---

fects on a particular child. Instead the research shows that a child exposed to lead is more at risk for adverse effects (Mendelsohn and others, 1998). Which child will develop problems and at what stage of development cannot be predicted. In general, any child with a history of lead poisoning has increased risk for experiencing the harmful effects of lead. Children with higher lead burdens for a prolonged period of time are most likely to develop cognitive or behavioral problems.

### Diagnostic Evaluation

A diagnosis of lead poisoning is based only on a venous blood specimen from a venipuncture. Identification of a child who may have lead poisoning is usually performed using a fingerstick blood specimen screening test for lead. The collection process is important. Blood must be collected carefully to avoid contamination by lead on the skin. Specimens are usually placed in a capillary tube and sent to a laboratory for the blood lead measure. If a specimen is free of contamination, capillary blood levels used for screening are reliable indicators of a child's lead status.

Acceptable blood lead values for children in the United States have dropped drastically in the past 40 years. The blood lead level of concern has been lowered as increasing evidence of the harmful effects of lead has become available. In 1950 a level of 80 µg/dl or greater was of concern. In 1985 the level was 25 µg/dl, and as of 2000, 10 µg/dl of lead or greater is the level of concern—a drop of 70 µg/dl since 1950 (American Academy of Pediatrics, 1998; Centers for Disease Control and Prevention, 2000).

The *erythrocyte protoporphyrin (EP)* test was the first blood test used for screening young children for lead poisoning. EP is an enzyme that increases as a child's body burden of lead rises. The EP test was a good indicator of the early toxic effects of lead on the heme synthesis in the hemoglobin of developing red cells.

As acceptable lead levels have become lower, the EP test cannot consistently identify those children with more moderate and lower blood leads. Therefore the *blood lead level (BLL) test* is currently used for screening and diagnosis. The EP remains useful as a clinical tool, along with the BLL test, to help estimate the potential body burden of lead in a child.

## Anticipatory Guidance

Childhood lead poisoning is entirely preventable. Teaching families how to protect their children from lead hazards is a major thrust of prevention efforts. Anticipatory guidance for families with young children is essential for achieving a goal of lead-free children. The Centers for Disease Control and Prevention (1997a) has made recommendations for when families should be taught about lead poisoning in children. During prenatal care, when a child is 3 to 6 months old, and at 1 year of age, the following topics should be discussed with families:

- Hazards of lead-based paint in older housing
- Ways to control lead hazards safely
- Hazards accompanying repainting and renovation of homes built before 1978
- Other exposure sources, such as traditional remedies, that might be relevant for a family

Ideally, there should be no lead-based paint in the home of a child, but this is not always possible. The current consensus is that lead paint presents a hazard only when it deteriorates or is disturbed. Families must be made aware of potential lead hazards when they live in older homes. Before beginning a repainting or renovation project on a home built before 1978, the family must be informed of the need to investigate the type of paint they may be disturbing. In addition, the public must become more aware about other sources of lead that can be harmful.

In older homes containing lead-based paint, ambient household dust may contain lead contaminants. Cleaning techniques are aimed at decreasing this potential exposure. In the past the Environmental Protection Agency (EPA) recommended trisodium phosphate as the lead dust clean-up agent. Because of the known negative effects of this chemical on the environment, the EPA now suggests the use of a regular household cleaner or one made specifically for lead. Of most importance is the amount of effort put into the cleaning procedure. To control lead dust hazards, the cleaning approach should include at least two buckets, one for the cleaning solution and one for rinsing the mop. Professional cleaners use three buckets, an additional one in which to wring the mop. Other hard surfaces, such as moldings and window sills and wells, should also be washed. Cleaning should occur approximately every 5 days in order to control the dust effectively (EPA, 1997).

## Screening for Lead Poisoning

Screening children for lead poisoning is an important secondary prevention activity. Although devastating effects are known to occur at high levels of lead, the evidence of impact on an individual child at lower levels is less clear. Screening does not prevent the initial exposure of a child to lead. However, identification can lead to intervention and prevention of the harmful effects before the exposure is prolonged and the lead burden increases to an extreme level. Nurses are in a position to advocate for and carry out screening activities.

Guidelines from the Centers for Disease Control and Prevention (1997b; 2000) recommend universal or targeted screening on the basis of each state's determination of need. This need is established using blood lead surveillance and other risk factor data collected over time to establish the status and risk of children throughout the state. In areas without available data, *universal screening* is recommended. The Guidelines indicate that universally, all children should have a BLL test at the ages of 1 and 2 years. Any child between 3 and 6 years of age who has not been screened should also be tested. Children at high risk should be screened earlier and more often. A mobile child in an environment containing lead dust hazards is at high risk, particularly when frequent hand-to-mouth behaviors are present.

*Targeted screening* is acceptable when an area has been determined by existing data to have less risk. At 1 and 2 years of age (or from 3 to 6 years if previously unscreened), a child may be targeted for screening for several reasons. Children should be screened if they live in a geographic area determined to be at risk, are members of a group determined to be at risk (e.g., Medicaid recipients), or if their family can answer "yes" to these *personal risk questions:*

- Does your child live in or regularly visit a house that was built before 1959?
- Does your child live in or regularly visit a house built before 1978 with recent or ongoing renovations or remodeling within the past 6 months?
- Does your child have a sibling or playmate who has or did have lead poisoning?

The American Academy of Pediatrics (1998) supports the new recommendations. In addition, the Health Care Financing Administration (HCFA) is expected to publish new rules on lead screening for children who are Medicaid recipients. Nurses should be aware of these recommendations and apply them to their practice when appropriate.

## Therapeutic Management

The degree of concern, urgency, and need for medical intervention changes as the lead level increases. Regardless of medical need and urgency, providing education to the family is the most important element of the treatment process. The Guidelines from the Centers for Disease Control and Prevention (1997a) have identified several areas that should be discussed with the family of a child with a BLL of 10 $\mu$g/dl or greater:

- The child's BLL and what it means
- Potential adverse health effects of the elevated BLL
- Sources of lead exposure and suggestions on how to reduce exposure
- Importance of wet cleaning to remove lead dust on floors, window sills, and other surfaces; the ineffectiveness of dry methods of cleaning, such as sweeping
- Importance of good nutrition in reducing the absorption and effects of lead; if there are poor nutritional patterns, discuss adequate intake of calcium and iron and encourage regular meals
- Need for follow-up BLL testing to monitor the child's BLL, as appropriate
- Results of environmental inspection, if applicable
- Hazards of improper removal of lead-based paint; particularly hazardous are open-flame burning, power sanding, water blasting, methylene chloride-based stripping, and dry sanding and scraping

Because education is an integral part of the nursing role, the nurse is in a prime position to provide and reinforce this teaching.

Management of a child with an elevated blood lead level is best approached by a team effort. This involves health care professionals, social services, and local health departments. Roles vary depending on the severity of lead poisoning. The Guidelines (Centers for Disease Control and Prevention, 1997b) recommend the following actions based on a diagnosis using a venous BLL:

| BLL ($\mu$g/dl) | Action |
| --- | --- |
| <10 | Reassess or rescreen in 1 year. If exposure status changes, do this sooner. |
| 10-14 | Provide family lead education, follow-up testing, and social service referral if necessary. |
| 15-19 | Provide family lead education, follow-up testing, social service referral as needed; if it persists, initiate actions for BLL of 20 to 44 $\mu$g/dl. |
| 20-44 | Provide coordination of care, clinical management, environmental investigation, and lead-hazard control. |
| 45-69 | Within 48 hours, provide coordination of care and clinical management, including treatment, environmental investigation, and lead hazard control. The child must not remain in a lead-hazardous environment if resolution is to occur. |
| ≥70 | *Immediately* provide medical treatment and begin coordination of care, clinical management, environmental investigation, and lead-hazard control. |

How quickly and effectively a lead poisoning case is identified and resolved depends an several factors. These include the child, the family, the community, the resources available, and the political climate surrounding the lead poisoning issue in the municipality and state. Of equal importance are the attitudes and health care policies regarding lead poisoning that have been established by local and state health agencies. A more positive climate prompts more lead screening activities and subsequent follow-up. State and local legislation supporting prevention and detection activities leads to more available resources. Community awareness and coordinated action can help to quickly eliminate cases of lead poisoning.

Lead poisoning in children with behavioral issues such as *pica* (the habitual, purposeful, and compulsive ingestion of nonfood substances) and profound mouthing activities tend to resolve more slowly. Families dealing with additional crises, such as lack of supports and resources and/or violence or substance abuse, sometimes find it difficult to appreciate the importance of housing that is safe from lead hazards. Thus these children may not recover as quickly. Nurses must be aware of these issues if they are to effectively advocate and care for children with lead poisoning.

**Acute Lead Poisoning.** A venous BLL greater than 20 $\mu$g/dl requires clinical management. It is also the level at which an environmental investigation should occur in order to determine the source of the lead poisoning. However, the most important treatment at this level is family education. Chelation therapy is usually not instituted until a child reaches a BLL of near 45 $\mu$g/dl or greater. The nurse must keep in mind that lead poisoning acuity follows an upward gradient, with higher lead levels demonstrating a more severe problem. When a child reaches a BLL that requires chelation, treatment may take place in a hospital or on an outpatient basis, depending on the drug used and the circumstance of the treatment.

**Chelation Therapy.** *Chelation* is the term used for removing lead from circulating blood and, theoretically, some lead from organs and tissues. It is unclear whether chelation affects lead stores in bones. Although not an antidote in the truest sense, it does serve a similar purpose in that the toxic substance or poison is removed from the body. However, chelation does not counteract any effects of the lead. Because lead in circulating blood (the compartment most readily accessed by the chelator) is such a small part of the total body burden, the equilibration process will cause blood lead to rise again after treatment. The greater the amount of lead in other parts of the body, the higher the rise in BLL expected postchelation (although not as high as the prechelation level). This is often termed the *rebound phenomenon* and occurs when a child has a very high body burden of lead. Because of this phenomenon, children with very high lead levels are sometimes chelated several times before the BLL stabilizes and begins a downward trend (Baldwin and Marshall, 1999).

Historically, two drugs have been used for chelation. One is *British antilewisite,* commonly referred to as *BAL* but also called *dimercaprol* or *dimercaptopropanol.* The other is *calcium disodium edetate (CaNa₂EDTA),* commonly called *EDTA* with the chemical name ethylenediaminetetraacetic acid. In the early 1990s an oral chelator, *succimer (Chemet),* with the chemical name meso-2,3 dimercaptosuccinic acid (sometimes referred to as *DMSA*), was introduced. Additional drugs may be used, but these three are typically used by nearly all practitioners who treat lead poisoning (American Academy of Pediatrics, 1998).

*Succimer* is administered orally. It comes in the form of small beads in a capsule, which can be opened and sprinkled on a small amount of food or liquid to be swallowed or the capsule may also be swallowed whole. Although this drug may be given on an outpatient basis, some practitioners may begin the initial treatment with a few days in an inpatient setting. This allows the child to receive direct observed therapy and be monitored for unexpected adverse effects and also allows the family to use the social services and other available resources to help address alternative housing needs. Adverse effects include nausea, vomiting, diarrhea, loss of appetite, rash, elevation in liver function tests, and neutropenia. Dosage is 10 mg/kg three times a day for 5 days, then twice a day for 14 days. Because the chelates are excreted via the kidneys, adequate hydration is essential. Periodic urinalysis and monitoring of blood urea nitrogen (BUN), creatinine, liver transaminases, alkaline phosphatase, complete blood count with differential, and platelets, as well as BLL, necessary during chelation.

*EDTA* may be administered through the intravenous (IV) or intramuscular (IM) route. It is most often given using the IV route. The IM route is recommended for instances in which fluid restriction is necessary, such as the occurrence of cerebral edema. Potential adverse effects include proteinuria, hematuria, nephrotoxicity with renal tubular necrosis, increased BUN and/or creatinine, headache, paresthesias, numbness, anorexia, nausea, vomiting, elevation in liver function tests, and electrocardiograph (ECG) changes such as T wave inversion. Untoward effects, sometimes seen several hours after IV infusion has begun, are sudden fever, chills, fatigue, excessive thirst, sneezing, and nasal congestion. This drug may be used as therapy for a BLL of 45 µg/dl and greater. It is often used in conjunction with BAL when the BLL is 70 µg/dl or greater or in place of succimer when that oral chelator is not considered appropriate. Parameters that should be monitored while receiving EDTA include BLL; electrolytes; BUN and creatinine; complete blood count with differential and platelets; liver transaminases; alkaline phosphatase; urine specific gravity and dipstick; urinalysis if dipstick shows increased blood, protein, or white blood cells; blood pressure; and intake and output (American Academy of Pediatrics, 1998).

*BAL* is given only by deep IM injection. Because significant adverse effects involving intravascular hemolysis have been reported, it should not be used in the presence of a glucose-6-phosphatase dehydrogenase deficiency (G6PD). Before beginning treatment, a G6PD screen should be performed to rule out the existence of such a deficiency. It is also contraindicated for a child with peanut allergy because it is prepared in a peanut oil solution. BAL may form a complex with iron that is potentially toxic; therefore iron supplementation is not recommended during treatment. BAL is used in conjunction with EDTA to treat children with a BLL of 70 µg/dl and higher; it is never used as a single agent therapy. Potential adverse effects include increased blood pressure; tachycardia; nausea; vomiting; burning sensation in lips, mouth, and throat; abdominal pain; dysuria; fever; headache; pain in the throat, chest, or hands; paresthesias; muscle pain or weakness; mild conjunctivitis; lacrimation; rhinorrhea; salivation; and elevations in liver function test. Necessary ongoing monitoring includes all of those parameters for EDTA plus ECG monitoring at least for the first 24 hours of BAL treatment. If the BLL is 100 µg/dl or greater, it is necessary to continue ECG monitoring and to perform neurologic assessments and observe for seizure activity for at least the first 24 hours (American Academy of Pediatrics, 1998).

Any child with a new or recent sharp rise in BLL should have an abdominal x-ray examination to determine the presence of lead chips. If lead chips are present in the stomach or small intestine, it is necessary to decontaminate the bowel using a cathartic such as magnesium citrate or polyethylene glycol solution before beginning chelation (McKinney, 2000).

**Prognosis.** Although most of the pathophysiologic effects of lead are reversible, the most serious consequences of both high and low lead exposure are the effects on the central nervous system. In children with lead encephalopathy, permanent brain damage can result in mental retardation, behavior changes, possible paralysis, and seizures. However, moderate- to low-dose exposure may also cause permanent neurologic deficits. Increased distractibility, short attention span, impulsivity, reading disabilities, and

school failure have been associated with lead exposure (Rice, 1996; Mendelsohn and others, 1998). There is some evidence that treatment of moderate levels of lead poisoning can result in cognitive improvement (American Academy of Pediatrics, 1998).

### Nursing Considerations

The primary nursing goal in lead poisoning is to prevent the child's initial or further exposure to lead. For children with low-level exposure, this often requires identifying the sources of lead in the environment. Careful history taking is one of the most useful and valuable tools and should concentrate on the personal risk questions (see p. 679). (See Critical Thinking Exercise box.) Suggestions for reducing lead in the child's environment are listed in the Community Focus box on p. 682.

If chelation therapy is required, compliance is paramount. Oral medications must be given according to schedule and this must be stressed to the family. Children who receive multiple injections deserve an explanation of the treatment and may benefit from medical play.

Chelating agents are administered deeply into a large muscle mass. (See Atraumatic Care box on p. 682.) To lessen the pain from CaNa$_2$EDTA, the local anesthetic procaine is injected with the drug. Rotation of sites is essential

## Critical Thinking Exercise

### Lead Poisoning

The clinic in which you practice has received funds to begin a program to reduce lead poisoning in children. As a member of the planning committee, which of the following initial projects is effective and easy to implement?

FIRST, THINK ABOUT IT . . .

- What concepts or ideas are central to your thinking?
- What conclusions are you reaching?

1. Screening for blood lead levels by heel or finger puncture in all children under age 6 years
2. Questioning parents about the age and condition of their home(s) since the child's birth, including recent renovations
3. Screening for blood lead levels by venipuncture in all children under age 6 years who are at risk for lead exposure
4. Questioning parents about hobbies, occupations, and ethnic remedies that may expose the child to lead

*The best response is two. Asking about the family's dwelling to identify instances in which lead, especially on painted surfaces, could be present is the single most important screening procedure. The idea of asking about hobbies, occupations, and ethnic remedies should be considered, but option four is not the priority question. An accurate conclusion is that screening for blood lead levels is expensive and time consuming. Option three is incorrect because collection of blood by venipuncture is not a recommended screening procedure, and all children, regardless of risk, should be screened.*

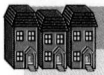

## COMMUNITY FOCUS
### Reducing Blood Lead Levels

Make sure child does not have access to peeling paint or chewable surfaces painted with lead-based paint, especially window sills and wells.

If a house was built before 1960 (possibly before 1980) and has hard-surface floors, wet mop them at least once a week. Wipe other hard surfaces (e.g., window sills, baseboards). If there are loose paint chips in an area, such as a window well, use a wet disposable cloth to pick up and discard them. Do not vacuum hard-surfaced floors or window sills or wells, because this spreads dust. Use vacuum cleaners with agitators to remove dust from rugs rather than vacuum cleaners with suction only. If a rug is known to contain lead dust and cannot be washed, it should be discarded.

Wash and dry child's hands and face frequently, especially before eating.

Wash toys and pacifiers frequently.

If soil around home is or is likely to be contaminated with lead (e.g., if home was built before 1960 or is near a major highway), plant grass or other ground cover; plant bushes around outside of house so that child cannot play there.

During remodeling of older homes, be sure to follow correct procedures. Be certain children and pregnant women are not in the home, day or night, until process is completed.

Modified from Centers for Disease Control and Prevention: *Preventing lead poisoning in young children,* Atlanta, 1991, CDC.

\*For more information, contact the county or state department of health or environment for information on local water quality. For general information on lead, call the EPA Safe Drinking Water Hotline, (800) 426-4791; *www.epa.gov;* National Lead Information Center (National Safety Council), 1025 Connecticut Ave NW, Suite 1200 Washington, DC, 20036, 202-293-2270, *www.nsc.org;* (800) LEAD-FYI; Water Quality Association (WQA), (630) 505-0160, *www.wqa.org,* or National Sanitation Foundation (NSF), (800) NSF-MARK, (734) 769-8010, *www.nsf.org.*

After deleading, thoroughly clean house using cleaning solution to damp mop and dust before inhabitants return.

In areas where lead content of water exceeds the drinking water standard and a particular faucet has not been used for 6 hours or more, "flush" the cold-water pipes by running the water until it becomes as cold as it will get (30 seconds to greater than 2 minutes). The more time water has been sitting in pipes, the more lead it may contain.

*Use only cold water* for consumption (drinking, cooking, and especially for making infant formula). Hot water dissolves lead more quickly than cold water and thus contains higher levels of lead. May use first-flush water for nonconsumption uses.

Have water tested by a competent laboratory. This action is especially important for apartment dwellers; flushing may not be effective in high-rise buildings or in other buildings with lead-soldered central piping

Do not store food in open cans, particularly if cans are imported.

Do not use pottery or ceramic ware that was inadequately fired or is meant for decorative use for food storage or service. Do not store drinks or food in lead crystal.

Avoid folk remedies or cosmetics that contain lead.

Make sure that home exposure is not occurring from parental occupations or hobbies. Household members employed in occupations such as lead smelting should shower and change into clean clothing before leaving work. Construction and lead abatement workers may also bring home lead contaminants.

Make sure child eats regular meals because more lead is absorbed on an empty stomach.

Make sure child's diet contains sufficient iron and calcium and not excessive fat.

---

## ATRAUMATIC CARE
### Lead Chelation Therapy

To lessen the pain from IM injection of CaNa$_2$EDTA, the local anesthetic procaine is injected with the drug. Apply EMLA cream over the puncture site 2½ hours before the injection of EDTA and BAL. Use IV EDTA whenever possible.

to prevent the formation of painful areas of fibrotic tissue. Because CaNa$_2$EDTA and lead are toxic to the kidneys, records are kept of intake and output, and the results of urinalysis are assessed to monitor renal functioning. Because of the risk of seizures, appropriate precautions are instituted at the bedside of children with high BLLs.

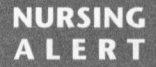

**NURSING ALERT** CaNa$_2$EDTA is never given in the absence of an adequate urinary output. Children receiving the drug intramuscularly must be able to maintain adequate oral intake of fluids.

Discharge planning for children with lead poisoning must include thorough education of families regarding safety from lead hazards, clear instructions regarding medication administration and needed follow-up, and confirmation that the child will be discharged to a home without

lead hazards. Although caution must be used to avoid alarming parents unnecessarily, it is important that they know the risk implications for their child's behavior and cognitive functions. Nurses are in a position to make observations about the development and behavior of a child who is hospitalized. Concerns that are identified should be more thoroughly evaluated. Referral to a child development or speech and language specialist may be indicated.

As in any situational crisis, parents need support and understanding if their child is treated for lead poisoning. Many of the families at highest risk for lead poisoning have the fewest resources to comply with measures such as relocation or deleading the home. Appropriate referrals are essential in locating assistance for parents. (See Nursing Care Plan: The Child with Lead Poisoning.\*)

The nature of childhood lead poisoning makes it not only a health issue but also a public policy issue. It is a condition that affects hundreds of children each year. Through education, prevention efforts, early identification, provision of care, and advocacy for the protection of children, nurses can contribute to the eventual control and elimination of this harmful but preventable condition.

---

\*In Wong DL, Hess CS: *Wong and Whaley's clinical manual of pediatric nursing,* ed 5, St Louis, 2000, Mosby.

# CHILD MALTREATMENT

The broad term *child maltreatment* includes intentional physical abuse or neglect, emotional abuse or neglect, and sexual abuse of children, usually by adults. It is one of the most significant social problems affecting children, and parent-child abuse may be only one type of violence in the family. The Child Abuse Prevention and Treatment Act (CAPTA), as amended and reauthorized in October 1996 (Public Law 104-235, Section 111; 42 USC 5106g), defines child abuse and neglect as, at a minimum, any recent act or failure to act that results in imminent risk of serious harm, death, serious physical or emotional harm, sexual abuse, or exploitation of a child (a person under the age of 18, unless the child protection law of the state in which the child resides specifies a younger age for cases not involving sexual abuse) by a parent or caretaker (including any employee of a residential facility or any staff person providing out-of-home care) who is responsible for the child's welfare.

CAPTA defines sexual abuse as employment, use, persuasion, inducement, enticement, or coercion of any child to engage in, or assisting any other person to engage in, any sexually explicit conduct or any simulation of such conduct for the purpose of producing any visual depiction of such conduct. The definition also includes rape, and in cases of caretaker or intrafamilial relationships, statutory rape, molestation, prostitution or other forms of sexual exploitation of children, or incest with children.

There are four major types of child maltreatment: (1) physical abuse (the infliction of physical injury as a result of punching, beating, kicking, biting, burning, shaking, or otherwise harming a child), (2) child neglect (characterized by failure to provide for the child's basic needs—physical, educational, or emotional), (3) sexual abuse (includes fondling a child's genitals, intercourse, incest, rape, sodomy, exhibitionism, and commercial exploitation through prostitution or the production of pornographic materials), and (4) emotional abuse (includes acts or omissions by the parents or other caregivers that have caused, or could cause, serious behavioral, cognitive, emotional, or mental disorders). Emotional abuse is almost always present when other forms are identified. The assessment of child neglect requires consideration of cultural values and standards of care, as well as recognition that the failure to provide the necessities of life may be related to poverty (Chiocca, 1998; Nester, 1998).

Violence between parents also often occurs; the abusing parent may also be the abused spouse (Chiocca, 1998). Family violence also increases the risk of physical and sexual abuse in youngsters who leave the home to avoid maltreatment. Ironically these "runaways" often encounter continued abuse "on the streets" as they try to survive.

Dentists, like physicians, have a responsibility to protect their patients and probably see many more cases than they realize. Almost three fourths of child abuse cases involve injuries to the head, face, mouth, and neck—exactly the area that dentists see closely when treating a patient. Unfortunately, most dentists are not taught to detect the signs of possible child abuse, and many are unaware of their legal responsibility to report abuse. All 50 states require health professionals, by law, to report child abuse. Many mouth injuries occur as a result of force-feeding. Most physical abuse is the result of a spontaneous loss of control rather than an act of premeditation (Jessee, 1996).

The number of children reported as abused or neglected declined from 900,000 in 1998 to an estimated 826,000 victims in 1999. More children suffer neglect than any other form of maltreatment. In 1999 approximately 58% of victims suffered neglect, 21% physical abuse, and 11% sexual abuse. The highest rates of maltreatment occurred in the 0 to 3 age group, and rates declined as age increased. Rates of abuse were similar for male and females, but the rate of sexual abuse for females was approximately four times that of males (Health and Human Services, 1999).

Nationally, approximately 1100 children are known to have died from abuse or neglect in 1999. Children less than 1 year old accounted for 42% of these deaths, and approximately 83% of these fatalities were in children younger than 6 years of age (Health and Human Services, 1999).*

## Child Neglect

Child neglect is the most common form of maltreatment. Approximately one half of all reported cases are associated with deprivation of necessities, and more than one third of deaths from maltreatment are in this group. *Neglect* is generally defined as the failure of a parent or other person legally responsible for the child's welfare to provide for the child's basic needs and an adequate level of care (Nester, 1998; Kaplan, Pelcoritz, and Labruna, 1999).

Little is known about the etiology of neglect, but it appears that many of the risk factors identified in physical abuse also apply to neglect (see the following discussion). Ignorance of the child's needs and a lack of resources are important contributing factors. For example, neglectful parents often demonstrate poor parenting skills. They may be unaware that an infant needs to be fed every 3 to 4 hours, may not know what to feed the child, and may have insufficient funds to buy food. The most serious lack of knowledge is failure to recognize emotional nurturing as an essential need of children. (See Failure to Thrive, Chapter 13.)

### Types of Neglect

Neglect takes many forms and can be classified broadly as physical or emotional maltreatment. *Physical neglect* involves the deprivation of necessities such as food, clothing, shelter, supervision, medical care, and education. *Emotional neglect* generally refers to failure to meet the child's needs for affection, attention, and emotional nurturance. It may also include lack of intervention for or fostering of maladaptive behavior, such as delinquency or substance abuse. *Emotional abuse,* an even more difficult aspect of maltreatment to define, refers to the deliberate attempt to destroy or significantly impair a child's self-esteem or competence. Emotional abuse may take the following forms: rejecting,

---

*Additional information is available from the **National Clearinghouse on Child Abuse and Neglect Information,** 330 C Street SW, Washington, DC, 20447; (703) 835-7565 or (800) FYI-3366; www.calib.com/nccanch.

isolating, terrorizing, ignoring, corrupting, verbally assaulting, and overpressuring the child (Nester, 1998).

## Physical Abuse

The deliberate infliction of physical injury on a child, usually by the child's caregiver, is termed *physical abuse.* Minor physical injury is responsible for more reported cases of maltreatment than major physical injury, but major physical abuse causes more deaths.

### Munchausen Syndrome by Proxy (MSBP)

One of the more unusual and perplexing types of abuse, usually physical, is MSBP, which refers to illness that one person fabricates or induces in another person (Hall and others, 2000; Paulk, 2001). Children as young as neonates and as old as 21 years of age have been seen clinically with factitious illness by proxy. The illness is usually dramatic and results in repeated visits to multiple health care providers and numerous diagnostic tests and therapeutic procedures. It is not uncommon for these children to demonstrate symptoms involving more than one organ system (Pasqualone and Fitzgerald, 1999). In children, it is usually the mother who fabricates the signs and symptoms of illness in her child (the proxy) to gain attention from the medical staff. Cases have been reported with adults as both perpetrators and as victims.

MSBP can take many forms, such as adding human blood to the child's urine to simulate hematuria, presenting a fictitious medical history, chronic poisoning of the child, or suffocating the child to cause apnea and seizures. Another form of MSBP is alleging that the child has been sexually abused by someone else to gain recognition as the child's protector (Hornor, 2001).

Such cases are often very difficult to confirm and require a high index of suspicion to protect the children. Warning signs of MSBP include (Table 16-6):

- Unexplained, prolonged, recurrent, or extremely rare illness
- Discrepancies between clinical findings and history
- Illness unresponsive to treatment
- Signs and symptoms occurring only in parent's presence
- Parent knowledgeable about illness, procedures, and treatments
- Parent very interested in interacting with health team members
- Parent very attentive toward child (refuses to leave hospital)
- Family members with similar symptoms

**TABLE 16-6**  Common presentations of Munchausen syndrome by proxy and the usual methods of deception

| Presentation | Mechanism |
| --- | --- |
| Apnea | Suffocation, drugs, poisoning |
| Seizures | Drugs, poisoning, asphyxiation |
| Bleeding | Adding blood to urine, vomit, etc.; opening intravenous line |
| Fevers, blood infection | Injection of feces, saliva, contaminated water into the child |
| Vomiting | Poisoning with drugs that cause vomiting |
| Diarrhea | Poisoning with laxatives, salt, mineral oil |

It is important to consider environmental and psychosocial factors when the clinical presentation does not seem medically plausible. Health care providers should consult the Child Protection Team when MSBP is suspected. The multidisciplinary team can provide concrete suggestions for confirming MSBP, help initiate the necessary legal action after the diagnosis has been established, formulate a treatment/intervention plan for the mother, outline a monitoring system to protect the child in the future, and establish criteria for reunification (Bryk and Siegel, 1997).

The consequences for children with MSBP can be serious. They often undergo needless and painful medical procedures and treatments. The parent's actions may induce a serious illness in children—one that is fatal in almost 10% of the cases (Souid, Keith, and Cunningham, 1998; Hall and others, 2000). Children may develop chronic invalidism, accepting the illness story and believing themselves to be ill. Finally, they may develop MSBP as an adult. Even when some of these children are removed from the home, they continue to suffer severe psychologic trauma. Other siblings remaining in the home may become substitute victims.

### Factors Predisposing to Physical Abuse

The exact cause of child abuse is not known, but three major criteria—parental characteristics, characteristics of the child, and environmental characteristics—influence the potential for abuse. However, no one factor or group of factors is predictive of abuse. Rather, an *interaction* between several factors appears to increase the risk of abuse occurring in a particular family; the greater the number of factors, the greater the risk. Different factors may be responsible for certain types of maltreatment. For example, poverty may be more strongly associated with neglect, whereas parental characteristics may be more strongly related to physical abuse.

**Parental Characteristics.** Extensive research has focused on parental characteristics that distinguish abusive parents from nonabusive parents.

Some studies provide conflicting evidence, but it is now generally recognized that parental history of abuse or neglect during childhood is a significant risk factor for child abuse (Behrman and Kliegman, 1998; Murry, Baker, and Lewin, 2000).

**NURSING ALERT**  Nurses must be careful to avoid stereotyping parents and children in an attempt to predict or diagnose abuse. No test has sufficient sensitivity to predict abuse without falsely accusing many individuals (false-positives) and missing some abusers (false-negatives).

Abusive parents who report receiving severe punishment as children are much more likely to injure their own children (Murry, Baker, and Lewin, 2000). If the abuse was not overt physical violence, abusive parents typically recall their punishment as unfair and severe, and they characterize their relationship with their parents as negative. Abusive parents tend to have difficulty controlling aggressive impulses, and the free expression of violence is one of the most consistent qualities of these families (Rodriguez and Green, 1997).

Another finding is that abusive families are often more socially isolated and have fewer supportive relationships than nonabusive parents. Children of teenage mothers are more at risk for abuse than children of older mothers (McCullough and Scherman, 1998; Murry, Baker, and Lewin, 2000). With little or no available support system and the presence of concurrent stresses imposed by the child or environment, these parents are extremely vulnerable to additional crises of any nature and literally strike out at the child as a method of releasing their increasing frustration and anxiety.

Other factors identified in abusive parents include low self-esteem and less adequate maternal functioning. Although inadequate knowledge of childrearing is often cited as a characteristic of abusive parents, research findings do not consistently support this belief. However, this does not mean that these parents cannot benefit from learning more constructive ways of rearing their children, especially nonviolent discipline methods (Nester, 1998).

**Characteristics of the Child.**  The child also unintentionally contributes to the abusive situation. In families of two or more children, usually only one child is the victim of abuse. This child's temperament, position in the family, additional physical needs if ill or disabled, activity level, or degree of sensitivity to parental needs all contribute to the potential for physical abuse. For example, one child may not be abused if he or she fits into the "easy-child pattern," whereas another sibling with a difficult temperament may add to the parent's stress sufficiently to precipitate an abusive act. However, temperament alone is not the critical factor; rather, it is the "fit" or compatibility between the child's temperament and the parent's ability to deal with that behavioral style.

Occasionally the abused child is illegitimate, unwanted, brain damaged (especially in situations in which the parents cannot accept the retardation), hyperactive, or physically disabled. Sometimes children are abused because they remind the parent of someone the parent dislikes, such as a younger brother or sister who received all the attention from their own parents. Premature infants may be at risk for maltreatment because of the failure of parent-child bonding during early infancy. A difficult pregnancy, labor, or delivery is often a predisposing factor in abuse, especially when the infant is born prematurely or with congenital anomalies.

Although one child is usually the victim in an abusive family, removing that child from the home often places the other siblings at risk for abuse. Child maltreatment usually is not confined to one child because of a disturbed parent-child relationship but is a result of a family in distress. Therefore no child is safe if left in the abusive environment unless the parents can be helped to learn new parenting skills and to meet their needs and release their frustration through outlets other than attacking their children.

**Environmental Characteristics.**  The environment plays a significant role in the potential abusive situation. Typically the environment is one of chronic stress, including problems of divorce, poverty, unemployment, poor housing, frequent relocation, alcoholism, and drug addiction. Increased exposure between children and parents, such as that which occurs in crowded living conditions, also increases the likelihood of abuse.

Although most reporting of abuse has been from lower socioeconomic populations, child abuse is by no means the problem of any one societal group. It spans all educational, social, and economic levels. Certainly, stresses imposed by poverty predispose lower socioeconomic families to abusive situations, and abuse in these groups is more apt to be reported. However, concealed crises can also be present in upper-class families. For example, a wealthy family experiencing major life changes (e.g., rehousing, the birth of an additional child, marital discord) may have sufficient environmental stressors imposed on them to produce a potentially abusive situation. Wealthy families may be so overinvolved with commitments outside the home that abuse may be inflicted by substitute caregivers. Nurses need to be aware of such factors in order to identify the less obvious examples of child abuse and neglect.

## Sexual Abuse

Sexual abuse is one of the most devastating types of child maltreatment, and current estimates indicate that it has increased significantly during the past decade. However, the increased rate of reporting may not reflect a true increase in prevalence of sexual abuse but may be a result of changes in legislation and in society's attitudes toward women and children (Wang and Daro, 1998). In 1997 the number of reported occurrences was approximately 8% of all child maltreatment cases, but many authorities believe this figure represents only a small percentage of the actual incidence (Wang and Daro, 1998).

As with all forms of child maltreatment, no universal definition for sexual abuse exists. The Child Abuse and Prevention Act (Public Law 100-235) defines *sexual abuse* as "the use, persuasion, or coercion of any child to engage in sexually explicit conduct (or any simulation of such conduct) for producing any visual depiction of such conduct, or rape, molestation, prostitution, or incest with children."

To be considered child abuse, these acts must be committed by a person responsible for the child's care, such as a parent or baby-sitter. If a stranger commits the act, it is considered sexual assault. Sexual abuse may include physical abuse, both as part of sexual arousal for the abuser and to force compliance from the child.

Sexual abuse includes several types of sexual maltreatment, including the following: (See Rape, Chapter 20.)

**Incest**—Any physical sexual activity between family members; blood relationship is not required (abusers can include stepparents, unrelated siblings, grandparents, uncles, and aunts); does not include sexual relations between legally sanctioned partners, such as spouses

**Molestation**—A vague term that includes "indecent liberties," such as touching, fondling, kissing, single or mutual masturbation, or oral-genital contact

**Exhibitionism**—Indecent exposure, usually exposure of the genitals by an adult to children or other adults

**Child pornography**—Arranging and photographing (in any media) sexual acts involving children, either alone or with adults or animals, regardless of consent by the child's legal guardian; also may denote distribution of such material in any form with or without profit

**Child prostitution**—Involving children in sex acts for profit and usually with changing partners

**Pedophilia**—Literally means "love of child" and does not denote a type of sexual activity but the preference for prepubertal children as the means of achieving sexual excitement

## Characteristics of Abusers and Victims

Anyone, including siblings and mothers, can be sexual abusers, but a typical abuser is a male that the victim knows. Offenders come from all levels of society. Some are prominent persons in the community; some, especially in the case of pedophiliacs (also called "child molesters"), are in positions that involve working closely with children, such as teaching and coaching. (See Community Focus box.)

Pornography and prostitution may involve strangers or the children's own parents. There are no typical characteristics of these offenders, although the abused children tend to be runaways—young adolescents who engage in these activities to obtain money for food, shelter, drugs, and alcohol. Incestuous relationships between father or stepfather and daughter are generally prolonged, and the victims are usually reluctant to report the situation because of fear of retaliation and fear that they will not be believed. The presence of a stepfather is the family feature most noted when families are at risk for incest. The eldest daughter is usually abused, but in her absence another sister is substituted. Sibling incest may also occur (Adler and Schultz, 1995). Sexual abuse by relatives who have a strong emotional bond with the victim is the most devastating to the child (Fischer and McDonald, 1998).

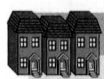

## COMMUNITY FOCUS
### Characteristics of Personality Disorders

Abusive individuals appear indifferent to emotional pain in others. Eighty-eight percent of families in which physical abuse and neglect occurred also had animals that were abused.

Hurting animals can be one of the earliest symptoms of conduct disorder, with a median onset age of 6.5 years. Conduct disorder is a label for disturbances of behavior contradictory to accepted social norms; there is a direct relationship between the antisocial tendency and deprivation. Conduct disorder or criminal behaviors in either parent or in both parents have been associated with psychiatric disturbances in children. Whether this effect is a result of inadequate parenting, modeling, or the greater likelihood of parental maltreatment—or to some combination of factors—remains unclear.

The essential feature of antisocial personality disorder (conduct disorder) is a pervasive pattern of disregard for and violation of the rights of others. An individual with an antisocial personality disorder does not exhibit any sense of guilt and often is very manipulative. To be diagnosed with antisocial personality disorder, the individual must be at least 18 years old and must have shown evidence of conduct disorder before the age of 15. Conduct disorder is often present across generations within families.

All health providers (human and animal) in a given community should be aware of these statistics and characteristics and should be morally and legally obligated to report their suspicions and clinical findings to the proper authorities (Carson and Arnold, 1996).

Boys are also victims of both intrafamilial and extrafamilial abuse. Males are much less likely to report abuse, and they may suffer much greater emotional harm from incestuous relationships, especially between mother and son, than do female victims. Boys are likely to be subjected to anal penetration and oral-genital contact, to have subtle physical findings, and to be abused by a father, stepfather, or mother's boyfriend.

## Initiation and Perpetuation of Sexual Abuse

The cycle of sexual abuse often starts innocently unless it involves an isolated attack such as rape. Offenders often spend time with the victims to gain their trust before initiating any sexual contact. Most victims are then pressured into being an accessory to the sexual activity through various means (Box 16-11) and may be unaware that sexual activity is part of the offer. Children may not reveal the truth for fear that their parents will not believe them, especially if the offender is a trusted member of the family. Some fear they will be blamed for the situation, and many young children with limited vocabulary have difficulty describing the activity when they do have the courage or the opportunity to reveal the abuse.

> **NURSING ALERT**
> Nonspecific behavior problems associated with sexual abuse include school dysfunction, phobias, acting out, eating disorders, and suicide attempts (Behrman and Kliegman, 1998).

Seductiveness by the child does not initiate incest. Most young girls experiment in seduction, especially during the preschool years, but the father's response normally differentiates this playfulness from overt sexual invitation. Although the reasons for incest are complicated and can occur in various family types, it does not occur in healthy families. Most incestuous relationships are directly tied to sexual maladjustment and estrangement between husband and wife. Most begin following the cessation of sexual relationships with the usual partner. Most fathers experience little guilt, and many wives at some level are aware of the incestuous affair. The wife may react by tolerating the situation or may resort to use of denial; some remain unaware of the activity. Consequently, the home offers little protection to young victims,

> **Box 16-11** ■ ■ ■
> **Methods Used to Pressure Children into Sexual Activity**
>
> The child is offered gifts or privileges.
> The adult misrepresents moral standards by telling the child that it is "okay to do."
> Emotionally and socially impoverished children are enticed by adults who meet their needs for warmth and human contact.
> The successful sex offender pressures the victim into secrecy regarding the activity by describing it as a "secret between us" that other people may take away if they find out.
> The offender plays on the child's fears, including fear of punishment by the offender, fear of repercussions if the child tells, and fear of abandonment or rejection by the family.

because abusers have easy access to their victims and the children believe they cannot reveal their secret to other family members. However, not all incestuous relationships follow this pattern of silence. Reports of father-daughter incest during child custody conflicts have become more common and have raised serious concerns regarding the possibility of false accusation. Rather than tolerating or denying the child's sexual abuse, the other parent (usually the mother) is typically the chief accuser.

## Nursing Care of the Maltreated Child

### ⚏ Assessment

One of the most critical responsibilities of all health professionals is identifying abusive situations as early as possible. (See Community Focus box.) The characteristics that may predispose members of some families to commit abuse can serve as a framework for assessing vulnerability but are never predictive of actual abuse. A thorough physical examination and a careful, detailed history are the diagnostic tools needed to identify abuse.* Nurses have a very special role because they may be the first person to see the child and parent and are the consistent caregivers if the child is hospitalized. (See Guidelines box.)

**Evidence of Maltreatment.** Recognition of abuse or neglect necessitates a familiarity with both the physical and the behavioral signs that suggest maltreatment (Box 16-12). No one indicator can diagnose maltreatment; rather, it is a pattern or combination of indicators that should arouse suspicion and further investigation. In addition, signs of possible abuse must be coupled with an understanding of diseases (e.g., bleeding disorders, osteogenesis imperfecta, or sudden infant death syndrome [SIDS]) and cultural practices such coin rubbing (see Health Practices, Chapter 2) that may mimic physical abuse. Unintentional injuries, such as burns from metal buckles on car seats, lacerations from seat belts, or retinal hemorrhage after cardiopulmonary resuscitation, may also be wrongly diagnosed as abuse. Normal variants, such as mongolian spots and congenital anomalies of genitalia, can be mistaken for abuse (Box 16-13).

---

*Child abuse diagnostic slide kits are available from the American Academy of Pediatrics, www.aap.org.

Not all forms of physical abuse demonstrate obvious signs. Violent shaking of children, especially infants under 6 months old *(shaken baby syndrome [SBS]),* can cause fatal intracranial trauma without signs of external head injury (Castiglia, 2001). Nurses should suspect SBS in infants less than 1 year of age who present with subdural and/or retinal hemorrhages in the absence of external signs of trauma (Box 16-14) (Castiglia, 2001). If MSBP is suspected, nurses play an important role in monitoring the parent's activities to identify instances of causing the children's symptoms. Using a hidden video camera to document the parent's behavior is becoming a more common diagnostic procedure, but the parent's right to privacy must be considered (Hall and others, 2000).

> **NURSING ALERT**
>
> Stress to parents the dangers of shaking infants (can cause "shaken baby syndrome"). Advise against:
> Shaking as a method of burping or waking infant
> Tossing infant in air
> Shaking infant when feeling angry or tense

*Neglect and emotional abuse.* Neglect from deprivation of necessities is easier to identify than emotional neglect or abuse because the physical signs are usually evident. Emotional maltreatment may be readily suspected but is very difficult to substantiate. The physical signs are often nonspecific, and nurses must rely on behavioral indicators that range from depression to acting-out behavior to help identify a possibly abusive situation. Any persistent and unexplained change in the child's behavior is an important clue to possible emotional abuse.

*Sexual abuse.* Identifying instances of sexual abuse is particularly difficult because often few if any obvious physical indications of the activity may exist. Also, many individuals are hesitant to believe children and unwilling to report incidents. Even health professionals are sometimes at fault when they perform cursory physical examinations of the genitalia and ignore behavior or verbal comments that suggest abuse. When sexual abuse is suspected, other children in the family should also be evaluated, because multiple victims are not uncommon.

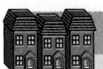

## COMMUNITY FOCUS
### Identifying Abuse

In assessing both adults and children, look for a history of animal abuse, torment, or torture. Look also for childhood or adolescent acts of violence toward other children and, possibly, adults. A history of destructiveness to property is also significant (Kaplan, Pelcovitz, and Labruna, 1999).

Cruelty to animals and cruelty to humans should be viewed as a continuum. These acts are not harmless ventings of emotions in healthy individuals; they are warning signs that these individuals need professional intervention. Abusing animals does not dissipate violent emotions; rather, the abuse may fuel them (Lockwood and Church, 1996).

## GUIDELINES
### Talking with Children Who Reveal Abuse

Provide a private time and place to talk.
Do not promise not to tell; tell them that you are required by law to report the abuse.
Do not express shock or criticize them or their family.
Use their vocabulary to discuss body parts.
Avoid using any leading statements that can distort their report.
Reassure them that they have done the right thing by telling.
Tell them that the abuse is not their fault and that they are not bad or to blame.
Determine their immediate need for safety.
Let the child know what will happen when you report.

## PHYSICAL NEGLECT
### Suggestive Physical Findings
Failure to thrive
Signs of malnutrition, such as thin extremities, abdominal distention, lack of subcutaneous fat
Poor personal hygiene
Unclean and/or inappropriate dress
Evidence of poor health care, such as delayed immunization, untreated infections, frequent colds
Frequent injuries from lack of supervision

### Suggestive Behaviors
Dull and inactive; excessively passive or sleepy
Self-stimulatory behaviors, such as finger-sucking or rocking
Begging or stealing food
Absenteeism from school
Drug or alcohol addiction
Vandalism or shoplifting

## EMOTIONAL ABUSE AND NEGLECT
### Suggestive Physical Findings
Failure to thrive
Feeding disorders
Enuresis
Sleep disorders

### Suggestive Behaviors
Self-stimulatory behaviors such as biting, rocking, sucking
During infancy, lack of social smile and stranger anxiety
Withdrawal
Unusual fearfulness
Antisocial behavior, such as destructiveness, stealing, cruelty
Extremes of behavior, such as overcompliant and passive or aggressive and demanding
Lags in emotional and intellectual development, especially language
Suicide attempts

## PHYSICAL ABUSE
### Suggestive Physical Findings
Bruises and welts (may be in various stages of healing)
  On face, lips, mouth, back, buttocks, thighs, or areas of torso
  Regular patterns descriptive of object used, such as belt buckle, hand, wire hanger, chain, wooden spoon, squeeze or pinch marks
Burns
  On soles of feet, palms of hands, back, or buttocks
  Patterns descriptive of object used, such as round cigar or cigarette burns, sharply demarcated areas from immersion in scalding water, rope burns on wrists or ankles from being bound, burns in the shape of an iron, radiator, or electric stove burner
  Absence of "splash" marks and presence of symmetric burns
  Stun gun injury—lesions circular, fairly uniform (up to 0.5 cm) and paired approximately 5 cm apart (Frechette and Rimsza, 1992)
Fractures and dislocations
  Skull, nose, or facial structures
  Injury may denote type of abuse, such as spiral fracture or dislocation from twisting of an extremity or whiplash from shaking the child
  Multiple new or old fractures in various stages of healing

Lacerations and abrasions
  On backs of arms, legs, torso, face, or external genitalia
  Unusual symptoms, such as abdominal swelling, pain, and vomiting from punching
  Descriptive marks such as from human bites or pulling out of hair
Chemical
  Unexplained repeated poisoning, especially drug overdose
  Unexplained sudden illness, such as hypoglycemia from insulin administration

### Suggestive Behaviors
Wariness of physical contact with adults
Apparent fear of parents or of going home
Lying very still while surveying environment
Inappropriate reaction to injury, such as failure to cry from pain
Lack of reaction to frightening events
Apprehensiveness when hearing other children cry
Indiscriminate friendliness and displays of affection
Superficial relationships
Acting-out behavior, such as aggression, to seek attention
Withdrawal behavior

## SEXUAL ABUSE
### Suggestive Physical Findings
Bruises, bleeding, lacerations or irritation of external genitalia, anus, mouth, or throat
Torn, stained, or bloody underclothing
Pain on urination or pain, swelling, and itching of genital area
Penile discharge
Sexually transmitted disease, nonspecific vaginitis, or venereal warts
Difficulty in walking or sitting
Unusual odor in the genital area
Recurrent urinary tract infections
Presence of semen
Pregnancy in young adolescent

### Suggestive Behaviors
Sudden emergence of sexually related problems, including excessive or public masturbation, age-inappropriate sexual play, promiscuity, or overtly seductive behavior
Withdrawn behavior, excessive daydreaming
Preoccupation with fantasies, especially in play
Poor relationships with peers
Sudden changes, such as anxiety, loss or gain of weight, clinging behavior
In incestuous relationships, excessive anger at mother for not protecting daughter
Regressive behavior, such as bed-wetting or thumb-sucking
Sudden onset of phobias or fears, particularly fears of the dark, men, strangers, or particular settings or situations (e.g., undue fear of leaving the house or staying at the daycare center or the baby-sitter's house)
Running away from home
Substance abuse, particularly of alcohol or mood-elevating drugs
Profound and rapid personality changes, especially extreme depression, hostility, and aggression (often accompanied by social withdrawal)
Rapidly declining school performance
Suicidal attempts or ideation

Unfortunately, there is no typical profile of the victim; there must be a high index of suspicion to identify such children. Physical signs vary and may include any of those listed for sexual abuse in Box 16-12. The victim may exhibit various behavioral manifestations but, unfortunately, none of these

behaviors is diagnostic of sexual abuse. When abused children exhibit these behaviors, the signs may be incorrectly attributed to the normal stresses of childhood, especially in older school-age children or adolescents. Even those signs considered most predictive of sexual abuse, such as certain genital

## Box 16-13 ■ ■ ■
### Conditions That Can Be Mistaken for Sexual Abuse

Accidental straddle injuries
Accidental impaling injuries
Waterskiing injuries
Vulvovaginitis and proctitis
Diaper dermatitis
Foreign bodies
Lower extremity girdle paralysis
Defects that cause chronic constipation, Hirschsprung disease, anteriorly displaced anus
Crohn disease
Labial adhesions
Anal fissures

Modified from Brodeur AE, Monteleone JA: *Child maltreatment: a clinical guide and reference*, St Louis, 1994, GW Medical.

## Box 16-14 ■ ■ ■
### Physical Findings in Shaken Baby Syndrome

Retinal hemorrhages
CNS (closed head) injury
    Bleeding (subdural, epidural, subarachnoid, subgaleal)
    Laceration
    Contusion
    Concussion
Bruises—facial, scalp, arms, abdomen, back
Soft tissue swelling
Skull fracture(s)
Other fracture(s) (long bones, ribs, metaphyseal)
Abdominal injuries
Chest injuries
Delayed capillary refill
Hypotension
Tense or bulging fontanel

Data from Brodeur AE, Monteleone JA: *Child maltreatment: a clinical guide and reference*, St Louis, 1994, GW Medical, and Castiglia R: Shaken baby syndrome, *J Pediatr Health Care* 15(2):78-80, 2001.

## EVIDENCE-BASED PRACTICE
### *Using Findings from the Genital Examination to Diagnose Sexual Abuse in Children*

Unlike physical abuse, in which signs of maltreatment are often apparent, little or no evidence of sexual activity may be found in sexual abuse. To help substantiate accusations of molestation, several investigators have attempted to define characteristics of genitalia in males and females that are "diagnostic" of sexual abuse. Of the many findings that have been reported as conclusive or "highly suspect," the following are often considered the most significant: vaginal opening greater than 4 mm (Cantwell, 1983; White, Ingram, and Lyna, 1989), hymenal tears and synechiae (tissue bands) inside the vagina (Emans and others, 1987), reflex and dilation (Hobbs and Wynne, 1989), and condylomata acuminata (anogenital or venereal warts) (Hanson and others, 1989).

However, most subjects in these studies were children suspected of sexual abuse; without a control group of nonabused children, it is impossible to be certain that the same findings are not present in all children. The few studies with control groups found the same genital signs in the nonabused children, although not as often. Surprisingly, little is known about the normal range of genital characteristics in children. What is known casts serious doubt on the diagnostic validity of any of the "highly suspect" signs. McCann and others (1990) conducted studies on prepubertal children who had been carefully screened to rule out sexual abuse. They found that the size of the vaginal opening varied greatly; an opening greater than 4 mm was not unusual. The size was influenced by the examination position, amount of traction applied to the labia, degree of relaxation during the examination, and the child's age. In examining the anal and vaginal areas, the researchers found that the findings often associated with sexual abuse, including reflex and dilation (opening of the anal sphincters during knee-chest position), hymenal tears, and vaginal synechiae, were not unusual in nonabused children (Berenson, Somma-Garcia, and Barnett, 1993; McCann and others, 1989, 1990).

One of the most controversial issues is the diagnostic importance of finding a sexually transmitted disease in a prepubertal child. For example, the American Academy of Pediatrics (1999) states that for a child with postperinatal condylomata acuminata, sexual abuse is "probable" and the case should be reported to the community agency for child abuse and neglect. Another issue is the possibility of sexual abuse in children with human immunodeficiency virus (HIV) who lack risk factors, such as acquiring the infection perinatally (American Academy of Pediatrics, 1990).

Obviously, the diagnosis of child sexual abuse is difficult, and *proof* of sexual abuse does not rest on the physical examination. The only definitive physical evidence of sexual assault is the presence of sperm (Aiken, 1990). However, the presence of sperm in a pubertal girl may not necessarily be there from sexual abuse, but from consensual intercourse (Gardner, 1993). In reviewing cases of sexual abuse with successful conviction of the perpetrator, experts contend that the most important evidence is the quality of the history (including the medical record) and the ability of children to tell their story (Lauritsen, Meldgaard, and Charles, 2000).

Nurses who are aware of these recent findings regarding normal genitalia can encourage practitioners to consider their findings on the genital examination very cautiously in terms of diagnosing sexual abuse. The use of a *colposcope* can improve the accuracy and reliability of the examination, and nurses are often responsible for assisting the practitioner with the colposcopic examination. The instrument consists of a pair of binoculars mounted on a tripod or a movable mechanical arm. It has a light for better visualization, magnifies the structure from 10 to 20 times, and is equipped with a special camera to take photographs (McClain and others, 2000).

findings, sexually inappropriate behavior for age, enactment of adult sexual activity, and intense focus on sexual activity (e.g., masturbation), do not always indicate that sexual abuse has occurred. (See Evidence-Based Practice box.) Conversely, abused children may not demonstrate more knowledge of sexual activity than nonabused children. However, one difference in abused children's explanation of sexual activity may be unusual affective responses. For example, abused children may relate stories that include a fear of going to sleep or of being with a parent (Calam and others, 1998).

**History Pertaining to the Incident.**　In addition to observable evidence of abuse, the type of history revealed by the parents or other caregiver, such as the baby-sitter or mother's boyfriend, is a significant factor. Areas of the history that should arouse suspicion of abuse are summarized in Box 16-15.

> **NURSING ALERT**
>
> Incompatibility between the history and the injury is probably the most important criterion on which to base the decision to report suspected abuse.

An important point to remember when taking a history is that maltreated children rarely betray their parents by admitting to the abuse they have received. If questioned, they repeat the same story as the parents and try to defend their parents' actions. If the interviewer directly accuses the parents of abuse, the child may accept responsibility for the act in an attempt to vindicate the parents. Whether children respond in this way out of fear is uncertain. However, children also fear losing whatever security and love they have. Between abusive acts children may receive some measure of attention and love from the parents. If they betray the parents, they believe they may lose this and are uncertain or fearful of the consequences, such as foster care. Preserving the present situation may be less frightening than facing an unknown future.

The *disclosure of sexual abuse* can occur in a variety of ways: the act is observed by others, resulting in a direct confrontation; the child tells someone, such as a teacher or parent of a friend; visible clues of the relationship are observed, such as an accumulation of coins, gifts, or candy; more obvious clues are seen, such as a child coming home disheveled or becoming pregnant; or physical or behavioral signs and symptoms are observed. Children usually describe the experience in terms of whether it was unpleasant or

hurt or was pleasurable (usually a response to hand-genital contact); some indicate no reaction. Young children often feel no guilt or shame because the act is pleasurable and they are unaware of its inappropriateness.

> **NURSING ALERT**
>
> When children report potentially sexually abusive experiences, their reports need to be taken seriously but also cautiously to avoid alarming the child or falsely accusing a person.

Children's reports may vary from contradictory stories to unwavering versions of the experience. Stories that sound contradictory may reflect the child's experiences in several instances of abuse. Children who repeatedly tell identical facts may have been prompted to do so. Increasing evidence suggests that children's thinking is shaped by the types of interrogation they are exposed to following reports of sexual abuse. In addition, a parent may persuade a child to believe that abuse occurred for a particular purpose, such as gaining custody in a divorce dispute (Hornor, 2001). Consequently, children may falsely accuse individuals of abuse, not because the children are lying but because they are affirming what the interviewer or parent wants to hear. Through the use of leading questions, closed questions (those requiring yes or no answers), intimidation, prodding, and selective reinforcement for certain answers, children begin to tell stories that never occurred. Eventually they may come to consider the fictitious experience as reality (Ceci and Bruck, 1995).

In preparation for the *interview,* every effort is made to make the child feel comfortable, with appropriate introductions, and to avoid duplicating the behaviors typically used by offenders, such as touching the child without permission. The interview is conducted in a quiet and private location, preferably a neutral place such as a school playroom or office, and not where the abuse occurred. Neutral questions are asked first, such as the child's reaction to the hospital (if appropriate). The incident is then discussed in general terms. The interview should include nonleading questions such as "Do you know why you were brought to the hospital?" "Do you know what will happen here?" or "How do you feel about being here?" Later the question "Can you tell me what happened?" and other questions may elicit an account of the incident. Sometimes the parents are able to help the child to describe the incident, and questions can then be directed to the circumstances of the assault. Questions should progress chronologically and proceed from the nonsexual to the more sexual content. If the child shows evidence of becoming too upset, the focus is redirected toward more neutral and less emotionally charged areas.

To avoid biasing the interaction, nurses must be very skillful interviewers when questioning children who may be victims of abuse. Courts may allow a hearsay declaration (an out-of-court statement or videotape) to be used as legal evidence. Medical records should include verbatim statements made by the child and interviewer that reflect appropriate nonleading questions and statements (Hornor, 2001; McClain and others, 2000). Nurses should clarify their role in the

---

> **Box 16-15**　■　■　□
>
> **Warning Signs of Abuse**
>
> Physical evidence of abuse and/or neglect, including previous injuries
> Conflicting stories about the "accident" or injury from the parents or others
> Cause of injury blamed on sibling or other party
> An injury inconsistent with the history, such as a concussion and broken arm from falling off a bed
> History inconsistent with child's developmental level; such as a 6-month-old turning on the hot water
> A complaint other than the one associated with signs of abuse (e.g., a chief complaint of a cold when there is evidence of first- and second-degree burns)
> Inappropriate response of caregiver, such as an exaggerated or absent emotional response; refusal to sign for additional tests or to agree to necessary treatment; excessive delay in seeking treatment; absence of the parents for questioning
> Inappropriate response of child, such as little or no response to pain; fear of being touched; excessive or lack of separation anxiety; indiscriminate friendliness to strangers
> Child's report of physical or sexual abuse
> Previous reports of abuse in the family
> Repeated visits to emergency facilities with injuries

child abuse investigation process. Some experts suggest that health professionals limit the interview to the child's physical and mental health concerns and leave the topics of the family's social, legal, or other problems to the police or CPS personnel (McClain and others, 2000).

Children are given the opportunity to ask questions, but are never pressured into talking if they are reticent. Young children in particular lack the verbal skills to describe body parts adequately. These children may benefit from play situations that provide opportunities for disclosure, such as drawing or using anatomically correct dolls and dollhouses.

Considerable controversy exists regarding the use of children's *drawings* as diagnostic tests for sexual abuse. Two studies that investigated the type of human figure drawings made by allegedly sexually abused and by nonsexually abused children found that those in the abuse group included more details about genitalia than the other group (Palmer and others, 2000). In these studies it is not known if the interview process with the sexual abuse group influenced the subsequent drawings. The authors caution that the presence of genitalia on a human figure drawing does not prove sexual abuse; the children's description and explanation of the drawing are more relevant than its content. Genitalia on drawings may raise suspicion of abuse but are not diagnostic. The use of drawings as an assessment technique is not supported by scientific research (Palmer and others, 2000).

The controversy regarding the validity of *anatomically correct dolls* is of even more concern, because some professionals use the dolls as diagnostic tools in the investigation of suspected sexual abuse. Research on the dolls' diagnostic value has yielded conflicting results, and their appropriate use is not yet clear (DeLoach and Marzolf, 1995). Although it appears the use of anatomically correct dolls is not diagnostic of sexual abuse, some professionals believe the dolls, when used in conjunction with direct questions help children communicate what happened (Katz and others, 1995).

In interviewing the child, every effort is made to coordinate the number of interviewers and to assign a primary professional to work with the child. Videotaping or audiotaping can be used to limit the number of traumatic events (McClain and others, 2000).

**Parental Behaviors.** Certain behavioral responses of the parents to their child and to the interviewer should alert the nurse to the possibility of maltreatment. Although no one pattern of behaviors is characteristic of these parents, some responses include the following. Abusive parents have difficulty in showing concern toward their child. They are unable to comfort the child and give no indication of realizing how the child may feel, physically or emotionally. Instead they are critical of and angry with the child for being injured. They maintain that the child is responsible for the injury and, if asked any question regarding their responsibility of protecting or supervising the child, become hostile and aggressive. They act as if the child's injury is an assault on them. Their entire perception of the incident is in terms of how it affects them, not the child, which is an indication of their preoccupation with their own needs and of their inability to give any support to others.

During the child's hospitalization they may not become involved in the child's care and may show little concern for his or her progress, eventual discharge, or need for follow-up care. However, if pressured during interrogation, they immediately demand to take the child home, regardless of the child's readiness for discharge.

Families respond to sexual abuse with a wide variety of emotional reactions ranging from not believing the child to being very supportive. Parents and other family members may display the same type of emotional responses as the victim (e.g., inability to eat or sleep) and somatic complaints (e.g., headache). In the acute emotional phase parents have a need to blame someone. The three common targets are the offender, the child, and themselves. The parents commonly express anger at the child for "the child's" behavior and may even restrict the child's privileges as punishment. When the victim is a girl, the parents may question her sexual provocation of the event. Self-blaming parents assume full responsibility, believing that they have been inadequate parents or should not have allowed the child to go out. When a baby-sitter or trusted relative is involved in the assault and the child's complaint has not been believed until gross evidence is presented, the parents are often devastated by guilt.

**Child Behaviors.** Abused children's responses to their parents or to the injury may also support the suspicion of abuse. Although no one pattern is typical, extremes of behavior may be observed. Children may be very unresponsive to the parent or excessively clinging and intolerant of separation. There may be overattachment to the abusive parent, possibly in the hope of preventing any upset that may precipitate anger and another attack. During care of the injury, children may be passive and accepting of the discomfort or uncooperative and fearful of any physical contact. Some children maintain a wary watchfulness of all strangers; some shy away from strangers as if frightened; others are unusually affectionate and outgoing.

## ⣿ Nursing Diagnoses

A number of nursing diagnoses are prominent in the nursing care of the maltreated child and family, and others specific to individual cases become evident. The most common nursing diagnoses are outlined in the Nursing Care Plan on pp. 694-695.

## ⣿ Planning

The main goals related to the child who is maltreated and the family are as follows:

1. Child will be protected from further abuse.
2. Child and family will receive adequate support.
3. Hospitalized child and family, including foster parents if appropriate, will be prepared for discharge.
4. Child will not experience any maltreatment.

## ⣿ Implementation

Interventions related to child maltreatment include immediate actions once a child is suspected of being abused, long-range care if the child is placed outside the home, and general strategies that may reduce the occurrence of abuse.

**Protect Child from Further Abuse.**  Initially, identification of instances of suspected abuse or neglect is essential. The nurse may come in contact with abused children in an emergency department, practitioner's office, home, daycare center, or school.

**NURSING ALERT**  The priority is to remove the child from the abusive situation to prevent further injury.

All states and provinces in North America have laws for mandatory reporting of child maltreatment. Suspected child abuse is reported to the local authorities.* Referrals usually come to the state child welfare department and are assigned to a caseworker in an agency such as the **Child Protective Services (CPS).** Once a referral has been made, a caseworker is assigned to investigate the report. Based on the findings, the child is left in the home or temporarily removed.

A court proceeding may be necessary when parental rights are to be terminated or before the child can be placed outside the home. When the courts are involved, they usually require firsthand testimony by the referring parties. Nurses may be subpoenaed to appear in court, or their notes may be introduced as evidence in court hear-

---

*Telephone numbers are usually listed under "Child Abuse" in the business white pages of the local directory, or call the emergency child abuse hotline (Childhelp USA, 15757 N 78th Street, Scottsdale, AZ, 85260) ([800] 4-A-CHILD, [800] 2-A-CHILD).

## GUIDELINES
### *Recording Assessment Data in Suspected Abuse*

**HISTORY OF INJURY**
1. Date, time, and place of occurrence
2. Sequence of events with recorded times
3. Presence of witnesses, especially person caring for child at time of incident
4. Time lapse between occurrence of injury and initiation of treatment
5. Interview with child when appropriate, including verbal quotations and information from drawing or other play activities
6. Interview with parent, witnesses, or other significant persons, including verbal quotations
7. Description of parent-child interactions (verbal interactions, eye contact, touching, parental concern)
8. Name, age, and condition of other children in home (if possible)

**PHYSICAL EXAMINATION**
1. Location, size, shape, and color of bruises; approximate location, size, and shape on drawing of body outline
2. Distinguishing characteristics, such as a bruise in the shape of a hand; round burn (possibly caused by cigarette)
3. Symmetry or asymmetry of injury; presence of other injuries
4. Degree of pain; any bone tenderness
5. Evidence of past injuries; general state of health and hygiene
6. Developmental level of child; perform screening test (see Developmental Assessment, Chapter 7)

---

ings. Accurate and factual documentation is essential. A suggested outline for recording pertinent assessment data is presented in the Guidelines box. Behaviors are described, not interpreted, and they are recorded daily to establish a progress record. Conversations between the nurse, child, and parent are recorded verbatim as much as possible.

**Support Child.**  Children suspected of abuse are often hospitalized for medical management of their injuries. When the sexually abused child has been physically harmed, the care is consistent with that provided to a rape victim. (See Chapter 20.) Regardless of the type of abuse, their needs are the same as those of any hospitalized child. The child should be treated as a child with the usual physical needs, developmental tasks, and play interests—not as a victim of abuse. The nurse is the child's advocate in this goal. The nurse also encourages the child's relationship with the parents. *The nurse does not become a substitute parent to the exclusion of the child's natural parents.* Such an intent only intensifies the parents' feelings of inadequacy, worthlessness, and isolation. It in no way helps them understand their child or promotes their trust in health professionals. The goal of the *consistent* nurse-child relationship is to provide a role model for the parents in helping them to relate positively and constructively to their child and to foster a therapeutic environment for the child in his or her reprieve from the abusing situation.

**Support Family.**  One of the most difficult, yet essential, components of success with abusive parents is the quality of the *therapeutic relationship.* It must be one of genuine concern and treatment, not one of accusation and punishment. Nurses must examine their personal feelings toward the parents, particularly when sexual abuse is present. A therapeutic approach is to view the parent as the patient and the child as the victim of abuse. Unless the nurse's attitude is positive, abusive parents will not be motivated to change because they will not be working with a trusting person who demonstrates the type of behavior that is being asked of them.

When parental ignorance of childbearing practices has played a part in the abuse, the nurse can educate the parent regarding *children's physical and emotional needs.* Parents and other adults need to be informed that patterns of childhood cruelty to animals should be of concern and not dismissed as typical childhood exploration or pranks.

Because of the parents' own upbringing, they may not be aware of nonviolent methods of discipline, such as time-out or consequences. They may also need help in dealing with their frustration so they do not vent anger on the child. Because these parents may be sensitive to criticism or domination and already possess a very low self-esteem, teaching is implemented through demonstration and example rather than through lecturing. Any *competent parenting abilities* they demonstrate are praised to promote their sense of parental adequacy.

Care of the family also depends on the circumstances of the *sexual abuse.* With a nonparent offender the family may be better able to support the child than if incest were involved. Family members are encouraged to express their feelings of anger, guilt, shame, and/or embarrassment but are also cautioned to avoid displacing such feelings on the child. For example, it is easy for parents to admonish the child with a statement such as "We told you never to go with strangers," which makes the child feel responsible.

Family members are advised to encourage the child to resume normal activities and to observe the child for signs of distress (see Posttraumatic Stress Disorder, Chapter 18). Children express their feelings primarily through behavior. Parents should be alert for changes in behavior that indicate distress resulting from the incident, such as remaining in the house, refusing to go to school, changes in sleeping patterns, and frequency of dreams and nightmares. Children are encouraged to talk about these feelings and nightmares, because the more they can talk about the experience, the more they are able to gain control over it.

Most abusive parents tend to live in poverty, and the daily stresses imposed by their lifestyle are overwhelming. *Referral* to appropriate agencies is also essential. Resources for financial aid, improved housing, and child care should be sought. Self-help groups also provide important services. Groups such as **Parents Anonymous\*** (a group for parents who have abused or fear they may abuse their child—but only in terms of physical abuse, not sexual abuse) and **Parents United International, Inc.†** (a group devoted to helping sexually abused families) are very accepting and nonjudgmental because everyone has been in the same position.

There is no way to predict which families will be successfully rehabilitated. With father-daughter incest, the best results occur when the father accepts full responsibility for the act, the mother acknowledges her role in failing to protect the child, and the child is able to understand and forgive the parents and develop a positive self-image despite the traumatic experience.

**Plan for Discharge.** Discharge planning should begin as soon as the legal disposition for placement has been decided, which may be temporary foster home placement, return to the parents, or permanent termination of parental rights. The latter is the most drastic solution but is necessary in situations of repeated, life-threatening abuse. Whenever children are remanded to a foster home or juvenile institution, they must be allowed the opportunity to express their feelings. No matter how severe the abuse, they usually mourn the loss of their parents. They need help to understand why they must not return home and that this new home is in no way a punishment. Whenever possible, foster parents are encouraged to visit in the hospital, and the nurse should take an active role in helping them understand the child. It is unfortunate that some abused children live in torment as they are sent from one foster home to another, sometimes enduring worse circumstances than those that existed in their original home. Only through constant evaluation of the placement residence and the child's adjustment to a new environment can the vicious circle of abuse, abandonment, and neglect be stopped.

**Prevent Abuse.** Prevention of child maltreatment has been an extremely difficult goal. Although there are no universal characteristics of offenders, programs aimed at identifying potential abusers and instituting supportive interventions before the occurrence of an abusive act have met with variable success (Flournoy, 1996). Nurses have played an important role in such programs. For example, home visiting by nurses to primiparas who were either teenagers, unmarried, or of low socioeconomic status is noted to be an effective preventative measure (McMillian, 2000; Eckenrode and others, 2000). The nurses provided information on normal child growth and development and routine health care needs, served as informal support persons, and referred families to appropriate services when a need for assistance was identified.

Such programs provide models that can be used to reduce factors known to increase the risk of abuse. However, nurses in a variety of settings can implement similar activities. Nurses in prenatal clinics can prepare expectant families for the adjustment of parenthood. Nursery and postpartum nurses can foster the attachment process by encouraging parents to hold and look at their infant. In neonatal intensive care units nurses can minimize the effects of separation by encouraging parents to visit and can help them become comfortable in the child's care. Those in ambulatory settings can stress the normal needs and developmental characteristics of children and can teach parents appropriate methods of bathing, feeding, toileting, disciplining, and preventing injuries. Nurses need to be sensitive to the parents' needs for attention, reassurance, and reinforcement. Nurses need to know what types of community services are available, including self-help groups, and make timely referrals.

Unlike preventive efforts for neglect and physical abuse, which have been aimed at the potential offender, *prevention of child sexual abuse* has centered on educating children to protect themselves. Currently there is much controversy regarding the effectiveness of these programs. The main issue is whether young children should be expected to participate in their own protection. Programs should not give parents and children a false sense of security and should not place ultimate responsibility for prevention on children. Clearly, sexual abuse prevention is more than teaching children to say "no" or to recognize their right not to be touched in "private places." It is equally important to teach children safety in terms of potential risk situations. Several suggestions for parents regarding protecting and educating children against possible molestation are presented in the Family Home Care box on p. 694.

The nurse is often in a position to discuss prevention with parents as part of health maintenance and to provide guidelines. Books that describe sexual abuse and its prevention are available for parents.\* Supporting respect, affection, empathy, boundaries, quality child care and education—all components of good parenting—comprise the true preventive approach to sexual abuse (Flournoy, 1996). Helpful

---

\*675 Foothill Blvd, Suite 220, Claremont, CA, 91711, (909) 621-6181 www.parentsanonymous/natl.org.
†615 15th Street, Modesto, CA, 95354, (209) 572-3446.

\*Sources of information are the **National Committee for Prevention of Child Abuse,** Publishing Department, 332 S Michigan Ave, Suite 1600, Chicago, IL 60604-4357, (312) 663-3520; **Kempe Children's Center,** 1825 Marion St, Denver, CO, 80218, (303) 864-5252, www.kempcenter.org; **American Association for Protecting Children, American Humane Association,** 63 Inverness, CO 80112, (800) 227-4645 (outside Colorado) or (303) 792-9900.

## FAMILY HOME CARE
### Preventing or Dealing with Sexual Abuse of Children

Sexual assault of children is much more common than most people realize. It may be preventable if children have good preparation. *To provide protection and preparation:*
Pay careful attention to who is around children. (Unwanted touch *may* come from someone liked and trusted.)
Back up a child's right to say "no."
Encourage communication by taking seriously what children *say.*
Take a second look at signals of potential danger.
Refuse to leave children in the company of those not trusted.
Include information about sexual assault when teaching about safety.
Provide specific definitions and examples of sexual assault.
Remind children that even "nice" people sometimes do mean things.
Urge children to tell about *anybody* who causes them to be uncomfortable.
Prepare children to deal with bribes and threats as well as possible physical force.
Virtually eliminate secrets between children and parents.
Teach children how to say "no," ask for help, and control who touches them and how.
Model self-protective and limit-setting behavior for children.
Should it ever become necessary to *help a child recover from a sexual assault:*
Listen carefully to understand children.
Support the child for telling by praise, belief, sympathy, and lack of blame.
Know local resources and choose help carefully.
Provide opportunities to talk about the assault.
Provide opportunities for the entire family to go through a recovery process.
Sexual assault affects everyone. *To help deal with this social problem:*
Provide care and support to those who have been victimized.
Recognize that offenders do not change without intervention.
Organize neighborhood programs to support each other's efforts to protect children.
Encourage schools to provide information about sexual assault as a problem of health and safety.
Organize law enforcement programs and community groups to support educational treatment.

Modified from Adams C, Fay J: *No more secrets: protecting your child from sexual assault,* San Luis Obispo, CA, 1981, Impact.

games such as "What if the baby-sitter wants to wrestle and hug but tells you to keep it a secret?" can be used to explore dangerous situations in advance and help children learn the importance of saying "no." They need reassurance that no matter what the other person says or does, the parents want to know about it and will not punish them. Even if children do participate in the activity before telling the parents, they must be reassured that it was not their fault.

In addition, parents need to be made aware that "nice" people, including friends and relatives, can be offenders; parents should carefully observe how others act toward the child. A sudden change in the child's behavior and a response such as "I don't like to go visit Uncle John anymore" are clues to investigate the relationship. In the event of any doubt, further solitary encounters with this person and the child should be prevented. It is sometimes to the child's great misfortune that parents do not take certain comments seriously, such as "He hugs me too tight" or "I don't want to go with him." Casual parental statements such as "He just loves you" or "You do whatever adults tell you to do" can place children in jeopardy. Health professionals can alert parents to such dangers and guide them toward an appreciation of the problem, providing concrete guidelines toward child education and protection. (See Family Home Care box.)

## ✣ Evaluation

The effectiveness of nursing interventions is determined by continual reassessment and evaluation of care based on the following observational guidelines:

1. Observe child for additional physical and behavioral evidence of abuse; observe child's reactions to health professionals; if child is hospitalized, check staffing patterns for schedule of consistent group of nurses caring for child.
2. Interview parents regarding their knowledge of children's physical and development needs.
3. Interview child regarding feelings about returning home or placement outside the home.
4. Investigate community programs aimed at preventing child maltreatment.

The **expected outcomes** are described in the Nursing Care Plan on pp. 694-695.

# *Nursing Care Plan*
## The Child Who Is Maltreated

**NURSING DIAGNOSIS:** Risk for trauma related to characteristics of child, caregiver(s), environment

**PATIENT GOAL 1:** Will experience no further abuse or neglect

• **NURSING INTERVENTIONS/*RATIONALES***
Implement measures *to prevent abuse:*
  Report suspicions to appropriate authorities
  Assist in removing child from unsafe environment and establishing a safe environment

Establish protective measures for the hospitalized child as indicated *to prevent continued abuse in hospital*
Refer family to social agencies for assistance with finances, food, clothing, housing, and health care *to help prevent neglect*
Keep factual, objective records *for documentation,* including:
  Child's physical condition
  Child's behavioral response to parents, others, and environment
  Interviews with family members
Collaborate efforts of multidisciplinary team *to continually evaluate progress of child in foster home or in return to own family*

## Nursing Care Plan
### The Child Who Is Maltreated—cont'd

Be alert for signs of continued abuse or neglect

Help parents identify those circumstances that precipitate an abusive act and alternative ways to deal with the release of anger other than attacking child

Refer for alternative placement when indicated *to prevent further injury or neglect*

- **EXPECTED OUTCOME**

Child experiences no further injury or neglect

---

**NURSING DIAGNOSIS:** Fear/anxiety related to negative interpersonal interaction, repeated maltreatment, powerlessness, potential loss of parents

---

**PATIENT GOAL 1:** Will experience reduction or relief of anxiety and stress

- **NURSING INTERVENTIONS/*RATIONALES***

Provide consistent caregiver and therapeutic environment during hospitalization *in order to relieve child's stress and to be a role model for family*

Demonstrate acceptance of child while not expecting same in return

Show attention while not reinforcing inappropriate behavior because *all children have this need*

Plan appropriate activities for attention with nurse, other adults, and other children; use play *to work through relationships*

Praise child's abilities *in order to promote self-esteem*

Treat child as one who has a specific physical problem for hospitalization, not as "abused" victim

Avoid asking too many questions *because this can upset child and interfere with other professionals' interrogations*

    Use play, especially family or dollhouse activity, *to investigate type of relationships perceived by child*

    Provide one consistent person to whom child relates regarding events of abuse *so that child is not overwhelmed*

    Help child grieve for loss of parents if their rights are terminated *because child may be very attached to parents despite abuse*

Encourage child to talk about feelings toward parents and future placement *to facilitate coping*

Encourage introduction to foster parents before placement if possible *to give child time to adjust*

- **EXPECTED OUTCOMES**

Child exhibits minimal or no evidence of distress

Child engages in positive relationships with caregivers

Child grieves for loss of parent(s)

---

**NURSING DIAGNOSIS:** Impaired parenting related to child, caregiver, or situational characteristics that precipitate abusive behavior

---

**PATIENT (FAMILY) GOAL 1:** Will exhibit evidence of positive interaction with children

- **NURSING INTERVENTIONS/*RATIONALES***

Identify families at risk for potential abuse *so that appropriate intervention is instituted*

Promote parental attachment to child *because all children have this need*

Emphasize childrearing practices, especially effective methods of discipline *because parents may lack knowledge about nonviolent discipline methods*

Increase parents' feeling of adequacy and self-esteem

Encourage support systems *that lessen stress and total responsibility of child care on one or both parents*

Teach children to recognize situations that place them at risk for sexual abuse, and teach assertive responses *to discourage abuse*

- **EXPECTED OUTCOME**

Families exhibit evidence of positive interaction with children

---

**PATIENT (FAMILY) GOAL 2:** Will receive adequate support

- **NURSING INTERVENTIONS/*RATIONALES***

Provide "mothering" by directing attention to parent, taking over child care responsibilities until parent feels ready to participate, and focusing on parent's needs *so that parents can eventually meet child's needs*

Convey an attitude of genuine concern, not one of accusation and punishment *because this serves only to further alienate family*

Refer parents to special support groups and/or counseling *for long-term support*

Help identify a support group for parents, such as extended family or nearby neighbors; help these significant others understand their important role in also preventing further abuse

Refer to social agencies that can provide assistance in areas such as financial support, adequate housing, and employment

- **EXPECTED OUTCOMES**

Parents demonstrate appropriate parenting activities

Parents seek group and individual support

Parents receive assistance with problems

---

**PATIENT (FAMILY) GOAL 3:** Will exhibit knowledge of normal growth and development

- **NURSING INTERVENTIONS/*RATIONALES***

Teach realistic expectations of child's behavior and capabilities

Emphasize alternate methods of discipline, such as time-out, consequences, and verbal disapproval, *so that parents learn nonviolent discipline methods*

Suggest methods of handling developmental problems or goals, such as toddler negativism, toilet training, and independence *because these situations may precipitate abuse*

Teach through demonstration and role modeling rather than lecture; avoid authoritarian approach *because family may be sensitive to criticism or domination and lack self-esteem*

- **EXPECTED OUTCOME**

Parents demonstrate an understanding of normal expectations for their child

## KEY POINTS

- Common disorders during early childhood include communicable diseases, intestinal parasitic infections, conjunctivitis, and stomatitis.
- Nursing goals in the treatment of communicable disease are identification, prevention of transmission, provision of comfort, and prevention of complications.
- Intestinal parasitic diseases constitute the most common infections in the world; giardiasis and enterobiases are the most widespread parasitic infections among children in the United States.
- Although the incidence of poisoning has decreased in the last 30 years as a result of more stringent packaging regulations, childhood poisoning remains a serious health concern.
- The most common accidentally ingested medications are analgesics (acetaminophen and ibuprofen), topical preparations, and cough/cold preparations.
- The major principles of emergency treatment for poisoning are assessment, supportive measures, gastric decontamination, family support, and prevention of recurrence.
- Ipecac is an effective and safe emetic for home use in poisonings but is being used less often. Activated charcoal and gastric lavage are common treatments for many toxic ingestions.
- Three simple measures that can reduce the severity of poisoning are knowing the telephone number of the poison control center, having ipecac in the home (two doses per child), and administering it correctly.
- The most important factor contributing to lead poisoning is its availability in the child's environment. Lead-based paint is the most toxic source of lead.
- With increasing awareness of the detrimental effects of low levels of lead on the developing nervous system, acceptable blood lead levels have been decreasing and now are at less than 10 µg/dl.
- Child maltreatment may take the form of physical abuse or neglect, emotional abuse or neglect, or sexual abuse.
- Parental, child, and environmental characteristics are criteria that may predispose children to maltreatment.
- Identification of abuse entails securing evidence of maltreatment, taking a history pertaining to the incident, and assessing parental and child behaviors.
- The reported incidence of sexual abuse has increased in the last decade; common forms are incest, molestation, rape, exhibitionism, child pornography, child prostitution, and pedophilia.

## REFERENCES

Adler NA, Schultz J: Sibling incest offenders, *Child Abuse Negl* 19(7):811-819, 1995.

Aiken MM: Documenting sexual abuse in prepubertal girls, *MCN* 15(3):176-177, 1990.

American Academy of Pediatrics, Committee on Environmental Health: Screening for elevated blood levels, *Pediatrics* 101(6): 1072-1078, 1998.

American Academy of Pediatrics: Guidelines for the evaluation of sexual abuse of children: a subject review, *Pediatrics* 103(1): 186-191, 1999.

American Academy of Pediatrics, Committee on Infectious Diseases, Pickering L, editor: *2000 Red book: report of the Committee on Infectious Diseases*, ed 25, Elk Grove Village, IL, 2000, The Academy.

Babcock N: Detection of poisoning by substances other than drugs: a neglected art, *Ann Clin Biochem* 37(2):146-157, 2000.

Baldwin D, Marshall W: Heavy metal poisoning and its laboratory investigation, *Ann Clin Biochem* 36(10):267-300, 1999.

Behrman R, Kliegman R: *Nelson essentials of pediatrics*, ed 3, Philadelphia, 1998, WB Saunders.

Berenson AB, Somma-Garcia A, Barnett S: Perianal findings in infants 18 months of age or younger, *Pediatrics* 91(4):838-840, 1993.

Bilgrami S and others: Varicella zoster virus infection associated with high-dose chemotherapy and autologous stem-cell rescue, *Bone Marrow Transplant* 23(5):469-474, 1999.

Binder S and others: Lead testing of children and homes: results of a national telephone survey, *Public Health Reports* 111(4):342-346, 1996.

Bryk M, Siegel PT: My mother caused my illness: the story of a survivor of Münchausen by proxy syndrome, *Pediatrics* 100(1):1-7, 1997.

Calam R and others: Psychological disturbances and child sexual abuse: a follow-up study, *Child Abuse Negl* 22(9):901-913, 1998.

Cantwell HB: Vaginal inspection as it relates to child sexual abuse in girls under thirteen, *Child Abuse Negl* 7(2):171-176, 1983.

Carson UB, Arnold EN: *Mental health nursing: the nurse-patient journey*, Philadelphia, 1996, WB Saunders.

Castiglia R: Shaken baby syndrome, *J Pediatr Health Care* 15(2):78-80, 2001.

Ceci SJ, Bruck M: *Jeopardy in the courtroom: a scientific analysis of children's testimony*, Washington, DC, 1995, American Psychological Association Publishing.

Centers for Disease Control and Prevention: *Preventing lead poisoning in young children*, Atlanta, 1997a, CDC.

Centers for Disease Control and Prevention: *Screening young children for lead poisoning: guidance for state and local public health officials*, Atlanta, 1997b, CDC.

Centers for Disease Control and Prevention: Recommendations for blood lead screening of young children enrolled in Medicaid: targeting a group at high risk, *MMWR* (RR-14):1-13, 2000.

Chapman S: Varicella in pregnancy, *Semin Perinatol* 22(4):339-346, 1998.

Chiocca E: Child abuse and neglect: (Part 1) a status report, *J Pediatr Nurs* 13(2):128-130, 1998.

Cody MM, Sottnek HM, O'Leary VS: Recovery of *Giardia lamblia* cysts from chairs and tables in child day-care centers, *Pediatrics* 94(6, pt 2):1006-1008, 1994.

DeLoache J, Marzolf D: The use of dolls to interview young children: issues of symbolic representation, *J Experimental Child Psychol* 60(1):155-175, 1995.

Diamant M and others: Beware the hazards of activated charcoal, *Am J Nurs* 12:10, 1994.

Douidar SM, Al-Khalil I, Habersang RW: Severe hepatotoxicity, acute renal failure, and pancytopenia in a young child after repeated acetaminophen overdosing, *Clin Pediatr* 33(1):42-45, 1994.

Eckenrode J and others: Preventing child abuse and neglect with a program of nurse home visitation: the limiting effects of domestic violence, *JAMA* 284(11): 1385-1391, 2000.

Emans S and others: Genital findings in sexually abused symptomatic and asymptomatic girls, *Pediatrics* 79(5):778-785, 1987.

Environmental Protection Agency, United States: *Laboratory study of lead-cleaning efficacy*, Washington, DC, 1997, The Agency.

Etzel R: The 'fatal four' indoor air pollutants, *Pediatr Ann* 29(6):344-350, 2000.

Feder H: Periodic fever; aphthous stomatitis, pharyngitis, adenitis: a clinical review of a new syndrome, *Curr Opin Pediatr* 12(3): 253-256, 2000.

Finkelstein Y, Markowitz ME, Rosen JF: Low-level lead induced neurotoxicity in children: an update on central nervous system effects, *Brain Res Brain Res Rev* 27(2):168-176, 1998.

Fischer DG, McDonald WL: Characteristics of intrafamilial and extrafamilial child sexual abuse, *Child Abuse Negl* 22(9):915-929, 1998.

Fisher AM, Vessey JA: Preventing lead poisoning and its consequences, *Pediatr Nurs* 24(4):348-350, 1998.

Flournoy J: Incest prevention: the role of the pediatric nurse practitioner, *J Pediatr Health Care* 10(6):246-254, 1996.

Frechette A, Rimsza ME: Stun gun injury: a new presentation of the battered child syndrome, *Pediatrics* 89(5):898-901, 1992.

Furness B, Beach M, Roberts J: Giardiasis surveillance—United States 1992-1997, *MMWR* 49(2207):1-13, 2000.

Gardner RA: Medical findings and child sexual abuse, *Issues Child Abuse Accus* 5(1):12-23, 1993.

Gulson B and others: Comparison of the rates of exchanges of lead in blood of newly born infants and their mothers with lead from their current environment, *J Lab Clin Med* 130(1):51-62, 1997.

Hall D and others: Evaluation of covert video surveillance in the diagnosis of Munchausen by proxy: lessons from 41 cases, *Pediatrics* 105(6):1305-1312, 2000.

Hanson R and others: Anogenital warts in childhood, *Child Abuse Negl* 13(2):225-233, 1989.

Health and Human Services: *Child maltreatment 1999*, Washington, DC, 1999, Administration on Children, Youth and Family.

Hobbs C, Wynne J: Sexual abuse of English boys and girls: the importance of anal examination, *Child Abuse Negl* 13(2):195-210, 1989.

Hornor G: Repeated sexual abuse allegations: a problem for primary care providers, *J Pediatr Health Care* 15(2):71-76, 2001.

Hughes L, Corbo-Richert B: Munchausen by proxy: literature review and implications for critical care nurses, *Crit Care Nurs* 19(3):71-78, 1999.

Jacob B and others: The effect of low level blood on hematological parameters in children, *Environ Res* 82(2):150-159, 2000.

Jessee S: Dental detectives can pinpoint child abuse, *UT Houston* (online newspaper), April, 1996.

Kakourou T and others: Herpes zoster in children, *J Am Acad Dermatol* 39(2, pt 1): 207-210, 1998.

Kaplan S, Pelcovitz D, Labruna V: Child and adolescent abuse and neglect research:

a review of the past 10 years. Part I: Physical and emotional abuse and neglect, *J Am Acad Child Adolesc Psychiatr* 38(10): 1214-1222, 1999.

Katz S and others: The accuracy of children's reports with anatomically correct dolls, *J Behav Pediatr* 16(2):71-76, 1995.

Lanphear BP and others: Environmental lead exposure during early childhood, *J Pediatr* 140(1):40-47, 2002.

Lauritsen A, Meldgaard K, Charles A: Medical examination of sexually abused children: medico-legal value, *J Foren Sci* 45(1):115-117, 2000.

Litovitz T and others: 1999 Annual Report of the American Association of Poison Control Centers Toxic Exposure Surveillance System, *Am J Emerg Med* 18(5):517-574, 2000.

Lockwood R, Church A: *Deadly serious: an FBI perspective on animal cruelty*, 1996, The Humane Society of the United States.

McCann J and others: Perianal findings in prepubertal children selected for nonabuse: a descriptive study, *Child Abuse Negl* 13(2):179-193, 1989.

McCann J and others: Genital findings in prepubertal girls selected for nonabuse: a descriptive study, *Pediatrics* 86(3):428-439, 1990.

McClain N and others: Evaluation of sexual abuse in the pediatric patient, *J Pediatr Health Care* 14(3):93-102, 2000.

McCullough M, Scherman A: Family-of-origin interaction and adolescent mothers' potential for child abuse, *Adolescence* 33(130): 375-384, 1998.

McDonough J: Acetaminophen overdose, *Am J Nurs* 98(3):52, 1998.

McKinney P: Acute elevation of blood lead levels within hours of injection of large quantities of lead shot, *J Toxicol Clin Toxicol* 38(4):435-440, 2000.

McMillian H: Child maltreatment; what we know in the year 2000, *Can J Psychiatr* 45(8):702-709, 2000.

Mendelsohn A and others: Low-level lead exposure and behavior in early childhood, *Pediatrics* 101(3):E10, 1998.

Moore T: Parovirus-associated arthritis, *Curr Opin Rheumatol* 12(4):289-294, 2000.

Morrissey-Ross M: Lead poisoning and its elimination: an opportunity for success, *Pub Health Nurs* 17(4):229-230, 2000.

Murry S, Baker A, Lewin L: Screening families with young children for child maltreatment potential, *Pediatr Nurs* 26(1):47-65, 2000.

Nester C: Prevention of child abuse and neglect in the primary care setting, *Nurs Prac* 22(9):61-73, 1998.

Olin BR and others: *Drug facts and comparisons*, St Louis, 2000, Facts and Comparisons.

Palmer L and others: An investigation of the clinical use of the house-tree-person projective drawings in the psychological evalua-

tion of child sexual abuse, *Child Maltreatment* 60(1):155-173, 2000.

Pasqualone G, Fitzgerald S: Munchausen by proxy syndrome: the forensic challenges of recognition, diagnosis, and reporting, *Crit Care Nurs Q* 22(10):55-64, 1999.

Paulk D: Munchausen syndrome by proxy, *Clin Rev* 11(8):51-56, 2001.

Perry H, Shannon M: Emergency department gastrointestinal decontamination, *Pediatr Ann* 25(1):19-26, 1996.

Porter E, Severton D: Potential effectiveness of parents' actions to reduce children's lead exposure, *J Pediatr Nurs* 15(5):282-291, 2000.

Powers K: Diagnosis and management of common toxic ingestions and inhalations, *Pediatr Ann* 29(6):330-342, 2000.

Rice D: Behavioral effects of lead: commonalities between experimental and epidemiological data, *Environ Health Perspect* 104(suppl 2):337-351, 1996.

Rodgers GC Jr, Tenenbein M: The role of adverse bittering agents in the prevention of pediatric poisonings, *Pediatrics* 93(1): 68-69, 1994.

Rodriquez CM, Green AJ: Parenting stress and anger expression as predictors of child abuse potential, *Child Abuse Negl* 21(4): 367-377, 1997.

Ruppert S: Different diagnosis of pediatrics conjunctivitis (red eye), *Nurs Pract* 21(7): 12-26, 1996.

Semba RD: Vitamin A as "anti-infective" therapy, 1920-1940, *J Nutr* 129(4):783-791, 1999.

Soud T, Rogers J: *Manual of pediatric emergency nursing*, St Louis, 1998, Mosby.

Souid AD, Keith DV, Cunningham AS: Munchausen syndrome by proxy, *Clin Pediatr* 37(8):497-503, 1998.

Stoeckle M: The spectrum of human herpesvirus 6 infection: from roseola infantum to adult disease, *Ann Rev Med* 51:423-430, 2000.

Verberk MM and others: Environmental lead and renal effects in children, *Arch Environ Health* 51(1):83-87, 1996.

Vernberg K, Culver-Dickinson P, Spyker DA: The deterrent effect of poison-warning stickers, *Am J Dis Child* 138:1018-1020, 1984.

Wang CT, Daro D: *Current trends in child abuse reporting and fatalities: the results of the 1997 annual fifty state survey*, Chicago, 1998, Prevent Child Abuse America.

White ST, Ingram DL, Lyna PR: Vaginal introital diameter in the evaluation of sexual abuse, *Child Abuse Negl* 13(2):217-224, 1989.

Yetman R, Coody D: Conjunctivitis; a practice guideline, *J Pediatr Health Care* 11(5):238-241, 1997.

# Chapter 17

# Health Promotion of the School-Age Child and Family

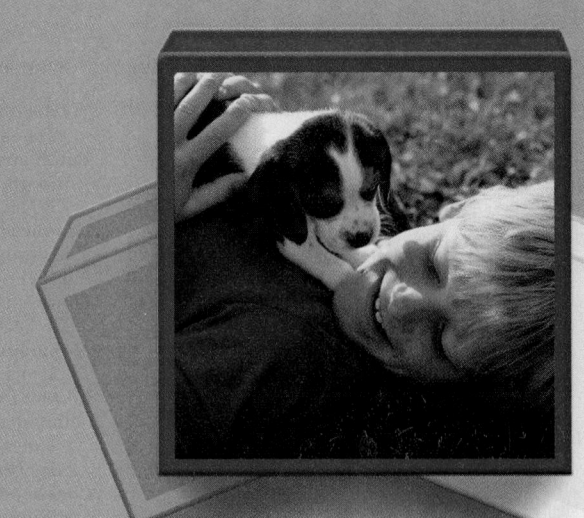

## Chapter Outline

**PROMOTING OPTIMUM GROWTH AND DEVELOPMENT, 698**
**Biologic Development, 699**
Proportional Changes, 699
Maturation of Systems, 699
Prepubescence, 700
**Psychosocial Development, 700**
Developing a Sense of Industry (Erikson), 700
**Temperament, 701**
**Cognitive Development (Piaget), 702**
**Moral Development (Kohlberg), 704**
**Spiritual Development, 705**
**Language Development, 705**
**Social Development, 706**
Social Relationships and Cooperation, 706
Relationships with Families, 707
**Development of Self-Concept, 708**
Body Image, 708
Self-Esteem, 709
**Development of Sexuality, 709**
Sex Education, 710

Nurse's Role in Sex Education, 710
**Play, 711**
Rules and Rituals, 711
Quiet Games and Activities, 712
Ego Mastery, 712
**COPING WITH CONCERNS RELATED TO NORMAL GROWTH AND DEVELOPMENT, 714**
**School Experience, 714**
Anticipatory Socialization, 714
Role of the Teacher, 715
Role of the Parents, 716
**Limit-Setting and Discipline, 716**
Dishonest Behavior, 717
**Coping with Stress, 717**
Fears, 719
Latchkey Children, 720
**PROMOTING OPTIMUM HEALTH DURING THE SCHOOL YEARS, 720**
**Health Behaviors, 720**
**Nutrition, 721**
Outside Influences, 721

School Programs, 722
**Sleep and Rest, 723**
Sleep Problems, 723
**Physical Activity, 724**
Physical Fitness, 724
Acquisition of Skills, 726
Television and Video Games, 726
**Dental Health, 727**
Brushing, 727
**School Health, 728**
Health Education, 728
School Nursing Services, 729
**Injury Prevention, 730**
Risk-Taking Behavior, 732
Motor Vehicle Injury, 732
Bicycle Injury, 733
Other Vehicles, 734
Injuries at School, 735
Farm Injuries, 735
Other Injuries, 735
Nurse's Role in Injury Prevention, 736
**Anticipatory Guidance—Care of Families, 736**

## Related Topics

Dental Health, Ch. 14
Eating Problems/Disorders, Ch. 21
Guidelines: Assessing Sleep Problems in Children, Ch. 6
Health Problems of Middle Childhood, Ch. 18

Injuries and Health Problems Related to Sports Participation, Ch. 39
Injuries—The Leading Killer, Ch. 1
Limit-Setting and Discipline, Ch. 3
Nutrition, Ch. 13

Physical and Developmental Assessment of the Child, Ch. 7
Psychosocial History, Ch. 6
Sleep Problems, Chs. 12 and 15
Television, Ch. 2

## PROMOTING OPTIMUM GROWTH AND DEVELOPMENT

The segment of the life span that extends from age 6 to approximately age 12 has a variety of labels, each of which describes an important characteristic of the period. The mid-

dle years are most often referred to as *school-age* or the *school years.* This period begins with entrance into the wider sphere of influence represented by the school environment, which has a significant impact on development and relationships.

Physiologically the middle years begin with the shedding of the first deciduous tooth and end at puberty with the acquisition of the final permanent teeth (with the exception

■ Marilyn L. Winkelstein, PhD, RN, revised this chapter.

of the wisdom teeth). During the preceding 5 to 6 years, children have progressed from helpless infants to sturdy, complicated individuals with the capacity to communicate, conceptualize in a limited way, and become involved in complex social and motor behavior. Physical growth has been equally rapid. In contrast, the period of middle childhood, between the rapid growth of early childhood and the prepubescent growth spurt, is a time of gradual growth and development, with more even progress in both physical and emotional aspects.

## Biologic Development

During middle childhood, growth in height and weight assumes a slower but steady pace as compared with the earlier years. Between ages 6 and 12, children will grow an average of 5 cm (2 inches) per year to gain 30 to 60 cm (1 to 2 feet) in height and will almost double in weight, increasing 2 to 3 kg (4½ to 6½ pounds) per year. The average 6-year-old child is about 116 cm (45 inches) tall and weighs about 21 kg (46 pounds); the average 12-year-old child stands about 150 cm (59 inches) tall and weighs approximately 40 kg (88 pounds). During this age period girls and boys differ very little in size, although boys tend to be slightly taller and somewhat heavier than girls. Toward the end of the school-age years both boys and girls begin to increase in size, although most girls begin to surpass boys in both height and weight, to the acute discomfort of both girls and boys.

### Proportional Changes

School-age children are more graceful than they were as preschoolers, and they are steadier on their feet. Their body proportions take on a slimmer look with longer legs, varying body proportion, and a lower center of gravity. Posture improves over that of the preschool period to facilitate locomotion and efficiency in using the arms and trunk. These proportions make climbing, bicycle riding, and other activities much easier. Fat gradually diminishes, and its distribution patterns change, contributing to the thinner appearance of children during the middle years.

Accompanying the skeletal lengthening and fat diminution is an increase in the percentage of body weight represented by muscle tissue. By the end of this age period, both boys and girls will double their strength and physical capabilities, and their steady and relatively consistent acquisition of refined coordination will increase their poise and skill. However, this increased strength can be misleading. Although strength increases, muscles are still functionally immature when compared with those of the adolescent, and they are more readily damaged by muscular injury caused by overuse.

The most pronounced changes and those that seem best to indicate increasing maturity in children are a decrease in head circumference in relation to standing height, a decrease in waist circumference in relation to height, and an increase in leg length related to height. These observations often provide a clue to a child's degree of maturity that has proved useful in predicting readiness for meeting the de-

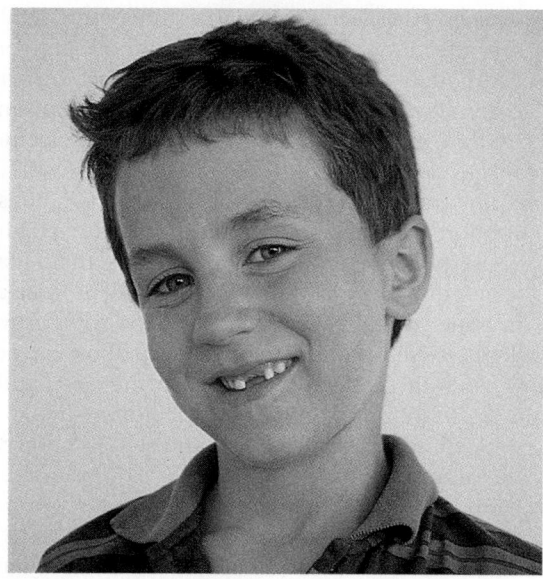

**Fig. 17-1**   Middle childhood is the stage of development when deciduous teeth are shed.

mands of school. There appears to be a correlation between physical indications of maturity and success in school.

**Facial Changes.**   Certain physiologic and anatomic characteristics are typical of children in middle childhood. Facial proportions change as the face grows faster in relation to the remainder of the cranium. The skull and brain grow very slowly during this period and increase little in size thereafter. Since all of the primary (deciduous) teeth are lost during this age span, middle childhood is sometimes known as the *age of the loose tooth* (Fig. 17-1) and the early years of middle childhood as the *ugly duckling stage,* when the new secondary (permanent) teeth appear to be much too large for the smaller face.

### Maturation of Systems

Maturity of the *gastrointestinal system* is reflected in fewer stomach upsets, better maintenance of blood sugar levels, and an increased stomach capacity, which permits retention of food for longer periods. The school-age child does not need to be fed as carefully, as promptly, or as frequently as before. Caloric needs are less than they were in the preschool years and less than they will be during the coming adolescent growth spurt.

Physical maturation is evidenced in other body tissues and organs. *Bladder capacity,* although differing widely among individual children, is generally greater in girls than in boys. There are individual variations in frequency of urination and differences in the same child according to circumstances such as temperature, humidity, time of day, amount of fluids ingested, and emotional state.

The *heart* grows more slowly during the middle years and is smaller in relation to the rest of the body than at any other period of life. Heart and respiratory rates steadily decrease, and blood pressure increases during ages 6 to 12 (see inside back cover).

The *immune system* becomes more competent in its ability to localize infections and produce an antibody-antigen response. Although children have several infections in the first 1 to 2 years of school because of increased exposure to other children, immunity to a wide variety of pathogenic microorganisms develops (Wilson, Lewis, and Penix, 1996).

*Bones* continue to ossify throughout childhood, but since mineralization is not completed until maturity, children's bones resist pressure and muscle pull less than mature bones. Consequently, care must be taken to prevent alterations in bone structure, and children should be provided with well-fitted shoes, chairs, and desks that allow correct sitting posture with the feet able to reach the floor and the hips able to fit well back in the seat. Children should have ample opportunity to move around and should observe appropriate caution in carrying heavy loads. For example, they should shift books and/or tote bags from one arm to the other. Back packs distribute weight more evenly.

Wider differences between children are observed at the end of middle childhood than at the beginning; such differences are sometimes striking. These differences become increasingly apparent and, if extreme or unique, may create emotional problems. The associated characteristics of height and weight relationships, rapid or slow growth, and other important features of development should be explained to children and their families. Physical maturity is not necessarily correlated with emotional and social maturity. Seven-year-old children who look like 10-year-old children will think and act like 7-year-old children. To expect behavior appropriate for 10-year-old children from them is unrealistic and can be detrimental to their development of competence and self-esteem. Conversely, to treat 10-year-old children as though they were 7 years old is an equal disservice to them.

### Prepubescence

*Preadolescence* is the period that begins toward the end of middle childhood and ends with the thirteenth birthday. Since puberty signals the beginning of the development of secondary sex characteristics, *prepubescence,* the 2-year period that precedes puberty, typically occurs during preadolescence.

Toward the end of middle childhood the discrepancies in growth and maturation between boys and girls become apparent. On the average, there is a difference of approximately 2 years between girls and boys in the age of onset of pubescence. Preadolescence is a period of rapid growth, especially for girls. For others, mostly boys, it is generally a period of continued steady growth in height and weight.

There is no universal age at which children assume the characteristics of preadolescence. The first physiologic signs appear at about 9 years (particularly in girls) and are usually clearly evident in 11- to 12-year-old children. Although preadolescent children do not want to be different, variability in physical growth and physiologic changes between children of the same sex, and between the two sexes, is often striking at this time. This variability, especially in relation to the onset of secondary sex characteristics, is of utmost concern to the preadolescent. Either early or late appearance of these characteristics is a source of embarrassment and un-

easiness to both sexes. Early appearance of secondary sex characteristics in girls may be associated with dissatisfaction with physical appearance, greater general unhappiness, and lower self-esteem. Late-developing boys often have a negative self-concept. Both early appearance of physical characteristics in girls and late appearance in boys have been linked to participation in risk-taking behaviors (early sexual activity, substance use, and reckless vehicle use).

Preadolescence is a time when considerable overlapping of developmental characteristics occurs, with elements of both middle childhood and early adolescence. However, there are sufficient unique characteristics to set this period apart as an age category. Generally, the earliest age at which puberty begins is 10 years in girls and 12 years in boys, although there has been an increase in the number of girls reaching puberty at age 9. The average age of puberty is 12 in girls and 14 in boys. Boys experience little sexual maturation during preadolescence.

## Psychosocial Development

Middle childhood is the period of psychosexual development that Freud described as the *latency period,* a time of tranquility between the Oedipal phase of early childhood and the eroticism of adolescence. During this time children experience relationships with same-sex peers following the indifference of earlier years and preceding the heterosexual fascination that occurs for most boys and girls in puberty.

### Developing a Sense of Industry (Erikson)

Successful mastery of Erikson's first three stages of psychosocial development is probably the most important accomplishment in terms of development of a healthy personality (Erikson, 1963). Successful completion of these stages requires a loving environment within a stable family unit that has prepared the child to engage in experiences and relationships beyond this intimate group. During childhood, children affiliate with agemates, receive the systematic instruction prescribed by their individual cultures, and develop the skills needed to become useful, contributing members of their social communities.

A *sense of industry,* or a *stage of accomplishment,* is achieved somewhere between age 6 and adolescence. The goal of this stage of development is to achieve a sense of personal and interpersonal competence through the acquisition of technologic and social skills. School-age children are eager to build skills and participate in meaningful and socially useful work. Interests expand, and, with a growing sense of independence, children want to engage in tasks that can be carried through to completion (Fig. 17-2). Failure to develop a sense of accomplishment may result in a sense of *inferiority.*

Many attributes of industry contribute to the child's sense of competence and mastery. Intrinsic motivation is associated with increased competence in mastering new skills and assuming new responsibilities. Children gain a great deal of satisfaction from independent behavior in exploring and manipulating their environment and from interaction with peers. Extrinsic sources of reinforcement in the form of grades, material rewards, additional privileges, and

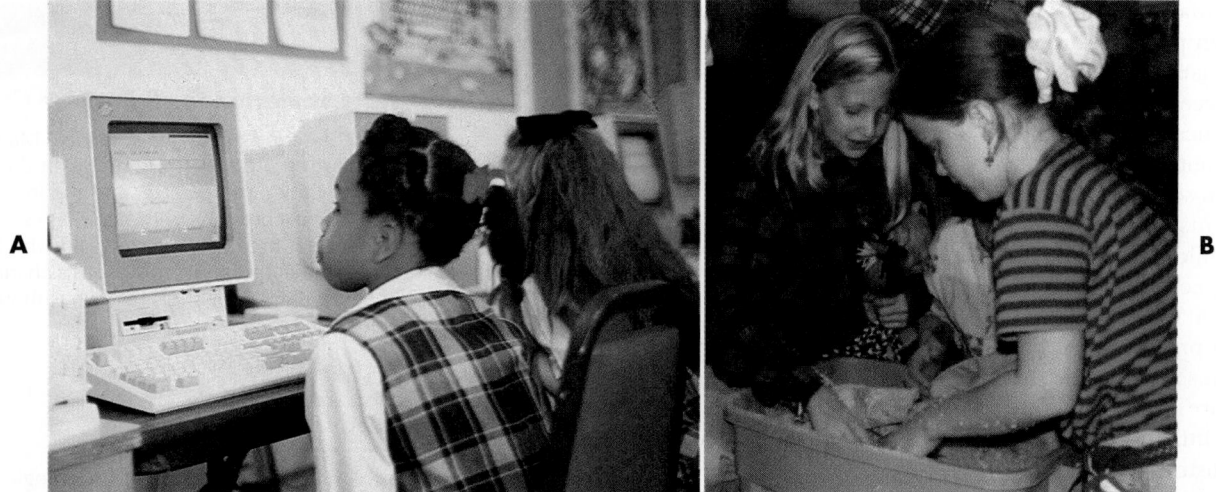

**Fig. 17-2**   School-age children are motivated to complete tasks. **A,** Working alone. **B,** Working with others.

recognition provide encouragement and stimulation. Often the acquisition of skills is a means for achieving success in special activities such as athletics or social organizations. Peer approval is a strong motivating power.

The danger inherent in this period of personality development is the occurrence of situations that might result in a sense of inadequacy or inferiority. This may happen if the previous stages have not been successfully achieved or if a child is incapable of or unprepared to assume the responsibilities associated with developing a sense of accomplishment. Feelings of inferiority or lack of worth can be derived from children themselves or from the social environment. Children with physical or mental limitations may be at a disadvantage for acquisition of certain skills. When the reward structure is based on evidence of mastery, children who are incapable of developing these skills are at risk for feeling inadequate and inferior.

Even children without chronic disabilities represent such a wide range of individual differences in capabilities and preferences that they will experience feelings of inadequacy in some areas. No child is able to do well in everything, and children must learn that they will not be able to master each skill that they attempt. All children, even children who in most instances have positive attitudes toward work and their own capabilities, will feel some degree of inferiority in regard to a specific skill that they cannot master.

For some children, success or aptitude in one area may compensate for failure or ineptitude in another. However, the differences in reinforcement provided for success in various areas have significant effects on feelings of adequacy. For example, in the United States, reading proficiency is more highly rewarded than the mechanical aptitude needed for tinkering with broken automobile engines. A higher social value is placed on success in team sports than on success in repairing a bicycle. Compensating for the inability to excel in more socially valued skills through mastery of other, less valued skills is difficult for children. If the social environment places a negative value on any failure,

feelings of inferiority may be increased in the less capable child. Repeated failures can generate such strong feelings that eventually the child is reluctant to attempt any new task or is fearful of not being able to perform as well as his or her peers. Thus, intrinsic motivation toward engaging in a task for the pleasure of the challenge conflicts with the external forces that cause feelings of doubt and inferiority. Consequently, the child may no longer try.

A child's concept of success or failure is important. Children who aspire for more than they are capable of will usually experience failure. In contrast, children who set their aspirations lower than their level of achievement are likely to experience success. Most accomplishments during the school years are very public. Success or failure in school is known to family, teachers, and peers. In school and sometimes at home, feelings of inferiority may be produced through comparison with others, suggesting that the child is not as good as a peer, sibling, or member of another group. This inadequacy becomes a source of embarrassment. The child may even be shamed for the failure. Earlier conflicts of doubt and guilt are very closely associated with feelings of inferiority.

A sense of accomplishment also involves the ability to cooperate, to compete with others, and to cope effectively with people. Middle childhood is the time when children learn the value of doing things with others and the benefits derived from division of labor in the accomplishment of goals. Children need and want real achievement. When they can accomplish tasks that need to be done and perform well despite individual differences in capacities and emotional development, and, when they are suitably rewarded, children develop a sense of industry and accomplishment that prepares them for establishing a stable identity later in life.

## Temperament

The reactivity patterns or temperamental traits identified in infancy may continue to influence behavior in middle childhood. Analyzing behavioral patterns observed in past situations can provide clues to the way that a child may react to new situations although long-range projections are not always successful. Through interaction with the environment, experiences, motives, and abilities, many children change. Major temperamental characteristics persist into adolescence in some children; in others they do not.

Parents and teachers are in an excellent position to assess a child's behavioral style and try to make their demands and expectations consonant with the individual child's temperamental characteristics. With *easy children* this rarely poses a problem. They adapt readily to many childrearing programs and new situations. School entry or other experiences are usually smooth and accomplished with minimal stress. Difficulties arise with slow-to-warm-up and difficult or easily distracted children.

*Slow-to-warm-up children* usually exhibit discomfort when introduced to new situations and need time to become accustomed to a new environment, authority figures, and expectations. These children may respond with tears, somatic complaints, or other maneuvers to avoid the event. They should be encouraged to try new experiences but should be allowed to adapt to their surroundings at their own speed. Pressure to move quickly into new situations only strengthens the tendency to withdraw. After-school activities can be a cause for reaction, but attending with a friend or contracting for permission to withdraw after a trial of a specified number of times may provide them with sufficient incentive to try. (See Critical Thinking Exercise box.)

*Difficult* or *easily distracted children* may benefit from "practice" sessions in which they are prepared for the event by role-playing, visiting the site, reading or listening to stories, or other methods of getting them acquainted with what to expect. Children who are very persistent need to know when they are expected to stop what they are doing so that the signal to stop will not come as a surprise or trigger a reaction. Children with difficult temperaments need to be handled with exceptional patience, firmness, and understanding so that they can learn appropriate behavior in their interactions with others. If possible, it is important to match teachers to the temperament of children to ensure a "good fit."

## Cognitive Development (Piaget)

When they enter the school years, children begin to acquire the ability to relate a series of events and actions to mental representations that can be expressed both verbally and symbolically. This is the stage that Piaget describes as *concrete operations,* when children are able to use their thought processes to experience events and actions. Because the term *operation* implies an action that is performed on an object or set of objects, a *mental operation* is an alteration or transformation that is carried out in thought rather than in action. Toddlers or preschool children can perform acts that involve ordering, such as correctly arranging a graduated set of circles from largest to smallest on a stick, or they can find their way to a friend's house, but they are unable to verbalize the actions involved in the process. School-age children are able to articulate the process and perform the actions mentally without the need to carry out the behaviors.

## Critical Thinking Exercise

### Temperament in the School-Age Child

Mary's teacher asks the school nurse for guidance. Mary is 8 years old and has just entered the third grade. In the classroom Mary is very quiet and passive, and she frequently cries when the teacher talks with her. Mary's mother describes her daughter as a healthy child who has always required more time and effort to adapt to changes in her routine. In counseling Mary's teacher, what should the nurse encourage the teacher to do?

FIRST, THINK ABOUT IT . . .

• What information are you using?
• How are you interpreting that information?

1. Send Mary to the health suite as soon as she begins to exhibit any withdrawal behaviors.
2. Appoint Mary as the leader for several class activities.
3. Include Mary in all classroom activities, but avoid giving her any specific responsibilities until she initiates active classroom participation.
4. Give Mary extra schoolwork to complete at home so that she does not fall behind in class.

*The best response is three. The nurse recognizes Mary as having a slow-to-warm-up temperament. When placed in new settings, children with this behavioral style need to be allowed to adjust at their own pace, which is the correct interpretation of the child's behavior. Pushing these children to accept leadership roles too quickly, allowing them to visit the nurse when stressed, or requiring extra homework will only cause them to increase their efforts to withdraw. However, if teachers can modify classroom routines and their responses to fit the temperament of these children, the coping strategies of these children will be facilitated.*

As children move from the preschool years into the school years, their conceptual abilities become increasingly more flexible. During the *concrete-operational period,* they acquire cognitive operations and apply these new skills when thinking about objects, situations, and events. Their rigid, egocentric outlook is replaced by thought processes that allow them to see things from another's point of view. They become aware of a variety of perspectives and become more sensitive to the fact that others do not always perceive events exactly as they do. They are able to delay an action until they have evaluated alternative responses to situations. Their steady reduction in egocentricity helps form the basis for logical thought and the development and maturation of morality.

The concrete-operational stage takes place between the years 7 and 11. During this stage children develop an understanding of relationships between things and ideas. They progress from making judgments based on what they see *(perceptual thinking)* to making judgments based on what they reason *(conceptual thinking)*. They are increasingly able to master symbols and to use their memory store of past experiences to evaluate and interpret the present.

One of the major cognitive tasks of school-age children is mastering the concept of *conservation*—that physical matter does not appear and disappear by magic. They learn that certain properties of the environment are not changed sim-

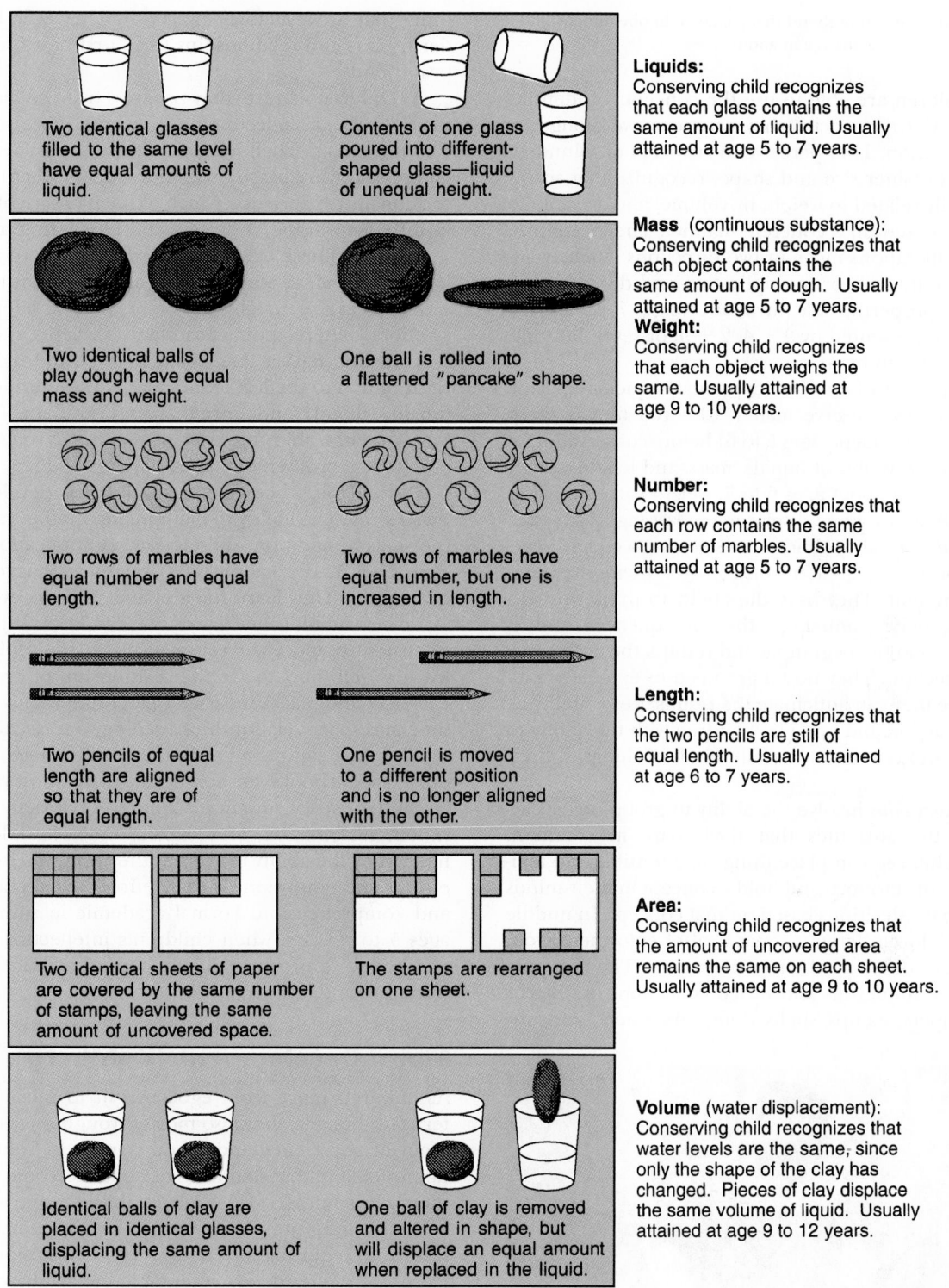

**Liquids:**
Conserving child recognizes that each glass contains the same amount of liquid. Usually attained at age 5 to 7 years.

Two identical glasses filled to the same level have equal amounts of liquid.

Contents of one glass poured into different-shaped glass—liquid of unequal height.

**Mass** (continuous substance):
Conserving child recognizes that each object contains the same amount of dough. Usually attained at age 5 to 7 years.
**Weight:**
Conserving child recognizes that each object weighs the same. Usually attained at age 9 to 10 years.

Two identical balls of play dough have equal mass and weight.

One ball is rolled into a flattened "pancake" shape.

**Number:**
Conserving child recognizes that each row contains the same number of marbles. Usually attained at age 5 to 7 years.

Two rows of marbles have equal number and equal length.

Two rows of marbles have equal number, but one is increased in length.

**Length:**
Conserving child recognizes that the two pencils are still of equal length. Usually attained at age 6 to 7 years.

Two pencils of equal length are aligned so that they are of equal length.

One pencil is moved to a different position and is no longer aligned with the other.

**Area:**
Conserving child recognizes that the amount of uncovered area remains the same on each sheet. Usually attained at age 9 to 10 years.

Two identical sheets of paper are covered by the same number of stamps, leaving the same amount of uncovered space.

The stamps are rearranged on one sheet.

**Volume** (water displacement):
Conserving child recognizes that water levels are the same, since only the shape of the clay has changed. Pieces of clay displace the same volume of liquid. Usually attained at age 9 to 12 years.

Identical balls of clay are placed in identical glasses, displacing the same amount of liquid.

One ball of clay is removed and altered in shape, but will displace an equal amount when replaced in the liquid.

**Fig. 17-3**   Common examples that demonstrate the child's ability to conserve (ages are only approximate).

ply by altering their disposition in space. They are able to resist perceptual cues that suggest alterations in the physical state of an object.

Conservation of liquid, mass, number, length, area, and volume can be demonstrated by the use of commonplace items (Fig. 17-3). To explain the observations that the mass has not been altered, children use one of three concepts:

**Identity**—Since nothing has been added and nothing has been taken away, the pancake is still the same clay. Nothing has changed but the shape.

**Reversibility**—The clay can be reshaped into its original form (a ball).

**Reciprocity**—Although the pancake appears larger in circumference, the ball is much thicker. In this instance the child demonstrates the ability to deal with two dimensions at the same time and comprehend that a change in one dimension compensates for a change in another.

When children are able to use the concepts of identity, reversibility, and reciprocity, they can conserve along any physical dimension. They perceive the concept of volume in relation to container size and shape, recognize that size is not necessarily related to weight or volume, and are able to manipulate or "see" in a concrete manner. They recognize that logical operations move in two directions (such as addition and subtraction or multiplication and division) and that certain properties are invariant (e.g., 7 remains 7 whether it is represented by 3 + 4, 2 + 5, or seven buttons, seven stars, or seven boys).

There appears to be a developmental sequence in children's capacity to conserve matter. Children usually grasp conservation of numbers (ages 5 to 6) before conservation of substance. Conservation of liquids, mass, and length usually is accomplished at about ages 6 to 7, weight sometime later (ages 9 to 10), and volume displacement last (ages 9 to 12).

*Reversibility* is used by children in selecting a course of action, thus providing greater control over themselves and their environment. They have the ability to think through an action sequence, anticipate the consequences, and, if needed, return to the beginning and rethink the action in a different direction. They no longer need to experience an action before they can anticipate the results. Reversibility allows mental action and provides children with the ability to disassemble and reassemble certain kinds of things in their thoughts.

*Classification skills* involve the ability to group objects according to the attributes that they share in common. School-age children can place things in a sensible and logical order, group and sort, and hold a concept in their minds while they make decisions based on that concept. In middle childhood children derive a great deal of enjoyment from classifying and ordering their environment. They become occupied with numerous and varied collections of objects, such as wrappers, stamps, shells, dolls, cars, stones, and anything that is classifiable (Fig. 17-4). They even begin to order friends and relationships (e.g., first best friend, second best friend).

As children mature, they progress from collecting simply for the sake of collecting and become more selective and discriminating. Their classification systems become more complex and are based on abstract ideas rather than on perception and experience. Much of the pleasure of collections is in the appraising, ordering, and reordering of the parts.

Schoolchildren are able to *serialize* (i.e., to arrange objects according to some ordinal scale or quantified dimension such as size, weight, or color). They develop the ability to understand relational terms and concepts, such as bigger and smaller; darker and paler; heavier and lighter; to the right of and to the left of; first, last, and intermediate (e.g., fourth, second); and more than and less than. They can see family relationships in terms of reciprocal roles. For example, to be a brother, one must have a sibling.

During the school-age years children develop *combinational skills*—the ability to manipulate numbers and to learn the skills of addition, subtraction, multiplication, and division. They learn to apply the basic operations to any object or quantity. They learn the alphabet and the ever-widening world of symbols called words that can be arranged in terms of structure and their relationship to the alphabet. They learn to tell time, to see the relationship of events in time (history) and places in space (geography), and to combine time and space relationships (geology and astronomy).

The most significant skill, the *ability to read,* is acquired during the school years and becomes the most valuable tool for independent inquiry. Children's capacity for exploration, imagination, and expansion of knowledge is enhanced by the ability to read as they progress from the repetition and confusion of early efforts to increasing facility and comprehension. Formal academic learning begins at ages 5 to 6 years, when children's intellectual capabilities and cognitive processes allow them to acquire intellectual achievements.

## Moral Development (Kohlberg)

As children move from egocentrism to more logical patterns of thought, they also move through stages in development of conscience and moral standards. Young children do not believe that standards of behavior come from within themselves but that rules are established and set down by others. During preschool years, rules are perceived as definite and requiring no reason or explanation. Children learn the standards for acceptable behavior, act according to these standards, and feel guilty when they violate the standards. Although children 6 or 7 years old know the rules and what they are supposed to do, they do not understand the reasons behind them. Young children usually judge an act by its consequences. Rewards and punishment guide their judgment; a "bad act" is one that breaks a rule or does harm. When a child and an adult differ in judging an act, the adult is right. Children may believe that what other people tell them to do is right and that what they themselves think is wrong. Consequently, children 6 or 7 years old are

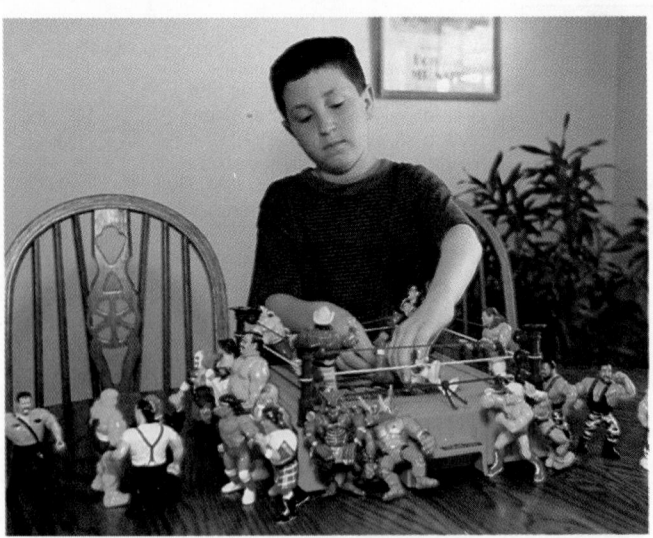

**Fig. 17-4** School-age children are often avid collectors.

more likely to interpret accidents and misfortunes as punishment for misdeeds or "bad" acts.

Older school-age children are able to judge an act by the intentions that prompted it rather than just by the consequences. Rules and judgments become less absolute and authoritarian and begin to be founded more on the needs and desires of others. Rules of conduct are more readily considered in terms of mutual agreement and are based on cooperation and respect for others. For older children a rule violation is apt to be viewed in relation to the total context in which it appears; reactions are influenced by the situation, as well as by the morality of the rule itself. However, it is not until adolescence or beyond that children are able to view morality on an abstract basis with sound reasoning and principled thinking. Although younger children can judge an act only according to whether it is right or wrong, older children take into account a different point of view to make a judgment. They are able to understand and accept the concept of treating others as they would like to be treated.

## Spiritual Development

Children at this age think in very concrete terms but are avid learners and have a great desire to learn about their God. They picture God as human and use adjectives such as "loving" and "helping" to describe their deity. They are fascinated by heaven and hell and, with a developing conscience and concern about rules, they fear going to hell for misbehavior. School-age children want and expect to be punished for misbehavior and, if given the option, tend to choose a punishment that "fits the crime." Often they view illness or injury as a punishment for a real or imagined misdeed. The beliefs and ideals of family and religious personages are more influential than those of their peers in matters of faith.

School-age children begin to learn the difference between the natural and the supernatural but have difficulty understanding symbols. Consequently, religious concepts must be presented to them in concrete terms. They try to relate phenomena in the world in a logical, systematic manner, which is at once both satisfying and occasionally disheartening. Religion affords a means whereby children can relate themselves to their deity in a direct and personal way.

Children are comforted by prayer or other religious rituals, and if these activities are a part of their daily lives, they can help children cope with threatening situations (Fig. 17-5). Their petitions to their God in prayers tend to be for very tangible rewards. Although younger children expect their prayers to be answered, as they get older they begin to recognize that this does not always occur and become less concerned when prayers are not answered. They are able to discuss their feelings about their faith and how it relates to their lives. (See Cultural Awareness box.)

## Language Development

Children enter middle childhood with remarkably efficient language skills, but they achieve many important linguistic accomplishments during the school-age years. During the elementary school years they learn to correct previous syntactic errors and begin to use more complex grammatical forms, such as correct past tenses for irregular verbs, correct plurals for irregular nouns, and correct use of personal pronouns.

Word usage, as well as the ability to find and retrieve words quickly when called on to produce what they know in a relatively short period of time, grows considerably during the school years. Children learn to apply the minimum-distance principle—the rule that the subject of a verb in an active sentence is the noun or pronoun that immediately precedes it. For example, a 6-year-old child will understand the sentence "Ask Mary her last name" but until age 9 or 10 years will be confused by the sentence "Ask Mary what to bring to the party."

Narrative skills improve markedly. School-age children are increasingly able to provide directives that others can correctly interpret without visual data (e.g., explaining directions over the telephone). By age 10 to 12 years the child should be able to use factive words (such as "know," "think," and "believe"), as well as complex pronouns and conjunctions, and be able to form grammatically correct sentences. School-age children gradually become more proficient at making inferences about meanings and learn the

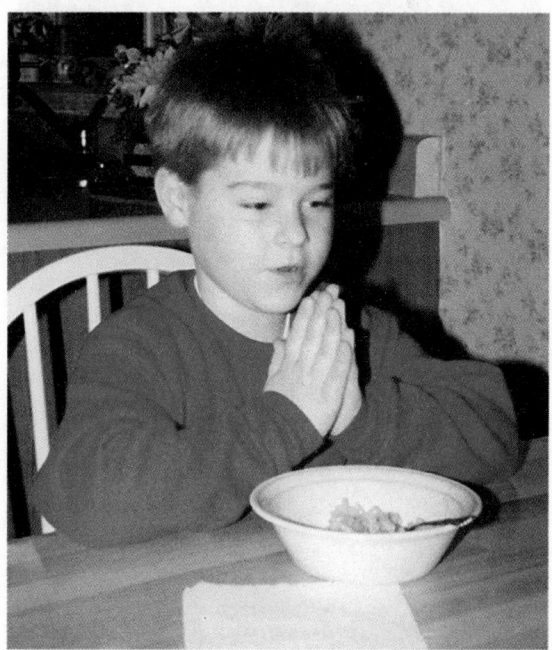

**Fig. 17-5** Children are comforted by prayer or other religious rituals.

---

### 🌐 CULTURAL AWARENESS
*Religious Orientation*

Many schools and communities have a Judeo-Christian orientation toward prayer, holidays, and values. This may result in conflict and discomfort for children of other religious/ethnic groups. Sensitivity must be exercised so as not to offend and confuse children from other religious backgrounds, such as the Buddhist, Hindu, and Muslim faiths.

subtle exceptions to grammatical rules. This makes them less likely to engage in literal interpretation of messages.

They rapidly develop *metalinguistic awareness*—an ability to think about language and to comment on its properties. This enables them to appreciate jokes, riddles, and puns because of their play on words, sounds, or double meanings. They are beginning to understand metaphors and figurative statements, such as "A stitch in time saves nine." The acquisition of cognitive skills enables them to think about the quality of their own and others' speech and to evaluate and clarify messages.

## Social Development

At the beginning of middle childhood, children enter a period of less intense emotions, secure in their dependency on their parents and family and with self-confidence tempered by a more realistic perspective. They have the energy to explore the environment beyond the family, to gradually increase the scope of interpersonal interactions, and to invest their curiosity in understanding the world.

Identification with peers is a strong influence in children's gaining independence from parents. The aid and support of peers provides children with enough security to risk the moderate parental rejection brought about by each small victory in their development of independence.

Questions of masculinity and femininity take on importance as sex-role learning assumes more prominence. Boys associate with boys, and girls with girls, each pursuing their own interests, with communication between the sexes confined to that which is necessary. Much of the child's concept of the appropriate sex role is acquired through relationships with peers. During the early school years there is little difference relative to sex in the play experiences of children. Games and many other activities are shared by both girls and boys. However, in the later school years the differences become marked.

## Social Relationships and Cooperation

Daily relationships with age-mates provide the most important social interactions for school-age children. For the first time, children are able to join in group activities with unrestrained enthusiasm and steady participation. Previously, interactions were limited to short periods under considerable adult supervision. With increased skills and wider opportunities, children become involved with one or several peer groups in which they can gain status as respected members.

Valuable lessons are learned from daily interaction with age-mates. First, children learn to appreciate the numerous and varied points of view that are represented in the peer group. As they play together, children discover that there are numerous occupations for fathers and mothers, more than one version of the same song, different rules for the same game, and different customs for celebrating the same holiday. As children interact with peers who see the world in ways that are somewhat different from their own, they become aware of the limits of their own point of view. Because age-mates are peers and are not forced to accept one another's ideas as they are expected to accept those of adults, other children have a significant influence on decreasing the egocentric outlook of the individual child. Consequently, they learn to argue, persuade, bargain, cooperate, and compromise in order to maintain friendships.

Second, children become increasingly sensitive to the social norms and pressures of the peer group. The peer group establishes standards for acceptance and rejection, and children may be willing to modify their behavior to be accepted by the group. They are judged by the physical impression they convey, the skills they can perform, and other abilities they can demonstrate. The need for peer approval becomes a powerful influence toward conformity. Children learn to dress, talk, and otherwise behave in a manner acceptable to the group. A variety of roles, such as class joker or class hero, may be assumed by the individual child to gain approval from the group. However, no child can adapt perfectly to all the requirements of the peer group. If some children find the discrepancies between the values of the peer group and the values of their families to be too great, they may be forced to relinquish the pleasure of interaction with the group to abide by the regulations established in the home. Thus, to diminish conflict within the family, some children may be forced into a position outside the peer group.

Third, the interaction among peers leads to the formation of intimate friendships between same-sex peers (Fig. 17-6). School age is the time when children have "best friends" with whom they share secrets, private jokes, and adventures; they come to one another's aid in times of trouble. In the course of these friendships, children also fight, threaten, break up, and reunite. These dyadic relationships, in which children experience love and closeness for a peer, seem to be impor-

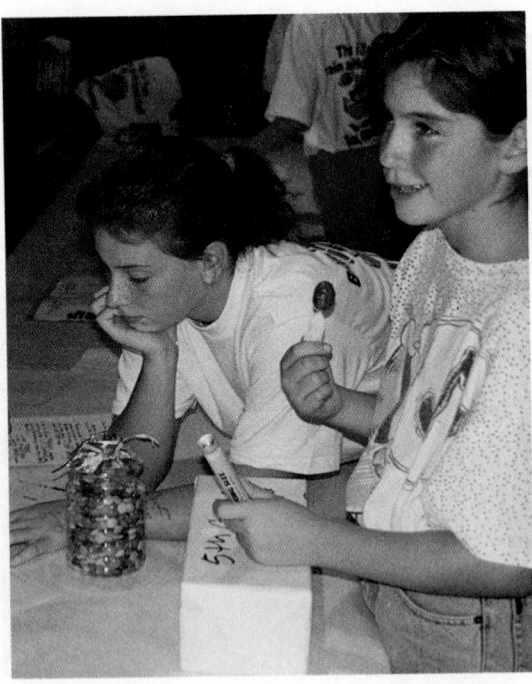

**Fig. 17-6**   School-age children enjoy engaging in activities with a "best friend."

tant as a foundation for heterosexual relationships in adulthood. The conflicts encountered in the relationship are usually resolved in terms that children are able to control. Since neither child has authority over the other, as in an adult-child relationship, children must work through their differences within the framework of their commitment to each other.

**Clubs and Peer Groups.**   One of the outstanding characteristics of middle childhood is the formation of formalized groups or clubs. Initially, children in the early middle years merely hang around the periphery of the formalized group, watching, learning, practicing various skills, and participating in group activities whenever the members of the group allow them to do so. As they advance in age, children eventually take their places as full-fledged participating group members.

A prominent feature of middle childhood groups is the code of rigid rules imposed on the members. There is an exclusiveness in the selection of persons who have the privilege of joining. They often adopt a "uniform" and special words that signify membership in the group. Acceptance in the group is often determined on a pass-fail basis according to social or behavioral criteria. Conformity is the core of the group structure. There are often secret codes, shared interests, and special modes of dress, and each child must abide by a standard of behavior established by the group. Conforming to the rules provides children with feelings of security and relieves them of the responsibility of making decisions.

Membership in the group provides children with a comfortable place in society. Many of the values of the group, such as physical strength, daring, ingenuity, and comradeship, have not been stressed in the family. However, these are values that contribute to an individual child's total personality. By merging their identity with the identities of their peers, children move from the family group to an outside group as a step toward seeking further independence. They substitute conformity to a peer-group pattern for conformity to a family pattern while they are still too shaky and insecure to function independently.

During the early school years, groups are rather small and loosely organized, with changing membership and little formal structure. They do not demonstrate the elements of give-and-take, cooperation, and order that are seen in groups of older children. As a rule, girls' groups are less formalized than boys' groups, and, although there may be a mixture of both sexes in the earlier school years, the groups of later school years are composed predominantly of children of the same sex. Common interests are a frequent basis around which a group is structured.

Children's strong desire not to be different creates problems for those who are, for various reasons, unable to meet the accepted standards of the peer group. Children with disabilities or those who are in some way unable to compete have a difficult time. Self-consciousness results when children are unable to dress as other children dress, do not have spending money like other children, or appear different from other children.

Children who have physical characteristics that are obviously different (such as birthmarks or "ears that stick out" or physical defects) may be set apart from the group and become a target for the criticism and ridicule of the peer group. Peer-group identification and association are essential to socialization.

Poor relationships with peers and a lack of group identification can also contribute to bullying behavior. *Bullying* is defined as one or more individuals inflicting physical, verbal, or emotional abuse on another. Bullying can involve the threat of bodily harm, weapon possession, gang activity, and assault and battery.* Bullying occurs at school, on playgrounds, in hallways, bathrooms, in classrooms before instruction, and in the cafeteria. Boys are more likely than girls to engage in bullying and to be the victims of bullies (Kumpulainen, Rasanen, Henttonen, 1999). Children who are bullies are often defiant, antisocial, and likely to break school rules. Children who bully may also be at risk for psychologic disturbances and psychiatric symptoms later in life (Kumpulainen, Rasanen, and Henttonen, 1999).

Bullying also has a negative effect on children who experience this behavior. An increase in common pediatric symptoms such as headache, stomachache, and sleep disturbances has been associated with increased bullying in school (Williams and others, 1996). In addition, victims of bullying are at risk for remaining involved in this behavior, either as bullies themselves or as victims for several years beyond childhood into adolescence (Kumpulainen, Rasanen, Henttonen, 1999; Sourander and others, 2000). Although peer-group identification and association are essential to a child's emergence into the world, there can be dangers inherent in strong peer-group attachment. Peer pressures may force children into taking risks, even against their better judgment. Peer-group activities that result in unacceptable, unlawful, or criminal **gang violence** are increasing in the United States and represent a significant challenge for health professionals and teachers who work with children. (See Community Focus box on p. 708.)

## Relationships with Families

Although the peer group is highly influential and necessary to normal child development, parents are the primary influence in shaping children's personalities, setting standards for behavior, and establishing value systems. Family values usually predominate when parental and peer value systems come into conflict. Although children may appear to reject parental values while testing the new values of the peer group, ultimately they will retain and incorporate into their own value systems the parental values they have found to be of worth. Peer associations seem to remain within the social class system, and not infrequently there may be discriminate membership on the basis of ethnic or racial origin.

---

*The following organizations all provide information on bullying and how to prevent it in the school setting: **ERIC Clearinghouse on Elementary and Early Childhood Education**, University of Illinois at Urbana-Champaign, Children's Research Center, 51 Gerty Drive, Champaign, IL 61820-7469, (800) 583-4135; e-mail: ericeece@uiuc.edu; www.ericeece.org; **NPIN (National Parent Information Network)** www.npin.org; **Educators for Social Responsibility,** 23 Garden Street, Cambridge, MA 01238, (617) 492-1764; www.esrnational.org; and **National Association for the Education of Young Children,** 1509 16th St, NW, Washington, DC 20036-1426, (800) 421-2460; www.naeyc.org.

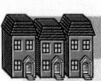

Parents of school-age children often worry about the informal and unstructured social groups that their children are attracted to and wish to join. Parents of boys seem particularly concerned about "boys only" groups and the possibility that such groups could become gangs and participate in violent activities.

To help parents cope with these fears, nurses can encourage parents to become aware of any gang-related activities in their community. Typically, activities of organized gangs are illegal, and children involved in gang activities may experience frequent accidents or trips to the emergency room or police station. In addition, gang members frequently have characteristics that parents can identify, such as graffiti, a particular clothing style, unique tattoos, hand signals, or violent illegal initiation rituals. Parents can also be encouraged to become acquainted with their child's friends and to become involved in providing positive recreational activities for their children.

The community's awareness of gangs that promote violence is essential to stop the spread of gang membership among youth. The media can inform the community of gang influx, identification, and activities to raise parents' awareness of the potential dangers to their children. Community services that promote a sense of belonging among children and offer structured recreational and social events can help youth find alternatives to being a gang member.

As children move into the wider world of peer-group relationships, parents are faced with the task of relinquishing their hold. They may find it difficult to face the rejection that is demonstrated as their children stand solidly with the peer group. Children may want to spend more time in the company of their peers, may seem eager to leave the house, and often prefer activities of the group to family activities. During this time parents can best serve the interests of their children through tolerant understanding and support even when there may be intolerance and criticism of the parents and their ways when those ways deviate from those of the group. In the child's eyes, the parents no longer assume the stature they previously enjoyed. Children discover that parents can be wrong, and they begin to question the knowledge and authority of the parents who previously were considered to be all-knowing and all-powerful.

Although increased independence is the goal of middle childhood, children are not yet prepared to abandon parental control. Children need and want restrictions placed on their behavior; they are not yet prepared to cope with all of the problems of their expanding environment. They feel more secure knowing that there is an authority greater than themselves to implement controls and restrictions. Children may complain loudly about the restrictions and try to break down parental barriers, but they are uneasy if they succeed in doing so. Children feel secure with reasonable, consistent controls. They respect the adults on whom they can rely to prevent them from acting on each and every urge. Children sense in this behavior an expression of love and concern for their welfare.

Children also need their parents as adults, not as "pals." Sometimes parents, hurt by their children's rejection, attempt to maintain their love and gratitude by assuming the role of pal. Children need the stable, secure strength provided by mature adults to whom they can turn during troubled relationships with peers or stressful changes in their world. During a disruption in their lives, such as times of failure, periods of illness, or a move that separates them from the security of friends, children need the firm, secure anchor of parental interest and concern. With a secure base in a loving family, children are able to develop the self-confidence and maturity needed to break loose from the group and stand independently.

Children's relationships with siblings change during the middle years. Siblings are viewed as equal in power and status. In earlier years, older siblings were influential in the younger siblings' learning. In the middle years the relationship becomes one of companionship. Positive emotional tone increases, but sibling conflict also increases as the siblings get older. Middle childhood is a period of transition for sibling relationships, a juncture between the open bickering of early childhood and the supportive relationship observed in adult siblings.

## Development of Self-Concept

Closely associated with developing a sense of industry is developing a concept of one's value and worth. With the emphasis on skill building and broadened social relationships, children are continually occupied in the process of self-evaluation. Children's self-concepts are composed of their own critical self-assessment plus their interpretations of the opinions of others. **Self-concept** refers to a conscious awareness of a variety of self-perceptions, such as one's physical characteristics, abilities, values, self-ideals, and one's idea of self in relation to others.

### Body Image

Body image is what children think about their bodies. School-age children are knowledgeable about the human body, and social development during this period focuses to a large extent on the body and its capabilities. School-age children can draw a recognizable human figure although individually their portrayal of body parts may vary considerably. They are acutely aware of their own bodies as well as those of their peers and those of adults. It is important that children know body functions and that adults correct any misinformation children have about the body (e.g., what is fat).

During the school years, children focus on peer relationships and conform to group norms. They evaluate how their physical appearance, body configuration, and coordination compares with their peers. The head is the most noticeable and, to them, important part of the body. They also model themselves after their parents and compare themselves to favored peers and images observed in the media.

Children are acutely aware of physical disabilities in others, and it is not unusual for them to believe that their own bodies are not the right size or the right shape or are in some way defective. They respond to such concerns in a variety of ways. For example, they will conceal perceived shortcomings of body or performance, such as the obese child who refrains from going swimming, the child who conveniently forgets a gym suit, the child who conceals an imagined defect, or the child with enuresis who declines invitations to slumber parties. Children seldom express these concerns to families. However, they need to be reassured about both the uniqueness and the sameness of their bodies while their privacy is respected and they are allowed appropriate protective strategies. Children who are different become acutely aware of the differences and may find themselves excluded from the group. When children are teased or criticized about being different, the effect can be lasting and remembered into adulthood.

### Self-Esteem

Self-esteem is children's pictures of their individual worth and consists of both positive and negative qualities. Children actively strive to achieve internalized goals or levels of attainment. At the same time, they continually receive feedback on the quality of their performance from individuals they consider to be authorities. By the time they reach school age, children have received messages regarding the extent to which they are able to accomplish tasks that have been delegated to them. For example, one child may have been given prestigious responsibilities at home or at school or received special commendation for an achievement. On the other hand, another child may have been sent to a special class for slow learners or may have been the last person chosen when children chose sides for a game. These and other signs serve as clues to social worth that children incorporate as part of their self-evaluation.

Children approach the process of self-evaluation from a framework of either self-confidence or self-doubt. Children who have mastered the maturational crises of autonomy and initiative are able to face the world with feelings of pride rather than shame. At first, children's self-concepts are formed exclusively from their perceptions of their parents' evaluation of them. During middle childhood the opinions of peers and teachers are important. Criticisms and peer approval are additional sources of data for evaluation. Parents and other adults are no longer the only persons who respond to their skills, talents, and abilities; peers also identify skills and capabilities. Each child soon begins to internalize these outside opinions. If children regard themselves as worthwhile or satisfactory persons, they are considered to have high self-esteem, self-confidence, or a positive self-concept. If they view themselves as worthless, they are said to have poor or low self-esteem.

Pets have also been observed to influence a child's self-esteem. Pets can have a positive effect on children's attitudes about themselves and can increase their ability to relate to others (Beck and Meyers, 1996).

Children encounter difficulties assessing their own abilities because they rely on their own expectations or on the expectations expressed by others regarding their performance. They depend almost entirely on external evidence of worth, such as school grades, teachers' comments, and parental and peer approval. Children do not yet have the capacity to develop their own independent criteria to evaluate their own accomplishments. It is especially difficult for them to assess their achievement in abstract skills.

Nothing succeeds like success. Significant adults in children's lives can often manage to manipulate the environment so that children meet with success. Each small success increases a child's self-image. The more positive children feel about themselves, the more confident they feel in trying again for success. All children profit from feeling that they are special to significant adults. A positive self-image makes them feel likable, worthwhile, and capable of valuable contributions. Such feelings lead to self-respect, self-confidence, and a general feeling of happiness. Parents can help their school-age children to develop self-esteem by being honest, by providing opportunities for creativity, by helping them succeed in activities, and by providing positive reinforcement. Nurses can enhance self-esteem by fostering supportive relationships between children and members of their families and by emphasizing children's strengths and positive aspects of their behavior. (See Community Focus box.)

## Development of Sexuality

Evidence indicates that many children experience some form of sex play during or before preadolescence as a response to normal curiosity not as a result of love or sexual urge. Children are experimentalists by nature, and this play is incidental and transitory. Adverse emotional consequences or guilt feelings depend on how the behavior is managed by the parents and whether children view their actions as wrong in the eyes of significant persons, particularly their parents.

Children's attitudes toward sex are acquired indirectly at a very early age and affect the way they respond to sexual information presented at a later time. Many parents discourage sex exploration, either through subtle substitution of activities that divert their children's attention from the genitalia or by expressions of anger or disgust at their children's behavior. These tactics clearly communicate to children that they should not engage in such activities, discourage questions about sex, and limit the sources of information.

In addition, parents may not teach young children the correct terminology for sexual organs or sexual feelings. Often the only vocabulary available to children is one that identifies sexual organs with excretory functions. If children learn that excretory organs and functions are dirty, they may associate "dirtiness" with the reproductive organs and functions. If children learn the correct terminology for the organs and their functions, this association should be reduced or eliminated.

## Sex Education

Because parents often either repress or avoid their children's sexual curiosity, sexual information received in childhood may be acquired almost entirely from peers. Such information is often transmitted in secret conversations and contains considerable misinformation. These communications can also create anxiety in children and inhibit spontaneous expressions or questioning of their parents.

Although middle childhood is an ideal time for formal sex education, this subject has created considerable controversy. Many parents and groups are unconditionally opposed to the inclusion of sex education in the schools. Others believe that information relating to sexual maturation and the process of reproduction should be presented as naturally as information about other natural phenomena, such as the growth of plants, the changing seasons, and the migratory habits of birds. When sex education is presented from a life span approach and treated as a normal part of growth and development, the information is less likely to contain overtones of uncertainty, guilt, or embarrassment that could in turn produce anxiety in children.

Sex education programs have been successfully incorporated into a number of elementary school curricula. In many of these programs, sexuality is presented in the context of its central role as a biologic mechanism for the survival of the culture. Children learn that sexual maturation and reproduction represent each individual's contribution to the natural order of things. This approach provides a natural entry into discussion of sexuality as a basis for family units, marriage, and attitudes toward children as well as an entry into a presentation of the biologic facts of sexuality. Many sex education programs also emphasize that sexual intimacy is part of a close, personal relationship and a means of conveying love, as well as a means for ensuring the survival of the species.

## Nurse's Role in Sex Education

No matter where nurses practice, they can provide information on human sexuality to both parents and children. To discuss the topic adequately, nurses must have an understanding of the physiologic aspects of sexuality, the common myths and misconceptions associated with sex and the re-

productive process, knowledge of cultural and societal values, and an awareness of their own attitudes, feelings, and biases.

When nurses present sexual information to children, they should treat sex as a normal part of growth and development. Questions should be answered honestly, matter-of-factly, and at the child's level of understanding. School-age children may be more comfortable when boys and girls are segregated for discussions; however, each group needs information about both sexes.

Children need help to differentiate sex and sexuality. Exercises on clarifying values, identifying role models, problem solving, and accepting responsibility are important to prepare school-age children for early adolescence and puberty. In addition, children need to have sexual information that is provided via the media or jokes explained and defused. Information concerning acquired immunodeficiency syndrome (AIDS) should be (1) presented in simple, accurate terms; (2) focus on how the AIDS virus is transmitted; (3) dispel myths regarding transmission; (4) explain the effects of AIDS on the body, and (5) identify resource personnel in the school who can answer children's questions about AIDS (American Academy of Pediatrics, 1998a).

Preadolescents need precise and concrete information that will allow them to answer questions such as "What if I start my period in the middle of class?" or "How can I keep people from telling I have an erection?" It is important to tell them what they want to know and what they can expect to happen as they mature sexually.

During encounters with parents, nurses can be open and available for questions and discussion. They can set an example by the language they use in discussing body parts and their function and by the way in which they deal with problems that have emotional overtones, such as exploratory sex play and masturbation. Parents need to be helped to understand normal behaviors and to view sexual curiosity in their children as a part of the developmental process. Assessing the parents' level of knowledge and understanding of sexuality provides cues to their need for supplemental information that will prepare them for the increasingly complex explanations that will be needed as their children grow older.

Parents of children with developmental disabilities may need special assistance and help with sex education. These parents often appreciate specific, concrete guidelines concerning how to teach their children about changes in their bodies, how and when to express physical affection, how to protect themselves from sexual abuse or exploitation, and how to assume independence in personal hygiene and self-care (American Academy of Pediatrics, 1996a).

Sometimes short classes or group discussions for parents are helpful for discussing disturbing behaviors and anticipating the questions and learning needs of their children. When possible, it is wise to include both parents. Sex education in the home should be assumed by both parents so that the children will not acquire a distorted view of either the male or the female role that may alter relationships with the opposite sex in later life.

## Play

As children enter the school years, their play takes on new dimensions that reflect a new stage of development. Not only does play involve increased physical skill, intellectual ability, and fantasy, but, as children form groups and cliques, they begin to evolve a sense of belonging to a team or club. To belong to a group is of vital importance. Clubs, societies, and organizations are important parts of the culture of childhood.

### Rules and Rituals

The need for conformity in middle childhood is strongly manifested in the activities and games so important in the life of school-age children. Up to this point, they have either played games they have invented themselves or have played in the company of a friend or an adult, and rules more or less evolved with the game. Now they begin to see the need for rules, and the games they play have fixed and unvarying rules that may be bizarre and extraordinarily rigid (especially those made up by the group). But part of the enjoyment of the game is knowing the rules because knowing means belonging. Once the rules are established and agreed on, the demand for conformity is vigorous (Fig. 17-7).

Conformity and ritual permeate the play of school-age children. Not only do they dominate in games, but they are also evident in much of the children's behavior and language. Childhood is full of chants and taunts, such as "Eeny, meeny, miney, mo," "Last one is a rotten egg," and "Step on a crack, break your mother's back." Children derive a great deal of pleasure and power from such sayings, which have been handed down with few changes through generations.

**Team Play.** A more complex form of group play that evolves from the need for peer interaction involves the team games and sports that are part of the school years. The rules of such games may require the presence of a referee, umpire, or person of authority so the rules can be followed more accurately. Team membership has several characteristics that promote child development during the middle years.

Children learn to subordinate personal goals to group goals. Team membership means that each child is accountable to the other team members and that each member's acts may affect the success or failure of the entire group. Each member's behavior is open to public evaluation, and children risk ostracism, ridicule, or being made a scapegoat if they contribute to a team loss. Although individual skills are recognized, team successes and failures are shared by all members. Children learn the concept of interdependence and that all players rely on one another.

Children learn that division of labor is an effective strategy for the attainment of a goal. Each position on a team has a specific function, and the team has a greater chance of winning if each person performs a specific function. Once children learn this concept, they can transfer the knowledge to other aspects of life. When they learn that certain goals are best accomplished by dividing tasks among several individuals, they begin to see a relationship to principles of organization in other social structures. Children

Sticker Riot
RULES
1. Keep club a secret.
2. Must come to as many meetings as posable.
3. Must bring sticker to every meeting and school ressec.
4. When in another house for meetings do not run in house unless told.
5. When at house don't touch or eat anything unless told.
6. If you don't come to a meeting you must make up the meeting at some one's house.
7. If you miss a meeting you can bet that the other members are still going to have the meeting.

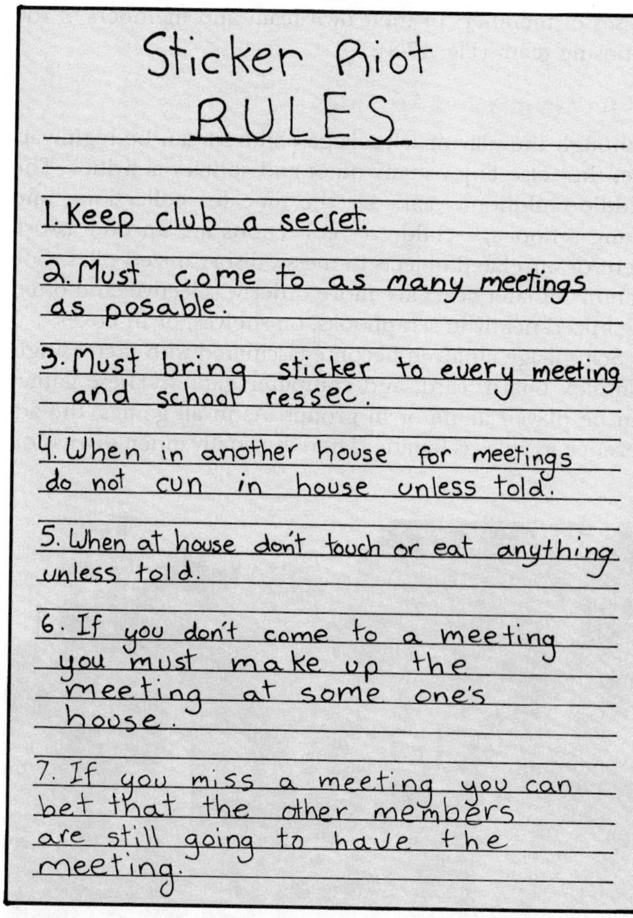

**Fig. 17-7** A list of club rules compiled by a group of 9-year-old children.

also learn that some children are best equipped to perform one part of the task, and other children are best suited to another aspect of the task.

Team play helps children to learn about the nature of competition. In all team play there is a winning side and a losing side. Because losing is often interpreted as failure, children will go to great lengths to avoid the public embarrassment and personal shame that accompany failure. The more a child identifies with the team and values membership in the group, the more distasteful losing becomes. Fear of losing and the failure it implies are strong incentives for group commitment. The importance of winning is not universally valued, however. Some cultures and subcultures place emphasis on the game and consideration for one's companions rather than on the outcome.

Team play also contributes to children's social, intellectual, and skill growth. Children will work hard to develop the skills needed to become members of a team, to improve their contribution to the group effort, and to anticipate the consequences of their behavior for the group. Team play helps stimulate cognitive growth as children are called on to learn many complex rules, make judgments about those rules, plan strategies, and assess the strengths and weaknesses of members of their own team and members of the opposing team (Fig. 17-8).

## Quiet Games and Activities

Although the play of school-age children can be highly active, they also enjoy many quiet and solitary activities. The middle childhood years are the time for collections, and young school-age children's collections are an odd assortment of unrelated objects in messy, disorganized piles. Collections of later years are more orderly, selective, and often organized neatly in scrapbooks, on shelves, or in boxes.

School-age children become fascinated with increasingly complex board, card, and computer games. These games can be played alone or in groups. As in all games, the adherence to rules is fanatic. There is usually much discussion

and argument, but disagreement is easily resolved by learning the appropriate rules of the game.

The newly acquired skill of reading becomes increasingly satisfying as school-age children begin to expand their knowledge of the world through books (Fig. 17-9). School-age children never tire of stories, and, just like preschool children, they love to have stories read aloud. Sewing, cooking, carpentry, gardening, and creative endeavors such as painting are other activities enjoyed. Many creative skills, such as music and art, as well as athletic skills, such as swimming, riding, hiking, dancing, and skating, are acquired during childhood and continue to be enjoyed into adolescence and adulthood (Fig. 17-10).

Hero worship is another characteristic of children and adolescents. The object of the adoration can be a number of persons, such as a friend, relative, teacher, or national sports or entertainment figure. The difficulty arises when the idol proves to be an inappropriate role model.

## Ego Mastery

Play also affords children the means to acquire representational mastery over themselves, their environment, and other persons. Through play, children can feel as big, as powerful, and as skillful as their imaginations will allow, and

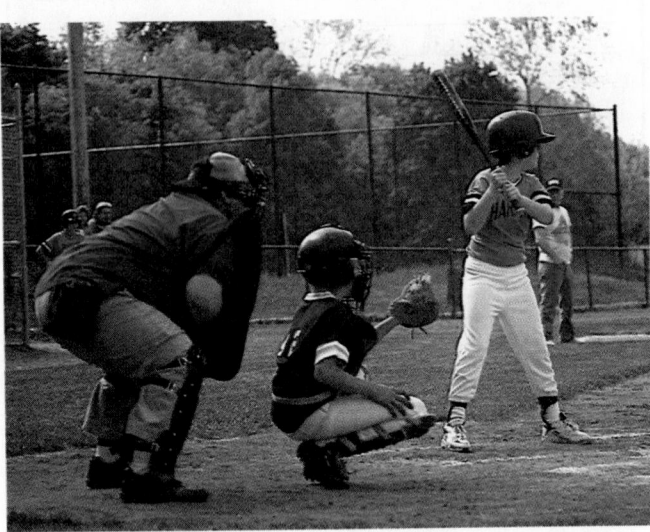

**Fig. 17-8** Activities engaged in by school-age children, such as Little League baseball, vary according to the child's interest and opportunity.

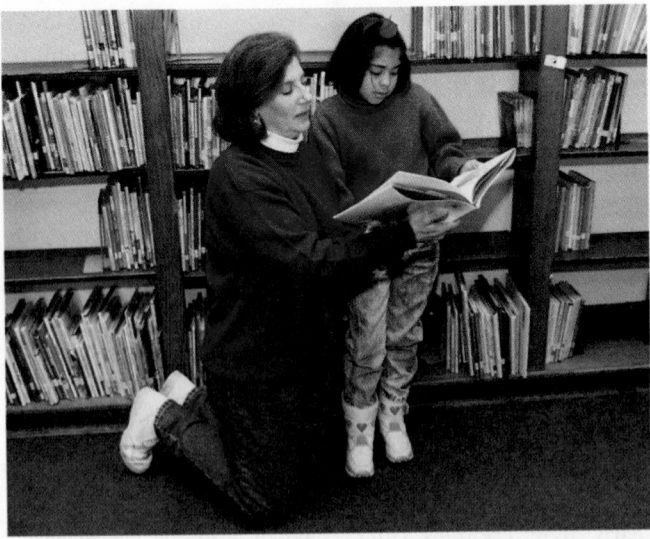

**Fig. 17-9** Selecting a book with the assistance of an adult.

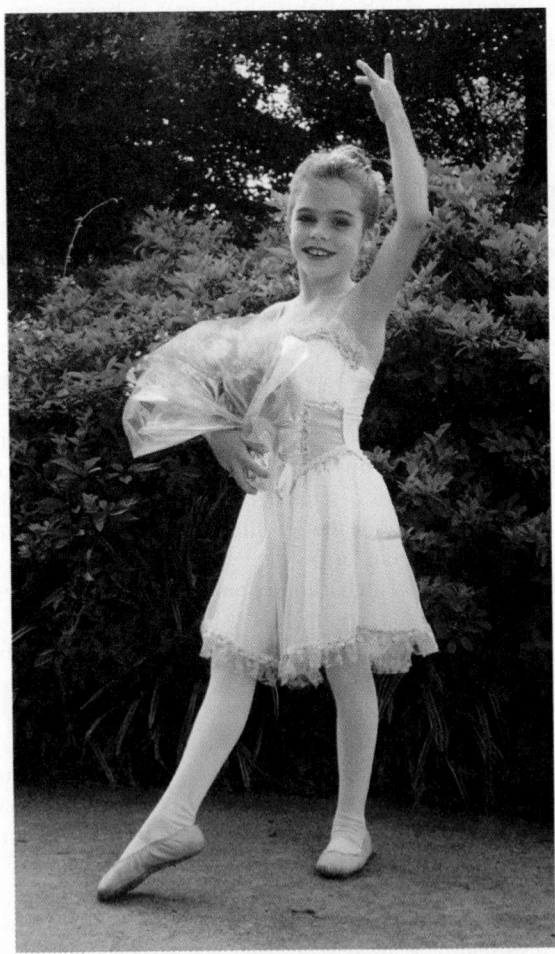

**Fig. 17-10** School-age children take pride in learning new skills.

they can attain vicarious mastery and power over whomever and whatever they choose. They need to feel in control in their play. Schoolchildren still need the opportunity to use large muscles in exuberant outdoor play and the freedom to exert their newfound autonomy and initiative. They need space in which to exercise large muscles and to work off tensions, frustrations, and hostility. Physical skills practiced and mastered in play help them develop a feeling of personal competence, which contributes to a sense of accomplishment and helps provide a place of status in the peer group. A summary of growth and development in middle childhood is presented in Table 17-1. Because each child has a unique developmental pattern, any attempt to describe the typical child of any age-group can only represent an average and should not be considered as absolute criteria for any given child.

**TABLE 17-1  Growth and development during school-age years**

| Age (years) | Physical and Motor | Mental | Adaptive | Personal-Social |
|---|---|---|---|---|
| 6 | Height and weight gain continues slowly<br>Weight: 16-23.6 kg (35½-53 pounds); height: 106.6-123.5 cm (42-48 inches)<br>Central mandibular incisors erupt<br>Loses first tooth<br>Gradual increase in dexterity<br>Active age; constant activity<br>Often returns to finger feeding<br>More aware of hand as a tool<br>Likes to draw, print, and color<br>Vision reaches maturity | Develops concept of numbers<br>Counts 13 pennies<br>Knows whether it is morning or afternoon<br>Defines common objects such as fork and chair in terms of their use<br>Obeys triple commands in succession<br>Knows right and left hands<br>Says which is pretty and which is ugly in a series of drawings of faces<br>Describes objects in a picture rather than simply enumerating them<br>Attends first grade | At table, uses knife to spread butter or jam on bread<br>At play, cuts, folds, pastes paper toys, sews crudely if needle is threaded<br>Takes bath without supervision; performs bedtime activities alone<br>Reads from memory; enjoys oral spelling game<br>Likes table games, checkers, simple card games<br>Giggles a lot<br>Sometimes steals money or attractive items<br>Has difficulty owning up to misdeeds<br>Tries out own abilities | Can share and cooperate better<br>Has great need for children of own age<br>Will cheat to win<br>Often engages in rough play<br>Often jealous of younger brother or sister<br>Does what adults are seen doing<br>May have occasional temper tantrums<br>Is a boaster<br>Is more independent, probably influence of school<br>Has own way of doing things<br>Increases socialization |
| 7 | Begins to grow at least 5 cm (2 inches) in height per year<br>Weight: 17.7-30 kg (39-66½ pounds); height: 111.8-129.7 cm (44-51 inches)<br>Maxillary central incisors and lateral mandibular incisors erupt<br>More cautious in approaches to new performances<br>Repeats performances to master them<br>Jaw begins to expand to accommodate permanent teeth | Notices that certain parts are missing from pictures<br>Can copy a diamond<br>Repeats three numbers backward<br>Develops concept of time; reads ordinary clock or watch correctly to nearest quarter hour; uses clock for practical purposes<br>Attends the second grade<br>More mechanical in reading; often does not stop at the end of a sentence, skips words such as "it," "the," and "he" | Uses table knife for cutting meat; may need help with tough or difficult pieces<br>Brushes and combs hair acceptably without help<br>May steal<br>Likes to help and have a choice<br>Is less resistant and stubborn | Is becoming a real member of the family group<br>Takes part in group play<br>Boys prefer playing with boys; girls prefer playing with girls<br>Spends a lot of time alone; does not require a lot of companionship |
| 8-9 | Continues to gain 5 cm (2 inches) in height per year<br>Weight: 19.6-39.6 kg (43-87 pounds); height: 117-141.8 cm (46-56 inches)<br>Lateral incisors (maxillary) and mandibular cuspids erupt<br>Movement fluid; often graceful and poised<br>Always on the go; jumps, chases, skips<br>Increased smoothness and speed in fine motor control; uses cursive writing | Gives similarities and differences between two things from memory<br>Counts backward from 20 to 1; understands concept of reversibility<br>Repeats days of the week and months in order; knows the date<br>Describes common objects in detail, not merely their use<br>Makes change out of a quarter<br>Attends third and fourth grades<br>Reads more; may plan to wake up early just to read<br>Reads classic books, but also enjoys comics | Makes use of common tools such as hammer, saw, or screwdriver<br>Uses household and sewing utensils<br>Helps with routine household tasks such as dusting, sweeping<br>Assumes responsibility for share of household chores<br>Looks after all of own needs at table<br>Buys useful articles; exercises some choice in making purchases<br>Runs useful errands<br>Likes pictorial magazines | Is easy to get along with at home<br>Likes the reward system<br>Dramatizes<br>Is more sociable<br>Is better behaved<br>Is interested in boy-girl relationships but will not admit it<br>Goes about home and community freely, alone or with friends<br>Likes to compete and play games<br>Shows preference in friends and groups |

*Continued*

**TABLE 17-1** Growth and development during school-age years—cont'd

| Age (years) | Physical and Motor | Mental | Adaptive | Personal-Social |
|---|---|---|---|---|
| 8-9— cont'd | Dresses self completely<br>Likely to overdo; hard to quiet down after recess<br>More limber; bones grow faster than ligaments | More aware of time; can be relied on to get to school on time<br>Can grasp concepts of parts and whole (fractions)<br>Understands concepts of space, cause and effect, nesting (puzzles), conservation (permanence of mass and volume)<br>Classifies objects by more than one quality; has collections<br>Produces simple paintings or drawings | Likes school, wants to answer all the questions<br>Is afraid of failing a grade; is ashamed of bad grades<br>Is more critical of self<br>Takes music and sport lessons | Plays mostly with groups of own sex but is beginning to mix<br>Develops modesty<br>Compares self with others<br>Enjoys organizations, clubs, and group sports |
| 10-12 | *Boys:* Slow growth in height and rapid weight gain; may become obese in this period<br>*Girls:* Pubescent changes may begin to appear; body lines soften and round out<br>Weight: 24.3-58 kg (54-128 pounds); height: 127.5-162.3 cm (50-64 inches)<br>Posture is more similar to an adult's; will overcome lordosis<br>Remainder of teeth will erupt and tend toward full development (except wisdom teeth) | Writes brief stories<br>Attends fifth to seventh grades<br>Writes occasional short letters to friends or relatives on own initiative<br>Uses telephone for practical purposes<br>Responds to magazine, radio, or other advertising<br>Reads for practical information or own enjoyment—stories or library books of adventure or romance, or animal stories | Makes useful articles or does easy repair work<br>Cooks or sews in small way<br>Raises pets<br>Washes and dries own hair<br>Is responsible for a thorough job of cleaning hair, but may need reminding to do so<br>Is sometimes left alone at home for an hour or so<br>Is successful in looking after own needs or those of other children left in his or her care | Loves friends; talks about them constantly<br>Chooses friends more selectively; may have a "best friend"<br>Enjoys conversation<br>Develops beginning interest in opposite sex<br>Is more diplomatic<br>Likes family; family really has meaning<br>Likes mother and wants to please her in many ways<br>Demonstrates affection<br>Likes father who is adored and may be idolized<br>Respects parents |

# COPING WITH CONCERNS RELATED TO NORMAL GROWTH AND DEVELOPMENT

## School Experience

The school serves as the agent for transmitting the values of the society to each succeeding generation of children and as the setting for many relationships with peers. As a socializing agent second only to the family, the school exerts a profound influence on the social development of children.

School entrance causes a sharp break in the structure of a child's world. For some children it is their first experience in conforming to a group pattern imposed by an adult who is not a parent and who has responsibility for too many children to be constantly aware of each child as an individual. Children want to go to school and usually adapt to the new condition with little difficulty. Successful adjustment is directly related to the child's physical and emotional maturity and the parent's readiness to accept the separation associated with school entrance. Cooperation among parents and support for the child are successful ways of coping with school entry stress. Unfortunately, some parents express their unconscious attempts to delay their child's maturity by clinging behavior, particularly with their youngest child.

## Anticipatory Socialization

By the time they enter school, most children have a fairly realistic concept of what school involves. They receive information regarding the role of pupil from parents, playmates, and the media. In addition, most children have had experience with daycare or preschool and kindergarten.

Children's attitudes toward school and the extent of their adjustment are strongly influenced by the attitudes of their parents. Middle-class children have fewer adjustments to make and less to learn about expected behavior because the school tends to reflect dominant middle-class customs and values, although this may be tempered by the school's location and predominant teachers and student body. Parents who view school as a place that they have helped to create and support and that is directed toward the same objectives for socialization as their own usually prepare their children with useful anticipatory socialization and furnish them with confidence to meet the challenge. Parents who view the school as an alien culture and one that they have little, if any, power to affect may unknowingly teach their children to be fearful and resentful toward school, even though they agree with its purposes and objectives.

Anticipatory socialization is also provided by television, which influences the acquisition of information and attitudes. Television viewing has the potential to increase a child's vocabulary, extend the child's horizons, and enrich

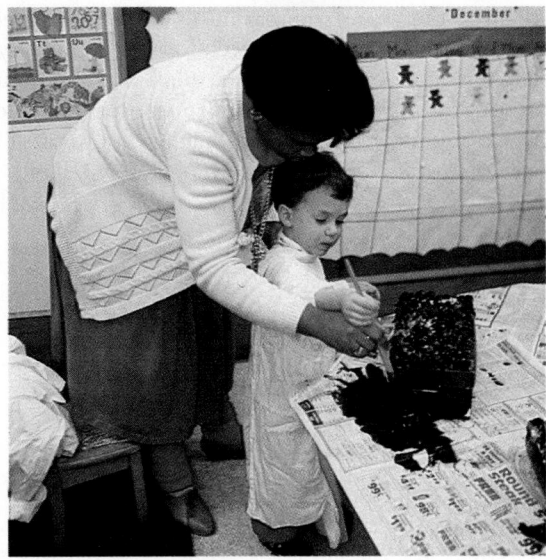

**Fig. 17-11** School represents an important change in a child's life, and teachers exert a significant influence on the child.

the school experience. However, television relies heavily on images to convey information. Consequently, difficult, complex issues are often not adequately explored by this medium. Extensive television viewing may also encourage children to seek simple answers to tough problems and to believe that violence is the most effective and quick solution to conflict.

Although most children have had some experience with schooling before they enter the first grade, the extent to which early childhood education prepares children for primary school varies. Some preschool programs provide custodial care; others emphasize emotional, social, and intellectual development as well. The type of early childhood programming that stresses a cognitive over a social emphasis appears to be more effective in facilitating later academic performance.

## Role of the Teacher

To facilitate the transition from home to school, teachers should have personality characteristics that allow them to deal with the needs of young children. Because they react to the teacher on the basis of past experience, children respond best to teachers with attributes that they would find

in a warm, loving parent. As a parental surrogate, teachers in the early grades perform many of the activities formerly assumed by the parents, such as recognizing the children's personal needs (e.g., a need to go to the bathroom or for help with clothing) and helping to develop their social behavior (e.g., manners).

Teachers, like parents, are concerned about the psychologic and emotional welfare of children. Although the functions of teachers and parents differ, both place constraints on behavior, and both are in a position to enforce standards of conduct. However, the teacher's primary responsibility is stimulating and guiding children's intellectual development as opposed to providing for their physical welfare beyond the school setting.

Teachers share the parental influence in shaping a child's attitudes and values. They serve as models with whom children can identify and whom they try to emulate. Teacher approval is sought; teacher disapproval is avoided. The teacher is a very significant person in the life of the early school-age child, and hero worship of a teacher may extend into late childhood and preadolescence. It is not uncommon for the first or second grader to be heartbroken and tearful at leaving a familiar teacher at the end of the school term or to be upset when faced with a substitute teacher for even a short period.

Children's interest in school and learning and much of their social interaction and self-concept are related to interactions with the teacher (Fig. 17-11). The differential systems of reward and punishment administered by teachers affect the emotional adjustment and self-concept of children as well as how they respond to school in general. (See Evidence-Based Practice box.) The interaction between the teacher and individual pupils affects the pupil's acceptance by other children, which in turn affects the child's self-concept. Behaviors praised by the teacher usually acquire a positive value, whereas those viewed negatively by the teacher are devalued by the children. In this way the teacher exerts considerable influence in a number of areas, such as attitudes toward minority groups, the disabled, or less favorably endowed children. Teacher approval of children and their self-acceptance are very closely related.

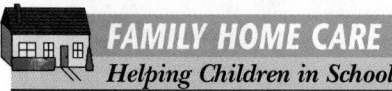

### FAMILY HOME CARE
*Helping Children in School*

**GENERAL GUIDELINES**

Be supportive—through companionship share ideas and thoughts.

Be positive—every child should experience some success each day.

Share an interest in reading—use the library, discuss books they are reading.

Support and encourage activity rather than passivity.

Encourage originality—help children make their own projects from discarded articles or other available materials.

Foster the development of hobbies and collections.

Encourage children to wonder and reflect during free time.

Encourage family experiences and trips to places of interest.

Encourage questions—help children discover sources for information or places in which to explore and investigate.

Stimulate creative thinking and problem solving—help children try out new solutions to problems without fear of making mistakes.

Use rewards rather than punishment.

**SPECIFIC GUIDELINES**

Meet the teacher at the beginning of school and plan to visit the school to see what is taught and expected.

Send the child to school every day—teachers are concerned when parents make other plans for their children; it conveys the impression that school is unimportant.

Demonstrate an interest in what the child is learning.

Demonstrate an interest in content and growth more than in grades.

Make it clear to the child that schoolwork is between the child and the teacher; teacher and child should set goals for better school performance to allow the child to feel responsible for school successes and failures.

Take advantage of situations that support and reinforce school learning.

Share information with teachers that will help them understand the child better.

Communicate with the teacher if there appears to be a problem—avoid waiting for a scheduled conference.

Provide a quiet, well-lighted area for study that is safe from interruption; do not allow television or radio.

Avoid dictating a study time, but do enforce rules, such as no television until homework is done; accept the child's word that work is complete.

Help with homework should focus on explaining the question, not giving the answer.

Teach the child to break large tasks (such as a report) into smaller, manageable tasks spread over the allotted time rather than attempt the entire project the night before it is to be completed.

Limit home tutoring to special circumstances, such as when the teacher requests parental assistance after a child's prolonged absence.

Request special help for children with learning problems.

Support the school staff by showing respect for both the school system and the teacher, at least in the child's presence.

The teacher sets the emotional tone of the classroom. Those who are able to establish a positive social climate are usually concerned about the mental health and social dynamics of children. Feeling a responsibility for personality development in their pupils, they are alert and sensitive to a child's anxieties, peer-group relationships, self-concepts, and general attitudes toward school. Learner-centered behaviors, such as supportive statements that reassure or commend children, accepting and clarifying statements that help them refine ideas and feelings to provide a sense of being understood, and constructive assistance that aids them with their own problem solving, contribute to the expansion and development of a positive self-concept.

### Role of the Parents

Parents share responsibility within the schools for helping children achieve their maximum potential. There are numerous ways in which parents can supplement the school program. (See Family Home Care box.) Cultivating responsibility is the goal of parental assistance. Being responsible for schoolwork helps children learn to keep promises, meet deadlines, and succeed at their jobs as adults. Responsible children may occasionally ask for help (e.g., with a spelling list), but usually they like to think through their work by themselves. Excessive pressure or lack of encouragement from parents may inhibit the development of these desirable traits.

## Limit-Setting and Discipline

Numerous factors influence the amount and manner of discipline and limit-setting imposed on school-age children: the psychosocial maturity of the parents, the childhood child-rearing experiences of the parents, the temperament of the children, the context of the children's misconduct, and the response of the children to rewards and punishments. Discipline serves many purposes: (1) to help the child interrupt or inhibit a forbidden action; (2) to point out a more acceptable form of behavior so that the child knows what is right in a future situation; (3) to provide some reason, understandable to the child, that explains why one action is inappropriate and another action is more desirable; and (4) to stimulate the child's ability to empathize with the victim of a misdeed.

As children are increasingly able to see a situation from the point of view of another, they are able to understand the effects of their reactions on others and themselves. Disciplinary techniques should help children control their own behavior.

To be effective, discipline should take place in an environment characterized by positive, supportive parent-child relationships and should involve strategies that teach and stengthen desired behaviors and eliminate undesired or ineffective behaviors (American Academy of Pediatrics, 1998b). Parenting practices that include punitive interactions and corporal punishment are of limited value and are associated with increasingly disruptive behavior in children. In particular, physically aggressive parenting practices that involve spanking are linked to aggression in young children and to substance abuse and increased risk of crime and violence in older children (American Academy of Pediatrics, 1998b; Stormshak and others, 2000). Reasoning, on the other hand, is an effective technique for schoolage children.

With advancing cognitive skills they are able to benefit from more complex disciplinary strategies. For example, withholding privileges, requiring recompense, imposing penalties, and contracting can be used with great success. Problem solving is the best approach to limit-setting, and children themselves can be included in the process of determining appropriate disciplinary measures.

### Dishonest Behavior

During middle childhood, children may engage in what is considered to be antisocial behavior. Lying, stealing, and cheating may become manifest in previously well-behaved children. It is especially disturbing to parents, who may have difficulty coping with this behavior.

*Lying* can occur for a number of reasons. Preschool children often have difficulty distinguishing between fact and fantasy. They do not have the cognitive capacity to deliberately mislead. Sometimes they misperceive or fail to remember an event. By the time they reach school age, they still tell stories but can distinguish between what is real and what is make-believe. If not, they need to be taught to distinguish between fantasy and reality. Often children will exaggerate a story or situation as a means to impress their family or friends.

Young children will lie to escape punishment or get out of some difficulty, even when the evidence of their misbehavior is before their eyes. Lying is more common in families in which punishment is severe. Honesty and veracity modeled by the parents is repeated in the children. If parents lie, the children will emulate their behavior. Older children may lie to meet expectations set by others to which they have been unable to measure up. They may also lie because of low self-esteem or as a means of getting ahead or acquiring something with little effort. However, most children are very concerned with the wrongfulness of lying and cheating—especially in their friends. They are quick to tell on others when they detect cheating.

Parents need to be reassured that all children lie sometimes and that they often have difficulty separating fantasy from reality. Parents should be helped to understand the importance of their own behavior as role models and of being truthful in their relationships with children. The issue can be discussed with the children directly to impress on them how much of their own security and respect is lost when they are not believed.

*Cheating* is most common in young children, ages 5 to 6. They find it difficult to lose at a game or contest, and they cheat to win. They have not yet acquired the full realization of the wrongfulness of this behavior and do it almost automatically. It usually disappears as they mature. However, when children observe parental behaviors such as boasting about cheating on income taxes, they assume this to be appropriate behavior. Parents need to be aware of the types of behaviors they model for their children. When they set examples of honesty, children are more likely to conform to these standards.

As with other ethically related behavior, *stealing* is not an unexpected event in the younger child. Between ages 5 and 8 years, children's sense of property rights is limited, and they tend to take something simply because they are attracted to it, or they take money for what it will buy. They are equally likely to give away something valuable that belongs to them. When young children are caught and punished, they are penitent—they "didn't mean to," and promise "never to do it again," but it is quite likely that they will repeat the performance the following day. Often they not only steal, but will lie about it as well or attempt to justify the act with excuses. It is seldom helpful to trap children into admission by asking directly if they did the offensive thing. Children do not take on such responsibility until nearer the end of middle childhood.

There are several reasons why children steal: lack of a sense of property rights, an attempt to acquire the means with which to bribe favors from other children, a strong desire to own the coveted item, or as a means for revenge in order to "get back at someone" (usually a parent) for what they consider to be unfair treatment. Older children may steal to supplement an inadequate income from other sources. Sometimes stealing is an indication that something is seriously wrong or lacking in the child's life. Children may steal to make up for love or another satisfaction that they feel is lacking.

In some settings where living arrangements are crowded and children have little privacy and much of the family property is communal, children may fail to develop a sense of property rights. Sometimes parents unintentionally confuse children with seemingly conflicting values. In an attempt to teach unselfishness, they may force children to share belongings with others, with the result that the children fail to develop a true sense of property rights.

If children are told not to take money from their mother's purse or their father's pocket but observe the parents doing the same thing, they receive conflicting messages. Parents may go through a child's pockets or other private areas at night and even discard, without explanation, items of which they do not approve. Children should have a place that is private to them alone and that is respected by other family members. If children's personal rights are respected, they are more likely to respect the rights of others.

It is difficult for many parents to cope with stealing by their children. In most situations it is best not to attempt to find a hidden or deep meaning to the stealing. An admonition, together with an appropriate and reasonable punishment, such as having the older child pay back the money or return the stolen items, will ordinarily take care of most cases. Most children can be taught to respect the property rights of others with little difficulty despite the temptations and opportunities presented to them. Some children simply need more time to learn the importance of the culture's rules regarding private property.

## Coping with Stress

Children today experience more stress than children in previous generations. This stress comes from a variety of sources. Some are discussed elsewhere in this book under specific types of stresses, especially those in which nurses assume a major role, such as hospitalization, illness, abuse, crippling injuries, and death or the threat of death.

In the normal course of growing up, children are pressured by their peers to identify with their friends; to eat, dress, and look like their friends; to talk about the same things that their friends talk about; to engage in the same activities as their friends; and yet to compete with them. They are pressured by parents to excel in school, in athletics, and socially at ever-younger ages. Children in the middle school years are often overprogrammed with activities such as ballet lessons, music lessons, athletics, and other activities until the cumulative effect is overwhelming.

Although children receive better treatment than in earlier times when beatings and child labor were common, their physical and emotional well-being is threatened by different stresses, especially *violence.* Children are stressed by conflict within the home. The high divorce rate and the number of single-parent families results in altered relationships and increasing responsibilities for children.

In recent years, increasing domestic violence has become a significant problem in many American homes. Such violence takes a toll on children who observe or experience it (Kerker and others, 2000; McCloskey and Walker, 2000). A study of school-age children and their mothers who lived in homeless shelters or facilities for battered women indicated that 54% of these children were exposed to some form of violence in their homes (McCloskey and Walker, 2000). Another study of 2245 public school students in grades 3 through 8 indicated that 11% to 18% of these children were beaten up at home, 38% to 45% were slapped, hit, or punched at home, and 19% to 29% were threatened (Singer and others, 1999). A small group of the boys (17%) in this study reported that they had experienced a gun being pointed directly at them in their home, at school, or in their neighborhood (Singer and others, 1999).

Exposure to violence in the family, school, or community affects children's ability to concentrate and function. Children exposed to violence often display symptoms associated with posttraumatic stress disorder such as nightmares, flashbacks, a fatalistic orientation to the future, depression, and anxiety (Kerker and others, 2000; Singer and others, 1999).

The school environment itself is stressful for many children. The shooting tragedy at a middle school in Jonesboro, Arkansas in 1998 indicates the potential for violence in the school environment (Skaug, 1999). A randomly selected sample of 2227 sixth through eighth grade students attending 53 middle schools also indicated that 14.1% of these children had carried a weapon such as a knife or club to school; 3% of the students had carried a gun (DuRant and others, 1999).

The school environment may also pose a threat to the middle schooler's self-image. Competing with classmates for grades and teacher recognition, failing an examination, being teased or made fun of in school, or being labeled as "stupid" or "learning disabled" all result in emotional distress. Teachers or parents may not always recognize or appreciate the worries or sources of stress for school-age children. A re-

cent study of 7- to 12-year-old children revealed that they were very worried about being asked to take drugs, being caught stealing, and losing a game, while their parents were either unaware or did not believe that these were problems for their children (Neff and Dale, 1996).

Children also become very distressed when teachers raise their voices, yell or scream, or use fear or physical punishment in the classroom (see Evidence-Based Practice box). Students exposed to such behavior may demonstrate symptoms of stress, expressions of excessive worry about school, negative self-perceptions, and verbalizations of fear of physical harm from the teacher. Although parents and nurses should be cautious in attempts to interpret such behaviors (they are in many ways similar to school phobia; see Chapter 18), a high degree of suspicion might be justified if the symptoms are not explained by other factors or if they represent a marked change from previous patterns.

Children are also encouraged to feel, think, and behave at a level of maturity far beyond what could reasonably be expected of persons their age (Elkind, 1981). They are expected to take on many adult-type responsibilities, to make decisions they are not really able to make, and to achieve more. They have little time for being *children* and enjoying the spontaneous activities of childhood.

When asked to describe sources of stress and worry, school-age children have identified such worries as being in a war, being lost and not able to see, being in a fire, and having a parent die (Neff and Dale, 1996). Stickler (1996) noted that fourth through sixth grade boys worried about issues concerning failure and criticism, while girls this age reported more danger-related worries. A study of school-age children ages 8 through 12 years indicated the most common fears related to categories of safety, animals, and natural phenomena (Carroll and Ryan-Wenger, 1999). Other potential sources of stress are listed in Box 17-1.

Children respond to stress by using coping mechanisms that include activities such as crying, screaming, physical aggression, avoidance behaviors, delaying tactics, daydreaming, and problem-solving activities such as seeking support from a parent, teacher, or friends (Ryan-Wenger, 1996). Variables that contribute to children's ability to cope with stress include socioeconomic status, family relationships, social support, gender, and previous life experiences.

**NURSING ALERT**   The nurse who observes the following signs of stress in a child should explore the situation further:

Stomach pains or headache
Sleep problems
Bed-wetting
Changes in eating habits
Aggressive or stubborn behavior
Reluctance to participate
Regression to earlier behaviors (e.g., thumb sucking)

To help children cope with the stresses in their lives, the parent, teacher, or health care worker must recognize signs that indicate a child is undergoing stress (see Box 17-1) and identify the source promptly. Children need to be taught

## Box 17-1
## Potential Sources of Stress in Middle Childhood*

### SOURCES OF STRESS FOR THE SIX-YEAR-OLD

**Expectations**—Parents, teachers, and other adults begin to demand more

**School**—First grade introduces the child to the more formal, academic setting; it may be the child's first experience away from home all day

**Activity level**—May find it difficult to sit still for long periods of time; may have frequent accidents, such as spilling milk

**Competition**—The child wants to be "first" or best

**Shyness**—May initially be shy in a new situation but usually recovers quickly

**Aggression**—May become hostile or aggressive; temper tantrums peak

**Sensitivity**—Begins to read body language or facial expressions and becomes upset when disapproval is sensed

**Teasing**—Engages in teasing but becomes upset when on the receiving end

**Decisions**—Has difficulty coping with increasing independence

**Jealousy**—Sibling rivalry is common

**Fears**—Usually center around newly found independence and might include fear of getting lost or fear of making an embarrassing social blunder

### SOURCES OF STRESS FOR THE SEVEN-YEAR-OLD

**Moodiness**—Is often moody, unhappy, or pensive

**Approval**—Continues to need praise and approval from peer group and parents

**Modesty**—Demands privacy when in the bathroom or dressing

**Organization**—Is comfortable with rules, regulations, routines, and order; becomes upset when they are disrupted

**Interruptions**—Hates to be disturbed when intensely involved in an activity

**Idols**—Has a desire to be more like an admired idol

**Friendship**—Becomes more selective about playmates

### SOURCES OF STRESS FOR THE EIGHT-YEAR-OLD

**Self-criticism**—Is very critical of personal ability and performance

**Parental authority**—Is beginning to resent parental authority

**Loneliness**—Likes frequent interaction with friends; may hate to miss school

**Praise**—Continues to seek approval but can identify when praise is not genuine

**Independence**—Many begin to stay alone for brief periods of time while parents run errands; with resulting feelings of uneasiness

### SOURCES OF STRESS FOR THE NINE-YEAR-OLD

**Rebelliousness**—Occasionally tests independence by rebelling

**Opposite sex**—Engages in sex-segregated play; expresses an aversion to the opposite sex

**Fair play**—Has a keen sense of what is fair and is vehement in demanding personal rights when a situation is perceived as unfair

**Interruptions**—Continues to dislike interruptions but will usually resume an activity after an interruption

**Propriety**—Has a sense of propriety and will often be upset if siblings or parents offend the child's notion of decorum or dignity

### SOURCES OF STRESS FOR THE TEN- TO TWELVE-YEAR-OLD

**Sexual maturation**—Girls, in particular, may become self-conscious regarding obvious signs of development

**Social issues**—A new level of awareness can generate concern regarding pressing societal problems

**Size**—Both boys and girls may be upset by the fact that the girls are taller; the extremely small or extremely large child may be concerned about his or her size

**Shyness**—If the child already has a problem in this area, it is likely to become more pronounced at this stage

**Opposite sex**—May become interested, yet shy, around members of the opposite sex

**Confusion**—Too much freedom can cause the child to flounder

**Health**—It is not uncommon for a child to become a hypochondriac during this period of development

**Money**—Child is anxious to earn and handle money but often uses poor judgment

**Competition**—Continues to be highly competitive and looks to peer group for prestige

**Burnout**—Child may become vigorously involved in so many activities that he or she finally becomes exhausted

**Self-concept**—May engage in teasing, scapegoating, or vicious attacks to temporarily boost his or her self-image; guilt often ensues; may be self-conscious about attempting a new skill

**Parents**—Often becomes highly critical or intolerant of parents

**Idols**—Continues hero worshipping

**Fair play**—Continues to have a highly developed sense of fair play

**Drugs and sex**—May be tempted to experiment with drugs or sex because "everyone" is doing it

**Peer pressure**—Becomes a powerful motivating force

**Self-criticism**—Child may be highly critical of personal performance

From Kuczen B: *Childhood stress: don't let your child be a victim*, New York, 1982, Delacorte Press.
*Violence is a universal stress at all ages (see text).

how to recognize signs of stress in themselves, such as a pounding heart, rapid breathing, or "butterflies" in the stomach. Once they are able to recognize that they are stressed, they can employ techniques for managing their stress. Probably the most useful technique is to help them plan a means for dealing with any stress through problem solving.

Children can learn relaxation techniques such as deep-breathing exercises, progressive relaxation of muscle groups, and positive imagery. Encouraging them to "blow off steam" through physical activity reduces tension and anxiety. They need to identify the problem. Those involving situations or actions of others are easy to identify. Feelings within themselves are sometimes more difficult. Alternative actions must be explored. Children should list all possibilities, including those that they know will not work. They

need to examine what might happen as a consequence of each alternative. The final step is to select what they perceive to be the best option. It is sometimes helpful to have children model their behavior after someone they know who has successfully coped with a similar problem. When children work through this process a few times, they are able to apply problem solving automatically.

### Fears

Several anxiety symptoms, including fear of the dark, excessive worry about past behavior, self-consciousness, social withdrawal, and an excessive need for reassurance, are considered normal developmental events for children. School-children are less fearful of body safety than they were as preschoolers, although they still fear being hurt, kidnapped, or having to undergo surgery. They also fear death

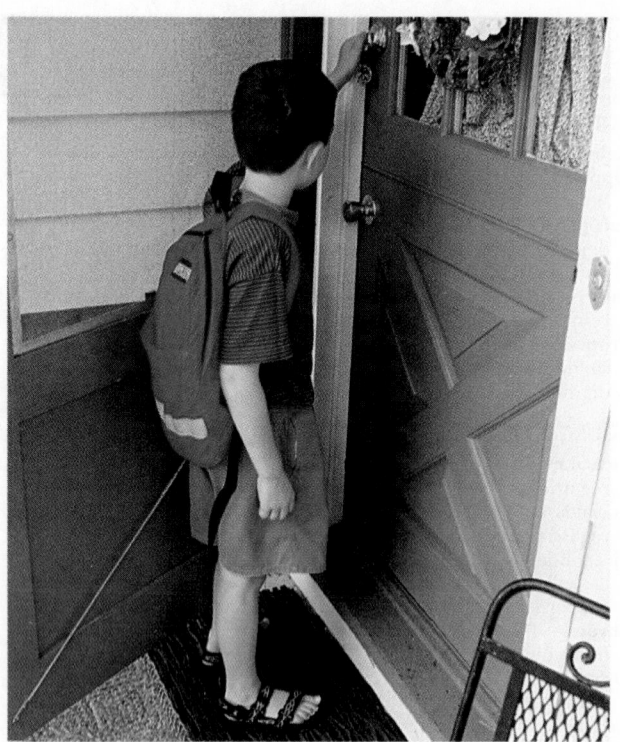

**Fig. 17-12**  A child unlocks the door to let himself into his home after school.

and are fascinated by all aspects of death and dying. There is less fear of noises, darkness, storms, and dogs. Most new fears that trouble school-age children are related to school and family (e.g., fear of failing, fear of teachers and bullies, or fear of something bad happening to their parents).

Parents and other persons involved with children should discuss children's fears with them individually or through group activities. Their viewpoints must be respected, and their need to communicate their concerns should be recognized. Sometimes school-age children are inclined to hide their fears to avoid being ridiculed or labeled as a "baby" or "chicken." Hiding fears does not end them, and children who are afraid to communicate their fears may develop displaced fears, or phobias. Children need to know that their concerns are heard and understood. Parents who convey this to their children without becoming overprotective help their children to feel less lonely and less frightened.

### Latchkey Children

The term *latchkey children* is used to describe children in elementary school who are left to care for themselves before or after school without supervision of an adult (Fig. 17-12). The increasing numbers of single-parent families and working mothers, together with a lack of available child care, have created a stress-provoking situation for many school-age children. Some latchkey children may have a chronic illness as well.

Inadequate adult supervision after school leaves children at greater risk for injury and delinquent behavior. Latchkey children feel more lonely, isolated, and fearful than chil-

dren who have someone to care for them. To cope with their fears and anxieties while alone, these children may devise strategies such as hiding (in a bathroom, closet, shower, or under a bed), playing the television at loud volume as a distraction to drown out noises, and using pets as a comfort.

Many communities and persons concerned about their welfare are trying to help children and their parents deal with this potentially serious problem. School-age care programs have been implemented by some communities and employers. Some guidelines appropriate for presentation to parents and/or children to help alleviate their stress and increase the children's safety are listed in the Family Home Care box. Other types of programs include those designed to teach self-help skills to children, "hotlines" that provide telephone check-in and reassurance programs for children, and programs that link latchkey children with reassuring older persons in their community.

Nurses should be aware of services in their communities designed to meet the needs of latchkey children and include this information in anticipatory guidance of school-age children and their families. It is vital that children have adequate supervision and companionship.

## PROMOTING OPTIMUM HEALTH DURING THE SCHOOL YEARS

### Health Behaviors

During the middle childhood years, children acquire increased cognitive skills that allow them to make decisions about health behaviors they will pursue and select. By the end of middle childhood, children should be able to assume personal responsibility for self-care in the areas of hygiene, nutrition, exercise, recreation, sleep, and safety.

Little is known about how school-age children acquire positive health behaviors. However, both boys and girls view themselves as healthy and can manage their own care in the areas of seat belt use, exercise, emergency situations, and dental health.

Health education is a primary component of comprehensive health care, and health education programs should be designed to promote desired health behavior through guided learning and modeling. An optimum program helps children learn about their bodies and how their behavior affects their health.

Health promotion projects teach middle school children that social decision making to promote health is important. Children who attain skills in self-control, social awareness, and problem solving through classroom discussions and practice may engage in fewer risk-taking behaviors.

Children can also be taught to take a more active role in relationships with health care providers. If asked what they would like to ask the health practitioner, most children can formulate several questions related to the reason for their visit. Children can also be taught how to ask these questions so they can learn about their health during well child visits to the pediatrician, nurse practitioner, or school nurse.

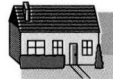

## FAMILY HOME CARE
### Latchkey Children

### SAFETY

Teach child not to display keys and to always lock doors.

Tell child not to enter the house after school if the door is ajar, a window is open, or anything appears unusual.

Talk through the after-school routine with the child.

Consult with public safety officials about burglar-proofing and fireproofing the home.

Teach child first-aid procedures.

Teach safety rules to the child who is expected to cook (microwave ovens are safest).

Emphasize fire safety rules and conduct practice fire drills.

Teach and reinforce traffic and bicycle safety.

Teach child weather-related safety (e.g., stay inside but do not take a bath during an electrical storm; go to and stay in a storm cellar during a tornado warning).

Teach and reinforce water safety practices (e.g., do not go swimming alone; caution about safe bathing methods and keeping the toilet lid down when infants or toddlers are in their care).

Keep firearms securely locked away and teach child that they are for adult use only.

Teach child not to open the door to anyone.

### TELEPHONE USE

Teach the child his/her home telephone number, address, and parents' names.

Teach child to tell callers that parents are "busy"; do not tell a caller that parents are not at home.

Teach child not to tell casual callers the home address. Tell the caller that the parent cannot come to the phone right now and will call back later.

Keep a list of emergency numbers by the telephone. Make certain that child knows how to report emergencies.

Have a list of telephone numbers of friends or neighbors who are available for help with emergencies.

Ask public safety officials to offer classes about when and how to call them.

If a "telephone hotline" for latchkey children exists, teach child how to use it.

### AFTER-SCHOOL ACTIVITIES

Arrange for child to spend some afternoons with friends.

Provide structured activities for the child.

Have the child attend a public library–sponsored activity rather than watch television at home.

Discuss with child things to do after school.

Emphasize positive aspects of independence and resourcefulness but do not demand too much from child.

Help child feel successful in self-care.

Counsel parents to consider the potential problems of an older child assuming care of younger ones before the child is developmentally ready.

### LONELINESS

Help child talk about experiences and feelings about being alone after school.

Consider a pet to help provide company for the child.

Be punctual in arriving home. A child's anxiety level accelerates when parents are not home when expected.

Call child if there is a delay in arriving home.

Leave a tape-recorded message for the child to play on arrival home from school.

Form a group of parents with flex-time so that children can be cared for by one of the group after school.

Modified from McClellan MA: On their own: latchkey children, *Pediatr Nurs* 10:198-202, 1983.

## Nutrition

Although calorie needs are diminished in relation to body size during middle childhood, resources are being laid down for the increased growth needs of the adolescent period. It is important to impress on children and their parents the value of a balanced diet to promote growth (Box 17-2). When children enter school, they develop an eating style that is increasingly independent of parental influence and scrutiny. Parents do not know what their children eat when they are away from home. A parent may pack a lunch to be eaten at school but be unaware of how much is eaten, traded, sold, or thrown away.

Mealtime continues to be a central issue in many families. Although it should be a pleasant part of a child's day, parents' concern and emphasis on manners often make it a battleground. Likes and dislikes established at an early age continue in middle childhood although the propensity for single food preferences begins to end and children acquire a taste for an increasing variety of foods. Because children usually eat as the family does, the quality of their diet depends to a large extent on their family's pattern of eating. Other interests and participation in outside activities often compete with mealtime.

### Outside Influences

Influenced by the mass media and the temptation of an immense variety of "junk food," it is all too easy for children to fill up on empty calories—foods that do not promote growth, such as sugars, starches, and excess fats. They have more freedom to move without parental supervision and often have small amounts of money to spend on candy, soft drinks, and other easily accessible treats. Midafternoon snacks are common, and it is wise to encourage fruit, nuts, and other wholesome finger foods to meet this need. Nutrition is a joint responsibility of both the child and the family.

The popularity of fast-food restaurants has aroused the interest of nutritionists and other health care professionals concerned with children's nutrition. The restaurants are fast, relatively inexpensive, and appealing to children, and their convenience is attractive to busy parents as an alternative to eating at home. Because the nutritional content of fast foods is usually known, it is easier for nutrition-conscious parents to help children select appropriate items from the available menu. Nurses can support consumer groups and parents in advocating that these restaurants offer items higher in nutritional value (such as skimmed milk,

## School-Based Interventions to Promote Nutrition Education

Have young children collect pictures of healthy foods and make a poster for display in the school cafeteria.

Make healthy foods (fruits, vegetables, whole grains, low-fat snacks) available in school vending machines and at school sporting events.

Discourage the use of high-fat foods (candy bars) as part of school fund-raising projects.

Avoid the use of food as rewards for behavior; use verbal praise and token gifts to reinforce healthy eating and physical activity.

Have teachers and school personnel model healthy eating habits.

Ask children to select foods from a fast-food restaurant menu and to identify those foods high in fat, cholesterol, and sodium.

Ask each child to keep a diary of foods eaten in 1 day; using the Food Guide Pyramid, evaluate these foods.

Incorporate nutrition education into other classes (such as using a computer to analyze the nutritional content of foods).

Have students keep a diary to identify cues for their eating behavior (e.g., hunger, stress, other people, social situations).

Teach students how to read and discuss the nutrition labels on foods.

Ask students to examine television commercials, magazine advertisements, and billboards to identify social influences on eating and physical activities.

Use role-playing to help students learn to cope with social and peer pressures to eat specific foods.

Have students identify environmental barriers to healthy eating.

Have students prepare nutritious foods, plan menus, and develop a recipe book of healthy foods.

Involve parents in nutrition education through homework assignments or by inviting parents to attend student-led nutrition fairs.

Modified from Center for Communicable Diseases: Guidelines for school programs to promote lifelong healthy eating, *J Sch Health* 67:9-26, 1996.

## Sample Menu for School-Age Children Based on Food Guide Pyramid*

| | |
|---|---|
| **Breakfast** | 2 four-inch waffles |
| | 2 tbsp syrup |
| | ½ cup orange juice |
| **Lunch** | 1 four-ounce cheeseburger and bun |
| | ½ cup raw carrot sticks |
| | ¾ cup apple juice |
| **Snack** | 1 cup frozen yogurt *or* |
| | 1 cup unsweetened cereal with low-fat milk |
| **Dinner** | 1 cup spaghetti with tomato sauce |
| | 1 piece garlic bread |
| | Green salad with romaine lettuce and dressing |
| | ½ cup broccoli |
| | 1 banana |
| | 1 cup low-fat milk |
| **Snack** | 2 cups plain popcorn |

**TOTAL SERVINGS**

| | |
|---|---|
| **Bread, cereal, rice, pasta** | 6-7 |
| **Vegetable** | 3 |
| **Fruit** | 3 |
| **Milk, yogurt, cheese** | 3 |
| **Meat, poultry, fish, dried beans, nuts** | 2 |

*Use fats, oils, and sweets sparingly. Increase fluids with servings of water. Serving sizes are minimums for nutritional adequacy. Many children eat more.

broiled meats, and fresh fruits and vegetables) and listing ingredients on the menu as required for packaged foods.

Childhood obesity is an increasingly prevalent health problem in school-age children. It is estimated that approximately 11% of American children are overweight (ADA, 1999). The easy availability of high-calorie foods, the tendency toward more sedentary activities (such as watching television and playing or working at a computer), and the trend away from walking or cycling and toward transportation by automobile and bus have reduced caloric expenditure. The consumption of a high-fat diet also contributes to obesity. The problem of childhood obesity is discussed further in Chapter 21. Given the threat of obesity and a diet-conscious society, many school-age children start to diet in an effort to prevent obesity or lose weight or to conform to peer behaviors and pressures. Children need education about food selection and the importance of body-building nutrients as opposed to empty caloric intake.

## School Programs

Working parents assume their children are sufficiently mature and frequently leave the responsibility of meal prepa-

ration to them. Although most older school-age children are capable of preparing simple fare, all too often breakfast and/or lunch may be inadequate, makeshift, or nonexistent. In recognition of this problem, the federal government has established the National School Lunch Program (NSLP) and the School Breakfast Program (SBP) in many areas. These meals must meet specified nutritional requirements and furnish one third of the daily recommended dietary allowance for children in the United States. Most schools subscribe to the programs, and, although it is difficult to measure directly, it is believed that these school meal programs positively influence the behavior and learning capacity of children. However, the average school lunch may also exceed the recommended dietary guidelines for saturated and total fat. In addition, children who purchase school lunches often select only the items they want.

Surveys of the eating habits of American children indicate that they are not eating recommended amounts of fruits, vegetables, grains and dairy foods. Food choices in general do not meet recommended intakes outlined in the Food Guide Pyramid (ADA, 1999).

**Nutrition Education.** Nutrition education should be integrated throughout the school years into classroom learning. In school, daily food choices, serving sizes, and the elements of a wholesome diet can be taught using the U.S. Department of Agriculture Food Guide Pyramid (Box 17-3). (See Nutrition, Chapter 13.) The American Dietetic Association recently updated their dietary guidelines for healthy

## Critical Thinking Exercise

### Physical Growth in the School-Age Child

Janie, an 8-year-old girl, has just received her annual school physical examination. Janie weighs 30 kg (66 pounds) and is 127 cm (50 inches) tall. Janie has gained 4.5 kg (10 pounds) since last year. Which of the following characteristics of physical growth in the school-age child should guide the nurse's health teaching concerning Janie's eating habits and nutritional status?

FIRST, THINK ABOUT IT . . .

- What information are you using?
- What are you taking for granted?

1. Janie's weight and height are at the 50th percentile for her age, and she should be advised to continue with her usual eating habits.
2. Because school-age children have a high metabolism, they need extra calories. Janie should be encouraged to eat as much as she wants.
3. The school-age child gains an average of 2.5 kg (5½ pounds) each year. Janie's weight gain is excessive; the nurse should assess Janie's eating habits in greater depth and determine the specific types of foods she is consuming.
4. School-age children often experience large weight gains in a single year. Janie's pattern of weight gain will probably slow down and level off when she approaches puberty.

*The best response is three. School-age children do not grow as quickly as they did in the preschool-age years. Growth is more even and steady, and the average weight gain per year is 5½ pounds. The 50th percentile for weight and height for an 8-year-old girl is 25.3 kg (55¾ pounds) and 127 cm (50 inches), respectively. In the school-age years, calorie needs are diminished in relation to body size, and children do not need as many feedings or snacks. Fast foods, which are high in sugar and fat, and snack foods with empty calories are tempting at this age. Childhood obesity is increasing, and the physical and mental effects should not be taken for granted. Many school-age children are sedentary and spend more time watching television than they do in active play or physical exercise.*

children 2 to 11 years of age (ADA, 1999). Current guidelines (Derelian, 1996) are:

1. Balance food eaten with physical activity to maintain an appropriate weight
2. Choose a diet with plenty of grain products, vegetables, and fruits
3. Choose a diet low in fat, saturated fat, and cholesterol
4. Eat a variety of foods
5. Choose a diet moderate in salt and sodium
6. Choose a diet moderate in sugars

The school nurse should take an active role in nutrition education and work with teachers to implement nutrition instruction that is relevant and interesting to children (see Box 17-2). (See Critical Thinking Exercise box.) The U.S. Department of Agriculture also maintains a web site called "Team Nutrition" that provides nutrition education infor-

mation and resources for schools, students, parents, and communities.*

## Sleep and Rest

The amount of sleep and rest required during middle childhood is highly individualized. There is no specific amount needed by a child at any given age. The amount depends on the child's age, activity level, and other factors such as health status. The growth rate has slowed; therefore, less energy is expended in growth than was expended during the preceding periods.

During the school years children usually do not require a nap, but they sleep approximately 9½ hours (Blum, Ditmar, and Charney, 1997). Fewer bedtime problems occur during these years, but occasional difficulties are still associated with the necessary bedtime ritual. Usually there is little problem for children 6 and 7 years old, and the task of going to bed can be facilitated by encouraging quiet activity before bedtime, such as coloring and reading.

Although most children in middle childhood must be reminded to go to bed, 8- to 9-year-old children and 11-year-old children are particularly resistant. Often children are unaware that they are tired; if they are allowed to remain up later than usual, they are fatigued the following day. Sometimes bedtime resistance can be resolved by allowing a later bedtime in deference to their advancing age. Twelve-year-old children usually offer no difficulty in relation to bedtime. Some even retire early in order to enjoy slow preparations for bed, to read, or to listen to music. A firm approach to bedtime is usually the most successful. Parents can help children by giving them a little advance warning, but children should realize that when **the final bedtime is announced, the parents mean it.**

### Sleep Problems

During middle childhood, nighttime sleep is usually continuous, and the child has developed a repertoire of tactics (such as reading or playing quietly without involving the parents) to deal with occasional difficulties in falling asleep. If a child has a sleep problem, a thorough assessment may be needed to plan appropriate interventions. (See Guidelines box on p. 157.)

The cause of **bedtime resistance** is not always clear. For some children it is related to normal fears of their age, such as fear of the dark, strange noises, intruders, or other imagined phenomena. Children who are subject to frightening dreams are hesitant to retire, and their sleep is more apt to be disturbed following emotional stimulation before bedtime. Sometimes children are loath to give up an exciting or interesting activity in which they are involved, or they are reluctant to leave the protective social circle of the family. Another factor associated with reluctance to go to bed is related to status. For example, older children are given the privilege of a later bedtime than younger children. Promotion to a later bedtime is highly prestigious, and age-mates

*USDA, Food and Nutrition Service, 3101 Park Center Drive, Room 1010, Alexandria, VA 22302; www.usda.gov/fcs/team.htm.

compare their bedtimes. This may explain why parental decisions are often strongly contested by children who believe that playmates enjoy a more privileged position. In some situations going to bed is used as a method of control. When going to bed early is imposed as a punishment or when staying up late is a reward, children may view bedtime as punitive or status degrading.

Some children resort to multiple "curtain calls," such as wanting a drink of water, one more story, needing to go to the bathroom, or wanting to watch television. Some children persist in coming out of their rooms repeatedly after being put back to bed. Some voice fears, such as someone being outside their window. Parents may have difficulty determining whether the fear is legitimate or whether the behavior is a bid for attention. Consistent reassurance and limit-setting usually resolve the problem. Children feel tense and insecure when limits are applied inconsistently, such as granting permission one night and punishing the next for the same behavior.

The night terrors of preschool children may be replaced by sleepwalking and sleep talking. Like night terrors, *sleepwalking* is associated with the transition from stage 4 to stage 1 of non-REM sleep. When children arouse from stage 4 sleep, it is often difficult for them to reach a fully alert, wakeful state rapidly. Consequently, the transitional period from the deep sleep of stage 4 to the next sleep cycle is marked by limited awareness and confusion (Ferber and Kryger, 1995).

Sleepwalking occurs in the first 3 to 4 hours of sleep. Children often have no memory of sleepwalking in the morning. The episodes begin when the child sits up abruptly and walks. During sleepwalking, movements are clumsy and repetitive; finger and hand movements are often observed. Most commonly, children move about restlessly, then lie down and return to sleep. However, they may get out of bed and engage in nonpurposeful walking. They rarely perform purposeful acts during sleepwalking. Any attempts to communicate with a child elicit only mumbled and slurred responses. *Sleep talking,* like sleepwalking, is not purposeful, and speech is usually incomprehensible and monosyllabic.

The best approach is to leave sleepwalking children alone unless they are in danger or may endanger others. However, clumsiness and stereotyped movements can make sleepwalking very dangerous. If the environment is not safe, a child can get hurt. If children must be wakened, it is best to call them by name slowly and softly, orient them to where they are, explain that they were walking in their sleep, and assure them that it will not happen when they are more relaxed. Preventive measures include avoiding overfatigue, getting adequate rest, employing relaxation techniques, and relieving any stress the children may be experiencing.

Sleepwalking is usually self-limiting and requires no treatment. Persistent sleepwalking occurs in some older children and adolescents who are well behaved and tend to repress strong emotions, such as anger. They may benefit from learning to express their feelings and from doing self-relaxation before bedtime.

*Nightmares* are a part of the normal developmental process although they are less common in children ages 6 to 12 than in younger children. However, nightmares at this more tranquil age may indicate a specific underlying conflict that strongly influences the child's behavior and thought. Resolving worries will often reduce nightmares. If nightmares become chronic, professional counseling should be considered (Ferber and Kryger, 1995).

A traumatic event will often produce *posttraumatic nightmares,* which are anxiety provoking and literal in their depiction of the trauma. As time goes on, the dreams of affected children may consist of "modified repetitions" that may add more current material to the recurrent dreams (e.g., involving others who were not a part of the traumatic event). Current external stresses, movies, or stories may also precipitate a nightmare by reactivating old traumas. (For a comparison of nightmares and night terrors, see Table 15-3.)

## Physical Activity

Exercise is essential for muscle development and tone, refinement of balance and coordination, gaining strength and endurance, and stimulating body functions and metabolic processes. Throughout middle childhood, children's increasing capabilities and adaptability permit greater speed and effort in motor activities. Larger, stronger muscles with greater efficiency and skill permit longer and increasingly strenuous play without exhaustion. During this period children acquire the coordination, timing, and concentration that are required to participate in adult-type activities, even though they may lack the strength, stamina, and control of the adolescent and adult. Consequently, a larger amount of physical activity should be expected and encouraged during the school years.

Children should be afforded opportunities that provide satisfying experiences to meet individual likes and dislikes. Children need ample space to run, jump, skip, and climb as well as safe facilities and equipment to use both inside and outside. Appropriate activities that promote coordination and development include running, skipping rope, swimming, roller skating, ice skating, in-line skating, and bicycle riding. Positive reinforcement achieved by experiencing increasingly smooth, rhythmic, and efficient use of the body conditions the child toward regular physical activity. However, it must be kept in mind that although school-age children are large and appear to be strong, they may not be prepared for strenuous competitive athletics.

Most children need little encouragement to engage in physical activity. They have so much energy that they seldom know when to stop. However, children with disabilities or those who hesitate to become involved in active play, such as obese children, require special assessment and help in determining activities that appeal to them, are compatible with their limitations, and meet their developmental needs. Parents also need to limit television viewing to encourage outside activities.

### Physical Fitness

The development of physical fitness is a goal for all children. This goal was easy to accomplish in the past when school-age children spent a considerable amount of time each day playing on playgrounds, walking to school, and participating in games or sports at school or in their communities. With the advent of technology and the information age, many children are less active physically and spend large portions of their day in front of a computer or television. School systems have contributed to the sedentary habits of children by devoting fewer resources to physical education programs, playgrounds, and after-school sports programs. From 1991 through 1997, there has been a 50% drop in required physical activity in school physical education programs; currently, only one state in the United States (Illinois) requires daily physical education from kindergarten through the twelfth grade (Clark and Ferguson, 2000). One objective of *Healthy People 2010* is to increase the proportion of the nation's public and private schools requiring daily physical education for all students by 47% (Clark and Ferguson, 2000). The American Academy of Pediatrics (2000b) has also issued recommendations for schools to include increased physical activity in the curriculum, has suggested ways in which schools can meet this goal, and has encouraged pediatricians to offer their assistance to schools. Nurses can also support efforts to include physical fitness in school programs and encourage children to engage in aerobic physical activities that provide cardiorespiratory benefits, maintain normal weight, and have the potential to contribute to lifelong fitness.

**Sports.**  Much controversy has surrounded the trend toward earlier participation in competitive athletics and the amount and type of competitive sports that are appropriate for children in the elementary grades. The current view is that virtually every child is suited for some type of sport, and authorities do not discourage participation if children are matched to the type of sport appropriate to their abilities and to their physical and emotional constitution. School-age children enjoy competition, and when teachers, parents, and coaches understand children's physical limitations and teach them the proper techniques and safety measures to avoid injury to developing bones and muscles, a safe and appropriate sport can be found for even the most unskilled and nonaggressive child.

During middle childhood, girls have the same basic structure as boys and thus have a similar response to systematic exercise training. At puberty, when boys become larger and have more muscle mass, it is usually recommended that girls compete only against other girls. Before puberty there is no essential difference in strength and size between girls and boys, making these precautions unnecessary.

Enjoyment of sports and fitness in childhood can be encouraged by well-organized extracurricular sports programs based in the community or school (Box 17-4). Preadolescence is a time to teach fundamental motor skills; develop fitness in a practical, safe, and gradual manner; and promote desired attitudes and values. Activities should include practice sessions and unstructured play; the actual game or event should be managed in a manner that stresses mastery of the sport and enhancement of self-image rather than winning or pleasing others. All children should have an opportunity to participate, and special ceremonies should recognize all participants rather than individuals.

In addition to ensuring the interest, suitability, and safety (Box 17-5) of the sport, parents must make certain that coaches (if involved in the sport) are skillful in managing children and do not engage in abusive types of behavior. Coaches, parents, and others involved in children's sports play critical roles in shaping children's self-esteem. Any sport for children should emphasize the pleasure of the activity. It is wise to expose children to a variety of individual sports. The overall emphasis of both team and individual sports should be on playing and learning. Parents who pressure their children to perform beyond their capabilities run the risk of the child being injured, developing a distaste for the activity, and developing a lowered self-image. (See Family Focus box on p. 726.)

The same principles described in the preceding paragraphs apply to children with chronic illnesses, such as diabetes, epilepsy, asthma, or allergies, if the disorder is mild and can be controlled with medication. Children with mental retardation need not be excluded from sports competition if they are matched evenly against other children of equal abilities and provided with skilled supervision and coaching. Some activities may need to be modified to accommodate the skills of these children.

---

**Box 17-4** ■ ■ ■
**Goals of Organized Athletics for Preadolescent Children**

Organized extracurricular athletic programs for preadolescent children should focus on helping children to develop:
Enjoyment of sports and fitness that will be sustained through adulthood
Physical fitness
Basic motor skills
A positive self-image
A balanced perspective on sports in relation to the child's school and community life
A commitment to the values of teamwork, fair play, and sportsmanship

Modified from American Academy of Pediatrics, Committee on Sports Medicine and Committee on School Health: Organized athletics for preadolescent children, *Pediatrics* 84:583-584, 1989.

---

**Box 17-5** ■ ■ ■
**Safeguards for Athletic Programs**

Every athletic program should require the following:
Participation physical examinations at least every 2 years
Warm-up procedures
The availability of a medically trained person who is competent in recognizing significant injuries during practices and games of contact sports
The establishment of policies for first aid, referral of injured participants, treatment, rehabilitation, and certification for return to participation
Suitable and well-maintained sports facilities
Appropriate protective equipment
Strict enforcement of rules concerning safety
A formal surveillance method to ensure that goals are met

Modified from American Academy of Pediatrics, Committee on Sports Medicine and Committee on School Health: Organized athletics for preadolescent children, *Pediatrics* 84:583-584, 1989.

## Acquisition of Skills

School-age children demonstrate increasing capacity in fine muscle facility and complex artistic skills. Handedness is well established by the beginning of the school years, and children make great strides in writing and drawing during this age period. It is a period of energetic and vibrant creative productivity. With the tools of language and reading, children can create poems, stories, and plays. With more advanced fine motor skills, they are able to master an unlimited variety of handicrafts, such as ceramics, needlework, wood carving, and beadwork. They avidly pursue these skills in solitude, with a friend, or in programs offered through organizations such as boys' or girls' clubs or special interest groups that use crafts as a means to occupy, entertain, and educate children.

Music is a favorite form of expression in middle childhood (Fig. 17-13). School-age children are stimulated and invigorated by music. They can sing in harmony, play in-struments in orchestras and bands, and manage music at a more complex level. They can compose original songs, learn lyrics almost effortlessly, and turn any empty moment into an occasion for singing.

School-age children are capable of assuming responsibility for their own needs although their distaste for soap and water and "dress" clothes is legendary. School-age children can and want to assume their share of household tasks, which usually are related to the male and female roles that have been defined by their culture (Fig. 17-14). Many also assume responsibility for tasks outside the home, such as baby-sitting, yard work, or paper routes.

### Television and Video Games

For some time, child development specialists and parents have been concerned about the effect that television has on child development and behavior.

Children spend a significant amount of time each day watching television. When 4063 children ranging in age from 8 to 16 years were interviewed for the third National Health and Nutrition Survey, 26% of these children reported that they watched television 4 or more hours a day; 67% spent at least 2 hours a day watching television (Andersen and others, 1998). A report by Nielsen Media (1998) indicated that children watched television at least 3 hours per day.

There is no doubt that children learn from television, but the values and attitudes depicted on television are not always realistic and may conflict with previous values that children have been taught. School-age children can distinguish fantasy from reality, and some have had sufficient life experience to view television programs with skepticism. However, television rarely depicts the reality of day-to-day situations that confront children.

In addition, there is now adequate evidence to show that exposure to violence on television and in the media is unhealthy for some children (Cantor, 2000; Grossman, 2000).

---

**FAMILY FOCUS**

*Athletic Stress in School-Age Children*

Participating in a competitive sport should be an enjoyable experience for school-age children. However, for some children this activity is associated with considerable stress and anxiety. It is their parents' reaction to their performance that serves as the source of this stress. Children state that they feel awful when they strike out or are unable to catch a "fly ball," or when their team loses a game. These children report that their parents often yell at them and are more upset over a lost game than their coach is. Children notice that their mothers and fathers consider themselves a failure if their child is not a star player.

Parents of children who participate in competitive sports need to praise and support their children regardless of whether games are won or lost. Parents need to avoid the temptation to identify with their child. Parental success and self-worth should not depend on whether their child wins. At the very minimum, parents should monitor their behavior at games and avoid criticizing their child, other players, the officials, or the coaches.

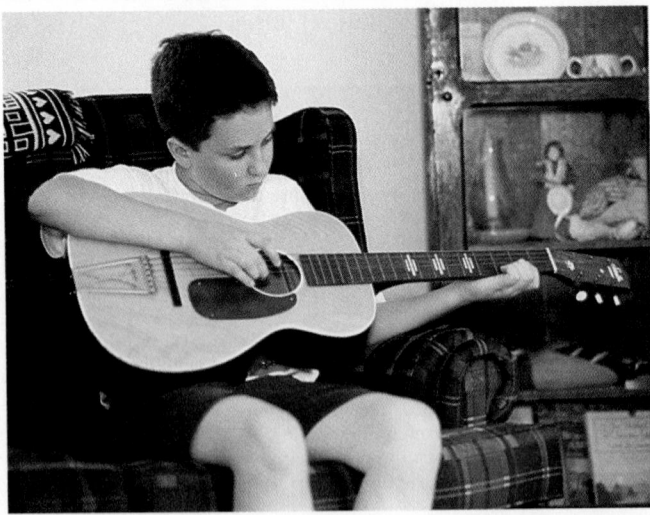

**Fig. 17-13** Music is a favorite form of expression for school-age children.

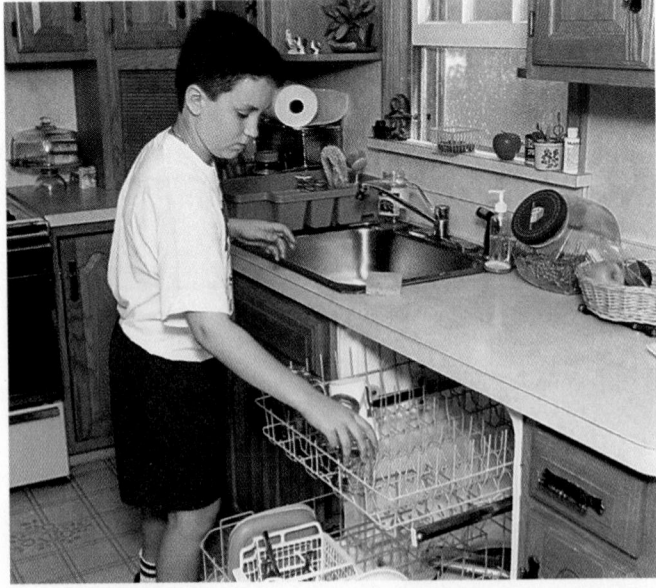

**Fig. 17-14** Children can assume responsibility for a variety of household tasks.

Research has consistently indicated that some children who view violent programming are more likely to become aggressive, to feel desensitized, and to experience fear on viewing (American Academy of Pediatrics, 2001a; Grossman, 2000). A tendency to be less likely to prevent or stop a fight and having repetitive nightmares, obsessive thoughts, and sleep disturbances have also been noted in children who watch violent television (Cantor, 2000). A random survey of parents of children in kindergarten through sixth grade noted that 37% of these children had been frightened or upset by a television program in the past year (Cantor and Nathanson, 1996).

Parents make the ultimate decisions about whether their children watch violent content. Therefore, to reduce exposure to violence and to maximize the beneficial effects of television, parents are advised to monitor program selection, view programs with their children, and discuss program content when the programs are finished (American Academy of Pediatrics, 2001a; Hamilton, 2000). (See Chapter 2 for a more in-depth discussion of children and television.)

Video games have been both criticized and supported in relation to their effect on children and adolescents. Critics maintain that videogames keep children from school work and cause tension, sleeplessness, and violence. Others support the activity as a means for improving eye-hand coordination and as a substitute for the inactivity of passive television viewing. Benefits may also include development of inductive reasoning (drawing generalizations from specific observations), improving spatial perception, and learning to handle multiple variables that interact simultaneously.

Research suggests that video games may affect physical and psychologic functioning. Physical effects may include triggering of epileptic seizures. (See Seizure Disorders, Chapter 37.) However, positive applications of videogames have been noted with language-learning–impaired children (Merzenich and others, 1996).

As with television, parent and teacher education relating to video games should include recommendations to limit playing time, monitor game selection and content, and increase access to games that are educational.

## Dental Health

The first permanent (secondary) teeth erupt at about 6 years of age. Before their appearance they have been developing in the jaw beneath the deciduous (primary) teeth. The roots of the latter are gradually absorbed, so that when a deciduous tooth is shed, only the crown remains. At 6 years of age, all of the primary teeth are present, and those of the secondary dentition are relatively well formed. Eruption of the permanent teeth begins, with the 6-year molar, which erupts posterior to the deciduous molars. The others appear in approximately the same order as eruption of the primary teeth and follow shedding of the deciduous teeth (Fig. 17-15).

The pattern of shedding of primary teeth and eruption of secondary teeth is subject to wide variation among children. To allow the larger permanent teeth to occupy the limited space left by shed primary teeth, a series of complicated changes must take place in the jaws. At this time many of the difficulties created by crowding of teeth become apparent. With the appearance of the second permanent (12-year) molars, most of the permanent teeth are present. The third permanent molars, or wisdom teeth, may erupt from 18 to 25 years of age or later. Permanent dentition is somewhat more advanced in girls than in boys.

Because permanent teeth erupt during the school-age years, good dental hygiene and regular attention to dental caries are vital parts of health supervision during this period. Children of this age tend to become lax about oral hygiene unless they are carefully supervised. Although children are assuming more responsibility for their own care, they are not as motivated by improved appearance and odor as they will be during adolescence. School nurses should be alert for opportunities to teach correct brushing and flossing techniques, to reinforce avoidance of fermentable carbohydrates and sticky sweets, and to be alert for problems of malocclusion, toothache, and mouth infections.

Comprehensive dental supervision should be an integral part of the health maintenance program. Regular dental prophylaxis (teeth cleaning) by a dentist or dental hygienist and continued fluoride supplementation are essential to decrease the susceptibility of the tooth enamel to acid breakdown. (See Chapter 14 for a discussion of fluoride and other aspects of dental care.)

### Brushing

The most effective means of preventing dental caries is a regimen of proper oral hygiene tailored to the individual child by the dentist. Children should be taught to carry out

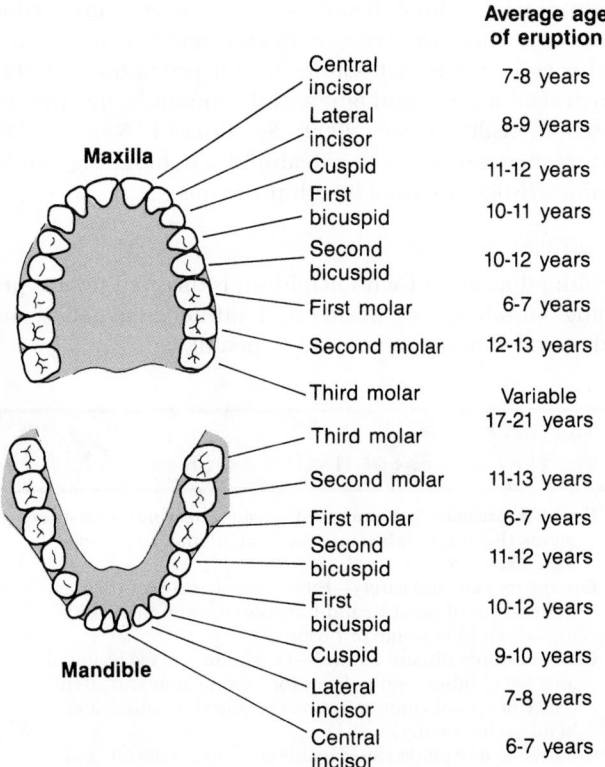

| | Average age of eruption |
|---|---|
| **Maxilla** | |
| Central incisor | 7-8 years |
| Lateral incisor | 8-9 years |
| Cuspid | 11-12 years |
| First bicuspid | 10-11 years |
| Second bicuspid | 10-12 years |
| First molar | 6-7 years |
| Second molar | 12-13 years |
| Third molar | Variable 17-21 years |
| **Mandible** | |
| Third molar | |
| Second molar | 11-13 years |
| First molar | 6-7 years |
| Second bicuspid | 11-12 years |
| First bicuspid | 10-12 years |
| Cuspid | 9-10 years |
| Lateral incisor | 7-8 years |
| Central incisor | 6-7 years |

**Fig. 17-15**   Sequence of eruption of secondary teeth. (Data from McDonald RE, Avery DR: *Dentistry for the child and adolescent*, ed 6, St Louis, 1994, Mosby.)

their own dental care with the supervision and guidance of parents. Parents should learn proper brushing technique along with their children and should inspect their children's efforts until the children can assume full responsibility for their own care.

Most practitioners believe that the majority of children do not possess the fine motor skills needed to brush their teeth properly until approximately second grade. Children under 10 years of age may need parental assistance to brush back teeth. Ideally, teeth should be brushed after meals, after snacks, and at bedtime. The bedtime brushing is especially important because there is more time for interaction between oral bacteria and unremoved substrate on the tooth substance. Children who brush their teeth frequently and become accustomed to the feel of a clean mouth at an early age usually maintain the habit throughout life.

The thoroughness of plaque removal (cleaning) can be checked using a plaque-disclosing agent that stains any remaining plaque red. The child should inspect the teeth closely with the aid of a mirror and under adequate light. The teeth are again cleansed with a fluoridated dentifrice to remove the remaining plaque and provide further protection. This procedure may be carried out regularly or occasionally, according to instructions from the child's dentist. Toothpastes recommended by the American Dental Association Council on Dental Therapeutics carry a seal of approval, which is easily identified on the package. They have been submitted to testing and demonstrate the ability to reduce the incidence of dental caries when used correctly.

For school-age children with mixed and permanent dentition, the best toothbrush is one with soft nylon bristles and an overall length of about 21 cm (6 inches). Numerous methods of brushing the teeth have been described and recommended for children, but no conclusive evidence indicates that one method is superior to another. The thoroughness of the cleaning is more important than the specific technique used. The dentist will assess all factors, such as manipulative skills and special needs of a child, and suggest the most appropriate brushing technique and regimen. Flossing follows brushing. Flossing is done by the parents until children acquire the manual dexterity needed. Most children are not able to floss properly until about 8 or 9 years of age.

## School Health

Child health maintenance is ultimately the responsibility of parents; however, public schools and health departments in the United States have contributed to the improvement of child health by providing a healthful school environment, health services, and health education functions that emphasize sound health practices. These functions constitute major components of community health services and involve large amounts of public funds and many health professionals, including nurses.

A safe and healthful school environment is an essential element of any school health program. Conditions within the school must contribute to the physical, mental, and social development and well-being of the children. One model that has been used to provide information about the essential components of school health is the Coordinated School Health Program (Marx and Wooley, 1998). The eight basic components of this program are a healthy school environment; school health services; health instruction; school nutrition services; school counseling, psychological, and social services; school-site health promotion for staff; physical education; and family and community involvement in school health (Vessey, 2000). See Boxes 17-6 and 17-7 for factors that contribute to a healthful school setting and for characteristics of school health programs.

### Health Education

Health education of schoolchildren is directed toward providing knowledge of health and influencing habits, attitudes, and conduct in relation to health.

---

**Box 17-6 ■ ■ ■**
**Components of a Coordinated School Health Program**

*Healthy School Environment:* A clean, safe environment that meets OSHA regulations, addresses sanitation measures, identifies environmental irritants, enforces disciplinary measures and monitors safety risks.

*School Health Services:* Services that provide health appraisals, prevention and control of communicable diseases, emergency care, educational counseling.

*Health Instruction:* A planned, sequential preK to grade 12 curriculum that addresses physical, mental, emotional, and social dimensions of health.

*School Nutrition Services:* Food service that reflects U.S. Department of Agriculture guidelines and ensures balanced diets and, when needed, special diets.

*School Counseling, Psychological, and Social Services:* Services to provide either on-site or referral to counseling services to meet psychosocial needs and guarantee adherence to individualized education prorams (IEPs) and other accommodations for students with chronic illnesses or speical needs.

*School-Site Health Promotion for Staff:* Services to promote health and wellness (e.g., blood pressure screening, stress reduction programs) among school staff.

*Physical Education:* Physical education for students in kindergarten to twelfth grade.

*Family and Community Involvement:* Dynamic partnerships with interested individuals and groups in the community.

From Vessey JA: Coordinated school health, *Pediatr Nurs* 26(3):303-307, 2000.

---

**Box 17-7 ■ ■ ■**
**Content of School Health Services**

**Health appraisal**—Screening tests (vision, hearing), measurements (height, weight), and medical, dental, and psychologic examinations

**Emergency care and safety**—Emergency treatment (first aid), notification of parents, and transportation of the ill or injured child to home or hospital

**Communicable disease control**—Detection and exclusion of affected children and policies for readmission and attendance at school (immunizations required in most states before school entry)

**Counseling and guidance**—Health guidance, referral, and follow-up for parents and children with special health needs Adjustment to individual student needs

A recent Gallup poll of Americans indicated the importance of health education in the school curriculum; 36% of the top 25 subjects in this survey were related to health topics that should be taught in schools (Doyen, Duffy, and Metz, 1999). Specific guidelines for health education programs in the school are outlined in Box 17-8.

A viable health education program is based on sound health concepts but should be adjusted to meet specific local needs, objectives, and legal requirements. Parents must understand and approve the health education curriculum so that its teaching will be reinforced at home. A comprehensive approach to health education is more successful in developing positive health practices than one in which the subjects are taught in isolation. Many topics presented in health education classes are associated with differing social and cultural attitudes and should be presented accurately and with sensitivity to these attitudes.

Health education concerning AIDS is a specific example. Most authorities agree that AIDS education should begin in the elementary grades to prevent high-risk behaviors. However, educational programs concerning AIDS must be developmentally appropriate and, to be effective, must be implemented with parental and community support. Young children need information on how the AIDS virus is transmitted, in simple, accurate terms without elaborate, unnecessary discussions of sex. Misconceptions that increase children's anxiety about contracting the virus should be corrected. Although many children have heard that sex and drugs cause AIDS, some children also have misconceptions about AIDS. Children need information on how AIDS is transmitted through infected blood on shared drug needles and that the virus is not spread through common forms of expressing affection such as hugging and holding hands.

## School Nursing Services

School nurses assume a major role in the school health program and can impact the lives of school-age children significantly. Working in collaboration with others in the school and community, school nurses provide health supervision, health counseling, and health education. These functions are not necessarily limited to the confines of the school environment but extend into the community in which the students live. As a health practitioner, the school nurse is in a position to promote and evaluate health services throughout the community as they affect children and to collaborate with agencies in planning for health and safety. For some children, especially those in poverty, the school nurse may be the only contact with illness prevention and health promotion. For children with chronic health conditions or children who depend on technologic devices, the school nurse not only performs essential skilled nursing tasks, such as gastrostomy feedings, suctioning, and catheterizations, but also manages and coordinates all the care that these children require to function in the school setting (Porter and others, 1996).

Traditionally, school nurses have been viewed from a limited perspective that placed them in the role of disease detector, applier of bandages, and official caregiver in cases of illness and injury. Although these are still important functions, this traditional role has acquired much broader dimensions. School nurses develop, implement, and evaluate health care plans and programs. In many settings the role of school health service has been enlarged into family health centers. These centers include school-based or school-linked health centers. Within these centers, school nurse practitioners provide primary health care that includes assessment of physical, psychomedical, psychoeducational, behavioral, and learning disorder problems, as well as comprehensive well-child care (American Academy of Pediatrics, 2001b).

In 1990 the National Association of School Nurses determined that the minimum preparation for entry into school nursing should be a baccalaureate degree from an accredited college or university (National Association of School Nurses, 1996). Despite this recommendation, some school districts have hired paraprofessionals or unlicensed assistive personnel (UAP) to meet school health needs. These paraprofessionals are trained to assist a professional but are not trained to recognize, assess, manage, or make appropriate referrals for the many health problems now being handled in schools. The competence of UAP must be determined and documented by the licensed school nurse. The licensed professional school nurse is also responsible for the super-

---

**Box 17-8**

### Recommendations for School Health Programs

Health education is a subject that should be taught as part of basic education and deserves the same priority in the curriculum as traditional subjects.

Planned integrated programs of comprehensive health education should be a requirement for students from kindergarten through grade 12 and should be taught by specially qualified teachers or those certified to teach health education.

Health education should include the active participation of students for the most effective learning of sound health concepts.

Financial support for health education programs must be ensured. Proper funding is critical to the development of effective programs, and the agencies responsible must be convinced to continue or increase funding.

Comprehensive health education programs should be directed by qualified health educators who function in consultation and cooperation with school personnel and administrators.

The programs should be monitored by a well-organized school health committee composed of representative parents, students, pediatricians, and health agencies (e.g., public health nurses) in the community.

Health education should be a part of every elementary school and secondary school teacher's training program.

School districts, other public agencies, the medical community, and private agencies should intensify their health education program for adults as part of a coordinated community health education effort, and pediatricians should make health education a regular component of the child health supervision and routine illness visits.

Research studies to evaluate the impact of such programs on students must be carried out at local and national levels.

From American Academy of Pediatrics, Committee on School Health: Health education and schools, *Pediatrics* 75:1160-1165, 1985.

vision of UAP and must use nursing assessment and professional judgment in deciding which procedures may be delegated to UAP (Delegation of School Health Services to Unlicensed Assistive Personnel, 1995; Rhodes, 1997).

**NURSING ALERT** In the delegation or transfer of responsibility for the performance of an activity to an assistant, the nurse remains accountable for the outcome.

The passage of Public Laws 94-142 and 99-457 required the integration of children with chronic illness or disability into the regular classrooms. School nurses are responsible for the medical and nursing needs of these children in the school setting. School nurses assess and monitor all health problems that come into the school and compile a health care list of all of these problems and their associated therapies. Nurses may call the parent of the child and arrange a visit to the home, made by either themselves or a public health nurse. After gathering information, a nursing care plan can be developed for use in the school. Nurses collaborate with the family and include their suggestions in the care plan. The plan is discussed with the child's teachers, and any needed education is provided. School nurses are the only ones in the school system qualified to deal with medical problems. However, there are many instances in which the school nurse can collaborate with teachers to provide atraumatic care. (See Community Focus box.)

Sometimes all that is required is an assessment and making the teacher aware that the child has a health problem.

## COMMUNITY FOCUS
### Collaboration Between School Nurse and Teachers

All students should have health cards completed by their parents.
All teachers should receive a list of students who have health problems.
Students with health needs should be coded in teacher grade books so that substitute teachers can recognize these students and intervene immediately if problems occur in the classroom.
Teachers should schedule students who miss physical education into an adaptive physical education class if possible.
All students with asthma should have their metered dose inhalers available to them for emergency use in physical education and all other classes.
Adult volunteers should serve as team captains for games; selections of team members should be supervised so that one team is not stacked with all the good players.
In physical education, a skill or activity should be rerun several times if some students score extremely high and others extremely low because every child has good and bad days.
A child's ability should never be questioned in front of other students.
Privacy should be maintained for height/weight checks and vision/hearing tests (students should be taken into the nurse's office individually so other students do not hear the test results).

Suggestions submitted by Linda L. Smith, Health/Physical Education Teacher.

In other cases more complex teaching is needed, such as how to observe for certain signs (e.g., insulin reaction), techniques that must be learned (e.g., tracheostomy suctioning, gastrostomy or nasogastric tube feedings), and management of emergencies (care of a child during a seizure). School nurses instruct teachers in the necessary procedures and review their performance.

The American Academy of Pediatrics (2001c) has established guidelines for emergency medical care of children in schools. Many schools require not only the school nurses, but also teachers and coaches to demonstrate competence in cardiopulmonary resuscitation (CPR). In some schools, emergency life saving courses can also be taught to students. One recommended curriculum is the "Basic Emergency Lifesaving Skills (BELS): A framework for teaching emergency lifesaving skills to children and adolescents" created and published by the Health Resources and Services Administration (Maternal and Child Health Bureau, 1999).

Children who must take medications at school need written authorization from the child's attending physician and/or written permission from the parents allowing the nurse to administer or supervise the administration of the medication. The medication must be brought to the school in a container appropriately labeled by the pharmacist or physician. Medications are kept locked up in the nurse's office; and usually the child is not allowed to carry medications at school. This may vary in some school districts or situations. For example, some children may be allowed to carry metered dose inhalers that contain their asthma medication. The children are allowed to do so provided that the physician and a parent provide the required authorization. Guidelines for administration of medications in schools can also be obtained from the **National Association of School Nurses, Inc.***

The preparation, qualifications, and utilization of school nurses and school nurse practitioners vary throughout the United States. Some communities consider the school nurse an essential member of the school organization with a full-time school commitment; in other communities school health practice is merely a part of the total community health program assumed by the health department.

## Injury Prevention

Because school-age children have developed more refined muscular coordination and control and can apply their cognitive capacities to a more judicious course of action, the incidence of unintentional injury is diminished in children in this age-group as compared with the incidence in early childhood. School-age children have exposure to more environments in which they need protection, they acquire skills and interests that expose them to new perils, they have less supervision, and they take more responsibility as they begin to participate in the adult world.

Injuries most prevalent in school-age children reflect their developmental stage. Table 17-2 outlines the develop-

*Lamplighter Lane, PO Box 1300, Scarborough, ME 04074, (207) 883-2117, e-mail: NASN@aol.com; www.vrmedia.com/nurses/.

**TABLE 17-2**   Injury prevention during school-age years

| Developmental Abilities Related to Risk of Injury | Injury Prevention |
|---|---|
| Is increasingly involved in activities away from home<br>Is excited by speed and motion<br>Is easily distracted by environment<br>Can be reasoned with | **Motor vehicles**<br>Educate child regarding proper use of seat belts while a passenger in a vehicle<br>Maintain discipline while a passenger in a vehicle (e.g., keep arms inside, do not lean against doors or interfere with driver)<br>Remind parents and children that no one should ride in the bed of a pickup truck<br>Emphasize safe pedestrian behavior<br>Insist on wearing safety apparel (e.g., helmet) where applicable, such as when riding a bicycle, motorcycle, moped, or all-terrain vehicle (see Family Home Care boxes on pp. 733-735) |
| Is apt to overdo<br>May work hard to perfect a skill<br>Has cautious, but not fearful, gross motor actions<br>Likes swimming | **Drowning**<br>Teach child to swim<br>Teach basic rules of water safety<br>Select safe and supervised places to swim<br>Check sufficient water depth for diving<br>Swim with a companion<br>Use an approved flotation device in water or boat<br>Advocate for legislation requiring fencing around pools<br>Learn cardiopulmonary resuscitation (CPR) |
| Has increasing independence<br>Is adventuresome<br>Enjoys trying new things | **Burns**<br>Make sure smoke detectors are in homes<br>Set water heaters to 48.9° C (120° F) to avoid scald burns<br>Instruct child in behavior in areas involving contact with potential burn hazards (e.g., gasoline, matches, bonfires or barbecues, lighter fluid, firecrackers, cigarette lighters, cooking utensils, chemistry sets); avoid climbing or flying kites around high-tension wires<br>Instruct child in proper behavior in the event of fire (e.g., fire drills at home and school) (see Chapter 29)<br>Teach child safe cooking (use low heat, avoid any frying, be careful of steam burns, scalds, or exploding foods, especially from microwaving) |
| Adheres to group rules<br>May be easily influenced by peers<br>Has strong allegiance to friends | **Poisoning**<br>Educate child regarding hazards of taking nonprescription drugs and chemicals, including aspirin and alcohol<br>Teach child to say "no" if offered illegal or dangerous drugs or alcohol<br>Keep potentially dangerous products in properly labeled receptacles, preferably out of reach |
| Has increased physical skills<br>Needs strenuous physical activity<br>Is interested in acquiring new skills and perfecting attained skills<br>Is daring and adventurous, especially with peers<br>Frequently plays in hazardous places<br>Confidence often exceeds physical capacity<br>Desires group loyalty and has strong need for friends' approval<br>Attempts hazardous feats<br>Accompanies friends to potentially hazardous facilities<br>Delights in physical activity<br>Is likely to overdo<br>Growth in height exceeds muscular growth and coordination | **Bodily damage**<br>Help provide facilities for supervised activities<br>Encourage playing in safe places<br>Keep firearms safely locked up except during adult supervision<br>Teach proper care of, use of, and respect for devices with potential danger (power tools, firecrackers)<br>Teach children not to tease or surprise dogs, invade their territory, take dogs' toys, or interfere with dogs' feeding<br>Stress eye, ear, or mouth protection when using potentially hazardous objects or devices or when engaged in potentially hazardous sports (e.g., baseball)<br>Teach safety regarding use of corrective devices (glasses); if child wears contact lenses, monitor duration of wear to prevent corneal damage<br>Do not permit use of trampolines except as part of supervised training<br>Stress careful selection, use, and maintenance of sports and recreation equipment such as skateboards and in-line skates (see Family Home Care box on p. 735)<br>Emphasize proper conditioning, safe practices, and use of safety equipment for sports or recreational activities<br>Caution against engaging in hazardous sports, such as those involving trampolines<br>Use safety glass and decals on large glassed areas, such as sliding glass doors<br>Use window guards to prevent falls.<br>Teach name, address, and phone number and emphasize that child should ask for help from appropriate people (cashier, security guard, policeman) if lost; have identification on child (sewn in clothes, inside shoe)<br>Teach stranger safety:<br>   Avoid personalized clothing in public places<br>   Caution child to never go with a stranger<br>Have child tell parents if anyone makes child feel uncomfortable in any way<br>Always listen to child's concerns regarding others' behavior<br>Teach child to say "no" when confronted with uncomfortable situations |

mental characteristics and accomplishments of middle childhood that predispose children to physical injury and offers guidelines for injury prevention.

The incidence of injury during middle childhood is significantly higher in school-age boys than in school-age girls, and their death rate is twice that of girls. (See Chapter 1.) Most injuries occur in or near the home or school. The prevalence of injury depends on the dangers present in the environment, protection offered by adults, and the behavior patterns of the children. Although school-age children are conscious of rules and frequently impose them in relationships with peers, they also tend to challenge established rules. It is often difficult to maintain a balance between the level of supervision and restriction needed by children and their need for freedom and independence.

The incidence of transportation-related injuries in school-age children is higher than that of younger children, and the incidence of non–motor vehicle–involved bicycle injury is higher than that of teenagers and preschool children. Injuries from burns and poisonings is lowest in school-age children. However, physically active school-age children are highly susceptible to cuts and abrasions, and the incidence of childhood fractures, strains, and sprains is impressive.

### Risk-Taking Behavior

Achieving social acceptance is a primary objective for school-age children. They often attempt dangerous acts (sometimes extreme behaviors) to prove themselves worthy of acceptance and improve their status in the peer group. Peer pressure is a normal part of psychologic development, but it is also a major contributor to risk-taking behaviors. Peer challenges often encourage problem behaviors that place children at risk for injury or hazardous habits. School-age children are in the process of moving from preoperational to concrete operational thinking and are only beginning to understand causal relationships. Therefore they may attempt certain activities without planning or evaluating the consequences.

Children who are risk takers may have inadequate self-regulatory behavior. These children need to learn the motivation or the incentives for such behavior and to visualize the consequences if the risk-taking behavior ends in a tragic outcome.

### Motor Vehicle Injury

As in all other age-groups, the most common cause of severe accidental injury and death in school-age children is motor vehicle accidents—either as a pedestrian or as a passenger. Pedestrian fatalities are two and a half times more frequent than occupant deaths in school-age children, and the peak incidence is in the 5- to 9-year-old age-group. Most of the injuries are caused by children who misinterpret traffic signs or disobey common traffic safety regulations, cross the street against a red light, cross in other-than-designated crosswalks, dart into the street, and walk in the same direction as the traffic. Parents consistently overestimate the street-crossing skills of young children ages 5 to 6 years and need education about their children's developmental abilities and compe-

tence as pedestrians. Nurses can help parents to develop more realistic expectations of their children's behavior and teach them to model safe street-crossing behaviors through pedestrian skills training programs.

Use of restraint systems, door-lock mechanisms, and appropriate passenger seating and behavior are simple but effective measures for eliminating noncrash injuries and reducing the severity of crash injuries. The importance of emphasizing the correct use of seat restraints cannot be overemphasized. Children in the school-age age-group do not usually require special car seats. However, despite evidence that safety belt use saves lives and prevents injury, estimates of seat belt use in school-age children are still discouragingly low.

Children have been critically injured by car air bags (Morbidity and Mortality Weekly Report, 1995). The National Highway Traffic Safety Administration (NHTSA) currently recommends that children under the age of 12 not ride in the front passenger seat of vehicles with air bags.* The American Academy of Pediatrics (2002) reiterates this view and strongly emphasizes that the rear seat of any vehicle is the safest place for children to ride. When in the car, school-age children should always be buckled properly in a weight- and age-appropriate seat. If the child weighs less than 40 pounds, a convertible safety seat that is positioned in the semi-upright and forward-facing position may be used if the child fits well. If the child has outgrown the convertible safety seat but is still too small for a regular lap/shoulder belt, a booster seat restraint device equipped with a combination lap/shoulder belt can be used.

Injuries to children ages 5 to 9 years restrained in adult-type seat belts are related to anatomic differences between adults and children. The child's sitting height is less than the adult's, and the center of gravity is located above the level of the lap belt. Consequently, the greater proportion of body mass above the belt may cause more forward motion and jackknifing over the belt, increasing the risk of head injury from impact with interior vehicle parts. The child's smaller and less developed iliac crests are not suited to serve as an anchor for belts designed to restrain adults, and their intraabdominal organs are less protected by the bony pelvis. The natural behavior of children, such as readjusting the seating position, moving about, and otherwise altering the fit of the restraint, influences its effectiveness.

When children use adult-type seat belts, parents should make certain that the restraints are fitted to their children and fastened correctly. To reduce the risk of sliding beneath the standard seat belt during a collision, children should sit up straight and well back in the seat, and the seat should be moved forward until the feet fit firmly against the toe board. Children should be cautioned against assuming alternate seating positions, such as tailor fashion, while riding in the car. (See Chapter 14 for a comprehensive discussion of safety restraints.*)

---

*Guidelines for car seat safety are also available in Wong DL, Hess CS: *Wong and Whaley's clinical manual of pediatric nursing*, ed 5, St Louis, 2000, Mosby. The Department of Transportation provides discussion of child safety seats at www.nhtsa.dot.gov.

Although it has been established that seat belts reduce motor vehicle injuries, most school buses are not equipped with seat restraints. The American Academy of Pediatrics (1996c) recommends that seat belts be installed in all newly purchased school buses. In addition, school districts that provide bus transportation for school-age children with assistive devices such as wheelchairs are encouraged to follow the guidelines outlined in the National School Bus Safety Standards (Twelfth National Conference on School Transportation, 1995). Seat belts in buses serve two purposes: they (1) reduce the risk of injury and (2) serve to teach and reinforce the importance of seat belt use while riding in any motor vehicle. Seat belts specifically designed for school buses also keep children from being ejected from their seats and colliding with hard interior surfaces.

*All-terrain vehicles (ATVs),* designed for off-road use by children and adolescents, are popular with children under 16 years of age but are responsible for a significant number of childhood injuries. These vehicles have a short wheelbase and low profile, which makes them relatively unstable and unable to be seen easily. The vehicles can also achieve substantial speed. Most injuries occur when the driver loses control of the vehicle, is thrown from the vehicle, or collides with fixed objects or other vehicles. Immature judgment and poorly developed motor skills also contribute to injury. The Committee on Injury and Poison Prevention of the American Academy of Pediatrics (2000c) views ATVs as a major hazard to the health of children and opposes their use by children less than 16 years of age. However, for parents who allow their use, the Committee provides safety guidelines. (See Family Home Care box.)

## Bicycle Injury

The majority of school-age children have bicycles, and their love of riding them increases the risk of injury on streets and byways. Bicycle injuries account for approximately 500,000 emergency room visits and more than 900 deaths annually

---

### FAMILY HOME CARE
#### Safe Use of All-Terrain Vehicles

Children under the age of 16 years should not operate an off-road vehicle.

Vehicles should be sturdy and stable; quality construction is essential.

Riders should receive instruction from a mature, experienced cyclist or a certified instructor.

Riding should be supervised and allowed only after the rider has demonstrated competence in handling the machine on familiar terrain (preferably require licensing).

Riders should wear approved helmets, eye protection and protective reflective clothing (e.g., trousers, boots, gloves).

Parents should prohibit street use of off-road vehicles.

Riding should be restricted to familiar terrain.

Nighttime riding should not be allowed.

Vehicle should not carry more than one person.

Based on and modified from American Academy of Pediatrics, Committee on Injury and Poison Prevention: All-terrain vehicle injury prevention: two-, three-, and four-wheeled unlicensed motorized vehicles, *Pediatrics* 105:1352-1354, 2000.

---

(Liller and others, 1998). Most of the bicyclists treated in emergency rooms are younger than 15 years of age.

Deaths are usually caused by head injuries and almost always are the result of bicycle–motor vehicle collision (American Academy of Pediatrics, 1995a). Many injuries are related to violations of traffic laws by the bicyclist, including wrong-way riding (facing traffic), failure to yield the right-of-way, and turning violations. Others have been related to road conditions described as hazardous—bumps, potholes, and gravel found on mountain bike trails. Injuries among young children using their bicycles occur among young children playing in their own neighborhood and older children using their bicycles for transportation on streets with heavy traffic.

In addition to major injuries, cuts and bruises from falls and collisions account for a large number of injuries. Other injuries include trauma to internal organs. These injuries initially seem to be trivial, but injured children develop serious symptoms (e.g., pain, vomiting, or collapse) hours later.

Many of the injuries to school-age children on bicycles can be attributed to their developmentally limited range of vision and their inability to process perceptions of road situations sufficiently well and quickly enough to ride safely in traffic. Other important factors are lack of instruction in use of the equipment, lack of safety equipment, and riders who are unfamiliar with the bicycle (e.g., having ridden their bicycle for less than a month).

To prevent bicycle injuries, both parents and children should learn and periodically review bicycle safety. Children need bicycles that are suited to their size and age—they should be able to stand with the balls of both feet on the ground when seated on the bicycle, be able to place both feet flat on the ground when straddling the center bar, and be able to grasp the brake lever comfortably and easily enough to apply sufficient pressure to brake the bicycle. Parents should be discouraged from buying their child a bicycle that the child can "grow into."

Because head injury is the major cause of bicycle-related fatalities, the single most important aspect of bicycle safety is to encourage the rider to wear a protective helmet (Fig. 17-16). Hard-shelled helmets lined with expanded polystyrene (Styrofoam) provide the best head protection. The helmet should be one that can be adjusted to the individual child's head, fits securely, and does not limit the child's vision or hearing. A brightly colored helmet improves visibility. The helmet should carry the seal indicating it is approved by the Snell Memorial Foundation or that it has passed the safety standards of the American National Standards Institute (ANSI). Since children's head sizes have nearly reached adult size before their full skeletal height is reached, a helmet purchased at age 7 or 8 may be worn through adolescence with a few alterations in the fitting pads.

National estimates of bicycle helmet use among children indicate that only 50% of children own a helmet and only half of these wear a helmet every time they ride (Liller and others, 1998). Although most young riders acknowledge that wearing a helmet is important for safety, reasons for not wearing them include the helmet design itself and lack of peer support for wearing a helmet (Liller and others, 1998).

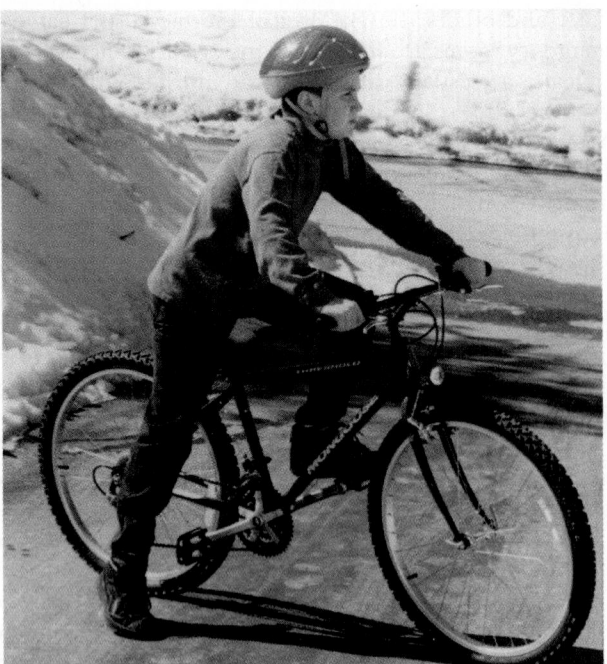

**Fig. 17-16** The right-size bike is important; the child should be able to sit on the bike and place balls of both feet on the ground. The foot should comfortably reach and manipulate the pedal in the down position. Wearing a protective helmet is mandatory for safe cycling. The helmet should sit on top of the head in a level position and should not rock back and forth or from side to side. The strap should always be fastened securely under the chin.

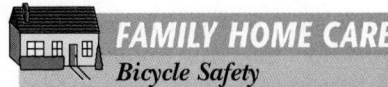

### FAMILY HOME CARE
#### Bicycle Safety

Always wear a properly fitted helmet that is approved by Snell or the American National Standards Institute (ANSI); replace a damaged helmet.
Ride bicycles with traffic and away from parked cars.
Ride single file.
Walk bicycles through busy intersections and only at cross-walks.
Give hand signals well in advance of turning or stopping.
Keep as close to the curb as practical.
Watch for drain grates, potholes, soft shoulders, and loose dirt or gravel.
Keep both hands on handlebars, except with signaling.
Never ride double on a bicycle.
Do not carry packages that interfere with vision or control; do not drag objects behind bike.
Watch for and yield to pedestrians.
Watch for cars backing up or pulling out of driveways; be especially careful at intersections.
Look left, right, then left before turning into traffic or roadway.
Never hitch a ride on a truck or other vehicle.
Learn rules of the road and respect for traffic officers.
Obey all local ordinances.
Wear shoes that fit securely while riding.
Wear light colors at night and attach fluorescent material to clothing and bicycle.
Be certain the bicycle is the correct size for the rider.
Equip bicycle with proper lights and reflectors.
Have the bicycle inspected to ensure good mechanical condition.
Children riding as passengers must wear appropriate-size helmets and sit in specially designed protective seats.

Modified from American Academy of Pediatrics, Committee on Injury and Poison Prevention: Bicycle helmets, *Pediatrics* 95(4):609-610, 1995.

Parental attitudes and behaviors also influence children's use of bicycle helmets. Parental nonuse of a helmet is strongly associated with lack of intention to require the children to use helmets. In contrast, sibling helmet use is a positive predictor of helmet use (Liller and others, 1998). Parents, as well as children, need to be educated on safety. The American Academy of Pediatrics (1995a) recommends that (1) parents be informed of the dangers of riding without a helmet, (2) retail outlets carry inexpensive helmets available at the time of bicycle purchase, (3) state and local governments enact legislation requiring helmet use by all bicyclists, (4) parents and community-based programs promote bicycle safety and helmet use, and (5) the media depict helmet use in all programs and promotional materials.

Numerous bicycle helmet promotion programs have been developed by schools, hospital emergency rooms, and communities. Programs that are most successful are those that address the cost of helmets and peer pressure and combine multimedia public education announcements with the support of community organizations. The University of California–Santa Cruz has also developed several videos on bicycle safety.* Guidelines for bicycle safety are listed in the Family Home Care box. (Bicycle helmets are discussed in the Critical Thinking Exercise box on p. 735.)

### Other Vehicles

After a short period of decline, *skateboards* are again assuming popularity, with an accompanying resurgence of related injuries. Although the majority of injuries involve the extremities, severe injuries involving the head and neck can occur and are more prevalent among children 9 years of age and younger (American Academy of Pediatrics, 1995b). School-age children often use their skateboards on streets and highways, increasing the likelihood of high-speed collisions with objects or vehicles. Recommendations for safe skateboard use are listed in the Family Home Care box on p. 735.

Like skateboard injuries, *roller skate* or *in-line skate injuries* involve predominantly the upper extremities (especially the wrist and forearm) as children attempt to break the fall with outstretched arms. Safety measures are basically the same as for skateboards. The skill level of the child should be carefully evaluated before the child is allowed to use these conveyances. Younger children sustain injuries more frequently than older children. Some authorities believe that children should not be encouraged to engage in these activities until their bone strength and skills are sufficiently mature to decrease the risk of fracture.

---

*Available from Transit Media Communication, 22-D Hollywood Ave, Hohokus, NJ 07423, (800) 343-5540, e-mail: tmcndy@aol.com; www.new-day.com.

## Critical Thinking Exercise

### Bicycle Helmets

During the past month in your school district, one child died and another sustained a serious head injury from bicycle-vehicle collisions. Neither child wore a bicycle helmet. As a school nurse, you are considering effective approaches to increase the students' use of bicycle helmets. Which of the following is most likely to achieve your goal?

FIRST, THINK ABOUT IT . . .
- What conclusions are you reaching?
- What would the consequences be if you put your thoughts into action?

1. Send home to every family an educational packet of material about bicycle safety.
2. Ask the local television station to report the details of the victims' injuries and the families' grief.
3. Invite local athletes engaged in sports, such as football, that require protective headgear to discuss being safe and acting "cool."
4. Organize other school nurses, faculty, and parents to petition the state legislature for mandatory bicycle helmet laws.

*The best response is three. All of the options are constructive ones, but the one most likely to influence the school children immediately is three. Issues of stylishness, comfort, and social acceptability are major determinants of compliance. Education by respected athletes provides a strong incentive for youngsters to wear helmets. Involving local athletes in a bicycle helmet campaign may have many positive consequences for the school and community.*

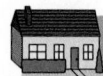

## FAMILY HOME CARE
### Skateboard and In-Line Skate Safety

Children younger than 5 years of age should not use skateboards or in-line skates. They are not developmentally prepared to protect themselves from injury.

Children who ride skateboards and in-line skates should wear helmets and protective padding, especially on wrists, knees, and elbows, to prevent injury.

Skateboards and in-line skates should never be ridden near traffic. Their use should be prohibited on streets and highways. Activities that bring skateboards or in-line skates and cars together (e.g., "catching a ride") are especially dangerous.

Some types of use, such as riding homemade ramps on hard surfaces, may be particularly hazardous.

Modified from American Academy of Pediatrics, Committee on Accident and Poison Prevention: Skateboard injuries, *Pediatrics* 95(4):611-612, 1995.

*Ride-on mower injuries* also occur among school age children. These injuries occur when children are allowed to operate the mower, when they are run over or backed over by another driver, or when they fall from the mower or from a trailer pulled by a mower. Similar injuries involve snowmobiles. Most deaths and injuries involving snowmobiles occur when the vehicle strikes a tree, cable, wire or another vehicle. The American Academy of Pediatrics (2000d) recommends that persons under 16 years of age be prohibited from the recreational operation of snowmobiles.

### Injuries at School

The risk of injury at school is relatively low, despite the amount of time children spend in that environment. Some injuries occur in the gyms, shops, and laboratories, as well as on the playground and playing fields. Most injuries occur on the way to and from school. Many are related to sports activities. (See Chapter 39.)

Trampolines have become popular with young children, and injuries on this piece of equipment have increased significantly. In 1996, 83,000 patients were treated for trampoline injuries in hospital emergency departments; 66% of these patients were between 5 and 14 years of age (Cassidy, 1996; Furnival, Street, and Schunk, 1999). Fractures, sprains, and head injuries have all been attributed to tram-

polines. The American Academy of Pediatarics (1999) recommends against the use of trampolines in the home, during physical education classes at school or on outdoor playgrounds. Persons concerned for child safety should be alert to hazards in the school environment and should become involved in efforts to make the environment safe from every aspect—physical facilities, equipment, training practices, and supervision.

### Farm Injuries

Many school-age children are involved in farm activities and play in the farm environment. They may be children of migrant workers, and as such, they constitute a significant proportion of agricultural workers. Most injuries take place during the summer when children are home from school and in the autumn when farming activity is brisk. Health facilities are also more scattered and less accessible for emergency treatment than they are in urban areas.

Health workers need to be aware of the problems and to emphasize to the farm family the hazards related to their environment and ways to prevent injuries, especially when children are present. Rural schools should provide safety education regarding operating machinery, safety procedures, and injury prevention. Nurses in rural areas can be advocates for farm safety programs and for revision of the current farm safety legislation.

### Other Injuries

Falls are still a source of injury but less so than in preschool children and toddlers. "Flipping," a popular activity in which children jump from an elevated surface and perform an aerial flip with the idea of landing upright, has resulted in several serious injuries to the face and head and places children at risk for back and spinal cord injury. Seasonal injuries such as sledding accidents are common and more likely to occur when children sled ride without adult supervision and in streets as opposed to parks. Horseback riding injuries are another source of concern for parents of school-age children. The most common cause of death from horseback riding activities is head injury, followed by injuries to the chest and abdomen. Before enrolling children for rid-

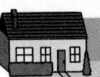

**FAMILY HOME CARE**
*Guidance During School Years*

### AGE 6 YEARS

Prepare parents to expect strong food preferences and frequent refusal of specific food items.

Prepare parents to expect increasingly ravenous appetite.

Prepare parents for emotionality as child experiences erratic mood changes.

Help parents anticipate continued susceptibility to illness.

Teach injury prevention and safety, especially bicycle safety.

Encourage parents to respect child's need for privacy and to provide a separate bedroom for child, if possible.

Prepare parents for child's increasing interests outside the home.

Help parents understand the need to encourage child's interactions with peers.

### AGES 7 TO 10 YEARS

Prepare parents to expect improvement in health with fewer illnesses, but warn them that allergies may increase or become apparent.

Prepare parents to expect an increase in minor injuries.

Emphasize caution in selecting and maintaining sports equipment and reemphasize safety.

Prepare parents to expect increased involvement with peers and interest in activities outside the home.

Emphasize the need to encourage independence while maintaining limit-setting and discipline.

Prepare mothers to expect more demands at 8 years.

Prepare fathers to expect increasing admiration at 10 years; encourage father-child activities.

Prepare parents for prepubescent changes in girls.

### AGES 11 TO 12 YEARS

Help parents prepare child for body changes of pubescence.

Prepare parents to expect a growth spurt in girls.

Make certain child's sex education is adequate with accurate information.

Prepare parents to expect energetic but stormy behavior at 11, to become more even tempered at 12.

Encourage parents to support child's desire to "grow up" but to allow regressive behavior when needed.

Prepare parents to expect an increase in masturbation.

Instruct parents that the amount of rest child needs may increase.

Help parents educate child regarding experimentation with potentially harmful activities.

### HEALTH GUIDANCE

Help parents understand the importance of regular health and dental care for child.

Encourage parents to teach and model sound health practices, including diet, rest, activity, and exercise.

Stress the need to encourage children to engage in appropriate physical activities.

Emphasize providing a safe physical and emotional environment.

Encourage parents to teach and model safety practices.

---

ing lessons, parents should determine the instructor's safety record with students and whether the instructor is certified by a recognized organization. Injuries at public playgrounds and amusement parks (especially water slides), as well as around the home (power tools, ladders, fireworks), are ongoing concerns of parents and health care providers.

Injuries to eyes and teeth are a constant threat to school-age children involved in rough play. (See Chapter 24 [eyes] and Chapter 18 [teeth].) The normally shallow bony orbit of children in this age-group makes them particularly vulnerable to eye trauma, especially during contact sports or activities, such as baseball or softball. Wearing protective eye and mouth gear is essential (American Academy of Pediatrics, 1996d.)

Injuries have been reported for a variety of toys (slingshots, water balloons, lawn darts, chemistry sets) and household equipment (mowers, lawn trimmers). Gunshot wounds have become a significant problem during past years. The overall rate of firearm deaths for US children younger than 15 years of age is nearly 12 times greater than that found for 25 other industrialized countries (Centers for Disease Control and Prevention, 1997). So-called toy firearms (air guns and air rifles) also cause frequent firearm injuries to children. Most of these injuries involve the face or eyes.

### Nurse's Role in Injury Prevention

Nurses are primary advocates for preventive care and guidance. Safety education and anticipatory guidance for both parents and school-age children can be incorporated in all nursing interventions. The most effective means of prevention is education of the child and family regarding the hazards of risk-taking behavior and improper use of equipment. No piece of equipment is safe unless a child is physically and mentally equipped to use it. A careful history and a knowledge of normal growth and development serve as guidelines for both planned and impromptu education.

Parents are often unaware of hazards to their children at various ages, especially those related to normal developmental progress. Susceptibility to injuries and understanding of safety issues are influenced by children's developmental level. Nurses who understand the growth and development of school-age children can provide effective safety education to parents and children and can correct misconceptions before injuries occur.

School nurses should be alert to hazards in the school and instrumental in evaluating safety risks and implementing safety programs. Characteristics of the school-age child and preventive measures are listed in Table 17-2.

## Anticipatory Guidance— Care of Families

The parents of the school-age child find themselves in the position of sharing their child's time and interests with the increasingly important peer group. As a child feels the need to fit into a peer group and gain a sense of industry through individual and cooperative production and performance, he or she moves away from the close, familiar relationships of the family group. It is through these early peer relationships that children prepare for moving from narrow, sheltered family relationships to a broader world of relationships and increased independence. Parents must learn to provide support as unobtrusively as possible without feeling rejected, hurt, or angry. The nurse can help parents of the school-age child by providing anticipatory guidance and reassurance throughout this period of child development and maturation. (See Family Home Care box.)

# KEY POINTS

- Middle childhood, also known as the school years, is a comfortable period of life that extends from 6 to 12 years of age.
- Although growth is slower than in previous years, there is a steady gain in height and weight with maturation of body systems; primary teeth are lost and replaced by permanent teeth.
- Skeletal lengthening, a higher ratio of muscle mass to fat, and maturation of the gastrointestinal system are major components of biologic development during middle childhood.
- Developing a sense of industry or accomplishment is a major task during the middle years (Erikson).
- Piaget's theory of concrete operations refers to the school-age period, when children are able to use their thought processes to experience events and actions and make judgments based on what they reason.
- Through identity, reversibility, and reciprocity, children master the cognitive task of conservation.
- The child develops a conscience and is able to understand and adhere to rules and standards set by others.
- Spiritual development entails a curiosity about deities, a knowledge of the difference between the natural and the supernatural, and reliance on prayers or other religious rituals.
- Entertaining different points of view, becoming sensitive to social norms of peers, and forming peer friendships are the most important features of social development in the middle years.
- Children develop a self-concept from their own self-assessment and feedback from others.
- Increased socialization, earlier pubertal development, and constant media exposure make the school years an ideal time for sex education.
- Cooperative play, team activities, and acquisition of skills are prime elements of play during the school years; rules and rituals assume greater importance.
- Optimum nutrition is often hampered by an affinity for and availability of junk foods, irregular family meals, and schedules of working parents.
- Typical parental concerns during middle childhood include dishonest behavior, lying, cheating, stealing, and school-related stress.
- The school years are an ideal time for children to begin to take responsibility for their own health.
- School health ideally offers programs that include health appraisal, emergency care, safety education, communicable disease control, counseling, guidance, and health education, with adjustment to individual student needs.
- The major sources of accidental injury during middle childhood involve a variety of conveyances, including motor vehicles, bicycles, skateboards, and in-line skates.
- Injury prevention is directed toward safety education, provision of safe play areas and equipment, and well-supervised sports activities.

# REFERENCES

American Academy of Pediatrics, Committee on Children with Disabilities: Sexuality education of children and adolescents with developmental disabilities, *Pediatrics* 97(2):275-278, 1996a.

American Academy of Pediatrics, Committee on Injury and Poison Prevention: All-terrain vehicle injury prevention: two-, three-, and four-wheeled unlicensed motor vehicles, *Pediatrics* 105(6):1352-1354, 2000c.

American Academy of Pediatrics, Committee on Injury and Poison Prevention: Bicycle helmets, *Pediatrics* 95(4):609-610, 1995a.

American Academy of Pediatrics, Committee on Injury and Poison Prevention: Selecting and using the most appropriate car safety seats for growing children: guidelines for counseling parents, *Pediatrics* 109(3):550-553, 2002.

American Academy of Pediatrics, Committee on Injury and Poison Prevention: Skateboard injuries, *Pediatrics* 95(4):611-612, 1995b.

American Academy of Pediatrics, Committee on Injury and Poison Prevention: Snowmobiling hazards, *Pediatrics* 106(5):1142-1144, 2000d.

American Academy of Pediatrics, Committee on Injury and Poison Prevention and Committee on Sports Medicine and Fitness: Trampolines at home, school, and recreational centers, *Pediatrics* 103(5):1053-1056, 1999.

American Academy of Pediatrics, Committee on Pediatric AIDS: Human immunodeficiency virus/acquired immunodeficiency syndrome education in schools, *Pediatrics* 101(5):933-935, 1998a.

American Academy of Pediatrics, Committee on Psychosocial Aspects of Child and Family Health: Guidance for effective discipline, *Pediatrics* 101(4):723-728, 1998b.

American Academy of Pediatrics, Committee on Public Education: Children, adolescents and television, *Pediatrics* 107(2):423-426, 2001a.

American Academy of Pediatrics, Committee on School Health: Corporal punishment in schools, *Pediatrics* 106(2):343, 2000a.

American Academy of Pediatrics, Committee on School Health: Guidelines for emergency medical care in school, *Pediatrics* 107(2):435-436, 2001c.

American Academy of Pediatrics, Committee on School Health: School health centers and other integrated school health services, *Pediatrics* 107(1):198-201, 2001b.

American Academy of Pediatrics, Committee on School Health and Committee on Injury and Poison Prevention: School transportation safety, *Pediatrics* 97(5):754-757, 1996c.

American Academy of Pediatrics, Committee on Sports Medicine and Fitness: Protective eyewear for young athletes, *Pediatrics* 98 (2 Pt 1):311-312, 1996d.

American Academy of Pediatrics, Committee on Sports Medicine and Fitness and Committee on School Health: Physical fitness and activity in schools, *Pediatrics* 105(5):1156-1157, 2000b.

American Dietetic Association: Position of the American Dietetic Association: dietary guidance for healthy children aged 2 to 11 years, *J Am Diet Assoc* 99(1):93-101, 1999.

Andersen RE and others: Relationship of physical activity and television watching with body weight and level of fatness among children: results from the third National Health and Nutrition Examination Survey, *J Am Med Assoc* 279(12):938-942, 1998.

Beck AM, Meyers NM: Health enhancement and companion animal ownership, *Ann Rev Public Health* 17:247-257, 1996.

Blum NJ, Ditmar MF, Charney EB: Behavior and development. In Polin RA, Ditmar MF, editors: *Pediatric secrets,* ed 2, St Louis, 1997, Mosby.

Cantor J: Media violence, *J Adolesc Health* 27S(2):30-34, 2000.

Cantor J, Nathanson AI: Children's fright reactions to television news, *J Communication* 46:139-152, 1996.

Carroll MK, Ryan-Wenger NA: School-age children's fears, anxiety, and human figure drawings, *J Pediatr Health Care* 13(1):24-31, 1999.

Cassidy SP: *United States Consumer Product Safety Commission (USCPSC), Trampolines, Memorandum, May 15, 1996 and National Electronic Injury Surveillance System(NEISS) data,* Washington, DC, 1991-1995; 1996, Consumer Product Safety Commission.

Centers for Disease Control and Prevention: Rates of homicide, suicide, and firearm-related death among children in 26 industrialized counties, *MMWR* 46:101-105, 1997.

Clark MMC, Ferguson SL: The physical activity and fitness of our nation's children, *J Pediatric Nurs* 15(4):250-252, 2000.

Delegation of school health services to unlicensed assisitve personnel: a position paper of the National Association of State School Nurse Consultants, *J Sch Nurs* 11(4):13-16, 1995.

Derelian D: *They're not little adults: children's nutrition and dietary guidelines,* Rosemont, IL, 1996, National Dairy Council.

Doyen MM, Duffy DK, Metz JR: Health ranks first among subjects Americans believe students should know, *Colorado School Health News* 14:1-2, 1999.

DuRant RH and others: Weapon carrying on school property among middle school students, *Arch Pediatr Adoles Med* 153(3):21-26, 1999.

Elkind D: *The hurried child, growing up too fast too soon,* Menlo Park, CA, 1981, Addison-Wesley.

Erikson EH: *Childhood and society,* ed 2, New York, 1963, WW Norton.

Ferber R, Kryger M: *Principles and practice of sleep medicine in the child,* Philadelphia, 1995, WB Saunders.

Furnival, RA, Street KA, Schunk, JE: Too many pediatric trampoline injuries, Pediatrics 103(5)e57, 1999.

Grossman D: Teaching kids to kill, *National Forum* 80(4):10-14, 2000.

Hamilton JT: The market for television violence, *National Forum* 80(4):15-18, 2000.

Kerker BD and others: Identification of violence in the home: pediatric and parental reports, *Arch Pediatr Adoles Med* 154(5): 475-462, 2000.

Kumpulainen K, Rasanen E, Henttonen I: Children involved in bullying: Psychological disturbance and the persistence of the involvement, *Child Abuse Negl* 23(12):1253-1262, 1999.

Liller KD and others: Middle school students and bicycle helmet use: knowledge, Attitudes, beliefs, and behaviors, *J School Health* 68(8):329-333, 1998.

Marx E, Wolley SF, editors: *Health is academic: a guide to coordinated school health programs,* New York, 1998, Teacher's College Press.

Maternal and Child Health Bureau: *Basic emergency lifesaving skills (BELS): a framework for teaching emergency lifesaving skills to children and adolescents,* Newton, MA, 1999, Children's Safety Network, Education Development Center.

McCloskey LA, Walker M: Posttraumatic stress in children exposed to family violence and single-event trauma, *J Am Acad Child Adolesc Psychiatr* 39(1):108-115, 2000.

Merzenich MM and others: Temporal processing deficits of language-learning impaired children ameliorated by training, *Science* 271:77-81, 1996.

Morbidity and Mortality Weekly Report: Airbag associated fatal injuries to infants and children riding in front passenger seats—United States, *MMWR* 44(45): 845-847, 1995.

National Association of School Nurses: School health nursing services: exploring national issues and priorities, *J Sch Nurs* 12(3):23-36, 1996.

Neff EJ, Dale JC: Worries of school-age children, *J Soc Pediatr Nurs* 1(1):27-32, 1996.

Porter S and others: *Children and youth assisted by medical technology in educational settings,* ed 2, Baltimore, 1996, Paul H Brookes.

Rhodes AM: Liability for unlicensed assistive personnel, Part I, *MCN* 22:269, 1997.

Ryan-Wenger NA: Children, coping and the stress of illness: a synthesis of research, *J Soc Pediatr Nurs* 1(3):126-138, 1996.

Singer MI and others: Contributors to violent behavior among elementary and middle school children, *Pediatrics* 104(4):878-884, 1999.

Skaug W: The Jonesboro school shootings: lessons for us all (commentaries), *Pediatrics* 103(1):156, 1999.

Sourander A and others: Persistence of bullying from childhood to adolescence—a longitudinal 8-year follow-up study, *Child Abuse Negl* 24(7):873-881, 2000.

Stickler GB: Worries of parents and their children, *Clin Pediatr* 35(2):84-90, 1996.

Stormshak EA and others: Parenting practices and child disruptive behavior problems in early elementary school, *J Clin Child Psychol* 29(1):17-29, 2000.

Twelfth National Conference on School Transportation: *National standards for school buses and school bus operations,* revised ed, Warrensburg, 1995, Missouri Safety Council, Central Missouri State University.

Vessey JA: Coordinated school health, *Pediatr Nurs* 26(3):303-304, 307, 2000.

Williams K and others: Association of common health symptoms with bullying in primary school children, *BMJ* 313(7048):17-19, 1996.

Wilson CB, Lewis DB, Penix LA: Immunodeficiency of immaturity. In Stiehm R, editor: *Immunologic disorders in infants and children,* ed 4, Philadelphia, 1996, WB Saunders.

# Chapter *18*

# Health Problems of Middle Childhood

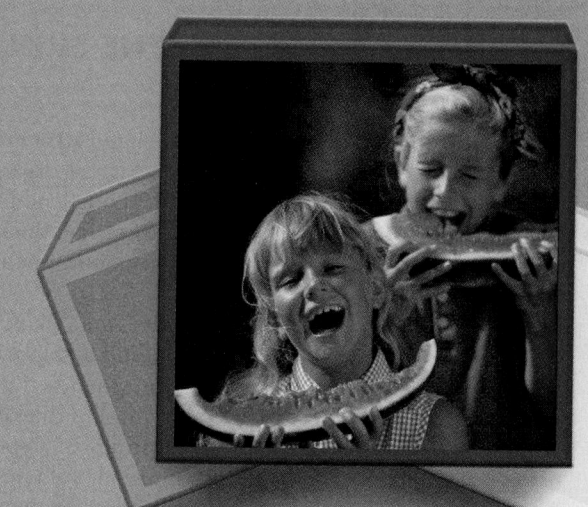

## Chapter Outline

**DISORDERS AFFECTING THE SKIN, 740**
**The Skin, 740**
Purposes of the Skin, 740
Skin Structure, 740
Skin of Younger Children, 742
**Skin Lesions, 742**
**Wounds, 745**
Process of Wound Healing, 745
Factors That Influence Healing, 748
**General Therapeutic Management, 749**
Dressings, 749
Topical Therapy, 749
Systemic Therapy, 749
**Nursing Care of the Child with a Skin Disorder, 751**
*Nursing Care Plan: The Child with a Skin Disorder, 756*

**INFECTIONS OF THE SKIN, 754**
**Bacterial Infections, 754**
**Viral Infections, 755**
**Dermatophytoses (Fungal Infections), 759**
**Scabies, 760**
**Pediculosis Capitis, 761**

**SYSTEMIC DISORDERS RELATED TO SKIN LESIONS, 763**
**Systemic Mycotic (Fungal) Infections, 763**
**Rickettsial Infections, 763**

Lyme Disease, 763
Cat Scratch Disease (CSD), 766

**SKIN DISORDERS RELATED TO CHEMICAL OR PHYSICAL CONTACTS, 767**
**Contact Dermatitis, 767**
**Poison Ivy, Oak, and Sumac, 767**
**Foreign Bodies, 768**
Cactus Spines, 769
**Sunburn, 769**
**Cold Injury, 770**
**Hypothermia, 771**

**SKIN DISORDERS RELATED TO DRUG SENSITIVITY, 772**
**Drug Reactions, 772**
**Erythema Multiforme, 772**
**Erythema Multiforme Exudativum (Stevens-Johnson Syndrome) (SJS), 773**
**Toxic Epidermal Necrolysis (TEN) (Lyell Disease), 773**

**MISCELLANEOUS AND CONGENITAL SKIN PROBLEMS, 773**
**Neurofibromatosis-1 (NF1), 773**

**BITES AND STINGS, 775**
**Arthropod Bites and Stings, 775**
Hymenoptera Stings, 775
Arachnid Bites, 776

Ticks, 777
**Animal Bites, 778**
**Snakebites, 779**
**Human Bites, 779**

**DENTAL DISORDERS, 780**
**Dental Caries, 780**
**Periodontal Disease, 781**
**Malocclusion, 781**
**Trauma, 782**

**DISORDERS OF CONTINENCE, 783**
**Enuresis, 783**
**Encopresis, 785**

**DISORDERS WITH BEHAVIORAL COMPONENTS, 786**
**Attention Deficit Hyperactivity Disorder (ADHD), 786**
**Learning Disability (LD), 791**
**Tic Disorders, 792**
**Tourette Syndrome (TS), 793**
**Posttraumatic Stress Disorder (PTSD), 794**
**School Phobia, 794**
**Recurrent Abdominal Pain (RAP), 796**
**Conversion Reaction, 797**
**Childhood Depression, 797**
**Childhood Schizophrenia, 799**

## Related Topics

Acne, Ch. 20
Autism, Ch. 13
"Birthmarks," Ch. 9
Bullous Impetigo, Ch. 9
Burns, Ch. 29
Candidiasis, Ch. 9
Communicable Diseases, Ch. 16

Dental Health: Infant, Ch. 12; Toddler, Ch. 14; Preschooler, Ch. 15; School-Age Child, Ch. 17
Maintaining Healthy Skin, Ch. 27
Pain Assessment; Pain Management, Ch. 26
Physical Assessment: Newborn, Ch. 8

Physical Examination: Skin, Ch. 7
Preparation for Procedures, Ch. 27
Restraints, Ch. 27
Sexually Transmitted Diseases, Ch. 20
Skin Disorders (Infancy), Ch. 13
Suicide, Ch. 21

# DISORDERS AFFECTING THE SKIN

## The Skin

The skin and its component and associated structures constitute the integumentary system. The largest organ in the body, the skin is a thin structure (only about 1 mm thick at birth, increasing to approximately twice that thickness at maturity) that serves primarily as an insulator, not as an organ of exchange.

Anatomically and physiologically the skin differs markedly in various areas of the body, and each variation is adapted to meet special stresses. Regions such as the soles of the feet, the eyelids, and the back vary in skin thickness and looseness and in the kinds and quantities of appendages they contain, such as sweat glands and hair follicles. These variations are the basis for the localization of many disorders to specific areas and for the distribution of certain eruptions in characteristic patterns.

### Purposes of the Skin

This functionally simple but morphologically complex structure serves several physical functions essential to life.

**Protection.** The skin serves as a protection against trauma, including mechanical, thermal, chemical, and radiant. The intact, tough outer layer is a mechanical barrier. Organisms and chemicals penetrate it with difficulty, and it is further protected by the oily and slightly acid secretions of its sebaceous glands, which limit the growth of bacteria. The acidic level of a pH of 4.5 to 5 is known as the skin's *acid mantle.*

**Impermeability.** Very few substances are able to penetrate the skin with ease. It seals the body from the environment. The outer side of the upper layer, with its low water content, is in equilibrium with the viable cells underneath. It protects against loss of essential body constituents to the environment. The effectiveness of this impermeable membrane is demonstrated by the profuse fluid loss that follows damage to the epidermis by burns, injury, poison ivy, or other agents. Loss of water and some electrolytes takes place only through pores in this effective barrier.

**Heat Regulation.** The skin adjusts heat loss to heat production to maintain the thermal balance of the body. This is accomplished primarily through functioning of cutaneous blood vessels and sweat glands. The vascular supply to the skin, much more extensive than needed for tissue nourishment, is regulated by way of central and local neural and hormonal processes.

**Sensation.** As a sensory organ, perceptions (touch, pain, heat, and cold) are transmitted through the nerves that permeate the skin. The skin may also betray strong feelings: blushing (shame or embarrassment), redness (anger), blanching (fear), and sweating (anxiety).

### Skin Structure

The skin consists of two layers: the epidermis and the dermis. Under the dermis is the subcutaneous tissue, or hypo-

dermis, which is composed primarily of fatty tissue of varying thickness. The activity of the skin is controlled by the autonomic nervous system and the endocrine glands (Fig. 18-1).

The efficiency with which the skin layers prevent evaporative loss of water (independent of sweat) increases with development. A transitional zone between the epidermal layers allows more of the larger fluid content (70%) of the lower layers to enter the outer, drier layers (15% water), where it is lost in greater or lesser amounts, depending on environmental temperature and humidity. In the young child the transitional zone is less effective than that in an older child or adult. The fluid loss is most marked in the preterm infant.

**Epidermis.** The epidermis, the outermost portion of relatively uniform thickness, consists of five layers. The lowest, the *stratum germinativum,* or "basal layer," is composed of specialized cells called *keratinocytes* or *basal cells* that are continually replacing the cell population. As they multiply, the older cells are displaced outward by the constant stream of new cells. The older cells progressively flatten and alter until they form dead, scalelike, or horny flakes with no cellular details and that are composed of *keratin.* These flakes are constantly sloughed off the surface of the body. This continual epidermal renewal is nourished by fluid from blood vessels in the dermis. The intact epidermis provides a relatively impenetrable barrier to the loss of body contents and the entrance of environmental hazards.

All layers of the epidermis consist of peaks and valleys. In the basal layer, the peaks that protrude downward into the dermis are called *rete pegs* or *rete ridges.* They help anchor the epidermis to the dermis. The epidermis also contains specialized cellular invaginations: the *glandular appendages* and *hair follicles.* Although they are situated mainly in the dermis, these structures are lined with epithelial cells and are derived from the epithelial skin layer. This has significance when a large area of epidermis is damaged. It is from the cells lining these structures that new epithelium is derived.

Diseases of the skin focus sharply on the epidermis, which is the site of many distinctive patterns, ranging from the vesiculation of contact dermatitis to common superficial tumors. Clearly visible, these morphologic changes produce the varied patterns on which a dermatologic diagnosis is made.

**Dermis.** The dermis, or *corium,* constitutes the bulk of the skin. It is a firm, fibrous, and elastic connective tissue network containing an elaborate system of blood vessels, lymphatics, and nerves and varies throughout the body from 1 to 4 mm in thickness. It is invaded by the epidermal downgrowth of hair follicles and glands. Functionally, the corium has a major protective role for these varied essential components of the skin.

More hidden than the epidermis, changes in the dermis are more difficult to interpret on inspection. Biopsy and histologic studies are often needed to confirm a diagnosis based on manifestations in the corium. Because it is composed predominantly of connective tissue, the dermis frequently permits an awareness and observation of many diffuse systemic disorders of connective tissue—the *collagen diseases.*

---

■ Marilyn L. Winkelstein, PhD, RN, revised this chapter.

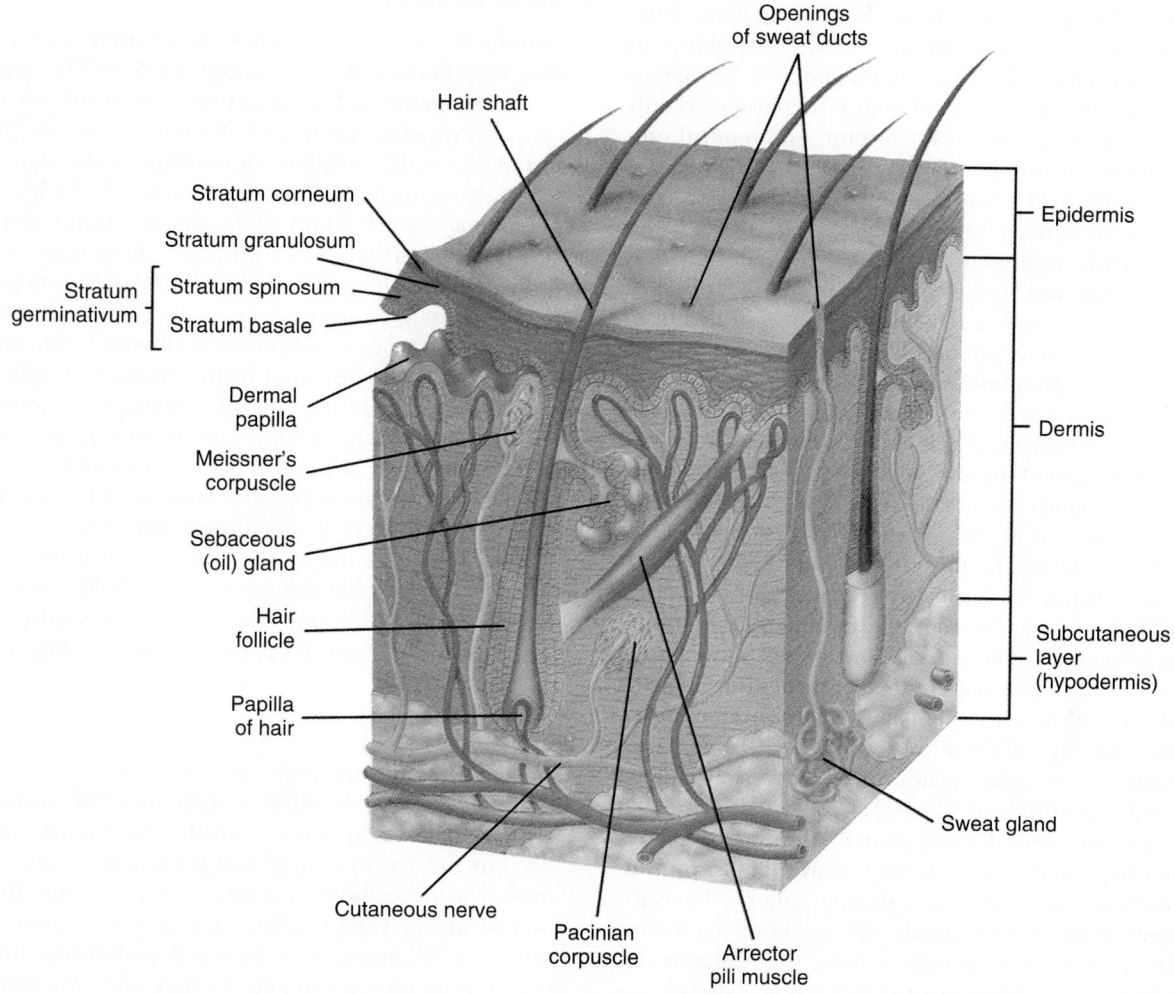

**Fig. 18-1** Microscopic diagram of the skin. Epidermis, shown in longitudinal section, is raised at one corner to reveal the ridges in the dermis. (From Thibodeau GA, Patton KT: *Anatomy and physiology*, ed 3, St Louis, 1996, Mosby.)

**Subcutaneous Tissue.** A thick layer of subcutaneous tissue lies beneath the dermis and is composed of a looser type of connective tissue that varies greatly in various parts of the body. In addition to larger blood vessels, lymph channels, and nerve trunks, the subcutaneous tissue serves as a depot for the storage of fat that acts as a cushion, insulates the body against cold, and largely determines its contours.

**Hair.** The various skin appendages develop at different times and at different rates. An extensive growth of fine body hair, *lanugo,* begins to appear at the end of the second intrauterine month, reaches its maximum development between the seventh and eighth months of fetal life, and begins to decrease before birth. It continues to regress steadily during early infancy and is replaced by a less extensive distribution of hair. *Hair follicles* are fully developed at birth, but the amount and texture of scalp hair vary among individual infants. The *scalp hair* is lost during the first few months after birth and then is slowly replaced by permanent hair, which gradually thickens and often darkens as the child grows.

At puberty the secretion of androgenic hormones stimulates an increase in the thickening and darkening of scalp hair, the growth of hair in the axilla and pubic regions of both sexes, and the growth of facial hair in boys. Late in adolescence some boys acquire additional amounts and distribution of body hair, such as on the chest.

**Sebaceous Glands.** The sebaceous glands form in connection with hair follicles. Their function is to produce a fatty secretion called *sebum* that helps keep the skin supple by decreasing water loss. The sebaceous activity is maintained at a relatively constant rate by the secretion of androgens; an increase in androgens causes an increase in sebum production. Sebaceous glands have a regional distribution and are most abundant on the scalp, the face, and the genitalia; are less numerous on the trunk; are sparse on the extremities; and do not appear on the palms and soles.

Sebaceous glands begin to form during the fifth month of fetal life and are very active during the month before birth, when they produce the protective *vernix caseosa* observed on newborn infants. The sebaceous activity slowly subsides after birth and continues to decrease throughout infancy. In the newborn period and early infancy, sebaceous secretion may cause minor problems such as "cradle cap" in some infants. The secretion remains low during early childhood, which contributes to dryness and susceptibility to chapping, especially during the winter months. Sebaceous secretion gradually rises in childhood to increase markedly at puberty, where it remains constant and contributes greatly to the disturbing skin problems of adolescence.

**Sweat Glands.** The sweat glands, both eccrine and apocrine, are present at birth. They appear between the fifth and seventh months of fetal life, but their activity is scant. The *eccrine sweat glands* function primarily as part of the body heat–regulating mechanism and to some extent in maintaining electrolyte balance. They produce a transparent, watery liquid (*perspiration* or *sweat*) that is composed of salts, ammonia, uric acid, urea, and other wastes. At birth the density of the eccrine glands is greater than at any other time of life (because of the smaller skin surface area and because no new glands are formed after birth). The sweat glands are equivalent in size, structural maturity, and position within the dermis in the full-term newborn and the adult. They function at birth but produce more sweat as childhood advances, to reach full potential at puberty. There are individual differences in the amount of sweat produced, and there are no sex differences until after puberty, when males sweat more than females. Numerous factors influence the amount and chemical content of the sweat (e.g., emotions and some disease states, such as congestive heart failure in infancy and cystic fibrosis).

*Apocrine sweat glands,* located primarily in the axilla, areola of the breast, and anal area, are inactive throughout infancy and childhood and mature during puberty. They are much larger than eccrine glands and are connected with hair follicles. When the secretions from these glands are acted on by bacteria, they cause the unpleasant odor associated with sweating.

## Skin of Younger Children

The major skin layers arise from different embryologic origins. Early in the embryonic period, a single layer of epithelium forms from the ectoderm, while simultaneously the corium develops from the mesenchyme. In the infant and small child the epidermis is still loosely bound to the dermis, partly because the rete pegs are flat. This poor adherence causes the layers to separate readily during an inflammatory process to form blisters. This is especially true in preterm infants, who have an even greater propensity to blister formation and separation during careless handling (such as removal of adhesive tape). The skin is thinner than in older children, and the cells of all strata are more compressed.

Several characteristics influence skin responses in infants and young children. Their skin is far more susceptible to superficial bacterial infection. They are more likely to have associated systemic symptoms with some infections and are more apt to react to a primary irritant than to a sensitizing allergen. Infants and young children are more frequently affected by chronic atopic dermatitis (eczema). The infant's skin is much more prone to develop a toxic erythema as a result of skin eruptions or drug reactions and is subject to maceration, infection, and the moisture retention associated with diaper rash.

# Skin Lesions

Lesions of the skin can result from a variety of etiologic factors. In general, skin lesions originate from (1) contact with injurious agents such as infectious organisms, toxic chemicals, and physical trauma; (2) hereditary factors; (3) an external factor that produces a reaction in the skin (e.g., allergens); or (4) a systemic disease in which the lesions are a cutaneous manifestation (e.g., measles, lupus erythematosus, nutritional deficiency diseases). Responses are highly individual. An agent that may be harmless to one individual may be damaging to another, and a single agent may produce various types of responses in different individuals.

Another factor involved in the etiology of skin manifestations is the age of the child. For example, infants are subject to "birthmark" malformations and atopic dermatitis that appear early in life, the school-age child is susceptible to ringworm of the scalp, and acne is a characteristic skin disorder of puberty. Contact dermatitis, such as poison ivy, is seen only where the noxious agent is a feature of the area. Similarly, insect bites are associated with life-cycle and seasonal activities. Although less common in children, tension and anxiety may produce, modify, or prolong many skin conditions.

## Pathophysiology of Dermatitis

Over half of dermatologic problems are various forms of dermatitis. This implies a sequence of inflammatory changes in the skin that are grossly and microscopically similar but diverse in course and causation. Acute responses produce intercellular and intracellular edema, the formation of intradermal vesicles, and an initial minimum infiltration of inflammatory cells into the epidermis. In the dermis there is edema, vascular dilation, and early perivascular cellular infiltration. The location and manner of these reactions produce the lesions characteristic of each disorder. The changes are reversible, and the skin ordinarily recovers without blemish and completely intact unless complicating factors such as ulceration from the primary irritant, scratching, and infection are introduced or underlying vascular disease develops. In chronic conditions permanent effects are seen that vary according to the disorder, the general condition of the affected individual, and available therapy.

## Clinical Manifestations and Diagnostic Evaluation

Although the history and subjective symptoms are explored first, objective findings are often noted simultaneously. One of the more advantageous aspects of skin lesions is that often the diagnosis is readily established after simple, careful inspection.

**History and Subjective Symptoms.**  Many cutaneous lesions are associated with local symptoms, the most common of which is itching (*pruritus*) that varies in kind and intensity. Pain or tenderness often accompanies some skin lesions, and other sensations may be described as burning, prickling, stinging, or crawling. Alterations in local feeling or sensation include absence of sensation (*anesthesia*), excessive sensitiveness (*hyperesthesia*), diminished sensation (*hypesthesia* or *hypoesthesia*), or abnormal sensation, such as burning or prickling (*paresthesia*). These symptoms may remain localized or may migrate, may be constant or intermittent, and may be aggravated by a specific activity or circumstance, such as exposure to sunlight.

It is also important to determine whether the child has had an allergic condition such as asthma or hay fever or has had previous skin disease. Atopic dermatitis, often associated with allergies, frequently begins in infancy. It should be determined when the lesion or symptom first became apparent, as well as whether it is related to ingestion of a food or other substance, including any medication the child might be taking. It should be kept in mind that the condition may be related to an activity such as contact with plants, insects, or chemicals.

**Objective Findings.**  Much can be determined by the distribution, size, morphology, and arrangement of the lesions. Extrinsic causes usually result from physical, chemical, or allergic irritants or from an infectious agent such as bacteria, fungi, viruses, or animal parasites. Skin manifestations can be produced by such intrinsic causes as a specific infection (such as measles or chickenpox), drug sensitization, or other allergic phenomena. Other diagnostic tools are subjective symptoms, the history, and medical and laboratory studies.

**Lesion.**  According to the nature of the pathologic process, lesions assume more or less distinct characteristics. Names that have been applied to these lesions are important for descriptive purposes in the processes of record keeping and communication. Nurses should also become familiar with the more common terms used to describe skin lesions seen in dermatologic conditions:

> **Erythema**—A reddened area caused by increased amounts of oxygenated blood in the dermal vasculature.
>
> **Ecchymoses (bruises)**—Localized red or purple discolorations caused by extravasation of blood into dermis and subcutaneous tissues.
>
> **Petechiae**—Pinpoint, tiny, and sharp circumscribed spots in the superficial layers of the epidermis.
>
> **Primary lesions**—Skin changes produced by some causative factor (Fig. 18-2). Common primary lesions in pediatric skin disorders are macules, papules, and vesicles.
>
> **Secondary lesions**—Changes that result from alteration in the primary lesions, such as those caused by rubbing, scratching, medication, or involution and healing (Fig. 18-3).
>
> **Distribution pattern**—The pattern in which lesions are distributed over the body, whether local or generalized, and specific areas associated with the lesions.
>
> **Configuration and arrangement**—The size, shape, and arrangement of a lesion or groups of lesions (e.g., *discrete* [individually distinct], *clustered* [appear close together], *diffuse* [scattered], *confluent* [running together], or *annular* [ringed] or *arciform* lesions).

**Laboratory Studies.**  When it is suspected that a skin problem might be related to a systemic disease, such as one of the collagen diseases or immunodeficiency disease, stud-

Macule—flat; nonpalpable; circumscribed; less than 1 cm in diameter; brown, red, purple, white, or tan in color
Examples: Freckles; flat moles; rubella; rubeola

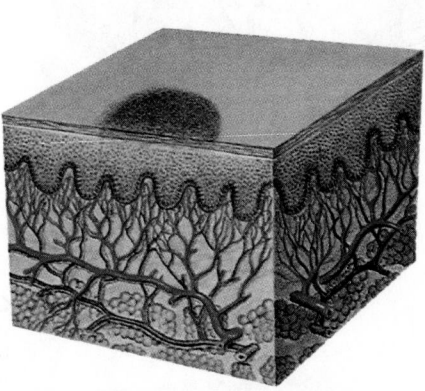

Plaque—elevated; flat topped; firm; rough; superficial papule greater than 1 cm in diameter; may be coalesced papules
Examples: Psoriasis; seborrheic and actinic keratoses

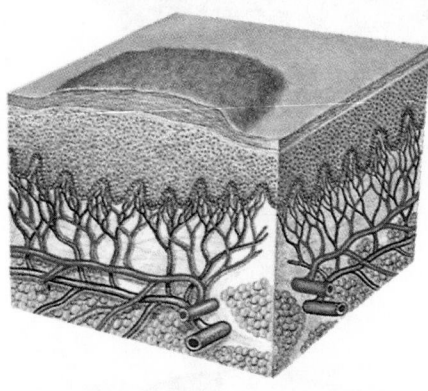

Patch—flat; nonpalpable; irregular in shape; macule that is greater than 1 cm in diameter
Examples: Vitiligo; port-wine marks

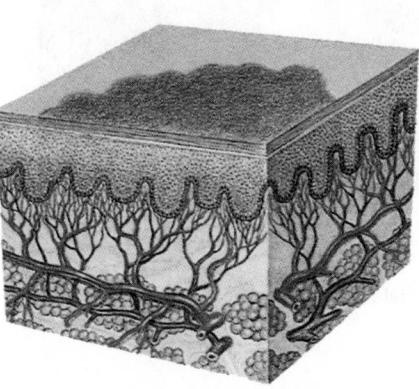

Wheal—elevated, irregularly shaped area of cutaneous edema; solid, transient, changing, variable diameter; pale pink with lighter center
Examples: Urticaria; insect bites

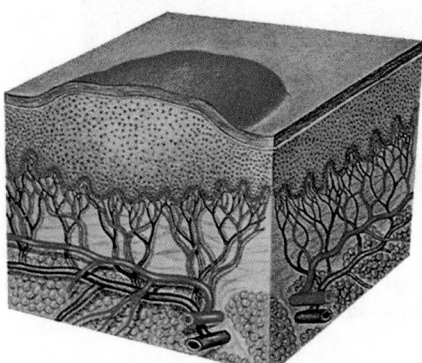

**Fig. 18-2**  Primary skin lesions. (From Seidel HM and others: *Mosby's guide to physical examination,* ed 4, St Louis, 1999, Mosby.)

*Continued*

Papule—elevated; palpable; firm; circumscribed; less than 1 cm in diameter; brown, red, pink, tan, or bluish red in color
Examples: Warts; drug-related eruptions; pigmented nevi

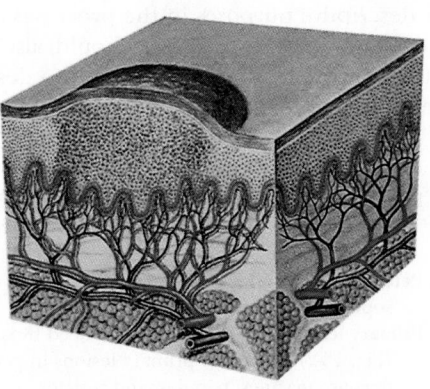

Nodule—elevated; firm; circumscribed; palpable; deeper in dermis than papule; 1 to 2 cm in diameter
Examples: Erythema nodosum; lipomas

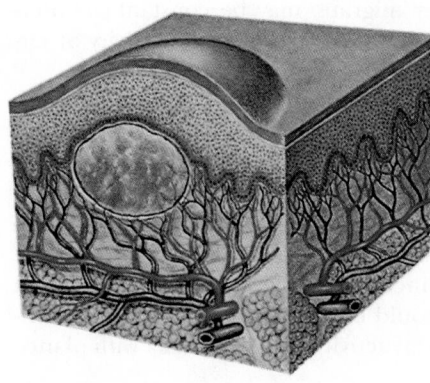

Vesicle—elevated; circumscribed; superficial; filled with serous fluid; less than 1 cm in diameter
Examples: Blister; varicella

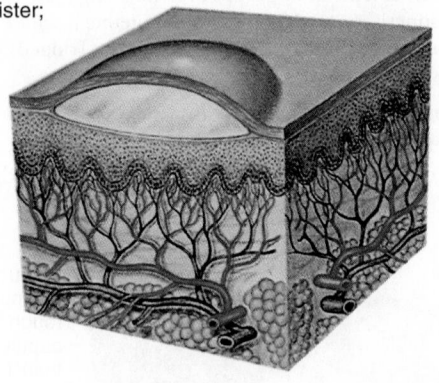

Pustule—elevated; superficial; similar to vesicle but filled with purulent fluid
Examples: Impetigo; acne; variola

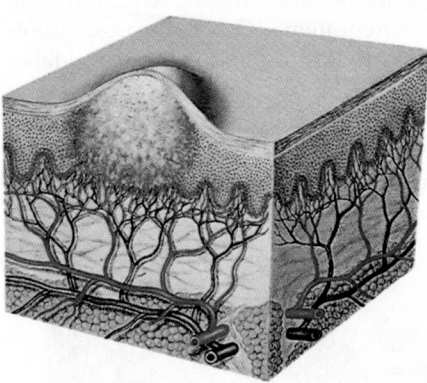

Bulla—vesicle greater than 1 cm in diameter
Examples: Blister; pemphigus vulgaris

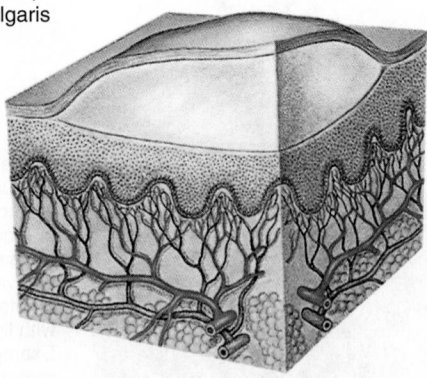

Cyst—elevated; circumscribed; palpable; encapsulated; filled with liquid or semisolid material
Example: Sebaceous cyst

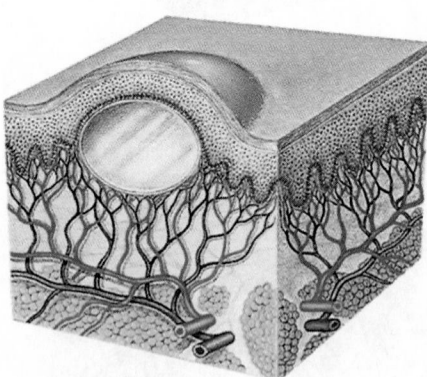

**Fig. 18-2, cont'd** Primary skin lesions. (From Seidel HM and others: *Mosby's guide to physical examination*, ed 4, St Louis, 1999, Mosby.)

ies are needed to rule out these possibilities. Diagnostic modalities include microscopic examination, cultures, skin scrapings or biopsy, cytodiagnosis, patch testing, and Wood light examination. Allergic skin testing and various other laboratory tests (blood count, sedimentation rate) are used when indicated.

## Wounds

Wounds are structural or physiologic disruptions of the integument that call for normal or abnormal tissue repair responses. All wounds can be classified as acute or chronic. *Acute wounds* are those that heal uneventfully within the usual time frame. *Chronic wounds* are those that do not heal in the expected time frame or are associated with many complications. In children most wounds are acute and can be prevented from becoming chronic through appropriate nursing care. Wounds are classified in the same manner as burns: partial-thickness, full-thickness, and complex wounds that include muscle and/or bone. Wounds that often become chronic are burns and *pressure ulcers,* localized areas of cellular necrosis that develop when soft tissue is compressed between a bony prominence and a firm surface. (See Burns, Chapter 29, and Maintaining Healthy Skin, Chapter 27.)

Some types of acute wounds include:

**Abrasion**—Removal of the superficial layers of skin by rubbing or scraping
**Evulsion**—Forcible pulling out or extraction of tissue
**Laceration**—Torn or jagged wound; accidental cut wound
**Incision**—Division of the skin made with a sharp object; cut
**Penetrating wound**—Disruption of the skin surface that extends into underlying tissue or into a body cavity
**Puncture**—Wound with relatively small opening compared with the depth

### Process of Wound Healing

**Epidermal Injuries.**  Abrasions are the most common epidermal wounds of childhood, usually in the form of a skinned knee or elbow. In most injuries the margins of the abraded area are superficial, involving only the outer layers of epidermis, although the central portion may extend into the dermis. Initially the defect is filled by a blood clot and necrotic debris, which subsequently dehydrate to form a scab. Epithelial tissue is composed of *labile cells,* which are constantly destroyed and replaced throughout life. Injury to these tissues results in *regeneration* (i.e., rapid replacement by similar cells).

The epithelial wound heals by migration and proliferation of epithelial cells from the wound margin and from cells surviving in transected skin appendages. This response

Scale—heaped-up keratinized cells; flaky exfoliation; irregular; thick or thin; dry or oily; varied size; silver, white, or tan in color
Examples: Psoriasis; exfoliative dermatitis

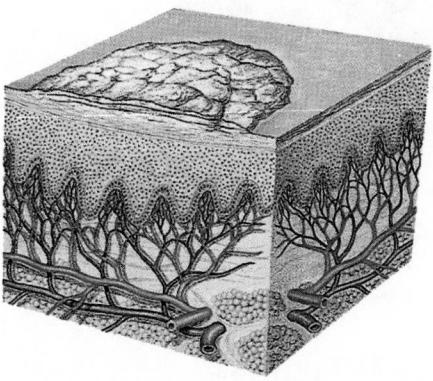

Crust—dried serum, blood, or purulent exudate; slightly elevated; size varies; brown, red, black, tan, or straw in color
Examples: Scab on abrasion; eczema

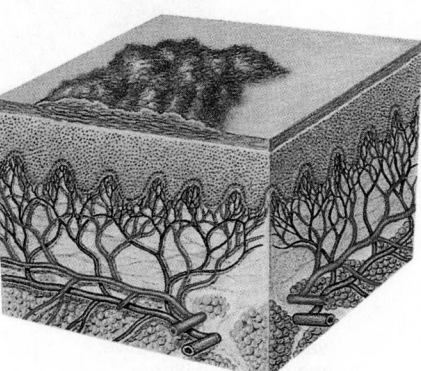

Lichenification—rough, thickened epidermis; accentuated skin markings caused by rubbing or irritation; often involves flexor aspect of extremity
Example: Chronic dermatitis

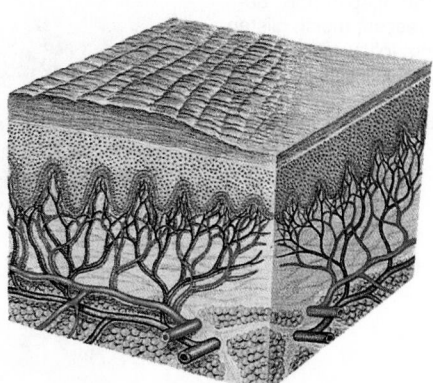

**Fig. 18-3**   Secondary skin lesions. (From Seidel HM and others: *Mosby's guide to physical examination,* ed 4, St Louis, 1999, Mosby.)

*Continued*

Scar—thin to thick fibrous tissue replacing injured dermis; irregular; pink, red, or white in color; may be atrophic or hypertrophic
Example: Healed wound or surgical incision

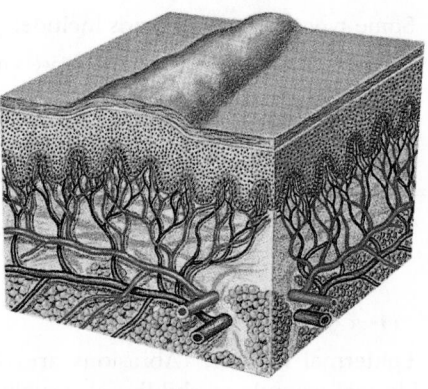

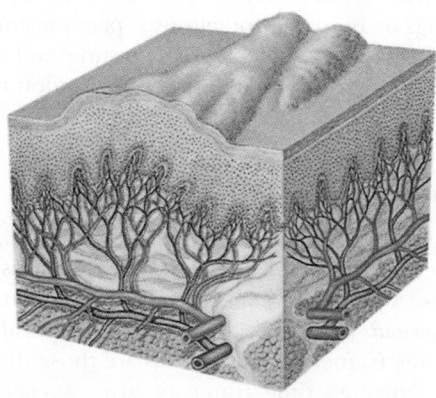

Keloid— irregularly shaped, elevated, progressively enlarging scar; grows beyond boundaries of wound; caused by excessive collagen formation during healing
Example: Keloid from ear piercing or burn scar

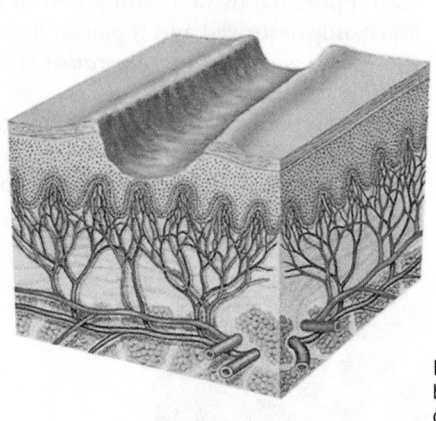

Excoriation—loss of epidermis; linear or hollowed-out crusted area; dermis exposed
Examples: Abrasion; scratch

Fissure—linear crack or break from epidermis to dermis; small; deep; red
Examples: Athlete's foot; cheilosis

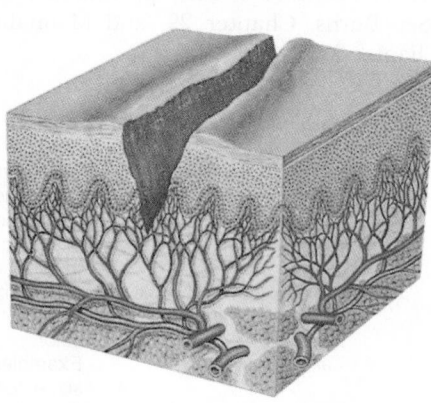

Erosion—loss of all or part of epidermis; depressed; moist; glistening; follows rupture of vesicle or bulla; larger than fissure
Examples: Varicella; variola following rupture

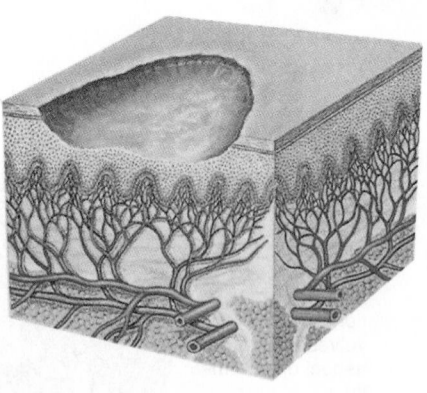

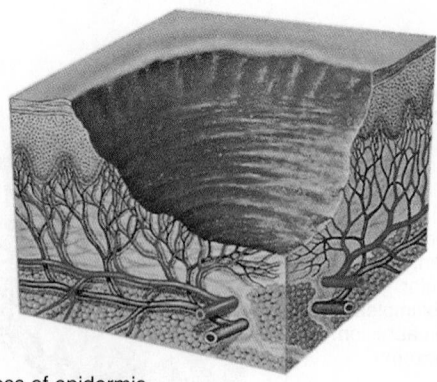

Ulcer—loss of epidermis and dermis; concave; varies in size; exudative; red or reddish blue
Examples: Decubiti; stasis ulcers

**Fig. 18-3, cont'd** Secondary skin lesions. (From Seidel HM and others: *Mosby's guide to physical examination*, ed 4, St Louis, 1999, Mosby.)

begins within 24 to 48 hours after the wound is incurred. Cell migration ceases when migrating cells make contact with epithelial cells migrating from all other sites. Fixed basal cells adjacent to the wound edge and in skin appendages begin to divide rapidly to replace the migrated cells. As resurfacing is accomplished, the migrated cells begin to divide and thicken the new epithelial layer.

Epithelial cells advance over the wound surface by "flowing." The first cell advances, anchors, and then moves no more. Instead, a cell from behind advances over it, anchors, and subsequently is overridden by other cells that advance over both of the primary cells—similar to a leapfrog movement. Epithelial cells move most rapidly in moist environments, such as those covered with a transparent or other occlusive-type dressing, and the rate of epithelization depends on a variety of elements, particularly the amount of oxygen supplied to the wound. Allowing the skin to dry and form an *eschar* or crust (scab) impedes the migration of epithelial cells (Fig. 18-4). In addition, fluid may collect and infection may occur under the eschar.

**Injury to Deeper Tissues.**   Tissues composed of *permanent cells,* such as muscle and some nerve cells, are unable to regenerate. Therefore these tissues repair themselves by substituting fibrous connective tissue for the injured tissue. This fibrous tissue, or *scar,* serves as a patch to preserve or restore the continuity of the tissue. Wounds involving permanent cells include surgical incisions, lacerations, ulcers, evulsions, and full-thickness burns. Injured cells of glandular organs and bones, composed of *stable* cells, multiply less vigorously and heal more slowly (see Bone Healing and Remodeling, Chapter 39). With some wounds an overgrowth of nerve endings may occur, resulting in *allodynia,* or sensation of pain from nonpainful stimuli, such as light touch.

**Process of Wound Healing.**   The nonspecific repair mechanism of wound healing with scar formation involves the processes of inflammation, fibroplasia, scar contraction, and scar maturation. The initial response at the site of injury is *inflammation,* a vascular and cellular response, which prepares the tissues for the subsequent repair process. There is a transient constriction of transected blood vessels, lasting 5 to 10 minutes, followed by active vasodilation of all local small vessels and increased blood flow to the area. This is accompanied by increased permeability of small venules, allowing plasma to leak into surrounding tissues *(edema).* A blood clot is formed along wound edges, forming a framework for future growth of capillaries *(angiogenesis)* and epithelial cells.

At the same time, vessel walls become lined with leukocytes, primarily neutrophils, which pass through the walls and concentrate at the injured site, where they ingest bacteria and debris *(phagocytosis).* The presence of neutrophils is superseded by macrophages, which continue phagocytosis, and also by growth factors needed for skin repair and angiogenesis. Fibroblasts attracted to the area from blood vessels deposit fibrin throughout the clot. Adjacent capillaries begin to form buds that stretch across the supporting fibrin threads, and epithelial cells secrete a fibrolytic enzyme that allows their advancement across the wound. This initial phase of wound healing takes place during the first 3 to 5 days following injury. The wound is weakest at this time.

*Fibroplasia (granulation* or *proliferation),* the second phase of healing, lasts from 5 days to 4 weeks. Fibroblasts, immature connective tissue cells, migrate to the healing site and begin to secrete collagen into the meshwork spaces. Granulation tissue is highly vascular, "beefy" red, and shiny connective tissue that organizes and restructures, forming thicker, stronger fibers arranged in orderly layers. A thin layer of epithelial tissue is regenerated over the surface of the wound, and leukocytes gradually disappear from the area. The wound is fragile at this time, and granulation tissue bleeds profusely if disturbed.

During *contraction* and *maturation,* the third and fourth phases of wound healing, collagen continues to be deposited and organized into layers, compressing the new blood vessels and gradually ceasing blood flow across the wound. Fibroblasts disappear as the wound becomes stronger. Fibroblast movement causes contraction of the healing area, helping to bring wound edges closer together. A mature scar is then formed. Initially the scar is pink and raised. With maturation, the scar becomes pale in color, does not tan when exposed to sunlight, will not sweat or produce hair, and may cause itching. The maturation process may continue for years, and the extent to which the scar remodels and matures varies among individuals.

Children heal aggressively with abundant scar tissue, especially during growth spurts. The highly elastic quality of children's skin pulls on wounds, which defend against the pull by aggressive scarring. Consequently, the child's skin heals with more scar tissue than the less elastic skin of the adult.

**Types of Wound Healing.**   Repair healing takes place in one of three ways: by primary, secondary, or tertiary intention (Fig. 18-5). *Primary intention* healing takes place when all layers of the wound (skin, subcutaneous tissue, and muscle) margins are neatly approximated, as in a surgical incision. Unless infection interferes or the wound edges separate, these wounds heal with a minimum of scarring.

Repair by *secondary intention* takes place in wounds that occur from ulceration and lacerations in which the edges

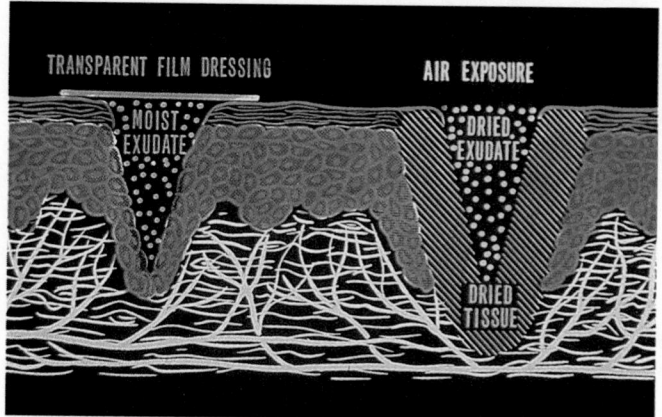

**Fig. 18-4**   Process of epithelialization is facilitated by maintaining a moist environment as opposed to a dry, open environment. In a moist environment, epithelial cells freely migrate across the wound surface. (Courtesy ConvaTec, Princeton, NJ.)

**First intention** (clean incision)

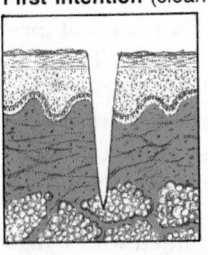 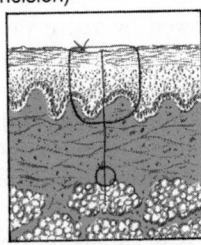 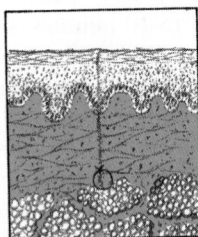

**Second intention** (wide, irregular wound)

Granulation

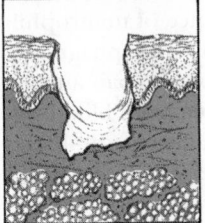 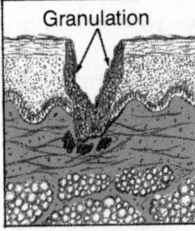 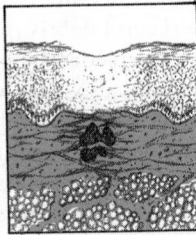

**Third intention** (puncture wound)

Granulation

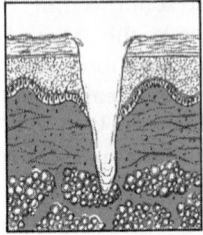 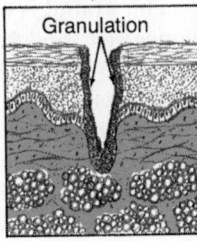 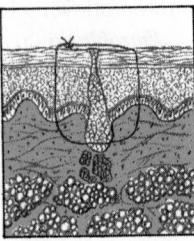

**Fig. 18-5** Types of wound healing.

| TABLE 18-1 | Factors that delay wound healing |
|---|---|
| **Factor** | **Effect on Healing** |
| Dry wound environment | Allows epithelial cells to dry out and die; impairs migration of epithelial cells across wound surface |
| **Nutritional deficiencies** | |
| Vitamin C | Inhibits formation of collagen fibers and capillary development |
| Protein | Reduces supply of amino acids for tissue repair |
| Zinc | Impairs epithelialization |
| Impaired circulation | Reduces supply of nutrients to wound area |
| | Inhibits inflammatory response and removal of debris from wound area |
| Stress (pain, poor sleep) | Releases catecholamines that cause vasoconstriction |
| **Antiseptics** | |
| Hydrogen peroxide | Toxic to fibroblasts; can cause subcutaneous gas formation (mimics gas-forming infection) |
| Povidone-iodine | Toxic to white and red blood cells and fibroblasts |
| Chlorhexidine | Toxic to white blood cells |
| Corticosteroids | Impair phagocytosis |
| | Inhibit fibroblast proliferation |
| | Depress formation of granulation tissue |
| | Inhibit wound contraction |
| Foreign bodies | Inhibit wound closure |
| | Increase inflammatory response |
| Infection | Increases inflammatory response |
| | Increases tissue destruction |
| Mechanical friction | Damages or destroys granulation tissue |
| Fluid accumulation | Accumulation in area inhibits tissues from approximating |
| Radiation | Inhibits fibroblastic activity and capillary formation |
| | May cause tissue necrosis |
| **Diseases** | |
| Diabetes mellitus | Inhibits collagen synthesis |
| | Impairs circulation and capillary growth |
| | Hyperglycemia impairs phagocytosis |
| Anemia | Reduces oxygen supply to tissues |

cannot be approximated, such as an evulsion or a third-degree burn. The inflammatory reaction may be greater, and the chance of infection is increased. Often debris, cells, and exudate must be cleaned away (debrided) before healing can take place. Healing takes place from the edges inward and from the bottom of the wound upward until the defect is filled. More granulation tissue and a larger scar are formed than in healing by primary intention.

Repair by *tertiary intention* takes place when suturing is delayed after injury or the wound later breaks down and is sutured or resutured when granulation is present. More granulation tissue is formed than in healing by primary intention, and there is a greater chance of microorganisms invading the wound. Frequently, suturing a contaminated wound is deliberately delayed to afford better removal of infection before closing. Wounds healed by tertiary intention result in a larger and deeper scar than those healed by primary intention.

### Factors That Influence Healing

During the last two decades understanding of wound healing has revolutionized the interventions used to promote healing. Emphasis has shifted from interventions directed at maintaining a dry environment that promoted eschar formation to those that promote a moist, crust-free environment that enhances the migration of epithelial cells across the wound and facilitates resurfacing.

An acute full-thickness wound kept in a moist environment usually reepithelializes in 12 to 15 days, whereas the same wound kept open to the air heals in approximately 25 to 30 days. A superficial wound covered with an occlusive dressing, rather than the typical adhesive bandage strip, heals faster and results in a better cosmetic appearance (Bonham, 2000; Skewes, 1996) (see Fig. 18-4).

Eschar (thick, fibrin-containing necrotic tissue) also interferes with healing by preventing wound contraction. In most situations it is best to remove eschar and other dead tissue from the wound. Repeated application of occlusive dressings mobilizes the body's own enzymes to lyse the eschar, a process known as *autolysis.*

Adequate nutrition is essential for wound healing. In particular, sufficient protein, calories, vitamin C, and zinc are needed for extensive wounds, such as burns; supplemental nutrition is an integral aspect of severe wound treatment.

Numerous factors delay healing (Table 18-1). Traditional practices, such as the use of antiseptics (hydrogen peroxide and povidone-iodine [Betadine] solutions) have a cytotoxic effect on healthy cells and minimal effect on controlling infections (Skewes, 1996). Povidone-iodine may be absorbed through the skin in neonates and young children and must be used with caution in patients with thyroid or renal disease.

> **NURSING ALERT**  Do not put anything in a wound that one would not put in the eye. The safest solution is normal saline.

## General Therapeutic Management

The human body tends to heal; therefore, treatment is directed toward eliminating or ameliorating influences that interfere with normal healing processes. Some disorders may demand aggressive therapy, but by and large the major aim of any treatment is to prevent further damage, eliminate the cause, prevent complications, and provide relief from discomfort while tissues undergo healing. Factors that contribute to the dermatitis and prolong the course of the disease must be eliminated when possible. The most common offenders in pediatrics are environmental factors (such as soaps, bubble baths, shampoos, rough or tight clothing, wet diapers, blankets, and toys) and the natural elements (such as dirt, sand, heat, cold, moisture, and wind). Dermatitis can also be aggravated by home remedies and medications.

### Dressings

Dressings serve the following functions: (1) provide a moist healing environment, (2) protect the wound from infection and trauma, (3) provide compression in the event of anticipated bleeding or swelling, (4) apply medication, (5) absorb drainage, (6) debride necrotic tissue, (7) reduce pain, and (8) control odor. To provide a moist environment, open wounds are covered with an occlusive ointment or dressing (Table 18-2).

Occlusive dressings can be classified according to their degree of permeability. The term *occlusive* is synonymous with *impermeable*, *semiocclusive* is synonymous with *semipermeable*, and *nonocclusive* is synonymous with *permeable* (McCulloch, Kloth, and Feedar, 1995). No one dressing meets the needs of all types of wounds. The traditional gauze dressing is a *permeable* dressing that reduces the moisture content in a wound by absorbing exudate and allowing it to evaporate. Traditional gauze dressings should not be used on open wounds because they allow wounds to dehydrate, are permeable to bacteria, increase the probability of wound sepsis, and adhere to the wound when removed, causing additional trauma to newly regenerating epithelial cells. In many situations traditional gauze dressings have been replaced with new "active occlusive" dressings, which allow for moist wound healing. Gauze dressings, however, may be the temporary dressing of choice during initial treatment of some wounds that are heavily exudative (both necrotic and infected) or when other dressings are contraindicated (McCulloch, Kloth, and Feedar, 1995).

### Topical Therapy

A variety of agents and methods are available for treatment of dermatologic problems. In selecting a therapeutic program, the practitioner considers (1) a choice of active ingredient, (2) a proper vehicle or base, (3) the cosmetic effect, (4) the cost, and (5) instructions for its use. In addition, several basic concepts are kept in mind. Overtreatment is avoided. For example, when the dermatitis is acute, the applications should be mild and bland to avoid further irritation. Broken or inflamed skin, especially in children, is more absorbent than intact skin, and chemicals that are nonirritating to intact skin may be quite irritating to inflamed skin.

Topical applications may be applied to treat the disorder, reduce the itching associated with many diseases, decrease external stimuli, or apply external heat or cold. The emollient action of soaks, baths, and lotions provides a soothing film over the skin surface that reduces external stimuli. Ordinarily, lukewarm, tepid, or cool applications offer the greatest relief.

> **NURSING ALERT**  Application of heat tends to aggravate most conditions, and its use is usually reserved for reducing specific inflammatory processes, such as folliculitis and cellulitis.

**Topical Corticosteroid Therapy.** The glucocorticoids are the therapeutic agents used most widely for skin disorders. Their local antiinflammatory effects are merely palliative, so that the medication must be applied until the disease state undergoes a remission or the causative agent is eliminated. Corticosteroids are applied directly to the affected area, and because they are essentially nonsensitizing and have only minor side effects, they can be applied over prolonged periods with continuing effectiveness. As with the use of any steroids, their use in large amounts may mask signs of infection, and symptoms may be exacerbated following termination of the drug. Families are cautioned that the medication cannot be used for all skin disorders. The concentrations available without prescription are not adequate for some stubborn conditions (e.g., psoriasis) and may cause worsening of inflammation caused by fungus or bacteria. It has also been found that users apply too much topical hydrocortisone; therefore, they should be counseled that it is both effective and economical to apply only a thin film and massage it into the skin.

**Other Topical Therapies.** Other topical treatments include chemical cautery (especially useful for warts), cryosurgery, electrodesiccation (chiefly used for warts, granulomas, and nevi), ultraviolet therapy (primarily used in psoriasis and acne), laser therapy (especially for birthmarks), and special acne therapies such as dermabrasion and chemical peels.

### Systemic Therapy

Therapeutic agents are often used as an adjunct to topical therapy in dermatologic disorders, and those most frequently used therapeutically are the corticosteroids and the antibiotics. The corticosteroid hormones, with their capacity to inhibit inflammatory and allergic reactions, are valuable in the treatment of severe skin disorders. Dosage is carefully adjusted and gradually tapered to the minimum that is effective and tolerated. In infants and children, dosage is

**TABLE 18-2** Properties of commonly used dressings and other products

| Examples | Indications | Advantages | Disadvantages | Considerations |
|---|---|---|---|---|
| **Polyurethane Films** | | | | |
| Op-Site, Tegaderm, Bioclusive, Blister-film, Acu-derm, Polyskin II, Transorb, Epi View | Protection of partial-thickness red wounds<br>Cover dressing for hydrophilic preparations and hydrogels<br>Autolytic debridement of wounds with dry eschar | Transparent; good adhesion; reduces pain, minimizes friction forces to wound; time-saving; easy to store; cost-effective<br>Moisture, vapor, and oxygen transmission<br>Impermeable to water and bacteria | Adhesive injury to intact and new skin; nonabsorbent; some products difficult to apply; variable barrier function; can promote wound infection<br>Unsuitable for electrical stimulation wound healing | Protect wound margins; avoid in wounds with infection, copious drainage, tracts or fragile skin surrounding lesion<br>Change only if dressing leaks<br>Contraindicated in third-degree burns |
| **Polymeric Foams** | | | | |
| Allevyn, Allevyn Adhesive, Allevyn Cavity, Nu-Derm, Lyofoam, PolyMem | Used when a nonadherent dressing is needed<br>Used for wounds with moderate to heavy exudate | Moisture is absorbed into foam; maceration is decreased<br>Removal does not cause reinjury to wound<br>Comfortable, easy to apply; cushions and protects wound | Requires an additional dressing to secure if the foam does not have an adhesive surface | Do not use on infected wounds<br>Contraindicated for third-degree burns |
| **Hydrocolloids** | | | | |
| Duoderm CGF, Duoderm Extra Thin, Comfeel, Restore, Tegasorb, SignaDress, Cutinova Hydro, Ultec, Actiderm, Replicare | Protection of superficial and small, deep red wounds<br>Autolytic debridement of small, noninfected yellow wounds*<br>Partial thickness, stages 2 and 3; shallow full thickness, granulating with minimal to moderate exudate, stage 4 | Absorbent; nonadhesive to healing tissue; waterproof; reduces pain; easy to apply; time-saving; easy to store<br>Moldable to area; occlusive; provides insulation; maintains moist wound surface; wet-to-dry adherence | Nontransparent; may soften and lose shape with heat or friction; odor and brown drainage on removal (melted dressing material) | Frequency of changes depend on amount of exudate (change as needed for leakage)<br>DO NOT USE for heavily exudative wounds, sinus tracts, or infected wounds; shape dressing to wound area<br>Contraindicated in third-degree burns |
| **Hydrogels/Sheets** | | | | |
| Vigilon, Elastogel, Aquasorb, Nu-Gel, Duoderm Gel, Second Skin, Hypergel, Intra-Site Gel, Carrasyn | Protection of superficial and moderately deep red wounds<br>Autolytic debridement of small, noninfected yellow or black wounds*<br>Delivery system for topical antimicrobial creams (increases penetration)<br>Partial and full thickness | Absorbent; nonadhesive; reduces pain; compatible with topicals; good conformity; easy to store<br>Maintains a moist wound surface, has a "cooling" effect | Poor barrier; semitransparent; requires cover dressing to secure; can promote growth of *Pseudomonas* and other gram-negative bacteria and yeast<br>Unused portion will dessicate<br>Not for weight-bearing ulcers<br>Expensive; nonadhesive<br>High water content can macerate surrounding skin | Avoid in infected wounds; change every 8 hr or as needed for leakage<br>Cut and shape to wound<br>DO NOT REMOVE poly backing<br>Monitor wound for over-hydration and skin maceration around wound edges |
| **Hydrocolloid Absorption Powders, Pastes, Beads, and Granules** | | | | |
| Bard absorption dressing, Comfeel Ulcus paste, Comfeel Ulcus powder, Multidex powder and gel, Debrisan | Used on uneven and exudating ulcers | Controls bacteria<br>Cleanses wound<br>Reduces odor<br>Cost-effective | | Cleanse with lukewarm water or saline to remove<br>Contraindicated in third-degree burns |
| **Alginates** | | | | |
| Sorbsan, Kaltostat, Curasorb, Algi Site, Restore, CalciCare | Used for leg ulcers, donor sites, infected traumatic or exudating wounds | Nonallergenic; biodegradable; little to no local tissue reaction<br>Decreases pain at wound site | Expensive; easily displaced by mechanical forces<br>Permeable to bacteria, urine | Change daily after proper cleansing if used on infected wounds<br>Requires a secondary cover dressing<br>Contraindicated in third-degree burns |

Modified from Bryant RA: *Acute and chronic wounds, nursing management,* St Louis, 2000, Mosby, and McCulloch JM, Kloth LC, Feedar JA: *Wound healing alternatives in management,* Philadelphia, 1995, FA Davis.
*NOTE: Users should read package inserts for any contraindications to use of these products. Some dressings, such as Duoderm CGF, have been approved for application to infected wounds, provided that wound is cultured and treated for infection. Many products should not be used on third-degree burns (see Chapter 29).

larger than is usually calculated from body weight ratios. However, prolonged use may temporarily suppress growth.

Antibiotics, which interfere with the growth of microorganisms, are used in severe or widespread skin infections. However, because they tend to produce a hypersensitivity in the patient, they are used with caution. Antifungal agents are the only means for treating systemic fungal infections.

## Nursing Care of the Child with a Skin Disorder

### ▉ Assessment

To help establish a diagnosis, it is important for nurses to accurately describe any deviation in the character of the skin, using both inspection and palpation. The color, shape, and distribution of the lesions or wounds are noted. The individual lesions are described according to the accepted terminology and may involve more than one type, such as a maculopapular rash. Wounds are assessed for depth of tissue damage, evidence of healing, and signs of infection.

> **NURSING ALERT**
>
> Signs of wound infection are:
> Increased erythema, especially beyond wound margin
> Edema
> Purulent exudate
> Pain
> Increased temperature

To confirm or amplify the findings made by inspection, the skin is gently palpated to detect characteristics such as temperature, moisture, texture, elasticity, and the presence of edema. It should be indicated whether the findings are restricted to the area of the lesion(s) or are generalized.

The child's subjective symptoms provide additional information. Older children are able to describe the condition as painful, itching, or tingling or in other descriptive terms. However, much can be determined by observing the younger child's behavior and the parents' account of these reactions. Does the child scratch? Is the child restless or irritable? Does the child favor or avoid using a body part? A careful history may provide clues. Has the child had access to chemicals or been in the woods or around a woodpile? Has the child eaten a new food? Is the child taking medication? Has the child any known allergy? Do any playmates have a similar lesion? A doubtful diagnosis is frequently confirmed on the basis of the history.

### ▉ Nursing Diagnoses

Nursing diagnoses are determined following an assessment of the child and the skin lesions. The major diagnoses identified for the child with a skin disorder are outlined in the Nursing Care Plan on pp. 756-757.

### ▉ Planning

The goals for the child with a skin condition and the family are as follows:

- Child will exhibit signs of skin healing.
- Child will not experience secondary damage, such as from infection, to the lesion.

> ## ATRAUMATIC CARE
> ### *Painless Suturing and Wound Cleansing*
>
> A variety of topical anesthetic solutions, such as lidocaine, adrenaline, tetracaine combined (LAT) and tetracaine-phenylephrine (tetraphen) applied to wounds, especially on the head, scalp, and face, provide anesthesia in 10 to 15 minutes (Smith and others, 1996). Tetracaine, adrenaline, and cocaine combined (TAC) or AC (without tetracaine) should not be used because of the potential for lethal cocaine intoxication. LAT is as effective, is safer, and is much less expensive than TAC. If further anesthesia is required or if the topical preparations are not available, using buffered lidocaine administered with a 30-gauge needle reduces the stinging and burning of the injection (see Pain Management, Chapter 26). The use of a noninvasive tissue adhesive (e.g., Derma Bond*) provides a faster and less painful method of facial laceration repair with cosmetic results comparable to suturing (Osmond, Klassen, and Quinn, 1995).
>
> *Manufactured by Closure Medical Corporation, Raleigh, NC.

- Child will demonstrate acceptable level of comfort, especially if pain or itching exists.
- Child and family will receive appropriate education and support.

### ▉ Implementation

Therapeutic programs are usually designed to provide general measures, such as rest, protection, and relief of discomfort, and specific treatments, such as a definitive medication or physical technique. Because only a few skin diseases are contagious, it is usually not necessary to isolate the affected child unless there is a danger of acquiring a secondary infection (e.g., the child who is receiving large doses of corticosteroids or other immunosuppressant drugs or the child with an immunologic deficiency disorder). If the skin manifestation is caused by a viral exanthem, such as measles or chickenpox, the child is prevented from exposing other susceptible children.

**Wound Care.** Small wounds to the skin are managed by the parents at home. The parents are instructed to wash their hands and then wash the wound gently with mild soap and water for several minutes, followed by thorough rinsing. To prevent possible tattooing, an abrasion from which the dirt cannot be removed will require wound cleaning with the patient receiving topical anesthesia, and those covering a very large area (over 15% of the body) will need medical attention with the child receiving conscious sedation/analgesia. (See Atraumatic Care box.) Open wounds are covered with a dressing, such as a commercial adhesive bandage, although larger wounds may benefit from the use of occlusive dressings (see Table 18-2). If occlusive dressings are applied, instruct the parents on their correct application and removal. For example, hydrocolloid dressings adhere best if a wide margin is left around the wound and the dressing is pressed against intact skin until it adheres.* The edges of the dressing can be secured to the skin with waterproof tape.

*Information on the use of the hydrocolloid dressing Duoderm is available from ConvaTec Professional Services, PO Box 5254, Princeton, NJ 08543, (800) 422-8811, fax: (908) 281-2405; www.convatec.com.

The dressings are removed if leakage occurs or after a specific time interval, usually 7 days. Dressings are removed carefully to protect intact skin from damage and the epithelial surface of the wound. To remove transparent or hydrocolloid dressings, raise one edge of the dressing and pull *parallel* to the skin to loosen the adhesive. The longer the dressings are left on, the easier they are to remove.

> **NURSING ALERT**   Advise parents that the yellow gel forming under hydrocolloid dressings may look like pus and has a distinct odor (somewhat fruity) but is normal leakage.

Lacerations present a special challenge. The injured child and family are usually very distressed by the bleeding and are in variable degrees of shock; parental guilt usually accompanies the injury. Because scalp lacerations bleed so profusely, they are especially frightening. The initial nursing intervention is to apply pressure to the area and attempt to calm the child before further examination. Unless there is bleeding from a severed artery, the wound can be cleansed with a forced jet of sterile tepid water or saline (via syringe) and examined for extent, depth, and presence of foreign material such as dirt, glass, or fabric fragments.

> **NURSING ALERT**   Hydrogen peroxide and povidone-iodine are contraindicated for cleaning fresh, open wounds. Hydrogen peroxide can cause formation of subcutaneous gas when applied under pressure.

The location of the wound also dictates assessment. For example, wounds over bony areas may contain bone chips, and clear fluid seeping from severe head wounds may indicate cerebrospinal fluid. A pressure dressing is applied for transfer to medical care; the child in a medical facility is prepared for suturing. (See Atraumatic Care box on p. 751.)

Puncture wounds that do not require a tetanus booster are soaked in warm water and soap for several minutes. Causing the wound to rebleed may be helpful. An adhesive bandage can be applied if desired. Puncture wounds of the head, chest, or abdomen or those that could still contain a portion of the puncturing object must be evaluated.

Parents are cautioned against opening blisters or kissing a wound "to make it better." The wound can easily become contaminated from germs in the human mouth. If scabs form, they are allowed to slough off without assistance; picking or early removal may cause scarring. Parents are advised to seek medical help if there is evidence of infection.

**Relief of Symptoms.**   Most of the therapeutic regimens are directed toward relief of pruritus, the most common subjective complaint. Itching is believed to result from stimulation of C-fibers at the dermoepidermal junction. These fibers are similar to but distinct from pain fibers. Substances released within the skin, histamine and endopeptidases, also elicit itching, although their release triggers are unknown (Barnett, 2001).

Cooling the affected area and increasing the skin pH with measures such as cool baths or compresses to reduce external stimuli to the area and alkaline applications, such as baking soda baths, to increase skin pH help to prevent scratch-

ing. Clothing and bed linen should be soft and lightweight to decrease the irritation from friction and stimulation.

During any type of treatment, both affected and unaffected skin is protected from damage and secondary infection. Preventing scratching is of primary importance. Older children will usually cooperate, although they may need to be reminded to stop scratching or rubbing; but in smaller and uncooperative children the use of techniques and devices such as mittens (especially during sleep) or special coverings is required. Keeping fingernails short, well trimmed, and clean helps reduce the chance of secondary infection.

Antipruritic medications, such as diphenhydramine (Benadryl) or hydroxyzine (Atarax), may be prescribed for severe itching, especially if it disturbs the child's rest. Pain and discomfort are usually managed with nonpharmacologic measures and mild analgesia; severe pain requires more potent medication. Occlusive dressings over wounds reduce pain. For suturing wounds a topical anesthetic, tissue adhesive, or intradermal buffered lidocaine can be used. (See Pain Management, Chapter 26.)

Topical therapy usually involves some type of topical treatment, and the mode of application depends on the nature and location of the lesion being treated. For example, soothing lotions, creams, and intermittent wet dressings or soaks help cool and dry; ointments, lotions, and creams soften and lubricate dry, scaling areas. Nurses and parents are responsible for the application of topical therapeutic agents.

It is especially important to wash the hands before and after application of topical therapies. The skin is assessed before the treatment or application of medication and reassessed after the treatment is completed. Any observed changes are noted and described.

Wet compresses or dressings cool the skin by evaporation, relieve itching and inflammation, and cleanse the area by loosening and removing crusts and debris. Any of a variety of ingredients, such as plain water or Burow solution (available without a prescription), can be applied on Kerlix gauze, plain gauze, or (preferably) soft cotton cloths such as freshly laundered handkerchiefs or strips from cloth diaper, sheeting, or pillowcase material.

Dressings immersed in the desired solution are wrung out slightly and applied to the affected area wet but not dripping. They are applied flat and smooth and in such a way that motion is not totally restricted—fingers are wrapped separately, and arms and legs are wrapped so that elbows and knees can bend. Dressings are kept in place by Kerlix or other cotton wrap, tubular stockinette, mittens, or socks (two pair—one to hold the dressings in place, the other to take up movement) but are left uncovered. When evaporation begins to dry them, the dressings are removed, rewet in the solution, and reapplied to the area using aseptic technique. The solution is not poured or syringed directly over the dressings. As fluid evaporates, the solution becomes increasingly concentrated and thus stronger, which may be damaging to sensitive lesions.

Fresh solution at room temperature is applied at 2-, 3-, or 4-hour intervals and is allowed to remain on the lesion from 30 minutes to 1½ hours. Wet dressings are seldom continued after about 48 hours. The child must be guarded against chilling during treatment, and no more than 20% of the body should be covered at one time to avoid the risk of hypothermia. After treatment, the skin is dried thoroughly by patting with a towel. Application of lotion or other medication may be ordered at this time.

When children are uncooperative in the use of wet dressings, *soaks* are often used for removal of crusts and for their mild astringent action, with the same solution as for wet compresses. Gaining young children's cooperation for hand or foot soaks is difficult unless the procedure is made attractive to them through play. Older infants and toddlers delight in playing with brightly colored objects or poker chips scattered over the bottom of the receptacle, and preschoolers can be challenged to hold a floating item beneath the water's surface. These activities require supervision; infants and small children will often place items in their mouths, and children can easily lose control with water play. Washing dishes, cars, dolls, or doll clothes will occupy many children for quite some time.

Although older children are able to cooperate, they need something to do during the procedure, such as listening to music or a story, or watching television or a video. A single extremity (a foot or a hand) can be easily soaked by placing the solution and the extremity in a plastic sealable bag. The closure is then zipped snugly around the limb.

Baths are especially useful in the treatment of widespread dermatitis by evenly distributing the soothing antipruritic and antiinflammatory effects of the solution, usually oatmeal or mineral oil preparations. The solution is added to a tub of water. The temperature of the bath is tepid, and the treatment usually lasts 15 to 30 minutes. Therapeutic baths are always more interesting when the child has toy boats or other items for water play.

Topical applications are applied to skin lesions to ease discomfort, prevent further injury, and facilitate healing. Most preparations are placed directly on the skin and left uncovered; others may be applied under an occlusive dressing. A thin application of the ointment or cream is covered with plastic film and anchored with adhesive or covered with a commercial transparent dressing. Occlusive dressings promote moisture retention and nonevaporation of the preparation, which increases the penetration of the medication. Regardless of the type of preparation used, parents need detailed information on how to apply it and how long the preparation should remain on the skin or under an occlusive dressing.

Apply topical applications systematically with the contour of the body surface (not simply up and down). Children love to be "painted." Therefore lotion applications can be fun when an ordinary paintbrush is used.

**NURSING ALERT** Provide written instructions and demonstrate to parents the correct amount of topical medication to apply (e.g., size of a pea; thin film to cover). If more than one preparation is applied, mark the containers 1 and 2 for parents to remember the correct order. Stress that more is not necessarily better with some medications, such as steroids.

Recombinant growth factors are the newest group of topical wound care products. These products are human platelet–derived growth factors that are engineered outside the body. They foster the formation of new granulation tissue by stimulating the migration of fibroblasts, macrophages, smooth muscle cells, and capillary endothelial cells to the wound site (Beaumont and Anderson-Dam, 1998). Becoplermin (Regranex) is the only recombinant growth factor currently approved by the Food and Drug Administration; however, safety of this product has not been established for children under age 16.

The vacuum-assisted closure device (VAC) is another new wound technology currently available for both acute and chronic wound care. Vacuum-assisted closure uses a sub-atmospheric technique, which involves placing an open-cell foam dressing into the wound, using an occlusive dressing and applying suction. The negative force of the suction is applied from the foam dressing to the wound surfaces. The mechanical force removes excess fluids from the wound, stimulates formation of granulation tissue, restores capillary flow and fosters closure of the wound (Patel and others, 2000). Vacuum-assisted closure has been used to prepare wounds for a skin graft and also to treat chronic pressure ulcers.

**Home Care and Family Support.** Dermatologic conditions always involve the family. Because few situations require hospitalization and children who are hospitalized will complete a therapy program at home, the family must carry out the treatment plan; therefore, their cooperation is essential. Regimens that are simple to accomplish in the hospital or office may be frustrating and baffling at home. The family often needs assistance in adapting equipment available in the home to the therapy.

It is important that the child and family be given as detailed explanations as possible about both the expected and the unexpected results of treatment, including any ill effects that might occur. If unexplained reactions do develop, the family is directed to discontinue treatment and report the reactions to the appropriate person(s). The use of over-the-counter medicines is discouraged unless they have first been discussed with the attending practitioner and received approval.

Because the skin is the most visible portion of the body, defects in its surface that alter its appearance are sometimes a source of distress to the child and a source of revulsion and rejection by others. Parents of other children may fear that their children will "catch" the disorder. Occasionally the affected child's own family members will reduce their interaction with him or her, especially close physical contact, or otherwise demonstrate a distaste for the condition, which the child may interpret as rejection. This is seldom a difficulty with dermatitis of short duration, but chronic conditions can create problems and affect the child's self-concept. (See Family Focus box on p. 754.)

The National Institute of Nursing Research has also recently established a laboratory and clinical center to study wound healing. This center will enroll patients in clinical studies and provide research training and clinical experiences for nurses interested in wound healing.*

---

*For more information contact Dr. Annette Wysocki at email: wysockia@mail.nih.gov; www.aw127w@nih.gov.

## ✂ Evaluation

The effectiveness of nursing interventions is determined by continual reassessment and evaluation of care based on the following observational guidelines:

- Observe whether reasonable care is used in performing nursing activities, and observe lesions and child's reactions to therapies.
- Observe signs of wound healing.
- Use assessment techniques to identify relief of discomfort as described in Chapter 26.
- Reassess skin lesions; observe and interview child and family regarding compliance with therapy.

The *expected outcomes* are described in the Nursing Care Plan on pp. 756-757.

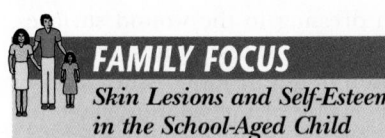

### FAMILY FOCUS
#### Skin Lesions and Self-Esteem in the School-Aged Child

When I was 8 years old, a lot of small, oval, tannish brown spots developed, especially around my neck and waist. The dermatologist said it was a rare condition and that it should disappear by the time I was 11 or 12. They actually disappeared when I was 10. Because the spots were kind of unusual, the dermatologist invited me to attend a dermatology meeting where people with strange skin problems were placed in private clinic rooms and doctors came in and looked at each person's skin. They were all nice, but I felt a little like an animal in the zoo. The thing I mostly remember about the spots was that I always tried to keep them covered. People stared, and kids made fun of me. The spots didn't hurt or itch, but I always knew they were there. I would not wear a two-piece swimsuit, even though my friends wore them. My mom and I tried to think of anything that might have caused the spots, but I never knew why they developed on me. I remember thinking it wasn't fair that it happened to me. I learned that many times, people cannot prevent the bad things that happen to them.

Marissa White, age 16
Tulsa, Oklahoma

## INFECTIONS OF THE SKIN
### Bacterial Infections

Normally, the skin harbors a variety of bacterial flora, including the major pathogenic varieties of staphylococci and streptococci. The degree of their pathogenicity depends on the invasiveness and toxigenicity of the specific organism, the integrity of the skin, the barrier of the host, and the immune and cellular defenses of the host. Children with congenital or acquired immunodeficiency disorders such as AIDS, children in a debilitated condition, those receiving immunosuppressive therapy, and those with a generalized malignancy such as leukemia or lymphoma are at risk for developing bacterial infections.

Because of the characteristic "walling-off" process of the inflammatory reaction (abscess formation), staphylococci are more difficult to attack, and the local infected area is associated with an increase in numbers of bacteria all over the skin surface that serve as a source of continuing infection. Staphylococcal infections occur most often in children in the younger age-groups, and the incidence decreases with advancing age. All of these factors emphasize the importance of careful handwashing and cleanliness when caring for infected children and their lesions to prevent spread of the infection and as an essential prophylactic measure when caring for infants and small children. Common bacterial skin disorders are outlined in Table 18-3.

### Nursing Considerations

The major nursing functions related to bacterial skin infections are to prevent the spread of infection and to prevent complications. Handwashing is mandatory before and after contact with an affected child. Handwashing is also emphasized to both the child and the family, and the child should be provided with towels separate from those of other family members. Impetigo contagiosa is easily spread by self-inoculation; therefore the child must be cautioned against

**Fig. 18-6** Impetigo contagiosa. (From Weston WL, Lane AT: *Color textbook of pediatric dermatology*, ed 2, St Louis, 1996, Mosby.)

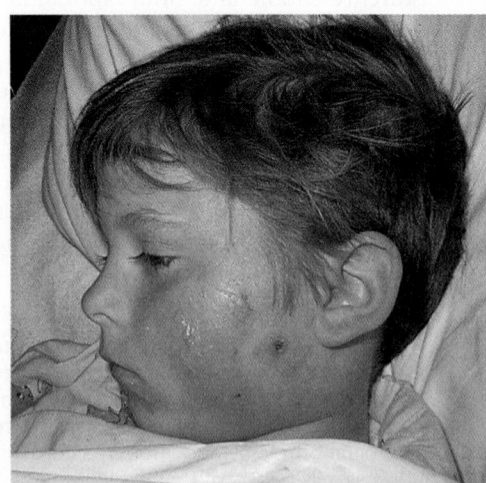

**Fig. 18-7** Cellulitis of cheek from puncture wound. (From Weston WL, Lane AT: *Color textbook of pediatric dermatology*, ed 2, St Louis, 1996, Mosby.)

**TABLE 18-3**   Bacterial infections

| Disorder/Organism | Manifestations | Management | Comments |
|---|---|---|---|
| **Impetigo contagiosa**—*Staphylococcus* (Fig. 18-6) | Begins as a reddish macule<br>Becomes vesicular<br>Ruptures easily, leaving superficial, moist erosion<br>Tends to spread peripherally in sharply marginated irregular outlines<br>Exudate dries to form heavy, honey-colored crusts<br>Pruritus common<br>Systemic effects: minimal or asymptomatic | Careful removal of undermined skin, crusts, and debris by softening with 1:20 Burow solution compresses<br>Topical application of bactericidal ointment<br>Systemic administration of oral or parenteral antibiotics (penicillin) in severe or extensive lesions | Tends to heal without scarring unless secondary infection<br>Autoinoculable and contagious<br>Very common in toddler, preschooler<br>May be superimposed on eczema |
| **Pyoderma**—*Staphylococcus, Streptococcus* | Deeper extension of infection into dermis<br>Tissue reaction more severe<br>Systemic effects: fever, lymphangitis | Soap and water cleansing<br>Wet compresses<br>Bathing with antibacterial soap as prescribed | Autoinoculable and contagious<br>May heal with or without scarring |
| **Folliculitis** (pimple), **furuncle** (boil), **carbuncle** (multiple boils)—*Staphylococcus aureus* | Folliculitis: infection of hair follicle<br>Furuncle: larger lesion with more redness and swelling at a single follicle<br>Carbuncle: more extensive lesion with widespread inflammation and "pointing" at several follicular orifices<br>Systemic effects: malaise, if severe | Skin cleanliness<br>Local warm, moist compresses<br>Topical application of antibiotic agents<br>Systemic antibiotics in severe cases<br>Incision and drainage of severe lesions, followed by wound irrigations with antibiotics or suitable drain implantation | Autoinoculable and contagious<br>Furuncle and carbuncle tend to heal with scar formation<br>A lesion should *never* be squeezed |
| **Cellulitis**—*Streptococcus, Staphylococcus, Haemophilus influenzae* (Fig. 18-7) | Inflammation of skin and subcutaneous tissues with intense redness, swelling, and firm infiltration<br>Lymphangitis "streaking" frequently seen<br>Involvement of regional lymph nodes common<br>May progress to abscess formation<br>Systemic effects: fever, malaise | Oral or parenteral antibiotics<br>Rest and immobilization of both affected area and child<br>Hot, moist compresses to area | Hospitalization may be necessary for child with systemic symptoms<br>Otitis media may be associated with facial cellulitis |
| **Staphylococcal scalded skin syndrome**—*S. aureus* | Macular erythema with "sandpaper" texture of involved skin<br>Epidermis becomes wrinkled (in 2 days or less), and large bullae appear | Systemic administration of antibiotics<br>Gentle cleansing with saline, Burow solution, or 0.25% silver nitrate compresses | Infant subject to fluid loss, impaired body temperature regulation, and secondary infection, such as pneumonia, cellulitis, and septicemia<br>Heals without scarring |

touching the involved area. This is difficult to accomplish; distraction or reminders are useful but are not helpful when the child is alone, such as at bedtime.

Children and parents are often tempted to squeeze follicular lesions. They must be warned that squeezing will not hasten the resolution of the infection and that there is a risk of making the lesion worse or spreading the infection. No attempt should be made to puncture the surface of the pustule with a needle or sharp instrument. A child with a stye may waken with the eyelids of the affected eye sealed shut with exudate. The child or the parents are instructed to gently wipe the lid from the inner to the outer edge with warm water and a clean washcloth until the exudate has been removed.

The child with limited cellulitis of an extremity is usually managed at home on a regimen of oral antibiotics and warm compresses. The parents are taught the procedures and instructed in administration of the medication. Children with more extensive cellulitis, especially around a joint with lymphadenitis or on the face, may be admitted to the hospital for parenteral antibiotics, with continued treatment at home. Nurses are responsible for teaching the family to administer the medication, and to apply compresses.

## Viral Infections

Viruses are intracellular parasites that produce their effect by using the intracellular substances of the host cells. Composed of only a DNA or RNA core enclosed in an antigenic protein shell, viruses are unable to provide for their own metabolic needs or to reproduce themselves. After a virus

# Nursing Care Plan
## The Child with a Skin Disorder

> **NURSING DIAGNOSIS:** Impaired skin integrity related to environmental agents, somatic factors, immunologic deficit

**PATIENT GOAL 1:** Will exhibit signs of skin healing

- **NURSING INTERVENTIONS/*RATIONALES***

Carry out therapeutic regimens as prescribed or support and assist parents in carrying out treatment plan *to promote skin healing*

Provide moist environment (dressing or ointment) *for optimum wound healing*

*Administer topical treatments and applications

*Administer systemic medications, if ordered

Prevent secondary infection and autoinoculation *because these delay healing*

Reduce external stimuli that aggravate condition, *causing delay in healing*

Encourage rest *to support body's natural defenses*

Encourage well-balanced diet *to support body's natural defenses*

Administer skin care and general hygiene measures *to promote skin healing*

- **EXPECTED OUTCOME**

Affected area exhibits signs of healing

> **NURSING DIAGNOSIS:** Risk for impaired skin integrity related to mechanical trauma, body secretions, increased susceptibility to infection

**PATIENT GOAL 1:** Will maintain skin integrity

- **NURSING INTERVENTIONS/*RATIONALES***

Keep intact skin clean and dry; cleanse skin at least once daily *to minimize risk of infection*

Inspect total skin area frequently for evidence of irritation or breakdown *so that appropriate therapy can be initiated*

Protect skinfolds and surfaces that rub together *to prevent mechanical trauma to skin*

Keep clothing and linen clean and dry *to prevent excoriation and infection of skin*

Apply protective lotion to anal and perineal areas, knees, elbows, ankles, and chin, *because excoriation is most likely to occur in these areas*

Carry out good perineal care under urine collection device when applicable *to prevent impaired skin integrity*

Remove adhesives and occlusive dressings carefully *to prevent skin trauma*

- **EXPECTED OUTCOME**

Skin remains clean, dry, and free of irritation

**PATIENT GOAL 2:** Will exhibit no evidence of secondary infection

- **NURSING INTERVENTIONS/*RATIONALES***

Maintain careful handwashing before handling affected child *to prevent infection*

---
*Dependent nursing action.

Wear surgical gloves when handling or dressing affected parts if indicated by nature of lesion *to prevent contamination of lesion(s)*

Teach child and family hygienic care and medical asepsis *to prevent secondary infection*

Devise methods to prevent secondary infection of lesion in small or uncooperative children

   Keep nails short and clean *to minimize trauma and secondary infection*

   Apply mittens or elbow restraints *to prevent child from reaching skin lesions(s)*

   Dress in one-piece outfit with long sleeves and legs *to keep lesion(s) covered and out of child's reach*

Observe skin lesions for signs of infection (increased erythema, edema, purulent exudate, pain, increased temperature) *so that appropriate therapy can be initiated*

- **EXPECTED OUTCOMES**

Skin lesions remain confined to primary sites

Skin lesions exhibit no signs of secondary infection

**PATIENT GOAL 3:** Will maintain integrity of healthy skin

- **NURSING INTERVENTIONS/*RATIONALES***

Teach and impress on child importance of keeping hands away from lesion(s) *to prevent spreading lesion(s) and secondary infection*

Help child determine ways of preventing autoinoculation *to increase compliance*

Keep healthy skin dry *to prevent maceration*

- **EXPECTED OUTCOMES**

Healthy skin remains clean and intact

Skin lesions remain confined to primary sites

> **NURSING DIAGNOSIS:** Risk for infection related to presence of infective organisms

**PATIENT GOAL 1:** Will not spread infection to self or others

- **NURSING INTERVENTIONS/*RATIONALES***

Implement standard precautions *to prevent spread of infection*

Isolate affected child from susceptible individuals if indicated *to prevent spread of infection*

Maintain careful handwashing after caring for child *to remove infective organisms*

Avoid unnecessary close contact with affected child during infective stage of disease *to prevent spread of infection to others*

Use correct technique for disposal of dressings, solutions, and other fomites in contact with lesion(s) *to safely dispose of infective organisms*

Teach and reinforce positive habits of hygienic care *to decrease risk of infection*

- **EXPECTED OUTCOMES**

Infection remains confined to primary site

Child and family comply with preventive measures

# Nursing Care Plan
## The Child with a Skin Disorder—cont'd

**NURSING DIAGNOSIS:** Risk for impaired skin integrity related to allergenic factors

**PATIENT GOAL 1:** Will experience no occurrence or recurrence of skin lesion(s)

- **NURSING INTERVENTIONS/*RATIONALES***

Avoid or reduce contact with agents or circumstances known to precipitate skin reaction *to prevent occurrence or recurrence of lesion(s)*

Teach child to recognize agents or circumstances that produce reaction *to prevent occurrence or recurrence of lesion(s)*

- **EXPECTED OUTCOME**

Child avoids precipitating agents

**NURSING DIAGNOSIS:** Pain related to skin lesions, pruritus

**PATIENT GOAL 1:** Will exhibit optimum comfort level

- **NURSING INTERVENTIONS/*RATIONALES***

Avoid or reduce external stimuli that aggravate the condition, such as clothing and bed linen, *to increase comfort*

Implement other appropriate nonpharmacologic pain reduction techniques (see Chapter 26)

*Apply soothing treatments and topical applications as ordered *to relieve pain or pruritus*

*Administer medications *to relieve discomfort and/or restlessness and irritability*

Advocate for child regarding appropriate topical anesthesia and/or sedation/analgesia for wound suturing or cleansing *to prevent unnecessary pain and emotional trauma*

- **EXPECTED OUTCOME**

Child remains calm and exhibits no evidence of discomfort or pruritus

**NURSING DIAGNOSIS:** Interrupted family processes related to having a child with a severe skin condition (e.g., eczema, psoriasis, ichthyosis)

**PATIENT GOAL 1:** Will demonstrate positive self-image

- **NURSING INTERVENTIONS/*RATIONALES***

Encourage child to express feelings about personal appearance and perceived reactions of others *to facilitate coping*

Discuss with child improvement in skin condition *to instill hope*

- **EXPECTED OUTCOME**

Child verbalizes feelings and concerns

**PATIENT GOAL 2:** Will receive tactile contact

- **NURSING INTERVENTIONS/*RATIONALES***

Hold child *to provide tactile stimulation;* remember there is no substitute for stimulation/comfort of human contact

Touch and caress unaffected area *to provide tactile contact without risk of spreading infection*

- **EXPECTED OUTCOMES**

Child exhibits signs of comfort

Child responds positively to tactile stimulation

**PATIENT GOAL 3:** Will receive adequate support

- **NURSING INTERVENTIONS/*RATIONALES***

Teach self-care where appropriate *to encourage sense of adequacy*

Involve child in planning treatment schedules *to give child some control*

Support and encourage child in efforts to deal with multiple problems that may be associated with disorder, including discomfort, rejection, discouragement, and feelings of self-revulsion *to facilitate coping*

Encourage child to maintain usual activities *so that child experiences normalcy in situation*

Help child improve appearance (e.g., attractive clothing) *to promote positive self-image*

- **EXPECTED OUTCOMES**

Child collaborates in determining means for improving appearance

Child maintains customary activities and relationships

Child participates in own care and treatment

**NURSING DIAGNOSIS:** Disturbed body image related to perception of appearance

**PATIENT (FAMILY) GOAL 1:** Will receive adequate support

- **NURSING INTERVENTIONS/*RATIONALES***

Teach family skills needed *to carry out therapeutic program*

Provide written instructions *to increase compliance*

Inform family of expected and unexpected results of therapy and a course of action to follow *to prevent noncompliance*

Help devise special techniques to carry out therapy *to increase compliance and cooperation*

Be aware of overprotectiveness and restrictiveness *to prevent stifling child's emotional growth*

Allow and encourage family members, particularly the one who cares for the child most of the time, to express negative feelings, such as anger, frustration, and perhaps guilt *to facilitate coping*

Stress that negative feelings are normal, acceptable, and expected *to provide support;* however, encourage family members to find outlets for negative feelings to remain healthy

Encourage family in efforts to carry out plan of care *to provide support*

Refer to agencies and services that assist with social, financial, and medical problems *to provide ongoing support*

- **EXPECTED OUTCOME**

Family demonstrates necessary skills (specify)

---

*Dependent nursing action.

penetrates a cell of the host organism, it sheds the outer shell and disappears within the cell, where the nucleic acid core stimulates the host cell to form more virus material from its intracellular substance. In a viral infection the epidermal cells react with inflammation and vesiculation (as in herpes simplex) or by proliferating to form growths (warts).

Most of the communicable diseases of childhood are associated with rashes, and each rash is characteristic. The type of lesion and the configuration of the viral exanthems of rubeola, rubella, and chickenpox are described in Table 16-1. Other common viral disorders of the skins are outlined in Table 18-4.

| **TABLE 18-4** Viral infections | | | |
|---|---|---|---|
| **Disease** | **Manifestations** | **Management** | **Comments** |
| **Verruca (warts)** Cause: human papillomavirus (various types) | Small, benign tumors<br>Usually well-circumscribed, gray or brown, elevated firm papules with a roughened, finely papillomatous texture<br>Occur anywhere, but usually appear on exposed areas such as fingers, hands, face, and soles<br>May be single or multiple<br>Asymptomatic | Not uniformly successful<br>Local destructive therapy, individualized according to location, type, and number—surgical removal, laser therapy, electrocautery, curettage, cryotherapy (liquid nitrogen), caustic solutions (lactic acid and salicylic acid in flexible collodion, retinoic acid, salicylic acid plasters), x-ray treatment<br>Hypnotherapy may be effective | Common in children<br>Tend to disappear spontaneously<br>Course unpredictable<br>Most destructive techniques tend to leave scars<br>Autoinoculable<br>Repeated irritation will cause to enlarge<br>Apply topical anesthetic, EMLA |
| **Verruca plantaris** (plantar wart) | Located on plantar surface of feet and, because of pressure, are practically flat; may be surrounded by a collar of hyperkeratosis | Apply caustic solution to wart, wear foam insole with hole cut to relieve pressure on wart; soak 20 min after 2-3 days; repeat until wart comes out | Destructive techniques tend to leave scars, which may cause problems with walking<br>Apply topical anesthetic, EMLA |
| **Herpes simplex virus** (Type I [cold sore, fever blister]; Type II [genital]) | Grouped, burning, and itching vesicles on inflammatory base, usually on or near mucocutaneous junctions (lips, nose, genitals, buttocks)<br>Vesicles dry, forming a crust, followed by exfoliation and spontaneous healing in 8-10 days<br>May be accompanied by regional lymphadenopathy | Avoidance of secondary infection<br>Burow solution compresses during weeping stages<br>Topical therapy (penciclovir) can shorten duration of cold sores<br>Oral antiviral (Acyclovir) for initial infection or to reduce severity in recurrence<br>Valacyclovir (Valtrex), an oral antiviral used for episodic treatment of recurrent genital herpes; reduces pain, stops viral shedding, and has a more convenient administration schedule than Acyclovir | Heal without scarring unless secondary infection<br>Type I cold sores can be prevented by using sunscreens protecting against ultraviolet A (UVA and ultraviolet B (UVB) light to prevent lip blisters<br>Aggravated by corticosteroids<br>Positive psychologic effect from treatment<br>May be fatal in children with depressed immunity |
| **Varicella zoster virus** (herpes zoster; shingles) | Caused by same virus that causes varicella (chickenpox)<br>Virus has affinity for posterior root ganglia, posterior horn of spinal cord, and skin; crops of vesicles usually confined to dermatome following along course of affected nerve<br>Usually preceded by neuralgic pain, hyperesthesias, or itching<br>May be accompanied by constitutional symptoms | Symptomatic<br>Analgesics for pain<br>Mild sedation sometimes helpful<br>Local moist compresses<br>Drying lotions may be helpful<br>Ophthalmic variety: systemic corticotropin (ACTH) and/or corticosteroids<br>Acyclovir<br>Lidoderm topical anesthetic | Pain in children usually minimal<br>Postherpetic pain does not occur in children<br>Chickenpox may follow exposure; isolate affected child from other children in a hospital or school<br>May occur in children with depressed immunity; can be fatal |
| **Molluscum contagiosum** Cause: pox virus | Flesh-colored papules with a central caseous plug (umbilicated)<br>Usually asymptomatic | Cases in well children resolve spontaneously in about 18 months<br>Treatment reserved for troublesome cases<br>Apply topical anesthetic, EMLA<br>Curettage or cryotherapy | Common in school-age children<br>Spread by skin-to-skin contact, including autoinoculation and fomite-to-skin contact |

# Dermatophytoses (Fungal Infections)

The dermatophytoses (ringworm) are infections caused by a group of closely related filamentous fungi that invade primarily the stratum corneum, hair, and nails. These are superficial infections that live on, not in, the skin. They are confined to the dead keratin layers and are unable to survive in the deeper layers. Because keratin is being shed constantly, the fungus must multiply at a rate that equals the rate of keratin production to maintain itself; otherwise the infection would be shed with the discarded skin cells. Common dermatophytoses are outlined in Table 18-5.

Three principal types of fungi are responsible for dermatophyte infections: *Trichophyton, Microsporum,* and *Epidermophyton.* They are designated by the Latin word *tinea,* with further designation related to the area of the body where they are found (e.g., tinea capitis [ringworm of the scalp]) (Fig. 18-8, *A*). Dermatophyte infections are most often transmitted from one person to another or from infected animals to humans. Atopic (tendency to develop allergy) individuals are more susceptible to dermatophyte infections. Fungi exert their effect by means of an enzyme that digests and hydrolyzes the keratin of hair, nails, and the stratum

## TABLE 18-5   Dermatophytoses (fungal infections)

| Disease/Organism | Manifestations | Management | Comments |
|---|---|---|---|
| **Tinea capitis**—*Trichophyton tonsurans, Microsporum audouini, Microsporum canis* (Fig. 18-8, *A*) | Lesions in scalp but may extend to hairline or neck<br>Characteristic configuration of scaly, circumscribed patches and/or patchy, scaling areas of alopecia<br>Generally asymptomatic, but severe, deep inflammatory reaction may occur that manifests as boggy, encrusted lesions (kerions)<br>Pruritic<br>Microscopic examination of scales is diagnostic | Oral griseofulvin<br>Oral ketoconazole for difficult cases<br>Selenium sulfide shampoos<br>Topical antifungal agents (e.g., clotrimazole, haloprogin, miconazole) | Person-to-person transmission<br>Animal-to-person transmission<br>Rarely, permanent loss of hair<br>*M. audouini* transmitted from one human being to another directly or from personal items; *M. canis* usually contracted from household pets, especially cats<br>Atopic individuals more susceptible |
| **Tinea corporis**—*Trichophyton rubrum, Trichophyton mentagrophytes, M. canis, Epidermophyton* (Fig. 18-8, *B*) | Generally round or oval, erythematous scaling patch that spreads peripherally and clears centrally; may involve nails (tinea unguium)<br>Diagnosis: direct microscopic examination of scales<br>Usually unilateral | Oral griseofulvin<br>Local application of antifungal preparation such as tolnaftate, haloprogin, miconazole, clotrimazole; apply 1 inch beyond periphery of lesion; continual application 1 to 2 weeks after no sign of lesion | Usually of animal origin from infected pets<br>Majority of infections in children caused by *M. canis* and *M. audouini* |
| **Tinea cruris** ("jock itch")—*Epidermophyton floccosum, T. rubrum, T. mentagrophytes* | Skin response similar to tinea corporis<br>Localized to medial proximal aspect of thigh and crural fold; may involve scrotum in males<br>Pruritic<br>Diagnosis: same as for tinea corporis | Local application of tolnaftate liquid<br>Wet compresses or sitz baths may be soothing | Rare in preadolescent children<br>Health education regarding personal hygiene |
| **Tinea pedis** ("athlete's foot")—*T. rubrum, Trichophyton interdigitale, E. floccosum* | On intertriginous areas between toes or on plantar surface of feet<br>Lesions vary:<br>  Maceration and fissuring between toes<br>  Patches with pinhead-sized vesicles on plantar surface<br>  Pruritic<br>  Diagnosis: direct microscopic examination of scrapings | Oral griseofulvin<br>Local applications of tolnaftate liquid and antifungal powder containing tolnaftate<br>Acute infections: compresses or soaks followed by application of glucocorticoid cream<br>Elimination of conditions of heat and perspiration by clean, light socks and well-ventilated shoes; avoidance of occlusive shoes | Most frequent in adolescents and adults; rare in children, but occurrence increases with wearing of plastic shoes<br>Transmission to other individuals rare despite general opinion to contrary<br>Ointments not successful |
| **Candidiasis** (moniliasis)—*Candida albicans* | Grows in chronically moist areas<br>Inflamed areas with white exudate, peeling, and easy bleeding<br>Pruritic<br>Diagnosis: characteristic appearance | Amphotericin B, nystatin ointment, or other antifungal preparations to affected areas | Common form of diaper dermatitis (see Chapter 13)<br>Oral form common in infants<br>Vaginal form in older females (see Chapter 20)<br>May be disseminated in immunosuppressed children |

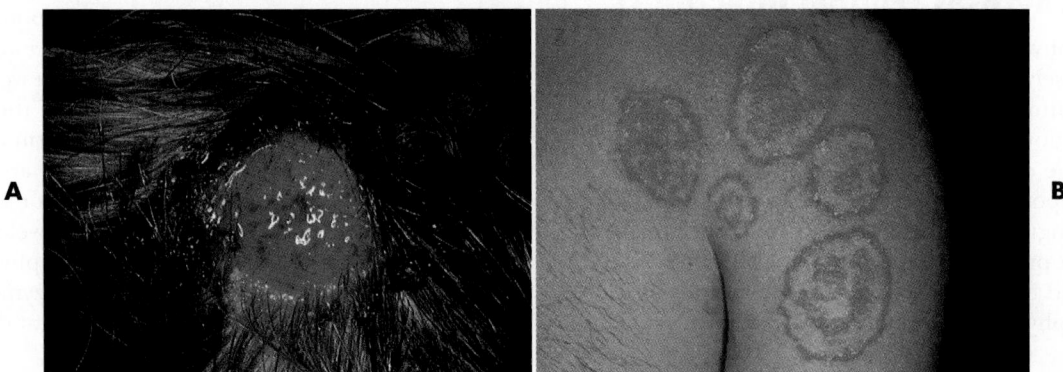

**Fig. 18-8** **A,** Tinea capitis. **B,** Tinea corporis. Both infections are caused by *Microsporum canis*, the "kitten" or "puppy" fungus. (From Habif TP: *Clinical dermatology: a color guide to diagnosis and therapy*, ed 3, St Louis, 1996, Mosby.)

corneum. Dissolved hair breaks off to produce the bald spots characteristic of tinea capitis. In the annular lesions the fungi are found principally in the edge of the inflamed border as they move outward from the inflammation. Diagnosis is made from microscopic examination of scrapings taken from the advancing periphery of the lesion, which almost always produces scale.

### Nursing Considerations

When teaching families about the care of children with ringworm, the nurse should emphasize good health and hygiene. Because of the infectious nature of the disease, infected children should not exchange any grooming items, headgear, scarves, or other articles of apparel that have been in proximity to the infected area with other children. Affected children are provided with their own towels and directed to wear a protective cap at night to avoid transmitting the fungus to bedding, especially if they sleep with another person. Because the infection can be acquired by animal-to-human transmission, all household pets should be examined for the presence of the disorder. Other sources of infection are seats with headrests (theater seats), seats in public transportation, helmets, and gymnasium mats.

Treatment with the drug griseofulvin frequently continues for weeks or months, and, because subjective symptoms subside, children or parents may be tempted to decrease or discontinue the drug. The nurse should emphasize to family members the importance of maintaining the prescribed dosage schedule and of taking the medication with high-fat foods for best absorption (Bradley and others, 1996). They are also informed about possible side effects from the drug, such as headache, gastrointestinal upset, fatigue, insomnia, and photosensitivity. For children who take the drug over many months, periodic testing is required to monitor leukopenia and assess liver and renal function.

## Scabies

Scabies is an endemic infestation caused by the scabies mite, *Sarcoptes scabiei*. Lesions are created as the impregnated female scabies mite burrows into the stratum corneum of the

epidermis (never into living tissue), where she deposits her eggs and feces.

### Clinical Manifestations

The inflammatory response causes intense pruritus that leads to punctate discrete excoriations secondary to the itching. Maculopapular lesions are characteristically distributed in intertriginous areas: interdigital surfaces (Fig. 18-9), the axillary-cubital area, popliteal folds, and the inguinal region. There is variability in the lesions. Infants often develop an eczematous eruption; therefore, the observer must look for discrete papules, burrows, or vesicles. A mite is identified as a black dot at the end of a minute, linear, grayish-brown threadlike burrow. In children over 2 years of age, most eruptions are found in the hands and wrists. In children less than 2 years, on the feet and ankles. Children with Down syndrome may not complain of itching; therefore, they can get a severe infestation before it is recognized.

The inflammatory response and itching occur after the host becomes sensitized to the mite, approximately 30 to 60 days following initial contact. (In persons previously sensitized to the mite, the inflammatory response occurs within 48 hours after exposure.) After this time, anywhere the mite has traveled will begin to itch and develop the characteristic eruption. Consequently, mites will not necessarily be located at all sites of eruption. A person needs prolonged contact with the mite to become infested. It takes about 45 minutes for the mite to burrow under the skin; consequently, transient body contact is less likely to cause transfer of the mite. The diagnosis is made by microscopic identification from scrapings of the burrow.

### Therapeutic Management

The treatment of scabies is the application of a scabicide. Permethrin 5% cream (Elimite) is safer and more effective than lindane and is the preferred treatment. Because of the length of time between infestation and physical symptoms (30 to 60 days), all persons who were in close contact with the affected child will need treatment. This may include boyfriends or girlfriends, baby-sitters, and grandparents as well as immediate family members. The objective is to treat

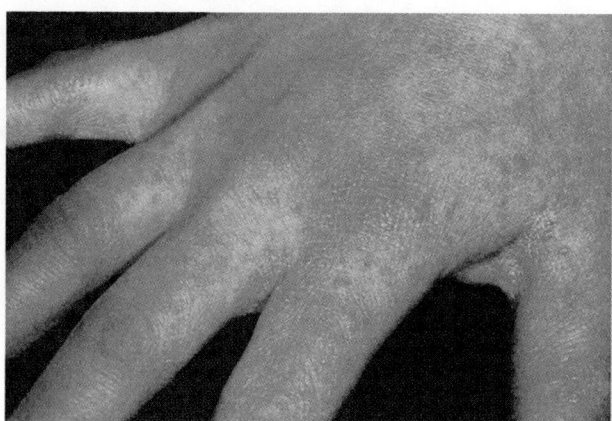

**Fig. 18-9**   Scabies. (From Habif TP: *Clinical dermatology; a color guide to diagnosis and therapy,* ed 3, St Louis, 1996, Mosby.)

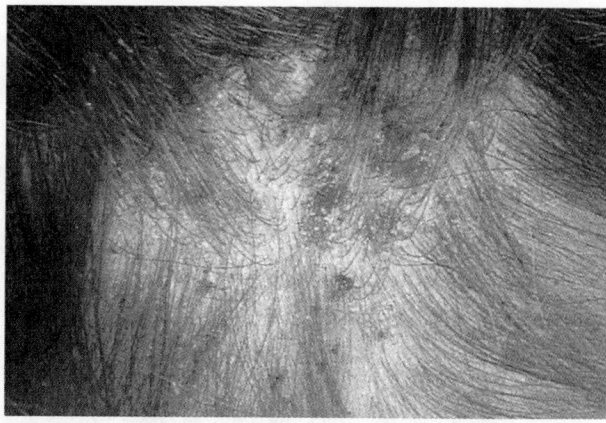

**Fig. 18-10**   Pediculosis capitis. (From Habif TP: *Clinical dermatology: a color guide to diagnosis and therapy,* ed 3, St Louis, 1996, Mosby.)

as thoroughly as possible the first time. Enough medication for the entire family should be prescribed, allowing 2 ounces for adults and 1 ounce for each child.

## Nursing Considerations

Nurses instructing families in use of the scabicide should emphasize the importance of following the directions carefully. If lindane lotion is prescribed, it is applied to cool, dry skin—not following a hot bath. It is applied over the entire cutaneous surface from the neck down and is left on for the recommended time, usually 4 hours for infants and 6 hours for older children and adults. Because scabies is a superficial skin disorder, penetration need not be promoted. One liberal application is sufficient.

When permethrin 5% (Elimite) is used, the cream should be thoroughly and gently massaged into all skin surfaces (not just the areas that have a rash) from the head to the soles of the feet. Skin surfaces between the fingers and toes, the folds of the wrist and waist, the umbilicus, and the cleft of the buttocks should not be missed. A toothpick can be used to apply Elimite cream beneath the fingernails and toenails. Care should be taken to avoid contact with the eyes. If Elimite cream accidentally gets into the eyes, they should be flushed immediately with water. Elimite cream should remain on the skin for 8 to 14 hours, after which time it can be removed by bathing and shampooing.

Touching and holding the child should be minimized until treatment is completed, and the hands are washed carefully after contact is made. Nurses wear gloves when caring for the child. Following treatment, freshly laundered bed linen and clothing are used, and bed clothes and previously worn clothing are washed in very hot water and dried at the high setting in the dryer. Aggressive house cleaning is not necessary. Families need to know that although the mite will be killed, the rash and the itch will not be eliminated until the stratum corneum is replaced, which takes approximately 2 to 3 weeks. Soothing ointments or lotions can be used for itching. Antibiotics may be given for secondary infection.

Ivermectin, an oral medication, may be used to treat scabies in patients with secondary excoriations for whom topical scabicides are irritating and not well tolerated (Dourmishev,

Serafimova, and Dourmishev, 1998; Offidani and others, 1999). However, the safety and efficacy of ivermectin for children less than 5 years of age or children weighing less than 15 kg (33 pounds) has not been established.

## Pediculosis Capitis

Pediculosis capitis (head lice) is an infestation of the scalp by *Pediculus humanus capitis,* a common parasite in school-age children. These lice infestations create embarrassment and concern in the family and community. They can also cause a child to be ridiculed by other children.

The *louse* is a blood-sucking organism that requires approximately five meals a day. The adult louse lives only about 48 hours when away from a human host, and the life span of the average female is 1 month. The female lays her eggs at night at the junction of a hair shaft and close to the skin because the eggs need a warm environment. The *nits,* or eggs, hatch in approximately 7 to 10 days.

### Clinical Manifestations and Diagnostic Evaluation

Itching, caused by the crawling insect and insect saliva on the skin, is usually the only symptom. Common sites of involvement are the occipital area, behind the ears, and at the nape of the neck. Diagnosis is made by observation of the white eggs (nits) firmly attached to the hair shafts. Because of their brief life span and mobility, adult lice are difficult to locate. Nits must be differentiated from dandruff, lint, hair spray, and other items of similar size and shape. On inspection, nits are seen attached to the hair shaft. Scratch marks and/or inflammatory papules caused by secondary infection may be found on the scalp in the vulnerable areas (Fig. 18-10).

### Therapeutic Management

Treatment consists of the application of pediculicides and manual removal of nit cases. The drug of choice for infants and children is permethrin 1% creme rinse (Nix), which kills adult lice and nits. This product and preparations of pyrethrin with piperonyl butoxide (RID or A-200 pyrinate) can be obtained without a prescription and are more effective and safer than lindane. However, pyrethrin products are contraindi-

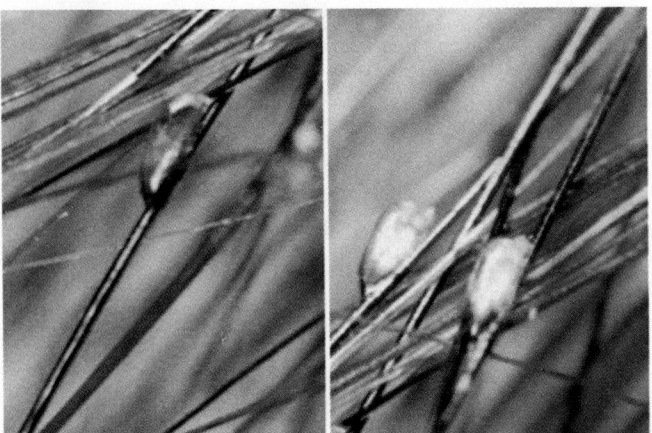

**Fig. 18-11** **A,** Empty nit case. **B,** Viable nits. (From *The contemporary approach to the control of head lice in schools and communities*, Pittsburg, 1991, SmithKline Beecham.)

cated for individuals with contact allergy to ragweed or turpentine. If neither permethrin or pyrethrin products are effective, the prescription drug, 0.5% malathion, has been approved for treatment of head lice. However, malathion contains flammable alcohol, must remain in contact with the scalp for 8 to 12 hours, and is not recommended for children less than 2 years of age. Because there are concerns that head lice may be developing resistance to chemical shampoos and that repeated exposure of children to strong chemicals on the scalp may be unwise, effective nonchemical control measures are essential. Daily removal of nits from a child's hair with a metal nit or flea comb is an essential control measure following treatment with the pediculicide. Complete combing of the child's entire head should be performed every day until no more nits are found. In most instances, a nit comb will remove most of the nits. However, in some instances, nits will need to be removed by scraping them off strands of hair with the examiner's fingernail. Several nit combs are currently available at community pharmacies. The National Pediculosis Association markets a metal comb with long teeth that is easy to use and effective. Electronic head lice detectors that comb the hair and kill adult lice with an electrical charge are also available (O'Brien, 1998).

Lice are small and grayish tan, have no wings, and are visible to the naked eye. The nits, or eggs, appear as tiny whitish oval specks adhering to the hair shaft about ¼ inch from the scalp. The adherent nature of the nits distinguishes them from dandruff, which falls off readily. *Empty nit cases,* indicating hatched lice, are translucent rather than white and are located more than ¼ inch from the scalp (Fig. 18-11).

If evidence of infestation is found, it is important to perform the treatment according to the directions described on the label of the pediculicide. Parents are advised to read the directions carefully before beginning treatment. Instructions indicate that dead lice and remaining nits are removed with an extra-fine-tooth comb. Many preparations include a comb to dislodge the firmly adhered nits. However, if a comb is ineffective, nits must be removed with tweezers or between the fingernails.

The child is made as comfortable as possible during the application process because the pediculicide must remain

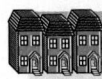

## COMMUNITY FOCUS

*Preventing the Spread and Recurrence of Pediculosis*

Machine wash all washable clothing, towels, and bed linens in hot water, and dry in a hot dryer for at least 20 minutes. Dry-clean nonwashable items.

Thoroughly vacuum carpets, car seats, pillows, stuffed animals, rugs, mattresses, and upholstered furniture.

Seal nonwashable items in plastic bags for 14 days if unable to dry-clean or vacuum.

Soak combs, brushes, and hair accessories in lice-killing products for 1 hour or in boiling water for 10 minutes.

In daycare centers, store children's clothing items such as hats and scarfs and other headgear in separate cubicles.

Discourage the sharing of items such as hats, scarfs, hair accessories, combs, and brushes among children in group settings such as daycare centers.

Avoid physical contact with infested individuals and their belongings, especially clothing and bedding.

Inspect children in a group setting regularly for head lice.

Provide educational programs on the transmission of pediculosis, its detection, and treatment.

From Benenson AS, editor: *Control of communicable diseases manual,* Washington, DC, 1995, American Public Health Association.

on the scalp and hair for several minutes. If eye irritation occurs, the eyes must be flushed well with tepid water.

Playing "beauty parlor" during the shampoo is a useful strategy. The child lies supine, with the head over a sink or basin, and covers the eyes with a dry towel or washcloth. This prevents medication, which can cause chemical conjunctivitis, from splashing into the eyes.

Live lice survive for up to 48 hours away from the host, but nits are shed into the environment and are capable of hatching in 7 to 10 days. Therefore measures must be taken to prevent further infestation. (See Community Focus box.) Spraying with insecticide is not recommended because of the danger to children and animals. Families should also be advised that the pediculicide is relatively costly, especially when several members of the household require treatment.

The psychologic effects of lice infestations are stressful to children. They are influenced by the reactions of others, including their parents, school nurses, and officials. Some children feel ashamed or guilty. Parents are strongly cautioned against cutting a child's hair or, worse, shaving a child's head. Lice infest short hair as readily as long hair, and these actions only compound the child's distress and serve as a continual reminder to peers who are prone to taunt children who have a different appearance.

**Prevention.** The increasing incidence of pediculosis in schoolchildren has become a serious concern for school nurses, parents, and community health agencies. School nurses usually coordinate school-community prevention control programs for pediculosis. The **National Pediculosis Association**\* offers education and advocates a "no nits" policy for treated children's reentry into school.

A recent study of 382 school nurses also indicated that 60% of these nurses supported a "no nit" rule of enforced

\*PO Box 610189, Newton, MA 02161, (617) 449-6487 or (800) 446-4NPA, fax: (781) 449-8129, www.headlice.org.

Pediculosis capitis is an infestation, not an infectious disease. School personnel and many health care providers seem to regard head lice as very contagious and transmissible. Parents associate head lice with a lack of cleanliness and feel stigmatized when told that their child has head lice. Part of the hysteria relating to head lice stems from the fact that many schools enforce a "no nit" policy for head lice. When a school nurse finds head lice in a child's hair, that child is promptly sent home from school with directions for the parents to shampoo the child's hair and remove the lice. Parents comply with these directions and send their children back to school after shampooing and meticulously combing their hair. If the school nurse finds a single egg or nit remaining in the child's hair, the school's "no nit" policy demands that the nurse exclude the child from school until the eggs or nits are completely removed. The problem is all nits are often not eliminated by treatment, but the nits left after treatment are inactive, dead, and harmless. Remnants of dead nits may remain attached to the hair for months or years. If the eggs are dead, there is no reason for a child to miss school. A "no nit" policy inflates the risks associated with lice infestations, increases the probability of overusing pediculicides, and may hinder academic performance by excluding children from school. In addition, a recent investigation has provided evidence that such policies are counterproductive.

To determine how often children were excluded from school inappropriately, health care providers as well as nonspecialists were invited to submit specimens to the Harvard School of Public Health that they found in children's hair when they suspected head lice (Pollack, Kiszewski, and Spielman, 2000). Analysis of 614 specimens indicated that lice and eggs were present in less than two thirds of these specimens; and only 53% of the specimens contained a live louse or viable eggs. Health professionals as well as nonspecialists overdiagnosed pediculosis capitis and failed to distinguish active from extinct infestations. Eighty-two percent of the schools involved in this study had a "no nits" policy, and noninfested children were excluded from school as often as infested children. Pediculicidal treatments are overapplied and ordered for noninfested children as often as for children with active infestations.

Several practice implications can be derived from this study: (1) school nurses should receive training and a microscope or magnifying glass to help them identify head lice correctly; (2) a diagnosis of head lice should be based on observation of live lice rather than dead eggs, dandruff, or other suspicious material in a child's hair; (3) a "no nit" policy should be invoked only as a last resort; and (4) repeated failure of parents to rid a child's hair of nits is not a sound basis for suspecting neglect or abuse or instituting legal action against parents.

---

absenteeism for any children with nits in their hair (Price and others, 1999). However, recently the "no nit" policy has become very controversial, and many school systems and some state associations of pediatricians have questioned its value. (See Evidence-Based Practice box.)

### Nursing Considerations

Nurses should emphasize that *anyone* can get pediculosis; it has no respect for age, socioeconomic level, or cleanliness. The louse does not jump or fly, but it can be transmitted from one person to another on personal items. Children are cautioned against sharing combs, hair ornaments, hats, caps, scarves, coats, and other items used on or near the hair. Children who share lockers are more

likely to contract an infestation, and slumber parties place children at risk. Lice are not carried or transmitted by pets.

Nurses or parents should carefully inspect a child who scratches the head more than usual for bite marks, redness, and nits. The hair is systematically spread with two flat-sided sticks or tongue depressors, and the scalp is observed for any movement that indicates a louse. Nurses should wear gloves when examining the hair and use new tongue depressors or examining sticks for each child (Bradley and others, 1996).

## SYSTEMIC DISORDERS RELATED TO SKIN LESIONS

### Systemic Mycotic (Fungal) Infections

Mycotic (systemic or deep fungal) infections have the capacity to invade the viscera as well as the skin. The best known of these are primarily lung diseases, which are usually acquired by inhalation of fungal spores. They produce a variable spectrum of disease, and some are quite common in certain geographic areas. They are not transmitted from person to person but appear to reside in the soil, from which their spores are airborne. The cutaneous lesions are granulomatous and appear as ulcers, plaques, nodules, fungating masses, and abscesses. The course of deep fungal diseases is chronic, with slow progression that favors sensitization (Table 18-6).

### Rickettsial Infections

Rickettsiae are intracellular parasites, similar in size to bacteria, that inhabit the alimentary tract of a wide range of natural hosts. With the exception of Q fever, mammals become infected only through the bites of infected insects (lice and fleas) or arachnids (ticks and mites), which serve as both infectors and reservoirs. Rickettsial diseases are more common in temperate and tropical climates and in areas where humans live in association with arthropods. Infection in humans is incidental (except epidemic typhus) and not necessary for the survival of the rickettsial species. However, once the organism invades a human, it causes a disease that varies in intensity from a benign self-limiting illness to a fulminating and frequently fatal one. Some rickettsial infections are outlined in Table 18-7.

### Lyme Disease

Lyme disease is the most common tick-borne disorder in the United States. It is caused by the spirochete, *Borrelia burgdorferi,* which enters the skin and bloodstream through the saliva and feces of ticks, especially the deer tick *Ixodes dammini* (also known as *Ixodes scapularis*) in the Midwest and Northeast and *Ixodes pacificus* in the Pacific Northwest regions of the United States. The ticks are clear to light brown and are very small, 2 to 4 mm in length (the size of a poppy seed), making detection difficult. The preferred hosts of *I. dammini* are white-tailed deer and white-footed mice (Siegel, 1997).

**TABLE 18-6** Systemic mycoses

| Disorder/Organism | Skin Manifestations | Systemic Manifestations | Treatment | Comments |
|---|---|---|---|---|
| **North American blastomycosis—** *Blastomyces dermatitidis* | Chronic granulomatous lesions and microabscesses in any part of body<br>Initial lesion is a papule; undergoes ulceration and peripheral spread | Pulmonary symptoms, such as cough, chest pain, weakness, and weight loss<br>May have skeletal involvement, with bone destruction and formation of cutaneous abscesses | Intravenous administration of amphotericin B | Usual portal of entry is lungs<br>Source of infection unknown<br>Noninfectious<br>Pulmonary infections may be mild and self-limiting and require no treatment<br>Progressive disease often fatal |
| **Cryptococcosis—** *Cryptococcus neoformans* (*Torula histolytica*) | Usually on face; acneiform, firm, nodular, painless eruption | Central nervous system (CNS) manifestations; headache, dizziness, stiff neck, and signs of increased intracranial pressure<br>Low-grade fever, mild cough, lung infiltration | Intravenous amphotericin B; may be administered intrathecally for CNS involvement<br>5-Flurocytosine for meningitis<br>Excision and drainage of local lesions | Acquired by inhalation of dust but may enter through skin<br>Prognosis serious<br>Noninfectious<br>Increased incidence in persons receiving corticosteroids with lymphoreticular malignancies, or with type 2 diabetes |
| **Histoplasmosis—** *Histoplasma capsulatum* | Not distinctive or uniform but most appear as punched-out or granulomatous ulcers | General systemic symptoms may include pallor, diarrhea, vomiting, irregular spiking temperature, hepatosplenomegaly, and pulmonary symptoms<br>Any tissue of body may be involved with related symptoms | Intravenous amphotericin B for severe cases<br>Oral ketoconazole | Organism cultured from soil, especially where contaminated with fowl droppings<br>Fungus enters through skin or mucous membranes of mouth and respiratory tract<br>Endemic in Mississippi and Ohio River valleys<br>Disseminated diseases most common in infants and children |
| **Coccidioidomycosis** (valley fever)— *Coccidioides immitis* | Erythema nodosum<br>Erythema multiforme<br>Erythematous maculopapular rash | Primary lung disease usually asymptomatic<br>May be sign of acute febrile illness<br>Disseminated disease is very serious | Intravenous amphotericin B<br>Intravenous miconazole (synthetic imidazole)<br>Intraventricular miconazole plus oral ketoconazole for CNS involvement<br>Surgical resection of persistent pulmonary cavities | Inhalation of aerospores from soil<br>Endemic in southwestern United States<br>Usually resolves spontaneously<br>Increased incidence in dark-skinned races (Filipino, African-American, Mexican, Asian) |

## Clinical Manifestations

The disease may present in any of three stages. *Stage 1* consists of the tick bite at the time of inoculation, followed in 3 to 32 days by the development of *erythema chronicum migrans (ECM)* at the site of the bite. The lesion begins as a small erythematous papule that enlarges radially over a period of days to weeks, resulting in a large circumferential ring with a raised, edematous doughnutlike border (Fig. 18-13). The thigh, groin, and axilla are common sites. The lesion is described as "burning," feels warm to the touch, and occasionally is pruritic.

Many patients develop multiple, smaller, secondary annular lesions without the indurated center. They may occur anywhere, except on the palms and soles, and in untreated patients they disappear in 3 to 4 weeks. Constitutional symptoms, including fever, headache, malaise, fatigue, anorexia, stiff neck, generalized lymphadenopathy, splenomegaly, conjunctivitis, sore throat, abdominal pain, and cough, are often observed.

*Stage 2,* the most serious stage of the disease, is characterized by systemic involvement of neurologic, cardiac, and musculoskeletal systems that appears 2 to 11 weeks after the cutaneous phase is completed. Headache is the most frequent symptom, but in early stages it is not associated with neurologic abnormalities. Later neurologic features include meningoencephalitis, cranial nerve palsies, and peripheral radiculoneuritis.

Cardiac complications, which may appear in a smaller number of persons 4 to 5 weeks after ECM, are commonly atrioventricular conduction abnormalities and may result in severe heart block (Hines, 2001). Patients may be asymptomatic but can develop syncope, palpitations, dyspnea, chest pain, and severe bradycardia.

*Stage 3,* or the late stage, includes musculoskeletal pains that involve the tendons, bursae, muscles, and synovia and which may develop months or years later. Chronic arthritis may also occur. In children the arthritis is characterized by intermittently painful swollen joints (primarily the knees),

**TABLE 18-7   Eruptions caused by rickettsiae**

| Disorder/Organism/Host | Manifestations | Management | Comments |
|---|---|---|---|
| **Rocky Mountain spotted fever—** *R. rickettsii* (Fig 18-12) Arthropod: tick Transmission: tick Mammal source: wild rodents; dogs | Gradual onset: fever, malaise, anorexia, myalgia Abrupt onset: rapid temperature elevation, chills, vomiting, myalgia, severe headache Maculopapular or petechial rash primarily on extremities (ankles and wrists) but may spread to other areas, characteristically on palms and soles | Control: protection from tick bite by wearing proper apparel, tick repellent Tetracycline or chloramphenicol Vigorous supportive therapy | Usually self-limited in children Onset in children may resemble any infectious disease Severe disease rare in children Children and dogs should be inspected regularly if they play in wooded areas See Table 18-10 for management of ticks |
| **Epidemic typhus—***R. prowazekii* Athropod: body louse Transmission: infected feces into broken skin Mammal source: humans | Abrupt onset of chills, fever, diffuse myalgia, headache, malaise Maculopapular rash becomes petechial 4 to 7 days later, spreading from trunk outward | Control: immediate destruction of vectors Tetracycline or chloramphenicol Supportive treatment | Patient should be isolated until deloused See discussion on p. 761 for management of pediculosis Excreta from infected lice also in dust—disinfect patient's clothing, bedding, and possessions and wash in hot water |
| **Endemic typhus—***R. typhi* Arthropod: rat fleas, or lice Transmission: flea bite; inhaling or ingesting flea excreta Mammal source: rats | Headache, arthralgia, backache followed by fever; may last 9-14 days Maculopapular rash after 1-8 days of fever; begins in trunk and spreads to periphery; rarely involves face, palms, soles | Control: eliminate rat reservoir, insect vectors, or both Tetracycline or chloramphicol Supportive treatment | Fairly common in United States Shorter duration than epidemic typhus A mild, seldom fatal illness Difficult to distinguish from epidemic typhus |
| **Rickettsialpox—***R. akari* Arthropod: mouse mite Transmission: mite Mammal source: house mouse | Maculopapular rash following primary lesion and eschar at site of bite, fever, chills, headache | Control: eradication of rodent reservoir and mite vector Tetracycline or chloramphenicol Supportive treatment | Self-limited, nonfatal disease Endemic in New York City Found in many cities in United States |

with spontaneous remissions and exacerbations. Late neurologic problems may include deafness, chronic encephalopathy, and keratitis.

## Diagnostic Evaluation

The diagnosis is based primarily on the history, observation of the lesion, and development of clinical manifestations. Laboratory diagnosis can be established in later stages through serologic testing, either by indirect immunofluorescence (IFA) or enzyme immunoassay (EIA). However, serologic testing for Lyme disease at the time of a recognized tick bite is not recommended (Fix, Strickland, and Grant, 1998). Serologic testing is not standardized. Many laboratories provide inaccurate results, and there is a high frequency of false-negative and false-positive results (Seltzer and Shapiro, 1996).

## Therapeutic Management

At the time the rash appears or shortly thereafter, children over 8 years of age are treated with oral doxycycline or amoxicillin, and children under 8 years of age are given amoxicillin or penicillin. For patients who are allergic to penicillin alternative drugs include cefuroxime or erythromycin (Wade, 2000).

The length of treatment depends on the clinical response and other disease manifestations but is usually from 14 to 21 days (American Academy of Pediatrics, 2000b). The treatment is effective in preventing second-stage mani-

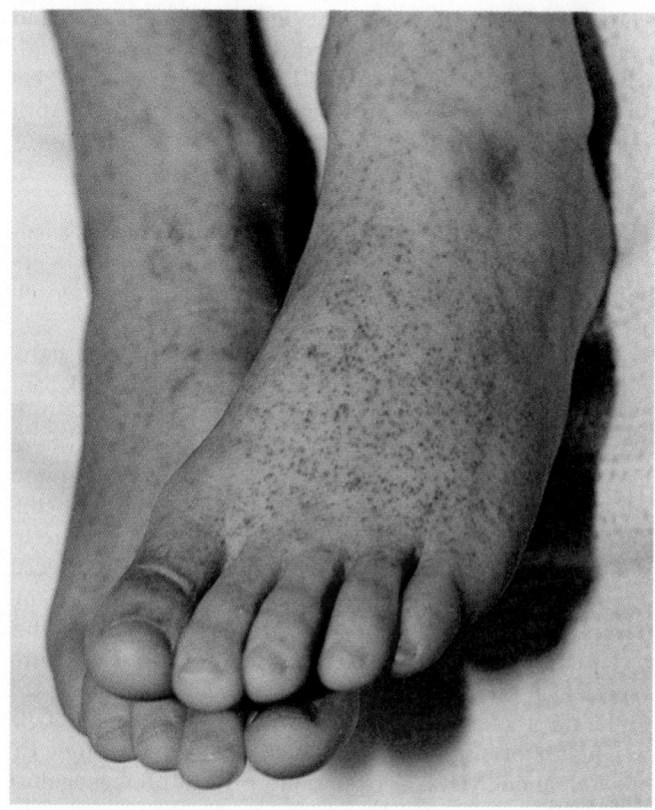

**Fig. 18-12**   Petechial rash of Rocky Mountain spotted fever.

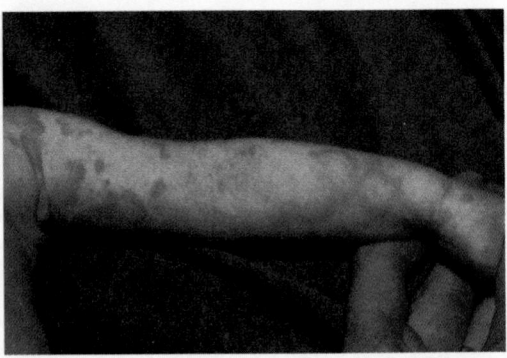

**Fig. 18-13** Lyme disease. Note annular red rings in erythema chronicum migrans. (From Weston WL, Lane AT: *Color textbook of pediatric dermatology*, St Louis, 1991, Mosby.)

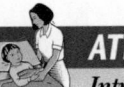

### ATRAUMATIC CARE
#### Intramuscular Ceftriaxone (Rocephin)

To decrease the pain of intramuscular Rocephin, apply EMLA to the site 2½ hours before the injection and/or use lidocaine—preferably buffered to reduce the stinging of the anesthetic—as the diluent rather than sterile water (Hayward and others, 1996).

festations in most cases. Neurologic, cardiac, and arthritic manifestations are managed with intravenous or intramuscular antibiotics, such as ceftriaxone or penicillin G (see Atraumatic Care box). For patients in whom tetracycline is contraindicated or who have allergies to penicillin, parenterally administered ceftriaxone is as effective as doxycycline in the treatment of acute disseminated Lyme disease (Dattwyler and others, 1997). Follow-up care is important in ensuring that treatment is initiated or terminated as needed.

A vaccine against Lyme disease, LYMErix, is available. The vaccine is recommended for individuals ages 15 to 70 years at high risk for Lyme disease from significant exposure to tick habitats in endemic areas (currently, the northeast and north central United States) and for those who have been infected with Lyme disease (Shapiro and Gerber, 2002). It is administered on a 0-, 1-, and 12-month schedule; doses 2 and 3 should be given several weeks before *B. burgdorferi* season, which usually begins in April (American Academy of Pediatrics, 2000a).

### Nursing Considerations

The major thrust of nursing care should be educating parents to protect their children from exposure to ticks. In endemic areas tick habitats can include yards and parks as well as wooded areas.

Children should avoid tick-infested areas or wear light-colored clothing so that ticks can be spotted easily, tuck pant legs into socks, and wear a long-sleeved shirt tucked into pants when in weeded areas. Grass and shrubbery where ticks may be lurking should be avoided, and children and adults should walk in the center of trails. Parents and children need to perform regular tick checks when they are in infested areas. After a hike, a bare skin check (with special attention to the scalp, neck, armpits and groin areas) is important to spot any ticks and remove them (see Table 18-10).

Parents should also be alert for signs of the skin lesion, especially if their children are known to have been exposed to the tick vector.

The use of insect repellents such as those containing diethyltoluamide (DEET) or permethrin can protect against insects. Parents should be advised to use them cautiously.

DEET is absorbed through the skin and can cause toxicity in infants and children. These preparations should not be used on children younger than 1 year of age. In older children the preparation should be sprayed on the child's clothing not directly on the skin.

Information about Lyme disease can be obtained from the **American Lyme Disease Foundation, Inc.***

## Cat Scratch Disease (CSD)

Cat scratch disease (CSD) is the most common cause of regional lymphadenitis in children and adolescents. It usually follows the scratch or bite of an animal (a cat or kitten in 90% of the cases) and is caused by *Bartonella henselai*, a gram-negative bacterium (Margileth, 2000; Rombaux and others, 2000). The disease is usually a benign, self-limiting illness that resolves spontaneously in 2 to 4 months.

The usual manifestations are a painless, nonpruritic erythematous papule at the site of inoculation, followed by regional lymphadenitis. The lymph nodes most commonly involved are axillary epitrochlear, cervical, submandibular, inguinal, and preauricular. The disease may persist for several months before gradual resolution. In some children, especially those who are immunocompromised, the adenitis may progress to suppuration. Some children may develop serious complications that include encephalitis, hepatitis, and Parinaud oculogandular syndrome. This syndrome is characterized by granulomatous lesions on the palpebral conjunctiva associated with swelling of the ipsilateral preauricular nodes. Diagnosis is made on the basis of (1) history of contact with a cat or kitten, (2) the presence of regional lymphadenopathy for several days, and (3) serologic identification of the causative organism by indirect fluorescent antibody assay or polymerase chain reaction test (St. Geme, Haslam, and Ditmar, 1997).

Treatment is primarily supportive. Antibiotics do not shorten the duration or prevent progression to suppuration, but antibiotics may be helpful in severe forms of the disease. Trimethoprim-sulfamethoxasole, ciprofloxacin, gentamicin, and rifampin have shown some benefit in uncontrolled clinical studies (St. Geme, Haslam, and Ditmar, 1997).

Activity is limited to prevent trauma to the large lymph nodes, and bed rest is indicated for children with fever. Analgesics are given for discomfort. Most children can continue normal activities during the disease. The animals are

*Mill Pond Offices 293, Route 100, Suite 204, Somers, NY 10589, (914) 277-6970, (800) 876-LYME, fax: (914) 277-6974; www.aldf.com.

not ill during the time they transmit the disease, and most authorities do not recommend disposal of a cherished pet.

# SKIN DISORDERS RELATED TO CHEMICAL OR PHYSICAL CONTACTS

## Contact Dermatitis

Contact dermatitis is an inflammatory reaction of the skin to chemical substances, natural or synthetic, that evoke a hypersensitivity response or to those agents that cause direct irritation. The initial reaction occurs in an exposed region, most commonly the face and neck, backs of the hands, forearms, male genitalia, and lower legs. There is characteristically a sharp delineation between inflamed and normal skin early in the reaction that ranges from a faint, transient erythema to massive bullae on an erythematous swollen base. Itching is a constant symptom.

The cause may be a primary irritant or a sensitizing agent. A *primary irritant* is one that irritates any skin. A *sensitizing agent* produces an irritation on those who have met the irritant or something chemically related to it, have undergone an immunologic change, and have become sensitized. A sensitizer irritates in relatively low concentrations only persons who are allergic to it.

The clinical course is relatively short (1 to 4 weeks) if the causative agent is eliminated, and whether or not there are complications from secondary invasion or reactions to topical therapy depends on the severity of the original reaction.

Sensitizing reactions are acquired by repeated or prolonged exposure, and the sensitizing capacity of different substances varies widely. Strong sensitizers require only one or two exposures and occur in a higher percentage of individuals; weak sensitizers require numerous exposures, and a smaller percentage of those exposed will be sensitized. The length of time from exposure to development of sensitivity varies and may be as short as a week or much longer. Sometimes with repeated exposure and reactions the skin loses its capacity to return to normal, or secondary factors become predominant to produce a chronic inflammatory process.

The major goal in treatment is to prevent further exposure of the skin to the offending substance. Provided there is no further irritation, the normal recuperative powers of the skin will produce satisfactory results without treatment. The most frequent offenders are plant and animal irritants, the prototype of which is poison ivy (see discussion following).

The most common contact dermatitis in infants occurs on the convex surfaces of the diaper area as a result of chemical irritation from putrefactive fecal enzymes acting on urine or laundry products. (See Diaper Dermatitis, Chapter 13.) Other agents that frequently produce dermatologic responses from contact are animal irritants such as wool, feathers, and furs; vegetable irritants such as oleoresins, oils, and turpentine; and chemicals of all kinds, including synthetic fabrics (e.g., shoe components), dyes, metals, cosmetics, perfumes, and soaps (including bubble baths). The list is endless.

Several cosmetic products advertised as safe for children may be responsible for skin irritation. These include a

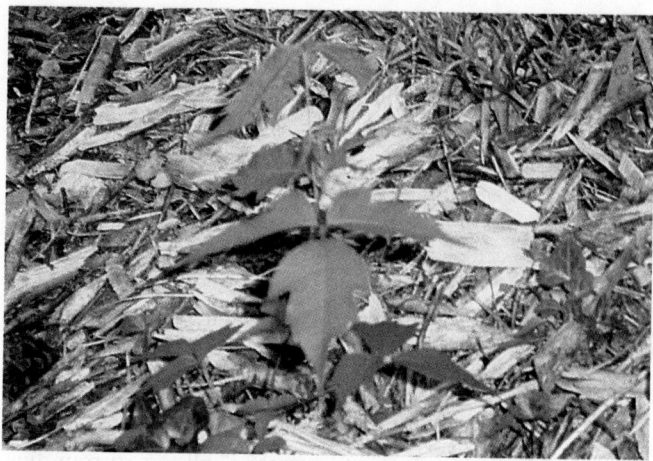

**Fig. 18-14**   Poison ivy.

cream hair relaxer marketed especially for children that contains lye and must be used with extreme care. Because children's hair is more resistant to artificial curling or straightening, pediatric preparations contain chemicals as strong as or stronger than those intended for use on adults.

### Nursing Considerations

Nurses frequently detect evidence of contact dermatitis during routine physical assessments. Skin manifestations in specific areas suggest limited contact, such as around the eyes (mascara), areas of the body covered by clothing but not protected by undergarments (wool), or areas of the body not covered by clothing (ultraviolet injury). Generalized involvement is more likely to be caused by bubble bath or soap. Often nurses are able to elicit the offending agent and counsel families regarding management. If the lesions persist, are extensive, or show evidence of infection, medical evaluation is indicated.

## Poison Ivy, Oak, and Sumac

Contact with the dry or succulent portions of any of three poisonous plants (ivy, oak, or sumac) produces localized, streaked or spotty, oozing, and painful impetiginous lesions. Poison ivy grows almost everywhere east of the Rockies, poison oak is found primarily west of the Rockies, and poison sumac is usually restricted to swamp areas of the Southeast. Only Nevada, Hawaii, and Alaska (and regions above 4000 feet) appear to be free of the plants (Fig. 18-14).

The offending substance in these plants is an oil, *urushiol,* that is extremely potent. Sensitivity to urushiol is not inborn but is developed after one or two exposures and may change over a lifetime. Repeated exposures appear to lower the reaction; exposure after long periods away from it may elicit a heightened response. Some highly sensitive persons may suddenly become resistant and vice versa. All parts of the plants contain urushiol; thus dried leaves and stems contain the irritant. Even smoke from burning brush piles can produce a reaction. There is widespread contact with the skin from the smoke of burning plants, and lung reactions from smoke inhalation can be life-threatening.

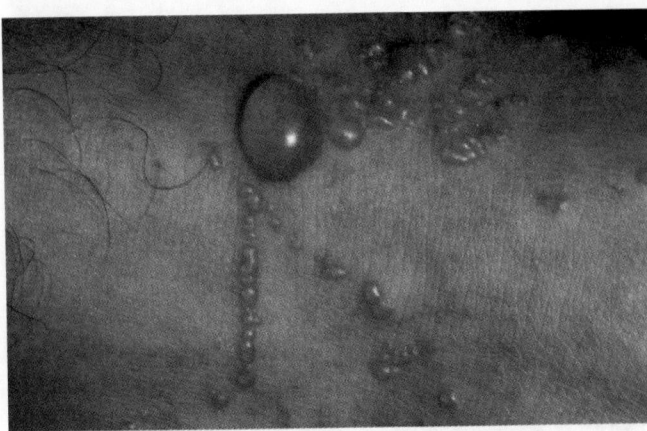

**Fig. 18-15** Poison ivy; note "streaked" blisters surrounding one large blister. (From Habif TP: *Clinical dermatology: a color guide to diagnosis and therapy*, ed 3, St Louis, 1996, Mosby.)

### Critical Thinking Exercise

#### Poison Ivy

While on an overnight camping trip, Billy, age 9, runs up to the camp nurse with some leaves he has picked on a trail in the woods. The nurse recognizes the leaves as poison ivy. What would be the best intervention for the camp nurse to implement?

FIRST, THINK ABOUT IT . . .
- What information are you using?
- What are you taking for granted, and what assumptions are you making?

1. Isolate Billy from his classmates and telephone his parents to pick him up immediately from the camp.
2. Scrub Billy's hands vigorously with a strong soap.
3. Rinse Billy's hands in the cool water of the nearby stream and apply calamine lotion.
4. Throw the poison ivy leaves into the camp fire and examine Billy's hands for any reddened areas.

*The best response is three. Poison ivy lesions are not contagious, which is important information. Also children who are exposed to poison ivy do not need to be isolated. However, the leaves of a poison ivy plant do contain an oil called urushiol, which begins to initiate an immune response as soon as the oil touches the human skin. Contact with the leaves should not be taken for granted. An effective way to remove this oil is by rinsing the skin with cold, running water; the cool water of a running stream is ideal. Calamine lotion will relieve the itching and discomfort. Harsh soaps dilute the urushiol and allow the oil to spread; vigorous scrubbing irritates the skin. Burning the leaves is dangerous because contact with the smoke can not only cause a skin reaction but is dangerous to the lungs if it is inhaled.*

Animals do not seem to be affected by the oil; dogs or other animals who have run or played in the plants may carry the sap on their fur, and animals who eat the plants can transfer the oil in saliva. Shoes, tools, and toys can transfer the oil. Golf balls that have been in the rough are sources of contact.

### Clinical Manifestations

Urushiol takes effect as soon as it touches the skin. It penetrates through the epidermis and bonds with the dermal layer, where it initiates an immune response. The full-blown reaction is evident after about 2 days, with redness, swelling, and itching at the site of contact. Several days later, streaked or spotty blisters oozing serum from damaged cells produce the characteristic impetiginous lesions (Fig. 18-15). The lesions dry and heal spontaneously, and itching stops by 10 to 14 days.

### Therapeutic Management

Treatment of the lesions includes calamine lotion, soothing Burow solution compresses, and/or Aveeno baths to relieve discomfort. Topical corticosteroid gel is very effective for prevention or relief of inflammation, especially when applied before blisters form. Oral corticosteroids may be needed for severe reactions, and a sedative such as diphenhydramine (Benadryl) may be ordered.

### Nursing Considerations

When it is known that the child has made contact with the plant, the area is immediately flushed (preferably within 15 minutes) with *cold* running water to neutralize the urushiol not yet bonded to the skin. If there is a stream nearby, an effective method is to have the child enter the water (clothes and all) and allow the water to rinse the oil from both skin and clothing. Harsh soap is contraindicated because it removes protective skin oils and dilutes the urushiol, allowing it to spread. Hard scrubbing irritates the skin. All clothing that has come in contact with the plant is removed with care and thoroughly laundered in hot water and detergent. Every effort is made to prevent the child from scratching the lesions. Although the lesions do not spread by contact with the blister serum or from scratching, the lesions can become secondarily infected. (See Critical Thinking Exercise box.)

**Prevention.** Prevention is best accomplished by avoiding contact and removing the plant from the environment. All children, especially those known to be sensitive, should be taught to recognize the plant. A cream that protects exposed skin is Stokogard.* Information regarding means for destroying plants can be obtained from the U.S. Department of Agriculture or Forestry Service. Home garden sprays that kill broad-leaf plants or all vegetation (i.e., Round Up or Spectracide) are ineffective. If poisonous plants are growing in public community areas, the local authorities should be contacted to remove the plants.

## Foreign Bodies

Small wooden splinters can be removed by parents with a needle and tweezers that have been sterilized with alcohol or a flame. The area around the sliver is washed with soap

---

*Distributed in the United States by Stockhausen, Inc, Greensboro, NC 27406, (800) 334-0242.

and water before removal is attempted. The sliver is exposed with the needle and then grasped firmly by the tweezers and pulled out. Some foreign bodies, such as a fishhook, a piece of glass, a difficult-to-see object, or a deeply embedded object (such as a needle in a foot or near a jont), require medical evaluation.

## Cactus Spines

Small cactus prickles or spines are troublesome to remove, and attempts are distressing to the child and family. Large spines or clumps can be removed with tweezers. Smaller prickles or spines may be removed by the following methods:

- Apply a thin layer of water-soluble household glue and cover with gauze; when the glue dries, peel off the gauze.
- Apply hair removal wax or body sugar (Aplon*), let dry, and remove.
- Place cellophane tape, sticky side down, over the spines and lift off.

## Sunburn

Sunburn is a very common skin injury caused by overexposure to ultraviolet (UV) light waves—either sunlight or artificial light in the UV range. The sun emits a continuous spectrum of visible and nonvisible light rays that range in length from very short to very long. The shorter, higher-frequency waves are more damaging than longer wavelengths, but much of the light is filtered out as it travels through the atmosphere. Of the light that does filter through, *ultraviolet A (UVA) waves* are the longest and cause only minimum burning but play a significant role in photosensitive and photoallergic reactions. They are also responsible for premature aging of the skin and potentiate the effects of *ultraviolet B (UVB)* waves, which are shorter and responsible for tanning, burning, and most of the harmful effects attributed to sunlight, especially skin cancer.

Numerous factors influence the amount of UVB exposure. Maximum exposure occurs at midday (10 AM to 3 PM) when the distance from the sun to a given spot on the earth is shortest. Solar intensity also varies with the seasons, time zones, and altitude. Exposure is greater at higher altitudes and near the equator, and less when the sky is hazy (although its effect is easily underestimated). Window glass effectively screens out UVB but not UVA. Fresh snow, water, and sand reflect UV rays, especially when the sun is directly overhead.

Some persons are more susceptible to sunburn than others. Protection from the sun is provided by the fibrous keratin of the outer epidermis and the pigment melanin, produced by the melanocytes of the innermost, or basal, layer of the epidermis. Areas of the body with thick keratin layers (palms and soles) offer the greatest protection. The protective pigment layer decreases the intensity of all UV light by physically blocking and scattering the radiation. UV rays stimulate the melanocytes to produce more melanin, turning the skin darker. After several days of exposure, the dark melanin absorbs most of the incoming UV radiation before the rays can cause further damage.

Persons with light skin and eyes produce melanin slowly and are more prone to burn, whereas those with very dark skin are able to tolerate more rays without damage. People with certain diseases (e.g., porphyria, lupus erythematosus) are more sensitive to the sun's rays. Some substances increase the skin's sensitivity, including numerous medications (e.g., barbiturates, oral contraceptives, sulfonamides, antiepileptics), topical products (e.g., retinoic acid [Retin-A], antiseptic soap, aftershave lotions, perfumes, colognes), and certain foods containing photosensitizing chemicals (e.g., carrots, parsley, limes).

UV rays penetrate the skin surface, precipitate a chemical change in the cell molecules, and produce toxic by-products that irritate surrounding tissues. The result is redness, tissue swelling, increased capillary permeability, and the tenderness characteristic of superficial (first-degree) burns and the coagulation, necrosis, and blistering of partial-thickness (second-degree) burns. (See Burns, Chapter 29.) Sunburned skin is exquisitely sensitive, and severe sunburn may be accompanied by nausea, chills, fever, abdominal cramping, and headache. Dehydration may occur.

Excessive or long-term exposure to the sun causes permanent damage to the skin. Ninety percent of skin cancers occur in areas that are exposed to sunlight, and rates of skin cancers are higher in parts of the world where sunlight is more intense. Studies have also shown that childhood is a crucial time for sun exposure. Children who immigrate to sunny climates after 10 years of age develop cancer at lower rates than native-born children. In general, children receive three times as much sun exposure as adults. Teenagers spend even more time in the sun than school-age children, and their desire for the "perfect tan" places their skin at high risk for sun damage. Only 9% of teens actually use sunscreens (Heffernan and O'Sullivan, 1998).

### Nursing Considerations

Treatment involves stopping the burning process, decreasing the inflammatory response, and rehydrating the skin. Local application of cool tap water soaks or immersion in a tepid water bath (temperature slightly below 36.7° C [98° F]) for 20 minutes or until the skin is cool limits tissue destruction and relieves the discomfort. After the cool applications, a bland oil-in-water moisturizing lotion can be applied, but petrolatum-based products that trap radiant heat in the tissues should be avoided. Acetaminophen is recommended for relief of discomfort. Partial-thickness burns are treated the same as those from any heat source.

**Prevention.**   Protection from sunburn is the major goal of management, and the harmful effects of the sun on the delicate skin of infants and children have been receiving increased attention. Protection can be achieved by physical means (i.e., protective clothing and a hat) or by chemical means. Two types of products are available for sun protection: *topical sunscreens,* which partially absorb UV light, and *sun blockers,* which block out UV rays by reflecting sunlight. The most frequently recommended sun blockers are zinc oxide and titanium dioxide ointments.

---

*Distributed by Corsa, Ltd, 555 N Lane, Suite 5025, Conshohocken, PA 19428, (610) 834-1555; www.corsa.com.

Sunscreens are products containing a *sun protective factor (SPF)* based on evaluation of effectiveness against UV rays. The SPF is indicated by a number, such as 15, which indicates that if individuals normally burn in 10 minutes without a sunscreen, use of a sunscreen with an SPF of 15 allows them to remain in the sun for 15 times 10, or 150 minutes (2½ hours) before acquiring the same degree of burn.

Most sunscreens have an SPF ranging from 2 to over 30; the higher the number, the greater the protection. Waterproof sunscreens with a minimum SPF of 15 are recommended. The SPF provides information primarily in relation to the effects of UVB, not UVA. Claims such as "broad-spectrum" or "UVA-UVB sunblock" are usually unsubstantiated. One product that affords protection against UVA is Parsol 1789, found in Photoplex and UVA Guard.

The most effective sunscreens against UVB contain *p-aminobenzoic acid (PABA)* and *PABA-esters*. PABA is more effective, penetrates the outer layer of skin, and may accumulate with repeated use, thus providing protection even when the child is swimming or sweating. PABA may stain clothing; PABA-esters are less likely to stain clothing but are less effective than PABA. However, PABA can cause an allergenic response in sensitive persons, manifested as redness and itching 24 hours after application. *Benzophenones* also offer protection against UVA but are less effective than the PABA preparations and wash off easily. For best results, the sunscreen should be effective against both UVA and UVB.

The range of sunscreens available offer the consumer access to a type and combination to meet any need. Sunscreens are applied evenly to all exposed areas, with special attention to skinfolds and areas that might become exposed as clothing shifts. The Federal Drug Administration recommends a layer of sunscreen that is 2 mg/cm². Parents are directed to read labels of sunscreen products carefully for the SPF and follow the manufacturer's directions for application.

**NURSING ALERT** Sunscreens are not recommended for infants under 6 months of age. However, infants under 6 months of age may have sunscreen applied over small areas of skin such as the back of the hands that may not be adequately covered by clothing when they are in the sun (American Academy of Pediatrics, 1999). Infants should be kept out of the sun or physically shaded from it. Fabric with a tight weave, such as cotton, offers good protection.

Individuals who work in the community, such as teachers, daycare workers, coaches, youth group leaders, and relatives, should all be made aware of sun safety for children. Sunscreens must be applied *liberally*.

It is wise to avoid direct sun exposure when solar radiation is at maximum intensity. The strongest radiation occurs when the sun is at its highest (directly overhead). Earlier or later in the day, with the sun at a 45-degree angle, the earth's atmosphere provides protection equivalent to an SPF of 2.4. Observe the length of one's shadow to assess the time when the sun's rays are most damaging. Seek protection from the sun when the shadow is shorter than one's height (Starr, 1999).

## COMMUNITY FOCUS
### Reducing Sun Exposure

Remember that tanning indicates sun injury, and risks of skin cancer begin in childhood.
Keep infants and children out of the sun as much as possible.
  Use carriage with hood when taking infants outdoors.
  Use canopy on stroller for older infants.
Schedule child's activities to avoid sun exposure between 10 AM and 3 PM whenever possible.
Take increased precautions when living or vacationing in the mountains or the tropics.
Protect child with clothing when outdoors (sun hat, long-sleeved shirt, long pants); avoid sandals (wear closed shoes).
Avoid sheer clothing or bathing suits that allow the sun's rays to penetrate the fabric.
Apply sunscreen with SPF of at least 15.
Apply sunscreen liberally to exposed areas.
  Before every exposure
  On cloudy as well as sunny days
  Even when child plays in shade; sun reflects from sand, snow, cement, and water
Reapply liberally every 2 to 3 hours and whenever child goes in the water or sweats heavily.
Check with child's practitioner regarding any medications the child is taking and observe for any evidence of side effects (rash, redness, swelling).
Examine skin regularly for signs of any change in pigmented nevi (rapid growth, crusting, ulceration, bleeding, change in pigmentation, development of inflamed satellite lesions, loss of normal skin lines) or subjective symptoms (tenderness, pain, itching).
Prohibit child from using sun lamps or tanning parlors.
Set a good example by following the above guidelines.

Modified from *For every child under the sun*, New York, The Skin Cancer Foundation.

Sun damage is cumulative. Although most long-term effects (cancer, wrinkling) are not evident until adulthood, skin care must begin in childhood. Nurses should teach skin care as a basic practice that becomes a part of the child's life, much the same as toothbrushing. (See Community Focus box.) Sun-protection behaviors should also be included as educational components in the school health curricula (Robinson, Rigel, and Amonette, 1998).

## Cold Injury

Cold injuries are most commonly seen in very cold regions. The nature of the heat-regulating mechanisms of the body are such that the inner portion of the body, or core, produces heat and the periphery, or outer area, conserves or dissipates the heat. When the body attempts to conserve heat, the outer tissues are subjected to low temperatures, and local trauma may result.

*Chilblain,* redness and swelling of the skin, occurs when extremities, usually the hands, are exposed intermittently to temperatures of 1.1° to 15.5° C (30° to 60° F). The response may vary but is characterized by intense vasodilation that increases the temperature of involved tissues above that of unaffected tissue and produces edematous, reddish blue patches that itch and burn. As warming takes place, the sensations become more intense but ordinarily subside in a few days.

**TABLE 18-8**    Physical effects of hypothermia

| Temperature | Characteristics |
| --- | --- |
| 35° C (95° F) | Increased respiratory rate, decreased intestinal motility; vigorous shivering; may be conscious and alert; task performance often impaired |
| 32° C (90° F) | May continue uncontrollable shivering or may begin to show muscular rigidity; decreased respiratory rate; atrial fibrillation; may still be conscious but sensorium changes evident; impaired cognition, reasoning, and speech; loss of manual skills and dexterity; brief vasodilation that causes flushes and warm sensation and possible confusion |
| 30° C (86° F) | Decreased cerebral blood flow; may show increased blood pressure (may be difficult to obtain), tachycardia, and tachypnea; may have supraventricular arrhythmia, PCVs, and T-wave inversion; usually conscious, but a loss of consciousness is preceded by irritability |
| 27° C (80° F) | Bradycardia and slowed respiratory rate; metabolic rate decreased by 50%; decreased oxygen uptake, $CO_2$ production; ventricular fibrillation; rigid extremities |
| 25° C (77° F) | Hypotension; glomerular filtration and blood flow to kidneys reduced by 30% |
| 20° C (68° F) | Unconscious; nonfunctioning reflexes; unresponsive pupils; respirations barely detectable or undetectable; extremities and trunk cold to touch; abnormal ECG; pulse may decrease to 4 per minute, progressing to cardiac standstill; flat EEG; dead appearance |
| 18° C (65° F) | Injury to peripheral tissue |

**Frostbite** is the term used to describe tissue damage caused when excessive heat loss to local tissues allows ice crystals to form in tissues. The mechanisms of slow and rapid freezing differ. Slow freezing causes ice crystals to form in the extracellular fluid, leading to increased osmolality and movement of water from the cells. This causes cellular dehydration and destruction. Rapid freezing produces both extracellular and intracellular freezing and immediate cellular destruction. Rapid freezing takes place at high altitudes or with high conductivity from cold water immersion.

When frozen tissues thaw, the tissue damage is like that from a high-temperature burn—red blood cell aggregation, stasis, venous thrombosis, tissue edema and ischemic damage, increased tissue pressure, and death and necrosis of surrounding tissues. The frostbitten part appears white or blanched, feels solid, and is without sensation.

Rapid rewarming is associated with less tissue necrosis than slow thawing. It restores blood flow and shortens the period of cellular damage. Rewarming produces a flush (sometimes deep purple) and a return of sensation, which is extremely painful. Large blisters may appear 24 to 48 hours after rewarming and begin to resorb within 5 to 10 days, followed by the formation of a hard black eschar. Superficial injury often heals satisfactorily.

### Therapeutic Management

Rewarming is accomplished by immersing the part in well-agitated water at 37.8° to 42.2° C (100° to 108° F). Discomfort is managed with analgesics and sedatives. Care of blistered skin is similar to that described for burns. It is seldom possible to estimate the extent of tissue loss until new skin layers are revealed after the eschar layer separates. Therefore amputation of extremities is usually delayed for 60 to 90 days unless there is evidence of gangrene.

### Nursing Considerations

The frostbite victim should be transferred to the nearest emergency treatment center. Injured parts are protected from trauma and handled gently. The patient is prevented from ambulating on injured feet. Rubbing injured tissues is contraindicated and can cause damage by rupture of crystallized cells. After rewarming, a loose dressing is applied. Dry heat is not applied. (See Burns, Chapter 29, and Pain Management, Chapter 26.)

## Hypothermia

Hypothermia is defined as the cooling of the body's core temperature (pulmonary artery or esophageal) to injurious levels, usually identified as below 35° C (95° F). Hypothermia occurs in environmental settings when heat production by exercise and metabolism is less than heat lost by convection, conduction, or radiation. There is a 6% drop in blood flow for each 1° C decrease in core temperature. Very young children with a large surface area relative to body mass and thin persons are at the greatest risk for hypothermia.

The body in positive heat balance conserves heat by alternating vasoconstriction and vasodilation in extremities. Threat of prolonged or severe cold exposure causes the body to conserve core temperature at the expense of the extremities by shunting warm blood to the core after passing through the muscles of the extremities. Shivering contributes to warming by raising the metabolic rate to increase the heat of blood before it returns to the core. Clinical manifestations related to degree of hypothermia are outlined in Table 18-8.

### Therapeutic Management

Rewarming is the major objective of therapy. For mild hypothermia (30° to 35° C [86° to 95° F]), only external application of heat lamps or immersion in water (38° to 42° C [100.4° to 107.6° F]) is necessary to restore core temperature with little risk of complications. Lower temperatures require core rewarming by any of several modalities—warm humidified oxygen, intravenous fluids, rectal lavage, peritoneal lavage (dialysis) with warm fluids, hemodialysis, application of external warmth to core circulation areas (groin, axilla, posterior neck region), and/or extracorporeal blood rewarming.

Supportive therapy includes maintenance of ventilation, cardiac monitoring, monitoring of renal function, and correction of fluid and acid-base imbalances. The prognosis is directly correlated with the degree of hypothermia, method of rewarming, and presence of underlying medical conditions.

### Nursing Considerations

Nursing care consists of monitoring vital functions and assisting with therapies. Obtaining a history from the family or other observers, including outside environmental temperature, length of exposure to elements, location of exposure site (e.g., outside or inside a vehicle or structure), and any care that may have been given, is essential. If trauma is associated with the hypothermia, the mechanism and circumstances of injury are ascertained.

**Prevention.** Anticipation of cold conditions and knowledge of cold survival techniques are the basis of prevention. Children living in cold climates should have adequate protection when outdoors. Multiple layers of warm clothing are more effective than a single heavy layer for reducing the rate of heat loss, although they do not prevent it. Families living in cold climates should take precautions against unexpected prolonged exposure to cold (e.g., store extra blankets, food rations, and other equipment in their vehicles in the event of an unexpected mechanical breakdown).

Loss of central core temperature can be reduced by 50% when an individual assumes the fetal position or when a person in water remains still. A person suspected of having hypothermia should be moved to a sheltered area, and wet clothing should be removed and replaced with dry, warm garments. Warm, high-calorie liquids are important if the person is conscious.

## SKIN DISORDERS RELATED TO DRUG SENSITIVITY

### Drug Reactions

Adverse reactions to drugs are seen more often in the skin than in any other organ, although any organ of the body can be affected. The reaction may be a result of toxicity related to drug concentration, individual intolerance to the average dosage of the drug, or an allergic or idiosyncratic response. The manifestations may be associated with side effects or secondary effects of a drug, either of which are unrelated to its primary pharmacologic actions.

Although any drug is capable of producing almost any form of reaction in the susceptible individual, some have a tendency to produce a particular reaction consistently, and some are more likely than others to produce an untoward effect. Many are allergenic responses following a prior administration of the drug, even a topical application. Other factors influence a drug response in a particular individual. For example, the incidence increases with the amount and the number of drugs given.

**NURSING ALERT**  Intravenous drugs are more likely to cause a reaction than oral drugs. Stop the drug but maintain the infusion with normal saline.

Manifestations of drug reactions may be delayed or immediate. A period of 7 days is usually required for a child to develop sensitivity to a drug that has never been administered previously. With prior sensitivity the manifestations appear almost immediately. Rashes—exanthematous, urticarial, or eczematoid—are the most common manifestation of adverse drug reactions in children. However, individual drug reactions may vary from a single lesion to extensive, generalized epidermal necrosis. Cutaneous manifestations can resemble almost any skin disease and can be seen in almost any degree of severity. With few exceptions, the distribution of a drug eruption is widespread because it results from a circulating agent, appears as an inflammatory response with itching, is sudden in onset, and may be associated with constitutional symptoms such as fever, malaise, gastrointestinal upsets, anemia, or liver and kidney damage.

Another common response is a *fixed eruption* (i.e., a recurrent eruption at the same site with each readministration of the drug). The lesion, a purplish red round or oval plaque with a sharp border seen most frequently on the extremities, disappears slowly, and the pigmentation deepens with each episode.

In most cases treatment for simple cutaneous reactions consists of discontinuation of the drug. Sometimes a decision is made to continue the drug (such as an antibiotic in an infant or small child) until the cause of the rash is clearly indicated. In urticarial-type eruptions, antihistamines may be ordered, and for widespread and severe lesions corticosteroids are beneficial. Severe anaphylactic reactions are a medical emergency. (See Anaphylaxis, Chapter 29.)

### Nursing Considerations

The most effective means of management is prevention. Parents always remember a severe response. A careful history will elicit evidence of a previous drug reaction. The history should include the name of the drug, nature of the reaction, drug dose, and how soon after administration the reaction occurred. (See Past History, Chapter 6.)

Nurses who suspect that a rash is caused by a medication should withhold any further dose and report the eruption to the practitioner. Frequent offenders in drug reactions are penicillin and sulfonamides, and nurses must be alert to this possibility. However, even commonplace drugs, including aspirin, barbiturates, chemical agents in some foods, flavoring agents, and preservatives, are capable of producing an undesired response. Persons who have severe reactions should wear an identification bracelet or chain in case of emergency or inadvertent administration of the offending drug.

## Erythema Multiforme

Erythema multiforme is an acute, cutaneous disorder that may be associated with infections (usually viruses) or ingestions of drugs. The characteristic lesion consists of an urticarial plaque with a dusky or vesicular center, which appears primarily on the palms, soles, and extensor surfaces.

Treatment involves discontinuing the drug, applying wet compresses for erosive lesions, and administering analgesics for discomfort. Antihistamines may be prescribed for pruritus.

## Erythema Multiforme Exudativum (Stevens-Johnson Syndrome) (SJS)

SJS is the severe form of erythema multiforme characterized by lesions of the skin and mucous membranes, fever, and multiple systemic symptoms. The disease is presumed to be a hypersensitivity reaction to certain drugs although the reaction may follow an upper respiratory tract infection. The disorder is relatively rare, occurs at any age, and is more common in males than in females.

The syndrome begins with flulike symptoms—malaise, sore throat, fever, and severe headache. Inflammation of the glans penis (balanitis), eyes (conjunctivitis), or mouth/pharynx (stomatitis) appears next, followed in a few days by an erythematous papular rash. The lesions can involve any cutaneous surface, including the palms and soles, but usually spare the scalp. They can be scattered or confluent. The initial lesions enlarge by peripheral expansion with a vesicular center that often becomes bullous (Fig. 18-16). Mucous membrane ulceration often becomes severe enough to interfere with eating, and many patients have pulmonary involvement.

Mild disease requires only symptomatic treatment. However, severe disease requires hospitalization. Fluid and nutritional requirements are high, and patients often respond to topical lidocaine to relieve oral pain and a liquid diet. Intravenous opioids, such as morphine, and parenteral feedings may be needed for extensive oral involvement. Meticulous mouth care is important, and skin care frequently requires management in a burn unit. (See Stomatitis, Chapter 16, and Burns, Chapter 29.) Daily ophthalmologic examination is advised. Dry eyes are a problem as well as risk of chronic mild symblepharon (adhesion of lids to the eyeball). Antibiotics are administered to patients with positive cultures, but the use of corticosteroids is controversial.

The mortality is estimated at 10% to 15% during the acute phase, especially in patients with pulmonary involvement. The disease is self-limiting, and the skin lesions gradually disappear without scarring in 2 to 3 weeks but may recur on reexposure to an offending drug. The family needs emotional support to cope with the life-threatening nature of the disease.

## Toxic Epidermal Necrolysis (TEN) (Lyell Disease)

TEN is a drug-induced injury to the skin characterized by a generalized erythematous rash that rapidly evolves into bul-

lae and peeling. It appears to be a hypersensitivity reaction with precipitating factors similar to those responsible for erythema multiforme. The more common offending drugs are phenobarbital, phenytoin, allopurinol, sulfonamides, and penicillin. In children, the clinical appearance is the same as that seen in *staphylococcal scalded skin syndrome (SSSS).*

The disease begins with a prodromal period of fever and malaise. Symptoms include a generalized erythematous rash that rapidly evolves into bullae and extensive epidermal peeling, and oral lesions similar to those observed in SJS. Treatment consists of withdrawal of the offending drug, fluid and electrolyte replacement, and skin management as for severe burns. The disease can be protracted, and mortality can range from 25% to 50%. It is essential that families of children receiving antiepileptics or sulfonamides be informed of the significance of a rash and the importance of reporting it to their health professional promptly.

## MISCELLANEOUS AND CONGENITAL SKIN PROBLEMS

A number of miscellaneous skin disorders also occur in children (Table 18-9). Psoriasis can occur in children less than 16 years of age, and photosensitivity eruptions associated with inherited diseases appear early in childhood. Ichthyoses are a heterogeneous group of disorders characterized by scaling that creates challenging treatment problems.

## Neurofibromatosis-1 (NF1)

NF1, or von Recklinghausen disease, is a relatively common disorder with an autosomal dominant inheritance pattern. It occurs in 1:3000 persons and has a high mutation rate. The manifestations are highly variable and appear to result from a defect that alters peripheral nerve differentiation and growth.

Initial clinical presentation involves small, discrete, flat, pigmented skin lesions with smooth edges (*café-au-lait spots, pigmented nevi*) (Fig. 18-17) and/or axillary or inguinal freckling that develops in early infancy or childhood. Slow-

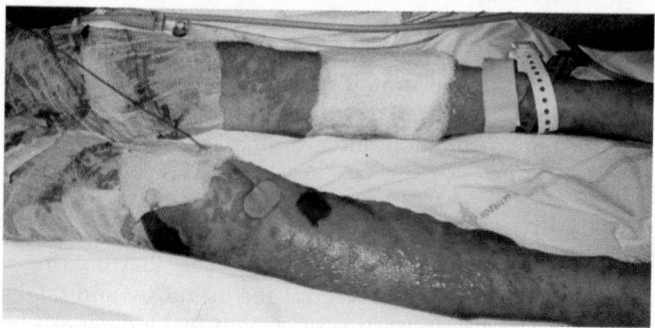

**Fig. 18-16**   Stevens-Johnson syndrome.

**Fig. 18-17**   Café-au-lait patches. (From Seidel HM and others: *Mosby's guide to physical examination,* ed 4, St Louis, 1999, Mosby.)

**TABLE 18-9**   Miscellaneous skin disorders

| Disease/Causative Agent | Local Manifestations | Management | Comments |
|---|---|---|---|
| **Urticaria**—Usually allergic response to drugs or infection | Development of wheals<br>Vary in size and configuration and tend to appear quickly, spread irregularly, and fade within a few hours<br>May be constant or intermittent, sparse or profuse, small or large, discrete or confluent<br>May be acute, chronic, or recurrent in acute attacks | Local soothing and antipruritic applications<br>Antihistamines<br>Epinephrine or ephedrine<br>Cortisone in severe cases<br>Severe upper respiratory involvement may require tracheostomy | Known etiologic agents should be avoided<br>May be accompanied by malaise, fever, lymphadenopathy<br>Severe cases may involve mucous membranes, internal organs, and joints<br>Obstruction to air passages constitutes medical emergency (see Chapter 31) |
| **Intertrigo**—Mechanical trauma and aggravating factors of excessive heat, moisture, and sweat retention | Red, inflamed, moist, partially denuded, marginated areas, the shape of which is determined by location<br>Appears where opposing skin surfaces rub together, such as intergluteal folds, groin, neck, and axilla<br>Excessive moisture and obesity are often factors | Affected areas kept clean and dry<br>Skinfolds kept separated with a generous supply of nonmedicated powder<br>Exposure to air and light<br>Removal of excess clothing | A form of diaper irritation<br>Prevent recurrence by keeping susceptible areas clean and dry<br>Frequently associated with overheating from too much clothing |
| **Psoriasis**—Unknown; hereditary predisposition; may be triggered by stress | Round, thick, dry, reddish patches covered with coarse, silvery scales over trunk and extremities; first lesions commonly appear in scalp; facial lesions more common in children than adults<br>Affected cells proliferate at a much more rapid rate than normal cells | Exposure to sunlight, ultraviolet light<br>Topical corticosteroids<br>Tar derivatives<br>Trihydroxyanthracine<br>Keratolytic agents (salicylic acid)<br>Psoralin—ultraviolet A (PUVA)*<br>Emollients may provide relief | Uncommon in children under age 6 years<br>Persons are otherwise healthy individuals<br>Coal tar and psoralin act synergistically with ultraviolet light<br>Keratolytic agents enhance absorption of corticosteroids<br>Humidifiers may help in winter |
| **Alopecia**<br>  Alopecia areata | Sudden onset of asymptomatic, noninflammatory, round, bald patches in hairy parts of body | Psychologic support<br>Inducement of allergic contact dermatitis to stimulate growth of hair<br>Minoxidil (peripheral vasodilator) | Family history in 10%-26% of cases<br>Some concern regarding drug therapy safety<br>Refer to support groups† |
|   Traumatic alopecia | Traction alopecia around scalp margins from tight hair styles (e.g., braids, pony tails, corn rows) | Counseling regarding hair styling, use of hair cosmetics, hot combs, rollers | More prevalent in black children and adolescents<br>Prolonged traction can produce fibrosis of hair root and permanent loss |
|   Trichotillomania | Compulsive hair pulling | Determine and treat cause | Chronic hair pulling may require psychologic therapy |
|   Tinea capitis | See Table 18-5 | See Table 18-5 | See Table 18-5 |

*Still considered investigational.
†**National Alopecia Areata Foundation,** 710 C St, Suite 11, San Rafael, CA 94901, (415) 456-4644, fax: (415) 456-4274; e-mail: 74301.1642@compuserve. com.

growing cutaneous and subcutaneous neurofibromas that grow along the course of a peripheral nerve appear in later childhood or adolescence and increase in number with age. *Lisch nodules,* dome-shaped clear-to-yellow or brown elevations on the iris surface, develop before puberty in most affected individuals. *Elephantiasis* (thickening and enfolding of the skin) may also occur.

Other characteristics include developmental delay, retardation, seizures, scoliosis or kyphosis, short stature, macrocephaly, speech defects, learning disabilities, and problems with fine and gross motor skills (Johnson and others, 1999). Severity varies within the same family. One family member may have only café-au-lait spots or axillary freckling, while another may have more severe manifestations.

Diagnosis is established by physical findings based on National Institutes of Health (NIH) Consensus Conference guidelines (Box 18-1). A family history is elicited to determine if the specific case is inherited or if it represents a new mutation. Risk for transmitting the disorder to offspring is 50%. Therapy is limited to excision of tumors that produce pain or impair function and symptomatic management of manifestations.

## Nursing Considerations

Nursing care involves recognition of signs that indicate a possibility of the disease, referral for diagnosis, and family counseling and support. It is important that a diagnosis be made, even when the only manifestations are a few café-au-

**Box 18-1**  ▪ ■ ▪
**Criteria for Diagnosis
of Neurofibromatosis-1**

An individual with two or more of the following clinical signs
meets the criteria for NF1:
Six or more café-au-lait spots larger than 5 mm in diameter
in prepubertal children and larger than 15 mm in postpu-
bertal individual
Two or more neurofibromas of any type or one plexiform
neurofibroma
Freckling in the axillary or inguinal region
Optic glioma
Two or more Lisch nodules
A distinctive osseous lesion (e.g., sphenoid dysplasia or thin-
ning of long bone cortex with or without pseudoarthrosis)
A first-degree relative with NF1 according to the criteria
listed above

lait spots. The family needs to know the genetic implications and be alert for signs that indicate the child is developing more serious characteristics of the disease. Cancer occurs in patients with the disorder although the rates vary widely. Other members of the family should be assessed for evidence of the disorder.

In addition, families need to know that children with NF1 have a significantly increased risk for social and emotional problems. Parents need to receive written materials about these problems that they can share with teachers and other adults who interact with the child. Children with NF1 should be screened with systematic standardized tests and more aggressive and intensive treatment should be provided for speech, motor, and cognitive deficits that may contribute to social and emotional problems (Johnson and others, 1999).

The **National Neurofibromatosis Foundation, Inc.*** is an organization dedicated to increasing public awareness of NF1, providing help and support to families affected by the disorder, and stimulating research.

# BITES AND STINGS
## Arthropod Bites and Stings

*Arthropods* include insects and arachnids (mites, ticks, spiders, and scorpions). Manifestations and management of skin lesions caused by arthropods are outlined in Table 18-10.

Some proteins in insect venom are species-specific; others are common to a number of species, and crossover reactivity is common. The usual local response to a sting is sharp pain, a local wheal (less than 2 inches in diameter), and erythema accompanied by intense itching at the site, lasting less than 24 hours. The reaction is produced by enzymes, cytotoxic proteins, and vasoactive compounds, primarily histamine and kinins.

Systemic reactions can occur and, in some instances, can be life-threatening. Non–life-threatening systemic reactions

begin several minutes to several hours after the sting and consist of simple urticaria, erythema, pruritus, and angioedema. Serious, life-threatening reactions usually begin within 5 to 10 minutes after the sting and include airway obstruction secondary to laryngeal edema, bronchospasm, hypotension, and cardiovascular collapse.

To prevent contact with stinging and biting insects, children should be taught behaviors that reduce the likelihood of injury. In addition, topical insect repellents generally provide safe and effective protection for several hours. The best all-purpose repellents contain the active ingredient *diethyltoluamide (DEET),* which is effective for a variety of insects, mosquitoes, chiggers, ticks, fleas, deerflies, and sand flies. Protection may last from 1 to several hours, but effectiveness is influenced by the concentration of active ingredients. The product must be reapplied after sweating, swimming, wiping, or exposure to rain. Because adverse effects have been reported in young children and because long-term effects of DEET are unknown, caution is advised against excessive application or prolonged use, especially of products with high concentrations of DEET. The insect repellent should not be applied to children's hands because it may be rubbed in the eyes. It should be removed with soap and water when the child is brought inside.

Most bites are managed by simple symptomatic measures such as cool compresses, calamine lotion, and prevention of secondary infection. Often treatment consists of application of a substance that relieves the swelling and discomfort and can be made from common household products.

### Hymenoptera Stings

When a hymenopteran (bees, in particular) stings, its barbed stinger penetrates into the skin. The stinger also contains a nerve ganglion, muscles, and a venom sac. As long as the stinger remains in the skin, the muscles push the stinger deeper and venom is pumped into the wound. A recent study of different methods of removing the stinger revealed that the method of removal did not influence the amount of venom injected into the wound. There was no difference in the amount of venom injected when the stinger was removed by external compression with forceps or when the stinger was flicked or scraped off the skin. The influencing factor was the amount of time from the bee sting to removal of the stinger; the longer the time interval, the greater the amount of venom injected (Visscher, Vetter, and Camazine, 1996). The best approach is to remove the bee sting as quickly as possible and to get away from the vicinity of other bees to prevent further injury.

Children are taught to avoid contact with bees and to recognize the insect (e.g., it is not part of the flower). For those who have become sensitized to hymenoptera stings and demonstrate a severe life-threatening systemic response, intramuscular administration of epinephrine provides immediate relief and must be available for emergency use. For hypersensitive children, a kit must be available that contains epinephrine, a hypodermic syringe, and perhaps ephedrine and an antihistamine preparation. Hypersensitive children should wear medical identification, such as a bracelet, and the families are reminded to check the expiration date on

---

*95 Pine St, 16th Floor, New York, NY 10005, (800) 323-7938, (212) 344-6633, fax: (212) 747-0004, e-mail: nnff@aol.com.

**TABLE 18-10**   Skin lesions caused by arthropods

| Mechanism/Characteristics | Manifestations | Management |
|---|---|---|
| **Insect Bites—Flies, Gnats, Mosquitoes, Fleas**<br>Mechanism:<br>  Foreign protein in insects' saliva introduced when skin is penetrated for a blood-sucking meal<br>Distribution:<br>  Almost everywhere—fleas, mosquitoes, ants<br>  Suburbs and rural areas—bees<br>  Urban areas—hornets, wasps, yellow jackets | Hypersensitivity reaction<br>  Papular urticaria<br>  Firm papules; may be capped by vesicles or excoriated<br>Little or no reaction in nonsensitized person | Treatment:<br>  Use antipruritic agents and baths<br>  Administer antihistamines<br>  Prevent secondary infection<br>Prevention:<br>  Avoid contact<br>  Remove focus, such as treating furniture, mattresses, carpets, and pets, where insects may live<br>  Apply insect repellent when exposure is anticipated |
| **Chiggers—Harvest Mite**<br>Mechanism:<br>  Attach with claws and secrete a digestive substance that liquefies the host's epidermis<br>Manifestations:<br>  Erythematous papules<br>  Intense itching | Same as insect bites<br>Favor warm areas of body, especially intertriginous areas and areas covered with clothing | Avoid contact, especially in areas of tall grass and underbrush<br>Apply insect repellent when exposure is anticipated; insecticides such as diazinon can also be sprayed in yards<br>May require systemic steroids for extensive bites |
| **Hymenopteran Stings—Bees, Wasps, Hornets, Yellow Jackets, Fire Ants**<br>Mechanism:<br>  Injection of venom through stinging apparatus<br>  Venom contains histamine, allergenic proteins, and often a spreading factor, hyaluronidase<br>  Severe reactions caused by hypersensitivity and/or multiple stings | Local reaction: small red area, wheal, itching, and heat<br>Systemic reactions: may be mild to severe, including generalized edema, pain, nausea and vomiting, confusion, respiratory embarrassment, and shock | Treatment:<br>  Carefully scrape off or pull out stinger as quickly as possible<br>  Cleanse with soap and water<br>  Apply cool compresses<br>  Apply common household product (e.g., lemon juice, paste made with aspirin or baking soda)<br>  Administer antihistamines<br>  Severe reactions: administer epinephrine, corticosteroids; treat for shock<br>Prevention:<br>  Teach child to wear shoes; to avoid wearing bright clothing, flowery prints, shiny jewelry, or perfumed grooming products (cologne, scented hairspray), which might attract the insect; and to avoid places where the insect may be contacted<br>Hypersensitive children should wear identifying tag to indicate allergy and therapy needed; family should keep emergency medication and be taught its administration |
| **Black Widow Spider**<br>Mechanism:<br>  Venom injected through a clawlike appendage; has neurotoxic action | Mild sting at time of bite<br>Area becomes swollen, painful, and erythematous | Treatment:<br>  Cleanse wound with antiseptic<br>  Apply cool compresses<br>  Administer antivenin |

the kit and replace an outdated one. Families should determine if a school nurse is available at the school; if not, someone at the school should be designated to inject the epinephrine in case of an emergency.

Children with a history of generalized reactivity to an insect sting should undergo skin testing with the radioallergosorbent test (RAST), and possibly immunotherapy with venous extract (desensitization) to prevent serious or fatal reactions. In the United States venous extracts are available for the honeybee, yellow jacket, yellow hornet, and wasp.

## Arachnid Bites

Most arachnids in the United States, including tarantulas, are relatively harmless. All spiders produce venom that is

**TABLE 18-10**   Skin lesions caused by arthropods—cont'd

| Mechanism/Characteristics | Manifestations | Management |
|---|---|---|
| **Black Widow Spider—cont'd**<br>Characteristics:<br>  Spider is shiny black, with a body about 1.25 cm (0.5 inches) long and a red or orange hourglass-shaped marking on underside<br>  Avoids light and bites in self-defense | Dizziness, weakness, and abdominal pain<br>May produce delirium, paralysis, seizures, and (if large amount of venom absorbed) death | Administer muscle relaxant, such as calcium gluconate; analgesics and/or sedatives; hydrocortisone or diazepam IV<br>Prevention:<br>  Teach children to avoid places that harbor the spider (e.g., woodpiles) |
| **Brown Recluse Spider**<br>Mechanism:<br>  Venom injected via fangs<br>  Venom contains powerful necrotoxin<br>Characteristics:<br>  Spider is slender, long legged, with body length of 1 to 2 cm; color is fawn to dark brown; recognized by fiddle-shaped mark on head<br>  Shy; bites only when annoyed or surprised<br>  Prefers dark areas where seldom disturbed | Mild sting at time of bite<br>Transient erythema followed by bleb or blister; mild to severe pain in 2-8 hours; purple, star-shaped area in 3-4 days; necrotic ulceration in 7-14 days (Fig. 18-18)<br>Systemic reactions may include fever, malaise, restlessness, nausea and vomiting, and joint pain<br>Generalized petechial eruption<br>Wounds heal with scar formation | Treatment:<br>  Apply cool compresses locally<br>  Administer antibiotics, corticosteroids<br>  Relieve pain<br>  Wound may require skin graft<br>Prevention:<br>  Teach children to avoid possible nesting sites |
| **Scorpions**<br>Mechanism:<br>  Sting by means of a hooked caudal stinger that discharges venom<br>  Venom of more venomous species contains hemolysins, endotheliolysins, and neurotoxins<br>Characteristics:<br>  Usual habitat is southwestern United States | Intense local pain, erythema, numbness, burning, restlessness, vomiting<br>Ascending motor paralysis with convulsions, weakness, rapid pulse, excessive salivation, thirst, dysuria, pulmonary edema, coma, and death<br>Some species produce only local tissue reaction with swelling at puncture site (distinctive)<br>Symptoms subside in a few hours<br>Deaths occur among children under 4 years of age, usually in first 24 hours | Treatment:<br>  Delay absorption of venom by keeping child quiet; place involved area in dependent position<br>  Administer antivenin<br>  Relieve pain<br>  Admit to pediatric intensive care unit for surveillance<br>Prevention:<br>  Teach children to avoid possible nesting sites |
| **Ticks**<br>Mechanism:<br>  In process of sucking blood, head and mouth parts are buried in skin<br>Characteristics:<br>  Feed on blood of mammals<br>  Significant in humans because of pathologic organism carried<br>  May be vectors of various infectious diseases, such as Rocky Mountain spotted fever, Q fever, tularemia, relapsing fever, Lyme disease, tick paralysis<br>  Must attach and feed 1-2 hours to transmit disease<br>  Usual habitat is very wooded area | Tick usually attached to skin, head embedded<br>Produce firm, discrete, intensely pruritic nodules at site of attachment<br>May cause urticaria or persistent localized edema | Treatment:<br>  Grasp tick with tweezers (forceps) as close as possible to point of attachment<br>  Pull straight up with steady, even pressure; if bare hands touch tick during removal, wash hands thoroughly with soap and water<br>  Remove any remaining part (e.g., head) with sterile needle<br>  Cleanse wounds with soap and disinfectant<br>Prevention:<br>  Teach children to avoid areas where prevalent<br>  Inspect skin (especially scalp) after being in wooded areas |

injected via fangs. Some are unable to pierce the skin; others produce a venom that is insufficiently toxic to be harmful. There is a local tissue reaction that is relieved by cool compresses or the methods described for hymenoptera stings.

Only scorpions and two spiders—the brown recluse and black widow—inject venom deadly enough to require im-

mediate attention. Children bitten by these arachnids must receive medical attention as soon as possible.

## Ticks

Ticks are troublesome because they become partially imbedded in the skin as they feed. The recommended method for their removal is to grasp the tick with curved

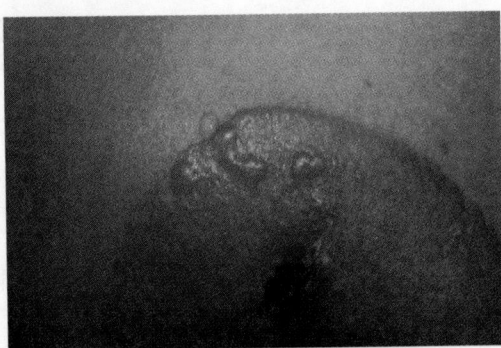

**Fig. 18-18** Brown recluse spider bite; note central necrosis surrounded by purplish area and blisters. (From Weston WL, Lane AT: *Color textbook of pediatric dermatology*, St Louis, 1991, Mosby.)

forceps as close as possible to the point of attachment and pull straight up with a steady, even pressure. If a portion of the body (e.g., the head) remains, it can be removed with a sterile needle in the same manner as a sliver. The bite is cleansed with soap and a disinfectant after removal. If the hands have touched the tick, they are washed thoroughly with soap and water.

To avoid ticks, children should wear long pants tucked into the socks and a long-sleeved shirt when walking in infested areas, especially in the spring and summer. Children should avoid grass and shrubbery where ticks may be lurking. Ticks can also be picked up by dogs and other household pets. Permethrin may be purchased in some pet stores and can be applied to the family dog to guard against tick infestation. Parents are advised to check their children carefully for the organisms when their children have been in areas where they might be acquired. Light clothing makes ticks more visible.

## Animal Bites

Animal bites are common injuries and include both wild and domestic animals. Wild animal bites are discussed in relation to rabies, and their wounds are treated the same as bites of domestic animals, such as dogs, cats, hamsters, and mice. This discussion is directed primarily toward dog bites.

Approximately half the victims of dog bites are less than 5 years of age; boys are bitten more frequently than girls (Bernardo and others, 2000). Stray dogs are seldom involved in attacks; most dogs are owned by the family of the victim or a neighbor. Most dog attacks occur in or adjacent to the owners' yards, and the attack is usually preceded by verbal or physical contact with the animal (Bernardo and others, 2000). This problem is increasing because there is a growing trend to acquire large, aggressive guard dogs. Large dogs account for most fatal dog wounds in children (Sacks and others, 1996).

Most animal bites are caused by dogs. Cat bites are less common, but cat scratches are extremely common (see Cat Scratch Disease, p. 766). Most dog or cat injuries are to the upper extremities. Small children are more likely to receive bites or scratches to the head, face, and neck because they tend to put their heads near the animal's head and flail their arms rather than protecting their heads.

Deaths from dog bite–related injuries in the United States occur predominantly in the pediatric age-group. Of the reported cases, 57% were in children less than 10 years of age (Sacks and others, 1996). Pit bulls were the most commonly reported breeds involved in fatal attacks. Fifty-nine percent of the deaths involved an unrestrained dog on the owner's property.

Animal bites are potentially serious because of the likelihood of significant infection. Injuries vary in intensity from small puncture wounds to complete evulsion of tissue that is associated with significant crush injury. Dog bites present as lacerations or evulsions; cats exert less biting force, but their sharp teeth penetrate more deeply, inoculating organisms deep into tissues.

The location of a bite influences the incidence of infection. Injuries to the arm and hand tend to become infected more often than those on the legs, scalp, and face. Redness, swelling, and tenderness develop around the site of injury, often accompanied by purulent or serosanguineous drainage. It may be difficult to assess hand infection because most lymphatic drainage is contained in the dorsal subcutaneous space, and swelling occurs in this area when the injury may be elsewhere.

### Therapeutic Management

General wound care consists of rinsing the wound with copious amounts of saline or Ringer's lactate delivered under pressure via a large syringe and of washing the surrounding skin with mild soap. A clean pressure dressing is applied, and the extremity is elevated if the wound is bleeding. Medical evaluation is advised because there is danger of tetanus and rabies although dogs in most urban areas are required to be immunized against rabies. Bites from wild animals, such as raccoons, skunks, foxes, and bats, are potentially dangerous (American Academy of Pediatrics, 2000b). (See Rabies, Chapter 37.)

Prophylactic antibiotics are indicated for puncture wounds and wounds in areas that may prove to be cosmetically or functionally impaired if infected. Extensive lacerations are debrided and loosely sutured to allow for drainage in the event of infection. Primary closure of jagged, irregular wounds with associated crush injury and devitalized tissue is contraindicated, except for facial wounds because of cosmetic reasons (Dinman and Jarosz, 1996). Tetanus toxoid is administered according to standard guidelines (see Chapter 12), and rabies protocol is followed. Injuries to poorly vascularized areas such as the hands are more likely to become infected than those in more vascularized areas such as the face; puncture wounds are more apt to become infected than lacerations.

### Nursing Considerations

The most important aspect related to animal bites is prevention. Children should understand animal behavior and develop respect for animals. (See Community Focus box.) It is vital that they learn how to treat animals and how to react to them. Parents should monitor their children's behavior with a dog and instruct them not to tease or surprise a dog, invade its territory, interfere with its feeding or sleeping, take its toy, or interact with a sick or injured dog or a dog with pups (Humane Society of United States, 1998).

Parents who are considering getting a pet, especially a dog, for themselves or their children should select a dog that is least likely to be a danger to their children. The level of sociability with children is the key to a selection, and dogs range from dangerous and unsuitable to tolerant of children and well behaved.

Parents should obtain dogs from a reputable source that breeds dogs for good temperament. After the dog is purchased, obedience training and socialization should begin to prevent the dog from developing behaviors that are undesirable to the family and neighborhood. Such training is often provided through veterinary services or animal shelters (Bernardo and others, 2000). Adequate socialization of puppies and basic obedience training in dogs could result in fewer dog bites (Wallace, 1998).

## Snakebites

Approximately 1600 venomous bites from domestic snakes were reported to the American Association of Poison Control Centers in 1998 (Litovitz and others, 1999). Asian and African snakes are far more dangerous than those in the United States and Europe. The major species in the United States are the *Crotalidae* (pit vipers), which include rattlesnakes, copperheads, and cottonmouths, and the *Elapidae*, which include coral snakes and cobras. Most bites are attributed to the *Crotalidae*.

The manifestations and morbidity are highly variable and depend on the species and size of the snake, the amount of venom injected, the time of year, the age and size of the child, and the location of the bite. Not every bite from a poisonous snake injects venom (Schexnayder and Schexnayder, 2000).

The initial action after snakebite is to move the victim away from the area, attempt to calm the child, and place the child at rest. A *loose* tourniquet applied proximal to the bite delays the flow of lymph, which can carry the venom to the systemic circulation. It should not be tight enough to occlude circulation; a pulse distal to the bite should be palpable. Any constricting items of clothing or jewelry should be removed from the affected limb. A splint should be applied to immobilize the limb, and the victim should be transported to the nearest medical facility.

**NURSING ALERT**   Do not apply ice to the snakebite because doing so decreases the blood supply to the envenomated site, thereby allowing the venom to work more destruction while decreasing the effect of antivenom on the natural immune mechanisms.

If the child has been bitten by a large snake, if less than 30 minutes (some authorities say 5 minutes) has elapsed since the child was bitten, and if medical help is more than 30 minutes away, suction may be beneficial. Suction should

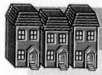

## COMMUNITY FOCUS
### Animal Safety

Teach children to avoid all strange animals, especially wild, sick, or injured ones, who may be carriers of rabies (use the same techniques employed in teaching children not to talk to strangers).

Teach children to avoid dangerous and nervous animals in the neighborhood.

Vaccinate your own dog against rabies.

Never permit children to break up an animal fight, even when their own pet is involved. Use a rake, broom, or garden hose to separate animals.

Teach children the danger of mistreating or teasing pets (animals will bite if mauled, annoyed, or frightened).

Spay or neuter your pets (spaying or neutering reduces aggression, not protectiveness).

Avoid direct eye contact with a threatening dog and remain motionless until a threatening dog leaves the area.

Never hold your face close to an animal.

Teach children not to disturb an animal that is eating, sleeping, or caring for young puppies, kittens, etc.

Never tease, pull the tail, or take away food, a bone, or a toy with which an animal is playing.

Never approach a strange dog who is confined or restrained; do not keep animals confined with short ropes or chains (this can make them aggressive or vicious, especially when teased).

Do not run, ride a bicycle, or skate in front of a dog (it will startle the dog); teach children the importance of avoiding bike routes where dogs are known to chase vehicles.

Do not allow an inexperienced child or adult to feed a dog (if the person pulls back when the animal moves to take the food, this can frighten and startle the animal).

If a dog is asleep or unaware of your presence, or has not seen you approach, speak to the animal to make it aware of your presence and to avoid startling the animal.

Allow a dog to see and sniff a child before attempting to pet the animal.

Do not permit a child to lead a large dog.

Train or socialize a dog for appropriate behavior; avoid aggressive play with pets.

Do not adopt pets for children until children demonstrate their maturity and ability to handle and care for pets.

From The Humane Society of the United States: *Preventing and avoiding dog bites*, Washington, D.C., 1998, The Society.

be applied by a suction device such as the Sawyer Extractor, which is very effective if used within 3 minutes.

If possible, the dead snake should be transported with the patient for identification. If there is any possibility that a child has been bitten by a coral snake, aggressive use of antivenom is indicated, because once symptoms occur, it is very difficult to stop the respiratory paralysis and death.

## Human Bites

Children often acquire lacerations from the teeth of other humans in rough play, during fights, or as victims of child abuse. Many preschool children bite others out of frustration or anger. Because human dental plaque and gingiva harbor pathogenic bacteria, all human bites should receive attention. Delayed treatment increases the risk of infection.

If the laceration is less than $\frac{1}{4}$ inch in length, the wound can be treated at home. The wound is washed vigorously with soap and water, and a pressure dressing is applied to stop bleeding. Ice applications minimize discomfort and swelling. Increased pain or redness at the wound site is an indication that the child should receive medical attention for antibiotic therapy. Tetanus toxoid is needed if the child is insufficiently immunized. Wounds greater than ¼ inch should receive medical attention.

# DENTAL DISORDERS
## Dental Caries

Dental caries (cavities) is one of the most common chronic diseases that affect individuals at all ages; it is the principal oral problem in children and adolescents. Although the overall incidence of dental caries in children has decreased since the introduction of fluoridation, reducing the incidence and consequences of the disorder remains important. Dental caries, if untreated, result in total destruction of involved teeth. The ages of greatest vulnerability are 4 to 8 years for the primary dentition and 12 to 18 years for the secondary or permanent dentition. (See Figs. 12-14 and 17-15 for sequence of tooth eruption.)

### Pathophysiology

Dental caries is a multifactorial disease. It involves a number of factors: (1) the host, (2) microorganisms, (3) substrate, and (4) time.

**Host.** The prevalence of caries is directly related to the tooth size and morphology and to the consistency, composition, and amount of saliva. Improperly developed, crowded, or deeply fissured teeth increase the incidence of caries. The areas most subject to attack by bacteria are: grooves and fissures, interdermal areas, gum margins, and other smooth surfaces. Newly erupted teeth that have not yet acquired sufficient surface minerals are more susceptible to decay than those that have been erupted for 2 or more years. Hereditary factors influence resistance and susceptibility, and similar patterns and anatomic characteristics are seen in successive generations. Salivary flow can mechanically clean away bacteria and food debris. It also contains buffering systems, lysozymes, peroxidases, and immunoglobulins that influence the development of caries.

**Microorganisms.** Certain types of microflora that produce different effects contribute to the formation of dental caries. *Acidogenic bacteria* act on fermentable carbohydrates in dental plaque to produce organic acids that decalcify hard surface tooth enamel. With the inner organic matrix exposed, proteolytic organisms and acids digest and destroy the inner tooth structure. These destructive organisms are harbored and protected in a gelatinous plaque formed on the tooth surface by another group of bacteria that are thought to play no primary role in production of decay.

**Substrates.** Caries formation is strongly influenced by the two concurrent processes that continually operate on enamel surfaces—*acid production* and *acid neutralization* by saliva. The material on which the acid-forming bacteria act consists essentially of carbohydrates. Among the fermentable carbohydrates, sucrose has been consistently implicated as the most cariogenic. Sucrose-containing substances, especially in forms that cling (such as chewy candy) or that promote prolonged contact with the teeth (such as hard candy and lollipops), when ingested between meals, contribute markedly to the development of dental caries. Saliva, some foods, and chewing gum after a meal tend to help neutralize much of the acid formed from sucrose.

**Time and Other Factors.** Bacterial enzymes act on salivary glycoproteins to produce a tenacious protein matrix on the tooth surface. This substance, along with the microorganisms, forms *dental plaque.* If plaque removal is inadequate or nonexistent for a significant length of time (a few days), the plaque is metabolized by the bacteria to form acid, which initiates the demineralization of enamel.

Other factors that contribute to caries formation are heredity, the amount of fluoride in drinking water, lack of or ineffectual oral hygiene, and the child's general state of health. Hereditary factors influence both resistance and susceptibility to dental caries. For example, structural defects, such as deep fissures on occlusive surfaces, predispose the teeth to decay, and individuals in whom acid formation exceeds neutralization are prone to caries. The effectiveness of the buffering action of saliva is highly variable among individuals.

*Fluoride* incorporated into the crystallites of the surface enamel increases the resistance to acid dissolution (Blum, Ditmar, and Charney, 1997). Poor oral hygiene that permits the accumulation of food debris on tooth surfaces allows acid-forming bacteria to thrive and proliferate. Removal of food particles and bacteria-laden plaque inhibits destructive acid formation.

The susceptibility to dental decay is also influenced by the general health of the child. Children who suffer from chronic debilitating disease show increased caries activity as do children with systemic conditions that alter the quality and quantity of saliva produced.

### Diagnostic Evaluation

Because the permanent teeth erupt during middle childhood, children are more susceptible to development of dental caries during this time than at any other age. Caries penetrate the vulnerable teeth rapidly at this age, as opposed to the slower, intermittent activity characteristic at later ages.

Caries on visible surfaces are easily detected by oral inspection. Large, extensive caries are apparent to the untrained eye, but small, beginning lesions are best identified by trained professionals. Caries between the teeth may not be located without x-ray examination. A common site of decay is the fissures of the molars.

### Therapeutic Management

Well-informed health care professionals can provide dental information and make periodic dental assessments. However, dentists are prepared to provide both of these services and are the only ones qualified to treat most dental problems. Prophylaxis is the major thrust of dental therapy, including hygiene and fluoride treatment. (See Chapter 14.) *Plasticized sealant,* applied to deep fissures and grooves of healthy teeth, is effective in blocking cavity formation (Blum, Ditmar, and Charney, 1997).

Treatment of dental caries involves removal of all carious portions of teeth as soon as detected, preparation of a retentive cavity, and replacement of the lost portion of the tooth with a material that is durable in the mouth environment. This restoration of involved teeth not only prevents progression of established caries but also reduces the number of bacteria in the oral cavity to decrease the danger to uninvolved teeth.

### Nursing Considerations

Oral inspection is an integral part of the nursing assessment of the child. If there is evidence of dental caries or other unhealthy state, the child is referred for dental services. Many families have a family dentist or a pedodontist who can provide needed care. However, an alarming number of children do not receive regular dental supervision, and a significant number reach adulthood without being examined or treated by a dentist. Nurses can be active members of preventive educational programs and serve as counselors to families regarding the importance of regular dental care, oral hygiene, and dietary management.

Nurses should encourage good oral hygiene and teach correct tooth cleaning to both children and their parents. The random brushing allowed during the early childhood years should be replaced by more careful and methodic cleaning techniques. Children should brush their teeth and use dental floss according to the method recommended by their dentist. (See Chapter 14.) Regular administration of fluoride is also important. (See Chapter 14.) Families should be aware of the fluoride content of the drinking water, including bottled water if this is the family practice. School-age children can usually manage the chewable tablets, which have both a topical and a systemic effect. If it is difficult for parents to give fluoride on a daily basis over a period of years, children are taught to assume responsibility for taking fluoride as part of their daily dental hygiene.

Restriction of cariogenic foods is important to prevent dental caries, but this should be viewed as an activity in which all family members are involved and not simply a directive for the child to obey. It should not be communicated in such a way that the child interprets the withholding of sweets as a punishment.

Concern has been generated about the sugar content of children's pharmaceutical products, especially because children with chronic conditions, such as seizure disorders, asthma, and recurrent urinary tract or ear infections, must take medications over a period of years. Children with chronic illness who regularly take medications containing sugar are cautioned to brush their teeth after taking the medication, just as they would after eating any carbohydrate substance. Children taking tricyclic antidepressants are also prone to develop dental caries.

The greatest task for nurses is counseling children and families to develop sound dental hygiene and nutritional practices. School nurses have an excellent opportunity to participate in community detection of dental needs, to educate children in dental hygiene, to make referrals, and motivate children to comply with prophylaxis and treatment.

Children should be prepared for dental services in such a way that visits to the dentist are a positive experience. Keeping appointments and following through on recommended treatments and practices are habits that extend beyond childhood.

## Periodontal Disease

Periodontal disease, an inflammatory and degenerative condition involving the gums and tissues supporting the teeth, often begins in childhood and accounts for a significant amount of tooth loss in adulthood. The more common periodontal problems are *gingivitis* (simple inflammation of the gums) and *periodontitis* (inflammation of the gums and loss of connective tissue and bone in the supporting structures of the teeth). An uncommon condition is *acute necrotizing ulcerative gingivitis* ("trench mouth").

The most prevalent periodontal disease, gingivitis, is a reversible inflammatory disease that begins very early in many children and is most often associated with the buildup of plaque on the teeth. Changes take place in the plaque bacteria, in both type and number of organisms, causing them to release a variety of destructive exotoxins, enzymes, and other noxious agents. They act to produce an inflammatory reaction in the gingival tissues, causing the gums to become red, edematous, tender, and subject to bleeding at slight irritation.

Management is directed toward prevention by conscientious brushing and flossing and by depriving the bacteria of the substrates required to produce the disease. The implementation and maintenance of preventive dental practice, including the use of fluoride, and conscientious brushing and flossing are effective in preventing both caries and periodontal disease.

### Nursing Considerations

Nursing care of the child with periodontal disease is primarily supportive and preventive; it includes education regarding dental hygiene and regular inspection of the gingival tissues for signs of early inflammation. The child is advised to see the dentist at any sign of inflammation or irritation.

Nurses caring for teenagers should observe for use of chewing tobacco. The easily detectable clinical lesions appear as tooth erosion, periodontal destruction, and red or white mucosal alterations. The primary site of lesions is the anterior mandibular mucobuccal fold region.

## Malocclusion

When teeth of the upper and lower dental arches do not approximate in the proper relationships, the physiologic function of mastication is less effective, and the cosmetic effect is less pleasing. Teeth that are uneven, crowded, or overlapping or are otherwise unable to meet their opponents in the opposite jaw in the appropriate relationships may be predisposed to dental disease. More than half of children 12 to 17 years of age suffer from malocclusions that could be corrected.

The most common cause of malocclusion is hereditary factors, but abnormal growth and habits such as thumb sucking and tongue thrusting also contribute to the disordered alignment and occlusion of the teeth. Treatment of malocclusion includes eliminating habits that aggravate the deformity and corrective therapy at the optimum time. Orthodontic treatment is usually most successful when it is started in the later school-age years or the early adolescent years, after the last primary teeth have been shed and before growth ceases. However, because some deformities can be corrected at an earlier age, referral should be made as soon as malocclusion is evident. For example, removal of extra teeth, impacted teeth, or prosthetic replacement of missing teeth can prevent problems from developing.

### Nursing Considerations

The nurse who detects malocclusion is obligated to recommend that the teeth be examined by a dentist. The sooner the child is evaluated, the sooner treatment can begin.

Although orofacial appearance is a subjective phenomenon, it can have an adverse effect on a child's self-esteem and body image. Poorly aligned teeth can be a source of psychologic as well as physical stress to affected children. Many children with malocclusion are teased by their peers or siblings if the irregularities are severe.

If fixed appliances, or braces are applied, the child is advised that there will be some discomfort for a few days. During the period of orthodontic treatments, which averages 18 to 30 months, proper oral hygiene is vital. Although the bands or brackets protect the teeth they cover, plaque can collect on the unprotected surfaces or under loose-fitting bands. The teeth should be brushed with a fluoride toothpaste after every meal and snack and at bedtime, using the method recommended by the dentist. Some orthodontists recommend using an oral irrigating device to remove food from between the teeth and around the braces. However, the device does not remove plaque and is not a substitute for thorough brushing. Some foods can damage the braces; others may be difficult to remove from the teeth during cleaning. Forbidden foods include chewing gum, ice, nuts, toffee, hard candy, corn-on-the-cob, uncut apples, hard taco shells, nachos, and popcorn.

Occasionally, tooth movement or poking at braces with a pencil or other object may cause an arch wire to break or protrude. If this happens, the child is instructed to cover the broken portion with a special wax provided by the dentist and schedule an appointment as soon as possible. Regular visits are usually scheduled every 3 to 6 weeks. After braces are removed, a removable or permanent retainer must be used to maintain the desired position of the teeth. A permanent wire placed behind the front teeth requires no compliance from the youngster.

Sometimes children need considerable reinforcement for orthodontic compliance. It may be difficult for some to relate the present barriers of discomfort, inconvenience, and embarrassment with the future reinforcers of improved appearance and dental health. Teenagers with a heightened awareness of body image and physical attractiveness are especially at risk for noncompliance. (See Chapter 27 for a discussion of compliance.)

## Trauma

Dental injury is not an uncommon occurrence in childhood. Most injuries occur following bicycle and playground mishaps and include fractures of varying degrees of severity, chipping, dislocation, or evulsion. All tooth injuries require prompt treatment by a competent dentist to prevent permanent displacement or loss. Delayed examination and diagnosis of tooth damage can result in infection or pulp involvement. Because it can affect the remaining teeth, loss of a permanent tooth requires professional attention to maintain normal alignment and position of teeth.

Trauma usually involves the maxillary incisors, and children with protruding teeth, craniofacial abnormalities, or neuromuscular disorders are more likely to sustain dental injuries.

### Nursing Considerations: Tooth Evulsion

A tooth that is evulsed (avulsed, exarticulated, or "knocked out") should be replanted by the child, parent, or nurse and stabilized as soon as possible so that the blood supply to the tooth can be reestablished and the tooth kept alive. (See Emergency Treatment box.) If the tooth is replaced within 30 minutes, there is a 70% chance that it will become reattached and the roots will not resorb or the crown exfoliate. Evulsed primary teeth are usually not reimplanted.

Before reimplantation it is important to carefully rinse a dirty tooth in milk, saline solution, or under running water to avoid disturbing the adhering periodontal membrane, which is essential to the success of the reimplantation. The tooth is held by the crown, not the root, while rinsing, with the drain plugged. The tooth is then fit back into its socket as atraumatically as possible (Troupe, 1995). If the tooth is reimplanted almost immediately, excessive pressure is not needed; however, it becomes extremely difficult after clot formation (in approximately 10 minutes). The tooth is held in place by the child during transportation to a dentist. Care is taken to avoid sudden stops or turns that might cause the child to swallow or aspirate the loose tooth.

If the child or parents are reluctant to reimplant the tooth, the next best alternative is to place the tooth in cold milk, contact lens solution, or saline for transport to the dentist. Cold milk has precisely the osmolality needed to maintain fluid balance within the tissues surrounding the tooth. Water is the least desirable storage medium because the hypotonic environment causes rapid cell lysis (Troupe, 1995).*

After implantation, the tooth will usually become firmly attached, although endodontic therapy is often required. If reimplantation is not permanent, the tooth may be retained anywhere from 6 months to 12 years and serves to facilitate normal development and occlusion, because loss of teeth during the period of permanent tooth eruption may adversely affect such development.

As with all mouth trauma, an evulsed tooth causes a large amount of bleeding, which is frightening to children and their families. The nurse or anyone faced with dental

---

*For more information on Save-a-Tooth, call (800) 537-2191.

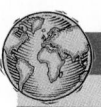

## CULTURAL AWARENESS
*Enuresis*

The age at which children attain urinary continence varies widely. For example, white children in the United States tend to achieve continence earlier than African-American children. In addition, children in Great Britain and Sweden appear to attain continence slightly earlier than children in the United States, and, in the extreme, the East African Digos often achieve bladder control by the age of 12 months. Therefore practitioners must be sensitive to the differences among groups before labeling a child enuretic (Rappaport, 1992).

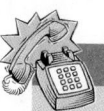

## EMERGENCY TREATMENT
*Avulsed Tooth*

Recover tooth.
Hold tooth by crown; avoid touching root area.
If tooth is dirty, rinse it gently under running water or saline; be sure to insert stopper in sink or basin (to avoid tooth loss).
Insert tooth into socket.
Have child maintain tooth in place.
Transport child to dentist immediately.
Avoid sudden stops or sharp turns to prevent dislodging tooth.

### IF RELUCTANT TO REIMPLANT TOOTH:

Place evulsed tooth in suitable medium for transport:
  a. Cold milk
  b. Saliva—under child's or parent's tongue
If child is holding tooth in the mouth, avoid sudden stops to prevent swallowing tooth.
**DON'T FORGET TO TAKE TOOTH**

trauma should be prepared to cope with the emotionality that accompanies tooth evulsion. Using a calm approach and providing gentle reassurance to the child is often successful in reducing anxiety.

## DISORDERS OF CONTINENCE

### Enuresis

Enuresis (bed-wetting) is a common and troublesome disorder that is defined as intentional or involuntary passage of urine into bed (usually at night) or into clothes during the day in children who are beyond the age when voluntary bladder control should normally have been acquired. The inappropriate voiding of urine must occur at least twice a week for at least 3 months, and the chronologic or developmental age of the child must be at least 5 years. (See Cultural Awareness box.) In addition, the urinary incontinence must not be related to the direct physiologic effects of a substance (e.g., diuretics) or a general medical condition (e.g., diabetes mellitus or insipidus, spina bifida, seizure disorder, or sickle cell disease).

Enuresis can also be defined as *primary* (bed-wetting in children who have never been dry for extended periods) or *secondary* (the onset of wetting after a period of established urinary continence). The passage of urine may occur only during nighttime sleep *(nocturnal)*, only during the waking hours *(diurnal)*, or during both times of the day. The nocturnal type is most common.

Enuresis is more common in boys, and nocturnal bedwetting usually ceases between 6 and 8 years of age (American Academy of Pediatrics, 1996a).

Although most children with enuresis do not have coexisting psychopathology, some children do have other developmental disorders, learning problems, or behavioral difficulties, such as increased motor activity and aggression. Enuresis can cause serious psychologic problems. The degree of impairment is related to the effect on the child's social life, such as not being able to attend overnight camps, and the effect on others, who may ostracize or ridicule the youngster. Adolescents with enuresis have described themselves as tense, having difficulty sleeping, and having bad dreams. Children state they are embarrassed about the disorder and are often hesitant to sleep at other children's homes. Avoiding overnight excursions can impede normal socialization or self-esteem. Self-esteem can be influenced if parental response to the disorder is harsh or punitive. In some instances, enuresis may serve as a trigger for child abuse. Although behavioral problems can be associated with these psychologic effects, research suggests that adults treated for enuresis as children have normal psychologic profiles.

### Etiology and Pathophysiology

No clear etiology for enuresis has been determined. However, predictive factors have been noted, including longer duration of sleep in infancy, a positive family history, and a slower rate of physical development in children up to 3 years of age. There is a high concordance rate of enuresis in monozygotic twins and an even higher one in dizygotic twins, suggesting more than a pure genetic link in the disorder. Approximately 75% of all children with functional enuresis have a first-degree relative who has, or has had, the disorder.

Enuresis is primarily an alteration of neuromuscular bladder functioning and as such is benign and self-limiting. The symptom may be influenced by emotional factors. Some children exhibit temporary regressive behavior resulting in enuresis after the birth of a sibling or other trauma. Other children, such as those with attention deficit hyperactivity disorder (ADHD), may have occasional "accidents" when they become so involved in play that they are unaware of a full bladder or "forget" to empty their bladder. In other children enuresis may be related to problems with toilet training, such as the age at which training began, the emotional atmosphere surrounding the training situation, or an excessive amount of emotional dependence on the parent, usually the mother. Occasionally enuresis can be a behavioral manifestation of a personality disorder.

Although several theories have been proposed, no one theory thoroughly explains enuresis. The *sleep theory* stems from parental reports that these children sleep more soundly and are difficult to arouse from sleep.

Another theory relates to *functional bladder capacity*, the volume of urine voided after maximum delay of micturition. Although there is evidence that some children with enuresis have a smaller bladder capacity than nonaffected children, other evidence suggests that this is not the cause. For example, children without enuresis but with a smaller bladder capacity awaken during the night to void, as opposed to children with enuresis who do not awaken.

The *nocturnal polyuria theory* currently offers the most promising etiology of nocturnal enuresis. It suggests that the kidneys of these children fail to concentrate urine during sleep because of insufficient *antidiuretic hormone (ADH)*. The ADH circadian rhythm may thus be a significant biologic marker in enuresis, but additional research must be conducted to clarify its role.

The *dysfunctional detrusor activity theory* suggests that an unstable bladder detrusor muscle spontaneously contracts, producing bed-wetting, either by abnormal innervation or as a result of other, unknown reasons. Studies of this theory have been contradictory and inconclusive; more research is needed to clarify these contradictions and to determine if there is a relationship between ADH production and detrussor activity.

## Clinical Manifestations

The predominant symptom of enuresis is urgency that is immediate and accompanied by acute discomfort, restlessness, and sometimes urinary frequency. With nocturnal enuresis, the child may or may not feel urgency. If awareness of the urgency is present, the child often reports difficulty awakening to urinate. Spontaneous voiding during sleep occurs, usually resulting in multiple nightly incidents. Spontaneous remission of nocturnal enuresis occurs in approximately 15% of cases. However, some cases continue into adolescence and adulthood.

## Diagnostic Evaluation

During initial phases of evaluation, a routine physical examination is performed to rule out physical etiologies, such as urinary tract infection, structural disorders, major neurologic deficits, nocturnal epilepsy, disorders that increase the normal output of urine (such as diabetes mellitus and diabetes insipidus), and disorders that impair the concentrating ability of the kidneys (such as chronic renal failure or sickle cell disease). The examination may include diagnostic evaluation of functional bladder capacity. Normal bladder capacity (in ounces) is the child's age plus 2; therefore, normal bladder capacity for a 6-year-old is 8 ounces. Functional bladder capacity is determined by having children hold off voiding until they feel the strongest urgency, at which time they void into a measured container. A bladder volume of 300 to 350 ml is sufficient to hold a night's urine.

If psychologic difficulties are evident or a personality disorder is suspected, a routine psychiatric evaluation should be sought.

A history of wetting behavior is obtained, including information about the toilet-training process and parental attempts at coping with the bed-wetting behavior. Parental attitudes are assessed by listening and asking parents how they have attempted to cope with the wetting. An important feature of assessment is a baseline count of enuretic incidents and the time of day when each occurs. This is necessary not only to establish diagnostic reliability, but also to establish outcome success after treatment. This baseline is gathered for 1 to 2 weeks by the child and family. It usually consists of a chart or calendar given to the family on which they indicate the date of the incident, the time of the incident, and the approximate volume of the urinary output.

## Therapeutic Management

Enuresis not resulting from known organic causes has been treated in several ways. No single method has achieved universal endorsement. Frequently, more than one technique is employed. In some cases, a spontaneous decrease in bed-wetting occurs with age and irrespective of the treatments used (American Academy of Pediatrics, 1996a). Successful treatment is defined as a specified period of dry nights, varying from 7 to 28 consecutive dry nights.

*Conditioning therapy* involves training the child to awaken to urinate after a stimulus is given, especially with a urine alarm. The device consists of a wire pad that is placed inside the underpants and is attached to a bell or buzzer that is sensitive to moisture. When the system detects urine, the bell or buzzer sounds, which fully awakens the child. The child is thus conditioned to awaken at the initiation of micturition or to the stimulus of the bell or buzzer and eventually learns to continue voiding in the toilet. The success rate of the urine alarm is approximately 60% to 90%, but children often relapse once they stop using the alarm (American Academy of Pediatrics, 1996a). Relapse is addressed by reinstituting the alarm during sleep. This method is inexpensive compared with drug therapy and has no side effects.

*Retention control training (RCT)* was initiated after the observation of reduced functional bladder capacity in children who were bed-wetters. The child drinks fluids and delays urination as long as can be tolerated in order to stretch the bladder to accommodate increasingly larger volumes of urine. The use of Kegel, or pelvic muscle, exercises may be helpful in children with daytime enuresis (Foreman, 1997).

With the *waking schedule* treatment, the child is awakened during the night at intervals to void. This method has been successful in reducing, but not eliminating, the incidents.

*Drug therapy* is increasingly being prescribed to treat enuresis. Three types of drugs are used: tricyclic antidepressants, antidiuretics, and antispasmotics. The selection depends on the interpretation of the cause. The drug used most frequently is the tricyclic antidepressant drug imipramine (Tofranil), which exerts an anticholinergic action in the bladder to inhibit urination. The dosage and time of administration are individualized, and the drug is given in amounts sufficient to lighten sleep but not to cause wakefulness. Some practitioners prescribe low doses, which result in a reduction in bed-wetting in two thirds of children. However, it is important to note that almost all children relapse when the medication is stopped. The suggested length of treatment is 6 to 8 weeks, followed by gradual withdrawal over 4 weeks. Because this drug is dangerous in overdosage, parents must be cautioned about safe use and keeping supplies of the drug from the reach of younger siblings.

Anticholinergic drugs, especially oxybutynin, reduce uninhibited bladder contractions and may be helpful for children with daytime urinary frequency. Success has also been achieved with *desmopressin (DDAVP)* nasal spray, an analog of vasopressin, which reduces nighttime urinary output to a volume less than functional bladder capacity. Typically, the child receives two sprays before bedtime. The medication is generally well tolerated but may cause nasal irritation or, rarely, headaches or nausea. A preparation of desmopressin acetate is also available in tablet form. This preparation is equally as effective and safe as the nasal spray while avoiding the problems of nasal irritation.

One of the challenges of using the drug therapeutically is the difficulty simulating the normal circadian rhythm of ADH secretion. Another concern is the cost of the treatment. DDAVP costs from $120 to $240 a month for daily doses of 20 to 40 μg. Although DDAVP is effective in reducing the number of wet nights, only about 25% of children become completely dry, and the relapse rate is high (Foreman, 1997).

Other therapies/treatment options include stream interruption, paired associations, overlearning, reinforcement systems, and self-monitoring (motivation therapy). Frequently these therapies are coupled with other treatment modalities. Counseling may be beneficial in helping the child, and sometimes the family, adjust to the bed-wetting.

It is imperative that punishment not be used to correct enuresis. Supportive therapy such as teaching the child to change pajamas and bed linens, as well as restriction of fluids before bedtime, should be used (American Academy of Pediatrics, 1996). Behavior-modification techniques, such as a chart with stars or stickers for each dry night and rewards for achieving a certain goal, are also helpful. Token or social reinforcement can also be used to enhance the rewards for success.

### Nursing Considerations

No matter what techniques are used, the nurse can help both children and parents to understand the problem of enuresis, the treatment plan, and the difficulties they may encounter in the process. Essential to the success of any method is the supportive management of parents and their children. Both need encouragement and patience. The problem is discussed with both the parent and the child because any treatment involves and requires the child's active participation. In some treatment interventions, the child is in charge of the intervention; therefore parents must be taught to support the child rather than intervene themselves.

Parents should also be taught to observe for side effects of the medications. All children with primary enuresis should be encouraged to void before bedtime. Diapering should be avoided. Positive reinforcement in the form of diaries to record dry nights have been effective in fostering motivation in children.

The most important predictor for the outcome of treatment is family difficulties. Family disturbances influence the initial arrest of the enuresis, the relapse rate, and the long-term success rate.

Many parents believe that enuresis is caused by an emotional disturbance and fear that they have somehow produced the situation by improper childrearing practices. They need reassurance that the bed-wetting is not a manifestation of emotional disturbance and does not represent willful misbehavior. Parents need to understand that punishment such as scolding, shaming, and threatening are contraindicated because of their negative emotional impact and limited success in reducing the behavior. Parents are encouraged to be patient, to be understanding, and to communicate love and support to the child.

Communication with children is directed toward eliminating the emotional impact of the problem; relieving feelings of shame, guilt, and the burden of parental disapproval; building self-confidence; and motivating them toward independent control. More important, the nurse can provide consistent support and encouragement to help children through the inconsistent and unpredictable treatment process. Children need to believe that they are helping themselves and to maintain feelings of confidence and hope.

## Encopresis

Encopresis is repeated voluntary or involuntary passage of feces of normal or near-normal consistency in places not appropriate for that purpose according to the individual's own sociocultural setting. The event must occur at least once a month for at least 3 months, and the chronologic or developmental age of the child must be at least 4 years. The fecal incontinence must not be caused by physiologic effects of a substance (e.g., laxatives) or a general medical condition except through a mechanism involving constipation. The consistency of the stool may vary from normal or near-normal to liquid, especially in individuals who have overflow incontinence secondary to fecal retention.

A child who has never achieved fecal continence by 4 years of age is said to have *primary encopresis.* This type is more frequently observed as a result of neglect, lax training methods, mental subnormalities, and familial causes. *Secondary encopresis* is fecal incontinence occurring in a child over 4 years of age after a period of established fecal continence. The disorder is more common in males than in females.

### Etiology

One of the most common causes of encopresis is constipation, which may be precipitated by environmental change, such as the birth of a new sibling, moving to a new house, changing schools, or even having to use new or unfamiliar toilet facilities. Chronic, severe constipation has a tendency to impair the usual movement and contractions of the colon, which can lead to fecal obstruction. Abnormalities in the digestive tract (i.e., Hirschsprung disease, anorectal lesions, malformations, and rectal prolapse) and medical conditions such as hypothyroidism, myelomeningocele, and cerebral palsy are also associated with constipation, which can lead to encopresis (Loening-Baucke, 1996). Voluntary retention of stool may also follow a painful incident of defecation (e.g., in a child with anal fissures). Involuntary retention may be produced by emotional problems caused by the encopresis, which sets up a fear-pain cycle and results in a learned process of abnormal defecation patterns. Psychogenic encopresis, in which the soiling is caused by emotional problems, is often related to a disturbed mother-child relationship.

Normally, children and adolescents have one or two soft-formed stools per day. Children with soiling problems tend to form large-bore stools, which are painful to excrete. Therefore they tend to avoid defecation and withhold stooling. Stool held in the rectum and sigmoid colon loses water and progressively hardens, causing successively more painful bowel movements. A pain-retention-pain cycle is established. Many children have diarrhea or loose leakage in their clothing and pass small amounts of hard stool, suggesting leakage around an impaction.

Children may experience exacerbations with transitions in the school setting. Some reasons for developing retentive tendencies at this time are fear of using school bathrooms, a busy schedule, and the interruption of an established time schedule for bowel evacuation. Children may also react to stress with bowel dysfunction.

## Clinical Manifestations

The manifestation of simple constipation is painful expulsion of hard, pelletlike stools. Voluntary retention is usually temporary, with a history of a painful precipitating episode and blood-streaked stools. Involuntary retention is associated with a history of abdominal pain, distention, moodiness, poor appetite, and accumulation of stools with periodic passage of voluminous stools. Children display a characteristic posturing during suppression of colonic signals to defecate—stiffening, standing in a corner with straight legs and a bright red face, "doing a little dance," "crawling," or hiding behind furniture or a tree when playing outdoors. They typically hide soiled underwear. It is not unusual for soiling to take place after bathing because of reflex stimulation.

The child with encopresis often feels ashamed and may wish to avoid situations (e.g., camp or school) that might lead to embarrassment. School performance and attendance are affected as the child's offensive odor becomes a target for scorn and derision from classmates. The child is not well liked by peers and may be severely rejected by the parents as a result of the symptom. Rejection by peers and parents causes further withdrawal and other behavioral manifestations.

## Therapeutic Management

Treatment is directed toward the cause of the soiling. To determine the cause, a complete physical examination should be performed. An abdominal x-ray film may be obtained to determine the severity of impaction. Diet, lubricants, and a toilet ritual that encourages the child to establish normal defecation are used. Fecal impaction is relieved by catharsis, suppositories, and/or mineral oil. Customary dosages are usually insufficient. Dietary changes may be helpful, such as elimination of milk and dairy products and increased amounts of high-fiber foods, such as fruits, vegetables, and cereals, as well as increased fluids. Behavior therapy may be indicated to eliminate any fear that has developed as a result of painful defecation. Frequently, psychotherapeutic intervention with the child and the family becomes necessary (Vogt and Schaffner, 1996).

## Nursing Considerations

A thorough history of the soiling is essential—when soiling began, how often it occurs, under what circumstances, and

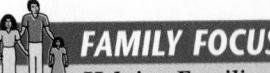

### FAMILY FOCUS
*Helping Families Understand Encopresis*

The prevailing attitude of nurses toward the family of a child with encopresis should be one of no fault, thus relieving the guilt of both parents and child. Because parents and children are often reluctant to volunteer information, direct questioning about the soiling is more successful. Family education about the condition can be very helpful. Parents are usually relieved to know that other families share this problem and are surprised to know that functional changes that take place as the condition develops make control of seepage impossible. Many parents complain that their children soil because they do not take time from play for a bowel movement. Actually, the children may be unaware of a prior sensation and unable to control the urge once it begins. They may be so accustomed to bowel accidents that they are unable to smell or feel it and even deny soiling when it occurs.

if the child uses the toilet successfully at all. Because the parents and child are reluctant to volunteer information, direct questioning about the soiling is more successful.

Education regarding the physiology of normal defecation, toilet training as a developmental process, and the treatment outlined for the particular family is prerequisite to a successful outcome. The regimen prescribed for stimulating elimination is explained to parents. Bowel "retraining" with mineral oil, a high-fiber diet, and a regular toileting routine is essential in treating encopresis or chronic constipation.

Sitting the child on the toilet at routine intervals is not recommended because it may intensify parent-child conflict. Enemas may be needed for impactions, but long-term use prevents the child from assuming responsibility for defecation. Initially lubricants are given liberally, but stimulant cathartics often cause abdominal cramps that can be frightening for a child. Biofeedback techniques such as teaching the child to relax the muscles of the pelvic floor during defecation have been associated with a short-term recovery from constipation but have not been associated with increased long-term recovery rates (Loening-Baucke, 1995).

Family counseling is directed toward reassurance that most problems resolve successfully, although the child may have relapses during periods of stress, such as vacations or illness. (See Family Focus box.) If encopresis persists beyond occasional relapses, the condition will need to be reevaluated. Behavior-modification techniques are explained, and the family is assisted with a plan suited to their particular situation.

# DISORDERS WITH BEHAVIORAL COMPONENTS

## Attention Deficit Hyperactivity Disorder (ADHD)

ADHD refers to developmentally inappropriate degrees of inattention, impulsiveness, and hyperactivity. Some hyperactive-impulsive or inattentive symptoms must have been present before age 7 years and must be present in at least two settings. ADHD affects 6% of school-age children and is diagnosed three times more frequently in boys than in girls (Law and Schachter, 1999). The symptoms of ADHD were first recognized in the early 1900s. Several different names have been applied to the disorder. ADHD was originally called "minimal brain damage," then "minimal brain dysfunction," and in the mid-1900s the term "hyperkinetic reaction of childhood" was given to the symptoms. Currently the term *attention deficit hyperactivity disorder* has been adopted by the American Psychiatric Association (1994).

Difficulties associated with ADHD are most often school related or academic. Family and social relationships can also be affected if aggressive behavior and mood lability interfere with peer relationships, cause difficulties in social interactions, or make disciplining difficult. An investigation by Biederman and others (1996) indicated that children with ADHD are at greater risk for conduct, mood, and anxiety disorders, as well as impairment in cognitive and interpersonal functioning, than are children without ADHD.

Early identification of affected children is important because the characteristics of ADHD significantly interfere with the normal course of emotional and psychologic development. Many children develop maladaptive behavior patterns that hinder psychosocial adjustment. Their behavior evokes negative responses from others, and repeated exposure to negative feedback adversely affects the child's self-concept.

Research has documented decreased self-perception and increased problems in scholastic competence, social acceptance, and behavioral conduct in children with ADHD (Dumas and Pelletier, 1999). ADHD affects children of all intelligence levels; many children have average or above-average intelligence and are often very creative.

## Etiology

The exact etiology of ADHD is unknown. A combination of organic, genetic, and environmental factors is probably involved. A variety of factors put a child at risk for symptoms of ADHD. ADHD is seen more often in children who have family members with ADHD, especially the father, a brother, or uncle (Biederman and others, 1996). There is also an increased incidence of substance abuse, conduct disorders, learning disabilities, depression, and antisocial personality disorder in families of ADHD children (Blum, Ditmar, and Charney, 2001). Chromosomal or genetic abnormalities such as fragile X syndrome have been implicated in ADHD. (See Chapter 24.) Girls with Turner syndrome have a high incidence of impaired spatial abilities and right-left directional sense, and a large number of boys with Klinefelter syndrome have learning, behavioral, or peer problems. A sex-linked factor may be operating because the disorder is much more common in boys than in girls.

Other risk factors include exposure to toxins, medications, perinatal complications, chronic otitis media, head trauma, meningitis, neurologic infections, and mental disorders such as the affective disorders.

Another popular theory is the concept of a **developmental lag.** Distractibility, short attention span, and impulsiveness are normal characteristics of children at a much younger developmental level. However, current research indicates that symptoms of ADHD do not diminish with age. Symptoms, such as inattentiveness and impulsivity, last into adolescence and young adulthood in many affected youngsters (King, 2000). In addition, hyperactivity may be a normal variant of innate temperament in some children who represent the extreme end of the normal distribution curve for activity.

Support for a neurochemical etiology is suggested by the fact that many children with ADHD respond to medications affecting the central nervous system. In some children, there may be an absence or insufficiency of norepinephrine, dopamine, and serotonin. These neurotransmitters normally occur in high concentrations in the brain and affect activity level, mood, and awareness. It is hypothesized that children who lack these neurotransmitters experience learning difficulties in reading, math, and language and are prone to impulsivity. Many of these children respond to psychostimulants, such as methylphenidate hydrochloride, that increase dopamine and norepinephrine (American Academy of Pediatrics, 2001). The fact that some children with ADHD manifest decreased symptoms in stressful situations (such as in the doctor's or principal's office) provides additional support for this theory because stress increases the level of norepinephrine.

Another neurochemical theory suggests that symptoms result from an excess of norepinephrine and/or an alteration in the reticular activating system of the midbrain, an area that controls consciousness and attention. This excess or abnormality interferes with the function of filtering out extraneous stimuli. Consequently, children are unable to focus on one stimulus and are compelled to respond to every stimulus in the environment. They demonstrate hyperactive behaviors that result from cognitive "flooding" and exaggerated arousal that overwhelms the attention filters and overrides inhibitory processes (O'Connell, 1996). Other theories maintain that symptoms of ADHD result from dysfunction in the brain circuits of the behavioral inhibition system; structural abnormalities in the prefrontal cortex, caudate, and thalamus; and a gene variant known to code for a receptor for dopamine (Castellanos and others, 1996).

Interest in diet as a factor in hyperactivity continues to generate controversy. There are those who believe that the observed behavioral patterns are related to an innate sensitivity to food items such as sucrose and/or food additives such as aspartame (Nutrasweet). This theory does not have widespread support and has not been validated by empirical studies (Wolraich, Wilson, and White, 1995). Nevertheless, some children do show improvement when certain foods are eliminated from their diet, particularly those that cause hyperallergic reactions, such as chocolate, cow's milk, and eggs.

## Clinical Manifestations

The behaviors exhibited by the child with ADHD are not unusual aspects of child behavior. The difference lies in the quality of motor activity and developmentally inappropriate inattention, impulsivity, and hyperactivity that the child displays. The manifestations may be numerous or few, mild or severe, and will vary with the developmental level of the child. Any given child will not have every manifestation that is characteristic of a syndrome, and the degree of severity is highly variable. Mild manifestations of the symptoms may not be apparent in some educational and family environ-

---

**Box 18-2** ▪ ▪ ▪
**Diagnostic Criteria for Attention Deficit Hyperactivity Disorder**

A. Either (1) or (2):
   (1) Six (or more) of the following symptoms of **inattention** have persisted for at least 6 months to a degree that is maladaptive and inconsistent with developmental level:
   *Inattention*
   (a) Often fails to give close attention to details or makes careless mistakes in schoolwork, work, or other activities
   (b) Often has difficulty sustaining attention in tasks or play activities
   (c) Often does not seem to listen when spoken to directly
   (d) Often does not follow through on instructions and fails to finish schoolwork, chores, or duties in the workplace (not because of oppositional behavior or failure to understand instructions)
   (e) Often has difficulty organizing tasks and activities
   (f) Often avoids, dislikes, or is reluctant to engage in tasks that require sustained mental effort (such as schoolwork or homework)
   (g) Often loses things necessary for tasks or activities (e.g., toys, school assignments, pencils, books, or tools)
   (h) Is often easily distracted by extraneous stimuli
   (i) Is often forgetful in daily activities
   (2) Six (or more) of the following symptoms of **hyperactivity-impulsivity** have persisted for at least 6 months to a degree that is maladaptive and inconsistent with developmental level:
   *Hyperactivity*
   (a) Often fidgets with hands or feet or squirms in seat
   (b) Often leaves seat in classroom or in other situations in which remaining seated is expected
   (c) Often runs about or climbs excessively in situations in which it is inappropriate (in adolescents

or adults, may be limited to subjective feelings of restlessness)
   (d) Often has difficulty playing or engaging in leisure activities quietly
   (e) Is often "on the go" or often acts as if "driven by a motor"
   (f) Often talks excessively
   *Impulsivity*
   (g) Often blurts out answers before questions have been completed
   (h) Often has difficulty awaiting turn
   (i) Often interrupts or intrudes on others (e.g., butts into conversations or games)

B. Some hyperactive-impulsive or inattentive symptoms that caused impairment were present before age 7 years.
C. Some impairment from the symptoms is present in two or more settings (e.g., at school [or work] and at home).
D. There must be clear evidence of clinically significant impairment in social, academic, or occupational functioning.
E. The symptoms do not occur exclusively during the course of a pervasive developmental disorder, schizophrenia, or other psychotic disorder and are not better accounted for by another mental disorder (e.g., mood disorder, anxiety disorder, dissociative disorder, or a personality disorder).

*Code* based on type:
   **314.01 Attention-Deficit/Hyperactivity Disorder, Combined Type:** if both Criteria A1 and A2 are met for the past 6 months
   **314.00 Attention-Deficit/Hyperactivity Disorder, Predominantly Inattentive Type:** if Criterion A1 is met but Criterion A2 is not met for the past 6 months
   **314.01 Attention-Deficit/Hyperactivity Disorder, Predominantly Hyperactive-Impulsive Type:** if Criterion A2 is met but Criterion A1 is not met for the past 6 months
**Coding note:** For individuals (especially adolescents and adults) who currently have symptoms that no longer meet full criteria, "in partial remission" should be specified.

From American Psychiatric Association: *Diagnostic and statistical manual of mental disorders (DSM-IV)*, ed 4, Washington, DC, 1994, The Association.

---

ments, whereas severe symptomatology will be recognizable in most environments. Every child with ADHD is different from all other children with ADHD (Box 18-2).

Most behavioral manifestations are apparent at an early age, but the learning disabilities may not become evident until the child enters school. The disorder is unpredictable; it may remit spontaneously at any age, and the number of years that a child will require treatment is unknown.

A major clinical manifestation is distractibility. The stimuli may come from external sources or internal sources. Children frequently demonstrate immaturity relative to chronologic age. Selective attention is often seen, in which the child has difficulty attending to "nonpreferred" tasks, such as completing chores or finishing homework. The child may not consider the consequences of behavior, may take excessive physical risks (often beginning early in life), and may demonstrate inappropriate social skills.

Children with ADHD demonstrate one of three subtypes (American Psychiatric Association, 1994):

1. **Combined type**—Six (or more) symptoms of inattention and six (or more) symptoms of hyperactivity-impulsivity have persisted for at least 6 months. Most children and adolescents with the disorder have the combined type.

2. **Predominantly inattentive type**—Six (or more) symptoms of inattention (but fewer than six symptoms of hyperactivity-impulsivity) have persisted for at least 6 months.

3. **Predominantly hyperactive-impulsive type**—Six (or more) symptoms of hyperactivity-impulsivity (but fewer than six symptoms of inattention) have persisted for at least 6 months. Inattention may often still be a significant clinical feature in such cases.

**Course of ADHD.** In the majority of children the disorder is relatively stable through early adolescence. Some children have decreased symptoms during late adolescence and adulthood. However, 50% to 80% continue to demonstrate symptoms in adolescence, and two thirds carry the symptoms into adulthood (O'Connell, 1996).

### Diagnostic Evaluation

The basic characteristics outlined in Box 18-2 are used to establish a clinical diagnosis of ADHD. It is important to emphasize the need for a complete and thorough multidisciplinary evaluation of the child, incorporating the efforts of the pediatrician (often a developmental pediatrician or pediatric neurologist), psychologist, pediatric nurse, classroom teacher, reading/math specialist, special education teacher, possibly a speech therapist, and the child's parents. The clinicians and professionals must first determine whether the child's behavior is age-appropriate or truly problematic.

A history, both medical and developmental, and description of the child's behavior should be obtained from as many observers of the child as possible, especially the parents and teachers, along with the observations of the health professionals involved. It should include descriptions of the child's behavior in home and school situations. In obtaining descriptive material, the interviewer must question the observers carefully, because some persons, especially parents, may be so concerned with gross behaviors that they overlook less distressing but equally important symptoms. For example, parents may report a "colicky" infant, a child who began to run soon after walking, a toddler who is compelled to touch everything in sight, and a child who resists sleep until exhausted. A pregnancy and birth history may provide clues to a situation that might have produced an episode of hypoxia.

A physical examination, including vision and hearing screening and a detailed neurologic evaluation, will help rule out any severe neurologic disorders. Psychologic testing, especially projective tests, is valuable in determining visual-perceptual difficulties, problems with spatial organization, and other phenomena that suggest cortical or diencephalic involvement, and it helps to identify the child's intelligence and achievement levels.

Behavioral checklists and adaptive scales are also helpful in measuring social adaptive functioning in children with ADHD. Recent investigations using the computer to provide objective measurements of body movement and attention in boys with ADHD who were engaged in a continuous performance task may provide another useful technique to be used in the diagnosis of ADHD (Teicher and others, 1996). Psychiatric disorders and medical problems as well as traumatic experiences are ruled out, including lead poisoning, seizures, partial hearing loss, psychosis, and witnessing sexual activity and/or violence.

## Therapeutic Management

Management of the child with ADHD involves many approaches including: family education and counseling, medication, proper classroom placement, environmental manipulation, and behavioral therapy and/or psychotherapy for the child.

The National Institute of Mental Health conducted a large multicenter randomized study of several of these approaches to the treatment of ADHD. This study, called the MTA study, examined the long-term effectiveness of (1) medication, (2) intensive behavioral treatment with a therapist, (3) a combination of medication plus behavioral therapy, and (4) routine community care for the treatment of ADHD in children (Jensen, 1999). Over 579 children with ADHD, aged 7 to 9 years, were randomly assigned to one of these four types of therapy and received the therapy for 14 months. Although all four approaches provided some improvement, the medication-only group and the combined treatment group had superior outcomes on the core symptoms of ADHD. How-

ever, the medication-only approach was superior to the behavioral therapy–only approach and the community approach (Jensen, 1999; MTA Study, 1999).

**Behavioral Therapy and Psychotherapy.**  Behavioral therapy focuses on the prevention of undesired behavior. Families are helped to identify new appropriate contingencies and reward systems to meet the child's developing needs. They may also receive instruction in effective parenting skills, such as positive reinforcement, rewarding small increments of desired behaviors, and age-appropriate consequences (e.g., time-out, response-cost). Through collaborative team work, parents learn techniques to help the child become more successful at home and in school. Organization charts for completing self-care activities and using a word processor instead of manually writing out assignments are emphasized.

**Pharmacologic Therapy.**  The most frequently used medications are the psychostimulants: methylphenidate hydrochloride (Ritalin), pemoline (Cylert), and dextroamphetamine sulfate (Dexedrine) (American Academy of Pediatrics, 2001). Seventy-five percent of ADHD cases are treated with the psychostimulant, methylphenidate (Law and Schachar, 1999). Psychostimulants cause an increase in dopamine and norepinephrine levels that leads to stimulation of the inhibitory system of the central nervous system. Children are given a small dose initially, and the dose is gradually increased until the desired response is achieved. Children who receive stimulants should be monitored carefully for the development of tics during initial treatment, and stimulants should be avoided in children who have a history of ticlike behaviors, a family history of Tourette syndrome, or ADHD combined with Tourette syndrome. On rare occasions, pemoline has been linked to a hypersensitivity reaction that results in jaundice and altered liver enzymes. Methylphenidate and pemoline are not recommended for children younger than 6 years of age.

Other medications used in the treatment of ADHD include the tricyclic antidepressants, primarily imipramine (Tofranil), desipramine (Norpramin), and nortriptyline (Pamelor). The tricyclic antidepressants block norepinephrine and serotonin at the nerve endings and increase the action of these substances in nerve cells. However, in some children, antidepressants have been noted to cause electrocardiographic changes (American Academy of Pediatrics, 1996b). Clonodine, used occasionally in the treatment of ADHD, has been recommended primarily for children with ADHD and coexisting conditions such as sleep disturbances (American Academy of Pediatrics, 2001).

Regularly scheduled reevaluation of the child is essential with all of these medications to determine medication effectiveness, detect and evaluate any side effects, monitor development and health status (especially growth and blood pressure), and assess family interaction.

## Nursing Considerations

Nurses, especially school nurses, are active participants in all aspects of management of the child with ADHD. Nurses in the community setting work with families in the home on a long-term basis to help plan and implement therapeutic regimens and to evaluate the effectiveness of therapy. They coordinate services and serve as a liaison between health and education professionals directly involved in the child's therapy program. School nurses have an understanding of the child's special needs and work with teachers. Nurses in any setting (community, school, hospital, practitioner's office) provide support and guidance to children and families during the difficult period of growing up with a disabling condition.

Management begins with an explanation to the parents and the child about the diagnosis, including the nature of the problem and the practitioner's concept of the underlying central nervous system basis for the disorder. Most parents are confused and feel some measure of guilt. To some parents, a diagnosis of ADHD is confirmation of the fear that their child has some irreversible, serious disease; to others it is a relief. They need the opportunity to vent their feelings and suspicions. A common complaint of parents is that health professionals do not listen to what they have to say about their child.

Parents need information about the prognosis and an understanding of the treatment plan. The greater their understanding of the disorder and its effects, the more likely they will be to carry out the recommended program of therapy. It is important that they understand that the therapy is not necessarily a panacea and that it will extend over a long period. This has particular significance for changes they need to make in environmental management. Reading material to help the child and family can be obtained from a variety of sources.

**Medication.** Psychostimulants are prescribed using a variety of schedules, but the most common schedule is twice daily, usually in the morning at breakfast and at noon. Many school-age children take their medication at home in the morning before going to school and at lunchtime in the school health suite. Both parents and school nurses should appreciate and be sensitive to the issue of peer stigma and the feelings that children have in relation to taking these medications at school. (See Family Focus box.)

Parents are reminded that some medications (pemoline) require 2 to 3 weeks to achieve an effect. Others are begun at low dosage and increased until the desired effect is attained. When evaluating the child's response to the medication, it is helpful to obtain reports from the teacher, as well as from the parents, because the parents may see the child when the effects of the drug are wearing off. Observing the child's behavior through visits to the home and school is useful for assessing attention span, interactional patterns with others at school, and performance on academic tasks. The nurse can consult with the teacher and analyze data needed to regulate dosage based on recorded, systematic observations of the child's behaviors.

Parents need to be informed of the possible side effects of medications. The psychostimulants have similar side effects that include weight loss, abdominal pain, headaches, decreased appetite, sleeplessness, increased crying and irritability, nervous stimulation, and cardiovascular stimulation (See Critical Thinking Exercise box.) The use of caffeine will decrease the efficacy of these drugs. Insulin requirements may also be altered, and stimulants should be used

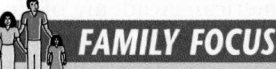

## FAMILY FOCUS
### A Child's Perception of Taking Ritalin at School

I feel embarrassed by having to leave class early to go take my medication. The other kids always ask where I'm going and why. It would be better if we could leave class at the same time as everyone else, go take the medication and then just be a little late to the next class. Students don't ask why people are late for class, only why they leave early. It also bothers me when kids tell other kids, "Go take a pill," and other mean things just because someone is acting up.

What could nurses and teachers do to help? Most kids do not understand why other kids have to take medication. I think it would help if a nurse or teacher talked with the other kids and explained why some children take the medication and how ADHD affects people. That way there would be more understanding among all kids.

Marissa White, age 16
Tulsa, Oklahoma

## Critical Thinking Exercise

### Attention Deficit Hyperactivity Disorder

Johnnie, age 8 years, is a third grader who was diagnosed with attention deficit hyperactivity disorder (ADHD) 1 year ago. Johnnie has been taking the drug methylphenidate (Ritalin) for the past year. Which of the following behaviors indicates that Johnnie may need to have the administration times of his medication changed?

FIRST, THINK ABOUT IT . . .

- What concepts or ideas are central to your thinking?
- What precise questions are you trying to answer?

1. For the past week, Johnnie has not eaten his lunch. He states he is not hungry.
2. During this school year Johnnie's math grade has increased from a letter grade of D to a grade of B.
3. Johnnie's mother told the school nurse that Johnnie has been sleeping very well at night.
4. During the past year, Johnnie's teacher has noted that Johnnie has been socializing more with his classmates and that he now has a "best friend."

*The best response is one. Children taking stimulant medications often experience positive effects such as improvement in schoolwork and increasing self-confidence in social skills. However, there are also negative side effects for some of the drugs used to treat ADHD. For example, side effects for methylphenidate include nervousness, decreased appetite, and insomnia. Recalling these side effects helps you to answer the question precisely. The absorption rate of methylphenidate is increased when this drug is taken with meals; therefore, side effects such as decreased appetite may become more pronounced when the medication is taken with meals. Side effects can be alleviated by changing the times that the drug is administered or by switching to a sustained time-release form of the drug that can be given once a day in the morning. When evaluating a child's response to the medication, it is important to obtain reports from the child's teacher, the school nurse, and the parents. Information concerning the child's behavior in at least two settings should be obtained before adjustments are made in the medication dosage or scheduling.*

cautiously in children with diabetes (O'Connell, 1996). If decreased appetite is a concern, giving the psychostimulants with or after meals rather than before, encouraging nutritious snacks in the evening when the effects of the medication are decreasing, and serving frequent small meals with healthy "on the go" snacks are helpful interventions. Sleeplessness is reduced by administering medication early in the day.

Children taking tricyclic antidepressants display a dramatic increase in the incidence of dental caries. The marked anticholinergic action of the drugs increases saliva viscosity and produces a dry mouth. Emphasis on rigorous dental hygiene, conscientious home fluoride treatments, regular visits to the dentist, limited intake of refined carbohydrates, and artificial saliva is an important nursing function. The child should be kept well hydrated.

The issue of continuous administration of psychostimulants and their relationship to growth suppression is another area of concern for parents. Although some practitioners have suggested "drug holidays" on the weekends and during summer vacations, research has not documented that growth suppression occurs with prolonged medication or that intermittent administration of these drugs increases or heightens their effects (American Academy of Pediatrics, 1996b). Children who respond well to medication often benefit from continuous therapy. For many children, the symptoms of ADHD do not disappear on the weekends or during vacations. For these children, continuous medication may provide an enhancement that allows them not only to succeed in school but also to function successfully in other social situations and to develop a positive self-image.

Parents often express concern that their child will become addicted to the psychostimulants or the antidepressant drugs. Both types of drugs have the potential for abuse, and all children taking these drugs should be monitored closely for psychologic dependence, tolerance, depression, and other adverse behavioral changes or idiosyncratic effects. Most children with ADHD are not interested in abusing their drugs because the effect of the drugs in these children is opposite that produced in normal individuals. However, parents are cautioned to keep these drugs safely stored away from young children who may inadvertently ingest them and adolescents who may abuse these drugs.

**Environmental Manipulation.** Families are encouraged to learn how to modify the environment to allow the child to be more successful. Consistency is especially important for children with ADHD. Consistency between families and teachers in terms of reinforcing the same goals is essential. Fostering improved organizational skills requires a more highly structured environment than most children require. The child should be encouraged to make more appropriate choices and to take responsibility for actions.

Other helpful interventions include teaching parents how to make organization charts (e.g., listing all activities preceding leaving for school), decreasing distractions in the environment while completing homework (e.g., television off, having a consistent study area equipped with needed supplies), and helping parents to understand ways to model

positive behaviors and problem solving. The focus is on strategies to help the child succeed and cope with deficits while emphasizing strengths.

**Appropriate Classroom Placement.** Children with ADHD need an orderly, predictable, and consistent classroom environment with clear and consistent rules. Homework and classroom assignments may need to be reduced, and more time may need to be allotted for tests to allow the child to complete the task. Verbal instructions should be accompanied by visual references such as written instructions on the blackboard. Schedules may need to be arranged so that academic subjects are taught in the morning when the child is experiencing the effects of the morning dose of medication. Low-interest and high-interest classroom activities should be intermingled to maintain the child's attention and interest. Regular and frequent breaks in activity are helpful because sitting in one place for an extended time may be difficult. Computers are helpful for children who have difficulty with written assignments and fine motor skills.

If learning disabilities exist, special training activities may be accomplished in self-contained classes with a limit of six to eight children, special resource rooms with equipment and teaching teams, mobile consultants who move from room to room to provide assistance to teachers and children, and special first grade programs in which high-risk children receive special attention to prevent or reduce the need for services as they progress. The purpose of programs for children with special learning disabilities is to assist them toward more successful achievement, personal adjustment, and retention in the regular classroom.

**Psychiatric, Psychologic, and Social Therapies.** Counseling or therapy can be very helpful for children who demonstrate signs of anxiety or depression. Therapy can help the child to develop a healthier self-esteem and practice problem-solving strategies. The adolescent may benefit from group work focusing on social skill development. Parenting stress among families of children with ADHD can be quite high, and therapy may be indicated for parents and other family members.

## Learning Disability (LD)

Learning disorders exist when the individual's achievement on individually administered, standardized tests in reading, mathematics, or written expression is substantially below that expected for age, schooling, and level of intelligence. The learning problems significantly interfere with academic achievement or activities of daily living that require reading, mathematics, or writing skills (American Psychiatric Association, 1994). They do not include learning problems that result primarily from visual, hearing, or motor disabilities; mental retardation; emotional disturbances; or environmental disadvantage. The types of disabilities include *dyslexia* (difficulty with reading, letter reversal), *dysgraphia* (difficulty with writing), *dyscalculia* (difficulty with calculation), right-left confusion, and short attention span.

A comprehensive battery of tests is needed to confirm a learning disability. These include intelligence tests (these children tend to have normal or above-average intelligence), hand-eye coordination tests, and measurements of auditory and visual perception, comprehension, and memory. Often there is a wide gap between verbal and performance scores on intelligence tests.

## Therapeutic Management

Special training activities in the schools are designed to offer assistance in such areas of deficit as visual perception, auditory perception, and other areas involving integration and coordination. The purpose of programs for children with special learning disabilities is to assist them toward more successful achievement, personal adjustment, and eventual retention in the regular classroom. According to Public Law 94-142, The Education for All Handicapped Children's Act, children with learning disorders must receive free public education in the least restrictive environment. (See Chapters 1 and 22.)

Nurses must understand which type of learning disability a child has in order to best provide direction for the child, parents, and teachers. Children with an auditory perceptual deficit appear unable to follow directions or to comprehend large amounts of verbal teaching. These children need to be taught with diagrams, pictures, demonstration, and written lists. Children with a visual perceptual deficit may have difficulty reading, lining up numbers for mathematical operations, or judging distance. These children may have dyslexia and do better with demonstration and a verbal approach. Children with an integrative deficit may have difficulty sequencing data or storing and retrieving sensory data. Multisensory techniques should be used, and comprehension should be checked frequently throughout instruction. Children with motor deficits may need to use computers or typewriters in the classroom because their handwriting will *not* improve. They may need to find alternatives to physical competition that requires coordination of movement (Selekman and Snyder, 2000). The **Learning Disabilities Association of America**\* provides information and support to families who have a child with a learning disability. An online interactive web site is also available for parents, teachers, and children with learning disabilities.†

Children with learning disorders grow up to be adults with learning disorders. The goal is to help them identify their area of weakness and to compensate for it.

---

\*4156 Library Rd, Pittsburgh, PA 15234, (412) 341-1515, fax: (412) 344-0224, e-mail: ldanatl@usaor.net; www.ldanatl.org.
†www.ldonline.org/index.html#top.

## Tic Disorders

A *tic* is an involuntary, recurrent, random, rapid, highly stereotyped movement or vocalization, occurring in 10% to 35% of all children (Table 18-11). Tics can be simple or complex and involve motor movements, eye movements, or vocalizations (Box 18-3). Tics decrease during concentration, are markedly diminished during sleep, and become more exaggerated when the affected children are experiencing stress or excitement. Obsessive-compulsive behaviors, in the form of ritualistic activities, may also be present and can occur in individuals free of tics. A number of medications can precipitate or exacerbate tics.

Almost all mild, transient tic disorders of childhood are self-limited and disappear within a few months, usually less than a year. The most common tics involve the eyes, head, and face, and treatment does not affect recovery. Tic disorders can begin at any time during childhood. Boys are affected at least three times as often as girls, and transient tic disorders are observed in other family members.

A recent study of Italian children points to a possible connection between Group A streptococcal infections and the development of tics (Cardona and Orefici, 2001). Results from this study indicated a relationship between severity of a tic disorder and the magnitude of serologic response to group A streptococcal antigens. The authors postulate that group A streptococcal infections may trigger a specific neurobehavioral disorder such as tics.

Tic disorders that persist beyond 1 year are considered chronic and consist of either motor or vocal manifestations, but not both (Scahill, Lynch, and Ort, 1995). The most severe of the chronic tics is Gilles de la Tourette syndrome. Diagnosis of a tic disorder is based on clinical observations.

Most tic disorders resolve by late childhood or adolescence without treatment and cause no physical harm to the child. Therapeutic management consists primarily of support to the child and family, reassurance about the prognosis, and education regarding expectations (of the child) for control. Although the child is able to suppress the manifestations to some degree, persistent pressure for control constitutes an additional stress to an affected child. Haloperidol, pimozide, and clonidine may provide relief of symptoms of chronic tics. Genetic counseling is also advised for families of children with chronic tics.

---

| **Box 18-3** |
|---|
| **Types of Tics** |

**Simple motor**—Eye blinking, grimacing, neck jerking, shoulder jerking
**Complex motor**—Jumping, squatting, stamping the foot, thrusting out an arm, hitting or biting self, ritualistic movements (smelling an object, touching own or another's body, obsessive or compulsive patterns of behavior), grooming behaviors
**Simple vocal**—Throat clearing, sniffing, grunting, coughing, snorting, lip noises
**Complex vocal**—Echolalia (repeating last-heard sound, word, or phrase of another), palilalia (repeating own sounds or words), coprolalia (use of socially unacceptable words, often obscene), shouting words out of context

---

| **TABLE 18-11** | **Spectrum of tic disorders** | | | |
|---|---|---|---|---|
| | **Mild** | ⟷ | | **Chronic** |
| Duration | Acute | Subacute | | Chronic |
| Motor tics | Simple | Complex | | Obscene gestures |
| | Few | | | Multiple |
| Vocal tics | None | | Noises | Coprolalia |
| Suppressible | Yes | | | No |

# Tourette Syndrome (TS)

TS is the most complex and severe of the tic disorders. It begins between ages 2 and 16, persists throughout life, and is characterized by rapidly repetitive multiple motor and vocal movements. The etiology is uncertain; most theories implicate abnormalities of various neurotransmitters or a dysregulation in brain circuits that connect the basal ganglia to the motor cortex (Leckman and others, 1997). Support for a genetic origin, based on family studies, suggests that TS follows a pattern of inheritance that involves a mixed genetic-environmental model (Walkup and others, 1996). Factors such as prenatal and perinatal hypoxic injuries may interact with genetic factors and influence the severity of TS.

The manifestations of TS wax and wane in intensity and exhibit a continuing pattern of change in which old tics disappear and new tics develop (Box 18-4). The onset is usually mild, and the initial tic is of brief duration. The minor tics then come and go, becoming more intense and lasting longer. Some tics may be severe from the onset, often with no symptom-free periods. A high percentage of children with TS have associated obsessive-compulsive symptoms (e.g., recurring thoughts; the need to arrange and rearrange objects, repeatedly turn the light switch off and on, tie and retie their shoes, and so on). Other problems associated with TS include ADHD, disruptive behavior, and learning disabilities (Scahill, Lynch, and Ort, 1995). For some children, these associated symptoms may be more disturbing than the tics.

Diagnosis is based on clinical observations, especially if other family members are affected. The tics do not lead to physical deterioration or affect the child's life expectancy.

## Therapeutic Management

Treatment of TS is primarily symptomatic and consists of child and family education and support. Children with more severe tics sometimes obtain symptomatic relief from medications. Dopamine-blocking agents, such as haloperidol or fluphenazine, are the most widely prescribed drugs. Clonidine, an $\alpha_2$-adrenergic drug, may also be prescribed (Bingham and Clancy, 1997).

---

### Box 18-4 ■ ■ ■
### Diagnostic Criteria for Tourette Syndrome

A. Both multiple motor and one or more vocal tics have been present at some time during the illness, although not necessarily concurrently. (A *tic* is a sudden, rapid, recurrent, nonrhythmic, stereotyped motor movement or vocalization.)
B. The tics occur many times a day (usually in bouts) nearly every day or intermittently throughout a period of more than 1 year, and during this period there was never a tic-free period of more than 3 consecutive months.
C. The disturbance causes marked distress or significant impairment in social, occupational, or other important areas of functioning.
D. The onset is before age 18 years.
E. The disturbance is not due to the direct physiologic effects of a substance (e.g., stimulants) or a general medical condition (e.g., Huntington disease or postviral encephalitis).

From *Diagnostic and statistical manual of mental disorders, (DSM-IV)*, ed 4, Washington, DC, 1994, American Psychiatric Association.

---

Psychostimulants and tricyclic antidepressants have been used to treat the coexisting symptoms of attention deficit hyperactivity disorder. Antidepressant medications such as clomipramine (Anafranil), fluoxetine (Prozac), and sertraline (Zoloft), which block the reuptake of serotonin in the brain, have also been used to treat obsessive-compulsive symptoms associated with TS. A pilot study of children and adolescents indicated that risperidone, another serotonin receptor antagonist, reduced the frequency and intensity of both motor and phonic tics in a small sample of children and adolescents (Lombroso and others, 1995). Genetic counseling is also advised.

## Nursing Considerations

Education of children, families, teachers, and others involved in children's everyday life is a major aspect of therapy. Punishment for the behaviors is inappropriate because they are involuntary. Affected children are often quick to anger, have a low frustration tolerance, and may engage in temper tantrums. These children need to be guided toward acceptable substitute behaviors in order to develop normally, socially and emotionally. For example, suggesting that a child retire to a quiet area to gain control of emotions or providing a pillow, stuffed toy, or punching bag on which to vent feelings is often helpful.

Influential persons in the children's lives must help foster feelings of self-esteem. Children with TS demonstrate a constant, ongoing battle to control their impulses and need positive relationships with their parents to become well-adjusted. A child's self-concept can be damaged if parents react to their disability with controlling behaviors, guilt, anger, or hostility.

School nurses can help children with TS cope with teasing from their classmates, can advocate to ensure that they are not barred from extracurricular activities, and can educate teachers and classmates about the effects of TS and which behaviors the child can and cannot control in the classroom. Many children with TS experience difficulty writing and benefit from using a tape recorder or computer in the classroom. Extra time may also be needed when taking standardized tests (Scahill, Lynch, and Ort, 1995).

Nurses can assist families in long-term monitoring of symptoms, which includes establishing the waxing and waning pattern and whether or not symptoms interfere with development and adaptation or require more intense therapy. Families of children taking medication need to be alert to possible side effects, including lethargy, personality change, increased appetite and overweight, depression, parkinsonian symptoms (tremor, muscle rigidity, shuffling gait, hypokinesia, and difficulty chewing, swallowing, and speaking), and anticholinergic symptoms (confusion, excitement, dilated pupils, blurred vision, dry mouth, and dysphagia).

The family may benefit from referral to health agencies such as the local health departments, social services, and parent groups. The **Tourette Syndrome Association**\* is ac-

---

\*42-40 Bell Blvd, Bayside, NY 11361, (718) 224-2999, fax: (718) 279-9596, e-mail: tourette@ix.netcom.com.

tive in research and education and provides services to affected children and their families.

## Posttraumatic Stress Disorder (PTSD)

PTSD refers to the development of characteristic symptoms following exposure to an extremely traumatic experience or catastrophic event. The traumatic experience or catastrophic event is typically life-threatening to self or a significant other and may involve grotesque mutilation or death, serious injury, or physical coercion. An accident; an assault or victimization; a natural disaster (earthquake, flooding, train wreck, plane crash); sexual abuse; or witnessing of a suicide, homicide, beating, shooting, or other act of violence can lead to PTSD. The response to the event must involve intense fear, helplessness, or horror. In children the response must involve disorganized or agitated behavior. The characteristic symptoms include persistent reexperiencing of the traumatic event, persistent avoidance of stimuli associated with the trauma, numbing of general responsiveness, and persistent symptoms of increased arousal. The full symptom picture must be present for more than 1 month, and the disturbance must cause clinically significant distress or impairment in social, educational, occupational, or other important areas of functioning (American Psychiatric Association, 1994).

The response to the event takes place in three stages. The *initial response* to the stressor is intense arousal, which usually lasts for a few minutes to 1 or 2 hours, depending on the stressor and the individual. The stress hormones are at the maximum as the individual prepares for "fight" or "flight." A prolonged arousal phase may indicate psychosis.

The *second phase,* which lasts approximately 2 weeks, is one in which defense mechanisms are mobilized. It is a period of quiescence in which the event appears to have produced no impression. The victims feel numb, and stress hormone secretion is absent. The reaction is outside their awareness, not well controlled, and involves some type of behavioral pattern. Defense mechanisms are less adaptive to specific situations and may not be what the situation demands. Denial that anything is wrong is a frequently observed defense mechanism.

The *third phase* is one of coping, which normally extends over 2 to 3 months. It is one of consciously directed inquiry. The victims want to know what happened and appear to be getting worse, when actually they are getting better. Numerous psychologic symptoms such as depression, repetitive phenomenon, phobic symptoms, anxiety symptoms, and conversion reactions may be apparent. Children frequently display repetitive actions. They play out the situation over and over again in an attempt to come to terms with their fear. Flashbacks are common. This phase can be self-perpetuating, and a prolonged reaction can develop into an obsession with the traumatic event. Some traumatic effects remain indefinitely.

### Nursing Considerations

Children need to deal with any traumatic event; much depends on the intensity of the event and their reaction to it. Their reactions depend heavily on their social environment and the way in which their caretaking adults react to the event. Children usually react in the same manner as their caregivers (contagious pathology); therefore it is important to be aware of these reactions. In the second, or defense, phase of the PTSD the appropriateness of the defense mechanism must be assessed, and children must be assisted in application of their defense. If children do not engage in some catharsis or if their defense phase is prolonged, they may need referral for special psychologic help.

Coping is a learned response, and children in the third phase can be helped to use their coping strategies to deal with their fear. Children usually are willing to accept reasoning. Those who are assisted in their catharsis and allowed expression will survive without serious lasting effects. They should be encouraged to play out the stress and/or discuss their feelings about the event. If they are unable to do this, they may become obsessed with the traumatic event and need professional help. Conversion reactions are common obsessive behaviors in children.

Children need professional help if any of the phases of PTSD are prolonged. Boys tend to have a prolonged defense phase more often than girls. Occasionally the event will be unrecognized, and the affected child will engage in what is considered to be unusual behavior. In the case of any sudden change in behavior, the child needs to be assessed for a traumatic event—"Did something happen?" When the change in behavior is determined to be caused by a traumatic event, treatment can be implemented.

## School Phobia

Children, other than beginning students, who resist going to school or who demonstrate extreme reluctance to attend school for a sustained period of time as a result of severe anxiety or a fear of school-related experiences are said to have school phobia. The terms "school refusal" and "school avoidance" are also used to describe this behavior. School phobia occurs in children of all ages, but it is more common in children 10 years of age and older. School avoidance behaviors occur in both boys and girls and in children from all socioeconomic levels.

Anxiety that frequently verges on panic is a constant manifestation, and children can develop symptoms as a protective mechanism to keep them from facing the situation that distresses them. Physical symptoms are prominent and may affect any part of the body—anorexia, nausea, vomiting, diarrhea, dizziness, headache, leg pains, or abdominal pains. They may even develop a low-grade fever. A striking feature of school phobia is the prompt subsiding of symptoms when it is evident that the child can remain at home. Another significant observation is absence of symptoms on weekends and holidays, unless they are related to other places such as Sunday school or parties. Occasional mild reluctance is not uncommon among schoolchildren, but if the fear continues for longer than a few days, it must be considered a serious problem—a warning of an important personality problem.

The onset is usually sudden and precipitated by a school-related incident. A poor attendance record for trivial reasons can be elicited by a careful history.

## Etiology

School phobia can be caused by a number of factors. Sometimes the complaints can be related to a transient, specific cause, such as fear of a mismatched or overcritical teacher, fear of failing an examination or giving an oral recitation for a painfully shy child, or discrimination based on race, dress, or physical defect. Sometimes it may be related to a school bully or threatening gang. An insecure home situation in which children fear that they may be deserted by a parent may be the basis of anxiety, especially if the parent has previously threatened to leave.

A frequent source of fear is separation anxiety based on a strong, dependent relationship between the mother and child in which the child is reluctant to leave the mother and she is equally reluctant (even though this may be unconscious) to have the child leave her. The intense need for closeness between mother and child is normal in infancy, but the persistence of this type of relationship into childhood is totally inappropriate.

Characteristically, these children are not afraid to go to school; rather, they are afraid to leave home. They fear something dreadful might happen while they are separated from their families. No event is required to trigger the associated behaviors. However, symptoms may be precipitated by a situation that intensifies the mutual dependency between the mother and the child, such as illness, arrival of a new baby, a move to a strange neighborhood or a new school, or parental discord.

In some instances children have an unrealistic, exaggerated view of their abilities and achievements. When they feel threatened by incidents that challenge their estimate of themselves, such as a minor episode that leads to embarrassment, return to school after an absence, transfer to another class, or even imagined social or academic failure, they become anxious and withdraw, frequently seeking proximity to the mother. Sometimes the step-up in expectations at school or change of important personnel at school (e.g., teacher or principal) is a contributing factor. Occasionally the child may be suffering from an undiagnosed learning disability.

## Therapeutic Management

The treatment for school phobia depends on the cause. If the cause of the problem is an examination, a relationship with a bully, or a mismatch between teacher and child, it can be dealt with accordingly. When the child is helped to understand and cope with the fear, the symptoms usually disappear. In severe cases when returning to school is unsuccessful, professional psychiatric consultation is usually desirable to help identify possible distorted family relationships or a personality disturbance in the child and to help both the child and the family understand the sources of the problem.

Some children with a moderately severe separation anxiety disorder and school refusal may be treated with a tricyclic antidepressant. Anxiolytic agents and/or benzodiazepines such as diazepam, alprazolam, and clonazepam have been used in children who display increased agitation and anxiety related to going to school (Greydanus and Pratt, 1995b). However, psychiatric evaluation is almost always required before anxiolytic agents are prescribed.

## Nursing Considerations

The primary goal for the child with school phobia is to *return the child to school*. The longer the child is permitted to stay out of school, the more difficult it is to reenter. Well-meaning parents or others who permit the child to stay away from school or who support the child's behavior with written excuses only confirm the child's feelings of worthlessness and inability to cope. Parents must be convinced gently but firmly that *immediate* return is essential and that they, the parents, must insist on the child's return for it to be effective.

A school reentry protocol may be necessary for the child with severe symptoms. In reentry programs, the child role-plays routines involved in getting ready for school and that occur during the school day itself. The child also learns to use relaxation techniques, such as progressive muscle relaxation and imagery. Finally, the child is slowly reintroduced into the school setting—usually going to school for a half day initially and then progressing to a full day. Children are rewarded with points for each period during the day that they are able to remain in school. These points are then redeemed for rewards (e.g., playing with favorite toys or social rewards). Often the school nurse can provide both the teacher and the parents with support in carrying out this plan.

**Prevention.**   Prevention of school phobia, as well as other dependency problems, can be developed by the encouragement of independence at appropriate times during infancy and early childhood. For example, by 6 months of age children can be left with a baby-sitter during a parents' night out. Two-year-olds can be left at home (while awake) with a sitter. By 3 years of age children should experience being left somewhere other than their home (e.g., grandparents' home). As soon as they are able, they are allowed to feed, dress, and wash themselves. By 3 to 4 years of age children can be allowed to play in the yard by themselves, and later they should be allowed to play in the neighborhood by themselves.

Specific clues indicate that a child may be experiencing first-time fear of school and may need help to cope. Extra preparation may be needed for children who are very fearful, have trouble adjusting to new situations, or are very clinging. Many individuals continue to manifest some form of fear throughout the school years. When the problem is identified early and effectively treated, negative emotions surrounding school are minimized, and a child is less likely to carry residual fears throughout life.

For most first-time school fears, simple reassurances and a little advance preparation are all that is necessary. Direct contact with the school and teachers is an excellent way to allay anticipatory anxiety. Parents can take children to visit the school about a month before school starts, introduce them to the teacher, and let them experience the classroom firsthand.

Bedtime is also an excellent time to help children resolve first-day jitters. Bedtime stories and books suited to the occasion are available from bookstores and libraries. Several videotapes and tape recordings are also available to help children cope with a variety of common fears (dark, nightmares, baby-sitters, doctors, dentists, monsters).

Parents who suspect that their child may be especially frightened may want to accompany the child to school and wait outside the classroom the first day. A gradual breakaway over succeeding days should relieve their child's and their own anxiety. If the distress extends over a long period of time, professional help may be needed.

## Recurrent Abdominal Pain (RAP)

RAP is a complaint of childhood that is often attributed to a psychogenic etiology although it can be a symptom of either psychosomatic or organic disease. RAP is traditionally defined as three or more separate episodes of abdominal pain during a 3-month period similar to the "spastic" or "irritable" colon syndrome of adulthood. The disorder affects mostly school-age children and is rarely seen in children less than 5 years of age. Girls are affected slightly more often than boys (Walker and others, 1998).

### Etiology and Pathophysiology

Only a minority of youngsters with RAP have an organic basis for their pain, which includes inflammatory bowel disease, peptic ulcer disease, lactose intolerance, pelvic inflammatory disease, urinary bladder infection, and pancreatitis. Psychogenic causes of abdominal pain, such as school phobia, depression, acute reactive anxiety, and conversion reaction, account for a small number of cases. The bulk of children with RAP suffer from functional abdominal pain.

If no organic cause can be identified, the functional abdominal pain of RAP has been attributed to dysfunctional causes (Smith, 2001). The dysfunctional category includes such etiologic factors as constipation, chronic stool retention, overeating, irritable colon, and intestinal gas with heightened awareness of intestinal motility or dysmotility. Normally, intestinal contents arrive at the distal portion of the intestine with a relatively high fluid content, and fluid is extracted in the distal colon and rectum. If the normally relaxed distal intestine fails to relax and prevents the flow of its contents toward the rectum, the resulting excessive distention and spasms of the distal intestinal musculature produce pressure on nerve endings, causing pain.

The symptoms of RAP may result from multiple causes, and it is important to assess a number of factors that could place a child at risk for this condition. These factors include (1) somatic predisposition, dysfunction, or disorder; (2) lifestyle and habit, including routines, diet, and life tempo; (3) temperament and learned response patterns, such as the child's behavior style, personality, and learned coping skills; and (4) milieu and critical events (i.e., the child's intimate surroundings [familial, social, and cultural norms] and unexpected sources of stress or gratification).

Children at risk for RAP tend to be high achievers who have extensive personal goals or whose parents have unusually high expectations. They are described as being more mature and sensitive than others or as worriers. At risk are children who are overly concerned about what others think about them but have difficulty meeting the expectations of parents, teachers, and others. They are uncomfortable with expressions of anger or argument, especially in those persons who are significant in their lives. School attendance is adversely affected, and these children generally exhibit poor learning performance. It is not uncommon for symptoms to be aggravated during school days.

### Clinical Manifestations

Children with RAP have real pain that is usually located in the periumbilical and/or epigastric area. On palpation the pain is more likely to be experienced in the epigastric area or in the lower right or left quadrant and is accompanied by vague tenderness without muscle guarding. The pain is irregular in time, duration, and intensity and is associated with either loose or pellet-formed stools. Other symptoms that may accompany the abdominal pain are headache, flushing, pallor, dizziness, and fatigue. Nausea, vomiting, diarrhea, and dysuria are sometimes part of the syndrome. The symptoms reflect the heightened intensity of response to stimulation of the autonomic bowel sites. The loose stools are a result of the exaggerated propulsive motility, and the pain is caused by the sharply increased mechanical tension in the gut.

### Diagnostic Evaluation

Diagnosis consists of a complete family history, the child's health history, physical examination, and laboratory tests. The family history may provide evidence of a hereditary disorder or mimicry of adult symptoms. The child is evaluated for evidence of an organic basis for symptoms such as pain that radiates to the back, pain that awakens the child from sleep, recurrent fever, and weight loss. The pain is assessed for location, quality, frequency, duration, any associated symptoms, alleviating factors, and exacerbating factors (Smith, 2001). (See Critical Thinking Exercise box.)

### Therapeutic Management

Treatment involves providing reassurance and reducing or eliminating symptoms (Hyams and Hyman, 1998). Hospitalization may be necessary, and the child frequently shows improvement in the hospital environment. Initial efforts are directed toward ruling out organic causes of the pain, relieving discomfort, and attempting to determine the situations that precipitate attacks.

A high-fiber diet, psyllium bulk agents, lubricants such as mineral oil, and bowel training are emphasized. When simple measures are ineffective, an antispasmodic drug such as propantheline bromide may be prescribed to relieve the muscle spasm.

### Nursing Considerations

The nurse can be instrumental in assessment and management of recurrent abdominal pain in children. Many techniques used in a routine assessment elicit information that might help identify factors that contribute to the child's symptoms. The child's social and psychologic adjustment should be evaluated, and details of the pain should be obtained directly from the child.

Questions that provide clues to parent-child relationships and how the family deals with angry feelings provide

## Critical Thinking Exercise

### Recurrent Abdominal Pain

Sharon is a 10-year-old child who has had four episodes of abdominal pain in the last 12 weeks. The nurse practitioner in the school-based clinic at Sharon's school is discussing Sharon's symptoms with her mother. Which of the following symptoms could indicate an organic cause for Sharon's pain?

FIRST, THINK ABOUT IT . . .

- What information are you using?
- How are you interpreting that information?

1. Vague abdominal pain in the epigastric area that comes and goes with no regularity or pattern
2. Complaints of nausea, especially on school days
3. Complaints of fatigue and headache
4. Pain that awakens Sharon from sleep and that is accompanied by an elevated temperature

*The best response is four. The majority of children with recurrent abdominal pain (RAP) have no identifiable organic cause for their pain. However, there are organic causes for recurrent abdominal pain. Therefore the nurse practitioner should conduct a thorough assessment of the characteristics of Sharon's pain. Pain that localizes away from the umbilicus; radiates to the back, shoulder, or lower extremities; or awakens the child from sleep is not typical in RAP and requires prompt and accurate interpretation. An elevated temperature could be a sign of an infection.*

information for diagnosis and management. Relationships with peers, school problems, and other concerns of the child need to be explored. Any evidence of depression should be noted.

Once the diagnosis has been established, the parents and the child need an explanation of the pain, which can be compared to a skeletal muscle cramp or "charley horse" for easier comprehension. Reassurance that the symptoms are not unique to their child and that the pain can be expected to subside is helpful in relieving parental fears and anxieties.

A high-fiber diet is discussed with the child and family (see Chapter 33), and bowel training is emphasized. The child is encouraged to establish a pattern of sitting on the toilet for 10 to 15 minutes immediately after breakfast to take advantage of the increased colonic activity following meals. If necessary, stimulatory suppositories can be used to induce early morning defecation.

When parents are reassured that there is no organic cause for the pain, they will need some guidance regarding what they can do during a pain episode. All too often, they feel helpless and anxious, which tends to compound the child's distress. The simple measure of having the child rest in a peaceful, quiet environment and providing comfort will often relieve the symptoms in a short time. A heating pad may also ease the discomfort. (See Nonpharmacologic [Pain] Management, Chapter 26.) If pain is not relieved by these simple measures, the parents are taught how to administer antispasmodics, if prescribed. For example, if pain

is precipitated by meals, having the child take the medication 20 to 30 minutes before mealtime may prevent an episode.

The most valuable assistance that the nurse can provide is support and reassurance to the family. When open communication is established and families are able to see a relationship between stress-provoking situations and the child's symptoms, the chance for remedial action is enhanced. Follow-up care and continued support are essential because the symptoms tend to remit and exacerbate; therefore, the availability of a supportive health professional can be a source of comfort to the child and family.

## Conversion Reaction

*Conversion reaction,* also known as *hysteria, hysterical conversion reaction,* and *childhood hysteria,* is a psychophysiologic disorder with a sudden onset that can usually be traced to a precipitating environmental event. The manifestations involve primarily the voluntary musculature and special senses and include abdominal pain, fainting, pseudoseizures, paralysis, headaches, and visual field restriction. Once considered rare in childhood, the diagnosis occurs more frequently than has generally been acknowledged. In childhood the disorder is observed with equal frequency in both sexes, but girls outnumber boys during adolescence. The most commonly observed symptom is seizure activity, which can be differentiated from symptoms of neurogenic origin by formal tests, the most useful of which is the finding of a normal electroencephalogram.

It has been observed that many children with conversion reaction have experienced a major family crisis before the onset of symptoms, such as loss of a parent or other significant person through death, divorce, or moving. It is not uncommon for the child to exhibit symptoms of the lost person. The families of children with conversion reaction characteristically display problems in communication, and depression or hypochondriasis in a parent.

Educating the child and family regarding the cause underlying emotional stresses or feelings and alternative approaches to coping with stress may alleviate the child's symptoms. If deep personality problems are evident, psychiatric consultation is indicated. Nursing care is similar to that for the child with recurrent abdominal pain.

## Childhood Depression

Depression in childhood is often difficult to detect because children may be unable to express their feelings and tend to act out their problems and concerns. Authorities agree that childhood depression exists, but, the manifestations of depression in children may differ from those of adults. The characteristics of depression are largely determined by parallel developments in symbolism, language, and cognitive development. Younger children demonstrate a more cause-and-effect relationship between the stressors and the depressive manifestations. In older children the relationships between stressful events and depression are less clear. Their reactions are less physiologic and more cognitively complex,

---

**Box 18-5** ■ ■ ■
**Criteria for Major Depressive Episode**

A. Five (or more) of the following symptoms have been present during the same 2-week period and represent a change from previous functioning; at least one of the symptoms is either (1) depressed mood or (2) loss of interest or pleasure. **Note:** Do not include symptoms that are clearly due to a general medical condition, or mood-incongruent delusions, or hallucinations.

  (1) Depressed mood most of the day, nearly every day, as indicated by either subjective report (e.g., feels sad or empty) or observation made by others (e.g., appears tearful). **Note:** In children and adolescents, can be irritable mood.
  (2) Markedly diminished interest or pleasure in all, or almost all, activities most of the day, nearly every day (as indicated by either subjective account or observation made by others)
  (3) Significant weight loss when not dieting or weight gain (e.g., a change of more than 5% of body weight in a month), or decrease or increase in appetite nearly every day. **Note:** In children, consider failure to make expected weight gains.
  (4) Insomnia or hypersomnia nearly every day
  (5) Psychomotor agitation or retardation nearly every day (observable by others, not merely subjective feelings of restlessness or being slowed down)
  (6) Fatigue or loss of energy nearly every day
  (7) Feelings of worthlessness or excessive or inappropriate guilt (which may be delusional) nearly every day (not merely self-reproach or guilt about being sick)
  (8) Diminished ability to think or concentrate, or indecisiveness, nearly every day (either by subjective account or as observed by others)
  (9) Recurrent thoughts of death (not just fear of dying), recurrent suicidal ideation without a specific plan, or a suicide attempt or a specific plan for committing suicide.

B. The symptoms do not meet criteria for a mixed episode, which includes symptoms of a manic episode, such as rapidly alternating moods (sadness, irritability, euphoria).
C. The symptoms cause clinically significant distress or impairment in social, occupational, or other important areas of functioning.
D. The symptoms are not due to the direct physiologic effects of a substance (e.g., a drug of abuse, a medication) or a general medical condition (e.g., hypothyroidism).
E. The symptoms are not better accounted for by bereavement; i.e., after the loss of a loved one, the symptoms persist for longer than 2 months or are characterized by marked functional impairment, morbid preoccupation with worthlessness, suicidal ideation, psychotic symptoms, or psychomotor retardation.

Slightly modified from American Psychiatric Association: *Diagnostic and statistical manual of mental disorders (DSM-IV)*, ed 4, Washington, DC, 1994, The Association.

---

and the observed behaviors tend to be age-specific. Depressed children exhibit a distinctive style of thinking characterized by low self-esteem, hopelessness, and a tendency to explain negative events in terms of personal shortcomings.

Some states of depression are of a temporary nature (e.g., acute depression precipitated by a traumatic event). This might include a period of hospitalization, loss of a parent through death or separation, or loss of a significant relationship with something (a pet), someone (a friend or family member), or a place (move from a familiar home, neighborhood, or city). The easily identified manifestations include a sad, downcast face, tearfulness, irritability, and withdrawal from previously enjoyed activities and relationships. The child tends to spend more time in solitary activities, especially television viewing. Schoolwork is impaired. Some children become more dependent and clinging; others become more aggressive and disruptive. Sleeplessness or hypersomnia, changes in appetite or weight (either increased or decreased), constipation, tiredness, and nonspecific complaints of not feeling well are common reactions. Responses are not sustained and can be modified with social and family support.

More serious and less common are depressive responses to more chronic stress and loss; these are frequently observed in children with chronic illness or disability. There is no apparent precipitating event, but there is often a history of frequent disruptions in important relationships. Commonly there is also a history of depressive illness in one or both parents during the child's lifetime. The manifestations are similar to responses to acute reactions. Some of the primary and associated symptoms that are observed in depressed children and the DSM-IV criteria currently used for establishing a diagnosis of major depression are outlined in Box 18-5. There are a number of similarities among major depressive disorders in childhood and several other psychologic disorders.

## Therapeutic Management

Depressed children are managed by a health team especially prepared in the care of children with mental disorders. Treatment is highly individualized and should be undertaken in the least constrictive environment, usually an outpatient setting. Suicidal children are admitted to the hospital for protection if the family is unable to provide constant monitoring. Hospitalization may also be advised for children with associated disruptive behavior, such as fighting with peers or family. Most therapeutic regimens focus on various combinations of counseling, psychotherapy, family therapy, cognitive therapy, education (teaching social and life skills that facilitate coping skills), environmental improvement, and pharmacotherapy.

Pharmacotherapy may involve tricyclic antidepressants such as desipramine, imipramine, nortriptyline, and amitriptyline. Serotoninergic-reuptake inhibitors (SRIs), second-generation antidepressants, do not have the anticholinergic, hypotensive, and sedative side effects of tricyclic antidepressants. SRIs include fluoxetine (Prozac), trazodone (Desyrel), sertraline (Zoloft), and paroxetine (Paxil) (Greydanus and Pratt, 1995a). Recently, a group of third- and fourth-generation antidepressant drugs that inhibit the uptake of serotonin and/or dopamine have been used to treat depression in children. These drugs include bupropion (Wellbutrin) and venlafaxine (Effexor).

## Nursing Considerations

Nurses should be aware that depression is a problem that can easily be overlooked in the school-age child and one that can interrupt normal growth and development. Recognizing depression and making appropriate referrals is an important nursing function. Identification of the depressed child requires a careful history (health, growth and development, social, and family health), interviews with the child, and observations by the nurse, parents, and teachers. If antidepressants are prescribed, the child and family need to know that antidepressants require between 2 and 4 weeks at a therapeutic level to achieve a beneficial effect. The child and family also need to be instructed to monitor the child for side effects of the specific drug prescribed and any interactions with other drugs. (See Chapter 21 for a definitive discussion of suicide because suicidal ideation is common during depression.)

## Childhood Schizophrenia

Childhood schizophrenia refers to severe deviations in ego functioning and is generally reserved for psychotic disorders that appear after the first 4 or 5 years of life. Schizophrenia in adults occurs with relative frequency, and, although childhood psychosis is not as common, it is by no means rare.

The cause of schizophrenia is unknown, but three risk factors have been identified: genetic characteristics, gestational and birth complications, and winter birth. Biologic relatives of affected individuals have an increased chance of developing the disorder. For example, the risk for the children if both parents are afflicted is 40%. The rate of concordance is 10% for dizygotic (nonidentical) twins and 40% to 50% for monozygotic (identical) twins. Current thinking supports altered development of the central nervous system as an etiologic factor. Psychosocial theories, especially in regard to the parent-child relationship, have not been supported, but certain social and environmental factors may play a role in a child's vulnerability to developing schizophrenia.

Childhood schizophrenia is characterized by a gradual onset of neurotic symptoms that show wide variation according to each affected child's developmental level, the age of onset, the nature of early childhood experiences, and the type of defense mechanisms used. However, the basic core disturbance is a lack of contact with reality and the subsequent development of a world of the child's own. Secondary characteristics represent impairment in a wide number of areas of development, including cognition, perception, emotion, language, and physical motor control. The most common manifestations involve language disturbances, impaired interpersonal relationships, and inappropriate affect (outward expression of emotion) (Box 18-6).

Treatment involves management of the symptoms, the prevention of a relapse, and the social and occupational rehabilitation of the young person. In some individuals drug therapy produces dramatic improvement in symptoms and social adjustment. Antipsychotic drugs that may be used include haloperidol, clozapine, chlorpromazine, and risperidone. Risperidone blocks receptors for subtypes of serotonin and dopamine and has fewer side effects than traditionally used antipsychotic drugs (Findling and

---

**Box 18-6**  ▪ ▪ ▫
### Some Characteristics of Childhood Schizophrenia

Bizarre behavioral patterns and stereotyped movements such as robotlike walking, whirling, or graceful gyrations

Periods of hypoactivity alternating with periods of hyperactivity

Inappropriate affect that ranges from flatness to explosiveness

Common occurrences of temper tantrums

Language disturbances such as speaking in fragmented sentences, parrotlike repetition of words, development of a private language, and altered tone of voice; some schizophrenic children are mute or will only utter a single word on rare occasions

Distorted time orientation with a blending of past, present, and future

Distorted sense of and use of their bodies

Apparent denial of the human quality in people, such as attempting to use a person as a step stool to reach an object

Conveying a nonhuman identity by action, sounds, or posture, such as barking or calling self a vacuum cleaner

Frequent occurrences of compulsive behavior and phobias

---

others, 1996; Lykes and Cueva, 1996). Olanzapine and quetiopine are other antipsychotic medications recently approved by the Food and Drug Administration (Citrome, 1997). Family interventions and family therapy have also resulted in improvements in psychotic symptoms, thought disorders, and social functioning among children with schizophrenia (Dixon and Lehman, 1995; Schooler and others, 1995).

### Nursing Considerations

Nursing of psychotic children is a highly specialized area, but, because such problems are occuring with increasing frequency, nurses should recognize children who consistently demonstrate abnormal behavior and refer them for evaluation.

Nurses should also instruct family members of children taking antipsychotic drugs to observe for possible side effects. Common side effects of both haloperidol and clozapine include dizziness, drowsiness, tachycardia, and hypotension. Extrapyramidal side effects, such as abnormal movements, have been reported with haloperidol. A small percentage of patients taking clozapine may have seizures. However, the most significant side effect of clozapine is lethal agranulocytosis, which has occurred in 1% to 2% of patients (Citrome, 1997). Therefore, a mandatory monitoring program requires that patients on clozapine have a white blood cell (WBC) count done every week for as long as they receive the drug and for 4 weeks after the drug is stopped. Pharmacies report the weekly WBC counts to the manufacturer of the drug and cannot release clozapine to the patient without evidence of a safe WBC count (Citrome, 1997). Risperidone has fewer extrapyramidal side effects than other antipsychotics, but possible adverse effects of this drug include orthostatic hypotension, sedation, and, less commonly, seizures (Citrome, 1997; de Oliveira and others, 1996).

## KEY POINTS

- Middle childhood is a relatively healthy period, and most problems encountered are not considered serious.
- The skin serves several important functions: protection, prevention of loss of body fluids, heat regulation, and sensation.
- It is important for nurses to be able to describe skin lesions accurately.
- The process of wound healing consists of inflammation, fibroplasia, scar contraction, and scar maturation.
- Wound healing occurs by primary, secondary, or tertiary intention.
- Bacterial, viral, and fungal infections are common in childhood.
- Prevention of infection or reinfection is the primary goal in management of pediculosis.

- Contact dermatitis may involve a reaction to a primary irritant or sensitization.
- Teaching prevention of thermal injury, especially sunburn, is an important nursing function.
- Adverse reactions to drugs occur more often in the skin than in any other organ.
- Dental care is essential in middle childhood; the most frequent problems that arise are dental caries and malocclusion.
- The behavioral disorders of childhood are primarily attention deficit hyperactivity disorder and tic disorders.
- Other major behavioral or mental disorders involving school-age children include school phobia, recurrent abdominal pain, conversion reaction, depression, and schizophrenia.

## REFERENCES

American Academy of Pediatrics: *Bedwetting: guidelines for parents*, Elk Grove Village, IL, 1996a, The Academy.

American Academy of Pediatrics: Clinical practice guidelines: treatment of the school-aged child with attention-deficit/hyperactivity disorder, *Pediatrics* 108(4):1033-1044, 2001.

American Academy of Pediatrics, Committee on Children with Disabilities and Committee on Drugs: Medication for children with attentional disorders, *Pediatrics* 98(2):301-304, 1996b.

American Academy of Pediatrics, Committee on Environmental Health: Ultraviolet light: a hazard to children, *Pediatrics* 104(2):328-333, 1999.

American Academy of Pediatrics, Committee on Infectious Diseases: Prevention of Lyme disease, *Pediatrics* 105(1):142-147, 2000a.

American Academy of Pediatrics, Committee on Infectious Diseases: *Red book: report of the Committee on Infectious Diseases*, ed 25, Elk Grove Village, IL, 2000b, The Academy.

American Psychiatric Association: *Diagnostic and statistical manual of mental disorders, (DSM IV)*, ed 4, Washington, DC, 1994, American Psychiatric Association.

Barnett NK: Pruritus. In Hoekelman RA and others, editors: *Primary pediatric care*, ed 4, St Louis, 2001, Mosby.

Beaumont E, Anderson-Dam M: Technology scorecard, wound care science at the crossroads, a guide for selecting from the latest wound care products, *Am J Nurs* 98(12):16-21, 1998.

Bernardo LM and others: Dog bites in children treated in a pediatric emergency department, *JSPN* 5(2):87-95, 2000.

Biederman J and others: A prospective 4-year follow-up study of attention-deficit hyperactivity and related disorders, *Arch Gen Psychiatry* 50:437-446, 1996.

Bingham P, Clancy RR: Neurology. In Polin RA, Ditmar MF, editors: *Pediatric secrets*, ed 2, Philadelphia, 1997, Mosby.

Blum NJ, Ditmar MF, Charney EB: Behavior and development. In Polin RA, Ditmar MF, editors: *Pediatric secrets*, ed 3, Philadelphia, 1997, Mosby.

Bonham P: Topical therapy tips: wound care with hydrocolloid dressings, *Advance Nurs* 22:6-7, 2000.

Bradley BJ and others: Tinea capitis today: what nurses need to know about identifying and managing fungal infections of the scalp in the school setting, *J Sch Nurs* (special suppl), Oct 1996.

Cardona F, Orefici G: Group streptococcal infections and tic disorders in an Italian pediatric population, *J Pediatr* 138:71-75, 2001.

Castellanos FX and others: Quantitative brain magnetic resonance imaging in attention-deficit hyperactivity disorder, *Arch Gen Psychiatry* 53:607-616, 1996.

Citrome L: New antipsychotic medications: what advantages do they offer? *Postgrad Med* 101(2):207-214, 1997.

Dattwyler RJ and others: Ceftriaxone compared with doxycycline for the treatment of acute disseminated Lyme disease, *N Engl J Med* 337(5):289-294, 1997.

de Oliveira IR and others: Risperidone versus haloperidol in the treatment of schizophrenia: a meta-analysis comparing their efficacy and safety, *J Clin Pharm Ther* 21:349-358, 1996.

Dinman S, Jarosz DA: Managing serious dog bite injuries in children, *Pediatr Nurs* 22:413-417, 1996.

Dixon LB, Lehman AF: Family interventions for schizophrenia, *Schizophr Bull* 21(4):631-643, 1995.

Dourmishev A, Serafimova D, Dourmishev L: Efficacy and tolerance of oral ivermectin in scabies, *J Europ Acad Dermatol Venereol* 11(3):247-251, 1998.

Dumas D, Pelletier L: Perception in hyperactive children, *MCN* 24(1):12-19, 1999.

Findling RL and others: Antipsychotic medications in children and adolescents, *J Clin Psychiatry* 57(suppl 9):19-23, 1996.

Fix AD, Strickland GT, Grant J: Tick bites and Lyme disease in an endemic setting: problematic use of serologic testing and prophylactic antibiotic therapy, *JAMA* 279:206-210, 1998.

Foreman JW: Nephrology. In Polin RA, Ditmar MF, editors: *Pediatric secrets*, ed 2, Philadelphia, 1997, Mosby.

Greydanus DE, Pratt HD: Emotional and behavioral disorders of adolescence, part 1, *Adolesc Health Update* (3):1-8, 1995a.

Greydanus DE, Pratt HD: Emotional and behavioral disorders of adolescence, part 2, *Adolesc Health Update* 8(1):1-8, 1995b.

Hayward CJ and others: Investigation of bioequivalence and tolerability of intramuscular ceftriaxone injections by using 1% lidocaine, buffered lidocaine, and sterile water diluents, *Antimicrob Agents Chemother* 40(2):485-487, 1996.

Heffernan AE, O'Sullivan A: Pediatric sun exposure, *Nurs Pract* 23(7):67-86, 1998.

Hines SE: Lyme disease: the debate continues, *Patient Care Nurs Practitioner* 38-54, 2001.

Humane Society of the United States: *Preventing and avoiding dog bites*, Washington, DC, 1998, The Society.

Hyams JS, Hyman PE: Recurrent abdominal pain and the biopsychosocial model of medical practice, *J Pediatr* 133:473-478, 1998.

Jensen PS: Fact versus fancy concerning the multimodal treatment study for attention deficit hyperactivity disorder, *Can J Psychiatry* 44(10):975-980, 1999.

Johnson NS and others: Social and emotional problems in children with neurofibromatosis type 1: evidence and proposed interventions, *J Pediatr* 134:767-772, 1999.

King DE: Attention deficit disorder isn't just for kids, *Nurs Spect* 10(25DC):24-25, December 11, 2000.

Law SF, Schachar RJ: Do typical clinical doses of methylphenidate cause tics in children treated for attention deficit hyperactivity disorder? *J Am Acad Child Adolescent Psychiatry* 38(8):944-951, 1999.

Leckman JF and others: Pathogenesis of Tourette's syndrome, *J Child Psychol Psychiatry* 38:119-142, 1997.

Litovitz TL and others: 1998 Annual Report of the American Association of Poison Control Centers Toxic Exposure Surveillance System, *Am J Emerg Med* 17:435-487, 1999.

Loening-Baucke V: Encopresis and soiling, *Pediatr Clin North Am* 43(1):279-298, 1996.

Loening-Baucke V: Biofeedback treatment for chronic constipation and encoporesis in childhood: long-term outcome, *Pediatrics* 96:105-110, 1995.

Lombroso PJ and others: Risperidone treatment of children and adolescents' chronic tic disorders: a preliminary report, *J Am Acad Child Adolesc Psychiatry* 34(9):1147-1152, 1995.

Lykes WC, Cueva JE: Risperidone in children with schizophrenia, *J Am Acad Child Adolesc Psychiatry* 35(4):405-406, 1996.

Margileth AM: Recent advances in diagnosis and treatment of cat scratch disease, *Curr Infect Dis Rep* 2(2):141-146, 2000.

McCulloch JM, Kloth LC, Feedar JA: *Wound healing alternatives in management,* ed 2, Philadelphia, 1995, FA Davis.

MTA Study: A 14-month randomized clinical trial of treatment strategies for attention-deficit/hyperactivity disorder. The MTA cooperative group multimodal treatment study of children with ADHD, *Arch Gen Psychiatry* 56(12):1097-1099, 1999.

O'Brien E: Detection and removal of head lice with an electronic comb: zapping the louse! *J Pediatr Nurs* 13(4):265-267, 1998.

O'Connell KL: Attention deficit hyperactivity disorder, *Pediatr Nurs* 22:30-33, 1996.

Offidani A and others: Treatment of scabies with ivermectin, *Europ J Dermatol* 9(2):100-101, 1999.

Osmond MH, Klassen TP, Quinn JV: Economic comparison of a tissue adhesive and suturing in the repair of pediatric facial lacerations, *J Pediatr* 126(6):892-895, 1995.

Patel CTC and others: Vacuum-assisted wound closure, changing atmospheric pressure assists wound healing, *Am J Nurs* 100(12):45-48, 2000.

Pollack RJ, Kiszewski AE, Spielman A: Over-diagnosis and consequent management of head louse infestations in North America, *Pediatr Infect Dis J* 19(8):689-693, 2000.

Price JH: School nurses' perceptions of and experiences with head lice, *J Sch Health* 69(4):153-158, 1999.

Rappaport LA: Enuresis. In Levine M and others: *Developmental-behavioral pediatrics,* ed 2, 1992, WB Saunders.

Robinson JK, Rigel DS, Amonette RA: Sun-protection behaviors used by adults for their children—United States, 1997, *MMWR Weekly* 47(23):480-482, 1998.

Rombaux P and others: Cervical lymphadenitis and cat scratch disease (CSD): an overlooked disease? *Acta Otorhinolaryngol Belg* 54(4):491-496, 2000.

Sacks JJ and others: Fatal dog attacks, 1989-1994, *Pediatrics* 97(6):891-895, 1996.

Scahill L, Lynch KA, Ort SI: Tourette syndrome: update and review, *J Sch Nurs* 11(2):26-32, 1995.

Schexnayder SM, Schexnayder RE: Bites, stings, and other painful things, *Pediatr Ann* 29(6):354-358, 2000.

Schooler NR and others: Maintenance treatment of schizophrenia: a review of dose reduction and family treatment strategies, *Psychiatr Q* 66(4):279-292, 1995.

Selekman J, Snyder M: Learning disabilities and/or attention deficit disorder. In Jackson PL, Vessey JA, editors: *Primary care of the child with a chronic condition,* ed 3, St Louis, 2000, Mosby.

Seltzer EG, Shapiro ED: Misdiagnosis of Lyme disease: when not to order serologic tests, *Pediatr Infect Dis J* 15:762-763, 1996.

Shapiro ED, Gerber MA: Lyme disease: fact versus fiction, *Pediatr Ann* 31(3):170-177, 2002.

Siegel DM: Lyme disease. In Hoekelman RA and others, editors: *Primary pediatric care,* ed 3, St Louis, 1997, Mosby

Skewes SM: Skin care rituals that do more harm than good, *Am J Nurs* 96(10):33-35, 1996.

Smith GA and others: Comparison of topical anesthetics without cocaine to tetracaine-adrenaline-cocaine and lidocaine infiltration during repair of lacerations: bupivacaine-norepinephrine is an effective new topical anesthetic agent, *Pediatrics* 97(3):301-307, 1996.

Smith JC: Abdominal pain. In Hoekelman RA and others, editors: *Primary pediatric care,* ed 4, St Louis, 2001, Mosby.

Starr NB: Sun smarts: the essentials of sun protection, *J Pediatr Health Care* 13:136-138, 1999.

St. Geme JW, Haslam DB, Ditmar MF: Infectious diseases. In Polin RA, Ditmar MF, editors: *Pediatric secrets,* ed 2, Philadelphia, 1997, Mosby.

Teicher MH and others: Objective measurement of hyperactivity and attentional problems in ADHD, *J Am Acad Child Adolesc Psychiatry* 35(3):334-342, 1996.

Troupe M: Clinical management of the avulsed tooth, *Dent Clin North Am* 39(1):93-112, 1995.

Visscher PK, Vetter RS, Camazine S: Removing bee stings, *Lancet* 348:301-302, 1996.

Vogt MA, Schaffner B: Pediatric management problems: what is your assessment? Constipation with encoporesis, *Pediatr Nurs* 22(5):444-445, 1996.

Wade CF: Keeping Lyme disease at bay, an integrated approach to prevention, *Am J Nurs* 100(7):26-31, 2000.

Walker LS and others: Recurrent abdominal pain: a potential precursor of irritable bowel syndrome in adolescents and young adults, *J Pediatr* 132:1010-1015, 1998.

Walkup JT and others: Family study and segregation analysis of Tourette syndrome: evidence for a mixed model of inheritance, *Am J Hum Genet* 59:684-693, 1996.

Wallace M: Injuries from dog bites (letter to the editor), *JAMA* 279:1174, 1998.

Wolraich ML, Wilson DB, White JW: The effect of sugar on behavior or cognition in children: a meta-analysis, *JAMA* 274(20):1617-1621, 1995.

# Chapter 19

# Health Promotion of the Adolescent and Family

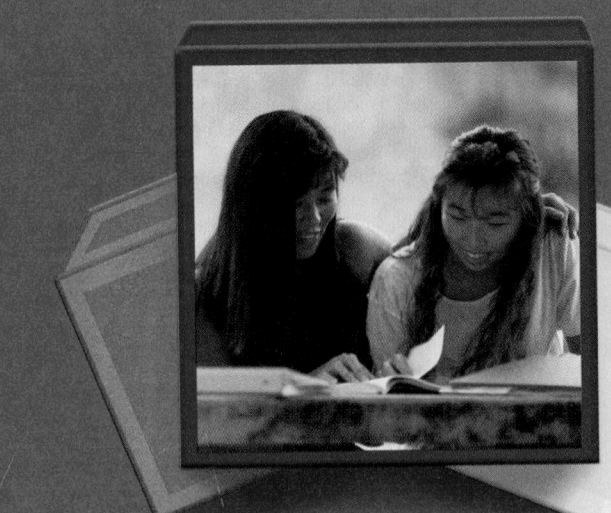

## Chapter Outline

**PROMOTING OPTIMUM GROWTH AND DEVELOPMENT, 802**
**Biologic Development, 803**
  Neuroendocrine Events of Puberty, 803
  Changes in Reproductive Hormones, 803
  Pubertal Sexual Maturation, 805
  Physical Growth During Puberty, 807
  Other Physiologic Changes, 809
**Cognitive Development, 809**
  Emergence of Formal Operational
    Thought (Piaget), 809
  Adolescent Conceptions of Self, 810
  Changes in Social Cognition, 810
**Development of Value Autonomy, 811**
  Moral Development, 811
  Spiritual Development, 811
**Psychosocial Development, 812**
  Identity Development, 812
  Development of Autonomy, 812
  Achievement, 813
  Sexuality, 814
  Intimacy, 816

Social Environments, 817
  Families, 817
  Peer Groups, 818
  Schools, 818
  Work, 819
  Community and Society, 819
**PROMOTING OPTIMUM HEALTH DURING ADOLESCENCE, 820**
**Adolescents' Perspectives on Health, 820**
**Factors That Promote Adolescent Health and
  Well-Being, 821**
  Contexts for Adolescent Health
    Promotion, 822
  Schools, 822
  School-Based and School-Linked Health
    Services, 822
  Communities, 823
  Health Care Settings, 823
  Adolescent Health Screening, 824
**Health Concerns of Adolescence, 826**
  Parenting and Family Adjustment, 826
  Psychosocial Adjustment, 827

Intentional and Unintentional Injury, 828
Dietary Habits, Eating Disorders, and
  Obesity, 829
Physical Fitness, 830
Sexual Behavior, Sexually Transmitted
  Diseases (STDs) and Unintended
  Pregnancy, 830
Use of Tobacco, Alcohol, and Other
  Substances, 831
Depression and Suicide, 832
Physical, Sexual, and Emotional Abuse, 832
School and Learning Problems, 833
Hypertension, 833
Hyperlipidemia, 833
Infectious Diseases/Immunizations, 833
**Health Promotion Among Special Groups of
  Adolescents, 834**
  Adolescents of Color, 834
  Gay, Lesbian and Bisexual
    Adolescents, 835
  Rural Adolescents, 836
**Nursing Considerations, 837**

## Related Topics

Adolescent Pregnancy, Ch. 20
Eating Problems/Disorders, Ch. 21
Health Problems of the Female Reproductive
  System, Ch. 20
Health Problems of the Male Reproductive
  System, Ch. 20

Health Problems Related to Sexuality, Ch. 20
Hyperlipidemia, Ch. 34
Immunizations, Ch. 12
Injuries and Health Problems Related to
  Sports Participation, Ch. 39
Injury Prevention, Ch. 17

Precocious Puberty, Ch. 38
Sexually Transmitted Diseases, Ch. 20
Substance Abuse, Ch. 21
Suicide, Ch. 21
Systemic Hypertension, Ch. 34

## PROMOTING OPTIMUM GROWTH AND DEVELOPMENT

Adolescence is a period of transition between childhood and adulthood, a time of profound biologic, intellectual,

psychosocial, and economic change. During this period individuals reach physical and sexual maturity, develop more sophisticated reasoning abilities, and make educational and occupational decisions that will shape their adult careers. The changes of adolescence have important implications for understanding the kinds of health risks to which young people are exposed, the health-enhancing and risk-taking

■ Elizabeth M. Saewyc, PhD, RN, PHN, revised this chapter.

behaviors in which they engage, and the major opportunities for health promotion among this population.

In the process of examining widely accepted theories of adolescent development, researchers have challenged many popular notions. For example, the belief was commonly held that teenagers' behaviors are overwhelmingly determined by "raging hormones" and that adolescence is a period when abnormal behavior is the norm. Both notions are misguided, but these mistaken beliefs are not benign. They may have detrimental effects on attitudes and interactions with individual adolescents and on policy and program development. Although current research supports a more positive view of this life period, it also confirms that adolescence involves a complex interplay of biologic, cognitive, psychologic, and social change, *perhaps more so than at any other time of life.* Unfortunately, the United States as a society has provided little help to individuals as they try to cope with the normal changes of adolescence.

Change during adolescence occurs on multiple levels. Individual level changes include biologic maturation, cognitive development, and psychologic development. Change also occurs in the social contexts of adolescents' families, peer groups, schools, and workplaces. Adolescence can be thought of as involving three distinct subphases: *early adolescence* (ages 11 to 14), *middle adolescence* (ages 15 to 17), and *late adolescence* (ages 18 to 20). The changes, opportunities, pressures, skills, and resources available to young people differ during these subphases. For example, early adolescence is characterized primarily by the changes of puberty and responses to those changes. Middle adolescence is characterized by transition to a dominant peer orientation, with all of the stereotypic adolescent preoccupations of music, dress and appearance, language, and behavior. Late adolescence involves transition into adulthood, including taking on adult work roles and developing adult relationships (Table 19-1).

## Biologic Development

### Neuroendocrine Events of Puberty

The fundamental biologic changes of adolescence are collectively referred to as *puberty.* Puberty involves a predictable sequence of hormonal and physical changes that occur universally over a defined period of time. It encompasses both sexual maturation and physical growth. It is generally accepted that the events of puberty are triggered by hormonal influences and are controlled by the anterior pituitary gland in response to a stimulus from the hypothalamus. Puberty begins as some not completely understood cluster of events triggers the production of *gonadotropin-releasing hormone (GnRH)* by the hypothalamus. GnRH travels through a network of capillaries to the anterior pituitary gland, where it stimulates the production and secretion of *follicle-stimulating hormone (FSH)* and *luteinizing hormone (LH).* Increasing levels of FSH and LH in the blood stimulate gonadal response. For females, FSH stimulates growth of ovarian follicles and production of estrogen. LH initiates ovulation, the formation of the corpus luteum, and progesterone production. For males, LH acts on testicular Leydig cells, prompting maturation of the testicles and testosterone production. FSH, acting with LH, stimulates sperm production. The sex steroids—estrogen, progesterone, and testosterone and other androgens—are released from the gonads and effect biologic changes in various organs, including muscles, bones, skin, and hair follicles. Increasing serum levels of sex steroids also provide feedback to the hypothalamus, causing decreases in GnRH secretion. When serum sex hormone levels decrease, the hypothalamus is stimulated to increase GnRH secretion, again initiating the sequence that produces the appropriate gonadal responses (Fig. 19-1).

**Initiation of Puberty.**   The precise mechanism that institutes the changes at puberty is not completely understood. Although the pituitary gland and gonads are capable of mature function and can respond to stimuli at any age, the *hypothalamic-pituitary-gonadal system* is maintained in a dormant state throughout childhood by some central nervous system inhibitory mechanism in the region of the hypothalamus. It is believed that the receptor sites in the hypothalamus are so highly sensitive that the most minute quantities of circulating sex hormones are sufficient to inhibit the secretion of GnRH during childhood. The hypothalamus loses this negative sensitivity at puberty, which allows the hypothalamic-pituitary-gonadal mechanism to attain full secretory function. As puberty progresses, the pituitary and gonads become increasingly sensitive to positive hormonal stimulation.

### Changes in Reproductive Hormones

**Females.**   The primary sex characteristic in females is the development and release of an egg, or *ovum,* from the ovaries approximately every 28 days. Beginning in *early pu-*

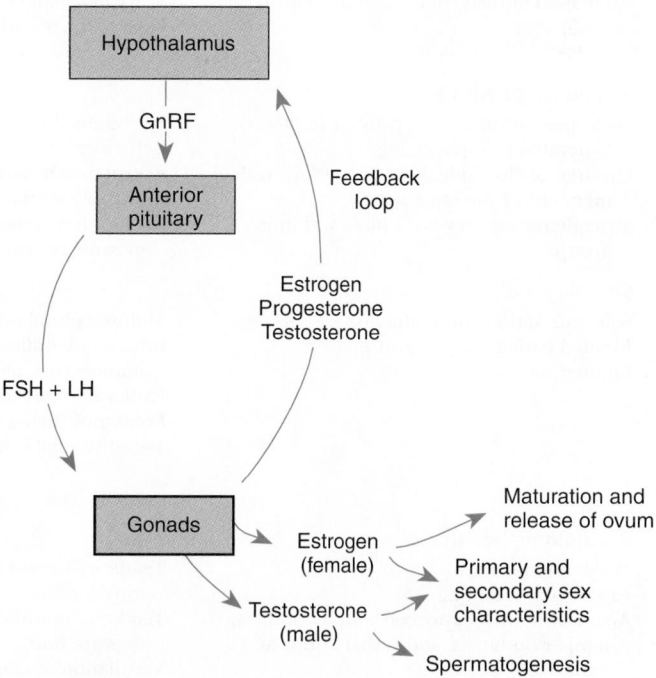

**Fig. 19-1**   Hormonal interaction between hypothalamus, pituitary, and gonads.

*berty,* FSH stimulates estrogen production by the ovaries. However, concentrations of estrogen do not reach levels high enough to cause ovulation. By the time girls reach *mid-puberty,* estrogen is generally produced in larger amounts. This quantity of estrogen production results in the building of an endometrial lining of the uterus and first menstruation, or *menarche.* At menarche, ova still do not generally mature enough to be released. However, as puberty progresses, one ovarian follicle becomes dominant during each menstrual cycle and produces increasing amounts of estro-

**TABLE 19-1** Growth and development during adolescence

| Early Adolescence (11-14 years) | Middle Adolescence (14-17 years) | Late Adolescence (17-20 years) |
|---|---|---|
| **Growth** | | |
| Rapidly accelerating growth | Growth decelerating in girls | Physically mature |
| Reaches peak velocity | Stature reaches 95% of adult height | Structure and reproductive growth almost |
| Secondary sex characteristics appear | Secondary sex characteristics well-advanced | complete |
| **Cognition** | | |
| Explores newfound ability for limited abstract thought | Developing capacity for abstract thinking | Established abstract thought |
| Clumsy groping for new values and energies | Enjoys intellectual powers, often in idealistic terms | Can perceive and act on long-range operations |
| Comparison of "normality" with peers of same sex | Concern with philosophic, political, and social problems | Able to view problems comprehensively |
| | | Intellectual and functional identity established |
| **Identity** | | |
| Preoccupied with rapid body changes | Modifies body image | Body image and gender-role definition nearly secured |
| Trying out of various roles | Very self-centered; increased narcissism | Mature sexual identity |
| Measurement of attractiveness by acceptance or rejection of peers | Tendency toward inner experience and self-discovery | Phase of consolidation of identity |
| Conformity to group norms | Has a rich fantasy life | Stability of self-esteem |
| | Idealistic | Comfortable with physical growth |
| | Able to perceive future implications of current behavior and decisions; variable application | Social roles defined and articulated |
| **Relationships with Parents** | | |
| Defining independence-dependence boundaries | Major conflicts over independence and control | Emotional and physical separation from parents completed |
| Strong desire to remain dependent on parents while trying to detach | Low point in parent-child relationship | Independence from family with less conflict |
| No major conflicts over parental control | Greatest push for emancipation; disengagement | Emancipation nearly secured |
| | Final and irreversible emotional detachment from parents; mourning | |
| **Relationships with Peers** | | |
| Seeks peer affiliations to counter instability generated by rapid change | Strong need for identity to affirm self-image | Peer group recedes in importance in favor of individual friendship |
| Upsurge of close, idealized friendships with members of the same sex | Behavioral standards set by peer group | Testing of romantic relationships against possibility of permanent alliance |
| Struggle for mastery takes place within peer group | Acceptance by peers extremely important—fear of rejection | Relationships characterized by giving and sharing |
| | Exploration of ability to attract opposite sex or same sex romantic partners | |
| **Sexuality** | | |
| Self-exploration and evaluation | Multiple plural relationships | Forms stable relationships and attachment to another |
| Limited dating, usually group | Internal identification of heterosexual, homosexual, or bisexual attractions. | Growing capacity for mutuality and reciprocity |
| Limited intimacy | Exploration of "self-appeal" | Dating as a romantic pair |
| | Feeling of "being in love" | May publicly identify as gay, lesbian, or bisexual |
| | Tentative establishment of relationships | Intimacy involves commitment rather than exploration and romanticism |
| **Psychologic Health** | | |
| Wide mood swings | Tendency toward inner experiences; more introspective | More constancy of emotion |
| Intense daydreaming | Tendency to withdraw when upset or feelings are hurt | Anger more apt to be concealed |
| Anger outwardly expressed with moodiness, temper outbursts, and verbal insults and name-calling | Vascillation of emotions in time and range | |
| | Feelings of inadequacy common; difficulty in asking for help | |

gen during the early-cycle, follicular phase. This follicle releases an ovum, a process termed *ovulation,* around day 14 of the menstrual cycle. After ovulation the follicle involutes and its estrogen production decreases; this leads to a drop in serum estrogen and progesterone. The pituitary gland responds to the drop in these hormone levels with increased production of FSH, initiating the start of a new menstrual cycle.

By direct action, estrogens cause growth and development of the vagina, uterus, and fallopian tubes. The skin of the labia majora, as well as that of the breast areola and nipples, grows and darkens under the influence of estrogen. Estrogen is responsible for breast enlargement. Estrogen also promotes the growth of pubic and axillary hair, pigmentation of genital skin, and widening of the hips. At low levels estrogen tends to stimulate skeletal growth in both boys and girls, but at higher levels it inhibits growth.

**Males.**   The primary male sex characteristic is the development of viable sperm. During puberty, FSH acts on testicular cells, which stimulates the production of viable sperm. FSH and LH also act on a different group of testicular cells, resulting in increased production and secretion of testosterone. In this process of sexual development, boys do not experience a discrete event analogous to menstruation or ovulation in girls. However, just as the production of a mature ovum tends to occur 1 year or more after menarche in girls, the production of viable sperm tends to follow boys' first ejaculations. The capacity to ejaculate appears relatively early in boys' sexual development, approximately 1 year after initial testicular enlargement and the appearance of pubic hair. From a clinical perspective, however, an adolescent should be considered potentially fertile with a first menstrual period or first ejaculation.

Testosterone and other androgens have a direct impact on growth of the penis, scrotum, prostate, and seminal vesicles of the testicles. The tremendous growth-promoting properties of these hormones also result in rapid increases in muscle mass, skeletal growth, bone age, and bone density. In both sexes androgens are responsible for the development of pubic, axillary, facial, and body hair. Clinically, increased activity of androgens is associated with pubertal conditions such as acne, body odor, deepening of the voice, a spurt in height, and an increase in red blood cell levels.

## Pubertal Sexual Maturation

Increases in reproductive hormones are responsible for dramatic changes in secondary sexual characteristics that occur during puberty. As with general growth, development of secondary sexual characteristics occurs in a predictable sequence. This sequence has been divided into a series of five phases termed the *Tanner stages* (Figs. 19-2 to 19-6). While the sequence of sexual development is predictable, the ages at which these changes occur and the rate of developmental progression vary considerably among individuals. Over the course of pubescence, many young people have questions about the timing, rate, and normalcy of their body changes. These concerns provide nurses with a prime opportunity to discuss health-related topics such as puberty, sexuality, birth control, prevention of sexually transmitted diseases, nutrition, exercise, and safe methods of weight control.

**Sexual Maturation in Girls.**   In four out of five girls, changes in the nipple and areola and development of a small bud of breast tissue *(thelarche)* are the earliest, most easily visible changes of puberty. The average age of thelarche is 11 years, with a range of 9 to 13½ years. The appearance of pubic hair *(adrenarche)* usually follows initial breast development by about 2 to 6 months; however, in a minority of normally developing girls, pubic hair may precede breast development. Early in puberty there is often an increase in normal vaginal discharge *(physiologic leukorrhea),* associated with uterine development. Girls or their parents may be concerned that this vaginal discharge is a sign of infection; they can be reassured that the discharge is normal and a sign that the uterus is preparing for menstruation. During midpuberty, breast enlargement occurs, and pubic hair progresses to adult-type sexual hair covering the mons pubis and labia majora. Most girls reach their peak height velocity and peak weight velocity in midpubescence. The hallmark of late puberty is the first menstrual period, or *menarche.* Initial menstrual periods are usually scanty and irregular and may not be accompanied by ovulation. Ovulation and regular menstrual periods usually begin 6 to 14 months after menarche. Menarche occurs about 2 years after the appearance of breast buds, approximately 9 months after attainment of peak height velocity and 3 months after attainment of peak weight velocity. The mean age of menarche in the United States is 12.8 years, with a normal age range of 10½ to 15 years. Menarche has been reported to occur at about 17% body fat, with 22% body fat reported to be required to maintain menstruation (Neinstein, 1996). Girls may be considered to have *pubertal delay* if breast development has not occurred by age 13 or if menarche has not occurred within 4 years of the onset of breast development.

In the United States the mean age of menarche has gradually decreased over the past century, corresponding to pop-

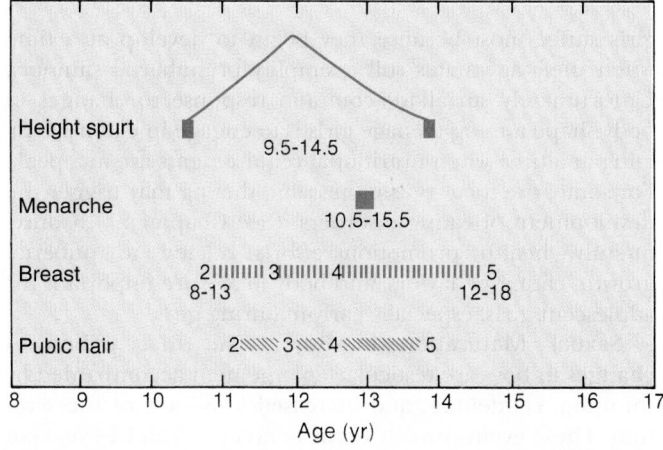

**Fig. 19-2**   Approximate timing of developmental changes in girls. Numbers indicate stages of development. Range of ages during which some of the changes occur is indicated by inclusive numbers below them. See Figs. 19-3 and 19-4 for explanation. (From Marshall WA, Tanner JM: *Arch Dis Child* 44:291, 1969.)

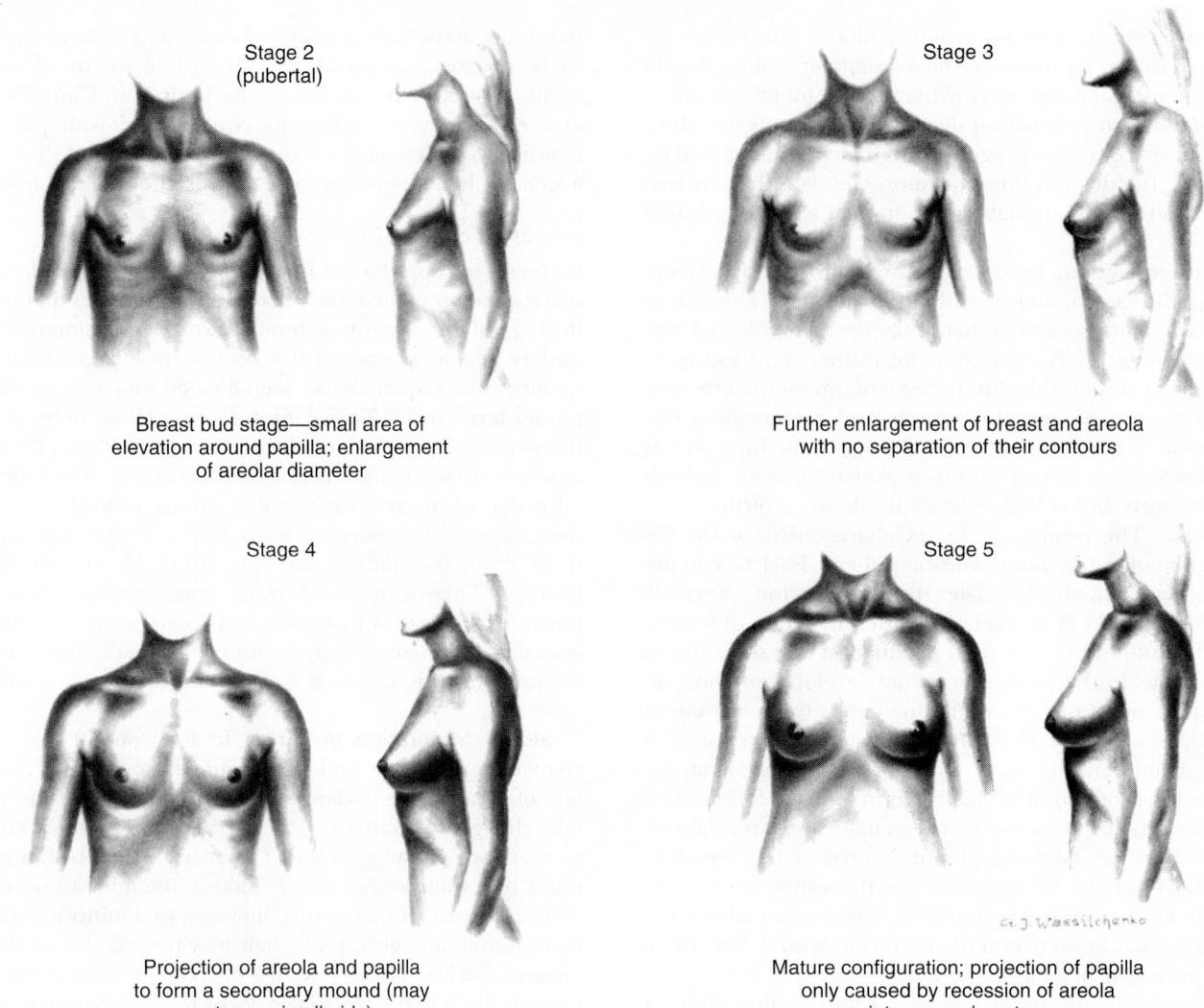

Stage 2
(pubertal)

Breast bud stage—small area of
elevation around papilla; enlargement
of areolar diameter

Stage 3

Further enlargement of breast and areola
with no separation of their contours

Stage 4

Projection of areola and papilla
to form a secondary mound (may
not occur in all girls)

Stage 5

Mature configuration; projection of papilla
only caused by recession of areola
into general contour

**Fig. 19-3** Development of the breast in girls—average age span, 11 to 13 years. Stage I (prepubertal—elevation of papilla only) is not shown. (Modified from Marshall WA, Tanner JM: *Arch Dis Child* 44:291, 1969; and Daniel WA, Paulshock BZ: *Patient Care*, May 13, 1979, pp 122-124.)

ulation improvements in nutrition, sanitation, and control of infectious diseases. This decline in the average age of menarche appears to have leveled off in recent years (Neinstein, 1996). Internationally, a decline in the average age at first menses has not been seen in countries where individuals are more likely to be malnourished and suffer from chronic illness.

Sexual maturation influences young peoples' satisfaction with their appearance, with the effects appearing to differ for girls and boys. For girls, physical maturation can lead to greater dissatisfaction with their appearance. For example, recent studies indicate that adolescent girls are more dissatisfied and significantly more likely to identify themselves as being overweight than adolescent boys (Centers for Disease Control and Prevention, 2000).

Normal increases in weight and fat deposition that accompany puberty among girls conflict with cultural norms that emphasize a slender look (Marsh, 1999). Early-maturing

girls suffer most because they begin to develop at a time when their age-mates still exemplify prepubertal slimness. Unfortunately, an all-too-common response to changes in body shape among teenage girls is to engage in extensive dieting at a time when nutritional requirements are at a peak. For some, the focus on slimness and dieting may trigger the development of eating disorders. (See Chapter 21). Consequently, health promotion efforts related to pubertal growth, eating behaviors, and body image are important for adolescent girls, especially early-maturing girls.

**Sexual Maturation in Boys.** The first pubescent changes in boys are testicular enlargement accompanied by thinning, reddening, and increased looseness of the scrotum. These events usually occur between 9½ and 14 years of age. Early puberty is also characterized by the initial appearance of pubic hair. Penile enlargement begins, and testicular enlargement and pubic hair growth continue throughout midpuberty. During this period there is also in-

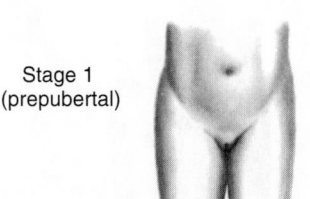

Stage 1
(prepubertal)

No pubic hair; essentially the same as
during childhood; no distinction between
hair on pubis and over the abdomen

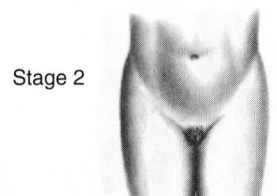

Stage 2

Sparse growth of long, straight, downy, and
slightly pigmented hair extending along labia;
between stages 2 and 3 begins to appear on pubis

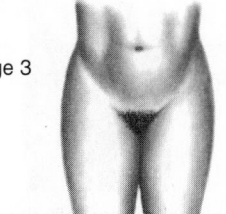

Stage 3

Hair darker, coarser, and curly and
spread sparsely over entire pubis in
the typical female triangle

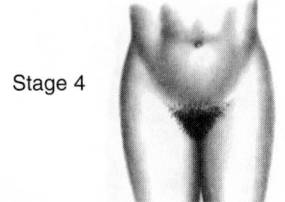

Stage 4

Pubic hair denser, curled, and adult in distribution
but less abundant and restricted to the pubic area

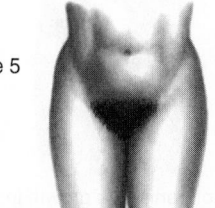

Stage 5

Hair adult in quantity, type, and pattern
with spread to inner aspect of thighs

**Fig. 19-4**   Growth in pubic hair in girls—average age span for stages 2 through 5, 11 to 14 years. (Modified from Marshall WA, Tanner JM: *Arch Dis Child* 44:291, 1969; and Daniel WA, Paulshock BZ: *Patient Care*, May 13, 1979, pp 122-124.)

creasing muscularity, early voice changes, and development of early facial hair. ***Gynecomastia,*** breast enlargement and tenderness, is common during midpuberty; it occurs in up to one third of boys and is usually temporary. The spurts in height and weight occur concurrently toward the end of midpuberty. For most boys, breast enlargement disappears within 2 years. By late puberty, there is a definite increase in the length and width of the penis, testicular enlargement continues, and first ejaculation occurs. Axillary hair develops, and facial hair extends to cover the anterior neck. Final voice changes occur secondary to the growth of the larynx. Concerns about ***pubertal delay*** should be considered for boys who exhibit no enlargement of the testes or scrotal changes by ages 13½ to 14, or if genital growth is not complete 4 years after the testicles begin to enlarge.

Changes in the size and shape of the penis and testicles and changes in genital functioning can be areas of great concern for adolescent boys. Although the ability for penile erection is present at birth, only with pubertal maturation do boys have seminal emissions. Ejaculation may occur spontaneously as a nocturnal emission or "wet dream," as a result of self-stimulation, or during sexual activity with others. Unless they are prepared in advance, spontaneous ejaculations are frequently puzzling, troublesome, and embarrassing events for boys. Pubertal changes and related concerns create important opportunities for health promotion among young teenage boys. Health care professionals can be a resource for boys and provide appropriate information and guidance around issues related to sexual maturation.

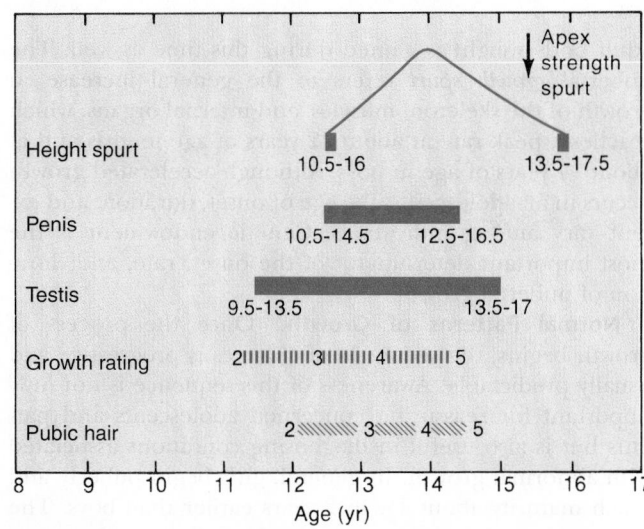

**Fig. 19-5**   Approximate timing of developmental changes in boys. Numbers indicate stages of development. Range of ages during which some of the changes occur is indicated by inclusive numbers below them. See Fig. 19-6 for explanation. (From Marshall WA, Tanner JM: *Arch Dis Child* 45:13, 1970.)

## Physical Growth During Puberty

Along with increases in reproductive hormones and sexual maturation, major changes in skeletal and lean body mass occur during puberty. The final 20% to 25% of linear growth is achieved during puberty, and up to 50% of ideal

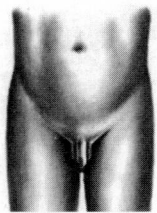

Stage 1
(prepubertal)

No pubic hair; essentially the same as
during childhood; no distinction between
hair on pubis and over the abdomen

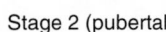

Stage 2 (pubertal)

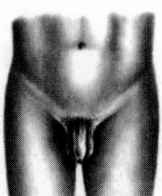

Initial enlargement of scrotum and testes;
reddening and textural changes of scrotal skin;
sparse growth of long, straight, downy, and
slightly pigmented hair at base of penis

Stage 3

Initial enlargement of penis, mainly in
length; testes and scrotum further enlarged;
hair darker, coarser, and curly and spread
sparsely over entire pubis

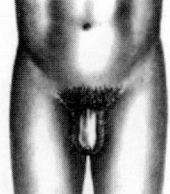

Stage 4

Increased size of penis with growth in diameter and
development of glans; glans larger and broader; scrotum
darker; pubic hair more abundant with curling but
restricted to pubic area

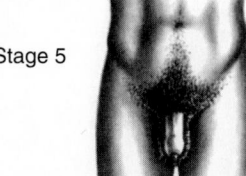

Stage 5

Testes, scrotum, and penis adult in size and shape;
hair  adult in quantity and type with spread to inner
surface of thighs

**Fig. 19-6**   Developmental stages of secondary sex characteristics and genital development
in boys—average age span, 12 to 16 years. (Modified from Marshall WA, Tanner JM: *Arch Dis Child*
45:13, 1970; and Daniel WA, Paulshock BZ: *Patient Care*, May 13, 1979, pp 122-124.)

adult body weight is gained during this time as well. The pubertal *growth spurt* refers to the general increase in growth of the skeleton, muscles, and internal organs, which reaches a peak rate at about 12 years of age in girls and at about 14 years of age in boys. Although accelerated growth occurs in all adolescents, the age of onset, duration, and extent vary among individuals. Genetic endowment is the most important determinant of the onset, rate, and duration of pubertal growth.

**Normal Patterns of Growth.**   Once the process of growth begins, the sequence of changes is progressive and usually predictable. Awareness of this sequence is not only important for reassuring concerned adolescents and parents but is also useful in diagnosing conditions associated with abnormal growth. In general, girls begin puberty and reach maturity about 1½ to 2 years earlier than boys. The pubertal growth spurt begins as early as 9½ years or as late as 14½ years in girls, and as early as 10½ years and as late as 16 years in boys.

General growth includes accumulation of body mass, along with increases in height and weight. *Lean body mass*, primarily muscle mass, increases in both girls and boys during early puberty. For girls, the rate of muscle mass growth peaks at menarche and then slows. For boys, muscle mass continues to increase throughout puberty, resulting in the attainment of significantly higher lean body mass in boys than in girls. In girls, gain in *fat mass* increases markedly early in puberty and continues to increase following menarche. In boys, there is a

peak deceleration in the rate of fat mass accumulation at the time of their growth spurt and thereafter a slower and much less dramatic increase than in girls.

The rate of *linear growth* (height) (Figs. 19-7 and 19-8) begins to increase in girls during early puberty, whereas in boys the rate does not increase until midpuberty. *Peak height velocity (PHV)* occurs at about 12 years of age in girls, around 6 to 12 months before menarche. PHV is used as a predictor of menarche; height at menarche is a predictor of ultimate adult height. Very few girls grow more than 2 inches in height following menarche. Growth in girls' height usually ceases 2 to 2½ years after menarche. Boys typically reach peak height velocity at about 14 years of age, following growth of the testicles and penis and the appearance of axillary and mature pubic hair. Among most boys, growth in height ceases at 18 or 20 years of age. Increases in leg length tend to precede growth of the trunk by about 6 to 9 months and that of the shoulders and chest by about 1 year. In short, teenagers tend to follow a linear growth pattern in which they outgrow their shoes first, then their pants, and finally their shirts. *Peak weight velocity* occurs about 6 months after PHV in girls. In contrast, weight and height spurts occur simultaneously for boys. On average, girls will gain 5 to 20 cm (2 to 8 inches) in height and 7 to 25 kg (15 to 55 pounds) in weight during adolescence, and boys will gain 10 to 30 cm (4 to 12 inches) in height and 7 to 30 kg (15 to 65 pounds) in weight during adolescence.

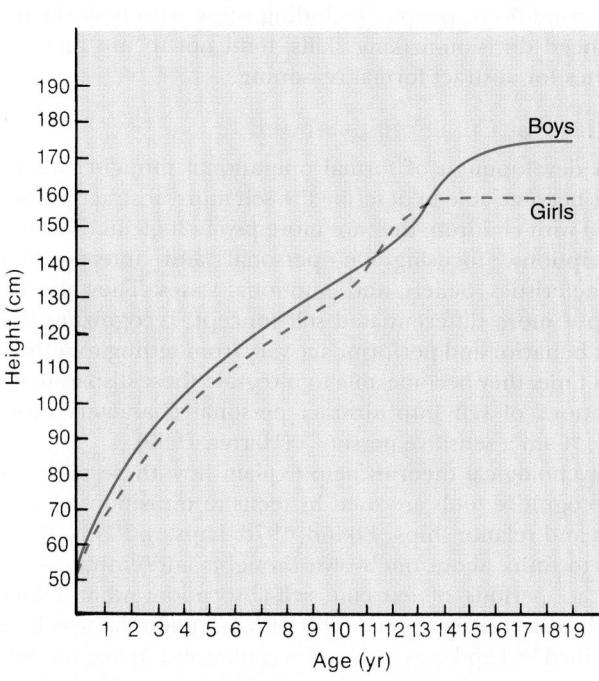

**Fig. 19-7**   Linear growth throughout childhood. (From Tanner JM, Whitehouse RH, Takaishi M: *Arch Dis Child* 41:454-471, 1966.)

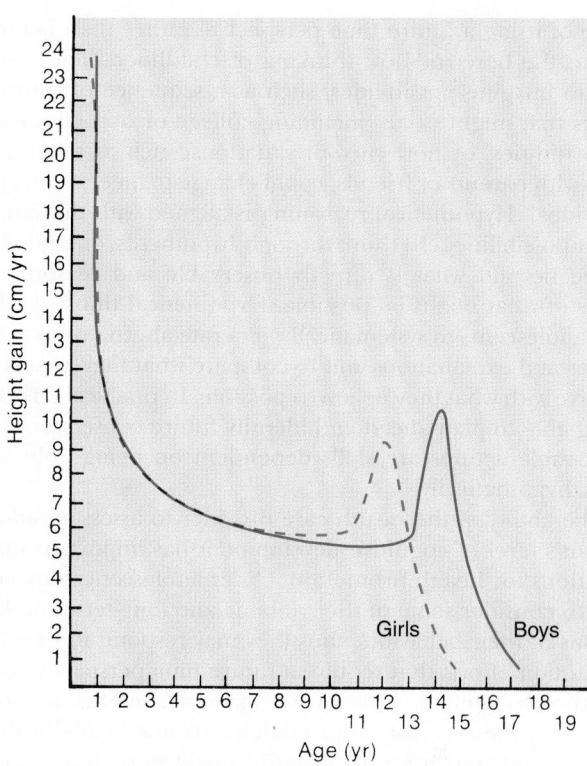

**Fig. 19-8**   Linear growth in centimeters per year. (From Tanner JM, Whitehouse RH, Takaishi M: *Arch Dis Child* 41:454-471, 1966.)

## Other Physiologic Changes

In addition to the characteristic changes of puberty already discussed, numerous others occur. The size and strength of the heart, blood volume, and systolic blood pressure increase, whereas the heart rate decreases. Consistent with the general developmental timetable, these changes appear earlier in girls, who establish a slightly higher pulse rate and a slightly lower systolic blood pressure than boys. Blood volume, which has increased steadily during childhood, reaches higher levels in boys than in girls, a fact that may be related to the increased muscle mass in pubertal boys. Adult values are reached for all formed elements of the blood; for instance, there is a marked increase in serum iron, the number of red blood cells, hemoglobin, and hematocrit in boys, but not in girls.

The lungs increase in both diameter and length during puberty. The respiratory rate, decreasing steadily throughout childhood, reaches the adult rate in adolescence. Respiratory volume, vital capacity, and other physiologic properties related to respiratory function are increased, and to a greater extent in boys than in girls. The differences between the sexes are a result of the greater lung growth associated with the increased shoulder and chest size in boys.

The rate of steady decline in basal metabolic rate from birth to adulthood slows during puberty, coinciding with the growth spurt in both sexes; this probably reflects the increase in physiologic activities. A slightly higher metabolic rate in boys than in girls is thought to be a function of differences in androgenic hormones. Basal body temperature gradually decreases with age in both sexes, reaching adult values by 12 years of age in girls and somewhat later in boys.

Adolescence is also a time of continued brain growth. Although the number of neurons does not increase, there is a proliferation of the support cells that brace and nourish the neurons. In addition, the growth of the myelin sheath around the nerve cells continues at least until puberty, enabling faster neural processing. This "fine tuning" of the neural system coincides with development of the more advanced cognitive capacities of youth.

## Cognitive Development

### Emergence of Formal Operational Thought (Piaget)

Jean Piaget (1972) described the shift from childhood to adolescence as a movement from concrete to formal operational thought. Children's thinking is oriented to things and events that they can observe directly. Unable to think in terms of abstract possibilities, they process information based on what is directly observable. For most young people, emergence of *formal operational thinking* occurs between the ages of 11 and 14. Formal operational thought includes being able to think in abstract terms, think about possibilities, and think through hypotheses. Young people become able to think about abstractions; thus they can symbolically associate behaviors with abstract concepts such as attractiveness, adult status, or happiness. Adolescents also become capable of using a future time perspective rather than being tied to the here-and-now thinking of childhood. They are able to imagine possibilities, such as a sequence of future events that might occur, including college or occupational opportunities, or how current situations, such as relationships with parents or friends, could change to meet an imagined ideal. Hypothetical reasoning is aligned with thinking about possibilities. To think through hypotheses, one needs to see beyond what is directly observable and reason in terms of what might be possible. Hypothetical thinking allows adolescents to systematically generate alternative possibilities and explanations and to compare what they actually observe with what they believe is possible. In practical terms, being able to plan ahead and identify future consequences of possible actions are skills dependent on being able to think hypothetically.

The ability of the health care provider to assess an adolescent's level of cognitive development has important implications for health promotion. Older adolescents may be able to consider some of the symbolic and long-term implications of their behaviors; thus they may respond to health promotion efforts that require a future time perspective or attention to symbolic rewards. For example, an effective antismoking message for older adolescents may symbolically associate tobacco use with negative qualities such as unattractiveness, lack of peer acceptance, or long-term health consequences. For young people who primarily use concrete thinking (i.e., younger teenagers), health promotion efforts should emphasize immediate risks or benefits of the behavior. For example, although younger adolescents may be unable to comprehend the long-range consequences of smoking, they can appreciate some of the short-term consequences of cigarette use, including resulting bad breath or the cost of purchasing cigarettes.

Along with cognitive development, decision-making abilities increase over the adolescent period. Young people develop the ability to consider hypothetical risks and benefits of possible behaviors, along with potential consequences of such behaviors. In addition, the likelihood of teenagers consulting with adult experts, mentors, and role models increases over the junior and senior high school years. By middle adolescence, most teenagers are able to reason as well as adults. Health promotion efforts, especially those aimed at younger adolescents, should offer learning strategies that enhance decision-making skills. Such efforts might include discussions emphasizing health-promoting norms for behavior among young people and alternatives to unhealthy behaviors, as well as practicing skills necessary to resist unhealthy behaviors.

Even with the best framework for health promotion, persons who are capable of formal operational thought and reasoned decision making do not use these processes all of the time. In the face of time pressures, overriding personal stress, or overwhelming peer pressures, young people are more likely to abandon rational thought processes. Thoughts about unfamiliar or emotionally arousing topics also tend to be less sophisticated and more vulnerable to the effects of stresses and pressures. Unfortunately, many of the health-related decisions adolescents confront, such as those related to substance use or sexual behavior, involve issues that are personally stressful, emotion laden, or new. Under such conditions, people, including those who typically use advanced decision-making skills, tend not to use their capacities for abstract formal reasoning.

## Adolescent Conceptions of Self

With development of formal operational thought, adolescents become able to describe the self more abstractly. Compared with children, they are more psychologic in their self-descriptions, focusing on personal and interpersonal characteristics, beliefs, and emotional states. They also develop a more differentiated self-concept, recognizing that their behavior and performance vary from setting to setting. With time, they become able to integrate these disparate observations of self into abstract personal characterizations (e.g., "I am a sensitive person") (Harter, 1990).

Psychological theories help explain how these powerful new cognitive tools are used by teens to transition to adult roles and relationships (Elkind, 1978; Lapsley, 1993). Being able to think about one's own thoughts and emotions can lead to periods of extreme self-absorption, what Elkind called *adolescent egocentrism.* This self-absorption has also been described by Lapsley as a way of imagining and "trying on" various personas and practicing hypothetical interactions in an attempt to develop a separate sense of self. Two common patterns of thinking help to explain some of the health-related beliefs and behaviors of youth. The first, the *imaginary audience,* involves having such a heightened sense of self-consciousness that an adolescent imagines that everyone notices and is focused on his or her behavior. For example, a teen who has diabetes may worry about injecting insulin at school because "everybody will notice." The second pattern of thinking, called the *personal fable,* is the belief that one's feelings and experiences are completely unique. For example, a sexually active adolescent may choose not to use condoms or other barrier methods for safe sex, truly believing that "other people can get sexually transmitted diseases, but not me," or an adolescent who has been drinking may choose to drive home after a party, believing that he or she could never be involved in a car crash.

## Changes in Social Cognition

Gains in cognitive abilities also have an impact on perspective-taking capacities of young people. Adolescents are better able than children to "step into the shoes" of others. During elementary school, children begin to realize that other people have thoughts and feelings; however, they have difficulty understanding that what affects their own thoughts and feelings can also influence the thoughts and feelings of others. Preadolescents develop limited perspective-taking skills, first learning to step into the shoes of best friends, then peers and family members, and finally people of other ages and backgrounds. However, perspective-taking capacities develop further during adolescence when an adolescent becomes able to engage in *mutual role taking* (Selman, 1976). In other words, teenagers can both understand the perspectives of others and see how the thoughts or actions of one person can influence those of others. Role-taking capabilities continue to expand throughout adolescence. Older teenagers are able to understand that people's perspectives are influenced by their social roles as well as by their cultural and ethnic backgrounds. They are able to discuss various issues highlighting points of importance to people in various social roles (e.g., "From a parent's perspective, having a curfew is important because . . ."). Older adolescents also realize that the perspectives people hold are complicated in that they are influenced by a range of intrapersonal, interpersonal, and sociocultural factors. Ultimately, gains in perspective-taking skills that take place during adolescence lead to an increased capacity to learn from the experiences of others. Older adolescents are able to consider the choices, behaviors, and outcomes experienced by others in making their own health-related choices. This newfound capacity significantly expands the opportunities to learn health-promoting behaviors, in that once perspective-taking skills reach this point, young people can learn from their own experiences, as well as from the life experiences of others.

## Development of Value Autonomy

With advances in cognitive development, adolescents' beliefs become more abstract and increasingly rooted in general ideologic principles. At the same time, young people are gaining increasing emotional independence from parents, relying less on their parents' beliefs and values than they did as children. Adolescents also progress toward greater behavioral independence, encountering situations and decisions they have not previously experienced. With these new capacities and experiences, young people face a variety of cognitive conflicts caused by having to compare the advice of parents and friends and having to deal with competing pressures to behave in given ways. These conflicts may prompt young people to consider, in serious and thoughtful terms, what it is that they themselves really believe. Whereas earlier in life they may have merely accepted the decisions or points of view of adults, adolescents begin to substitute a set of values distinct from those of significant adults in their lives. This struggle to clarify values, created in part by an expanded behavioral independence, is a large part of the process of developing a sense of what has been termed *value autonomy* (Steinberg, 1989). The development of a personal value system is a gradual process, with evidence that value autonomy occurs relatively late in adolescence, between the ages of 18 and 20 (Steinberg, 1989).

### Moral Development

Moral development parallels advances in reasoning and social cognition. With the attainment of abstract thought and the realization that people's perspectives and opinions may differ, the ways adolescents approach moral issues change. According to one theory of moral development (Kohlberg and Gilligan, 1972), older children and young adolescents function at a *conventional level of moral reasoning* in which absolute moral guidelines are seen to emanate from authorities such as parents or teachers. Thus judgments of right and wrong are made according to a set of concrete rules. A major concern is to act or behave in ways that will gain or maintain the approval of others. The correctness of society's

rules is not questioned—one "does one's duty" by upholding and respecting the social order.

Elements of *principled moral reasoning* emerge during adolescence. With this level of reasoning, absolutes and rules come to be questioned as moral standards are seen as subjective and based on points of view that are subject to disagreement. One may have a moral duty to abide by social standards for behavior—but only insofar as those standards support and serve human ends. Thus occasions arise in which social conventions ought to be questioned and when principles such as justice, caring, or quality of life take precedence over established social norms. Empirical research on Kohlberg's theory has demonstrated that aspects of both conventional and principled reasoning are present during adolescence, and different levels of reasoning are used at different times and in different situations.

Kohlberg's scheme of moral development focuses on an orientation to justice. This orientation holds as its ideal a morality based on reciprocity and equal respect. From this orientation the most important consideration in making moral decisions would be whether the individuals involved were treated "fairly" by the ultimate decision. Gilligan (1982) proposes that an equally valid alternative to the justice orientation is one that emphasizes caring. From this perspective, the ideal is a morality of attention to others and responses to human need. As opposed to the justice orientation, which assumes that moral decisions are best made from a detached position of "objectivity," the caring orientation is rooted in the belief that moral decisions should be shaped by attachments and responsiveness to others. Studies (Gilligan, 1986; Walker, de Vries, and Trevethan, 1987) have found that while both men and women are capable of approaching moral problems from the perspectives of justice and caring, women may be more likely to give caring-oriented responses before justice-oriented ones, whereas men are more likely to follow the opposite pattern.

### Spiritual Development

Religious beliefs also become more abstract and principled during the adolescent years. Specifically, adolescents' beliefs become more oriented toward spiritual and ideologic matters and less oriented toward rituals, practice, and the strict observance of religious customs. Compared with children, adolescents place more emphasis on the internal aspects of religious commitment, such as what a person believes, and less on the external manifestations, such as whether an individual attends religious worship (Elkind, 1978).

Generally speaking, the stated importance of participation in organized religion declines somewhat during the adolescent years. More high school students than post-secondary school young people attend religious services regularly; and, not surprisingly, the younger the adolescents, the more likely they are to view religion as being important to them. Among older adolescents, there is more decline in the importance of organized religion among college students than among young people not in college. Late adolescence appears to be a time when individuals reexamine and reevaluate many of the beliefs and values of their childhood. Consistent with developmental changes in the value autonomy, the religious beliefs of young people are likely to become more personalized and less bound to the traditional religious practices they may have been exposed to when they were younger.

Although religious cults and dramatic religious conversion have attracted a great deal of attention in the media, they remain rare phenomena among American adolescents and often reflect nonreligious concerns. Membership in a religious cult is often associated with a preceding period of psychologic stress, identity diffusion, rootlessness, and dissatisfaction with mainstream societal values.

## Psychosocial Development

### Identity Development

The task of identity formation is to develop a stable, coherent picture of oneself that includes integrating one's past and present experiences with a sense of where one is headed in the future. Before adolescence the child's identity is like pieces of a puzzle scattered about on a table. Both cognitive development and social situations encountered during adolescence push individuals to combine puzzle pieces—to reflect on their place in society, on the way others view them, and on their options for the future. For most individuals, puzzle pieces first form a coherent whole sometime during late adolescence and early adulthood. Erik Erikson, one of the most influential theorists in the area of psychosocial development, describes identity achievement as one of the main psychosocial tasks of the adolescent years. According to Erikson (1968), "from among all possible and imaginable relations (the adolescent) must make a series of ever-narrowing selections of personal, occupational, sexual, and ideological commitments."

Social forces play a large role in shaping an adolescent's sense of self. Erikson (1968) argues that the key to identity achievement lies in adolescents' interactions with others. The people with whom a young person interacts serve as mirrors that reflect information back to the adolescent about who she or he is and who she or he ought to be. During the period of identity formation, adolescents also learn from others what it is they ought to keep doing and what it is they ought not to do. Society also plays an important role in determining the range of available alternatives open to young people involved in identity formation. Optimally, adolescents have the opportunity to explore a range of possible options related to ideologic, occupational, and interpersonal roles before making an identity commitment.

Progress toward identity achievement can be measured by the status of personal commitments in occupational, social, and ideologic domains. The status of personal commitments has four proposed levels: achievement, moratorium, foreclosure, and diffusion (Marcia, 1966). Individuals who demonstrate *identity achievement* have established a coherent identity after actively exploring possible alternatives; individuals currently engaged in this exploration are in *moratorium*. *Foreclosure* refers to making identity commitments without a period of exploration or experimentation, and *identity diffusion* refers to a lack of firm identity commitments, along with a lack of effort to make those commit-

ments. During adolescence, many individuals progress from diffusion to moratorium to identity achievement, or alternatively, from diffusion to foreclosure.

Experiences and opportunities within one's social environment influence both the content of identity and progression toward identity achievement. Among minority adolescents identity foreclosure may be more common than among teenagers from the majority culture because of restricted opportunities to explore alternative roles. Identity diffusion also appears to be more common among minority males than among other groups. Possible barriers to identity formation among minority youth may include conflicting values between the minority reference group and the broader society, a lack of adult role models who exemplify positive ethnic identity, and inadequate preparation for stereotyping and prejudice that are frequently experienced.

### Development of Autonomy

Becoming an autonomous, self-governing person is another of the fundamental psychosocial tasks of adolescence. Autonomy includes emotional, cognitive, and behavioral components. *Emotional autonomy* is that aspect of independence related to changes in an individual's close relationships, and *behavioral autonomy* is the capacity to make independent decisions and follow through with them. Generally, emotional and behavioral autonomy are likely to surface as psychosocial concerns somewhat earlier during adolescence than *value autonomy,* which usually does not become a prominent concern until middle or late adolescence.

Individuals generally begin the process of emotional autonomy during early adolescence by becoming more emotionally independent from their parents but less separate from their friends. In the process of separating from their parents, younger adolescents often shift a portion of their emotional ties to other adults, often developing "crushes" on teachers, coaches, nationally known media figures, or the parent of a best friend. By the end of adolescence, individuals are less emotionally dependent on their parents than they were as children. This emotional autonomy can be seen in several ways. First, older adolescents do not generally rush to their parents when they are worried or upset. Second, they no longer see their parents as all-knowing or all-powerful. Third, teenagers often have increasing amounts of emotional energy invested in relationships outside of their families. Finally, older adolescents are able to see and interact with their parents as people—not just as their parents.

As adolescents increasingly find themselves in situations where adults are not present and where they must make decisions and take responsibility for their own actions, the extent to which they are capable of independent decision making and autonomous behavior takes on added importance. An individual who is behaviorally autonomous is able to turn to others for advice when it is appropriate, weigh alternative courses of action based on his or her own judgment and the suggestions of others, and reach an independent conclusion about how to behave. Behavioral autonomy includes the ability to make independent decisions based on one's own choices rather than conforming to the opinions of others. Decision-making abilities improve over the adolescent years, with older adolescents being more likely than younger adolescents to be aware of risks involved with a particular decision, to consider future consequences, to turn to "experts" for advice, and to realize when vested interests may influence the advice of others. Conformity to parents' opinions declines during early adolescence; however, conformity to peer influence increases during this time. During middle and late adolescence, conformity to *both* parents and peers declines, allowing for genuine behavioral autonomy. Subjective feelings of self-reliance increase steadily over the adolescent years.

In contrast to popular stereotypes, the development of autonomy during adolescence does not typically involve rebellion, nor is it usually accompanied by strained or tense family relationships. Especially in households where guidelines for adolescent behavior are clear and consistently enforced, where changes in guidelines are open to discussion, and where an atmosphere of interpersonal warmth, concern, and fairness exists, family relationships nurture a gradual and smooth maturational process over the course of the adolescent years. Problems in the development of autonomy are often understandable reactions to excessively controlling circumstances or to growing up in the absence of clear standards. In addition to dispelling the myths that major parent-child conflicts and adolescent rebellion are essential to the development of autonomy, research has shown that parent and peer influences are not necessarily opposing forces but can play complementary roles in the development of a healthy degree of individual independence.

### Achievement

Another set of psychosocial tasks encountered during adolescence centers around achievement. Broadly speaking, achievement concerns the development of motives, capabilities, interests, and behaviors related to performance in evaluative situations. The study of the development of achievement during adolescence has focused almost exclusively on young people's performance in educational settings and on the development and implementation of plans for future scholastic and occupational careers. Various theories have attempted to explain why some young people achieve at higher levels in school. Some have focused on differences in individuals' motivations to succeed. Others have examined young people's beliefs about success and failure. Still others have pointed to differences in adolescents' opportunities for success and to the roles of important adults and peers in their lives. Various indicators of achievement are highly interrelated. For example, success in school during the early elementary years leads to later success in school; doing well in school generally leads to higher levels of educational attainment, which in turn lead to more challenging forms of employment with greater earning power.

Although there are distinct differences, the actual process leading toward occupational achievement can be a lengthy one in contemporary society. Because career options have expanded and changed so dramatically, and because increasing numbers of individuals enter college after completing high school, many adolescents do not decide on a career until well into early adulthood. (See Critical Thinking Exercise box.)

There is a definite relationship between social class and both educational and occupational achievement. A significant problem facing those interested in promoting achievement during adolescence is socioeconomic disparities in educational and occupational achievement. Beginning in early childhood, through no action of their own, many individuals find themselves on an educational course that directs them toward low levels of academic achievement, curtailed schooling, and limited occupational mobility. They reach adulthood with little hope and few dreams for their future. Understanding how this course is set in motion and identifying factors that help individuals from economically disadvantaged backgrounds to succeed despite tremendous odds are necessary steps in building interventions that promote the development and health of young people from lower socioeconomic populations.

 *Critical Thinking Exercise*

### Discussing the Future

Jeremy, age 17, will be graduating from high school in the spring. His mother, a single parent, tells you that she is concerned because graduation is quickly approaching and Jeremy has made no plans for what he will do with his life after graduation. Whenever Jeremy mentions the topic, his mother tells him, "This is what you must do," and begins to outline the steps he must take. Jeremy just walks away. She asks, "What should I do?" Which of the following would be the most appropriate advice for Jeremy's mother?

FIRST, THINK ABOUT IT . . .
- Within what point of view are you thinking?
- What conclusions are you reaching?

---

1. "Think about Jeremy's interests and what he has been successful doing in the past. Arrange for him to speak to someone whose career builds on those interests."
2. "Continue to tell him what he must do. Eventually you will get through to him, and he will listen."
3. "Be open and available to him. Tell him what you think, but not what to do."
4. "You are wise to be concerned. We need to arrange some counseling for Jeremy."

---

*The best response at this stage is three. Most adolescents want adult guidance and help, and messages are more likely to be heard if they are presented in an open-ended, nonjudgmental, nondictatorial fashion. Teenagers are unlikely to discuss their concerns on a timetable, and it is important to respect their point of view. Parents create the time and space and then wait. Parents who are available and willing to listen generally find that their adolescents are eager to talk. Answer one could be a good second step if Jeremy and his mother explore his interests together. Answer two is disrespectful of Jeremy, has not worked in the past, and is not likely to work in the future. Answer four may be necessary at a later time if other strategies fail.*

## Sexuality

Adolescence represents a critical time in the development of sexuality. Hormonal, physical, cognitive, and social changes that occur during adolescence all have an impact on sexual development.

Of all the developmental changes that affect adolescent sexuality none is more obvious than the impact of puberty. Adolescents must come to terms with hormonal influences, physiologic manifestations such as menstruation and ejaculation, and physical changes such as breast and genital development. All of these changes have a profound impact on the way teenagers perceive their bodies (i.e., *body image*). In addition to transitions in body image, increasing levels of pubertal hormones contribute to increased levels of sexual motivation among both boys and girls. Evidence also suggests that early development of secondary sex characteristics is associated with early sexual activity. For example, some early-maturing girls begin dating earlier and initiate sexual intercourse at younger ages than same-age peers (Doswell and others, 1998). Even when physical development occurs at an average onset and pace, the degree to which adolescents feel comfortable with their bodies may affect sexual behaviors.

Changes in sexual motivations and feelings, happening at the same time as shifts in cognitive skills, contribute to painful conjectures ("Is what I'm feeling normal?"), self-

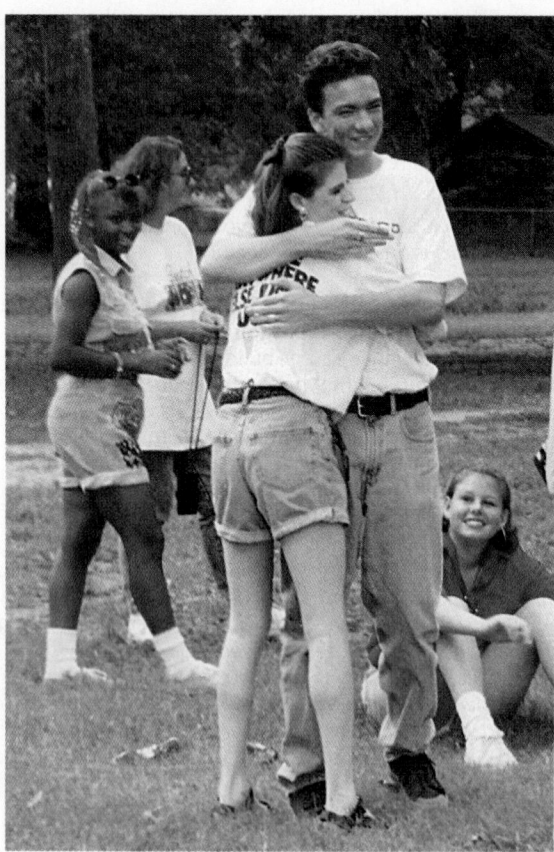

**Fig. 19-9** Romantic relationships are an important part of adolescence.

conscious concern ("Am I good-looking enough?"), and hypothetical thinking ("What if she wants to have sex?"). The emergence of formal operational thinking also increases adolescents' decision-making capabilities concerning sexual issues. As they mature, teenagers become better able to think through potential risks and benefits of sexual behaviors before they engage in any behavior. Older adolescents may also be able to conceptualize more long-term consequences of present behaviors. One of the important tasks of adolescence is to incorporate sexuality successfully into close, intimate relationships (Sullivan, 1953). This task is made possible by the advanced cognitive abilities that emerge over the course of adolescence.

Part of adolescent identity formation involves the development of *sexual identity*. As they begin to integrate changes involved with puberty, young adolescents also develop emotional and social identities separate from their families. For young adolescents, the process of sexual identity development usually involves forming close friendships with same-sex peers, with whom they may experiment sexually, often to satisfy curiosity. Sexual activity among young teenagers varies by gender. Masturbation provides an opportunity for sexual self-exploration; participation in this behavior is influenced by learned cultural attitudes, as well as sex-role expectations. Boys typically begin masturbating during early adolescence; the age of first masturbation is extremely variable for girls. Although some girls begin masturbating during early adolescence, many do not masturbate until after they have had intercourse. About one third of males and one fourth of females have had sexual intercourse by age 15; these young people are at high risk for sexually transmitted diseases and pregnancy.

Many teenagers begin to make a shift from relationships with same-sex peers to intimate relationships with members of the opposite sex during middle adolescence (Fig. 19-9). Opposite-sex relationships typically begin with peer activities involving both boys and girls. Pairing off as couples becomes more common as middle adolescence progresses. The type and degree of seriousness of partner relationships vary. Initial relationships are usually noncommittal, extremely mobile, and seldom characterized by any deep romantic attachments. Sexual activity becomes more common during middle adolescence. Nationally, approximately 45% of ninth-grade males and 33% of females report having had sexual intercourse. By twelfth grade, 64% of males and 66% of females report having had intercourse (Centers for Disease Control and Prevention, 2000). The relationship between love and sexual expression is brought into focus during middle adolescence. Most young people oppose exploitation, pressure, or force in sex as well as sex solely for the sake of physical enjoyment without a personal relationship. Adolescents find it hard to believe that sex can exist without love; therefore, each relationship is viewed as real love.

An integrated sexual identity often emerges during late adolescence as individuals incorporate sexual experiences, feelings, and cognitions. For most, this identity is consistent with their own physical and mental capacities and with societal limits and expectations. Most older adolescents identify themselves as being predominantly heterosexual or bisexual, with a smaller number self-identifying as homosexual and an even smaller group still unsure of their sexual orientation, although this varies somewhat by ethnicity (Saewyc and others, 1998; Russell, Seif, and Truong, 2001). Whatever their sexual orientation, most older teenagers possess the capacity to have intimate relationships that satisfy the emotional and sexual needs of both partners.

The meaning and implication of sexual activity as it affects psychosocial development may be quite different for adolescent boys and girls; that is, sexual socialization differs for males and females in our society. Typically, adolescent boys' first sexual experiences are in early adolescence through masturbation. Before adolescent boys begin dating, they have generally already experienced orgasm and know how to arouse themselves sexually. For males, the development of sexuality during adolescence revolves around efforts to integrate the forming of close relationships into an already existing sense of sexual capability. Girls' first sexual experiences are likely to be very different and to carry very different meanings. Masturbation is a less prevalent activity among girls, and it is less regularly practiced. The adolescent girl, in contrast to the adolescent boy, is more likely to experience sexual intercourse for the first time in a perceived close relationship. For girls, the development of sexuality involves the integration of sexual activity into an existing capacity for emotional involvement.

*Sexual orientation* is an important aspect of sexual identity. Sexual orientation is defined as a pattern of sexual arousal or romantic attraction toward persons of the opposite gender (heterosexual), of the same gender (homosexual, often called gay or lesbian) or of either or both genders (bisexual). Sexual orientation encompasses several dimensions, including attraction, fantasy, actual sexual behavior, and self-labeling or group affiliation. In individuals, the direction and intensity of each dimension is not necessarily consistent with any of the others. For example, individuals may be attracted most strongly to their same gender, fantasize about both genders, have sexual activity only with the opposite gender, and identify as gay or lesbian. Other individuals may engage in same-gender sexual behavior, fantasize about both genders, but identify as heterosexual. As with all aspects of sexual identity, the dimensions of sexual orientation are influenced by cultural meaning and expectation, by gender, by peer groups and by other environmental contexts. Recent research has suggested that the trajectory of developing sexual orientation may be different for boys and girls (Diamond, 1998).

Adolescence is the period during which individuals commonly begin to identify their sexual orientation as part of their developing sexual identity. However, this identification process can be profoundly influenced by cultural beliefs and values, by societal and family pressures, or by a lack of similar peers. The majority of adolescents eventually report an orientation toward exclusively heterosexual relationships. For adolescents whose orientation encompasses any same-gender dimensions, the identity process during adolescence can be complicated, especially when community norms disapprove of orientations other than heterosexual.

Adolescents who have witnessed harassment or violence directed at gay, lesbian, and bisexual people, for example, may be reluctant to self-identify, even when their attractions and behaviors are exclusively same-gender or bisexual. In contrast, in some American Indian cultures, there is a positive, highly respected role for tribal members who exhibit same-gender sexual attraction and behavior; as a result, reservation-based American Indian adolescents may be less likely to feel pressured to identify as heterosexual (Saewyc and others, 1998). In several population-based studies throughout the 1990s, researchers have found approximately 1% to 5% of adolescents identify as gay, lesbian, or bisexual, while 3% to 12% report same-gender or bisexual orientation in one or more of the other dimensions of sexual orientation (Reis and Saewyc, 1999).

The development of sexual orientation as part of sexual identity includes several developmental milestones during late childhood and throughout adolescence. These milestones do not necessarily occur in the same order for everyone nor are they completed in the same amount of time (Rosario and others, 1996). They include (1) the realization of romantic or erotic attraction to people of one (or both) genders, (2) erotic daydreaming about one or more genders, (3) romantic partners or dates without sexual activity, (4) sexual activity with people of the preferred gender or genders (also, for some teens, sexual activity with a non-preferred gender, out of curiosity or through social pressure), (5) self-identification of the orientation that best fits one's current circumstances and understanding, (6) publicly self-identifying that orientation, usually to intimate friends and family first, then the wider social group, and (7) an intimate, committed, sexual relationship with a person of the gender appropriate to one's orientation. Although only a few European countries legally recognize same-gender marriages at present, some religious faiths and social groups do celebrate committed same-gender couples' relationships. There is no evidence that gay, lesbian, or bisexual adults are more or less likely to create long-term, stable relationships than are heterosexual couples. It should be noted that bisexual adolescents and adults do not generally engage in sexual relationships with both genders concurrently; self-identification as bisexual usually refers to the ability to be attracted to either gender but does not imply that such a person requires partners of both genders, or that one must be equally attracted to and have sexual experience with both genders in order to be bisexual.

Although the order of these milestones varies greatly among adolescents, adolescents who will identify as gay, lesbian, or bisexual tend to publicly self-identify later than heterosexual peers. Without positive gay, lesbian, or bisexual role models or a supportive peer group, sexual minority teens can feel isolated, and they may not share their orientation with anyone for fear of rejection or violence. (See Critical Thinking Exercise box on p. 816.) When adolescents who would otherwise identify as bisexual can only find a peer group of gay and lesbian teens, they may focus on their same-gender dimensions of orientation and adopt the label of lesbian or gay; later, they may self-label as bisexual. Likewise, some gay and lesbian adolescents may first identify as heterosexual, then bisexual, before identifying as gay or lesbian. In recent studies among self-identified gay, lesbian, and bisexual adolescents, many of the adolescents report changing their self-labels one or more times during their adolescence (Rosario and others, 1996; Diamond, 1998).

### Intimacy

Intimate relationships are emotional attachments between two people characterized by concern for each other's well-being; a willingness to disclose private, possibly sensitive topics; and a sharing of common interests and activities. Intimate relationships are distinct from sexual relationships. It is possible for individuals to have close relationships without becoming sexually involved. At the same time, people can be involved in sexual relationships that are not particularly intimate.

It is not until adolescence—a time characterized by pubertal changes, advances in social cognitive abilities, and broadening of social worlds—that truly intimate relationships first emerge. Although children have important friendships, these relationships are activity oriented. To a child, a friend is someone who likes to do the same things he or she does. Adolescents' close friendships are more likely to include a strong emotional foundation in which individuals understand and care about each other. The development of intimacy during adolescence involves changes in the adolescent's needs for intimacy, as well as changes in the capacity and opportunities to have intimate friendships. Puberty and its resultant changes in sexual impulses often raise new issues and concerns requiring serious, intimate discussions. Over the course of the adolescent years, individuals become more capable of emotional closeness, and they become more interested in seeking it in their relationships with other people. The greater degree of behavioral independence often accompanying the transition into adolescence provides more opportunities for teenagers to be alone with friends and to come into meaningful contact with adults outside of their families. Although research on intimacy during adolescence has focused on peer friendships, intimate relationships are by no means limited to peers. In addition to forming close friendships with peers, teenagers may also have intimate relationships with parents, siblings, and adults who are not part of their immediate families.

Harry Stack Sullivan (1953) was among the first to describe the developmental course of intimacy. Usually adolescents develop the capacity for intimacy through preadolescent and early adolescent relationships with same-sex peers. Intimate relationships with opposite-sex peers develop relatively late during adolescence. Opposite-sex friendships may play a more important role in the development of intimacy among boys than among girls, who may develop and experience intimacy earlier during the course of adolescence with same-sex peers.

Individuals move through a series of stages in their close relationships with others. Children most often function at a *self-focused* level with friends, still wrapped up in their own needs and perspectives. They tend to react to friends' actions in simplistic ways—either by trying to hold on to the friendship at all costs or by trying to flee from it. During adolescence, many individuals move into *role-focused* friendships, behaving in ways that are dominated by conventional norms. In their close relationships, individuals at this level attempt to avoid controversy and control their emotions. Role-focused persons are generally more concerned with conforming to the appropriate roles and norms in a relationship (e.g., what the "good" girlfriend does) than with a friend as an individual. It is not until later in adolescence that people develop the capacity for having *individuated-connected* friendships. With this level of friendship, individuals are able to form close, intimate relationships with others that acknowledge the complexity and contradictions in close relationships. Differences in outlook between individuals are not only tolerated but encouraged as part of what makes the relationship vital.

Although teenagers may begin dating during early adolescence, these early dating relationships are not usually very psychosocially intimate. Early dating relationships typically follow highly ritualized "scripts," in which adolescents are more likely to play stereotypic roles than to really be themselves. Participating in mixed-sex group activities—such as going to parties or other events—may have a positive impact on the well-being of young teenagers. A moderate degree of dating, with serious relationships delayed until late adolescence, may be the most ideal pattern of interpersonal involvement.

# Social Environments

Although all adolescents experience similar biologic and cognitive changes and face similar psychosocial tasks, the health-related effects of these changes are not the same for all people. Why aren't individuals affected in the same ways by puberty, by changes in thinking patterns, and by changes in social and legal status? The answer lies in the fact that biologic, cognitive, and social changes of adolescence are shaped by the social environment in which the changes take place (Bronfenbrenner, 1979). The social environment provides the opportunities, barriers, role models, and support for individuals' development and health. Systems within the social environment, including family, peers, schools, community, and the larger society, all contribute uniquely to an adolescent's development and health.

An *ecologic model* can be used as a way of understanding adolescents' social environments (Bronfenbrenner, 1979). In this model, the social environment is divided into proximal and more distal systems. The social environment includes microsystems, mesosystems, exosystems, and macrosystems.

*Microsystems* are the most proximal social contexts in which adolescents participate directly, such as family, peer groups, school, and the workplace. All of these contexts have substantial influences on the development and health-related behaviors of adolescents (Perry, Kelder, and Komro, 1993).

The next layer of social environment, *mesosystems,* is formed by linkages between microsystems. The extent to which individuals in one microsystem are involved in other systems determines the strength or "richness" of the mesosystem. For example, regular interactions between family members and school personnel, which have positive effects on student achievement and school performance, reflect a rich mesosystem.

The third layer of social environment, *exosystems,* consists of settings that influence adolescent behavior and development but in which they do not directly participate. Many community-level influences fall within this layer. These include opportunities within a community for health-enhancing or health-compromising behaviors, such as the availability of age-appropriate activities for young people that do not include alcohol, tobacco, or drugs.

The most distal social environment, *macrosystems,* consists of culturally based belief systems as well as economic and political systems. These systems can have profound effects on young people's health-related behaviors and development, mostly through their influences on more proximal systems.

Social systems are embedded within each other, and what happens within one system can influence what happens in others. To have the most impact on adolescent health promotion, interventions must address multiple environmental systems (Perry, Kelder, and Komro, 1993).

## Families

Over the past several decades, changes that have taken place within the family microsystem have important implications for adolescent health. High rates of divorce, increasing numbers of single-parent families, and greater percentages of working mothers have become characteristic of contemporary U.S. society. The "ideal" family consisting of an employed father, an at-home mother, and two or more school-age children is no longer the norm for American society. Higher rates of divorce and the decisions of single women to have children have increased the number of U.S. children spending at least part of their childhood in a single-parent family. Correspondingly, many young people find themselves in blended families, thus developing relationships with stepparents during their adolescent years. Changes in family structure have been accompanied by changes in parent work patterns and a dramatic increase in the percentage of mothers who work outside the home (Gottfried and Gottfried, 1994). (See Family Structure, Chapter 3.)

Changes in family structure and parent employment have resulted in young people having more time unsupervised by adults. The result is increased time alone or with peers. Although for mature adolescents there may be little risk involved with minimal supervision, for less competent teenagers, decreased adult supervision may result in more risk-taking behaviors, such as substance use and sexual intercourse. Poorly monitored teenagers may also socialize with deviant peers. Lack of adult supervision also decreases adolescents' opportunities for communication and intimacy with a parent or other supportive adults. Although quantity of time does not guarantee quality, sufficient quantity is necessary for communication and the development of intimate relationships.

Consistently, adolescents who feel close to their parents show more positive psychosocial development and behavioral competence, less susceptibility to negative peer pressure, and lower tendencies to be involved in risk-taking behaviors (Resnick and others, 1997). In many situations lack of direct adult supervision may be counterbalanced by parent monitoring and communication about adolescents' activities during parental absence.

On the other hand, in dysfunctional or abusive families spending greater amounts of time with parents may compromise the health of teenagers. In these situations the type and content of communication may be the most important factors to address (Perry, Kelder, and Komro, 1993).

In addition to adult supervision, the overall parenting style affects adolescent development. Both effective conflict resolution within families and family cohesion create environments conducive to healthy adolescent development. These two characteristics, along with parent expectations for mature behavior on the part of the adolescent and the practice of setting and enforcing reasonable limits for behavior, form the basis of effective parenting. This parenting style, termed *authoritative parenting,* is related to greater psychosocial maturity and school performance and less substance abuse among young people.

Adolescents from low-income households spend less supervised time with adults, are more likely to have parents working at more than one job, are more likely to drop out of high school, and are more likely to experience violence in their homes and communities (Perry, Kelder, and Komro, 1993). While disorder within their larger social environments often creates a need for a buffer that could include spending quality time with adults, poor adolescents often experience fewer of these types of health-enhancing activities.

Nurses should be cautious in attributing differences in adolescent risk behaviors to racial or ethnic group membership, socioeconomic status, or family structure. A recent national longitudinal study of adolescent health among seventh to twelfth graders in the United States examined the effects of race/ethnicity, income, and family structure on risk behaviors (Blum and others, 2000). The risk behaviors included emotional distress, suicide attempts, smoking, drinking, weapon-related violence, and sexual intercourse. Study results indicated that, while there were some differences in behaviors by ethnic group, income, or family structure, these three elements together explained only about 10% of the variation in behaviors for seventh and eighth grade students, and only 7% among ninth through twelfth grade students.

## Peer Groups

One hallmark of adolescence is the increasing value young people place on friendships and relationships with peers (Fig. 19-10). Adolescents spend more time with their peers than do children. Compared with children, their peer groups are more autonomous and are more likely to include peers of the opposite sex. Because of the changes that have taken place within family systems in contemporary society, peer groups play a very significant role in the socialization of adolescents.

Peers serve as credible sources of information, role models of new social behaviors, sources of social reinforcement, and bridges to alternative lifestyles. Close and supportive peer friendships have beneficial effects for young people. However, adolescents with greater peer identification than parental identification, especially when peers model and support problem behaviors, are more prone to deviant and health-compromising behaviors. Thus, the transition to greater peer involvement, like other developmental transitions of adolescence, is a process requiring guidance, skills, and, to be accomplished optimally, a prolonged time to complete the transitions. At a time when they are develop-

ing interpersonal skills to deal with peer pressure, young adolescents who lack adult supervision and opportunities for communication with adults may be more susceptible to peer influences and at a higher risk for poor peer-group selection than teenagers who have close relationships with caring adults (Perry, Kelder, and Komro, 1993).

The heightened value placed on adolescent peer relationships leads to questions about the quality and nature of peer influence. Rather than thinking of all peer influence as either good or bad, it is important to recognize that the influence of peers varies from one adolescent to another, from one peer group to another, and across different societies and cultures. Adolescents' selection of peer groups seems to be most strongly influenced by sociodemographic factors and by common patterns of behavior, including, for example, substance use, school achievement, and religious participation. Peers can have either positive or negative effects on adolescent behavior. Negative effects include increased substance use, gang membership, and violent behaviors. Positive effects include an orientation supporting academic achievement, an environmental commitment, or a commitment to religious youth groups (Perry, Kelder, and Komro, 1993). Peers can also be a positive force in health promotion. Same-age and older adolescents can encourage healthy behavior by serving as positive role models and promoting prohealth norms in the peer group (Rosenfeld and others, 2000; Tuttle and others, 2000). For most adolescents, prosocial pressures from peers are greater than antisocial ones, and they are influenced more by prosocial or neutral pressures than by pressures toward misconduct.

## Schools

In contemporary society, schools play an increasingly important role in preparing young people for adulthood (Fig. 19-11). Schooling is essential for a successful future for both boys and girls. Failure to complete high school reduces employment opportunities and the probability of

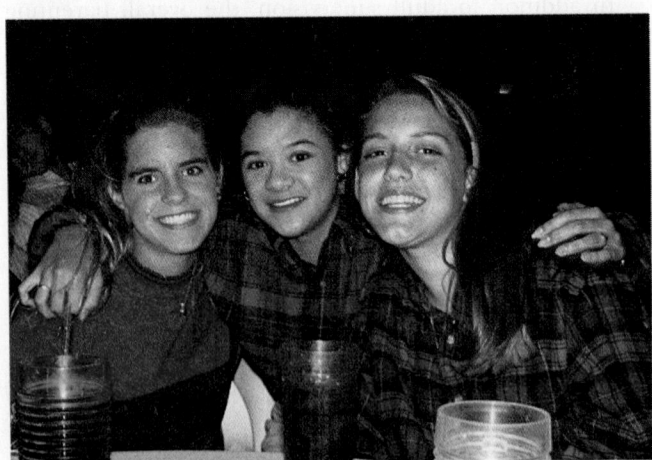

**Fig. 19-10** The peer group is a major influence in adolescent development.

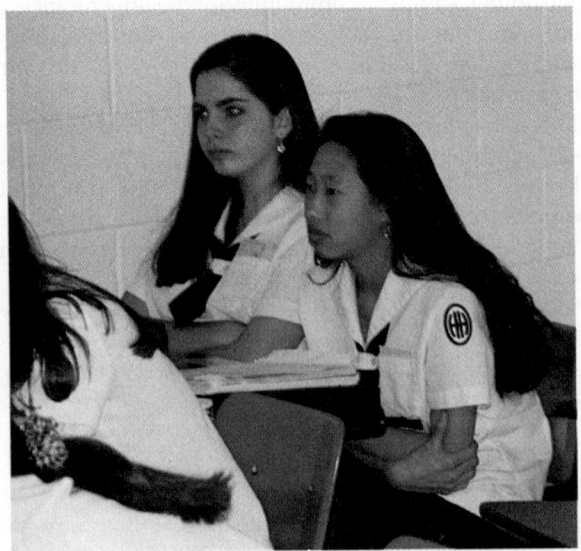

**Fig. 19-11** School is an important part of adolescents' life.

earning an adequate income. Yet, many schools in the United States are not meeting the developmental needs of all young people.

Many minority-group members are not at appropriate grade levels for their age, and the dropout rate among minority groups is higher than among nonminority students. Dropout rates are highest among Hispanic and American Indian adolescents (Blum and others, 1992).

Another important problem is the lack of parental involvement in schools. Parental involvement increases the effectiveness of schools at all levels. However, with the larger number of single-parent and two-working parent families, parents have less time for involvement in schools.

There is also evidence that the transition from elementary school can have negative effects on youth. The timing of school transition is critical, especially in cases where the school environment is not appropriate to the developmental needs of the adolescent. In particular, the transition into a junior high school at age 12 or 13 typically occurs at the same time as the rapid physical changes of puberty. Relatively few kindergarten-through-eighth-grade schools exist in the United States, and the trend is toward earlier rather than later transition out of primary school. Earlier transition may be advantageous if it precedes the changes of puberty and allows young adolescents to become accustomed to the change in school environment before having to cope with pubertal events.

Another characteristic of school that may have negative effects is a system of grading that acknowledges few young people for their academic successes. Teenagers whose grades fall below average may spend a high proportion of their time in environments in which they perceive negative evaluations by adult authorities. Students' reactions to such environments may include alienation from school; then, subgroups of adolescents may unite and develop counter-cultures or exhibit antisocial behavior. This process may be most intense for young people from poorer families who attend schools that include students from a broad range of socioeconomic classes.

In addition, students who repeat one or more grades exhibit greater emotional distress (Resnnick and others, 1997). Students with below-average grades are more likely to be engaged in health-compromising behaviors such as tobacco and alcohol use, unprotected sexual intercourse, and suicide attempts (Neinstein, 1996).

The social environment of schools has an impact on student outcomes. Small classroom size and small school size are both related to higher-quality social environments within schools. Safety and respect for all students are critical issues because students have difficulty learning in unsafe environments. In some schools, violence and harassment of students on the basis of race, gender, or sexual orientation is common, affecting more than half of all students (Saewyc and others, 2000). Students targeted for repeated teasing and harassment are more likely to skip school, are more likely to report symptoms of depression, and are more likely to attempt suicide. Equally troubling, teens who are regularly harassed are also more likely to bring weapons to school in order to feel safe. In the 1999 Youth Risk Behavior Survey in the United States, 11% of adolescent boys and 2.8% of adolescent girls nationwide reported carrying a weapon at school one or more days of the month before the survey (Centers for Disease Control and Prevention, 2000). School practices and conditions that lead to better student outcomes stress the importance of supportive environments that foster positive peer group relationships, promote health and fitness, encourage family involvement in school, and strengthen connections between schools and communities.

## Work

For the majority of young people in the United States, the workplace becomes a fourth microsystem. Most teenagers are employed in a relatively restricted array of jobs as restaurant workers, cashiers, sales clerks, clerical assistants, and unskilled laborers. The jobs tend to be monotonous, require little initiative or decision making, and rarely use skills learned in school; furthermore, some are highly stressful, requiring work under extreme time pressures. Adolescent work as it exists today may negatively affect development. The typical teenager's job provides neither continuity to adult employment nor links to adults who could serve as vocational mentors. In addition, the monotonous nature of many adolescent jobs is neither intellectually stimulating nor related to role experimentation involved in identity development. Rather, involvement in work may take time away from other activities that could contribute to identity development. Greater involvement in work can also lead to fatigue, decreased interest in school, reduced extracurricular involvement, and poorer grades. Detrimental effects are especially likely for adolescents who work more than 20 hours a week (Resnick and others, 1997). Although much work done by teenagers may not contribute to healthy development, jobs that allow young people to develop intellectual and social skills, to have some autonomy, or to feel that their contributions matter can prove to be positive experiences. Jobs that provide adolescents with experiences relevant to future employment or that link them to adults who can serve as vocational mentors may be especially valuable.

## Community and Society

Society influences adolescent health and development indirectly through the structures of social institutions, division of economic wealth, and construction and implementation of public policies. Society also provides a dominant set of values and expectations for behavior to which adolescents are exposed. These values and expectations are transmitted through the mass media as well as through local institutions and social networks.

In the United States, adolescence is a time during which individuals are expected to make the transition from childhood to adulthood. Adolescents are given more autonomy than children and are also expected to show more responsible behavior. Young people are given more personal control over health-related behaviors but often fail to receive necessary guidance, support, or access to positive adult role models. At the same time, society seeks to limit adolescents' involvement in some risk-taking behaviors that may convey adult status, such as alcohol and tobacco use or sexual behaviors. Many of these same behaviors are glamorized through media programming and advertising campaigns directed at teenagers. For some teenagers faced with societal expectations to "grow up," risk-taking behaviors take on specific functional meanings. Behaviors such as substance use or unsafe sex may offer adolescents opportunities to challenge social authority, demonstrate autonomy, or gain social approval.

Local communities, as part of the broader societal context, also influence adolescents' capacity for healthy development. The local community has a more proximal influence on adolescents' motivations and opportunities to engage in health-enhancing or risk-taking behaviors. For example, adults within the community serve as direct role models, affecting adolescents' expectations concerning their likely roles and activities as adults. Communities with a high proportion of employed, well-educated, financially successful adults provide a different array of models than impoverished neighborhoods where poor households predominate as well as chronic illness and drug abuse, and the financially successful adults are those involved in illicit activities. Such environmental characteristics affect young people's expectations for the future, their perceptions of how current behavior could jeopardize future chances, and, consequently, their motivation to avoid high-risk behavior (Schorr, 1997).

A community's economic resources play a significant role in the health and well-being of young people. Resources affect opportunities for health promotion (e.g., by influencing the quality of local schools and health-related services). Schools in wealthy areas can provide high-quality education that will enhance students' interest in school and their chances of future success. Wealthy communities also provide opportunities for alternative, health-enhancing activities through community clubs and organizations. Thus community resources influence the type and number of health risks young people face as well as the local capacity for health promotion.

## PROMOTING OPTIMUM HEALTH DURING ADOLESCENCE

Health promotion involves empowering individuals, families, and communities to take developmentally and contextually appropriate actions toward realizing their potential; it includes physical, cognitive, emotional, and social dimensions. For adolescents, health promotion involves helping youth acquire the power (including knowledge, attitudes, and skills), authority (permission to use their power), and opportunities to make choices that increase the likelihood of their creating positive expressions of health for themselves in their contexts.

A comprehensive approach to health promotion combines activities aimed at individuals with interventions focused on changing norms, attitudes, and behaviors of peer groups, families, communities, and society at large. For example, prevention of tobacco use involves more than a teacher's lecture on the consequences of cigarette and smokeless tobacco use, a ban on tobacco use in schools, a parent's admonition not to smoke, or a nurse's question to an adolescent about smoking history. In reality, it requires all of these components and more. Effective health promotion requires the support of many individuals and institutions that affect the lives of adolescents.

By some measures, adolescents are a relatively healthy group. If health is limited to physical illness, adolescents fare quite well. However, if the definition of health includes physical fitness, psychologic health, and social well-being, unmet needs of this age-group become apparent (*Healthy People 2010*, 1999). In *Healthy People 2010* (see Chapter 1), adolescent goals include risk reduction efforts in the areas of mental health, substance use, sexual behavior, violence, unintentional injury, nutrition, physical activity and fitness, and oral health.

The rationale for focusing on these health issues becomes obvious when one examines the major sources of mortality and morbidity during adolescence. The primary causes of mortality during adolescence are injuries, homicide, and suicide; together these three causes are responsible for 75% of all adolescent deaths. Major causes of adolescent morbidity include injury and disability associated with the use of motor and recreational vehicles the sequelae of sexual and physical abuse, the consequences of sexual activity such as pregnancy and sexually transmitted diseases, and the outcomes of substance use. Mental disorders, chronic illness, eating disorders, and oral health problems are other important sources of morbidity (Centers for Disease Control and Prevention, 2000). Chapters 20 and 21 provide further information about threats to adolescent health and well-being.

The goals of *Healthy People 2010* also target inequities in health status that exist among subsets of the U.S. population; adolescents are one subgroup that experiences health inequities. For example, a substantial gap in life expectancy exists between African-American and white adolescents. African-American and Native American males have a higher risk of premature mortality than any other racial/ethnic group. Adolescent males die at a rate more than twice that of females. Mortality rates increase by more than 200% between early and late adolescence. There are also age differences in the causes of death, with a shift toward more violent deaths occurring in late adolescence. Among white adolescents a dramatic increase in suicide occurs during later adolescence, making it the second leading cause of death in this group. For older African-American adolescents homicide ranks as the most likely cause of death. Similar to mortality, patterns of morbidity vary within the adolescent population. For example, rates of vehicular injury are high among males, whereas for females morbidities associated with "quietly disturbed" behaviors such as eating disorders and emotional distress are common (Centers for Disease Control and Prevention, 2000).

### Adolescents' Perspectives on Health

To be most effective, adolescent health promotion efforts must incorporate adolescents' perspectives on what health means. It also must focus on their concerns and priorities related to health and health care services. From a positive perspective, adolescents' developmentally based sense of curiosity and movement toward autonomy provide opportunities for health promotion that should not be wasted.

One 13-year-old girl, when asked what health meant to her, responded: "You want to do things . . . to live . . . to get out, have fun, be active. You have to be healthy to work hard . . . to survive in this world. If you're not, you might as well be put out on a mountain like they used to do to babies in the ancient myths and let the wolves eat you 'cause you're not going to get anywhere" (Irwin, 1976). Adolescents define health in much the same way as adults: health means being able to live up to one's potential; being able to function physically, mentally, and socially; and experiencing positive emotional states. The content of their definitions often goes beyond an "absence of illness" perspective and includes what can be done to maintain and enhance health.

Adolescents' health-related interests and concerns include stress and anxiety, relationships with adults and peers, weight, acne, and feeling down or depressed. Health concerns are often consistent with the immediate developmental tasks that teenagers face. For example, younger adolescents—in the midst of the physical changes of puberty—have a particular interest in issues related to growth and development. In the process of making transitions from middle or junior high school to senior high school, middle adolescents have questions and concerns related to peer-group acceptance, relationships with friends, and physical appearance. Older adolescents' focus increasingly on school performance as well as on future career/employment plans and emotional health issues.

Among the behaviors that adolescents view as risky are substance use, sexual activity, and risks related to the use of recreational and motor vehicles. Adolescents also identify health threats that primarily involve psychologic issues, such as clinical depression and eating/weight problems. Other perceived health threats include violence and pollution as well as threats within the more immediate social environment, including school problems and conflicts with parents, teachers, and friends. When adolescents are asked about general threats to youth, they respond differently than if asked about how their own personal behaviors produce certain risks. Like adults, adolescents tend to underestimate the potentially negative consequences of their own behaviors.

Although young people identify health risks and concerns that are primarily social and psychologic in nature, many are reluctant to seek health services for problems they do not consider to be organic in nature, despite the fact that they indicate they would like help with these problems. An adolescent's reluctance to seek health care is influenced by many factors, including perceived availability of confidential services, characteristics of health care providers, geographic access, and financial limitations (Ginsburg, Menapace, and Slap, 1997).

The availability of confidential services is particularly important to adolescents, especially when they have concerns related to sensitive issues such as sexual or substance use behaviors. Many teenagers are unwilling to seek health care related to sensitive topics if their parents will know about the visit. Although most states have provisions for confidential care related to problems such as substance abuse and sexual health, adolescents demonstrate significant misperceptions about whether and where they can receive confidential health care.

Adolescents may be more likely to participate in health care services when they are delivered by caring, respectful providers. In a study that explored the factors that influenced ninth graders' decisions to seek care, researchers found that teens were more concerned about provider characteristics than about site or system characteristics (Ginsburg, Menapace, and Slap, 1997). Students wanted providers who were honest and respectful, competent, kept confidentiality, and did not treat them "like children." Their definitions of honesty included providing accurate, factual information, without evasiveness or false reassurances, especially around painful procedures. Students felt respected when providers were nonjudgmental, demonstrated genuine caring, acknowledged the teen's illness or discomfort, were sensitive to modesty issues, thoroughly explained procedures in advance, and did not make teens wait long before being seen. Adolescents felt disrespected when providers had condescending or impatient attitudes, used biomedical jargon and unfamiliar terms, and did not stop painful procedures when requested. Students recommended that health care providers conduct health histories and talk with them while they were still clothed before they had changed into a hospital gown for any examinations. Teens wanted their provider to be competent and to demonstrate competence by displaying their diplomas or certificates prominently in the clinic. In addition to concerns about provider characteristics, adolescents were deeply concerned about disease transmission in the clinical setting. They ranked provider and site cleanliness and precautions as more important than confidential care or respect because they viewed these issues as life and death matters. Study adolescents believed HIV transmission via routine health care was common. They felt providers should wash their hands in full view of the adolescent before beginning the exam and that providers should keep sterile instruments in the sterile package and unwrap them in the adolescent's presence before the examination (Ginsburg, Menapace, and Slap, 1997).

## Factors That Promote Adolescent Health and Well-Being

Despite being exposed to risk factors such as poverty, high rates of neighborhood violence, parental abuse, parental neglect, or divorce of parents, many adolescents become competent, healthy adults. It is important to understand how this group of young people succeed despite odds against them. Important questions for nurses and other professionals involved in health promotion are "Who doesn't experience adverse health outcomes (e.g., teenage pregnancy, sexually transmitted diseases, school failure, delinquency, depression, suicide, or substance abuse)?" and "Why?" Answers to these questions lead to identification of personal and environmental factors that protect adolescents from experiencing high-risk health outcomes. Future health promotion efforts with adolescents should focus on nurturing such protective factors.

Protective factors that characterize children and youth who cope successfully when faced with adverse life situations such as poverty, parental alcoholism or psychopathology, or poor relationships between parents include individual personal attributes, attributes of families, and attributes of the larger social environment (Resnick and others, 1997). One protective personal factor is the ability to adapt to new persons and situations. A recent prospective study of infants born into inner-city disadvantaged families identified several other characteristics that fostered or hindered favorable outcomes in these children later in life at 27 to 33 years of age (Hardy and others, 1997). Personal characteristics that fostered success or self-sufficiency in later years included satisfactory cognitive and academic development in the early school years (particularly, competence in language and reading skills), being on the honor roll, participating in extracurricular activities, having a summer job, and going to the library. Characteristics associated with unfavorable outcomes later in life included being retained in a grade in school, using drugs or alcohol, regular cigarette smoking, problems with the criminal justice system, or becoming pregnant before 18 years of age.

Adolescents who cope successfully in the midst of adverse circumstances are often supported by caring, cohesive families in which the parents are concerned with the well-being of their children. This "family" support can also be provided by some other caring adult—such as a grandparent—in the absence of a supportive parent. Protective factors within the community include connections with adults outside the family, with the school, or with a church group (Resnick and others, 1997). For example, health care providers who are able to connect with adolescents help to support successful coping. Schools that are small, comfortable, safe, and intellectually engaging can make a difference in the health and well-being of young people. Involvement with healthy peer groups, guided by caring and culturally appropriate adults, has also been shown to prevent poor outcomes.

The potential positive impact of social interactions suggests guidelines for making changes in adolescent environments that support overall health and well-being. Nurses involved with adolescents can develop interventions that shift the balance for young people from vulnerability to resilience either by decreasing exposures to health risks or stressful life events (such as the impact of parental alcoholism or the threats of violence) or by increasing the number of protective factors (such as communication and problem-solving skills or sources of emotional support) available to them.

## Contexts for Adolescent Health Promotion

There is a growing consensus that the most effective adolescent health promotion efforts involve multiple systems and address multiple issues. Interventions integrating programs and expertise from health care, school, and community-based settings can effectively increase adolescents' prevention skills, improve their access to health care services, build adult motivation and support for adolescent prevention

practices, and change physical environments and social norms to support healthy behavior (Schorr, 1997). Such a comprehensive approach to health promotion requires a great deal of cooperation and coordination on the part of complex institutions. On the other hand, by not limiting the responsibility for adolescent health to one person or one setting, multiple opportunities for health promotion occur. Individual efforts reinforce important themes and become an integral part of an overall health promotion strategy. For example, a plan for smoking cessation devised by a teenager with the help of a nurse is most likely to be successful if the teenager is encouraged by peers and family members to abstain, and if use and access to tobacco products are discouraged through policy interventions such as "smoke-free" schools and bans on cigarette vending machines.

### Schools

Schools are a primary site for adolescent health promotion and disease prevention. Large numbers of young people can be affected by school-based health promotion efforts, because virtually all teenagers attend school at least through the early adolescent years. Group interventions offer adolescents a sense of anonymity, which they prefer when obtaining information about sensitive topics. School personnel often have special expertise and experience with health education. Through daily contact, school staff can develop supportive relationships with a limited number of students. Parent-teacher associations and school boards also link schools with the larger community in ways that can be used to expand the scope of adolescent health promotion efforts.

School-based health promotion interventions include classroom health education as well as school-level policies and environmental changes. Classroom programs often include components that focus on building students' knowledge and skills and establishing peer support for health-enhancing behaviors. Some programs have effectively used classroom peer leaders as positive role models and social support for healthy behaviors. Out-of-class assignments often involve parents or other admired adults, emphasizing the roles that adults play as resources regarding health issues. Classroom programs have been designed to address health-related issues, including healthy eating and exercise habits (Fig. 19-12), nonviolent conflict resolution, substance use and abuse prevention, and promotion of responsible sexual behavior. Other school-level interventions involve changing the school environment itself. Examples of this type of intervention include efforts to improve physical education and food service programs or to adopt tobacco-free school policies. School-wide environmental changes serve to reinforce classroom programs aimed at promoting health-enhancing behavior.

### School-Based and School-Linked Health Services

Another avenue for health promotion is school-based and school-linked clinics. *School-based clinics (SBCs)* are located on school grounds and serve adolescents within a specific school. *School-linked clinics (SLCs)* may be located off school grounds or on school campuses but serve more than one school. Originally designed to address issues related to adolescent pregnancy, SBCs and SLCs have expanded to include services that

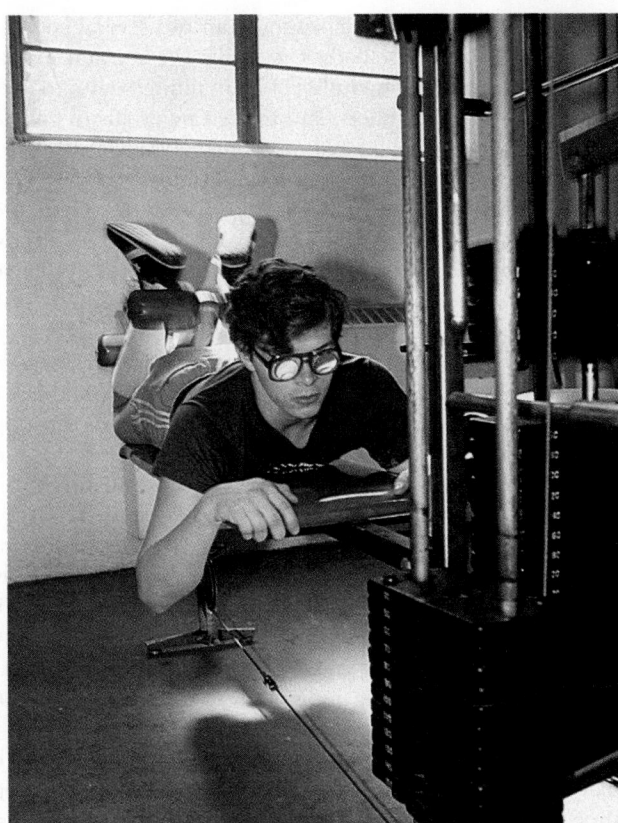

**Fig. 19-12** Adolescents should be encouraged to participate in activities that contribute to lifelong physical fitness.

address a broad range of health problems and psychosocial issues. In combination, school-linked health services and traditional school-based health promotion efforts provide a comprehensive approach to health promotion that integrates health care, education, and environmental support.

Several private foundations, as well as state and local governments, have provided considerable resources to initiate school-linked health services in which adolescents are offered confidential services at minimal cost. Parental consent for services is usually obtained on a blanket basis before adolescents seek services. These services increase adolescents' access to preventive and primary care services, a fact that may be related to their highly visible locations, convenient hours, affordability, and ability to provide confidential care. SLCs have made a concerted effort to provide the services of a multidisciplinary team of health professionals—which may include nurses, nurse practitioners, health educators, medical assistants, physicians, psychologists, nutritionists, and social workers—skilled in meeting both the mental and physical health needs of adolescents. Adolescents are receptive to services offered by SLCs, especially when emotionally charged issues such as depression are addressed.

Among the potential barriers to the use of schools as sites for health promotion are a lack of resources and community-level resistance to program implementation. Some schools may be reluctant to commit resources to health promotion activities that may decrease the time available to pursue more traditional educational goals. Other schools may be faced with vocal groups of parents or community members who express concern for

schools becoming involved in issues that they consider should be taught at home. Barriers, including inadequate funding, community and provider resistance, limitations in the numbers of trained personnel, and lack of systematic data on effectiveness, have interfered with the successful implementation of SLCs in some communities. Political influences and variations in the resources available within any particular community result in a lack of uniformity in the scope, depth, and quality of health education and health services offered to students across school systems.

## Communities

Community-level approaches to adolescent health promotion, involving both media campaigns and initiatives on the part of community groups, offer the advantage of reaching a broad audience. Specifically, community-based approaches can reach adolescents who do not attend school or have no source of preventive health care. This type of approach directly addresses changing social environments where risk behaviors occur. For example, violence prevention may be more effectively addressed by changing community-wide standards related to issues such as conflict resolution than by focusing on the individual. Community-level approaches have the potential to be most effective when they involve various sectors of the community (including adolescents) and include persons representing a variety of youth-serving agencies. With the involvement of multiple sectors, adolescents have the opportunity to hear consistent health messages across a variety of social contexts.

The media is commonly used in community-level health promotion efforts. Adolescents receive considerable information from sources such as television, radio, and magazines. Media campaigns can be an effective way to reach adolescents with health promotion messages. Messages can also be targeted to appeal to parents and other adults who have an impact on the health-related behavior of youth. Information delivered by media campaigns uses brief images and provides short, superficial coverage of specific issues. Typically, the goal of media campaigns involves increasing knowledge and changing attitudes around a single issue. However, if used alone, media campaigns have little direct influence on changing health behaviors.

The goal of initiatives launched by parent and community groups is to build climates within communities that support health-enhancing behaviors. Such initiatives create social contexts in which teenagers encounter more health-promoting messages and norms. An example of a community-level initiative is a task force developed to address issues related to adolescent alcohol use. Goals of this task force may include educating community members about the extent and consequences of adolescent alcohol use, developing strategies that decrease the availability of alcohol to young people within the community (such as better enforcement of age-of-alcohol-sales laws), and sponsoring alcohol-free social events for community youth.

## Health Care Settings

Consistent, supportive, one-on-one interactions over time between adolescents and members of the health care team provide significant opportunities for health promotion.

These relationships can create "safe environments" in which adolescents can disclose sensitive information related to health risk. In turn, this information should be incorporated into preventive interventions specific to individual adolescent needs.

Health care settings offer the advantage of being able to provide confidential services, which are especially important in sensitive situations such as those involving substance use and sexual behavior. Interventions provided through health care settings can include parents and help to create social environments that support adolescents' health-enhancing behaviors. Another advantage of health promotion efforts within health care settings is the resources available to address various components of health, including physical, emotional, and social needs.

There are limitations to health promotion interventions provided in health care settings. Individual care is time-consuming, limiting the number of adolescents who can be reached through one-on-one encounters. While one-on-one interventions can foster health-enhancing attitudes and behaviors of individual adolescents, they do not address changes in social environments, such as peer groups and communities, that may be necessary to support these attitudes and behaviors.

To be effective, health care services for adolescents must be accessible and appropriate. To be *accessible,* services must be available, affordable, and approachable. Services must include outreach to adolescents and their parents, informing them of the availability of services. Mechanisms for low or no-cost services must be developed because cost is a major barrier to adolescents receiving appropriate care. Locating health care services in places such as schools, youth services centers, shopping malls, and detention facilities and offering convenient clinical hours are two strategies that increase accessibility among teenagers who may not use traditional services.

Research has shown that adolescent-focused care can be cost-effective and improve health outcomes (Bensussen-Walls and Saewyc, 2001). To be *appropriate,* services must take into consideration the cultural contexts, as well as adolescents' needs for confidential, developmentally appropriate care that addresses their specific health concerns. For example, appropriate health services for urban Latino teenagers may be very different from services for a rural population of white teenagers.

## Adolescent Health Screening

One vehicle for health promotion used by nurses and other professionals in health care settings is one-on-one health screening. Through information gained during a *health screening interview,* both assets and threats to an adolescent's health and well-being can be identified. The health screening interview also offers an opportunity for health professionals to build trusting relationships with adolescents. This sense of trust may be critical for adolescents to act on information, attitudes, and skills, which are shared to help them successfully negotiate particular stressors.

In addition, the health screening interview provides an opportunity for teaching adolescents self-advocacy skills.

Nurses in schools and clinic settings can use several specific strategies to promote self-advocacy skills (Vessey and Miola, 1997). These strategies include (1) maintaining an up-to-date file of handouts, pamphlets, and written materials to give to adolescents during "teachable moments"; (2) directing adolescents to resources in their community and to appropriate, accurate sources of health information on the Internet; and (3) teaching adolescents how the health care system works, how to schedule their health care appointments, and how to keep their own personal health records of immunizations, allergies, and health care encounters (Vessey and Miola, 1997).

**Interview Process.**   The development of trust between the adolescent and the health professional is vital to a health screening interview. Within the context of trusting relationships, adolescents are able to disclose sensitive and personal information, and nurses are able to transmit information, attitudes, and/or skills necessary for adolescents to take health-promoting actions. Three critical elements in establishing trusting relationships are active listening, responding to the adolescent's emotions, and ensuring confidentiality and privacy.

*Active listening* involves seeking to understand what is being said without imposing judgment. It includes paying attention to teenagers' nonverbal cues and noting inconsistencies between verbal and nonverbal communication. Finally, active listening requires listening for understanding rather than truth. For example, when an adolescent states, "My mother hates me," a nurse who is listening for understanding may reply, "That must be very hard for you," rather than "What does your mother do to make you think that?" Listening in order to understand the psychoemotional context of situations can be a difficult skill to master because the cultural milieu in which health care services are provided often encourages "getting just the facts." However, in noncrisis situations this approach is a critical element in encouraging communication and establishing trusting relationships.

*Responding to an adolescent's emotions* includes verbalizing concern about nonverbal cues that are observed. It also involves expressing empathy and support. Furthermore, it includes respecting adolescents' rights and abilities to make decisions and acknowledging potential issues related to developmental stage, cultural and religious values, beliefs and practices, gender, and sexual orientation.

A third critical element in establishing trusting relationships is *ensuring confidentiality and privacy.* (See Critical Thinking Exercise box.) In general, adolescents have the right to confidential communication with providers unless they are being abused or a life-threatening situation arises. Health care providers need to become familiar with the legal rights of adolescent patients in their state as well as their obligations to adolescent patients and families (Center for Continuing Education in Adolescent Health, 1995).

The boundaries around confidentiality and privacy should be established at the beginning of the interview so that adolescents feel that they can discuss sensitive topics. A brief, clear explanation of confidentiality can clarify that most things discussed during the interview will not be shared with others and that life-threatening issues that need to be shared (e.g., report of ongoing abuse, suicidal or

## Critical Thinking Exercise

### Respecting Privacy

Jamie S., a 17-year-old, arrives with her mother for a routine history and physical examination for college entrance. As you are taking Jamie to the examination room, her mother whispers to you, "I need to speak with you in private." What would be your most appropriate response?

FIRST, THINK ABOUT IT . . .

• What concepts or ideas are central to your thinking?
• What precise question are you trying to answer?

1. Ask Jamie to undress to prepare for the examination while you take her mother to another room to find out what's on her mind.
2. Say to Jamie's mother in Jamie's presence, "Mrs. S., whatever you have to say to me, you need to say in front of Jamie."
3. Say to Jamie and her mother. "I would like to begin by speaking with both of you together, then spend some time with just you, Mrs. S., and then with just you, Jamie."
4. Say to Jamie and her mother, "I would like to begin by speaking with both of you together, then spend some time with just you, Jamie, and then with just you, Mrs. S."

*The best response is four. Jamie and her mother need to know ahead of time that they will each have an opportunity to express their concerns in private. Since Jamie is your patient, she should be first, which is a central concept in your thinking. Knowing that her mother will also have an opportunity to express concerns, Jamie will likely be more open and may even say, "I know that my mother will tell you . . ." and address the issue herself. Option one is disrespectful of Jamie, and option two is disrespectful of Jamie's mother and her concerns. Option one is poor for two reasons. First, an explanation of what will occur and the interview should precede getting undressed for an examination. Second, Jamie likely will be aware that you are speaking with her mother, feel that her privacy is being violated, and become defensive and distrustful of both you and her mother. Although response three gives both mother and daughter an opportunity to express concerns, if Mrs. S. goes first, Jamie is likely to spend time trying to draw from you what her mother said and/or become defensive.*

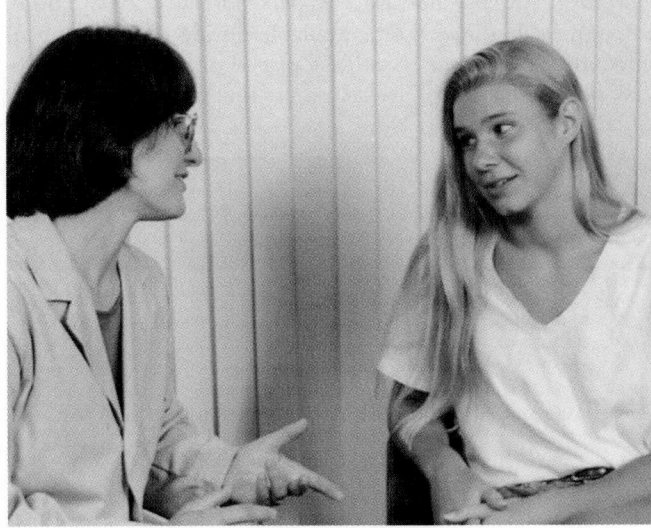

**Fig. 19-13** Most of the health screening interview with the adolescent can be completed with parents out of the room. (From Barkauskas VH and others: *Health and physical assessment,* ed 2, St Louis, 1998, Mosby.)

## GUIDELINES
### Interviewing Adolescents

Ensure confidentiality and privacy; interview adolescent without parents.
Show concern for adolescent's perspective: "First, I'd like to talk about your main concerns" and "I'd like to know what you think is happening."
Offer a nonthreatening explanation for the questions you ask: "I'm going to ask a number of questions to help me better understand your health."
Maintain objectivity; avoid assumptions, judgments, and lectures.
Ask open-ended questions when possible; move to more directive questions if necessary.
Begin with less sensitive issues and proceed to more sensitive ones.
Use language that both the adolescent and you understand.
Restate: reflect back to adolescents what they have said, along with feelings that may be associated with their descriptions.

homicidal plans) will not be shared without the adolescent's prior knowledge. To allow for private conversation, most of the health screening interview can be completed with parents out of the room (Fig. 19-13).

Several other considerations related to the interview process are listed in the Guidelines box. To convey an interest in adolescents' perspectives, interviews can begin by asking teenagers to explain their reasons for the visit. At the beginning of the interview, adolescents should be given a nonthreatening explanation of why questions are asked, such as "I'll be asking you questions, including some that some people find personal or even embarrassing, so that I can better understand your health." To increase adoles-

cents' comfort in disclosing sensitive information, lectures and questions that convey judgmental attitudes should be avoided. Asking open-ended questions and avoiding assumptions (e.g., all teenagers have supportive families, all teenagers are heterosexual) give adolescents opportunities to share more of their psychosocial contexts. Any medical language used during the interview should be clarified, and adolescents should be asked to explain any terms they use that are unfamiliar. Restating issues that adolescents may verbalize during an interview allows for a mutual understanding of their concerns.

**Interview Content.** Reviewing the major morbidities and mortalities of youth reveals that many threats to adolescent health are psychosocial and behavioral in nature. Therefore, given the limited time available during routine clinical encounters, emphasis should be placed on assessment of social, personal, and behavioral factors that underlie the major

threats to the health and well-being of adolescents (Blum and others, 1996). This approach to assessment will help to identify the majority of adolescents who are coping well, those who require simple health information and/or counseling, and those who have significant psychosocial problems requiring referral to appropriate resources.

The mnemonic device **SAFE TIMES** can be used to guide interview questions. As shown in Box 19-1, each letter of this mnemonic device represents an important issue in preventive care. The less sensitive issues are toward the bottom (i.e., safety, education). It is best to begin the interview with less sensitive topics, ending with more sensitive areas such as sexuality.

## Health Concerns of Adolescence

In 1994 the American Medical Association (AMA) issued a comprehensive set of recommendations—*The Guidelines for Adolescent Preventive Services (GAPS)*—intended to provide a framework for providers who have one-on-one contact with adolescents in clinical settings (Elster and Kuznets, 1994). The GAPS recommendations are directed at 14 health topics (Box 19-2). The following discussion is an overview of the GAPS topics and provides specific recommendations related to screening, guidance, and immunizations.

### Parenting and Family Adjustment

Having family members who are emotionally available and appropriately involved in their lives has proved to be a key factor in the well-being of adolescents (Resnick and others, 1997). On the other hand, family dysfunction can be a strong contributor to many adolescent problems, including depression, alcohol and other drug abuse, eating disorders, and school failure. A wide variety of family disorders, including parental discord, alcohol or drug abuse, mental illness, sexual and physical abuse, can lead to additional stresses in teenagers coping with the tasks of adolescence.

Screening questions such as "Who is in your family?" "How are things going at home?" and "Who in your family could you talk with about problems you are having?" help to

---

### Box 19-1 ■ ■ □
### Safe Times: A Method for Health-Screening Interviews with Adolescents

**Note:** In clinical interviewing, SAFE TIMES is best used in reverse order.

**S  SEXUALITY**
  a. Pubertal development, menstrual history (girls)
  b. Extent of sexual activity, type of relationships, symptoms of STDs
  c. Pregnancy and STD prevention methods
  d. Orientation issues (attractions, behaviors)
  e. History of sexual abuse

**A  AFFECT**
  a. Symptoms of depression ("feeling down or blue") or hopelessness ("discouraged about the future")

  **ABUSE**
  a. Use of tobacco, alcohol, marijuana, cocaine, other drugs

**F  FAMILY**
  a. Who the patient lives with and if there are any family conflicts or problems
  b. Family history—medical, psychiatric

**E  EXAMINATION**
  a. Self-breast or self-testicular examination (middle to late adolescence)
  b. Explain pelvic examination (if indicated)

**T  TIMING OF DEVELOPMENT**
  a. For younger adolescents, "Is your development going too fast, too slow, or at about the right speed?" and "Do you feel too tall, too short, or about the right height?"
  b. For all, "Do you feel too thin, too heavy, or about the right weight?"

**I  IMMUNIZATION**
  a. Tetanus-diphtheria (Td) needed every 10 years
  b. Measles-mumps-rubella (MMR) unless two vaccines given during childhood or pregnancy
  c. Hepatitis B if engaging in risk behavior
  d. PPD yearly for high-risk groups
  e. Pneumovax, influenza if chronic disease

**M  MINERALS**
  a. Iron—supplementation required if less than two servings of meats daily or low hemoglobin
  b. Calcium—supplementation required (especially in females) for those who drink less than 2 to 3 glasses of milk daily (e.g., Tums, 3 to 4 tablets daily)
  c. Cholesterol—intake of fats, lipid levels

**E  EDUCATION, EMPLOYMENT**
  a. If in school, what grades attained; any problems?
  b. Work history and future plans

**S  SAFETY**
  a. Especially car safety, use of seat belts, drinking and driving, or accepting rides from drivers using drugs
  b. Motorcycles, mopeds, all-terrain vehicles
  c. Handguns in the home, handgun availability

Modified from Schubiner H: Preventive health screening in adolescent patients, *Prim Care* 16:211-230, 1989.

---

### Box 19-2 ■ ■ □
### Topics for Preventive Health Care of Adolescents

Parenting and family adjustment
Psychosocial adjustment
Risk for intentional and unintentional injury
Dietary habits, eating disorders, and obesity
Physical fitness
Sexual development, sexual orientation, and sexual intercourse
Use of tobacco products
Use of alcohol and other substances
Severe or recurrent depression and suicide
Physical, sexual, and emotional abuse
Learning and school problems
Hypertension
Hyperlipidemia
Infectious diseases

Data from Elster AB, Kuznets NJ: *AMA guidelines for adolescent preventive services (GAPS)*, Baltimore, 1994, Williams & Wilkins.

give a general sense of family relationships. More directed questions that give insight into family functioning include "How does your family generally solve disagreements?" "What are some of the rules in your family related to (areas such as underage drinking, curfew, friends)?" "Who sets these rules?" and "Are you currently having conflicts with your family?"

Many parents are interested, concerned, and involved in the lives of their adolescent. Parents who are appropriately involved serve as an important protective factor in the lives of adolescents, and efforts to exclude parents from adolescent health services are both unrealistic and unwise. What must be sought in providing health care is a balance between the individual adolescent's growing autonomy and the parents' diminishing control over, and responsibility for, the adolescent.

Parents should be offered health guidance at least once during their child's early adolescence, once during middle adolescence, and once during late adolescence (American Medical Association, 1996). Such guidance can include information about normative adolescent development, along with signs and symptoms of troubled adolescents. Parents can be engaged in discussion of parenting behaviors that promote healthy adolescent adjustment, including maintaining open communication, employing age-appropriate limit-setting, monitoring their child's social and recreational activities, and acting as role models for health-enhancing behaviors. Parents should be encouraged to discuss health-related behaviors with their adolescents. (See Family Focus and Community Focus boxes as well as Family Home Care Box on p. 836.)

Generally, if an adolescent is doing well in school, relates well to peers, and is able to resolve areas of conflict with family members, family intervention is not necessary. Nurses can support positive conflict resolution around minor issues between adolescents and their families, such as curfew hours

and appropriate limit-setting. Families dealing with major conflicts or dysfunctional relationships should be referred to a family therapist or other mental health professional.

### Psychosocial Adjustment

As adolescents experience the many changes of adolescence, they redefine who they are and what they want out of life. Most individuals progress through the changes of their adolescent years with minimal amounts of emotional upheaval, countering the belief that this period in life is one of "storm and stress." Some adolescents, however, do have difficulty coping and exhibit emotional distress, especially when multiple normative events happen simultaneously and are combined with nonnormative life events.

Adolescence is characterized by change within multiple domains. Changes associated with pubertal development typically take place during the early adolescent years. Early- and late-maturing adolescents, who feel they are "out of synch" with their age-mates' growth patterns, may have a more difficult time emotionally than those who develop "on time" with their peers. Another normative change, typically occurring during middle adolescence, is the transition from middle or junior high school to high school. With this transition, adolescent concerns often have an increasing emphasis on same- and opposite-sex peer relationships. School transitions may also expose teenagers to social environments that are larger, less individualized, and less capable of providing adult support and supervision. During the period of older adolescence, psychosocial concerns are focused on school achievement and future career plans.

Questions such as "Do you feel that your development is going too fast, too slow, or at about the right speed?" may allow young adolescents to discuss issues related to physical development. Questions about feeling cared for and connected to teachers, counselors, students, and/or other school people, along with questions about their level of involvement in school-related activities, give teenagers an opportunity to talk about strengths and deficits they experience within their school environments. Questions about the quality of peer relationships may help to identify teenagers who feel socially isolated. Finally, questions about future

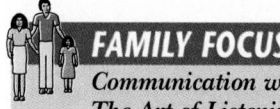

### FAMILY FOCUS
*Communication with Teens: The Art of Listening*

Conflicts between parents and their adolescents are often a result of a very natural characteristic of parenthood: the desire to protect one's offspring—from harm or from simply doing something "stupid," embarrassing, or something they may later regret. Teens sometimes "bounce" their thoughts and ideas off adults. At times they really want some feedback; at other times they simply want to elicit a reaction.

I found it easy to listen openly, thoughtfully, and without interrupting when my teenager's friends discussed troublesome topics. However, one day, when one of my own teenagers had a similar conversation with me, the parent part kicked in. I felt responsible and spoke my piece on the spot. This brought communication to a halt and resulted in defensiveness. It was a long time before my child tried to talk to me about anything controversial again.

The next time one of my teenagers started a similar conversation, I decided to try to trick myself. Throughout the entire conversation, I told myself over and over again to act as if this were not my teenager, but rather someone else's child. I found this actually worked quite well, and I was able to listen without interrupting. I continue to use the system, sometimes with more success than at other times.

Mother of four

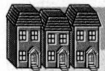

### COMMUNITY FOCUS
*Rules for Adolescents*

U.S. society does little to help adolescents mature and separate. Americans have remarkably few rites of passage that mark the stages of life. Few ceremonies and tests are practiced to determine eligibility for specific adult privileges. Obtaining a driver's license, graduating from high school, and reaching legal age for drinking are among the few that exist. U.S. society also does not have many generally agreed-on social dictums. When is the right age to begin dating? What is a reasonable curfew? Should an 18-year-old be allowed to stay out all night? There are few areas of general agreement. Every family makes up its own rules, influenced, but uninstructed, by the society at large. Many families have great difficulty with this process.

Modified from Prothrow-Stith D: *Deadly consequences: how violence is destroying our teenage population and a plan to begin solving the problem,* New York, 1993, HarperCollins.

plans related to education and employment/career choices may give older youth the chance to talk through significant sources of stress.

As sources of credible information, support, and encouragement, nurses can help adolescents cope with the changes and challenges they face. To promote both emotional health and psychosocial adjustment, nurses and other health care professionals can encourage adolescents to develop (1) skills to cope with stress and change and (2) skills to become involved in personally meaningful activities.

## Intentional and Unintentional Injury

Injuries kill more U.S. adolescents than any other single cause, with unintentional injury, homicide, and suicide accounting for 72% of deaths in teenagers and young adults in 1997 (Centers for Disease Control and Prevention, 2000). (See Childhood Mortality, Chapter 1.) Motor vehicle crashes are the single greatest source of unintentional injury, accounting for 78% of all unintentional injuries in young people (Sells and Blum, 1996). The majority of fatal and nonfatal motor vehicle crashes involve alcohol (Neinstein, 1996). Homicide, a form of intentional injury, is the second leading cause of death (after motor vehicle crashes) among all U.S. adolescents; for African-American teenagers it is the most likely cause of death (Sells and Blum, 1996; National Safety Council, 2000).

In the United States, homicides among teenagers are most likely to involve firearms and to occur among friends or gangs. In 1997, 85.2% of all homicides for persons 15 through 19 years of age were firearm-related (American Academy of Pediatrics, 2000a). In addition to being the leading cause of death, injuries also account for substantial morbidity among youth. The leading causes of injury-related morbidity include vehicular crashes, firearms, drownings, poisonings, burns, and falls (Table 19-2).

---

**TABLE 19-2  Injury prevention during adolescence**

| Developmental Abilities Related to Risk of Injury | Injury Prevention |
|---|---|
| Need for independence and freedom<br>Testing independence<br>Age permitted to drive a motor vehicle (varies)<br>Inclination for risk taking<br>Feeling of indestructibility<br>Need for discharging energy, often at expense of logical thinking and other control mechanisms<br>Strong need for peer approval<br>May attempt hazardous feats<br>Peak incidence for practice and participation in sports<br>Access to more complex tools, objects, and locations<br>Can assume responsibility for own actions | **Motor/nonmotor vehicles**<br>*Pedestrian*—Emphasize and encourage safe pedestrian behavior<br>At night, walk with a friend<br>If someone is following you, go to nearest place with people<br>Do not walk in secluded areas; take well-traveled walkways<br>*Passenger*—Promote appropriate behavior while riding in a motor vehicle<br>*Driver*—Provide competent driver education; encourage judicious use of vehicle, discourage drag racing, "playing chicken"; maintain vehicle in proper condition (brakes, tires, and so on)<br>Teach and promote safety and maintenance of two-wheeled vehicles<br>Promote and encourage wearing of safety apparel such as helmet, long trousers<br>Reinforce the dangers of drugs, including alcohol, when operating a motor vehicle<br>**Drowning**<br>Teach nonswimmer to swim<br>Teach basic rules of water safety<br>    Judicious selection of place to swim<br>    Sufficient water depth for diving<br>    Swimming with companion<br>**Burns**<br>Reinforce proper behavior in areas involving contact with burn hazards (gasoline, electric wires, fires)<br>Advise regarding excessive exposure to natural or artificial sunlight (ultraviolet burn)<br>Discourage smoking<br>Encourage use of sunscreen<br>**Poisoning**<br>Educate in hazards of drug use, including alcohol<br>**Falls**<br>Teach and encourage general safety measures in all activities<br>**Bodily damage**<br>Promote acquisition of proper instruction in sports and use of sports equipment<br>Instruct in safe use of and respect for firearms and other devices with potential danger (e.g., power tools, firecrackers)<br>Provide and encourage use of protective equipment when using potentially hazardous devices<br>Promote access to and/or provision of safe sports and recreational facilities<br>Be alert for signs of depression (potential suicide)<br>Discourage use of and/or availability of hazardous sports equipment (trampoline, surfboards)<br>Instruct regarding proper use of corrective devices such as glasses, contact lenses, hearing aids<br>Encourage and foster judicious application of safety principles and prevention |

In terms of behaviors that increase the risk of unintentional injury, 16% of high school students nationwide report rarely or never using safety belts when riding in a vehicle driven by someone else. When asked about their practices over the past 30 days, one third (33%) of U.S. high school students reported riding with a driver who had been drinking; around 13% of students had driven a vehicle after drinking alcohol. Among students who ride bicycles and motorcycles, 85% and 38%, respectively, stated that they rarely or never wear a helmet (Centers for Disease Control and Prevention, 2000).

Behaviors that contribute to intentional injury are also quite prevalent among young people. For example, 17% of U.S. high school students reported carrying a weapon (e.g., a gun, knife, or club) at some point during the previous month, with 6.9% noting that they carried a weapon on school property during that same time period. Nationwide, 38% of students reported being in a physical fight during the previous year (Centers for Disease Control and Prevention, 2000). Many adolescents have easy access to a gun in their home, and such accessibility is significantly associated with involvement in violent behavior and suicidal thoughts and attempts among adolescents.

During an interview, the segment addressing injury prevention should include screening and counseling related to motor vehicle crashes, firearm use, and suicide. In relation to prevention of motor vehicle injury, one might initially ask how the adolescent "gets around town." Further questions and health education might focus on seat belt and/or helmet use and the practice of drinking and driving or riding with drivers who have been drinking. Adolescents should be asked whether they have access, at home or elsewhere, to firearms; whether they carry a gun; and whether they ever use alcohol or other substances in combination with handling guns.

Health education related to firearm injury prevention should include advising parents to limit their children's household access to firearms, counseling on nonviolent ways to resolve conflicts, and discouraging use of weapons (American Medical Association, 1996).

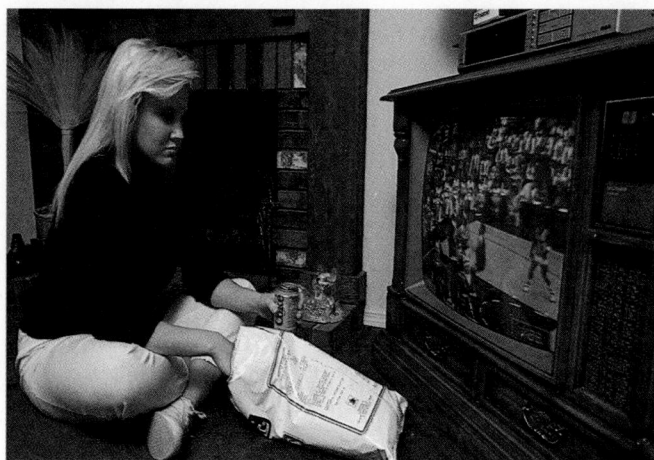

**Fig. 19-14** Snacking on empty calories is common among adolescents, especially during inactivity.

## Dietary Habits, Eating Disorders, and Obesity

Puberty marks the beginning of accelerated physical growth, which can as much as double adolescents' nutritional requirements for iron, calcium, zinc, and protein. At the same time, growing independence, the need for peer acceptability, concern with physical appearance, and an active lifestyle may affect eating habits, food choices, nutrient intake, and thus nutritional status. Although problems related to overt nutritional deficiencies (excluding iron deficiencies) have decreased since the 1940s, they have been replaced by problems of dietary imbalances and excess. Excess intake of calories, sugar, fat, cholesterol, and sodium is common among adolescents and is found in all income and racial/ethnic groups and both genders (Fig. 19-14). Inadequate intake of certain vitamins (folic acid, vitamin $B_6$, vitamin A) and minerals (iron, calcium, zinc) is also evident, particularly among girls and teenagers of low socioeconomic status. In combination with other factors, these dietary patterns could result in increased risk for chronic diseases such as heart disease, osteoporosis, and some types of cancer later in life.

Girls, in particular, may be susceptible to iron deficiency at menarche. Maximum bone mass is also acquired during adolescence; therefore, the calcium deposited during these years determines the risk of osteoporosis.

In terms of weight concerns and weight control behaviors, nearly one third (30%) of U.S. high school students thought they were overweight, with female students (36%) more likely than male students (24%) to describe themselves as overweight. Female students (59%) were also more likely to be currently attempting to lose weight than were male students (26%). Overall, 7.6% of female students and 2.2% of male students reported taking laxatives or vomiting to lose weight (Centers for Disease Control and Prevention, 2000).

Currently in the United States, approximately 18% to 22% of all adolescents are obese, and 22% of adolescent girls and 20% of adolescent boys are considered overweight based on measures of *body mass index (BMI)* (Keller and Stevens, 1996; Neinstein, 1996). Adolescent obesity poses both immediate and long-term problems for adolescents. Anorexia nervosa and bulimia nervosa also commonly occur during the adolescent and young adult years. If left untreated, these disorders, like obesity, can lead to considerable morbidity and mortality. (See Chapter 21 for discussion of obesity and the eating disorders commonly seen in adolescence.)

Routine nutrition screening for all adolescents should include questions about meal patterns, dieting behaviors, consumption of high-fat and high-salt foods, and recent changes in weight. Healthy dietary habits should be discussed with all adolescents, including the benefits of a healthy diet; ways to consume foods rich in calcium, iron, and other vitamins and minerals; and safe weight management.

A screening hemoglobin or hematocrit is recommended at the first encounter with an adolescent, at the end of puberty, or at both screening visits and at the end of pubertal development (Neinstein, 1996). The American Medical Association (1996) recommends annual measures of weight and height, along with calculation and plotting of BMI

| **TABLE 19-3** | Adolescent body mass index percentile rankings | | | | | | | | | |
|---|---|---|---|---|---|---|---|---|---|---|
| | **Males** | | | | | **Females** | | | | |
| Age | 5th | 15th | 50th | 85th | 95th | 5th | 15th | 50th | 85th | 95th |
| 11 | 15 | 16 | 17 | 20 | 24 | 15 | 16 | 18 | 21 | 25 |
| 12 | 15 | 16 | 18 | 21 | 25 | 15 | 16 | 18 | 22 | 26 |
| 13 | 16 | 17 | 19 | 22 | 26 | 15 | 16 | 19 | 23 | 27 |
| 14 | 16 | 17 | 19 | 23 | 27 | 16 | 17 | 19 | 24 | 28 |
| 15 | 17 | 18 | 20 | 24 | 28 | 16 | 17 | 20 | 24 | 29 |
| 16 | 17 | 18 | 21 | 24 | 29 | 16 | 18 | 20 | 25 | 29 |
| 17 | 17 | 19 | 21 | 25 | 29 | 17 | 18 | 20 | 25 | 30 |
| 18 | 18 | 19 | 21 | 26 | 30 | 17 | 18 | 21 | 26 | 30 |

Data from Must A, Dallal G, Deitz W: Reference data for obesity: 85th to 95th percentiles of body mass index (wt/ht$^2$) and triceps skinfold thickness, *Am J Clin Nutr* 53:839-846, 1991.

(BMI equals weight in kilograms divided by the height in meters squared). Reference BMI values for adolescent males and females are listed in Table 19-3. Along with height and weight measurements, an appropriate screening or interview question related to obesity and eating disorders might be "Do you feel that you are too heavy, too thin, or about the right weight?"

Adolescents with a BMI equal to or greater than the 95th percentile for age and gender are overweight and should have an in-depth dietary and health assessment to determine psychosocial effects and risk for future cardiovascular disease. (See Chapter 21 for a comprehensive discussion of the management of obesity.) Adolescents with a BMI between the 85th and 94th percentiles are at risk for becoming overweight. A dietary and health assessment should be performed to determine the risk for psychosocial and physical morbidity if (1) the BMI has increased by 2 or more units during the previous 12 months; (2) there is a family history of premature heart disease, obesity, hypertension, or diabetes mellitus; (3) the adolescent is concerned about weight; or (4) the adolescent has an elevated serum cholesterol level or blood pressure (American Medical Association, 1996). If any of the following risk factors are present, the adolescent should be referred for further assessment of organic disease, anorexia nervosa, or bulimia nervosa: weight loss greater than 10% of previous weight; recurrent dieting when not overweight; use of self-induced emesis, laxatives, starvation, or diuretics to lose weight; distorted body image; or BMI below the 5th percentile for gender and age-group (American Medical Association, 1996).

### Physical Fitness

Nationwide, nearly two thirds (65%) of all high school students reported that they had participated in activities that made them "sweat and breathe hard for at least 20 minutes" (i.e., vigorous physical activity) during 3 or more of the past 7 days. Male students (72%) were more likely than female students (57%) to engage in vigorous physical activity. About 56% of students were enrolled in a school physical education (PE) class; nearly 76% of students enrolled in PE reported exercising for at least 20 minutes during an average PE class (Centers for Disease Control and Prevention, 2000).

High levels of physical activity and fitness may reduce cardiovascular disease risk factors during adolescence, including obesity, high blood pressure, and hyperlipidemia. In addition, routine exercise may reduce adolescents' risk for depression and emotional distress. While only some evidence supports a positive relationship between a person's level of physical activity and fitness during adolescence and this level as an adult, the association between exercise and physical fitness and reduced risk for cardiovascular disease during adulthood is well documented.

Routine screening related to exercise should include questions about frequency, intensity, and type of physical activity. The GAPS recommend that the emotional, social, and physical benefits of exercise be discussed annually with all adolescents. Furthermore, all adolescents should be encouraged to engage in safe exercise on a regular basis (American Medical Association, 1996).

Nurses should encourage all adolescents to be physically active daily, or nearly every day, as part of play, games, sports, work, transportation, recreation, physical education, or other planned exercise. One of the goals of *Healthy People 2010* is to have 85% of adolescents engage in three or more sessions of moderate to vigorous physical activity per week, with each session lasting for 20 minutes (*Healthy People 2010*, 1999).

### Sexual Behavior, Sexually Transmitted Diseases (STDs), and Unintended Pregnancy

Sexual activity has increased among U.S. youth. At the same time, rates of STDs, unintended pregnancy, and human immunodeficiency virus (HIV) infection have also increased among adolescents. Nationwide, half (49.9%) of ninth through twelfth graders reported having had sexual intercourse at some time, and 36% of students reported having had sexual intercourse in the previous 3 months (Centers for Disease Control and Prevention, 2000).

Many sexually active young people are engaging in behaviors that put them at risk for STDs and/or pregnancy, such as having sex with multiple partners and having sex without the use of condoms or other forms of contraception. Approximately 16% of U.S. high school students reported having had four or more sexual partners during their lifetime. Among the sexually active students, slightly over half (58%) reported using a condom during their most recent experience of intercourse, and 16% reported using birth control pills at the time of their most recent experience of intercourse (Centers for Disease Control and Prevention, 2000). The high prevalence of risky sexual behaviors among teenagers contributes to high rates of STDs and pregnancy in this age-group. *Each year* 3 million U.S. adolescents—1 in 6—acquire an STD. About 1 million U.S. adolescents become pregnant each year; about half of these adolescents obtain abortions, and about half of them give birth (Centers for Disease Control and Prevention, 2000).

Obtaining a sexual history can be an important step in promoting sexual health and preventing sexually transmitted infections and unintended pregnancies among young people. Given their sensitive nature, questions about sexuality should be prefaced by an explanation of their purpose and the limits of confidentiality. Initial questions can cover less sensitive topics, such as milestones in pubertal development and, for girls, the menstrual history (including the age at menarche, timing of menstrual cycles, duration of menstrual flow, and symptoms of dysmenorrhea). Questions should also address dating behavior, same- and opposite-gender attractions, and same- and opposite-gender sexual behavior (e.g., "There are many ways people can be sexual with others, such as kissing, touching, and having oral, vaginal, and rectal intercourse. In what ways have you been sexual with others?"). Adolescents should be asked about a history of uninvited or nonconsensual sexual contact (e.g., "Has anyone ever touched you in a way that felt uncomfortable or wrong to you?"). Sexually active youth should be asked about their consistency and motivation to use condoms, oral contraceptives, or other forms of contraception; the number of sexual partners they have had over the past 6 months; and the use of alcohol or other substances in connection with sexual activity. Sexually active adolescents should also be asked about any history of pregnancies or STDs. Sexually active teenagers who reveal a history of physical or sexual abuse, who admit to heavy use of alcohol or other drugs, or who have unstable social or economic support systems should be asked whether they have ever exchanged sex for money, shelter, or drugs.

Sexually active adolescents should be screened for sexually transmitted infections with laboratory tests for gonorrhea, chlamydial infection, and, for females, a Papanicolaou (Pap) test to detect human papilloma virus (HPV) infection or other cervical dysplasia. Both males and females should be evaluated for HPV by visual inspection. Sexually active teenagers should have a serologic test for syphilis if they have lived in an area endemic for syphilis, have had other STDs, have had more than one sexual partner within the last 6 months, have exchanged sex for drugs or money, or are males who have had sex with other males. Adolescents at risk for HIV infection should be offered confidential HIV screening tests. HIV risk status includes a history of injecting drug use (including anabolic steroid injections), having had sexual intercourse in an area with high prevalence of HIV infection, having had other STDs, having had more than one sexual partner in the last 6 months, having exchanged sex for drugs or money, being a male and having

engaged in sex with other males, or having had a sexual partner who is at risk for HIV infection. The frequency of laboratory screening for STDs and HIV will depend on the sexual practices and STD history of individual adolescents (American Medical Association, 1996).

All adolescents should receive health guidance regarding responsible sexual behaviors, including abstinence. Adolescents should receive information on how STDs, including HIV, are transmitted and on possible consequences of infection. Sexually active adolescents should be counseled about ways to reduce their risk of STDs and pregnancy, including limiting the number of sexual partners, using condoms consistently, using appropriate methods of birth control, and avoiding substance use in connection with sexual activity. Counseling should include instruction on how to use condoms and other methods of birth control effectively. Adolescents should receive positive reinforcement for responsible sexual behaviors, including abstinence, consistent condom use, and appropriate use of birth control. Adolescents should also be counseled on ways to reduce their risk of sexual exploitation. Techniques for counseling adolescents to reduce risky sexual behaviors are discussed in detail in Chapter 20.

Gay, lesbian, and bisexual teens are as likely to be sexually active as their heterosexual peers although the age of sexual debut is more likely to be during early adolescence, in part because of a higher risk for sexual abuse (Saewyc and others, 1999; Tonkin, 1999). These youths may engage in heterosexual intercourse in an attempt to "cure" themselves, or as a way to blend in with their peers. This strategy can even include pregnancy and teen parenting, in an attempt to avoid detection as gay, lesbian, or bisexual. Recent studies have found sexual minority teens more likely to be involved in a pregnancy during their adolescent years than their heterosexual peers (Saewyc and others, 1999; Reis and Saewyc, 1999). Nurses need to acknowledge the possibilities of same-gender and bisexual attractions and relationships in their work with adolescents. Screening questions regarding sexual attractions and experiences should be phrased in ways that allow adolescents to discuss same- and opposite-gender attractions, such as using the term "partner" rather than "boyfriend" or "girlfriend." Gay, lesbian, and bisexual adolescents need the same sexuality education and information on pregnancy prevention and STD transmission and prevention that is appropriate for all other adolescents.

## Use of Tobacco, Alcohol, and Other Substances

Statistically, experimentation with substances is common among U.S. adolescents. By the twelfth grade, 80% to 90% of students have used alcohol, 62% have tried cigarettes, and 35% have tried marijuana. Heavy use of alcohol and tobacco is not uncommon; one third of high school seniors report having had five or more drinks in a row over the previous 2 weeks, and 17% to 26% report smoking at least one cigarette per day (Johnston, O'Malley, and Bachman, 1995).

In contemporary U.S. society, tobacco, alcohol, and marijuana may be used by adolescents because these substances provide the adolescent with an opportunity to challenge authority, demonstrate autonomy, gain entry into a peer group, or simply relieve the stresses of growing up. While use may be common among U.S. teenagers, there are substantive, documented consequences of early experimentation with alcohol, tobacco, and other drugs. Drinking and driving is the leading cause of death among teenagers. Persons who begin smoking at younger ages are more likely to become heavier smokers and are at increased risk for illness and death attributable to smoking (Rojas and others, 1998). Substance use has also been implicated with other problem behaviors, such as delinquency, absenteeism, dropping out of school, lower academic achievement, and precocious sexual behavior.

In terms of health screening, adolescents can be asked whether they or their friends have ever used tobacco, alcohol, marijuana, or other substances. They should also be asked about their own current use as well as current use patterns among peers. Practices of drinking and driving or riding with someone who has been drinking should be assessed. If answers to these initial questions indicate some level of problem use, an adolescent should be asked about the amount and frequency of use, frequency of getting "high" or "wasted," use in relation to sexual activity, and difficulties with peers, school, parents, and/or the law in relation to use.

Adolescents who have begun experimenting or who engage in low-level use need to be made aware of other options that can help them achieve the same goals, and of the risks of higher-level use. Furthermore, they need to know the short-term effects of alcohol, tobacco, or other drugs, partic-

ularly in relation to driving and school or work performance. Cessation plans should be discussed with adolescents who use tobacco products. Adolescents whose substance use patterns endanger their health should be referred to an appropriate mental health provider. Chapter 21 includes an in-depth discussion of etiology, prevention strategies, and nursing considerations related to adolescent substance use.

## Depression and Suicide

A national survey of ninth through twelfth grade students found that 36% of the girls and 21% of the boys reported feeling "sad or hopeless almost every day for greater than or equal to 2 weeks in a row" in the past year (Centers for Disease Control and Prevention, 2000) (Fig 19-15). Nearly 20% of ninth through twelfth grade students reported seriously considering suicide during the past year, with female students (25%) being more likely than male students (14%) to have considered a suicide attempt. Around 8% of U.S. high school students reported actually having attempted suicide during the previous 12 months, with girls (11%) being more likely than boys (5.7%) to have attempted suicide (Centers for Disease Control and Prevention, 2000).

A brief psychologic screening is warranted during the course of a routine health visit. Screening for depression or suicidal risk should be done with adolescents who note declining school grades, chronic melancholy, family dysfunction, alcohol or other drug use, gay, lesbian, or bisexual orientation, a history of abuse, or previous suicidal attempts. Most adolescents who are depressed will respond affirmatively to the question "Have you been feeling down or blue lately?" although they may not necessarily "look" depressed. Nonsuicidal adolescents who report commonly feeling "blue," "down," or "depressed" should be referred to a psychologist, psychiatrist, or other mental health professional who works with young people (Elster and Kuznets, 1994).

It is crucial to explore thoughts about and possible plans for suicidal acts with all troubled adolescents. Once an assessment of the immediate risk of suicide is completed, a management scheme can be constructed. If the adolescent has a specific plan, immediate referral for acute intervention with a psychiatrist or other mental health professional is indicated. (See Chapter 21 for further discussion of suicide.)

## Physical, Sexual, and Emotional Abuse

Adolescents who have been physically, sexually, and emotionally abused during childhood or adolescence face challenges to healthy development. In the past two decades, reported cases of physical and sexual abuse have increased dramatically. It is not clear whether this change represents an actual increase in abuse rates or is the result of better reporting. In anonymous school-based surveys of adolescents, the proportion of teens reporting abuse appears to be relatively stable. Approximately 25% of adolescents report having been physically abused by family members. While girls are more likely than boys to report a history of sexual abuse in such surveys, approximately 3% to 5% of boys and 10% to 15% of girls report experiencing sexual abuse by someone outside the family, incest (sexual abuse by a family member), or both types of abuse (Magee and others, 2001).

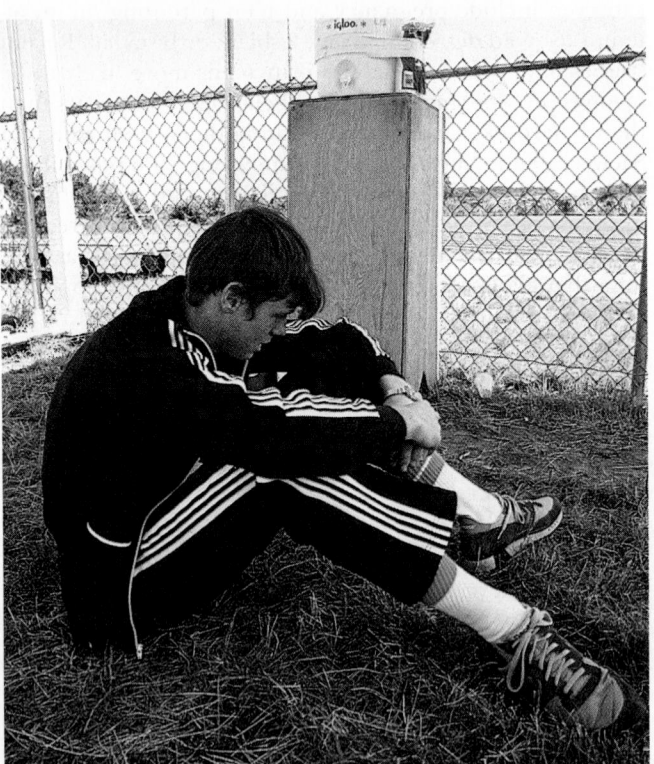

**Fig. 19-15** Adolescents use being alone as a method of coping with stress. Health care professionals need to assess whether this method also indicates an attempt to cope with depression.

Certain groups of adolescents may be especially vulnerable to abuse, such as gay, lesbian, or bisexual youth (Saewyc and others, 1998), or those who are developmentally delayed (Elster and Kuznets, 1994).

A common constellation of symptoms among adolescents who have been victims of sexual abuse includes substance abuse, depression, withdrawn mood, suicidal ideation, and somatic complaints (Frederickson, 1999). Adolescents who have been abused are more likely than non-abused adolescents to engage in health-compromising behaviors such as self-mutilation, suicide attempts, injection drug use, early sexual activity, and prostitution (Neinstein, 1996; Widom and Kuhns, 1996). Adolescents with a history of sexual abuse are more likely to become pregnant or father a child during their teen years (Pierre and others, 1998).

Early identification of abuse can protect adolescents who have been victims of physical, sexual, and emotional trauma. For this reason, questions about abuse should be part of routine adolescent health visits. Privacy should be ensured before inquiring about abuse. If an adolescent reports a history of sexual or physical abuse, further questions should be directed toward assessing for the occurrence of any ongoing abuse, the circumstances surrounding the abuse incident, and the presence of physical, emotional, or behavioral sequelae, including involvement in risk-taking behaviors. Once a history of maltreatment is suspected or proved, health care providers have a legal responsibility to report the case to the appropriate child protection agency (American Medical Association, 1996). The more acute the nature of the problem, the more quickly the report must be made. Adolescents reporting abuse must always be informed about steps in the reporting process before information is disclosed to local authorities.

## School and Learning Problems

In 1996, 10% of U.S. youth dropped out of school before completing high school. Dropout rates vary by ethnicity. In 1990 only 42% of Hispanic teenagers graduated from high school by age 19 years, compared with 61% of black teenagers and 73% of white teenagers (Annie E. Casey Foundation, 1999). Among in-school adolescents, a low grade point average has been associated with higher levels of emotional distress; cigarette, alcohol, and marijuana use; and earlier onset of sexual activity (Neinstein, 1996). School problems and dropping out of school can also be markers for difficulties such as learning disabilities, language barriers, family problems, lack of supportive relationships at school, and employment needs (American Medical Association, 1996). In contemporary U.S. society, education is critical to economic self-sufficiency. Teenagers who drop out of school can expect to earn approximately one third less income each year than those who graduate (Annie E. Casey Foundation, 1999).

Specific questions about recent grades, school absences, suspensions, and any history of repeating a grade in school can be used to screen for school-related problems. Specific management plans for youth who note school problems should be coordinated with school personnel and with the adolescent's parents or caregivers if possible.

## Hypertension

As adolescents experience sexual maturation, along with increases in height and weight, blood pressure increases from the onset of adolescence and continues to rise until the end of pubertal growth. This trend is especially apparent among males (Elster and Kuznets, 1994). Approximately 1% of adolescents have sustained hypertension, defined as a blood pressure greater than the 95th percentile of standards. (See inside back cover and Chapter 34 for an in-depth discussion of hypertension in children and adolescents.) Although sustained hypertension is relatively uncommon, the detection of hypertension during adolescence is important because hypertension is one of the major preventable risk factors for adult cardiovascular disease. To detect early hypertension, blood pressure should be taken on all adolescents annually (American Medical Association, 1996).

## Hyperlipidemia

Along with hypertension, smoking, and obesity, elevated serum cholesterol and triglyceride levels are major risk factors for the development of adult cardiovascular disease. Results of several studies suggest that 23% to 35% of young adolescents have at least one cardiovascular disease risk factor; approximately 5% to 10% have two or more risk factors. Results from other studies indicate that approximately 20% to 30% of children and adolescents have serum cholesterol levels greater than 170 mg/dl, generally considered the upper limit of normal (Elster and Kuznets, 1994; Fox, 2002).

The American Medical Association (1996) recommends that all adolescents over 19 years of age be screened for total blood cholesterol level (nonfasting) at least once. In addition, the GAPS recommend that selected adolescents be screened to determine their risk of developing hyperlipidemia and adult coronary heart disease. These selected categories include (1) adolescents whose parents have a serum cholesterol level greater than 240 mg/dl; (2) adolescents with an unknown family history or adolescents who have a family history of multiple risk factors, such as smoking, hypertension, obesity, diabetes mellitus, and excessive consumption of dietary saturated fats and cholesterol; and (3) adolescents who have a parent or grandparent with coronary artery disease, peripheral vascular disease, cerebrovascular disease, or sudden cardiac death at age 55 or younger.

## Infectious Diseases/Immunizations

Preventable infectious diseases such as measles, mumps, rubella, and hepatitis B can cause significant morbidity and mortality when contracted by adolescents. Adolescents become susceptible to measles, mumps, and rubella if (1) they do not receive the recommended vaccinations, (2) they fail to respond to vaccines administered at the appropriate ages, (3) they receive appropriate vaccines but at too young an age (e.g., measles vaccine before 12 months), or (4) they receive an incomplete series of immunizations (American Academy of Pediatrics, 2000b).

An immunization update is an important part of adolescent preventive care. With the exception of pregnant teenagers, all adolescents should receive a second dose of the *measles-mumps-rubella (MMR) vaccine* unless they have documentation of two MMR vaccinations following the first 12 months of life. All adolescents who have not previously completed the three-dose series of the **hepatitis B (HBV) vaccine** should initiate or complete the series at age 11 to 12 years. The second dose of HBV should be administered at least 1 month after the first dose, and the third dose should be administered at least 4 months after the first dose and at least 2 months after the second dose. (See Immunizations, Chapter 12.) **Hepatitis A vaccine** should be given to adolescents who are traveling or living in countries where the hepatitis A virus is endemic, or in communities with high rates of hepatitis A, those with chronic liver disease, intravenous drug users, or males who have sex with other males. Ideally, all vaccinations should be reviewed, and the necessary vaccines administered at the 11- to 12-year visit (American Academy of Pediatrics, 2000b; American Medical Association, 1996).

Adolescents ages 11 to 12 years and no older than 16 years should receive a booster dose of **diphtheria-tetanus (Td) vaccine** if they have received the primary series of vaccinations and if no dose has been received during the previous 5 years. All subsequent routine Td boosters (i.e., those given in the absence of tetanus-prone injury) should be administered at 10-year intervals. Finally, unvaccinated adolescents who lack a reliable history of chickenpox should receive the **varicella virus vaccine** (American Academy of Pediatrics, 2000b). For adolescents over 13 years, the varicella vaccine is given in two doses 4 or more weeks apart (American Academy of Pediatrics, 2000c).

Adolescents should receive a Mantoux tuberculin skin test if they have been exposed to active **tuberculosis (TB)**, have lived in a homeless shelter, have been incarcerated, have lived in or come from an area with a high prevalence of TB, or currently work in a health care setting. Among adolescents who are at high risk for infection, an induration of 10 mm or more at the skin test site is considered positive. Adolescents with a positive skin test should be referred for evaluation of active TB. The frequency of TB testing depends on the risk factors for the individual adolescent (American Medical Association, 1996).

Adolescents who have chronic disorders or underlying medical conditions that place them at high risk for complications associated with influenza should receive the **influenza vaccine** annually. The **pneumococcal polysaccharide vaccine** should be administered to those adolescents who have chronic illnesses that are associated with an increased risk for pneumococcal disease or its complications (American Academy of Pediatrics, 2000b).

## Health Promotion Among Special Groups of Adolescents

Certain groups of adolescents—including adolescents of color, gay, lesbian, and bisexual youth, and adolescents living in rural areas—experience health problems at disproportionate rates and face barriers to health care because of a lack of financial resources, limited availability of appropriate resources, or other factors.

### Adolescents of Color

Children of color (i.e., children of African-American, Latino-Hispanic, Asian, Native-American, and Alaskan Native descent) are the fastest-growing population within the United States. By 2020 roughly 40% of the U.S. child population will be made up of minorities (Isaacs, 1993). Currently, almost half of African-American children and more than a third of Hispanic children live in families with incomes below the poverty level (Annie E. Casey Foundation, 1999). Large numbers of Native-American children also live in poverty; unemployoment on some reservations is estimated at 80%. The disproportionate levels of health problems experienced by adolescents from these racial, ethnic, and tribal groups can be attributed, at least in part, to the effects of poverty and the lack of access to health care that is associated with being poor.

It must be recognized that most of these children grow and develop normally and successfully meet the challenges of adolescence and young adulthood. Research has begun to identify factors that promote resiliency among minority adolescents from disadvantaged backgrounds, including those who grow up in poverty. Often these young people have come from families and communities that provide nurturing, supportive, and culturally rich environments (Isaacs, 1993). To be most effective, future health promotion interventions must include strategies that increase these protective factors in the lives of other adolescents growing up in high-risk environments.

However, too many minority adolescents experience predictable outcomes associated with living in environments where risk factors disproportionately outweigh protective factors. Higher percentages of minority children and adolescents have learning, emotional, and/or physical disabilities; have higher school dropout rates and fewer opportunities for higher education; become parents at an early age; are incarcerated in youth detention facilities; or die as a result of homicide or unintentional injuries before reaching adulthood. The increase in health risk behaviors during adolescence, in combination with limited access to health care and effective preventive services, places these adolescents at significantly higher risk for adolescent pregnancy, STDs, HIV infection and acquired immunodeficiency syndrome (AIDS), chronic or other infectious diseases (such as hypertension, tuberculosis, and hepatitis), substance abuse, emotional problems, and violence. All of these health problems, which often lead to premature death or chronic disorders, are preventable.

Effective health promotion programs can make important contributions to the prevention of health problems among minority adolescents. There is a growing consensus that health promotion programs will be most effective if they are culturally competent. A **culturally competent approach** is one that both recognizes the importance of culture and incorporates—at all levels—the assessment of relations across cultures, vigilance toward dynamics that result from cultural differences, the expansion of cultural knowledge, and the adaptation of programs to meet culture-specific needs (Schorr, 1997). Nurses, working with other health

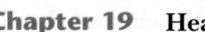

care professionals and community leaders, can develop or adapt culture-specific health promotion interventions. (See Cultural Awareness box.) Several basic principles can be used to guide the development of culturally appropriate health promotion efforts (Isaacs, 1993):

- Health promotion messages can be most effective when they are conveyed through multiple community institutions. The content of these messages should be consistent across agencies, culturally appropriate, and couched in terms that deal with health destructive behaviors in a pragmatic rather than a judgmental manner.
- Health promotion efforts should include involvement of peer groups, schools, communities, and families. In particular, families must be recognized as a positive source of cultural strength, as well as a primary source of information, education, and support for young people. Because "family" is defined differently by different cultures, a culture-specific definition of family must be the basis of developing interventions involving families. For example, prevention strategies that involve concerned relatives and friends have proved to be a highly successful approach to reaching Hispanic youth involved in high-risk behavior. The willingness of family and friends to be involved is rooted in Hispanic values of familialism and community.
- Those who develop strategies for minority adolescents and communities must draw on community-based values, traditions, and customs and work with knowledgeable persons from the community in developing focused interventions and communication channels. The challenge for professionals, many of whom are from other cultures, is to develop collaborative relationships with community members that enable communities to identify health problems and their underlying causes and to design and evaluate programs that address identified needs.
- Health promotion interventions focused on minority adolescents may be most effective if they provide a generic framework and skills for developing relationships and problem solving that can be applied to any health-related decision. There is an emerging belief that this type of generic approach can be more effective than interventions focused on problem-specific entities (such as STDs, pregnancy, and substance use) because the behaviors that lead to many adolescent health problems are highly interrelated.
- Health promotion and prevention strategies must be developed and implemented in places where these adolescents are found.

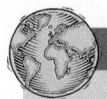

## CULTURAL AWARENESS
### The Adolescent Years

Other societies in which adolescence is seen as part of the life cycle may have ideas very different from American culture about how the adolescent years are to be spent. For example, some societies discourage contact between adolescent males and females. Sexual experimentation is outlawed, and all grown children, males and females, remain in the homes of their parents until they wed. In America we tend to believe that the way our culture is organized is the way all cultures are or should be organized, but, of course, this is not so. Each society is unique. The way we describe adolescence, the way we experience it, and the predisposition of our adolescents toward violence are peculiar to our American culture.

Modified from Prothrow-Stith D: *Deadly consequences: how violence is destroying our teenage population and a plan to begin solving the problem,* New York, 1993, HarperCollins.

Adolescents who have left the school system are often at greater risk for health problems than those who remain in school. Health promotion messages must be incorporated into shelters for homeless and runaway youth, detention centers, residential programs, and community recreation centers to reach young people at highest risk.

To date, there has been little systematic evaluation of the effectiveness of health promotion interventions among minority adolescents. Interventions that work must be documented so that these efforts can be disseminated and adapted for other communities of color.

### Gay, Lesbian, and Bisexual Adolescents

The population of gay, lesbian, and bisexual adolescents has unique developmental issues and health challenges. Although adolescents may participate in same-gender sexual activity or have same-gender attractions, they do not necessarily become gay, lesbian, or bisexual adults. Assigning sexual orientation labels to adolescents is complex and should be approached cautiously, but most studies conclude that between 3% and 10% of adolescents are lesbian or gay and a larger percentage are bisexual in orientation (Bidwell, 1997). Most of the health challenges of sexual minority teens are responses to negative societal attitudes and messages about homosexual or bisexual orientation. The stigma associated with gay, lesbian, or bisexual identity makes adolescents reluctant to acknowledge or identify their orientation to themselves and others. For those who try to manage this stigma by keeping their same-gender attractions hidden, the isolation and fear of disclosure can create emotional distress. They may use alcohol and other substances to escape their anxieties, and they are at much greater risk for suicidal behaviors than their heterosexual peers. In several population-based studies, nearly one third of gay, lesbian, and bisexual adolescents report attempting suicide one or more times (Saewyc and others, 1998; Reis and Saewyc, 1999; Resnick, Borowski, and Ireland, 2000). While nurses should screen all youth about suicidal thoughts and history of suicide attempts, it is especially critical for an adolescent who identifies as gay, lesbian, or bisexual, or one who is questioning his or her orientation.

Publicly disclosing a gay, lesbian, or bisexual orientation during adolescence, "coming out," brings additional challenges. Many adolescents face hostility and even violence from their families when they first come out. Some families physically or sexually assault the adolescent, while others seek psychological counseling or treatment to "change" their teen's orientation (D'Augelli, Hershberger, and Pilkington, 1998). The American Psychological Association and the American Academy of Pediatrics have both issued statements that "reparative therapy," or treatment designed to alter sexual orientation, shows no evidence of effectiveness but does show evidence of psychological harm and is therefore unethical. Some families are so distressed and angry by their teen's disclosure of a homosexual or bisexual identity that they throw the adolescent out of the house. A disproportionate number of homeless and street youth are gay, lesbian, or bisexual (Tonkin, 1999).

Nurses should not encourage teens to disclose their sexual orientation to their families without first forming a safety plan in case the reaction is not supportive. Teenagers who question their sexual orientation should not be reassured that these feelings are only a passing phase. For the majority of young people, referral to an agency providing support services or social opportunities for gay, lesbian, and bisexual adolescents is appropriate. In addition, parents who seek assistance in adjusting to their son or daughter's disclosure can be referred to a local chapter of Parents and Friends of Lesbians and Gays (PFLAG), which provides information and support for parents and family members.

Teens who acknowledge same-gender attractions or relationships are also at risk for violence and harassment from schoolmates, neighbors, and even strangers. Gay, lesbian, and bisexual adolescents who are homeless face additional risks of physical and sexual violence. They may be forced to exchange sex for shelter, food, or to avoid assault and may not be able to negotiate safe sex practices. As a result, they may be at increased risk for sexual abuse, STDs, and pregnancy.

Given their pervasive experiences of negative attitudes and potential violence, sexual minority adolescents may fear similar uncaring attitudes among health care providers and might avoid disclosing their orientation during health assessments. Many gay, lesbian, and bisexual adolescents have experienced insensitive behaviors from health care providers, and they may avoid needed health care as a result (Ryan and Futterman, 1997). In order to provide sensitive, professional care for gay, lesbian, and bisexual adolescents, nurses should be sensitive to their choice of language and be nonjudgmental and caring in their communication. Placing a poster or brochure about local services for gay, lesbian, and bisexual youth in a prominent position in the clinic setting sends the message it is safe to talk about such issues at the clinic. Health professionals who work with teenagers regarding sexual orientation issues are encouraged to seek out additional information and resources that address health needs and services for gay, lesbian, and bisexual adolescents (Ryan and Futterman, 1997).

## Rural Adolescents

Outside of higher rates of accidental injuries (caused in part to farm injuries) and lower rates of delinquency, there are few known differences in the health problems of rural and urban adolescents. Research on the health status of rural adolescents is limited, but rural adolescents experience many of the same health problems as adolescents in metropolitan areas. However, rural adolescents face barriers to health promotion, because they have more limited access to appropriate health care services.

Rural adolescents' access to health care is limited by shortages of professionally staffed mental and physical health services, inadequately trained providers, transportation problems, and less access to Medicaid in rural states. Rural communities often lack adequately trained nurses, physicians, dentists, psychologists, social workers, and allied health professionals, in addition to modern equipment. Rural health professionals often feel inadequately prepared to address physical and psychosocial health issues of adolescents.

In metropolitan areas providers who are unwilling or unable to address adolescents' concerns can refer to colleagues with expertise in adolescent health issues. The absence of adolescent health specialists, combined with a limited network of agencies focused on adolescent health promotion, exacerbates rural youth's problems concerning access to appropriate services. Finally, rural adolescents who live in poverty are less likely than their urban low-income counterparts to be covered by Medicaid and to have financial coverage for health care services.

In addition to health promotion topics addressed with other populations of adolescents, prevention efforts focused on rural adolescents must include efforts to improve the safety of farm machinery and farming practices. Innovative efforts are needed to increase rural adolescents' access to health care services, including development and funding for school-linked health services, improvements in transportation, use of nonprofessionals and adult community members, better dissemination of information about avail-

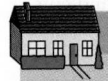

## FAMILY HOME CARE
### Guidance During Adolescence

**ENCOURAGE PARENTS TO:**

Accept adolescent as a unique individual.
Respect adolescent's ideas, likes and dislikes, and wishes.
Be involved with school functions and attend adolescent's performances, whether it be a sporting event or a school play.
Listen and try to be open to adolescent's views, even when they disagree with parental views.
Avoid criticism about no-win topics.
Provide opportunity for choosing options and accept natural consequences of these choices.
Allow young person to learn by doing, even when choices and methods differ from those of adults.
Provide adolescent with clear, reasonable limits.
Clarify house rules and consequences for breaking them.
Let society's rules and consequences teach responsibility outside the home.
Allow increasing independence within limitations of safety and well-being.
Be available but avoid pressing teen too far.
Respect adolescent's privacy.
Try to share adolescent's feelings of joy or sorrow.
Respond to feelings as well as words.
Be available to answer questions, give information, and provide companionship.
Try to make communication clear.
Avoid comparisons with siblings.
Assist adolescent in selecting appropriate career goals and preparing for adult role.
Welcome adolescent's friends into the home and treat them with respect.
Provide unconditional love.
Be willing to apologize when mistaken.

**BE AWARE THAT ADOLESCENTS:**

Are subject to turbulent, unpredictable behavior.
Are struggling for independence.
Are extremely sensitive to feelings and behaviors that affect them.
May receive a different message than what was sent.
Consider friends extremely important.
Have a strong need "to belong."

ability of local health services, and access to further education in adolescent health for health care providers.

## Nursing Considerations

With continued increases in the numbers of adolescents in the United States and rising rates of health-related problems of youth, there is an unprecedented need for adolescent health promotion. Nursing professionals can make significant contributions to health promotion among adolescents and their families. Because nurses understand the biologic, cognitive, psychosocial, and social transitions of adolescence and their impact on health behavior, they can address the developmental and health needs of adolescents. Working with colleagues from other disciplines, community members, parents, and adolescents themselves, nurses must be-

come part of comprehensive approach that delivers consistent messages across clinical, school, and community-based settings. Nurses should be at the forefront of developing and disseminating culturally appropriate health promotion interventions among special populations, including adolescents of color, gay, lesbian, and bisexual youths, and rural teenagers.

The parents of the adolescent are often confused and perplexed about the changes and behaviors of adolescence. They need support and guidance to help them through this time. They need to understand the changes taking place and to accept the expected behaviors that accompany the process of detachment, to be prepared to "let go," and to promote the changed relationship from one of dependency to one of mutuality. Suggestions for anticipatory guidance of parents of adolescents are listed in the Family Home Care box.

## KEY POINTS

- Adolescence is characterized by important biologic, cognitive, psychologic, and social change.
- The biologic events of puberty result in hormonal changes; changes in height, weight, strength and endurance; and development of secondary sex characteristics.
- During adolescence most individuals move from patterns of concrete thinking to abstract, hypothetical thinking.
- Major psychologic tasks of adolescence involve establishing a sense of identity along with behavioral, emotional, and value autonomy.
- According to Kohlberg's theory of moral development, adolescents begin to question existing moral values and learn to make choices. Gilligan observed differences in the way males and females make moral decisions.
- Spiritual development is characterized by the questioning of family values and ideals, a move to more philosophical thinking, and emphasis on personal religion.
- As adolescents establish identities separate from parents and families, relationships with peers often become more important.

- Biologic cognitive and psychosocial changes all affect sexual activity and sexual identity development of adolescents.
- Gay, lesbian, and bisexual youth have unique issues to cope with in identity formation.
- The three primary causes of death during adolescence are injuries, homicide, and suicide.
- Motor vehicle injuries and drowning are the greatest causes of mortality from unintentional injuries in this age-group.
- Major causes of adolescent morbidity include injury, sexually transmitted diseases, unintended pregnancy, and mental health problems, including depression, chronic illness, and eating disorders.
- To be most effective, adolescent health promotion efforts must actively involve teenagers at all stages.
- The availability of confidential health services is particularly important to adolescents.
- Certain groups of adolescents, including youth of color, rural youth, and gay, lesbian, and bisexual youth, experience health problems at disproportionate rates and face barriers to health care because of limited access to appropriate affordable resources.

## REFERENCES

American Academy of Pediatrics, Committee on Infectious Diseases: Recommended childhood immunization schedule—United States, January—December 2000, *Pediatrics* 105(1):148, 2000c.

American Academy of Pediatrics, Committee on Infectious Diseases: *Red book: report of the Committee on Infectious Diseases,* ed 25, Elk Grove Village, IL, 2000b, The Academy.

American Academy of Pediatrics, Committee on Injury and Poison Prevention: Firearm-related injuries affecting the pediatric population, *Pediatrics* 105(4):888-895, 2000a.

American Medical Association: *Guidelines for adolescent preventive services,* ed 3, Chicago, 1996, The Association.

Annie E Casey Foundation and the Center for the Study of Social Policy: *KIDS COUNT data book: state profiles of child well-being,* Washington, DC, 1999, Center for the Study of Social Policy.

Bensussen-Walls W, Saewyc, EM: Teen-focused vs adult-focused prenatal care models for high-risk pregnant adolescents *Public Health Nurs* 18(6):424-435, 2001.

Bidwell RJ: Homosexuality: challenges of treating lesbian and gay adolescents. In

Hoekelman RA and others, editors: *Primary pediatric care,* ed 3, St Louis, 1997, Mosby.

Blum RW and others: American Indian–Alaska Native youth health, *JAMA* 267(12):1637-1644, 1992.

Blum RW and others: Don't ask, they wouldn't tell: the quality of adolescent health screening in five practice settings, *Am J Pub Health* 86(12):1767-1772, 1996.

Blum RW and others: The effects of race/ethnicity, income, and family structure on adolescent risk behaviors, *Am J Pub Health* 90(12):1879-1884, 2000.

Bronfenbrenner U: *The ecology of human development,* Cambridge, MA, 1979, Harvard University Press.

Centers for Disease Control and Prevention: Youth Risk Behavior Surveillance—United States, 1999, *MMWR* 49(SS-5):1-94, 2000.

Center for Continuing Education in Adolescent Health: *National state minor consent statutes: a summary,* Cincinnati, 1995, Division of Adolescent Medicine, Children's Hospital Medical Center.

D'Augelli AR, Hershberger SL, Pilkington NW: Lesbian, gay, and bisexual youth and their families: disclosure of sexual orientation and its consequences, *Am J Orthopsychiat* 68(3):361-371, 1998.

Diamond LM: Development of sexual orientation among adolescent and young adult women. *Dev Psychol* 34(5):1085-1095, 1998.

Doswell WM and others: Self-image and self-esteem in African-American preteen girls: implications for mental health, *Issues Mental Health Nurs* 19(1):71-94, 1998

Elkind D: Understanding the young adolescent, *Adolescence* 13:128-134, 1978.

Elster AB, Kuznets NJ: *AMA guidelines for adolescent preventive services,* Baltimore, 1994, Williams & Wilkins.

Erikson E: *Identity: youth in crisis,* New York, 1968, WW Norton.

Fox JA: *Primary health care of infants, children, and adolescents,* St Louis, 2002, Mosby.

Frederickson D: Maltreatment of children, *Child Family Nurs* 2(6):393-401, 1999.

Gilligan C: *In a different voice,* 1982, Cambridge, MA, 1982, Harvard University.

Gilligan C: *Adolescent development reconsidered,* Paper presented at the Invitational Conference on Health Futures of Adolescents, Daytona Beach, FL, 1986.

Ginsburg KR, Menapace AS, Slap GB: Factors affecting the decision to seek health care: the voice of adolescents, *Pediatrics* 100(6):922-930, 1997.

Gottfried AE, Gottfried AW: *Redefining families: implications for children's development.* New York, 1994, Plenum Press.

Hardy JB and others: Self-sufficiency at ages 27 to 33 years: factors present between birth and 18 years that predict educational attainment among children born to inner-city families, *Pediatrics* 99(1):80-87, 1997.

Harter S: Self and identity development. In Feldman S, Elliott G, editors: *At the threshold: the developing adolescent,* Cambridge, MA, 1990, Harvard University Press.

*Healthy People 2010, Fed Register* 64(44):11011-11012, 1999.

Irwin CE: *Toward a new health behavior model for adolescents,* Chicago, 1976, Society for Adolescent Medicine.

Isaacs M: Developing culturally competent strategies for adolescents of color. In Elster A, Panzarine S, Holt K, editors: *American Medical Association State of the Art Conference on Adolescent Health Promotion: proceedings,* Arlington, VA, 1993, National Center for Education in Maternal and Child Health.

Johnston LD, O'Malley PM, Bachman JG: *National survey results on drug use from Monitoring the Future study, 1975-1994,* NIH Pub No 95-4026, Washington, DC, 1995, National Institutes of Health.

Kann L and others: Youth risk behavior surveillance—United States, 1995, *J Sch Health* 66(10):365-377, 1996.

Keller C, Stevens KR: Assessment, etiology and intervention in obesity in children, *Nurse Pract* 21(9):31-42, 1996.

Kohlberg L, Gilligan C: The adolescent as philosopher: the discovery of the self in a post-conventional world. In Kagan J, Coles R, editors: *Twelve to sixteen: early adolescence,* New York, 1972, WW Norton.

Lapsley, DK: Toward an integrated theory of adolescent ego development: the "new look" at adolescent egocentrism, *Am J Orthopsychiat* 63(4):562-571, 1993.

Magee LL and others: *Family environment correlates of sexually abused adolescents in a school-based population,* Paper presented at Society for Adolescent Medicine, San Diego, March 21, 2001.

Marcia J: Development and validation of ego identity status, *J Pers Soc Psychol* 3(5):551-558, 1966.

Marsh CL: To be thin is in: or is it? Recognizing and measuring adolescent eating disorders, *J Child Fam Nurs* 2(6):447-452, 1999.

National Safety Council: *Injury facts,* Itaska, Il, 2000, The Council.

Neinstein L: *Adolescent health care: a practical guide,* ed 3, Baltimore, 1996, Williams & Wilkins.

Perry C, Kelder S, Komro K: The social world of adolescents: family, peers, schools, and the community. In Millstein S, Petersen A, Nightingale E, editors: *Promoting the health of adolescents: new directions for the twenty-first century,* New York, 1993, Oxford University Press.

Piaget J: Intellectual evolution from adolescence to adulthood, *Hum Dev* 15:1-12, 1972.

Pierre N and others: Adolescent males involved in pregnancy: associations of forced sexual contact and risk behaviors, *J Adoles Health* 23(6):362-369, 1998.

Reis E, Saewyc EM: *83,000 youth: selected findings of eight population-based studies as they pertain to anti-gay harassment and the safety and well-being of sexual minority students,* Seattle, WA, 1999, Safe Schools Coalition of Washington.

Resnick MD and others: Protecting adolescents from harm: findings from the National Longitudinal Study of Adolescent Health, *JAMA* 278(10):823-831, 1997.

Resnick MD, Borowski I, Ireland M: Suicide risk and protective factors in youth reporting same-gender attractions, *J Adoles Health* 25:86, 2000.

Rojas NL and others: Nicotine dependence among adolescent smokers, *Arch Pediatr Adoles Med* 152(2):151-156, 1998.

Rosario M and others: The psychosexual development of urban lesbian, gay, and bisexual youth, *J Sex Res* 33:113-126, 1996.

Rosenfeld SL and others: Youth perceptions of comprehensive adolescent health services through the Boston HAPPENS program, *J Pediatr Health Care* 14(2):60-67, 2000.

Russell ST, Seif H, Truong N: School outcomes of sexual minority youth in the United States: evidence from a national study, *J Adoles Health* 24(1):111-127, 2001.

Ryan C, Futterman D: *Lesbian and gay youth: care and counseling,* New York, 1997, Columbia University Press.

Saewyc EM and others: The intersection of racial, gender and orientation harassment in school and health risk behaviors among adolescents, *J Adoles Health* 25:148, 2000.

Saewyc EM and others: Gender differences in health and risk behaviors among bisexual and homosexual adolescents, *J Adoles Health* 23(3):181-188, 1998.

Saewyc EM and others: Sexual intercourse, abuse and pregnancy among adolescent women: does sexual orientation make a difference? *Family Plan Persp* 31(3):127-131, 1999.

Schorr LB: *Common purpose: strengthening families and neighborhoods to rebuild America,* New York, 1997, Anchor Books.

Sells CW, Blum RW: Morbidity and mortality among US adolescents: an overview of data and trends, *Am J Public Health* 86(4):513-519, 1996.

Selman R: Toward a structural analysis of developing interpersonal relations concepts: research with normal and disturbed preadolescent boys. In Pick A, editor: *Minnesota symposia of child psychology,* vol 10, Minneapolis, 1976, University of Minnesota Press.

Steinberg L: Autonomy, conflict and harmony in the family relationship. In Feldman S, Elliot G, editors: *At the threshold: the developing adolescent,* Cambridge, MA, 1989, Harvard University Press.

Sullivan H: *The interpersonal theory of psychiatry,* New York, 1953, WW Norton.

Tonkin R: *Being out—lesbian, gay, bisexual, and transgender youth in BC: an adolescent health survey,* Burnaby, British Columbia, 1999, McCreary Centre Society.

Tuttle J and others: Teen club: a nursing intervention for reducing risk-taking behavior and improving well-being in female African-American adolescents, *J Pediatr Health Care* 14(3):103-108, 2000.

Vessey JA, Miola ES: Teaching adolescents self-advocacy skills, *Pediatr Nurs* 23(1):53-56, 1997.

Walker L, de Vries B, Trevethan S: Moral stages and moral orientations in real-life and hypothetical dilemmas, *Child Dev* 58:842-858, 1987.

Widom C, Kuhns J: Childhood victimization and subsequent risk for promiscuity, prostitution and teen pregnancy: a prospective study, *Am J Public Health* 86(11):1607-1611, 1996.

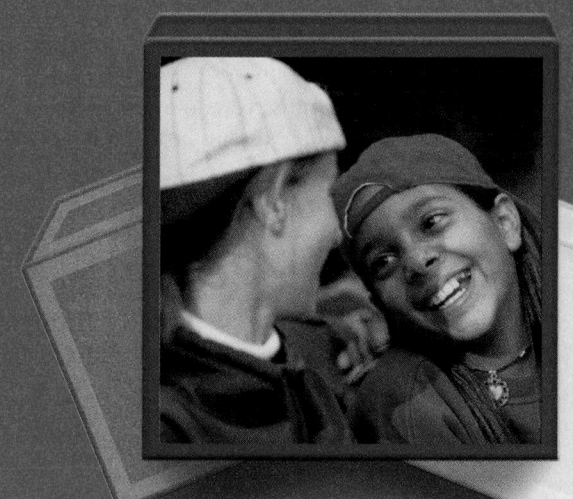

# Chapter 20

# Physical Health Problems of Adolescence

## Chapter Outline

COMMON HEALTH CONCERNS OF ADOLESCENCE, 839
Acne, 839
Vision Changes, 842
HEALTH PROBLEMS OF THE MALE REPRODUCTIVE SYSTEM, 842
Penile Problems, 842
Testicular Tumors, 843
Varicocele, 843
Epididymitis, 844
Testicular Torsion, 844
Gynecomastia, 844
HEALTH PROBLEMS OF THE FEMALE REPRODUCTIVE SYSTEM, 844
Gynecologic Examination, 844
Menstrual Disorders, 845
 Primary Amenorrhea, 845
 Secondary Amenorrhea, 845

Menstrual Irregularities in the Female
 Athlete, 846
Dysmenorrhea, 846
Endometriosis, 847
Premenstrual Syndrome (PMS), 847
Dysfunctional Uterine Bleeding (DUB), 848
Vaginitis and Vulvitis (Vulvovaginitis), 848
HEALTH PROBLEMS RELATED TO SEXUALITY, 849
Adolescent Pregnancy, 850
 Medical Aspects, 850
 Complications of Pregnancy, 850
 Causal Factors, 851
 Social and Economic Aspects, 851
 Mother-Infant Relationship, 851
 Adolescent Fathers, 852
Adolescent Abortion, 853
Contraception, 854

Contraceptive Methods, 854
Use of Contraception, 855
Rape, 858
 Assailants, 858
SEXUALLY TRANSMITTED DISEASES (STDs), 860
Gonorrhea, 861
Chlamydial Infection, 862
Pelvic Inflammatory Disease (PID), 863
Human Papillomavirus (HPV), 864
Human Immunodeficiency Virus (HIV) Infection and Acquired Immunodeficiency Syndrome (AIDS), 864
Hepatitis B Virus (HBV), 865
Other Sexually Transmitted Genital Lesions, 865
Nursing Considerations, 866

## Related Topics

Behavioral Health Problems of Adolescence,
 Ch. 21
Disorders Affecting the Skin, Ch. 18

Genitalia (Examination), Ch. 7
Health Promotion of the Adolescent and
 Family, Ch. 19

Infection Control, Ch. 27
Precocious Puberty, Ch. 38

## COMMON HEALTH CONCERNS OF ADOLESCENCE

### Acne

Adolescents are subject to the same skin conditions that affect the school-age child, such as bacterial, viral, and fungal infections; contact dermatitis; and drug reactions. However, one skin disorder, although not limited to the adolescent age-group, appears predominantly at this time—acne vulgaris (common acne). Acne is the most common skin problem treated by physicians (Laude, 2000). Acne involves

anatomic, physiologic, biochemical, genetic, immunologic, and psychologic factors of significant importance.

Over half of the adolescent population will have had acne by the end of the teenage years, and many children have evidence of the disorder before the age of 10. The peak incidence is in mid to late adolescence, at age 16 to 17 in females and 17 to 18 in males. The disorder is more common in males than in females. After this age period the disease usually decreases in severity, but it may persist well into adulthood. Early acne occurs in the midface region (midforehead, nose, and chin) and later spreads to the lateral cheeks, lower jaw, back, and chest. The degree to which an individual is affected may range from nothing more than a few iso-

■ Linda M. Kollar, MSN, RN, revised this chapter.

lated comedones to a severe inflammatory reaction. Although the disease is self-limited and is not life-threatening, its significance to the affected adolescent is great, and it is a mistake to underestimate the impact that it has on teens.

### Etiology

Numerous factors affect the development and course of acne. Research has shown a familial aspect to acne vulgaris, with a high concordance of severe acne and increased sebum secretion among monozygotic twins. Forty-five percent of adolescent males with acne have a positive family history, as compared with only 8% of adolescent males exhibiting no acne with a positive family history. Premenstrual flares of acne occur in nearly 70% of females, suggesting a hormonal cause. Scientific studies do not demonstrate a clear association between stress and acne; however, adolescents commonly cite stress as a cause for acne outbreaks. Cosmetics containing lanolin, petrolatum, vegetable oils, lauryl alcohol, butylstearate, and oleic acid can increase comedone production. Exposure to oils in cooking grease can be a precursor to acne in adolescents working over fast-food restaurant hot oils. There is no known link between dietary intake and the development or worsening of acne lesions (Kaminer and Gilchrest, 1995).

### Pathophysiology

Acne is a disease that involves the *pilosebaceous unit,* which consists of the sebaceous glands and hair follicles. Acne is most commonly found on the face, chest, upper back, and neck because of the large quantity of sebaceous glands located on these skin areas. There are nearly 900 glands per square centimeter on the skin surfaces of the face, chest, neck, and upper back as compared with 100 glands per square centimeter on the rest of the body (Leyden, 1995). There are three pathophysiologic factors that have the greatest influence on acne development: excessive sebum production, comedogenesis, and the overgrowth of *Propionibacterium acnes* (Mancini, 2000).

Increased sebum production begins at the time of adrenocortical maturation and subtly continues to increase

until the late teens. Acne severity is proportional to the sebum secretion rate, which is genetically determined.

Comedogenesis (formation of comedones) results in a noninflammatory lesion that may be either an open comedone (blackhead) or a closed comedone (whitehead). Inflammation occurs with the proliferation of *P. acnes*, which draws in neutrophils causing inflammatory papules, pustules, nodules, and cysts (Fig. 20-1). The traditional ice pick scarring results from macrophages that digest the inflamed skin as well as the normal dermis in the process.

### Psychosocial Ramifications

Adolescents are acutely aware of their physical appearance, and their cognitive development results in the feeling that they are constantly on stage. In a recent survey, one third of the teenagers reported that pimples were the first thing people noticed about them when looking at them. Even mild acne can result in significant concern for the adolescent; moderate to severe acne lesions can result in negative effects on self-esteem. A 1998 survey of teens with noncystic acne revealed high rates of clinical depression with a 5.6% rate of suicidal ideation (Gupta and Gupta, 1998).

### Therapeutic Management

Successful management of acne depends on a cooperative effort between the care provider, the adolescent, and the parents. The care provider must understand the adolescent's goals and their understanding of the cause of acne. Unlike many dermatologic conditions, the acne lesions resolve slowly, and improvement may not be apparent for at least 6 weeks. Individual comedones may take several weeks to months to resolve, and papules and pustules usually resolve in about 1 week.

The multifactorial causes of acne necessitate a combined approach for successful treatment. Treatment consists of general measures of care and specific treatments determined by the type of lesions involved.

**General Measures.** An overall explanation of the disease process and the plan of care is given to the adolescent, with emphasis on the requirements of the adolescent. Parents should be present at the time of the initial discussion to ensure their cooperation, understanding, and support. Adolescents should be reminded that acne occurs, to some degree, in almost all teenagers.

Improvement of the adolescent's overall health status is part of the general management. Adequate rest, moderate exercise, a well-balanced diet, reduction of emotional stress, and elimination of any foci of infection are all part of general health promotion.

**Cleansing.** Acne is not caused by dirt or oil on the surface of the skin. Gentle cleansing with a mild cleanser once or twice daily is usually sufficient. Antibacterial soaps are ineffective and may be drying when used in combination with topical acne medications. For some adolescents, hygiene of the hair and scalp appears to be related to the clinical activity of acne. Acne on the forehead may improve with brushing the hair away from the forehead and more frequent shampooing.

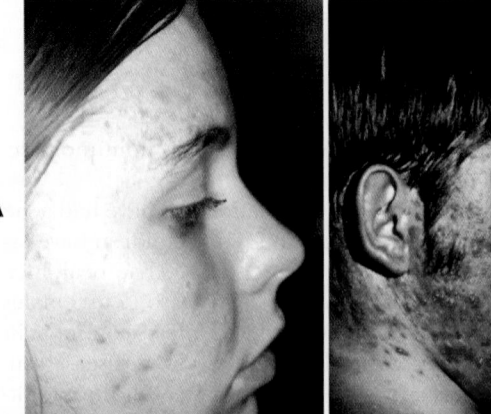

**A**　　　　　　　　　　　　　　　　　　　　　　**B**

**Fig. 20-1**　Acne vulgaris. **A,** Comedones with a few inflammatory pustules. **B,** Papulopustular acne. (From Weston WL, Lane AT: *Color textbook of pediatric dermatology,* St Louis, 1991, Mosby.)

## Medications

Treatment success depends on commitment from the adolescent. Before prescribing treatment, the adolescent's level of comfort and readiness to begin treatment should be determined. Discussion about acne treatment should begin in early puberty. In young girls, the early development of acne is the best predictor of future severe acne (Lucky and others, 1997). Early intervention, most often with topical medications, may prevent the development of more severe acne.

*Tretinoin (Retin-A)* is the only drug that effectively interrupts the abnormal follicular keratinization that produces microcomedones, the invisible precursors of the visible comedones. Tretinoin alone is usually sufficient for management of comedonal acne (Russell, 2000). Tretinoin is available as a cream, gel, or liquid. The cream is less irritating than the gel, which is less irritating than the liquid. Tretinoin can be extremely irritating to the skin and requires careful patient education for optimum product usage. The patient should be instructed to begin with a pea-sized dot of medication, which is divided into the three main areas of the face and then gently rubbed into each area. The medication should not be applied until at least 20 to 30 minutes after washing to decrease the burning sensation. The avoidance of sun and the need for daily use of a sunscreen must be emphasized, because sun exposure may easily result in severe sunburn. Adolescents should be advised to apply the medication at night and to use a sunscreen with a sun protective factor (SPF) of at least 15 in the daytime. Affected teenagers are also instructed to employ other measures to minimize sun exposure, such as wearing a hat or sun visor, to reduce exposure to potentially harmful ultraviolet rays. (See Sunburn, Chapter 18.)

Topical *benzoyl peroxide* is an antibacterial agent that inhibits the growth of *P. acnes*. Benzoyl peroxide is effective against both inflammatory and noninflammatory acne and is an effective first-line agent. The medication is available as a cream, lotion, gel, or wash. Using benzoyl peroxide is less likely to result in the development of antibiotic-resistant strains of *P. acnes*. The convenient dosing increases patient compliance with the regimen (Laude, 2000). Patient education should include information regarding the bleaching effect on sheets, bedclothes, and towels. The adolescent can be reassured that skin bleaching will not occur. Accommodation to the medication can be gained with gradual increases in strength and frequency of application.

When inflammatory lesions accompany the comedones, a *topical antibacterial agent* may be prescribed. These treatments are used to prevent new lesions, as well as to treat pre-existing acne. Clindamycin, erythromycin metronidazole, azelaic acid, and the combination of either benzoyl peroxide and erythromycin (Benzamycin) or benzoyl peroxide and glycolic acid are all choices for topical therapy (Leyden, 1997). The combination of 5% benzoyl peroxide and 3% erthromycin (Benzamycin) is especially beneficial in the treatment of acne although the exact mechanism of action is not clearly understood (Burkhart, Specht, and Neckers, 2000). Tretinoin improves the penetration of these topical agents. Combination therapy with tretinoin and an antibacterial treatment is the only means to address three of the pathogenic causes of acne: keratinization, *P. acnes,* and inflammation (Laude, 2000).

*Systemic antibiotic therapy* is initiated when moderate to severe acne does not respond to topical treatments. The foundation for using systemic antibiotics in acne treatment has been the elimination of the inflammatory effects of *P. acnes* by suppressing the bacteria. Researchers have established that the inflammatory potential may be eradicated through nonlethal means at the cellular level (Webster, 1995). Oral antibiotics are considered extremely safe even when given for years as part of acne treatment. Tetracycline, erythromycin, minocycline, doxycycline, clindamycin, and trimethoprim-sulfamethoxazole are all successful oral antibiotics used to treat acne (Leyden, 1997). They are relatively free of side effects with the exception of occasional gastrointestinal upset or vaginal candidiasis. Minocycline is more expensive but is less likely to cause gastrointestinal side effects and is very effective against severe inflammatory acne. Resistance to antibiotics may develop, especially with tetracycline and erythromycin. Resistance can be prevented with judicious use of oral antibiotics. Providers should avoid use of multiple antibiotic classes and shorten the course by using the full dose of systemic antibiotics for 1 month and then begin a taper. The adolescent can then be maintained on topical treatment (Mancini, 2000).

Females with mild to moderate acne may respond to topical treatment and the addition of an *oral contraceptive pill (OCP)*. Oral contraceptive pills reduce the endogenous androgen production and decrease the bioavailability of the woman's circulating androgens. Studies have indicated that combination oral contraceptive pills containing levonorgestrel, gestodene, and desogestrel as the progestin have decreased acne in women (Stevenson, 1998). Ethinyl estradiol with norgestimate (Ortho Tri-Cyclen) has been approved by the FDA for the treatment of acne in women over 14 years of age.

*Isotretinoin 12-cis-retinoic acid (Accutane),* a very potent and effective oral agent, is reserved for severe, cystic acne that has not responded to other treatments. Isotretinoin is the only agent available that affects all factors in the development of acne (Laude, 2000). However, treatment with isotretinoin should be managed *only* by a dermatologist. Adolescents with multiple, active, deep dermal, or subcutaneous cystic and nodular acne lesions are treated for 20 weeks. Long-term remissions occur with this highly effective drug (Berson and Shalita, 1995). However, multiple cutaneous side effects can occur; these effects vary from mild to moderate in severity. Dry skin, dry eyes, dry mucous membranes, nasal irritation, decreased night vision, photosensitivity, arthralgia, headaches, mood changes, depression, and suicidal ideation may occur. Adolescents on this drug should be monitored for depression, depressive symptoms, and suicidal ideation (Jacobs, Deutsch, and Brewer, 2001). Recent research has not found any detrimental effects on bone mineralization with the use of isotretinoin (Margolis, Attie, and Leyden, 1996). The most significant side effects are the teratogenic effects. Isotretinoin is absolutely contraindicated in pregnant women. Sexually active young women must be using an effective contraceptive method during treatment and for 1 month after treatment (Mitchell, VanBennekom, and Louik, 1995). Patients receiving isotretinoin should also be carefully monitored for elevated cholesterol and triglyceride levels. Significant elevation may require discontinuation of the medication (Orfanos and Zouboulis, 1998; Rodondi and others, 2002).

Scarring begins early in all types of acne, from papulopustular to nodulocystic. Most of the scarring is a result of loss of tissue rather than thickening. Chemical peels have been traditionally used for the treatment of scarring in acne. Only the mildest acne scarring will actually resolve with chemical peels. Pulsed and scanned $CO_2$ lasers have achieved success in resurfacing of acne scarring (Goodman, 2000).

### Nursing Considerations

The health screening interview should contain questions regarding the adolescent's concern about acne. Because acne is so common and its appearance may seem so mild, the health care provider may underestimate the relative importance of the disease to the adolescent. The nurse should assess the individual adolescent's level of distress, current management, and perceived success of any regimen before initiating a referral. If the adolescent does not perceive the acne to be a problem, motivation to follow the treatment plan may be absent. Most cases of acne can be managed by the primary care provider without referral to a dermatologist.

The nurse can provide ongoing support for the adolescent when a treatment plan has been initiated. The family is also encouraged to support the adolescent in his or her efforts. (See Family Home Care box.) Use of the medications and basic skin care information should be discussed in detail with the adolescent. Written information to accompany the discussion is helpful. (See Critical Thinking Exercise box.) Information to dispel myths regarding the use of abrasive cleansing products as a means of removing blackheads can prevent unnecessary costs and trauma to the skin.

Teenagers also need to be educated about factors that may aggravate acne and damage skin, such as too vigorous scrubbing. Picking, squeezing, and manual expression with fingernails breaks down ductal walls and causes acne to worsen. Mechanical irritation, such as vinyl helmet straps that rub areas predisposed to acne, can cause the development of lesions. (See Nursing Care Plan: The Adolescent with Acne.*)

---

*In Wong DL, Hess: *Wong and Whaley's clinical manual of pediatric nursing*, ed 5, St Louis, 2000, Mosby.

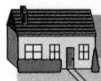

### FAMILY HOME CARE
*Acne*

Effective acne therapy requires long-term consistent use of the recommended treatment. The nurse can help the family learn skills to support the adolescent with compliance. During middle and late adolescence, parental supervision of daily skin care may result in struggles for independence. Parents should be encouraged to take a supportive role, giving positive reinforcement for compliance and noticeable improvements in skin appearance. To assist the parents, the nurse should review normal adolescent psychosocial development and the pathophysiology of acne.

## Vision Changes

Vision changes are common during the teenage years. The onset of refractory errors or worsening of previous errors peaks in adolescence as a result of the growth spurt. Other than myopia, new eye problems in this age-group are rare. Vision screening is usually performed in the school by nurses. The main goal is to detect new refractive errors. Adolescents with vision changes are referred for contacts or glasses as appropriate.

# HEALTH PROBLEMS OF THE MALE REPRODUCTIVE SYSTEM
## Penile Problems

Common congenital anomalies of the penis are almost always detected and corrected in infancy or early childhood, although some boys who need several operative procedures to repair a hypospadias (the most common congenital deformity of the penis) reach adolescence with a penis that looks different from those of their friends. A few who have received no medical care have uncorrected deformities that can cause serious psychologic problems during this sensitive

### Critical Thinking Exercise

*Acne*

Kim, who is 16 years old, recently started "breaking out." During her visit to the nurse practitioner, she was diagnosed as having a mild form of acne and was told to cleanse her face twice a day and apply Retin-A and benzoyl peroxide daily. Which instructions describe the correct skin care schedule?

First, Think About It . . .
• What precise questions are you trying to answer?
• What information are you using?

1. Use a mild facial scrub in the morning and apply the Retin-A; at night use an astringent to remove makeup and apply benzoyl peroxide.
2. Wash the face with soap in the morning and at night; wait 30 minutes after the night cleansing to apply Retin-A, followed by benzoyl peroxide.
3. Wash the face with soap in the morning and apply benzoyl peroxide; wash the face before bedtime and apply Retin-A.
4. Wash the face with soap in the morning and apply benzoyl peroxide; wash the face in the evening and apply Retin-A about 30 minutes later.

*The best response is four. Precisely, the most important aspects of the skin care regimen are to apply the topical preparation at different times of the day, because it is less effective when applications are close together. Also, the face should be completely dry before applying Retin-A to reduce skin irritation. Although either preparation can be used first, it is preferable to suggest applying Retin-A at night, when the teenager has time to wait after cleansing the skin. The information that you need to recall is that facial scrubs and astringents are not used, because they increase skin dryness.*

period of development. These young boys need to be identified for surgical repair of the defect.

Uncircumcised males may encounter some problems during adolescence. Some young men have tight foreskins that cannot be retracted over the enlarging glans; some may not cleanse the area properly. These boys are at risk for more frequent infections. Penile carcinoma is associated with human papilloma virus (HPV) types 16 and 18 (HPV 16, 18). Although HPV is a common sexually transmitted infection among American males, penile carcinomas are rare in the United States and most Western countries.

Trauma to the penis may occur in various ways, including burns and accidental injuries. The frenulum (the fold on the lower surface of the glans that connects it with the prepuce) can be torn after retraction of the foreskin, masturbation, or coitus. It can be frightening to the young boy but usually heals spontaneously with minimum care. However, any extensive bleeding may require suturing of the tissues.

## Testicular Tumors

Tumors of the testes are not a common condition, but when they are manifested in adolescence, they are generally malignant. Testicular cancer is the most common solid tumor in males 15 to 34 years of age. The usual presenting symptom is a heavy, hard, painless mass that is palpable on the anterior or lateral aspect of a testis. The tumor may be smooth or nodular and does not transilluminate unless accompanied by a hydrocele. The involved testicle hangs lower and is therefore more susceptible to trauma. Although not all scrotal masses are malignant, any firm swelling of the testes demands immediate evaluation. If a firm swelling is noted, the youth should be evaluated by ultrasonography and immediately referred for direct biopsy if the mass is found to be solid.

Treatment for testicular cancer consists of surgical removal of the affected testicle (orchiectomy) and the adjacent lymph nodes if they are affected. If metastases are evident in more distant nodes or organs, chemotherapy and radiation therapy are implemented. (See Chapters 23 and 36.)

### Nursing Considerations

To supplement routine health assessment, every adolescent male should be taught to perform monthly *testicular self-examination (TSE)*. This provides an opportunity for the adolescent to familiarize himself with his own anatomy and to ensure early detection of any abnormality. Each testicle is examined individually, preferably after a warm bath or shower, when scrotal skin is more relaxed, using the thumbs and fingers of both hands and applying a small amount of firm, gentle pressure. The normal testicle is a firm organ with a smooth, egg-shaped contour. The epididymis can be palpated as a raised swelling on the superior aspect of the testicle and should not be confused with an abnormality. The nurse can play an important role in providing anticipatory guidance to all adolescent males. This guidance includes an explanation of the rationale for TSE and how to perform this procedure. (See Critical Thinking Exercise box.)

## Varicocele

Varicocele usually presents as an asymptomatic scrotal mass or as scrotal aching after physical exercise in approximately 15% of all adolescent males (Skoog and others, 1997). A varicocele is characterized by elongation, dilation, and tortuosity of the veins of the spermatic cord superior to the testicle. The finding is rare in prepubertal children, but there is a dramatic increase in incidence at the onset of puberty. Varicoceles are found most often on the left side because of the greater length of the left spermatic vein and its entry into the left renal artery; the right spermatic vein enters the vena cava directly and at a lesser angle, which may be a source of future difficulty. A varicocele can be palpated as a wormlike mass, situated above the testicle, that decreases in size when the male is recumbent and becomes distended and tense when he is upright. There may be discomfort during sexual stimulation in some males.

In pubertal males the left testicle is usually larger than the right. However, when there is an associated varicocele, the left testicle is usually smaller than the right. Testicular size and levels of dihydrotestosterone in seminal plasma decrease with increasing duration of the varicocele. Varicocelectomy is thought to be indicated when a man is found to have abnormal spermatogenesis, a normal partner, and a

### Critical Thinking Exercise

#### Testicular Self-Examination

At a recent faculty meeting, the school nurse presented plans for a class on testicular self-examination (TSE) to be delivered to the sophomore boys. Several faculty members questioned the value of providing such a class when there is limited time to deliver content relating to "routine academic subjects." Which of the following responses could the nurse use to justify including the TSE class in the curriculum?

FIRST, THINK ABOUT IT . . .

• What assumptions are you making?
• What is the purpose of your thinking?

1. TSE provides an opportunity for adolescent males to pick up early cases of epididymitis, a common infection in this age-group.
2. TSE allows adolescent boys to determine if they have an asymptomatic sexually transmitted disease (STD).
3. TSE permits detection of any tumors of the testes, which are not common in adolescence, but which are often malignant and demand immediate attention when they occur.
4. TSE allows easy identification of malignant testicular tumors, which occur in 5% of adolescent males

*The best response is three. TSE is an easily learned technique that allows the adolescent male to become familiar with his own anatomy and to determine any abnormalities. Although testicular tumors are not common in adolescence, when they do occur, they are often malignant, and early detection is essential, which is an important assumption. Although TSE is easily learned by adolescents, the method does not allow the adolescent male to determine if he has an STD or epididymitis.*

varicocele. The adolescent with a varicocele is not likely to undergo infertility evaluation; therefore the management is controversial. Numerous research studies have identified varicoceles as a major cause of male infertility; however, none have shown that the effects of varicoceles are progressive over time. Pediatric urologists do not recommend routine prophylactic varicocele repair to protect future fertility (Jarow, Coburn, and Sigman, 1996).

## Epididymitis

Epididymitis is an inflammatory reaction of the epididymis of the testicle as a result of an infection (bacterial or viral), a chemical irritant (urine), or a nonspecific cause (local trauma). The clinical presentation is an insidious (slow) onset of unilateral scrotal pain, redness, and swelling. Associated symptoms include urethral discharge, dysuria, fever, and pyuria. Epididymitis is not associated with gastrointestinal symptoms as found in testicular torsion. The causative factors in males less than 35 years of age are predominantly *Chlamydia trachomatis* and *Neisseria gonorrhoeae* (Adelman and Joffe, 2000). Mild presentation of symptoms may mimic testicular torsion, which requires immediate surgical intervention. Therefore immediate evaluation by a practitioner is indicated. Treatment consists of analgesics, scrotal support, bed rest, and initiation of appropriate antibiotic therapy.

## Testicular Torsion

Intravaginal torsion of the testicle is a condition in which the tunica vaginalis, which normally encases the testicle, fails to do so and the testis hangs free from its vascular structures. This condition can result in partial or complete venous occlusion with rotation around this vascular axis. In severe torsion the organ can become swollen and painful; the scrotum becomes red, warm, and edematous and appears to be immobile or fixed as a result of spasm of the cremasteric fibers.

Testicular torsion occurs in 1 in every 4000 males, with a peak onset at 13 years of age. Testicular torsion is the most common cause of testicular loss in young males (Adelman and Joffe, 2000). Typically, the adolescent will complain of pain that was either acute or insidious in onset and that has radiated to the groin. Nausea, vomiting, and abdominal pain may accompany the pain. Fever and urinary symptoms are generally not present. The history will often reveal that similar painful episodes have occurred previously, resolving spontaneously. This is a surgical emergency to preserve the testicle.

### Nursing Considerations

Nurses should be alert to the possibility of testicular torsion in adolescents who complain of scrotal pain. Because torsion often results from trauma to the scrotum, school nurses are likely to encounter such injuries and should refer the adolescent for medical evaluation immediately.

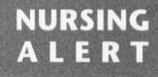 **NURSING ALERT**  Refer any male with signs of testicular torsion (red, painful, swollen scrotum) for immediate medical evaluation.

## Gynecomastia

Some degree of bilateral or unilateral breast enlargement occurs frequently in young boys during puberty. Approximately half of adolescent boys have transient gynecomastia, which usually lasts less than 1 year. When the onset of gynecomastia is prepubertal or at Tanner stage 5 (see Fig. 19-3), the adolescent should be evaluated for rare adrenal or gonadal tumors, liver disease, or Klinefelter syndrome. Gynecomastia may also be drug induced; calcium channel blockers, cancer chemotherapeutic agents, histamine-2 receptor blockers, and oral ketoconazoles have all been shown to cause the disorder. Marijuana has also been thought to cause gynecomastia.

If gynecomastia persists or is extensive enough to cause embarrassment, plastic surgery is indicated for cosmetic and psychologic considerations. Administration of testosterone has no effect on breast development or regression and may even aggravate the condition.

### Nursing Considerations

Treatment usually consists of assurance to the adolescent and his parents that this situation is benign and temporary. The adolescent may benefit from the knowledge that it occurs in more than 50% of his peers.

# HEALTH PROBLEMS OF THE FEMALE REPRODUCTIVE SYSTEM
## Gynecologic Examination

Whether it is her first experience or one of many, adolescent females are often apprehensive before a pelvic examination. Adolescents are self-conscious about their bodies and the changes taking place. The adolescent needs anticipatory guidance regarding what to expect and what she can do to help herself relax during the procedure. Many of the fears and apprehensions are a result of information she has obtained from family members and friends. The discussion should begin by addressing these anxieties.

The ideal time to begin to prepare the young women for the pelvic examination is as she is entering puberty. External genitalia examination should always be included as part of a routine physical assessment; excluding the genitalia reinforces the attitude that sexuality is something to be avoided. During this time the girl in early adolescence and her parents are informed that a pelvic examination should be performed during late adolescence.

The timing of the initial pelvic examination is controversial, but examination and early assessment have several advantages. Some health care providers recommend that the first pelvic examination take place 1 year after menarche; others recommend waiting until sexual activity or age 18. The ultimate decision will depend on the adolescent and the health care provider. Indications for a pelvic examination during adolescence are listed in Box 20-1.

The pelvic examination provides an excellent opportunity for teaching about hygiene, body functions, and sexuality. The adolescent and her parents can be assured that her body is normal, which contributes to a positive body image. The girl is encouraged to ask questions about her changing body and its implications. The pelvic examination also allows opportunity for discussion about practicing safe sex, prevention of sexually transmitted diseases (STDs), and postponing sexual involvement (Muscari, 1999). Lack of knowledge is a factor in risky sexual experimentation in adolescence. The pelvic examination should be as non-stressful as possible. Nurses should attempt to make the initial pelvic exam a positive experience for the adolescent because this can increase the likelihood of compliance with annual visits (Muscari, 1999).

The teenager should have the option of choosing a supportive person to be present during the pelvic examination. Suggested individuals might include a parent, best friend, boyfriend, or other health professional. The use of models and drawings and a display of equipment to be used facilitate understanding. Allowing the adolescent to handle the speculum may help to decrease some of the fear. The adolescent is given the choice of wearing a gown or her own clothing during the examination. A description of the examination, including information about the procedure and words that describe anticipated feelings and sensations experienced during the examination, has reduced anxiety. Of major concern to the adolescent is fear of discovery of pelvic pathology. Reassurance regarding normal physical findings is extremely important. A Danish study of 1500 adolescents demonstrated the importance of careful education, information sharing, and reassurance; 32% of the girls reported that the examination was a negative experience. The girls with negative feelings reported pain, embarrassment, a feeling of lack of control, lack of knowledge before the examination, and learning nothing about the examination at completion (Larsen and Kragstrup, 1995).

Most girls favor a semisitting position, which has the additional advantage of allowing eye contact during the procedure. Sometimes a pillow will help the patient feel more comfortable and less vulnerable. The provision of a mirror for the girl to see what is taking place if she so desires helps the examiner explain various aspects of anatomy. When possible, it is important to respect the adolescent's request for a female provider.

Numerous techniques have been described to teach women to relax during a pelvic examination, including breathing exercises, imagery, and other strategies for reducing stress. (See Pain Management, Chapter 26.) However, these techniques are not effective with all individuals. When the examination is finished, the findings are discussed with the adolescent, and necessary referrals are made if indicated. Written materials are useful educational materials.

## Menstrual Disorders

The average age of menarche is about 12½ years, with a normal range of 9 to 16 years. In an evaluation for amenorrhea, an accurate history of the timing of development of secondary sexual characteristics is necessary. ***Primary amenorrhea*** is defined as no menses by age 17. An evaluation is necessary at age 15 if there are no secondary sexual characteristics or if menarche does not follow within 2 years of the onset of secondary sexual characteristics. ***Secondary amenorrhea*** is no menses for 6 months in a previously menstruating female when pregnancy has been excluded. Secondary amenorrhea is much more common than primary amenorrhea.

It is not unusual for an adolescent to have irregular menses when establishing ovulatory cycles. This is a result of an immature hypothalamic-pituitary-ovarian axis. In general, the later menarche occurs, the longer the period of anovulation. Two thirds of adolescent females will establish regular menstrual cycles by 2 years after menarche. Oligomenorrhea (abnormally light or infrequent menstruation) early after menarche is of little concern unless it creates undue anxiety on the part of the adolescent or her parents, which can ordinarily be allayed by explanation and reassurance. A careful examination should be done to reveal any congenital defects of the genital tract (a rare cause).

### Primary Amenorrhea

Primary amenorrhea may be a result of absence or malformation of the female genital structures or the inability of normal structures to respond to hormonal stimulation. This can be of hypothalamic, pituitary, ovarian, or uterine origin and can include hypopituitarism, Turner syndrome, tumors, polycystic ovary disease, and infections. Primary amenorrhea in an adolescent complaining of periodic (usually monthly) lower abdominal pain with evidence of estrogen production and sexual maturation may be an imperforate hymen, closed hymen from female circumcision, or transverse vaginal septum. The treatment is simple surgical perforation and drainage.

A group of systemic disorders that may affect the functions of the reproductive tract are thyroid hypofunction or hyperfunction, prolonged or severe infections, adrenal hyperplasia, diabetes mellitus, and other chronic diseases. Obesity or malnutrition (including protein, vitamin, or iron deficiencies) may also delay the onset of menstruation. The age of menarche is significantly later in adolescents involved in intensive physical exercise, especially those sports requiring low weight, such as gymnastics, ballet, and distance running (Gidwani, 1997).

### Secondary Amenorrhea

Secondary amenorrhea is defined as absence of menses for at least three cycles or 6 months in females who have established cycles. The most common cause of secondary amenorrhea in adolescence is pregnancy. Other factors, which

---

**Box 20-1** ■ ■ ■

### Indications for Pelvic Examination of Adolescent Females

Menstrual disorders:
  Amenorrhea
  Irregular uterine/vaginal bleeding
  Dysmenorrhea unresponsive to therapy
Undiagnosed abdominal pain
Any sexually active adolescent
Request for a prescription contraceptive method
Suspected pelvic mass
Rape
Request by patient
Virginal 18-year-old

disturb the hypothalamic-pituitary-gonadal axis and cause secondary amenorrhea, include physical or emotional stress, sudden environmental change, hyperthyroidism or hypothyroidism, polycystic ovary disease, chronic illness, extreme weight loss or gain, intensive exercise, anorexia nervosa, bulimia, ovarian disturbance, and extrinsic pharmacologic agents, especially phenothiazines, contraceptive steroids, and heroin (Neinstein, 1996; Selzer and others, 1996).

## Menstrual Irregularities in the Female Athlete

The most common clinical indications of potentially adverse effects of exercise on an adolescent's reproductive cycle include (1) delayed menarche, (2) anovulation associated with dysfunctional uterine bleeding, and (3) oligomenorrhea or amenorrhea with hypoestrogenic states. Researchers have not been able to identify the exact mechanism of these menstrual changes. The most probable cause is at the hypothalamus level, including changes in the endogenous opiates and the gonadotropin-releasing hormones (Gidwani, 1997).

Adolescents who exercise regularly and have menstrual bleeding more frequently than every 21 days or at intervals of 35 to 120 days are likely to have chronic anovulation. They usually produce estrogen but have inadequate levels of progesterone. Unopposed estrogen can lead to endometrial hyperplasia and theoretic risk of endometrial adenocarcinoma.

Sometimes a trial of decreasing the intensity or duration of exercise and improving nutrition will relieve irregularities. If no improvement in symptoms is seen, cyclic progesterone or low-dose oral contraceptive pills (OCPs) may be prescribed. OCPs will protect the endometrium and provide sufficient estrogen for bone density while providing contraception for the sexually active adolescent.

> **NURSING ALERT** Female athletes are at risk for menstrual dysfunction. In addition, they also may be at risk for eating disorders and decreased bone mineral density (American Academy of Pediatrics, 2000).

## Dysmenorrhea

Dysmenorrhea is defined as painful menstrual flow. *Primary dysmenorrhea* is painful menses without any identifiable pathologic disorder. Primary dysmenorrhea is the most common cause of painful menses in adolescents. *Secondary dysmenorrhea* is defined as painful menses with a pathologic condition such as endometriosis, salpingitis, or congenital anomalies of the mullerian system. The incidence of dysmenorrhea is as high as 92%, with 15% experiencing pain that inhibits participation in daily activities. The condition is highly underreported to health care providers (Schroeder and Sanfilippo, 1999).

### Etiology

The factor present in all instances of primary dysmenorrhea is the onset of ovulatory cycles. Although it is not invariable, the symptoms do not occur during the first few postmenarchal months or during months of irregular anovulatory

menses. Estrogen production alone does not appear to be related to the level of discomfort, and progesterone is associated with diminished uterine contractility.

There is a relationship between uterine contractility and the secretion of prostaglandins. Prostaglandins of the $F_2$alpha class cause myometrial contraction, vasoconstriction, and ischemia; prostaglandin $E_2$ causes vasodilation and hypersensitivity of pain nerve terminals in the myometrium (Neinstein, 1996). The secretion of prostaglandins increases at about the twenty-fifth to the twenty-eighth day of the menstrual cycle and follows the decrease in progesterone secretion. The degree of discomfort may be related to vascular changes in the endometrial bed during menstruation caused by alterations in vasoconstriction and vasodilation of endometrial vessels that induce local ischemia, edema, necrosis, and slough. Nerve terminals also become sensitive to prostaglandins by lowering the threshold of these nerve terminals to the action of chemical and physical stimuli. Most of the prostaglandin release occurs in the first 48 hours of menstruation; therefore, pain is greater during the first 2 days. Nausea, vomiting, diarrhea, headache, and emotional changes that are associated with primary dysmenorrhea are also related to release of prostaglandins.

The presence and severity of dysmenorrhea is increased in smokers as compared with nonsmokers. The severity increases significantly with the number of cigarettes per day. The exact mechanism remains unclear but may be related to decreased endometrial blood flow in girls who smoke.

Long-held beliefs that behavioral and psychologic factors may be a cause of primary dysmenorrhea have now been abandoned. There is strong evidence of a physiologic basis for the pain (Golomb, Solidum, and Warren, 1998).

### Clinical Manifestations

Typical complaints of the adolescent with dysmenorrhea are lower abdominal cramping and pain or discomfort. About 50% of females also have systemic symptoms, including nausea and vomiting, fatigue, nervousness, diarrhea, and headache. The pain usually begins several hours before the appearance of visible vaginal bleeding, is most severe on the first day of menstruation, and may last from a few hours to a day or more but seldom exceeds 2 to 3 days. The symptoms and degree of discomfort vary considerably from one individual to another and from one period to another in the same woman. The pain may be only a mild fleeting discomfort or so severe as to be incapacitating, requiring absence from school. After adolescence the menstrual discomfort decreases with age and may resolve completely after childbirth.

### Therapeutic Management

A careful history, including a menstrual and sexual history, is necessary. In addition, a careful review of gastrointestinal and genitourinary systems is necessary to rule out problems. A thorough gynecologic examination is carried out to exclude any pelvic abnormalities. The pelvic examination may not be indicated in an adolescent who is not sexually active and who responds to medical therapy.

The treatment of choice for adolescents is the administration of nonsteroidal antiinflammatory drugs (NSAIDs). These drugs block the formation of prostaglandins, leading to a reduction in uterine activity and the prevention of pain (Schroeder and Sanfilippo, 1998). Antiprostaglandins are taken for only 2 to 3 days of the menstrual cycle. Prophylactic use of NSAIDs has proved effective when begun a few days before the onset of the menses, approximately 11 days after ovulation. The relief appears to be a result of prostaglandin inhibition rather than analgesic effect.

A variety of drugs that are taken at the onset of symptoms are available without prescription, such as ibuprofen and naproxen. The fenamates have the additional benefit of antagonizing the action of already-formed prostaglandins. If NSAIDs are unsuccessful in relieving the pain or if the adolescent desires contraception, cyclic estrogen therapy to prevent ovulation can provide dramatic and predictable relief from pain. Oral contraceptives are effective in approximately 90% of cases. Further evaluation to rule out causes of secondary dysmenorrhea should be undertaken when the pain does not respond to four to six cycles of compliant medical therapy with NSAIDs and OCPs (Banerjee and Laufer, 1998).

Transcutaneous electrical nerve stimulation (TENS), which hampers the perception of pain, has been found to be an effective nonpharmacologic source of relief of pain associated with dysmenorrhea. Acupuncture is also effective. Exercise is widely believed to alleviate dysmenorrhea, but careful research studies are not currently available to show a definitive relationship (Golomb, Solidum, and Warren, 1998).

### Nursing Considerations

The nurse may be the person to whom a young woman turns for advice regarding menstrual problems. Anticipatory guidance concerning menstrual physiology and hygiene and the importance of a well-balanced diet, exercise, and general health maintenance should be provided. Adolescents need information regarding availability of effective treatment for dysmenorrhea. Only about 50% of females with dysmenorrhea take medication to relieve the symptoms, even though effective treatment is available.

Most of the prostaglandin inhibitors are available without prescription. Whatever drug the adolescent chooses to use, she needs to be told how the drug produces its effect, how to take the drug for maximum effect, and the side effects. The drug should be taken with food and a full glass of water. If no satisfactory relief is achieved, the adolescent is referred for further evaluation.

## Endometriosis

Dysmenorrhea that is not substantially relieved after three cycles of oral contraceptive pills and NSAIDs requires an evaluation with laparoscopy to rule out endometriosis. The disease is much more common in adolescents than was previously thought. Research has demonstrated that 70% of adolescents evaluated with laparoscopy after treatment failure with NSAIDSs and oral contraceptives have endometriosis (Banerjee and Laufer, 1998).

Endometriosis is defined as the presence of endometrial glands and stroma outside of the normal intrauterine endometrial cavity. The etiology is still unclear. The presentation of endometriosis is variable and includes dysmenorrhea, chronic pelvic pain, dyspareunia, uterosacral ligament nodularity, and adnexal mass (Lapp, 2000). Treatment is medical, surgical, or a combination of both. The goal of treatment is pain control and suppression of the disease. The patient and family need to understand that recurrence is high and that there is currently no cure for the disease.

### Nursing Considerations

Adolescents require careful counseling about the use of the medications prescribed. The hormonal treatments have common side effects that are not well tolerated by adolescents, requiring education and support throughout the course of treatment.

## Premenstrual Syndrome (PMS)

Although PMS was first described in 1931, after several decades of research it remains poorly defined. The natural history of PMS is not known, there are over 150 reported symptoms, and, with no confirmatory laboratory test, providers are hesitant to initiate treatment (Frye and Silverman, 2000). The symptoms are stable across cycles and occur regularly in the late luteal phase and resolve within days of onset of menstrual bleeding. The manifestations most frequently cited are headache, backache, increased fatigue, weight gain, and breast congestion. PMS is very common, occurring at some point in most women's reproductive lives; 2%-10% of women have severe enough symptoms to disrupt productivity, interpersonal relationships, and quality of life (Freeman and others, 2000).

Accurate diagnosis of PMS requires a thorough history and careful physical examination to exclude other medical or psychiatric conditions. A daily report form will allow the young woman to pinpoint symptoms, which will allow for monitoring during treatment. There are currently few well-controlled studies that demonstrate effective treatment. Treatment options vary depending upon the type and severity of symptoms.

Nutritional supplements have long been recommended as a treatment for PMS. Supplementation with 1200 mg/day of calcium has been demonstrated to reduce water retention, food craving, and pain (Ward and Holimon, 1999). Although widely used, there is no clear evidence that supplementation with vitamin $B_6$ is effective in the treatment of PMS. Recent small preliminary studies are showing promising results with supplements of magnesium and Vitamin E for mood changes. There is not enough evidence to refute or reinforce the claims that primrose oil is effective in relieving physical symptoms (Bendich, 2000).

The serotonin reuptake inhibitors (SSRIs) have been shown to be effective in the severe cases of PMS. Benefits are seen immediately, and recent studies are exploring the use of the medications only during the luteal phase of the

cycle (Schatzberg, 2000). The medications are usually effective at lower doses than necessary for treatment of depression, allowing for fewer side effects.

The nurse helps adolescents and their families experience the process of health. The nurse can provide information regarding direct-care measures, adequate rest, good nutrition, and regular exercise. Families often have questions about the myriad of treatment options available. The nurse can provide information about current recommended therapies. Coping with the psychosocial aspect of the syndrome can be taught through stress reduction techniques, counseling, and support groups.

## Dysfunctional Uterine Bleeding (DUB)

DUB is abnormal vaginal bleeding that occurs in the absence of pregnancy, infection, neoplasms, or any other demonstrable pathologic condition or disease. DUB is usually associated with anovulation. Up to 95% of abnormal menstrual bleeding in adolescents is caused by DUB (Bravender and Emans, 1999). During adolescence, abnormalities in the timing (intervals of less than 20 days or greater than 40 days), length (greater than 8 days' duration), and amount (more than 80 ml) of menstrual flow can occur frequently. This irregularity is usually attributed to immaturity of the positive feedback mechanism between the hypothalamic-pituitary-gonadal axis and absence of the luteinizing hormone (LH) surge late in the menstrual cycle. The result is anovulatory cycles in which the production of estrogen is unopposed because of a lack of progesterone. The effect of the estrogen is an increase in the thickness of the endometrial lining without structural integrity. Without progesterone, menstrual flow is not limited. Not all anovulatory females have DUB. One contributing factor is the amount of endogenous estrogen.

A comprehensive health history and physical examination, including a pelvic examination, is indicated to ascertain the cause of bleeding. The initial assessment should evaluate the amount of blood loss and the possible need for hospitalization. Common causes of vaginal bleeding need to be ruled out before the diagnosis of DUB can be established. The most common reason for vaginal bleeding in adolescence is pregnancy. Other causes of vaginal bleeding can be related to anatomic anomalies, foreign bodies, endocrine disease, STDs, chronic illness, or previously undetected familial bleeding disorders (e.g., von Willebrand disease).

Treatment of vaginal bleeding depends on determination of the underlying mechanism. The initial management depends on the amount of blood lost and the patient's symptoms. If the bleeding is infrequent and not associated with anemia, reassurance and a menstrual calendar for follow-up are often sufficient.

In persistent cases hormonal therapy, in the form of OCPs or cyclic medroxyprogesterone, has been beneficial. The adolescent needs to know that at the completion of the recommended regimen there will probably be a heavy flow with cramping for 3 to 4 days. Without this information, she may believe that her condition is worse and assume that the

treatment was ineffective. Untreated patients are at increased risk for endometrial hyperplasia and adenocarcinoma from the persistent unopposed estrogen stimulation of the endometrium. The OCPs are continued for several months, after which bleeding irregularities seldom recur. DUB may persist for up to 2 years in more than half of the cases.

Dilation and curettage may be necessary to control hemorrhage in severe cases or in those that do not respond to more conservative management. Supplemental iron is sometimes needed to correct anemia.

### Nursing Considerations

Ordinarily, only reassurance and attention to general health status are needed, with emphasis on a well-balanced diet, adequate rest, and moderate exercise. When OCPs are prescribed, the adolescent and her parents need careful explanation of the use of these medications. The high-dose estrogen OCPs can result in nausea and vomiting. Anticipatory supportive care includes preparation for procedures if these are a possibility.

## Vaginitis and Vulvitis (Vulvovaginitis)

A small quantity of vaginal mucus is normal and in adolescent girls usually increases at the time of ovulation and before the onset of menstruation. It is characteristically clear and, except in rare instances when it appears in large amounts, causes no discomfort. However, some teenagers mistakenly believe that the discharge is a sign of vaginal infection. After an examination the girl can generally be reassured and given anticipatory guidance about hygiene and the increased secretions associated with sexual excitement.

*Leukorrhea* is the term used to describe a glutinous, gray-white discharge, which can be caused by physical, chemical, or infectious agents. Physical causes include foreign bodies such as a forgotten tampon. Leukorrhea can also be caused by irritation from pinworms, bubble bath, douching, deodorant pads or tampons, or improper wiping after defecation. The resulting discharge may be purulent, blood tinged, or brown with an offensive odor. Removal of the offending material is usually all that is necessary.

The normal vaginal flora is composed of predominantly *lactobacillus acidophilus,* which produces lactic acid and hydrogen peroxide to maintain an acidic environment. *Vaginitis* occurs when pathogens or changes in the environment disrupt this balance. Oral antibiotics, oral and vaginal contraceptive agents, sexual intercourse, douching, and stress may allow pathogen proliferation and the development of vaginitis (Egan and Lipsky, 2000). The availability of over-the-counter anti-fungal creams has resulted in high levels of self-diagnosis and self-treatment for vaginal infections. However, only about 20% of vaginitis is caused by a fungal infection (Nyirjesy, 1999).

*Vulvovaginal candidiasis* results when *Candida* begins to proliferate, resulting in overgrowth and infection. The most common organism is *Candida albicans,* accounting for 80% to 90% of infections (Egan and Lipsky, 2000). Many factors can increase the susceptibility to candidiasis, including pregnancy, broad-spectrum antibiotics, oral contraceptives, diabetes, receptive oral sex, and depressed cellular immunity. Recurrent yeast infections are not uncommon and may be a result of shorter treatment courses that do not completely eradicate the fungus (Carr, Felsenstein, Friedman, 1998). The nurse should be alert to risk factors for human immunodeficiency virus (HIV) because recurrent or persistent vulvovaginal candidiasis may be the first symptom of the infection.

The adolescent with vulvovaginal candidiasis will generally have vaginal pruritus and sometimes dysuria. The presence of the classic thick "cottage cheese–like" discharge is seen in a minority of patients. Most females have a minimal amount of an uncharacteristic discharge. The diagnosis is easily confirmed with microscopic evaluation.

First-line treatment of candidiasis remains the administration of over-the-counter topical antifungal drugs. The medications are available in cream, lotion, suppository, and tablet formulations. Shorter treatment regimens are associated with increased compliance but higher rates of recurrence. Oral 1-day treatment regimens are safe and as effective as topical treatments but may result in more systemic side effects. Treatment of the male partner in sexually active adolescents is not necessary unless there is inflammation of the glans penis.

*Trichomonas vaginalis* is an anaerobic parasitic protozoan involved in 20% to 30% of all cases of vaginitis. *T. vaginalis* is sexually transmitted and can be recovered from 60% to 100% of female partners of infected men and 30% to 85% of male partners of infected women (Egan and Lipsky, 2000). The protozoan may act as a vector for other sexually transmitted infections.

The infection is often asymptomatic and self-limiting in men. Women may be asymptomatic, but many have a vaginal discharge and vulvovaginal soreness. Dysuria and an odor often accompany the symptoms. The diagnosis is confirmed with microscopic examination of a specimen from the vaginal flora.

Metronidazole is used for the treatment of trichomoniasis, in either a 2-g single dose or 500 mg b.i.d. for 7 days. Single-dose treatment is ideal in the adolescent population. Sexual partners should also be treated.

*Bacterial vaginosis (BV)* is the most common vaginal infection in young women. The infection is non-inflammatory and caused by an overgrowth of a variety of organisms. The symptoms include a thin, homogeneous, malodorous vaginal discharge. The diagnosis is confirmed by identification of clue cells with the microscope. BV is associated with abnormal pap smears, pelvic inflammatory disease (PID), premature rupture of membranes, and pre-term labor. Bacterial vaginosis is not a sexually transmitted disease; however, sexual transmission occurs as a result of disruption of normal vaginal flora. Other associated factors are pregnancy, use of intrauterine devices, and douching.

The most effective treatment is metronidazole 500 mg b.i.d. for 7 days, single-dose therapy is not recommended for this infection. Treatment of the male sexual partner is not necessary. The adolescent should be instructed to abstain from sexual intercourse while taking the medication.

### Nursing Considerations

The adolescent presenting with vaginal discharge provides an opportunity for health teaching. The young woman should be taught how to differentiate normal vaginal discharge from a potential infection. The discussion may elicit questions and concerns the adolescent has regarding other aspects of her developing body and sexuality. The nurse should stress the importance of an evaluation whenever the adolescent notices a change in her normal vaginal discharge.

When an infection is identified, the adolescent will need an explanation of how the etiologic agents produced the irritation and the principles behind management. The prescription of a vaginal cream will require a careful explanation and demonstration of use. Girls who have never used a tampon will be less familiar with insertion of the vaginal applicator.

Health teaching should include the prevention of future infections. Girls should be taught at an early age to wipe front to back after toileting. Douching is not an uncommon practice among adolescents and should be discouraged because it leads to changes in the normal vaginal microflora. Bacterial vaginosis, PID, and ectopic pregnancies are associated with douching (Merchant, Oh, and Klerman, 1999). The use of condoms for prevention of trichomoniasis and other sexually transmitted infections should also be stressed.

## HEALTH PROBLEMS RELATED TO SEXUALITY

The biologic maturation that forms the foundation of adolescent development and the transition to adulthood is accompanied by conflicting feelings, attitudes, and social practices related to developing sexuality. During adolescence the sexual drive emerges, and adolescents begin to explore their ability to attract a partner. The physical urges often precede emotional maturity.

Approximately 50% of high school students report having had sexual intercourse by their senior year in high school. Eight percent of high school students report having engaged in sex before the age of 13 (Division of Adolescent and School Health, 2000).

The causes of adolescent sexual risk-taking are multifactorial. There is great social pressure to experiment with sex, and enticements by the media to enhance physical attractiveness conflict with traditional religious and societal expectations for chastity. Easy access to cars, unsupervised time at home, and changing family composition have also contributed to the incidence of sexual experimentation among the adolescent population. Egocentrism and the concept of the personal fable (feelings of omnipotence, invulnerability, and immortality) lead to risk-taking and experimentation. A recent study found that self-esteem may influence intercourse at an early age (Spencer and others, 2002).

Family influences can delay the initiation of sexual activity. Adolescents who have at least one warm and supportive parent engage in less risky behavior. Effective parent-child communication about sexuality topics can delay the onset of first sexual intercourse. In addition, supervision of the adolescent's social activities and peer group, frequently referred to as parental monitoring, has consistently been shown to postpone sexual involvement (Blythe and Rosenthal, 2000).

The social environment also has an effect on sexual risk-taking behavior. Adolescents who attend schools where they feel connected and involved in the programming are more likely to postpone sexual involvement (Resnick and others, 1997). Community support, resources, and supervision will also decrease risk-taking among adolescents.

Prevention strategies must be comprehensive to decrease high-risk sexual behaviors. Delaying sexual intercourse, using condoms, choosing partners carefully, limiting sexual partners, and using reliable contraception help to reduce the impact of sexual activity on the adolescent. Instruction in the skills needed to resist sexual intercourse has a stronger influence on reducing sexual activity than simply providing information on acquired immunodeficiency syndrome (AIDS) or birth control methods.

## Adolescent Pregnancy

In recent years, the teenage pregnancy rate has shown a continual downward trend. Between 1990 and 1998, birth rates for teenagers 15 to 19 years of age declined nationally for all age groups, races, and Hispanic origin populations. The steepest declines were recorded for African-American women. Birth rates fell in all states; overall declines ranged from 9% to 32% (Ventura, Mathews, and Curtin, 1999). The decline was largely the result of a drop in the number of repeat pregnancies, and an increase in the use of long-term hormonal contraceptive methods among adolescents (Henshaw and Feivelson, 2000). However, adolescent birth rates still remain high in the United States compared to other developed countries (American Academy of Pediatrics, 1999a).

The rate of contraceptive use at first intercourse is 78% among adolescents. The method most frequently used at first intercourse is a condom. Condom use drops off in older adolescents. Among sexually active teens, the oral contraceptive pill remains the most commonly used method (48%), followed by the condom (38%), injectable contraceptives (10%), and withdrawal (4%). Among heterosexual teens, condoms are used more frequently to prevent pregnancy than to prevent sexually transmitted diseases. After a hormonal contraceptive method is initiated, condom use decreases. Only about 1 in 6 teens uses both a condom and another contraceptive method (Alan Guttmacher Institute, 1999).

In most cases, with early prenatal care, teenage pregnancy is no longer considered to be biologically disadvantageous to the child. However, teenage parenting is still regarded as socially, educationally, psychologically and economically disadvantageous to both the mother and the child. Poverty is often the result of teenage childbearing (Aquilino and Bragadottir, 2000). Only 7 out of 10 adolescent mothers complete high school, and the likelihood of adolescent mothers going to college is much less than for their non-childbearing peers (Alan Guttmacher Institute, 1999). Many of these social risk factors can be decreased or

ameliorated if a second pregnancy is prevented during the adolescent years or if the second pregnancy does not occur until 26 months postpartum (Brown, Saunders, and Dick, 1999). Other predictors of maternal success include participation in a program for pregnant teens, a social support system and a sense of control over one's life (American Academy of Pediatrics, 2001a).

### Medical Aspects

Early comprehensive prenatal care is still not provided to most teenage mothers. Lacking adequate care, adolescent mothers and their unborn infants are at greater risk for complications of both pregnancy and delivery (Quint, 1996). The most frequent complications are premature labor and low-birth-weight infants, high neonatal mortality, iron deficiency anemia, fetopelvic disproportion, and prolonged labor. The pregnancies of adolescents less than 15 years old are more frequently complicated by obstetric problems and neonatal morbidity and mortality than those of adolescents ages 15 to 19. The increased risk has traditionally been thought to be related to incomplete growth and physiologic immaturity. Pregnancy can take place only after the girl has achieved an advanced state of growth and sexual maturity. Therefore concerns are dietary habits, substance use (especially cigarettes), STDs, the effects of poverty, and the onset of prenatal care.

Adolescents often receive delayed or inadequate prenatal care. The reasons prenatal care is delayed may be related to the adolescent not realizing she is pregnant or denial of the pregnancy until the second or third trimester. Misinformation is another cause; adolescents often do not understand the importance of early prenatal care.

The obstetric risk and risk to the infant during a second pregnancy for the teenager is much higher. An adolescent with a poor outcome in the first pregnancy has a threefold risk of repeating the poor outcome in the second pregnancy. The risk for a preterm delivery recurring is double the rate in older women. However, the mean birth weight for second deliveries is higher, related to an increase in the maternal prepregnancy body mass index.

**Developmental Factors.** It does not necessarily follow that early biologic development is accompanied by early emotional and psychologic development. The physically mature young girl is still a teenager who must cope with the developmental tasks of adolescence. When the tasks of motherhood are superimposed on adolescent needs, the girl may be ill prepared to deal appropriately with either.

### Complications of Pregnancy

Bleeding is common in early pregnancy (20% to 25%) and about half of these pregnancies end in spontaneous abortion. Most spontaneous abortions occur in the first trimester as a result of abnormal chromosomal complement, uterine or cervical abnormalities, maternal systemic illness, or infection. Bedrest is usually recommended when bleeding occurs; however, no treatment has been found to alter a threatened abortion (Polaneczky and O'Connor, 1999).

When a young woman presents with bleeding and abdominal pain, an ectopic pregnancy must be ruled out. The incidence of ectopic pregnancy is on the increase. Fortunately, because of early diagnosis and treatment, death and serious complications from ectopic pregnancies are decreasing. Adolescents continue to have the highest mortality rates from ectopic pregnancy. Risk factors for an ectopic pregnancy include a history of pelvic inflammatory disease (PID), use of an intrauterine device (IUD), and history of pelvic surgery, or previous ectopic pregnancy (Lyon, 2000). When ectopic pregnancy is suspected, prompt evaluation and treatment are necessary.

**Structural Factors.**   Labor may be prolonged in younger teenagers; this is directly related to fetopelvic incompatibility and is a reflection of the teenager's smaller stature and incomplete growth process. This is particularly true in girls 12 to 16 years of age. The incidence of prolonged labor is highest in girls younger than age 14. Girls who are 12 and 13 years old have the highest rate of cesarean births, primarily because of cephalopelvic disproportion. However, older adolescents, 15 to 21 years of age, and especially those who have previously delivered a baby, often have labors that are shorter than average. The critical point between pelvic disproportion and adequacy appears to occur around 15 years of age in the average adolescent.

**Nutritional Needs.**   Caloric requirements during adolescence closely parallel the growth curve, and the need for protein, calcium, and iron is increased. Young adolescents tolerate caloric restriction poorly, and the anabolic need for calories during pregnancy places an added burden on their bodies. The preconception weight is a major determinant of birth weight for infants born to adolescents. Weight gain recommendations for pregnant women should be based on their weight-for-height percentile or body mass index and not on their age.

Because there is marked variation in the dietary needs of individual teenagers, no hard-and-fast rule can be laid down to describe an adequate diet for all pregnant girls. The diet must provide sufficient nutrients to meet growth needs of both the prospective mother and the unborn child without the threat of obesity or evidence of malnutrition. The best guide for determining nutritional needs is the Recommended Dietary Allowances (RDAs) of the Food and Nutrition Board for adolescents plus the additional 300 calories per day needed during the second and third trimesters of pregnancy (Worthington-Roberts and Rees, 1997). However, these do not take into consideration deviations and deficiencies. Pregnant teenagers exhibit food preferences, eating behaviors, and lifestyle habits that are similar to those of their nonpregnant peers. Frequent snacking on foods high in fat and sugar and low in essential nutrients results in intakes of calcium, iron, zinc, folic acid, and vitamins $B_6$, A, and C—nutrients of special concern during pregnancy— that are below recommended intakes.

> **NURSING ALERT**
> All pregnant women should take a vitamin/ mineral supplement to ensure the RDA for folic acid to help prevent neural tube defects.

**Infants.**   There is a higher incidence of prematurity and low birth weight in infants born to teenagers. It is difficult to determine if this is a result of the developmental stage of the mother or a reflection of multiple factors associated with teenage pregnancies, including poor nutrition, lower socioeconomic status, concomitant disease, and late or no prenatal care. Bacterial infections within the uterus are associated with early (less than 30 weeks) preterm delivery (Goldenberg, Hauth, and Andrews, 2000). Several factors demonstrate a high degree of association with prematurity, such as first birth, immaturity, illegitimacy, and the young age of the mother, and can create an accumulative effect that places the pregnant teenager in a perilously high-risk situation.

## Causal Factors

The causes of teenage pregnancy are complex, and attempts to disentangle the many facets have not been successful. Several factors contribute to premarital births to teenagers. First, the trend toward earlier initiation of sexual activity, which started in the 1970s, continues. Second, only about 1 in 3 sexually active adolescents uses a reliable method of contraception consistently. Approximately 7 in 10 births to adolescents under age 20 are outside of marriage. However, teenagers account for a smaller proportion of births outside of marriage than they did in the 1970s (Alan Guttmacher Institute, 1999).

Clearly, youth who delay childbearing until they have completed their own development and education are socially and economically better prepared to become parents.

## Social and Economic Aspects

Poor school performance usually precedes adolescent pregnancy. Unable to achieve academically, the girl views motherhood as a rite of passage into adult status. Adolescents with high educational expectations are less likely than others to become pregnant. Another significant aspect of school dropout and accelerated maturity is the girl's alienation and isolation from her peers during a stage of development when identity formation is closely allied with peer identification. She is deprived of the interrelationship with the adolescent social system that is so essential to the development of a sense of identity. The girl may believe that she no longer "belongs" to the peer group and does not qualify for membership in the older peer group of mothers. On the other hand, the pregnancy may give the adolescent an entrance into a peer group.

## Mother-Infant Relationship

Adolescents often have unrealistic expectations for the child. The young mother may view the infant as a plaything or a love object for herself. Children of adolescent mothers experience more developmental problems than children of adult mothers. The amount of cognitive stimulation in the child's early home environment is associated with the child's level of cognitive attainment. Many children of adolescents are raised by a grandparent. Although living with a grandparent may have positive effects on child outcomes, co-residence with the grandmother may have negative effects if the mother and grandmother are in conflict. The best outcome for both the adolescent and the child appears to occur when the adolescent lives separately but has her mother's support (Black and Bentley, 1995). Nurses need to stress the importance of the adolescent caring for the child even when other adults (e.g., mother or grandmother) are involved. The other adults present need education and support to allow optimal development of the infant and adolescent mother (American Academy of Pediatrics, 2001a).

Several factors influence the mother-infant relationship. Maternal stresses, including changes in circumstances, influence coping ability and sensitivity to the needs of the infant. Teenage mothers may consider an argument with a parent, boyfriend, or husband stressful, whereas adult mothers focus on problems directly involving the infant. Vocational and educational disadvantages to both teenage mothers and fathers further impinge on their coping abilities. It is important to recognize that not all adolescent mothers are alike. Some teenagers adjust well to the stresses and responsibilities of parenting, whereas others may lack the maturity or confidence to nurture optimally.

When socioeconomic status is controlled for, it has been found that younger adolescent mothers have lower acceptance of their children as compared with older adolescent mothers. Studies in the literature indicate that specific family variables, including the age of the mother (less than 19 years of age), are risk indicators for child abuse and neglect (Murray, Baker, and Lewin, 2000).

There is a positive correlation between the total amount of social support and the frequency of appropriate maternal behavior. An assessment of whom the adolescent feels she receives the most support from (family, her partner, his family, or a close friend) allows the nurse to help the young mother access this support to her benefit. (See Family Home Care box.)

The cognitive development of the adolescent influences the development of attitudes and realistic expectations regarding childbearing. To cope effectively and solve situational dilemmas, pregnant teenagers must be able to use the problem-solving approach to assess and evaluate consequences. The concrete thought and egocentrism of early adolescence can influence the mother's ability to evaluate

## FAMILY HOME CARE
### Adolescent Pregnancy

Ninety-seven percent of adolescent girls who make the decision to continue a pregnancy will choose to parent the infant rather than release the newborn for adoption (Neinstein, 1996). Recent research has demonstrated that many of these young mothers have successful childrearing skills. One key factor is the amount of assistance the mother receives from her family of origin. This assistance may be in the form of financial support and/or child care assistance. Family support allows the young mother to complete her education and acquire vocational skills while still meeting the needs of her child.

Nurses can increase the young mother's sense of competence by providing feedback about positive parenting skills and referring the teenager to community resources, such as parenting classes and infant stimulation programs. Nurses can also initiate and lead support groups for adolescent parents to foster self-confidence and parenting skills.

the needs of the infant. Adolescent mothers lack knowledge of normal infant growth and development. This deficit may directly affect their perception, interpretation, and responsiveness to infant cues.

Infant characteristics also influence parental behavior. Teenage parents view their children as more temperamentally difficult than do adult parents. Temperamentally difficult infants have an adverse effect on sensitivity and responsiveness of parents. Parent-infant interaction that is not mutually satisfying can alter the parents' feelings of effectiveness and self-worth as well as their sensitivity and relationship with the infant.

### Adolescent Fathers

There is little information available about adolescent fathers; most studies have small sample sizes and rely on reporting from the mother rather than the young man himself. Most teen fathers are involved and interested in their children. This involvement has positive effects on the self-esteem of the mother as well as decreasing her level of distress and depression (American Academy of Pediatrics, 2001a). The teen mother and her mother largely influence the level of participation a teen father has with his children. A high rate of involvement in substance use is another contributing factor that leads to decreased involvement on the part of the father (Rhein and others, 1997).

### Nursing Considerations

It is evident from the preceding discussion that nurses play a central role in meeting the needs of pregnant teenagers. It may be the nurse to whom the young girl turns for help and guidance in her dilemma and on whom she relies for support and reassurance.

The first goal in nursing care of the pregnant teenager is to help her obtain health care whether she elects to continue or terminate the pregnancy. Typically, adolescents are reluctant to seek medical help, in part because of anxiety but more often because of a tendency to deny the pregnancy. Early prenatal care is essential for the welfare of both mother and infant. For guidelines, teaching, and general support measures during pregnancy, the reader is directed to the excellent textbooks available on nursing care throughout the maternity cycle.

Basic to the implementation of any program of care is communication and the establishment of a trusting relationship. Initially the adolescent may appear apathetic and display little interest in discussing her pregnancy. The nurse must make every effort to put the adolescent at ease and avoid undue pressure. The young girl may have encountered rejection and open criticism from authority figures and peers. Conveying a nonjudgmental and genuine caring acceptance of the adolescent and her goals will assist the nurse in gaining the adolescent's confidence and trust.

Communication takes time and patience. Asking open-ended questions and listening for cues will help identify physical, emotional, social, and cultural influences that might affect the adolescent's progress through the maternity cycle. Factors that might affect her physical status, such as smoking, drug use, and nutritional state and habits, need to be explored and confronted. Each teenager presents a unique situation in relation to background, lifestyle, support structure, and coping mechanisms. Listening to the teenager is key to the development of the relationship. Understanding the situation from the adolescent's perspective is essential for a trusting relationship and effective communication.

Nutrition assessment should focus on the dietary adequacy of iron and calcium; multivitamins with folic acid are prescribed. The adolescent is referred for food supplement programs and other financial assistance, such as Women, Infants, and Children (WIC); Medicaid; Aid to Families with Dependent Children (AFDC); housing; and food stamps. Social work referral for thorough psychosocial assessment and planning may be initiated. Programs that have been most successful are comprehensive in approach and use an interdisciplinary team concept.

The adolescent needs to know what is happening to her, what is expected of her, and how she can help in developing a plan of care. Adolescents have their own ideas about the type of help they need and the support that they would find most beneficial. They should be consulted and provided with an opportunity to share their ideas. It is important to jointly choose goals that the adolescent believes are personally beneficial, attainable, and able to be maintained over time.

The adolescent will need help to improve her altered self-image, a crucial factor in adolescence. Giving her as much individual attention as possible; being a sympathetic listener; providing the opportunity for her to know, support, and be supported by other girls in the same situation; and helping her to experience success will facilitate progress toward achieving this goal.

The nurse should involve the family whenever possible. The parents of the adolescent mother and the father of the child need to express feelings and attitudes about the situation. The nurse should not make assumptions about whether or not the girl wishes to have these persons involved in her decisions and care.

Education regarding child care begins during pregnancy, and preparations should be made for continued education and assistance after the birth. Educational programs alone are probably not enough for high-risk youth. Home visiting programs have been helpful in the prevention of maltreatment of children with adolescent parents (Wurtele, 1999). Recognizing and referring high-risk teenage parents for additional services is crucial. Referral should target adolescents with low self-esteem, adolescents less than 14 years of age, and those without a social support network in place. The adolescent and her labor partner should attend childbirth education classes designed to meet the developmental level of the adolescent.

Postpartum care of adolescents should be directed toward the goal of preventing subsequent pregnancies. Health care programs that provide contraceptive services for the young mother at the time of her child's appointment are important. Merely dispensing contraception is not enough. Comprehensive programs to promote positive parenting, self-esteem, career goals, and family cohesiveness are necessary.

## Adolescent Abortion

In 1973 the landmark Supreme Court case of *Roe v. Wade* concluded that the right to an abortion rested within the rights of the individual. This right was not absolute but subject to certain state restrictions. Abortion is one of the most controversial moral issues in the United States. For example, most Americans believe that a pregnant woman should be able to obtain an abortion if her own life is endangered, if there is a strong chance that the fetus has a serious defect, or if the pregnancy is a result of a rape. However, some Americans do not believe that a woman should be able to have an abortion for any reason. The right to an abortion is also legally determined by the stage of pregnancy.

Among pregnant adolescents, many young women are choosing to continue their pregnancies and parent the child. The abortion rate has fallen more quickly than the drop in the pregnancy rate for adolescents. There are many possible explanations for this trend, including the possibility that access to abortion services for teens has decreased, that those who truly do not want to parent are abstaining or using more effective methods of contraception, and that there is more social support for parenting among adolescents (Henshaw and Feivelson, 2000).

Under current federal constitutional law, minors have the right to obtain abortions without parental consent unless otherwise specified by state law (American Academy of Pediatrics, 1996). (See the concept of "mature minor" and informed consent in Chapter 27.) Legislation that mandates parental involvement as a requirement for adolescents who seek an abortion has generated considerable controversy. Recent Supreme Court rulings have held that it is not unconstitutional for states to impose a parental notification requirement as long as pregnant adolescents who feel that this involvement would not be in their best interest are allowed to go to court without involving their parents and are legally permitted to make their own decisions (American Academy of Pediatrics, 1996). The American Academy of Pediatrics (1996) and several other health organizations have all reached a consensus that minors should not be compelled or required to involve their parents in this decision but should be encouraged to discuss their pregnancies with their parents and other responsible adults.

Currently, over 30 states have laws in place requiring one or both parents to be notified before the abortion is performed on the minor (Borgman and Jones, 2000). A study evaluating the outcome of parental notification laws found that they have no significant impact on the probability of abortions for minors because of parental involvement (Joyce and Kaestner, 1996).

Although abortion is a controversial and emotional issue, health care professionals involved in delivery of services to pregnant adolescents are confronted with this reality frequently. Because the law in this area is unsettled, is changing rapidly, and varies by state, nurses must stay abreast of legal changes as they relate to reproductive rights of minors in the state in which they practice.

Other barriers to receiving an abortion include distance to the clinic, cost, and antiabortion harassment. Abortion services in the United States are offered primarily at freestanding abortion clinics, usually in major population centers. Abortions are not covered by insurance, and the cost may be prohibitive to many women, especially adolescents.

The medical safety of a legal abortion has been well established. The mortality rate associated with teenage full-term pregnancy is much higher than the rate with abortion. A discussion of surgical procedures available is beyond the scope of this discussion. First-trimester abortions are performed as an outpatient procedure and require local anesthesia or mild sedation only. Complication rates have been reported to be 1% or less. Problems that arise after abortion are endometritis, hemorrhage, Rh sensitization, genital tract injury, retained fetal elements, and (in rare cases) pulmonary embolism or death. Second-trimester abortions are more complicated and are associated with greater risk from hemorrhage. Women who have an induced abortion are no more likely than other women to experience problems in bearing a healthy baby in subsequent pregnancies.

In 2000, the Food and Drug Administration approved mifepristone for medical abortion. This oral medication provides women with the option of a nonsurgical abortion procedure at 49 days or less of pregnancy. The drug prevents receptor binding of endogenous or exogenous progesterone, which causes an abortion. The cervix is softened and the myometrium is sensitized to the contraction-inducing activity of prostaglandins. The medication can be used from the time of detection of pregnancy up to 49 days since the last menstrual period (Meier, 2000). The abortion completion rate is 92% to 95% in pregnancies less than 49 days (Grimes, 2000a).

At the time of the diagnosis of pregnancy, the American Academy of Pediatrics (1998) recommends that the adolescent should be counseled about all three options which include (1) continue the pregnancy and parent the child, (2) continue the pregnancy and put the child up for adoption, or (3) obtain a medical or surgical abortion. The adolescent needs information about state laws for parental notification and/or consent for abortion. This is often the first time an adolescent is faced with such an important decision. Time and support are necessary to allow the adolescent to make the best decision for her current situation. The provider should voice unconditional support of the adolescent no matter what choice she makes. The adolescent should be discouraged from making an immediate decision and should be provided time and encouragement to discuss the options with her support system.

Numerous studies have examine the mental health risks associated with obtaining an abortion. There is no empirical evidence that women of any age who choose to have a legal first trimester abortion experience psychologic problems or regret. Most of the studies have examined the effects up to 2 years after the abortion (Major and others, 2000).

### Nursing Considerations

Early identification of pregnancy is essential, and nurses are in an optimum position to provide counseling on pregnancy options. Whatever option is chosen by the adolescent, referral should be initiated as quickly as possible to eliminate risk. Pelvic ultrasound may be indicated to assess gestational age correctly for those adolescents who cannot recall the date of their last menstrual period and when a bimanual examination is inconclusive.

Patient education regarding the medical aspects of the abortion should be conducted verbally, and the patient should be provided with written instructions before the procedure. Reviewing relaxation strategies that can be used during the procedure is helpful. Parents or other significant adults are encouraged to be present during the medical procedure.

Discussions about future contraceptive needs should be conducted before the abortion. The adolescent may be started on a hormonal method of contraception immediately after the abortion. The young woman should be seen 3 weeks after an abortion to receive medical, contraceptive, and psychologic follow-up care.

## Contraception

Family planning services have developed and expanded during recent years. In the mid-1980s, contraceptive use among adolescents increased significantly, with about 60% to 67% of adolescents reporting that some form of contraception was used at first intercourse (Neinstein, 1996). Although all teenagers need sexuality education, not all of them are candidates for contraception. Among the large adolescent population, there are those who have made the decision to postpone sexual involvement, and there are also those who may wish to have a child.

Confidentiality is a critical issue when discussing contraception with adolescents. Privacy is important to adolescents as they struggle to forge a personal identity and establish social relationships. Adolescents are particularly concerned about the judgments of others. The American Medical Association (AMA), the Society of Adolescent Medicine (SAM), the American Academy of Pediatrics (AAP), and the American College of Obstetrics and Gynecology (ACOG) have all written policy statements in support of a minor's right to confidential health care. All agree that although parental involvement is desirable, confidentiality may be central to encouraging teens to access needed health advice and treatment. Health delivery systems must be structured to allow confidentiality, including methods for appointment scheduling, billing, record keeping, and follow-up that ensure privacy rights for adolescents. Family-centered care and parental involvement in contraceptive choice are ideal for patient compliance. However, there are adolescents who need confidential care. The predominant feeling among health professionals is that parental notification is important but that the "parents' rights" view is not necessarily sensitive to the health needs and basic rights of youth. There is no evidence to substantiate the belief that providing contraceptive guidance contributes to sexual irresponsibility and promiscuity. Actually, a request for contraceptive information indicates a responsible effort on the part of the teenager to avoid an unplanned pregnancy.

### Contraceptive Methods

To be safe and effective a contraceptive method must be suited to the individual. The choice is based on the adolescent's preference after being informed of all the benefits and disadvantages of the methods available. The adolescent must be motivated to use whatever method is chosen. Factors associated with use of contraception include education, expectations, availability, cost of methods, parent education level, perception of high likelihood of pregnancy, perception of disadvantages of having a pregnancy, and low rate of disadvantages of birth control methods. Providing a birth control device is only part of a comprehensive sex education program. Partner involvement, when possible, is important to enhance user compliance. To make truly informed choices about contraception, adolescents need to know not only the efficacy of methods as they are actually used but also their efficacy when used consistently. The advantages and disadvantages of various contraceptive methods recommended for use in adolescents are outlined in Table 20-1.

**Nonprescription Methods.**   Sometimes, despite the effectiveness of prescription methods, teenagers use less effective methods to avoid the necessity for medical screening and supervision inherent in the use of prescription methods. Adolescents may report the use of withdrawal and reliance on "safe" periods in the menstrual cycle as their current method of contraception. Using the method of periodic abstinence, or the rhythm method, is very risky. When the rules are broken in this method, the couple is having unprotected sexual intercourse at times during the menstrual cycle when pregnancy is most likely to occur. Providing factual information about condoms and clarifying myths and misinformation about pregnancy prevention helps to reduce the incidence of unwanted pregnancy.

Because of the high incidence of STDs in the adolescent population, condom use should be discussed with all adolescents seeking contraceptive advice. The adolescent can then be assisted in choosing an *additional* method to prevent pregnancy.

The lack of female-controlled barrier methods known to protect against infection with STDs has led to the development of the female condom. The contraceptive efficacy of the female condom during typical use is similar to that of the diaphragm, sponge, or cervical cap. The female condom is nearly as effective in preventing pregnancy as the male condom without spermicidal lubricant. The female condom appears to have great potential for giving a woman control in reducing her risk of HIV infection (Trussell and others, 1994).

There is a growing body of research to evaluate the possibility that the spermicide nonoxynol-9 may actually increase the risk of HIV transmission. The Centers for Disease Control (CDC) is reassessing HIV prevention guidelines. The current policy is to recommend against the use of spermicides with nonoxynol-9 but not against condoms lubricated with the chemical (Hollander, 2000).

**Prescription Methods.**   The recommendation of a prescription method of contraception requires a careful medical history and understanding of the method by the adolescent. A discussion of the pros and cons of each method will assist the adolescent to dispel myths and help her to find the right method for her current situation. The clinician should provide accurate unbiased information about the benefits and risks, effectiveness, and return to fertility for each contraceptive method.

Intrauterine devices (IUDs) are not commonly recommended in the adolescent population. IUDs increase the risk of pelvic inflammatory disease (PID) and its consequences, and nulliparous females are more likely to have difficulty during insertion of the device, to suffer cramping and bleeding, and to expel the IUD.

IUDs are usually reserved for adolescents who cannot use other contraceptive methods and whose sexual behavior does not put them at risk for sexually transmitted diseases (American Academy of Pediatrics, 1999b). Sterilization is contraindicated for adolescents, especially those who have not borne children (Hatcher and others, 1998).

## Use of Contraception

In adolescents who are using contraception, the oral contraceptive pill (OCP) and the condom are the most popular methods. Delay in seeking contraceptive information is common in adolescence. The typical interval from onset of sexual intercourse until the first visit for contraception is 1 year. A pregnancy scare is usually the precipitating event for the contraception appointment. Reasons adolescents give for not making better use of contraception are listed in Box 20-2.

Recently, combinations or oral contraceptive or progestin-only oral contraceptives have been used as a form of emergency contraception (ECP) to prevent pregnancy after unprotected intercourse (Glasier, 1997) (see Table 20-1). It is estimated that the use of OCPs for emergency contraception could reduce the number of unintended pregnancies and abortions by 50% each year (Morris and Young, 2000).

Compliance in contraceptive use is related to many factors, including those discussed in the following sections.

**Lack of Information.**   Sometimes health professionals have a tendency to confuse a teenager's sophistication with knowledge. Although adolescents are acutely aware of their sexuality, their understanding of reproductive anatomy and physiology is often incomplete. If they are using contraception, they often do so with little or no instruction and with only vague understanding. Misinformation is commonplace. Lacking a fundamental understanding of fertility,

---

**Box 20-2** ■ ■ ■
**Reasons for Not Seeking or Using Birth Control**

Responses of teenagers at initial interview for contraception in order of frequency:
   Dangerous to use
   Waiting for closer relationship with partner
   Afraid family would find out
   Not having sex
   Afraid of examination
   Did not think had sex often enough for pregnancy
   Did not expect to have sex
   Thought wanted pregnancy
   Thought too young to get pregnant
   Partner objected
   Thought it cost too much
   Thought had to be older to get birth control

Modified from Zabin LS, Stark HA, Emerson MR: Reasons for delay in contraceptive clinic visit: adolescent clinic and nonclinic populations compared, *J Adolesc Health* 12:225-232, 1991.

**TABLE 20-1**   Advantages and disadvantages of contraceptive methods in the adolescent

| Method | Advantages | Disadvantages |
|---|---|---|
| **Abstinence** | • Increased popularity among adolescents<br>• No risk for pregnancy or STD | • Perceptions of peer sexual activity may stigmatize |
| **Withdrawal**<br>(coitus interruptus) | • No monetary cost<br>• No devices or chemicals<br>• Available in any situation<br>• No medical side effects | • No protection from STDs<br>• Unforgiving with incorrect use<br>• Requires self-control and self-awareness on the part of the male |
| **Fertility awareness**<br>Abstain from intercourse or use barrier method during times of cycle | • Increases user knowledge of reproductive potential<br>• Minimal cost | • Risk for STD transmission<br>• Adolescent females often have irregular cycles<br>• Complicated; limits spontaneity |
| **Condom**<br>Male: Thin sheath over penis to act as barrier to semen<br>Female: Polyurethane sheath that lines the vagina to block the passage of semen | • Inexpensive (female condom more expensive)<br>• No hormonal influence<br>• Rare side effects<br>• Easily available, no prescription<br>• STD protection | • Reduced sensitivity<br>• Limits spontaneity<br>• May be embarrassing to buy<br>• Female condom may be complicated to insert |
| **Spermicides**<br>A chemical barrier (foam, jelly, cream, suppository) inserted into the vagina before sexual intercourse | • Readily available<br>• Some STD protection<br>• Rare side effects<br>• Provides lubrication during intercourse | • Limits spontaneity<br>• Skin irritation may develop<br>• Messy |
| **Diaphragm**<br>A dome-shaped rubber cup with a flexible rim, coated with spermicide and inserted into the vagina to provide a protective barrier over the cervix | • No systemic side effects<br>• Decreased rates of cervical cancer | • Increased rates of urinary tract infections<br>• Requires a health visit for fitting<br>• Female must be comfortable with touching herself<br>• Limits spontaneity |
| **Combination**<br>**Oral Contraceptive Pill (OCP)**<br>Prevent pregnancy by suppressing ovulation, thickening cervical mucus, and thinning the endometrial lining | • Very effective when taken correctly<br>• Well studied method with minimal risk in the adolescent age group<br>• Noncontraceptive benefits include decreased acne, menstrual regulation, decreased dysmenorrhea<br>• Decreased risk of PID | • Hormonal changes<br>• Expensive<br>• Require office visit and prescription<br>• Nausea<br>• Daily involvement<br>• No STD protection |
| **Emergency Contraceptive Pill (ECP)**<br>Regimen of combined or progestin-only OCP administered within 72 hours after sexual intercourse to prevent implantation if fertilization were to occur | • May be used as a back up method for condom breakage, slippage of the diaphragm, or for unprotected intercourse<br>• Easy to use | • Requires prescription<br>• No STD protection<br>• Nausea with some regimens<br>• Change in next menses |
| **Depo Provera**<br>Injectable progestin-only contraceptive method that inhibits ovulation, thickens cervical mucus, and thins endometrial lining; injection given every 12-14 weeks | • Use is separate from act of intercourse<br>• No estrogen complications<br>• Scanty or no menses<br>• Effective long-term contraceptive method | • No STD protection<br>• Requires visit and injection every 12 weeks<br>• Expensive<br>• Change in menstrual pattern<br>• Weight gain<br>• Decreased libido<br>• Bone density decrease |
| **Combination Contraceptive Injection**<br>Lunelle™<br>Monthly injectable combined hormonal contraceptive (progestin and estrogen) that prevents ovulation, thins endometrium, and thickens cervical mucus | • Rapid return to ovulation after discontinuation<br>• Use is separate from act of intercourse<br>• Regular menstrual patterns and decreased menstrual cramping | • Monthly injection (women cannot go longer than 33 days between injections without a pregnancy test)<br>• No STD protection<br>• Expensive<br>• Nausea<br>• Breast tenderness |
| **Norplant**<br>Levonorgesterol implants inserted beneath the skin in the upper arm; prevents ovulation in at least half the cycles, thickens cervical mucus, and thins the endometrial lining | • No estrogen effects<br>• Use is separate from act of intercourse<br>• Immediate return to fertility at removal<br>• 5 years of pregnancy protection | • Expensive<br>• Requires clinician insertion and removal<br>• Bleeding pattern changes<br>• Weight gain<br>• No STD protection<br>• Removal may be difficult |
| **Intrauterine Device (IUD)**<br>Copper IUD prevents sperm from meeting ovum and prevents implantation; the progestin IUDs have a hormonal action thickening cervical mucus, thinning the endometrial lining | • Progestin IUDs decrease menstrual blood loss<br>• Easy to use after insertion<br>• Use is separate from act of intercourse<br>• No systemic side effects | • Risk of spontaneous expulsion<br>• Requires office visit for insertion and removal<br>• Risk of infection at time of insertion<br>• Change in menstrual patterns<br>• Dysmenorrhea with copper IUD<br>• No STD protection |

they often believe they are too young or have sex too infrequently to become pregnant. A majority of girls mistakenly believe that maximum fertility begins with menses and that the safe period occurs midway between menstrual periods.

**Anxiety Regarding Contraception.**   Some adolescents are concerned that their parents will be notified. Many have exaggerated ideas about the hazards of prescription methods, which correlates with misguided fears in the adult population. Myths about undesirable side effects prevail even after educational courses about contraception. Other teens are fearful of the pelvic examination and delay seeking contraception to avoid the procedure.

**Conflict About Sexual Activity.**   Many teenagers feel ambivalent regarding their sexual activity and avoid many contraceptives because their use seems too premeditated and implies that sex is planned rather than a spontaneous activity. Most of these girls believe that sex is all right if it is not planned. This may often play a role in those adolescents who delay contraception, waiting for a relationship that is "close enough." A close relationship would allow the adolescents to accept and acknowledge their sexual activity.

**Desire for Pregnancy.**   Some teens are seeking pregnancy and will fail to use an effective method of contraception or use a prescribed method improperly. Some adolescents seek pregnancy as a legitimate rite of passage into adulthood or as a misdirected attempt to have someone to love them. Careful counseling and assistance with decision-making skills are essential when counseling the adolescent desiring pregnancy.

## Nursing Considerations

Much of contraceptive education and service is assumed by nurses as part of sex education programs, family planning services, or postpartum health services. The introduction of contraceptive methods should ideally be associated with ongoing sex education. When they are included in this education process, the sexually active adolescent will consider contraceptives as a natural and logical part of intercourse. Education about sexuality, conception, and contraception should be accurate, straightforward, and presented in a nonjudgmental manner.

While sexual abstinence is highly desirable as a form of contraception, it is difficult for many adolescents to "just say no." Postponing sexual involvement requires effective communication and decision-making skills. Adolescents benefit from role-playing refusal skills in a safe environment. The nurse should also discuss with the adolescent how to introduce condoms into an existing relationship as well as into new relationships. Young women who have requested a partner to use a condom are more likely to use a condom consistently than women who have never made the request. The nurse plays an important role in offering appropriate education, helping build confidence in adolescents' ability to make requests of their partners, and providing social support to the sexually active adolescent.

To make an informed decision, the adolescent needs a careful review of all methods available, including their advantages and disadvantages. When possible, this counseling should include the parent(s) and/or partner.

Discontinuation rates of prescription methods are high among all women and particularly for adolescents. A critical aspect of counseling about a contraceptive method is education about use, non-contraceptive benefits and the expected side effects. (See Atraumatic Care box.) Clear oral explanations and demonstrations with the actual methods will assist the concrete thinker to understand the complicated instructions. Whenever possible, the parent should be included in the teaching. Written instructions and a phone number for questions should be provided. When hormonal methods are chosen, condom use should be reinforced for the prevention of sexually transmitted diseases. (See Community Focus box.) The nurse should demonstrate the correct use of condoms to all sexually active adolescents. Frequent follow-up with a review of side effects, usage patterns, and an opportunity to voice concerns increases the likelihood that the adolescent will continue to use contraception effectively.

An organization that provides education and services for adolescents, including both individual and group counseling, is the **Planned Parenthood Federation of America.*** It has branches in most cities in the United States.

---

*810 7th Ave, New York, NY 10019, (800) 230-PLAN; www.plannedparenthood.org.

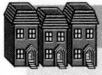

## COMMUNITY FOCUS
### Steps for Condom Use*

1. Be careful when opening the package, handle the condom gently, and check for breaks or holes in the condom.
2. Squeeze a dab of contraceptive jelly or cream with nonoxynol-9 into the tip of the condom.
3. Put on the condom as soon as erection occurs and before any vaginal, anal, or oral contact with the penis.
4. Unroll the condom on the erect penis, leaving about ½ inch of space at the tip of the condom.
5. Apply some of the contraceptive cream or jelly around the vagina or anus before entry.
6. Hold the rim of the condom in place when withdrawing the penis.
7. Take the condom off away from the partner's genitalia.
8. Throw the used condom away. **Never reuse a condom.**

Modified from *Entering adulthood: preventing sexually transmitted diseases,* Santa Cruz, CA, 1989, Network Publications.
*For additional information on AIDS/HIV, contact **CDC National AIDS Clearinghouse,** PO Box 6003, Rockville, MD 20849, (800) 458-5231, e-mail: hivmail@cdc.gov; **CDC National AIDS Hotline:** (800) 342-AIDS, Spanish: (800) 344-7432, Deaf: (800) 243-7889; and **National Center for HIV, STD, and TB Prevention (NCHSTP),** e-mail: hivmail@cidhivl.em.cdc.gov, *www.cdc.gov.*

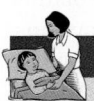

## ATRAUMATIC CARE
### Norplant and Depo-Provera

Apply EMLA over the site for the implant or injection 2½ hours before the procedure. A prescription should be given to the female for EMLA to be applied at home. When time does not permit the use of the topical anesthetic, use intradermal *buffered* lidocaine for insertion and removal of the implant.

# Rape

The adolescent girl is particularly vulnerable to sexual assault. It is estimated that more than 50% of rape victims are less than 18 years old; the peak age for victimization is age 16 to 19 years (Neinstein and others, 1996). Females are more likely to report these experiences than males (Neinstein and others, 1996). Adolescents and children with a physical or developmental disability are also more vulnerable to sexual abuse than their peers. In each instance the victim is potentially subjected to serious physical and/or emotional harm. There is no typical victim. Sexual assault victims are of all ages, ethnic groups, and economic groups and are of either gender.

Legal definitions of rape vary from state to state but include the following categories: completed rape, attempted rape, and statutory rape. Many current definitions of rape have been expanded to include all forms of sexual victimization, including anal and oral, as well as genital, penetration. Sexual assault is not restricted to vaginal or anal penetration but includes every form of sexual activity, including voyeurism.

Statutory rape may be charged when the victim is unable to give consent legally by virtue of age (age varies from state to state but is usually less than 16 years), mental deficiency, psychosis, or an altered state of consciousness caused by sleep, drugs, or illness.

## Assailants

Three relationships are identified for assault: stranger, nonstranger, and incest. Although all can have serious and long-lasting effects, they are presumed to be different in a number of important ways: in the nature of the dominant psychologic and cognitive behaviors they provoke, in the issues they raise for service providers and other potential helpers, and in the techniques that may be helpful for treating existing and new cases.

**Nonstranger Rapist.** The majority of rapes are committed by a nonstranger. This is often referred to as *acquaintance rape.* The acquaintance may be a date, someone who lives near the adolescent, someone who has contact with the victim through recreational activities, or someone in an official association with the teenager. Some assailants wait for an opportunity when the victim is defenseless, such as the teenager at home alone with an uncle or cousin or the baby-sitter being driven home.

The assailant may be another teenager known through social activity. The nature of sex-role learning in most cultures associates females with softness, nonassertiveness, and dependence on men. Young women are socialized to be alluring yet sexually unavailable and to assume the role of pacesetter in sexual situations. Males are conditioned to be strong, powerful, and aggressive (measures of masculinity) and to be aggressors in sexual situations.

Most studies on the relationship between sex-role attitudes and violence indicate that the determinants of dating violence are different for males and females. However, more research is needed to determine the nature of these differences. Some studies indicate an association between traditional gender-role attitudes in the female and an early onset of dating violence in a relationship. Other studies indicate that sex-role attitudes do not predict courtship violence but may explain an individual's response to violence (Rhynard, Krebs, and Glover, 1997).

One frequent research finding relating to acquaintance rape is the association between alcohol and drug consumption and forcible intercourse. A recent study of high school students indicated that 53% of the students who were forced into sexual intercourse had used alcohol or drugs as compared with 15% of those who did not use alcohol or drugs (Rhynard, Krebs, and Glover, 1997). When drugs or alcohol are involved, the adolescents' recall of events and their ability to distinguish between blame and responsibility is blurred (Slaughter, 2000).

Recently there has been a reported increase in the use of drug-facilitated sexual assaults. Older adolescents and young adults at parties, bars, and raves are at risk for having a drug slipped into their beverage when they are not looking. Substances most often referred to as "date rape" drugs are flunitrazepam (Rohypnol), a sedative-hypnotic benzodiazepine; gammahydroxybutyric acid (GHB), a sleep aid; and ketamine, an anesthetic agent (Smith, 1999). These fast-acting drugs cause disinhibition, passivity, relaxation of muscles, and lasting amnesia. The victim wakes up in strange surroundings and realizes she has been sexually assaulted. She may not report the crime for days, weeks, or may never report.

Prevention efforts for drug-facilitated sexual assault must focus on limiting alcoholic beverages. Alcohol not only potentiates the effects of the drugs, it remains the most widely used "date rape" drug (Schwartz and Milteer, 2000). Young women should be instructed to never accept already opened beverages of any kind at bars or parties and not to drink anything that has an unusual odor or taste.

Acquaintance rape is frequently underreported because the victim may believe she contributed to the act in some way. The victim may not identify the experience as rape because it does not fit the standard concept of rape.

Findings also indicate that not only are teenagers at risk for rape by peers, but they may also face multiple assailants or "gang rapes." These variations on teenage rape include multiple assailants and a single victim, multiple assailants and multiple victims, and peer rape in tandem (e.g., offenders who group together specifically to rape).

**Stranger Rapist.** It is believed that stranger rapes probably account for nearly 50% of all rapes reported to the police. Victims are frequently selected at random because they are apparently helpless.

**Incest.** The most commonly reported incestuous relationships are between a daughter and a father or stepfather (or other man in a caretaking role). The victim's participation is gained through the application of authority, subtle pressure, persuasion, or misrepresentation of moral standards. (For a further discussion of sexual abuse, see Child Maltreatment, Chapter 16.)

## Clinical Manifestations

Adolescents who have been raped arrive at the emergency room or practitioner's office under a variety of circumstances. They are usually brought in by parents, friends, or the police, but some girls may seek medical help on their own. They may display a variety of manifestations, such as hysterical crying or giggling; agitation; feelings of degradation, anger or rage, or helplessness; nervousness; and rapid mood swings. Adolescents may alternately appear calm and controlled, masking inner turmoil; they may be angry, confused, and filled with self-blame.

The rape victim may present with evidence of physical force, including roughness, nonbrutal beating (slapping), brutal beating (slugging, kicking), and choking or gagging. The predominant reaction of the victim is fear of the rape and of injury. Thus the victim is faced with the dilemma of submission or resistance. Resistance increases the victim's chance of escape but also increases the likelihood of violence against the victim.

## Therapeutic Management

It is advisable to obtain parental consent for examination, but the examination may be performed without consent if the adolescent is legally mature or the parents are unavailable. A female observer should be present during the history taking and examination of female victims who are examined by a male practitioner. Whether a parent should be present during the examination is determined on an individual basis. The parent's presence is usually encouraged, but only if the parent is supportive. Often the presence of a parent or a police officer inhibits the person's ability to describe the incident.

Because rape is a legal matter to be determined by the courts, medical examination merely provides evidence of penetration, ejaculation, and, when possible, use of force. However, many young women are left unmarked after sexual assault and have no evidence of physical trauma. A recent study of adolescent girls who reported sexual assault revealed abnormal genital findings in only 32% (Adams and Knudson, 1996).

**Initial Contact.** The circumstances of the initial medical evaluation may be frightening and stressful. The initial contact with the rape victim must be supportive, and the fundamental goal is to do no further harm. The interrogating and associated activities have the potential to add to the trauma of the sexual assault. The victim needs to know that she is (1) all right and (2) not being blamed for the situation. The first approach is not one of repeated interrogation but an attempt to reduce the victim's stress.

**History.** Although it is important to obtain a clear account of the circumstances of an alleged rape, it is also essential to minimize any further psychologic trauma that might occur if the adolescent is forced to relive a very painful experience. The adolescent will in all likelihood have been questioned by family and the police. If the person is too upset, the detailed history may be delayed. The adolescent should not be further victimized by insensitive care and unnecessary trauma.

The history should be as complete as possible and must be taken and presented in the patient's own words, including any account of force or threats. Information includes the date, time, location, and an accurate description of all types of sexual contact. All related activities are included. For example, evidence can be altered if the victim has bathed, urinated, defecated, douched, or changed clothing; therefore these activities are recorded. Use of a condom by the alleged assailant can alter evidence. For adequate care, other important data include the date of the last menstrual period, the date of last intercourse, use of contraception, and any possibility of a preexisting pregnancy or STD. The victim's behavior and emotional state are also recorded.

**Examination.** The physical examination and collection of evidence is carried out as soon as possible because physical evidence deteriorates rapidly. Practitioners specially trained for rape examination should be used when possible. Nurses are often members of this group and are known as *sexual assault nurse examiners (SANE).* The adolescent is always told in advance in understandable terms exactly what to expect in the way of tests and procedures, and the explanation is accompanied by emotional support. The victim is examined thoroughly, including nongenital areas, for evidence of injury that might substantiate the use of force. Photographs are taken of bruises, lacerations, or scratches for evidence, and rips or tears in clothing and the presence of dirt or grass stains are noted and recorded. Perineal, vaginal, or rectal lacerations suggest rape.

Specimens are obtained from the vaginal cul-de-sac and are examined immediately to assess sperm mobility. A cervical smear is prepared and sent to the laboratory. Vaginal secretions are also tested for acid phosphatase because this enzyme is not normally present in the female genital tract but is found in high concentrations in semen. This is especially important if the assailant has had a vasectomy or is infertile. Prostatic acid phosphatase has been found up to 22 hours after the alleged assault. The Papanicolaou (Pap) smear is the most reliable test for documentation of sexual intercourse from 14 to 26 hours after the event. Forensic materials should be turned over to law enforcement officials promptly after collection. A baseline serology for syphilis and hepatitis B is drawn, and a culture for chlamydial and gonococcal infection is obtained to prove that the victim did not have a preexisting infection. HIV testing should also be discussed with the victim. The adolescent is reexamined at appropriate intervals (4 to 6 weeks for syphilis; 2 to 3 days for gonorrhea) to determine if a disease was acquired from the assailant.

**Treatment.** Any injuries sustained by the victim that require surgical treatment are repaired. Most care providers prescribe prophylactic administration of antibiotics at the time of initial examination. Pregnancy prophylaxis with high-dose estrogen is offered to the victim who is not pregnant or using a contraceptive method.

## Nursing Considerations

Many of the approaches described for the sexually abused child apply to the adolescent. (See Chapter 16.) Sexual assault is a devastating experience with long-lasting effects. The primary goal of nursing care is to not inflict further stress on the victim, who is often angry, confused, frightened, embarrassed, and filled with self-blame. Young rape victims fear pregnancy, bodily injury, and the reactions of their parents and peers. Some believe that their bodies are permanently damaged and may even fear death as a consequence of the experience.

The nurse must do everything possible to reduce the stress of the interrogation and examination. Application of stress reduction techniques during the process can help the adolescent manage the immediate experience. Although most health professionals and law enforcement officers are sensitive to the needs of the victim and attempt to make the process as nonstressful as possible, the nurse acts as the advocate for the adolescent and is alert for cues that the victim is being overstressed.

Follow-up care of the rape victim is essential and extends over a long period of time. Rape victims typically show very high levels of distress within the first week, which peaks in severity by 3 weeks following the assault, continues at high levels for the next month, and then begins to decrease by 2 to 3 months after the assault. Referral to a public health agency and/or mental health agency should be made as soon as possible. Victims who live in areas with established rape crisis centers are referred to these facilities.*

Issues related to substance abuse must be addressed at the time of the assault, with continued monitoring at follow-up visits. Future alcohol and drug use by the victim of an assault is increased even when there is no history of prior use. The continued use of drugs places adolescent in a vicious cycle of increased risk for future assaults, which results in increased drug usage (Slaughter, 2000).

Aside from the universal need for emotional support, there are no firm guidelines for meeting the needs of rape victims. Their needs vary widely and depend on the nature of the incident, when it took place, the physical and emotional injuries sustained by the victim, the actions being considered as a result, the resources available for informal support, and the anticipated reactions of persons in the informal support network. (See Family Focus box.) Posttraumatic stress disorder (PTSD) occurs in many victims of rape. (See Chapter 18.) Acquaintance rape is as devastating to the victim as stranger rape. There are few reliable predictors of positive readjustment among rape survivors. In general, a young age at the time of assault is associated with increased distress. Women victimized in childhood are more likely than nonvictims to be assaulted as adults.

**Prevention.** With the increasing incidence of rape, many professionals are looking for additional means for preventing rape at all ages. Many schools and organizations arrange for classes on how to avoid an attack and how to behave in the event of an attempted rape. Rape trauma centers and most law enforcement agencies provide this service to groups. Every effort should be made to protect children and adolescents from injury and to teach them how to avoid situations that may promote an attack and how to behave in a threatening situation.

Nurses can be advocates for improving the community environment and street lighting, providing safe housing and transportation, and improving the effectiveness of the criminal justice system. They can work toward educating adolescents about the relationship of risk-taking behaviors and sexual attack. These behaviors include drinking, taking drugs, and hitchhiking.

The nurse can also play a role in identifying intimate partner violence. Only a small percentage of victims will initiate a discussion about partner violence with their health care provider. One step toward increasing safety is to begin to ask adolescents about safety in their current relationship. Young men should be offered antiviolence information as routinely as other messages about pregnancy prevention, driving safety, and prevention of sexually transmitted diseases.

Information about dating violence should be displayed in the waiting room, examining room, and bathroom. Awareness of local resources for adolescents who experience violence will allow the nurse to assist in referring those teens in need of help. At a broader level, nurses can also provide community education about intimate partner violence, including antiviolence presentations that target young men.

## SEXUALLY TRANSMITTED DISEASES (STDs)

STDs represent one of the major causes of morbidity during adolescence and young adulthood and annually afflict approximately 10 million persons under the age of 25 years. Teenagers represent one of the groups at highest risk. The actual prevalence rates among adolescents is underestimated, because the most prevalent STDs in adolescents—chlamydial infection and human papilloma virus (HPV) infection—are not required to be reported to the Centers for Disease Control and Prevention.

Several unique characteristics—biologic, developmental, and environmental—place adolescents at risk for acquisition of STDs. Biologically, the immature adolescent female cervix is composed of columnar epithelium on the exocervix (cervical ectopy). The thin layer of columnar cells appears to favor attachment of infectious agents (especially *Chlamydia trachomatis* and HPV), which accounts in part for the increased prevalence of these infections in adolescents. The unchallenged immune system does not provide local-

---

*For information about local organizations contact the **National Organization for Victim Assistance,** 1730 Park Rd, NW, Washington, DC 20010, (800) TRY-NOVA, (202) 232-6682, e-mail: NOVA@try-nova.org; www.try-nova.org.

### FAMILY FOCUS
*Supporting the Rape Victim's Parents*

In addition to the needs of the adolescent rape victim, the nurse should also be sensitive to the needs and reactions of the youngster's parents. Some will be angry and blame the adolescent; others will feel guilty and embarrassed. Many reactions can be expected at the time of the incident, ranging from despair to extreme agitation. Frequently the parents require as much support and reassurance as the victim. Agitated, angry, or incapacitated parents are unable to provide support for their youngster. Meeting parental needs can facilitate their ability to support the teenager during the crisis.

ized antibody response at the cervical level when exposed repeatedly to infectious agents. During anovulatory cycles estrogen predominates, as demonstrated by the clear and watery cervical discharge. This may facilitate the transport of pathogens to the upper genital tract (Vermillion, Holmes, and Soper, 2000).

Developmentally, teenagers experience biologic discontinuities when pubertal maturation precedes psychologic and cognitive maturity. For example, the average age of menarche has declined to 12½ years, and the age of sexual debut has also declined. An earlier age at sexual initiation results in increased numbers of sexual partners; 16% of high school–age adolescents report having had four or more partners in their lifetime (Centers for Disease Control and Prevention, 1998). The absence of future planning is often evident in the failure to see the implications of current behavior on future outcome, such as condom use to prevent an STD or pregnancy or the need to return for follow-up visits for contraceptive refill or STD treatment.

Adolescents lack the knowledge that many STDs can be asymptomatic or fail to recognize the symptoms when they occur. Rosenthal and others (1995) found that even among girls with a history of an STD, 42% believed that their partner could always (or most of the time) tell if he had a disease. During this time of evolving identity and emerging sexuality, the outcome is teenagers who have reproductive capabilities but insufficient maturity to make safe decisions and communicate effectively with their partner.

Studies have shown that as young women have more sexual partners, their use of hormonal contraception increases; at the same time, the use of condoms declines. Adolescents diagnosed with an STD have a 40% risk of acquiring another STD in the same year (Fortenberry and others, 1999). While knowledge alone does not change behavior, some AIDS education programs have been effective in increasing the use of condoms and prescription contraceptive methods at the same time (Stanton and others, 1996). (See Community Focus box on p. 865.)

Designing health care systems and providing in-service education for all health care personnel are essential to providing services that meet the needs of adolescents. Environmental barriers to health care use by teenagers include high cost, lack of insurance, inconvenient timing of appointments, and inconvenient location of health facilities. Services need to be easily accessible and sensitive to the adolescent's developmental needs and desire for confidentiality. State statutes vary regarding the right to confidential testing and treatment for STDs. States without specific statutes outlining treatment can offer confidential care based on common law precedent. Nurses should review the guidelines in the state in which they are practicing.

## Gonorrhea

### Epidemiology

Several demographic factors have been described for persons who are at risk for acquiring gonorrhea. Adolescents 15 to 19 years of age have the highest overall incidence of gonococcal infection compared with any other age-group when rates are adjusted for sexual activity. Gonorrhea among nonwhites is 10 times more frequent than among whites. Part of this discrepancy can be explained by the fact that nonwhites are more likely to attend public health clinics, where reporting of the disease is better than in the private sector. Other known risk factors are low socioeconomic status, urban residence, early onset of sexual activity, single marital status, previous history of gonorrhea, and multiple sexual partners.

**NURSING ALERT**   Prior infection is an important marker and should alert the clinician that the individual is at risk for reinfection.

Epidemiologic evidence suggests that there is a core group, or clustering of individuals, who are never treated or are inadequately treated and thus serve as a reservoir for reinfection. This emphasizes the need for partner identification and appropriate treatment to interrupt this cycle of reinfection.

Gonorrhea is almost always sexually transmitted, except when it appears in the conjunctiva. Vertical transmission from the maternal cervix to the newborn's conjunctiva is the usual mode of infection. The incidence of gonococcal ophthalmia has decreased in developed countries as a result of the routine application of prophylactic antibiotics to the eyes of newborn infants. (See Chapter 8.) Gonococcal infections do not confer lifelong immunity; therefore, individuals are subject to reinfection.

### Pathophysiology

The causative organism is *Neisseria gonorrhoeae,* a gram-negative diplococcus. The organisms have very specific survival requirements. A moist, alkaline environment (pH 7.2 to 7.6) and a temperature of 35° to 36° C (95° to 96.8° F) are preferred. The gonococci survive only on the columnar and transitional epithelium; stratified epithelium is resistant to the onslaught. The organism spreads along the mucosa from the point of entry. It penetrates between the epithelial cells and, when dead, liberates an irritant that produces the inflammatory response, characterized by localized capillary dilation, edema, and leukocytosis. This process accounts for the purulent discharge and erosive balanitis and cervicitis sometimes observed in affected persons.

### Clinical Manifestations

Symptoms can appear as early as 1 day or as late as 2 weeks after sexual contact. Gonococcal infection can present in many diverse ways, with four basic presentations: asymptomatic, uncomplicated symptomatic, complicated symptomatic, and disseminated disease. The infection can involve a number of organs and a wide range of manifestations (Table 20-2). Pelvic inflammatory disease (PID) in females simulates the inflammatory process caused by other bacterial infections, and differential diagnosis is made for more definitive medical treatment. Because a large percentage of affected persons are asymptomatic, gonorrhea should be considered in the evaluation of all sexually active adoles-

**TABLE 20-2** Comparison between gonorrhea and chlamydial infection

| Characteristics | Gonorrhea | Chlamydia |
|---|---|---|
| Incubation period | 2-6 days; rare cases 10-16 days | 8-21 days |
| Major site of infection | Urethritis (males) | Urethritis (males) |
| | Cervicitis (females) | Cervicitis (females) |
| Local complications | Epididymitis, bartholinitis, salpingitis, prostatitis, PID, conjunctivitis, pharyngitis, proctitis | Epididymitis, bartholinitis, salpingitis, postpartum endometritis, PID, conjunctivitis (trachoma), proctitis |
| Systemic complications | Septicemia with resulting arthritis, dermatitis, endocarditis, meningitis, perihepatitis, peritonitis | Arthritis, perihepatitis, chronic conjunctivitis |
| Carrier state | Recognized, especially in women; can last for months; primary reservoir is cervix; male urethra is a minor site | Recognized, especially in women; can last for months; primary reservoir is cervix; male urethra is a minor site |
| Effects of maternal infection on newborn | Less well-established | Well-known; inclusion conjunctivitis and pneumonia |
| | Ophthalmia neonatorum | |
| Treatment | Ceftriaxone or cefixime | Azithromycin single-dose treatment |
| | Single-dose treatment | Doxycycline b.i.d. for 7 days |
| | Treat for possible chlamydial infection as well | Treat sexual contacts |
| | Treat sexual contacts | |

cents. Lack of clinical symptoms is especially characteristic of the rectal and pharyngeal infections.

### Diagnostic Evaluation

Diagnosis is made by culture from the urethra in males or the cervix in females. Other diagnostic techniques for females include rapid antigen tests or polymerase or ligase chain reaction (PCR, LCR) tests from endocervical swabs or urine specimens. Diagnosis of urethritis in the male can be made with the use of leukocyte esterase activity in a urine specimen. Identification of the pathogen can also be made with cell culture, or PCR, or LCR from urethral or urine specimens.

Proper urine collection techniques are necessary for accurate diagnosis. When collecting urine specimens from females from LCR/PCR, the perineum should not be cleansed before collection as it is for urine bacterial culture. The adolescent should be instructed to collect the urine from the beginning of the stream, not mid-stream. Males should also be instructed to collect the first part of the urine stream (Blake and Woods, 2001).

### Therapeutic Management

The emergence of gonococcal strains resistant to penicillin has changed treatment recommendations. Uncomplicated gonorrhea is treated with a single dose of cefixime 400 mg PO plus azithromycin 1 g PO one time. Azithromycin is added to cover the high incidence of co-existent chlamydial infection. Treatment failure is rare, and a test of cure after completion of antibiotics is not necessary. Sexual partners must be treated, and the teen is instructed to abstain from sexual intercourse for 7 days following treatment (Centers for Disease Control and Prevention, 1997).

### Prevention

Until a genuine prophylaxis against gonorrheal infections is available, preventive efforts must be directed toward finding and treating affected persons, locating and examining contacts of affected persons, and educating young people regarding the facts of the disease and its spread. The use of latex condoms helps prevent transmission of the infection.

## Chlamydial Infection

Chlamydia is the most common bacterial STD in the United States. Rates among adolescents range from 5% to 12% with rates as high as 40% in some high-risk populations (Lahoti and others, 2000). The sequelae of untreated chlamydial infections include pelvic inflammatory disease, ectopic pregnancy, epididymitis, and infertility. Infants born to infected mothers may be born prematurely and develop conjunctivitis and pneumonia.

### Pathophysiology

The disease is caused by the bacterium *C. trachomatis*. Like viruses, chlamydiae are intracellular parasites during part of their life cycle. The organisms consist of alternating forms: the extracellular, or elementary, body and the intracellular, or initial, body. The elementary body attaches to the host cell, where it induces active phagocytosis and is ingested in a vesicle that serves as a setting for the next stage of the cycle.

Unlike other phagocytosed organisms, *C. trachomatis* is able to circumvent host cell defenses and become a part of the cell. Within the host cell the elementary body reorganizes into the larger initial body, which uses the cell's synthetic functions and energy sources for its own metabolic needs. It divides to produce microcolonies of chlamydiae. After 18 to 24 hours the initial bodies again reorganize into elementary bodies and exit from the disrupted host cell to infect new cells. The entire process takes about 40 hours, and the result is a slow, steady accumulation of intracellular inclusions that are diagnostic of the infection.

### Clinical Manifestations

The incidence of asymptomatic chlamydia infections is as high as 50% of men and 75% of women (Grimes, 2000b).

**TABLE 20-3**   Sensitivity and specificity for chlamydia tests

| Test | Sensitivity | Specificity |
|------|-------------|-------------|
| Culture | 70%-85% | 100% |
| Ligase chain reaction (LCR) | 94% | 99%-100% |
| Polymerase chain reaction (PCR) | 90% | 99%-100% |
| DNA probe | 85% | 98%-99% |

From Black CM: Current methods of laboratory diagnosis of *Chlamydia trachomatis* infections, *Clin Microbiol Rev* 10(1):160-184, 1997.

The most common symptoms for females are vaginal discharge or dysuria. As the infection ascends to the endometrium and fallopian tubes, menstrual irregularities and lower abdominal pain may develop. Symptomatic males have a urethral discharge or dysuria. Rectal infections are generally asymptomatic; however, symptoms of proctitis may occur.

### Diagnostic Evaluation

The diagnosis is confirmed in females by endocervical cultures, rapid antigen tests, or polymerase or ligase chain reaction (PCR, LCR) tests. Table 20-3 gives specificity/sensitivity data on available tests for chlamydia. Diagnosis of urethritis in the male can be made with the use of leukocyte esterase (LE) activity in a urine specimen. Identification of the pathogen is made with cell culture, PCR, or LCR from urethral or urine specimens.

### Therapeutic Management

The recommended treatment for uncomplicated chlamydial infections is azithromycin 1 g PO as a single dose. The alternate therapy is doxycycline 100 mg PO b.i.d for 7 days. The single-dose treatment is preferred for compliance. A test of cure is not necessary. All sexual partners must be treated, and the adolescent should abstain from sexual intercourse for 7 days following treatment (Centers for Disease Control and Prevention, 1997).

## Pelvic Inflammatory Disease (PID)

PID is an infection of the upper genital tract (endometrium, fallopian tubes, and ovaries), most commonly caused by sexually transmitted bacteria, such as *N. gonorrhoeae*, *C. trachomatis*, and a variety of other anaerobic bacteria.

Only 10% to 15% of women with *C. trachomatis* or *N. gonorrhoeae* will develop an upper tract infection (Wald, 1996). Menstruation at the time of initial infection can increase the risk for the development of PID. The loss of the mucous plug allows the infecting organism to ascend to the upper tract more readily. The blood itself acts as a culture medium for the growth of the infecting organisms. Other mechanical factors that may increase the risk of PID development include the presence of an IUD and douching; sperm and motile trichomonas may also carry other infections up the genital tract (Wald, 1996).

PID can have acute complications, such as tubo-ovarian abscess and the *Fitz-Hugh–Curtis syndrome.* This syndrome occurs in about 5% to 20% of women who have acute **salpingitis** (infection of the fallopian tubes). The same organisms that cause the salpingitis produce an acute inflammation of the covering surrounding the liver (the hepatic capsule) and the peritoneum in contact with the hepatic capsule. The Fitz-Hugh–Curtis syndrome causes acute or chronic right upper quadrant abdominal pain and can lead to chronic adhesions between the hepatic capsule and the peritoneum. In some individuals the pain and tenderness associated with this syndrome may be more pronounced than the pelvic signs and symptoms (Neinstein, 1996).

The long-term effects of PID include infertility because of tubal scarring, ectopic pregnancy, and chronic abdominal pain. It is estimated that each year 1 million females of reproductive age experience an episode of PID, with approximately 20% of cases occurring in teenagers. Women under the age of 25 years have a 1-in-8 chance of experiencing PID compared with those over age 25 years, whose risk is 1 in 80. Previously discussed biologic and behavioral risk factors account for the increased rate.

Symptoms in the adolescent may be generalized, with lower abdominal pain, urinary tract symptoms, and vague influenza-like manifestations, such as malaise, nausea, diarrhea, or constipation. A pelvic examination to evaluate the possibility of PID is indicated for every sexually active female who complains of lower abdominal pain.

The diagnosis of PID is based on clinical findings. The 1998 STD guidelines (Centers for Disease Control and Prevention, 1997) list the minimum criteria for diagnosis as lower abdominal tenderness, adnexal tenderness, and cervical motion tenderness. Additional supportive evidence for the diagnosis of PID includes oral temperature 101° F, abnormal cervical discharge, elevated erythrocyte sedimentation rate, elevated C-reactive protein, and laboratory documentation of chlamydia or gonorrhea.

The potential for sequelae even after one episode of PID is as high as 25%. The adolescent with PID is at increased risk for infertility, ectopic pregnancy, and recurrent PID. Chronic pelvic pain and dyspareunia are not uncommon after an episode of PID (Lawson and Blythe, 1999).

The risk of sequelae requires aggressive management of PID in the adolescent. The severity of the disease at presentation does not predict the incidence of undesirable sequelae (Wald, 1996). Outpatient therapy includes a single dose of cefoxitin or ceftriaxone given intramuscularly plus doxycycline 100 mg given orally b.i.d. for 14 days. Inpatient therapy may be necessary for adolescents who are unable to tolerate an outpatient regimen, adolescents who are pregnant, or adolescents who have a suspected abscess or uncertain diagnosis. Inpatient therapy includes intravenous antibiotics such as cefoxitin, cefotetan, doxycycline, clindamycin, or gentamicin. On discharge, the adolescent receives a 14-day course of oral doxycycline or metronidazole (Centers for Disease Control and Prevention, 1997).

Adolescents with PID need counseling to prevent future infections. Partner notification and treatment is necessary to avert recurrent infection. The adolescent should be instructed to abstain from sexual intercourse while taking the medication and until after her partner is treated. A discussion of negotiating condom usage is beneficial for the prevention of future infections.

## Human Papillomavirus (HPV)

Anogenital warts, caused by HPV infection, are the most common STD in the United States. There is strong evidence linking HPV to the development of cervical dysplasia and carcinoma (Walboomers and others, 1999; Yacobi and others, 1999).

Individuals with HPV are more likely to develop carcinoma in situ; the highest rates for HPV infection are found in sexually active women under the age of 25 (Koutsky, 1997). Risk factors for HPV infection include sexual behavior (multiple partners), lack of condom use, age at first sexual intercourse, and history of prior infection (Koutsky, 1997; Kahn and others, 2002).

HPV may remain asymptomatic or present as exophytic condyloma on the genitals or cervical dysplasia and carcinoma. The rates of cervical dysplasia have increased significantly over the past decade (Mangan and others, 1997). Most of the more than 70 identified types of HPV that infect the genital tract have been divided into low and high oncogenic risk categories. Types 6 and 11 are categorized as low oncogenic risk. Types 16, 18, 31, 45, and 56 are higher risk and are associatead with high-grade cervical changes and invasive carcinomas of the anus, cervix, and penis.

The most visible type of wart is *condyloma acuminatum,* a raised, polypoid mass with an irregular fingerlike surface and fissures, commonly described as having a "cauliflower" appearance. In females these warts are most commonly seen on the external genitalia or the vagina, cervix, or rectum. The shaft of the penis is the most common site in males, but warts may also appear on the meatus, anus, and scrotum. The presence of warts on the rectum or anus of males is frequently associated with anal intercourse; anal warts in females can be associated with autoinoculation.

Subclinical genital HPV infection is much more common than the warts that are exophytic (grows outward from surface). The previously common practice of treating areas that give a white appearance after application of acetic acid is no longer recommended. Acetowhitening is not a specific test for HPV. Subclinical infections often regress spontaneously without treatment (Centers for Disease Control and Prevention, 1997).

Annual Pap smear screening is essential for sexually active adolescent females to detect the presence of cervical cell changes. DNA testing for HPV is becoming more widely used to assist with identification of high-risk categories. Patients with warts and/or cervical dysplasia should be counseled that they may infect sexual partners. Female partners should receive a Pap smear if sexually active with a male partner with warts.

### Therapeutic Management

The treatment of external warts on females and males consists of both patient-applied and provider-administered options. The *patient-applied* option includes (1) podofilox 0.5% solution applied with a cotton swab twice daily for 3 days followed by 4 days without therapy; this cycle is repeated as needed for a total of 4 cycles; or (2) imiquimod 5% cream applied every day for 3 days a week for 16 weeks (McClain and others, 2000). The *provider-administered* option includes (1) cryotherapy with liquid nitrogen every 1 to 2 weeks, (2) podophyllinresin 10% to 25% in benzoin repeated weekly, or (3) 80% to 90% trichloroacetic acid (TCA) applied weekly (Centers for Disease Control and Prevention, 1997).

Patient education regarding the use of medication and the importance of follow-up is essential and should be ongoing. When parents are aware of the infection, their participation in the education may be beneficial to the adolescent. The concrete aspects of HPV and cervical dysplasia may be more easily understood by the adolescent; however, the abstract concepts of asymptomatic infections and the relationship of cigarette smoking to cervical cancer are more difficult to comprehend (Gerhardt and others, 2000). The nurse plays an important role in educating the adolescent about the disease process, assisting with smoking cessation, as well as providing information regarding procedures and treatments.

## Human Immunodeficiency Virus (HIV) Infection and Acquired Immunodeficiency Syndrome (AIDS)*

As of June 2000, 3865 adolescents 13 to 19 years of age and 26,518 young people from 20 to 24 years of age had been diagnosed with AIDS. Although this only accounts for 4% of the cumulative total of AIDS cases in the United States, HIV infection is the ninth leading cause of death in the United States for all races 15 to 24 years of age and the sixth leading cause of death for African-Americans 15 to 24 years of age (Murphy, 2000).

Half of all new HIV infections in the United States occur in persons between the ages of 13 and 24. Sexual transmission accounts for most cases of HIV during adolescence (American Academy of Pediatrics, 2001b).

Sexual partners of female adolescents are often several years older and may have already been infected. The known high prevalence rates of other STDs and pregnancy among adolescents document that adolescents are sexually active, and the high incidence of STDs in the adolescent population puts the adolescent at risk for the transmission of AIDS.

Several years may elapse between infection and the development of clinical AIDS. Because the greatest number of reported AIDS cases occur among young adults in their twenties, it can be inferred that many of these infections were acquired in adolescence. Adolescents infected with the virus can continue to spread the infection without knowing they have the disease.

■ *Nancy Kline, PhD, RN, CPNP, revised this section.

Many adolescents do not perceive that they are at risk for HIV infection or AIDS. In a study of sexually active adolescent females attending a hospital-based clinic, 81% of these teenagers reported that they had never done anything to place themselves at risk for AIDS. The reasons these teenagers gave for low personal risk included current monogamy, belief in their partner's safety and fidelity, and their ability to choose partners carefully (Overby and Kegeles, 1994). (See Community Focus box. (See Acquired Immunodeficiency Syndrome, Chapter 35.)

## Hepatitis B Virus (HBV)

HBV is an infection of the liver that affects 300,000 persons annually, 10,000 of whom require hospitalization (see Chapter 33). Major concerns have been voiced because of the increased rate of infection, particularly among high-risk populations: intravenous drug users, sexual partners of HBV-infected individuals, homosexual males, and infants of HBV-infected pregnant women. It is estimated that infants whose mothers are positive for HBV will have a 70% to 90% chance of becoming infected, and nearly all of these infants will develop chronic HBV carrier status. Another area of concern is transmission of HBV through contaminated body fluids to health care workers.

Many potential negative outcomes can be avoided through immunization. Current immunization guidelines recommend beginning the hepatitis B vaccine series at birth or, in unimmunized children, at 11 to 12 years of age (U.S. Department of Health and Human Services, 1996). The immunization consists of a series of three intramuscular injections. (See Atraumatic Care box.) The goal of universal immunization is to target noninfected infants and adolescents before the onset of high-risk behaviors. (See Immunizations, Chapter 12.)

## Other Sexually Transmitted Genital Lesions

Many sores or lesions that appear on the genitalia are the result of STDs. Experienced clinicians can correctly diagnose these lesions by visual examination only 60% of the time. A complete health history, physical examination, and appropriate diagnostic cultures are needed to determine the causative factors. Nurses who interact with adolescents are in a primary position to obtain a health history and refer any sexually active adolescent for appropriate evaluation. Follow-up health education regarding any treatment regimen and prevention strategies is a major nursing role. Because many of the lesions are viral in nature, the nurse can assist the adolescent with communication techniques to inform future sexual partners about the potential for infection with an STD. A summary of the most common genital lesions seen in adolescents is given in Table 20-4.

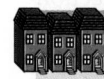

### COMMUNITY FOCUS
#### HIV Prevention Programs

HIV prevention programs aim to reduce sexual activity and substance use and reduce adolescents' HIV risk. Some examples of HIV prevention strategies include ensuring access to health care and HIV testing, encouraging employment, and providing general social skills training. Providing HIV education programs at key development points (e.g., preadolescence, during pregnancy) and community settings (e.g., school-based clinics, afterschool programs) may prove to be a good approach (Rotheran-Borus, 2000). A program titled "Safer Choices" encourages HIV, STD, and pregnancy prevention in adolescents. Safer Choices has been shown to enhance knowledge, self-efficacy for condom use, HIV risk perceptions, and parent-child interactions (Coyle and others, 1999).

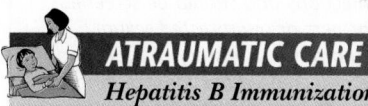

### ATRAUMATIC CARE
#### Hepatitis B Immunization

Apply EMLA cream to the deltoid site 2½ hours before administering the injection to *anesthetize* the area.

| TABLE 20-4 | Genital lesions in adolescents | | | |
| --- | --- | --- | --- |
| **Disease** | **Manifestations** | **Therapy** | **Nursing Considerations** |
| Herpes simplex (viral) | Prodrome: intense burning or itching at site of outbreak; often flulike symptoms <br> Painful, enlarged inguinal lymph nodes <br> First lesions; clear, raised vesicles, very painful <br> Recurrent lesions resolve more quickly and are less painful | Acyclovir (oral) or Famciclovir <br> Shortens clinical course in first episode <br> Prophylaxis decreases recurrence rate | Immunocompromised patient at risk for overwhelming infection <br> Sex partner only treated if lesion present <br> Infection can be transmitted to infant during birth <br> Adolescent needs education and support <br> Increased risk for HIV with open lesion |
| Primary syphilis | Chancre: a hard, nontender, red, sharply defined lesion with indurated base, raised border, eroded surface, and scanty yellow discharge <br> Nonpainful, enlarged lymph nodes | Penicillin | Affected person more infectious during first year of disease <br> May be transmitted to fetus <br> Partner treatment necessary <br> Increased risk for HIV with open lesion |
| Molluscum (viral) | Solitary clusters of raised, pearly white, firm, nontender papules <br> Umbilicated dimpled lesions | Excision and expression of core material <br> Cryotherapy | No known complications <br> Sex partner only treated if lesions present |

## Critical Thinking Exercise

### Sexually Transmitted Diseases

Jane, age 15 years, comes in for a refill of oral contraceptive pills (OCPs). During the sexual history, Jane reveals that she is using condoms 50% of the time. She has had 2 new sexual partners since last seen 3 months ago and has a lifetime history of 10 male partners. She has a past history of gonorrhea, chlamydial infection, and trichomoniasis. Jane reports no vaginal discharge, no abdominal pain, and no urinary symptoms today. Her last gynecologic examination with a Pap smear was 3 months ago.

Which of the following would be the best plan for Jane's visit today?

FIRST, THINK ABOUT IT . . .

• Within what point of view are you thinking?
• What would the consequences be if you put your thoughts into action?

1. Obtain a prescription for another 3 months' supply of OCPs and encourage 100% condom usage.
2. Perform a screening examination for sexually transmitted diseases (STDs), discuss HIV testing, encourage STD prevention, and obtain a prescription for another 3 months' supply of OCPs.
3. Call Jane's mother and discuss Jane's high-risk sexual behavior.
4. Lecture Jane that she was lucky this time and does not have an STD. However, remind her that if she does not change her sexual behavior, she will become infected again and possibly become infertile.

*The best response is two. Adolescents with multiple sex partners are at risk for the transmission of STDs. Females often have asymptomatic infections and should be screened when they have new sex partners or unprotected sexual intercourse. Adolescents with a previous history of STDs and multiple sexual partners are at increased risk for acquiring HIV. The availability of anonymous and confidential testing should be discussed with Jane. Scare tactics have not been shown to be effective in initiating changes in adolescent behavior and reflect a very narrow point of view. Jane has a legal right to receive confidential care for STDs and contraception; parental notification requires the adolescent's knowledge and may bear many consequences. The nurse should assess the barriers to condom usage for Jane. Role-playing the negotiation of condom usage will assist Jane in developing new communication skills.*

## Nursing Considerations

Nursing responsibilities encompass all aspects of STD education, prevention, and treatment. Primary prevention by avoiding exposure is the least expensive and most effective approach. The nurse can play a role in offering this education to young people before they initiate sexual intercourse. Sexuality education should include information about these diseases, such as their symptoms or lack of symptoms and treatment, as well as information dispelling the myths associated with their mode of transmission. These diseases are not contracted from toilet seats, drinking glasses, or bath towels. Most teens are uninformed or misinformed about STDs.

The promotion of the inclusion of STD information, access to care, and interpersonal and social skills building in school sexuality education programs is an important function of the nurse. (See Critical Thinking Exercise box.) No matter what their area of practice, nurses are in a position to disseminate information, identify probable cases of STDs, and refer these cases for treatment.

The increasing incidence of STDs in young people is influenced to a great extent by the larger numbers of teens who engage in sexual activity at younger ages and with more partners. In addition, the changing pattern of contraceptive use is a contributing factor to more risky sexual activity. The hormonal contraceptive methods provide no protection against STDs. Unfortunately, many girls using these methods mistakenly believe they are also protected against STDs. To decrease the likelihood of infection, sexually active adolescents are encouraged to *always* use a condom.

Essential measures for control of the disease include treating the disease, reporting it promptly, and tracking and treating contacts. When working with adolescents, nurses need highly developed interviewing skills and a nonjudgmental approach to elicit an accurate sexual history. Several characteristics of teenagers influence the way health professionals address specific issues related to STDs. Teenagers are often concrete thinkers, which affects the way they process information. Teenagers also have limited coping mechanisms to draw on to assist in dealing with such information. To gain the adolescent's cooperation, the nurse must convey acceptance, gain the adolescent's trust, and assure the adolescent of confidentiality. The nurse should always consider the early involvement of parents with permission from the adolescent. Family support may make access to health services easier and decrease the emotional stressors associated with acquiring an STD.

## KEY POINTS

■ Adolescent health-seeking behaviors center on skin problems, abdominal discomfort, menstrual symptoms, and anxieties about physical development and sexual changes.

■ Acne is prevalent in the adolescent years; medication and gentle facial cleansing are the treatments of choice.

■ The most frequent problems related to the male reproductive system are infections, scrotal conditions, and gynecomastia.

■ The most frequent problems of the female reproductive system involve menstruation delays, irregularities, discomfort, and infections.

■ Adolescent pregnancy has profound social, educational, psychologic, and economic ramifications. The pregnancy necessitates special attention to nutrition as well as psychologic and emotional support for the mother and father.

- Abortion as an alternative to birth is a highly controversial issue; there is evidence that it has no long-term psychologic sequelae for most women.
- Contraception is often not used because of lack of information, anxiety regarding use, conflict over sexual activity, and desire for pregnancy.
- Rape is a serious problem among adolescents; common forms are rape by a nonstranger, rape by a stranger, and incest.

- Sexually transmitted diseases are the most frequently occurring infectious diseases and a major cause of adolescent morbidity. Human immunodeficiency virus (HIV) infection is an increasingly important adolescent health problem.

# REFERENCES

Adams JA, Knudson S: Genital findings in adolescent girls referred for suspected sexual abuse, *Arch Pediatr Adolesc Med* 150(8):850-857, 1996.

Adelman WP, Joffe A: The adolescent with a painful scrotum, *Contemp Pediatr* 17(3): 111-127, 2000.

Alan Guttmacher Institute: *Teen sex and pregnancy, facts in brief,* New York, 1999, The Institute.

American Academy of Pediatrics: Care of adolescent parents and their children, *Pediatrics* 107(2):429-434, 2001a.

American Academy of Pediatrics, Committee on Adolescence: Adolescent pregnancy—current trends and issues: 1998, *Pediatrics* 103(2):516-520, 1999a.

American Academy of Pediatrics, Committee on Adolescence: Contraception and adolescents, *Pediatrics* 104(5):1161-1166, 1999b.

American Academy of Pediatrics, Committee on Adolescence: The adolescent's right to confidential care when considering abortion, *Pediatrics* 97(5):746-751, 1996.

American Academy of Pediatrics, Committee on Pediatric AIDS and Committee on Adolescence: Adolescents and human immunodeficiency virus infection: the role of the pediatrician in prevention and intervention, *Pediatrics* 107(1):188-190, 2001b.

American Academy of Pediatrics, Committee on Sports Medicine and Fitness: Medical concerns in the female athlete, *Pediatrics* 106(3):610-613, 2000.

American Academy of Pediatrics: Counseling the adolescent about pregnancy options, *Pediatrics* 101(5):938-940, 1998.

Aquilino ML, Bragadottir H: Adolescent pregnancy, *MCN* 25(4):192-197, 2000.

Banerjee R, Laufer MR: Reproductive disorders associated with pelvic pain, *Semin Pediatr Surg* 7(1):52-61, 1998.

Bendich A: The potential for dietary supplements to reduce premenstrual syndrome (PMS) symptoms, *J Am Coll Nutrit* 19(1): 3-12, 2000.

Berson DS, Shalita AR: The treatment of acne: the role of combination therapies, *J Am Acad Dermatol* 32(5):S31-S41, 1995.

Black MM, Bentley MF: Adolescent parenthood: a family centered culturally based perspective, *Pediatr Basics* 73:2-9, 1995.

Blake DR, Woods ER: The future is here: noninvasive diagnosis of STDs, *Contem Pediatr* 18(2):71-87, 2001.

Blythe MJ, Rosenthal SL: Female adolescent sexuality, promoting healthy sexual development, *Obstet Gynecol Clin* 27(1):125-141, 2000.

Borgmann JD, Jones BS: Early medical abortion, *Am J Obstet Gynecol* 183(2 suppl): 84-94, 2000.

Bravender T, Emans SJ: Adolescent gynecology, part I—common disorders, *Pediatr Clin North Am* 46(3):543-553, 1999.

Brown HN, Saunders RB, Dick MJ: Preventing secondary pregnancy in adolescents: a model program, *Health Care Women Intern* 20(1):5-11, 1999.

Burkhart CN, Specht K, Nechers D: Synergistic activity of benzoyl peroxide and erythromycin, *Skin Pharmacol Appl Skin Physiol* 13(5):292-296, 2000.

Carr PH, Felsenstein D, Friedman RH: Evaluation and management of vaginitis, *JGIM* 13(5):335-346, 1998.

Centers for Disease Control and Prevention: 1998 guidelines for trreatment of sexually transmitted diseases, *MMWR* 47(RR-1): 1-118, 1997.

Centers for Disease Control and Prevention: Trends in sexual risk behaviors among high school students, United States, 1991-1997, *MMWR* 47(36):749, 1998.

Coyle K and others: Short-term impact of safer choices: a multicomponent, school-based HIV, other STD, and pregnancy prevention program, *J Sch Health* 69(5): 181-188, 1999.

Division of Adolescent and School Health, National Center for Chronic Disease Prevention and Health Promotion: Youth risk behavior surveillance—United States, 1999, *MMWR* 49(SS05):1-96, 2000.

Egan ME, Lipsky MS: Diagnosis of vaginitis, *Am Fam Physician* 62(5):1095-1104, 2000.

Fortenberry JD and others: Subsequent sexuallly transmitted infections among adolescent women with genital infection due to *Chlamydia trachomatis, Neisseia gonorrhoae,* or *Trichomonas vaginalis, Sex Transm Dis* 26(1): 26-35, 1999.

Freeman EW and others Predictors of response to sertraline treatment of severe premenstrual syndromes, *J Clin Psychiatr* 61(8):579-584, 2000.

Frye GM, Silverman SD: Is it premenstrual syndrome? *Postgrad Med* 107(5):151-155, 2000.

Gerhardt CA and others: Adolescents' knowledge of human papillomavirus and cervical dysplasia, *J Pediatr Adolesc Gynecol* 13(1):15-20, 2000.

Gidwani GP: Menstruation and the athlete, *Contemp Pediatr* 14(1):27-48, 1997.

Glasier A: Emergency postcoital contraception, *N Engl J Med* 337(15):1058-1064, 1997.

Goldenberg RL, Hauth JC, Andrews WW: Intrauterine infection and preterm delivery, *N Engl J Med* 342 (20):1500-1507, 2000.

Golomb LM, Solidum AA, Warrren MP: Primary dysmenorrhea and physical activity, *Med Sci Sports Exerc* 30(6):906-909, 1998.

Goodman GJ, Postacne scarring: a review of its pathophysiology and treatment, *Dermatol Surg* 26(9):857-871, 2000.

Grimes DA: FDA approval of mifepristone: an overview, *Contracep Report* 11(4):4-11, 2000a.

Grimes DA: STD Update: Incidence, trends and new screening test, *Contracep Report* 11(3):4-10, 2000b.

Gupta MA, Gupta AK: Depression and suicidal ideation in dermatology patients with acne, alopecia areata, atopic dermatitis and psoriasis, *Br J Dermatol* 139(5):846-853, 1998.

Hatcher RA and others: *Contraceptive technology,* ed 17, New York, 1998, Irvington.

Henshaw SK, Feivelson DJ: Teenage abortion and pregnancy statistics by state, 1996, *Fam Plan Perspect* 32(6):272-280, 2000.

Hollander D: Nix to nonoxynol-9 to prevent HIV, *Fam Plan Perspect* 32(6):266, 2000.

Jacobs DG, Deutsch NL, Brewer M: Suicide, depression, and isotretinoin: is there a causal link? *J Am Acad Dermatol* 45(5):S168-175, 2001.

Jarow JP, Coburn M, Sigman M: Incidence of varicoceles in men with primary and secondary infertility, *Urology* 47(1):73-76, 1996.

Joyce T, Kaestner R: State reproductive policies and adolescent pregnancy resolution: the case of parental involvement laws, *J Health Econ* 15(5):579-607, 1996.

Kahn JA and others: Mediators of the association between age of first sexual intercourse and subsequent human papillomavirus infection, *Pediatrics* 109(1):e5, 2002.

Kaminer MS, Gilchrest BA: The many faces of acne, *J Am Acad Dermatol* 32(5):S6-S14, 1995.

Koutsky L: Epidemiology of genital human papillomavirus infection, *Am J Med* 102(5A):3-8, 1997.

Lahoti S and others: Screening and treatment of sexually transmittted diseases,

Part 1: Chlamydia, gonorrhea, and bacterial vaginosis, *J Pediatr Health Care* 14(1):34-36, 2000.

Lapp T: ACOG issues, recommendations for the management of endometriosis, *Am Fam Physician* 62(6):1431-1432, 2000.

Larsen SB, Kragstgrup J: Experiences of the first pelvic examination in a random sample of Danish teenagers, *Acta Obstet Gynecol Scand* 74(2):137-141, 1995.

Laude TA: Acne in childhood and adolescence: update on treatment choices, *Consultant* 3:457-465, 2000.

Lawson MA, Blythe MJ: Pelvic inflammatory disease in adolescents, *Pediatr Clin North Am* 46(4):767-782, 1999.

Leyden JJ: New understandings of the pathogenesis of acne, *J Am Acad Dermatol* 32(5): S15-S25, 1995.

Leyden JJ: Therapy for acne vulgaris, *N Engl J Med* 336(16):1156-1162, 1997.

Lucky AW and others: Predictors of severity of acne vulgaris in young adolescent girls: results of a five-year longitudinal study, *J Pediatr* 130(1):30-39, 1997.

Lyon DS: First trimester bleeding and pain, *Female Patient* 25:80-84, 2000.

Major B and others: Psychological responses of women after first-trimester abortion, *Arch Gen Psychiatr* 57(8):777-784, 2000.

Mancini AJ: Acne vulgaris: a treatment update, *Contemp Pediatr* 17(12):122-133, 2000.

Mangan SA and others: Increased prevalence of abnormal Papanicolaou smears in urban adolescents, *Arch Pediatr Adolesc Med* 151(5):481-488, 1997.

Margolis DJ, Attie M, Leyden J: Effects of isotretinoin on bone mineralization during routine therapy with isotretinoin for acne vulgaris, *Arch Dermatol* 132(7):769-774, 1996.

McClain N and others: Screening and treatment of sexually transmitted diseases, Part 2: Trichomonas, human papillomavirus infection, and herpes simplex virus, *J Pediatr Health Care* 14(3):130-132, 2000.

Meier E: RU-486 and implications for use among adolescents seeking an abortion, *Pediatr Nurs* 26(1):93-94, 2000.

Merchant JS, Oh MK, Klerman LV: Douching: a problem for adolescent girls and young women, *Arch Pediatr Adolesc Med* 153(8):834-837, 1999.

Mitchell AA, Van Bennekom CM, Louik C: A pregnancy-prevention program in women of childbearing age receiving isotretinoin, *N Engl J Med* 333(2):101-106, 1995.

Morris BJ, Young C: Emergency contraception, *AJN* 100(9):46-48, 2000.

Murphy SL: Deaths: final data for 1998. In Centers for Disease Control and Prevention: *National Vital Statistics Reports*, Hyattsville, MA, 2000, National Center for Health Statistics.

Murray SK, Baker AW, Lewin L: Screening families with young children for child maltreatment potential, *Pediatr Nurs* 26(1): 47-54, 65, 2000.

Muscari ME: The first gynecologic exam: make it a positive experience for your teenage patients, *AJN* 99(1):66-67, 1999.

Neinstein LS: *Adolescent health care: a practical guide*, ed 3, Baltimore, 1996, Williams & Wilkins.

Neinstein LS and others: Rape and sexual abuse. In Neinstein LS, editor: *Adolescent health care*, ed 3, Baltimore, 1996, Williams & Wilkins.

Nyirjesy P: Vaginitis in the adolescent patient, *Pediatr Clin North Am* 46(4):733-745, 1999.

Orfanos CE, Zouboulis C: Oral retinoids in the treatment of seborrhea and acne, *Dermatology* 196(1):148-152, 1998.

Overby KJ, Kegeles SM: The impact of AIDS on an urban population of high-risk female minority adolescents: implications for intervention, *J Adolesc Health* 15(3):216-227, 1994.

Polaneczky M, O'Connor K: Pregnancy in the adolescent patient, screening, diagnosis and initial management, *Pediatr Clin North Am* 46(4):649-668, 1999.

Quint EH: Adolescent pregnancy: an update, *Female Patient* 21:15-21, 1996.

Resnick MD and others: Protecting adolescents from harm: findings from the National Longitudinal Study of Adolescent Health, *JAMA* 278(10):823-831, 1997.

Rhein LM and others; Teen father participation in child rearing: family perspectives, *J Adolescent Health* 21(4):244-252, 1997.

Rhynard J, Krebs M, Glover J: Sexual assault in dating relationships, *J Sch Health* 67(3): 89-93, 1997.

Rodondi N and others: High risk for hyperlipidemia and the metabolic syndrome after an episode of hypertriglyceridemia during 13-cis retinoic acid therapy for acne: a pharmocogentic study, *Ann Intern Med* 136(8):582-589, 2002.

Rosenthal SL and others: Parents, peers, and the acquisition of an STD, *J Adolesc Health* 16(1):45-49, 1995.

Rotheram-Borus MH: Expanding the range of interventions to reduce HIV among adolescents, *AIDS* 14(suppl 1):S33-40, 2000.

Russell JJ: Topical therapy for acne, *Am Fam Physician* 61(2):357-366, 2000.

Schatzberg AF: New indications for antidepressants, *J Clin Psychiatr* 61(suppl 1):9-17, 2000.

Schroeder B, Sanfilippo JS: Dysmenorrhea and pelvic pain in adolescents, *Pediatr Clin North Am* 46(3):555-571, 1999.

Schwartz RH, Milteer R: Drug facilitated sexual assault ("date rape"), *Southern Med J* 93(6):558-561, 2000.

Selzer R and others: The association between secondary amenorrhea and common eating disordered weight control practices in an adolescent population, *J Adolesc Health* 19(1):56-61, 1996.

Skoog SJ and others: The adolescent varicocele: what's new with an old problem in young patients, *Pediatrics* 100(1):112-122, 1997.

Slaughter L: Involvement of drugs in sexual assault, *J Reprod Med* 45(5):425-430, 2000.

Smith KM: Drugs used in acquaintance rape, *J Am Pharm Assoc* 39(3):519-581, 1999.

Spencer JM and others: Self-esteem as a predictor of intiation of coitus in early adolescents, *Pediatrics* 109(4):581-584, 2002.

Stanton BF and others: Sexually transmitted diseases, human immunodeficiency virus, and pregnancy prevention: combined contraceptive practices among African-American early adolescents, *Arch Pediatr Adolesc Med* 174(1):17-24, 1996.

Stevenson AM: Advantages of the new progestins, *MCN* 23(1):56, 1998.

Trussell J and others: Comparative contraceptive efficacy of the female condom and other barrier methods, *Fam Plan Perspect* 26(2):66-72, 1994.

US Department of Health and Human Services: Immunization of adolescents, *MMWR* 45(RR-13):202-203, 1996.

Ventura SJ, Matthews TJ, Curtin SC: Declines in teenage birth rates, 1991-1998: update of national and state trends. In Centers for Disease Control and Prevention: *National Vital Statistics Reports*, Hyattsville, MA, 1999, National Center for Health Statistics.

Vermillion ST, Holmes MM, Soper DE: Adolescents and sexually transmitted diseases, *Obstet Gynecol Clin North Am* 27(1):163-179, 2000.

Verschoore M and others: Topical retinoids, their uses in dermatology, *Dermatol Clin* 11(1):107-116, 1993.

Walboomers JMM and others: Human papillomavirus is a necessary cause of invasive cervical cancer, *J Pathol* 189(1):12-19, 1999.

Wald E: Pelvic inflammatory disease in adolescents, *Curr Probl Pediatr* 26(3):86-97, 1996.

Ward MW, Holimon TD: Calcium treatment for premenstrual syndrome, *Ann Pharmacother* 33(12):1356-1358, 1999.

Webster GF: Inflammation in acne vulgaris, *J Am Acad Dermatol* 33(2):247-253, 1995.

Worthington-Roberts BS, Rees JM: The pregnant adolescent: special concerns. In Worthington-Roberts BS, Williams SR, editors: *Nutrition in pregnancy and lactation,* ed 6, Madison, 1997, Brown & Benchmark.

Wurtele SK: Preventing child maltreatment: multiple windows of opportunity in the health care system, *Child Health Care* 28:151-165, 1999.

Yacobi E and others: University students' knowledge and awareness of HPV, *Prevent Med* 28:535-541, 1999.

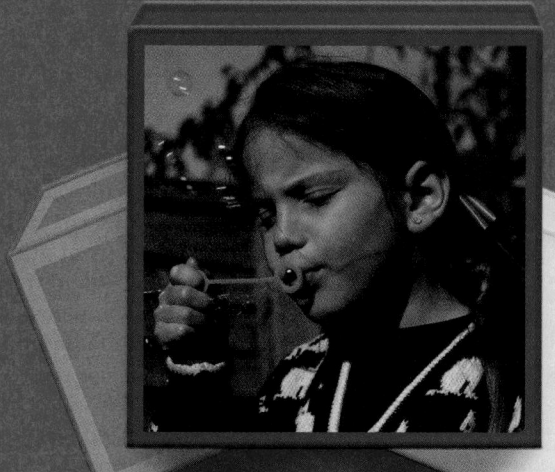

# Chapter 21

# Behavioral Health Problems of Adolescence

## Chapter Outline

**EATING PROBLEMS/DISORDERS, 869**
**Adipose Tissue, 869**
**Obesity, 870**
  Obesity in Adolescence, 872
  Complications of Adolescent Obesity, 873
**Anorexia Nervosa (AN), 876**
*Nursing Care Plan: The Adolescent with Anorexia*
  *Nervosa, 881*
**Bulimia, 882**
**"Fear of Fat" Syndrome, 883**
**SUBSTANCE ABUSE, 884**
**Overview, 884**
  Definitions, 884

Patterns of Drug Use, 884
Types of Drugs Abused, 884
**Tobacco, 885**
  Process of Becoming a Smoker, 887
  Smokeless Tobacco, 887
**Alcohol, 888**
**Additional Drugs, 890**
**Therapeutic Management, 892**
**Nursing Considerations, 893**
  Long-Term Management, 894
  Prevention, 895
**SUICIDE, 895**
**Incidence, 896**

**Factors Associated with Suicide Risk, 897**
  Individual Factors, 897
  Family Factors, 899
  Social/Environmental Factors, 899
**Methods, 899**
  Completed Suicide, 899
  Suicide Attempt, 899
**Precipitating Factors, 899**
**Nursing Considerations, 899**
  Prevention, 899
  Screening for Suicidality, 901
  Care of the Suicidal Adolescent, 902

## Related Topics

Childhood Depression, Ch. 18
Childhood Mortality, Ch. 1
Cocaine Exposure, Ch. 10
Communicating with Children, Ch. 6

Drug-Exposed Infants, Ch. 10
Fetal Alcohol Syndrome, Ch. 11
Health Promotion of the Adolescent and
  Family, Ch. 19

Infants of Mothers Who Smoke, Ch. 10
Nutritional Assessment, Ch. 6
Obesity, Ch. 13
Passive Smoking, Ch. 32

## EATING PROBLEMS/DISORDERS*

### Adipose Tissue

Fat is contained in connective tissue cells that are usually referred to as adipose tissue. Fat is characteristically found in subcutaneous tissues (except those of the eyelids, external ear, nose, scrotum, and backs of hands and feet, which contain very little), in the omentum, and in close relation to some viscera, such as the heart and kidneys. Fat contributes substantially to body weight, and fat deposits function primarily as a means for storing energy. Another important role of adipose tissue is the production and regulation of hormones, most notably testosterone and estrogen. Abnormalities in body fat levels can have profound effects on the

regulation of these hormones, thus affecting menstrual regularity and reproductive capabilities.

Normal fat distribution during childhood follows a definite pattern. Fat first appears in the subcutaneous tissues of the fetus at approximately the sixth month of prenatal life. There is a rapid accumulation from the seventh month of prenatal life through the first six months of postnatal life; the amount of subcutaneous fat present in the newborn correlates with the weight of the infant. However, by the end of the first year the infant who was lean at birth has approximately the same length and muscle mass as infants who were fatter initially. The significance of subcutaneous fat in relation to both the specialized brown fat and gestational age is discussed in relation to problems of prematurity and temperature regulation in the newborn. (See Chapters 8 and 10.)

---

■ *Marilyn L. Winkelstein, PhD, RN, revised this section.

After 6 months of age the rate of fat accumulation declines rapidly and decreases steadily in both sexes until 6 to 8 years of age. All children slim down soon after their first birthday, but the decrease is less in girls than in boys; at any age girls have slightly more fat than boys. From the ages of 6 to 8 years fat begins to accumulate slowly. During this period obesity may develop in some children. Many children also put on excess fat before the adolescent growth spurt.

Until the onset of puberty there is little difference in fat accumulation and distribution in boys and girls. During the adolescent growth spurt the amount of fat in boys decreases sharply (especially in the limbs) and is not reestablished until early adulthood. The increase in body weight and mass in boys is primarily the result of accelerated bone and muscle growth. In many boys a preadolescent period of fat growth, often a source of social concern to both the child and his parents, precedes the general changes of adolescence. In girls the fat accumulation continues but assumes the typical feminine distribution pattern of the mature female.

The amount and distribution of fat also correlate with a genetically controlled body build that appears to be unrelated to caloric intake. In addition, culturally determined diets, amount of exercise, and emotions influence caloric consumption and are reflected in increased fat deposits. It is now believed that the number of fat cells is established at an early age and that overfeeding during this time may have a significant influence on the development of obesity at a later age.

## Obesity

Few health problems in adolescence are so obvious to others, so difficult to treat, and have such long-term effects on psychologic and physical health status as obesity. It is the most common nutritional disturbance of children and one of the most challenging contemporary health problems at all ages. Current estimates of childhood obesity in the United States range from 22% to 33% (Troiano and others, 1995) with 13.7% of children between the ages of 6 and 11 being above the 95th percentile for body mass index (BMI) (MMWR, 1997). During the past decade the number of obese children has doubled and the number of overweight children has increased by 40% (Troiano and others, 1995). The greatest increases have occurred among children 6 to 11 years of age (Moran, 1999).

Obesity in childhood and adolescence has been related to elevated blood cholesterol, high blood pressure, respiratory disorders, orthopaedic conditions, cholelithiasis, some types of adult-onset cancer (MacKenzie, 2000), and an increase in type 2 diabetes mellitus (Ehtisham, Barrett, and Shaw, 2000). Being obese as a child and adolescent is also a significant risk factor for adult obesity. Freedman and others (2002) found increased height to be associated with the onset of obesity in later life. After the age of 3 years the probability that obesity will persist into adulthood increases with advancing age. The more obese the child is, the greater the probability (Whitaker and others, 1997). Because adult obesity is associated with increased mortality and morbidity from a variety of complications, both physical and psychologic, the presence of adolescent obesity is a serious condition.

Several different definitions have been proposed for obesity and overweight. *Obesity* has been defined as an increase in body weight resulting from an excessive accumulation of body fat relative to lean body mass (Keller and Stevens, 1996). *Overweight* refers to the state of weighing more than average for height and body build. In the past, most clinicians considered children obese if their weight exceeded the 95th percentile for their age, gender, and height on the National Center for Health Statistics (NCHS) growth charts. Children were considered overweight if their weight fell in the 90th to 95th percentile for age, gender, and height on the NCHS growth charts. However, recently the International Task Force on Obesity (Dietz and Robinson, 1998), the Expert Committee on Pediatric Obesity (Barlow and Dietz, 1998) and the Expert Committee on Clinical Guidelines for Overweight in Adolescent Preventive Services (Himes and Dietz, 1994) recommended that the BMI measurement be used to screen for childhood obesity. (See Appendix C.) The BMI measurement is strongly associated with subcutaneous and total body fat and also with skinfold thickness measurements. It is also highly specific for children with the greatest amount of body fat (MacKenzie, 2000). It has been proposed that the 95th percentile of the BMI be used to define overweight. Children above this cutoff are very likely to be obese, to be at risk for remaining obese, and to be obese as adults (MacKenzie, 2000). Children with a BMI between the 85th and 95th percentile should be considered at risk for overweight (Troiano and others, 1995).

### Etiology/Pathophysiology

Obesity results from a caloric intake that consistently exceeds caloric requirements and expenditure and may involve a variety of interrelated influences, including metabolic, hypothalamic, hereditary, social, cultural, and psychologic factors. Birth weight offers no clue in the detection and prediction of childhood obesity; obese children do not have higher birth weights than nonobese children. There is, however, a high correlation between childhood adiposity and parental adiposity (Ehrman, 2001).

**Genetic Factors.** The incidence of obese children born to obese parents (80%) is significantly higher than the incidence of obese children born to parents of normal weight (14%). A comparison of natural and adopted children shows a positive correlation for weight between children and their natural parents. Identical twins reared apart tend to resemble their natural parents to a greater extent than they do their adoptive parents.

General body build seems to have some effect on obesity. Children who are inclined toward a rounded body build, with soft body contours and larger amounts of subcutaneous fat, are somewhat predisposed to the accumulation of fat. Some individuals may inherit a metabolic defect that interferes with the breakdown of fat once it has been stored in adipose tissue. This defect makes maintaining an ideal weight more difficult for them than for others.

It is almost impossible to distinguish between hereditary and environmental factors because both may be operative in any situation, especially when other family members are also obese. Family and cultural eating patterns, as well as psychologic factors, play an important role; fat is considered by many persons to be an indication of good health. The tendency toward obesity is manifested whenever environmental conditions are favorable toward excessive caloric intake, such as an abundance of food, limited access to low-fat foods, reduced or minimal physical activity, and snacking combined with excessive television viewing.

**Diseases.** Fewer than 5% of the cases of childhood obesity can be attributed to an underlying disease. Such diseases include hypothyroidism, adrenal hypercorticoidism, hyperinsulinism, and dysfunction or damage to the central nervous system as a result of tumor, injury, infection, or vascular accident. Obesity is a frequent complication of muscular dystrophy, paraplegia, Down syndrome, spina bifida, and other chronic illnesses that limit mobility.

Several congenital syndromes have obesity as a feature: Laurence-Moon-Biedl, Prader-Willi, Alström syndromes, and pseudohypoparathyroidism. The most common is Prader-Willi syndrome, a disorder characterized by hypogonadism, slow intellectual development, short stature, and dysmorphic facial features, including a narrowed bifrontal diameter, almond-shaped eyes, and triangular-shaped mouth. These children are hypotonic and hyperphagic. They lack the internal mechanism that regulates satiety and as a result go to great lengths to obtain food.

**Metabolic and Endocrine Factors.** The complex interrelationships between hunger, satiety, the central nervous system, and the metabolism of carbohydrates, fats, and proteins continue to be investigated. Theories advanced to explain individual variability in energy requirements include increased metabolic efficiency in obese persons that facilitates fat storage, enhanced adipose tissue triglyceride synthesis, and retarded adipocyte lipolysis that facilitates fat retention:

**Brown fat theory.** Obese people have less heat-producing brown fat than normal persons, and their brown fat works less efficiently. The body's heat production influences food intake. This may explain why some individuals are able to overeat and remain slim.

**Adipose cell theory.** Adipose tissue is hyperplastic, hypertrophic, or a combination of the two. *Hyperplastic, or hypercellular, obesity* occurs when the number of cells in adipose tissue is increased, producing lifelong and intractable obesity. Hyperplastic obesity is associated with earlier onset. *Hypertrophic obesity* is associated with an increase in cell size and therefore is more likely to be responsive to treatment. Obese children have larger cells that stay the same size once they reach a maximum, and their fat cells appear to increase in number during childhood.

**Set point theory.** Individuals have a programmed level, or set point, for body weight that remains relatively stable during adulthood. With increased caloric intake the metabolic rate increases to burn the excess; when intake is reduced, metabolism decreases to conserve energy.

**Sodium (Na)/potassium (K) pump theory.** A basal enzyme is used to keep potassium in and sodium out of body cells. Obese persons have less of the required substance and therefore use less energy to maintain equilibrium.

**Lipoprotein lipase theory.** This enzyme on fat cells is responsible for depositing globules in fat cells. When weight is lost, the body increases production of the enzyme to grasp and store fat. Obese persons are unable to inhibit this process during normal fat intake.

**Caloric Equilibrium.** Obese children are less active than lean children, but it is uncertain whether inactivity creates the obesity or obesity is responsible for the inactivity. Obesity in adolescents and children can be caused by overeating, low activity levels, or both. The rate of energy expenditure in obese children may be as high as or higher than that of children of average weight and the same height. This is due in part to the increase in lean body tissue that accompanies the increase in body fat during weight gain. Caloric expenditure above and beyond that of children with average weight is required to mobilize excess energy stores and reduce body fat levels. In childhood, overeating is the dominant feature, whereas in adult life, reduced physical activity with normal intake is more likely.

Although the intake of obese persons who are inactive may be lower than that of leaner persons, obese persons eat more at a given sitting and tend to eat more rapidly than nonobese persons. Delany (1998) has reported that, as a group, obese children consume more than lean children. They may respond to other cues, as well as to the hunger stimulus. Eating habits and frequency of food ingestion may produce alterations in enzyme activities in both adipose cells and muscle cells. A comparison of individuals who consume similar amounts of calories—ingested either as one meal (gorging) or intermittently over a period of time (nibbling or grazing)—shows an increase of body fat in the "gorgers." It appears that lipogenesis is accelerated following "gorging" patterns of food intake as compared with "nibbling" patterns. Obese adolescents are characteristically night eaters and often skip meals, particularly breakfast.

**Sociocultural Factors.** Cultural and social eating patterns play a role in weight gain. Some cultures consider plumpness a sign of health and see obesity as evidence of well-being. In other cultures obesity is a status symbol or an indication of affluence. It is not uncommon for obese children to have families in which large meals are emphasized or children are admonished for leaving food on their plates. Parents may have an exaggerated concept of the amount of food children require and expect them to eat more than they need.

In countries such as the United States and western Europe, there is a marked difference in the prevalence of obesity between upper- and lower-class children, with differences often becoming apparent before 6 years of age. Lower socioeconomic groups have a greater prevalence of obesity, especially in girls.

Physical activity may also be influenced by sociocultural factors. Results of the National Longitudinal Study of Adolescent Health indicate that activity and inactivity patterns differ by ethnicity and minority adolescents (non-Hispanic African-Americans, Hispanics, and Filipinos) engage in less physical activity and more inactivity than their non-Hispanic white counterparts (Gordon-Larsen, McMurray, and Popkin, 1999).

**Psychologic Factors.** Psychologic factors also affect eating patterns. In infancy, children experience relief from discomfort through feeding and learn to associate eating with a sense of well-being, security, and the comforting presence of the nurturing person. Eating is soon associated with the feeling of being loved. In addition, the pleasurable oral sensation of sucking provides a connection between emotions and early eating behavior. Many parents use food as a positive reinforcer for desired behavior. This practice may become a habit, and the child may continue to use food as a reward, a comfort, and a means to deal with feelings of depression or hostility.

Many individuals eat when they are not hungry or in response to boredom, loneliness, sadness, depression, or tiredness. Difficulty in determining feelings of satiety can lead to weight problems and may compound the factor of eating in response to emotional rather than physical hunger cues.

In some children overweight may be the normal state and may simply represent the upper end of the normal distribution curve. These children are comfortable when they are overweight and may or may not have emotional problems. Others may begin overeating in response to traumatic or upsetting events, such as the death of a parent or sibling, separation from a parent, parental divorce, school failure, or physical, sexual, or emotional abuse.

**Decreased Physical Activity.** Decreased physical activity among children is clearly related to body fatness and increased risk of obesity. There is little doubt that physical activity has decreased in elementary and secondary schools in the United States. Currently less than 36% of elementary and secondary schools offer daily physical education classes (Sothern and others, 1999). Consequently, most of a child's or adolescent's physical activity must occur within the family or outside of school. Decreased physical activity within the family is a powerful influence on children because children model their parents and other adults. Parental obesity and low levels of physical activity are correlated with decreased physical activity in children (Strauss, 1999).

**Television Viewing.** Increased television viewing has been consistently identified as a factor associated with higher rates of childhood obesity. In fact, there is a dose-reponse relationship between the number of hours of television watched and the incidence of obesity with the odds of becoming overweight 8.3 times greater for individuals who watch more than 5 hours of television a day (Gortmaker and others, 1996). Recent studies indicate that 33% of children watch more than 5 hours a day (Gortmaker and others, 1996).

## Obesity in Adolescence

Obesity in adolescence may appear simultaneously with the onset of adolescence, or it may have existed before puberty. Although there may be differences in the psychophysiologic factors involved in its development, the effects of the obesity remain the same. Obesity is a serious deterrent to the social life of a child and, for a teenager, obesity can be devastating. Common emotional sequelae of obesity in adolescence are poor body image, low self-esteem, social isolation, and feelings of rejection and depression.

Adolescent-onset obesity may be related to an inability to master the developmental tasks of adolescence; as a result, young people regress to the self-satisfying tactic of overeating to compensate. Unfortunately, this mechanism creates an additional obstacle to achieving developmental goals. For some adolescents, obesity may ward off the pressures engendered by the internal changes of puberty and the outside world. As long as they remain fat, adolescents have a vehicle for avoiding repressed emotional material. They may come to view obesity as the cause of all their disappointments. Consequently, they avoid taking the steps necessary for maturation. Eating is their means of coping with the normal drives of adolescence and more closely binds them to the family, who provides the food. They become increasingly dependent on food as a means of gratification. This dependence impedes the normal processes of separation and individuation because obese adolescents may shy away from interactions with their peers.

**Vulnerable Personality.** Obesity has also been found in some passive-dependent, compliant adolescents who are controlled by guilt and shame. They are easily influenced by outside forces that they consider to be more powerful than themselves (e.g., parents, peers, and school). When faced with internal or external stress, these adolescents react with helplessness, ambivalence, and a tendency to seek support from someone they see as stronger than themselves, either an adult or peer.

There are many psychologic implications in the development and perpetuation of obesity. It may represent aggression directed at the self, an attempt (in younger children) to grow bigger to physically deal with a hated person, or a means of bringing shame and embarrassment to another (often the mother). Many overweight adolescents use obesity as a means of revenge. However, they easily become a scapegoat for the frustrations and anger of parents and a source of embarrassment and shame. A common problem is the ambivalence of parents who like to see their children eat but at the same time desire them to be slim.

**Self-Concept and Obesity.** Obese adolescents score higher on depression-measurement tests than thinner teens and significantly lower on body-image tests, indicating a less positive or more impaired body concept. Unlike other disorders, an adolescent's obesity is continually on display for others to see. Some of the personality characteristics reflecting the psychologic effects of obesity have been compared to those of ethnic and racial minorities who have been subjected to ongoing discrimination. These traits include passivity, obsessive concern with self-image, expectation of rejection, and progressive withdrawal. This sets into motion a cyclic pattern in which adolescents expect rejection, feel awkward and out of place in social situations, isolate themselves from social contacts, and then experience actual rejection. Decreased opportunities for activity outside the home provide increased exposure to food, leading to an increase in obesity.

Obese adolescents, particularly obese girls, often consider obesity undesirable and intensely dislike their figures and physical characteristics. They are concerned about their obesity, are self-deprecating, and judge other people in terms of weight. They may express contempt for fat persons and admiration for thin ones. Stylish, age-appropriate clothing is difficult to find and, when available, is restricted to special shops or departments. Sexual attractiveness is severely impaired or nonexistent; obese adolescents are much less likely to date than their nonobese peers.

Three major factors contribute to the development of a disturbed body image:

1. **Age of onset of the obesity.** Body-image disturbances are found primarily in persons who were obese as children and adolescents or as adolescents alone.
2. **Presence of emotional disturbances or neuroses.** A stable personality and a secure childhood appear to prevent body-image distortion, whereas emotional disturbances caused by the effects of a disturbed family invite the development of a distorted body image.
3. **A negative evaluation of the obesity by others.** The child internalizes the attitudes conveyed by significant others.

During adolescence, when the teen is establishing a sense of identity, derogatory views by peers and parents are incorporated into enduring views of the self. Fig. 21-1 shows interrelated factors that contribute to adolescent obesity. However, obesity does not always imply low self-esteem (Kim and others, 1995).

## Complications of Adolescent Obesity

The most prevalent complication of adolescent obesity is its persistence into adulthood, with remarkable resistance to treatment. Adults with long-standing obesity are at risk for medical complications that include hypertension, diabetes, coronary heart disease, stroke, and colorectal cancer.

The most serious physical effect of severe obesity in childhood is pickwickian syndrome, named after the Charles Dickens character who was continually falling asleep. Although the mechanism is unknown, narcolepsy associated with an obese state is thought to be caused by carbon dioxide narcosis from a decreased ventilatory capacity. There is an increased incidence of orthopaedic problems in obese children, especially Legg-Calvé-Perthes disease and genu valgum (knock-knee). However, the most destructive complications are the psychosocial problems that occur as a result of teasing, ridicule, and rejection by peers and family.

## Diagnostic Evaluation

A careful history is obtained regarding the development of obesity, and a physical examination is performed to differentiate simple obesity from increased fat that results from organic causes. A psychologic assessment, accomplished via interviews with the teen and standardized personality tests, provides insight into the personality and emotional problems that contribute to obesity and that might interfere with therapy. Appropriate diagnostic tests rule out suspected metabolic and endocrine disorders.

It is useful to obtain an estimation of the degree of obesity to determine the component of body weight that can be modified. All of the following methods have been used to assess obesity: body mass index, body weight, weight-height ratios, weight-age ratios, hydrostatic (underwater) weight, skinfold measurements, bioelectrical analysis, computed tomography, magnetic resonance imaging, and neu-

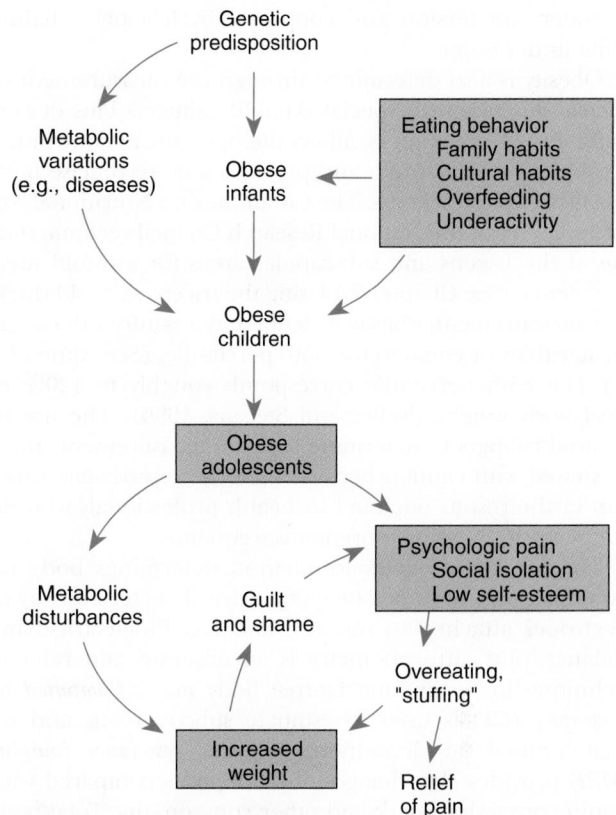

**Fig. 21-1** Complex relationships in adolescent obesity.

tron activation. Each of these methods has advantages and disadvantages.

The **body mass index (BMI),** measurement expresses the relationship between height and weight (e.g., kilograms divided by meters squared [$kg/m^2$]). BMI is easily calculated, or the ratio can be found on BMI charts. Using the BMI technique, a child is classified as overweight when the BMI index is equal to or exceeds the 85th percentile. BMI percentiles are age- and gender-specific. The National Center for Health Statistics has released new BMI-for-age charts that allow practitioners to track a child within a percentile range over time. (See Appendix C.) The new BMI growth charts were designed to allow health care providers to detect at early ages children who are showing signs of being at risk for overweight and obesity. The new charts are also considered more accurate than the older weight-for-stature charts.

*Hydrostatic,* or *underwater, weighing* provides the most accurate measurement of lean body weight. However, this method is not practical in clinical settings. In hydrostatic weighing, total body density is determined indirectly by application of Archimedes' principle, which states that the loss of weight of a body in water is equal to the weight of the water displaced by the body. The child or adolescent is totally submerged in a water-filled tank. The child forcibly exhales as much air as possible, and measurements are obtained to calculate the density of fat and lean body tissues. This method can be used only in children who can tolerate underwater submersion and cooperate by forcibly exhaling while under water.

Obesity is also determined through the measurement of *skinfold thickness* with special skinfold calipers. This device, calibrated in millimeters, allows the operator to control the pressure on the skinfold and provides a more precise measurement of its thickness. The Committee on Nutritional Anthropometry of the National Research Council recommends use of the triceps and subscapular areas for skinfold measurements. (See Chapter 7.) Using the triceps skinfold thickness measurement, obesity is defined as a skinfold thickness greater than or equal to the 85th percentile. (See Appendix C.) The 85th percentile corresponds roughly to 120% of ideal body weight (Keller and Stevens, 1996). The use of skinfold calipers to determine body fat measurements must be viewed with caution because there is considerable variation in the results obtained by health professionals who do not perform these measurements frequently.

The *bioelectric impedance* method determines body fat from measures of impedance of electrical current by way of electrodes attached to the arm and leg. Bioelectrical impedance plus anthropometry is an accurate and reliable technique for estimating fat-free body mass. *Computed tomography (CT)* is used to estimate subcutaneous and intraabdominal fat deposition. *Magnetic resonance imaging (MRI)* provides clear images of fat deposits compared with tissues containing water and other components. Total-body *neutron activation* provides an estimation of water and fat, as well as calcium, protein, and other components. These techniques are expensive and are typically used in specialized clinical settings (Keller and Stevens, 1996).

## Therapeutic Management

The self-perpetuating nature of obesity makes treatment disappointing because many approaches do not achieve long-term success. The best approach is a preventive one. Early recognition and control measures are essential before the adolescent reaches an obese state. Some degree of success has been achieved with weight-reduction techniques that include diet, exercise, behavior modification, and psychologic support in a family-based approach.

**Diet.** Diet modification is an essential part of weight reduction programs. The ideal diet for children and adolescents should include the components listed in Box 21-1. Formal calorie-limited diets are difficult to maintain, and long-term maintenance is usually unsuccessful. The adop-

tion of healthier eating habits—increasing fiber and complex carbohydrates, modifying fat intake (especially saturated fats), and eating only in response to physical hunger cues—can lead to gradual weight control and the development of desirable, lifelong dietary habits. Significant caloric restriction, especially for children and adolescents who are still growing, is never recommended (Table 21-1). The restriction of calories and nutrients can cause delayed or stunted growth and is effective for only short periods of time. It is also important to emphasize the undesirable nature of fad diets and crash programs that continually appear in the media.

**Physical Activity.** Regular physical activity is incorporated into all weight-reduction programs. In the absence of exercise, both fat and lean body mass are lost. Lean body mass is a site of high energy expenditure, and any loss in lean body mass affects the resting metabolic rate and weight loss (Roberts, 2000). Decreases in the percentage of overweight are more likely to occur in children who exercise in conjunction with diet than in children who follow a diet regimen alone. Exercise activities should be those that emphasize self-improvement rather than competition.

**Behavior Modification.** Behavior-modification approaches to weight loss are based on the observation that obese individuals have abnormal eating practices that can be altered. Attention is focused not on food but on the social and behavioral aspects surrounding food consumption.

Successful behavior-modification weight programs help adolescents to identify and eliminate inappropriate eating habits and include a problem-solving component that enables adolescents to identify problems and determine solutions.

**Drugs.** The use of appetite-suppressant drugs is not supported by most practitioners. These drugs are no more effective than diet and exercise in maintaining long-term weight loss. There is also concern that many appetite-suppressant drugs are habit-forming and have dangerous side effects.

**Surgical Techniques.** Surgical techniques that bypass portions of the intestine or occlude a segment of the stomach to produce a marked diet restriction and weight loss are hazardous and cause many metabolic complications. These

---

**Box 21-1** ■ ■ ■
### Essentials of an Ideal Weight Management Program

Weight maintenance or steady slow weight loss
Nutrient, energy, and growth needs met
Feelings of hunger avoided
Preservation of lean body mass
Increased physical activity
Absence of metabolic complications
Absence of psychiatric reactions

---

**TABLE 21-1** Average calorie requirements for maintenance from age 5 years

| Age | Boys | Girls |
|-----|------|-------|
| 5 | 1350 | 1300 |
| 6 | 1400 | 1370 |
| 7 | 1600 | 1450 |
| 8 | 1650 | 1500 |
| 9 | 1750 | 1600 |
| 10 | 1800 | 1700 |
| 11 | 1900 | 1800 |
| 15 | 2400 | 2100 |
| 18 | 2500 | 2200 |

Data from Merritt RJ and others: Consequences of modified fasting in obese pediatric and adolescent patients. I. Protein-sparing modified fast, *J Pediatr* 96:13-19, 1980.

complications include severe water and electrolyte depletion, persistent diarrhea, vitamin deficiency, internal herniation, and fatty infiltration and degeneration of the liver. They should not be considered an easy or cosmetic approach to weight control in children or adolescents.

### Nursing Considerations

Nurses play a key role in the adherence and maintenance phases of many weight reduction programs. Nurse practitioners assess, manage, and evaluate the progress of many overweight adolescents. They also play an important role in recognizing potential weight problems and assisting parents and adolescents in preventing obesity.

The presence of obesity is obvious from appearance and a comparison of height and weight or body mass index measurements with standard growth charts. Children with a BMI greater than or equal to the 95th percentile for age and sex should receive an in-depth medical assessment. Children with a BMI in the 85th to 95th percentile range should be evaluated for secondary complications such as hypertension and hyperlipidemia (Barlow and Dietz, 1998). Evaluation includes a height and weight history of the adolescent and family members, as well as eating habits, appetite and hunger patterns, and physical activities. A psychosocial history is also helpful in understanding the impact that obesity has on the child's life.

The reasons behind the desire to lose weight need to be explored with adolescents because motivation to lose weight is the key to success. Adolescents need to take personal responsibility for dietary habits and physical activity. Teens who are forced by their parents to seek help are seldom motivated, become rebellious of parental nagging, and are unwilling to control their dietary intake.

**Nutrition Counseling.**   The most realistic approach, especially during growth, is simply to prevent an increase in body fat. This is often accomplished by adjusting three aspects of eating: (1) reducing the *quantity* eaten by purchasing, preparing, and serving smaller portions; (2) altering the *quality* consumed by substituting low-calorie, low-fat foods for high-calorie foods (especially for snacks); and (3) altering *situations* by severing associations between eating and other stimuli, such as eating while watching television.

The most successful diets are those that use ordinary foods in controlled portions rather than diets that require the avoidance of specific foods. Adolescents and parents are taught how to incorporate favorite foods into their diet and to select substitutes that are satisfying. The dieting teen should eat what the rest of the family eats, but less of it. When parents buy and prepare smaller amounts, tempting second helpings and leftovers are eliminated. To maintain a healthy diet, it is necessary to encourage the consumption of high-nutrient foods such as fruits, vegetables, whole grains, and low-fat dairy and protein products. Calories and fat should be kept to a healthy level without being significantly restricted. The family should avoid focusing on the fat or caloric content of foods or meals; doing so can cause the child or adolescent to become "fat phobic" or "calorie conscious" to the point of believing that fat and calories are bad and, as a result, trying to avoid all calories or fat.

For most teenagers, snacking is an integral part of the daily routine. Adolescents who are serious about dieting should be helped to eliminate or select snack foods wisely. Getting rid of high-calorie junk foods and placing snack foods out of sight helps divert attention away from eating. Typically, snacking involves eating a large quantity of one type of snack food; therefore substituting several items with lower caloric value can be more satisfying while avoiding the high caloric impact. Foods containing complex carbohydrates are more satisfying than those containing simple sugars. Many schools are providing more wholesome "snacks" such as fruit, juices, and raw vegetables in cafeteria vending machines. However, favorite gathering places for children and teens are the fast-food establishments, which are often located near large schools.*

No adolescent should initiate a reduction diet without a health assessment, evaluation, and counseling. It is important to emphasize the undesirable nature of fad diets and crash programs that continually appear in the media. Exotic diets have not been successful, and their unbalanced nature makes them potentially dangerous for growing children or adolescents. To be successful, a dietary program should be nutritionally sound with sufficient satiety value, produce the desired weight loss, and be accompanied by nutrition education and continued support.

**Behavior Therapy.**   Altering eating behavior and eliminating inappropriate eating habits are essential to weight reduction, especially in maintaining long-term weight control. Most behavior-modification programs include the following concepts:

- A description of the behavior to be controlled, such as eating habits
- Attempts to modify and control the stimuli that govern eating
- Development of eating techniques designed to control speed of eating
- Positive reinforcement for these modifications through a suitable reward system

Specific strategies used to modify eating habits are included in Box 21-2.

**Group Involvement.**   Commercial groups or diet workshops composed primarily of adults may be helpful to some teenagers; however, a group composed of other adolescents is often more effective. Teenage groups include summer camps designed for obese young people and conducted by health professionals, school groups organized and led by a school nurse, and groups associated with special clinics.

These groups are concerned not only with weight loss but also with the development of a positive self-image and the encouragement of physical activity. Nutrition education, diet planning, and the improvement of social skills are essential components of these groups. Improvement is determined by positive changes in all aspects of behavior.

**Family Involvement.**   There is a definite connection between family environment, interaction, and obesity. Parents

---

*Information on the nutrient value of name-brand foods, including several fast-food restaurants, is available from the **Nutrition Coordinating Center,** 1300 South 2nd St, Suite 300, Minneapolis, MN 55454, (612) 626-9450, e-mail: nccservice@epi.umn.edu; www.ncc.umn.edu.

## Box 21-2 ■ ■ ■
## Strategies Used to Modify Eating Habits

Identify eating patterns and behaviors.
   Keep a record of everything eaten, including:
      All solids and liquids, including alcohol
      Time eaten
      Amount eaten
      Where food was consumed (e.g., at dinner table, at school,
        in front of television)
      Activity engaged in while eating
      With whom food was eaten
      Feelings at time food was eaten (e.g., angry, depressed,
        lonely, happy)
   Analyze record for patterns and relationships to other
      factors as a basis for making changes.
Control eating patterns.
   Eat only at specific times.
   Eat only in a specific place.
   Do not engage in other activities while eating.
   Prepare low-calorie, low-fat foods in attractive ways.
   Get rid of junk foods.
   Place snacks out of sight.
   Avoid purchasing problem foods.
   If tempted to eat (e.g., from watching a television commer-
      cial), substitute an activity other than eating as a distraction.
Change the act of eating.
   Slow down the pace of eating.
   Use smaller plates to make food portions appear larger.
   Leave a small amount of food on the plate at the end of a
      meal.
   Serve foods from the stove or an inconvenient area to make
      obtaining second helpings more difficult.
Use methods other than eating to deal with emotional stress,
   boredom, and fatigue.
   Substitute a hobby, walking, listening to music, talking on
      the phone, dusting, cleaning a room, or reading a book in
      response to feelings that usually lead to eating.
Provide positive reinforcements for accomplishments.
   Establish a system of rewards for changes in eating behavior,
      exercise, and weight loss.
   Use tangible rewards such as new CDs, a movie, a concert, or
      new clothes.
   Think positively.
   Have a family member provide positive support and praise
      daily.

## Critical Thinking Exercise

### Obesity in Adolescence

Jane is an obese 13-year-old girl who visits the office of the school nurse. Jane states that she wants to lose weight. In addition to assessing Jane's dietary intake and physical activity, what should the school nurse do?

FIRST, THINK ABOUT IT . . .

- What precise questions are you trying to answer?
- Within what point of view are you thinking?

1. Help Jane plan and follow a low-calorie, low-protein diet.
2. Obtain information concerning Jane's birth weight.
3. Assess Jane's home environment and involve the entire family in efforts to help Jane lose weight.
4. Encourage Jane to follow one of the new "fat-burning" diets.

*The best response is three. The knowledge that hereditary and environmental factors influence obesity is essential to precisely answering the question. Family eating habits can contribute significantly to obesity in children. The most successful adolescent weight loss programs involve an approach that enlists the family's cooperation in planning healthy, balanced meals and snacks and enjoyable physical activity for all members of the family. Nurses who work with adolescents who are obese need to enlist the cooperation and support of family members. Because there is no relationship between birth weight and obesity, the nurse does not need to obtain Jane's birth weight. Most authorities on weight loss do not recommend limiting calories or protein during adolescence; such limitations can cause delays in growth and produce only short-term weight loss. Fad diets should be avoided because they are often very expensive, are rarely successful, and can be dangerous for growing adolescents.*

---

need education in the purposes of the therapeutic measures and their role in management. The family needs nutrition education and counseling regarding the reinforcement plan, altering the food environment, and maintaining proper attitudes. They can support their child in efforts to change eating behaviors, food intake, and physical activity. (See Critical Thinking Exercise box.)

**Prognosis.** Lifelong eating habits and psychologic problems make weight reduction difficult. Weight reduction is more successful in older adolescents who have lean parents, a good academic performance, no affective disorder, and no recent stressful life event (such as parents' divorce or a death).

**Prevention.** Weight loss programs do not enjoy the success of therapeutic interventions for other disorders. Gradual accumulation of adipose tissue during childhood establishes a pattern of eating that is difficult to reverse in adolescence. Prevention of obesity should begin in early childhood with the development of healthy eating habits,

regular exercise patterns, and a positive relationship between parents and children. Prevention of adolescent obesity is best accomplished by early identification of obesity in the preschool age, school-age, and preadolescent periods. Health care professionals should encourage frequent health visits for children who are overweight or obese and incorporate a dietary history and counseling into each well-infant, well-child, and well-adolescent visit. (See Nursing Care Plan: The Child Who Is Obese.*)

## Anorexia Nervosa (AN)

AN is an eating disorder characterized by a refusal to maintain a minimally normal body weight and by severe weight loss in the absence of obvious physical causes (American Psychiatric Association, 2000).

In *anorexia nervosa (AN)*, individuals experience hunger but deny its existence. Emaciation is the result of this self-inflicted starvation. AN occurs predominantly in middle-

---

*In Wong DL, Hess CS: *Wong and Whaley's clinical manual of pediatric nursing,* ed 5, St Louis, 2000, Mosby.

and upper-class white females; the incidence is 0.5% to 1%. However, young school-age children also admit a preoccupation with diet and atypical eating habits. Fewer than 10% of persons with AN are males.

## Etiology/Pathophysiology

The mean age of onset of AN is 13.75 years, but the age range is from 10 to 25 years (MacKenzie and Neinstein, 1996). Individuals with this disorder are described as perfectionists, academically high achievers, conforming, and conscientious. Typically, they have high energy levels, even when there is marked emaciation. There is a psychologic component, and the diagnosis is based primarily on psychologic and behavioral criteria. However, the physical manifestations of AN lend support to possible organic factors in the etiology. A strong extrinsic motive has, for some reason, suppressed the vital function of eating.

**Psychologic Aspects.** Dominating the psychologic aspects of AN are a relentless pursuit of thinness and a fear of fatness, which are usually preceded by a period of mood disturbances and behavior changes. The weight loss is usually triggered by a traumatic interpersonal incident or a typical adolescent crisis (e.g., the onset of menstruation), which precipitates serious dieting that continues out of control. Often there is an exaggerated misinterpretation of the normal fat deposition characteristic of the early adolescent period. The weight loss may be a response to teasing, changing schools, going to college, or an incident that requires an independent decision that the teen is unprepared to make, such as a career choice. Childhood sexual abuse may be a factor in some cases of AN.

The current emphasis on slimness is a significant factor contributing to the increasing incidence among girls and young women. The standard for beauty is one exemplified by models in advertising. Consequently, the pressure to diet and be slim is relentless. Young girls entering puberty, when biologic fat accumulation is the normal course of development, are particularly vulnerable. Young people involved in competitive sports or activities such as ballet and gymnastics are also at risk for unsafe weight control practices and eating disorders such as AN.

Some studies suggest that AN is a symptom of family psychopathology. Girls are usually strongly dependent on their parents; an ambivalent mother-daughter relationship is often present with AN. There is often a history of family strife, with AN being a symptom of the family's problems. Families are usually rigid, overly enmeshed, excessively controlling, unable to display their feelings, and lacking in skills for resolving conflict.

Vulnerable girls are model daughters who are afraid to assume adult responsibilities. They find it difficult to formulate an identity and feel ineffective in their personal lives, even if they appear successful and capable. They feel out of control in all aspects of their lives and choose control of food intake to express their autonomy. Interventions are viewed as attempts to remove this control.

**Organic Etiology.** Evidence of organic etiology may be indicated by abnormalities of hypothalamic-pituitary and end-organ function in individuals with AN. Secondary

---

> **Box 21-3** ■ ■ ■
> **Clinical Findings Associated with Anorexia Nervosa**
>
> | | |
> |---|---|
> | Amenorrhea | Dryness of skin |
> | Constipation | Bradycardia |
> | Abdominal pain | Peripheral edema |
> | Cold intolerance | Yellowing of skin |
> | Lethargy | Hypertrophy of the salivary |
> | Excess energy | glands |
> | Emaciation | |

---

amenorrhea is a common finding. Appetite and satiety are hypothalamic functions. Associated symptoms of AN that relate to hypothalamic dysfunction include abnormalities of thermoregulation, water conservation, and secretion of catecholamines.

A biologic or biochemical vulnerability has also been suggested because cases of AN have been associated with depression and addiction in several family studies. The same biochemical predeterminant may be responsible for both the depression or addiction and the anorexia nervosa (Schneider and Fisher, 2001). Familial factors are also involved in AN (Strober and others, 2000). AN has been found to be eight times higher in female relatives of anorexic persons than in the general population (Bryant-Waugh and Lask, 1995).

## Clinical Manifestations

The most obvious manifestation of AN is the severe and profound weight loss induced by self-imposed starvation (Box 21-3). The adolescents identify with this skeleton-like appearance and do not regard it as abnormal or ugly. Adolescents with AN will often eat small amounts of food or play with food on their plates to give the impression that they are eating adequately and not experiencing disturbances in their eating habits. This can lead friends and family to disregard the possibility of AN. The adolescents can display a marked preoccupation with food—preparing meals for others, talking about food, and hoarding food. Some become obsessed with fasting and engage in frequent strenuous exercise, self-induced vomiting, and/or taking laxatives to speed up the weight-loss process (Muscari, 1998).

These young people tend to withdraw from peer relationships and engage in self-imposed social isolation. They continually strive for perfection, which may be demonstrated in other compulsive behaviors. They are usually overachievers, and their schoolwork is very important to them.

In the wake of the severe weight loss, these girls and young women exhibit physical signs of altered metabolic activity. They develop secondary amenorrhea, bradycardia, lowered body temperature, decreased blood pressure, and cold intolerance. They have dry skin and brittle nails and develop lanugo hair. The changes are usually reversible with adequate weight gain and improved nutritional status. Table 21-2 lists the differences between AN and bulimia.

**TABLE 21-2** Some characteristics of eating disorders

| Factors | Anorexia Nervosa | Bulimia |
|---|---|---|
| Food | Turns away from food to cope | Turns to food to cope |
| Personality | Introverted | Extroverted |
| | Avoids intimacy | Seeks intimacy |
| | Negates feminine role | Aspires to feminine role |
| Behavior | "Model" child | Often "acts out" |
| | Obsessive/compulsive | Impulsive |
| School | High achiever | Variable school performance |
| Control | Maintains rigid control | Loses control |
| Body image | Body distortion | Less frequent body distortion |
| Health | Denies illness | Recognizes illness |
| | | Fluctuates |
| Weight | Body weight less than 85% of expected norm | Within 5 to 15 lb of normal body weight or may be overweight |
| Sexuality | Usually not sexually active | Often sexually active |

**Box 21-4** ■ ■ ■
**Diagnostic Criteria for Anorexia Nervosa**

1. Refusal to maintain body weight at or above a minimally normal weight for age and height (e.g., weight loss leading to maintenance of body weight less than 85% of that expected; or failure to make expected weight gain during period of growth, leading to body weight less than 85% of that expected)
2. Intense fear of gaining weight or becoming fat, even though underweight
3. Disturbance in the way in which one's body weight or shape is experienced, undue influence of body weight or shape on self-evaluation, or denial of the seriousness of the current low body weight
4. In postmenarcheal females, amenorrhea (i.e., the absence of at least three consecutive menstrual cycles). A woman is considered to have amenorrhea if her periods occur only following hormone (e.g., estrogen) administration.

*Specify type:*

**Restricting type:** During the current episode of anorexia nervosa, the person has not regularly engaged in binge-eating or purging behavior (i.e., self-induced vomiting or the misuse of laxatives, diuretics, or enemas).

**Binge-eating/purging type:** During the current episode of anorexia nervosa, the person has regularly engaged in binge-eating or purging behavior (i.e., self-induced vomiting or the misuse of laxatives, diuretics, or enemas).

From American Psychiatric Association: *Diagnostic and statistical manual of mental disorders,* ed 4 (DSM-IV TR), Washington, DC, 2000, The Association.

## Diagnostic Evaluation

Diagnosis is made on the basis of clinical manifestations and conformity to the criteria established by the American Psychiatric Association (2000) (Box 21-4).

## Therapeutic Management

The treatment and management of AN involve three major thrusts: (1) reinstitution of normal nutrition or reversal of the severe state of malnutrition, (2) resolution of disturbed patterns of family interaction, and (3) individual psychotherapy to correct deficits and distortions in psychologic functioning. Because of the psychogenic nature of the disorder, the treatment period may be long.

Most adolescents with AN are treated on an outpatient basis. However, adolescents who have severe malnutrition, electrolyte disturbances, vital sign abnormalities, or psychiatric disturbances (e.g., severe depression or suicidal ideation) may require hospitalization. Therapy for the adolescent with AN requires interventions delivered by an interdisciplinary team that includes dietitians, physicians, nurses, counselors, and psychologists or psychiatrists.

**Nutrition.** The initial goal is to treat the life-threatening malnutrition with strict adherence to dietary requirements, which may necessitate intravenous or tube feedings. These methods are usually reserved for severe situations. Dietary interventions are combined with family psychotherapy to improve the underlying psychologic misconceptions about the weight loss. Weight gain alone cannot be considered a cure for the disease and is an unreliable sign of progress. Relapses are frequent as the person reverts to previous eating patterns when removed from the therapeutic environment.

An adjunct to therapy is deconditioning by producing a mild euphoria incompatible with maintaining an anxiety about eating. There is a relationship between AN and depression. Decreasing the individual's consciousness of and vigilance about eating reduces anxiety and increases atten-

tion to other suggestions. Interventions may include the administration of antianxiety or antidepressant drugs such as fluoxetine (Prozac). When these drugs are used, patients should be carefully monitored for adverse effects, especially cardiovascular side effects.

**Psychotherapy.** Psychotherapy is essential for adolescents with anorexia. Patients need to be active participants in the treatment process and become aware of their impulses, feelings, and needs. It is essential that adolescents rely on their own thinking, become more realistic in self-appraisal, and become capable of living as self-directed, competent individuals who enjoy life without manipulating the body and its functions. Psychotherapy is aimed at helping the young person resolve the adolescent identity crisis, particularly as it relates to a distorted body image. Adolescents whose illness can be clearly related to a dysfunctional family situation need a combination of family therapy plus individual and group therapy to maintain the desired weight.

**Prognosis.** Complete recovery rates for AN are less than ideal. Approximately 25% of affected individuals attain full recovery; 50% improve substantially but may relapse during times of stress, and 25% do poorly despite adequate treatment (Schneider and Fisher, 2001). Deaths from AN are almost always associated with long-standing symptoms and other associated factors such as depression, bulimia, and vomiting. Adolescents with AN are also at risk for suicide because of the strong association between depression and AN (Muscari, 1998). Although the changes associated with AN are often reversible, the physical complications can involve every organ system in the body, and the effects of severe malnutrition are often obvious for many years. Long-term studies of these patients indicate that as many as 20% have died from complications of AN (Sullivan, 1995). More recent studies have indicated that brain abnormalities associated with AN are present in adolescents with relatively short durations of illness (Katzman and others, 1996). Further investigation is necessary to determine the functional significance of these abnormalities and the extent to which they return to normal after nutritional rehabilitation.

For many, AN will be a lifelong problem. The prognosis is best for teenagers in whom the disorder is diagnosed at a relatively early age, before abnormal eating patterns and other weight-loss techniques are established and emaciation has set in.

Many patients restored to normal weight still demonstrate low self-esteem, are highly sensitive to social interactions, and remain "obsessoid" (MacKenzie and Neinstein, 1996).

### Nursing Considerations

### ✷ Assessment

Because AN is becoming increasingly prevalent in younger age-groups, pediatric nurses should be alert to the possibility of the disorder when weight loss becomes evident during a routine assessment. The health interview and nutritional assessment often provide clues and guidelines for further investigation.

### ✷ Nursing Diagnoses

Several nursing diagnoses are identified through a thorough assessment. The more common diagnoses for the adolescent with AN are included in the Nursing Care Plan on pp. 881-882. Others may apply in specific situations.

### ✷ Planning

The goals for the adolescent with AN and the family include the following:

1. Adolescent will normalize eating behaviors.
2. Adolescent will develop realistic perceptions of the body and food.
3. Adolescent will develop adaptive ways to cope with the distorted body image and interpersonal relationships.
4. Adolescent and family will receive support and guidance.

### ✷ Implementation

Nurses need to adopt and maintain a kind and supportive yet firm manner in managing the care of a teen with AN without creating a passive-dependent attitude. The adolescent requires sustained support and reassurance to cope with ambivalent feelings related to body concept and the desire to be seen as cooperative, reliable, and worthy of receiving kindness. Encouraging the adolescent with education and activities that strengthen self-esteem facilitates the resocialization process and promotes social acceptance among peers.

**Diet.** Rapid weight gain should be avoided because it has been associated with severe metabolic abnormalities in

## Critical Thinking Exercise

### Anorexia Nervosa

Jane is a 13-year-old whose grades have been excellent and whom the teachers describe as a "model student." Recently some of Jane's friends have expressed concern to the school nurse practitioner that Jane has begun to "jog" at lunch time and seldom eats with them. Jane has told her friends that she gained weight over the winter months and that she is "jogging" because she wants to qualify for the track team this spring. In addition to severe weight loss, which of the following symptoms of anorexia nervosa is the school nurse practitioner likely to observe when she interviews Jane and performs a sports physical?

FIRST, THINK ABOUT IT. . .
- What conclusions are you reaching?
- If you accept the conclusions, what are the implications?

1. Decreased body temperature
2. History of dysmenorrhea
3. Tachycardia
4. Heat intolerance

*The best response is one. A correct conclusion is that anorexia nervosa is a condition in which several alterations in metabolic activity can occur following excessive weight loss. Also, you may conclude that these alterations include lowered body temperature, bradycardia, secondary amenorrhea, decreased blood pressure, and cold intolerance. When the nutritional status improves and normal body weight has been restored, these metabolic changes are usually reversed.*

some patients. Deaths associated with AN have also occurred during rehabilitation as a result of cardiovascular overload. Restoration of body weight to a target weight or end point within 10% of the patient's ideal body weight should be one of the main goals of nutritional rehabilitation (Schneider and Fisher, 2001).

Establishing a "maintenance weight range" of 1 kg over or under the target weight helps the adolescent to feel in control, encourages maintenance of weight through healthy dietary habits, and teaches the adolescent that uncontrollable weight gain is not inevitable when a normal diet is consumed.

It is important that nurses be aware of the physical side effects of AN. Patients with AN often limit their fluid intake. Urinary tract problems are frequent, and ketones and proteins are commonly detected in the urine as a result of fat and protein breakdown. Vital sign instability can be severe and can include orthostatic hypotension; the pulse becomes irregular and may decrease markedly. Bradycardia and hypothermia can result in cardiac arrest. (See Critical Thinking Exercise box.)

**Behavior Therapy.** The use of behavioral modification in the treatment of AN has met with varying degrees of success. Providing privileges or activities for weight gain or positive eating behaviors may be successful, but treatment should also address the conflict precipitating the disorder. A clearly defined behavior-modification plan is communicated to the young person and maintained through a unified team approach by all persons involved in care.

The team responsible for the management of young people with AN arranges a carefully structured environment. First, there must be consistency. The team decides on an approach and adheres to it. The plan is structured with reality testing regarding caloric intake and body-image perception as an essential component. The team members provide a unified front to avoid any possibility of manipulation or inconsistency. Second, all members of the team are involved; the responsibility of the program cannot be left to one person. The role and boundaries of each member are clearly spelled out. Third, continuity of team members is important, and it is helpful to have the same team members all the time.

Fourth, communication among team members is essential. Communication with the patient regarding what is expected is also important. Sometimes the limit-setting may seem unreasonable; if the rationale for the limits is not understood, the adolescent may sabotage the entire program. It is also important to communicate with the family. Fifth, the plan must provide for support of the adolescent, the family, and team members. The adolescent's efforts should be supported, and positive feedback should be provided for accomplishments made in normalizing eating habits. Meetings are held to discuss the feelings and concerns of the patient, immediate caregivers, and team members.

All individuals involved in therapy must remember that the adolescent's distorted sense of body image and self-awareness, feelings of self-doubt, ineffectiveness, helplessness, and lack of control prompt the self-damaging behavior. The underlying principle in many behavior-modification programs for hospitalized adolescents is to grant privileges only as a reward for weight gain. Adolescents who view these programs as coercive and become depressed by this approach seldom maintain weight gain outside the hospital environment.

A *behavioral contract,* an agreement that the adolescent makes with others to change a maladaptive behavior, has proved to be effective in some cases. The written contract is constructed by the therapeutic team and approved and signed by the adolescent. Unless the adolescent agrees to its terms, the contract can become the source of a power struggle. However, it can be an effective tool that places the responsibility for weight gain or other behavioral change on the adolescent.

**Family Support.** Family therapy is effective when begun soon after the onset of illness but is less successful when the condition has existed for some time. Therapy is directed toward disengagement and redirection of malfunctioning processes in the family. Individual psychotherapy may also be needed for family members.

Nurses, patients, and families can find assistance and information from several organizations. The **American Anorexia/Bulimia Association, Inc. (AABA)** provides in-

---

### Box 21-5 ◼ ◼ ◻
### Early Signs of Anorexia Nervosa

The adolescent:
Consumes an inappropriate diet (excessively strict) or may refuse to eat altogether
Develops peculiar eating habits such as toying with food, food "rituals," preparing and forcing food on family members without eating any herself
Engages in excessive exercise, such as compulsive jogging, running up and down stairs, rigorous calisthenics to burn off calories—often to the point of exhaustion
Withdraws from social interaction—starts to spend all her time in her room studying, exercising, or otherwise occupied
Ceases to have menstrual periods after sudden or excessive weight loss—sometimes almost as soon as dieting begins
Takes laxatives, diuretics, or enemas to speed intestinal transit time, to lose added weight, and to empty intestines to flatten abdomen
Vomits deliberately—may go to bathroom after a meal and turn on faucets to avoid being heard
Denies hunger even after eating practically nothing for days or even weeks
Develops a distorted body image—states she "feels fat" as she becomes increasingly thinner
Loses weight—growing girls fail to achieve the 25th percentile on normal growth curves

---

formation, referrals, counseling, and activities aimed at combating eating disorders. The **National Association of Anorexia Nervosa and Associated Disorders, Inc. (ANAD)** provides counseling, referral, and self-help programs for young people with AN. The **National Eating Disorders Association**† provides information and support services for both patients and families.

**Prevention.** There are no easy ways to prevent AN. However, public and professional awareness of signs and symptoms can facilitate early identification and treatment to prevent or reduce the long-term adverse consequences. The early signs of AN are outlined in Box 21-5.

### ◼ Evaluation

The effectiveness of nursing interventions is determined by continual reassessment and evaluation of care based on the following observational guidelines:

1. Perform nutritional assessment; measure weight; review diet and nutritional intake (e.g., log); interview adolescent regarding food and eating behaviors; observe eating behaviors.
2. Interview adolescent regarding self-perceptions; observe behavior; confer with psychologist and other members of the health team regarding evidence of progress.
3. Observe adolescent's behavior and interview young person regarding attitudes, concerns, and behaviors.
4. Interview family and confer with team members regarding progress; observe interpersonal interactions between adolescent and others, especially family members.

The *expected outcomes* are described in the Nursing Care Plan on pp. 881-882.

---

*165 West 46th St, Suite 1108, New York, NY 10036, (212) 575-6200, e-mail: info@aaba.inc; www.aabainc.org .

*PO Box 7, Highland Park, IL 60035, (847) 831-3438, e-mail: info@anad. org; www.anad.org .
†603 Stewart St, Suite 803, Seattle, WA 98101, www.nationaleatingdisorders. org .

# Nursing Care Plan
## The Adolescent with Anorexia Nervosa

| **NURSING DIAGNOSIS:** Imbalanced nutrition: less than body requirements related to self-starvation |
| --- |

**PATIENT GOAL 1:** Will consume nourishment adequate for weight gain

- **NURSING INTERVENTIONS/*RATIONALES***

Implement high-calorie diet as prescribed *to ensure nourishment adequate for gradual weight gain*

Explain nutritional plan to adolescent and family *to encourage compliance*

With dietitian and patient, select balanced diet with the prescribed incremental increase in calories; *rapid weight gain is avoided because it can cause cardiovascular overload and give child an overwhelming sense of being out of control*

Help patient prepare an eating-habits diary *to assess adequacy of nutrition*

- **EXPECTED OUTCOME**

Adolescent evidences gradual weight gain

**PATIENT GOAL 2:** Will follow behavior-modification plan (if implemented)

- **NURSING INTERVENTIONS/*RATIONALES***

Ensure that all members of the health care team determine an approach, understand the plan, and adhere to it consistently

Involve all team members, including the patient

Ensure continuity of caregivers (team members)

Provide for clear communication among team members and with the patient *so that patient understands precisely what is expected*

Consult with patient regarding progress

Avoid coercive techniques *because coercion is usually ineffective for long-term success*

Support patient in efforts (e.g., positive feedback for accomplishments)

- **EXPECTED OUTCOME**

Expectations are met consistently (specify)

**PATIENT GOAL 3:** Will reduce energy expenditure

- **NURSING INTERVENTIONS/*RATIONALES***

Monitor physical activity *to evaluate appropriateness for child's condition*

Supervise selection and performance of activity

Be alert to evidence of secretive exercising *because child may use exercising as a weight loss strategy*

- **EXPECTED OUTCOME**

Adolescent engages in quiet and specified activities

| **NURSING DIAGNOSIS:** Disturbed body image related to altered perception |
| --- |

**PATIENT GOAL 1:** Will express self in acceptable ways

- **NURSING INTERVENTIONS/*RATIONALES***

Channel need for control and feeling of effectiveness in appropriate directions (rather than control of weight)

Obtain psychiatric referral as indicated *because psychotherapy is essential in treatment*

Encourage patient to monitor own care as appropriate *to provide a sense of control*

- **EXPECTED OUTCOME**

Adolescent expresses self in acceptable ways

**PATIENT GOAL 2:** Will receive adequate support

- **NURSING INTERVENTIONS/*RATIONALES***

Maintain open communications with adolescent *so that adolescent is able to express feelings and concerns*

Convey an attitude of caring and protection to adolescent

Avoid conveying an attitude of intrusion

Encourage participation in own care *so that adolescent has an appropriate sense of control*

- **EXPECTED OUTCOMES**

Adolescent expresses feelings and concerns

Adolescent becomes actively involved in own care and management

**PATIENT GOAL 3:** Will receive assistance in altering distorted self-image

- **NURSING INTERVENTIONS/*RATIONALES***

Support psychiatric plan of care *because this is essential in helping adolescent alter distorted self-image*

- **EXPECTED OUTCOMES**

Adolescent receives appropriate psychiatric care

Adolescent displays evidence of developing a positive self-image

| **NURSING DIAGNOSIS:** Ineffective coping related to unrealistic perceptions |
| --- |

**PATIENT/FAMILY GOAL 1:** Will conform to therapeutic program

- **NURSING INTERVENTIONS/*RATIONALES***

Maintain consistency in therapeutic approach selected

Maintain vigilance to detect signs of sabotaging the therapeutic plan, such as self-induced vomiting, laxative or enema use, hoarding food, disposing of food, placing weighted material in clothing for weigh-in, *because adolescent may use these methods to prevent weight gain*

Provide positive reinforcement for progress

Be alert for signs of depression

Support psychotherapeutic measures

Help arrange for follow-up care *because treatment requires long-term care*

*Continued*

## *Nursing Care Plan*
### The Adolescent with Anorexia Nervosa—cont'd

- **EXPECTED OUTCOME**
Adolescent and family conform to therapeutic program (specify behaviors)

> **NURSING DIAGNOSIS:** Readiness for enhanced family coping related to ambivalent family relationships

**PATIENT/FAMILY GOAL 1:** Will recognize disturbed pattern of family interaction

- **NURSING INTERVENTIONS/*RATIONALES***
Observe family interaction *for assessment of coping patterns*
Explore feelings and attitudes of family members
Support psychotherapeutic measures for redirecting malfunctioning family processes
Help arrange for referral to individuals and groups that further therapeutic goals

- **EXPECTED OUTCOME**
Family patterns of interaction are recognized and evaluated

**PATIENT/FAMILY GOAL 2:** Will be prepared for home care

- **NURSING INTERVENTIONS/*RATIONALES***
Make certain both patient and family understand therapeutic plan
Arrange for follow-up care *because treatment needs to be long-term*
Refer to special agencies for additional information and support

- **EXPECTED OUTCOMES**
Family demonstrates an understanding of the etiology of the disorder and conforms to therapeutic program
Family uses available resources

## Bulimia

Bulimia (from the Greek meaning "ox hunger") refers to an eating disorder similar to AN. Bulimia is characterized by repeated episodes of binge eating followed by inappropriate compensatory behaviors, such as self-induced vomiting; misuse of laxatives, diuretics, or other medications; fasting; or excessive exercise (American Psychiatric Association, 2000). The binge behavior consists of secretive, frenzied consumption of large amounts of high-calorie (or "forbidden") foods during a brief period of time (usually less than 2 hours). The binge is counteracted by a variety of weight control methods (purging), including self-induced vomiting, diuretic and laxative abuse, and rigorous exercise. These binge/purge cycles are followed by self-deprecating thoughts, a depressed mood, and an awareness that the eating pattern is abnormal.

### Clinical Manifestations

Bulimia is observed more commonly in older adolescent girls and young women; males with bulimia are uncommon. Although persons with bulimia have many issues in common with other eating disorders, impulse control and satiety regulation are important problems in bulimia. Many individuals with bulimia begin with only occasional binges and purges "just for fun," enjoying the control over their weight while eating amounts of food that would normally produce obesity. As the disease progresses, the frequency of binges increases, the amount of food consumed increases, and there is a gradual loss of control over the binge/purge cycle. The binge/purge cycle provides relief from feelings of guilt resulting from the enormous amounts of food consumed. The family becomes angry, and the individual with bulimia becomes frightened, frustrated, and increasingly guilt-ridden, which only increases the symptoms in the self-destructive cycle.

The frequency of bingeing can be anywhere from once per week to seven or eight times per day. Because persons with bulimia usually binge on high-calorie foods, especially sweets, ice cream, and pastries, insulin production is stimulated to cope with the added carbohydrates. When the food is vomited, the unused insulin stimulates hunger and the desire to eat. An intake of 20,000 to 30,000 calories per day is not unusual.

Bulimia appears in all socioeconomic levels. Adolescents most at risk are those who aspire to careers or sports that require low weight, those who have been sexually abused, and those who have a family history of eating disorders, affective disorders, and substance abuse (Muscari, 1998). Males with eating disorders often have a history of dieting related to sports activities.

### Therapeutic Management

Therapy is similar to the management of AN. Hospitalization may be required, especially for complications, which are treated symptomatically. Intravenous fluids and potassium replacement are the essential elements of care, and cardiac monitoring is indicated. The integration of medical, psychologic, behavioral, and nutritional approaches to eating disorders is essential in effective treatment programs. Each component provides a unique perspective to the individual, and therapy should be individualized to the person's needs.

Several studies have indicated deficient serotonergic function in bulimic patients (Halmi, 1999). Recent studies have indicated that antidepressants, especially selective serotonin-reuptake inhibitors (SSRIs) such as fluoxetine (Prozac) or sertraline (Zoloft), diminish the obsessive-compulsive urge to binge and vomit in some patients who have bulimia (Kotler and Walsh, 2000).

Persons with bulimia are characteristically individuals who have been unsuccessful dieters, have low impulse con-

**Box 21-6** ▪ ▪ ▫
### Diagnostic Criteria for Bulimia Nervosa

1. Recurrent episodes of binge eating. An episode of binge eating is characterized by both of the following:
   a. Eating, in a discrete period of time (e.g., within any 2-hour period), an amount of food that is definitely larger than most people would eat during a similar period of time and under similar circumstances
   b. A sense of lack of control over eating during the episode (e.g., a feeling that one cannot stop eating or control what or how much one is eating)
2. Recurrent inappropriate compensatory behavior in order to prevent weight gain, such as self-induced vomiting; misuse of laxatives, diuretics, enemas, or other medications; fasting; or excessive exercise.
3. The binge eating and inappropriate compensatory behaviors both occur, on average, at least twice a week for 3 months.
4. Self-evaluation is unduly influenced by body shape and weight.
5. The disturbance does not occur exclusively during episodes of anorexia nervosa.

*Specify type:*
   **Purging type:** During the current episode of bulimia nervosa, the person has regularly engaged in self-induced vomiting or the misuse of laxatives, diuretics, or enemas.
   **Nonpurging type:** During the current episode of bulimia nervosa, the person has used other inappropriate compensatory behaviors, such as fasting or excessive exercise, but has not regularly engaged in self-induced vomiting or the misuse of laxatives, diuretics, or enemas.

From American Psychiatric Association: *Diagnostic and statistical manual of mental disorders*, ed 4 (DSM-IV TR), Washington, DC, 2000, The Association.

trol, and may have been self-conscious about being overweight in childhood. They may consciously or unconsciously suppress their feelings and have a strong desire to fit into the group.

Individuals with bulimia fall into two types: (1) those who purge and (2) those who do not purge (Box 21-6). Some women with bulimia are of normal or (more often) slightly above normal weight; others become as underweight as individuals with AN. This latter type of bulimia, wherein individuals have a tendency to restrict intake, is also called **bulimarexia.** (See Table 21-2 for a comparison of AN and bulimia.)

**Complications.** Adolescents with bulimia suffer from several medical complications as a result of the frequent vomiting. As with any disorder characterized by gastrointestinal losses, the loss of fluids and electrolytes can occur rapidly. Potassium depletion causes diminished reflexes, fatigue and, if severe, possible cardiac arrhythmias. Potassium losses are more likely to occur with diuretic abuse. Laxative abuse can interfere with absorption of fat, protein, and calcium and can produce abdominal complaints such as cramping, constipation, steatorrhea, and gastrointestinal bleeding. Anemia is common.

Frequent vomiting and irritation from stomach acid causes erosion of tooth enamel, an increase in dental caries, chronic esophagitis, chronic sore throat, difficulty swallowing, inflammation, and parotitis. Vomiting may be so severe

that the patient suffers esophageal tears, hiatal hernia, and spontaneous bleeding in the eye.

### Diagnostic Evaluation

A diagnosis of bulimia may be first suspected from the presence of complications. Final diagnosis is made on the basis of criteria established by the American Psychiatric Association (2000) (see Box 21-6). Distinctive hand lesions (Russell's sign) have also been observed; the backs of the hands are often scarred and cut from repeated abrasion of the skin against the maxillary incisors during self-induced vomiting (Muscari, 1998). Other aspects to note in the physical examination include skin, salivary gland, and dental changes and signs of self-mutilation.

### Nursing Considerations

Nursing care is similar to care of the patient with AN. Acute care involves careful monitoring of fluid and electrolyte alterations and observation for signs of cardiac complications. Nutritional consultation and follow-up are essential. The nurse should encourage the adolescent and family members to structure the environment to reduce the bingeing behavior. Getting rid of binge foods, restricting eating to one room of the house, not engaging in other activities while eating, and substituting exercise, crafts, visualization, and relaxation techniques for bingeing are helpful interventions. Telephone support networks are also effective (Muscari, 1996).

## "Fear of Fat" Syndrome

Another phenomenon that affects some preteens and teenagers is the fear of becoming fat. In their enthusiasm to avoid becoming overweight, these young people restrict their caloric intake to the degree that they stop growing normally and pubertal changes do not take place. The disorder is distinct from AN, in which adolescents have a distorted body image. Adolescents who are afraid of obesity worry that being overweight will make them physically unattractive, jeopardize their health, and shorten their life span.

The desire for thinness in these adolescents is often triggered by the normal weight gain and fat accumulation of adolescent growth and development. Dissatisfaction with their appearance often causes them to resort to fad diets and severely reduce their intake below the recommended daily allowances for nutrients. Many underweight adolescents describe themselves as extremely fearful of being overweight and preoccupied with body fat. Unfortunately, to achieve low-calorie, low-fat diets, teenagers eliminate many basic foods such as milk, cheese, eggs, and meat without replacing them with other nutritious items such as cereal and bread. Their diets are lacking in iron, calcium, and zinc, a mineral closely tied to growth and the onset of puberty.

Many children worry about their weight long before adolescence, even when there is no reason for concern. Society's emphasis on thinness and the prevention of obesity may be detrimental to this vulnerable age-group.

Nurses encountering young people who self-impose unwarranted dieting need to focus their approach on education regarding normal body changes and the hazards of dieting. The risks of dieting are more serious than the risks associated with unwanted weight gain.

# SUBSTANCE ABUSE*
## Overview

Although experimentation with drugs during adolescence is widespread, the majority of teens do not become high-risk users. National and statewide surveys indicate that although there is a steady increase in the incidence of adolescents using tobacco, alcohol, and marijuana between the ages of 12 and 18, experimentation is limited to 1 adolescent in 5 for stimulants and inhalants and to less than 1 adolescent in 10 for "hard" drugs such as hallucinogens, sedatives, and crack. Adolescents at greatest risk are not the estimated 80% to 90% of high school students who have tried alcohol or the 45% to 55% who have tried marijuana, but rather the estimated 4% who report daily use of alcohol during the past 30 days and the 1% to 2% who use "hard" drugs regularly (U.S. Department of Health and Human Services, 1999).

The etiology of substance abuse is poorly understood. Current research focuses on biopsychosocial risk and protective factors (Weinberg and others, 1998). For the majority of adolescents, experimentation with drugs occurs during a period in which a variety of behaviors are tried on for size and then discarded when the fit is not right. There are a number of theories about pathways leading to the abuse of substances (Bauman and Phongsavan, 1999). Although research has identified risk factors such as the presence of an enzyme (aldehyde dehydrogenase [ALDH]) that makes decomposition of ethanol in the body possible (Patton, 1995), family history of drug abuse and dependence (Baer and others, 1998; Kosterman and others, 2000), and individual psychopathology (Angold, Costello, and Erkanli, 1999), no single factor explains the cause of adolescent substance abuse. The enormous impact of poverty and greater availability of substances, combined with biogenetic predispositions for abuse, are likely factors to consider in understanding etiology. Although there is much to learn about what leads an adolescent to abuse substances, most experts agree with a *diathesis-stress model*, which presumes a biologic predisposition accompanied by psychosocial risk factors.

An adolescent abusing drugs has often adopted the use of substances as a means of coping with feelings of depression, anxiety, restlessness, or chronic feelings of boredom or emptiness. Because denial is often associated with substance abuse, nurses, other health care professionals, and parents may not be aware of the abuse problem.

## Definitions

Considerable misinformation and confusion are related to the terms applied to drug use. The most important differences among these terms is the distinction between voluntary and involuntary behavior and between culturally defined and physiologically identified events. *Drug abuse,*

*misuse,* and *addiction* are culturally defined and are voluntary behaviors. *Drug tolerance* and *physical dependence* are involuntary physiologic responses to the pharmacologic characteristics of drugs, such as opioids and alcohol. Consequently, an individual can be addicted to a narcotic with or without being physically dependent, and a person may be physically dependent on a narcotic without being addicted (e.g., patients who use opioids to control pain).

The broad term "drug abuse," which is often applied to all forms of drug misuse, is confusing and does not necessarily define the problem related to drug use. Many substances are controlled by law and involve severe penalties for their illegal use; others are sanctioned from a legal, social, and medical standpoint. Problems concerning drug use are defined as follows:

**Legal**. The drug being taken is strictly controlled by law and is accompanied by severe penalties for its use or possession.

**Social**. Use of a substance leads to disruptive or bizarre behavior that alienates the user from the rest of society; this results in a social problem.

**Medical**. Current or continued use of a substance may adversely affect the physical or mental health of an adolescent.

**Individual**. Focuses on the role that drug use plays in the individual's life and factors that contribute to the individual's need for the drug.

### Patterns of Drug Use

Many factors influence the extent to which drugs are used by teenagers. The type of drug used, mode of administration, duration of use, frequency of use, and single- or multiple-drug use must be considered in determining the severity of the individual drug problem. Most drug use begins with experimentation. The drug may be tried only once, may be used occasionally, or may become an integral part of a drug-centered lifestyle. Identification of the pattern of drug use in an individual facilitates the formulation of an approach to the problem. Patterns have been observed based on dose and frequency of use.

There are two broad categories of adolescents who use drugs: the *experimenters* and the *compulsive users.* Between these groups on opposite ends of a continuum there is a wide range in terms of degree of abuse. Between the experimenters and compulsive users is a broad range of *recreational users,* principally of drugs such as marijuana, cocaine, alcohol, and prescription drugs. For many the goal is typically peer acceptance; these users fit more closely with the experimenting, intermittent users. For others the goal is intoxication; these users resemble the compulsive users. These users may engage in periodic heavy use or "binges." The groups of greatest concern to health care workers are those whose patterns of use involve high doses or mixed drugs with the danger of overdose and those compulsive users with the threat of dependence, withdrawal syndromes, and altered lifestyle.

### Types of Drugs Abused

Any drug can be abused, and most are potentially harmful to adolescents still going through formative life experiences. Although rarely considered drugs by society, the chemically active substances most commonly used are the

---

■ *Kevin Krull, PhD, ABPP, revised this section.

xanthines and theobromines contained in chocolate, tea, coffee, and colas. Ethyl alcohol and nicotine are others that, although recognized as drugs, are sanctioned by society. Any of these substances can produce mild to moderate euphoric and/or stimulant effects and can lead to physical or psychologic dependence.

Many factors determine personal preferences for gratification. Many drugs are not harmful for all teenagers, and some, used intermittently, will probably not produce ill effects or result in dependence. Reactions vary according to the drug used, its purity, the expectations of the user, the route of administration, and the context in which the drug is used. These factors determine to a great extent whether the experience is viewed as pleasant or unpleasant. The type of drugs used also varies according to geographic location, socioeconomic status, urban vs suburban areas, and various historical periods.

A drug that is popular with one "generation" of adolescents may not be attractive to another. Changing trends are influenced by the adolescent's search for new and different experiences. The present concern is the rising use of alcohol, tobacco, marijuana, heroin, hallucinogens, inhalants, prescription drugs, and cocaine.

Drugs with mind-altering capacity that are available on the black market and are of medical and legal concern are the hallucinogenic, narcotic, hypnotic, and stimulant drugs. In addition, health care professionals are concerned about the use of various volatile substances such as gasoline, model airplane cement, and organic solvents; these substances are inhaled by the user to achieve an altered sensation. More recently, abuse of prescription and synthetic drugs have become of great concern. Drugs available on the street are often mixed with other compounds and fillers so that the purity of the drug, its strength, and the nature of the additives are highly variable. Many of the hazards associated with drug use are related to driving a car or operating equipment that may be harmful when carelessly used while under the influence of the drug. Some of the more commonly abused substances and their general manifestations are outlined in Table 21-3.

# Tobacco

An alarming number of teens smoke. By 1999 the rate of daily smoking for adolescents had increased to 16.8% (Centers for Disease Control and Prevention, 1999). The percentage of senior high school students who reported smoking in the past 30 days was approximately 45.2% for boys and 40.5% for girls (Centers for Disease Control and Prevention, 1999). Recent reports of smoking among youths between ages 12 and 17 years indicate that males have slightly higher smoking rates than females although females display an earlier peak in rates of abuse (by tenth grade) than males (twelfth grade) (Centers for Disease Control and Prevention, 1999).

Although the number of adult smokers has declined in recent years, cigarette smoking is still considered the chief avoidable cause of death. Unfortunately, cigar smoking is increasing and is as deadly as cigarette smoking.

The hazards of smoking at any age are undisputed; however, a preventive approach to teenage smoking is especially important. There is a high probability that regular smoking in childhood and adolescence leads to a lifetime habit, with concomitant increases in morbidity and mortality. Smoking has also been related to health risk and deviant behaviors. Approximately three times as many adolescents who smoke report carrying weapons and drinking alcohol compared with adolescents who do not smoke (Willard and Schoenborn, 1995). There is also a clear association between the use of tobacco and the use of other drugs (Torabi, Bailey, and Majd-Jabbari, 1993).

## Etiology

Teenagers begin smoking for a variety of reasons. Factors related to the onset of smoking can be categorized as social, sociodemographic, psychosocial, and biologic. Once smoking behavior is established, smoking itself produces enough reinforcement to sustain the practice without the initial pressure.

**Social Factors.** Social pressures to smoke include imitation of the smoking behavior and attitudes of parents and other adults, the association of smoking with maturity or "mature" behavior, pressures from peers who view smoking as the popular thing to do, and the use of smoking as an outlet for real or imagined school, social, or home pressures. Other pressures come from advertisements aimed directly at teens although moves to limit such advertisements have recently begun.

Previous research did not indicate a definite parental influence on tobacco use in children (Institute of Medicine, 1994). Recent findings, however, indicate parent disapproval of smoking may influence adolescents not to smoke (Sargent and Dalton, 2001). The 1994 Surgeon General's report of 15 prospective studies investigating parental smoking indicated that parental smoking was a predictive factor for both boys and girls in 7 out of 15 studies and a predictive factor only for girls in 2 studies. In 6 studies, parental smoking was not a predictor of smoking in children (Centers for Disease Control and Prevention, 1994a). The influence of same-sex family members is important, but maternal smoking has been found to be a more important long-term predictor of daily smoking in young adults (Oygard and others, 1995).

Parental attitudes and reactions to tobacco use may have a stronger influence on adolescent smoking than the actual smoking status of parents. When parents disapprove of smoking and consistently reinforce the expectation that their children will not use tobacco, adolescents are less likely to begin smoking regardless of their parent's smoking status (Institute of Medicine, 1994).

The influence of peers or friends on smoking initiation has been documented in several studies (Bertrand and Abernathy, 1993; Flay and others, 1994). In particular, the effects of friends' smoking have been found to be greater for females than for males, leading to greater peer pressure for young girls to start smoking (Hu and others, 1995).

Another social factor that can influence the initiation of smoking is the belief that cigarette smoking controls weight gain. Several studies have indicated a relationship between

**TABLE 21-3** Major drugs abused by adolescents

| Chemical Agent/Route | Physical Signs | Behavior | Complications |
|---|---|---|---|
| **Opiates** | | | |
| **Heroin, morphine, meperidine, hydromorphone, fentanyl, methadone**—injected subcutaneously or intravenously (IV), intranasal (sniffing), oral | Constricted pupils, respiratory depression, cyanosis<br>Needle marks | Initial euphoria, tranquilization, lethargy, coma | Overdose: coma, respiratory arrest, death<br>Injection site infection, hepatitis, abscesses, septicemia, tetanus, pulmonary complications, acquired immunodeficiency syndrome (AIDS)<br>Withdrawal: muscle/stomach cramps, diarrhea, runny nose/eyes, restlessness, seizures, death<br>Dental caries |
| **Depressants** | | | |
| **Barbiturates**—secobarbital, amobarbital, pentobarbital, amobarbital/secobarbital—oral, IV | Slurred speech, ataxia, slowed reflexes, constricted pupils (barbiturates); dilated pupils (glutethimide) | Short attention span, impaired judgment, combativeness, violence | Overdose: respiratory depression, coma, death<br>Injection site infection, hepatitis, septicemia, AIDS<br>Withdrawal: hyperreflexia, irritability, seizures, death |
| **Nonbarbiturates**—methaqualone (Quaalude), ethchlorvynol (Placidyl)—oral | Poor coordination, tremors, ataxia, confusion, slurred speech, hyperreflexia, diplopia, general muscle weakness | Hyperexcitability; euphoria of methaqualone similar to opiate experience | Overdose: delirium and coma, convulsions, hepatic damage, respiratory arrest, death<br>Withdrawal: similar to barbiturates and alcohol |
| **Alcohol (ethanol)**—oral | Poor coordination | Impaired judgment and perception, loss of inhibitions, emotional lability, quarrelsomeness, aggressiveness, hostility<br>Lethargy | Hazards related to impaired judgment (e.g., automobile accidents, fights)<br>Nutritional deficiencies<br>Gastritis<br>Overdose: coma, death, especially when used in combination with barbiturates<br>Withdrawal: anxiety, tremors, hallucinations, hyperreflexia, seizures, death |
| **Minor Tranquilizers** | | | |
| **Chlordiazepoxide (Librium), diazepam (Valium), meprobamate**—oral | Nonspecific | Decreased anxiety and tension<br>Occasional disinhibition | Similar to barbiturates but with reduced intensity |
| **Organic Solvents** | | | |
| **Hydrocarbons and fluorocarbons**—glue, cleaning fluid, lighter fluid, aerosol sprays, nail polish, gasoline, paint thinner, butane, varnish—sniffed | Nonspecific (may include sore throat, cough, runny nose) | Euphoria, dysphoria, confusion, impaired perception and coordination, restlessness<br>Loss of consciousness | Asphyxia from plastic bags used to inhale fumes<br>Lead poisoning<br>Possible irreversible damage to central nervous system, kidneys, liver, and bone marrow |
| **Stimulants** | | | |
| **Amphetamines**—amphetamine sulfate, dextroamphetamine, methamphetamine—oral, subcutaneous, IV | Hypertension, weight loss, dilated pupils<br>Sweating (when injected) | Psychologic and motor stimulation<br>Hyperactivity, false bravado, euphoria, increased alertness, insomnia, anorexia, irritability, personality change | Injection site infection<br>Paranoia, severe depression with suicidal tendency when drug stopped |
| **Cocaine**—intranasal, IV, smoke | Hypertension, tachycardia, hyperreflexia | Restlessness, hyperactivity, intense euphoria | Nausea/vomiting, inflammation/perforation of nasal septum |
| **Hallucinogens** | | | |
| **Cannabis**—marijuana, hashish—smoke, oral | Occasionally tachycardia, delayed response time, poor coordination | Simple euphoria, mild intoxication, heightened sensory awareness, drowsiness | Occasionally depressive or anxiety reactions |
| **LSD, PCP, DMT, STP, THC, mescaline**—oral | Dilated pupils, reddened eyes, occasionally hypertension, hyperthermia, piloerection | Euphoria, heightened sensory awareness, increased appetite, hallucinations, confusion, paranoia | Primarily psychiatric: may intensify latent psychotic tendencies, panic, suicide possible, flashbacks |

smoking and concerns about weight among adolescent females (Klesges and Robinson, 1995; Tomeo and others, 1999; Strauss, 2000). Some individuals do gain weight after they quit smoking and resume the habit to lose the weight.

The mass media have contributed to the incidence of smoking in adolescents. In advertisements smokers are engaged in activities and dressed in clothes suitable for adolescents, and smoking is associated with fun, risk taking, and sexual adventure, maturity, and autonomy. The ads also imply an association between smoking and youthful vigor, a slim figure, good looks, and personal, social, and professional acceptance and success. Children also seem to respond to the use of cartoon characters in cigarette advertising. An increase in the smoking of Camel cigarettes among underage children and teens was noted after the introduction of the Joe Camel ad campaign (U.S. Department of Health and Human Services, 1994).

Some uses of the media have been helpful in increasing adolescent exposure to antismoking messages. Unfortunately, these mass media antismoking campaigns have had little effect on smoking-related beliefs or on the smoking behaviors of adolescents (Murray, Prokhorov, and Harty, 1994).

**Sociodemographic Factors.**   Sociodemographic factors that relate to levels of smoking include socioeconomic status, sex, and performance in school. A consistent, negative association has been observed between socioeconomic status and smoking (especially among boys), and there is a positive correlation between low academic goals and performance and smoking. Smoking among college students has dramatically increased in recent years (Rigotti, Lee, and Wechsler, 2000). Although cigarette use is still most prominent (28.5% of college students), regular cigar use has also become common (8.5% of college students). Rates of smoking are still highest among adolescents who do not complete high school. Students who focus on schoolwork and who have high educational goals for themselves are significantly less likely than their peers to develop a long-term smoking habit (Johnston, O'Malley, and Bachman, 1995).

**Psychosocial Factors.**   Although theories explaining the relationship between personality and smoking behavior have been suggested, research has not documented any significant differences between adolescents who smoke and those who do not smoke. Rather than discriminating between smokers and nonsmokers, personality traits such as anxiety have been shown to predict *how much* adolescents will smoke once they begin the habit. Although depression does not seem to be related to heavy cigarette smoking in adolescents, current use is a determinant to the development of depressive symptoms (Goodman and Capitman, 2000).

Recent research has examined the development of different personality characteristics of adolescents at the time of the onset of tobacco use and with continued use. Youthful smokers (seventh grade) have been found to be extroverted and involved with their peers, whereas older smokers are often depressed and withdrawn (Stein, Newcomb, and Bentler, 1996). This research supports the hypothesis that smoking takes on different psychosocial meanings with continued use.

**Biologic Factors.**   Biologic factors serve both to encourage and to deter further experimentation by would-be smokers. The initial harshness, nausea, and irritation may influence many youngsters not to try smoking again. For others, however, such symptoms are a challenge to overcome. Smoking has been found to lower endurance by decreasing breathing capacity or ventilatory muscle endurance. Cigarette smoking is also associated with mild airway obstruction and slowed growth of lung function in adolescents. The detrimental effects of smoking on growth of lung function may be more pronounced in adolescent girls (Gold and others, 1996). Cigarette smoking showed a dose-response relationship with the development of sleep problems in a group of greater than 3000 adolescents (Patten and others, 2000).

Dependence is a result of nicotine, the primary alkaloid in tobacco. Nicotine exerts both stimulating and sedating effects on the central and peripheral nervous systems and on several organ systems. Attempts to stop smoking are accompanied by severe craving and withdrawal symptoms.

## Process of Becoming a Smoker

The process of becoming a smoker involves three stages: initiation (trying the first cigarette), experimental smoking (less than weekly), and regular smoking (at least weekly). Some researchers also recognize a preparation stage in which psychosocial, environmental, and possibly biologic factors prepare some youngsters to be smokers. Regardless of reason, the fact remains that 75% of teenage smokers will smoke regularly as adults (Moolchan, Ernst, and Henningfield, 2000).

## Smokeless Tobacco

The term *smokeless tobacco* refers to tobacco products that are placed in the mouth but not ignited (e.g., snuff and chewing tobacco). This increasingly popular substitute for cigarettes is now posing a serious hazard to school-age children, adolescents, and young adults (U.S. Department of Health and Human Services, 1994). Significantly more boys (46%) than girls (4.7%) have tried smokeless tobacco by the twelfth grade. Many children and adolescents believe that smokeless tobacco is a safe alternative to cigarette smoking and is not addictive, and they believe they can stop using it at any time. However, among adolescents who have tried smokeless tobacco, an alarming rate of 17% report that they are addicted to this substance (Riley and others, 1996). These products have also been proved to be carcinogenic, and regular use can cause dental problems, foul-smelling breath, and tooth erosion or loss.

In a 1994 Surgeon General's report (U.S. Department of Health and Human Services, 1994), two conclusions were drawn concerning the use of smokeless tobacco by adolescents: (1) smokeless tobacco use is associated with early indicators of periodontal degeneration and with lesions in the oral soft tissue, and (2) adolescent smokeless tobacco users are more likely than nonusers to become cigarette smokers.

## Nursing Considerations

Prevention of regular smoking in teenagers is the most effective way to reduce the overall incidence of smoking. A variety of methods have been employed. Posters, charts, displays, statistics, and the use of examples of actual damaged lungs to communicate the hazards of smoking all have their supporters and doubters. Presentation of films and demonstrations in science classes have also been used in some schools.

For the most part, smoking-prevention programs that focus on the negative, long-term effects of smoking on health have been ineffective. Youth-to-youth programs and those

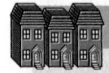

## COMMUNITY FOCUS
### Nonsmoking Strategies

Nurses who work in schools, hospitals, managed care organizations, and other community agencies can take advantage of all opportunities to provide education concerning the dangers of smoking, to discourage smoking initiation by children and adolescents, to encourage smoking cessation, and to promote smoke-free community environments. In particular, school nurses need to be alert to the vulnerability of young preteens when they enter junior high school. These nurses are in an ideal position to assess the degree of stress, personal conflict, concerns about weight, peer pressures, and other factors that place these preteens at risk for smoking initiation (Winkelstein, 1992). Nurses can also serve as consultants and counselors to student, teacher, and parent groups and as advocates for antismoking legislative efforts. Several additional strategies are recommended*:
- Provide only a cursory mention of long-term health consequences (e.g., cardiovascular and cancer risks).
- Discuss immediate physiologic consequences in some detail (e.g., changes in heart rate and blood pressure, minor respiratory symptoms, and blood carbon monoxide concentrations).
- Mention alternatives to smoking for establishing a self-image that appears tough, independent, mature, or sophisticated (e.g., establishing a weight-lifting regimen, jogging, dancing, joining a Boys and Girls Club or a Girls Club, engaging in volunteer work for a hospital or political or religious group).
- Mention the negative effects of smoking (e.g., earlier wrinkling of skin, yellow stains on teeth and fingers, tobacco odor on breath and clothing).
- Mention the increasing ostracism of smokers by nonsmokers, both legal and informal, in the workplace and in public places.
- Mention the increasing evidence that second-hand smoke is injurious to the health of nonsmokers who are regularly exposed, especially small children.
- Acknowledge that many adults once believed that important social benefits were associated with smoking, but point out that the vast majority of adult smokers would now quit smoking if they could.
- Arm the cooperative adolescent with arguments for dealing with peer pressure (e.g., by not smoking, a teenager demonstrates independence and nonconformity, traits normally prized by youth).
- Request posters and pamphlets from local voluntary agencies (e.g., American Cancer Society, American Heart Association, and American Lung Association) to display prominently.

*For information on smoking cessation, nurses can contact the **Nursing Center for Tobacco Intervention**, 1585 Neil Ave, Columbus, Ohio 43210-1216, (614) 292-0653, fax: (614) 292-7976, *www.con.ohio-state.edu/tobacco/*.
Information can also be obtained from **Stop Teenage Addiction to Tobacco (STAT)**, a national organization devoted to educating the public and professionals, at Northeastern University, 360 Huntington Ave., 241 Cushing Hall, Boston, MA 02115, (617) 373-7828, email: info@stat.org.

emphasizing the immediate effects are more effective but are effective primarily in improving the teenagers' attitudes toward smoking. Because smoking and smoking-related behaviors are social symbols, antismoking campaigns must address the norms of potential smokers. Anything that ridicules or threatens the social norms of the peer group can be unproductive or counterproductive. Investigators have found that teaching resistance to peer pressure to smoke is effective in early adolescence. Although the effects of these programs may decrease with time, the effects can be enhanced in older adolescents when using a curriculum compared with simply handing out written material to the students (Adelman and others, 2001).

Two areas of focus for antismoking programs are peer-led programming and use of media in smoking prevention (i.e., videotapes and films). Peer-led programs emphasizing the social consequences of smoking have proved most successful. If a significant number of influential peers can "sell" their classmates on the idea that the habit is not popular, the followers will imitate their behavior. Short-term rather than long-term consequences are emphasized (e.g., the effects of smoking on personal appearance, such as the unattractive stains on teeth and hands and the unpleasant odor that smoking gives to the breath and clothing).

The impact of school-based antismoking programs can be strengthened by expanding these programs to include parents, mass media, youth groups, and community organizations. For example, mass media efforts that involve antismoking radio campaigns have been identified as the most cost-effective mass media intervention.

Smoking bans in schools also accomplish several goals: (1) they discourage students from starting to smoke, (2) they reinforce knowledge of the health hazards of cigarette smoking and exposure to environmental tobacco smoke, and (3) they promote a smoke-free environment as the norm. (See Community Focus box.)

## Alcohol

Acute or chronic abuse of alcohol (ethanol), a socially accepted depressant, is responsible for many acts of violence, suicide, accidental injury, and death. Ethanol reduces inhibitions against aggressive and sexual acting out. Abrupt withdrawal is accompanied by severe physical and psychologic symptoms, and long-term use leads to slow tissue destruction, especially of the brain and liver cells.

Teenage drinking is not a new phenomenon. Because of its social acceptance, peer pressure, and easy accessibility, alcohol is the drug of choice for many adolescents. It is the most widely accepted drug, can be purchased legally by adults, is relatively inexpensive, is often part of a meal (wine, beer), is approved by adults throughout the world when used in moderation, and is even promoted as a health benefit under certain circumstances. Young people may be afraid of hard drugs, but they feel comfortable with alcohol. Many have been exposed to alcohol all their lives.

Although there are racial, ethnic, and gender differences, the pattern of frequent, heavy drinking is likely to begin in the middle school years. Drinking increases with age.

By age 18 years, alcohol has been used by 80% to 90% of all adolescents. In 1995 the monthly prevalence of alcohol use was 50% among high school seniors; with more than 30% of these youths reporting episodic heavy drinking (Centers for Disease Control and Prevention, 1999). These rates have apparently leveled off and slightly decreased over the past several years (U.S. Department of Health and Human Services, 1999).

Although the majority of adolescents who experiment with alcohol are not heavy users, social drinking remains a great concern primarily because of the disturbing rates of morbidity and mortality related to drinking. Alcohol-related motor vehicle incidents result in 8000 adolescent deaths and 45,000 injuries each year. Alcohol use is also involved in 40% of the 10,000 annual nonautomotive accidental deaths of adolescents and in the 5500 suicides and 5000 homicides of adolescents each year (Neinstein and Pinsky, 1996).

The most noticeable effects of alcohol occur within the central nervous system and include changes in cognitive and autonomic functions such as judgment, memory, learning ability, and other intellectual capacities. Marked mood changes are characteristic of adolescent drinkers, who are described as hard to live with and unable to make up their minds. They can be identified by the way in which they use alcohol. Adolescent alcoholics often drink alone, cannot predictably control their use of alcohol, and protect their supply, afraid that they will be caught without anything to drink.

Teenage alcoholics often rely on alcohol as a defense against depression, anxiety, fear, and anger. They become increasingly tolerant to the drug, and there is an increased use of sedatives with alcohol. Some alcoholics have difficulty remembering things done while intoxicated and often intend to swear off the drug or cut down on its use. Not all of these characteristics are observed in the alcoholic, but if several of the signs are evident, individuals should be considered at risk and detoxification therapy should be initiated.

Answers to questions and information about alcohol can be obtained by calling the **Alcohol Hotline.*** Several support groups such as **Al-Anon, Ala-Teen,** and **Ala-Tot** also exist to help children and families who have an alcoholic family member. Information about these groups can be obtained from **Alcoholics Anonymous** listings in local telephone directories.

## Etiology

**Social Factors.**   Parents, siblings, and peers have a significant impact on adolescent alcohol use. Adolescents who develop drinking problems tend to come from families with negative communication patterns, inconsistent parental discipline, marital discord, and an absence of parent-child closeness. Parental and older sibling drinking practices and parental attitudes about alcohol influence adolescent alcohol use, especially during early adolescence (Hoffman and Su, 1998). Several studies assessing family structure have found a relationship between adolescent substance abuse and the overinvolvement of one parent, accompanied by distancing from the other. (See Family Focus box.)

Although the family environment may provide the kindling for adolescent alcohol abuse, peers provide the spark. An association with substance-using peers is the strongest predictor of an adolescent's continued use (Hoffman and Su, 1998). Peer association does not cause adolescent substance abuse, but in most cases adolescents who drink have friends who also drink. The impact of peers on drug use has also been demonstrated among African-Americans, Asians, and Hispanics (Warheit and others, 1995).

**Sociodemographic Factors.**   Frequency of alcohol use is influenced by several sociodemographic factors. Adolescents in urban areas drink more than their rural or suburban peers. Girls and boys report a similar onset and course of experimentation with alcohol although boys more often become heavy users. A commitment to education reduces risk; in contrast, school failure is associated with alcohol abuse. School dropouts are at particularly high risk and have been shown to drink more than high school graduates (Neinstein and Pinsky, 1996). However, "binge" drinking is reported to be highest among college students.

**Psychosocial Factors.**   Research on personality and alcohol abuse in adolescence has investigated the interplay of complex factors that determine risk for alcohol abuse. Although aggressiveness early in life predicts subsequent alcohol use, only one third of boys with aggressive behavior continue to be aggressive into adulthood (White, Brick, and Hansell, 1993). Children with hyperactivity, particularly when combined with conduct problems, are at risk for drug abuse, including alcohol. Personality traits associated with alcohol abuse include excessive and consistent rebelliousness and rejection of social norms.

In his research, Jessor (1991) examined several psychosocial factors and developed the Problem Behavior Theory for understanding adolescent drug and alcohol use. This theory identified several domains of psychosocial variation: the personality system, the perceived environmental system, the social system, and the behavior system. These systems are interrelated and constitute the risk of occurrence of problem behaviors. A common dimension within these systems that distinguishes drug users from nonusers is conventionality vs unconventionality. In reference to the personality system, for example, an adolescent who lacks interest in conventional

---

*800-ALCOHOL.

## FAMILY FOCUS
### Adolescent Alcohol Abuse

The two primary tasks of parenting an adolescent are to provide nurturing and to set appropriate limits (Green, 1994). Research on families with alcohol-abusing adolescents reveals serious deficiencies in one or both of these areas. There is nothing to be gained by explicitly or implicitly blaming the parents. In fact, further assessment often reveals the parents' own history of neglect and substance abuse. One of the most difficult yet important challenges for health care professionals is to establish a trusting relationship with families when attempting to help the adolescent who is struggling with a substance abuse problem. The services and referrals provided must be determined by the unique needs and circumstances of the individuals whom nurses are serving.

institutions such as the church and school is at greater risk for involvement with drugs and alcohol. Conversely, adolescents who embrace conventional values such as academic achievement and community involvement are less likely to engage in drug use. Jessor also identified protective factors that enable at-risk adolescents to resist pressures to use drugs and alcohol. Protective factors include a cohesive family, peer models for conventional behavior, church attendance, and participation in school activities.

Newcomb and Felix-Ortiz (1992) also analyzed risk factors and protective factors from an epidemiologic approach and defined protective factors as those influences that buffer, neutralize, and interact with risk factors to prevent, limit, or reduce drug use. Protective factors do not imply the absence of risk but are viewed as distinctly different from risk factors (Scheier, Newcomb, and Skager, 1994). Strong attachment to parents, a commitment to schooling, regular involvement in church activities, and a belief in the generalized expectations, norms, and values of society serve as protective factors (Hawkins, Catalano, and Miller, 1992). Research has also identified the development of resiliency as another important protective factor against alcoholism (Patton, 1995).

**Biologic Factors.** Research on the association between biochemical and genetic factors and adolescent alcohol abuse is important. Twin studies comparing the concordance of alcoholism in monozygotic (identical) and dizygotic (nonidentical) twins indicate a significantly higher rate of alcoholism in monozygotic twins than in dizygotic twins (Morrison, Rogers, and Thomas, 1995). This finding holds true even if the twins were reared separately early in life.

Aldehyde dehydrogenase (ALDH) is an enzyme that assists with the breakdown of ethanol in the body. The absence of ALDH significantly reduces the likelihood that alcoholism will develop (Patton, 1995). Other genetic studies have indicated an association between the dopamine D2 receptor gene (DRD2) and alcoholism; this gene may confer susceptibility to at least one form of alcoholism (Blum and others, 1990; Patton, 1995). Furthermore, a strong family history of alcoholism is associated with increased rates of cognitive delays and learning difficulties. This cognitive pattern may predispose adolescents to school failure and in turn alcohol abuse.

Research has also documented a relationship between early sexual maturation and cigarette and alcohol use, especially among adolescent girls (Wilson and others, 1994). This association may be an external manifestation of the emotional reaction that occurs in girls who feel physically different because of early biologic maturation. (See Community Focus box.)

## Additional Drugs

The majority of adolescents limit their experimentation with drugs to alcohol, tobacco, and marijuana. A smaller proportion try other drugs that have serious consequences, including cocaine, inhalants, barbiturates, narcotics, and hallucinogens. Adolescent abuse of inhalants and prescription drugs has substantially increased over recent years, with current lifetime reports being 14.6% (Centers for Disease Control and Prevention, 1999). In fact, in a recent survey conducted by the National Institute on Drug Abuse, 12 to 14-year-old adolescents reported psychotherapeutic drugs as some of the most frequently abused substances (U.S. Department of Health and Human Services, 2001).

Drug users have developed a specialized terminology for abused substances (Box 21-7). The vocabulary varies in different localities, and new descriptive terms arise spontaneously wherever drugs are part of the environment.

*Cocaine* is the most potent antifatigue agent known. Although pharmacologically not a narcotic, it is legally categorized as such. Cocaine is available in two forms: (1) water-soluble cocaine hydrochloride administered by insufflation (snorting) and intravenous injection, and (2) a nonsoluble alkaloid (freebase) used primarily for smoking. Crack, or rock, is a purer and more menacing form of the drug; it can be produced cheaply and smoked in either water pipes or mentholated cigarettes. Cocaine taken by injection is associated with the highest levels of dependence, "crack" smoking has intermediate levels, and intranasal forms of cocaine have the lowest levels of dependence (Gossip and others, 1994). The increased use of cocaine is related to its availability and affordability, the false perception that it is safe, its association with persons in glamorous occupations, its snob appeal, its reputation as a sexually enhancing drug, and peer pressure.

Cocaine creates a sense of euphoria, or an indefinable high. Withdrawal does not produce the dramatic symptoms

### COMMUNITY FOCUS
#### Early Sexual Maturation, Alcohol, and Cigarettes

Cigarette smoking and the drinking of alcohol among adolescents are complex behaviors that cannot be explained by any single causative factor. However, theorists and investigators have looked at the relationship between biologic maturation and these behaviors. A young girl who is sexually mature at the age of 12 years may be attracted to a group of 14- to 16-year-old girls and boys who smoke and drink. If these teens have not been in any motor vehicle accidents while drinking, the young girl reasons that she, too, will be safe if she smokes, drinks, or is in an automobile with friends who are drinking.

Although parents and nurses cannot influence the time of biologic maturation, they can identify young girls who are at risk for the initiation of smoking and drinking because of early puberty. Parents needs to understand that an early-maturing daughter might be uncomfortable with her body, and they should take advantage of all opportunities to build her self-esteem. Parental sensitivity to the importance of peer-group acceptance is crucial. Parents need to be very supportive of a teenage daughter who feels left out or different. School nurses are in an excellent position to provide anticipatory guidance to girls who enter puberty early and to help them role-play responses they can use to cope with situations that involve offers to smoke and drink. In addition, school nurses can provide information on the bodily changes that accompany puberty and can emphasize the fact that not all teens enter puberty at the same time.

Teachers, coaches, and church leaders can provide opportunities for these girls to "fit in" with their same-age peers through activities that stress mutual goals. For example, an early-maturing girl is typically taller than her age-mates and can be an asset in sports such as basketball and track-and-field events.

## Box 21-7
## Glossary of Drug Jargon

### AMPHETAMINES

| | | |
|---|---|---|
| Bams | Dice | Orange hearts |
| Beans | Doe | Peaches |
| Benn | Drives | Pep pills |
| Bennies | Eyeopeners | Rippers |
| Black beauties | Fives (5 mg) | Roses |
| Black cadillacs | Footballs | Speed |
| Black dex | Goofballs | Splash |
| Bombido | Green hearts | Thrusters |
| (injectable) | Greenies | Truck drivers |
| Browns | Greens | Wake-up |
| Cartwheels | Heart(s) | White crosses |
| Chalk | Horse hearts | White dexies |
| Co-pilots | Jolly babies | Whites |
| Cranks | Leapers | Yellow bams |
| Cross | Lid rollers | Zeeters |
| Crystal | Lightning | Zip |
| Dexies | Meth | |

### BARBITURATES (GENERAL)

| | | |
|---|---|---|
| Barbs | Goofers | Nimbles |
| Courage pills | Idiot pills | Peanuts |
| Downers | Nimbie | Sleepers |
| Golf balls | | |

### BARBITURATES (SPECIFIC)

| | |
|---|---|
| Blue birds (amobarbital) | Pink ladies (secobarbital) |
| Blue devils (amobarbital) | Pinks (secobarbital) |
| Blue heaven (amobarbital) | Rainbow (secobarbital; |
| Canary (pentobarbital) | amobarbital) |
| Christmas trees (mixtures) | Red birds (secobarbital) |
| Downers (amobarbital) | Red devils (secobarbital) |
| F-40s (secobarbital) | Reds (secobarbital) |
| F-66s (amobarbital sodium | Roofies (Rohypnol) |
| and secobarbital sodium) | Seggy, seccy (secobarbital) |
| (gorilla pills) | Tooies (tuinal) |
| Mexican yellows (pentobarbital) | Yellow jackets (pentobarbital) |
| Nemmies (pentobarbital) | Yellows (pentobarbital) |

### COCAINE

| | |
|---|---|
| Bernies flake | Leaf (the) |
| C | Movie star drug |
| Candy | Nose |
| Cecil | Nose candy |
| Charlie | Pimp |
| Coca-cola | Pimp's drug |
| Coke | Rich man's drug |
| Cokomo (Kokomo) | Rock |
| Crack | Schoolboy |
| Dust | Snow |
| Flake | Society high |
| Gift of the Sun God | Stardust |
| Gold dust | Star-spangled powder |
| Happy trails | White horse |
| Incentive | White stuff |
| Lady snow | |

### HEROIN

| | | |
|---|---|---|
| Big Harry | Dust | Smack |
| Blanco | H | Stuff |
| Boy | Harry; hairy | Sugar |
| Caballo | Horse | Ticata |
| Chiva | Joy powder | White lady |
| Deuce (a $2 packet) | Scag | White stuff |
| Doojee | Scat | |

### LSD (LYSERGIC ACID DIETHYLAMIDE)

| | | |
|---|---|---|
| Acid | Cube (the) | Royal blue |
| Blotter acid | D (big) | Sugar |
| (on paper) | Heavenly blue | Wedding bells |
| Blue microdot | Purple haze | Windowpane |

### MARIJUANA

| | |
|---|---|
| **General terms:** Da-kind, Herb, Ganga | Kind buds (highly potent flowers from female plants) |
| Acapulco gold (potent) | Mary Jane |
| Blunt (large marijuana cigarette rolled in outer leaves of a cigar) | Mohasky |
| | Mooters |
| | Mu |
| Buds (highly potent flowers from female plants) | Mutah |
| | Nugs (highly potent flowers from female plants) |
| Bush | |
| Butter | Panama red |
| Flower | Pot |
| Golden Nuggets (highly potent flowers from female plants) | Reefer (cigarette) |
| | Rockets |
| Grass | Smoke |
| Griffo | Spleaf |
| Hemp | Splimi |
| Hooch | Stick (cigarette) |
| Hooter | Straw |
| Indian hay | Superjoint |
| J | Texas tea |
| Jive | Tie stick (mixed with opium and tied to a popsicle stick) |
| Joint | |
| Kif | Weed |

### MISCELLANEOUS

| | |
|---|---|
| Alcohol: mountain dew, alley juice (methyl alcohol), moonshine (ethyl alcohol), sauce, hootch, booze, juice | Methadone: dolls, dollies fizzies (tablets) |
| | Methaqualone (Quaalude): 714, ludes, sopors, westcoast, lemons |
| Amyl nitrite: aimes, snappers | |
| Chloral hydrate: joy juice | Opium for smoking: black stuff |
| Ethchlorvynol (Placidyl): dyls, plastic red, K-H, K-N | Paregoric: licorice, bitter |
| | Peyote: button, cactus, Hikori, Kikuli, Huatari, Wokouri, seni, tops |
| Meperidine hydrochloride: Diane | |
| Mescaline: chief, mesc, mescalito, mescal beans | Tobacco: coffin, deck (pack), fag |

### MIXED SUBSTANCES

| | |
|---|---|
| Chicago green (marijuana/opium) | In-betweens (barbiturates/amphetamines) |
| Double trouble (amobarbital/secobarbital) | Mickey Finn (chloral hydrate/alcohol) |
| Fours (acetaminophen with 60 mg codeine) | Speedball (heroin/cocaine; Percodan/methedrine) |
| Fuel (marijuana/insecticide) | Star-spangled powder (heroin/cocaine) |
| Hog (phencyclidine/vegetable material [veterinary drug]) | |

### MORPHINE

| | | |
|---|---|---|
| Dreamer | Hard stuff | Morf |
| Dust | Hocus | Morpho |
| Emma (Miss) | M | Unkie |
| Emsel | Monkey | White stuff |

### OTHER HALLUCINOGENS

| | |
|---|---|
| DMT (dimethyltryptamine): businessman's special | STP (dimethoxymethyl-amphetamine), DOM (syndicate acid, tranquility) |
| DMZ (benactyzine) | |
| DOM 2,5-dimethoxy-4-methyl-amphetamine, STP | |
| Hashish; black hash; black Russian (potent) | THC (tetrahydrocanna-binol): hallucinogen in marijuana and hashish |

### PCP (PHENCYCLIDINE)

| | | |
|---|---|---|
| Angel dust | Hog (also chloral hydrate) | Rocket fuel |
| Busy bee | | Sherman's |
| DOA | Horse tranquilizer | White horizon |
| Elephant | Magic mist | Wobble |
| Goon | Peace pills | |

observed during withdrawal from other substances. The effects are those more commonly seen in depression, including a lack of energy and motivation, irritability, appetite changes, psychomotor retardation, and irregular sleep patterns. More serious symptoms include cardiovascular manifestations and seizures. Physical withdrawal is not to be confused with the so-called crash after a cocaine high, which consists of a long period of sleep. In 1999, 9.5% of high school seniors reported having tried cocaine (Centers for Disease Control and Prevention, 1999). Answers to questions about the health risks of cocaine can be obtained by calling the **National Cocaine Hotline.*** It also provides referrals to support groups and treatment centers.

*Narcotics* include opiates, such as heroin and morphine, and opioids (opiate-like drugs), such as hydromorphone (Dilaudid), fentanyl, meperidine (Demerol), and codeine. The narcotics produce a state of euphoria by removing painful feelings and creating a pleasurable experience of a specific quality and a sense of success accompanied by clouding of consciousness and a dreamlike state. Physical signs of narcotic abuse include constricted pupils, respiratory depression and often cyanosis. Needle marks may be visible on the arms or legs of chronic users. Physical withdrawal from opiates is extremely unpleasant unless controlled with supervised tapering doses of the opioid or substitution of methadone.

Perhaps more important are the indirect consequences related to the illegal status of narcotic use and the problems associated with securing the drug—time-consuming searches and methods used to meet the high cost. Health problems result from self-neglect of physical needs (nutrition, cleanliness, dental care), overdose, contamination, and infection, including human immunodeficiency virus (HIV) and hepatitis B.

*Central nervous system depressants* include a variety of hypnotic drugs that produce physical dependence and withdrawal symptoms on abrupt discontinuation. They create a feeling of relaxation and sleepiness but impair general functioning. Drugs in this category include barbiturates and nonbarbiturates (e.g., methaqualone [Quaalude]) and alcohol. Barbiturates combined with alcohol produce a profound depressant effect.

Barbiturates and other sedatives have also been associated with attempted and successful suicides (Mendelson and Rich, 1993). Flunitrazepam (Rohypnol), known as the "date rape drug," is a recent hypnotic drug abused by adolescents. Many women report being raped after unknowingly being given Rohypnol in a drink. Rohypnol is 10 times more powerful than diazepam (Valium). It produces prolonged sedation, a feeling of well-being, and short-term memory loss. The drug is being illegally imported into the United States at an alarming rate. Since 1990, over 1000 federal, state and local investigations have been initiated regarding flunitrazepam.†

The *central nervous system stimulants,* amphetamines and cocaine, do not produce strong physical dependence and can be withdrawn without much danger. However, psycho-

logic dependence is strong, and acute intoxication can lead to violent, aggressive behavior or psychotic episodes manifested by paranoia, uncontrollable agitation, and restlessness. When combined with barbiturates, the euphoric effects are particularly addictive.

Methamphetamine can be snorted, injected, swallowed, or smoked and produces a burst of energy along with intense, alternating attacks of boldness and paranoia. It provokes an excitement far more intense than that caused by crack and cocaine. The drug, with the street names "crank," "meth," and "crystal," is inexpensive and has a longer period of action than cocaine. Instead of the short (few minutes) high achieved with crack, a user can remain "up" for hours on a similar dose of crank.

*Inhalants* include glue "sniffing" and the inhalation of plastic cement, spray paint, and other volatile substances (e.g., gasoline, nitrous oxide, and air "dusters" used to remove dust from computers and camera lenses). These dusters contain chemical solvents, usually a form of freon, that can cause fatal cardiac arrhythmias. Inhalant abuse is increasing rapidly and is most common in the early teenage years. A recent survey noted that 14.6% of adolescents in the United States had abused inhalants at least once in their lives (Centers for Disease Control and Prevention, 1999). Inhalants are becoming a gateway drug for young children, who often progress to other harder drugs such as marijuana, heroin, and cocaine. Young children are often completely unaware of the inherent dangers of "sniffing" or "huffing." They breathe the inhalants directly or place them in paper or plastic bags or soda cans from which they rebreathe the fumes, which produces an immediate euphoria and altered consciousness. Although these substances give the child an inexpensive euphoric or "high" feeling, they are also extremely dangerous and can cause rapid loss of consciousness and respiratory arrest. In addition, visual-spatial difficulties, visual scanning problems, language deficiencies, motor instability, memory deficits, and attention and concentration problems may occur.

*Mind-altering drugs* or hallucinogens (psychedelic, psychotomimetic, psychotropic, or illusionogenic) are drugs that produce vivid hallucinations and euphoria. These drugs do not produce physical dependence and therefore can be abruptly withdrawn without ill effect. However, the acute and long-term effects are variable, and in some individuals the dissociative behavior may be unduly protracted. This category includes cannabis (marijuana, hashish) and lysergic acid diethylamide (LSD).

Marijuana is the third most widely used drug by teens, after alcohol and tobacco. In 1996, 36% of high school seniors reported using marijuana in the past year, with 5% reporting use in the past 30 days (Johnston, O'Malley, and Bachman, 1996).

## Therapeutic Management

Adolescents experiencing toxic drug effects or withdrawal symptoms are commonly seen in emergency departments. Experienced emergency department personnel are familiar with the management of acute drug toxicosis; the signs,

---

*800-COCAINE.
†U.S. Drug Enforcement Administration, www.dea.gov

symptoms, and behavioral characteristics of a variety of substances; and the differences and similarities among them. When the drug is questionable or unknown, knowledge of these factors facilitates handling of the youngster and implementation of a treatment regimen.

The treatment for drug toxicity or withdrawal varies according to the drug and the method used. Every effort should be made to determine the type and amount of drug taken, the time it was taken, the mode of administration, and factors related to the onset of presenting symptoms.

It is helpful to know the patient's pattern of use. For example, if two types of drugs are involved, they may require different treatments. Gastric lavage may be employed when the drug has been ingested recently and the cough reflex is intact but would be of little value when the drug has been administered by the intravenous ("mainlined") or intranasal ("sniffed") route. Because the actual content of most street drugs is highly questionable, other pharmaceutical agents are administered with caution, except perhaps the narcotic antagonists in cases of suspected opiate overdose. It is necessary to assess for possible trauma sustained while the patient was under the influence of the drug.

Rehabilitation from hard drug use may require withdrawing the adolescent from both the environment and the chemical agent. Programs must be suited to the individual and may involve foster home placement or a residential treatment setting, although many youngsters are handled in an ambulatory setting. Programs often include group sessions with other troubled adolescents. Information regarding help can be obtained from the **Center for Substance Abuse Treatment** hotline.*

## Nursing Considerations

Nurses in almost every setting are increasingly likely to have contact with adolescent drug abusers or to be in a position to serve as educator and patient advocate. Nurses can serve as listener, confidant, and counselor to troubled teens. They are essential members of health care teams whose efforts are directed toward short-term and long-term therapy for drug abusers.

Observation or a description of the behavior often is more valuable than a report by patients or friends as to the chemical agent taken (Box 21-8). For example, aggressive behavior and disorientation are often seen in barbiturate, alcohol, stimulant, or hallucinogen intoxication but not in opiate intoxication. Overdose from barbiturates, inhalants, or opiates can result in respiratory failure and coma. Pinpoint pupils are seen only in opiate toxicity. Nurses must be alert for life-threatening consequences of drug toxicity; equipment and personnel should be available, or the patient should be transferred to facilities that are prepared to provide supportive measures for physiologic depression and psychogenic phenomena.

Stimulation should be kept to a minimum for agitated, frightened youngsters. Treatments or tests not immediately required are postponed. These teens primarily need psy-

*(800) 662-HELP.

---

> ### Box 21-8
> ### Diagnostic Criteria for Substance Dependence
>
> A maladaptive pattern of substance use, leading to clinically significant impairment or distress, as manifested by three (or more) of the following, occurring at any time in the same 12-month period:
> 1. **Tolerance,** as defined by either of the following:
>    a. A need for markedly increased amounts of the substance to achieve intoxication or desired effect
>    b. Markedly diminished effect with continued use of the same amount of the substance
> 2. **Withdrawal,** as manifested by either of the following:
>    a. The characteristic withdrawal syndrome for the substance
>    b. The same (or a closely related) substance taken to relieve or avoid withdrawal symptoms
> 3. The substance is often taken in larger amounts or over a longer period than was intended.
> 4. There is a persistent desire or unsuccessful efforts to cut down or control substance use.
> 5. A great deal of time is spent in activities necessary to obtain the substance (e.g., visiting multiple doctors or driving long distances), use the substance (e.g., chainsmoking), or recover from its effects.
> 6. Important social, occupational, or recreational activities are given up or reduced because of substance use.
> 7. The substance use is continued despite knowledge of having a persistent or recurrent physical or psychological problem that is likely to have been caused or exacerbated by the substance (e.g., current cocaine use despite recognition of cocaine-induced depression, or continued drinking despite recognition that an ulcer was made worse by alcohol consumption).
>
> *Specify if:*
> **With physiological dependence:** Evidence of tolerance or withdrawal (i.e., either item 1 or 2 is present)
> **Without physiological dependence:** No evidence of tolerance or withdrawal (i.e., neither item 1 nor 2 is present)
> *Course specifiers*
> **Early full remission**
> **Early partial remission**
> **Sustained full remission**
> **Sustained partial remission**
> **On agonist therapy**
> **In a controlled environment**
>
> From American Psychiatric Association: *Diagnostic and statistical manual of mental disorders, (DSM-IV TR),* ed 4, Washington, DC, 2000, The Association.

chologic support in a nonthreatening environment and close contact with a caring, understanding person who can stay with them and help them maintain social contact.

School nurses play an essential role because they may be the only health care professionals with an opportunity to identify many adolescents with substance abuse problems who appear anxious, depressed, or angry. Assessment of potential substance abuse problems is an important part of evaluation. By ensuring confidentiality within appropriate limits and in a straightforward manner, nurses enable many adolescents to discuss problems involving substance abuse openly. (See Critical Thinking Exercise box on p. 894.)

Obstetric and nursery personnel encounter drug dependence and withdrawal in newborn infants or in a compulsive drug-using mother. Affected infants are at risk and require special surveillance for complications of withdrawal; there-

## Critical Thinking Exercise

### Problem Behaviors in Adolescents

Harry is a 14-year-old freshman in high school. In the past month his math teacher has observed that Harry has marked mood swings, is loud and aggressive in class, is abusive toward his classmates, and has difficulty concentrating on math problems.

Harry's physical education teacher states that Harry "dropped off" the baseball team after becoming very clumsy in his outfield position. Before leaving the team, Harry started to "hang out" with a different group of friends. Now he is no longer interested in sports, his old friends, or any other school activities.

The school nurse, who has a trusting relationship with Harry, remembers that his parents have recently separated and that Harry is very angry at his father for leaving the family. She also remembers that Harry has been to the health suite five times in the past month because of a stomachache. At the last visit, Harry was very lethargic, his pupils were dilated, his eyes were "bloodshot," and his clothes smelled "funny." Harry stated that he was up late studying the night before and forgot to do his laundry. In responding to concerns about Harry's behavior, what should the school nurse do?

First, Think About It . . .

- What are you taking for granted, and what assumptions are you making?
- If you accept the conclusions, what are the implications?

1. Do nothing, because Harry is demonstrating normal adolescent rebellion.
2. Talk with Harry (ensuring confidentiality) and determine whether he is using alcohol, inhalants, or other drugs.
3. Refer Harry for evaluation of an emotional disorder.
4. Determine whether Harry is depressed or at risk for suicide.

*Both two and four are correct. Poor coordination, marked mood swings, aggression, hostility, lethargy, and stomach pain (due to gastritis) are all common signs of alcohol abuse. Dilated pupils are seen with the abuse of some barbiturates and also some hallucinogens. Reddened or "bloodshot eyes" occur with alcoholism and with the abuse of hallucinogens and alcohol. The funny smell on Harry's clothes could be from either inhalants or alcohol. Selecting new friends and changing a peer group commonly occur when adolescents become involved with drugs. The strong association between substance abuse and depression and suicide necessitates assessment for both suicide and depression and is not to be taken for granted. Harry has experienced a recent loss and may be struggling to cope with the absence of his father. He could be depressed and using alcohol or drugs to cope. The school nurse should screen Harry for any thoughts of suicide and should make an immediate referral if necessary. Although rebellion is a feature of adolescence and has been identified in children who do not abuse drugs, the implications of Harry's behavior suggest that he has undergone a dramatic change in the last month. Therefore the current changes in his behavior should be investigated and not just assumed to be a normal part of adolescence or dismissed by a referral before interviewing the teen.*

fore nurses should be aware of the possibility of drug dependence in mothers who come to the hospital for delivery. (See Chapter 10.)

### Long-Term Management

A major factor in the treatment and rehabilitation of young drug users is careful assessment in the nonacute stage to determine the function that the drug plays in these teens' lives. Several standardized instruments can be used to identify and screen for substance abuse. These instruments include the HEADSS interview questions, which assess the topics of home, education, activities, drugs, sex, and suicide; and the CAGE questionnaire, which assesses alcohol use and abuse (Neinstein and Pinsky, 1996). Before they can embark on a rehabilitation program, adolescents need help in identifying the issues that motivated them to use drugs and in recognizing their own role in self-destructive, inappropriate drug-abuse behavior.

The motivation phase of treatment is directed toward exploring the factors that influence drug use. It also involves establishing in the teen a feeling of self-worth and a commitment to self-help. It requires a trusting relationship between the adolescent and the health care team and involves a thorough physical examination and assessment of psychologic, educational, and vocational status. A realistic appraisal of the adolescent's potential and efforts aimed at short-term goals, along with building self-esteem, lays the groundwork for a successful rehabilitation program.

Rehabilitation begins when teens decide that they can and are willing to change. Rehabilitation involves fostering healthy interdependent relationships with caring and supportive adults and exploring alternate mechanisms for problem solving while simultaneously reducing or eliminating drug use. Persons working with troubled young people must be prepared for recidivism, or the tendency to relapse, and maintain a plan for reentry into the treatment process.

The majority of treatment programs for adolescent substance abusers are based on adult 12-step models such as Alcoholics Anonymous. Research is needed to determine whether applying adult models to adolescents is warranted. **Toughlove\*** is one such program. The Toughlove philosophy, first employed by Alcoholics Anonymous and Al-Anon, is based on the conviction that parents have the right and the responsibility to be the policymakers in the family, set limits on the behavior of their children, and take control of the household from out-of-control teenagers. The premise is that allowing teenagers to experience the negative consequences of their behavior will bring them closer to accepting help and changing their behavior. Adolescents are offered the choice of (1) getting treatment for their mental health or drug problem or (2) finding another place to live.

Pieper and Pieper (1992) criticize the Toughlove approach, contending that the uncompromising position adopted by parents is harmful to both the parents and the child. In contrast, treatment emphasizing self-caretaking is

---

*PO Box 1069, Doylestown, PA 18901, (215) 348-7090, www.toughlove.com.

described as more useful as a long-term approach. The fact remains that effective approaches to the treatment of adolescent substance abuse are not clearly understood. Treatments sensitive to the developmental transitions of adolescence and the variety of biopsychosocial factors affecting substance use need to be developed and evaluated. One group that provides support and counseling for families experiencing crises with their children is **Parents Anonymous.**\*

### Prevention

Given the difficulty of treating substance abusers, prevention is the most effective policy. In recent years, a variety of programs have been applied with promising results. Successful programs reducing substance abuse risk have promoted parenting skills, social skills among distractible children, academic achievement, and skills to resist peer influence (Patton, 1995).

Peer pressure has been used effectively in prevention efforts. For example, **Students Against Driving Drunk (SADD)**† is an organization of young people who work to eliminate teenage drunk driving. Techniques used by this group include peer counseling, the development of parental guidelines for teenage parties, and community awareness efforts. Nurses should encourage the formation of a SADD chapter in high schools in their communities.

Nurses can also play an important role in other preventive efforts. Young people need to be educated regarding the appropriate use of chemicals. Health care professionals associated with adolescents should listen to what they are saying, determine what is bothering them, and try to help them meet their needs before they resort to drugs.

Prevention programs carry the implicit assumption that poor outcomes facing children at risk can be forestalled or at least reduced. In the past, prevention research has focused on the identification of risk factors and their relationship to drug use. Less research has investigated the protective forces that contribute to resisting drug use. It is important for nurses to consider the multiple factors of risk and protection and their interactions in influencing drug use and abuse. Preventive and clinical interventions should attempt to increase the protective factors and reduce the risk factors.

Children need to feel they are loved. Parents need to provide love while setting appropriate limits. Substance abuse is only one of the many outcomes facing young people for whom the basic needs are consistently neglected. Nurses in a variety of settings are in a position to identify emerging risk factors, to refer problems for assessment and management, and to foster those parenting skills and interpersonal skills that may be protective against substance abuse.

---

\*675 W Foothill Blvd, Suite 220, Claremont, CA 91711, (909) 621-6184. Another source of information: **National Clearinghouse for Alcohol and Drug Abuse Information,** PO Box 2345, Rockville, MD 20852, (800) 729-6686, e-mail: info@health.org; www.health.org.

†PO Box 800, Malboro, MA 01752, (508) 481-3568, (800) 886-2972; www.saddonline.com.

## SUICIDE\*

*Suicide* is defined as the deliberate act of self-injury with the intent that the injury result in death. Most experts distinguish between suicidal ideation, suicide attempt (or *parasuicide*), and suicide. *Suicidal ideation* involves a preoccupation with thoughts about committing suicide and may be a precursor to suicide. Although it is not uncommon for adolescents to experience occasional suicidal thoughts, expressions of suicidal preoccupation should be taken seriously and an assessment should be conducted for appropriate referral. A *suicide attempt* is intended to cause injury or death but is unsuccessful.

Some researchers and clinicians prefer to use the term *parasuicide* to refer to behaviors ranging from gestures to serious attempts to kill oneself. It is a deliberate act that might inflict self-harm but results in a nonfatal outcome. Parasuicide is a preferred term because it makes no reference to intent and because a person's motive may be too difficult or complex to ascertain. All parasuicidal activity should be taken seriously.

**NURSING ALERT** A history of a previous suicide attempt is a serious indicator for possible suicide completion in the future. Studies of adolescent suicides have found that as many as half had made previous attempts.

A recent survey of U.S. high school students indicated that 10.9% of females and 5.7% of males had attempted suicide in the previous 12 months. However, 18.3% of females and 10.9% of males had serious suicide ideation during the 12 months preceding the survey and had made a specific plan to attempt suicide (Centers for Disease Control and Prevention, 2000). In the United States the suicide rate for adolescents has increased dramatically in the last few decades. Suicide is currently the third leading cause of death for adolescents 15 to 19 years of age (Centers for Disease Control and Prevention/National Center for Health Statistics, 1999). This increase in the suicide rate may reflect the difficulties that some adolescents face as they encounter the cognitive, physical, psychosocial, and spiritual changes that accompany puberty.

The major tasks of adolescence are (1) developing a coherent sense of personal identity, (2) establishing a clear gender identity, (3) establishing autonomy from parents, (4) beginning to master the ability to be in intimate relationships, (5) acquiring coping skills, (6) consolidating values, and (7) developing educational or vocational goals. It is quite likely that the rise in suicide and depression during adolescence is due to cognitive development and the newly developed capacity for self-observation and future orientation. Some young people experience a pervasive sense of despair when they look into the future and are faced with a discrepancy between what they have been led to anticipate and what they are truly able to obtain. Self-hate and hopelessness may

---

■ \*Marilyn Winkelstein, RN, PhD, wrote this section.

result. In part, the despair is a consequence of adolescents' newly developed cognitive ability to consider the abstract and hypothetical, which may paint a bleak picture of their lives in the future. As adolescents struggle to establish their sense of self, they constantly seek external validation and confirmation of who they are. Introspection becomes a prominent part of this process. Social experiences and peer relationships become more important during the adolescent years, and the increased need to belong and conform leads to an increased vulnerability to depression and suicidal thought. In the context of this intrapersonal and interpersonal searching, self-esteem becomes pivotal, moderating hopelessness and developing a strong sense of self.

Young people also focus on mastering empathy during the teen years. The ability to truly empathize with others creates a new awareness of the suffering of others. The capacity to passionately feel both joy and sorrow is exciting, yet frightening. For some, the pain seems overwhelming. Because they most likely have not lived through intensely painful experiences, they have not developed the means to cope with deep emotions. They may feel alone in experiencing pain and sorrow and unable to recognize or express their need for support. For adolescents who have not had guidance and experience in problem solving and coping with sorrow, suicide may represent a means of escape and seem the only option.

Today the electronic media expose young people to countless deaths. Young people have been desensitized to death by constantly viewing it on television, in the movies, and in video games. Suicide may be romanticized and inaccurately portrayed. The frequency of **contagion,** or **copycat, suicides** among young people (i.e., an increase in youth sui-

cides after the suicide of one teenager is publicized) is disturbing and may indicate an adolescent perception of suicide as "glamorous." Simultaneously, changes in families have insulated teens from death experiences. Improvements in health care and geographic mobility in the United States isolate family members from one another, and young people are not as likely to participate in the painful emotional realities of sickness and death among older family members.

Over several decades the increasing youth suicide rate has paralleled increasing rates of child poverty, violence, parental divorce, and decreasing parental involvement and support. As adolescents strive for healthy autonomy from their parents and master the skills required for interdependence with others, they begin to question and criticize their parents. They attempt to discover their own identity and discern which qualities of their parents they want to incorporate into their lives. This questioning and criticizing process can generate a sense of guilt, insecurity, fear, and conflict. Even though they may rebel against their parents, young people need to feel needed, wanted, and loved by their families. Studies indicate that young people who believe that their families care about them are less likely to show suicidal behaviors (Resnick and others, 1997).

The changing roles of young people in society have also had an impact on adolescent suicidality. The period of adolescence is prolonged in the United States, and roles for young people are unclear and difficult to formulate. The earlier onset of puberty and the growing need for higher educational attainment has increased the period of adolescence from 6 years to potentially 14 years. The extended time "in limbo" between childhood and adulthood has created greater role confusion. Today the majority of parents are employed at jobs away from home; consequently, young people do not have the opportunity to see their parents as vocational role models. The higher percentage of adolescents within the total population and the increased difficulties adolescents have in obtaining jobs and being admitted to college also contribute to a higher youth suicide rate.

Although most people emerge from adolescence with a healthy sense of who they are and where they are headed, the widespread belief that adolescence is a time of turmoil—of storm and stress—has created a sense that hopelessness and despair are a normal part of the second decade of life. *This is not so.* Most young people do not experience adolescence as a time of despair. However, depressive symptoms, acting-out behaviors, and talk of suicide need to be taken seriously. They are *not* a common "phase" of adolescence; they are a call for help that requires the response of nurses and other professionals.

## Incidence

The suicide rate in the United States for children ages 10 to 24 years has more than doubled in recent years. For individuals between 15 and 24 years of age, the rate was 11.1 per 100,000 population in 1998 (Murphy, 2000).

The incidence of youth suicide varies greatly by gender and racial/ethnic background (Fig. 21-2). In 1998, for every 100,000 persons ages 15 to 24, suicide rates were 18.5 for all

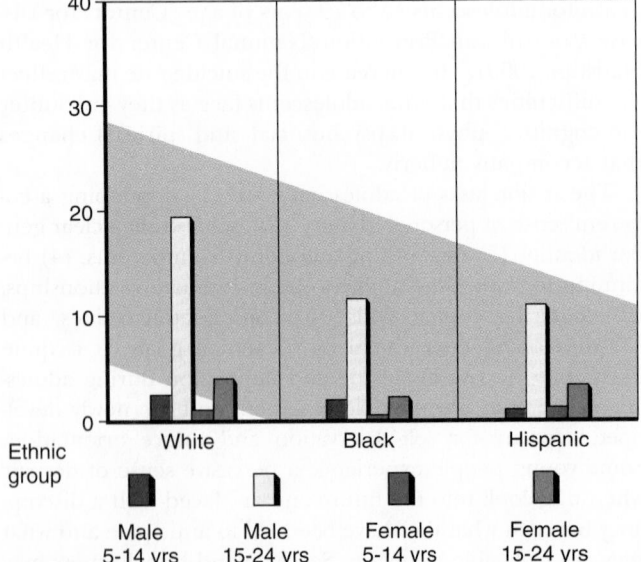

**Fig. 21-2** U.S. suicide rates (per 100,000 population) in 1998 by age, race, ethnicity, and gender. (Redrawn from Murphy SL: Deaths: final data for 1998, *Nat Vital Stat Rep* 48(11):1-105, 2000.)

males and 3.3 for all females. The rates per 100,000 were lower for black adolescents as compared with white adolescents: 15 for black males and 2.2 for black females, and 19.3 for white males and 3.5 for white females (Murphy, 2000).

Although Native Americans have a high rate of suicide compared to other racial/ethnic groups in the United States, there is great variation among tribes. Tribes with less social integration, less adherence to tribal traditions, and a high degree of individuality generally have higher suicide rates than tribes that are tightly integrated and adhere to traditional values and practices. Family, school, and tribal connectedness has been shown to be a protective factor associated with lower rates of hopelessness and suicidality among high-risk Native American adolescents (Dexheimer-Pharris, Resnick, and Blum, 1997). The suicide rate (per 100,000) for Hispanic youth ages 15 to 24 is 13.4 for males and 2.8 for females. (See Cultural Awareness box.)

Incarcerated youths in public correctional facilities have a higher suicide rate than adolescents in the general population. Minors detained in adult jails are at especially high risk for suicide.

Even though the statistics reveal hopelessness and despair among young people, the true incidence of completed suicides in children and adolescents is not known because of general underreporting. Deaths by suicide often are reported as accidental because of pressures exerted by the family and society to avoid the cultural and religious stigma associated with self-destruction. The high accident rate in this age-group may reflect suicides masked by accidental death or homicide.

In the United States, the mortality patterns for suicide and homicide among youths follow similar trends. Both the numbers and the yearly trends over the past six decades are remarkably similar (Holinger and others, 1994). It is quite possible that these forms of violent death in youths share common antecedents.

The true incidence of suicide attempts is difficult to measure. There is no national reporting system for suicide attempts. Although more males than females complete suicide, suicide attempts are far more common in females than in males (American Academy of Pediatrics, 2000). The major difference between suicide attempts and suicide completions is whether or not a lethal weapon is available. There is also a higher likelihood of successful suicide when alcohol and firearms are involved. Thus a higher incidence of youth suicide occurs in societies in which alcohol and lethal weapons are readily available to youths. Firearms were more likely to be present in the homes of suicide completers than in those of youths who had attempted suicide or who had suicidal ideation (American Academy of Pediatrics, 2000).

## Factors Associated with Suicide Risk

An effective research methodology that studies the risk factors associated with suicide is psychologic autopsy, which involves data collection from the deceased person's family, friends, teachers, counselors, spiritual advisors, and educational and health care records. Psychologic autopsies reveal

several factors associated with adolescent suicide: depression or other affective disorders, drug and alcohol abuse, family conflict, prior suicide attempt, antisocial or aggressive behavior, a family history of suicidal behavior, and the availability of a firearm (Box 21-9).

### Individual Factors

The single most important individual factor associated with an increased risk of suicide is the presence of an active psychiatric disorder (namely, affective disorders such as depression and bipolar disorder, substance abuse, and conduct disorder).

The relationship between psychiatric illness and suicide has been documented in several studies. Shaffer and others (1996) found that more than 90% of the children and adolescents who committed suicide were retrospectively found

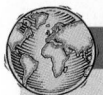

## CULTURAL AWARENESS
### *International Trends in Youth Suicide*

International trends in youth suicide are difficult to accurately assess, because fewer than one third of the almost 180 member states of the United Nations are listed as reporting suicide mortality statistics to the World Health Organization (1995). There is also wide variation by country in the sensitivity and specificity of the vital records and reporting systems. Existing data suggest an increase during most of this century among the white urban adolescent and young adult populations of North America and Europe. In these countries the suicide rate has increased along with the rate of depressive disorders, substance abuse, access to firearms, social stressors, models of suicide, and psychobiologic changes caused in part by the dramatic lowering of the age of puberty (Diekstra and Garnefski, 1995).

Youth suicide rates increase in some countries as the proportion of youth in the country increases. Holinger and colleagues (1994) report the results of a 30-year longitudinal study that compared the effect of *relative cohort size (RCS)*, or the proportion of youth in the general population, to youth suicide rates in 12 different countries—5 capitalist countries, 3 welfare capitalist countries, and 4 communist nations. In the capitalist countries the RCS was positively correlated with youth suicide; in the communist countries it was equally likely to be related or unrelated; in the welfare capitalist countries RCS was not significantly related to youth suicide. The researchers concluded that RCS declines in importance in explaining youth suicide when economic welfare is determined more by central planning and policies such as full employment and redistributive measures, which act as a potential cushion against the potentially harsh effects of RCS. This study suggests that the amount of social support available to young people can counter the effects of other social factors that set the stage for an increased youth suicide rate.

Looking only at children age 14 and under in 26 industrialized countries, the Centers for Disease Control and Prevention (1997) concluded that the suicide rate for children in the United States was two times higher than in the 25 other countries combined (0.55 per 100,000 compared with 0.27 per 100,000). Suicide rates for 15- to 24-year-old youths vary greatly—from a high of 50.9 per 100,000 for males in Finland to a low of 1.2 for females in Mexico (Holinger and others, 1994). Finland has the highest male youth suicide rate but a relatively low male youth homicide rate. Conversely, Mexico has the lowest youth suicide rate for 15- to 24-year-old males but the highest youth homicide rate for males. These potential cultural differences in internal vs. external directions of aggression warrant further research.

---

**Box 21-9** ■ ■ □
## Factors Associated with Suicide Risk

### PAST HISTORY

Previous suicide attempt
Family member, friend has made a suicide attempt
History of child abuse or neglect
Past psychiatric hospitalization
Death of a parent when child was young

### INDIVIDUAL FACTORS

Hopelessness
Marked, persistent depression
Alcohol or drug abuse
Impulsive
Difficulty tolerating frustration
Feelings of self-hatred or excessive guilt, feelings of humiliation
Thinking disorder (wishes to join a deceased person, hears voices telling to kill self)
Physical/body image problems (delayed puberty, chronic illness, disability, attention-deficit hyperactivity disorder, learning disorders)
Gender identity concerns; gay or lesbian in an unsupportive environment
Sees self as totally helpless—a victim of fate
A need to do things perfectly

### FAMILY FACTORS

Difficult home situation—long, bitter parent-child conflict
Hostile parents
Overt rejection by one or both parents
Divorce or separation of parents
Recent or impending move
Family breakup or parental loss
Exposure to unrealistically high parental expectations
Parental indifference with very low expectations

### SOCIAL/ENVIRONMENTAL FACTORS

Firearms in the home
Incarceration
Lack of effective social support system
Isolation
Exposure to suicide of another
Few social, vocational, educational opportunities

---

## FAMILY FOCUS
### Suicide, Sexual Identity, and Sexual Orientation

Approximately four times as many gay, lesbian, and bisexual teens attempt suicide as other teens (Ryan and Futterman, 1998). Gay or lesbian adolescents who live in families or communities that do not accept homosexuality are likely to suffer low self-esteem, self-loathing, depression, and hopelessness as a result of lack of acceptance from their family or community. Such internalization, without treatment and support, can lead to substance abuse and eventually suicide. Youths most at risk are those who struggle with gender atypicality, gay identity formation at a young age, intrapersonal conflict regarding sexuality, and nondisclosure of orientation to others (Remafedi and others, 1998).

Supportive parents, friends, or relationships serve as protective factors against suicide. However, many gay, lesbian, and transgender adolescents do not feel supported, understood, or accepted by their friends, parents, and families. Nurses who interact with adolescents must be aware of the association between suicide and adolescent homosexuality and gender nonconformity. School nurses may be the first individuals to discuss issues of sexual identity and orientation with adolescents and their families. In their professional capacity, nurses can also serve as support persons for adolescents who are homosexual or transgender and provide the supportive relationship so important to these teens. Nurses can also provide guidance and resources to families so that they know and understand how best to nurture and support their child.

Nurses must also capitalize on those opportunities or experiences that promote the healthy development of self-esteem in gay, lesbian, bisexual, and transgender youths. Educational programs to raise the level of consciousness about the risk factors for and warning signs of suicide are one example. Another possibility could be programs conducted in or outside of school that are designed to foster peer relationships and competency in social skills among high-risk adolescents and young adults, such as support groups and social organizations for gay, lesbian, bisexual, and transgender youths.

---

to meet the criteria for at least one major psychiatric diagnosis. Depression is the predominant affective disorder that represents a major risk for suicide. Psychiatric illness is also associated with an increased potential for suicidal ideation or suicide attempts. In a random sample of 1285 children and adolescents, Gould and others (1998) noted that the rate of suicide attempts was 22% among children with one psychiatric illness (major depression). For children with two or more psychiatric disorders, the rate of suicide attempts was 18 times higher and the rate of suicidal ideation was 8 times higher than in healthy children. Comorbidity of an affective disorder and substance abuse also increases the risk for suicide (Jellineck and Synder, 1998). Alcohol use in particular has been associated with more than 50% of suicides (American Academy of Pediatrics, 2000) and 25% of suicide attempts (Gould and others, 1998). For some teens, suicide becomes the final pathway for release from their psychiatric and social problems (Jellineck and Synder, 1998). Childhood and adolescent suicide victims are reported to have higher rates not only of depression but also conduct

disorders; bipolar disorders; substance abuse; interpersonal problems with parents; and a family history of depression, substance abuse, and suicidal behavior.

Gay and lesbian adolescents are at particularly high risk for suicide completion, especially if raised in an environment where they are denied support systems. When gay or lesbian young persons grow up in a community and family that does not accept homosexuality, they are likely to internalize the homophobia and feel self-hate, which often turns into suicidal feelings. In this alienating social context, self-esteem is challenged. Youths most at risk are those who struggle with gender issues, such as gay identity formation at a young age, intrapersonal conflict regarding sexuality, and nondisclosure of orientation to others. In assessing for level of risk, the youths' knowledge, feelings, and experience in the area of sexual orientation and identity are important. The amount of accurate knowledge and the level of support youths feel directly affect their risk for depression, substance abuse, and suicidality.

By providing care that enhances support systems and nurtures opportunities for the healthy development of self-esteem in gay, lesbian, and bisexual adolescents and their families, nurses can play a significant role in reducing youth suicide rates in the United States. (See Family Focus box.)

Additional individual risk factors for suicidal behavior include poor academic progress, a history of being a victim of sexual abuse, learning disabilities, attention-deficit disorder, chronic illness, disability, and antisocial behavior (especially assaultive behavior, which when experienced with suicidal feelings provides a strong risk indicator for suicide potential).

In the context of these major risk factors, adolescents' maturity, particularly their cognitive development, may determine the likelihood of suicidal behavior. Adolescents who have developed and mastered problem-solving and social skills, have an internal locus of control, and a positive sense of their future will be less likely to turn to suicide, even when faced with extreme stressors. In contrast, youths who see themselves as totally helpless, as victims of fate, or who are impulsive, unable to tolerate frustration, filled with self-hatred, experiencing excessive guilt, suffering from humiliation, withdrawn and aloof, or aggressive and impulsive will be more likely to take their own life.

### Family Factors

Families hold the greatest potential for protecting young people from suicidal behavior. Families who respect individuality, are cohesive and caring, balance discipline with a supportive and understanding relationship, have good systems of communication, and have at least one attentive and caring parent available to the child protect adolescents from suicidal outcomes. In contrast, family risk factors for suicide include parental loss; family disruption; a family history of suicidality, substance abuse, or emotional disturbance; child abuse or neglect; unavailable parents; poor communication; isolation within an inflexible family system; family conflict; unrealistically high parental expectations; and parental indifference with low expectations.

Nursing interventions should be designed to enhance family cohesiveness (Box 21-10). However, in working with families who have experienced the loss of a child through suicide, nurses should remember that although there is a higher risk of suicide in families who are under stress and less cohesive, youth suicide can and does happen in the context of a very caring and cohesive family environment.

### Social/Environmental Factors

Important social/environmental influences that protect adolescents from suicidal behavior include good peer relationships, regular participation in regligious services, strong social support within the community or school system, and available options for vocational and educational development. In contrast, factors associated with increased suicide risk include incarceration, isolation, acute loss of a boyfriend or girlfriend, lack of future options, increased size of the adolescent population, and the availability of firearms in the home.

## Methods

### Completed Suicide

Firearms are by far the most commonly used instruments in completed suicides among male and female adolescents (American Academy of Pediatrics, 2000). For adolescent males the second and third most common means of suicide are hanging and overdose, respectively; for adolescent females the second and third most common means are overdose and strangulation (Centers for Disease Control and Prevention, 1995).

### Suicide Attempt

The most common method of suicide attempt is overdose or ingestion of a potentially toxic substance, such as drugs. The second most common method of suicide attempt is self-inflicted laceration.

## Precipitating Factors

Although suicide is often an impulsive act, it takes place against a backdrop of individual, family, and social risk factors and is often carried out in response to an exacerbation of long-standing stressors or in reaction to an acute precipitating factor. The most common factors precipitating adolescent suicide are a fight with a close friend, the breakup of an important relationship, failure in an important area (e.g., school activities), changing schools or moving, involvement in the legal system, discovery of pregnancy plus family crisis or rejection by boyfriend, and the death of a close friend, relative, or pet.

Fig. 21-3 presents a model for understanding the dynamics of the pathway from risk factors to completed suicide. This model incorporates multiple factors related to individual differences, as well as family and social contexts (Box 21-11).

## Nursing Considerations

### Prevention

Nurses play a pivotal role in reducing youth suicide. Nurses have the opportunity to provide anticipatory guidance to parents and adolescents. They can teach parents to be supportive and to develop positive communication patterns that help teens feel connected with and loved by their fam-

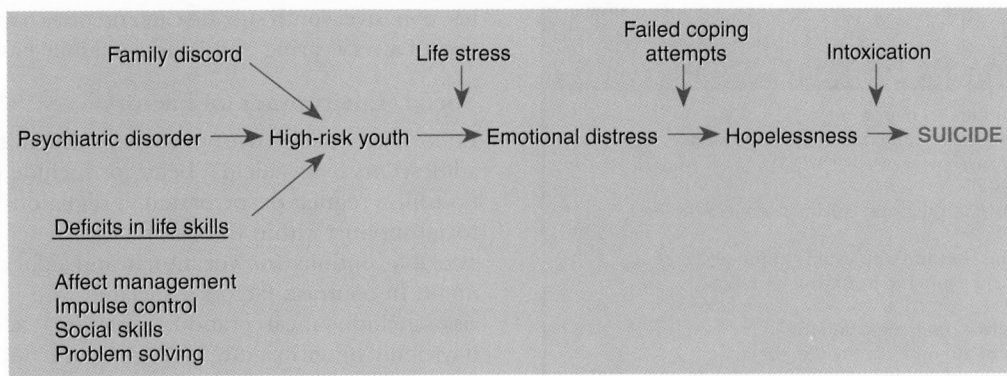

**Fig. 21-3** Pathway from risk factors to completed suicide. (From Hoberman H: Completed suicide in children and adolescents: a review, *Resid Treat Child Youth* 7:61-88, 1989.)

---

**Box 21-11 ▪ ▪ ▪**
**Precipitating Factors for Suicide**

Increased depression and hopelessness
Fight with close friend
Failure to achieve specific goals in school, job, personal life
Breakup of important relationship
Friend moved away
Relocated to new community or school
Discovery of pregnancy combined with family stress or rejection by boyfriend
Death of close friend, relative, or pet
Argument within family
Shameful or humiliating experience
Trouble with police

---

ilies. To foster healthy development, parents can be encouraged to provide teens with creative outlets and to assist young people in accepting strong emotions—pain, anger, frustration—as a normal part of the human experience.

**NURSING ALERT** Given what is known about youth suicide, nurses should ask parents, especially those of at-risk teenagers, if firearms are available in the house and, if so, recommend their removal. Parents must ensure that their children—especially children who are depressed, have poor problem-solving skills, or use drugs or alcohol—do not have access to firearms. Parents must be educated on the warning signs of suicide (Box 21-12).

Nurses working in the community are in a strategic position to conduct educational programs in schools, places of worship, and community centers to help young people develop healthy, effective coping mechanisms and problem-solving skills. Nurses can teach parents, teachers, and youth workers about youth depression and stress. Informed parents are more likely to seek help in the form of psychologic evaluation and treatment for young people who report persistent, deep feelings of sadness, hopelessness, and suicidal feelings. Those who work with teens should keep in mind that depression in adolescents is manifested differently from that in adults. In teens it may be masked by impulsive,

aggressive behaviors. Defiance, disobedience, and behavior problems can be indicative of underlying depression, suicidal ideation, and impending suicide attempts.

Prevention of youth suicide also involves advocating for social programs that reduce social isolation among young people, enhance opportunities for social support, and promote interaction with peers, youth leaders, and community workers. Young people need to be meaningfully involved in society. As adolescents become involved in their schools and communities and experience a sense of competence and confidence in these roles, they become capable of coping with feelings of sadness and despair and stressful life events.

The clustering of suicides ("copycat" suicides) requires a specific response from television and newspaper reporters. Suicide needs to be portrayed as a poor means of coping with life's stressors and, at times, a response to underlying psychiatric disorders. (See Community Focus box.) In addition, to reduce "copycat" suicides, schools and communities must provide programs when a suicide has occurred. Information can be obtained from the **American Association of Suicidology.***

Health care professionals must be alert to the warning signs of adolescent suicide. No threat of suicide should be ignored. Too often, suicidal threats or minor attempts are confused with bids for attention. It is a mistake to be lulled into a false sense of security when an adolescent's depression is apparently relieved. The improvement in attitude may mean that the adolescent has made the decision and found the method to carry out the threat.

In educating youth, nurses should include the following in their teaching plan: the importance of seeking help when feeling sad or depressed, sources of available help for depression, warning signs of suicide (see Box 21-12), the importance of informing a responsible adult if a friend is talking about suicide, and how to access local suicide prevention services. Peers or other confidants are valuable observers and excellent sources of information. They are able to sense when a friend has undergone a marked personality change. It is important to emphasize that the peer

---

*Suite 408, 4201 Connecticut Ave NW, Washington, DC 20008, (202) 237-2280, www.suicidology.org.

## COMMUNITY FOCUS
### *Working With the Media to Prevent Youth Suicide Clustering*

A small percentage of adolescent suicides occur in clusters after the suicide of another adolescent has been highly publicized. Excessive media coverage after the suicide of an adolescent is believed to contribute to *copycat* or *contagion* suicides, particularly if the suicide is romanticized and the good points of the person's life are overemphasized while their struggles are not mentioned.

In the face of this tendency to sensationalize youth suicide, nurses, public health professionals, teachers, and community officials can work with the media to ensure responsible reporting. Responsible reporting of suicides should include the following elements (Centers for Disease Control and Prevention, 1994b):

- Minimizing sensationalism by limiting the morbid details of the suicide
- Refraining from describing the technical details regarding the method of suicide and from displaying dramatic photos related to the suicide
- Minimizing the reporting of public expressions of grief (e.g., memorial services, public eulogies, creation of memorials at the site)
- Not overemphasizing the positive aspects of the person's life while deleting mention of his or her problems
- Emphasizing that the precipitating event was not the only cause of the suicide
- Including information on identifying persons at risk for suicide and resources for adolescents who are feeling depressed or suicidal

### Box 21-12 ■ ■ ■
### Warning Signs of Suicide

- Preoccupation with themes of death—focuses on morbid thoughts
- Wants to give away cherished possessions
- Talks of own death, desire to die
- Loss of energy—loss of interest, listlessness
- Exhaustion without obvious cause
- Changes in sleep patterns—too much or too little
- Increased irritability, argumentativeness, or stubbornness
- Physical complaints—recurrent stomachaches, headaches
- Repeated visits to doctor, nurse practitioner, or emergency department for treatment of injuries
- Reckless behavior
- Antisocial behavior—engages in drinking, uses drugs, fights, commits acts of vandalism, runs away from home, becomes sexually promiscuous
- Sudden change in school performance—lowered grades, cutting classes, dropping out of activities
- Resists or refuses to go to school
- Remains distant, sad, remote—flat affect, frozen facial expression
- Describes self as worthless
- Sudden cheerfulness following deep depression
- Social withdrawal from friends, activities, interests that were previously enjoyed
- Impaired concentration
- Dramatic change in appetite

who detects any change in a friend is a "potential rescuer" and should not remain quiet about the observations. All youths should be taught that, when a peer talks of suicide, they must alert someone who is in a position to help—a parent, teacher, guidance counselor, or other person. Suicide prevention education should be incorporated into a comprehensive adolescent health curriculum.

### Screening for Suicidality

Routine assessment of adolescents should include questions that assess the presence of suicidal thought or intent. The following questions can be asked (Greydanus and Pratt, 1995):

1. Do you consider yourself more a happy person, an unhappy person, or somewhere in the middle?
2. Have you ever been so unhappy or upset that you felt like being dead?
3. Have you ever thought about hurting yourself?
4. Have you ever developed a plan to hurt yourself or kill yourself?
5. Have you ever attempted to kill yourself?

If adolescents answer "yes" to questions 2, 3, or 4, they should be asked if they feel that way now to assess for current suicidality. If teens say they have attempted suicide in the past, assess the number of times and ask them to describe what they were feeling, which method they used, what happened, if they would make a similar attempt, and how they would handle their despair now. Any previous suicide attempt indicates an increased risk for a future attempt. The risk of a suicide attempt in the near future increases as the

frequency of suicidal ideation increases (Lewinsohn, Rohde, and Seely, 1996).

Adolescents who do not currently have a plan for suicide but who struggle with frequent thoughts of suicide should be asked what they would do if they felt suicidal. They should have a plan to access immediate help. Many nurses contract with such youths, asking them to sign an agreement that they will not attempt suicide during an agreed-upon period of time and that they will call the 24-hour crisis line immediately if they feel they cannot keep the contract. The amount of time for which a youth feels comfortable contracting may be an indication of his or her level of risk and stability.

For youths who have suicidal thoughts, are depressed, and abuse substances, the nurse should discuss safety issues with the parent or guardian. Clear instructions should be given to remove any firearms from the home (not just locking them up, because adolescents are adept at unlocking gun cabinets) and to remove all prescription medications and over-the-counter medications such as acetaminophen and aspirin. Parents should be encouraged to contract with their children, asking them to inform the parents if they are feeling suicidal. Youths will usually honor such contracts and welcome the support and monitoring by parents.

Youths who are actively suicidal need inpatient care, monitoring, and treatment. Medications for depression and bipolar disorder often take several weeks to reach therapeutic doses. The time until medications and therapy begin to take effect can be trying for the adolescent and the family. Youths who are suffering from psychiatric disorders (major depression, bipolar disorder, and psychoses) and substance abuse need a comprehensive treatment referral that incorporates mental health and chemical dependency treatment.

### Care of the Suicidal Adolescent

In caring for young persons who express suicidal feelings, the nurse's first responsibility is to ensure their safety. Any suicidal remarks must be taken seriously, and the young persons should not be left alone until the degree of suicidality is assessed. An acronym for the assessment process is **SLAP** (*specificity, lethality, accessibility,* and *proximity*). The first step (*specificity*) is to ask adolescents if they feel suicidal or feel as though they would like to take their own life. If so, what is their plan? Have they chosen a means of suicide, and do they have a specific plan? The second stage of assessment (*lethality*) involves determining the lethality of the methods available to them. Do they plan to use a gun or knife? Have they chosen highly lethal medications, hanging, or carbon monoxide poisoning? The third stage (*accessibility*) involves determining the availability of the means of suicide, and the fourth stage (*proximity*) involves assessing whether they have determined a time to commit suicide and when.

> **NURSING ALERT** Adolescents who express suicidal feelings and have a specific plan should be monitored at all times. They should not have access to belts, scarves, weapons, shoestrings, sharp objects, matches, or lighters. If they are intoxicated, they must be restrained or placed in a protective environment until they can be assessed by a psychiatrist or psychologist.

Confidentiality cannot be honored in the case of self-destructive behaviors. Suicidal behaviors must be reported to the family and other professionals, and the adolescent should be informed that this will be done. Such action conveys an important message to an attempter—that the nurse understands and cares.

Understanding and caring demonstrated by the nurse to the adolescent is extremely therapeutic. Adolescents have a deep need to be *normal* and will only feel more depressed and suicidal if they are stigmatized. Expressing a commitment to keep them safe until they no longer feel so terribly sad and assuring them that they will indeed feel better with time are helpful nursing actions. A person who feels extremely suicidal will welcome the security of being restrained if it is presented as an act of care, not punishment. Feeling actively suicidal is a very frightening experience, and the adolescent should not be left alone. By demonstrating care, open communication, and understanding, the nurse is modeling appropriate behavior for the young person's family. Time spent listening to family members and helping them understand will reduce the incidence of future suicidal actions.

The attempted and, especially, the completed suicide of an adolescent is a major family crisis. In an attempted suicide there is an opportunity for the family and teenager to obtain help. Because these families are often already in conflict and at risk, nurses play an important role in referring them to appropriate mental health services. They should stress to parents the seriousness of the attempt and that this crisis offers the opportunity to avoid the tragedy of completed suicide. (See Care of the Family Experiencing Unexpected Childhood Death, Chapter 23.)

## KEY POINTS

- Obesity in adolescence is a significant risk factor for adult obesity.
- Diet, exercise, and behavior modification are the hallmarks of treatment for obesity.
- The nurse's involvement in obesity control includes nutritional counseling, behavior therapy, group programs, and family counseling.
- Anorexia nervosa, a disorder characterized by severe weight loss in the absence of obvious physical cause, consists of three areas of disordered psychologic functioning: disturbed body image and body concept of delusional proportions, inaccurate and confused perception and interpretation of inner stimuli, and a paralyzing sense of ineffectiveness that pervades all aspects of daily life.
- Therapeutic management of anorexia involves reinstitution of normal nutrition, resolution of the disturbed patterns of family interaction, and individual psychotherapy to correct deficits and distortions in psychologic functioning.

- Individuals with bulimia can be classified into two categories: (1) those who consume vast quantities of food followed by purging but who, if unable to purge, still consume large amounts, and (2) those who restrict their caloric intake, especially when unable to purge.
- Smoking is a widespread problem among teenagers. Reasons for smoking include social pressure, mass media influence, and a need to develop a self-concept.
- Substance abuse is a severe problem in adolescence; abusers include experimenters and compulsive users.
- Common types of drugs abused include alcohol, hydrocarbons and fluorocarbons, mind-altering drugs, narcotics, central nervous system depressants, and central nervous system stimulants.
- Suicide, the deliberate act of self-injury with the intent to kill, may occur in adolescents because of psychiatric disorders—primarily depression, family discord, and difficulties in coping with stress.
- Suicide is much more likely to occur if the adolescent has access to a firearm or has been drinking or using drugs.

# REFERENCES

Adelman WP and others: Effectiveness of a high school smoking cessation program, *Pediatrics* 107(4):E50, 2001.

American Academy of Pediatrics, Committee on Adolescence: Suicide and suicide attempts in adolescents, *Pediatrics* 105(4): 871-874, 2000.

American Psychiatric Association: *Diagnostic and statistical manual of mental disorders,* ed 4 (DSM-IV TR), Washington, DC, 2000, The Association.

Angold A, Costello EJ, Erkanli A: Cormorbidity, *J Child Psychol Psychiatr* 40(1):57-87, 1999.

Baer JS and others: Prenatal alcohol exposure and family history of alcoholism in the etiology of adolescent alcohol problems, *J Stud Alcohol* 59(5):533-543, 1998.

Barlow SE, Dietz WH: Obesity evaluation and treatment: expert committee recommendations, *Pediatrics* 102(3):e29, 1998.

Bauman A, Phongsavan P: Epidemiology of substance use in adolescence: prevalence, trends and policy implications, *Drug Alcohol Depend* 55(3):187-207, 1999.

Bertrand LD, Abernathy TJ: Predicting cigarette smoking among adolescents using cross-sectional and longitudinal approaches, *J Sch Health* 63(2):98-103, 1993.

Blum K and others: Allelic association of human dopamine D2 receptor gene in alcoholism, *JAMA* 263(15):2055-2060, 1990.

Bryant-Waugh R, Lask B: Annotation: eating disorders in children, *J Child Psychol Psychiatr* 30(2):191-200, 1995.

Centers for Disease Control and Prevention: *Preventing tobacco use among young people: a report of the Surgeon General,* S/N 017-001-004901-0, Washington, DC, 1994a, US Department of Health and Human Services.

Centers for Disease Control and Prevention: Programs for the prevention of suicide among adolescents and young adults: suicide contagion and the reporting of suicide, *MMWR* 43(RR-6):1-18, 1994b.

Centers for Disease Control and Prevention: Rates of homicide, suicide and firearm-related death among children—26 industrialized countries, *MMWR* 46(5):101-105, 1997.

Centers for Disease Control and Prevention: *Suicide in the United States 1980-1992,* Atlanta, 1995, National Center for Injury Prevention and Control.

Centers for Disease Control and Prevention: Youth risk behavior surveillance—United States, 1999, *MMWR* 49(SS05):1-96, 2000.

Centers for Disease Control and Prevention/National Center for Health Statistics: *Death rates from 72 selected causes by 5-year age groups, race and sex: United States, 1979-1997,* Atlanta, 1999, Centers for Disease Control and Prevention/National Center for Health Statistics.

Delaney JP: Role of energy expenditure in the development of pediatric obesity, *Am J Clin Nutr* 68 (Suppl):950S-955S, 1998.

Dexheimer-Pharris M, Resnick MD, Blum RW: Protecting against hopelessness and suicidality in sexually abused American Indian adolescents, *J Adolesc Health* 21(6):400-406, 1997.

Diekstra RF, Garnefski N: On the nature, magnitude, an causality of suicidal behaviors: an international perspective, *Suicide Life Threat Behav* 25(1):36-57, 1995.

Dietz WH, Robinson TN: Use of the body mass index (BMI) as a measure of overweight in children and adolescents, *J Pediatr* 132(2):191-193, 1998.

Ehrman WG: Obesity. In Hoekelman RA, editor: *Primary pediatric care,* ed 4, St. Louis, 2001, Mosby.

Ehtisham S, Barrett TG, Shaw NJ: Type 2 diabetes mellitus in UK children—an emerging problem, *Diabetes Med* 17(12):867-871, 2000.

Flay BR and others: Differential influence of parental smoking and friends' smoking on adolescent initiation and escalation of smoking, *J Health Soc Behav* 35(3):248-265, 1994.

Freedman DS and others: Relation of childhood height to obesity among adults: the Bogalusa Heart Study, *Pediatrics* 109(2):e 23, 2002.

Gold DR and others: Effects of cigarette smoking on lung function in adolescent boys and girls, *N Engl J Med* 335(13):931-937, 1996.

Goodman E, Capitman J: Depressive symptoms and cigarette smoking among teens, *Pediatrics* 106(4):748-755, 2000.

Gordon-Larsen P, McMurray RG, Popkin BM: Adolescent physical activity and inactivity vary by ethnicity: The National Longitudinal Study of Adolescent Health, *J Pediatr* 135:301-306, 1999.

Gortmaker SL and others: Television viewing as a cause of increasing obesity among children in the United States, *Arch Pediatr Adolesc Med* 150:536-562, 1996.

Gossip M and others: Cocaine: patterns of use, route administration, and severity of dependence, *Br J Psychiatr* 164(5):660-664, 1994.

Gould MS and others: Psychopathology associated with suicidal ideation and attempts among children and adolescents, *J Am Acad Child Adolesc Psychiatr* 37:915-923, 1998.

Green M, editor: *Bright futures: guidelines for health supervision of infants, children and adolescents,* Arlington, VA, 1994, National Center for Education in Maternal and Child Health.

Greydanus DE, Pratt HD: Emotional and behavioral disorders of adolescence. II. *Adolesc Health Update* 8(1):1-8, 1995.

Halmi KA: Eating disorders: defining the phenotype and reinventing the treatment, *Am J Psychiatr* 156:1673-1675, 1999.

Hawkins JD, Catalano RF, Miller JY: Risk and protective factors for alcohol and other drug problems in adolescence and early adulthood: implications for substance abuse prevention, *Psychol Bull* 112:44-105, 1992.

Himes J, Dietz WH: Guidelines for overweight in adolescent preventive services: recommendations from an expert committee, *Am J Clin Nutr* 59:307-316, 1994.

Hoffmann JP, Su SS: Parental substance use disorder, mediating variables and adolescent drug use: a non-recursive model, *Addiction* 93(9):1351-1364, 1998.

Holinger PC and others: *Suicide and homicide among adolescents,* New York, 1994, The Guiliford Press.

Hu FB and others: The influences of friends' and parental smoking on adolescent smoking behavior: the effects of time and prior smoking, *J Appl Soc Psychol* 25(22):2018-2047, 1995.

Institute of Medicine, Committee on Preventing Nicotine Addiction in Children and Youths: Lynch BS, Bonnie RJ, editors: *Growing up tobacco free,* Washington, DC, 1994, National Academy Press.

Jellinek MS, Snyder JB: Depression and suicide in children and adolescents, *Pediatr Rev* 19(8):255-264, 1998.

Jessor R: Risk behavior in adolescence: a psychosocial framework for understanding and action, *J Adolesc Health* 12:597-605, 1991.

Johnston LD, O'Malley PM, Bachman JG: *National survey results on drug use from the Monitoring the Future study 1975-1994,* NIH Publication No. 95-4026, Washington, DC, 1995, National Institutes of Health.

Johnston LD, O'Malley PM, Bachman JG: *Monitoring the Future study,* Ann Arbor, December 19, 1996, News and Information Services of the University of Michigan.

Katzman DK and others: Cerebral gray matter and white matter volume deficits in adolescent girls with anorexia nervosa, *J Pediatr* 129:794-803, 1996.

Keller C, Stevens KR: Childhood obesity: measurement and risk assessment, *Pediatr Nurs* 22(6):494-499, 1996.

Kim S and others: Self-concept measures, and childhood obesity: a descriptive analysis, *J Dev Behav Pediatr* 12(1):19-24, 1995.

Klesges RC, Robinson LA: Predictors of smoking onset in adolescent African-American boys and girls, *J Health Educ* 26(2):85-89, 1995.

Kosterman R and others: The dynamics of alcohol and marijuana initiation: patterns and predictors of first use in adolescence, *Am J Public Health* 90(3):360-366, 2000.

Kotler LA, Walsh BT: Eating disorders in children and adolescents: pharmacological therapies, *Euro Child Adolesc Psychiatr* 9(suppl 1):1108-1116, 2000.

Lewinsohn PM, Rohde P, Seely JR: Adolescent suicidal ideation and attempts: prevalence, risk factors, and clinical implications, *Clin Psychol Sci Pract* 3(1):25-46, 1996.

MacKenzie NR: Childhood obesity: strategies for prevention, *Pediatr Nurs* 26(5):527-530, 2000.

MacKenzie R, Neinstein LS: Anorexia nervosa and bulimia. In Neinstein LS, editor: *Adolescent health care,* ed 3, Baltimore, 1996, Williams & Wilkins.

Mendelson WB, Rich CL: Sedatives and suicide: the San Diego study, *Acta Psychiatr Scand* 88(5):337-341, 1993.

MMWR: Update: prevalence of overweight among children, adolescents, and adults—United States, 1988-1994, *MMWR* 46: 199-202, 1997.

Moolchan ET, Ernst M, Henningfield JE: A review of tobacco smoking in adolescents: treatment implications, *J Am Acad Child Adolesc Psychiatr* 39(6):682-693, 2000.

Moran R: Evaluation and treatment of childhood obesity, *Am Fam Physician* 59:861-868, 1999.

Morrison SF, Rogers PD, Thomas MH: Alcohol and adolescents, *Pediatr Clin North Am* 42(2): 371-387, 1995.

Murphy SL: Deaths: final data for 1998, *Nat Vital Stat Rep* 48(11):1-105, 2000.

Murray DM, Prokhorov AV, Harty KC: Effects on a statewide anti-smoking campaign on mass media messages and smoking beliefs, *Prev Med Int J Pract Theory* 23(1):54-60, 1994.

Muscari ME: Primary care of adolescents with bulimia nervosa, *J Pediatr Health Care* 10: 17-25, 1996.

Muscari ME: Screening for anorexia and bulimia, *Am J Nurs* 98(11):22-24, 1998.

Neinstein LS, Pinsky D: Alcohol. In Neinstein LS, editor: *Adolescent health care: a practical guide*, ed 3, Baltimore, 1996, Williams & Wilkins.

Newcomb MD, Felix-Ortiz MF: Multiple protective and risk factors for drug use and abuse: cross-sectional and prospective findings, *J Pers Soc Psychol* 63(2):280-296, 1992.

Oygard L and others: Parental and peer influences on smoking among young adults: ten-year follow up of the Oslo youth study participants, *Addiction* 90(4):561-569, 1995.

Patten CA and others: Depressive symptoms and cigarette smoking predict development and persistence of sleep problems in US adolescents, *Pediatrics* 106(2):E23, 2000.

Patton LH: Adolescent substance abuse, *Pediatr Clin North Am* 42(2):283-293, 1995.

Pieper MH, Pieper WJ: It's not tough, it's tender love: problem teens need compassion that the "tough love" approach to childrearing doesn't offer them, *Child Welfare* 71:369-377, 1992.

Remafedi G and others: The relationship between suicide risk and sexual orientation: results of a population-based study, *Am J Public Health* 88(1):57-60, 1998.

Resnick MD and others: Protecting adolescents from harm: findings from the National Study on Adolescent Health, *JAMA* 278: 823-832, 1997.

Rigotti NA, Lee JE, Wechsler H: US college students' use of tobacco products: results of a national survey, *JAMA* 284(6):699-705, 2000.

Riley WT and others: Perceived smokeless tobacco addiction among adolescents, *Health Psychol* 15(4):289-292, 1996.

Roberts SO: The role of physical activity in the prevention and treatment of childhood obesity, *Pediatr Nurs* 26(1):33-41, 2000.

Ryan CC, Futterman D: *Lesbian and gay youth: care and counseling*, New York, 1998, Columbia University Press.

Sargent JD, Dalton M: Does parental disapproval of smoking prevent adolescents from becoming established smokers? *Pediatrics* 108(6):1256-1262, 2001.

Scheier LM, Newcomb MD, Skager R: Risk protection, and vulnerability to adolescent drug use: latent-variable models of three age groups, *J Drug Educ* 24(1);49-82, 1994.

Schneider MB, Fisher MM: Anorexia and bulimia nervosa. In Hoeckelman RA, editor: *Primary pediatric care*, ed 4, St Louis, 2001, Mosby.

Shaffer D and others: Psychiatric diagnosis in child and adolescent suicide, *Arch Gen Psychiatr* 53:339-348, 1996.

Sothern MS and others: Motivating the obese child to move: the role of structured exercise in pediatric weight management, *South Med J* 92:577-584, 1999.

Stein JA, Newcomb MD, Bentler PM: Initiation and maintenance of tobacco smoking: changing personality correlates in adolescence and young adulthood, *J Appl Soc Psychol* 26(2):160-187, 1996.

Strauss R: Childhood obesity, *Curr Prob Pediatr* 29:4-29, 1999.

Strauss RS: Childhood obesity and self-esteem, *Pediatrics* 105(1):E15, 2000.

Strober M and others: Controlled family study of anorexia nervosa and bulimia nervosa: evidence of shared liability and transmission of partial syndromes, *Am J Psychiatr* 157:393-401, 2000.

Sullivan PF: Mortality in anorexia nervosa, *Am J Psychiatr* 152:1073-1074, 1995.

Tomeo CA and others: Weight concerns, weight control behaviors, and smoking initiation, *Pediatrics* 104(4):918-924, 1999.

Torabi MR, Bailey WJ, Majd-Jabbari M: Cigarette smoking as a predictor of alcohol and other drug use by children and adolescents: evidence of the "gateway drug effect," *J Sch Health* 63:302-306, 1993.

Troiano RP and others: Overweight prevalence and trends for children and adolescents, *Arch Pediatr Adolesc Med* 149:1085-1091, 1995.

US Department of Health and Human Services: *National household survey on drug abuse, 1999,* Washington, DC, 1999, Substance Abuse and Mental Health Services Administration.

US Department of Health and Human Services: NIDA and partners announce national initiative on prescription drug misuse and abuse, *NIH News Release,* Washington, DC, April 10, 2001.

US Department of Health and Human Services: *Preventing tobacco use among young people: a report of the Surgeon General,* Atlanta, 1994, US Department of Health and Human Services, Public Health Services, Centers for Disease Control and Prevention, National Center for Chronic Disease Prevention and Health Promotion and Health Promotion, Office on Smoking and Health.

Warheit GJ and others: Self rejection/derogation, peer factors, and alcohol, drug, and cigarette use among a sample of Hispanic, African-American and white non-Hispanic adolescents, *Int J Addict* 30(2):97-116, 1995.

Weinberg NZ and others: Adolescent substance abuse: a review of the past 10 years, *J Am Acad Child Adolesc Psychiatr* 37(3): 252-261, 1998.

Whitaker RC and others: Predicting obesity in young adulthood from childhood and parental obesity, *New Engl J Med* 337:869-873, 1997.

White HR, Brick J, Hansell S: Longitudinal investigation of alcohol use and aggression in adolescence, *J Stud Alcohol* 11:62-77, 1993.

Willard JC, Schoenborn CA: Relationship between cigarette smoking and other unhealth behaviors among our nation's youth: United States, 1992, *Adv Data* 24(263):1-11, 1995.

Wilson DM and others: Timing and rate of sexual maturation and the onset of cigarette and alcohol use among teenager girls, *Arch Pediatr Adolesc Med* 148:789-795, 1994.

Winkelstein ML: Adolescent smoking: influential factors, past preventive efforts and future nursing implications, *J Pediatr Nurs* 7(2):120-127, 1992.

World Health Organization: *World health statistical annual,* 1994, Geneva, 1995, The Organization.

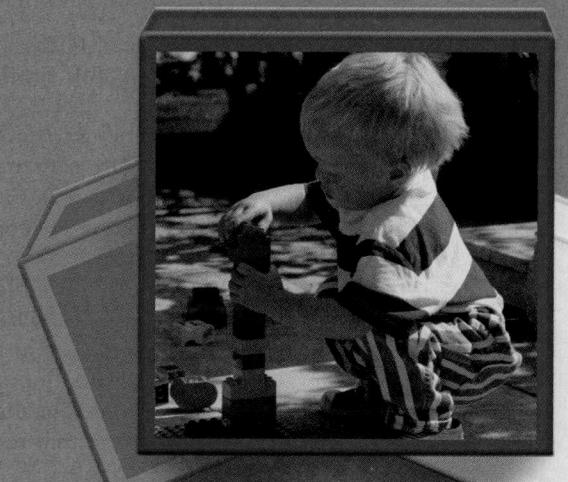

# Chapter 22

# Family-Centered Care of the Child with Chronic Illness or Disability

## Chapter Outline

**PERSPECTIVES IN THE CARE OF CHILDREN WITH SPECIAL NEEDS, 905**
**Scope of the Problem, 905**
**Trends in Care, 907**
   Developmental Focus, 907
   Family Development, 907
   Family-Centered Care, 907
   Normalization, 908
   Home Care, 908
   Mainstreaming, 908
   Early Intervention, 909
   Managed Care, 909
**Cultural Issues, 910**

**IMPACT OF CHRONIC ILLNESS OR DISABILITY ON THE CHILD, 910**
**Promoting Normal Development, 910**
   Infant, 910
   Toddler, 912
   Preschooler, 913
   School-Age Child, 914
   Adolescent, 916

**Helping the Child to Cope, 917**
   Coping Mechanisms, 917
   Normalization, 917
   Hopefulness, 918
   Health Education/Self-Care, 918
   Realistic Future Goals, 919

**THE FAMILY OF THE CHILD WITH SPECIAL NEEDS, 920**
**Assessing Family Strengths and Adjustment, 921**
**Accepting the Child's Condition/Support at the Time of Diagnosis, 921**
**Managing the Condition on an Ongoing Basis, 923**
   Special Information Needs, 923
   Family Management Styles, 924
**Meeting the Child's Normal Developmental Needs, 925**
**Meeting Developmental Needs of Other Family Members, 925**
   Parents, 925

   Sibling Issues, 928
   Extended Family Members and Friends, 929
**Coping with Ongoing Stress and Periodic Crises, 931**
   Concurrent Stresses Within the Family, 931
   Coping Mechanisms, 931
   Parental Empowerment, 932
**Assisting Family Members in Managing Their Feelings, 933**
   Shock and Denial, 933
   Adjustment, 933
   Reintegration and Acknowledgment, 934
**Establishing a Support System, 935**
   Intrafamilial Resources, 935
   Social Support Systems, 936
   Parent-to-Parent Support, 936
   Parent-Professional Partnerships, 937
   Community Resources, 938
*Nursing Care Plan: The Child with Chronic Illness or Disability, 939*

## Related Topics

Birth of a Child with a Physical Defect, Ch. 11
The Child with Cognitive, Sensory, or Communication Impairment, Ch. 24
Childhood Morbidity, Ch. 1
Communicating with Families, Ch. 6
Developmental Assessment, Ch. 7
Discharge Planning and Home Care (High-Risk Newborn), Ch. 10

Facilitating Parent-Infant Relationships (High-Risk Newborn), Ch. 10
Family Assessment, Ch. 6
Family-Centered Care, Ch. 1
Family-Centered Care of the Child During Illness and Hospitalization, Ch. 26
Family-Centered End-of-Life Care, Ch. 23
Family-Centered Home Care, Ch. 25

Health Promotion: Infant, Ch. 12; Toddler, Ch. 14; Preschooler, Ch. 15; School-Age Child, Ch. 17; Adolescent, Ch. 19
Recommendations for Health Supervision, Ch. 7
School Phobia, Ch. 18
Social, Cultural, and Religious Influences on Child Health Promotion, Ch. 2

## PERSPECTIVES IN THE CARE OF CHILDREN WITH SPECIAL NEEDS

### Scope of the Problem

Significant budget reductions in Medicaid benefits, implementation of managed care, and other changes in the health care system have increased the need for services and benefits to children with chronic illness or disability (Westbrook, Silver, and Stein, 1998). A major impediment to the effort to provide these services has been the issue of how best to define populations of children with chronic

■ Nancy Gerhard, RN, MN, WS, and Nancy Kline, PhD, RN, CPNP, revised this chapter.

conditions. For many years a number of terms have been used to classify and describe children with special health care needs (Box 22-1).

More recently there has been an impetus to develop a definition of children with special health care needs that could be used by federal and state programs to facilitate planning of comprehensive, family-centered, community-based services for this population (Jackson, 2000). To date, children with special health care needs, as defined by the federal Maternal and Child Health Bureau (McPherson and others, 1998), are "Children who have or are at increased risk for a chronic physical, behavioral, developmental, or emotional condition and who also require health and related services of a type or amount beyond that required by children in general."

Patterns of childhood mortality have changed considerably over the past 20 years, attributable to advances in medical technology, improved management of infectious diseases, identification of children with previously unrecognized illnesses, and implementation of preventive and public health measures (Jackson, 2000).

For example, the median life expectancy of children with cystic fibrosis today is more than 30 years, in contrast to 5 years in 1955. In 1955, 90% of children born with spina bifida died in infancy; today 90% survive infancy and have a normal life expectancy if they are provided with appropriate and timely medical intervention. The life expectancy of children with spina bifida has increased because of im-

proved surgical advances and management of urinary tract infections (Jackson, 2000).

Advances in combination antiretroviral therapy have resulted in a decreased mortality rate for children with human immunodeficiency virus (HIV) (Fahrner and Mario, 2000; Peters, Kochanek, and Murphy, 1998). Infants with very low birth weight and extreme prematurity are living longer (Jackson, 2000), and an estimated 80% of children diagnosed with cancer today will be cured of their disease (Harvey and others, 1999).

The dramatic decline seen in mortality rates has resulted in increased numbers of children with special health care needs and has implications for provision of comprehensive, long-term health care services for these patients (Jackson, 2000). Chronic illness has surpassed acute illness as the major health concern for children (Curtin and Lubkin, 1995). In the United States an estimated 18% of children (12.6 million) have a chronic illness or disability that warrants health care services beyond those usually required by children (Newacheck and others, 1998).

Data from the 1992-1994 National Health Interview Survey (Newacheck and Halfon, 1998) revealed that the most common chronic childhood conditions causing disability are respiratory diseases (primarily asthma) and impairments of speech, sensory functions, and intelligence (primarily mental retardation). Asthma is the single most prevalent cause of disability in children and has been largely responsible for much of the recent increase in childhood disability. Mental and nervous system disorders account for about one sixth of all childhood disability. The prevalence of disability increases among boys, children over the age of 5 years, and children from single-parent and low-income families (Newacheck and Halfon, 2000).

The impact of chronic illness and disability on children's health and functional status is profound. The National Health Interview Survey revealed that 18% of children with disabilities were in fair or poor health, in contrast to 2% of children without disabilities (Newacheck and Halfon, 1998). Children with disabilities spent three times as many days ill in bed and days absent from school as other children. They had more than twice the number of physician contacts and five times as many days hospitalized as other children (Newacheck and others, 1998). They were limited in their daily activities for slightly more than 2 weeks each year, and one tenth of all children with disabilities were unable to play or attend school (Newacheck and Halfon, 1998). In addition, children with disabilities are more likely to be a victim of emotional or sexual abuse, have behavioral problems, drop out of school, and be involved in the juvenile justice system than their peers without disabilities (Center for the Future of Children, 1997).

Chronic illness and disability have substantial effects on family functioning (Patterson and Blum, 1996). Chronic conditions present most families with additional tasks, responsibilities, and concerns such as the additional caretaking needs of the child, finding and accessing educational and medical services, paying for services, uncertainty about the future, emotional grieving, stigmatizing reactions from the community, social isolation, and lost social opportuni-

---

**Box 22-1** ■ ■ ■
### Key Terms Regarding Children with Special Health Care Needs

**Chronic illness**—A condition that interferes with daily functioning for more than 3 months in a year, causes hospitalization of more than 1 month in a year, or (at time of diagnosis) is likely to do either of these

**Congenital disability**—A disability that has existed since birth but is not necessarily hereditary

**Developmental delay**—An abnormal, slower rate of development in which a child demonstrates a functioning level below that observed in normal children of the same age

**Developmental disability**—Any mental and/or physical disability that is manifested before age 22 years and is likely to continue indefinitely

**Disability**—A long-term reduction in the child's ability to engage in day-to-day activities (e.g., playing, attending school) because of a chronic condition

**Handicap**—A condition or barrier imposed by society, the environment, or one's own self; not a synonym for disability

**Impairment**—A loss or abnormality of structure or function

**Technology-dependent child**—A child between the ages of birth and 21 years with a chronic disability that requires the routine use of a medical device to compensate for the loss of a life-sustaining bodily function; daily ongoing care and/or monitoring is required by trained personnel

Modified from Westbrook LE, Silver EJ, Stein RE: Implications for estimates of disability in children: a comparison of definitional components, *Pediatrics* 101(6):1025-1030, 1998; and Newacheck PW, Halfon N: Prevalence and impact of disabling chronic conditions in childhood, *Am J Public Health* 88(4):610-617, 1998.

ties. These demands can be grouped according to their personal impact on a parent, the financial impact on the family, and the impact on social and family relationships.

Parents are caught in a juggling act of meeting their child's normal growth and development needs and dealing with the consequences of the chronic illness (Clawson, 1996). Parents of children with disabilities are twice as likely to report depression than parents of children without disabilities—30% vs 15%, respectively (Singer and Yovanoff, 1996). Family members of children with disabilities are more likely to experience behavioral and psychologic symptoms. Parents may miss days from work, experience financial strain, and be challenged both physically and emotionally while they deal with caring for a child with a chronic illness or disability. Siblings experience a wide range of emotional reactions to having a "different" brother or sister, and frequently their lives reflect the routines imposed by the affected child's chronic condition (Curtin and Lubkin, 1995).

The heightened prevalence of chronic illness and disability in children and its far-reaching effects on the affected child and family members have many implications for nursing. Nurses need to take an active role in early screening, case finding, and assessment and provide supportive and educational interventions that decrease the disruptive effects of the chronic condition on the child and family members. In addition, nurses should attempt to prevent disabling conditions by removing their known causes by encouraging compliance with immunization programs, identifying infants and mothers at risk, recognizing the disability early, fostering injury prevention programs and policies, and providing innovative health education programs. Skilled case management is necessary to ensure that families of children with special needs have the support to successfully adapt to the consequences of the child's chronic condition. This includes providing community-based, comprehensive, and culturally appropriate care to the child with special needs (Patterson and Blum, 1996).

# Trends in Care

Prompted by advances in technology, economic ramifications, and the demand for more meaningful models of care, trends in care not only show changes in the types of services and care children receive, but also reveal shifts in where services are provided and who provides that care.

## Developmental Focus

Using a developmental approach rather than chronologic age when caring for children with special health care needs helps the nurse to determine where children are at present and to understand their response to the chronic illness or disability. Developmental changes in the child continue despite the added stress of coping with a chronic illness. Having a chronic condition imposes a dimension of behavioral and developmental risk (Patterson and Blum, 1996). Because children with chronic conditions are more alike than different, a noncategorical approach emphasizing the commonalities of these children, rather than solely the illness, is beneficial (Stein, 1996). Referring to children by the name

of their disability or illness affects both professional and parental attitudes, as well as the assessment of the child's present abilities and future expectations (Perrin and Shonkoff, 2000). Therefore parents and the health care team should work jointly for the benefit of the child who has an illness rather than having the illness define the child. Knowledge of the developmental theory perspective is paramount in providing the support necessary for children to successfully adjust to a stressful life experience such as a chronic illness or disability.

## Family Development

A developmental approach also includes an assessment of family development (Hymovich and Hagopian, 1992). Duvall (1977) defined an eight-stage family life cycle that focuses on the changing ages and developmental tasks of both children and adults and on the changing external demands as the family grows older. Families are expected to achieve certain tasks at various stages throughout their life span (e.g., finding, furnishing, and maintaining their first home during the married couple stage). A diagnosis of chronic illness in a family member has a profound effect on every member of the family unit (Peters, 1998). As with individual development, family development may be interrupted or even regress to a previous level of functioning. For example, having a child with a chronic illness may impose an added stress on the newly married couple who are in the midst of establishing a family identity. Nurses can apply family developmental theory when planning interventions for families of children with special health care needs. (See Developmental Assessment, Chapter 19.)

## Family-Centered Care

Family-centered care is paramount in the care of children with special health care needs. Over the past 40 years significant changes have emerged in parents' responsibility for providing and coordinating the care of their ill child. Today families of chronically ill children have comprehensive and complex caretaking responsibilities in the hospital or at home (Bruce and Ritchie, 1997).

The increasing numbers of chronically ill children and the families who are assuming the major burden of coordinating their child's care have reinforced the demand for new approaches in the health care system. The outcome has been the emergence of family-centered care to reflect, recognize, and facilitate the changing roles of families in care delivery. Because a cure is not likely for a number of chronic conditions, health care professionals must focus their efforts on care.

The federal 99-457 legislation, which affords states the opportunity to continue benefits of Public Law 94-142 (the Education for All Handicapped Children Act of 1975) to children from birth to age 2, targets family-centered care. This legislation establishes a process whereby families become active participants in decision making about the care of their children.

The goal of family-centered care is to minimize the manifestations of the illness and maximize the child's cognitive, physical, and psychosocial potential. Attainment of this goal is facilitated by advocating a family-centered approach to care (Vessey and Mebane, 2000). (See Family-Centered Care, Chapter 3.) Integrating family-centered care in practice requires health professionals to do the following: (a) to acknowledge and respect a family's individuality and strengths, (b) to foster a family's competence and confidence in caring for the child, and (c) to empower a family to advocate for their child when dealing with the health care system (Vessey and Mebane, 2000). In the family-centered framework, consistent attention is given to the effects of the child's chronic illness on all family members, not only on the affected child. This is paramount because the best predictors of the well-being of children with special health needs include factors associated with family functioning (Perrin and Shonkoff, 2000).

As parents become knowledgeable about their child's special health needs, they frequently become experts in providing care. As part of the health care team, nurses are adjuncts to the child's care and need to build alliances with parents, respecting and drawing on their expertise. One of the key principles in family-centered care is the involvement of family members in decision making about their child's physical care. Collaboration, consistent sharing of information about the illness, responsibility, and decision making, is necessary in establishing effective and trusting partnerships with parents.

Care conferences with the child's family and members of the health care team, including nurses, offer opportunities for mutual sharing of thoughts and concerns about the child's care. Being attentive to observations made by parents helps assure them that their role is valued and that their opinions are important.

In fostering effective family-centered care the nurse not only acknowledges that the family is a key component of the child's care and illness experience, but also recognizes and respects the expertise of the family in caring for the child within and outside of the hospital milieu. In the absence of the child's family during hospitalization, the nurse should try to maintain routines established by the family. In the family's presence, the nurse, child, and parent form a relationship in which the process of care negotiation occurs. This relationship is pivotal to the needs of the child and family and is where roles are defined and guidelines are developed. Through open communication the nurse *values* the parents' roles by perceiving them as the ultimate experts in caring for their child. Simultaneously the family looks to the nurse for empowerment, support, education, and expertise in caring for their child (Knight, 1995).

## Normalization

Normalization refers to establishing a normal pattern of living. (See Guidelines box on p. 918.) Normalization occurs on several levels. It implies child and family access to services in as usual a fashion and environment as possible, placing a focus on home and community. Through application of the principles of normalization, daily routines for the child with illness or disability should be fitted to the family's schedule, rather than vice versa. Age-appropriate expectations for the child's behavior should be applied. As neces-

sary, the environment should be structured to encourage the child's engagement in age-appropriate activities. Thus consequences of the illness are minimized, and the child and family live as normal a life as possible given the disability.

Nurses can facilitate the normalization process for families of children with special needs by acknowledging their normalcy, strengths, and weaknesses. Being supportive of the child's illness and treatment and actively including the family in all aspects of the care will improve their self-esteem and promote further development (Shepard and Mahon, 2000).

## Home Care

Concurrent with the trend towards normalization has been the earlier discharge of children from acute or chronic care facilities to the family and community. Home care refers to the return to a system and set of priorities whereby family values are as salient in the care of a child with a chronic illness as they are in the care of healthy children. The primary incentive for home care for children with special health needs originated from a parental need to keep these children at home and from professionals' willingness to work with families to attain this goal.* As proposed by Stein (1985), the goal of home care is to achieve goals that are consistent with the developmental model:

- Normalize the life of a child with special needs, including those with technologically complex care, in a community and family setting and context.
- Lessen the disruptive impact of the child's condition on the family.
- Promote the child's maximum growth and development.

With appropriate support and training, families today can provide complex treatments and procedures in the home. Parents are challenged to maintain a homelike setting in the midst of ventilators, monitors, and other sophisticated equipment. Throughout this text home care is discussed as appropriate for specific conditions. Chapter 25 focuses on family-centered home care, and the process of transition from the hospital to the home setting is described in Chapter 26.

## Mainstreaming

Mainstreaming refers to a process of integrating children with special needs into regular classrooms and child care centers. School allows these children to acquire a sense of self and understanding of their place with respect to their peers and provides important opportunities for socialization with nondisabled children, enabling the latter group to develop attitudes of respect for and acceptance of their peers with special needs. A crucial developmental task for children 5 years of age and older is to move beyond the family environment into the school community, where social competence, academic achievement, and regular attendance are important goals (Vessey and Jackson, 2000). A va-

---

*For additional information, please view "Family-Centered Care" in *Whaley and Wong's Pediatric Nursing Video Series*, St. Louis, 1996, Mosby; (800) 426-4545; www.mosby.com.

riety of supplemental programs exist in the school system to accommodate children with special needs, thereby affording them an equal education opportunity. For the most part this change facilitating normalization for these children has resulted from passage of Public Law (PL) 94-142, the *Education for All Handicapped Children Act of 1975,* which provides children with "free and appropriate public education" inclusive of special education and related services rendered at public expense, under public supervision, without charge, which meet the standards of the state educational agency (Vessey and Jackson, 2000). Its 1990 amendment, PL 101-476, changed the name of the act to the *Individuals with Disabilities Education Act (IDEA).* Passage of PL 101-476, along with current federal child care mandates and increasing public concern about child care, demonstrates a considerable national commitment to the concept that early services are crucial if children with disabilities are to achieve their full potential.

Public Law 94-142 requires states to identify, diagnose, teach, and provide related services for children age 5 to 18 years. In 1977 the age range was expanded to include children ages 3 to 21 years, with services for children ages 3 to 5 years optional. In accordance with this law, a multidisciplinary team writes an Individualized Education Program (IEP), which includes specific therapeutic and educational goals and strategies for each eligible child referred for special education. Parents may intervene in educational decisions and have the right to a hearing when the team's decision is seen as harmful or inappropriate. Because many parents are unaware of this or other laws advocating rights for disabled children, it is imperative that nurses inform them of the laws and where to obtain information. Nurses may also be involved in formulating individualized educational programs.

## Early Intervention

Early intervention includes any systematic and sustained effort to assist young, disabled, and developmentally vulnerable children from birth to 3 years of age. *Public Law 99-457, the Education of the Handicapped Act Amendments of 1986,* directs states to develop and enact statewide coordinated, comprehensive, multidisciplinary interagency programs of early intervention services for infants and toddlers with disabilities, in addition to support services for their families.

An important component of the law's implementation is the *Individualized Family Service Plan (IFSP).* As an outcome of collaboration between professionals and families, the IFSP consists of information relating to the infant or toddler's current level of development, family needs and strengths for improving development, main outcomes anticipated, services required, designation of a case manager, and transition steps to preschool services. All outcomes and services concern the needs of the child and family. The IFSP represents a commitment to families and children that their strengths will be acknowledged and built on, that their needs will be satisfied in a manner that respects their values and beliefs, and that their aspirations will be fostered and empowered.

Nurses can provide many services for children covered by PL 99-457. Implementation of family-centered care and

clinical expertise in practice provide nurses with a role in early identification and assessment of children at risk for disability, multidisciplinary assessment, and case management. Nurses can assess children in preschool settings, implement ongoing staff and patient education, coordinate care with the heath care team, become actively involved in community nursing networks, and develop health promotion programs for school personnel and family members. Because many families may not be cognizant of the value or availability of early intervention, marketing and other public relations strategies may be employed to aid them in realizing the need for services (Fugate and Fugate, 1995, 1996).

## Managed Care

Managed care health plans are rapidly becoming the primary form of health care coverage in the United States (Jackson, 2000). Initially managed care plans were developed to provide services for adults, whose care depleted 86% of health care dollars; thus the plans paid little attention to the needs of children (Deal, Shiono, and Behrman, 1998). Along with the rapid expansion of managed care, particularly for Medicaid-eligible patients, the roles and responsibilities of state Title V programs for children with special health needs changed as well (McManus and others, 1996). Provision of direct services by specialty clinics funded through Title V were reduced while managed care systems attempted to provide services to children within the managed care organization.

Implementing managed care for children with disabilities differs from providing care for adults with disabilities in three ways (American Academy of Pediatrics, 1998): (1) the changing dynamics of child development affect the needs of these children at various developmental stages and change their anticipated outcomes; (2) the prevalence and epidemiology of childhood disabilities, with few common conditions and many low-incidence or rare ones, vary considerably from those of adults, for whom there are many common conditions and few rare ones; and (3) due to children's need for adult guidance and protection, their development and health rely heavily on their families' socioeconomic status and health. These differences have implications for monitoring care provided to children with chronic conditions in managed care settings. The diverse effects of managed care on these children are seen in seven major domains: access to care, use of services, quality of care, satisfaction with care, costs for care, health outcomes, and family impact (Newacheck and others, 1996).

Families offer four basic suggestions for improving services for their children with chronic conditions: (1) reduce barriers to programs and services; (2) improve the quality of services; (3) improve the training given to families, health care professionals, and the community relating to chronic conditions and their management; and (4) increase the availability and quality of community-based services (Garwick and others, 1998). All of these suggestions are based on two factors: universality of care and adequate funding (Vessey and Jackson, 2000). Health care providers play an important role in working jointly with the leadership of managed care programs to ensure quality of care for children with chronic conditions.

## Cultural Issues

Increasing migration around the world in the past 10 years has been responsible for the heterogeneity of many nations, including the United States, which does not have a generalized culture. For this reason cultural competence is an important goal of nursing practice.

For many minority and ethnic populations, cultural understanding of disability and illness, social roles for disabled individuals, the structure of family life, and other factors associated with the perception of children vary from those of "mainstream" American culture. These may affect family choices regarding the care of their child with special needs.

Although culture cannot fully define how an individual will act and think, knowledge of cultural perspectives can assist nurses in anticipating and understanding why families make certain decisions. Cultural attributes, including beliefs and values about disability or illness and its causes, family structure, social roles for the disabled, the role of children, childrearing practices, spirituality, and time orientation also influence a family's reaction to a chronic condition. Although eliciting health beliefs and negotiating interventions can be challenging, it is necessary for compliance, collaboration, gratification, and optimal care. (See Guidelines box.)

When parents are informed of their child's chronic illness, interpreters familiar with both culture and language should be used. Children, family members, and friends of the family should not be used as translators because their presence may prevent parents from an open discussion of the issues (Purnell and Paulanka, 1998).

Recognizing the growing presence of cultural diversity in our society, nurses must incorporate cultural competence in their clinical practice to promote delivery of effective and sensitive care to children with chronic illness and their families. Care should be consistent with the cultural practices and beliefs of the child's family whenever possible; increasing cultural competence will improve communication and promote respect for human diversity (Rehm, 2000). In a study by Garwick and others (1998) citing recommendations of Hispanic, African-American, and European-American families for improving the care of children with chronic con-

ditions, no distinctive differences in families' recommendations on the basis of ethnicity alone were found. These families emphasized the importance of individualizing care to meet the specific needs of the child and family, rather than providing culturally specific care for certain ethnic groups.

# IMPACT OF CHRONIC ILLNESS OR DISABILITY ON THE CHILD

A child's reaction to chronic illness or disability depends largely on his or her developmental level. Knowledge of developmental stages is essential for nurses in understanding how children interpret events. Because children's understanding adheres to a usual growth pattern in cognitive abilities, they require varied explanations of their chronic illness as they grow older (Perrin, 2000). Normal development should be fostered in the context of the child's temperament, intelligence, motor skills, and relationships with family and friends. Identifying the child's coping strategies and promoting successful adaptation to the illness are essential. Factors influencing coping include the developmental stage, age and gender, type and duration of illness, and family cohesion (Amer, 1999). Caring for the child involves health education efforts, normalization principles, and assisting the growing child in planning realistic future goals. (See Nursing Care Plan on pp. 939-944.)

## Promoting Normal Development

The impact of a chronic illness or disability on a child is affected by the age of onset (Vessey and Mebane, 2000). Children of all ages are affected by chronic illness, although each age-group poses its own specific challenges. Children redefine their illness and its implications as they develop and grow. Accordingly, nurses must plan and implement care that promotes the child's successful progression from one stage of development to the next.

In addition to learning about the illness and its effects on the child's abilities, the family needs to be taught strategies promoting appropriate development in their child. Even though there may be a delay in acquisition of developmental milestones, nurses need to be instrumental in teaching parents how best to help their child reach his or her developmental potential (Vessey and Mebane, 2000). Table 22-1 describes developmental aspects of chronic illness or disability in children and accompanying supportive interventions.

### Infant

During infancy the child is establishing trust and learning about the environment through sensorimotor exploration (Vessey and Mebane, 2000). However, the diagnosis of a chronic illness, accompanied by a disruption in routines and physical discomfort, may compromise the dependability and consistency of an infant's environment and hinder the development of basic trust. Disability or chronic illness frequently impairs the child's motor abilities, restricting the child to a crib and decreasing contact with the environ-

---

**GUIDELINES**

*Identifying Cultural Influences on Health Beliefs*

Asking parents about the following perceptions can help determine cultural health beliefs:
  Perception of the cause of the illness
  Understanding of what the illness does to the child
  Perception of the seriousness or severity of the illness/disability
  How long the illness is expected to last
  Type(s) of treatment that the family would prefer to have used
  Results to be expected from the type(s) of treatment preferred
  Concerns or worries about the condition

Modified from Carrillo JE, Green AR, Betancourt JR: Cross-cultural primary care: a patient-based approach, *Ann Intern Med* 130(10): 829-834, 1999.

**TABLE 22-1**   Developmental aspects of chronic illness or disability in children

| Developmental Tasks | Potential Effects of Chronic Illness or Disability | Supportive Interventions |
|---|---|---|
| **Infancy** | | |
| Develop a sense of trust | Multiple caregivers and frequent separations, especially if hospitalized | Encourage consistent caregivers and care by parent in hospital or other care settings |
| | Deprived of consistent nurturing | Encourage parents to visit frequently or "room in" during hospitalization and to participate in care |
| Attach to parent | Delayed because of separation, parental grief for loss of "dream" child, parental inability to accept the condition, especially a visible defect | Emphasize healthy, perfect qualities of infant |
| | | Help parents learn special care needs of infant for them to feel competent |
| Learn through sensorimotor experiences | Increased exposure to painful experiences over pleasurable ones | Expose infant to pleasurable experiences through all senses (touch, hearing, sight, taste, movement) |
| | Limited contact with environment from restricted movement or confinement | Encourage age-appropriate developmental skills (e.g., holding bottle, finger feeding, crawling) |
| Begin to develop a sense of separateness from parent | Increased dependency on parent for care | Encourage all family members to participate in care to prevent overinvolvement of one member |
| | Overinvolvement of parent in care | Encourage periodic respite from demands of care responsibilities |
| **Toddlerhood** | | |
| Develop autonomy | Increased dependency on parent | Encourage independence in as many areas as possible (e.g., toileting, dressing, feeding) |
| Master locomotor and language skills | Limited opportunity to test own abilities and limits | Provide gross motor skill activity and modification of toys or equipment, such as modified swing or rocking horse |
| Learn through sensorimotor experience, beginning preoperational thought | Increased exposure to painful experiences | Give choices to allow simple feeling of control (e.g., choice of what book to look at or what kind of sandwich to eat) |
| | | Institute age-appropriate discipline and limit-setting |
| | | Recognize that negative and ritualistic behavior are normal |
| | | Provide sensory experiences (e.g., water play, sandbox, finger paint) |
| **Preschool** | | |
| Develop initiative and purpose | Limited opportunities for success in accomplishing simple tasks or mastering self-care skills | Encourage mastery of self-help skills |
| Master self-care skills | | Encourage socialization, such as inviting friends to play, daycare experience, trips to park |
| Begin to develop peer relationships | Limited opportunities for socialization with peers; may appear "like a baby" to age-mates | Provide age-appropriate play, especially associative play opportunities |
| | Protection within tolerant and secure family may cause child to fear criticism and withdraw | Emphasize child's abilities; dress appropriately to enhance desirable appearance |
| Develop sense of body image and sexual identification | Awareness of body may center on pain, anxiety, and failure | Encourage relationships with same-sex and opposite-sex peers and adults |
| | Sex-role identification focused primarily on mothering skills | Help child deal with criticisms; realize that too much protection prevents child from mastering realities of world |
| Learn through preoperational thought (magical thinking) | Guilt (thinking he or she caused the illness/disability or is being punished for wrongdoing) | Clarify that cause of child's illness or disability is not his or her fault or a punishment |
| **School Age** | | |
| Develop a sense of accomplishment | Limited opportunities to achieve and compete (e.g., many school absences or inability to join regular athletic activities) | Encourage school attendance; schedule medical visits at times other than school; encourage to make up missed work |
| | | Educate teachers and classmates about child's condition, abilities, and special needs |
| | | Encourage physical activity |
| Form peer relationships | Limited opportunities for socialization | Encourage socialization (e.g., Girl Scouts, Campfire, Boy Scouts, 4-H Clubs) |
| Learn through concrete operations | Incomplete comprehension of the imposed physical limitations or treatment of the disorder | Provide child with knowledge about his or her condition |
| | | Encourage creative activities |
| **Adolescence** | | |
| Develop personal and sexual identity | Increased sense of feeling different from peers and less able to compete with peers in appearance, abilities, special skills | Realize that many of the difficulties the teenager is experiencing are part of normal adolescence (rebelliousness, risk taking, lack of cooperation, hostility toward authority) |

*Continued*

**TABLE 22-1** Developmental aspects of chronic illness or disability in children—cont'd

| Developmental Tasks | Potential Effects of Chronic Illness or Disability | Supportive Interventions |
|---|---|---|
| **Adolescence—cont'd** | | |
| Develop personal and sexual identity | Increased dependency on family; limited job/career opportunities | Provide instruction on interpersonal and coping skills |
| Achieve independence from family | Limited opportunities for heterosexual friendships; less opportunity to discuss sexual concerns with peers | Encourage socialization with peers, including peers with special needs and those without special needs |
| Form personal relationships | Increased concern with issues such as why did he or she get the disorder, can he or she marry and have a family | Provide instruction on decision making, assertiveness, and other skills necessary to manage personal plans |
| Learn through abstract thinking | Decreased opportunity for earlier stages of cognition may impede achieving level of abstract thinking | Encourage increased responsibility for care and management of the disease or condition, such as assuming responsibility for making and keeping appointment, planning stages of health care delivery, contacting resources |
| | | Encourage activities appropriate for age, such as attending parties, sports activities, driving a car |
| | | Be alert to cues that signal readiness for information regarding implications of condition on sexuality and reproduction |
| | | Emphasize good appearance |
| | | Discuss planning for future and how condition can affect choices |

ment. Illness may influence the infant's growth and developmental parameters by its effects on mobility, sleeping, feeding, and sensory functions (Perrin, 2000). Separation of infant and parent as a result of frequent hospitalizations may prevent attachment and the emergence of a trusting relationship for the infant.

For the infant with a painful illness, exploration of his or her environment is restricted, which further curtails development (Vessey and Mebane, 2000). Messages transmitted to infants about their body are affected by the amount of pain and discomfort they experience. Associating pain with touch can lessen the infant's ability to give and receive affection. Lack of pleasant sensations can result in an irritable and unhappy child. Parents may interpret this behavior as indicative of their inadequacy in satisfying the child's emotional and physical needs, which further affects the parent-child relationship and the development of trust. Indeed, an illness may threaten the parents' confidence and competence in their newly acquired parenting roles.

The presence of a visible or serious defect can hinder parental attachment while the parents mourn the loss of the perfect child. They may derive little comfort in trying to satisfy their child's basic needs despite their best efforts. Physical deformity or fatigue may influence a child's responsiveness to his or her parents, who may in turn react differently to their child. A poor prognosis for the child may cause some parents to emotionally detach themselves from their infants to protect themselves from future emotional pain (Vessey and Mebane, 2000).

Nurses can be pivotal in helping parents care for their infant with special needs. They may need assistance in learning how best to meet their infant's needs, for example, how to hold a flaccid or rigid infant, how to comfort an irritable infant, how to feed a child with dyspnea or tongue thrust, or how to stimulate a child unable to attain common skills.

Nurses should advocate for practices and policies that support the developmental needs of the infant and the family. Twenty-four hour visitation in the neonatal intensive care unit (NICU) and other infant units is paramount and lessens the infant's experience of separation. In addition, nurses need to limit the number of caregivers for the infant to enhance consistency and continuity of care. Showing parents how to hold and touch their infant will foster their competence and confidence. Kangaroo care has demonstrated to be both beneficial and safe to the infant. (See Chapter 10.) Mothers who want to breast-feed should be encouraged and provided with a private room to pump or nurse and storage facilities for breast milk. Sibling visitation should be promoted.

### Toddler

The toddler is acquiring a sense of autonomy, developing self-control, and forming symbolic representation through language acquisition. The need for parental involvement in managing the child's illness may interfere with the toddler's need for increasing independence and impede his or her sense of autonomy and self-control. Mobility is possibly the primary tool used by the toddler to experiment with attaining control. For the toddler who is incapacitated, a sense of helplessness results that is difficult to overcome at a later time (Peters, 1998).

If a child's chronic illness warrants curtailing daily activities and setting limits, autonomy in such tasks as feeding, toileting, and building larger social networks may be impeded. Developmental tasks that have just been achieved are often easily lost in the toddler suffering from an acute exacerbation of the illness. Regression of behavior causes the child to revert to earlier, once-abandoned stages when they lack the energy needed to function at developmental levels previously attained (Freud, 1966). Behavioral regression, commonly seen in toddlers, is worsened by stress related to pain and separation.

Because of the toddler's desire for autonomy, the need for mastery of language and locomotor skills is very important. The child learning to talk and walk progresses toward being a separate individual, both psychologically and physically. A toddlers' limited ability to verbally communicate thoughts and feelings makes it especially difficult for the child to cope with the stresses imposed by a chronic illness. In the presence of disability or illness, mobility to explore and master the environment is impeded and the child is prevented from acquisition of this skill. Within the confines of the illness or disability, the nurse should help parents provide safe opportunities that foster independence in these and other areas for their toddler, both at home and in the hospital.

Illness can impose separations that cause anxiety in the toddler. A disability or chronic illness can entail frequent painful procedures and hospitalizations. The latter may hinder the normal development of trusting relationships within the family. If the need to maintain the parent-child relationship is not supported in the hospital, the child may become depressed and eventually detach from parents. Children appear to have a great ability to withstand stress as long as their attachment to the parent is maintained.

Toddlers are especially sensitive to changes in familiar routines, in addition to hospitalizations. They may perceive disruption of normal daily activities and hospitalization as punishment. If invasive and painful medical procedures are included in the treatment of the child's illness, this perception is further validated. Therefore parents should be encouraged to bring in familiar toys for the toddler during hospitalization, and routines should be established so the child can become acclimated.

Parents of toddlers may seek out daycare or respite care, which can be difficult to find for the child with special needs.* They need time away from caring for their child to allow for their own growth and development. The *Americans with Disabilities Act (ADA)* requires that daycare providers make "reasonable modifications" for equal access to program participation (Siegel, 1995). Special medical daycare facilities are emerging in some areas (Ahmann and Scher, 1996; Monical, 1995).

## Preschooler

The preschooler is focused on acquiring a sense of initiative to successfully meet the challenges of his or her growing world. Preschoolers with a chronic illness may lack the resources or energy to plan and engage in such activities; thus opportunities for building social relationships, learning about the environment, and developing a sense of purpose and self-confidence are curtailed. Illness may restrict the preschooler to the home and cause the child to fall behind in social skills beneficial in school or group settings.

The preschooler is also forming a sexual identity, and this may be accomplished by imitation of gender-related activities. The child with special needs may have few opportunities to participate in these activities and may see the parent mostly in the caregiving role because this may be the focus of their relationship. It may be difficult for preschoolers to build a healthy sexual identity and body image, especially if the majority of their body awareness is linked with pain and disability.

The preschooler begins to develop a body image. Children's understanding of their body image is confined to what they see, feel, and use. In the presence of a chronic illness, their body awareness may be focused on the anxiety and pain elicited. The chronically ill child may lose control over newly acquired bowel and bladder function, resulting in feelings of embarrassment and inferiority. The child with a disability may find it difficult to form a mental image of impaired body parts, for example, paralyzed extremities. This poorly developed sense of body integrity causes children to be particularly fearful of mutilating or intrusive experiences, which can occur frequently during a lengthy illness. Thus before any medical procedure children should be given a short, honest explanation of what the procedure is, how it will be performed, and the duration and intensity of any accompanying pain.

When the young child has a disability that affects motor development, there is the potential risk of shifting to development of compensatory intellectual pursuits before the child is ready. If this occurs, attainment of initiative and autonomy may be compromised, and the child may be at risk for emotional problems. Thus intervention must focus on providing activities that allow maximum motor development. For example, if a child has paraplegia, it is not enough to strengthen the upper extremities to compensate for the lower ones. Rather, the activity must consider the child's need for a sense of control over the body, social interaction, feeling of achievement and competence, and an outlet for aggression. Appropriate activities may include ball throwing; building blocks; water and swimming activities such as bubble blowing, splashing, and racing; or pounding with a hammer.* With minor changes, children with disabilities may be able to ride a tricycle with the use of self-adhering straps to protect the hands or feet (Fig. 22-1).

One of the more crucial effects of chronic illness or disability on preschoolers is the feeling of guilt that they "caused" the illness through an imagined or real misdeed. This is less of an issue if the child is born with the condition than if it occurs during the preschool period. Such guilt can significantly affect the child's developing but fragile self-esteem. In contrast to the child with a temporary physical disability who has added opportunities for attaining mastery

---

*Access to Respite Care and Help (ARCH)** is a national information center on respite programs: ARCH, c/o Chapel Hill Training Outreach Project, 800 Eastowne Dr, Chapel Hill, NC 27514, (919) 490-5577 or (888) 671-2594 (toll-free), fax:(919) 490-4905; www.chtop.com (look for ARCH icon).

*Information on individual toy selection and on a toy library system for children with sensory deficits, motor disabilities, and developmental delay is available from the **National Lekotek Center,** 2100 Ridge Ave, 2nd floor, Evanston, IL 60201, (847) 328-0001 or (800) 366-7529, e-mail: lekotek@lekotek.org; www.lekotek.org. *Toy Guide for Differently Abled Kids!* is published by Toys-R-Us. The October 1996 issue of *Exceptional Parent* focuses on the issue of toy selection. For information about this excellent magazine, call (877) 372-7368; www.eparent.com.

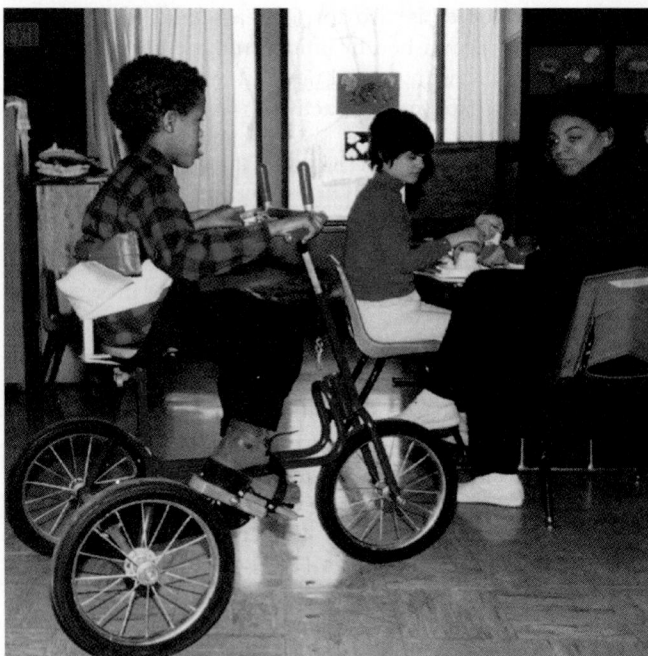

**Fig. 22-1** Modified tricycle with block pedals, self-adhering straps for support, and a modified seat and handlebars can help a child with disabilities gain mobility.

## Critical Thinking Exercise

### Self-Care Skills

You want to encourage self-care skills in children with chronic illness. A preschooler with asthma needs a peak flow reading and receives nebulizer treatments three times daily. You can reasonably suggest which of the following self-care activities as options to the family?

FIRST, THINK ABOUT IT . . .
- What is the purpose of your thinking?
- What conclusions are you reaching?

1. Gather the supplies needed for the treatment.
2. Put medication in a nebulizer cup.
3. Record the peak flow reading on the chart.
4. Turn on the peak flow meter.

*The best response is one. The purpose of your thinking is to focus on the developmental stage of the preschooler, who is old enough to be instructed to gather the needed supplies for the treatment. Also, some preschoolers may be ready to put premeasured medication into the nebulizer cup with parental supervision. Accuracy in measuring medication or recording peak flow readings would not be expected at this age. A peak flow meter is not a powered device.*

and therefore overcoming feelings of inferiority and guilt, the child with a chronic illness or disability may experience frequent insults. Structuring situations to foster success can assist a child in developing a sense of confidence and competence. (See Critical Thinking Exercise box.)

Another critical component for normal child development is discipline. Discipline is essential to the child's sense of security because boundaries are necessary for the child to test behavior; it also teaches the child socially acceptable behavior. Applying appropriate discipline to the child who is chronically ill or disabled can also limit the resentment and hostility that can develop among siblings if different standards are applied to each child. The nurse's responsibility is to help parents learn successful methods of guiding the child. (See Chapter 14.)

When a chronic illness imposes restrictions that cause difficulty with mastery, it can inflict a lasting sense of failure as well. Preschoolers are egocentric and have naive reasoning, which may affect their interpretation and understanding of their illness.

Because preschoolers need to explore and acquire experience with pretend situations and objects before they really experience them, nurses need to facilitate opportunities for imaginative play (e.g., using dolls and syringes) and to give simple answers to their questions about their illness and treatment.

### School-Age Child

School-age children focus on increasing mastery over their environment and independence. A lack of physical stamina may prevent the child with a chronic illness from engaging in school and extracurricular activities and result in feelings of inferiority or inadequacy. These activities influence acquisition of social skills, developing a sense of achievement, gaining the skills resulting in self-sufficiency, and learning to effectively deal with stress. School-age children should be involved as much as possible in their own care and in decision making about their treatment to facilitate their sense of control and mastery.

School-age children are mostly concerned with learning to take initiative (Peters, 1998). School initiates the processes of working toward independence from parents, gaining academic skills, and building peer relationships. Concomitantly with the family, school is the major context in which children develop their sense of self and understanding of their place relative to their peers.

During the school-age period, the child has an increasing ability to distinguish fantasy from reality and self from others, and important advances in reasoning and conceptual abilities occur (Piaget, 1952). Coupled with this limited sense of causality comes a deeper understanding of difference. Children with an illness that is not very obvious may try to hide its existence until forced to admit otherwise when they realize that it differentiates them from their peers (Vessey and Mebane, 2000).

Active inquiry is manifested in the school-age period. School-age children are usually verbal regarding their condition and ask for information about all phases of the illness and treatment. In addition, they experience pride after they learn the correct label for the illness, treatment, and medication. From the beginning, nurses should respond to the child's questions in a simple, direct manner.

The school-age child separates from parents more easily and becomes more active in peer relationships. Peers

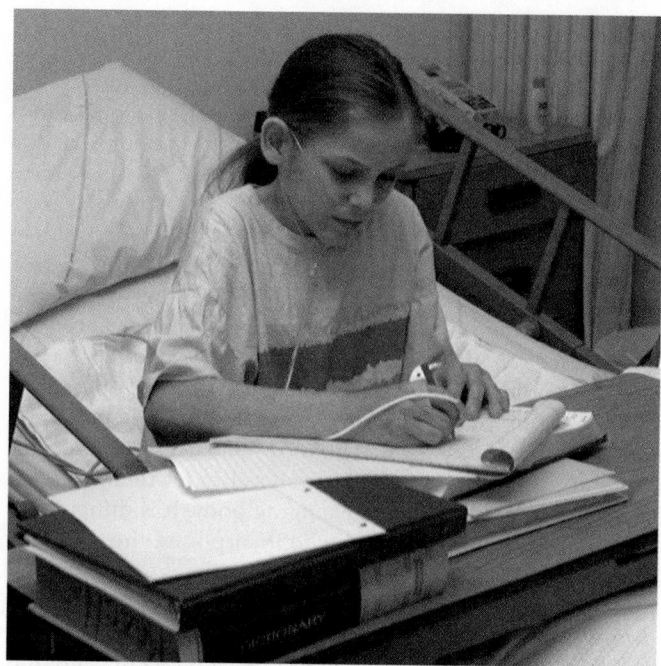

**Fig. 22-2** Children with special needs should continue their schooling as soon as their condition allows.

scription of the child's condition, prepared for any visible changes in the child, and allowed an opportunity to ask questions. The child should have the option to attend this session. As the child's condition changes, particularly if the illness is potentially fatal, school personnel, including the students, need periodic appraisal of the child's status and preparation for what to expect.* (See Chapter 23.)

Children with special needs are encouraged to maintain or reestablish relationships with peers and to participate according to their capabilities in any age-appropriate activities. Alternative activities may be substituted for those that are impossible or that place a strain on their health. It is important for these children to have the opportunity to interact with healthy peers, as well as to engage in activities with groups or clubs composed of similarly affected age-mates. Such organizations as ostomy clubs, diabetic clubs, and cerebral palsy groups share information and provide support related to the special problems the members face.

Programs such as the **Special Olympicst**† offer children with physical disabilities an opportunity to compete with their peers and to achieve athletic skill.‡ Summer camps§ also provide children with unique opportunities to associate with similarly affected peers and develop a wide variety of skills, including increased independence in activities of daily living and self-care associated with their condition. With innovation, many adaptations can be implemented in children's environments to increase their mobility and independence.‖ Technologic advances are mushrooming, especially in the application of computers, and parents should be directed to the latest developments that may help their child.

Children with special needs derive enormous benefits from expressive activities, such as art, music, poetry, dance, and drama. With adaptive equipment and imagination, children can participate in a variety of activities. Organizations such as **VSA arts**¶ offer children an opportunity to celebrate and share their accomplishments.

strongly influence school-age children's opinions of themselves and their self-esteem (Murray, 2000). If not provided with the required skills to disseminate information about their illness to peers, school-age children may withdraw with a diminished self-concept (Vessey and Mebane, 2000).

The number of children with chronic illnesses who return to school has increased in the last decade (Kliebenstein and Broome, 2000). Children need preparation before entering or resuming school. Having a tutor in the hospital or home as soon as children are physically able helps them realize that school will continue and gives them time to consider this prospect (Fig. 22-2). They need to investigate possible answers to the many questions others will ask. One method of anticipatory preparation is to role-play, with the child as the "returned pupil" and the nurse as "other schoolmates." The nurse asks questions about the reason for the child's absence, the name of the disease, and so on. The child is provided with a safe opportunity to explore possible answers and to experience some of the possible reactions of others. If the child returns to school with some obvious physical change, such as hair loss, an amputation, or a visible scar, the nurse might also ask questions about these alterations to prompt preparatory responses from the child.

Initially the child may find it easier to attend half-day school sessions or to participate in a limited number of activities. It is preferable to plan the school program with as much participation and leadership from the child as possible. Once children return, regular assessments of their progress in various areas (academic, social, physical) are essential to ensure a satisfactory adjustment.

Classroom peers also need preparation, and a joint plan involving the schoolteacher, nurse, parents, and child is best. At a minimum the classmates should be given a de-

*Several publications available to help prepare school personnel, health care professionals, and families for the child's return to school are listed at the end of this chapter.
†**Special Olympics, Inc,** 1325 G St, NW, Suite 500, Washington, DC 20005, (202) 628-3630, (800) 700-8585, fax: (202) 824-0200; www.specialolympics.org.
‡The May 1996 issue of *Exceptional Parent* focuses on recreation and fitness for the child with a disability.
§A directory of camps for children with a variety of chronic illnesses or general physical disabilities is available for a fee from **American Camping Association,** Publications Service, 5000 State Rd, 67 N Martinsville, IN 46151-7902, (765) 342-8456 or (800) 428-CAMP, fax: (765) 342-2065; www.aca-camps.org. A camp list is also available from the **Candlelighter's Childhood Cancer Foundation,** 3910 Warner St, Kensington, MD 20895, (301) 962-3520 or (800) 366-2223, fax: (301) 962-3521; www.candlelighters.org. Information on choosing camps for children with disabilities is available from the **National Easter Seal Society,** 230 W Monroe, Suite 1800, Chicago, IL 60606-4802, (312) 726-6200, fax: (312) 726-1494, (800) 221-6827; www.easterseals.com.
‖Excellent publications on adapting the environment for children with disabilities are available from the **National Rehabilitation Information Center,** 1010 Wayne Ave, Suite 800, Silver Spring, MD 20910, (800) 346-2742, fax: (301) 562-2401; www.naric.com.
¶**VSA arts,** an international organization that creates learning opportunities through the arts for individuals with disabilities (VSA-Vision, Strength, and Artistic Expression), has affiliate chapters throughout the United Sates and in selected sites internationally; festivals are held worldwide. Information is available from **VSA arts,** 1300 Connecticut Ave, Suite 700, Washington, DC 20036, (202) 628-2800 or (800) 933-8721, fax: (202) 737-0725; info@vsarts.org.

## Adolescent

Adolescence marks the transitional period from childhood to adulthood and is characterized by important changes in intellectual, physical, social, and psychologic growth and development (Betz, 1998). During this period, adolescents build their ego identity, establish intimate relationships, form a value and belief system that integrates their own and their family's, seek further training and education, and formulate career goals and future plans (Kohlberg, 1969; Piaget and Inhelder, 1958). Acquisition of these crucial developmental tasks may be influenced greatly by a diagnosis of chronic illness (Sands and Wehmeyer, 1996).

Chronic illness may impose the additional burden of hospitalization, pain, surgery, extensive diagnostic testing, medications, school absences, and activity restrictions on the adolescent. Such stressors may provoke many anxieties, fears, and grief reactions (Woodgate, 1998). Illness-related fears include loss of physical integrity, not being able to separate successfully from one's parents, loss of control, being different from peers, and death. Thus adolescents with chronic illness experience a "dual crisis" (Woodgate, 1998). They must cope with not only complex normative developmental tasks, but the stress related to the diagnosis and treatment of life-threatening or long-term illness as well.

The adolescent is striving for autonomy, which is threatened by the forced dependence, compliance, and loss of control associated with an illness and treatment. In addition, the adolescent becomes increasingly independent of his or her parents. Consequently, dealing with the illness may be more difficult and adolescents may be at greater risk for depression, anxiety, and adjustment problems. Many adolescents wish to assume total responsibility for their care despite their inexperience; however, their extensive care needs may prevent this from occurring (Vessey and Miola, 1997). If the chronic illness is associated with mobility limitations forcing dependence on caregivers for basic needs, it may compromise the emergence of a secure sexual and physical identity and peer relationships. (Peters, 1998).

Adolescence is a time for achieving independence from the family and planning for future goals and responsibilities. Adolescents with long-term chronic illness may be less future directed and less independent than well peers. Enforced dependency from physical impairment can exacerbate the parent-child conflicts surrounding independence. Lack of understanding by both parties can result in bitter feelings and intrafamilial turmoil. The tendency toward rebellion may be directed at the disorder and reflected in decreased compliance with treatment, denying the disorder to preserve a sense of normalcy with peers, and risk-taking behavior that can place the teenager in jeopardy, such as driving a car despite a disorder that increases the chance of an accident. Such behaviors can further strain an already tense parent-child relationship.

On the other hand, parents can promote independence by giving the adolescent a greater role in his or her own treatment regimen, encouraging the adolescent to develop a relationship with the physicians and nurses that is not mediated by parents, and promoting normalization principles.

During adolescence hormonal changes elicit the onset of puberty and simultaneously preoccupation with body image (Faro, 1999). The major task of adolescents is to develop their own identity. Hormonal changes must be integrated into the self-image while the adolescent is gaining mastery and control over sexuality and increased physical abilities. During early adolescence this occurs mostly within the peer group. Puberty, a period of rapid uncertainty and change for the adolescent, makes this time more confusing for teenagers with chronic illnesses. Delayed puberty is associated with many illnesses, underscoring the differences between affected and unaffected teenagers.

Most adolescents are embarrassed by their appearance and emerging sexuality. For chronically ill adolescents the illness or its treatment may be most embarrassing and may influence their body image, as well as hinder their sense of mastery and control over a changing body. It is difficult for the adolescent with a disability to incorporate the disability into a changing self-concept and body image. The young person who has a disability or is diagnosed with an illness during the critical adolescent years has more difficulty achieving these tasks than does the adolescent who has been affected since childhood. The earlier the onset of a limiting illness, the better the individual is able to adjust to it. The youngster with a newly acquired condition has the added task of grieving the loss while adapting to the changes occurring as a natural course of events. The adolescent often feels rejected because of personal appearance or inability to participate in activities expected of a healthy teenager. However, during middle adolescence the adolescent has less energy available to deal with illness because emotional resources are being used to meet the normal demands of this developmental period.

Adolescence is a most difficult period to be seen as different by one's peers, and some adolescents may withdraw from social relationships and activities that foster healthy psychosexual development. Appearance, abilities, and skills are highly regarded by peers; an adolescent who is limited in any of these qualities is subject to rejection by this influential group. A sense of feeling different from peers can cause isolation, loneliness, and depression for the adolescent. Some adolescents may decide to participate in risky behaviors, such as unprotected sex and smoking, despite the possible harmful effects, to be accepted by peers. Participation in groups of teenagers with chronic illnesses or disabilities can alleviate feelings of isolation and ease the transition to a meaningful relationship with one person in adulthood.*

The topic of sexuality related to the effects of the illness is an important concern of adolescents, although they seldom initiate a discussion of this sensitive subject. Any likely interference in sexual function due to the disability should be discussed candidly and openly with the adolescent. Un-

---

*Lasting Impressions, a well-developed psychosocial support program for adolescent cancer patients and their parents, provides an excellent model for supporting adolescents with cancer and other chronic conditions. For information about the program, contact Linda Wells, BS, Center for Cancer Treatment and Research, Seven Richland Medical Park, Columbia, SC 29203, (803) 434-3533.

fortunately, many nurses are reluctant to discuss sexual issues with teenagers. Adults often underestimate the degree to which adolescents participate in unrealistic fantasies about sexual activities and related matters, or even in sexual activity itself.

Nurses can facilitate the adolescent's striving for autonomy by allowing and encouraging his or her participation in medical decisions, including cosigning informed consents. Within the confines of the specific treatment center, the adolescent can be given control over the scheduling of procedures and treatments, allowed to view test results or radiographs, and included in discussions of alternative therapies. Adolescents should assume increasing responsibility for management of their illness consistent with their developmental stage, level of maturity, and understanding of their illness. Areas of responsibility may include monitoring their condition, assessing indicators of exacerbation and change, self-medication, and asking for assistance (Perrin, 2000).

## Helping the Child to Cope

Through ongoing contact with the child, the nurse (1) observes the child's reactions to chronic illness or disability, ability to function, and adaptive behaviors within the environment and with significant others; (2) explores the child's own understanding of the nature of his or her illness; and (3) provides support while the child learns to cope with his or her feelings. Children are encouraged to verbalize their concerns rather than allowing others to verbalize for them because open discussions may lessen anxiety.

Parents often express concern because their child cannot communicate the anxieties he or she is feeling. If the child will not or cannot speak, the child may need to play out his or her feelings. Toys can be provided to facilitate the meaning of stressful or threatening emotions. The nurse may realize that the child responds best to telling stories or drawing pictures. (See Chapter 6.)

### Coping Mechanisms

Children's innate and learned coping mechanisms are very crucial in their ability to cope with their conditions. Children with special needs are likely to use distinct coping patterns (Box 22-2). Children with more accepting and positive attitudes about their chronic illness use a more adaptive coping style, characterized by competence, optimism, and

compliance. They display fewer behavior problems at school and at home.

Because it is often easier to recognize children who cope poorly with illness or disability, it is helpful to describe those behaviors typical of well-adjusted children. Well-adapted children gradually learn to accept their physical limitations (Box 22-3).

### Normalization

One of the most important interventions to promote coping is alleviating the child's feeling of being different and normalizing his or her life as much as possible. The principles in the Guidelines box on p. 918 are fundamental in implementing the normalizing process. The nurse can help parents to assess the child's daily routine for indications of

---

**Box 22-2** ■ ■ ☐
### Coping Patterns of Chronically Ill Children

Using family and friends as resources
Developing patterns of coping with their parents
Utilizing the hospital environment to promote coping
Relying on health care professionals for gentle, supportive, and competent care

Modified from Boyd JR, Hunsberger M: Chronically ill children coping with repeated hospitalizations: their perceptions and suggested interventions, *J Pediatr Nurs* 13(6):330-342, 1998.

---

**Box 22-3** ■ ■ ☐
### Individual Characteristics That Affect Coping in Children

**GENDER**
Males are more vulnerable to stress than females.
Females are more likely to use emotional sensory and emotional expression responses than males.
Males are more likely to use physical aggression in coping.

**AGE**
Children between ages 6 months and 4 years are considered most vulnerable.

**TEMPERAMENT**
The "difficult child" is considered more vulnerable than the easy child.
The more active, strong-willed child seems to cope better than the passive child.

**PREEXISTING CONDITIONS**
The child with preexisting anxiety is considered at greater risk for coping poorly.

**SELF-CONCEPT**
The child with low self-esteem and/or a low sense of self-direction is at greater risk for coping poorly.

**SOCIAL SKILLS**
The child with few social skills is at greater risk for coping poorly.

**GENETIC FACTORS**
Inborn traits influence the overall ability to adapt (e.g., vulnerability to alcoholism, sociopathy, mood disorders).

**INTELLIGENCE**
Children with above-average intelligence tend to have fewer psychiatric problems than children with lower intelligence.

**HARDINESS/RESILIENCE**
Positive behavioral patterns and favorable outcomes can be affected by a combination of temperament, familial traits, and support factors.

Data from Adams P, Fras I: *Beginning child psychiatry*, New York, 1988, Brunner/Mazel; Garmezy N: Resilience in children's adaptation to negative life events and stressed environments, *Pediatr Ann* 20(9):459-466, 1991; and Sorensen E: Children's coping responses, *J Pediatr Nurs* 5(4):259-267, 1990.

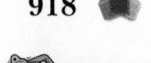

## GUIDELINES
### *Promoting Normalization*

**Preparation.** Prepare the child in advance for changes that may occur from the illness or disability; for example, the child is told in advance of the possible side effects of drug therapy.

**Participation.** Include the child in as many decisions as possible, especially those relating to his or her care regimen; for example, the child is responsible for taking medications or scheduling home treatments.

**Sharing.** Allow both family members and the child's peers to be a part of the care regimen whenever possible; for example, the child is given his or her medication when the other siblings receive their vitamins; the parent cooks the same menu for the whole family; and if the child is invited to another's home, the parent advises the family of the child's dietary restrictions.

**Control.** Identify areas where the child can be in control so that feelings of uncertainty, passivity, and helplessness are decreased; for example, the child identifies activities that are appropriate to his or her energy level and chooses to rest when fatigued.

**Expectations.** Apply the same family rules to the child with a chronic illness or disability as to the well siblings or peers; for example, the child is disciplined, expected to fulfill household responsibilities, and attends school in accordance with abilities.

**Positive attitude.** Focus, and help the child to focus, on areas of ability and competence to build self-esteem.

## GUIDELINES
### *Facilitating Hopefulness*

Give honest reports of conditions or events.

Encourage and participate with the child in physical activities (e.g., arrange activities, play games, or go for walks together).

Convey a fond, personal interest in the child (give hugs, ask follow-up questions from previous discussions).

Introduce conversations on neutral, non–disease-related or less sensitive topics (discuss child's favorite sports, tell stories).

Convey competence and gentleness when delivering care.

Provide information about other children in similar situations who are doing well.

Encourage the child to think ahead to more comfortable and preferred natural times.

Be lighthearted and initiate or respond to teasing or other playful interactions with the child.

Modified from Hinds P, Martin J, Vogel RJ: Nursing strategies to influence adolescent hopefulness during oncologic illness, *J Assoc Pediatr Oncol Nurs* 4(1/2):14-22, 1987.

normalizing practices. For example, the child who remains in a bedroom all day needs a restructured daily routine to provide activities in different parts of the house, such as eating in the kitchen with the family, and the inclusion of social, recreational, and academic activities in the plan of care.

Children who are concerned that their condition detracts from their physical attractiveness need attention focused on the normal aspects of appearance and capabilities. Health professionals can help parents strengthen and consolidate the child's self-image by emphasizing the normal, while at the same time allowing children to express anger, isolation, fear of rejection, feelings of sadness, and loneliness. Anything that might improve attractiveness and contribute to a positive self-image is encouraged, such as makeup for a teenager with a scar, clothing that disguises a prosthesis, or a hairstyle or wig to cover a deformity or lost hair.

The parent's behavior, particularly in relation to childrearing, is one of the most critical influences in the child's adaptation to chronic illness. For example, children who are reared by parents who establish reasonable limits are likely to develop independence that is appropriate for their age and achievement commensurate with their limitations. They frequently exhibit confidence and pride in their ability to cope successfully with the challenges resulting from their condition. On the contrary, children whose parents are overprotective are likely to have fearfulness, marked dependency, inactivity, and few outside interests. Using anticipatory guidance and encouragement of normalizing practices, the nurse may assist parents in facilitating positive adaptation in their children. Normalization is important because it focuses on the child, not the condition.

Nurses can demonstrate the process of normalization to the child's family by acknowledging the strengths and weaknesses of the family unit, by being supportive and open about the child's condition and treatment, and by actively including the family in all aspects of care (Shepard and Mahon, 2000). If the child's family adopts a normalized view of management of the chronic illness, the child may be more confident in the home, as well as in social and community situations. Thus the family's perception of the impact and the integration of the chronic illness may directly or indirectly improve the child's adaptation (Amer, 1999).

Nurses also can assist parents by identifying and building on family strengths, promoting family and child competence, and fostering the development of a nurturing environment that addresses the needs of siblings and parents, as well as the child with special needs.

### Hopefulness

Children, especially adolescents, are sensitive to the presence or absence of hope. From a psychologic perspective, Erikson's theory of psychosocial growth and development proposes that hope is a basic ego quality that is initially experienced in infancy and is the positive outcome of the developmental task of trust vs mistrust (Ritchie, 2001).

Hopefulness has two functions: (1) to protect the adolescent from incapacitating despair and (2) to assist the adolescent in coping with a situation wherein personal needs are unmet (Lazarus, 1981). A sense of hopefulness can result in increased participation in health-seeking behaviors and an improved sense of well-being. Nurses can be instrumental in facilitating hopefulness through environmental and interpersonal means. (See Guidelines box above.)

### Health Education/Self-Care

Health education prepares children in self-care behaviors and development of self-advocacy skills for dealing with the health care community. These are important skills for children and adolescents with chronic conditions to master because they are likely to use the health care system frequently throughout their lives (Vessey and Mebane, 2000). Active participation in care requires comprehensive family and patient education. Empowerment of individuals with disabilities is the philosophy that is currently advocated for provision of services. Targeting adolescents, this patient population can be empowered with the information needed to make responsible choices. Gaining access to information helps the individual make informed decisions and acquire some control over the environment (Hauser and Dorn, 1999).

Children need information about how their body works, characteristics of their condition, the treatment plan, the impact of illness or therapy, and when age-appropriate, the intricacies of the health care system. Education is a primary component of self-care, and teaching methods must be modified to meet the child's developmental age. In addition, children near puberty need to understand the maturation process and how their disability may change this event. For example, the child with Crohn disease should know that this illness is linked with delayed puberty and growth failure; the child with diabetes needs to understand that increased growth needs and hormonal changes will change insulin and food requirements at this time; and the sexually active girl with systemic lupus erythematous or sickle cell anemia needs to be aware of the risks of pregnancy. The information should not be provided during a single teaching session, but rather timed appropriately to meet the changing needs of the child, and it should be de-

scribed and repeated as frequently as the situation warrants. (See Evidence-Based Practice box.)

For young children the information presented needs to be concise, simple, and honest, even if the news is not positive. Questions should be answered openly because children need answers to questions they are able to ask. If they have no confidence in the answer provided or are ignored, the only alternative left to them is to relate their experience to something fantasized or seen on television (Peters, 1998). If young children verbalize that they do not want to learn more, then their wishes should be respected.

Developing the judgment and expertise for participating in self-care of chronic illness or disability is a process that occurs gradually. Self-care necessitates negotiation between child and parents. Nurses can be instrumental in providing information on strategies for teaching children of various ages in self-care (Faulkner, 1996).

## Realistic Future Goals

Concomitant with prolonged survival for many chronic illnesses, these individuals are confronted with new decisions and problems such as employment,* marriage, and insurance coverage. (See Evidence-Based Practice box on p. 920.) Adolescents usually look forward to what their lives will be like in the future.

One of the most difficult adjustments to some chronic illnesses or severe disabilities is establishing realistic goals for the child and for those involved in his or her continual care. Occasionally the impact of this decision does not surface until the child graduates from school or the parents move toward retirement, when a crisis can arise because all the family roles and relationships that maintained stability are now disrupted.

For those children with severe disabilities, preparing for the future should be a gradual process. All along the child and parents should consider realistic vocational options. For example, children with physical disabilities can be directed to artistic, intellectual, or musical pursuits. Children with developmental disabilities can be instructed in manual skills. Thus the child's development progresses to self-support through gainful employment.

Unfortunately, vocational pursuits and independence are not realistic goals for all persons. Persons with multiple or severe disabilities may require lifelong care and assistance. In these situations parents must look to the time when they will no longer be able to care for their child. Advance financial planning should be considered (Rosenfeld, 1994). Residential placement may be very difficult unless the family mutually participates in the decision-making and planning process. Care outside the home should not be

*Information about employment is available from the **Office of Disability Employment Policy (ODEP) for the Department of Labor,** 1331 F St NW, Suite 300, Washington, DC 20004-1107, (202) 376-6200, fax: (202) 376-6219; www.pcepd.gov. The Americans with Disabilities Act ensures that most employers can neither ask questions related to health and disability nor discriminate based on disability; more information can be obtained from the **ADA Center** at (800) 949-4232; www.adainfo.org. The **Job Accommodation Network** provides information about job accommodations and the employability of individuals with disabilities (800) 526-7234; www.jan.wvu.edu.

## EVIDENCE-BASED PRACTICE
*Issues Facing Survivors of a Chronic Illness*

Chronically ill adolescents are faced with a number of serious dilemmas as they enter adulthood. For example, should they share the truth of their condition with dating partners, prospective spouses, or potential employers? Should they seek a job with good health insurance rather than pursue a career with fewer employee benefits?

Employment-related discrimination has improved because of better legal regulations and education. However, rates of unemployment for individuals with chronic conditions are 50% to 71%, compared with the general population rates of 3% to 5% (Sawin, Cox, and Metzger, 2000). Only 1 in 500 individuals receiving Supplemental Security Insurance (SSI) ever permanently discontinue their coverage (U.S. General Accounting Office, 1998). A U.S. General Accounting Office (GAO) survey of unemployed adults in 1998 cited many viewpoints about employment disincentives, including (a) uncertainty about their health situation, (b) their fear of losing health insurance, (c) lack of job site stability, (d) negative employer attitudes, and (e) limited workplace accommodations. Personal motivation factors and quality of family and social support network were found to be psychosocial factors having an influence on employment status. Nurses can discuss with adolescents the appropriateness of career and employment choices and the impact of their chronic illness (Betz, 1999).

For those whose conditions are genetic in origin, there is a need for counseling about future offspring. Future spouses often benefit from an opportunity to discuss their feelings about marriage to an individual with continued health needs and possibly, a limited life span.

Until recently, health insurance coverage was a crucial issue because some private carriers no longer insured a young person who left home or might be reluctant to reinsure the person who is no longer a dependent. Federal legislation now mandates continuing coverage. Life insurance is another dilemma, particularly when children have serious defects (e.g., congenital cardiac anomalies).

Consent and confidentiality are frequent dilemmas in providing care to any minor adolescent and are often made more complex by the teenager's health problem. Two principles may be used when making consent and confidentiality decisions: the principle of **autonomy,** which states that a person should have a say in any action that will affect him or her, and the principle of **benevolence,** which states that whenever something beneficial can be done, it should be done.

---

- Knowledge of the condition and its management
- Readiness to assume responsibility for treatment management
- Prior involvement and compliance with the treatment regimen
- Demonstration of responsible and independent judgment
- Prior response to emergency situations
- Coping ability
- Attitude of pediatric provider to transition

Nurses can take steps to help the adolescent prepare for the transition. These include presenting the idea of transfer; assessing the readiness of the adolescent and parent; coordinating a meeting with the adolescent, the family, and both pediatric and adult care providers; and formally, acknowledging the transfer (Russell, Reinbold, and Maltby, 1996).

Nurses can be instrumental in assisting and supporting adolescents in assuming responsibility for managing their own care as much as possible. Adolescents should be encouraged to actively participate in the planning and decision-making processes for transition to adult care. In addition, nurses can foster continuity of care by providing information to adult health care providers about the needs of the adolescent relating to disease management and the adolescent's compliance with the treatment regimen. The ultimate goal of transition care to adulthood for the adolescent with a chronic illness is to promote the achievement of responsible self-care and linkages to adult health care services, thus enabling the best prospects for educational options, social networks and relationships, community living, and employment (Betz, 1998, 1999).

## THE FAMILY OF THE CHILD WITH SPECIAL NEEDS

A major goal in working with the family of a child with special needs is to support the family's coping and foster their optimum functioning throughout the child's life. Long-term, comprehensive, family-centered approaches extend beyond supporting the child and family during the crucial periods of diagnosis and hospitalization. Comprehensive care involves building parent-professional partnerships that can support a family's adaptation to the many changes that may be necessary in everyday life, defining expectations of and for the child, and providing a long-term perspective (Box 22-4).

---

viewed as abandonment. Not infrequently it is the only way to preserve the family unit. The nurse should help the family investigate suitable placements, discuss their feelings regarding this decision, and explore measures to maintain meaningful communication with the member who has a disability. The nurse can take a larger, advocacy role to educate the public regarding persons with special needs and help normalize the experience for the child, the family, and the community.

Determining readiness for transfer to adult providers is a primary consideration. Arbitrary transfer to adult services based solely on age criterion can compromise both psychosocial and physical care for some young adults. Many adolescents have received care in the same medical setting since birth and have established a trusting relationship with practitioners and staff. Moreover, age is not an indicator of adolescent readiness for transfer to an adult care provider. Important factors include the following (Betz, 1999):

**TABLE 22-2**   Assessment of factors affecting family adjustment

| Factors Affecting Adjustment | Assessment Questions |
|---|---|
| **Available support system** | |
| Marital or other partner relationship | Are you and your spouse (partner) able to discuss your child's condition and care? |
| Alternate support systems | When something is worrying you, what do you do? |
| | What helps you most when you are upset? |
| Ability to communicate | Does talking seem to help when you feel upset? |
| | Do you have people you can talk to about your child's condition? |
| **Perception of the illness/disability** | |
| Previous knowledge of disorder | Have you ever heard the word (name of diagnosis) before? Tell me about it (if answer is yes). |
| Influence of religion | Has your religion or faith been of help to you? Tell me how (if answer is yes). |
| Influence of culture | In your culture, what do people think about this condition? Are there special treatments used? |
| Imagined cause of disorder | What are your thoughts about the causes of the disorder? |
| Effects of illness or disability on family | How has your child's illness or disability affected you and your family? |
| | How has your lifestyle changed? |
| **Coping mechanisms** | |
| Reactions to previous crises | Tell me one time you've had another serious problem in your family. How did you solve that problem? |
| Reactions to the child | Do you find yourself being a little more cautious with this child than with your other children? |
| Childrearing practices | Do you feel as comfortable disciplining this child as compared with your other children? |
| Attitudes | How is this child different from the siblings or other children of similar age? |
| | Describe your child's personality. Is it easy, difficult, or in-between? |
| | When you think of your child's future, what thoughts come to mind? |
| **Available resources** | What parts of your child's care are the most difficult for you and your family? |
| | What services are available to help? |
| | What services do you need that presently are not available? |
| **Concurrent stresses** | What other problems are you facing now? (Be specific—ask about employment, financial, family issues). |

## Assessing Family Strengths and Adjustment

The purpose of a family assessment is to determine what assistance a family may need or want in managing the care of their child. Ideally an assessment should be initiated as soon as the family learns the diagnosis. Integral in the family-centered care philosophy, the family should be an active participant in the process. Sample questions designed to elicit information for assessing the family's adjustment are listed in Table 22-2. Family members should always be informed of the purpose of the assessment, including the rationale for personal questions. They should be afforded the opportunity to participate or not as they choose.

A number of instruments can be used to assess the family's overall functioning and support system. (See Chapter 6.) In addition, specific tools have been developed for families of children with chronic illness or disability. For example, the *Coping Health Inventory for Parents (CHIPS)* is an 80-item checklist that provides self-report information about how parents perceive their overall response to the management of family life with a child with a chronic illness. Coping behaviors (e.g., "believing that my child[ren] will get better" or "talking with the hospital staff [nurses, social workers] when we visited the medical center") are listed, and parents are asked to rate "how helpful" (0 to 3) the coping items are to them in managing the home situation (McCubbin and others, 1993). Tools that a family can use to assess their home environment and resources are described in Chapter 25.

Regardless of the approach, assessment should be a continual process. Because support systems may change and the perception of events may be altered at any time during an illness, nurses must assist families on an ongoing basis in evaluating the effectiveness of changes and interventions in support needs.

## Accepting the Child's Condition/ Support at the Time of Diagnosis

The impact of a child's developmental or medical condition is often experienced as a crisis at the time of diagnosis, which may be during birth, following a long period of psychologic and/or physical testing, or soon after a tragic injury. It may also begin before the diagnosis, when parents know that something is wrong with their child but there has been no medical confirmation (Cohen, 1995).

Interventions facilitating parental adjustment to the diagnosis of their child's chronic illness or disability and their ability to care for their child include planning the setting for informing parents, assessing the family's prior knowledge and experience about chronic conditions (see Family Focus box on p. 922), selecting strategies that best meet the family's needs and situation, evaluating the family's understanding of the information presented, and ongoing follow-up. Effectively "discussing the diagnosis" provides a vital foundation for a strong collaborative relationship between parents and health care providers that will be needed in the future.

The physician or advanced practice nurse usually informs the family of the child's diagnosis. Nurses are also responsible for providing follow-up information and coordinating services with other agencies. Whatever role the nurse assumes, some guidelines can be used during the dis-

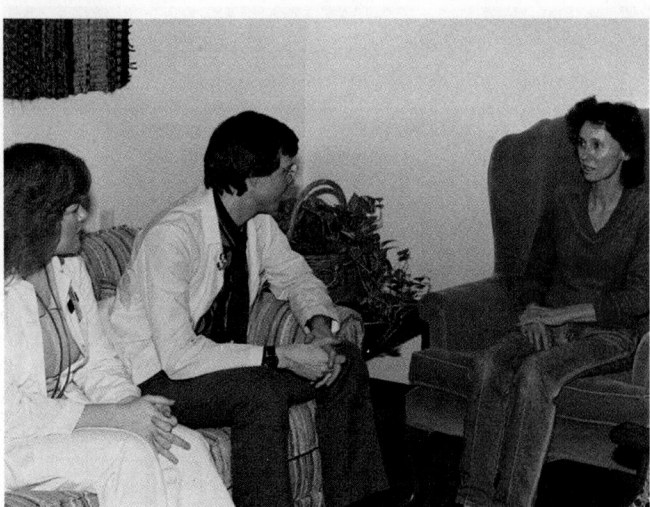

**Fig. 22-3** Informing sessions should take place in a private, comfortable setting free of distractions and interruptions.

closure of the diagnosis to offer the family support at this crucial time. (See Guidelines box.)

The informing conference should take place in a private, comfortable setting free of interruptions and distractions. (Fig. 22-3.) The environment should be one in which parents feel free to show their emotions. If their emotions can be expressed and acknowledged, parents can be helped to deal openly with them, and their need for additional counseling can be determined. Parents often sense a certain attitude of rejection, acceptance, hope, or despair that may affect their ability to assimilate the shock and begin adapting to the implications the illness has for their future.

The emotional needs of parents at the time of diagnosis are acknowledged by exhibiting acceptance of such expressions as sadness, crying, disappointment, and anger. Emotional support is provided by having tissues available if a family member cries and showing through body and facial language that indeed this is a painful and difficult time. Even though touching is a strong expression of empathy, it must be used cautiously. For example, it can prematurely terminate free expression of feelings, particularly when combined with statements such as "Everything will be all right." Nurses should also be cognizant of cultural sensitivity regarding touching. (See Chapter 2.)

Nurses should observe the responses of family members upon hearing the diagnosis. Their facial expressions, their ability to maintain eye contact with the nurse, the times they look down, their behaviors that demonstrate that they are avoiding what the nurse is saying (such as turning their heads, looking away, or looking around), and any other activities that demonstrate that they are dealing with a very difficult matter are observed.

One of the most supportive interventions is to accept the family's emotional reactions to the diagnosis in a nonjudgmental manner. Even though all families react differently and in varying degrees of intensity, three reactions are common and frequently poorly managed: guilt, denial, and anger.

Parents should receive the kind of information they want. Most parents prefer a simple, clear explanation of the diag-

## FAMILY FOCUS
### Meaning of the Chronic Illness or Disability

The meaning and significance of the child's condition to the family are influenced by individual perceptions of the diagnosis. Nurses can help families evaluate the influence of their previous knowledge about and imagined causes of the disorder, religious beliefs, and culture on their perceptions. These beliefs will influence coping strategies.

Although family members may be shocked to learn that their child has a serious illness or disability, they usually have some prior knowledge about the disorder from previous reading or associations. Nurses can help families explore the accuracy and completeness of their previous knowledge. Some people, for example, think that a diagnosis of cancer is always terminal.

While the causes of many disorders are unknown, people commonly feel a need to supply a reason for an illness or disability. Sometimes reasons are associated with cultural or religious beliefs, but they may also be influenced by previous events. Children, for example, may interpet the illness as a punishment for disobedience. Parents may be convinced that the condition was inherited or due to behaviors during pregnancy. Once the fantasy cause is revealed, family members can be helped to consider the implications of that thinking and to move beyond feelings of guilt, blame, or anger.

Religious beliefs and spirituality are a source of meaning and support for many people. For some, healing and faith are synonymous, and any criticism of the family's spirituality can weaken their trust in medical care. For others, religious beliefs may intensify feelings of guilt, shame, or punishment. Some may ask: "What have I done to deserve this?" or "God, why are you punishing me in this way?" Such statements should be taken seriously; the person should be helped to explore the reason why he or she believes the condition is a punishment.

Culture influences the understanding of illness or disability and appropriate treatment strategies. Families can be helped to express their culturally related beliefs about causes and severity of the condition and treatments that may be culturally specific or that may conflict with cultural beliefs. A respectful approach has the goal of both explaining the beliefs and approaches of health care providers and supporting the family's culturally determined needs.

nosis, including what is and is not known about the diagnosis, a prediction of possible prospects for the child, advice on what to do next, an opportunity to ask questions, a sympathetic and warm listener, and, most important, time. The family's level of understanding and expectations should be determined. Clarification of explanations is elicited with such questions as "Is this clear to you?" or "Do you see what I mean?" Notes can be taken for the family to refer to in the future. Parents can be provided with supplemental written information or a written summary of the diagnosis congruent with the emotional readiness of the family.

A crucial task for parents is to decide when, what, and how to tell their child about the diagnosis. Like parents, children later remember vividly what happened when the diagnosis was disclosed. Ideally the parents should be responsible for sharing this information with their child. However, they need much guidance in communicating information about the nature of the illness and changes imposed on physical appearance and energy using a calm and honest approach. This is because parents frequently use euphemisms and try to protect their child from the harsh realities of the diagnosis and illness. Nurses can promote

## GUIDELINES
*Informing the Family of a Serious Condition*

**INITIAL DISCUSSION**

Discuss suspicions of a problem with parents when waiting for a definite diagnosis to help prepare them for a potentially serious diagnosis.

Have both parents present or have a friend or family member accompany a single parent.

Let the practitioner who knows the family best present the diagnosis with the primary nurse present.

Share information about the child's diagnosis:

Use the correct terminology for the diagnosis.

Avoid names of symptoms to define the disorder that immediately have negative connotations. For example, instead of saying "Down syndrome is retardation," say, "Down syndrome is a chromosome abnormality." Once the dialogue has begun, tell parents other characteristics of the condition (e.g., "A characteristic of Down syndrome is mental retardation").

Mention alternative names for the condition.

Discuss the possible range of functioning.

Explain other medical problems and how these are or are not related to the child's diagnosis.

Be willing to repeat information if necessary.

Convey kindness and understanding by sitting down near the parents, touching the parent's hand or shoulder, having tissues available, calling the child by name, and saying the parent's name during the conversation.

Stress the personhood of the child by showing love, concern, and respect for the child as an individual.

Allow parents to express emotion and to work through feelings naturally.

Encourage parents to ask questions, and provide a telephone number for them to call with questions later or if they just want to talk more.

Be patient if the parents continue to ask the same questions.

Help parents feel competent and in control:

Assure parents that they will be kept informed to enable them to participate effectively in decision making regarding their child's treatment and care.

Provide parents with information about parent support groups or family resource centers, as well as knowledge about services and resources and financial assistance programs.

Ask for permission to call and give their name and phone number to a parent self-help organization, enabling the organization to reach out to them.

Discuss the siblings and assure parents that siblings tend to do well, especially if kept informed and included in the child's care.

**ONGOING INFORMATION**

Share complete information with parents on an ongoing basis.

Share information in manageable doses. Ask parents what information they want to receive at a given time to determine readiness and to avoid overload.

Be sensitive to parents' reactions.

Listen carefully when parents identify their needs, remembering that they may not always know the level of service they require (e.g., that respite service is having someone else take over for a while so they can get some rest).

Provide technical information in understandable terms, yet link these explanations with medical terminology.

Explain why certain questions are being asked.

Offer to share information with the child or with others involved in the child's care (e.g., brothers, sisters, grandparents, other extended family members, teachers, caregivers).

Provide information on family support programs, referrals for specialty consultations and intervention programs, and opportunities to meet other parents whose child has a similar condition.

---

open communication between parents and their ill child by providing them with information about how young children think and respond to illness and to changes in their parents (crying or increased concern).

**NURSING TIP** Develop a glossary of commonly used technical, medical, or discipline-specific terms and acronyms to give to parents. The list can stand alone or be included in patient or parent handbooks.

Lastly, the informing conference should not conclude with the presentation of devastating news. Rather, the child's appealing behaviors, strengths, and potential for development need to be emphasized, as well as available treatment or rehabilitation. The parents are also assured that the nurse will be available to answer questions and to provide further assistance as needed in the future. Due to the need for long-term follow-up of chronic conditions, the initial informing conference is only one in a series of ongoing discussions. In all interactions the family's input is requested and included in the plan of care. (See Guidelines box on p. 937.)

## Managing the Condition on an Ongoing Basis

Promoting the family's adaptation to the day-to-day management of the child's condition involves education about the child's condition, general health care, developmental needs of the child, and realistic goal setting. Emotional support and assessment of the family also play a pivotal role in adaptation. Encourage families to articulate their goals and approaches to managing their children's condition, thus providing vital information on how to intervene more thoughtfully with families based on their treatment approach.

Because the majority of mothers and fathers of children with special needs have little or no experience with children who have chronic or disabling conditions, the nurse can remind them of their child's many strengths and normal traits. Mothers and fathers need to experience happiness, success, and pride in their children. The nurse can model appropriate interventions with the child. Most importantly, the nurse should ensure that the siblings and parents learn to perceive the child as a child first, with unique and individual needs and characteristics. The nurse needs to convey an accepting, humanistic attitude toward the child so that the parents can observe this acceptance. This attitude of having concern for, liking, and demonstrating acceptance of the child should begin in early infancy and continue throughout the child's life.

### Special Information Needs

Educating the family about the child's condition is actually a continuation of the diagnostic talk. (See Guidelines box above.)

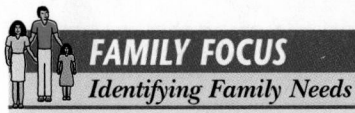

Education involves providing technical information regarding management of the condition, such as how to administer insulin injections, and assessing both parental skills and understanding. In childhood cancer, educational components may include facilitating understanding and adherence to a chemotherapy protocol, administering chemotherapy medications at home, anticipating and treating side effects, managing the child's adjustment to the illness, and provision of support and care from home health agencies and community resources (Clarke-Steffen, 1997). Discussions with parents must also address the impact of the condition on the child. For example, children who have lost a limb require more than an explanation about the prosthetic leg. They need to know the restrictions it imposes on their activity level and how to function with it.

Parents also need guidance on how the child's condition may interfere with activities of daily living (ADLs), such as dressing, eating, toileting, and sleeping.* (See Family Focus box.) Common nutritional problems include overnutrition, resulting from a caloric intake in excess of energy expenditure or boredom and lack of stimulation in other areas, and undernutrition, usually caused by food being inappropriately restricted, vomiting, loss of appetite, increased metabolic needs, or motor deficits that interfere with feeding. Even though the child has the same basic needs as other children, the daily requirements may vary. Special nutritional considerations appropriate in this situation are discussed throughout the text.

Another major area in which modifications may be warranted is car safety. Children with conditions such as orthopaedic, respiratory, or neuromuscular problems or low birth weight often cannot safely use conventional car restraints. For example, children with hip spica casts are unable to sit properly in child safety seats. (See Developmental Dysplasia of the Hip, Chapter 11). Alterations can be made to some commercial models,† and for older children a special vest‡ is available that secures the child in a lying-down position to the back seat. Children in wheelchairs present special challenges because the wheelchair should be anchored with four points of attachment to the vehicle (two in front and two behind) and should always face forward. The family should contact the wheelchair manufacturer for specific instructions to ensure safe car transportation.

Children with special needs require the usual primary health care recommended for any child. Anticipatory guidance, including attention to immunizations, injury prevention, dental health, and regular physical examinations, is important. Nurses play a pivotal role in reminding parents regarding these issues that are so frequently neglected when the concern is focused on the child's specific illness or disability. (See Recommendations for Health Supervision in Chapter 7 for assessing the general aspects of health maintenance.) Specific discussions of sleep and activity, nutrition, dental health, and injury prevention are presented in the chapters on health promotion for particular age groups. See Chapter 12 for a discussion of immunizations.

Parents also need to be aware of the importance of communicating the child's condition in the event of an emergency. Young children are unable to give information regarding their condition, and older children may be unable or unwilling to speak following an accident. Thus all children with any type of chronic condition that may affect medical care should carry some type of identification, such as a Medic-Alert bracelet,* which lists the medical condition and a collect telephone number for access to emergency medical records and other vital information.

### Family Management Styles

Families who have a child with a chronic illness are confronted with multiple challenges, such as making sense of the illness in regard to its meaning for their life, mastering demanding treatment regimens, accommodating the family budget and routine to the demands of the illness, creating a normal life for the child despite the illness, and negotiating with school and health care professionals.

Family management style is the configuration formed by individual family members, the management behaviors they engage in with regard to the chronic condition, and the sociocultural context in which these behaviors occur (Shepard and Mahon, 2000). Five distinct family management styles have been identified: thriving, accommodating, enduring, struggling, and floundering.

Thriving and accommodative families perceive the condition and the child as "normal." Parents are confident in their ability to manage the illness; children see themselves as "healthy." Accommodative families differ from thriving families by perceiving their situation as essentially normal, but somewhat more negatively. They also take a more compliant approach to illness management. Enduring families view having a child with a chronic illness as difficult, having major consequences for family life, and describe illness management as a burden. In contrast to the thriving and accommodating management styles, these families perceive their child as a tragic figure, someone whose life chances have been irreparably compromised because of the illness, and are more protective of the child. Struggling families are

---

*Home care instruction sheets, which may be copied and given to families, are available in Wong DL, Hess CS: *Wong and Whaley's clinical manual of pediatric nursing,* St Louis, ed 5, 2000, Mosby.

†Information on restraints for children with special needs is available from **Automotive Safety for Children Program,** Riley Hospital for Children, 575 West Dr, Room 004, Indianapolis, IN 46202, (317) 274-2977 or (800) KID-N-CAR (in Indiana), fax: (317) 278-0399.

‡E-Z-On Vest is available from E-Z-On Products, 605 Commerce Way West, Jupiter, FL 33458, (561) 747-6920 or (800) 323-6598 (outside Florida), fax: (561) 747-8779; www.ezonpro.com.

---

*2323 Colorado Ave, Turlock, CA 95382, (800) 432-5378, fax: (209) 669-2450.

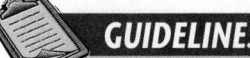

characterized by conflict over how best to manage their child's condition. Struggling parents perceive less support and mutuality from one another, especially mothers who feel they receive inadequate support from their spouses in illness management. Lastly, in floundering families the overriding theme is confusion. Parents view the illness negatively and perceive the child as a tragic figure. They are uncertain about the best management approaches, and illness management is viewed as burdensome and difficult (Shepard and Mahon, 2000).

Understanding the various ways in which families may respond to a chronic illness, specifically how they define the situation, manage daily life, handle conflict, and work jointly can help nurses develop interventions tailored to the unique problems and strengths individual families encounter in managing the illness. Tailored interventions may best foster optimal adaptation (see discussion of coping strategies on p. 931).

## Meeting the Child's Normal Developmental Needs

General strategies for meeting a child's normal developmental needs in both the home and school settings include normalizing practices such as emphasizing abilities, deemphasizing limitations, structuring the environment to promote age-appropriate development, and providing appropriate discipline. (See earlier discussion of these issues under Impact of Chronic Illness or Disability on the Child.)

For parents the task of meeting the child's normal developmental needs is integrally related to accepting the child's condition. (Garwick and others, 1998). Thus helping a family become aware of their reactions to the diagnosis and their reactions to managing the condition can help them evaluate their readiness to support the child's needs (see Table 22-2 for assessment questions).

While questioning parents about their reactions and understanding, the nurse can help them to focus on the child's and sibling's knowledge of the condition. It is not uncommon for parents who appear knowledgeable and well-adjusted to acknowledge that they have never told the children the truth about the illness. Conflict arises when the siblings or child learn of the diagnosis from nonparental sources. Parents may need assistance in deciding how best to explain a condition to children of various ages. (See Informing Children of a Life-Threatening Diagnosis, Chapter 23.)

Special challenges are present when assessing children's feelings about having a disability. The discussion on communication techniques in Chapter 6 focuses on a number of approaches to encourage children to discuss feelings regarding their diagnosis and future. For example, using play and drawing as a method of communication is appropriate for any child dealing with difficult feelings or the child who may lack verbal skills.

School is the second most important setting for a child. Teachers have a profound influence on the child's developmental progress, learning ability, feelings of self-esteem, and formation of social relationships. Whenever possible, nurses should ask parents for permission to visit the school to ob-

### GUIDELINES
#### Assessing Child's Home and School Environment

Observe the child's home and classroom behaviors, such as the ability to sit, follow directions, and comply with requests; determine appropriate responses to questions; and determine the child's independence in functioning.

Gather data on reported behavioral problems such as "hyperactivity," "noncompliance," or "stubbornness."

Observe the child's interactions with siblings and peers.

Observe the child's behaviors in structured and nonstructured activities.

Observe the parents' and teacher's appropriate and nonappropriate interactions with the child.

Observe the parents' and teacher's teaching strategies with the child. (Are school strategies consistent with home teaching?)

Observe the child's relationships with adults.

Determine the parents' and teacher's concerns and expectations of the child.

Administer standardized screening tools with the parent or teacher.

Observe the child's energy level and any illness-related symptoms in relation to the daily schedule.

Observe the child's behavior before, during, and following a medication regimen.

Observe the child's eating patterns at home and at school.

Collaborate with the parents and teacher in future planning for the child.

Determine the effectiveness of programs of care for the child.

Coordinate parents, teachers, and others' plans for the child.

Assess the teacher's and school nurse's understanding of the child's disorder.

serve the child's interaction and behavior with classmates and teachers. A summary of objectives for home and school visits is presented in the Guidelines box.

## Meeting Developmental Needs of Other Family Members

Each family who has a child with special needs is affected by the experience. The effects on the parents and their responses are so critical that they directly influence the other members' reactions and the child's own coping.

### Parents

Grieving for the loss of a perfect child and managing the demands of caregiving can place many strains on parents. Box 22-5 contains a list of stresses faced by families. In addition, parents may or may not receive positive feedback from interactions with their child. Many parents of children with special needs feel satisfaction and fulfillment from the parenting role. Adequate information, parent-to-parent support, collaboration with health care providers, and other resources can support and empower many parents. However, for others, parenting a child with a disability or chronic illness may be a series of unrewarding experiences that continually undermine the parents' feelings of adequacy and competence. These responses may be most evident in parents who are responsible for the child's care. For example, they may become preoccupied with

## Box 22-5 ■ ■ ■
### Stresses of Families with a Child with Special Needs

**DAY-TO-DAY STRESSES**

Constant attention required by the child
Reactions of other children and the larger community
Social relations
Effect on siblings
Marital relations

**LIFE MAINTENANCE STRESSES**

Financial stress, insurance
Housing
Transportation
Clothing and appliances

**WORRIES ABOUT THE FUTURE**

Future children
Schooling and vocational training
Residential care

**ANTICIPATED PARENTAL STRESS**

Diagnosis of the condition—requires considerable education, as well as dealing with emotional response
Developmental milestones—may be delayed or not attained
Starting school—situations in which appropriate learning will not take place in a regular classroom
Adolescence—addressing issues such as sexuality and independence
Future placement—decisions about placement must be made when the child becomes an adult or when the parents can no longer care for the child
Death of the child

**ANTICIPATED SIBLING STRESS**

Birth of another child—may be the affected sibling or the subsequent birth of an unaffected child
Diagnosis of condition—times of remission or exacerbations
Starting school—particularly stressful if friends reject the child with special needs
Adolescence—may be embarrassed to bring peers home
Future placement—may worry about responsibility for the affected sibling, especially if the parents are ill or die
Death of the child

their ability to carry out certain procedures, perhaps overlooking the child's personal comfort and satisfaction or failing to offer praise for anything less than perfect cooperation or performance. For these parents several strategies may be helpful: education regarding what can reasonably be expected of their child, assistance in identifying the child's strengths, praise for a parental job well-done, and finding respite care so that the parent can renew his or her own energies.

**Parental Roles.** Tremendous demands may be placed on the parents' energy, time, and financial resources to care for a child with chronic illness or disability. Depending on the roles assumed by each parent, the mother often performs the bulk of the traditional child care and household responsibilities and the father shoulders the financial responsibilities. However, with changing gender roles these responsibilities may be shared, and parents may divide the tasks according to their level of comfort or skills. For example, the parent with patience for waiting may be the logical person to bring the child for tests, procedures, and examinations. In contrast, the parent who deals best with the illness and side effects of therapy can prepare the home for the child's return. On the other hand, involving both parents in decision making and in education regarding the care of the child with special needs can decrease some of the burden of care often placed inadvertently on mothers.

In some families, changing gender roles signify additional responsibilities for one parent. For example, the working mother may feel the need to remain employed to help defray expenses, but she incurs the added burden of increased home and child responsibilities. This may result in conflict because one parent may perceive an unequal sharing of tasks with the partner.

In addition, the parent who is not involved in the caregiving activities may feel neglected, because much attention is directed toward the child, and resentful that he or she is not adequately informed to be competent in the care. Without active participation in the care of the child, the parent may have little understanding of the time and energy needed to perform those activities. When the less competent parent makes an effort to become involved, the other parent often criticizes the less skillful efforts. As a result, communication may break down, and neither is able to support the other.

Nurses can assist the parents in avoiding role conflict by providing anticipatory guidance early in the child's diagnosis. Teaching should address the stressors often identified as having an impact on marriage: (a) home care with the burden assumed primarily by one parent, (b) the financial burden, (c) fear of the child dying, (d) pressure from relatives, (e) the hereditary nature of the illness (if applicable), and (f) fear of pregnancy. Other causes of marital stress may focus on the inconveniences related to care, for example, long waiting times for appointments, lack of overnight accommodations, and lack of parking near health care facilities. These stressors are certainly within the realm of health care professionals to minimize, if not eliminate, for parents.

**Mother/Father Differences.** Although mothers and fathers in the same family appear to experience similar stressors, including concerns regarding the child's health, finances, and the child's future, studies have revealed some differences in how mothers and fathers cope as parents of a child with special needs. The results of a study examining the differences between mothers and fathers of a child with a life-threatening illness suggested that mothers and fathers had very different coping styles at diagnosis. Mothers coped by using emotional release and perceived they were coping poorly, whereas fathers were more likely to cope by using a "practical" approach or withdrawing. These coping styles were not always viewed as effective by the parents themselves, with just 50% feeling they had coped well at diagnosis (Mastroyannopoulou and others, 1997).

Leonard, Kratz, and Skay (1997) showed that mothers and fathers have differences in perceptions of their child's self-management of diabetes. Areas of significant differences included how parent support groups, social activities, and the child's temperament influenced how much responsibility the child should assume in self-management. In con-

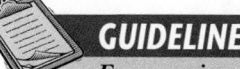

trast to fathers, mothers viewed social activities and the child's temperament as being strongly influential.

To foster communication between parents during adjustment to their child's chronic illness, the nurse can encourage them to recognize and accept differences in coping behaviors. This may increase mutual support and effect positive outcomes for their child's care.

**Fathers.** There is a paucity of research regarding the role and responses of fathers of chronically ill children. How fathers cope with their child's illness and treatment regimen is relatively unknown (Sterken, 1996).

In a study of father's of children with cancer the child's future, the child's health, their spouse's health, and the lack of time spent with their spouse were identified as the most common stressors during their child's illness. These fathers coped with stress by seeking information and through emotion-focused strategies, for example, prayer (Cayse, 1994).

Some fathers escape into their work as a way of dulling the pain. Others perceive having a child with special needs as a challenge to overcome and are not fearful of pushing the limits and being assertive to obtain the services needed for the child (May, 1996).

Sterken (1996) explored uncertainty and consequential coping patterns in fathers of children with cancer. The findings suggested that the age of the child, the age of the father, and the length of time since diagnosis were directly correlated with paternal uncertainty and coping. Younger fathers found the information provided regarding the treatment plan, system of care, and seriousness of their child's illness to be ill-defined and vague and were likely to use optimistic, evasive, and emotive coping styles to deal with uncertainty. Fathers with evasive coping styles used avoidant activities such as drugs, alcohol, food, driving alone, yard work, and putting increased energy into work. Those with optimistic coping styles used positive comparisons, positive thinking, and positive outlooks. Lastly, fathers with emotive coping styles included expression and release of emotions, as well as ventilation of feelings.

Fathers of children with chronic illness or disability are faced with formidable challenges that are very distinct from those of mothers. Fathers must reexamine priorities, come to terms with losses, and develop and strengthen caretaking abilities. Men quickly learn that they can neither safeguard their families from the problems nor control the outcomes (May, 1996). Many fathers experience feelings of guilt and failure and may suffer from isolation because of fewer social supports available for men than women. Feelings of isolation can be intensified by a health care system that frequently excludes, disenfranchises, and disregards men (May, 1996). Nurses can be instrumental in helping fathers of children with special needs overcome these challenges by addressing their concerns and engaging them in becoming supportive and important figures in the lives of their children. (See Guidelines box.)

As the traditional paternal role, particularly with sons, emphasizes joint recreation over caregiving, fathers appear to have more difficulty adjusting to a son with special needs than to a daughter with special needs. With today's increasing emphasis on fathers' involvement in the lives of their

> **GUIDELINES**
> *Encouraging the Involvement of Fathers in Caring for Children*
>
> - Have a willingness to include men, in the care of the child even when it appears they are not interested.
> - Include the father in education regarding the illness.
> - Provide flexible clinic schedules.
> - Foster the father's strengths.
> - Provide opportunities for men to embrace their children.
> - Encourage men to talk with their own fathers, if possible.
> - Provide a private place for men to grieve their loss.
> - Encourage men to speak with other men.

children, this loss is felt more profoundly than in the past. However, fearful of losing control or being perceived as ineffectual or weak, a father may hide his feelings and exhibit an outward confidence that can lead others to believe that everything is fine (May, 1996).

Traditionally the mother and child have actively participated and received professional care, while the father and siblings have been excluded. However, for the family unit to achieve optimum functioning each member must be included. This entails scheduling home and office visits at times when other family members can be present and may dictate early morning, early evening, or late afternoon hours. Fathers will often adjust their work schedule to meet with a health care professional once an invitation is offered.

The task of including other members of a family in a visit is approached positively. If they have not been included in the past, they may view such an invitation as a sign of more bad news or an indication of their own problems. One approach of welcoming others to participate in a visit is to verbalize that after hearing so often about the father and the other siblings, the nurse wishes to meet them. This implies a friendly connotation and is nonthreatening.

**Single-Parent Families.** Single-parent families of children with special needs are of particular concern. The absence of a parent may be due to death or divorce, or the parents may never have married. Special efforts should be made to assist the single parent in obtaining support and financial services that can lessen the burden of care. Nurses can also be advocates for the single parent by suggesting helping roles to enlist the support of friends and relatives. Some single parents are reluctant to join support groups because they feel out of place if the group is largely composed of married couples. Nurses need to assist single parents in mobilizing a positive social support network and need to be empathetic to the concerns of single parents by obtaining appropriate resources to meet their needs.

**Foster/Adoptive Families.** Foster or adoptive families may benefit from information and support to encourage effective early adaptation to a child with chronic illness or developmental disability. Information on the child's condition, unique needs, available services, warning signs of problems, and sources of both respite and support care can assist families in coping. Supporting foster families may promote longer-term placements or adoption for children with special needs.

## Sibling Issues

Many parents express concern regarding when and how to inform the other children in the family about the birth of a child who is disabled. The answer depends on each child's level of understanding and sophistication. Adolescents and even younger siblings routinely use the Internet to obtain information. What siblings piece together or overhear is often much worse than the truth. Oftentimes they imagine gruesome things regarding the experiences related to the illness, treatment, and hospitalization (Shepard and Mahon, 2000). Health care professionals need to anticipate questions and provide answers to children about the medical condition of their siblings in an age-appropriate manner that respects their constant need for information. Children need to be informed throughout the course of their sibling's illness. Parents are usually in the best position to impart this information, although they are often overwhelmed with the medical crisis at hand (Fleitas, 2000). Nurses can encourage parents to talk with the siblings about how they perceive their sick brother or sister and to be accepting of the siblings' feelings. Provisions should be made to allow siblings to visit the child in the hospital.

Nurses can demonstrate that they perceive the parents as being capable by their own unique style of discussing the child's condition. The nurse also can provide information to parents about teaching children of various ages and developmental stages. If the parents are unable to talk to the siblings, it is essential to find someone else who can speak to the siblings in an appropriate manner. Nurses are ideal individuals to educate and counsel siblings during the course of their brother's or sister's illness (Shepard and Mahon, 2000).

Siblings must be prepared for the physical changes that their brother or sister will experience and for the possible role changes occurring in the family. Siblings must realize that their concerns, thoughts, and questions are important and acceptable; this includes jealousy towards the sick child and feelings of anger toward their parents. Siblings need to be reassured that they will be kept abreast of their brother's or sister's treatment progress and, when possible, be involved in the care. When treatment necessitates parental absence from home or hospitalization of the sick child is warranted, a regularly scheduled time should be arranged for the siblings and parents to speak by telephone. This will help to decrease separation anxiety and allows the sibling a sense of consistency, belonging, and involvement in the sick child's care.

Some siblings develop behavior or adjustment difficulties, particularly younger male or older female siblings. Younger children tend to become irritable and withdrawn, whereas older siblings tend to act out. Some common difficulties include bed-wetting, headaches and other physical complaints, school phobia, changes in school performance, proneness to injury, sleep problems, depression, and severe separation anxiety.

Some problems for siblings arise from demands imposed by the child's condition. For example, at diagnosis the child with special needs by necessity becomes the focus of parental concern and attention. Frequent visits to a health care facility or hospitalizations disrupt the family routine.

## Critical Thinking Exercise

### Siblings' Feelings

Siblings of children with chronic illness or disability are likely to have which of the following feelings?

FIRST, THINK ABOUT IT . . .
- What conclusions are you reaching?
- How are you interpreting that information?

1. Jealousy and anger
2. Guilt
3. Embarrassment, worry, sadness
4. Pride and affection

*An accurate conclusion is that any or all of the above are, in fact, possible feelings for siblings. Siblings may be jealous or angry because of extra attention received by the child with special needs. They may feel guilty, thinking that something they did or wished caused the problem. Aspects of the child's condition, especially if visible, may embarrass siblings. Worry about the child's health and sadness about the child's missing out on events or opportunities can occur. Pride in the child's achievements and affection are other sibling experiences.*

Siblings are pushed to the background, often staying at the homes of friends and relatives. The child's condition may interfere with vacations, holiday celebrations, and other special events. Siblings may resent these intrusions, which often require self-sacrifice. (See Critical Thinking Exercise box.) For a while parents may miss the siblings' ball games, school functions, or other activities and at times may be emotionally and physically unavailable for them. The family's emotional and financial resources may be directed toward the child with special needs. When this happens, there is often not only a decrease in normal family activities but a decrease in personal items and attention for the other children as well. Feelings of jealousy, anger, and resentment are not uncommon. Siblings may worry about "catching" the condition or worry that playing rough with their brother or sister or even thinking bad thoughts about the sibling caused the condition. Nurses need to reassure siblings that their emotions are acceptable, but misconceptions must be clarified.

Fleitas (2000) compiled data from interviews conducted with siblings of hospitalized children and comments from other siblings who responded on a Web site entitled "Band-Aides and Blackboards: When Chronic Illness . . . or Some Other Medical Problem . . . Goes to School." Feelings reported by siblings in response to having a brother or sister with medical problems were loneliness, responsibility, fear, jealousy, guilt, and resentment.

Feelings of resentment are also reported by siblings when their brother or sister with special needs becomes the focus of parental attention or is overprotected, indulged, or permitted to exhibit unacceptable behaviors. Parents may not realize that they are treating their children with different standards, or they may feel that the child's condition calls for leniency.

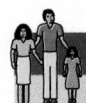

## FAMILY FOCUS
### Helping Parents Establish Expectations

Parents whose children have had prolonged or chronic illnesses sometimes have difficulty setting limits with the child. They do not know how to set the boundaries of acceptable behavior with the child who is ill. The nurse has an opportunity to model behavior for the parent as care is delivered. For example, the nurse can establish a level of expectation that the child will perform age-appropriate self-care activities. It is important that expectations are established within an environment of respect for the child and the parent. For a child who has been acutely ill, it is often a signal to the family that the nurse thinks the child is getting better if he or she is expected to wash his or her face, brush his or her teeth, or pick up the toys in the room.

Chronically ill children can and should have age-appropriate assigned chores for which they are held responsible. Further, children should be knowledgeable and participative in the management of their own health care regimen. Parents can learn what parts of the regimen to delegate to the child and where the parent must maintain control. The nurse can be a model for this type of parental behavior and a mentor as the parent learns where the boundaries need to be.

Teresa L. Hall, MS, RN
Hathaway Children's Services
Sylmar, CA

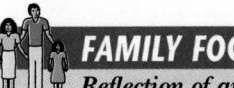

## FAMILY FOCUS
### Reflection of an Older Brother

My youngest sister, Kerry, was on an apnea monitor 3 years ago, when I was 15. I was never embarrassed about Kerry being on the monitor, except for the time it went off in church and everyone turned around to look at us.

Joey Bellino
Oldest sibling of an infant
on an apnea monitor
Washington, DC

Discipline provides structure, and limits and should be consistent between siblings and within families. (See Family Focus box.) When a child becomes seriously ill or disabled, the entire family is affected and role changes occur. Siblings, particularly older sisters, are often asked to assume increased responsibilities.

Foremost among the fears identified by children when their brothers or sisters are chronically ill or disabled are the fears that they will develop the illness. Siblings often acknowledge feelings of guilt arising from a belief that they caused disability or illness (Fleitas, 2000).

When children have complex disabilities or medical needs, particularly those that involve some degree of physical difference (e.g., hair loss), siblings must cope with the responses of others to differences in appearance or behavior. This causes embarrassment for the siblings; however, at the same time they want to protect their brother or sister from the sarcastic remarks or stares of others (Fleitas, 2000). Having a child in the family who is disfigured, ill, or disabled labels the family as "different." (See Family Focus box.) When siblings perceive an illness to be life-threatening, the power of the unspoken sibling bond is manifested. Feelings of sadness are manifested when their future together as siblings is threatened. Lastly, siblings report confusion arising from lack of information and poor communication with them about their brother's or sister's condition (Fleitas, 2000).

Often overlooked is the positive caring that exists between children with special needs and their brothers and sisters. Siblings feel pride and satisfaction in their own contributions to the family, happiness and excitement in their brother's or sister's achievements, and genuine love. Some siblings express that they sense more closeness in their families.

Research has supported the assertion that there are positive aspects of sibling resilience when a child is ill. Children in families where a sibling has a disability exhibit greater independence and maturity than do their peers. These children acknowledge feeling good about themselves and are proud of their patience and sense of responsibility. Their also have a great appreciation of family closeness and health (Fleitas, 2000). Parental attitudes about the child and efforts promoting normalization are crucial in the development of positive reactions in siblings.

Nurses must be aware of and responsive to the reactions of siblings to their brother's or sister's illness or disability. Williams and others (1997) evaluated the outcomes of a structured, educational, and support group intervention for siblings of children with chronic illness, including a session with parents about sibling needs. Results of the study suggested that sibling and parent perceptions were congruent, confirming the sources of potential sibling adjustment problems. Screening for sibling social support, mood, and self-esteem at the time of diagnosis and over time, may be conducive to the prevention of mental health problems among siblings.

Focusing on strengths rather than problems requires nurses to impart an appreciation of how family members proceed with their lives despite having a child with a chronic illness. Whenever possible, nurses need to intervene to foster positive adaptation. Siblings often state that they are expected to assume additional responsibilities to help parents care for the child. It is not unusual for them to display a positive reaction to taking on the extra duties but a negative reaction to feeling unappreciated for doing so. Such feelings can often be minimized by encouraging the siblings to discuss this with the parents and by advocating ways of showing gratitude, such as an increase in allowance, special privileges, and, most importantly, verbal praise. (See Family Home Care box on p. 930.)

### Extended Family Members and Friends

In addition to parents and siblings, significant family members or friends may be affected by a child's chronic illness or disability. Even though extended family relationships are often helpful to parents in rearing a child with special needs, they may also be sources of stress. For example, grandparents or other well-meaning relatives may attempt to reassure the parents that the child "will grow out of" his or her slowness at a time when parents are struggling to accept reality.

The nurse must be aware of the family's cues concerning sources of stress from extended members, such as grandparents. Parents can be encouraged, if appropriate, to pro-

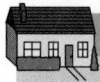

## FAMILY HOME CARE
### Supporting Siblings of Children with Special Needs

### PROMOTE HEALTHY SIBLING RELATIONSHIPS

Value each child individually and avoid comparisons. Remind each child of his or her positive qualities and contribution to other family members.

Help siblings see the differences and similarities between themselves and a child with special needs. Create a climate in which children can achieve successes without feeling guilty.

Teach siblings ways to interact with the child.

Seek to be fair in terms of discipline, attention, and resources; require the affected child to do as much for himself or herself as possible.

Let siblings settle their own differences; intervene only to prevent siblings from hurting one another.

Legitimize reasonable anger. Even children with special needs behave badly sometimes.

Respect a sibling's reluctance to be with or to include the child with special needs in activities.

### HELP SIBLINGS COPE

Listen to siblings to let them know that their thoughts and suggestions are valued.

Praise siblings when they have been patient, have sacrificed, or have been particularly helpful. Do not expect siblings to always act in this manner.

Modified from Powell T, Ogle P: *Brothers and sisters—a special part of exceptional families*, Baltimore, 1985, Paul H Brooks; Spokane Washington Deaconess Medical Center, Pediatric Oncology Unit: Tips for dealing with siblings, *Candlelighters Childhood Cancer Found Quart Newsletter* 11(3,4):7, 1987; and Carlson J, Leviton A, Mueller M: Services to siblings: an important component of family-centered practice, *ACCH Advocate* 1(1):53-56, 1993.

Acknowledge the personal strengths siblings have and their ability to cope with stress successfully.

Provide age-appropriate information about the child's condition, and update when appropriate.

Let teachers know what is happening so they can be understanding and helpful.

Recognize special stress times for siblings and plan to minimize negative effects.

Schedule special time with siblings; have a friend or family member substitute when parent is unavailable.

Encourage siblings to join or help establish a sibling support group.

Use the services of professionals when needed. If parent feels that such a service is necessary, it should be provided in as vigorous a manner as a service for the child with special needs.

### INVOLVE SIBLINGS

Seek out ways to realistically include siblings in the care and treatment of the child with special needs.

Limit caregiving responsibilities and give recognition when siblings perform them.

Develop a library of children's books on special needs.

Invite siblings to attend meetings to develop plans for the child with special needs (e.g., IEP, IFSP).

Discuss future plans with them.

Solicit their ideas on treatment and service needs.

Have them visit professionals who work with the child.

Help them develop competencies to teach the child new skills.

Provide opportunities for siblings to advocate for the child.

Allow siblings to set their own pace for learning and involvement.

---

vide literature or to invite the grandparents to be present during one of the child's visits to the outpatient health care facility, during the diagnostic period, or during a conference with the health care team. Including grandparents in a discussion in which they can share their concerns may assist them in coping with their feelings, thereby lessening stress on the entire family. Grandparents may adapt even less well than parents because they lack adequate information, have limited involvement in decision making, and have less responsibility for the child's care. Often they feel helpless to provide assistance. Grandparents' feelings of anger and blame should be openly discussed. Grandparents can be helped to understand the impact of their behavior on the family with an appropriate statement such as "Your son is presently experiencing a lot of pain and anguish. We realize that this is difficult for you, as well as your son; however, you can be of great help by being supportive of him."

Most grandparents experience some ambivalence because they love their grandchild yet feel personal disappointment when a diagnosis is made. They often experience two types of grief: for their grandchild who is ill, and for their child, the parent, who is suffering. The future is now unpredictable, not only for the grandchild, but for the child's parents as well. Behavioral disturbances such as poor decision making, disorganization, and disorientation, already seen in some older adults, may be intensified during grief. Grandparents do not often admit these emotions, and

they are left to adjust on their own. Although uncommon, support groups for grandparents can be helpful. Special support may be needed for the grandparent assuming the role of a primary caregiver for the child.

Significant stress can also arise from nonfamilial sources, such as neighbors, friends, or strangers. Neighbors display various reactions to the child's diagnosis. Some turn away, some pry, and some ask inappropriate questions or make insensitive remarks. Inability to deal with comments about the condition or curious stares by others may promote the tendency to protect and isolate the child in the home. The family needs guidance in preparing for these inevitable encounters. One approach is encouraging parents to dress the child as much as possible like his or her peers. Good grooming is extremely important in minimizing differences in appearance. Through role-playing, parents can rehearse responses to comments such as "Is your child retarded?" or "Has he always been crippled?" Parent groups can allow family members to share experiences and learn from each other about dealing with unkind remarks or probing questions. They also provide a type of support parents cannot obtain from relatives, friends, and neighbors.

Some neighbors and friends will not allow their children to play with the child or siblings for fear of contagion or becoming close to a child who might die. For some parents friendships may be difficult to maintain because they have little time and energy for social gatherings. Friends may withdraw for a number of reasons, such as being uncomfortable with the situation and feeling unable to help.

Parents have to decide how much and what to tell relatives, friends, baby-sitters, and teachers. Concerns regarding discrimination are very real for parents and must be balanced with the need to share information so that the child receives proper care.

Nurses can address the issue of discrimination by asking parents if they have worries about how to inform others of the child's condition. Intervention strategies must focus not only on problems confronting children and families but must also discreetly consider the many sources from which discrimination may develop. Nurses may also be able to provide suggestions regarding essential education for others who will care for the child.

## Coping with Ongoing Stress and Periodic Crises

Families of children with chronic conditions confront the potential for ongoing stress associated with factors such as the child's condition and financial concerns (see Box 22-5 on p. 926). They also confront periodic crises that may include uncertainty regarding the diagnosis and coping with recurrent hospitalizations. Some families are strengthened by being able to deal with these stressors. Others become overwhelmed when stressors exceed resources. The family needs to prevent increasing stress that can overwhelm family resources and result in crisis (Clawson, 1996). Concurrent stresses unrelated to the chronic condition pose additional challenges.

Health care professionals can assist families in coping with stress by providing anticipatory guidance, providing emotional support, helping the family to assess and recognize specific stressors, assisting the family in developing problem-solving strategies and coping mechanisms, continuing efforts to meet developmental needs, using spiritual beliefs to provide hope and meaning, and working collaboratively with parents so they become empowered in the process.

### Concurrent Stresses Within the Family

The ability to cope with the overwhelming stresses of a life-long illness or disability is challenged further when additional stresses are present. Ongoing stresses and strains in the family "accumulate," increasing the family's vulnerability and lessening its ability to adapt to a child with special needs. For some family members, non–illness-related stressors are perceived as more stressful than those related to a child's chronic condition.

Stressors may be developmental or situational. They may be associated with sibling needs, marital discord, homelessness, or social isolation. Even the more minor stresses, such as managing the home, arranging care for siblings, and commuting to distant treatment centers, can challenge a family's ability to cope successfully (see Box 22-5 on p. 926).

Family or child developmental stressors exacerbate situational stresses. For example, a common developmental stressor in the family life cycle is the birth of a child, an event that necessitates adjustment by the parents. The birth of a child with a congenital health problem adds situational stress to the equation.

For the majority of families, regardless of their insurance coverage or income, financial concerns exist. The costs of caring for a child with special needs can be overwhelming. Children with functional limitations constitute one third of child hospital days, and their hospital stays are twice as long; they also visit physicians twice as often as children without limitations. Direct medical expenses, transportation costs, nonprescription medication, wigs or cosmetics to conceal the effects of the illness or treatment, parking, meals, housing, and child care can consume a high percentage of a family's income.

Additional loss of family income occurs when parents take time off work or quit a job to care for a child.* The family breadwinner may also have to sacrifice career opportunities to remain close to the child's treatment center.

Nurses can make appropriate referrals to case managers and social workers to assist a family in reviewing various options for financial assistance, including insurance; health maintenance organization (HMO) or managed care policies; Medicaid; Supplemental Security Income (SSI); Woman, Infants, and Children program (WIC); the state program for Children with Special Health Needs; disease-related associations, and local philanthropic organizations (Scher and Ahmann, 1996).

### Coping Mechanisms

Coping mechanisms are those behaviors directed at reducing the tension elicited by a crisis. Approach behaviors are those coping mechanisms resulting in movement toward adjustment and resolution of the crisis. Avoidance behaviors result in movement away from adjustment or maladaptation to the crisis. Several approach and avoidance behaviors utilized in coping with a chronic illness or disability are listed in the Guidelines box on p. 932. None of the indexes can be utilized alone to assess the possible success or failure in resolving the crisis. Each behavior must be seen in the context of all of the variables influencing the family. For example, the observation of many avoidance behaviors in an emotionally healthy family may indicate significantly less risk to the successful resolution of the crisis than an equal number of avoidance behaviors in an individual who has few available supports.

Two long-term coping strategies of familial adaptation to severe and chronic childhood illness have been significantly related to a high level of family functioning. The first is the parent's ability to assign the illness meaning within an existing medical/scientific or spiritual philosophy of life. There is an optimistic belief that things work out for the good and an emphasis on the positive qualities of the situation. Statements such as "God has chosen our family to care for this special child" reflect the religious philosophy.

---

*Information regarding financial issues is available from **Family Voices**, PO Box 769, Algodones, NM 87001, (505) 867-2368, fax: (505) 867-6517 or (888) 835-5669; www.kidshealth@familyvoices.org and the **Federation for Children with Special Needs,** 1135 Tremont St, Suite 420, Boston, MA 02120, (617) 236-72100, (800) 331-0688, (617) 572-2094; www.fcsn.org.

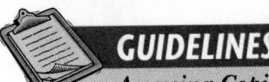

## GUIDELINES
### Assessing Coping Behaviors

**APPROACH BEHAVIORS**

Asks for information regarding diagnosis and present condition

Seeks help and support from others

Anticipates future problems; actively seeks guidance and answers

Shares burden of disorder with others

Plans realistically for the future

Acknowledges and accepts child's awareness of diagnosis and prognosis

Expresses feelings, such as sorrow, depression, and anger, and realizes reason for the emotional reaction

Realistically perceives child's condition; adjusts to changes

Recognizes own growth through passage of time, such as earlier denial and nonacceptance of diagnosis

Verbalizes possible loss of child

**AVOIDANCE BEHAVIORS**

Fails to recognize seriousness of child's condition despite physical evidence

Refuses to agree to treatment

Intellectualizes about the illness, but in areas unrelated to child's condition

Is angry and hostile to members of the staff, regardless of their attitude or behavior

Avoids staff, family members, or child

Entertains unrealistic future plans for child, with little emphasis on the present

Is unable to adjust to or accept a change in progression of disease

Continually looks for new cures with no perspective toward possible benefit

Refuses to acknowledge child's understanding of disease and prognosis

Uses magical thinking and fantasy, may seek "occult" help

Places complete faith in religion to point of relinquishing own responsibility

Withdraws from outside world; refuses help

Punishes self because of guilt and blame

Makes no change in lifestyle to meet needs of other family members

Resorts to excessive use of alcohol or drugs to avoid problems

Verbalizes suicidal intention

Is unable to discuss possible loss of child or previous experiences with death

The second long-term coping strategy of family adaptation is an ability to share the burdens imposed by the illness with individuals both inside and outside the family network. Intrafamilial relationships promote togetherness of the family members and support a mutual recognition that all members are vital contributors to the family unit. Extrafamilial supports help preserve meaningful external contacts and provide needed assistance to the family.

Two theories provide some insight into family coping. The *chronic illness trajectory model* recognizes that chronic conditions have a course that changes over time (Corbin and Strauss, 1995). The course of the illness is influenced by several psychologic and medical factors, including resources (interpersonal, intrapersonal, and instrumental), technology, motivation, past experience, the type and severity of illness, lifestyle, and the social climate. Most chronic illness management occurs in the home, not in the hospital. This model advocates that the goal of nursing care in chronic illness is to assist the family in shaping the course of

the illness medically while maintaining quality of life for the child and family. This is achieved through assessment, teaching, monitoring, and initiating referrals.

A second theory is associated with family management styles. This theory, described by Knafl and Deatrick (1990) underscores the family's role in actively responding to childhood chronic illness. Aspects of family management style include the following:

- How the family members define the illness situation—what it means to them
- Management behaviors that the family employs with regard to chronic illness, including restructuring family member roles and adapting lifestyle choices
- The sociocultural context in which these behaviors and values occur

Knafl and Deatrick (1990) suggest that coping techniques and patterns can be learned. When nurses move toward understanding a family's management style, interventions can be targeted most appropriately to foster the growth of individual family members and the family as a whole.

Teaching the family to cope with the child's chronic illness or disability can foster positive adaptation. Cognitive, behavioral, and emotional tasks are components of the adaptive coping process (Clarke-Steffen, 1997):

- Cognitive tasks include learning about the disability, its management, and prognosis.
- Behavioral tasks include the actual management of the child's condition—monitoring treatment, performing daily therapies, and teaching self-care.
- Emotional tasks include mourning the loss of normal functioning in the child, processing anger, and addressing limitations the condition imposes on all family members.

Fostering normalization, teaching coping skills, and assisting the family in using or further defining their social support networks are other nursing interventions that can encourage and empower the parents and promote positive adaptation in the family and optimum mental health for the child.

### Parental Empowerment

Empowerment can be viewed as a personal process in which individuals develop and use the necessary knowledge, confidence, and competence for making their voices heard. Participatory competence, the ability to be heard by those in power, is the outcome of the process of empowerment (Gibson, 1995).

In addition, nurses can provide resources and support to parents of chronically ill children based on their individual level of empowerment. Nurses can also encourage parent membership on staff, boards, and committees and include parents in presentations at conferences and meetings. Nurses can help keep parents abreast of pending legislation on child health issues and take action when appropriate.*

---

*An excellent resource for becoming involved in political action is the *Public Affairs Public Issues Handbook*, available from the **American Cancer Society**, Government Relations Department, 701 Pennsylvania Ave, NW, Suite 650, Washington, DC, 20004, (202) 661-5700 or (800) ACS-2345, fax: (202) 661-5750; www.cancer.org. **Family Voices**, PO Box 769, Algodones, NM 87001 (888) 835-5669 or (505) 867-2368, fax: (505) 867-6517, www.kidshealth@familyvoices.org, is a grassroots advocacy network of parents and professionals.

# Assisting Family Members in Managing Their Feelings

Although some earlier research has postulated stages of adaptation to a chronic illness or disability, there is considerable individual variation in reactions to the diagnosis, use of defense mechanisms, and time frames for coming to terms with a diagnosis. It is imperative that professionals recognize and respect a vast range of reactions and coping mechanisms. In fact, members of a family of a child with chronic illness or disability may experience many difficult emotions, such as guilt, fear, anger, resentment, and anxiety. (See Guidelines box.) Support from health professionals, extended family members, and friends can help the family deal with their feelings. When parents are able to cope successfully with the stress of caring for their disabled child, positive outcomes are accrued by all family members in the sense of increased love and warmth within the family, finding meaning for one's life, a strong sense of having done a good job parenting, a sense of pride in the disabled child's achievements no matter how small, and finding meaning in the presence of a disabled child in the family.

## Shock and Denial

The initial diagnosis of a chronic illness or disability is often met with intense emotion and is characterized by shock, disbelief, and sometimes denial, especially if the disorder is not obvious, such as in chronic illness. Denial as a defense mechanism is a necessary cushion to prevent disintegration and is a normal response to grieving for any type of loss. Probably all family members experience various degrees of adaptive denial as they learn of the impact that the diagnosis has on their lives.

Shock and denial can last from days to months, sometimes even longer. Examples of denial that may be exhibited at the time of diagnosis include (1) physician shopping; (2) attributing the symptoms of the actual illness to a minor condition; (3) refusal to believe the diagnostic tests; (4) delay in agreeing to treatment; (5) acting very happy and optimistic despite the revealed diagnosis; (6) refusing to tell or talk to anyone about the condition; (7) insisting that no one is telling the truth, regardless of others' attempts to do so; (8) denying the reason for admission; and (9) asking no questions about the diagnosis, treatment, or prognosis. Generally these mechanisms should be respected as short-term responses that allow individuals to distance themselves from the onslaught of a tremendous emotional impact and to collect and mobilize their energies toward goal-directed, problem-solving behaviors.

In some instances, various indicators of denial can actually be adaptive behaviors. Searching for another professional opinion may mean that parents cannot obtain answers to their questions or that they are looking for a different approach to treatment that better meets the needs of their child and family. When parents discuss their strengths and the benefits they derive from caring for their child with special needs, it does not necessarily reflect refusal to accept their difficult circumstances. Sometimes a delay in making decisions or a failure to ask questions simply reflects a lack of information.

Families with children who have life-threatening conditions commonly exhibit partial denial, such as seeking additional professional consultations or occasionally acting as if nothing were wrong. Without such a temporary protective mechanism, few people could survive the constant emotional drain of anticipating their own death or the death of a family member. Partial denial allows the child and family to absorb stressful information—or "dose" themselves—in amounts they can personally manage at the time.

In children the importance of denial has repeatedly been demonstrated as a factor in their positive coping with the diagnosis. Denial allows the child to maintain hope in the face of overwhelming odds and to function adaptively and productively. Like hope, denial may be an adaptive mechanism for dealing with loss that persists until a family or patient is ready or needs other responses.

Denial is probably the reaction that is least understood and most poorly coped with. Health care professionals commonly label denial as "maladaptive" and act inappropriately by attempting to strip it away by repeated and oftentimes blunt explanations of the prognosis. Because denial is based on fear, nurses need to address parental feelings of inadequacy. It is imperative that health professionals understand that denial is a necessary coping mechanism, and until one has met the parents' psychologic needs that result in denial, one cannot help the child (Luterman, 1999).

Denial becomes maladaptive only when it impedes recognition of treatment or rehabilitative goals essential for the child's optimum development or survival. For example, protracted denial may be evident in the response of a family to mental retardation; as long as the family can maintain a fiction of normality and manage the difference within the present familial values and roles, there may exist no recognition of the diagnosis. Rather, the problem is explained as an easily treated condition or as slow maturation. The denial may be strengthened by the child's social development, which belies the degree of speech and motor retardation. Not uncommon, this ability to rationalize delayed development is successful until the child begins school and is compared with other children, making his or her differences very apparent. At this point the family may start to perceive the illness as a crisis and respond with shock and disbelief. Denial is no longer beneficial to the family, and other coping mechanisms must be used.

## Adjustment

For most families, adjustment gradually follows shock and is usually characterized by an open admission that the condition exists. Adjustment may be accompanied by a number of

## Critical Thinking Exercise

### Parental Anger

A mother of a child recently diagnosed with diabetes begins arguing with you over the child's correct insulin dose. She raises her voice. Which of the following responses would *not* be appropriate?

FIRST, THINK ABOUT IT . . .

• What information are you using?
• If you accept the conclusions, what are the implications?

1. "You sound angry about this."
2. "Perhaps my supervisor should talk to you."
3. "Let me understand what you are saying here . . . "
4. "Perhaps we have a misunderstanding."

*The best response is two. You are using information that anger in the parent of a child with a newly diagnosed illness is not uncommon. The implications are that reflecting feelings (option one), trying to understand the parent's point of view (option three), and calmly trying to defuse the situation (option four) would all be appropriate actions. Although a supervisor might need to intervene (option two) in a hostile or dangerous situation, this situation does not pose such a threat.*

responses, which are normal components of the adaptation process. Perhaps the most universal of these feelings are **guilt** and **self-accusation.** Guilt is often greatest when the cause of the condition is directly linked to the parent, such as in genetic disorders or from accidental injury. However, it can arise even without any realistic or scientific basis for parental responsibility. Often the guilt develops from a false assumption that the disability is a result of personal wrongdoing or failing, such as not doing something correctly during the pregnancy or the birth. Guilt may be associated with religious or cultural beliefs as well. Some parents are convinced that they are being punished for some earlier misdeed. Others may perceive the condition as a sacrifice required by God to test their religious faith and strength. With appropriate information, support, and time, most parents deal with self-accusation and guilt. The ability to cope with resentful and self-accusatory feelings of having "caused" the child's condition is a critical factor in determining the parents' acceptance of their child.

Children may perceive their serious illness as retribution for past misbehavior as well. The nurse should be particularly cognizant of the child who passively accepts all painful procedures. This child may believe that such acts are inflicted because of deserved punishment. It is always best to assure children that the goal during diagnosis or treatment is to make them feel better.

Other normal and common reactions to a diagnosis of chronic illness or disability are **anger** and **bitterness.** Anger is a normal and expected reaction to chronic illness that arises when an individual realizes that certain needs, wishes, and plans for the future can no longer be satisfied due to limitations imposed by an illness. An intense feeling of unfairness

consequently leads to feelings of frustration and anger. Anger directed inward may be manifested as punitive or self-reproaching behavior, such as verbally degrading oneself and neglecting one's health. In contrast, anger directed outward may be revealed in either open arguments or withdrawal from communication with several individuals, such as the child, siblings, and spouse. Passive anger toward the child may be manifested in refusal to believe how sick the child is, inability to provide comfort, or decreased visiting. Among the most common targets for parental anger are members of the health care team. Parents may complain about the lack of time physicians spend with them, the nursing care, or the lack of qualified individuals to draw blood or start intravenous infusions. (See Critical Thinking Exercise box.)

Children are likely to respond with anger, and this includes the ill child and the healthy siblings. Children are cognizant of the loss provoked by their illness or disability and may react angrily to the feelings of being different from their peers or to the limitations instituted. Siblings may also feel resentment and anger toward the ill child and parents for the loss of parental attention and daily routines in the home. It is difficult for older children and almost impossible for younger children to understand the plight of the ill child. Their perception is of a sister or brother who has the undivided attention of their parents, is showered with toys and other gifts, and is the focus of everyone's concern.

Children of various ages exhibit anger differently. Young children may display their uncooperativeness by screaming, yelling, and physically fighting off the adversary. In contrast, older children use abusive language. Passive anger, expressed in such statements as "I don't know" or "I don't care," usually elicits anger in others and may be misconstrued as an obnoxious, sullen, or hostile response. As a result, these statements are effective in keeping people at a distance, when the hidden message really is "I need to talk. Please help me understand what is happening."

During the period of adjustment, four types of parental reactions to the child affect the child's eventual response to the condition: (1) overprotection, in which the parents fear allowing the child to achieve any new skill, avoid all discipline, and cater to every desire to impede frustration; (2) rejection, in which the parents detach themselves emotionally from the child but usually constantly nag and scold the child and provide adequate physical care; (3) denial, in which the parents act as if the condition does not exist or attempt to have the child overcompensate for it; and (4) gradual acceptance, in which the parents place realistic and necessary limitations on the child, foster reasonable social and physical activities, and promote self-care. Overprotection (Box 22-6) is such a common parental reaction that it behooves the nurse to assess for its presence and to begin anticipatory guidance with the family when appropriate. Many of these characteristics are also seen in the vulnerable child syndrome and could occur or persist should the child recover from injury or illness. (See Chapter 10.)

### Reintegration and Acknowledgment

For many families the adjustment process culminates in the development of realistic expectations for the child and rein-

---

**Box 22-6** ■ ■ □
### Characteristics of Parental Overprotection

Sacrifices self and rest of family for the child
Continually helps the child, even when the child is capable
Is inconsistent with regard to discipline or employs no discipline; frequently different rules apply to the other siblings
Is dictatorial and arbitrary, making decisions without considering the child's wishes, such as keeping the child from attending school
Hovers and offers suggestions; calls attention to every activity, overdoing praise
Protects the child from every possible discomfort
Restricts play, often because of fear that the child will be injured
Denies the child opportunities for growing up and assuming responsibility, such as learning to give own medications or perform treatments
Does not understand the child's capabilities and sets goals too high or too low
Monopolizes the child's time, such as sleeping with the child, permitting few friends, or refusing participation in social or educational activities

---

**Box 22-7** ■ ■ □
### Concept of Functional Burden

**IMPACT OF CHILD WITH SPECIAL NEEDS**

The child's need for medical and nursing care
The child's fixed deficits
The child's age-appropriate dependency in activities of daily living
The disruptions in the family routine caused by the care
The psychologic burden of the prognosis on the family

**FAMILY RESOURCES AND ABILITY TO COPE**

The family's physical resources
The family's emotional resources
The family's educational resources
The family's social supports and available help
The competing demands for family members' time and energy

Data from Stein REK: Home care: a challenging opportunity, *Child Health Care* 14(2):90-95, 1985.

---

tegration of family life with the disability or illness in a manageable perspective. Because as a significant portion of this phase is one of grief for a loss, total resolution is not possible until the child dies or leaves home as an independent adult. Thus one can regard adjustment as "increased comfort" with day-to-day living rather than a complete resolution.

This adjustment phase also involves social reintegration in which the family broadens its activities to include relationships outside the home, with the child as a participating and acceptable member of the group. This latter criterion often distinguishes the reaction of gradual acceptance during the adjustment period from total acceptance or possibly is more descriptive of the acknowledgment process.

During the acknowledgment phase of adjustment, individuals take stock of what remains rather than focusing on what is lost and begin to establish new goals for their life. It is a time when the family is particularly motivated to learn about the restrictions imposed by the child's illness and to decide how they want to function within those confines. Nursing interventions that emphasize self-control are particularly beneficial because they promote the highest level of function possible and increase a sense of self-worth.

Many parents of children with special needs will experience some *chronic sorrow*, an emotional reaction exhibited throughout the life span of the parent-child interaction. Olshansky (1962) first described this phenomenon as a pattern of sadness in response to a child's differences that is an ongoing process distinguishable from grief. Chronic sorrow is not static (Gravelle, 1997) but includes elements of permanence with episodic surges in the presence of developmental or situational crisis. Chronic sorrow occurs while parents redefine parental expectations and the parameters for appraising the child's achievements. External events, such as the passage of a child's expected date of graduation, trigger resurgences of chronic sorrow when the parent is again reminded of what could have been.

## Establishing a Support System

The diagnosis of a child with a serious health problem or disability is a major situational crisis affecting the entire family. However, families can experience positive outcomes while they successfully cope with the many challenges that accompany a child with chronic illness or disability. One nursing goal is to assess which families are at lesser or greater risk for succumbing to the effects of the crisis. A number of variables—available support system, reactions to the child, perception of the event, coping mechanisms, available resources, and concurrent stresses within the family—affect the resolution of a crisis. Even though most families do cope, the needs of families at risk are considerable. If they receive guidance and emotional support early in the crisis, there is an increased possibility that they will cope successfully.

Even though it is easy to assume that families of children with the most severe illnesses or disabilities would have the poorest adjustment, the severity of the condition reflects only one part of the overall picture. The level of adjustment is greatly influenced by the *functional burden* on the individual family (Stein, 1985). This concept considers the issues associated with caring for and living with the child in relation to the family's resources and coping ability (Box 22-7). The family of a child with multiple disabilities warranting complex care—yet having many coping strategies and resources—may adjust more successfully to the child's situation than the family of a child with a less serious condition and few resources to counter balance it.

Intrafamilial resources, social support from friends, parent-to-parent support, parent-professional partnerships, and community resources intertwine to provide a flexible web of support for the family of a child with a chronic condition.

### Intrafamilial Resources

Family members' ages, education, intelligence, ability and willingness to learn the child's care, sense of humor, and sense of optimism are resources they can bring to a situation. Resources within the family, such as adaptability, cohesion, a sense of coherence, and hardiness, are aspects of the family system that can greatly facilitate the family's adjustment.

The marital relationship is a primary source of potential support and overall is considered the best predictor of coping behavior and adjustment. Conflicts in parental role definition and differences in paternal and maternal coping patterns can place a strain on the marital relationship. Most health care professionals assume that the rate of family dissolution is greater due to increased familial stress from the presence of a chronic condition in a family. These families may experience more conflict and strain over the roles of their members, as well as fewer exchanges of affection. Parents of chronically ill children, however, are not more likely to experience higher levels of marital dissatisfaction or depression than families of healthy children (Quittner and others, 1998). When partners can openly discuss their feelings, there appears to be much less guilt, blame, anger, and indecision. Each crisis during the lengthy period of chronic illness is successfully resolved, reducing the overlapping and accumulation of multiple stresses.

## Social Support Systems

The significant others who are available to individuals for emotional strength during periods of crisis constitute their support system. Support systems may be available through various relationships and may include one significant other, such as a spouse, or a group of significant others, such as the health care team or the extended family. The amount and type of social support received by families is a crucial factor in their adjustment to the child's chronic condition (Frankel and Wamboldt, 1998).

Research has revealed that the source of support is a determining factor in the effectiveness of certain forms of support. For example, emotional or expressive support is best provided by individuals with whom one has strong ties and who are like oneself. The ability to verbalize feelings such as guilt, anger, fear, or anxiety helps individuals deal with the particular emotion. Verbalization allows for the validation of thoughts and feelings. When professionals develop a strong therapeutic relationship with the family, they also can be appropriate sources of emotional support (see discussion on parent-professional partnerships on p. 937).

On the other hand, instrumental support can often be provided by those to whom the family has weaker ties and can link the family to a more diverse and broader social network. For example, the most appropriate sources of informational support may include both professionals, who have practical and theoretic knowledge, and nonprofessionals—parents—whose experience makes them experts.

Coping with illness or disability may be a new experience for a family and their support system, and families may benefit from recommendations on effective ways to use their support system to meet their needs. Providing parents with written information they can share with extended family can often help them in reaching out to others during a stressful time. In addition, helping family members to identify members of their support system and consider practical tasks to request assistance with (e.g., laundry, care of siblings, and transportation) can mobilize resources.

Even though studies have shown that lack of support negatively influences individual and family adjustment to chronic illness and disability (Schaefer, McCaul, and Glasgow, 1986; Wallander and Varni, 1989), little is known about which behaviors parents perceive as hurtful or nonsupporting. Garwick and others (1998) identified parents' perceptions of helpful vs unhelpful types of support received in managing the care of preadolescents with chronic conditions. They found that both mothers and fathers reported that other family members were the major source of helpful tangible and emotional support, whereas health care providers were the major support of helpful informational support. Extended family, school, health care, and community systems were important sources of social support for families of preadolescents.

Health care providers should assess the type of support needed before planning interventions. They may assist families early in the diagnostic and treatment process by encouraging them to plan for and use helpful resources. Parents may also benefit from the suggestion that it is okay to refuse certain types of "well-intended" support from friends and family (Shepard and Mahon, 2000). Families often express needing assistance with finding recreational activities and community resources for their children with chronic conditions, and health care providers can facilitate family support by identifying the types of support that may be most helpful to the family and by being culturally sensitive and informed about parents' groups and community resources.

Because of withdrawal and social isolation, some individuals may not be able to reach out to others for practical or emotional support. These individuals are more likely to feel overwhelmed and may benefit from a social worker or therapist.

## Parent-to-Parent Support

The support a parent receives from another parent is unique and cannot be obtained from any other source. Veteran parents provide something that other support systems cannot—shared experiences. They have intimately known the stress related to diagnosis, weathered the many transitional times, such as moving from one program to another, and have sifted through services so that they have a practical knowledge of resources (Santelli, Turnbull, and Higgins, 1997). A growing number of clinics and hospitals now have on staff a parent with a child who is chronically ill or disabled. The services these parents provide are invaluable for parents of children with special needs who are likely to experience lengthy and repeated hospitalizations, as well as many routine outpatient visits.

Just being with another parent who has shared similar experiences can be beneficial. A parent of a child with the same diagnosis is not always necessary, for parents in the process of adjusting to a child with special needs—or finding respite services, rehabilitative or educational services, special equipment vendors, or financial counseling—walk a common path. Because veteran parents have "been there" and have both experienced the many intense emotional reactions associated with disability in the family and also adjusting to the disability, they are in a unique position to establish a bond with referred parents and to provide helpful emotional and informational support (Santelli, Turnbull, and Higgins, 1997).

A national survey of parent-to-parent program coordinators examined referral sources, program descriptions and demographics, program supports, and examples of best practices. Findings revealed that parents ranked "having someone listen" and "getting information about their child's disability" as the two most important supports. Examples of emotional support that parents received included (1) help in seeing hope for the future, (2) feeling less alone, (3) seeing the positive, (4) coping with the diagnosis, (5) seeing family strengths, and (6) coping with stress. Best program practices identified for culturally diverse families were developing materials in languages other than English, using alternate media to reach families, supporting long-distance phone calls between parents, having a respected community member as a program coordinator, having support groups for specific populations, and adding parent-to-parent programs to an existing family resource center. Parent-to-parent programs can complement health care services by empowering parents through support and information and should be included in a comprehensive family support system (Santelli, Turnbull, and Higgins, 1997).

If the child's treatment center does not have a parent staff position, the nurse can contact parent groups, who will usually send a representative. Another intervention is to ask another parent with a chronically ill or disabled child to talk with the parents. The nurse should seek out a parent who has a nonjudgmental approach to differences in families, is a good listener, and has good problem-solving and advocacy skills.

The parent self-help group is another approach to foster parent-to-parent support.* Group members feel less alone and have the opportunity to observe both mastery role modeling and coping from other members. Parents' groups are rich resources for information seeking. Even if parents cannot attend meetings, they can still benefit from group newsletters and other literature that often accompany membership. The nurse can promote parent participation in self-help groups by serving as a group advisory board member, a referral agent, a resource person, or an assistant in finding a group. Oftentimes all that is necessary in starting a group is identifying one or two parents as leaders; sharing with them the names, addresses, and telephone numbers of other families; and guiding them in how to organize a first meeting.

---

*Information about self-help groups, as well as books and pamphlets, is available from the **National Self-Help Clearinghouse**, 365 5th Ave, Suite 3300, New York, NY 10016, (212) 817-1822, fax (212) 817-2990.

## Parent-Professional Partnerships

One important component of family-centered care is parent-professional collaboration. By their nature collaborative relationships show respect for families and therefore support. Collaboration reflects a change from the traditional models of care. For this reason nurses must examine their attitudes to determine their ability to participate in parent-professional partnerships. A basic characteristic is the belief that parents are experts concerning their child. The partnership is based on trust and is built on comunication. The Guidelines box offers strategies for developing successful partnerships with parents.

Throughout the lengthy process of caring for a child with special needs, family members become experts in management of their child's care. Unfortunately, this expertise is not always acknowledged by health care providers who tend to be directive, rather than collaborative, in their ap-

---

### GUIDELINES
#### Developing Successful Parent-Professional Partnerships

Promote primary nursing; in nonhospital setting designate a case manager.

Acknowledge the parents' overall competence and their unique expertise with their child.

Respect the parents' time as having equal value to that of other members of the child's health care team.

Explain or define any medical, technical, or disciplinary-specific terms.

Tell families, "I am not sure" or "I don't know" when appropriate.

Facilitate the family's effectiveness in team meetings:

Provide families with the opportunity to decide on the appropriate family members and professionals to include in assessment conferences and other meetings.

Provide information to parents in a face-to-face meeting before convening any formal decision-making meeting about their child.

Distribute meeting agendas to all participants, including the family, before the date of the meeting. Families, like all other team members, should always be made aware of why a meeting is being held, who will be there, and what to expect.

Introduce other professionals who may be involved with the child to the parents before any group meeting.

Provide parents with the same information as other participants so that they can contribute to any decision about their child (e.g., child development checklist, copies of assessment reports).

Invite parents to speak first and often throughout any information-giving or decision-making meetings, to give their perspectives and describe their observations before professionals give theirs.

Be open with families and with other professionals when there is disagreement about any aspect of assessment or programming.

---

Data from Bruder M: Parent and professional partnerships under PL 99-457, *Early Child Update* 5(2):1-2, 1989; Johnson B, McGonigel M, Kaufmann R, editors: *Guidelines and recommended practices for the Individualized Family Service Plan*, Washington, DC, 1989, Association for the Care of Children's Health; and Johnson BH, Jeppson ES, Redburn L: *Caring for children and families: guidelines for hospitals*, Bethesda, MD, 1992, Association for the Care of Children's Health.

proach to the family. This is particularly common during periods of hospitalization, when role confusion occurs. At home parents are expected to care for their child, yet in the hospital they may be disregarded as participants in care. Providing a supportive atmosphere must include respect for their knowledge, coordination of care with family members, and willingness to include their suggestions in the treatment plan.

Partnership depends on good communication. Research has suggested that these are factors that influence nurse-family communication. A family whose child is ill responds along what health care providers may perceive as a continuum from the "good" to the "difficult" family stereotype. Nurses readily establish relationships with the "good" family, who perceives staff as having control or power and accepts this hierarchy. However, this is often not the case with a family that is considered "difficult" and is characterized as being overinvolved or underinvolved in the child's care (Table 22-3).

**NURSING TIP**   Use cards and a file box to store information about parent self-help groups. The system facilitates adding new groups, updating old ones, and keeping cards in easy-to-retrieve alphabetic order.

Nurses also display patterns of behavior with regard to parents of ill children. First, facilitative nurses acknowledge the parents' crucial roles and attempt to remove barriers to their involvement in care. Second, nurses who desire a high degree of control over their work may become "rule enforcers" with parents. Third, nurses may establish collegial relationships with parents over time, in which there is respect for the parents as experts regarding their child. Lastly, nurses may avoid a parent whose values differ from their own or a parent who is overly demanding from the nurses' perspective.

The nurse and family come to share explicit and implicit expectations of one another, form views of one another, and negotiate roles about the child's care. Levels of trust and control are central to their interactions. (See Family Focus box.)

Parents who mistrust professionals act differently than those who have faith in the health care team. Nurses trust parents differently as well, based on the judgment of the parenting they observe. Strategies for managing parent-nurse interactions are described in Table 22-3.

## Community Resources

In the past if coping strategies could not be used to reduce the disruption and stress of maintaining the child in the home, the seriously affected child may have been permanently placed outside the home in a residential facility. Such placements are increasingly difficult to secure. Options vary from one location to another; however, many possibilities

| **TABLE 22-3**   Strategies for facilitating parent-nurse interaction | |
|---|---|
| **Parent Characteristics** | **Strategies** |
| **Silent in Care** | |
| Have trust and mistrust | Do not force participation |
| May not accompany child; prefer to wait outside | Avoid authoritarian stance |
| Are very uncertain, quiet | Use simple terms and demystify surroundings |
| Use little verbal communication | Explain what will happen |
| Visit on limited or irregular basis | Point out how their presence helps child |
| **Recipient of Care** | |
| Have total trust | Offer/provide information; elicit feedback to ensure their understanding |
| Want nurse to make decisions | |
| Offer numerous positive comments | Allow unlimited contact with child |
| Are easily impressed with information | Engage them in gaining child's cooperation |
| Are prone to misunderstandings | |
| Comply with rules | |
| Focus on child while visiting | |
| **Monitor of Care** | |
| Have high levels of mistrust | Believe that you can build trust |
| Have attitude that "mistakes can happen" | Negotiate, negotiate, negotiate! |
| Monitor everyone's performance | Be flexible regarding rules |
| Involved in all decisions | Avoid issues of control |
| Want high levels of information | Ask their opinion and use their suggestions |
| Know agency's hierarchy | |
| Seek care from nurses | |
| Ask for rule changes | |
| **Manager of Care** | |
| Are similar to monitors, but less angry | Recognize them as experts about their child |
| Achieve complex coordination of child's chronic care | Recognize need for respite |

Developed by Donna M Dixon, Memorial Medical Center, Springfield, IL, 1993. Modified from Knafl KA, Cavallari KA, Dixon DM: *Pediatric hospitalization: family and nurse perspectives*, Glenview, IL, 1988, Scott, Foresman.

## FAMILY FOCUS
### Respect for Parents' Intuitive "Sixth Sense"

I have great admiration for parents of children with chronic disorders and their ability to manage complex medical and nursing problems. Parents who receive education regarding the nature of the disorder and who are encouraged to practice the skills necessary to care for their child during the diagnostic period often achieve acceptance and have a shortened period of grieving.

Parents can achieve mastery over many of the skills needed to care for their child and can in turn teach the child to perform self-care as the child matures. Parents often develop a "sixth sense" about impending problems related to their child's disorder. I have found that accessing this "sixth sense" and facilitating the parent's ability to solve problems based on this intuitive knowledge has averted many health-related crises in the child. The greatest gift we as nurses can give to patients and families is to respect their independence and their ability to manage self-care with input as needed from the health care team.

A pediatric nurse

can be considered: in-home care by nursing personnel, medical daycare, respite care, transitional/long-term care, and medical or specialized foster care (Ahmann and Scher, 1996).

A family's acknowledgment that caring for their child is burdensome is not necessarily maladjustment. Alternative placements may be the only option that will maintain the integrity of the family. Aging parents may be forced to accept such alternatives because of progressive inability to meet the demands of a severe disability. When most of the child's care is given to others, abandoning the role of primary caregiver may be followed by an initial sense of loss, guilt, relief, and ambivalence; a pattern of reactions not unlike that seen after the death of a terminally ill child. (See Chapter 23.)

Besides out-of-home placement options, several community resources, such as parent support groups, health care resources, availability of funding, rehabilitation, respite care, alternatives for schooling, equipment, and educational facilities and recreational programs,* are major elements in family adjustment. These kinds of resources are better developed in some areas than in others, meaning that what is available to a family largely depends on where they reside.

Local and national disease-oriented organizations may provide needed support and assistance to families that qualify. Many of these are identified elsewhere in the text under the diagnosis. Federal and state departments of health, social service, mental health, and labor may be able to help locate appropriate regional resources. For example, state *Pro-*

*grams for Children with Special Health Needs* (formerly Crippled Children's Services) offer financial assistance for children with various disabling conditions. Nurses should become familiar with those in their communities and with vocational programs for special groups.

Even though community resources may exist, it is often very difficult for parents to find appropriate services, and coordination among many agencies many be lacking. Fragmented care is a key complaint from families, with specific problems of delayed referral and negative experiences with agency personnel identified as other concerns. Therefore community networking for improved services is essential.*

Case management is a crucial service for families of children with special needs. Effective case management can result in both the use of more community services and improved financial assistance for families. (See Case Management in Chapter 1.) See the Nursing Care Plan on pp. 939-944.

> **NURSING ALERT**
>
> Be aware that many families may not have a telephone. Other families may have telephones but are reluctant to reveal the telephone number. To overcome these difficulties, use the following strategies:
> 1. Help family identify telephone access close to home (e.g., neighbor's home, nearby store).
> 2. Explore methods to obtain telephone service for family (e.g., social service agencies, charitable organizations).
> 3. Be sensitive to family's concern for privacy when asking for a telephone number; explain reason for needing number and to whom it will be given.

---

*A general source of information is the **National Information Center for Children and Youth with Disabilities,** PO Box 1492, Washington, DC 20013, (202) 884-8200 or (800) 695-0285, fax: (202) 884-8441; e-mail: nichcy@aed.org; www.nichcy.org. A comprehensive list of books and pamphlets for parents and teachers is available from the **National Easter Seal Society,** 230 W Monroe St, Suite 1800, Chicago, IL 60606, (312) 726-6200, (800) 221-6827, fax: (312) 726-1494; www.easter-seals.org.

*__Georgetown University Child Development Center__ publishes workbooks and other texts pertinent to community services for children with disabilities—3307 M St NW, Suite 401, Washington, DC 20007-3935, (202) 687-8635, fax: (202) 687-8899; website/e-mail: gvcdc.georgetown.edu.

# *Nursing Care Plan*
## The Child with Chronic Illness or Disability

| |
|---|
| **NURSING DIAGNOSIS:** Delayed growth and development related to chronic illness or disability, parental reactions (overbenevolence), repeated hospitalization |

**PATIENT GOAL 1:** Will attain maximum expected growth and developmental potential

- **NURSING INTERVENTIONS/*RATIONALES***
See Table 22-1

- **EXPECTED OUTCOME**
Child attains appropriate physical, psychosocial, and cognitive development for age and abilities

| |
|---|
| **NURSING DIAGNOSIS:** Risk for interrupted family processes related to situational crisis (child with a chronic disease or disability) |

**PATIENT (FAMILY) GOAL 1:** Will exhibit positive adjustment to the diagnosis

- **NURSING INTERVENTIONS/*RATIONALES***
Provide opportunity for family to adjust to discovery of diagnosis
Anticipate grief reaction to loss of the "perfect" child *because this usually occurs in the adjustment process*

*Continued*

## Nursing Care Plan
## The Child with Chronic Illness or Disability—cont'd

### PATIENT (FAMILY) GOAL 1—cont'd

- **NURSING INTERVENTIONS/*RATIONALES*—cont'd**

Explore family's feelings regarding child and their ability to cope with the disorder

Encourage family to express their concerns

Repeat information as often as necessary *to reinforce family's understanding*

Serve as a role model regarding attitudes and behavior toward child

- **EXPECTED OUTCOMES**

Parents verbalize feelings and concerns regarding implications of the disease

Family demonstrates an attitude of acceptance and adjustment

### PATIENT (FAMILY) GOAL 2: Will demonstrate understanding of disorder and treatment options

- **NURSING INTERVENTIONS/*RATIONALES***

Help family to understand the disorder, its therapies, and implications

Reinforce information given by others *to promote better understanding*

Clarify misconceptions

Provide accurate information at a rate family can absorb *because information given too rapidly will not be learned*

Discuss advantages and limitations of therapeutic plan

Encourage family to ask questions and express concerns

- **EXPECTED OUTCOME**

Family demonstrates an understanding of the disease (specify) and treatment options

### PATIENT (FAMILY) GOAL 3: Will experience reduction of fear and anxiety

- **NURSING INTERVENTIONS/*RATIONALES***

Explore family's concerns and feelings of irritation, guilt, anger, disappointment, inadequacy, and other feelings

Help family distinguish between realistic fears and unfounded fears; address unfounded fears

Discuss with parents their fears regarding:
    Dealing with child's anxiety about condition
    Fear of dreadful developments
    Fear of death
    Fear of tests and procedures
    Child's ability to compete with peers

Explore their feelings regarding prescribed therapies

- **EXPECTED OUTCOME**

Family members discuss their fears and concerns

### PATIENT (FAMILY) GOAL 4: Will exhibit positive adaptation to child's condition

- **NURSING INTERVENTIONS/*RATIONALES***

Explore family's reaction to child and the disorder

Assess family's coping skills, abilities, and resources *so that these can be reinforced*

Help family to achieve a realistic view of child's capabilities and limitations

Foster positive family relationships *so that their ability to cope is maximized*

Assess interpersonal relationships within family, especially behaviors that reflect family's attitudes toward affected child

Intervene appropriately if there is evidence of maladaptation; refer for counseling if appropriate

Encourage parents in their attempts to promote child's development

Emphasize positive aspects of child's abilities or attributes

Help family gain confidence in their ability to cope with child, the disorder, and its impact on other family members

- **EXPECTED OUTCOME**

Family verbalizes feelings and concerns regarding special needs of child and their effect on the family process

Family members demonstrate an attitude of confidence in their ability to cope

### PATIENT (FAMILY) GOAL 5: Will exhibit ability to care for child

- **NURSING INTERVENTIONS/*RATIONALES***

Help family develop a thorough plan of care

Teach skills needed *to provide optimum care*

Interpret child's behavior to parents (e.g., anger, depression, regression, physical modifications as a result of disorder) *to prevent any unwarranted negative reaction (e.g., punishment) to child*

Help family plan for the future

- **EXPECTED OUTCOME**

Family sets realistic goals for selves, child, and others

### PATIENT (FAMILY) GOAL 6: Will have needs as family unit met

- **NURSING INTERVENTIONS/*RATIONALES***

With family, identify family support systems (immediate family, extended family, friends, health service providers, parent-to-parent support groups)

With family, assess the number, affiliation, and interrelationships (if any) of persons the family sees as important

Help family to assign specific tasks to specific people *so that family receives support they need*

Reinforce positive coping mechanisms

Encourage family members to discuss their feelings with each other

Impress on parents the importance of providing as normal a life as possible for the affected child

Emphasize the growth and developmental progress of their child *to help family feel adequate in their maternal-paternal roles*

Help family foster child's development by stimulating child to achieve age-appropriate goals consistent with activity tolerance

- **EXPECTED OUTCOMES**

Family demonstrates positive, growth-promoting behaviors

Family avails itself of support

# Nursing Care Plan
## The Child with Chronic Illness or Disability—cont'd

**PATIENT (FAMILY) GOAL 7:** Will receive adequate support

- **NURSING INTERVENTIONS/RATIONALES**

Be available to family *to provide support*

Listen to family members—singly or collectively

Allow for expression of feelings, including feelings of guilt, helplessness, and their perception of the impact that the condition may have (or does have) on the family

Refer to community agencies or special organizations providing assistance—financial, social, and support

Refer to genetic counseling if appropriate

Help family learn to expect feelings of frustration and anger toward child; reassure them that it is not a reflection on their parenting

Assist family in problem solving

Encourage interaction with other families who have a similarly affected child

   Introduce to families

   Provide information regarding support groups

Help families learn when to accept and when to "fight" for the care and services they feel are needed

- **EXPECTED OUTCOMES**

Family maintains contact with health care providers

Family demonstrates an understanding of the needs of the child and the impact the condition will have on them

Problems are dealt with early

Family becomes involved with local agencies and support groups as needed

**PATIENT (FAMILY) GOAL 8:** Will be prepared for home care

- **NURSING INTERVENTIONS/RATIONALES**

Teach skills needed *to ensure optimum home care*

With family, assess home situation, including family's strengths, weaknesses, and support systems

Help devise an individualized plan of care based on assessment of family's needs and resources

Encourage family involvement in care while still in the hospital *so that they are better prepared to assume child's care*

Encourage family to ask questions regarding posthospital care

Explore family's attitudes toward child's entry (or reentry) into the home

Help family acquire needed drugs, supplies, and equipment

Refer to special agencies, based on needs assessment, *for ongoing support and assistance*

Arrange for regular follow-up care *to assess effectiveness of home management*

- **EXPECTED OUTCOMES**

Family demonstrates competence with needed skills (specify skills and method of demonstration)

Family members avail themselves of resources within their community (specify)

Family complies with home care program

**PATIENT (FAMILY) GOAL 9:** Will participate in ongoing care

- **NURSING INTERVENTIONS/RATIONALES**

Participate in follow-up care *to ensure continuity of care*

Coordinate team management of child and family

Be alert to comments by child or family members that indicate possible problems *so that problems are identified early*

Assess interpersonal relationships within family, especially behaviors that reflect family's attitudes toward child

Be alert for cues that signal undue anxiety and guilt: preoccupation with causative factors, constant analysis of effects of therapies, experimentation with diets and folk remedies, seeking magical cures

Be alert for overprotective behaviors such as assuming self-care activities for child, restricting child's activities or interaction with peers

Allow family to express discouragement at interference with activities and what appears to be slow progress

- **EXPECTED OUTCOMES**

Family participates in follow-up care

Family expresses both positive and negative reactions to child's progress

Signs that may indicate family's difficulty in adjusting to child's condition are identified early

**PATIENT (SIBLINGS) GOAL 10:** Will exhibit positive attachment behaviors with child

- **NURSING INTERVENTIONS/RATIONALES**

Assess siblings *to identify areas of concern*

Communicate honestly with siblings about child's disease or disability in accord with parental wishes

Provide opportunity for siblings to ask questions and express feelings, but avoid lengthy explanations before they ask *so that they are not overwhelmed*

Help parents talk to siblings about child's condition and interpret siblings' needs and questions

Encourage parents to spend special time with their children who are not ill or disabled

Help siblings and family understand that it is normal for them to sometimes have negative feelings about child

Prepare siblings in advance for any household changes *because preparation encourages coping*

Encourage parents to allow sibling(s) to participate in child's care and therapy as appropriate

Help siblings learn how to explain child's condition to their peers and others

Acknowledge siblings' strengths and abilities to cope

Refer to sibling groups and networks composed of siblings of children with same or similar conditions *for ongoing support*

Assess siblings periodically *to determine their adjustment to the family situation*

- **EXPECTED OUTCOMES**

Siblings verbalize or otherwise demonstrate their feelings and concerns

Parents include siblings in discussions about affected child

Parents make an effort to spend time with other children

Siblings exhibit an understanding of household changes

*Continued*

# Nursing Care Plan
## The Child with Chronic Illness or Disability—cont'd

**PATIENT (SIBLINGS) GOAL 10—cont'd**

• **EXPECTED OUTCOMES—cont'd**
Siblings assist with affected child's care (specify)
Siblings become involved in support groups (specify)

---

**NURSING DIAGNOSIS:** Anxiety/fear related to tests, procedures, hospitalization, and so on (specify)

---

**PATIENT GOAL 1:** Will demonstrate understanding of hospitalization, procedures, and so on (specify)

• **NURSING INTERVENTIONS/RATIONALES**
See Preparation for Diagnostic and Therapeutic Procedures, Chapter 27
See Nursing Care Plan: The Child in the Hospital, Chapter 26

• **EXPECTED OUTCOME**
Child copes with stresses of procedures, tests, etc. (specify)

---

**NURSING DIAGNOSIS:** Risk for injury (specify)

---

**PATIENT GOAL 1:** Will experience no injury

• **NURSING INTERVENTIONS/RATIONALES**
Assess environment for hazards if indicated
Teach safety precautions *to decrease risk of injury*
Encourage activities that are compatible with the disease or disability

• **EXPECTED OUTCOME**
Child remains free of injury and complications

**PATIENT GOAL 2:** Will cope with limitations positively

• **NURSING INTERVENTIONS/RATIONALES**
Help devise alternatives for restricted activities and help child cope with physical limitations *so that child's ability to cope is maximized*

• **EXPECTED OUTCOME**
Child demonstrates appropriate adaptation to limitations (specify)

**PATIENT GOAL 3:** Will experience no complications

• **NURSING INTERVENTIONS/RATIONALES**
Stress importance of sound health practices and frequent health supervision *so that complications are less likely to develop*
Make certain child and family understand the therapeutic measures prescribed *to promote optimum health*
Encourage older child to choose activities but take responsibility for own safety
Plan with allied personnel (e.g., teachers, coaches, counselors) appropriate activities
Confer with school nurse (or other person) regarding any special needs of child
Discuss with parents any indicated limit-setting

• **EXPECTED OUTCOME**
Child maintains optimum health

---

**NURSING DIAGNOSIS:** Deficient diversional activity related to environmental lack of diversion, physical limitations (specify), hospitalization

---

**PATIENT GOAL 1:** Will have opportunity to participate in diversional activities

• **NURSING INTERVENTIONS/RATIONALES**
Provide appropriate stimulation
Encourage activities appropriate to age, interest, and capabilities of child
Encourage physical exercise that does not overtax child (if indicated)
Incorporate therapeutic needs in play activities as appropriate
Supervise and encourage activities of daily living
Encourage child's natural tendency to be active
Encourage interaction with family and peers
Include child in planning and scheduling care *to ensure adequate time for diversional activities*

• **EXPECTED OUTCOME**
Child engages in age-appropriate activities within limits of capabilities

**PATIENT GOAL 2:** Will engage in appropriate exercise

• **NURSING INTERVENTIONS/RATIONALES**
Encourage child to participate in normal childhood activities commensurate with interests and capabilities
Encourage and reinforce age-appropriate behaviors, experiences, and socialization with peers
Discourage physical inactivity *so that child receives needed exercise*

• **EXPECTED OUTCOME**
Child engages in nonsedentary activities within limits of disability or condition

---

**NURSING DIAGNOSIS:** Impaired social interaction related to hospitalization, confinement to home, frequent illness, activity intolerance, fatigue (specify)

---

**PATIENT GOAL 1:** Will experience positive interpersonal relationships

• **NURSING INTERVENTIONS/RATIONALES**
Encourage child to maintain usual activities
Arrange for continued interpersonal contacts while hospitalized or otherwise confined
Provide opportunities for interaction with others, especially peers, *for optimum growth and development*
Encourage regular school attendance (including daycare, beginning school, return to school)
Arrange for rest periods at school if needed *so that child is better able to attend school*

# Nursing Care Plan
## The Child with Chronic Illness or Disability—cont'd

Promote peer contact whenever possible *so that relationships can develop and be maintained*

Encourage recreational outlets and after-school activities appropriate to child's interests and capabilities

Discourage activities that increase isolation from others

- **EXPECTED OUTCOMES**

Child engages in appropriate activities

Child associates with peers and family

Child attends school with reasonable regularity

> **NURSING DIAGNOSIS:** Self-care deficit (specify) related to specific impairment (specify)

**PATIENT GOAL 1:** Will engage in self-care activities

- **NURSING INTERVENTIONS/***RATIONALES*

Teach child about the disease and therapies *to ensure optimum understanding, cooperation, and safety*

Encourage child to assist in own care as age and capabilities permit

Provide or help devise methods to facilitate maximum functioning

Incorporate play that encourages desired behavior *to encourage cooperation and compliance*

Select toys and activities that allow maximum participation by child

Modify environment if needed (specify) *so that child can assume self-care activities*

Assist with self-care activities where needed (specify)

Avoid undue persistence to accomplish a goal

Provide incentives *to achieve desired behavior*

Instruct when to seek assistance from family or health care providers

- **EXPECTED OUTCOME**

Child engages in self-help activities commensurate with capabilities (specify activities and extent of involvement)

**PATIENT GOAL 2:** Will achieve sense of competence and mastery

- **NURSING INTERVENTIONS/***RATIONALES*

Capitalize on child's assets; help child compensate for liabilities

Praise child for accomplishments and "near" accomplishments, such as partial completion of a task, *to encourage sense of competency*

Ensure adequate rest before attempting energy-expending activities

Emphasize child's abilities and focus on realistic endeavors

Emphasize positive coping behaviors

Discourage activities that are beyond child's capabilities; promote and reinforce successful endeavors

Encourage participation in own care to the extent that child is able

Teach and encourage responsibility for use of equipment, appliances, testing, medication (specify)

Help child become adept at self-management to maximum capabilities

- **EXPECTED OUTCOMES**

Child takes responsibility for self-care according to age and capabilities (specify)

Child engages in appropriate activities without undue fatigue

> **NURSING DIAGNOSIS:** Disturbed body image related to perception of disability (self and others), feeling of differentness, inability to participate in specific activities (specify)

**PATIENT GOAL 1:** Will maintain positive attitude

- **NURSING INTERVENTIONS/***RATIONALES*

Convey an attitude of understanding, caring, and acceptance *to encourage positive attitude and self-image*

Maintain open communications with child

Relate to child on appropriate cognitive level

Serve as a role model for others *so that they are more accepting*

- **EXPECTED OUTCOME**

Child maintains a positive attitude (specify behaviors)

**PATIENT GOAL 2:** Will express feelings and concerns

- **NURSING INTERVENTIONS/***RATIONALES*

Encourage verbalization of feelings and perceptions, especially feelings of "differentness"

Explore feelings concerning disease or disability and its implications: stress of being "different," physical limitations, difficulty competing, relationships with peers, self-image

Encourage child to discuss feelings about how he or she thinks others feel about the disorder

- **EXPECTED OUTCOME**

Child openly discusses feelings and concerns about the condition, therapies, and perceived reactions of others

**PATIENT GOAL 3:** Will cope with actual or perceived changes caused by illness

- **NURSING INTERVENTIONS/***RATIONALES*

Acknowledge feelings and facilitate sharing feelings with family and other health professionals

Clarify misconceptions child may have acquired

Help child to identify positive aspects of situation *to facilitate coping*

- **EXPECTED OUTCOME**

Child discusses the disorder and feelings regarding limitations imposed by it

**PATIENT GOAL 4:** Will cope with disorder and its effects

- **NURSING INTERVENTIONS/***RATIONALES*

Help child assess own strengths and assets; emphasize strengths

Identify coping behaviors *so that they can be reinforced*

Support positive coping mechanisms and extinguish negative ones

*Continued*

# Nursing Care Plan
## The Child with Chronic Illness or Disability—cont'd

**PATIENT GOAL 4—cont'd**

- **NURSING INTERVENTIONS/**RATIONALES**—cont'd**

Help child set realistic goals *to facilitate coping*

Encourage as much independence as condition allows

Introduce child to other children who have adjusted well to this or a similar disorder

Suggest involvement with special groups and facilities for children with similar problems

- **EXPECTED OUTCOMES**

Child identifies own assets and strengths realistically

Child verbalizes positive suggestions for adjusting to the disability

Child becomes involved with special group activities

**PATIENT GOAL 5:** Will exhibit improved self-esteem and self-concept

- **NURSING INTERVENTIONS/**RATIONALES**

Encourage an appealing physical appearance: good body hygiene; clean straight teeth; good grooming; stylish hair and clothing; makeup for teenage girls

Assist with improving appearance and grooming

Point out positive aspects of own coping, appearance, and other capabilities

Promote constructive thinking in child; encourage child to maximize strengths

Reinforce positive behaviors

Help child to determine and engage in activities that foster self-esteem

Promote independence, *because this is an important part of self-esteem*

- **EXPECTED OUTCOMES**

Child demonstrates a positive appearance and good body image (specify)

Child appears clean, well-groomed, and attractively dressed

Child exhibits behaviors that indicate elevated self-esteem (specify)

**PATIENT GOAL 6:** Will exhibit appropriate sense of control

- **NURSING INTERVENTIONS/**RATIONALES**

Channel need for control and feeling of effectiveness in appropriate directions

Encourage child to monitor own care as appropriate

Provide opportunities for child to make choices and participate in care when appropriate *to ensure sense of control*

Assess child for vocational planning when appropriate

- **EXPECTED OUTCOME**

Child becomes actively involved in own care and management

**PATIENT GOAL 7:** Will be prepared for discharge

- **NURSING INTERVENTIONS/**RATIONALES**

Begin early in hospitalization to discuss "going home"

Help child develop independence and self-help capabilities

Encourage visits from friends *to help child assess the impact of any change in appearance or behavior that might interfere with returning to previous environments*

- **EXPECTED OUTCOME**

Child verbalizes and otherwise demonstrates interest in going home

See also:

Nursing Care Plan: The Child in the Hospital, Chapter 26

Nursing Care Plan: The Family of the Child Who Is Ill or Hospitalized, Chapter 26

Nursing Care Plan: The Child Who Is Terminally Ill or Dying, Chapter 23

## KEY POINTS

- Trends in the care of children with chronic illness or disability have focused on developmental stages, family development, family-centered care, normalization, mainstreaming, early intervention, and managed care.

- Promoting normal development in the child with a chronic condition or disability involves a variety of individualized strategies of support, normalization, and problem solving at each developmental stage.

- Providers and parents can play an active role in helping the child with a chronic condition or disability to cope. Acknowledging positive and negative coping strategies, applying principles of normalization, fostering hope, providing age-appropriate health education, and assisting the older child in setting realistic future goals are some key strategies.

- The family should play an active role in assessing needs and strengths.

- Supporting the family at the time of diagnosis includes observation of the setting, cognizance of the family's past experiences and background, individualizing support strategies, and ensuring that the family receives the information they want and need.

- Family tasks in adjusting to the child's condition include managing the child's condition on a daily basis, meeting developmental needs of all family members, coping with stress, managing a wide range of feelings stemming from the diagnosis and other stresses, and developing personal and professional supports.

- While families confront the challenges of caring for a child with a chronic condition, nurses can help families realize their abilities and strengths, identify problems, develop problem-solving strategies, and identify new coping strategies. The goal is optimal family functioning, as defined by the family.

- A family-centered approach to care that strengthens parent-professional collaboration enables and empowers parents and provides the best opportunity for appropriate intervention strategies that meet the unique needs of all family members.

# REFERENCES

Ahmann E, Scher A: Alternatives to home care for medically fragile children. In Ahmann E, editor: *Home care for the high risk infant: a family centered approach*, Gaithersburg, MD, 1996, Aspen.

Amer KS: A conceptual framework for studying child adaptation to type 1 diabetes, *Issues Compr Pediatr Nurs* 22(1):13-25, 1999.

American Academy of Pediatrics, Committee on Children with Disabilities: Managed care and children with special health care needs: a subject review, *Pediatrics* 102(3): 657-660, 1998.

Betz CL: Adolescent transitions: a nursing concern, *Pediatr Nurs* 24(1):23-26, 1998.

Betz CL: Adolescents with chronic conditions: linkages to adult service systems, *Pediatr Nurs* 25(5):473-476, 1999.

Bruce B, Ritchie JR: Nurses' practices and perceptions of family-centered care, *J Pediatr Nurs* 12(4):214-222, 1997.

Cayse L: Fathers of children with cancer: a descriptive study of their stressors and coping strategies, *J Pediatr Oncol Nurs* 11:102-108, 1994.

Center for the Future of Children, The David and Lucille Packard Foundation: Children and poverty, *Future Child* 7(2), 1997.

Clarke-Steffen L: Reconstructing reality: family strategies for managing childhood cancer, *J Pediatr Nurs* 12(5):278-287, 1997.

Clawson JA: A child with chronic illness and the process of family adaptation, *J Pediatr Nurs* 11(1):52-61, 1996.

Cohen MH: The stages of the prediagnostic period in chronic life-threatening childhood illness: a process analysis, *Res Nurs Health* 18(1):39-48, 1995.

Corbin JS, Strauss A: A nursing model for chronic illness management based upon the trajectory framework, *Sch Inq Nurs Pract* 3(3):155-174, 1995.

Curtin M, Lubkin I: What is chronicity? In Lubkin IL, editor: *Chronic illness*, ed 3, Boston, 1995, Jones & Bartlett.

Deal LW, Shiono PH, Behrman RE: Children and managed health care: analysis and recommendations, *Future Child* 8(2):4-24, 1998.

Duvall E: *Marriage and family development*, ed 5, New York, 1977, JB Lippincott.

Fahrner R, Mario EB: HIV infection and AIDS. In Jackson PL, Vessey JA: *Primary care of the child with a chronic condition*, ed 3, St Louis, 2000, Mosby.

Faro B: The effect of diabetes on adolescents' quality of life, *Pediatr Nurs* 25(3):247-253, 1999.

Faulkner MS: Family responses to children with diabetes and their influence on self-care, *J Pediatr Nurs* 11(2):82-93, 1996.

Fleitas J: When Jack fell down . . . Jill came tumbling after: siblings in the web of illness and disability, *MCN Am J Matern Child Nurs* 25(5):267-273, 2000.

Frankel K, Wamboldt MZ: Chronic childhood illness and maternal mental health: why should we care? *J Asthma* 35:621-630, 1998.

Freud A: *The ego mechanism of defense*, New York, 1966, International Universities Press.

Fugate DL, Fugate JM: Helping parents of young children with disabilities become consumers of early intervention: a marketing approach, *Infants Young Child* 8(2):71-80, 1995.

Fugate DL, Fugate JM: Putting the marketing plan to work: practical suggestions for early intervention programs, *Infants Young Child* 8(4):70-79, 1996.

Garwick AW and others: Parents' perceptions of helpful vs unhelpful types of support in managing the care of preadolescents with chronic conditions, *Arch Pediatr Adolesc Med* 152(7):665-671, 1998.

Gibson CH: The process of empowerment in mothers of chronically ill children, *J Adv Nurs* 21:1201-1210, 1995.

Gravelle AM: Caring for a child with a progressive illness during the complex phase: parents' experience of facing adversity, *J Adv Nurs* 25:738-745, 1997.

Harvey and others: Providing quality care in childhood cancer survivorship: learning from the past, looking to the future, *J Pediatr Oncol Nurs* 16(3):117-125, 1999.

Hauser ES, Dorn L: Transitioning adolescents with sickle cell disease to adult-centered care, *Pediatr Nurs* 25(5):479-488, 1999.

Hymovich DP, Hagopian GA: *Chronic illness in children and adults: a psychosocial approach*, Philadelphia, 1992, WB Saunders.

Jackson PL: The primary care provider and children with chronic conditions. In Jackson PL, Vessey JA: *Primary care of the child with a chronic condition*, ed 3, St. Louis, 2000, Mosby.

Kliebenstein MA, Broome ME: School re-entry for the child with chronic illness: parent and school personnel perceptions, *Pediatr Nurs* 26(6):579-583, 2000.

Knafl KA, Deatrick JA: Family management style: concept analysis and development, *J Pediatr Nurs* 5(1):4-14, 1990.

Knight L: Negotiating care roles, *Nurs Times* 91:31-33, 1995.

Kohlberg L: *Stages in the development of moral thought and action*, New York, 1969, Holt, Rinehart, & Winston Publishers.

Lazarus RS: The costs and benefits of denial. In Spinetta JJ, Deasy-Spinetta P, editors: *Living with childhood cancer*, St Louis, 1981, Mosby.

Leonard BJ, Kratz BJ, Skay CL: Comparison of mother-father perceptions of their child's self-management of diabetes, *Issues Compr Pediatr Nurs* 20:69-87, 1997.

Luterman D: Counseling families with a hearing impaired child, *Otolaryngol Clin North Am* 32(6):1037-1050, 1999.

Mastroyannopoulou K and others: The impact of childhood non-malignant life-threatening illness on parents: gender differences and predictors of parental adjustment, *J Child Psychol Psychiatry* 38(7):823-829, 1997.

May J: Fathers: the forgotten parent, *Pediatr Nurs* 22(3):243-271, 1996.

McCubbin HI and others: Culture, ethnicity, and the family: critical factors in childhood chronic illness and disabilities, *Pediatrics* 91(5):1063-1070, 1993.

McManus MA and others: *Strengthening partnerships between state programs for children with special health needs and managed care organizations*, Washington, DC, March 1996, US Department of Health and Human Services, Public Health Service, Health Resources and Services Administration, Maternal and Child Health Bureau.

McPherson M and others: A new definition of children with special needs, *Pediatrics* 102(1):137-140, 1998.

Monical W: Daycare for children who are medically fragile, *Except Parent* 25(2):27-31, 1995.

Murray JS: Understanding sibling adaptation to childhood cancer, *Issues Compr Pediatr Nurs* 23:39-47, 2000.

Newacheck PW, Halfon N: Prevalence and impact of disabling chronic conditions in childhood, *Am J Public Health* 88(4): 610-617, 1998.

Newacheck PW, Halfon N: Prevalence, impact, and trends in childhood disability due to asthma, *Arch Pediatr Adolesc Med* 154:287-293, 2000.

Newacheck PW and others: Monitoring and evaluating managed care for children with chronic illnesses and disabilities, *Pediatrics* 98:952-958, 1996.

Newacheck PW and others; An epidemiologic profile of children with special health care needs, *Pediatrics* 102:117-123, 1998.

Olshansky S: Chronic sorrow: a response to having a mentally defective child, *Soc Casework* 43:190-193, 1962.

Patterson J, Blum RW: Risk and resilience among children and youth with disabilities, *Arch Pediatr Adolesc Med* 150:692-698, 1996.

Perrin JM: Chronic illness in childhood. In Nelson WE and others: *Nelson textbook of pediatrics*, Philadelphia, 2000, WB Saunders.

Perrin JM, Shonkoff JP: Developmental disabilities and chronic illness: an overview. In Nelson WE and others: *Nelson textbook of pediatrics*, Philadelphia, 2000, WB Saunders.

Peters D: Individual and family growth and development. In Lubkin IM: *Chronic illness: impact and interventions*, ed 4, Boston, 1998, Jones & Bartlett.

Peters KD, Kochanek KD, Murphy SL: Deaths: final data for 1996, *Natl Vital Stat Rep* 47(9):1-100, 1998.

Piaget J: *The origins of intelligence in children*, New York, 1952, International Universities Press.

Piaget J, Inhelder B: *The growth of logical thinking from children to adolescence*, New York, 1958, Basic Books.

Purnell LD, Paulanka BJ: Purnell's model for cultural competence. In Purnell LD, Paulanka BJ, editors: *Transcultural health care: a culturally competent approach*, Philadelphia, 1998, FA Davis.

Quittner AL and others: Role strain in couples with and without a child with chronic illness: associations with marital satisfaction, intimacy, and daily mood, *Health Psychol* 17(2):112-124, 1998.

Rehm RS: Family culture and chronic conditions. In Jackson PL, Vessey JA: *Primary care of the child with a chronic condition*, ed 3, St Louis, 2000, Mosby.

Ritchie, MA: Self-esteem and hopefulness in adolescents with cancer, *J Pediatr Nurs* 16(1):35-42, 2001.

Rosenfeld L: *Your child and healthcare: a "dollars and sense" guide for families with special needs,* Baltimore, 1994, Paul H Brookes.

Russell MT, Reinbold J, Maltby HJ: Transferring to adult health care: experiences of adolescents with cystic fibrosis, *J Pediatr Nurs* 11(4):262-268, 1996.

Sands D, Wehmeyer M, editors: *Self-determination across the life span: independence and choice for people with disabilities,* Baltimore, 1996, Paul H Brookes.

Santelli B, Turnbull A, Higgins C: Parent to parent support and health care, *Pediatr Nurs* 23(3):303-306, 1997.

Sawin KJ, Cox AW, Metzger SG: Transition to adulthood. In Jackson PL, Vessey JA: *Primary care of the child with a chronic condition,* ed 3, St Louis, 2000, Mosby.

Schaefer L, McCaul K, Glasgow R: Supportive and unsupportive family behaviors: relationships to adherence and metabolic control in persons with type 1 diabetes, *Diabetes Care* 9:179-185, 1986.

Scher A, Ahmann E: Community resources for the family. In Ahmann E, editor: *Home care for the high risk infant: a family centered approach,* Gaithersburg, MD, 1996, Aspen.

Shepard MP, Mahon MM: Chronic conditions and the family. In Jackson PL, Vessey JA: *Primary care of the child with a chronic condition,* ed 3, St Louis, 2000, Mosby.

Siegel RD: Child care and the ADA, *Except Parent* 25(2):34, 1995.

Singer GHS, Yovanoff P: *A meta analysis and critical report of research on depression in parents of children with developmental disabilities on chronic illness.* Paper presented at American Association on Mental Retardation Annual Meeting, San Antonio, TX, May, 1996.

Stein REK: Home care: a challenging opportunity, *Child Health Care* 14(2):90-95, 1985.

Stein REK: To be or not to be . . . noncategorical, *J Dev Behav Pediatr* 17:36-37, 1996.

Sterken DJ: Uncertainty and coping in fathers of children with cancer, *J Pediatr Oncol Nurs* 13(2):81-88, 1996.

US General Accounting Office (USGAO), Report to the Chairman, Subcommittee on Employer-Employee Relations, Committee on Economic and Educational Opportunities, House of Representatives: *People with disabilities: federal programs could work together more efficiently to promote employment,* Pub No GAO/HEHS 96-126, Washington, DC, 1998, USGAO.

Vessey JA, Jackson PL: School and the child with a chronic condition. In Jackson PL, Vessey JA: *Primary care of the child with a chronic condition,* ed 3, St Louis, 2000, Mosby.

Vessey JA: *Primary care of the child with a chronic condition,* ed 3, St Louis, 2000, Mosby.

Vessey JA, Mebane DJ: Chronic conditions and child development. In Jackson PL, Vessey JA: *Primary care of the child with a chronic condition,* ed 3, St Louis, 2000, Mosby.

Vessey JA, Miola ES: Teaching adolescents self-advocacy skills, *J Pediatr Nurs* 23:53-56, 1997.

Wallander J, Varni J: Social support and adjustment in chronically ill and handicapped children, *Am J Community Psychol* 17:185-201, 1989.

Westbrook LE, Silver EJ, Stein REK: Implications for estimates of disability in children: a comparison of definitional components, *Pediatrics* 101(6):1025-1030, 1998.

Williams PD and others: Outcomes of a nursing intervention for siblings of chronically ill children: a pilot study, *J Soc Pediatr Nurs* 2(3):127-137, 1997.

Woodgate R: Adolescents' perspectives of chronic illness: "It's hard," *J Pediatr Nurs* 13(4):210-223, 1998.

Yoos HL: Children's illness concepts: old and new paradigms, *Pediatr Nurs* 20(2):134-140, 1994.

**Chapter** **23**

# Family-Centered End-of-Life Care

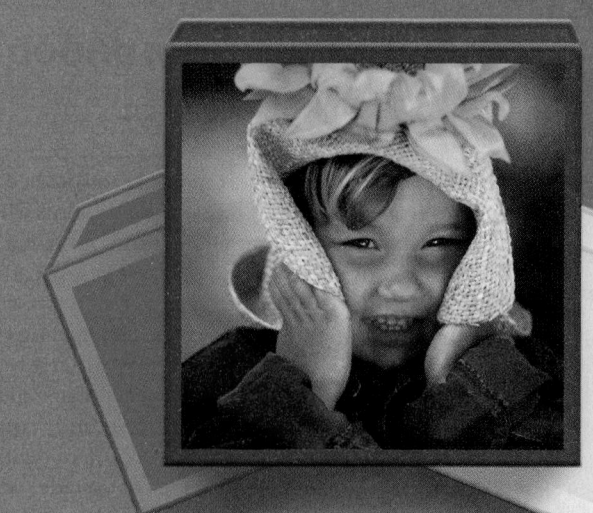

## Chapter Outline

**PALLIATIVE CARE IN CHILDHOOD TERMINAL ILLNESS, 948**
**Scope of the Problem, 948**
**Principles of Palliative Care, 948**
**Decision Making at the End of Life, 948**
Ethical Considerations in End-of-Life Decision Making, 949
Physician/Health Care Team Decision Making, 949
Parental Decision Making, 950
**Awareness of Dying in Children with Life-Threatening Illness, 950**
Developmental Age, 951
Previous Knowledge, 951
Honesty, 952
**Children's Understanding of and Reactions to Dying, 953**
Infants and Toddlers, 953
Preschool Children, 953
School-Age Children, 954
Adolescents, 954
**Delivery of Palliative Care Services, 955**
Hospital, 955
Home Care, 955
Hospice Care, 955

**NURSING CARE OF THE CHILD AND FAMILY AT THE END OF LIFE, 956**
**Management of Pain and Suffering, 956**
Pain and Symptom Management, 956
**Parents' and Siblings' Need for Education and Support Through the Caregiving Process, 958**
Educational Needs, 958
Emotional Support, 958
Religious and Spiritual Support, 958
Sibling Support, 958
Caregiver Support, 959
**Care at the Time of Death, 960**
Physical Changes, 960
Emotional Changes, 961
**Postmortem Care, 961**
*Nursing Care Plan: The Child Who Is Terminally Ill or Dying, 962*
**Care of the Family Experiencing Unexpected Childhood Death, 964**
Community-Based Follow-up, 965
**SPECIAL DECISIONS AT THE TIME OF DYING AND DEATH, 966**
**Right to Die/Do Not Resuscitate (DNR), 966**
**Viewing of the Body, 966**

Organ or Tissue Donation/Autopsy, 966
Siblings' Attendance at Funeral Services, 967
**CARE OF THE GRIEVING FAMILY, 968**
**Grief, 968**
Parental Grief, 969
Sibling Grief, 969
**Mourning, 970**
Shock and Disbelief, 970
Expression of Grief, 970
Disorganization and Despair, 971
Reorganization, 971
**Bereavement Programs, 971**
**THE NURSE AND THE CHILD WITH LIFE-THREATENING ILLNESS, 972**
**Nurses' Reactions to Caring for Children with Life-Threatening Illness, 972**
Denial, 972
Anger and Depression, 972
Guilt, 972
Ambivalence, 972
**Coping with Stress, 973**
Self-Awareness, 973
Knowledge and Practice, 973
Support Systems, 973
Other Strategies, 974

## Related Topics

The Child with Cancer, Ch. 36
Communicating with Families, Ch. 6
Compliance, Ch. 27
Ethical Decision Making, Ch. 1
Family-Centered Care, Ch. 1

Family-Centered Care of the Child with Chronic Illness or Disability, Ch. 22
Family-Centered Home Care, Ch. 25
Human Immunodeficiency Virus Infection and Acquired Immunodeficiency Syndrome, Ch. 35

Long-Term Sequelae of Treatment, Ch. 36
Neonatal Loss, Ch. 10
Neonatal Pain, Ch. 10
Pain Assessment; Pain Management, Ch. 26
Sudden Infant Death Syndrome, Ch. 13

# PALLIATIVE CARE IN CHILDHOOD TERMINAL ILLNESS

## Scope of the Problem

In 1998 over 55,000 children from birth to 19 died in the United States from all causes. Of the 28,371 infants who died, 67% died within the first month of life, most often in a neonatal intensive care unit (Murphy, 2000). These deaths were most often related to complications of prematurity, congenital birth defects, and infectious illnesses. The leading cause of death in toddlers and preschool children was largely related to accident or trauma. Children 5 to 14 years of age died most frequently from injuries/trauma, cancer, and congenital anomalies. In children older than 15 over 50% of deaths were related to accidents/trauma, homicide, or suicide, with cancer being the most common disease-related cause of death (Minino and Smith, 2001).

In addition to the number of children who die each year, it is estimated that approximately another 400,000 children in the United States are living with a serious, chronic, or life-threatening illness (Newacheck and Halfon, 1998, Newacheck and others, 1998). The numbers of children living with chronic, life-limiting illnesses has increased exponentially as advances in technology and pharmacology lead to improved treatments. These conditions often result in substantial health care needs and increase the possibility of death during childhood (Box 23-1). Although the number of children who die of any one illness is small, there is a significant amount of care needed for those children who do not survive their illness. The majority of these children die

◼ Melody Brown-Hellsten, MSN, RN, CPNP, revised this chapter.

---

### Box 23-1 ◼ ◼ ◼
### Medical Conditions Contributing to Childhood Death

Cancer
Complications of prematurity
Congenital anomalies
   Trisomy 13, 18
   Anencephaly
   Holoprosencephaly
   Lissencephaly
   Inborn errors of metabolism
Cystic fibrosis
Human immunodeficiency virus (HIV)/acquired immunodeficiency syndrome (AIDS)
Major organ dysfunction/failure
   Congenital heart defects
   Liver defects
   Renal failure
Neurodegenerative diseases
   Muscular dystrophy
   Spinal muscular atrophy
   Adrenoleucodystrophy
   Ataxia-telangiectasia
Severe neurologic/physical disability
Trauma
   Accidents
   Homicide/legal interventions
   Suicide

---

in a hospital setting, most frequently in an intensive care unit (ICU) (McCallum, Byrne, and Bruera, 2000) and often with some degree of pain or suffering in the hours to days before death (Wolfe and others, 2000).

Fortunately, there has been increasing attenton in recent years to the needs of children experiencing irreversible trauma or who have incurable diseases or disorders. The American Academy of Pediatrics (2000) recently released a statement on the necessity of incorporating principles of palliative care in pediatric practice. In addition, a number of international specialty groups have published suggested guidelines for care of children with life-threatening and terminal illnesses (Masera and others, 1999; World Health Organization, 1998; National Hospice and Palliative Care Organization, 2000). Unfortunately, there is currently a lack of clinical education of health care professionals in the principles of transitioning children from curative to palliative care or how to adequately manage the pain and suffering experienced by children and their families during the dying process. It is clear, however, that as our ability to treat disease, disability, and trauma advances, we must also improve our care of those children who live with the specter of chronic, life-threatening illness and premature death.

## Principles of Palliative Care

Palliative care involves a multidisciplinary approach to the management of a terminal illness or the dying process that focuses on symptom control and support rather than on cure or life prolongation in the absence of the possibility of a cure (Billings, 1998). The World Health Organization (WHO) (1990) defines *palliative care* as the "active total care of patients whose disease is not responsive to curative treatment." Palliative care interventions do not serve to hasten death; rather, they provide pain and symptom management, attention to issues faced by the child and family with regard to death and dying, and promotion of optimal functioning and quality of life during the time the child has remaining. There are several principles that are the hallmark of palliative care.

The child and family are considered the unit of care. The death of a child is an extremely stressful event for a family because it is out of the natural order of things. Children represent health and hope, and their death calls into question the understanding of life. A multidisciplinary team of health care professionals consisting of social workers, chaplains, nurses, personal care aids, and physicians skilled in caring for dying patients assist the family by focusing care on the complex interactions between physical, emotional, social, and spiritual issues.

Palliative care seeks to create a therapeutic environment, as homelike as possible, if not in the child's own home. Through education and support of family members, an atmosphere of open communication is provided regarding the child's dying process and its impact on all members of the family.

## Decision Making at the End of Life

Discussions concerning the possibility that a child's illness or condition is not curable and that death is an inevitable outcome causes everyone involved a great deal of stress. Physicians, other members of the health care team, and families must consider all information regarding the child's situation and make decisions that all parties agree to and that will have a profound impact on the child and family.

## Ethical Considerations in End-of-Life Decision Making

A number of ethical concerns arise when parents and health care professionals are deciding on the best course of care for the dying child (Table 23-1). Many parents and health care providers are concerned that not offering treatment that would cause potential pain and suffering, but might extend life, would be considered euthanasia or assisted suicide. To eliminate such concerns, it is necessary to understand the various terms. *Euthanasia* involves an action carried out by a person other than the patient to end the life of the patient suffering from a terminal condition. The intent of this action is based on the belief that the act is "putting the person out of his or her misery," and this action has also been called *mercy killing. Assisted suicide* occurs when someone provides the patient with the means to end his or her life and the patient uses that means to do so. The important distinction between these two actions involves who is actually acting to end the person's life.

The American Nurses Association (ANA) Code for Nurses (1995) does not support the active intent on the part of a nurse to end a person's life. However, it does permit the nurse to provide interventions to relieve symptoms in the dying patient even when the interventions involve substantial risks of hastening death. When the prognosis for a patient is poor and death is the expected outcome, it is ethically acceptable to withhold or withdraw treatments that may cause pain and suffering and provide interventions that promote comfort and quality of life. Therefore providing palliative care for patients is the ethically correct choice in such a circumstance.

## Physician/Health Care Team Decision Making

Decisions by physicians regarding care are often made on the basis of the progression of the disease or amount of trauma, the availability of treatment options that would provide cure from disease or restoration of health, the impact of such treatments on the child, and the child's overall prognosis (Davis and Eng, 1998). Often the main determinants prompting physicians to discuss end-of-life issues and options for children with critical illnesses include the child's age, premorbid cognitive condition and functional status,

---

| **TABLE 23-1**    Common ethical dilemmas in caring for terminally ill children | |
| --- | --- |
| **Rationale in Providing to Patient** | **Rationale in Withholding from Patient** |
| **Pain Control** | |
| Comfort is primary goal. | Side effects of opioids. |
| Improved quality of life. | Decreased level of cognition. |
| Easier dying process if child is pain free. | Fear of addiction (unfounded in terminally ill patients). |
| **Chemotherapy or Experimental Therapy** | |
| Prolonged life span. | Decreased blood counts, increased risk of infection, bleeding. |
| Possible increase in quality of life. | Side effects of treatment may be painful, uncomfortable. |
| Provides sense that family has done everything they can to save the child. | |
| **Supplemental Nutrition and Hydration (Intravenous, Nasogastric, G-Tube)** | |
| Belief that the child is hungry/thirsty. | Supplemental feedings beyond what child can ingest may actually cause nausea/vomiting. |
| Child cannot or will not eat. | Increase in tumor growth (feeding the tumor). |
| Fear that child will "starve" to death. | Increase in fluid volume may result in congestive heart failure, increased respiratory secre- |
| Primary role of parent to feed and nourish child. | tions and/or pulmonary congestion, which leads to questions of whether or not to imple- |
| Parental guilt. | ment diuretic. |
| | Increased urine output leads to increased risk of skin breakdown if child is incontinent. |
| | Risk of third spacing. |
| | Death is more comfortable and natural. |
| | Complaint of thirst is associated with dying process, not level of hydration (Zerwekh, 1997). |
| **Resuscitation** | |
| Family does not want to give up. | Allowing nature to take its course. |
| Conflicts with cultural or religious beliefs. | Family believes child has suffered enough, does not want aggressive intervention. |
| Denial that child is actually going to die. | Relieves family of responsibility to stop interventions that might prolong life. |
| **Autopsy** | |
| Research to help other children. | Religious, cultural belief. |
| Ability to check genetic link. | Family feelings. |
| | Desecrates body for funeral viewing (an unfounded fear). |

Modified from Hockenberry-Eaton M and others: *Essentials of pediatric oncology nursing: a core curriculum*, Glenview, IL, 1998, Association of Pediatric Oncology Nurses.

pain or discomfort, probability of survival, and quality of life (Masri and others, 2000). When the physician discusses this information openly with families, a shared decision-making process can occur and decisions can be made regarding *"do not resuscitate" (DNR) orders* and care that is focused on the comfort of the child and family during the dying process (see Table 23-1).

Unfortunately, many families are not given the option of shifting the focus of treatment to the child's comfort and quality of life when cure is unlikely. Currently there are no clear standards for determining the precise time that these discussions should take place, and results of studies of physician decision making regarding when to change the focus of care to palliation and comfort continue to be highly variable across physicians and settings (Randolph and others, 1999). This occurs for a number of reasons, including the belief that not being able to "save" a child is a "failure." Also, the physician and other members of the health care team may lack knowledge of and experience with the principles of palliative care.

### Parental Decision Making

Rarely are families prepared to cope with the numerous decisions that must be made when a child is dying. When the death is unexpected, as in the case of an accident or trauma, the confusion of emergency services and possibly an intensive care setting presents challenges to parents as they are asked to make very difficult choices. If the child has experienced either a life-threatening illness such as cancer or lived with a chronic illness that has now reached its terminal phase, parents are often unprepared for the reality of their child's impending death. (See Family Focus box.) Numerous studies have found that families facing the impending death of a child depend on information provided to them by the health care team, particularly an honest appraisal of the child's prognosis, to make difficult decisions regarding care options for their child (Hinds and others, 1997; James and Johnson, 1997; Kirschbaum, 1996).

As the group of health professionals who are most involved with families, nurses are in an excellent position to ensure that families are presented with the options available to them (Box 23-2). The nurse's first responsibility is to explore the family's wishes. This is best done in concert with the physician but at times they need to be initiated by the nurse. When initiating discussion around difficult issues, the nurse should be open to the child or family's indirect comments that communicate uncertainty or concerns about the course of care. Nurses should answer questions honestly, and if they do not know the answer, reassure the family that they will arrange for a discussion with the physician. It is important for the nurse caring for the child and family to address any fantasies or misunderstandings by seeking to clarify what the family has heard. Lastly, it is very important for the nurse to remain neutral and avoid giving personal opinions or experiences. The goal of communication should always be to assist the family to identify *their wishes,* based on their unique values and beliefs (Table 23-2).

## Awareness of Dying in Children with Life-Threatening Illness

One of the initial reactions of parents (and some health care professionals) to the discovery of a life-threatening illness is to protect the child from the impact of the diagnosis. However, it is now widely understood that terminally ill children develop an awareness of the seriousness of their diagnosis, even when protected from the truth. Anxiety may not always be attributable to fear of death but may be demonstrated in

---

### FAMILY FOCUS
#### Family of the Dying Child

No matter whether you have a PhD or many children, when your child dies, it is a new experience and nothing can prepare you for it. Like so many things in life, experience is the best teacher.

Three of our children have died, and by the time the third was dying, we handled many things differently. We learned a lot about dignity and the rights of the child and family. For example, at first, we didn't know that we had a right to have our child die at home. We also didn't understand pain medications and that if children are taking these medicines and are still in agony, they have not overdosed on the medication.

We learned a lot about case management. With our first two children, lots of different people were making decisions and disagreeing about what was best and what should be done. No one had primary authority. With our third child, one doctor took a primary role. Any questions and problems were handled by one person. I could call him 24 hours a day. It made a lot of difference, and I felt our concerns and needs were better heard and respected.

The nurses caring for our third child at home enabled me to step back and just be his mommy. When I could do this, I realized that we were fighting so hard for his life that we weren't really letting him die. His nurses had worked with him for a long time and really loved him. It was hard for them when we decided to let him die. In his last several days we wanted a lot of family time with our son, and I think the nurses felt left out. Something about their reaction to our increased time with him in the last few days made us feel guilty. If we had all been able to communicate a little more openly, I would have understood that they needed more time with him at the end, too. Everyone's needs could have been met.

Jeni Stepanek
Mother
Upper Marlboro, MD

---

### Box 23-2 ■ ■ □
#### Communicating with Families

Listen for an "invitation" to talk about the situation.
"Sometimes I wonder if I am doing the right thing."
"What have other parents done in this situation?"
"Do you know of other children who have survived this?"
"I think the doctor is not telling me everything."
Use open-ended, nonjudgmental questions to explore families' wishes.
"Can you tell me more about how you are feeling?"
"What questions do you (or your child) have that I can have answered for you?"
"What are your concerns (or worries, fears) right now?"
"What is important to you (your child/family) at this time?"

relationship to separation, pain, intrusive procedures, bodily change or mutilation, loneliness, immobilization, and punishment. Children as young as 2 or 3 years of age perceive and act in relation to their parents' emotions.

Children need honest and accurate information about their illness, treatments, and prognosis; this information needs to be given in clear, simple language. In most situations this best occurs as a gradual process over time, characterized by increasingly open dialogue between parents, professionals, and the child (Hockley, 2000; Lee and Johann-Liang, 1999). Providing an atmosphere of open communication early in the course of an illness facilitates answering difficult questions as the child's condition worsens. Providing appropriate literature about the disease, as well as the experience of illness and possible death, is also helpful.

Exactly how and when to involve children in decisions regarding care during their dying process and death is a very individual matter. In general, parents should be asked how they would like their child to be told of their prognosis and should be included in their care. Some parents may request that their child not be told that he or she is dying, even if the child asks. This often places health care providers in a difficult situation. Children, even at a young age, are very perceptive. Despite not being "told" outright that they are dying, they realize that there is something seriously wrong and that it involves them. Often, helping parents understand that honesty and shared decision making between them and their child at this time is very important to the child's emotional health, as well as the emotional health of the family, will encourage parents to allow discussion of dying with their child. Parents may require professional support and guidance in this process from a nurse, social worker, or child life specialist who has a good relationship with the child and family. Certain principles and guidelines can assist nurses and families in determining how to present facts about possible death and hope to a child in a way that fosters trust, enhances meaningful communication, and offers emotional support (Table 23-3 and Box 23-3).

## Developmental Age

A primary concern in any relationship with children is their age; the level of comprehension is a function of children's cognitive development. As discussed in detail on pp. 953-955, children at various ages have different understandings and fears of death. The younger child fears separation, which can be imposed by any number of circumstances, only one of which is death or illness. The older child fears the results of illness, particularly pain or bodily injury, as well as death itself. Anyone working with children must be aware of such developmental variations and be sensitive to their verbal and nonverbal language. Sharing with parents any information and observations relevant to the child's experience is important.

## Previous Knowledge

Another essential principle is finding out what the child is thinking and feeling. Before any explanations (true or false) are offered to children, they have already invented their own. Answers to questions such as "What do you think is wrong with you?" or "What have you heard others say?" provide information on which to structure further explanations. Very often a child will respond with an answer of such detailed, accurate information that the only element lacking is the name of the disease. Other answers may reveal possible areas of misconception, which can then be clarified or refocused.

Sometimes health care professionals, parents, and others hear the children's words but fail to comprehend their

| TABLE 23-2   Communicating bad news to families | |
|---|---|
| **Approach** | **Effective Techniques** |
| Provide a setting conducive to communication | Ensure privacy; use appropriate body language; make eye contact. Have parents choose who will attend. |
| Determine what the parent knows | Ask questions. ("What have you made of all this?" or "What were you told?") Listen to the vocabulary and comprehension of the parents. Recognize denial but do not acknowledge it at this stage. |
| Determine what the parent wants to know | Obtain a clear invitation to share information (if this is what the parent wants). Use questions such as "Are you the sort of person who likes to know every detail, or just the basic facts?" |
| Give information (aligning and educating) | Start at level of parent's comprehension and use the same vocabulary. Give information slowly, concisely, and in simple language. Avoid medical jargon. Check regularly to be certain that content is understood. |
| Respond to parents' reactions | Acknowledge all reactions and feelings, particularly using the empathic response technique (identifying emotion, identifying cause of emotion, and responding appropriately). Expect tears, anger, and other strong emotions. |
| Close | Briefly summarize major areas discussed. Ask parents if they have other important issues to discuss at this time. Make an appointment for the next meeting. |

Modified from Buchman R, Baile W: *How to break bad news to patients with cancer: a practical protocol for clinicians,* Spring Education Book, Alexandria, VA, 1998, American Society of Clinical Oncology.

**TABLE 23-3** Communicating with dying children

| Approach | Effective Techniques |
|---|---|
| Discuss at the child's level | Gear information to the developmental age of the child, remembering that younger children tend to be concrete thinkers, whereas older children are capable of abstract thought. <br> Begin with the child's experiences; "You've told us how tired you've been lately." |
| Let the child's questions guide | Begin the conversation with basic information, and let the child's questions direct the conversation. |
| Provide opportunities for the child to express feelings | Look for clues that child is open to communication. <br> Be accepting of whatever emotion is expressed. |
| Encourage feedback | Ask the child to summarize what has been heard. This provides the opportunity to clarify misunderstandings. |
| Use other resources | Books and movies can encourage dialogue. <br> Ask the child to name the people whom he or she can discuss problems with. |
| Use the child's natural expressive means to stimulate dialogue | Use books, games, art, play, and music to provide a means of expression. |

Modified from Doka KJ: *Living with life-threatening illness: a guide for patients, their families, and caregivers,* Lexington, MA, 1993, Lexington Books.

---

**Box 23-3** ■ ■ ■

**Themes That May Assist Parents in Discussing Possible Death with Children**

The following themes may be useful to parents as they communicate with their children about their possible death. They should be used with cautious judgment, generally at the child's lead.

1. Death, like birth, is part of the natural order of things. It happens sooner for some, later for others.
2. Death has social significance. We have special feelings for the people with whom we share our lives.
3. Death is a separation. The child loses family and friends, and they lose the child.
4. The child will not be alone at death and after death. Parental presence and support are important to the child. (Cultural and religious beliefs will influence the interpretation of this point.)
5. Even a young child has touched others and influenced the world in some way. Children can be assured that they have contributed and have led full, happy lives.
6. The child should be reassured that all feelings are normal: sadness, tears, anger, and resentment are all OK.
7. The child should be reassured that it is all right not to want to discuss his or her illness. When the child wants to talk, adults will be ready to listen.
8. Silence is acceptable if the child prefers. So are confused or silly-sounding expressions of feelings.
9. Although some of the experience leading to death may be painful, doctors will do what is necessary to minimize pain. Death itself will not hurt. After death the pain will never return.
10. When a loved one dies, people want a chance to say good-bye. Sometimes the person who is going to die will want to say good-bye to friends. Afterward, a funeral is a way many friends and relatives will say good-bye and gather to talk about how much they loved the child. People do not need to fear funerals.
11. Adults do not know much about death either and sometimes cry because they love the child and do not want to lose him or her. However, if a child has to die, parents, family, and friends will remember the happy times. The child's memory will live on in mind and spirit.

Modified from Deasy-Spinetta P, Spinetta J, Kung FH: *Emotional aspects of childhood leukemia: a handbook for parents,* New York, 2000, Leukemia Society of America.

---

meaning. They erroneously assume that because children can recite all the facts, they understand the implications or have dealt with all their fears. This may not be so; intellectualizing about one's condition can be a powerful defense mechanism. For example, an adolescent who was undergoing serious open-heart surgery knew precisely every detail of the operation, preoperative and postoperative care, and involved risks. The medical and nursing staff considered her exceptionally well prepared. However, everyone had failed to ask her how she felt. When the nurse asked her this before her surgery, the child answered, "I fear that I may die." Once this was verbalized, the girl, her parents, and the nurse focused on her fears instead of on the facts of the illness.

### Honesty

The last principle in explaining events such as death to children is honesty. Although the truth is usually the most difficult answer to give, in the long run it lessens many of the conflicts or problems that arise from lies, half-truths, or conspiracies. The truth provides answers for future questions and fosters trust. Children adeptly perceive the maxim: Do as I say, not as I do. It is very difficult to encourage children to be honest, confide in others, and openly discuss their fears if parents refuse to do the same.

Honesty is certainly not the easiest solution; the truth may prompt children to ask other distressing questions. The question many parents and health professionals dread the most is "Am I going to die?" When children have the answer to this question, the next question is "When?" Children need answers that are straightforward, yet caring. In telling children that a cure is no longer possible, one must also leave room for hope. The hope is redirected from cure to quality of life and comfort.

Adults need to be prepared to assist children in understanding and coping with the emotions of dealing with their own death and to reassure children that it is all right to express their feelings as they choose. There should be opportunity for the child to ask questions. If given the opportunity, children will tell others how much they want to know.

Asking questions such as "If the disease came back, would you want to know?" or "Do you want others to tell you everything, even if the news is not good?" helps children set the limits of how much truth they can accept and cope with.

Children need time to process feelings and information so that they can assimilate and hopefully accept the inevitable fact of mortality. As the child and family move through the dying process, it is important for the family to share their beliefs about the importance of the child and what they believe happens after death and to reassure the child that he or she will not be alone at the time of death and that the child will always be loved and remembered (Stevens, 1998).

# Children's Understanding of and Reactions to Dying

To effectively assist a child and family facing expected or unexpected death, nurses first need to learn about the child's understanding and experience of death. In addition, nurses need to understand how children generally perceive death, the fears associated with death in each age-group, and the personal meanings of death and bereavement during various stages of development. The concept of death is acquired through the sequential development of cognitive abilities and closely follows Piaget's stages. Although the abstract adult meaning of death as irreversible, inevitable, and universal is not understood by many children until preadolescence, throughout childhood the concept of death is greatly influenced by children's personal experiences with it and by the explanations and attitudes offered by others.

## Infants and Toddlers

Exactly how preverbal children view death is a mystery, because there is no way of reliably assessing their views of death. On the basis of their cognitive abilities, it is quite likely that they have no concept of death. The egocentricity of toddlers and their vague separation of fact and fantasy make it impossible for them to comprehend absence of life. Although they may repeat what initially sounds like a correct definition of death, such as "Grandpa is dead; he went to heaven," they may later refer to Grandpa as if he still exists. They can perceive events only in terms of their own frame of reference—living.

**Reactions to Dying.** Immobilization, regression to less independent levels of behavior, separation, intrusive or painful procedures, and alterations in ritualistic routine represent the greatest threats to seriously ill toddlers. They may perceive the seriousness of their condition from the parents' reactions of anxiety, sadness, depression, or anger. Although the children are unaware of the reason for such emotions, they are disturbed and upset by their parents' behavior. Helping parents deal with their feelings allows them more emotional reserve to meet the needs of their children. Encouraging parents to stay in the hospital as much as possible and to participate in the child's care promotes the parents' and children's adjustment to a serious, potentially fatal illness or accident.

## Preschool Children

Several characteristics of preschoolers' cognitive and psychologic development affect their concept of death. Because of their sense of precausality, they are unable to differentiate physical cause from logical or psychologic motivation. In addition, their egocentricity implies a tremendous sense of self-power and omnipotence. Therefore they believe that their thoughts are sufficient to cause events. The consequence of such magical thinking is the burden of guilt, shame, and punishment.

**Concept of Death.** Children between ages 3 and 5 years have usually heard the word "death" and have some connotation of its meaning. They see death as a departure, possibly as a type of sleep. They may recognize the fact of physical death but do not separate it from living abilities. The dead person in the coffin still breathes, eats, and sleeps. Death is temporary and gradual; life and death can change places with one another. Because of their immature concept of time, there is no real understanding of the universality and inevitability of death. Words such as "forever" and "everyone" have meaning only in the child's egocentric thinking. Waiting until Christmas may be "forever," and anybody the child denotes is "everyone."

**Reactions to Dying.** If preschoolers become seriously ill during this time, they may conceive of the illness as punishment for their thoughts or actions. The usual diagnostic and treatment procedures, in combination with enforced hospitalization, can confirm their belief that they are being punished. If their parents do not stay with them during hospitalization or prevent the traumatic procedures, they may be convinced that the parents are retaliating for previous misdeeds or bad thoughts.

The same principles of magical thinking and omnipotence affect preschoolers when a sibling becomes critically ill or dies. One of the most significant types of death is sudden infant death syndrome (SIDS). Because it occurs unexpectedly to a healthy infant (who may have been rejected and unwanted by a jealous sibling), preschoolers find no evidence to support a physical cause of death. Indeed, the parents often are unaware of the reason for the fatality and may question any possible cause. If preschoolers are in any way accused or suspected of having harmed the infant, they may feel extremely guilty and responsible for the tragedy. On observing their parents' acute grief, they may interpret the anger or depression as a rejection of them.

When a child becomes ill, the healthy siblings experience the loss of routine and parental attention. It is natural for them to resent such disruptions and blame the changes on the ill child. However, preschoolers have less ability than older children to understand the reasons for the parents' prolonged absence from home. Even though parents may explain how ill the sibling is, what the hospital is like, and why they must be there, preschoolers see only the special attention and material rewards that the ill sister or brother is receiving. Because they are also unable to differentiate causes for separation of the parents and ill child, they may fear that the parents will never return. If they should learn that the ill child may not get well or come home, they may interpret this to mean that the parents will also never return. Their greatest fear concerning death is separation from parents.

## School-Age Children

Although school-age children have a better understanding of causality, less egocentricity, and an advanced perception of time, they still associate misdeeds or bad thoughts with causing death and feel intense guilt and responsibility for the event. However, because of their higher cognitive abilities, they respond well to logical explanations and comprehend the figurative meaning of words better than children in younger age-groups. Although they are less likely to interpret explanations in a purely literal sense, they are still prone to self-referenced definitions. For this reason, it is important for adults to clarify the meanings of statements and to repeatedly ask the children what they think.

**Concept of Death.** Much of what pertains to the preschool period regarding the understanding of death also relates to school-age children, particularly those near 6 or 7 years of age. However, these children have a deeper understanding of death in the concrete sense. According to Nagy (1948), children of this age attempt to ascribe a more comprehensible meaning to the event by personifying death as a devil, God, ghost, or "bogeyman." Naturalistic-physiologic explanations of why death occurs and what happens to the dead body may also be a preoccupation in this age-group. Factual explanations, such as "When you die, your body decays in the ground," are consistent with their concrete thinking.

By age 9 or 10 years, most children have an increasingly adult concept of death. They realize that it is inevitable, universal, and irreversible. Their attitudes toward death are greatly influenced by the reactions and attitudes of others, particularly their parents.

**Reactions to Dying.** The increased ability of school-age children to comprehend and reason poses additional risks for them. They may fear the reason for the illness, communicability of the disease to themselves or others, consequences of the disease on their functioning and relationships with others, and the process of dying and death itself. They tend to fear the expectation of the event more than its realization. Their fear of the unknown is greater than that of the known; like preschoolers, their fantasy explanations for the unexpected or the unknown are usually much more frightening and extreme than the actual situation. For this reason, anticipatory preparation is both necessary and effective. These children respond well to explanations of the disease, names of drugs, and so on. The developmental task of this age is industry; thus helping children who may be facing their own death to maintain control over their body—by understanding what is happening to them and participating in what is done to them—allows them to achieve independence, self-worth, and self-esteem and to avoid a sense of inferiority.

Because dying is loss of control over every aspect of living, the realization of impending death or failure to recover is a tremendous threat to school-age children's sense of security and ego strength. These children are likely to exhibit their fear more through verbal uncooperativeness than actual physical aggression. Health care professionals may erroneously interpret this behavior as rude, impolite, insolent, or stubborn. In reality the words are conveying the same meaning as physical attempts to run away or fight off others. This verbal "flight or fight" reaction to stress is a plea for some control and power. Encouraging children to talk about their feelings, allowing control where possible and appropriate, and providing outlets for aggression through play are means of dealing with this expression of anger and fear.

## Adolescents

By the time most children reach adolescence, they have a mature understanding of death. As abstract thinking develops, there is more questioning of death and related topics, such as the religious meaning of afterlife. However, other developmental needs, especially identity, make this an exceptionally difficult time for young people to cope with the loss of a loved one or with their own impending death.

**Concept of Death.** Although adolescents have a mature understanding of death, they are still very much influenced by "remnants" of magical thinking and are subject to feelings of guilt and shame. Adolescents are exploring many new areas of interpersonal relationships and are likely to see deviations from accepted behavior as reasons for illness. It is important to clarify that thoughts and activities, especially sexual experimentation, do not cause diseases such as cancer. The background environment and prior experience of the adolescent may also influence perceptions of death (Morin and Welsh, 1996).

**Reactions to Dying.** Adolescents may have a great deal of difficulty in coping with death. Although they have reached the level of adult comprehension of the concept of death, they are least likely to accept cessation of life, particularly their own. Developmentally, the rejection of death is understandable because the adolescents' tasks are to establish an identity by finding out who they are, what their purpose is, and where they belong. Any suggestion of being different or of not being is a tremendous threat to this task.

Adolescents strive for group acceptance and independence from parental constraints. As a result, they rely on peer rules and beliefs for personal direction and reject opposing parental demands. However, when faced with the crisis of serious illness, they may consider themselves alienated from peer associations and unable to communicate with their parents for emotional support. Therefore they may feel virtually alone in their struggle. Support groups or other means of networking adolescents facing death may be useful.

Healthy adolescents must deal with several maturational crises, such as the acceptance of bodily changes and socialization of intensifying sexual impulses. Any threat to either task increases the vulnerability of adolescents to the stress of coping with such crises. The ravages of a terminal illness and the deleterious effects of chemotherapy may be greater concerns than the prospect of dying. Adolescents' orientation to the present compels them to worry about physical changes even more than the prognosis for future recovery.

Nurses are in a most advantageous position in working with terminally ill adolescents; in the hospital setting they

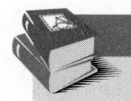

spend the greatest amount of time with them. They can structure the hospital admission to allow for maximum self-control and independence while allowing the adolescent the opportunity to get to know the nurse. Answering adolescents' questions honestly, treating them as mature individuals, and respecting their needs for privacy, solitude, and personal expressions of emotions such as anger, sadness, or fear convey to adolescents the adult's true concern for their physical and emotional welfare. Nurses can help parents to communicate with adolescents by providing information on typical adolescent responses and coping patterns, acting as role models, avoiding alliances with either parent or child, and allowing parents the opportunity to vent their feelings of frustration, incompetence, or failure in an atmosphere of acceptance and nonjudgment. (See Evidence-Based Practice box.)

## Delivery of Palliative Care Services

Once the health care team and family have discussed the likelihood of death as the outcome of a child's medical condition or illness, it is necessary to determine how and where palliative care will be provided. The circumstances of the child's illness will influence the location in which palliative care will be provided. For instance, traumatic injury/illness often leads to death in the emergency department or ICU setting. Children with progressive chronic illnesses or disability may initially receive palliative care services as a coordination of services between outpatient visits to their primary physician and care provided by a community agency (home health or hospice) in the home. As the illness progresses, the family may cease to come to the clinic or hospital and depend solely on care provided at home by the community agency as directed by their primary physician. Despite the circumstance of the illness or location of care, it is important to focus on interventions that address all aspects of the child and family's comfort. This requires attention to the child's physical comfort and the social, emotional, and spiritual needs of the child and family. Based on the outcome of the decision by the child and family regarding their wishes for care, there are several options for care that the family may choose.

### Hospital

Families may choose to remain in the hospital to receive care if the child's illness or condition is unstable and home care is not an option, or the family is uncomfortable with providing care at home. If a family chooses to remain at the hospital for terminal care, the setting should be made as homelike as possible. Families should be encouraged to bring familiar items from the child's room at home. In addition, there should be a consistent and coordinated plan of care for the child and family's comfort.

### Home Care

Some families may prefer to take their child home and receive services from a home care agency. Generally these services entail periodic nursing visits to administer a treatment or provide medications, equipment, or supplies. The child's

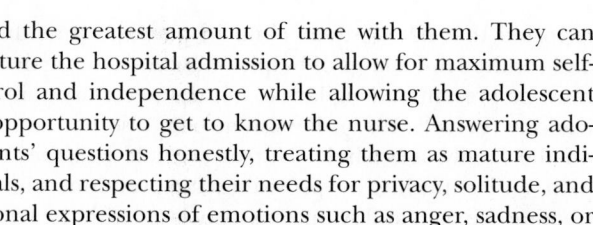

## EVIDENCE-BASED PRACTICE
### The Dying Child's Right to Refuse Further Treatment

Traditionally, minor children (age of minority varies with state law) have not had the legal right to give informed consent for treatment or to refuse treatment. However, there is a growing concern for children in the end stage of fatal disease to have a voice in their care during the terminal phase. One of the major issues is the age at which children have the cognitive ability to understand the medical information, consider and comprehend the consequences of the decision—death, and choose freely among the options (Leikin, 1989). According to children's development of the death concept, a mature understanding of death does not occur until approximately 9 years of age. Experience with death and an awareness of one's own impending death may affect the ability to understand (Martinson, 1995). Centers that have developed protocols for allowing informed choice by children document that youngsters as young as 6 years of age understand the implications of their disease as incurable and death as irreversible (Nitschke and others, 1982). These findings are consistent with those of Bluebond-Langner (1978, 1989), who found that fatally ill children progress through a series of stages that shape their understanding of their disease and death.

Other issues raised by opponents include the concern for dispelling hope in the child once death is pronounced as imminent, parents' guilt if they later question the decision, and possible conflict between the child's and parents' wishes (Shumway, Grossman, and Sarles, 1983; Stanfill and Strong, 1985). Although there is insufficient research to answer these concerns, it seems unlikely that they will occur if the family is allowed to choose therapeutic alternatives in an atmosphere of professional support and with sufficient information. In addition, staff members need to assess each child's capacity to understand the implications of refusing treatment, with documentation of the child's words and actions that support their conclusions (Foley, 1985).

care continues to be directed by the primary physician. Home care is often the option chosen by physicians and families because of the traditional view that a child must be considered to have a life expectancy of less than 6 months to be referred to hospice care. Fortunately, a number of hospice organizations are expanding their services to children based on the presence of a life-limiting disease process for which cure is not possible, rather than on the sole criteria of a limited 6-month prognosis.

### Hospice Care

Parents should be offered the option of caring for their child at home during the final phases of an illness with the assistance of a hospice organization. *Hospice* is a community health care organization that specializes in the care of dying patients by combining the hospice philosophy with the principles of palliative care. Hospice philosophy regards dying as a natural process and care of dying patients as including management of the physical, psychologic, social, and spiritual needs of the patient and family. Care is provided by a multidisciplinary group of professionals in the patient's home or an inpatient facility that employs the hospice philosophy. Hospice care for children was introduced in the 1970s (Martinson, 1993), and a number of community hospice organizations now accept children into their care

(Faulkner and Armstrong-Daily, 1997).* Collaboration between the child's primary treatment team and the hospice care team is essential to the success of hospice care. Families may continue to see their primary care physicians as they choose.

Hospice care is based on a number of important concepts that significantly set it apart from hospital care. First, family members are the principal caregivers and are supported by a team of professional and volunteer staff. Second, the priority of care is comfort. The child's physical, psychologic, social, and spiritual needs are considered. Pain and symptom control are primary concerns, and no extraordinary efforts are used to attempt a cure or prolong life. Third, the needs of the family are considered to be as important as those of the patient. Fourth, hospice is concerned with the family's postdeath adjustment, and care may continue for a year or more.

The goal of hospice care is for children to live life to the fullest without pain, with choices and dignity, in the familiar environment of their home, and with the support of their family. Hospice care is covered under state medicaid programs, as well as by most insurance plans. The service provides home nursing visits and visits from social workers, chaplains, and, in some cases, physicians. Medications, medical equipment, and any necessary medical supplies are all coordinated by the hospice organization providing care.

With children, the home has been the more common environment for implementing the hospice concept; it benefits the family in a variety of ways. Children who are dying are allowed the opportunity to remain with those they love and with whom they feel secure. Many children who were thought to be in imminent danger of death have gone home and lived longer than expected. Siblings can feel more involved in the care and often have more positive perceptions of the death. Parental adaptation is often more favorable, as is shown by their perceptions of how the experience at home affected their marriage, social reorientation, religious beliefs, and views on the meaning of life and death.

If the home is chosen for hospice care, the child may or may not die in the home. Reasons for final admission to a hospital vary but may be related to the parents' or siblings' wish to have the child die outside the home; exhaustion on the part of the caregivers; and physical problems such as sudden, acute pain or respiratory distress.

# NURSING CARE OF THE CHILD AND FAMILY AT THE END OF LIFE
## Management of Pain and Suffering

The presence of unrelieved pain and symptoms in a terminally ill child can have very detrimental effects on the quality of life experienced by the child and family. Parents have

reported that having their child in pain was unendurable and resulted in feelings of helplessness and a sense that they must be present and vigilant to get the necessary pain medications (Ferrell, 1995). Persistent pain also has an impact on the family as a whole. Nurses can alleviate the fear of pain and suffering by providing interventions aimed at treating the pain and symptoms associated with the terminal process in children.

### Pain and Symptom Management

When managing pain and symptoms experienced by dying children, it is important to clearly communicate the intent of any interventions proposed. For example, many children with progressive cancer may be given "palliative chemotherapy" or "palliative radiation." It is important that the health care team and family understand that the goal of these treatments is either to increase comfort by slowing the progression of an incurable tumor (palliative chemotherapy) or to reduce swelling or pressure from a tumor that is causing pain (palliative radiation). The family should understand that these treatments would not ultimately change the outcome of death for the child. This understanding reduces the chance of confusion among family members and health care providers regarding the focus of care being aimed toward palliation. In addition, the benefit vs risk of any suggested interventions in relation to the child's current quality of life should be considered.

The child and family's view of quality of life, religious and cultural values, and level of acceptance of the terminal prognosis will shape the types of interventions considered as symptoms occur. One family may choose to continue blood-product support if the child is otherwise comfortable and active but has fatigue and shortness of breath related to anemia. Another child and family may choose to forgo transfusions to avoid having to return to the hospital or clinic. The child and family should be aware of potential side effects of any proposed treatments and consequences of choosing not to intervene and should be provided with options that are consistent with their values and goals for the child's comfort. Health care practitioners must respect each individual families choice regarding their child's care.

A holistic approach to symptom management that includes pharmacologic and nonpharmacologic interventions should be used when possible to optimize treatment. For instance, in addition to giving lorazepam for anxiety, the child and family should be instructed in nonpharmacologic techniques such as distraction or relaxation breathing and encouraged to explore and communicate fears to further help alleviate feelings of anxiety.

The route of medication administration used for pain and symptom management should be carefully considered. Generally the least traumatic method of administration should be used. Children present a special challenge in administering medication depending on their age, level of cooperation, and temperament. If taking medicine becomes a struggle, children and parents may underreport the severity of pain and symptoms to avoid the trauma of administering the medication. Most medications can be administered orally, sublingually, transdermally, or by intravenous (IV) or

*National Hospice and Palliative Care Organization, 1700 Diagonal Rd, Suite 300, Arlington, VA 22314, (703) 243-5900, fax: (703) 525-5762; www.nhpco.org; and Children's Hospice International, Alexandra, VA 22301, (703) 684-0330 or (800) 24-CHILD, fax: (703) 684-0226, (800) 2-4-child; www.chionline.org.

subcutaneous (SC) infusion. Compounding pharmacists can be helpful in making medications in palatable form or providing them in a form that can be delivered with less distress.

Pain control for children in the terminal stages of illness or injury must be given the highest priority. Despite ongoing efforts to educate physicians and nurses on pain management strategies in children, studies have reported that children continue to be undermedicated for their pain (Wolfe and others, 2000). Nearly all children experience some amount of pain in the terminal phase of their illness. The current standard for treating children's pain is according to the World Health Organization's analgesic stepladder (1998) (Fig. 23-1). This approach promotes tailoring the pain interventions to the child's level of reported pain. Children's pain should be assessed frequently, and medications adjusted as necessary. Pain medications should be given on a regular schedule, and extra doses for "breakthrough pain" should be available to maintain comfort. Opioid drugs such as morphine should be given for severe pain, and the dose should be increased as necessary to maintain optimum pain relief. Techniques such as distraction, relaxation techniques, and guided imagery (Lambert, 1999) should be combined with drug therapy to provide the child and family with strategies to control pain. (See Chapter 26 for further discussion of pain assessment and management strategies.)

Occasionally children require very high doses of opioids to control pain. There are several reasons why this occurs. The child on long-term opioid pain management can become *tolerant* of the drug, meaning that it is necessary to give more drug to maintain the same level of pain relief. This should not be confused with *addiction,* which is a psychologic dependence on the side effects of opioids. Addiction is not a factor in managing terminal pain in children. Other obvious reasons for requiring increased doses of opi-

oids include progression of disease and other physiologic experiences of pain. It is important to understand that there is no maximum dose that can be given to control pain. However, nurses often express concern that administering doses of opioids that exceed what they are familiar with will hasten the child's death. The principle of double effect (Box 23-4) addresses such concerns. It provides an ethical standard that supports the use of interventions that have the intention of relieving pain and suffering even though there is a foreseeable possibility that death may be hastened (Siever, 1994). However, in cases where the child is terminally ill and in severe pain, using large doses of opioids and sedatives to manage pain is justified when there are no other treatment options are available that would relieve the pain but make the risk of death less likely (Fleischman, 1998). (See Chapter 26 for an extensive discussion of pain assessment and management.)

In addition to pain, children experience a variety of symptoms during their terminal course either as a result of their disease process or as a side effect of medicines used to maintain their comfort (Box 23-5). The underlying disease and previous treatment history will contribute to the types

---

**Box 23-4** ■ ■ ☐
**Ethical Principle of Double Effect**

An action that has one good (intended) and one bad (unintended but foreseeable) effect is permissible if the following conditions are met:
The action itself must be good or indifferent. Only the good consequences of the action must be sincerely intended.
The good effect must not be produced by the bad effect.
There must be a compelling or proportionate reason for permitting the foreseeable bad effect to occur.

---

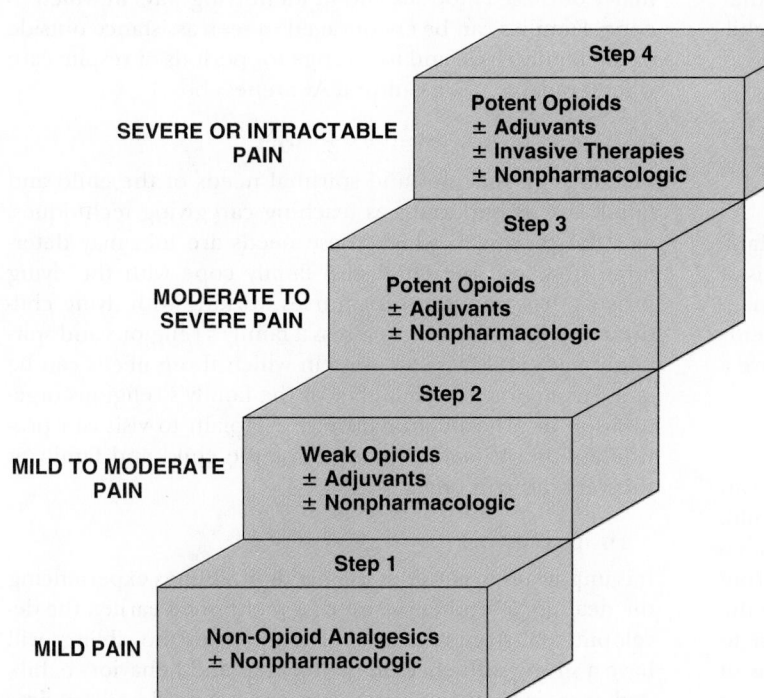

**Fig. 23-1** Therapeutic ladder for pain management. (From the World Health Organization in conjunction with IASP: *Cancer pain relief and palliative care in children,* Geneva, 1998, WHO. Adapted with permission.)

**Box 23-5** ■ ■ ▢
### Common Symptoms Experienced by Dying Children

**PAIN**
Visceral
Bone
Neuropathic

**GASTROINTESTINAL**
Anorexia
Nausea/vomiting
Constipation
Diarrhea

**GENITOURINARY**
Urinary tract infections
Urinary retention

**HEMATOLOGIC**
Anemia
Bleeding

**RESPIRATORY**
Cough
Congestion
Shortness of breath
Wheezing

**CENTRAL NERVOUS SYSTEM**
Fevers/chills
Sleep disturbance
Restlessness/agitation
Seizures

**INTEGUMENTARY**
Dry skin
Rash/itching
Pressure sores
Edema

**EMOTIONAL**
Fear
Anxiety
Depression

## CULTURAL AWARENESS
### Cultural Considerations in Dying and Death

Culture influences perceptions, coping styles, and family dynamics in every arena of life. A death in the family is no exception. When language and cultural barriers influence help seeking by families, there may be less support sought during the process of dying, death, and bereavement. This can result in unfortunate outcomes. For example, in relationship to grief resolution in children, more severe symptoms (e.g., posttraumatic stress disorder and depression) can result. When health care providers have a poor understanding of cultural influences on family dynamics and the family's perception of an illness, death, and grief, optimum support cannot be provided when help is sought. To provide comprehensive care, health care professionals must take both language differences and cultural influences seriously.

Data from Prong LL: Childhood bereavement among Cambodians: cultural considerations, *Hospice* 10(2):51-64, 1995; and Saiki SC, Martinson IM, Inano M: Japanese families who have lost children to cancer: a primary study, *J Pediatr Nurs* 9(4):239-250, 1994.

and severity of symptoms the individual child experiences during the dying process. Nurses caring for children who are receiving palliative care for a terminal condition or illness must frequently assess for any symptoms that are causing the child physical distress. Assessment should include information regarding the symptom's onset, severity, duration, and effect on the child's quality of life.

These symptoms should be consistently managed with appropriate medications or treatments and interventions such as repositioning, relaxation, massage, and other measures to maintain the child's comfort and quality of life. (For further information on pain and symptom management for children see *www.childcancerpain.org* and *www.childendoflife.org*.)

## Parents' and Siblings' Need for Education and Support Through the Caregiving Process

Often, as the child's illness worsens, parents and other family members are the primary caregivers while the child is at home. This role can create physical, emotional, and financial strain on the larger family system. Therefore parents and other family members caring for dying children have a number of educational and support needs.

### Educational Needs

Family caregivers need comprehensive education about various aspects of care that they will be providing to their child. This preparation can ease feelings of helplessness and anxiety and provide a sense of competence as they move from caring for an ill child to caring for a dying child. This education should begin early in the transition from curative to palliative care. Table 23-4 provides some common areas of educational needs of family caregivers and suggestions on

how nurses can assist families in meeting these needs. Education about physical care is best provided as the need arises. Instructing parents too early in the signs and symptoms of respiratory distress or how to stop a nosebleed can increase the parents' anxiety.

### Emotional Support

Members of the family can be overwhelmed by powerful emotions that can threaten their ability to cope. Anger, guilt, anxiety, and helplessness are normal feelings that many parents experience and often project onto other members of the family or health care team. Nurses assisting these families cannot prevent parents from feeling this way; however, they can assist the family in recognizing the normalcy of these emotions and in identifying ways in which to cope. Families can be encouraged to seek assistance outside of the family circle and to arrange for periods of respite care when available. (See Cultural Awareness box.)

### Religious and Spiritual Support

Meeting the religious and spiritual needs of the child and family are as important as teaching caregiving techniques, and the success to which these needs are met may determine how well the child and family cope with the dying process. It is important for nurses working with dying children and their families to assess a family's religious and spiritual needs and facilitate ways in which those needs can be met. Arranging for a member of the family's religious organization or a hospital or hospice chaplain to visit can provide another valuable resource for the child and family at this very difficult time.

### Sibling Support

It is important to consider the needs of siblings experiencing the death of a brother or sister. As mentioned earlier, the developmental stage and level of maturity of the siblings will have a strong influence on the feelings and behaviors exhibited as their brother or sister becomes more ill and requires

**TABLE 23-4   Preparation and education of family caregivers**

| Needs of Family Caregivers | Professional Interventions |
| --- | --- |
| **Practical Needs** | |
| Is home care, hospice care or care in the hospital appropriate for my child?<br>How will we pay for end of life care at home, in the hospital, or in hospice?<br>How will we pay our other bills?<br>Where do I get equipment and supplies?<br>How does the equipment work?<br>Who do I call if equipment malfunctions?<br>How should we arrange our house to best meet the needs of our child?<br>Will there be help available to us at home?<br>Who do I call for medical questions? | Explore family's preferences for home care or hospice as appropriate.<br>Evaluate family's funding source and provide resources and assistance as necessary.<br>Provide family with appropriate telephone numbers and contact people for questions about equipment and medical care.<br>Plan for availability of caregiver's family (i.e. parents, family, friends, professionals) and help coordinate a schedule for provision of care.<br>Provide contact person for family to call with concerns or questions. |
| **Personal Care** | |
| How do I give my child a bath?<br>How do I give my child a bed bath?<br>How do I wash my child's hair in bed?<br>How do I change linen with my child in bed?<br>How do I perform skin care?<br>How do I perform mouth care?<br>How do I administer medications?<br>What do I do if my child does not want to eat?<br>Is there something I can do to get my child to eat?<br>Does my child need supplements or a special diet? | Instruct all caregivers about providing daily care to the child.<br>Provide written instructions and reference material for caregivers to review.<br>Assess the child's nutritional status and parent's view on supplemental nutrition.<br>Educate family on decreased nutritional needs and potential complications with over-feeding or over-hydration. |
| **Physical Care** | |
| How do I assess my child's pain?<br>When should I give pain medications?<br>What do I do when pain management is ineffective?<br>What should I do when our child is constipated or has diarrhea?<br>How do I control nausea and vomiting?<br>What do I do if my child has a fever?<br>What do I do if my child has seizures?<br>What do I do if my child has trouble breathing? | Assess the child's current comfort status and educate family on current interventions.<br>Educate family about assessing the child's comfort level.<br>Instruct the family that the child may be uncomfortable for a variety of reasons (i.e., constipation, anxiety, fever, headache, muscle cramp, disease) and educate the family about the appropriate interventions for particular circumstances.<br>Provide an accessible supply of medications that can help alleviate discomfort (i.e., laxative, sedative, antipyretic).<br>Encourage caregiver to telephone contact person for questions or ineffective interventions. |
| **Activity and Social Interactions** | |
| Can we safely travel and enjoy family gatherings with our child?<br>In which activities can we engage our child?<br>Should friends and family be encouraged to visit?<br>What interventions can I do to help my child relax and rest comfortably? | Encourage family to engage in fun and memorable activities with the child.<br>Encourage visitors when appropriate.<br>Encourage family to employ relaxation techniques that have previously been beneficial to the child. |

From Brown-Hellsten M and others: *End of life care for children*, Austin, TX, 1999, Texas Cancer Council, with permission.

more care. Siblings may feel isolated and displaced during the time that a brother or sister is dying. Parents devote the majority of their time to the care and comfort of the dying child, causing siblings to feel left out of the parent–sick child relationship. Siblings may become resentful of their sick sibling and begin to feel guilty or shameful about such feelings (Murry, 1999). Nurses can assist the family by helping the parents identify ways to involve the siblings in the caring process, perhaps by bringing some supply or favorite toy, game, or food item. Parents should be encouraged to schedule some time to spend with the other children where the focus is on them; nurses can assist the parents by helping them

identify a trusted friend or family member who can sit with the ill child for a short period of time.

## Caregiver Support

As the care of the dying child becomes the primary focus of the parent, personal and household needs often take on secondary significance. These tasks, however, can become burdensome and increase the family's stress if not attended to. Nurses should help the family identify ways for friends, community service organizations, and extended family members to assist with such tasks as household chores, shopping, meal preparation, and laundry.

## Care at the Time of Death

Very few parents have cared for a dying child, and thus parents are not prepared to lead their child through the dying process (Fig. 23-2). Awareness that the child's death is near allows the parents and family to determine the location and circumstance of the child's death. This allows the family to create a meaningful death for their child, facilitating improved coping in the difficult days, weeks, and years after the child has died. Nurses have an important role in helping parents recognize the changes in their child that signal that death may be near. (See Guidelines Box.)

### Physical Changes

These changes are more often seen in children dying of prolonged illness or disability and can vary widely among children. Generally as the child progresses through the dying process there will be an overall decline in the child's physical condition. This decline may be interspersed with brief spurts of energy or periods of alertness and can cause parents to become exhausted and overwhelmed in "waiting for the inevitable." Often parents may ask "how long" their child has to live. Initially this question may be an attempt by the parent to determine what special activities or events the family should try to accomplish. As the dying process progresses, this question may be a search for how long they and their child will have to endure the dying process.

As the child moves closer to his or her actual death, there are some general physical changes that occur. Initially the

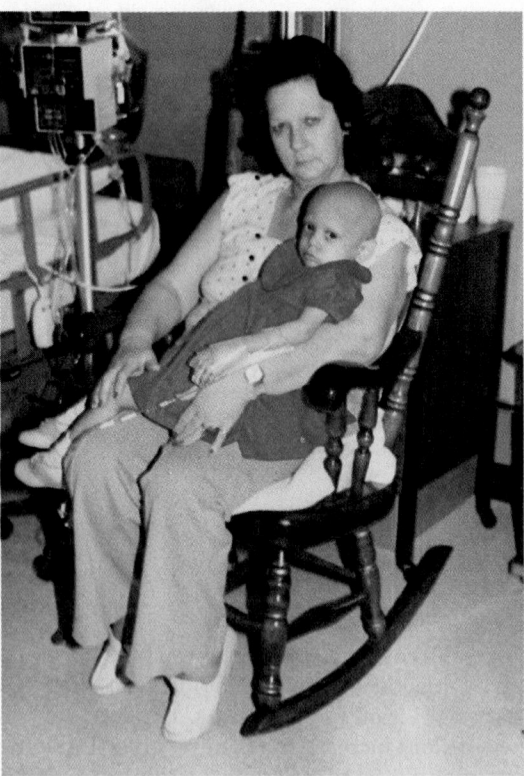

**Fig. 23-2** For the dying child there is no greater comfort than the security and closeness of a parent.

child may begin to sleep more. Appetite will decrease, and the child will begin to take only small bites of favorite foods or sips of fluids. As the child begins to eat and drink less, urinary frequency will decline and the urine will become more concentrated. (Box 23-6 includes additional signs of approaching death.) In the final few days before death, the child will most likely become less responsive. Breathing may

## GUIDELINES
### *Supporting Grieving Families\**

**GENERAL**

Stay with the family; sit quietly if they prefer not to talk; cry with them if desired.

Accept the family's grief reactions; avoid judgmental statements (e.g., "You should be feeling better by now").

Avoid offering rationalizations for the child's death (e.g., "You should be glad your child isn't suffering anymore").

Avoid artificial consolation (e.g., "I know how you feel," or "You are still young enough to have another baby").

Deal openly with feelings such as guilt, anger, and loss of self-esteem.

Focus on feelings by using a feeling word in the statement (e.g., "You're still feeling all the pain of losing a child").

Refer the family to an appropriate self-help group or for professional help if needed.

**AT THE TIME OF DEATH**

Reassure the family that everything possible is being done for the child, if they wish lifesaving interventions.

Do everything possible to ensure the child's comfort, especially relieving pain.

Provide the child and family the opportunity to review special experiences or memories in their lives.

Express personal feelings of loss or frustrations (e.g., "We will miss him so much," or "We tried everything; we feel so sorry that we couldn't save him").

Provide information that the family requests and be honest.

Respect the emotional needs of family members, such as siblings, who may need brief respites from the dying child.

Make every effort to arrange for family members, especially parents, to be with the child at the moment of death, if they wish to be present.

Allow the family to stay with the dead child for as long as they wish and to rock, hold, or bathe the child.

Provide practical help when possible, such as collecting the child's belongings.

Arrange for spiritual support, such as clergy; pray with the family if no one else can stay with them.

**AFTER THE DEATH**

Attend the funeral or visitation if there was a special closeness with the family.

Initiate and maintain contact (e.g., sending cards, telephoning, inviting them back to the unit, or making a home visit).

Refer to the dead child by name; discuss shared memories with the family.

Discourage the use of drugs or alcohol as a method of escaping grief.

Encourage all family members to communicate their feelings rather than remaining silent to avoid upsetting another member.

Emphasize that grieving is a painful process that often takes years to resolve.

---

\*"Family" refers to all significant persons involved in the child's life, such as parents, siblings, grandparents, or other close relatives or friends.

become slow and shallow, with periodic deep sighs. Urine output may decrease or stop. As the child nears the final hours before death, the breathing will become more irregular, deep, and gasping, with long periods of apnea (Cheyne-Stokes respirations). The skin may have a pale, grayish-blue color and may be cool to the touch. The child's eyes may be slightly open, with a fixed gaze. It is important to prepare the family for these changes, and provide them with caregiving activities that promote a loving presence in the child's care (Box 23-7). Reassure parents that this is a normal process and that the child is not suffering.

### Emotional Changes

As children approach death, they may begin to recall events that were important with their family. They may want to draw pictures or leave messages for important friends and family. Often children begin to reassure their parents and other significant people that they are not afraid and are ready to die.

During the final few days to hours of death, children may experience visions of "angels" or people and talk with them. They may mention that they are not afraid and that someone is waiting for them. Often these visions are of family members or friends who have preceded them in death. In most instances these visions provide a comforting presence and reassurance for the child and family. Again, these experiences are highly individual, and not all children will have them.

As the child's death approaches, the family may begin the "death vigil," which is a natural phenomenon in which family and friends gather at the bedside. Rarely is the child left alone for any length of time. During this time families may read favorite books, recite prayers, light candles, or play music that is special to the child. Religious or family rituals surrounding the time of death are important, and nurses involved with the care of the family at this time should be sensitive to such needs. See Nursing Care Plan on pp. 962-964.

## Postmortem Care

The final moments of a child's life are often extremely stressful as the family waits for the child to die. Families often depend on trusted health care professionals, particularly nurses, to help them recognize the exact moment of the child's death. Once the nurse (if RN pronouncement is allowed by the state practice act) has observed that the child is no longer showing signs of life, the child is pronounced dead. Initially the family may show joy and relief that the child is no longer struggling. There may be many varied emotions in the immediate moments after the child's death, and the nurse must be prepared for a range of reactions. Generally all that is necessary is a supportive presence at this time, as the family begins their grief process. In rare instances, particularly in more conflicted families, there may be strong outbursts of anger. It is important for the nurse to be aware of families in which this situation may occur and respond by assuring them that appropriate resources (social worker, chaplain, security personnel) are readily available to ensure that the situation does not escalate.

Once the initial reaction to the moment of death has occurred, the family often moves away from the bedside and enters a phase of relaxation. One or both of the parents may stay with the child while others in attendance make brief visits to view the child. Nursing care at this time is to facilitate the parents' wishes with regard to time with their child. The family should be allowed the time needed to say good-bye.

When the parents are ready, the nurse should offer to bathe and dress the body for removal from the home or hospital room. The parents may wish to undertake this task, participate with the nurse, or ask the nurse to do the bathing for them. If the death was at home and the body is prepared for removal, and the parents are ready, the funeral home can be contacted. Often hospice organizations have arrangements with the medical examiners in their area that allow the body to be directly removed by a funeral director.

---

**Box 23-6** ■ ■ ■
**Physical Signs of Approaching Death**

Loss of sensation and movement in the lower extremities, progressing toward the upper body
Sensation of heat, although body feels cool
Loss of senses:
  Tactile sensation decreases
  Sensitive to light
  Hearing is last sense to fail
Confusion, loss of consciousness, slurred speech
Muscle weakness
Loss of bowel and bladder control
Decreased appetite/thirst
Difficulty swallowing
Change in respiratory pattern:
  Cheyne-Stokes respirations (waxing and waning of depth of breathing with regular periods of apnea)
  "Death rattle" (noisy chest sounds from accumulation of pulmonary and pharyngeal secretions)
Weak, slow pulse; decreased blood pressure

---

**Box 23-7** ■ ■ ■
**Care During the Terminal Phase**

**PHYSICAL SUPPORT**
Provide frequent mouth care to prevent drying, cracking, and bleeding of lips and mucous membranes.
Maintain good hygiene by giving bed baths, using skin lotion, and giving frequent diaper changes.
Continue necessary medications to manage symptoms and maintain comfort using IV (if access is easily established) or SC infusion. Discontinue unnecessary medications and procedures.

**EMOTIONAL SUPPORT**
Encourage family to discuss impending death openly with child and other family members.
Encourage family to continue to speak to child in calm, reassuring voice.
Provide familiar surroundings or objects.
Encourage caregivers to provide each other with periods of respite.
Allow family time with child after the death and participation in the preparation of the body if they choose.

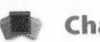

# Nursing Care Plan
## The Child Who Is Terminally Ill or Dying

NURSING DIAGNOSIS: Delayed growth and development related to terminal illness or impending death

**PATIENT GOAL 1:** Will receive adequate support during terminal phase

- **NURSING INTERVENTIONS/RATIONALES**

Encourage family to remain near child as much as possible *to provide support through their presence*

Encourage child to talk about feelings; help family as they encourage child to express feelings

Provide safe, acceptable outlets for aggression

Answer questions honestly while maintaining a positive, hopeful approach

Explain all procedures and therapies, especially the physical effects child will experience

Help child distinguish between consequences of therapies and manifestations of disease process

Structure hospital environment to allow for maximum self-control and independence within the limitations imposed by child's developmental level and physical condition

Respect child's need for privacy without neglecting child

Provide for presence of customary support systems

- **EXPECTED OUTCOMES**

Child expresses feelings freely

Child demonstrates an understanding of symptoms

Child feels supported by family and caregivers

Child is free to exert self-control and independence as desired and appropriate for age

**PATIENT GOAL 2:** Will exhibit minimal or no evidence of physical discomfort

- **NURSING INTERVENTIONS/RATIONALES**

Appreciate that pain control is an essential component of physical and emotional care during terminal stage

Provide pain relief around the clock *to prevent recurrence of pain*

Encourage family to provide comfort measures child prefers (e.g., rocking, stroking)

Avoid excessive noise or light *that may irritate child*

Place all commodities within easy reach *to increase child's control and lessen need for excessive movement*

Use gentle, minimal physical manipulation

Avoid pressure (bedclothes, sheets) on painful areas

Experiment with using heat or cold on painful areas (*use cautiously because of easy skin breakdown*)

Whenever possible, make use of procedures (e.g., noninvasive temperature monitoring) *to minimize discomfort*

Change position frequently; if difficult for child, coordinate with pain relief from analgesics *to make moving easier and less distressing*

Avoid pressure on bony prominences or painful sites (water bed, flotation mattress); ensure good body alignment *to prevent skin breakdown*

Keep fresh air circulating in room (open window, use small fan)

Use pillows or other supports to prop child in comfortable position

Carry child (if possible) to other areas for diversion if desired

Place absorbent pads under hips *because child may be incontinent*

Help child to toilet if desired

Limit care to essentials

May need to forego usual hygienic measures such as bath or clothing change, but provide comfort measures (e.g., mouth care, wiping forehead, gentle back rub)

*Administer anticholinergic drugs (atropine or scopolamine) *to reduce secretions (lessens "death rattle," which can be distressing to family)*

- **EXPECTED OUTCOME**

Child exhibits minimal or no evidence of physical discomfort

**PATIENT GOAL 3:** Will receive adequate emotional support at time of dying

- **NURSING INTERVENTIONS/RATIONALES**

Preserve child's physical closeness with family members (e.g., parent may want to rock child in chair or lie next to child in bed)

Teach family about supportive interventions

Talk to child even though child may not appear to be awake

Position self and others where child can easily see face (e.g., sit at head of bed)

Speak to child in clear, distinct voice; avoid whispering

Avoid conversation about child in child's presence *to reduce anxiety/fear*

Offer calm reassurance and orient child to surroundings when awake

Phrase questions for "yes" or "no" answers *to conserve energy*

Avoid repeated measurements of vital signs, *which only disturb child*

Play favorite music (*may soothe child*)

- **EXPECTED OUTCOME**

Child appears calm and relaxed

NURSING DIAGNOSIS: Imbalanced nutrition: less than body requirements related to loss of appetite, disinterest in food

**PATIENT GOAL 1:** Will receive optimum nutrition

- **NURSING INTERVENTIONS/RATIONALES**

Offer any food and fluids child desires

Provide small meals and snacks several times a day

Avoid excessive encouragement to eat or drink

Avoid foods with strong odors *because they may cause nausea*

Provide pleasant environment for eating

Serve foods that require the least energy to eat (soups, shakes)

Feed slowly *to conserve energy*

*Administer antiemetic as prescribed if nausea/vomiting is a problem

Provide mouth care before and after eating; lubricate lips with petrolatum *to prevent cracking and promote comfort*

- **EXPECTED OUTCOME**

Child consumes some nutrients and fluids

---

*Dependent nursing action.

## Nursing Care Plan
### The Child Who Is Terminally Ill or Dying—cont'd

> **NURSING DIAGNOSIS:** Fear/anxiety related to diagnosis, tests, therapies, and prognosis

**PATIENT GOAL 1:** Will experience reduction of anxiety

- **NURSING INTERVENTIONS/*RATIONALES***

Explain all procedures and other aspects of care to child *to reduce anxiety and fear*

Remain with child or provide for constant attendance

Determine what child has been told about prognosis *so this information can be reinforced*

Determine what family wishes child to know about prognosis

Emphasize importance of honesty

Encourage child to express feelings

Answer child's questions openly and honestly while maintaining a hopeful approach

Involve parents in child's care

Remain nonjudgmental regarding child's behavior

- **EXPECTED OUTCOME**

Child discusses fears without evidence of stress

> **NURSING DIAGNOSIS:** Anticipatory grieving related to potential loss of a child

**PATIENT (FAMILY) GOAL 1:** Will receive adequate support

- **NURSING INTERVENTIONS/*RATIONALES***

Discuss the grieving process with family *so that family better understands normalcy of feelings*

Provide opportunities for family to express emotions

Help parents deal with their feelings, *allowing them more emotional reserve to meet the needs of their children*

Encourage parents to remain as near to child as possible, yet be sensitive to parents' needs

Provide information regarding child's status and anticipated reactions *to decrease anxiety/fear*

Help parents to understand behavioral reactions of their child, especially that child's concern for present crisis, such as loss of hair, may be much greater than for future crises, including possible death

Facilitate family's assistance with child's care

Provide comfort measures for child and family

Encourage family to address own health care needs

Provide as much privacy as possible

Assist family in assessing their need for referral services (e.g., hospice services, specific organizations for grieving families)

Encourage parents to honestly answer child's questions about dying rather than avoiding questions or using euphemisms

Encourage parents to share their moments of sorrow with child

Discuss with parents appropriate involvement of siblings

Identify religious and cultural beliefs related to death (e.g., prayer, rites, rituals)

Provide preparation for postdeath services

Discuss with family their preferences for care if death is imminent

Arrange for appropriate spiritual care in accordance with family's beliefs and/or affiliations

Maintain contact with family

Provide support for families who choose home care/hospice for their child

See Guidelines box on p. 960.

- **EXPECTED OUTCOMES**

Family expresses fears, concerns, and any special desires for child

Family demonstrates an understanding of child's needs (specify)

Family members avail themselves of services as desired

See also:

Nursing Care Plan: The Child in the Hospital, Chapter 26

Nursing Care Plan: The Family of the Child Who Is Ill or Hospitalized, Chapter 26

**PATIENT GOAL 2:** Will exhibit no evidence of loneliness

- **NURSING INTERVENTIONS/*RATIONALES***

Offer calm reassurance to child

Reassure child of the love of others

Continue to set some limits for child *to provide a sense of security*

Spend time with child when not directly involved in care

Reinforce to child that what is happening is not child's fault *to decrease feelings of guilt*

Involve child in routine activities as tolerated

Maintain a "normal" atmosphere

Talk to child even though child may not appear to be awake

Situate self and others where easily visible to child

Speak to child in clear, distinct voice; avoid whispering

Avoid conversation about child's condition in presence of child *to decrease anxiety/fear*

Play favorite music and read stories to child

Orient child to surroundings when child is awake

Phrase questions for "yes" or "no" answers when possible *to conserve child's energy*

Instruct/encourage parents in above interventions

- **EXPECTED OUTCOME**

Child exhibits no evidence of loneliness

> **NURSING DIAGNOSIS:** Anticipatory grieving related to imminent death of a child

**PATIENT (FAMILY) GOAL 1:** Will receive adequate support

- **NURSING INTERVENTIONS/*RATIONALES***

Be available to family

Inform family of what to expect at time of death

Convey an attitude of caring for both child and family

Encourage at least one family member to stay with child

Help family to provide care of child as they desire without forcing involvement

*Continued*

## Nursing Care Plan
### The Child Who Is Terminally Ill or Dying—cont'd

**PATIENT (FAMILY) GOAL 1—cont'd**

- **NURSING INTERVENTIONS/*RATIONALES*—cont'd**

*Administer medications or other agents as prescribed *to reduce unpleasant manifestations*
  Oxygen *for respiratory distress*
  Anticonvulsants *for seizures*
  Anticholinergic drugs *to reduce secretions ("death rattle")*
  Analgesics *for pain*
  Stool softeners/laxatives *for constipation*
  Antiemetics *for nausea/vomiting*

Help and encourage family to express feelings appropriately

Encourage family to meet their own physical needs

Provide privacy

Provide for physical comfort of family

Provide emotional support and comfort to family

Encourage family to talk to child

Involve family and other children in decision making whenever possible, especially regarding alternatives for terminal care (hospital, home, hospice)

Support and assist family in giving explanations to other family members regarding child's status

Maintain nonjudgmental attitude toward behavior of family members

---

*Dependent nursing action.

- **EXPECTED OUTCOMES**

Family members discuss their feelings

Family members are actively involved in child's care

**PATIENT (FAMILY) GOAL 2:** Will receive adequate support for home care/hospice

- **NURSING INTERVENTIONS/*RATIONALES***

Teach family physical care of child

Provide family with means for contacting health care professionals at any time (e.g, phone numbers)

Maintain daily contact with family (e.g., telephone call, home visit)

Refer to community agencies as appropriate *for ongoing support*

Reassure family that they can readmit child to the hospital at any time

Help plan with family what to do and what to expect when the child dies

- **EXPECTED OUTCOMES**

Family demonstrates ability to provide care for child

Family is in contact with appropriate support groups as desired

---

In some instances it may be necessary for the police to make a report before the release of the child's body. It is important for the nurse to explain to the parents the requirements of their local area for removal of a body. This allows the parents to be prepared for questions or necessary information that may be required. Hospital deaths require the parents to leave the child, and the body is taken to the morgue. Some parents may ask to go with the body to the morgue, and nurses should work within their institutions' regulations to try to honor such requests if possible.

The final separation of the child's body from the parents and family is often the most emotional and traumatic time. The nurse should be prepared to offer support to the parents and ensure that there are other family members or friends available in the coming hours to continue to provide support and assistance to the parents and siblings.

### Care of the Family Experiencing Unexpected Childhood Death

In long-term, potentially fatal illnesses, families may experience anticipatory grief. The parents mourn the loss of their child long before the death. They are reminded of their child's uncertain future each time they see the pain the child must endure or experience the sudden loss of hope during a relapse. This prolonged period of chronic anticipatory grief provides families with the precious opportunity to complete all "unfinished business," such as helping child and siblings understand and cope with a fatal prognosis. Many families reflect on their changed perspective of

time after learning of the diagnosis, particularly their heightened awareness of the value and worth of each day.

With sudden, unexpected death, the family is deprived of any of the advantages of anticipatory grief. There is no opportunity to prepare oneself or others for the death, and the initial denial may be very strong. Because of this lack of time to prepare, many families feel great guilt and remorse for not having done something additional or different with the child. For example, they may berate themselves for depriving the child of some desired material object or privilege or, more painfully, for not having prevented the sudden death in some way. "If only I'd been a better parent" is a common feeling at this time. Without proper support, the risk of pathologic grief responses may be high (Oliver and Fallat, 1995).

Death resulting from accident or trauma, or acute illness in settings such as the emergency department or intensive care unit often requires the active withdrawal of some form of life-supporting intervention, such as a ventilator or bypass machine. These situations often raise difficult ethical issues (Savage, 1997), and parents are often less prepared for the actual moment of death (Box 23-8). Nurses can assist these parents by providing detailed information about what will happen as supportive equipment is withdrawn, ensuring that appropriate pain medications are administered to prevent pain during the dying process, and allowing the parents time before the start of the withdrawal to be with and speak to their child. It is important that the nurse attempt to control the environment around the family at this time by providing privacy, asking if they would like to play music,

## Box 23-8 ■ ■ □
### Strategies for Intervention with Survivors of Sudden Childhood Death

**ARRIVAL OF THE FAMILY**

Meet the family immediately and escort to a private area.

A health care worker with bereavement training should remain with the family.

Provide information about the extent of illness or injury and treatment efforts.

If the health care worker must leave the family or if the family requests privacy, return in 15 minutes so the family does not feel forgotten.

Provide tissues, telephone, coffee, and a Bible.

**PRONOUNCEMENT OF DEATH**

When available, the family's own physician should inform them of the child's death.

Alternatively, the physician or nurse should introduce himself or herself and establish calm, reassuring eye contact with the parents.

Honest, clear communication that avoids misinterpretation is essential.

Nonverbal communication such as hugging, touching, or remaining with the family in silence may be most empathetic.

Acknowledge the family's guilt, attempt to alleviate it, and deal openly and nonjudgmentally with anger.

Provide information, answer questions, and offer reassurance that everything possible was done for the child.

**VIEWING THE BODY**

Offer the parents the opportunity to see the body; repeat the offer later if they decline.

Before viewing, inform the parents of bodily changes they should expect (tubes, injuries, cold skin).

A single staff member should accompany the family but remain inconspicuous.

Offer the opportunity to hold the child.

Allow the family as much time as they need.

Offer parents the opportunity for siblings to view the body.

**FORMAL CONCLUDING PROCESS**

Discuss and answer questions concerning autopsy and funeral arrangements; obtain signatures on the body release and autopsy forms.

Provide anticipatory guidance regarding symptoms of grief response and their normalcy.

Provide written materials about grief symptoms.

Escort the family to the exit or to their car if necessary.

Provide a follow-up phone call in 24 to 48 hours to answer questions and provide support.

Provide referral for community health nursing visit.

Provide referrals to local support and resource groups (e.g., bereavement groups, bereavement counselors, SIDS groups, Parents of Murdered Children, Mothers Against Drunk Driving).

Modified from Back K: Sudden, unexpected pediatric death: caring for the parents, *Pediatr Nurs* 17(6):571-574, 1991.

---

softening lights and monitoring noises, and arranging for any religious or cultural rituals that the family may want performed. After the child's death, the family should be allowed to remain with the body and hold or rock the child if they desire. Once the nurse has removed all tubes and equipment from the body, parents should be given the option of assisting with the preparation of the body, such as bathing and dressing.

At some point the nurse should discuss if the family has made preparations for the burial service and if the staff can help in any way. Parents often have concerns about the funeral, such as siblings' involvement in the death rituals. Although no absolute answers exist regarding the question of siblings attending the funeral or burial services, the general consensus is that the surviving children benefit from being involved in these events. However, children need preparation for postdeath services. They should be told what to expect, particularly how the deceased person will look if the coffin is open; allowed their private time to say good-bye; and permitted to stay as long as they wish. Ideally, the parents should prepare the siblings. If the parents' grief prevents this communication, a significant family member or friend should substitute. (See Family Focus box.)

**NURSING TIP** Reviewing with parents at a follow-up visit the circumstances of a child's sudden and traumatic death can be a very important nursing intervention. Clarifying any misconceptions is important. For example, parents of children who have head injuries commonly confuse coma and "brain death" and may feel guilty, thinking they should have waited longer for their brain dead child to recover from a coma (Oliver and others, 2001).

### FAMILY FOCUS
#### Children Need to Say Good-Bye

As a nurse/grief counselor, I conduct grief workshops with children who have experienced the death of someone special. Children often communicate their feelings of being excluded through drawings. They may draw a picture of the dying person in a hospital bed that is raised too high for them to see the person's face clearly. Sometimes children reveal that they did not get to say good-bye because a family member told them, for example, "You don't want to see your grandma this way. She is too sick for you to visit." If the special person died at home, the children had to stay in their room when the funeral home staff took away the body.

I have learned never to underestimate the importance of allowing children to be involved with the dying person and the significance of a child's loss. Once, when I asked a 6-year-old girl to draw a picture with the theme. "This is what I was doing when my _____ died," she drew a picture and completed the sentence with "when my *home* died." Her grandmother had been like her mother; to the child, her home was gone. We need to give children the choice of being included in the family's activities of saying good-bye.

Barbara Bilderback, MS, MA, RN
Bereavement Supervisor
Saint Francis Hospice
Tulsa, OK

### Community-Based Follow-Up

A community health or visiting nurse referral may be helpful after a sudden, unexpected pediatric death. Some families have reported that this was a missing piece in their care (Dent and others, 1996). Several home visits by a nurse can be instrumental in ensuring that the families' questions are answered, information about the grief process is provided, coping is assessed and supported, and appropriate referrals to support groups are provided (Box 23-9) (Buckalow and Esposito, 1995).

Families who experience a child's sudden death may experience recurrent memories of both the child and the death experience and may long grieve over missed opportunities. Support and resource groups that may be useful to families include the **Sudden Infant Death Syndrome Alliance,*** **National Sudden Infant Death Syndrome Resource Center,†** **American Sudden Infant Death Syndrome Institute,‡** **Mothers Against Drunk Driving,§** and **National Organization of Parents of Murdered Children, Inc.‖**

## SPECIAL DECISIONS AT THE TIME OF DYING AND DEATH

Rarely are people prepared to cope with the numerous decisions that must be made when a loved one is dying or dies. When the death is expected, there is the opportunity to make plans in advance, such as where the child should spend the last days or what type of funeral arrangements are desired. When death is unexpected, the shock is sufficient to render the survivors incapable of making even simple decisions. Those in attendance at the death and those caring for the dying child can be instrumental in initiating decisions that may facilitate the grief resolution process. The following is a brief review of selected instances in which nurses

*1314 Bedford Ave, Suite 210, Baltimore, MD 21208, (800) 221-7437 or (410) 653-8226, fax: (410) 653-8709; e-mail: sidshq@charm.net.
†2070 Chain Bridge Rd, Suite 450, Vienna, VA 22182, (703) 821-8955, fax: (703) 821-2098; www.sidscenter.org.
‡6065 Roswell Rd, Suite 876, Atlanta, GA 30328, (404) 843-1030 or (800) 232-SIDS; www.sids.org.
§511 E John Carpenter Frwy, #700, Irving, TX 75062, (800) 438-6233; www.madd.org.
‖100 E 8th St, Rm B41, Cincinnati, OH 45202, (513) 721-5683, fax: (513) 345-4489.

can guide parents in making decisions related to the expected or unexpected death.

## Right to Die/Do Not Resuscitate (DNR)

One of the benefits of hospice has been the recognition of patients' right to die as they wish, with emphasis on the *quality* of life. Unfortunately, this is not always the focus of care, especially in the traditional hospital setting. Many families are not given the option of terminating treatment when cure is unlikely, and staff may be reluctant to raise the question of "no code" or do not resuscitate (DNR) orders (withholding cardiopulmonary resuscitation in response to cardiac arrest). Some situations affecting quality of life, such as the dying child's right to refuse additional treatment, often pose difficult ethical questions.

If parents choose "DNR," they must be aware of exactly what will and will not be done for the child and assured that this does not mean "no care." For example, the family may wish that oxygen be given to the child for difficult breathing but not want active resuscitation. Once a decision is made, it must be communicated to all members of the health team and include a *written* medical order for the use or withholding of lifesaving measures. An order of "slow" or "delay" code is not legal. Because the child's condition or the family's wishes may change, DNR orders are reviewed regularly. Orders should be respected even if difficult at the moment of death (Martinson, 1995).

## Viewing of the Body

Although most institutions recognize the need for parents to hold and spend time with the dead child, a dilemma may arise when the body is mutilated. Although the memory of the child's disfigurement can be extremely upsetting and generate concern for how much the child suffered, not seeing the body can leave the parents with imagined ideas of how their child looked, which can be worse than the reality and can delay the acceptance of the death. When family members choose to view the body, they need preparation for this upsetting experience. They should be told what to expect and why certain parts of the body are covered or bandaged. It is desirable to place the body in a private room, without medical apparatus, and make it as presentable as the situation allows. Some people appreciate the presence of a nurse in the room with them; others desire privacy. Regardless of how badly the body is harmed, parents may want to hold the child. Such options are offered and respected. Family members should be given as much time as they need to say good-bye; for many, viewing the body is a sign of closure—an opportunity to finish their good-byes and leave the hospital.

## Organ or Tissue Donation/Autopsy

Many states have legislated a mandatory request for organ/tissue donation when a child dies. For some families this may be a meaningful act—one that benefits another human being despite the loss of their child. Unfortunately, initiating a discussion about tissue donation is often very stressful for staff, and there may be confusion regarding whose responsibility this is. In centers in which transplants are performed, a full-time transplant coordinator is usually available to inform the family about organ donation and to take care of details. If such services are not available, the staff needs to determine which members should discuss this topic with the family. Ideally the person who knows the family best, knows when the death is expected, or has the opportunity to spend time with the family when the death is unexpected takes the role. Often nurses are in an optimum position to suggest tissue donation after consultation with the attending physician. When possible, the topic should be raised before death occurs. The request should be made in a private and quiet area of the hospital and should be simple and direct, with questions such as "Are you a donor family?" or "Have you ever considered organ donation?"

Most states have "required request" laws that mandate that the hospital make a request for tissue donation from the family of the deceased, especially if the patient is brain dead. A written consent from the family is required before donation can proceed. When requests for organ donation are made, health care practitioners must address common misunderstandings families have about brain death and organ donation (Franz and others, 1997). Training health care professionals on sensitive approaches to request for organ donation has been shown to increase families' willingness to consent to organ donation (Evanisko and others, 1998). The option to donate organs should always be separate from the communication of impending or actual death.

Nurses need to be aware of common questions about organ donation to help families make an informed decision. Healthy children who die unexpectedly are excellent candidates for organ donation. Children with cancer, chronic disease, or infection or who have suffered prolonged cardiac arrest may not be suitable candidates, although this is individually determined. The nurse should inquire if organ donation was discussed with the child or if the child ever expressed such a wish. Any number of body tissues or organs can be donated (skin, corneas, bone, kidney, heart, liver, pancreas), and their removal does not mutilate or desecrate the body or cause any suffering. The family may have an open casket, and there is no delay in the funeral. There is no cost to the donor family, but organ donation does not eliminate funeral or cremation responsibilities. Most religions permit organ donation as long as the recipient benefits from the transplant, although Orthodox Judaism forbids it.

In cases of unexplained death, violent death, or suspected suicide, autopsy is required by law. In other instances it may be optional, and parents should be informed of this choice. The procedure, as well as forms that require signing, should be explained. The family should know that the child can be in an open casket following an autopsy.

## Siblings' Attendance at Funeral Services

One of the most frequent concerns of parents is whether young or school-age children should attend funeral or burial services. (See Evidence-Based Practice box.) Sharing mo-

ments of deep significance with parents helps children understand the experience and deal with their own feelings of shock, sorrow, and grief; depriving them of this opportunity may leave children with lifelong regrets (Fig. 23-3). However, children need preparation for postdeath services. They should be told what to expect, particularly how the deceased person will look if the coffin is open. Ideally the parent should explain the details to the child; if the parent's grief prevents this communication, a significant family member or friend should substitute.

It is often helpful to bring children to the funeral service before many visitors arrive. They are allowed private time to say good-bye but are spared some of the unpredictable emotional reactions of others, which can be very distressing to them. Allowing children to stay as long as they wish, but respecting their need to leave, provides maximum control for them over their ability to grieve comfortably.

## EVIDENCE-BASED PRACTICE
### Children Attending the Funeral or Burial Service of a Loved One

This question generates much controversy among the general public and professionals. Many lay people feel it is too frightening for children to be exposed to the dead and that it is better for them to remember the loved person as he or she was when alive. There is a general attitude of protecting children from unhappy or distressing events. However, among health care professionals involved with children, there is a fairly general consensus that children should attend such services, and some authors suggest that no child is too young merely by virtue of age (Foley, 1986). Some suggest that children can be involved in planning a funeral (Martinson, 1995). Others recommend that the parents make the decision regarding attendance until children are 6 or 7 years of age, at which time children should choose (Zelauskas, 1981). Several retrospective studies indicate that attendance at funerals is both meaningful and useful to children (Dickinson, 1992; Silverman and Warden, 1992). Attendance at funerals helps children acknowledge the death, honor the deceased, and receive support and comfort. In addition, children, like adults, have "unfinished business," and visiting the dead person may represent an opportunity to complete those affairs. For example, the child may wish to say good-bye (verbally or written) or to leave a memento.

Unfortunately, little research has focused on the difference in adjustment between children who do and those who do not attend postdeath services. However, one study indicated substantial evidence of the benefit of involving children in the experience of their dying sibling. Lauer and others (1985) compared children's perceptions of their sibling's death at home vs in the hospital. The home care group (ages 5 to 23 years) reported they were prepared for the impending death, received consistent information and support from their parents, were involved in most activities, found the funeral experience comforting, and viewed their own involvement as the most important aspect of the experience. The non–home care group (ages 2 to 26 years) had opposite perceptions. Another study found that greater participation in the child's care and death, including funeral attendance, was associated with higher self-esteem in the siblings (Michael and Lansdown, 1986). Among adolescents, Kuntz (1991) found that seeing a parent who had died and being involved with the rituals surrounding the death promoted adaptive grieving. Thus it appears that increased involvement with the death, rather than isolation and "protection," benefits children.

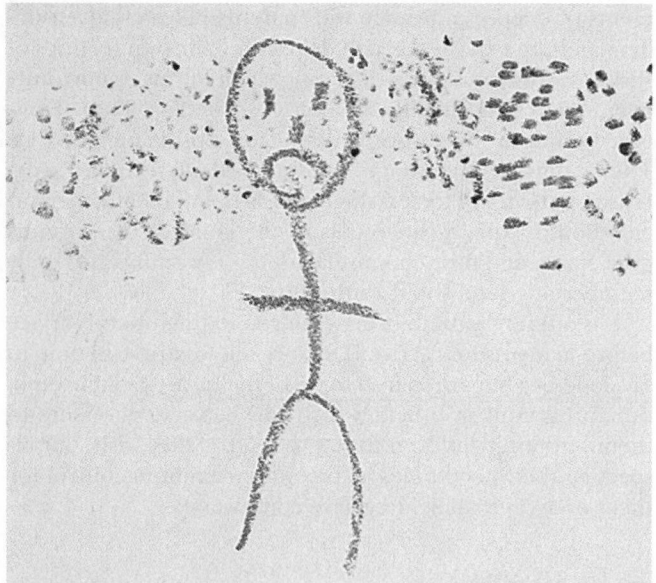

**Fig. 23-3** Drawing made by a 7-year-old child whose sister died in a car crash. The drawing shows the boy sad and crying (dots are tears) because he was not allowed to see his dead sibling.

### Critical Thinking Exercise

**Talking with Parents at the Time of Death**

Which of the following statements would **not** be a therapeutic approach to communicating with parents at the time of a child's death?

First, Think About It . . .

• Within what point of view are you thinking?
• What would be the consequences if you put your thoughts into actions?

1. You can touch her and hold her if you wish.
2. I will miss her.
3. Don't worry, everything will work out.
4. Have you made arrangements for a funeral?

*The best response is three, because offering reassurance to the bereaved parents is too simplistic and would not be therapeutic. Also, this action may bear negative consequences in the near future and interfere with trust in the nurse-family relationship. Answer one (a simple explanation of options), answer two (validating the loss), and answer four (asking a nonjudgmental question) are all appropriate therapeutic communications.*

## CARE OF THE GRIEVING FAMILY

No event is more devastating for families than the threatened or actual loss of a child. Families, especially parents, are deprived of the joy and fulfillment of watching a child grow. All family members are affected by the loss, and their needs must be recognized to resolve their grief.

In expected death the child and family are generally involved in the plan for intervention both before and after the death. In unexpected death the survivors face the tremendous task of integrating the loss into their lives, with no opportunity for anticipatory grief. In either situation nurses can facilitate the grief process by having a basic understanding of the process, being aware of expected psychologic and somatic reactions, and talking with family members, ascertaining their needs, and supporting their efforts to cope, adapt, and grieve. (See Critical Thinking Exercise box and Guidelines box.) Applying the principles of family-centered care is as important at this time as any other.

### Grief

The crisis of loss does not end with the child's death. In many ways it only begins. Unfortunately, the child's death often marks the close of the family's contacts with health professionals involved in the care. Consequently, many of these families never receive the support and guidance that could assist them in resolving the loss. Fortunately, hospice programs recognize this need and provide regular follow-up after the death.

When death is the expected or possible outcome of a disorder, the child and family members experience the behavioral reactions of anticipatory grief. Anticipatory grief may be manifested in varying behaviors and intensities and may include denial, anger, depression, and other psychologic and somatic symptoms.

When death occurs—whether expected or unexpected—acute grief develops within hours to days. Acute grief is a definite syndrome with psychologic and somatic symptoms that cause intense distress. Anticipatory guidance may assist grieving family members. Health care professionals should emphasize that grief reactions such as hearing the dead person's voice, feeling distant from others, or seeking reassurance that they did everything possible for the lost person are normal, necessary, and expected. They in no way signify poor coping, insanity, or an approaching mental breakdown. On the contrary, such behaviors signify that the survivor is working through the acute grief. They are a necessary part of satisfactory resolution of the loss. These reactions are part of the process of resuming or restructuring a meaningful role in the social environment.

After the death the lengthy process of grief work or mourning begins and extends into a period of adjustment to the loss, with eventual attachment to new people and the development of new interests. Contrary to the common belief that mourning is completed in a year, research indicates that resolution of grief may take years and that there may be an *intensification* of grief during the early years. The time since a child's death is not necessarily a factor in reducing the intensity of grief for families (Davis and Eng, 1998). Anticipatory guidance regarding the mourning process may be helpful to families so that they can recognize the normalcy of their experiences.

It is important to recognize that some family members may experience "complicated" grief. Complicated grief reactions (more than a year after the loss) include such symptoms as intense intrusive thoughts, pangs of severe emotion, distressing yearnings, feeling excessively alone and empty, unusual sleep disturbance, and maladaptive levels of loss of interest in personal activities (Horowitz and others, 1997). Bereaved persons experiencing such prolonged and complicated grief should be referred to an expert in grief and bereavement counseling.

Another important aspect of grief is the individual nature of the grief experience. Each member of the family will experience the grief of the child's death in their own way based on their particular relationship with that child. This can create potential conflict for families because each member of the family has expectations that the other members of the family should feel and grieve as they do. Nurses caring for families experiencing grief should be aware of the different grieving styles and help the family learn to recognize and support the uniqueness of each other's grief.

## Parental Grief

The death of a child leaves a vast emptiness within the family. For the parents it is not only the present loss of a dearly loved child, but also the loss of future joys with the child. There will be no graduations, marriages, or grandchildren by this child. It is for this reason that parental grief can extend over a lifetime.

Parental grief can be very stressful on a marriage. As parents become lost in their grief, they are unable to perform many of their roles within the family. For instance, a mother who is generally the nurturing parent now finds herself immobilized by grief and unable to nurture and support her husband and surviving children. Her husband functions in the family as the provider and protector; however, he could not "fix" his dying child. He may now feel the need to "fix" the other members of his family. In addition, he may not have the resources to express his grief, leading to postponing his grief by keeping busy at work or around the house. This "tabling" of emotion can lead to outbursts of anger and emotional distancing. Parents must be guided in understanding each other's needs during their grief process. In addition to the parents' unavailability to each other, they may also be so lost in their own grief that they cannot easily respond to their children's grief.

## Sibling Grief

Children, even adolescents, grieve very differently than adults. Children of all ages grieve the loss of a loved one, and their understanding and reactions to death will depend on their age and developmental level (Table 23-5). In addition, children will revisit their grief as they grow and develop new understanding of the effect of their sibling's death on the family. However, they do not grieve 100% of the time. They grieve in spurts and can be emotional and sad in one instance and then, just as quickly, off and playing (see Critical Thinking Exercise box on p. 971). Children can be exquisitely attuned to their parents' grief and will try to protect them by not asking questions or by trying not to upset them. This can set the stage for the sibling to try to become the "perfect child." The other side of this is the child who is so in need of his or her parents' attention that the child begins to act out. Again, nurses should be attentive for

---

### GUIDELINES
#### Communicating with the Bereaved Family

**EXAMPLES OF NONTHERAPEUTIC STATEMENTS**

| | |
|---|---|
| Advice | You should get out more. |
| | Stop feeling sorry for yourself. |
| | You need to be strong for your family. |
| Cheerfulness | Now, now, don't cry; cheer up. |
| | Cheer up, you can always have another baby. |
| Interpretation | It was God's will. |
| | It's better now because she is at peace. |
| Reassurance | I know how you feel. |
| | God never gives us more than we can handle. |
| | Don't worry, everything will work out. |
| | At least you still have the rest of your family. |
| Argument | How can you say that? |
| | It's wrong to blame anyone. |
| | You should be glad his suffering is over. |
| Ignoring loss | Remember, you're young and can still have another baby. |
| | It could be worse; he could have lived with severe brain damage. |

**EXAMPLES OF THERAPEUTIC STATEMENTS**

| | |
|---|---|
| Feeling-focused | You seem confused and angry. |
| | You are still feeling the pain. |
| | Tell me more about how you are feeling. |
| Nonjudgmental questions | Can I be of any help? |
| | Have you decided who the pallbearers will be? |
| Clarification | Correct me if I'm wrong, but you intend to make all the arrangements. |
| | You feel the accident was your husband's fault? |
| | I'm not sure I understand. Tell me more about . . . . |
| Explanations | You can touch her and hold her if you wish. |
| Concern | Your daughter's birthday is near. That must be painful to deal with. |
| Support, empathy | It's OK to cry. |
| | It sounds like you have been doing some painful thinking. |
| Support, silence | I'm here if you want to talk. (Silence) |
| | Hello. (Touch, silence) |
| Assessing coping and support | Do you have friends and family who can help you now? |
| | You have been through a lot. How are you doing now? |
| | Is there someone who can drive you home? |
| Validating loss | You have been through a very tough time. |
| | He was a special boy to all the staff. I will miss him. |

Data from Davidowitz M, Myrick R: Responding to the bereaved: an analysis of "helping statements," *Death Educ* 8:1-10, 1984; Johnson L, Mattson S: Communication: the key to crisis prevention in pediatric death, *Crit Care Nurs*, pp 23-27, Dec 1992; and Segal S, Fletcher M, Meekison W: Survey of bereaved parents, *Can Med Assoc J* 134(1):38-42, 1986.

**TABLE 23-5** Children's reactions to death

| Reactions to Death | Interventions |
| --- | --- |
| **Infants and Toddlers** | |
| With the death of someone else, they may continue to act as though the person is alive | Help parents deal with their feelings, allowing them more emotional reserve to meet the needs of their children |
| As children grow older, they will be increasingly able and willing to let go of the dead person | Encourage parents to remain as near to child as possible, yet be sensitive to parents' needs |
| Ritualism is important; a change in lifestyle could be anxiety producing | Maintain as normal an environment as possible to retain ritualism |
| This age-group also reacts to parental anxiety and sadness | If a parent has died, encourage having consistent caregiver for child |
| | Promote primary nursing |
| **Preschool Children** | |
| May feel guilty and responsible for the death of a sibling | Help parents deal with their feelings, allowing them more emotional reserve to meet the needs of their children |
| Greatest fear concerning death is separation from parents | Help parents to understand behavioral reactions of their children |
| May engage in activities that seem strange or abnormal to adults | Encourage parents to remain near the child as much as possible, to minimize the child's great fear of separation from parents |
| Because of their fewer defense mechanisms to deal with loss, young children may react to a less significant loss with more outward grief than to the loss of a very significant person | If a parent has died, encourage having a consistent caregiver for child |
| The loss is so deep, painful, and threatening that the child must deny it for the present in order to survive its overwhelming impact | Promote primary nursing |
| Behavior reactions such as giggling, joking, attracting attention, or regressing to earlier developmental skills indicate children's need to distance themselves from tremendous loss | |
| **School-Age Children** | |
| Because of their increased ability to comprehend, they may have more fears, for example: | Help parents deal with their feelings, allowing them more emotional reserve to meet the needs of their children |
|   The reason for the illness | Encourage parents to remain near child as much as possible, yet be sensitive to parents' needs |
|   Communicability of the disease to themselves or others | Because of children's fear of the unknown, anticipatory preparation is very important |
|   Consequences of the disease | Because the developmental task of this age is industry, interventions of helping children maintain control over their bodies and increasing their understanding allow them to achieve independence, self-worth, and self-esteem and avoid a sense of inferiority |
|   The process of dying and death itself | Encourage children to talk about their feelings and provide aggressive outlets |
| Their fear of the unknown is greater than their fear of the known | Encourage parents to honestly answer questions about dying rather than avoiding or fabricating euphemisms |
| The realization of impending death is a tremendous threat to their sense of security and ego strength | Encourage parents to share moments of sorrow with their children |
| Likely to exhibit fear through verbal uncooperativeness rather than actual physical aggression | Provide preparation for postdeath services |
| Very interested in postdeath services | |
| May be inquisitive about what happens to the body | |
| **Adolescents** | |
| Straddle transition from childhood to adulthood | Help parents deal with their feelings, allowing them more emotional reserve to meet the needs of their children |
| Have the most difficulty in coping with death | Avoid alliances with either parent or child |
| Least likely to accept cessation of life | Answer adolescents' questions honestly, treating them as mature individuals and respecting their needs for privacy, solitude, and personal expressions of emotions |
| Concern is for the present much more than for the past or the future | Help parents understand their child's reactions to death/dying, especially that concern for present crises, such as loss of hair, may be much greater than for future ones, including possible death |
| May consider themselves alienated from their peers and unable to communicate with their parents for emotional support, feeling alone in their struggle | |
| Because of their idealistic view of the world, they may criticize funeral rites as barbaric, money making, and unnecessary | |

signs that siblings are struggling with their grief and provide guidance to parents when possible.

## Mourning

### Shock and Disbelief

Shock, numbness, and disbelief are seen during the immediate phase of grief. As one parent described, "We were as prepared for our son's death as anyone could be, but it was a shock when in a moment his life was finished. I just can't get over the rapidity with which life ends." This temporary numbness protects the survivors from the overwhelming pain associated with grief. Decisions are often made automatically, and only certain details are remembered.

### Expression of Grief

When the numbness fades, a period of intense grief begins, characterized by a yearning and loneliness for the deceased. During this stage many of the signs of acute grief are evident, and physical complaints such as appetite changes and an inability to sleep are common. There is a tendency to review the events of the deceased's life and to evaluate the relationship with the loved one. Feelings of guilt and anger at this time are common.

## Critical Thinking Exercise

### Preschool Siblings and Death

Parents consult you about the preschool-age sibling of an infant who recently died. Which of the following concerns, expressed by the parents, are normal responses?

FIRST, THINK ABOUT IT . . .

- What are you taking for granted?
- What assumptions are you making?

1. "Our daughter cut her knee and said it was because the baby died."
2. "Our daughter used to enjoy preschool but now clings to us every morning and doesn't want to go."
3. "Our daughter sometimes asks where the baby is and when she'll come home."
4. "Our daughter lost a stuffed rabbit at the park and was distraught."

*Any of the above reactions of a preschool child may be normal responses to the death of a sibling and reflect correct assumptions. Young children may feel guilty and responsible for a sibling's death or may interpret illness or injury as a punishment for their thoughts about the sibling (answer one). Regression to earlier behaviors is common, and separation from parents is a particular concern (answer two). Preschoolers are not as likely as toddlers to think a person who has died is still alive, but they may deny the loss for a time (answer three). After a significant loss, a young child may express more outward grief at small losses because of their fewer defense mechanisms (answer four).*

## Critical Thinking Exercise

### Bereavement Programs

A family with a terminally ill child has seen a flyer about a bereavement program sponsored by the hospital. They ask you for information about the purpose of the program. Which of the following is the best reply?

FIRST, THINK ABOUT IT . . .

- What information are you using?
- How are you interpreting that information?

1. The bereavement program helps the family who wishes to have the child die at home.
2. The bereavement program helps you to plan the funeral.
3. The bereavement program provides information and support for the grieving process.
4. The bereavement program settles concerns you may have about whether your child is receiving appropriate treatment during the hospital stay.

*The best response is three. Bereavement programs provide information and support for the grieving process. Although a bereavement program might have some information about funeral planning, that is not its purpose. A social worker, chaplain, and funeral home director would be possible appropriate persons to assist in funeral planning. The hospital ethics committee would be an appropriate forum in which to raise concerns about appropriate treatment if discussions with nursing and medical staff fail to bring resolution. Some hospice programs, but not bereavement programs, may provide important information and support for a family who wishes to have their child die at home.*

### Disorganization and Despair

During this stage the pain of the loss is replaced primarily by emptiness, apathy, and deep depression. There is a feeling that life has no meaning and that the pain will never end. This is particularly relevant for parents. For example, mothers often comment that they feel they have suffered a double loss—loss of their child and loss of the mothering role. Feelings of estrangement from other loved ones are common, and social isolation may foster the depression.

### Reorganization

Reorganization refers to recovery from the loss. During this very gradual process the survivors again find meaning in living, readjust to life without the deceased, develop new or renewed relationships, and learn to live with the memory of the deceased with much less pain. It never means that the loved one is forgotten and the pain is gone. There always remains a deep ache that is never totally replaced with happiness and one that returns more intensely, for example, on holidays or anniversaries.

Resolution of grief may not always result in "letting go" of the loved one. Many survivors describe the pressure of an "empty space" in their lives years after the death of a child. Families attempt to fill the emptiness by keeping busy, often through altruistic involvements in self-help groups or by maintaining the connection with the lost child through recalling cherished memories.

## Bereavement Programs

Part of the difficulty in helping the bereaved family is lack of opportunity for follow-up in the traditional health care system. Consequently, many families never receive the support and guidance that could help them resolve the loss. At a minimum, one follow-up phone call or meeting with the family should be arranged, possibly 1 month after the child's death, to give the family time to overcome the phase of shock and disbelief. Families can also be referred to self-help groups, such as **The Compassionate Friends,*** an international organization for bereaved families, parents, and siblings. When such groups are not available, nurses can be instrumental in networking families or facilitating parent and sibling groups.

The ability of family members to work through their grief may be facilitated by a formal bereavement program or bereavement counseling. Comprehensive bereavement programs begin at the time of the child's death and continue for as long as is desired by the family. (See Critical Thinking Exercise box.) The purpose of a bereavement program is to assist and support families in the process of coping with the devastating impact of the loss of a child and hopefully with grief resolution. The components of such a program in-

*PO Box 3696, Oak Brook, IL 60522-3696, (630) 990-0010, fax: (630) 990-0246; www.compassionatefriends.org.

clude initial contact and support by knowledgeable staff, information and reading materials relevant to the grief process, follow-up contacts by phone or mail, parent and sibling support groups, and referrals for counseling if indicated (Stewart, 1995).* Parents should be given the option of participating in such a program, when available, but the desire not to participate should not be judged adversely by staff, because grief work is an individual process.

# THE NURSE AND THE CHILD WITH LIFE-THREATENING ILLNESS

## Nurses' Reactions to Caring for Children with Life-Threatening Illness

Nurses experience reactions to fatal illness that are very similar to the responses of family members. Some common reactions help nurses provide care by protecting them from the emotional impact of the event. Other reactions interfere with the establishment of a therapeutic relationship with family members. Analysis and understanding of these reactions are as important in providing effective care to the dying child as the recognition of specific responses in the family.

### Denial

When children are admitted to a pediatric unit with a suspected diagnosis of a serious illness, the initial response from some nurses is shock and denial. However, their behavioral reaction may be withdrawal from the child and family. They choose the "cure" philosophy over the "care" philosophy as a method of distancing themselves from the implications of emotional involvement. Because of their own dependency on denial, some nurses may inappropriately support denial in parents. There are several methods of conveying this message, such as emphasizing only optimistic "survival statistics," negating the seriousness of the illness, focusing on "cheering up" the family, and engaging in casual conversation to avoid meaningful dialogue. Although this increases nurses' comfort in caring for the dying child, it does little to provide family members an opportunity to progress beyond denial and begin anticipatory grieving.

Some denial is as important for nurses as it is for the child or parents; it protects nurses from the overwhelming reality of death. It would be extremely difficult to participate in the treatment plan without some expectation of a cure. Denial is also necessary to prevent feelings of failure. In general, nursing and medical goals emphasize curing illness and saving lives, not allowing patients to die. However, denial loses its beneficial functions when nurses refuse to admit the failure of treatment efforts and insist on adhering to the "curing" regimen, regardless of its effectiveness or value. Failure of treatment should not be equated with personal failure or failure to provide optimum nursing care.

---

*A manual that can be useful in the development of a family-centered bereavement program is *Whispers of Hope: A Hospital-Based Program for Bereaved Parents and Their Families* by T. Rose and E.S. Stewart, available from Duke University Pediatric Brain Tumor Family Support Program, Durham, NC, (919) 684-5301.

### Anger and Depression

Some nurses may be angry for having been assigned to the "leukemia case" because the very exposure to potential failure in a fatal illness is extremely threatening. Others may feel angry for having to subject the child to painful procedures or for being unable to relieve the child's physical and emotional suffering. Instead of anger, some nurses may feel depression for any of these reasons.

However, without an understanding of the reason for the emotion, nurses may project the anger onto others, particularly family members. They may be unable to tolerate the child's uncooperative behavior or the parents' continual requests for information. Anger fuels more anger, and parents react with hostility and think the members of the nursing staff are rejecting them. A vicious circle of resentment, mistrust, and frustration results.

Depression also has adverse effects on a therapeutic relationship because nurses may withdraw from the child and parents as a method of controlling their sadness. Unaware of the reason for the avoidance, family members interpret it as evidence of inadequate care. This reaction also fosters a nonsupportive cycle of avoidance, withdrawal, resentment, and frustration. However, the messages are usually more covert than when the nurses' reaction is anger and may prevent a climax that could result in a solution to the problem.

### Guilt

Nurses who feel unable to deal with fatal illness in a child often experience guilt. Nurses who become angry or depressed when caring for a dying child often reveal that they are very uncomfortable with this response but are unable to choose a more direct and constructive approach. They express guilt for having been intolerant of the child's or parents' behavior and, even more important, realize the missed opportunity to provide these individuals with professional support and guidance.

Nursing staff may experience guilt even when they can deal effectively with the family. There is often a feeling that the family's needs are never completely met. Such nurses tend to set expectations that are beyond anyone's ability to meet, such as the expectation that they are supposed to save lives, not let people die.

The one important difference between a dying child and an ill child is that there may be no second chance to meet the needs of the dying child. This finality is difficult to comprehend but can be a catalyst toward better understanding one's own responses to dying. For example, when guilt makes an individual uncomfortable enough to seek alternate behavior patterns, there is an opportunity for change to occur, provided the individual is given some assistance and support.

### Ambivalence

One of the most universal reactions of nurses is ambivalence in their feelings toward a dying child. There is the fluctuating adherence to hope for a cure and fear of a relapse. Sometimes the motivations for either are more for personal needs. For example, they may hope that the child recovers to avoid readmissions. Or they may wish for a remission so that discharge is ensured. Such thoughts are certainly understandable in light of the emotional toll of nursing a dying child.

Ambivalence may be demonstrated in a particular type of bargaining. Rather than bargaining for extra time, nurses may hope that their colleagues are assigned to the patient or that a death may occur on a shift other than their own. Bargaining for a temporary absence from the dying child is a healthy response, because it denotes nurses' awareness of their own emotional limits. Nurses who are unable to recognize their personal emotional limits are in danger of seeking from the professional relationship their own needs for gratification, achievements, and fulfillment. This results in the loss of an objective evaluation of therapeutic interventions and the increased potential for subjective overinvolvement with the family.

## Coping with Stress

Pediatric critical care and oncology nurses surveyed about work stresses rank patient death as most stressful (Kushnir, Rabin, and Azulai, 1997). The less experienced the nurse, the more likely that death is rated as a stressor. Furthermore, nurses overestimated the percentage of deaths on their unit, which suggests that the experience overwhelms them.

One stress-related behavior that can result from caring for dying children is *burnout*—a state of physical, emotional, and mental exhaustion. It occurs as a result of prolonged involvement with individuals in situations that are emotionally demanding. Nurses working in intensive care units are particularly prone to this occupational hazard, but staff nurses also can experience it when dealing with certain groups of children, such as those who may die. To avoid burnout and cope constructively, effectively, and therapeutically with children who are dying requires a deliberate and concerted effort on the part of the nurse.

### Self-Awareness

The initial step in effectively caring for a dying child is making a deliberate choice to become involved. Many nurses react negatively to the word "involvement" because they believe that professionals must remain uninvolved to maintain objectivity. Involvement does not displace objectivity. On the contrary, allowing oneself to feel with the other person expands one's ability to comprehend the meaning and depth of that emotion. (See Family Focus box.) Ideally the nurse achieves *detached concern,* which allows sensitive, understanding care as a result of being sufficiently detached to make objective, rational decisions.

Involvement does have the potential risk of clouding objectivity, but awareness of one's reactions and investments in the care of a dying child minimizes this hazard. Developing awareness requires the willingness to investigate one's motivations for choosing to work in such an area and an understanding of the stresses inherent in the role, to review one's resolution of past losses, and to contemplate one's own fears of death. Often nurses who have a cold, impersonal reaction to dying patients come to realize that their reaction stems from previous unresolved conflicts or losses. Once they are

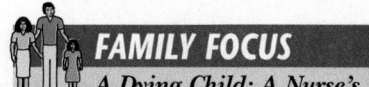

**FAMILY FOCUS**
*A Dying Child: A Nurse's Perspective*

Claire was unresponsive with slow, gasping breathing. Her mother asked me what I thought was happening. I replied honestly, "Your baby is dying because of her brain tumor." The mother put her arms around me and cried. We arranged for Claire to be baptized.

Honesty. Painful as the loss of a child is, my job is to assist the family through this experience. Although I usually wait until a private moment, such as driving home, I found tears streaming down my face as family and friends gathered for Claire's baptism. I went into the kitchen to compose myself, only to find several of my colleagues crying as well. Saying good-bye to a dying child will always be a difficult but shared experience.

Jeanne O'Connor Egan, RN, MSN
Pediatric Clinical Specialist
Children's Hospital, Washington, DC

able to talk about such experiences, they are usually able to gain insight into their behavior and begin to form alternative methods of reacting.

### Knowledge and Practice

Intervening therapeutically with terminally ill children and their families requires more than self-awareness. It also necessitates basing nursing practice on sound theoretic formulations and empirical observations that serve as a general, concise analysis of the typical reactions of families.

Nurses also must explore ethical issues surrounding the definition of death, the use of extraordinary and lifesaving measures vs passive or active euthanasia, and patients' rights to know and choose their own destiny. Once they have soundly formulated the principles by which to practice, they need opportunities for decision making. When a team approach is used, nurses can be valuable members of the group if their own values are clarified and they have critically assessed the family's responses. (See Ethical Decision Making in Chapter 1.)

### Support Systems

Support systems are essential to continued functioning in a high-stress environment. They allow for regeneration of energies by sharing feelings and concerns with others. Dealing with feelings about death in isolation can lead to repressed feelings such as denial, anger, depression, and grief. These feelings may be manifested in poor interactions between staff, inappropriate or unsupportive interactions with families, an inability to evaluate care plans or advocate for families, and a need to control (Hammer, Nichols, and Armstrong, 1992). Support is an important catalyst for processing feelings about death.

Social supports may be personal family members such as parents or spouses, extended relatives, and friends. Professional supports include colleagues, consultants, teachers, and supervisors. Peers may be sources of technical and practical advice. Because less-experienced nurses experience death as more stressful, a mentoring relationship between a senior nurse and the less-experienced nurse may provide

---

**Box 23-10** ■ ■ □

**Nurses Experiencing the Stress of Caregiving—Strategies That Help**

1. *Recognize the inevitability of the child's death*—One's own unrealistic expectations can cause the greatest grief, due to the belief that something more should or could have been done to prevent the child's death. Shift the focus of care to providing guidance and comfort for the child and family to increase a sense of accomplishment. Avoid self-blame for situations over which one has no control.

2. *Develop knowledge and apply it*—Increase personal knowledge about caring for dying children and their families. Apply this knowledge to provide the best possible care to the patient and family.

3. *Identify ways the work setting can provide support*—Ask for relief from highly emotional or conflicted situations, take time off and vacation, seek mentorship, make use of institutional support services such as multidisciplinary team meetings or employee assistance personnel.

4. *Briefing*—Inform others involved in the child's care about the child's condition and changes as they occur. After the death, notify caregivers who were closely involved to allow them the opportunity to grieve for the child.

5. *Debriefing*—Organize staff remembrance services to share experiences and feelings, "bereavement" rounds, multidisciplinary team review of care.

6. *Find meaning*—Accept that even the death of a child is a part of life, and find meaning in the caregiving experience with the child and family. Reflect on the experience, what it meant, how it influenced one's view on nursing care.

7. *Separate work and personal life*—Develop strategies to leave work behind when at home with family. Avoid trips to the hospital on off days.

8. *Take care of yourself*—Recognize the stress of caring for dying children and find healthy activities to help manage that stress. Exercise, good nutrition, and rest are important when work stress is high.

9. *Say good-bye*—Identify comfortable ways to say good-bye to the dead child. Attending memorial or funeral services, keeping a memento, journaling, plantings, and so on are all individual ways to acknowledge the importance of the child to the caregiver.

Modified from Brown-Hellsten M and others: *End of life care for children*, Austin, Texas, 1999, Texas Cancer Council.

---

support and role modeling and assist in the development of effective coping strategies (Gardner, 1999).

## Other Strategies

Any number of other strategies may be used to reduce stress. These include maintaining good general health practices, especially regular exercise, and diversionary activities that are of personal interest beyond the workplace. Distancing techniques are also effective, such as leaving work at work, informing other staff not to contact them on their days off, periodically assuming less demanding assignments, and taking time off when needed.

A final technique is to focus on the positive aspects of the caregiving role. Despite the difficult times in caring for these children and families, there are many rewarding experiences that must be remembered. Dedicated efforts reap numerous rewards, and these must not be forgotten or minimized. Reflection on positive feedback from appreciative families can revitalize self-esteem and job satisfaction.

Some nurses find shared remembrance rituals useful in resolving grief. Similarly, attending the funeral services can be a supportive act for both the family and the nurse and in no way detracts from the professionalism of care. For the family it conveys a sense of worth and caring by the nurse. For the nurse it can provide a sense of "closure" with the family and assist in the resolution of personal grief (Box 23-10).

---

## KEY POINTS

- A family-centered approach to care of the child and family facing life-threatening illness or death respects the central role of the family and emphasizes communication, collaboration, and cultural sensitivity.

- There are common phases of family reactions to a life-threatening illness such as cancer. These phases correspond to the progression of the disease and the status of treatment.

- Special decisions at the time of dying and death may involve hospital or hospice care, the child's right to die/do not resuscitate (DNR), viewing the body, organ/tissue donation/autopsy, and siblings' attendance at the funeral.

- Special needs of the family facing the unexpected death of a child include support while awaiting news of the child's status; a sensitive pronouncement of death; acknowledgement of feelings of denial, guilt, and anger; an opportunity to view the body; closure; and referrals for support.

- To counsel families and children regarding death, nurses need to understand children's perceptions of death, the fears in each age-group, and personal meanings of death and bereavement during developmental stages.

- Toddlers' egocentricity and vague separation of facts from fantasy make death incomprehensible; they may still refer to a dead person as though the person exists.

- Because of their sense of precausality and self-power, preschoolers may believe that their thoughts actually cause another person's death.

- With their reasoning power and fear of the unknown, school-age children may feel intense guilt and responsibility about someone's death.

- Adolescents have difficulty accepting death because of their preoccupation with developing a sense of identity.

- Nurses may offer the following assistance in education about death: counseling parents about children's age-specific understanding of death, encouraging parents to help children become familiar and comfortable with loss, taking part in organized death education in schools, and serving as a resource to answer families' and children's questions.

- What children are told about their serious illness is the family's decision and can be based on several general principles regarding developmental age, previous knowledge, and honesty.
- Siblings have special needs, including the need for information, reassurance about their own health status, assurance that they are not responsible for the illness or death, and support for their own grieving process.
- Acute grief is a syndrome with psychologic and somatic symptomatology that may appear after the crisis or be delayed, exaggerated, or apparently absent. "Distorted" re-

actions may represent one aspect of the syndrome and can be transformed into normal grief work.

- Mourning, or grief work, consists of four phases that do not necessarily proceed in sequence and may recur at any time: shock and disbelief, expression of grief, disorganization and despair, and reorganization.
- Formal bereavement programs may assist families in coping with the loss of a child and in the process of grief resolution.
- In dealing with stress related to the dying patient, the nurse can cope successfully through self-awareness, knowledge and practice, available support systems, maintaining general good health, and focusing on the positive rewards of involvement with dying children and their families.

# References

American Academy of Pediatrics, Committee on Bioethics and Committee on Hospital Care: Palliative care of children, *Pediatrics* 106(2):351-357, 2000.

American Nurses Association: *Nursing's social policy statement,* Washington, DC, 1995, American Nurses' Publishing.

Billings JA: What is palliative care? *J Palliat Med* 1(1):73-81, 1998.

Bluebond-Langner M: *The private worlds of dying children,* Princeton, NJ, 1978, Princeton University Press.

Bluebond-Langner M: Worlds of dying children and their well siblings, *Death Stud* 13:1-16, 1989.

Buckalow PG, Esposito CM: The role of the home health nurse in sudden infant death syndrome, *Home Health Care Pract* 7(3):36-45, 1995.

Davis B, Eng B: Special issues in bereavement and staff support. In Doyle D, Hanks GWC, MacDonald N, editors: *Oxford textbook of palliative medicine,* ed 2, New York, 1998, Oxford University Press.

Dent A and others: A study of bereavement care after a sudden and unexpected death, *Arch Dis Child* 74(6):522-526, 1996.

Dickinson GE: First childhood death experiences, *Omega J Death Dying* 2(3):169-182, 1992.

Evanisko MJ and others: readiness of critical care physicians and nurses to handle requests for organ donation, *Am J Crit Care* 7(1):4-12, 1998.

Faulkner KW, Armstrong-Dailey A: Care of the dying child. In Pizzo PA, Poplack DG, editors: *Principles and practice of pediatric oncology,* ed 3, Philadelphia/New York, 1997, Lippincott-Raven.

Ferrell B, Virani R, Grant M: Analysis of end-of-life content in nursing textbooks, *Oncol Nurs Forum* 26(5):869-876, 1999.

Ferrell BR: The impact of pain on quality of life: a decade of research, *Nurs Clin North Am* 30(4):609-624, 1995.

Fleischman AR: Commentary: ethical issues in pediatric pain management and terminal sedation, *J Pain Symptom Manage* 15(4):260-261, 1998.

Foley GV: Conflicts in practice: the argument, *J Assoc Pediatr Oncol Nurses* 2(3):22-24, 1985.

Foley KM: The treatment of pain in the patient with cancer, *CA Cancer J Clin* 36(4):194-215, 1986.

Franz HG and others: Explaining brain death: a critical feature of the donation process, *J Transpl Coord* 7(1):14-21, 1997.

Gardner JM: Perinatal death: uncovering the needs of midwives and nurses and exploring helpful interventions in the United States, England, and Japan, *J Transcult Nurs* 10(2):120-130, 1999.

Hammer M, Nichols DJ, Armstrong L: A ritual of remembrance, *MCN Am J Matern Child Nurs* 17(6):310-313, 1992.

Hinds PS and others: Decision making by parents and healthcare professionals when considering continued care for pediatric patients with cancer, *Oncol Nurs Forum* 24(9):1523-1528, 1997.

Hockley J: Psychosocial aspects in palliative care—communicating with the patient and family, *Acta Oncol* 39(8):905-910, 2000.

Horowitz MJ and others: Diagnostic criteria for complicated grief disorder, *Am J Psychiatry* 154(7):904-910, 1997.

James L, Johnson B: The needs of parents of pediatric oncology patients during palliative care phase, *J Pediatr Oncol Nurs* 14(2):83-95, 1997.

Kirshbaum MS: Advances in nursing science, *Adv Nurs Sci* 19(1):51-71, 1996.

Kuntz B: Exploring the grief of adolescents after death of a parent, *J Child Adolesc Psychiatr Ment Health Nurs* 4(3):105-109, 1991.

Kushnir T, Rabin S, Azulai S: A descriptive study of stress management in a group of pediatric oncology nurses, *Cancer Nurs* 20(6):414-421, 1997.

Lambert S: Distraction, imagery, and hypnosis techniques for management of children's pain, *J Child Fam Nurs* 2(1):5-15, 1999.

Lauer ME and others: Children's perceptions of their sibling's death at home or hospital: the precursors of differential adjustment, *Cancer Nurs* 8(1):21-27, 1985.

Lee CL, Johann-Liang R: Disclosure of the diagnosis of HIV/AIDS to children born of HIV-infected mothers, *AIDS Patient Care* 13(1):41-45, 1999.

Leikin S: A proposal concerning decisions to forego life-sustaining treatment for young people, *J Pediatr* 115(1):17-22, 1989.

Martinson IM: Hospice care for children: past, present, and future, *J Pediatr Oncol Nurs* 10(3):93-98, 1993.

Martinson IM: Improving care of dying children, *West J Med* 163:258-262, 1995.

Masera G and others: Guidelines for assistance to terminally ill children with cancer: a report of the SIOP working committee on psychosocial issues in pediatric oncology, *Med Pediatr Oncol* 32:44-48, 1999.

Masri C and others: Decision making and end-of-life care in critically ill children, *J Palliat Care* 16(suppl):S45-S52, 2000.

McCallum DE, Byrne P, Bruera E: How children die in hospital, *J Pain Symptom Manage* 20(6):417-423, 2000.

Michael S, Lansdown R: Adjustment to the death of a sibling, *Arch Dis Child* 61:278-283, 1986.

Minino AM, Smith BL: Deaths: preliminary data for 2000, *National Vital Statistics Reports,* vol 49, no 12, Hyattsville, MD, 2001, National Center for Health Statistics.

Morin SM, Welsh LA: Adolescents' perceptions and experiences of death and grieving, *Adolescence* 31(123):585-595, 1996.

Murphy SL: Deaths: final data for 1998, *Nat Vital Stat Rep* 48(11), 2000.

Murray JS: Siblings of children with cancer: a review of the literature, *J Pediatr Oncol Nurs* 16(1):25-34, 1999.

Nagy M: The child's view of death, *J Genet Psychol* 73:3-27, 1948.

National Hospice and Palliative Care Organization's Children's International Project on Palliative/Hospice Services: *Compendium of pediatric palliative care,* Alexandria, VA, 2000, National Hospice and Palliative Care Organization.

Newacheck PW, Halfon N: Prevalence and impact of disabling chronic conditions in childhood, *Am J Public Health* 88(4): 610-617, 1998.

Newacheck PW and others: An epidemiologic profile of children with special health care needs, *Pediatrics* 102(1):117-123, 1998.

Nitschke R and others: Therapeutic choices made by patients with end-stage cancer, *J Pediatr* 101(3):471-476, 1982.

Oliver and others: Beneficial effects of a hospital bereavement intervention program after traumatic childhood death, *J Trauma* 50(3):440-446, 2001.

Oliver, Fallat ME: Traumatic childhood death: how well do parents cope? *J Trauma* 39(2):303-307, 1995.

Randolph AG and others: Variability in physician opinion on limiting pediatric life support, *Pediatrics* 103:e46, 1999.

Savage TA: Ethical decision making for children, *Crit Care Nurs Clin North Am* 9(1): 97-105, 1997.

Shumway CN, Grossman LS, Sarles RM: Therapeutic choices by children with cancer, *J Pediatr* 103(1):168, 1983 (letter).

Siever BA: Pain management and potentially life-shortening analgesia in the terminally ill child: the ethical implications for pediatric nurses, *J Pediatr Nurs* 9(5):307-312, 1994.

Silverman PR, Warden JW: Children's understanding of funeral ritual, *Omega J Death Dying* 25(4):319-331, 1992.

Stanfill P, Strong C: Conflicts in practice: the argument against, *J Assoc Pediatr Oncol Nurs* 2(3):25-26, 1985.

Stevens MM: Care of the dying child and adolescent: family adjustment and support. In Doyle D, Hanks GWC, MacDonald N, editors: *Oxford textbook of palliative medicine*, ed 2, New York, 1998, Oxford University Press.

Stewart ES: Family-centered care for the bereaved, *Pediatr Nurs* 21(2):181-184, 1995.

Wolfe J and others: Symptoms and suffering at the end of life in children with cancer, *N Engl J Med* 342(5):326-333, 2000.

World Health Organization, Expert Committee: Cancer pain relief and palliative care, *World Health Organ Tech Rep Ser* 804:1-75, 1990.

World Health Organization: *Cancer pain relief and palliative care*, Geneva, Switzerland, 1998, The Organization.

World Health Organization in conjunction with IASP: *Cancer pain relief and palliative care in children*, (order no. 1150459), WHO Publications Center USA, 1998, WHO.

Zelauskas B: Siblings: the forgotten grievers, *Issues Compr Pediatr Nurs* 5(1):45-52, 1981.

Zerwekh JV: Do dying patients really need IV fluids? *Am J Nurs* 3:26-30, 1997.

Chapter

# Chapter 24

# The Child with Cognitive, Sensory, or Communication Impairment

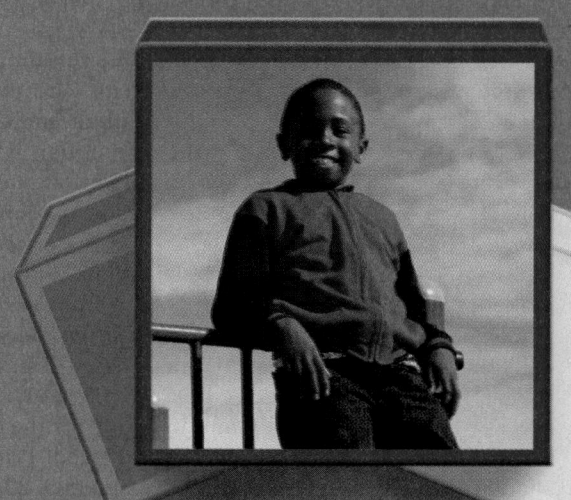

## Chapter Outline

**COGNITIVE IMPAIRMENT, 977**
**General Concepts, 977**
**Nursing Care of Children with Cognitive Impairment, 979**
*Nursing Care Plan: The Child with Mental Retardation, 988*
**Down Syndrome, 987**

Fragile X Syndrome, 993
**SENSORY IMPAIRMENT, 994**
**Hearing Impairment, 994**
**Visual Impairment, 1000**
**The Deaf-Blind Child, 1006**
**COMMUNICATION IMPAIRMENT, 1007**

General Concepts, 1007
    Language Impairment, 1007
    Speech Impairment, 1007
**Nonspeech Communication, 1007**
**Autism, 1008**
**Nursing Care of Children with Communication Impairment, 1010**

## Related Topics

Auditory Testing, Ch. 7
Autism, Ch. 13
Defects Caused by Chemical Agents, Ch. 11
Dental Health: Toddler, Ch. 14; School-Age Child, Ch. 17
Developmental Assessment, Ch. 7
Family-Centered Care of the Child with Chronic Illness or Disability, Ch. 22
Family-Centered Home Care, Ch. 25

Fetal Alcohol Syndrome, Ch. 11
Hereditary Influences on Health Promotion of the Child and Family, Ch. 5
Human Immunodeficiency Virus Encephalopathy, Ch. 37
Infant, Ch. 12; Toddler, Ch. 14; Preschooler, Ch. 15
Limit-Setting and Discipline, Ch. 3

Optic, Otic, and Nasal Administration (of Medication), Ch. 27
Otitis Media, Ch. 32
Play: Infant, Ch. 12; Toddler, Ch. 14; Preschooler, Ch. 15; School-Age Child, Ch. 17
Preparation for Hospitalization, Ch. 26
Toilet Training, Ch. 14
Vision Testing, Ch. 7

# COGNITIVE IMPAIRMENT

## General Concepts

*Cognitive impairment* is a general term that encompasses any type of mental difficulty or deficiency. In this chapter the term is used synonymously with *mental retardation (MR)*. Although the needs and concerns of the family are a primary focus throughout the chapter, the reader is encouraged to review Chapter 22, which details the family's adjustment to disabilities in general.

The definition of MR developed by the American Association of Mental Retardation (AAMR) includes three diagnostic criteria that place increased emphasis on the child's functional strengths and weaknesses and the environmental supports the child needs. The AAMR definition requires a delineation of intellectual functioning, functional strengths and weaknesses in a number of real-world adaptive skills, and onset before 18 years of age. The child must manifest subaverage intellectual functioning, which in practical terms means an intelligence quotient (IQ) of 70 to 75 or below. In addition, the child must demonstrate functional impairment in at least 2 of 10 adaptive skill domains, including communication, self-care, home living, social skills, community use, self-direction, health and safety, functional academics, leisure, and work (Fredericks and Williams, 1998; Schalock and others, 1994).

It is critical to note that low IQ alone is not the sole criterion for MR. For example, individuals with IQ scores near 75 may not be classified as retarded if deficits in everyday adaptive behavior skills are not present. Or, if cognitive impairment accompanied by adaptive limitations occurs from injury and disease after age 18, the person is not considered retarded.

■ Nancy Kline, PhD, RN, CPNP, and Douglas Bloom, PhD, revised this chapter.

The AAMR definition of MR emphasizes abilities, environments, supports, and empowerment. The intensity of needed support is classified as intermittent, limited, extensive, or pervasive. The underlying assumption is that with appropriate supports over a prolonged period, the ability of the person with MR to function each day will generally improve. For educational purposes the terms *educable mentally retarded,* which corresponds to the mildly retarded group (about 85% of all people with MR), and *trainable mentally retarded,* which corresponds to children with moderate levels of MR (about 10% of the MR population), may be used (First, McQueen, and Pincus, 1996) (Table 24-1).

The central role of the family in caring for the child with cognitive impairment cannot be overlooked. Principles of family-centered care are key. (See Chapters 6, 22, and 25.) Nurses can be instrumental in helping to socialize families of children with MR toward a collaborative model of care, which is critical in regard to efforts to teach these children functional skills.

## Diagnosis

The diagnosis of MR is usually made after a period of suspicion by professionals or the family that the child's developmental progress is delayed. In some cases it is made at birth because of recognition of distinct syndromes, such as Down syndrome, or when severe to profound delays in development are apparent. At the other extreme, it is made after the child begins school and does poorly. In all cases a high index of suspicion for developmental delay is necessary for early diagnosis, and routine developmental screening can assist in early identification. (See Chapter 7.) Delays are most commonly seen in language and cognitive skills, although delays in fine and gross motor skills are also typically noted. MR must be distinguished from other causes of developmental delay, some of which may occur in conjunction with MR in an individual.

Results of standardized tests are helpful in making the diagnosis of MR. The most commonly used test for infants is the Bayley Scales of Infant Development, Second Edition, although the Mullen Scales of Early Learning is also used for this population. (See Chapter 7.) During the school years the Wechsler Intelligence Scale for Children-III (WISC-III) is most often used. The Differential Ability Scales (DAS), Stanford-Binet Intelligence Scale, Fourth Edition, and Kaufman Assessment Battery for Children (KABC) are additional tests that can be used with toddlers through school age. Specialized tests such as the Leiter International Performance Scale—Revised can be useful for assessing children with language differences, nonverbal children, or those with significant language or motor impairment. All of these tests are individually administered (never given as a group test) in a standardized manner under favorable conditions by specially trained clinicians, such as psychologists, psychometrists, or child development specialists. Tests for assessing adaptive behavior functioning include the Vineland Adaptive Behavior Scales and the AAMR Adaptive Behavior Scale. Informal appraisal of adaptive behavior may be made by those fully acquainted with the child (e.g., teachers, parents, or other care providers). Frequently these observations lead parents to seek a developmental evaluation.

When a family suspects a diagnosis of MR, it can be devastating. Care should be taken to provide support from sensitive professionals at the time of diagnosis. (See Chapter 22.) Information should be provided to address any misconcep-

| **TABLE 24-1** Classification of mental retardation | | | |
|---|---|---|---|
| Level (IQ)* | Preschool (Birth-5 Years)—Maturation and Development | School Age (6-21 Years)—Training and Education | Adult (21 Years and Older)—Social and Vocational Adequacy |
| **Mild**—50-55 to approximately 70-75 | Often not noticed as retarded by casual observer but is slower to walk, feed self, and talk than most children; follows same sequence in development as normal children | Can acquire practical skills and useful reading and arithmetic to a third to sixth grade level with special education; can be guided toward social conformity; achieves mental age of 8 to 12 years | Can usually achieve social and vocational skills adequate to self-maintenance; may need occasional guidance and support when under unusual social or economic stress; can adjust to marriage but not childrearing |
| **Moderate**—35-40 to 50-55 | Noticeable delays in motor development, especially in speech; responds to training in various self-help activities | Can learn simple communication, elementary health and safety habits, and simple manual skills; does not progress in functional reading or arithmetic; achieves mental age of 3 to 7 years | Can perform simple tasks under sheltered conditions; participates in simple recreation; travels alone in familiar places; usually incapable of self-maintenance |
| **Severe**—20-25 to 35-40 | Marked delay in motor development; little or no communication skills; may respond to training in elementary self-care (e.g., self-feeding) | Usually walks, barring specific disability; has some understanding of speech and some response; can profit from systematic habit training; achieves mental age of toddler | Can conform to daily routines and repetitive activities; needs continuing direction and supervision in protective environment |
| **Profound**—below 20-25 | Gross retardation; minimum capacity for functioning in sensorimotor areas; needs total care | Obvious delays in all areas of development; shows basic emotional responses; may respond to skillful training in use of legs, hands, and jaws; needs close supervision; achieves mental age of young infant | May walk; needs complete custodial care; has primitive speech; usually benefits from regular physical activity |

*Data from First MB, McQueen LE, Pincus HA: *DSM-IV coding update,* Washington, DC, 1996, American Psychiatric Association.

tions and answer parental questions and concerns. Referrals can be made for counseling or additional information if appropriate or desired. Nurses can be an important resource as parents sort through an often bewildering array of educational, health, and therapeutic services to determine how best to meet the needs of their child.

### Etiology

The etiology of MR includes familial, social, environmental and organic causes. Among individuals with severe retardation, chromosome disorders and prenatal toxins are common, with Down syndrome, fragile X syndrome, and fetal alcohol syndrome accounting for a sizable proportion of cases. Other identifiable disorders or syndromes, such as severe cerebral palsy, microcephaly, or infantile spasms, are also associated with MR. The prenatal, perinatal, and postnatal causes of MR are listed in Box 24-1.

### Prevention

Currently there is much concern with prevention of MR. *Primary prevention strategies*—those designed to preclude the occurrence of the condition that causes retardation—include rubella immunization; genetic counseling, especially in terms of Down or fragile X syndrome; use of folic acid supplements during pregnancy to prevent neural tube defects; education regarding the dangers of ingesting alcohol during pregnancy and lead during childhood; adequate prenatal care and childhood nutrition; and reduction of head injuries. In the future, gene therapy for selected conditions will probably be a significant advance in preventing genetic disorders, such as phenylketonuria.

*Secondary prevention activities*—those designed to identify the condition early and institute treatment to avert cerebral damage—include prenatal diagnosis or carrier detection of disorders, such as Down syndrome, and newborn screening for treatable inborn errors of metabolism, such as congenital hypothyroidism, phenylketonuria, and galactosemia.

*Tertiary prevention strategies*—those concerned with treatment to minimize long-term consequences—include early identification of conditions and appropriate therapies and rehabilitation services. These include medical treatment of coexisting problems, such as hearing and visual impairment in Down syndrome, and programs for infant stimulation, parent training, preschool education, and counseling services to preserve the integration of the family unit.

## Nursing Care of Children with Cognitive Impairment

The goal of caring for children with MR is to promote their optimum social, physical, cognitive, and adaptive development as individuals within a family and community. General guidelines for coping with and adjusting to the child with special needs are discussed extensively in Chapter 22.

### ▐▐ Assessment

Nurses play a major role in identifying children with cognitive impairment. In the newborn and early infancy period, few signs are present, with the exception of various syndromes that have distinctive features, such as Down syndrome. After this age, delayed developmental milestones are the major clues to MR. In addition, nurses must have a high index of suspicion for early behavioral patterns that may suggest cognitive impairment (Box 24-2) and be aware of stereotypes that may delay diagnosis, such as "retarded children have to look dumb." Parental concerns, such as delayed development compared with siblings, need to be taken seriously. All children should receive regular developmental assessment, and the nurse is often the person responsible for performing such developmental screening tests. (See Chapter 7.) When delays are found, the nurse must use sensitivity and discretion in revealing this finding to parents and refer the child for diagnostic testing.

---

**Box 24-1** ▪ ▪ ▫
**Causes of Mental Retardation**

**Infection and intoxication**—Any agent associated with abnormalities or malformations, such as rubella, syphilis, toxoplasmosis, maternal drug consumption (including alcohol), exposure to industrial chemicals, increased blood levels of lead; Rh incompatibility resulting in kernicterus; or maternal disorders, such as eclampsia

**Trauma or physical agent**—Injury to brain suffered during prenatal, perinatal, or postnatal period, including physical injury, lack of oxygen, or exposure to radiation

**Metabolism or nutrition**—Imbalances in fat, carbohydrates, and amino acids; inadequate nutrition; and metabolic or endocrine disorders, such as phenylketonuria or congenital hypothyroidism

**Gross postnatal brain disease**—Diseases characterized by skin eruptions, lesions, and tumors, such as neurofibromatosis and tuberous sclerosis

**Unknown prenatal influence**—Cerebral, spinal, and craniofacial malformations, such as microcephaly, hydrocephalus, meningomyelocele, and craniostenosis

**Chromosome abnormalities**—Chromosome aberrations resulting from radiation, viruses, chemicals, parental age, and genetic mutations, such as Down syndrome and fragile X syndrome

**Gestational disorders**—Prematurity, low birth weight, and postmaturity

**Psychiatric disorders with onset during child's developmental period**—For example, autism

**Environmental influences**—Evidence of a deprived environment associated with a history of mental retardation among parents and siblings

---

**Box 24-2** ▪ ▪ ▫
**Early Behavioral Signs Suggestive of Cognitive Impairment**

Nonresponsiveness to contact
Poor eye contact during feeding
Diminished spontaneous activity
Decreased alertness to voice or movement
Irritability
Slow feeding

From Crocker A, Nelson R: Mental retardation. In Levine MD, Carey WB, Crocker AC, editors: *Developmental-behavioral pediatrics*, ed 3, Philadelphia, 1999, WB Saunders.

## Nursing Diagnoses

A number of nursing diagnoses are prominent in the nursing care of the child with cognitive impairment and the child's family; other diagnoses specific to individual cases become evident. The most common nursing diagnoses are outlined in the Nursing Care Plan on p. 988.

## Planning

The goals for the child with MR and family are as follows:

1. Child will be educated using effective teaching strategies.
2. Child's optimum development will be promoted.
3. Child will learn self-care skills.
4. Family will plan for future care.
5. Child will be cared for appropriately during hospitalization.

## Implementation

Nurses play a role in developing and implementing the Individualized Education Plan (IEP) for each child with special

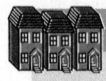

### COMMUNITY FOCUS
*Key Terms to Know in Special Education and Early Intervention*

**ADA–Americans with Disabilities Act (PL 101-336)** prohibits discrimination against individuals with disabilities. The act applies to adults and children and affects many businesses and services, including stores, hotels, public transportation terminals, parks, museums, employers, schools, and daycare centers.

**IDEA–Individuals with Disabilities Education Act (PL 101-476)** is based on the Education for All Handicapped Children Act (PL 94-142). Children enrolled in special education (criteria vary by state) may be eligible to receive special education and related services mandated by IDEA. Covered disabilities range widely and include severe visual and hearing impairments, speech impairment, mental retardation, emotional problems, learning disabilities, physical disabilities, and other health impairments.

**IEP–Individualized Education Plan** is required under IDEA. Based on a multidisciplinary evaluation and shared with parents, the IEP outlines special education and other related services to be received by the child with special needs. Related services can include transportation, developmental services (speech, audiology, physical therapy, occupational therapy, and others), supportive services (psychologic services, social work), and medical services as required to assist a child in benefitting from special education.

**IFSP–Individualized Family Service Plan,** called for in PL 99-457, is based on the IEP concept but has components including a developmental assessment, identification of family strengths, plan for supporting the child's development, early intervention services to be provided for the child and the family, expected outcomes, a designated case manager, and a plan for transition to school services.

**Part H–Title I (Part H) of PL 99-457** addresses early intervention services for children with special needs from birth to age 2 years 11 months.

**PL 99-457 (The Education of the Handicapped Act Amendments of 1986)–PL 99-457** was passed to address the needs of young children with disabilities. Title I (Part H) asks states to coordinate early intervention services for children from birth through age 2 years 11 months. Title II extends the provisions of PL 94-142, a special education law, to children 3 to 5 years of age and notes that the services can be provided in the home or in other settings.

Copyright Elizabeth Ahmann, ScD, RN.

needs in the school system and the Individualized Family Service Plan (IFSP) designed for the family and child with special needs in an early intervention program (American Academy of Pediatrics, 2000). (See Community Focus box.)

Standards of care have been developed for nurses working with persons with developmental disabilities or MR (Aggen and Moore, 1994; Ardito and others, 1997; Ridenour, 1999) and for nurses working in early intervention programs. Nursing organizations related to developmental disabilities are listed in Box 24-3.

**Educate Child and Family.** To teach children with cognitive impairment, it is necessary to investigate their learning abilities and deficits. This is important for the nurse who may be involved in a home care type of program or who may be caring for the child in a school or health care setting. The nurse who understands how these children learn can effectively teach them basic skills or prepare them for various health-related procedures.

Children with cognitive impairment have a marked deficit in their ability to discriminate between two or more stimuli because of difficulty in recognizing the relevance of specific cues. However, these children can learn to discriminate if the cues are presented in an exaggerated, concrete form and if all extraneous stimuli are eliminated. For example, the use of colors to emphasize visual cues or the use of singing or rhymes to stress auditory cues can help them learn. Their deficit in discrimination also implies that concrete ideas are learned much more effectively than abstract ideas. Therefore demonstration is preferable to verbal explanation, and learning should be directed toward mastering a skill rather than understanding the scientific principles underlying a procedure.

Another cognitive deficit is in short-term memory. Whereas children of average intelligence can remember several words, numbers, or directions at one time, these children are less able to do so. Therefore they need simple one-step directions. Learning through a step-by-step process

### Box 24-3 ■ ■ ■
### Nursing Organizations for Developmental Disabilities

**American Association on Mental Retardation (Nursing Division)**
444 North Capitol St NW
Suite 846
Washington, DC 20001-1512
(202) 387-1968
(800) 424-3688
Fax: (202) 387-2193
Web site: *www.aamr.org*

**Developmental Disabilities Nurses Association**
1720 Willow Creek Circle, Suite 515
Eugene, OR 97402
(541) 485-0477
(800) 888-6733
Fax: (541) 485-7372

Modified from Nehring WM: The nurse whose specialty is developmental disabilities, *Pediatr Nurs* 20(1):78-81, 1994.

requires a *task analysis,* in which each task is separated into its necessary components and each step is taught completely before proceeding to the next activity (see Box 24-4). Considerable repetition and review of new instructional information is important for long-term retention.

One critical area of learning that has had a tremendous impact on education for cognitively impaired individuals is *motivation,* employing positive reinforcement for specific tasks or behaviors. Two techniques are especially important with this group of learners: *fading* (physically taking the child through each sequence of the desired activity and gradually fading out physical assistance so that the child becomes more independent) and *shaping* (waiting for the child to give a response that approximates the desired behavior, then reinforcing successive approximations of the end goal through the use of praise or tangible reinforcers). Repetition plays an important part in learning. As the child gains mastery, reinforcement can gradually be decreased. Such principles can easily be implemented in the home in teaching self-help skills. Maintaining feelings of success in accomplishing specified goals also promotes a feeling of self-esteem in the child. If a learning program does not move forward successfully, both parent and nurse can reevaluate the last sequence the child mastered to see if they are expecting too much too soon.

When behavior modification is employed, it is crucial not only to reinforce desirable behavior, but also to consistently ignore undesirable behavior. Ignoring the child may be particularly difficult for many parents, because they may equate ignoring their child with being a "bad parent." Therefore support and encouragement of the parents' efforts will be beneficial.

Advances in technology have greatly assisted in providing reinforcement, especially in children who are severely retarded and may have physical disabilities that limit their range of capabilities. For example, with the use of specially designed switches, children are given control of some event in the environment, such as turning on the computer (Fig. 24-1). The computer becomes reinforcement for activating the switch. Repetitive use of these switches provides an early, simplistic association with a technical device that may progress to the use of increasingly complex aids.

*Early intervention programs* have been widely promoted for children with developmental disabilities, and there is considerable evidence that these programs are valuable for children with cognitive impairment. Nurses working with the families need to be aware of the types of programs available in their community. Early intervention programs are provided by a number of organizations. Under Public Law 101-476, The Individuals with Disabilities Education Act of 1990, states are encouraged to provide full early intervention services* and are required to provide educational opportunities for all children with disabilities from birth to 21 years of age. Early intervention services may be provided by each state, such as **Programs for Children with Special Health Needs** (formerly **Crippled Children's Program**) or **Head Start,** or by private organizations, such as the **National Easter Seal Society**† and the **Association for Retarded Citizens of the United States.**‡ Educational services that begin when the child reaches age 3 are provided by local school districts. Parents should inquire about these programs by contacting the appropriate agencies. To promote optimum outcomes, education should begin as soon as possible, not at 5 or 6 years of age. As children grow older, their education can be directed toward vocational training that prepares them for as independent a lifestyle as possible within their scope of abilities (American Academy of Pediatrics, 2000).

**Promote the Child's Optimum Development.** Optimum development requires appropriate guidance for establishing acceptable social behavior and personal feelings of self-esteem, worth, and security. These attributes are not simply learned through a stimulating program, but must arise from the genuine love and caring that exists among family members. However, families may need guidance in providing an environment that fosters optimum development. Often it is the nurse who can provide assistance in these areas of childrearing.

Another important area for promoting optimum development and self-esteem is ensuring the child's physical well-being. Any congenital defects, such as cardiac, gastrointestinal, or orthopaedic anomalies, should be repaired. Plastic surgery may be considered when the child's appearance may be substantially improved. Dental health is very significant, and orthodontic and restorative procedures can immensely improve facial appearance.

*Communication.* Verbal skills are often delayed more than other physical skills. Speech requires adequate hearing and interpretation of sounds (receptive skills) and facial muscle coordination (expressive skills). Both receptive and

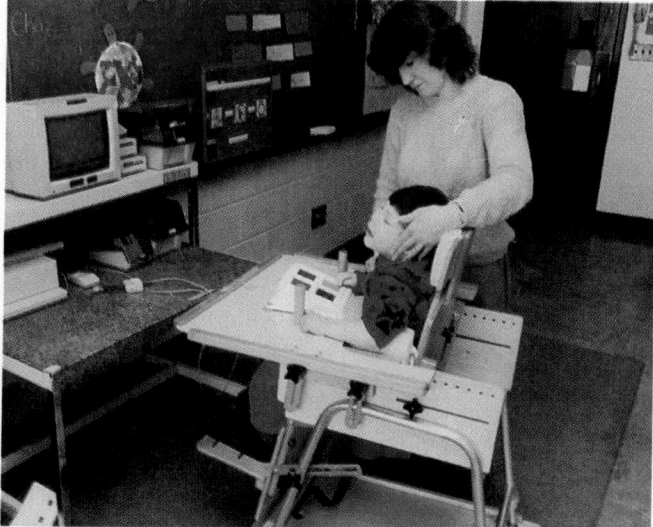

**Fig. 24-1** A push panel allows a child with cognitive impairment to turn a computer on and off.

*Information on early intervention programs in each state is available from the **National Down Syndrome Society,** 666 Broadway, 8th floor, New York, NY 10012, (800) 221-4602, fax: (212) 979-2873, e-mail: info@ndss.org; www.ndss.org.
†230 W Monroe, Suite 1800, Chicago, IL 60606-4802, (800) 221-6827, TTY: (312) 726-4258, fax: (312) 726-1494, e-mail: nessinfo@seals.com; www.seals.org.
‡500 E Border St, Suite 300, Arlington, TX 76010, (800) 433-5255, fax: (817) 277-3491; www.thearc.org.

expressive skills may be significantly impaired, so frequent audiometric testing should be conducted with hearing aids provided when needed. Other children may require training in controlling their facial muscles. For example, some children may need tongue exercises to correct tongue thrust or gentle reminders to keep the lips closed.

For some of these children, nonverbal methods of communication should be employed. The choice of an assistive device will often depend on the child's cognitive level and physical abilities. For the child without associated physical disabilities, a talking picture board is helpful. For children with physical limitations, several adaptations or types of communication devices are available to facilitate selection of the appropriate picture or word. Some children may be taught sign language or Blissymbols, a system of graphic symbols representing words, ideas, and concepts. The symbols are typically arranged on a board, and the individual points or uses a selector to communicate a message.

*Discipline.* Discipline must begin early. Limit-setting measures must be simple, consistent, and appropriate for the child's mental age. Control measures are based primarily on teaching a specific behavior, rather than on an understanding of the reasons behind it. Stressing moral lessons is of little value to a child who lacks the cognitive skills to learn from self-criticism and evaluation of previous mistakes. Behavior modification, especially reinforcement of desired actions and the use of time-out procedures, are appropriate forms of behavior control. (See Chapter 3.) Aversive strategies should be avoided.

*Socialization.* Acquiring social skills is complex; active rehearsal with role-playing and practice sessions, and positive reinforcement for desired behavior are successful approaches. Parents should be encouraged early to teach their child socially acceptable behavior: waving good-bye, saying "hello" and "thank you," responding to his or her name and greeting visitors. The teaching of socially acceptable sexual behavior is especially important to minimize sexual exploitation. Parents also need to expose the child to strangers so that manners can be practiced because transfer of learning from one situation to another is not automatic.

Social acceptance and self-esteem are enhanced when a child is appropriately dressed and well-groomed. Clean, stylish, well-fitting clothing that has self-adhering fasteners and elastic openings will facilitate self-dressing and social acceptance.

Opportunities for social interaction and training should begin at an early age. Parents should be encouraged to enroll their child in infant stimulation programs and other appropriate preschool programs as soon as possible. These programs provide education and training, as well as opportunities for social interaction with other children and adults.

As children grow older, they should have peer experiences similar to those of other children, including group outings, sports, and organized activities, such as Boy Scouts, Girl Scouts, or Special Olympics. These children often experience greater success in individual and dual sports than in team sports and enjoy themselves with children of the same developmental age (American Academy of Pediatrics,

2000). A close relationship with a best friend can be encouraged. Vacations, family outings, dances, and dating are important social opportunities.

*Sexuality.* Adolescence may be a particularly difficult time for parents, especially in terms of the child's sexual behavior, possibility of pregnancy, future plans to marry, and ability to be independent. Often, minimal anticipatory guidance has been offered to parents to prepare the child for physical and sexual maturation, and the degree of the adolescent's interest in and experience with sex has been underestimated.

The question of contraceptive protection for female adolescents is often a parental concern. Permanent contraception through sterilization is a special dilemma because of moral and ethical questions, as well as psychologic effects on the adolescent. State laws vary; some allow no sterilization, whereas others permit review of requests. Intramuscular injections of medroxyprogesterone acetate (Depo-Provera) is a contraceptive choice that provides long-term protection, requires little compliance, and often produces amenorrhea.

Parents of these adolescents are often very concerned about the advisability of marriage between two individuals with significant cognitive impairment. There is no conclusive answer; each situation must be judged individually. In many instances marriage would help the couple achieve a mutually satisfying and supportive relationship, meaningful companionship, and a more normal social/sexual adjustment. Every individual has the right to marry and have a family, regardless of his or her mental capacity, but violations of these rights occur worldwide (Gostin, 2000). The nurse should discuss this topic with parents and with the prospective couple, stressing suitable living accommodations and contraceptive methods to prevent pregnancy. If children are conceived, these parents require specialized assistance in learning to meet the needs of their offspring (Shaughnessy and others, 1996).

Nurses can help in this area by providing parents with information about sex education that is geared to the child's developmental level. For example, the adolescent female needs a *simple* explanation of menstruation and instructions on personal hygiene during the menstrual cycle.*

These adolescents also need practical sexual information regarding anatomy, physical development, and conception. Because of their easy persuasion and lack of judgment, they need a well-defined, concrete code of conduct with specific instructions for handling certain situations. Girls should know never to go alone anywhere with any person they do not know well. Boys should be warned of intimate advances from other males. Sexual assault of a cognitively impaired adolescent should be treated and investigated by law enforcement personnel (McNally, 2000).

*Play/exercise.* Children who are cognitively impaired have the same need for play as any other children. Exercise is beneficial for development of coordination, cardiovascu-

---

*Sources of information on sexuality and conception include **Planned Parenthood Federation of America,** 810 7th Ave, New York, NY 10019, (212) 541-7800 or (800) 829-7732; www.plannedparenthood.org; and the **Association for Retarded Citizens of the United States,** 500 E Border St, Suite 300, Arlington, TX 76010, (800) 433-5255, fax: (817) 277-3491; www.thearc.org.

lar fitness, and weight management. However, because of the child's slower development, parents may be less aware of the need to provide for such activities. They may also feel inadequate in playing with the child because the usual reciprocal interaction and resulting satisfaction between child and parent may be slower in developing.

In addition, children who are mentally retarded may not be able to institute appropriate play activities on their own. As a result of boredom, they may resort to self-stimulatory behavior, such as rocking, twirling, masturbating, or finger sucking, and self-injurious behaviors, such as head banging or biting, hitting, or scratching themselves (Symons, Koppekin, and Wehby, 1999). Such behaviors limit developmental progress and impede social acceptance. Therefore the nurse may guide parents toward selection of suitable toys and interactive activities.

The type of play is based on the child's developmental age, although the need for sensorimotor play may be prolonged. Parents should use every opportunity to expose the child to as many different sounds, sights, and sensations as possible. Appropriate toys include musical mobiles, stuffed toys, floating toys, a rocking chair or horse, a swing, bells, and rattles. The child should be taken on outings, such as trips to the grocery store or shopping center; other people should be encouraged to visit in the home; and the child should be related to directly, through such means as cuddling, holding and talking to the child in the face-to-face position.

Toys are selected for their recreational and educational value. For example, a large inflatable beach ball is a good water toy, encourages interactive play, and can be used to learn motor skills, such as balance, rocking, kicking, and throwing. Attractive toys encourage a child to reach, thus assisting in the development of motor skills (Fig. 24-2). Musical toys that mimic animal sounds or respond with social phrases are excellent ways of encouraging speech. A doll with removable clothes and different types of closures can help the child learn dressing skills. Toys should be simple in design so that the child can learn to manipulate them without help. For children with severe cognitive or physical impairment, electronic switches can be used to allow them to operate toys (Fig. 24-3).

Suitable activities for physical activity are based on the child's size, coordination, physical fitness and maturity, motivation, and health. Some children may have physical problems that prevent certain sports, such as atlantoaxial instability in children with Down syndrome. Children with mental impairment often have greater success in individual and dual sports than in team sports and enjoy themselves most with children of the same developmental level. The **Special Olympics*** provide a unique competitive opportunity.

Safety is a major consideration in selecting recreational and exercise activities. Some toys that may be appropriate developmentally may present dangers to a child who is strong enough to break them or use them incorrectly.

**Promote Independent Self-Help Skills.**   When a child with cognitive impairment is born, parents often need assistance in promoting normal developmental skills that are more easily learned by other children. There is no way to predict when a child should be able to master self-help skills, and studies demonstrate that wide variability exists in the ages at which these children accomplish such functions (see Table 24-3). Parents must be supported, included as the primary caretaker and teacher of the child, and provided with detailed written descriptions of a jointly devel-

---

*1325 G St NW, Suite 500, Washington, DC 20005, (202) 628-3630, (800) 700-8585, fax: (202) 824-0200; www.specialolympics.org (web site includes listing of state offices). In Canada: **Canadian Special Olympics,** 60 St Clair Ave E, Suite 70, Toronto, Ontario M4T 1N5, Canada, (416) 927-9050, fax: (416) 927-8475; www.cso.on.ca

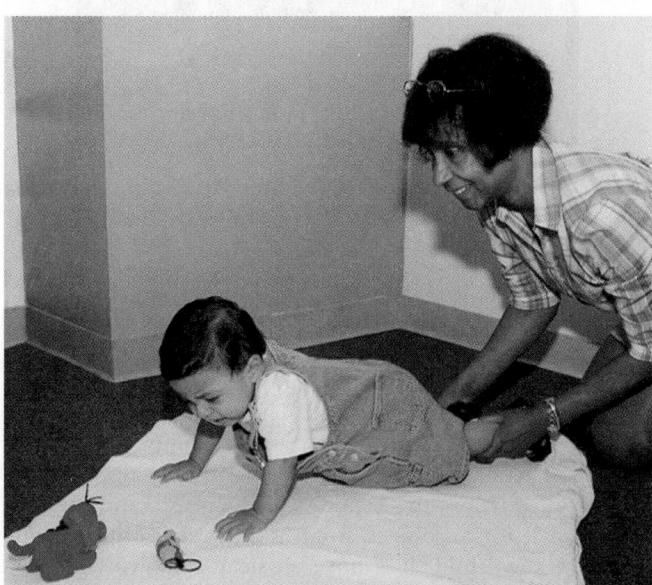

**Fig. 24-2**   Placing an attractive object outside of the child's reach encourages crawling movements. (Courtesy James DeLeon, Texas Children's Hospital.)

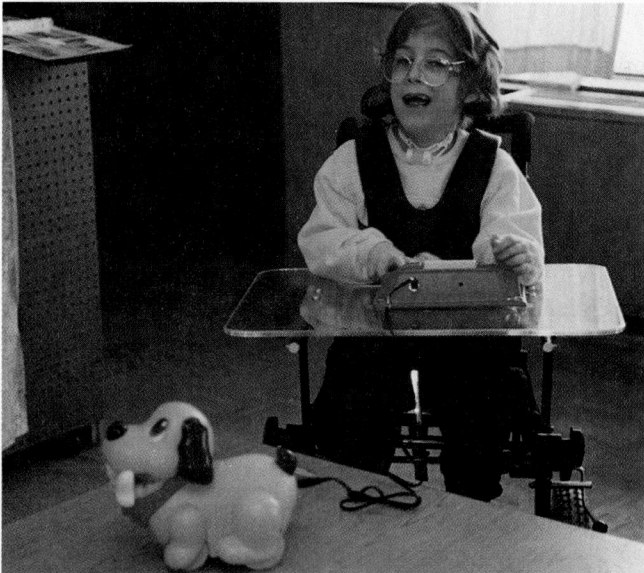

**Fig. 24-3**   An electric switch allows a child with physical impairment to play with a battery-operated toy.

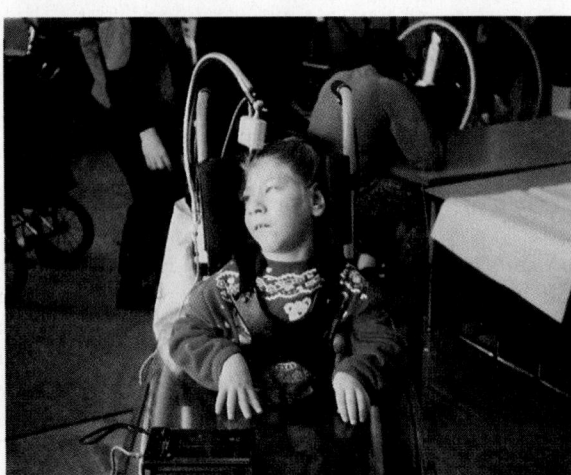

**Fig. 24-4** A child with cognitive and physical impairments can play a tape recorder by moving a device near her head.

---

**Box 24-4** ■ ■ ■
**Sample Task Analysis: Spoon Feeding**

1. Orients to the food by looking at it
2. Delivers the spoon to the bowl
3. Lowers it into the food
4. Scoops food onto the spoon
5. Lifts it
6. Delivers the spoon to the mouth
7. Opens the mouth
8. Inserts the spoon into the mouth
9. Moves the tongue and mouth to receive the food
10. Closes the lips
11. Swallows the food
12. Returns the spoon to the bowl

---

oped training program. Parents should also be given information about commercially available devices that can aid in achievement of independence (Fig. 24-4).*

*Feeding.* Self-feeding is recognized as the first major self-help skill that children learn. It involves the integration of fine and gross motor skills and visual perception. Most parents take for granted that they will be successful in teaching their children to feed themselves. Therefore the nurse and other team members must be especially sensitive to the needs of the parent, as well as the child, if assistance is offered.

Before beginning a self-feeding program, the nurse and parent should do a task analysis, breaking the process of feeding into its smallest components (Box 24-4). It is important to observe the child in an eating situation to determine whether any self-feeding skills have been mastered.

In addition to a task analysis, a number of other factors are assessed, such as the shape of the child's mouth and control of mouth, lip, and tongue movements (whether the

*A resource for a wide variety of equipment, including self-help devices, is Sammons/Preston, Inc, PO Box 5071, Bolingbrook, IL 60440, (800) 323-5547. In Canada: (800) 665-9200, fax: (800) 547-4333; www.sammonspreston.com.

**A**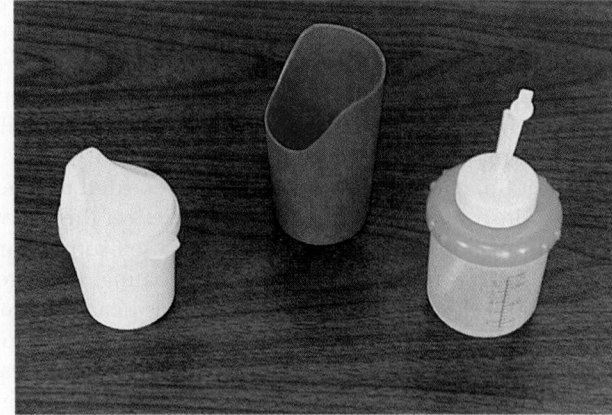

**B**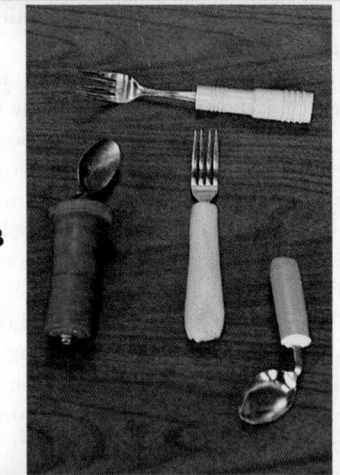

**C**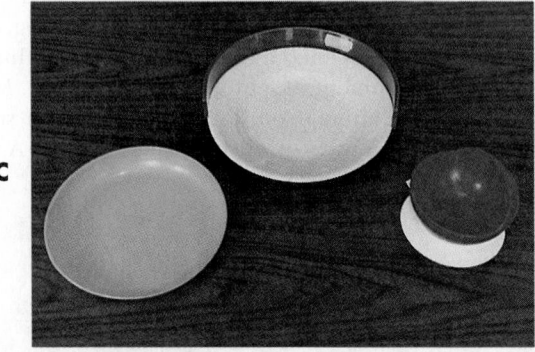

**Fig. 24-5** Self-help aids for feeding. **A,** Modified drinking cups. **B,** Modified utensils. **C,** Modified dishes.

---

tongue moves forward and backward or from side to side, whether there are rotary movements). The presence of teeth determines the textures and consistencies of foods that may be offered to the child. The child's developmental readiness for self-feeding, such as the ability to maintain head and trunk support and to sit without support, eye-hand coordination, the firmness of the grasp, and the ability to reach for an object, hold it, and release it, is examined. If the child has any physical impairments that interfere with holding or grasping the utensil, specially designed utensils can be substituted (Fig. 24-5) or homemade modifications can be used, such as building the handle up with a sponge or piece of wood or bending it to accommodate arm movement.

Further data are obtained from the parent by asking specifically about the family's approach to feeding. For example, who feeds the child regularly? Is the child fed when hungry or according to a prescribed schedule? What are the child's appetite patterns? Does the parent know when the child is full? What foods does the child like? How long does feeding take? A short feeding time, such as 10 minutes, might indicate that the child is being deprived of sensory experiences or appropriate interactions; a long time might indicate frustration and fatigue on the parent's part. Is the feeding environment described as quiet and nondistracting? What is the best time to begin teaching this new task? If the family is going on vacation, if someone is visiting, or if there has been a major stress in the family, this may not be the ideal time to begin a teaching program.

Preparation for the feeding activity is also considered, such as proper placement of the child at the table and protection of the area against spills. The principle of normalization is employed to make feeding fit in with family life. (See Chapter 22.) For example, the child is fed in the kitchen, at the table, or in a high chair in a sitting position, and with other family members whenever possible. Food should be offered in separate servings, not pureed or mixed together; be served at the appropriate temperature; and be of sufficient variety and texture from each of the basic food groups.

Once the feeding program is begun, the nurse is in an important position to give parents supportive feedback. The parents' observational skills and their ability to share observations, keep records of the child's progress, and establish goals that are appropriate and realistic for both the child and the parents are acknowledged.

*Toileting.*   Independent toileting is another major self-help skill that can be taught using behavior-modification principles. It is usually started after self-feeding because this is the normal sequence of development. Plans for a toileting program begin by assessing the child's physical and psychologic readiness. (See Chapter 14.) Because of physical or developmental limitations, certain signals may not be possible. For example, children who cannot walk can be trained once they are able to sit with good balance, and children with poor speech may need to rely on hand gestures to signal their toileting needs.

Parents are interviewed regarding their readiness to pursue a toilet-training program that is characterized by a positive, consistent, individualized, nonpunitive, nonpressured style of teaching. It is important to explore with parents the time they have to invest in the program, the advantages they see, the inconveniences that toilet training may cause them, the reason they wish to start, and whether this is the best time for both the parents and the child to begin.

Any past attempts at toilet training the child are reviewed: When and why did the parents start training? What methods did they use? Did they experience feelings of frustration, indifference, or discomfort? How long did they attempt training, and what were their reasons for discontinuing training efforts? Were their efforts consistent? Looking back, how did they view the experience for themselves and the child? If the parents acknowledge using punishment in any form, including spanking, scolding, withholding privileges, using suppositories, withholding fluid, or getting the child up in the middle of the night, the nurse offers positive alternatives.

As part of the procedure for determining the readiness of both parents and child to become involved in a successful toilet-training program, parents are asked to keep detailed records for 7 days. They should be cautioned to discontinue record keeping if the child becomes ill or if fluid intake is changed. Record keeping includes the following events:

- Oral intake.
- Behavioral indicators (e.g., the child was noticeably quieter or louder, started fussing or tugging at clothes, pointed toward the bathroom, cried, or squirmed).
- Positive parenteral feedback related to toileting behaviors only, in the form of praise, concrete rewards, affection, or approval.
- Parental criticism in the form of scolding, threatening, or spanking if the child had wet or soiled the underclothes or did not tell them before eliminating.
- The child indicated the need to go to the toilet by either gestures or words.
- The child was noted to have dry underclothes.
- The child was noted to have wet underclothes.

If possible, a toilet-training program should begin after such records are completed, because they show how parents are responding to the child's behaviors and at what times the child is most likely to eliminate.

The goal of any toilet-training program is to help the child achieve small goals and experience comfort and success and to help the parents simultaneously experience feelings of adequacy, minimum tension, and success. Parents should understand that they will be capitalizing on the times the child is most likely to eliminate and that they should respond immediately to any cues indicating this need.

A task analysis of toileting includes the same discrete steps as outlined for feeding (see Box 24-4). A positive and relaxed attitude toward toilet training is important and differs little from the approach used with other children. (See Chapter 14.)

*Dressing.*   Although dressing skills develop without special training in most children, special training is necessary to promote this skill in children with cognitive impairment. Factors that interfere with spontaneous learning include immature motor skills, lack of motivation, physical impairments, and lack of opportunity.

The level of independence in dressing varies according to the degree of retardation. Children with mild to moderate retardation and no accompanying physical limitations can become independent in all dressing skills, except for more complex tasks such as color coordination. Those who are severely retarded can achieve most dressing skills, except the ability to fasten complicated closures such as buttons or ties. Those who are profoundly retarded are usually able to assist in undressing and dressing but achieve no independent skills.

Children are considered mentally ready for dressing training if they can sit quietly for 3 to 5 minutes while working on a task, can watch what they are doing while working on a task, can follow physical gestures or cues, can follow verbal commands, and can relate clothing with the appropriate body part, such as socks with feet. As with other self-help skills, the child may not be able to master every task but should be evaluated for evidence of willingness to participate at his or her level of readiness. The use of teaching devices, such as dolls with mock closures, and reinforcement for success in managing the fasteners can increase the child's manipulative skills, which may be transferred to ready-to-wear clothing.

Choice of clothing is an important aspect of the training program. Clothes should be clean, up-to-date, and well fitting. They should be easy to put on and take off, easy to fasten, comfortable and nonrestricting, capable of disguising a physical disability, and easy to maintain. Suggested clothing includes undershirts with large neck openings; bras that have front fasteners; slip-on polo shirts with large armholes and wide neck openings (not tight turtleneck sweaters); front-buttoning shirts or dresses; pants with elastic waistbands or large, side hook fasteners; wool or cotton ankle socks (not tight nylon knee socks); slip-on shoes; and apparel or shoes with self-adhering (Velcro) closures.

*Grooming.*   Self-grooming is usually learned along with other independent skills, such as washing hands during toilet training. As with self-dressing, a major factor in learning independent grooming is the opportunity to practice the skills.

Special mention must be made of dental hygiene. An odor-free mouth and clean teeth are essential in promoting a positive image. In addition, healthy teeth are necessary for proper chewing and speech. Missing teeth interfere with proper tongue positioning for clear speech. Most dental problems are preventable with the dental hygiene practices discussed in Chapter 14.

If the child has physical impairments that limit the ability to brush, special devices may be necessary, such as a larger handle or a curved toothbrush, to reach all surfaces of the teeth. Any strategies that help motivate the child to brush are used. For example, the parent can place a special calendar on the wall and mark each date with stars to represent the number of brushings per day. At the end of a specified number of stars, the child can receive a special reward.

The child should be routinely taken to a dentist. It is important to prepare the child for such visits, since it is much more difficult to change an unsatisfactory experience than to prevent one. The nurse can assist families by locating dentists who are familiar with treating children with cognitive impairment and discussing with parents procedures for preparing their child.

**Help Families Adjust to Future Care.**   Not all families are able to cope with home care of children who are mentally retarded, especially those who are severely or profoundly retarded or have multiple disabilities. Older parents may not be able to continue with care responsibilities once they reach retirement or old age. The decision regarding residential placement is difficult for families, and the availability of such facilities varies widely. The nurse's role includes assisting parents in investigating and evaluating programs and helping parents in adjusting to the decision for placement. Guidelines for assessing out-of-home care facilities are listed in the Guidelines box. (See Community Focus box and Critical Thinking Exercise box.)

**Care for the Child During Hospitalization.**   Caring for the child during hospitalization can be a special challenge. Frequently nurses are unfamiliar with children who are cognitively impaired, and they may cope with their feelings of insecurity and fear by ignoring or isolating the child. Not only is this approach nonsupportive, it may also be destructive to the child's sense of self-esteem and optimum development and may impair the parents' ability to cope with the stress of the experience. To prevent use of this nontherapeutic approach, nurses can use the mutual participation model in planning the child's care. Parents are encouraged to stay with their child and assist with care, but they should not be made to feel as if the responsibility is totally theirs. Ideally the family should make a visit to the hospital before admission. A visit minimizes the unfamiliarity of the hospital setting and is an opportunity for staff members to allay

## GUIDELINES
### Assessing Out-of-Home Care Facilities

Assess the environment for adequacy of stimuli for the residents.

Determine the appropriateness of amounts of stimuli in the environment.

Observe care provider–to–resident ratios.

Observe care personnel interacting with residents in a variety of teaching and learning experiences.

Determine the appropriateness of the setting for the person being considered for placement.

Observe the quality of physical care administered.

See if the residents are attended to regularly and consistently, instead of when inappropriate behaviors occur.

Determine if activities are age-appropriate for the residents.

Determine the existence of structured and nonstructured activities.

Determine if individual plans of care are available and implemented.

Determine the functional levels of those who reside in settings (e.g., are they ambulatory and is speech encouraged?).

Determine if speech, physical, and occupational therapies are available.

Determine if each person is perceived as unique and distinct and if care is given to residents according to their needs.

Determine if and to what degree official standards of care are met.

Meet with parents of those who reside in special settings to hear their comments, both positive and negative.

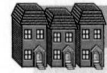

## COMMUNITY FOCUS
### Long-Term Care

Long-term care for a dependent with cognitive impairment is a concern for many parents, particularly those who are aging. Some parents have concerns about quality of care in institutions and group homes. Changes in the health care system, human service systems, and the disability field may leave parents wondering what the future holds. Many organizations recommend that parents write a detailed plan, outlining their preferences in each area of their child's life, to be followed after the parents die. Parents may also be interested in building a network of relationships to provide ongoing support to the child with cognitive impairment. This process is described in *Laying Community Foundations for Your Child with a Disability* by L.J. Stengle (1996, Woodbine House).

any fears the parents or child may have. When the child is admitted, a detailed history is taken, especially in terms of all self-care abilities. (See Chapter 26.) During the interview the child's developmental age is assessed.

Questions about the child's abilities are approached positively. For example, rather than asking, "Is your child toilet trained yet?" the nurse may state, "Tell me about your child's toileting habits." The assessment should also focus on any special devices the child uses, effective measures of limit-setting, unusual or favorite routines, and any behaviors that may require intervention. For example, if the parent states that the child engages in self-stimulatory or self-injurious activities, the nurse inquires about events that precipitate them and techniques the parents use to manage them. Once the child's functional level is known, he or she is encouraged to be as independent as possible in the hospital setting.

The nurse can help the child feel less lonely during the hospital stay by making certain that the child is provided with toys and other activities and has a roommate with approximately the same developmental age. The nurse should treat the child with dignity and respect in a manner that promotes acceptance and understanding of the child by children, parents, or others with whom the child comes into contact in the hospital.

Procedures are explained to the child using methods of communication that are at the appropriate cognitive level. Generally explanations should be simple, short, and concrete, emphasizing what the child will *physically* experience.

## Critical Thinking Exercise

### Future Planning

Mr. and Mrs. Tilden are the aging parents of Gina, an 18-year-old with moderate cognitive impairment. They are beginning to consider long-term planning for her care on their death. They ask you for advice. In your first conversation with them, which of the following would be the *least* appropriate question to ask them?

FIRST, THINK ABOUT IT . . .

• What is the purpose of your thinking?
• What precise question are you trying to answer?

1. Have you discussed this with Gina?
2. Does Gina have any siblings?
3. Have you considered institutionalization?
4. What options have you considered?

*Question three is the best response; it would be the least appropriate of these considerations in an initial discussion of long-term planning for someone with moderate cognitive impairment (see Table 24-1). Institutionalization would be inconsistent with promoting optimum development. The other questions would be better choices in an initial conversation. Gina's preferences about long-term plans should be taken into consideration, because her ultimate well-being is the precise question that you are trying to answer. Also, Gina certainly needs to be prepared for any transitions. Siblings are an important part of a family's network in long-term planning. Finally, it is essential to learn of the options being considered by the family before advice can be offered.*

Demonstration either through actual practice or with visual aids is preferable to verbal explanation. Parents are included in preprocedural teaching to aid in the child's learning and to help the nurse learn effective methods of communicating with the child.

During hospitalization the nurse should also focus on growth-promoting experiences for the child. For example, hospitalization may be an excellent opportunity to emphasize to parents abilities the child does have but has not had the opportunity to practice, such as self-dressing. It may also be an opportunity for social experiences with peers, group play, or new educational/recreational activities. For example, one child who had the habit of screaming and kicking demonstrated a definite decrease in these behaviors after learning to pound pegs and use a punching bag. Through social services the parents may become aware of specialized programs for the child. Nutritional counseling is available if the child is overweight or has evidence of specific deficiencies, such as iron deficiency. Hospitalization may also offer parents a respite from everyday care responsibilities and an opportunity to discuss their feelings with a concerned professional.

## Evaluation

The effectiveness of nursing interventions is determined by continual reassessment and evaluation of care based on the following observational guidelines:

1. Observe techniques used to teach child and child's success in learning; inquire if child is enrolled in early intervention program.
2. Interview family regarding provision of appropriate socialization, discipline, and play for child; observe child's ability to communicate with others; if possible, interview child regarding feelings of self-worth.
3. Observe those activities of daily living that child can completely or partially perform.
4. Interview family regarding any plans for future care and their awareness of community services.
5. Check patient record for evidence of nursing admission history, especially for self-help activities; observe parent's involvement in child's care; observe social interaction of child and family with other patients.
6. Investigate community programs aimed at preventing retardation and inquire as to nursing involvement in these efforts.

The *expected outcomes* are described in the Nursing Care Plan on p. 988.

## Down Syndrome

Down syndrome (DS) is the most common chromosome abnormality of a generalized syndrome, occurring in 1 in 800 to 1000 live births (Stoll and others, 1998). It occurs slightly more often in whites than in blacks, although the incidence is unchanged in various socioeconomic classes.

### Etiology

The cause of DS is not known. A number of theories, including genetic predisposition to nondisjunction, radiation before conception, immunologic problems, and infection, have been proposed, but none of the hypotheses has been substantiated. Recent reports in cytogenetic and epidemiologic studies support the concept of multiple causality.

# Nursing Care Plan
## The Child with Mental Retardation

---

**NURSING DIAGNOSIS:** Delayed growth and development related to impaired cognitive functioning

**PATIENT GOAL 1:** Will achieve optimum growth and development potential

- **NURSING INTERVENTIONS/RATIONALES**

Involve child and family in an early infant stimulation program *to help maximize child's development*

Assess child's developmental progress at regular intervals; keep detailed records to distinguish subtle changes in functioning *so that plan of care can be revised as needed*

Help family determine child's readiness to learn specific tasks, *because readiness may not be easily recognized*

Help family set realistic goals for child *to encourage successful attainment of goals and to support self-esteem*

Employ positive reinforcement for specific tasks or behaviors *because this improves motivation and learning*

Encourage learning of self-care skills as soon as child is ready

Reinforce self-care activities *to facilitate optimum development*

Encourage family to investigate special daycare programs and educational classes as soon as possible

Emphasize that child has same needs as other children (e.g., play, discipline, social interaction)

Before adolescence, counsel child and parents regarding physical maturation, sexual behavior, marriage, and child-rearing

Encourage optimum vocational training

- **EXPECTED OUTCOMES**

Child and family are actively involved in infant stimulation program

Family applies developmental concepts and continues activities in home care of child

Child performs activities of daily living at optimum capacity

Family investigates special educational programs

Appropriate limit-setting, recreation, and social opportunities are provided

Adolescent issues are explored as appropriate

**PATIENT GOAL 2:** Will achieve optimum socialization

- **NURSING INTERVENTIONS/RATIONALES**

Emphasize that child has same need for socialization as other children

Encourage family to teach child socially acceptable behavior (e.g., saying "hello" and "thank you," manners, appropriate touch)

Encourage grooming and age-appropriate dress *to encourage acceptance by others and self-esteem*

Recommend programs that provide peer relationships and experiences (e.g., mainstreaming, Boy Scouts, Girl Scouts, Special Olympics) *to promote optimum socialization*

Provide adolescent with practical sexual information and a well-defined, concrete code of conduct *because child's easy persuasion and lack of judgment may place child at risk*

- **EXPECTED OUTCOMES**

Child behaves in socially acceptable manner

Child has peer relationships and experiences

Child does not experience social isolation

---

**NURSING DIAGNOSIS:** Risk for interrupted family processes related to having a child with MR

**PATIENT (FAMILY) GOAL 1:** Will receive adequate information and support

- **NURSING INTERVENTIONS/RATIONALES**

Inform family at or as soon as possible after birth, *because family may suspect a problem and need immediate support*

Have both parents present at informing conference *to avoid problem of one parent having to relay complex information to the other parent and deal with the initial emotional reaction of the other*

Give family written information about the condition, when possible (e.g., a specific syndrome or disease), *for family to refer to later*

Discuss with family members pros and cons of home care and other placement options; allow them opportunities to investigate all residential alternatives before making a decision

Encourage family to meet other families having a child with a similar diagnosis *so that they can receive additional support*

Refrain from giving definitive answers about the degree of retardation; stress the potential learning abilities of each child, especially with early intervention, *to encourage hope*

Demonstrate acceptance of child through own behavior *because parents are sensitive to the affective attitude of the professional*

Emphasize normal characteristics of child *to help family see child as an individual with strengths, as well as weaknesses*

Encourage family members to express their feelings and concerns *because this is part of the adaptation process and effective collaboration*

- **EXPECTED OUTCOMES**

Family members' needs for information and support are met

Family expresses feelings and concerns regarding the birth of a child with MR and its implications

Family members make realistic decisions based on their needs and capabilities

Family members demonstrate acceptance of child

**PATIENT (FAMILY) GOAL 2:** Will be prepared for long-term care of child

- **NURSING INTERVENTIONS/RATIONALES**

As child grows older, discuss with parents alternatives to home care, especially as parents near retirement or old age, *so that appropriate long-term care can be provided*

Encourage family to consider respite care as needed *to facilitate family's ability to cope with child's long-term care*

Help family investigate residential settings, *because this may be needed for child's optimum care*

Encourage family to include affected member in planning and to continue meaningful relationships after placement

Refer to agencies that provide support and assistance

- **EXPECTED OUTCOMES**

Family identifies realistic goals for future care of child

Family avails themselves of supportive services as desired

See also Nursing Care Plan: The Child with Chronic Illness or Disability, Chapter 22

Although the etiology is unclear, the cytogenetics of the disorder are well established. Approximately 92% to 95% of all cases of DS are attributable to an extra chromosome 21 (group G), hence the name *trisomy 21.* Although children with trisomy 21 are born to parents of all ages, there is a statistically greater risk in older women, particularly those over 35 years of age (Table 24-2). For example, in women 30 years of age the incidence of Down syndrome is about 1 in 952 live births, but in women age 40 it is about 1 in 100. However, the majority (about 80%) of infants with Down syndrome are born to women under age 35. In about 5% of cases the extra chromosome is from the father (Hixon and others, 1998). Paternal age is a factor.

About 3% to 6% of the cases may be caused by *translocation of chromosome 21.* This type of genetic aberration is usually hereditary and is not associated with advanced parental age. From 1% to 3% of affected persons demonstrate *mosaicism,* which refers to cells with both normal and abnormal chromosomes. The degree of physical and cognitive impairment is related to the percentage of cells with the abnormal chromosome makeup. (For a discussion of the genetics involved in DS, see Chapter 5.)

Except for mosaicism, the mechanism by which the syndrome occurs has little effect on the characteristics displayed by the affected child and the management of the disorder. However, it is significant for purposes of genetic counseling. Whereas nondisjunction is usually a sporadic event associated with a low risk of recurrence (0.5% to 1%), a translocation is more often hereditary, with a recurrence risk of 10% to 15% if the mother is the carrier and 5% to 8% if the father is the carrier (Vessey, 1996). In DS caused by translocation, testing of the parents is necessary to identify the carrier and offer genetic counseling.

## Clinical Manifestations

DS can usually be diagnosed by the clinical manifestations alone, although no one physical feature is diagnostic (Box 24-5 and Fig. 24-6), and there is considerable varia-

**TABLE 24-2** Relation between maternal age and the estimated risk of Down syndrome*

| Age | Risk of Down Syndrome |
|-----|----------------------|
| 20 | 1/1667 |
| 25 | 1/1250 |
| 30 | 1/952 |
| 35 | 1/385 |
| 40 | 1/106 |
| 45 | 1/30 |
| 49 | 1/11 |

Modified from D'Alton ME, DeCherney AH: Prenatal diagnosis, *N Engl J Med* 328(2):114-120, 1993.
*Ages are at the expected time of delivery.

---

**Box 24-5** ■ ■ ■
## Clinical Manifestations of Down Syndrome

**HEAD**
*Separated sagittal suture
Brachycephaly
Skull rounded and small
Flat occiput
Enlarged anterior fontanel
Sparse hair (variable)

**FACE**
Flat profile

**EYES**
*Oblique palpebral fissures (upward, outward slant)
Inner epicanthal folds
Speckling of iris (Brushfield spots)
Short, sparse eyelashes
Blepharitis

**NOSE**
*Small
*Depressed nasal bridge (saddle nose)

**EARS**
Small
Short pinna (vertical ear length)
Overlapping upper helixes
Narrow canals

**MOUTH**
*High, arched, narrow palate
Small osseous orbit
Protruding tongue, may be fissured at lip and furrowed on the surface
Hypoplastic mandible
Downward curve (especially noted when crying)
Mouth kept open

**TEETH**
Delayed eruption
Alignment abnormalities common
Microdontia
Periodontal disease

**CHEST**
Shortened rib cage
12th rib anomalies
Pectus excavatum/carinatum

**NECK**
*Skin excess and lax
Short and broad

**ABDOMEN**
Protruding
Muscles lax and flabby
   Diastasis recti abdominis
   Umbilical hernia

**GENITALIA**
Small penis
Cryptorchidism
Bulbous vulva

**HANDS**
Broad, short
Stubby fingers
Incurved little finger (clinodactyly)
Transverse palmar crease
Characteristic dermal ridge patterns
   Distally located axial triradius
   Increased ulnar loops on fingers

**FEET**
*Wide space between big and second toes
*Plantar crease between big and second toes
Broad, stubby, short

**MUSCULOSKELETON**
*Hyperflexibility
*Muscle weakness
Hypotonia
Atlantoaxial instability

**SKIN**
Dry, cracked, and frequent fissuring
Cutis marmorata (mottling)

**OTHER**
Reduced birth weight

*Most common findings (Pueschel, 1999).

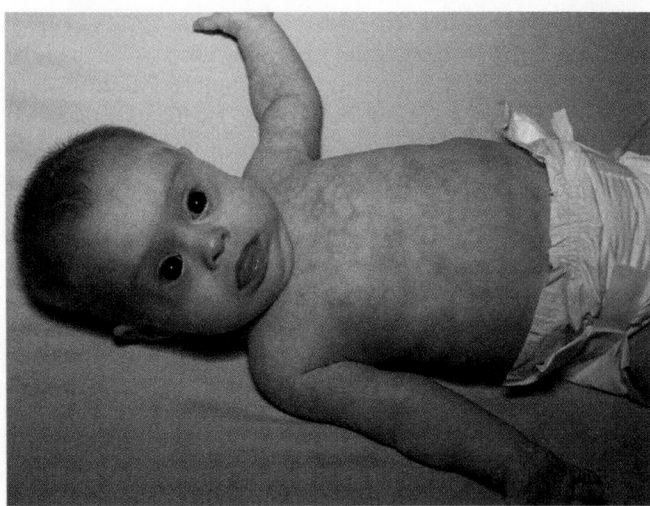

**Fig. 24-6** Down syndrome in infant. Note small square head with upward slant to eyes, flat nasal bridge, protruding tongue, mottled skin, and hypotonia.

tion in phenotypic expression. In addition, some infants may have characteristics of DS, such as epicanthal folds, a narrow palate, short broad hands, and a transpalmar crease, but may be cytologically normal. A chromosome analysis is therefore done to confirm the genetic abnormality. The following are other outstanding features of the syndrome:

Intelligence—Varies from severely retarded to low-average intelligence but is generally within the mild to moderate range of retardation and may be related to parental intelligence (Pueschel, 1999). Initial development may appear near normal. Although there can be considerable variation in abilities, relative strengths are often seen in visual over auditory processing, with relative weaknesses in grammar and expressive language and delays in motor development (Hodapp and others, 1996).

Social development—May be 2 to 3 years beyond the mental age, especially during early childhood. Temperamental characteristics show the same range as those found in unaffected peers. However, there is a relative strength in sociability (Kasari and Freeman, 2001) and a trend toward the easy-child pattern that may facilitate parent-child attachment and assist in integration with peers at school and in the community.

Congenital anomalies—About 40% to 45% have congenital heart disease (CHD), especially septal defects. Other structural defects include renal agenesis, duodenal atresia, Hirschsprung disease, and tracheoesophageal fistula. Skeletal defects include patella dislocation, hip subluxation, and atlantoaxial instability (instability of the first and second cervical vertebrae) in some children.

Sensory problems—Ocular problems include strabismus, nystagmus, astigmatism, myopia, hyperopia, head tilt, excessive tearing, and cataracts. Hearing loss occurs in a large percentage of children with DS. Conductive, mixed, or sensorineural losses each account for approximately one third of the diagnoses. Frequent otitis media, narrow canals, and impacted cerumen contribute to the problem (Kanamori and others, 2000).

Other physical disorders—These children have altered immune function, possibly as a result of early senescence (aging) (Cuadrado and Barrena, 1996), which contributes to numerous other conditions. Respiratory infections are very prevalent; when combined with cardiac anomalies, they are the chief cause of death, particularly during the first year. The incidence of leukemia is several times more frequent than expected in the general population, and in about half of the cases the type is acute megakaryoblastic leukemia. Thyroid dysfunction, including Graves disease, goiter, chronic lymphocytic thyroiditis, and hypothyroidism, is common. Acquired thyroid dysfunction also occurs frequently. Acquired cardiac disease, primarily valve dysfunction, has also been reported in adolescents (Geggel, O'Brien, and Feingold, 1993).

Growth—Growth in both height and weight is reduced, but weight gain is more rapid than growth in stature, often resulting in overweight by 36 months of age. Deficient growth is most marked during infancy and adolescence. Growth of children with moderate or severe CHD is more affected than growth of those with mild or no CHD.

Sexual development—May be delayed, incomplete, or both. Male genitalia, as well as secondary sex characteristics such as facial hair, may be underdeveloped. Breast development in females is mild to moderate. Menstruation usually occurs at the average age, and postpubertal women can be fertile; a small number have had offspring, the majority of whom were born with some type of abnormality. Men with DS are infertile.

## Therapeutic Management

Although there is no cure for DS, these children may require surgery to correct serious congenital anomalies, and they benefit from regular health care. Evaluation of sight and hearing is essential, and treatment of otitis media is required to prevent hearing problems, which can influence cognitive function. Neonatal and subsequent periodic testing of thyroid function is recommended, especially if growth is delayed. Special growth charts are available to monitor nutrition, height, weight, and general aspects of well-child care. Growth hormone therapy may be considered to increase height. Plastic surgery to alter phenotypic stigma is performed in some cases.

Fifteen to twenty percent of children with DS have *atlantoaxial instability*. Symptoms of the disorder include neck pain, weakness, and torticollis; however, most affected children are asymptomatic. Screening of children with DS for atlantoaxial instability after their second birthday and before they engage in physically active exercise or sports or undergo surgical or rehabilitative procedures has been recommended but is controversial (Taylor and Walter, 1996). If children are diagnosed with atlantoaxial instability, surgery may be required, and they should refrain from participating in activities that may involve stress on the head and neck. If children become symptomatic, they should receive prompt attention because they are at risk for spinal cord compression.

**NURSING ALERT** Report immediately any child with the following signs of spinal cord compression:
Persistent neck pain
Loss of established motor skills and bladder/bowel control
Changes in sensation

**Prognosis.** Life expectancy for those with Down syndrome has improved in recent years but remains lower than for the general population. Over 80% of individuals with DS survive to age 30 and beyond. As the prognosis continues to improve for these individuals, it will be important to provide for their long-term health care, social, and leisure needs.

## Nursing Considerations

**Support Family at Time of Diagnosis.** Because of the distinctive physical characteristics, the infant with DS is usually diagnosed at birth. Generally parents wish to know the diagnosis as soon as possible. Most parents prefer that both of them be present during the informing interview so that they can support each other emotionally.

Parental responses to the child may greatly influence decisions regarding future care. (See Cultural Awareness box.) Whereas some families willingly plan to take the child home, others consider foster care or adoption. Institutionalization is no longer an option. The nurse must carefully answer questions regarding developmental potential be-

cause the responses may influence the parents' decision. It is obvious from ranges such as those in Table 24-3 that potential for developmental achievement varies greatly. Therefore it would be inaccurate and unfair to predict the child's intellectual capacity at birth. It is important to stress that a decision regarding placement will affect all of the family members' lives and need not be made at the time of diagnosis. (See Critical Thinking Exercise box.) The nurse should emphasize every available source of assistance, such as parent groups, professional counseling, and literature, to help the family learn about Down syndrome and deal with childrearing problems.*

It may also be helpful for parents to know that studies of families who chose to rear the child at home report many favorable responses. Parental feelings toward the child usually are very positive; parents believe the experience of having this special child makes them stronger and more accepting of others. Behavioral problems among the siblings are similar to those found among families without children with DS.

**Assist Family in Preventing Physical Problems.** Many of the physical characteristics of DS present challenges. The hypotonicity of muscles and hyperextensibility of joints

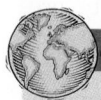

## CULTURAL AWARENESS
### *Importance of Cultural Factors in Coping*

The importance of cultural factors in parental coping with a child's disability cannot be overstated. Perceptions of illness/disability and its meaning are culturally influenced. Styles of interacting with health care professionals may have cultural determinants. Approaches to treatment and intervention, including the use of "alternative or adjunctive" therapies, may be influenced by cultural values and practices. Finally, coping styles are often influenced by cultural background. Awareness of these variables, appreciation of and respect for cultural diversity, and learning about the values and practices of different cultural groups can augment nursing practice in any setting.

---

*Sources of information include the **Association for Retarded Citizens of the United States,** 500 E Border St, Suite 300, Arlington, TX 76010, (800) 433-5255, fax: (817) 277-3491; www.thearc.org; **National Down Syndrome Society,** 666 Broadway, 8th floor, New York, NY 10012, (800) 221-4602, fax: (212) 979-2873, e-mail: info@ndss.org; www.ndss.org; **American Association on Mental Retardation,** 444 N Capitol St NW, Suite 846, Washington, DC 20001, (202) 387-1968 or (800) 424-3688, fax: (202) 387-2198; www.aamr.org; and the **National Down Syndrome Congress,** 1370 Center Dr, Suite 102, Atlanta, GA 30338, (770) 604-9500 or (800) 232-6372, fax (770) 604-9898; e-mail: NDSC center@aol.com, www.ndsccenter.org.

**TABLE 24-3** Developmental milestones and skills in children with Down syndrome

| Milestone | Average (months) | Range (months) |
|---|---|---|
| Smiling | 2 | 1½ to 3 |
| Rolling over | 6 | 2 to 12 |
| Sitting | 9 | 6. to 18 |
| Crawling | 11 | 7 to 21 |
| Creeping | 13 | 8 to 25 |
| Standing | 10 | 10 to 32 |
| Walking | 20 | 12 to 45 |
| Talking, words | 14 | 9 to 30 |
| Talking, sentences | 24 | 18 to 46 |
| Skill | | |
| Eating | | |
| Finger feeding | 12 | 8 to 28 |
| Using spoon/fork | 20 | 12 to 40 |
| Toilet training | | |
| Bladder | 48 | 20 to 95 |
| Bowel | 42 | 28 to 90 |
| Dressing | | |
| Undressing | 40 | 29 to 72 |
| Putting clothes on | 58 | 38 to 98 |

From Pueschel SM: The child with Down syndrome. In Levine MD, Carey WB, Crocker AC, editors: *Developmental-behavioral pediatrics,* ed 3, Philadelphia, 1999, WB Saunders.

### *Critical Thinking Exercise*

#### *Diagnosis of Down Syndrome*

The parents of Melissa, a newborn diagnosed as having Down syndrome, ask you, "What are we supposed to do with her?" They further state that they already have three other children at home. How should you respond?

FIRST, THINK ABOUT IT . . .
- Within what point of view are you thinking?
- What are you taking for granted, and what assumptions are you making?

1. Encourage the parents to consider placement arrangements.
2. Actively listen to the parents' concerns.
3. Refer the parents to their pediatrician.
4. Ask the social worker to see the parents.

---

*The best response is two. The general point of view is that the parents of a newborn with Down syndrome need time to process information given to them. The best choice for the nurse is not to take anything for granted and to listen. Then the nurse is able to guide them to appropriate resources, not simply give them suggestions that would affect their family's future. Options three and four are appropriate interventions but should not replace the nurse's role with the family.*

complicate positioning. The limp, flaccid extremities resemble the posture of a rag doll; as a result, holding the infant is difficult and cumbersome. Sometimes parents perceive this lack of molding to their bodies as evidence of inadequate parenting. The extended body position promotes heat loss because more surface area is exposed to the environment. Parents are encouraged to swaddle or wrap the infant tightly in a blanket before picking up the infant to provide security and warmth. The nurse also discusses with parents their feelings concerning attachment to the child, emphasizing that the child's lack of clinging or molding is a physical characteristic, not a sign of detachment or rejection.

Decreased muscle tone compromises respiratory expansion. In addition, the underdeveloped nasal bone causes a chronic problem of inadequate drainage of mucus. The constant stuffy nose forces the child to breathe by mouth, which dries the oropharyngeal membranes, increasing the susceptibility to upper respiratory tract and ear infections. Measures to lessen infection include clearing the nose with a bulb-type syringe,* rinsing the mouth with water after feedings, increasing fluid intake and using a cool-mist vaporizer to keep the mucous membranes moist and the nasal secretions liquefied, changing the child's position frequently, and practicing good handwashing technique. If antibiotics are ordered, the importance of completing the full

---

*Home care instructions for using a bulb syringe are available in Wong DL, Hess CS: *Wong and Whaley's clinical manual of pediatric nursing,* ed 5, St Louis, 2000, Mosby.

## Critical Thinking Exercise

### Down Syndrome in the Classroom

Johanna, an 8-year-old with Down syndrome, has been mainstreamed into a regular second grade class. Johanna's teacher thinks Johanna is a behavior problem because she frequently leaves her seat in the back of the room, comes to the front, and then sits quietly on the floor. As the school nurse, what do you think is a likely explanation for this behavior?

FIRST, THINK ABOUT IT . . .
• What concepts or ideas are central to your thinking?
• What conclusions are you reaching?

1. The class content is too advanced for Johanna, and she is bored.
2. Johanna is socially retarded, and she cannot be expected to behave like other children her age.
3. Johanna is having trouble hearing or seeing.
4. Johanna wants extra attention.

*The best response is three. A central concept is that children with Down syndrome frequently have vision and hearing problems. Johanna's behavior suggests that she cannot see or hear what is happening in the class. The other answers are incorrect because Johanna's movement about the classroom is not disruptive. The nurse should do hearing and vision screening on Johanna as soon as possible.*

---

course of therapy for successful eradication of the infection and prevention of growth of resistant organisms is stressed. Because hearing impairment is common and can interfere with development, the nurse should emphasize the importance of auditory testing.

Feeding difficulties may occur. The large, protruding tongue and hypotonia interfere with breast-feeding, bottle-feeding, and introduction of solid foods. Parents need to know that the tongue thrust does not indicate refusal to feed but is a physiologic response. Parents are advised to use a small but long, straight-handled spoon to push the food toward the back and side of the mouth. If food is thrust out, it should be refed. At times the family may require the assistance of a specially trained individual, such as a lactation expert or occupational therapist, to guide them in dealing with feeding problems.

Dietary intake needs supervision, especially of solid foods. Decreased muscle tone affects gastric motility, predisposing the child to constipation. Dietary measures such as increased fiber and fluid promote evacuation. The child's eating habits need careful monitoring to prevent obesity. Height and weight measurements should be obtained on a serial basis and plotted on specialized growth charts, especially during infancy, because excessive weight gain can impede motor development. The child receives calories in accordance with height and weight, not chronologic age.

During infancy the child's skin is pliable and soft. However, it gradually becomes rough and dry and is prone to cracking and infection. Skin care involves the use of minimum soap and application of lubricants. Lip balm should be applied to the lips, especially when the child is outdoors, to prevent excessive chapping.

**Promote Child's Developmental Progress.** Hypotonicity affects muscular development. Supporting skills, such as rolling over, sitting up, standing, or pulling oneself to a sitting or standing position, may be delayed. These children should be involved in an early stimulation program that provides physical therapy to help them learn motor skills.

At regular intervals the child's developmental progress is assessed and therapeutic adherence to a stimulation program is encouraged. Developmental screening tests are inadequate to evaluate indications of progress such as increased strength, balance, coordination, or muscle tone. Therefore detailed written records of the child's motor abilities can be kept to distinguish subtle changes in functioning. Periodic formal testing should also be conducted.

Parents can be encouraged to investigate appropriate daycare programs for the child as soon as possible. They should also investigate the public school system for special education classes, including early intervention programs and preschools. (See Critical Thinking Exercise box.) In essence, attention should be given to preventing the problems of overprotection and including family members, especially the father and siblings, in the caring role.

**Assist in Prenatal Diagnosis and Genetic Counseling.** Prenatal diagnosis of DS is possible through chorionic villus sampling and amniocentesis, because chromosome analysis of fetal cells can detect the presence of trisomy or translocation. There will be sporadic cases in young women who will not be identified when there is no indication for prenatal testing. However, testing for low maternal serum alpha-fetoprotein, high chorionic gonadotropin, and low unconjugated estriol levels may identify affected young women, who can then undergo amniocentesis (Yankowitz and others, 1998).

Prenatal testing and genetic counseling should be offered to women of advanced maternal age or those who have a family history of DS. Although many women will elect to have testing, some will not. If testing is conducted and the fetus is affected, the nurse must allow the parents to express their feelings concerning elective abortion and support their decision to terminate or proceed with the pregnancy. It is important for nurses to be aware of their own attitudes regarding testing and related decisions. (See Nursing Care Plan: The Child with Down Syndrome.*)

## Fragile X Syndrome

Fragile X syndrome is the most common inherited cause of MR and the second most common genetic cause of MR after DS. It has been described in all ethnic groups and races. The incidence of affected males is 1 in 1250; 1 in 2000 females are affected, and 1 in 259 females are carriers (Hagerman and Cronister, 1996). Because its identification as a disorder is relatively rare, many health care professionals and educators lack the necessary familiarity with the manifestations for appropriate referral and management once it is diagnosed.

The syndrome is caused by an abnormal gene on the lower end of the long arm of the X chromosome. Chromosome analysis may demonstrate a *fragile site* (a region that fails to condense during mitosis and is characterized by a nonstaining gap or narrowing) in the cells of affected males and females and in carrier females. Since 1991, however, direct DNA analysis for the gene mutation causing fragile X syndrome has greatly increased the accuracy of diagnostic testing of both affected and carrier individuals as well as permitted prenatal diagnosis. However, when mentally impaired individuals without an established family history of fragile X syndrome are being evaluated, cytogenetic and DNA studies should be performed to rule out another chromosome abnormality as the cause of the mental impairment (Murray and others, 1997).

This fragile site has been determined to be caused by a gene mutation that results in excessive repeats of nucleotide base pairs in a specific DNA segment of the X chromosome. The number of repeats in a normal individual is between 6 and 52. An individual with 50 to 200 base pair repeats is said to have a *premutation* and is therefore a carrier. When passed from a parent to a child, these base pair repeats can expand from 200 to 2000 or more, which is termed a *full mutation*. This expansion occurs only when a carrier mother passes the mutation to her offspring; it does not occur when a carrier father passes the mutation to his daughters. Males with a full mutation are usually affected (80%) (i.e., have the physical and behavioral features and mental impairment); however, only 30% of females with a full mutation

are affected. Interestingly, even females with a full mutation who do not appear to be affected, as well as carrier males and females with normal intelligence, may exhibit some learning disabilities and psychosocial disorders. This inheritance pattern has been termed *X-linked dominant with reduced penetrance.* It is in distinct contrast to the classic X-linked recessive pattern, wherein all carrier females are normal, all affected males have symptoms of the disorder, and no males are carriers. Consequently, genetic counseling of affected families is more complex than that for families with a classic X-linked disorder, such as hemophilia. Prenatal diagnosis of the fragile X gene mutation is possible with direct DNA testing in a family with an established history, using amniocentesis or chorionic villus sampling (Murray and others, 1997). Both affected sexes are fertile and capable of transmitting the disorder.

### Clinical Manifestations

The classic pattern of physical findings in adult males with fragile X syndrome consists of a long face with a prominent jaw (prognathism); large, protruding ears; and large testes (macro-orchidism). However, in prepubertal children (Fig. 24-7) these features may be less obvious, and behavioral manifestations may initially suggest the diagnosis (Box 24-6). Developmental delay and language delay are common. Rapid, perseverative speech with greater delays in acquisition of expressive than receptive language, have been reported (Roberts and others, 2001; Belser and

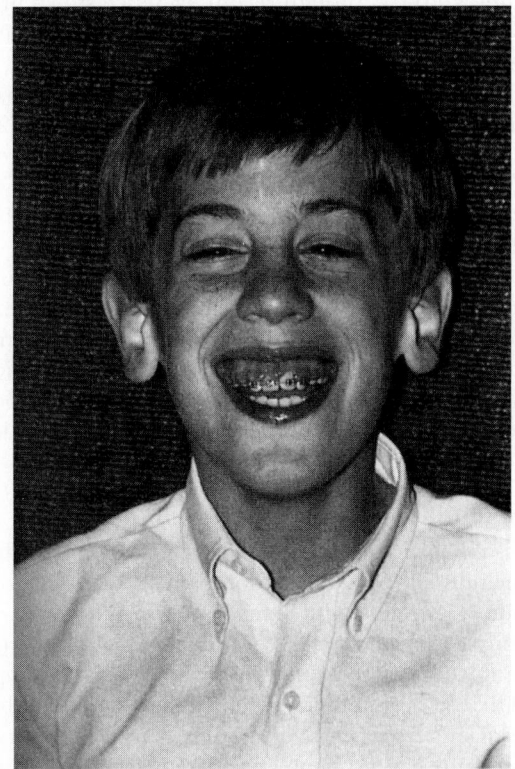

**Fig. 24-7** Prepubertal fragile X male. (From Silverman AC, Hagerman RJ: Fragile X syndrome. In Jackson PL, Vessey JA, editors: *Primary care of the child with a chronic condition,* ed 3, St Louis, 2000, Mosby.)

---

*In Wong DL, Hess CS: *Wong and Whaley's clinical manual of pediatric nursing,* ed 5, St Louis, 2000, Mosby.

---

### Box 24-6
### Clinical Manifestations of Fragile X Syndrome

**PHYSICAL FEATURES**

Long, wide, or protruding ears
Long, narrow face with prominent jaw
In postpubertal males, enlarged testicles
Long palpebral fissures
High, arched palate
Strabismus
Increased head circumference
Mitral valve prolapse/aortic root dilation
Hypotonia
Hyperextensible finger joints
Transpalmar crease
Pes planus (flat feet)

**BEHAVIORAL FEATURES**

Mild to severe MR (occasional normal IQ with learning disabilities)
Expressive language may be more delayed than receptive language; this pattern may increase with age
Speech delay; speech may be rapid, with stuttering and repetition of words
Short attention span, hyperactivity
Mouthing beyond expected age for behavior
Hypersensitivity to taste, sounds, touch
Intolerance to change in routine
Autistic-like behaviors; social anxiety; gaze aversion; sensitivity to sensory stimulation
May exhibit aggressive behavior

---

Sudhalter, 2001). Although recent evidence shows little association between autism and fragile X syndrome, autistic-like behavior (e.g., rocking, talking to self, spinning, hand flapping, hand biting, poor eye contact, echolalia) is seen in some affected individuals (Belser and Sudhalter, 2001). Some individuals also show social anxiety, whereas others have appropriate social skills and adaptive behavior, which means they may function or appear to function at a higher level than their IQ scores would predict.

In carrier females the clinical manifestations are extremely varied. Carrier and affected females may exhibit psychosocial deficits such as anxiety, withdrawal, and depression (Roberts and others, 2001). In fact, some evidence suggests that low-expressing fragile X may be associated with personality changes in the absence of cognitive deficits (Turk, 1995).

### Therapeutic Management

There is no cure for fragile X syndrome. Medical treatment may include the use of serotonin agents such as carbamazepine (Tegretol) or fluoxetine (Prozac) to control violent temper outbursts and central nervous system (CNS) stimulants to improve attention span and decrease hyperactivity. The use of folic acid, which affects the metabolism of CNS transmitters, is controversial. Medical treatment also addresses physical problems associated with the syndrome, which may include musculoskeletal concerns, mitral valve prolapse, recurrent otitis media, and seizures.

All affected children require early speech and language therapy, occupational therapy, and special education assis-

tance. Without appropriate intervention, a progressive decline in IQ can occur. Children with fragile X syndrome mimic the behavior of other children; therefore mainstreaming them with similar-age children may improve their behavior.

**Prognosis.** Individuals with fragile X syndrome are expected to live a normal life span. Their cognitive impairment may be ameliorated by behavioral and educational interventions, which should be begun in preschool.

### Nursing Considerations

Because cognitive impairment is a fairly consistent finding in individuals with fragile X syndrome, the care afforded to these families is the same as for any child with MR. Because the disorder is hereditary, genetic counseling is important to inform parents and siblings of the risks of transmission. In addition, any male or female with unexplained or nonspecific mental impairment should be referred for chromosome analysis and DNA testing, as well as appropriate genetic counseling. Families with a member affected by the disorder should be referred to the **National Fragile X Foundation.***

## SENSORY IMPAIRMENT
### Hearing Impairment

Hearing impairment is one of the most common disabilities in the United States. The incidence of infants who are born with permanent hearing loss is estimated to be 2 in 1000 (Appelbaum, 1999). For infants admitted to the neonatal intensive care unit, the incidence rises sharply to approximately 2 to 4 per 100 neonates (American Academy of Pediatrics, 1999). There are about 1 million children with hearing impairment ranging in age from birth to 21 years in the United States, and almost a third of these children have other disabilities, such as visual or cognitive deficits.

### Definition and Classification

*Hearing impairment* is a general term indicating disability that may range in severity from mild to profound and includes the subsets of deaf and hard-of-hearing. *Deaf* refers to a person whose hearing disability precludes successful processing of linguistic information through audition, with or without a hearing aid. *Hard-of-hearing* refers to a person who, generally with the use of a hearing aid, has residual hearing sufficient to enable successful processing of linguistic information through audition. Other terms, such as "deaf and dumb," "mute," or "deaf-mute," are unacceptable. Hearing-impaired persons are not "dumb" and, if mute, have no physical speech defect other than that caused by the inability to hear.

Hearing defects may be classified according to etiology, pathology, or symptom severity. Each is important in terms of treatment, possible prevention, and rehabilitation.

**Etiology.** Hearing loss may be caused by a number of prenatal and postnatal conditions. These include a family

---

*1441 York St, Suite 303, Denver, CO 80206, (303) 333-6155 or (800) 688-8765, fax: (303) 333-4369, e-mail: natlfx@aol.com.

**TABLE 24-4** Intensity of sounds expressed in decibels

| Decibels (dB) | Representative Sound |
|---|---|
| 0 | Softest sound normal ear can hear |
| 10 | Heartbeat, rustling of leaves |
| 20 | Whisper at 1.8 m (5 feet) |
| 30-45 | Normal conversation |
| 60 | Noise in average restaurant |
| 70-80 | Street noises |
| 80 | Loud radio in home |
| 90-100 | Train |
| 120 | Thunder, rock music |
| 140 | Jet airplane during departure |
| >140 | Pain threshold |

**TABLE 24-5** Classification of hearing loss based on symptom severity

| Hearing Level (dB) | Effect |
|---|---|
| Slight—16-25 (hard-of-hearing) | Has difficulty hearing faint or distant speech |
| | Usually is unaware of hearing difficulty |
| | Likely to achieve in school but may have problems |
| | No speech defects |
| Mild to Moderate—26-55 (hard-of-hearing) | Understands conversational speech at 3 to 5 feet but has difficulty if speech is faint or if not facing speaker |
| | May have speech difficulties |
| Moderately Severe—56-70 (hard-of-hearing) | Unable to understand conversational speech unless loud |
| | Considerable difficulty with group or classroom discussion |
| | Requires special speech training |
| Severe—71-90 (deaf) | May hear a loud voice if nearby |
| | May be able to identify loud environmental noises |
| | Can distinguish vowels but not most consonants |
| | Requires speech training |
| Profound—>91 (deaf) | May hear only loud sounds |
| | Requires extensive speech training |

history of childhood hearing impairment, anatomic malformations of the head or neck, low birth weight, severe perinatal asphyxia, perinatal infection (cytomegalovirus, rubella, herpes, syphilis, toxoplasmosis, and bacterial meningitis), maternal prenatal substance abuse, chronic ear infection, cerebral palsy, Down syndrome, or administration of ototoxic drugs (Billings and Kenna, 1999; Berrettini and others, 1999).

In addition, high-risk neonates who are surviving formerly fatal prenatal or perinatal conditions may be susceptible to hearing loss from the disorder or its treatment. For example, sensorineural hearing loss may be a result of continuous humming noises or high noise levels associated with incubators, oxygen hoods, or intensive care units, especially when combined with the use of potentially ototoxic antibiotics.

Environmental noise is a special concern. Sounds loud enough to damage sensitive hair cells of the inner ear can produce irreversible hearing loss. Very loud, brief noise, such as gunfire, can cause immediate, severe, and permanent loss of hearing. Longer exposure to less intense but still hazardous sounds can also produce hearing loss (LePage and Murray, 1998; Roizen, 1999). The exact sound level that produces hearing loss is unknown.

**Pathology.**   Disorders of hearing are divided according to location of the defect. *Conductive* or *middle-ear hearing loss* results from interference of transmission of sound to the middle ear. It is the most common of all types of hearing loss and most frequently is a result of recurrent serous otitis media. Conductive hearing impairment mainly involves interference with loudness of sound.

*Sensorineural hearing loss,* also called *perceptive* or *nerve deafness,* involves damage to the inner ear structures or the auditory nerve. The most common causes are congenital defects of inner ear structures or consequences of acquired conditions, such as kernicterus, infection, administration of ototoxic drugs, or exposure to excessive noise. Sensorineural hearing loss results in distortion of sound and problems in discrimination. Although the child hears some of everything going on around him or her, the sounds are distorted, severely affecting discrimination and comprehension.

*Mixed conductive-sensorineural hearing loss* results from interference with transmission of sound in the middle ear and along neural pathways. It frequently results from recurrent otitis media and its complications.

*Central auditory imperception* includes all hearing losses that do not demonstrate defects in the conductive or sensorineural structures. They are usually divided into organic or functional losses. In the *organic type* of central auditory imperception, the defect involves the reception of auditory stimuli along the central pathways and the expression of the message into meaningful communication. Examples are *aphasia,* the inability to express ideas in written or verbal form; *agnosia,* the inability to interpret sound correctly; and *dysacusis,* difficulty in processing details or in discriminating among sounds.

In the *functional type* of hearing loss there is no organic lesion to explain a central auditory loss. A functional hearing loss may be seen in a conversion disorder (an unconscious withdrawal from hearing to block remembrance of a traumatic event).

**Symptom Severity.**   Hearing impairment is expressed in terms of a *decibel (dB),* a unit of loudness (Table 24-4); it is measured at various frequencies, such as 500, 1000, and 2000 cycles per second, the critical listening speech range. Hearing impairment can be classified according to *hearing-threshold level* (the measurement of an individual's hearing threshold by means of an audiometer) and the degree of symptom severity as it affects speech (Table 24-5). These classifications offer only general guidelines regarding the effect of the impairment on any individual child, because children differ greatly in their ability to use residual hearing.

## Therapeutic Management

Treatment of hearing loss depends on the cause and type of hearing impairment. Many conductive hearing defects respond to medical or surgical treatment, such as antibiotic therapeutic management. When conductive loss is permanent, hearing can be improved with the use of a hearing aid to amplify sound.

Treatment for sensorineural hearing loss is much less satisfactory. Because the defect is not one of intensity of sound, hearing aids are of less value in this type of defect. The use of cochlear implants (a surgically implanted prosthetic device) provides a sensation of hearing for children with severe bilateral hearing loss or profound deafness (Slattery and Fayad, 1999). Children with sensorineural hearing loss have damage to the tiny hair cells lining the cochlea or to nerve cells that transmit auditory stimuli to the brain. Therefore hearing aids often provide little benefit because even amplified sounds cannot be processed as a result of damage to the inner ear. A cochlear implant bypasses the damage and directly stimulates undamaged auditory nerve fibers that transmit signals to the brain, where they can be perceived as sound. Technologic refinements have produced multichannel cochlear implants that stimulate the auditory nerve at multiple locations. This produces improved processing of different pitches represented in speech sounds so the individual can better understand and develop oral speech (Allen, Nikolopoulos, and O'Donoghue, 1998). Implantation of cochlear devices as early as possible in children with congenital or prelingual deafness appears to facilitate development of speech (Nikolopoulos, O'Donoghue, and Archbold, 1999; Cheng, Grant, and Niparko, 1999).

## Nursing Considerations

**Assess for Hearing Concerns.** Assessment of children for hearing impairment is a critical nursing responsibility. Identification of a hearing loss within the first 3 to 6 months of life is essential to facilitate language and educational development for children with hearing impairments (Yoshinago-Itano and others, 1998). Assessment involves (1) identifying those children who by virtue of their history are at risk (Box 24-7), (2) observing for behaviors that indicate a hearing loss, and (3) screening all children for auditory function. This discussion focuses on development/behavior associated with hearing impairment. There is controversy regarding who should be assessed and when they should be assessed. The American Academy of Pediatrics (1999) has issued guidelines on auditory screening of newborns and infants to standardize practice.

*Infancy.* At birth the nurse can observe the neonate's response to auditory stimuli as evidenced by the startle reflex, head turning, eye blinking, and cessation of body movement. The infant may vary in the intensity of the response, depending on the state of alertness. However, a consistent absence of a reaction should lead to suspicion of hearing loss. Other clinical manifestations of hearing impairment in the infant are summarized in Box 24-8.

*Childhood.* The child who is profoundly deaf is much more likely to be diagnosed during infancy than the child who is less severely affected. If the defect is not detected during early childhood, the likelihood is that it will surface during entry into school, when the child has difficulty in learning. Unfortunately, some children with hearing im-

---

**Box 24-7** ■ ■ ▫
**Risk Criteria for Sensorineural Hearing Impairment in Young Children**

**NEONATES (BIRTH TO 28 DAYS)**
1. Family history of congenital or delayed-onset childhood sensorineural impairment
2. Congenital infection known or suspected to be associated with sensorineural hearing impairment, such as toxoplasmosis, syphilis, rubella, cytomegalovirus, and herpes
3. Craniofacial anomalies, including morphologic abnormalities of the pinna and ear canal, absent philtrum, low hairline, etc.
4. Birth weight less than 1500 g (<3.3 pounds)
5. Hyperbilirubinemia at a level exceeding indication for exchange transfusion
6. Ototoxic medications including but not limited to the aminoglycosides used for more than 5 days (e.g., gentamicin, tobramycin, kanamycin, streptomycin), and loop diuretics used in combination with aminoglycosides
7. Bacterial meningitis
8. Severe depression at birth, which may include infants with Apgar scores of 0 to 3 at 5 minutes and those who fail to initiate spontaneous respiration by 10 minutes or those with hypotonia persisting to 2 hours of age
9. Prolonged mechanical ventilation for a duration equal to or greater than 10 days (e.g., persistent pulmonary hypertension)
10. Stigmata or other findings associated with a syndrome known to include sensorineural hearing loss (e.g., Waardenburg or Usher syndrome)
11. Maternal prenatal alcohol abuse

**RISK CRITERIA: INFANTS (29 DAYS TO 2 YEARS)**
1. Parent/caregiver concern regarding hearing, speech, language, and/or developmental delay
2. Bacterial meningitis
3. Neonatal risk factors that may be associated with progressive sensorineural hearing loss (e.g., cytomegalovirus, prolonged mechanical ventilation, and inherited disorders)
4. Head trauma, especially with either longitudinal or transverse fracture of the temporal bone
5. Stigmata or other findings associated with syndromes known to include sensorineural hearing loss (e.g., Waardenburg or Usher syndrome)
6. Ototoxic medications including but not limited to the aminoglycosides used for more than 5 days (e.g., gentamicin, tobramycin, kanamycin, streptomycin) and loop diuretics used in combination with aminoglycosides
7. Children with neurodegenerative disorders such as neurofibromatosis, myoclonic epilepsy, Werdnig-Hoffmann disease, Tay-Sachs disease, Niemann-Pick disease, any metachromatic leukodystrophy, or any infantile demyelinating neuropathy
8. Childhood infectious diseases known to be associated with sensorineural hearing loss (e.g., mumps, measles)

From American Speech-Language Hearing Association: Joint Committee on Infant Hearing 1990 position statement, *ASHA* 33 (suppl 5):3-6, 1991.

---

pairments are erroneously placed in special classes for students with learning disabilities or mental retardation. Therefore it is essential that the nurse suspect a hearing impairment in any child who demonstrates the behaviors listed in Box 24-8.

Of primary importance is the effect of hearing impairment on speech development. A child with a mild conductive hearing loss may speak fairly clearly but in a loud, mo-

## Box 24-8
## Clinical Manifestations of Hearing Impairment

### INFANTS

Lack of startle or blink reflex to a loud sound
Failure to be awakened by loud environmental noises
Failure to localize a source of sound by 6 months of age
Absence of babble or inflections in voice by age 7 months
General indifference to sound
Lack of response to the spoken word; failure to follow verbal directions
Response to loud noises as opposed to the voice

### CHILDREN

Use of gestures rather than verbalization to express desires, especially after age 15 months
Failure to develop intelligible speech by age 24 months
Monotone quality, unintelligible speech, lessened laughter
Vocal play, head banging, or foot stamping for vibratory sensation
Yelling or screeching to express pleasure, annoyance (tantrums), or need
Asking to have statements repeated or answering them incorrectly
Responding more to facial expression and gestures than to verbal explanation
Avoidance of social interaction; often puzzled and unhappy in such situations; prefer to play alone
Inquiring, sometimes confused facial expression
Suspicious alertness, sometimes interpreted as paranoia, alternating with cooperation
Frequently stubborn because of lack of comprehension
Irritable at not making themselves understood
Shy, timid, and withdrawn
Often appear "dreamy," "in a world of their own," or markedly inattentive

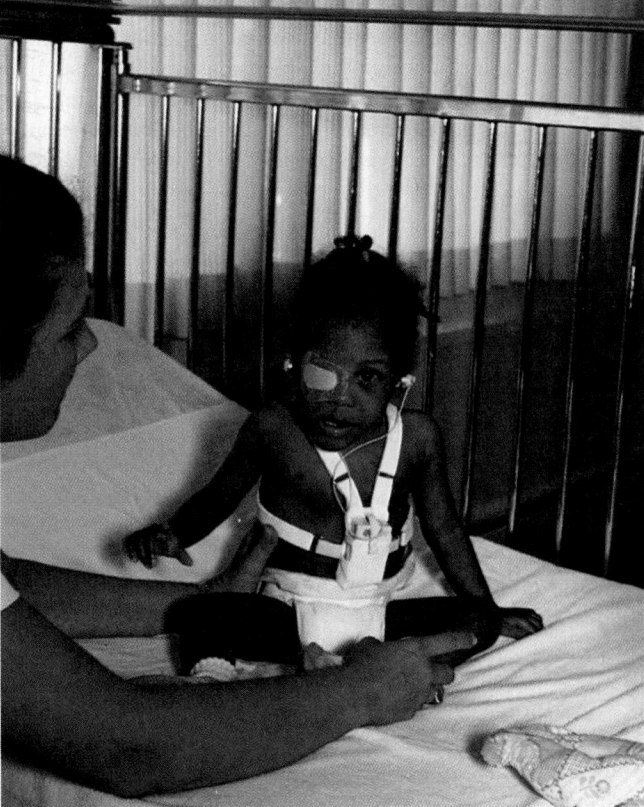

**Fig. 24-8** On-the-body hearing aids are convenient for young children, such as this child with severe bilateral hearing loss. Note eye patch for strabismus.

notone voice. A child with a sensorineural defect usually has difficulty in articulation. For example, inability to hear higher frequencies may result in the word "spoon" being pronounced "poon." Children with articulation problems need to have their hearing tested.

**NURSING ALERT** When parents express concern about their child's hearing and speech development, refer the child for a hearing evaluation. Absence of well-formed syllables ("da," "na," "yaya") by 11 months of age should result in immediate referral.

**Promote the Communication Process.**   The nurse's initial role in rehabilitation is to encourage the family to participate in an auditory training program.* Rehabilitation training provides assistance in learning appropriate methods for improv-

*Home training correspondence programs are sponsored by the **John T. Tracy Clinic,** 806 W Adams Blvd, Los Angeles, CA 90007, (800) 522-4582, TTY: (213) 747-2924; www.johntracyclinic.org. Other sources of information on several aspects of hearing loss and on the International Parents' Organization are the **Alexander Graham Bell Association for the Deaf,** 3417 Volta Place NW, Washington, DC 20007, (202) 337-5220, TTY: (202) 337-5221, fax: (202) 337-8314, e-mail: agbell2@aol.com; www.agbell.org; and the **Canadian Hearing Society,** 271 Spadina Rd, Toronto, Ontario M5R 2V3, (416) 964-9595, TTY: (416) 964-0023; www.chs.ca. Another resource for parents is the *Make a Joyful Noise* parent kit, (877) 672-5332, www.oraldeafed.org.

ing communication, such as use of hearing aids, lipreading, sign language, and speech and language therapy.

*Hearing aids.*   The nurse should be familiar with the types, basic care, and handling of hearing aids, especially when the child is hospitalized.* Types of aids include those worn in or behind the ear, models that are incorporated into an eyeglass frame, or types worn on the body with a wire connection to the ear (Fig. 24-8). One of the most common problems with a hearing aid is *acoustic feedback,* an annoying whistling sound usually caused by improper fit of the ear mold. Sometimes the whistling may be at a frequency that the child cannot hear but that is annoying to others. In this case, if children are old enough, they are told of the noise and asked to readjust the aid.

**NURSING TIP**   To reduce or eliminate whistling from a hearing aid, try removing and reinserting the aid, making certain that no hair is caught between the ear mold and canal, cleaning the ear mold or ear, or lowering the volume of the aid.

As children grow older, they may be self-conscious about the device. Every effort is made to make the aid inconspicu-

*Information about hearing aids is available from the **International Hearing Society,** 16880 Middlebelt Rd, Suite #4, Livonia, MI 48154, (800) 521-5247, fax: (734) 522-0200.

ous, such as an appropriate hairstyle to cover behind-the-ear or in-the-ear models, attractive frames for glasses, and placement of the on-the-body type where it is not seen, such as under a blouse or sweater. Children are given responsibility for the care of the device as soon as they are able, because fostering independence is a primary goal of rehabilitation.

> **NURSING ALERT**   Stress to parents the importance of storing batteries for hearing aids in a safe location out of reach of children and of teaching children (or supervising young children) not to remove the battery from the hearing aid. Battery ingestion requires immediate emergency management.

*Lipreading.*   Even though the child may become an expert at lipreading, only about 40% of the spoken word is understood, and less if the speaker has an accent, mustache, or beard. Exaggerating pronunciation or speaking in an altered rhythm further lessens comprehension. Parents can help the child understand the spoken word by using the suggestions in the Guidelines box. The child learns to supplement the spoken word with sensitivity to visual cues, primarily body language and facial expression (e.g., tightening the lips, muscle tension, and eye contact).

*Cued speech.*   This method of communication is an adjunct to straight lipreading. It uses hand signals to help the hearing-impaired child distinguish between words that look alike when formed by the lips (e.g., "mat," "bat"). It is most commonly used by hearing-impaired children who are using speech rather than those who are nonverbal.

*Sign language.*   Sign language, such as **American Sign Language (ASL),** or **British Sign Language (BSL),** is a visual-gestural language that uses hand signals that roughly correspond to specific words and concepts in the English language. Family members are encouraged to learn signing because using or watching hands requires much less concentration than lipreading or talking. Also, a symbol method enables some deaf children to learn more and to learn faster.

*Speech and language therapy.*   The most formidable task in the education of a child with profound hearing impairment is learning to speak. Speech is learned through a multisensory approach, using visual, tactile, kinesthetic, and auditory stimulation. Since the usual mechanism for learning language (imitation and reinforcement) is not available to the deaf child, systematic formal education is required. Parents are encouraged to participate fully in the learning process.

*Additional aids.*   Everyday activities present problems for older children with hearing impairment. For example, they may not be able to hear the telephone, doorbell, or alarm clock. Several commercial devices are available to help them adjust to these dilemmas. Flashing lights can be attached to a telephone or doorbell to signal its ringing. Trained hearing ear dogs can provide great assistance to deaf individuals because they alert the person to sounds, such as someone approaching, a moving car, a signal to wake up, or a child's cry. Special teletypewriters or **telecommunications devices for the deaf** (**TDD** or **TTY**) help deaf people communicate with each other over the telephone; the typed message is conveyed via the telephone lines and displayed on a small screen.*

Any audiovisual medium presents dilemmas for these children, who can see the picture but cannot hear the message. However, with **closed captioning,** a special decoding device is attached to the television, and the audio portion of a program is translated into subtitles that appear on the screen.

As children learn to compensate for their lack of hearing, they become extremely perceptive to visual and vibratory changes. They often know when another person wishes to talk to them because the person will walk close by but not pass. They learn to be alert to other people approaching them by seeing their shadows or feeling the vibrations of their footsteps. They are acutely aware of facial expressions and may comprehend the unspoken word more quickly than the spoken word.

*Socialization.*   Socialization is extremely important to the child's development. If children attend a special school for the deaf, they are able to socialize with peers in that setting. Classmates become a potential source of close friendships because they communicate more easily among themselves. Parents are encouraged to promote these relationships whenever possible.

Children with a hearing impairment may need special help in school or social activities. For those children wearing hearing aids, background noise should be kept to a minimum. Because many of these children are able to attend regular classes, the teacher may need assistance in adapting methods of teaching for the child's benefit. The school nurse is often in an optimum position to emphasize methods of facilitated communication, such as lipreading. (See Guidelines box.) Because group projects and audiovisual teaching aids may hinder the deaf child's learning, the use of these educational methods should be carefully evaluated.

---

## GUIDELINES
### Facilitating Lipreading

Attract child's attention before speaking; use light touch to signal speaker's presence.
Stand close to child.
Face child directly or move to a 45-degree angle.
Stand still; do not walk back and forth or turn away to point or look elsewhere.
Establish eye contact and show interest.
Speak at eye level and with good lighting on speaker's face.
Be certain nothing interferes with speech patterns, such as chewing food or gum.
Speak clearly and at a slow and even rate.
Use facial expression to assist in conveying messages.
Keep sentences short.
Rephrase message if child does not understand the words.

---

*Directory listings stating "TDD or TTY only" before a phone number indicate that regular telephone use is not possible; "TDD or TTY and voice" indicates that both TDD/TTY users and speaking/hearing people can use the telephone number. Additional information is available from the **National Captioning Institute, Inc,** 1900 Gallows Rd, Suite 3000, Vienna, VA 22182, (703) 917-7600; fax: (703) 917-9878; www.ncicap.org.

In a group setting, it is helpful for the other members to sit in a semicircle in front of the child. Because one of the difficulties in following a group discussion is that the deaf child is unaware of who will speak next, someone should point out each speaker. Speakers can also be given numbers, or their names can be written down as each person talks. If one person writes down the main topic of the discussion, the child is able to follow lipreading more closely. Such suggestions can increase the child's ability to participate in sports, clubs such as Boy Scouts or Girl Scouts, and group projects.

**Support Child and Family.** Once the diagnosis of hearing impairment is made, parents may need extensive support to adjust to the shock of learning about their child's disability and an opportunity to realize the extent of the hearing loss. If the hearing loss occurs during childhood, the child also requires sensitive, supportive care during the long and often difficult adjustment to this sensory loss. Early rehabilitation is one of the best strategies for fostering adjustment. However, progress in learning communication may not always coincide with emotional adjustment. Depression or anger is common, and such feelings are a normal part of the grieving process. Parent support groups are often very helpful because other parents have dealt with the same issues and can offer practical advice and emotional support.* (See Chapter 22 for an extensive discussion of the emotional support of the child and family.)

**Care for Child During Hospitalization.** The needs of the hospitalized child with a hearing impairment are the same as those of any other child, but the disability presents special challenges to the nurse. (See Critical Thinking Exercise box.) For example, verbal explanations must be supplemented with tactile and visual aids, such as books or actual demonstration and practice. Children's understanding of the explanation needs to be constantly reassessed. If their verbal skills are poorly developed, they can answer questions through drawing, writing, or gesturing. For example, if the nurse is attempting to clarify where a spinal tap is done, the child is asked to point to where the procedure will be done on the body. Because deaf children often need more time to grasp the full meaning of an explanation, the nurse needs to be patient, allowing ample time for understanding.

When communicating with the child, the nurse should use the same principles as those outlined for facilitating lipreading. Ideally nurses without foreign accents should be assigned to the child. The child's hearing aid is checked to ensure that it is working properly. If it is necessary to awaken the child at night, the nurse should gently shake the child, or turn on the hearing aid before waking the child. The nurse should always makes sure that the child can see him or her before any procedures, even routine ones such as changing a diaper or regulating an infusion, are performed. It is important to remember that the child may not be aware of one's presence until alerted through visual or tactile cues.

Ideally parents are encouraged to room with the child. However, it must be conveyed to them that this is not to serve as a convenience to the nurse but as a benefit to the child. Although the parents' aid can be enlisted in familiarizing the child with the hospital and explaining procedures, the nurse also talks directly to the youngster, encouraging expression of feelings about the experience. If there is difficulty in understanding the child's speech, an effort is made to become familiar with his or her pronunciation of words. Parents often can be helpful by explaining the child's usual speech habits. Nonverbal communication devices that employ pictures or words that the child can point to are also available. Such boards can also be made by drawing pictures or writing the words of common needs on cardboard, such as *parent, food, water,* or *toilet*.

The nurse has a special role as child advocate with the deaf and is in a strategic position to alert other health care team members and other patients to the child's special needs regarding communication. For example, the nurse

## Critical Thinking Exercise

### Hearing Impairment

Five-year-old Jason has a severe congenital hearing impairment. You have been assigned to care for him in the outpatient surgery postanesthesia care unit (PACU), where he has just been admitted following a herniorrhaphy. As he emerges from anesthesia, he becomes more and more agitated. The most likely cause for his behavior is which of the following?

FIRST, THINK ABOUT IT . . .

- What precise question are you trying to answer?
- What would the consequences be if you put your thoughts into actions?

1. This is a normal reaction to anesthesia.
2. He is experiencing separation anxiety.
3. He is unable to communicate properly.
4. He is in pain.

*The best response is three. Precisely, the focus of the question is on the expected behaviors associated with the emergence from anesthesia. Because Jason became increasingly more agitated as he emerged from anesthesia, his behavior does not suggest the transitory confusion associated with the initial emergence from anesthesia. Rather, it suggests that as he became more aware of his surroundings and tried to communicate with the staff, Jason became increasingly frustrated. Reasons for this might include (a) not having his hearing aid in place; (b) having his arms restrained by intravenous lines, pulse oximetry monitors, and a blood pressure cuff, thus restricting his use of sign language; (c) being unable to read the nurse's lips from a prone position; or (d) not having a nurse who could understand his speech or know or recognize his attempts to use sign language. Although pain is a possibility and needs to be evaluated, regional blocks are typically given during the surgery to keep children comfortable until after they are discharged home. It is unlikely that Jason is having separation anxiety, because this usually is a consequence experienced in younger children.*

---

*The **Oral Deaf Education Film and Information Office** has a free resource kit designed for parents of newly identified deaf and hard-of-hearing infants or toddlers. The kit is available at (877) 672-5332 (voice), (877)-672-5889 (TTY), or www.oraldeafed.org.

should accompany other practitioners on visits to the child's room to ensure that they speak to the child and that the child understands what is said. Not infrequently, caregivers forget that the child has the ability to perceive and learn despite a hearing loss, and consequently they communicate only with the parents. As a result, the child's needs and feelings remain unrecognized and unmet.

Because children with hearing impairment may have difficulty in forming social relationships with other children, the child is introduced to roommates and encouraged to engage in play activities. The hospital setting can provide growth-promoting opportunities for social relationships. With the assistance of a child-life specialist, the child can learn new recreational activities, experiment with group games, and engage in therapeutic play. The use of puppets, dollhouses, role-playing with dress-up clothes, building with a hammer and nails, finger painting, playing with syringes, and water play can help the child express feelings that previously were suppressed.

**Assist in Measures to Prevent Hearing Impairment.**  A primary nursing role is prevention of hearing loss. Because the most common cause of impaired hearing is chronic otitis media, it is essential that appropriate measures be instituted to treat existing infections and prevent recurrences. (See Chapter 32.) Children with a history of ear or respiratory infections or any other condition known to increase the risk of hearing impairment should receive periodic auditory testing.

To prevent the causes of hearing loss that begin prenatally and perinatally, pregnant women need counseling regarding the necessity of early prenatal care, including genetic counseling for known familial disorders; avoidance of all ototoxic drugs, especially during the first trimester; tests to rule out syphilis, rubella, or blood incompatibility; medical management of maternal diabetes; strict control of alcoholism; and adequate dietary intake. The necessity of routine immunization during childhood to eliminate the possibility of acquired sensorineural loss from rubella, mumps, or measles (encephalitis) is stressed.

Exposure to excessive noise pollution is a well-established cause of sensorineural hearing loss. The nurse should routinely assess the possibility of environmental noise pollution and advise children and parents of the potential danger. When individuals engage in activities associated with high-intensity noise, such as flying model airplanes, target shooting, or snowmobiling, they should wear ear protection such as earmuffs or earplugs (not ordinary dry cotton). However, any protection is better than none. Even common household equipment, such as lawn mowers and power vacuum cleaners, can be harmful. (See Nursing Care Plan: The Child with Hearing Impairment.*)

**NURSING ALERT**  Suspect hazardous noise if the listener experiences (1) difficulty in communication while hearing the sound, (2) ringing in the ears (tinnitus) after exposure to the sound, or (3) muffled hearing after leaving the sound.

*In Wong DL, Hess CS: *Wong and Whaley's clinical manual of pediatric nursing,* ed 5, St Louis, 2000, Mosby.

## Visual Impairment

Visual impairment is a common problem during childhood. In North America the prevalence of blindness and serious visual impairment in the pediatric population is estimated to be between 30 and 64 children per 100,000 population. Another 100 children per 100,000 have less serious impairment (Davidson, 1999). The nurse's role is one of assessment, prevention, referral, and sometimes rehabilitation.

### Definition and Classification

*Legal blindness* is defined as visual acuity of 20/200 or less or a visual field of 20 degrees or less in the better eye. *Partially sighted* (also termed *school vision*) is defined as visual acuity better than 20/200 but worse than 20/70 in the better eye with correction. These children can generally use normal-sized print because near vision is nearly always better than distance vision. *Visual impairment* is a general term that includes both of these categories. Children who are visually impaired, including those who are legally blind, often have considerable useful vision and are able to use printed material, such as large-print books, as their major method of learning. It is important to keep in mind that legal blindness is not a medical diagnosis but used as a legal definition. As such, educational and governmental agencies in the United States use the legal definition of blindness to determine eligibility for services in regard to taxes, entrance into special schools, eligibility for aid, and other benefits.

### Etiology

Visual impairment can be caused by a number of genetic and prenatal or postnatal conditions. These include perinatal infections (herpes, chlamydial infection, gonorrhea, rubella, syphilis, or toxoplasmosis), retinopathy of prematurity, trauma, postnatal infections (meningitis), and disorders such as sickle cell disease, juvenile rheumatoid arthritis, Tay-Sachs disease, albinism, and retinoblastoma. In many instances, such as with refractive errors, the cause of the defect is unknown.

Refractive errors are the most common types of visual disorders in children. The term *refraction* means bending and refers to the bending of light rays as they pass through the lens of the eye. Normally light rays enter the lens and fall directly on the retina. However, in refractive disorders the light rays either fall in front of the retina (*myopia*) or beyond it (*hyperopia*). Other eye problems, such as strabismus, may or may not include refractive errors, but they are very important because, if untreated, they result in blindness from amblyopia. These along with other, less frequent visual disorders are summarized in Box 24-9. In addition to these disorders, other visual problems can be a result of infection or trauma.

**Trauma.**  Trauma is a common cause of blindness in children. Injuries to the eyeball and adnexa (supporting or accessory structures, such as eyelids, conjunctiva, and lacrimal glands) can be classified as penetrating or nonpenetrating. *Penetrating wounds* are most often the result of sharp instruments, such as sticks, knives, or scissors; propulsive objects, such as firecrackers, guns, bows and arrows, or slingshots; or a powerful contusion by a blunt object, which

## Box 24-9
## Types of Visual Impairment

### REFRACTIVE ERRORS

### Myopia

*Nearsightedness*—Ability to see objects clearly at close range but not at a distance

*Pathophysiology*

Results from eyeball that is elongated, causing image to fall in front of retina

*Clinical manifestations*

Rubs eyes excessively
Tilts head or thrusts head forward
Has difficulty in reading or other close work
Holds books close to eyes
Writes or colors with head close to table
Clumsy; walks into objects
Blinks more than usual or is irritable when doing close work
Is unable to see objects clearly
Does poorly in school, especially in subjects that require demonstration, such as arithmetic
Dizziness
Headache
Nausea following close work

*Treatment*

Corrected with biconcave lenses that focus rays on retina

### Hyperopia

*Farsightedness*—Ability to see objects at a distance

*Pathophysiology*

Results from eyeball that is too short, causing image to focus beyond retina

*Clinical manifestations*

Because of accommodative ability, child can usually see objects at all ranges
Most children normally hyperopic until about 7 years of age

*Treatment*

If correction is required, use convex lenses to focus rays on retina

### Astigmatism

Unequal curvatures in refractive apparatus

*Pathophysiology*

Results from unequal curvatures in cornea or lens that cause light rays to bend in different directions

*Clinical manifestations*

Depends on severity of refractive error in each eye
May have clinical manifestations of myopia

*Treatment*

Corrected with special lenses that compensate for refractive errors

### Anisometropia

Different refractive strength in each eye

*Pathophysiology*

May develop amblyopia as weaker eye is used less

*Clinical manifestations*

Depends on severity of refractive error in each eye
May have clinical manifestations of myopia

*Treatment*

Treated with corrective lenses, preferably contact lenses, to improve vision in each eye so they work as a unit

### AMBLYOPIA

*Lazy eye*—Reduced visual acuity in one eye

*Pathophysiology*

Results when one eye does not receive sufficient stimulation
Each retina receives different images, resulting in diplopia (double vision)
Brain accommodates by suppressing less intensive image
Visual cortex eventually does not respond to visual stimulation, with loss of vision in that eye

*Clinical manifestations*

Poor vision in affected eye

*Treatment*

Preventable if treatment of primary visual defect, such as anisometropia or strabismus, begins before 6 years of age

### STRABISMUS

*"Squint" or cross-eye*—Malalignment of eyes
  *Esotropia*—Inward deviation of eye
  *Exotropia*—Outward deviation of eye

*Pathophysiology*

May result from muscle imbalance or paralysis, poor vision, or congenital defect
Since visual axes are not parallel, brain receives two images, and amblyopia can result

*Clinical manifestations*

Squints eyelids together or frowns
Has difficulty in focusing from one distance to another
Inaccurate judgment in picking up objects
Unable to see print or moving objects clearly
Closes one eye to see
Tilts head to one side
If combined with refractive errors, may see any of the manifestations listed for refractive errors
Diplopia
Photophobia
Dizziness
Headache
Cross-eye

*Treatment*

Treatment depends on cause of strabismus
May involve occlusion therapy (patching stronger eye) or surgery to increase visual stimulation to weaker eye
Early diagnosis is essential to prevent vision loss

### CATARACTS

Opacity of crystalline lens

*Pathophysiology*

Prevents light rays from entering eye and refracting on retina

*Clinical manifestations*

Gradually less able to see objects clearly
May lose peripheral vision
Nystagmus (with complete blindness)
Gray opacities of lens
Strabismus
Absence of red reflex

*Treatment*

Requires surgery to remove cloudy lens and replace lens (intraocular lens implant, removable contact lens, prescription glasses)
Must be treated early to prevent blindness from amblyopia

*Continued*

**Box 24-9**
## Types of Visual Impairment—cont'd

### GLAUCOMA
Increased intraocular pressure

*Pathophysiology*
Congenital type results from defective development of some component related to flow of aqueous humor
Increased pressure on optic nerve causes eventual atrophy and blindness

*Clinical manifestations*
Mostly seen in acquired types—loses peripheral vision
May bump into objects not directly in front
Sees halos around objects

May complain of mild pain or discomfort (severe pain, nausea, vomiting, if sudden rise in pressure)
Redness
Excessive tearing (epiphora)
Photophobia
Spasmodic winking (blepharospasm)
Corneal haziness
Enlargement of eyeball (buphthalmos)

*Treatment*
Requires surgical treatment (goniotomy) to open outflow tracts
May require more than one procedure

---

may occur during a fight or from a serious car accident. *Nonpenetrating injuries* may be a result of foreign objects in the eyes, lacerations, a blow from a blunt object such as a ball (baseball, softball, basketball, and racquet sports) or fist, or thermal or chemical burns.

Treatment is aimed at preventing further ocular damage and is primarily the responsibility of the ophthalmologist. It involves adequate examination of the injured eye (with the child sedated or anesthetized in cases of severe injury); appropriate immediate intervention, such as removal of the foreign body or suturing of the laceration; and prevention of complications, such as administration of antibiotics or steroids and complete bed rest to allow the eye to heal and blood to reabsorb. (See Emergency Treatment box.) The prognosis varies according to the type of injury. It is usually guarded in all cases of penetrating wounds because of the high risk of serious complications.

**Infections.**  Infections of the adnexa and the structures of the eyeball or globe are not infrequent in children. The most common eye infection is conjunctivitis. (See Chapter 16.) Treatment is usually with ophthalmic antibiotics. Severe infections may require systemic antibiotic therapy. Steroids are used cautiously because they exacerbate viral infections such as herpes simplex, increasing the risk of damage to the involved structures.

## Nursing Considerations

Nursing care of visually impaired children is a specialized area requiring additional training in vision testing and habilitation. However, general goals that focus on assessment, prevention, and rehabilitation of the child with visual impairment are every nurse's responsibility. In addition, nurses may have to care for a visually impaired child who is hospitalized and must know how to best meet the child's and family's special needs.

**Assessment.**  Assessment of children for visual impairment is a critical nursing responsibility. Discovery of a visual impairment as early as possible is essential to prevent social, physical, and psychologic damage to the child. Assessment involves (1) identifying those children who by virtue of their history are at risk, (2) observing for behaviors that indicate

a vision loss, and (3) screening all children for visual acuity and signs of other ocular disorders, such as strabismus. Clinical manifestations of various types of visual problems are given in Box 24-9. Vision testing is discussed in Chapter 7.

*Infancy.*  At birth the nurse should observe the neonate's response to visual stimuli, such as following a light or object and cessation of body movement. The intensity of the response may vary, depending on the infant's state of alertness.

Of special importance in detecting visual impairment during infancy are parental concerns regarding visual responsiveness in their child. Their concerns, such as lack of eye contact from the infant, must be taken seriously. During infancy the child should be tested for strabismus. Lack of binocularity after 4 months of age is considered abnormal and must be treated to prevent amblyopia.

> **NURSING ALERT**
> Suspect blindness if the infant does not react to light and in a child of any age if parents express concern.

*Childhood.*  Since the most common visual impairment during childhood is refractive errors, testing for visual acuity is essential. The school nurse usually assumes major responsibility for vision screening in schoolchildren. Besides refractive errors, the nurse should be aware of signs and symptoms that indicate other ocular problems. If a referral is made to the family requesting further eye testing, the school nurse is responsible for follow-up concerning the recommendation.

**Support of Child and Family.**  The shock of learning that their child is blind or only partially sighted is an immense crisis for families. Of all types of disabilities, many people fear loss of sight the most. Vision is involved in almost every activity of daily living. Parents need support during the initial phase of learning about the diagnosis and help to gain a realistic understanding of their child's abilities. The family is encouraged to investigate appropriate early intervention and educational programs for their child as soon as possible. Sources of information include state **Commissions for the Blind;** local schools for the blind; and the **American Foundation for the Blind,*** **National Federation for the Blind,†** **National Association for Parents of the Visually Impaired, Inc.,‡** **National Association for the Visually Handicapped,§** and **American Council of the Blind.‖**

When blindness is not congenital but acquired, newly blind children need a great deal of support to help them adjust to the disability. They are usually frightened and confused by the sudden or progressive loss of sight and benefit from an environment that provides security and familiarity.

**Promotion of Parent-Child Attachment.**   A crucial time in the life of blind infants is when they and their parents are getting acquainted with each other. Pleasurable patterns of interaction between the infant and parents may be lacking if there is not enough reciprocity. For example, if the parent gazes fondly at the infant's face and seeks eye contact but the infant fails to respond because he or she cannot see the parent, a troubled cycle of responses may occur. The nurse can help parents learn to look for other cues that indicate the infant is responding to them, such as whether the eyelids blink; whether the activity level accelerates or slows; whether respiratory patterns change, such as faster or slower breathing when the parents come near; and whether the infant makes throaty sounds when they speak to the infant. In time parents learn that the infant has unique ways of relating to them. They are encouraged to show affection using nonvisual methods, such as talking or reading, cuddling, and walking the child.

**Promotion of Child's Optimum Development.**   Promoting the child's optimum development requires rehabilitation in a number of important areas. These include learning self-help skills and appropriate communication techniques to become independent. Although nurses may not be directly involved in such programs, they can provide direction and guidance to families regarding the availability of programs and the importance of promoting these activities in their child.

***Development and independence.***   Motor development depends on sight almost as much as verbal communication depends on hearing. From earliest infancy, parents are encouraged to expose the infant with any sight to as many visual-motor experiences as possible, such as sitting supported in an infant seat or swing and being given opportunities for holding up the head, sitting unsupported, reaching for objects, and crawling.

Despite visual impairment, a child can become independent in all aspects of self-care. The same principles used for

---

*11 Pennsylvania Plaza, Suite 300, New York, NY 10001, (212) 502-7600, (800) 232-5463, TTY: (212) 502-7662, fax: (212) 502-7777; www.afb.org.
†1800 Johnson St, Baltimore, MD 21230, (410) 659-9314, fax: (410) 685-5653; www.nfb.org.
‡PO Box 317, Watertown, MA 02471, (617) 972-7441 or (800) 562-6265, fax: (617) 972-7444; www.spedex.com/NAPVI.
§22 W 21st St, 6th Floor, New York, NY 10010, (212) 889-3141, fax: (212) 727-2931; www.navh.org.
‖1155 15th St NW, Suite 1004, Washington, DC 20005, (202) 467-5081 or (800) 424-8666, fax: (202) 467-5085, e-mail: info@acb.org; www.acb.org.
Sources of information in Canada include the **Canadian National Institute for the Blind,** 1931 Bayview Ave, Toronto, Ontario M4G 4C8; **Low Vision Association of Canada,** 145 Adelaide St W, Toronto, Ontario M5H 3H4; and **Blind Organization of Ontario,** 597 Parliament St, Suite B-3, Toronto, Ontario M4X 1W3.

---

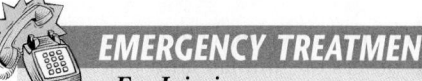

## EMERGENCY TREATMENT
### *Eye Injuries*

**FOREIGN OBJECT**

Examine eye for presence of a foreign body (evert upper lid to examine upper eye).
Remove a freely movable object with pointed corner of gauze pad lightly moistened with water.
Do not irrigate eye or attempt to remove a penetrating object (see below).
Caution child against rubbing eye.

**CHEMICAL BURNS**

Irrigate eye copiously with tap water for 20 minutes.
Evert upper lid to flush thoroughly.
Hold child's head with eye under tap of running lukewarm water.
Take to emergency room.
Have child rest with eyes closed.
Keep room darkened.

**ULTRAVIOLET BURNS**

If skin is burned, patch both eyes (make sure lids are completely closed); secure dressing with Kling bandages wrapped around head rather than tape.
Have child rest with eyes closed.
Refer to an ophthalmologist.

**HEMATOMA ("BLACK EYE")**

Use a flashlight to check for gross hyphema (hemorrhage into anterior chamber; visible fluid meniscus across iris; more easily seen in light-colored than in brown eyes).
Apply ice for first 24 hours to reduce swelling if no hyphema is present.
Refer to an ophthalmologist immediately if hyphema is present.
Have child rest with eyes closed.

**PENETRATING INJURIES**

Take child to emergency department.
Never remove an object that has penetrated eye.
Follow strict aseptic technique in examining eye.
Observe for:
  Aqueous or vitreous leaks (fluid leaking from point of penetration)
  Hyphema
  Shape and equality of pupils, reaction to light
  Prolapsed iris (not perfectly circular)
Apply a Fox shield if available (not a regular eye patch) and apply patch over unaffected eye to prevent bilateral movement.
Maintain bed rest with child in 30-degree Fowler position.
Caution child against rubbing eye.

---

promoting independence in sighted children apply, with additional emphasis given to nonvisual cues. For example, the child may need help in dressing, such as special arrangement of clothing for style coordination and braille tags to distinguish colors and prints.

The blind child also must learn to become independent in navigational skills. The two main techniques are the ***tapping method*** (use of a cane to survey the environment for direction and to avoid obstacles) and ***guides,*** such as a human sighted guide or a dog guide, such as a Seeing Eye dog. Partially sighted children may benefit from ocular aids, such as a monocular telescope.

***Play and socialization.***   Blind children do not learn to play automatically. Because they cannot imitate others or actively explore the environment as sighted children do, they depend much more on others to stimulate and teach them how to play. Parents need help in selecting appropriate play materials, especially those that encourage fine and gross motor development and stimulate the senses of hearing, touch, and smell. Toys with educational value are especially useful, such as dolls with various clothing closures.

Blind children have the same needs for socialization as sighted children. Because they have little difficulty in learning verbal skills, they are able to communicate with age-mates and participate in suitable activities. The nurse discusses with parents opportunities for socialization outside of the home, especially regular preschools. The trend is to include these children with sighted children to help them adjust to the outside world for eventual independence.

To compensate for inadequate stimulation, these children may develop *blindisms* (self-stimulatory activities, such as body rocking, finger flicking, or arm twirling). Such habits retard the child's social acceptance and are discouraged. Behavior modification is often successful in reducing or eliminating blindisms.

*Education.* The main obstacle to learning is the child's total dependence on nonvisual cues. Although the child can learn via verbal lecturing, he or she is unable to read the written word or to write without special education. Therefore the child must rely on *braille,* a system that uses raised dots to represent each letter and number. The child can then read the braille with the fingers and can write a message using a small typewriter-like device called a *braillewriter.* However, unless others read braille, this type of communication is not useful for communicating with others. A more portable system for written communication is the use of a *braille slate* and *stylus* or a microcassette tape recorder. A recorder is especially helpful for leaving messages for others and for taking notes during classroom lectures. For mathematic calculations, portable calculators with voice synthesizers are available.*

Records and tapes are significant sources of reading material other than braille books, which are large and cumbersome. The **Library of Congress**† has talking books, braille books, and a special records program, which are available at many local and state libraries and directly from the Library of Congress. The talking book machine and tape player are provided at no cost to families, and there is no postage fee for returning the materials. **Recording for the Blind and Dyslexic**‡ also provides texts and tapes of books, which are very helpful for secondary and college students who are blind.

Learning to use a regular typewriter is another form of writing but has the disadvantage of the blind person's being unable to check the accuracy of the typing. Computers eliminate this drawback; a home computer with a voice synthesizer can be adapted to speak each letter or word that has been typed.

The child with partial sight benefits from specialized visual aids, which produce a magnified retinal image. The basic devices are accommodation, such as bringing the object closer, special plus lenses, handheld and stand magnifiers, telescopes, video projection systems, and large print. Special equipment is available to enlarge print. Information about services for the partially sighted is available from the **National Association for the Visually Handicapped** and **American Foundation for the Blind.** Children with diminished vision often prefer to do close work without their glasses and compensate by bringing the object very near to their eyes. This should be allowed. The exception is the child with vision in only one eye, who should always wear glasses for protection. Information on job opportunities for the blind can be obtained from the **National Federation for the Blind.***

**Care for Child During Hospitalization.**   Because nurses are more likely to care for children who are hospitalized for procedures that involve temporary loss of vision than for children who are blind, the following discussion concentrates primarily on the needs of such children. The nursing care objectives in either situation are to (1) reassure the child and family throughout every phase of treatment, (2) orient the child to the surroundings, (3) provide a safe environment, and (4) encourage independence. Whenever possible, the same nurse should care for the child to ensure consistency in the approach. These same principles also apply to a blind child who requires hospitalization.

When sighted children temporarily lose their vision, almost every aspect of the environment becomes bewildering and frightening. They are forced to rely on nonvisual senses for help in adjusting to the blindness without the benefit of any special training. Nurses have a major role in minimizing the effects of temporary loss of vision. They need to talk to the child about everything that is occurring, emphasizing aspects of procedures that are felt or heard. They should approach the child by always identifying themselves as soon as they enter the room. Since unfamiliar sounds are especially frightening, these are explained. Parents are encouraged to room with their child and participate in the care. Familiar objects, such as a teddy bear or doll, should be brought from home to help lessen the strangeness of the hospital. As soon as the child is able to be out of bed, he or she is oriented to the immediate surroundings. If the child is able to see on admission, this opportunity is taken to point out significant aspects of the room. The child is encouraged to practice ambulating with the eyes closed to become accustomed to this experience.

The room is arranged with safety in mind. For example, a stool or chair is placed next to the bed to help the child climb in and out of bed. The furniture is always placed in the same position to prevent collisions. Cleaning personnel are reminded of the need to keep the room in order. If the child

*A catalog of numerous products for people with vision problems is available from **The Lighthouse, Inc,** (800) 829-0500; www.lighthouse.org.
†The National Library Service for the Blind and Physically Handicapped, Library of Congress, 1291 Taylor St NW, Washington, DC 20542, (202) 707-5100, (800) 424-8567, TTY: (202) 707-0744, fax: (202) 707-0712; www.loc.gov/nls. (A state-by-state listing of libraries for blind and physically handicapped readers, as well as other reference circulars, is available from this office.)
‡20 Roszel Rd, Princeton, NJ 08540, (609) 452-0606 or (800) 221-4792; www.rfbd.org.

*(800) 638-7518.

has difficulty navigating by feeling the walls, a rope can be attached from the bed to the point of destination, such as the bathroom. Attention to details such as well-fitting slippers or robes that do not hang on the floor is important in preventing tripping. Unlike the child who is blind, these children are not familiar with navigating with a cane.

The child is encouraged to be independent in self-care activities, especially if the visual loss may be prolonged or potentially permanent. For example, during bathing, the nurse sets up all the equipment and encourages the child to participate. At mealtime the nurse explains where each food item is on the tray, opens any special containers, and prepares cereal or toast, but encourages the child in self-feeding. Favorite finger foods, such as sandwiches, hamburgers, hot dogs, or pizza, may be good selections. The child is praised for efforts at being cooperative and independent. Any improvements made in self-care, no matter how small, are stressed.

Appropriate recreational activities are provided, and if a child-life specialist is available, such planning is done jointly. Since children with temporary blindness have a wide variety of play experiences to draw on, they are encouraged to select activities. For example, if they like to read, they may enjoy books on tape or having someone read to them. If they prefer manual activity, they may appreciate playing with clay or building blocks or feeling different textures and naming them. Simple board and card games can be played with a "seeing partner" or if the opponent helps with the game. They should have familiar toys from home to play with, because familiar items are more easily manipulated than new ones. If parents wish to bring presents, they should be objects that stimulate hearing and touch, such as a radio, music box, or stuffed animal.

Occasionally children who are blind come to the hospital for procedures to restore their vision. Although this is an extremely happy time, it also requires intervention to help them adjust to sight. They need an opportunity to take in all that they see. They should not be bombarded with visual stimuli. They may need to concentrate on people's faces or their own to become accustomed to this experience. They often need to talk about what they see and to compare the visual images with their mental ones. The child may also go through a period of depression, which must be respected and supported. The child should be encouraged to discuss how it feels to see, especially in terms of seeing himself or herself.

Newly sighted children also need time to adjust to the ability to engage in activities that were impossible before. For example, they may prefer to use braille to read, rather than learning a new "visual approach," because of familiarity with the touch system. Eventually, as they learn to recognize letters and numbers, they will integrate these new skills into reading and writing. However, parents and teachers must be careful not to push them before they are ready. This applies to social relationships and physical activities, as well as learning situations.

**Prevention.**   An essential nursing goal is to prevent visual impairment. This involves many of the same interventions discussed under hearing impairment: (1) prenatal screening for pregnant women at risk, such as those with rubella or syphilis infection and family histories of genetic disorders associated with visual loss; (2) adequate prenatal and perinatal care to prevent prematurity and iatrogenic damage from excessive administration of oxygen; (3) periodic screening of all children, especially newborns through preschoolers, for congenital blindness and visual impairments caused by refractive errors, strabismus, and other disorders; (4) rubella immunization of all children; and (5) safety counseling regarding the common causes of ocular trauma. Safety counseling should include safe practices when working with, playing with, or carrying objects such as scissors, knives, and balls.

> **NURSING ALERT**
>
> A helmet with a face mask should be required for children playing baseball, hockey, or football.

Following detection of eye problems, the nurse should encourage the family to prevent further ocular damage by ensuring that corrective treatment is employed. For the child with strabismus, this often necessitates occlusion patching of the stronger eye. Compliance with the procedure is greatest during the early preschool years. It is more difficult to encourage young school-age children to wear the occlusive patch because the poor visual acuity of the uncovered weaker eye interferes with schoolwork and the patch sets them apart from their peers. In school they benefit from being positioned favorably (closer to the chalkboard or primary instructional area) and being allowed extra time to read or complete an assignment. If treatment of the eye disorder requires instillation of ophthalmic medication, the family is taught the correct procedure.* (See Chapter 27.)

Children who need glasses to correct refractive errors will need time to adjust to wearing these. Young children, who often pull glasses off, may benefit from temporal pieces that wrap around the ears or from an elastic strap attached to the frames and around the back of the head to hold the glasses on securely. Once children appreciate the value of clear vision, they are more likely to wear the corrective lenses.

Glasses should not interfere with activity. Special protective guards are available to prevent accidental injury during contact sports, and all corrective lenses should be made from safety glass, which is shatterproof. Often corrective lenses improve visual acuity so dramatically that children are able to compete more effectively in sports. This in itself is a tremendous inducement to continue wearing glasses.

*Contact lenses* are a popular alternative to conventional glasses. Several types are available, such as gas-permeable and soft lenses, which may be designed for daily or extended wear. Contact lenses offer several advantages over glasses, such as greater visual acuity, total corrected field of vision, convenience (especially with the extended wear

---

*Home care instructions for giving eye medications are available in Wong DL, Hess CS: *Wong and Whaley's clinical manual of pediatric nursing,* ed 5, St Louis, 2000, Mosby.

type), and optimum cosmetic benefit. Unfortunately, they are usually more expensive and require much more care than glasses, including considerable practice to learn techniques for insertion and removal. If they are prescribed, the nurse can be very helpful in teaching parents or older children how to care for the lenses.

Because trauma is the leading cause of blindness, the nurse has the major responsibility of preventing further eye injury until the specific treatment is instituted. The major principles to follow when caring for an eye injury are outlined in the Emergency Treatment box on p. 1003. Since patients with a serious eye injury fear blindness, the nurse should stay with the child and family to provide support and reassurance. (See Nursing Care Plan: The Child with Visual Impairment.*)

## The Deaf-Blind Child

The most traumatic sensory impairment is loss of both sight and hearing. One of the chief causes of deaf-blindness was congenital rubella syndrome, but immunization has decreased its incidence. Other causes are usually the result of one congenital sensory impairment combined with an acquired impairment, such as congenital blindness and acquired deafness from meningitis, or congenital deafness and acquired blindness from an eye injury. Most children with multisensory impairments have some residual hearing and vision to supplement the senses of touch, smell, and taste.

Auditory and visual impairments have profound effects on the child's development. They interfere with the normal sequence of physical, intellectual, and psychosocial growth. Although the child often achieves the usual motor milestones, they are delayed. Children only learn communication with specialized training. *Finger spelling* is one desirable method often taught to these children. The letters are spelled into the deaf-blind child's hand, and the child spells out ideas to the other person. Another type of tactile communication, the *Tadoma method,* involves the child placing the hand over the speaker's face and neck to monitor facial movements associated with speech production (Tan and others, 1999). Some children with residual hearing or vision can learn to speak. Whenever possible, speech is encouraged because it allows communication with individuals not familiar with the preceding approaches.

Programs for these children vary. The **John Tracy Clinic†** offers a home correspondence course for parents, and the **American Foundation for the Blind,‡ Helen Keller National Center,§ Perkins School for the Blind,‖** and **Foundation for**

the **Junior Blind*** provide publications and various special services. The **Library of Congress National Library Service for the Blind and Physically Handicapped†** publishes a reference circular titled *Deaf-Blindness: National Organizations and Resources.*

### Nursing Considerations

One of the major concerns of families with children who are deaf-blind is helping them establish communication. The nurse is in a vital position to help parents with this goal. Because infants may not coo, laugh, or make directed eye movements, they are limited in the cues they can send and receive. Therefore initiating and maintaining communication is the caregiver's responsibility. The nurse discusses with parents behaviors that signal the infant's recognition of them, such as quieting behavior, blinking, and change in respiration. The parents are encouraged to find ways of increasing stimulation for the child, especially cues that help the child identify each parent. For example, each person involved with the child should choose something that only he or she does, such as a kiss on the forehead or a stroke on the cheek. In this way the infant learns to discriminate among people in the environment.

As many sensory experiences as possible are provided, such as placing children in different positions during the day in relation to light and providing variation in stimuli so that they will be motivated to move toward, reach, touch, and explore the environment. Changing position also encourages muscle development and movement patterns. Sounds should be brought near and made interesting to these children. For example, they can participate in hearing by placing the hand on a radio or on a person's throat. Consistent tactile cues should be associated with a change of position and activities so that the movement is experienced as a positive, nonthreatening experience.

Children who are deaf and blind need secure, safe experiences while learning to walk and gain confidence. Once ambulatory, they need help in exploring the environment on a gradual, *planned* basis. After they succeed in becoming well oriented to the environment, they are ready for a plan of locomotion. Sighted guide, trailing (movement directed by touching objects, such as the wall), and cane walking are three methods. An individually planned mobility program is based on the child's age, needs, and functional status and is shared with the child's therapist, teachers, parents, and siblings.

The future prospects for deaf-blind children are at best unpredictable. Sometimes congenital blindness or deafness is accompanied by other physical or neurologic handicaps, which further lessen the child's learning potential. The most favorable prognosis is often for children who have acquired deaf-blindness and have few, if any, associated disabilities. Their learning capacity is greatly potentiated by their developmental progress before the sensory impairments and the assistance of a trained companion. Al-

*In Wong DL, Hess CS: *Wong and Whaley's clinical manual of pediatric nursing,* ed 5, St Louis, 2000, Mosby.

†806 W Adams Blvd., Los Angeles, CA 90007, (213) 748-5481, (800) 522-4582, TTY: (213) 747-2924; johntracyclinic.org.

‡11 Pennsylvania Plaza, Suite 300, New York, NY 10001, (212) 502-7600, (800) 232-5463, TTY: (212) 502-7662; www.afb.org.

§111 Middle Neck Rd, Sands Point, NY 11050, (516) 944-8900 (voice/TTY), TTY: (516) 944-8637, fax: (516) 944-7302 (also regional offices); www.helenkeller.org.

‖175 N. Beacon St, Watertown, MA 02472-2790, (617) 924-3434, (800) 852-3133, TTY: (516) 994-8637; www.perkins.pvt.k12.ma.us.

*5300 Angeles Vista Blvd, Los Angeles, CA 90043, (213) 295-4555 or (800) 352-2290.

†1291 Taylor St NW, Washington, DC 20542, (202) 707-5100, (800) 424-8567, TTY: (202) 707-0744, fax: (202) 707-0712; www.loc.gov/nls.

though total independence, including gainful vocational training, is the goal, some deaf-blind children are unable to develop to this level. They may require lifelong parental or residential care. The nurse working with such families helps them deal with future goals for the child, including possible alternatives to home care during the parents' advancing years.

# COMMUNICATION IMPAIRMENT

## General Concepts

Communication impairment is a broad term that refers to the inability to (1) receive or process symbol systems for the spoken word, (2) represent concepts or symbol systems, or (3) transmit and use symbol systems. With severe communication impairment, other symbol systems, such as nonverbal methods (e.g., gestures, sign language, braille), may be needed to substitute for the spoken word.

Because of the complexity of communication, various classification systems are available and there is no universal agreement on one system. Basically a communication impairment may occur in language, speech, or hearing or any combination of these. The problems encountered when hearing is affected are discussed earlier in this chapter. *Language* primarily refers to the symbol system used to convey thoughts or feelings to others. The two major types are *receptive language,* or understanding the spoken word, and *expressive language,* or speaking verbal symbols. *Speech* is the oral production of language, including articulation of sounds, rhythm, and tone. *Pragmatics* involves the rules for the use of language (including nonverbal communication), as in social contexts.

Delayed development of language and speech is the most common symptom of developmental disability in children. Speech problems are more prevalent than language disorders, and both impairments decline as children grow older. Communication impairment often occurs in conjunction with impairment in other developmental realms. In the absence of other affected domains, the term *developmental language disorder* may be used.

### Etiology

The most common causes of communication impairment are mental retardation, followed by hearing impairment. Other causes include (1) central nervous system dysfunction or injury, such as learning disabilities or traumatic brain injury; (2) autism; (3) childhood schizophrenia; (4) organic problems, such as cerebral palsy, cleft palate, vocal cord injury, and paralysis or foreshortening of the soft palate and uvula; and (5) some genetic disorders, such as cri-du-chat syndrome and Gilles de la Tourette syndrome. In some instances, such as in stuttering, the cause is unknown or speculative.

### Language Impairment

Language disorders include impairment in:

- Assigning meaning to words (vocabulary)
- Organizing words into sentences
- Altering word forms to indicate tense, possession, and plurality

Examples of language disorders are failure to develop vocabulary at the expected age, a reduced vocabulary for age, poor sentence structure, such as "Me see dog," or omitting words from the sentence, such as "Me fun." Such short or "telegraphic" phrases are normal during the first 2 years but should be replaced by more complete statements during the preschool years. Clinical manifestations of language disorders are presented in Box 24-10.

### Speech Impairment

Speech impairments include differences from normal in articulation, fluency, and voice production. *Articulation* errors refer to those speech sounds that a child makes incorrectly or inappropriately. For example, the child tends to distort or substitute a few consonants or blends, especially those that are learned last—*s, l, r,* and *th*—or the child omits many consonants, usually at the end of words, and substitutes the letters *t, d, k,* or *y* for them (Figs. 24-9 and 24-10).

*Dysfluencies,* or *rhythm disorders,* usually consist of repetitions of sounds, words, or phrases. One of the most common and potentially serious dysfluencies is stuttering. *Stuttering,* describes dysfluent speech characterized by tense repetition of sounds or complete blockages of sounds or words. A stutter is sometimes referred to as a *block* when no sound comes out when the person tries to speak.

*Voice disorders* are characterized by differences in pitch, loudness, or quality. Clinical manifestations of speech disorders are presented in Box 24-11.

## Nonspeech Communication

Many individuals who have severe disabilities, such as cerebral palsy, mental retardation, or multiple physical impairments, comprehend language but are unable to speak. Consequently, they benefit from communication methods that

---

**Box 24-10** ■ ■ ■
**Clinical Manifestations of Language Disorders**

**ASSIGNING MEANING TO WORDS**

First words not uttered before second birthday
Vocabulary size reduced for age or fails to show steady increase
Difficulty in describing characteristics of objects, although may be able to name them
Infrequent use of modifier words (adjectives or adverbs)
Excessive use of jargon past 18 months

**ORGANIZING WORDS INTO SENTENCES**

First sentences not uttered before third birthday
Short and incomplete sentences
Tendency to omit words (articles, prepositions)
Misuse of the "be," "do," and "can" verb forms
Difficulty understanding and producing questions
Plateaus at an early developmental level; uses easy speech patterns

**ALTERING WORD FORMS**

Omission of endings for plurals and tenses
Inappropriate use of plurals and tense endings
Inaccurate use of possession words

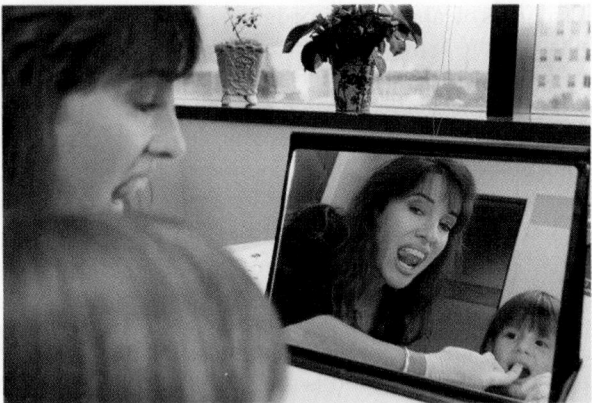

**Fig. 24-9** Using visual and tactile cues, the clinician demonstrates tongue placement for production of the *L* sound. (Courtesy Paul Vincent Kuntz, Texas Children's Hospital.)

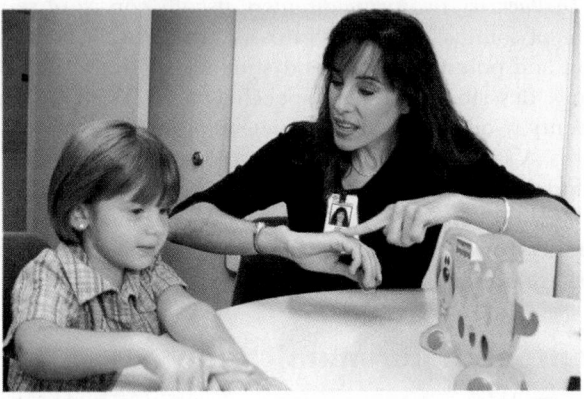

**Fig. 24-10** Child practices a gestural cue to elicit sustained airflow for the *S* sound. (Courtesy Paul Vincent Kuntz, Texas Children's Hospital.)

employ nonverbal symbols, such as sign language. Besides the use of hand or body gestures, numerous other communication systems exist. For example, *Blissymbols* are a highly stylized system of graphic symbols that represent words, ideas, and concepts. Although Blissymbols require education for their use, no reading skill is needed. These symbols or other self-explanatory graphics are usually arranged on a board, and the person points to the symbol(s) to convey a message; more sophisticated devices employ voice synthesizers that "speak" the symbol's meaning. For children with physical limitations that prevent fine hand movements, numerous devices are available that facilitate isolating a symbol. Nonverbal communication systems are allowing individuals with severe communication disorders a much more meaningful life; many children are able to learn more and faster.* The *situated approach* is a shift from an emphasis on repairing the disabilities to supporting those disabilities so

*Information about communication aids for children is available from Crestwood Communication Aids, Inc, 6625 N Sidney Pl, Milwaukee, WI 53209, (414) 352-5678, fax: (414) 352-5679, e-mail: crestcomm@aol.com; www.communicationaids.com.

---

> ### Box 24-11 ■ ■ ■
> ### Clinical Manifestations of Speech Disorders
>
> **DYSFLUENCY (STUTTERING)**
>
> Disturbance in the normal fluency and time patterning of speech (inappropriate for the individual's age), characterized by frequent occurrences of one or more of the following:
> Sound and syllable repetitions
> Sound prolongations
> Interjections
> Broken words (e.g., pauses within a word)
> Audible or silent blocking (filled or unfilled pauses in speech)
> Circumlocutions (word substitutions to avoid problematic words)
> Words produced with an excess of physical tension
> Monosyllabic whole-word repetitions (e.g., "I-I-I see him")
> The disturbance in fluency interferes with academic or occupational achievement or with social communication.
> If a speech-motor or sensory deficit is present, the speech difficulties are in excess of those usually associated with these problems.
>
> **ARTICULATION DEFICIENCY**
>
> Intelligibility of conversational speech absent by age 3 years
> Omission of consonants at beginning of words by age 3 and at end of words by age 4
> Persisting articulation faults after age 7
> Omission of a sound where one should occur
> Distortion of a sound
> Substitution of an incorrect sound for a correct one
>
> **VOICE DISORDERS**
>
> Deviations in pitch (too high or too low, especially for age and sex); monotone
> Deviations in loudness
> Deviations in quality (hypernasality or hyponasality)

they can achieve more. The goals of a situated approach are to increase opportunities for the children to participate in everyday life activities (Duchan, 1997).

## Autism

Autism is a complex developmental disorder of brain function accompanied by a broad range and severity of intellectual and behavioral deficits. It is manifested during early childhood primarily from 24 to 48 months of age. It occurs in 1:500 children, is about four times more common in males than in females (although females are more severely affected), and is not related to socioeconomic level, race, or parenting style.

### Etiology

The etiology of autism is an unknown. However, considerable evidence supports multiple biologic causes. Individuals with autism may have abnormal electroencephalograms, epileptic seizures, delayed development of hand dominance, persistence of primitive reflexes, metabolic abnormalities (elevated blood serotonin), and cerebellar vermal hypoplasia (part of the brain involved in regulating motion and some aspects of memory).

There is also strong evidence for a genetic basis that in twins is consistent with an autosomal-recessive pattern of in-

## Box 24-12 ■ ■ ■
## Diagnostic Criteria for Autistic Disorder

A. A total of six (or more) items from (1), (2), and (3), with at least two from (1), and one each from (2) and (3):
  (1) Qualitative impairment in social interaction, as manifested by at least two of the following:
    (a) Marked impairment in the use of multiple nonverbal behaviors such as eye-to-eye gaze, facial expression, body postures, and gestures to regulate social interaction
    (b) Failure to develop peer relationships appropriate to developmental level
    (c) A lack of spontaneous seeking to share enjoyment, interests, or achievements with other people (e.g., by a lack of showing, bringing, or pointing out objects of interest)
    (d) Lack of social or emotional reciprocity
  (2) Qualitative impairments in communication as manifested by at least one of the following:
    (a) Delay in, or total lack of, the development of spoken language (not accompanied by an attempt to compensate through alternative modes of communication such as gesture or mime)
    (b) In individuals with adequate speech, marked impairment in the ability to initiate or sustain a conversation with others
    (c) Stereotyped and repetitive use of language or idiosyncratic language
    (d) Lack of varied, spontaneous make-believe play or social imitative play appropriate to developmental level
  (3) Restricted repetitive and stereotyped patterns of behavior, interests, and activities, as manifested by at least one of the following:
    (a) Encompassing preoccupation with one or more stereotyped and restricted patterns of interest that is abnormal either in intensity or focus
    (b) Apparently inflexible adherence to specific, nonfunctional routines or rituals
    (c) Stereotyped and repetitive motor mannerisms (e.g., hand or finger flapping or twisting, or complex whole-body movements)
    (d) Persistent preoccupation with parts of objects
B. Delays or abnormal functioning in at least one of the following areas, with onset prior to age 3 years: (1) social interaction, (2) language as used in social communication, or (3) symbolic or imaginative play.
C. The disturbance is not better accounted for by Rett's Disorder or Childhood Disintegrative Disorder.

From American Psychiatric Association: *Diagnostic and statistical manual of mental disorders (DSM-IV-TR)*, ed 4, Washington, DC, 2000, The Association.

ported in association with a number of conditions such as fragile X syndrome, tuberous sclerosis, metabolic disorders, fetal rubella syndrome, *Haemophilus influenzae* meningitis, and structural brain anomalies (Williams, Dalrymple, and Neal, 2000). Recent reports have retrospectively tied autism to perinatal events such as a high incidence of uterine bleeding during pregnancy, lower incidence of vaginal infections during pregnancy, a decreased maternal use of contraceptives, and a higher incidence of neonatal hyperbilirubinemia (Juul-Dam, Townsend, and Courchesne, 2001). These same researchers, however, urge caution in interpreting these findings.

### Clinical Manifestations and Diagnostic Evaluation

Children with autism demonstrate several peculiar and often seemingly bizarre characteristics, primarily in social interactions, communication, and behavior. One hallmark characteristic is the inability to maintain eye contact with another person. Children with autism also display limited functional play and may interact with toys in an unusual manner (Williams, Dalrymple, and Neal, 2000). Other clinical manifestations typically seen in children with autism are described in Box 24-12. Studies of these children at play suggest that deficits in social development are a primary feature of the illness. Children with autism do not always have the same manifestations; there is a range in severity of clinical manifestations from mild forms, requiring minimal supervision, to severe forms in which self-abusive behavior is common. The majority (50% to 70%) of children with autism have some degree of mental retardation, with scores typically in the moderate to severe range. More females than males tend to have very low intelligence scores. Despite their relatively moderate to severe disability, some children with autism (known as **savants**) excel in particular areas, such as art, music, memory, mathematics, or perceptual skills such as puzzle building.

**NURSING TIP**   The therapeutic management of autism with the hormone secretin is controversial. One recent study failed to demonstrate significant improvement when autistic children were given one dose of synthetic human secretin (Sandler and others, 1999).*

Speech and language delays are also common in autistic children. The new Practice Parameter Report of the American Academy of Neurology (AAN) (2000) recommends immediate evaluation of any child who does not display such language skills as babbling or gesturing by 12 months, no single word by 16 months, and lack of two-word phrases by 24 months. A sudden deterioration in extant expressive speech is also a red-flag event for further evaluation.

This report emphasizes early recognition, referral, diagnosis, and intensive early intervention to improve outcomes for children with autism. Unfortunately, diagnosis is often

heritance. Twin studies demonstrate a very high concordance (96%) for monozygotic (identical) twins and a 24% concordance for dizygotic (nonidentical) twins. In addition, between 5% and 16% of males with autism are positive for the fragile X chromosome.

There is a 10% to 20% risk of recurrence of autism in families with one affected child (Filipek and others, 2000). Although the serotonin-transporter gene has been suggested as a possible causative factor in autism, no specific gene for the disorder has been identified (Rapin, 1997).

Contrary to previous reports, autism does not appear to be caused by the measles-mumps-rubella (MMR) vaccine (Dales, Hammer, and Smith, 2001). Autism has been re-

*Additional information on secretin may be found at www.autism.org/secretin.html; **Autism Society of America,** 7910 Woodmont Ave, Suite 300, Bethesda, MD 20814, (800) 3AUTISM or (301) 657-0881; www.autism-society.org.

not made until 2 to 3 years after symptoms are first recognized. The Academy of Neurology report has a comprehensive set of suggested diagnostic criteria to be used to either rule out or establish the diagnosis of childhood autism (Filipek and others, 2000) (see Box 24-12).*

## Prognosis

Autism is usually a severely disabling condition. However, some children improve with acquisition of language skills and communication with others (Rapin, 1997). Some ultimately achieve independence, but most require lifelong adult supervision. Aggravation of psychiatric symptoms occurs in about half of the children during adolescence, with girls having a tendency for continued deterioration.

Early recognition of behaviors associated with autism is critical to implement appropriate interventions and family involvement. The prognosis is most favorable for children with communicative speech development by age 6 years and an intelligence quotient above 50 at the time of diagnosis.

## Nursing Considerations

Therapeutic intervention for the child with autism is a specialized area involving professionals with advanced training. Although there is no cure for autism, numerous therapies have been used. The most promising results have been through highly structured and intensive behavior-modification programs. In general the objective in treatment is to promote positive reinforcement, increase social awareness of others, teach verbal communication skills, and decrease unacceptable behavior. Providing a structured routine for the child to follow is a key in the management of autism.

When these children are hospitalized, the parents are essential to planning care and ideally should stay with the child as much as possible. Nurses should recognize that not all children with autism are the same and will require individual assessment and treatment. Decreasing stimulation by using a private room, avoiding extraneous auditory and visual distraction, and encouraging the parents to bring in possessions the child is attached to may lessen the disruptiveness of hospitalization. Because physical contact often upsets these children, minimum holding and eye contact may be necessary to avoid behavioral outbursts. Care must be taken when performing procedures on, administering medicine to, or feeding these children, because they are either fussy eaters who may willfully starve themselves or gag to prevent eating or indiscriminate hoarders, swallowing any available edible or inedible items, such as a thermometer. Eating habits of autistic children may be particularly problematic for families and may involve food refusal, mouthing objects, eating nonedibles, and smelling and throwing food (Williams, Dalrymple, and Neal, 2000).

They need to be introduced slowly to new situations, with visits with staff caregivers kept short whenever possible. Because these children have difficulty organizing their behavior and redirecting their energy, they need to be told directly what to do. Communication should be at the child's developmental level, brief, and concrete.

**Family Support.** Autism, like so many other chronic conditions, involves the entire family and often becomes "a family disease." Nurses can help alleviate the guilt and shame often associated with this disorder by stressing what is known from a biologic standpoint, as well as how little is known about the cause of autism. It is imperative to help parents understand that they are not the cause of the child's condition.

Parents need expert counseling early in the course of the disorder and should be referred to the **Autism Society of America (ASA).*** ASA provides information about education, treatment programs and techniques, and facilities such as camps and group homes. There is also a siblings group called **SHARE (Siblings Helping Persons with Autism Through Resources and Energy).** Other helpful resources for parents of children with autism are the local and state departments of mental health and developmental disabilities; these organizations provide important programs for autistic children and in-school programs throughout the United States.

As much as possible, the family is encouraged to care for the child in the home. With the help of family support programs in many states, families are often able to provide home care and assist with the educational services the child needs. As the child approaches adulthood and parents become older, the family may require assistance in locating a long-term placement facility. (See Chapter 22).

# Nursing Care of Children with Communication Impairment

## Prevention

The primary intervention for communication disorders is prevention. Much of prevention directly relates to factors that predispose to causes of language/speech impairment, namely, mental retardation and hearing loss. Infants at risk for either condition (see Boxes 24-1 and 24-7) should be referred for audiologic evaluation within the first 3 to 6 months of age so that audiologic and speech therapy can be initiated immediately, when required.

Prevention also involves early recognition of children at risk for language delays and involves timely intervention to promote adequate language development. Nurses are often able to provide education for families that fosters the child's communication skills.

One area that is particularly important in terms of preventing communication impairment through appropriate parental guidance is *stuttering*. This hesitancy or dysfluency in speech pattern is a *normal* characteristic of language development during the preschool years. It occurs because children know what they want to say but hesitate or repeat words or sounds as they try to find the vocabulary to express themselves. Eventually their language skills parallel their other abilities, and speech becomes fluent.

---

*At the time of this writing the AAN report is available online at www.aan. com/public/practiceguidelines/autism.pdf.

*7910 Woodmont Ave, Suite 300, Bethesda, MD 20814-3067, (800) 3AUTISM or (301) 657-0881; www.autism-society.org.

However, when parents or other significant persons place undue emphasis or stress on this pattern of dysfluency, an abnormal speech pattern may result. Chances for reversal of stuttering are good until about 5 years of age. Therefore prevention must begin early. The nurse discusses with parents the normal dysfluencies in children's speech. When stuttering does occur, parents are advised to use the suggestions listed in the Family Home Care box to prevent inadvertently reinforcing the dysfluent pattern. If excessive concern of the parent or frustration and struggling behavior from the child are noted, the child is referred for speech and language evaluation.*

**NURSING ALERT** Dysfluency must be arrested before the child develops an awareness or anticipation of the difficulty and begins to mistrust his or her speech skills.

## Assessment

Communication disorders can occur at any age but are most often found during childhood. The preschool period is considered critical to language development and therefore is a prime age for assessment and intervention. Failure to detect communication disorders during early childhood affects the development of social relationships and emotional interactions, increases difficulty in developing academic skills, and lessens the chances for successful correction of deficient skills.

Assessment of abnormalities requires knowledge of normal speech and language development. Awareness of when

*Information about sources of assistance is available from the **Stuttering Foundation of America,** PO Box 11749, Memphis, TN 38111-0749, (901) 452-7343 or (800) 992-9392, fax: (901) 452-3931, e-mail: stuttersfa@aol.com; www.stuttersfa.org.

children achieve such milestones enables nurses to distinguish when specific communication characteristics are expected and when they are considered deviations (Table 24-6). Nurses must also be aware of clinical manifestations of speech and language impairment (see Boxes 24-10 and 24-11) and cognitive or hearing deficits (see Boxes 24-2 and 24-8 and Cognitive Impairment, p. 977).

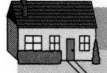

### FAMILY HOME CARE
#### Stuttering in Young Children

**TO BE ENCOURAGED**

Viewing hesitancy and dysfluency as a normal part of speech development

Giving the child plenty of time and the impression that you are not rushed or in a hurry

Looking directly at the child while he or she is talking; being patient and never ridiculing or criticizing

Setting a good example by speaking clearly and articulating well

Identifying situations when stuttering increases and avoiding them or ignoring the hesitancy

Minimizing stress, such as talking at the child's eye level; avoiding frequent questioning; and preventing interruptions while the child is speaking

Capitalizing on periods of fluent speech with positive reinforcement, such as singing songs or repeating nursery rhymes

**TO BE AVOIDED**

Practicing the natural tendency to finish the sentence for the child by supplying the word when the child has a block

Telling the child to stop and start over, to think before speaking, or to take it easy and go slowly

Showing great concern, embarrassment, or disapproval for hesitancy

Doing *anything* that emphasizes stuttering and calls the child's attention to speech skills

Promising a reward for proper speech

| **TABLE 24-6** | Normal speech/language development during early childhood | |
|---|---|---|
| **Age (years)** | **Development** | **Intelligibility** |
| 1 | Says two to three words with meaning<br>Imitates sounds of animals<br>Omits most final and some initial consonants | Usually no more than 25% intelligible to unfamiliar listener<br>Height of unintelligible jargon at age 18 months |
| 2 | Uses two- to three-word phrases<br>Has vocabulary of about 300 words<br>Uses "I," "me," and "you"<br>Articulation lags behind vocabulary | 50% intelligible in context |
| 3 | Says four- to five-word sentences<br>Has vocabulary of about 900 words<br>Uses "who," "what," and "where" in asking questions<br>Uses plurals, pronouns, and prepositions<br>Often repeats and hesitates | 75% intelligible |
| 4-5 | Has vocabulary of 1500 to 2100 words<br>Able to use most grammatical forms correctly, such as past tense of verb with "yesterday"<br>Uses complete sentences with nouns, verbs, prepositions, adjectives, adverbs, and conjunctions | At age 4 years, speech is 100% intelligible, although some sounds are still imperfect |
| 5-6 | Has vocabulary of 3000 words<br>Comprehends "if," "because," and "why"<br>Masters most sounds; still distorts *s, z, sh, ch,* and *j* | |

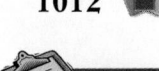

## GUIDELINES
*Assessing Communication Impairment*

### KEY QUESTIONS FOR LANGUAGE DISORDERS

1. How old was your child when he (or she) began to speak his (or her) first words?
2. How old was your child when he (or she) began to put words into sentences?
3. Does your child have difficulty in learning new vocabulary words?
4. Does your child omit words from sentences (i.e., do sentences sound telegraphic?) or use short or incomplete sentences?
5. Does your child have trouble with grammar, such as the verbs "is," "am," "are," "was," and "were"?
6. Can your child follow two or three directions given at once?
7. Do you have to repeat directions or questions?
8. Does your child respond appropriately to questions?
9. Does your child ask questions beginning with "who," "what," "where," and "why"?
10. Does it seem that your child has made little or no progress in speech and language in the last 6 to 12 months?

### KEY QUESTIONS FOR SPEECH IMPAIRMENT

1. Does your child ever stammer or repeat sounds or words?
2. Does your child seem anxious or frustrated when trying to express an idea?
3. Have you noticed certain behaviors, such as blinking the eyes, jerking the head, or attempting to rephrase thoughts with different words, when your child stammers?
4. What do you do when any of these occur?
5. Does your child omit sounds from words?
6. Does it seem like your child uses *t, d, k,* or *g* in place of most other consonants when speaking?
7. Does your child omit sounds from words or substitute the correct consonant with another one (such as "rabbit" with "wabbit")?
8. Do you have any difficulty in understanding your child's speech? How much of it is intelligible?
9. Has anyone else ever remarked about having difficulty in understanding your child?
10. Has there been any recent change in the sound of your child's voice?

---

Three methods are available for assessing speech and language development. *Direct observation* necessitates spontaneous language interaction between the child and the nurse. Suggestions for initiating conversation include showing children an object and asking them to describe it. The word-imitative procedure may also be used by having children repeat sentences or words. This approach is valid because children are not able to reproduce statements using correct grammatical forms that they have not previously learned to use. Whenever possible, the child's conversation should be tape-recorded for serial documentation of progressive speech/language development and further evaluation by or consultation with a speech and language therapist.

*Indirect assessment* relies on parental information obtained through a history. Key questions that reflect problems in language or speech are listed in the Guidelines box. Information obtained from the history is critically impor-

tant, and parental concerns must be taken seriously. However, caution must also be exercised in evaluating parental comments. Parents may be unaware of the child's difficulties because of lack of comparison with normal language development. Also, they may not realize the degree of unintelligible speech because of familiarity with the child's approximation of words. Conversely, parents may have unrealistic expectations regarding verbal development and may exaggerate the degree of dysfluency, misarticulation, or word usage.

Consequently, *screening tests* are a very important component of objective measurement of speech development. The *Denver Articulation Screening Examination (DASE)* employs the word-imitative procedure and is one of the most frequently used tests. (See Appendix B.) The child repeats 22 words but pronounces 30 different sound elements. The raw score, or the number of correctly pronounced sounds, is then compared with the percentile rank for children in that age-group. The examiner must be careful to evaluate the specific sound rather than the quality of the entire word. For beginning examiners, it is helpful to validate the final score by comparing the results with a different examiner, ideally a speech therapist. The child is also scored on intelligibility by selection of one of four possible categories: (1) easy to understand, (2) understandable half of the time, (3) not understandable, or (4) cannot evaluate. The DASE is a reliable, effective screening tool because it requires only 10 minutes for the examiner to perform and is designed to discriminate between significant speech delay and normal variations in the acquisition of speech sounds. It also detects common abnormal physical conditions such as hyponasality, hypernasality, tongue thrust, and lateral lisp.

The *Early Language Milestone Scale (ELM)\** is a standardized screening instrument for assessing language development in children less than 3 years of age. The test focuses on expressive, receptive, and visual language, and the revised form includes intelligibility (Coplan and Gleason, 1988; Coplan and others, 1982; Coplan and others, 1998). The ELM relies primarily on the parent's report, with occasional direct testing of the child, and takes 1 to 4 minutes to administer.

A number of other tests are available to screen children for impaired language development. The *Denver II,* a revision of the Denver Developmental Screening Test, includes an expanded section on language items, and delays in that area provide an early indication for those children who require further evaluation. (See Chapter 7.) For children ages 2½ to 18 years, the *Peabody Picture Vocabulary Test—III* is a useful screening instrument for single word comprehension (Dunn and Dunn, 1997).

### Referral

Following assessment and detection of language or speech problems, the nurse can assist the family in making a decision regarding appropriate referral. Waiting and watching for progession of symptoms is often to the detriment of the

---

*The complete testing kit can be purchased from Pro-Ed, Inc, (800) 897-3702, fax: (800) 397-7633; www.proedinc.com.

## GUIDELINES
### Referral Regarding Communication Impairment

**AGE 2 YEARS**

Failure to speak any meaningful words spontaneously
Consistent use of gestures rather than vocalizations
Difficulty in following verbal directions
Failure to respond consistently to sound

**AGE 3 YEARS**

Speech largely unintelligible
Failure to use sentences of three or more words
Omission of initial consonants
Frequent omission of final consonants
Use of vowels rather than consonants

**AGE 5 YEARS**

Stutters or has any other type of dysfluency
Sentence structure noticeably impaired
Substitutes easily produced sounds for more difficult ones
Omits word endings (e.g., plurals, tenses of verbs)

**SCHOOL AGE**

Poor voice quality (monotonous, loud, or barely audible)
Vocal pitch inappropriate for age
Any distortions, omissions, or substitutions of sounds after age 7 years
Connected speech characterized by use of unusual confusions or reversals

**GENERAL**

Any child with signs suggesting a hearing impairment (see Boxes 24-7 and 24-8)
Any child who is embarrassed or disturbed by his or her speech
Parents who are excessively concerned or who pressure the child to speak at a level above that appropriate for the child's age

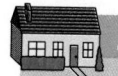

## FAMILY HOME CARE
### Helping a Child Learn Language

Provide listening opportunities:
Select a small group of words connected to a specific activity (e.g., say "open" each time a door is opened). Repeat the word with the activity several times, then repeat the word but wait for the child to initiate the activity.
Choose vocabulary that is useful, easy to pronounce, and understandable to the child.
Encourage vocabulary development by having the child say the word rather than gesture before fulfilling a request (e.g., expect the child to say all or part of the word "drink" before giving a beverage).
Speak at a level slightly above the child's level (e.g., if the child speaks two words, use three- or four-word phrases).
Substitute questions with statements about an observed activity (e.g., rather than asking, "What's that?" say, "Look at the kitty").
Reinforce the child's attempt to use language with verbal praise and affection.

**Exceptional Children\*** (see p. 977 for organizations devoted to hearing impairment).

### Education

When a child has delayed language development, it becomes very important to try to structure the parents' communication to expand the child's language, including new words, new sentence construction, and rules of grammar. The underlying principle is not to bombard children with words so that they learn more language, but to plan what will be said to them, what responses will be expected, and how they will be reinforced. Suggestions to help parents foster their child's attainment of language skills are presented in the Family Home Care box.

Parents should also be aware that children learn language through imitation. Therefore serving as role models by speaking clearly, fluently, and with proper grammar is essential to children's mastery of language and speech. Parents need guidance regarding normal language and speech development so that they expect neither too little nor too much from their child.

child's future development. Because children normally vary greatly in their development of verbal skills, the nurse needs guidelines for determining abnormal development. The Guidelines box lists general recommendations for referring children for specialized audiologic and language evaluations. Information regarding available services for language, speech, and hearing can be obtained from the **American Speech-Language Hearing Association\*** and the **Council for**

*10801 Rockville Pike, Rockville, MD 20852, (800) 638-8255 (voice/TTY); www.asha.org.

*Division for Children's Communication Development, 1110 North Glebe Rd, Suite 300, Arlington, VA 22201-5704, (703) 620-3660 or (888) 232-7733, TTY: (703) 264-9446; www.cec.sped.org.

## KEY POINTS

■ The American Association on Mental Retardation (AAMR) defines mental retardation as significantly subaverage intellectual functioning existing concurrently with related limitations in two or more adaptive skill areas (communication, self-care, home living, social skills, leisure, health and safety, self-direction, functional academics, community use, and work), and manifested before age 18 years.

■ Diagnosis of cognitive impairment is based on standard developmental tests and an accurate history, and no child is too young to be assessed.

■ Causes of severe mental retardation are primarily genetic, biochemical, and infectious. Mild retardation is associated primarily with familial, social, and environmental causes, whereas severe retardation is more likely to be associated with specific syndromes.

- Primary prevention efforts focus on support for the premature neonate and other high-risk newborns, rubella immunization, genetic counseling, education regarding alcohol, adequate prenatal nutrition, and reduction of nonintentional and intentional cerebral injuries.
- Secondary prevention activities include prenatal diagnosis or carrier detection.
- Tertiary prevention is aimed at minimizing long-term consequences through medical treatment.
- Education of children with cognitive impairment emphasizes sensory and verbal discrimination, improvement of short-term memory, motivation, and technologic support.
- Promoting optimum development may be achieved through family guidance regarding play, communication, discipline, socialization, and sexuality.
- Promotion of independent self-help skills is aimed at feeding, toileting, dressing, and grooming.
- For the hospitalized child with mental retardation, nurses must be aware of the child's abilities and needs, provide a familiar setting, and support families.
- Down syndrome, a chromosome abnormality, is characterized by subnormal intelligence, numerous physical stigmata, slowed social development, congenital anomalies, sensory problems, diminished growth and sexual development, and reduced life expectancy.
- Fragile X syndrome is characterized by mental retardation and phenotypic findings in affected males. It is considered the most common hereditary form of mental retardation and the second most common genetic cause after Down syndrome.
- Hearing defects may be categorized according to etiology, pathology, or symptom severity; prevention, treatment, and rehabilitation are based on these factors.
- Hearing disorders may be classified according to the location of the defect: conductive, sensorineural, mixed conductive sensorineural, or central auditory imperception.
- Some of the effects of hearing loss on growth and development are impaired knowledge of objects, impaired academic learning, and decreased socialization.
- Prevention of hearing loss is the nurse's major responsibility. Efforts include treatment of infection, auditory testing, immunization, pregnancy and genetic counseling, and reduction of excessive noise.
- Rehabilitation for hearing loss involves parent education and support, hearing aids, lipreading, sign language, cued speech, speech therapy, and promotion of socialization.
- Common visual impairments in childhood are refractive errors, amblyopia, strabismus, cataracts, glaucoma, trauma, and infections.
- Effects of serious visual impairment on development include impaired motor function, reduced stimulation, and greater challenges in academic learning.
- Prevention of visual impairment focuses on prenatal screening, prenatal and perinatal care, periodic vision screening of all children, immunization, and safety counseling.
- Nursing goals in visual rehabilitation include helping the family and child adjust to the child's visual impairment, promoting parent-child attachment, fostering optimum development and independence, providing for play and socialization, and being aware of educational facilities.
- For the child undergoing ocular surgery, nursing care is aimed at reassuring the child and family throughout treatment, orienting the child to the surroundings, providing a safe environment, and encouraging independence.
- Communication impairment is a broad term that refers to the inability to (1) receive or process symbol systems for the spoken word, (2) represent concepts or symbol systems, or (3) transmit and use symbol systems. With severe communication impairment, other symbol systems, such as nonverbal methods (e.g., gestures, sign language, braille), may be needed to substitute for the spoken word.
- Language refers to the symbol system involved in communication. Speech is the oral production of language.
- The primary intervention for communication disorders is prevention, which involves early recognition of children at risk for language delays and timely intervention to promote adequate language development. Nurses are often able to provide education for families that fosters the child's communication skills.
- Hesitancy or dysfluency in speech patterns is a normal characteristic of language development. Speech problems, such as stuttering, can be magnified when a child is anxious or pressured, such as when adults express excessive concern about this pattern.
- Autism is a disabling, permanent condition characterized by a broad range and severity of deficits in social interaction, communication, and behavior.

## REFERENCES

Aggen RL, Moore NJ: *Standards of nursing practice in mental retardation/developmental disabilities*, Albany, NY, 1994, Office of Mental Retardation and Developmental Disabilities.

Allen MC, Nikolopoulos TP, O'Donoghue GM: Speech intelligibility in children after cochlear implantation, *Am J Otol* 19(6): 742-746, 1998.

American Academy of Pediatrics, Committee on Children with Disabilities: Provision of educationally-related services for children and adolescents with chronic diseases and disabling conditions, *Pediatrics* 105(2): 448-451, 2000.

American Academy of Pediatrics, Task Force on Newborn and Infant Hearing: Newborn and infant hearing loss: detection and intervention, *Pediatrics* 103(2):527-530, 1999.

Appelbaum E: Detection of hearing loss in children, *Pediatr Ann* 28(6):351-356, 1999.

Ardito M and others: Delivering home-based case management to families with children with mental retardation and developmental disabilities, *J Case Manage* 6(2):56-61, 1997.

Belser RC, Sudhalter V: Conversational characteristics of children with fragile X syndrome: repetitive speech, *Am J Ment Retard* 106(1):28-38, 2001.

Berrettini S and others: Progressive sensorineural hearing loss in childhood, *Pediatr Neurol* 20(2):130-136, 1999.

Billings KR, Kenna MA: Causes of pediatric sensorineural hearing loss: yesterday and today, *Arch Otolaryngol Head Neck Surg* 125(5):517-521, 1999.

Cheng AK, Grant GD, Niparko JK: Meta-analysis of pediatric cochlear implant literature, *Ann Otol Rhinol Laryngol Suppl* 177:124-128, 1999.

Coplan J, Gleason J: Unclear speech: recognition and significance of unintelligible speech in preschool children, *Pediatrics* 82(3, pt 2):447-452, 1988.

Coplan J and others: Validation of an early language milestone scale in a high-risk population, *Pediatrics* 70(5):677-683, 1982.

Coplan J and others: Early language development in children exposed to or infected with human immunodeficiency virus, *Pediatrics* 102(1):e8, 1998.

Cuadrado E, Barrena MJ: Immune dysfunction in Down's syndrome: primary immune deficiency or early sensescence of the immune system? *Clin Immunol Immunopathol* 78(3):209-214, 1996.

Dales L, Hammer SJ, Smith NJ: Time trends in autism and in MMR immunization coverage in California, *JAMA* 285(9):1183-1185, 2001.

Davidson PW: Visual impairment and blindness. In Levine MD, Carey WB, Crocker AC, editors: *Developmental-behavioral pediatrics,* ed 3, Philadelphia, 1999, WB Saunders.

Duchan JF: A situated pragmatics approach for supporting children with severe communication disorders, *Top Lang Disord* 17(2):1-18, 1997.

Dunn L, Dunn L: *The Peabody Picture Vocabulary Test—III,* Circle Pines, MN, 1997, American Guidance Service.

Filipek PA and others: Practice parameter: screening and diagnosis of autism: report of the Quality Standards Subcommittee of the American Academy of Neurology and the Child Neurology Society, *Neurology* 55(2 of 2):468-479, 2000.

First MB, McQueen LE, Pincus HA: *DSM-IV coding update,* Washington, DC, 1996, American Psychiatric Association.

Fredericks DW, Williams WL: New definition of mental retardation for the American Association of Mental Retardation, *Image J Nurs Sch* 30(1):53-56, 1998.

Geggel RL, O'Brien JE, Feingold M: Development of valve dysfunction in adolescents and young adults with Down syndrome and no known congenital heart disease, *J Pediatr* 122:821-823, 1993.

Gostin LO: Human rights of persons with mental disabilities: The European Convention of Human Rights, *Int J Law Psychiatry* 23(2):125-159, 2000.

Hagerman RJ, Cronister A: Fragile X syndrome. In Jackson PL, Vessey JA, editors: *Primary care of the child with a chronic condition,* ed 2, St. Louis, 1996, Mosby.

Hixon M and others: FISH studies of the sperm of fathers of paternally derived cases of trisomy 21: no evidence for an increase in aneuploidy, *Hum Genet* 103(6):654-657, 1998.

Hodapp RM and others: Down syndrome: developmental, psychiatric, and management issues, *Child Adolesc Psychiatr Clin North Am* 5:881-894, 1996.

Juul-Dam N, Townsend J, Courchesne E: Prenatal, perinatal, and neonatal factors in autism, pervasive developmental disorder-not otherwise specified, and the general population, *Pediatrics* 107(4):e63, 2001.

Kanamori G and others: Otolaryngologic manifestations of Down syndrome, *Otolaryngol Clin North Am* 33(6):1285-1292, 2000.

Kasari C, Freeman SF: Task-related social behavior in children with Down syndrome, *Am J Ment Retard* 106(3):253-264, 2001.

LePage EL, Murray NM: Latent cochlear damage in personal stereo users: a study based on click-evoked otoacoustic emissions, *Med J Aust* 169(11-12):588-592, 1998.

McNally S: Caring for people with a learning disability who are victims of crime, *Br J Nurs* 9(8):493-496, 2000.

Murray J and others: Screening for fragile X syndrome, *Health Technol Assess* 1(4):i-iv,1-71, 1997.

Nickolopouls TP, O'Donoghue GM, Archbold S: Age at implantation: its importance in pediatric cochlear implantation, *Laryngoscope* 109(4):595-599, 1999.

Pueschel SM: The child with Down syndrome: In Levine MD, Carey WB, Crocker AC, editors: *Developmental-behavioral pediatrics,* ed 3, Philadelphia, 1999, WB Saunders.

Rapin I: Autism, *N Engl J Med* 337(2):97-103, 1997.

Ridenour N: Challenges for nurse practitioners: realistic health outcomes for developmentally disabled individuals, *Nurse Pract Forum* 10(4):191-194, 1999.

Roberts JE and others: Receptive and expressive communication development of young males with fragile X syndrome, *Am J Ment Retard* 106(3):216-230, 2001.

Roizen NJ: Etiology of hearing loss in children: nongenetic causes, *Pediatr Clin North Am* 46(1):49-64, 1999.

Sandler AD and others: Lack of benefit of a single dose of synthetic human secretin in the treatment of autism and pervasive developmental disorder, *N Engl J Med* 341(24):1801-1806, 1999.

Schalock RL and others: The changing conception of mental retardation: implications for the field, *Ment Retard* 32(3):181-193, 1994.

Shaughnessy M and others: *Teaching the mentally retarded parenting skills: international perspectives,* EDRS microfiche report, 1996.

Slattery WH, Fayad, JN: Cochlear implants in children with sensorineural inner ear hearing loss, *Pediatr Ann* 28(6):359-363, 1999.

Stoll C and others: Study of Down syndrome in 238,942 consecutive births, *Ann Genet* 41(1):44-51, 1998.

Symons FJ, Koppekin A, Wehby JH: Treatment of self-injurious behavior and quality of life for persons with mental retardation, *Ment Retard* 37(4);297-307, 1999.

Tan HZ and others: Information transmission with a multifinger tactual display, *Percept Psychophys* 61(6):993-1008, 1999.

Taylor TK, Walters WL: Screening of children with Down syndrome for atlantoaxial (C1-2) instability: another contentious health question, *Med J Aust* 165(8):448-450, 1996.

Turk J: Fragile X syndrome, *Arch Dis Child* 72(1);3-5, 1995.

Vessey JA: Down syndrome. In Jackson PL, Vessey JA, editors: *Primary care of the child with a chronic condition,* ed 2, St. Louis, 1996, Mosby.

Williams PG, Dalrymple N, Neal J: Eating habits of children with autism, *Pediatr Nurs* 26(3):259-264, 2000.

Yankowitz J and others: Prospective evaluation of prenatal maternal serum screening for trisomy 18, *Am J Obstet Gynecol* 178(3):446-450, 1998.

Yoshianga-Itano C and others: Language of early- and later-identified children with hearing loss, *Pediatrics* 102(5):1161-1171, 1998.

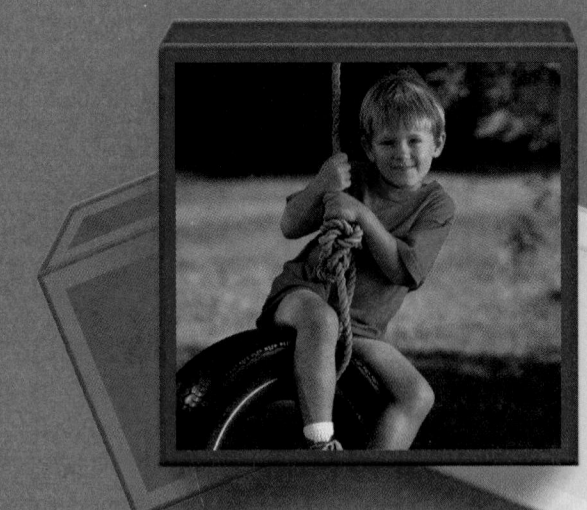

## Chapter 25

# Family-Centered Home Care

## Chapter Outline

**GENERAL CONCEPTS OF HOME CARE, 1016**
Home Care Trends, 1017
Effective Home Care, 1017
Discharge Planning and Selection of a Home Care Agency, 1018

Case Management, 1019
Role of the Nurse, Training, and Standards of Care, 1020
**FAMILY-CENTERED HOME CARE, 1021**
Respect for Diversity, 1021
Parent-Professional Collaboration, 1022

The Nursing Process, 1023
Promotion of Optimum Development, Self-Care, and Education, 1024
Safety Issues in the Home, 1028
Family-to-Family Support, 1028

## Related Topics

Communicating with Families, Ch. 6
Discharge Planning and Home Care, Chs. 10 and 26
Family Assessment, Ch. 6
Family-Centered Care of the Child with Chronic Illness or Disability, Ch. 22

Family-Centered Care of the Child During Illness and Hospitalization, Ch. 26
Family Influences on Child Health Promotion, Ch. 3
Parenteral Fluid Therapy, Ch. 28

Pediatric Variations of Nursing Interventions, Ch. 27
Respiratory Therapy, Ch. 31
Social, Cultural, and Religious Influences on Child Health Promotion, Ch. 2

## GENERAL CONCEPTS OF HOME CARE

Home care nursing has become a routine option for the pediatric patient in today's health care environment. Advances in medical technology have produced a large population of children with a variety of health care needs. The growing demand for home care services came in part as the result of increasing health costs of institutionalized care. More importantly, home-based health care recognizes the value of the contribution of the family to the overall health of the child in his or her most natural environment. As a result, pediatric home care nursing is one of the fastest growing segments of the health care community (Balinsky and Marié, 2001, Dittbrenner, 1999; *Ensuring access,* 1999).

Nursing education is shifting to incorporate a broader focus on community and home health nursing. In addition, nurses wishing to work in the home care setting will need to develop pertinent skills for this rapidly growing sub-

specialty (Betz, 2000; Petit de Mange, 1998; Pignatello and others, 1998; Woodring, 2000).

Home care is not a new concept in pediatrics. Over time the term has referred to parents caring for mildly ill children at home, to nursing home visits after children are discharged from the hospital, to hospice care, and to care at home for children with more serious chronic illness and dependence on medical technology. As discussed in this chapter, **home care** refers to care provided for children with complex health care needs and their families in their places of residence for the purpose of promoting, maintaining, or restoring health or for maximizing the level of independence while minimizing the effects of disability and illness, including terminal illness. It differs from **hospice care**—a program of palliative and supportive care services that provides physical, psychologic, social, and spiritual care for dying persons, their families, and other loved ones. Hospice services are available both in the home and in inpatient settings (Carlin, 1999) and are discussed more fully in Chapter 23.

---

■  Bonnie L. Minter, MS, RN, CPNP, wrote this chapter.

# Home Care Trends

The shift towards home-based health care is propelled by numerous factors. Providing quality home health care for children generally requires parental desire and ability, professional assistance, and community preparedness to achieve this goal. A natural family environment optimizes growth and development when stress is minimal and support is maximized.

Advances in medical technology have resulted in increased survival for children with congenital and acquired illnesses. Premature infants or children who are ventilator dependent were once cared for indefinitely in an intensive care unit or long-term care facility. These children are now able to live with their families in their own home.

Children with cancer, kidney disorders, cystic fibrosis, spina bifida, cardiac anomalies, gastrointestinal disorders, neurodegenerative diseases, and human immunodeficiency virus (HIV) infection may have ongoing health care needs as a result of the disease, its treatment, or side effects of treatment. Parents frequently have ongoing stressors after a child's hospitalization for diagnosis and treatment. Subsequent needs may include reinforcement about the disease process, addressing the physical care needs of the child, emotional support during this change in parental role, and learning in a low-stress environment (Snowdon and Kane, 1995; Stephenson, 1999).

The *cost of care* is an important factor in the health care delivery system today. Shorter inpatient stays are due in part to the overwhelming cost of lengthy hospitalizations. Children are either not admitted to the hospital at all or are returned home as soon as possible after their illness. Shifting the financial burden to home care agencies is an attractive alternative to third-party reimbursers. Likewise, a portion of the financial burden is shifted to the family. The family may be forced to absorb the costs of certain medications, supplies, transportation, shelter, utilities, food, laundry, housekeeping, and a portion of the nursing care. Over time chronically ill children can cause a financial burden to the family. Lifetime insurance benefits may be used up quickly, the primary caregiver may be unable to work, and many costs of health care are simply not covered by other means (Capen and Dedlow, 1998; Dittbrenner, 1999).

# Effective Home Care

Providing home-based care for children gives the nurse an opportunity to assess and interact with the family in their environment. This assessment can provide the health care team with valuable information about safety, support systems, nutrition, parental ability, and actual health care practices. This valuable information will determine future decisions for individualized care and realistic outcomes (Engel, 1997; Thompson, 2000).

There are two distinct areas of implementation of care for the pediatric home care nurse. Nurses who perform *intermittent skilled nursing visits* may see many different types and numbers of patients each day. These nurses typically have a caseload assigned to them and accept responsibility for implementing the plan of care.

---

## Box 25-1 ■ ■ □
### Intermittent Skilled Nursing and Private Duty Nursing

**INTERMITTENT SKILLED NURSING**
*Health Care Need*
- ☐ Child at risk: parental substance abuse, nonorganic failure to thrive
- ☐ Chronically ill, but medically stable child with multiple skilled nursing needs

*Intervention*
- ☐ Regular scheduled visits to assess patient status, evaluate home environment, teach parenting skills, determine status of growth and development, goal setting with family for positive health outcomes
- ☐ As-needed home visits during illness exacerbation to assess physical status and determine appropriate intervention

*Health Care Need*
- ☐ Skilled procedures: regularly scheduled injections/infusions, dressing changes, phototherapy

*Intervention*
- ☐ Regular visits of limited duration to perform skilled nursing intervention, assess parental ability/desire to perform procedure, teach procedure technique, supervise parental performance of procedure

**PRIVATE DUTY NURSING**
*Health Care Need*
- ☐ Technology-dependent child (e.g., ventilator or oxygen use)
- ☐ Chronically ill child with multiple skilled nursing needs

*Intervention*
- ☐ Provide direct nursing care for specified time to accomplish activities of daily living, respite for parental caregiver
- ☐ Provide assessment of patient status, evaluate home environment, teach parenting skills, determine status of growth and development, goal setting with family for positive health outcomes

---

Nurses who perform *private duty nursing* or block nursing are usually assigned individual patients, and they remain in the home for a predetermined amount of time (e.g., 8- or 12-hour block of time). The plan of care is implemented over the course of the time in the home.

Required nursing skills will be determined by patient need, parental ability, complexity of family, and the home environment. In both types of home care, the pediatric nurse is responsible for patient and family assessment, evaluating the appropriateness of the plan of care (Petit de Mange, 1998) (Box 25-1).

From technology dependence to pain management to failure to thrive, pediatric nurses are appropriate professionals to affect a child's health care needs at home. Quality interdisciplinary care can create a significant, positive impact on family coping and child outcomes (Box 25-2) (Betz, 2000; Bilodeau, 1995; Black and others, 1995; Reifsnider, 1996; Chan and Filippone, 1998; Cuthbert-Allman and Burrows, 1998; Mahony and Murphy, 1999).

Adequate family training and preparation
Primary care physician willing to oversee medical aspects of care
Professional caregivers trained in relevant nursing and communication skills
Developmental intervention (e.g., physical, occupational, and speech therapy, early intervention)
Appropriately designed and well-maintained equipment
Supportive therapies (e.g., respiratory therapy, parenteral therapy, nutritional support)
Adequate social and psychologic support services
High-quality respite care
Appropriate home renovation
Telephone service in the home
Appropriate transportation
Appropriate locally available emergency facilities
Competent case management services

Modified from Office of Technology Assessment (OTA), Congress of the United States: *Technology dependent children: hospital v. home care—a technical memorandum* (OTA-TM-H-38), Washington, DC, 1987, U.S. Government Printing Office; and Bakewell-Sachs S, Porth S: Discharge planning and home care of the technology-dependent infant, *J Obstet Gynecol Neonat Nurs* 24(1):77-83, 1995.

## Discharge Planning and Selection of a Home Care Agency

Identifying appropriate local community resources is critical to a successful transfer to home care. The ultimate goal of discharge planning is for the family to become familiar with the child's needs and to be competent in providing that care. A discharge plan should include emergency management and provision of social and emotional support (Neal and Kieffer, 1998; Townsend, 1997). General guidelines for discharge that allow for family individuality provide for ideal outcomes (Barnes, 1997) (Box 25-3).

The American Academy of Pediatrics Committee on Children with Disabilities (1995b) states that "the goal for a home health care program for infants, children, or adolescents with chronic conditions is the provision of comprehensive, cost-effective health care within a nurturing home environment that maximizes the capabilities of the individual and minimizes the effects of the disabilities. This may be established to prevent hospitalization or reduce the length of hospitalization."

**NURSING TIP**  If home care equipment is different than hospital equipment, deliver portable equipment to the hospital to allow family use before discharge.

Much of the success of home care, particularly for the child who is dependent on medical technology or has complex medical problems, depends on careful planning and preparation. General principles of discharge planning and the transition to home care are presented in Chapter 26. Discharge planning must begin early, should be based on criteria of child and family readiness (AWHONN, 1993), must be a multidisciplinary process and include representatives from inpatient and home care/community settings, and must in-

Fully trained pediatric staff to provide for all aspects of care (nursing, rehabilitation therapies, pharmacy, dietitian, social worker, home medical equipment)
Prompt responsive staff with 24-hour availability
Family-centered care
Comprehensive continuing education programs
Certification of local, state, and federal regulatory agencies
Accreditation by Joint Commission on Accreditation of Healthcare Organizations (JCAHO) or Community Health Accreditation Program (CHAP)

Data from Dittbrenner H: Pediatric home care as a viable new service, *Caring*, 18(2):12-15, 1999; and Lovejoy D: *Making the transition to home health nursing: a practical guide*, New York, 1997, Springer Publishing.

volve the family. Predischarge assessment (Box 25-4) and planning should include the following areas:

- The child's medical, nursing, educational, and other therapeutic needs
- Family members' (including siblings') education and training, coping skills, and adjustment needs
- Community readiness in areas such as availability of equipment, appropriate nursing and other personnel, educational and developmental services, respite care, and emergency plans
- Financial arrangements

Creative financial planning, including negotiating arrangements with the insurance company, health maintenance or managed care organization, and public programs may be required.

Early involvement of the home care agency in the discharge planning process promotes continuity of care and a smooth transition from hospital to home. Before discharge, a general plan, sometimes called an *Individualized Home Care Plan (IHCP)*, should be developed with multidisciplinary input (American Academy of Pediatrics, 1995b). This plan should address the range of needs identified as part of the comprehensive predischarge assessment.*

**NURSING TIP**  An excellent method of providing home care instructions is with video recordings. Once the family masters the procedures, consider video recording their performance. Visual learning is most helpful for people who cannot read or who are not fluent in English (Bryant, Davis, and Lagrone, 1997).

The plans for transition from hospital to home should include family members (ideally two persons) both learning and demonstrating all aspects of the child's care in the hospital. An in-hospital trial period, during which parents provide total care for the child, is generally beneficial. After a successful trial, the family may benefit from taking the child home on a brief pass before making final discharge plans. (This arrangement may need to be negotiated with the insurance company.) The home care nurse plays an important

---

*Numerous care plans and home care instruction sheets, which may be copied and given to families, are available in Wong DL, Hess CS: *Wong and Whaley's clinical manual of pediatric nursing*, ed 5, St Louis, 2000, Mosby.

## Box 25-4

### Example of Predischarge Assessment for Technology-Dependent Infant

1. **The child's family**
   Identification and training of primary caretakers
   Identification and training of caretakers for respite and emergency care
   Parent employment status while caring for child at home
   Family financial picture, especially if one parent must stop working
   Sibling preparation
   Availability of psychosocial support services
2. **Technical equipment and supplies for the home**
   Home care company's availability and experience
   Home care company's coordination of services with local health care provider and others
   24-hour availability and coverage for unexpected situations
3. **Community nursing and support services**
   Availability, training, and experience
   Adequacy of number of personnel to meet needs
   Additional training of staff, if needed
   24-hour availability of ambulance services
4. **Physical environment of the home**
   Adequacy of space for equipment and supplies
   Heavy equipment (e.g., ventilator, $O_2$ tanks, compressor) accessibility
   Layout of home (e.g., number of floors, stairways, room accessibility, room sizes)
   Location and layout of bedrooms
   Adequacy of apartment building elevator and fire escape
   Telephone access
   Type of transportation family uses
   Possibility of modifying living space to minimize invasiveness of technology without isolating child
   Adequacy of heating and cooling systems
   Adequacy of electrical system to accommodate equipment
5. **Emergency plan**
   Identification and training of those involved
   Written implementation plan: who, what, where, when, how (include telephone numbers)
   Notification of utility companies for priority repairs and maintenance
   Notification of emergency medical unit (911)
   Emergency drill
6. **Primary care provider**
   Identification of local primary provider/pediatrician able to assume direct care responsibility and coordinate other care providers
   Inclusion of local provider in discharge planning
   Needs of local provider before child's discharge

From Bakewell-Sachs S, Porth S: Discharge planning and home care of the technology-dependent infant, *J Obstet Gynecol Neonat Nurs* 24(1):77-83, 1995.

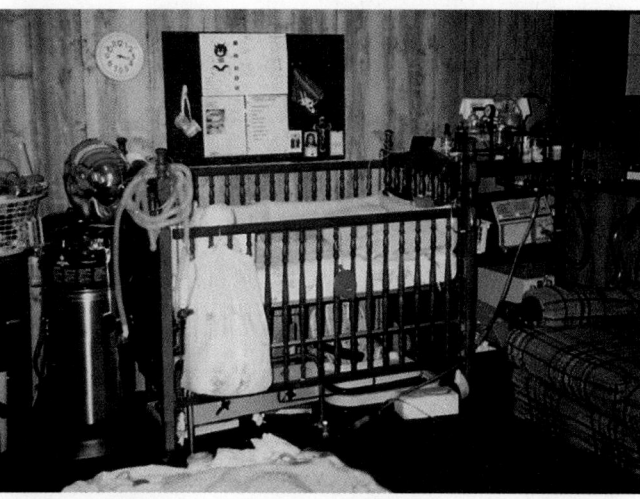

**Fig. 25-1** An essential aspect of preparation for home care is the arrangement of equipment and supplies.

## Box 25-5

### Critical Home Care Referral Information

Scheduled medications
Durable medical equipment (DME)
Medical supplies
Transportation needs
Adaptive equipment
Rehabilitation therapies (occupational therapy [OT], physical therapy [PT], speech)
Psychologic counseling
Social work referral
Nursing care
Respite plans
Key family members
Demographic information
Reimbursement information

Modified from Townsend JL: Assessment of the child and family. In Votroubek WL, Townsend JL, editors: *Pediatric home care*, ed 2, Gaithersburg, MD, 1997, Aspen.

role in assessing this experience with the family. Whether or not the child is taken home on a pass, a predischarge home visit offers the home care nurse the opportunity to meet the family, help them assess their preparedness and the preparedness of the home environment, discuss plans for arranging the child's equipment at home (Fig. 25-1), reinforce prior discharge teaching, and implement any additional teaching that may be necessary (American Academy of Pediatrics, 1998; Bakewell-Sachs and others, 2000; Gamblian, Hess, and Kenner, 1998).

A comprehensive discharge plan includes the IHCP, specific written instructions to facilitate continuity, and detailed information about home care expectations (Box 25-5).

## Case Management

Traditional definitions of **case management** generally focus on cost control, attainment of desired clinical outcomes, and the monitoring and evaluation of care provided. However, for optimum home care of the child who is technology-dependent, case management—or **care coordination**—should be viewed more broadly.

Care coordination has several purposes. Its primary goal is ensuring continuity for the child and family across hospital, home, educational, therapeutic, and other settings. Care should be coordinated among multiple providers to reduce the complexity of care for the child, reduce fragmentation of care, and decrease the burden of care for the family. Care coordination should ensure that the medical, nursing, and health maintenance needs of the child, as well as the financial issues, psychosocial concerns, and educational needs of the child and family, are addressed (American Academy of Pediatrics, 1999; Dittbrenner, 1999).

> **Box 25-6**
> ### Care Coordination for Children with Special Health Care Needs
>
> Facilitate timely access to services and resources
> Promote continuity of care
> Provide family support and enhance family well-being
> Improve health, developmental, educational, vocational, psychosocial, and functional outcomes
> Maximize efficient, effective use of resources
>
> ---
>
> Modified from Presler B: Care coordination for children with special health care needs, *Orthop Nurs* 17(25 suppl):45-51, 1998.

> **Box 25-7**
> ### Qualities of a Pediatric Home Care Nurse
>
> Demonstrates flexibility in skills and case management
> Recognizes that the nurse is a guest in the home
> Respects family culture and adapts appropriately
> Works as an interdisciplinary team member
> Demonstrates expertise in pediatric care

Care coordination is most effective if a single person works with the family to accomplish the many tasks and responsibilities involved (Box 25-6). The *nurse case manager* should have a minimum of a baccalaureate degree in nursing and 3 years' experience (American Nurses Association, 1988). The nurse should also be knowledgeable about community resources, including the following: primary, secondary, and tertiary health care services; speech, language, hearing, and vision resources; respite care services; financial assistance programs; parent groups; advocacy groups; local, state, and federal public officials; transportation services; and private sector individuals with an interest in children with disabilities (Thompson, 2000).

Although professionals must always see part of their role as ensuring that integrated, coordinated care is provided, care coordination should promote the family's role as primary decision maker and enhance the family's capability to meet the special needs of the child and the family unit (Petit de Mange, 1998; Townsend, 1997). Families may choose to be involved to varying degrees in the tasks constituting coordination of their child's care. Many parents will take on increasing responsibility for care coordination over time; they should be encouraged and supported in this role. Home care nurses and case managers should be aware that the termination of private duty or home care nursing can be a difficult transition for which families may need preparation (Agazio, 1997).

## Role of the Nurse, Training, and Standards of Care

The home care nurse must share a level of technical expertise with the critical care nurse while being able to adapt equipment, procedures, and the nursing process to the home setting. (See Chapters 27, 28, and 31 and many citations in the references for specific technical skills that may be required in home care practice.) The need for technical expertise must be matched by a knowledge of child development and the ability to work creatively with the child who is challenged by chronic illness and technology dependence. When practicing in the home, the nurse must be comfortable making independent nursing judgments and problem solving with no immediate assistance. At the same time the nurse must have excellent interpersonal skills, an ability to work with other professionals and the family, and,

most important, an ability to respect family autonomy. Patient outcomes are more readily achieved with a balance of nursing skills that demonstrate clinical excellence, adaptability, accountability, and the ability to develop positive relationships with patients and families (Petit de Mange, 1998) (Box 25-7).

When working with a home care agency, nurses should expect to receive patient placements appropriate to their expertise. They should also expect to receive orientation to the skills and knowledge base of the home health care nursing specialty and subsequent continuing education to develop as expert practitioners (Chan and Filippone, 1998; Pignatello and others, 1998). The minimum initial orientation should include the following areas: the individual patient's care plan and equipment needs; the agency's policies and procedures, including procedures for addressing any problems that may occur when care is provided in the home; legal liability issues; and documentation procedures.

Stronger emphasis should be placed on issues specific to home care. For example, the nursing care plan should be based on information obtained about the environment, family dynamics, and health-related behaviors (Petit de Mange, 1998; Slack and McEwen, 1999; Weber, 1998; Zerull, 1999).

In addition, reimbursement-driven documentation in home care differs from documentation practices in the hospital setting; increasingly, documentation must be written in specific ways to qualify for reimbursement (Lovejoy, 1997).

Supervision of practice, including occasional site visits by a nursing supervisor, should be provided. Mentoring or precepting is ideal. Because of the unique practice environment of home health nurses, it is important for an agency to facilitate sharing among peers to decrease work-related stress, increase job satisfaction, and support quality patient care (Moore and Katz, 1996).

Public or private home care agencies that participate in the Medicare or Medicaid programs must be certified by a federally designated state certifying body and abide by federal and state regulations. Additionally, the **American Nurses' Association (ANA)** has developed standards of nursing practice for both community health and home health nurses (ANA, 1986a,b). Generalist and clinical specialist certification in both home health and community health is offered by the **American Nurses Credentialing Center (ANCC),*** a subsidiary of ANA (Wilson, 1996). **The Hospice**

---

*c/o ANA, 600 Maryland Ave SW, Suite 100-W, Washington, DC 20024-2571, (202) 651-7000, (800) 284-2378, fax: (202) 651-7001; www.nursingworld.org/ancc.

**Nurses Association** offers certification in hospice nursing. Despite important differences between pediatric and adult care in the home, as of this writing no national standards specific to pediatric home care practice have been developed. Nursing practice in pediatric home care should be guided by published guidelines, books, and articles related to pediatric home care.

## FAMILY-CENTERED HOME CARE

Technology dependence, chronic illness, and complex care requirements cross social, cultural, and economic boundaries. Regardless of a family's background, family values must be respected in the provision of home care services. *The home is the family's domain,* and the child is at home because the family's central role is to nurture and raise their child. The ultimate responsibility for managing the child's health, developmental, and emotional needs lies with the family. The nurse must respect the family's central role in the care of the child and must work in collaboration with the family in efforts to care for the child. Family-centered nursing practice is essential in the home setting (Hostler, 1999; Townsend, 1997).

The philosophic basis for family-centered practice is the recognition that the family is the constant in the child's life, whereas the service systems and personnel within those systems fluctuate. Professionals working with families of children with complex chronic problems must respect the family's central, caring role, their knowledge, and their particular and unique expertise. Families have the most intimate knowledge of the child's strengths and abilities, the challenges of providing care, and the abilities and needs of other family members (Messinger and Dolan, 1997; Newton, 2000). *Believing that no one knows the child better than the family* is critical to the success of any health care plan.

### Respect for Diversity

Respect for varied family structures and for racial, ethnic, cultural, and socioeconomic diversity among families is essential in home care. Home care nurses work in close relationship with family members. (See Family Focus box.) The nurse shares in these relationships, participating in care throughout the course of illness. The nurse must assess and respect the family's background and lifestyle choices. Particular attention is given to *communication.* The meaning of the words used and the way in which they are said may affect various cultural groups in different ways. Volume of speech and language style must be taken into consideration as part of a family cultural assessment.

**NURSING TIP** Color-coded medication bottles, written schedules, and pillboxes or oral syringes may aid compliance with prescription administration. Do not assume that everyone who speaks English can read the language.

In addition, the nurse must pay particular attention to nonverbal communication. Body language, eye contact, and degree of physical contact have different meanings within a particular culture.

**FAMILY FOCUS**

*Developing a Relationship with Culturally Diverse Families*

I work in the inner city, and my home care patients come from a variety of racial and ethnic backgrounds. I am Caucasian, from Australia. Often, when I first visit a family, there is an initial coolness or apprehension toward me. This is understandable because I am a stranger, and perhaps families think I'll judge them in one way or another. By the end of the first visit, however, there is usually a smile as I leave; by the second visit they often greet me with a smile at the door; and by the third visit we usually have a friendship, a trust, and an ease of communication.

If I'm working on a case for an extended time, I use a holistic nursing approach. This involves being aware of how the illness of the child affects the entire family. As I listen over many weeks to their fears and questions, and often as I share faith perspectives, a bond begins to form. I find it a privilege to share in their joys and their pain, and I feel rewarded by the trust that they invest in me.

Julie Edgerton, RN
Home Care Nurse
Children's National Medical Center
Washington, DC

Families may also differ in their cultural view of children, in childrearing practices, and in their view of illness, its causes, and its meaning. The family's **health care practices and beliefs** may influence the level of investment a family will make in the child's care. The family's health care beliefs and folk and healing practices may be foreign to the nurse's background and experience (Cuthbert-Allman and Burrows, 1998; McNeal, 1998).

*Religion* is another area that can have a major influence on a family's response to their child with special needs. The family will often look for spiritual meaning and purpose for illness. In other instances, the family may reject past religious ties. This is particularly true if the impact of illness causes prolonged grief. In either case, the religious background of individuals within the family will influence coping with the illness.

A variety of cultural assessment tools are available (Davidhizar, Havnes, and Bechtel, 1999; Spruhan, 1996). The home care nurse, aware that **personal values** drive behavior, needs to learn about the family's culture, ask questions without implying judgment, interpret the mainstream medical culture, and help families design interventions that meet their preferences (Davidhizar, Havnes, and Bechtel, 1999; McNeal, 1998). When possible, culture-specific teaching materials should be used (Spruhan, 1996).

Respect for family diversity and an awareness of family developmental stages and the stages of a family's adjustment to a child's illness (Newby, 1996) will assist the home care nurse in recognizing and promoting family strengths and in respecting various coping mechanisms. Labels such as "dysfunctional," "difficult," and "noncompliant" can reinforce negative expectations and shape the behaviors of both parents and professionals (Hostler, 1999; MacPhee, 1995). On the other hand, identifying, emphasizing, and building on family strengths and coping mechanisms are strategies that promote a central goal in nursing care of the child and family: family empowerment. The nurse working with families should remain flexible and open-minded because new family strengths may emerge over time and coping mechanisms may wax and wane with the stresses of caring for a child with serious or multiple problems (Hart, 1999).

## Parent-Professional Collaboration

Family-centered nursing practice is built on a foundation of parent-professional collaboration, which represents a shift from the traditional unidirectional relationships between health care providers and families. The **Collaborative Family Health Care Coalition** has developed core competencies for professionals collaborating with families (McDaniel and Campbell, 1996). *Collaborative caring* allows the nurse and family to work together and share outcomes in a deep and meaningful way. This approach, essential in the home care setting, is characterized by the following (Gaudet, 1997; Kellet and Mannion, 1999):

- Encouraging activities to develop self-confidence and self-esteem
- Displaying increased awareness and respect for family caregivers
- Recognizing that families vary in defining their role
- Demonstrating an ability to understand the family's approach to caregiving

- Sharing perspectives, not just tasks and functions
- Supporting family in their primary, irreplaceable role as caregiver
- Exchanging expertise in providing care to the child
- Assisting family in recognizing their contributions as worthwhile
- Identifying strengths and resources of child and family
- Negotiating options, priorities, and preferences
- Assisting coping by allowing family to find meaning in caring

Communication with the family should not be invasive. There is no need to collect information from the family that can be obtained from the child's records. The nurse should explain to the family the reason for questions, particularly those that the family may perceive as intrusive, and should tell families who will have access to the information. (See Critical Thinking Exercise Box.) The nurse must also assure families that they have a right to expect confidentiality in regard to the data collected. When working in the home, the nurse must respect the privacy of family communications that may be overheard.

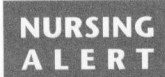 **NURSING ALERT**  Home care nurses should restrict their communications with other professionals to clinically relevant information about the family.

---

 *Critical Thinking Exercise*

### Family-Centered Home Care and Conflicts

After the family agreed to learn how to administer intravenous (IV) antibiotics, Patricia, a 4-year-old with cystic fibrosis, was discharged home. The family has been supervised by the home care nurse and has been performing the medication administration quite well. On day 3 of home care, the nurse reminds the parents that it is policy that the IV site be changed. The IV site is without redness, and the child denies pain or discomfort during infusion or flushing. The parents and child become very upset and refuse the procedure.

FIRST, THINK ABOUT IT . . .

- What conclusions are you reaching?
- If you accept your conclusions, what are the implications?

1. Refuse to alter the plan because infection and phlebitis are potential outcomes in keeping a peripheral IV in place longer than 3 days. Try to persuade the family toward restarting the IV today.
2. Allow the parents to assume responsibility for any adverse outcomes of not changing the peripheral IV. Agree that the child has been through enough.
3. Don't change the IV. Watch for signs and symptoms of infiltration and infection.
4. Acknowledge the child and family's desire. Explore specific reasons for not wanting to change the IV. Explore options with the family.

*The best response is four. The basis of a good nurse-child-family relationshp is to engage in nonbiased communication. Engaging the family in this way encourages trust. The process of negotiation over this issue builds the foundation for future interactions.*

*The family may have legitimate reasons for wanting their daughter spared from unnecessary IV starts. The nurse should*

*inquire about these reasons. The parents may feel that this most recent hospitalization, as well as previous hospitalizations, may have affected the child's emotional well-being because of multiple painful IV starts. Health care professionals may have overlooked the importance of anticipatory anxiety that a child experiences before a painful procedure. The family may be striving to maintain as much normalcy as possible. This is an admirable goal, making option one not the best choice.*

*Option two is not the best choice. The home care nurse must work with the parents to determine the best outcome for their child. The parent probably does not have the complete knowledge base to accept total responsibility for their decision. The nurse should be certain that the family understands the possible risks of not changing the peripheral IV as suggested by policy.*

*Likewise, option three is not the best choice. Professional expertise can provide valuable guidance on approaching a painful procedure. Suggestions such as EMLA cream or guided imagery may change the adverse experience of a painful IV start. This approach is perfect for a preschool-age child. The topical anesthetic can be described as "magic cream" and may make the procedure more tolerable.*

*Option four encourages the nurse and the family to discuss the issue, to plan for consultations and evaluation with the practitioner, and to meet the family's goals of decreasing emotional stress. Communication between the nurse and the child and family may also lead to other approaches for decreasing stress. For example, include the child in the procedure by having her hold the band-aid or swab the tubing injection site with alcohol. The home care nurse can teach the parents how to comfort their child during these stressful events. Finally, the nurse may assist the family in planning for the placement of a long-term infusion device such as a percutaneously inserted central catheter (PICC) line.*

Communication with family members should include sharing with the family, in a supportive manner, complete and unbiased information about all aspects of the child's condition and care (Chapman, 1998). Parents often feel overwhelming frustration related to obtaining accurate information about their child's illness and its management. Parents want information given slowly and repeated as necessary over time; they want explanations in terms they can understand; and they want the opportunity to ask questions, which should be answered in a straightforward manner. Stating "I don't know" or "I'll find out" is better than pretending to know or giving excuses. A plan can be made with the parents to gather relevant information when necessary (Hanson and Randall, 1999; Newton, 2000). Information should be shared with families in a way that has meaning in their cultural context (Davidhizar, Havnes, and Bechtel, 1999). Many parents report a preference for interactions with professionals who communicate empathy and concern. Families will vary in the amount and delivery of information they can tolerate regarding the status of their child.

On occasion, disagreements may arise between parents and nurses over proper procedures for care of the child. Nurses should respect parental preferences in any situation that does not pose danger or risk for the child. (See Family Focus box.) If parents wish to alter a plan of treatment that is part of medical orders, the nurse should ask that they negotiate the change with the practitioner because the nurse must follow the written medical orders. If disagreements cannot be resolved, a home care supervisor or case manager should be contacted to assist with problem solving. Increasingly, home care agencies are developing ethics committees and policies for managing difficult situations such as treatment refusal (Salladay, 1995). (See Critical Thinking Exercise box.)

## The Nursing Process

In the home the family is a partner in each step of the nursing process. Assessment should address family strengths and

---

 **FAMILY FOCUS**
*Knowledgeable Parents*

It is not unusual for parents, particularly those whose children have chronic illnesses or complex care regimens, to be more knowledgable about their child's condition than a nurse who is assigned to the child's care. This can be disconcerting for both the parent(s) and the nurse. It is important to remember and reinforce that, regardless of the condition, parents will always know more about their child than the professional caring for the child. The nurse and parents can set goals for care in an atmosphere of mutual respect. If the parents' goal is respite from prolonged caregiving, they are less likely to want to give long explanations about the child's care, and assistance from an experienced peer may be more appropriate for the nurse to seek. If the parents wish to maintain maximum participation in care delivery, the nurse and the parents can negotiate the collaboration.

When teaching parents to perform complex chronic care regimens at home, include teaching them to expect to know more about their child's care than professionals who may come to assist them, whether that be home health, hospital, or outpatient personnel. At the same time, assure them that what various professionals who work with them *will have* from working with a multitude of families is a scientific knowledge base and a wealth of options for addressing and solving care problems.

Teresa L. Hall MS, RN
Hathaway Children's Services
Sylmar, CA

---

## Critical Thinking Exercise

### *Medical Neglect*

An 8-year-old child experienced a burn to her left arm. After a lengthy hospitalization the child was discharged home. The discharge orders included a home care referral with orders for the child to receive a twice-daily dressing change. The home care nurse visits in the morning for the first dressing change and for assessment of wound status. The parent has been instructed to change the dressing approximately 12 hours later. The nurse returns the next day and finds that the mother did not change the dressing as instructed. The nurse is responsible for all of the following actions *except* which?

FIRST, THINK ABOUT IT . . .

• What conclusions are you reaching?
• If you accept your conclusions, what are the implications?

---

1. Educating and counseling the family about the importance and reasons for twice-daily dressing changes.
2. Reporting the family for medical neglect.
3. Assessing the wound for any signs of infection.
4. Documenting the missed dressing change and corrective measures taken.

---

*The best answer is two. It is correct to conclude that some behaviors that might be considered medical neglect may actually be the result of other issues. The nurse should question the family about reasons for the missed dressing change. The family may feel overwhelmed with the responsibility of the dressing change. This may be the first time the mom has actually been alone, without professional assistance in changing the dressing. Also the child may have had a different reaction during the dressing change during the attempt the previous evening. Assess for pain and the need for premedication and other behavioral interventions before and during the dressing change. Role model parenting techniques for the mother to use for the dressing change. Allow the child to assist with preparation or holding dressing supplies during the procedure. On the other hand, the family may not understand the process of wound healing and need the information presented to them again. Always consider the frequency and severity of noncompliance. Missing a dressing change once may be handled with counseling and documentation. On the other hand, frequently missed dressing changes may result in infection or readmission to the hospital. The practitioner should be notified soon after the home care nurse recognizes repeated noncompliance. The point where these instances cross the line into mandated reporting depends in part on the definitions of abuse or neglect in the state in which services are provided.*

**Box 25-8** ■ ■ ■
**Sample Family Assessment Questions**

☐ What are the child and family's past experiences, expectations of disease/illness?
☐ How does that affect the current situation?
☐ Is the current coping status a reflection of a new condition? Same chronic condition? Or new phase in chronic condition?
☐ How can the nurse address family needs and promote health among all family members?
☐ What specific nursing interventions will facilitate a healthy response to child and family limitations caused by the illness?

Modified from Gedaly-Duff V, Heims ML: Family child health nursing. In Hanson SMH, Boyd ST, editors: *Family health care nursing*, Philadelphia, 1996, FA Davis.

**FAMILY FOCUS**
*What I Learned About Home Care*

I learned many things as a result of having home care for four children over a period of 8 years. Two of the major areas I learned about were communication and families' rights. It took a long time to learn some of these things.

Initially I tried very hard to be sensitive to the professionals and often put my own feelings and needs aside. It took a while to learn that I could stand up for myself and my family and that my child could continue to receive good care. One area important to me was to have nurses withhold judgment on our parenting style, even if they might have parented differently.

Communication needs to be open and two-way. Families and nurses ought to tell each other what is going well. For example, "Thanks for keeping the room so neat while you're here" can help a nurse see a family's appreciation. There was so little I could do as just "Mommy" that it really meant a lot to me when nurses would say, "That's such a cute outfit you picked out for him today." Communicating about little things, even inconsequential topics such as favorite TV shows, makes it easier to communicate about more important things and about problems. Communication has to be open about problems, too.

Jeni Stepanek
Mother
Upper Marlboro, MD

resources.* (See Family Assessment, Chapter 6.) The principles of communication discussed previously guide data collection. The nurse's observations are shared neutrally, without value judgment, and in a way that preserves the family's own role in decision making (Townsend, 1997).

All information gathered as part of the assessment process is shared with the family. The nurse should recognize that the family's perception of their most important need will generally guide their behavior and consume their attention and energy (Box 25-8). Family priorities should guide the planning process (Ross, 1997).

Both short- and long-term goals should be outlined and agreed on by the child, family, and professionals involved. The plan of care should integrate various disciplines that may be involved with the child to minimize duplication and consolidate care requirements. Cross-training of professionals and a transdisciplinary mode of treatment can also be useful when a child has multiple and complex care requirements (Rothkopf and Rothkopf, 1997). For example, certain physical or occupational therapy routines may be incorporated into the child's morning nursing procedures, or speech therapy interventions may be conducted by the parent or nurse around eating times so that the entire day is not occupied by procedures. A written schedule of daily routines should be developed and followed by all caregivers.

**NURSING TIP** At each visit physically handle and look at all medications. Check them against the medical orders. Read the labels. There may be discrepancies, duplications, or changes between hospitalizations. Clear up confusions for the family.

Goals of care are supported by intervention strategies that reflect normalization (see Chapter 22) and the interests and abilities of the child and family. Nurses can help the family explore a range of alternative strategies, services, and resources so that the family can choose the best match for their situation.

Family participation in evaluating a home care plan can occur on several levels. Families and care providers should regularly review the goals of care and update the care plan as required. The nurse can ask the family open-ended questions at regular intervals to assess their opinions on the effectiveness of care (Townsend, 1997). As part of the evaluation process, families should be acknowledged for their successes and accomplishments. Finally, families should be given an opportunity to evaluate the home care agency and other service providers periodically. The evaluations should be used by the agency to improve quality of care. (See Family Focus box.)

In addition to maintaining a sense of control over their child's care, families need to control their home and personal lives (Messinger and Dolan, 1997). For this reason, nurses should discuss "house rules" with the family and address issues such as the physical environment, private areas in the home, responsibility for maintaining the child's environment, and interactions with siblings. (See Guidelines box.)

Home care nursing encourages a close and rewarding relationship with the family. One of the most important aspects of this relationship is maintaining professional boundaries and a therapeutic role that is supportive but not intrusive (McKlindon and Barsteiner, 1999). (See Critical Thinking Exercise box.)

## Promotion of Optimum Development, Self-Care, and Education

There is little question that living at home offers most children with complex medical problems great social and emotional advantages over living in the hospital or other institutional setting. (See Evidence-Based Practice box on p. 1026.) However, in infancy and throughout the developmental

*Self-report instruments to help families identify concerns, priorities, resources, and sources of support include *Family Needs Survey*, available from **Frank Porter Graham Child Development Center**, CB No 8180, 105 Smith Level Rd, University of North Carolina, Chapel Hill, NC 27599, (919) 966-2622; www.fpg.unc.edu.

## GUIDELINES
### *Negotiating "House Rules" for Home Care*

**HOUSE RULES**

**Parking:** Where to park and community regulations.
**Access:** Where to enter the home. Is knocking preferred or ringing the bell?
**Personal belongings:** Where does the nurse store own coat, boots, etc.? Does the family prefer slippers to shoes in the home?
**Meals:** Where may the nurse store own food? NOTE: This is very important given cultural diversity of clients.
**Radio and television:** Identify preferences regarding usage. Remember, this may help nurses to remain awake at night.
**Patient room:** The nurse is responsible for the child's immediate environment. Maintaining a clean working area and cleaning up the room at the end of the shift is the nurse's responsibility.
**Telephone:** Agency policy may dictate that all personal calls be limited to very brief time periods and be charged to the nurse making them. NOTE: Many nurses do need to check in with home at some interval during the evening.
**Visitors:** Identify who may enter the home when the parents are away (that is, child's friends or grandparents). A list of names should be available.
**Privacy:** Describe what parts of the home are off-limits to the nurse and at what times.

**CHILD**

**Routine:** Specify times for playtime, bathtime, and bedtime. What does the parent want to participate in regarding these routines?
**Mealtime:** Specify where the family wants the child fed; if tube fed, specify a preference as to how and where it is done.
**Clothing:** Identify who picks out the child's clothes. Identify where the laundry is and who is responsible for washing the sick child's clothing.
**Discipline:** Discuss specific guidelines for discipline.
**Homework:** Discuss when it should be done and who is responsible for it being completed.

**SIBLINGS**

**Discipline:** Establish guidelines regarding how parents should be informed of siblings' conflicts and how discipline should be handled. NOTE: Parents or another caregiver must be in the home when siblings are home.
**Patient care:** Be specific regarding how children have helped with the child's care. Discuss any concerns regarding behavior that may compromise the child's or siblings' safety.

**NURSING**

**Parental notification:** Specify what information the family wishes to be aware of immediately and what can wait until they are home.
**Limits of responsibility:** Specify duties the nurse may not perform, such as transportation of the child to care facilities.
**Environment:** Discuss the need to have adequate lighting and a comfortable working area.

***

Modified from Klug R: Clarifying roles and expectations in home care, *Pediatr Nurs* 19(4):375, 1993.

## *Critical Thinking Exercise*

### *Maintaining Therapeutic Boundaries*

You are a home care nurse and have been working with a 3-year-old child who is ventilator dependent. You have been visiting the Jones family several days a week for the last 5 months. You notice that the parents are arguing increasingly. Some of the arguments are about whether Mr. Jones helps enough with the child's care. Mrs. Jones approaches you to complain about her husband. Depending on your relationship with the family, you might do any of the following *except* which?

FIRST, THINK ABOUT IT . . .

• What concepts or ideas are central to your thinking?
• If you accept the conclusions, what are the implications?

***

1. Mention that home care can be stressful for a family.
2. Indicate that you can provide referrals for counseling should the parents want them.
3. Agree with Mrs. Jones that her husband is not contributing enough to the child's care.
4. Listen and reflect with Mrs. Jones about her feelings.

***

*The best response is three. The concept of therapeutic boundaries supports the idea that they are not rigid and fixed. They must be responsive to the relationship preferred by the family and the style in which the family operates. For this reason, depending on the family, options one, two, or four (or a combination) might be most appropriate. For any conclusion you may arrive at, it would be inappropriate to agree with Mrs. Jones that her husband is not helping enough with the child's care. Such an action implies a judgment that is not within the nurse's role to make and undermines rather than supports the family system.*

***

regression can occur in response to stress; fatigue may result from an underlying pathologic condition, the flare of an illness, or medication side effects; and equipment requirements may impede mobility, exploration, and independence. The challenge of providing support for normal development in a child who is chronically ill and technology dependent is to optimize the opportunities for developmentally appropriate experiences within the constraints posed by the medical condition and the equipment requirements (Jaffe and others, 1998).

Home care plans are designed to promote optimum child development through assessment, planning, and referrals and by interventions that address normalization issues and self-care (Box 25-9). General principles for a family-centered assessment and planning process have been addressed earlier in this chapter and are also applied in developmental assessment and planning.

Some parents may not pursue developmental intervention because they do not believe their child needs the services. In this case professionals need to explain the child's developmental needs to parents in ways that are meaningful from the parents' own cultural and socioeconomic perspectives. Only then can parents make truly informed decisions.

stages, a child's medical condition(s) and the dependence on medical technology can place constraints on and pose challenges to *normal development.* For example, the child may have lengthy and repeated hospitalizations; developmental

## EVIDENCE-BASED PRACTICE
### *High-Risk Children and Nurses' Roles and Responsibilities*

Caring for special needs children at home is commonplace in today's health care environment. Children who are chronically ill or technology dependent generally have a predictable, well-defined plan of care. Intervention and outcome goals are typically concrete and easily measured. On the other hand, children who are at high risk for poor outcomes may have more difficulty accessing home care services. This may be due to lack of incentives for third-party reimbursement or a poorly defined nursing intervention. The following demonstrates the importance of home care nursing and the impact it can have on this high-risk population.

1. Who are high-risk children, and how might home care nursing make a difference? This category of children may include infants born to mothers with little or no prenatal care, drug/alcohol-exposed infants, children diagnosed with nonorganic failure to thrive (NOFTT), children with suspected abuse/neglect, children with developmental delay, and children of parents with poor parenting skills. Home care pediatric nurses are in a perfect position to evaluate the family and child in their own living environment. This allows the nurse to see exactly what health care and parenting practices are actually occurring in the home. For example, teaching or role modeling a desired behavior can be implemented in an informal, less threatening environment. In addition, the nurse can assess alterations in growth and development and intervene in a timely manner (Reifsnider, 1996).
2. How has pediatric home care nursing been shown to effect a positive outcome for high-risk children? Several studies have been conducted to evaluate the effectiveness of home care programs in children with NOFTT. Black and others (1995) compared children who were followed with weekly home care visits plus multidisciplinary clinic evaluations vs clinic visits only. The study evaluated physical growth; cognitive, motor, and language

development; parent-child behavior during feeding; and the home environment. The data collection and intervention occurred over the period of 1 year. Both sets of children had positive weight gain, but the home care intervention group demonstrated fewer developmental delays. The results suggest that early intervention can promote a nurturant home environment and can reduce developmental delays. Home care referral may be ideal if transportation or multidisciplinary growth and development clinics are not available.

In addition, Mahony and Murphy (1999) evaluated a visiting nurse program that provided services to alcohol- and drug-exposed infants over a 7-year period. The most frequent problems noted were poor maternal-infant attachment, altered sleep patterns, infant feeding difficulty, and delayed infant development. Pediatric nursing interventions included regular physical assessment, nutrition management, monitoring growth and development, and education about parenting skills. When looking at the outcome criteria of infant weight gain, more than 50% of infants gained at least 1 percentile and 31% gained at least 2 percentiles in weight for age. The authors of the study concluded that visiting nurses' interventions were effective to improve the health of alcohol- and drug-exposed infants.

Clearly nursing research is highly valuable in demonstrating the effectiveness of home care nursing for this vulnerable population of children. Positive outcomes are generally attributed to (1) the collaborative and supportive relationship developed with the home care nurse and (2) clinical expertise in skill, knowledge, and training of pediatric home care nurses (Behrman, 1999; Reifsnider, 1996; Woodring, 2000). The search for quality, cost-effective health care for children with special needs may need to go no further than the child's own home. Who better than pediatric home care nurses to prove this point?

---

### Box 25-9 ■ ■ ■
### Incorporating Developmental Support into the Home Care Plan

**Example:** 6-month-old infant: history of 24-week prematurity, currently uses cardiorespiratory monitor and oxygen per nasal cannula and nasogastric feeding tube

#### OUTCOME CRITERIA
☐ Age-appropriate growth: developmental activities promoted with normal parameters achieved
☐ Absence of growth and development deficits for age within limits imposed by illness

#### INTERVENTION
☐ Assess growth and development with the Denver-II
☐ Reassess growth and development every 4 weeks
☐ Provide consistent caregiver
☐ Instruct parents in normal growth and development for child's age, reasons for delay, and anticipated outcomes
☐ Inform of age-related play and other activities that enhance growth and development and provide stimulation
☐ Consult with PT, OT, speech therapy to incorporate recommendations in daily routines
☐ Provide visual, auditory, tactile stimulation, including mobiles with or without color, music, toys, books, television
☐ Hold, rock, pat, and talk to child

Modified from Klijanowicz AS: Care of high-risk infant. In Votroubek WL, Townsend JL, editors: *Pediatric home care*, ed 2, Gaithersburg, MD, 1997, Aspen; and Jaffe M and others: *Pediatric nursing care plans*, ed 2, Englewood, CO, 1998, Skidmore-Roth.

---

Once parents have been fully informed of the child's condition, likely developmental sequelae, and the expected benefits of intervention, developmental goals outlined by the child and family should guide planning and intervention (Jaffe and others, 1998; Pokorni, 1997).

Each family is entitled to an ***Individualized Family Service Plan (IFSP)*** to help ensure early intervention. All U.S. states have agencies that develop IFSPs (American Academy of Pediatrics, 1995a). Several principles underlie the appropriate developmental intervention plans for children with complex medical problems (Jaffe and others, 1998). First, understanding a child's medical condition ensures that the nurse and family can plan to maximize developmental opportunities at times when the child has the most energy and endurance and when stress signals that determine the child's tolerance for type, intensity, and duration of activity will be noted (Ahmann and Klockenbrink, 1996; Glass and Blinkoff, 1996). Second, plans for developmental support must be flexible and tailored to the individual child's abilities, interests, and needs. Third, familiarity with the child's medical equipment facilitates the planning of creative ways to meet the child's developmental needs. For example, the use of lengthy oxygen tubing allows the active toddler freedom of movement during the day (Fig. 25-2); portable equipment of any type facilitates family outings; and mounting a ventilator to a wheelchair allows the adolescent greater independence.

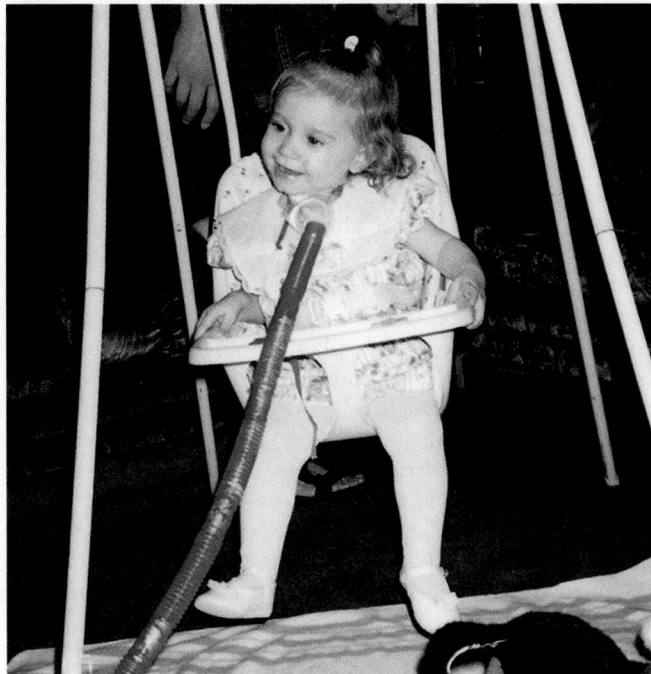

**Fig. 25-2** The use of lengthy tubing facilitates a child's freedom of movement.

The impact of chronic illness on development is discussed in Chapter 22. Behaviors that may be observed in children receiving home care that need to be addressed by the nurse include the following (Jaffe and others, 1998):

- Infants—crying, withdrawal, detachment, inability to achieve/maintain milestones
- Toddlers—inactive, sad, screaming, regressive behavior, delays in motor, speech, social skills
- Preschoolers—temper tantrums, refusal to comply with routines, refusal to eat or participate in self-care
- School-age children—expression of loneliness, boredom, isolation, depression, worry about school absences, altered physical growth
- Adolescents—dependency, uncooperativeness, withdrawal, fear of loss of peer status or acceptance at school, altered image

Promoting coping and capability can buffer stress and contribute to mental health and self-esteem in a child with chronic illness (Jaffe and others, 1998). The extent to which a child is involved in his or her own care depends on many factors, including parental comfort and support and the child's developmental age, level of interest, and physical ability.

Beyond infancy, almost every child can participate in the health care regimen. Toddlers can participate in simple ways such as holding equipment and discarding used supplies. School-age children may be able to clean medical equipment, restock supplies, and administer their own medications with supervision. Adolescents may be able to perform many of their own procedures, participate in decision making, and assume responsibility for scheduling caregivers' visits and out-of-home appointments. (See Critical

 **Critical Thinking Exercise**

### Home Care and the Adolescent

A 13-year-old girl has been diagnosed with ulcerative colitis following a 2-month period of bloody diarrhea, abdominal pain, and significant weight loss. Because of the chronic malabsorption and weight loss, continuous nasogastric tube feedings for 12 hours per night have been recommended as nutritional support therapy. In preparation for home care, which of the following nursing interventions should you question?

FIRST, THINK ABOUT IT . . .

- What precise question are you trying to answer?
- What conclusions are you reaching?

1. Providing education regarding symptoms or problems to be reported to the health care professionals.
2. Educating the girl regarding nasogastric tube insertion and administration of formula.
3. Providing emotional support regarding the new diagnosis and therapy.
4. Arranging for home care supplies and nursing visits at home as needed.

*The best response is two. Although an essential component of the nursing plan of care includes patient education and preparation for home care, there is no mention of including other family members in the teaching. Although it is a correct conclusion that the adolescent should know how to insert the tube and administer the formula, she should not be expected to have sole responsibility for this procedure. Adolescents newly diagnosed with a chronic disease require emotional support regarding their prognosis, medical or nutritional care, and body image. Many children and adolescents with ulcerative colitis have gastrointestinal symptoms, extraintestinal symptoms, and growth delay, all of which can cause anxiety. Many adolescents will benefit from support from other patients their age with the same disease, as well as support and assistance from family members. Education should include the rationale for therapy, symptoms and problems to be monitored and reported, nasogastric tube insertion, administration of formula, and use of a feeding pump. Supplies for nasogastric tube feedings will need to be obtained, and a visiting nurse will likely be needed to monitor care and assist and educate the patient at home.*

Contributed by Lynn Mattis, RN, MSN.

Thinking Exercise box.) Most adolescents should not be left completely without supervision, because adolescent developmental issues, including denial and a sense of invulnerability and rebellion, may interfere with appropriate care. Effective teaching for self-care is focused at the child's own level of conceptual understanding and may be augmented by the use of dolls, models and diagrams, simple explanations, and repetition.

Educational planning is important for the child who has a chronic medical condition. Federal laws ensure that all children receive a public education. Before age 3, children with developmental delays are eligible for an ***early intervention program.*** The child can receive rehabilitation therapies as appropriate (PT/OT/speech therapy). After age 3, the local school system is responsible for providing this education. Some children may be eligible for special education preschools. The home care nurse should refer the family to local county programs.

When a child requiring special medical care is to be placed in an educational setting, the parents, child, school health coordinator, educational evaluation team, and education and administrative staff should meet to determine safe and appropriate placement, as well as the necessary services and personnel to enable the child to attend school in the least restrictive environment. Training of education staff and caregivers is essential to ensuring the child's safety in the educational setting. Special assistance can also be beneficial in reintegrating previously schooled children, such as those with cancer, into the school setting. The home care nurse may need to assist parents in developing the skills necessary to advocate effectively for their child in the educational system.

## Safety Issues in the Home

Safety is an important consideration in pediatric home care and should be addressed in the home care plan.

**NURSING TIP** If the family does not have a telephone, arrangements may be made with the telephone company to supply service. Alternatively, one or two nearby neighbors may agree to let the family use their services. In rural areas a local pharmacy or police or ranger station may be willing to receive messages and relay them to the family.

The telephone and electric companies (if the use of medical equipment requires electricity) must be notified that the family needs to be placed on a priority service list. In this way the family will learn of any anticipated interruptions in service and will receive priority in reinstatement of interrupted services. Prior contact with rescue squad and local emergency facility personnel can help ensure prompt and appropriate interventions if required (Ahmann, 1996).

Before hospital discharge, emergency protocols are developed and reviewed with the parents and professional caregivers. Cardiopulmonary resuscitation (CPR) guidelines, if appropriate, should be posted near the child's bedside or in another accessible location. A list of emergency telephone numbers can be placed near each home phone and should include those of the rescue squad, emergency department, managing physician(s), nursing agency, and equipment vendor(s) (Neal and Kieffer, 1998).

Another aspect of safety relates to the provision of care by appropriately trained individuals. Family members should receive thorough training in the child's care requirements and have the opportunity to demonstrate knowledge and confidence before hospital discharge. Professional staff caring for the child should have the appropriate background and training for the child's particular care needs. Because of the child's body size, special skill and caution are required in both the performance of procedures (e.g., gastrostomy feedings, suctioning) and in moni-

toring the use of equipment (e.g., ventilator settings, intravenous flow rates, and total fluid volumes) (see Chapters 27, 28, and 31).

The activity level and curiosity of young children raise additional safety considerations in the provision of home care. All medications, needles, syringes, and contaminated materials must be securely stored well out of the reach of curious hands. Arrangements for the disposal of sharp items or contaminated materials can be made with the home health agency or hospital. Special attention is paid to childproofing the control panels on ventilators, pumps, monitors, and other equipment. The use of clear plastic tape, covers, or panels to cover control knobs or buttons reduces the risk of accidental changes in settings. Electrical cords are kept short and out of reach, and safety covers are used on any open outlets. Equipment is unplugged when not in use, and any wires (e.g., lead wires for an apnea monitor) are stored out of reach. (See Chapter 13 for use of apnea monitors in the home.)

Care at night poses other safety concerns. Parents or other caregivers need to be able to clearly hear monitor, ventilator, or pump alarms at night; an inexpensive intercom system or baby monitor can be used. Steps must be taken to prevent accidental strangulation by apnea, oximeter, or cardiac monitor wires or lengthy intravenous tubing during sleep.

**NURSING TIP** Coiling extra tubing and taping it at the exit site, as well as running wires or tubes out the bottoms of pajamas, is a precaution against strangulation.

Safe transportation is a vitally important concern. Wheelchairs and large equipment must be properly secured to the vehicle, including vans and buses. Appropriate child restraints must be used. If necessary, an extra adult should be present to monitor the child while in transit.

## Family-To-Family Support

Family-to-family support networks can be an important source of emotional and instrumental support and empowerment for families of children with chronic health problems. (See Establishing a Support System, Chapter 22.) Family-to-family support does not replace professional sources of support but rather is a unique resource that promotes family strengths through shared experience.

Families will most likely experience increased emotional stress as the result of living with and caring for a child with special needs. Identifying meaningful sources of support can make a difference in coping abilities. The nurse can assist the family in increasing their involvement in community social networks. For example, a referral to a parent support group may meet an individual family's needs. The nurse should inform the parents of the group's goals so that the family can determine if they might benefit from this connection. In addition, informal support networks can be extremely beneficial. A link to a family in the same or similar situation allows the sharing of common experiences. This in itself may decrease the sense of isolation and provide a connection with someone who can really identify with family struggles. Positive outcomes can include understanding, empathy, problem solving, or just talking to someone who will listen. The nurse should remember that the needs of each family member differ. The care plan should acknowledge each family member's needs (mother, father, siblings, grand-parents). Peer support for school-age children and adolescents with complex care needs may be beneficial. These connections can be expanded to include letter writing, e-mails, telephone calls, or specialty camping programs (Patterson and Blum, 1996; Johnson, Ravert, and Everton, 2001).

## KEY POINTS

- Effective home care depends on many factors, including the child's relative medical stability; the family's willingness, training, and ability to accommodate the child's care requirements; and professional, financial, and community support.
- Comprehensive, multidisciplinary discharge planning should begin early and should include the family and a home care representative in addition to hospital personnel.
- Thorough training of the family—including a trial of care, a predischarge pass to home, and a predischarge home visit—can ease the transition to home.
- Care coordination ensures continuity of care and reduces fragmentation of services. The family may assume varying degrees of care coordination over time.
- The home care nurse must share a level of technical expertise with the critical care nurse while being able to adapt equipment, procedures, and the nursing process to the home setting.
- Federal standards apply to agencies that participate in Medicare or Medicaid; standards of practice by the American Nurses Association can guide nurses in the home setting.
- Family-centered nursing practice is applied in the home setting; diversity in family structures, cultural backgrounds, strengths, and coping mechanisms is respected.
- Collaborative relationships are characterized by communication, dialogue, active listening, awareness and acceptance of difference, and negotiation.
- The nursing process is adapted to involve the family in each step and to preserve the family's central role in decision making.
- House rules agreed on by the nurse and family allow the family to maintain a feeling of control over their own environment when professionals are present.
- Home care plans are designed to promote optimum development of the child and to focus on normalization, the impact of the child's medical condition and technologic requirements on development, self-care, and educational needs.
- Safety in the provision of home care services involves emergency preparations and protocols, appropriate training of family and home care personnel, and the safe use and childproofing of medical equipment.
- Family-to-family support networks can provide emotional and instrumental support and encourage family empowerment.

## REFERENCES

Agazio JZ: Family transition through the termination of private duty home care nursing, *J Pediatr Nurs* 12(2):74-84, 1997.

Ahmann E: *Home care for the high risk infant: a family centered approach*, Gaithersburg, MD, 1996, Aspen.

Ahmann E, Klockenbrink KL: Developmental assessment and intervention in the home. In Ahmann E: *Home care for the high risk infant: a family-centered approach*, Gaithersburg, MD, 1996, Aspen.

American Academy of Pediatrics: *Care coordination: integrating health and related systems of care for children with special health care needs*, Elk Grove Village, IL, 1999, The Academy.

American Academy of Pediatrics, Committee on Children with Disabilities: Guidelines for home care of infants, children and adolescents with chronic disease, *Pediatrics* 96(1):161-164, 1995b.

American Academy of Pediatrics: *Hospital discharge of the high-risk neonate—proposed guidelines*, Elk Grove, Village, IL, 1998, The Academy.

American Academy of Pediatrics: *The medical home and early intervention*, Elk Grove Village, IL, 1995a, The Academy.

American Nurses' Association: *Standards of community health nursing practice*, Washington, DC, 1986a, The Association.

American Nurses' Association: *Standards of home health nursing practice*, Washington, DC, 1986b, The Association.

American Nurses' Association: *Nursing case management*, Washington DC, 1988, The Association.

AWHONN Practice Resource: *Preparation for home care of technology-dependent infants*, Washington, DC, 1993, AWHONN.

Bakewell-Sachs S and others: Home care considerations for chronic and vulnerable populations, *Nurse Pract Forum* 11(1):65-72, 2000.

Balinsky W, Marié J: Pediatric home care: a cost benefit and cost effectiveness update, *Caring* 20(6):16-19, 2001.

Barnes LP: Critical pathways: linking discharge planning and family teaching, *MCN Am J Matern Child Nurs* 22(2):103, 1997.

Behrman R, editor: *Executive summary: the future of children—home visiting—recent program evaluation*, Los Altos, CA, 1999, The David and Lucille Packard Foundation.

Betz CL: Children and youth in out-of-home placements: nursing care opportunities for pediatric nurses, *J Pediatr Nurs* 15(1):1-2, 2000.

Bilodeau JA: A home parenteral nutrition program for infants, *J Obstet Gynecol Neonat Nurs* 24(1):72-76, 1995.

Black MM and others: A randomized clinical trial of home intervention for children with failure to thrive, *Pediatrics* 95(6): 807-814, 1995.

Bryant K, Davis C, Lagrone C: Streamlining discharge planning for the child with a new tracheotomy, *J Pediatr Nurs* 12(3): 191-192, 1997.

Capen CL, Dedlow ER: Discharging ventilator-dependent children: a continuing challenge, *J Pediatr Nurs* 13(3):175-184, 1998.

Carlin MC: Hospice nursing: more than a job, *Caring* 18(1):8-9, 1999.

Chan JSL, Filippone AM: High-tech pediatric home care: a collaborative approach, *Caring* 17(5):30-36, 1998.

Chapman D: Family-focused pediatric home care, *Caring* 17(5):12-15, 1998.

Cuthbert-Allman C, Burrows K: Overcoming obstacles: challenges of caring for an urban pediatric population, *Caring* 17(5):44-47, 1998.

Davidhizar R, Havnes R, Bechtel G: Assessing culturally diverse pediatric clients, *Pediatr Nurs* 25(4):371-376, 1999.

Dittbrenner H: Pediatric home care as a viable new service, *Caring* 18(2):12-15, 1999.

Engel J: *Pocket guide to pediatric assessment,* ed 3, St Louis, 1997, Mosby.

Ensuring access and adequate reimbursement for pediatric care, *Caring* 18(2): 42-43, 1999.

Gamblian V, Hess DJ, Kenner C: Early discharge from the NICU, *J Pediatr Nurs* 13(5):296-301, 1998.

Gaudet L: Stress tolerance. In Votroubek WL, Townsend JL, editors: *Pediatric home care,* ed 2, Gaithersburg, MD, 1997, Aspen.

Glass P, Blinkoff R: Overview of developmental issues. In Ahmann E: *Home care for the high risk infant: a family-centered approach,* Gaithersburg, MD 1996, Aspen.

Hanson JL, Randall VF: Evaluating and improving the practice of family-centered care, *Pediatr Nurs* 25(4):445-449, 1999.

Hart D: Assessing culture: pediatric nurses' beliefs and self-reported practices, *J Pediatr Nurs* 14(4):255-262, 1999.

Hostler SL: Pediatric family-centered rehabilitation, *J Head Trauma Rehabil* 14(4):384-393, 1999.

Jaffe M and others: *Pediatric nursing care plans,* ed 2, Englewood, CO, 1998, Skidmore-Roth.

Johnson KB, Ravert RD, Everton A: Hopkins Teen Central: assessment of an internet-based support system for children with cystic fibrosis, *Pediatrics* 107(2):e24, 2001.

Kellett UM, Mannion J: Meaning in caring: reconceptualizing the nurse–family carer relationship in community practice, *J Adv Nurs* 29(3):697-703, 1999.

Lovejoy D: *Making the transition to home health nursing: a practical guide,* New York, 1997, Springer.

MacPhee M: The family systems approach and pediatric nursing care, *Pediatr Nurs* 21(5):417-423, 437, 1995.

Mahony DL, Murphy JM: Neonatal drug exposure: assessing a specific population and services provided by visiting nurses, *Pediatr Nurs* 25(1):27-34, 108, 1999.

McDaniel SH, Campbell TL: Training for collaborative family healthcare, *Fam Syst Health* 14(2):147-150, 1996.

McKlindon D, Barsteiner JH: Therapeutic relationships, *MCN Am J Matern Child Nurs* 24(5):237-243, 1999.

McNeal GJ: Diversity issues in the homecare setting, *Crit Care Nurs Clin North Am* 10(3):357-368, 1998.

Messinger R, Dolan MK: The parent's perspective on pediatric home care. In Votroubek WL, Townsend JL, editors: *Pediatric home care,* ed 2, Gaithersburg, MD, 1997, Aspen.

Moore S, Katz B: Home health nurses: stress, self-esteem, social intimacy and job satisfaction, *Home Health Nurs* 14(12):963-969, 1996.

Neal W, Kieffer S: Preparing pediatric home care patients for a medical emergency, *Caring* 17(5):48-50, 1998.

Newby NM: Chronic illness and the family life cycle, *J Adv Nurs Pract* 23(4):786-791, 1996.

Newton MS: Family-centered care: current realities in parent participation, *Pediatr Nurs* 26(2);164-168, 2000.

Patterson J, Blum RW: Risk and resilience among children and youth with disabilities, *Arch Pediatr Adolesc Med* 150(7):692-698, 1996.

Petit de Mange EA: Pediatric considerations in homecare, *Crit Care Nurs Clin North Am* 10(3):339-346, 1998.

Pignatello CH and others: Expanding the role of the pediatric nurse from inpatient to community health, *Nurs Adm Q* 22(4): 48-54, 1998.

Pokorni JL: Promoting the overall development of infants and young children receiving home health services, *Pediatr Nurs* 23(2):187-190, 1997.

Reifsnider E: Helping children grow: a home-based intervention protocol, *J Community Health Nurs* 13(2):93-106, 1996.

Ross BJ: Nursing process and family health care. In Votroubek WL, Townsend JL, editors: *Pediatric home care,* ed 2, Gaithersburg, MD, 1997, Aspen.

Rothkopf MM, Rothkopf GS: The home care team. In Rothkopf MM, editor: *Standards and practice of homecare therapeutics,* ed 2, Baltimore, MD, 1997, Williams & Wilkins.

Salladay S: Ethical problems: refusing treatment, *Nursing 95* 25(9):28, 1995.

Slack M, McEwen M: The impact of interdisciplinary case management on client outcomes, *Fam Community Health* 22(3):30-48, 1999.

Snowdon AW, Kane DJ: Parental needs following the discharge of a hospitalized child, *Pediatr Nurs* 21(5):425-428, 1995.

Spruhan JB: Beyond traditional nursing care: cultural awareness and successful home healthcare nursing, *Home Health Nurs* 14(6):445-449, 1996.

Stephenson C: Well-being of families with healthy and technology-assisted infants in the home: a comparative study, *J Pediatr Nurs* 14(3):164-176, 1999.

Thompson J: Pediatric assessment in the home, *Home Health Nurs* 18(10):639-646, 2000.

Townsend JL: Assessment of the child and family. In Votroubek WL, Townsend JL, editors: *Pediatric home care,* ed 2, Gaithersburg MD, 1997, Aspen.

Weber MM: Neonates making the transition from intensive care to home care, *Caring* 17(5):26-29, 1998.

Wilson JS: National certification for home health care nurses: bird by bird, *Home Health Nurs* 14(10):817-821, 1996.

Woodring B: Home visits: should they remain a significant component of today's pediatric-healthcare continuum? *J Child Fam Nurs* 3(3):232-233, 2000.

Zerull L: Community nurse case management: evolving over time to meet new demands, *Fam Community Health* 22(3): 12-29, 1999.

## Selected Resources on Home Care

**American Academy of Pediatrics**
141 Northwest Point Blvd.
Elk Grove Village, IL 60007-1098
(847) 434-4000
Fax: (847) 434-8000
*www.aap.org*

**Association of Maternal and Child Health Programs**
1220 19th St., NW
Suite 801
Washington, DC 20036
(202) 775-0436
Fax: (202) 775-0061
*www.amchp.org*

**Children's Hospice International**
2202 Mt. Vernon Ave., Suite 3C
Alexandria, VA 22301
(800) 2-4-CHILD
Fax: (703) 684-0226
*www.chionline.org*

**National Association for Home Care**
228 7th St., SE
Washington, DC 20003
(202) 547-7424
Fax: (202) 547-3540
*www.nahc.org*

**National Fathers' Network**
16120 NE 8th St.
Bellevue, WA 98008-3937
(206) 747-4004, ext 218
*www.fathersnetwork.org*

**National Information Center for Children and Youth with Disabilities**
PO Box 1492
Washington, DC 20013-1492
(202) 884-8200 (voice/TTY) or (800) 695-0285 (voice/TTY)
Fax: (202) 884-8441
*www.nichcy.org*

**Pediatric Home Care Association of America**
Division of National Association for Home Care
228 Seventh St., SE
Washington, DC 20003
(202) 547-7424
Fax: (202) 547-3540
*www.nahc.org*

**Sibling Support Project**
Children's Hospital and Medical Center, CL-09
PO Box 5371
Seattle, WA 98105-0371
*www.chmc.org/departmt/sibsupp*

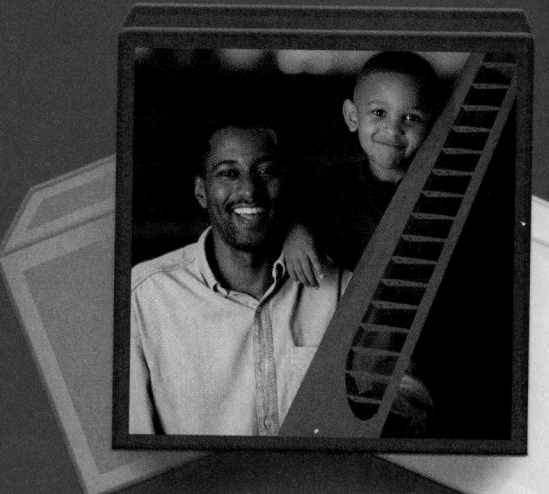

# Chapter 26

# Family-Centered Care of the Child During Illness and Hospitalization

## Chapter Outline

**STRESSORS OF HOSPITALIZATION AND CHILDREN'S REACTIONS, 1032**
**Separation Anxiety, 1032**
Early Childhood, 1033
Later Childhood, 1033
**Loss of Control, 1034**
Infants, 1034
Toddlers, 1034
Preschoolers, 1034
School-Age Children, 1035
Adolescents, 1035
**Bodily Injury and Pain, 1036**
Infants, 1036
Toddlers, 1037
Preschoolers, 1037
School-Age Children, 1038
Adolescents, 1039
**Effects of Hospitalization on the Child, 1039**
Individual Risk Factors, 1039
Changes in the Pediatric Population, 1040
Beneficial Effects of Hospitalization, 1040

**STRESSORS AND REACTIONS OF THE FAMILY OF THE CHILD WHO IS HOSPITALIZED, 1040**
**Parental Reactions, 1040**
**Sibling Reactions, 1041**
**Altered Family Roles, 1041**

**NURSING CARE OF THE CHILD WHO IS HOSPITALIZED, 1041**
**Preventing or Minimizing Separation, 1041**

Parent Participation, 1042
Strategies to Minimize the Effects of Separation, 1043
**Minimizing Loss of Control, 1044**
Promoting Freedom of Movement, 1044
Maintaining the Child's Routine, 1045
Encouraging Independence, 1045
Promoting Understanding, 1046
**Preventing or Minimizing Bodily Injury, 1046**
**Pain Assessment, 1046**
Fallacies and Facts, 1048
Principles of Pain Assessment in Children, 1049
**Pain Management, 1057**
Nonpharmacologic Management, 1057
Pharmacologic Management, 1057
**Providing Developmentally Appropriate Activities, 1068**
**Using Play/Expressive Activities to Minimize Stress, 1069**
Diversional Activities, 1070
Expressive Activities, 1071
**Maximizing Potential Benefits of Hospitalization, 1072**
Fostering Parent-Child Relationships, 1072
Providing Educational Opportunities, 1073
Promoting Self-Mastery, 1073
Providing Socialization, 1073
**Supporting Family Members, 1073**
Providing Information, 1074

*Nursing Care Plan: The Child in the Hospital, 1075*
*Nursing Care Plan: The Family of the Child Who Is Ill or Hospitalized, 1080*

**PREPARATION FOR HOSPITALIZATION, 1083**
**Guidelines in Preparing for Hospitalization, 1084**
Group Size and Timing of Preparation, 1084
Setting of the Tour, 1085
Preparatory Materials, 1085
Opportunity for Discussion, 1085
Prehospital Counseling by Parents, 1086
**Hospital Admission Procedure, 1086**
Nursing Admission History, 1086
Physical Assessment, 1089
Placing the Child, 1090
Adolescent Unit, 1090
**Nursing Care During Special Hospital Situations, 1091**
Ambulatory/Outpatient Setting, 1091
Isolation, 1092
Emergency Admission, 1093
Intensive Care Unit (ICU), 1093
**Discharge Planning and Home Care, 1095**
Assessment, 1096
Planning, 1096
Transitional Care, 1097
Evaluation and Continuing Support, 1097

## Related Topics

Administration of Medication, Ch. 27
Communication and Health Assessment of the Child and Family, Ch. 6
Compliance, Ch. 27
Family-Centered Care of the Child with Chronic Illness or Disability, Ch. 22

Family-Centered End-of-Life Care, Ch. 23
Family-Centered Home Care, Ch. 25
Neonatal Pain, Ch. 10
Nursing Care of the Surgical Neonate, Ch. 11
Physical and Developmental Assessment of the Child, Ch. 7

Preparation for Diagnostic and Therapeutic Procedures, Ch. 27
Social, Cultural, and Religious Influences on Child Health Promotion, Ch. 2
Surgical Procedures, Ch. 27

The recent trends of shortened hospital stays, increased use of outpatient surgery, and managed care have had a direct impact on the practice of pediatric nursing. Many aspects of psychosocial care were developed during an era of extended inpatient stays; however, many of the principles and issues remain relevant in today's changing health care environment. The challenge for nurses is to adapt practices by supporting the physical, emotional, and developmental needs of the child and family while reducing costs without negatively influencing the quality of care provided.

## STRESSORS OF HOSPITALIZATION AND CHILDREN'S REACTIONS

Often illness and hospitalization are the first crises children must face. Especially during the early years, children are particularly vulnerable to the crises of illness and hospitalization because (1) stress represents a change from the usual state

■ Chris Algren, EdD, MSN, RN, revised this chapter.

---

of health and environmental routine and (2) children have a limited number of coping mechanisms to resolve *stressors* (those events that produce stress). Major stressors of hospitalization include separation, loss of control, bodily injury, and pain. Children's reactions to these crises are influenced by their developmental age; their previous experience with illness, separation, or hospitalization; their innate and acquired coping skills; the seriousness of the diagnosis; and the support system available.

### Separation Anxiety

The major stress from middle infancy throughout the preschool years, especially for children ages 16 to 30 months, is separation anxiety, also called *anaclitic depression.* The principal behavioral responses of these children to the three phases of separation anxiety are summarized in Box 26-1.

During the phase of *protest,* children cry loudly, scream for the parent, refuse the attention of anyone else, and are inconsolable in their grief (Fig. 26-1). They may continue this behavior for a few hours to several days. Some children may protest continuously, ceasing only from physical exhaustion. If a stranger approaches them, children will initially protest even louder.

During the phase of *despair,* the crying stops. The child is much less active, is disinterested in play or food, and withdraws from others. The child looks sad, lonely, isolated, and apathetic (Fig. 26-2). The major behavioral characteristic is depression, a result of increasing hopelessness, grief, and mourning.

The third phase, *detachment,* sometimes also called *denial,* is uncommon and occurs only after lengthy separations from the parent or guardian (days or weeks). Superficially, the child appears to have finally adjusted to the loss. The child becomes more interested in the surroundings, plays with others, and seems to form new relationships. However,

---

### Box 26-1 ■ ■ ■
### Manifestations of Separation Anxiety in Young Children

**PHASE OF PROTEST**
Observed behaviors during later infancy
  Cries
  Screams
  Searches for parent with eyes
  Clings to parent
  Avoids and rejects contact with strangers
Additional behaviors observed during toddlerhood
  Verbally attacks strangers (e.g., "Go away")
  Physically attacks strangers (e.g., kicks, bites, hits, pinches)
  Attempts to escape to find parent
  Attempts to physically force parent to stay
Behaviors may last from hours to days
Protest, such as crying, may be continuous, ceasing only with physical exhaustion
Approach of stranger may precipitate increased protest

**PHASE OF DESPAIR**
Observed behaviors
  Inactive
  Withdraws from others
  Depressed, sad
  Uninterested in environment
  Uncommunicative
  Regresses to earlier behavior (e.g., thumb sucking, bed-wetting, use of pacifier, use of bottle)
Behaviors may last for variable length of time
Child's physical condition may deteriorate from refusal to eat, drink, or move

**PHASE OF DETACHMENT**
Observed behaviors
  Shows increased interest in surroundings
  Interacts with strangers or familiar caregivers
  Forms new but superficial relationships
  Appears happy
Detachment usually occurs after prolonged separation from parent; rarely seen in hospitalized children
Behaviors represent a superficial adjustment to loss

---

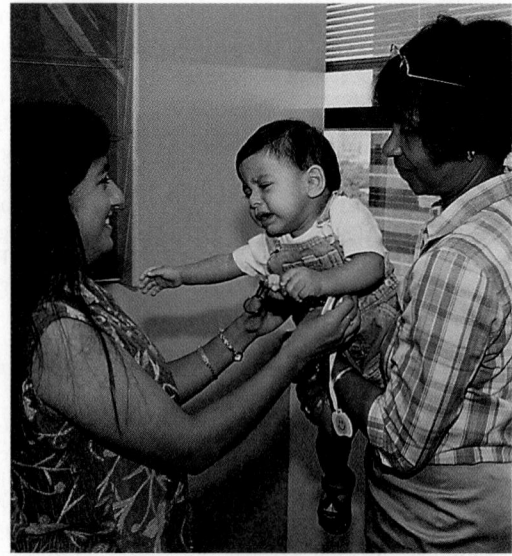

**Fig. 26-1** In the protest phase of separation anxiety, children cry loudly and are inconsolable in their grief for the parent. (Courtesy James DeLeon, Texas Children's Hospital.)

this behavior is a result of resignation and is not a sign of contentment. The child detaches from the parent in an effort to escape the emotional pain of desiring the parent's presence. The child copes by forming shallow relationships with others, becoming increasingly self-centered, and attaching primary importance to material objects. This is the most serious phase because reversal of the potential adverse effects is less likely to occur once detachment is established. However, in most situations the temporary separations imposed by hospitalization do not cause such prolonged parental absences that the child enters into detachment. In addition, considerable evidence suggests that, even with stresses such as separation, children are remarkably resilient, and permanent ill effects are rare.

Although progression to detachment is uncommon, the initial phases are frequently observed even with very brief separations from either parent. Without an understanding of the meaning of each stage of behavior, health team members may erroneously label the behaviors as positive or negative. In the phase of protest, they may view the loud crying as "bad" behavior. Because the protesting increases if a stranger approaches, staff may interpret the reaction as evidence of their need to stay away. During the quiet, withdrawn phase of despair, they regard the child as finally "settling in" to the new surroundings and see the detachment behaviors as proof of a "good adjustment." The faster a child reaches this stage, the more likely it is that the child will be regarded as the "ideal patient."

Because children seem to react "negatively" to visits by their parents, uninformed observers feel justified in restricting parental visiting privileges. For example, during

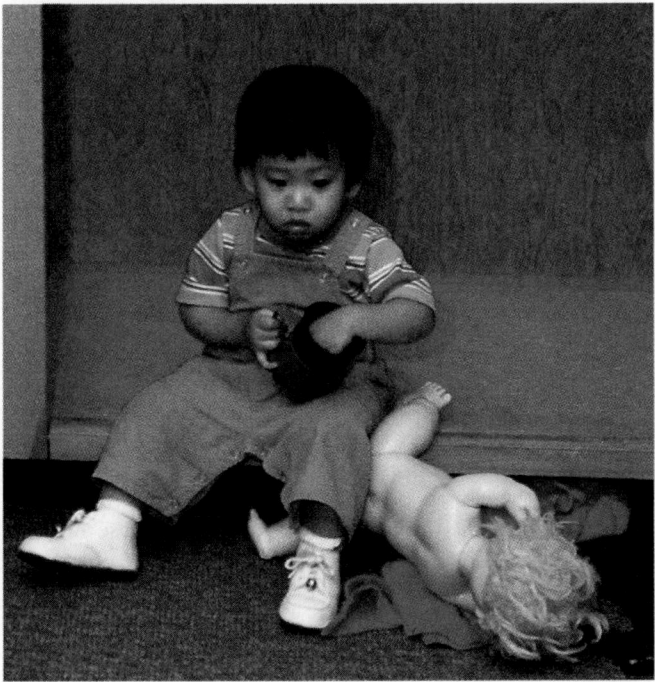

**Fig. 26-2**   During the despair phase of separation anxiety, children are sad, lonely, and uninterested in play or food.

the protest phase, children outwardly do not appear happy to see their parents. Instead, they may cry louder than before the parents' visit. If children are depressed, they may reject their parents or begin to protest once more. Often they cling to their parents in an effort to ensure their continued presence. Consequently, the parents' visits may be regarded as "disturbing" the child's adjustment to the surroundings. If the separation has progressed to the phase of detachment, children will respond no differently to their parents than to any other person.

Such reactions are distressing to parents, who may be unaware of their meaning. If they are regarded as intruders, parents will view their absence as "beneficial" to the child's adjustment and recovery. They may respond to the child's behavior by staying for short periods, decreasing the frequency of visits, or deceiving the child when it is time to leave. Consequently, a destructive cycle of misunderstanding and unmet needs results.

### Early Childhood

If separation is avoided, young children have a tremendous capacity to withstand any other stress. Separation anxiety is most evident during the ages of 6 to 30 months and is the greatest stress imposed by hospitalization. During this time the typical reactions just described are seen. However, children in the toddler stage demonstrate more goal-directed behaviors. For example, they may verbally plead for their parents to stay and physically attempt to secure or find them. They may demonstrate displeasure on the parents' return or departure by having temper tantrums; refusing to comply with the usual routines of mealtime, bedtime, or toileting; or regressing to more primitive levels of development. However, temper tantrums, bed-wetting, or other behaviors may also be explained as expressions of anger or even a physiologic response to stress.

Since preschoolers are much more secure interpersonally than toddlers, they can tolerate brief periods of separation from their parents and are more inclined to develop substitute trust in other significant adults. However, the stress of illness usually renders them less able to cope with separation; as a result, they manifest many of the behaviors of separation anxiety. In general, the protest behaviors are more subtle and passive than those seen in younger children. Preschoolers may demonstrate separation anxiety through refusing to eat, difficulty in sleeping, crying quietly for their parents, continually asking when they will visit, or withdrawing from others. They may express anger indirectly by breaking their toys, hitting other children, or refusing to cooperate during usual self-care activities. Nurses need to be sensitive to these less obvious signs of separation anxiety to intervene appropriately.

### Later Childhood

Previous research, usually based on adult recollections, indicated that the family does not play as important a role for school-age children as it does during the toddler and preschool years. However, in a study wherein children were asked about their fears when hospitalized, children ranked "being away from my family" higher than any other fear associated with hospitalization (Wilson and Yorker, 1997). Although school-age children are better able to cope with separation in general, the stress and often accompanying regression imposed by illness or hospitalization may increase their need for parental security and guidance. This is particularly true for young school-age children who have only recently left the safety of the home and are struggling with the crisis of school adjustment. Middle and late school-age children may react more to the separation from their usual activities and peers than to absence of their parents. Their high level of physical and mental activity frequently finds no suitable outlets in the hospital environment. Even when they dislike school, they admit to missing its routine and associated activities and worry that they will not be able to compete or "fit in" with their classmates on returning to school. Feelings of loneliness, boredom, isolation, and depression are common. It is important to recognize that such reactions may occur more as a result of separation than from concern over the illness, treatment, or hospital setting.

School-age children may need and desire parental guidance, or support from other adult figures, but be unable or unwilling to ask for it. Because the goal of attaining independence is so important to them, they are reluctant to seek help directly for fear that they will appear weak, childish, or dependent. Cultural expectations to "act like a man" or to "be brave and strong" bear heavily on these children, especially males, who tend to react to stress with stoicism, withdrawal, or passive acceptance. Often the need to express hostile, angry, or other negative feelings finds alternate outlets, such as irritability and aggression toward parents, withdrawal from hospital personnel, inability to relate to peers, rejection of siblings, or subsequent problems in school.

For adolescents, separation from home and parents may be difficult. However, loss of peer-group contact may be a severe emotional threat because of loss of group status, inability to exert group control or leadership, and loss of group acceptance. Deviations within peer groups are poorly tolerated, and although members may express concern for the adolescent's illness or need for hospitalization, they continue their group activities, quickly filling the gap of the absent member. During the temporary separation from their usual group, ill adolescents may benefit from group associations with hospitalized peers.

## Loss of Control

One of the factors influencing the amount of stress imposed by hospitalization is the amount of control that children perceive themselves as having. Lack of control increases the perception of threat and can affect children's coping skills. Many hospital situations decrease the amount of control a child feels. Although the usual sensory stimulations are lacking, the additional hospital stimuli of sight, sound, and smell may be overwhelming. Without an insight into the type of environment conducive to children's optimum growth, the hospital experience can at best temporarily slow development and at worst permanently retard it. Because the needs of children vary greatly depending on their age, the major areas of loss of control in terms of physical re-

striction, altered routine or rituals, and dependency are discussed for each age-group.

### Infants

Infants are developing the most important attribute of a healthy personality—trust. Trust is established through consistent, loving care by a nurturing person. Infants attempt to control their environment through emotional expressions, such as crying or smiling. In the hospital setting, cues may be missed or misinterpreted, and routines may be established to meet the hospital staff's needs instead of the infant's needs. Inconsistent care and deviations from the infant's daily routine may lead to mistrust and a decreased sense of control (Wells and others, 1994).

### Toddlers

Toddlers are striving for autonomy, and this goal is evident in most of their behaviors—motor skills, play, interpersonal relationships, activities of daily living, and communication. When their egocentric pleasures meet with obstacles, toddlers react with negativism, especially temper tantrums. Any restriction or limitation of movement, such as the simple act of laying toddlers on their backs, can cause forceful resistance and noncompliance.

Loss of control also results from altered routines and rituals. Toddlers rely on the consistency and familiarity of daily rituals to provide a measure of stability and control in their life. The hospitalization or illness severely limits their sense of expectation and predictability because most details of the hospital environment differ from those at home.

Toddlers' rituals include eating, sleeping, bathing, toileting, and play. When the routines are disrupted, difficulties can occur in any or all of these areas. The principal reaction to such change is regression. For example, when mealtime and food choices differ from those at home, toddlers often refuse to eat, demand a bottle, or request that others feed them. Although regression to earlier forms of behavior may seem to increase toddlers' security and comfort, in reality it is very threatening for them to relinquish their most recently acquired achievements.

Enforced dependency is a chief characteristic of the sick role and accounts for the numerous instances of toddler negativism. For example, rigid schedules, altered caregiving activities, unfamiliar surroundings, separation from parents, and medical procedures usurp toddlers' control over their world. Although most toddlers initially react negatively and aggressively to such dependency, prolonged loss of autonomy may result in passive withdrawal from interpersonal relationships and regression in all areas of development. Therefore the effects of the sick role are most severe in instances of chronic, long-term illnesses or in those families who foster the sick role despite the child's improved state of health.

### Preschoolers

Preschoolers also suffer from loss of control caused by physical restriction, altered routines, and enforced dependency. However, their specific cognitive abilities, which make them feel omnipotent and all-powerful, also make them feel out of control. This loss of control in the context of their sense of self-power is a critical influencing factor in their perception of and reaction to separation, pain, illness, and hospitalization.

Preschoolers' egocentric and magical thinking limits their ability to understand events because they view all experiences from their own self-referenced perspective. Without adequate preparation for unfamiliar settings or experiences, preschoolers' fantasy explanations for such events are usually more exaggerated, bizarre, and frightening than the facts. One typical fantasy to explain the reason for illness or hospitalization is that it represents punishment for real or imagined misdeeds. The response to such thinking is usually feelings of shame, guilt, and fear.

Preschoolers' cognitive ability is also concrete. Explanations are understood only in terms of real events. Purely verbal instructions are often inadequate for them because of their inability to abstract and synthesize beyond what their senses tell them. When combined with their egocentric and magical powers, they can interpret any message according to their particular past experiences. Even with the best preparation for a procedure, they may misconstrue the details.

Transductive reasoning implies that preschoolers deduce from the particular to the particular, rather than from the specific to the general, or the general to the specific. For example, if preschoolers' concept of nurses is that they inflict pain, preschoolers will think that every nurse or caregiver will also inflict pain.

## School-Age Children

Because of their striving for independence and productivity, school-age children are particularly vulnerable to events that may lessen their feeling of control and power. In particular, altered family roles; physical disability; fears of death, abandonment, or permanent injury; loss of peer acceptance; lack of productivity; and inability to cope with stress according to perceived cultural expectations may result in loss of control.

Because of the nature of the patient role, many routine hospital activities usurp individual power and identity. For these children, dependent activities such as enforced bed rest, use of a bedpan, inability to choose meals, lack of privacy, help with a bath, or transport by a wheelchair or stretcher can be a direct threat to their security. Although all of these procedures seem routine and inconsequential, they allow no freedom of choice to children who want to "act grown-up." However, when children are allowed to exert a measure of control, regardless of how limited it may be, they generally respond very well to any procedure. For example, some of the most cooperative, satisfied, and contented patients are school-age children who help make their beds, choose their schedule of activities, and assist in procedures. An increased sense of control usually results from a feeling of usefulness and productivity.

In addition to the hospital environment, illness may also cause a feeling of loss of control. One of the most significant problems of children in this age-group is boredom. When physical or enforced limitations curtail their usual abilities to care for themselves or to engage in favorite activities, school-

age children generally respond with depression, hostility, or frustration. Keeping a normally active child on bed rest is difficult. However, emphasizing areas of control and capitalizing on quiet activities, particularly hobbies such as building models, promote their adjustment to physical restriction.

## Adolescents

Adolescents' struggle for independence, self-assertion, and liberation centers on the quest for personal identity. Anything that interferes with this poses a threat to their sense of identity and results in a loss of control. Illness, which limits one's physical abilities, and hospitalization, which separates one from usual support systems, constitute major situational crises. (See Family Focus box.)

The patient role fosters dependency and depersonalization. Adolescents may react to dependency with rejection,

## FAMILY FOCUS
### *Reflections on Hospitalization from an Adolescent*

July 1997 will always be a significant date to me. It was a time when my life took an unexpected turn. I was diagnosed with osteosarcoma—a type of bone cancer. I was 14 years old at the time. I knew cancer was not a good thing, but, other than that, I knew nothing else about it.

After the doctors verified that I had cancer, it was time to talk about treatment. At first I thought that I would only need to have surgery and then I could go back to my normal life in a few weeks. When the doctors discussed treatment with me, I realized it wasn't going to be that easy. Looking back, I think I was not fully aware of what I was dealing with. The doctors talked about chemotherapy, surgery, and many possible side effects such as hearing loss, heart damage, nausea, vomiting, and hair loss.

The first chemotherapy was awful. I couldn't stop vomiting. I received methotrexate, cisplatin, and doxorubicin. Those medicines cause a lot of nausea and vomiting. The doctors and nurses tried giving me all sorts of medicines for nausea, but nothing seemed to work. Some of the medicines made me sleepy. Anything was better than feeling sick and throwing up. From then on, I knew what to expect the next time and all the times after that.

The chemotherapy also caused me to get many mouth sores, so many that on the few times I felt like eating, I couldn't because of the mouth sores. Sometimes the mouthwashes I was given worked and I didn't get that many sores, but sometimes I forgot to use them. It always helped when the nurses reminded me though.

When I went home, I wasn't there for too long. I would be home for about 2 days and then I would have to go back to the hospital. I would start to dehydrate from not eating or drinking enough, or I would develop a fever. I didn't like being hospitalized for a long time because I couldn't spend very much time at home with my family. I practically felt like I lived in the hospital; I felt trapped and incarcerated being there. It was very hard and depressing to be in the hospital for so long. The only good thing about feeling like I lived in the hospital was that I also felt as if I had a second family there.

The nurses and doctors were great. Diane and Julie were two of my favorite daytime nurses; they would always cheer me up and keep me company. Tiffany and Carrie were two of my favorite night nurses. When I wasn't sleepy, they would talk or play a game with me. All of the nurses helped me feel better and made me forget about everything else for a while.

Modified from Fuentes S: Looking back, looking forward, *J Pediatr Oncol Nurs* 17(3):188-190, 2000.

**TABLE 26-1** Children's developmental concepts of illness and pain

| Concept of Illness* | Concept of Pain† |
|---|---|
| **Preoperational Thought (2-7 Years)** | |
| *Phenomenism:* Perceives an external, unrelated, concrete phenomenon as the cause of illness (e.g., "being sick because you don't feel well") | Relates to pain primarily as physical, concrete experience |
| *Contagion:* Perceives cause of illness as proximity between two events that occurs by "magic" (e.g., "getting a cold because you are near someone who has a cold") | Thinks in terms of magical disappearance of pain |
|  | May view pain as punishment for wrongdoing |
|  | Tends to hold someone accountable for own pain and may strike out at person |
| **Concrete Operational Thought (7-10+ Years)** | |
| *Contamination:* Perceives cause as a person, object, or action external to the child that is "bad" or "harmful" to the body (e.g., "getting a cold because you didn't wear a hat") | Relates to pain physically (e.g., headache, stomachache) |
| *Internalization:* Perceives illness as having an external cause but as being located inside the body (e.g., "getting a cold by breathing in air and bacteria") | Is able to perceive of psychologic pain (e.g., someone dying) |
|  | Fears bodily harm and annihilation (body destruction and death) |
|  | May view pain as punishment for wrongdoing |
| **Formal Operational Thought (13 Years and Older)** | |
| *Physiologic:* Perceives cause as malfunctioning or nonfunctioning organ or process; can explain illness in sequence of events | Is able to give reason for pain (e.g., fell and hit nerve) |
| *Psychophysiologic:* Realizes that psychologic actions and attitudes affect health and illness | Perceives several types of psychologic pain |
|  | Has limited life experiences to cope with pain as adult might cope despite mature understanding of pain |
|  | Fears losing control during painful experience |

*From Bibace R, Walsh ME: Development of children's concepts of illness, *Pediatrics* 66(6):912-917, 1980.
†From Hurley A, Whelan EG: Cognitive development and children's perception of pain, *Pediatr Nurs* 14(1):21-24, 1988.

uncooperativeness, or withdrawal. They may respond to depersonalization with self-assertion, anger, or frustration. Regardless of which response they manifest, hospital personnel generally tend to regard them as difficult, unmanageable patients. Parents may find this challenging because these behaviors serve to further isolate them from understanding the adolescent. Although peers may visit, they may not be able to offer the type of support and guidance needed. Sick adolescents often voluntarily isolate themselves from age-mates until they feel they can compete on an equal basis and meet group expectations. As a result, ill adolescents may be left with virtually no support systems.

Loss of control also occurs for many of the reasons discussed for school-age children. However, adolescents are more sensitive than younger children to potential instances of loss of control and dependency. For example, both groups seek information about their physical status and rely heavily on anticipatory preparation to decrease fear and anxiety. Adolescents, however, react not only to what information is supplied, but also to how it is conveyed. They may feel very threatened by others who relate facts in a derogatory manner. Adolescents want to know that others can relate to them on their own level. This necessitates a careful assessment of their intellectual abilities, previous knowledge, and present needs. It may also require the nurse's willingness to learn the adolescent's language.

## Bodily Injury and Pain

Fears of bodily injury and pain are prevalent among children. The consequences of these fears can be far-reaching; adults who experience more medical fear and pain in childhood are more fearful of medical pain as adults and tend to avoid medical care (Pate and others, 1996). Research documents that young children, including newborns, react to painful stimuli. In caring for children, nurses must appreciate the concerns related to bodily harm and children's reactions to pain at different developmental periods.

Developmental considerations related to children's understanding of illness and pain are summarized in Table 26-1. Developmental characteristics of children's reactions to pain are also important (see Box 26-9). Although the piagetian structuralist perspective argues that changes in *cognitive structure* enable children to reach higher levels of reasoning, others argue that changes in *content* drive the system to higher levels. Thus illness experiences can produce child "experts" who may be better able to see underlying principles and connections about their particular illness or condition than a "novice" adult.

### Infants

Infants' response to pain after the neonatal period is quite similar to earlier reactions, although there is marked variability in measures of distress, especially initial cry and heart rate, which may decrease in some infants. The most consistent indicator of distress is a facial expression of discomfort (Fig. 26-3). Infants may express pain by assuming certain postural positions, such as squirming, writhing, jerking, and flailing (Franck, Greenberg, and Stevens, 2000). Some infants may cry loudly following the procedure, whereas others are easily calmed by a gentle hug. It is important to recognize and respect such early signs of individuality and to realize that children who react less intensely may still be experiencing significant discomfort.

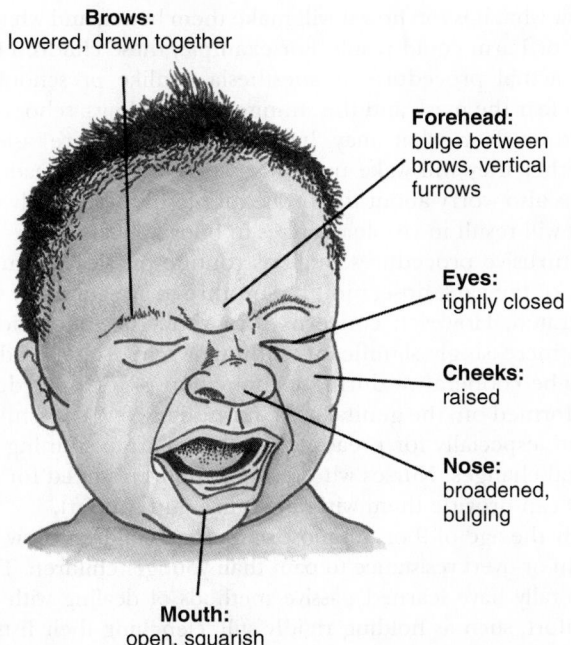

**Brows:**
lowered, drawn together

**Forehead:**
bulge between brows, vertical furrows

**Eyes:**
tightly closed

**Cheeks:**
raised

**Nose:**
broadened, bulging

**Mouth:**
open, squarish

**Fig. 26-3**   Facial expression of physical distress is the most consistent behavioral indicator of pain in infants.

Infants less than 6 months of age seem to have no obvious memory of previous painful experiences and react to a potentially stressful situation with less apprehension and fear than older children. However, after this time, children's response to pain is influenced by their recall of prior painful experiences and the emotional reaction of parents during the procedure. Older infants react intensely with physical resistance and uncooperativeness. They may refuse to lie still, attempt to push the person away, or try to escape with whatever motor activity they have achieved. Distraction does little to lessen their immediate reaction to pain, and anticipatory preparation, such as showing them the equipment, tends to increase their fear and resistance.

### Toddlers

Toddlers' concept of body image, particularly the definition of body boundaries, is very poorly developed. Intrusive experiences, such as examining the ears or mouth or taking a rectal temperature, are very anxiety producing. Toddlers may react to such painless procedures as intensely as they do to painful ones.

Toddlers' reactions to pain are similar to those seen during infancy, except that the variables influencing the individual response are highly complex and varied. Memory, physical restraint, separation from the parent or guardian, emotional reactions of others, and lack of preparation partially determine the intensity of the behavioral response. In general, children in this age-group continue to react with intense emotional upset and physical resistance to any actual or perceived painful experience. Behaviors indicating pain include grimacing, clenching the teeth/lips, opening the eyes wide, rocking, rubbing, and aggressiveness, such as

biting, kicking, hitting, or running away. Unlike adults, who usually decrease their activity when in pain, young children typically become restless and overly active; frequently this response is not recognized as a consequence of pain.

By the end of this age period, toddlers usually are able to communicate about their pain. Although they have not developed the ability to describe the type or intensity of the pain, they usually are able to localize it by pointing to a specific area.

### Preschoolers

Concepts of illness begin during the preschool period and are influenced by the cognitive abilities of the preoperational stage. Preschoolers differentiate poorly between themselves and the external world. Their thinking is focused on externally perceived events, and causality is based on the proximity of two events. Consequently, children define illness according to what they are told or are given external evidence of, such as "You are sick because you have a fever." The cause of illness is seen as a concrete action the child does or fails to do, such as "Catching a stomach virus because you don't wash your hands." Consequently, it implies a degree of responsibility and self-blame. Another explanation may be based on contagion, that the proximity of two objects or persons causes the illness (e.g., "A person gets a cold when someone else with a cold gets near him").

The psychosexual conflicts of children in this age-group make them very vulnerable to threats of bodily injury. Intrusive procedures, whether painful or painless, are threatening to preschoolers, whose concept of body integrity is still poorly developed. Preschoolers may react to an injection with as much concern for withdrawal of the needle as for the actual pain. They fear that the intrusion or puncture will not reclose and that their "insides" will leak out.

Concerns of mutilation are paramount during this age period. Loss of any body part is threatening, but preschool boys' fears of castration complicate their understanding of surgical or medical procedures associated with the genital area, such as circumcision, repair of hypospadias or epispadias, cystoscopy, or catheterization. Their limited comprehension of body functioning also increases their difficulty in understanding how or why body parts are "fixed." For example, telling preschoolers that their tonsils are to be removed may be interpreted as "taking out their voice," or having the penis "fixed" may be understood as cutting it off. Words such as "dye," "cut off," "take out," or "draw" (e.g., "draw some blood") are understood literally and can lead to confusion and fear. (See Communicating with Children, Chapter 6.)

Reactions to pain tend to be similar to those seen during toddlerhood, although some differences become apparent. For example, preschoolers respond more favorably to preparatory interventions, such as explanation and distraction, than younger children. Physical and verbal aggression are more specific and goal directed. Instead of showing total body resistance, preschoolers may push the offending person away, try to secure the equipment, or attempt to lock themselves in a safe place. Much more thought is evident in their plan of attack or escape.

Verbal expression in particular demonstrates their advanced development in response to stress. They may verbally abuse the attacker by stating, "Go away" or "I hate you." They may also use the more cunning approach of trying to persuade the person to delay the intended activity. A common plea is "I have to go to the bathroom." Some statements are not only attempts to avoid the event but also evidence of children's perceptions about the experience.

Attempts to be comforted may also be evident through behaviors such as clinging to a parent, wanting to be held, or refusing to be left alone. A typical expression denoting the need for dependency is "Help me." It is important to recognize such requests as the need for support from others during a time of stress. Admonishing children to act grown-up or encouraging them to do things by stating, "I know you can do it yourself," deprives them of the temporary support they are requesting and increases their own feelings of inadequacy.

### School-Age Children

Fears of the physical nature of the illness surface at this time. School-age children may be less concerned with pain than with disability, uncertain recovery, or possible death. Children with chronic illness are more likely to identify intrusive procedures as stressful, whereas children who are acutely ill are more likely to indicate physical symptoms (Boyd and Hunsberger, 1998). Girls tend to express more and stronger fears than boys, and previous hospitalizations may have no effect on the frequency or intensity of these fears. Because of their developing cognitive abilities, school-age children are aware of the significance of different illnesses, the indispensability of certain body parts, potential hazards in treatment, lifelong consequences of permanent injury or loss of function, and the meaning of death. A major concern of hospitalized school-age children is their fear of being told that something is wrong with them (Hart and Bossert, 1994). They generally take a very active interest in their health or illness. Even those children who rarely ask questions usually reveal detailed knowledge of their condition by attentively listening to all that is said around them. They request factual information and quickly perceive lies or half-truths. Seeking information tends to be one way of their maintaining a sense of control despite the stress and uncertainty of illness.

The school-age child defines illness by a set of multiple concrete symptoms, such as signs of a cold, and views the cause as primarily germs or bacteria. The germs have a powerful, almost magical quality, so that in the child's mind, illness can be prevented by avoiding people with the germs. There is also the idea of contamination, which is similar to that seen in the younger age-group; for example, the illness occurs because of physical contact or because the child engaged in a harmful action and became contaminated. Consequently, feelings of self-blame and guilt may be associated with the reason for becoming ill.

School-age children begin to show concern for the potential beneficial and hazardous effects of procedures. Besides wanting to know if a procedure will hurt, they want to know what it is for, how it will make them better, and what injury or harm could result. For example, these children fear the actual procedure of anesthesia. Unlike preschoolers, who fear the mask and the strange surroundings, school-age children fear what may happen while they are asleep, whether they will wake up, and if they may die. Preadolescents also worry about the procedure itself, particularly one that will result in visible changes in body appearance.

Intrusive procedures, such as routine physical examination of the ears, nose, mouth, and throat, are generally well tolerated. However, concerns for privacy become evident and increasingly significant. Although school-age children may be cooperative during examination of, or procedures performed on, the genital area, it is usually very stressful for them, especially for preadolescents who are beginning pubertal changes. Nurses who respect children's need for privacy can provide them with assurance and support.

By the age of 9 or 10, most school-age children show less fright or overt resistance to pain than younger children. They generally have learned passive methods of dealing with discomfort, such as holding rigidly still, clenching their fists or teeth, or trying to act brave. If they display signs of overt resistance, such as biting, kicking, pulling away, trying to escape, crying, or plea bargaining, they may deny such reactions later, especially to their peers, for fear of embarrassment.

School-age children verbally communicate about their pain in respect to its location, intensity, and description. Unlike younger children, who may have difficulty choosing words to describe pain, children 8 years and older use a wide variety of words and phrases, similar to adults, such as "hurting," "sore," "burning," "stinging," and "aching" (Franck, Greenberg, and Stevens, 2000).

School-age children also use words as a means of controlling their reactions to pain. For example, these children may ask the nurse to talk to them during a procedure. Some prefer to participate in a procedure, whereas others choose to distance themselves by not looking at what is happening. Most appreciate an explanation of the procedure and seem less fearful when they knew what to expect. Others try to gain control by attempting to postpone the event. A typical request is "Start the IV when I am finished with this." Although the ability to make decisions does increase their sense of control, unlimited procrastination results in heightened anxiety. When choices are allowed, such as arm for the intravenous (IV) line, it is best to structure the number of possible sites and to limit the number of "procrastination" techniques.

Similar to their more passive acceptance of pain is their nondirective request for support or help. School-age children will rarely initiate a conversation about their feelings or ask someone to stay with them during a lonely or stressful period. Their visible composure, calmness, and acceptance often mask their inner longing for support. It is especially important to be aware of nonverbal clues, such as a serious facial expression, a halfhearted reply of "I am fine," silence, lack of activity, or social isolation, as signs of the need for help. Usually when someone identifies the unspoken messages and offers support, they readily accept it.

## Adolescents

Although the development of body image begins early in life, its relevance is paramount during adolescence. Injury, pain, disability, and death are viewed primarily in terms of how each affects adolescents' views of themselves in the present. Any change that differentiates the adolescent from peers is regarded as a major tragedy. For example, diseases such as diabetes mellitus often present a more difficult adjustment period for children in this age-group than for younger children because of the necessary changes in the adolescent's lifestyle. Conversely, serious, even life-threatening illnesses that entail no visible bodily changes or physical restrictions may have less immediate significance for the adolescent. Therefore the nature of bodily injury may be more important in terms of adolescents' perception of the illness than its actual degree of severity.

Adolescents' rapidly changing body image during pubertal development often makes them feel insecure about their bodies. Illness, medical or surgical intervention, and hospitalization increase their existing concerns for normalcy. They may respond to such events by asking numerous questions, withdrawing, rejecting others, or questioning the adequacy of care. Frequently their fear for loss of control and body image change is demonstrated as overconfidence.

Because of the development of secondary sex characteristics, adolescents are very concerned about privacy. Lack of respect for this need can cause greater stress than physical pain. In addition, adolescents look for signs that indicate that they are developing normally and according to acceptable standards. When illness occurs, they fear that growth may be retarded, leaving them behind their peers. Although they may not voice this concern, they may demonstrate it by carefully observing others' reactions to them.

Adolescents typically react to pain with much self-control. Physical resistance and aggression are unusual at this age, unless the adolescents are unprepared for a procedure. As with older school-age children, they are very concerned with remaining composed and feel embarrassed and ashamed of losing control. They are able to describe their pain experience and to use the pain assessment tools developed for adults. However, they may be reluctant to disclose their pain, and the nurse may have to closely assess for physical indications, such as limited movement, excessive quiet, or irritability. They may also believe that the nurse knows how they feel; thus they may see no need to ask for analgesia.

# Effects of Hospitalization on the Child

Children may react to the stresses of hospitalization before admission, during hospitalization, and after discharge (Box 26-2). A child's conception of illness is even more important than age and intellectual maturity in predicting the level of adjustment before hospitalization (Clatworthy, Simon, and Tiedeman, 1999). This may or may not be affected by the duration of the condition or prior hospitalizations. Therefore nurses should avoid overestimating the illness concepts of children with prior medical experience.

## Individual Risk Factors

A number of risk factors make certain children more vulnerable than others to the stresses of hospitalization (Box 26-3). It has also been noted that rural children exhibit significantly greater degrees of psychologic upset than urban children, possibly because urban children have opportunities to become familiar with a local hospital (Gillis, 1990). Perhaps because separation is such an important issue surrounding hospitalization for young children, children who are active and strong willed tend to fare better when hospitalized than youngsters who are passive. Consequently, nurses should be alert to children who passively accept all changes and requests; these children may need more support than the "oppositional" child.

The stressors of hospitalization may cause young children to experience short-term and long-term negative outcomes. Adverse outcomes may be related to the length and number of admissions, multiple invasive procedures, and the anxiety of parents. Common responses include regression, separation anxiety, apathy, fears, and sleep disturbances, especially for children younger than 7 years of age (Melnyk, 2000). Supportive practices, such as family-centered care, frequent

---

**Box 26-2** ■ ■ ■
**Posthospital Behaviors in Children**

**YOUNG CHILDREN**

Initial aloofness toward parents; may last from a few minutes (most common) to a few days
Tendency to cling to parents
Demand parents' attention
Vigorously oppose any separation (e.g., staying at preschool or with a baby-sitter)
New fears (e.g., nightmares)
Resistance to going to bed, night waking
Withdrawal and shyness
Hyperactivity
Temper tantrums
Food finickiness
Attachment to blanket or toy
Regression in newly learned skills (e.g., self-toileting)

**OLDER CHILDREN**

Emotional coldness, followed by intense, demanding dependence on parents
Anger toward parents
Jealousy toward others (e.g., siblings)

---

**Box 26-3** ■ ■ ■
**Risk Factors That Increase Children's Vulnerability to the Stresses of Hospitalization**

"Difficult" temperament
Lack of fit between child and parent
Age (especially between 6 months and 5 years)
Male gender
Below-average intelligence
Multiple and continuing stresses (e.g., frequent hospitalizations)

family visits, and mothers who know exactly how they can be involved in their child's care, may lessen the detrimental effects of hospitalization. Research also indicates that the child's pain experience determines how the overall hospitalization is experienced (Woodgate and Kristjanson, 1996).

## Changes in the Pediatric Population

Children are hospitalized for different reasons today than two decades ago. Although there is a growing trend toward shortened hospital stays and outpatient surgery, a greater percentage of the children hospitalized today have more serious and complex problems than those hospitalized in the past. Many of these children are fragile newborns and children with severe injuries or disabilities who survived because of incredible technologic advances, yet were left with chronic or disabling conditions that require frequent and lengthy hospital stays. The nature of their conditions increases the likelihood that this group of children will experience more invasive and traumatic procedures while they are hospitalized. These factors make them more vulnerable to the emotional consequences of hospitalization and result in their needs being significantly different from those of short-term patients. (See Chapter 22 for further discussion on children with special needs.) The majority of these children are infants and toddlers, the age-group most vulnerable to the effects of hospitalization.

Concern in recent years has focused on the increasing length of hospitalization because of complex medical and nursing care, elusive diagnoses, and complicated psychosocial issues. Without special attention devoted to meeting the child's psychosocial and developmental needs in the hospital environment, the detrimental consequences of prolonged hospitalization may be severe.

## Beneficial Effects of Hospitalization

Although hospitalization can be and usually is stressful for children, it can also be beneficial. The most obvious benefit is the recovery from illness, but hospitalization also can present an opportunity for children to master stress and feel competent in their coping abilities. The hospital environment can provide children with new socialization experiences that can broaden their interpersonal relationships. The psychologic benefits need to be considered and maximized during hospitalization. Appropriate nursing strategies to achieve this goal are presented on pp. 1072-1073.

---

**Box 26-4** ◼ ◼ ◻

**Factors Affecting Parents' Reactions to Their Child's Illness**

Seriousness of the threat to the child
Previous experience with illness or hospitalization
Medical procedures involved in diagnosis and treatment
Available support systems
Personal ego strengths
Previous coping abilities
Additional stresses on the family system
Cultural and religious beliefs
Communication patterns among family members

---

# STRESSORS AND REACTIONS OF THE FAMILY OF THE CHILD WHO IS HOSPITALIZED

The crisis of childhood illness and hospitalization affects every member of the family. The stressors and reactions of families have been discussed in detail in Chapter 22 in relation to chronic illness and in Chapter 23 in relation to life-threatening illness. In many respects they differ little regardless of the diagnosis except for their intensity and persistence, which are proportional to the degree of severity. Consequently, when a child is admitted to an intensive care unit, the family members' reactions and needs are typically greater than when a child is admitted with a less serious condition to the regular pediatric unit.

## Parental Reactions

Parents' reactions to illness in their child depend on a variety of influencing factors. Although one cannot predict which factors are most likely to influence their response, a number of variables have been identified (Box 26-4).

Almost all parents respond to their child's illness and hospitalization with remarkably consistent reactions. Initially parents may react with *disbelief,* especially if the illness is sudden and serious. Following the realization of illness, parents react with *anger, guilt,* or both. They tend to search for self-blame regarding why the child became ill or to project anger at others for some wrongdoing. Even in the mildest of illnesses, parents question their adequacy as caregivers and review any actions or omissions that could have prevented or caused the illness. When hospitalization is indicated, parental guilt is intensified because the parents feel helpless in alleviating the child's physical and emotional pain.

*Fear, anxiety,* and *frustration* are common feelings expressed by parents. Fear and anxiety may be related to the seriousness of the illness and the type of medical procedures involved. Often a great deal of anxiety is related to the trauma and pain inflicted on the child from the various procedures. Feelings of frustration are often related to lack of information about procedures and treatments, unfamiliarity with hospital rules and regulations, unfriendly staff, or fear of asking questions. Much frustration can be alleviated in a pediatric unit where parents are aware of what to expect and what is expected of them, are encouraged to participate in their child's care, and are regarded as the most significant contributors to the child's total health.*

Parents eventually may react with some degree of *depression.* Mothers often comment on their feeling of physical and mental exhaustion after all the other family members have adapted to the crisis. Parents may also worry about and miss their other children, who may be left in the care of family, friends, or neighbors. Other reasons for anxiety and depression are related to concerns for the child's future well-being, including negative effects produced by the hos-

---

*An excellent resource for parents is *Your Child in the Hospital: A Practical Guide for Parents* by N. Keene, R. Prentice, and L. Lamb, editors (1999, O'Reilly).

pitalization and any subsequent financial burden incurred from the hospitalization.

## Sibling Reactions

Siblings' reactions to a sister's or brother's illness or hospitalization are discussed in Chapters 22 and 23 and differ little when a child becomes temporarily ill. Siblings experience loneliness, fears, and worry. Their main reactions are anger, resentment, jealousy, and guilt. Various factors have been identified that influence the effects of the child's hospitalization on siblings. Although these factors are similar to those seen when a child has a chronic illness, Craft (1993) reported that the following factors are related specifically to the hospital experience and have been found to increase the effects on the sibling:

- Being younger and experiencing many changes
- Being cared for outside the home by care providers who are not relatives
- Receiving little information about their ill brother or sister
- Perceiving their parents to be treating them differently as compared with before their sibling's hospitalization

Simon (1993) asked 45 siblings of children who were hospitalized their perceptions of the stress of the hospitalization of a brother or sister. The siblings' perceptions of the stress they experienced were equal to the level of stress of hospitalized children. No relationship between age or sex of the sibling was found. However, the perception of stress varied significantly in relation to the type of sibling relationship and frequency of sibling visitation, with those siblings who visited daily demonstrating a higher degree of perceived stress.

Parents are often unaware of the number of effects that siblings experience during the sick child's hospitalization and of the benefit of simple interventions to minimize such effects, such as explicit explanations about the illness and provisions for the siblings to remain at home. Sibling visitation is advocated and is usually advantageous.* However, unless siblings are prepared for what they may see, their visits may confuse them, leaving room for greater anxiety and worry when they are at home, away from their hospitalized brother or sister (Murray, 1998). In one study, one third of the siblings reported that being unprepared for the changes in physical appearance of their hospitalized brother or sister with cancer was their worst experience, and that the image remained in their minds long after the visit (Havermans and Eiser, 1994).

## Altered Family Roles

In addition to the effects of separation on family roles, loss of the parent and sibling roles may affect each family member differently. One of the most common reactions of parents is specialized and intensified attention toward the sick

child. The other siblings may regard this as unfair and interpret the parents' attitude toward them as rejection. Although such responses are usually unconscious and unintended, they place unique burdens on ill children. For example, the ill child may feel obligated to play the sick role to meet parents' expectations, especially in the case of children who have had limited physical ability and regain normal health status, such as following corrective heart surgery. Parents, as well, may have difficulty perceiving the child's recovery and therefore continue the pattern of overprotection and indulgent attention.

Ill children may also feel jealousy and resentment from other siblings. Because of their singular position in the family, they may be denied the companionship of their brothers and sisters. Rivalry between siblings tends to be greatest in the sibling who is nearest the ill child's age. Without an understanding of the interpersonal dynamics between siblings, parents are likely to blame the well children for antisocial behavior. Illness may also result in children's loss of status within either their family or peer group. For example, illness in the oldest child may temporarily terminate special privileges as "big" brother or sister.

## NURSING CARE OF THE CHILD WHO IS HOSPITALIZED

Children and their families require competent and sensitive care to minimize the potential negative effects of hospitalization and also to promote positive benefits from the experience. Interventions should focus on (1) eliminating or minimizing the stressors of separation, loss of control, and bodily injury and pain for children (see Nursing Care Plan: The Child in the Hospital, pp. 1075-1080) and (2) providing specific supportive strategies for family members, such as fostering family relationships and providing information (see Nursing Care Plan: The Family of the Child Who Is Ill or Hospitalized, pp. 1080-1083).

### Preventing or Minimizing Separation

A primary nursing goal is to prevent separation, particularly in children under 5 years of age. Hospitals no longer consider parents "visitors" and welcome their presence at all times throughout the child's hospitalization. Many hospitals have adopted a philosophy of *family-centered care*. This philosophy of care recognizes the integral role of the family in a child's life and acknowledges the family as an essential part of the child's care and illness experience. In the broadest sense the family is considered to be partners in the care of the child (Smith and Conant Rees, 2000). Emphasis is placed on providing services that demonstrate the value of collaboration between the health care provider, the child, and the family. Many provide facilities such as a chair or bed for at least one person per child, unit kitchen privileges, and other amenities that create a welcoming atmosphere for parents. The parents' own schedules may prevent them from being present. In such instances, strategies to minimize the effects of separation must be implemented.

---

*A very useful book for preparing young (4 to 9 years of age) siblings before the hospital visit is *When Molly Was in the Hospital: A Book for Brothers and Sisters of Hospitalized Children* by D. Duncan (1994, Rayve Productions).

## Parent Participation

Although some health facilities provide special accommodations for parents, the concept of family-centered care can be instituted anywhere. The first requirement is the staff's positive attitude toward parents. A negative attitude toward parent participation can create barriers to collaborative working relationships (Smith and Conant Rees, 2000). Unfortunately, although nurses often express explicit support for the concept of family-centered care, some of their practices and beliefs suggest otherwise (Newton, 2000).

Hospital staff who genuinely appreciate the importance of continued parent-child attachment foster an environment that encourages parents to be active caregivers. When parents are included in the care planning and are assured that they are a contributing factor to the child's recovery, they are more inclined to remain with their child and have more emotional reserves to support themselves and the child through the crisis. An empowerment model of helping allows the nurse to focus on parents' strengths and to seek ways to promote growth and family functioning so that parents become empowered in caring for their child (Fig. 26-4).

Because the mother tends to be the usual family caregiver, she spends more time in the hospital than the father (Fig. 26-5). However, not all mothers feel equally comfortable in assuming responsibility for their child's care. Some

may be under such great emotional stress that they need a temporary reprieve from caregiving activities. Others may feel insecure in participating in specialized care. On the other hand, some mothers may feel a great need to have control of their child's care. Individual assessment of each parent's preferred involvement is necessary to prevent the effects of separation while supporting parents in their needs as well. Parents and other family members should be prepared and supported for the roles they choose.

With lifestyles and gender roles changing, some fathers may assume all or some of the usual mothering roles in the household. In this case it may be the father-child relationship that requires preservation. Fathers need to be included in the plan of care and respected for their parental role. For some fathers the child's hospitalization may represent an opportunity to alter their usual caregiving role and increase their involvement. In single-parent families the caregiver may not be a parent but an extended family member, such as a grandparent or aunt.

One of the potential problems with continuous parent visiting is that the parent often neglects the need for sleep, nutrition, and relaxation. (See Family Focus box.) The sleeping accommodations may be limited to a chair, and sleep is disrupted by nursing procedures. After a few days parents may become exhausted but feel obligated to stay.

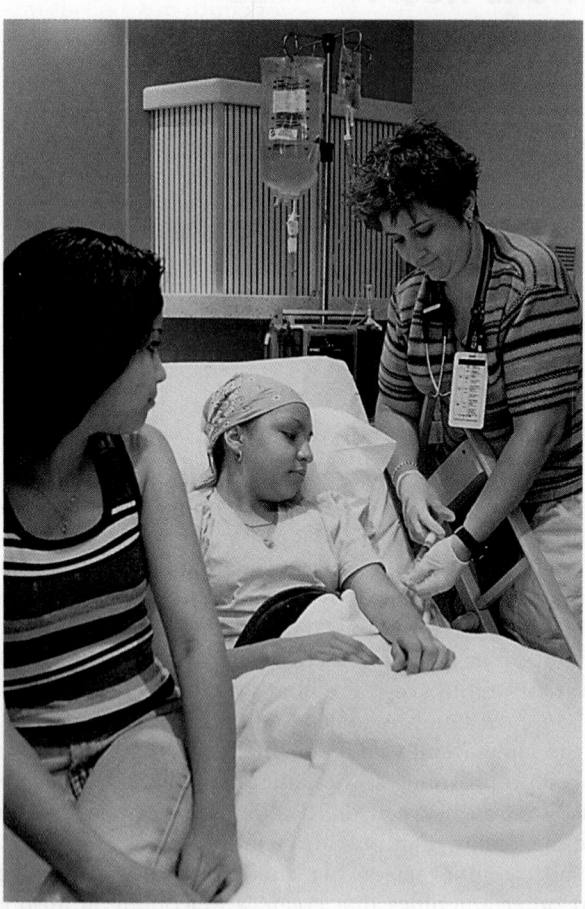

**Fig. 26-4** Family presence during hospitalization, including during procedures, provides emotional support. (Courtesy Paul Vincent Kuntz, Texas Children's Hospital.)

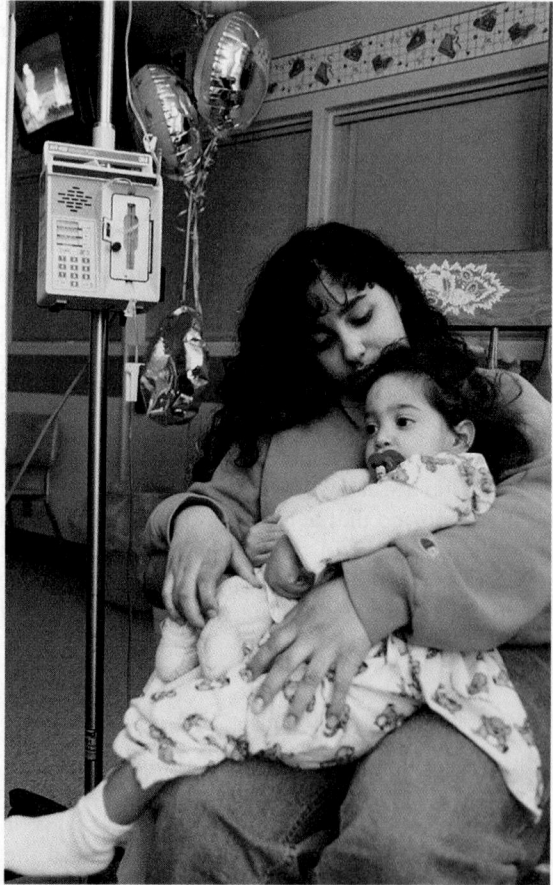

**Fig. 26-5** Despite changing lifestyles and gender roles, mothers tend to be the usual family caregiver and spend more time at the hospital than fathers.

Encouraging them to leave for brief periods, arranging for sleeping quarters on the unit but outside the child's room, and planning a schedule of alternating visiting with the other parent or with a family member can minimize the stresses for the parent.

All too often, nurses respond to parental participation by abandoning their patient responsibilities. Nurses need to restructure their roles to complement and augment the caregiving functions of parents. Even in units structured to promote care by parents, parents frequently feel anxiety in their caregiving responsibilities; those more involved in direct care may feel greater anxiety than those less involved in direct care. A moderate amount of visiting and participation may be optimal for many. Assistance by nursing personnel should always be available to these families.

## Strategies to Minimize the Effects of Separation

When separation cannot be prevented, numerous strategies can be employed to minimize the effects of temporary separation on children. Ideally, a primary nurse is assigned to meet the child's needs. The nurse should obtain a thorough, detailed history that specifically identifies the child's established daily routine (see Box 26-14). Usual daily activities such as meal preparation and method of feeding help establish a complementary schedule of caregiving practices. It also helps the parent feel as if he or she is participating in the child's care but through another person. A consistent staff member can also keep the family informed of the child's condition and support the family's concerns and priorities.

The nurse caring for the child must be aware of the child's separation behaviors. As discussed earlier, phases of protest and despair are normal. The child is allowed to cry. Even if the child rejects strangers, the nurse provides support through physical presence. This includes spending time being physically close to the child, using a quiet tone of voice, appropriate choice of words, eye contact, and touch in ways that establish rapport and communicate empathy. If detachment behaviors are evident, the nurse maintains the child's contact with the parents by frequently talking with them, encouraging the child to remember them, and stressing the significance of their visits, telephone calls, or letters.

Separation may be equally as difficult for parents, especially when they do not understand the behaviors of separation anxiety. To avoid the immediate protest, parents may sneak out or lie to the child about leaving. As a result, the child does not learn that absence is associated with a guaranteed return because there is an element of uncertainty. Helping parents recognize that separation behaviors are normal and expected can decrease anxiety and may ease their fears about leaving the child. Explaining to parents how the child reacts after they leave may also be helpful. Many parents think the child cries for hours after they leave, whereas in reality the child may cry for a few minutes but then settle down when comforted by someone else.

Toddlers and preschoolers have a very limited concept of time. Time is measured in associations, such as "Eating dinner when daddy comes home." Therefore, when helping parents with their fears of separation, nurses need to suggest ways of explaining leaving and returning. For example, if parents must leave to go to work or to make meals for the other family members, they should tell the hospitalized child the reason for leaving. They also need to convey the expected time of return in terms of anticipated events. For example, if the parents return in the morning, they can tell the child that they will see him or her "After the sun comes up" or "When [a favorite program] is on television."

The young child's ability to tolerate parental absence is very limited. Therefore parental visits should be frequent. For example, it is better for parents to visit three times a day for short periods than once a day for an extended time. This may necessitate that each parent visit at different times to lessen the length of separation. When parents cannot visit, the presence of other significant people may be comforting for the child (Fig. 26-6).

If parents leave after the child is asleep, they still need to communicate their absence. The parents of a 5-year-old boy solved this problem by devising a sign; on one side they drew a picture of a telephone and on the other a hamburger. Before they left, they turned the sign to the appropriate side to tell the child when he awoke that they were out using the telephone or eating.

For older children who know how to tell time, it is helpful to give them a clock or watch. However, these children have the same needs for honesty from their parents regarding visiting schedules. Because peer groups are also important, adolescents often appreciate planning visiting hours to provide them with some private time for friends.

Familiar surroundings also increase the child's adjustment to separation. If parents cannot stay with the child, they should leave favorite articles from home, such as a blanket, toy, bottle, feeding utensil, or article of clothing. Because young children associate such objects with signifi-

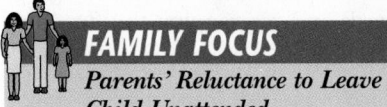

## FAMILY FOCUS

### Parents' Reluctance to Leave Their Child Unattended

Parents are often very reluctant to leave their child who is hospitalized or to ask the nurse to watch their child while they take a break. In his research on the experiences of nurses and parents when parents room-in, Darbyshire (1994) found that many parents did not eat properly or, in some cases, at all. The following are two mothers' experiences:

I just about starved to death the first couple of days . . . just . . . I mean, it was my own fault really, 'cos I wouldn't leave the wee one. There was always going to be something else happening and I thought . . . if he gets upset, I'd better be there when it finishes.

There was one day I couldn't get any of the visitors to look after the wee chap so I could go for something to eat, and it was about 6 o'clock at night, and nurse said, "You look awful, are you OK?" and I said, "No, actually I feel awful and I think I'm going to pass out," and she said, "Oh, you've just gone a funny colour," and I said, "What time is it?" and I said, "It's OK, it's just because I haven't eaten all day"—because none of my family had come to take the child from me, and I didn't think to say to a nurse, "Could you watch him till I go for something to eat?"

Modified from Darbyshire P: *Living with a sick child in a hospital*, London, 1994, Chapman & Hall.

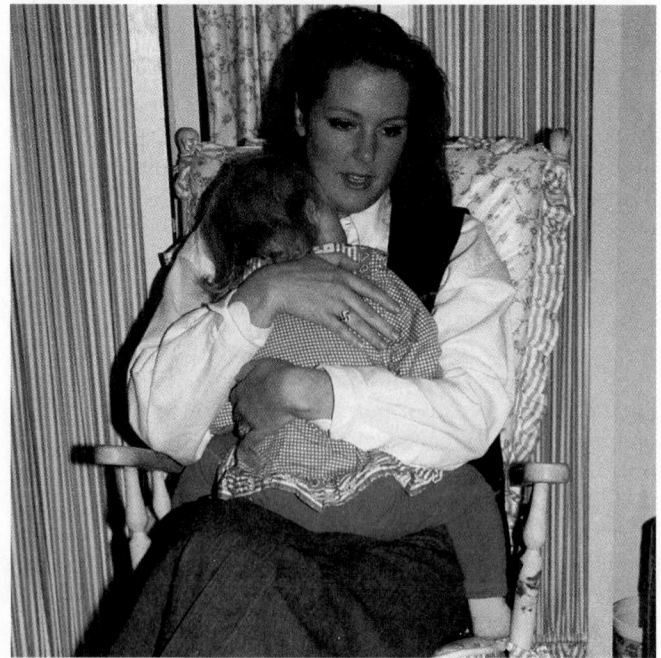

**Fig. 26-6** When parents cannot visit, other significant persons can provide comfort to the hospitalized child.

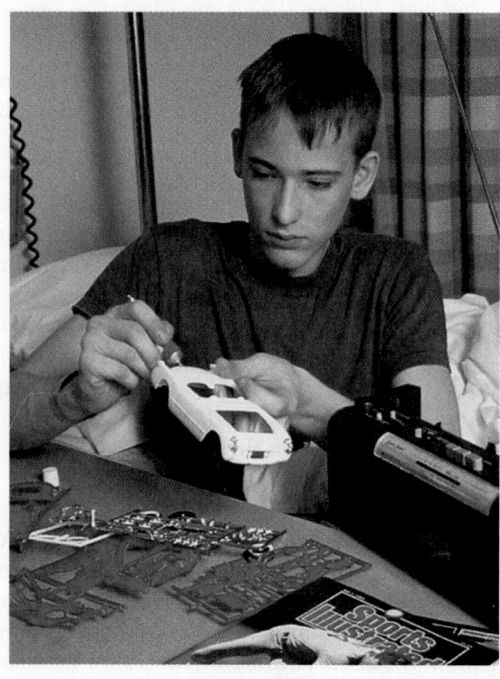

**Fig. 26-7** For extended hospitalizations, children enjoy having projects to occupy time. (Courtesy St Louis Children's Hospital.)

cant people, they gain comfort and reassurance from these possessions. They make the association that if the parent left this, the parent will surely return. Other mementos of home include photographs and tape recordings of family members reading a story, singing a song, or relating events at home. Some units allow pets to visit, which can be a special event for a child and can have therapeutic benefits.

Older children also appreciate familiar articles from home, particularly photographs, a radio, a favorite toy or game, and their own pajamas. The importance of treasured objects for school-age children may be overlooked or criticized. However, approximately half of school-age children have a special object to which they formed an attachment in early childhood. This is a normal and healthy phenomenon. Therefore such treasured or transitional objects can help even older children feel more comfortable in a strange environment.

The sights and sounds in the hospital that are commonplace for the nurse can be strange, frightening, and confusing for children. It is important for the nurse to try to evaluate stimuli in the environment from the child's point of view (considering also what the child may see or hear happening to other patients) and to make every effort to protect the child from frightening and unfamiliar sights, sounds, and equipment. The nurse should offer explanations or prepare the child for those experiences that are unavoidable. Combining familiar or comforting sights with the unfamiliar can relieve much of the harshness of medical care.

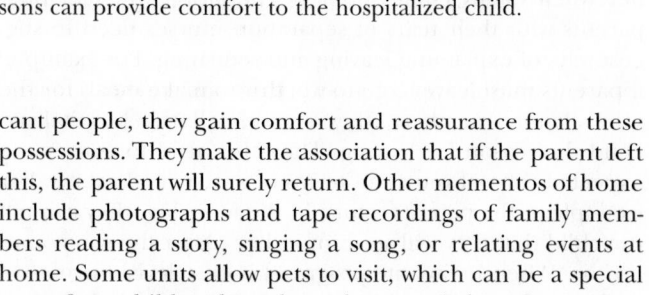

**NURSING TIP** Soften medical equipment (e.g., clip a bear or other animal to a stethoscope; use decorations to transform an IV pump into a friendly animal) to create a pleasant and more familiar environment for children.

Helping children maintain their usual contacts also minimizes the effects of separation imposed by hospitalization. This includes continuing school lessons during the illness and confinement; visiting with friends either directly or through letter writing, telephone calls, or e-mail; and participating in stimulating projects whenever possible (Fig. 26-7). For extended hospitalizations, youngsters enjoy personalizing the hospital room to make it "home" by decorating the walls with posters and cards and rearranging the furniture (when possible).

## Minimizing Loss of Control

Feelings of loss of control result from separation, physical restriction, changed routines, enforced dependency, magical thinking, and altered roles within the family or peer group. Although some of these cannot be prevented, most of them can be minimized through individualized nursing care.

### Promoting Freedom of Movement

Younger children react most strenuously to any type of physical restriction or immobilization. Although some restraint, such as immobilizing an extremity for maintenance of an intravenous (IV) line, is frequently necessary, most physical restriction can be prevented if the nurse gains the child's cooperation.

For young children, particularly infants and toddlers, preserving parent-child contact is the best means of decreasing the need for or stress of restraint. For example, almost the entire physical examination can be done in a parent's lap, with the parent hugging the child for procedures such as otoscopy. For painful procedures the parents' preferences for assisting, observing, or waiting outside the room are assessed.

Environmental factors, may restrict movement. Keeping children in cribs or playpens may not represent immobilization in a concrete sense, but it certainly limits sensory stimulation. Increasing mobility by transporting children in carriages, wheelchairs, carts, or wagons provides them with a sense of freedom.

In some cases physical restraint or isolation is necessary. Whenever possible, restraints should be removed to allow the child some period of supervised freedom, such as during the bath or when parents visit. When restraints or isolation cannot be discontinued, such as with severe burns, the environment can be manipulated to increase sensory freedom. For example, moving the bed toward the door or window; opening window shades; providing musical, visual, or tactile toys; and increasing interpersonal contact can substitute mental mobility for the limitations of physical movement.

## Maintaining the Child's Routine

Altered daily schedules and loss of rituals are particularly stressful for toddlers and early preschoolers and may increase separation anxiety. As stated previously, the nursing admission history provides a baseline for planning care around the child's usual home activities.

Children's response to loss of routine and ritualism is often demonstrated in problems with activities such as eating, sleeping, dressing, bathing, toileting, and social interaction. Although some regression is to be expected, sensitivity to the special needs of children can minimize the negative effects. For example, loss of appetite and marked food preferences are common in children who are ill or hospitalized. In addition, the food selections on hospital menus may differ greatly from preferred cultural or ethnic food preparation. Encouraging the child to eat is often a challenge, yet it is an essential nursing responsibility. Suggestions for feeding sick children are discussed in Chapter 27.

A frequently neglected aspect of altered routines is the change in the child's daily activities. A nonhospitalized child's day, especially during the school years, is structured with specific times for eating, dressing, going to school, playing, and sleeping. However, this time structure vanishes when the child is hospitalized. Although the nurses have a set schedule, the child is frequently unaware of it; new schedules are imposed that may be rigid. For example, some units have uniform nap and bedtimes for all children, whereas others allow children to stay up very late. Many children obtain significantly less sleep in the hospital than at home; the primary causes are delay in sleep onset and early termination of sleep because of hospital routines. Not only are hours of sleep disrupted, but waking hours are spent in passive activities. For example, few institutions impose any regulation on the amount of time children spend watching television, which tends to be considerably more time than they spend watching at home.

One technique that can minimize the disruption in the child's routine is establishing a daily schedule. This approach is most suitable for the noncritically ill school-age and adolescent child who has mastered the concept of time. It involves scheduling the child's day to include all necessary

| ERIC'S DAILY SCHEDULE: | | | |
|---|---|---|---|
| 7:30 AM | – Breakfast, Morning Bath | 3:00 PM | – Tutor (M, W, F) Study Time (T, Th) |
| 9:00 | – Medications, Dressing Change | 4:00 | – Physical Therapy |
| 11:00 | – Physical Therapy | 5:30 | – Dinner |
| 12:00 PM | – Lunch | 9:00 | – Medications, Dressing Change |
| | | 9:15 | – Bedtime |

**Fig. 26-8**  A daily schedule helps to normalize the hospital environment and increases the child's sense of control.

activities that are important to patient care procedures, activities of daily living, mealtimes, and medications. Together, the nurse, parent, and child then plan a daily schedule with times and activities written down, with blocks of free time available for playroom activities, hobbies, and television viewing (Fig. 26-8). This is left in the child's room, and a clock is available for the child's use. For lengthy hospitalizations, a calendar may be constructed with special events such as favorite television programs, visits by friends or relatives, events in the playroom, and holidays or birthdays identified. If specific changes in treatment are expected (e.g., "beginning physical therapy in 2 days"), these are added.

**NURSING TIP**  Ask the young child to select or draw pictures or symbols to represent daily or weekly fun activities (e.g., favorite TV programs, family visits, playroom times). Next to the child's representation, draw a clock face with the hands of the clock depicting the time each event will occur. Have the child compare the clock on the schedule with a clock or watch in the room. When the two match, the child knows that it is time for a favorite activity and exactly what that activity is.

## Encouraging Independence

The dependent role of the hospitalized child imposes feelings of loss on older children. Principal interventions should focus on respect for individuality and the opportunity for decision making. Although these sound simple, their efficacy lies with nurses who are flexible and tolerant. It is also very important to empower the patient and not be threatened by a sense of lessened control.

Promoting children's control involves maintaining independence and promoting self-care. *Self-care* refers to the practice of activities that individuals initiate and perform on their own behalf to maintain life, health, and well-being (Orem, 1995). Although self-care is limited by the child's age and physical condition, most children beyond infancy can perform some activities with little or no help. Whenever possible, these activities are encouraged in the hospital. Other approaches include jointly planning care, time structuring, wearing street clothes, making choices in food selections and bedtime, continuing school activities, and rooming with an appropriate age-mate. For example, adolescents generally prefer a roommate their own age or, ideally, quarters separate from the pediatric unit (see p. 1090).

### Promoting Understanding

Loss of control can occur both from feelings of having too little influence on one's destiny and from sensing overwhelming control or power over fate. Although preschoolers' cognitive abilities predispose them most to creative thinking and self-power, all children are vulnerable to misinterpreting causes for stresses such as illness and hospitalization.

Most children feel more in control when they know what to expect, because the element of fear is reduced. Anticipatory preparation and providing information help greatly to lessen stress and prevent lack of understanding. (See Preparation for Procedures, Chapter 27.)

Informing children of their rights while hospitalized fosters greater understanding and may relieve some of the feelings of powerlessness they experience. Standards used to accredit hospitals recommend that hospitals providing services to children have a hospital-wide policy on the rights and responsibilities of these patients and of their parents or guardians (Joint Commission on Accreditation of Healthcare Organizations, 1999). An increasing number of hospitals and organizations have developed a "Bill of Rights" that is prominently displayed throughout the hospital or is presented to children and their families on admission (see Box 26-5 for an example).

## Preventing or Minimizing Bodily Injury

Beyond early infancy all children fear bodily injury either from mutilation, intrusion, body image change, disability, or death. In general, preparation of children for painful procedures decreases their fears. Manipulating procedural techniques for children in each age-group also minimizes fear of bodily injury. For example, since toddlers and young preschoolers are traumatized by insertion of a rectal thermometer, axillary or tympanic electronic temperature probes can effectively be substituted. Whenever procedures are performed on young children, the most supportive intervention is to do them as quickly as possible and maintain parent-child contact.

Due to the toddler's and preschooler's poorly defined body boundaries, the use of bandages may be particularly helpful. For example, telling children that the bleeding will stop after the needle is removed does little to relieve their fears, whereas applying a Band-Aid usually provides much reassurance. The size of bandages is also significant to children in this age-group. The larger the bandage, the more importance is attached to the wound. Successively smaller surgical dressings is one of their ways of measuring healing and improvement. Removing a dressing may cause them concern for their well-being.

In children who fear mutilation of body parts, repeatedly stressing the reason for a procedure and evaluating their understanding are essential to minimize fear. For example, explaining cast removal to preschoolers may seem simple enough, but the child's comprehension of the details may vary considerably from the explanation. Asking them to draw a picture of what they think will happen provides substantial evidence of how they perceive events.

Children may fear bodily injury from a great variety of sources. Diagnostic imaging machines, use of strange equipment for examination, unfamiliar rooms, or awkward positions can be perceived as potentially hazardous. In addition, thoughts and actions can be imagined sources of bodily damage. Therefore it is important to investigate imagined reasons, particularly of a sexual nature, for illness. Because children may fear revealing such thoughts, using techniques such as drawing or doll play may demonstrate previously undisclosed misconceptions.

Older children fear bodily injury of both internal and external origins. For example, school-age children are aware of the heart's significance and may fear the actual procedure as much as the pain, the stitches, and the possible scar. Adolescents may express concern for the surgery but be much more anxious over the resulting scar. An appreciation of each child's special concerns helps nurses focus on critical areas during preparation for procedures or when explaining the disease processes.

Children can grasp information only if it is presented on or close to their level of cognitive development. This necessitates an awareness of the words used to describe events or processes. For example, young children told that they are going to have a CAT scan may wonder, "Will there be cats? Or something that scratches?" It is clearer to describe the procedure in simple terms and explain what the letters of the common name stand for.

When children are upset about their illness, their perception can be changed by (1) providing a somewhat different and less negative account of the disease or (2) offering an explanation that is characteristic of the next stage of cognitive development. An example of the first strategy is reassuring a preschool child who, after a tonsillectomy, fears that another sore throat means a second operation. Explaining that once tonsils are "fixed," they do not need fixing again can help relieve the fear. An example of the second strategy is to explain that germs made the tonsils sick and even though germs can cause another sore throat, they cannot cause the tonsils to ever be sick again. This higher-level explanation is based on the school-age child's concept of germs as a cause of disease.

## Pain Assessment*

Pain assessment is a critical component of the nursing process. Unfortunately, health professionals, including nurses, tend to

---

> **Box 26-5** ■ ■ ■
> ### Bill of Rights for Children and Teens
>
> In this hospital you and your family have the right to:
> Respect and personal dignity
> Care that supports you and your family
> Information you can understand
> Quality health care
> Emotional support
> Care that respects your need to grow, play, and learn
> Make choices and decisions

---

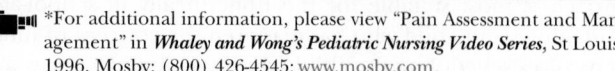

*For additional information, please view "Pain Assessment and Management" in *Whaley and Wong's Pediatric Nursing Video Series*, St Louis, 1996, Mosby; (800) 426-4545; www.mosby.com.

underestimate the existence of pain in children (Boughton and others, 1998; Broome, Rehwaldt, and Fogg, 1998). (See Evidence-Based Practice box.) One of the reasons for inadequate management of pain is a lack of understanding of what pain is—a personal phenomenon that *cannot* be experienced by any other individual. Therefore defining pain in terms of another's perceptions is inappropriate and inaccurate. An operational definition that is useful in clinical practice is: ***pain is whatever the experiencing person says it is, existing whenever the person says it does*** (McCaffery and Pasero, 1999). This defini-

## EVIDENCE-BASED PRACTICE
### *Undermedication of Pain in Children*

Several studies have examined the pattern of pain medication for children as compared with adults and have found remarkably consistent findings—that children have been undermedicated for pain. Eland and Anderson (1977) investigated the incidence of administration of analgesics to 25 hospitalized children for postoperative pain. Twelve of the children received a total of 24 doses of analgesics; the remaining 13 children were never given any medication for pain relief. In contrast, 18 adults with identical diagnoses received 372 opioid analgesic doses and 299 nonopioid analgesic doses for a total of 671 doses. One of the saddest findings was that more than twice as many children had pain medication ordered as received it. This lack of response to the need for pain medication directly relates to the nurses who failed to administer the analgesic.

Another study investigating analgesic prescriptions given to children and adults after open heart surgery found that all of the adults received medication, for a total of 564 doses, but only three-fourths of the children were given medication, for a total of 237 doses during the first 3 postoperative days. This difference was even greater on the fifth postoperative day, when 83% of the adults continued to receive analgesics (a total of 136 doses) but only 12% of the children were medicated (a total of 10 doses) (Beyer and others, 1983).

Another study on postoperative pain found that 75% of the children reported pain on the day of surgery, and if orders for opioid or nonopioid analgesics were written, the nonopioid was given exclusively. In addition, the doses ordered were usually too small or too infrequent to be maximally effective. Most orders were written "PRN," which was often interpreted by nursing staff to mean "as little as possible" (Mather and Mackie, 1983).

A review of analgesic use in the emergency department reported significantly low use in children with mild to moderate trauma, including children with painful fractures. Head injury was associated with especially low use of analgesics (Friedland and Kulick, 1994).

Johnston and others (1992) studied 150 randomly selected hospitalized children and found that 87% reported pain, with 19% stating that their pain was severe. Of the 150 children, only 38% had received analgesics during the previous 24 hours.

An even sadder and more disappointing finding is that two decades after Eland's seminal research, some nurses may neither have knowledge about appropriate analgesic medications for children nor appreciate the consequences of undermedication. In Boughton and others' study (1998), 25% of 36 patients were given no pain medication, and 25% of the patients stated that their pain intervention was only partially effective. *All* patients had PRN orders for analgesics. Clearly the responsibility for inadequate pain control rested with the nurses.

The situation is even more serious with infants. One analysis of anesthetic practices with newborns undergoing surgical ligation of patent ductus arteriosus found that 76% of the infants received only nitrous oxide and a paralyzing agent. These infants could not move during surgery but could feel all the pain of a thoracotomy (Anand and Aynsley-Green, 1985). In a survey of nurses working in neonatal intensive care units, 79% believed that infants were undermedicated for pain. The same study found that more than half of the medications used for pain relief had no analgesic properties (Franck, 1987). A study comparing premedication for procedures, such as arterial line or chest tube placement, found that infants in neonatal intensive care units received no premedication much more often than children in pediatric intensive care units (Bauchner, May,

and Coates, 1992). In the United States the use of analgesia and anesthesia for newborn circumcision is not routine. A survey of pediatric, obstetric, and family practice residents showed that training in the use of pain reducers during this painful procedure was inadequate (Howard and others, 1998). Unfortunately, discussion of pain in nursing curricula is also inadequate, and some of the textbooks contain inaccurate information (Davis, 1998; Ferrell, McCaffery, and Rhiner, 1992).

Much research has been done examining the stress response in premature infants, and the results support the belief that unrelieved pain has detrimental physiologic, anatomic, and behavioral effects. (See Neonatal Pain, Chapter 10.) Much less research has been done on the long-term effects of pain on children, from both a psychologic and a physiologic point of view. Stuber and others (1997) examined the psychologic effects on survivors of childhood cancer. Many children reported long-term sequelae that resembled posttraumatic stress syndrome. (See Chapter 18.) Children's fears were related to their perception of the intensity of treatment, not the illness itself. Symptoms included stomachaches and bad dreams. Another study found that memory of a painful experience may cause anxiety about subsequent procedures. Weisman, Bernstein, and Schechter (1998) showed that children who had a placebo, rather than oral transmucosal fentanyl, before a painful procedure were more anxious than the medicated group for the subsequent procedure *even when the analgesic was given*. Based on their results, the authors argue strongly for aggressive pain control beginning with the first noxious procedure.

On a positive note, Schechter (1997) outlines the growth in research and published literature (33 articles in 1974 to 2966 articles from 1980 to 1991) in pediatric pain management that comprises many topics such as oncology, sickle cell disease, acute pain, and chronic pain. One outcome of the large number of research studies has been the development of pain teams or pain specialists. Unfortunately, when these services exist, other health care professionals may abandon any responsibility for pain control to the pain experts or neglect to consult the pain team. Although pain teams play a very important role in treating pain adequately (Ferrell and others, 1994), in a survey of 35 pediatric pain services only 17% had written guidelines (Tyc and others, 1998).

Guidelines are available to help practitioners assess and manage pain using methods based on the published scientific literature. In the United States the Agency for Healthcare Research and Quality (AHRQ) (formerly the agency for Health Care Policy and Research [AHCPR]) has published guidelines developed by pain experts that focus on the issues of postoperative, procedure-related or trauma, and cancer pain. Other national and international organizations, including the Joint Commission on the Accreditation of Healthcare Organizations, have also contributed research-based recommendations that nurses can use to improve pain control (Box 26-6, p. 1048).

If these references are not readily available to your staff, order them, especially the AHRQ publications, and distribute them, stressing that they provide state-of-the-art information. As you practice, carry your copy of the guidelines; mark sections, such as those discussing addiction and listing drug dosages, for quick reference. Compare your pain assessment and management interventions with those in the published guidelines and make a commitment to increase your knowledge. *Remember: to relieve pain effectively, pain management must be based on scientific research, not personal opinion or belief.*

tion implies a very important attitude toward patients—*that they are believed.* It includes both verbal and nonverbal expressions of pain.

## Fallacies and Facts

Children are undertreated for pain for a number of complex and interrelated reasons, including professionals' mis-

conceptions about pain and pain management; the complexities of pain assessment, particularly in nonverbal children; and the lack of awareness of the detrimental consequences of unrelieved pain. A number of fallacies continue to flourish because of incorrect knowledge about pain in infants and children, despite these fallacies having been disproved by current research and other excellent resources

---

**Box 26-6 ■ ■ ▫**
## Selected Resources on Pain

**Epidural Analgesia for Acute Pain Management: a Self-Directed Learning Program and Pre and Post Tests/Answers and Explanations.** By Chris Pasero, MS, RN. The objectives for the program are to identify the nurse's role in assessing and managing acute pain of adult patients and to identify how to care for adult patients who are receiving epidural analgesia. Available from the American Society of Pain Management Nurses (ASPMN), 7794 Grow Dr., Pensacola, FL 32514-7022, (888) 34ASPMN; fax: (805) 484-7862; e-mail: aspmn@puetzamc.com; *www.aspmn.org.*

**Guidelines for Treatment of Cancer Pain: the Pocket Edition of the Final Report of the Texas Cancer Council's Workgroup on Pain Control in Cancer Patients.** By C. Stratton Hill, Jr., MD (1997). Available free from the Texas Cancer Council, PO Box 12097, Austin, TX 78711, (512) 463-3190; fax: (512) 475-2563; *www.texascancercouncil.org.*

**Managing Pain Before It Manages You.** By Margaret A. Caudill, MD, PhD (1995). Available from The Guilford Press, A Division of Guilford Publications, Inc., 72 Spring St., New York, NY 10012.

**McCaffery: Contemporary Issues in Pain Management.** Four videotapes: *Pain Management in the Elderly; Improving the Quality of Pain Management; Epidural Analgesia for Chronic Pain;* and *Preventing and Managing Opioid-Induced Respiratory Depression.* Also **McCaffery on Pain: Nursing Assessment and Pharmacological Intervention in Adults.** Four videotapes: *Nursing Assessment of the Patient with Pain; The Three Analgesic Groups: Practical Considerations; Use of Opioid Analgesic;* and *Undertreatment of Pain.* A resource manual also accompanies the videotapes. Available for purchase from Lippincott Williams & Wilkins, (800) 527-5597; *www.lww.com.*

**No Fears, No Tears: Children with Cancer Coping with Pain.** Videotape demonstrates the use of distraction and imagery to reduce distress from various procedures. Available from the Candian Cancer Society, (416)961-7223; fax (416) 961-4189. For information on **No Fears, No Tears—13 Years Later,** contact Burness Communications directly online: *www. burnessc.com/nofears.*

**No More Crying: Reducing Distress During Venipuncture.** Videotape describes distraction, limit-setting, and positive reinforcement to reduce the distress associated with procedures. Available for rental or purchase from Leo Media, 110 W. Main St., Urbana, IL 61801-2715, (800) 421-6999; *www.leomedia.net.*

**Pain Management in Children with Cancer.** By Marilyn Hockenberry-Eaton, PhD, RN-CS, PNP, CPON, FAAN, and others. Published by the Texas Cancer Council (1999). Booklet provides information on treating pain in children with cancer but provides guidelines that apply generally to acute pain management as well; *www. childcancerpain.org.*

**Pain Relief: How to Say No to Acute, Chronic, and Cancer Pain!** By Jane Cowles (1993). Book written for consumers that focuses on the prevention, assessment, and individualized treatment of pain in children and adults. Available from MasterMedia Pub., PO 1117, Sandy, OR 97055, (800) 334-8232.

**Pain Resource Center.** Serves as a clearinghouse to disseminate information and resources to improve the quality of pain management. Contact City of Hope National Medical Center, Pain/Palliative Care Resource Center, 1500 E. Duarte Rd., Duarte, CA 91010, (626) 359-8111, ext. 3829; fax: (626) 301-8941; e-mail: prc@coh.org; *www.mayday.coh.org.*

**Pediatric Pain Letter.** By Patrick J. McGrath, PhD, and G. Allen Finley, MD, FRCPC. Quarterly review of the literature on pain in infants, children, and adolescents that presents a series of struc-

tured abstracts accompanied by critical commentaries. Questions and subscriptions may be addressed to Julie Goodman, Managing Editor, *Pediatric Pain Letter,* Psychology Department, Dalhousie University, Halifax, Nova Scotia, B3H 4J1; e-mail: jgoodman@is2.dal.ca.

**Perioperative Analgesia, Approaching the 21st Century.** Study guide and audiocassette reviews current and emerging approaches, such as preemptive analgesia, for surgery. Available from the American Pain Society, 4700 W. Lake Dr., Glenview, IL 60025-1485, (847) 375-4715; fax (877) 734-8758, e-mail: info@ampainsoc.org; *www.ampainsoc.org.*

**Prevention and Management of Pain and Stress in the Neonate.** Committee on Fetus and Newborn, Committee on Drugs Section on Anesthesiology, and Section on Surgery of the American Academy of Pediatrics. This statement is intended for health care professionals caring for neonates (preterm to 1 month of age), *Pediatrics* 105(2):454, 2000; *www.aap.org* or *www.pediatrics.org.*

**Quality of Mercy: A Case for Better Pain Management.** Videotape highlights problems in infant pain control and cancer and burn pain. Available for rental or purchase from Filmakers Library, 124 E. 40th St., New York, NY 10016, (212) 808-4980; fax: (212) 808-4983; e-mail: info@filmakers.com; *www.filmakers.com.*

**Questions Parents and Concerned Professionals Might Ask of Their Local Health Care Institutions.** A one-page sheet that addresses questions to effectively raise awareness about infant pain control. In Butler NB: How to raise professional awareness of the need for adequate pain relief for infants, *Birth* 12(1): 38-41, 1988.

**Reducing the Anxiety and Pain of Injections.** Guide based on a composite of research data, clinical studies, and expert opinion. Available from Becton Dickinson Media Center, (800) ALL MEDIA; fax: (201) 847-4963; *www.bd.com* (reorder number BDM#01). Another excellent article: Reis EC and others: Taking the sting out of shots: control of vaccination-associated pain and adverse reactions, *Pediatr Ann* 27(6):376-386, 1998.

**Whaley and Wong's Pediatric Pain Assessment and Management.** By Donna Wong, PhD, RN. Videotape focuses on process of QUESTT for pain assessment and Six Rights for Pharmacologic Pain Relief. Available from Mosby, an affliate of Elsevier Health Sciences, 11830 Westline Industrial Dr., St. Louis, MO 63146, (800) 325-4177; fax: (800) 535-9935; *www.mosby.com.*

**Wong-Baker FACES Pain Rating Scale Reference Manual.** Describes development and research of the scale. Available from the City of Hope National Medical Center, Pain/Palliative Care Resource Center, 1500 E. Duarte Rd., Duarte, CA 91010, (626) 359-8111, ext. 3829; fax: (626) 301-8941; e-mail: prc@coh.org. To obtain permission to use the scale, contact Julie Lawley, W.B. Saunders, The Curtis Center, Independence Square W., Philadelphia, PA 19106, (800) 523-1649, ext. 8302; fax: (215) 238-8483; *www.mosby.com/WOW/.* A compilation of many pain scales, including the FACES, is available free from Purdue Frederick Company, 100 Connecticut Ave., Norwalk, CT 06850-3950, (800) 733-1333 or (203) 853-0123, ext. 7378 or 7314; *www.partnersagainstpain.com.*

**Wong-Baker FACES Pain Rating Scale Pins.** Pins may be purchased in gold, red, or blue and with coding of 0 to 5 for all colors and 0 to 10 for red only. For information contact Linda Toth, PO Box 2984, Sanford, NC 27331, (919) 498-1158; fax: (919) 498-3993.

on pediatric pain (Boxes 26-6 and 26-7). Two fallacies that exist among nurses and probably most commonly promote undertreatment of pain are unrealistic fears about respiratory depression and concern about addiction to opioids* (Schmidt, Eland, and Weiler, 1994).

**Fear of Addiction.** A major concern that prevents health professionals from adequately using opioids to relieve pain is an unwarranted fear of addiction. Children treated appropriately for pain rarely if ever become addicted (Yaster and others, 1997). The Acute Pain Manage-

---

*The term *opioid* refers to natural or synthetic analgesics with morphine-like actions. It is preferred to the term *narcotic*, which in a legal context refers to any substance that causes psychologic dependence, such as cocaine, which is not an opioid. The word "narcotic" also engenders fears of addiction in older children and parents that are unwarranted when opioids are used for pain control.

---

### Box 26-7 ■ ■ ■
#### Fallacies and Facts About Children and Pain

**Fallacy:** Infants do not feel pain.
**Fact:** Infants demonstrate behavioral, especially facial, and physiologic, including hormonal, indicators of pain. Neonates have the neural mechanisms to transmit noxious stimuli by 20 weeks of gestation (Anand and Hickey, 1987; Marshall, 1989; Shapiro, 1989; Stevens, Johnston, and Horton, 1993). (See Neonatal Pain, Chapter 10.)
**Fallacy:** Children tolerate pain better than adults.
**Fact:** Children's tolerance for pain actually *increases* with age (Haslam, 1969; Lander and Fowler-Kerry, 1991). Younger children tend to rate procedure-related pain higher than older children (Fradet and others, 1990; Humphrey and others, 1992; Wong and Baker, 1988).
**Fallacy:** Children cannot tell you where they hurt.
**Fact:** By 4 years of age, children can accurately point to the body area or mark the painful site on a drawing (Savedra and others, 1993; Van Cleve and Savedra, 1993); children as young as 3 years old can use pain scales, such as FACES (Beyer, Denyes, and Villarruel, 1992; Wong and Baker, 1988).
**Fallacy:** Children always tell the truth about pain.
**Fact:** Children may not admit having pain to avoid an injection; because of constant pain, they may not realize how much they are hurting; children may believe that others know how they are feeling and not ask for analgesia (Favaloro and Touzel, 1990; Hester, 1989).
**Fallacy:** Children become accustomed to pain or painful procedures.
**Fact:** Children often demonstrate *increased* behavioral signs of discomfort with repeated painful procedures (Dolgin and others, 1989; Fitzgerald, Millard, and MacIntosh, 1988; Katz, Kellerman, and Siegel, 1980; Lander and Fowler-Kerry, 1991).
**Fallacy:** Behavioral manifestations reflect pain intensity.
**Fact:** Children's developmental level, coping abilities, and temperament, such as activity level and intensity of reaction to pain, influence pain behavior (Beyer, McGrath, and Berde, 1990; Wallace, 1989; Young and Fu, 1988). Children with more active, resisting behaviors may rate pain lower than children with passive, accepting behaviors (Broome and others, 1990).
**Fallacy:** Narcotics are more dangerous for children than they are for adults.
**Fact:** Narcotics (opioids) are no more dangerous for children than they are for adults. Addiction to opioids used to treat pain is extremely rare in children (Brozovic and others, 1986; Morrison, 1991; Rodgers and others, 1988; Rogers, 1990). Reports of respiratory depression in children are also uncommon (Berde and others, 1991; Billmire, Neale, and Gregory 1985; Dilworth and MacKellar, 1987). By 3 to 6 months of age healthy infants can metabolize opioids like other children (Hertzka and others, 1989; Koren and others, 1985).

---

ment Guideline Panel (1992) has made the following statement regarding addiction from opioid use in pain management for children: *There is no known aspect of childhood development or physiology that indicates any increased risk of physiologic or psychologic dependence from the brief use of opioids for acute pain management.*

One of the reasons for the unfounded and prevalent fear regarding addiction is confusion among three terms: physical dependence, tolerance, and addiction. Health care professionals erroneously equate all three terms with addiction, when in reality these terms reflect completely different behavioral and physiologic actions. (See Community Focus box on p. 1050)

**Fear of Respiratory Depression.** Respiratory depression is the most serious side effect of opioids; however, it is a rare occurrence in children. Several studies document the safety of appropriately dosed opioids in infants and children (Jacobson and others, 1997; Kennedy and others, 1998; Zernikow and Lindena, 2001). Evidence suggests that in children over 3 months of age (and possibly younger) opioids cause no greater respiratory depression than in adults (Kart, Christrup, and Rasmussen, 1997; Sabatino and others, 1997). Respiratory depression is most likely to occur when the opioid is administered with other sedating drugs, such as promethazine (Phenergan), chlorpromazine (Thorazine), midazolam (Versed), or diazepam (Valium) (Gibbons and others, 1998). Unlike many sedatives, opioids have the advantage of the antidote naloxone (Narcan), which rapidly reverses the respiratory depressant effect. The benzodiazepines, such as diazepam and midazolam, have the drug flumazenil (Romazicon) to treat respiratory depression. (See Community Focus box on p. 1050)

In addition, as tolerance to the analgesic effect of opioids occurs, tolerance to the respiratory depressant effect also occurs. Pain acts as a natural antagonist to the action of opioids. With increased pain, a patient can receive increased opioids and, except for constipation, will not experience increased side effects. Respiratory depression is rare in children receiving long-term opioid therapy even when large doses are needed (Collins, 1996).

### Principles of Pain Assessment in Children

The American Pain Society (2000) created the phrase "pain: the fifth vital sign" to increase awareness of pain assessment among health care professionals. The rationale is that if pain were assessed with the same seriousness as other vital signs, it would more likely be treated properly. Thus one principle of pain assessment is to assess patients for pain every time you check for pulse, blood pressure, temperature, and respiratory rate (Federwisch, 1999). Because pain is both a sensory and an emotional experience, using several assessment strategies provides qualitative and quantitative information about pain. One approach to pain assessment in children is *QUESTT* (Baker and Wong, 1987):

> **Q**uestion the child.
> **U**se pain rating scales.
> **E**valuate behavior and physiologic changes.
> **S**ecure parents' involvement.
> **T**ake cause of pain into account.
> **T**ake action and evaluate results.

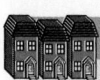

## COMMUNITY FOCUS
*Fear of Opiod Addiction*

One of the reasons for the unfounded but prevalent fear of addiction to opioids used to relieve pain is a misunderstanding of the differences among the concepts of physical dependence, tolerance, and addiction. Health care professionals and the community often confuse addiction with the physiologic effects of opioids, when in reality the events are unrelated.

The American Society of Addiction Medicine (1997) defines the three terms as follows:

*Physical dependence* on an opioid is a physiologic state that often includes tolerance in which abrupt cessation of the opioid, rapid dose reduction, or administration of an opioid antagonist results in a withdrawal syndrome. Physical dependency on opioids is an expected occurrence in all individuals in the presence of continuous use of opioids for therapeutic or for nontherapeutic purposes. It does not, in and of itself, imply addiction.

*Tolerance* is a form of neuroadaption to the effects of chronically administered opioids (or other medications) that is indicated by the need for increasing or more frequent doses of the medication to achieve the initial effects of the drug. Tolerance may occur both to the analgesic effects of opioids and to some of the unwanted side effects, such as respiratory depression, sedation, or nausea. The occurrence of tolerance is variable, but it does not, in and of itself, imply addiction.

*Addiction* in the context of pain treatment with opioids is characterized by a persistent pattern of dysfunctional opioid use that may involve any or all of the following:

☐ Continued use despite adverse reactions
☐ Loss of control over the use of opioids
☐ Preoccupation with obtaining opioids, despite the presence of adequate analgesia

Behaviors suggestive of addiction include inability to take medication on the prescribed schedule, taking multiple doses at one time, frequent reports of lost or stolen prescriptions, doctor shopping, and isolation from family or friends.

Unfortunately, individuals who have severe, unrelieved pain may become intensely focused on finding relief for their pain. Sometimes behaviors such as "clock watching" make patients appear to others to be preoccupied with obtaining opioids. However, this preoccupation focuses on finding relief of pain, not on using opioids for reasons other than pain control. This phenomenon has been termed *pseudoaddiction* and must not be confused with real addiction.

Nurses must educate older children, parents, and health care professionals about the extremely low risk of real addiction (less than 1%) from the use of opioids to treat pain. Infants, young children, and comatose or terminally ill children simply cannot become addicted because they are incapable of a consistent pattern of drug-seeking behavior such as stealing, drug dealing, prostitution, and use of family income to obtain opioids for nonanalgesic reasons.

*Data from American Society of Addiction Medicine: *Public policy statement on definitions related to the use of opioids for the treatment of pain,* February 2001; *www.asam.org.*

---

**Question the Child.** Children's verbal statements of pain are the *most* reliable indicators of pain (Acute Pain Management Guideline Panel, 1992). However, young children may not know what the word "pain" means and may need help in describing it using familiar language. Using a variety of words to describe pain, such as "owie," "boo-boo," "hurt," "ouch," or words in the child's native language, such

---

---

as the Spanish words "dolor," "duele," "le le," or "ai ai," is often necessary. Older children also benefit from using simple words to describe pain. Questions for obtaining a history of children's experiences with pain are presented in Box 26-8. Asking children to locate the pain is also helpful, and play can provide other means for helping children to reveal discomfort.

**NURSING TIP** Ask child to point to where it hurts; have child mark or color the painful area on a drawing of a human figure (Fig. 26-9); ask child to tell how a puppet, doll, or stuffed animal is feeling or to point out areas on these models that "hurt" or "don't feel good."

When asking children about pain, the nurse must remember that they may deny pain because they fear receiving an injectable analgesic or because they believe they deserve to suffer as punishment for some misdeed. They may also deny pain to a stranger but readily admit it to a parent. This behavior should not be interpreted as seeking attention from the parent, but as a valid indication of pain.

**Use a Pain Rating Scale.** Pain rating scales (instruments) provide a subjective quantitative measure of pain. Although various pain scales exist (Table 26-2), not all of them are appropriate for young children. For the most valid and reliable pain intensity rating, a scale is selected that is suitable to the child's age, abilities, and preference. Nurses frequently state that assessment is the first step toward alleviating pain in children. A study of pediatric nurses in eight hospitals, however, demonstrated that it was not evident in their documentation that developmentally appropriate

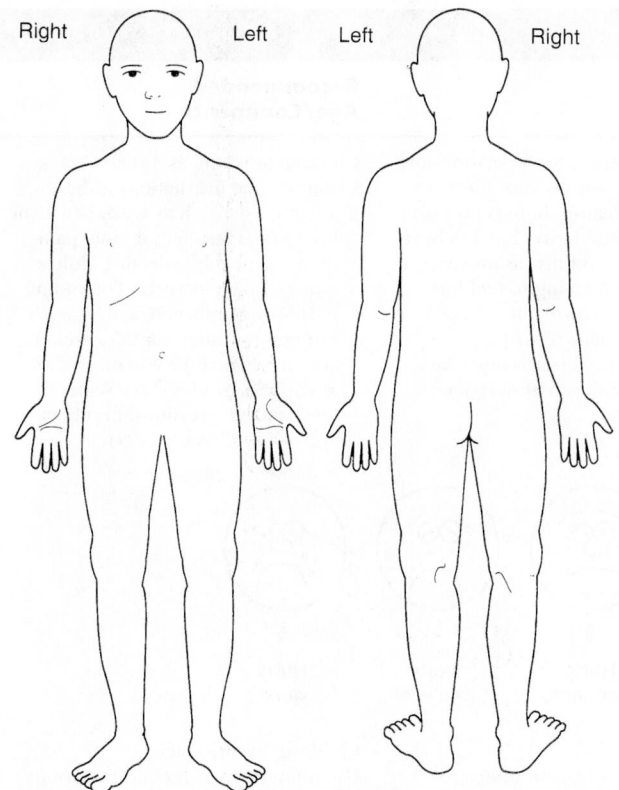

Right   Left   Left   Right

**Fig. 26-9**   Adolescent Pediatric Pain Tool (APPT): body outlines for pain assessment. Instructions: "Color in the areas on these drawings to show where you have pain. Make the marks as big or as small as the place where the pain is." (From Savedra MC, Tesler MD, Holzemer WL, and Ward JA, School of Nursing, University of California—San Francisco, San Francisco, CA. Copyright 1989, 1992.)

tools were used for pain assessment (Jacob and Puntillo, 1999).

This phenomenon is not unique to the United States. In Finland a survey of 303 nurses revealed that they relied on observation of the child's behavior and physiologic changes to assess pain. Pain measurement scales were not recognized as an important part of pain assessment (Salantera and others, 1999a). However, research has consistently demonstrated that scales using expressions of actual children (Oucher) or of cartoon drawings are readily accepted and can be used with children as young as 3 years of age.

Several cartoon-type facial scales exist. Bieri and others (1990) developed a pain intensity scale that uses seven oval-shaped cartoon faces for a coding system of 0 to 6. The faces range from a neutral expression to various degrees of distressed pain expressions. McGrath, de Veber, and Hearn (1985) constructed the Pain Affect Scale to measure how badly a child feels about having pain rather than pain intensity. The scale includes nine faces ranging from a very happy face to a very sad, tearful face. The coding system is from 0.04 to 0.97. The Wong-Baker FACES Pain Rating Scale consists of six cartoon-type faces. A smiling face represents "no hurt," and the faces range from this smiling face to a tearful face that represents "the worst hurt you could

imagine." The pictures in between these faces represent varying degrees of facial grimaces (Wong and Baker, 1988).

The Wong-Baker FACES Pain Rating Scale has been studied for validity and reliability, ease of use for nurses and patients, and preference among nurses, parents, and patients. Wong and Baker (1988) compared six assessment scales (simple descriptive scale, Numeric Scale, Glasses Rating Scale, modified Poker Chip Tool, modified Color Tool, and FACES Scale) in 150 children; the FACES Scale was preferred in all three age-groups tested (3 to 7 years, 8 to 12 years, and 13 to 18 years). In a study involving pediatric oncology patients ages 5 to 13 years, nurses, patients, and parents preferred the FACES Scale over the Poker Chip Tool (West and others, 1994). The FACES Scale was also preferred over the Numeric Scale, Word-Graphic Rating Scale, and Word Description Scale by 118 children in all age-groups (3 to 7 years, 8 to 12 years, and 13 to 18 years). The researchers also believed that the FACES Scale met criteria for ease of use among nurses and children (Keck and others, 1996). In a study conducted among 100 African-American children, the FACES Scale was compared with the Visual Analogue Scale (VAS) and the African-American Oucher (Luffy, 1997). The FACES Scale was chosen by 56% of the children as their first preference, Oucher by 26%, and VAS by 18%. Another study compared the FACES Scale to the Oucher, using the culturally appropriate version, and found that 71% of the children and 80% of the nurses preferred the FACES (Razmus and Lammert, 1998). The FACES Scale has also been shown to be preferred by adults (Carey and others, 1997).

One criticism of the Wong-Baker FACES Pain Rating Scale is that children may perceive that they are being asked to rate how they are "feeling" rather than their amount of pain. The use of smiling faces and affective words such as "happy," "sad," and "ask the person how he/she is feeling" in the original instructions raises the concern that the scale may address affect rather than pain intensity (Champion and others, 1998). Therefore children feeling anxious about an upcoming event may choose a face other than the "no hurt face" even if they are not in pain (Robertson, 1993). Studies have addressed this issue. One hundred 4- and 5-year-old children were randomly assigned to one of two instruction groups. One of the groups was given the original FACES instructions, and the other group was given a modified version without affective or feeling-related words. There were no significant differences in the groups' pain rating scores for immunization injections (Nix, Clutter, and Wong, 1998). Another study showed that pain ratings of same-age children using brief descriptive words placed under each face did not differ significantly from pain ratings obtained with the original instructions (Lefkowicz and others, 1998). To increase the reliability and ease of use of the FACES Scale, only the instrument with simple words is recommended (see Table 26-2). Numerous studies have also demonstrated good correlation between the FACES Scale and other scales purported to measure pain intensity (Keck and others, 1996; Oakes and others, 1993; West and others, 1994; Wilson, Cason, and Grissom, 1995; Wong and Baker, 1988).

**TABLE 26-2** Pain rating scales for children

| Pain Scale/Description | Instructions | Recommended Age/Comments |
|---|---|---|
| **FACES Pain Rating Scale\*** (Wong and Baker, 1988, Wong, 1996): Consists of six cartoon faces ranging from smiling face for "no pain" to tearful face for "worst pain" | *Original Instructions:* Explain to child that each face is for a person who feels happy because there is no pain (hurt) or sad because there is some or a lot of pain. FACE 0 is very happy because there is no hurt. FACE 1 hurts just a little bit. FACE 2 hurts a little more. FACE 3 hurts even more. FACE 4 hurts a whole lot, but FACE 5 hurts as much as you can imagine, although you don't have to be crying to feel this bad. Ask child to choose face that best describes own pain. Record the number under chosen face on pain assessment record.<br>*Brief word instructions:* Point to each face using the words to describe the pain intensity. Ask the child to choose face that best describes own pain and record the appropriate number. | Children as young as 3 years<br>Using original instructions without affect words, such as *happy* or *sad*, or brief words resulted in same pain rating, probably reflecting child's rating of pain intensity. For coding purposes, numbers 0, 2, 4, 6, 8, 10 can be substituted for 0-5 system to accommodate 0-10 system.<br>The FACES provides three scales in one: facial expressions, numbers, and words (Pasero, 1997). |

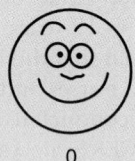 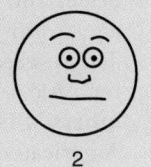 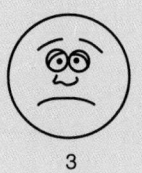  

| 0 | 1 | 2 | 3 | 4 | 5 |
|---|---|---|---|---|---|
| No hurt | Hurts little bit | Hurts little more | Hurts even more | Hurts whole lot | Hurts worst |

| Pain Scale/Description | Instructions | Recommended Age/Comments |
|---|---|---|
| **Oucher** (Beyer, Denyes, and Villarruel, 1992): Consists of six photographs of child's face representing "no hurt" to "biggest hurt you could ever have"; also includes a vertical scale with numbers from 0 to 100; scales for African-American and Hispanic children have been developed (Villarruel and Denyes, 1991) | *Numeric scale*<br>Point to each section of scale to explain variations in pain intensity: "0 means no hurt." "This means little hurts" (pointing to lower part of scale, 1 to 29). "This means middle hurts" (pointing to middle part of scale, 30 to 69). "This means big hurts" (pointing to upper part of scale, 70 to 99). "100 means the biggest hurt you could ever have." Score is actual number stated by child.<br>*Photographic scale*<br>Point to each photograph on Oucher and explain variations in pain intensity using following language: first picture from the bottom is "no hurt," second is "a little hurt," third is "a little more hurt," fourth is "even more hurt than that," fifth is "pretty much or a lot of hurt," and the sixth is the "biggest hurt you could ever have." Score pictures from 0 to 5, with the bottom picture scored as 0.<br>*General*<br>Practice using Oucher by recalling and rating previous pain experiences (e.g., falling off a bike). Child points to number or photograph that describes pain intensity associated with experience. Obtain current pain score from child by asking, "How much hurt do you have right now?" | Children 3 to 13 years<br>Use numeric scale if child can count to 100 by ones and identify larger of any two numbers, or by tens (Jordan-Marsh and others, 1994).<br>Determine whether child has cognitive ability to use photographic scale; child should be able to seriate six geometric shapes from largest to smallest.<br>Determine which ethnic version of Oucher to use. Allow the child to select a version of Oucher, or use version that most closely matches physical characteristics of child. |
| **Poker Chip Tool†** (Hester and others, 1998): Uses four red poker chips placed horizontally in front of child | Say to the child: "I want to talk with you about the hurt you may be having right now." Align the chips horizontally in front of the child on the bedside table, a clipboard, or other firm surface.<br>Tell the child, "These are pieces of hurt." Beginning at the chip nearest the child's left side and ending at the one nearest the right side, point to the chips and say, "This [first chip] is a little bit of hurt and this [fourth chip] is the most hurt you could ever have." For a young child or for any child who may not fully comprehend the instructions, clarify by saying, "That means this [one] is just a little hurt, this (two) is a little more hurt, this [three] is more yet, and this [four] is the most hurt you could ever have."<br>Do not give children an option for zero hurt. Research with the Poker Chip Tool has verified that children without pain will so indicate by responses such as "I don't have any." | Children as young as 4 years |

---

\**Wong-Baker FACES Pain Rating Scale Reference Manual* describing development and research of the scale is available from the Mayday Pain Resource Center, City of Hope National Medical Center, 1500 East Duarte Rd, Duarte, CA 91010, (626) 359-8111, ext. 3829, fax: (626) 301-8941; *www.mosby.com/WOW/*. Translations of the FACES are in Appendix F. A compilation of many pain scales, including the FACES, is available free from Purdue Frederick Company, 100 Connecticut Ave, Norwalk, CT 06850-3950, (800) 733-1333 or (203) 853-0123, ext. 7378 or 7314; *www.partnersagainstpain.com*. The use of FACES with children is demonstrated in **Whaley and Wong's Pediatric Nursing Video Series**, "Pain Assessment and Management," narrated by Donna Wong, PhD, RN. Available from Mosby, 11830 Westline Industrial Dr, St Louis, MO 63146, (800) 426-4545; fax: (800) 535-9935; *www.mosby.com*.
†Developed in 1975 by N.O. Hester, University of Colorado Health Sciences Center, School of Nursing, Denver, CO 80262. Also available in Spanish and French.

**TABLE 26-2**   Pain rating scales for children—cont'd

| Pain Scale/Description | Instructions | Recommended Age/Comments |
|---|---|---|
| **Poker Chip Tool—cont'd** | Ask the child, "How many pieces of hurt do you have right now?" After initial use of the Poker Chip Tool, some children internalize the concept "pieces of hurt." If a child gives a response such as "I have one right now," *before* you ask or before you lay out the poker chips, record the number of chips on the Pain Flow Sheet. Clarify the child's answer by words such as "Oh, you have a little hurt? Tell me about the hurt." | |
| **Word-Graphic Rating Scale‡** (Tesler and others, 1991): Uses descriptive words (may vary in other scales) to denote varying intensities of pain | Explain to child, "This is a line with words to describe how much pain you may have. This side of the line means no pain and over here the line means worst possible pain." (Point with your finger where "no pain" is, and run your finger along the line to "worst possible pain," as you say it.) "If you have no pain, you would mark like this." (Show example.) "If you have some pain, you would mark somewhere along the line, depending on how much pain you have." (Show example.) "The more pain you have, the closer to worst pain you would mark. The worst pain possible is marked like this." (Show example.) "Show me how much pain you have right now by marking with a straight, up-and-down line anywhere along the line to show how much pain you have right now." With a millimeter rule, measure from the "no pain" end to the mark and record this measurement as the pain score. | Children 4 to 17 years |

```
No          Little      Medium      Large       Worst
pain        pain        pain        pain        possible pain
```

| Pain Scale/Description | Instructions | Recommended Age/Comments |
|---|---|---|
| **Numeric Scale** Uses straight line with end points identified as "no pain" and "worst pain" and sometimes "medium pain" in the middle; divisions along line are marked in units from 0 to 10 (high number may vary) | Explain to child that at one end of the line is a 0, which means that a person feels no pain (hurt). At the other end is usually a 5 or a 10, which means the person feels the worst pain imaginable. The numbers 1 to 5 or 10 are for a very little pain to a whole lot of pain. Ask child to choose a number that best describes own pain. | Children as young as 5 years, as long as they can count and have some concept of numbers and their values in relation to other numbers. Scale may be used horizontally or vertically. Number coding should be same as other scales used in a facility. |

```
No pain                      Worst pain
|___|___|___|___|___|
 0   1   2   3   4   5
```

| Pain Scale/Description | Instructions | Recommended Age/Comments |
|---|---|---|
| **Visual Analogue Scale** (Cline and others, 1992): Defined as a vertical or horizontal line that is drawn to a certain length, such as 10 cm, and anchored by items that represent the extremes of the subjective phenomenon, such as pain, that is measured | Ask child to place a mark on line that best describes amount of own pain. With a centimeter ruler, measure from the "no pain" end to the mark and record this measurement as the pain score. | Children as young as 4½ years, preferably 7 years. Vertical or horizontal scale may be used. |
| **Color Tool** (Eland, 1993): Uses markers for child to construct own scale that is used with body outline | Present eight markers to child in a random order. Ask child, "Of these colors, which color is like . . .?" (the event identified by the child as having hurt the most). Place the marker (represents severe pain) away from the other markers. Ask child, "Which color is like a hurt, but not quite as much as . . .?" (the event identified by the child as having hurt the most). Place the marker with the marker chosen to represent severe pain. Ask child, "Which color is like something that hurts just a little?" Place the marker with the other colors. Ask child, "Which color is like no hurt at all?" Show the four marker choices to child in order from the worst to the no-hurt color. Ask child to show on the body outlines where they hurt, using the markers chosen. After child has colored the hurts, ask if they are current hurts or hurts from the past. Ask if child knows why the area hurts if it is not clear to you why it does. | Children as young as 4 years, provided they know their colors, are not color blind, and are able to construct the scale if in pain |

‡Instructions for Word-Graphic Rating Scale from Acute Pain Management Guideline Panel: *Acute pain management in infants, children, and adolescents: operative and medical procedures; quick reference guide for clinicians,* ACHPR Pub No 92-0020, Rockville, MD, 1992, (now the Agency for Healthcare Research and Quality [AHRQ]), Public Health Service, US Department of Health and Human Services. Word-Graphic Rating Scale is part of the Adolescent Pediatric Pain Tool and is available from Pediatric Pain Study, University of California, School of Nursing, Department of Family Health Care Nursing, San Francisco, CA 94143-0606, (415) 476-4040.

It is best to use the same scale each time with the child to avoid confusing him or her with different instructions and to use the pain assessment scale for pain only. Multiple uses of the scale (e.g., as a general measure of the child's feelings) can cause the child to lose interest in the scale. In introducing the pain scale, nurses should explain that this is one way for children to let nurses know how they are feeling. Ideally, children should be taught to use the scale before pain is expected, such as preoperatively. Familiarizing children with the scale facilitates its use when children are actually in pain.

---

### Box 26-9 ▪ ▪ ▫
### Developmental Characteristics of Children's Responses to Pain

**YOUNG INFANTS**

Generalized body response of rigidity or thrashing, possibly with local reflex withdrawal of stimulated area

Loud crying

Facial expression of pain (brows lowered and drawn together, eyes tightly closed, mouth open and squarish) (See Fig. 26-3.)

Demonstrates no association between approaching stimulus and subsequent pain

**OLDER INFANTS**

Localized body response with deliberate withdrawal of stimulated area

Loud crying

Facial expression of pain or anger (same facial characteristics as pain but eyes may be open)

Physical resistance, especially pushing the stimulus away *after* it is applied

**YOUNG CHILDREN**

Loud crying, screaming

Verbal expressions of "Ow," "Ouch," or "It hurts"

Thrashing of arms and legs

Attempts to push stimulus away *before* it is applied

Uncooperative; needs physical restraint

Requests termination of procedure

Clings to parent, nurse, or other significant person

Requests emotional support, such as hugs or other forms of physical comfort

May become restless and irritable with continuing pain

All these behaviors may be seen in anticipation of actual painful procedure

**SCHOOL-AGE CHILDREN**

May see all behaviors of young child, especially *during* painful procedure but less in anticipatory period

Stalling behavior, such as "Wait a minute" or "I'm not ready"

Muscular rigidity, such as clenched fists, white knuckles, gritted teeth, contracted limbs, body stiffness, closed eyes, wrinkled forehead

**ADOLESCENTS**

Less vocal protest

Less motor activity

More verbal expressions, such as "It hurts" or "You're hurting me"

Increased muscle tension and body control

Data from Craig KD and others: Developmental changes in infant pain expression during immunization injections, *Soc Sci Med* 19(12):1331-1337, 1984; and Katz E, Kellerman J, Siegel S: Behavioral distress in children with cancer undergoing medical procedures: developmental considerations, *J Consult Clin Psychol* 48(3):356-365, 1980.

---

**Evaluate Behavioral and Physiologic Changes.** Behavioral changes are common indicators of pain and are especially valuable in assessing pain in nonverbal children. Children's behavioral responses to pain change with age and follow a developmental trend (Box 26-9). However, children vary widely in their responses and may exhibit behaviors at one age that are more typically seen at a different age. Children with more positive moods may appear to be in less pain than they actually are. Children who use passive coping behaviors (offering no resistance, cooperating) may rate pain as more intense than children who use active coping behaviors (resisting, attacking). (See Critical Thinking Exercise box.)

Recent evidence, however, indicates that temperament does not seem to be a useful predictor of response to pain (Broome, Rehwaldt, and Fogg, 1998). Cultural background may also play a role in children's pain responses (Lipson, Dibble, and Minarik, 1996). (See Cultural Awareness box.) In addition, cultural and linguistic differences may hinder assessment. Unfortunately, making judgments about pain based solely on behavior may lead to underestimation of its severity and inadequate pain management (McCaffery and Pasero, 1999; Tesler, Holzemer, and Savedra, 1998).

> **NURSING ALERT** If children's behaviors appear to differ from their rating of pain, believe their pain rating.

---

### Critical Thinking Exercise

#### Pain Assessment

Stacy is 14 years old, and this is her second day following abdominal surgery. As you enter her room, she smiles at you and continues to talk and joke with her visitor. Stacy rates her pain a 4 on a scale of 0 to 5 (no to worst pain), respectively. Her roommate, Jill, is 12 years old, and this is her third day following scoliosis surgery. She does not smile and is lying very still in bed. Jill rates her pain a 4 on the same scale. Based on your assessment, which of the following would you write in their charts (choose two items)?

FIRST, THINK ABOUT IT . . .

• What information are you using?
• How are you interpreting that information?

_____

1. Stacy: In no acute distress and appears comfortable, talking and joking with a visitor.
2. Jill: Rates her surgical pain a 4 on a 0 to 5 scale and is unable to move because of pain; she appears depressed.
3. Stacy: Rates her surgical pain a 4 on a 0 to 5 scale.
4. Jill: Rates her surgical pain a 4 on a 0 to 5 scale.

_____

*The best responses are three and four. The best estimate of pain is the person's self-report. Responses one and two are based on subjective impressions. In response one the adolescent's report of pain is disregarded. In response two there are no assessment data to support that Jill's behavior indicates inability to move or depression.*

Depending on the characteristics of pain, children may display behaviors that indicate localized pain, such as pulling the ears for ear pain; lying on the side with legs flexed for abdominal pain; limping for leg or foot pain; and refusing to move a body part. Children who experience chronic or repeated pain often develop effective behavioral coping strategies, such as squeezing a hand, talking, counting, relaxing, or distraction (watching TV, listening to music). Once these coping skills are identified, the child can be encouraged to use them in future experiences with pain.

Physiologic responses indicating acute pain include flushing of the skin; diaphoresis, hypertension, tachycardia, and tachypnea; decreases in oxygen saturation; restlessness; and dilation of the pupils. However, these signs vary considerably from patient to patient and also may be produced by emotions such as fear, anger, or anxiety. They occur primarily in acute pain from stimulation of the sympathetic nervous system. If pain persists, the body begins to adapt, and these responses decrease or stabilize. Consequently, if nurses rely primarily on observing for physiologic indications and not asking patients whether they are having pain, many instances of pain will go unrecognized (Van Cleve, Johnson, and Pothier, 1996).

Several scales have been developed that use changes in behavioral and physiologic parameters to measure pain in nonverbal children. The most common items assessed in these instruments are facial expression, cry, activity, heart rate, respiratory rate, oxygen saturation, and body movements. One example of such a tool is the **FLACC Postoperative Pain Scale** (Table 26-3). Facial expression, leg position, activity, cry, and consolability are assessed (Merkel and others, 1997). Unfortunately, many of these signs can be affected by events other than pain (e.g., anxiety and fear) and are subject to misinterpretation. Other scales that are designed for nonverbal children are summarized in Table 26-3. (For a discussion of pain scales for newborns, see Neonatal Pain, Chapter 10.)

The issue of assessing pain in children with developmental or physical disabilities or children in a coma, on a ventilator, or pharmacologically paralyzed remains challenging and largely unexplored. Researchers are investigating parents' description of recognizing pain in the child with serious cognitive and physical impairment (Fanurik and others, 1999; McGrath and others, 1998; Oberlander, O'Donnell, and Montgomery, 1999).

One of the most valuable clues to pain is a change in behavior and vital signs after administration of an analgesic. Behaviors such as decreased irritability, cessation of crying, and decreased pulse, respirations, and blood pressure provide important evidence for pain management. Often the change in vital signs, especially respiratory rate, is attributed to the depressant effect of opioids, and the return to more normal physiologic functioning is due to pain relief.

**Encourage Parents' Involvement.** Parents are often the primary source of information about how their child exhibits pain and should play a key role in the assessment of their child's pain. They are sensitive to changes in behavior and typically want to be involved in their child's pain relief. However, parents' ability to recognize pain in their children varies. In a recent study researchers report that parents may be able to identify the presence of pain but may have difficulty assessing its severity. Thus they underestimate their child's pain, which may contribute to inadequate pain control (Chambers and others, 1998).

To better assess the child's pain, the nurse can interview the parents about their child's previous pain experiences (see Box 26-8). Ideally, this questioning should occur before the child is in pain, such as on admission to the hospital. When obtaining a parent's rating of pain, the nurse should inquire about specific behavior rather than how severe the parent believes the pain is (Merkel and Malviya, 2000). Parents need to realize, however, that their knowledge of their child is important in managing their child's pain. They sometimes leave the assessment of pain up to the nurse because "nurses are more experienced," and they expect the nurse to know when their child is in pain (Woodgate and Kristjanson, 1996). Parents need to be taught about pain behaviors and encouraged to inform the staff when they think their child is in pain. Educational activities such as watching a videotape can change parental knowledge concerning pediatric pain and can be useful in preventing inadequate pain management (Greenberg and others, 1999).

Parents usually know what comforts their children when they are in pain and want to be involved in pain relief. Encouraging their participation gives them control and a sense of helping. More importantly, 99% of children state that the supportive presence of a parent provides the most comfort when in pain (Broome, 2000).

**Take Cause of Pain into Account.** When children exhibit behaviors or other clues that suggest pain, reasons for discomfort should be investigated. Pathology may give clues to the expected intensity and type of pain. For example, pain associated with vaso-occlusive crises in sickle cell disease is severe. Pain caused by bone marrow puncture is greater than the discomfort associated with a venipuncture. However, it is a mistake to believe that certain conditions or procedures always produce a standard amount of pain. For example, sore throat pain may be mild or severe—only the child knows the intensity.

## CULTURAL AWARENESS
### Traditional Ethnic Treatments

Many traditional ethnic treatments are used to relieve pain and other symptoms. Although they are widely available in the United States, they are not marketed as drugs and have not been tested for safety and effectiveness. One recent alert from the Food and Drug Administration asked for a recall of 13 herbal products because of the potential health risk. The products contained aristolochic acid, which can cause serious kidney damage, and products containing this substance have been associated with kidney failure. It is important for nurses to inquire about the use of alternative products for pain or symptom relief and advise the family regarding potential adverse events.*

*www.fda.gov. Consumer inquiries: (888) INFO-FDA.

**TABLE 26-3** Summary of selected behavioral pain assessment scales for young children

| Tools and Authors/ Ages of Use | Reliability and Validity | Variables and Scoring Range |
|---|---|---|
| **Objective Pain Score (OPS)** (Hannallah and others, 1987) Ages of use: 4 months-18 years | No testing in original publication Later tested by original authors: 1988-concurrent validity with Linear Analogue Pain Scale, Spearman's r = 0.721 with scores ≥6 and 0.419 with scores < 6 1991-interrater agreement, coefficient alpha = 0.986 for one rater and 0.983 for the other 1991-concurrent validity with CHEOPS, Pearson correlation coefficient = 0.88 and 0.94 | Blood pressure (0-2) Crying (0-2) Moving (0-2) Agitation (0-2) Verbal evaluation/body language (0-2) **Scoring range:** 0 = no pain; 10 = worst pain |
| **Children's Hospital of Eastern Ontario Pain Scale (CHEOPS)** (McGrath and others, 1985) Ages of use: 1-5 years | Interrater reliability = 90%-99.5% Internal correlation = significant correlations between pairs of items Concurrent validity between CHEOPS and VAS = .91; between individual and total scores of CHEOPS and VAS = 0.50-0.86 Construct validity with preanalgesia and postanalgesia scores = 9.9-6.3 | Cry (1-3) Facial (0-2) Child verbal (0-2) Torso (1-2) Touch (1-2) Legs (1-2) **Scoring range:** 4 = no pain; 13 = worst pain |
| **Nurses Assessment of Pain Inventory (NAPI)** (Stevens, 1990) Ages of use: newborn-16 years | Not tested by original author. Later tested by Joyce and others (1994) Interrater agreement: weighted kappa 0.37-0.80 Discriminant validity: statistically significant differences between preanalgesia and postanalgesia scores (p < .0001) Reliability: Cronbach's alpha = 0.35-0.69 | Body movement (0-2) Facial (0-3) Touching (0-2) **Scoring range:** 0 = no pain; 7 = worst pain |
| **Behavioral Pain Score (BPS)** (Robieux and others, 1991) Ages of use: 3-36 months | Original article stated, "reliability of the VAS and BPS scores was tested by a k test"; no further testing of reliability or validity was mentioned | Facial expression (0-2) Cry (0-3) Movements (0-3) **Scoring range:** 0 = no pain; 8 = worst pain |
| **Modified Behavioral Pain Scale (MBPS)** (Taddio and others, 1995) Ages of use: 4-6 months | Concurrent validity between MBPS and VAS scores = correlation coefficient 0.68 (p < 0.001) and 0.74 (p < 0.001) Construct validity using prevaccination and postvaccination scores with EMLA vs placebo: significantly lower scores with EMLA (p < 0.01) Internal consistency of items = significant correlations between items Interrater agreement: ICC = 0.95, p < 0.001 Test-retest reliability: r 0.95, p < .001 | Facial expression (0-3) Cry (0-4) Movements (0, 2, 3) **Scoring range:** 0 = no pain; 10 = worst pain |
| **Riley Infant Pain Scale (RIPS)** (Schade and others, 1996) Ages of use: <36 months and children with cerebral palsy | Interrater agreement using Intraclass Correlation Coefficient = 0.53-0.83, p < 0.0001 Discriminant validity using Mann-Whitney U test with preanalgesia and postanalgesia scores = statistically significant (p < 0.001) Sensitivity = 0.31-0.23 Specificity = 0.86-0.90 Interrater reliability using two-way cross tabulations and kappa statistics (r[87] = 0.94; p < 0.001) and kappa values above 0.50 for each category | 0-Neutral face/smiling, calm, sleeping quietly, no cry, consolable, moves easily 1-Frowning/grimace, restless body movements, restless sleep, whimpering, winces with touch 2-Clenched teeth, moderate agitation, sleeps intermittently, pain crying, difficult to console, cries with touch 3-Full cry expression, thrashing/flailing, sleeping prolonged periods interrupted by jerking or no sleep, screaming/high-pitched cry, inconsolable, scream when touched/moved **Scoring range:** 0 = no pain; 3 = worst pain |
| **FLACC Postoperative Pain Scale** (Merkel and others, 1997) Ages of use: 2 months-7 years | Validity using ANOVA for repeated measures to compare FLACC scores before and after analgesia; pre-analgesia FLACC scores were significantly higher than postanalgesia scores at 10, 30, and 60 minutes (p < 0.001 for each time) Correlation coefficients used to compare FLACC pain scores and OPS pain scores; significant positive correlation between FLACC and OPS scores (r = 0.80; p < 0.001); positive correlation also found between FLACC scores and nurses' global ratings of pain (r[47] = 0.41; p < 0.005) | Face (0-2) Legs (0-2) Activity (0-2) Cry (0-2) Consolability (0-2) **Scoring range:** 0 = no pain; 10 = worst pain |

**TABLE 26-3**   Summary of selected behavioral pain assessment scales for young children—cont'd

FLACC SCALE*

| | 0 | 1 | 2 |
|---|---|---|---|
| Face | No particular expression or smile | Occasional grimace or frown, withdrawn, disinterested | Frequent to constant frown, clenched jaw, quivering chin |
| Legs | Normal position or relaxed | Uneasy, restless, tense | Kicking, or legs drawn up |
| Activity | Lying quietly, normal position, moves easily | Squirming, shifting back and forth, tense | Arched, rigid, or jerking |
| Cry | No cry (awake or asleep) | Moans or whimpers, occcasional complaint | Crying steadily, screams or sobs, frequent complaints |
| Consolability | Content, relaxed | Reassured by occasional touching, hugging, or "talking to"; distractable | Difficult to console or comfort |

*From Merkel S and others: The FLACC: a behavioral scale for scoring postoperative pain in young children, *Pediatr Nurs* 23(3):293-297, 1997. Used with permission of Jannetti Publications, Inc and the University of Michigan Health System. Can be reproduced for clinical and research use.

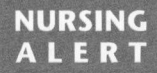

**NURSING ALERT**   A good rule to follow in pain assessment is whatever is painful to an adult is painful to an infant or child until proved otherwise.

**Take Action and Evaluate Results.**   The reason for assessing pain is to relieve it. Complete pain relief, with the use of both pharmacologic and nonpharmacologic interventions, should be the goal. Regardless of the type of pain intervention, evaluation of the results is essential. No one pain reduction technique is effective for all children. Therefore a *pain assessment record* is used to monitor the effectiveness of the interventions. With nonverbal children, behavioral and physiologic signs are evaluated for evidence of pain relief. With verbal children, their statements about pain relief and pain ratings are also recorded. Changes in the medication regimen are made as needed to provide maximum pain relief with minimum side effects. Family members are often excellent allies for keeping a pain assessment record for the nurse (Fig. 26-10).

## Pain Management

Effective pain management requires that health professionals be willing to try a number of interventions to achieve optimum results. Pain reduction methods can be grouped into two categories: nonpharmacologic and pharmacologic. Whenever possible, both should be used; however, nonpharmacologic measures should not be considered substitutes for analgesics.

### Nonpharmacologic Management

Pain is often associated with fear, anxiety, and stress. A number of nonpharmacologic techniques, such as distraction, relaxation, guided imagery, and cutaneous stimulation, provide coping strategies that may help reduce pain perception, make pain more tolerable, decrease anxiety, and enhance the effectiveness of analgesics or reduce the dosage required (Rusy and Weisman, 2000). (See Guidelines box on p. 1059.) In addition, these techniques decrease the perceived threat of pain, provide a sense of control, enhance comfort, and promote rest and sleep

(McCaffery and Pasero, 1999). Although there is a paucity of research on the effectiveness of many of these interventions, the strategies are safe, noninvasive, and inexpensive, and most are independent nursing functions.

If the child cannot identify a familiar coping technique, the nurse can describe several strategies and let the child select the most appealing one. Experimentation with several strategies that are suitable to the child's age, pain intensity, and abilities is often necessary to determine the most effective approach. Parents should be involved in the selection process; they may be familiar with the child's usual coping skills and can help identify potentially successful strategies. Involving parents also encourages their participation in learning the skill with the child and acting as coach. If the parent cannot assist the child, other appropriate persons may include a grandparent, older sibling, nurse, or child-life specialist.

Children should learn a specific strategy before pain occurs or before it becomes severe. To reduce the child's effort, instructions for a strategy, such as distraction or relaxation, can be audiotaped and played during a period of comfort. However, children often need help using the intervention during the procedure after they have learned it. The intervention can also be used after the procedure. This gives the child a chance to recover, feel mastery, and cope more effectively (Fanurik and others, 1997).

### Pharmacologic Management

Using pharmacologic methods to control pain requires attention to four "rights": right drug, right dose, right route, and right time. Although nurses may not prescribe the medication, knowledge of these essential principles assists in optimally implementing analgesic orders and discussing with other practitioners possible strategies to improve pain control. In addition, observing for side effects of the drugs and using supportive approaches with children when administering the drug are important nursing interventions.

**Right Drug.**   *Nonopioids,* including acetaminophen (Tylenol, paracetamol) and nonsteroidal antiinflammatory drugs (NSAIDs), are suitable for mild to moderate pain; *opioids* are needed for moderate to severe pain. A combination of the two analgesics attacks pain on two levels: nonopioids

**Pain Assessment Record**

Directions for each column:

1. Record date and time of administering analgesic; assess analgesic effect _____ minutes later and then _____

2. Use a pain rating scale if child understands its use. Name of scale

   _____

   Ratings: No pain = ____ Worst pain = ____ Comfort/function goals* ____

3. Record analgesic, dose, and route

4. Record possible indications of effects of pain, such as shallow breathing due to incisional pain, parental request for pain relief; record indications or effect of pain relief, such as "moves easily, playing"

5. Record any other side effects (e.g., nausea, itching)

6. Record LOS (see inset) R (respiratory function); record breaths per minute and/or other observations of respiratory status (e.g., depth of respiration, change in color of skin)

7. Signature or initials of person recording information

| Level of Sedation (LOS) Scale† |
|---|
| S = Sleeping, easily aroused Requires no action |
| 1 = Awake and alert Requires no action |
| 2 = Occasionally drowsy, easy to arouse Requires no action |
| 3 = Frequently drowsy, arousable, drifts off to sleep during conversation Notify practitioner and decrease dose |
| 4 = Somnolent, minimal or no response to stimuli Notify practitioner and stop opioid |

| 1 Date/time | 2 Pain rating | 3 Analgesic | 4 Possible effects/indications of pain or relief of pain | 5 Side effects | 6 LOS/R | 7 Signature |
|---|---|---|---|---|---|---|
| | | | | | | |
| | | | | | | |
| | | | | | | |
| | | | | | | |
| | | | | | | |
| | | | | | | |
| | | | | | | |
| | | | | | | |
| | | | | | | |
| | | | | | | |
| | | | | | | |
| | | | | | | |
| | | | | | | |
| | | | | | | |
| | | | | | | |

*Ask the child what pain rating would be acceptable in terms of usual function (e.g., activities of daily living, playing, attending school, and so on). From McCaffery M, Pasero C, editors: *Pain: a clinical manual*, ed 2, St Louis 1999, Mosby.

†From Pasero C, McCaffery M: Providing epidural analgesia: how to maintain a delicate balance, *Nurs 99* 29(8):34-39, 1999.

**Fig. 26-10** Pain assessment record.

## GUIDELINES
*Nonpharmacologic Strategies for Pain Management*

### GENERAL STRATEGIES

Use nonpharmacologic interventions to supplement, not replace, pharmacologic interventions, and use for mild pain and pain that is reasonably well controlled with analgesics.

Form a trusting relationship with child and family.

Express concern regarding their reports of pain, and intervene appropriately.

Take an active role in seeking effective pain management strategies.

Use general guidelines to prepare child for procedure. (See Chapter 27.)

Prepare child before potentially painful procedures, but avoid "planting" the idea of pain. For example, instead of saying, "This is going to (or may) hurt," say, "Sometimes this feels like pushing, sticking, or pinching, and sometimes it doesn't bother people. Tell me what it feels like to you."

Use "nonpain" descriptors when possible (e.g., "It feels like heat" rather than "It's a burning pain"). This allows for variation in sensory perception, avoids suggesting pain, and gives child control in describing reactions.

Avoid evaluative statements or descriptions (e.g., "This is a terrible procedure" or "It really will hurt a lot").

Stay with child during a painful procedure.

Allow parents to stay with child if child and parent desire; encourage parent to talk softly to child and to remain near child's head.

Involve parents in learning specific nonpharmacologic strategies and assisting child in their use.

Educate child about the pain, especially when explanation may lessen anxiety (e.g., that pain may occur after surgery and does not indicate something is wrong; reassure that child is not responsible for the pain).

For long-term pain control, give child a doll, which represents "the patient," and allow child to do everything to the doll that is done to the child; pain control can be emphasized through the doll by stating, "Dolly feels better after the medicine."

Teach procedures to child and family for later use.

### SPECIFIC STRATEGIES

#### Distraction

Involve parent and child in identifying strong distractors.

Involve child in play; use radio, tape recorder, CD player or computer game; have child sing or use rhythmic breathing.

Have child take a deep breath and blow it out until told to stop (French, Painter, and Coury, 1994).

Have child blow bubbles to "blow the hurt away."

Have child concentrate on yelling or saying "ouch" by focusing on "yelling loud or soft as you feel it hurt: that way I know what's happening."

Have child look through kaleidoscope (type with glitter suspended in fluid-filled tube) and encourage to concentrate by asking, "Do you see the different designs?" (Vessey, Carlson, and McGill, 1994).

Use humor, such as watching cartoons, telling jokes or funny stories, or acting silly with child.

Have child read, play games, or visit with friends.

#### Relaxation

With an infant or young child:

Hold in a comfortable, well-supported position, such as vertically against the chest and shoulder.

Rock in a wide, rhythmic arc in a rocking chair or sway back and forth, rather than bouncing child.

Repeat one or two words softly, such as "Mommy's here."

With a slightly older child:

Ask child to take a deep breath and "go limp as a rag doll" while exhaling slowly; then ask child to yawn (demonstrate if needed).

Help child assume a comfortable position (e.g., pillow under neck and knees).

Begin progressive relaxation: starting with the toes, systematically instruct child to let each body part "go limp" or

"feel heavy"; if child has difficulty with relaxing, instruct child to tense or tighten each body part and then relax it.

Allow child to keep eyes open, since children may respond better if eyes are open rather than closed during relaxation.

#### Guided Imagery

Have child identify some highly pleasurable real or pretend experience.

Have child describe details of the event, including as many senses as possible (e.g., "feel the cool breezes," "see the beautiful colors," "hear the pleasant music").

Have child write down or tape record script.

Encourage child to concentrate only on the pleasurable event during the painful time; enhance the image by recalling specific details through reading the script or playing the tape.

Combine with relaxation and rhythmic breathing.

#### Positive Self-Talk

Teach child positive statements to say when in pain (e.g., "I will be feeling better soon," "When I go home, I will feel better, and we will eat ice cream").

#### Thought Stopping

Identify positive facts about the painful event (e.g., "It does not last long").

Identify reassuring information (e.g., "If I think about something else, it does not hurt as much").

Condense positive and reassuring facts into a set of brief statements and have child memorize them (e.g., "Short procedure, good veins, little hurt, nice nurse, go home"). Have child repeat the memorized statements whenever thinking about or experiencing the painful event.

#### Cutaneous Stimulation

Includes simple rhythmic rubbing; use of pressure or electric vibrator; massage with hand lotion, powder, or menthol cream; application of heat or cold, such as vapocoolant spray on the site before giving injection or application of ice to the site opposite the painful area (e.g., if right knee hurts, place ice on left knee).

A more sophisticated method is *transcutaneous electrical nerve stimulation (TENS)* (use of controlled low-voltage electricity to the body via electrodes placed on the skin).

Another method is the use of *Pain Relief Therapeutic Electro-Membrane (PREM)*, a high-technology membrane electron reservoir fabricated from a nonwoven, nonallergenic dressing that when placed in contact with the skin, releases the stored electrons in the form of microcurrent impulses.*

#### Behavioral Contracting

*Informal*—May be used with children as young as 4 or 5 years of age:

Use colorful stickers or tokens as rewards.

Give uncooperative or procrastinating children (during a procedure) a limited time (measured by a visible timer) to complete the procedure.

Proceed as needed if child is unable to comply.

Reinforce cooperation with a reward if the procedure is accomplished within specified time.

*Formal*—Use written contract, which includes:

Realistic (seems possible) goal or desired behavior

Measurable behavior (e.g., agrees not to hit anyone during procedures)

Contract written, dated, and signed by all persons involved in any of the agreements

Identified rewards or consequences that are reinforcing

Goals that can be evaluated

Commitment and compromise from both parties (e.g., while timer is used, nurse will not nag or prod child to complete procedure)

*For more information contact Helio Medical Supplies, Inc, 606 Charcot Ave, San Jose, CA 95131, (408) 433-3355; e-mail: eileen@heliomed.com.

**Box 26-10** ■ ■ ■
### Selected Combination Opioid and Nonopioid Oral Analgesics—Nonaspirin Products*

| | | | |
|---|---|---|---|
| Fioricet with Codeine | 30 mg codeine | Percocet 7.5/500† | 7.5 mg oxycodone |
| | 325 mg acetaminophen | | 500 mg acetaminophen |
| | 50 mg butalbital | Percocet 10/650† | 10 mg oxycodone |
| | 40 mg caffeine | | 650 mg acetaminophen |
| Hydrocet | 5 mg hydrocodone | Tylenol with Codeine | 7.5 mg codeine |
| | 500 mg acetaminophen | No. 1 | 300 mg acetaminophen |
| Lorcet-HD | 5 mg hydrocodone | Tylenol with Codeine | 15 mg codeine |
| | 500 mg hydrocodone | No. 2 | 300 mg acetaminophen |
| Lorcet Plus | 7.5 mg hydrocodone | Tylenol with Codeine | 30 mg codeine |
| | 650 mg acetaminophen | No. 3 | 300 mg acetaminophen |
| Lorcet 10/650 | 10 mg hydrocodone | Tylenol with Codeine | 60 mg codeine |
| | 650 mg acetaminophen | No. 4 | 300 mg acetaminophen |
| Lortab 2.5/500 | 2.5 mg hydrocodone | Tylenol and Codeine | 12 mg codeine |
| | 500 mg acetaminophen | Elixir (each 5 ml) | 120 mg acetaminophen |
| Lortab 5/500 | 5 mg hydrocodone | | 7% alcohol |
| | 500 mg acetaminophen | Tylox† | 5 mg oxycodone |
| Lortab 10/500 | 10 mg hydrocodone | | 500 mg acetaminophen |
| | 500 mg acetaminophen | Vicodin | 5 mg hydrocodone |
| Lortab Elixir | 7.5 mg hydrocodone | | 500 mg acetaminophen |
| (each 15 ml) | 500 mg acetaminophen | Vicodin ES | 7.5 mg hydrocodone |
| Percocet 2.5/325† | 2.5 mg oxycodone | | 750 mg acetaminophen |
| | 325 mg acetaminophen | Vicodin HP | 10 mg hydrocodone |
| Percocet-5/325† | 5 mg oxycodone | | 650 mg acetaminophen |
| | 325 mg acetaminophen | Vicoprofen | 7.5 mg hydrocodone |
| | | | 200 mg ibuprofen |

*Aspirin is not recommended for children because of its possible association with Reye syndrome. Analgesic compounds with aspirin include Darvon Compound, Darvon with ASA, Percodan, and Percodan-Demi. Darvon or Darvocet (propoxyphene) is not recommended; its analgesic effect is no greater than that from aspirin, acetaminophen, or other NSAIDs. Propoxyphene, an opioid, can depress respirations, and its major metabolite is cardiotoxic and is a central nervous system (CNS) stimulant that can produce seizures (Dahl, 1998).

†All medications require a prescription, but these are classified as schedule II drugs (like morphine), and each filling requires a written prescription that includes the patient's name and address, the practitioner's DEA (Drug Enforcement Agency) number, and the date. In case of emergency, verbal prescriptions for schedule II substances may be filled; however, the practitioner must provide a signed prescription within 72 hours. Schedule II prescriptions cannot be refilled but require a new prescription.

primarily at the peripheral nervous system and opioids primarily at the central nervous system (CNS). This approach provides increased analgesia without increased side effects. Several combinations, such as acetaminophen (Tylenol) with codeine, may have increasing doses of the opioid but a constant dose of the nonopioid (Box 26-10). Therefore, before increasing the opioid, it may be preferable to increase the nonopioid component, for example, adding one regular-strength acetaminophen tablet (325 mg) to acetaminophen with codeine No. 3 before advancing to acetaminophen with codeine No. 4. However, if this approach is not successful, the pain management will require a stronger opioid.

Oxycodone is available without a nonopioid in an immediate release and controlled release preparation (Oxy-Contin) (Olin and others, 1998). The oxycodone dose can be safely increased without the risk of toxicity from excessive acetaminophen use.

Actions of various opioids differ. Morphine is considered the gold standard for the management of severe pain. When morphine is not a suitable opioid, drugs such as hydromorphone (Dilaudid) and fentanyl (Sublimaze) are effective substitutes. Although fentanyl is used as an anesthetic in the operating room, it is classified as an analgesic. It can be safely administered by nurses by the IV, intramuscular (IM), subcutaneously (SC), transmucosal, and transdermal routes (Algren and Algren, 1998; Golianu and others, 2000).

Several drugs, known as **coanalgesics** or **adjuvant analgesics,** may be used alone or with opioids to control pain symptoms. Drugs frequently used to relieve anxiety, cause sedation, and provide amnesia are diazepam (Valium) and midazolam (Versed); however, these drugs are not analgesics. Other adjuvants include tricyclic antidepressants

**NURSING ALERT** Meperidine (Demerol, pethidine) is not recommended as a first line opioid analgesic for the management of any type of pain (American Pain Society, 1999; McCaffery and Pasero, 1999). A major drawback in the use of meperidine is its metabolic, normeperidine. Normeperidine is a CNS stimulant that can produce restlessness, irritability, twitching, jerking, agitation, tremors, and seizures (American Pain Society, 1999). When meperidine is administered for longer than 24 hours or in patients with renal insufficiency, seizures may occur (Yaster and others, 1997). Research shows that meperidine is more likely than other opioids to cause emergence delirium in children (Kussman and Sethna, 1998). Assess the child for early signs of toxicity, such as tremors, twitching or jerking, or increased excitation or irritability. If normeperidine toxicity is suspected, discontinue the meperidine immediately and notify the practitioner. Adverse drug reaction reports should be sent to the U.S. Food and Drug Administration (FDA).*

*The FDA Safety Information and Adverse Event Reporting Program, Food and Drug Administration, 5600 Fishers Lane, Rockville, MD 20857-0001, (888) 463-6332; www.fda.gov/medwatch.

**TABLE 26-4** Nonsteroidal antiinflammatory drugs (NSAIDs) approved for children*

| Drug (Trade Name) | Dose | Comments |
|---|---|---|
| Acetaminophen (Tylenol and other brands) | 10-15 mg/kg/dose every 4-6 hours not to exceed 5 doses in 24 hours or 75 mg/kg/day, orally | Available in numerous preparations<br>Nonprescription<br>Higher dosage range may provide increased analgesia |
| Choline magnesium trisalicylate (Trilisate)† | Children 37 kg or less: 50 mg/kg/day divided into 2 doses<br>Children over 37 kg: 2250 mg/day divided into 2 doses | Available in suspension 500 mg/5 ml<br>Prescription |
| Ibuprofen‡<br>Children's Motrin<br>Children's Advil | Children 6 months and older: 5-10 mg/kg/dose every 6-8 hours not to exceed 40 mg/kg/day | Available in numerous preparations<br>Available in suspension 100 mg/5 ml and drops 100 mg/2.5 ml<br>Nonprescription |
| Naproxen (Naprosyn) | Children over 2 years: 10 mg/kg/day divided into 2 doses | Available in suspension 125 mg/5 ml and several different dosages for tablets |
| Tolmetin (Tolectin) | Children over 2 years: 20 mg/kg/day divided into 3 or 4 doses | Prescription<br>Available in 200-mg, 400-mg, and 600-mg tablets<br>Prescription |

Data from Olin BR and others: *Drug facts and comparisons*, St Louis, 2000, Facts and Comparisons.
NOTE: Newer formulations of NSAIDs, such as celecoxib (Celebrex) or rofecoxib (Vioxx), selectively inhibit one of the enzymes of cyclooxygenase (COX-2, which is responsible for pain transmission) but do not inhibit the other (COX-1). Inhibition of COX-1 decreases prostaglandin production, which is necessary for normal organ function. For example, prostaglandins help maintain gastric mucosal blood flow and barrier protection, regulate blood flow to the liver and kidneys, and facilitate platelet aggregation and clot formation. Theoretically, the COX-2 NSAIDs provide similar analgesic and antiinflammatory benefits with fewer side effects than the nonselective agents. Celebrex and Vioxx are approved for use in patients over 18 years of age.
*All NSAIDs in the table (except acetaminophen) have significant antiinflammatory, antipyretic, and analgesic actions. Acetaminophen has a weak antiinflammatory action, and its classification as an NSAID is controversial. Patients respond differently to various NSAIDs; therefore changing from one drug to another may be necessary for maximum benefit.
†Acetylsalicylic acid (aspirin) is also an NSAID but is not recommended for children because of its possible association with Reye syndrome. The NSAIDs in the table have no known association with Reye syndrome. However, caution should be exercised in prescribing any salicylate-containing drug (e.g., Trilisate) for children with known or suspected viral infection.
‡Side effects of ibuprofen, naproxen, and tolmetin include nausea, vomiting, diarrhea, constipation, gastric ulceration, bleeding nephritis, and fluid retention. Acetaminophen and choline magnesium trisalicylate are well tolerated in the gastrointestinal tract and do not interfere with platelet function. NSAIDs (except acetaminophen) should not be given to patients with allergic reactions to salicylates. All the NSAIDs should be used cautiously in patients with renal impairment.

(e.g., amitriptyline, imipramine) and antiepileptics (e.g., gabapentin, carbamazepine, clonazepam) for neuropathic pain; stool softeners, laxatives, and antiemetics for constipation and nausea/vomiting; steroids for inflammation and bone pain; and dextroamphetamine and caffeine for possible increased analgesia and decreased sedation (McCaffery and Pasero, 1999).

The use of placebos to determine whether the patient is having pain is unjustified and unethical; a positive response to a placebo, such as a saline injection, is common in patients who have a documented organic basis for pain. Therefore the deceptive use of placebos does not provide useful information about the presence or severity of pain. The use of placebos can cause side effects similar to those of opioids, can destroy the patient's trust in the health care staff, and raises serious ethical and legal questions. The **American Society of Pain Management Nurses** has issued a position statement against the use of placebos to treat pain (1998).

**Right Dosage.** The optimum dosage is one that controls pain without causing severe side effects. This usually requires *titration,* the gradual adjustment of drug dosage (usually by increasing the dose) until optimum pain relief without excessive sedation is achieved. Dosage recommendations, such as those in Tables 26-4 and 26-5 are only safe initial dosages, not optimum dosages. Children (except infants younger than about 3 to 6 months of age) metabolize drugs more rapidly than adults; younger children may require higher doses of opioids to achieve the same analgesic effect. Therefore the therapeutic effect and duration of

analgesia vary. Children's dosages are usually calculated according to body weight, except in children with a weight greater than 50 kg (110 pounds), where the weight formula may exceed the average adult dose. In this case the adult dose is used.

A reasonable starting dose of opioid for infants under 6 months who are *not* mechanically ventilated is one fourth to one third of the recommended starting dose for older children. The infant is monitored closely for signs of pain relief and respiratory depression. The dose is titrated to effect. Because tolerance can develop rapidly, large doses may be needed for continued severe pain (American Pain Society, 1999).

If pain relief is inadequate, the initial dose is increased (usually by 25% to 50% if pain is moderate, or by 50% to 100% if pain is severe) to provide greater analgesic effectiveness. Decreasing the interval between doses may also provide more continuous pain relief. A major difference between opioids and nonopioids is that nonopioids have a *ceiling effect,* which means that doses higher than the recommended dose will not produce greater pain relief. Opioids do not have a ceiling effect other than that imposed by side effects; therefore larger dosages can be safely given for increasing severity of pain. (See Critical Thinking Exercise box on p. 1063.)

**NURSING ALERT** A frequent error in attempts to improve pain control is to change to another analgesic. If an opioid, such as morphine, hydromorphone, or fentanyl, is used, rarely is the problem one of drug choice. Rather, the problem is usually one of inadequate dosage.

**TABLE 26-5** Selected opioids for children

| Drug | Approximate Equianalgesic Oral Dose | Approximate Equianalgesic Parenteral Dose | Recommended Starting Dose (Children Less Than 50-kg Body Weight)[a] | |
|---|---|---|---|---|
| | | | Oral | Parenteral[b] |
| Morphine[c] | 30 mg every 3-4 hours (around-the-clock dosing) | 10 mg every 3-4 hours | 0.2-0.4 mg/kg every 3-4 hours 0.3-0.6 mg/kg time released every 12 hours | 0.1-0.2 mg/kg IM every 3-4 hours 0.02-0.1 mg/kg IV bolus every 2 hours 0.015 mg/kg every 8 minutes PCA 0.01-0.02 mg/kg/hr IV infusion (neonates) 0.01-0.06 mg/kg/hr IV infusion (child) |
| Fentanyl (Sublimaze) (oral mucosal form— Fentanyl Oralet)[d] | Not available | 0.1 mg IV | 5-15 μg/kg; maximum dose 400 μg | 0.5-1.5 μg/kg IV bolus every ½ hour 1-2 μg/hr IV infusion |
| Codeine[e] | 200 mg every 3-4 hours | 130 mg every 3-4 hours | 1 mg/kg every 3-4 hours | Not recommended |
| Hydromorphone[c] (Dilaudid) | 7.5 mg every 3-4 hours | 1.5 mg every 3-4 hours | 0.04-0.1 mg/kg every 4-6 hours | 0.02-0.1 mg/kg IM every 3-4 hours 0.005-0.2 mg/kg IV bolus every 2 hours |
| Hydrocodone (in Lorcet, Lortab, Vicodin, others) | 30 mg every 3-4 hours | Not available | 0.2 mg/kg every 3-4 hours[g] | Not available |
| Levorphanol (Levo-Dromoran) | 4 mg every 6-8 hours | 2 mg every 6-8 hours | 0.04 mg/kg every 6-8 hours | 0.02 mg/kg every 6-8 hours |
| Meperidine (Demerol)[f] | 300 mg every 2-3 hours | 100 mg every 3 hours | Not recommended | 0.75 mg/kg every 2-3 hours |
| Methadone (Dolophine, others) | 20 mg every 6-8 hours | 10 mg every 6-8 hours | 0.2 mg/kg every 6-8 hours | 0.1 mg/kg every 6-8 hours |
| Oxycodone (Roxicodone, Oxycontin; also in Percocet, Percodan, Tylox, others) | 20 mg every 3-4 hours | Not available | 0.2 mg/kg every 3-4 hours[g] | Not available |

Data from Acute Pain Management Guideline Panel: *Acute pain management: operative or medical procedures and trauma: clinical practice guideline,* AHCPR Pub No 92-0032, Rockville, MD, 1992, Agency for Health Care Policy and Research, Public Health Service, US Department of Health and Human Services; and Berde C and others: Report of the subcommittee on disease-related pain in childhood cancer, *Pediatrics* 86(5, pt 2):820, 1990.

*IV,* Intravenous; *IM,* intramuscular; *PCA,* patient-controlled analgesia.

**Note:** Published tables vary in the suggested doses that are equianalgesic to morphine. Clinical response is the criterion that must be applied for each patient; titration to clinical response is necessary. Because there is not complete cross-tolerance among these drugs, it is usually necessary to use a lower than equianalgesic dose when changing drugs and to retitrate to response. **Caution:** Recommended doses do not apply to patients with renal or hepatic insufficiency or other conditions affecting drug metabolism and kinetics.

[a]**Caution:** Doses listed for patients with body weight less than 50 kg cannot be used as initial starting doses in infants less than 6 months of age. For nonventilated infants under 6 months of age, the initial opioid dose should be about one fourth to one third of the dose recommended for older infants and children. For example, morphine could be used at a dose of 0.03 mg/kg instead of the traditional 0.1 mg/kg.

[b]IM injections should not be used.

[c]For morphine, hydromorphone, and oxymorphone, rectal administration is an alternate route for patients unable to take oral medications, but equianalgesic doses may differ from oral and parenteral doses because of pharmacokinetic differences.

[d]Fentanyl Oralet is indicated for use in a hospital setting only (1) as an anesthetic premedication in the operating room setting or (2) to induce conscious sedation before a diagnostic or therapeutic procedure in other monitored anesthesia care settings in hospital; is contraindicated in children who weigh less than 15 kg (33 lb).

[e]**Caution:** Codeine doses above 65 mg often are not appropriate because of diminishing incremental analgesia with increasing doses but continually increasing constipation and other side effects. Dosages are from McCaffery M, Pasero C: *Pain: a clinical manual,* ed 2, St Louis, 1999, Mosby.

[f]Meperidine is not recommended for continuous pain control (i.e., postoperatively) because of risk of normeperidine toxicity (see p. 1060).

[g]**Caution:** Doses of aspirin and acetaminophen in combination with opioid/NSAID preparations must also be adjusted to patient's body weight.

Parenteral and oral dosages of opioids are not the same. Because of the *first-pass effect,* an oral opioid is rapidly absorbed from the gastrointestinal tract and in the liver is partially metabolized before reaching the central circulation. Therefore oral dosages must be larger to compensate for the partial loss of analgesic potency to achieve *equianalgesia* (equal analgesic effect). Conversion factors for selected opioids, when a change is made from IV (preferred) or IM to oral, are listed in Tables 26-5 and 26-6. Immediate conversion from IM or IV to the suggested equianalgesic oral dose may result in a substantial error. For example, the dose may be significantly more or less than what the child requires. Small changes ensure small errors.

**Right Route.** Several routes of administration can be used (Box 26-11 on pp. 1064-1065). Children should not have to endure pain, such as from IM injections, to achieve pain relief. Therefore the most effective and least traumatic route of administration should be selected.

A significant advance in the administration of IV, epidural, or SC analgesics is the use of *patient-controlled analgesia (PCA).* As the name implies, the patient controls the amount and frequency of the analgesic, which is typically delivered through a special infusion device. Children who are physically able to "push a button," (i.e., 5 to 6 years of age) and who can understand the concept of "pushing a button" to obtain pain relief can use PCA (Maxwell and Yaster, 2000). Although it is controversial, parents and nurses have used the IV-PCA system for the child. Nurses can efficiently use the infusion device on a child of any age to administer analgesics to avoid signing for and preparing

## Critical Thinking Exercise

### Pain Management—Patient-Controlled Analgesia

Juan, 9 years old, is hospitalized for a fractured pelvis and multiple other injuries as a result of a motor vehicle accident. Since admission he has been receiving patient-controlled analgesia (PCA) ordered as "morphine, 1.0 to 1.5 mg/hr, lock-out 10 minutes; bolus dose 1.5 mg, not to exceed one dose per hour." In assessing his pain, you note that he rates the pain a 4 on a scale of 0 to 5 (no to worst pain), respectively, and he has been pushing the PCA button an average of 15 times an hour. What should be the first action you take?

FIRST, THINK ABOUT IT . . .

- What assumptions are you making?
- What conclusions are you coming to?

1. Tell Juan that he is pushing the button too often; he should wait 10 minutes before using the PCA machine.
2. Administer the bolus dose of morphine and reassess pain in 10 minutes.
3. Increase the hourly dose of morphine from 1.0 to 1.5 mg and reassess pain in 1 hour.
4. Contact the surgeon about Juan's inadequate pain management.

*The best response is two. The conclusion that Juan's pain is inadequately treated is correct, and your first intervention is to give the ordered bolus dose. If the bolus dose relieves the pain to an acceptable level for Juan, the next step is to increase the hourly dose of 1.5 mg. Because the PCA order allows titrating (adjusting) the dosage upward, this action precedes calling the surgeon. It is absolutely inappropriate to tell Juan to push the PCA button less often; this response disregards his need for improved pain control and eliminates a valuable assessment parameter, the number of PCA uses.*

**TABLE 26-6**   Selected analgesics (equianalgesia)

| Drug* | Equal to Oral Morphine (mg) | Equal to IM/IV Morphine (mg) |
|---|---|---|
| Hydromorphone (Dilaudid) 1 mg | 4 | 1.3 |
| Codeine 30 mg | 4.5 | 1.5 |
| Meperidine (Demerol) 50 mg | 4.8 | 1.6 |
| Codeine 30 mg + 300 mg acetaminophen (Tylenol No. 3) | 7.2 | 2.4 |
| Oxycodone 5 mg + 325 mg acetaminophen (Percocet) | 7.2 | 2.4 |
| Oxycodone 5 mg + 325 mg aspirin (Percodan) | 7.2 | 2.4 |
| Hydrocodone 5 mg + 500 mg acetaminophen (Vicodin, Lortab) | 9 | 3 |
| Oxycodone 5 mg + 500 mg acetaminophen (Tylox) | 9 | 3 |
| Dolophine (Methadone) 10 mg | 15 | 7.5 |
| Acetaminophen (Tylenol) 325 mg | 2.7 | 0.9 |
| Aspirin 325 mg | 2.7 | 0.9 |
| Acetaminophen (Tylenol Extra Strength) 500 mg | 4 | 1.3 |
| Codeine 60 mg + acetaminophen 300 mg (Tylenol No. 4) | 11.7 | 3.9 |
| Transdermal fentanyl patch (Duragesic) (based on 25 μg/hr patch applied every 3 days = 50 mg oral morphine every 24 hours or divided into 6 doses = 8.3 mg) | 8.3 | 2.77 |

Courtesy Betty R. Ferrell, PhD, FAAN, 1999. Used with permission.
*Oral medication with exception of fentanyl.
NOTE: When converting to oral oxycodone from oral morphine, an appropriate conservative estimate is 15 to 20 mg of oxycodone per 30 mg of morphine; however, when converting to oral morphine from oral oxycodone, an appropriate conservative estimate is 30 mg of morphine per 30 mg of oxycodone (McCaffery and Pasero, 1999).

opioid injections every time one is needed. When used as "nurse"- or "parent"-controlled analgesia, the concept of patient control is negated, and the inherent safety of PCA may be compromised. Nevertheless, recent research reported safe and effective analgesia in children when the PCA was controlled by patient, parent, or nurse (Algren and others, 1998; Maxwell and Yaster, 2000).

PCA infusion devices typically allow for three methods or modes of drug administration to be used alone or in combination:

1. **Patient-administered boluses** that can only be infused according to the preset amount and *lockout interval* (time between doses); more frequent "attempts at self-administration" usually means the patient may need the dose and time adjusted for better pain control
2. **Nurse-administered boluses** that are typically used to give an initial loading dose to increase blood levels rapidly and to relieve *breakthrough pain* (pain not relieved with the usual programmed dose)
3. **Continuous basal rate infusion** that delivers a constant amount of analgesic and prevents pain from returning during those times, such as sleep, when the patient cannot control the infusion; may decrease safety of PCA

However, as with any type of analgesic management plan, continued assessment of the child's pain relief is essential for the greatest benefit from PCA. (See Critical Thinking Exercise box.) Typical uses of PCA are for controlling pain from surgery, sickle cell crisis, trauma, and cancer.

Morphine is the drug of choice for PCA and is usually prepared in a concentration of 1 mg/ml. Other options are hydromorphone (0.2 mg/ml) and fentanyl (0.01 mg/ml) (Table 26-7). Hydromorphone is often used when pruritis and nausea are side effects of morphine PCA treatment (Maxwell and Yaster, 2000). Because PCA is typically used for continuous and extended pain control, meperidine should not be administered. (See Nursing Alert, p. 1060.)

Recently there has been increased use of **epidural analgesia** for postoperative pain management in pediatric patients. Epidural analgesia may also be used to manage pain in other selected cases. Although a catheter may be inserted at any vertebral level, it is usually placed into the epidural space of the spinal column at the lumbar or caudal level. The thoracic level is usually reserved for older children or adolescents who have had an upper abdominal or thoracic procedure, such as a lung transplant (Houck, 1998). An opi-

## Box 26-11 ■ ■ ■
## Routes and Methods of Analgesic Drug Administration

### ORAL

Preferred because of convenience, cost, and bioavailability

Higher dosages of oral form of opioids required for equivalent parenteral analgesia

Peak drug effect occurs after 1½ to 2 hours for most analgesics

Delay in onset is disadvantage when rapid control of severe pain or of fluctuating pain is desired

### SUBLINGUAL/BUCCAL/TRANSMUCOSAL

Tablet or liquid placed between cheek and gum (buccal) or under tongue (sublingual)

Highly desirable because more rapid onset than oral route

Less first-pass effect through liver than oral route, which normally reduces analgesia from oral opioids (unless sublingual/buccal form swallowed, which occurs often in children)

Few drugs commercially available in this form

Many drugs can be compounded into a sublingual troche or lozenge*

*Fentanyl Oralet*—Oral transmucosal fentanyl citrate in hard confection base on a plastic holder; used for preoperative or preprocedural sedation/analgesia

*Actiq*—Same formulation as Fentanyl Oralet; indicated only for management of breakthrough cancer pain in patients with malignancies who are already receiving and are tolerant to opioid therapy

### INTRAVENOUS (IV) (BOLUS)

Preferred for rapid control of severe pain

Provides most rapid onset of effect, usually in about 5 minutes

Advantage for acute pain, procedural pain, and breakthrough pain

Initial bolus dose is controversial; one recommendation is one half intramuscular (IM) dose

Needs to be repeated hourly for continuous pain control

Drugs with short half-life (morphine, fentanyl, hydromorphone) are preferred, to avoid toxic accumulation of drug

### INTRAVENOUS (CONTINUOUS)

Preferred over bolus and IM for maintaining control of pain

Provides steady blood levels

Easy to titrate dosage

Amount of initial dose is controversial; one approach to calculating hourly infusion rate is to divide IM dose by drug's expected duration for IM route

Peak effect is delayed; for rapid pain relief, begin with initial IV bolus dose (see preceding section)

### SUBCUTANEOUS (SC) (CONTINUOUS)

Used when oral and IV routes not available

Provides equivalent blood levels to continuous IV infusion

Suggested initial bolus dose to equal 2-hour IV dose; total 24-hour dose usually equal to total IV or IM 24-hour dose

### PATIENT-CONTROLLED ANALGESIA (PCA)

Generally refers to self-administration of drugs, regardless of route

Typically uses programmable infusion pump (IV, epidural, or SC) that permits self-administration of boluses of medication at preset dose and time interval (*lockout interval* is time between doses)

PCA bolus administration may be combined with initial bolus and continuous (basal or background) infusion of opioid

Optimum lockout interval not known, but must be at least as long as time needed for onset of drug

Should effectively control pain during movement or procedures

Longer lockout requires larger dose

### FAMILY-CONTROLLED ANALGESIA

A responsible family member (usually a parent) or significant other is designated child's primary pain manager and has responsibility of pressing PCA button

Guidelines for selecting a primary pain manager for family-controlled analgesia:

Spends a significant amount of time with the patient

Is willing to assume responsibility of being primary pain manager

Is willing to accept and respect patient's reports of pain (if able to provide) as best indicator of how much pain the patient is experiencing; knows how to use and interpret a pain rating sale

Understands the purpose and goals of patient's pain management plan

Understands concept of maintaining a steady analgesic blood level

Recognizes signs of pain and side effects and adverse reactions to opioid

### NURSE-ACTIVATED DOSING

Child's nurse is designated primary pain manager and is only person who presses PCA button during that nurse's shift

Guidelines for selecting primary pain manager for family-controlled analgesia apply to nurse-activated dosing

May be used in addition to a basal rate to treat breakthrough pain with bolus doses; patients are assessed q 30 min for the need for a bolus dose

May be used without a basal rate as a means of maintaining analgesia with around-the-clock (ATC) bolus doses

### INTRAMUSCULAR (IM)
### *Not Recommended for Pain Control*

Painful administration

Some drugs (e.g., meperidine) can cause tissue damage

Wide fluctuation in absorption of drug from muscle

Faster absorption from deltoid than from gluteal sites

Shorter duration and more expensive than oral drugs

Data primarily from American Pain Society: *Principles of analgesic use in the treatment of acute pain and chronic cancer pain*, ed 4, Skokie, IL, 1999, The Society; and McCaffery M, Pasero C: *Pain: a clinical manual*, ed 2, St Louis, 1999, Mosby.

*For further information about compounding drugs in troche or suppository form, contact: Professional Compounding Centers of America (PCCA), Inc, 9901 South Wilcrest Dr, Houston, TX 77009, (800) 331-2498; *www.thecompounders.com*.

**TABLE 26-7** Suggested intravenous patient-controlled analgesia-opioid infusion orders

| Drug | Basal Rate ($\mu$g/kg/hr) | Bolus Rate ($\mu$g/kg/dose) | Lockout Period (min) | Maximum Dose/Hour (mg/kg) |
|---|---|---|---|---|
| Morphine | 10-30 | 10-30 | 6-10 | 0.1-0.15 |
| Hydromorphone | 3-5 | 3-5 | 6-10 | 0.015-0.02 |
| Fentanyl | 0.5-1.0 | 0.5-1.0 | 6-10 | 0.002-0.004 |

From Yaster M and others: *Pediatric pain management and sedation handbook*, St Louis, 1997, Mosby.

## Box 26-11 ■ ■ ■
### Routes and Methods of Analgesic Drug Administration—cont'd

#### INTRANASAL

*Midazolam (Versed)* has been used as nasal spray
   Although effective, route may be traumatic for children
Available commercially as Stadol NS (butorphanol); approved for those over 18 years of age; should not be used in patient receiving morphine-like drugs because butorphanol is partial antagonist

#### INTRADERMAL

Used primarily for skin anesthesia (e.g., for lumbar puncture, bone marrow aspiration, arterial puncture, skin biopsy)
Local anesthetics (such as lidocaine) cause stinging, burning sensation
To avoid stinging sensation associated with lidocaine:
   Buffer the solution by adding 1 part sodium bicarbonate (1 mEq/ml) to 10 parts 1% or 2% lidocaine (see Guidelines box on p. 1067)

#### TOPICAL/TRANSDERMAL

*EMLA (eutectic mixture of local anesthetics [lidocaine/prilocaine]) cream and Anesthetic Disc*
   Eliminates or reduces pain from most procedures involving skin puncture
   Must be placed over puncture site and covered by occlusive dressing or as anesthetic disc for 1 hour or more before procedure (see Guidelines box on p. 1066)
*LAT (lidocaine/adrenaline/tetracaine)* or *tetracaine/phenylephrine (tetraphen)*
   Provides skin anesthesia about 15 minutes after application
   Gel (preferable) or liquid placed on wounds for suturing (nonintact skin)
   Cocaine should no longer be used because of the risk of systemic absorption and toxicity
   Adrenaline must not be used on distal arterioles (fingers, toes, tip of nose, penis, earlobes) because of vasoconstriction
*Numby Stuff*
   Uses iontophoresis to rapidly transport lidocaine 2% and epinephrine 1:100,000 *(Iontocaine)* into the skin
   A small battery-powered device delivers current via an electrode with Iontocaine and a ground electrode
   Produces local dermal anesthesia in about 10 minutes to a depth of approximately 10 mm at maximum setting
   May be frightening to young children when they see the device and feel the mild current
   Child should be observed during iontophoresis
*Transdermal Fentanyl (Duragesic)*
   Available as "patch" for continuous cancer pain control
   Safety and efficacy not established in children under 12 years
   Not appropriate for initial relief of acute pain because of long interval to peak effect (from 12 to 24 hours); for rapid onset of pain relief, an immediate-release opioid must be given
   Orders for "rescue doses" of an immediate-release opioid should be available for **breakthrough pain,** a flare of severe

pain that "breaks through" the medication being administered at regular intervals for persistent pain
   Has duration of up to 72 hours for prolonged pain relief
   If respiratory depression occurs, several doses of naloxone may be needed

*Vapocoolant*
   Use of spray coolant, such as fluori-methane or ethyl chloride; placed on the skin immediately before the needle puncture
   Some children dislike the cold; spraying the coolant on a cotton ball and then applying this to the skin may be less uncomfortable
   Application of ice to the skin for 30 seconds was found to be ineffective

#### RECTAL

Alternative to oral or parenteral routes
Variable absorption rate
Generally disliked by children
Many drugs can be compounded into rectal suppositories*

#### REGIONAL NERVE BLOCK

Use of long-acting anesthetic (bupivacaine or ropivacaine) injected into nerves to block pain at site
Provides prolonged analgesia postoperatively, such as after inguinal herniorrhaphy
May be used to provide local anesthesia for surgery, such as dorsal penile nerve block for circumcision or for reduction of fractures

#### INHALATION

Use of anesthetics, such as nitrous oxide or halothane, to produce partial or complete analgesia for painful procedures
Occupational exposure to high levels of nitrous oxide may cause side effects

#### EPIDURAL/INTRATHECAL

Involves catheter placed into epidural, caudal, or intrathecal space for continuous infusion or single or intermittent administration of opioid with or without a long-acting anesthetic (e.g., bupivacaine or ropivacaine)
Analgesia primarily from drug's direct effect on opioid receptors in spinal canal
Respiratory depression is rare but may have slow and delayed onset; can be prevented by checking level of sedation and respiratory rate and depth hourly for initial 24 hours and decreasing dose when excessive sedation is detected
Nausea, itching, and urinary retention are common dose-related side effects from the epidural opiod
Mild hypotension, urinary retention, and temporary motor or sensory deficits are common unwanted effects of epidural local anesthetic

---

*For further information about compounding drugs in troche or suppository form, contact: Professional Compounding Centers of America (PCCA), Inc, 9901 South Wilcrest Dr, Houston, TX 77009, (800) 331-2498; *www.thecompounders.com.*

---

oid (usually fentanyl, hydromorphone, or preservative-free morphine, which is often combined with a long-acting local anesthetic such as bupivacaine or ropivacaine) is instilled via single or intermittent bolus, continuous infusion, or patient-controlled epidural analgesia (PCEA). Analgesia results from the drug's effect on opiate receptors in the dorsal horn of the spinal cord, rather than the brain. As a result, respiratory depression is rare, but if it occurs, it

develops slowly, typically 6 to 8 hours after administration (Golianu and others, 2000).

Properly securing the epidural catheter with an occlusive dressing decreases the possibility of soiling or inadvertently displacing the catheter. Careful monitoring of sedation level and respiratory status is critical to preventing opioid-induced respiratory depression. Assessment of pain and the skin condition around the catheter site are important aspects of nursing care (Golianu and others, 2000; McCaffery and Pasero, 1999).

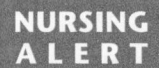

**NURSING ALERT** When the epidural or intrathecal route is used, check the child's level of consciousness and respiratory rate and depth hourly for the first 24 hours to detect delayed-onset respiratory depression (Pasero, 1999).

Other routes that have benefitted from new products for pain control are the *oral transmucosal* and *transdermal routes.* Oral transmucosal *fentanyl* (Fentanyl Oralet) provides nontraumatic preoperative and preprocedural analgesia and sedation (Golianu and others, 2000). (See Surgical Procedures, Chapter 27.) Fentanyl is also available as a transdermal patch (Duragesic). Although contraindicated for acute pain management, it may be used for older children and adolescents who have cancer or sickle cell pain or for opioid-tolerant patients.

One of the most significant improvements in the ability to provide atraumatic care to children is the anesthetic cream, *EMLA,** a eutectic mixture of local anesthetics (lidocaine 2.5% and prilocaine 2.5%). The eutectic mixture, whose melting point is lower than that of the two anesthetics alone, permits effective concentrations of the drug to penetrate *intact* skin. (See Guidelines box.)

Another transdermal option is *Numby Stuff,* which uses iontopheresis (mild electrical current) to actively push the drug into the skin. This preparation of Iontocaine (lidocaine HCl 2% with epinephrine 1:100,000 topical solution) provides dermal anesthesia to a depth of 10 mm in approximately 10 minutes. It can be used for IV placement, insertion of percutaneously inserted central catheters (PICC) lines, lumbar punctures, implantable port needle insertion, and pulsed dye laser therapy (IOMED, 1996). It is important to provide explanations and let the child become familiar with the equipment. Some children may find the tin-

---

*For additional information about EMLA, contact Astra Pharmaceuticals, (800) 228-EMLA.

---

## GUIDELINES
### Using EMLA (Eutectic Mixture of Local Anesthetics—Lidocaine 2.5% and Prilocaine 2.5%)

Explain to child that EMLA is like a "magic cream that takes the hurt away." Tap or lightly scratch site of procedure to show child that "skin is now awake."

Apply the "peel-and-stick" Anesthetic Disc or a thick layer of EMLA cream over normal intact skin to anesthetize site (about one half of a 5-g tube; can use one third of tube if puncture site is localized and superficial) (e.g., intradermal injection or heel/finger puncture).

For venous access, apply to two sites; place enough cream on antecubital fossa to cover medial and lateral veins. Do not rub the cream into the skin.

If using the cream, place transparent occlusive dressing (e.g., Tegaderm) over EMLA. Make sure cream remains in a thick layer.

To make the dressing less accessible, cover it loosely with a self-adhering Ace-type bandage (such as Coban) or an IV protector (such as I.V. House*). Label the dressing with "EMLA applied" the date and the time to distinguish it from other types of dressings. Instruct older children not to disturb the dressing. Supervise younger or cognitively compromised children throughout the application time.

Leave EMLA on skin for at least 60 minutes for venipuncture and 2½ hours for deep penetration (e.g., lumbar puncture, biopsy). EMLA may need to be kept on longer in persons with dark and/or thicker skin. Anesthesia may last up to 4 hours after EMLA is removed.

The availability of the disc makes home use of EMLA very convenient.† In a recent study of application of EMLA at home, parental application was as effective as application by health care professionals. In addition, the anxiety of children 5 to 12 years was decreased by applying EMLA at home in preparation for IV placement (Koh and others, 1999).

Remove Anesthetic Disc or dressing before procedure and wipe cream from skin. For transparent dressing, grasp opposite sides, and while holding dressing *parallel* to skin,

pull sides away from each other to stretch and loosen. An adhesive remover may be used.

Observe skin reaction (e.g., either blanched or reddened). If there is no obvious skin reaction, EMLA may not have penetrated adequately. Test skin sensitivity and reapply if needed.

After procedure, assess behavioral response. If child was upset, use pain scale (e.g., FACES) to help child distinguish between pain and fear (see FACES Pain Rating Scale in Table 26-2).

In the United States, EMLA is approved for use in infants born at 37 weeks of gestation and older. It should not be used in those patients with congenital or idopathic methemoglobinemia and in infants under the age of 12 months who are receiving treatment with methemoglobin-inducing agents such as sulfonamides, phenytoin (Dilantin), phenobarbital, and acetaminophen (Tylenol). Methemoglobin, a dysfunctional form of hemoglobin, reduces the blood's oxygen-carrying capacity, causing cyanosis and hypoxemia. The use of IV methylene blue promptly eliminates the methemoglobinemia.

NOTE: Although the package insert lists under "Warnings" that patients taking drugs associated with drug-induced methemoglobinemia, such as acetaminophen, are at greater risk for developing methemoglobinemia, there have been no reported cases of this complication occurring in children taking acetaminophen and using EMLA.

Follow the manufacturer's guidelines for MAXIMUM RECOMMENDED APPLICATION AREA TO INTACT SKIN FOR INFANTS AND CHILDREN:

| AGE AND BODY WEIGHT REQUIREMENTS | MAXIMUM TOTAL DOSE OF EMLA | MAXIMUM APPLICATION AREA |
|---|---|---|
| 1 to 3 months or <5 kg | 1 g | 10 cm² (1.25 × 1.25 in) |
| 4 to 12 months and >5 kg | 2 g | 20 cm² (1.75 × 1.75 in) |
| 1 to 6 years and >10 kg | 10 g | 100 cm² (4 × 4 in) |
| 7 to 12 years and >20 kg | 20 g | 200 cm² (5.5 × 5.5 in) |

---

*For more information, contact I.V. House, 7400 Foxmont Dr, Hazelwood, MO 63042-2198, (800) 530-0400, fax: (314) 831-3683, e-mail: ivhouse@ivhouse.com; *www.ivhouse.com.*

†Community and home care instructions on applying EMLA are available in Wong DL, Hess CS: *Wong and Whaley's clinical manual of pediatric nursing,* ed 5, St Louis, 2000, Mosby.

NOTE: If a patient over 3 months old does not meet the minimum weight requirement, the maximum total dose of EMLA should be restricted to that which corresponds to the patient's weight.

gling sensation uncomfortable or frightening while the drug is administered (McCaffery and Pasero, 1999).

In some situations where there is not ample time for preparations like EMLA to take effect, refrigerant sprays such as ethyl chloride and fluori-methane can be used (Reis and Holubkov, 1997). When sprayed on the skin, these sprays vaporize, rapidly cool the area, and provide superficial anesthesia.

The *intradermal route* is often used to inject a local anesthetic, typically lidocaine (Xylocaine), into the skin to reduce the pain from a lumbar puncture, bone marrow aspiration, or venous or arterial access. One problem with the use of lidocaine is the stinging and burning that initially occur. However, the used of *buffered lidocaine* (with sodium bicarbonate) reduces the stinging sensation (Wong and Pasero, 1997). (See Guidelines box.) Warming the lidocaine to 37° C (98.6° F) may also accomplish the same effect (McCaffery and Pasero, 1999).

**Right Time.** The right timing for administering analgesics depends on the type of pain. For continuous pain control, such as for postoperative or cancer pain, a preventive schedule of medication *around the clock (ATC)* is effective. The ATC schedule avoids the low plasma concentrations that permit breakthrough pain. If analgesics are administered only when pain returns (a typical use of the PRN, or "as needed," order), pain relief may take several hours. This may require higher doses, leading to a cycle of undermedication of pain alternating with periods of overmedication and drug toxicity. This cycle of erratic pain control also promotes "clock watching," which may be erroneously equated with "addiction." Nurses can effectively use PRN orders by giving the drug at regular intervals because "as needed" can be interpreted to mean "as needed to prevent pain."

Preventive pain control is best provided through continuous IV infusion rather than intermittent boluses. If intermittent boluses are given, the intervals between doses should not exceed the drug's expected duration of effectiveness. For extended pain control with fewer administration times, drugs that provide longer duration of action

(e.g., some NSAIDs, time-released morphine or oxycodone, methadone, levorphanol) can be used.

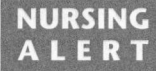 **NURSING ALERT** Because breakthrough pain can occur even with optimum ATC scheduling, there should be an order for PRN "rescue" doses of an analgesic.

Continuous analgesia is not always appropriate, because not all pain is continuous. Frequently, temporary pain control or conscious sedation is needed to provide analgesia before a scheduled procedure. When pain can be predicted, the drug's peak effect should be timed to coincide with the painful event. For example, with opioids the peak effect is approximately ½ hour for the IV route; with nonopioids the peak effect occurs about 2 hours after oral administration. For rapid onset and peak of action, opioids that quickly penetrate the blood-brain barrier (e.g., IV fentanyl) provide excellent pain control. (See Surgical Procedures, Chapter 27.)

**Observe for Side Effects.** Both NSAIDs and opioids have side effects, although the major concern is with those from opioids (Box 26-12). *Respiratory depression* is the most serious complication and is most likely to occur in sedated patients. The respiratory rate may decrease gradually or may cease abruptly; lower limits of normal are not established for children, but any significant change from a previous rate calls for increased vigilance. A slower respiratory rate does not necessarily reflect decreased arterial oxygenation; an increased depth of ventilation may compensate for the altered rate (Rowbotham and others, 1989). If respiratory depression or arrest occurs, the nurse must be prepared to intervene quickly (Pasero and McCaffery, 1994). (See Guidelines box on p. 1068.)

Although respiratory depression is the most feared side effect, *constipation* is a common, and sometimes serious, side effect of opioids, which decrease peristalsis and increase anal sphincter tone. Prevention with stool softeners and laxatives is more effective than treatment once constipation occurs. Dietary treatment, such as increased fiber, is usually

---

## GUIDELINES
### Using Buffered Lidocaine (BL)

**Supplies:** 8.4% sodium bicarbonate (1 mEq/ml), 1% to 2% lidocaine with or without epinephrine, syringe with removable needle, and a 30-gauge needle

**Instructions**

Use 1 part sodium bicarbonate to 10 parts lidocaine (i.e., draw up 1 ml of lidocaine and 0.1 ml of sodium bicarbonate).

Change needle used to withdraw BL to 30-gauge needle for intradermal injection.

For venipuncture or port access, inject 0.1 ml or less BL intradermally directly over intended puncture site; anesthesia occurs almost immediately.

Suggested maximum dose of lidocaine for local anesthesia is 4.5 mg/kg.

If buffering lidocaine vial (e.g., 20 ml lidocaine with 2 ml sodium bicarbonate), use solution for 7 days unrefrigerated or 14 days refrigerated.

---

### Box 26-12 ■ ■ ▢
### Side Effects of Opioids

| GENERAL | SIGNS OF TOLERANCE |
|---|---|
| Constipation (possibly severe) | Decreasing pain relief |
| Respiratory depression | Decreasing duration of pain relief |
| Sedation | |
| Nausea and vomiting | **SIGNS OF PHYSICAL DEPENDENCE** |
| Agitation, euphoria | |
| Mental clouding | Initial signs of withdrawal: |
| Hallucinations |   Lacrimation |
| Orthostatic hypotension |   Rhinorrhea |
| Pruritus |   Yawning |
| Urticaria |   Sweating |
| Sweating | Later signs: |
| Miosis (may be sign of toxicity) |   Restlessness |
| Anaphylaxis (rare) |   Irritability |
| |   Tremors |
| |   Anorexia |
| |   Dilated pupils |
| |   Gooseflesh |

not sufficient to promote regular bowel evacuation. However, dietary measures, such as increased fluid and fruit intake, as well as physical activity, are encouraged.

*Pruritus* from epidural or IV infusion can be treated with low doses of IV naloxone, nalbuphine, or diphenhydramine. *Nausea, vomiting,* and *sedation* usually subside after 2 days of opioid administration, although oral or rectal antiemetics may be necessary.

Both tolerance and physical dependence can occur with prolonged use of opioids. Treatment of *tolerance* involves increasing the dose or decreasing the duration between doses. Treatment of *physical dependence* involves gradually reducing the dose over several days to prevent occurrence of withdrawal symptoms (similar to tapering of steroid dosages after chronic steroid therapy). The following are guidelines for treating physical dependence from morphine (American Pain Society, 1999):

- Gradually reduce dose (similar to tapering of steroids): Give one half of previous daily dose every 6 hours for first 2 days. Then reduce dose by 25% every 2 days.
- Continue this schedule until total daily dose of 0.6 mg/kg/day of morphine (or equivalent) is reached.
- After 2 days on this dose, discontinue opioid.
- May also switch to oral methadone, using one fourth of equianalgesic dose as initial weaning dose and proceeding as described above.

**Use Supportive Statements When Administering Analgesics.** The effectiveness of analgesics can be enhanced by a supportive attitude toward the child. By reinforcing the cause and effect of the medication and analgesia, the nurse can condition the child to expect pain relief, provided the regimen is likely to be effective. Although IM injections

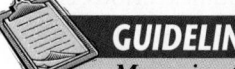

## GUIDELINES

*Managing Opioid-Induced Respiratory Depression*

**If respirations are depressed:**
  Assess sedation level.
  Reduce infusion by 25% when possible.
  Stimulate patient (shake gently, call by name, ask to breathe).
**If patient cannot be aroused or is apneic** (American Pain Society, 1999):
  Administer naloxone (Narcan):
    For children less than 40 kg, dilute 0.1 mg of naloxone in 10 ml of sterile saline to make 10 µg/ml solution and give 0.5 µg/kg.
    For children over 40 kg, dilute 0.4-mg ampule in 10 ml of sterile saline and give 0.5 ml.
    Administer bolus slow IV push every 2 minutes until effect is obtained.
  Closely monitor patient. Naloxone's duration of antagonist action may be shorter than that of opioid, requiring repeated doses of naloxone

NOTE: Respiratory depression caused by benzodiazepines (e.g., diazepam [Valium] or midazolam [Versed]) can be reversed with flumazenil (Romazicon). Pediatric dosing experience suggests 0.01 mg/kg (0.1 ml/kg); if no (or inadequate) response after 1 to 2 minutes, administer same dose and repeat as needed at 60-second intervals for maximum dose of 1 mg (10 ml) (Yaster and others, 1997).

should *not* be given, when they are, older children need an explanation of why the injection is being given. However, toddlers and preschoolers do not have the cognitive ability to understand. All they know is that when they admit having pain, someone gives them an injection with a needle.

Parents and older children may fear addiction when opioids are prescribed. These concerns should be addressed with assurance that any such risk is extremely low. It may be helpful to ask the question, "If you did not have this pain, would you want to take this medicine?" The answer is invariably no, which reinforces the solely therapeutic nature of the drug. It is also important to avoid making statements to the family such as "We don't want you to get used to this medicine" or "By now you shouldn't need this medicine," which may reinforce the fear of becoming addicted.

## Providing Developmentally Appropriate Activities

A primary goal of nursing care for the child who is hospitalized is to minimize threats to the child's development. Many strategies (e.g., minimizing separation) have been discussed and may be all that the short-term patient requires. However, children who experience prolonged or repeated hospitalization are at greater risk for developmental delay or regression. The nurse who provides opportunities for the child to participate in developmentally appropriate activities further normalizes the child's environment and helps reduce interference with the child's ongoing development. (See Normalization, Chapter 22.)

Play assumes a critical role in the child's development. Because of its other important purposes in the hospital setting, play is discussed in the next section.

Interference with normal development may have long-term implications for the rapidly developing infant and toddler. The nurse plays a primary role in identifying children at risk and helping to plan, implement, and evaluate developmental intervention. (See Chapters 12 and 14.)

School is an integral part of the school-age child's and adolescent's development. Accreditation standards for hospitals serving children consider access to appropriate educational services a key factor in the accreditation decision process when a child's treatment requires a significant absence from school (Joint Commission on Accreditation of Healthcare Organizations, 1999). The nurse can encourage children to resume schoolwork as quickly as their condition permits it, help them schedule and protect a selected time for studies, and help the family coordinate hospital educational services with their children's schools. Children should have the opportunity to continue to progress through art and music classes, as well as their academic subjects.

Although regression is expected and normal, nurses have the responsibility of fostering the child's growth and development. Hospitalization can become a significant opportunity for learning and advancing. Extended hospitalizations for long-term chronic illness or situations of failure to thrive, abuse, or neglect represent instances in which regression must be seen as an adjustment period, to be followed by plans for promoting appropriate developmental skills.

## Using Play/Expressive Activities to Minimize Stress

Play is one of the most important aspects of a child's life and one of the most effective tools for managing stress. Because illness and hospitalization constitute crises in the child's life and often involve overwhelming stresses, the acting out of fears and anxieties gives the child a means to cope with these stresses. Children who play are coping positively; children who cannot play are waiting, testing, holding back, or making some inner decisions about the setting (Bolig, 1997).

Play is essential to children's mental, emotional, and social well-being. As with their developmental needs, the need for play does not stop when children are ill or when they enter the hospital. On the contrary, play in the hospital serves many functions (Box 26-13). Of all hospital facilities, no room probably does more to alleviate the stressors of hospitalization than the playroom. In this room children temporarily distance themselves from the fears of separation, loss of control, and bodily injury. They can work through their feelings in a nonthreatening, comfortable atmosphere and in the manner most natural for them. They also know that the boundaries of this room are safe from intrusive or painful procedures, strange faces, and probing questions. The playroom becomes a sanctuary of peace and safety in an otherwise frightening environment. (See Critical Thinking Exercise box.)

Engaging in play activities puts children in charge, removing them for a time from the usual passive role of recipients of a constant stream of procedures and hospital routines. In the hospital environment most decisions are made for the child; play and other expressive activities offer the child much-needed opportunities to make choices. Even if a child chooses not to participate in a particular activity, the nurse has offered the child a choice, perhaps one of but a few real choices the child has had that day.

Children who are ill and hospitalized typically have lower energy levels than healthy children. Therefore, although children may not appear very enthusiastic when participating in an activity, they may be enjoying the experience (Rollins and Mahan, 1996). Rather than assuming otherwise, the nurse can observe for subtle signs—such as a fleeting smile or intent concentration—or simply ask children if they are enjoying themselves.

Children in various age-groups require different types of play facilities. Infants and toddlers need maximum safety, whereas school-age children and adolescents benefit most from group activities. Providing space for special needs of children in each age-group can be difficult in institutions where space availability is limited, but innovative solutions can ensure practical answers. Playroom schedules can be structured to allow one age-group at a time; for example, adolescents can use the facility in the evening when younger children are asleep. Older children can also congregate in one patient's room and listen to music, play games, or just talk. If the location of the session is rotated each evening, older children can look forward to arranging or setting up for the activities.

## Critical Thinking Exercise

### The Playroom

You are watching 7-year-old Hannah play Candyland with her brother, sister, and several other children in the playroom. A laboratory technician enters the playroom and says, "Hannah, I need to take some blood. I can see that you are playing a game, so I'll just do it while you play. It will just take a minute." Your most appropriate response would be which of the following?

FIRST, THINK ABOUT IT . . .
- What is the purpose of your thinking?
- If you accept the conclusions, what are the implications?

1. "Go right ahead. It's silly to have to interrupt her game."
2. "Let me help you so that you can finish sooner."
3. "Hannah, is this okay with you?"
4. "We don't allow any procedures in the playroom."

*The best response is four. The playroom should be considered a safe place—a sanctuary—and therefore off-limits for procedures. In many hospitals the child's bed is accorded the same status; children are taken to a treatment room for such procedures. Even if you accept the conclusion that it is "okay" with Hannah (number three), it is important to consider the possible negative implications for the other children in the room, who may be confused about even a simple procedure (e.g., checking blood pressure) or the sanctuary status of the playroom for themselves.*

*An exception is sometimes made when all the children present are older and the procedure is a quick, painless one (e.g., checking blood pressure or giving oral medication) that all the children present have experienced. In such cases the patient is asked if it is okay and give permission before the procedure is undertaken.*

---

**Box 26-13** ■ ■ ☐
### Functions of Play in the Hospital

Provides diversion and relaxation
Helps the child feel more secure in a strange environment
Helps to lessen the stress of separation and feelings of homesickness
Provides a means for release of tension and expression of feelings
Encourages interaction and development of positive attitudes toward others
Provides an expressive outlet for creative ideas and interests
Provides a means for accomplishing therapeutic goals (See Use of Play in Procedures, Chapter 27.)
Places the child in active role and provides opportunity to make choices and be in control

## Diversional Activities

Almost any form of play can be used for diversion and recreation, but the activity should be selected on the basis of the child's age, interests, and limitations (Fig. 26-11). Children do not necessarily need special direction for using play materials. All they require are the materials with which to work and adult approval and supervision to help keep their natural enthusiasm or expression of feelings from getting out of control. Small children enjoy a variety of small, colorful toys they can play with in bed or in their room or more elaborate play equipment, such as playhouses, sandboxes, rhythm instruments, and large boxes and blocks, that may be a part of the hospital playroom.

Games that can be played alone or with another child or an adult are popular with older children, as are puzzles; reading material; quiet individual activities such as sewing, stringing beads, and weaving; and Tinker-Toys, Lego blocks, and other building materials. Assembling models is an excellent pastime, and developmentally appropriate books are of infinite value to the child. To have someone read aloud provides endless hours of pleasure and is of special value to the child who has limited energy to expend in play.

A radio, videocassette recorder (VCR), electronic games, and television, included among most hospital room equipment, are useful tools for entertaining a child. Computers with modems providing access to the Internet and World Wide Web are popular features in hospital playrooms and offer a window to the world for children who are hospitalized. A child can talk electronically with others and share experiences or even join a virtual support group.* Today's sophisticated technology also provides the opportunity for children to explore every imaginable interest. As with television and other types of electronic entertainment, parents and nurses should monitor both the content and the time that a child spends engaging in these activities to avoid their becoming a substitute for social interaction or therapeutic play.

When supervising play for children who are ill or convalescing, it is best to select activities that are simpler than would normally be chosen according to the child's developmental level. Children may not have the energy to cope with more challenging activities. Other limitations also influence the type of activities. Special consideration must be given to the child who has limited movement, has a restricted extremity, or is isolated. Toys for children on isolation must be disposable or be disinfected after use. For this reason stuffed animals are not recommended for use as community toys on a hospital unit.

**Toys.**   Parents of hospitalized children often ask nurses about the types of toys that would be best to bring for their child. Most want to bring new ones to cheer and comfort the child and assuage their own guilt feelings regarding the child's need for hospitalization. The nurse should tell the parents that although wanting to provide these things for their child is natural, it is often better to wait awhile to bring new things, especially for younger children. Small children need the comfort and reassurance of familiar things, such as the stuffed animal the child hugs for comfort and takes to bed at night. These are a link with home and the world outside the hospital. The nurse is responsible for assessing the safety of the toys brought to the child.

Large numbers of toys often confuse and frustrate a small child. A few small, well-chosen toys are also usually preferred to one large, expensive one. Children who are hospitalized for an extended time benefit from changes. Rather than a confusing accumulation of toys, older toys should be replaced periodically as interest wanes.

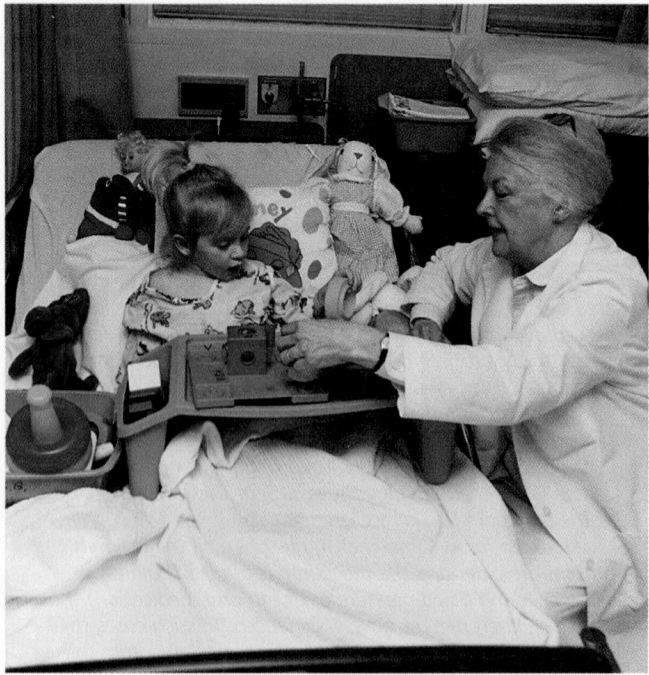

**Fig. 26-11**   Play materials for children in the hospital need to be appropriate for their age, interests, and limitations.

---

*One such group children can access through the Internet is called SICKKIDS. This listserve is an open, unmoderated discussion list for children with chronic or life-threatening illnesses. The list is for children only, ages 18 and under. They can talk about their illness, their feelings and frustrations, their families and friends, and what they do in their spare time; and they can share poems or jokes. Because no adults are allowed, the adults who manage the list do not participate in the discussions; the direct management of the list is handled by several teenage "discussion managers" who are also subscribers. A team of adult, professionally trained counselors are available to provide guidance in difficult situations. Archives of SICKKIDS are kept in monthly files but are not available to the public to preserve the privacy of the children's conversations. Children who wish to subscribe can e-mail at LISTSERV@SJUVM. STJOHNS.EDU, with the following command as the message: SUB SICKKIDS YourFirstName YourLastName.

A highly successful diversion for a child who is hospitalized for a length of time is a box with small, inexpensive, and brightly wrapped items with a different day of the week printed on the outside. The child will eagerly anticipate the time for opening each one. When the parents know when their next visit will be, they can provide the number of packages that corresponds to the days between visits. In this way the child knows that the diminishing packages also represent the anticipated visit from the parent.

## Expressive Activities

Play provides one of the best opportunities for encouraging emotional expression, including the safe release of anger and hostility. Nondirective play that allows children freedom for expression can be very therapeutic. Therapeutic play, however, should not be confused with the psychologic technique of play therapy. *Play therapy* is reserved for use by trained and qualified therapists who use the technique as an interpretative method with emotionally disturbed children. *Therapeutic play,* on the other hand, is a very effective nondirective modality for helping children deal with their concerns and fears; at the same time, it often helps the nurse to gain insights into their needs and feelings.

Tension release can be facilitated through almost any activity. With younger ambulatory children, large-muscle activity, such as the use of tricycles and wagons, is especially beneficial. Much aggression can be safely directed into games and activities that involve pounding and throwing. Beanbags are often thrown at a target or open receptacle with surprising vigor and hostility. A pounding board is employed with enthusiasm by young children; clay and play dough are beneficial at any age.

**Creative Expression.**   Although all children derive physical, social, emotional, and cognitive benefits from engaging in art or other creative activities, children's need for such activities is intensified when they are hospitalized (Rollins, 1995). Drawing and painting are excellent media for expression (Fig. 26-12). Children are more at ease expressing their thoughts and feelings through art, because humans think first in images and later learn to translate these images into words. The child needs only to be supplied with the raw materials, such as crayons and paper. Children usually require little direction for self-expression; however, older children may be given some direction in what to paint or draw. For example, they may be asked to draw the hospital room or draw what they like or do not like about the hospital. Groups of children can enjoy this creative activity either working individually or, with older children, collaborating on a group project such as a mural painted on a long piece of paper. For children confined to bed, an old sheet spread over the bed provides protection for clean linen.

Although interpretation of children's drawing requires special training, observing changes in a series of the child's drawings over time can be helpful in assessing psychosocial adjustment and coping. The nurse can use children's drawings, stories, poetry, and other products of creative expression as a springboard for discussion of thoughts, fears, and understanding of concepts or events. A child's drawing before surgery or chemotherapy, for example, will often reveal unvoiced concerns about mutilation, body changes, and loss of self-control.

Nurses can incorporate opportunities for musical expression into routine nursing care. For example, simple musical instruments, such as bracelets with bells, can be placed on infants' legs for them to shake to accompany mealtime music or dressing changes. Dance/movement suggestions may encourage a child to ambulate.

Holidays provide stimulus and direction for unlimited creative projects. Making pictures and decorations for their rooms gives the children a sense of pride and accomplishment. This is especially beneficial for immobilized and isolated children. Making gifts or decorations for someone at home helps to maintain interpersonal ties.

**Dramatic Play.**   Dramatic play is a well-recognized technique for emotional release, allowing children to reenact frightening or puzzling hospital experiences. Through use of puppets and replicas or actual hospital equipment, children can act out the situations that are a part of their hospital experience (Fig. 26-13). Dramatic play enables children to learn about procedures and events that are of concern to them and to assume the roles of the adults in the hospital environment.

Puppets are universally effective for communicating with children. Most children view them as peers and readily communicate with them. Children will tell the puppet feelings that they hesitate to express to adults. Puppets dressed to represent figures in the child's environment (e.g., a physician, nurse, child patient, therapist, and members of the child's own family) are especially useful. Small, appropriately attired dolls are also effective in encouraging the child to play out situations, although puppets are usually best for direct conversation.

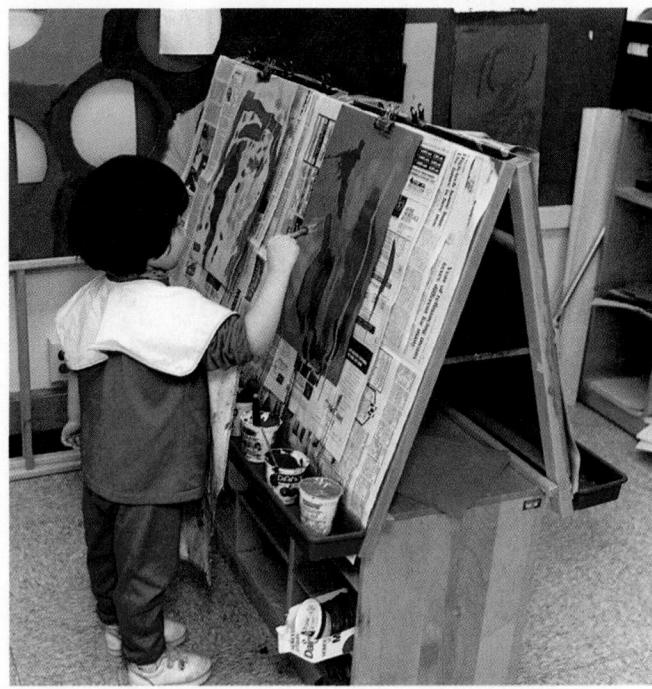

**Fig. 26-12**   Drawing and painting are excellent media for expression.

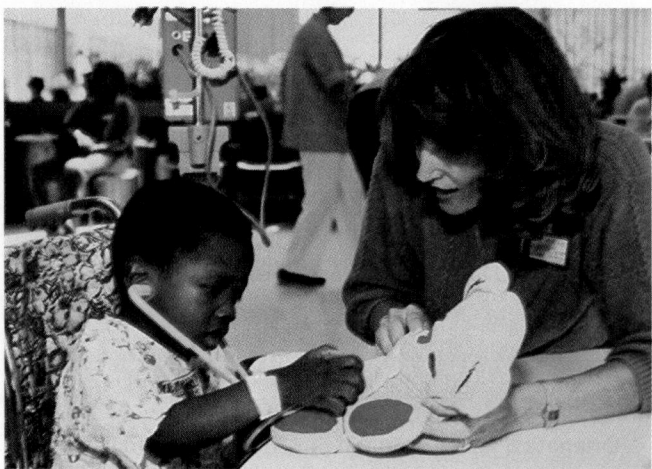

**Fig. 26-13** Playing with miniature hospital equipment allows children to explore feelings and concerns and achieve mastery over hospital situations. (Courtesy St. Louis Children's Hospital.)

**NURSING TIP** Make a simple puppet using a large handkerchief. Place some cotton balls in the center of the cloth and wrap a rubber band over the handkerchief and cotton balls to form a "head." Place the head over the index finger so that the rubber band secures it to the finger. Let the cloth drape over the front and back of the hand. The cloth forms four parts of the puppet: the index finger is the head, the thumb and other fingers are the arms, and the draped cloth is the body. Decorate the head by drawing features on it (Wong, 1993).

Play must consider medical needs, but at times a procedure can be postponed for a short time to allow the child to complete a special activity. (See Critical Thinking Exercise box.) Play must consider any limitations imposed by the child's condition. For example, small children may eat paste and other creative media; therefore a child who is allergic to wheat should not be given finger paint made from wallpaper paste or play dough made with flour. A child with restricted salt intake should not play with modeling dough, because salt is one of its major components.*

## Maximizing Potential Benefits of Hospitalization

Although hospitalization generally represents a stressful time for children and families, it also presents an opportunity for facilitating positive change within the child and among family members. For some families the stress of a child's illness, hospitalization, or both can lead to strengthening of family coping behaviors and the emergence of new coping strategies (Kirkby and Whelan, 1996). Therefore nursing interventions must also focus on maximizing the potential benefits of the experience.

*Information about art materials can be obtained from the Glassell School of Art, 5101 Montrose Blvd, Houston, TX 77006, (713) 639-7500.

### Critical Thinking Exercise

**Scheduling Procedures**

Robert, 5 years old, is recovering from abdominal surgery. You enter his room to check his dressing. His mother is reading him a story. Your most appropriate response would be which of the following?

FIRST, THINK ABOUT IT . . .
• What concepts or ideas are central to your thinking?
• What conclusions are you coming to?

1. To Robert's mother: "I need to check Robert's dressing."
2. "Robert, I need to check your dressing, but I can see that you are in the middle of a story right now. I'll check back in about 10 minutes and do it then."
3. "It's time to check your dressing, Robert. Let's get started."
4. "Robert, I need to check your dressing. It should take about 5 minutes. Would you like me to check it now, or to come back in about 10 minutes when you have finished hearing the story?"

*The best response is four, although number two would also be acceptable. The ideas presented in number four not only indicate that you value and respect the activity Robert is engaged in, but also offer him an opportunity to make a choice: to interrupt the story and complete the procedure, or to finish the story and wait for your return. If, because of your own schedule, you conclude that you are unable to offer such choices, express your desire to come back later, but explain that this time it is not possible. Number one ignores Robert's presence; number three fosters a passive role.*

### Fostering Parent-Child Relationships

The crisis of illness or hospitalization can mobilize parents into more acute awareness of their children's needs. For example, hospitalization provides opportunities for parents to learn more about their children's growth and development. When parents are helped to understand children's usual reactions to stress, such as regression or aggression, they not only are better able to support the child through the hospital experience, but also may extend their insight into childrearing practices following discharge.

Difficulties in parent-child relationships that may result in feeding problems, negative behavior, and enuresis may decrease during hospitalization. The temporary cessation of such problems sometimes alerts parents to the role they may be playing in propagating the negative behavior. With assistance from health professionals, parents can restructure ways of relating to their children to foster more positive behavior.

On occasion, hospitalization may represent a temporary reprieve or refuge from a disturbed home. Typically, abused or neglected children's dramatic physical and social improvement during hospitalization is proof of the growth potential of this experience. Hospitalized children temporarily are able to seek support, reassurance, and security from new relationships, particularly with nurses, hospitalized peers, and others.

### Providing Educational Opportunities

Illness and hospitalization represent excellent opportunities for children and other family members to learn more about their bodies, each other, and the health professions. For example, during a child's admission for a diabetic crisis, the child may learn about the disease; the parents may learn about the child's needs for independence, normalcy, and appropriate limits; and each of them may find a new support system in the hospital staff.

Illness or hospitalization can also help older children in choosing a vocational career. Frequently children have pre-existing impressions of physicians or nurses that are either positive or negative. Experience with different health professionals can influence the child's decision regarding a career in health care.

### Promoting Self-Mastery

The experience of facing a crisis such as illness or hospitalization, coping successfully with it, and maturing as a result of it constitutes an opportunity for self-mastery. Younger children have the chance to test out fantasy vs reality. They realize that they were not abandoned, mutilated, castrated, or punished. In fact, they were loved, cared for, and treated with respect for their individual concerns. It is not unusual to hear children who have undergone hospitalization or surgery to tell others that "it was nothing" or to proudly display their scars or bandages. For older children, hospitalization may represent an opportunity for decision making, independence, and self-reliance. They are proud of having survived the experience and may feel a genuine self-respect for their achievements. Nurses can facilitate such feelings of self-mastery by emphasizing aspects of personal competence in the child and not acknowledging uncooperative or negative behavior.

### Providing Socialization

Hospitalization may offer children a special opportunity for social acceptance. Lonely, asocial, and even delinquent children find a sympathetic environment in the hospital. Children who are physically deformed or in some other way "different" from their age-mates may find an accepting social peer group. Although this does not always spontaneously occur, nurses can structure the environment to foster a supportive child group. For example, judicious selection of a roommate can help children gain a new friend and learn more about themselves. Forming relationships with significant members of the health care team, such as the physician, nurse, child-life specialist, or social worker, can greatly enhance the child's adjustment in many areas of life.

Parents may also encounter a new social group in other parents who have similar problems. They meet while in the hospital or clinic and discuss their children's illnesses and treatment. Nurses can capitalize on this informal gathering by encouraging parents to discuss collectively their concerns and feelings. They can also refer parents to organized

parent groups or can use the help and support of parents of recovered hospitalized patients. It is important that nurses emphasize that each child responds differently to certain aspects of the disease or treatment and that parents should clarify questions or concerns that are raised with other parents with a nurse or doctor. (See discussion of parent-to-parent support in Chapter 22.)

## Supporting Family Members

The term *family-centered care* defines the focus of pediatric care because nursing care of children cannot be optimally performed unless the family as a whole is designated the "client." (See Family-Centered Care, Chapter 1.) Family-centered care supports the family by prioritizing their values and needs, developing collaborative relationships, and empowering the family unit.

Other types of support include emotional and instrumental support. Providing emotional support involves the willingness to stay and listen to parents' verbal and nonverbal messages. Sometimes the support is not given directly by the nurse. For example, the nurse may offer to stay with the child to allow the parents time alone or may discuss with other family members the parents' need for extra relief. Often, extended relatives and friends want to help but do not know how. The nurse can suggest baby-sitting, preparing meals, cleaning the house, doing laundry, or transporting the siblings to school and activities as ways to lessen the parents' responsibilities. An ongoing parent support group held on the pediatric unit has also proved effective in helping parents share emotions and concerns related to hospitalization.

Support may also be provided through the clergy. Parents with deep religious beliefs may appreciate the counsel of a clergy member, but because of their stress they may not have sufficient energy to initiate the contact. Nurses can be supportive by arranging for clergy to visit and by respecting and upholding parents' religious beliefs.

Support involves an acceptance of cultural, socioeconomic, and ethnic values. For example, health and illness are defined differently by various ethnic groups. For some, disorders that have few outward manifestations of illness, such as diabetes or cardiac problems, are not viewed as a sickness. Consequently, following a prescribed treatment may be seen as unnecessary. Nurses who appreciate the influences of culture are more likely to intervene therapeutically. (See Chapter 21 for an extensive discussion of cultural/religious influences on health care.)

Parents may need help in accepting their own feelings toward the ill child. If given the opportunity, parents often disclose their feelings of loss of control, anger, and guilt. They often resist admitting to such feelings because they expect others to disapprove of behavior that is less than perfect. Unfortunately, health personnel, including nurses, sometimes show little tolerance for deviation from the expected norm. This only increases the psychologic impact of a child's illness on family members. Helping parents identify the specific reason for such feelings and emphasizing that each is a normal, expected, and healthy response to stress provides them with an opportunity to lessen their emotional burden. Support may also include preparing siblings for hospital visits, assessing their adjustment, and providing appropriate interventions or referrals when needed.

## Providing Information

One of the most important nursing interventions is to provide information regarding (1) the disease, its treatment, and prognosis; (2) the child's emotional, as well as physical, reaction to illness and hospitalization; and (3) the probable emotional reactions of family members to the crisis.

For many families the child's illness is their first contact with hospitalization. Often parents are not prepared for the child's behavioral reactions to hospitalization, such as separation anxiety, regression, aggression, and hostility. Providing the parents with information about these normal and expected behavioral responses can decrease the parents' stress during the hospital admission. The family is equally unfamiliar with hospital rules, which often adds to feelings of confusion and anxiety. Therefore the family needs clear explanations about what to expect and what is expected of them. Nurses can also help family members become more adept at seeking information about their child's condition by asking questions that elicit meaningful information. (See Guidelines box.) In giving information, nurses need to be alert to information overload. Repetition of information can be helpful.

Parents also need to be aware of the effects of illness on the family and strategies that prevent negative changes. Specifically, parents should keep the family informed and communicating as much as possible. They should treat all of the children as equally and as normally as before the illness occurred. Discipline, which initially may be lessened for the ill child, should be continued to provide a measure of security and predictability. When ill children know that their parents expect certain standards of conduct from them, they feel certain that they will recover. When all limits are removed, they fear that something catastrophic will happen.

Helping parents to understand and accept the meaning of posthospitalization behaviors in the sick child is necessary in order for them to tolerate and support such behaviors. Consequently, they should be forewarned of the common reactions following discharge. Parents who do not expect such reactions may misinterpret them as evidence of the child's "being spoiled" and demand perfect behavior at a time when the child is still reacting to the stress of illness and hospitalization. If the behaviors, especially the demand for attention, are dealt with in a supportive manner, most children are able to relinquish them and assume precrisis levels of functioning.

Nurses should also forewarn parents of the common reactions of siblings to the ill child—particularly anger, jealousy, and resentment. Older siblings may deny such reactions because they provoke feelings of guilt. However, everyone needs outlets for emotions, and the repressed feelings may surface as problems in school, with age-mates, as psychosomatic illnesses, or in delinquent behavior.

Probably one of the most neglected areas involves giving information to siblings. Age frequently becomes the primary factor that leads to an awareness of this need, because older children may begin to ask questions or request explanations. However, even in this situation the information may be seriously inadequate. Children in every age-group deserve some explanation of the child's illness or hospitalization, preferably appropriate written information for older children. Although the exact wording may differ, the answer should focus on the following concerns: (1) "Will I get sick and have to go to the hospital?" (2) "Did I cause the illness?" (for actual or imagined reasons), and (3) "Will my parents abandon me if my brother or sister doesn't recover?" If parents or nurses address the explanations to these three questions, the siblings' own fears of illness, guilt, and abandonment will be minimized.

Nursing approaches with siblings can be direct or indirect. Direct services might include (1) incorporating siblings into hospital admission programs; (2) liberalizing visiting regulations; (3) extending parent participation programs to include sibling involvement, such as through family dining or group play sessions; and (4) developing programs designed specifically for siblings, such as group sessions to discuss their concerns or posthospital discharge visits to evaluate the siblings' adjustment. Older siblings may not wish to attend a group; the nurse can be available for casual talks or for a tour, which may encourage the youngster to talk.

Indirect services (which can be influenced by any existing nursing role) involve helping parents understand, cope with, and support the siblings' reactions to the experience. Siblings do best with as little disruption in their lives as possible. Other interventions include helping well siblings maintain contact with the child who is hospitalized through telephone calls or sending tape recordings, letters, or postcards. (See Family Home Care box on p. 1084.) See Nursing Care Plans on pp. 1075-1083.

## GUIDELINES

### Helping Families Elicit Information

Find out what the family wants to know.

Teach them to avoid general questions, such as "Why is my child sick?"

Help them prepare specific questions, such as "What is causing my child's pain?" or "What does this drug do?"

Encourage the use of short and open-ended questions.

Have the family write down the questions, preferably in a diary or journal that is kept in an accessible area, such as a pocket, to have available when needed.

Encourage the family to speak up when they do not understand an answer and to ask to have it explained in clearer or easier language.

Have the family repeat the information to be certain they understand it and record unfamiliar terms.

Modified from Norris L: Coaching the question, *Nursing 86* 16(5): 100, 1986.

*Text continued on p. 1083*

## *Nursing Care Plan*
## The Child in the Hospital

> **NURSING DIAGNOSIS:** Anxiety/fear related to separation from accustomed routine and support system; unfamiliar surroundings

**PATIENT GOAL 1:** Will experience minimized separation.

- **NURSING INTERVENTIONS/*RATIONALES***

Assign same nursing personnel as much as possible and a primary nurse *to provide the consistency that builds trust*

Arrange workload and schedule to allow personal contact with child

Encourage parents to room-in whenever possible *to prevent separation*

Provide an atmosphere of warmth and acceptance for both child and parents

Encourage parents and others to demonstrate affection for child

Recognize child's separation behaviors as normal

Allow child to cry, *because this is a normal response to separation*

Provide support through physical presence

Maintain child's contact with parents and siblings and home

Talk about child's family frequently

Encourage child to talk about and remember family members, pets

Stress significance of parents' and siblings' visits, telephone calls, or letters

Help parents understand the behaviors of separation anxiety (see Box 26-1) and suggest ways of supporting the child

Explain to child when parents leave and when they will return

Tell hospitalized child the reason for leaving

Convey the expected time of return in terms of anticipated events. For example, if the parents will return in the morning, they can say they will see the child, "After the sun comes up," or, "When (a favorite program) is on television"

Use a clock or calendar for an older child *so child can anticipate next family visit*

Visit for short but frequent times rather than one long time; encourage parents and relatives to take turns visiting

Encourage siblings, grandparents, and other significant persons to visit

Leave favorite articles from home, such as a blanket, toy, bottle, feeding utensil, or article of clothing, with child, *because this helps child tolerate separation*

Respect treasured objects of children, such as a stuffed animal

Encourage family to provide photographs of family members and recordings of the parents' voices (e.g., reading a story, singing a song, saying prayers before bedtime, or relating events at home) *to familiarize the unfamiliar environment and to provide comfort during times of separation*

Play family recordings at lonely times, such as before sleep

Suggest that the family leave small gifts for the child to open each day: if the parents know when their next visit will be, have them leave the number of packages that corresponds to the days between visits

Assign a "foster grandparent" or consistent volunteer to be with child if available

- **EXPECTED OUTCOMES**

Child has consistent caregivers

Parents visit as much as possible

Parents cooperate in care (specify)

Child accepts and responds positively to comforting measures

Child discusses family members, including pets

Parents demonstrate an understanding of separation behaviors

Siblings, grandparents, and other significant persons visit as much as possible

Family provides child with familiar or cherished articles from home

Assigned person spends time with child (specify amount)

**PATIENT GOAL 2:** Will express feelings

- **NURSING INTERVENTIONS/*RATIONALES***

Accept expression of feelings *so that child continues these expressions*

Provide an atmosphere that encourages free expression of feelings

Provide opportunities for the child to verbalize, "act out," or otherwise express feelings without fear of punishment

Encourage drawing and other expressive activities *because children often find it easier to express themselves in images instead of words*

Encourage keeping a journal or diary *to allow child to express feelings and review progress and changes in feelings*

- **EXPECTED OUTCOME**

Child verbalizes or plays out feelings or concerns

**PATIENT GOAL 3:** Will remain calm

- **NURSING INTERVENTIONS/*RATIONALES***

Do nothing to make child more anxious, remembering that what may not provoke anxiety in an adult may make a child very anxious

Maintain calm, relaxed, and reassuring manner

Spend time with child and family *to establish rapport*

Give competent, consistent nursing care *to instill confidence in both parents and child*

Explain intrusive procedures in a developmentally appropriate manner

- **EXPECTED OUTCOMES**

Child exhibits no signs of apprehension

Child rests quietly and calmly

**PATIENT GOAL 4:** Will exhibit trusting behaviors

- **NURSING INTERVENTIONS/*RATIONALES***

Be positive in approach to child

Be honest with child *to encourage child to trust*

Convey to the child the behavior expected

Be consistent in expectations and relationships with child *because consistency is an important component of the development of trust*

Treat child fairly

*Continued*

## Nursing Care Plan
### The Child in the Hospital—cont'd

Encourage parents to maintain a truthful relationship with the child

Make certain child has call light or other signal device within reach

- **EXPECTED OUTCOMES**

Child develops rapport with primary nurse

Child maintains trusting feelings toward family

**PATIENT GOAL 5:** Will experience feelings of security

- **NURSING INTERVENTIONS/***RATIONALES*

Maintain child's identity

Address child by name or nickname

Avoid assigning a nickname to child or converting a given name to its counterpart in another language (e.g., using Joe instead of José)

Avoid communicating any signals of rejection, distaste, or other negative feelings to child

When necessary, communicate disapproval of unacceptable *behavior,* not disapproval of the *child*

Communicate (verbally and nonverbally) that the child is a valued person

Discourage treatments or procedures in the child's room or playroom *to maintain these areas as "safe places"*

- **EXPECTED OUTCOMES**

Child interacts with staff

*Staff demonstrates respect for child

**PATIENT GOAL 6:** Will experience reduction of fear or no fear

- **NURSING INTERVENTIONS/***RATIONALES*

Explain routines, items, procedures, and events in a language and method appropriate to the child's developmental level; use simple language, drawings, and play *to facilitate understanding and mastery*

Reassure child and repeat reassurance as necessary

Ask child to explain reason for hospitalization and correct if necessary *to help absolve child from any guilt about being hospitalized*

Encourage parent(s) to participate in child's care

Encourage child to handle items that may seem strange or threatening *to reduce fear of the unknown*

Give encouragement and positive feedback for cooperation in care

- **EXPECTED OUTCOMES**

Child exhibits understanding of information presented (specify information and means of demonstration)

Child discusses procedures and activities without evidence of anxiety

**PATIENT GOAL 7:** Will be allowed to express regressive behavior

- **NURSING INTERVENTIONS/***RATIONALES*

Inform parents that regressive behavior is a feature of illness *so that it is not viewed as abnormal*

Accept regressive behavior and help child with dependency

Assist child in reconquering the negative counterpart of the psychosocial stage to which child has regressed (e.g., overcome mistrust; facilitate development of trust)

- **EXPECTED OUTCOME**

*Staff and parents exhibit an attitude of acceptance of regressive behaviors

**PATIENT GOAL 8:** Will experience adequate comfort level

- **NURSING INTERVENTIONS/***RATIONALES*

Provide pacifier, if appropriate, *to meet oral needs and to provide comfort*

Hold infant or young child when this does not interfere with therapy

Touch, talk, and otherwise comfort child who cannot be held

Provide sensory stimulation and diversion appropriate to child's level of development and need for rest

Encourage family members to visit and allow them to comfort and care for child to the extent possible

- **EXPECTED OUTCOMES**

Infant or young child engages in nonnutritive sucking

Child exhibits no signs of distress

Family is involved in care

---

**NURSING DIAGNOSIS:** Anxiety/fear related to distressing procedures, events

---

**PATIENT GOAL 1:** Will be prepared for hospitalization

- **NURSING INTERVENTIONS/***RATIONALES*

Prepare child as needed *to reduce fear of the unknown and to promote cooperation*

Select appropriate preparatory materials

Involve parents *to enable them to serve as effective resources for their child*

Modify preparation in special situations (e.g., day hospital, emergency admission, intensive care unit [ICU]) (see Guidelines box on p. 1087)

- **EXPECTED OUTCOME**

Child is prepared for hospital experience

**PATIENT GOAL 2:** Will exhibit decreased fear of bodily injury

- **NURSING INTERVENTIONS/***RATIONALES*

Recognize developmental fears associated with illness and procedures *to ensure appropriate intervention*

Provide age-appropriate explanations for procedures, especially those that are intrusive or involve the genitals, and include information about what body parts will not be affected, as well as those that will

Provide age-appropriate explanations for procedures the child may see or hear performed on other patients *to decrease child's fears*

Reassure child that certain body parts can be removed without producing harm (e.g., blood, tonsils, appendix)

---

*Nursing outcome.

*Nursing Care Plan*
## The Child in the Hospital—cont'd

### PATIENT GOAL 2—cont'd

- **NURSING INTERVENTIONS/**RATIONALES**—cont'd**

Provide privacy for any procedure that exposes the body

Use interventions that preserve child's concept of body integrity (e.g., bandages over puncture sites)

- **EXPECTED OUTCOME**

Child displays minimum fear of bodily injury

### PATIENT GOAL 3: Will receive support during tests and procedures

- **NURSING INTERVENTIONS/**RATIONALES**

Prepare child for procedures according to age and level of understanding, including strategies for coping

Remain with child *to provide support by physical presence*

Prepare child and family for surgery if appropriate

Answer questions and explain purposes of activities

Keep child (and family) informed of progress

- **EXPECTED OUTCOME**

Child remains calm and cooperative during procedures

Child feels supported by others during procedure

---

**NURSING DIAGNOSIS:** Acute pain related to (specify)

---

### PATIENT GOAL 1: Will perceive less pain by using appropriate strategies

- **NURSING INTERVENTIONS/**RATIONALES**

Employ nonpharmacologic strategies to help child manage pain *because techniques such as relaxation, rhythmic breathing, and distraction can make pain more tolerable*

Use strategy that is familiar to child or describe several strategies and let child select one (see Guidelines box, p. 1059) *to facilitate child's learning and use of strategy*

Involve parent in selection of strategy *because parent knows child best*

Select appropriate person(s), usually parent, to assist child with strategy

Teach child to use specific nonpharmacologic strategies before pain occurs or before it becomes severe, *because these approaches appear to be most effective for mild pain*

Assist or have parent assist child with using strategy during actual pain *because coaching may be needed to help child focus on required actions*

- **EXPECTED OUTCOMES**

Child exhibits acceptable pain level

Child learns and implements effective coping strategies

Parent learns coping skills and is effective in assisting child to cope

### PATIENT GOAL 2: Will experience no pain or reduction of pain to level acceptable to child when receiving analgesics

- **NURSING INTERVENTIONS/**RATIONALES**

Plan to administer prescribed analgesic before procedure *so that its peak effect coincides with painful event*

Plan preventive schedule of medication around the clock (ATC) or "PRN as needed to prevent pain" when pain is continuous and predictable (e.g., postoperatively) *to maintain steady blood levels of analgesic*

Administer analgesia by least traumatic route whenever possible *to avoid causing additional pain;* avoid intramuscular or subcutaneous injections (see Box 26-11)

Prepare child for administration of analgesia by using supportive statements (e.g., "This medicine I am putting in the IV will make you feel better in a few minutes")

Reinforce effect of analgesic by saying that child will begin to feel better in (fill in appropriate amount of time, according to drug use); use clock or timer to measure onset of relief with child; reinforce cause and effect of pain and analgesic *so that child becomes conditioned to expecting relief*

If injection must be given, provide a developmentally appropriate explanation

Avoid statements such as "By now you shouldn't need so much pain medicine" *because they convey a judgmental and belittling attitude*

Give child control whenever possible (e.g., using patient-controlled analgesia, choosing which arm for a venipuncture, taking bandages off, holding tape or other equipment)

*Administer prescribed analgesic; nonopioids, including acetaminophen (Tylenol, paracetamol) and nonsteroidal antiinflammatory drugs (NSAIDs), are suitable for mild to moderate pain (see Table 26-4); opioids are needed for moderate to severe pain (see Table 26-5); combination of the two analgesics (see Table 26-6) attacks pain at peripheral nervous system and at central nervous system and provides increased analgesia without increased side effects

Titrate dosage for maximum pain relief

Begin with recommended dosage for age and weight

Increase dosage or decrease dose interval between dosages if pain relief is inadequate

If using parenteral route, change to oral route as soon as possible using equianalgesic dosages (see Tables 26-5 and 26-6) *because of first-pass effect (oral opioid is rapidly absorbed from gastrointestinal tract and enters portal circulation, where it is partially metabolized before reaching central circulation; therefore oral dosages must be larger)*

*Avoid combining opioids with so-called "potentiators," *because combining drugs such as promethazine (Phenergan) and chlorpromazine (Thorazine) adds risk of sedation and respiratory depression without increasing analgesia*

Do not use placebos in the assessment or treatment of pain, *because deceptive use of placebos does not provide useful information about presence or severity of pain, can cause side effects similar to those of opioids, can destroy child's and family's trust in health care staff, and raises serious ethical and legal questions*

- **EXPECTED OUTCOMES**

Child exhibits absence or minimal evidence of pain

Child accepts administration of analgesia with minimal distress

---

*Dependent nursing action.

*Continued*

# Nursing Care Plan
## The Child in the Hospital—cont'd

> **NURSING DIAGNOSIS:** Risk for poisoning or injury from medications related to sensitivity, excessive dose, decreased gastrointestinal motility

**PATIENT GOAL 1:** Will exhibit normal respiratory function

- **NURSING INTERVENTIONS/RATIONALES**

Monitor rate and depth of respirations and level of sedation

Have emergency drugs and equipment in case of respiratory depression from opioids (see Guidelines box on p. 1068) to begin therapy as soon as needed

- **EXPECTED OUTCOME**

Child's respirations and sedation level remain within acceptable limits (see inside back cover for normal variations)

**PATIENT GOAL 2:** Will not develop constipation and will receive treatment for other opioid-related side effects

- **NURSING INTERVENTIONS/RATIONALES**

*Administer stool softener or laxative *to prevent constipation*

Stop or decrease medication if evidence of rash

*Administer antipruritic *for itching*

*Administer antiemetic *for nausea and vomiting*

Encourage child to lie quietly *because movement increases nausea and vomiting*

Recognize signs of tolerance: decreasing pain relief, decreasing duration of pain relief

Recognize signs of withdrawal after discontinuation of drug (physical dependence) (see Box 26-12)

†Help treat tolerance and physical dependence appropriately *because these are involuntary, physiologic responses that occur from prolonged use of opioids*

Never refer to child who is tolerant or physically dependent as "addicted"

- **EXPECTED OUTCOMES**

Child has regular bowel movements

Child exhibits no evidence of rash or itching

Child receives appropriate therapy for tolerance/dependency

See also Preparation for Diagnostic and Therapeutic Procedures, Chapter 27

See also Administration of Medication, Chapter 27

> **NURSING DIAGNOSIS:** Powerlessness related to the health care environment

**PATIENT GOAL 1:** Will experience "homelike" atmosphere in the hospital environment

- **NURSING INTERVENTIONS/RATIONALES**

Determine from parents or other caregiver the child's customary routine and the usual manner of handling the child (see Box 26-14)

Maintain a routine similar to the one the child is accustomed to at home

Minimize a hospital-like environment as much as possible; allow child to sit at table to eat and wear own pajamas or street clothes

Use terms familiar to child, such as those for body functions

Encourage patients with extended hospitalizations to decorate room (e.g., pictures, bedspread from home) *to make it more "homelike"*

Encourage sibling visitation

Explore the possibility of pet visitation for children with extended hospitalizations

Advocate for appropriate hospital signs that assist the child in moving freely throughout the unit and hospital with confidence

- **EXPECTED OUTCOME**

Child's routines and environment are similar to those at home (specify)

Child feels relatively at ease in hospital environment

**PATIENT GOAL 2:** Will experience opportunities to exert control

- **NURSING INTERVENTIONS/RATIONALES**

Allow child choices whenever possible, such as food selection, clothing, options for time of basic care (bath, play, bedtime), selection of television channels, choice of activities *to give child some measure of control*

Use time structuring with an older child (a jointly planned and written schedule of daily activities)

Permit freedom on the unit within defined and enforced limitations

Explain the reason for physically restraining a child to both child and parents

Encourage self-care according to child's abilities

Assign tasks to an older child, especially in extended hospitalization (e.g., making the bed, supervising younger children, distributing menus)

Respect child's need for privacy

- **EXPECTED OUTCOMES**

Child participates in planning care (specify)

Child moves about the unit but respects limits

Child participates in care activities (specify activities)

Child assumes responsibility for tasks (specify)

Child's need for privacy is maintained

> **NURSING DIAGNOSIS:** Deficient activity related to impaired mobility, musculoskeletal impairment, confinement to hospital, effects of illness

**PATIENT GOAL 1:** Will have opportunity to participate in activities

- **NURSING INTERVENTIONS/RATIONALES**

Schedule therapies and periods of rest to allow for activities

Involve child in planning care to the extent of capabilities

Arrange for and encourage interaction with others as feasible

Encourage visits from family and friends

Provide opportunity to socialize with noninfectious children

- **EXPECTED OUTCOMES**

Child helps plan care and schedule

Child interacts with family and other children

---

*Dependent nursing action.
†Nursing outcome.

## Nursing Care Plan
## The Child in the Hospital—cont'd

**PATIENT GOAL 2:** Will have opportunity to participate in diversional activities

- **NURSING INTERVENTIONS/*RATIONALES***

Spend time with child

Query child and parents regarding child's favorite diversional activities

Change position of bed in room periodically *to alter sensory stimuli* if child is confined to bed

Provide activities appropriate to child's condition, physical limitations, and developmental level

Encourage family to caress and hold infant or child

Maintain accustomed routine when possible

Consult with a child-life specialist *to provide diversional activities*

Encourage interaction with other children

Choose a roommate compatible in age, sex, and physical abilities

Monitor time spent watching television or playing electronic games vs interactive or creative activities

Allow ample time for play

Make play, art, music, and other expressive materials available to child

Encourage play activities and diversions appropriate to child's age, condition, and capabilities

Help facilitate an activity by acting under the child's instructions to perform tasks the child is unable to do

Use play as a teaching strategy and an anxiety-reducing technique

Promote the use of a separate activity room or area for adolescents

- **EXPECTED OUTCOMES**

Child engages in activities appropriate for age, interests, and physical limitations (specify activities)

Child receives attention and comfort

Child engages in age-appropriate play (specify)

---

**NURSING DIAGNOSIS:** Activity intolerance related to generalized weakness, fatigue, imbalance between oxygen supply and demand, pain or discomfort

---

**PATIENT GOAL 1:** Will maintain adequate energy levels

- **NURSING INTERVENTIONS/*RATIONALES***

Assess child's level of physical tolerance

Anticipate child's need for rest, as evidenced by irritability and short attention span; assist child in activities of daily living that may be beyond tolerance

Provide entertainment and quiet diversional activities appropriate to child's age and interest *to conserve energy*

Provide diversional play activities

Instruct child to rest when feeling tired

Balance rest and activity when ambulatory

- **EXPECTED OUTCOMES**

Child plays and rests quietly and engages in activities appropriate to age and capabilities (specify)

Child tolerates increasingly more activity

**PATIENT GOAL 2:** Will receive optimum rest

- **NURSING INTERVENTIONS/*RATIONALES***

Provide quiet environment *to promote rest*

Organize activities for maximum sleep time

Schedule visiting to allow for sufficient rest

Keep visiting periods with friends and family short

Encourage parents to remain with child *to decrease separation and anxiety*

*Administer sedatives and analgesics as indicated if ordered for restlessness and pain

Encourage frequent rest periods

Enforce regular sleep times

Follow child's usual routine for bedtime, nap time

Implement measures to ensure sleep, such as quiet, darkened room

Be alert to signs that child is tired or overstimulated *to allow flexibility in scheduling or enforcing rest and sleep periods*

- **EXPECTED OUTCOMES**

Child remains calm, quiet, and relaxed

Child gets a sufficient amount of rest (specify)

---

**NURSING DIAGNOSIS:** Risk for injury/trauma related to unfamiliar environment, therapies, hazardous equipment

---

**PATIENT GOAL 1:** Will experience no injury

- **NURSING INTERVENTIONS/*RATIONALES***

Employ environmental safety measures

Report any potential hazards (e.g., slippery floors, poor illumination, electrical hazards, damaged or malfunctioning furniture or equipment, unprotected windows, stairwells)

Dispose of breakable items appropriately (thermometers, bottles)

Keep potentially hazardous articles out of child's reach

Check bathwater for temperature before bathing infant or child *to prevent burns*

Do not leave children unsupervised in bathtub/shower

Keep crib sides up and securely fastened; use side rails for children who may fall out of bed

Use safety restraints only when absolutely necessary

    Remove as often as possible

    Discontinue as soon as possible

    Check regularly for adequate circulation to the restrained area and any pressure points, and that restraint is applied properly

Maintain hand contact while caring for a child in a crib with side rails down *to prevent falls*

Transport infants and children appropriately

    Hold with proper support

    Fasten safety belt on gurney, wheelchair

Alert parents and ancillary hospital personnel regarding child's physical tolerance and need for assistance during activity

Fasten safety belts in high chairs, swings

- **EXPECTED OUTCOME**

Child remains free of injury

---

*Dependent nursing action.

*Continued*

## Nursing Care Plan
### The Child in the Hospital—cont'd

> **NURSING DIAGNOSIS:** Bathing/hygiene and dressing/grooming self-care deficit related to physical or cognitive disability, mechanical restrictions

**PATIENT GOAL 1:** Will engage in self-help activities

- **NURSING INTERVENTIONS/*RATIONALES***

Allow child to help plan own daily routine and choose from alternatives when appropriate *to promote sense of control*

Encourage participation in self-care activities according to developmental level and capabilities *to promote mastery and decrease regression*

Provide devices, equipment, and methods to assist child in self-care

Advocate for child-sized features (e.g., bathroom door handles low enough for children to reach)

Assist with dressing, grooming, bathing as indicated

- **EXPECTED OUTCOME**

Child engages in self-help activities to maximum capabilities

> **NURSING DIAGNOSIS:** Toileting self-care deficit related to physical or cognitive disability, mechanical restrictions

**PATIENT GOAL 1:** Will exhibit normal elimination patterns

- **NURSING INTERVENTIONS/*RATIONALES***

Solicit information from child and parents regarding child's normal patterns and procedures of elimination

Sit child in upright position when possible *to encourage elimination*

Employ special devices where appropriate (e.g., fracture pan, commode, elevated toilet seat)

Carry out bowel-training program with hydration, high-fiber diet, stool softeners, and mild laxatives if needed

Provide privacy

- **EXPECTED OUTCOME**

Child has regular bowel movements

> **NURSING DIAGNOSIS:** Impaired urinary elimination related to discomfort, positioning

**PATIENT GOAL 1:** Will exhibit normal voiding

- **NURSING INTERVENTIONS/*RATIONALES***

Solicit information from child and parents regarding child's normal patterns and procedures of elimination

Position child as upright as possible to void

Hydrate child *to ensure adequate urinary output for age*

Stimulate bladder emptying with running water

Catheterize as needed

- **EXPECTED OUTCOME**

Child exhibits normal frequency and volume of urinary voiding with minimal discomfort

See also:

Nursing Care Plan: The Child with Chronic Illness or Disability, Chapter 22

Nursing Care Plan: The Child Undergoing Surgery, Chapter 27

Nursing Care Plan: The Child Who Is Terminally Ill or Dying, Chapter 23

Nursing Care Plan for specific health problem(s)

## Nursing Care Plan
### The Family of the Child Who Is Ill or Hospitalized

> **NURSING DIAGNOSIS:** Anxiety/fear related to situational crisis, threat to role functioning, change in environment

**FAMILY GOAL 1:** Will adjust to hospital environment

- **NURSING INTERVENTIONS/*RATIONALES***

Introduce family to significant staff members

Describe hospital routine that affects child

Acclimate family to the new and strange surroundings (e.g., physical layout of unit, including playroom, unit kitchen, toilet, telephone

Direct family to areas they may need to use outside the unit (e.g., dining room, laundry facility)

Provide an atmosphere that promotes questioning, expression of doubts and feelings

Be available to family *for questions or concerns*

Be alert to signs of tension in family members

Provide privacy

- **EXPECTED OUTCOMES**

Family demonstrates familiarity with hospital environment

Family members ask questions

**FAMILY GOAL 2:** Will feel a part of the health care team

- **NURSING INTERVENTIONS/*RATIONALES***

Employ a polite, respectful approach and demeanor

Greet family by name when they arrive on the unit

Encourage family's presence

Include family in planning patient care

Encourage family to select and assume specific roles in child's care, as comfortable for them

Offer encouragement for their efforts

## Nursing Care Plan
### The Family of the Child Who Is Ill or Hospitalized—cont'd

**FAMILY GOAL 2—cont'd**

• **NURSING INTERVENTIONS**/*RATIONALES*—cont'd
Ask family to share with staff what they know about child's
care and needs
Convey an attitude of collegiality with family, not competition

• **EXPECTED OUTCOME**
Family becomes involved in planning and carrying out care
for the child to extent they desire

**FAMILY GOAL 3:** Will experience reduced apprehension

• **NURSING INTERVENTIONS**/*RATIONALES*
Allow for expression of feelings about child's hospitalization
and illness
Provide needed information *to alleviate fear of the unknown*
Prepare family for what to expect (e.g., procedures, behaviors)
Explore family's expectations
Explore family's concerns and feelings of irritation, guilt,
anger, disappointment, inadequacy
Explore family's fears and anxieties regarding child's status
and expectations of results of procedures or therapy
Introduce parents to other families who have a child in the
hospital, especially a child who is similarly affected, *to
facilitate family-to-family support*
Provide something constructive and meaningful for family to
focus on (e.g., keeping record of intake and output, pain
relief record, ensuring a specified amount of fluid intake,
collecting a specimen) as comfortable for them

• **EXPECTED OUTCOMES**
Family members verbalize feelings and concerns
Family demonstrates an understanding of procedures and
behaviors (specify manner of demonstration and learning)
Family interacts with other families, as desired

**FAMILY GOAL 4:** Will be prepared for special
procedures (e.g., radiology, diagnostic tests, surgery)

• **NURSING INTERVENTIONS**/*RATIONALES*
Assess family's understanding of the procedure and its purpose
Provide needed information; clarify misconceptions
Explain special preparation needed (e.g., nothing by mouth
[NPO], shaving, preprocedure medication or equipment)
Describe
  Where child will be during the procedure
  Whether family can be with child
  Where family can wait
  Approximate length of time procedure requires
Reassure family that they will be notified regarding progress
of the procedure

• **EXPECTED OUTCOME**
Family demonstrates an understanding of procedures and
tests (specify)

**FAMILY GOAL 5:** Will receive support during child's
absence

• **NURSING INTERVENTIONS**/*RATIONALES*
Provide a comfortable place for family to wait
Suggest activities to help reduce anxiety (e.g., go to the
dining room, take a short walk [specify activity])
Be available to family *for support*

Make contact with family at frequent intervals *to relay information, provide comfort*

• **EXPECTED OUTCOME**
Family feels a sense of support

**FAMILY GOAL 6:** Will adjust to child's appearance and
behavior following procedure(s) or in special care unit

• **NURSING INTERVENTIONS**/*RATIONALES*
Remain calm *to decrease family's anxiety*
Explain the environment, if appropriate (e.g., intensive care
unit [ICU])
Apply principles of learning to explanations
  Begin with small amounts of information
  Begin with very general information
  Allow ample time for family to absorb information and to
    ask questions
  Use age-appropriate explanations and techniques for
    siblings
Explain how child will look and the reasons for the child's
appearance and equipment
Explain what child is experiencing
Prepare child and surroundings *to lessen the impact of the first
impression*
  Tidy the bed
  Personalize the bed and bedside with a toy or other item(s)
  Provide chairs for family
  Be prepared for possible adverse reaction (e.g., fainting)
Convey an attitude of caring *about*, as well as *for*, the child
Accompany the family to the child's bedside
Allow time for follow-up discussion of questions and concerns

• **EXPECTED OUTCOME**
Family feels prepared before coming to child's bedside

**FAMILY GOAL 7:** Will experience reduction of fear or
no fear

• **NURSING INTERVENTIONS**/*RATIONALES*
Help family distinguish between realistic and unfounded fears
Help eliminate unfounded fears
Discuss with family their fears regarding
  Child's signs and symptoms
  Child's anxiety
  Consequences of disease or therapy
  Deterioration of child's condition
  Tests and procedures
  Death
Answer questions honestly and compassionately

• **EXPECTED OUTCOME**
Family members verbalize fears and explore nature and ramifications of these fears

---

**NURSING DIAGNOSIS:** Powerlessness related to
health care environment

---

**FAMILY GOAL 1:** Will experience a sense of control

• **NURSING INTERVENTIONS**/*RATIONALES*
Encourage family's presence at times convenient for them;
consider variations (e.g., cultural, occupational) in visiting
Encourage expression of concerns regarding child's care and
progress

*Continued*

## Nursing Care Plan
## The Family of the Child Who Is Ill or Hospitalized—cont'd

Explore family's feelings regarding prescribed therapies
Encourage family to assume as much control as possible in child's management
  Encourage participation in child's care
  Include family in setting goals for care
  Involve family in scheduling and other aspects of care
  Explain what family can do for child and how to handle child to maintain therapy (e.g., how to pick up the child who has an IV line)
  Employ family's suggestions regarding child's care whenever possible

• **EXPECTED OUTCOMES**
Family schedules time to be with child
Family discusses feelings and concerns
Family contributes to care and management of child, as desired
*Family's suggestions are incorporated into plan of care

---

> **NURSING DIAGNOSIS:** Interrupted family processes related to situational crisis (threat to role functioning, hospitalization of a child)

---

**FAMILY GOAL 1:** Will demonstrate knowledge of child's illness

• **NURSING INTERVENTIONS/RATIONALES**
Recognize family's concern and need for information, support
Assess family's understanding of diagnosis and plan of care
Reinforce and clarify health professional's explanation of child's condition, suggested procedures and therapies, and the prognosis
Use every opportunity to increase family's understanding of the disease and its therapies
Repeat information as often as necessary *to facilitate understanding*
Interpret technical information, *because family may not understand*
Help family interpret infant's or child's behaviors and responses
Set and keep an appointed time for patient/family education and discussion of questions and concerns

• **EXPECTED OUTCOME**
Family demonstrates an understanding of the disease and its therapies (specify knowledge)

**FAMILY GOAL 2:** Will experience reduction of guilt feelings or no guilt feelings

• **NURSING INTERVENTIONS/RATIONALES**
Acknowledge feelings of guilt as normal
Provide accurate and specific information regarding the cause of the illness
Clarify misconceptions and false assumptions

• **EXPECTED OUTCOME**
Family verbalizes their understanding of the cause of the illness (specify)

**FAMILY GOAL 3:** Will receive adequate support

• **NURSING INTERVENTIONS/RATIONALES**
Respect parental rights
Convey an attitude of respectful caring for both child and family
Support and emphasize family's strengths and abilities
Provide feedback and praise
Refer to other professionals (e.g., social service, clergy) as needed

• **EXPECTED OUTCOMES**
Family exhibits behaviors that indicate a feeling of self-respect
Family uses supportive services

**FAMILY GOAL 4:** Will demonstrate positive coping behaviors toward child

• **NURSING INTERVENTIONS/RATIONALES**
Determine family's understanding of the normal childhood responses to the stress of illness and hospitalization
Explain child's regression, magical thinking, egocentricity, separation anxiety, fears
Explain behavioral reactions generally expected of child (specify according to age and developmental level)
Reinforce family's endeavors to support child

• **EXPECTED OUTCOME**
Family demonstrates an understanding of child's unfamiliar behaviors (specify manner of demonstration—verbalization, physical attitude, behaviors with child)

**FAMILY GOAL 5:** Will assist child in coping effectively with hospitalization

• **NURSING INTERVENTIONS/RATIONALES**
Help parents determine the best way to prepare child for hospitalization, procedures
Provide family with precise information about what will take place so they know what child is likely to experience
Encourage family to trust child's capacity to cope
Impress on family the need for honesty in relating to child
Encourage family to use play as a coping strategy
Suggest appropriate items to bring to child (e.g., pajamas, favorite toys)
See also Nursing Care Plan: The Child in the Hospital, pp. 1075-1080

• **EXPECTED OUTCOMES**
Family helps in planning strategies
Family is honest with child
Family uses play as a tool for relating with child

**FAMILY GOAL 6:** Will experience positive relationships

• **NURSING INTERVENTIONS/RATIONALES**
Recognize that family members know child best and are in tune with child's needs
Welcome unlimited family presence *to promote family relationships*
Encourage family to bring other significant family members to visit (e.g., siblings, grandparents, and [where permitted] pets)

---

*Nursing outcome.

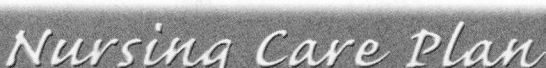

## *Nursing Care Plan*
## The Family of the Child Who Is Ill or Hospitalized—cont'd

Encourage family to provide child with significant items from home *to provide security*

Arrange for family members to have a meal together, if possible

- **EXPECTED OUTCOMES**

Child and family exhibit behaviors that indicate positive coping

Family is with child as often as desired

Child demonstrates an attitude of security with familiar persons and things

**FAMILY GOAL 7:** Will exhibit evidence of optimum health

- **NURSING INTERVENTIONS/*RATIONALES***

Stress importance of maintaining family members' health during child's illness and hospitalization

Encourage adequate rest

    Provide sleeping facilities where possible

    Encourage members to alternate visiting with child to allow some time at home

    Explore means for respite care of dependent family members

Assure family that child will receive optimum care in their absence

Provide relief for family from direct care of child as needed

Promote adequate nutrition

    Provide meals for parents if possible

    Direct family to nutritious resources for meals

    Encourage regular mealtimes

    Provide access to unit kitchen to store and prepare snacks

- **EXPECTED OUTCOMES**

Family shows no evidence of illness

Family members appear well rested

Family members eat regularly

**FAMILY GOAL 8:** Will experience smooth transition from hospital to home

- **NURSING INTERVENTIONS/*RATIONALES***

Assess family's learning needs

Outline and carry out a teaching plan

Determine services needed and make necessary referrals

Include family in planning and problem solving

Maintain open communication between family and health care providers

- **EXPECTED OUTCOME**

Child and family demonstrate the ability to provide needed care in the home

Family has support during transition to home care

**FAMILY GOAL 9:** Will demonstrate knowledge of home care

- **NURSING INTERVENTIONS/*RATIONALES***

Assess family's knowledge to facilitate planning

Teach family the skills needed to carry out the therapeutic program (specify)

    Allow ample time for preparation

    Teach necessary techniques and observations

    Help family by demonstration

    Distribute appropriate home care instructions or other educational materials

    Encourage questions/expression of feelings and concerns

    Allow sufficient time for family to perform procedures under supervision

Inform parents of

    Signs of progress to observe for

    Any unfavorable signs to be alert for

    Problems that can be anticipated (e.g., care of equipment or devices)

    Behaviors that indicate special needs (e.g., pain medication, imminent seizures)

    A course of action to follow (e.g., seizure care)

    Make certain family knows how to contact appropriate persons if or when needed

Prepare family for possible posthospital behaviors of the child (see Box 26-2)

Ensure family's comprehension of child's needs before discharge

- **EXPECTED OUTCOMES**

Family demonstrates procedures needed to care for child in the home (specify learning and method of demonstration)

Family is aware of how to seek help

**FAMILY GOAL 10:** Will demonstrate understanding of continuity of care

- **NURSING INTERVENTIONS/*RATIONALES***

Inform family of community resources available

Refer to agencies as appropriate (specify)

Help identify support group(s) for family, as desired

Be available to family by telephone or other means

Schedule follow-up appointments as needed

Ensure coordination of home care, if needed

- **EXPECTED OUTCOMES**

Family seeks appropriate assistance

Family keeps appointments

See also:

    Nursing Care Plan: The Child in the Hospital, pp. 1075-1080

    Nursing Care Plan: The Child with Chronic Illness or Disability, Chapter 22

    Nursing Care Plan: The Child Who Is Terminally Ill or Dying, Chapter 23

## PREPARATION FOR HOSPITALIZATION

The rationale for preparing children for the hospital experience and related procedures is based on the principle that fear of the unknown exceeds fear of the known. Therefore decreasing the elements of the unknown results in less fear. When children do not have paralyzing fears to cope with, they can direct their energies toward dealing with the other unavoidable stresses of hospitalization and benefit optimally from the growth potential of the experience.

For children past infancy and early toddlerhood, in-hospital or home preparation for hospitalization reduces their stress. Even when children are too young to benefit from direct preparation, parents benefit from prehospital counseling to lessen their fears and thus increase their ability to support the child psychologically. Prehospital counseling has two major goals:

1. To make the hospital less strange and frightening to parents and children
2. To establish a positive atmosphere and trusting relationship with hospital staff and family members

Although preparation may create stress for children initially, eventually the process results in greater trust in parents and staff, increased integration of information, and greater ability to cooperate and participate in treatment (Petrillo and Azarnoff, 1997).

## Guidelines in Preparing for Hospitalization

Although preparation for hospitalization is a common practice, there is no universal standard or program that is advocated in both general and children's hospitals. Some hospital admission programs focus on group preparation before actual admission, whereas others prepare each child either before or on the day of admission. The preparation process may include tours, puppet shows, or therapeutic play with toy or real medical equipment. Other strategies for preparation may include books, photograph albums, videos, or films; or it may be a simple description of the major aspects of a hospital stay (Lancaster, 1997; Stewart, Algren, and Arnold, 1994). The primary audience of most hospital preparation programs is children and families who are experiencing an initial hospitalization. Subsequent readmissions, however, may also be stressful and anxiety provoking. Children's fear and fantasies may not subside with repeated hospital stays but may intensify. Also, concerns change as children develop and grow. These children need preparation as well, although the type of program needs to be individualized and may differ from the following guidelines for planning prehospital tours for groups or individual families who have not yet experienced hospital admission.

Ideally, preparatory procedures should be:

- Planned by hospital staff before child's admission to the hospital
- Appropriately designed for each child's developmental age
- Sufficiently individualized to account for different children's previous experience with hospitalization, present reason for admission, and available support system

Child-life programs have become the standard in pediatric settings to address the psychosocial concerns that hospitalization and other health care experiences precipitate. Child-life programs facilitate coping and the adjustment of children and families by presenting developmentally appropriate information about events and procedures, providing therapeutic play experiences, and establishing therapeutic relationships with children and parents.

*Child-life specialists* are health care professionals with extensive knowledge of child growth and development and

## FAMILY HOME CARE
### Supporting Siblings During Hospitalization

Trade off staying at the hospital with spouse or have parent surrogate who knows siblings well stay in the home.

Offer information about the child's condition to young siblings, as well as older siblings; respect the sibling who avoids information as a means of coping with the situation.

Arrange for children to visit their brother or sister in the hospital if possible.

Encourage phone visits and mail between brothers and sisters; provide children with phone numbers, writing supplies, and stamps.

Help each sibling identify an extended family member or friend to be their support person and provide extra attention during parental absence.

Make or buy inexpensive toys or trinkets for siblings, one gift for each day the child will be hospitalized.

Wrap each gift separately and place in a basket, box, or other container at each child's bedside.

Instruct siblings to open one gift each night at bedtime and to remember that he or she is in the parent's thoughts.

If the child's condition is stable and distance is not prohibitive, plan a special time at home with the siblings or have spouse or another relative or friend bring the children to meet parent(s) at a restaurant or other location near the hospital.

Have extended family members or friends schedule a visit to child in hospital during parental absence.

Arrange a pass for the child to leave the hospital to join the family if the child's condition permits it.

Modified from Craft M, Craft J: Perceived changes in siblings of hospitalized children: a comparison of sibling and parent reports, *Child Health Care* 18(1):42-48, 1989; and Rollins J: *Brothers and sisters: a discussion guide for families,* Landover, MD, 1992, Epilepsy Foundation of America.

the special psychosocial needs of children who are hospitalized and their families. They help prepare children for hospitalization, surgery, and procedures. Although all members of the health care team share these responsibilities, this is the primary role of the child-life specialist. A collaborative effort between the nurse, child-life specialist, and other members of the child's health care team will help ensure the best possible hospital experience for the child and family (American Academy of Pediatrics, 2000). (In addition to the following discussion, the reader should review Preparation for Procedures, Chapter 27.)

### Group Size and Timing of Preparation

If group preparation is used, group size should be small (about 10 children to a group) to provide individualized attention and to facilitate discussion. If tours are arranged for each child, the parents should be included and possibly the well siblings.

Prehospital admission programs should be scheduled for the time of day when staff members are most available and after most treatment procedures are completed. They should occur before actual admission. For young children, who may begin to fantasize about what they observed, 1 or 2 days before admission is usually considered sufficient time for anticipatory preparation. Some authorities recommend preparing children 4 to 7 years of age about 1 week in

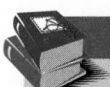

## EVIDENCE-BASED PRACTICE
### *Preparation for Short-Stay Hospitalization*

The mid-1960s ushered in a flurry of research on the issue of preparing children for hospitalization and procedures, resulting in the general consensus that all children benefit from some form of prior behavioral preparation. By 1980 an estimated 70% of hospitals routinely offered preoperative behavioral programs to children (Peterson and Ridley-Johnson, 1980). Most studies suggest that behavioral preparation for the child reduces stress and enhances coping, yet other reports indicate that such behavioral programs have no effect on some children and may actually "sensitize" younger children (Field, 1992; Robinson and Kobayashi, 1991). This is often attributed to the younger child's inability to distinguish fantasy from reality, a developmental task that most children have accomplished by the age of 6 years.

However, the need to consider the age of the child is but one part of the issue when planning preparation interventions. Research findings from a study of 143 children ages 2 to 10 years who underwent elective outpatient surgery and general anesthesia at a children's hospital highlight the complexities in assuming that a behavior-based preparation program is effective for *all* children (Kain, Mayes, and Caramico, 1996). Investigators found that children older than 6 years were least anxious on separation from their parents if they participated in the preparation program more than 5 to 7 days before surgery, moderately anxious if they did not receive preparation, and most anxious if they received the preparation 1 day before surgery. Although the preparation program itself was not a predictor of a child's behavior on separation to the operating room, the interaction between the child's age and the timing of the program, and the child's previous hospitalization were predictors of children's anxiety response. Also, in the preoperative holding area, independent predictors of anxiety included the timing of the preparation program, the age of the child, and the child's baseline temperament characteristics.

The investigators caution that the study findings should be viewed in light of several methodologic issues, such as a nonrandomized sample. Yet they conclude from these findings that children who are 6 years old or older should receive preparation at least 1 week before surgery. They further suggest that if this is not possible and the options are either not to receive the preparation or to receive the preparation 1 or 2 days before surgery, *no preparation* is more advantageous. Further research is needed, because these findings, methodologic issues aside, have serious implications when one considers the prevalence of outpatient surgery and the trend to prepare children the day before the event.

special areas, such as the group dining room. Other areas that may be visited are the radiology department and laboratory area, the preoperative area, and the recovery room. Different hospitals may tailor this tour to include special rooms, such as the "OR playroom," where children and parents first go before any induction is administered. Children who are undergoing serious surgery requiring special postoperative care may be taken to visit the intensive care unit (ICU). Children scheduled for special tests, such as cardiac catheterization or cystoscopy, are sometimes shown these areas. Young children may respond better to shorter tours that concentrate on the areas of most concern, such as the pediatric unit, playroom, and recovery room. In any case, throughout the tour, the nurse (or other guide) must be alert to signs of concern or fear in the children. Strange noises, sights, sounds, and smells that are routine to hospital personnel can be frightening to children.

### Preparatory Materials

The most suitable type of presentation for children includes a variety of preparatory materials, including films, lecture, demonstration, and play. The following discussion explores some of the typical methods that may be used in preparing children for elective surgery.

A puppet show may reenact the basic steps of hospitalization—admission procedures; preparation for surgery, the operating room, and the recovery room; and postsurgical treatment. The main focus of each scene is the use of concrete actions and models to familiarize the family members with what will occur. The puppets talk about children's common fears—pain, anesthesia, and parent separation. Although the sophistication of the materials varies, the basic characters should include a puppet family (mother, father, child) and hospital staff (physician, nurse) that are racially representative of the patient and hospital population. For example, both black and white dolls are required in many urban areas. Hospital equipment includes mask, cap, gloves, gown, IV equipment, syringes, thermometer, blood pressure machine, stethoscope, scale, oxygen mask, suture removal set, bandages, bed, and sheets. If children are routinely admitted for diagnostic evaluations, miniature replicas of equipment (e.g., diagnostic imaging machines) or slides may be used as visual aids. The use of scaled-down models is especially beneficial for young children, who may be frightened by the actual proportions of some equipment. However, the *intent* of what is conveyed greatly surpasses the sophistication of the materials used.

### Opportunity for Discussion

Any type of preparatory program needs to provide ample opportunity for discussion both before and after the tour. During the tour family members are encouraged to ask questions and to familiarize themselves with the environment by sitting on a bed, using the electric bed controls, riding in a wheelchair, or handling the equipment in the special rooms. Ideally, the tour should also be an opportunity for meeting the child's primary nurse. Although this is not always possible because of staffing schedules, the nursing staff should be introduced to the children by name. Intro-

advance so they can assimilate the information and ask questions. For older children the time may be longer. (See Evidence-Based Practice box.)

Because standardized programs cannot adequately meet the needs of the full age range of pediatric patients, some hospitals have developed preparation programs that target a specific age-group, such as toddlers or adolescents. The length of the session should be suited to the children's attention span—the younger the child, the shorter the program. The optimum approach is one that is individualized for each child and family.

### Setting of the Tour

The setting of the hospital tour should avoid any frightening aspects of the environment and should typically include an inpatient room, the playroom (a highlight of the tour), the parents' waiting room, the nurses' station, and other

ducing them to one specific nurse, such as the head nurse, clinical specialist, or nurse practitioner, helps them feel more comfortable in knowing who is available for questions or concerns during the hospital stay.

Following the tour there should be a question-and-answer period, monitored by a nurse. Sometimes the group is reticent about asking questions. In this case the nurse can stimulate discussion by posing a question to the audience or inviting the children to see and touch the puppets and equipment. Allowing children to play with the equipment and having them draw pictures about what they observed are excellent methods of evaluating the learning process and clarifying any misconceptions.

The tour may conclude with serving refreshments, which helps people relax and gather their thoughts and often stimulates discussion. By informally visiting each table, the nurse has an excellent opportunity to discuss individual concerns. The parents also are encouraged to call the pediatric unit before admission, because questions or concerns may arise during this interval.

### Prehospital Counseling by Parents

In many situations the preparation of children for hospitalization is left up to parents. Parents may abdicate this responsibility for a variety of reasons. For example, they sometimes think the child is too young to understand or is better off not knowing beforehand; often they are unable to prepare the child because of their own lack of knowledge and understanding.

Professionals can help parents prepare their children by adequately informing them of the specific details of hospitalization and related procedures, through both direct discussion and written material. Responsibility for such guidance often rests with office and clinic nurses. They can discuss with parents the appropriate timing of the preparation and the methods, such as picture books about going to the hospital.* Many hospitals develop their own books and photograph albums for this purpose. Nurses working with these parents should also assess their level of anxiety regarding the impending hospitalization. A parent who is at ease will convey that feeling to the child.

## Hospital Admission Procedure

The preparation that children require on the day of admission depends on their prehospital counseling. If they have been prepared in a formalized program, they will usually know what to expect in terms of initial medical procedures, inpatient facilities, and nursing staff. However, prehospital counseling does not preclude the need for support during procedures such as drawing blood, x-ray tests, or physical examination. For example, undressing young children before they feel comfortable in their new surroundings can be very

---

*Several educational books to prepare children for hospitalization include *Going to the Hospital* by A. Civardi, S. Cartwright, (1993, EDCP publications) for toddlers and preschoolers; *Franklin Goes to the Hospital* by S. Jennings and others (2000, Scholastic Trade) and *Good-Bye Tonsils!* by C. Hatkoff, M. Mets, J.L. Hatkoff (2001, Viking Children's Books) for 4- to 8-year-old children.

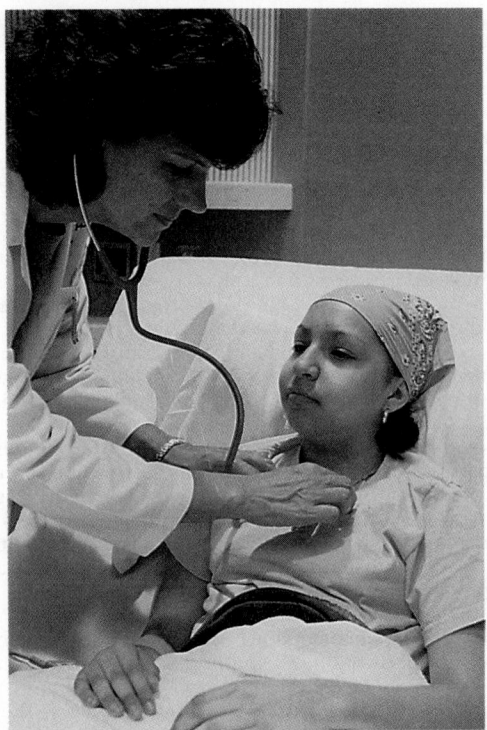

**Fig. 26-14** The initial admission procedures may be coordinated by a nurse practitioner who examines the child on admission. (Courtesy Paul Vincent Kuntz, Texas Children's Hospital.)

upsetting. Causing needless anxiety and fear during admission may adversely affect the nurse's establishment of trust with these children. Therefore nursing assistance during the admission procedure is vital, regardless of how well prepared any child is for the hospitalization. In addition, spending this time with the child gives the nurse an opportunity to evaluate understanding of subsequent procedures, such as surgery (Fig. 26-14). The usual admission procedures for children are outlined in the Guidelines box on p. 1087.

### Nursing Admission History

The nursing admission history refers to a systematic collection of data about the child and family that allows the nurse to plan individualized care. The nursing admission history presented in Box 26-14 is organized according to the Functional Health Patterns outlined by Gordon (1994), which facilitates the formulation of nursing diagnoses. (See Nursing Diagnosis, Chapter 1.) One of the main purposes of the history is to assess the child's usual health habits at home to promote a more normal environment in the hospital. Therefore questions related to activities of daily living are a major part of the assessment. The questions found under the health perception–health management pattern are directed toward evaluation of the child's preparation for hospitalization and are key factors in determining if additional preparation is needed.

As with any history form, the questions are only guidelines; for maximum communication, nurses should ask these questions as a part of conversation, not as a direct questionnaire. Answers to questions that are broad and

## GUIDELINES

*Supporting the Child and Family During Hospital Admission*

### PREADMISSION

Assign a room based on developmental age, seriousness of diagnosis, communicability of illness, and projected length of stay.

Prepare roommate(s) for the arrival of a new patient; when children are too young to benefit from this consideration, prepare parents.

Prepare room for child and family, with admission forms and equipment nearby

### ADMISSION

Introduce primary nurse to child and family.

Orient child and family to inpatient facilities, especially to assigned room and unit; emphasize positive areas of pediatric unit.

    Room: Explain call light, bed controls, television; show bathroom, telephone

    Unit: Direct to playroom, desk, dining area, other areas

Introduce family to roommate and his or her parents.

Apply identification band to child's wrist, ankle, or both (if not done).

Explain hospital regulations and schedules (e.g., visiting hours, mealtimes, bedtime, limitations [give written information if available]).

Perform nursing admission history. (See Box 26-14.)

Take vital signs, blood pressure, height, and weight.

Obtain specimens as needed and order required laboratory studies.

Support child and perform or assist practitioner with physical examination (for purposes of nursing assessment).

### EMERGENCY ADMISSION

Lengthy preparatory admission procedures are often impossible and inappropriate for emergency situations.

Unless an emergency is life-threatening, children need to participate in their care to maintain a sense of control.

Focus on essential components of admission counseling, including:

    Appropriate introduction to the family

    Use child's name, not terms such as "honey" or "dear"

    Determination of child's age and some judgment about developmental age (if the child is of school age, asking about the grade level will offer some evidence for concurrent intellectual ability)

    Information about child's general state of health, any problems that may interfere with medical treatment (e.g., sensitivity to medication), and previous hospitalizations or surgeries

    Information about the chief complaint from both the parents and the child

### ADMISSION TO INTENSIVE CARE UNIT (ICU)

Prepare child and parents for elective ICU admission, such as for postoperative care after cardiac surgery.

Prepare child and parents for unanticipated ICU admission by focusing primarily on the sensory aspects of the experience and on usual family concerns (e.g., persons in charge of child's care, schedule for visiting, area where family can stay).

Prepare parents regarding child's appearance and behavior when they first visit child in ICU.

Accompany family to bedside to provide emotional support and answer questions.

Prepare siblings for their visit; plan length of time for sibling visitation; monitor siblings' reactions during visit to prevent them from becoming overwhelmed.

Encourage parents to stay with their child:

    If visiting hours are limited, allow flexibility in schedule to accommodate parental needs.

    Give family members a written schedule of visiting times.

    If visiting hours are liberal, be aware of family members' needs and suggest periodic respites.

    Assure family they can call the unit at any time.

Prepare parents for expected role changes and identify ways for parents to participate in child's care without overwhelming them with responsibilities:

    Help with bath or feeding.

    Touch and talk to child.

    Help with procedures.

Provide information about child's condition in developmentally appropriate language:

    Repeat information often.

    Seek clarification of understanding.

    During bedside conferences, interpret information for family members and child or, if appropriate, conduct report outside room.

Prepare child for procedures, even if this involves explanation while procedure is performed.

Assess and manage pain; recognize that a child who cannot talk, such as an infant or child in a coma or on a ventilator, can be in pain.

Establish a routine that maintains some similarity to daily events in child's life whenever possible:

    Organize care during normal waking hours.

    Keep regular bedtime schedules, including quiet times when television or radio is lowered or turned off.

    Provide uninterrupted sleep cycles (60 minutes for infant, 90 minutes for older child).

    Close and open drapes and dim lights to allow for day/night.

    Place curtain around bed for privacy as needed.

    Orient child to day and time; have clocks or calendars in easy view for older children.

Schedule a time when child is left undisturbed (e.g., during naps, visit with family, playtime, or favorite program).

Provide opportunities for play.

Reduce stimulation in environment:

    Refrain from loud talking or laughing.

    Keep equipment noise to a minimum:

        Turn alarms as low as safely possible.

        Perform treatments requiring equipment at one time.

        Turn off bedside equipment that is not in use, such as suction and oxygen.

    Avoid loud, abrupt noises.

---

nonspecific, such as "What does your child know about this hospitalization?" need to be followed by more specific questions, such as "Tell me what you told him." Children may respond to questions regarding their knowledge of hospitalization with statements such as "I don't know why I am here." Although this may be correct, frequently they have been given some explanation concerning the reason for hospitalization. Such an answer may mean that the explanation was inadequate, their anxiety blocked the recall, or they are testing out the explanation by prompting the nurse to supply additional information.

The nurse should also inquire about the use of any complementary or alternative medicine practices. In a study of children with cancer, 42% had used alternative or complementary therapies, simultaneously with or following conventional treatments (Fernandez, Pyesmany, and Stutzer,

---

**Box 26-14** ■ ■ ■
## Nursing Admission History According to Functional Health Patterns*

### HEALTH PERCEPTION–HEALTH MANAGEMENT PATTERN

Why has your child been admitted?

How has your child's general health been?

What does your child know about this hospitalization?

  Ask the child why he or she came to the hospital.

  If answer is "For an operation or for tests," ask the child to tell you about what will happen before, during, and after the operation or tests.

Has your child ever been in the hospital before?

  How was that hospital experience?

  What things were important to you and your child during that hospitalization? How can we be most helpful now?

What medications does your child take at home?

  Why are they given?

  When are they given?

  How are they given (if a liquid, with a spoon; if a tablet, swallowed with water; or other)?

  Does your child have any trouble taking medication? If so, what helps?

  Is your child allergic to any medications?

What, if any, forms of alternative or complementary medicine are being used?

### NUTRITION-METABOLIC PATTERN

What are the family's usual mealtimes?

Do family members eat together or at separate times?

What are your child's favorite foods, beverages, and snacks?

  Average amounts consumed or usual size portions

  Special cultural practices, such as family eats only ethnic food

What foods and beverages does your child dislike?

What are your child's feeding habits (bottle, cup, spoon, eats by self, needs assistance, any special devices)?

How does your child like the food served (warmed, cold, one item at a time)?

How would you describe your child's usual appetite (hearty eater, picky eater)?

  Has being sick affected your child's appetite?

Are there any known or suspected food allergies? Is your child on a special diet?

Are there any feeding problems (excessive fussiness, spitting up, colic); any dental or gum problems that affect feeding?

What do you do for these problems?

### ELIMINATION PATTERN

What are your child's toilet habits (diaper, toilet trained—day only or day and night, use of word to communicate urination or defecation, potty chair, regular toilet, other routines)?

What is your child's usual pattern of elimination (bowel movements)?

Do you have any concerns about elimination (bed-wetting, constipation, diarrhea)?

What do you do for these problems?

Does your child sweat a lot?

### SLEEP-REST PATTERN

What is your child's usual hour of bedtime and awakening?

What is your child's schedule for naps; length of naps?

Is there a special routine before sleeping (bottle, drink of water, bedtime story, nightlight, favorite blanket or toy, prayers)?

Is there a special routine during sleep time, such as waking to go to the bathroom?

What type of bed does your child sleep in?

What are the home sleeping arrangements (alone or with others, e.g., sibling, parent, other person)?

What is your child's favorite sleeping position?

Are there any sleeping problems (falling asleep, waking during night, nightmares, sleep walking)?

Are there any problems awakening and getting ready in the morning?

What do you do for these problems?

### ACTIVITY-EXERCISE PATTERN

What is your child's schedule during the day (preschool, daycare center, regular school, extracurricular activities)?

What are your child's favorite activities or toys (both active and quiet interests)?

What is your child's usual television viewing schedule at home?

  What are your child's favorite programs?

  Are there any TV restrictions?

Does your child have any illness or disabilities that limit activity? If so, how?

What are your child's usual habits and schedule for bathing (bath in tub or shower, sponge bath, shampoo)?

What are your child's dental habits (brushing, flossing, fluoride supplements or rinses, favorite toothpaste); schedule of daily dental care?

Does your child need help with dressing or grooming?

Are there any problems with the above (dislike of or refusal to bathe, shampoo hair, or brush teeth)?

What do you do for these problems?

Are there special devices that your child requires help in managing (eyeglasses, contact lenses, hearing aid, orthodontic appliances, artificial elimination appliances, orthopedic devices)?

NOTE: Use the following code to assess functional self-care level for feeding, bathing/hygiene, dressing/grooming, toileting:

  **O:** Full self-care

  **I:** Requires use of equipment or device

  **II:** Requires assistance or supervision from another person

  **III:** Requires assistance or supervision from another person and equipment or device

  **IV:** Is dependent and does not participate

### COGNITIVE-PERCEPTUAL PATTERN

Does your child have any hearing difficulty?

  Does the child use a hearing aid?

  Have "myringotomy tubes" been placed in your child's ears?

Does your child have any vision problems?

  Does the child wear glasses or contact lenses?

---

*The focus of the admission history is the child's psychosocial environment. Most of the questions are worded in terms of parental responses. Depending on the child's age, they should be addressed directly to the child when appropriate.

---

1999). Widespread use of complementary medicine is often explored, however, without discussion with the primary care physician or nurse (Moenkhoff and others, 1999; Spiegel, Stroud, and Fyfe, 1998). It is important for the use of any herbal therapy to be noted in a preoperative assessment because of possible anesthesia and/or surgical complications related to herbal products (Flanagan, 2001). (See Critical Thinking Exercise box and Box 26-15 on p. 1090.)

Once the data are collected as part of the nursing admission history, they must be applied to the nursing process and communicated to other staff. It makes little sense to assess a child's home routine if none of this knowledge is integrated into the plan of care. Most nursing units have provisions for care plans in which specific information about the child's habits and needs are recorded.

## Box 26-14 ■ ■ ■
## Nursing Admission History According to Functional Health Patterns—cont'd

Does your child have any learning difficulties?
What is the child's grade in school?

### SELF-PERCEPTION–SELF-CONCEPT PATTERN

How would you describe your child (e.g., shy, friendly, quiet, talkative, serious, playful, stubborn, easygoing)?
What makes your child angry, annoyed, anxious, or sad? What helps?
How does your child act when annoyed or upset?
What have been your child's experiences with and reactions to temporary separation from you (parent)?
Does your child have any fears (places, objects, animals, people, situations)? How do you handle them?
Do you think your child's illness has changed the way he or she thinks about self (e.g., shy, embarrassed, less competitive with friends, stays at home more)?

### ROLE-RELATIONSHIP PATTERN

Does your child have a favorite nickname?
What are the names of other family members or others who live in the home (relatives, friends, pets)?
Who usually takes care of your child during the day/night (especially if other than parent, such as baby-sitter, relative)?
Which members of your family/extended family participate in childrearing/health decisions? To what extent?
What are the parents' occupation and work schedules?
Are there any special family considerations (adoption, foster child, stepparent, divorce, single parent)?
Have any major changes in the family occurred lately (death, divorce, separation, birth of a sibling, loss of a job, financial strain, mother beginning a career, other)? Describe child's reaction.
Who are your child's play companions or social groups (peers, younger or older children, adults, prefers to be alone)?
Do things generally go well for your child in school or with friends?
Does your child use "security" objects at home (pacifier, thumb, bottle, blanket, stuffed animal or doll)? Did you bring any of these to the hospital?
How do you handle discipline problems at home? Are these methods always effective?
Does your child have any condition that interferes with communication? If so, what are your suggestions for communicating with your child?
Will your child's hospitalization affect the family's financial support or care of other family members, (e.g., other children)?
What concerns do you have about your child's illness and hospitalization?
Who will be staying with your child while hospitalized?
How can we contact you or another close family member outside of the hospital?

### SEXUALITY-REPRODUCTIVE PATTERN

(Answer questions that apply to your child's age-group.)
Has your child begun puberty (developing physical sexual characteristics, menstruation)? Have you or your child had any concerns?

Does your daughter know how to do breast self-examination?
Does your son know how to do testicular self-examination?
How have you approached topics of sexuality with your child?
Do you feel you might need some help with some topics?
Has your child's illness affected the way he or she feels about being a boy or a girl? If so, how?
Do you have any concerns with behaviors in your child, such as masturbation, asking many questions or talking about sex, not respecting others' privacy, or wanting too much privacy?
Initiate a conversation about an adolescent's sexual concerns with open-ended to more direct questions and using the terms "friends" or "partners" rather than "girlfriend" or "boyfriend":
Tell me about your social life.
Who are your closest friends? (If one friend is identified, could ask more about that relationship, such as how much time they spend together, how serious they are about each other, if the relationship is going the way the teenager hoped.)
Might ask about dating and sexual issues, such as the teenager's views on sex education, "going steady," "living together," or premarital sex.
Which friends would you like to have visit in the hospital?

### COPING–STRESS TOLERANCE PATTERN

(Answer questions that apply to your child's age-group.)
What does your child do when tired or upset?
If upset, does your child want a special person or object? If so, explain.
If your child has temper tantrums, what causes them and how do you handle them?
Whom does your child talk to when worried about something?
How does your child usually handle problems or disappointments?
Have there been any big changes or problems in your family recently?
How did you handle them?
Has your child ever had a problem with drugs or alcohol or tried suicide?

### VALUE-BELIEF PATTERN

Do you practice organized religion?
How is religion or faith important in your child's life?
What religious practices would you like continued in the hospital (e.g., prayers before meals/bedtime; visit by minister, priest, or rabbi; prayer group)?
What religious practices do you follow that affect childrearing/health practice (fasting/herbal remedies)?
What do you believe caused your child's illness/condition?
When illness/injury occurs, do you use any herbs, medicines, healer, rituals, or ceremonies?
What are your family's prior health care experiences?
What are your concerns with this health care system?
What do you do when your child is sick? What person do you go to first?
What generation immigrant are you—first? Second? Third?
What languages does your child speak/understand? What languages do you and other family members speak/understand?
With whom do you discuss child-related concerns or problems?

## Physical Assessment*

Although physical examinations by practitioners are a required part of the admission procedure, nurses should also use the valuable information gained from physical assessments in their planning of care. (See Chapter 7.) Subjecting children to two separate examinations is unnecessary if the nurse and other practitioners cooperate during the procedure. For example, the opportunity can also be used to observe the child's body for any bruises, rashes, signs of neglect, deformities, or physical limitations. Collaboration also prevents the often frustrating and needless waste of the family's time in repeating histories and examinations, espe-

 *For additional information, please view "Pediatric Assessment" in *Whaley and Wong's Pediatric Nursing Video Series*, St Louis, 1996, Mosby; (800) 426-4545; www.mosby.com.

## Critical Thinking Exercise

### Complementary Medicine Practices

Maria, a 10-year-old Hispanic girl, has had severe nose-bleeds. She is admitted to the hospital for a complete workup in an attempt to determine the cause. Her parents and grandparents have gathered around her bed. When you enter her room to begin admitting procedures, you notice an unusual scent. Maria's mother is rubbing the contents from an unfamiliar bottle of liquid on Maria. Meanwhile, the grandmother is rubbing Maria's head. She is startled at your entry and drops something on the floor near your feet. You bend over to pick it up and discover that it is a penny. After introducing yourself and explaining the purpose of your visit, your most appropriate response would be which of the following?

FIRST, THINK ABOUT IT . . .

- Within what point of view are you thinking?
- What would the consequences be if you put your thoughts into action?

1. "Here is your penny."
2. "I need to take this bottle and have the lab examine its contents."
3. "Many families tell me that they use certain medicine practices that are traditional in their families. Can you tell me about yours?"
4. "What is going on here?"

*The best response is three. The third-person technique gives families permission to share information. (See Chapter 6.) What you have probably observed is Santeria, the African-Caribbean religion that was brought to the New World by slaves from West Africa. Although it is common among immigrants from Cuba, Puerto Rico, Brazil, and Santo Domingo, it is believed that a majority of Latin immigrants will have contact with Santeria sometime in their lives. Answer one avoids the issue, which could have negative consequences. Although at some point you may need to take action and have the contents of the bottle examined (answer two), it is an inappropriate initial response. Answer four is confrontational and disrespectful.*

---

**Box 26-15 ■ ■ ■**

### Complementary or Alternative Medicine Practices and Examples

**Nutrition, diet, and lifestyle/behavioral health changes**—Macrobiotics, megavitamins, diets, lifestyle modification, health risk reduction/health education, wellness

**Mind/body control therapies**—Biofeedback, relaxation, prayer therapy, guided imagery, hypnotherapy, music/sound therapy, education therapy

**Traditional and ethnomedicine therapies**—Acupuncture, ayurvedic medicine, herbal medicine, homeopathic medicine, Native American medicine, natural products, traditional Asian medicine

**Structural manipulation and energetic therapies**—Acupressure, chiropractic medicine, massage, reflexology, rolfing, therapeutic touch, Qi Gong

**Pharmacologic and biologic therapies**—Antioxidants, cell treatment, chelation therapy, metabolic therapy, oxidizing agents

**Bioelectromagnetic therapies**—Diagnostic and therapeutic application of electromagnetic fields (e.g., transcranial electrostimulation, neuromagnetic stimulation, electroacupuncture)

---

Although there are no absolute rules to govern room selection, in general, placing children of the same age-group and with similar types of illness in the same room is both psychologically and medically advantageous. However, there are many exceptions. For example, a child in traction may be very therapeutic for another child confined to bed because of a serious illness. A child who is very independent despite physical disabilities may help another child with similar or different limitations and the parents achieve deeper insight and acceptance of the disorder.

### Adolescent Unit

To meet the unique needs of adolescents, special units have been developed that provide privacy, increased socialization, and appropriate activities. Typically these units are set apart from the general pediatric facility so that the teenagers do not share space with younger children, who are often perceived as a threat to their maturity. These units also provide more flexible routines and activities, such as more group activity, provisions to leave the adolescent unit temporarily, and access to the items important to teenagers—telephones, computers, compact disc (CD) and tape players, VCRs, and televisions (Fig. 26-15). Because adolescents' food habits are rarely limited to the three traditional meals a day, a supply of snacks should be available. One of the most important benefits of these units is increased socialization with peers. In addition, many staff members usually enjoy working with this age-group and are well suited to establishing the trust that is essential for communication.

Despite the advantages of adolescent units, all young people require preparation for the experience. They need orientation to the unit, introduction to staff and other patients, and an atmosphere of warmth and welcome. Just as teenagers form "cliques" in normal social relationships, this also occurs in the hospital. Staff must be aware of exclusiveness of group membership, especially when new patients are admitted. Scheduled and supervised group meetings are effective in preventing feelings of "nonbelonging" and

cially when the child has a chronic condition that requires many hospitalizations.

The nurse should listen to the heart and lungs or do other target assessments pertinent to the illness or reason *for* hospitalization. It is impossible to evaluate improvement in respiratory function in a child admitted with pulmonary disease unless there are baseline data with which to compare subsequent findings.

### Placing the Child

Room assignments are usually made before the child is admitted to the pediatric unit. The minimum considerations for room assignment are age, sex, and nature of the illness. Ideally, however, room selection should be based on a variety of developmental and psychobiologic needs. Determining compatible roommates, both for the children and for parents, greatly influences satisfaction with hospital experience.

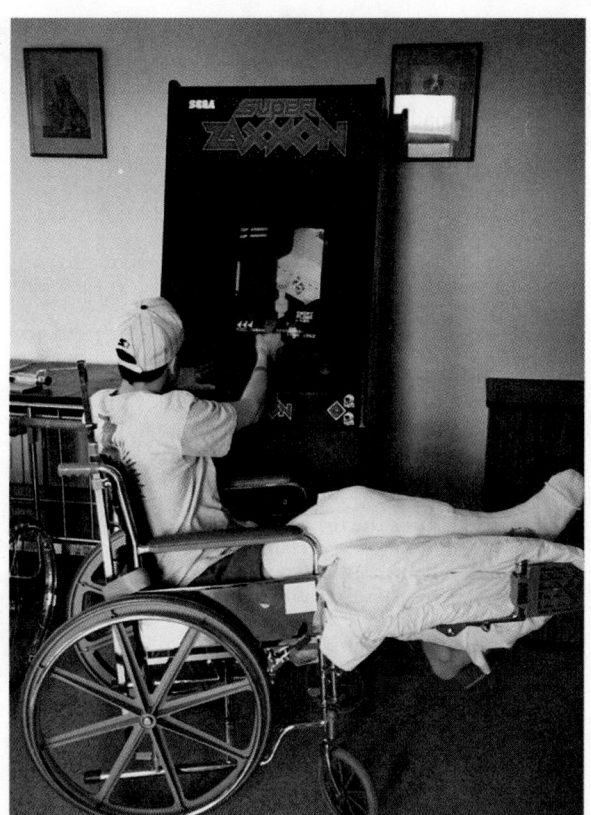

**Fig. 26-15** Adolescent units include recreational activities that adolescents enjoy.

in facilitating introductions and new friendships. They also provide an excellent opportunity for discussions about typical adolescent concerns (e.g., sexuality, drugs, drinking, parental relations) and special illness-related concerns of adolescents (e.g., peer rejection for being different).

## Nursing Care During Special Hospital Situations

In addition to a general pediatric unit, children may be admitted to special facilities, such as an ambulatory/outpatient setting, an isolation room, or an ICU. Some admissions are unexpected and frequently constitute medical emergencies. Such situations require special preparation of the child and family and nursing care interventions based on an awareness of the child's needs and the unique stressors associated with these hospital facilities.

### Ambulatory/Outpatient Setting

The ambulatory/outpatient setting provides needed medical services for the child while eliminating the necessity of overnight admission. Among the benefits of ambulatory/outpatient care are (1) minimization of the stressors of hospitalization, especially separation from the family; (2) reduced risk of infection; and (3) cost savings. Admission to the ambulatory/outpatient hospital setting usually is for surgical or diagnostic procedures, such as insertion of myringo-

tomy tubes, hernia repair, adenoidectomy, tonsillectomy, cystoscopy, or bronchoscopy. In addition, expanded roles of pediatric nurse specialists in areas such as children newly diagnosed with diabetes have resulted in fewer overnight hospitalizations and increased use of ambulatory/outpatient settings for management of chronic conditions and other special health care needs (Lowes and Davis, 1997).

Because of limited contact with the child in an ambulatory setting, adequate preparation is particularly challenging (Stewart, Algren, and Arnold, 1994). Ideally, the child and parents should receive preadmission preparation, including a tour of the facility and a review of the day's events (Brewer and Lambert, 1997). When this is not possible, surgery should be scheduled to allow time for children to become acquainted with their surroundings and for nurses to assess, plan, and complement appropriate teaching.

Parents need information in advance, not only to help them to prepare the child and themselves for the event, but also to help them plan for afterward. For example, families who rely on public transportation may need help making or paying for other arrangements to transport their child home after surgery or other procedures. Others may need to arrange time off work to enable one person to drive and one to assist the child during the trip home. Families a considerable distance from home may need help making arrangements to stay overnight nearby. Knowing in advance what kind of diet the child will likely be on immediately after discharge will provide parents the opportunity to purchase items ahead of time to avoid having to make a shopping trip right after the child's discharge. Parents also appreciate suggestions for items to bring for the child's trip home, such as a blanket, pillow, cup with a cap and straw for the child to drink fluids, and an emesis basin.

The need for creating a welcoming environment for children and families often may be overlooked in the ambulatory/outpatient setting, particularly in day surgery centers or settings that are not exclusively focused on pediatric patients. A small number of toys, books, and other play materials can be made available to children while they wait.

Waiting is usually inevitable in ambulatory/outpatient settings, a factor families often report as the most stressful part of the hospitalization experience. Providing a pager allows the family (and in many instances, the child) to leave the area and then be paged to return when needed (Ashenberg and others, 1996).

Discharge instructions must also be explicit after outpatient surgery. (See Family Home Care box on p. 1092.) Parents need guidelines on when to call their practitioner regarding a change in the child's condition. Nurses often make a follow-up telephone call after discharge to the family to assess the child's progress. A short length of stay challenges the nurse to provide accurate and complete discharge teaching within a brief time frame. Parents may be apprehensive about having enough information to care for their child after discharge. A telephone follow-up system, with nurses telephoning families within 48 to 72 hours after discharge, provides an opportunity for the nurse to review disease/condition–specific criteria and discharge information, and to answer questions. If problems are identified,

## FAMILY HOME CARE
### *Discharge from Ambulatory Settings*

1. Before beginning, explain that all instructions will also be presented in writing for the family to refer to later.
2. Provide an overview of the typical trajectory (expected pattern) of recovery.
3. Discuss expected progression of the child's activity level during the postdischarge period (e.g., "Mary will probably sleep for the rest of the day, feel tired most of tomorrow, but be back to her usual activities the next day.").
4. Explain which activities the child is allowed and what is not permitted (e.g., bed rest, bathing).
5. Discuss dietary restrictions, being very specific and giving examples of "clear fluids" or what is meant by a "full liquid diet."
6. Discuss nausea and vomiting, if applicable, explaining how much is "normal" and what to do if more occurs (e.g., "Juan may be sick to his stomach and vomit. This is normal. However, if he vomits more than three times, please call us at this number right away.").
7. Discuss fever and the comfort measures to use, explaining how much fever is considered "normal," and specifically what to do if the child goes beyond the range.
8. Explain the amount, location, and kind of pain or discomfort the child may experience.
   Give any prescribed medication before leaving the facility.
   Send a pain scale home with the family. (See Fig. 26-10.)
   Explain how much pain and discomfort is "normal" and what to do if the child surpasses that level or if pain management interventions are unsuccessful.
   Discuss pain management, including dosage for pain medications and details on how to administer them.
   Describe appropriate nonpharmalogic comfort measures, such as holding, rocking, or distraction techniques.
9. Provide information about each medication that the child will be taking at home.
   Review the details, including dose, route, and side effects.
   Demonstrate how to administer medications, if necessary (e.g., how to use suppositories).
10. Make certain the family has all of the equipment and supplies (e.g., gauze and tape for dressing changes) they will need at home.
11. Discuss complications that may occur and the steps to take if they do.
12. Ensure that appropriate measures are in place for safe transport home.
    Remind family to use a seat belt or car seat for the child.
    Determine if there will be one person whose sole responsibility is helping ensure the child's safety and comfort during transport.
    Discuss measures the driver may need to take if this is impossible (e.g., be certain a basin is within the child's reach should vomiting occur; take a route that permits slower traffic and has places along the roadside to stop if necessary).
    Determine the availability of a blanket, pillow, and cup with a cap and straw for the child's use in the car.
    Provide a basin or plastic bag in case of vomiting.
13. Provide emergency phone numbers for the family to call.
14. Explain that the family will be contacted to follow-up on the child but that they should not hesitate to call if concerns arise before then.
15. Ask the family and child, if appropriate, if they have any questions, and problem solve with family members to meet any needs.

parents can contact the practitioner to report symptoms and possibly avoid rehospitalization (Lancaster, 1997).

## Isolation

Children with infectious diseases or impaired immune systems may require isolation. Isolation precautions increase all of the stressors typically associated with hospitalization, particularly for the young child who has not developed the cognitive ability to understand the purpose. In addition to the separation from familiar persons, loss of control, and the appearance of people in strange attire, the use of physical barriers such as masks, gloves, gowns, and closed doors add to the confusion and anxiety in the child. Children may suffer from a lack of stimulation from reduced interaction with the environment. The negative effects are particulary evident for children who have undergone bone marrow transplants and must be kept in organism-free environments for extended periods of time (Kuntz and others, 1996). A limited amount of research is available on the effects of isolation on children.

When a child is placed in isolation, preparation is essential for the child to feel in control. All children, but especially younger ones, need preparation in terms of what they will see, hear, or feel in isolation. If possible, they are shown the mask, gloves, and gown before being placed in isolation. Playing with the equipment lessens the fear when they see persons in isolation walk into the room. Before entering the room, nurses and other health care personnel should intro-

duce themselves and let the child see their face before donning a mask. In this way the child associates them with significant experiences and gains a sense of familiarity in an otherwise strange and lonely environment. In addition, it is imperative that the parents understand the rationale for isolation precautions so that isolation is properly maintained.

Appropriate play activities are provided to minimize boredom, stimulate the senses, provide a real or perceived sense of movement, orient the child to time and place, provide social interaction, and reduce depersonalization.* For example, the environment can be manipulated to increase sensory freedom by moving the bed toward the door or window. Opening window shades; providing musical, visual, or tactile toys; and increasing interpersonal contact can substitute mental mobility for the limitations of physical movement. Rather than dwelling on the negative aspects of isolation, the child can be encouraged to view this experience as challenging and positive. For example, the nurse can help the child look at isolation as a method of keeping others out and letting only special people in. Children often think of devising intriguing signs for their doors, such as "Enter at your own risk" or "Many have entered, but few have left." These signs also encourage people "outside the room" to

---

*An excellent resource for providing environmental stimulation with music is *Music Therapy for Hospitalized Children* by M. Froehlich (1996, MMB Music).

talk with the child about the ominous greetings if the child's condition permits.

## Emergency Admission

One of the most traumatic hospital experiences for the child and parents is an emergency admission. The sudden onset of an illness or the occurrence of an injury leaves little time for preparation and explanation. Sometimes the emergency admission is compounded by admission to an ICU or the need for immediate surgery. However, even in those instances requiring outpatient treatment, the child is exposed to a strange, frightening environment and to experiences that may cause pain. Thus every medical emergency requires psychologic intervention to reduce the fear and anxiety frequently associated with the experience. Although underutilized, child-life specialists may provide teaching and support (Krebel, Clayton, and Graham, 1996).

There is a wide discrepancy between what constitutes a medically defined emergency and a client-defined emergency. In pediatric populations most visits are for respiratory infections, with skin conditions, gastrointestinal disorders, and trauma such as poisoning accounting for the remainder of the cases. The most common reason parents give for bringing the child to the emergency department is concern about the illness worsening. However, practitioners may not consider the progressive symptoms as necessitating emergency care. One of nursing's primary goals is to assess the parents' perception of the event and their reasons for considering it serious or life-threatening.

Lengthy preparatory admission procedures are often inappropriate for emergency situations. In such instances nurses must focus their nursing interventions on the essential components of admission counseling (see Guidelines box on p. 1087) and complete the process as soon as the child's condition is stabilized.

Unless an emergency is life-threatening, children need to participate in their care to maintain a sense of control. Because emergency departments are frequently hectic, there is a tendency to rush through procedures in order to save time. However, the extra few minutes needed to allow children to participate may save many more minutes of useless resistance and uncooperativeness during subsequent procedures. Other supportive measures include ensuring privacy, accepting various emotional responses to fear or pain, preserving parent-child contact, explaining all events before or as they occur, and remaining calm.

At times, because of the child's physical condition, little or no preparatory counseling for emergency hospitalization can be done. In such situations the implementation of **postvention,** or counseling subsequent to the event, has therapeutic value. The process of postvention involves evaluating children's thoughts regarding admission and related procedures. It is similar to precounseling techniques; however, instead of supplying information, the nurse listens to the explanations offered by the child. Projective techniques such as drawing, doll play, or storytelling are especially effective. The nurse then bases additional teaching on what has already been revealed. (See Critical Thinking Exercise box.)

### Critical Thinking Exercise

#### Postvention Counseling

David, 4 years old, is admitted to the hospital for an emergency appendectomy. The following day you ask him to describe his experiences. He describes the usual admission and preoperative procedures correctly but has no understanding of why they were done. His most prominent recollection focuses on all the needles he has received (blood tests, IV fluid, sedation).

When David tells you he thinks he got so many needles because he did not tell his mother about his stomachache soon enough, what would be your most appropriate response?

FIRST, THINK ABOUT IT . . .

- What is the purpose of your thinking?
- What would the consequences be if you put your thoughts into action?

1. "Everyone who has an appendectomy needs to have blood tests, a tube in the hand because you can't drink right after surgery, and medicine to make you sleepy before surgery."
2. "You would still have had to have an appendectomy and those shots, even if you had told your mommy about your stomachache sooner."
3. "There were reasons for all of the needles. Your stomach probably didn't hurt badly in the beginning, so you didn't say anything until it hurt a lot. You didn't do anything wrong; that is not why you had to get shots."
4. I wish you didn't have to get any shots, but you were a good boy."

*The best answer is three. Although some of the other answers give the child good information, they do not fully answer his fear that he did something wrong and is being punished. Children who have little or no preparation before surgery often come to this conclusion. Without any other explanation, a young child will resort to magical thinking and provide his or her own explanation for the event, which can lead to negative consequences. You should reassure the child that he did not cause bad things to happen.*

*Also refrain from labeling him a "good boy" or "big boy" for undergoing difficult procedures. If he is unable to do as well for another procedure, he may assume he is bad or is being a baby. Praise a child for doing well, trying hard to follow directions, or for any positive aspect of his behavior.*

## Intensive Care Unit (ICU)

Admission to an ICU can be a particularly traumatic event for both the child and the parents (Fig. 26-16). The nature and severity of the illness and the circumstance surrounding the admission are major factors, especially for parents. Parents experience significantly more stress when the admission is unexpected rather than expected. A recent study shows that parental anxiety levels reach near panic levels initially (Huckabay and Tilem-Kessler, 1999). Stressors for the child and parent are described in Box 26-16. Although several studies have described what parents perceive as most stressful, the most effective strategy may be to simply ask

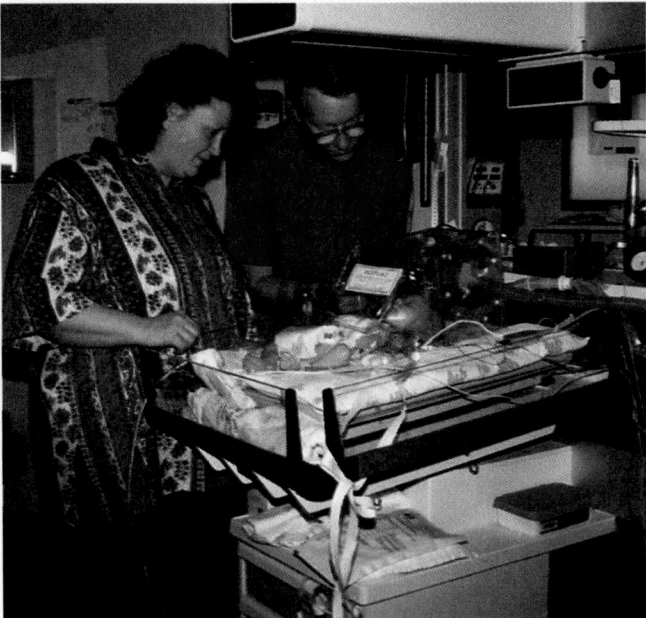

**Fig. 26-16** Parents can be overwhelmed when their child is critically ill and requires care in an ICU.

parents what is stressful and implement interventions that will enhance coping outcomes (Melnyk and Alpert-Gillis, 1998). Assessment should be repeated periodically to account for changes in perceptions over time.

The emotional needs of the family are important when a child is admitted to an ICU. Although the same interventions discussed earlier for separation anxiety, loss of control, and bodily injury and pain apply here, additional interventions may also benefit the family and child. (See Guidelines box on p. 1087 and Family Focus box on p. 1095.) Critical care must be family centered, and visiting hours should be liberal and flexible enough to accommodate parental needs (Giganti, 1998; Hazinski, 1999).

Critically ill children become the focus of the parents' lives, and the parents' most pressing need is for information (Scott, 1998). They want to know if their child will live, and if so, whether the child will be the same as before. They need to know why various interventions are being done for the child, that the child is being treated for pain and/or is comfortable, and that the child may be able to hear them even though not awake.

When an ICU admission is expected, such as for postoperative care after cardiac surgery, the child and parents should be prepared for the event. Some units advocate a tour, whereas others use picture books of the unit to familiarize the family with the environment and usual equipment. Dolls can be used to demonstrate the types of tubes that the child may have. Special care or effects of the tubes are discussed, such as the need to move despite the presence of chest tubes and inability to talk with an endotracheal tube. As much reassurance as possible should accompany the introduction of stressful information. For example, children should be reassured that they will be able to speak again after the tube is removed and that in the meantime they can use a communication board to convey their needs.

---

**Box 26-16** ■ ■ □
## Neonatal/Pediatric ICU Stressors for the Child and Family

**PHYSICAL STRESSORS**

Pain and discomfort (e.g., injections, phlebotomy, intubation, suctioning, dressing changes, other invasive procedures)
Immobility (e.g., use of restraints, bed rest)
Sleep deprivation
Inability to eat or drink
Changes in elimination habits

**ENVIRONMENTAL STRESSORS**

Unfamiliar surroundings (e.g., crowding)
Unfamiliar sounds
    Equipment noise (e.g., monitors, telephone, suctioning, mechanical ventilator)
    Human sounds (e.g., talking, laughing, crying, coughing, moaning, retching, walking)
Unfamiliar people (e.g., health care professionals, patients, visitors)
Unfamiliar and unpleasant smells (e.g., alcohol, adhesive remover, body odors)
Constant lights (disturb diurnal rhythms)
Activity related to other patients
Sense of urgency among staff

**PSYCHOLOGIC STRESSORS**

Lack of privacy
Inability to communicate (if intubated)
Inadequate knowledge and understanding of situation
Severity of illness
Parental behavior (expression of concern)

**SOCIAL STRESSORS**

Disrupted relationships (especially with family and friends)
Concern with missing school/work
Play deprivation

---

Data primarily from Tichy AM and others: Stressors in pediatric intensive care units, *Pediatr Nurs* 14(1):40-42, 1988.

---

When parents first visit the child in the ICU, they need preparation for how the child will look and what the child is experiencing if awake. Ideally, the nurse should accompany the family to the bedside to provide emotional support and answer any questions. If siblings visit, they need the same preparation as parents. Whether they should visit soon after the child is admitted or after the child's condition has stabilized is controversial. Early visiting minimizes the opportunity for siblings to fantasize about the experience and imagine fears that are probably greater than the actual situation. However, visiting early may be frightening, especially when the child is in pain or unresponsive and attached to numerous tubes and equipment. However, if there is a concern that the child may not survive the illness, an early visit may be the only option. The length of time for sibling visitation should be planned ahead and monitored during the visit to prevent the well child from becoming overwhelmed.

Children admitted to the ICU need their parents' comfort and security, and parents are encouraged to stay with their child. If visiting hours are limited, the schedule should be flexible to accommodate parental needs. Family members should be given a schedule of the visiting times permitted and assured that they can call the unit at any time. With liberalization of visiting hours, many parents think they must

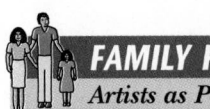

**FAMILY FOCUS**
*Artists as Partners in Care*

A teenage boy with a rare genetic disorder, having made steady progress after awakening from a coma, relapsed and seemed very depressed. When told that a musician was visiting the pediatric intensive care unit (PICU), he immediately perked up and asked to have his room lights turned on. He whispered endless song requests to the musician. Family members and staff were treated to some of his first smiles in days; his biggest came when the musician held his hand and guided it across the guitar strings while they sang "Born to Be Wild" together at the boy's request. His dad was misty eyed as he thanked the musician for the visit.

A few weeks later the boy's condition worsened and he again lapsed into a coma. There was nothing more to be done. His parents began the necessary preparations to take their son home to die.

We continued to visit our friend and his family, offering a song, a story, or just simply to say hello. I hold a vivid picture of our final visit. We stood around the boy's bed with his parents singing together songs they remembered from their youth, from more carefree times. Song and laughter filled the boy's room.

Perhaps the boy heard his parents' laughter and knew then that they would be okay. He died a few days later on the morning he was to have been discharged.

Judy Rollins, MS, RN
Washington, DC

Modified from Rollins J: *Placed in our keeping*, 1995, Unpublished.

stay; nurses need to be sensitive to their needs, suggesting periodic respites from the stressful ICU environment.

Because altered parental roles are a major stress for parents, nurses need to implement interventions to minimize this concern, such as (1) educating and preparing parents for the expected role changes; (2) identifying ways in which parents can continue to fulfill parenting functions, such as helping with the bath or feeding and touching and talking to the child; and (3) determining new roles, such as helping with procedures. Information sharing can increase parents' sense of control and responsibility, but facts must be conveyed simply, repeated often, and monitored to prevent overwhelming family members. Because medical jargon abounds in a complex environment such as the ICU, unfamiliar terms need to be clarified and simpler terms substituted. (See Guidelines box under Preparation for Procedures: Psychologic Preparation, Chapter 27.)

As in emergency admissions, there is a tendency in the ICU to perform procedures quickly and without attention to the child's preparational needs. Therefore nurses need to remember the special concerns of children in each age-group about bodily injury. Explaining each procedure, altering it whenever possible to decrease the child's fears, and supporting the child are essential. Giving children an object that symbolizes their coping, such as a "hero badge" or an "ICU diploma," provides a positive memento of an otherwise stressful experience. Because of the numerous procedures performed on the child and the nature of the illness, pain management needs to receive a high priority.

Of particular importance in decreasing fear is ensuring that discussions that do not directly include the family are held where the child and family cannot overhear them. Casual conversation in the nursing station or in the halls can often be overheard and taken out of context. When discussions are held at the bedside, it is very easy to forget the patient and make remarks that are misunderstood. Usually a quiet reminder of how frightened the child can become from listening to these discussions is sufficient. If bedside conferences are necessary, the nurse interprets them for family members in language they can comprehend.

Extensive monitoring makes a usual day-night cycle difficult in an ICU. However, some schedule should be established that maintains a similarity to daily events in the child's life. These include organizing care during normal waking hours, keeping regular bedtime schedules, including quiet times when televisions and radios are lowered or turned off, closing and opening drapes as appropriate, dimming lights, placing a curtain around the bed for privacy and decreased stimulation, and having clocks or calendars in easy view for older children. In particular, staff members must realize the need for quiet and refrain from loud talking or laughing. Equipment noise should be kept to a minimum by turning alarms as low as safely possible, scheduling nursing care in blocks of time to minimize interruptions, turning off bedside equipment not in use (e.g., suction, oxygen), and avoiding loud, abrupt noises. Such measures can reduce the sensory overload and the sleep deprivation commonly associated with ICU admissions.

Play opportunities should be provided for every child. Although children who are critically ill may be unable to initiate spontaneous play, others (e.g., nurse, social worker, child-life specialist, parent, sibling) can structure play interactions in which children watch and direct as the person plays for them.

Despite the stresses normally associated with ICU admission, a special security develops from being carefully monitored and receiving individualized care. Therefore planning for transition to the regular unit is essential and should include (1) assignment of a primary nurse on the regular unit who visits before the transfer; (2) continued visits by the ICU staff to assess the child's and parents' adjustment and to act as a temporary liaison with the nursing staff; (3) explanation of the differences between the two units and the rationale for the change to less intense monitoring of the child's physical condition; and (4) selection of an appropriate room, such as one close to the nursing station, and a compatible roommate. In one study of parents whose children were being transferred from the ICU to the regular pediatric unit, parents who received a transfer preparation letter and verbal explanation of the process had significantly lower anxiety scores than the parents who did not receive this information (Bouve, Roozmus, and Giordano, 1999).

## Discharge Planning and Home Care

Most hospitalizations necessitate some type of discharge planning. Often this involves education of the family for continued care and follow-up in the home. Depending on the diagnosis, this may be relatively simple or considerably complex. With the current concern for cost containment and recognition of children's emotional needs, home care for children with technologically complex care, such as youngsters on ventilators, has become increasingly common. Preparing the family for home care demands a high degree of competence in planning and implementing discharge instruction. (See Chapter 25.) This usually is best accomplished using an *interdisciplinary team approach,* which requires a shift from the *multidisciplinary team approach* that hospital teams use during an acute phase of a child's illness (Hornick, 1996). Leadership and decision-making functions differ. A physician or nurse practitioner is often both leader and chief decision maker of the multidisciplinary

team; however, interdisciplinary team members typically share leadership and make decisions by consensus.

Nurses are often key individuals in initiating the discharge process and collaborating with others in the planning and implementing stages. Although it is not possible to discuss all of the details needed for effective discharge planning and home care, this section presents a brief overview of the more critical aspects. More specific details are discussed throughout the text for conditions such as home apnea monitoring, tracheostomy care, or hyperalimentation, and numerous sources of information exist in the literature.

### Assessment

Discharge planning for home care must begin with an assessment of the family's desire and capability in assuming care responsibilities. Ideally, at least two individuals should be committed to learning the skills needed for home care. The family should participate in a thorough assessment of their needs and the home environment to ensure that the family's emotional and physical resources are sufficient to manage the tasks of home care (Dokken and Sydnor-Greenberg, 1998). (For a discussion of family and home assessment strategies, see Chapters 22 and 25.) In addition to adequate family resources, an investigation of community services, including respite care, is needed to ensure that appropriate support agencies are available, such as emergency facilities, home health agencies, and equipment vendors. To coordinate the immense task of assessment and to plan implementation, a discharge planning coordinator should be appointed early in the process (Jacob, 1999).

### Planning

Ideally, preparation for hospital discharge and home care begins during the admission assessment with the establishment of short- and long-term goals. These goals are concerned with the child's physical needs, as well as the psychologic needs of the child and family. For children who require complex care, discharge planning focuses on obtaining appropriate equipment and health care personnel for the home and on the skills that parents or children are expected to continue at home* (Jacob, 1999). In planning appropriate teaching, nurses need to assess (1) the actual and perceived complexity of the skill, (2) the parents' or child's ability to learn the skill, and (3) the parents' or child's previous or present experience with such procedures. (See Compliance, Chapter 27, for guidelines for effective teaching.)

The teaching plan should incorporate levels of learning, such as observing, participating with assistance, and finally acting without help or guidance. Each skill should be divided into discrete steps, and each step taught to the family member. Return demonstration of the skill should be requested before new skills are introduced. A record of teaching and performance provides an efficient checklist for evaluation. All families should receive detailed *written in-*

---

## Critical Thinking Exercise

### Discharge Planning and Home Care

Two-year-old Rhonda comes from a rural home 150 miles from the medical center. Last month she suffered a severe case of meningitis that left her profoundly cognitively impaired. During her hospitalization her parents have called infrequently and have never visited because they do not have a telephone or car. Rhonda is now ready to be discharged from the tertiary care center. As the nurse who is responsible for Rhonda's discharge planning, which of the following activities would you initiate?

FIRST, THINK ABOUT IT . . .

• What are you taking for granted, what assumptions are you making?
• What would the consequences be if you put your thoughts into action?

1. Arrange for Rhonda to be institutionalized because her family will be unable to care for her.
2. Give to the transport team a list of local services with an encouraging note about the importance of arranging follow-up care to give to her parents.
3. Call and arrange for the public health nurse from Rhonda's district to make a home visit shortly after her return.
4. Arrange for a multidisciplinary care conference to implement Rhonda's discharge.

*The best response is four. Making the arrangements for a multidisciplinary care conference, including the parents, will require some planning. Transportation assistance may be necessary for the parents to attend the care conference. The discharge planning coordinator will advise the interdisciplinary team regarding services available in Rhonda's community. Because Rhonda will need care from a variety of professionals, this conference will help ensure that there are no gaps or overlaps in services.*

*Providing Rhonda's parents with a list of agencies is inappropriate. First, they do not own their own phone. Second, the parents are not in the position of knowing what services they will need. Third, dealing with professional agencies is often an arduous task and one that parents should not be expected to do while adjusting to the child's disability. Any agency providing home health care will need to be notified well in advance of discharge. This way the nurse could perform a home assessment to help arrange for appropriate services. Institutionalization of children with cognitive impairment is considered a last resort. All other options should be explored first.*

---

*Home care instructions for a wide variety of technical skills are available in Wong DL, Hess CS: *Wong and Whaley's clinical manual of pediatric nursing,* ed 5, St Louis, 2000, Mosby.

structions about home care before they leave the hospital, as well as telephone numbers should they require assistance. (See Critical Thinking Exercise box on p. 1096.)

### Transitional Care

Once the family is competent in performing required skills, they should be given responsibility for the care. Whenever possible, the family should have a transition or trial period to assume care with minimum supervision. This may be arranged on the unit, during a home pass, or in a facility (e.g., a motel or Ronald McDonald House) near the hospital. Some programs incorporate a hospital trial into their discharge criteria, necessitating that the family successfully manage this phase before discharge to home. Such transitions provide a safe practice period for the family, with assistance readily available when needed, and are especially valuable when the family lives far from the hospital.

### Evaluation and Continuing Support

Evaluation is a critical part of any discharge plan and assumes even more importance in home care of children with complex needs. Factors to consider in home care planning include need for subsequent hospitalization, child's developmental and physical progress, effects of home care on the family, actual vs expected use of resources by the family and home care team, and financial costs and savings.

In most instances parents need only simple instructions and understanding of follow-up care. However, the often overwhelming care assumed by some families necessitates continued professional support after discharge. A follow-up home visit or telephone call gives the nurse a better opportunity to individualize care and provide information in perhaps a less stressful learning environment than the hospital (Snowdon and Kane, 1995). Appropriate referrals and resources may include visiting nurse or home health agencies, private nurse services, the school system, physical therapist, mental health counselor, social worker, and various community agencies, including special organizations. Sharing the important issues surrounding the child's and family's needs is essential. Referral summaries should be concise, specific, and factual. When numerous support services are involved, periodic collaboration among the professionals involved and the family is an excellent strategy to ensure efficient implementation and comprehensive delivery of services.

## KEY POINTS

- Children are particularly vulnerable to the stresses of illness and hospitalization because stress represents a change from the usual state of health and routine and because they possess limited coping mechanisms.
- The three phases of separation anxiety are protest, despair, and detachment.
- Feelings of loss of control are caused by unfamiliar environmental stimuli, physical restriction, altered routine, and dependency.
- Fear of pain may be manifested in the following ways: infants—expressions, body movements; toddlers—intense emotional upset, physical resistance; preschoolers—aggression, verbal expression, dependency; school-age children—precise verbalization of pain, passive requests for support or help, procrastination technique; adolescents—self-control, irritability, limited movement.
- Because of their separation from significant people, children who are hospitalized may lack the opportunity to form new attachments in the strange environment and may exhibit negative behaviors after discharge.
- Family reactions are influenced by the seriousness of illness, experience with illness or hospitalization, diagnostic or therapeutic procedures, available support systems, personal ego strengths, coping abilities, additional stresses, cultural and religious beliefs, and family communication patterns.
- The following increase the negative effects of a brother's or sister's illness/hospitalization on siblings: fear of contracting the illness, their age, a close relationship with the ill sibling, substitute child care, minimum explanation of the illness, and perceived changes in parenting.
- Nursing care of children who are hospitalized is aimed at preventing or minimizing separation, decreasing loss of control, minimizing bodily injury and pain, using play

and other expressive activities to lessen stress, maximizing potential benefits of hospitalization, and supporting family members.
- Pain assessment includes questioning the child, using pain rating scales, evaluating behavior and physiologic changes, securing parents' involvement, taking the cause of pain into account, and taking action.
- Pain management should incorporate both pharmacologic and nonpharmacologic methods. Pharmacologic methods focus on four "rights:" right drug, right dose, right route, and right time.
- Play and other expressive activities are effective tools in minimizing stress.
- The nurse can maximize potential benefits of hospitalization by fostering parent-child relations, providing educational opportunities, promoting self-mastery, and encouraging socialization.
- Supporting family members involves listening to parents' verbal and nonverbal messages; providing social and spiritual support; accepting cultural, socioeconomic, and ethnic values; and giving information to families and siblings.
- The major goals of prehospital counseling are to make the hospital less strange and frightening to parents and children and to establish a positive atmosphere and trusting relationships with staff and family members.
- In preparing families for hospitalization, the nurse should consider small group size and timing of the event, setting of the tour, inclusion of preparatory materials, time for discussion, and prehospital counseling for parents.
- Emergency admission or admission to an ambulatory/outpatient setting, isolation room, or intensive care unit requires additional intervention strategies to meet the child's and family's needs.

# REFERENCES

Acute Pain Management Guideline Panel: *Acute pain management in infants, children and adolescents,* AHCPR Pub No 92-0019, Rockville, MD, 1992, Agency for Health Care Policy and Research, Public Health Service, US Department of Health and Human Services.

Algren JT, Algren CL: Management of procedural and perioperative pain in children. In Weiner R, editor: *Pain management: a practical guide for clinicians,* Boca Raton, FL, 1998, St Lucie Press.

Algren JT and others: Efficacy and safety of morphine administered by patient-, parent-, or nurse-controlled analgesia in children (abstract), *Anesthesiology* 89:A1003, 1998.

American Academy of Pediatrics Committee on Hospital Care: Child life services, *Pediatrics* 106(5):1156-1159, 2000.

American Pain Society: *Principles of analgesic use in the treatment of acute pain and chronic cancer pain,* ed 4, Skokie, IL, 1999, The Society.

American Pain Society: [On-line]. Available: *www.ampainsoc.org,* 2000.

American Society of Addiction Medicine: *Public policy statement on the rights and responsibilities of physicians in the use of opioids for the treatment of pain,* Chevy Chase, MD, April 16, 1997, The Society.

American Society of Pain Management Nurses: ASPMN position statement: use of placebos for pain management, *Ostomy Wound Manage* 44(2):56-57, 1998.

Anand K, Aynsley-Green A: Metabolic and endocrine effects of surgical ligation of patent ductus arteriosus in the human preterm neonate: are there implications for further improvement of postoperative outcome? *Mod Probl Paediatr* 23:143-157, 1985.

Anand KJS, Hickey P: Pain and its effects in the human neonate and fetus, *N Engl N Med* 317(21);1321-1329, 1987.

Ashenberg MD and others: Easing the wait: development of a pager program for families, *Pediatr Nurs* 22(2):103-107, 1996.

Baker C, Wong D: Q.U.E.S.T.: a process of pain assessment in children, *Orthop Nurs* 6(1):11-21, 1987.

Bauchner H, May A, Coates E: Use of analgesic agents for invasive medical procedures in pediatric and neonatal intensive care units, *J Pediatr* 121(4):647-649, 1992.

Berde C and others: Patient-controlled analgesia in children and adolescents: a randomized, prospective comparison with intramuscular administration of morphine for postoperative analgesia, *J Pediatr* 118(3):460-466, 1991.

Beyer J and others: Patterns of postoperative analgesic use with adults and children following cardiac surgery, *Pain* 17:71-81, 1983.

Beyer JE, Denyes MJ, Villarruel AM: The creation, validation and continuing development of the Oucher: a measure of pain intensity in children, *J Pediatr Nurs* 7(5): 335-346, 1992.

Beyer JE, McGrath PJ, Berde CB: Discordance between self-report and behavioral pain measures in children aged 3-7 years after surgery, *J Pain Symptom Manage* 5(6):350-356, 1990.

Bieri D and others: The FACES Pain Scale for the self-assessment of the severity of pain experienced by children: development, initial validation, and preliminary investigation for ratio scale properties, *Pain* 41(2): 139-150, 1990.

Billmire DA, Neale HW, Gregory RO: Use of IV fentanyl in the outpatient treatment of pediatric facial trauma, *J Trauma* 25(11): 1079-1080, 1985.

Bolig R: No play permitted: indicator of psychological abuse. In Azarnoff P, Lindquist P, editors: *Psychological abuse of children in health care: the issues,* ed 2, Tarzana, CA, 1997, Pediatric Projects.

Boughton K and others: Impact of research on pediatric pain assessment and outcomes, *Pediatr Nurs* 24(1):31-35, 62, 1998.

Bouve LR, Roozmus CL, Giordano P: Preparing parents for their child's transfer from the PICU to the pediatric floor, *Appl Nurs Res* 12(3):114-120, 1999.

Boyd, J, Hunsberger M: Chronically ill children coping with repeated hospitalizations: their perceptions and suggested intervention, *J Pediatr Nurs* 13(6):330-342, 1998.

Brewer S, Lambert C: Preparing children for same day surgery: innovative approaches, *J Pediatr Nurs* 12(4):257-259, 1997.

Broome M, Rehwaldt M, Fogg L: Relationships between cognitive behavioral techniques, temperament, observed distress, and pain reports in children and adolescents during lumbar puncture, *J Pediatr Nurs* 13:48-54, 1998.

Broome M and others: Children's medical fears, coping behaviors, and pain perceptions during a lumbar puncture, *Oncol Nurs Forum* 17(3):361-367, 1990.

Broome ME: Helping parents support their child in pain, *Pediatr Nurs* 26(3):315-317, 2000.

Brozovic M and others: Pain relief in sickle cell crises, *Lancet* 2(8507):624-625, 1986.

Carey SJ and others: Improving pain management in an acute care setting, *Orthop Nurs* 16(4):29-36, 1997.

Chambers CT and others: Agreement between child and parent reports of pain, *Clin J Pain* 14(4):336-342, 1998.

Champion GD and others: Measurement of pain by self-report. In Finley GA, McGrath PJ, editors: *Measurement of pain in infants and children,* Seattle, 1998, IASP Press.

Clatworthy S, Simon K, Tiedeman ME: Child drawing: hospital—an instrument designed to measure the emotional status of hospitalized school-aged children, *J Pediatr Nurs* 14(1):2-9, 1999.

Cline ME and others: Standardization of the visual analogue scale, *Nurs Res* 41(6): 378-380, 1992.

Collins J: Intractable cancer pain in children, *J Palliat Care* 12(3):29-34, 1996.

Craft MJ: Siblings of hospitalized children: assessment and intervention, *J Pediatr Nurs* 8(5):289-297, 1993.

Dahl JL: Darvon: a drug with dubious distinction, *Cancer Pain Update* 48:3, 6, Summer, 1998.

Davis GC: Nursing's role in pain management across the health care continuum, *Nurs Outlook* 46(1):19-23, 1998.

Dilworth NM, MacKellar A: Pain relief for the pediatric surgical patient, *J Pediatr Surg* 22:264-266, 1987.

Dokken DL, Sydnor-Greenberg N: Helping families mobilize their personal resources, *Pediatr Nurs* 24:66-69, 1998.

Dolgin M and others: Behavioral distress in pediatric patients with cancer receiving chemotherapy, *Pediatrics* 84(1):103-110, 1989.

Eland J: Children with pain. In Jackson OB, Saunders RB, editors: *Child health nursing,* Philadelphia, 1993, JB Lippincott.

Eland JM, Anderson JE: The experience of pain in children. In Jacox A, editor: *Pain: a source book for nurses and other health professionals,* Boston, 1977, Little, Brown.

Fanurik D and others: Pharmacobehavioral intervention: integrating pharmacologic and behavioral techniques for pediatric procedures, *Child Health Care* 26(1):1-13, 1997.

Fanurik D and others: Children with cognitive impairment: parent report of pain and coping, *J Dev Behav Pediatr* 20(4):228-234, 1999.

Favaloro R, Touzel B: A comparison of adolescents' and nurses' postoperative pain ratings and perceptions, *Pediatr Nurs* 16(4): 414-417, 424, 1990.

Federwisch A: Complete assessment: making pain the fifth vital sign, *Health Week* 4(14):18, 1999.

Fernandez C, Pyesmany A, Stutzer C: Alternative therapies in childhood cancer, *N Engl J Med* 340(7):569-570, 1999.

Ferrell BR, McCaffery M, Rhiner M: Pain and addiction: an urgent need for change in nursing education, *J Pain Symptom Manage* 7:48-55, 1992.

Ferrell BR and others: The experience of pediatric cancer pain. I. Impact of pain on the family, *J Pediatr Nurs* 9:368-379, 1994.

Field T: Infants' and children's responses to invasive procedures. In La Greca A, editor: *Stress and coping in child health,* New York, 1992, Guilford.

Fitzgerald M, Millard C, MacIntosh N: Hyperalgesia in premature infants, *Lancet* 6(8580): 292, 1988.

Flanagan K: Preoperative assessment: safety considerations for patients taking herbal products, *J Perianesth Nurs* 16(1):19-26, 2001.

Fradet C and others: A prospective survey of reactions to blood tests by children and adolescents, *Pain* 40(1):53-60, 1990.

Franck L: A national survey of the assessment and treatment of pain and agitation in the neonatal intensive care unit, *J Obstet Gynecol Neonat Nurs* 16:387-395, 1987.

Franck LS, Greenberg CS, Stevens B: Pain assessment in infants and children, *Pediatr Clin North Am* 47:487-512, 2000.

French GM, Painter EC, Coury DL: Blowing away shot pain: a technique for pain management during immunization, *Pediatrics* 93(3):384-388, 1994.

Friedland LR, Kulick RM: Emergency department analgesic use in pediatric trauma victims with fractures, *Ann Emerg Med* 23(2):203-207, 1994.

Gibbons J and others: Opiate-induced respiratory depression in young pediatric burn patients, *J Burn Care Rehabil* 19:225-229, 1998.

Giganti AW: Families in pediatric critical care: the best option, *Pediatr Nurs* 24(3):261-265, 1998.

Gillis A: Hospital preparation: the children's story, *Child Health Care* 19(1):19-27, 1990.

Golianu B and others: Pediatric acute pain management, *Pediatr Clin North Am* 47(3):559-587, 2000.

Gordon M: *Nursing diagnosis: process and application*, ed 3, St Louis, 1994, Mosby.

Graff KJ, Kennedy RM, Jaffe DM: Conscious sedation for pediatric orthopaedic emergencies, *Pediatr Emerg Care* 12(1):31-35, 1996.

Greenberg RS and others: Videotape increases parental knowledge about pediatric pain management, *Anesth Analg* 89(4):899-903, 1999.

Hannallah RS and others: Comparison of caudal and ilioinguinal/iliohypogastric nerve blocks for control of post-orchiopexy pain in pediatric ambulatory surgery, *Anesthesiology* 66:832-834, 1987.

Hart D, Bossert E: Self-reported fears of hospitalized school-age children, *J Pediatr Nurs* 9(2):83-90, 1994.

Haslam DR: Age and the perception of pain, *Psychosom Sci* 15:86, 1969.

Havermans T, Eiser C: Sibling of a child with cancer, *Child Care Health Dev* 20:309-322, 1994.

Hazinski MF: *Manual of pediatric critical care*, St Louis, 1999, Mosby.

Hertzka R and others: Fentanyl-induced ventilatory depression: effects of age, *Anesthesiology* 70:213-218, 1989.

Hester NO: Comforting the child in pain. In Funk SG and others, editors: *Key aspects of comfort*, New York, 1989, Springer.

Hester NO and others: Putting pain measurement into clinical practice. In Finley GA, McGrath PJ, editors: *Measurement of pain in infants and children*, vol 10, Seattle, 1998, International Association for the Study of Pain Press.

Hornick R: Discharge teams. In Gunter K, Manago R, editors: *Beyond discharge: interdisciplinary perspectives for transitioning children with complex medical needs from hospital to home*, Bethesda, MD, 1996, Association for the Care of Children's Health.

Houck CS: The management of acute pain in the child. In Ashburn MA, Rice LJ, editors: *The management of pain*, Philadelphia, 1998, Churchill Livingstone.

Howard CR and others: Neonatal circumcision and pain relief: current training practices, *Pediatrics* 101(3):423-428, 1998.

Huckabay LMD, Tilem-Kessler D: Patterns of parental stress in PICU emergency admission, *Dimens Crit Care Nurs* 18(2):36-42, 1999.

Humphrey BG and others: The occurrence of high levels of acute behavioral distress in children and adolescents undergoing routine venipunctures, *Pediatrics* 90(1):87-91, 1992.

IOMED, Inc: *Iontocaine package insert*, Salt Lake City, 1996, IOMED, Inc.

Jacob E: Making the transition from hospital to home: caring for the newly diagnosed child with cancer, *Home Care Provid* 4:62-73, 1999.

Jacob E, Puntillo KA: Pain in hospitalized children: pediatric nurses' beliefs and practices, *J Pediatr Nurs* 14(6):379-391, 1999.

Jacobson SJ and others: Randomised trial of oral morphine for painful episodes of sickle-cell disease in children, *Lancet* 350(9088):1358-1364, 1997.

Johnston CC and others: A survey of pain in hospitalized patients aged 4-14 years, *Clin J Pain* 8(2):154-163, 1992.

Joint Commission on Accreditation of Healthcare Organizations: *AMH92 accreditation manual for hospitals*, Chicago, 1999, The Commission.

Jordan-Marsh M and others: Alternate Oucher form testing: gender, ethnicity, and age variations, *Res Nurs Health* 17:111-118, 1994.

Joyce BA and others: Reliability and validity of preverbal pain assessment tools, *Issues Compr Pediatr Nurs* 17:121-135, 1994.

Juhlin L, Evers H: EMLA: a new topical anesthetic, *Adv Dermatol* 5:75-92, 1990.

Kain Z, Mayes L, Caramico LA: Preoperative preparation in children: a cross-sectional study, *J Clin Anesth* 8(6):508-514, 1996.

Kart T, Christrup LL, Rasmussen M: Recommended use of morphine in neonates, infants and children based on a literature review. I. Pharmacokinetics, *Paediatr Anaesth* 7(1):5-11, 1997.

Katz E, Kellerman J, Siegel S: Behavioral distress in children with cancer undergoing medical procedures: developmental considerations, *J Consult Clin Psychol* 48(3):356-365, 1980.

Keck J and others: Reliability and validity of the FACES and Word Descriptor scales to measure procedural pain, *J Pediatr Nurs* 11(6):368-374, 1996.

Kennedy RM and others: Comparison of fentanyl/midazolam with ketamine/midazolam for pediatric orthopedic emergencies, *Pediatrics* 102:956-963, 1998.

Kirkby R, Whelan T: The effects of hospitalization and medical procedures on children and their families, *J Fam Stud* 2(1):65-77, 1996.

Koh JL and others: Efficacy of parental application of eutectic mixture of local anesthetics for intravenous insertion, *Pediatrics* 103(6):79, 1999.

Koren G and others: Postoperative morphine infusion in newborn infants: assessment of disposition characteristics and safety, *J Pediatr* 107(6):963-967, 1985.

Krebel MS, Clayton C, Graham C: Child life programs in the pediatric emergency department, *Pediatr Emerg Care* 12(1):13-15, 1996.

Kuntz N and others: Therapeutic play and bone marrow transplantation, *J Pediatr Nurs* 11(6):359-367, 1996.

Kussman BD, Sethna NF: Pethidine-associated seizure in a healthy adolescent receiving pethidine for postoperative pain control, *Paediatr Anaesth* 8:349-352, 1998.

Lancaster KA: Care of the pediatric patient in ambulatory surgery, *Nurs Clin North Am* 32(1):441-455, 1997.

Lander J, Fowler-Kerry S: Assessment of sex differences in children's and adolescents' self-reported pain from venipuncture, *J Pediatr Psychol* 16(6):783-793, 1991.

Lefkowicz AB and others: Young children's pain rating using the FACES Pain Rating Scale with original vs abbreviated word instructions. In Wong DL, Baker CM, editors: *Reference manual for Wong-Baker FACES Pain Rating Scale*, 1998, Duarte, CA, City of Hope Mayday Fund.

Lipson J, Dibble S, Minarik P: *Culture and nursing care: a pocket guide*, San Francisco, 1996, UCSF Nursing Press.

Lowes L, Davis R: Minimizing hospitalization: children with newly diagnosed diabetes, *Br J Nurs* 6(1):28-33, 1997.

Luffy RI: The validity, reliability, and preference of three pediatric pain assessment tools. In Wong DL, Baker CM, editors: *Reference manual for Wong-Baker FACES Pain Rating Scale*, Duarte, CA, 1997, City of Hope Mayday Fund.

Marshall RE: Neonatal pain associated with caregiving procedures, *Pediatr Clin North Am* 36(4):885-903, 1989.

Mather L, Mackie J: The incidence of postoperative pain in children, *Pain* 15:271-282, 1983.

Maxwell LG, Yaster M: Perioperative management issues in pediatric patients, *Anesthesiol Clin North Am* 18(3):601-632, 2000.

McCaffery M, Pasero CL: When the physician prescribes a placebo, *Am J Nurs* 98(1):52-53, 1998.

McCaffery M, Pasero C: *Pain: a clinical manual*, ed 2, St Louis, 1999, Mosby.

McGrath PA, de Veber L, Hearn M: Multidimensional pain assessment in children. In Fields HL, Dubner R, Cervero F, editors: *Advances in pain research and therapy*, New York, 1985, Raven.

McGrath PJ and others: The Children's Hospital of Eastern Ontario Pain Scale (CHEOPS): a behavioral scale for rating post-operative pain in children. In Fields HL, Dubner R, Cervero F: *Advances in pain research and therapy*, New York, 1985, Raven.

McGrath PJ and others: Behaviours caregivers use to determine pain in non-verbal, cognitively impaired individuals, *Dev Med Child Neurol* 40:340-343, 1998.

Melnyk B, Alpert-Gillis L: The COPE Program: a strategy to improve outcomes of critically ill young children and their parents, *Pediatr Nurs* 24(6):521-527, 1998.

Melnyk BM: Intervention studies involving parents of hospitalized young children: an analysis of the past and future recommendations, *J Pediatr Nurs* 15(1):4-13, 2000.

Merkel S, Malviya S: Pediatric pain, tools, and assessment, *J Perianesth Nurs* 15(6):408-414, 2000.

Merkel SI and others: The FLACC: a behavioral scale for scoring postoperative pain in young children, *Pediatr Nurs* 23:293-297, 1997.

Moenkhoff M and others: Parental attitude towards alternative medicine in the paediatric intensive care unit, *Eur J Pediatr* 158(1):12-17, 1999.

Morrison R: Update on sickle cell disease: incidence of addiction and choice of opioid in pain management, *Pediatr Nurs* 17(6):503, 1991.

Murray JS: The lived experienced of childhood cancer: one sibling's perspective, *Issues Compr Pediatr Nurs* 21:217-227, 1998.

Newton MS: Family-centered care: current realities in parent participation, *Pediatr Nurs* 26(2):164-168, 2000.

Nix K, Clutter L, Wong DL: The influence of the type of instructions in measuring pain intensity in young children using the FACES Pain Rating Scale. In Wong DL, Baker CM, editors: *Reference manual for Wong-Baker FACES Pain Rating Scale*, 1998, Duarte, CA, City of Hope Mayday Fund.

Oakes L and others: Chest tube stripping in pediatric oncology patients: an experimental study, *Am J Crit Care* 2(4):293-301, 1993.

Oberlander TF, O'Donnell ME, Montgomery CJ: Pain in children with neurological impairment, *J Dev Behav Pediatr* 20(4):234-243, 1999.

Olin BR and others: *Drug facts and comparisons*, ed 1998, St Louis, 1998, Facts and Comparisons.

Orem D: *Nursing concepts of practice*, ed 5, St Louis, 1995, Mosby.

Pasero C: Pain control, epidural analgesia in children, *Am J Nurs* 99(5):20, 1999.

Pasero CL, McCaffery M: Avoiding opoid-induced respiratory depression, *Am J Nurs* 94(4):25-31, 1994.

Pasero CL: Using the FACES scale to assess pain, *Am J Nurs* 97(7):19, 1997.

Pate J and others: Childhood medical experience and temperament as predictors of adult functioning in medical situations, *Child Health Care* 25(4):281-298, 1996.

Peterson L, Ridley-Johnson R: Pediatric hospital responses to survey on pre-hospital preparation for children, *J Pediatr Psychol* 5:1-7, 1980.

Petrillo M, Azarnoff P: Preparation programs and new strategies. In Azarnoff P, Lindquist P, editors: *Psychological abuse of children in health care: the issues*, ed 2, Tarzana, CA, 1997, Pediatric Projects.

Razmus I, Lammert D: *A description of rating scale preference among children ages 4-18 years in the self-report of pain*. Presented at the Society of Pediatric Nurses, Poster Presentation, Orlando, FL, April 26-28, 1998.

Reis EC, Holubkov R: Vapocoolant spray is equally effective as EMLA cream in reducing immunization pain in school-aged children, *Pediatrics* 100(6):e5, 1997.

Robertson J: Pediatric pain assessment: validation of a multidimensional tool, *Pediatr Nurs* 19(3):209-313, 1993.

Robieux I and others: Assessing pain and analgesia with a lidocaine-prilocaine emulsion in infants and toddlers during venipuncture, *J Pediatr* 118(6):971-973, 1991.

Robinson P, Kobayashi K: Development and evaluation of a presurgical preparation program, *J Pediatr Psychol* 16:193-212, 1991.

Rodgers BM and others: Patient-controlled analgesia in pediatric surgery, *J Pediatr Surg* 23(3):259-262, 1988.

Rogers A: The ABC of pediatric pain, *Prim Care Cancer* 10:7-8, 1990.

Rollins J: Art: helping children meet the challenges of hospitalization, *Interacta* 15(3):36-41, 1995.

Rollins J, Mahan C: *From artist to artist-in-residence: preparing artists to work in pediatric healthcare settings*, Washington, DC, 1996, Rollins & Associates.

Rowbotham D and others: Transdermal fentanyl for the relief of pain after upper abdominal surgery, *Br J Anaesth* 63:56-59, 1989.

Rusy LM, Weisman SJ: Complementary therapies for acute pediatric pain management, *Pediatr Clin North Am* 47(3):589-599, 2000.

Sabatino G and others: Hemodynamic effects of intravenous morphine infusion in ventilated preterm babies, *Early Hum Dev* 47(3):263-270, 1997.

Salantera S and others: Nurses' knowledge about pharmacological and nonpharmacological pain management in children, *J Pain Symptom Manage* 18(4):289-299, 1999.

Savedra MC and others: Assessment of postoperative pain in children and adolescents using the adolescent pediatric pain tool, *Nurs Res* 42(1):5-9, 1993.

Schade JG and others: Comparison of three preverbal scales for postoperative pain assessment in a diverse pediatric sample, *J Pain Symptom Manage* 12(6):348-359, 1996.

Schechter NL: The need for premedication for painful procedures in children, *Am J Anesthesiol* 24(1, suppl):10-12, 1997.

Schmidt K, Eland J, Weiler K: Pediatric cancer pain management: a survey of nurses' knowledge, *J Pediatr Oncol Nurs* 11(1):4-12, 1994.

Scott LD: Perceived needs of parents of critically ill children, *J Soc Pediatr Nurs* 3(1):4-12, 1998.

Shapiro C: Pain in the neonate: assessment and intervention, *Neonatal Network* 8(1):7-21, 1989.

Simon K: Perceived stress of nonhospitalized children during the hospitalization of a sibling, *J Pediatr Nurs* 8(5):298-304, 1993.

Smith T, Conant Rees HL: Making family-centered care a reality, *Sem Nurs Manage* 8(3):136-142, 2000.

Snowdon A, Kane D: Parental needs following the discharge of a hospitalized child, *Pediatr Nurs* 21(5):425-428, 1995.

Spiegel D, Stroud P, Fyfe A: Complementary medicine, *West J Med* 168(4):241-247, 1998.

Stevens B: Development and testing of a pediatric pain management sheet, *Pediatr Nurs* 16(6):543-548, 1990.

Stevens BJ, Johnston CC, Horton L: Multidimensional pain assessment in premature neonates: a pilot study, *J Obstet Gynecol Neonat Nurs* 26(5):531-541, 1993.

Stewart E, Algren C, Arnold S: Preparing children for a surgical experience, *Todays OR Nurse* 16(2):9-14, 1994.

Stuber M and others: Predictors of posttraumatic stress symptoms in childhood cancer survivors, *Pediatrics* 100(6):958-964, 1997.

Taddio A and others: A revised measure of acute pain in infants, *J Pain Symptom Manage* 10(6)456-463, 1995.

Tesler M, Holzemer W, Savedra M: Pain behaviors: postsurgical responses of children and adolescents, *J Pediatr Nurs* 13(1):41-47, 1998.

Tesler MD and others: Children's words for pain. In Funk SG and others, editors: *Key aspects of comfort: management of pain, fatigue, and nausea*, New York, 1991, Springer.

Tyc V and others: A survey of pain services for pediatric oncology patients: their composition and function, *Pediatr Oncol Nurs* 15(4):207-215, 1998

Van Cleve L, Johnson L, Pothier P: Pain responses of hospitalized infants and children to venipuncture and intravenous cannulation, *J Pediatr Nurs* 11:161-168, 1996.

Vessey JA, Carlson KL, McGill J: Use of distraction with children during an acute pain experience, *Nurs Res* 43(6):369, 1994.

Villarruel AM, Denyes MJ: Pain assessment in children: theoretical and emprical validity, *Adv Nurs Sci* 14(2):32-41, 1991.

Wallace M: Temperament: a variable in children's pain management, *Pediatr Nurs* 15(2):118-121, 1989.

Weisman SJ, Bernstein B, Schechter NL: Consequences of inadequate analgesia during painful procedures in children, *Arch Pediatr Adolesc Med* 132(2):147-149, 1998.

Wells PW and others: Growing up in the hospital. I. Let's focus on the child, *J Pediatr Nurs* 9(2):66-73, 1994.

West N and others: Measuring pain in pediatric patients in the ICU, *J Pediatr Oncol Nurs* 11(2):64-68, 1994.

Wilson J, Cason C, Grissom N: Distraction: an effective intervention for alleviating pain during venipuncture, *J Emerg Nurs* 21:87, Feb 1995.

Wilson A, Yorker B: Fears of medical events among school-age children with emotional disorders, parents and health care providers, *Issues Ment Health Nurs* 18:57-71, 1997.

Wong DL: Practice pointers, *School Healthwatch* 5(1):2, 1993.

Wong DL: The Wong-Baker FACES pain rating scale, *Home Health Focus* 2(8):62, 1996.

Wong DL, Baker C: Pain in children: comparison of assessment scales, *Pediatr Nurs* 14(1):9-17, 1988.

Wong DL, Pasero CL: Pain control: reducing pain of lidocaine, *Am J Nurs* 97(1):17-18, 1997.

Woodgate R, Kristjanson L: "Getting better from my hurts": toward a model of the young child's pain experience, *J Pediatr Nurs* 11(4):233-242, 1996.

Yaster M and others: *Pediatric pain management and sedation handbook*, St Louis, 1997, Mosby.

Young M, Fu V: Influence of play and temperament on the young child's response to pain, *Child Health Care* 16(3):209-215, 1988.

Zernikow B, Lindena G: Long-acting morphine for pain control in pediatric oncology, *Med Pediatr Oncol* 36:451-458, 2001.

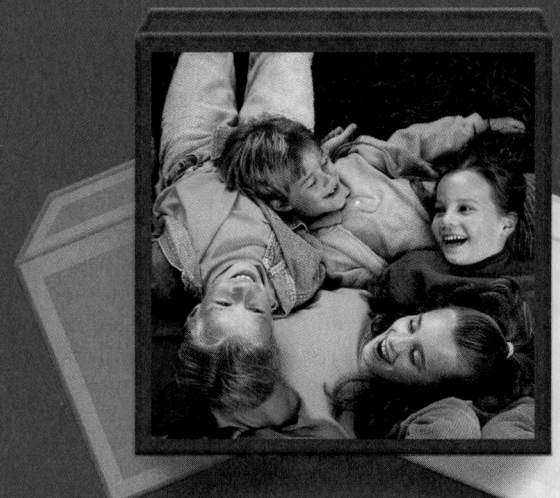

# Chapter 27

# Pediatric Variations of Nursing Interventions

## Chapter Outline

**GENERAL CONCEPTS RELATED TO PEDIATRIC PROCEDURES, 1102**
**Informed Consent, 1102**
  Requirements for Obtaining Informed
    Consent, 1102
  Eligibility for Giving Informed
    Consent, 1102
**Preparation for Diagnostic and Therapeutic
  Procedures, 1103**
  Psychologic Preparation, 1103
  Physical Preparation, 1108
  Performance of the Procedure, 1109
  Postprocedural Support, 1109
  Use of Play in Procedures, 1110
**Surgical Procedures, 1110**
  Preoperative Care, 1110
  Postoperative Care, 1113
*Nursing Care Plan: The Child Undergoing
  Surgery, 1114*
**Compliance, 1118**
  Assessment, 1118
  Compliance Strategies, 1120
**GENERAL HYGIENE AND CARE, 1121**
**Maintaining Healthy Skin, 1121**
**Bathing, 1125**
**Oral Hygiene, 1127**
**Hair Care, 1128**
**Feeding the Sick Child, 1128**
**Controlling Elevated Temperatures, 1130**
**Family Teaching and Home Care, 1131**

**SAFETY, 1132**
**Infection Control, 1132**
**Environmental Factors, 1135**
**Toys, 1136**
**Limit-Setting, 1136**
**Transporting Infants and Children, 1136**
**Restraining Methods and Therapeutic
    Holding, 1136**
  Mummy Restraint or Swaddle, 1138
  Jacket Restraint, 1140
  Arm and Leg Restraints, 1140
  Elbow Restraint, 1140
**POSITIONING FOR PROCEDURES, 1140**
**Jugular Venipuncture, 1140**
**Femoral Venipuncture, 1141**
**Extremity Venipuncture, 1141**
**Lumbar Puncture, 1141**
**Bone Marrow Aspiration/Biopsy, 1142**
**Other Procedures, 1142**
**COLLECTION OF SPECIMENS, 1142**
**Urine Specimens, 1143**
  Clean-Catch Specimens, 1144
  Twenty-Four-Hour Collection, 1144
  Bladder Catheterization and Other
    Techniques, 1144
**Stool Specimens, 1146**
**Blood Specimens, 1147**
**Respiratory Secretion Specimens, 1148**
**ADMINISTRATION OF MEDICATION, 1149**
**Determination of Drug Dosage, 1149**

**Preparation for Safe Administration, 1150**
  Checking Dosage, 1150
  Identification, 1151
  Parents, 1151
  Child, 1151
**Oral Administration, 1151**
  Preparation, 1151
  Administration, 1153
**Intramuscular (IM) Administration, 1153**
  Selecting the Syringe and Needle, 1153
  Determining the Site, 1154
  Administration, 1155
**Subcutaneous and Intradermal
    Administration, 1157**
**Intravenous (IV) Administration, 1158**
**Nasogastric, Orogastric, or Gastrostomy
    Administration, 1159**
**Rectal Administration, 1159**
**Optic, Otic, and Nasal Administration, 1160**
**Family Teaching and Home Care, 1161**
**ALTERNATIVE FEEDING TECHNIQUES, 1162**
**Gavage Feeding, 1162**
  Preparations, 1162
  Procedure, 1162
**Gastrostomy Feeding, 1164**
**PROCEDURES RELATED TO
ELIMINATION, 1165**
**Enema, 1165**
**Ostomies, 1166**
**Family Teaching and Home Care, 1167**

## Related Topics

Communicating with Families, Ch. 6
Dental Health: Infant, Ch. 12; Toddler,
  Ch. 14; Preschooler, Ch. 15; School-Age
  Child, Ch. 17
Family-Centered Home Care, Ch. 25
Febrile Seizures, Ch. 37
Feeding Resistance, Ch. 10

Injury Prevention: Infant, Ch. 12; Toddler,
  Ch. 14; Preschooler, Ch. 15; School-Age
  Child, Ch. 17; Adolescent, Ch. 19
Limit-Setting and Discipline, Ch. 3
Neonatal Pain, Ch. 10
Nursing Care of the Surgical Neonate, Ch. 11
Nutritional Assessment, Ch. 6
Pain Assessment; Pain Management, Ch. 26

Parenteral Fluid Therapy, Ch. 28
Preparation for Hospitalization, Ch. 26
Skin Care (Neonatal), Ch. 10
Temperature (Measurement), Ch. 7
Using Play/Expressive Activities to Minimize
  Stress, Ch. 26
Venous Access Devices, Ch. 28
Wounds, Ch. 18

# GENERAL CONCEPTS RELATED TO PEDIATRIC PROCEDURES

## Informed Consent

*Informed consent* refers to the legal and ethical requirement that the patients or his or her surrogate clearly, fully, and completely understand the proposed medical treatment to be performed, including significant risks associated with the treatment. The patient must also be informed of alternative treatments that could be offered, including their benefits and risks and the risks of nontreatment, before giving informed consent. To obtain valid informed consent, the following three conditions must be met:

1. The person must be capable of giving consent; he or she must be over the age of majority (usually age 18 years) and must be considered competent (i.e., possess the mental capacity to make choices and understand their consequences).
2. The person must receive the information needed to make an intelligent decision.
3. The person must act voluntarily when exercising freedom of choice without force, fraud, deceit, duress, or other forms of constraint or coercion.

Because of the numerous variations of the laws and institutional policies within the United States, the following discussion of informed consent is presented in general terms and is not to be interpreted as legal advice. Although informing patients of the risks, benefits, and alternatives of a procedure is the physician's responsibility, nurses frequently are responsible for securing the person's signature on a written consent form. In caring for children, special dilemmas may arise regarding who may sign the consent for treatment when parental consent is not available. The **age of majority competence** is a key issue in decisions involving minors who are retarded or otherwise mentally incapacitated. Also, the judicial system may intervene in cases where the parents' views and the child's best interests conflict (Guertler, 1997; Moskop, 1999). Consequently, nurses need to be familiar with the issues involved in this highly significant and complex subject and must keep current on legal aspects of practice within their community.

### Requirements for Obtaining Informed Consent

Written informed consent of the parent or legal guardian is usually required for medical or surgical treatment, including many diagnostic procedures. One blanket consent is not sufficient. Separate informed permissions must be obtained for each surgical or diagnostic procedure, including the following:

- Major surgery
- Minor surgery (e.g., cutdown, biopsy, dental extraction, suturing a laceration [especially one that may have a cosmetic effect], removal of a cyst, closed reduction of a fracture)
- Diagnostic tests with an element of risk (e.g., bronchoscopy, needle biopsy, angiography, ECG, lumbar puncture, cardiac catheterization, ventriculography, bone marrow aspiration)

- Medical treatments with an element of risk (e.g., blood transfusion, thoracentesis/paracentesis, radiation therapy, shock therapy)

Situations such as the following are not directly related to medical treatment but also require parental consent:

- Taking photographs for medical, educational, or other public use
- Removal of the child from the health care institution against the advice of the physician
- Postmortem examinations, except in unexplained deaths, such as sudden infant death, violent death, or suspected suicide
- Examination of medical records by unauthorized persons, such as attorneys or insurance representatives (family members have a legal right to medical records)

The need for informed consent is also an issue with proposed treatments or research involving children with a mental age of 7 years or older. **Assent** (usually verbal agreement) requires that the child be informed about the proposed treatment or research and agree or concur with the decisions made by the person(s) who can give informed consent. Multiple methods should be used to explain the study, including age-appropriate methods (e.g., videotapes, peer discussion, diagrams, and written materials). An assent form should be provided to each child to sign, and the child should keep a copy (Broome, 1999). By including children in the decision-making process and gaining their acceptance, children are treated with respect. Assent is not a legal requirement but an ethical one to protect the rights of children. The nurse, whether acting as a researcher, assisting in research, or caring for the child, must ultimately have the best interest of the child in mind (Algren and Schwartz, 1998).

### Eligibility for Giving Informed Consent

In most situations the parent or legal guardian gives informed consent. However, problems may arise when parents are not available to give informed consent, the child is a borderline or emancipated minor, or the parents neglect or refuse care for their minor children. Consent from either divorced parent is sufficient; the consent of both parents is generally not required (Bernardo and Lesniak, 1998).

**Informed Consent of Parents or Legal Guardians.** Parents have full responsibility for the care and rearing of their minor children, including legal control over them. Therefore, as long as children are minors, their parents or legal guardians are required to give informed consent before medical treatment is rendered or any procedure is performed. Parents also have a right to withdraw consent later.

**Evidence of Consent.** Whether consent is written or verbal depends on local, state, or institutional requirements. A signed consent form is only evidence that the process of informed consent has occurred; it is not legally required. Verbal consent is also evidence of the process (Selbst, 1999). For example, when parents are unavailable to sign consent forms, verbal consent may be obtained via telephone. Verbal consent may also be obtained from parents who are unable to sign (e.g., because of injury). It is good risk management to have a witness to a parent's or guardian's verbal consent. Another nurse may be present or listening on a telephone extension. Both nurses record that informed consent was given and the name, address, and re-

---

▮ Chris Algren, Ed, MSN, RN, and Debra Arnow, MSN, RN, CNA, revised this chapter.

lationship of the person giving consent, together with their signatures indicating that they witnessed the consent.

**Informed Consent of Mature and Emancipated Minors.** State laws differ with regard to the so-called age of majority. Although some variation still exists, children become adults on their eighteenth birthday in most states. Competent adults can give informed consent on their own behalf. Nonetheless, some courts have permitted minors to consent to their treatment based on the *mature minors' doctrine,* which permits minors to give consent even though they are not technically adults as long as they understand the consequences of their decisions (Moskop, 1999; Guertler, 1997). For example, statutes in many states permit minors to give consent on their own behalf to certain treatments, such as for sexually transmitted diseases, contraceptive services, pregnancy, or drug or alcohol abuse. (See Evidence-Based Practice box.)

An *emancipated minor* is one who is legally under the age of majority but is recognized as having the legal capacity of an adult under circumstances prescribed by state law, such as pregnancy, marriage, high school graduation, living independently, or military service.

Consent to abortion is more complex. The issue of parental notification before or after an abortion is still undecided, although several states have enacted laws stating that minors seeking abortions must involve their parents or obtain court permission (Johannsen, 1995). A woman's right to abortion is an extremely controversial legal and moral issue in the United States.

**Treatment Without Parental Consent.** Exceptions to requiring parental consent before treating minor children occur in situations in which children need prompt medical or surgical treatment and a parent is not readily available to give consent or refuses to give consent. In the absence of parents or legal guardians, some providers permit persons in charge of the child to give informed consent for treatment. In emergencies consent is not needed; it is implied according to the law (Selbst, 1999). Emergencies include danger to life or the possibility of permanent injury.

Refusal to give consent can occur when the treatment, such as blood transfusions, conflicts with the parents' religious beliefs. All states recognize such exceptions and have statutory procedures to permit treatment if the life or health of such a minor is in jeopardy or if delayed treatment would create a risk to the minor's health. The state is also able to intervene in situations that jeopardize the health and welfare of children, as in cases in which parents neglect or impose excessive or improper punishment on a child. Most communities have procedures by which custody of the child can be transferred to a governmental or private agency when parental neglect or abuse can be proved.

## Preparation for Diagnostic and Therapeutic Procedures

Technologic advances and changes in health care have resulted in more pediatric procedures being performed in a variety of settings. Many procedures are both stressful and painful experiences for children and their parents. For most procedures the focus of care is psychologic preparation of the child and family. However, some procedures require the administration of sedatives/analgesics.

### Psychologic Preparation

Preparing children for procedures decreases their anxiety, promotes their cooperation, supports their coping skills and may teach them new ones, and facilitates a feeling of mastery in experiencing a potentially stressful event. Many institutions have developed preadmission teaching programs designed to educate the pediatric patient and family by offering hands-on experience with hospital equipment, the procedure performed, and departments they will visit (Algren, Ireland, and Stewart, 1998). Preparatory methods may be formal, such as group preparation for hospitalization. Most preparation strategies used by nurses are informal, focus on providing information about the experience, and are directed at stressful or painful procedures.

General guidelines for preparing children for procedures are described and age-specific guidelines that consider children's developmental needs and cognitive abilities are presented in the Guidelines boxes on pp. 1104-1105. In addition to these suggestions, nurses should consider the child's temperament, existing coping strategies, and previous experiences in individualizing the preparatory process. Children who are distractible and highly active, as well as those who are "slow to warm up," may need individualized sessions that are shorter for the active child but more slowly paced for the shy child. Youngsters who tend to cope well may need more emphasis on using their present skills, whereas those who appear to cope less adequately can benefit from more time devoted to simple coping strategies, such as relaxing, breathing, counting, squeezing a hand, or singing. Children with previous health-related experiences still need preparation for repeat or new procedures; however, the nurse must assess what they know, correct misconceptions, supply new information, and introduce new coping skills as indicated by their previous reactions. Especially

---

## EVIDENCE-BASED PRACTICE

### Informed Consent and Parental Right to the Child's Medical Chart

Does the right to certain types of information before giving valid informed consent include the right to review medical records? Because the process of consent continues throughout the patient's treatment, is there an ongoing right of parents to see their children's medical charts?

The answer to these questions varies depending on state law. Some state statutes give parents the unrestricted right to a copy of children's medical records. Other states have no statutes that address this point. In these states the best practice is to allow parents to review or have a copy of minors' charts under reasonable circumstances. That is, records should be available in a reasonable time. In addition, practitioners should avoid restrictive requirements such as review permitted only in the presence of a clinician. Rather, an appropriate practitioner should be available to answer any questions that parents may have during their reviews.

## GUIDELINES
*Preparing Children for Procedures*

Determine the details of the exact procedure to be performed.

Review the parents' and child's present level of understanding.

Plan the actual teaching based on the child's developmental age and existing level of knowledge.

Incorporate parents in the teaching if they desire, especially if they plan to participate in the care.

Inform parents of their role during the procedure, such as standing near the child's head or in the line of vision and talking softly to the child.

While preparing the child and family, allow for ample discussion to prevent information overload and ensure adequate feedback.

Use concrete, not abstract, terms and visual aids to describe the procedure. For example, use a simple line drawing of a boy or girl (Fig. 27-1), and mark the body part that will be involved in the procedure.

Emphasize that no other body part will be involved.

If the body part is associated with a specific function, stress the change or noninvolvement of that ability (e.g., following tonsillectomy, the child can still speak).

Use words appropriate to the child's level of understanding (a rule of thumb for the number of words is the age in years plus 1).

Avoid words/phrases with dual meanings (see Guidelines box on p. 1108) unless the child understands such words.

Clarify all unfamiliar words (e.g., "Anesthesia is a *special* sleep").

Emphasize the sensory aspects of the procedure—what the child will feel, see, smell, and touch and what the child can do during the procedure (e.g., lie still, count out loud, squeeze a hand, hug a doll).

Allow the child to practice those procedures that will require cooperation (e.g., turning, deep breathing, using an incentive spirometer or mask).

Introduce anxiety-laden information last (e.g., an injection).

Be honest with the child about the unpleasant aspects of a procedure but avoid creating undue concern. When discussing that a procedure may be uncomfortable, state that it feels different to different people.

Emphasize the end of the procedure and any pleasurable events afterward (e.g., going home, seeing the parent). Stress the benefits of the procedure to the child (e.g., "After your tonsils are fixed, you won't have as many sore throats").

## GUIDELINES
*Preparing Children for Procedures Based on Developmental Characteristics*

### INFANCY: DEVELOPING A SENSE OF TRUST AND SENSORIMOTOR THOUGHT

#### Attachment to Parent

*Involve parent in procedure if desired.

Keep parent in infant's line of vision.

If parent is unable to be with infant, place familiar object with infant (e.g., stuffed toy).

#### Stranger Anxiety

*Have usual caregivers perform or assist with procedure.

Make advances slowly and in nonthreatening manner.

*Limit number of strangers entering room during procedure.

#### Sensorimotor Phase of Learning

During procedure use sensory soothing measures (e.g., stroking skin, talking softly, giving pacifier).

*Use analgesics (e.g., local anesthetic, intravenous opioid) to control discomfort.

Cuddle and hug child after stressful procedure; encourage parent to comfort child.

#### Increased Muscle Control

Expect older infants to resist.

Restrain adequately.

Keep harmful objects out of reach.

#### Memory of Past Experiences

Realize that older infants may associate objects, places, or persons with prior painful experiences and will cry and resist at the sight of them.

*Keep frightening objects out of view.

*Perform painful procedures in a separate room, not in crib (or bed).

*Use nonintrusive procedures whenever possible (e.g., axillary or tympanic temperatures, oral medication).

#### Imitation of Gestures

Model desired behavior (e.g., opening mouth).

---
*Applies to any age.

### TODDLER: DEVELOPING A SENSE OF AUTONOMY AND SENSORIMOTOR TO PREOPERATIONAL THOUGHT

Use same approaches as for infant in addition to the following:

#### Egocentric Thought

Explain procedure in relation to what child will see, hear, taste, smell, and feel.

Emphasize those aspects of procedure that require cooperation (e.g., lying still).

Tell child it's okay to cry, yell, or use other means to express discomfort verbally.

#### Negative Behavior

Expect treatments to be resisted; child may try to run away.

Use firm, direct approach.

Ignore temper tantrums.

Use distraction techniques (e.g., singing a song *with* a child).

Restrain adequately.

#### Animism

Keep frightening objects out of view (young children believe objects have lifelike qualities and can harm them).

#### Limited Language Skills

Communicate using behaviors.

Use a few, simple terms familiar to child.

Give one direction at a time (e.g., "Lie down," then "Hold my hand").

Use small replicas of equipment; allow child to handle equipment.

Use play; demonstrate on doll but avoid child's favorite doll, since child may think doll is really "feeling" procedure.

Prepare parents separately to avoid child's misinterpreting words.

#### Limited Concept of Time

Prepare child shortly or immediately before procedure.

Keep teaching sessions short (about 5 to 10 minutes).

Have preparations completed before involving child in procedure.

## GUIDELINES
*Preparing Children for Procedures Based on Developmental Characteristics—cont'd*

Have extra equipment nearby (e.g., alcohol swabs, new needle, adhesive bandages) to avoid delays.
Tell child when procedure is completed.

### *Striving for Independence*

Allow choices whenever possible but realize that child may still be resistant and negative.
Allow child to participate in care and to help whenever possible (e.g., drink medicine from a cup, hold a dressing).

### PRESCHOOLER: DEVELOPING A SENSE OF INITIATIVE AND PREOPERATIONAL THOUGHT

#### *Egocentric*

Explain procedure in simple terms and in relation to how it affects child (as with toddler, stress sensory aspects).
Demonstrate use of equipment.
Allow child to play with miniature or actual equipment.
Encourage "playing out" experience on a doll both before and after procedure to clarify misconceptions.
Use neutral words to describe the procedure (see Guidelines box on p. 1108).

#### *Increased Language Skills*

Use verbal explanation but avoid overestimating child's comprehension of words.
Encourage child to verbalize ideas and feelings.

#### *Concept of Time and Frustration Tolerance Skill Limited*

Implement same approaches as for toddler but may plan longer teaching session (10 to 15 minutes); may divide information into more than one session.

#### *Illness and Hospitalization May Be Viewed as Punishment*

Clarify why each procedure is performed; a child will find it difficult to understand how medicine can make him or her feel better and can taste bad at the same time.
Ask child thoughts regarding why a procedure is performed.
State directly that procedures are never a form of punishment.

#### *Animism*

Keep equipment out of sight, except when shown to or used on child.

#### *Fears of Bodily Harm, Intrusion, and Castration*

Point out on drawing, doll, or child where procedure is performed.
Emphasize that no other body part will be involved.
Use nonintrusive procedures whenever possible (e.g., axillary temperatures, oral medication).
Apply an adhesive bandage over puncture site.
Encourage parental presence.
Realize that procedures involving genitalia provoke anxiety.
Allow child to wear underpants with gown.
Explain unfamiliar situations, especially noises or lights.

#### *Striving for Initiative*

Involve child in care whenever possible (e.g., hold equipment, remove dressing).
Give choices whenever possible but avoid excessive delays.
Praise child for helping and attempting to cooperate; never shame child for lack of cooperation.

### SCHOOL-AGE CHILD: DEVELOPING A SENSE OF INDUSTRY AND CONCRETE THOUGHT

#### *Increased Language Skills; Interest in Acquiring Knowledge*

Explain procedures using correct scientific/medical terminology.

Explain reason for procedure using simple diagrams of anatomy and physiology.
Explain function/operation of equipment in concrete terms.
Allow child to manipulate equipment; use doll or another person as model to practice using equipment whenever possible (doll play may be considered "childish" by older school-age child).
Allow time before and after procedure for questions and discussion.

#### *Improved Concept of Time*

Plan for longer teaching sessions (about 20 minutes).
Prepare in advance of procedure.

#### *Increased Self-Control*

Gain child's cooperation.
Tell child what is expected.
Suggest ways of maintaining control (e.g., deep breathing, relaxation, counting).

#### *Striving for Industry*

Allow responsibility for simple tasks (e.g., collecting specimens).
Include in decision making (e.g., time of day to perform procedure, preferred site).
Encourage active participation (e.g., removing of dressings, handling equipment, opening packages).

#### *Developing Relationships with Peers*

May prepare two or more children for same procedure or encourage one to help prepare another peer.
Provide privacy from peers during procedure to maintain self-esteem.

### ADOLESCENT: DEVELOPING A SENSE OF IDENTITY AND ABSTRACT THOUGHT

#### *Increasingly Capable of Abstract Thought and Reasoning*

Supplement explanations with reasons why procedure is necessary or beneficial.
Explain long-term consequences of procedure.
Realize that adolescent may fear death, disability, or other potential risks.
Encourage questioning regarding fears, options, and alternatives.

#### *Conscious of Appearance*

Provide privacy.
Discuss how procedure may affect appearance (e.g., scar) and what can be done to minimize it.
Emphasize any physical benefits of procedure.

#### *Concerned More with Present Than with Future*

Realize that immediate effects of procedure are more significant than future benefits.

#### *Striving for Independence*

Involve in decision making and planning (e.g., choice of time; place; individuals present during procedure, such as parents; clothing to wear).
Impose as few restrictions as possible.
Suggest methods of maintaining control.
Accept regression to more childish methods of coping.
Realize that adolescent may have difficulty in accepting new authority figures and may resist complying with procedures.

#### *Developing Peer Relationships and Group Identity*

Same as for school-age child but assumes even greater significance.
Allow adolescent to talk with other adolescents who have had the same procedure.

for painful procedures, the most effective preparation includes provision of sensory-procedural information and helping the child develop coping skills, such as imagery or relaxation (Algren and Algren, 1998; Broome, Rehwaldt, and Fogg, 1998).

**NURSING TIP** Prepare a basket (toy or treasure chest or cart) to keep near the treatment area. Items ideal for the basket include a Slinky; a sparkling "magic" wand (clear, acrylic tube sealed on both ends and partially filled with liquid in which is suspended metallic confetti); a soft foam ball; bubble solution; party blowers; pop-up books with fold-out, three-dimensional scenes; real medical equipment, such as a syringe, adhesive bandages, and alcohol packets; toy medical supplies or a toy medical kit; marking pens; a note pad; and stickers. Have the child choose an item to use during a procedure, such as a party blower to help distract and relax the youngster. After the procedure, allow the child to choose a small gift, such as a sticker, or to play with items, such as medical equipment.

Children differ in their "information-seeking dimension." Some actively solicit information about the intended procedure, whereas others characteristically avoid information. Parents can often guide nurses in deciding how much information is enough for the child, because parents know whether the child is typically inquisitive or satisfied with short answers. Asking older children their preferences about the amount of explanation is also important. Drawings may also be helpful in preparing children for procedures (Fig. 27-1).

The exact timing of the preparation for a procedure varies with the child's age and the type of procedure. There are no exact guidelines to govern timing, but in general the younger the child, the closer the explanation should be to the actual procedure to prevent undue fantasizing and worrying. With complex procedures, more time may be needed for assimilation of information, especially with older children. For example, the explanation for an injection can immediately precede the procedure for all ages, but preparation for surgery may begin the day before for young children and a few days before for older children, although older children's preferences should be elicited. (See Preparation for Hospitalization, Chapter 26.)

**Establish Trust and Provide Support.** The nurse who has spent time with and who has established a positive relationship with a child will usually find it easier to gain cooperation. If the relationship is based on trust, the child will associate the nurse with caregiving activities that give comfort and pleasure most of the time and not as someone who brings discomfort and stress. If the nurse does not know the child, it is best if the nurse is introduced by another staff person whom the child trusts. The first visit with the child should not include any painful procedure and ideally should focus on the child first and then on explanation of the procedure. (When talking with the child, the nurse uses the same guidelines for communicating with children that are discussed in Chapter 6.)

**Parental Presence and Support.** Children need support during procedures, and for young children the greatest source of support is the parents. They represent security, safety, and comfort. However, controversy exists regarding the role parents should assume during the procedure, especially if discomfort is involved. (See Evidence-Based Practice

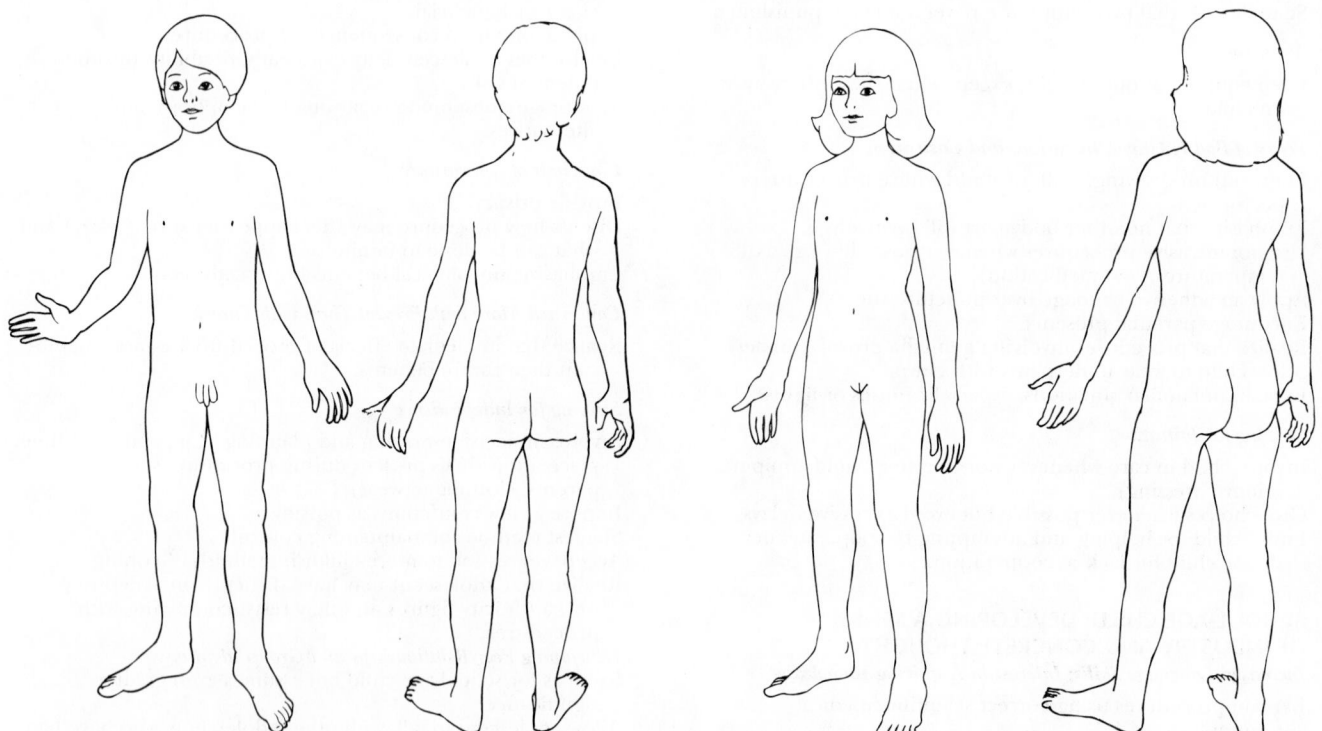

**Fig. 27-1** Examples of line drawings to be used in preparing child for procedures.

box.) Parental presence is preferable, however, because it can reduce patient and parent anxiety and decrease the need for sedation (Nelson, 1999). The parents' preferences for assisting, observing, or waiting outside the room should be assessed, as well as the child's preference for parental presence. The child's and parents' choices should be respected. Parents who wish to stay should be given appropriate explanation about the procedure and coached about what to do, where to sit or stand, and what to say to help the child through the procedure. Parents who do not want to be present are supported in their decision and encouraged to remain close by so that they can be available to support the child immediately following the procedure. Parents should also know that someone will be with their child to provide support. Ideally, this person should inform the parents after the procedure about how the child did.

**Provide an Explanation.**   Age-appropriate explanations are one of the most widely used interventions for reducing anxiety in children undergoing procedures. Before performing a procedure, the nurse explains to children what is to be done and what is expected of them. The explanation should be short, simple, and appropriate to the child's level of comprehension. Long explanations are not necessary and may only increase anxiety in a small child. This is especially true regarding painful procedures. When explaining the procedure to parents with the child present, the nurse uses language appropriate to the child because unfamiliar words can be misunderstood. (See Guidelines box on p. 1108.) If the parents

## EVIDENCE-BASED PRACTICE
### *Parental Presence During Their Child's Stressful Procedure*

A major source of stress for parents of a hospitalized child is the loss of the parental role. Parents often discuss their frustrations with not knowing how to help their child and not being able to protect them from pain (Melnyk, 2000). Over the years numerous studies have established the positive effects of parent involvement during the child's hospitalization. In recent years this involvement has expanded to include parental presence during invasive, often painful procedures. Researchers have found that parents want to participate, are cooperative, and even when the experience is difficult and stressful, are able to support their child (Giganti, 1998; LaRosa-Nash and Murphy, 1996; Melnyk, 2000). Changes in hospital policies to allow parental involvement in previously restricted areas such as operating rooms, intensive care settings, and emergency departments have occurred in many hospitals because previous fears and concerns have been addressed. These concerns include the following:

1. *Concern for infection:* Research found in the literature involved visitation policies in neonatal intensive care units. These studies revealed no increased infection rates when 24-hour visitation policies vs restricted hours were implemented (Giganti, 1998).
2. *Parents are perceived to be in the way:* Hospital staff frequently forget that the parent is granting permission for treatment and that staff are providing a service. Parental rights are often not considered.
3. *Confidentiality:* Health care providers may feel uncomfortable discussing details of the procedure in the presence of the parents because of concern that they may frighten the parent or appear unprofessional. Studies have found that parents can comfort their children during frightening events even when they are concerned and stressed. In addition, staff may act more professional when parents are present (Giganti, 1998; Melnyk, 2000).

In a study of parental presence during procedures in the emergency department, parents who were present reported less anxiety than absent parents, and clinicians did not find that parental presence interfered with their ability to perform the procedure (Bauchner and others, 1996). Boie and others (1999) evaluated the interest of parents in being present when invasive procedures were performed in the emergency department. This study used a written survey consisting of five pediatric scenarios of painful procedures. Four hundred parents waiting for their child to be seen in the emergency department completed the survey. The number of parents who desired to be present during a procedure was 387 (97.5%) for venipuncture, 375 (94%) for laceration repair, 341 (86.5%) for lumbar puncture, and 317 (80.9%) for endotracheal intubation. Eighty percent of the parents wished to be present during cardiopulmonary resuscitation (CPR). An important finding indicated that nearly all parents wanted to participate in the decision about their presence during the procedures (Boie and others, 1999).

Zain and others (1996) found that measures of anxiety did not differ significantly between parents who were either absent or present for induction of general anesthesia. However, serum cortisol levels (a marker for stress) were lower in children over 4 years of age when parents were present during induction. An interesting finding in this study was that parents rated their presence as being helpful to their child and the anesthesiologist, whereas the anesthesiologists rated parental presence as not being helpful. Blesch and Fisher (1996) found no significant differences in parental anxiety between parents attending during their child's anesthesia induction and parents not attending. Parents who were present during the induction expressed satisfaction with being there and having clear explanations of the procedure given to them. A well-coordinated parental presence during induction anesthesia program offers several benefits for the child and parents. Parents can maintain a role as comforter and supporter. They are able to see that their child is safe and may worry less about anesthesia. The child's stress may be reduced because of the parent is present (LaRosa-Nash and Murphy, 1996; Stephens, Barkey, and Hall, 1999).

Parental presence during invasive procedures in the pediatric intensive care unit also has been explored (Powers and Rubenstein, 1999). Invasive procedures included intubation and placement of central lines or chest tubes. This study used surveys given to parents of 16 children undergoing one or more invasive procedures. Results showed that parental presence significantly reduced parent anxiety related to the procedures but did not reduce anxiety related to the medical condition.

Parental participation in distraction and comfort measures during invasive procedures has been shown to be effective in decreasing the child's anxiety. Blount and others (1994) found that parents who were trained to use distraction methods such as toys, coloring books, and party blowers during the procedure helped reduce the child's severity of anxiety during bone marrow aspirations or lumbar punctures. One study examining the level of stress experienced by 57 parents observing a lumbar puncture found that parents who were present during the procedure experienced no difference in the level of anxiety than those who were not present (Haimi-Cohen and others, 1996).

Although there continues to remain considerable resistance to parental presence during CPR, the Emergency Nurses Association (1998) supports the option of family presence during resuscitation efforts. (This is further explored in Chapter 31.) The rights of parents who may lose a child during CPR or a life-threatening procedure should be considered when establishing all hospital "visiting" policies.

**GUIDELINES**

*Selecting Nonthreatening Words or Phrases*

| WORDS/PHRASES TO AVOID | SUGGESTED SUBSTITUTIONS | WORDS/PHRASES TO AVOID | SUGGESTED SUBSTITUTIONS |
|---|---|---|---|
| Shot, bee sting, stick | Medicine under the skin | Deaden | Numb, make sleepy |
| Organ | Special place in body | Cut, fix | Make better |
| Test | See how [specify body part] is working | Take (as in "take your temperature or blood pressure") | See how warm you are Check your pressure; hug your arm |
| Incision | Special opening | Put to sleep, anesthesia | Special sleep |
| Edema | Puffiness | Catheter | Tube, straw |
| Stretcher, gurney | Rolling bed | Monitor | TV screen |
| Stool | Child's usual term | Electrodes | Stickers, ticklers |
| Dye | Special medicine | Specimen | Sample |
| Pain | Hurt, discomfort, "ouch," "owie," "boo-boo" | | |

need additional preparation, this is done in an area away from the child. Teaching sessions are planned at times most conducive to the child's learning (e.g., after a rest period).

Special equipment is not necessary for preparing a child, but for young children who cannot yet think conceptually, using objects to supplement verbal explanation is important. Allowing children to handle actual items that will be used in their care, such as a stethoscope, sphygmomanometer, or oxygen mask, helps them to develop familiarity with these items and to reduce the threat often associated with their use. Miniature versions of hospital items such as gurneys and x-ray and intravenous (IV) equipment can be used to explain what the children can expect and permit them to safely experience situations that are unfamiliar and potentially frightening. Written and illustrated materials are also valuable aids to preparation.*

**NURSING TIP** Use photographs of children in different areas of the hospital (e.g., radiology department, operating room) to give children a more realistic idea of equipment they may encounter.

### Physical Preparation

For many diagnostic and therapeutic procedures, no special physical preparation is needed. However, some do require physical preparation. One area of special concern is the administration of appropriate sedation and analgesia before stressful procedures. The drug is given before the procedure to allow time for the medication to reach its peak effect. Whenever possible, the IV (through an existing infusion), oral, or transdermal route is used rather than the intramuscular (IM) or rectal route because children dislike injections and body intrusions. Buffering lidocaine with sodium bicarbonate (10:1, 1% or 2% lidocaine/NaHCO$_3$)

---

*Sources of preparatory materials include *Going to the Hospital* and *Going to the Doctor*, available from **Family Communications, Inc**, 4802 5th Ave, Pittsburgh, PA 15213, (412) 687-2990; www.fci.org; *Hospital Friends*, available from the **Centering Corporation**, 1531 N Saddle Creek Rd, Omaha, NE 68104, (402) 553-1200; www.centering.org; and *Health, Illness, and Disability: A Guide to Books for Children and Young Adults*, available from **Pediatric Projects, Inc**, PO Box 571555, Tarzana, CA 91357-1555, (800) 947-0947. Other resources include *Berenstein Bears Go to the Doctor* and *Berenstein Bears Visit the Dentist* (New York, Random House), available in most bookstores.

will reduce pain caused by the injection of local anesthetic. EMLA, a eutectic mixture of local anesthetics, may be used to reduce the pain of venipunctures. It should be applied 1 to 2 hours before the procedure to intact skin. Another option for local anesthesia is Numby Stuff, which uses iontophoresis to increase absorption of lidocaine. Some institutions are using short-acting anesthetics (e.g., propofol or ketamine), general anesthetics, or potent analgesics (e.g., fentanyl) to eliminate the pain and trauma associated with treatments such as bone marrow aspirations, lumbar punctures, burn debridement, and suturing (see Preoperative Sedation, p. 1112). (See Pain Management, Chapter 26.)

The safety of sedated children can be facilitaed by performing a detailed presedation assessment, carefully selecting patients for sedation, and using drugs with a wide margin of safety. Once sedatives are administered, stringent monitoring will permit early recognition of untoward drug effects (Malviya and others, 2000). The use of sedating drugs for procedures has serious associated risks, such as hypoventilation, apnea, airway obstruction, and cardiopulmonary impairment. In a recent study, adverse events were associated with all routes and all classes of drugs, even those thought to have minimal effect on respiration (Coté and others, 2000).

It is recommended that sedation be viewed as a continuum, ranging from conscious to deep sedation. ***Conscious sedation*** is a medically controlled state of depressed consciousness that (1) allows protective reflexes to be maintained, (2) retains the patient's ability to maintain a patent airway independently, and (3) permits appropriate response by the patient to physical stimulation or verbal command (e.g., "Open your eyes"). ***Deep sedation*** is a medically controlled state of depressed consciousness or unconsciousness from which the patient is not easily aroused. This state may be accompanied by (1) partial or complete loss of protective reflexes, (2) loss of the ability to maintain an independent patent airway, and (3) loss of the ability to respond to physical stimulation or verbal command. The loss of these capabilities may progress to general anesthesia (Algren and Algren, 1997).

Reports of adverse events have led to the development of guidelines and standards of care to ensure the safety of sedated children. The American Society of Anesthesiologists

(1996) and the American Academy of Pediatrics (1992) have developed policies and guidelines for sedation. These guidelines emphasize provision of emergency equipment, such as a positive-pressure oxygen delivery system, airway management and breathing equipment, and an emergency cart. The patient's level of consciousness and responsiveness, heart rate, blood pressure, respiratory rate, and oxygen saturation (via pulse oximetry) must be monitored during the procedure by an individual present for this purpose. In all cases the patient's condition after the procedure is also documented.

The use of *nitrous oxide* for conscious sedation (defined as the administration of nitrous oxide—50% or less, with the balance as oxygen, without any other sedative, opioid, or other depressant drug before or concurrent with the nitrous oxide) does not require pulse oximetry monitoring, although it is strongly encouraged. The patient is able to maintain verbal communication throughout, and a second individual whose responsibility is to monitor the patient may also assist with the procedure. In all cases the patient's condition after the procedure is also documented.

## Performance of the Procedure

Supportive care continues during the procedure and can be a major factor in a child's ability to cooperate. Ideally, the same nurse who explains the procedure should perform or assist with the procedure. Before beginning, all equipment is assembled and the room is readied to prevent unnecessary delays and interruptions that only serve to increase the child's anxiety.

**NURSING TIP**   To avoid a delay during a procedure, have extra supplies handy. For example, have tape, bandages, alcohol swabs, and an extra needle in your pocket when giving an injection or performing a venipuncture.

If at all possible, procedures should be performed in a special treatment room rather than the child's hospital room. Traumatic procedures should never be performed in "safe" areas, such as the playroom. If the procedure is lengthy, conversation that could be misinterpreted by the child is avoided. As the procedure is nearing completion, the nurse should inform the child that it is almost over in language the child understands.

**Expect Success.**   Nurses who approach children with confidence and who convey the impression that they expect to be successful are less likely to encounter difficulty. It is best to approach a child as though cooperation is expected. Children sense anxiety and uncertainty in an adult and will respond by striking out or actively resisting. Although it is not possible to eliminate such behavior in every child, a firm approach with a positive attitude from the nurse tends to convey a feeling of security to most children.

**Involve the Child.**   As in any other aspect of care, involving children helps to gain their cooperation. Permitting them to make choices gives them some measure of control. However, a choice is given only in situations in which one is available. Asking children, "Do you want to take your medicine now?" or "I'm going to give you an injection now, okay?" leads them to believe that there is an option and pro-

vides them with the opportunity to legitimately refuse or delay the medication. This places the nurse in an awkward, if not impossible, position. It is much better to state firmly, "It's time to drink your medicine now." Children usually like to make choices, but the choice must be one that they do indeed have (e.g., "It's time for your medicine. Do you want to drink it plain or with a little water?"). When giving instructions, describe the expected behavior, such as "Keep your leg still," rather than giving orders, such as "Don't move your leg."

Many children respond to tactics that appeal to their maturity or courage. This also gives them a sense of participation and achievement. For example, preschool children will be proud that they can hold the dressing during the procedure or remove the tape. The same is true for the school-age child, who often cooperates with minimal resistance.

**Provide Distraction.**   Distraction is a powerful coping strategy during painful procedures (Algren and Algren, 1998). It is accomplished by focusing the child's attention on something other than the procedure. Singing favorite songs, listening to music with a headset, counting aloud, or blowing bubbles to "blow the hurt away" are effective techniques. (For other nonpharmacologic interventions, see Chapter 26.)

**NURSING TIP**   Help the child to select and practice a coping technique before the procedure. Consider having the parent or some other supportive person, such as a child-life specialist, "coach" the child in learning and using the coping skill.

**Allow Expression of Feelings.**   The child should be allowed to express feelings of anger, anxiety, fear, frustration, or any other emotion. It is natural for children to strike out in frustration or to try to avoid stress-provoking situations. The child needs to know that it is all right to cry. Whatever the response, the nurse must accept the behavior for what it is. Telling a child with limited verbal skills, such as a toddler, to stop kicking, biting, or otherwise expressing frustration conveys to the child that he or she is not being understood. Behavior is children's primary means of communication and coping and should be permitted unless it inflicts harm on them or those caring for them.

## Postprocedural Support

After the procedure the child continues to need reassurance that he or she performed well and is accepted and loved. If the parents did not participate, the child is united with them as soon as possible so that they can provide comfort.

**Encourage Expression of Feelings.**   Planned activity after the procedure is helpful in encouraging constructive expression of feelings. For verbal children, reviewing the details of the procedure can clarify misconceptions and provide feedback for improving the nurse's preparatory strategies. Play is an excellent activity for all children. Infants and young children are given the opportunity for gross motor movement. Even older children are able to vent their anger and frustration in acceptable pounding or throwing activities. Play dough is a remarkably versatile medium for pounding and shaping. Dramatic play provides

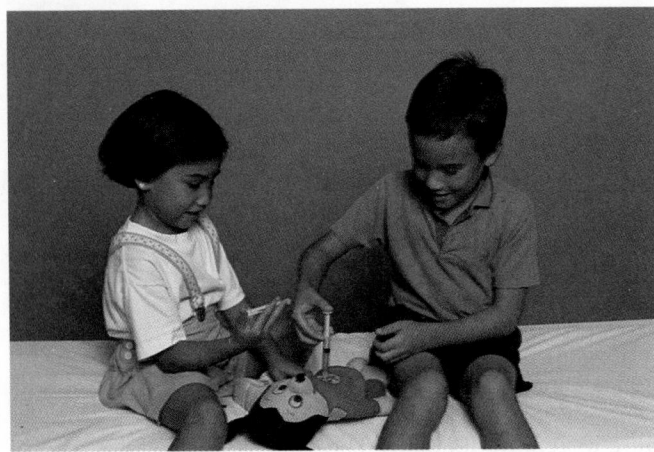

**Fig. 27-2** Playing with syringes provides children with the opportunity to play out fears and concerns.

an outlet for anger and places the child in a position of control, in contrast to the position of helplessness in the real situation. Puppets may also be used to allow the child to communicate feelings in a nonthreatening way. One of the most effective interventions is therapeutic play, which includes well-supervised activities such as permitting the child to give an injection to a doll or stuffed toy to reduce the stress of injections (Fig. 27-2). (See next section and Using Play/Expressive Activities to Minimize Stress, Chapter 26.)

**Positive Reinforcement.** Children need to hear from adults that they did the best they could in the situation—no matter how they behaved. For example, a child may be praised for holding still during a procedure even if they screamed. It is important for children to know that their worth is not being judged on the basis of their behavior in a stressful situation. Reward systems, such as earning stars, stickers, or a badge of courage are often helpful.

Returning to the child a short while after the procedure helps the nurse to strengthen a supportive relationship. Relating with the child in a relaxed and nonstressful period allows him or her to see the nurse not only as someone associated with stressful situations but as someone with whom to share pleasurable experiences as well.

### Use of Play in Procedures

The use of play is an integral part of relationships with children. As such, its value in specific situations is discussed throughout this book, such as in Chapter 26 in relation to hospitalization. Many institutions have very elaborate and well-organized play areas and programs under the direction of child-life specialists; other institutions have limited facilities. However, no matter what the institution provides for children, nurses can still include play activities as part of nursing care. Play can be used to teach, for expression of feelings, or as a method to achieve a therapeutic goal. Consequently, it should be included in preparing children for and encouraging their cooperation during procedures. Play sessions after procedures can be structured, such as directed toward needle play, or general, with a wide variety of equipment available for children to play with.

**NURSING TIP** Play can also be spontaneous at the bedside and does not always require many supplies or much nursing time. Small items, such as finger puppets or a small bottle of bubbles, can be kept in the nurse's pocket for immediate use.

Even "routine" procedures such as measuring blood pressure and oral administration of medication may be of concern to children. Suggestions for incorporating play into nursing procedures and activities for the hospitalized child that facilitate learning and adjustment to a new situation are described in Box 27-1.

## Surgical Procedures

### Preoperative Care

Children experiencing surgical procedures require both psychologic and physical preparation. In general, psychologic preparation is similar to that discussed earlier for any procedure and employs many of the same techniques used in preparing a child for hospitalization, such as films, books, brochures, play, and tours. (See Chapter 26.) However, some important differences exist. Even though children are asleep for the actual surgical intervention, they are subjected to numerous preoperative and postoperative procedures. Stress points before and after surgery include the admission, the blood test, injection of preoperative medication (if prescribed), the period before and during transport to the operating room, and the return from the postanesthesia care unit (PACU).

Psychologic intervention consisting of systematic preparation, rehearsal of the forthcoming events, and supportive care at each of these points has been shown to be more effective than a single-session preparation (which is a common method of preoperative preparation) or consistent supportive care without systematic preparation and rehearsal. Play is always an effective strategy in preparing children, and increased familiarity with medical procedures decreases anxiety.

Surprisingly little research has been conducted on children's perception of the surgical experience and their fears of the event. Although fear of anesthesia is thought to be a major concern among children, little evidence of this exists. One study of school-age children reported few remembered events and even fewer fears. Those events recalled most often were the ride to and arriving in the operating room, the preoperative or induction injection, waking up in pain, and not being allowed to eat or drink. The most feared events were the injection and the mask on the face.

**Parental Presence.** Parent-present induction (PPI) grew out of the trend to increase parental participation in the care of the child and thus decrease separation anxiety. Parental presence during induction of anesthesia is becoming a more common practice. Although few institutions endorse the policy (Fig. 27-3), reports from parents who attend the induction are very favorable. Even though some may become anxious, most parents control their anxiety, do not disrupt the induction, and support the child (Hall and others, 1995; LaRosa-Nash and Murphy, 1997; Munro and

## Box 27-1 ■ ■ ■
### Play Activities for Specific Procedures

**FLUID INTAKE**

Make freezer pops using child's favorite juice.
Cut gelatin into fun shapes.
Make game of taking sip when turning page of book or in games such as "Simon Says."
Use small medicine cups; decorate the cups.
Color water with food coloring or powdered drink mix.
Have a tea party; pour at small table.
Let child fill a syringe and squirt it into mouth or use it to fill small, decorated cups.
Cut straws in half and place in small container (much easier for child to suck liquid).
Decorate straw: cut out small design with two holes and pass straw through; place small sticker on straw.
Use a "crazy" straw.
Make a "progress poster"; give rewards for drinking a predetermined quantity.

**DEEP BREATHING**

Blow bubbles with bubble blower.
Blow bubbles with straw (no soap).
Blow on pinwheel, feathers, whistle, harmonica, balloons, toy horns, party blowers.
Practice band instruments.
Have blowing contest using balloons, boats, cotton balls, feathers, marbles, Ping-Pong balls, pieces of paper; blow such objects on a table top over a goal line, over water, through an obstacle course, up in the air, against an opponent, or up and down a string.
Suck paper or cloth from one container to another using a straw.
Use blow bottles with colored water to transfer water from one side to the other.
Dramatize stories, such as "I'll huff and puff and blow your house down" from the Three Little Pigs.
Do straw-blowing painting.
Take a deep breath and "blow out the candles" on a birthday cake.
Use a little paint brush to "paint" nails with water and blow nails dry.

**RANGE OF MOTION AND USE OF EXTREMITIES**

Throw beanbags at fixed or movable target; toss wadded paper into wastebasket.
Touch or kick Mylar balloons held or hung in different positions (if child is in traction, hang balloon from trapeze).
Play "tickle toes"; wiggle them on request.
Play Twister game or "Simon Says."
Play pretend and guess games (e.g., imitate a bird, butterfly, horse).
Have tricycle or wheelchair races in safe area.
Play kick or throw ball with soft foam ball in safe area.
Position bed so that child must turn to view television or doorway.
Climb wall like a "spider."
Pretend to teach "aerobic" dancing or exercises; encourage parents to participate.

Encourage swimming if feasible.
Play video games or pinball (fine motor movement).
Play "hide and seek" game: hide toy somewhere in bed (or room if ambulatory) and have child find it using specified hand or foot.
Provide clay to mold with fingers.
Paint or draw on large sheets of paper placed on floor or wall.
Encourage combing own hair; play "beauty shop" with "customer" in different positions.

**SOAKS**

Play with small toys or objects (cups, syringes, soap dishes) in water.
Wash dolls or toys.
Bubbles may be added to bathwater if permissible; move bubbles to create shapes or "monsters."
Pick up marbles, pennies* from bottom of bath container.
Make designs with coins on bottom of container.
Pretend a boat is a submarine by keeping it immersed.
Read to child during soaks, sing with child, or play game, such as cards, checkers, or other board game (if both hands are immersed, move the board pieces for the child).
Sitz bath: give child something to listen to (music, stories) or look at (Viewmaster, book).
Punch holes in bottom of plastic cup, fill with water, and let it "rain" on child.

**INJECTIONS**

Let child handle syringe, vial, alcohol swab and give an injection to doll or stuffed animal.
Use syringes to decorate cookies with frosting, squirt paint, or target shoot into a container.
Draw a "magic circle" on area before injection; draw smiling face in circle after injection, but avoid drawing on puncture site.
Allow child to have a "collection" of syringes (without needles); make "wild" creative objects with syringes.
If child is receiving multiple injections or venipunctures, make a "progress poster"; give rewards for predetermined number of injections.
Have child count to 10 or 15 during injection or "blow the hurt away."

**AMBULATION**

Give child something to push.
    Toddler: push-pull toy
    School-age child: wagon or decorated IV stand
    Adolescent: a baby in a stroller or wheelchair
Have a parade; make hats, drums, etc.

**EXTENDING ENVIRONMENT (PATIENTS IN TRACTION, ETC.)**

Make bed into a private ship or airplane with decorations.
Put up mirrors so patient can see around room.
Move patient's bed frequently, especially to playroom, hallway, or outside.

*Small objects such as marbles or coins, as well as gloves or balloons, are unsafe for young children because of possible aspiration. Latex products also produce the risk of an allergic reaction.

---

D'Errico, 2000). Clinical observations show parental presence decreases anxiety in the child and reduces the need for heavy doses of preoperative sedation (Fennell, 1999).

Some concern exists regarding the appropriateness of this practice for all parents. Some parents may become upset by the rapid succession of induction events, by observing their child becoming limp, and by leaving the child in the care of strangers. Parents who are very anxious before

surgery tend to become even more anxious after the induction, whereas the reverse is true of parents with little anxiety.

However, based on the parents' favorable response to the practice and most children's desire to have their parents with them during any stressful procedure, parents should have the option of attending the induction. (See Evidence-Based Practice box, p. 1107.) Appropriate education is essential, however, to help parents understand the stages of

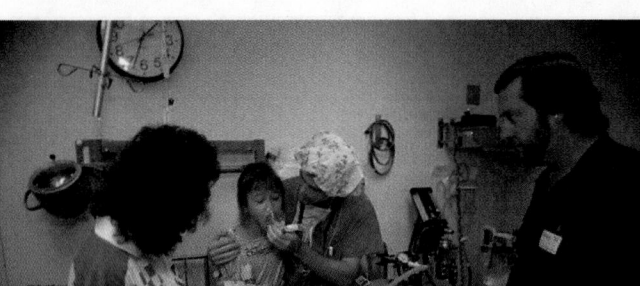

**Fig. 27-3** Parental presence during induction of anesthesia can minimize the child's and parents' anxiety during the preoperative period.

## GUIDELINES
### Preoperative Checklist

☐ Signed informed consent on chart and properly witnessed.
☐ Child receives nothing by mouth (NPO) for appropriate length of time.
☐ Child's medication orders changed as needed because of NPO status.
☐ Results of laboratory tests and vital signs reviewed for abnormal findings, such as elevated temperature, and reported to practitioner.
☐ Any specific physical preparation of surgical area, such as shaving or administration of enemas, performed.
☐ Child appropriately attired and any personal items (e.g., underwear or favorite toy) labeled.
☐ Dental appliances (e.g., retainers) contact lenses, prosthesis, hearing aid, nail polish, and makeup removed.
☐ Loose teeth and appliances remaining with child noted on chart.
☐ Child voided before preoperative sedation administered.
☐ Child wearing correct patient identification.
☐ Child's identification charge card on chart.
☐ Child and family adequately prepared for surgery experience (e.g., where family can wait for surgeon's report; whether parents can accompany child to perioperative suite, induction area, or PACU).
☐ Any special circumstances, such as allergies, skin problems, respiratory or cardiac conditions, paralysis, or family history of malignant hyperthermia, clearly displayed on front of chart.
☐ History and physical examination, including child's weight and laboratory test results, indicated on chart.

anesthesia, what to expect, and how to support their child (Fennell, 1999). When parents choose not to or are not allowed to attend the induction, leaving a favorite possession with the child and uniting the child and parents as soon as possible after surgery (preferably in the PACU) are important interventions. During surgery the family should have a designated place to wait and should be kept informed of the child's progress. They also should know where and when they can visit the child after surgery.

Aside from possibly being separated from the parents before and after surgery, children also may be cared for by a number of unfamiliar practitioners (e.g., 7 to 12 staff during a 24-hour period), which promotes fear and uncertainty (Kristensson-Hallstrom, 2000). Although the same supportive nurse should remain with the child through as many of the procedures as possible, the child may have other nurses, especially if the patient returns to a special care unit postoperatively. However, joint planning of care between the various nursing staffs, such as in pediatrics and the PACU, can overcome some of the disadvantages of unfamiliar nurses caring for the child. Many hospitals have surgical tours for children and parents to familiarize them with the strange environment and to introduce them to other individuals who will be involved in their care (Stewart, Algren, and Arnold, 1994).

**Physical Care.** Besides psychologic preparation, children usually require various types of physical care before surgery, such as those listed in the Guidelines box and in the Nursing Care Plan on pp. 1114-1117. Traditionally, solid food and nonclear liquids were withheld from the midnight before surgery, with clear liquids withheld from 4 to 8 hours before the procedure, depending on the child's age. However, research indicates that clear liquids given up to 2 hours before surgery for children of any age do not present any additional risk for pulmonary aspiration in those undergoing elective surgery. New guidelines can be summarized as 8-6-4-2 (i.e., 8 hours solids, 6 hours formula, 4 hours breast milk, 2 hours clear liquids). This results in children who are less anxious, better hydrated, and have

fewer headaches and nausea postoperatively* (Maxwell and Yaster, 2000.) (See Guidelines box.)

Although most preoperative care procedures are routine, nurses should keep in mind that they can be anxiety provoking for children and parents. For example, for young children, having to wear a hospital gown without the security of underpants or pajama bottoms can be traumatic. Therefore these articles of clothing should be allowed. They can be removed after induction of anesthesia.

**Preoperative Sedation.** Historically the most upsetting event for children has been the preoperative injection. Unfortunately, little research has been done on the necessity of this practice. If children have no preoperative pain, are well prepared psychologically for surgery, and have their parents nearby, preanesthetic medication may be unnecessary. When drugs are used, administration should be "atraumatic" by using oral or IV routes.

Numerous preanesthetic drug regimens are used with children, and no consensus exists on the optimum method. The goals for using preoperative medications include (1) anxiety reduction, (2) amnesia, (3) sedation, (4) antiemetic effect, and (5) reduction of secretions (Landsman and Cook, 1998; Manworren and Fledderman, 2000) (Box 27-2). Midazolam (Versed) provides excellent preoperative anxiety reduction, amnesia, and sedation. It is popular because of its short duration, predictable onset, and rare occurrence of respiratory depression. Oral transmucosal fentanyl (OTFC), or Fentanyl Oralet, is available

---

*http://asahq.org/Practice/NPO/NPOguide.html

## GUIDELINES

### Summary of Fasting Recommendations to Reduce the Risk of Pulmonary Aspiration*

| INGESTED MATERIAL | MINIMUM FASTING PERIOD (HOURS)† |
|---|---|
| Clear liquids‡ | 2 |
| Breast milk | 4 |
| Infant formula | 6 |
| Nonhuman milk§ | 6 |
| Light meal‖ | 6 |

From American Society of Anesthesiologists: Practice guidelines for preoperative fasting and the use of pharmacologic agents to reduce the risk of pulmonary aspiration: application to healthy patients undergoing elective procedures, *Anesthesiology* 90(3):896-905, 1999; *www.ASAhq.org/practice/NPO/NPOguide.html.*
*These recommendations apply to healthy patients who are undergoing elective procedures. They are not intended for women in labor. Following the guidelines does not guarantee a complete gastric emptying has occurred.
†The fasting periods noted above apply to all ages.
‡Examples of clear liquids include water, fruit juices without pulp, carbonated beverages, clear tea, and black coffee.
§Since nonhuman milk is similar to solids in gastric emptying time, the amount ingested must be considered when determining an appropriate fasting period.
‖A light meal typically consists of toast and clear liquids. Meals that include fried or fatty foods or meat may prolong gastric emptying time. Both the amount and type of foods ingested must be considered when determining an appropriate fasting period.

### Box 27-2 ■ ■ ■
### Suggested Medications for Sedation

**OPIOIDS***

Morphine sulfate, 0.05 to 0.10 mg/kg IV over 1 to 2 minutes given 5 minutes before procedure
Fentanyl, 1 to 2 μg/kg (0.001 to 0.002 mg/kg) IV 3 minutes before procedure
Fentanyl Oralet, 5 to 15 μg/kg, maximum to 400 μg, orally 20 to 40 minutes before procedure†
Hydromorphone (Dilaudid), 0.015 to 0.02 mg/kg IV over 1 to 2 minutes given 5 minutes before procedure.
Meperidine (if morphine sulfate or fentanyl is not available), 0.5 to 1 mg/kg IV over 1 to 2 minutes given 2 to 5 minutes before procedure or 1.5 mg/kg orally 45 to 60 minutes before procedure

**SEDATIVES‡**

Midazolam (Versed), 0.25 to 0.5 mg/kg (children 6 months to less than 6 years of age and less cooperative children may require a higher dose of up to 1 mg/kg), maximum to 20 mg, using oral preparation, 10 to 20 minutes, or 0.05 mg/kg IV 3 minutes before procedure
Diazepam (Valium), 0.2 to 0.3 mg/kg, maximum to 10 mg, orally 45 to 60 minutes before procedure
Pentobarbital (Nembutal), 1 to 3 mg/kg IV boluses to maximum of 100 mg until asleep
Chloral hydrate, 50 to 75 mg/kg, to maximum of 100 mg/kg or 2.5 g, orally or rectally 60 minutes before procedure

Modified from Zeltzer LK and others: Report of the subcommittee on the management of pain associated with procedures in children with cancer, *Pediatrics* 86(suppl):826-831, 1990; and Coté CJ: Sedation for the pediatric patient, *Pediatr Clin North Am* 41(1):31-58, 1994; and Yaster M and others: *Pediatric pain management and sedation handbook*, St Louis, 1997, Mosby.
*Provide analgesia and sedation.
†Not recommended for children less than 15 kg. Lozenge should be sucked, not chewed and swallowed. If chewed, drug is less effective because part of it is metabolized by liver before entering bloodstream. Swallowing drug rapidly does not increase risk of respiratory depression during first 15 to 30 minutes, period of greatest risk for decreased respiration.
‡Provide sedation but no analgesia.

as a sweetened lozenge on a plastic stick. When first approved, this appeared to be an excellent, atraumatic route of administration. However, associated nausea and vomiting, respiratory depression, and the need for more intensive monitoring and observation than with other oral sedatives have limited its popularity to date (Cravero, Manzi, and Rice, 1998).

Anesthesia induction of the pediatric patient is commonly accomplished by administering inhalation agents in combination with nitrous oxide and oxygen by mask. Children may fear induction of anesthesia by mask. Practices that can minimize anxiety related to inhalation anesthesia are (1) disguising the unpleasant odor of anesthetic gases by applying a pleasant-smelling substance on the mask; (2) using a transparent plastic mask rather than an opaque black mask and gradually bringing it toward the face; (3) directing a stream of gas toward the child's face from the bare tube until the child becomes drowsy, then using the mask; (4) allowing the child to sit up rather than lie down for anesthesia induction; and (5) allowing preoperative play with a mask and a doll or mannikin.

### Postoperative Care

Immediately following surgery, the child is admitted to the PACU. Various psychologic and physical interventions and observations are required to prevent or minimize possible untoward effects from anesthesia and the surgical procedure. (See Nursing Care Plan on pp. 1114-1117.) Although the incidence of serious postoperative complications in healthy children undergoing surgery is less than 1% (Maxwell and Yaster, 2000), continuous monitoring of the child's cardiopulmonary status is essential during the immediate postoperative period. Postanesthesia complications

such as airway obstruction, postextubation croup, laryngospasm, and bronchospasm make maintaining a patent airway and maximum ventilation critical.

Monitoring of the patient's oxygen saturation and providing supplemental oxygen as needed, maintaining body temperature, and promoting fluid and electrolyte balance are important aspects of immediate postoperative care. Vital signs are continuously monitored, and each vital sign is evaluated in terms of side effects from anesthesia, shock, or respiratory compromise (see Table 27-1).

A change in vital signs that demands immediate attention in the perioperative period is caused by *malignant hyperthermia (MH)*, a potentially fatal genetic myopathy. In susceptible children anesthetics such as succinylcholine and halothane trigger the disorder, producing hypermetabolism, muscle rigidity, and an elevated temperature. Early symptoms of the disorder include tachycardia and tachyarrhythmias, tachypnea, hypercarbia, and metabolic and respiratory acidosis. An elevated temperature is considered by many to be a late sign of the disorder (Miranda and others, 1997; Noble and others, 1997). Early screening and identification of patients at risk for developing MH before surgery is imperative. Children with a family or previous history of sud-

# Nursing Care Plan
## The Child Undergoing Surgery

### PREOPERATIVE CARE

> **NURSING DIAGNOSIS:** Risk for injury related to surgical procedure, anesthesia

**PATIENT GOAL 1:** Will receive fully informed consent and sign appropriate documents

- **NURSING INTERVENTIONS/RATIONALES**

Inquire whether parents have any questions about procedure *to determine their level of understanding and to provide for additional information (from nurse or other professional)*

Check chart for signed informed consent form or obtain informed consent

Contact physician to determine if parents have been informed of procedure *because informed consent is physician's responsibility*

Obtain and witness signature if not obtained earlier

- **EXPECTED OUTCOMES**

Family receives fully informed consent

Family signs appropriate documents

**PATIENT GOAL 2:** Will receive proper hygiene measures

- **NURSING INTERVENTIONS/RATIONALES**

Bathe child, groom hair

Provide mouth care *to promote comfort while NPO*

Cleanse operative site according to prescribed method, if ordered, *to minimize risk of infection*

- **EXPECTED OUTCOME**

Child is cleansed and prepared appropriately (specify)

**PATIENT GOAL 3:** Will receive proper preparation

- **NURSING INTERVENTIONS/RATIONALES**

Carry out special procedure as prescribed (e.g., colonic enemas)

*Administer antibiotics as ordered, observing for known side effects

Order or assist with special tests such as radiographs

Consult with practitioner for appropriate change in schedule or route of administration of any medication child ordinarily receives

Attire child appropriately (e.g., special operating room gown)

Allow child to wear underwear or pajama bottoms, if possible, *to provide privacy*

Label personal articles and clothing

Remove any makeup and nail polish *to observe for cyanosis*

Remove jewelry and prosthetic devices (e.g., mouth retainers) *because they may be lost or interfere with anesthesia/surgery*

Check for loose teeth

Inform anesthesiologist, if detected, *to prevent aspiration of teeth during anesthesia*

- **EXPECTED OUTCOME**

Child is prepared appropriately (specify)

---
*Dependent nursing action.

**PATIENT GOAL 4:** Will experience no complications

- **NURSING INTERVENTIONS/RATIONALES**

Maintain child NPO (nothing by mouth) as ordered *to prevent aspiration during anesthesia (clear liquids up to 2 hours before surgery for children at any age pose no additional risk for pulmonary aspiration during elective surgery)*

Be sure child is well hydrated before NPO begins, especially infants *who are more at risk for dehydration*

Take and record vital signs

Report any deviations from admission readings, especially elevated temperature, *which may indicate infection*

Have child void before preoperative medication is administered *to prevent bladder distention or incontinence during anesthesia*

Record time of last voiding if unable to void

Be certain allergies are clearly indicated on chart *to decrease risk of adverse reaction*

Check laboratory values for any sign of systemic abnormality, such as infection (increased white blood cells), anemia (decreased hemoglobin and/or hematocrit), or bleeding tendencies (reduced platelets or prolonged bleeding or clotting time)

Keep small infants warm during transport and waiting time

- **EXPECTED OUTCOMES**

Child is NPO for designated time preoperatively

Child voids

Pertinent information about child is visible

**PATIENT GOAL 5:** Will experience no injury

- **NURSING INTERVENTIONS/RATIONALES**

Check that identification band is securely fastened

Check identification band with surgical personnel *to ensure correct identification*

Fasten side rails of bed or crib *to prevent falls*

Use restraints during transport by stretcher (or other conveyance) *to prevent falls*

Do not leave child unattended

- **EXPECTED OUTCOMES**

Child is safe from immediate harm

Child is clearly and correctly identified

> **NURSING DIAGNOSIS:** Anxiety/fear related to separation from support system, unfamiliar environment, knowledge deficit

**PATIENT GOAL 1:** Will demonstrate optimum sense of security

- **NURSING INTERVENTIONS/RATIONALES**

Institute preoperative teaching *to reduce anxiety/fear*

Orient child to strange surroundings

Explain where parents will be while child is in operating room

Have someone stay with child *to provide increased sense of security*

- **EXPECTED OUTCOME**

Child demonstrates minimum insecurity or anxiety

## *Nursing Care Plan*
## The Child Undergoing Surgery—cont'd

**PATIENT/FAMILY GOAL 2:** Will demonstrate understanding of surgery and postoperative care

**• NURSING INTERVENTIONS/*RATIONALES***

Prepare for postoperative procedures, as indicated (e.g., nasogastric tube, IV fluids, nothing by mouth, dressing changes, wound drains if necessary)

Explain reason for surgery; if special operative procedure is to be performed, explain basic principles and briefly outline care if needed *to reinforce information given by practitioner*

Explain all preoperative procedures (e.g., blood work, any other laboratory test)

In emergency situation, explain most essential components of surgery (e.g., where child will be before and after surgery, anesthesia, dressing)

Accept behavioral reactions of parents and child *because these can be highly variable*

**• EXPECTED OUTCOMES**

Child and family demonstrate an understanding of forthcoming events (specify methods of learning and evaluation)

Family's behavioral reactions are accepted and supported

**PATIENT GOAL 3:** Will exhibit signs of optimum relaxation, sedation, and support before arriving in operating room

**• NURSING INTERVENTIONS/*RATIONALES***

*Administer preoperative sedation (preferably oral), if ordered, *to promote relaxation and sleep*

Place unfamiliar equipment out of child's view *to decrease anxiety/fear*

Place child in quiet room with minimum distraction *to promote relaxation and encourage sleep*

Do not leave child unattended

Explain what is happening, unless child is asleep

Encourage parents to stay with child as long as permitted and according to their wishes

Permit parent to hold child until child falls asleep, if desired

Encourage parents to accompany child as far as possible, preferably through induction of anesthesia

Allow significant objects to accompany child (e.g., a favorite toy) *to provide comfort and sense of security*

**• EXPECTED OUTCOMES**

Child falls asleep or lies quietly

Child is not left alone

> **NURSING DIAGNOSIS:** Interrupted family processes related to a surgical procedure

**PATIENT (FAMILY) GOAL 1:** Will receive adequate support and reassurance

**• NURSING INTERVENTIONS/*RATIONALES***

Reinforce and clarify information given by practitioner

Explain associated diagnostic tests and procedures (e.g., x-ray examinations)

Explain child's schedule
  When child will receive premedication
  Time child will leave for surgery
  Where parents can wait for child to return
  Room to which child will return
  Postprocedural care and routines

Explore family's feelings regarding the procedure and its implications *to assess need for further intervention*

Include parents in preparation of child

Be available to family *to provide support and reassurance as needed*

See also Nursing Care Plan: The Family of the Child Who Is Ill or Hospitalized, Chapter 26

**• EXPECTED OUTCOMES**

Family demonstrates an understanding of procedure (specify demonstration) and related information (specify)

Family complies with directives (specify)

## POSTOPERATIVE CARE

> **NURSING DIAGNOSIS:** Risk for injury related to surgical procedure, anesthesia

**NURSE GOAL 1:** Receive child on return from surgery

**• NURSING INTERVENTIONS/*RATIONALES***

Place child in bed (unless transported in own bed or crib) using techniques appropriate to type of surgery *to prevent injury*

Hang IV apparatus and connect any needed equipment (e.g., suction apparatus, traction)

Place child in position of comfort and safety in accordance with surgeon's orders

Perform stat (immediate) activities

**• EXPECTED OUTCOME**

Child is transferred to bed without injury and with minimum stress

**PATIENT GOAL 2:** Will exhibit signs of wound healing without evidence of wound infection

**• NURSING INTERVENTIONS/*RATIONALES***

Use proper handwashing techniques and other universal precautions, especially if wound drainage is present

Employ careful wound care *to minimize risk of infection*
  Keep wound clean and dressings intact
  Apply dressings *that promote moist wound healing* (i.e., hydrocolloid dressings [e.g., Duoderm])
  Change dressings if indicated, whenever soiled; carefully dispose of soiled dressings
  Carry out special wound care as prescribed (e.g., irrigation, drain care)
  Cleanse with prescribed preparation (if ordered)
  *Apply antibacterial solutions and/or ointments as ordered *to prevent infection*
  Report any unusual appearance or drainage *for early detection of infection*

Place diapers below abdominal dressing *if appropriate to prevent contamination*

When child begins oral feedings, provide nutritious diet as ordered *to promote wound healing*

---

*Dependent nursing action.

*Continued*

## Nursing Care Plan
### The Child Undergoing Surgery—cont'd

- **EXPECTED OUTCOME**
Child exhibits no evidence of wound infection

**PATIENT GOAL 3:** Will exhibit no evidence of complications

- **NURSING INTERVENTIONS/*RATIONALES***
Ambulate as prescribed *to decrease complications associated with immobility*
Maintain child NPO until fully awake *to prevent aspiration*
Encourage to void when awake
　Offer bedpan
　Boys may be allowed to stand at bedside
Notify practitioner if child is unable to void *to ensure appropriate intervention*
Maintain abdominal decompression, chest tubes, or other equipment, if prescribed
Provide diet as prescribed; advance as appropriate

- **EXPECTED OUTCOME**
Child exhibits no evidence of complications

> **NURSING DIAGNOSIS:** Anxiety/fear related to surgery, unfamiliar environment, separation from support systems, discomfort

**PATIENT GOAL 1:** Will experience reduced anxiety

- **NURSING INTERVENTIONS/*RATIONALES***
Maintain calm, reassuring manner
Encourage expression of feelings *to facilitate coping*
Explain procedures and other activities before initiating
Answer questions and explain purposes of activities
Keep informed of progress
Remain with child as much as possible
Give encouragement and positive feedback for cooperation in care
Encourage parental presence as soon as permitted *to decrease stress of separation*
If emergency procedure, review child's memory of previous events *so that misconceptions can be clarified*

- **EXPECTED OUTCOMES**
Child rests quietly and calmly
Child discusses procedures and activities without evidence of anxiety

> **NURSING DIAGNOSIS:** Acute pain related to surgical incision

**PATIENT GOAL 1:** Will experience no pain or reduction of pain to level acceptable to child

- **NURSING INTERVENTIONS/*RATIONALES***
*Administer analgesics prescribed for pain around the clock
Do not wait until child experiences severe pain to intervene *in order to prevent pain from occurring*

Avoid palpating operative area unless necessary
Insert rectal tube, if indicated, *to relieve gas*
Encourage to void, if appropriate, *to prevent bladder distention*
Administer mouth care *to provide comfort*
Lubricate nostril *to decrease irritation* from nasogastric tube if present
Allow child position of comfort if not contraindicated
Perform nursing activities and procedures (e.g., dressing change, deep breathing, ambulation) after analgesia
*Administer antiemetics as ordered *for nausea and vomiting* and laxatives *to prevent constipation*
Monitor effectiveness of analgesics

- **EXPECTED OUTCOME**
Child rests quietly and exhibits minimal or no evidence of pain (specify)

> **NURSING DIAGNOSIS:** Risk for fluid volume deficient related to NPO status before and after surgery, loss of appetite, vomiting

**PATIENT GOAL 1:** Will receive adequate hydration

- **NURSING INTERVENTIONS/*RATIONALES***
Monitor IV infusion at prescribed rate *to ensure adequate hydration*
　Attach pediatric IV apparatus if not done in operating room
Offer fluids as soon as ordered or child tolerates
　Start with small sips of water or ice chips and advance as tolerated
　Encourage to drink
　Tempt with favorite fluids, ice chips, or flavored ice pops

- **EXPECTED OUTCOMES**
Child exhibits no evidence of dehydration
Child takes and retains fluid when allowed (specify)

> **NURSING DIAGNOSIS:** Risk for infection related to weakened condition, presence of infective organisms

**PATIENT GOAL 1:** Will maintain normal respiratory function

- **NURSING INTERVENTIONS/*RATIONALES***
Assess need for pain medication before respiratory therapy
Help to turn, deep breathe
　Splint operative site with hand or pillow if possible before coughing (if coughing prescribed) *to minimize pain*
Assist with use of incentive spirometer or blow bottle
Perform percussion and vibration if indicated
Suction secretions if needed
Assess respirations, including breath sounds

- **EXPECTED OUTCOME**
Lungs remain clear

---

*Dependent nursing action.

## Nursing Care Plan
### The Child Undergoing Surgery—cont'd

> **NURSING DIAGNOSIS:** Interrupted family processes related to situational crisis (emergency hospitalization of child), knowledge deficit

**PATIENT/FAMILY GOAL 1:** Will receive adequate support and reassurance

- **NURSING INTERVENTIONS/*RATIONALES***

Explain all procedures *to reduce anxiety/fear*
Keep family informed of child's progress
Encourage expression of feelings *to facilitate coping*
Refer to public health nurse if indicated *for follow-up care*
Refer to appropriate agency or persons for specific help (e.g., social service, clergy)
See also Nursing Care Plan: The Child in the Hospital, Chapter 26
See also Nursing Care Plan: The Family of the Child Who Is Ill or Hospitalized, Chapter 26

- **EXPECTED OUTCOMES**

Family discusses child's condition and therapies comfortably
Family demonstrates an awareness of child's progress (specify method of evaluation)
Family members avail themselves of appropriate assistance

**PATIENT (FAMILY) GOAL 2:** Will demonstrate understanding of home care

- **NURSING INTERVENTIONS/*RATIONALES***

If dressing changes are required at home, teach parents sterile or aseptic procedures; provide written list of necessary equipment and instructions *for referral at home*
Instruct parents regarding administration of medications (if ordered), including possible side effects and untoward reactions, *to ensure adequate home care*
Instruct parents in care and management of special procedures (e.g., ostomy care, irrigations) *to ensure adequate home care*

- **EXPECTED OUTCOME**

Family demonstrates an understanding of instructions (specify methods of learning and evaluation)

---

den high fever associated with a surgical procedure and those with certain neuromuscular disorders are at a higher risk for the development of MH; children who have successfully undergone prior surgery without adverse effects may still be considered susceptible for the occurrence of MH (Dunn, 1997). Treatment includes immediate discontinuation of the triggering agent and surgical procedure, hyperventilation with 100% oxygen, and IV dantrolene sodium. The patient's elevated core temperature is managed with IV infusions of cool saline, topical cooling blankets, gastric or perineal lavage, packed ice bags in the axillae and groin and, possibly, cardiopulmonary bypass (Dunn, 1997; Miranda and others, 1997). The patient is transferred to an ICU and is closely monitored for stabilization of vital signs, metabolic state, and possible recurrence of symptoms.

> **NURSING ALERT**   When taking the preoperative history, ask the family if any relatives have had anesthetic difficulties suggesting malignant hyperthermia; report findings immediately.

Providing pain control is a major nursing responsibility after surgery. Pain is assessed, and analgesics are administered to provide comfort and facilitate the child's cooperation with postoperative care such as ambulation and deep breathing. Opioids are the most commonly used analgesic drugs for this purpose. Routinely scheduled IV analgesics, patient-controlled analgesia, and epidural infusions, rather than as-needed (PRN) orders, provide excellent analgesia in postoperative pediatric patients.

When vital signs are stable and airway obstruction is not a threat, parents are allowed in some postanesthesia care units. Little information is available regarding parental presence on emergence from anesthesia, and policies on parental visitation in the PACU vary among hospitals. One study, however, showed that children cried significantly less, were less restless, and more comfortable during parental visits in the PACU (Fina and others, 1997). According to a recent study, when given the choice, 100% of parents chose to be with their child in the PACU. The age of the child had no bearing on the parents' views. Almost all parents (98%) believed they and their child benefited from their presence (Turner, 1997). As with induction of anesthesia, parents should receive instructions on what to expect when they visit their child in terms of appearance, level of consciousness, pain, monitoring equipment, and what their role can be (Munro and D'Errico, 2000).

Because respiratory infections are a potential complication, every effort is taken to aerate the lungs and remove secretions. The lungs are auscultated regularly to identify abnormal sounds or any areas of diminished or absent breath sounds. To prevent hypostatic pneumonia, respiratory movement can be encouraged with incentive spirometers or other motivating activities (see Box 27-1). If these measures are presented as games, the child is more likely to comply. The child's position is changed every 2 hours, and deep breathing is encouraged.

> **NURSING TIP**   Because deep breathing is usually painful after surgery, be sure the child has received analgesics. Have the child splint the operative site (depending on its location) by hugging a small pillow or a favorite stuffed animal.

> **NURSING ALERT**   Early signs of respiratory involvement are abnormal rate, shallow depth, and cough. These findings are reported immediately.

During the recovery period, some time should be spent with children to assess their perceptions of surgery. Play, drawing, and storytelling are excellent methods of discovering their thoughts. With such information the nurse can support or correct their perceptions and assist children in achieving mastery for having endured a stressful procedure.

With the changing trends of outpatient surgery and shortened stays in the hospital, many pediatric patients are discharged shortly after surgery. Preparation for discharge actually begins with the preadmission preparation visit. Instructions for postoperative care should be discussed and reviewed throughout the perioperative visit. Following discharge, phone calls are often made by the nursing staff to check the status of the patient. Patient education and compliance with discharge instructions can also be assessed during this phone call (Barnes, 2000). (See Guidelines box.)

## Compliance

One of the most significant nursing interventions concerning procedures that must be repeated in the hospital or continued at home is related to compliance. *Compliance,* also termed *adherence,* refers to the extent to which the patient's behavior in terms of taking medication, following diets, or executing other lifestyle changes coincides with the prescribed regimen. Because nurses are frequently responsible for teaching families about treatment protocols, they must have knowledge of factors that influence compliance, methods to measure compliance, and strategies to enhance adherence to prescribed treatment.

### Assessment

In developing strategies to improve compliance, the nurse must first assess the patient's level of compliance. Because many children are too young to assume partial or total responsibility for their care, parents are usually the primary caregivers in terms of home management. Consequently, the nurse needs to assess their ability to carry out instructions. The first approach to assessment is knowledge of those factors that influence compliance. The second is to apply methods to assess more objectively the child's and parents' levels of compliance.

**Factors That Influence Compliance.** Research on compliance has identified several factors that influence compliance (Box 27-3). The first area relates to factors about the patient. Contrary to what might be expected, no typical characteristics of noncompliers exist, and even education is not correlated with compliance. Some evidence suggests that higher levels of self-esteem and increased autonomy favorably affect adolescent compliance (Kyngas, Kroll, and Duffy, 2000). However, family factors are important, and characteristics associated with good compliance include family support, family reminders, good communication, and expectations for successful completion of the therapeutic regimen (Kyngas, Kroll, and Duffy, 2000).

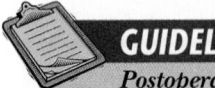

## GUIDELINES
### Postoperative Care

Ensure that preparations are made to receive child.
  Bed or crib is ready.
  Intravenous equipment, such as pumps, and any other
    relevant equipment, such as suction apparatus, oxygen
    flow meter, or Gomco suction, is at bedside.
Obtain baseline information:
  Take vital signs, including blood pressure (BP); keep BP
    cuff in place, deflated to lessen amount of disturbance
    to child.
  Assess pain level as part of "fifth" vital sign. (See Pain
    Assessment, Chapter 26.)
  Take and record more frequently if any value fluctuates
    (Table 27-1).
  Inspect operative area.
    Check dressing if present.
    Outline any bleeding area on dressing or cast with pen.
    Reinforce, but do not remove, loose dressing.
    Observe areas below surgical site for blood that may
      have drained toward bed.
    Assess for bleeding and other symptoms in areas not
      covered with a dressing, such as throat following
      tonsillectomy.
  Assess skin color and characteristics.
  Assess level of consciousness, activity.
Notify practitioner of any irregularities in child's condition.
Review surgeon's orders after completing initial assessment,
  and check that any preoperative orders, such as seizure
  or cardiac medications, have been reordered and can be
  given by available routes (oral preparations may be con-
  traindicated).
Monitor vital signs as ordered and more often if indicated.
Check dressings for bleeding or other abnormalities.
Check bowel sounds.
Observe for signs of shock, abdominal distention, bleeding.
Assess for bladder distention.
Observe for signs of dehydration.
Detect presence of infection:
  Take vital signs every 2 to 4 hours, as ordered.
  Collect or request needed specimens.
  Inspect wound for signs of infection—redness, swelling,
    heat, pain, purulent drainage.

---

**Box 27-3** ■ ■ ■
**Factors That Positively Influence Compliance**

**INDIVIDUAL/FAMILY FACTORS**

High self-esteem
Positive body image
High degree of autonomy (increased locus of control)
Supportive and well-adjusted family
Effective family communication
Family expectation for successful completion of therapy

**CARE SETTING FACTORS**

Perceived satisfaction with care
Positive interactions with practitioners
Continuity of care
Individualized care
Minimum waiting time for appointments
Convenient care setting

**TREATMENT FACTORS**

Simple regimen
Minimum disruption in usual lifestyle
Short duration
Inexpensive
Visible benefits
Tolerable side effects

Factors relating to the care setting are very important in determining compliance and provide useful guidelines in planning strategies to improve compliance. Basically, any aspect of the health care setting that increases the family's satisfaction with the physical setting and the relationship with the practitioner positively influences adherence to the treatment regimen. In addition, the type of care required to manage the disorder is important. The more complex, expensive, inconvenient, longer, and disruptive the treatment protocol, the less likely the family is to comply. During long-term conditions that involve multiple treatments and considerable rearrangement of lifestyle, compliance is most severely affected.

**Measurement of Compliance.** Although it is helpful to know those factors that influence compliance, especially in assessing the likelihood of compliance in a family, assessment must include more direct measurement techniques. A number of methods exist, each with its advantages and disadvantages. The most successful approach includes a combination of at least two of the following methods:

**Clinical judgment.** The nurse judges family compliance. This method is subject to bias and inaccuracy unless the nurse carefully evaluates the criteria used in evaluation.

**Self-reporting.** The family is asked about their ability to carry out the prescribed treatments. Although this is a simple method, most people overestimate their compliance by about 20%, even when they admit to lapses in treatment.

**Direct observation.** The nurse directly observes the patient or family perform the treatment. Although this approach is very effective in identifying errors related to the correct procedure, it is difficult to employ outside the health care setting. Also, the family's awareness of being observed frequently affects their performance.

**TABLE 27-1** Potential causes of postoperative vital sign alterations in children

| Alteration | Potential Cause | Comments |
|---|---|---|
| **Heart Rate** | | |
| Increase | Decreased perfusion (shock) | Heart rate may increase to maintain cardiac output |
| | Elevated temperature | |
| | Pain | |
| | Respiratory distress (early) | |
| | Medications (atropine, morphine, epinephrine) | |
| Decrease | Hypoxia | Bradycardia is of more concern in the young child than tachycardia |
| | Vagal stimulation | |
| | Increased intracranial pressure | |
| | Respiratory distress (late) | |
| | Medications (prostigmine) | |
| **Respiratory Rate** | | |
| Increase | Respiratory distress | Body responds to respiratory distress primarily by increasing rate |
| | Fluid volume excess | |
| | Hypothermia | |
| | Elevated temperature | |
| | Pain | |
| Decrease | Anesthetics, opioids | Decreased respiratory rate from opioids may be compensated for by increased depth of respiration |
| | Pain | |
| **Blood Pressure** | | |
| Increase | Excess intravascular volume | Serious in premature infants because it increases risk of intraventricular hemorrhage |
| | Increased intracranial pressure | |
| | Carbon dioxide retention | |
| | Pain | |
| | Medications (ketamine, epinephrine) | |
| Decrease | Vasodilating anesthetic agents (halothane, isoflurane, enflurane) | Decreased blood pressure is late sign of shock because of elasticity and constriction of vessels to maintain cardiac output |
| | Opioids (e.g., morphine) | |
| **Temperature** | | |
| Increase | Shock (late sign) | Fever associated with infection usually occurs later than fever of noninfectious origin |
| | Infection | |
| | Environmental causes (warm room, excess coverings) | Absence of fever does not rule out infection, especially in infants |
| | Malignant hyperthermia | Malignant hyperthermia requires immediate treatment |
| Decrease | Vasodilating anesthetic agents (halothane, isoflurane, enflurane) | Neonates are especially susceptible to hypothermia, with serious or fatal consequences |
| | Muscle relaxants | |
| | Environmental causes (cool room) | |
| | Infusion of cool fluids/blood | |

From Smith DP and others, editors: *Comprehensive child and family nursing skills,* St Louis, 1991, Mosby.

**Monitoring appointments.** The family's attendance at scheduled appointments is recorded. Keeping appointments indicates general levels of compliance but only indirectly indicates compliance with the prescribed care.

**Monitoring therapeutic response.** The child's response in terms of benefit from treatment is monitored and preferably recorded on a graph or chart. Unfortunately, few treatments yield directly measurable results (e.g., decreased blood pressure, weight loss), making this a less satisfactory method for most types of therapies. Also, adherence does not ensure clinical improvement, and less than 100% compliance may achieve therapeutic results, reinforcing partial compliance.

**Pill counts.** The nurse counts the number of pills remaining in the original container and compares the number missing with the number of days the medication should have been taken. Although this is a simple method, families may forget to bring the container or deliberately alter the number of pills to avoid detection. This method is also poorly suited to liquid medication, which is so often prescribed in pediatrics. Another technique is the use of pill container caps that record every opening as a presumptive dose.

**Chemical assay.** For certain drugs, such as digoxin, theophylline, and phenytoin, measurement of plasma drug levels provides information on the amount of drug recently ingested. However, this method is expensive, indicates only short-term compliance, and requires precise timing of the assay for accurate results.

## Compliance Strategies

Strategies to improve compliance are concerned with those interventions that encourage families to follow the prescribed treatment regimen. Ideally, such strategies should be implemented before or concurrent with the initiation of

---

### GUIDELINES
#### Effective Teaching of Family Members

Establish rapport; reduce anxiety and fear.
Assess what family knows and expects to learn, especially if they have concerns, and address their concerns before beginning teaching.
Assess family's learning style; ask if they prefer having everything explained in detail or knowing only the major facts.
Direct teaching to family decision maker or primary caregiver.
Use a variety of teaching materials (lecture, demonstration, video or slide presentation, written material).
Speak family's language, avoid jargon, and clarify all terms.
Be specific when giving information; divide information into small steps.
Keep information short, simple, and concrete.
Introduce most important information first.
Use verbal "headings" to organize information, such as, "There are two things you need to learn: how to give the medicine and what side effects to look for. First, how to give. . . . Second, what side effects. . . ."
Stress importance of instructions and expected benefits; explain detrimental effects of inadequate treatment but avoid fear tactics.
Evaluate teaching by eliciting feedback to ensure that family understands information.
Repeat information as needed.
Reward family for learning through verbal praise.
Use "teachable" moments—times when family is most likely to accept new information (e.g., when symptoms are present).

---

therapy to avoid compliance problems. When compliance problems are suspected, however, the nurse should assess why the child or family is having difficulty adhering to the treatment plan. A number of strategies have been found to be effective, but, as with measurement methods, no one approach is always successful, and the best results occur when at least two strategies are employed.

*Organizational strategies* refer to those interventions concerned with the care setting and the therapeutic plan. They include manipulating the factors listed in Box 27-3 that positively affect compliance. Depending on the individual situation, this may involve increasing the frequency of appointments, designating a primary practitioner, reducing the cost of medication by purchasing generic brands, reducing the disruption of the treatment on the family's lifestyle, and the use of "cues" to minimize forgetting. Numerous devices are available commercially or can be improvised for cueing, such as pill dispensers, watches with alarms, charts to record completed therapy, reminders such as messages on the refrigerator or morning coffee pot, and treatment schedules that incorporate the treatment plan into the daily routine, such as physical therapy after the evening bath.

*Educational strategies* are concerned with instructing the family about the treatment plan. Although education is an important component in enhancing compliance and patients who are more knowledgeable about their condition are more likely to comply, education alone does not ensure compliant behavior. Also, for education to be effective, it must incorporate teaching principles known to enhance understanding and retention of material. (See Guidelines box.) Written materials are essential, especially in any regimen requiring multiple or complex treatments, and need to be readable by the average individual, which appears to be at the fourth grade level. One study found that 30% to 50% (depending on the educational level) of mothers failed to understand basic medical terms that residents presumed the mother would understand, such as *asthma, vitamin, fever, development,* and *virus* (Gablehouse and Gitterman, 1990). Including the culturally significant decision maker (e.g., maternal grandmother) in teaching sessions may help improve compliance.

*Treatment strategies* are related to the child's refusal or inability to take the prescribed medication. The family may also have difficulty following a prescribed treatment regimen. They may remember and understand the instructions but may not be able to give the medicine as prescribed. It is essential to assess the reason for refusal. For example, the child may not be able to swallow pills. In this case, perhaps they could be crushed or a liquid medication substituted. The opposite also may occur; the child may have difficulty drinking a liquid medication but be able to swallow pills. (See Nursing Tip on p. 1152.)

Also assess the treatment/medication schedule to determine if it is reasonable for a home situation. While an every-6-hour or every-8-hour schedule is reasonable for hospitals, a parent would have difficulty getting up one or two times in the night, and it may be possible to give the medication during the day at times that would be easy to remember. (See Critical Thinking Exercise box.)

*Behavioral strategies* encompass those interventions designed to modify behavior directly. Several strategies are effective in encouraging the desired behavior and are very useful with children. Ideally, positive reinforcement should be employed to strengthen the behavior and may consist of earning stars or tokens, which gains the child a special privilege or gift. A more formal method is the use of contracting (see following discussion). However, at times, disciplinary techniques, such as time-out for young children (see p. 87) or withholding privileges for older children, may be needed to reduce noncompliance.

**NURSING TIP**   To encourage a child to perform a treatment for a certain time frame (e.g., soaking a foot), ask the child to soak during a favorite TV show, including commercials. This technique also helps evaluate compliance by asking the child what show was watched.

*Contracting* is a process in which the exact elements of desired behavior are explicitly outlined in the form of a written contract. Based on behavior modification, it is a very effective method of shaping behavior, especially with older children who are involved in the process of defining the rules of the agreement. Ideally, it should involve tangible rewards but may include negative consequences, such as demerits or "checks" for failing to comply. In deciding whether to use positive or negative reinforcers, the nurse should question parents about their opinion regarding powerful motivators for the child. Often the contract includes a commitment from the parent, such as agreeing to stop nagging the child about taking medication.

An effective contract includes the following:

- The goal or desired behavior is realistic and seems possible.
- The behavior is measurable (e.g., agreeing to take the drug before leaving for school without being reminded).
- The contract is written and signed by all those involved in any of the agreements.
- The contract is dated, and if appropriate, a date is specified when a goal should be reached (e.g., taking medication until the container is empty).
- The identified rewards or consequences are reinforcing.
- The goal can be evaluated (e.g., counting number of tablets).

More informal arrangements can be used with young children, such as rewarding desired behavior with stars, stickers, or other small novelties. Once the contract is implemented, it is evaluated at the end of the time specified in the agreement and revisions are made, such as extending the time or terminating the contract. If the contract has not been successful, every effort is made to ascertain if the goals were realistic, the time period was sufficient for accomplishing the goal, and the rewards or consequences were motivating. A successful contract may or may not work the next time.

# GENERAL HYGIENE AND CARE
## Maintaining Healthy Skin

Skin, the largest organ of the body, is a complex structure that serves many functions, the most important of which is the interface between the human internal and external environment. The skin provides protection, sensation, thermoregulation, biochemical, and metabolic functions, and immune function (Wysocki, 1999). Many routine nursing activities—maintaining an IV line, removing a dressing, po-

### Critical Thinking Exercise

#### Discharge Instructions

Ms. Jordan is preparing to take 2-month-old Brittany home from the hospital after a 4-day admission for a severe ear infection and eye infection. Brittany will be going home taking an antibiotic that you have been giving every 8 hours and eye drops that you have been giving every 6 hours. The infant is fed about every 4 hours. Choose the appropriate home schedule.

FIRST, THINK ABOUT IT . . .

- What precise question are you trying to answer?
- What are you taking for granted, and what assumptions are you making?

1. 12 AM—Feed and give antibiotic and eye drops
   4 AM—Feed
   6 AM—Give eye drops
   8 AM—Feed and give antibiotic
   12 PM—Feed and give eye drops
   4 PM—Feed and give antibiotic
   6 PM—Give eye drops
   8 PM—Feed
2. 12 AM—Feed and give antibiotic
   4 AM—Feed
   8 AM—Feed and give eye antibiotic and eye drops
   12 PM—Feed and give eye drops
   4 PM—Feed and give antibiotic and eye drops
   8 PM—Feed and give eye drops
3. 12 AM—Feed and give antibiotic and eye drops
   6 AM—Feed and give antibiotic and eye drops
   10 AM—Feed and give eye drops
   2 PM—Feed and give antibiotic
   6 PM—Feed and give eye drops
   9 PM—Feed

*The best response is two. Even though you followed the every-6-hour schedule for the eye drops in the hospital, the precise question is whether the parent could manage this at home. It is sometimes difficult getting eye drops into an infant's eyes, and giving the parent a schedule in which they must be given twice during the night would be difficult. Reducing the number of times the parent and infant must awaken during the night decreases the likelihood of a missed dose because the parent forgot to awaken.*

*If this were an older child, the antibiotic schedule could also be altered to waking hours only so the child and parent would not have to awaken at night for medication.*

*Although the assumption exists that not every medication can be given on a more flexible schedule, most can. Ask the practitioner if the medication can be given three times a day instead of every 8 hours or four times a day instead of every 6 hours, etc. Medications or treatments given at unusual times are more likely to be missed. Discharge instructions should always be given while keeping in mind the parent's ability to be compliant with them.*

sitioning a child in bed, changing a diaper, using electrode patches, or maintaining restraints—have the potential to contribute to skin injury. Skin care must go beyond the daily bath and become a part of each nursing intervention. General guidelines for skin care are listed in the Guidelines box. (Specific guidelines for skin care of neonates are provided in Chapter 10 under Skin Care.)

Assessment of the skin is most easily accomplished during the bath, but often the nurse is not the one who bathes the child. In this case the nurse needs to plan a time to observe the child's skin and to request feedback from the caregiver. Developmental changes are also considered. A newborn's skin and nails are thinner than an adolescent's skin. In adolescence hormones stimulate sebaceous gland activity and hair growth (Calianno, 1999). The skin is examined for any early signs of injury, especially in the child who is at risk. Risk factors include impaired mobility, protein malnutrition, edema, incontinence, sensory loss, anemia, and infection.

Identification of risk factors helps to determine those children who need a more thorough skin assessment (Fig. 27-4).

When capillary blood flow is interrupted by pressure, the blood flows back into the tissue when the pressure is relieved. As the body attempts to reoxygenate the area, a bright red flush appears. This *reactive hyperemia*, or flush, is the earliest sign of tissue compromise and pressure-related ischemia. If the pressure is prolonged, reactive hyperemia will not be sufficient to revitalize ischemic tissue (Calianno, 1999).

Staging of pressure ulcers is used to classify the amount of tissue damage that has occurred. Necrotic tissue must be removed so that the tissue depth can accurately be assessed (Box 27-4). Accurate documentation of redness or obvious skin breakdown is essential. Color, size (diameter and depth), location, presence of sinus tracts, odor, exudate, and response to treatment are observed and recorded at least daily. (For treatment of wounds, see Chapter 18). (See Critical Thinking Exercise box.)

The nurse must also have an understanding of the types of mechanical damage that can occur, such as pressure, friction, shearing, and epidermal stripping. When a combination of risk factors and mechanical injury is present, skin breakdown can occur.

When a child is identified as being at risk for skin breakdown, nursing interventions are directed toward prevention

## GUIDELINES
### Skin Care

Cleanse skin with mild, nonalkaline soap or soap-free cleaning agents for routine bathing. Mild, nonalkaline cleansers prevent dryness and preserve the skin's natural pH (Calianno, 1999).

Provide daily cleansing of eyes, oral, diaper or perianal areas, and any areas of skin breakdown.

Apply moisturizing agents after cleansing to retain moisture and rehydrate skin. Commonly used agents include lactic acid, glycolic acid, mineral oil, glycerin, and petrolatum. Moisturizing agents are most effective when applied during or immediately after bathing.

Use minimum tape/adhesive. On very sensitive skin, use a protective, pectin-based or hydrocolloid skin barrier between skin and tape/adhesives.

Use water or possibly adhesive remover (if skin is not fragile) when removing tape/adhesives.

Place pectin-based or hydrocolloid skin barriers directly over excoriated skin. Leave barrier undisturbed until it begins to peel off. With wet, oozing excoriations, place a small amount of stoma powder (as used in ostomy care) on site, remove excess powder, and apply skin barrier. Hold barrier in place for several minutes to allow barrier to soften and mold to skin surface.

Alternate electrode placement and thoroughly assess skin underneath electrodes at least every 24 hours.

Be certain fingers or toes are visible whenever extremity is used for IV or arterial line.

Reduce friction by keeping skin dry (may apply absorbent powder, such as cornstarch) and using soft, smooth bed linen and clothes.

Use a draw sheet to move a child in bed or onto a stretcher to reduce friction and shearing injuries; do not drag the child from under the arms.

Identify children who are at risk for skin breakdown before it occurs. Employ measures, such as pressure-reducing devices, to prevent breakdown.

Do not massage reddened bony prominences because it can cause deep tissue damage; provide pressure relief to those areas instead.

Keep skin free of excess moisture (i.e., urine or fecal incontinence, wound drainage, excessive perspiration).

Routinely assess the child's nutritional status. A child who is NPO for several days and is only receiving IV fluid is nutritionally at risk, which can also affect the skin's ability to maintain its integrity. Parental nutrition should be considered for these children before they are at risk.

### Critical Thinking Exercise

#### Risk of Skin Breakdown

You work on a pediatric surgical unit. In a recent continuous quality improvement report, it was noted that 10% of the patients developed some type of skin breakdown, most often stage II wounds. Which of the following variables identified about this patient population should be investigated further?

FIRST, THINK ABOUT IT . . .

- What precise questions are you trying to answer?
- How are you interpreting the information?

1. Average age of the child is 6 years, and sex is more often male.
2. Major reason for surgery is orthopaedic repair, especially as a result of trauma.
3. Average length of surgery is 4 hours; average duration until appearance of wound is 24 to 48 hours.
4. All children receive adequate pain medication.

*The best response is three. Precisely, the questions are, how prolonged was the surgery and was the patient placed on an adequately padded surface? The excessive pressure on bony prominences causes redness and deeper tissue damage that may not be apparent until hours or days later. An accurate interpretation of the information reveals the fact that these children are most likely to need orthopaedic surgery (members of this age-group and sex-group are at risk for injuries), and it may also be a risk factor if mobility is impaired. However, with good pain control, these children should be able to move quite easily. If pressure ulcers develop postoperatively from immobility, they are most likely to develop later than during the first 2 days.*

of mechanical injury. Wounds caused by pressure can be prevented by using current technology and resources (Bryant, 1998). *Pressure ulcers* can develop when the pressure on the skin and underlying tissues is greater than the capillary closing pressure, causing capillary occlusion. If the pressure remains unrelieved, vessels can collapse, resulting in tissue anoxia and cellular death. Pressure ulcers most often occur over bony prominences. These lesions are usually

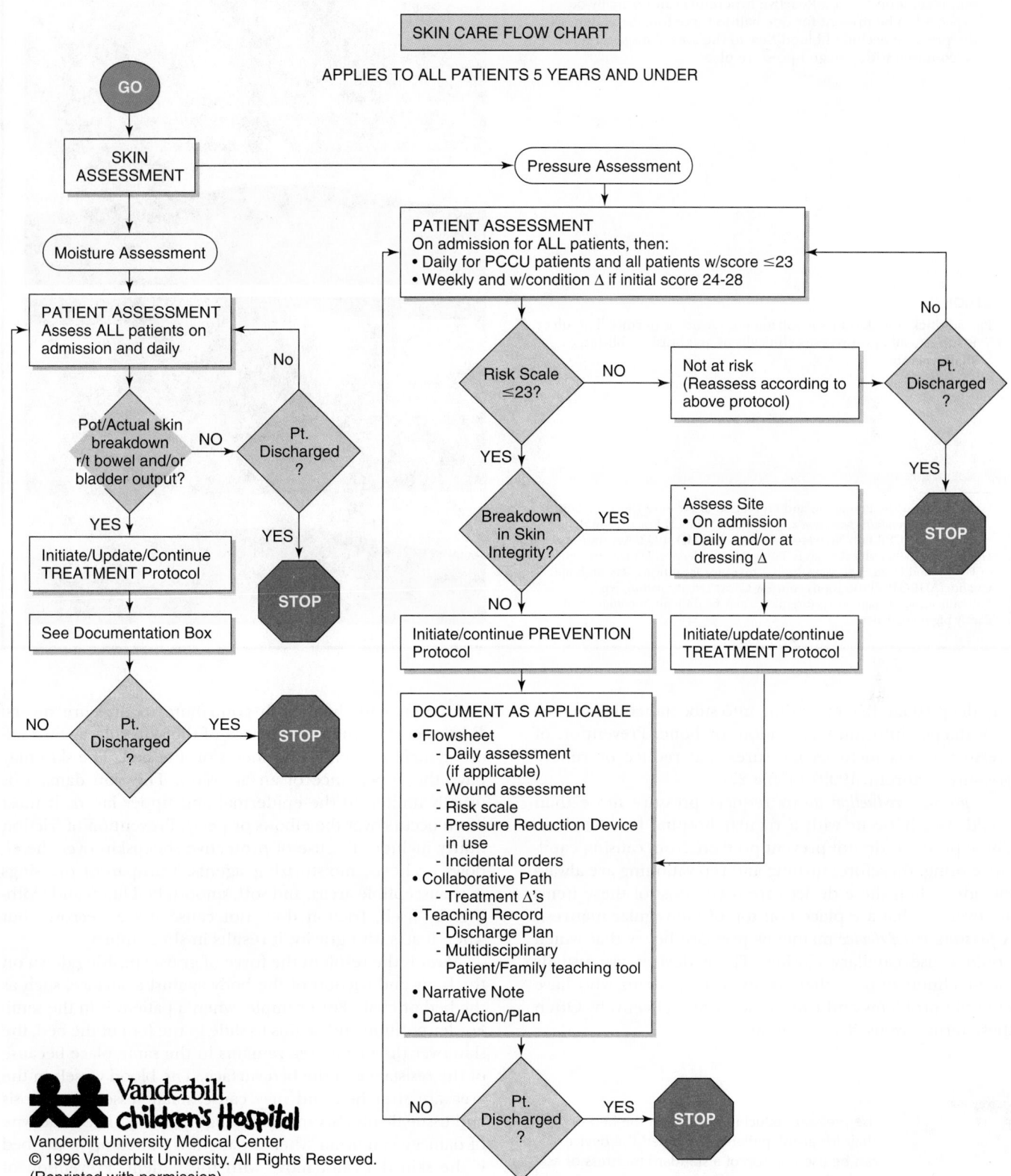

**Fig. 27-4** Skin care flow chart. (Courtesy Vanderbilt University Medical Center. Reprinted with permission.)

## Box 27-4
### Staging of Pressure Ulcers

**STAGE I**

Nonblanchable erythema of intact skin; the heralding lesion of skin ulceration.* NOTE: Reactive hyperemia can normally be expected to be present for one half to three fourths as long as the pressure occluded blood flow to the area. This should not be confused with a stage I pressure ulcer.

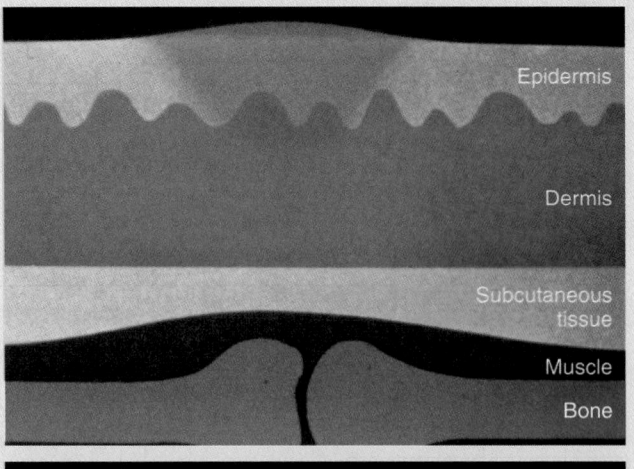

**STAGE II**

Partial-thickness skin loss involving epidermis or dermis. The ulcer is superficial and presents clinically as an abrasion, blister, or shallow crater.

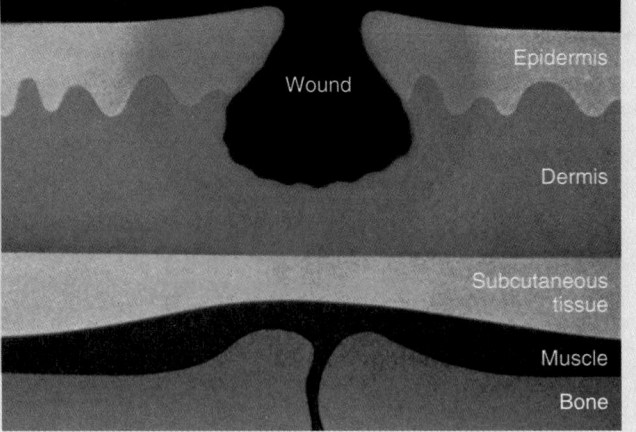

From Panel for the Prediction and Prevention of Pressure Ulcers in Adults: *Pressure ulcers in adults: prediction and prevention,* Clinical Practice Guideline Number 3, AHCPR Pub No 92—0047, Rockville, MD, 1992, Agency for Health Care Policy and Research, Public Health Service, US Department of Health and Human Services (now Agency for Healthcare Research and Quality [AHRQ]). Illustrations courtesy ConvaTec, Princeton, NJ. *Identification of stage I pressure ulcers may be difficult in patients with darkly pigmented skin.

---

very deep (stage IV), extending into subcutaneous tissue or even deeper into muscle, tendon, or bone. Prevention of pressure ulcers includes measures that reduce or relieve pressure (Laurent, 1999) (Table 27-2).

A ***pressure reduction device*** reduces pressure more than would usually occur with a regular hospital bed or chair. These products do not prevent pressure from causing capillary closing; therefore, turning and repositioning are always included when these devices are used. Most of these items are overlays that are placed on top of the regular mattress. A ***pressure relief device*** maintains pressure below that which would cause capillary closing. These devices are usually high-technology beds that are used for patients who have multiple problems and cannot be turned effectively. Often these terms are used synonymously.

**NURSING ALERT**　Use pressure-reducing devices on the bed or chair for at-risk patients. On a bed the device can be used on top of a standard mattress or as a mattress replacement system; or it can be a pressure-reducing bed (Calianno, 1999).

Friction and shear both contribute to pressure ulcers. ***Friction*** occurs when the surface of the skin rubs against another surface, such as the sheets on the bed. The skin may have the appearance of an abrasion. The skin damage is usually limited to the epidermal and upper layers. It most often occurs over the elbows or heels. Prevention of friction injury includes the use of protective sheepskin over the elbows or heels, moisturizing agents, transparent dressings over susceptible areas, and soft, smooth bed linen and clothing. By itself, friction does not cause tissue necrosis, but when it acts with gravity, it results in shear injury.

***Shear*** is the result of the force of gravity pushing down on the body and friction of the body against a surface, such as the bed or chair. For example, when a patient is in the semi-Fowler position and begins to slide to the foot of the bed, the skin over the sacral area remains in the same place because of the resistance of the bed surface. The blood vessels in the area are stretched and may cause small vessel thrombosis and tissue death (Bryant and Doughty, 2000). The same type of damage can occur when a patient is pulled up in the bed if the skin does not move with the patient. Prevention of shear injury includes using "lift sheets" when repositioning a patient, elevating the bed no more than 30 degrees for short

**Box 27-4** ■ ■ ■
**Staging of Pressure Ulcers—cont'd**

**STAGE III**

Full-thickness skin loss involving damage or necrosis of subcutaneous tissue that may extend down to, but not through, underlying fascia. The ulcer presents clinically as a deep crater with or without undermining of adjacent tissue.*

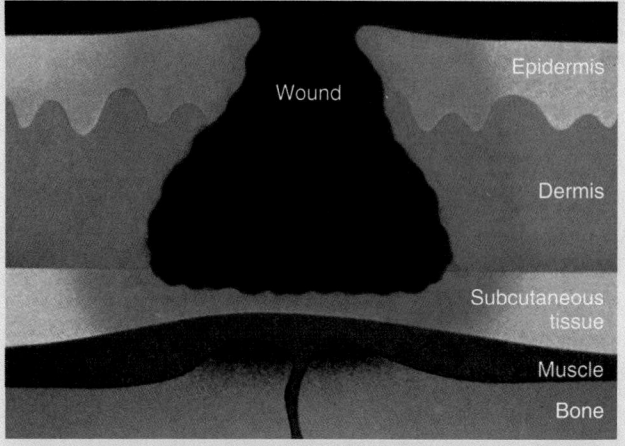

**STAGE IV**

Full-thickness skin loss with extensive destruction, tissue necrosis or damage to muscle, bone, or supporting structures (e.g., tendon or joint capsule). NOTE: Undermining and sinus tracts may also be associated with stage IV pressure ulcers.

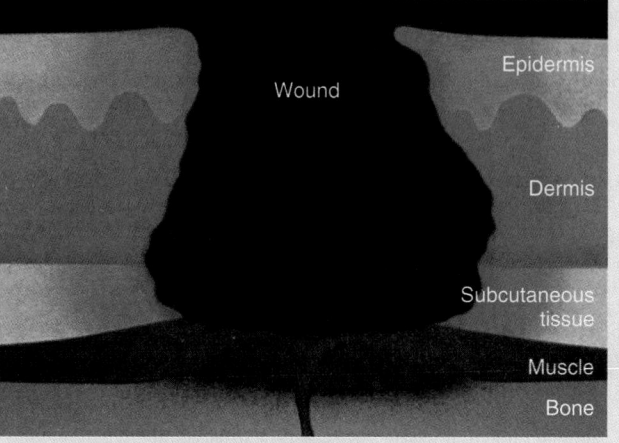

*When eschar is present, accurate staging of the pressure ulcer is not possible until the eschar has sloughed or the wound has been debrided.

---

periods, and using the knee gatch to interrupt the pull of gravity on the body toward the foot of the bed.

*Epidermal stripping* results when the epidermis is unintentionally removed with tape removal. These lesions are usually shallow and irregularly shaped. Prevention of epidermal stripping includes recognizing fragile skin, such as in neonates; using minimum tape; using solid-wafer skin barriers, transparent dressings, or laced binders to secure dressings (Montgomery straps) on areas in which tape must be changed frequently; using skin sealants under adhesives unless skin is fragile; and using porous tapes. Tape is placed so that there is no tension, traction, or wrinkling on the skin. To remove tape, slowly peel the tape away while stabilizing the underlying skin. Adhesive remover may be used to break the adhesive bond but may be drying to the skin (Bryant, 1998); adhesive removers should be avoided in preterm neonates, since absorption rates vary and toxicity may occur. Adhesive may also be removed with warm water and cotton balls, mineral oil, or an emollient. (See Atraumatic Care box.)

Chemical factors can also lead to skin damage. Fecal incontinence, especially when mixed with urine; wound drainage; or gastric drainage around gastrostomy tubes can

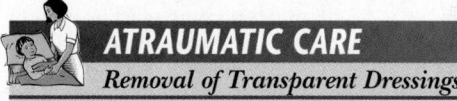

## ATRAUMATIC CARE
### Removal of Transparent Dressings

To remove the dressing, lift the opposite corners and pull apart, keeping the film parallel with the skin. Stretch the other corners apart until the adhesive lifts off the skin.

erode the epidermis. The skin can very quickly progress from redness to denudement if exposure continues. Moisture barriers, gentle cleansing as soon after exposure as possible, and skin barriers can be used to prevent damage caused by chemical factors.

## Bathing

Unless contraindicated, most infants and children can be bathed in a basin at the bedside or on the bed, or in a standard bathtub located on the unit, which is often conveniently adapted for pediatric use. For infants and young children confined to bed, the towel method can be used. Two towels are immersed in a dilute soap solution and wrung damp. With the child lying supine on a dry towel,

**TABLE 27-2** Pressure reduction/relief devices

| Description | Advantages | Disadvantages | Examples* |
|---|---|---|---|
| **Overlay†** | | | |
| **Gel/water filled:** Pressure reduction; water or gel conforms to patient's contours | One-time charge; low cost for water; gels are expensive; relieves pressure and shear; nonpowered, easy cleaning | Mattress is a dense collection of viscous fluid cells; there have been reports that the mattress is cold to the touch; can patients spare the vital calories needed to warm the mattress? Heavy | Aqua-Pedics (water and gel), Tender Gel and Water, Theracare (water and gel), RIK mattress |
| **Alternating-pressure mattress:** An overlay with rows of air cells and pump; pump cycles air to provide inflation and deflation over pressure points | The intent is to relieve pressure points to create pressure gradients that enhance blood flow | Studies show inconsistent results; some have reported very low deflation interface pressures, but only the deflation pressures were used for analysis; tissue interface pressures during inflation are consistently higher and must be incorporated into the statistical analysis; clinical trials indicate higher pressure ulcer incidence rates when compared with other products | AeroPulse, AlphaBed, AlphaCare, BetaBed, Bio Flote, Dyna-CARE, Lapidus, PCA Systems, Pillo-Pump, Tenderair |
| **Static air:** Designed with interlocking air cells that provide dry flotation; inflated with a blower | Mattress overlays that are designed with multiple chambers, allowing air exchange between the compartments | Pressure reduction is contingent on adequate air volume and periodic reinflation | DermaGard, K-Soft, Koala-Kair, Roho, Sof-Care, Tenderair |
| **Low-air-loss specialty overlay:** Multiple air-flow cushions that cover the entire bed; pressures can be set and controlled by a blower | Surface materials are constructed to reduce friction and shear and to eliminate moisture; pressure relief; can be used for prevention or treatment of ulcers | Surface mattress and pump are a rental item; cost of electricity used is incurred by family; not available for cribs | Acucair, Bio Therapy, CLINI-CARE, CRS 4000, RibCor Therapeutic Mattress Pad, TheraPulse, Select Firstep®,Dynapulse® |
| **Specialty Beds‡** | | | |
| **Low-air-loss beds:** Bed surface consists of inflated air cushions; each section is adjusted for optimum pressure relief for patient's body size; some models have built-in scales | Provides pressure relief in any position; treatment for stages III and IV pressure ulcers; available in pediatric crib sizes | Bed is more bulky than a hospital bed, and some homes may not be able to accommodate its size; reimbursement is questionable; family incurs electric bill | Air Plus, Flexicair, KinAir III® Mediscus; Cribs: Pedcare, PNEU-CARE/PEDI, Clinitron, TheraPulse,® KCI's PediDyne,™ BariKare,® with FirstStep,® Select Heavy Duty™ |
| Low-air-loss mattress replacements | Provides pressure relief in any position; fits on hospital frame | Requires mattress storage | Flexicair Eclipse SilkAir—home use |
| **Air-fluidized beds:** Air is blown through beads to "float" patient | Provides pressure relief for oncology patients and for treatment of full-thickness pressure ulcers, postoperative flaps, burns; lighter weight home care units available | Can be difficult to transfer patient | Clinitron At Home, Clinitron Elexis, Clinitron Fluid Air, Skytron, Elite,™ Clinitron Uplift Fluid Air |
| **Kinetic therapy:** Therapy surfaces that provide continuous gentle side-to-side rotation of 40 degrees or more on each side; table based or cushion based | Has been demonstrated to improve mucus transport, redistribute pulmonary blood flow, and mobilize pulmonary interstitial fluid; has been utilized for trauma victims and unstable spinal cord injuries (should use table based; once stabilized, may use cushion based) | Can only be used in acute care setting | *Cushion Based* **With air loss:** BioDyne II, Effica CC, Pulmonex, Triadyne,™ Pro-Turn, Synergy, Pneu-Care Plus, Pediadyne™  *Table Based* **Without air loss:** RotoRest,® Delta, Keane Mobility bed |
| **Continuous lateral rotation beds (CLRT):** Less than 40 degrees side-to-side rotation | Helps reposition unstable spinal cord injury patient; promotes comfort and shifts pressure points | | BariAir,™ Q2Plus,® Effica Pulmonex |

Modified from Hagelgans NA: Pediatric skin care issues for the home care nurse, *Pediatr Nurs* 19(5):499-507, 1993.
Table revised by Debra Arnow, MSN, RN, CNA.
*This list is a representative sampling of products that is not intended to be all inclusive. No endorsement of any product is intended. Within each category, products must be individually evaluated on their efficacy as comfort, pressure-reducing, or pressure-relieving devices. All products within a category do not necessarily perform equally.
†A device that is made to fit over a regular hospital mattress.
‡"High-tech" beds used in place of the standard hospital bed. These are usually used on a rental basis and are intended for short-term use. They usually provide pressure relief and eliminate shear, friction, and maceration.

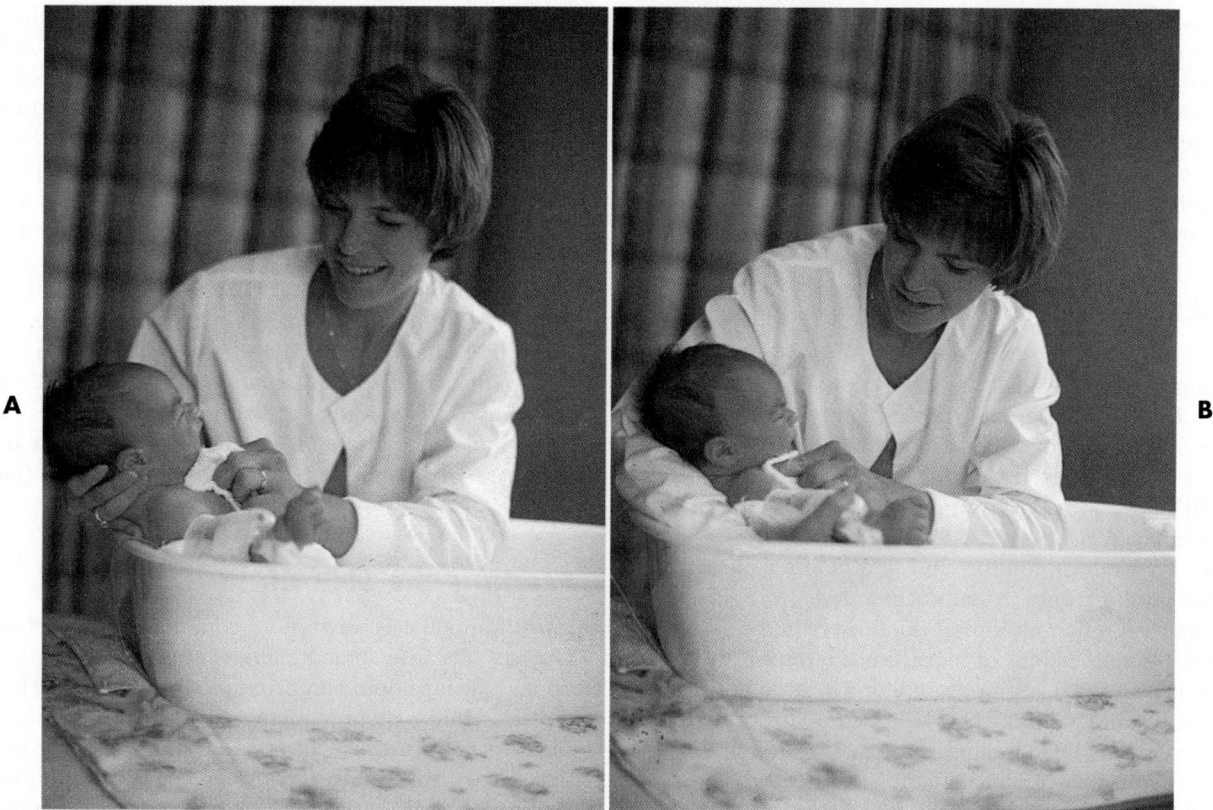

**Fig. 27-5** Two methods of supporting infant during tub bath. **A,** Using hand to support neck and head. **B,** Using arm to support neck and head.

one damp towel is placed on top of the child and used to gently clean the body. This towel is discarded, and the child is dried and turned prone. The procedure is repeated using the second damp towel.

Infants and small children are *never* left unattended in a bathtub, and infants who are unable to sit alone are securely held with one hand during the bath. The infant's head is supported securely with one hand, or the farther arm is firmly grasped in the nurse's hand while the head rests comfortably on the arm. This provides secure control of the infant while the other hand is free to wash the infant's body (Fig. 27-5). Infants or children who are able to sit without assistance need only close supervision and a pad placed in the bottom of the tub to prevent slipping and loss of balance, which could result in a bumped head or submersion of the face.

Older children may enjoy a shower if it is available. School-age children may be reluctant to bathe, and many are not accustomed to a daily bath. However, most children who feel well require little encouragement to participate in their daily care. Nurses will need to use judgment regarding the amount of supervision the child requires. Some can be trusted to assume this responsibility unaided, whereas others will need someone in constant attendance. Children with cognitive impairments, physical limitations such as severe anemia or leg deformities, or suicidal or psychotic problems (who may commit bodily harm) require close supervision.

Areas that require special attention during bed baths and for children performing their own care are the ears, between skinfolds, the neck, the back, and the genital area. The genital area should be carefully cleansed and dried, with particular care given to skinfolds. In uncircumcised boys, usually those over 3 years of age, the foreskin should be gently retracted, the exposed surfaces are cleansed, and the foreskin is then replaced. If the condition of the glans indicates inadequate cleaning, such as accumulated smegma, inflammation, phimosis, or foreskin adhesions, teaching proper hygiene is indicated. In the Vietnamese and Cambodian cultures the foreskin is traditionally not retracted until adulthood. Older children have a tendency to avoid the genitalia; therefore they may need a gentle reminder.

Children who are ill or debilitated will need more extensive assistance with bathing and other aspects of hygienic care, but they should be encouraged to perform as much of their care as they are able without overtaxing their energies. Increasing involvement can be expected with improved strength and endurance. Children with limited capacity for self-help but no other contraindications benefit greatly from tub baths. They can be transported to the tub and, with the aid of lifting devices or an appropriate number of persons to assist, gain the advantages of a tub bath.

## Oral Hygiene

Mouth care is an integral part of daily hygiene and should be continued in the hospital. Infants and debilitated children will require the nurse or a family member to perform mouth care. Although young children can manage a toothbrush and are encouraged to use it, most will need assistance to perform a satisfactory job. Older children, although capable of brushing and flossing without assistance, sometimes need to be reminded that this is a part of their hygiene care. Most hospitals have equipment available for those children who do not have a toothbrush or toothpaste of their own.

## Hair Care

Brushing and combing hair are a part of the daily care for all persons in the hospital, including infants and children. If the child does not have a brush or comb, many hospitals provide one as part of the usual admission kit. If not, the parents should be asked to bring hair care equipment for the child's use. Both boys and girls are helped to comb or brush their hair, or it is done for them, at least once daily. The hair is styled for comfort and in a manner pleasing to the child and parents. A satisfactory style for girls with longer hair is French braiding, which is created by starting with three equal portions of hair from the top of the scalp; as the hair is braided, segments of hair are added at successive intervals until all of the hair has been incorporated into one or more neat, head-hugging braids. The ends are firmly anchored with an elastic hair band or barrette. The hair should not be cut without parental permission, although shaving hair to provide access to a scalp vein for IV needle insertion may be necessary.

If children are hospitalized for more than a few days, the hair may need shampooing. With infants, the hair may be washed during the daily bath or less frequently. For most children, washing the hair and scalp once or twice weekly is sufficient, unless there is an indication to wash it more frequently, such as following a high fever and profuse sweating. Some hospitals have shampoo basins, but almost any child can be conveniently transported by a stretcher to an accessible sink or washbasin for shampooing. Those who are unable to be transported can receive a shampoo in their beds with adequate protection and specially adapted equipment or positioning. A convenient method involves positioning the child near the edge of the bed, placing towels under the shoulders, and draping a large plastic garbage bag at the edge of the bed with one open end under the shoulders and the hair placed inside the opening. The other end is opened and placed in a collection container. Water can be transported in a basin.

**NURSING TIP**   For a convenient source of water, fill an empty enema bag with warm water and hang the bag from an IV pole; use the clamp on the bag's tubing to adjust the flow of water.

Teenagers, with their normally increased oily sebaceous secretions, are particularly in need of frequent hair care and usually require more frequent shampoos. Commercial "dry shampoo" products may also prove useful on a short-term basis.

African-American children require special hair care, and this need is frequently neglected or inadequately managed.

For the child with curly hair, most standard combs are inadequate and may cause hair breakage and discomfort to the child. If a special comb with widely spaced teeth is not available on the unit, the parent can be reminded to bring a comb, for the child's use. It is also much easier to comb the hair after shampooing, when it is wet. This type of hair requires a special hair dressing or pomade, which usually has a coconut oil base. The preparation is rubbed on the hands and then transferred to the hair to make it more pliable and manageable. The child's parents should be consulted regarding the preparation they wish to be used on their child's hair and asked if they can provide some for use during the child's hospitalization. Petroleum jelly should *not* be used. If braiding or plaiting the hair is desired, the hair should be damp and loosely woven. The hair tightens as it dries, which could result in tension folliculitis (Jackson, 1998).

## Feeding the Sick Child

Loss of appetite is a symptom common to most childhood illnesses. Because an acute illness is usually short, the nutritional state is seldom compromised. In fact, urging foods on the sick child may precipitate nausea and vomiting and in some cases even cause an aversion to the feeding situation that can extend into the convalescent period and beyond. In most cases children can be permitted to determine their own need for food.

Refusing to eat may also be one way children can exert power and control in an otherwise helpless situation. For young children, loss of appetite may be related to depression caused by separation from their parents. Parents' concern with eating can intensify the problem. Forcing a child to eat only meets with rebellion and reinforces the behavior as a control mechanism. Parents are encouraged to relax any pressure during an acute illness. Although it is best to encourage high-quality nutritious foods, the child may desire foods and liquids that contain mostly calories. Some well-tolerated foods include gelatin, diluted clear soups, carbonated drinks, flavored ice pops, dry toast, and crackers. Even though these substances are not nutritious, they can provide necessary fluid and calories.

Dehydration is always a hazard when children are febrile or anorexic, especially when this condition is accompanied by vomiting or diarrhea. An adequate fluid intake is encouraged by offering small amounts of favored fluids at frequent intervals and by providing salty foods if allowed. If diarrhea is present, high-carbohydrate liquids (e.g., carbonated beverages, gelatin, flavored ice pops) are avoided because they may aggravate the diarrhea through an osmotic effect. Replacing abnormal losses with plain water or undiluted broth may worsen the electrolyte imbalance. Fluids should not be forced, and the child is not awakened from rest to take fluids. Forcing fluids may create the same difficulties as urging unwanted food. Gentle persuasion with preferred beverages will usually meet with success. Using play techniques can also be very effective (see Box 27-1).

In general, hamburgers, peanut butter and jelly sandwiches, fruit yogurt, milkshakes, spaghetti, tacos, macaroni and cheese, and pizza are favorite foods of most children. Although alone they may not typify well-balanced diets, they can be adjusted to include sufficient amounts from the basic four food groups. It is better to work with preferred food choices than with selections that children rarely eat. Approaches to food preparation that can increase the child's interest in eating are presented in the Guidelines box.

An understanding of children's feeding habits can also increase food consumption. For example, if children are given all of their food at one time, they will generally eat the dessert first. Likewise, if they are presented with large portions, they often push the food away because the amount overwhelms them. If young children are not supervised during mealtime, they tend to play with the food rather than eat it. Therefore nurses should present food in the usual order, such as soup first, followed by small portions of meat, potatoes, and vegetables, and ending with dessert. The principles of conservation can also be used to increase food consumption. (See Cognitive Development, Chapter 15.)

Once the child is feeling better, appetite usually begins to improve. It is also best to take advantage of any hungry period by serving high-quality foods and snacks. If the child still refuses to eat, nutritious fluids, such as prepared breakfast drinks, should be encouraged. Parents can be very helpful by bringing in these food items from home. This is especially important if the family's cultural eating habits differ from the hospital's food services. A clinical dietician in the hospital may also be consulted for alternative food choices.

When children are placed on special diets, such as clear liquids after surgery or during episodes of diarrhea, assessment of their intake and readiness to advance to more complex foods is essential.

### NURSING ALERT

Evidence of lack of readiness to advance the diet:
Vomiting or diarrhea
Decrease in appetite
Abdominal cramping or distention
Absence of bowel sounds
Dehydration or weight loss

Regardless of the type of diet, charting the amount consumed is an important nursing responsibility. Descriptions need to be detailed and accurate, such as "4 ounces of orange juice, one pancake, and 8 ounces of milk." Comments such as "ate well" or "ate poorly" are inadequate. Charting the percentage of the meal eaten is also inadequate unless food is measured before serving.

### NURSING ALERT

Ask the parent if the child ate all of the food from the tray. Occasionally a parent may eat something from the tray because the child did not eat or want it. The fact that a family member has eaten some of the food makes a marked difference in the report of how much the child ate.

If parents are involved in the child's care, they are encouraged to keep a list of everything eaten. Using a pre-

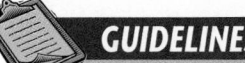

### GUIDELINES
#### Feeding the Sick Child

Take a dietary history (see Chapter 6) and use information to make eating time as much like home as possible.
Encourage parents or other family members to feed child or to be present at mealtimes.
Make mealtimes pleasant; avoid any procedures immediately before or after eating; make sure child is rested and pain free.
Serve small, frequent meals rather than three large meals or serve three meals and nutritious between-meal snacks.
Bring in foods from home, especially if food preparation is very different from hospital's; consider cultural differences.
Provide finger foods for young children. Avoid foods that pose a choking hazard for the infant, toddler, and preschool-age child (i.e., hot dogs, grapes, peanuts, and popcorn).
Involve children in food selection and preparation whenever possible.
Serve small portions, and serve each course separately, such as soup first, followed by meat, potatoes, and vegetables, and ending with dessert; with young children, offer second helpings; ensure a variety of foods, textures, and colors.
Provide food selections that are favorites of most children, such as peanut butter and jelly sandwiches, hot dogs, hamburgers, macaroni and cheese, pizza, spaghetti, tacos, fried chicken, corn on the cob, and fruit yogurt.
Avoid foods that are highly seasoned, have strong odors, are served hot, or are all mixed together, unless typical of cultural practices.
Provide fluid selections that are favorites of most children, such as fruit punch, cola, ginger ale, sweetened tea, ice pops, sherbet, ice cream, milk and milkshakes, pudding, gelatin, clear broth, or creamed soups.
Offer nutritious snacks, such as frozen yogurt or pudding, ice cream, oatmeal or peanut butter cookies, hot cocoa, cheese slices, pieces of raw vegetable or fruit, and dried fruit or cereal.
Make food attractive and different, for example:
  Serve a "picnic lunch" in a paper bag.
  Pack food in a Chinese-food container; decorate container.
  Put a "face" or a "flower" on a hamburger or sandwich with pieces of vegetable.
  Use a cookie cutter to shape a sandwich.
  Serve pudding, yogurt, or juice frozen as a flavored ice pop.
  Make slurpies or snowcones by pouring flavored syrup on crushed ice.
  Serve fluids through brightly colored or unusually shaped straws.
  Make "bowtie" sandwiches by cutting them in triangles and placing two points together.
  Slice sandwiches into "fingers."
  Grate mounds of cheese.
  Cut apples horizontally to make circles.
  Put a banana on a hot dog bun and spread with peanut butter.
Praise children for what they do eat.
Do *not* punish children for not eating by removing their dessert or putting them to bed.

measured cup for fluids ensures a more accurate estimate of intake. A comparison of the intake at each meal can isolate food deficiencies, such as insufficient intake of meat or vegetables. Behaviors associated with mealtime also identify possible factors influencing appetite. For example, the observation, "Child eats well when with other children but plays with food if left alone in room," helps the nurse plan mealtime activities that stimulate the child's appetite.

## Controlling Elevated Temperatures

An elevated temperature, most frequently from fever but occasionally caused by hyperthermia, is one of the most common symptoms of illness in children. This manifestation is a great concern to parents. To facilitate an understanding of fever, the following terms are defined:

*Set point*—The temperature around which body temperature is regulated by a thermostat-like mechanism in the hypothalamus
*Fever (hyperpyrexia)*—An elevation in set point such that body temperature is regulated at a higher level; may be arbitrarily defined as temperature above 38° C (100.4° F)
*Hyperthermia*—A situation in which body temperature exceeds the set point, which usually results from the body or external conditions creating more heat than the body can eliminate, such as in heat stroke, aspirin toxicity, or hyperthyroidism

Body temperature is regulated by a thermostat-like mechanism in the hypothalamus. This mechanism receives input from centrally and peripherally located receptors. When temperature changes occur, these receptors relay the information to the thermostat, which either increases or decreases heat production to maintain a constant set point temperature. However, during an infection, pyrogenic substances cause an increase in the body's normal set point, a process that is mediated by prostaglandins. Consequently, the hypothalamus increases heat production until the core temperature reaches the new set point (Connell, 1997).

During the fever (febrile) state, shivering and vasoconstriction generate and conserve heat during the *chill phase* of fever, raising central temperatures to the level of the new set point. The temperature reaches a *plateau* when it stabilizes in the higher range. When the temperature is greater than the set point or when the pyrogen is no longer present, a crisis, or *defervescence,* of the temperature occurs.

Most fevers in children are of brief duration with limited consequences and are viral in origin. When fever is caused by bacteria, endotoxins are produced that activate the inflammatory process and produce fever (Rote, Huether, and McCance, 2000). Contrary to popular belief, neither the rise

in temperature nor its response to antipyretics indicates the severity or etiology of the infection, which casts doubt on the value of using fever as a diagnostic or prognostic indicator.

### Therapeutic Management

Treatment of elevated temperature depends on whether it is due to a fever or hyperthermia. Because the set point is normal in hyperthermia but increased in fever, different approaches must be used to lower body temperature successfully. An unusual presentation of elevated temperature is malignant hyperthermia. Management of this emergency condition differs from the usual measures for fever or hyperthermia (see p. 1113).

**Fever.** The principal reason for treating fever is the relief of discomfort. Relief measures include pharmacologic and environmental intervention. The most effective intervention is the use of antipyretics to lower the set point.

Antipyretic drugs include acetaminophen, aspirin, and nonsteroidal antiinflammatory drugs (NSAIDs). Acetaminophen is the preferred drug. Aspirin should not be given to children because of the possible association between aspirin use in children with influenza virus or chickenpox and Reye syndrome. One nonprescription NSAID, ibuprofen, is approved for fever reduction in children as young as 6 months of age (Table 27-3). Dosage is based on the initial temperature level: 5 mg/kg of body weight for temperatures less than 39.2° C (102.5° F) or 10 mg/kg for temperatures greater than 39.2° C (102.5° F). The recommended dosage for pain is 10 mg/kg every 6 to 8 hours, and the recommended maximum daily dose for pain and fever is 40 mg/kg. The duration of fever reduction is generally 6 to 8 hours and is longer with the higher dose.

The recommended dosages of acetaminophen are listed in Table 27-4. It should be given every 4 hours, but no more than five times in 24 hours. Because body temperature normally decreases at night, three to four doses in 24 hours will usually control most fevers. The temperature is usually retaken 30 minutes after the antipyretic is given to assess its effect but should not be repeatedly measured. The child's level of discomfort is the best indication for continued treatment.

Environmental measures to reduce fever may be used if tolerated by the child and if they do not induce shivering.

---

**TABLE 27-3** Dosage recommendations for ibuprofen* (children's Motrin)

| Weight Pounds | kg | Age | Oral Drops (50 mg/1.25 ml) | Suspension (100 mg/5 ml) | Chewable Tablets (50 mg†) | Caplets (100 mg) |
|---|---|---|---|---|---|---|
| 12-17 | 5.4-7.7 | 6-11 months | 1 dropper | ¼ tsp | | |
| 18-23 | 8.2-10.4 | 12-23 months | 1½ droppers | ½ tsp | | |
| 24-35 | 10.9-15.9 | 2-3 years | | 1 tsp | 2 | 1 |
| 36-47 | 16.3-21.3 | 4-5 years | | 1½ tsp | 3 | 1½ |
| 48-59 | 21.8-26.8 | 6-8 years | | 2 tsp | 4 | 2 |
| 60-71 | 27.2-32.2 | 9-10 years | | 2½ tsp | 5 | 2½ |
| 72-95 | 32.7-43.1 | 11 years | | 3 tsp | 6 | 3 |

Modified from *Physician's Desk Reference*, Monvale, NJ, 2001, Medical Economics.
*Dosages based on fever <39.2° C using 5 mg/kg. For fever ≥39.2° may use 10 mg/kg.
Doses administered every 6 to 8 hours. Another nonprescription ibuprofen is children's Advil.
†Also available in 100-mg tablets.

Shivering is the body's way of maintaining the elevated set point by producing heat. Compensatory shivering greatly increases metabolic requirements above those already caused by the fever.

> **NURSING ALERT**
>
> Treatment of shivering is directed at modifying or interfering with the rate of heat loss by warming the body with increased clothing (especially on the extremities), higher environmental temperature, and warm baths.

Traditional cooling measures, such as minimum clothing, exposing the skin to the air, reducing room temperature, increasing air circulation, and cool moist compresses to the skin (e.g., the forehead), are effective if employed approximately 1 hour *after* an antipyretic is given so that the set point is lowered. Cooling procedures such as sponging or tepid baths are ineffective in treating *febrile* children (these measures are used for hyperthermia) either when used alone or in combination with antipyretics, and they cause considerable discomfort (Sharber, 1997).

Seizures associated with a fever occur in 3% to 4% of all children, usually in those between 3 months and 5 years of age. Although most children never have febrile seizures after the first occurrence, a younger age at onset and a family history of febrile seizures are associated with recurring episodes (Berg and others, 1999; Shinnar and others, 2001). There is little evidence to support the use of antipyretic drugs to prevent febrile seizures, nursing intervention should focus on ways in which care and comfort can be provided during a febrile illness (Purssell, 2000). (See Febrile Seizures, Chapter 37.)

**Hyperthermia.** Unlike in fever, antipyretics are of no value in hyperthermia, because the set point is already normal. Consequently, cooling measures are used. Cool applications to the skin help to reduce the core temperature. Cooled blood from the skin surface is conducted to inner organs and tissues, and warm blood is circulated to the surface, where it is cooled and recirculated. The surface blood vessels dilate as the body attempts to dissipate heat to the environment and facilitate this cooling process.

Commercial cooling devices, such as cooling blankets or mattresses, are available to reduce body temperature. They are placed on the bed and covered with a sheet or lightweight blanket. Frequent temperature monitoring is essential to prevent excessive cooling of the body.

Traditionally, cool compresses have been used to decrease high temperature. However, no particular water temperature is agreed on as being optimum. For tepid tub baths, it is usually best to start with warm water and gradually add cool water until the desired water temperature of 37° C (98.6° F) is reached to accustom the child to the lower water temperature. Generally the temperature of the water only has to be 1° to 2° (usually a warm temperature) less than the child's temperature to be effective (Kinmonth, Fulton, and Campbell, 1992). The child is placed directly in the tub of tepid water for 20 to 30 minutes while water is gently squeezed from a washcloth over the back and chest or gently sprayed over the body from a sprayer. In the bed or crib, cool washcloths or towels are used, exposing only one area of the body at a time. The sponging is continued for approximately 30 minutes.

> **NURSING ALERT**
>
> Isopropyl alcohol should *never* be used for sponging; neurotoxic effects such as stupor, coma, and even death have been reported.

After the tub or sponge bath, the child is dried and dressed in lightweight pajamas, a nightgown, or a diaper and is placed in a dry bed. The temperature is retaken 30 minutes after the tub or sponge bath. The child is dried by gently rubbing the skin surface with a towel to stimulate circulation. The tub or sponge bath should not be continued or restarted until the skin surface is warm or if the child feels chilled. Chilling causes vasoconstriction, which defeats the purpose of the cool applications. In this condition little blood is carried to the skin surface; the blood remains primarily in the viscera to become heated.

Whether a temperature elevation in the critically ill child is caused by fever or hyperthermia, it should be treated more aggressively. The metabolic rate increases 10% for every 1° C increase in temperature and three to five times during shivering, increasing oxygen, fluid, and caloric requirements. If the child's cardiovascular or neurologic system is already compromised, these increased needs are especially hazardous. In all children with an elevated temperature, attention to adequate hydration is essential. Most children's needs can be met through additional oral fluids.

## Family Teaching and Home Care

Nurses have a unique opportunity for teaching the family about health care practices while the child is hospitalized. Although most children have learned self-care and hygiene in the home or at school, many have not. For some young children, this is their first introduction to the use of a toothbrush. Much health teaching can be accomplished even when the child is hospitalized for only a short time. The

**TABLE 27-4** Dosage recommendations for acetaminophen (Tylenol)*

| Age | Weight (pounds) | Dose (mg) |
|---|---|---|
| Under 3 months | 6-11 | 40 |
| 4-11 months | 12-17 | 80 |
| 12-23 months | 18-23 | 120 |
| 2-3 years | 24-35 | 160 |
| 4-5 years | 36-47 | 240 |
| 6-8 years | 48-59 | 320 |
| 9-10 years | 60-71 | 400 |
| 11 years | 72-95 | 480 |
| 12 years and above | 96+ | 640 |

*Doses should be administered four or five times daily but should not exceed five doses in 24 hours.

daily bath, handwashing before meals and after bowel and bladder evacuation, and conscientious dental hygiene are taught by example during routine care. Clean hair, nails, and clothing, as well as good grooming, are emphasized as being essential to a pleasing appearance. Positive reinforcement of good hygiene practices helps to create a positive body image, promote the development of self-esteem, and prevent health problems (e.g., teaching girls to wipe the genital area from front to back after toileting).

Although sick children's appetites may be poor and not characteristic of their home eating habits, the hospital stay provides numerous opportunities for nurses to assess the family's knowledge of good nutrition and to implement teaching as needed to improve nutritional intake. Creative games can be employed that not only teach but provide diversion as well.

Fever is one of the most common problems in pediatrics for which parents seek health care. Parental anxiety levels are increased with temperature elevation and its management (Liebman and Barnsteiner, 2001). Nurses have the opportunity to provide parents information regarding the recognition of fever and the appropriate measures to manage it. Parents need to know that sponging is indicated for elevated temperatures from hyperthermia rather than fever and that ice water and alcohol are inappropriate, potentially dangerous, solutions (Axelrod, 2000). Parents should know how to take the child's temperature, read the thermometer accurately, and have guidelines for seeking

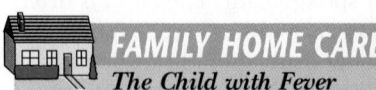

## FAMILY HOME CARE
### The Child with Fever

**CALL OUR OFFICE IMMEDIATELY IF:**

Your child is less than 3 months old, unless the fever is
    caused by a diphtheria-pertussis-tetanus (DPT) shot.
The fever is over 40.5° C (105° F).
Your child is crying inconsolably or whimpering.
Your child is difficult to awaken.
Your child cries if you touch or move him or her.
Your child's neck is stiff.
Any purple spots are present on the skin.
Breathing is difficult *and* no better after you clear the nose.
Your child is unable to swallow anything and is drooling
    saliva.
Your child looks or acts very sick (if possible, check your
    child's appearance 1 hour after he or she has taken
    acetaminophen).
Your child has a history of febrile seizures.
You have other questions or concerns.

**CALL WITHIN 24 HOURS IF:**

Your child is 3 to 6 months old, unless the fever is due to a
    DPT shot.
The fever is 40° to 40.5° C (104° to 105° F), especially if
    your child is less than 2 years old.
Burning or pain occurs with urination.
Your child has had a fever for more than 24 hours without
    an obvious cause or location of infection.

Modified from Schmitt BD: *Instructions for pediatric patients*, ed 2, Philadelphia, 1999, WB Saunders.

professional care. (See Family Home Care box.) Some of the newer temperature-measuring devices, such as plastic strip or digital thermometers, may be better suited for home use. (See Temperature, Chapter 7.) If the use of antipyretics (acetaminophen or ibuprofen) is indicated, the parents need instruction in administering the drug.* It is important to emphasize accuracy in both the amount of drug given and the time intervals at which the drug is administered.

**NURSING ALERT**    The nurse must be certain of the type of acetaminophen being used in the home. For example, the chewable tablets come in *two* strengths (80 mg and 160 mg). The infant liquid form contains 80 mg/0.8 ml (one dropperful), whereas the elixir has 160 mg/5 ml. Using the wrong preparation can underdose or overdose the child. As children grow the dose needs to be recalculated (10 to 15 mg/kg).

## SAFETY

Safety is an essential component of any patient's care, but children have special characteristics that require an even greater concern for safety. Because small children are separated from their usual environment and do not possess the capacity for abstract thinking and reasoning, it is the responsibility of everyone who comes in contact with them to maintain protective measures throughout their hospital stay. Nurses need a good understanding of the age level at which each child is operating and should plan for safety accordingly.

Identification bands, a part of hospital safety practices, are particularly important for children in the pediatric age-group. Infants and unconscious patients are unable to tell or respond to their names. Toddlers may answer to any name or to a nickname only. Older children may exchange places, give an erroneous name, or choose not to respond to their own names as a joke, unaware of the hazards of such practices.

### Infection Control

According to the **Centers for Disease Control and Prevention (CDC),** approximately 2 million patients each year develop nosocomial (hospital-acquired) infections. These infections occur when there is interaction among patients, health care personnel, equipment, and bacteria (Russell, 1999). Nosocomial infections are preventable if caregivers practice meticulous cleaning and disposal techniques.

The CDC and the **Hospital Infection Control Practices Advisory Committee (HICPAC)** have revised the "CDC Guideline for Isolation Precautions in Hospitals," which was published in 1983. The guideline was revised to meet the following objectives: (1) to be epidemiologically

---

*Home care instructions for measuring temperature and giving medications are available in Wong DL, Hess CS: *Wong and Whaley's clinical manual of pediatric nursing*, ed 5, St Louis, 2000, Mosby.

sound; (2) to recognize the importance of all body fluids, secretions, and excretions in the transmission of nosocomial pathogens; (3) to contain adequate precautions for infections transmitted by the airborne, droplet, and contact routes of transmission; (4) to be as simple and user friendly as possible; and (5) to use new terms to avoid confusion with existing infection control and isolation systems (Garner, 1997).

The revised guideline contains two levels of precautions. *Standard precautions* synthesize the major features of universal (blood and body fluid) precautions (UP) (designed to reduce the risk of transmission of blood-borne pathogens) and body substance isolation (BSI) (designed to reduce the risk of transmission of pathogens from moist body substances). Standard precautions involve the use of *barrier protection,* such as gloves, goggles, gown, and mask, to prevent contamination from (1) blood; (2) all body fluids, secretions, and excretions *except sweat,* regardless of whether or not they contain visible blood; (3) nonintact skin; and (4) mucous membranes. Standard precautions are designed for the care of *all* patients to reduce the risk of transmission of microorganisms from both recognized and unrecognized sources of infection.

*Transmission-based precautions* are designed for patients documented or suspected to be infected or colonized with highly transmissible or epidemiologically important pathogens for which additional precautions beyond standard precautions are needed to interrupt transmission in hospitals. There are three types of transmission-based precautions: airborne precautions, droplet precautions, and contact precautions. They may be combined for diseases that have multiple routes of transmission (Box 27-5). When used either singularly or in combination, they are to be used in addition to standard precautions.

*Airborne precautions* are designed to reduce the risk of airborne transmission of infectious agents. Airborne transmission occurs by dissemination of either airborne droplet nuclei (small-particle residue [5 $\mu$m or smaller in size] of evaporated droplets that may remain suspended in the air for long periods of time) or dust particles containing the infectious agent. Microorganisms carried in this manner can be dispersed widely by air currents and may become inhaled by or deposited on a susceptible host within the same room or over a longer distance from the source patient, depending on environmental factors. Therefore *special air handling* and *ventilation* are required to prevent airborne transmission. Airborne precautions apply to patients known or suspected to be infected with epidemiologically important pathogens that can be transmitted by the airborne route. Examples of such illnesses include measles, varicella (chickenpox), and tuberculosis.

*Droplet precautions* are designed to reduce the risk of droplet transmission of infectious agents. Droplet transmission involves contact of the conjunctivae or the mucous membranes of the nose or mouth of a susceptible person with large-particle droplets (larger than 5 $\mu$m in size) containing microorganisms generated from a person who has a clinical disease or who is a carrier of the microorganism. Droplets are generated from the source person primarily during coughing, sneezing, or talking and during the performance of certain procedures such as suctioning and bronchoscopy. Transmission via large-particle droplets re-

---

### Box 27-5 ■ ■ ▢
## Summary of Types of Precautions and Patients Requiring Them

**STANDARD PRECAUTIONS**

Use standard precautions for the care of all patients.

**AIRBORNE PRECAUTIONS**

In addition to standard precautions, use airborne precautions for patients known or suspected to have serious illnesses transmitted by airborne droplet nuclei. Examples of such illnesses include measles, varicella (including disseminated zoster), and tuberculosis.

**DROPLET PRECAUTIONS**

In addition to standard precautions, use droplet precautions for patients known or suspected to have serious illnesses transmitted by large-particle droplets. Examples of such illnesses include the following:

Invasive *Haemophilus influenzae* type b disease, including meningitis, pneumonia, epiglottitis, and sepsis

Invasive *Neisseria meningitidis* disease, including meningitis, pneumonia, and sepsis

Other serious bacterial respiratory infections spread by droplet transmission, including diphtheria (pharyngeal), mycoplasmal pneumonia, pertussis, pneumonic plague, streptococcal pharyngitis, pneumonia, or scarlet fever in infants and young children

Serious viral infections spread by droplet transmission, including adenovirus, influenza, mumps, parvovirus B19, rubella

**CONTACT PRECAUTIONS**

In addition to standard precautions, use contact precautions for patients known or suspected to have serious illnesses easily transmitted by direct patient contact or by contact with items in the patient's environment. Examples of such illnesses include the following:

Gastrointestinal, respiratory, skin, or wound infections or colonization with multidrug-resistant bacteria judged by the infection control program, based on current state, regional, or national recommendations, to be of special clinical and epidemiologic significance

Enteric infections with a low infectious dose or prolonged environmental survival, including *Clostridium difficile.* For diapered or incontinent patients: enterohemorrhagic *Escherichia coli* O157:H7, *Shigella,* hepatitis A, or rotavirus

Respiratory syncytial virus, parainfluenza virus, or enteroviral infections in infants and young children

Skin infections that are highly contagious or that may occur on dry skin, including diphtheria (cutaneous); herpes simplex virus (neonatal or mucocutaneous); impetigo; major (noncontained) abscesses, cellulitis, or decubiti; pediculosis; scabies; staphylococcal furunculosis in infants and young children, zoster (disseminated or in the immunocompromised host)

Viral/hemorrhagic conjunctivitis

Viral hemorrhagic infections (Ebola, Lassa, or Marburg)

Modified from Garner JS: Guideline for isolation precautions in hospitals, *Infect Control Hosp Epidemiol* 17(1):66, 1996.

quires close contact between source and recipient persons because droplets do not remain suspended in the air and generally travel only short distances, usually 3 feet or less, through the air. Because droplets do not remain suspended in the air, special air handling and ventilation are not required to prevent droplet transmission. Droplet precautions apply to any patient known or suspected to be infected with epidemiologically important pathogens that can be transmitted by infectious droplets (see Box 27-5).

*Contact precautions* are designed to reduce the risk of transmission of epidemiologically important microorganisms by direct or indirect contact. *Direct-contact transmission* involves skin-to-skin contact and physical transfer of microorganisms to a susceptible host from an infected or colonized person, such as occurs when personnel turn patients, bathe patients, or perform other patient care activities that require physical contact. Direct-contact transmission also can occur between two patients (e.g., by hand contact), with one serving as the source of infectious microorganisms and the other as a susceptible host. *Indirect-contact transmission* involves contact of a susceptible host with a contaminated intermediate object, usually inanimate, in the patient's environment. Contact precautions apply to specified patients known or suspected to be infected or colonized (presence of microorganism in or on patient but without clinical signs and symptoms of infection) with epidemiologically important microorganisms that can be transmitted by direct or indirect contact.

Nurses caring for young children are frequently in contact with body substances, especially urine, feces, and vomitus. Nurses need to exercise judgment concerning those situations when gloves, gowns, or masks are necessary. For example, gloves and possibly gowns should be worn for changing diapers when there are loose or explosive stools. Otherwise, the plastic lining of disposable diapers provides a sufficient barrier between the hands and body substances. The type of diaper may be an important aspect of infection control. Superabsorbent disposable diapers with elastic legs contain urine and feces better than cloth diapering systems, and their use can reduce fecal contamination in the environment (Kubiak and others, 1993).

Antimicrobial-resistant organisms are causing increasing numbers of nosocomial infections. Nearly 70% of nosocomial infections can be attributed to seven pathogens: the gram-positive organisms *Staphylococcus aureua*, coagulase-negative staphylococci, and enterococci; and the gram-negative organisms *Escherichia coli, Pseudomonas aeruginosa, Enterobacter,* and *Klebsiella pneumonia.* In hospitals, patients are the most significant sources of methicillin-resistant *S. aureus* (MRSA), and the main mode of transmission is patient to patient via the hands of a health care provider (Russell, 1999). Therefore handwashing is the most critical infection control practice.

During feedings, gowns should be worn if the child is likely to vomit or spit up, which often occurs during burping. When gloves are worn, the hands are washed thor-

---

### EVIDENCE-BASED PRACTICE
*The Effects of Fingernail Polish and Gloves on Hand Contamination*

Clean hands, with a minimum presence of microorganisms, have always been the most important measure for controlling infection.

One controversy has been whether to allow surgical staff members to wear nail polish. The argument against polish has been that microorganisms could be harbored in nail polish once it cracks, chips, or peels. However, a study compared microorganism counts on personnel's hands with or without nail polish. Twenty-six healthy volunteer subjects were compared over a period of time in groups randomly assigned to have polished or unpolished nails. Their results indicated that "nail polish did not pose a microbial risk under . . . test conditions. . . . In fact, the data are consistent with the hypothesis that polish, because of the hard, smooth surface, may actually seal crevices in which microorganisms could be harbored" (Baumgardner and others, 1993).

The study did raise two concerns about the use of polish: (1) the possibility that more seriously damaged nails could be adversely affected by nail polish and (2) the possibility that the presence of polish might have an effect on behavior in the surgical scrub; that is, the individual might be protective of the manicure and be "less inclined to perform a vigorous surgical scrub to protect the nails." Either of these cases, researchers asserted, could prove detrimental by fostering bacterial growth on the hands, although neither would reflect the direct effects of the polish itself. In conclusion, keeping nails short, clean, and healthy is probably more important than the effects of wearing nail polish.

In another study, researchers examined the efficacy of gloves as barriers to hand contamination during endotracheal tube care, digital rectal stimulation, and dental examination.

Of the 135 gloves that were cultured, 86 were contaminated with gram-negative rods or enterococci on the outside of the gloves. In 11 of the 86 events, the health care worker's hands were contaminated, an event that occurred more frequently with vinyl (10 of 42) than with latex (1 of 44) gloves. Likewise, glove leaks occurred more frequently with vinyl (26 of 61) than with latex (6 of 70) gloves. However, there was not a strong correlation between glove leaks and contaminated hands; leaky gloves kept hands clean 77% of the time. Interestingly, health care workers were aware of the leaks in only 7 of the 32 instances. These results indicate that the absence of visible leaks cannot be used by personnel to assume that gloves are intact.

This study supported conclusions similar to those of the nail polish study. Although gloves provide "substantial protection," their use does not decrease the importance of routine handwashing after each patient contact (Olsen and others, 1993).

Two additional studies focused on the incidence of handwashing and contamination of latex examination gloves. Researchers found that health care workers washed their hands only 27% of the time before putting on gloves and changed gloves only 16% of the time after patient interaction (Thompson and others, 1997). Hannigan and Shields (1998) found that the diversity of glove parts presenting from the box contributes to contamination and that examination gloves could not be extracted from the box by health care workers with unwashed hands without contaminating the external surfaces with common skin-borne bacteria. It is recommended that in order to minimize nonsocomial infections, health care workers should wash their hands before gloving and after examination, and only sterile gloves should be supplied in critical areas of patient care (Hannigan and Shields, 1998).

oughly after removing the gloves because both latex and vinyl gloves fail to provide complete protection. The absence of visible leaks does not indicate that gloves are intact. (See Evidence-Based Practice box.) An additional consideration is that some people are allergic to latex. (See Latex Allergy, Chapter 11.)

> **NURSING ALERT** Patients and staff may be sensitive to latex and demonstrate allergic reactions ranging from hives, wheezing, and localized swelling to anaphylaxis. Latex is present in numerous health care products, including gloves, tourniquets, airway equipment, catheters, IV supplies, and dressings.

Another essential practice of infection control is that all needles (uncapped and unbroken) are disposed of in a rigid, puncture-resistant container located near the site of use. Consequently, these containers are installed in patients' rooms. Because children are naturally curious, extra attention is needed in selecting a suitable type of container and a location that discourages access to the disposed needles (Fig. 27-6). The use of needleless systems allows secure syringe or IV tubing attachment to vascular access devices without the risk of needle-stick injury to the child or nurse.

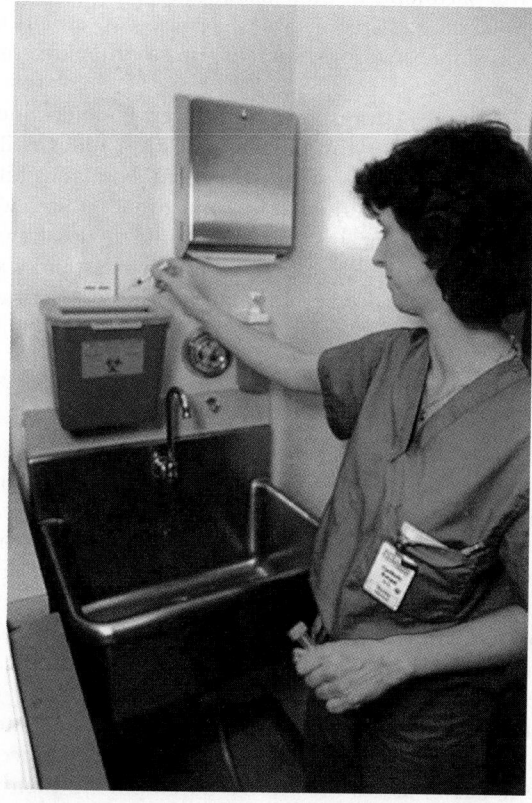

**Fig. 27-6** To prevent needle-stick injuries, used needles (and other sharp instruments) are not capped or broken and are disposed of in a rigid, puncture-resistant container located near the site of use. Note placement of the container to prevent children's access to the contents.

## Environmental Factors

All of the environmental safety measures for the protection of adults apply to children as well, such as good illumination, floors clear of fluid or other objects that might contribute to falls, and nonskid surfaces in showers and tubs. Electrical equipment is maintained in good working order, is used only by personnel familiar with its use, and is not in contact with moisture or near tubs, where it could prove to be a shock hazard. Beds of ambulatory patients are locked in place and at a height that allows easy access to the floor. A special hazard for children is the danger of entrapment under an electronically controlled bed when it is activated to descend. Staff members should practice proper care and disposal of small objects such as temperature probes and needle covers. All staff members should be familiar with the area-specific fire plan.

All windows should be securely screened, and elevators and stairways should be made safe. Ideally, electrical outlets should be provided with covers to prevent burns in small children, whose exploratory activities may extend to inserting objects into the small openings. Bathwater is carefully checked before placing the child in it, and children must never be left alone in a bathtub. Infants are helpless in water, and small children (and some older ones) may turn on the hot water faucet and be severely burned. All windows should be secured. Blind and curtain cords should be out of reach.

Furniture is safest when it is scaled to the child's proportions, is sturdy, and is well-balanced to prevent its being easily tipped over. Infants and small children must be securely strapped into infant seats, feeding chairs, and strollers. Baby walkers should be discouraged because they provide access to hazards, resulting in burns, falls, and poisonings. Infants, young children, and those who are weak, paralyzed, agitated, confused, sedated, or cognitively impaired are never left unattended on treatment tables, on scales, or in treatment areas. Even premature infants are capable of surprising mobility; therefore portable incubators must be securely fastened when not in use.

Crib sides are kept up and fastened securely unless an adult is at the bedside. It is safer to leave crib sides up, regardless of the child's ability to get out, even when the crib is unoccupied, to remove the temptation to climb in. Anyone attending an infant or small child in a crib with the sides down should never turn away without maintaining hand contact with the child; that is, one hand is kept on the child's back or abdomen to prevent rolling, crawling, or jumping from the open crib (Fig. 27-7). Children in beds may fall despite raised siderails by climbing over them. A child who tends or seems inclined to climb over the sides of the crib is safest when placed in a specially constructed crib with a cover over the top. (See Injury Prevention, Chapter 12.)

> **NURSING ALERT** Do not place cribs within reach of heating units, appliances, dangling cords, outlets, or other objects that can be reached by curious hands.

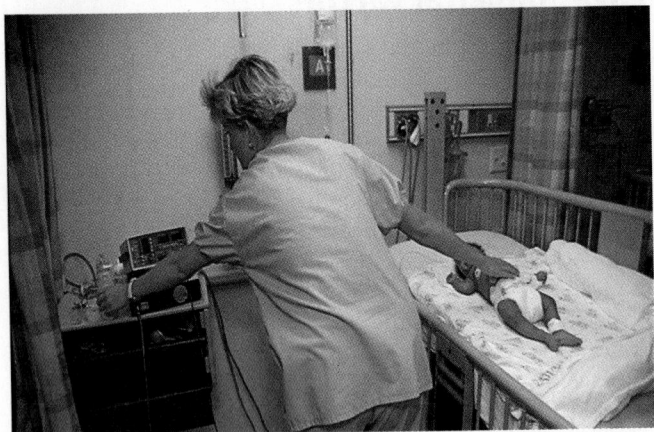

**Fig. 27-7** Nurse maintains hand contact when back is turned.

Plants and flowers harbor gram-negative bacteria and molds that may be of risk to the immunocompromised child. These items may also pose the danger of poisoning to curious toddlers.

## Toys

Toys play a vital role in the everyday life of children, and they are no less important in the hospital setting. However, nurses are responsible for assessing the safety of toys brought to the hospital by well-meaning parents and friends. Toys should be appropriate to the child's age, condition, and treatment. For example, if the child is in an oxygen tent, electrical or friction toys or equipment cannot be placed in the tent, because sparks can cause oxygen to ignite. Toys are inspected to make certain that they are non-allergenic, washable, and unbreakable and that they have no small, removable parts that can be aspirated or swallowed or that can otherwise inflict injury on a child. Latex balloons pose a serious threat to children of all ages. If the balloon breaks, a child may put a piece of the latex in his or her mouth. If it is aspirated or swallowed, the latex piece is difficult to remove, resulting in choking. Latex balloons should **never** be permitted in the hospital setting.

## Limit-Setting

Setting limits is essential to a child's safety. Children must understand where they are permitted to go and what they are permitted to do in the hospital. These limitations are made clear to them, are consistently enforced, and are repeated as frequently as necessary to make certain that they are understood. The nurse is responsible for where children are at all times. Children can easily wander off unnoticed, and their access to tubs, laundry chutes, medication rooms/carts, and elevators must be prevented. Normally active older children often become restless when their activity is restricted and may resort to pillow fights, water fights, and other rough play that might endanger the safety of other children, staff, or visitors. Children in the hospital require surveillance, and appropriate tension-reducing activities

can be planned and supervised by nurses or by a child life specialist. A useful discipline technique is time-out. (See Limit-Setting and Discipline, Chapter 3.)

## Transporting Infants and Children

In the course of a hospital stay, infants and children usually need to be transported within the unit and to areas outside the pediatric unit. It is ordinarily safe to carry infants and small children for short distances within the unit, but for more extended trips the child should be securely transported in a suitable conveyance.

Small infants can be held or carried in the horizontal position with the back supported and the thigh grasped firmly by the carrying arm (Fig. 27-8, *A*). In the football hold, the infant is carried on the nurse's arm with the head supported by the hand and the body held securely between the nurse's body and elbow (Fig. 27-8, *B*). Both these holds leave the nurse's other arm free for activity. The infant can be held in the upright position with the buttocks on the nurse's forearm and the front of the body resting against the nurse's chest. The infant's head and shoulders are supported by the nurse's other arm to allow for any sudden movement by the infant (Fig. 27-8, *C*). Older infants are able to hold their heads erect but are still subject to sudden movements.

Infants can be transported to other areas, such as the radiology department, in their bassinet or crib. Strollers and wheeled feeding chairs or tables are also convenient transporters in some situations, such as trips to the playroom, or nurse's station.

The method of transporting children is determined by their age, condition, and destination. Most older children are safe in wheelchairs or on stretchers. Younger children can be transported in their crib, on a stretcher, in a wagon with raised sides, or in a wheelchair with a safety belt. Stretchers should be equipped with high sides and a safety belt, both of which are kept in place during transport.

## Restraining Methods and Therapeutic Holding

Some type of restraining method may be necessary during the course of caring for an infant or child. The reasons for the restraining methods may vary from ensuring the child's safety to facilitating examination. An alternative approach for temporary restraint is *therapeutic holding*. Therapeutic holding is the use of a secure, comfortable, temporary holding position that provides close physical contact with the parent or caregiver (Fig. 27-9). The use of restraint can often be avoided with adequate preparation of the child, parental or staff supervision of the child, or adequate protection of a vulnerable site, such as an infusion device. The nurse needs to assess the child's development, mental status, potential to hurt others or self, and safety. Alternative measures to using restraints should be a careful consideration of the nurse. Some examples of alternative measures include bringing a child to the nurses' station for continuous observation, providing diversional activities such as music, or encouraging the participation of the parents.

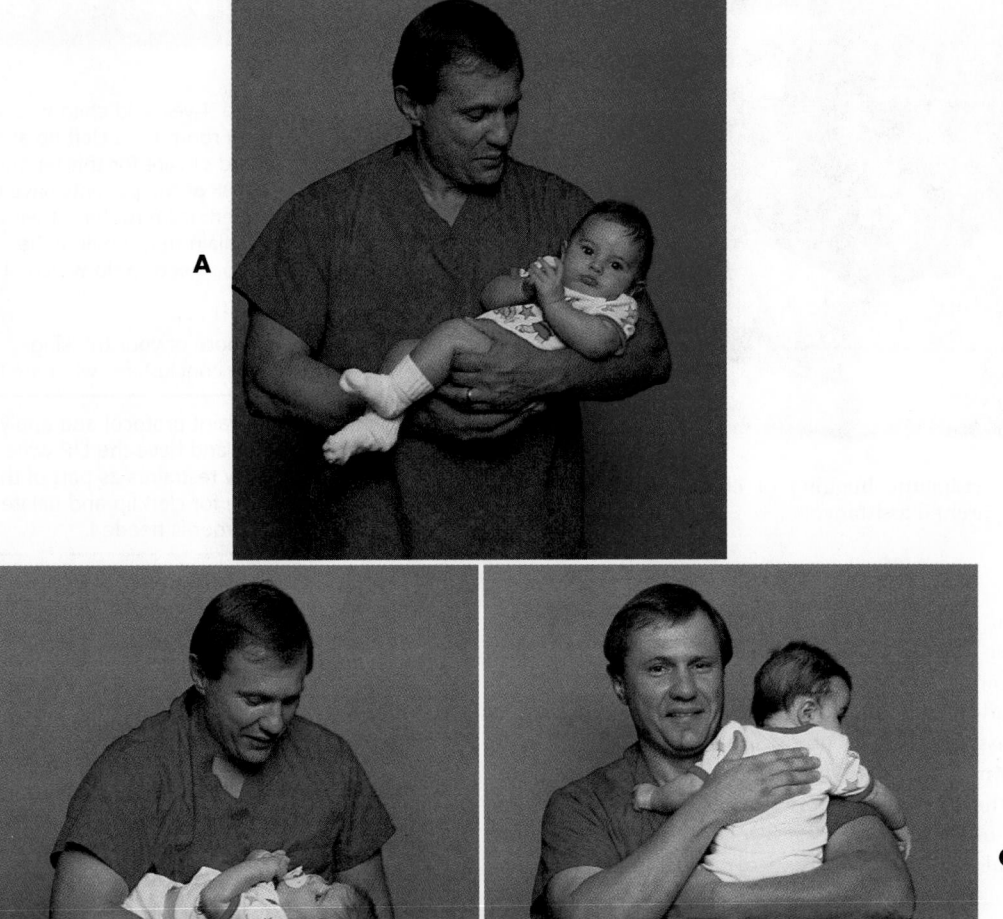

**Fig. 27-8**   Transporting infants. **A,** Infant's thigh firmly grasped in nurse's hand. **B,** Football hold. **C,** Back supported.

---

**NURSING ALERT**   Physical restraint should never be used as a substitute for good nursing care, for punishment, or as a convenience to the staff.

The **Health Care Financing Administration (HCFA)** and the **Joint Commission on Accreditation of Healthcare Organizations (JCAHO)** have developed standards to guide acute care hospitals in the use of restraints. JCAHO defines restraint as "any method, physical or mechanical which restricts a person's movement, physical activity, or normal access to his or her body" (JCAHO, 2001). Their standards mandate that a policy be in effect that is clear and consistent and includes the assessment of the patient's need for restraint (reason for restraint); at least one alternative method must be attempted before restraint application; and, when restraints are applied, the least restrictive method is used. An order must be be written and an evaluation performed by a licensed independent practitioner (LIP) within 1 hour of applying the restraint. The LIP order must include the start and stop time, date, reason for restraint, type of restraint used, and signature of the LIP. An initial verbal order can be obtained by the RN (Krozek and Scoggins, 2001).

Some standards of care or protocols have been developed for specific diagnoses and include restraint application. When a standard or protocol states that a restraint is required 100% of the time, the above standards do not apply (Krozek and Scoggins, 2001). For example, use of elbow restraints postoperatively after a cleft lip repair written in

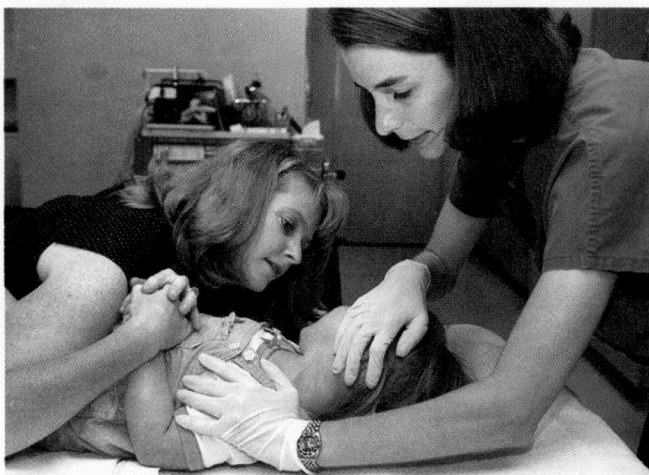

**Fig. 27-9** Therapeutic hugging of child for jugular vein puncture with parental assistance.

*Critical Thinking Exercise*

### Use of Restraints

You are caring for a 4-year-old child who just returned from the operating room for a cleft lip and palate repair. Part of the standard of care for this type of surgical patient is that 100% of the patients have elbow restraints applied to keep them from rubbing their lip. The child is beginning to complain that the lip itches. To apply the elbow restraints, you need to do which of the following?

FIRST, THINK ABOUT IT . . .

• What is the purpose of your thinking
• If you accept the conclusions, what are the implications?

1. Initiate the restraint protocol and apply the restraints.
2. Apply restraints and have the LIP write an order.
3. Apply the elbow restraints as part of the postoperative standard of care for cleft lip and palate procedures. No additional LIP order is needed.

*The best response is two. When applying a restraint, a LIP must evaluate and write an order within 1 hour of application.*

*When a child is restrained, it is important to explain to the child the reason for the restraint. Reassure the child that the restraint is not a punishment. Parents also need to know the purpose of restraints, how to remove them, and the signs of complications from their use. Document parental consent for the restraints. Explain to parents ways in which they can help to ensure maximum benefit and minimum stress (e.g., have the parent emotionally support the child by staying near the child). Position the parent at the head of the bed so that the parent can soothe or calm the child by talking softly, singing, or stroking the child's skin.*

the protocol or standard of care in 100% of patients would not fall under the JCAHO or HCFA mandates. In *all* restraints, ongoing assessment, evaluation, and documentation must be addressed. The RN must remove the restraining devices, assess, and document findings *at least every 2 hours.* Documentation includes circulation status and condition of the limb, hydration status, feeling and toilet needs, range-of-motion needs, level of consciousness, and emotional status. (See Critical Thinking Exercise box.)

The nurse is responsible for selecting the least restrictive type of restraint. For example, arm boards are less restrictive than two-point extremity restraint. Using less restrictive restraints is often possible by gaining the cooperation of the child and parents.

Restraining devices are not without risk, which is the reason for the JCAHO and HCFA strict mandates on the use of restraints. Restraining devices must be checked every 1 to 2 hours to ensure that they are accomplishing their purpose; that they are applied correctly; and that they do not impair circulation, sensation, or skin integrity. Restraints with ties must be secured to the bed or crib *frame,* not the siderails. Suggestions for increasing safety and comfort while the child is in a restraint include the following: leaving one finger breadth between skin and the device; tying knots for quick release; ensuring the restraint does not tighten as the child moves; decreasing wrinkles or bulges in the restraint; placing jacket restraints over an article of clothing; placing limb restraints below the level of the waist, below the knee level, or distal to the IV; and tucking in dangling straps (Selekman and Synder, 1997).

### Mummy Restraint or Swaddle

When an infant or small child requires short-term restraint for examination or treatment that involves the head and neck (e.g., venipuncture, throat examination, gavage feeding), a papoose board with straps or a mummy wrap effectively controls the child's movements. A blanket or sheet is opened on the bed or crib with one corner folded to the center. The infant is placed on the blanket with shoulders at the fold and feet toward the opposite corner (Fig. 27-10, *A*). With the infant's right arm straight down against the body, the right side of the blanket is pulled firmly across the infant's right shoulder and chest and secured beneath the left side of the body (Fig. 27-10, *B*). The left arm is placed straight against the infant's side, and the left side of the blanket is brought across the shoulder and chest and locked beneath the infant's body on the right side (Fig. 27-10, *C*). The lower corner is folded and brought over the body and tucked or fastened securely with safety pins. Safety pins can be used to fasten the blanket in place at any step in the process.

To modify the mummy restraint for chest examination, the folded edge of the blanket is brought over each arm and under the back, after which the loose edge is folded over and secured at a point below the chest to allow visualization and access to the chest (Fig. 27-10, *D*).

**NURSING ALERT** Papoose boards or mummy wraps are not substitutes for use of sedation and analgesia during painful procedures. They should be used only when no other options exist.

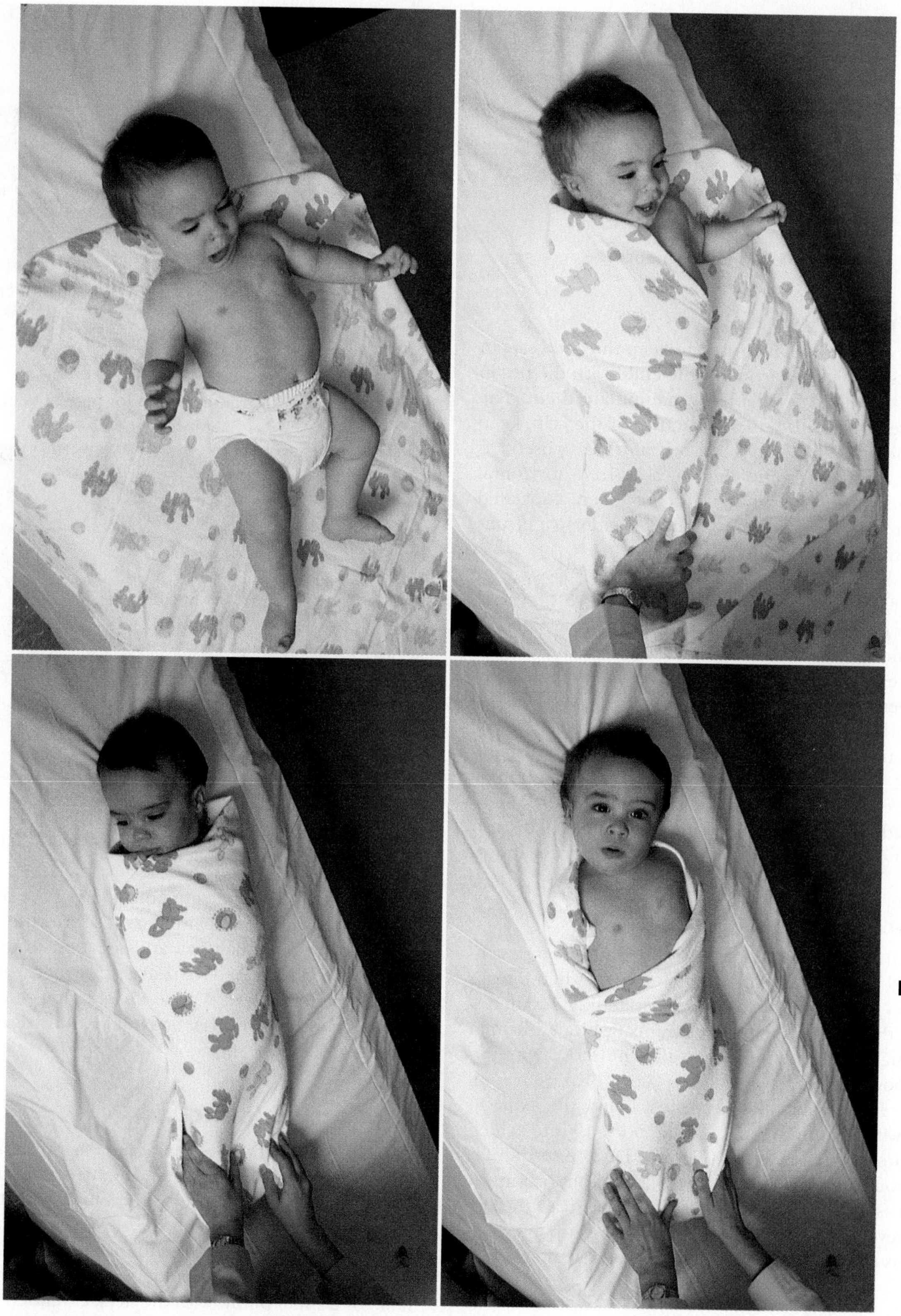

**Fig. 27-10** Application of mummy restraint. **A,** Infant placed on folded corner of blanket. **B,** One corner of blanket brought across and secured beneath the body. **C,** Second corner brought across body and secured, and lower corner folded and tucked or pinned in place. **D,** Modified mummy restraint with chest uncovered.

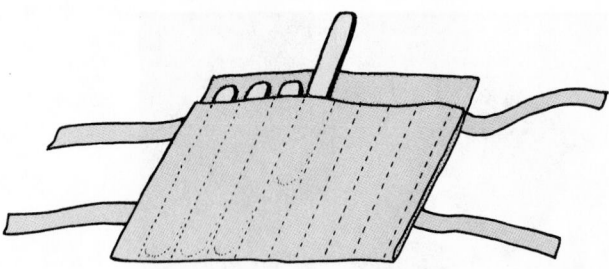

**Fig. 27-11** Elbow restraints.

## Jacket Restraint

A jacket restraint is sometimes used to keep the child safe in various chairs. The jacket is put on the child with the ties in back so that the child is unable to manipulate them. The long tapes, secured to the understructure of the crib, keep the child inside the crib. The jacket restraint is also useful as a means for maintaining the child in a desired horizontal position. The jacket type of restraint has been associated with accidental strangulation deaths in elderly persons (U.S. Department of Agriculture, 1992).

## Arm and Leg Restraints

Occasionally one or more extremities must be restrained or limited in motion. Several commercial restraining devices are available, including disposable wrist and ankle restraints. When this type of restraint is used, it must be appropriate to the child's size; it must be padded to prevent undue pressure, constriction, or tissue injury; and the extremity must be observed frequently for signs of irritation or impaired circulation. The ends of the restraints are never tied to the siderails, because lowering of the rail will disturb the extremity, frequently with a jerk that may hurt or injure the child.

## Elbow Restraint

Sometimes it is important to prevent the child from reaching the head or face (e.g., after lip surgery or when a scalp vein infusion is in place) or to prevent scratching in skin disorders. For this purpose, elbow restraints fashioned from a variety of materials function very well. The most common form of elbow restraint consists of a piece of muslin long enough to reach comfortably from just below the axilla to the wrist, with a number of vertical pockets into which tongue depressors are inserted (Fig. 27-11). The restraint is wrapped around the arm and secured with tapes or pins. It may be necessary to pin the top of the restraint to the undershirt sleeve to prevent the restraint from slipping. Similar restraints can be made from readily available items.

## POSITIONING FOR PROCEDURES

Infants and small children are unable to cooperate for many procedures; therefore the nurse is responsible for minimizing their movement and discomfort with proper positioning. Older children usually need only minimal, if any, restraint. Careful explanation and preparation beforehand

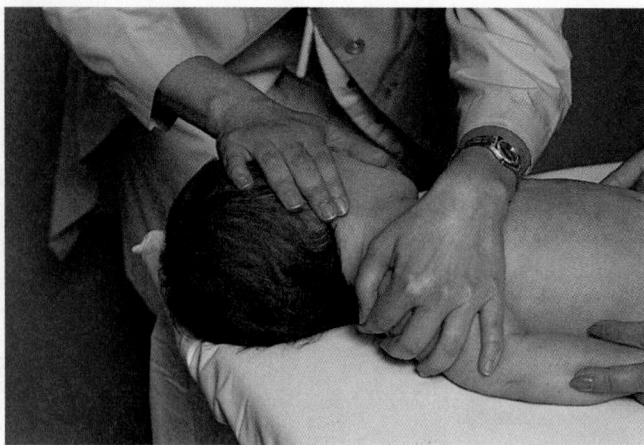

**Fig. 27-12** Restraining child for jugular vein puncture.

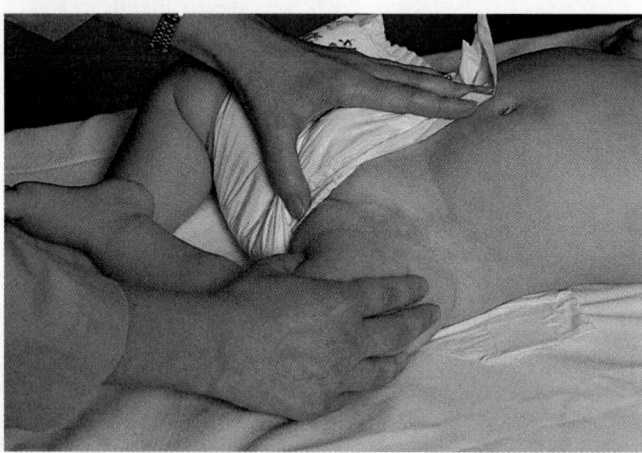

**Fig. 27-13** Restraining infant for femoral vein puncture.

and support and simple guidance during the procedure are usually sufficient. For painful procedures the child should receive adequate analgesia and sedation to minimize pain and the need for excessive restraint. For local anesthesia use buffered lidocaine to reduce the stinging sensation or the topical anesthetic EMLA or Numby Stuff. (See Pain Management, Chapter 26.)

## Jugular Venipuncture

The large, superficial external jugular vein may be used to obtain blood specimens from infants and young children. For easy access to the vein, the child is first placed in a mummy restraint in which the top edge of the restraint is low enough to permit access to the vein. The child is placed so that the head and shoulders extend over the edge of a table or a small pillow with the neck extended and the head turned sharply to the side. An alternate method for restraining the arms and legs is for the nurse to hold the child's arms and legs at the same time that the child's head is restrained and positioned (Fig. 27-12). It is important for the nurse holding the infant to maintain control of the infant's head without interfering with the operator's approach to the vein. Following venipuncture, digital pressure

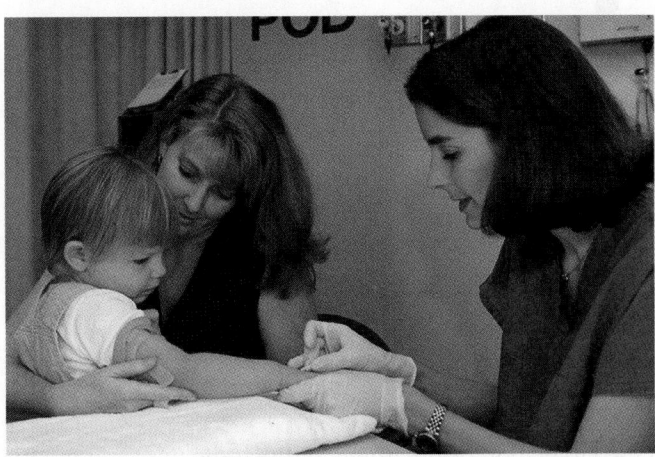

**Fig. 27-14** Therapeutic hugging of child for extremity vein puncture with parental assistance.

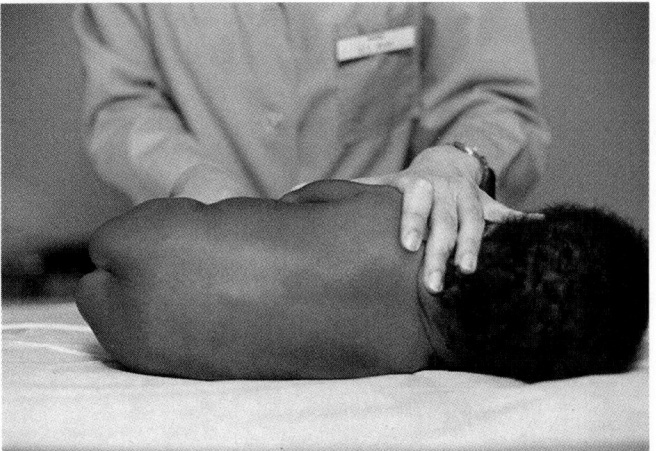

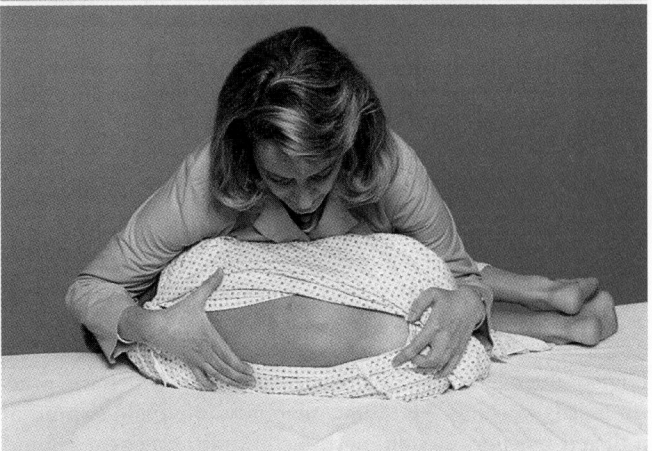

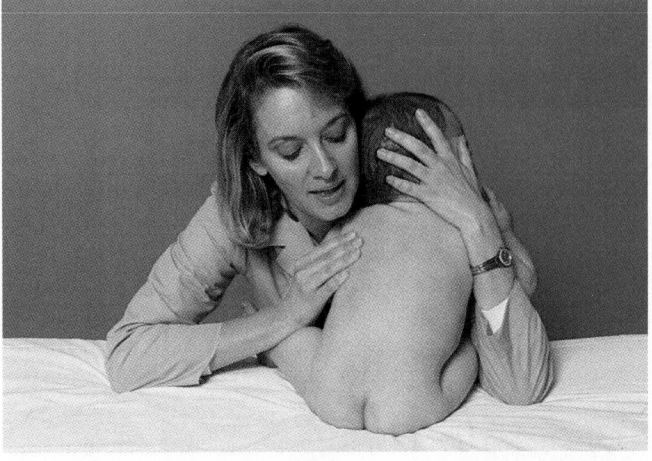

**Fig. 27-15** **A,** Modified side-lying position for lumbar puncture. **B,** Older child in side-lying position. **C,** Infant sitting position allows for flexion of lumbar spine.

is applied to the site with a dry gauze square for 3 to 5 minutes or until bleeding stops. Care must be taken not to apply excessive pressure that might compromise circulation or breathing during or following the procedure.

## Femoral Venipuncture

Other frequently used sites for venipuncture are the large femoral veins. The nurse restrains the infant by placing the child supine with the legs in a frog position to provide extensive exposure of the groin area. The legs of the infant can then be effectively controlled by the nurse's forearms and hands (Fig. 27-13). Only the side used for the venipuncture is uncovered so that the operator is protected should the child urinate during the procedure. Pressure is applied after the withdrawal of blood to prevent oozing from the site.

## Extremity Venipuncture

The most common sites of venipuncture are the veins of the extremities, especially the arm and hand. A convenient position for restraint is having one person on either side of the bed. The child's outstretched arm is partially stabilized by the technician drawing the blood. The other person hugs the child's upper body, preventing movement, and uses an arm to immobilize the venipuncture site. This type of restraint also comforts the child because of the close body contact and allows each person to maintain eye contact (Fig. 27-14).

## Lumbar Puncture

The technique for lumbar puncture (LP) in infants and children is similar to that in the adult, although modifications are suggested in neonates, who have less distress in a side-lying position with modified neck extension than in flexion or a sitting position (Fig. 27-15, *A*). Pediatric lumbar puncture sets contain smaller spinal needles, but sometimes

the practitioner will specify a particular size or type of needle that the nurse should make certain is placed on the tray.

Children are usually controlled best in the side-lying position, with the head flexed and the knees drawn up toward the chest. Even cooperative children need to be held gently to prevent possible trauma from unexpected, involuntary movement. They can be reassured that, although they are trusted, holding will serve as a reminder to maintain the de-

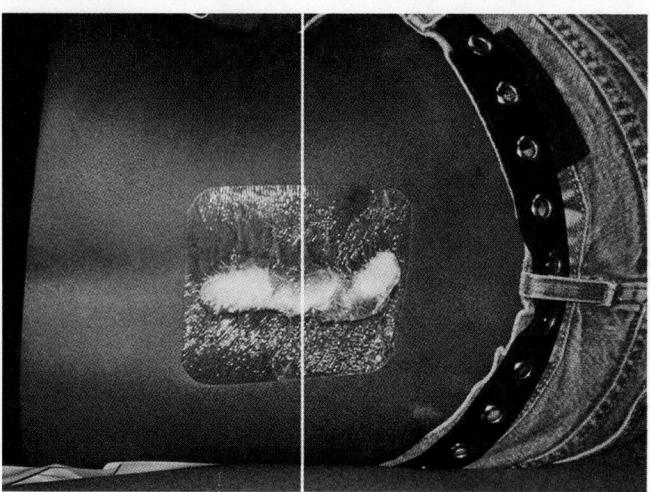

**Fig. 27-16** EMLA, a local anesthetic cream, is placed under an occlusive dressing to decrease pain of lumbar puncture. The site is located by drawing an imaginery line from the top of the iliac crest to cross the spine at the approximate needle insertion site.

sired position. It also provides a measure of support and reassurance to them.

The child is placed on the side with the back close to the edge of the examining table on the side from which the practitioner is working. The nurse maintains the child's spine in a flexed position by holding the child with one arm behind the neck and the other behind the thighs (Fig. 27-15, *B*). The flexed position enlarges the spaces between the lumbar vertebral spines, which facilitates access to the spinal fluid space. It is helpful to wrap the legs before positioning to decrease leg movement.

An alternate position used with small infants and some older children is the sitting position. The child is placed with the buttocks at the edge of the table and with the neck flexed so that the chin rests on the chest or on the nurse's arm. Before starting the procedure, ensure that the infant's airway is not compromised by the position chosen for restraint. The infant's arms and legs are immobilized by the nurse's hands (Fig. 27-15, *C*).

> **NURSING ALERT**
> The sitting position may interfere with chest expansion and diaphragm excursion, and in infants the soft, pliable trachea may collapse. Therefore observe the child for difficulty with breathing.

Another position that employs close and comforting contact for the child involves holding the child upright against the nurse's (or parent's) chest with the child's legs wrapped around the adult's waist. The adult's arms are used to hug and restrain the child. For ease of the examiner, the adult should be standing. A small pillow is placed between the child's abdomen and the adult to help arch the child's back. If the pillow proves unsuccessful, a third person can place an arm in this space to achieve the desired position. Care should be taken that excessive pressure does not compro-

### ATRAUMATIC CARE
*Lumbar Puncture and Bone Marrow Test*

Apply EMLA to the puncture site at least 60 minutes before the procedure. To identify the LP site, draw an imaginary line from the posterior iliac crest across the spine to the opposite iliac crest. The puncture site is intersected by the line at approximately L4 (Fig. 27-16). For additional anesthesia, buffered lidocaine with a 30-gauge needle can be used. *Unconscious sedation* with agents such as propofol (Diprivan) or ketamine is recommended for bone marrow biopsy and aspiration. Conscious or unconscious sedation is recommended for LP.

mise circulation or breathing and that the nose and mouth are not covered by the restrainer's body.

Specimens and spinal fluid pressure are obtained, measured, and sent for analysis in the same manner as for the adult patient. Vital signs are taken as ordered, and the child is observed for any changes in level of consciousness, motor activity, or other neurologic signs. Post–lumbar puncture headache may occur and is related to postural changes; this is less severe when the child lies flat. Headache is seen much less frequently in young children than in adolescents.

## Bone Marrow Aspiration/Biopsy

The position for a bone marrow aspiration or biopsy depends on the location of the chosen site. In children the posterior or anterior iliac crest is most frequently used, although in infants the tibia may be selected because of easy access to the site and holding of the child. The sternum, which is the most frequent site in adults, is generally avoided in children because the bone is more fragile and adjacent to vital organs.

If the posterior iliac crest is used, the child is positioned prone. Sometimes a small pillow or folded blanket is placed under the hips to facilitate obtaining the bone marrow specimen. Children should receive adequate analgesia or anesthesia to relieve pain. If the child may awaken, holding may be needed and is best done with two people—one person to immobilize the upper body and a second person to immobilize the lower extremities. (See Atraumatic Care box.)

## Other Procedures

For subdural puncture through a fontanel or burr hole, the infant is wrapped in a mummy restraint and placed in the supine position with the head accessible to the examiner. To control the head, the nurse uses a firm hold on each side of it. (Procedures for immobilizing the head are discussed in Chapter 7 under Ears; Nose; Mouth and Throat.)

## COLLECTION OF SPECIMENS

Many of the specimens needed for diagnostic examination of children are collected in much the same way as they are for adults. Older children are able to cooperate if given proper instruction regarding what is expected of them. Infants and small children, however, are unable to follow directions or control body functions sufficiently to help in collecting some specimens.

## Urine Specimens

Children admitted to the hospital or seen in a clinic or office may require a urine specimen. Older children and adolescents will readily use the bedpan or urinal or can be trusted to follow directions for collection in the bathroom. However, they may have special needs. School-age children are cooperative but curious. They are concerned about the reasons behind things and are likely to ask questions regarding the disposition of their specimen and what one expects to discover from it. Self-conscious adolescents may be reluctant to carry a specimen bottle through a hallway or waiting room and appreciate a paper bag or other means for disguising the container. The presence of menses may be an embarrassment or a concern to teenage girls; therefore it is a good idea to ask them about this and make adjustments as necessary. The specimen can be delayed or a notation made on the laboratory slip to explain the presence of red blood cells.

Preschoolers and toddlers are less cooperative, primarily because they are usually unable to void on request. It is often best to offer them water or other liquids that they enjoy and wait about 30 minutes until they are ready to void voluntarily.

**NURSING TIP**   Wipe the abdomen with an alcohol pad and fan it dry; the cooling effect often causes voiding within 2 minutes. Apply pressure over the suprapubic area or stroke the paraspinal muscles (along the spine) to elicit the Perez reflex; in infants 4 to 6 months of age, this reflex causes crying, extension of the back, flexion of the extremities, and urination.

Children will better understand what is expected if the nurse uses familiar terms for the function, such as "pee-pee," "wee-wee," or "tinkle." Some will have difficulty voiding in an unfamiliar receptacle. Potty chairs or a "potty hat" placed on the toilet are usually satisfactory. Toddlers who have recently acquired bladder control may be especially reluctant, since they undoubtedly have been admonished for "going" in places other than those approved by parents. A useful approach is to enlist the help of parents; they are likely to be successful, and this helps them to feel a part of the child's care.

For infants and toddlers who are not toilet trained, special urine collection devices are used. These devices are clear plastic, single-use bags with self-adhering material around the opening at the point of attachment. To prepare the infant, the genitalia, perineum, and surrounding skin are washed and dried thoroughly, because the adhesive will not stick to a moist, powdered, or oily skin surface. The collection bag is easiest to apply if attached first to the perineum, progressing to the symphysis pubis (Fig. 27-17). With little girls the perineum is stretched taut during application to that area to ensure a leakproof fit. With small boys the penis and sometimes the scrotum are placed inside the

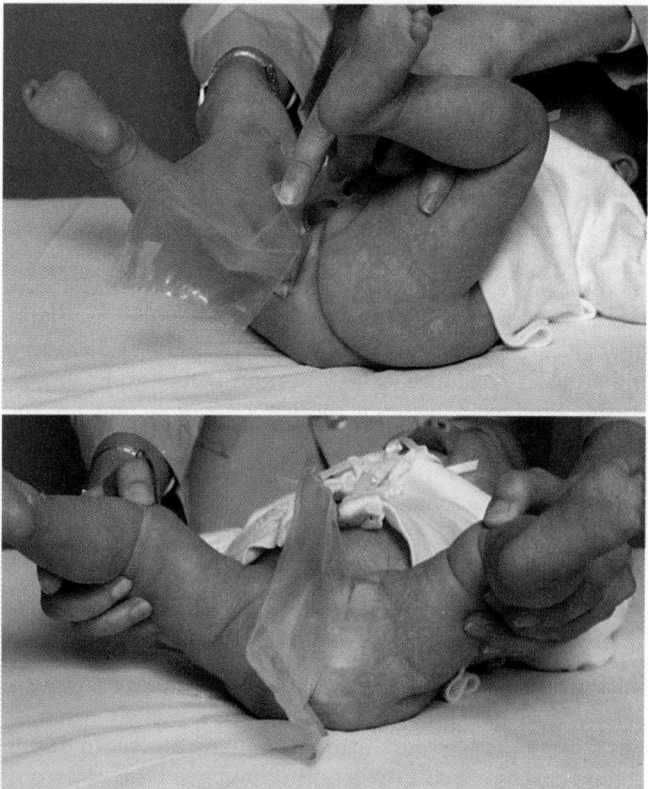

**Fig. 27-17**   Application of urine collection bag. **A,** On female infant, adhesive portion is applied to exposed and dried perineum first. **B,** Bag adheres firmly around perineal area to prevent urine leakage.

bag. The adhesive portion of the bag must be firmly applied to the skin all around the genital area to avoid possible leakage. The diaper is carefully replaced. For low–birth-weight infants, small bags with adhesive that is gentle to the skin are available.* Anatomically correct urine collection bags are also available.† The bag is checked frequently and removed as soon as the specimen is available, because the moist bag may become loosened on an active child. For some types of urine testing, such as checking specific gravity, ketones, sugar, and protein, urine can be aspirated directly from the diaper.

**NURSING TIP**   When using a urine collection bag, cut a small slit in the diaper and pull the bag through to allow room for urine to collect and to facilitate checking on the contents. To obtain small amounts of urine, use a syringe without a needle to aspirate urine directly from the diaper; if diapers with absorbent gelling material that trap urine are used, place a small gauze dressing, some cotton balls, or a urine collection device‡ inside the diaper to collect urine and aspirate the urine with a syringe.

---

*Available from Hollister, Inc, 2000 Hollister Dr, Libertyville, IL 60048, (800) 323-4060.
†Available from ConvaTec, CN 5254, Princeton, NJ 08543-5254, (800) 422-8811; www.convatec.com.
‡The Bard Infant Urine Collector is available from Bard Urological Division, CR Bard, Inc, Covington, GA 30209, (800) 526-4455.

Urine obtained from disposable diapers can be tested accurately for glucose, ketones, proteins, blood, and urea. In one study, urine obtained from a disposable diaper provided a valid sample for diagnosing urinary tract infections (Cohen Reis and Holubkov, 1997). Erythrocyte and leukocyte counts may be low. Superabsorbent disposable diapers may produce a false crystalluria. Specific gravity measurements are accurate for up to 4 hours provided that the disposable diapers are kept folded. Urine samples collected by the cotton ball method were accurate for pH and specific gravity and were atraumatic to the skin of newborns (Burke, 1995). Traditionally, specific gravity refractometers have been used on nursing units to measure specific gravity. One study showed strong agreement between the use of a refractometer and regeant strip to test urine specific gravity (Barton and Holmes, 1998). However, current regulations have limited use of the refractometer to the laboratory. Urine dipsticks can be used on the nursing unit with reasonable accuracy. When urine is collected for culture, the bag is removed immediately. If the urine is not tested within 30 minutes, the specimen is refrigerated or placed in a sterile container with a preservative.

At times parents may be asked to bring a urine sample to a health care facility for examination, especially when infants are unable to void during an outpatient visit. In this instance parents need instruction on applying the collection device and storage of the specimen.* Ideally, the specimen should be brought to the designated place as soon as possible; if there is a delay, the sample should be refrigerated and the lapsed time reported to the examiner.

### Clean-Catch Specimens

Clean-catch specimens traditionally refer to urine samples obtained for culture after the urethral meatus is cleaned and the first few millimeters of urine are voided before the urine is collected (midstream specimen). The procedure consists of cleaning the perineum in females and the tip of the penis in males using a soap or antiseptic solution. In females the perineum is wiped with a soaked cotton ball or pad from front to back at least three times using a new cotton ball or pad each time. In males the tip of the penis is cleansed. The area may be wiped with sterile water to prevent accidental contamination of the urine with a solution that may destroy pathogens. Although this traditional cleansing procedure is often practiced, studies have found that it does not significantly reduce contamination rates in infants, circumcised or uncircumcised males, or toilet-trained prepubertal children. Also midstream collection does not significantly reduce contamination rates over non-midstream specimens (Lohr, Donowitz, and Dudley, 1989; Prandoni and others, 1996; Saez-Llorens and others, 1989).

### Twenty-Four-Hour Collection

The need to collect urine voided over a 24-hour period creates a special challenge in infants and children. Collection

bags are required in infants and small children. Older children require special instruction about notifying someone when they need to void or have a bowel movement so that urine can be collected separately and is not discarded. Some older school-age children and adolescents can be trusted to take responsibility for collection of their own 24-hour specimens. They can keep output records and transfer each voiding to the 24-hour collection container if this is permitted.

As in any 24-hour urine collection, the collection period always starts and ends with an empty bladder. At the time the collection begins, the child is instructed to void and the specimen is discarded. All urine voided in the subsequent 24 hours is saved in a container with a preservative or is placed on ice. Twenty-four hours from the time the precollection specimen was discarded, the child is again instructed to void, the specimen is added to the container, and the entire collection is taken to the laboratory for examination.

Infants and small children who are bagged for 24-hour urine collection require a special collection bag; frequent removal and replacement of adhesive collection devices can produce skin irritation. A thin coating of sealant, such as Skin-Prep, applied to the skin helps to protect it and aids adhesion unless its use is contraindicated, such as in a premature infant or a child with irritated skin. Plastic collection bags with collection tubes attached are ideal when the container must be left in place for a time. These can be connected to a collecting device or emptied periodically by aspiration with a syringe. When such devices are not available, a regular bag with a feeding tube inserted through a puncture hole at the top of the bag serves as a satisfactory substitute. However, care is taken to empty the bag as soon as the infant urinates to prevent leakage and loss of contents. An indwelling catheter may also be placed for the collection period.

### Bladder Catheterization and Other Techniques

*Bladder catheterization* or *suprapubic aspiration* is employed when a specimen is urgently needed or when the child is unable to void or otherwise provide an adequate specimen. Catheterization is used to obtain a sterile urine specimen and when urethral obstruction or anuria caused by renal failure is believed to be the cause of the child's failure to void. Suprapubic aspiration is useful in clarifying the diagnosis of suspected urinary tract infection in acutely ill infants.

The anxiety, fear, and discomfort experienced during catheterization can be significantly alleviated by adequate preparation of the child and parents, by selection of the correct catheter, and by appropriate technique of insertion. Specifically, generous lubrication of the urethra before catheterization and use of a lubricant containing 2% lidocaine (Xylocaine) may significantly reduce or eliminate the burning and discomfort frequently associated with this invasive procedure.

Preparation for catheterization includes instruction on pelvic muscle relaxation whenever possible. The toddler, preschooler, or younger child is taught to blow a pinwheel and to press the hips against the bed or procedure table during catheterization in order to relax the pelvic and peri-

---

*Home care instructions for obtaining a urine sample are available in Wong DL, Hess CS: *Wong and Whaley's clinical manual of pediatric nursing,* ed 5, St Louis, 2000, Mosby.

urethral muscles. The location and function of the pelvic muscles are described briefly to the older child or adolescent. The patient is then taught to contract and relax the pelvic muscles, and the relaxation procedure is repeated during catheter insertion. If the patient vigorously contracts the pelvic muscles when the catheter reaches the striated sphincter (proximal urethra in boys and midurethra in girls), catheter insertion is temporarily stopped. The catheter is neither removed nor advanced; instead, the child is helped to press the hips against the bed or examining table and relax the pelvic muscles. The catheter is then gently advanced into the bladder (Gray, 1996).

> **NURSING ALERT**
>
> Use an appropriate-length urinary catheter to prevent knotting of the catheter in the bladder and urethral trauma. Feeding tubes for intermittent catheterization have been associated with a high incidence of catheter knotting in the bladder. The catheter's extra length coils around its end as bladder decompression occurs, causing subsequent catheter knotting. Surgical removal of a knotted catheter may be required (Carlson and Mowery, 1997).

Children and adolescents will experience some discomfort and anxiety during this procedure. Assistance and gentle holding may be necessary, especially in the younger child. Most children prefer to have the parents remain with them during the procedure. Encourage the parent to talk softly and hold the child's hand as the catheter is inserted. Using distractions such as reading a book, singing a favorite song, or playing with small toys may assist the child in decreasing anxiety. Older children and adolescents may wish to listen to music with headphones. Adolescent patients should be asked if they would like a parent to remain with them during the procedure. The decision should be made before the perineum is exposed, and the sterile field is prepared (Gray, 1996).

Catheterization is a sterile procedure, and standard precautions for body substance protection should be followed. When placing a catheter for a sterile urine specimen or to check for residual urine, a sterile feeding tube may be used. If the catheter is to remain in place, a Foley catheter is used. Table 27-5 gives guidelines for choosing the appropriate-size catheter and length of insertion. The supplies needed for this procedure include sterile gloves, sterile lubricant anesthetic, the appropriate-size catheter, povidone-iodine (Betadine) swabs or an alternative cleansing agent and 4 × 4 inch gauze squares, a sterile drape, and a syringe with sterile water if a Foley catheter is being used. Test the balloon of the Foley catheter by injecting sterile water before catheter insertion.

> **NURSING ALERT**
>
> Identify patients who have allergies to povidone-iodine or latex before using these items in catheterization.

Adolescent boys and children with a history of urethral surgery may be catheterized with a coudé-tipped catheter. The child with myelodysplasia or one who has been identified as being sensitive or allergic to latex is catheterized

**TABLE 27-5** Straight catheter or Foley catheter*

| | Female (Length of Insertion [cm]) | Male (Length of Insertion [cm]) |
|---|---|---|
| Term neonate | 5-6 (5) | 5-6 (6) |
| Infant—3 years | 5-8 (5) | 5-8 (6) |
| 4-8 years | 8 (5-6) | 8 (6-9) |
| 8 years—prepubertal | 10-12 (6-8) | 8-10 (10-15) |
| Pubertal | 12-14 (6-8) | 12-14 (13-18) |

*Foley catheters are approximately 1 French size larger because of circumference of balloon. Example 10 French Foley = approximately 12 French calibration.

with a catheter or feeding tube manufactured from an alternative material. When an indwelling catheter is indicated for urinary drainage, a lubricious coated or silicone catheter is selected because these materials produce less irritation of the urethral mucosa as compared with a Silastic or latex catheter when the catheter is left in place for more than 72 hours.

A 2% lidocaine lubricant with applicator is assembled according to the manufacturer's instructions,* and several drops of the lubricant are placed at the meatus. The child is advised that the lubricant is used to reduce any discomfort associated with inserting the catheter and that introduction of the catheter into the urethra will produce a sensation of pressure and a desire to urinate (Gray, 1996).

In male patients the tip of the applicator is gently introduced into the urethra 1 to 2 cm so that the lubricant flows only into the urethra; 5 to 10 ml of 2% lidocaine lubricant is slowly inserted into the urethra and held in place for 2 to 3 minutes by gently squeezing the distal penis. This maneuver allows the mucosa to absorb the active ingredient. Additional lubricant is placed on the catheter tip, which is inserted into the urethra without allowing the intraurethral lubricant to exit the urethral meatus. Using this technique of retaining the lubricant as the catheter is inserted provides lubrication of the urethra and promotes opening of the sphincter mechanism.

In female patients 1 to 2 ml of 2% lidocaine lubricant is placed on the periurethral mucosa, and 1 to 2 ml is inserted into the urethral meatus. Catheterization is delayed for 2 to 3 minutes to maximize absorption of the anesthetic into the periurethral and intraurethral mucosa. Additional lubricant is added to the catheter, which is gently inserted into the urethra until urine returns. This additional lubrication, combined with the mild anesthetic effects of the 2% lidocaine lubricant, greatly reduces the discomfort frequently associated with insertion of a catheter.

Because the use of lidocaine jelly can increase the volume of intraurethral lubricant, urine return may not be as rapid as when minimum lubrication is used. However, with

---

*Lidocaine hydrochloride 2% jelly is available in 5-, 10-, and 20- ml (20 mg/ml) glass prefilled sterile syringes from International Medication Systems, Ltd, (IMS), South El Monte, CA 91733, (818) 913-4660. Lidocaine hydrochloride 2% jelly is available in 10- and 20- ml (20 mg/ml) plastic prefilled sterile syringes from Astra USA, Inc, Westborough, MA 01581-4500, (800) 225-4803.

## ATRAUMATIC CARE
### Bladder Catheterization or Suprapubic Aspiration

Use distraction to help the child relax (blowing bubbles, deep breathing, singing a song).
Use lidocaine jelly to anesthetize the area before insertion. EMLA cream may lessen an infant's discomfort as the needle passes through the skin, but care should be taken that the site is thoroughly cleaned and prepped before the procedure. Children often become agitated at being restrained for either procedure. Comfort measures through touch and voice, both during and after the procedure, should be used to help reduce the child's distress.

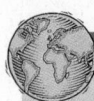

## CULTURAL AWARENESS
### Bladder Catheterization

Parents may be upset when their child is catheterized. Aside from the trauma the child experiences, some parents, especially those from different cultures, may fear that the procedure affects the daughter's virginity. To clarify this misconception, the family may benefit from a detailed explanation of the genitourinary anatomy, preferably with a model that shows the separate vaginal and urethral openings. The nurse can also indicate that catheterization has no effect on virginity.

patience, a urine return will occur, and the discomfort and anxiety commonly associated with catheterization will be avoided.

Gather the appropriate equipment and place onto a sterile field; don sterile gloves. Place a sterile drape under the buttocks of the female patient.

In female patients gently separate and pull up the labia minora to visualize the meatus. Use the nondominant hand for this action (which is now unsterile), and hold the labia open throughout the entire procedure. Swab the meatus from front to back three times, using a different povidone-iodine swab each time. Lubricate the sterile catheter and insert it into the urethra until urine is obtained. Advance the catheter an additional 1 to 2 inches. Inflate the balloon with the sterile water when using a Foley catheter, and gently pull back to test balloon inflation. Connect the Foley catheter to a closed drainage system. Gently remove a straight catheter once the desired amount of urine is obtained; cleanse the meatus and labia of povidone-iodine and lubricant with water. Praise the patient for her cooperation.

In male patients grasp the penis with the nondominant hand and retract the foreskin. In uncircumcised newborns and infants the foreskin may be adhered to the shaft; use care when retracting. If the penis is pendulous, place a sterile drape under the penis. Using the sterile hand, swab the glans and meatus three times with povidone-iodine. The remainder of the procedure is performed with the foreskin retracted. Hold the penile shaft just under the glans to prevent the foreskin from contaminating the area. Lubricate and insert the catheter while gently stretching the penis and lifting it to a 90-degree angle to the body. Resistance may occur when the catheter meets the urethral sphincter. Ask the patient to inhale deeply and advance the catheter at that time. *Do not force* a catheter that does not easily enter the meatus, particularly if the child has had corrective surgery. Once urine is obtained, advance the catheter to the hub or fork of the catheter (in indwelling catheters). For intermittent catheterization, insert only to the recommended length to avoid complications (Carlson and Mowery, 1997). Inflate the balloon with sterile water, pull it back gently to test inflation, and connect it to the closed drainage system. Cleanse the glans and meatus with water to prevent skin irritation, and replace the retracted foreskin in the uncircumcised patient.

If at any time during the procedure blood is seen, discontinue the procedure and notify the practitioner.

Suprapubic aspiration is mainly used when the bladder cannot be accessed through the urethra (such as with some congenital urologic birth defects) or to reduce the risk of contamination that may be present when passing a catheter. In general, with the advent of small-sized catheters (5 and 6 French straight catheters), the need for suprapubic aspiration has decreased. Access to the bladder via the urethra has a much higher success rate than suprapubic aspiration, where success depends on the practitioner's skill at assessing the location of the bladder and the amount of urine in the bladder (Pollack, Pollack, and Andrew, 1994).

Suprapubic aspiration, which is performed by a practitioner skilled in the procedure, involves aspirating bladder contents by inserting a 20- or 21-gauge needle in the midline approximately 1 cm above the symphysis pubis and directed vertically downward. The skin is prepared as for any needle insertion, and the bladder should contain an adequate volume of urine. This can be assumed if the infant has not voided for at least 1 hour, or the bladder can be palpated above the symphysis pubis. This technique is useful for obtaining sterile specimens from young infants, because the bladder is an abdominal organ and is easily accessed. Suprapubic aspiration is painful, and therefore pain management during the procedure is important. (See Atraumatic Care and Cultural Awareness boxes.)

## Stool Specimens

Stool specimens are frequently collected in children to identify parasites and other organisms that cause diarrhea, to assess gastrointestinal function, and to check for occult (hidden) blood. Ideally, stool should be collected without contamination with urine, but in children wearing diapers, this is difficult unless a urine bag is applied. Children who are toilet trained should urinate first, flush the toilet, and then defecate into the toilet or a bedpan (preferably one that is placed on the toilet to avoid embarrassment) or a commercial "potty hat."

**NURSING TIP** To obtain a stool specimen, place plastic wrap over the toilet bowl to collect the stool. Use a tongue depressor or disposable spoon or knife to collect the stool.

An ample amount of stool is collected and placed in the appropriate container, which is covered and labeled. If sev-

## ATRAUMATIC CARE
### *Drawing Blood from Central Lines*

Central lines can be used for obtaining blood specimens rather than performing a venipuncture. If laboratory personnel routinely draw blood for specimens, a sign placed on the door stating "Lab: Please check with the nurse before entering room" will eliminate unnecessary trauma because of venipunctures. Educating the parents and child (if age appropriate) with this alternative will reinforce atraumatic care.

eral specimens are needed, the containers are marked with the date and time and kept in a specimen refrigerator. Special care is exercised in handling the specimen because of the risk of contamination.

## Blood Specimens

Although most blood specimens are obtained by the laboratory staff or physicians, nurses are becoming increasingly responsible for specimen collection, especially if the child has an arterial or venous access device. Whether the specimen is collected by the nurse or by others, the nurse is responsible for making certain that specimens, such as serial examinations and fasting specimens, are collected on time and that the proper equipment is available. Collecting, transporting, and storing of specimen can have a major impact on laboratory results (Frizzell, 1998).

Venous blood samples can be obtained by venipuncture or by aspiration from a peripheral or central access device. Withdrawing blood specimens through peripheral lock devices (also known as intermittent infusion devices, PRN adapters, and heparin locks) in small peripheral veins has met with varying degrees of success. Although it avoids an additional venipuncture for the child, attempting to aspirate blood from the peripheral lock may shorten the life of the device. However, central lines may be used to withdraw blood samples (Fig. 27-18). (See Atraumatic Care box.) When using an IV infusion site for specimen collection, it is important to consider the type of fluid being infused. For example, a specimen collected for glucose determination would be inaccurate if removed from a catheter through which glucose-containing solution was being administered.

**NURSING TIP** To obtain a blood specimen from a central venous line or peripheral lock when the infusion solution may interfere with the test results, first aspirate a quantity of blood equal to the volume of fluid in the catheter and discard; then aspirate the blood sample. For a blood culture, use the first sample of blood, because organisms are most likely to collect within the catheter itself.

**NURSING ALERT** On small or anemic children, keep track of the amount drawn and discarded over time. Frequent blood sampling can rapidly decrease a child's blood volume. Coordinate blood samples as much as possible to reduce the frequency and withdraw only the amount needed for the test. (See Atraumatic Care box.)

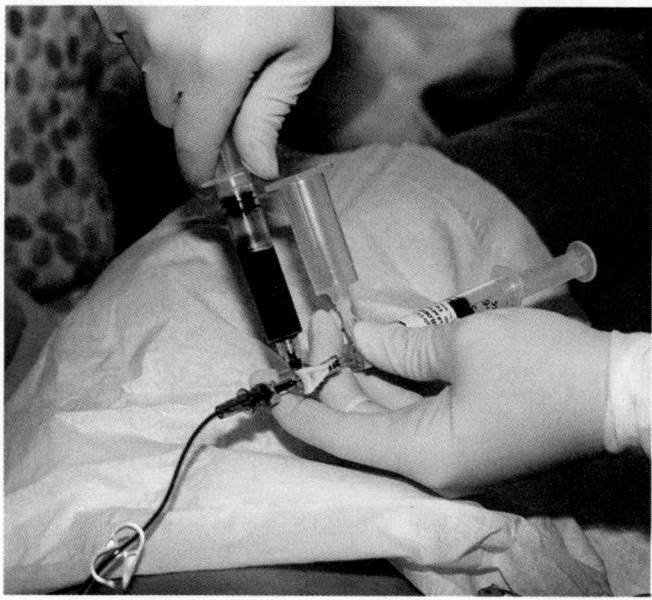

**Fig. 27-18** Drawing blood from a central line.

Arterial blood samples are sometimes needed for blood gas measurement, although noninvasive techniques, such as transcutaneous oxygen monitoring and pulse oximetry, are being used more frequently. Arterial samples may be obtained by arterial puncture using the radial, brachial, or femoral arteries; by deep heel puncture; or from indwelling arterial catheters (Harrison and others, 1997). Adequate circulation should be assessed before arterial puncture by observing capillary refill or performing the *Allen test,* a procedure that assesses the circulation of the radial, ulnar, or brachial arteries. (See Blood Gas Determination, Chapter 31.) Because unclotted blood is required, only heparinized collection tubes are used. In addition, no air bubbles should enter the tube, because they can alter blood gas concentration. Crying, fear, and agitation also affect blood gas values; therefore every effort is made to comfort the child. The blood samples are packed in ice to reduce blood cell metabolism and are taken to the laboratory for immediate analysis.

Capillary blood samples are taken from children by finger or earlobe puncture (stick), just as in the adult patient. A common method for taking peripheral blood samples from infants is by a heelstick. Before the blood sample is taken, the heel is warmed with warm, moist compresses for 5 to 10 minutes to dilate the vessels in the area. In a study of healthy full-term infants, warming the heel with a warm gel pack (40° C [104° F]) for 10 minutes before capillary blood sampling with an automated device (Autolet) did not significantly decrease the sampling time required (Barker and others, 1996). The researchers suggest that skin temperature is not a significant factor in heel blood sampling and that more research should be directed toward improving capillary sampling devices and technique.

The area is cleansed with alcohol, and with the infant's foot firmly restrained with the free hand, the heel is punctured with an automatic lancet device. An automatic device, such as

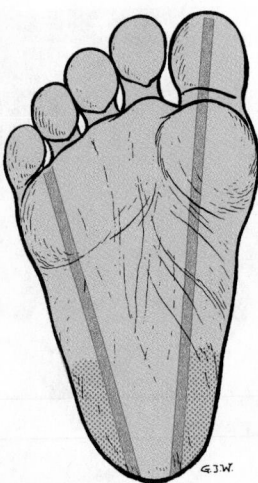

**Fig. 27-19** Puncture site (*pink stippled area*) on sole of infant's heel.

Tenderfoot* (available in various sizes) or Autolet, delivers a more precise puncture depth and is a less painful procedure than that achieved with a blade or lance (Vertanen and others, 2001; Paes and others, 1993). Meehan (1998) has provided a comprehensive review of available manual/mechanical lancing devices. Although obtaining capillary blood gases is a common practice, these measures may not accurately reflect arterial values.

The most serious complications of infant heel puncture are necrotizing osteochondritis from lancet penetration of the underlying calcaneus bone and infection or abscess of the heel (Meehan, 1998). To avoid osteochondritis, the puncture should be no deeper than 2.4 mm and should be made at the outer aspect of the heel. The boundaries of the calcaneus can be marked by an imaginary line extending posteriorly from a point between the fourth and fifth toes and running parallel with the lateral aspect of the heel and another line extending posteriorly from the middle of the great toe and running parallel with the medial aspect of the heel (Fig. 27-19). In addition, repeated trauma to the walking surface of the heel can cause fibrosis and scarring that may interfere with locomotion. Frequent heel punctures have been associated with development of plantar warts at a later age.

The needed specimens are quickly collected, and pressure is applied to the puncture site with a dry gauze square until bleeding stops. The arm is kept extended, not flexed, while pressure is applied for a few minutes after venipuncture in the antecubital fossa to reduce bruising. The site is then covered with an adhesive bandage. In young children, "spot" adhesive bandages pose an aspiration hazard; their use should be avoided, or the adhesive bandage should be removed as soon as the bleeding stops. Applying warm compresses to ecchymotic areas increases circulation, helps remove extravasated blood, and decreases pain.

No matter how or by whom the specimen is collected, children, even some older ones, fear the loss of their blood.

*Available from International Technidyne Corp, 23 Nevsky St, Edison, NJ 08820, (800) 631-5945.

This is particularly true for children whose condition requires frequent blood specimens. They mistakenly believe that blood removed from their body is a threat to their lives. Explaining to them that their blood is continually being produced by their body provides them with a measure of reassurance regarding this aspect of the stress-provoking procedure. When the blood is drawn, a simple comment such as, "Just look how red it is. You're really making a lot of nice red blood," confirms this information and affords them an opportunity to express their concern. An adhesive bandage gives them added assurance that the vital fluids will not leak out through the puncture site.

Children also dislike the discomfort associated with venous, arterial, or capillary punctures. In fact, children have identified these procedures as the ones most frequently causing pain during hospitalization and an arterial puncture as being one of the most painful of all procedures experienced (Van Cleve, Johnson, and Pothier, 1996). Toddlers are most distressed by venipunctures, followed by school-age children and then adolescents (Fradet and others, 1990; Humphrey and others, 1992). Consequently, nurses need to institute pain reduction techniques to lessen the discomfort of these procedures. (See Atraumatic Care box and Pain Management, Chapter 26.)

## Respiratory Secretion Specimens

Collection of sputum or nasal discharge is sometimes required for diagnosis of respiratory infections, especially tuberculosis and respiratory syncytial virus (RSV). Older children and adolescents are able to cough as directed and supply sputum specimens when given proper directions. It must be made clear to them that a coughed specimen, not mucus cleared from the throat, is needed. It is helpful to demonstrate a deep cough so that communication is clear. Infants and small children are unable to follow directions to cough and will swallow any sputum produced when they do; therefore **gastric washings (lavage)** may be used to collect a specimen. Sometimes a satisfactory specimen can be obtained by using a suction device such as a mucus trap if the catheter is inserted into the trachea and the cough reflex elicited. A catheter inserted into the back of the throat is not sufficient. For children with a tracheostomy, a specimen is easily aspirated from the trachea or major bronchi by attaching a collecting device to the suction apparatus.

**Nasal washings** are usually obtained to diagnose an infection of RSV. The child is placed supine, and 1 to 3 ml of sterile normal saline is instilled with a sterile syringe (without a needle) into one nostril. The contents are aspirated using a small, sterile bulb syringe and are placed in a sterile container. Another method uses a syringe with 2 inches of 18- to 20-gauge tubing. The saline is quickly instilled and then aspirated to recover the nasal specimen. To prevent any additional discomfort to the child, all of the equipment should be ready before beginning the procedure. Other respiratory secretion collection methods include nasopharyngeal swabs to diagnose *Bordetella pertussis* and throat cultures. The nurse swabs both the tonsils and the posterior pharynx when obtaining a throat culture. Because obtain-

## ATRAUMATIC CARE
### Guidelines for Skin/Vessel Punctures

**TO REDUCE THE PAIN ASSOCIATED WITH HEEL, FINGER, VENOUS, OR ARTERIAL PUNCTURES:**

Apply EMLA topically over the site if time permits (at least 60 minutes). To remove the Tegaderm dressing atraumatically, grasp opposite sides of the film and pull the sides away from each other to stretch and loosen the film. After the film begins to loosen, grasp the other two sides of the film and pull. Use iontophoresis (Numby Stuff) over the site if time permits (8 to 20 minutes, depending on the amount of current), a vapocoolant spray, or buffered lidocaine (injected intradermally near the vein with a 30-gauge needle) to numb the skin.

Use nonpharmacologic methods of pain and anxiety control (e.g., ask child to take a deep breath when the needle is inserted and again when the needle is withdrawn; have child exhale a large breath or blow bubbles to "blow hurt away"; ask child to count slowly and then faster and louder if pain is felt).

Keep all equipment out of sight until used.

Enlist parents' presence or assistance if they wish to participate.

Restrain child *only as needed* to perform the procedure safely; use therapeutic hugging (see p. 1136).

Allow the skin preparation to dry completely before penetrating the skin.

Use the smallest-gauge needle (e.g., 25 gauge) that permits free flow of blood; a 27-gauge needle can be used for obtaining 1 to 1.5 ml of blood and for prominent veins (needle length is only ½ inch).

Avoid putting an intravenous (IV) line in the dominant hand or the hand the child uses to suck the thumb.

Use an automatic lancet device for precise puncture depth of the finger or heel; press the device lightly against the skin and avoid steadying the finger against a hard surface.

Emphasize that blood entering the syringe or tube does not hurt and reassure young children that you did not "take their blood" away and that they have a lot more inside.

---

*Contrary to popular belief, a study of children ages 3 to 6 years found that asking them not to look at the finger stick to avoid the sight of blood or applying a decorated bandage did not lessen their rating of pain intensity (Johnston, Stevens, and Arbess, 1993).

†For an example of one hospital's guidelines for reducing excessive IV insertion attempts, see Catudal (1999).

Place a small bandage over the puncture site to make removal easy and less painful to reassure young children that "their blood will not leak out."*

Have a "two-try"–only policy to reduce excessive insertion attempts—two operators each have two insertion attempts; if insertion is not successful after four punctures, consider alternative venous access, such as a peripherally inserted central catheter (PICC); have a policy for identifying children with difficult access and appropriate interventions (e.g., most experienced operator for the first attempt).†

**FOR MULTIPLE BLOOD SAMPLES:**

Use an intermittent infusion device ("saline or heparin lock") to collect additional samples from an existing IV line; consider PICC lines early, not as a last resort. Preferably use a saline flush for a catheter larger than 24 gauge (less painful, compatible with drugs, and less costly).

Coordinate care to allow several tests to be performed on one blood sample using micromethods of testing.

Anticipate tests (e.g., drug levels, chemistry, immunoglobulin levels) and ask the laboratory to save blood for additional testing.

**FOR HEEL LANCING IN NEWBORNS:**

Heel lancing has been shown to be more painful than venipuncture (Larsson and others, 1998); consider venipuncture when the amount of blood from the heel would require much squeezing (e.g., genetic screening tests).

The effectiveness of EMLA is controversial, although application of 0.5 g for 30 minutes four times a day in preterm infants was found to be safe (Essink-Tebbes and others, 1999).

Place diapered newborn against mother's bare chest in skin-to-skin contact 10 to 15 minutes before and during heel lance (Gray, Watt, and Blass, 2000).

During the procedure, allow newborn to suck a pacifier coated with a slurry of sugar and water: to make an approximate 24% sucrose solution, add 1 teaspoon of table sugar to 4 teaspoons of sterile water. Use this solution to coat the pacifier or administer 2 ml to the tongue 2 minutes before the procedure (Blass and Watt, 1999).

---

ing throat and nasopharyngeal cultures may be traumatic to the child, using a gentle technique is important.

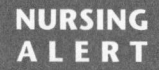 **NURSING ALERT**  Do not attempt to obtain a throat culture if acute epiglottitis is suspected. The trauma from the swab may increase edema, possibly occluding the airway.

# ADMINISTRATION OF MEDICATION
## Determination of Drug Dosage

Nurses must have an understanding of the safe dosage of medications they administer to children, as well as the expected action, possible side effects, and signs of toxicity.

Factors related to growth and maturation significantly alter an individual's capacity to metabolize and excrete drugs, and deficiencies associated with immaturity become more important with decreasing age. Immaturity or defects in any

or all of the important processes of absorption, distribution, biotransformation, or excretion can significantly alter the effects of a drug. Newborn and premature infants with immature enzyme systems in the liver, lower plasma concentrations of protein for binding with drugs, and immaturely functioning kidneys are particularly vulnerable to the harmful effects of drugs. Beyond the newborn period, many drugs are metabolized more rapidly by the liver, necessitating larger doses or more frequent administration. This is particularly important in pain control, when the dosage may need to be increased or the interval between administering analgesics may need to be decreased.

Other factors that create problems in drug dosages in children include the difficulty in evaluating drug response. For example, how is a toxic manifestation such as ringing in the ears assessed in a preverbal child? In disease states, particularly in children, water losses and water requirements are both increased, whereas the fluid intake decreases. Because water is required to excrete the drug, dehydration poses the danger of toxic accumulation.

Various formulas involving age, weight, and *body surface area (BSA)* as the basis for calculations have been devised to determine children's drug dosages from a standard adult dose. Because the administration of medication is a nursing responsibility, nurses need to have not only a knowledge of drug action and patient responses, but also some resources for estimating safe dosages for children.

The most reliable method for determining children's dosages is to calculate the proportional amount of BSA to body weight. The ratio of BSA to weight varies inversely with length; therefore the infant who is shorter and weighs less than an older child or adult has relatively more BSA than would be expected from the weight.

The usual determination of BSA requires the use of the *West nomogram* (Fig. 27-20). BSA is estimated from the

child's height and weight. Then this information is applied to a formula for dosage, such as either of the following formulas, which require different types of information:

$$\frac{\text{BSA of child}}{\text{BSA of adult}} \times \text{Adult dose} = \text{Estimated child's dose}$$

$$\text{BSA of child (m}^2) \times \text{Dose/m}^2 = \text{Estimated child's dose}$$

## Preparation for Safe Administration
### Checking Dosage

Administering the correct dosage of a drug is a shared responsibility between the practitioner who orders the drug and the nurse who carries out that order. Children react with unexpected severity to some drugs, and ill children

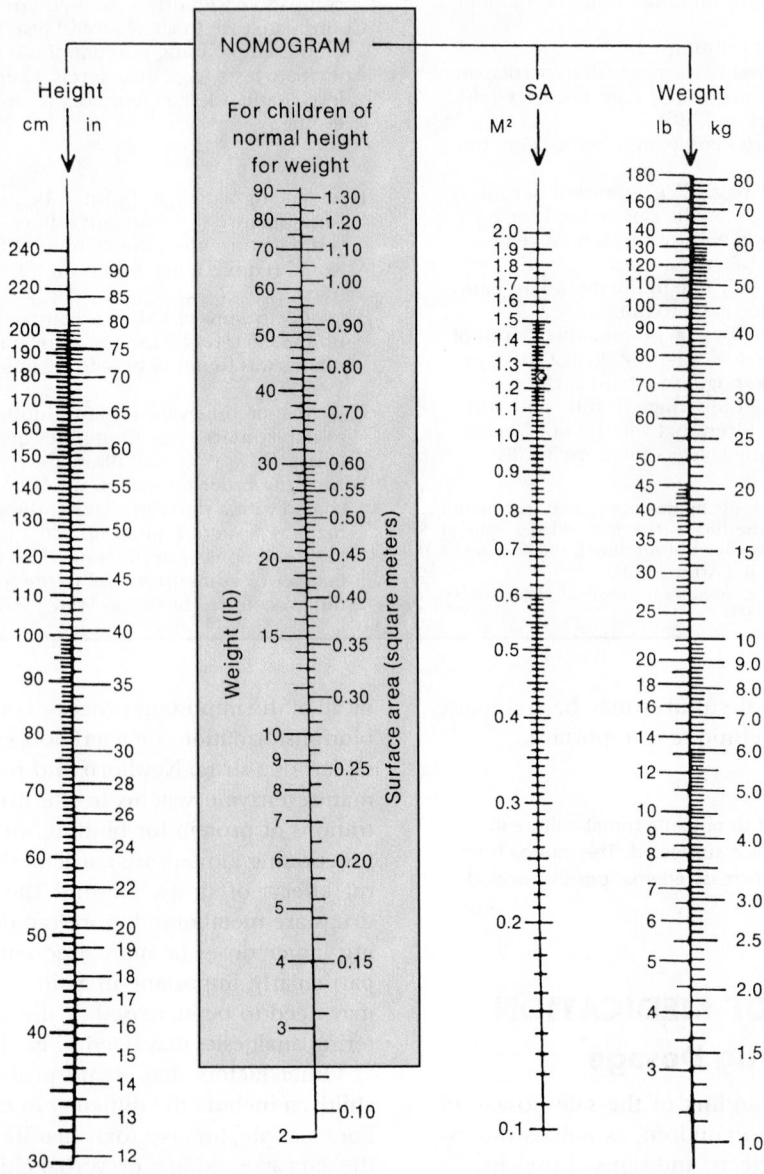

**Fig. 27-20** West nomogram (for estimation of surface areas). Surface area is indicated where a straight line connecting height and weight intersects surface area (SA) column or, if patient is approximately of normal proportion, from weight alone *(tinted area)*. (From Behrman RE, Vaughan VC, Jenson HB, editors: *Nelson textbook of pediatrics,* ed 16, Philadelphia, 2000, WB Saunders; modified from data of E Boyd by CD West.)

may be especially sensitive to drugs. Therefore checking the accuracy of the dose is a professional responsibility.

> **NURSING ALERT**
>
> When a dose is ordered that is outside the usual range or if there is some question regarding the preparation or the route of administration, the nurse always checks with the practitioner before proceeding with the administration because the nurse is legally liable for any drug administered.

Administering some medications requires added safeguards. Even when it has been determined that the dosage is correct for a particular child, many drugs are potentially hazardous or lethal. Most hospital units or other facilities where medications are given to children have regulations requiring that specified drugs be double-checked by another nurse before they are given to the child. Among those drugs that require such safeguards are digoxin, heparin, chemotherapy drugs, and insulin. Others that are frequently included are epinephrine, opioids, and sedatives. Even if this precaution is not mandatory, nurses are wise to take such precautions for their own sense of security. Errors in decimal point placement may easily occur and may result in a tenfold or more dosage error. For example, a milligram is 1000 times larger than a microgram.

### Identification

Before the administration of any medication, the child must be correctly identified, because children are not totally reliable in giving correct names on request. Infants are unable to give their name, toddlers or preschoolers may admit to any name, and school-age children may deny their identity in an attempt to avoid the medication. Parents may be present to identify their child, but the only safe method for identifying children is to check their hospital identification bands with the medication label.

### Parents

Parents are useful sources of information regarding the child and his or her capabilities. Nearly all parents have given some type of medication to their child and can describe the approaches that they have found to be successful. They can also provide information regarding the child's reaction to similar experiences if the child has been hospitalized before or has been given medication in a practitioner's office or clinic. In some cases it is less traumatic for the child if a parent gives the medication, provided that the nurse prepares the medication and supervises its administration. Children being given daily medications at home are accustomed to the parent's functioning in this capacity and are less apt to fuss than they would if the medication were administered by a stranger. Individual decisions need to be made regarding parental presence and participation, such as holding the child during injections. (See Evidence-Based Practice box on p. 1107.)

### Child

Every child requires psychologic preparation for parenteral administration of medication and supportive care during the procedure (see pp. 1103-1108). Even if children have re-

ceived several injections, they rarely become accustomed to the discomfort and have as much right to understanding and patience from those involved in giving the injection as any other child. Safe administration of any drug requires meticulous attention to the safeguards discussed here.

## Oral Administration

The oral route is preferred for administering medications to children whenever possible. Because of the ease of administration of oral medications, most are dissolved or suspended in liquid preparations. Although some children are able to swallow or chew solid medications at an early age, solid preparations are not recommended for young children. There is danger of aspiration in any oral preparation, but solid forms (pills, tablets, capsules) are especially hazardous if their administration causes extreme resistance or crying.

Most pediatric medications come in palatable and colorful preparations for added ease of administration. Some have a slightly unpleasant aftertaste, but most children will swallow these liquids with little if any resistance. The nurse can taste a minute amount of an oral preparation to ascertain if it is palatable or bitter. In this way, legitimate complaints of dislike from the child can be accepted and the taste camouflaged whenever possible. Most pediatric units have preparations available for this purpose. (See Atraumatic Care box.)

### Preparation

Selecting a vehicle to measure and administer a medication requires careful consideration. The devices available to measure medicines are not always sufficiently accurate for measuring the small amounts needed in pediatric nursing practice (Fig. 27-21). Although molded plastic cups offer reasonable accuracy in measuring moderate or large doses of liquids, paper cups are likely to have irregularly shaped

> **ATRAUMATIC CARE**
> *Encouraging a Child's Acceptance of Oral Medication*
>
> Give the child a flavored ice pop to suck to numb the tongue before giving the drug.
> Mix the drug with a small amount (about 1 tsp) of sweet-tasting substance, such as flavored syrups, jam, fruit purees, sherbet, or ice cream; avoid essential food items, such as formula or milk, because the child may later refuse to eat them.
> Give a "chaser" of water, juice, soft drink, or flavored ice pop or frozen juice bar after the drug.
> If nausea is a problem, give a carbonated beverage poured over finely crushed ice before or immediately after the medication.
> When medication has an unpleasant taste, have the child pinch the nose and drink the medicine through a straw. Much of what we taste is associated with smell.
> Another alternative is to have the pharmacist prepare the drug in a flavored, chewable troche or lozenge.
> Infants will suck medicine from a needleless syringe or dropper in small increments (0.25 to 0.5 ml) at a time. Use a nipple or special pacifier with a reservoir for the drug (see Fig. 27-21).

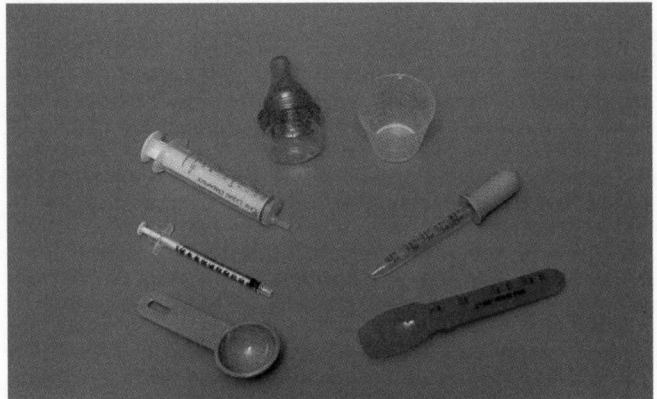

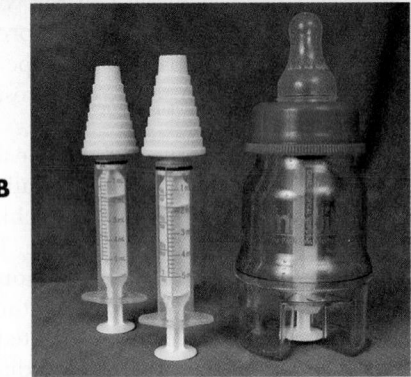

**Fig. 27-21** **A,** Acceptable devices for measuring and administering oral medication to children *(clockwise):* measuring spoon, plastic syringes, calibrated nipple, plastic medicine cup, calibrated dropper, hollow-handled medicine spoon. **B,** Medibottle used to deliver oral medication via a syringe. (**B,** Courtesy Paul Vincent Kuntz, Texas Children's Hospital.)

or crumpled bottoms. Calibrations on the cups (especially the teaspoon mark) and the personal equation or interpretation of a given measure are highly variable. Measures less than a teaspoon are impossible to determine accurately with a medicine cup.

Many liquid preparations are prescribed in measurements of teaspoons. However, teaspoons and soup spoons are inaccurate measuring devices and are subject to error from a number of variables. For example, teaspoons vary greatly in capacity, and different persons using the same spoon will pour different amounts. This variability is also influenced by the adequacy of available light, the color of the liquid, and the size of the bottle from which it is poured. Therefore a drug ordered in teaspoons should be measured in milliliters—the established standard is 5 ml per teaspoon. A convenient hollow-handled medicine spoon is available to accurately measure and administer the drug (see Fig. 27-21, *A*). A new device called the Medibottle has been shown to be more effective in delivering oral medication to infants than the oral syringe (Kraus and others, 2001).

Another unreliable device for measuring liquids is the drop, which varies to a greater extent than the teaspoon or measuring cup. The volume of a drop will vary according to the viscosity (thickness) of the liquid measured. Viscid fluids produce much larger drops than thin liquids. Many

medications are supplied with caps or droppers designed for measuring each specific preparation. These are accurate when used to measure that specific medication but are not reliable for measuring other liquids. Emptying dropper contents into a medicine cup invites additional error. Because some of the liquid clings to the sides of the cup, a significant amount of the drug can be lost.

**NURSING ALERT** Many pediatric medications are given by drops or dropper. A misunderstanding of these terms by parents can result in a potential overdose. In addition, many droppers that come with medications are marked in tenths of cubic centimeters. If a parent were to use a syringe instead of the dropper, 0.4 cc may be thought to be the same as 4 cc. Provide education to parents on correct methods for giving medication. Demonstrate the technique.

The most accurate means for measuring small amounts of medication is the plastic disposable (never glass) syringe, especially the tuberculin syringe for volumes less than 1 ml. Not only does the syringe provide a reliable measure, but it also serves as a convenient means for transporting and administering the medication. The medication can be placed directly into the child's mouth from the syringe. For added safety, a short length of flexible tubing can be placed on the tip of the syringe to prevent mouth injury, although the tubing must be completely emptied of medication.

Young children and some older children have difficulty in swallowing tablets or pills. Because a number of drugs are not available in pediatric preparations, the tablet will need to be crushed before it can be given to these children. Commercial devices are available, or simple methods can be employed for crushing tablets. Not all drugs can be crushed (e.g., medication with an enteric or protective coating or formulated for slow release).

**NURSING TIP** To minimize loss of the drug, crush the tablet between two spoons or place the tablet either in a medicine cup or between two small paper soufflé cups and use a pestle for crushing; collect the bits of pulverized medication that tend to cling to the sides of the cup or spoon and mix the crushed tablet with a palatable substance.

Another alternative is to have the pharmacist prepare the drug in a flavored, chewable troche or lozenge, lollipop (sucker), or flavored ice pop (Wong and Redding, 1987). Some oral or rectal medications can be prepared in a cream or gel and applied on the skin for topical absorption.

Children who must take solid oral medication for an extended period can be taught to swallow tablets or capsules. Training sessions include using verbal instruction, demonstration, reinforcement of progressively swallowing larger candy/capsules, no attention for inappropriate behavior, and gradual withdrawal of guidance once children can swallow their medication.

Because pediatric doses often require dividing adult preparations of medication, the nurse may be faced with the dilemma of accurate dosage. With tablets, only those that are scored can be halved or quartered accurately. If the medication is soluble, the tablet or contents of a capsule can be mixed in a small, premeasured amount of liquid and the appropriate portion given. If half a dose is required, the tablet is dissolved in 5 ml of water and 2.5 ml is given.

### Administration

Although administering liquids to infants is relatively easy, care must be observed to prevent aspiration. With the infant held in a semireclining position, the medication is placed in the mouth from a spoon, plastic cup, plastic dropper, or plastic syringe (without needle). The dropper or syringe is best placed along the side of the infant's tongue, and the liquid is administered slowly in small amounts, waiting for the child to swallow between deposits.

**NURSING TIP** In infants up to 11 months of age and children with neurologic impairments, blowing a small puff of air in the face frequently elicits a swallow reflex (Orenstein and others, 1988).

Medicine cups can be used effectively for older infants who are able to drink from a cup. Because of the natural outward tongue thrust in infancy, medications may need to be retrieved from the lips or chin and refed. Allowing the infant to suck the medication that has been placed in an empty nipple or inserting the syringe or dropper into the side of the mouth, parallel to the nipple, while the infant nurses are other convenient methods for giving liquid medications to infants. Medication is not added to the infant's formula feeding because the child may subsequently refuse the formula.

The young child who refuses to cooperate or resists consistently despite explanation and encouragement may require mild physical coercion. If so, it is carried out quickly and carefully. Every effort is made to determine why the child resists, and the reasons for this alternative are explained in such a way that the child will know that it is being carried out for his or her well-being and is not a form of punishment. There is always a risk in using even mild forceful techniques. A crying child can aspirate a medication, particularly when lying on the back. If the nurse holds the child in the lap with the child's right arm behind the nurse, the left hand firmly grasped by the nurse's left hand, and the head securely cradled between the nurse's arm and body, the medication can be slowly poured into the mouth (Fig. 27-22).

## Intramuscular (IM) Administration

### Selecting the Syringe and Needle

The volume of medication prescribed for small children and the small amount of tissue available for injection require that a syringe be selected that can measure very small amounts of solution (Table 27-6). For volumes less than 1 ml, the tuberculin syringe, calibrated in one-hundredth increments, is appropriate. Very minute doses may require the use of a 0.5-ml, low-dose syringe. These syringes, along with specially constructed needles, minimize the possibility of inadvertently administering incorrect amounts of a drug because of **dead space,** which allows fluid to remain in the syringe and needle after the plunger is pushed completely

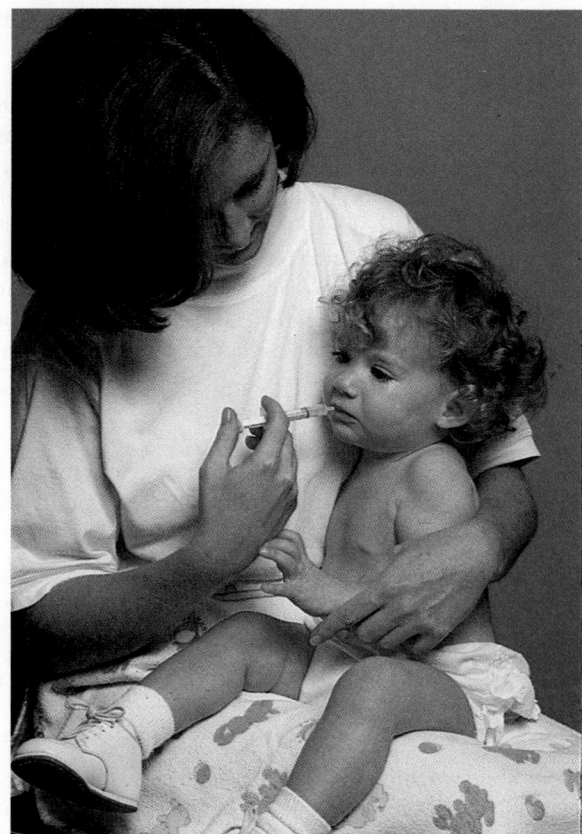

**Fig. 27-22** Nurse partially restrains child for easy and comfortable administration of oral medication.

forward. A minimum of 0.2 ml of solution remains in a standard needle hub; therefore, when very small amounts of two drugs are combined in the syringe, such as mixtures of insulin, the ratio of the two drugs can be altered significantly. Measures that minimize the effect of dead space follow: (1) when two drugs are combined in the syringe, always draw them up in the same order to maintain a consistent ratio between the drugs; (2) use the same brand of syringe (dead space may vary between brands); and (3) use one-piece syringe units (needle permanently attached to the syringe).

Dead space is also an important factor to consider when injecting medication because flushing the syringe with an air bubble adds an additional amount of medication to the prescribed dose. This can be hazardous when very small amounts of a drug are given.

Consequently, flushing is not recommended, especially when less than 1 ml of medication is given. Syringes are calibrated to deliver a prescribed drug dose, and the amount of medication left in the hub and needle is not part of the syringe barrel calibrations. Certain drugs such as iron dextran and diphtheria and tetanus toxoid may cause irritation when tracked into the subcutaneous tissue. In these cases the Z-track method is recommended for use in infants and children rather than an air bubble. Changing the needle after withdrawing the fluid from the vial is another technique to minimize tracking.

The needle length must be sufficient to penetrate the subcutaneous tissue and deposit the medication into the body of the muscle (see Table 27-6). Limited research is available on adequate needle length for children, although some traditional methods may be used. One study found that a 1-inch needle is necessary to adequately penetrate the vastus lateralis muscle in 4-month-old infants and probably is needed for 2-month-old infants (Hicks and others, 1989).

The needle gauge should be as small as possible to deliver the fluid safely. Smaller-diameter (25- to 30-gauge) needles cause the least discomfort, but larger gauges are needed for viscous medication and prevention of accidental bending of longer needles.

## Determining the Site

Factors that are considered when selecting a site for an IM injection on an infant or child include the following:

- The amount and character of the medication to be injected
- The amount and general condition of the muscle mass
- The frequency or number of injections to be given during the course of treatment
- The type of medication being given
- Factors that may impede access to or cause contamination of the site
- The child's ability to assume the required position safely

Older children and adolescents usually pose few problems in selecting a suitable site for IM injections, but infants, with their small and underdeveloped muscles, have fewer available sites. It is sometimes difficult to assess the amount of fluid that can be safely injected into a single site. Usually 1 ml is the maximum volume that should be administered in a single site to small children and older infants. The muscles of small infants may not tolerate more than 0.5 ml. As the child approaches adult size, volumes approaching those given to adults may be used. However, the larger the amount of solution, the larger must be the muscle into which it is injected.

Injections must be placed in muscles large enough to accommodate the medication, but major nerves and blood vessels must be avoided. There is no universal agreement regarding the best IM injection site for children. The preferred site for infants is the vastus lateralis (see Table 27-6). The ventrogluteal site is relatively free of major nerves and blood vessels, is a relatively large muscle with less subcutaneous tissue than the dorsal site, has well-defined landmarks for safe site location, and is easily accessible in several positions. These advantages make it a preferred site over the dorsogluteal muscle and challenge the recommendation that the ventrogluteal site not be used until children have been walking.

Beecroft and Kongelbeck's research (1994) into IM injection sites in children indicates that the ventrogluteal site has not been associated with complications and is therefore the preferred site for IM injections in children of all ages (see Table 27-6). In clinical practice this site has been safely used in children as young as newborns. The deltoid muscle, a small muscle near the axillary and radial nerves, can be used for small volumes of fluid in children

---

| **TABLE 27-6**  Intramuscular administration: location, needle length, gauge, and fluid administration amount | | | |
|---|---|---|---|
| | **Location of Injection** | **Needle Length** | **Needle Gauge (G)** | **Suggested Maximum Amount** |
| **Infant** (less than 4 months) | Vastus lateralis (not rectus femoris— anterior thigh) Ventrogluteal | ⅝ inch | 25 G most common for immunizations<br>23 G may be required for viscous medications | 1 ml<br><br>1 ml |
| **Infant** (4 months and older) | Vastus lateralis (not rectus femoris— anterior thigh) Ventrogluteal | 1 inch | 25 G most common for immunizations<br>23 G for all other injections<br>22 G may be required for viscous medications | 1 ml<br><br>1 ml |
| **Toddler** | Deltoid Ventrogluteal Vastus lateralis (not rectus femoris— anterior thigh) | ⅝ inch for deltoid and 1 inch for ventrogluteal and vastus lateralis | 25 G most common for immunizations<br>23 G for all other injections<br>22 G may be required for viscous medications | ½-1 ml<br><br>2 ml |
| **Preschool and older children** | Deltoid Ventrogluteal | ⅝ inch to 1 inch for deltoid and 1 inch for ventrogluteal | 25 G most common for immunizations<br>23 G for all other injections<br>22 G may be required for viscous medications | ½-1 ml<br><br>2-3 ml |
| **Adolescent** | Deltoid Ventrogluteal | ⅝ inch to 1 inch for deltoid and 1 inch for ventrogluteal | 25 G most common for immunizations<br>23 G for all other injections<br>22 G may be required for viscious medications | 1-1½ ml<br><br>2-5 ml |

Modified from Becton-Dickson Media Center: *A guide for managing the pediatric patient: reducing the anxiety and pain of injections,* 1 Becton Dr, Franklin Lakes, NJ, 1998, Becton-Dickson.

as young as 18 months of age. Its advantages are less pain and fewer side effects from the injectate (as observed with immunizations), compared with the vastus lateralis (Ipp and others, 1989). Table 27-7 summarizes the four major injection sites and illustrates the location of the preferred IM injection sites for children.

## Administration

Although injections that are executed with care seldom cause trauma to the child, there have been reports of serious disability related to IM injections in children. Repeated use of a single site has been associated with fibrosis of the muscle with subsequent muscle contracture. Injections

---

**TABLE 27-7   Intramuscular injection sites in children**

| Site | Discussion |
|---|---|
| **Vastus Lateralis**<br>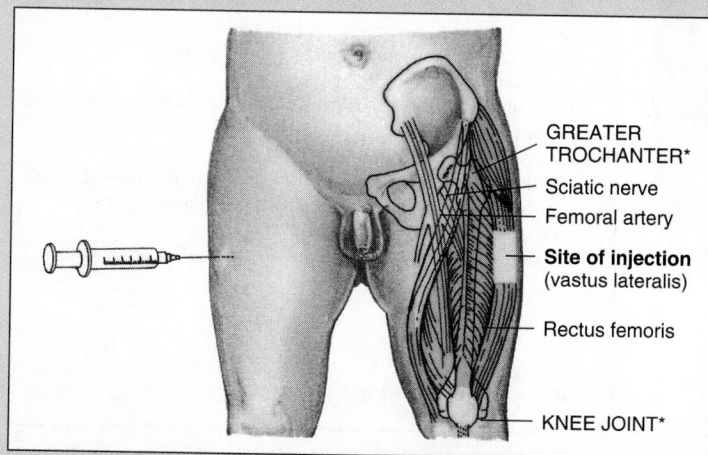 | **Location***<br>Palpate to find greater trochanter and knee joints; divide vertical distance between these two landmarks into thirds; inject into middle one third<br>**Needle insertion and size**<br>Insert needle at 90-degree angle between syringe and upper thigh in infants and in young children<br>22 to 25 gauge, ⅝ to 1 inch†<br>**Advantages**<br>Large, well-developed muscle that can tolerate larger quantities of fluid (0.5 ml [infant] to 2.0 ml [child])<br>Easily accessible if child is supine, side lying, or sitting<br>**Disadvantages**<br>Thrombosis of femoral artery from injection in midthigh area (rectus femoris muscle)<br>Sciatic nerve damage from long needle injected posteriorly and medially into small extremity<br>More painful than deltoid or gluteal sites |
| **Ventrogluteal**<br>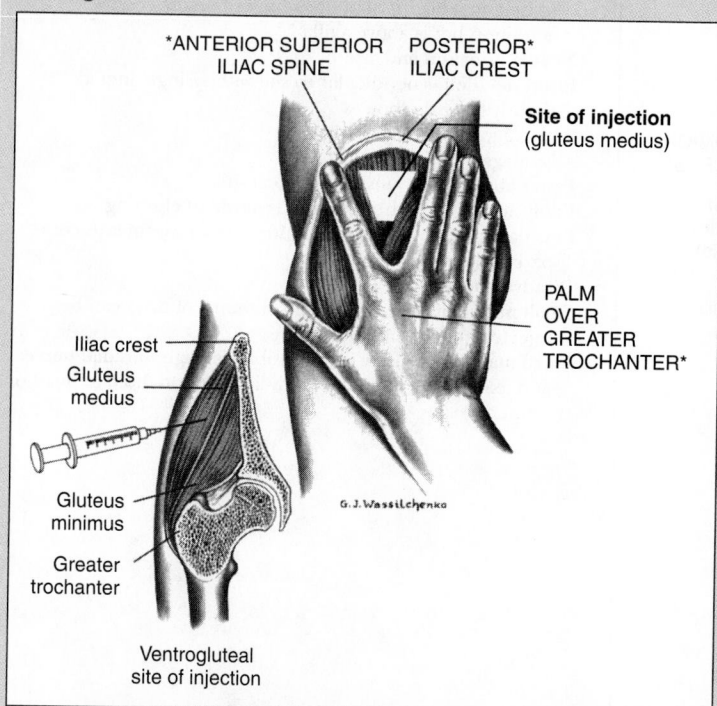 | **Location***<br>Palpate to locate greater trochanter, anterior superior iliac tubercle (found by flexing thigh at hip and measuring up to 1 to 2 cm above crease formed in groin), and posterior iliac crest; place palm of hand over greater trochanter, index finger over anterior superior iliac tubercle, and middle finger along crest of ilium posteriorly as far as possible; inject into center of V formed by fingers<br>**Needle insertion and size**<br>Insert needle perpendicular to site but angled slightly toward greater trochanter<br>22 to 25 gauge, ½ to 1 inch<br>**Advantages**<br>Free of important nerves and vascular structures<br>Easily identified by prominent bony landmarks<br>Thinner layer of subcutaneous tissue than in dorsogluteal site, thus less chance of depositing drug subcutaneously rather than intramuscularly<br>Can accommodate larger quantities of fluid (0.5 ml [infant] to 2.0 ml [child])<br>Easily accessible if child is supine, prone, or side lying<br>Less painful than vastus lateralis<br>**Disadvantages**<br>Health care professionals' unfamiliarity with site |

*Locations are indicated by asterisks on illustrations.
†Research has shown that a 1-inch needle is needed for adequate muscle penetration in infants 4 months old and possibly in infants as young as 2 months (Hicks and others, 1989). One of the most important features of injecting vaccines is adequate penetration of the muscle for the deposition of the drug intramuscularly and not subcutaneously. Based on ultrasonography, two injection techniques have been studied to determine the best needle length for the deltoid and vastus lateralis sites. If the muscle is grasped or bunched, a needle length of 25 mm (1 inch) is recommended. If the muscle is stretched or flattened, a needle length of 16 mm (⅝ inch) is adequate (Groswasser and others, 1997). Unfortunately, the conclusions of the study fail to address whether these lengths apply to both muscles. From the data, it appears more likely that the recommendations apply to the thigh muscle only. Other recommendations for needle size and volume of fluid are based on traditional practice and have not been verified by research.

*Continued*

**TABLE 27-7**    Intramuscular injection sites in children—cont'd

| Site | Discussion |
|---|---|
| **Dorsogluteal** 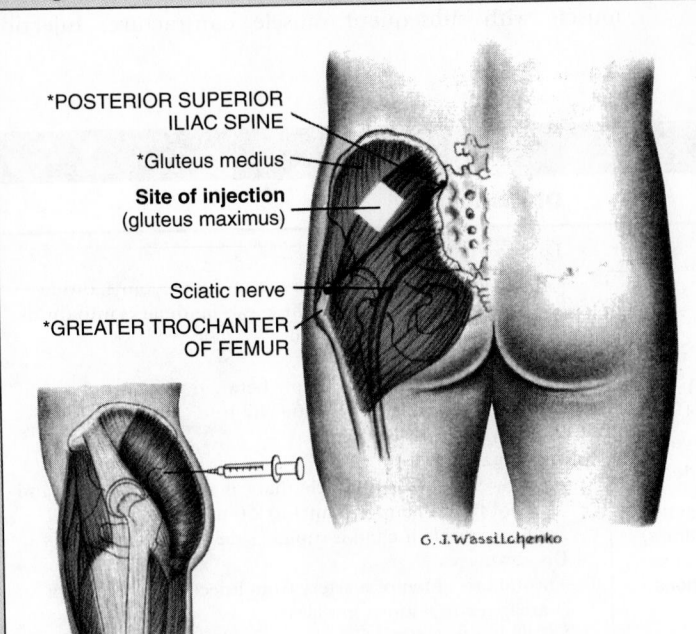 | **Location***<br>Locate greater trochanter and posterior superior iliac spine; draw imaginary line between these two points and inject lateral and superior to line into gluteus maximus or medius muscle<br>**Needle insertion and size**<br>Insert needle perpendicular to surface on which child is lying when prone<br>20 to 25 gauge, ½ to 1½ inches<br>**Advantages**<br>In older child, large muscle mass; well-developed muscle can tolerate greater volume of fluid (up to 2.0 ml)<br>Child does not see needle and syringe<br>Easily accessible if child is prone or side lying<br>**Disadvantages**<br>Contraindicated in children who have not been walking for at least 1 year<br>Danger of injury to sciatic nerve<br>Thick, subcutaneous fat, predisposing to deposition of drug subcutaneously rather than intramuscularly<br>Inaccessible if child is supine<br>Exposure of site may cause embarrassment in older child |
| **Deltoid** 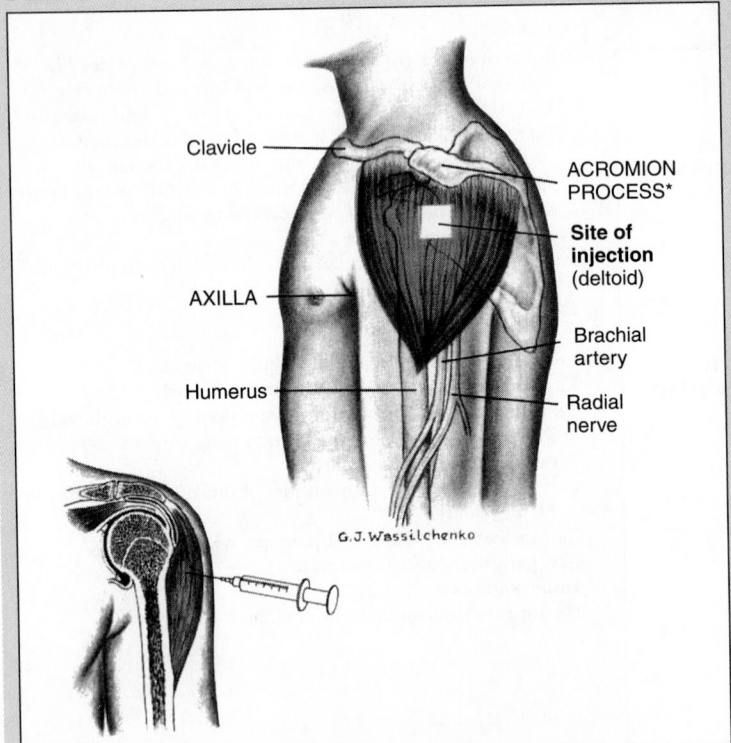 | **Location***<br>Locate acromion process; inject only into upper third of muscle that begins about two finger breadths below acromion but is above axilla<br>**Needle insertion and size**<br>Insert needle perpendicular to site with syringe angled slightly toward elbow<br>22 to 25 gauge, ½ to 1 inch<br>**Advantages**<br>Faster absorption rates than gluteal sites<br>Easily accessible with minimum removal of clothing<br>Less pain and fewer local side effects from vaccines as compared with vastus lateralis<br>**Disadvantages**<br>Small muscle mass; only limited amounts of drug can be injected (0.5 to 1.0 ml)<br>Small margins of safety with possible damage to radial nerve and axillary nerve (not shown, lies under deltoid at head of humerus) |

*Locations are indicated by asterisks on illustrations.

close to large nerves, such as the sciatic nerve, have been responsible for permanent disability, especially when potentially neurotoxic drugs are administered. There are several reports of tissue damage from penicillin; one of the difficulties in administering the opaque preparations, such as Bicillin, is that aspirated blood cannot be detected at the bottom of the syringe, thus increasing the risk of injecting into a blood vessel. When such drugs are injected, great care must be used in locating the correct site. When aspirating, the nurse should look for blood at the *top* of the syringe near the plunger, because blood may be drawn up through the column of penicillin.

A recent study of IM injection techniques revealed that the straighter the path of needle insertion (e.g., 90-degree angle), the less displacement and shear to tissue. Minimizing tissue shear and displacement causes less discomfort (Katsma and Smith, 1997) (see Table 27-7).

A reported potential hazard with medication in glass ampules is the presence of glass particles in the ampule after the container is broken. When the medication is withdrawn into the syringe, the glass particles are also withdrawn and are subsequently injected into the patient. As a precaution, medication from glass ampules is only drawn through a needle with a filter or injected intravenously through a site in the tubing that is distal to an IV filter. (Safety precautions for administering chemotherapeutic drugs are discussed in Chapter 36.)

Most children are unpredictable, and few are totally cooperative when receiving an injection. Even children who appear to be relaxed and constrained can lose control under the stress of the procedure. It is advisable to have someone available to help hold the child if needed. Because children often jerk or pull away unexpectedly, it is a good idea to carry an extra capped needle to exchange for a contaminated one so that delay is minimized. The child, even a small one, is told that he or she is receiving an injection (preferably using a phrase such as "putting the medicine under the skin"), and then the procedure is carried out as quickly and skillfully as possible to avoid prolonging the stressful experience. Invasive procedures such as injections are especially anxiety provoking in young children, who may associate any assault to the "behind" area with punishment. Because injections are painful, the nurse should employ excellent injection techniques and effective pain reduction measures to reduce discomfort. (See Guidelines box on p. 1158)

Small infants offer little resistance to injections. Although they squirm and may be difficult to hold in position, they can usually be restrained without assistance. The body of a larger infant can be securely restrained between the nurse's arm and body (Fig. 27-23). To inject into the body of a muscle, the muscle mass is firmly grasped between the thumb and fingers to isolate and stabilize the site. However, in obese children it is preferable to first spread the skin with the thumb and index finger to displace subcutaneous tissue and then grasp the muscle deeply on each side.

If medication is given around the clock, the nurse must be careful to wake the child before giving the injection. Although it may seem easier to surprise the sleeping child and

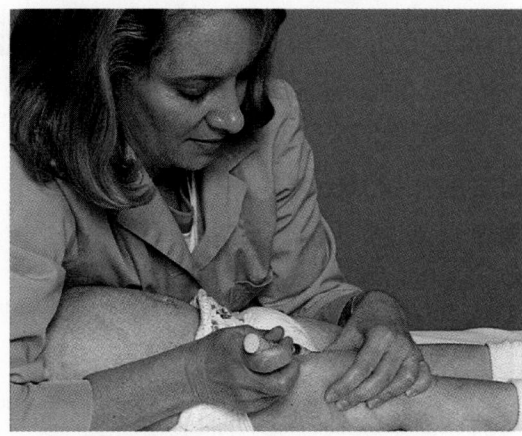

**Fig. 27-23**   Holding small child for intramuscular injection. Note how nurse isolates and stabilizes muscle.

do it as quickly as possible, performing the procedure in this way can cause the child to fear going back to sleep. If they are awakened first, children will know that nothing will be done to them unless they are forewarned. The Guidelines box summarizes administration techniques that maximize safety and minimize the discomfort often associated with injections.

A *needleless injection system* (i.e., *Biojector*) delivers IM or subcutaneous injections without the use of a needle and eliminates the risk of accidental needle puncture. This needle-free injection system is powered by a carbon dioxide cartridge that provides the power to deliver the medication through the skin. While it is not painless, it may reduce pain and also the anxiety of seeing the needle (Polillio and Kiley, 1997; Schultz and others, 1995).

## Subcutaneous and Intradermal Administration*

Subcutaneous and intradermal injections are frequently administered to children, but the technique differs little from the method used with adults. Examples of subcutaneous injections include insulin, hormone replacement, allergy desensitization, and some vaccines. Tuberculin (TB) testing, local anesthesia, and allergy testing are examples of frequently administered intradermal injections.

Techniques to minimize the pain associated with these injections include changing the needle if it pierced a rubber stopper on a vial, using 26- to 30-gauge needles (only to inject the solution), and injecting small volumes (up to 0.5 ml). The angle of the needle for the subcutaneous injection is typically 90 degrees. In children with little subcutaneous tissue, some practitioners insert the needle at a 45-degree angle. However, the benefit of using the 45-degree angle rather than the 90-degree angle remains controversial.

---

*Home care instructions for giving subcutaneous injections are available in Wong DL, Hess CS: *Wong and Whaley's clinical manual of pediatric nursing*, ed 5, St Louis, 2000, Mosby.

## GUIDELINES

### Intramuscular Administration of Medication

Use safety precautions in administering medication (e.g., check child's identification).

Select a method to anesthetize the puncture site:

Apply EMLA on site 2½ hours before IM injection.

Use a vapocoolant spray (e.g., Fluori-Methane or ethyl chloride)* just before injection (Abbott and Fowler-Kerry, 1995; Cohen Reis and Holubkov, 1997).

Prepare medication.

Select needle and syringe appropriate to the following:

Amount of fluid to be administered (syringe size)

Viscosity of fluid to be administered (needle gauge)

Amount of tissue to be penetrated (needle length)

Maximum volume to be administered in a single site is 1 ml for older infants and small children.

Determine the site of injection (see Tables 27-6 and 27-7); make certain muscle is large enough to accommodate volume and type of medication.

Older children: select site as with adult patient; allow child some choice of site, if feasible.

Following are acceptable sites for infants and small or debilitated children:

Vastus lateralis muscle

Ventrogluteal muscle

Dorsogluteal muscle is insufficiently developed to be a safe site for infants and small children.

Administer medication.

Provide for sufficient help in holding child; children are often uncooperative, and their behavior is usually unpredictable.

Explain briefly what is to be done and, if appropriate, what child can do to help.

Expose injection area for unobstructed view of landmarks.

Select a site where skin is free of irritation and danger of infection; palpate for and avoid sensitive or hardened areas. With multiple injections, rotate sites.

Place child in a lying or sitting position; child is not allowed to stand because:

Landmarks are more difficult to assess.

Restraint is more difficult.

Child may faint and fall.

Use a new, sharp needle with smallest diameter that permits free flow of the medication.

Grasp muscle firmly between thumb and fingers to isolate and stabilize muscle for deposition of drug in its deepest

part; in obese children, spread skin with thumb and index finger to displace subcutaneous tissue and grasp muscle deeply on each side.

Allow skin preparation to dry completely before skin is penetrated.

Have medication at room temperature.

Decrease perception of pain:

Distract child with conversation.

Give child something on which to concentrate (e.g., squeezing a hand or bed rail, "blowing" hurt away, counting, yelling "Ouch!").

Say to child, "If you feel this, tell me to take it out."

Have child hold a small adhesive bandage and place it on puncture site after IM injection is given.

Insert needle quickly, using a dartlike motion.

Avoid tracking any medication through superficial tissues:

Replace needle after withdrawing medication, or wipe medication from needle with sterile gauze.

If withdrawing medication from an ampule, use a needle equipped with a filter that removes glass particles; then use a new, nonfilter needle for injection.

Use the Z track or air-bubble technique as indicated.

Avoid any depression of the plunger during insertion of the needle.

Aspirate for blood.

If blood is seen, remove syringe from site, change needle, and reinsert into new location.

If no blood is seen, inject into a relaxed muscle:

Dorsogluteal—place child on abdomen with legs and toes rotated inward.

Ventrogluteal—place child on side with upper leg flexed and placed in front of lower leg.

Inject medication slowly.

Remove needle quickly; hold gauze firmly against skin near needle when removing it to avoid pulling on tissue.

Apply firm pressure to site after injection; massage site to hasten absorption unless contraindicated, as with irritating drugs.

Place a small adhesive bandage on puncture site; with young children decorate adhesive bandage by drawing a smiling face or other symbol of acceptance.

Hold and cuddle young child, and encourage parents to comfort child; praise older child.

Allow expression of feelings.

Discard syringe and uncapped, uncut needle in puncture-resistant container located near site of use.

Record time of injection, drug, dose, and injection site.

*Manufactured by Gebauer Company, Cleveland, OH 44104, (216) 271-5252.

---

Although *subcutaneous injections* can be given anywhere there is subcutaneous tissue, common sites include the center third of the lateral aspect of the upper arm, the abdomen, and the center third of the anterior thigh. Some practitioners believe it is not necessary to aspirate before injecting subcutaneously; however, this is not universally accepted. For example, not aspirating is an acceptable practice in the administration of insulin. Automatic injector devices do not aspirate before injecting.

When giving an *intradermal injection* into the volar surface of the forearm, the nurse should avoid the medial side of the arm, where the skin is more sensitive.

**NURSING TIP** Families often need to learn injection techniques to administer medications, such as insulin, at home. Begin teaching as early as possible to allow the family the maximum amount of practice time possible.

## Intravenous (IV) Administration

The IV route for administering medications is frequently used in pediatric therapy. For some drugs it is the only effective route of administration. This method is used for giving drugs to children who have poor absorption as a result of diarrhea, dehydration, or peripheral vascular collapse; children who need a high serum concentration of a drug; children who have resistant infections that require parenteral medication over an extended time; children who need continuous pain relief; and children who require emergency treatment.

Insertion sites and observation of the IV infusion are discussed in Chapter 28 under Parenteral Fluid Therapy and Venous Access Devices. However, several factors need to be considered in relation to IV medication. When a drug is administered intravenously, the effect is almost instantaneous and further control is limited. Most drugs for IV administration require a specified minimum dilution and/or rate of flow, and many are highly irritating or toxic to tissues outside the vascular system. In addition to the precautions and nursing observations related to IV therapy, factors to consider when preparing and administering drugs to infants and children by the IV route include:

- Amount of drug to be administered
- Minimum dilution of drug and if child is fluid restricted
- Type of solution in which drug can be diluted
- Length of time over which drug can be safely administered
- Rate of infusion that child and vessels can tolerate
- IV tubing volume capacity
- Time that this or another drug is to be administered
- Compatibility of all drugs that child is receiving intravenously and compatibility with infusion fluids

Before any IV infusion, the site of insertion is checked for patency. Medications are never administered with blood products. Only one antibiotic should be administered at a time.

IV infusion is suitable for children who can tolerate the necessary infusion rate and the extra fluid needed to administer the medication. For the very small infant or fluid-restricted child who is not able to tolerate the increased rate of fluids, special delivery systems, such as syringe pumps, are used. Regardless of the technique used, the nurse must know the minimum dilutions for safe administration of IV medications to infants and children.

> **NURSING ALERT**
>
> An often unrecognized source of contamination for vascular access lines (peripheral and central) is stopcock ports. Unaccessed ports should be covered at all times with a sterile cap or syringe, which is changed if contaminated during access for medication administration or blood collection.

Several methods of long-term venous access are available and include the peripheral lock device, central venous catheters, and implanted infusion ports. (See Venous Access Devices, Chapter 28.)

## Nasogastric, Orogastric, or Gastrostomy Administration

When a child has an indwelling feeding tube or a gastrostomy, oral medications are usually given via that route. An advantage of this method is the ability to administer oral medications around the clock without disturbing the child. A disadvantage is the risk of occluding or "clogging" the tube, especially when giving viscous (thick) solutions through small-bore feeding tubes. The most important preventive measure is adequate flushing after the medication is instilled. (See Guidelines box for administration guidelines.)

> **NURSING ALERT**
>
> Sprinkle-type medication should be avoided. However, if there is no other option and the tube is large gauge (18 French or greater), it may be given by mixing the sprinkles with a small amount of pureed fruit and thinning with water. The fruit keeps the sprinkles suspended so they do not float to the top. Flush well. This procedure is not recommended for skin-level gastrostomy devices.

## GUIDELINES
### Nasogastric, Orogastric, or Gastrostomy Medication Administration in Children

Use elixir or suspension (rather than tablets) preparations of medication whenever possible.
Dilute viscous medication or syrup if possible with a small amount of water.
If administering tablets, crush tablet to a very fine powder and dissolve drug in a small amount of warm water.
  Never crush enteric-coated or sustained-release tablets or capsules.
Avoid oily medications because they tend to cling to side of tube.
Do not mix medication with enteral formula unless fluid is restricted. If adding a drug:
  Check with pharmacist for compatibility.
  Shake formula well and observe for any physical reaction (e.g., separation, precipitation).
  Label formula container with name of medication, dosage, date, and time infusion started.
Have medication at room temperature.
Measure medication in calibrated cup or syringe.
Check for correct placement of nasogastric or orogastric tube.
Attach syringe (with adaptable tip but without plunger) to tube.
Pour medication into syringe.
Unclamp tube and allow medication to flow by gravity.
Adjust height of container to achieve desired flow rate (e.g., increased height for faster flow).
As soon as syringe is empty, pour in water to flush tubing.
  Amount of water depends on length and gauge of tubing.
  Determine amount before administering any medication by using a syringe to completely fill an unused nasogastric or orogastric tube with water. The amount of flush solution is usually 1½ times this volume.
  With certain drug preparations (e.g., suspensions), more fluid may be needed.
If administering more than one drug at the same time, flush the tube between each medication with clear water.
Clamp tube after flushing, unless tube is left open.

## Rectal Administration

The rectal route for administration is less reliable but sometimes used when the oral route is difficult or contraindicated. It is also used when oral preparations are unsuitable to control vomiting. Some of the drugs available in suppository form are acetaminophen, aspirin, sedatives, analgesics (morphine), and antiemetics. The difficulty in using the rectal route is that unless the rectum is empty at the time of insertion, the absorption of the drug may be delayed, diminished, or prevented by the presence of feces. Sometimes the drug is later evacuated, securely surrounded by stool.

The wrapping on the suppository is removed, and the suppository is lubricated with water-soluble jelly or warm water. Using a glove or finger cot, the suppository is quickly but gently inserted into the rectum, making certain that it is placed beyond both of the rectal sphincters. The buttocks are then held or taped together firmly to relieve pressure on the anal sphincter until the urge to expel the suppository has passed—which occurs within 5 to 10 minutes. Sometimes the amount of drug ordered is less than the dose available. The irregular shape of most suppositories makes the process of dividing them into a desired dose difficult if not dangerous. If it must be halved, it should be cut lengthwise.

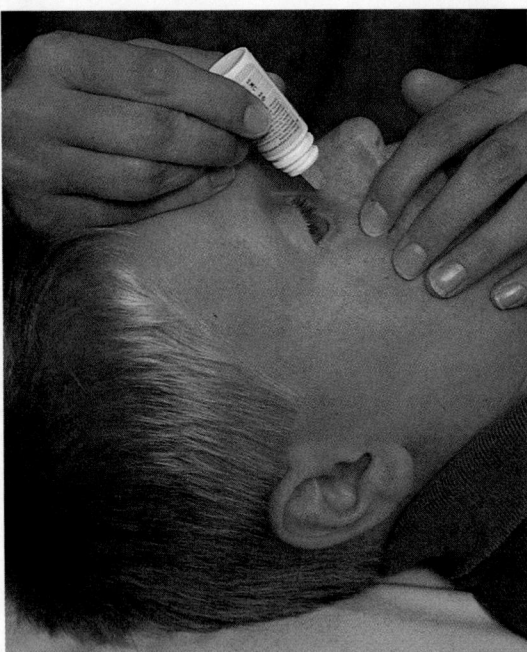

**Fig. 27-24** Administering eye drops.

However, there is no guarantee that the drug is evenly dispersed throughout the petrolatum base.

Rectal suppositories are traditionally inserted with the apex (pointed end) foremost. One study demonstrated easier insertion and a lower expulsion rate when the suppository was inserted with the base (blunt end) first. Reverse contractions or the pressure gradient of the anal canal may help the suppository to slip higher into the canal (Moppett and Parker, 1999).

If medication is administered via a retention enema, the same procedure is used. Drugs given by enema are diluted in the smallest amount of solution possible to minimize the likelihood of being evacuated.

## Optic, Otic, and Nasal Administration

There are few differences in administering eye, ear, and nose medication to children and to adults. The major difficulty is in gaining children's cooperation. The infant's or young child's head is immobilized in the same manner as described in Fig. 7-31, *B.* Older children need only explanation and direction. Although the administration of optic, otic, and nasal medication is not painful, these drugs can cause unpleasant sensations, which can be eliminated with various techniques.

To instill eye medication, the child is placed supine or sitting with the head extended and is asked to look up. One hand is used to pull the lower lid downward; the hand that holds the dropper rests on the head so that it may move synchronously with the child's head, thus reducing the possibility of trauma to a struggling child or dropping medication on the face (Fig. 27-24). As the lower lid is pulled down, a small conjunctival sac is formed; the solution or ointment

is applied to this area, rather than directly on the eyeball. Another effective technique is to pull the lower lid down and out to form a cup effect, into which the medication is dropped.

**NURSING TIP** To reduce unpleasant sensations:
**Eye**—Apply finger pressure to the lacrimal punctum at the inner aspect of the lid for 1 minute to prevent drainage of medication to the nasopharynx and the unpleasant "tasting" of the drug.
**Ear**—Allow medications stored in the refrigerator to warm to room temperature before instillation.
**Nose**—Position the child with the head hyperextended to prevent strangling sensations caused by medication trickling into the throat rather than up into the nasal passages.

The lids are gently closed to prevent expression of the medication. Excess medication is wiped from the inner canthus outward to prevent contamination to the contralateral eye.

Instilling eye drops in infants can be difficult because they often clench the lids tightly closed. One approach is to place the drops in the nasal corner where the lids meet. The medication pools in this area, and when the child opens the lids, the medication flows onto the conjunctiva. For young children, playing a game can be helpful, such as instructing the child to keep the eyes closed until the count of three and then open them, at which time the drops are quickly instilled. Ointment can be applied when the child is sleeping by gently pulling down the lower lid and placing the ointment in the lower conjunctival sac.

**NURSING ALERT** If both eye ointment and drops are ordered, give drops first, wait 3 minutes, then apply the ointment to allow each drug to work. When possible, administer eye ointments before bedtime or nap time, because the child's vision will be blurred for a while.

Ear drops are instilled with the child in the supine position and the head turned to the appropriate side. For children younger than 3 years of age, the external auditory canal is straightened by gently pulling the pinna downward and straight back. The pinna is pulled upward and back in children older than 3 years of age. (See Fig. 7-25.) To place the drops deep into the ear canal without contaminating the tip of the dropper, place a disposable ear speculum in the canal and administer the drops through the speculum. After instillation, the child should remain lying on the opposite side for a few minutes. Gentle massage of the area immediately anterior to the ear facilitates the entry of drops into the ear canal. The use of cotton pledgets prevents medication from flowing out of the external canal. However, they should be loose enough to allow any discharge to exit from the ear. Premoistening the cotton with a few drops of medication prevents the wicking action from absorbing the medication instilled in the ear.

Nose drops are instilled in the same manner as in the adult patient. Unpleasant sensations associated with medicated nose drops are minimized when care is taken to position the child with the head extended well over the edge of the bed or pillow (Fig. 27-25). Depending on their size, infants can be positioned in the football hold (see Fig. 27-8, *B*); in the nurse's arm with the head extended and stabilized between the nurse's body and elbow, and the arms and hands immobilized with the nurse's hands; or with the head extended over the edge of the bed or a pillow. Following instillation of the drops, the child should remain in position for 1 minute to allow the drops to come in contact with the nasal surfaces.

## Family Teaching and Home Care

The nurse usually assumes the responsibility for preparing families to administer medications at home. The family should have an understanding of why the child is receiving the medication and the effects that might be expected, as well as the amount, frequency, and length of time the drug is to be administered. Instruction should be carried out in an unhurried, relaxed manner, preferably in an area away from a busy ward or office, following the same guidelines for teaching outlined in the Guidelines box on p. 1120.

The caregiver is carefully instructed regarding the correct dosage. Some persons have difficulty in understanding or interpreting medical terminology, and just because they nod or otherwise indicate an understanding, it cannot be assumed that the message is clear. It is important to ascertain their interpretation of a teaspoon, for example, and to be certain they have acceptable devices for measuring the drug. If the drug is packaged with a dropper, syringe, or plastic cup, the nurse should show the point on the device that indicates the prescribed dose and demonstrate how the dose is drawn up into a dropper or syringe and measured and the bubbles eliminated. If the nurse has any doubts about the parent's ability to administer the correct dose, the parent should give a return demonstration. This is essential when the drug has potentially serious consequences from incorrect dosage, such as insulin or digoxin, or when more complex administration is required, such as parenteral injections. When teaching a parent to give an injection, adequate time for instruction and practice must be allotted.

Home modifications are often necessary because the availability of equipment or assistance can differ from the hospital setting. For example, the parent may need guidance in devising methods that allow for one person to hold the child and safely give the drug. One successful method is described here.

**NURSING TIP** To administer oral, nasal, or optic medication when only one person is available to hold the child, use the following procedure:
 Place child supine on a flat surface (bed, couch, floor).
 Sit facing child so that child's head is between operator's thighs and child's arms are under operator's legs.
 Place lower legs over child's legs to restrain lower body, if necessary.
 To administer oral medication, place a small pillow under child's head to reduce risk of aspiration.
 To administer nasal medication, place a small pillow under child's shoulders to aid flow of liquid through nasal passages.

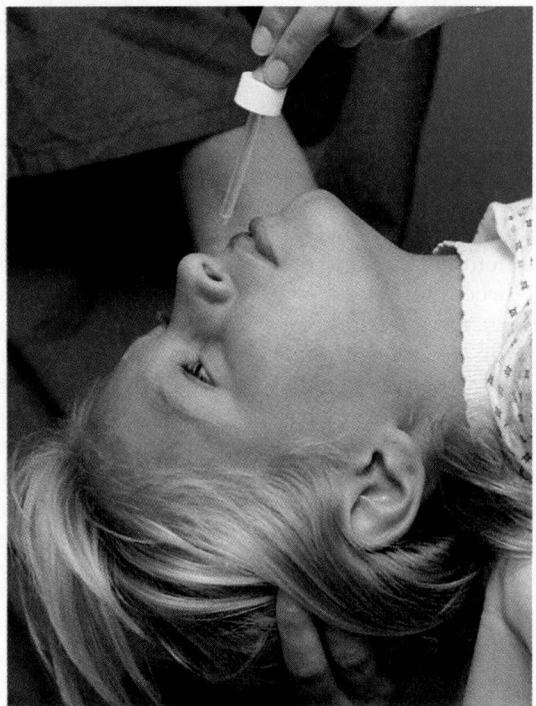

**Fig. 27-25** Proper position for instilling nose drops.

The time that the drug is to be administered is clarified with the parents. For instance, when a drug is prescribed in association with meals, the number of meals that the family is accustomed to eating influences the amount of drug the child receives. Does the family have meals twice a day or five times a day? When a drug is to be given several times during the day, together the nurse and parents can work out a schedule that accommodates the family's routine. Occasionally a drug must be given at equal intervals throughout a 24-hour period. However, telling parents that the child needs 1 teaspoon of medicine four times a day is subject to misinterpretation, since the parents may routinely schedule the doses at incorrect times. Instead, a preplanned schedule based on 6-hour intervals should be set up with the number of days required for the therapeutic dosage listed. Written instructions should accompany all drug prescriptions.*

**NURSING TIP** If parents have difficulty reading or understanding English, use colors to convey instructions. For example, mark each drug with a color and place the appropriate color on a calendar chart or on a drawing of a clock to identify when the drug needs to be given. If a liquid medication and syringe are used, also mark the syringe at the place the plunger needs to be with color-coded tape.

**NURSING ALERT** Dispose of any plastic covers that may be on the ends of syringes. These covers are small enough to be aspirated by young children.

---

*Home care instructions for giving medications are available in Wong DL, Hess CS: *Wong and Whaley's clinical manual of pediatric nursing*, ed 5, St Louis, 2000, Mosby.

# ALTERNATIVE FEEDING TECHNIQUES

Some children are unable to take nourishment by mouth because of conditions such as anomalies of the throat, esophagus, or bowel; impaired swallowing capacity; severe debilitation; respiratory distress; or unconsciousness. These children are frequently fed by way of a tube inserted orally or nasally into the stomach (*orogastric* or *nasogastric gavage*) or duodenum/jejunum (*enteral gavage*) or by a tube inserted directly into the stomach (*gastrostomy*) or jejunum (*jejunostomy*). Such feedings may be intermittent or by continuous drip. Feeding resistance, a problem that may result from any long-term feeding method that bypasses the mouth, is discussed in Chapter 10. During gavage or gastrostomy feedings, infants are given a pacifier. Nonnutritive sucking has been shown to have several advantages, such as increased weight gain and decreased crying. However, only pacifiers with a safe design can be used to prevent the possibility of aspiration. Using improvised pacifiers made from bottle nipples is not a safe practice.

When a child is concurrently receiving continuous-drip gastric or enteral feedings and parenteral (IV) therapy, the potential exists for inadvertent administration of the enteral formula through the circulatory system. The possibility for error increases when the parenteral solution is a fat emulsion, a milky-appearing substance. Safeguards to prevent this potentially serious error include (Garvin and Franck, 1989):

- Use a separate, specifically designed enteral feeding pump mounted on a separate pole for continuous-feeding solutions.
- Label all tubing of continuous enteral feeding with brightly colored tape or labels.
- Use specifically designed continuous-feeding bags to contain the solutions instead of parenteral equipment, such as a burette.

## Gavage Feeding

Infants and children can be fed simply and safely by a tube passed into the stomach through either the nares or the mouth. The tube can be left in place or inserted and removed with each feeding. In older children it is usually less traumatic to tape the tube securely in place between feedings. When this alternative is used, the tube should be removed and replaced with a new tube according to hospital policy, specific orders, and the type of tube used. Meticulous handwashing is practiced during the procedure to prevent bacterial contamination of the feeding, especially during continuous-drip feedings.

### Preparations

The equipment needed for gavage feeding includes:

- A suitable tube selected according to the size of the child and the viscosity of the solution being fed. Feeding tubes are available in silicone rubber, polyurethane, polyethylene, or polyvinylchloride. Polyurethane and silicone rubber tubes are smaller in diameter and more flexible than the others and are often referred to as small-bore tubes.
- A receptacle for the fluid; for small amounts a 10- to 30-ml syringe barrel or Asepto syringe is satisfactory; for larger amounts a 50-ml syringe with a catheter tip is more convenient.

- A syringe to aspirate stomach contents or to inject air after the tube has been placed.
- Water or water-soluble lubricant to lubricate the tube; sterile water is used for infants.
- Paper or nonallergenic tape to mark the tube and to attach the tube to the infant's or child's cheek (and nose, if placed through the nares).
- A stethoscope to determine the correct placement in the stomach.
- The solution for feeding.

Not all feeding tubes are the same. Polyethylene and polyvinylchloride types lose their flexibility and need to be replaced frequently, usually every 3 to 4 days. The polyurethane and silicone rubber tubes are indwelling and remain flexible so that they can remain in place longer and afford more patient comfort. Use of these small-bore tubes for continuous feeding has reduced the incidence of complications, such as pharyngitis, otitis media, and incompetence of the lower esophageal sphincter. Although the increased softness and flexibility of the tubes are advantages, they also cause disadvantages, such as difficult insertion (may require a stylet or metal guide wire), collapse of the tube during aspiration of gastric contents to test for correct placement, dislodgment during forceful coughing, and unsuitability for thick feedings. Traditional methods for verifying placement are less reliable with the small-bore tubes.

### Procedure

Infants will be easier to control if they are first wrapped in a mummy restraint (see Fig. 27-10). Even tiny infants with random movements can grasp and dislodge the tube. Preterm infants do not ordinarily require restraint, but, if they do, a small blanket folded across the chest and secured beneath the shoulders is usually sufficient. Care must be taken so that breathing is not compromised.

Whenever possible, the infant should be held and provided with a means for nonnutritive sucking during the procedure to associate the comfort of physical contact with the feeding. When this is not possible, gavage feeding is carried out with the infant or child on the back or toward the right side and the head and chest elevated. Feeding the child in a sitting position helps maintain the placement of the tube in the lowest position, thus increasing the likelihood of correct placement in the stomach.

The feeding tube can be passed through either the nose or the mouth. Because most young infants are obligatory nose breathers, insertion through the mouth causes less distress and helps to stimulate sucking. A tube passed through one of the nares in older infants and children is satisfactory once the tube is in place. An indwelling tube is almost always placed through the nose; the tube is alternated between the nares with each insertion to minimize irritation, the chance of infection, and possible breakdown of mucous membranes from pressure that occurs over time.

Two important issues remain unresolved regarding gavage feeding: measuring the insertion distance and checking the tube placement. Two standard methods of measuring tube length for insertion are (1) measuring from the nose to the bottom of the earlobe and then to the end of the xiphoid process and (2) measuring from the nose to the earlobe and then to a point midway between the xiphoid process and umbilicus (Fig. 27-26, *A*).(See Guidelines box.)

Ellett and Beckstrand (1999) found significant tube placement errors (43.5%) in a study of 39 hospitalized children. Children who were comatose or semicomatose, were inactive, had swallowing difficulty, or had Argyle tubes had

## GUIDELINES
### *Nasogastric Tube Feedings in Children*

Place the child supine with head slightly hyperflexed or in a sniffing position (nose pointed toward ceiling).

Measure the tube for approximate length of insertion, and mark the point with a small piece of tape.

Insert the tube that has been lubricated with sterile water or water-soluble lubricant through either the mouth or one of the nares to the predetermined mark. Because most young infants are obligatory nose breathers, insertion through the mouth causes less distress and helps to stimulate sucking. In older infants and children the tube is passed through the nose and alternated between nostrils.

An indwelling tube is almost always placed through the nose.

When using the nose, slip the tube along the base of the nose and direct it straight back toward the occiput.

When entering through the mouth, direct the tube toward the back of the throat (Fig. 27-26, *B*).

If the child is able to swallow on command, synchronize passing the tube with swallowing.

Check the position of the tube by using *both* of the following:

Attach the syringe to the feeding tube and apply negative pressure. Aspiration of stomach contents indicates proper placement, but aspiration of respiratory secretions may be mistaken for stomach contents. However, absence of fluid is not necessarily evidence of improper placement. The stomach may be empty, the tube may not be in contact with stomach contents, or a small-bore flexible tube may collapse. Note the amount and character of any fluid aspirated and return the fluid to the stomach.

With the syringe, inject a small amount of air (0.5 to 1 ml in preterm or very small infants to 5 ml in larger children) into the tube while simultaneously listening with a stethoscope over the stomach area. Sounds of gurgling or growling will be heard if the tube is properly situated in the stomach, although it is possible to hear the air entering the stomach even when the tube is positioned above the gastroesophageal sphincter.

Stabilize the tube by holding or taping it to the cheek, not to the forehead, because of possible damage to the nostril. To maintain correct placement, measure and record the amount of tubing extending from the nose or mouth to the

distal port when the tube is first positioned. Recheck this measurement before each feeding.

Warm the formula to room temperature. Do not microwave! Pour formula into the barrel of the syringe attached to the feeding tube. To start the flow, give a gentle push with the plunger, but then remove the plunger and allow the fluid to flow into the stomach by gravity. The rate of flow should not exceed 5 ml every 5 to 10 minutes in preterm and very small infants and 10 ml/minute in older infants and children to prevent nausea and regurgitation. The rate is determined by the diameter of the tubing and the height of the reservoir containing the feeding and is regulated by adjusting the height of the syringe. A usual feeding may take from 15 to 30 minutes to complete.

Flush the tube with sterile water (1 or 2 ml for small tubes to 5 to 15 ml or more for large ones) or see discussion of flushing for administering medication through nasogastric tubes in the Guidelines box on p. 1159 to clear the tube of formula.

Cap or clamp indwelling tubes to prevent loss of feeding.

If the tube is to be removed, first pinch it firmly to prevent escape of fluid as the tube is withdrawn. Withdraw the tube quickly.

Position the child on the right side for at least 1 hour in the same manner as following any infant feeding to minimize the possibility of regurgitation and aspiration. If the child's condition permits it, bubble the youngster after the feeding.

Record the feeding, including the type and amount of residual, the type and amount of formula, and how it was tolerated. For most infant feedings, any amount of residual fluid aspirated from the stomach is refed to prevent electrolyte imbalance, and the amount is subtracted from the prescribed amount of feeding. For example, if the infant is to receive 30 ml and 10 ml is aspirated from the stomach before the feeding, the 10 ml of aspirated stomach contents is refed plus 20 ml of feeding. Another method can be used in children. If residual is more than one fourth of the last feeding, return the aspirate and recheck in 30 to 60 minutes. When residual is less than one fourth of the last feeding, give scheduled feeding. If high aspirates persist and the child is due for another feeding, notify the practitioner.

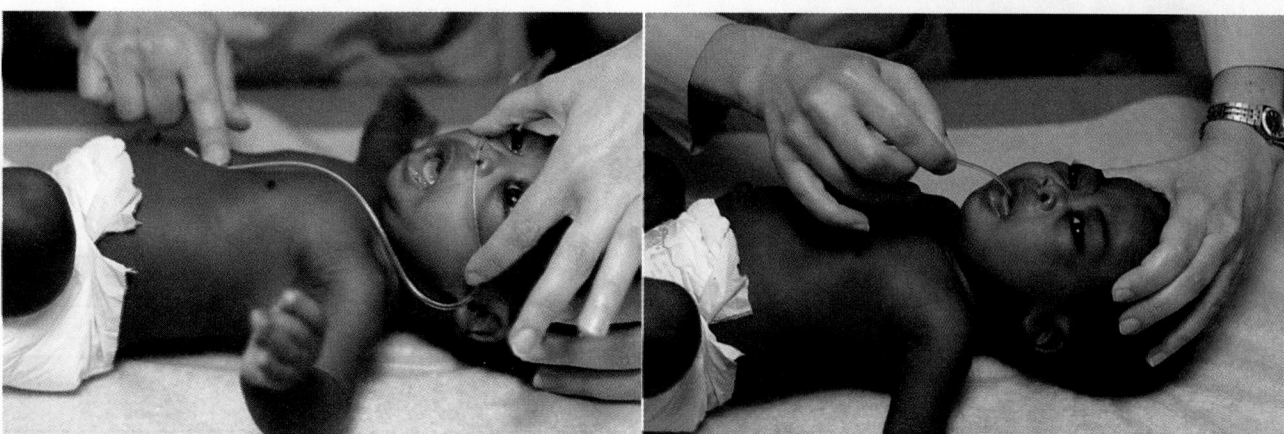

**Fig. 27-26** Gavage feeding. **A,** Measuring tube for orogastric feeding from tip of nose to earlobe and to midpoint between end of ziphoid process and umbilicus. **B,** Inserting tube.

increased tube placement errors. Findings supported radiographs to document tube placement. Although the most accurate method for testing tube placement is radiography, this practice is not feasible before each feeding. Research indicates that concentrations of the enzymes pepsin and trypsin in gastric and intestinal fluid are higher than in respiratory fluids, thus aiding in the prediction of feeding tube placement without the use of radiography (Metheny and others, 1997). Later studies demonstrated a simple bedside assessment of gastrointestinal aspirate color, pH, and bilirubin concentration was useful in predicting feeding tube placement (Metheny, Smith, and Steward, 2000). The use of auscultation, gastric pH determination, and presence of enzymes may assist in decreasing the uncertainty of gastric tube placement and reduce the incidence of accidental placement in the respiratory tract. Further studies are needed to be able to apply these findings to small children. If doubt exists regarding correct placement, the practitioner should be consulted. The procedure for gavage feeding is described in the Guidelines box on p. 1163.

In a survey of 113 level II and III nurseries, 98% of the nurseries measured from the nose or mouth to the earlobe and then to the xiphoid process to calculate the length of feeding tube placement in preterm infants. Auscultation was used to verify tube placement by 82% of the nurseries surveyed (Shiao and Difiore, 1996). For very-low-birth-weight infants, daily weight can be used to predict insertion length (Table 27-8). Until more definitive data are available, no method that results in a shorter distance than these methods should be used.

## Gastrostomy Feeding

Feeding by way of gastrostomy or a "G" tube is often used for children in whom passage of a tube through the mouth, pharynx, esophagus, and cardiac sphincter of the stomach is contraindicated or impossible. It is also used to avoid the constant irritation of a nasogastric tube in children who require tube feeding over an extended period. Placement of a gastrostomy tube may be performed with the child under general anesthesia or percutaneously using an endoscope and local anesthesia. The tube is inserted through the abdominal wall into the stomach about midway along the greater curvature and secured by a purse-string suture. The stomach is anchored to the peritoneum at the operative site. The tube used can be a Foley, wing-tipped, or mushroom catheter. Immediately after surgery the catheter may be left open and attached to gravity drainage for 24 hours or more.

Postoperative care of the wound site is directed toward prevention of infection and irritation. The area is cleansed at least daily or as often as needed to keep the area free of drainage. After healing occurs, meticulous care is needed to keep the area surrounding the tube clean and dry to prevent excoriation and infection. Daily applications of antibiotic ointment or other preparations may be prescribed to aid in healing and prevent irritation (see p. 1166). Care is exercised to prevent excessive pull on the catheter that might cause widening of the opening and subsequent leakage of highly irritating gastric juices. Securely tape the tube to the abdomen, leaving a small loop of tubing at the exit site to prevent tension on the site.

Granulation tissue may grow around a gastrostomy site (Fig. 27-27). This moist, beefy red tissue is not a sign of infection. However, if it continues to grow, the excess moisture can cause irritation of the surrounding skin.

For children on long-term gastrostomy feeding, a ***skin-level device*** (i.e., MIC-KEY, Bard Button, Gastroport) offers several advantages. The small, flexible silicone device protrudes slightly from the abdomen, is cosmetically pleasing in appearance, affords increased comfort and mobility to the child, is easy to care for, and is fully immersible in water. The one-way valve at the proximal end minimizes reflux and eliminates the need for clamping. However, the skin-level device requires a well-established gastrostomy site and is more expensive than the conventional tube. In addition, the valve may become clogged. When functioning, the valve prevents air from escaping; therefore the child may require frequent bubbling. With some devices, during feedings the child must remain fairly still because the tubing easily disconnects from the opening if the child moves. With other devices, extension tubing can be securely attached to the opening (Fig. 27-28). The feeding is instilled at the other end of the tubing in a manner similar to that for a regular gastrostomy. The extension tubing may also have a separate

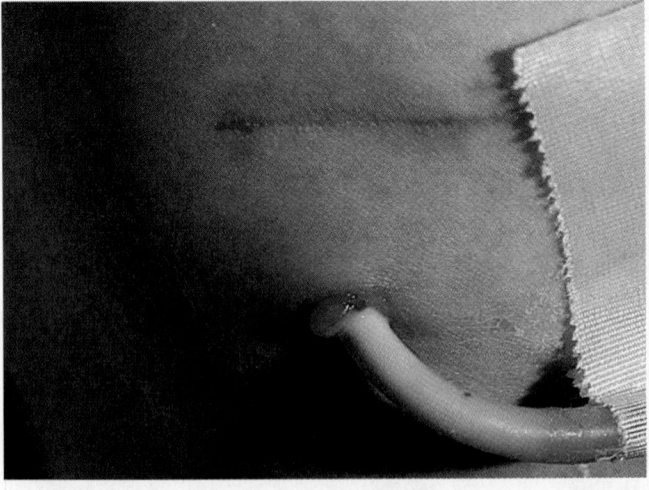

**Fig. 27-27** Appearance of healthy granulation tissue around stoma.

| TABLE 27-8 Recommended minimum insertion lengths for orogastric tubes in very-low-birth-weight infants | | | | |
|---|---|---|---|---|
| | **Daily Weight (g)** | | | |
| | **<750** | **750-999** | **1000-1249** | **1250-1499** |
| Insertion length (cm) | 13 | 15 | 16 | 17 |

From Gallaher KJ and others: Orogastric tube insertion length in very-low-birth-weight infants (<1500 grams), *J Perinatol* 13(2):128-131, 1993.

medication port. Both the feeding and the medication ports have plugs attached. Some skin-level devices require a special tube to be able to decompress the stomach (check residual or decompress air), and some do not.

Feeding of water, formula, or pureed foods is done in the same manner (including positioning) and rate as for gavage feeding. A mechanical pump may be used to regulate the volume and rate of feeding. Syringe pumps provide a more consistent rate of flow than peristaltic-type pumps and may be a better choice for infants with reflux. After feedings the infant or child is positioned on the right side or in the Fowler position, and the tube may be clamped or left open and suspended between feedings, depending on the child's condition. A clamped tube allows more mobility but is only appropriate if the child can tolerate intermittent feedings without vomiting or prolonged backup of feeding into the tube. Sometimes a Y tube is used to allow for simultaneous decompression during feeding. If a Foley catheter is used as the gastrostomy tube, very slight tension is applied and the tube is securely taped to maintain the balloon at the gastrostomy opening and prevent leakage of gastric contents and the tube's progression toward the pyloric sphincter, where it may occlude the stomach outlet. As a precaution, the length of the tube is measured postoperatively and then remeasured each shift to be sure it has not slipped. A mark can be made above the skin level to further ensure its placement. When the gastrostomy tube is no longer needed, it is removed; the skin opening usually closes spontaneously by contracture.

## PROCEDURES RELATED TO ELIMINATION

### Enema

The procedure for giving an enema to an infant or child does not differ essentially from that for an adult, except for the type and amount of fluid administered and the distance for inserting the tube into the rectum. (See Guidelines box.) Depending on the volume, a syringe with rubber tubing, an enema bottle, or an enema bag should be used.

> **NURSING ALERT** Proper insertion of the catheter tip, especially in infants, is essential to prevent rectal damage and perforation. (See Fig. 7-7, *B*.) If insertion of the enema tip causes discomfort, remove the tip and notify the practitioner.

### GUIDELINES
#### Administration of Enemas to Children

| AGE | AMOUNT (ML) | INSERTION DISTANCE (CM/INCHES) |
|---|---|---|
| Infant | 120-240 | 2.5 (1) |
| 2-4 years | 240-360 | 5.0 (2) |
| 4-10 years | 360-480 | 7.5 (3) |
| 11 years | 480-720 | 10.0 (4) |

An isotonic solution is used in children. Plain water is not used because, being hypotonic, it can cause rapid fluid shift and fluid overload. The Fleet enema (pediatric or adult sized) is not advised for children because of the harsh action of its ingredients (sodium biphosphate and sodium phosphate). Commercial enemas can be dangerous to patients with megacolon and to dehydrated or azotemic children. The osmotic effect of the Fleet enema may produce diarrhea, which can lead to metabolic acidosis. Other potential complications are extreme hyperphosphatemia, hypernatremia, and hypocalcemia, which may lead to neuromuscular irritability and coma (Walton and others, 2000).

> **NURSING TIP** If prepared saline is not available, it can be made by adding 1 teaspoon of table salt to 500 ml (1 pint) of tap water.

Because infants and young children are unable to retain the solution after it is administered, the buttocks must be held together for a short time to retain the fluid. The enema is administered and expelled while the child is lying with the buttocks over the bedpan and with the head and back supported by pillows. Older children are ordinarily able to hold the solution if they understand what to do and if they are not expected to hold it for too long. The nurse should have the bedpan handy or, for the ambulatory child, ensure that the bathroom is readily available before beginning the procedure. An enema is an intrusive procedure and thus threatening to the preschool child; therefore a careful explanation is especially important to ease possible fear.

A preoperative bowel preparation solution given orally or through a nasogastric tube is increasingly being used instead of an enema. The polyethylene glycol-electrolyte lavage solution (GoLYTELY) mechanically flushes the bowel without significant absorption, thereby avoiding po-

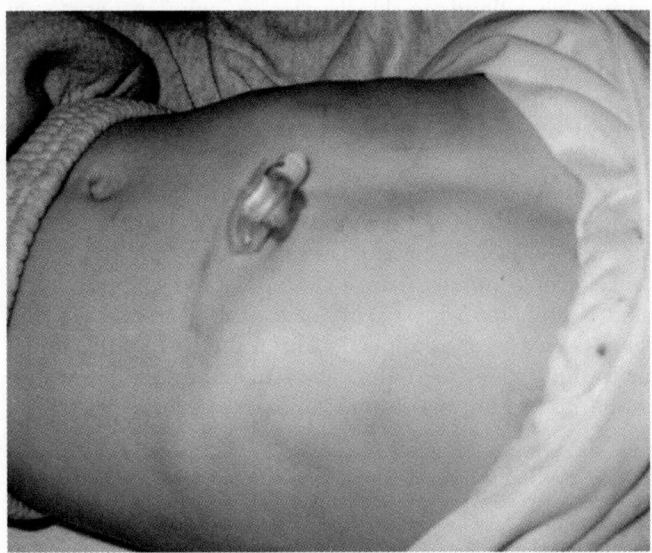

**Fig. 27-28** Child with skin-level gastrostomy device (MICKEY), which provides for secure attachment of extension tubing to gastrostomy opening.

tential fluid and electrolyte imbalances.* Another effective oral cathartic is magnesium citrate solution.

## Ostomies

Children may require stomas for various health problems. The most frequent causes are necrotizing enterocolitis and imperforate anus in the infant, and, less often, Hirschsprung disease. In the older child the most frequent causes are inflammatory bowel disease, especially Crohn disease (regional enteritis), and ureterostomies for distal ureter or bladder defects.

Care and management of ostomies in the older child differ little from the care of ostomies in the adult patient. The major emphasis in pediatric care is the preparation of the child for the procedure and teaching care of the ostomy to the child and family. The basic principles of preparation are the same as for any procedure (see p. 1103). Simple, straightforward language is most effective, together with the use of illustrations and a replica model (e.g., drawing a picture of a child with a stoma on the abdomen and explaining it as "another opening where bowel movements [or any other term the child uses] will come out"). At another time the nurse can draw a pouch over the opening to demonstrate how the contents are collected. Using a doll to demonstrate the process is an excellent teaching strategy, and special books are available.†

Children with ileostomies are fitted immediately after surgery with an appliance to protect the skin from the proteolytic enzymes in the liquid stool. Infants may not be fitted with a pouch in the immediate postoperative period. When stomal drainage is minimal, as is often the case in small or preterm infants, a gauze dressing will suffice. Parents are usually given a choice of caring for the colostomy with or without an appliance. Pediatric appliances are available in a variety of sizes to ensure an adequate fit.‡

Ostomy equipment consists of a one- or two-piece system with a hypoallergenic skin barrier to maintain peristomal skin integrity. The pouch should be large enough to contain a moderate amount of stool and flatus but not so large as to overwhelm the infant or child. A backing helps minimize the risk of skin breakdown from moisture trapped between the skin and pouch. Small clips or rubber bands should be avoided to prevent choking in the young child.

Protection of the peristomal skin is a major aspect of stoma care. Well-fitting appliances are important to prevent leakage of contents. Before the appliance is applied, the skin is prepared with a skin sealant that is allowed to dry. Then stoma paste is applied around the base of the stoma or to the back of the wafer. The sealant and paste work together to prevent peristomal skin breakdown.

In infants with a colostomy left unpouched, skin care is similar to that of any diapered child. However, the peristomal skin is protected with a wafer barrier, such as a hydrocolloid dressing (e.g., Duoderm) or a barrier substance (e.g., zinc oxide ointment [Desitin] or a mixture of zinc oxide ointment and stoma [Stomahesive]* powder). A gauze dressing may then be applied over the stoma and wafer to absorb stomal drainage. If the skin becomes inflamed, denuded, or infected, the care is similar to the interventions used for diaper dermatitis. (See Chapter 13.) A product that helps protect healthy skin, heal excoriated skin, and minimize pain associated with skin breakdown is Proshield Plus.† The skin protectant adheres to denuded, weeping skin. It can be applied over topical antifungal and antibacterial agents if infection is present.‡ "No-sting barrier film"§ is a skin sealant that has no alcohol base and can be used on open skin without stinging.

With young children, protection of the pouch from being pulled off is also an important consideration. One-piece outfits keep exploring hands from reaching the pouch, and the loose waist prevents any pressure on the appliance. Keeping the child occupied with toys during the pouch change is also helpful. As children mature, their participation in ostomy care is encouraged. Even preschoolers can assist by holding supplies, pulling paper backings from the appliance, and helping clean the stoma area. Toilet training for bladder control needs to begin at the appropriate time, as for any other child.

Older children and adolescents should eventually have total responsibility for ostomy care just as they would for usual bowel function. During adolescence, concerns for body image and the ostomy's impact on intimacy and sexuality emerge. The nurse should stress to teenagers that the presence of a stoma need not interfere with their activities. These youngsters can choose which ostomy equipment is best suited to their needs. Attractively designed and decorated pouch covers are well liked by teenagers.

Children with *familial adenomatous polyposis (FAP)* may require a colectomy with *ileoanal reservoir* to prevent or treat carcinoma of the colon. Peristomal skin care for these children is particularly challenging because of increased liquid stools, increased digestive enzymes that may cause skin breakdown, and the stoma being at skin level rather than raised. Additional care with this condition includes close monitoring of fluid and electrolyte status and increased incidence of bowel obstruction.

An enterostomal therapy nurse specialist is an important member of the health care team and will have additional suggestions and assistance with skin care information and ostomy pouching options. Further information and resources for ostomy and skin care may be obtained by con-

---

*Home care instructions for giving an enema are available in Wong DL, Hess CS: *Wong and Whaley's clinical manual of pediatric Nursing*, ed 5, St Louis, 2000, Mosby.
†*Chris Has an Ostomy* is available from the **United Ostomy Association, Inc,** 36 Executive Park, Suite 120, Irvine, CA 92714-6744, (800) 826-0826.
‡Little Ones Ostomy Products, ConvaTec, CN 5254, Princeton, NJ 08543-5254, (800) 422-8811; www.convatec.com.

---

*ConvaTec, (800) 422-8811.
†Healthpoint Medical, San Antonio, TX, (800) 441-8227.
‡Parents may find the following pamphlets helpful: *A Parent's Guide to Necrotizing Enterocolitis* or *Parent's Guide to Ostomy Care for Children;* available from ConvaTec (800) 422-8811.
§3M, St Paul, MN (800) 228-3957.

tacting the **Wound, Ostomy, and Continence Nurses Society (WOCN).***

## Family Teaching and Home Care

Because these children are almost always discharged with a functioning colostomy, preparation of the family should begin as early as possible in the hospital. The family is instructed in the application of the device (if used), care of

---

*(888) 224-WOCN; www.wocn.org.

the skin, and instructions regarding appropriate action in case skin problems develop. Early evidence of skin breakdown or stomal complications, such as ribbonlike stools, excessive diarrhea, bleeding, prolapse, or failure to pass flatus or stool, is brought to the attention of the physician, nurse, or stoma specialist. The same principles are applied as discussed earlier in this chapter for compliance, especially in terms of education (see Guidelines box on p. 1120), and in Chapter 26 for discharge planning and home care.*

---

*Home care instructions on caring for a colostomy are available in Wong DL, Hess CS: *Wong and Whaley's clinical manual of pediatric nursing,* ed 5, St. Louis, 2000, Mosby.

## KEY POINTS

- Informed consent is valid when the person is capable of giving consent (is over the age of majority and is competent), the person is supplied with information needed to make an intelligent decision, and the person acts voluntarily when exercising freedom of choice.
- Informed consent is needed for major surgery, minor surgery, and diagnostic tests and medical treatments with an element of risk.
- The major principles in psychologic preparation of the child for surgery are to establish trust, provide support, and give an explanation in easy-to-understand terms.
- Preparation for procedures should be based on developmental characteristics of the child and family, emphasizing the importance of the role of the parent when possible.
- Most parents and children want to be together during stressful procedures and should be offered this opportunity, with guidance on how the parent can comfort the child.
- The use of play activities to provide teaching about necessary nursing and medical interventions is an effective tool for use with children.
- In the performance of a procedure, the nurse should expect success, involve the child when possible in the procedure, provide distraction, and allow for expression of feelings.
- Proper positioning of infants and small children for procedures is essential to minimize movement and discomfort.
- In giving postprocedural support, the nurse should encourage children to express their feelings and praise them for completion of the procedure.
- Stressful times before and after surgery that produce anxiety in children are admission, blood tests, the day before surgery, injection of preoperative medication, transportation to the operating room, and return from the postanesthesia care unit.
- Assessment of compliance entails measuring factors that affect compliance (through clinical judgment, self-reporting, and direct observation), monitoring thera-

peutic response, taking pill counts, and performing chemical assay.
- Compliance strategies may be classified as organizational, educational, and behavioral.
- Knowledge of the ill child's eating habits and favorite foods can help in maintaining adequate nutrition.
- Skin care is an essential aspect of nursing care for the hospitalized child to prevent skin breakdown.
- Control of fever may be accomplished by pharmacologic means (administration of antipyretics); hyperthermia is controlled by environmental means (minimum clothing, increased air circulation, hypothermia mattress, or cool compresses).
- Infection control is based on two systems. Standard precautions provide protection when the infected person is undiagnosed. Transmission-based precautions add extra interventions for patients diagnosed with or suspected to have an infection.
- The revised CDC guideline for isolation precautions contains two levels of precautions: standardized precautions and transmission-based precautions.
- Ensuring safety in the hospital setting is a major concern and can be achieved through environmental measures, infection control measures, limit-setting, and safe transportation.
- Restraints are used cautiously and require a medical order. Therapeutic "hugging" can avoid the use of restraints.
- Factors that affect drug dosage determination are growth and maturation, difficulty in evaluating drug response, and body surface area.
- Family teaching regarding medication administration includes telling parents why the child is receiving the drug, its possible effects, and the amount, frequency, and length of time the drug is to be administered.
- The major forms of gastric feeding for children are gavage feeding and gastrostomy feeding.
- In the care of children with ostomies, nurses play an important role in family support and instruction in care of the stoma site.

# REFERENCES

Abbott K, Fowler-Kerry S: The use of a topical refrigerant anesthetic to reduce injection pain in children, *J Pain Symptom Manage* 10(8):584-590, 1995.

Algren C, Algren J: Pediatric sedation essentials for the preoperative nurse, *Nurs Clin North Am* 32(1):17-30, 1997.

Algren C, Ireland D, Stewart E: Perioperative and perianesthesia care of the child. In Albers AC and others, editors: *Comprehensive care of the pediatric patient: prehospital through rehabilitation,* Park Ridge, IL, 1998, Emergency Nurses Association.

Algren C, Schwartz P: The application of nursing research to the child, In Albers AC and others, editors: *Comprehensive care of the pediatric patient: prehospital through rehabilitation,* Park Ridge, IL, 1998, Emergency Nurses Association.

Algren JT, Algren CL: Management of procedural and perioperative pain in children, In Weiner R, editor: *Pain management: a practical guide for clinicians,* Boca Raton, FL, 1998, St Lucie Press.

American Academy of Pediatrics, Committee on Drugs: Guidelines for monitoring and management of pediatric patients during and after sedation for diagnostic and therapeutic procedures, *Pediatrics* 86(6):1110-1115, 1992.

American Pain Society: *Principles of analgesic use in the treatment of acute pain and cancer pain,* ed 3, Skokie, IL, 1992, The Society.

American Society of Anesthesiologists: Practice guidelines for sedation and analgesia by nonanesthesiologists, *Anesthesiology* 84:459-471, 1996.

Arditi M, Killner M: Coma following use of rubbing alcohol for fever control, *Am J Dis Child* 141(3):237-238, 1987.

Axelrod P: External cooling in the management of fever, *Clin Infect Dis* 31(suppl 5): S224-229, 2000.

Banco L, Powers A: Hospitals: unsafe environments for children, *Pediatrics* 82(5): 794-797, 1988.

Barker DP and others: Capillary blood sampling: should the heel be warmed? *Arch Dis Child Fetal Neonatal Ed* 74(1):F139-F140, 1996.

Barnes S: Not a social event: the follow-up phone call, *J Perianesth Nurs* 14(4):223-255, 2000.

Barton SJ, Holmes SS: A comparison of reagent strips and the refractometer of urine specific gravity in hospitalized children, *Pediatr Nurs* 24(5):480-482, 1998.

Bauchner H and others: Parents and procedures: a randomized controlled trial, *Pediatrics* 98(5):861-867, 1996

Baumgardner CA and others: Effects of nail polish on microbial growth of fingernails, *AORN J* 58(1):85-88, 1993.

Beecroft PC, Kongelbeck SR: How safe are intramuscular injections? *AACN Clin Issues* 5(2):207-215, 1994.

Berg AT and others: Predictors of recurrent febrile seizures: a metaanalytic review, *J Pediatr* 116(3):329-337, 1990.

Berg AT and others: Childhood-onset epilepsy with and without preceding febrile seizures, *Neurology* 53(8):1742-1748, 1999.

Bernado L, Lesniak D: Ethical and legal issues in pediatric nursing. In Albers AC and others, editors: *Comprehensive care of the pediatric patient: prehospital through rehabilitation,* Park Ridge, IL, 1998, Emergency Nurses Association.

Blass EM, Watt LB: Suckling- and sucrose-induced analgesia in human newborns, *Pain* 83(3):611-623, 1999.

Blesch P, Fisher M: The impact of parental presence on parental anxiety and satisfaction, *AORN J* 63(4):761-768, 1996.

Blount RL and others: Making the system work: training pediatric oncology patients to cope and their parents to coach them during BMA/LP procedures, *Behav Modif* 18(1):6-31, 1994.

Boie ET and others: Do parents want to be present during invasive procedures performed on their children in the emergency department? A survey of 400 parents, *Ann Emerg Med* 34(1):70-74, 1999.

Broome M: Consent (assent) for research with pediatric patients, *Semin Oncol Nurs* 15(2):96-103, 1999.

Broome M, Rehwaldt M, Fogg L: Relationship between cognitive behavioral techniques, temperament, observed distress, and pain reports in children and adolescents during lumbar puncture, *J Pediatr Nurs* 13(1):48-54, 1998.

Bryant RA, editor: *Acute and chronic wounds: nursing management,* ed 2, St Louis, 1998, Mosby.

Bryant RA, Doughty D, editors: *Acute and chronic wounds: nursing management,* ed 2, St Louis, 2000, Mosby.

Burke N: Alternative methods for newborn urine sample collection, *Pediatr Nurs* 21(6): 546-549, 1995.

Calianno C: Patient hygiene. II. Skin care: keeping the outside healthy, *Nursing* 29(12)(suppl):1-11, 1999.

Carlson D, Mowery BD: Standards to prevent complications of urinary catheterization in children: should and should-knots, *J Soc Pediatr Nurs* 2(1):37-41, 1997.

Catudal R: Pediatric IV therapy: actual practice, *J Vasc Access Devices* 4(1):27-29, 1999.

Cohen Reis E, Holubkov R: Vapocoolant spray is equally effective as EMLA cream in reducing immunization pain in school-aged children, *Pediatrics* 100(6):E5, 1997.

Connell F: The causes and treatment of fever: a literature review, *Nurs Stand* 12(11):40-43, 1997.

Cooke R, Werkman S, Watson D: Urine output measurements in premature infants, *Pediatrics* 83(1):116-118, 1989.

Coté CJ and others: Adverse sedation events in pediatrics: analysis of medications used for sedation, *Pediatrics* 106(4):633-644, 2000.

Cravero JP, Manzi DJA, Rice LJ: The management of procedure-related pain in the child. In Ashburn MA, Rice LJ, editors: *The management of pain,* Philadelphia, 1998, Churchill-Livingstone.

Dunn D: Malignant hyperthermia, *AORN J* 65(4):728-753, 1997.

Ellet ML, Beckstand J: Examination of gavage tube placement in children, *J Soc Pediatr Nurs* 4(2):51-60, 1999.

Emergency Nurses Association: *Position statement: family presence at the bedside during invasive procedures and/or resuscitation,* Park Ridge, IL, 1998, The Association.

Essink-Tebbes CM and others: Safety of lidocaine-prilocaine cream application four times a day in premature neonates: a pilot study, *Eur J Pediatr* 158(5):421-423, 1999.

Fennell ME: Parents in the OR? You bet! *RN* 62(12):38-40, 1999.

Fina DK and others: Parent participation in the postanesthesia care unit: fourteen years of progress at one hospital, *J Perianesth Nurs* 12(3):152-162, 1997.

Fradet C and others: A prospective survey of reactions to blood tests by children and adolescents, *Pain* 49(1):53-60, 1990.

Frizzell J: Avoiding lab test pitfalls, *Am J Nurs* 98(2):34-37, 1998.

Gablehouse BL, Gitterman BA: Maternal understanding of commonly used medical terms in a pediatric setting, *Am J Dis Child* 114:419, 1990.

Garner JS: What's in a name? The evolution of universal precautions to standard precautions: a guide to the latest recommendation in isolation practices, *Today's Surg Nurs* 19(1):14-21, 1997.

Garvin G, Franck L: Preventing delivery of enteral formula via parenteral route, *Pediatr Nurs* 15(1):17-18, 1998.

Giganti AW: Families in pediatric critical care: the best option, *Pediatr Nurs* 24(3): 261-265, 1998.

Gray L, Watt L, Blass EM: Skin-to-skin contact is analgesic in healthy newborns, *Pediatrics* 105(1):110-111, 2000; *www.pediatrics.org/ cgi/content/full/105/1/E14.*

Gray M: Atraumatic urethral catheterization of children, *Pediatr Nurs* 22(4):306-310, 1996.

Groswasser J and others: Needle length and injection technique for efficient intramuscular vaccine delivery in infants and children evaluated through an ultrasonographic determination of subcutaneous and muscle layer thickness, *Pediatrics* 99 (3, pt 1):400-402, 1997.

Guertler AT: Pearls, pitfalls, and updates: the clinical practice of emergency medicine, *Emerg Med Clin North Am* 15(2):303-313, 1997.

Haimi-Cohen Y and others: Parental presence during lumbar puncture: anxiety and attitude toward the procedure, *Clin Pediatr* 35(1):2-4, 1996.

Hall PA and others: Parents in the recovery room: survey of parental and staff attitudes, *BMJ* 310(6973):163-164, 1995.

Hannigan P, Shields JW: Handwashing and use of examination gloves, *Lancet* 351:571, 1998.

Harrison A and others: Comparison of simultaneously obtained arterial and capillary blood gases in pediatric intensive care unit patients, *Crit Care Med* 25(1):1904-1908, 1997.

Hicks JF and others: Optimum needle-length for diphtheria-tetanus-pertussis inoculation of infants, *Pediatrics* 84(1):136-137, 1989.

Hooker E and others: Subjective assessment of fever by parents: comparison with measurement by noncontact tympanic thermometer and calibrated rectal glass mercury thermometer, *Ann Emerg Med* 28(3):313-317, 1996.

Howland M, Goldfrank L: Meperidine usage in patients with sickle cell crisis, *Ann Emerg Med* 15(12):1506-1507, 1986.

Humphrey G and others: The occurrence of high levels of acute behavioral distress in children and adolescents undergoing routine venipunctures, *Pediatrics* 90(1): 87-91, 1992.

Ipp MM and others: Adverse reactions to diphtheria, tetanus, pertussis-polio vaccination at 18 months of age: effect of injection site and needle length, *Pediatrics* 83(5): 679-682, 1989.

Jackson F: The ABC's of black hair and skin care, *ABNF J* 9(5):100-104, 1998.

Johannsen L: Adolescent abortion and mandated parental involvement, *Pediatr Nurs* 21(1):82-84, 1995.

Johns Hopkins Hospital Department of Pediatrics: *The Harriet Lane handbook*, ed 14, edited by Barone M, St Louis, 1996, Mosby.

Johnston CC, Stevens B, Arbess G: The effect of the sight of blood and use of decorative adhesive bandages on pain intensity ratings by preschool children, *J Pediatr Nurs* 8(13): 147-151, 1993.

Joint Commission on Accreditation of Healthcare Organizations: Care of the patient: Restraint and seclusion standards, *Comprehensive accreditation manual for hospitals*, TX.7.1-TX.7.5.5, 2001.

Katsma D, Smith G: Analysis of needle path during intramuscular injection, *Nurs Res* 46(5):288-292, 1997.

Kinmonth AL, Fulton Y, Campbell MJ: Management of feverish children at home, *BMJ* 305(6862):1134-1136, 1992.

Kraus D and others: Effectiveness and infant acceptance of the Rx medibottle versus the oral syringe, *Pharmacotherapy* 21(4):416-423, 2001.

Kristensson-Hallstrom I: Parental participation in pediatric surgical care, *AORN J* 71(5):1021-1029, 2000.

Krozek J, Scoggins A: Restraints and seclusion policy . . . amended to comply with 2001 JCAHO standards, *Cinahl Information Systems* (9p), 2001.

Kubiak M and others: Comparison of stool containment in cloth and single-use diapers using simulated infant feces, *Pediatrics* 91(3):632-636, 1993.

Kyngas H, Kroll T, Duffy M: Compliance in adolescents with chronic diseases: a review, *J Adolesc Health* 26:379-388, 2000.

Landsman IS, Cook DR: Pediatric anesthesia. In O'Neill J and others, editors: *Pediatric Surgery*, St Louis, 1998, Mosby.

LaRosa-Nash PA and others: Implementing a parent-present induction program, *AORN J* 61(3):526-531, 1995.

LaRosa-Nash PA, Murphy JM: A clinical case study: parent-present induction of anesthesia in children, *Pediatr Nurs* 22(2):109-111, 1996.

LaRosa-Nash PA, Murphy JM: An approach to pediatric perioperative care: parent-present induction, *Nurs Clin North Am* 32(1):183-199, 1997.

Larsson BA and others: Alleviation of the pain of venepuncture in neonates, *Acta Paediatr* 87(7):774-779, 1998.

Laurent C: And so to beds, *Nurs Times* 95(3):7-8, 1999.

Liebman M, Barnsteiner J: Fever education: does it reduce parent fever anxiety? *Pediatr Emerg Care* 17(1):47-51,2001.

Lohr J, Donowitz L, Dudley S: Bacterial contamination rates in voided urine collections in girls, *J Pediatr* 114(1):91-93, 1989.

Lybrand M, Medoff-Cooper B, Monro B: Periodic comparisons of specific gravity using urine from a diaper and collecting bag, *MCN Am J Matern Child Nurs* 15(4): 238-239, 1990.

Malviya S and others: Sedation/analgesia for diagnostic and therapeutic procedures in children, *J Perianesth Nurs* 15(6):415-422, 2000.

Manworren R, Fledderman M: Preparation of the child and family for surgery. In Wise BV and others, editors: *Nursing care of the general pediatric surgical patient*, Gaithersburg, MD, 2000, Aspen.

Maxwell LG, Yaster M: Perioperative management issues in pediatric patients, *Anesthesiol Clin North Am* 18(3):601-632, 2000.

McCaffery M, Pasero C: *Pain: clinical manual for nursing practice*, ed 2, St Louis, 1999, Mosby.

Meehan RM: Heelsticks in neonates for capillary blood sampling, *Neonatal Network* 17(1):17-24, 1998.

Melnyk BM: Intervention studies involving parents of hospitalized young children: an analysis of the past and future recommendations, *J Pediatr Nurs* 15(1):4-13, 2000.

Metheny NA, Smith L, Steward BJ: Development of a reliable and valid bedside test for bilirubin and its utility for improving prediction of feeding tube location, *Nurs Res* 49(6):302-309, 2000.

Metheny and others: pH and concentrations of pepsin and trypsin in feeding tube aspirates as predictors of tube placement, *J Parenter Enteral Nutr* 21(5):279-285, 1997.

Miranda A and others: Malignant hyperthermia, *Am J Crit Care* 6(5):368-374, 1997.

Moppet S, Parker M: Insertion of a suppository, *Nurs Times* 95(23):suppl 1-2, 1999.

Moskop JC: Ethical issues in emergency medicine: informed consent in the emergency department, *Emerg Med Clin North Am*, 17(2):327-340, 1999.

Munro H, D'Errico FC: Parental involvement in perioperative anesthetic management, *J Perianesth Nurs* 15(6):397-400, 2000.

Nahata MC, Clotz MA, Krogg EA: Adverse effects of meperidine, promethazine, and chlorpromazine for sedation in pediatric patients, *Clin Pediatr* 24:558-560, 1985.

Nelson D: Procedural sedation in the emergency department. In Krauss B, Brustowicz RM, editors: *Pediatric procedural sedation and analgesia*, Philadelphia, 1999, Lippincott Williams & Wilkins.

Noble RR and others: Perioperative considerations for the pediatric patient: a developmental approach, *Nurs Clin North Am* 32(1):1-16, 1997.

Olsen RJ and others: Examination gloves as barriers to hand contamination in clinical practice, *JAMA* 270(3):350-353, 1993.

Orenstein S and others: The Santmyer swallow: a new and useful infant reflex, *Lancet* 1(8581):345-346, 1988.

Paes B and others: A comparative study of heelstick devices for infant blood collection, *Am J Dis Child* 147:346-348, 1993.

Polillio AM, Kiley J: Does a needleless injection system reduce anxiety in children receiving intramuscular injections? *Pediatr Nurs* 23(1):46-49, 1997.

Pollack CV, Pollack ES, Andrew ME: Suprapubic bladder aspiration versus urethral catheterization in ill infants: success, efficiency, and complication rates, *Ann Emerg Med* 23(2):225-230, 1994.

Powers KS, Rubenstein JS: Family presence during invasive procedures in the pediatric intensive care unit: a prospective study, *Arch Pediatr Adolesc Med* 153(9):955-958, 1999.

Prandoni D and others: Assessment of urine collection techniques for microbial culture, *Am J Infect Control* 24(3):219-221, 1996.

Purssell E: The use of antipyretic medications in the prevention of febrile convulsions in children, *J Pediatr Nurs* 9(4):473-480, 2000.

Ros S: Outpatient pediatric analgesia: a tale of two regimens, *Pediatr Emerg Care* 3(4): 228-230, 1987.

Rote N, Huether S, McCance K: Hypersensitivities, infaction, and immunodeficiencies. In Huether S, McCance K, editors: *Understanding pathophysiology*, ed 2, St Louis, 2000, Mosby.

Russell B: Nosocomial infections, *Am J Nurs* 99(6):24J-24P, 1999.

Saez-Llorens X and others: Bacterial contamination rates for non-clean catch and clean catch midstream urine collections in uncircumcised boys, *J Pediatr* 114(1):93-95, 1989.

Schlager TA and others: Bacterial contamination rate of urine collected in a urine bag from healthy non-toilet-trained male infants, *J Pediatr* 116(5):738-739, 1990.

Schultz WH and others: *Use of the Biojector 2000 for lidocaine prior to lumbar puncture and bone marrow aspiration/biopsy in the pediatric patient with cancer*, Durham, NC, 1995, Duke University Medical Center.

Selbst S: Risk management and medicolegal aspects of procedural sedation. In Krauss B, Brustowicz RM, editors: *Pediatric procedural sedation and analgesia*, Philadelphia, 1999, Lippincott Williams & Wilkins.

Selekman J, Snyder B: Institutional policies on the use of physical restraints on children, *Pediatr Nurs* 23(5):531-537, 1997.

Sharber J: The efficacy of tepid sponge bathing to reduce fever in young children, *Am J Emerg Med* 15:188-192, 1997.

Shiao SPK, Difiore TE: A survey of gastric tube practices in level II and level III nurseries, *Issues Compr Pediatr Nurs* 19(3):209-220, 1996.

Shinnar S and others: Short-term outcomes of children with febrile status epilepticus, *Epilepsia* 42(1):47-53, 2001.

Snodgrass WR, Dodge WF: Lytic/"DPT" cocktail: time for rational and safe alternatives, *Pediatr Clin North Am* 36(5):1285-1291, 1989.

Stebor A: Posturination time and specific gravity in infant's diapers, *Nurs Res* 38(4): 244-245, 1989.

Stephens BK, Barkey ME, Hall HR: Techniques to comfort children during stressful procedures, *Accid Emerg Nurs* 7(4):226-236, 1999.

Stewart EJ, Algren C, Arnold S: Preparing children for a surgical experience, *Todays OR Nurs* 16(2):9-14, 1994.

Sullivan D: Minors and emergency medicine, *Emerg Med Clin North Am* 11(4):841-851, 1993.

Thompson BL and others: Handwashing and glove use in a long-term care facility, *Infect Control Hosp Epidemiol* 18(2):97-103, 1997.

Turner P: Establishing a protocol for parental presence in recovery, *Br J Nurs* 6(14):794-799, 1997.

US Department of Agriculture: Potential hazards with protective restraint devices, *FDA Med Bull* 21(3), 1992.

Van R and others: The effect of diaper type and overclothing on fecal contamination in day-care centers, *JAMA* 265(14):1840-1844, 1991.

Van Cleve L, Johnson L, Pothier P: Pain responses of hospitalized infants and children to venipuncture and intravenous cannulation, *J Pediatr Nurs* 11:169-174, 1996.

Vertanen H and others: An automatic incision device for obtaining blood samples from the heels of the preterm infants causes less damage than a conventional manual lancet, *Arch Dis Child Fetal Neonatal Ed* 84:F53-F55, 2001.

Vessey J, Caserza L, Bogetz M: In my opinion . . . another Pandora's box? Parental participation in anesthetic induction, *Child Health Care* 19(2):116-118, 1990.

Walton DM and others: Morbid hypocalcemia associated with phosphate enema in a six-week-old infant, *Pediatrics* 106:e37, 2000.

Wlody GS: Malignant hyperthermia, *Crit Care Nurs Clin North Am* 3(1):129-134, 1991.

Wong DL, Redding B: Lozenges can be "life-savers," *Am J Nurs* 87(9):1129-1130, 1987.

Wong DL: DPT or pedi-cocktail: not a good mix, *Am J Nurs* 94(6):15, 1994.

Wysocki A: Skin anatomy, physiology, and pathophysiology, *Nurs Clin North Am* 34(4):777-797, 1999.

Zain ZN and others: Parental presence during induction of anesthesia: a randomized controlled trial, *Anesthesiology* 84:1060-1067, 1996.

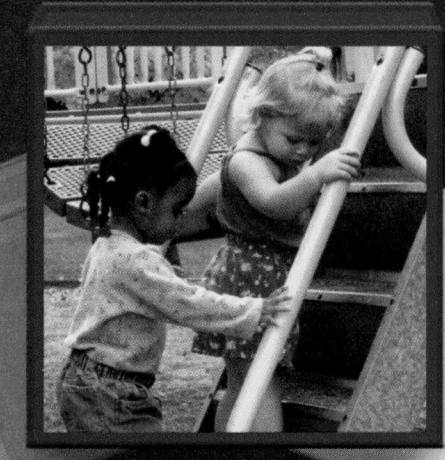

Chapter **28**

# Balance and Imbalance of Body Fluids

## Chapter Outline

**DISTRIBUTION OF BODY FLUIDS, 1171**
**Water Balance, 1172**
   Mechanisms of Fluid Movement, 1172
   Changes in Fluid Volume Related to
     Growth, 1173
   Water Balance in Infants, 1173
**DISTURBANCES OF FLUID AND
ELECTROLYTE BALANCE, 1174**
**Dehydration, 1174**
   Types of Dehydration, 1176
   Degree of Dehydration, 1178
**Water Intoxication, 1180**
**Edema, 1180**
   Mechanisms of Edema Formation, 1180
**DISTURBANCES OF ACID-BASE
BALANCE, 1181**
**Acid-Base Imbalance, 1182**
   Hydrogen Ion Concentration, 1182
   Compensatory Mechanisms, 1182

Laboratory Measurements, 1183
Associated Disturbances in Acid-Base
   Balance, 1183
**Respiratory Acidosis, 1183**
**Respiratory Alkalosis, 1184**
**Metabolic Acidosis, 1184**
**Metabolic Alkalosis, 1184**
**NURSING RESPONSIBILITIES IN FLUID
AND ELECTROLYTE DISTURBANCES,
1185**
**Assessment, 1185**
   History, 1185
   Clinical Observations, 1185
   Intake and Output (I & O)
     Measurement, 1186
**Oral Fluid Intake, 1186**
   The Child Who Is NPO, 1188
**Parenteral Fluid Therapy, 1188**
   Intravenous Infusion, 1188
   Intraosseous Infusion, 1191

Preparing the Child and Parents, 1192
The Procedure, 1192
Securing a Peripheral Intravenous (PIV)
   Line, 1194
Removal of a Peripheral Intravenous
   Line, 1196
Complications, 1196
**Venous Access Devices (VADs), 1198**
   Peripheral Intermittent Infusion
     Device, 1198
   Peripherally Inserted Central Catheters
     (PICCs), 1198
   Long-Term Central VADs, 1200
   Complications, 1201
   Parent/Child Teaching, 1202
**Total Parenteral Nutrition (TPN), 1203**
   Complications, 1203
   Home Total Parenteral Nutrition
     (HTPN), 1204

## Related Topics

Alternative Feeding Techniques, Ch. 27
Burns, Ch. 29
The Child with Gastrointestinal Dysfunction,
   Ch. 33
The Child with Renal Dysfunction, Ch. 30
Collection of Specimens, Ch. 27

Diarrhea, Ch. 29
Family-Centered Home Care, Ch. 25
Intravenous Administration (of Medication),
   Ch. 27
Oral Hygiene, Ch. 27

Pain Management, Ch. 26
Preparation for Diagnostic and Therapeutic
   Procedures, Ch. 27
Shock States, Ch. 29
Vomiting, Ch. 29

## DISTRIBUTION OF BODY FLUIDS

The distribution of body fluids, or **total body water (TBW)**, involves the presence of **intracellular (ICF)** and **extracellular (ECF)** fluids. Water is the major constituent of body tissues, and the TBW in an individual ranges from 45% to 75% of total body weight.

■ Nancy Rabin, RN, MN, CPNP; Theresa Reed, RN; and Lisa M. Vallino, BSN, RN, revised this chapter.

The ICF refers to the fluid contained within the cells, whereas the ECF is the fluid outside the cells. The ECF is further broken down into several components: **intravascular** (contained within the blood vessels), **interstitial** (surrounding the cell and the location of most ECF), and **transcellular** (contained within specialized body cavities such as cerebrospinal, synovial, pleural, and so on). In the newborn about 50% of the body fluid is contained within the ECF, whereas 30% of the toddler's body fluid is contained within the ECF.

The importance of body water to body function is related not only to its abundance but also to the fact that it is the medium in which body solutes are dissolved and all metabolic reactions take place. Because these metabolic processes are affected by even small alterations in fluid composition, precise regulation of the volume and composition of the fluid is essential. In healthy individuals, body water remains singularly constant, but marked alterations in either its volume or distribution, which occur in many disease states, can produce severely damaging physiologic consequences.

## Water Balance

Under normal conditions the amount of water ingested closely approximates the amount of urine excreted in a 24-hour period, and the water in food and from oxidation approximates the amount lost in feces and through evaporation. In this way, equilibrium is maintained.

### Mechanisms of Fluid Movement

Water is retained in the body in a relatively constant amount and, with few exceptions, is freely exchangeable among all body fluid compartments. The proximity of the extravascular compartment to the cells allows for continual change in volume and distribution of fluids, largely determined by solutes (especially sodium) and physical forces (Box 28-1). Transport mechanisms are the basis for all activity within the cells, and because they have limited ability to store materials, movement in and out of cells must be rapid. Internal control mechanisms are responsible for distribution and maintenance of fluid balance (Box 28-2).

**Maintaining Water Balance.** Maintenance water requirement is the volume of water needed to replace obligatory fluid loss such as that from *insensible water loss* (through the skin and respiratory tract), evaporative water loss, and losses through urine and stool formation. The amount and type of these losses may be altered by disease states such as fever (with increased sweating), diarrhea, gastric suction, and pooling of body fluids in a body space (often referred to as *third-spacing*).

Basal maintenance calculations for required body water are based on the body's requirements for water in a normometabolic state, at rest; estimated fluid requirements are then increased or decreased from these parameters based on increased or decreased water losses, such as with elevated body temperature or congestive heart failure. Daily maintenance fluid requirements are outlined in Table 28-1.

---

**NURSING ALERT** Nurses need to be alert for altered fluid requirements in various conditions:

Increased requirements:
- Fever (add 12% per rise of 1° C)
- Vomiting, diarrhea
- High-output renal failure
- Diabetes insipidus
- Burns
- Shock
- Tachypnea

Decreased requirements:
- Congestive heart failure
- Syndrome of inappropriate antidiuretic hormone (SIADH)
- Mechanical ventilation
- Postoperatively
- Oliguric renal failure
- Increased intracranial pressure

---

### Box 28-1 ■ ■ ■
### Physical Forces Influencing Fluid Balance

**Hydrostatic pressure**—The pumping action of the heart increases fluid pressure in the arterial portion of the circulatory system, forcing fluid through the capillary walls into the interstitial spaces and from glomerular capillaries into the collecting tubules of the kidneys; it is the pressure created by the weight of fluid.

**Osmotic pressure**—The physical force, or "pull," created by a solution of higher concentration across a semipermeable membrane. Fluid in the solution of lesser concentration moves to the solution of greater concentration to equalize the concentration on each side of the membrane. Major osmotic forces in body fluids are sodium and intravascular proteins.

**Diffusion**—Random movement of molecules from a region of greater concentration to regions of lesser concentration. Rate of diffusion is influenced by the size and the distance across which the particle mass must diffuse (small particles move more rapidly than large ones), temperature (heat increases the rate of movement), and agitation (stirring hastens movement). **Facilitated diffusion** employs a carrier substance to assist solute movement across a membrane.

**Active transport**—A substance is transported by way of a carrier substance *against* a pressure gradient, from a region of lesser or equal concentration to a region of equal or higher concentration; examples include solutes such as sodium, potassium, and glucose.

**Vesicular transport**—A portion of a membrane engulfs a large molecule and releases it on the other side of the membrane. Substances move into cells by *pinocytosis* and out of cells by *exocytosis*.

---

### Box 28-2 ■ ■ ■
### Internal Control Mechanisms Influencing Fluid Balance

**Thirst**—The impetus to ingest water is stimulated by increased solute concentration (osmolality) of extracellular fluid and/or diminished intravascular volume.

**Antidiuretic hormone (ADH)**—Released from the posterior pituitary gland in response to increased osmolality and decreased volume of intravascular fluid; promotes water retention in the renal system by increasing the permeability of renal tubules to water.

**Aldosterone**—Secreted by the adrenal cortex; enhances sodium reabsorption in renal tubules, thus promoting osmotic reabsorption of water.

**Renin-angiotensin system**—Diminished blood flow to the kidneys stimulates renin secretion, which reacts with plasma globulin to generate angiotensin, a powerful vasoconstrictor. Angiotensin also stimulates the release of aldosterone.

Maintenance fluids contain both water and electrolytes and can be estimated from the child's age, body weight, degree of activity, and body temperature. ***Basal metabolic rate (BMR)*** is derived from standard tables and adjusted for the child's activity, temperature, and disease state. For example, for afebrile patients at rest, the maintenance water requirement is approximately 100 ml for each 100 kilocalorie expended. Children with fluid losses or other alterations require adjustment of these basic needs to accommodate abnormal losses of both water and electrolytes as a result of a disease state. For example, insensible losses are increased when basal expenditure is increased by fever or hypermetabolic states. Hypometabolic states, such as hypothyroidism and hypothermia, decrease the BMR.

### Changes in Fluid Volume Related to Growth

The percentage of TBW varies among individuals and in adults and older children is related primarily to the amount of body fat. Consequently, females, who have more body fat than males, and obese persons tend to have less water content in relation to weight.

The embryo is composed primarily of water, with little tissue substance. As the organism grows and develops, a progressive decrease occurs in TBW, with the fastest rate of de-

| TABLE 28-1   Daily maintenance fluid requirements | |
|---|---|
| **Body Weight (kg)** | **Amount of Fluid per Day** |
| 1-10 | 100 ml/kg |
| 11-20 | 1000 ml plus 50 ml/kg for each kg >10 kg |
| >20 | 1500 ml plus 20 ml/kg for each kg >20 kg |

cline taking place during fetal life. The changes in water content and distribution that occur with age reflect the changes that take place in the relative amounts of bone, muscle, and fat making up the body. At maturity the percentage of total body water is somewhat higher in the male than in the female and is probably a result of the differences in body composition, particularly fat and muscle content (Fig. 28-1).

Another important aspect of growth change as it corresponds to water distribution is related to the ICF and ECF compartments. In the fetus and prematurely born infant, the largest proportion of body water is contained in the ECF compartment. As growth and development proceed, the proportion within this fluid compartment decreases as the ICF and cell solids increase. The ECF diminishes rapidly from approximately 40% of body weight at birth to 30% at 1 year of age (McEntee, 1997). The different effects on males and females become apparent at puberty.

### Water Balance in Infants

Because of several characteristics, infants and young children have a greater need for water and are more vulnerable to alterations in fluid and electrolyte balance. Compared with older children and adults, they have a greater fluid intake and output relative to size. Water and electrolyte disturbances occur more frequently and more rapidly, and children adjust less promptly to these alterations (Rabin, 2000).

The fluid compartments in the infant vary significantly from those in the adult, primarily because of an expanded extracellular compartment. The ECF compartment constitutes more than half of the TBW at birth and has a greater relative content of extracellular sodium and chlo-

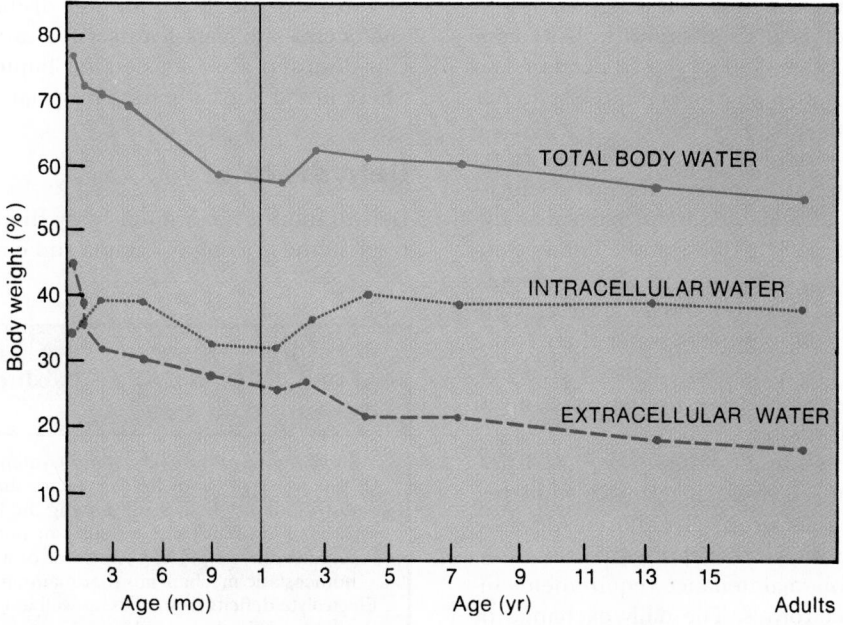

**Fig. 28-1**  Changes in total body water, extracellular water, and intracellular water in percentages of body weight. (Based on data from Fris-Hansen B: *Pediatrics* 28:169, 1961.)

ride. The infant loses a large amount of fluid at birth and still maintains a larger amount of ECF than the adult until about 2 years of age. This contributes to greater and more rapid water loss during this age period.

Fluid losses create compartment deficits that reflect the duration of dehydration. In general, approximately 60% of fluid is lost from the ECF, and the remaining 40% comes from the ICF (Finberg, Kravath, and Hellerstein, 1993). The amount of fluid lost from the ECF increases with acute illness and decreases with chronic loss.

Fluid losses may be divided into insensible, urinary, and fecal losses and vary with the patient's age. Approximately two thirds of insensible losses occur through the skin, and the remaining one third is lost through the respiratory tract (Ganong, 1995). Insensible fluid loss is influenced by heat and humidity, body temperature, and respiratory rate. Infants and children have a much greater tendency to become highly febrile than do adults. Fever increases insensible water loss by approximately 7 ml/kg/24 hours for each 1° F rise in temperature above 37.2° C (99° F). Fever and increased surface area relative to volume are both factors that contribute to greater insensible fluid losses in young patients.

**Body Surface Area (BSA).** The infant's relatively greater BSA allows larger quantities of fluid to be lost through the skin. It is estimated that the BSA of the premature neonate is five times as great, and that of the newborn is two to three times as great, as that of the older child or adult. The proportionately longer gastrointestinal tract in infancy is also a source of relatively greater fluid loss, especially from diarrhea.

**Metabolic Rate.** The rate of metabolism in infancy is significantly higher than in adulthood because of the larger BSA in relation to the mass of active tissue. Consequently, there is a greater production of metabolic wastes that must be excreted by the kidneys. Any condition that increases metabolism causes greater heat production, with its concomitant insensible fluid loss and an increased need for water for excretion. The BMR in infants and children is higher to support growth (Ganong, 1995).

**Kidney Function.** The kidneys of the infant are functionally immature at birth and are therefore inefficient in excreting waste products of metabolism. Of particular importance for fluid balance is the inability of the infant's kidneys to concentrate or dilute urine, to conserve or excrete sodium, or to acidify urine. Therefore the infant is less able to handle large quantities of solute-free water than is the older child and is more apt to become dehydrated when given concentrated formulas or overhydrated when given excessive water or dilute formula.

**Fluid Requirements.** As a result of these characteristics, infants ingest and excrete a greater amount of fluid per kilogram of body weight than do older children. Because electrolytes are excreted with water and the infant has limited ability for conservation, maintenance requirements include both water and electrolytes. The daily exchange of ECF in the infant is greatly increased over that of older children, which leaves the infant little fluid volume reserve in dehydrated states (Ganong, 1995). Fluid requirements de-

pend on hydration status, size, environmental factors, and underlying disease.

## DISTURBANCES OF FLUID AND ELECTROLYTE BALANCE

Disturbances of fluids and their solute concentration are closely interrelated. Alterations in fluid volume affect the electrolyte component, and changes in electrolyte concentration influence fluid movement. Because intracellular water and electrolytes move to and from the ECF compartment, any imbalance in the ICF is reflected by an imbalance in the ECF. Disturbances in the ECF involve either an excess or a deficit of fluid or electrolytes; of these, fluid loss occurs more frequently.

Depletion of ECF, usually caused by gastroenteritis, is one of the most common problems encountered in infants and children. (See Chapter 29.) Until modern techniques for fluid replacement were perfected, it was one of the chief causes of infant mortality. Fluid and electrolyte problems related to specific diseases and their management are discussed throughout the book where appropriate. The major fluid disturbances, their usual causes, and clinical manifestations are outlined in Table 28-2; the most common disturbances, dehydration and edema, are elaborated further. Problems of fluid and electrolyte disturbance always involve both water and electrolytes; therefore replacement includes administration of both, calculated on the basis of ongoing processes and laboratory serum electrolyte values.

In problems that involve alterations in the amount and composition of body fluid compartments, many areas are considered when planning management (Box 28-3). The following discussion is concerned with the general concepts of two common fluid volume disturbances—dehydration and edema—that are features of a variety of conditions. Specific disorders are discussed in Chapters 29 and 30 and elsewhere in the book where appropriate.

### Dehydration

Dehydration is a common body fluid disturbance encountered in the nursing of infants and children; it occurs when-

---

**Box 28-3** ■ ■ □
**Areas of Concern in Planning Management of Fluid Problems**

Volume of body fluids (i.e., water content of the patient)
Osmolality of the body fluids, a factor that has an effect on the distribution of body water among the various compartments
Hydrogen ion status (i.e., whether or not there has been a disturbance in the pH of body fluids or a disturbance in the homeostatic mechanisms that maintain the pH)
Electrolyte deficits from cells, as well as extracellular water
Disturbances in the equilibrium between the mineral skeleton and body fluids
Length of time alteration in fluid status has existed

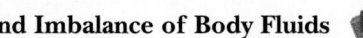

ever the total output of fluid exceeds the total intake, regardless of the underlying cause. Although dehydration can result from lack of oral intake (especially in elevated environmental temperatures), more often it is a result of abnormal losses, such as those that occur in vomiting or diarrhea, when oral intake only partially compensates for the abnormal losses. Other significant causes of dehydration are diabetic ketoacidosis and extensive burns.

**TABLE 28-2**   Disturbances of fluid and electrolyte balance

| Mechanisms/Situations | Manifestations | Management/Nursing Care |
|---|---|---|
| **Water Depletion** | | |
| Failure to absorb or reabsorb water | General symptoms: | Provide replacement of fluid losses commensurate with volume depletion |
| Complete sudden cessation of intake or prolonged diminished intake: | Thirst | |
| Neglect of intake by self or caregiver—confused, psychotic, unconscious, or helpless | Variable temperature—increased (infection) | Provide maintenance fluids and electrolytes |
| | Dry skin and mucous membranes | Determine and correct cause of water depletion |
| Loss from gastrointestinal tract—vomiting, diarrhea, nasogastric suction, fistula | Poor skin turgor | |
| | Poor perfusion (decreased pulse, slowed capillary refill time) | Measure intake and output |
| Disturbed body fluid chemistry: inappropriate ADH secretion | Weight loss | Monitor vital signs |
| | Fatigue | Monitor urine specific gravity |
| Excessive renal excretion: glycosuria (diabetes) | Diminished urinary output | |
| Loss through skin or lungs: | Irritability and lethargy | |
| Excessive perspiration or evaporation—febrile states, hyperventilation, increased ambient temperature, increased activity (basal metabolic rate [BMR]) | Tachycardia | |
| | Tachypnea | |
| | Altered level of consciousness, disorientation | |
| | Symptoms depend to some extent on proportion of electrolytes lost with water | |
| Impaired skin integrity—transudate from injuries | Laboratory findings: | |
| Hemorrhage | High urine specific gravity | |
| Iatrogenic: | Increased hematocrit | |
| Overzealous use of diuretics | Variable serum electrolytes | |
| Improper postoperative fluid replacement | Variable urine volume | |
| Use of radiant warmer or phototherapy | Increased blood urea nitrogen (BUN) | |
| | Increased serum osmolality | |
| **Water Excess** | | |
| Water intake in excess of output: | Edema: | Limit fluid intake |
| Excessive oral intake | Generalized | Administer diuretics |
| Hypotonic fluid overload | Pulmonary (moist rales or crackles) | Monitor vital signs |
| Plain water enemas | Intracutaneous (noted especially in loose areolar tissue) | Determine and treat cause of water excess |
| Failure to excrete water in presence of normal intake: | Elevated venous pressure | Analyze laboratory electrolyte measurements frequently |
| Kidney disease | Hepatomegaly | |
| Congestive heart failure | Slow, bounding pulse | |
| Malnutrition | Weight gain | |
| | Lethargy | |
| | Increased spinal fluid pressure | |
| | Central nervous system manifestations (seizures, coma) | |
| | Laboratory findings: | |
| | Low urine specific gravity | |
| | Decreased serum electrolytes | |
| | Decreased hematocrit | |
| | Variable urine volume | |
| **Sodium Depletion (Hyponatremia)** | | |
| Prolonged low-sodium diet | Associated with water loss: | Determine and treat cause |
| Decreased sodium intake | Same as with water loss—dehydration, weakness, dizziness, nausea, abdominal cramps, apprehension | Administer intravenous (IV) fluids with appropriate saline concentration |
| Fever | | |
| Excess sweating | Mild—apathy, weakness, nausea, weak pulse | |
| Increased water intake without electrolytes | Moderate—decreased blood pressure, lethargy | |
| Tachypnea (infants) | Laboratory findings: | |
| Cystic fibrosis | Sodium concentration <130 mEq/L (may be normal if volume low) | |
| Burns and wounds | Urine specific gravity depends on water deficit or excess | |
| Vomiting, diarrhea, nasogastric suction, fistulas | | |
| Adrenal insufficiency | | |
| Renal disease | | |
| Diabetic ketoacidosis (DKA) | | |
| Malnutrition | | |

*Continued*

**TABLE 28-2** Disturbances of fluid and electrolyte balance—cont'd

| Mechanisms/Situations | Manifestations | Management/Nursing Care |
|---|---|---|
| **Sodium Excess (Hypernatremia)** | | |
| High salt intake—enteral or IV<br>Renal disease<br>Fever<br>High insensible water loss:<br>    Increased temperature<br>    Increased humidity<br>    Hyperventilation<br>Diabetes insipidus<br>Hyperglycemia | Intense thirst<br>Dry, sticky mucous membranes<br>Flushed skin<br>Temperature may be increased<br>Hoarseness<br>Oliguria<br>Nausea and vomiting<br>Possible progression to disorientation, convulsions, muscle twitching, nuchal rigidity, lethargy at rest, hyperirritable when aroused<br>Lethargy findings:<br>    Serum sodium concentration ≥150 mEq/L<br>    High plasma volume<br>    Alkalosis | Determine and treat cause<br>Administer fluids as prescribed<br>Measure intake and output<br>Monitor laboratory data<br>Monitor neurologic status |
| **Potassium Depletion (Hypokalemia)** | | |
| Starvation<br>Clinical conditions associated with poor food intake<br>Malabsorption<br>IV fluid without added potassium<br>Gastrointestinal losses—diarrhea, vomiting, fistulas, nasogastric suction<br>Diuresis<br>Administration of diuretics<br>Administration of corticosteroids<br>Diuretic phase of nephrotic syndrome<br>Healing stage of burns<br>Potassium-losing nephritis<br>Hyperglycemic diuresis (e.g., diabetes mellitus)<br>Familial periodic paralysis<br>IV administration of insulin in DKA<br>Alkalosis | Muscle weakness, cramping, stiffness, paralysis, hyporeflexia<br>Hypotension<br>Cardiac arrhythmias, gallop rhythm<br>Tachycardia or bradycardia<br>Ileus<br>Apathy, drowsiness<br>Irritability<br>Fatigue<br>Laboratory findings:<br>    Decreased serum potassium concentration ≤3.5 mEq/L<br>    Abnormal ECG—notched or flattened T waves, decreased ST segment, premature ventricular contractions | Determine and treat cause<br>Monitor vital signs, including electrocardiogram (ECG)<br>Administer supplemental potassium<br>Assess for adequate renal output before administration<br>IV: administer K+ slowly<br>Oral: offer high-potassium fluids and foods<br>Evaluate acid-base status |
| **Potassium Excess (Hyperkalemia)** | | |
| Renal disease<br>Renal failure<br>Adrenal insufficiency (Addison disease)<br>Associated with metabolic acidosis<br>Too rapid administration of IV potassium chloride<br>Transfusion with old donor blood | Muscle weakness, flaccid paralysis<br>Twitching<br>Hyperreflexia<br>Bradycardia<br>Ventricular fibrillation and cardiac arrest<br>Oliguria<br>Apnea—respiratory arrest | Determine and treat cause<br>Monitor vital signs, including ECG<br>Administer exchange resin, if prescribed<br>Administer IV fluids as prescribed<br>Administer IV insulin (if ordered) to facilitate movement of potassium into cells |

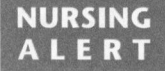 **NURSING ALERT** Whenever a child has a history of dehydration, nursing assessment should be geared toward the possibility of impending shock.

In early dehydration (during the first 2 days), fluid loss is derived from both the ECF and the ICF because the increased osmolality of the diminished ECF volume causes fluid from the ICF compartment to move into the ECF compartment. As dehydration becomes chronic, the cellular losses become greater (Ganong, 1995).

### Types of Dehydration

Because sodium is the primary osmotic force that controls fluid movement between the major fluid compartments, dehydration is often described according to plasma sodium concentrations (i.e., isonatremic, hyponatremic, or hyper-

natremic). Other osmotic forces, however, such as glucose in diabetic dehydration and protein in nephrotic syndrome, may also play a dominant role. Consequently, dehydration is conventionally classified as (1) isotonic, (2) hypotonic, or (3) hypertonic (Fann, 1998; Ledwith, 1997).

*Isotonic (isosmotic or isonatremic) dehydration* occurs in conditions in which electrolyte and water deficits are present in approximately balanced proportions. This is the primary form of dehydration occurring in children. The observable fluid losses are not necessarily isotonic, but losses from other avenues make adjustments so that the sum of all losses, or the net loss, is isotonic. Because no osmotic force is present to cause a redistribution of water between the ICF and ECF, the major loss is sustained from the ECF compartment. This significantly reduces the plasma volume and thus the circulating blood volume, with its effect on the skin, muscles, and kidneys. Shock is the greatest threat to

**TABLE 28-2**   Disturbances of fluid and electrolyte balance—cont'd

| Mechanisms/Situations | Manifestations | Management/Nursing Care |
|---|---|---|
| **Potassium Excess (Hyperkalemia)—cont'd** | | |
| Severe dehydration | Laboratory findings: | Monitor serum potassium levels |
| Crushing injuries | High serum potassium concentration | Evaluate acid-base status |
| Burns | ≥5.5 mEq/L | |
| Hemolysis | Variable urine volume | |
| Dehydration | Flat P wave on ECG, peaked T waves, widened | |
| Potassium-sparing diuretics | QRS complex, increased PR interval | |
| Increased intake of potassium (e.g., salt substitutes) | | |
| **Calcium Depletion (Hypocalcemia)** | | |
| Inadequate dietary calcium | Neuromuscular irritability | Determine and treat cause |
| Vitamin D deficiency | Tingling of nose, ears, fingertips, toes | Administer calcium supplements as |
| Rapid transit through gastrointestinal tract | Tetany | prescribed; administer slowly |
| Advanced renal insufficiency | Laryngospasm | Monitor IV site; calcium may cause vas- |
| Administration of diuretics | Generalized convulsions | cular irritation |
| Hypoparathyroidism | May be changes in clotting | Monitor serum calcium levels |
| Alkalosis | Positive Chvostek and Trousseau signs | Monitor serum protein levels |
| Trapped in diseased tissues | Hypotension | |
| Increased serum protein (albumin) | Cardiac arrest | |
| Cow's milk formula—tetany of the newborn | Laboratory findings: | |
| Exchange transfusion with citrated blood | Decreased serum calcium concentration | |
| Inadequate parenteral administration in diseased states | ($N = 8.8$-$10.8$ mEq/L) or Increased serum protein levels Prolonged QT interval | |
| **Calcium Excess (Hypercalcemia)** | | |
| Acidosis | Constipation | Determine and treat cause |
| Prolonged immobilization | Weakness, fatigue | Monitor serum calcium levels |
| Conditions associated with increased bone catabolism | Nausea, vomiting | Monitor ECG |
| Hypoproteinemia | Anorexia | |
| Kidney disease | Dryness of mouth (thirst) | |
| Hypervitaminosis D | Muscle hypotonicity | |
| Hyperparathyroidism | Bradycardia/cardiac arrest | |
| Hyperthyroidism | Increased calcium concentration in urine may | |
| Excessive IV or oral administration | cause formation of kidney stones | |
| | Laboratory findings: | |
| | Increased serum calcium levels or | |
| | Decreased serum protein levels | |
| | Prolonged QRS complex or PR interval, shortened QT interval | |

life in isotonic dehydration, and the child with isotonic dehydration displays symptoms characteristic of hypovolemic shock. Plasma sodium remains within normal limits, between 130 and 150 mEq/L (Fann, 1998).

*Hypotonic (hyposmotic* or *hyponatremic) dehydration* occurs when the electrolyte deficit exceeds the water deficit. Because ICF is more concentrated than ECF in hypotonic dehydration, water transfers from the ECF to the ICF to establish osmotic equilibrium. This movement further increases the ECF volume loss, and shock is a frequent result. Because there is a greater proportional loss of ECF in hypotonic dehydration, the physical signs tend to be more severe with smaller fluid losses than in isotonic or hypertonic dehydration. Plasma sodium concentrations are typically less than 130 mEq/L (Behrman, Kliegman, and Jenson, 2000).

*Hypertonic (hyperosmotic* or *hypernatremic) dehydration* results from water loss in excess of electrolyte loss and is usu-

ally caused by a proportionately larger loss of water or a larger intake of electrolytes. This type of dehydration is also the most dangerous and requires much more specific fluid therapy. This sometimes occurs in infants with diarrhea who are given fluids by mouth that contain large amounts of solute or in children receiving high-protein nasogastric tube feedings that place an excessive solute load on the kidneys. In hypertonic dehydration, fluid shifts from the lesser concentration of the ICF to the ECF. Plasma sodium concentration is greater than 150 mEq/L (Behrman, Kliegman, and Jenson, 2000).

Because the ECF volume is proportionately larger, hypertonic dehydration consists of a greater degree of water loss for the same intensity of physical signs. Shock is less apparent in hypotonic dehydration. However, neurologic disturbances, such as seizures, are more likely to occur. Cerebral changes are serious and may result in permanent damage. These include disturbance of consciousness, poor ability to focus attention, lethargy, increased muscle tone with hyperreflexia, and hyperirritability to stimuli (tactile, auditory, bright light).

## Degree of Dehydration

Traditionally the magnitude of fluid loss has been described as a percentage (5%, 10%, 15%) and ascertained by a comparison of preillness weight and current weight, because any weight loss is substantially equivalent to the amount of water lost. However, water constitutes only 60% to 70% of infant weight, and adipose tissue, which contains little water, is highly variable in individual infants and children. Rather than using a percentage, a more accurate means of describing dehydration is to reflect acute loss (over 48 hours or less) in milliliters per kilogram of body weight (Jospen, and Forbes, 1996). For each 1% weight loss, 10 ml/kg of fluids have been lost (Fann, 1998). For example, a loss of 50 ml/kg is considered to be a mild fluid loss, whereas a loss of 100 ml/kg produces severe dehydration.

Clinical signs provide clues to the extent of dehydration (Table 28-3). The earliest detectable sign is usually tachycardia, followed by dry skin and mucous membranes, sunken fontanels, signs of circulatory failure (coolness and mottling of extremities), loss of skin elasticity, and delayed capillary filling time (Held, 1995) (see Table 28-4 for clini-

cal manifestations of dehydration and Fig. 28-2 for signs of dehydration).

Compensatory mechanisms attempt to maintain fluid volume by adjusting to these losses. Interstitial fluid moves into the vascular compartment to maintain the blood volume in response to hemoconcentration and hypovolemia, and vasoconstriction of peripheral arterioles helps maintain pumping pressure. When fluid losses exceed the body's ability to sustain blood volume and blood pressure, circulation is seriously compromised and the blood pressure falls. This results in tissue hypoxia with accumulation of lactic acid, pyruvate, and other acid metabolites, which contributes to the development of metabolic acidosis (Ganong, 1995).

Renal compensation is impaired by reduced blood flow through the kidneys, and little urine is formed. Increased serum osmolality stimulates the secretion of antidiuretic hormone (ADH) to conserve fluid and initiates the renin-angiotensin mechanisms in the kidney, causing further vasoconstriction (Aker and O'Sullivan, 1998). Aldosterone is released to promote sodium retention and conserve water in the kidneys (Noble, 1998). If dehydration increases in severity, urine formation is greatly diminished and metabolites and hydrogen ions that are normally excreted by this route are retained.

Shock, a common manifestation of severe depletion of ECF volume, is preceded by tachycardia and signs of poor

---

**TABLE 28-3** Intensity of clinical signs associated with varying degrees of isotonic dehydration in infants

| | Degree of Dehydration | | |
| | Mild | Moderate | Severe |
| --- | --- | --- | --- |
| Fluid volume loss | <50 ml/kg | 50-90 ml/kg | ≥100 ml/kg |
| Skin color | Pale | Gray | Mottled |
| Skin elasticity | Decreased | Poor | Very poor |
| Mucous membranes | Dry | Very dry | Parched |
| Urinary output | Decreased | Oliguria | Marked oliguria and azotemia |
| Blood pressure | Normal | Normal or lowered | Lowered |
| Pulse | Normal or increased | Increased | Rapid and thready |
| Capillary filling time | <2 seconds | 2-3 seconds | >3 seconds |

---

**TABLE 28-4** Clinical manifestations of dehydration

| | Isotonic (Loss of Water and Salt) | Hypotonic (Loss of Salt in Excess of Water) | Hypertonic (Loss of Water in Excess of Salt) |
| --- | --- | --- | --- |
| Skin | | | |
|   Color | Gray | Gray | Gray |
|   Temperature | Cold | Cold | Cold or hot |
|   Turgor | Poor | Very poor | Fair |
|   Feel | Dry | Clammy | Thickened, doughy |
| Mucous membranes | Dry | Slightly moist | Parched |
| Tearing and salivation | Absent | Absent | Absent |
| Eyeball | Sunken | Sunken | Sunken |
| Fontanel | Sunken | Sunken | Sunken |
| Body temperature | Subnormal or elevated | Subnormal or elevated | Subnormal or elevated |
| Pulse | Rapid | Very rapid | Moderately rapid |
| Respirations | Rapid | Rapid | Rapid |
| Behavior | Irritable to lethargic | Lethargic to comatose; convulsions | Marked lethargy with extreme hyper-irritability on stimulation |

perfusion and tissue oxygenation (by pulse oximeter readings). Peripheral circulation is poor as a result of reduced blood volume; therefore the skin is cool and mottled, with decreased capillary filling after blanching. Impaired kidney circulation often leads to oliguria and azotemia. Although low blood pressure may accompany other symptoms of shock, in infants and young children it is usually a late sign and may herald the onset of cardiovascular collapse.

## Diagnostic Evaluation

To initiate a therapeutic plan, several factors must be determined: the degree of dehydration based on physical assessment; the type of dehydration based on the pathophysiology of the specific illness responsible for the dehydrated state; specific physical signs other than general signs; initial plasma sodium concentrations; and associated electrolyte (especially serum potassium) and acid-base imbalances. Initial and regular ongoing evaluations are carried out to assess the patient's progress toward equilibrium and the effectiveness of therapy.

When examining an infant or younger child, one of the most important determinants is the weight, because this can assist in determining the percentage of total body fluid lost. Other important clinical manifestations include changing sensorium (irritability to lethargy), response to stimuli, integumentary changes (decreased elasticity and turgor), capillary refill (prolonged), heart rate (increased), sunken eyes, and in infants, sunken fontanels (Held, 1995). The presence of any two of the following four factors—capillary refill of 2 seconds, absent tears, dry mucous membranes, and ill general appearance—are good predictors of a deficit of at least 5% (Gorelick, Shaw, and Murphy, 1997).

## Therapeutic Management

Medical management is directed at correcting the fluid imbalance and treating the underlying cause. When the child is alert, awake, and not in shock, correction of dehydration may be attempted with oral fluid administration. Most cases of dehydration are mild and can be managed at home by this method. Several commercial rehydration fluids are available for use. (See Table 29-2.) Oral rehydration management consists of rapid replacement of fluid loss over 4 to 6 hours, replacement of continuing losses, and providing for maintenance fluid requirements (Dillon-Dolan, 1997; Holliday, 1996; Meyers, 1995; Jospen and Forbes, 1996). Amounts and rates are determined from body weight and are increased if rehydration is incomplete or if excess losses continue, until the child is well hydrated and the basic problem is under control. (See Diarrhea, Chapter 29, for a complete discussion of fluid replacement therapy for dehydration.)

**Parenteral Fluid Therapy.** Parenteral fluid therapy is initiated whenever the child is unable to ingest sufficient amounts of fluid and electrolytes to (1) meet ongoing daily physiologic losses, (2) replace previous deficits, and (3) replace ongoing abnormal losses. Patients who usually require intravenous (IV) fluids are those with severe dehydration, those with uncontrollable vomiting, those who are unable to drink for any reason (e.g., extreme fatigue, coma), or those with severe gastric distention.

Because dehydration constitutes a great threat to life, the first priority is the restoration of circulation by rapid expansion of the ECF volume to treat shock or prevent its occurrence. IV administration of fluid is begun immediately, even though the exact nature of the dehydration and the serum electrolyte values are not known. The solution selected is based on what is known regarding the probable type and cause of the dehydration. This usually involves an isotonic solution such as 0.9% sodium chloride or lactated Ringer's, both of which are very close to the body's serum osmolality of 285 to 300 and do not contain dextrose (which is contraindicated in the early treatment stages of diabetic ketoacidosis) (Finberg, Kravath, and Hellerstein, 1993).

Parenteral rehydration therapy has three phases. The initial therapy is used to expand ECF volume quickly and to improve circulatory and renal function (Behrman, Kliegman, and Jenson, 2000). During initial therapy, an isotonic electrolyte solution is used at a rate of 20 to 30 ml/kg, given as an IV bolus and repeated a second and sometimes a third time. Subsequent therapy is used to replace deficits, provide maintenance water and electrolyte

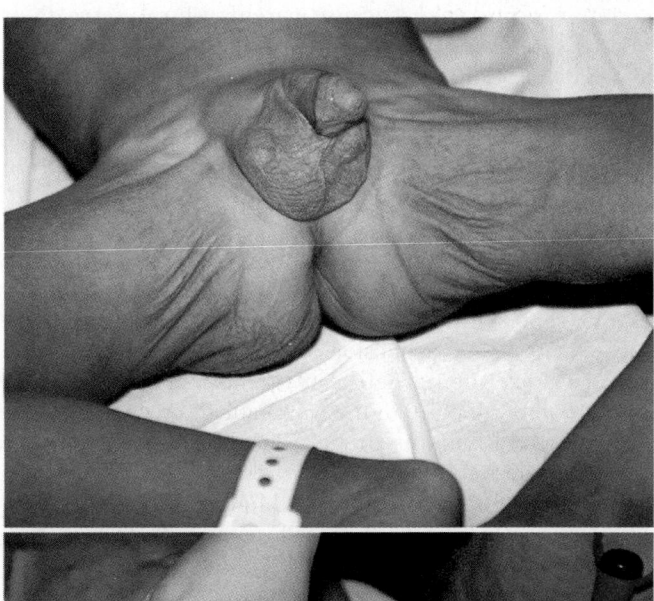
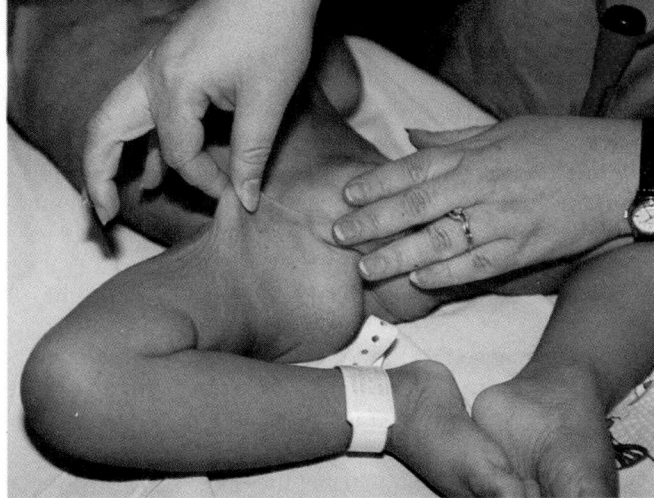

**Fig. 28-2**   Loss of skin elasticity because of dehydration.

requirements, and catch up with ongoing losses. Water and sodium requirements for the deficit, maintenance, and ongoing losses are calculated at 8-hour intervals, taking into consideration the amount of fluids given with the initial boluses and the amount administered during the first 24-hour period. With improved circulation during this phase, water and electrolyte deficits can be evaluated, and acid-base status can be corrected either directly through the administration of fluids or indirectly through improved renal function. Sodium bicarbonate may be added to the solution during this time, because acidosis is often associated with severe dehydration. Potassium is withheld until kidney function is assessed and circulation has improved.

The final phase of therapy allows the patient to return to normal and begin oral feedings, with a gradual correction of total body deficits. The potassium loss in ICF is replaced slowly by way of the ECF. The body fat and protein stores are replaced through diet. If the child is unable to eat or if feeding aggravates the condition (e.g., diarrhea), IV hyperalimentation is provided to prevent malnourishment.

Although the initial phase of fluid replacement is rapid in both isotonic and hypotonic dehydration, it is contraindicated in hypertonic dehydration because of the risk of water intoxication, especially in the brain cells. There is an apparent lag time for sodium to reach a steady state when diffusing in and out of brain cells, whereas water diffuses almost instantaneously. Consequently, rapid administration of fluid will cause equally rapid diffusion of water into the dehydrated brain cells, causing marked cerebral edema. Because ECF volume is maintained relatively well in hypertonic as opposed to the other types of dehydration, shock is not a usual manifestation.

## Water Intoxication

Water intoxication, or water overload, is observed less often than dehydration. However, it is important that nurses and others who care for children are aware that this can occur and are alert to the possibility in certain situations. Patients who ingest excessive amounts of fluid develop a concurrent decrease in serum sodium accompanied by central nervous system (CNS) symptoms. There is a large urinary output and, because water moves into the brain more rapidly than sodium moves out, the child may also exhibit irritability, somnolence, headache, vomiting, diarrhea, or generalized seizures. The affected child usually appears well hydrated but may be edematous or even dehydrated.

Fluid intoxication can occur during acute IV water overloading, too rapid dialysis, tap water enemas, feeding of incorrectly mixed formula, or excess water ingestion, or with too rapid reduction of glucose levels in diabetic ketoacidosis (Fann, 1998; Metheny, 2000). Patients with central nervous system infections occasionally retain excessive amounts of water. Administration of inappropriate hypotonic solutions (e.g., 0.45% sodium chloride) may cause a rapid reduction in sodium and result in symptoms of water overload.

Infants are especially vulnerable to fluid overload. Their thirst mechanism is not well developed; therefore they are unable to "turn off" fluid intake appropriately. A decreased glomerular filtration rate does not allow for repeated excretion of a water load, and ADH levels may not be maximally reduced. Consequently, infants are unable to excrete a water overload effectively.

Administration of inappropriately prepared formula is one of the more common causes of water intoxication (Centers for Disease Control and Prevention, 1994). Families who cannot afford to buy enough formula may dilute the formula to increase the volume or even substitute water for the formula. A family may run out of formula and dilute the remaining amount to make it last until they are able to purchase more. In addition, water is sometimes used for pacification. Water intoxication can also occur in infants who receive overly vigorous hydration during a febrile illness.

A number of clinicians have reported water intoxication in infants following swimming lessons (Fann, 1998; Metheny, 2000). Although they hold their breath, some infants apparently swallow a large amount of water during repeated submersion (Fann, 1998). This is probably not a common occurrence because parents who observe their infants swallowing water tend to keep the infant's head above water (Phillips, 1987). Anticipatory guidance to parents should include a discussion of swimming instruction and advice to stop a lesson if the child is observed to swallow unusual amounts of water or exhibit any symptoms of hyponatremia.

## Edema

Edema represents an abnormal accumulation of fluid and subsequent tissue expansion within the interstitial tissue and develops when a defect in the normal cardiovascular circulation or a failure in the lymphatic drainage to remove the increased amounts occurs. The processes responsible for fluid removal include venous hydrostatic pressure, oncotic pressure of intravascular and interstitial spaces, an intact semipermeable capillary wall, tissue tension, and lymphatic flow.

### Mechanisms of Edema Formation

A defect of any of the homeostatic mechanisms maintaining fluid balance can cause accumulation of interstitial fluid. Disequilibrium results from anything that (1) alters the retention of sodium, such as renal disease or hormonal influences; (2) affects the formation or destruction of plasma proteins, such as starvation or liver disease; or (3) alters membrane permeability, such as nephrotic syndrome or trauma.

Edema may be localized to a small or large area, such as that occurring in urticaria, infection, and pulmonary congestion, or it can be generalized, as in the hypoproteinemia of the nephrotic syndrome and starvation. A severe, generalized accumulation of great amounts of fluid in all body tissues is termed *anasarca*.

**Increased Venous Pressure.** The *colloidal osmotic pressure (COP)* of the plasma proteins draws fluid back into the vascular system as long as this force is greater than the venous hydrostatic pressure. However, when the venous pressure is increased, fluid tends to be retained in the interstitial spaces. This can occur when an individual remains in the same position for a long time, such as swollen ankles and feet after standing or sitting for long periods. Constrictive dressings or restraints applied too tightly to extremities will obstruct venous return, increase venous and capillary pressure, and cause edema. The most graphic pathologic illustrations are pulmonary edema caused by pulmonary circulation overload in cardiac defects with a left-to-right shunt and ascites caused by portal hypertension. Edema from any cause is increased in dependent areas because of this added factor of increased venous hydrostatic pressure and the gravitational effects in these areas.

**Capillary Permeability.** Damage to capillary walls or alteration in their permeability permits exudation of plasma protein into the interstitial space. Most often this occurs as local edema, such as that manifested in inflammatory and hypersensitivity reactions. Capillary damage from burns allows extensive exudation of protein-rich fluid into the interstitial spaces to compound edema formation.

**Diminished Plasma Proteins.** A fall in plasma protein levels hampers the osmotic pull back into the vessels. Consequently, fluid remains in the interstitial spaces. Although other factors play a role, such as hydrostatic pressure of both the arterial vascular system and the tissues and sodium concentration, significantly low protein levels (below 4.5 mg/dl) are associated with edema (Ganong, 1995). Examples of this are the massive albumin losses of the nephrotic syndrome, diminished serum protein from insufficient dietary protein, and (sometimes) hemodilution of plasma proteins from IV fluid administration in chronic dehydration.

**Lymphatic Obstruction.** Obstruction of lymph flow creates edema high in protein content. This occurs infrequently in childhood but can result from trauma to the lymphatic glands or from removal of lymph nodes.

**Tissue Tension.** Tissue hydrostatic pressure is ordinarily of little consequence. However, it plays a significant role in determining distribution of edema fluid in certain pathologic conditions. Loose tissues allow a greater amount of fluid accumulation than tissues that are tightly bound by dense fibrous bands in which tissue pressure rapidly increases to limit further extravasation of fluid. Edema appears earlier and more readily in loose structures such as those in the periorbital and genital tissues. The alveolar structure of lung tissue is probably a contributing factor in pulmonary edema, as well as in increased hydrostatic pressure in the pulmonary vessels.

**Other Factors in Edema Formation.** Any factor that causes sodium retention by the kidneys will produce or augment edema formation. This includes stimulation of the renin-angiotensin-aldosterone mechanisms for sodium reabsorption created by the diminished plasma volume in edema, which resulted from primary causes. The salt-retaining property of steroids is responsible for the edema associated with their administration.

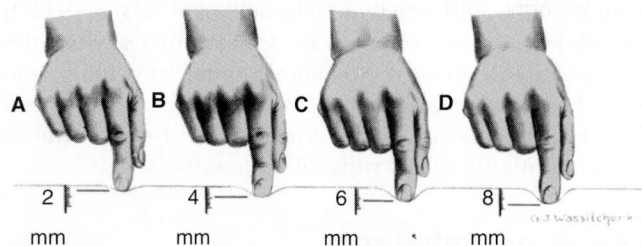

**Fig. 28-3** Assessment of pitting edema. **A,** +1, **B,** +2, **C,** +3, **D,** +4. (From Lowdermilk DL, Perry SE, Bobak IM: *Maternity and women's health care,* ed 6, St Louis, 1997, Mosby.)

Several types of edema exist, all of which can provide a palpable swelling of the interstitial space that is either localized or generalized. These include the following:

**Peripheral edema,** or localized or generalized palpable swelling of the interstitial space

**Ascites,** or the accumulation of fluid in the abdominal cavity (usually associated with renal or liver abnormalities)

**Pulmonary edema,** which occurs when there is an increase in the interstitial volume

**Cerebral edema,** which is a particularly threatening form of edema caused by trauma, infection, or other etiologic factors, including vascular overload or injudicious IV administration of hypotonic solutions

**Overall fluid gain,** especially seen in patients with kidney disease

### Assessment

Generalized edema resulting from any of the above types can occur and is manifested by swelling in the extremities, face, perineum, and torso. Loss of normal skin creases may be assessed. Daily weights are more sensitive indicators of water gain or loss and should be obtained. Abdominal girth measurement changes may also be an indicator of edema in children. Pitting edema may occur and can be assessed by pressing the fingertip against a bony prominence for 5 seconds. If the tissue rebounds immediately on removing the finger, the patient does not have pitting edema. A quick way to determine the severity is to measure the degree of pitting edema, as seen in Fig. 28-3.

### Therapeutic Management

The primary goal in the management of edema is treatment of the underlying disease process, which is discussed in relation to the specific disorder. However, an essential aspect in the management of any fluid overload is early recognition, in which nurses play a vital role.

## DISTURBANCES OF ACID-BASE BALANCE

The ability of the body to regulate the acid-base status is one of the most crucial physiologic functions. Many disease states, such as diarrhea, vomiting, or febrile conditions, are complicated by disturbances in the acid-base balance, which are often more hazardous to the child's survival than the primary disease process. Sometimes simply providing adequate hydration, replacing electrolytes, and correcting acid-base disturbances are all that is needed to sustain an infant or child until the primary disorder has stabilized.

## Acid-Base Imbalance

A disturbance of acid-base equilibrium in the direction of acidosis or alkalosis may come about in a variety of ways. However, very simply stated, *acidosis (acidemia)* results from either accumulation of acid or loss of base, and *alkalosis (alkalemia)* results from either accumulation of base or loss of acid.

### Hydrogen Ion Concentration

The *pH* represents the *concentration of hydrogen ($H^+$)* in solution and indicates only whether the imbalance is more acidic or more alkaline. It does not reflect the nature of the imbalance (i.e., whether it is of metabolic or respiratory origin). Body metabolism affects primarily the *base bicarbonate ($HCO_3^-$)*; therefore alterations in the concentration of $HCO_3^-$ are termed *metabolic* disturbances of acid-base balance. Also, because the amount of carbon dioxide ($CO_2$) exhaled through the lungs affects the *carbonic acid ($H_2CO_3$)*, changes in $H_2CO_3$ concentration are referred to as *respiratory* disturbances. Consequently, the simple disturbances (those with a single primary cause) are categorized as metabolic acidosis or alkalosis and respiratory acidosis or alkalosis (Ferri and Alario, 1997).

It is also significant that the major signs and symptoms of $H^+$ ion imbalances—acidosis and alkalosis—reflect central nervous system involvement. Depression of the CNS, manifested by lethargy, diminished mental capacity, delirium, stupor, and coma, is observed in acidosis of either metabolic or respiratory origin. On the other hand, alkalosis produces clinical manifestations of nervous system stimulation and excitement, including overexcitability, nervousness, tingling sensations, and tetany that may progress to seizures. Persons

with epilepsy are particularly susceptible to seizures, which can be precipitated by hyperventilation.

It is also important to note that eventually all body systems will become dysfunctional if the "normal" limits of pH are violated for very long. The extent and severity of signs and symptoms depend on the length of time the imbalance has existed and the magnitude or degree of the deviation from normal. A rapid, severe imbalance will seriously compromise the compensatory mechanisms to the point where it is incompatible with life, whereas the body will be able to compensate adequately for a mild, gradual distortion and produce few if any observable signs or symptoms.

### Compensatory Mechanisms

Respiratory regulation in acid-base balance involves $CO_2$ regulation; that is, the rate and depth of alveolar ventilation will determine the concentration of $CO_2$ that is eliminated or retained. Renal processes, however, involve the regulation of $HCO_3^-$ via reabsorption, regeneration, and secretion of $H^+$ ions (Noble, 1998). When the fundamental acid-base ratio is altered for any reason, the body attempts to correct the deviation. In a simple disturbance, a single *primary* factor affects one component of the acid-base pair and is usually accompanied by a *compensatory* or *secondary* change in the component that is not primarily affected. For example, increased formation of metabolic acid rapidly reduces the $HCO_3^-$ in the formation of $H_2CO_3$. The respiratory mechanism immediately attempts to compensate for the imbalance by eliminating the $H_2CO_3$ through exhaled $CO_2$ and water. The imbalance is corrected when the kidneys excrete hydrogen and ammonium ions in exchange for reabsorbed sodium bicarbonate.

When the secondary changes (the hyperventilation and renal excretion of $H^+$ in the preceding example) succeed in preventing a distortion of the acid-base ratio and the pH is restored to normal, the disturbance is described as *compensated*. The *uncompensated* state exists when there is no compensatory effect and the pH remains uncorrected. The imbalance is said to be *corrected* when physiologic mechanisms fully correct the primary abnormality.

| TABLE 28-5 | Laboratory tests employed in assessment of acid-base status | | | |
|---|---|---|---|---|
| **Abbreviation** | **Test** | | **Normal Values*** | **Description** |
| pH | Partial pressure of hydrogen | | Birth: 7.11-7.36<br>1 day: 7.29-7.45<br>Child: 7.35-7.45 | Expression of hydrogen ion concentration |
| $P_{CO_2}$ | Partial pressure of carbon dioxide or carbon dioxide tension | | Newborn: 27-40<br>Infant: 27-41<br>Girls: 32-45<br>Boys: 35-48 | Measure of carbon dioxide tension; reflects carbonic acid ($H_2CO_3$) concentration of plasma |
| $HCO_3^-$ (serum) arterial | Carbon dioxide content or carbon dioxide combining power | | Infant: 21-28 mEq/L<br>Thereafter: 22-26 mEq/L | Concentration of base bicarbonate |
| BE | Base excess (whole blood) | | Newborn: −2 to −10<br>Infant: −1 to −7<br>Child: +2 to −4<br>Thereafter: +3 to −3 | Used to express extent of deviation from normal buffer base concentration; indicates quantity of blood buffers remaining after hydrogen ion is buffered |

*Data from Behrman RE, Kliegman RM, Jenson HB, editors: *Nelson textbook of pediatrics*, ed 16, Philadelphia, 2000, WB Saunders.

## Laboratory Measurements

Several laboratory tests are employed to assess the nature and extent of acid-base disturbances. The importance of these data is readily apparent when a clinical observation such as hyperventilation can represent either the primary factor in respiratory alkalosis or a secondary or compensatory factor in metabolic acidosis. The laboratory tests of value in the assessment of acid-base status are outlined in Table 28-5. To determine the acid-base status, three variables—the respiratory component ($PCO_2$), the metabolic component (arterial $HCO_3^-$ or serum $CO_2$), and the serum pH—must be determined. Measurement of any two will allow computation of the third. A summary of relationships between these and other variables is outlined in Table 28-6.

## Associated Disturbances in Acid-Base Balance

Physiologic functions of the body take place optimally when the pH is maintained within a normal range. The disequilibrium created by moderately altered pH can produce disordered function of physiologic and enzyme systems, but great divergences are incompatible with life. In addition, electrolyte shifts that take place in response to changes in pH alter the electrolyte concentration in the fluid compartments to disturb the normal concentrations. For example, cell membrane permeability is affected by changes in pH. A lowered pH allows potassium ($K^+$) to move from the ICF to the ECF. Serum $K^+$ levels increase with acidosis and decrease with alkalosis.

**Serum Potassium.** One of the disturbances that complicates both fluid losses and acid-base imbalance is an alteration of $K^+$ levels. During dehydration, fluid moves out of the ICF compartment into the ECF compartment in an attempt to balance the fluid losses. In doing so, $K^+$ also moves out, creating a total body $K^+$ depletion. Because renal function is drastically reduced in dehydration, normal excretion of $K^+$ does not take place. This causes elevated serum levels that can produce all the signs and symptoms of hyperkalemia. During rapid rehydration therapy for gastrointestinal losses and diabetic ketoacidosis, the ECF $K^+$ moves back into the ICF compartment, thereby posing the risk of hypokalemia unless there is an anticipated replacement (Ganong, 1995). However, $K^+$ is not replaced until the ICF is sufficient to restore adequate renal function.

**Serum Calcium.** Disturbed ECF calcium ($Ca^{++}$) levels may occur in various types of dehydration. Usually the disturbance is in the form of reduced serum $Ca^{++}$ levels, especially where there is a concomitant potassium loss. Although hypocalcemia is a common finding, it rarely reaches a point of tetany in current practice, which includes adequate replacement of potassium losses. Immediate effects of $Ca^{++}$ imbalance associated with acidosis or alkalosis are tetany of metabolic alkalosis; long-term effects of chronic acidosis are related to bone resorption from renal disturbances.

**Oxygen Combination.** The capacity of oxygen ($O_2$) to combine with hemoglobin is also affected by changes in pH. The affinity of hemoglobin for $O_2$ decreases with a decrease in pH so that, in a state of acidosis, less $O_2$ will be picked up by the hemoglobin as blood travels through the lungs (Guyton and Hall, 2000). However, $O_2$ is more easily released to the tissues when the pH is lowered. The opposite effects operate during an increase in pH.

**Blood Flow.** Blood flow in various areas is altered by changes in pH. Pulmonary circulation constricts in acidosis, whereas decreased pH (acidosis) causes vasodilation in systemic vessels.

## Respiratory Acidosis

Respiratory acidosis results from diminished or inadequate pulmonary ventilation that causes an elevation in plasma $PCO_2$ and thus an increased concentration of dissolved $H_2CO_2$, which leads to elevated $H_2CO_3$ and $H^+$ concentration. Conditions that produce respiratory acidosis can originate at three levels in the respiratory system and result in inadequate gas exchange (Box 28-4).

Compensation is mediated through the kidneys, which are stimulated to conserve and thus increase the plasma $HCO_3^-$ concentration and to excrete hydrogen ions. Laboratory findings in respiratory acidosis include elevated plasma $HCO_3^-$ concentration (Lewis and Nocton, 1997).

The treatment of respiratory acidosis is aimed at correcting the primary defect and improving gas exchange at the alveolar level to provide more efficient removal of $CO_2$. $O_2$ therapy is usually indicated, as well as mechanical ventilation if the condition warrants it. Administration of buffers such as sodium bicarbonate to reduce $H^+$ concentration is usually not indicated, because it can result in fluid volume excess by causing an osmolar fluid shift from the blood to the intravascular space, which would only further compromise respiratory function and aggravate the acidosis. Sodium bicarbonate may be indicated with a pH 7.0 if the

---

**TABLE 28-6** Summary of simple acid-base disturbances (partially compensated)

| Disturbance | Plasma pH | Plasma $PCO_2$ | Plasma $HCO_3^-$ |
|---|---|---|---|
| Respiratory acidosis | ↓ | ↑ | ↑ |
| Respiratory alkalosis | ↑ | ↓ | ↓ |
| Metabolic acidosis | ↓ | ↓ | ↓ |
| Metabolic alkalosis | ↑ | ↑ | ↑ |

---

**Box 28-4** ■ ■ ■
**Origins of Inadequate Gas Exchange**

Factors that depress the respiratory center, such as head injury, depressant or narcotizing drugs, and infections of the central nervous system

Factors that affect the lung proper, such as obstructive pulmonary disease, pneumonia, cystic fibrosis, acute pulmonary edema, atelectasis, and occlusion of respiratory passages

Factors that interfere with the bellows action of the chest wall, including trauma to the chest wall, skeletal diseases or deformities, and diseases of the thoracic muscles or their innervation (e.g., muscular dystrophy or muscular atrophy)

cause is bronchial asthma or bronchospasm (Heitz and Horne, 2001).

## Respiratory Alkalosis

Conversely, respiratory alkalosis is caused by a primary increase in the rate and depth of pulmonary ventilation, resulting in unusually large amounts of $CO_2$ being exhaled or "blown off." This reduces the plasma $P_{CO_2}$, and raises the pH (Behrman, Kliegman and Jenson, 2000). Conditions that cause stimulation of the respiratory center to produce hyperventilation are listed in Box 28-5.

A frequent cause of hyperventilation in children is voluntary hyperventilation before underwater swimming. It is also a consideration in the care of persons having assisted ventilation. Incorrectly set mechanical ventilators can cause respiratory rates and tidal volumes in excess of physiologic needs.

Compensation of respiratory alkalosis takes place in the kidneys and consists of excretion of $H_2CO_3$ in association with sodium ($Na^+$) and $K^+$ to conserve $H^+$. Laboratory findings include elevated plasma pH (greater than 7.43), depressed plasma $H_2CO_3$ concentration (less than 23 mEq/L in older children, less than 20 mEq/L in young children), and lowered $P_{CO_2}$ (less than 35 mm Hg).

Treatment of respiratory alkalosis consists of correction of the primary defect and prevention of lost anions and the associated $K^+$ deficit. Rebreathing $CO_2$ slows respirations and provides rapid relief, as does $O_2$ therapy.

## Metabolic Acidosis

Metabolic acidosis is a lowered plasma pH caused by any process that reduces the $HCO_3^-$ concentration. Metabolic acidosis can be produced by the gain of nonvolatile acids or the loss of $HCO_3^-$. Strong acid is gained, and $HCO_3^-$ is lost by several specific mechanisms and routes (Box 28-6).

Compensation of metabolic acidosis is respiratory, with alveolar hyperventilation occurring immediately as the decrease in pH is sensed by the respiratory center. Strong acids are immediately buffered to generate the weaker $H_2CO_3$, which the respiratory system attempts to eliminate through increased alveolar ventilation. In this respiratory effort the breathing is deep and rapid—the *Kussmaul* or *air-hunger* type of respirations. $HCO_3^-$ conservation and excretion by the kidneys is a slower mechanism. Laboratory findings of uncompensated metabolic acidosis include lowered plasma pH (less than 7.33) and diminished plasma $HCO_3^-$ concentration (Behrman, Kliegman, and Jenson, 2000).

Treatment is directed at correcting the basic defect and replacing the excessive losses of $HCO_3^-$ with sodium or potassium bicarbonate or sodium lactate.

---

**Box 28-5** ■ ■ ■
### Conditions That Produce Hyperventilation

Primary central nervous system stimulation resulting from emotions, including hysteria, fear, apprehension, pain, anxiety; central nervous system infection (encephalitis); certain drug reactions, such as early salicylate intoxication (a primary respiratory stimulant); and mechanical ventilation

Reflex central nervous system stimulation from peripheral chemoreceptors as a result of hypoxia, which provides the stimulus for hyperventilation at high altitudes; fever or high environmental temperatures; congestive heart failure; and anemia

Reflex central nervous system stimulation from intrathoracic stretch receptors, which is believed to be the cause of hyperventilation in localized pulmonary disease

Pulmonary disorders: inhalation of irritants, asthma, pneumonia, and pulmonary edema

---

**Box 28-6** ■ ■ ■
### Metabolic Acidosis

Strong acid is gained by:
　Gain of exogenous acid (e.g., ammonium chloride) by ingestion or infusion (e.g., salicylates, methanol, ethylene glycol)
　Incomplete oxidation of fatty acids, which occurs in conditions such as diabetic ketoacidosis, starvation (including patients receiving nothing by mouth for therapeutic purposes)
　Incomplete oxidation of carbohydrate that produces large amounts of lactic acid as a result of primary lactic acidosis (rare) or secondary to tissue hypoxia from excessive exercise, serious trauma, and severe infection
　Inability of the renal system to excrete the normal, ongoing volume of inorganic acid metabolites, which results from the azotemic acidosis of advanced renal failure, renal tubular acidosis, and potassium-sparing diuretics
Base bicarbonate is lost by:
　Losses from the gastrointestinal tract—secretions distal to the pyloric sphincter contain large amounts of bicarbonate, which may be lost during conditions that produce diarrhea or vomiting, fistula drainage, and suction
　Losses as a result of inappropriate bicarbonate excretion in the kidneys because of renal tubular acidosis

---

## Metabolic Alkalosis

Metabolic alkalosis is represented by an elevated plasma pH that occurs when there is a reduction in $H^+$ concentration and an excess of $HCO_3^-$. This can be caused by a gain in base or a loss of acid (Box 28-7).

---

**Box 28-7** ■ ■ ■
### Metabolic Alkalosis

Loss of acid can result from the following:
　In children the most common cause of hydrogen ion depletion is loss of hydrochloric acid (HCL) incident to hypertrophic pyloric stenosis. The infant produces large amounts of HCL, which is vomited with repeated feedings. HCL is also lost in gastric tube drainage.
　Less often, hydrogen ions are lost through the kidneys in diuretic therapy, potassium depletion, or administration of adrenocortical hormones.
A gain in base is usually iatrogenic and relatively uncommon in children but can result from the following:
　Gain of exogeneous bicarbonate from ingestion or infusion
　Oxidation of salts or organic acid from infusion or ingestion of lactate, citrate, or acetate

Compensation in metabolic alkalosis theoretically should be respiratory; however, such compensation is irregular and unpredictable. In addition, renal correction is complicated by losses of $Na^+$, $K^+$, and $Cl^-$, which are lost in pyloric stenosis through vomiting. The kidneys will attempt to conserve the $Na^+$ and $K^+$ concentration at the expense of $H^+$ concentration and acid-base balance. Laboratory findings include elevated urine pH, elevated plasma pH, elevated plasma $HCO_3^-$, and, if in conjunction with chloride deficit, reduced $Cl^-$ concentration (Behrman, Kliegman, and Jenson, 2000).

Treatment of metabolic alkalosis is aimed at preventing further losses of acid and replacing lost electrolytes.

# NURSING RESPONSIBILITIES IN FLUID AND ELECTROLYTE DISTURBANCES

Nursing observation and intervention are essential to the detection and therapeutic management of disturbances in fluid and electrolyte balance. Imbalances may be precipitated in a variety of circumstances, and the balance is so precarious, especially in infants, that changes can take place in a very short time. Therefore an important nursing responsibility is anticipation and perceptive observation for any signs of imbalance, particularly in those situations and conditions in which imbalance is likely to occur. Conditions in which changes can develop with surprising rapidity in young children include diarrhea; vomiting; sweating; fever; disorders such as diabetes, renal disease, and cardiac anomalies; administration of certain drugs such as diuretics and steroids; and trauma, such as major surgery, burns, and other extensive injury.

Nurses must be comfortable with equipment used to deliver fluids to infants and children and be familiar with the knowledge and techniques for assessment. An understanding of normal serum levels provides additional data on which to base assessments and interventions and to validate observations. Data that are helpful in assessment related to fluid and electrolyte balance are the medical diagnosis, the treatment that the child is receiving (especially medications and fluid therapies), laboratory reports, history, and records of intake and output. An important nursing role is teaching parents to recognize early signs of dehydration.

## Assessment

Whether the child is at home, in the practitioner's office or clinic, or in the hospital, nursing assessment is an essential part of the nursing care plan. The assessment of suspected or potential fluid and electrolyte disturbance begins with the observation of general appearance. Ill children usually have drawn, flaccid expressions, and their eyes lack luster. Loss of appetite is one of the first behaviors observed in most childhood illnesses, and the infant's or child's activity level is diminished. The cry of an ill infant is less vigorous, often whining, and higher pitched than usual. The child is irritable, seeks the comfort and attention of the parent, and displays purposeless movements and inappropriate responses to people and familiar things. As the child's illness and level of dehydration become more severe, the irritability progresses to lethargy and even unconsciousness.

### History

Much of the information regarding the child's behavior can be elicited from the parent. In addition to initial observations, a good history is extremely valuable to the assessment. The amount and type of intake and output (especially abnormal output) are important. An accurate estimate of fluid losses is beyond the capacity of history givers, but rough estimates of excessive fluid losses or diminished output can usually be obtained from information such as the number and consistency of stools the child has passed in the past 24 hours, the number of times the child voided, and the type and amount of food and fluid ingested or vomited. If the child is an infant, ask about the number of wet diapers in the past 24 hours. Parents frequently omit this information from their discussion with the health professional. They tell how much has been taken but not how much was excreted unless asked specifically for this information.

Both the type and the amount of intake provide valuable information. The quality and quantity can be determined—is intake sustained, excessive, or curtailed? Loss early in diarrheal illness progresses rapidly, and the water losses can exceed sodium losses, leading to hypernatremia. Hypernatremic dehydration indicates a significant interference with water intake. Also important is a history of normal or increased intake of an unusual fluid, such as one containing sugar, tea, athletic hydration fluid (e.g., Gatorade), or other solute-containing fluids, which can contribute to hyponatremic dehydration in the face of abnormal losses (Meyers, 1995).

A history of gradual weight gain and observations of any puffiness, especially in areas with less dense tissues (periorbital, scrotal), or "clothes fitting tighter" offer early clues to edema. A history of excessive intake, especially when associated with diminished output, is important in assessing edema and water intoxication.

### Clinical Observations

Tachycardia, the earliest manifestation of dehydration, can also be produced by fever and infection; therefore these are considered in the assessment of dehydration. Dry skin and mucous membranes usually appear early. A sunken fontanel is a useful observation if the configuration of the fontanel is known when the infant is healthy. Signs of circulatory failure usually indicate severe dehydration, since compensatory mechanisms are able to sustain blood pressure in the low normal range for some time. Loss of skin elasticity, generally manifested in children less than 2 years of age, is measured by the time it takes for pinched abdominal skin to recoil. This sign is also observed in undernourished children. Also, in hypertonic dehydration the skin has a smooth, velvety feel before it develops disturbed elasticity.

Capillary filling time is assessed by pinching the abdominal skin, a toe, or a thumb and estimating the time it takes for the blood to return. Capillary filling time in mild dehydration is less than 2 seconds, increasing to more than 3 seconds in severe dehydration. The technique is effective in children of all ages. However, it can be altered in the presence of heart failure, which affects circulation time, and hypertonic dehydration, in which fluid loss is primarily intracellular.

The observations outlined in Table 28-7 are also used to arrive at a meaningful assessment. When caring for the ill child, vital signs are assessed as often as every 15 to 30 minutes, and weight is recorded frequently during the initial phase of therapy. It is important to use the same scale each time the child is weighed and to predetermine the weight of any equipment or devices that must remain attached during the weighing process, including arm boards and sandbags, as well as any clothing the child might be wearing. Routine weights should be taken at the same time each day.

### Intake and Output (I & O) Measurement

One of the most important roles of the nurse in fluid and electrolyte disturbance is related to I & O. Accurate measurements are essential to the assessment of fluid balance. Measurements from all sources—including both gastrointestinal and parenteral I & O from urine, stools, vomitus, fistulas, nasogastric suction, sweat, and drainage from wounds—must be taken and considered. Although the practitioner usually indicates when I & O are to be recorded, it is a nursing responsibility to keep an accurate I & O record on certain children, including those:

- Receiving IV therapy
- After major surgery
- With severe thermal burns or injuries
- With renal disease or damage
- With congestive heart failure
- With dehydration
- With diabetes mellitus
- With oliguria
- Receiving diuretic therapy
- Receiving corticosteroid therapy
- In respiratory distress

Infants or small children who are unable to use a bedpan or those who have bowel movements with every voiding will require the application of a collecting device. (See Urine Specimens, Chapter 27.) Collecting bags may not be suitable for all infants (e.g., preterm and other infants whose fragile skin does not tolerate some types of self-adhesive appliances). If collecting bags are not used, wet diapers or pads are carefully weighed to ascertain the amount of fluid lost. This includes liquid stool, vomitus, and other losses. The volume of fluid in milliliters is approximately equivalent to the weight of the fluid measured in grams. The specific gravity as a measure of osmolality is determined with a refractometer or urine dipsticks and assists in assessing the degree of hydration.

**NURSING TIP**    1 g wet diaper weight = 1 ml urine.

Disadvantages of the weighed diaper method of fluid measurement include (1) inability to differentiate one type of loss from another because of admixture; (2) loss of urine or liquid stool from leakage or evaporation, especially if the infant is under a radiant warmer; and (3) additional fluid in the diaper (superabsorbent disposable type) from absorption of atmospheric moisture (high-humidity incubators) (Metheny, 2000). Evaporative losses render measurements inaccurate unless the diaper is weighed and measured for specific gravity at least every 30 minutes when critical values are needed. Evaporative losses are greater in infants under radiant warmers or being treated with phototherapy. However, research indicates that accurate specific gravity measurements can be made for up to 2 hours on urine obtained from a diaper that has been removed from an infant, folded, and stored in a utility room (Kee and Paulanka, 2000; Metheny, 2000).

It is important to measure and record all intake, oral and parenteral, and output from all sources, including urine, stool, emesis, drainage tubes, fistulas, and wounds from which appreciable amounts of fluid are lost.

At home, parents are advised to observe the number of times and how much the child voids. Infants younger than 1 year of age normally void every 1 to 2 hours; toddlers urinate approximately every 3 hours. As children get older, they void less frequently. The parents are instructed to notify the nurse or clinician if the child appears to be voiding an insufficient amount or persistently losing fluid through vomiting or diarrhea.

## Oral Fluid Intake

Under ordinary circumstances an adequate oral intake is no problem in children who are able to respond to thirst cues. Hydration becomes a nursing problem when infants or children are unable to respond to the thirst mechanism and when fatigue or discomfort makes them reluctant to swallow. Children with elevated temperatures, those with continued gastrointestinal losses, those with labile diabetes, and those with cystic fibrosis are especially prone to dehydration. Occasionally dehydration caused by inadequate intake has been observed in breast-fed infants.

*Oral rehydration therapy* is recommended for mild to moderate dehydration. An *oral rehydration solution (ORS)* containing 75 to 90 mMol sodium and 111 to 139 mMol glucose (e.g., World Health Organization solution, Pedialyte RS, Rehydralyte) is most commonly recommended for the first 4 to 6 hours. If this is tolerated, then oral fluids containing 30 to 60 mMol sodium and 111 to 139 mMol glucose (e.g., Pedialyte, Lytren, Resol, Infalyte) can be given for the next 18 to 24 hours at a dose of 1 to 2 ounces per pound divided into frequent feedings consisting of 3 to 4 ounces for young children. Older children can be given 1 to 2 ounces every hour (Dillon-Dolan, 1997).

The American Academy of Pediatrics no longer advises withholding food and fluids for 24 hours after the onset of diarrhea, or administration of the BRAT diet (bananas, rice, applesauce, and toast) (Behrman, Kliegman, and Jenson, 2000; Dillon-Dolan, 1997).

Persuading a reluctant child to drink fluids can be a nursing challenge and is not uncommon in the care of infants and children. Older children will often respond to the challenge of meeting a specific goal for fluid intake (or de-

**TABLE 28-7**   Significance of clinical observations related to fluid and electrolyte effects

| Observation | Significant Variation | Possible Imbalance | Comments |
|---|---|---|---|
| **Temperature** | Elevated | Early water depletion<br>Sodium excess<br>Fluid volume deficit | Elevated temperature will increase rate of water loss<br>Caused by reduced energy output<br>Shock is outcome of severe fluid deficit |
| **Pulse** | Lowered<br>Rapid, weak, thready, easily obliterated<br><br>Bounding, easily obliterated<br><br>Bounding, not easily obliterated<br><br>Weak, irregular, rapid<br>Weak, irregular, slowing<br>Increased<br><br>Decreased | Circulatory collapse may result from fluid deficit, hemorrhage, plasma-to-interstitial fluid shift<br>Impending circulatory collapse<br>Sodium deficit<br>Fluid volume excess<br>Interstitial fluid-to-plasma shift<br>Severe potassium deficit<br>Severe potassium excess<br>Sodium excess<br>Magnesium deficit<br>Magnesium excess | Pulse rate should include assessment of volume and quality, as well as rate<br>Compare central with peripheral pulses<br>Pulse may be influenced by activity or emotions |
| **Respiration** | Slow, shallow<br>Rapid, deep<br>Dyspnea<br><br>Moist crackles<br><br>Shallow<br>Stridor | Respiratory alkalosis<br>Metabolic acidosis<br>Fluid volume excess either general or pulmonary<br>Fluid volume excess<br>Pulmonary edema<br>Potassium excess or deficit<br>Severe calcium deficit | Rapid respirations increase water loss<br>Not a reliable sign of respiratory alkalosis in infants |
| **Blood pressure** | Increased<br>Decreased | Fluid volume excess<br>Sodium deficit<br>Diminished vascular volume (loss of plasma-to-interstitial fluid shift)<br>Severe potassium excess or deficit | Blood pressure not a reliable sign in young children<br>Elasticity of blood vessels may keep blood pressure stable |
| **Skin** | | | |
| Color | Pallor<br><br><br>Flushed | Protein deficit<br>Fluid deficit<br>Fluid compartment shifts<br>Sodium excess | Environmental influences such as a cool room, uncovered infant, and fever may change skin color |
| Temperature | Cold, mottled extremities | Severe fluid volume deficit, even with fever<br>Severe sodium depletion | Caused by decreased peripheral blood flow |
| Feel | Dry<br><br>Clammy, cold | Fluid depletion<br>Sodium excess<br>Sodium deficit<br>Plasma-to-interstitial fluid shift<br>Hypotonic dehydration | |
| | Poor capillary filling | Fluid volume deficit | |
| Elasticity | Poor to very poor | Fluid depletion | Pinch of skin from abdomen or inner thigh is lifted and remains raised for several seconds |
| Pitting edema | Slight to severe | Fluid volume excess<br>Plasma-to-interstitial fluid shift | Obese infants may appear normal; loss of foot creases may occur |
| **Mucous membranes** | Dry<br>Longitudinal wrinkles on tongue<br>Sticky; rough, red, dry tongue | Fluid volume depletion<br><br><br>Sodium excess<br>Hypertonic dehydration | Elevated temperature and dehydration will cause dryness of mucous membranes |
| **Salivation and tearing** | Absent | Fluid volume deficit | |
| **Fontanels** | Sunken<br>Bulging | Fluid volume deficit<br>Fluid volume excess | Occurs with increased intracranial pressure |
| **Eyeballs** | Sunken<br>Soft | Fluid volume deficit | |

*Continued*

**TABLE 28-7**   Significance of clinical observations related to fluid and electrolyte effects—cont'd

| Observation | Significant Variation | Possible Imbalance | Comments |
|---|---|---|---|
| **Sensory alterations** | Tingling in fingers and toes | Calcium deficit<br>Alkalosis | Sensory alterations unreliable in infants and young children who are unable to communicate symptoms |
| | Abdominal cramps | Sodium deficit<br>Potassium excess | |
| | Muscle cramps | Calcium deficit<br>Potassium deficit | |
| | Light-headedness | Respiratory alkalosis | |
| | Nausea | Calcium excess<br>Potassium excess<br>Potassium deficit | |
| | Thirst | Fluid deficit<br>Sodium excess<br>Calcium excess | May be difficult to assess in infants<br>May be masked by nausea<br>Any condition that reduces intravascular volume will stimulate thirst receptors |
| **Neurologic signs** | Hypotonia | Potassium deficit<br>Calcium excess | |
| | Flaccid paralysis | Severe potassium deficit<br>Severe potassium excess | |
| | Weakness<br>Hypertonia | Metabolic acidosis | |
| |   Positive Chvostek sign | Calcium deficit | Children may develop calcium deficit easily, because growing bones do not readily relinquish calcium to circulation |
| |   Tremors, cramps, tetany | Alkalosis with diminished calcium ionization<br>Calcium deficit | |
| |   Twitching | Magnesium deficit | |
| **Behavior** | Lethargy | Fluid volume deficit overload | Behavioral changes are among first indications of dehydration as reported by parents |
| | Irritability | Fluid volume deficit | |
| | Comatose condition | Hypotonic fluid deficit<br>Profound acidosis of alkalosis | |
| | Lethargy with hyperirritability on stimulation | Hypertonic fluid deficit | |
| | Extreme restlessness | Potassium excess | |

privation) and can be active participants in planning an intake schedule. Contracts and rewards are effective strategies. However, young children require more creative tactics. Suggestions for encouraging children to drink fluids are discussed in Chapter 27. (See Chapter 27 for a discussion of nasogastric alimentation.)

## The Child Who Is NPO

Infants or children who are unable or not permitted to take fluids by mouth (NPO) have special needs. To ensure that they do not receive fluids, a sign can be placed in some obvious place, such as over their beds or pinned to their shirts, to alert others to the NPO status. Fluids are removed from the bedside to reduce the temptation. Drinking fountains and wash basins are monitored.

Oral hygiene, a part of routine hygienic care, is especially important when fluids are restricted or withheld. (See Chapter 27.) For young children who cannot brush their teeth or rinse their mouth without swallowing fluid, the mouth and teeth can be cleaned and kept moist by swabbing with a saline-moistened gauze. Judicious administration of ice chips provides moist, cool relief (if permitted by

the practitioner). A thin layer of petrolatum (Vaseline) or other commercial lip aid helps to keep lips soft and prevents cracking and caking. To meet the need to suck, infants should be provided a safe commercial pacifier.

**NURSING TIP**   Water sprayed into the mouth from an atomizer is refreshing and relieves a dry mouth.

The child on restricted fluids provides an equal challenge. Having fluids limited is often more difficult for the child than being NPO, especially when IV fluids are also eliminated. To make certain the child does not drink the entire amount allowed early in the day, the daily allotment is calculated to provide fluids at periodic intervals throughout the child's waking hours. Serving the fluids in small containers gives the illusion of larger servings. No extra liquid is left at the bedside if compliance is a problem.

## Parenteral Fluid Therapy

### Intravenous Infusion

Before an IV infusion is started, several preparatory activities must take place. All needed equipment is gathered so

**TABLE 28-7**   Significance of clinical observations related to fluid and electrolyte effects—cont'd

| Observation | Significant Variation | Possible Imbalance | Comments |
|---|---|---|---|
| **Weight** | Loss | Fluid deficit | See Table 28-2 |
| | Up to 5% (50 ml/kg) | Mild | |
| | 5% to 9% (75 ml/kg) | Moderate | |
| | 10% or higher (100 ml/kg) | Severe | |
| | | Protein or calorie deficiency | |
| | Gain | Edema—general or pulmonary | Check for hepatomegaly; children sequester |
| | | Ascites | excess fluid in liver |
| **Urine** | Increased (polyuria) | Interstitial fluid-to-plasma shift | Normal range: |
| | | Increased renal solute load | Infant: 2-3 ml/kg/hr |
| | Diminished | Mild fluid deficit | Toddler/preschooler: 2 ml/kg/hr |
| | | Moderate to severe fluid deficit | School-age child: 1-2 ml/kg/hr |
| | Oliguria | Moderate to severe fluid deficit | Adolescent: 0.5-1 ml/kg/hr (varies with |
| | | Plasma-to-interstitial fluid shift | intake and other factors) |
| | | Sodium deficit | |
| | | Potassium excess | |
| | | Severe sodium excess | |
| | | Renal insufficiency | |
| | Specific gravity | Adequate hydration | Used to monitor hydration status in infants |
| | Low (≤1.010) | Fluid excess | Fixed low reading occurs in renal disease |
| | | Renal disease | |
| | | Sodium deficit | |
| | High (≥1.030) | Fluid deficit | |
| | | Sodium excess | |
| | | Glycosuria | |
| | | Proteinuria | |
| | pH | | |
| | Acid | Acidosis—metabolic or respiratory | |
| | | Alkalosis accompanied by severe potassium deficit | |
| | | Fluid deficit | |
| | Alkaline | Alkalosis, metabolic or respiratory | |
| | | Hyperaldosteronism | |
| | | Acidosis accompanied by chronic renal infection and renal tubular dysfunction | |
| | | Diuretic therapy with carbonic anhydrase inhibitors | |

that the operator can proceed without interruption. More important, the child and the family must be prepared for this stressful procedure.

**Solution.** The composition of the IV solution is based on patient history and the diagnosis, or the type of fluid volume deficit being treated and is selected on the basis of tonicity (osmolarity) and electrolyte content. A solution that is *isotonic* has the same osmolality, or tonicity, as body fluids such as plasma. A *hypertonic* solution is one that has a greater concentration of solutes than plasma; a *hypotonic* solution has a lower concentration. Examples of isotonic solutions are 0.9% normal saline solutions, lactated Ringer's, and 5% dextrose in water; 10% glucose in water is a hypertonic solution; plain water and 0.2% sodium are hypotonic solutions. Although it is larger, one molecule of glucose has only half the osmolality of one molecule of sodium chloride (NaCl) because the NaCl ionizes in solution into two particles, the $Na^+$ and the $Cl^-$ ions. Thus one molecule of NaCl exerts twice the osmotic pressure of one molecule of glucose.

Most common pediatric maintenance solutions include a combination of dextrose (usually 5% or 10%) and NaCl (usually 0.22% to 0.3%). The hypotonic solution is necessary for children, because their daily turnover of "free" water exceeds that of adults. Because infants and young children are subject to rapid fluid shifts, any IV solution given to them contains at least 0.2% NaCl to prevent brain edema, a disorder to which they are susceptible if given plain water. Glucose is rapidly metabolized; therefore the osmolality of 5% glucose is further diminished.

To prevent the risk of infusing too much of the IV solution, the volume of the solution container should be based on the age and size of the child and the child's 24-hour volume needs. Bags containing 500 ml are commonly used as opposed to the 1000-ml bags used in adults (Frey, 2001).

For most IV infusions in children, an over-the-needle 24- to 22-gauge catheter may be used if therapy is expected to last less than 5 days. The smallest-gauge and shortest-length catheter that will accommodate the prescribed therapy should be chosen when evaluating the placement of a peripheral IV line. The length of the catheter may be directly related to infection or embolus formation—the shorter the catheter, the fewer the complications (Maki, 1994). The guage of the catheter should maintain adequate flow of the infusate into the cannulated vein while allowing adequate blood flow around the catheter walls to promote proper hemodilution of the infusate. Because stainless steel needles tend to dislodge and infiltrate more frequently than catheters, the use of these should be limited to short-term or single-dose administration (Infusion Nurses Society, 2000a, 2000b).

The goal of IV therapy is to deliver the prescribed fluids or medications without complications. Determining the best catheter for the patient early in the therapy provides the best chance of avoiding catheter-related complications (Moureau, 1999). As the length of therapy increases, decisions regarding the type of infusion device (short peripheral, midline, peripherally inserted central catheter, or central venous catheter) should be explored. Guidelines such as flow charts or algorithms are available to help in these decisions (Catudal, 1999).

**NURSING TIP**    The introduction of chlorhexidine as an antiseptic to be used for cleaning the site before initiating a peripheral IV is under way in the United States, and its use is listed in *Policies and Procedures for Infusion Nursing* (Infusion Nurses Society, 2000a, 2000b). Several clinical trials have demonstrated enhanced skin antisepsis when using chlorhexidine-containing products (Crosby and Mares, 2001). Chlorhexidine has been used in Europe for 30 years and in Canada since 1995. A published study in 1991 demonstrated that aqueous chlorhexidine was superior to povidine-iodine and alcohol-based products for preventing catheter-related bacteremia (Maki, Ringer, and Alvarado, 1991). Recent U.S. Food and Drug Administration (FDA) approval, *for patients above the age of 2 months*, has led to the introduction of one such product, Chloraprep.* It is a sterile applicator composed of 2% chlorhexidine gluconate and 70% isopropyl alcohol.

Other equipment needed includes gloves (if latex, check for patient latex sensitivity), chlorhexidine (Crosby and Mares, 2001), alcohol, and povidone-iodine swabs to clean the site, buffered lidocaine or EMLA to anesthetize the area, a tourniquet (again, check for patient latex sensitivity), rolled towels or small blankets for maintaining position of head or extremity, tape (or dressing and bacteriostatic ointment if hospital dictates), sterile transparent occlusive dressing, a T or J connector (an extension tube that decreases tension and movement of the catheter hub at the site, provides a port for piggyback medications, and makes changing the dressing and tubing easier) (Wilson, 2000), blood collection tubes and syringes for collecting blood (blood samples should be collected at the time of IV insertion whenever possible to avoid an additional needle stick), prefilled normal saline syringes to test patency of IV site before attaching the IV fluids, and an IV shield to protect the IV site after insertion. The prescribed solution is flushed or primed through the T or J connector (if blood samples will not be collected), tubing, filter, and infusion pump in advance, ready to connect to the catheter hub after insertion of the IV catheter. A sharps container should be within

reach if the IV cathether needle does not retract into a safety shield after the catheter is in place.

**NURSING TIP**    Applying the tourniquet over a piece of clothing or wrapping the area with a washcloth before applying the tourniquet will reduce the pain caused by pressure or pinching of the tourniquet.

**Safety Catheters and Needleless Systems.**    One of the main causes for change in IV therapy is the concern of needle-stick injuries. To provide safer care for the patient and health care worker, manufacturers have developed safety catheters and needleless IV systems (National Association of Vascular Access Networks, 2000).

Over-the-needle IV catheters with hollow-bore needles carry a high risk for transmission of blood-borne pathogens from needle-stick injuries. Safety catheters such as Insyte Autoguard* and Protectiv† prevent accidental needle sticks with the use of over-the-needle IV catheters (Hadaway, 1998). The ***Insyte Autoguard*** has a white activation button, located just beyond the catheter hub, which retracts the needle into a safety barrel. The button is depressed after the catheter has been threaded into the vein and the tourniquet has been removed. The ***Protectiv*** has a primary push-off tab, located on the needle guard, that allows one-finger catheter threading once the vein has been accessed. As the catheter is threaded, the needle guard begins to cover the needle, and when the catheter is completely threaded, a simple retraction of the needle housing completely locks the needle into the needle guard, confirming this with a click. Another improvement of these over-the-needle safety catheters is a sharper needle, which increases the ease of penetrating the skin when inserting the IV. Both manufacturers caution to never reinsert the needle into the catheter, as this could shear the catheter and cause a catheter fragment embolus. Safety catheters are discarded in "sharps" containers according to manufacturers' directions.

Needleless IV systems, which are designed to prevent needle-stick injuries during administration of IV push medications and IV piggyback medications, may vary from manufacturer to manufacturer, but the concept is essentially the same. Some needleless systems are universal, whereas others require complete use of the entire IV delivery system for compatibility. Needleless IV systems rely on prepierced septa that are accessed by blunted plastic cannulas or systems that use valves that open and close a fluid path when activated by insertion of a syringe.

Blunt plastic cannulas and preslit injection port sites found in Interlink IV access systems‡ (Fig. 28-4) eliminate the need for steel needles and conventional injection port sites

---

*Available from Medi-Flex Hospital Products, Inc, 8717 W 110 St, Suite 750, Overland Park, KS 66210-2129, (800) 523-0502; www.medi-flex.com; www.chloraprep.com.

*Available from Becton Dickinson & Co, 1 Becton Dr, Franklin Lakes, NJ 07417, (888) 237-2762; www.bd.com. In Canada: Becton Dickinson Canada, Inc, 2771 Bristol Circle, Oakville, ON, L6H 6R5, (905) 822-4820.
†Available from Johnson & Johnson Medical, 2500 E Arbrook Blvd, Arlington, TX 76014, (800) 433-5170; www.jnjmedical.com. In Canada: Johnson & Johnson Medical Products Inc, 200 Whitehall Dr, Markham, ON, L3R 0T5.
‡Available from Baxter Healthcare Corporation, IV Systems Division, Route 120 and Wilson Rd, Round Lake, IL 60073; www.bacter.com; or Becton Dickinson & Co, 1 Becton Dr, Franklin Lakes, NJ 07417, (888) 237-2762; www.bd.com. In Canada: Becton Dickinson Canada, 2771 Bristol Circle, Oakville, ON, L6H 6R5, (905) 822-4820.

but remain accessible via hypodermic needles, a drawback except in emergent situations. Systems that do not permit needled access enhance safety by preventing health care workers from attempting to use needles; however, such systems are limited by the lack of needled access, especially in emergency situations (Orenstein, 1999). A syringe with a blue spike is avavailable to access a single-dose vial (Fig. 28-4, *A*). The preslit injection port sites are identified by a white ring surrounding the port; this ring alerts users that the system is needleless (Fig. 28-4, *B*). Syringes are available with the blunt plastic cannula for accessing these sites (Fig. 28-4, *C*). A lever lock (Fig. 28-4, *D*) or threaded lock cannula (Fig. 28-4, *E*) attaches to an IV line, IV Y site, or peripheral intermittent infusion device. A preslit universal vial adapter (not pictured) provides access to standard multiple-dose vials, and syringe cannulas are then used to access the adapter.

**Infusion Pumps.**  There are several modifications in equipment used for IV infusion for children. A gravity drainage apparatus used for children is much the same as that for adults except that it is designed to deliver a reduced drop size (60 drops/ml) and contains a calibrated volume control chamber (e.g., a Buretrol or Solu-set) that regulates the amount of fluid that can be infused. A microdropper greatly facilitates calculation of flow rate because a prescribed number of milliliters per hour equals the number of drops per minute. For example, if the solution is to infuse at a rate of 30 ml per hour, the infusion is regulated to deliver 30 drops per minute.

A variety of infusion pumps are available. The IV solution is refillable from the bag, bottle, or Solu-set above or contained in a syringe pump to minimize the possibility of overloading the circulation. Infusion pumps are almost always used in pediatrics because they can accurately infuse fluids (especially the syringe pumps, which infuse very small amounts of fluids) as well as accurately provide the prescribed amount of IV solution. It is an important nursing responsibility to understand and follow manufacturer's directions for use, calculate the amount to be infused in a given length of time, set the infusion rate, and monitor the apparatus frequently (at least every 1 to 2 hours) to make certain that the desired rate is maintained, the integrity of the system remains intact, the site remains intact (free of redness, edema, infiltration, or irritation), and the infusion does not stop.

Continuous infusion pumps, although convenient and efficient, are not without risks. Overreliance on the accuracy of the machine can cause either too much or too little fluid to be infused; therefore its use does not eliminate careful periodic assessment by the nurse. Excess pressure can build up if the machine is set at a rate faster than the vein is able to accommodate (or continues to pump when the needle is out of the lumen). This is especially true in very small infants. No matter what device is used, a thorough understanding of the apparatus is essential for safe fluid administration.

### Intraosseous Infusion

Situations may occur in which rapid establishment of a systemic access is vital and venous access may be hampered by peripheral circulatory collapse, hypovolemic shock (sec-

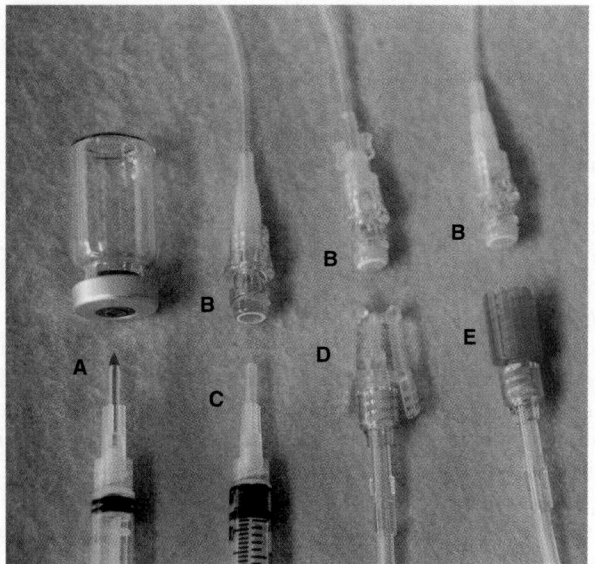

**Fig. 28-4**   Interlink IV access systems: **A,** Blue spike syringe. **B,** Preslit injection port (needleless). **C,** Blunt plastic cannula syringe. **D,** Lever lock cannula. **E,** Threaded lock cannula.

ondary to vomiting or diarrhea, burns, or trauma), cardiopulmonary arrest, or other conditions (Dubick and Holcomb, 2000). Intraosseous infusion provides a rapid, safe, and lifesaving alternate route for administration of fluids and medications until intravascular access can be attained, especially in children 6 years old and younger. Intraosseous cannulation can be secured within 30 to 60 seconds by health care providers, including physicians, nurses, and paramedics. Some hospitals suggest Pediatric Advanced Life Support (PALS) training before performing this procedure. This procedure is usually reserved for children who are unconscious or for those receiving analgesia because the procedure is painful. Local anesthesia should be used for a semiconscious patient.

A large-bore needle such as a bone marrow aspiration needle (e.g., Jamshidi) or an intraosseous needle (e.g., Cook) is inserted into the medullary cavity of a long bone. The anteromedial aspect of the tibia—1 to 3 cm below the tibial tuberosity—is the preferred site for children of all ages because it is flat and has a large marrow cavity. In newborns the distal one third of the femur may be used. The distal tibia is an alternative site.

The extremity is observed closely for swelling or oozing of fluid at the insertion site. Particular attention must be given to the dependent tissue of the leg. Extravasation of fluid from the bone marrow may be hidden under the leg. Check for swelling of the entire lower leg when the intraosseous bone marrow needle is in the tibia or ankle, and check the entire upper leg when the intraosseous needle is in the femur. Compartment syndrome has resulted from an infiltrated intraosseous line. Other complications, although rare, include fractures, skin necrosis, and osteomyelitis.

Once the bone marrow needle is in place, the needle should stand alone and feel very secure. Tape and gauze should be used to secure the needle to the leg. Gauze should be built up around the needle leaving the skin. Drugs may be pushed and fluids delivered via an infusion pump. The intraosseous line may be discontinued after intravenous access has been achieved.

### Preparing the Child and Parents

Children of any age are anxious and fearful of injections, and unless the IV infusion is implemented as an emergency procedure, there will be time to prepare them. (See Preparation for Diagnostic and Therapeutic Procedures, Chapter 27). Many children have never undergone the procedure, and those who have will remember the experience. It is useful to ask them what they think about the procedure and why it is needed for them specifically. Children's perceptions of the anticipated experience furnish information on misconceptions that need to be clarified and help the nurse prepare children for what they can expect. In addition, children's observations provide some insight into how to cope with a child's reactions during the insertion procedure and throughout the course of the IV therapy. For children who have repeated venipunctures, it is helpful to ask them or their parents which vein has been successfully accessed in the past.

Play, always an excellent stress reduction technique, can be employed during the preparation process. Allowing children to handle the equipment and to "start" an IV infusion on a toy animal or doll helps familiarize them with the frightening aspects of the procedure. In some instances it may be helpful to introduce a child to another child who is coping well in the same situation.

It is best to arrange for a quiet, private setting for the child during the insertion. Avoid "safe places," such as the playroom or the child's hospital room when possible. The assurance of privacy relieves the child of some anxieties concerning loss of control in front of others. It also avoids subjecting other children to the potentially stress-provoking scene. The child should be provided with some distracting activity, such as those described for injections, and perhaps be allowed to "help" by holding supplies such as a gauze square, helping to clean the site with alcohol, and assisting in taping the site after the procedure.

Children will usually cooperate better and feel more in command if they are allowed to sit up during the process, although this may not be possible even in some older, normally cooperative children. Toddlers and young children can be held on a parent's lap, with the child's leg tucked between the parent's leg, and the child's arm (not being used for the venipuncture) behind the parent. A hug should both restrain the child and provide comfort. The torso of the patient is held against the parent with the same hug. It is a mistake to assume that children will not lose control even after they promise to cooperate. It is wise to have ample assistance available in the event that a child cannot control anxiety. The child need not be restrained until necessary, but the assistant should be prepared to grasp a child gently but firmly during the insertion. Explaining to children what is being done during each step of the procedure and how they can participate helps to obtain their cooperation and reduce their stress. Every effort is made to reduce the pain of the needle insertion. (See Atraumatic Care box.)

Parents are told about the procedure, including the reasons for the procedure, how long the catheter must remain in place, and what they can expect during and after the insertion. They should be offered the option of remaining with their child or leaving. (See Evidence-Based Practice box on p. 1107.) Parents who remain should be encouraged to kiss, hug, and distract the child during the procedure.

### The Procedure

The site selected for peripheral IV infusion depends on accessibility and convenience (Box 28-8). Although it is possible to use any accessible vein in older children, attention must be directed toward the child's developmental, cognitive, and mobility needs when selecting a site. Whenever possible, it is best to avoid the child's favored hand in order to reduce the disability related to the procedure. Foot veins should be avoided in children learning to walk and in children already walking. A site is chosen that restricts the child's movements as little as possible—a site over a joint in an extremity is avoided, such as the antecubital fossa. An older child can help to select the site and thereby maintain some measure of control.

For veins in the extremities, it is best to start with the most distal sites. If the vein is damaged, using distal sites initially preserves access to the vein in proximal sites (Fig. 28-5). A

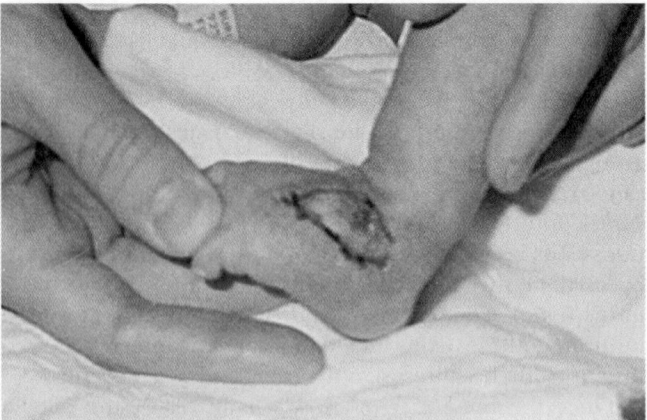

**Fig. 28-5** IV infiltration in an infant's foot.

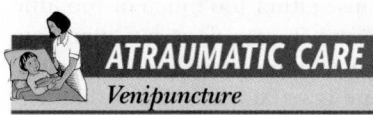

### ATRAUMATIC CARE
#### Venipuncture

To minimize or prevent the pain of the needle puncture for an IV (or blood sample or implanted port access), apply EMLA to the site 60 minutes before the procedure. Cover at least two sites in case the first attempt is not successful. Although some practitioners believe that EMLA causes vasoconstriction and vasospasm, there are no well-controlled studies to support this concern.

Another option for pain management is the use of intradermal buffered lidocaine or Numby Stuff. (See Pain Management, Chapter 26.)

scalp vein or a superficial vein of the wrist may also be used if larger veins are not accessible (Fig. 28-6). Arteries are avoided for peripheral IV therapy.

---

**NURSING ALERT**

- Never reinsert a stylet back into the catheter. This can damage the catheter and cause catheter fragment embolus.
- If unsuccessful, always obtain a new catheter for the second attempt.
- Some parents count the number of times the catheter is moved in, out, and around the area of insertion while trying to locate the vein (probing) as sticks their child receives as opposed to counting the number of IV insertion attempts. Limit the amount of probing because it is painful.
- When setting up the supplies for the IV insertion, use caution in determining where to affix the precut tape. Keep in mind that the precut tape should be affixed to a clean surface.

---

Most infants have one or two possible IV sites on each hand, arm, and foot and four to eight sites on the scalp. Because superficial veins of the scalp have no valves, fluid can be infused in either direction. Because insertion is easy, they are sometimes used for IV therapy in infants less than 9 months of age but should be used only when attempts at other sites have failed. The temporal and forehead areas are suitable and do not interfere with side-to-side head movements. The use of a scalp vein site may require removing the hair from the area around the site to better visualize the vein and provide a smoother surface on which to tape the tubing. Clipping off a portion of the infant's hair is very upsetting to parents; therefore they should *always* be told what to expect and be reassured that the hair will grow in again rapidly (save the hair because parents often wish to keep it). Remove as little hair as possible directly over the insertion site and taping surface. To avoid

---

**Box 28-8** ▪ ▪ ▫

### Procedure for Inserting and Taping a Peripheral Intravenous Catheter

- Verify physician order and confirm patient identity.
- Follow manufacturer's directions for all devices used.
- Wash hands and observe aseptic technique throughout procedure.
- Choose catheter insertion site and an alternative site in case the initial attempt is unsuccessful
- Prepare insertion site by applying with friction an antiseptic solution in a circular motion, working from the center of the insertion site to the exterior edge, approximately 2 inches. Allow solution to dry completely but do not blow, blot dry, or fan the area.
- Don gloves.
- Apply tourniquet when site is ready for catheter insertion.
- Stretch the skin taut downward below the point of insertion, upward above the site of insertion, or from underneath level with the point of insertion. This technique helps stabilize veins that roll or move away from the catheter as attempts are made to enter the vein.
- Inspect catheter, looking for damage [e.g., bent stylet, shavings on the catheter, or frayed catheter tip (follow employer's policy for reporting defective devices]). If stylet and catheter are intact, break the seal between the two (if recommended by manufacturer) by gently twisting the two pieces and separating them a minuscule amount. This allows easy advancement of the catheter from the stylet after entering the vein.
- Insert catheter through the skin, bevel up, at a 30-degree angle and enter the vein. This direct approach is best for large veins and enters the skin and vein in one step. The indirect approach for smaller veins enables the catheter to enter the vein from the side perpendicularly. It is sometimes helpful with short veins to start the catheter below the intended site and advance through the superficial layers of skin so that the advancement of the catheter in the vein is a shorter distance. In infants or children with very small veins insert the catheter bevel down, which prevents the needle from puncturing the back wall of the vein and provides an earlier flashback of blood as the vein is entered.
- Watch for blood return in the flashback chamber. Some 24-gauge catheters provide visualization of the flashback within the catheter so immediate vein entrance is recognized before the needle punctures the back of the vessel or goes through the other side of the vessel.
- Once the flashback is seen, lower the angle between the skin and catheter to 15 degrees. Advance the catheter another 1/16 to 1/8 inch to ensure that both the metal stylet and catheter are inside the vein. Look closely at the IV catheter before inserting

it and notice that the stylet tip is slightly longer than the catheter. It is necessary to have both pieces inside the vein before advancing the catheter. Holding the stylet steady, push the catheter off the stylet and into the vein until the catheter hub is situated against the skin at the insertion site. Activate safety mechanism if necessary (some safety catheters are passive and activate automatically), remove the stylet, and discard into sharps container. Apply pressure to catheter within the vein to prevent backflow of blood before attachment of extension tubing.
- Connect the extension tubing and reinforce connection with a junction securement device (Luer-Lok, clasping device, threaded device) to prevent accidental disconnection and subsequent air embolism or blood loss.
- Collect blood if ordered. Remove the tourniquet. Flush the IV line with normal saline to check for patency (ease of flushing fluid and lack of resistance while flushing), complaints of pain, or swelling to the site. If line flushes easily, proceed to secure the catheter to the skin.
- Place transparent dressing across catheter hub, up to but not including the junction securement device, and surrounding skin.
- Further secure the catheter to the skin using tape or adhesive securement devices (also known as adhesive anchors). Follow manufacturer's directions for adhesive anchors.
- Place a $\frac{1}{4}$- to $\frac{1}{2}$-inch strip of clear tape across the width of the transparent dressing and the catheter hub but avoid the insertion site. This will serve as an anchor tape strip, and all other tape will be affixed to this strip (tape-on-tape method). This strip will not compromise the transparent dressing properties or interfere with visual inspection of the catheter–skin insertion site.
- To stabilize the catheter and junction securement device attach 1 to $1\frac{1}{2}$ inches of clear tape that is $\frac{1}{4}$ to $\frac{1}{2}$ inch wide, adhesive side up, to the underneath side of the catheter hub and junction securement device at their connection. Wrap the ends of the tape around the connections and meet on top to form a V-shape (sometimes referred to as a chevron); secure the overlapping ends onto the anchor tape strip.
- Loop the IV tubing away from the catheter hub and toward the IV fluid source. Secure the looped tubing with a piece of tape on the anchor tape strip.
- Secure a commercial protective device over the catheter hub and looped tubing. Bending one corner of the tape over and onto itself provides a free tab to lift the tape easily for site visualization.

microabrasions, do not shave the site, which increases potential introduction of microorganisms into the vascular system (Infusion Nurses Society, 2000a, 2000b). A rubber band slipped onto the head from brow to occiput will usually suffice as a tourniquet, although if the vessel is visible, a tourniquet may not be necessary in some infants.

**NURSING TIP**   A tab of tape should be placed on the rubber band to help grasp it when removing it from the infant's head. The rubber band should be cut to avoid accidentally dislodging the catheter when moving the rubber band over the IV insertion site. The tape tab will lift the rubber band and allow it to be cut. Hold the rubber band in two places, and cut between these areas to prevent the rubber band from snapping on the head.

The extremity or head should be carefully restrained by an assistant for easier venipuncture and to minimize trauma resulting from the child's inadvertent movement. (See Chapter 27 for additional restraining methods.) For a scalp site it is helpful to visualize the way in which the needle will be secured following insertion.

Locating an extremity vein may be difficult because the veins are smaller and children have a significant amount of subcutaneous fat. When veins are not readily visible, ap-

plying a warm compress to the site, running warm water over the extremity, or, when using an extremity, holding the limb in a dependent position below body level will help fill the veins for better visualization. Gentle tapping sometimes causes the veins to stand out. A flashlight held against the skin below the intended site sometimes assists in locating vessels. A commercial vein transilluminator is very helpful in locating veins and assessing the depth and patency of the vessels.* If these measures do not help, a tourniquet applied with light pressure medially to the site may be needed. Although the tourniquet makes the veins more visible and provides a more rapid blood return, the added venous pressure may cause fragile veins to "blow" when punctured, producing a hematoma. Before beginning the procedure, it is important to prepare the materials needed to secure the IV. Tape should be precut and easily reached. All other necessary equipment should be set up in an orderly fashion, allowing the venipuncture to be performed in a timely manner.

**NURSING TIP**   A blood pressure cuff can also be used as a tourniquet and can give more control over the pressure needed to make the veins visible.

The needle or catheter must be placed in the direction of the blood flow, which creates no problem when an extremity is used. Scalp veins are easy to visualize but difficult to assess and may actually be an artery. Therefore palpation for a pulse on scalp sites is recommended but again may be difficult because the veins may be hidden within the suture lines (Frey, 2001). In general the venous blood flows from the top of the head toward the neck, so the catheter should be pointed downward toward the heart. To test the direction before insertion, the forefinger is placed on the vein at the site chosen for venipuncture. While the finger gently presses the vein, a second finger is used to "strip" the vein in the direction of the top of the head. The pressure from the second finger is released. If the vein fills distal to the compressing finger, the direction of flow is toward the stationary finger (Box 28-9).

### Securing a Peripheral Intravenous (PIV) Line

To maintain the integrity of the IV line, adequate protection of the site is required. The catheter hub is firmly secured at the puncture site with a transparent dressing or clear, non-allergenic tape. Transparent dressings are ideal because the insertion site is easily observed. Minimal tape should be used at the puncture site and on about 1 to 2 inches of skin beyond the site to avoid obscuring the insertion site for every detection of infiltration.

A protective cover is applied directly over the catheter insertion site to protect the infusion site (Intravenous Nurses Society, 2000b). Easy access to the IV site for frequent (1- to 2-hour) assessments must be considered. Improvised plastic cups that are cut in half with the ridged edges covered with

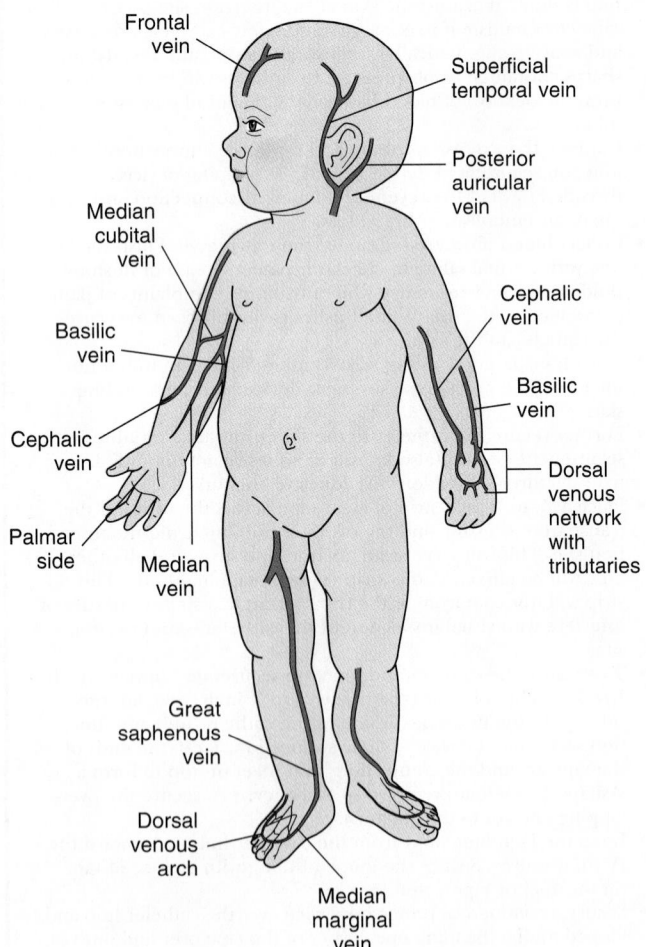

**Fig. 28-6**   Preferred sites for venous access in infants.

Frontal vein

Superficial temporal vein

Posterior auricular vein

Median cubital vein

Basilic vein

Cephalic vein

Cephalic vein

Basilic vein

Palmar side

Median vein

Dorsal venous network with tributaries

Great saphenous vein

Dorsal venous arch

Median marginal vein

---

*Venoscope Transilluminator Vein Finder is available from Applied Biotech Products, Inc, PO Box 52073, Lafayette, LA 70505-2073, (800) 284-7655; www.venoscope.com.

tape should not be used, because they have caused injury to patients (*Morris v Children's Medical Center,* 1992). A commercial site protector, *I.V. House,** is available in different sizes (Fig. 28-7). Its ventilation holes prevent moisture from accumulating under the dome (Lee and Vallino, 1996). This device is designed to protect the IV site; allow for visibility of the site; minimize use of padded boards, splints, or other restraints and tape; and maintain skin integrity. The connector tubing or extension tubing can be looped to make it small enough to fit under the protective cover to prevent accidental snagging of the catheter. It is important to safely secure the IV tubing to prevent infants and children from becoming entangled in the tubing or from accidentally pulling the catheter or needle out. This securement also eliminates movement of the catheter hub at the insertion site (mechanical manipulation). A colorful and interesting sticker can be applied to the protecting device to add a positive note to the procedure.

**NURSING TIP** I.V. House may be used to protect surgical insertion sites, such as jugular, femoral, or subclavian lines; implanted ports; or peripherally inserted central catheter lines; and for the application of EMLA.

*Available from I.V. House, 7400 Foxmont Dr, Hazelwood, MO 63042, (800) 530-0400; fax: (314) 831-3863; e-mail: ivhouse@ivhouse.com; www.ivhouse.com.

Finger or toe areas are left unoccluded by dressings or tape to allow for assessment of circulation. The thumb is never immobilized because of the danger of contractures with limited movement later on. An extremity should never be encircled with tape. The use of roll gauze, self-adhering stretch bandages (Coban), and Ace bandages can cause the same constriction and hide signs of infiltration (Infusion Nurses Society, 2000a).

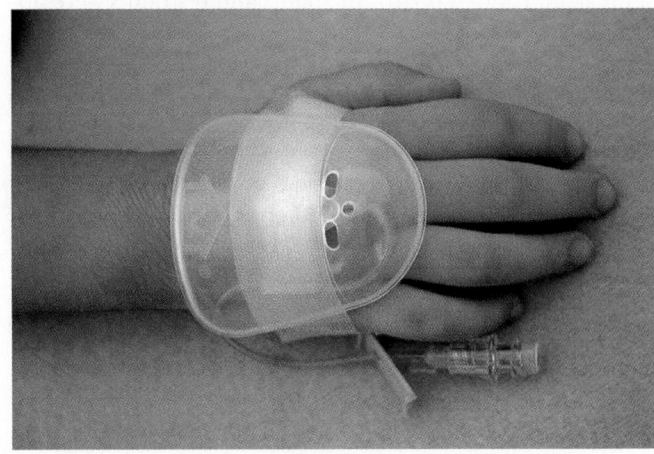

**Fig. 28-7** I.V. House used to protect the IV site.

---

**Box 28-9** ■ ■ ■
## Documentation of a Peripheral Intravenous Catheter

The entire procedure for inserting and taping a peripheral intravenous catheter should be documented in the patient's medical record. Important information includes but is not limited to the following:

### IV INSERTION DOCUMENTATION

Normally part of the patient's medical record)

- The date and time of insertion; name or initials of clinician inserting IV
- Preparation of site, including antiseptic solution used
- Manufacturer, gauge, and length of catheter
- Site of insertion (e.g., "right ankle," or more specifically "right saphenous vein")
- Number of attempts (e.g., "24 gauge, 1 inch, Insyte initiated in right saphenous vein in first attempt," or "24 gauge, 1 inch, Insyte initiated in right saphenous vein after one unsuccessful attempt to left saphenous vein")
- Presence of blood return and name of samples drawn and sent to laboratory if applicable
- Activation of junction securement devices (Luer-Lok) and explanation of taping (e.g., "IV catheter secured with transparent dressing and transpore tape")
- Use of arm board
- Appearance of site (e.g., site is soft without redness or edema, flushes easily)
- Flushing solution, amount used
- Connection to IV solution, naming the fluid and amount in the bag
- Tolerance of procedure; it is best to describe specific behaviors displayed by the patient or use quotes (e.g., "patient cried during insertion but quieted easily and fell asleep in mom's arms after procedure," or "patient stated, 'That hurt but it feels better now'")

### IV SITE DOCUMENTATION

Can be done on a piece of tape at the site

- Date, time, gauge, and length of catheter and initials of nurse initiating

### IV FLUID DOCUMENTATION

Frequently achieved on an IV flow sheet

- Date and time of fluid initiation
- Type and volume of bag hung; (e.g., "500-ml bag of normal saline")
- Type of delivery system used and rate of infusion (e.g., "IV connected to Baxter pump and infusing at a rate of 25 ml/hr")
- Any additives, type and dose, in the primary solution (e.g., "potassium chloride (KCl 2 mEq/100 ml")

### ONGOING IV SITE ASSESSMENT

Follow hospital's policy, but recommended at least every 2 hours (can be done in medical record or on the IV flow sheet)

- Appearance (e.g., site is soft without redness or edema" [any protective device needs to be lifted to see the entire site])
- Any patient comments regarding IV

### DISCONTINUATION OF IV THERAPY

(Can be done in medical record)

- Reason for discontinuing IV (e.g., "end of therapy, infiltration, or accidentally removed")
- Integrity of device, including length and condition of catheter
- Appearance of site
- Dressing applied
- Patient tolerance; again direct quotes from patient are best

Traditionally, padded boards or splints have been used to partially immobilize the IV site. Some institutions have even used rigid elbow restraints that do not allow the arm to bend at all. Padded boards or splints and restraints were appropriate when metal needles were inserted into the vein to prevent the sharp end from puncturing the vessel, especially at a joint. With the more recent use of soft, pliable catheters, arm or leg boards may not be necessary and have several disadvantages. They obscure the IV site, can constrict the extremity, may excoriate the underlying tissue and promote infection, can cause a contracture of a joint, restrict useful movement of the extremity, and are uncomfortable. Unfortunately, no research has been conducted to demonstrate their proposed benefit of increasing dwell time (patency of the IV line). Adequate taping and protection with a commercial device should eliminate the need for padded boards in most circumstances. Older children who are alert and cooperative can usually be trusted to protect the IV site.

Immobilization is intolerable to the naturally active child, and every effort is made to reduce the use of restraints. To relieve the stress of immobilization, frequent removal of the restraints provides the child with the opportunity to move the extremities. Whenever possible, the infant or child is held and cuddled to help meet emotional needs during this trying time (Fig. 28-8). Range-of-motion exercises are employed on infants and children who are too ill or unable to move their extremities, but others should be encouraged to move their arms and legs. Most infants or small children will instinctively move their extremities when released. If not, a toy or other stimulus can provide incentive.

### Removal of a Peripheral Intravenous Line

When it comes time to discontinue an IV infusion, many children are distressed by the thought of *catheter removal.* Therefore they need a careful explanation of the process and suggestions for helping. Encouraging children to remove or help remove the tape from the site provides them with a measure of control and often encourages their cooperation. The procedure consists of turning off any pump apparatus, occluding the IV tubing, removing the tape, pulling the catheter out of the vessel in the opposite direction of insertion, and exerting firm pressure at the site after the catheter is removed until bleeding stops. (It is painful to apply pressure on the catheter while pulling it out.) A dry dressing (adhesive bandage strip) is placed over the puncture site. The use of adhesive removal pads can decrease the pain of tape removal, but the skin should be washed off after use because the skin can become irritated. To remove transparent dressings (e.g., Op-Site or Tegaderm), pull the opposing edges parallel to the skin to loosen the bond. If a catheter was used for the IV infusion, the tip is inspected to make certain the catheter is intact and no portion remains in the vein.

### Complications

The same precautions regarding maintenance of asepsis, prevention of infection, and observation for infiltration are carried out with patients of any age. However, infiltration is more difficult to detect in infants and small children than in adults. The increased amount of subcutaneous fat and the amount of tape used to secure the catheter hub obscure the

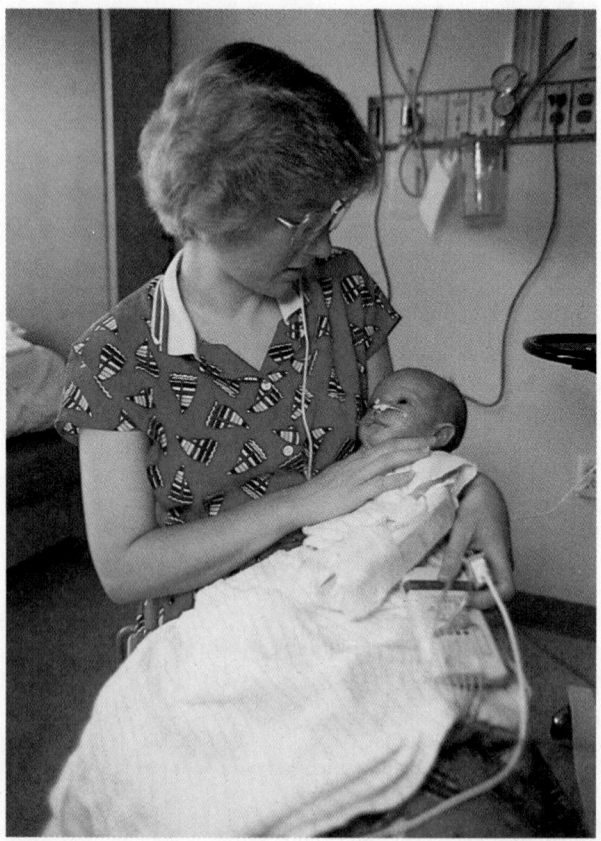

**Fig. 28-8** Intravenous infusion, as well as other equipment, does not prevent the infant from being picked up and cuddled.

signs of early infiltration. When the fluid appears to be infusing too slowly or ceases, the usual assessment for obstruction within the apparatus (i.e., kinks, screw clamps, shutoff valve, and positioning interference, such as a bent elbow) often locates the difficulty. When these actions fail to detect the problem, it may be necessary to carefully remove some of the tape and other material that obscure a clear view of the venipuncture site. Dependent areas, such as the palm and undersides of the extremity or the occiput and behind the ears, are examined.

Whenever possible, the IV infusion should be placed in an extremity to which the identification band (or bracelet) is not attached. Serious circulatory impairment can result from infiltrated solution distal to the band, which acts as a tourniquet preventing adequate venous return. To check for return blood flow through the catheter, the solution bag is lowered below the level of the infusion site. A good blood return, or lack thereof, is not always an indicator of infiltration in small infants. Flushing the catheter and observing the site for discoloration (i.e., blanching or redness), pain, tenderness, and edema or noting any exudate or drainage and increase in skin or basal temperatures is an appropriate assessment of the IV site (Infusion Nurses Society, 2000a, 2000b). If the tubing is connected to an infusion pump, it must be removed from the pump before lowering.

> **NURSING ALERT**
> Different infusion pumps have preset pressures for infusion, delivery, and occlusion; therefore the pump's occlusion alarm is not entirely reliable to detect infiltrations.

IV therapy in pediatrics tends to be difficult to maintain because of mechanical factors that may predispose the IV infusion to shortened dwell times. Such factors include vascular trauma due to PIV device selection (gauge and length of the catheter), the insertion site, the length of catheter dwell, the size of vessel, vessel fragility, the activity level of the patient, operator skill and insertion technique, forceful administration of boluses of fluid, and infusion of irritants or vesicants through a small vessel (Pettit and Hughes, 1999). These factors cause infiltration and extravasation injuries, which are reported with relative frequency. *Infiltration* is defined as inadvertent administration of a nonvesicant solution/medication into surrounding tissue. *Extravasation* is defined as inadvertent administration of vesicant solution/medication into surrounding tissue (Infusion Nurses Society, 2000a, 2000b). A *vesicant* or *sclerosing agent* causes varying degrees of cellular damage when even minute amounts escape into surrounding tissue. Guidelines for determining the severity of tissue injury by staging characteristics, such as the amount of redness, blanching, the amount of swelling, pain, the quality of pulses below infiltration, capillary refill, and warmth or coolness of the area, are available (Infusion Nurses Society, 2000a, 2000b;* Montgomery and others, 1999).

Treatment of an infiltration/extravasation varies according to the type of vesicant. Guidelines are available outlining the sequence of interventions and specific treatment of infiltration/extravasation with antidotes (Montomgery and others, 1999; Oncology Nursing Society, 1998*).

> **NURSING ALERT**
> When an infiltration/extravasation is observed (signs may include erythema, pain, edema, blanching, streaking on the skin along the vein, and darkened area at the insertion site), immediately stop the infusion, elevate the extremity, notify the practitioner, and initiate the ordered treatment as soon as possible. Dry heat may be applied, except if the infused solution is sclerosing. Remove the IV line when it is no longer needed (e.g., after infusing an antidote).

PIV catheters are the most commonly used intravascular device. Heavy cutaneous colonization of the insertion site is the single most important predictor of catheter-related infection with all types of short-term, percutaneously inserted catheters. Phlebitis, largely a mechanical rather than infectious process, remains the most important complication associated with the use of peripheral venous catheters.† (See Community Focus box.)

> **NURSING ALERT**
> Prevention of insertion site infection can be decreased by strict adherence to the following guidelines (Pearson, 1996):
> Practice good handwashing before starting an IV infusion.
> Rigorously cleanse the skin with an appropriate antiseptic, including alcohol, chlorhexidine, or povidone-iodine, before catheter insertion.
> When cleansing the insertion site, use a circular motion starting from the center and working outward.
> Allow the antiseptic to dry for 30 to 60 seconds before inserting the catheter.
> Do not palpate the insertion site after the skin has been cleansed with the antiseptic.

Proper education of the patient and family regarding signs and symptoms of an infected site can help prevent infections from going unnoticed. When an IV infusion continues for several days, the tubing and solution are changed at regular intervals according to hospital policy, most often every 72 hours (Pearson, 1995). The dressing, whether

---

*Guidelines on interventions for infiltration/extravasation are available from the **Oncology Nursing Society,** 501 Holiday Dr, Pittsburgh, PA 15220-2749, (412) 921-7373; fax: (412) 921-2131; www.ons.org.
†Guidelines for prevention of intravascular device–related infections are available from the Centers for Disease Control and Prevention, 1600 Clifton Rd NE, Atlanta, GA 30333, (404) 639-3311; www.cdc.gov/ncidod/hip/iv/iv.htm.

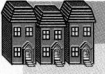

### COMMUNITY FOCUS
#### *Preventing IV Site Infections*

With the increasing use of IV therapy in the community, preventing infection is essential. The most effective ways to prevent infection of an IV site are to wash hands between each patient, wear gloves when inserting an IV catheter, closely monitor the date of IV placement, and inspect the insertion site and physical condition of the IV dressing. Proper education of the patient and family regarding signs and symptoms of an infected IV site can help prevent infections from going unnoticed.

---

*Guidelines for determining tissue injury severity are available from the **Infusion Nurses Society,** Fresh Pond Square, 10 Fawcett St, Cambridge, MA 02138, (617) 441-3008; fax: (617) 441-3009; www.nsl.org.

transparent dressing or sterile gauze and tape, can be left in place for the duration of the IV infusion (Maki, 1994) unless the integrity has been compromised. To ensure that the equipment is changed regularly, it is labeled with the date and time that the new bag and tubing are attached. Any signs of inflammation, such as redness or pain, are reported immediately. This usually requires removal of the infusion and restarting it at another site or administering the medication by another route.

## Venous Access Devices (VADs)

VADs have several different characteristics. The practitioner has to consider the best type of catheter for the individual patient's needs. Factors that can influence the decision include the reason for placement of the catheter (diagnosis), age of the patient, length of therapy, risk to the patient in placement of the catheter, and availability of resources to assist the family in maintaining the catheter (Reed and Phillips, 1996).

Central catheters can be categorized into three types:

1. Short-term or nontunneled catheters (subclavian, femoral, and jugular)
2. Peripherally inserted central catheters (see Table 28-8)
3. Long-term, tunneled catheters and implanted ports (see Table 28-9)

*Short-term* or *nontunneled catheters* are used in acute, emergency, and intensive care units. These catheters are made of polyurethane and are placed in large veins such as the subclavian, femoral, or jugular. A chest x-ray film should be taken to verify placement of the catheter tip before administration of fluids or medications. The other types are discussed in the following sections.

### Peripheral Intermittent Infusion Device

The *peripheral lock,* also known as an *intermittent infusion device, saline well,* or *heparin lock* is used as an alternative for a keep-open infusion when extended access to a vein is required without the need for continuous fluid. It is most frequently employed for intermittent infusion of medication into a peripheral venous route. A short, flexible catheter (or occasionally a steel butterfly needle) is used as the lock device, and a site is selected where there

will be minimum movement, such as the forearm. The needle/catheter is inserted and secured in the same manner as any IV infusion device, but the hub is occluded with a stopper or injection cap.

The type of device used may vary, and the care and use of the peripheral lock are carried out according to the specific protocol of the institution or unit. However, the general concept is the same. The needle or catheter remains in place and is flushed with saline or heparin (1:10 units/ml) after infusion of the medication. The flush solution prevents blood from clotting in the device between infusions. Because heparin is incompatible with many drugs, the peripheral lock must also be flushed with saline before and after administering medication. Controversy exists over saline vs heparin flush. (See Evidence-Based Practice box.) Children may be discharged with a peripheral lock in place in order to continue receiving medications without hospitalization; this is usually reserved for children who require medications on a short-term basis and are referred to a home-based infusion company. Those with chronic illnesses who require repeated blood sampling or medications, long-term chemotherapy, or frequent hyperalimentation or antibiotic therapy are best managed with a central venous catheter.

**NURSING TIP** There is controversy concerning the need to flush with heparin in any vascular access device, peripheral or central. A more important issue is the technique of flushing. The use of the turbulent-flow flush has proven to be successful in preventing clot formation in the device. It is described as the forward flushing motion on the syringe with a flush-stop-flush-stop technique. This causes a swirling and vigorous fluid movement that clears the catheter better than the continuous flush motion most commonly used. This procedure is combined with the positive pressure technique. As you complete the flush, hold the syringe stopper down, clamp the catheter, then remove the syringe. This prevents blood from backing into the tip of the catheter (Moureau, 2000).

### Peripherally Inserted Central Catheters (PICCs)

PICCs can be used for short-term to moderate-length therapy (Table 28-8). Researchers have shown catheter longevity

| **TABLE 28-8** Peripherally inserted central catheters | | |
|---|---|---|
| **Description** | **Benefits** | **Care Considerations** |
| Made of silastic or polyurethane material | Do not require operating room placement | Sometimes difficult to thread into SVC |
| Single or double lumen available | Can be inserted by specially trained RNs | Reports of resistance to removal |
| Inserted into antecubital fossa and passed through basilic or cephalic vein into superior vena cava (SVC) | Can use small insertion needles | Not suitable for rapid fluid replacement because of small lumen size |
| Positioning of tip in SVC maximizes hemodilution and reduces likelihood of vessel wall damage, phlebitis, or thrombus formation | Fast placement | 5- to 10-ml syringe is used for flushing to prevent catheter wall rupture |
| Can be placed as a "midline" catheter, also known as a halfway catheter, ending near axillary vein (not suitable for total parenteral nutrition [TPN], hyperosmolar solutions, or vesicant chemotherapy) | Sepsis rates are ≤2% | |

## EVIDENCE-BASED PRACTICE

### Saline vs Heparin to Flush Peripheral Intermittent IV Infusions in Children

Several pediatric studies have investigated the use of NS vs. heparinized saline (HS) (10 units/ml) as a flush solution in intermittent IV infusions in children. The main outcome measure was the length of dwell times or patency. Other factors that were considered were the type and gauge of the IV catheters, the subjective and objective cues of discomfort, the age of the child, the effect of the medication to be infused, and the frequency of line entry. Additional studies have evaluated the efficacy of NS vs. HS specifically in neonates.

Danek and Noris (1992) randomly assigned children from birth to 18 years of age to receive either NS or HS flush. They studied 160 infusion devices: 40 were 22 gauge, and 120 were 24 gauge. There were no significant differences in catheter patency for either flush for 22-gauge catheter. However, in 24-gauge catheters, patency was longer with HS.

Hanrahan, Kleiber, and Fagan (1994) conducted an evaluation of a policy change based on a previous study that compared HS and NS flushes (Kleiber and others, 1993). In the first study, no significant difference was found between the two flushes in the areas of IV duration, patient age, number of flushes, site location, or complications. The incidence of pain, however, was significantly higher in the patients who received HS flushes. The study resulted in a change of hospital policy from HS to NS flushes. To evaluate the policy change, the researchers divided a total of 126 children over 28 days old into two groups. The randomly selected children in group 1 were those who had received a saline flush in the 1993 study. The children in group 2 received the saline flush after the policy change was made. The study's results showed no significant differences between the two NS groups as far as age, site locations, dwell times (60.86 hours for group 1 and 60.03 hours for group 2), number of flushes, number and types of medications, and site complications. Catheter size was not considered. The study concluded that saline is a safe and effective flush solution for maintaining IV patency in children.

Graves and others (1997) studied the efficacy of NS flushes vs. HS flushes for peripheral IV lines with 24-gauge catheters in 58 preterm and term infants. The infants were randomly divided into two groups; group 1 received NS flushes, and group 2 received HS flushes. Results showed no statistically significant differences between the two groups in dwell time or patient response when considering body weight, medications used, site location, duration, or reason for discontinuing the IV infusion. However, IV lines that were flushed with NS lasted 4.5 hours longer than lines flushed with HS. Nurses reported a patient response of pain only when the lines were flushed with HS.

Paisley and others (1997) evaluated the duration of patency of HS and NS flushes in peripheral intravenous catheters in neonates. Subjects included term and preterm infants, with a range of 33 to 42 weeks' gestational age at birth. Eighty-seven infants were evaluated, with 33 receiving HS and 54 NS. A total of 159 catheter starts were evaluated in the infants, with the majority of catheters being 24 gauge (99.4%) and (57%) being started in the scalp. No statistical difference was found in duration of patency in the catheters locked with HS vs NS (chi-square 0.2). The researchers did find that gestational age and the site of catheter placement were predicting variables in relation to duration of catheter patency. Results showed that catheters in term infants remained patent longer than those placed in preterm infants. Also catheters placed in the scalp, arm, or hand remained patent longer than those placed in the leg or foot.

Gyr and others (1995) found significantly longer patency in the HS group as compared with the NS group in a group of 53 patients ranging from age 1 month to 19 years. There were also more instances of nonpatency for 16- to 20-gauge catheters than for 22-gauge catheters. Increased antibiotic administration was associated with shorter IV dwell times. They concluded

that there is insufficient evidence to support the use of NS. However, their sample included 11 children with cystic fibrosis who received antibiotic infusions. The inclusion of these subjects could have biased the results. In light of the findings from the earlier studies that support NS, this study should be replicated with a general pediatric population. Gyr and others (1995) also found more clotting problems in catheters flushed at 8-hour, rather than 4-hour, intervals. To evaluate the effectiveness of 4-, 6-, and 8-hour heparin flush times, Crews and others (1997) studied 83 children with 22- and 24-gauge catheters. The dwell times were significantly longer for lines flushed at 6- and 8-hour intervals that for those flushed at 4-hour intervals, regardless of catheter size. These findings are in contrast to those of Gyr and others (1995).

Heilskov and others (1998) evaluated the efficacy of HS vs NS flush solutions and found no statistical difference in catheter duration of IV locks. Ninety neonates hospitalized at birth were evaluated in this randomized, double-blind study. Study inclusion criteria established that infants had to weigh at least 800 g, had received no anticoagulants within the previous 48 hours, and had English-speaking parents. Only one IV site per subject was evaluated, and all locks were flushed at least every 6 hours. Infants were randomized to one of three groups in which catheters were flushed with either normal saline, heparinized saline 2 U/ml, or heparinized saline 10 U/ml. No statistically significant differences were found for the duration of IV catheter patency among the different groups.

A study conducted by Mudge, Forcier, and Slattery (1998) that looked specifically at the effectiveness of HS vs. NS flush solutions in maintaining the patency of 24-gauge infusion devices found greater patency with the use of HS. Study inclusion criteria included children less than 2 years of age, presence of a 24-gauge catheter, and the absence of medications affecting coagulation. Subjects were given one of two flush solutions, heparinized saline (10 U/ml) or normal saline. The flushes were rotated on a monthly basis by the hospital pharmacy, and catheters lasting over 1 month were only flushed with one solution for the life of the catheter. No control was made for flushing frequency, but all catheters were flushed every 8 to 12 hours, based on institutional policy. A total of 134 catheters were evaluated in 61 patients, with 124 being placed in neonates. Chi-square analysis showed no significant differences for variables such as age, catheter site, irritating substances infused, and whether the catheter was started as a continuous infusion before conversion to a peripheral intermittent infusion device. Findings were similar to those found in earlier studies by Danek and Noris (1992) and Gyr and others (1995). In this study, catheters flushed with NS had a median duration of 35 hours compared with 42 hours in catheters flushed with HS. Catheters flushed with NS developed more complications and had to be removed (71%) compared with those flushed with HS (52%).

Le Duk (1997) supported the use of NS over HS in emergency department pediatric patients. One hundred twenty three subjects, 1 to 22 years of age were enrolled in this prospective, randomized, double-blind study in the emergency department setting. Patients in the control group (N = 77) received 3 ml of 10 U/ml HS, and patients in the experimental group (N = 73) received 3 ml of NS. No significant differences were found in the occurrence of IV complications between the groups. A savings of $9.45 per patient when using NS flushes led to an annual cost savings of $27,594 with this group of patients.

Obviously, many factors influence the outcome measure of dwell time. Considering the cost, compatibility, and atraumatic benefits of using saline rather than heparin, more research is needed to clarify other factors influencing catheter patency. However, for catheters larger than 24 gauge, research supports the use of saline flushes.

ranging to over 200 days (Donaldson and others, 1995; Frey, 1995). These catheters consist of silicone or polymer material and are placed by specially trained nurses (Goodwin and Carlson, 1993). The most common insertion site is the antecubital area using the median, cephalic, or basilic vein. The catheter is threaded either with or without a guide wire into the superior vena cava. PICCs can be trimmed before insertion, and the decision can be made to insert the catheter "midline," which is considered between the insertion site and the axilla. The "midline" has a recommended dwell time of 2 to 4 weeks. Catheters with the terminal tip from above the axilla to the tip of the subclavian vein are considered a "midclavicular line." Numerous articles have been published on increased risks with this type of place-

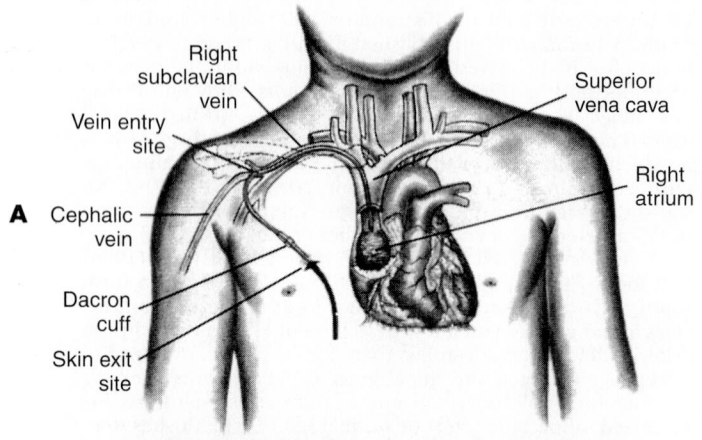

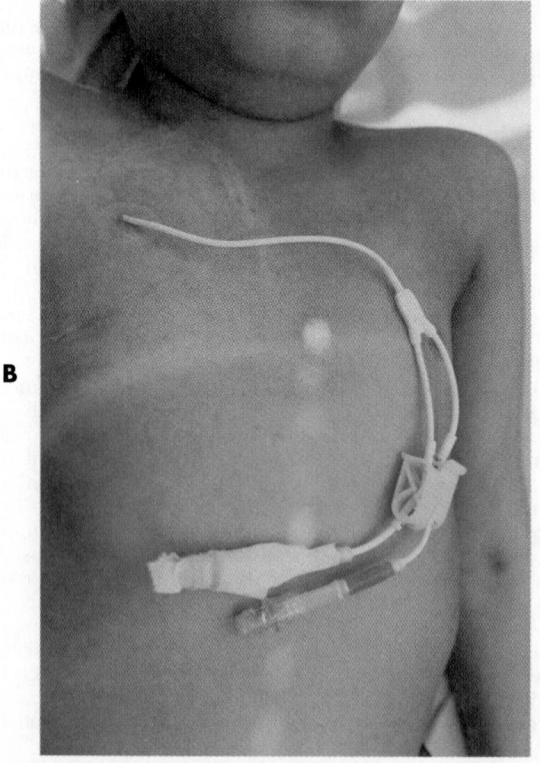

**Fig. 28-9**  **A,** Central venous catheter insertion and exit site. **B,** External venous catheter (note redness from dressing site).

ment. This placement location remains controversial because of the terminal tip location and is not used as optimal placement (Racadio and others, 2001).

If the catheter is threaded midline, total parenteral nutrition (TPN) should not be administered, because the high concentration of glucose makes it irritating to the vessel and it should be infused through a central catheter.

The decision to insert a PICC needs to be made before several attempts at IV insertions are done. Once the antecubital veins have been punctured repeatedly, they are not considered to be candidates for this type of catheter. Because this catheter is the least costly and has less chance of complications than other central VADs, it is an excellent choice for many pediatric patients. This catheter is also usually inserted in the unit's treatment room.

> **NURSING ALERT**   Most PICC lines are not sutured into place, so care needs to be maintained when changing the dressing.

PICCs can create problems with removal. Causes for this resistance in removal include infectious processes, fibrin formation, and endothelial thrombosis (Masoorli, 1998). Methods to free the catheter include gentle traction to the catheter, taping the catheter to create tension on the line, and warm soaks to the site. Aggressive pulling of the catheter is contraindicated.

### Long-Term Central VADs

Long-term central VADs include tunneled and implanted infusion ports. They may have single, double, or triple lumens. Several lumens (multilumen catheters) allow more than one therapy to be administered at the same time. Reasons to use multilumen catheters include repeated blood sampling, TPN, administration of blood products or infusion of large quantities or concentrations of fluids, ability to administer incompatible drugs or fluids at the same time (through different lumens), and central venous pressure (CVP) monitoring (Table 28-9).

With the patient under local or general anesthesia, the long-term catheter of choice is placed with aseptic technique. A vein, such as the jugular or subclavian, is entered through a small cutdown site, and the catheter is threaded to the junction of the superior vena cava and right atrium, confirmed by fluoroscopic dye injection, and then sutured in place. To stabilize the catheter and reduce the risk of infection, the remainder is tunneled beneath the skin to exit through a small incision at a convenient location on the anterior aspect of the chest or upper abdomen (Fig. 28-9). One or two Dacron cuffs or Vitacuffs on the catheter remain in the subcutaneous tunnel; as tissue adheres to the cuff, the cuff provides a barrier to infection (Weiner and Albanese, 1998). The cutdown site is surgically closed, the catheter is sutured to the skin at the exit site, and a sterile dressing is applied.

With any of the central venous catheters, instilling medication through the injection cap is easily accomplished. With the implanted device, the port must be palpated for placement and stabilized, the overlying skin cleansed, and only special noncoring Huber needles used to pierce the port's diaphragm on the top or side, depending on the style. To avoid repeated skin punctures, a special infusion set with a Huber needle and extension tubing with Luer connection can be used (Fig. 28-10). With this attached the injection procedure is the same as for the venous catheters. To prevent infection, meticulous aseptic technique must be used anytime the devices are entered, including instillation of heparin or saline to prevent clotting (Harris and Maguire, 1999).

## Complications

Central venous line bacteremia can be of major concern in a child. The mean incidence of catheter-related blood stream infection varies in the literature, but it averages around 2.4 episodes per 1000 hospital days (Jones, 1998). Centrally placed catheters are associated with fewer complications than are peripherally placed catheters (Racadio and others, 2001). The use of central line catheters for parenteral alimentation significantly increases the risk of infection (Tacconelli and Tumbarello, 2000). Prevention of catheter-related infections requires measures to eliminate the potential for microbial contamination of the skin at the catheter site, hub, tubing connectors, and any inline devices that may be present (Schierholz and others, 2000). Line connections should be wrapped with tape to prevent accidental disconnection. The number of line breaks for blood withdrawal or medication administration should be minimized. Central line dressing protocols should be developed, and nurses experienced in dressing change techniques should be responsible for line care. Family teaching must include how to care for the line, what to do if the line becomes disconnected or broken, and how to flush the line using aseptic technique.

Catheter-related central venous thrombosis can also be a serious problem in children (Kenney, David, and Bensoussan,

---

**TABLE 28-9** Comparison of long-term central venous access devices

| Description | Benefits | Care Considerations |
|---|---|---|
| **Tunneled Catheter (e.g., Hickman/Broviac Catheter)** | | |
| Silicone, radiopaque, flexible catheter with open ends<br>One or two Dacron cuffs or Vitacuffs (biosynthetic material impregnated with silver ions) on catheter(s) enhance tissue ingrowth<br>May have more than one lumen | Reduced risk of bacterial migration after tissue adheres to Dacron cuff or Vitacuff<br>Easy to use for self-administered infusions | Requires daily heparin flushes<br>Must be clamped or have clamp nearby at all times unless using positive-flow injection caps<br>Must keep exit site dry<br>Heavy activity restricted until tissue adheres to cuff<br>Risk of infection still present<br>Protrudes outside body; susceptible to damage from sharp instruments and may be pulled out; may affect body image<br>More difficult to repair<br>Patient/family must learn catheter care |
| **Groshong Catheter** | | |
| Clear, flexible, silicone, radiopaque catheter with closed tip and two-way valve at proximal end<br>Dacron cuff or Vitacuff on catheter enhances tissue ingrowth<br>May have more than one lumen | Reduced time and cost for maintenance care; no heparin flushes needed<br>Reduced catheter damage—no clamping needed because of two-way valve<br>Increased patient safety because of minimum potential for blood backflow or air embolism<br>Reduced risk of bacterial migration after tissue adheres to Dacron cuff or Vitacuff<br>Easily repaired<br>Easy to use for self-administered IV infusions | Requires weekly irrigation with normal saline<br>Must keep exit site dry<br>Heavy activity restricted until tissue adheres to cuff<br>Risk of infection still present<br>Protrudes outside body; susceptible to damage from sharp instruments and may be pulled out; can affect body image<br>Patient/family must learn catheter care |
| **Implanted Ports (Port-A-Cath, Infus-A-Port, Mediport, Norport, Groshong Port)** | | |
| Totally implantable metal or plastic device that consists of self-sealing injection port with top or side access with preconnected or attachable silicone catheter that is placed in large blood vessel | Reduced risk of infection<br>Placed completely under the skin; therefore cannot be pulled out or damaged<br>No maintenance care and reduced cost for family<br>Heparinized monthly and after each infusion to maintain patency (Groshong port only requires saline)<br>No limitations on regular physical activity, including swimming<br>Dressing only needed when port is accessed with Huber needle that is not removed<br>No or only slight change in body appearance (slight bulge on chest) | Must pierce skin for access; pain with insertion of needle; can use local anesthetic (EMLA) or intradermal buffered lidocaine before accessing port<br>Special noncoring needle (Huber) with straight or angled design must be used to inject into port<br>Skin preparation needed before injection<br>Hard to manipulate for self-administered infusions<br>Catheter may dislodge from port, especially if child "plays" with port site (twiddler syndrome)<br>Vigorous contact sports generally not allowed |

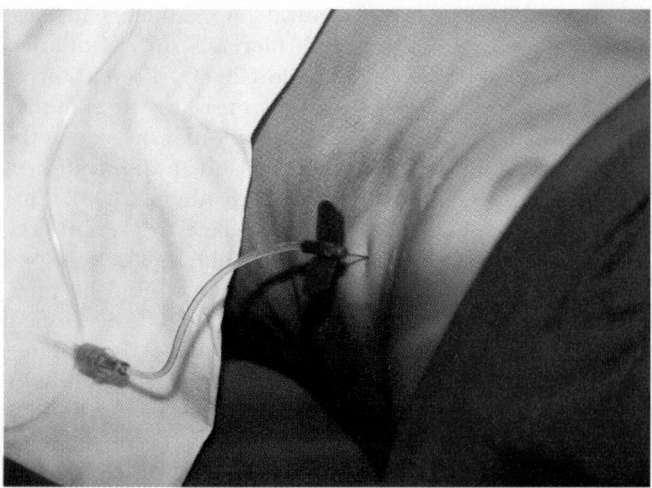

**Fig. 28-10** Implanted venous access device with Huber needle placement.

1996). Incidence rates vary, ranging from 7% to greater than 30% in some studies (Andrew and others, 1995; Kenney, David, and Bensoussan, 1996; Korones and others, 1996). Small thrombi at the tip of the catheter can usually be prevented with regular heparin flushes and, if present, lysed with a thrombolytic solution. The most common drug used to treat catheter-related thrombi was urokinase. In 1999 the FDA issued a mandate that ceased its distribution and found a significant risk of contamination. Tissue plasminogen activator, or t-PA (alteplase), is used for the treatment of thrombus-related catheter occlusions (Haire and Herbst, 2000).

Small thrombi can usually be detected if the nurse cannot easily flush or draw blood from the line. When there is a possibility of thrombus, fluoroscopy should be performed.

Larger thrombi outside of the catheter may require removal and anticoagulant therapy (Moureau, 2000). Symptoms of large thrombi include signs of superior vena cava occlusion, such as facial swelling and cyanosis, distended neck veins, and swelling of the upper arm.

### Parent/Child Teaching

Regardless of which catheter is used, the child and family are taught the care and management of the device with practice under supervision. It can be frightening to both child and parents to know that the catheter tip is situated near the heart. They need reassurance that with reasonable care they will do no harm to the apparatus. It is often useful to introduce the family to other children and families who are using central venous catheters successfully and with whom they can share concerns and helpful tips regarding care and management. This sharing is especially valuable for teenage patients. Because teenagers usually have a positive attitude toward use of the catheter, it is beneficial for them to share their experiences with adolescents who face the prospects of catheter placement.

Parents of children who engage in outside activities, go to school, or are otherwise under the supervision of another adult should inform the teacher, school nurse, coach, and baby-sitter about the presence of the central venous catheter. Vigorous contact sports, such as football, soccer, and hockey, are generally not allowed. A written information sheet concerning the VAD, including its purpose, pertinent facts about any restrictions for the child, and directions related to management of the device, should be provided for their reference. Grandparents and other family members who care for the child are taught the care and management of the catheter by the nurse or the parents.

Procedures and published standards for catheter care vary widely among organizations, and there is no evidence that one method is superior over another. For example, some advocate covering the healed catheter site with a dressing; others do not. All companies that manufacture central catheters have patient and professional teaching kits. The user should become thoroughly familiar with the specific device selected for use.*

The catheter is not a deterrent to most activities, including showers or tub bathing. However, the practitioner is consulted before activities such as swimming or physical contact sports are attempted. Swimming is usually prohibited but may be allowed in certain situations. If the exit site is healed and the cuff adheres to the tissue, a transparent dressing can be placed over the catheter and exit site, and swimming may be permitted for a limited time, such as 1 hour or less, in a chlorinated pool. Most contact sports are prohibited because of the possibility of the catheter being hit or pulled. A protective vest can prevent active children from accidentally dislodging the catheter.†

**NURSING TIP** A pocket sewn on the inside of a T-shirt provides a place in which to coil the catheter line while the child is at play if a dressing is not used. A commercial elastic vest is also available.†

Family members need to know the signs of infection and an occluded catheter. Signs of a localized infection are redness, swelling, and pain at the vein entry site. Bacteremia is a serious complication that produces fever, chills, general malaise, and an ill appearance. Uncapping can be prevented by taping the cap securely to the catheter and the clamped line to the dressing. Leaks can be prevented by using a smooth-edged clamp only. Parents are cautioned to keep scissors away from the child to prevent accidental cutting of the catheter. If the catheter leaks, they are instructed to tape it above the leak and then clamp the catheter at the taped site. The child should be taken to the practitioner as soon as possible to prevent infection or clotting following a catheter leak.

**NURSING ALERT** If a central venous catheter is accidentally removed, apply pressure to the *entry* site to the vein, not the exit site on the skin (Marcoux, Fisher, and Wong, 1990).

---

*Home care instructions for caring for a central venous catheter or an intermittent infusion device are available in Wong DL, Hess CS: *Wong and Whaley's clinical manual of pediatric nursing*, ed 5, St Louis, 2000, Mosby.
†The Security Vest is available from Advanced Patient Devices, 3564 Sabaka Trail, Verona, WI 53593, (800) 547-6412, fax: (608) 833-6694; www.cathetervest.com.

Children may benefit from the implanted ports, which consist of a small, circular "port of entry" that is placed under the skin (while the patient is under local or general anesthesia) over a bony prominence to provide a stable surface, usually under the distal third of the clavicle. A tunnel is created from the port to the point where the catheter enters a central vein leading to the entrance to the right atrium. Medication or other solution is injected with a special needle through the skin into the port. The device can remain situated indefinitely. Adolescents who are highly concerned about body image and may be troubled by the visible central venous catheter often prefer this method of venous access. One care consideration of an infusion port is that it requires repeated skin punctures, which may make it less acceptable to children. The use of a topical anesthetic, EMLA, can make the puncture painless (Miser and others, 1994). (See Atraumatic Care box on p. 1149.)

## Total Parenteral Nutrition (TPN)

TPN, also known as intravenous alimentation or hyperalimentation, provides for the total nutritional needs of infants or children whose lives are threatened because feeding by way of the gastrointestinal tract is impossible, inadequate, or hazardous. Common conditions for which TPN is used therapeutically include chronic intestinal obstruction from peritoneal sepsis or adhesions, bowel fistulas, inadequate intestinal length, chronic nonremitting severe diarrhea, extensive body burns, and abdominal tumors treated by surgery, irradiation, and chemotherapy. TPN may also be initiated prophylactically when prolonged starvation is expected.

Hyperalimentation therapy involves IV infusion of highly concentrated solutions of protein, glucose, and other nutrients. The hyperalimentation solution is infused through conventional tubing with a special filter attached to remove particulate matter or microorganisms that may have contaminated the solution. A solution of glucose, lipids, and other nutrients can be mixed together in a bag and delivered through a volumetric pump. The highly concentrated solutions require infusion into a vessel with sufficient volume and turbulence to allow for rapid dilution. The wide-diameter vessels selected are the superior vena cava and innominate or intrathoracic subclavian veins approached by way of the external or internal jugular veins. In some situations the inferior vena cava from a femoral vein serves as an alternative route. Central VADs are ideal for long-term and home TPN (HTPN).

The highly irritating nature of concentrated glucose precludes the use of the small peripheral veins in most instances. However, dilute glucose-protein hydrolysates that are appropriate for infusing into peripheral veins are being used with increasing frequency.

The major nursing responsibilities are the same as for any IV therapy: control of sepsis, monitoring of infusion rate, and assessment of the patient. The TPN solution must be prepared under rigid aseptic conditions best accomplished by specially trained technicians. In some institutions the solution and tubing are changed and the infusion site is redressed by specially trained nurses using meticulous aseptic precautions.

General assessments such as vital signs, intake and output measurements, daily weights, and checking results of laboratory tests facilitate early detection of infection or fluid and electrolyte imbalance. Additional amounts of $K^+$ and $Na^+$ are often required in hyperalimentation; therefore observation for signs of $K^+$ or $Na^+$ deficit or excess is part of nursing care. This is rarely a problem except in children with reduced renal function or metabolic defects.

The infusion is maintained at a constant rate by means of an infusion pump to ensure a continuous rate of infusion. This requires accurate calculation of the rate required to deliver a measured amount in a given length of time. The hyperalimentation infusion rate should not be increased or decreased without the practitioner being made aware, because alterations can cause hyperglycemia or hypoglycemia.

Hyperglycemia may occur during the first day or two as the child adapts to the high-glucose load of the hyperalimentation solution. Although it occurs infrequently, insulin may be required to assist the body's adjustment to the hyperglycemia. When this occurs, nursing responsibilities include blood glucose testing. To prevent hypoglycemia at the time hyperalimentation is discontinued, the rate of infusion is decreased gradually. The high concentration of glucose may produce an osmotic diuresis with the risk of hypertonic dehydration.

Some children will use cyclic TPN after they are stable on the formulation. This procedure allows for TPN to be administered a certain number of hours during the day, then cycle off for a prescribed amount of time. This process allows the child to be off the machines for a number of hours. It is usually done during waking hours so that the patient and family can enjoy the freedom of being off the pumps. Cycling also allows the liver to rest for a period of time and is believed to prevent TPN-induced liver damage (Hwang, Lue, and Chen 2000).

Because many children are treated with hyperalimentation regimens for long periods, it is especially important to be attuned to developmental needs. An infant stimulation program is initiated as early as feasible to prevent developmental delays. (See Developmental Intervention and Care, Chapter 10.) Delays in the areas of gross motor and language skills are observed most frequently in infants receiving long-term TPN (greater than 3 months), which may be caused by reduced mobility and social interaction. (See Feeding Resistance, Chapter 10.) The program is maintained throughout the hospital stay and extended into the home, where home hyperalimentation is implemented. In most instances, children achieve a satisfactory developmental level by 2 years of age.

### Complications

Complications from TPN are numerous, and a major nursing responsibility is to prevent these when possible and to be alert to signs of their development. Complications either (1) are related to the infusate (metabolic complications) or (2) result from the presence of the indwelling catheter.

Metabolic complications are associated with the infant's or child's capacity for the various components of the hyperalimentation solution. Excessive intake of any of the components will create an imbalance, such as hyperglycemia, azotemia, acid-base disorders, anemia, bone demineralization, vitamin and mineral deficiencies, hyperosmotic dehydration and coma, fluid overload, and a variety of electrolyte imbalances.

Liver disease is the most important gastrointestinal complication in pediatric populations. The cause is obscure, but liver disease appears to be more prevalent in preterm infants who have minimum enteral feedings and who were begun on TPN at an early age. Affected children develop cholestasis, hepatocellular necrosis, and, in advanced disease, cirrhosis or hepatic failure. Manifestations include hepatomegaly, jaundice, and elevated serum transaminase, bilirubin, and alkaline phosphatase levels, which become evident approximately 2 weeks after initiation of TPN. Cholelithiasis is an uncommon but possible occurrence in pediatric patients. Therefore children receiving TPN should be assessed periodically for signs and symptoms of cholelithiasis or cholecystitis.

Catheter-related complications include those involving catheter placement, such as pneumothorax, hemothorax, perforation, catheter dislodgment, and thrombus formation. However, the major complication associated with the catheter is infection: infection at the catheter entrance site, catheter "seeding" sepsis, venous thrombosis with infection and embolization, and endocarditis.

Pediatric TPN generally has a higher concentration of calcium and phosphorus. This makes some TPN solutions more susceptible to precipitation. Fibrinolytic agents, such as t-PA (alteplase), have no effect on precipitate (Hooke, 2000). Nonthrombolytic occlusions such as precipitations can be cleared successfully using hydrochloric acid (pH less than 7) and sodium hydroxide (pH greater than 7) (Reed and Phillips, 1996).

### Home Total Parenteral Nutrition (HTPN)

Some children require total parenteral nutrition over an extended period, often weeks or months. For many children, HTPN is an alternative for long-term hospitalization. The child must be one who is unable to maintain adequate enteral alimentation, has no medical problems requiring hospitalization, has a parent who is able to manage the home care (or is an older child who can participate in his or her own care), and has the potential to benefit from the treatment (Forchielli, Paolucci, and Lo, 1999; Puntis, 1995).

Before a home care program can be implemented, a thorough assessment is made of the family and the home situation. The parents must be capable of performing the technical aspects of the procedure and be able to adapt to the changes inherent in the home program. Psychosocial readiness of the family, family support systems, and practical considerations are investigated, including availability of a pharmacy to prepare the hyperalimentation solution, a practitioner to handle day-to-day emergency needs, and a cooperating insurance company or agency (because of the exorbitant cost of maintaining long-term parenteral feeding). In most areas home health care agencies are able to assume the major management of HTPN for families.

Before beginning HTPN, the parents are prepared for taking over the child's total care. Teaching may occur in the hospital or at home, depending on the policies of insurance companies and the home health care agency following the family. The parents assume full responsibility for the child's care, with help being readily available when needed.

The emotional and economic benefits of this approach are readily apparent. The familiar environment and the atmosphere of normality are enormously therapeutic, and the stress of separation is avoided. With support from health professionals, a home care program can be the ideal alternative to hospitalization of a capable, motivated family of a child who requires TPN.

The family is encouraged to make the home life as normal as possible for the child within the limits imposed by the therapy. For example, having the infant or child at the table during mealtimes and including the child in family activities contribute to a normal family atmosphere (Barks, 1996). Quiet play should be encouraged during the HTPN, and it may be helpful to have a potty chair available at the bedside. Toddlers who may crawl out of a crib may need to be protected from becoming tangled or catching IV tubing on the rail. It is also important to make certain the child's dental care is not neglected.

The family is referred to community agencies that provide support and practical assistance. The ***Oley Foundation,**** a nonprofit research and education organization, maintains a national registry of persons receiving HTPN and publishes a bimonthly newsletter for consumers, families, clinicians, and home care services.

---

\*214 Hun Memorial, A28, Albany Medical Center, Albany, NY 12208, (800) 776-6539 (USA), (518) 262-5079 (Outside USA); www.wizrak.net/oleyfdn/.

---

## KEY POINTS

- Water distribution and maintenance are determined by solutes, physical forces, internal control mechanisms, and boundary organs through which external exchanges occur.
- Infants are subject to fluid depletion because of their relatively greater surface area, their high rate of metabolism, and their immature kidney function.

- Management of fluid volume disturbances focuses on the following areas: volume of body fluids, osmolality, hydrogen ion status, electrolyte deficits, and disturbances in mineral skeleton and body fluid equilibrium.
- Fluid disturbances experienced by children are dehydration, water intoxication, and edema.
- Dehydration may be classified as isotonic, hypotonic, or hypertonic.

- Parenteral fluid therapy is initiated to meet ongoing daily physiologic losses, restore previous deficits, and replace ongoing abnormal losses.
- Fluid gains or losses from the interstitial spaces depend on the following factors: venous hydrostatic pressure, colloidal osmotic pressure, semipermeable capillary wall, tissue tension, and lymphatic flow.
- Edema formation is caused by increased venous pressure, capillary permeability, diminished plasma proteins, lymphatic obstruction, or decreased tissue tension.
- Disturbances in acid-base balance are respiratory acidosis, respiratory alkalosis, metabolic acidosis, and metabolic alkalosis.
- Respiratory acidosis may result from factors that depress the respiratory center, factors that affect the lungs, and factors that interfere with the bellows action of the chest wall.
- Respiratory alkalosis results primarily from central nervous system stimulation.
- Metabolic acidosis is a lowered plasma pH caused by any process that reduces base bicarbonate concentration or increases metabolic acid formation.
- Metabolic alkalosis is an elevated plasma pH that occurs when there is a reduction of hydrogen ion concentration or an excess of base bicarbonate.
- Nursing assessment of fluid and electrolyte disturbances entails observation of general appearance, vital signs, daily weights, intake and output measurement, and review of relevant laboratory results.
- Long-term venous access is accomplished by intermittent intravenous devices; central venous catheters, including short-term (subclavian, femoral, and jugular), short-term to moderate-term (peripherally inserted central catheters), and long-term (tunneled) catheters and ports; or implanted ports.
- Intravenous alimentation provides for total nutritional needs when feeding via the gastrointestinal tract is impossible, inadequate, or hazardous.
- Before initiating home total parenteral nutrition, the following factors are assessed: parents' ability to perform the procedure, existence of family support systems, availability of nearby pharmacies, and insurance coverage.

# REFERENCES

Aker J, O'Sullivan C: The selection and administration of perioperative intravenous fluids for the pediatric patient, *J Perianes Nurs* 13(3):172-181, 1998.

Andrew M and others: A cross-sectional study of catheter-related thrombosis in children receiving total parenteral nutrition at home, *J Pediatr* 126(3):358-363, 1995.

Barks L: Enteral nutrition. I. When a child needs to get meals by tube, *Except Parent* 26(8):63-65, 1996.

Behrman RE, Kliegman RM, Jenson HB, editors: *Nelson textbook of pediatrics*, ed 16, Philadelphia, 2000, WB Saunders.

Catudal R: Pediatric IV therapy: actual practice, *J Vascular Access Devices* 42:27-29, 1999.

Centers for Disease Control and Prevention: Hyponatremic seizures among infants fed with commercial bottled drinking water: Wisconsin, 1993, *MMWR* 43(35):641-643, 1994.

Crews BE and others: Effects of varying intervals between heparin flushes on pediatric catheter longevity, *Pediatr Nurs* 23(1):87-91, 1997.

Crosby CT, Mares A: Skin antisepsis: past, present, and future, *J Vascular Access Devices* 6(1):26-31, 2001.

Danek GD, Noris EM: Pediatric IV catheters: efficacy of saline flush, *Pediatr Nurs* 18(2):111-113, 1992.

Dillion-Dolan CJD: Diarrhea/loose stool. In Fox JA, editor: *Primary health care of children*, St Louis, 1997, Mosby.

Donaldson JS and others: Peripherally inserted central venous catheters: US-guided vascular access in pediatric patients, *Radiology* 197(2):542-544, 1995.

Dubick MA, Holcomb JB: A review of intraosseous vascular access: current status

and military application, *Mil Med* 165(7):552-559, 2000.

Fann B: Fluid and electrolyte balance in the pediatric patient, *J Intraven Nurs* 21(3):153-159, 1998.

Ferri F, Alario A: Acid-base disturbances. In Alario A, editor: *Practical Guide to the care of the pediatric patient*, St Louis, 1997, Mosby.

Finberg L, Kravath RE, Hellerstein S: *Water and electrolytes in pediatrics: physiology, pathology, and treatment*, Philadelphia, 1993, WB Saunders.

Forchielli MS, Paolucci G, Lo CW: Total parenteral nutrition and home nutrition: an effective combination to sustain malnourished children with cancer, *Nutr Rev* 57(1):15-20, 1999.

Frey AM: Pediatric peripherally inserted central catheter program report, *J Intraven Nurs* 18(6):280-291, 1995.

Frey AM: Intravenous therapy in children. In Hankins J and others, editors: *Infusion therapy in clinical practice*, ed 2, Philadelphia, 2001, WB Saunders.

Ganong WF: *Review of medical physiology*, East Norwalk, CT, 1995, Appleton & Lange.

Goodwin ML, Carlson I: The peripherally inserted central catheter, *J Intraven Nurs* 16(2):92-103, 1993.

Gorelick MH, Shaw KN, Murphy KO: Validity and reliability of clinical signs in the diagnosis of dehydration in children, *Pediatrics* 99(5):724, 1997.

Graves SM and others: Saline replaces heparin as capping solution, *Child Nurs* spring, 1997.

Guyton AC, Hall JE: *Textbook of medical physiology*, ed 10, Philadelphia, 2000, WB Saunders.

Gyr P and others: Double blind comparison of heparin and saline flush solutions in

maintenance of peripheral infusion devices, *Pediatr Nurs* 21(4):383-389, 1995.

Hadaway L: Vascular access in home care: 1998 update, *Infusion* 5(1):20-28, 1998.

Haire WB, Herbst SL: Use of alteplase (T-PA) for the management of thrombotic catheter dysfunction: guidelines from a consensus conference of the National Association of Vascular Access Networks, *Nutr Clin Pract* 15:265-275, 2000.

Hanrahan KS, Kleiber C, Fagan C: Evaluation of saline for IV locks in children, *Pediatr Nurs* 20(6):549-552, 1994.

Harris JL, Maguire D: Developing a protocol to prevent and treat pediatric central venous catheter occlusions, *J Intraven Nurs* 22(4):194-198, 1999.

Heilskov MA and others: A randomized trial of heparin and saline for maintaining intravenous locks in neonates, *J Soc Pediatr Nurs* 3(3):111-116, 1998.

Heitz U, Horne M: *Pocket guide to fluid, electrolyte, and acid-base balance*, ed 4, St Louis, 2001, Mosby.

Held JL: Correcting fluid and electrolyte imbalances, *Nursing* 25(4):71, 1995.

Holliday M: The evolution of therapy for dehydration: should deficit therapy still be taught? *Pediatrics* 98(2):171-177, 1996.

Hooke C: Recombinant tissue plasminogen activator for central venous access device occlusion, *J Pediatr Oncol Nurs* 17(3):174-178, 2000.

Hwang TL, Lue MC, Chen LL: Early use of cyclic TPN prevents further deteriorations of liver functions for the TPN patients with impaired liver function, *Hepatogastoenterology* 47(35):1347-1350, 2000.

Infusion Nurses Society: *Policies and procedures for infusion nursing*, Norwood, MA, 2000a,

The Society, pp 15-16, 25, 56, 58, 67, 98-99, 124-126.

Infusion Nurses Society: Revised infusion nursing standards of practice, *J Intraven Nurs* 23(6, suppl):S17, S39, S41, S45, S49-50, S60, 2000b.

Jones GR: A practical guide to evaluation and treatment of infections in patients with central venous catheters, *J Intraven Nurs* 21(5S):S134-S142, 1998.

Jospen N, Forbes G: Fluids and electrolytes: clinical aspects, *Pediatr Rev* 17(11):395-404, 1996.

Kee J, Paulanka B: *Handbook of fluid, electrolyte and acid-base imbalances,* Albany, 2000, Delmar.

Kenney BD, David M, Bensoussan AL: Anticoagulation without catheter removal in children with catheter-related central vein thrombosis, *J Pediatr Surg* 31(6):816-818, 1996.

Kleiber C and others: Heparin vs saline for peripheral IV locks in children, *Pediatr Nurs* 19(4):405-409, 1993.

Korones DN and others: Right atrial thrombi in children with cancer and indwelling catheters, *J Pediatr* 128:841-846, 1996.

Ledwith C: Fluids and electrolytes. In Merenstein G, Kaplan D, Rosenberg A, editors: *Handbook of pediatrics,* Stamford, CT, 1997, Appleton & Lange.

Le Duk K: Efficacy of normal saline solution versus heparin solution for maintaining patency of peripheral intravenous catheters in children, *J Emerg Nurs* 23(4):306-309, 1997

Lee WE, Vallino LM: Intravenous insertion site protection: moisture accumulation in intravenous site protectors, *J Intraven Nurs* 29(4):194-197, 1996.

Lewis DA, Nocton JJ: *On call pediatrics,* Philadelphia, 1997, WB Saunders.

Maki DG: Infections caused by intravascular devices used for infusion therapy: pathogenesis, prevention, and management. In Bisno AL, Waldvogel FA, editors: *Infections associated with indwelling medical devices,* ed 2, Washington, 1994, American Society for Microbiology.

Maki DG, Ringer M: Risk-factors for infusion-related phlebitis with small peripheral venous catheters: a ranodmized controlled

trial, *Ann Intern Med* 114(10):845-854, 1991.

Maki DG, Ringer M, Alvarado CJ: Prospective randomized trial of providone-iodine, alcohol, and chorhexidine for prevention of infection associated with central venous and arterial catheters, *Lancet* 338(8763): 339-343, 1991.

Marcoux C, Fisher S, Wong D: Central venous access devices in children, *Pediatr Nurs* 16:123-133, 1990.

Masoorli S: Removing a PICC?: proceed with caution, *Nursing* 28(3):56-57, 1998.

McEntee M: 1997. *Fluids and electrolytes,* Albany, NY, 1997, Delmar.

Metheny N: *Fluid and electrolyte balance,* ed 4, Philadelphia, PA, 2000, Lippincott.

Meyers A: Modern management of acute diarrhea and dehydration in children, *Am Fam Physician* 51(5):1103-1115, 1995.

Miser AW and others: Trial of a topically administered local anesthetic (EMLA cream) for pain relief during central venous port accesses in children with cancer, *J Pain Symptom Manage* 9(4): 259-264, 1994.

Montgomery LA and others: Guidelines for IV infiltrations in pediatric patients, *Pediatr Nurs* 25(2):167-180, 1999.

*Morris v Children's Hospital Medical Center,* 1992, Medica Press.

Moureau N: Practical access: a back-to-basics review of intravenous therapy, *J Vascular Access Devices* 4(2 suppl):1-4, 1999.

Moureau NL: Training for turbulence, *J Vascular Access Devices* 5(3):S2, 2000.

Mudge B, Forcier D, Slattery MJ: Patency of 24-gauge peripheral intermittent infusion devices: a comparison of heparin and saline flush solutions, *J Pediatr Nurs* 24(2):142-149, 1998.

National Association of Vascular Access Networks: Position paper: use of safety devices and sharps injury prevention, *J Vascular Access Devices* 5(1):7-8, 2000.

Noble M: Fluid and electrolyte imbalances. In Soud T, Rogers J, editors: *Manual of pediatric emergency nursing,* St Louis, 1998, Mosby.

Oncology Nursing Society: *Cancer chemotherapy guidelines and recommendations for practice,* ed 2, Pittsburgh, 1998, Oncology Nursing Press.

Orenstein R: The benefits and limitations of needle protectors and needleless intravenous systems, *J Intraven Nurs* 22(3): 122-127, 1999.

Paisley MK and others: The use of heparin and normal saline flushes in neonatal intravenous catheters, *J Pediatr Nurs* 23(5):521-527, 1997.

Pearson M: The Hospital Infection Control Practices Advisory Committee: Guidelines for prevention of intravascular-device-related infections, *Infect Control Hosp Epidemiol* 17:438-473, 1995.

Pearson M: Special Communication: Guidelines for prevention of intravascular device-related infections. I. Intravascular device-related infections: an overview; II. Recommendations for the prevention of nosocomial intravascular device-related infections, *Am J Infect Control* 24(4): 262-293, 1996.

Petit J, Hughes K: Neonatal intravenous therapy practices, *J Vascular Access Devices* 4(2):7-16, 1999.

Phillips KG: Swimming and water intoxication in infants, *Can Med Assoc J* 1136-1147, 1987 (letter).

Puntis JW: Home parenteral nutrition, *Arch Dis Child* 72(2):186-190, 1995.

Rabin N: Fluid and electrolyte management of the pediatric surgical patient. In Wise B and others, editors: *Nursing care of the general pediatric surgical patient,* Gaithersburg, MD, 2000, Aspen.

Racadio JM and others: Pediatric peripherally inserted central catheters: complication rates related to catheter tip location, *Pediatrics* 107(2):E28, 2001.

Reed T, Phillips S: Management of central venous catheter occlusions and repairs, *J Intraven Nurs* 19(6):289-294, 1996.

Schierholz J and others: Central venous catheters and bloodstream infection, *JAMA* 26(4):477-478, 2000.

Tacconelli E, Tumbarello MCR: Central venous catheter blood stream infection, *JAMA* 26(4):478-479, 2000.

Wiener ES, Albanese CT: Venous access in pediatric patients, *J Intraven Nurs* 21(5S): S122-S131, 1998.

Wilson D: Starting neonatal IVs: practical tips, *Mother Baby J* 5(1):11-19, 2000.

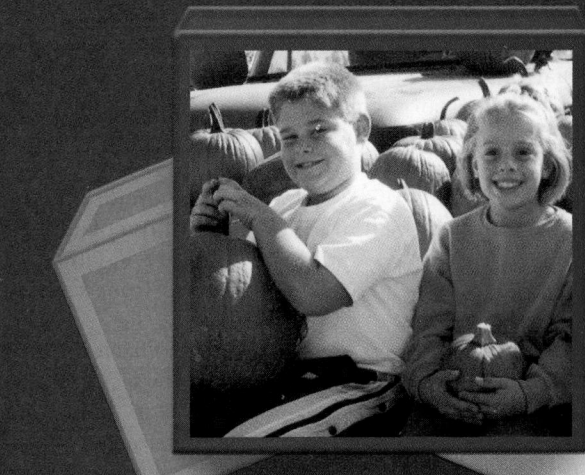

# Conditions That Produce Fluid and Electrolyte Imbalance

## Chapter Outline

GASTROINTESTINAL (GI)
DISORDERS, 1207
Diarrhea, 1207
Acute Diarrheal Disease, 1208
*Nursing Care Plan: The Child with Acute*
*Diarrhea (Gastroenteritis), 1215*
Chronic Diarrheal Disease, 1216
Intractable Diarrhea of Infancy, 1216
Chronic Nonspecific Diarrhea (CNSD), 1216
Vomiting, 1217
SHOCK STATES, 1219
Shock, 1219
Septic Shock, 1222

Anaphylaxis, 1224
Toxic Shock Syndrome (TSS), 1226
BURNS, 1227
Overview, 1227
Burn Wound Characteristics, 1228
    Extent of Injury, 1228
    Depth of Injury, 1228
    Severity of Injury, 1229
Pathophysiology, 1230
    Local Response, 1230
    Systemic Responses, 1231
    Complications, 1233
Therapeutic Management, 1234

Emergency Care, 1234
Management of Minor Burns, 1235
Management of Major Burns, 1236
Management of the Burn Wound, 1238
Nursing Considerations, 1242
    Acute Phase, 1243
    Management and Rehabilitative
        Phases, 1243
    Prevention of Burn Injury, 1248
*Nursing Care Plan: The Child with Burns:*
    *Management and Rehabilitative*
    *Stages, 1249*
Future Research Needs, 1253

## Related Topics

The Child with Cardiovascular Dysfunction,
    Ch. 34
The Child with Gastrointestinal Dysfunction,
    Ch. 33
Diaper Dermatitis, Ch. 13

Disorders Affecting the Skin, Ch. 18
Family-Centered Care of the Child During
    Illness and Hospitalization, Ch. 26
Family-Centered Care of the Child with
    Chronic Illness or Disability, Ch. 22

Family-Centered Home Care, Ch. 25
Injury Prevention: Infant, Ch. 12; Toddler,
    Ch. 14; School-Age Child, Ch. 17
Intestinal Parasitic Diseases, Ch. 16
Pain Assessment; Pain Management, Ch. 26

## GASTROINTESTINAL (GI) DISORDERS

### Diarrhea

It is estimated that 1.3 billion episodes of diarrhea occur worldwide each year in children. Approximately 24% of all deaths in children living in developing countries are related to diarrhea and dehydration (Endsley and Galbraith, 1998). Diarrhea is classified as acute or chronic. *Acute diarrhea* is the leading cause of illness in children younger than 5 years of age; each year 400 children die from complications of diarrhea in the United States, and in 1998 diarrhea was asso-

ciated with approximately 220,000 hospitalizations for children under 5 years of age (Endsley and Galbraith, 1998). Most cases of acute diarrhea are caused by infectious agents, including viral, bacterial, and parasitic pathogens.

*Chronic diarrhea* is usually caused by conditions such as malabsorption syndromes, inflammatory bowel disease, immune deficiency, food allergy, lactose intolerance, and chronic, nonspecific diarrhea. It may also be a result of inadequate management of acute infectious diarrhea.

Diarrhea is difficult to define because stool frequency and consistency vary among individuals. Generally diarrhea is present when there is an increase in stool frequency and an increased water content. Diarrhea varies by severity, duration, presence of blood or mucus, the age of the child, and the child's nutritional status.

■ Nicole M. Sevier, MSN, RN, CPNP, and Nancy E. Kline, PhD, RN, CPNP, revised this chapter.

## Pathophysiology

Diarrhea is caused by abnormal intestinal water and electrolyte transport. The transport of fluid and electrolytes in the developing GI tract is related to the child's age. The intestinal mucosa of the young infant is more permeable to water than that of an older child. Therefore in young infants with increased intestinal luminal osmolality due to diarrhea, more fluid and electrolytes are lost than in older children (Box 29-1). Diarrhea results from several pathophysiologic processes.

*Secretory diarrhea* is generally due to bacterial enterotoxins that stimulate fluid and electrolyte secretion from the mucosal crypt cell, the principal secretory cells of the small intestine. *Cytotoxic diarrhea* is characterized by viral destruction of the mucosal cells of the villi of the small intestine. This results in a smaller intestinal surface area, with a decreased capacity for fluid and electrolyte absorption. *Osmotic diarrhea* is commonly seen in malabsorption syndromes, such as lactose intolerance, because the intestine cannot absorb nutrients or electrolytes. *Dysenteric diarrhea* is associated with an inflammation of the mucosa and submucosa in the ileum and colon caused by infectious agents such as *Campylobacter, Salmonella,* or *Shigella.* Edema, mucosal bleeding, and leukocyte infiltration occur.

## Acute Diarrheal Disease

Acute diarrhea, a sudden increase in frequency and a change in consistency of stools, is often caused by an infectious agent in the GI tract. It may also be associated with upper respiratory or urinary tract infections. Antibiotic therapy or laxative use can also lead to acute diarrhea in children (Box 29-2). Acute diarrhea is usually self-limited (less than 14 days). Specific treatment is not required if dehydration does not create a serious complication.

*Acute infectious diarrhea (infectious gastroenteritis)* is caused by a wide variety of viral, bacterial, and parasitic pathogens. In the United States it is estimated that diarrhea results in 2.1 to 3.7 physician visits per year (Waters and others, 2000). Infants and young children are at a high risk for the development of dehydration and malnutrition—the two major consequences of diarrhea.

## Etiology

Most pathogens that cause diarrhea are spread by the fecal-oral route through contaminated food or water, or they are spread from person to person, especially where there is close contact (e.g., daycare centers). Lack of clean water, crowding, poor hygiene, nutritional deficiency, and poor sanitation are major risk factors, especially for bacterial or parasitic pathogens. The increased frequency and severity of diarrheal disease in infants is also related to age-specific alterations in susceptibility to pathogens. The immune system of infants has not previously been exposed to many pathogens and has not acquired protective antibodies (Box 29-3).

In the United States, *rotavirus* is the most common pathogen identified in young children who are hospitalized for diarrhea and dehydration; each year it accounts for up to 55,000 hospitalizations and causes 20 to 40 deaths (Zimmerman and others, 2001). In addition, rotavirus is a sig-

---

**Box 29-2** ■ ■ ■
**Causes of Acute Diarrhea**

**INFECTION AND PARASITIC INFESTATION**
**Bacteria:** *Salmonella, Shigella, Campylobacter, Escherichia coli, Yersinia, Aeromonas, Clostridium difficile, Staphylococcus aureus*
**Viruses:** Rotavirus, Norwalk virus, small and round viruses, adenovirus, Pestivirus, Astrovirus, Calicivirus, parvovirus
**Parasites:** *Giardia lamblia, Cryptosporidium, Isospora belli, Microsporidium, Strongyloides, Entamoeba histolytica*

**ASSOCIATED WITH:**
Upper respiratory tract infections
Urinary tract infections
Otitis media

**DIETARY CAUSES**
Overfeeding
Introduction of new foods
Reinstituting milk too soon after diarrheal episode
Osmotic diarrhea from excess sugar in formula or juice
Excessive ingestion of sorbitol or fructose

**MEDICATIONS**
Antibiotics
Laxatives

**TOXIC CAUSES**
Ingestion of:
Heavy metals (arsenic, lead, mercury)
Organic phosphates

**FUNCTIONAL CAUSES**
Irritable bowel syndrome

**OTHER CAUSES**
Necrotizing enterocolitis
Hirschsprung enterocolitis

---

**Box 29-1** ■ ■ ■
**Consequences of Fluid and Electrolyte Loss**

**DEHYDRATION**
Voluminous losses of fluid in frequent, watery stools
Losses when there is also vomiting
Reduced fluid intake resulting from nausea or anorexia
Increased insensible losses from fever, hyperpnea, and, sometimes, high environmental temperature
Continued (although diminished) obligatory renal losses

**ELECTROLYTE IMBALANCE**
Losses of sodium, chloride, potassium, and, in some cases, bicarbonate
Inadequate replacement of electrolytes when hypotonic or hypertonic solutions are used

**METABOLIC ACIDOSIS**
Increased absorption of short-chain fatty acids produced in the colon from bacterial fermentation of unabsorbed dietary carbohydrates
Accumulation of lactic acid from tissue hypoxia secondary to hypovolemia
Loss of bicarbonate in stools
Ketosis from fat metabolism when glycogen stores are depleted in untreated diarrheal dehydration or inadequate carbohydrate intake; may result in malnutrition

nificant nosocomial pathogen. *Salmonella, Shigella,* and *Campylobacter* are the most commonly isolated bacterial pathogens, and *Giardia* and *Cryptosporidium* are the parasites that most commonly produce acute, infectious diarrhea (Table 29-1). (See Intestinal Parasitic Diseases, Chapter 16.)

**Other Causes of Acute Diarrhea.** In addition to enteropathogens, acute diarrhea in children may be associated with other diseases (e.g., human immunodeficiency virus [HIV] infection). Ingestion of laxatives will also produce acute diarrhea, and excessive ingestion of sorbitol and fructose in common foods such as apple juice or in gum or candy can cause osmotic dietary diarrhea from the poorly absorbed carbohydrate.

Antibiotics commonly cause diarrhea because they alter the normal intestinal flora; the decreased colonic bacteria

---

**Box 29-3 ■ ■ ■**
**Factors That Predispose to Diarrhea**

**Age.** As a general rule, the younger the child, the greater the susceptibility and the more severe the diarrhea. Diarrhea occurs more commonly in infancy, is a lesser threat in early childhood, and usually constitutes only a minor problem in older children.

**Impaired health.** Malnourished or immunocompromised children are more susceptible and tend to have more severe diarrhea.

**Environment.** Diarrhea occurs with greater frequency where there is crowding, substandard sanitation, poor facilities for preparation and refrigeration of food, and generally inadequate health care education. The frequency of diarrhea in infancy is closely related to the ingestion of contaminated milk; there is a lower incidence of diarrhea in breast-fed infants.

---

**TABLE 29-1**    Infectious causes of acute diarrhea

| Organism | Pathology | Characteristics | Comments |
|---|---|---|---|
| **Viral Agents** | | | |
| Rotavirus<br>  Incubation period:<br>    1-3 days | Invasion of epithelium of small bowel mucosa<br>Severely distorted mucosal architecture with atrophic mucosa and severe inflammatory changes<br>Decreased absorption of salt and water | Abrupt onset<br>Fever (38° C or above) lasting approximately 48 hours<br>Nausea/vomiting<br>Abdominal pain<br>Associated upper respiratory tract infection<br>Diarrhea may persist for more than a week | Incidence higher in cool weather (80% in winter)<br>Affects all age-groups; 6- to 24-month-old infants more vulnerable<br>Usually mild and self-limited<br>Important cause of nosocomial infections in hospitals and gastroenteritis in children attending daycare centers |
| Norwalk-like organisms<br>  Incubation period:<br>    1-3 days | Mechanism of effect unknown<br>Blunting of villi and inflammatory changes in lamina propria<br>Reduced enzymes | Fever<br>Loss of appetite<br>Nausea/vomiting<br>Abdominal pain<br>Diarrhea<br>Malaise | Source of infection: drinking water, recreation water, food (including shellfish)<br>Affects all ages<br>Self-limited (2-3 days) |
| **Bacterial Agents** | | | |
| Pathogenic *Escherichia coli*<br>  Incubation period:<br>    highly variable;<br>    depends on strain | Usually caused by enterotoxin production (small bowel)<br>Reduced absorption and increased secretion of fluids and electrolytes | Onset gradual or abrupt<br>Variable clinical manifestations<br>Most—green, watery diarrhea with blood and mucus; becomes explosive<br>Vomiting may be present from onset<br>Abdominal distention<br>Diarrhea<br>Fever, appears toxic | Incidence higher in summer<br>Usually interpersonal transmission but may transmit via inanimate objects<br>A cause of nursery epidemics<br>With symptomatic treatment only, may continue for weeks<br>Full breast-feeding has a protective effect<br>Symptoms generally subside in 3-7 days<br>Relapse rate approximately 20% |
| *Salmonella* groups (nontyphoidal)—gram-negative, nonencapsulated, nonsporulating<br>  Incubation period:<br>    6-72 hours for gastroenteritis (usually less than 24); 3-60 days for enteric fever (usually 7-14) | Penetration of lamina propria (small bowel and colon)<br>Local inflammation—no extensive destruction<br>Stimulation of intestinal fluid excretion<br>Systemic invasion of other sites | Rapid onset<br>Variable symptoms—mild to severe<br>Nausea, vomiting, and colicky abdominal pain followed by diarrhea, occasionally with blood and mucus<br>Fever<br>Hyperactive peristalsis and mild abdominal tenderness<br>Symptoms usually subside within 5 days<br>May have headache and cerebral manifestations (e.g., drowsiness, confusion, meningismus, or seizures)<br>Infants may be afebrile and nontoxic<br>May result in life-threatening septicemia and meningitis | Two thirds of patients are younger than 20 years of age; highest incidence in children younger than age 5 years, especially infants<br>Highest incidence occurs from July through October, lowest from January through April<br>Transmission primarily via contaminated food and drink—most from animal sources, including fowl, mammals, reptiles, and insects<br>Most common sources are poultry and eggs<br>In children—pets (e.g., dogs, cats, hamsters, and especially pet turtles)<br>Communicable as long as organisms are excreted |

*Continued*

**TABLE 29-1**   Infectious causes of acute diarrhea—cont'd

| Organism | Pathology | Characteristics | Comments |
|---|---|---|---|
| **Bacterial Agents—cont'd** | | | |
| *Salmonella typhi* | Rapid invasion of bloodstream from minor sites of inflammation<br>Marked inflammation and necrosis of intestinal mucosa and lymphatics | Variable in infants<br>Older children—irregular fever, headache, malaise, lethargy<br>Diarrhea occurs in 50% at early stage<br>Cough is common<br>In a few days fever rises and is consistent; fatigue, cough, abdominal pain, anorexia, and weight loss develop; diarrhea begins | Acute symptoms may persist for a week or more<br>Transmitted by contaminated food or water (primary), infected animals (e.g., pet turtles) |
| *Shigella* groups—gramnegative, nonmotile anaerobic bacilli<br>Incubation period: 1-7 days, usually 2-4 | Enterotoxin<br>Stimulates loss of fluids and electrolytes<br>Invasion of epithelium with superficial mucosal ulcerations<br>*Shigella dysenteriae* forms exotoxin | Onset variable but usually abrupt<br>Fever and cramping abdominal pain initially<br>Fever—may reach 40.5° C<br>Convulsions in approximately 10%—usually associated with fever<br>Patient appears sick<br>Headache, nuchal rigidity, delirium<br>Watery diarrhea with mucus and pus starts approximately 12-48 hours after onset<br>Stools preceded by abdominal cramps; tenesmus and straining follow<br>Symptoms usually subside in 5-10 days | Approximately 60% of cases in children younger than age 9 years, with more than one third between ages 1 and 4 years<br>Peak incidence in late summer<br>Transmitted directly or indirectly from infected persons<br>Communicable for 1-4 weeks<br>Self-limited disease<br>Treat with antibiotics<br>Severe dehydration and collapse can affect all patients<br>Acute symptoms may persist for a week or more |
| *Yersinia enterocolitica*<br>Incubation period: dose-dependent; 1-3 weeks | Oxidase−, urease+, nonlactase-fermenting, gram− rods | Diarrhea—may be bloody<br>Fever (>38.7° C)<br>Abdominal pain in right lower quadrant (RLQ)<br>Vomiting, diarrhea | Seen more commonly in winter<br>Majority in first 3 years of life<br>Transmitted by food and pets<br>Can resemble appendicitis<br>May be relapsing and last for weeks |
| *Campylobacter jejuni*<br>Incubation period: 1-7 days or longer | Precise mechanism unclear<br>Jejunum, ileum, and colon involvement<br>Extensive ulceration with hemorrhagic ileitis<br>Broadening and flattening of mucosa | Fever<br>Abdominal pain—often severe, cramping, periumbilical<br>Watery, profuse, foul-smelling diarrhea with blood<br>Vomiting | Person-to-person transmission<br>May be transmitted by pets (e.g., cat, dog, hamster)<br>Food (especially chicken) and waterborne transmission<br>Relapse possible<br>Most patients recover spontaneously<br>Antibiotics may speed recovery<br>Peak incidence in summer |
| *Vibrio cholerae* (cholera) groups<br>Incubation period: usually 2-3 days; range from few hours to 5 days | Enterotoxin causes increased secretion of chloride and possibly bicarbonate<br>Intestinal mucosa congested with enlarged lymph follicles<br>Intact mucosal surface | Sudden onset of profuse, watery diarrhea without cramping, tenesmus, or anal irritation, although children may complain of cramping<br>Stools are intermittent at first, then almost continuous<br>Stools are bloody with mucus | Rare in infants younger than 1 year old<br>Mortality high in both treated and untreated infants and small children<br>Transmitted via contaminated food and water<br>Attack confers immunity |
| *Clostridium difficile* | Toxin stimulates colonic secretion by damaging epithelium | Diarrhea with blood in stools | May cause pseudomembranous colitis<br>Follows antibiotic therapy |
| **Food Poisoning** | | | |
| *Staphylococcus*<br>Incubation period: 4-6 hours | Produces heat-stable enterotoxin | Nausea, vomiting<br>Severe abdominal cramps<br>Profuse diarrhea<br>Shock may occur in severe cases<br>May be a mild fever | Transferred via contaminated food—inadequately cooked or refrigerated (e.g., custards, mayonnaise, creamfilled or cream-topped desserts)<br>Self-limited; improvement apparent within 24 hours<br>Excellent prognosis |
| *Clostridium perfringens*<br>Incubation period: 8-24 hours, usually 8-12 | Produces heat-resistant and heat-sensitive toxins | Moderate to severe crampy, midepigastric pain | Self-limited illness<br>Transmission by commercial food products, most often meat and poultry |
| *Clostridium botulinum*<br>Incubation period: 12-26 hours (range, 6 hours to 8 days) | Highly potent neurotoxin | Nausea, vomiting<br>Diarrhea<br>Central nervous system (CNS) symptoms with curare-like effect<br>Dry mouth, dysphagia | Transmitted by contaminated food products<br>Variable severity—mild symptoms to rapidly fatal within a few hours<br>Antitoxin administration |

result in excessive malabsorbed carbohydrate and osmotic diarrhea (Vanderhoof and others, 1999). Antibiotics can also lead to colonization and toxin production by *Clostridium difficile,* which may cause diarrhea and pseudomembranous colitis (Levy and others, 2000).

## Clinical Manifestations

The severity of the diarrhea, including the frequency and consistency of stools, is variable and depends on the etiology and the patient. The most serious consequences of acute diarrheal disease are dehydration, electrolyte disturbances, and malnutrition. Dehydration may be mild, moderate, or severe. (See Chapter 28 for clinical signs of dehydration.) Metabolic acidosis may be present with severe diarrhea and dehydration. Malnutrition may contribute to the severity of the diarrhea or may be a consequence of diarrheal disease due to decreased dietary intake, malabsorption, and the catabolic response to infection. The metabolic rate in infants and children is higher than that of the adult, a difference that predisposes the younger patient to more rapid depletion of nutritional reserves during periods of malabsorption or diminished intake. Prolonged withholding of feeding or hypocaloric diets contribute to malnutrition in diarrheal disease.

## Diagnostic Evaluation

The history provides valuable information regarding the duration, severity, associated symptoms, and potential cause of the diarrhea. A complete history should include present drugs the child is taking, possible ingestions, family history, and recent travel history. Specific questions include the onset and duration of diarrhea, presence of fever and other symptoms, frequency of vomiting, frequency and character of the stool (e.g., watery, bloody), urinary output, and the child's dietary habits and recent food and fluid intake.

Extensive laboratory evaluation is not indicated in a child with uncomplicated diarrhea and no evidence of dehydration. Laboratory tests are indicated when a child is moderately to severely dehydrated. Stool specimens should be examined in all children with diarrhea that persists for more than a few days and in children who have been internationally adopted.

Watery, explosive stools suggest sugar intolerance, and foul-smelling, greasy, bulky stools suggest fat malabsorption. Diarrhea that develops after the introduction of cow's milk, fruits, or cereals may be related to an enzyme deficiency or protein intolerance (Savilahti, 2000). Neutrophils or red blood cells in the stool indicate bacterial gastroenteritis or inflammatory bowel disease. The presence of eosinophils suggests protein intolerance or parasitic infection.

Cultures of the stool should be performed when blood or mucus is present in the stool, when symptoms are severe, when there is a history of travel to a developing country, and when polymorphonuclear leukocytes are found in the stool. An enzyme-linked immunosorbent assay (ELISA) may be used to confirm the presence of rotavirus, and the stool may be tested for the presence of *C. difficile* toxin if there is a history of recent antibiotic use. The stool may need to be examined for ova and parasites when bacterial and viral cultures are negative and when diarrhea persists for more than a few days.

A stool pH of less than 6 and the presence of reducing substances may indicate the presence of carbohydrate malabsorption or secondary lactase deficiency. Measurement of stool electrolytes may help identify children with secretory diarrhea.

The urine specific gravity should be determined if dehydration is suspected. A complete blood count, serum electrolytes, creatinine, and blood urea nitrogen (BUN) may also be obtained. The hemoglobin, hematocrit, creatinine, and BUN are often elevated in acute diarrhea and normalize with rehydration.

## Therapeutic Management

Therapeutic management is directed at correcting the fluid and electrolyte imbalances and preventing or treating malnutrition. The major goals in the management of acute diarrhea include (1) assessment of the fluid and electrolyte imbalance, (2) rehydration, (3) maintenance fluid therapy, and (4) reintroduction of adequate diet. Infants and children with acute diarrhea and dehydration should be treated first with *oral rehydration therapy (ORT).* In cases of severe dehydration and shock, parenteral fluids may be necessary. (See Chapter 28.) Early reintroduction of food is an important aspect of treating acute diarrhea in children. Antimicrobial agents are indicated for a few specific pathogens.

ORT is one of the major worldwide health care advances of the past decade. ORT is effective, safer, less painful, and less costly than intravenous rehydration. As a result of studies conducted in the United States, the American Academy of Pediatrics, World Health Organization, and Centers for Disease Control and Prevention recommend the use of ORT as the treatment of choice for most cases of dehydration caused by diarrhea (Endsley and Galbraith, 1998; Nappert and others, 2000).

*Oral rehydration solutions (ORSs)* are successful in treating the great majority of infants with isotonic, hypotonic, or hypertonic dehydration. Table 29-2 shows the most commonly used solutions for oral rehydration. Glucose-mediated, enhanced sodium absorption forms the physiologic basis for the composition of these solutions. Recently, a rice-based ORS has been developed as an alternative to the standard glucose ORS. These nutrient-based solutions may reduce vomiting, decrease diarrheal volume loss, and shorten the duration of disease (Endsley and Galbraith, 1998; Nappert and others, 2000; Sullivan, 1998). Table 29-3 includes ORT guidelines for rehydration, replacement of stool losses, and maintenance therapy in dehydrated infants and children.

After rehydration in infants, an ORS may be used during maintenance fluid therapy by alternating the solution with a low-sodium fluid such as water, breast milk, lactose-free formula, or half-strength lactose-containing formula. For older children, an ORS can be given and a regular diet continued.

Ongoing stool losses should be replaced on a 1:1 basis with ORS. If the stool volume is not known, approximately 10 ml/kg or ½ to 1 cup of ORS should be given for each diarrheal stool.

**TABLE 29-2** Composition of some oral rehydration solutions (ORSs)

| Formula | Na⁺ (mEq/L) | K⁺ (mEq/L) | Cl⁻ (mEq/L) | Base (mEq/L) | Glucose (g/L) |
|---|---|---|---|---|---|
| Pedialyte (Ross)* | 45 | 20 | 35 | 30 (citrate) | 25 |
| Rehydralyte (Ross) | 75 | 20 | 65 | 30 (citrate) | 25 |
| Infalyte (Mead Johnson) | 50 | 25 | 45 | 34 (citrate) | 30 |
| WHO (World Health Organization)† | 90 | 20 | 80 | 30 (bicarbonate) | 20 |

*Note that there are many generic products available with compositions identical to Pedialyte.
†Must be reconstituted with water.

**TABLE 29-3** Treatment of acute diarrhea

| Degree of Dehydration | Signs/Symptoms | Rehydration Therapy* | Replacement of Stool Losses | Maintenance Therapy |
|---|---|---|---|---|
| Mild (5%-6%) | Increased thirst Slightly dry buccal mucous membranes | ORS 50 ml/kg within 4 hr | ORS 10 ml/kg (for infants) or 150-250 ml at a time (for older children) for each diarrheal stool | Breast-feeding, if established, should continue; regular infant formula if tolerated If lactose intolerance suspected, give undiluted lactose-free formula (or half-strength lactose-containing formula for brief period only); infants and children who receive solid food should continue their usual diet |
| Moderate (7%-9%) | Loss of skin turgor, dry buccal mucous membranes, sunken eyes, sunken fontanel | ORS 100 ml/kg within 4 hr | Same as above | Same as above |
| Severe (>9%) | Signs of moderate dehydration plus one of following: rapid thready pulse, cyanosis, rapid breathing, lethargy, coma | Intravenous fluids (Ringer's lactate), 40 ml/kg/hr until pulse and state of consciousness return to normal; then 50 to 100 ml/kg of ORS | Same as above | Same as above |

*If no signs of dehydration are present, rehydration therapy is not necessary. Proceed with maintenance therapy and replacement of stool losses.

Solutions for oral rehydration are useful in most cases of dehydration, and vomiting is not a contraindication. A child who is vomiting should be given an ORS at frequent intervals and in small amounts. For young children, the fluid can be given in a spoon or small syringe in 5- to 10-ml increments every 1 to 5 minutes by the child's caregiver. ORSs may also be given by nasogastric or gastrostomy tube infusion in children who were feeding with this modality for other reasons.

Infants without clinical signs of dehydration do not need ORT. They should, however, receive the same fluids recommended for infants with signs of dehydration in the maintenance phase and for ongoing stool losses.

Early reintroduction of nutrients is desirable and is gaining more widespread acceptance. Continued feeding or early reintroduction of a normal diet is beneficial because of an improved nutritional outcome and because it may reduce the number of stools, reduce weight loss, and shorten the duration of illness (Endsley and Galbraith, 1998; Sullivan, 1998).

Infants who are breast-feeding should continue breast-feeding; ORSs should be used to replace ongoing losses.

**NURSING ALERT**

Diarrhea is not managed by encouraging intake of clear fluids by mouth, such as fruit juices, carbonated soft drinks, and gelatin. These fluids usually have a high carbohydrate content, a very low electrolyte content, and a high osmolality (Hugger, Harkless, and Rentschler, 1998). Caffeinated soda is avoided because caffeine is a mild diuretic and may lead to increased loss of water and sodium. Chicken or beef broth is not given because it contains excessive sodium and inadequate carbohydrate. A BRAT diet (bananas, rice, apples, and toast or tea) is contraindicated for the child, and especially for the infant, with acute diarrhea because this diet has little nutritional value (low in energy and protein), is too high in carbohydrates, and is low in electrolytes.

### Acute Diarrhea

An 8-month-old infant is evaluated in the primary care clinic because of fever, vomiting, and diarrhea of 12 hours' duration. The caregivers report that the infant had three times as many stools as usual, and the stools are watery in consistency. After the initial examination of the infant, it is apparent that the child is mildly dehydrated because of stool losses secondary to acute infectious diarrhea. Which of the following interventions would be indicated in this situation?

FIRST, THINK ABOUT IT . . .
- What is the purpose of your thinking?
- If you accept the conclusions, what are the implications?

1. Recommend that the caregivers offer fruit juice only and delay reintroduction of food for 48 hours.
2. Administer antidiarrheal medications.
3. Educate the infant's caregivers regarding administration of oral rehydration solution (ORS).
4. Administer intravenous (IV) fluids and provide nothing by mouth for several hours.

*The best response is three. The purpose of your thinking is to establish the goals of management of acute diarrhea, which include assessment of hydration, provision of fluids for rehydration and maintenance, and reintroduction of an adequate diet. In this case, because the infant is mildly dehydrated, oral rehydration therapy (ORT) should be attempted. ORT is effective, safer, less painful, and less costly than IV rehydration. If ORS is administered at frequent intervals, vomiting can be minimized and IV hydration probably avoided.*

*Early reintroduction of normal nutrients is desirable, because delayed introduction of food may be harmful in terms of nutritional status and duration of illness. Breast-feeding generally should be continued, and most infants who receive cow's milk formulas may resume their usual feedings as soon as they are rehydrated. Occasionally the implications may be that a soy formula is recommended after an episode of acute infectious diarrhea if the infant demonstrates evidence of lactose malabsorption. Use of antidiarrheal medications should not be recommended for acute infectious diarrhea. These drugs may be harmful, because adverse effects such as slowed motility and ileus may occur.*

Available evidence indicates that continued human milk feeding during diarrheal illness results in reduced severity and duration of illness (Sullivan, 1998). Tolerance to human milk may result from its low osmolality and its antimicrobial, enzymatic, and hormonal factors.

The use of nonhuman milk for infants and children with diarrhea remains controversial. Cow's milk and cow's milk formulas are of concern because maldigestion of lactose can occur in children with infectious diarrhea. Studies indicate that well-hydrated infants and children may resume full-strength nonhuman milk feeding immediately without adverse reactions (Hugger, Harkless, and Rentschler, 1998). Many infants and children can be safely managed with a diet containing cow's milk. Some health care providers advocate

the use of a lactose-free formula in infants only if milk or regular formula is not tolerated.

For older children a regular diet can generally be offered once rehydration has been achieved. In toddlers there is no contraindication to continuing soft or pureed foods of all groups. A diet of easily digestible foods such as cereals, cooked vegetables, and meats is adequate for the older child.

Intravenous fluids are required for severe dehydration and vomiting. A saline solution containing 5% dextrose in water is usually administered. The initial volume should be 20 to 30 ml/kg and should be administered as a bolus. Therapy during the remainder of the first 24 hours should be aimed at completely correcting the remaining fluid and sodium deficits and replacing ongoing abnormal losses. (See Chapter 28.)

Enteric infections are generally self-limited conditions. Antimicrobial therapy is not indicated in the majority of children with acute diarrhea and is not available for enteric viruses. Specific antimicrobial therapy is indicated only for culture-proven bacterial or parasitic infections in which this therapy can reduce the duration of the illness, the severity of the symptoms, or the shedding and secondary spread of organisms. Antibiotics may be warranted before culture results are available in the febrile, ill-looking infant with dysenteric diarrhea (blood and polymorphonuclear cells in the stool). Indiscriminate use of antibiotics may lead to pseudomembranous colitis.

Antidiarrheal drug therapy with agents such as loperamide (Imodium A-D), diphenoxylate hydrochloride/atropine (Lomotil), Kaopectate, or Diasorb is not indicated in acute infectious diarrhea in infants and young children. Toxicity and adverse side effects may occur, such as worsening of the diarrhea because of slowing of motility and ileus or a decrease in diarrhea with continuing fluid losses and dehydration.

The treatment of antibiotic-associated diarrhea is discontinuation of the antibiotic if possible and investigation for the presence of *C. difficile*. If laxatives or certain foods are the cause of diarrhea, their use should be discontinued. (See Critical Thinking Exercise box.)

## Nursing Considerations

### ▓ Assessment

The nursing assessment of diarrhea begins with observation of the infant's or child's general appearance and behavior. The physical assessment includes all the parameters described for assessment of dehydration, such as decreased urinary output and weight, dry mucous membranes, poor skin turgor, sunken fontanel in the infant, and pale, cool, dry skin. With more severe dehydration, increased pulse and respiration, decreased blood pressure, and a prolonged capillary refill time (≥2 seconds) may indicate impending shock.

A history provides valuable information regarding probable etiologic agents, such as introduction of a new food, exposure to infectious agents, travel to an area of high susceptibility, contact with foods that might be contaminated, and contact with pets known to be sources of enteric infections. An allergy, drug, and dietary history may indicate food allergies, use of laxatives or antibiotics, and sources of excess sorbitol and fructose, such as apple juice.

## Nursing Diagnoses

Several nursing diagnoses become apparent on the basis of a thorough physical assessment. The major diagnoses appropriate for the infant or child are described in the Nursing Care Plan on pp. 1215-1216. Other diagnoses will be evident depending on the age and condition of the child and the etiology of the diarrhea.

## Planning

The goals for the dehydrated infant or child and for the family are as follows:

1. Infant or child will maintain adequate hydration.
2. Infant or child will maintain appropriate nutrition for age.
3. Infant or child will not spread infection (if etiologic agent) to others.
4. Family will receive appropriate support and education, especially regarding home care.

## Implementation

The management of most cases of acute diarrhea can take place in the home with proper education of the child's caregivers regarding the cause of diarrhea, potential complications, and appropriate therapy. Because most infections that cause acute diarrhea are spread by the fecal-oral route, personal hygiene, water supply, and food preparation are important considerations. Meticulous attention to perianal hygiene, disposal of soiled diapers, proper handwashing technique, hygienic food preparation, and isolation of infected persons will minimize the transmission of infectious agents.

Caregivers are taught to monitor the child for signs of dehydration, especially the number of wet diapers or voidings, and to monitor fluids taken by mouth and the frequency and amount of stool losses. They need to be informed about ORT, including the administration of maintenance fluids and replacement of ongoing losses. ORT is time-consuming for the caregiver, but the benefits include safety, (possibly) cost, and less discomfort for the child as compared with intravenous therapy. ORT is administered in small quantities at frequent intervals. Vomiting is not a contraindication to ORT unless it is severe. Many parents and health care providers still follow the earlier practices of withholding feedings, providing clear fluids (e.g., juices, broth, or gelatin), or a BRAT (bananas, rice, applesauce, and tea or toast) diet. These practices are discouraged, and parents are educated about the appropriate administration of fluids and a normal diet. A slightly higher stool output initially occurs with continuation of a normal diet and with ongoing replacement of stool losses. The stool pattern is outweighed by the benefits of a better nutritional outcome with fewer complications and a shorter duration of illness. The concerns and priorities of the parents should be explored in order to gain compliance with therapeutic management.

If the child with acute diarrhea and dehydration is hospitalized, nursing responsibilities include the same interventions often administered in the home. Appropriate precautions should be implemented to prevent possible spread of the infection. For example, everyone caring for the child must be aware of "clean" areas and "dirty" areas, especially in the hospital, where the sink in the child's room is used for many purposes. Food, eating and drinking utensils, toothbrushes, pacifiers, toys, and other personal items are stored away from the sink, diaper-changing surface, and scale used to weigh diapers. The containment of feces is also a key factor in infection control. Research indicates that superabsorbent paper diapers with elastic legs permit less fecal leakage than cloth diapers with plastic coverings (Centers for Disease Control and Prevention, 1997).

**NURSING TIP** To remind caregivers to keep diapers and other soiled articles away from clean areas, place signs identifying "clean" (e.g., the bed table) and "dirty" (e.g., the sink or bathroom) areas in the room. List on each sign what articles should be stored in each area.

Strict assessment of hydration status, daily weights, and measurement of intake and output and urine specific gravity are essential. The stools should be examined and tested for blood, pH, and reducing substances to determine carbohydrate malabsorption. Specimens may need to be collected for laboratory examination. Parenteral fluids may be required, and specialized nutritional support, such as semi-elemental formulas, continuous tube feedings, or parenteral nutrition, may be needed when oral nutrition is not tolerated.

Because diarrheal stools are highly irritating to the skin, extra care is needed to protect the skin in the perianal area from becoming excoriated. The skin is cleansed gently, and protective ointments such as zinc oxide may be applied. (See Diaper Dermatitis, Chapter 13.) Rectal temperatures are avoided because they can stimulate the bowel, increasing the passage of stool.

Support for the child and family involves the same care and consideration as for all hospitalized children. (See Chapter 26.) Parents are kept informed of the child's progress and are instructed in special care techniques such as feeding, handwashing, and proper disposal of soiled diapers, clothes, and bed linen. Soiled diapers and linen should be discarded in receptacles close to the bedside.

## Evaluation

The effectiveness of nursing interventions is determined by continued reassessment according to the following observational guidelines:

1. Monitor fluid losses with careful intake and output measurements and daily weights.
2. Monitor food intake, especially calories.
3. Observe for evidence of complications from underlying disease (specify) or therapy.
4. Observe and interview family to determine extent and effectiveness of care.

The *expected outcomes* are described in the Nursing Care Plan on pp. 1215-1216.

# Nursing Care Plan
## The Child with Acute Diarrhea (Gastroenteritis)

> **NURSING DIAGNOSIS:** Deficient fluid volume related to excessive GI losses in stool or emesis

**PATIENT GOAL 1:** Will exhibit signs of rehydration and maintain adequate hydration

- **NURSING INTERVENTIONS/***RATIONALES*

*Administer oral rehydration solutions (ORS) *for both rehydration and replacement of stool losses* (see Table 29-2)

> Give ORS frequently in small amounts, especially if child is vomiting *(vomiting, unless severe, is not a contraindication to using ORS)*

*Administer and monitor IV fluids as prescribed *for severe dehydration and vomiting*

*Administer antimicrobial agents as prescribed *to treat specific pathogens causing excessive GI losses*

After rehydration, offer child regular diet as tolerated *(studies show that early reintroduction of normal diet is beneficial in reducing number of stools and weight loss and shortening duration of illness)*

Alternate ORS with a low-sodium fluid such as water, breast milk, lactose-free formula, or half-strength lactose-containing formula *for maintenance fluid therapy* (See Table 29-3.)

Maintain strict record of intake and output (urine, stool, and emesis) *to evaluate effectiveness of interventions*

Monitor urine specific gravity every 8 hours or as indicated *to assess hydration*

Weigh child daily *to assess for dehydration*

Assess vital signs, skin turgor, mucous membranes, and mental status every 4 hours or as indicated *to assess hydration*

Discourage intake of clear fluids such as fruit juices, carbonated soft drinks, and gelatin *(these fluids usually are high in carbohydrates, low in electrolytes, and have a high osmolality)*

Instruct family in providing appropriate therapy, monitoring intake and output, and assessing for signs of dehydration *to ensure optimum results and improve compliance with the therapeutic regimen*

- **EXPECTED OUTCOME**

Child exhibits signs of adequate hydration (specify)

> **NURSING DIAGNOSIS:** Imbalanced nutrition: less than body requirements related to diarrheal losses, inadequate intake

**PATIENT GOAL 1:** Will consume nourishment adequate to maintain appropriate weight for age

- **NURSING INTERVENTIONS/***RATIONALES*

After rehydration, instruct breast-feeding mother to continue feeding breast milk *(this tends to reduce severity and duration of illness)*

Avoid giving BRAT diet (bananas, rice, applesauce, and toast or tea) *(this diet is low in energy and protein, too high in carbohydrates, and low in electrolytes)*

Observe and record response to feedings *to assess feeding tolerance*

Instruct family in providing appropriate diet *to gain compliance with therapeutic regimen*

Explore concerns and priorities of family members *to improve compliance with therapeutic regimen*

- **EXPECTED OUTCOME**

Child takes prescribed nourishment and exhibits a satisfactory weight gain

> **NURSING DIAGNOSIS:** Risk for infection related to microorganisms invading GI tract

**PATIENT (OTHERS) GOAL 1:** Will not exhibit signs of gastrointestinal infection

- **NURSING INTERVENTIONS/***RATIONALES*

Implement enteric isolation or other hospital infection control practices, including appropriate disposal of stool and laundry and appropriate handling of specimens *to reduce risk of spreading infection*

Maintain careful handwashing *to reduce risk of spreading infection*

Use superabsorbent disposable diapers *to contain feces and decrease chance of diaper dermatitis*

Attempt to keep infants and small children from placing hands and objects in diaper area

Teach children, when possible, protective measures such as handwashing after using toilet, and so on, *to prevent spread of infection*

Instruct family members and visitors in isolation practices, especially handwashing, *to reduce risk of spreading infection*

- **EXPECTED OUTCOME**

Infection does not spread to others

> **NURSING DIAGNOSIS:** Impaired skin integrity related to irritation caused by frequent, loose stools

**PATIENT GOAL 1:** Skin will remain intact

- **NURSING INTERVENTIONS/***RATIONALES*

Change diaper frequently *to keep skin clean and dry*

Cleanse buttocks gently with bland, nonalkaline soap and water or immerse child in a bath for gentle cleansing *(diarrheal stools are highly irritating to skin)*

Apply ointment such as zinc oxide *to protect skin from irritation* (type of ointment may vary for each child and may require a trial period)

Expose slightly reddened intact skin to air whenever possible *to promote healing;* apply protective ointment to very irritated or excoriated skin *to facilitate healing*

Avoid using commercial baby wipes containing alcohol on excoriated skin *because they will cause stinging*

Observe buttocks and perineum for infection, such as *Candida, so that appropriate therapy can be initiated*

*Apply appropriate antifungal medication *to treat fungal infection of skin*

- **EXPECTED OUTCOME**

Child has no evidence of skin breakdown

---

*Dependent nursing action.

*Continued*

## Nursing Care Plan
### The Child with Acute Diarrhea (Gastroenteritis)—cont'd

---

**NURSING DIAGNOSIS:** Anxiety/fear related to separation from parents, unfamiliar environment, distressing procedures

---

**PATIENT GOAL 1:** Will exhibit signs of comfort

- **NURSING INTERVENTIONS/*RATIONALES***

Provide mouth care and pacifier for infants *to provide comfort*

Encourage family visitation and participation in care as much as the family is able, *to prevent stress associated with separation*

Touch, hold, and talk to child as much as possible *to provide comfort and relieve stress*

Provide sensory stimulation and diversion appropriate for child's developmental level and condition *to promote optimum growth and development*

- **EXPECTED OUTCOMES**

Child exhibits minimal signs of physical or emotional distress

Family participates in child's care as much as possible

---

**NURSING DIAGNOSIS:** Interrupted family processes related to situational crisis, deficient knowledge

---

**PATIENT (FAMILY) GOAL 1:** Family will understand about child's illness and its treatment and will be able to provide care

- **NURSING INTERVENTIONS/*RATIONALES***

Provide information to family about child's illness and therapeutic measures *to encourage compliance with therapeutic regimen, especially at home*

Assist family in providing comfort and support to child

Permit family members to participate in child's care as much as they desire, *to meet needs of both child and family*

Instruct family regarding precautions *to prevent spread of infection*

Arrange for posthospitalization health care *for continued assessment and treatment*

Refer family to a community health care agency *for supervision of home care as needed*

- **EXPECTED OUTCOME**

Family demonstrates ability to care for child, especially at home

---

## Chronic Diarrheal Disease

Chronic diarrhea is defined as an increase in stool frequency and increased water content with a duration of more than 14 days. It is often caused by chronic conditions such as malabsorption syndromes, inflammatory bowel disease, immune deficiency, food allergy, lactose intolerance, and chronic nonspecific diarrhea (Box 29-4). Chronic diarrhea may also be a result of inadequate management of acute diarrhea. (The etiology, pathophysiology, clinical manifestations, therapeutic management, and nursing considerations of many of these chronic conditions are discussed in Chapter 33.)

## Intractable Diarrhea of Infancy

Intractable diarrhea of infancy is a syndrome defined as diarrhea that occurs in the first few months of life, persists for longer than 2 weeks with no recognized pathogens, and is refractory to treatment. The most common cause is acute infectious diarrhea that was not managed adequately where nutrition is concerned. This condition is sometimes referred to as postenteritis diarrhea or protracted diarrhea of infancy. The original etiologic agent has disappeared, but the diarrhea persists.

Dehydration, electrolyte disturbances, and malnutrition occur with this condition. The diarrhea rapidly becomes intractable due to a combination of secondary consequences: malnutrition deprives the infant of essential nutrients necessary for mucosal regeneration; the villi of the small intestine atrophy; and secondary digestive and absorptive disorders develop as a result of malnutrition, dysmotility, and overgrowth of bacteria. Significant mucosal injury leads to severe intolerance of most nutrients that perpetuates the cycle of malabsorption, diarrhea, and malnutrition and may result in death.

Treatment consists primarily of nutritional support with oral feedings of a formula containing a protein hydrolysate, glucose polymers, and medium-chain triglycerides (MCT) to maximize tolerance and nutrient absorption. Occasionally, continuous tube feedings or parenteral nutrition is necessary.

## Chronic Nonspecific Diarrhea (CNSD)

CNSD, also known as irritable colon of childhood and toddlers' diarrhea, is a common cause of chronic diarrhea in children between 6 and 54 months of age. These children have loose stools, often with undigested food particles, with diarrhea of greater than 2 weeks' duration. Children with CNSD are growing normally and have no evidence of malnutrition, no blood in the stool, and no enteric infection.

The history often reveals certain prior events, including a viral infection, the institution of dietary restrictions (e.g., avoidance of milk and dairy products), and previous antibiotic use. These events may either be related to the origin of CNSD or influence the course of this disorder. The potential causes of CNSD include disordered small intestine motility, excessive fluid intake, dietary fat restriction, and carbohydrate malabsorption. Children with CNSD may have impaired intestinal motility, which causes rapid intestinal transit and impaired fluid absorption. In some children, excessive fluid intake may contribute to the initiation and perpetuation of CNSD.

It is apparent that specific dietary factors contribute to CNSD. Ingestion of a large quantity of osmotically active carbohydrates, which are poorly absorbed by the small intestine, contributes to diarrhea in many children with CNSD. Carbohydrates that are poorly absorbed include sorbitol and fructose. Sorbitol is found in significant concentrations in common foods such as prunes, prune juice, pears, pear juice, peaches, apple juice, and sugar-free gum and candy. Fructose is found in significant quantities in many soft drinks, fruit juices, honey, figs, dried dates, prunes, and prune juice. Although fruit juice is considered a nutritious snack and is a fluid staple for children, excessive fruit juice ingestion may cause chronic diarrhea. A low-fat diet may contribute to diarrhea by causing an increase in the rate of gastric emptying and faster intestinal transit

time, which contributes to malabsorption of fluid and nutrients. Many children with CNSD ingest low-fat diets with restricted milk and dairy products, for which large quantities of fruit and fruit juice are substituted. This pursuit of a healthful diet may contribute to CNSD.

The diagnosis of CNSD is one of exclusion. A history of prior illnesses and antibiotic use should be obtained. A dietary history, including fluid intake and quantities of fruit and fruit juice ingested, is important. The physical examination of the child with CNSD usually reveals normal growth, no blood in the stools, and no evidence of enteric infection. Chronic conditions such as pancreatic insufficiency, small bowel mucosal injury, and food allergy need to be excluded, often on the basis of the history and specific laboratory examinations (Vanderhoof, 1998).

The therapeutic management of CNSD may include the following measures: (1) avoidance of foods and liquids containing sorbitol and fructose, (2) increased fiber in the diet, (3) increased fat content in the diet, and (4) limitation of total fluid intake (Vanderhoof, 1998). CNSD often causes anxiety and frustration in the parents and affected child, but most cases resolve spontaneously or with simple treatment measures before the age of 4 or 5 years. The family needs reassurance that no significant morbidity is associated with CNSD.

## Vomiting

Vomiting is the forceful ejection of gastric contents through the mouth. It is a well-defined, complex, coordinated process that is under central nervous system control and is usually accompanied by nausea and retching. In contrast, regurgitation is a simpler, more passive, and effortless phenomenon. There are many causes of vomiting, including acute infectious diseases, increased intracranial pressure (ICP), toxic ingestions, food intolerances and allergies, mechanical obstruction of the GI tract, metabolic disorders, and psychogenic problems. Vomiting is common in childhood, is usually self-limited, and requires no specific treatment. However, complications can occur in children, including dehydration and electrolyte disturbances, malnutrition, aspiration, and Mallory-Weiss syndrome (small tears in the distal esophageal mucosa).

### Etiology

The child's age, pattern of vomiting, and duration of symptoms help to determine the etiology. For example, chronic and intermittent episodes of vomiting may indicate malrotation, whereas vomiting on a specific day at the same time before school is not likely to be a result of organic disease. The color and consistency of the emesis vary according to the etiology. Green, bilious vomiting suggests bowel obstruction. Curdled stomach contents, mucus, or fatty foods that are vomited several hours after ingestion suggest poor gastric emptying or high intestinal obstruction. Gastric irritation by certain medicines, foods, or toxic substances may cause vomiting.

Associated symptoms also help to identify the etiology. Fever and diarrhea accompanying vomiting suggest an infection. Constipation associated with vomiting suggests an anatomic or functional obstruction. Localized abdominal pain and vomiting often occur with appendicitis, pancreatitis, or peptic ulcer disease. A change in the level of consciousness or a headache associated with vomiting indicates a central nervous system or metabolic disorder. Forceful vomiting is associated with pyloric stenosis.

## Pathophysiology

The act of vomiting, including nausea and retching, is under control of the central nervous system. Two areas of the medulla are involved as the vomiting center. The medullary center is also activated by impulses from a second center, the chemoreceptor trigger zone, which is located in the floor of the fourth ventricle (Box 29-5). Nausea is a sensation that may be induced by visceral, labyrinthine (inner ear), or emotional stimuli. It is characterized by the desire to vomit, with discomfort felt in the throat or abdomen. Nausea is often associated with autonomic symptoms such as salivation, pallor, sweating, and tachycardia. Retching may occur with or without vomiting. Retching involves a series of spasmodic movements during inspiration, creating a negative intrathoracic pressure, and contraction of the abdominal muscles. Projectile vomiting is preceded and accompanied by vigorous peristaltic waves.

Vomiting is a well-recognized response to psychologic stress. During stress, adrenaline levels rise and may stimulate the chemoreceptor trigger zone. Nausea and vomiting is likely a protective mechanism to remove toxins from the system. Vomiting may follow GI infection or toxic ingestion, or it can be a learned behavioral response.

## Diagnostic Evaluation

The diagnostic evaluation includes a thorough history and physical examination. The description of the vomitus, relationship to meals or specific foods, behavior, and presence of pain, constipation, diarrhea, or jaundice are important components of the history. Physical examination should include an assessment of the hydration status and an abdominal examination.

Further evaluation may include analysis of urine for protein or blood, serum electrolytes, and radiographic studies. A plain radiograph of the chest or abdomen or ultrasonography may reveal anatomic abnormalities. Brain scans are used to detect tumors. Endoscopy of the upper GI tract may be a valuable diagnostic procedure if esophagitis is suspected. A psychiatric evaluation may be indicated if cyclic vomiting, anorexia nervosa, bulimia, or self-poisoning is present. Self-induced vomiting and rumination may be a self-stimulation or gratification activity.

## Therapeutic Management

The management of vomiting is directed toward detection and treatment of the cause of the vomiting and prevention of complications such as dehydration and malnutrition. Vomiting is often a symptom of a common infectious illness that is self-limited and resolves with no specific treatment. Further investigation is indicated if there is dehydration, progressively severe vomiting, or persistent vomiting for more than 24 hours, or when the history and physical examination fail to suggest a diagnosis. If vomiting leads to dehydration, oral rehydration or parenteral fluids may be required.

Antiemetic drugs may be indicated when the vomiting can be anticipated, is of limited duration, and has a known cause. Antiemetic drugs may block the receptors in the chemoreceptor trigger zone (ondansetron [Zofran] or trimethobenzamide [Tigan]), enhance gastroduodenal peristalsis (metoclopramide [Reglan]), or compete for $H_1$-receptor sites (promethazine [Phenergan]). For children who are prone to motion sickness, it is often helpful to administer an appropriate dose of dimenhydrinate (Dramamine) before a trip.

## Nursing Considerations

The major emphasis of nursing care of the vomiting infant or child is on observation and reporting of vomiting behavior and associated symptoms and on the implementation of measures to reduce the vomiting. Accurate assessment of the type of vomiting, appearance of the vomitus, and the child's behavior in association with the vomiting greatly aids in establishing a diagnosis of disorders that have vomiting as a clinical feature.

Nursing interventions are determined by the cause of the vomiting. When the vomiting is identified as a manifestation of improper feeding methods, establishing proper techniques through teaching and example ordinarily corrects the situation. If the vomiting is assessed as a probable sign of a GI obstruction, food is usually withheld or special feeding techniques are implemented. When vomiting is related to concurrent infection, dietary indiscretion, or emotional factors, efforts are directed toward maintaining hydration or preventing dehydration.

The thirst mechanism is the most sensitive guide to fluid needs, and ad libitum administration of a glucose-electrolyte solution to an alert child restores water and electrolytes satisfactorily. It is important to include carbohydrates in order to spare body protein and to avoid ketosis resulting from exhaustion of glycogen stores. Small, fre-

---

**Box 29-5** ■ ■ □
**Sources of Vomiting Stimuli**

**Higher cortical centers**—Either deep-seated or superficial psychologic disturbances. Stimuli include those associated with unpleasant sights, repugnant odors, and fright.

**Chemoreceptor trigger zone**—Transmits impulses to cortical center; located on the floor of the fourth ventricle. Stimuli include chemical stimulation by drugs (e.g., apomorphine, morphine, ipecac, and some digitalis derivatives), toxins (e.g., from uremia, infections, or radiation), cerebral hypoxia, increased ICP, and disturbances of the semicircular canals of the inner ear.

**Reflex excitement** (vagal and sympathetic afferent nerves)—Results from disturbed GI and other viscera. Stimuli include irritation, inflammation, or mechanical disturbance in GI tract (e.g., distention or obstruction); irritation of other viscera (e.g., heart, renal pelvis, bladder); and pain.

quent feedings of fluids or foods are preferable and more effective. Once vomiting has abated, more liberal amounts of fluids can be offered, followed by gradual resumption of the regular diet.

The infant or child who is vomiting is positioned to prevent aspiration and is observed for evidence of dehydration. It is important to emphasize the need for the child to brush the teeth or rinse the mouth after vomiting to dilute the hydrochloric acid that comes in contact with the teeth. Careful monitoring of fluid and electrolyte status must be exercised to avoid the possibility of hyperelectrolytemia.

# SHOCK STATES
## Shock

Shock, or circulatory failure, is a complex clinical syndrome characterized by tissue perfusion that is inadequate to meet the metabolic demands of the body, which results in cellular dysfunction and eventual organ failure. Although the causes are different, the physiologic consequences are the same: hypotension, tissue hypoxia, and metabolic acidosis.

### Etiology

The most common type of circulatory failure in children is *hypovolemic shock,* which follows a reduction in circulating blood volume related to blood loss (e.g., trauma, major bleeding), plasma losses (e.g., burns, peritonitis), or extracellular fluid losses (e.g., diarrhea, dehydration) beyond the child's physiologic ability to compensate. *Cardiogenic shock* results from impaired cardiac muscle function that leads to decreased cardiac output. It is uncommon in children but may be seen following cardiac surgery and in children with acute dysrhythmias, congestive heart failure, or cardiomyopathy. *Distributive shock,* or *vasogenic shock,* results from a vascular abnormality that produces maldistribution of blood supply throughout the body. This term includes (1) *neurogenic shock,* characterized by massive vasodilation due to the loss of sympathetic nervous system tone, which can occur with spinal cord injuries; (2) *anaphylactic shock,* which is characterized by a hypersensitivity reaction that causes massive vasodilation and capillary leak and may occur with drug or latex allergy, insect stings, or blood transfusion; and (3) *septic shock,* characterized by a decreased cardiac output and derangements in the peripheral circulation in response to a severe, overwhelming infection. The types of shock are listed in Box 29-6.

### Pathophysiology

The circulatory system of the healthy child is able to transport oxygen and nutrients to meet the essential needs of body tissues and can respond to increased demands resulting from an elevated metabolic rate. The cardiac output and distribution to the various body tissues can change very rapidly in response to intrinsic (myocardial and intravascular) or extrinsic (neuronal) control mechanisms. In shock states these mechanisms are altered or challenged.

Reduced blood flow, as in hypovolemic shock, causes diminished venous return to the heart, low central venous pressure (CVP), low cardiac output, and hypotension. The reduced intravascular volume triggers a chain of compensatory mechanisms. Fluid is mobilized from the extracellular compartment. Vasomotor centers in the medulla are signaled, causing depressed vagal activity and increased sympathetic activity, which increase the force and rate of cardiac contraction and constrict the arterioles and veins, thereby increasing peripheral vascular resistance.

Simultaneously the lowered blood volume also leads to the release of large amounts of catecholamines, antidiuretic hormone, adrenocorticosteroids, and aldosterone in an effort to conserve body fluids. The catecholamines augment the vasomotor activity to produce vasoconstriction and reduce blood flow to the skin, kidneys, muscles, and splanchnic viscera in order to shunt the available blood to the brain and heart. Consequently, the skin feels cold and clammy,

---

**Box 29-6**
**Types of Shock**

**HYPOVOLEMIC SHOCK**
*Characteristics*

Reduction in size of vascular compartment
Falling blood pressure
Poor capillary filling
Low central venous pressure (CVP)

*Most Common Causes*

Blood loss (hemorrhagic shock)—trauma, GI bleeding, intracranial hemorrhage
Plasma loss—increased capillary permeability associated with sepsis and acidosis, hypoproteinemia, burns, peritonitis
Extracellular fluid loss—vomiting, diarrhea, glycosuric diuresis, sunstroke

**DISTRIBUTIVE SHOCK**
*Characteristics*

Reduction in peripheral vascular resistance
Profound inadequacies in tissue perfusion
Increased venous capacity and pooling
Acute reduction in return blood flow to the heart
Diminished cardiac output

*Most Common Causes*

Anaphylaxis (anaphylactic shock)—extreme allergy or hypersensitivity to a foreign substance
Sepsis (septic shock, bacteremic shock, endotoxic shock)—overwhelming sepsis and circulating bacterial toxins
Loss of neuronal control (neurogenic shock)—interruption of neuronal transmission (spinal cord injury)
Myocardial depression and peripheral dilation—exposure to anesthesia or ingestion of barbiturates, tranquilizers, narcotics, antihypertensive agents, or ganglionic blocking agents

**CARDIOGENIC SHOCK**
*Characteristic*

Decreased cardiac output

*Most Common Causes*

Following surgery for congenital heart disease
Primary pump failure—myocarditis, myocardial trauma, biochemical derangements, congestive heart failure
Dysrhythmias—paroxysmal atrial tachycardia, atrioventricular block, and ventricular dysrhythmias; secondary to myocarditis or biochemical abnormalities

there is poor capillary filling, and glomerular filtration and urinary output are significantly reduced.

Impaired perfusion to the peripheral tissues also produces metabolic alterations. Oxygen depletion causes the cells to revert to anaerobic glycolytic metabolism, forming pyruvic acid; pyruvic acid is then converted to lactic acid, producing lactic acidosis. The acidosis places an extra burden on the lungs as they attempt to compensate for the metabolic acidosis by increasing the respiratory rate. Impaired cellular uptake and metabolism of glucose create an early, transient hyperglycemia. When plasma fluid is lost, hemoconcentration and diminished blood flow increase the viscosity of the blood and further impair perfusion.

Prolonged vasoconstriction results in fatigue, and the release of vasodilator substances such as histamine leads to vasodilation. Venules, which are less sensitive to vasodilator substances, remain constricted for a time. This causes massive pooling in the capillary and venular beds and transudation of plasma fluid into the tissues, which further depletes blood volume.

Complications of shock create further hazards. Central nervous system (CNS) hypoperfusion may eventually lead to cerebral edema, cortical infarction, or intraventricular hemorrhage. Renal hypoperfusion causes renal ischemia with possible tubular or glomerular necrosis and renal vein thrombosis. Reduced blood flow to the lungs can interfere with surfactant secretion and result in *shock lung,* or *adult respiratory distress syndrome (ARDS).* ARDS is characterized by sudden pulmonary congestion and atelectasis with formation of a hyaline membrane. (See Chapter 32.) GI tract bleeding and perforation are always a possibility following splanchnic ischemia and necrosis of intestinal mucosa. Metabolic complications of shock may include hypoglycemia, hypocalcemia, and other electrolyte disturbances.

Shock syndromes characterized by vascular abnormalities (distributive shock) have a somewhat different pathophysiologic pattern of hemodynamic collapse. In neurogenic shock, the sympathetic nervous system mechanisms that maintain vascular tone are interrupted, causing reduced vascular resistance and peripheral pooling of blood; with this increased vascular capacity there is loss of effective circulating blood volume. Septic shock produces a hyperdynamic state in which there is often an elevated plasma volume and reduced peripheral resistance that leads to widespread vasodilation. In many cases there is a high cardiac output caused by the vasodilation in infected tissues and elsewhere plus a high metabolic rate resulting from the elevated body temperature. Degenerating tissues cause aggregation of red blood cells and sludging of the blood. Development of *disseminated intravascular coagulation,* triggered by either the degenerating tissue or bacterial toxins, consumes the clotting factors and produces widespread hemorrhages. (See Chapter 35.)

### Clinical Manifestations

Shock can be regarded as a form of compensation for circulatory failure and, because of its progressive nature, can be divided into three stages or phases: compensated, uncompensated, and irreversible. At all stages the principal differentiating signs are observed in the (1) degree of tachycardia and perfusion to extremities, (2) level of consciousness, and (3) blood pressure (BP). Additional signs or modifications of these more universal signs may be present depending on the type and cause of the shock.

**Compensated Shock.** When vital organ function is maintained by intrinsic mechanisms and the child's ability to compensate is effective, cardiac output and systemic arterial BP are usually normal or increased. However, blood flow is generally uneven or maldistributed in the microcirculation. Early clinical signs are subtle and include apprehension, irritability, normal BP, narrowing pulse pressure, thirst, pallor, and diminished urinary output.

**NURSING ALERT** Unexplained mild tachycardia and a decrease in perfusion of the hands and feet are differentiating features of compensated shock.

**Decompensated Shock.** As shock progresses, perfusion in the microcirculation becomes marginal despite compensatory adjustments, and the signs are more obvious and indicate early decompensation. These signs are tachypnea, moderate metabolic acidosis, oliguria, and cool, pale extremities with decreased skin turgor and poor capillary filling. The outcomes of circulatory failure that progress beyond the limits of compensation are tissue hypoxia, metabolic acidosis, and eventual dysfunction of all organ systems.

**NURSING ALERT** In decompensated shock, tachycardia is pronounced; BP is maintained, but pulse pressure (difference between systolic and diastolic BP) becomes narrowed. There is poor capillary filling, and the child exhibits confusion, sleepiness, and decreased responsiveness.

**Irreversible Shock.** Irreversible, or terminal, shock implies damage to vital organs (e.g., the heart or brain) of such magnitude that the entire system is disrupted regardless of therapeutic intervention. There is pronounced systemic vasoconstriction and hypoxia of visceral and cutaneous circulations with hypotension, acidosis, lethargy or coma, and oliguria or anuria. The child is totally obtunded. A thready and weak pulse, hypotension, periodic breathing or apnea, anuria, and stupor or coma are signs of impending cardiopulmonary arrest. Death occurs even if cardiovascular measurements return to normal levels with therapy.

### Diagnostic Evaluation

The cause of shock can be discerned from the history and physical examination. The extent of the shock is determined by measurement of vital signs, including CVP and capillary filling. Laboratory tests that assist in assessment are blood gas measurements, pH, and sometimes liver function tests. Coagulation status (prothrombin time [PT], partial thromboplastin time [PTT], platelet count, fibrinogen, fibrin) is evaluated when there is evidence of bleeding, such as oozing from a venipuncture site, bleeding from any orifice, petechiae, or purpura. Cultures of blood and other sites are indicated when there is a high suspicion of sepsis. Renal function tests are performed when impaired renal function is evident.

## Therapeutic Management

Treatment of shock consists of three major thrusts: (1) ventilation, (2) fluid administration, and (3) improvement of the pumping action of the heart (vasopressor support). The first priority is to establish an airway and administer oxygen. Once the airway is ensured, circulatory stabilization is the major concern. Placement of one or more multilumen central lines, preferably above the diaphragm (to deliver drugs closer to the heart and limit tissue injury from caustic medications) is a priority in shock (Jindal, Hollenberg, and Dellinger, 2000). These lines are needed for rapid volume replacement, administration of vasoactive drugs, and hemodynamic monitoring. An alternative is rapid surgical cutdown cannulation of the saphenous vein. The vein is anatomically accessible, can accommodate the volumes of fluid needed, and is situated where it does not interfere with any necessary resuscitation procedures. Another effective emergency method is intraosseous administration of fluids. (See Chapter 28.)

**Ventilatory Support.** The lung is the organ most sensitive to shock. The decrease in or redistribution of blood flow to respiratory muscles plus the increased work of breathing can rapidly lead to respiratory failure. Critically ill patients are unable to maintain an adequate airway. To place the lung at rest and improve ventilation, endotracheal intubation is initiated early with positive-pressure ventilation and supplemental oxygen. Blood gases, oxygen saturation (using pulse oximetry), and pH are monitored frequently.

Increased extravascular lung water caused by edema—both hydrostatic and permeable—contributes to the development of respiratory complications. *Hydrostatic edema* occurs from the elevation of pulmonary microvascular pressure as a result of left ventricular dysfunction; *permeable edema* occurs when damage to alveolar cell and pulmonary capillary epithelium causes fluid to leak into the interstitial space, resulting in ARDS. (See Chapter 32.) Therapy is directed toward maintaining normal arterial blood gas measurements, normal acid-base balance, and circulation. Efforts are made to remove fluid and prevent its accumulation by increasing oncotic pressure and decreasing microvascular hydrostatic pressure. Elevated oncotic pressure is promoted by diuresis with furosemide or mannitol, colloid administration, or both.

**Cardiac Support.** In many cases rapid restoration of blood volume is the main therapy needed in the resuscitation of the child in shock. An *isotonic crystalloid solution* (normal saline or lactated Ringer's solution) is usually the first choice for fluid replacement. Crystalloid is given in intravenous boluses of 10 to 20 ml/kg over 10 to 15 minutes and repeated as necessary. The child's response is assessed after each bolus. Successful resuscitation will be reflected by an increase in BP and a decrease in heart rate. An increased cardiac output results in improved capillary circulation and skin color. *Colloids,* protein-containing fluids, are often administered to children in shock; albumin is the most com-

mon. Because albumin is a protein solution, it remains in the vascular space much longer than crystalloid fluids. A smaller volume of albumin can be given to increase intravascular volume and support cardiac output; with crystalloid fluids, a larger volume is needed to achieve the same effect. In general, blood administration is used only in situations of known blood loss, active bleeding, or markedly decreased hematocrit because of the infectious risks. Fresh-frozen plasma is used to correct coagulopathies, not as volume replacement.

For the critically ill child with shock and multisystem organ dysfunction, more aggressive monitoring is needed. Central venous measurements of right atrial pressure or pulmonary wedge pressure help guide fluid therapy. In children with persistent shock, a Swan-Ganz catheter should be placed for more accurate monitoring. Determination of arterial blood gases, hematocrit, serum electrolytes, glucose, and calcium concentrations provides additional information concerning composition of circulating blood. Correction of acidosis, hypoxemia, and any metabolic derangements is mandatory.

**Vasopressor Support.** Temporary pharmacologic support may be required to enhance myocardial contractility, reverse metabolic or respiratory acidosis, and maintain arterial pressure. The principal agents used to improve cardiac output and circulation are the exogenous catecholamines administered by constant infusion pump. Dopamine is the preferred drug in most situations because it also improves renal perfusion. Other agents used to improve cardiac output (e.g., dobutamine, isoproterenol, epinephrine) may also be used, depending on the situation.

*Vasodilator medications* are often used in combination with vasopressors. Common vasodilators are nitroprusside, amrinone, and hydralazine. It is important that the patient have adequate circulating blood volume before vasodilators are administered.

Metabolic acidosis is usually corrected with adequate tissue perfusion and improved renal function. This is accomplished with adequate ventilatory support, including oxygen, and restoration of blood volume and peripheral circulation. The administration of **sodium bicarbonate** may also be needed to correct acidosis resulting from shock. It should be given in small boluses that are diluted to avoid acute changes in osmolality. The major complications of bicarbonate administration are sodium overload and hyperosmolality.

*Calcium chloride* may be administered to improve cardiac function and to offset the reduced ionized calcium associated with large amounts of albumin, whole blood, or freshfrozen plasma. *Diuretics,* such as furosemide (Lasix), cause a reduction in ventricular filling pressures without changing cardiac output or heart rate and promote sodium and water excretion by the kidney in cases in which pulmonary congestion is a problem.

**Other Therapies.** Peritoneal dialysis may be necessary if hyperkalemia, acidosis, hypervolemia, or altered mental status occurs. Nutritional support is provided by both enteral and parenteral routes. Prevention of infection is a primary concern because host resistance is depressed in patients in shock. Other complicating disorders, such as disseminated intravascular coagulation and GI problems (e.g., paralytic ileus, stress ulceration), are managed appropriately. The *intraaortic balloon pump (IABP)* may be used for a child with low cardiac output who is refractory to conventional medical management. *Extracorporeal membrane oxygenation (ECMO)*, where available, is used occasionally as a last resort.

### Nursing Considerations

The child in shock requires observation and care, preferably in an intensive care environment.

> **NURSING ALERT**
>
> When shock is a likely complication, the child is observed carefully for any early signs, such as irritability, unexplained increase in heart rate, thirst, pallor, or diminished urinary output. The appearance of any of these signs requires further evaluation and initiation of therapy.

The initial action in caring for the child in shock is ensuring adequate tissue oxygenation. (See Emergency Treatment box.) The nurse should be prepared to administer oxygen by the appropriate route and to assist with any indicated intubation and ventilation procedures. Other procedures and activities that require immediate attention are establishing an intravenous line, estimating body weight, (weight is needed to calculate drug dosages), obtaining baseline vital signs, placing an indwelling urinary catheter, obtaining blood gas and other measurements, and administering medications as indicated.

The child is best positioned flat with the legs elevated. Hypotensive patients show no benefit from the traditional Trendelenburg position. Head-down positioning tends to increase ICP, decrease diaphragmatic excursion and lung volume, and decrease venous return to the heart because of the altered thoracic pressure. Elevating the lower extremities decreases pooling in the extremities, thereby returning blood supply to the heart.

The nurse's responsibilities are to monitor vital signs (BP in particular), monitor intake and output, and perform a general assessment of the level of consciousness, circulatory perfusion, and parenteral infusion sites. Intravenous medications are titrated according to patient responses, and vital signs are obtained every 15 minutes during the critical periods and thereafter as needed. Urinary output is measured hourly, and blood gases, hematocrit, pH, and electrolytes are monitored frequently to assess the status of the child and the efficacy of therapy. Apnea and cardiac monitors are attached and monitored continuously. Oxygen saturation monitors provide continuous measurement of oxygenation. In the initial stages of acute shock, care of the child often requires the attendance of more than one nurse to manage all necessary activities that must be carried out simultaneously.

**Family Support.** Throughout the intense activity the parents must not be overlooked. A member of the staff, such as a nurse, social worker, or clergy, may be called to help provide comfort and support. If the family is not at the hospital, someone should contact them at frequent intervals to inform them about what is being done and whether there is any improvement. Ideally, someone should remain with the parents to serve as a liaison between them and the intensive care team. However, this is not always feasible in such a critical situation. As soon as possible, the parents should be allowed to see the child.

## Septic Shock

Sepsis and septic shock are caused by an infectious organism. Normally an infection triggers an inflammatory response in a local area, which results in vasodilation, increased capillary permeability, and eventually elimination of the infectious agent. The widespread activation and systemic release of these inflammatory mediators is called the *systemic inflammatory response syndrome (SIRS)*. SIRS can occur in response to both infectious and noninfectious (e.g., trauma, burns) causes. When caused by infection, it is called *sepsis. Septic shock* is defined as sepsis with organ dysfunction and hypotension. Most of the physiologic effects of shock occur because the exaggerated immune response triggers more than 30 different mediators, which results in diffuse vasodilation, increased capillary permeability, and maldistribution of blood flow. This impairs oxygen and nutrient delivery to the cells, resulting in cellular dysfunction. If the process continues, multiple organ dysfunction occurs and may result in death. Fig. 29-1 outlines this framework for pediatric patients.

The incidence of septic shock is increasing in adults and children (Balk, 2000), possibly as a result of greater numbers of immunosuppressed patients, more widespread use of invasive devices in the seriously ill increased awareness for diagnosis, and a growing number of resistant microorganisms.

Three stages have been identified in septic shock. In early septic shock there are chills, fever, and vasodilation with increased cardiac output, which results in warm, flushed skin that reflects vascular tone abnormalities and *hyperdynamic, warm,* or *hyperdynamic-compensated responses.* BP and urine output are normal. The patient has the best chance for survival in this stage. The second stage—the *normodynamic, cool,* or *hyperdynamic-decompensated stage*—lasts only a few hours. The skin is cool, but pulses and BP are still normal. Urine output diminishes and the mental state becomes depressed. With advancing disease, certain signs of circulatory decompensation that deteriorate to signs of circulatory collapse are indistinguishable from late shock of any cause. In the *hypodynamic,* or *cold stage,* of *shock,* cardiovascular function progressively deteriorates, even with aggressive therapy. There is hypothermia, cold extremities, weak pulses, hypotension, and oliguria or anuria. Patients are severely lethargic or comatose. Multiorgan failure is common. This is the most dangerous stage of shock.

Management of septic shock involves measures to provide hemodynamic stability and adequate oxygenation to the tissues and the use of antimicrobials to treat the infectious organism. As with other forms of shock, hemodynamic stability is achieved with fluid volume resuscitation and inotropic agents as needed. Providing adequate oxygenation often requires intubation and mechanical ventilation, supplemental oxygen, sedation, and paralysis to decrease the work of breathing. Septic shock involves activation of complement proteins that promote clumping of the granulocytes in the lung. The granulocytes can release chemicals that can cause direct lung injury to the pulmonary capillary endothelium. This causes a fluid leak into the alveoli, which causes stiff, noncompliant lungs. Disseminated intravascular coagulation (DIC) and multiorgan dysfunction (MOD) may also occur and require prompt assessment and management.

Newer therapies are being developed to modify the host immune response by attempting to block various mediators, thereby interrupting the inflammatory cascade. It is likely that a combination of drugs and approaches will be needed because so many mediators and biochemical processes are involved. Although some therapies have been tried experimentally, none are yet available for widespread use in septic shock (Cohen and others, 2001; Leclerc and others, 2000).

## Nursing Care

Early identification of the symptoms of septic shock is critical to patient survival. A high index of suspicion is required in all critically ill patients who are at greater risk for sepsis because of multiple invasive lines and devices, poor nutrition, and impaired immune function. Subtle alterations in tissue perfusion and unexplained tachypnea and tachycardia often are early warning signs. Identification of the infectious agent and prompt treatment are also critical to patient survival. Broad-spectrum antibiotics should be given, and the site of infection should be removed if possi-

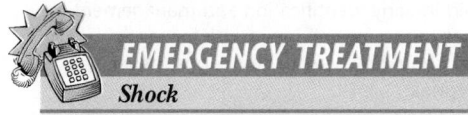

**EMERGENCY TREATMENT**

*Shock*

**VENTILATION**

Establish airway—be prepared for intubation.
Administer oxygen, usually 100% by mask.

**FLUID ADMINISTRATION**

Restore blood or fluid volume as ordered.

**CARDIOVASCULAR SUPPORT**

Administer vasopressors, (epinephrine 1:1000 0.01 mg/kg subcutaneously; maximum dose of 0.5 ml; may repeat if needed).

**GENERAL SUPPORT**

Keep child flat with legs raised above level of heart.
Keep child warm and calm.

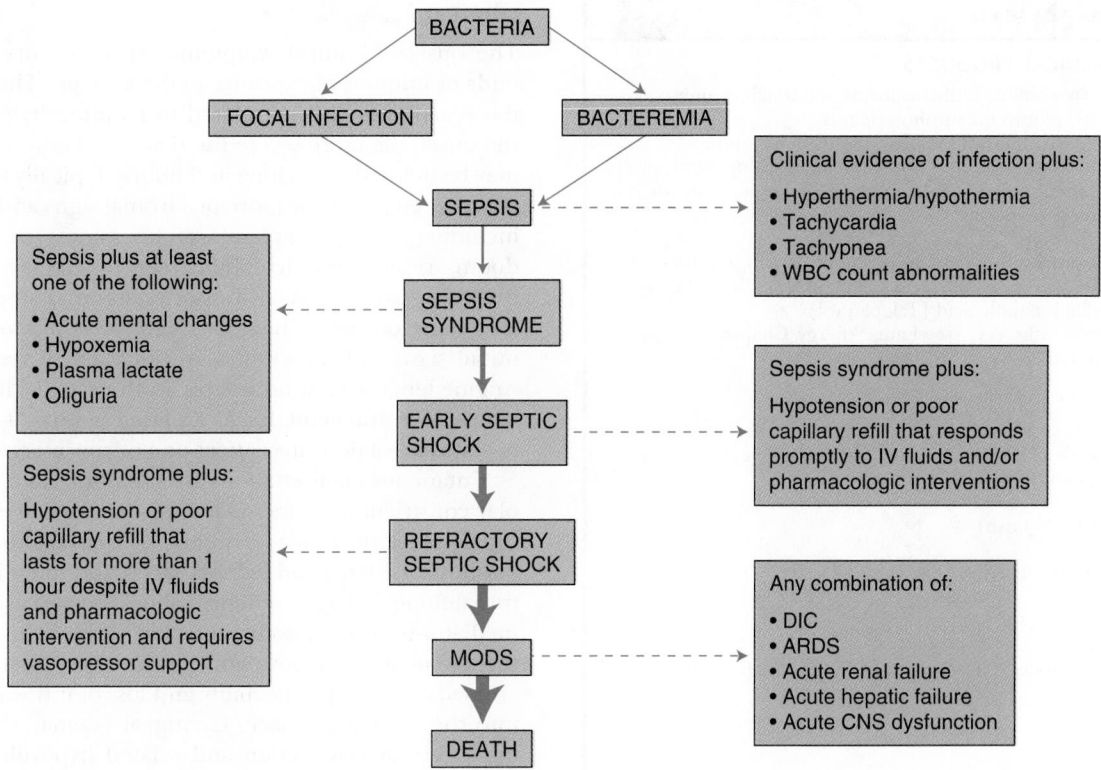

**Fig. 29-1** Proposed terminology of the septic process (systemic inflammatory response syndrome) in children. In general the risk of dying increases as one moves down the spectrum from sepsis to multiorgan dysfunction syndrome (MODS). *WBC,* white blood cell; *IV,* intravenous; *DIC,* disseminated intravascular coagulation; *ARDS,* adult respiratory distress syndrome; *CNS,* central nervous system. (Modified from American College of Chest Physicians and Society of Critical Care Medicine Consensus Conference Committee: Definitions for sepsis and organ failure and guidelines for the use of innovative therapies in sepsis, *Chest* 101:1644-1655, 1992.)

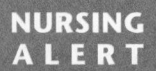

ble (e.g., drain abscesses, remove indwelling lines). Patients should be managed in an intensive care unit (ICU) setting, in which continuous monitoring and sophisticated cardiac and respiratory support are available. Multidisciplinary collaboration is essential in managing these critically ill patients.

> **NURSING ALERT**  To aid in early identification and management, nurses caring for children at risk for septic shock should be alert to early signs—fever, tachycardia, and tachypnea.

## Anaphylaxis

Anaphylaxis is the acute clinical syndrome resulting from the interaction of an allergen and a patient who is hypersensitive. This antigen-antibody (IgE) reaction stimulates the release of chemical substances, primarily histamine, from mast cells. Histamine release causes vasodilation and increases capillary permeability, allowing fluid to leak into the interstitial space. Severe reactions are immediate in on-set, are often life-threatening, and often involve multiple systems, primarily the cardiovascular, respiratory, GI, and integumentary systems. Exposure to the antigen can be through ingestion, inhalation, skin contact, or injection (Beck and Burks, 1999). The most common allergens are listed in Box 29-7.

Prevention of a reaction is the primary goal. Preventing exposure is more easily accomplished in children known to be at risk, including those with (1) a history of a previous allergic reaction to a specific antigen, (2) a history of allergy (atopy), (3) a history of severe reactions in immediate family members, and (4) a reaction to a skin test (although skin tests are not available for all allergens).

### Pathophysiology

An anaphylactic reaction occurs as a result of an interaction between an allergen and preexisting specific immunoglobulin E (IgE). When the antigen enters the circulatory system, a generalized reaction rapidly occurs. Vasoactive amines (principally histamine or histamine-like substances) are released from mast cells and cause vasodilation, bronchoconstriction, and increased capillary permeability. Consequently, there is increased venous capacity and pooling, reduced arterial pressure, and rapid loss of fluid into interstitial spaces, causing a marked decrease in venous return to the heart.

### Clinical Manifestations

The onset of clinical symptoms usually occurs within seconds or minutes of exposure to the antigen. The rapidity of the reaction is directly related to its intensity—the sooner the onset, the more severe the reaction. However, the onset may be delayed for as long as 2 hours. Typically the reaction is preceded by one or more prodromal signs and symptoms, including vague complaints of uneasiness or impending doom, restlessness, irritability, severe anxiety, headache, dizziness, paresthesia, and disorientation. The patient may lose consciousness. Cutaneous signs are the most common initial sign, and the child may complain of feeling warm. Angioedema is most noticeable in the eyelids, lips, tongue, hands, feet, and genitalia. As outlined in Box 29-8, any or all of several reactions may affect one or more organ systems.

Cutaneous manifestations are often followed by bronchiolar constriction. Bronchiolar constriction causes a narrowing of the airway, dilated pulmonary circulation produces pulmonary edema and hemorrhages, and there is often life-threatening laryngeal edema. Shock occurs as a result of mediator-induced vasodilation and sudden inadequacy of the circulation. Hypovolemia is further enhanced by increased capillary permeability and loss of intravascular fluid into the interstitial space. Laryngeal edema, with its acute upper airway obstruction and related hypovolemic shock, carries a more ominous prognosis.

### Therapeutic Management

Successful outcome of anaphylactic reactions depends on rapid recognition of their severity and prompt institution of treatment (Tuite, 1997). The goals of treatment are provid-

> **Box 29-7** ■ ■ ■
> ### Common Allergens Associated with Anaphylaxis
>
> **DRUGS/MEDICAL PRODUCTS**
> Antibiotics (penicillin, cephalosporins, tetracycline, aminoglycosides, streptomycin, amphotericin B)
> Analgesics (aspirin, indomethacin, phenylbutazone)
> Local anesthetics (lidocaine, procaine, bupivacaine, tetracaine)
> Chemotherapeutic agents (bleomycin, cisplatin, carboplatin, L-asparaginase, etoposide)
> Antiepileptic drugs
> Diagnostic contrast media (sulfobromophthalein sodium [BSP] dye, dehydrocholic acid [Decholin], iodinated contrast media, iopanoic acid [Telepaque])
> Latex (gloves, catheters) (see Latex Allergy, Chapter 11)
> Blood products
>
> **FOODS**
> Milk and milk products
> Nuts and seeds
> Legumes (peanuts, soybeans, beans, lentils)
> Eggs
> Seafood (fish, shellfish)
> Wheat
> Citrus fruits, strawberries
> Chocolate
>
> **VENOMS**
> Hymenoptera (bee, yellow jacket, hornet, wasp, fire ant)
> Snake
> Jellyfish
> Spider
>
> **BIOLOGIC AGENTS**
> Allergen extracts
> Antisera (snake, tetanus, diphtheria)
> Enzymes
> Hormones
> Immune globulin (gammaglobulin, blood, plasma)

ing ventilation, restoring adequate circulation, and preventing further exposure by identifying and removing the cause when possible (Beck and Burks, 1999).

A mild cutaneous reaction with no evidence of respiratory distress or cardiovascular compromise can be managed with antihistamines, such as diphenhydramine (Benadryl) and epinephrine (Beck and Burks, 1999). Moderate or severe distress presents a life-threatening emergency and requires immediate intervention. Severely unresponsive patients are transferred to hospital intensive care units when possible.

As in any shock state, the airway is the first concern. The most important drug is aqueous epinephrine 1:1000. The dose is 0.01 ml/kg to a maximum of 0.5 ml administered subcutaneously. With epinephrine 1:1000, the dose corresponds to 0.01 mg/kg. If the intravenous route is accessible, epinephrine 1:10,000 is used (0.1 ml/kg). Usually a single dose is effective, but additional doses are given if needed. The child should be observed for at least 6 hours because late deterioration may occur. Other routes of epinephrine administration are intramuscular and via an airway, either nebulized or by injection through an endotracheal tube.

Other drugs that may be used are aminophylline and diphenhydramine. Vasopressors may be required for severe shock from any cause. Corticosteroids are controversial, but some authorities advocate their use for control of persistent or recurrent symptoms (Beck and Burks, 1999). The time required for them to achieve their effect diminishes their value for emergency therapy.

The child is positioned and monitored in the same way as for any shock patient. If this is the initial anaphylactic reaction, it is especially important to identify the allergen and implement measures to prevent any future reaction. Medical identification should be carried by the patient at all times. Desensitization may be recommended in certain cases.

### Nursing Considerations

The major nursing responsibility in anaphylaxis is anticipating which children are likely to develop a reaction, recognizing the early signs, and intervening appropriately. When an anaphylactic reaction is suspected, both immediate intervention and preparation for medical therapy are nursing responsibilities. Help will be needed and the practitioner should be notified, but the nurse must not leave the patient. The child is placed in a head-elevated position (unless contraindicated by hypotension) to facilitate breathing, and oxygen is administered. If the child is not breathing, cardiopulmonary resuscitation (CPR) is initiated.

If the cause can be determined, measures are implemented to slow the spread of the offending substance. For example, an intravenous medication or dye infusion is discontinued. If an intravenous infusion line is not in place, one is established immediately, and the flow rate is monitored carefully. Vital signs are monitored every 15 minutes, and urinary output is measured at regular intervals. Medications are administered as prescribed, with regular assessment to monitor their effectiveness and to detect signs of the side effects of the medication and fluid overload.

To prevent an anaphylactic reaction, parents are always asked about possible allergic responses to foods, medications, products such as latex, and environmental conditions. (See Guidelines box on p. 156.) These are displayed prominently on the patient's chart. The specific allergen and the type and severity of the reaction are noted. Parents are excellent historians, especially when the child has displayed a dramatic reaction to a substance. Drugs, including related drugs (e.g., penicillin, nafcillin), that have produced a previous reaction are *never* given.

> **NURSING ALERT** Families should always inform other caregivers (e.g., daycare staff) and school personnel, especially the school nurse, of allergies in their children. These individuals should be prepared to respond immediately to a severe reaction.

The child and the parents need as much reassurance as can be provided without giving false hope. They are kept informed of the child's progress, the reasons for the therapies, and what they can reasonably expect. This is a frightening experience and one that the family will remember and make every effort to prevent from recurring. The use of medical information in a convenient and visible form, such as a bracelet or necklace, is reinforced. For the child who is allergic to insect venom, the family is prescribed an emergency kit to be kept with the child at all times (e.g., EpiPen Auto-Injector, or EpiPen Jr. Auto-Injector). Both the family and the child, if the child is old enough and is likely to be

---

**Box 29-8** ■ ■ □
**Possible Manifestations of Anaphylactic Reaction**

**CARDIOVASCULAR**
Tachycardia
Dysrhythmia
Hypotension
Relative hypovolemia

**RESPIRATORY**
Rhinitis—sneezing, nasal itching, rhinorrhea
Laryngeal edema—stridor
Bronchospasm—cough, wheezing

**GASTROINTESTINAL**
Nausea and vomiting
Abdominal pain
Diarrhea

**CUTANEOUS (SKIN)***
Diffuse flushing, feeling of warmth
Urticaria (itching of skin and raised rash [hives])
Angioedema—periorbital, perioral

**CENTRAL NERVOUS SYSTEM/OTHER**
Sense of impending doom, sometimes loss of consciousness*
Headache*
Seizures

―――――
*Early signs.

away from the family (e.g., at school), are taught how to use the equipment. (See Chapter 27.)

## Toxic Shock Syndrome (TSS)

TSS is a relatively rare condition caused by the toxins produced by the staphylococcus bacteria. First described in 1978, it can cause acute multisystem organ failure and a clinical picture that resembles septic shock. TSS became well known in 1980 because of the striking relationship between the disease and tampon use (Nakase, 2000). An aggressive health education campaign about the dangers of prolonged tampon use and a change in the chemical composition of tampons has markedly reduced the incidence of TSS in menstruating women. Cases of TSS have also been reported in men, older women, and children.

### Pathophysiology

Evidence from several sources suggests that TSS occurs secondary to infection with phage group-1 *Staphylococcus aureus*. The organism is believed to produce an epidermal toxin, but the precise mode of transmission is not known.

In approximately half the cases, TSS is seen in menstruating women and is usually associated with tampon use. The tampon may carry the organism from the fingers or vulva into the vagina during insertion, may traumatize the vaginal wall, or may provide a favorable environment for growth of the organism. TSS has also been associated with other bacterial infections, such as sinusitis or pneumonia, catheter site infections, skin infections, postoperative wound infections, and infection related to foreign bodies such as nasal packing or contraceptive diaphragms (Nakase, 2000).

---

**Box 29-9 ■ ■ ■**
**Criteria for Definition of Toxic Shock Syndrome**

Fever of 38.9° C (102° F) or higher
Presence of diffuse macular erythroderma
Desquamation, particularly of palms and soles, 1 to 2 weeks after onset of illness
Hypotension, defined as a systolic blood pressure of 90 mm Hg or less for adults and below the 5th percentile for children younger than 16 years of age; or an orthostatic drop in diastolic blood pressure of 15 mm Hg or more with a change from lying to sitting; or orthostatic syncope; or orthostatic dizziness
Involvement of three or more of the following organ systems: gastrointestinal, muscular, mucous membrane, renal, hepatic, hematologic, and central nervous system
Toxic shock syndrome is probable when four of the five major criteria are fulfilled.
In addition, if blood and cerebrospinal fluid cultures are obtained, they must be negative for any organisms other than *Staphylococcus aureus*. Serologic tests for Rocky Mountain spotted fever, leptospirosis, and measles also must be negative.

Modified from American Academy of Pediatrics, Committee on Infectious Diseases: *2000 Red book: report of the Committee on Infectious Diseases*, ed 25, Elk Grove Village, IL, 2000, The Academy.

---

### Clinical Manifestations

The sudden development of high fever, vomiting and diarrhea, profound hypotension, shock, oliguria, and an erythematous macular rash with subsequent desquamation are characteristic manifestations of TSS. Other manifestations include headache, blurred vision, purulent conjunctivitis, abdominal guarding, and purulent vaginal discharge. Because various signs and symptoms are associated with the disease and affected individuals seldom exhibit all of them, the American Academy of Pediatrics has published a case definition of TSS (Box 29-9).

Complications of TSS include respiratory distress, cardiac dysfunction, hematologic changes (particularly disseminated intravascular coagulation), and abnormal liver function. Impaired perfusion to the extremities may become severe, with eventual necrosis and loss of extremities.

### Diagnostic Evaluation

The diagnosis is established on the basis of criteria in the TSS case definition of the Centers for Disease Control and Prevention. A history of tampon use contributes to the diagnosis. Additional laboratory tests may include cultures from blood, vagina, cervix, and discharge from any suspected source of infection. Other laboratory tests are those that facilitate the management of shock.

### Therapeutic Management

The management of TSS is the same as management of shock of any cause. Because the disease is highly varied in intensity, therapy is directed toward supportive care in mild cases to hospitalization and intensive care in severe cases. Appropriate parenteral antibiotics are usually administered after cultures are obtained. Preventing complications of impaired circulation demands constant observation and immediate therapeutic intervention for hypotension, pulmonary dysfunction, acidosis, hematologic changes, and renal impairment.

### Nursing Considerations

Nursing care and observation of the acutely ill patient are the same as those described for shock of any cause. Because the disease is relatively rare, the major efforts of nursing are directed toward prevention. The association between TSS and the use of tampons provides some direction for education. Adolescent girls who use tampons can be taught general hygiene measures, such as handwashing before insertion of the tampon and not using a tampon that has been dropped or otherwise soiled. Tampons should be inserted carefully to avoid vaginal abrasion. Also it is wise to modify their use. For example, tampons may be used intermittently during the menstrual cycle, alternating with sanitary napkins—perhaps

**NURSING ALERT** Patients who use tampons need to understand that they should remove the tampon and consult their health care professional if they develop a sudden high fever, vomiting, diarrhea, muscle pain, dizziness, fainting or near-fainting when standing up, or a rash that resembles a sunburn.

using napkins during the night, when at home during the day, and when flow is light. Young girls are advised not to use superabsorbent tampons and not to leave any tampon in the body for more than 4 to 6 hours.

# BURNS*

## Overview

Burn injuries are usually attributed to extreme heat sources but may also result from exposure to cold, chemicals, electricity, or radiation. Most burns are relatively minor and do not require definitive medical treatment. However, burns involving a large body surface area, critical body parts, or the geriatric or pediatric population often benefit from treatment in specialized burn centers. The American Burn Association has established criteria to guide decisions regarding the severity of injury and the need for transfer for specialized care.

### Epidemiology and Etiology

Burn injuries represent one of the most severe traumas a body can sustain. Ongoing efforts toward education, burn prevention, a safer home and work environment, and new methods of firefighting have significantly decreased burn injuries. The death rate from fire and flame injury among children 14 years of age and under declined by 50% from 1987 to 1997. Fire and burns remain the third leading cause of unintentional injury-related death among children 14 years of age and under. Children, particularly those 5 years of age and under are at greatest risk because of their limited control of their environment and limited ability to act promptly and properly (National Safe Kids Campaign, 2001).

Another source of burn injury is child abuse. The most common victims are 2 years of age and younger, with the injury commonly inflicted by parents, siblings, and child care personnel (Herndon and others, 1996). Immersion in hot water is the most commonly seen injury, followed by contact burns with hot objects such as cigarettes. A high index of suspicion for abuse is raised by a burn distribution inconsistent with the reported incident, a delay in seeking treatment, and a history of family instability and inability to deal with stress in crisis situations. Laws now exist in all states requiring health care workers to report suspected child abuse.

The use of alternative heating devices such as kerosene heaters and wood-burning stoves has increased the risk of contact burns in all age-groups. Most contact burns result from the lack of shielding to prevent contact with hot surfaces. Flame burns involving flammable liquids such as gasoline account for approximately 30% of injuries seen in the pediatric population, especially over 8 years of age. The ignition of clothing is the second leading cause of burn injury. In the past, girls were more susceptible, but the incidence has decreased significantly as clothing fabric has improved (Herndon and others, 1996).

Children playing with matches or other ignition devices account for 1 in 10 house fires. Boys 2 to 5 years of age have the highest rate of nonfatal burns and incidence of house fire death (Herndon and others, 1996). Cigarettes are associated with the majority of fatal house fires and outnumber other causes by a factor of 2 to 1. The use of alternative heating sources is another common cause of house fires. The source of ignition is often a combustible material stored near the device, the buildup of creosote in the chimney, spillage of fuel, or use of the wrong fuel. Many of these fires result in multiple deaths and injuries, especially in rural areas. The majority of fatal house fires occur from October through March. The single most important element in the decrease in fire-related deaths seen since 1978 is the use of smoke detectors.

The majority of burns result from contact with thermal agents such as a flame, hot surfaces, or hot liquids. Electrical injuries caused by household current have the greatest incidence in young children, who insert conductive objects into electrical outlets and bite or suck on connected electrical cords (Herndon and others, 1996). They occur most commonly during the spring and summer months and are also associated with risk-taking behaviors in young males. Direct contact with high- or low-voltage current, as well as lightning strikes, is the most frequent mechanism of injury. The resistance of the tissue and the path of the electric current are responsible for the damage incurred. Electric current travels through the body on the path of least resistance—tissue, fluid, blood vessels, and nerves. A more localized burn is produced if skin resistance is high at the area of contact, whereas a more systemic pattern of injury is produced if the skin resistance is low. Often compared to a crush injury, serious electrical trauma results from current passing through vital organs, muscle compartments, and nerve or vascular pathways. Loss of limbs, cardiac fibrillation, respiratory collapse, and burns are common sequelae following exposure to electrical energy.

Chemical burns can cause extensive injury. The severity of injury is related to the chemical agent (acid, alkali, or organic compound) and the duration of contact. The mechanism of injury differs from other burns in that there is a chemical disruption and alteration of the physical properties of the exposed body area. Noxious agents exist in many cleaning products commonly found in the home. In addition to concern for localized damage, the potential for systemic toxicity must also be addressed. Of particular concern is the exposure of the eyes to chemical agents and the ingestion of caustic substances.

Although radiation injuries are rare, the most common sources in pediatrics are related to radiation exposure from medical therapies and ultraviolet light.

The causative agent in all burns has important implications for the treatment and prognosis of the pediatric patient. The nurse uses knowledge of the pathophysiologic processes of each type of injury in assessing the trauma and in planning, implementing, and evaluating care. Psychosocial issues are also important considerations in planning for the optimum long-term outcome.

■ *Rose A. Urdiales Baker, MSN, RN, CS, and Mary Mondozzi, MSN, RN, CS, revised this section.

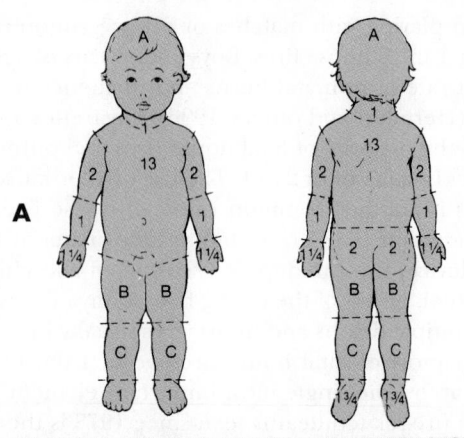

**RELATIVE PERCENTAGES OF AREAS AFFECTED BY GROWTH**

| AREA | BIRTH | AGE 1 YR | AGE 5 YR |
|---|---|---|---|
| A = ½ of head | 9½ | 8½ | 6½ |
| B = ½ of one thigh | 2¾ | 3¼ | 4 |
| C = ½ of one leg | 2½ | 2½ | 2¾ |

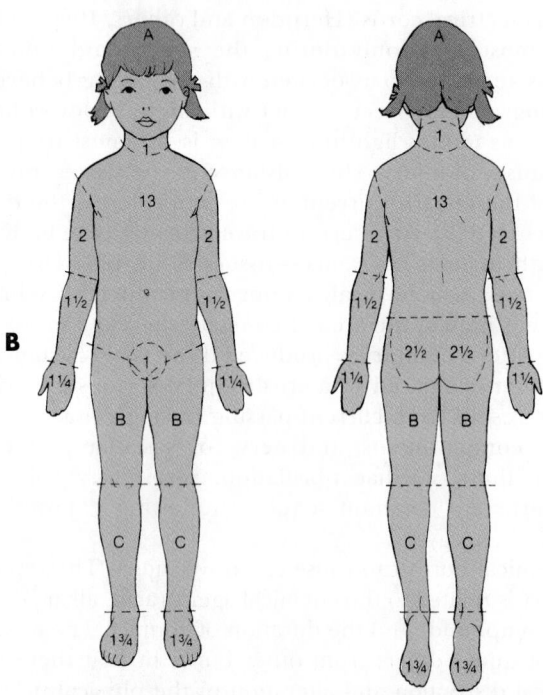

**RELATIVE PERCENTAGES OF AREAS AFFECTED BY GROWTH**

| AREA | AGE 10 YR | AGE 15 YR | ADULT |
|---|---|---|---|
| A = ½ of head | 5½ | 4½ | 3½ |
| B = ½ of one thigh | 4½ | 4½ | 4¾ |
| C = ½ of one leg | 3 | 3¼ | 3½ |

**Fig. 29-2**  Estimation of distribution of burns in children. **A,** Children from birth to age 5 years. **B,** Older children.

## Burn Wound Characteristics

The physiologic responses, therapy, prognosis, and disposition of the injured child are directly related to the amount of tissue destroyed; therefore the severity of the burn injury is assessed on the basis of the percentage of body surface area burned and the depth of the burn. Also important in

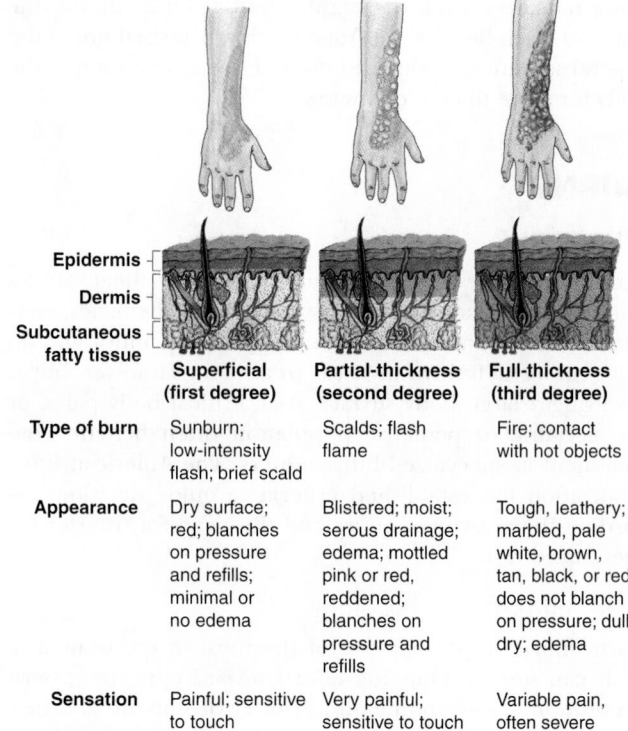

| | Superficial (first degree) | Partial-thickness (second degree) | Full-thickness (third degree) |
|---|---|---|---|
| **Type of burn** | Sunburn; low-intensity flash; brief scald | Scalds; flash flame | Fire; contact with hot objects |
| **Appearance** | Dry surface; red; blanches on pressure and refills; minimal or no edema | Blistered; moist; serous drainage; edema; mottled pink or red, reddened; blanches on pressure and refills | Tough, leathery; marbled, pale white, brown, tan, black, or red; does not blanch on pressure; dull, dry; edema |
| **Sensation** | Painful; sensitive to touch | Very painful; sensitive to touch | Variable pain, often severe |

**Fig. 29-3**  Classification of burn depth. (Redrawn from Grant HD, Murray RH: *Emergency care*, ed 7, Upper Saddle River, NJ, 1995, Prentice-Hall.)

determining the seriousness of injury are the location of the wounds, the age of the child, the causative agent, the presence of respiratory involvement, the general health of the child, and the presence of concomitant injuries.

### Extent of Injury

The extent of the burn is expressed as a percentage of *total body surface area (TBSA)* injured. The child has different body proportions than the adult, resulting in inaccurate estimation of injury if the standard adult rule of nines is used. The proportions of the child's trunk and arms are roughly the same as those of the adult. However, the infant's head and neck make up 18% of the TBSA, and each lower extremity accounts for 14% of the TBSA. As the child grows, percentages are deducted from the head and assigned to the legs. A *modified rule of nines* for the pediatric population proposes that for each year of life after age 2, 1% is deducted from the head and 0.5% is added to each leg (Helvig, 1993). It is generally more efficient to use any of a variety of charts designed to assign body proportions to children of different ages (Fig. 29-2).

### Depth of Injury

A thermal injury is a three-dimensional wound and is also assessed in relation to the depth of injury. Traditionally the terms "first-," "second-," "third-," and "fourth-degree" have been used to describe the depth of tissue injury. However, with the current emphasis on wound healing, this traditional terminology is being replaced by more descriptive

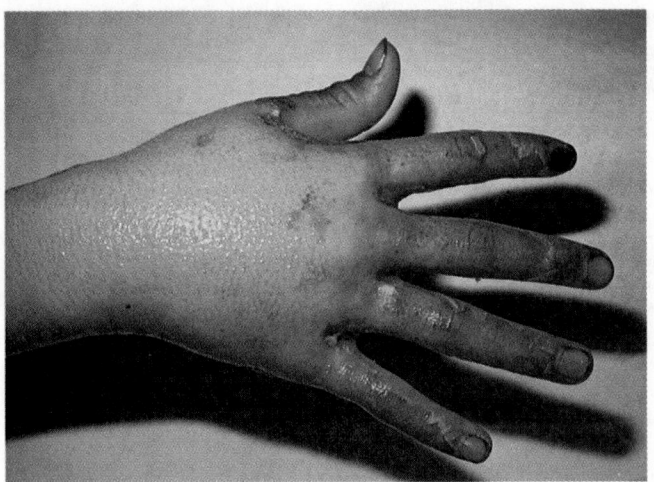

**Fig. 29-4** Deep partial-thickness burn.

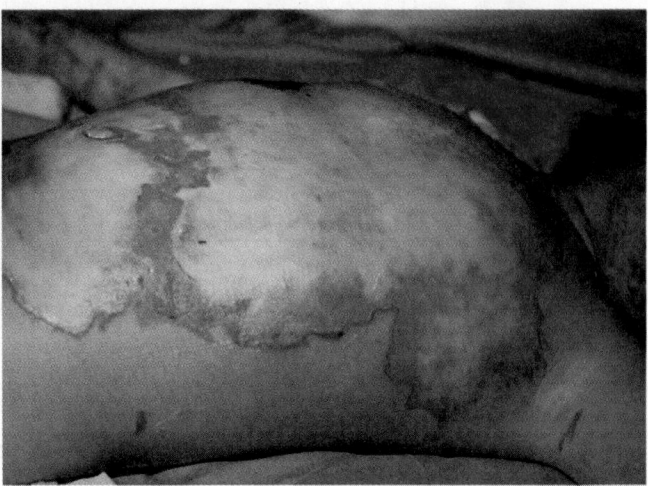

**Fig. 29-5** Full-thickness thermal injury.

terms related to the extent of destruction to the epithelializing elements of the skin. First- and second-degree burns are classified as partial-thickness injuries, and third- and fourth-degree wounds are classified as full-thickness wounds. Partial-thickness wounds are further classified as superficial or deep in relation to the time required for healing to occur and the functional and cosmetic results anticipated. Because both terminologies are often used interchangeably, they are presented concomitantly in Fig. 29-3, which describes the characteristics of burn wounds.

*Superficial (first-degree) burns* are usually of minor significance. There is often a latent period followed by erythema. Tissue damage is minimal, the protective functions of the skin remain intact, and systemic effects are rare. Pain is the predominant symptom, and the burn heals in 3 to 6 days without scarring (Carrougher, 1998). A mild sunburn is an example of a superficial first-degree burn.

*Partial-thickness (second-degree) injuries* involve the epidermis and varying degrees of the dermis. These wounds are painful, moist, red, and blistered. Superficial partial-thickness burns involve the epidermis and part of the dermis. Dermal elements are intact, and the wound should heal in approximately 14 days with variable amounts of scarring. The wound is extremely sensitive to temperature changes, exposure to air, and light touch. Although classified as second-degree or partial-thickness burns, deep dermal burns resemble full-thickness injuries in many respects. Sweat glands and hair follicles remain intact. The burn may appear mottled, with pink, red, or waxy white areas exhibiting blisters and edema formation (Fig. 29-4). Systemic effects are similar to those encountered with full-thickness burns. Although these wounds heal spontaneously in approximately 30 days, they do so with extensive scarring.

*Full-thickness (third-degree) burns* are serious injuries that involve the entire epidermis and dermis and extend into subcutaneous tissue. Thrombosed vessels can be seen beneath the surface of the wound, and nerve endings, sweat glands, and hair follicles are destroyed. The burn varies in color from red to tan, waxy white, brown, or black and is distinguished by a dry, leathery appearance (Fig. 29-5). Nor-

mally, full-thickness burns lack sensation in the area of injury because of the destruction of nerve endings. However, most full-thickness burns have superficial and partial-thickness burned areas at the periphery of the burn, where nerve endings are intact and exposed. Also, excised eschar and donor sites cause exposed nerve fibers. Finally, as peripheral fibers regenerate, painful sensation returns. Consequently, children often experience severe pain related to the size and depth of the burn. Full-thickness wounds are not capable of reepithelialization and require surgical excision and grafting to close the wound.

*Fourth-degree burns* are also full-thickness injuries and involve underlying structures such as muscle, fascia, and bone. The wound appears dull and dry, and ligaments, tendons, and bone may be exposed.

### Severity of Injury

Burns are classified as minor, moderate, or major, which is useful in determining the disposition of the patient for treatment. Burn patients can usually be distinguished as (1) those with a *major burn injury,* who require the services and facilities of a specialized burn center; (2) those with a *moderate burn,* who may be treated in a hospital with expertise in burn care; and (3) those with *minor injuries,* who are able to be treated on an outpatient basis (Table 29-4). The severity of the injury is determined by the extent and depth of the burn, the causative agent, the body area involved, the patient's age, and concomitant injuries and illnesses.

Initial assessment to estimate the extent of skin damage is made by observation and simple diagnostic techniques. The extent of body surface area involvement is readily calculated, and the appearance of the wound provides clues to whether the injury involves the full thickness of the skin or only a portion of the skin layers. Touching injured surfaces to test for blanching and capillary refill indicates if circulation to the area is intact.

It is important to consider the cause of injury, as well as the duration of contact with the burning agent. In general, the more intense the heat source and the longer the con-

| **TABLE 29-4** Severity grading system adopted by the American Burn Association | | | |
|---|---|---|---|
| | **Minor*** | **Moderate** | **Major** |
| Partial-thickness burns | <10% of TBSA | 10%-20% of TBSA | >20% of TBSA |
| Full-thickness burns | | | All |
| Treatment | Usually outpatient; may require 1-2 days admission | Admission to hospital, preferably one with expertise in burn care | Admission to a burn center |

From Vaccaro P, Trofino RB: Care of the patient with minor to moderate burns. In Trofino RB, editor: *Nursing care of the burn-injured patient*, Philadelphia, 1991, FA Davis.
*Minor burns exclude any burn involving the face, hands, feet, perineum, or crossing joints; electrical burns; any injury complicated by the presence of inhalation injury or concomitant trauma; and children with psychosocial factors impacting the injury.

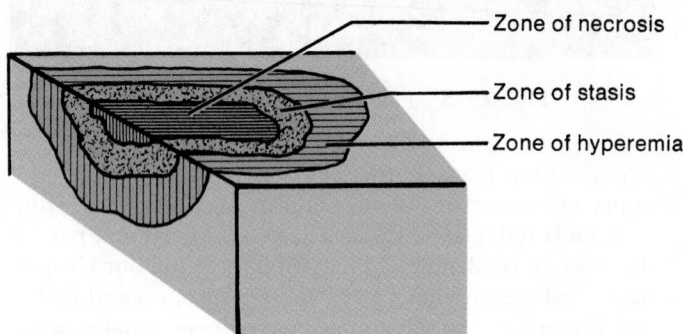

**Fig. 29-6** Zones of injury in burn. (Modified from Zawacki B: *Ann Surg* 180:98-102, 1974.)

tact, the deeper the resulting injury. Hot liquids may result in partial-thickness burns, whereas full-thickness injuries are associated with flame burns. This may vary with the age of the child. Very young children are likely to sustain deeper injuries because of the thin nature of infant skin. This makes estimation of burn depth difficult in young children, especially following scald injuries. Inflicted injuries tend to be more severe than accidental burns because contact with the burning agent is prolonged. Electrical injuries may also be difficult to assess initially. Visible tissue destruction may appear minimal, and damage to underlying structures may be masked. The circumstances of the burn may also suggest the presence of associated injuries.

Certain areas of the body carry a higher risk of complications and therefore require specialized care. Burns of the hands and feet and across joints may not necessarily involve a large body surface area, but injury and scar formation may interfere with normal growth and development. Specialized care is required to preserve maximum function. Burns to the face and neck, along with a history of the injury occurring in an enclosed space, raise a high index of suspicion of inhalation injury. In addition, airway compromise and hypoxia may result from edema formation, as well as pulmonary injury. Damage to the delicate cartilage of the nose and ears results in facial deformities. Facial burns may also involve the eyes and have long-term consequences for vision. Perineal burns are prone to infection and maceration in all patients, especially in young children who are not toilet trained. Scar bands and contractures in the perineal area may interfere with hygiene and mobility.

Children younger than 2 years of age have a significantly higher mortality than older children with burns of a similar magnitude. The infant has minimal protein stores, which are rapidly depleted during burn shock; an immature immune response, which increases the risk of infection and sepsis; and a greater amount of body water in proportion to size that is intolerant of rapid fluid shifts. In addition, the child has not achieved mature renal function. This negatively impacts the ability to retain sodium and water. These considerations, combined with the previously discussed fragility of the skin in the very young, increase the severity of injury.

Many patients sustaining thermal injuries may also suffer associated trauma. The circumstances of the accident may offer clues to related trauma. Children involved in house fires may have jumped from a window, sustaining fractures. Motor vehicle accidents and electrical injuries often result in concomitant injuries. Any suspicion of child abuse should alert the health care team to rule out other injuries.

## Pathophysiology

A burn injury represents a catastrophic insult that involves all organ systems. An understanding of the pathophysiology underlying thermal trauma is essential to provide appropriate nursing care to the pediatric burn victim.

### Local Response

Damage to human skin by heat results in two types of injury: an immediate direct cellular response and a delayed response due to dermal ischemia. Irreversible cellular damage from protein denaturation occurs at temperatures exceeding 45° C (113° F). Three zones of injury demonstrate the evolution of local tissue damage (Fig. 29-6). The unstable area of injured cells, which may survive under ideal conditions, is designated as the zone of *stasis*. Progressive injury due to dermal ischemia may occur in this zone (Box 29-10).

**Edema Formation.** Thermal injury to the vessels in the two outer zones results in increased capillary permeability. At the same time, vasodilation causes an increase in hydrostatic pressure within the capillaries. The increased hydrostatic pressure, combined with the increased capillary permeability, causes loss of water, protein, and electrolytes from the circulating volume into the interstitial spaces. This shift is further enhanced by a diminishing intravascular oncotic pressure as protein and sodium are lost to the interstitial spaces. Although the edema involves both burned and unburned areas, the accumulation of edema fluid beneath and around the site of injury can reach extreme proportions until the extravasation of fluid is limited by tissue tension.

In addition, there are changes in the permeability of cells in and around the burned area that result in an abnormal exchange of electrolytes between cells and the interstitial fluid; specifically, sodium enters the cells in exchange for potassium, resulting in further depletion of intravascular sodium. Edema forms rapidly and with extensive burns is generalized to nonburn tissue (Carrougher, 1998).

**Fluid Loss.** Burn-injured skin is more permeable to fluid, and evaporative water loss can be calculated (approximately 4000 ml/m² total body surface area) (Nguyen and others, 1996). This loss is maximum at approximately the fourth day after injury but continues to pose problems until the denuded surfaces are grafted or healed.

**Circulatory Status.** Significant circulatory alterations take place in the zone of stasis located around the dead coagulated tissue. Heated red blood cells become spherical in shape. These heat-damaged cells, together with hemoconcentration from fluid shifts, depressed cardiac output, and tissue edema, reduce the blood flow in the burned area, resulting in capillary stasis. Thrombi develop, which further impedes circulation and produces tissue ischemia and necrosis. Hyperviscosity and impaired blood flow are also attributed to the release of substances such as thromboplastin and clot-activating factors from damaged cells. These substances cause the production of microemboli, platelet adhesion and aggregation, and increased pain and edema. Circulation in the area around partial-thickness wounds ceases immediately after injury but is usually restored within 24 to 48 hours. In full-thickness burns, however, the vascular supply is completely occluded, and no appreciable circulation is reestablished until granulation takes place at the interface between burned and unburned skin.

**Burn Wound.** In superficial first-degree injuries, tissue damage is minimal. Protein loss is insignificant, and edema is barely perceptible. The burning sensation and pain resolve in 48 to 72 hours, and in 3 to 6 days the damaged epithelium peels off in small scales or sheets, leaving no scar (Carrougher, 1998).

Considerable edema and more severe capillary damage occur in partial-thickness burns. With reasonable care, su-

perficial partial-thickness injuries heal spontaneously and uneventfully through the generative capacity of the stratum germinativum and epithelial cells of the lining of skin appendages. The wound should heal in approximately 14 days with minimal scarring.

Deep dermal burns heal more slowly by regeneration from the epithelial lining of skin appendages, sweat glands, and hair follicles. A thin epithelial covering develops in 25 to 35 days, but this type of burn may require several months to heal. Scarring is common. Infection, trauma, or severe hypothermia easily converts a partial-thickness wound to a full-thickness injury, especially in the normally thinner skin of young children. Fluid loss and metabolic consequences may be considerable.

Cell destruction by coagulation necrosis occurs in full-thickness burns. Dead tissue and exudate convert to a thick, leathery eschar in 48 to 72 hours; the eschar liquefies and begins to separate in 12 to 21 days if not surgically excised. This process is a result of autolysis, leukocyte digestion, and disintegration of collagen fibers. The dead avascular tissue provides an ideal environment for bacterial growth. If tissue is not grafted, new granulation tissue forms on the wound bed. The wound heals slowly by proliferation from the edges, with a high risk of infection and severe scarring. Full-thickness burns result in severe edema with fluid and electrolyte shifts and extensive metabolic changes.

### Systemic Responses

**Cardiovascular System.** The immediate postburn period is marked by dramatic alterations in circulation, known as **burn shock.** There is a precipitous drop in cardiac output that precedes any change in circulating blood or plasma volumes. This initial decrease in cardiac output (approximately 50% of normal resting values) is attributed to a circulating myocardial depressant factor that is associated with severe burn injury and directly affects the contractility of the heart muscle. As a result of fluid losses through denuded skin, increased capillary permeability, and vasodilation, the circulating volume decreases rapidly; cardiac output is reduced even further, usually leveling off at approximately 20% of normal resting values. Following adequate fluid resuscitation, cardiac output returns to normal spontaneously in 24 to 36 hours. If fluid is not replaced, cardiac output continues to decrease, resulting in inadequate perfusion, organ dysfunction, and ultimately death.

Capillary permeability with leakage of fluid takes place both in uninjured areas and in the burn wound. Together with the shrinkage of drying eschar, severe edema due to the rapid fluid shift to the interstitial spaces may produce a tourniquet effect, resulting in a **compartment syndrome.** Compartments are composed of groups of muscles in the extremities and are surrounded by fibrous tissue. The inability of the fascia to expand in the presence of massive edema increases the pressure in the compartment, compromising circulation and entrapping nerves. Treatment is required during the acute phase and consists of surgical incision of the burned tissue **(escharotomy)** to restore distal circulation. If the escharotomy is not sufficient, an incision of the muscle sheath **(fasciotomy)** is performed (Fig. 29-7).

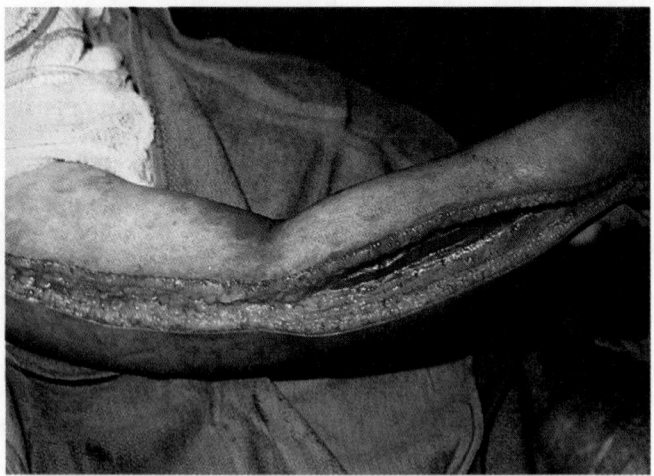

**Fig. 29-7** Escharotomy/fasciotomy in a severely burned arm.

Edema fluid accumulates rapidly in the first 18 hours after injury and reaches a maximum in approximately 48 hours. Capillary permeability returns to normal, and fluid is reabsorbed, chiefly by way of the lymphatics. Reabsorption usually proceeds at the rate of fluid accumulation, although it may persist longer. Redistribution of fluid is often complex and unpredictable and is marked by diuresis.

In most children the cardiovascular system is able to withstand the demands placed on it, although shock is a prominent feature of large thermal injuries. Some children are prone to congestive heart failure and pulmonary edema. In addition, peripheral circulation in infants is less efficient and more labile, which complicates the burn response and therapy in this age-group.

**Renal System.** Loss of fluid from the intravascular compartment causes renal vasoconstriction that in turn leads to reduced renal plasma flow and depressed glomerular filtration. When adequate fluids are provided, the glomerular filtration rate returns to normal, and by the third or fourth postburn day, urinary output increases as edema fluid is mobilized and eliminated. In the first few days oliguria is more commonly the result of inadequate fluid replacement than of acute renal failure. If the child does not respond to treatment or if there is inadequate fluid resuscitation, acute renal failure may develop, with significant kidney damage.

Blood urea nitrogen and creatinine levels are elevated as a result of tissue breakdown, decreased circulating volume, and oliguria. Hematuria may also be evident from the hemolysis of red blood cells, and oliguria may develop as a consequence of the increased pigment load. *Myoglobinuria* is especially common following extensive electrical injury. Cell destruction releases large amounts of *myoglobin,* which occludes the kidney tubules and places the victim of electrical trauma at high risk for renal failure.

**Gastrointestinal System.** Perfusion of the GI tract and liver are decreased as a result of alterations in blood flow. Ischemia of the GI tract has been found to initiate and aggravate erosion and necrosis. Gastric acid production is initially suppressed for 43 to 72 hours after injury and then surpasses normal levels. Catecholamines may be a factor in

the suppression. The accelerated acid production and autolysis of pepsin significantly increase the risk of erosion and ulceration.

Following a major burn injury, gastric *ileus* may occur—the stomach dilates, with digestion virtually ceasing. Ileus of the large intestine may also occur, but the small intestine usually maintains motility and absorptive capacity (Herndon and others, 1996).

With the placement of a nasogastric tube, gastric decompression empties the stomach to control aspiration of gastric contents until motility is reestablished. Care must be taken to observe for signs of aspiration of gastric contents into the lung as a result of incompetence of the gastroesophageal junction. With GI function intact, enteral feedings with a nasogastric tube are begun immediately after acute resuscitation (Andrews, 1994).

**Metabolism.** The greatly accelerated metabolic rate in burn patients is supported by protein and lipid catabolism. The child has limited glycogen stores to provide energy, which therefore accelerates the protein and lipid breakdown. No other disease state produces as great a hypermetabolism as the burn injury. Therefore the child is vulnerable to prolonged starvation (Herndon and others, 1996). When the burn injury is extensive (>50% of TBSA), energy needs may approach twice the predicted basal requirements.

The stress of injury places high demands on the body. Stress-invoked glycogen breakdown depletes the energy stores in 12 to 24 hours, after which the body resorts to glyconeogenesis for high-energy needs. Blood glucose levels may be elevated as a result of insulin resistance. Rapid protein breakdown and muscle wasting occur if sufficient protein replacement is not provided.

Body temperature reflects the net balance between heat production and heat loss. As a result of the accelerated metabolism, children with burn injuries typically exhibit an elevated body temperature, even in the absence of infection. Heat is lost as a result of the energy-consuming process of water evaporation from the damaged skin surface. Each milliliter of water evaporated uses 0.58 calories of heat energy (Herndon and others, 1996). Infants and young children are especially vulnerable because of the large surface area relative to metabolically active tissue. Burning destroys a lipid layer and converts skin that is normally impermeable to water to a state that transmits water vapor at least four times as rapidly as unburned skin. In partial-thickness burns this loss is greatest on the day of injury; in full-thickness burns it rises slowly at first and rapidly increases to reach a peak approximately the fourth day after the burn. Evaporative losses continue until partial-thickness wounds are healed and full-thickness burns are grafted. Therefore body stores of energy are rapidly depleted unless sufficient replacement is provided or losses are reduced.

Medications that affect metabolic rate may be used to prevent loss of body protein stores, which protects immunity, wound healing, muscle integrity, and organ function. Oxandrolone is an anabolic steroid that works to maintain and restore muscle mass, increase weight gain, and promote wound healing. Supplements of essential amino acids such as glutamine and arginine provide an anticatabolic effect, support wound healing, indirectly preserve lean body mass, improve immune function, and provide an antioxidant quality (Demling and DeSanti, 1996).

**Neuroendocrine System.** As a response to stress of any origin, the hypothalamic-hypophyseal mechanism restores equilibrium by secreting trophic hormones, which stimulate various target organs of the neuroendocrine system. Adrenal activity is markedly increased. The medulla responds by secreting additional amounts of the catecholamines epinephrine and norepinephrine. Adrenocortical hormones reach a peak immediately after injury and remain elevated for some time. Aldosterone secretion, as well as a release of antidiuretic hormone, is sustained at a high level throughout hospitalization. Despite this increased adrenal activity, adrenal insufficiency is a rare complication.

**Anemia and Metabolic Acidosis.** The hematocrit is initially elevated because of hemoconcentration resulting from fluid shifts to the interstitial spaces and red blood cell destruction. In addition, a reduced red blood cell half-life results from increased cell fragility. A significant loss of circulating red blood cell mass is predominantly associated with major burns.

Most burn patients exhibit some degree of metabolic acidosis as a result of the disruption of the body's buffering action because of the fluid shift to the extravascular spaces and the altered concentrations of potassium, sodium, chloride, and bicarbonate ions. Reduced blood volume and cardiac output result in diminished perfusion and tissue hypoxia, with a shift to anaerobic metabolism. The resultant formation of metabolic acids is usually sufficiently compensated by respiratory mechanisms. Renal compensatory activities are impaired by the decreased blood flow.

**Growth and Development.** Children may demonstrate postburn growth retardation. Severe growth delays in height and weight have been shown in children who sustained a greater than 40% TBSA burn. This growth lag lasted as long as 3 years postburn for some children, without any "catch up" growth spurt (Herndon and others, 1996). Children with this same level of burn injury also demonstrate reduced bone mass and may develop early onset osteoporosis (Klein and others, 1995). Regular height and extremity assessment are necessary to detect subtle deformities until development is normalized.

## Complications

Thermally injured children are subject to a number of serious complications, both from the wound and from systemic alterations resulting from the injury. The immediate threat to life is related to airway compromise and profound shock. During healing, infection—both local and systemic sepsis—is the primary complication. Mortality associated with thermal trauma in children increases with the severity of injury and decreases as age advances. In children older than 3 years, mortality rate is similar to that of adults. Below this age, rate of survival of the burn and its associated complications lessens considerably.

**Pulmonary System.** The impact of thermal injury on pulmonary function includes a full range of respiratory dysfunctions, including inhalation injury, aspiration of gastric contents, bacterial pneumonia, pulmonary edema and insufficiency, and emboli. Pulmonary complications remain the leading cause of death following thermal trauma. In every age and burn size category, mortality approaches 56% when inhalation injury accompanies surface burns, as compared with 4.1% without inhalation injury.

Inhalation injuries result from trauma to the tracheobronchial tree following inhalation of the heated gases and toxic chemicals produced during combustion. Although direct thermal injury to the upper airway may occur, heat damage below the vocal cords is rare. Inspired heated air is cooled in the upper airway before reaching the trachea. Reflex closure of the cords and laryngeal spasm prevent full inhalation. Evidence of direct thermal injury to the upper airway includes burns of the face and lips, singed nasal hairs, and laryngeal edema. Clinical manifestation may be delayed as long as 24 to 48 hours. Wheezing, increasing secretions, hoarseness, wet rales, and carbonaceous secretions are signs of respiratory tract involvement. Upper airway obstruction is often associated with burn shock and fluid resuscitation. In such situations endotracheal intubation may be necessary to preserve a patent airway.

Inhalation of carbon monoxide is suspected when the injury has occurred in an enclosed space. (See Smoke Inhalation Injury, Chapter 32, for a discussion of carbon monoxide inhalation.) Inhalation of other products of combustion, such as smoke and toxic chemicals, can produce varying degrees of pulmonary damage. Smoke from burning wood is extremely irritating; smoke from burning plastic materials, especially polyvinyl chloride, releases gases containing chlorine, sulfuric acid, and cyanide. Respiratory injury is manifested by mucosal erythema and edema followed by sloughing of the mucosa. A mucopurulent membrane replaces the mucosal lining and seriously compromises respiration and ventilation.

A common etiologic factor in respiratory failure in the pediatric population is bacterial pneumonia, which may be secondary to airway injury or contamination from intubation or may be acquired through hematogenous spread of bacteria. Early in the postburn period the largest percentage of pulmonary infections result from nosocomial exposure, immobility, and abdominal distention. The hematogenous variety occurs later and is related to the septic burn wound or other foci, such as phlebitis at the site of an invasive intravenous line. A 30% to 90% increase in mortality has been observed when inhalation injury and pneumonia are present concomitantly (Carrougher, 1998).

A less common complication is pulmonary edema resulting from fluid overload or ARDS in association with gram-negative sepsis. (See Chapter 32.) This syndrome results from pulmonary capillary damage and leakage of fluid into the interstitial spaces of the lung. A loss of compliance and interference with oxygenation are the consequences of pulmonary insufficiency in conjunction with systemic sepsis.

Deep burns, especially those circling the thorax, may cause restriction of chest excursion as a result of edema and inelastic eschar formation. Young children are particularly at risk because of the pliability of the skeletal structure. Hypoxia is relieved by an escharotomy of longitudinal incisions along the anterior axillary lines combined with a transverse incision at the costal level. This procedure allows expansion of the chest wall to facilitate ventilation.

**Wound Sepsis.** Sepsis is a critical problem in the treatment of burns and is an ever-present threat following the shock phase. Initially, burn wounds are relatively pathogen-free unless contaminated with potentially infectious material such as dirt or polluted water. However, dead tissue and exudate provide a fertile field for bacterial growth. On approximately the third postburn day, early colonization of the wound surface by a preponderance of gram-positive organisms (primarily staphylococcus) changes to predominantly gram-negative opportunistic organisms, particularly *Pseudomonas aeruginosa*. By the fifth postburn day, bacterial invasion is well underway beneath the surface of the burn wound.

Characteristics of the burn wound contribute to the proliferation of pathogenic organisms. Vascular supply to full-thickness burns is occluded immediately, and no appreciable blood is supplied to the area for approximately 3 weeks after the injury. In partial-thickness wounds the circulation to the injured area is suspended for 24 to 48 hours; circulation is then restored unless infection supervenes. Thrombosis from bacterial invasion will impair circulation sufficiently to convert partial-thickness wounds to full-thickness injuries. These large amounts of nonviable tissue also provide an excellent medium for the growth of microorganisms.

Occlusion of the local blood supply is believed to impair the delivery of both humoral and cellular defense mechanisms to the burned area. Initially there is a decrease in inflammatory and phagocytic cells to the wound, but the number of phagocytes gradually increases until they are present in abundance by the third postburn week, when granulation tissue is forming. Granulation tissue, with its rich blood supply, affords increasing resistance to infection. Organisms are normally a part of skin flora; therefore cultures with an organism concentration of $10^5$ per gram of tissue have been arbitrarily chosen as the level of burn wound invasion.

The microflora present at any institution are influenced by the treatment modalities and choice of antibiotics. During the past 30 years there has been a reduction in the percentage of specific bacteria and fungi recovered from burn wounds. This reduction reflects improvements in patient management, nutritional support, aggressive excision and grafting of wounds, and improved topical antimicrobial therapy. The incidence of wound sepsis is decreasing with the early excision of burns. Deaths in burned patients are more often due to pneumonia than sepsis (Herndon and others, 1996).

> **NURSING ALERT**
>
> Disorientation in the burned patient is one of the first signs of overwhelming sepsis. A spiking fever and diminished bowel sounds accompanied by paralytic ileus are noted and progressively increase over 48 to 72 hours, after which the temperature falls to subnormal limits. At this time the wound deteriorates, the white blood cell count is depressed, and septic shock becomes manifest.

**Gastrointestinal System.** Impaired gastric and large bowel motility is a common complication following burns greater than 20% TBSA. Most often following a burn injury, a gastric feeding may be used if the gag reflex and GI function remain intact. When gastric ileus is present, a nasoenteric tube allows the feeding to be delivered into the duodenum or jejunum. As long as gastric decompression is maintained, enteral nutrition can be safely supplied to the duodenum during periods of ileus. This transpyloric route is safe during resuscitation, surgery, anesthesia for major dressing changes, or septic ileus (Herndon and others, 1996).

If enteral feedings are begun early (as soon as 4 hours after burn care is initiated), increased protein requirements for wound healing and nitrogen loss in wound exudate and urine are supported. Albumin levels can be kept within the normal range to maintain a positive colloid oncotic pressure (Herndon and others, 1996). GI motility is usually restored following adequate fluid resuscitation. Recurrence of an ileus later in the hospital course suggests developing sepsis.

The precise pathogenesis of gastroduodenal erosion remains undefined. However, certain factors are known to contribute to mucosal damage. There is an increasing incidence of Curling ulcers with increasing size of injury. Altered submucosal blood flow in the immediate postburn period and atrophy of the intestinal microvilli due to lack of enteral nutrition have also been implicated in the development of GI erosion. Impaired blood flow during septic episodes results in the progression of existing lesions. Prophylactic administration of antacids, histamine $H_2$-antagonists, or sucralfate, as well as early initiation of enteral support, usually prevents the development of serious bleeding.

**Central Nervous System.** Encephalopathy in the burn patient is a relatively common occurrence. Autopsies often show edema, loss of neurons, and other lesions associated with toxic-hypoxic alteration (Herndon and others, 1996).

The manifestations of encephalopathy include hallucinations, personality changes, delirium, seizures, and coma. Postburn seizures appear to be unique to the pediatric burn patient. In most cases burn encephalopathy can be attributed to hypoxemia, hyponatremia, hypovolemia, septicemia, and drug administration. Although the cause is unidentified in one third of all cases, there is usually full neurologic recovery, even with prolonged and serious manifestations.

## Therapeutic Management

### Emergency Care

The initial management of the burn patient begins at the scene of injury. The first priority is to stop the burning process. (See Emergency Treatment box.) The child should then be transported immediately to the nearest medical facility for definitive treatment and evaluation for transfer to a burn center. The child and the family will be extremely frightened and anxious; sensitivity to their emotional state provides reassurance during the transport process.

**Stop the Burning Process.** The chief aim of rescue in flame burns is to smother the fire, not fan it. Children tend to panic and run, which serves only to spread the flames and make assistance more difficult. The injured child should be placed in a horizontal position and rolled in a blanket, rug, or similar article, with care taken not to cover the head and face because of the danger of inhaling toxic fumes. If nothing is available, the victim should lie down, cover the mouth with the hands, and roll over slowly to extinguish the flames. Remaining in the vertical position may cause the hair to ignite or may lead to the inhalation of flames, heat, or smoke.

Major burns with large amounts of denuded skin should not be cooled. Heat is rapidly lost from burned areas, and additional cooling leads to a drop in core body temperature and potential circulatory collapse. Wet dressings or the application of ice also promote vasoconstriction because of cooling, resulting in impaired circulation to the burned area and increased tissue damage. Chemical burns present special circumstances and require flushing with copious amounts of water during transport to a medical facility. The use of neutralizing agents on the skin is contraindicated because a chemical reaction is initiated and further injury may result. If the chemical is in powder form, the addition of water may spread the caustic agent. The powder should be brushed off if possible. If the chemical burn produces a blister, it is advisable to open the blister with a sterile object to remove any chemical present.

Burned clothing is removed to prevent further damage from smoldering fabric and hot beads of melted synthetic materials. Jewelry is also removed to eliminate the transfer of heat from the metal and constriction due to edema formation. These steps also provide better access to the wound and preclude more painful removal later on.

**Assess the Victim's Condition.** As soon as the flames are extinguished, the condition of the victim is assessed. Airway, breathing, and circulation are the priority concerns. Cardiopulmonary and cerebral emergencies are always a consideration following trauma. Cardiopulmonary complications may result from exposure to electric current, inhalation of toxic fumes and smoke, hypovolemia, and shock. Emergency measures are instituted as appropriate.

**Cover the Burn.** The burn wound should be covered with a clean cloth to prevent contamination and alleviate pain by eliminating air contact. The child with extensive burns is covered to prevent hypothermia. No attempt should be made to treat the burn. The application of topical ointments, oils, or other home remedies is contraindicated.

**Transport the Child to Medical Aid.** The child with an extensive burn is not given anything by mouth to avoid aspiration in the presence of paralytic ileus and upper airway edema and to prevent water intoxication. The child is transported to the nearest medical facility. If this cannot be accomplished within a relatively short period of time, intravenous (IV) access should be established if possible with a large-bore catheter. Oxygen, if available, is administered at 100%. A report of the initial assessment and any interventions implemented is given to the medical facility assuming responsibility for the child's care.

**Provide Reassurance.** Providing reassurance and psychologic support to both the family and the child helps immeasurably during postinjury crisis. Reducing anxiety helps

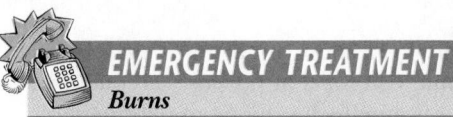

## EMERGENCY TREATMENT
### Burns

**MINOR BURNS**

Stop the burning process:
  Apply cool water to the burn or hold the burned area
    under cool running water. Do not use ice.
Do not disturb any blisters that form.
Do not apply anything to the wound.
Cover with a clean cloth if there is risk of damage or
  contamination.
Remove burned clothing and jewelry.

**MAJOR BURNS**

Stop the burning process:
  Flame burns—smother the fire.
  Place victim in the horizontal position.
  Roll victim in a blanket or similar object; avoid covering
    the head.
Assess for an adequate airway and breathing.
If not breathing, begin mouth-to-mouth resuscitation.
Remove burned clothing and jewelry.
Cover wound with a clean cloth.
Keep victim warm.
Transport to medical aid.
Begin IV and oxygen therapy.

to conserve the energy needed to cope with the physiologic and emotional stress of a traumatic injury.

### Management of Minor Burns

Treatment of burns classified as minor can usually be managed adequately on an outpatient basis when it is determined that the caregiver can be relied on to carry out instructions for care and observation. Patients with less than optimal circumstances may require close follow-up to ensure compliance with the treatment program.

The wound is cleansed with mild soap and tepid water. Debridement of the wound includes removal of any embedded debris, chemicals, and devitalized tissue. Removal of intact blisters remains controversial. Some authorities argue that blisters provide a barrier against infection; others maintain that blister fluid is an effective medium for the growth of microorganisms (Smith, 2000). Most practitioners favor covering the wound with an antimicrobial ointment to reduce the risk of infection and provide some form of pain relief. The dressing consists of a fine-mesh gauze placed over the ointment and a light wrap of gauze dressing that avoids interference with movement. This helps to keep the wound clean and protect it from trauma. The caregiver is instructed to wash the wound, reapply the dressing, and return the child to the office or clinic as directed for wound observation. The frequency of dressing changes can vary from every other day to twice a day.

Other practitioners prefer an occlusive dressing, such as a hydrocolloid, which is placed over the wound after cleansing. This method eliminates the discomfort associated with frequent dressing changes but impairs visualization of the wound surface.

If there is a high probability of infection or other complications or if there is doubt about the ability to carry out instructions, the parents may be directed to return daily for dressing changes and inspection, or a nurse may be assigned to make a home visit for that purpose. Frequent removal of the dressing is an effective mode of debridement. Soaking the dressing in tepid water before removal helps loosen the dressing and debris and reduces discomfort. Burns of the face and ears are usually treated by an open method (Carrougher, 1998). The wound is washed and debrided in the same manner, and a thin film of antimicrobial ointment is applied twice a day.

A tetanus history is obtained on admission. Tetanus prophylaxis is administered if there is no history of immunization or if more than 5 years have passed since the last immunization. Administration of antibiotics for minor burns is controversial. A mild analgesic such as acetaminophen is usually sufficient to relieve discomfort; the antipyretic effect of the drug also alleviates the sensation of heat.

Most minor burns heal without difficulty, but hospitalization is indicated if the wound margin becomes erythematous, gross purulence is noted, or the child develops evidence of systemic reaction (e.g., fever or tachycardia). The child should be evaluated for functional impairment, and the caregiver should be instructed in the exercise and ambulation program. Following wound healing, an evaluation of scar maturation and range of motion will indicate any need for further therapy.

## Management of Major Burns

When a child with extensive burns is admitted to the hospital for treatment, a variety of assessments are conducted and therapies initiated. Of these, the priority concerns include the establishment and maintenance of an adequate airway, initiation of fluid administration, and evaluation and treatment of the wound. Although the order of implementation may vary from institution to institution, a number of procedures and activities are generally initiated on admission. Some are carried out simultaneously (Box 29-11).

Other therapies, including nutritional support, positioning and splinting to prevent contractures, treatment of anemia and hypoproteinemia, psychosocial support, and rehabilitative aspects of burn management, are initiated as appropriate throughout the course of treatment.

**Establishment of an Adequate Airway.** The first priority of care is airway maintenance. Thermal injuries to the face, nares, and upper torso; a history of injury in an enclosed space; an examination of the oral and nasal membranes that reveals edema, hyperemia, and blisters; or evidence of trauma to the upper respiratory passages all suggest inhalation of noxious agents or respiratory burns. If there is evidence of respiratory involvement, 100% oxygen is administered and blood gas values, including carbon monoxide levels, are determined.

If the child exhibits changes in sensorium, air hunger, or other signs of respiratory distress, an endotracheal tube is inserted to maintain the airway. When severe edema of the face and neck is anticipated, intubation is performed before swelling makes tube placement difficult or impossible. A controlled intubation is preferred to an emergency procedure. Intubation allows for the delivery of humidified oxygen, the removal of secretions from respiratory passages, and the provision of ventilatory support.

Treatment may include bronchodilators to reduce bronchospasm. Bronchopulmonary hygiene to prevent atelectasis and pooling of secretions is used to reduce the risk of pneumonia. Therapies include percussion and postural drainage, frequent position changes, and suctioning to remove secretions. Placing the child in a semi-Fowler position with high-flow oxygen and maximum humidity is often sufficient to relieve bronchospasm produced by trauma to the bronchial mucosa.

When full-thickness burns encircle the chest, constricting eschar may limit chest wall excursion. The child becomes increasingly difficult to ventilate. Escharotomy of the chest relieves this pressure and improves ventilation.

**Fluid Replacement Therapy.** The objectives of fluid therapy are compensation for water and sodium losses to the traumatized area and the interstitial spaces, replenishment of sodium deficits, restoration of circulating volume, provision of adequate perfusion, correction of acidosis, and improvement of renal function. Treatment for burn shock should be initiated in children with burns in excess of 15% to 20% TBSA.

Types of fluid and electrolyte therapy in the first 24 hours after injury remain controversial. The controversy centers primarily around whether colloid solution should be a part of the resuscitation phase of fluid therapy. Those who favor crystalloid solutions believe that during this time the altered capillary membrane is unable to provide a structural barrier and that colloid solutions are of questionable value in restoring plasma oncotic pressure. However, others state that for the pediatric patient with extensive burns, plasma-like colloid solutions, administered intravenously in the re-

---

### Box 29-11 ■ ■ ■
### Outline of Major Burn Management

Ascertain the adequacy of the airway, and provide oxygen, intubation, and ventilatory support as indicated.

Insert a large-bore intravenous line, preferably through unburned skin, to deliver fluids at a sufficiently rapid rate to effect resuscitation.

Remove clothing and jewelry, and examine for secondary trauma.

Obtain an admission weight.

Insert a nasogastric tube to empty stomach contents and maintain gastric decompression.

Insert an indwelling Foley catheter to obtain specimens and monitor hourly output.

Evaluate the burn wound, and determine the extent and depth of injury.

Calculate fluid requirements, and establish the appropriate regimen.

Provide IV medication for control of pain and anxiety only after adequate oxygenation is ensured and fluid resuscitation is initiated.

Obtain baseline laboratory studies.

Perform escharotomy or fasciotomy to the chest and extremities for constricting circumferential eschar or elevated compartment pressures and for impaired circulation.

Apply topical antimicrobials and dressings to the burn wounds.

Obtain a history regarding the injury and other pertinent data.

Administer appropriate tetanus prophylaxis.

suscitative phase, decrease edema and reduce fluid volume (Shirani and others, 1996).

The composition of the fluid administered varies with the philosophy of the individual practitioner and may consist of an isotonic saline solution, a near-isotonic solution, or even a hypertonic saline solution. A decreased tolerance of children to hypertonic solutions may result in hypernatremia, hyperosmolality, and intracellular dehydration. Many formulas have been proposed as guidelines for fluid administration following burn injury. Perhaps the most commonly employed regimen is the Parkland formula. It is important to remember that any formula used during resuscitation serves only as a guideline; individual adjustments must be made on the basis of the patient's response to therapy. Fluid replacement is maintained at a rate that provides an hourly urinary output of 30 ml in older children and 1 to 2 ml/kg in children weighing less than 30 kg. Other parameters monitored during fluid resuscitation include vital signs, capillary refill, and sensorium.

Some common reasons for patients to require fluids well in excess of the calculated volume include underestimation of burn size (particularly in pediatric patients), pulmonary injury that sequesters resuscitation fluid in the lung, electrical injury with greater tissue destruction than is visible, and delay in the initiation of fluid resuscitation (Smith, 2000). Irreversible burn shock that persists despite aggressive fluid resuscitation remains a significant cause of death in the immediate postburn period. Exchange transfusion consisting of the replacement of circulating volume by banked whole blood provides a therapeutic modality that may benefit the patient who fails to respond to conventional resuscitation. Inflammatory response factors, thought to be important in burn shock, are removed, thus lowering the concentration present in the body, restoring capillary integrity, and substantially reducing fluid requirements.

> **NURSING ALERT**
>
> Capillary refill and alterations in sensorium and urinary output are the most reliable indicators for assessing the adequacy of fluid resuscitation in burned children. Blood pressure can remain normotensive even in a state of hypovolemia.

After the initial 24 to 48 hours, the capillary seal is restored. Fluid requirements decrease to a constant that persists until wound coverage is achieved. Colloid solutions such as albumin or plasma are useful to maintain plasma volume. Fluid balance may continue to be a problem throughout the course of treatment; especially during periods of increased evaporative loss from the burn wound. Approximately 48 to 72 hours after injury, interstitial fluid returns to the vascular compartment and diuresis occurs to eliminate excess fluids. During this phase, increasing intake to match urinary output can result in circulatory overload.

**Nutrition.** Burn injury is a severe insult that increases metabolism significantly. Well-planned nutritional support is necessary to prevent the depletion of body energy and protein stores. Energy requirements can increase according to the size of the burn—up to twice the normal to maintain metabolism. Because of the hypermetabolic state, protein

breakdown and gluconeogenesis increase. Fat metabolism increases as well, causing fatty infiltration of the liver, resulting in liver dysfunction (Cortiella and Marvin, 1997). Nutritional support, particularly the use of enteral feedings, recently has become more aggressive. The continuity of these feedings is very important.

Many burn patients are able to eat; a high-protein, high-calorie diet is encouraged as soon as possible after resolution of paralytic ileus. However, many have poor appetites and are unable to meet energy requirements solely by oral feeding. Most children with burns in excess of 25% TBSA require supplementation with tube feeding. An absence of bowel sounds does not preclude enteral nutrition. Because the small bowel maintains motility and absorptive capabilities, the placement of a small-bore feeding tube into the duodenum allows for the safe delivery of enteral nutrition during periods of paralytic ileus associated with trauma, sepsis, and anesthesia. Protection from aspiration is achieved by means of a nasogastric tube to decompress the stomach.

Burn patients with gastrointestinal dysfunction can be supported with total parenteral nutrition. However, enteral feeding increases blood flow in the intestinal tract, preserves GI function, and minimizes bacterial translocation by decreasing mucosal atrophy of the intestines. This makes enteral feeding the preferred route of nutritional support (Herndon and others, 1996). Specific guidelines for vitamin and micronutrient supplementation for the burn patient have no definitive basis in research. The needs and metabolic changes following a burn injury make it difficult to identify these requirements as they relate to protein and energy use.

**Medication.** Antibiotics are usually not administered prophylactically. The administration of systemic antibiotics to control wound colonization is not indicated, because decreased circulation to the injured area prevents delivery of the medication to areas of deepest injury. Surveillance cultures and monitoring of the clinical course provide the most reliable indicators of developing infection. Appropriate antibiotics can then be instituted to treat the identified organism. β-Streptococcus cultured from the throat or wounds is particularly destructive to grafted tissue. Otitis media should not be overlooked as a source of fever in the pediatric population.

Some form of sedation and analgesia is required in the care of burned children (Henry and Foster, 2000). Morphine sulfate is the drug of choice for severe burn injuries. Morphine has extensive distribution but is eliminated rapidly; continuous infusion or frequent administration is needed for pain management in burns. Morphine is administered intravenously and titrated to individual need. When combined with midazolam (Versed), fentanyl (Sublimaze) provides excellent analgesia for procedural pain. Morphine administered before a procedure is effective in controlling pain. Be sure to time the administration so that the morphine is in effect during the procedure (Cortiella and Marvin, 1997).

Anesthetic agents such as nitrous oxide, propofol, and ketamine also are used to control procedural pain. When ketamine is used, endotracheal intubation may not be needed. The gag reflex may be partially retained, but ketamine does

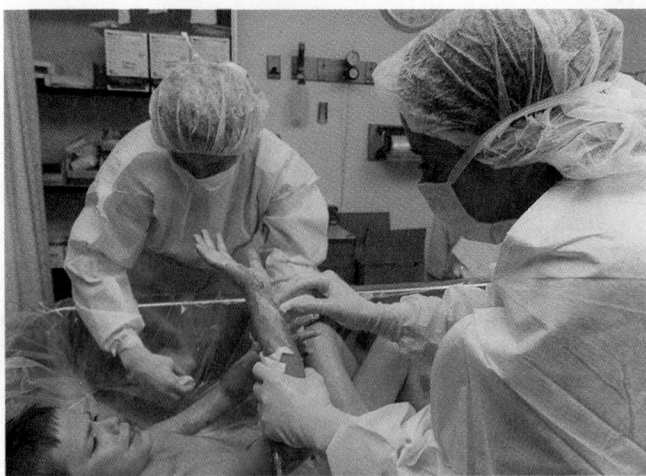

**Fig. 29-8** Removal of dressing during hydrotherapy. (Courtesy CR Boeckman Regional Burn Center, Akron, OH.)

---

**Box 29-12 ■ ■ ■**
**Methods of Burn Wound Management**

**Exposure.** Wounds are left open to air; crust forms on partial-thickness wounds, and eschar forms on full-thickness burns.
**Open.** Topical antimicrobial agent is applied directly to the wound surface, and the wound is left uncovered.
**Modified.** Antimicrobial is applied directly or impregnated into thin gauze and applied to the wound; gauze or net secures the area (Fig. 29-10).
**Occlusive.** Antimicrobial is impregnated in gauze or applied directly to the wound; multiple layers of bulky gauze are placed over the primary layer and secured with gauze or net.

---

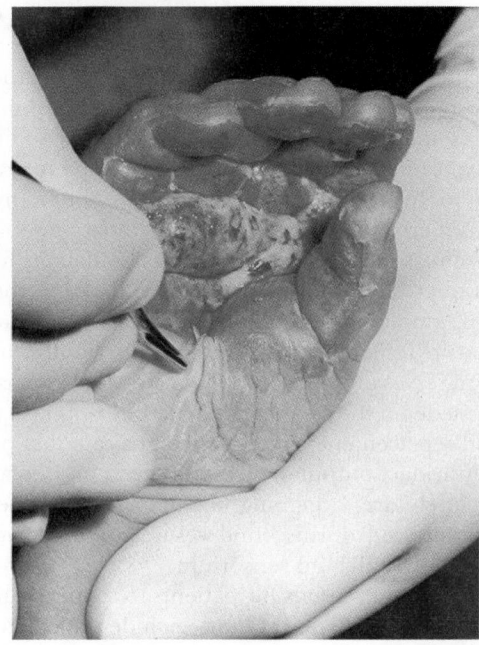

**Fig. 29-9** Dead skin and debris are carefully trimmed away before dressing is applied. (Courtesy CR Boeckman Regional Burn Center, Akron, OH.)

---

not prevent aspiration and may cause unpleasant hallucinations. To avoid volatile anesthetics, a combination of midazolam and fentanyl can be given intravenously (Herndon and others, 1996).

Entonox is a useful short-term analgesic mixture of gases in a fixed ratio of 50% nitrous oxide and 50% oxygen. Initiation of action is approximately 1 minute, with a peak effect reached in 3 to 5 minutes. It is eliminated from the body, mostly via the lungs, within 2 to 5 minutes. Entonox is useful for alleviating anxiety and raising the threshold of pain during procedures. The child must be able to follow instructions and may self-administer the gas with assistance. No treatment should last longer than 30 minutes, and the child should be monitored continuously during the procedure. Side effects of nitrous oxide administration may include excitability, shortness of breath, nausea, or vomiting. It is not recommended for children who are sedated, hypotensive, unconscious, pregnant, or intoxicated, or for those with abdominal distension or chest injuries (Selbst, 1993).

### Management of the Burn Wound

After the initial period of shock and restoration of fluid balance, the primary concern is the burn wound. The objectives of wound management include prevention of infection, removal of devitalized tissue, and closure of the wound. The application of dressings and topical antimicrobial therapy reduce pain by minimizing air exposure.

**Primary Excision.** In children with large, full-thickness burn wounds, excision is performed as soon as the patient is hemodynamically stable after initial resuscitation. Because the burn wound is precipitating the exaggerated physiologic response, many associated complications do not resolve until the eschar is excised and the wound is closed. Early wound excision has significantly decreased the incidence of infection, which can lead to sepsis and death (Nguyen and others, 1996).

**Debridement.** Hydrotherapy is used to cleanse the wound and involves soaking in a tub or showering once or twice a day for no more than 20 minutes. Hydrotherapy helps to cleanse not only the wound but the entire body and also aids in maintenance of range of motion.

Partial-thickness wounds require debridement of devitalized tissue to promote healing. Debridement is very painful and requires some type of analgesia before the procedure. The water acts to loosen and remove sloughing tissue, exudate, and topical medications. Mesh gauze entraps the exudative slough and is readily removed during hydrotherapy (Fig. 29-8). Any loose tissue is carefully trimmed away before the wound is redressed (Fig. 29-9).

**Topical Antimicrobial Agents.** Several methods are used for covering the burn wound (Box 29-12) (Fig. 29-10). All meet the objective of preparation for permanent wound coverage, and all use some type of topical agent. Before the development of effective topical agents for reducing the incidence of invasive organisms, wound sepsis was the major cause of mortality from burn injury. Topical agents do not eliminate organisms from the wound but can effectively inhibit bacterial growth. To be effective a topical application

**TABLE 29-5**   Comparison of common topical preparations

| Agent | Dressings | Advantages | Disadvantages |
|---|---|---|---|
| Silver nitrate 0.5% (AgNO₃) | Open, modified or occlusive; impedes joint movement; dressings changed twice daily; keep dressing moist, rewet at least every 2 hours | Greatly reduces evaporative losses; does not interfere with wound healing; bacteriostatic action against major burn flora, including *Pseudomonas* and *Staphylococcus;* inexpensive | Does not penetrate eschar; ineffective on established burn wound infections; little effect on *Klebsiella* and *Aerobacter* groups; stains skin, clothing, linens; makes assessment of the wound difficult because of staining; hypotonicity pulls electrolytes from the wound, depleting sodium, potassium, chloride, and magnesium; stings on application |
| Silver sulfadiazine 1% | Occlusive; motion of joints maintained; applied twice daily; do not use with a history of allergy to sulfa | Little pain on application; bactericidal by altering DNA and cell metabolism; effective against gram-positive and gram-negative bacteria; easy to apply; nontoxic | Transient neutropenia; does not penetrate eschar; forms proteinaceous gel on wound surface that is painful to remove; occasional rashes and pruritus; decreases granulocyte formation |
| Mafenide acetate 10% (Sulfamylon) | **Cream:** Usually open; do not apply to face; apply twice daily<br>**Solution:** Occlusive; keep dressing moist (rewet at least every 2 hours); protect solution from light | Penetrates eschar and diffuses rapidly into burn wound and underlying tissues; effective in deep flame, electrical, and infected wounds; biostatic against many gram-positive and gram-negative organisms, including *Pseudomonas* and *Clostridium* | Difficult and painful to remove cream; pain on application; metabolic acidosis, hypercapnia, and carbonic anhydrase inhibition; inhibits wound healing; hypersensitivity in some patients |
| Bacitracin | Open, modified; motion of joints maintained; change dressing twice daily | Bactericidal and bacteriostatic against gram-positive organisms; low toxicity; painless application; ease of application | Limited activity against gram-negative organisms; allergic reaction in sensitive individuals |

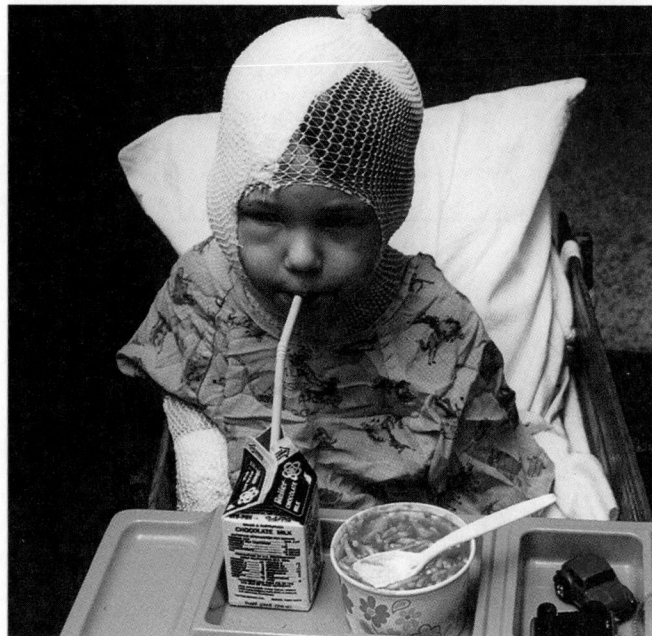

**Fig. 29-10**   Burn wound covered with gauze dressings and secured with tabular elastic netting. (Courtesy CR Boeckman Regional Burn Center, Akron, OH.)

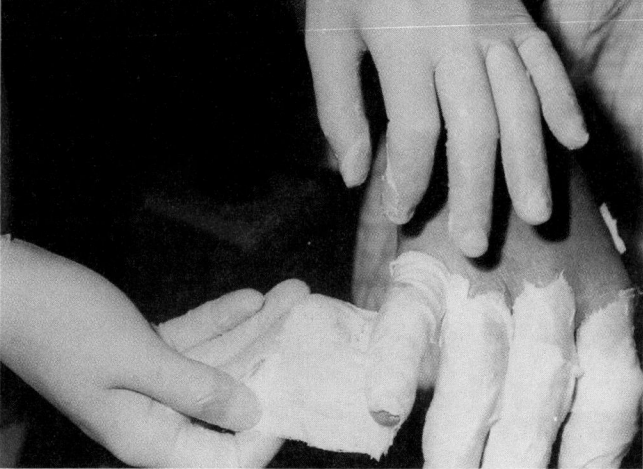

**Fig. 29-11**   Gauze impregnated with ointment applied to burn wound. Note how each finger is wrapped separately. (Courtesy CR Boeckman Burn Center, Akron, OH.)

must be nontoxic, capable of diffusing through eschar, harmless to viable tissue, inexpensive, and easy to apply. It should not encourage the development of resistent strains of bacteria and should produce minimum electrolyte de-

rangement (Fig. 29-11). The significant properties of commonly used agents are summarized in Table 29-5.

Some topical agents are packaged and prepared on a fine-mesh gauze, which allows ease of application. The gauze provides necessary protection for the wound, maximizes patient comfort, increases the rate of healing, reduces the necessity for frequent dressing changes, and is cost-effective. Daily dressing changes of the burn wound are recommended to allow for inspection (Herndon and others, 1996). Most often these gauzes are used on superficial second-degree burns, donor sites, and for graft care, except for Acticoat, which can also be used for full-thickness wounds. Refer to Table 29-6 for a comparative list.

**Biologic Skin Coverings.** Permanent coverage of extensive burns is a prolonged process that requires repeated operations for debridement and grafting. Early closure shortens the period of metabolic stress and decreases the likelihood of burn wound sepsis (Mlcak and others, 1998). In addition, biologic dressings markedly reduce pain and facilitate movement of joints to retain range of motion.

Allograft (homograft) skin is obtained from human cadavers and processed by commercial skin banks (see Box 29-13). Donors are screened for communicable diseases, and the skin is tracked much like blood transfusions. Homograft is particularly useful in the coverage of surgically excised, deep partial-thickness and full-thickness wounds in extensive burns when available donor sites are limited. Severe immunosuppression occurs in massively burned children, and the allograft becomes adherent (Fig. 29-12). The homograft can remain in place until suitable donor sites become available. Typically rejection is seen approximately 14 days after application. The use of a homograft is limited by the availability of tissue banks and the supply of suitable donors.

Xenograft from a variety of species, most notably pigs, is commercially available. In large burns the porcine xenograft is commonly applied when extensive early debridement is indicated to cover a partial-thickness burn; this allows available autograft to be applied to the full-thickness areas (Still and others, 1996). Pigskin dressings are replaced daily or every 2 to 3 days. They are particularly effective in children with partial-thickness scald burns of the hands and face because they allow relatively pain-free movement, which reduces contracture formation and has the added benefit of improving appetite and morale (Fig. 29-13).

| TABLE 29-6 | Common impregnated-gauze preparations | |
|---|---|---|
| **Product** | **Description** | **Use** |
| Acticoat* | Absorbent rayon/polyester core and upper and lower layer of silver-coated high-density polyethylene mesh | Partial- and full-thickness wounds, decubitus ulcers, second-degree burns, and donor sites; may be used over debrided and grafted partial-thickness wounds |
| Adaptic/ Aquaphor | Nonmedicinal white petrolatum–impregnated fine-mesh or porous-mesh gauze | Small superficial partial-thickness burns devoid of epithelium; may be used with bacitracin ointment to enhance comfort and add a topical antibiotic property |
| Scarlet Red† | 5% scarlet red in a nonmedicinal blend of lanolin, olive oil, and petrolatum on a fine-mesh absorbent gauze | Healing burns, often to dry them, and donor sites; helps promote epithelial cell proliferation and can protect the wound from contamination |
| Xeroflo | 3% bismuth tribromophenate in a nonmedicinal bland oil emulsion on fine-mesh absorbent gauze | Superficial second-degree wounds, grafts, and donor sites; allows healing wounds to dry without becoming cracked and prevents the tissue from becoming macerated by more wet types of dressings |
| Xeroform | 3% bismuth tribromophenate in a nonmedicinal petrolatum blend on fine-mesh absorbent gauze | A "greasy" texture |

*Contraindicated for third-degree burns.
†Contraindicated on patients with a hypersensitivity to lanolin or olive oil. May stain the skin.

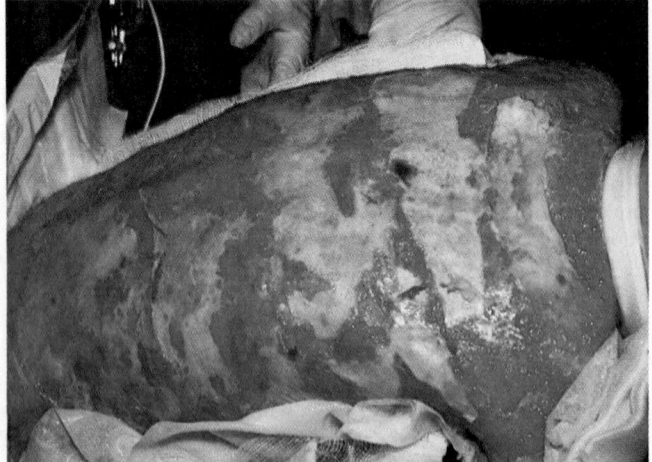

**Fig. 29-12** Adherent homograft applied to excised full-thickness wound.

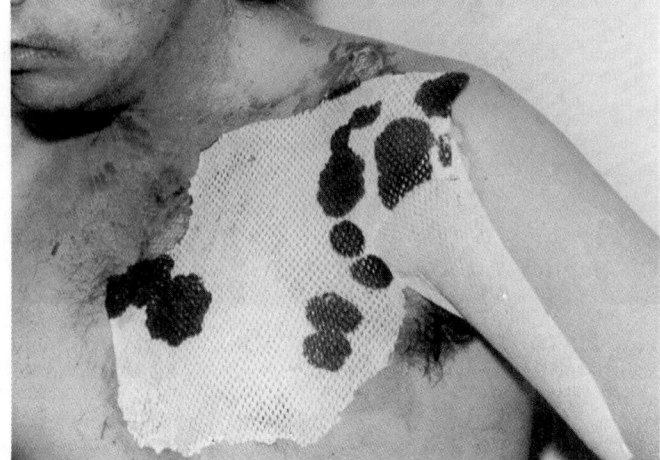

**Fig. 29-13** Porcine xenograft applied to partial-thickness burn. (Courtesy CR Boeckman Regional Burn Center, Akron, OH.)

When applied early to a superficial partial-thickness injury, biologic dressings appear to accelerate wound healing. They create an environment at the wound surface that is conducive to epithelial growth; this is in contrast to topical antimicrobial agents, which may slow epithelialization. Biologic dressings must be applied to clean wounds. If the dressing covers areas of heavy microbial contamination, infection occurs beneath the dressing. In the case of partial-thickness burns, such an infection may convert the wound to a full-thickness injury. It is important to observe the wound daily for any signs of an infectious process.

**Synthetic Skin Coverings.** A number of satisfactory skin substitutes are available for the management of partial-thickness burn wounds. Ideally, the dressing should provide many of the properties of human skin: adherence, elasticity, durability, and hemostasis. Synthetic skin substitutes are readily available, have varied shelf lives, and are relatively expensive.

Synthetic dressings are composed of a variety of materials and can be used very successfully in the management of superficial partial-thickness burns and donor sites. Examples include adherent elastic films, hydroactive materials, or colloidal suspensions that are usually permeable to air, vapor, and fluids. BCG Matrix* consists of a film-backed, mesh-reinforced, hydrocolloid dressing. Biobrane† is a flexible silicone-nylon membrane bonded to collagenous peptides of porcine skin. Calcium alginate is another treatment for donor sites.

As with biologic dressings, it is important that the wound be free of debris before the dressing is applied. Body temperature elevation or evidence of purulence, erythema, or cellulitis around the wound edges may indicate that the wound has become infected beneath the dressing. Prompt discontinuance of the synthetic dressing is indicated. All synthetic dressings are reputed to hasten wound healing and reduce discomfort.

---

*Brennan Medical Inc, (800) 328-9105.
†Dow Hickham Pharmaceuticals Inc, (800) 231-3052; www.dowhickham.com.

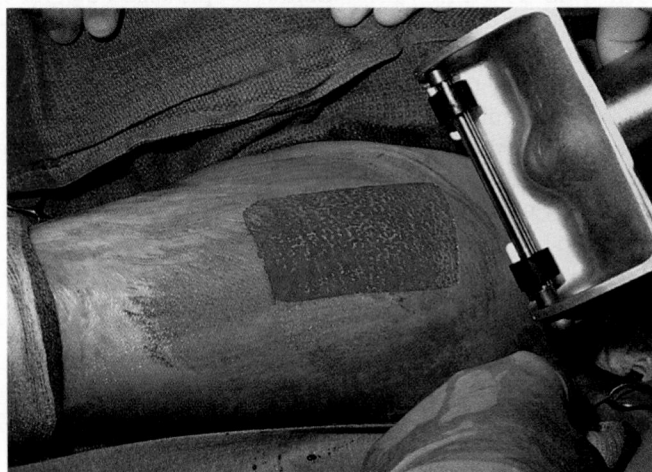

**Fig. 29-14** Removal of split-thickness skin graft with a dermatome.

**Artificial Skin.** The development of Integra,* a biologic two-layer product that allows the dermis to regenerate, has produced a significant improvement in burn wound healing and a decrease in scar formation. It is applied to partial-thickness and full-thickness burns. The inner layer is porous woven fiber made of a pure form of collagen (a fibrous protein taken from animal tendons and cartilage) and other materials designed to induce better regeneration of the patient's normal tissue. The outer layer is a soft silicone (i.e., Silastic) membrane that holds moisture for 2 to 3 weeks. The Silastic layer is peeled off after the dermis is formed. The application of artificial skin does not replace the grafting procedure, but it prepares the burn wound to accept an ultrathin autograft. Advantages include faster healing of the burn wound when integrity of the dermis is restored, faster healing of donor sites with the use of ultrathin grafts, and the restoration of sweat glands and hair follicles. A disadvantage is its high cost.

**Permanent Skin Coverings.** Permanent coverage of deep partial-thickness and full-thickness burns is usually accomplished with a split-thickness skin graft. This graft consists of the epidermis and a portion of the dermis removed from an intact area of skin by a special instrument—the dermatome (Fig. 29-14). If all of the wounds cannot be grafted at once, there are priority areas for coverage: the face, hands, joint surfaces, and neck. These preferential sites are chosen to hasten healing, establish function, and improve the patient's sense of well-being.

With extensive burns it is often difficult to find enough viable skin to cover the wounds; therefore available donor sites are used to the best advantage by special techniques. The various types of split-thickness skin grafts are described in Box 29-13. Sheet grafts are used in areas where

---

*Integra Life Sciences Corporation, Plainsboro, NJ, 1996, (609) 275-0500; www.integra-ls.com.

---

> **Box 29-13** ■ ■ ■
> **Types of Skin Grafts**
>
> **TEMPORARY GRAFTS**
>
> **Allografts (homografts)**—Skin that is obtained from genetically different members of the same species who are free of disease.
> **Xenografts (heterografts)**—Skin that is obtained from members of a different species, primarily pigskin.
>
> **PERMANENT GRAFTS**
>
> **Autografts**—Tissue obtained from undamaged areas of the patient's own body.
> **Isografts**—Histocompatible tissue obtained from genetically identical individuals.
>
> **METHODS OF APPLYING SPLIT-THICKNESS GRAFTS**
>
> **Sheet graft**—A sheet of skin, removed from the donor site, is placed intact over the recipient site and sutured in place (Fig. 29-15).
> **Mesh graft**—A sheet of skin is removed from the donor site and passed through a mesher, which produces tiny slits in the skin. The meshing allows the expansion of the skin to cover $1\frac{1}{2}$ to 9 times the area of the sheet graft (Fig. 29-16).

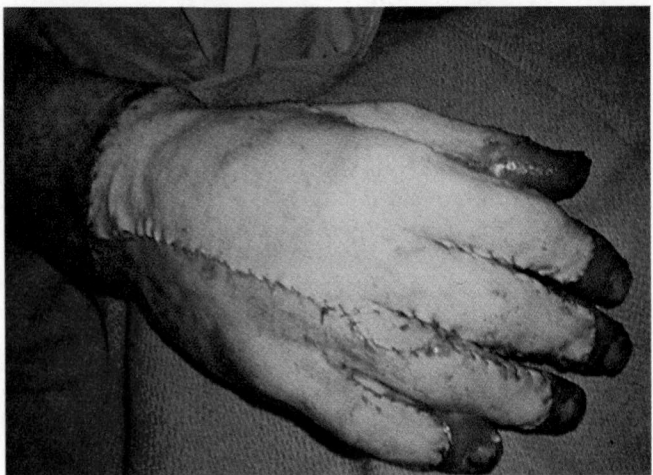

**Fig. 29-15** Sheet graft.

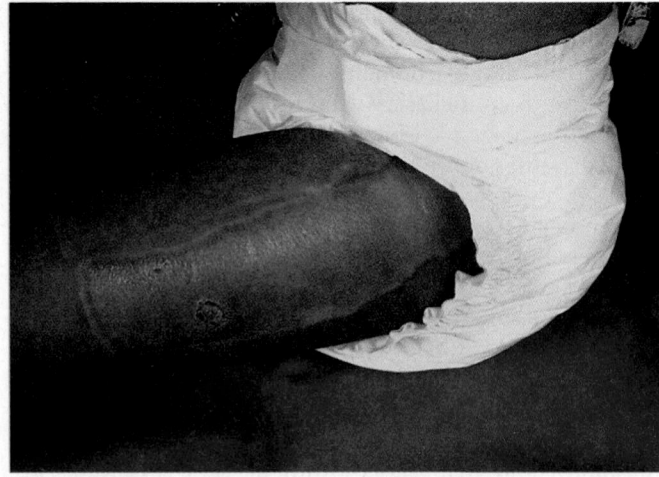

**Fig. 29-17** Healed donor site.

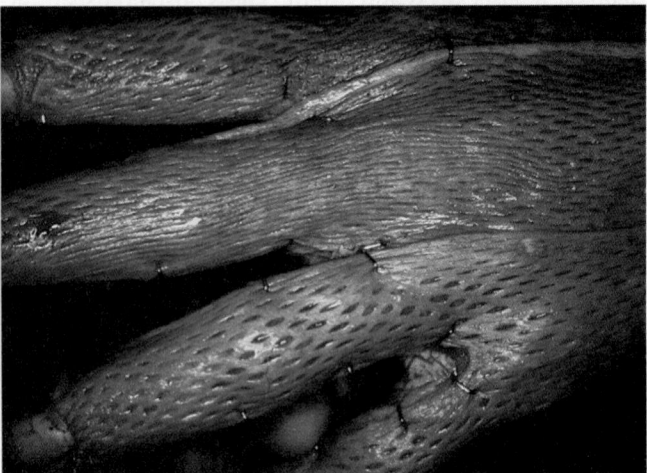

**Fig. 29-16** Mesh graft.

### Box 29-14 ■ ■ □
### Requirements for a Successful Graft

Sufficient nourishment until the new blood supply is established from the base of the recipient bed

Primary tissue contact (i.e., actual contact between the surface of the graft and a recipient bed that is free of bacteria and necrotic skin)

Avoidance of bleeding, hematoma formation, and fluid accumulation beneath the graft

Prevention of infection

Prevention of mechanical trauma

cosmetic results are most visible; mesh grafts result in a less desirable cosmetic and functional outcome. Requirements for the successful vascularization of any graft are listed in Box 29-14.

Until blood supply to the grafted skin is established, it is nourished by osmotic interchange with the recipient bed. Wound healing occurs as the area releases fibrin, which attaches the graft to the bed. The fibrin is infiltrated by leukocytes, fibroblasts, and the capillary buds of the granulation tissue. This process begins within hours of grafting, and vascularization is established after 3 days. Within 2 weeks the graft is attached to the recipient bed by connective tissue.

The donor site is dressed with synthetic wound coverings or fine-mesh gauze until the dressing separates at 10 to 14 days, when the wound is healed. Dressings are not changed on donor sites to avoid damage to newly healed, delicate epithelium. Healed donor sites are available for reharvesting in patients with extensive burns and limited undamaged skin. The quality of skin from donor sites is decreased when multiple grafts are taken (Fig. 29-17).

**Cultured Epithelium.** When burns are extensive and donor sites for split-thickness skin grafting are limited, it is possible to culture cells from a full-thickness skin biopsy and produce coherent sheets that can be applied to clean, excised full-thickness wounds. Epithelial cell culture grafts offer the possibility of an unlimited source of autografts in patients with extensive burns. Cultured epithelial autografts are effective in early wound closure. The child's own skin is fractionated and cultured in a porcine media to form a thin epithelial layer that is applied to the burn wound. The application of cultured epithelium on newly formed dermis generated by the use of artificial skin on the burn wound is under study (Nguyen and others, 1996). High cost is a disadvantage of using both applications.

## Nursing Considerations

Nursing care of the pediatric burn patient represents a challenge to the nurse's knowledge of anatomy and physiology, the behavioral sciences, and pathophysiology. Patient outcome following thermal injury is the result of the collaboration of a professional multidisciplinary team using a family-centered care approach. In addition to providing nursing care, the nurse coordinates the efforts of a multidisciplinary burn team (Henry and Foster, 2000).

Because the care of burned children encompasses such a broad range of skills and foci, it has been divided into segments that correspond with the major phases of burn treatment. The acute phase, also referred to as the emergent or resuscitative phase, involves the first 24 to 48 hours. The management phase extends from the completion of adequate resuscitation through wound coverage. The rehabilitative phase begins once the majority of the wounds have healed and rehabilitation has become the predominant focus of the plan of care. This phase continues until all reconstructive procedures and corrective measures have been accomplished and often extends over a period of months or years.

## Acute Phase

The primary emphasis during the emergent phase is the treatment of burn shock and management of pulmonary status. Monitoring vital signs, output, fluid infusion, and respiratory parameters are ongoing activities in the hours immediately following injury. Intravenous infusion is begun immediately and is regulated to maintain a urinary output of at least 1 to 2 ml/kg in children weighing less than 30 kg; an output of 30 to 50 ml/hr is expected in children weighing more than 30 kg. Urinary output and specific gravity, vital signs, laboratory data, and objective signs of adequate hydration guide the rate of fluid administration.

> **NURSING ALERT**
> Level of consciousness is another important indicator of the adequacy of hydration.

Children are observed for changes in all parameters. They require constant observation and assessment, with special attention given to signs of respiratory, cardiac, and renal complications. Alterations in electrolyte balance can produce clinical symptoms of confusion, weakness, cardiac irregularities, and seizures. Changes in respiratory function and gas exchange are reflected clinically by restlessness, irritability, and increased work of breathing, as well as by alterations in blood gas values. The loss of the protective function of the skin exposes burned children to an increased risk of hypothermia.

Care of the burn wound is secondary to the more critical problems of respiratory and cardiac failure. When transfer to a special burn care facility is anticipated, it is important to cover the wounds with clean sheets and wrap the child in blankets to maintain body temperature during transfer. The burn wound can be evaluated and dressed following arrival at the burn center. If no burn unit is available, the wound is cleansed and dressed in the emergency department. Many burn units maintain a pictorial record of the wound to record progress and for legal purposes, especially in cases of suspected child abuse. The burn wound is treated according to the protocol of the specific burn facility. Baseline cultures are obtained on admission. The burn team monitors infection control procedures and ensures that staff and visitors comply with established protocols to prevent cross-contamination in the burn unit.

Throughout the acute phase of care the psychosocial needs of the children and their families should not be overlooked. The child is frightened, uncomfortable, and often confused. Children may be isolated from familiar persons and surroundings; the often overwhelming physical needs at this time are the primary focus of the staff and parents. In addition to feeling concern for their child, the family experiences guilt, which has nothing to do with the burn injury. This guilt is instead related to the fact that the parents did not or could not protect their child. Consistency in the information presented and the attitude of the staff creates a sense of familiarity and stability during the emergent phase.

### Management and Rehabilitative Phases

After the patient's condition is stabilized, the management phase begins. The multidisciplinary team concentrates on preventing wound infections, closing the wound as quickly as possible, and managing the numerous complications that may occur. Although the rehabilitative phase begins when permanent wound closure has been achieved, rehabilitation issues are identified on admission and are included in the plan of care throughout the hospital course.

## Assessment

Wound assessment and comprehensive assessment of the child's general condition and behaviors are of major importance. Observation for signs of complications, especially infection, and assessment of the need for and effectiveness of pain management are important nursing functions.

## Nursing Diagnoses

Several nursing diagnoses are identified on the basis of a thorough assessment. The more common diagnoses for the child with burns are included in the Nursing Care Plan on pp. 1249-1252. Others may apply in specific situations.

## Planning

The age-specific goals for the child with a burn injury and the family are as follows:

1. Child will experience reduction of pain.
2. Child will exhibit evidence of wound healing.
3. Child will receive adequate nutrition and will achieve reduction in metabolic losses.
4. Child will not experience acute complications during the management phase.
5. Child will not experience long-term complications during the rehabilitative phase.
6. Child and family will receive emotional support.

## Implementation

The management phase of burn care involves intensive nursing care, which can be difficult for the patient, family, and nursing staff. Except for minor burn injuries, care usually takes place in a burn unit and involves members of a variety of disciplines, such as physical therapy, nutrition, social services, and respiratory care.

**Comfort Management.** The severe pain of the wound and resultant therapies, the anxiety generated by these experiences, sleep deprivation, itching related to wound heal-

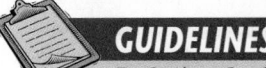

Have all materials ready before beginning.
Administer appropriate analgesics.
Remind the child of the impending procedure to allow sufficient time to prepare.
Allow the child to test and approve the temperature of the water.
Allow the child to select the area of the body on which to begin.
Allow the child to request a short rest period during the procedure.
Allow the child to remove the dressings if desired.
Provide something constructive for the child to do during the procedure (e.g., holding a package of dressings or a roll of gauze).
Inform the child when the procedure is near completion.
Praise the child for cooperation.

ing, and the conscious and unconscious interpretations of traumatic events contribute to the psychologic reactions and behaviors commonly observed in children with burns. It is always difficult to deal with a child in pain, and to inflict pain on a helpless child is contrary to the empathetic nature of nursing. A careful nursing history that includes the child's past experiences with pain and ways that caregivers successfully handled those events may provide clues to the control of current pain. Caregiver involvement is especially important for a child (Herndon and others, 1996). Interventions may include medications (including intravenous morphine and short-term anesthetics such as propofol or ketamine), relaxation techniques, distraction therapy, cutaneous stimulation by touching, and family participation. Nonpharmacologic therapies may be used as adjuncts to the treatment of pain. In young children, distraction and imagery work very well (Carrougher, 1998; Henry and Foster, 2000).

To reduce the anxiety associated with an unfamiliar environment and frightening treatments, it is important to offer thorough, age-appropriate explanations to the child before procedures. Compounding the pain is the child's interpretation of it and of the procedure; this is closely related to the developmental level of the child. There are often feelings of anger, guilt, and depression; as in all illnesses, there is also regressive behavior. When children appear to accept pain with little or no response, psychologic consultation is in order.

**Care of the Burn Wound.** The nurse has a major responsibility for cleansing, debriding, and applying topical medications and dressings to the burn wound. Because dressing removal is a painful procedure, children should receive adequate analgesia before the scheduled dressing change. Medication should be administered so that the peak effect of the drug coincides with the procedure. Children who have an understanding of the procedure to be performed and some perceived control demonstrate less maladaptive behavior. Children respond well to participating in decisions and the actual procedure as their condition allows. (See Guidelines box.)

With some children, nonpharmacologic interventions are effective means of coping with pain. Distraction therapy, deep breathing, and relaxation techniques may facilitate the procedure. Most children also benefit from parental participation. Medical play is often effective in helping the younger child to gain some mastery over the procedure. Those techniques that work best for the individual patient are incorporated into the plan of care and consistently implemented during the dressing change procedure.

Outer dressings are removed; any dressings that have adhered to the wound can be more easily removed by applying tepid water. Loose or easily detached tissue is also debrided during the cleansing process. Children can be encouraged to participate in dressing removal. Providing something constructive for them to do helps them to focus on something other than the procedure. In dressing the wound, it is important that all areas be clean, that medication be amply applied, and that no two burned surfaces touch each other (e.g., fingers or toes, or ears touching the side of the head). If touching, the burned surfaces will heal together, causing deformity or dysfunction.

Topical medications may be applied directly to the wound with a clean gloved hand or impregnated into fine-mesh gauze before application. Dressings are then applied to assist in exudate absorption, wound debridement, and increased patient comfort. All dressings applied circumferentially should be wrapped in a distal-to-proximal manner. The dressing is applied with sufficient tension to remain in place but not so tightly as to impair circulation or limit motion. Elastic bandages are applied over dressings to prevent epithelial breakdown, decrease edema formation, stimulate circulation, and improve mobility. The bandage is applied in a figure-8 to promote optimum circulation. A stable dressing is especially important when the child is ambulatory.

Burns that involve the eyelids require special care to prevent corneal ulceration. No solution other than saline should come in contact with the eyes during the cleansing process. Vigorous debridement is avoided in this area of thin, delicate tissue. The patient is assessed throughout the healing process for the ability to close the eyes. Inability to close the eyes because of contracture formation, administration of paralytic agents, or corneal burns requires instilling ophthalmic ointment and covering the eyes with a patch to prevent further corneal damage (Achauer and Adair, 2000).

Standard precautions, including the use of protective garb and barrier techniques, should be followed when caring for all patients with thermal injuries. Frequent hand and forearm washing is the single most important element of the infection control program. Strict policies for cleaning the environment and patient care equipment should be implemented to minimize the risk of cross-contamination. All visitors and members of other departments should be oriented to the infection control policies, including the importance of hand and forearm washing and use of protective garb. All visitors should be screened for infection and contagious diseases before patient contact.

**Nutrition.** Oral feedings are usually encouraged unless the child is intubated or paralytic ileus persists. Because

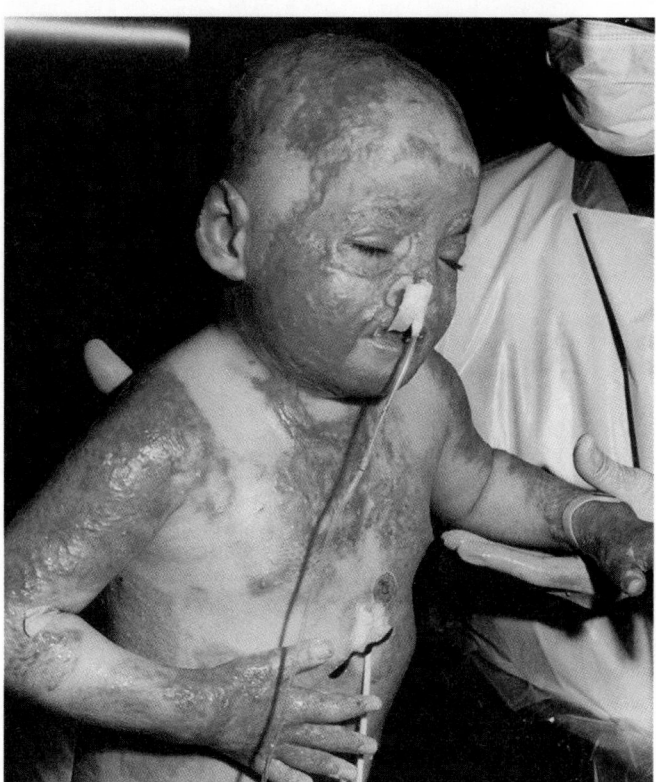

**Fig. 29-18** Extensive scars from flame burn. (Courtesy CR Boeckman Regional Burn Center, Akron, OH.)

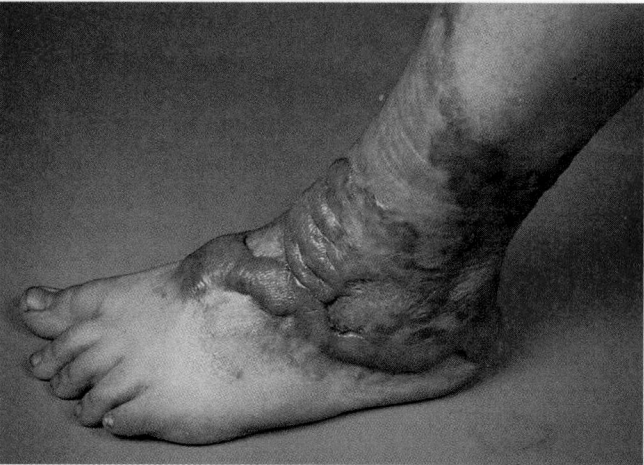

**Fig. 29-19** Hypertrophic immature scar.

children often lack an appetite, a great deal of encouragement, help, and patience is required of the nursing staff. Consultation between the parent and dietitian helps to determine food preferences. Children who are old enough to participate should be included in meal planning.

Nourishing snacks are provided between scheduled meals. Painful procedures should not be scheduled around meals; most children are too physically exhausted and emotionally upset to eat at this time. Many children eat better in an atmosphere more nearly like what they are accustomed to at home. When their condition allows, children enjoy sitting at a table for meals and interacting with other children.

Children who require enteral supplementation by tube feeding must be monitored on an ongoing basis for intolerance and tube malposition. The nurse should monitor and record any indications of abdominal distention, diarrhea, or electrolyte and metabolic derangement. Accurate documentation of oral, parenteral, and enteral nutritional intake is essential to evaluate the adequacy of nutritional support.

**Prevention of Complications: Acute Care.** The maintenance of body temperature is important to the child with burns. Reduction of heat loss is imperative to decrease energy demands and evaporative water loss. Ambient temperatures and humidity should be maintained at 28° to 33° C and 80%, respectively, to control heat loss (Herndon and others, 1996). Large areas of the body should not be exposed simultaneously during dressing changes. Warmed solutions, linens, occlusive dressings, heat shields, a radiant warmer, and warming blankets assist in preventing hypothermia. The

optimum environment for the child with burns can be very uncomfortable for persons attending the child.

The chief danger during acute care is infection—wound infection, generalized sepsis, or bacterial pneumonia. The burn wound should be assessed for changes indicative of wound infection, which include conversion of a partial-thickness to a full-thickness burn injury, early eschar separation, subeschar hemorrhage, degeneration of granulation tissue, discoloration of unburned skin at the wound margins, or green discoloration of subcutaneous fat (indicative of *Pseudomonas* and other gram-negative organisms). In addition to the signs of developing wound infection, the child with systemic sepsis may demonstrate hyperventilation, temperature lability, stupor, vasomotor instability, and ileus (Shirani and others, 1996).

Children are reluctant to move when doing so causes pain, and they are likely to assume a position of comfort. Unfortunately, the most comfortable position is often one that encourages the formation of contractures and loss of function. Ongoing efforts to prevent contractures include the positioning and splinting of involved extremities in extension, active and passive physical therapy, and the encouragement of spontaneous movement when feasible. In addition to maintenance of proper body alignment, frequent position changes are important to improve bronchopulmonary hygiene and capillary perfusion to common pressure areas. Low–air loss beds are beneficial for the morbidly obese or for children with posterior grafts. Areas of particular concern for pressure area development in the pediatric population are the posterior scalp, heels, and areas exposed to mechanical irritation from splints and dressings.

**Prevention of Complications: Long-Term Care.** The rehabilitative phase of care begins once wound coverage has been achieved. Scar formation becomes a major problem as burn wounds heal (Fig. 29-18). The scar tissue is metabolically active and highly vascular; collagen is deposited in an undefined pattern. Contractile properties of the scar tissue can result in disabling contractures, deformity, and disfigurement. As long as the scar is raised, red, and firm, it is considered to be active (Fig. 29-19). Hypertrophic scarring

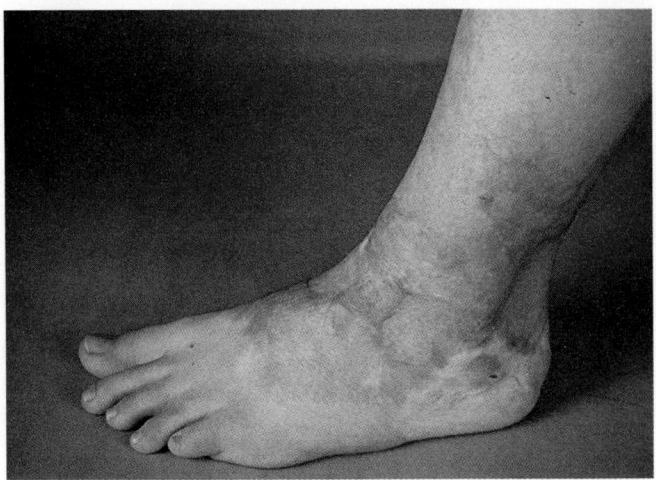

**Fig. 29-20** Flat, mature scar after pressure.

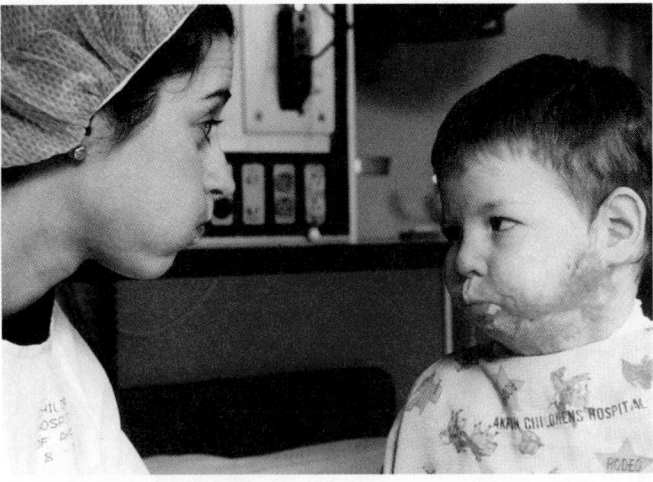

**Fig. 29-22** Daily physical therapy to prevent contracture deformity is continued at home or in an outpatient setting. Note how the nurse encourages the child to imitate her facial action. (Courtesy CR Boeckman Regional Burn Center, Akron, OH.)

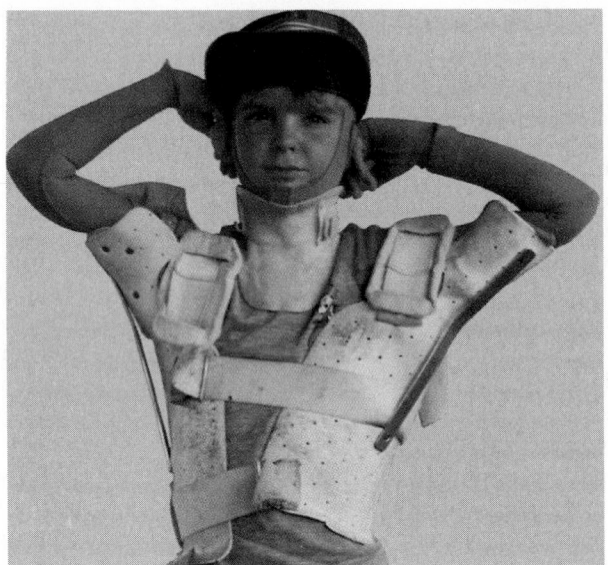

**Fig. 29-21** Child in elasticized (Jobst) garment and "airplane" splints.

typically reaches a peak approximately 4 to 6 months after wound healing, and most scars mature or become inactive in 1 to 2 years. The mature scar is characterized by pigmented color, flattening, and an increase in suppleness of the tissue (Fig. 29-20).

Uniform pressure applied to the scar decreases the blood supply and forces the collagen into a more normal alignment. When pressure is removed, blood supply to the scar is immediately increased; therefore periods without pressure should be brief to avoid nourishment of the hypertrophic tissue. Continuous pressure to areas of scarring can be achieved by elastic bandages or commercially available pressure garments. Because these custom-made garments are often worn for months, revision may be required as the child grows. It is much easier to prevent scarring and contracture of the wound than to resolve an existing problem. Splints and appliances may also be needed until wound maturation

is achieved (Fig. 29-21). Part of outpatient and home care often includes the continuation of regular physical therapy (Fig. 29-22).

Scar tissue has certain significant properties, particularly for growing children. Intense itching occurs in healing burn wounds and scar tissue until the scar is no longer active. Itching is usually treated with hydroxyzine (Atarax) or diphenhydramine (Benadryl) and frequent applications of a moisturizer, such as Eucerin, cocoa butter, or Nivea. Massage therapy during the application of moisturizers is also beneficial to stretch scar tissue and aid in contracture prevention. Scar tissue has no sweat glands, and children with extensive scarring may experience difficulty during hot weather. Caregivers should be alerted to this possibility and be prepared to institute alternate methods of cooling when necessary.

Scar tissue does not grow and expand as does normal tissue, which may create difficulties, especially in functional areas such as the hands and over joints. Additional surgery is sometimes required to allow independent functioning in daily activities, to improve cosmetic appearance, or to restore anatomic integrity. Reconstructive surgery employs various techniques, including local or distant flaps, full- or partial-thickness grafts, tissue expanders, or pedicle flaps.

The nursing activities in the rehabilitative phase of treatment focus on the child's and family's adaptation to the burn injury and their ability to reintegrate into the community. The multidisciplinary team approach remains the model for support of the child and family (Fig. 29-23).

The psychologic pain and sequelae of severe burn injury are as intense as the physical trauma. The impact of severe burns taxes the capabilities at all ages. Very young children, who suffer acutely from separation anxiety, and adolescents, who are developing an identity, are probably the most affected psychologically. Toddlers cannot understand why the parents they love and who have protected them can leave them in such a frightening and unfamiliar place. Adoles-

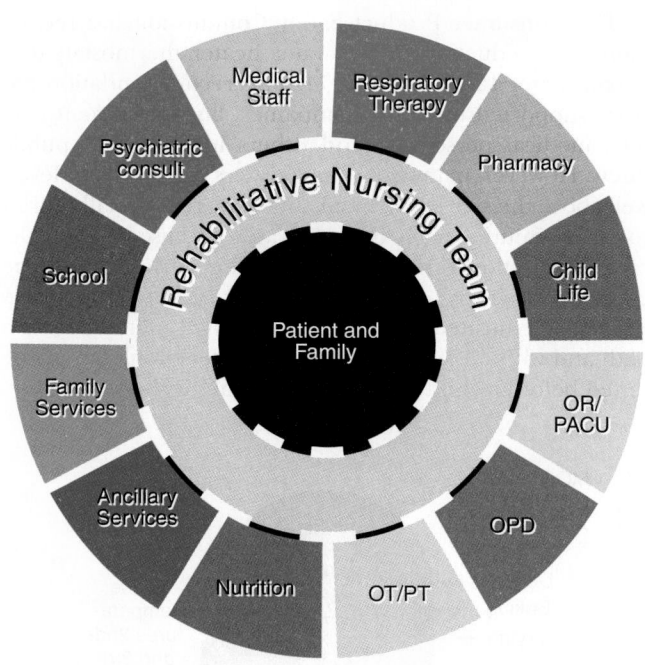

**Fig. 29-23**  Multidisciplinary approach to rehabilitation of the pediatric burn patient.

cents, in the process of achieving independence from the family, find themselves in a dependent role with a damaged body. Being different from others at a time when conformity with peers is so important is difficult to accept.

Anticipation of the return to school can be an overwhelming and frightening prospect. It is essential that health care professionals recognize the importance of preparing teachers and classmates for the child's return. Teachers need to be provided with information to assist the child and family and to promote the child's optimum adjustment. Hospital-sponsored school reentry programs use a variety of methods to provide education and information about the implications of the injury, the garments and appliances, and the need for support and acceptance. Telephone calls, videotapes, information packets, and visits by members of the health care team offer opportunities to help with reintegration into the school environment—a focal point of the child's life.

**Psychosocial Support of the Child.**  Children should begin early to do as much for themselves as possible and to be active participants in their care. Loss of control and perceived helplessness may result in acting-out behaviors. Nurses should be sensitive to these feelings and allow the child the opportunity for choices and decision making as the condition allows. At the same time, it is important to set boundaries and establish a daily schedule to provide a sense of predictability, security, and control. During illness, children regress to a previous developmental level that allows them to deal with stress. As children begin to participate in their care, they gain confidence and self-esteem. Fears and anxieties diminish with accomplishment and self-confidence. If the child demonstrates nonadherence in the

rehabilitative phase, a behavior modification program can be initiated to promote or reward the child's accomplishment in care.

Activities are selected and encouraged on the basis of each child's developmental level and interest. Quiet activities such as reading, coloring, and games are always appropriate. Critically ill children enjoy tapes and stories, even though they may not be able to actively participate in play. Television is a satisfactory diversion but should not replace contact with others. Play that encourages the expression of anger, frustration, and guilt is especially therapeutic. Medical play is a valuable tool to teach children what to expect and their role in the treatment process. School-age children benefit by continuing study activities as they are able.

Children need to feel they look nice. The burns, dressings, and medical equipment do little to foster a positive self-image. Small things, such as careful hair combing, a bright ribbon or pajamas, a pretty blanket, or colorful stickers will help them feel better about themselves and feel worthwhile to others.

Children need to know that their injury and the treatments are not punishment for real or imagined transgressions and that the nurse understands their fear, anger, and discomfort. They also need body contact. This is often difficult to arrange for the child with massive burns; stroking areas of unburned skin is comforting. Even older children enjoy sitting on the nurse's or parent's lap and being cuddled and hugged. This can be a reward or a comfort in times of stress, but most of all it should be kept in mind that it is a natural part of childhood.

**Psychosocial Support of the Family.**  There is a growing recognition that trauma affects not only the victim but also those closest to the child. Severe trauma challenges the belief that the world is safe and predictable. Parents and other family members are concerned about the child's survival, recovery, and future potential. Recognizing and respecting each family's strengths, differences, and methods of coping allows the nurse to respond to their unique needs by implementing a family-centered approach to care. It is the family, particularly the parents, who are the most significant persons in the child's life.

As in any emergency situation, all attention is focused on the child, and the parents feel powerless and ineffectual. Most parents feel overwhelming guilt, whether or not the guilt is justified. They feel responsible for the injury. These feelings may impede the child's rehabilitation. Parents may indulge the child and allow nonadherent behaviors that affect physical and emotional recovery.

Nurses have the opportunity to assist parents in coping with the stresses of the child's illness and with their own feelings of guilt and helplessness. The parents need to be informed of the child's progress and helped in their efforts to cope with their feelings while providing support to their child. The nurse can help them understand that it is not selfish to look after themselves and their own needs in order to better meet the needs of their child. Definitive professional help may be needed for parents whose response to the injury is severe or whose response to stress is manifested in destructive behavior.

The parents are members of the multidisciplinary team and participate in the development of the plan of care. It is important to address their input in order to consider all aspects of the physical, emotional, social, and cultural factors impacting the child and family and to establish a realistic home therapy program. The family's willingness to assume responsibility for care and their ability to implement the therapeutic regimen are assessed. Home, school, and other environmental factors are explored; financial concerns and available community resources are discussed; and a specific plan of care for the child, with an anticipated follow-up program, is developed.

**Caring for the Caregiver.**  Burn care is a very complex and demanding specialty. Nurses who choose this field of nursing reap many rewards and endure many stresses. Ongoing support from peers, the multidisciplinary team, and nursing management is important to assist burn nurses in caring for themselves and to continue to render quality care to their patients.

## ■ Evaluation

The effectiveness of nursing interventions is determined by the continual reassessment and evaluation of care based on the following observational guidelines:

1. Observe child's behavior during all aspects of care; listen for verbal cues; use a pain assessment tool to evaluate the effectiveness of the analgesics.
2. Observe the burn wound and child's general condition.
3. Observe child's eating behavior and the amount of food consumed; weigh weekly or as indicated.
4. Inspect the burn wound for signs of infection; measure vital signs; observe for evidence of respiratory complications, gastric bleeding, altered hemoglobin, and neurologic signs.
5. Observe for evidence of healing, scar formation, and contracture; assess the effectiveness of physical therapy and appliances (splints, pressure garments).
6. Observe child's and family's behaviors; interview child and family regarding concerns.

The *expected outcomes* are described in the Nursing Care Plan on 1249-1252.

### Prevention of Burn Injury

Burn prevention is the responsibility of all members of the community. Nurses have an obligation to participate in educational efforts directed at parents, children, and others regarding the prevention of burn injuries and fire-related deaths. The best cure is prevention.

Infants and toddlers are most commonly injured by hot liquids in the kitchen and bathroom. These injuries often occur as a result of inadequate supervision of this curious and energetic age-group. Prevention efforts are targeted at parents and other caregivers; education includes the importance of adequate supervision and the establishment of safe play areas in the home. Hot liquids should be kept out of reach; tablecloths and dangling appliance cords are often pulled by toddlers, spilling hot grease and liquids on them. Electrical cords and outlets represent a potential risk to small children, who may chew on accessible cords and insert objects into outlets.

The Consumer Product Safety Commission has recommended a reduction of hot water heater thermostats to a maximum of 120° F since 1974. This recommendation has been supported by utility companies, burn treatment centers, medical personnel, and others interested in public safety. However, many hot water heaters remain set at levels well above the safe level. Small children are especially at risk for scald injuries from hot tap water because of their decreased reaction time and agility, their curiosity, and the thermal sensitivity of their skin (Fig. 29-24). Caregivers should be educated never to leave a child unattended in a bath and without adult supervision. Water should always be tested before a child is placed in the tub or shower.

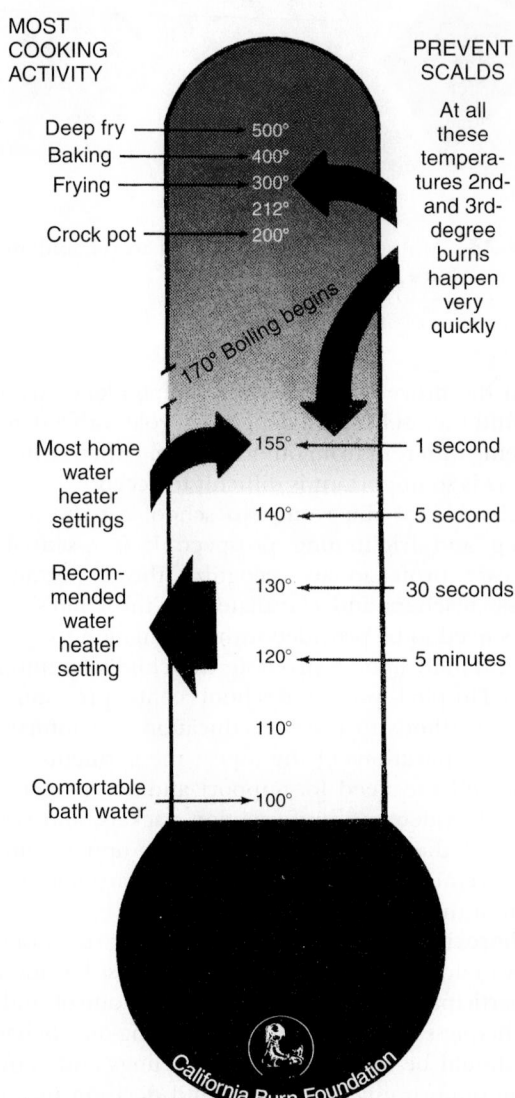

NOTE: Microwave cooking presents special hazards. Fillings in doughnuts, pies, tarts, etc., become super heated (600° or more) and may explode when moved.

**Fig. 29-24**  Temperatures associated with common burn injuries in the home. NOTE: Most authorities recommend that water heaters be kept at the lowest safe setting of 120° F. (Courtesy California Burn Foundation, Canoga Park, CA.)

## Nursing Care Plan

# The Child with Burns: Management and Rehabilitative Stages

---

**NURSING DIAGNOSIS:** Impaired skin integrity related to thermal injury

---

**PATIENT GOAL 1:** Will exhibit evidence of wound healing

- **NURSING INTERVENTIONS/*RATIONALES***

Shave hair to a 2-inch margin from the wound and area immediately surrounding the burn *to remove a reservoir for infection*

Thoroughly cleanse the wound and surrounding skin *to decrease the risk of infection;* debride devitalized tissue *to promote healing*

Keep child from scratching and picking at the wound
   Provide distraction appropriate to child's age
   Older child: Explain reasons to encourage cooperation
   Young child: Supervise as needed

Maintain care in handling the wound *to avoid damaging epithelializing and granulating tissues*

Offer high-calorie, high-protein meals and snacks *to meet augmented protein and calorie requirements caused by increased metabolism and catabolism*

Prevent infection, which can delay healing and convert partial-thickness wounds to full-thickness wounds

Administer supplementary vitamins and minerals—vitamins A, B, C, iron, and zinc—*to facilitate wound healing and epithelialization*

Pad burned ears *to prevent tissue necrosis due to minimal blood flow to cartilage*

Monitor for signs/symptoms of wound infection *to ensure prompt recognition and treatment*

Wrap fingers and toes separately *to avoid tissue adherence from prolonged contact*

- **EXPECTED OUTCOME**

Wounds heal without evidence of damage or inflammation

---

**PATIENT GOAL 2:** Will maintain integrity of skin graft

- **NURSING INTERVENTIONS/*RATIONALES***

Position for minimal mechanical disturbance of graft site

Restrain if necessary *to prevent graft from being dislodged*

Maintain splints or dressings *if needed for protection of the graft*

Observe grafts for evidence of hematoma/fluid accumulation; aspirate or express fluids *to ensure contact of the graft with the base*

- **EXPECTED OUTCOME**

Skin graft remains intact

---

**NURSING DIAGNOSIS:** Risk for ineffective tissue perfusion related to circumferential burns

---

**PATIENT GOAL 1:** Will retain optimal circulation to distal regions of the affected extremity

- **NURSING INTERVENTIONS/*RATIONALES***

Monitor closely for signs/symptoms of circulation compression related to edema *to ensure adequate circulation perfusion* (assess numbness, tingling, color, or temperature changes q 1-2 hr × 72 hours)

Assess diminished Doppler pulses and prolonged capillary refill *to indicate diminished distal perfusion* (Doppler checks q 1-2 hr × 72 hours)

Position extremity to elevate above the level of the heart *to prevent decreased circulation to the extremity*

Avoid restrictive dressings over the injured extremity *to prevent decreased circulation to the extremity*

- **EXPECTED OUTCOME**

Adequate distal perfusion to the affected extremity is maintained

---

**NURSING DIAGNOSIS:** Chronic pain related to skin trauma, therapies

---

**PATIENT GOAL 1:** Will experience reduction of pain to a level acceptable to the child

- **NURSING INTERVENTIONS/*RATIONALES***

Assess need for medication (see Pain Assessment, Chapter 26)

Recognize that burn pain is often overwhelming, engulfing, and irrepressible

Position in extension *to minimize pain resulting from exercising to regain extension*

Implement passive and active exercising *to minimize contracture formation*

Reduce irritation *to prevent increased pain*

Touch/stroke unburned areas *to provide physical contact and comfort*

Employ appropriate nonpharmacologic pain-reduction techniques (see Pain Management, Chapter 26)

Promote control and predictability during painful procedures (see Guidelines box on p. 1244)

Anticipate the need for pain medication and administer before the onset of severe pain and at regular intervals *to prevent recurrence* (see Pain Management, Chapter 26)

- **EXPECTED OUTCOME**

Child exhibits reduction of pain to level acceptable to child

---

**NURSING DIAGNOSIS:** Risk for infection related to denuded skin, presence of pathogenic organisms, and altered immune response

---

**PATIENT GOAL 1:** Will exhibit no evidence of wound infection

- **NURSING INTERVENTIONS/*RATIONALES***

Implement and maintain infection control precautions according to unit policy

Maintain careful handwashing by members of staff and visitors *to minimize exposure to infectious organisms*

Wear clean or sterile gown, cap, mask, and gloves when handling wound area *to minimize exposure to infectious organisms*

Debride eschar, crust, and blisters *to eliminate the reservoir for organisms*

Avoid patient contact with persons who have upper respiratory, skin, or gastrointestinal infection

Cover the wound or patient according to the protocol of the unit *to provide a barrier to organisms*

*Continued*

# Nursing Care Plan
## The Child with Burns: Management and Rehabilitative Stages—cont'd

### PATIENT GOAL 1—cont'd

• **NURSING INTERVENTIONS**/*RATIONALES*—cont'd
Provide good oral hygiene
*Apply prescribed topical antimicrobial preparation and dressings to the wound *to control bacterial proliferation*
Obtain baseline and serial wound cultures *to ascertain any increase or changes in wound flora*
Monitor closely for signs of sepsis and infection (disorientation, tachypnea, temperature above 38.4° C [101.1° F], hypothermia, delayed capillary refill, distention of the abdomen or intestinal ileus, change in wound appearance)

• **EXPECTED OUTCOMES**
Possible sources of infection are eliminated
Wound displays minimal or no evidence of infection

> **NURSING DIAGNOSIS:** Risk for ineffective thermoregulation related to heat loss and disruption of skin's defense mechanism to maintain body temperature

### PATIENT GOAL 1: Will maintain normal thermal regulation as evidenced by normal body temperatures ranging from 37.0° to 38.1° C (98.6° to 100.5° F)

• **NURSING INTERVENTIONS**/*RATIONALES*
Assess patient skin for coolness, color changes, and capillary refill (acrocyanosis, nail bed color, and mottling) *to identify vascular accommodation of heat loss*
Monitor vital signs, especially temperature, *to identify significant trends*
Observe for chilling and shivering *to identify fever*
Avoid exposure to cold stress procedures *to maintain body temperature* (limiting tubbing to 20 minutes, bundling child, covering the head of a child <6 months of age, artificial heat)

• **EXPECTED OUTCOME**
Child's temperature remains within normal limits for age

> **NURSING DIAGNOSIS:** Risk for deficient fluid volume related to normal fluid loss from tissues because of burn insult

### PATIENT GOAL 1: Will maintain adequate fluid hydration status during the acute postburn period

• **NURSING INTERVENTIONS**/*RATIONALES*
Administer crystalloid or colloid fluid as ordered, monitoring effect and maintaining IV *to replace fluid loss related to burn injury*
Assess fluid replacement status: inadequate (skin turgor, increased pulse, decreased urine output, decreased circulation status, or change in mental status [restlessness, disorientation]) or excessive (pulmonary congestion or pulmonary edema) *to recognize appropriate fluid balance*

Monitor daily weights *to evaluate status of fluid retention or diuresis*
Observe and monitor peripheral perfusion in relation to hypovolemia or overload *(change in blood pressure is a late sign)*
Monitor laboratory results *to identify fluid and electrolyte imbalance* (Hbg, Hct, glucose, serum potassium, serum sodium, serum protein, phosphorus, and magnesium)
Administer potassium-rich or potassium-restricted fluids or foods if child is hypokalemic or hyperkalemic, respectively, *to supplement IV therapy*

• **EXPECTED OUTCOME**
Adequate fluid resuscitation is maintained as evidenced by adequate tissue perfusion and maintenance of urine output

> **NURSING DIAGNOSIS:** Imbalanced nutrition: less than body requirements related to increased catabolism and metabolism, loss of appetite

### PATIENT GOAL 1: Will receive optimum nourishment

• **NURSING INTERVENTIONS**/*RATIONALES*
Encourage oral feeding (see Feeding the Sick Child, Chapter 27)
Provide high-calorie, high-protein meals and snacks *to avoid protein breakdown and meet augmented caloric requirements*
Provide foods child likes *to stimulate appetite*
Provide attractive meals and surroundings *to encourage eating*
Provide companionship at meals *to create a more homelike environment*
Administer supplemental enteral feedings as prescribed *to meet calculated needs*
Obtain daily weight *to monitor nutritional status and hydration*
Record accurate intake and output *to evaluate sufficiency of intake*
Monitor for diarrhea/constipation and institute prompt treatment *to avoid anorexia*

• **EXPECTED OUTCOME**
Child consumes a sufficient amount of nutrients (specify) and maintains preburn weight

> **NURSING DIAGNOSIS:** Risk for constipation and risk for diarrhea related to opioid administration, inadequate intake of nutrients, and the need for tube feedings

### PATIENT GOAL 1: Will have routine bowel patterns

• **NURSING INTERVENTIONS**/*RATIONALES*
Monitor for diarrhea/constipation and institute prompt treatment
Record amount and consistency of stool daily
Administer antidiarrhea agents
Administer bulk laxative, stool softener, or cathartic *to avoid anorexia*
Assess hydration status to correlate dehydration with development of constipation

---

*Dependent nursing action.

## Nursing Care Plan
### The Child with Burns: Management and Rehabilitative Stages—cont'd

Monitorserum electrolytes, replacing lost electrolytes via IV or tube feeding

Increase activity and ambulation *to increase peristalsis and motility when constipated*

- **EXPECTED OUTCOME**

Normal bowel elimination pattern returns as evidenced by soft, formed stools q 1-2 days

---

**NURSING DIAGNOSIS:** Impaired physical mobility (specify level) related to pain, impaired joint movement, scar formation

---

**PATIENT GOAL 1:** Will achieve optimum physical functioning

- **NURSING INTERVENTIONS/** *RATIONALES*

Carry out range-of-motion exercises *to maintain optimum joint and muscle function*

Encourage mobility if child is able to move extremities

Ambulate as soon as feasible

Splint involved joints in extension at night and during rest periods *to minimize contracture formation*

Encourage and promote self-help activities *to increase mobility*

Administer analgesia before painful activity (e.g., physical therapy) *so that child is more likely to cooperate and be mobile*

Encourage participation in activities of daily living and play activities *to incorporate exercise into enjoyable events*

- **EXPECTED OUTCOME**

Child achieves functioning to level of ability

**PATIENT GOAL 2:** Will exhibit minimal scarring

- **NURSING INTERVENTIONS/** *RATIONALES*

Position in a functional attitude for minimal deformity and optimum functioning

Apply splints as ordered and designed *to minimize contracture*

Wrap healing tissue with elastic bandage or dress in elastic garments as ordered *to help reduce scar hypertrophy by compressing collagen and decreasing vascularity*

Carry out physical therapy *to minimize deformity related to scar contracture formation*

Provide treatment for pruritus *to minimize scratching and irritation of newly healed tissue*

- **EXPECTED OUTCOME**

Wound heals with minimal scar formation; joints remain flexible and functional

---

**NURSING DIAGNOSIS:** Disturbed body image related to perception of appearance and mobility

---

**PATIENT GOAL 1:** Will receive adequate emotional support

- **NURSING INTERVENTIONS/** *RATIONALES*

Convey positive attitude toward child *so that child expects to get better*

Encourage parents to participate in care *to prevent the stress of separation*

Encourage as much independence as condition allows *to give child a sense of control*

Arrange for continued schooling *to encourage optimum development and sense of normalcy*

Promote peer contact where possible *to decrease isolation*

Be honest with child and family *to create a trusting nurse-patient relationship*

Encourage activities appropriate to age and capabilities *to promote normalcy and increase self-esteem*

Prepare peers for child's appearance *to encourage acceptance and support*

Provide opportunities for child and family to discuss the impact of the change in appearance and lifestyle *to increase coping*

Support behaviors suggesting adaptation *to build on strengths*

- **EXPECTED OUTCOMES**

Child accepts efforts of family and caregivers

Child engages in activities with others according to age and capabilities

**PATIENT GOAL 2:** Will demonstrate improved body image

- **NURSING INTERVENTIONS/** *RATIONALES*

Explore feelings concerning physical appearance *to facilitate coping with body image changes*

Discuss feelings about returning to home, family, school, and friends *to build coping mechanisms*

Provide reinforcement of positive aspects of appearance and capabilities *to recognize and build on strengths*

Point out evidence of healing *to encourage a sense of hope*

Discuss aids that camouflage disfigurement *to facilitate coping*
   Wigs
   Clothing
   Makeup

Provide recreational and diversional activities *to promote a sense of normalcy*

Promote constructive thinking in child *to encourage positive coping*

Help child devise a plan to address and cope with the reactions of others *to increase the sense of control*

- **EXPECTED OUTCOMES**

Child discusses feelings and concerns regarding appearance and the perceived reactions of others

Child verbalizes positive suggestions for adjusting to appearance and community/peer response

**PATIENT GOAL 3:** Will engage in self-care activities

- **NURSING INTERVENTIONS/** *RATIONALES*

Assist with self-care activities as needed

Encourage self-care according to capabilities

Begin to discuss "hospital discharge" early in hospitalization *so that child expects to get better*

Help child develop independence and self-help capabilities *to increase self-esteem*

- **EXPECTED OUTCOMES**

Child verbalizes and otherwise demonstrates interest in going home

Child engages in self-help activities

*Continued*

## *Nursing Care Plan*
### The Child with Burns: Management and Rehabilitative Stages—cont'd

> **NURSING DIAGNOSIS:** Interrupted family processes related to situational crisis (child with a serious injury)

**PATIENT/FAMILY GOAL 1:** Will be prepared for discharge and home care

- **NURSING INTERVENTIONS/***RATIONALES***

Teach wound care to caregiver *to achieve proficiency and increase confidence*

Discuss diet, rest, and activity *to assist in planning for a home care regimen*

Explore attitudes toward child's reentry into the family *to facilitate coping and identify a possible need for intervention*

Explore family's concept regarding child's capabilities and the possible restrictions and freedom they will allow *to assist them in planning realistically for an altered lifestyle*

Help family set realistic goals for themselves, the child, and other family members *to clarify and validate the plan of home care*

Help family acquire needed equipment and supplies *to reduce anxiety*

- **EXPECTED OUTCOMES**

Family demonstrates an understanding of child's needs and the impact child's condition will have on them

Family sets realistic goals for selves, child, and others

**PATIENT/FAMILY GOAL 2:** Will participate in follow-up care

- **NURSING INTERVENTIONS/***RATIONALES***

Coordinate team management of child and family for ongoing care *to provide continuity*

Arrange for return visits

Assess the needs of the family *to determine appropriate plan of care*

Arrange for referral agencies based on needs assessment

Collaborate with school nurse *to help with child's reintegration into school*

Visit the school, if possible, to prepare teacher and peers *to encourage acceptance of child*

- **EXPECTED OUTCOMES**

Family maintains contact with health providers

Child attends school regularly and interacts with age-mates

See also:

Nursing Care Plan: The Child in the Hospital, Chapter 26

Nursing Care Plan: The Family of the Child Who Is Ill or Hospitalized, Chapter 26

---

> ### Box 29-15 ◼ ◼ ◻
> #### Microwave Safety
>
> Place microwave ovens at a safe height (but higher than children's faces) and within easy reach to avoid spills.
> Never heat baby formula or milk in a plastic bottle liner because it may burst.
> Before adding a cold liquid to a liquid heated in the microwave, insert a spoon to prevent bubbling over of the hot liquid.
> For baby formula or milk in bottles, shake well to blend "hot spots."
> For containers, puncture plastic wrap, use vented lids, or wait 1 minute before removing a sealed covering, then lift the covering from the corner farthest away from face or arm.

Microwave ovens, although perceived by many as safer than conventional ovens and stoves, heat foods and liquids to very high temperatures that can result in burns from spills, splashes, and the release of steam (Box 29-15).

As children mature, risk-taking behaviors increase. Matches and lighters are very dangerous in the hands of the young. In 1998 approximately 2400 residential structure fires were caused by children younger than 5 years of age playing with cigarette lighters (U.S. Consumer Product Safety Commission, 2000). Adults must remember to keep potentially hazardous items out of the reach of children; a lighter, like a match, is a tool for adult use.

Education related to fire safety and survival should begin with the very young. "Stop, drop, and roll" to extinguish a fire can be practiced. The fire escape route, including a safe meeting place away from the home in case of fire, also should be practiced. Materials such as coloring books are available from many fire departments and burn foundations. Community burn prevention programs also provide opportunities to educate children and parents about fire, burn hazards, and prevention behaviors.

Community activities are very helpful in the effort to support burn survivors and prevent burns. The Aluminum Cans for Burned Children (ACBC) is an exemplary effort based in the Clifford R. Boeckman Regional Burn Center, Akron, Ohio.* Activities funded by ACBC include Burn Survivors Support Group, Burn Camp, and meetings of Juvenile Firestoppers (for children with fire-setting behavior). Adult weekend retreats and school and family education sessions are a part of this program. Burn center staff and fire department staff provide the personnel to present programs.

Additional information on burn care and prevention can be obtained from the **American Burn Association**† and the

---

*Children's Hospital Medical Center of Akron, One Perkins Square, Akron, OH 44308-1062, (330) 543-8224, fax: (330) 543-8152.

†625 North Michigan Ave, Suite 1530, Chicago, IL 60611, (312)642-9260, (800) 548-2876, fax: (312)642-9130, e-mail: aba@ameriburn.org.

**National Safety Council.*** The **Alisa Ann Ruch Burn Foundation**† provides assistance to burn victims and burn centers. The **Shriners Burn Institutes** are staffed to treat pediatric patients following acute burn injuries and those requiring rehabilitative and reconstructive services as a result of scarring and functional impairment. Information can be obtained from local Shrine Temples and Clubs, from Shriners Hospitals, or by contacting the **International Shrine Headquarters.‡** The Alisa Ann Ruch Foundation and Shriners Hospitals for Crippled Children support re-

---

*1121 Spring Lake Dr, Itasca, IL 60143-3201, (800) 621-7615; www.nsc.org.
†20944 Sherman Way, Suite 115, Canoga Park, CA 91303, (818) 883-7700; www.aarbf.org.
‡2900 Rocky Point Dr, Tampa, FL 33607, (800) 237-5055, in Florida: (800) 282-9161, International Shrine Headquarters web site: www.shrinershq.org, Shriners Burn Institutes web site: www.shrinershq.org/Hospitals/ BurnInst/.

search to improve burn care and treatment and promote public education in burn prevention.

## Future Research Needs

Many advances in burn prevention have reduced the occurrence of burn injury. Early excision and grafting of the burn wound, with control of infection, has improved survival rates for burn injury. Areas for future research include studies on the rate of wound healing, the characteristics of the healed wound, support techniques for inhalation injury, the effect of hypothermia immediately after burn injury, nursing interventions that promote healing of donor sites and skin grafts, and what is the most effective wound-cleansing protocol. Evidence for improvement of burn nursing care is best organized with research findings (Carrougher, 1998).

## KEY POINTS

- Gastrointestinal disorders of childhood that commonly cause fluid depletion and electrolyte disturbance are diarrhea and vomiting.
- The four general types of mechanisms of diarrhea are secretory, cytotoxic, osmotic, and dysenteric diarrhea.
- The treatment for acute diarrhea consists primarily of oral rehydration and provision of an adequate diet.
- Burns are caused by thermal, electrical, chemical, or radioactive agents.
- The severity of burn injury is assessed on the basis of the percentage of body surface area burned, depth, location, age, etiologic agent, concomitant injuries, and general health.

- Emergency measures for severe burns include stopping the burning process; assessing for airway, breathing, and circulation; covering the burn; transporting the child to the hospital; and providing reassurance to the child and family.
- Management of minor burns consists of facilitating wound healing, relieving discomfort, and preventing complications.
- Management of major burn injuries involves facilitating wound healing, relieving pain, replacing destroyed skin, preventing or treating complications, and providing rehabilitation.
- Active participation by the child and family is important in the care of the child with thermal trauma.

## REFERENCES

Achauer BM, Adair SR: Acute and reconstructive management of the burned eyelid, *Clin Plast Surg* 27(1):87-96, 2000.

Andrews DA: Management of the burned child, *Prob Gen Surg* 11(4):662-665, 1994.

Balk R: Severe sepsis and septic shock, *Crit Care Clin* 16(2):179-192, 2000.

Beck SA, Burks AW: Taking action against anaphylaxis, *Contemp Pediatr* 16(8):87-96, 1999.

Carrougher G: *Burn care and therapy*, St Louis, 1998, Mosby.

Centers for Disease Control and Prevention: Diarrheal diseases in the child care setting, *Center for Disease Prevention Division of Healthcare Quality Promotion* (on line), January 1997.

Cohen J and others: New strategies for clinical trials in patients with sepsis and septic shock, *Crit Care Med* 29(4):880-886, 2001.

Cortiella J, Marvin J: Management of the pediatric burn patient, *Nurs Clin North Am* 32(2):311-329, 1997.

Demling R, DeSanti, L: Use of anticatabolic agents for burns, *Curr Opin Crit Care* 2: 482-491, 1996.

Endsley S, Galbraith A: Are you overlooking oral rehydration therapy in childhood diarrhea? *Postgrad Med* 103(4):159-171, 1998.

Helvig E: Pediatric burn injuries, *AACN Clin Issues* 4(2):433-442, 1993.

Henry DB, Foster RL: Burn pain management in children, *Pediatr Clin North Am* 47(3):681-698, 2000.

Herndon DN and others: *Total burn care,* London, 1996, WB Saunders.

Hugger J, Harkless G, Rentschler D: Oral rehydration therapy for children with acute diarrhea, *Nurs Pract* 23(12):52-62, 1998.

Jindal N, Hollenberg SM, Dellinger RP: Pharmacologic issues in the management of septic shock, *Crit Care Clin* 16(2):233-249, 2000.

Klein GL and others: Long-term reduction in bone mass after severe burn injury in children, *J Pediatr* 126(2):252-256, 1995.

Leclerc F and others: Do new strategies in meningococcemia produce better outcomes? *Crit Care Med* 28(9):60-63, 2000.

Levy D and others: Antibiotics and *Clostridium difficile* diarrhea in the ambulatory care setting, *Clin Ther* 22(1):91-102, 2000.

Mlcak R and others: Emergency management of pediatric burn victims, *Pediatr Emerg Care* 14(1):51-54, 1998.

Nakase J: Update on emerging infections from the Centers for Disease Control and Prevention, *Ann Emerg Med* 36(3):268-270, 2000.

Nappert G and others: Oral rehydration solutions therapy in the management of children with rotavirus diarrhea, *Nutr Rev* 58(3):80-87, 2000.

National SAFE KIDS Campaign: Fire, 2001. *www.safekids.org.*

Nguyen K and others: Update on current therapeutic approaches in burns, *Ann Surg* 223(1):14-25, 1996.

Savilahti E: Food-induced malabsorption syndromes, *J Pediatr Gastroenterol Nutr* 30(S1): S61-S66, 2000.

Selbst SM: Pain management in the emergency department. In Schechter N, Berde C, Yaster M: *Pain in infants, children, and adolescents,* Baltimore, 1993, Williams & Wilkins.

Shirani K and others: Update on current therapeutic approaches to burns, *Shock* 5(1):4-16, 1996.

Smith ML: Pediatric burns: management of thermal, electrical, and chemical burns and burn-like dermatologic conditions, *Pediatr Ann* 29(6):367-378, 2000.

Still JM Jr and others: Decreasing length of hospital stay by early excision and grafting of burns, *South Med J* 89(6): 578-582, 1996.

Sullian P: Nutritional management of acute diarrhea, *Nutrition* 14(10):758-762, 1998.

Tuite P: Recognition and management of shock in the pediatric patient, *Crit Care Nurs Q* 20(1):52-61, 1997.

US Consumer Product Safety Commission: *Fires caused by children playing with lighters: an evaluation of the CPSC standard for cigarette lighters,* Russ Rader Release No 01-026, November 2000.

Vanderhoof J: Chronic diarrhea, *Pediatr Rev* 19(12):418-422, 1998.

Vanderhoof J and others: *Lactobacillus* GG in the prevention of antibiotic-associated diarrhea in children, *J Pediatr* 135(5):564-568, 1999.

Waters V and others: Etiology of community-acquired pediatric viral diarrhea: a prospective longitudinal study in hospitals, emergency departments, pediatric practices and child care centers during the winter rotavirus outbreak, 1997 to 1998, *Pediatr Infect Dis J* 19(9):843-848, 2000.

Zimmerman C and others: Cost of diarrhea-associated hospitalizations and outpatient visits in an insured population of young children in the United States, *Pediatr Infect Dis J* 20(1):14-19, 2001.

# Chapter 30

# The Child with Renal Dysfunction

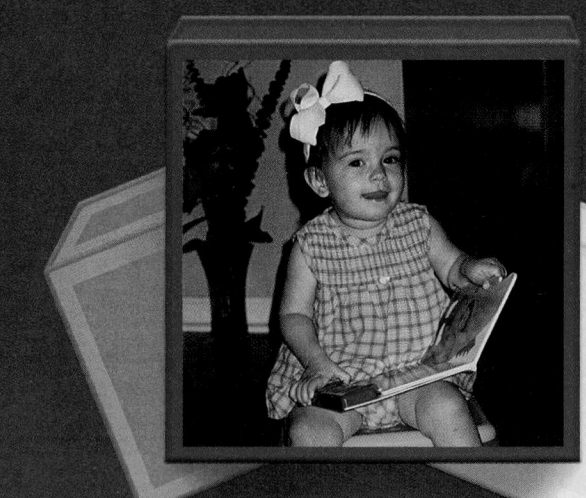

## Chapter Outline

**RENAL STRUCTURE AND FUNCTION, 1255**

**Renal Physiology, 1256**
Glomerular Filtration, 1256
Tubular Function, 1257
Renal Development and Function
in Early Infancy, 1258
**Renal Pelvis and Ureters: Structure
and Function, 1258**
**Urethrovesical Unit: Structure
and Function, 1259**

**GENITOURINARY TRACT DISORDERS, 1262**
**Urinary Tract Infection (UTI), 1262**
**Vesicoureteral Reflux (VUR), 1269**

**GLOMERULAR DISEASE, 1270**
**Acute Glomerulonephritis (AGN), 1270**
**Chronic or Progressive
Glomerulonephritis, 1274**

Nephrotic Syndrome, 1274
Types of Nephrotic Syndrome, 1274

**RENAL TUBULAR DISORDERS, 1279**
**Tubular Function, 1279**
**Renal Tubular Acidosis, 1279**
Proximal Tubular Acidosis (Type II), 1279
Distal Tubular Acidosis (Type I), 1280
**Nephrogenic Diabetes Insipidus (NDI), 1280**

**MISCELLANEOUS RENAL DISORDERS, 1281**
**Hemolytic Uremic Syndrome (HUS), 1281**
**Familial Nephritis (Alport Syndrome), 1282**
**Unexplained Proteinuria, 1282**
**Renal Trauma, 1282**

**RENAL FAILURE, 1283**
**Acute Renal Failure (ARF), 1283**
**Chronic Renal Failure (CRF), 1287**

*Nursing Care Plan: The Child with Chronic Renal
Failure (CRF), 1294*

**RENAL REPLACEMENT THERAPY, 1293**
**Hemodialysis, 1293**
Procedure, 1294
Home Hemodialysis, 1296
**Peritoneal Dialysis (PD), 1297**
Procedure, 1297
Home Dialysis, 1297
**Continuous Venovenous Hemofiltration
(CVVH), 1298**
**Transplantation, 1298**
Procedure, 1299
Selection of Donor Tissue, 1299
Suppression of the Immune
Response, 1299
Rejection, 1300

## Related Topics

Administration of Medication, Ch. 27
Collection of Specimens, Ch. 27
Defects of the Genitourinary Tract, Ch. 11

Family-Centered Care of the Child with
Chronic Illness or Disability, Ch. 22

Family-Centered Home Care, Ch. 25
Physical Examination: Genitalia, Ch. 7

## RENAL STRUCTURE AND FUNCTION

The primary responsibility of the kidney is to maintain the composition and volume of the body fluids in equilibrium. To maintain this constant internal environment, the kidney must respond appropriately to alterations in the internal environment caused by variations in dietary intake and extrarenal losses of water and solutes. This is accomplished by the formation of urine (the product of glomerular filtration), tubular reabsorption, and tubular secretion. *Reabsorption* is the transport of a substance from the tubular lumen to the blood in surrounding vessels. *Secretion* is transport in the opposite direction (i.e., from the blood to the lumen). These processes can be active or passive. *Excretion* is the elimination of a substance from the body, in this case urine.

A secondary function of the kidney is the production of certain humoral substances. One such substance is an enzyme, *erythropoietin-stimulating factor* (*ESF,* or *erythrogenin*), which acts on a plasma globulin to form erythropoietin, which in turn stimulates erythropoiesis in the bone marrow. Its production is increased in the presence of hypoxia and androgens. Few red blood cells are formed in the absence of erythropoietin, which accounts somewhat for the anemia

■ Barbara Montagnino, MS, RN, and Helen Currier, CNN, RN, revised this
chapter.

associated with advanced renal disease. Another enzyme, **renin,** is also secreted by the kidney in response to reduced blood volume, decreased blood pressure, or increased secretion of catecholamines. Renin stimulates the production of the angiotensins, which produce arteriolar constriction and an elevation in blood pressure and stimulate the production of aldosterone by the adrenal cortex.

## Renal Physiology

The structural and functional unit of the kidney is the **nephron,** which is composed of a complex system of tubules, arterioles, venules, and capillaries (Fig. 30-1). The nephron consists of the **Bowman capsule,** which encloses a tuft of capillaries and is joined successively to the **proximal convoluted tubule,** the **loop of Henle,** the **distal convoluted tubule,** and the **straight** or **collecting duct** (Fig. 30-2). Collecting tubules join larger ducts, and all of the larger collecting ducts of one renal pyramid join to form a single duct that opens into a **minor calyx.** A number of calyces empty into one of several **major calyces** that converge into the **renal pelvis.** The renal pelvis narrows after it leaves the kidney and forms what then becomes a **ureter,** through which urine drains into the **urinary bladder.**

The blood supply to the kidneys constitutes approximately one fifth of the total cardiac output; therefore profuse bleeding can accompany renal trauma. Because interstitial tissue is sparse, individual nephrons with their blood vessel component are closely packed together. Each nephron is supplied by a sizable **afferent arteriole,** which separates into capillary loops that constitute the glomerular tuft. Blood leaves by a smaller **efferent arteriole.** From there the efferent arterioles branch into a **peritubular capillary** network and hairpin loops called the **vasa recta,** which parallel the Henle loops and collecting ducts. The total surface area of the renal capillaries is approximately equal to the total surface of the tubules.

The **Bowman capsule** is composed of two cellular layers that separate the blood from the glomerular filtrate—the capillary endothelium and a layer of tubular epithelial lining cells. Situated between these layers is the basal lamina, or basement membrane. The permeability of this glomerular membrane is a result of its structure; the capillary endothelium is fenestrated with pores, or **fenestrae;** the outer surface of the glomerular epithelium consists of fingerlike projections (**pseudopodia,** or **podocytes**), which cover the entire surface to form slits called **slit pores.** The basement membrane has no visible openings but behaves as though it contains pores or channels. Consequently, the glomerular filtrate (which has essentially the same composition as plasma except for the large protein molecules and cellular elements) passes through these three layers and does so at a very rapid rate. The structure of these layers becomes altered in kidney disease.

### Glomerular Filtration

Filtration through the glomerular capillaries is governed by the same mechanism as filtration across other capillaries in the body (i.e., the size of the capillary bed, the permeability

of the capillaries, and the hydrostatic and osmotic pressure gradients across the capillaries). The filtration capacity of the glomerulus is the product of permeability of the glomerular capillaries and three pressure forces—**glomerular hydrostatic pressure, colloidal osmotic (oncotic) pressure (COP),** and **intracapsular pressure.**

Blood enters the nephron at a substantial pressure. This hydrostatic pressure forces plasma fluid and solutes through the capillary membrane and into the collecting apparatus of the unit. As this filtrate travels through the renal tubules, water and solutes are selectively reabsorbed back into the vascular compartment. That which is not reabsorbed is excreted as urine. Filtration takes place as long as hydrostatic pressure within the glomerular capillaries exceeds the opposing COP of the plasma proteins. If the pressure becomes equal through decreased hydrostatic pressure or decreased COP, no further filtration takes place. In a state of dehydration, more water is reabsorbed; when water

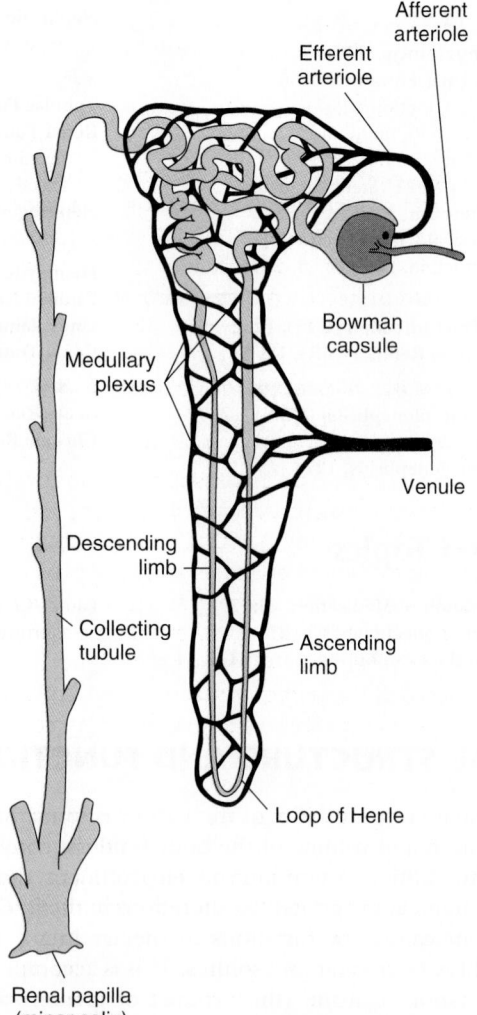

**Fig. 30-1**    The nephron, the functional unit of the kidney. (Redrawn from Tanagho EA: Anatomy of the genitourinary tract. In Tanagho EA, McAninch, JW, editors: *Smith's general urology,* ed 13, Norwalk, CT, 1992, Appleton & Lange.)

intake is increased, more is excreted as urine. In conditions that produce osmotic diuresis (i.e., when large solutes, such as glucose, are filtered through the capillaries in such excessive amounts that they cannot be reabsorbed), the osmotic attraction of the solute causes less water to be reabsorbed, resulting in water being excreted in the urine with the solute.

## Tubular Function

The function of the renal tubules is to modify the glomerular filtrate. Tubular cells may add more of a substance to the filtrate *(tubular secretion),* remove some or all of a substance from the filtrate *(tubular reabsorption),* or both. The reabsorption is selective and discriminating for substances essential to body processes and equilibrium, whereas nonessential substances are eliminated as waste. The substances are secreted or reabsorbed in the tubules by **osmosis, passive diffusion** down a chemical or electric gradient, or **actively transported** against these gradients. These processes operate throughout the length of the tubules, but there are variations in the types, amounts, and mechanisms by which substances are secreted or reabsorbed in the different tubular segments; these variations are caused in large part by the cellular characteristics of each segment (see Fig. 30-2).

Active transport mechanisms move vital substances both inward and outward from the tubular filtrate. For example, essential substances such as glucose, amino acids, and sodium ions are reabsorbed in the proximal tubule and returned directly to the blood. Active transport mechanisms here, as elsewhere, have a limited capacity, or threshold, for moving the solute. When the maximum of the transport mechanism is reached, no more substance is reabsorbed, and the remainder is excreted in the urine. For example, when blood glucose concentrations exceed their transport capacity, the surplus remains in the filtrate to be excreted in the urine (glycosuria). When two substances share a common transport mechanism, the first substance may be blocked by the addition of a second substance (selective inhibition). The effect of many therapeutic agents (e.g., diuretics) depends on this process.

Electrolytes are moved by both active transport and diffusion; the transport of certain electrolytes, particularly sodium, has important effects on other substances. For example, sodium is actively transported from all parts of the nephron. The movement of sodium ions produces both an electric and an osmotic gradient, which causes chloride ions and water to diffuse from the tubules in an effort to establish equilibrium. This is the obligatory water reabsorption in the kidneys. There is a limit to the concentration gradient against which sodium can be transported out; therefore when larger than normal amounts of sodium ions remain in the tubules, water is obliged to remain with the sodium.

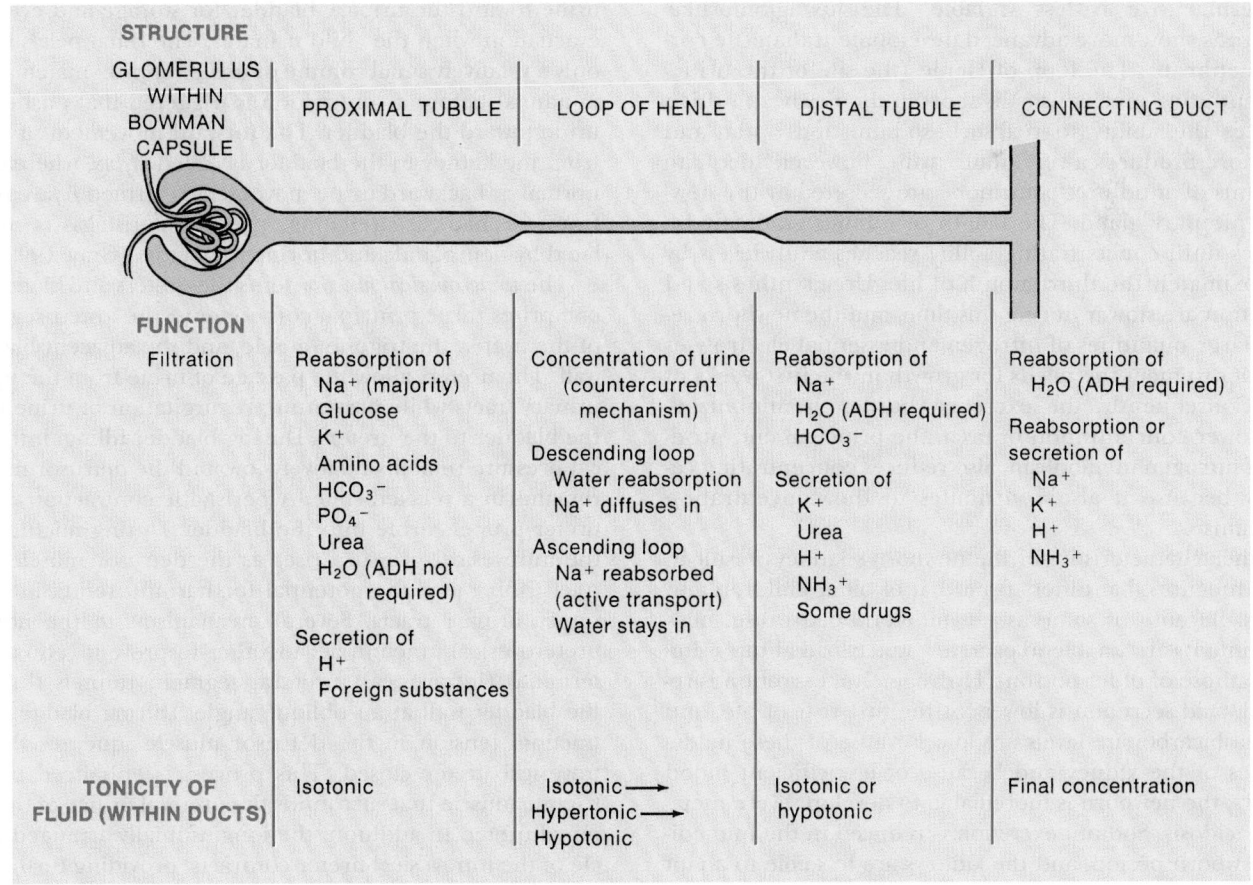

**Fig. 30-2**   Major functions of nephron components.

Under normal conditions the kidneys are able to adjust the urine and solute excretion in response to the requirements for body water and electrolyte balance. They are able to excrete or conserve both water and most electrolytes in addition to excreting the end products of protein metabolism, principally urea. The volume of urine excreted by the kidneys in a given period of time depends on the water balance (including intravascular filtration pressure), the quantity of solutes presented to the kidneys, and the capacity of the kidneys to dilute or concentrate the filtrate.

### Renal Development and Function in Early Infancy

Development of the kidney begins within the first weeks of embryonic life but is not completed until about the end of the first year after birth. The nephrons increase in number throughout gestation and reach their full complement by birth. However, at this point they are immature and less efficient than at later ages. Many of the tubular sections are not fully formed, and the glomeruli enlarge considerably after birth.

Glomerular filtration and absorption are relatively low and do not reach adult values until between 1 and 2 years of age. This appears to be related to a barrier imposed by more cuboidal-shaped glomerular epithelial cells and higher afferent arteriole resistance. Consequently, the newborn is unable to dispose of excess water and solutes rapidly or efficiently.

The tubular length of nephrons is highly variable; glomerular size is less variable. The juxtaglomerular nephrons show more advanced development than the cortical nephrons. The loop of Henle (the site of the urine-concentrating mechanism) is short in the newborn, which reduces the ability to reabsorb sodium and water and therefore produces a very dilute urine; however, adequate amounts of antidiuretic hormone are secreted by the newborn pituitary gland. The length of tubules gradually increases until concentrating ability reaches adult levels by approximately the third month of life. Urea synthesis and excretion are slower during this time, and the newborn retains large quantities of nitrogen and essential electrolytes in order to meet the needs for growth in the first weeks of life. Consequently, the excretory burden is minimized. The lower concentration of urea, the principal end product of nitrogen metabolism, also reduces concentrating capacity because it also contributes to the concentration mechanism.

Other characteristics of the newborn's kidneys result in renal function that differs from that of older children and adults. Because of some as yet undetermined cause, newborn infants are unable to excrete a water load at rates similar to those of older persons. Hydrogen ion excretion is reduced, acid secretion is lower for the first year of life, and plasma bicarbonate levels are low. Because of these inadequacies of the kidney and because of less efficient blood buffers, the newborn is more liable to develop severe metabolic acidosis. Sodium excretion is reduced in the immediate newborn period, and the kidneys are less able to adapt to sodium deficiencies and excesses. For example, an isotonic saline infusion may produce edema because of impaired ability to eliminate excess. Conversely, inadequate reabsorption of sodium from the tubules may increase sodium losses in disorders such as vomiting or diarrhea. Moreover, infants have a diminished capacity to reabsorb glucose and, during the first few days, to produce ammonium ions.

The kidney functions during fetal life and produces urine that contributes to the amniotic fluid volume. The 24-hour urine volume is low at birth, rapidly increases in the neonatal period, and steadily increases with normal growth. (See Appendix D.) The kidneys continue to grow in size until body growth is complete in adolescence.

## Renal Pelvis and Ureters: Structure and Function*

The *renal pelvis* is a funnel-shaped structure that originates at the major calyces and terminates in the funnel-shaped ureteropelvic junction. The *ureter* is a thin mucomuscular tube that extends from the ureteropelvic to the ureterovesical junction in the base of the bladder. Three areas—the ureteropelvic junction, the ureterovesical junction, and the segment nearest the sacroiliac junction—are particularly narrow and prone to obstruction when a solid body (such as a urinary calculus ["stone"]) passes.

The principal function of the renal pelvis and ureter is the transport of urine from the kidney to the bladder. Urine is moved via a process called *peristalsis,* whereby muscular movements originating in the renal pelvis propel a bolus of urine toward the urinary bladder for storage and eventual evacuation when the child urinates. The renal pelvis stores only a relatively small volume of urine (approximately 15 ml in adults) before a contraction is triggered that pushes the urine toward the bladder. The forward movement of urine from the kidney to the bladder is called *efflux,* whereas abnormal or backward urine movement is termed *reflux.* Aside from mechanical stretching, ureteral peristalsis is modulated by neurogenic and hormonal factors (Gray, 1992).

The *ureterovesical junction* joins the ureters and bladder. It comprises three principal components: the lowest segment of the ureter, the trigone muscle, and the adjacent bladder wall. The ureters allow the passage of urine from the upper urinary tracts while preventing regurgitation of urine from the bladder to the ureters. During bladder filling, intravesical pressure remains relatively low and the detrusor muscle remains in a relaxed state. A peristaltic contraction of the ureter propels urine into the bladder. During micturition, the intravesical pressure rises as the detrusor muscle contracts; this raises the potential for harmful reflux into the upper urinary tracts. Several mechanisms in the normal ureterovesical junction act together to prevent reflux. The terminal (intravesical) ureteral segment tunnels through the bladder wall at an oblique angle. During bladder contraction, tension in the detrusor muscle squeezes the intravesical ureter closed. This process is enhanced by the trigone muscle that surrounds the ureteral orifice of the terminal ureter. In addition, the longitudinally arranged muscle of the intravesical ureter contracts, providing further re-

---

■ *Mikel Gray, PhD, CUNP, CCCN, FAAN, originally wrote this section.

sistance to reflux. Anatomic defects of the ureterovesical junction, such as lateral displacement of the ureter or reduced length of the intravesical ureter, predispose the child to primary reflux. Voiding dysfunction associated with infections and high bladder pressures predisposes the child to secondary reflux (Greenfield and Wan, 2000; Soygur and others, 1999).

## Urethrovesical Unit: Structure and Function*

The *urethrovesical unit* consists of the bladder, urethra, and pelvic muscles; it is also called the *lower urinary tract* (Gray, 1992). The *urinary bladder* is a muscle-lined sac that stores and empties itself of urine. In the infant the bladder lies entirely in the abdomen. The bladder assumes its place in the true pelvis shortly before puberty. This change in position is caused by maturation of the pelvic bone rather than migration of the bladder and urethra.

The bladder is characterized by two inlets, the *ureteral orifices*, and a single outlet, the *urethral orifice*. The base of the bladder is a relatively fixed, triangular area consisting of the bladder neck and trigone. In contrast, the body of the bladder is distensible, changing from a tetrahedron (four-sided) shape when relatively empty to a nearly spherical shape as the bladder fills.

One of the four layers of the bladder wall consists of smooth muscle bundles that promote bladder evacuation via micturition. Collectively this muscular tunic is called the *detrusor*. The muscular tunic of the bladder wall also contains *collagen*, a tough, nonelastic substance that maintains the integrity of the bladder wall while also preventing overdistention. Certain pathologic factors, including denervation of the bladder and obstruction of the outlet, may cause an overabundance of collagen in the detrusor muscle. This causes a loss of bladder compliance (distensibility), abnormally high filling pressures, and trabeculation of the bladder wall.

The *urethra* is a mucomuscular tube that connects the external meatus and the bladder. The *male urethra* originates at the bladder neck, piercing the prostate and pelvic floor before tunneling through the posterior portion of the penis and terminating at the glans penis. The proximal portion of the urethra comprises the sphincter mechanism, whereas the distal portion serves as a conduit for the passage of urine or semen. The urethral meatus is a vertical slit located at the summit of the glans penis.

The *female urethra* follows a relatively short, straight course compared with the male. It originates at the bladder base and terminates at an external meatus located immediately superior to (in front of) the vaginal orifice. The distal two thirds of the female urethra is fused with the vaginal wall.

The primary responsibilities of the bladder are to store urine manufactured by the kidneys and to evacuate this urine at regular intervals via the process of micturition. During infancy, the bladder is expected to empty spontaneously; by the fourth year of life (or earlier), the child is expected to gain control of detrusor and urethral sphincter function. Control of the urethrovesical unit is referred to as *urinary continence*. Continent individuals are expected to hold their urine for a period of at least 2 hours while awake. During sleeping hours they may arise once to urinate, although many children and young adults sleep for 8 hours or more without interruption. Three factors—anatomic integrity of the lower urinary tract, detrusor control, and competence of the urethral sphincter mechanism—must function normally for continence to be achieved and maintained (Gray, 1992).

*Detrusor control* requires successful integration of neurologic structures in the brain, spinal cord, and peripheral nervous systems. The *brain* influences bladder function via its inhibitory role on detrusor contractions. The *stable detrusor* contracts only when its owner gives permission. Several areas of the brain act together to control detrusor stability. Pathology of one of these areas is known to produce *detrusor instability,* or the loss of control over detrusor contractions.

The *spinal cord* influences lower urinary tract function because it transmits messages between the brain and the target organ. Two areas in the spinal cord are particularly significant. The *thoracolumbar cord* (spinal levels T10 to L2) influences bladder and urethral sphincter function. Sympathetic impulses from the brain travel to the bladder body and smooth muscle of the urethra, causing relaxation of the detrusor muscle and contraction of urethral smooth muscle. This combination of actions promotes bladder filling and storage of urine. The *sacral spinal cord* (spinal segments S2 to S4) influences the bladder muscle, promoting micturition. Parasympathetic impulses travel from these nuclei, causing contraction of the detrusor muscle and indirectly promoting relaxation of smooth muscle in the urethra.

Two *peripheral nerve plexuses* directly influence control of the detrusor muscle. The pelvic plexus provides parasympathetic innervation to the bladder and urethra, and the inferior hypogastric plexus provides sympathetic innervation (Sugarman, 2000).

The final mechanism responsible for the attainment and maintenance of continence is the *urethral sphincter mechanism.* Traditionally two sphincters are described. The *internal sphincter* consists of the smooth muscle of the bladder and proximal urethra, and the *external sphincter* consists of the periurethral striated muscle. However, more recent explanations of the components of the sphincter mechanism have challenged this conception, and it is better to describe a single mechanism consisting of elements of compression and elements of tension.

*Elements of compression* are necessary for the urethra to form a watertight seal between episodes of urination. The softness (collapsibility) of the urethral wall is important for continence, particularly when urethral integrity is altered by placement of a catheter. The watertight seal of the urethra is further enhanced by the mucus produced by the epithelium. The mucus reduces surface tension, promoting collapse of the walls and sealing the microscopic fissures against urinary leakage.

---

■ *Mikel Gray, PhD, CUNP, CCCN, FAAN, originally wrote this section.

The vascular cushion also acts as an element of compression (in addition to producing tension), contributing to urethral closure during physical stress. The vascular cushion or network of the arterioles, venules, and arteriovenous communications in the urethra promotes urethral compression by transmitting pressure from the muscles surrounding the urethra and those intrinsic to its walls. The vascular cushion contributes to urethral closure pressure because it is filled with an incompressible fluid that has its own intrinsic pressure.

The *elements of tension* in the urethral sphincter mechanism consist of the vascular cushion, intrinsic smooth and skeletal muscles, and periurethral striated muscle. These muscles are specially innervated to maintain the tension needed for urethral closure between episodes of micturition and to provide an extra measure of urethral tension, which is needed when significant physical exertion stresses sphincter closure. The pelvic muscles receive somatic innervation, which allows voluntary interruption of the urinary stream and provides added protection against precipitous rises in abdominal pressure.

## Clinical Manifestations

As in most disorders of childhood, the incidence and type of kidney or urinary tract dysfunction change with the age and maturation of the child. In addition, the presenting complaints and their significance vary with maturation. For example, a complaint of enuresis has greater significance at age 8 years than at age 4. In the newborn, urinary tract disorders are associated with a number of obvious malformations of other body systems, including the curious and unexplained but frequent association between malformed or low-set ears and urinary tract anomalies. Important signs and symptoms that suggest possible renal or genitourinary tract disease in children at different ages are outlined in Box 30-1.

Many clinical manifestations are common to a variety of childhood disorders, but their presence is an indication to obtain further information from the past history, family history, and laboratory studies as part of a complete physical examination. Suspected renal disease can be further evaluated by means of radiographic studies and renal biopsy.

## Laboratory Tests

Both urine and blood studies contribute vital information for the detection of renal problems. The single most important test is probably routine urinalysis. Specific urine and blood tests provide additional information.

*Glomerular filtration rate* is a measure of the amount of plasma from which a given substance is totally cleared in 1 minute. Clearance is calculated from the ratio of substance excreted to the concentration of that substance in the plasma. A number of substances can be used, but the most useful clinical estimation of glomerular filtration is the clearance of *creatinine,* an end product of protein metabolism in muscle and a substance that is freely filtered by the glomerulus and secreted by renal tubular cells. The production and secretion of creatinine remain relatively constant from day to day, and its appearance in the urine is determined by the serum level. When the collection is complete and accurately timed, the results are fairly reliable and compare favorably with clearance of other substances (e.g., inulin) that require special equipment and long immobilization of the child to evaluate.

Any significant degree of renal disease can diminish the glomerular filtration rate, but renal vascular disease and diseases of the glomerulus have the most immediate effect. The nurse's responsibility in this test is collection of urine, usually a 12- or 24-hour specimen.

The major urine and blood tests are outlined in Tables 30-1 and 30-2. Special tests and nursing responsibilities are briefly described in Table 30-3.

## Nursing Considerations

Nursing responsibilities in the assessment of renal disorders and diseases begins with observation of the child for any

---

**Box 30-1** ◼ ◼ ◻
### Signs and Symptoms of Urinary Tract Disorders or Disease at Different Ages

**NEONATAL PERIOD (BIRTH TO 1 MONTH)**
Poor feeding
Vomiting
Failure to gain weight
Rapid respiration (acidosis)
Respiratory distress
Spontaneous pneumothorax or pneumomediastinum
Frequent urination
Screaming on urination
Poor urinary stream
Jaundice
Seizures
Dehydration
Other anomalies or stigmata
Enlarged kidneys or bladder

**INFANCY (1 TO 24 MONTHS)**
Poor feeding
Vomiting
Failure to gain weight
Excessive thirst
Frequent urination
Straining or screaming on urination
Foul-smelling urine
Pallor
Fever
Persistent diaper rash
Seizures (with or without fever)
Dehydration
Enlarged kidneys or bladder

**CHILDHOOD (2 TO 14 YEARS)**
Poor appetite
Vomiting
Growth failure
Excessive thirst
Enuresis, incontinence, frequent urination
Painful urination
Swelling of face
Seizures
Pallor
Fatigue
Blood in urine
Abdominal or back pain
Edema
Hypertension
Tetany

**TABLE 30-1** Urine tests of renal function

| Test | Normal Range | Deviations | Significance of Deviations |
|------|--------------|------------|----------------------------|
| **Physical Tests** | | | |
| **Volume** | Age related Newborn: 30-60 ml | Polyuria | Osmotic factors (urinary glucose level in diabetes mellitus) |
| | Children: Bladder capacity (oz) = age (years) + 2 | Oliguria | Retention caused by obstructive disease |
| | | | Inadequate bladder emptying caused by neurogenic bladder or obstructive disorder |
| | | Anuria | Obstruction of urinary tract; acute renal failure |
| **Specific gravity** | With normal fluid intake: 1.016-1.022 | High | Dehydration |
| | | | Presence of protein or glucose |
| | Newborn: 1.001-1.020 | | Presence of radiopaque contrast medium after radiologic examinations |
| | Others: 1.001-1.030 | Low | Excessive fluid intake |
| | | | Distal tubular dysfunction |
| | | | Insufficient antidiuretic hormone |
| | | | Diuresis |
| | | Fixed at 1.010 | Chronic glomerular disease |
| **Osmolality** | Newborn: 50-600 mOsm/L | High or low | Same as for specific gravity |
| | Thereafter: 50-1400 mOsm/L | | More sensitive index than specific gravity |
| **Appearance** | Clear, pale yellow to deep gold | Cloudy | Contains sediment |
| | | Cloudy reddish pink to reddish brown | Blood from trauma or disease |
| | | | Myoglobin following severe muscle destruction |
| | | Light | Dilute |
| | | Dark | Concentrated |
| | | Red | Trauma |
| **Chemical Tests** | | | |
| **pH** | Newborn: 5-7 | Weak acid or neutral | If associated with metabolic acidosis, suggests tubular acidosis |
| | Thereafter: 4.8-7.8 | | If associated with metabolic alkalosis, suggests potassium deficiency |
| | Average: 6 | | Urinary infection |
| | | | Metabolic alkalosis |
| | | Alkaline | Metabolic alkalosis |
| **Protein level** | Absent | Present | Abnormal glomerular permeability (e.g., glomerular disease, changes in blood pressure) |
| | | | Most kidney disease |
| | | | Orthostatic in some individuals |
| **Glucose level** | Absent | Present | Diabetes mellitus |
| | | | Infusion of concentrated glucose-containing fluids |
| | | | Glomerulonephritis |
| | | | Impaired tubular reabsorption |
| **Ketone levels** | Absent | Present | Conditions of acute metabolic demand (stress) |
| | | | Diabetic ketoacidosis |
| **Leukocyte esterase** | Absent | Present | Can identify both lysed and intact white blood cells via enzyme detection |
| **Nitrites** | Absent | Present | Most species of bacteria convert nitrates to nitrites in the urine |
| **Microscopic Tests** | | | |
| **White blood cell count** | Less than 1 or 2 | More than 5 polymorphonuclear leukocytes/field | Urinary tract inflammatory process |
| | | Lymphocytes | Allograft rejection |
| | | | Malignancy |
| **Red blood cell count** | Less than 1 or 2 | 4-6/field in centrifuged specimen | Trauma |
| | | | Stones |
| | | | Glomerular injury |
| | | | Infection |
| | | | Neoplasms |
| **Presence of bacteria** | Absent to a few | More than 100,000 organisms/ml in centrifuged specimen | Urinary tract infection |
| **Presence of casts** | Occasional | Granular casts | Tubular or glomerular disorders |
| | | | Degenerative process in advanced renal disease |
| | | Cellular casts | Pyelonephritis |
| | | White blood cell | Glomerulonephritis |
| | | Red blood cell | Proteinuria; usually transient |
| | | Hyaline casts | |

**TABLE 30-2** Blood tests of renal function

| Test | Normal Range (mg/dl) | Deviations | Significance of Deviations |
|---|---|---|---|
| Blood urea nitrogen (BUN) | Newborn: 4-18<br>Infant, child: 5-18 | Elevated | Renal disease—acute or chronic<br>  (the higher the BUN, the more severe the disease)<br>Increased protein catabolism<br>Dehydration<br>Hemorrhage<br>High protein intake<br>Corticosteroid therapy |
| Uric acid | Child: 2.0-5.5 | Increased | Severe renal disease |
| Creatinine | Infant: 0.2-0.4<br>Child: 0.3-0.7<br>Adolescent: 0.5-1.0 | Increased | Severe renal impairment |

**Box 30-2** ■ ■ ■
### Classifications of Urinary Tract Infections or Inflammations

**Bacteriuria**—Presence of bacteria in the urine
**Asymptomatic bacteriuria**—Significant bacteriuria with no evidence of clinical infection (usually defined as greater than 100,000 colony-forming units [CFU])
**Symptomatic bacteriuria**—Bacteriuria accompanied by physical signs of urinary infection (dysuria, suprapubic discomfort, hematuria, fever)
**Recurrent UTI**—Repeated episode of bacteriuria or symptomatic UTI
**Persistent UTI**—Persistence of bacteriuria despite antibiotic treatment
**Febrile UTI**—Bacteriuria accompanied by fever and other physical signs of urinary infection; presence of a fever typically implies pyelonephritis
**Cystitis**—Inflammation of the bladder
**Urethritis**—Inflammation of the urethra
**Pyelonephritis**—Inflammation of the upper urinary tract and kidneys
**Urosepsis**—Febrile urinary tract infection coexisting with systemic signs of bacterial illness; blood culture reveals presence of urinary pathogen

manifestations that might indicate dysfunction. The most significant ongoing assessments in children with renal conditions are accurate measurement and recording of *weight, intake* and *output,* and *blood pressure.* (See Chapter 7.) These assessments are necessary not only for children with known renal dysfunction but also for those children at risk for developing renal complications (e.g., children in shock, postoperative patients).

In addition to the general manifestations of renal conditions (see Box 30-1), many conditions have specific characteristics that distinguish them from other disorders. These are discussed as appropriate throughout the chapter.

The nurse is generally the one responsible for preparing infants, children, and parents for tests and collection of urine and (sometimes) blood specimens. (See Preparation for Diagnostic and Therapeutic Procedures, Chapter 27, and Collection of Specimens, Chapter 27.) Nurses observe the characteristics of the urine collected, often perform any

of a number of tests on urine specimens (e.g., urine specific gravity, protein, blood, glucose, ketones), and assist with more complex diagnostic tests (e.g., radiography, cystoscopy). Nurses must be familiar with significant laboratory tests, their implications, and preprocedural care.

**NURSING ALERT** Use of Fleet enemas in children with acute or chronic renal failure is potentially lethal because of hyperphosphatemia. Requests for Fleet enemas in this situation should not be implemented without careful investigation.

## GENITOURINARY TRACT DISORDERS
### Urinary Tract Infection (UTI)

UTI is a clinical condition that may involve the urethra, bladder *(lower urinary tract),* and the ureters, renal pelvis, calyces, and renal parenchyma *(upper urinary tract).* Because it is often impossible to localize the infection, the broad designation "UTI" is applied to the presence of significant numbers of microorganisms anywhere within the urinary tract (except the distal one third of the urethra, which is usually colonized with bacteria).

Infection of the urinary tract may be present with or without clinical symptoms. As a result, the site of infection is often difficult to pinpoint with accuracy. The various terms used to describe urinary tract disorders are listed in Box 30-2.

The peak incidence of UTI not caused by structural anomalies occurs between 2 and 6 years of age. Except for the neonatal period, females have a 10 to 30 times greater risk for developing UTI than males. It is estimated that 5% to 6% of girls will have had at least one episode of bacteriuria between the time they enter first grade and graduate from high school. The likelihood of recurrence is 50% or greater in girls; the recurrence rate is lower in boys (Kunin, 1997).

UTI in newborns differs in some respects from infections occurring in older children. In this age-group, males outnumber females. The prevalence of bacteriuria in infants is 3.7% in boys and 2% in girls (Rushton, 1997). At all ages asymptomatic bacteriuria is more common than sympto-

**TABLE 30-3** Radiologic and other tests of urinary system function

| Test | Procedure | Purpose | Comments and Nursing Responsibilities |
|---|---|---|---|
| Urine culture and sensitivity | Collection of sterile specimen | Determines presence of pathogens and the drugs to which they are sensitive | Does not require specific parental permission<br>Send specimen to laboratory immediately after collection<br>Catheterization, clean-catch, or suprapubic specimen |
| Renal/bladder ultrasound | Transmission of ultrasonic waves through renal parenchyma, along ureteral course, and over bladder | Allows visualization of renal parenchyma, renal pelvis without exposure to external beam radiation or radioactive isotopes<br>Visualization of dilated ureters and bladder wall also possible | Noninvasive procedure |
| Testicular (scrotal) ultrasound | Transmission of ultrasonic waves through scrotal contents and testis | Allows visualization of scrotal contents, including testis<br>Testicular ultrasound is used to identify masses, and Doppler-enhanced ultrasound is used to differentiate hyperemia of epididymo-orchitis from ischemia of torsion | Noninvasive procedure |
| Scout film | Flat plate roentgenogram of abdomen and pelvis for kidney, ureters, bladder (KUB) | Detects and establishes renal outlines, presence of calculi, or opaque foreign bodies in bladder | Prepare as for routine x-ray film |
| Voiding cystourethrography | Contrast medium injected into bladder through urethral catheter until bladder is full; films taken before, during, and after voiding | Visualizes bladder outline and urethra, reveals reflux of urine into ureters, and shows complications of bladder emptying | Prepare child for catheterization |
| Radionuclide (nuclear) cystogram | Radionuclide-containing fluid injected through urethral catheter until bladder is full; images generated before, during, and after voiding | Alternative to voiding cystourethrography in children with allergy to intravesical contrast material<br>Allows evaluation of reflux, although visualization of anatomic details is relatively poor | Prepare child for catheterization<br>Reassure patient and parents that allergic response to contrast materials is avoided by use of radionuclide |
| Radioisotope imaging studies | Contrast medium injected intravenously; computer analysis to measure uptake or washout (excretion) for analysis of organ function | *DTPA* radioisotope used to measure glomerular filtration rate; estimate of differential renal function and renal washout to determine presence and location of upper urinary tract obstruction<br>*DMSA* radioisotope allows visualization of renal scars and differential renal function; ureters and bladder are not visualized<br>*MAG 3* radioisotope combines features of DTPA (evaluation of upper urinary tract obstruction) with features of DMSA radioisotope (differential renal function) | Insert or assist with insertion of intravenous infusion<br>Monitor intravenous infusion<br>Urethral catheterization may accompany DTPA radioisotope scan; prepare child for catheterization when indicated |
| Intravenous pyelography (IVP) (intravenous urogram; excretory urogram) | Intravenous injection of a contrast medium<br>Medium secreted and concentrated by tubules<br>X-ray films made 5, 10, and 15 minutes after injection; delayed films (30, 60 minutes), etc.) are obtained if obstruction suspected | Defines urinary tract<br>Provides information about integrity of kidneys, ureters, and bladder<br>Retroperitoneal masses visualized when they shift position of ureters | Preparation for test:<br>Infants less than 2 years of age—no solid food, omit one bottle on morning of examination; studies should be performed early to avoid withholding of fluids<br>Children age 2-14 years—give cathartic evening before examination, nothing orally after midnight,* enema (Fleet [See Nursing Alert, p. 1262] or soapsuds) morning of examination |

*Current research supports oral intake of clear fluids up to 2 hours before test. (See Surgical Procedures, Chapter 27.)

*Continued*

**TABLE 30-3  Radiologic and other tests of urinary system function—cont'd**

| Test | Procedure | Purpose | Comments and Nursing Responsibilities |
|---|---|---|---|
| Computed tomography (CT) | Narrow-beam x-rays and computer analysis provide precise reconstruction of area | Visualizes vertical or horizontal cross section of kidney<br>Especially valuable to distinguish tumors and cysts | Noncontrast scan is noninvasive<br>Contrast-enhanced CT scan preparation is similar to IVP |
| Cystoscopy | Direct visualization of bladder and lower urinary tract through small scope inserted via urethra | Investigation of bladder and lower tract lesions; visualizes ureteral openings, bladder wall, trigone, and urethra | Give nothing orally after midnight*<br>Carry out preoperative preparations |
| Retrograde pyelography | Contrast medium injected through ureteral catheter | Visualizes pelvic calyces, ureters, and bladder | Prepare the child for cystoscopy |
| Renal angiography | Contrast medium injected directly into renal artery via catheter placed in femoral artery (or umbilical artery in newborn) and advanced to renal artery | Visualizes renal vascular system, especially for renal arterial stenosis | Give cathartic if ordered<br>Give preoperative medication if ordered<br>Observe for reaction to contrast medium<br>Monitor vital signs following procedure |
| Whitaker perfusion test | Injection of contrast material through renal pelvis and ureters<br>Pressures are measured in renal pelvis and urinary bladder | Determine presence of obstruction causing upper urinary tract dilation | Prepare child for insertion of a spinal needle or perfusion catheter in renal pelvis (anesthetic often required) |
| Renal biopsy | Removal of kidney tissue by open or percutaneous technique for study by light, electron, or immunofluorescent microscopy | Yields histologic and microscopic information about glomeruli and tubules; helps to distinguish between types of nephrotic syndromes<br>Distinguishes other renal disorders | Give nothing orally 4-6 hours before test*<br>Premedicate as ordered<br>Prepare setup for procedure<br>Assist with procedure<br>Take vital signs<br>Apply pressure to area with pressure dressing and, if feasible, a sandbag<br>Bed rest for 24 hours<br>Observe for abdominal pain, tenderness<br>Monitor input and output; surgical incision may be required in infants |
| Urodynamics | Set of tests designed to measure bladder filling, storage, and evacuation functions<br>Uroflowmetry is a test to determine efficiency of urination<br>Cystometrogram is a graphic comparison of bladder pressure as a function of volume<br>Sphincter electromyogram is a test of pelvic muscle function during bladder filling and evacuation<br>Voiding pressure study is a comparison of detrusor contraction pressure, sphincter EMG, and urinary flow | Determine characteristics of voiding dysfunction<br>Used to identify type (cause) of incontinence or urinary retention<br>Especially valuable for voiding dysfunction complicated by urinary infection, urinary retention, or neurogenic bladder dysfunction | Prepare child for catheterization<br>Insertion of a rectal tube will produce feelings of rectal fullness or pressure<br>Insertion of needles may be required for sphincter electromyography |

matic disease, and recurrence is not uncommon, especially in girls. The overall recurrence rate in young girls is much greater than for young boys or neonates (Walsh and others, 1998). An increased incidence of UTI is observed in adolescents, especially those with evidence of sexual activity.

## Etiology

A variety of organisms can be responsible for UTI. *Escherichia coli* (80% of cases) and other gram-negative enteric organisms are most commonly implicated; all are common to the anal, perineal, and perianal region. Other organisms associated with UTI include *Proteus, Pseudomonas, Klebsiella, Staphylococcus aureus, Haemophilus,* and coagulase-negative *Staphylococcus.* A number of factors contribute to the development of UTI, including anatomic, physical, and chemical conditions or properties of the host's urinary tract.

**Anatomic and Physical Factors.** The structure of the lower urinary tract is believed to account for the increased incidence of bacteriuria in females. The short urethra, which measures approximately 2 cm (¾ inch) in young females and 4 cm (1½ inches) in mature women, provides a ready pathway for invasion of organisms. In addition, the closure of the urethra at the end of micturition may return contaminated bacteria to the bladder.

The longer male urethra (as long as 20 cm [8 inches] in an adult) and the antibacterial properties of prostatic secretions inhibit the entry and growth of pathogens. Reports indicate an increased incidence of UTI in uncircumcised infants less than 1 year of age as compared with infants who are circumcised (Schoen, Colby, and Ray, 2000). The presence of a foreskin is associated with a greater quantity of periurethral bacteria that can ascend the urethra easily (Wiswell, 2000). The incidence of renal scarring is greatest in patients whose first infection occurs during infancy.

The single most important host factor influencing the occurrence of UTI is urinary stasis. Ordinarily urine is sterile, but at 37° C (98.6° F) it provides an excellent culture medium. Under normal conditions the act of completely and repeatedly emptying the bladder flushes away any organisms before they have an opportunity to multiply and invade surrounding tissue. However, urine that remains in the bladder allows bacteria from the urethra to rapidly become established in the rich medium.

Incomplete bladder emptying (stasis) may result from reflux (see p. 1269 for a discussion of reflux), anatomic abnormalities (especially those involving the ureters), or extrinsic ureteral or bladder compression. The pressure of overdistention within the bladder may increase the risk of infection by decreasing host resistance, probably as a result of lessened blood flow to the mucosa. This often occurs in a neurogenic bladder or as a consequence of voluntarily holding back urine despite the urge to void.

Urinary stasis may also occur because of dysfunctional voiding. Dysfunctional voiding describes a constellation of symptoms that are closely associated with the development of urinary tract infection and vesicoureteral reflux (Plachter, Schulman, and Canning, 1999) (Box 30-3).

Extrinsic factors that may be responsible for functional bladder neck obstruction are pregnancy and chronic and intermittent constipation. In both conditions the full uterus or rectum displaces the bladder and posterior urethra in the fixed and limited space of the bony pelvis, causing obstruction, incomplete micturition, and urinary stasis. Treating constipation and administering antibiotic therapy for UTI reduces the recurrence of infection; failure to relieve the fecal retention in spite of adequate treatment of the UTI may result in recurrence.

Other extrinsic factors that can contribute to UTI include catheters, especially short-term indwelling catheters,

---

**Box 30-3** ■ ■ □
### Symptoms of Dysfunctional Voiding

Urinary tract infection without fever
Changes in urinary frequency
Constipation
Squatting or holding to stay dry
Daytime or nighttime wetting
Straining to void
Urgency to void

Modified from Plachter NB, Schulman SL, Canning DA: Identification and management of urinary tract infection in the preschool child, *J Pediatr Health Care* 13(6 Part 1):268-272, 1999.

---

and administration of antimicrobial agents. Antimicrobials alter the host's normal perineal flora, allowing easier colonization of uropathogens. Tight clothing or diapers, poor hygiene, and local inflammation, such as from vaginitis, masturbation, or pinworm infestation, may also increase the risk of ascending infection. The essential oils in bubble baths and shampoos can irritate the urethra of both boys and girls, causing painful and frequent urination. Therefore bubble baths are discouraged. There is no evidence that plain tub baths increase the risk of UTI, but infections have been related to the use of hot tub or whirlpool baths. Sexual intercourse may produce transient bacteriuria in females and is associated with an increased risk of UTI.

**Altered Urine and Bladder Chemistry.** Several mechanical and chemical characteristics of the urinary tract promote urine sterility. Adequate fluid intake promotes urinary transport and lowers the concentration of pathogens (and nutrients) in the urine. Diuresis also enhances the antibacterial properties of the renal medulla, probably as a result of increased blood flow, which hastens leukocytosis, and diuresis promotes the mechanical removal of pathogens.

Much has been reported about the use of cranberry juice for the prevention of UTI. This mechanism was thought to result from increased urine acidity and inadherence of bacteria to the bladder lining. However, a recent study done on children with neurogenic bladder shows ingestion of cranberry juice results in a median pH of only 6.0. Urine is bacteriostatic to *E. coli* at a pH of 5.0 (attainable only by ingestion of pure hippuric acid). Further findings from this study suggest the antiadherence properties of cranberries are more often observed in UTI caused by fimbriated *E. coli* strains, which are more common in healthy patients with UTI and less common in patients with chronic medical illnesses or urinary tract anomalies (Schlager and others, 1999).

## Pathophysiology

Following invasion by bacteria, the first line of defense in the lower urinary tract is complete evacuation by voiding. Inflammation in the bladder and urethral walls is apparent within 30 minutes of invasion by a bacterial pathogen. Polymorphonucleocytes rapidly migrate to the bladder wall, which becomes completely injected within 2 hours. Complete evacuation of the bladder is particularly important for the eradication of bacteria from the urine. Urination not only removes bacteria and associated toxins contained in the urine, it also allows more efficient destruction of the bacteria remaining on the thin film of urine that is closely adherent to the vesical wall.

Recurrent infection of the urinary bladder predisposes the individual to transient episodes of vesicoureteric reflux. Following resolution of the infection, the reflux is not detectable on a voiding cystourethrography. Although it is known that certain adherent bacteria promote urinary system dilation, the relationship between bladder wall inflammation and utereovesical junction competence remains unclear (Walsh and others, 1998).

## Clinical Manifestations

The clinical manifestations of UTIs depend on the age of the child. In newborn infants and children less than 2 years of age the signs are characteristically nonspecific. They more nearly resemble gastrointestinal tract disorders: failure to thrive, feeding problems, vomiting, diarrhea, abdominal distention, and jaundice. Newborns may have fever, hypothermia, or sepsis. Other evidence that may be observed includes frequent or infrequent voiding, constant squirming and irritability, strong-smelling urine, and an abnormal stream. A persistent diaper rash may also be a helpful clue.

The classic symptoms of UTI are often observed in children more than 2 years of age. These include enuresis or daytime incontinence in the child who has been toilet trained, fever, strong- or foul-smelling urine, increased frequency of urination, dysuria, or urgency. They may also complain of abdominal pain or costovertebral angle tenderness (flank pain). Some will present with hematuria; preschoolers may vomit. There is a high frequency of obstructive uropathy in young infants and boys, which is characterized by dribbling of urine, straining with urination, or a decrease in the force and size of the urinary stream. High fever and chills accompanied by flank pain, severe abdominal pain, and leukocytosis suggest pyelonephritis. However, flank pain and tenderness may be the only indication of pyelonephritis on physical examination.

Manifestations in adolescents are more specific. Symptoms of lower tract infections include frequency and painful urination of a small amount of turbulent urine that may be grossly bloody. Fever is usually absent. Upper tract infection is characterized by fever, chills, flank pain, and lower tract symptoms, which may appear 1 or 2 days after the upper tract symptoms.

Many UTIs in children are asymptomatic or atypical in clinical presentation, and many complaints may be unrelated to the urinary tract. Many are treated as respiratory or gastrointestinal infections. It is important that these children be identified so that treatment can be initiated. Significant scarring can occur, especially in infants and very young children.

## Diagnostic Evaluation

The diagnosis of UTI depends on a high degree of suspicion, evaluation of the history and physical examination,

and urinalysis and culture. Urine with a possible infection appears cloudy, hazy, or thick with noticeable strands of mucus and pus; it also smells fishy and unpleasant, even when fresh. A presumptive UTI diagnosis can be made on the basis of microscopic examination of the urine, which often reveals pyuria (5 to 8 white blood cells/ml of uncentrifuged urine) and the presence of at least one bacterium in a Gram stain. However, a normal urinalysis may also be present in conditions of asymptomatic bacteriuria.

The diagnosis of UTI is confirmed by the detection of bacteria in a urine culture, but urine collection is often difficult, especially in infants and very small children. (See Collection of Specimens, Chapter 27.) Several factors may alter a urine specimen. Contamination of a specimen by organisms from sources other than the urine is the most common cause of false-positive results. Bag urine specimens are commonly contaminated by perineal and perianal flora and are usually considered inadequate for a definitive diagnosis. Clean-catch urine specimens have been determined to be no better than a regular midstream specimen. Unless the specimen is a first morning sample, a recent high fluid intake may indicate a falsely low organism count. Therefore children should not be encouraged to drink large volumes of water in an attempt to obtain a specimen quickly.

**NURSING TIP** Clean-catch urine specimen collection from a young girl is more easily done when the child sits on the toilet facing the tank. In this position the child (especially the toddler) is more stable and relaxed. The labia are naturally separated, decreasing the likelihood of contamination. This position is also useful for older girls who perform clean, intermittent self-catheterization.

The most accurate tests of bacterial content are suprapubic aspiration (children less than 2 years of age) and properly performed bladder catheterization (as long as the first few milliliters are excluded from collection). Care of a urine specimen obtained for culture is an important nursing aspect related to diagnosis. The specimen should be taken to the laboratory for culture immediately. If culture is delayed, the sample can be placed in a refrigerator for up to 24 hours, but storage can result in a loss of formed elements, such as blood cells and casts (Froom and others, 2000).

Tests to detect bacteriuria are being used with increased frequency in UTI screening. The plastic dipstick and agar-coated slide tests are quick and inexpensive methods for detecting infection before obtaining final culture results. The presence of nitrites on dipstick analysis of urine has been shown to have a predictive value of as much as 100% (identifies infected urine) (Raymond and Sauvestre, 1998). The absence of nitrites and leukocyte esterase in combination has been shown to have 92% negative predictive value (identifies uninfected urine) (Raymond and Sauvestre, 1998) (see Table 30-1). The agar-coated slides have a positive predictive value (identifies infected urine) of 96% and negative predictive value (identifies uninfected urine) of 99.8% (Colodner and Keness, 2000). These test results are used to initiate treatment of UTI while culture results are pending. It is important to remember that some organisms that cause UTI are non–nitrite producing (e.g., *Pseudomonas* organisms).

Localization of the infection site may involve more specific tests, including ureteral catheterization, bladder washout procedures, and radioisotope renography. Other tests, such as ultrasonography, voiding cystourethrogram (VCUG), intravenous pyelogram (IVP), and dimercaptosuccinic acid (DMSA) scan may be performed after the infection subsides to identify anatomic abnormalities contributing to the development of infection and existing kidney changes from a recurrent infection.

### Therapeutic Management

The objectives of treatment of children with UTI are to (1) eliminate the current infection, (2) identify contributing factors to reduce the risk of recurrence, (3) prevent urosepsis, and (4) preserve renal function (AAP Committee on Quality Improvement, Subcommittee on Urinary Tract Infections, 1999). Antibiotic therapy is guided by laboratory culture and sensitivity tests. Nonetheless, empiric therapy on the basis of the child's past history and presenting symptoms may be necessary when fever or systemic illness complicates UTI. Common antiinfective agents used for UTI include the penicillins, sulfonamide (including trimethoprim and sulfisoxazole in combination), the cephalosporins, nitrofurantoin, and the tetracyclines. All antibiotics may cause side effects or prove ineffective because of bacterial resistance (Table 30-4).

Children with suspected pyelonephritis and fever are admitted to the hospital and given appropriate antibiotics intravenously for a minimum of 48 hours. Blood and urine cultures are obtained on admission and following therapy. Urine cultures are usually repeated at monthly intervals for 3 months and at 3-month intervals for another 6 months.

Renal scarring can develop during the initial infection, especially in younger children. Therefore some practitioners believe that the first UTI in childhood necessitates radiologic evaluation, regardless of the age and sex of the patient (Goldman and others, 2000; Lama and others, 2000).

Anatomic defects such as primary reflux or bladder neck obstruction may require surgical correction to prevent recurrent infection or may indicate the need for prophylactic antibiotics and careful follow-up. Follow-up study is an important component of medical management, because the relapse rate is high and recurrent infection tends to occur 1 to 2 months after termination of treatment. The aim of therapy and careful follow-up in such cases is to prevent morbidity and reduce the chance of renal scarring.

**Prognosis.**   With prompt and adequate treatment at the time of diagnosis, the long-term prognosis for UTIs is usually excellent. The hazard of progressive renal injury is greatest when infection occurs in young children (especially under 2 years of age) and is associated with congenital renal malformations and reflux. Therefore early diagnosis of children at risk is particularly important during infancy and toddlerhood.

### Nursing Considerations

Objectives of nursing care include identification of children with UTI and education of parents and children regarding prevention and treatment of infection. Aside from the influence of renal abnormalities, females between the ages of 2 and 6 years are in general a high-risk group. Because they are not a captive population, mass screening is difficult. However, the annual health examination should include a routine urinalysis. In addition, nurses should instruct parents to observe regularly for clues that suggest UTI. Unfortunately, the signs of UTI are not as evident as those of upper respiratory tract infection. Therefore many cases go undetected because no one thought to investigate this very common problem.

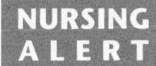 **NURSING ALERT**   A child who exhibits the following should be evaluated for UTI:
Incontinence in a toilet-trained child
Strong-smelling urine
Frequency or urgency

Because infants and young children are unable to express their feelings and sensations verbally, it is difficult to detect any discomfort they may be experiencing from dysuria. A careful history regarding voiding habits, stooling pattern, and episodes of unexplained irritability may assist

| TABLE 30-4   Common side effects of urinary antiinfective agents | | |
| --- | --- | --- |
| **Drug** | **Side Effects** | **Nursing Interventions** |
| Trimethoprim/sulfamethoxazole (Bactrim, Septra) | Rash, urticaria, photosensitivity, nausea, bone marrow depression (long-term use) | Maintain adequate fluid intake; use sunscreen; perform complete blood count (CBC) every 3 months (long-term use). |
| Amoxicillin (Amoxil, Polymox, Trimox) | Nausea, vomiting, diarrhea | Refrigerate suspension; discard suspension after 14 days. |
| Nitrofurantoin (Macrodantin, Furadantin) | Nausea, pneumonitis or pulmonary fibrosis (long-term use) | Administer with milk or food. |
| Cephalexin (Keflex) | Nausea, diarrhea | Administer with milk or food. |
| Carbenicillin (Geocillin, Geopen) | Nausea, diarrhea, urticaria | Take tablets with juice to mask foul taste. |
| Ceftazidime (Fortaz) | Renal toxicity | Do not use if allergic to penicillin. |
| Gentamicin (Garamycin) | Renal toxicity, ototoxicity | Keep well hydrated, monitor urine output, blood urea nitrogen (BUN), creatinine; monitor serum levels especially in infants. |

in detecting less obvious cases of UTI. Parents should be encouraged to observe for specific clues of UTI in suspected cases. (See Critical Thinking Exercise box.)

Collecting an appropriate specimen is essential when infection is suspected. It is the nurse's responsibility to take every precaution to obtain acceptable, clean-voided specimens in order to avoid using other collecting procedures except when absolutely indicated.

**NURSING TIP** To detect UTI in infants and toddlers, check the diaper every ½ hour; frequent observations increase the opportunity for observing the stream for such findings as straining or fretting before voiding begins, signs of discomfort before and during urinating, intermittent starting and stopping of the stream, and frequent dripping of small amounts of urine.

Other tests are often performed to detect anatomic defects. Children are prepared for these tests as appropriate for their age. Children who are old enough to understand

## Critical Thinking Exercise

### Urinary Tract Infection and Constipation

During your assessment of Elizabeth, a 4-year-old admitted to the hospital for severe UTI, her mother tells you that Elizabeth has bowel movements every third to fourth day. They are usually large, hard-formed stools, and Elizabeth sometimes has trouble evacuating the stool. What should you do?

FIRST, THINK ABOUT IT . . .

• What assumptions are you making?
• If you accept the conclusions, what are the implications?

1. Explain to the mother that this may be normal for Elizabeth, and she will have less trouble as she gets older.
2. Explain to the mother the relationship of diet to constipation as you develop a line of inquiry to elicit the fat content of Elizabeth's diet.
3. Explain to the mother that the diarrhea associated with the antibiotics Elizabeth is now receiving should correct the constipation.
4. Explain to the mother the relationship between chronic constipation and urinary tract infections as you move into a complete elimination history.

*The best response is four. Although Elizabeth may have an elimination pattern similar to her mother's, 3 to 4 days is a long interval between stools, even for an adult. In this instance the presence of a large stool mass within the colon is likely to cause pressure on the bladder and urethra and not allow the bladder to empty completely. The implications of stasis of urine within the bladder can then lead to infection. Although a diet and fluid intake history is part of the assessment of children with urinary tract infections and constipation, the fat content of Elizabeth's diet is not the most critical information at this time. Finally, Elizabeth may or may not develop diarrhea secondary to her antibiotic regimen. However, one bout of diarrhea will not eliminate the constipation, which has been present over a long period of time.*

need an explanation of the procedure, its purpose, and what they will experience. (See Preparation for Diagnostic and Therapeutic Procedures, Chapter 27.) Sometimes a simple description of the urinary system is helpful. For children under 3 to 4 years of age, the procedure can be explained on a doll. For those who are older, a simple drawing of the bladder, urethra, ureters, and kidneys makes the explanation more understandable. Especially with preschool children, the nurse must clarify that the urinary tract is separate from any sexual function and that the test is for a problem that they did not cause. It is not uncommon for children to associate blame for perceived wrongdoing (e.g., masturbation) or unacceptable thoughts with the reason for the illness or tests.

Children may be treated as outpatients to avoid overnight separation from home. In such cases nurses must be careful not to overlook the need for adequate preparation. If surgery is subsequently indicated, the child will be able to encounter the impending operation with these facts and an understanding of these procedures, which helps to decrease fear and anxiety regarding more extensive medical-surgical intervention.

Because antiinfective drugs are indicated in the treatment of UTI, the nurse teaches the patient and parents the appropriate dosage and scheduling and provides suggestions for administration of the agent.* Certain drugs are available in liquid form; others are available only in capsule or pill form. In general, capsules can be separated and pills can be crushed, with their contents mixed into a small volume of food or chilled liquid to mask a disagreeable taste. A simple suggestion is to introduce a medicine in divided doses and mixed with a flavored gelatin in an ice cube tray. Other medications are best tolerated with a small portion of partially frozen grape or apple juice.

Adequate fluid intake is always indicated during an acute UTI. It is recommended that a person drink 100 ml/kg, or approximately 50 ml/lb of body weight daily (Miller, 1996). The patient should primarily drink clear liquids. Caffeinated or carbonated beverages are avoided because of their potentially irritative effect on the bladder mucosa. The child who is febrile and unable to drink liquids is given intravenous (IV) hydration until the fever resolves and oral liquids are tolerated.

**Prevention.** Prevention is the most important goal in both primary and recurrent infection; most preventive measures are simple, ordinary hygienic habits that should be a routine part of daily care. Any signs of intestinal parasites (e.g., scratching between the legs and around the anal area) should be investigated and treated appropriately. Sexually active adolescent females are advised to urinate as soon as possible after intercourse to flush out bacteria introduced during sex play. Parents and older children are taught health practices that prevent UTI. (See Guidelines box.)

Children who experience recurrent febrile UTIs or recurrent infections complicated by vesicoureteric reflux may

*Home care instructions for giving medications to children are available in Wong DL, Hess CS: *Wong and Whaley's clinical manual of pediatric nursing*, ed 5, St Louis, 2000, Mosby.

be given a suppressive or prophylactic antibiotic for a period of months or several years. The medication is commonly administered once a day; the patient and parents are advised to give the antibiotic before sleep because this represents the longest period without voiding. A sulfonamide/trimethoprim, nitrofurantoin, or cephalosporin is often used for antibiotic prophylaxis.

## Vesicoureteral Reflux (VUR)

VUR refers to the retrograde flow of bladder urine into the ureters. Reflux increases the chance for and perpetuates infection, because with each void urine is swept up the ureters and then allowed to empty after voiding. Therefore the residual urine from the ureters remains in the bladder until the next void. The International Classification System describes the degree of reflux from the bladder into upper genitourinary tract structures (Fig. 30-3).

*Primary reflux* results from a congenital anomaly that affects the ureterovesical junction. Ectopic or orthotopic implantation of the ureter, abnormal tunneling of the intramural ureteral segment, and defects in the configuration of the ureter orifice are associated with primary reflux. Primary reflux has a significant familial pattern; the incidence of reflux in siblings of affected children has been reported as 36%. Siblings 24 months of age or younger had the highest incidence (46%) and the highest risk of bilateral reflux. Screening for reflux in siblings through 72 months of age is recommended to prevent renal damage, which can occur in the absence of symptomatic UTI (Connolly and others, 1997).

*Secondary reflux* occurs as a result of an acquired condition. UTI can produce transient reflux, and children with reflux are at greater risk for recurrent (and febrile) urinary infections. Neuropathic bladder dysfunction, particularly when poor bladder compliance coexists with bladder outlet obstruction, may produce reflux as urine seeks to escape the high pressures of the lower urinary tract.

Reflux with infection is the most common cause of pyelonephritis in children. Refluxed urine ascending into the collecting tubules of the nephrons allows the microorganisms to gain access to the renal parenchyma, initiating renal scarring. The shape of renal papillae and the angle of entry of the collecting ducts change with advancing age, making intrarenal reflux difficult. Therefore most renal scars associated with reflux occur at a very young age and are present at the time of diagnosis; few develop after 5 to 6 years of age. Between 30% and 60% of children with VUR have evidence of renal scarring, and scarring is almost always found in association with reflux. Careful routine follow-up is a critical part of management of children with UTIs; children with reflux as documented by voiding cystoureterography are assessed repeatedly during ensuing years.

### Therapeutic Management

In most cases of VUR, conservative, nonoperative therapy is effective in controlling infection. There is a high incidence of spontaneous resolution over time—approximately 20% to 30% for each 2-year period throughout childhood. An

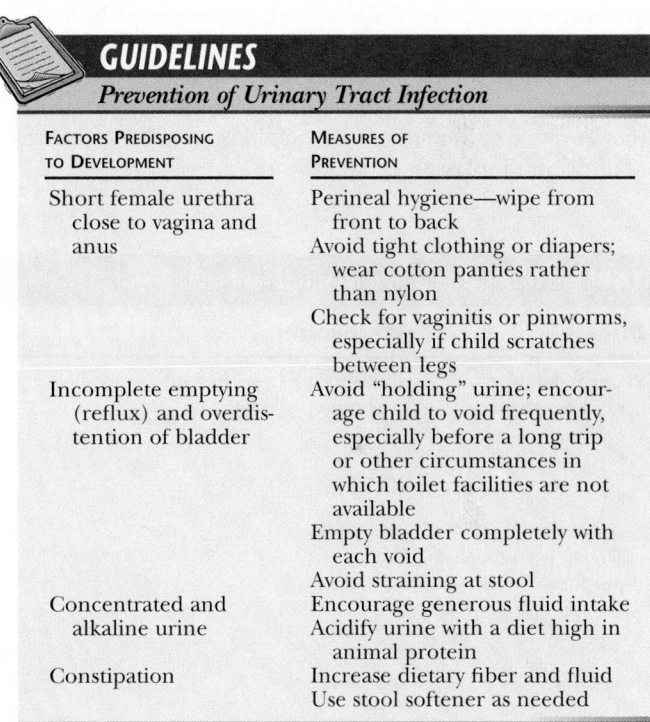

## GUIDELINES
### *Prevention of Urinary Tract Infection*

| FACTORS PREDISPOSING TO DEVELOPMENT | MEASURES OF PREVENTION |
| --- | --- |
| Short female urethra close to vagina and anus | Perineal hygiene—wipe from front to back |
| | Avoid tight clothing or diapers; wear cotton panties rather than nylon |
| | Check for vaginitis or pinworms, especially if child scratches between legs |
| Incomplete emptying (reflux) and overdistention of bladder | Avoid "holding" urine; encourage child to void frequently, especially before a long trip or other circumstances in which toilet facilities are not available |
| | Empty bladder completely with each void |
| | Avoid straining at stool |
| Concentrated and alkaline urine | Encourage generous fluid intake |
| | Acidify urine with a diet high in animal protein |
| Constipation | Increase dietary fiber and fluid |
| | Use stool softener as needed |

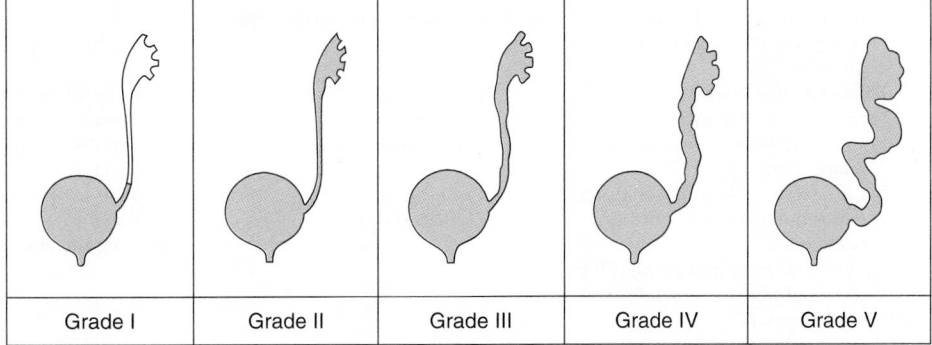

| Grade I | Grade II | Grade III | Grade IV | Grade V |

**Fig. 30-3**  Grades of reflux. (From Retik AB, Cukier J, editors: *Pediatric urology,* Baltimore, 1987, Williams & Wilkins.)

80% probability of remission may occur in grades I and II reflux when managed medically (Koff, 1997). Therapy consists of continuous low-dose antibacterial therapy with frequent urine cultures, which can usually be performed at home by the dip slide or dipstick methods. This long-term therapy requires medical supervision and reliable, cooperative parents. Surgical correction of reflux may be required for grades IV and V reflux. Grade III is managed conservatively unless there are complications.

The major indications for surgical intervention include significant anatomic abnormality at the ureterovesical junction, recurrent UTIs, high grades of VUR, noncompliance with medical therapy, intolerance to antibiotics, and VUR after puberty in females. Antireflux surgery consists of reimplantation of the ureters.

Renal ultrasonography is performed 1 month postoperatively to check for ureteral obstruction. If no obstruction is seen, antibiotic therapy is discontinued. A renal ultrasound and voiding cystourethrogram are recommended 6 months after surgery. Because of the anxiety experienced by some children undergoing catheterization for cystography and the high success rate of antireflux surgical procedures, some practitioners may omit the voiding cystogram at this time. Two years after surgery, the child is seen for a final renal ultrasound to assess renal growth.

### Nursing Considerations

The primary nursing goal in children receiving medical therapy is encouraging compliance. The importance of maintaining the medical regimen should be emphasized to parents and older children. The medications prescribed are usually well tolerated by children, but parents may need help in encouraging children to take the medication. The methods described in Chapter 27 provide some guidelines for administration and encouraging compliance. The importance of hygiene and a frequent voiding schedule are also discussed.

Because siblings are at risk for VUR, nurses should encourage parents to have their other children screened using renal ultrasonography and cystography. All children require age-appropriate preparation for the tests. Atraumatic care includes using lidocaine jelly before catheterization. (See Collection of Specimens, Chapter 27.)

## GLOMERULAR DISEASE
### Acute Glomerulonephritis (AGN)

AGN as a classification includes a number of distinct entities. It may be a primary event or a manifestation of a systemic disorder (Table 30-5), and the disease can range from

---

**TABLE 30-5** Renal involvement associated with a systemic disease process

| Disease | Mechanism | Renal Manifestation | Comments |
|---|---|---|---|
| Systemic lupus erythematosus (SLE) | Deposition of autoantibody-antigen complexes in kidney | Variable degrees of hematuria and proteinuria<br>More severe—nephrotic syndrome, hypertension, renal insufficiency | Responsive to corticosteroid and antimetabolite therapy<br>Renal failure most common cause of death from SLE<br>Rare before adolescence but may occur in school-age children |
| Anaphylactoid (Henoch-Schönlein) purpura | Unknown | Hematuria (gross or microscopic)<br>Less common—edema, hypertension<br>Nephrotic syndrome with oliguria and hypertension indicates severe involvement<br>Rarely—acute renal failure | Incidence from 20% to 70% of cases<br>Renal involvement most serious manifestation of the disease<br>More common in children over age 6 years<br>Responsive to corticosteroid therapy<br>Management similar to that for persistent glomerulonephritis |
| Sickle cell disease | Infarction of renal vessels by sickled cells (especially medullary)<br>Results in decreased circulation in vasa recta and impaired sodium and chloride ion reabsorption in collecting ducts | Hematuria<br>Nephrotic syndrome<br>Defective urine collection<br>Progressive glomerulonephritis | Irreversible with increasing age<br>Severe urinary tract infections with bacteremia not uncommon |
| Polyarteritis nodosa | Fibroid necrosis of arterial walls<br>Large vessels—patchy renal infarction<br>Microscopic vessels—necrotizing glomerulitis | Proteinuria<br>Hematuria<br>Severe hypertension | Kidney involvement of secondary importance in infancy<br>Variable course<br>Long-term prognosis guarded |
| Bacterial endocarditis | Focal or diffuse, immune-complex deposition related to chronic bacteremia<br>Some embolization of glomeruli by bacteria and fibrin from endocardial vegetations | Proteinuria<br>Hematuria | Seen in approximately 50% of cases<br>Renal involvement seldom of major significance |
| Prolonged bacteremia (infected atrioventricular shunts) | Immune-complex deposition with exudation and cellular proliferation | Variable degrees of persistent nephrotic syndrome | Vigorous antibiotic therapy or removal of infected shunt required |

minimal to severe. The common features include oliguria, edema, hypertension and circulatory congestion, hematuria, and proteinuria. Most cases are postinfectious and have been associated with pneumococcal, streptococcal, and viral infections. All postinfectious diseases are presumed to result from immune complex formation and glomerular deposition, and the clinical presentations may be indistinguishable.

*Acute poststreptococcal glomerulonephritis (APSGN)* is the most common of the noninfectious renal diseases in childhood and the one for which a cause can be established in the majority of cases. APSGN can occur at any age but affects primarily early school-age children, with a peak age of onset of 6 to 7 years. It is uncommon in children younger than 2 years of age (Milford, 1995).

## Etiology

It is now generally accepted that APSGN is an immune-complex disease (i.e., a reaction that occurs as a by-product of an antecedent streptococcal infection with certain strains of the group A β-hemolytic streptococcus). Most streptococcal infections do not cause APSGN. A latent period of 10 to 14 days occurs between the streptococcal infection of the throat or skin and the onset of clinical manifestations. The peak incidence of disease corresponds to the incidence of streptococcal infections. Disease secondary to streptococcal pharyngitis is more common in the winter or spring. However, when associated with pyoderma (principally impetigo), it may be more prevalent in later summer or early fall, especially in warmer climates. Multiple cases tend to occur in families. Second attacks are rare.

## Pathophysiology

The mechanism by which the reaction takes place is still speculative. The most popular proposal to explain the pathologic process is that the streptococcal infection is followed by the release of a membranelike material from the specific organism into the circulation. Because it is antigenic, antibodies are formed; an immune-complex reaction occurs after the appropriate period of time. These immune complexes become trapped in the glomerular capillary loop.

The kidney itself appears normal or moderately enlarged, but microscopic examination reveals a diffuse proliferative and exudative process. Glomerular capillary loops are almost obliterated by swelling, and infiltration with polymorphonuclear leukocytes adds to the appearance of increased cellularity. Consequently, the glomeruli appear dense and lobulated. Examination with the electron microscope reveals discrete nodules or "humps" in the basement membrane, which are identified as deposits of immune complexes. These deposits are not evident after approximately 6 weeks.

Endothelial cell proliferation and edema occlude the capillary lumen of affected glomeruli, and the afferent arteriole is probably constricted by vasospasm, both of which significantly reduce the glomerular filtration rate. This occurs without a proportional decrease in renal blood flow and results in a reduced capacity to form filtrate from the glomerular plasma flow. Vascular and tubular changes are mild and nonspecific; therefore tubular function is less severely impaired.

The decreased filtration of plasma results in an excessive accumulation of water and retention of sodium. These cause expanded plasma and interstitial fluid volumes that lead to circulatory congestion and edema. It is unclear whether a decreased glomerular filtration rate, increased capillary permeability, or vascular spasm is responsible for these various manifestations. The cause of the hypertension associated with acute glomerulonephritis is also unexplained. Plasma renin activity is low during the acute phase, but the hypervolemia may be a factor.

## Clinical Manifestations

Typically, affected children are in good health until they experience the antecedent infection. In some instances there is no history of an infection, or it is described only as a mild cold. The onset of nephritis appears after an average latent period of approximately 10 days. Because the child appears well during this time, the association is not recognized by parents.

Initial signs of nephrotic reaction include puffiness of the face, especially around the eyes (periorbital edema); anorexia; and the passage of dark-colored urine. The edema is more prominent in the face in the morning but spreads during the day to involve the extremities and abdomen. The edema is only moderate and may not be appreciated by someone unfamiliar with the child's normal appearance. The urine is cloudy, smoky brown, or what parents describe as resembling tea or cola, and it is severely reduced in volume.

> **NURSING ALERT**
>
> A child who exhibits the following should be evaluated for possible acute glomerulonephritis:
> Periorbital edema, which parents may report is worse in the morning
> Loss of appetite
> Decreased urinary output
> Dark-colored urine revealed by examination
> Antecedent streptococcal infection

The child is pale, irritable, and lethargic, and appears unwell but seldom expresses specific complaints. Older children may complain of headaches, abdominal discomfort, and dysuria. On examination there is usually a mild to moderate elevation in blood pressure compared with normal values for age. Occasionally a child will have an onset with severe symptoms such as seizures from hypertensive encephalopathy, pulmonary and circulatory congestion, or hematuria in the absence of hypertension and edema. Table 30-6 provides a comparison between APSGN and minimal-change nephrotic syndrome.

**Clinical Course.** The acute edematous phase of glomerulonephritis usually persists from 4 to 10 days but may persist for 2 or 3 weeks, during which time the child remains listless, anorexic, and apathetic. The weight fluctuates, the urine remains smoky brown in color, and the blood

**TABLE 30-6** Comparison of poststreptococcal glomerulonephritis and nephrotic syndrome

| Manifestations | Acute Poststreptococcal Glomerulonephritis | Minimal-Change Nephrotic Syndrome |
|---|---|---|
| Streptococcal antibody titers | Elevated | Normal |
| Blood pressure | Elevated | Normal or decreased |
| Edema | Primarily periorbital and peripheral | Generalized, severe |
| Circulatory congestion | Common | Absent |
| Proteinuria | Mild to moderate | Massive |
| Hematuria | Gross or microscopic | Microscopic or none |
| Red blood cell (RBC) casts | Present | Absent |
| Azotemia | Present | Absent |
| Serum potassium levels | Normal or increased | Normal |
| Serum protein levels | Minimal reduction | Markedly decreased |
| Serum lipid levels | Normal | Elevated |
| Peak age at onset (years) | 5-7 | 2-3 |

pressure may suddenly reach dangerously high levels at any time during this phase.

The first sign of improvement is a small increase in urinary output with a corresponding decrease in body weight. With diuresis the child begins to feel better, the appetite improves, and the blood pressure decreases to normal with the reduction of edema. Gross hematuria diminishes, in part because of dilution of the red blood cells in the more dilute urine, but microscopic hematuria may persist for weeks or months. Blood urea nitrogen and creatinine levels decrease during diuresis and usually return to normal. A slight to moderate proteinuria may persist for several weeks.

**Prognosis.** Almost all children correctly diagnosed as having APSGN recover completely, and specific immunity is conferred so that subsequent recurrences are uncommon. Deaths from complications still occur but fortunately are rare. A few of these children may develop chronic disease, but many of these cases are believed to be (probably) different glomerular diseases misdiagnosed as poststreptococcal disease.

**Complications.** The major complications that may develop during the acute phase of glomerulonephritis are hypertensive encephalopathy, acute cardiac decompensation, and acute renal failure. Normally, cerebral blood flow responds to acute arterial hypertension by vasoconstriction. However, acute and severe hypertension may cause this protective autoregulation of cerebral blood flow to fail, leading to hyperperfusion of the brain and cerebral edema. The premonitory signs of encephalopathy are headache, dizziness, abdominal discomfort, and vomiting. If the condition progresses there may be transient loss of vision or hemiparesis, disorientation, and generalized tonic-clonic seizures.

Cardiac decompensation during the acute edematous phase of nephritis is caused by hypervolemia and not by cardiac failure. However, signs of circulatory congestion are evident. The heart is enlarged, and increased pulmonary vascular markings are evident on roentgenographic examination. Increased pulmonary capillary permeability is also believed to be an important factor in the development of pulmonary edema.

Acute renal failure with persistent oliguria or anuria is an uncommon complication but one that requires an appropriate treatment regimen.

### Diagnostic Evaluation

Urinalysis during the acute phase characteristically shows hematuria, proteinuria, and increased specific gravity. The specific gravity is moderately elevated and seldom exceeds 1.020. Proteinuria generally parallels the hematuria, and the content usually shows 3+ or 4+ but is not the massive proteinuria seen in nephrotic syndrome. Gross discoloration of urine reflects its red blood cell and hemoglobin content. Microscopic examination of the sediment shows many red blood cells, leukocytes, epithelial cells, and granular and red blood cell casts. Bacteria are not seen, and urine cultures are negative.

Unless the disease has progressed to renal failure, the blood examination reveals normal electrolyte (sodium, potassium, and chloride ions) and carbon dioxide levels. Azotemia resulting from impaired glomerular filtration is reflected in elevated blood urea nitrogen and creatinine levels in at least 50% of cases. When proteinuria is heavy, there may be changes associated with nephrotic syndrome (i.e., transient hypoproteinemia and hyperlipidemia).

Cultures of the pharynx are positive for streptococci in only a few cases, and the numbers are not significantly greater than the normal carrier incidence in many communities. Positive cultures help to establish a diagnosis. Cultures should be obtained from other household members, and persons positive for group A streptococci should receive a course of antistreptococcal therapy.

Serologic tests are necessary for diagnosis. Antibody responses to the extracellular products of the streptococci provide indirect evidence of previous streptococcal infection. These include antistreptolysin O (ASO), antistreptokinase (ASKase), antihyaluronidase (AHase), antideoxyribonuclease-B (ADNase-B), and antinicotyladenine dinucleotidase (ANADase). The ASO titer is the most familiar and readily available test for streptococcal antibodies. ASO appears in the serum approximately 10 days after the initial infection; however, there is no correlation between the degree of elevation and the severity or prognosis of the glomerulonephritis. It is a useful diagnostic tool when nephritis follows a pharyngeal infection but is of less value after pyoderma. An ASO titer of 250 Todd units or higher is of diagnostic significance, as is a rising titer in two samples taken 1 week apart. More consistent and reliable antibody tests following streptococcal skin infections are elevated AHase and ADNase-B titers.

Of more importance for clinical serologic diagnosis is measurement of the serum complement level (C3). Serum C3 level is decreased initially but returns to normal 8 to 10 weeks after onset of the glomerulonephritis.

Other studies include a chest x-ray examination, which shows characteristic generalized cardiac enlargement, pulmonary congestion, and pleural effusion during the edematous phase of acute disease. Renal biopsy for diagnostic purposes is seldom required but may be useful in the diagnosis of atypical cases.

## Therapeutic Management

No specific treatment is available for acute glomerulonephritis, but recovery is spontaneous and uneventful in most cases. Management consists of general supportive measures and early recognition and treatment of complications. Children who have normal blood pressure and a satisfactory urinary output can generally be treated at home. Those with substantial edema, hypertension, gross hematuria, or significant oliguria should be hospitalized because of the unpredictability of complications. Short hospitalization is the rule in uncomplicated cases; prolonged hospitalization is required only for children with severely impaired renal function.

**General Measures.** Bed rest is no longer recommended during the acute phase because ambulation does not seem to have an adverse effect on the course of the disease once the gross hematuria, edema, hypertension, and azotemia have abated. Because they are generally listless and experience fatigue and malaise, most children voluntarily restrict their activities during the most active phase of the disease.

**Fluid Balance.** Regular measurement of vital signs, body weight, and intake and output is essential in order to monitor the progress of the disease and to detect complications that may appear at any time during the course of the disease. A record of daily weight is the most useful means to assess fluid balance and should be kept for children treated at home and for those who are hospitalized. Sodium and water restriction is useful when the output is significantly reduced (less than 2 to 3 dl/24 hr). In these children the water allowed is equivalent to the calculated insensible loss plus the volume of urine excreted.

Diuretics are of limited value when severe renal failure is present, because very little sodium reaches the distal tubules as a result of the reduced filtration rate. However, when renal failure is not severe, diuretic therapy (usually furosemide) is helpful if significant edema and fluid overload are present. Rarely, children with acute glomerulonephritis develop acute renal failure with oliguria that significantly alters the fluid and electrolyte balance. These children require careful management that may include peritoneal dialysis or hemodialysis.

Loss of glomerular filtration may produce electrolyte imbalances in children with severe forms of APSGN, especially hyperkalemia, acidosis, hypocalcemia, and hyperphosphatemia. Management of these electrolyte disturbances is described under acute renal failure.

**Hypertension.** Acute hypertension must be anticipated and identified early. Blood pressure measurements are taken every 4 to 6 hours. Significant but not severe hypertension is controlled with loop diuretics. Other antihypertensive drugs, such as calcium channel blockers, beta blockers, or angiotensin-converting enzyme (ACE) inhibitors, may be needed in severe cases. Seizure activity associated with hypertensive encephalopathy requires anticonvulsant therapy and antihypertensive agents (see Renal Failure, p. 1283, for management of severe hypertension).

**Nutrition.** Dietary restrictions depend on the stage and severity of the disease, especially the extent of edema. A regular diet is permitted in uncomplicated cases, but sodium intake is usually limited (no salt is added to foods). Moderate sodium restriction is usually instituted for children with hypertension or edema. Foods with substantial amounts of potassium are generally restricted during the period of oliguria. Protein restriction is reserved only for children with severe azotemia resulting from prolonged oliguria. The loss of appetite associated with the disease usually limits the protein intake sufficiently.

**Antibiotics.** Antibiotic therapy is indicated only for those children with evidence of persistent streptococcal infections. Antibiotics do not alter the course of the disease but are often recommended to prevent transmission of nephritogenic streptococci to other family members (Behrman, Kliegman, and Jenson, 2000). Authorities are divided in the use of prophylactic antimicrobials for other family members.

## Nursing Considerations

Nursing care of the child with glomerulonephritis involves careful assessment of the disease status, with regular monitoring of vital signs (including frequent measurement of blood pressure), fluid balance, and behavior. Vital signs provide clues to the severity of the disease and early signs of complications. They are carefully measured, and any abnormalities are reported and recorded. The volume and character of urine are noted, and the child is weighed daily. Assessment of the child's appearance for signs of cerebral complications is an important nursing function because the severity of the acute phase is variable and unpredictable. The child with edema, hypertension, and gross hematuria may be subject to complications, and anticipatory preparations such as seizure precautions and IV access are included in the nursing care plan.

For most children a regular diet is allowed but should contain no added salt. Foods high in sodium and salted treats are eliminated, and parents and friends should be advised not to bring items such as potato chips or pretzels. However, the total amount of salt ingested is usually less than prescribed because of poor appetite. Fluid restriction, if prescribed, is more difficult; the amount permitted should be evenly divided throughout the waking hours and served in small cups to give the illusion of larger servings. Meal preparation and service require special attention because the child has a poor appetite and is indifferent to meals during the acute phase. Again, collaboration with parents and the dietitian and special consideration for food preferences will facilitate meal planning.

During the acute phase children are generally quite content to lie in bed. As they begin to feel better and their symptoms subside, they will want to be up and about. Activities should be planned to allow for frequent rest periods and avoidance of fatigue.

Children with mild edema and no hypertension, as well as convalescent children being treated at home, need follow-up care. Parents are instructed regarding general measures, including activity, diet, and prevention of infection. Strenuous activity is usually restricted until there is no evidence of proteinuria or macroscopic hematuria.

Health supervision is continued with weekly, followed by monthly, visits for evaluation and urinalysis. Parent education and support in preparation for discharge and home care include education in home management and the need for follow-up care and health supervision.

## Chronic or Progressive Glomerulonephritis

The majority of cases of renal glomerular disease are acute glomerulonephritis, minimal-change nephrotic syndrome, and glomerulonephritis associated with systemic diseases. These pose relatively few problems of diagnosis, and their natural course is fairly predictable. A few cases present a prolonged course and a poor ultimate prognosis. They are a rather heterogeneous group and are defined by correlating the clinical manifestations, pathologic conditions, and natural course of the individual diseases.

*Chronic glomerulonephritis (CGN)* describes a variety of different disease processes that may be distinguished from each other by renal biopsy. These include membranoproliferative glomerulonephritis, membranous glomerulonephritis, focal segmental glomerulosclerosis, and IgA nephropathy. *Rapidly progressive glomerulonephritis* is used to describe an acute illness with severe, acute onset that causes rapidly progressive deterioration of renal function in weeks to months. Renal biopsy of these patients shows a variety of diseases with the common feature of greater than 50% glomerular crescents found in the biopsy section.

### Pathophysiology

In most cases of CGN, immunologic mechanisms can be implicated either through direct attack on the kidney or secondary to the accumulation of immune complexes in the glomerular filter or fibrin deposition from previously damaged glomeruli. Either can contribute to further glomerular damage and can initiate chronic changes in the glomerular structure. In many cases there is no history of an attack of acute glomerular disease. In other cases it may represent one of a succession of exacerbations of a preexisting disease. CGN that is not associated with other diseases may go undetected for years and be relatively asymptomatic until kidney destruction produces marked reduction in renal function. Consequently, the disease is more common in adolescents than in younger children. Renal insufficiency with all its manifestations occurs as the ultimate event.

### Clinical Manifestations

The clinical manifestations and laboratory findings reflect deteriorating renal function. Nephrotic syndrome often develops. Hypertension, edema, proteinuria, cardiac failure, dyspnea, osteodystrophy, and anemia are common manifestations of progressive disease.

### Diagnostic Evaluation

Laboratory findings may include proteinuria, with casts and red and white blood cells. Failing renal function is evidenced by elevated blood urea nitrogen, creatinine, and uric acid levels. Electrolyte alterations include metabolic acidosis, elevated potassium, elevated phosphorus, and decreased calcium levels. The renal insufficiency may extend from 5 to 15 years and even longer, or rapid deterioration may progress to end-stage renal disease.

### Therapeutic Management

Early in the course of the disease, treatment is appropriate to the underlying disease and is largely symptomatic in most cases. Efforts are directed toward providing optimum conditions for the child's physical, psychologic, and social development. As few restrictions as feasible are imposed, and the child is allowed to live as normal a life as possible for as long as possible. Some forms of CGN are treated with corticosteroids or cytotoxic agents. Marked hypertension is controlled with antihypertensive agents, and anemia may require recombinant erythropoietin and iron supplements. Ultimately, dialysis and transplantation may be needed to restore relatively good health; however, these alternatives are reserved until renal failure is far advanced (see Chronic Renal Failure, p. 1287, for more detailed management of specific problems). Children with rapidly progressive glomerulonephritis are usually referred to a center specializing in renal disease.

### Nursing Considerations

The problems of CGN and those encountered in chronic renal insufficiency from any cause are discussed in association with chronic renal failure.

## Nephrotic Syndrome

Nephrotic syndrome is the most common presentation of glomerular injury in children. It is defined as massive proteinuria, hypoalbuminemia, hyperlipemia, and edema, but the disorder is a clinical manifestation of a large number of distinct glomerular disorders in which increased glomerular permeability to plasma protein results in massive urinary protein loss. Following a description of the three major forms of nephrotic syndrome, the remainder of the discussion is devoted to minimal-change disease.

### Types of Nephrotic Syndrome

Nephrotic syndrome can be classified as primary, when the syndrome is restricted to glomerular injury, or secondary, when it develops as part of a systemic illness. Although it may have several different histologic variations, the most common form of the primary disease is minimal-change nephrotic syndrome. A congenital form is also recognized.

**Minimal-Change Nephrotic Syndrome (MCNS).** Approximately 80% of cases of nephrotic syndrome in children result from MCNS. MCNS can present at any age but is predominantly a disease of the preschool child. The disease is rare in children younger than 6 months of age, uncommon in infants younger than 1 year of age, and unusual after the age of 8. The incidence of the disease in North America is approximately 2:100,000 children per year, and males outnumber females 2:1. In adolescence the ratio is 1:1.

The cause of MCNS (also known as idiopathic nephrosis, "minimal-lesion" nephrosis, nil disease, childhood nephrosis, lipoid nephrosis, or uncomplicated nephrosis) remains obscure. A nonspecific illness, usually a viral upper respiratory tract infection, often precedes the manifestations by 4 to 8 days but is considered to be a precipitating factor rather than a cause.

**Secondary Nephrotic Syndrome.** Nephrotic syndrome may occur after or in association with glomerular damage of known or presumed etiology. Prominent among causes of glomerular damage is acute or chronic glomerulonephritis. Less commonly, secondary nephrotic syndrome occurs during the course of collagen vascular diseases (such as disseminated lupus erythematosus and anaphylactoid purpura) or as a result of toxicity to drugs (such as trimethadione and heavy metals), stings, or venom. Nephrotic syndrome is the major presenting symptom of renal disease in pediatric patients with acquired immunodeficiency syndrome (AIDS). Diverse, rare causes are sickle cell disease, hepatitis, malaria, cyanotic heart disease, tuberculosis, infected ventriculojugular shunts, renal vein thrombosis, or malignancies.

**Congenital Nephrotic Syndrome.** The hereditary form of nephrotic syndrome is caused by a recessive gene on an autosome. Infants who have nephrotic syndrome are small for gestational age, and proteinuria and edema are manifested early. The disease does not respond to the usual therapy, and death in the first year or two of life is the rule if the infant does not receive dialysis or a successful renal transplant.

## Pathophysiology

The pathogenesis of MCNS is not understood. There may be a metabolic, biochemical, or physiochemical disturbance in the basement membrane of the glomeruli that leads to increased permeability to protein, but the causes and mechanisms are only speculative.

The glomerular membrane, which is normally impermeable to albumin and other large proteins, becomes permeable to proteins, especially albumin, which leak through the membrane and are lost in urine *(hyperalbuminuria)*. This reduces the serum albumin level *(hypoalbuminemia)*, which decreases the colloidal osmotic pressure in the capillaries. As a result, the hydrostatic pressure exceeds the pull of the colloidal osmotic pressure, and fluid accumulates in the interstitial spaces and body cavities, particularly the abdomi-

nal cavity *(ascites)*. The shift of fluid from the plasma to the interstitial spaces reduces the vascular fluid volume *(hypovolemia)*, which in turn stimulates the renin-angiotensin system and the secretion of antidiuretic hormone and aldosterone. Tubular reabsorption of sodium and water is increased in an attempt to increase intravascular volume. The elevation of serum cholesterol, phospholipids, and triglycerides is unexplained. The sequence of events in nephrotic syndrome is diagrammed in Fig. 30-4.

## Clinical Manifestations

A previously well child begins to gain weight, which progresses insidiously over a period of days or weeks. Puffiness of the face, especially around the eyes, is apparent on arising in the morning but subsides during the day, when swelling of the abdomen and lower extremities is more prominent. The generalized edema develops so slowly that parents may consider it a sign of healthy growth. Although an acute infection may precipitate severe generalized edema *(anasarca)*, the usual course is one of progressive weight gain until either a rapid or a gradual increase in edema prompts the family to seek medical evaluation. Usually present are periorbital edema, abdominal swelling from ascites, and labial or scrotal swelling. Edema of the intestinal mucosa may cause diarrhea, loss of appetite, and poor intestinal absorption. The volume of urine is decreased, and it appears darkly opalescent and frothy.

Extreme skin pallor is often present, and the child has a tendency toward skin breakdown during periods of edema. The child is irritable and may be more easily fatigued or lethargic but does not appear seriously ill. Weight loss from poor appetite and loss of protein is not uncommon, although it is often obscured by edema. Changes in the nails appear as white (Muercke) lines parallel to the lunula, which are caused by prolonged hypoalbuminemia. The blood pressure is usually normal or slightly decreased. The child is more susceptible to infection, especially cellulitis, pneumonia, peritonitis, or sepsis.

> **NURSING ALERT**
>
> A child who exhibits the following should be evaluated for the possibility of nephrotic syndrome:
> Periorbital or ankle edema
> Weight gain over that expected based on previous pattern
> Parent observation that the child's clothes fit tightly
> Decreased urinary output
> Pallor, fatigue

In children with MCNS in rare instances there is significant or persistent hypertension, gross or persistent hematuria, significant or persistent azotemia (presence of increased nitrogenous products in the blood), or depression of serum $\beta 1_c$ globulin.

## Diagnostic Evaluation

The diagnosis of MCNS is made on the basis of the history and clinical manifestations (edema, proteinuria, hypoalbuminemia, and hypercholesterolemia in the absence of hematuria and hypertension) in children between the ages of 2 and 4 years. Massive proteinuria is reflected in urinary

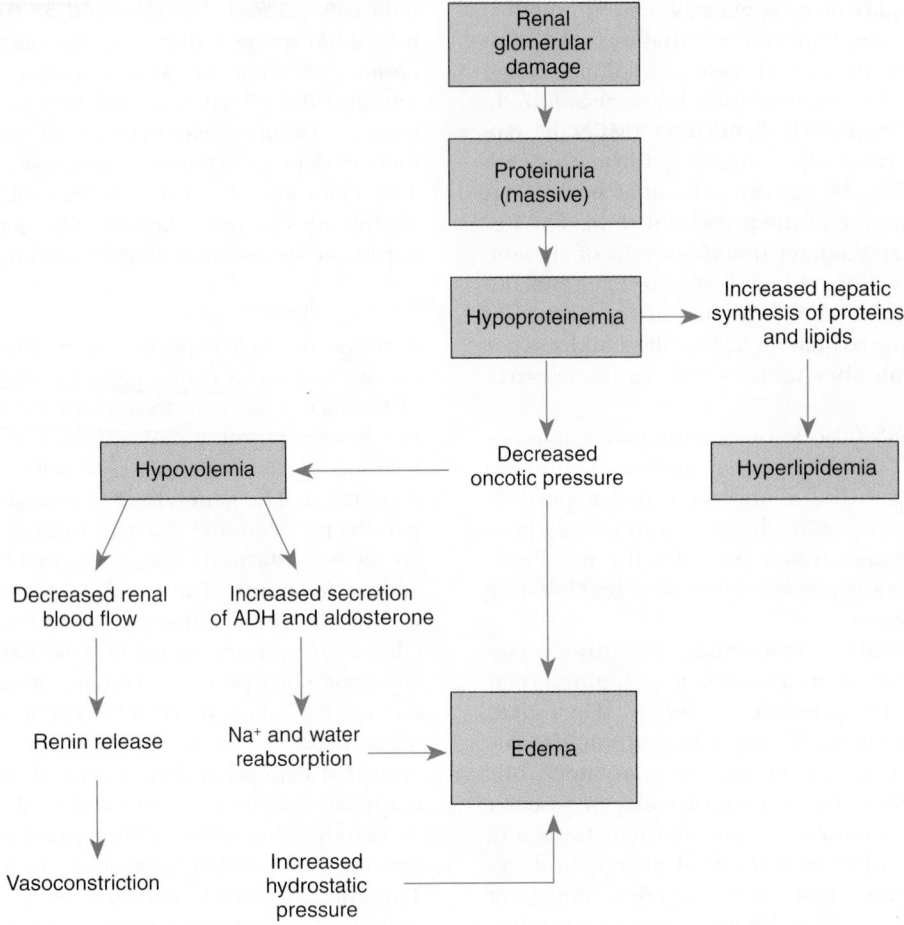

**Fig. 30-4**   Sequence of events in nephrotic syndrome.

excretion of protein that often reaches levels in excess of 2 g/m²/day of body surface, with relatively greater clearance of low–molecular-weight proteins. Hyaline casts from high protein and sluggish flow and oval fat bodies, as well as a few red blood cells, can be found in the urine of most affected children, although there is seldom gross hematuria. Specific gravity is high and proportionate to the amount of protein concentration. If hypovolemia is not significant and the child is well hydrated, the glomerular filtration rate is usually normal.

Total serum protein concentrations are reduced, with the albumin fractions significantly reduced (less than 2 g/dl) and plasma lipids elevated. Serum cholesterol may be as high as 450 to 1500 mg/dl. Hemoglobin and hematocrit are usually normal or elevated, and the platelet count is high (500,000 to 1,000,000) as a result of hemoconcentration. Serum sodium concentration is usually low, approximately 130 to 135 mEq/L.

If renal biopsy is performed, it provides information regarding the glomerular status and type of nephrotic syndrome, the response to drugs, and the probable course of the disease. Under the microscope the foot processes of the basement membrane appear fused. The major focuses in differential diagnosis are to establish the edema as renal in

origin and to distinguish minimum-change nephrotic syndrome from other glomerulopathies with nephrotic syndrome as a manifestation.

### Therapeutic Management

Medical management consists of both general and specific measures. The primary objective is to reduce the excretion of urinary protein and maintain a protein-free urine. Additional objectives include prevention or treatment of acute infection, control of edema, establishment of good nutrition, and readjustment of any disturbed metabolic processes. Children with severe symptoms or whose disease is newly recognized are hospitalized for assessment and observation for evidence of infection, response to therapy, and parental education.

**General Measures.**   General treatment is principally supportive. During the edema phase the child is often placed on bed rest, but activity is not restricted during remission. Children can be remarkably active with no evidence that restriction affects the ultimate outcome. Acute and intercurrent infections are treated with appropriate antibiotics, and efforts are made to eliminate possible infection.

**Diet.**   The child in remission is allowed a regular diet; however, salt is restricted during periods of massive edema—there is no salt added at the table, and foods with very high salt content are excluded. This diet is usually tolerated by the child for a time but should be adjusted to the child's appetite and must not interfere with nutrient intake. Although edema cannot be removed by a low-sodium diet, its rate of increase may be reduced. Water is seldom restricted. A diet generous in protein is logical, but there is no evidence that it is beneficial or alters the outcome of the disease. The presence of azotemia and renal failure is a contraindication for high-protein intake.

**Corticosteroid Therapy.** The response of most affected children to corticosteroids has established these drugs as prime therapeutic agents in the management of nephrotic syndrome. Corticosteroid therapy is begun as soon as the diagnosis has been determined and is administered orally in a dosage of 2 mg/kg of body weight or 60 mg/m²/day in evenly divided doses. Prednisone, the safest and least expensive drug, is the steroid of choice. The drug is continued until the urine is free from protein and remains normal for 10 days to 2 weeks.

The course of the disease is fairly predictable. There is little change during the first few days of therapy. In most patients diuresis occurs as the urinary protein excretion diminishes within 7 to 21 days after the initiation of steroid therapy. Other clinical manifestations stabilize or return to normal shortly thereafter. Almost 95% of patients between 1 and 10 years of age who have satisfactory laboratory measurements of C3 complement and a renal clearance of IgG, as well as no hypertension, hematuria, or renal insufficiency, will have complete resolution of proteinuria with therapy.

If the child has not responded to therapy within 28 days of daily steroid administration, the likelihood of subsequent response diminishes rapidly. When the child is free of proteinuria and edema, the total daily dose of prednisone is usually given for a time as a single dose every 48 hours. The dose is gradually tapered to discontinuation over a variable period, from several weeks to months depending on the medical philosophy. Once a satisfactory response is achieved, steroid therapy is reduced to every other day (q.o.d.). This dosage is less likely to depress pituitary-adrenal function and produces fewer side effects during prolonged therapy. If a tendency to relapse is demonstrated, the number of relapses can be reduced with administration of a low-dose, q.o.d. schedule of prednisone therapy that continues for 6 months to 1 year (provided remission is achieved and successful tapering to low-dose q.o.d. therapy occurs).

Children with MCNS are often described according to their response to corticosteroid therapy (Box 30-4). Children with MCNS typically relapse one to three times per year. Steroid-dependent children tend to have frequent relapses over many years and receive large amounts of steroids, which results in cushingoid features and growth retardation. They also require supportive treatment (diuretics, diet). The prognosis for steroid-unresponsive children is less predictable than for steroid-responsive children.

Children who require frequent courses of steroid therapy are highly susceptible to complications of steroids, such

---

**Box 30-4** ■ ■ □
**Classification of Nephrotic Syndrome According to Steroid Response**

1. **Steroid-sensitive** (20% to 40%)—Respond to a single short course of steroids without evidence of relapse after cessation of therapy
2. **Frequent relapsers** or **steroid-dependent** (60% to 80%)—Respond to steroids and can be tapered off completely; have three or more relapses in a 6- to 12-month period; remit when placed on steroids but tend to relapse on lowered dosage
3. **Steroid-unresponsive** or **steroid-resistant**—Never respond to steroids, or become resistant to steroids at some point during the course of disease

Modified from McEnery PT, Strife CF: Nephrotic syndrome in childhood, *Pediatr Clin North Am* 89:875-894, 1982.

---

as growth retardation, cataracts, obesity, hypertension, gastrointestinal bleeding, bone demineralization, infections, and hyperglycemia. Children who do not respond to steroid therapy, those who have frequent relapses, and those in whom the side effects threaten their growth and general health may be considered for a course of therapy using other immunosuppressant medications.

**Immunosuppressant Therapy.** It is often possible to reduce the relapse rate and induce long-term remission with administration of an oral alkylating agent, usually cyclophosphamide (Cytoxan), in conjunction with prednisone. Both drugs are administered for up to 2 to 3 months, after which cyclophosphamide is discontinued abruptly and the prednisone is decreased by decrements. Chlorambucil has also proved to be effective when given with corticosteroids. The two drugs share many characteristics, and the response to both appears to depend on dose, duration of therapy, age, and duration of the disease.

Significant side effects of cyclophosphamide must be considered and discussed with parents of children for whom this drug is contemplated. Leukopenia must be anticipated, and evidence suggests that cyclophosphamide may cause azoospermia with potential sterility in males treated for more than 2 to 3 months and may cause variable effects on gonadal function in females.

**Diuretics.** One characteristic of the edema of nephrotic syndrome is its usual lack of responsiveness to diuretic agents. However, loop diuretics, usually furosemide in combination with metolazone, are sometimes useful in cases in which edema interferes with respiration or there is hypotension, hyponatremia, or evidence of skin breakdown. In addition, plasma expanders such as salt-poor human albumin may be administered to severely edematous children requiring prompt control; however, they must be administered frequently because the glomeruli are readily permeable to albumin in the acute stage.

**Prognosis.** The prognosis for ultimate recovery in most cases is good. MCNS is a self-limiting disease, and in children who respond to steroid therapy the tendency to relapse decreases with time. With early detection and prompt implementation of therapy to eradicate proteinuria, progressive basement membrane damage is minimized so that renal function is usually normal or near normal when the tendency to exacerbations is past. It is estimated that approximately 80% of affected children have this favorable prognosis, although half the children have relapses even after 5 years, and 20% after 10 years (Warshaw, 1994).

## Nursing Considerations

Daily monitoring of intake and output is an important nursing function. Strict and accurate measurement is essential

## Critical Thinking Exercise

### Nephrotic Syndrome

Reese is an 8-year-old boy with relapsing nephrotic syndrome who has become steroid-dependent. During your initial assessment in the outpatient clinic you identify the following: (1) weight has increased 2 kg in the last 2 weeks; (2) blood pressure is 100/70 mm Hg; (3) mother reports that Reese is not urinating very much, and she does not know how much he has been drinking; (4) while you are measuring Reese's abdominal girth, he guards his abdomen and complains of stomachache; and (5) his temperature is 38° C (100.4° F) orally. You should first do which of the following correct actions?

FIRST, THINK ABOUT IT . . .

• What concepts or ideas are central to your thinking?
• If you accept the conclusions, what are the implications?

1. Examine Reese's abdomen more thoroughly while eliciting a 24-hour recall of illness symptoms from his mother.
2. Elicit a 24-hour recall of food and fluid intake from Reese and his mother together.
3. Obtain a clean-catch urine specimen. Divide the specimen so that you can perform a dipstick analysis immediately and retain the other specimen for possible urinalysis and culture after consultation with the primary health practitioner.
4. Explore the mother's understanding of Reese's illness and its relationship to his current condition to begin outlining your teaching plan for this family.

*The best response is one. One of the complications of severe nephrotic syndrome is peritonitis, which can occur secondary to migration of intestinal bacteria across the bowel wall and into the protein-rich acidic fluid. Reese's mother has already said that she does not know what he has been drinking. Therefore the idea may occur to you that your only possibility of assessing his intake is to elicit the recall while they are together. Although his weight gain and reduced urine output are major concerns, they are secondary to peritonitis. (It should be recognized that children on strict fluid restrictions are prone to obtain fluids from unauthorized sources.) Obtaining a urine specimen for dipstick analysis is part of the initial assessment for Reese. Also, you may initially conclude that the fever and abdominal pain are the first priority. As with option three, the fourth choice must be addressed, along with evaluation of the current stress level in the home, after the implications of fever and pain have been addressed.*

but may be difficult in very young children, but it can be done by methods such as weighing diapers. Other methods of monitoring progress include examination of the urine for albumin, daily weight, and measurement of abdominal girth. Assessment of edema such as increased or decreased swelling around the eyes and dependent areas, the degree of pitting (if noted), and the color and texture of the skin are part of nursing care. Vital signs are monitored to detect any early signs of complications such as shock or an infectious process.

In children hospitalized with MCNS, elevating most edematous parts may be helpful to shift fluid to more comfortable distributions, but diuresis with medications and salt and water restriction to remove edema fluid are the best therapy. Areas that are particularly edematous, such as the scrotum, abdomen, and legs, may require support; skin surfaces should be cleaned and separated with clothing, cotton, or antiseptic powder to prevent intertrigo.

Infection is a constant source of danger to edematous children and those receiving corticosteroid therapy. Because these children are particularly vulnerable to upper respiratory tract infection, they must be protected from contact with infected roommates, family, or visitors. Spontaneous peritonitis can occur secondary to migration of intestinal bacteria across the bowel wall and into the peritoneum. Vital signs are monitored to detect any early signs of an infectious process.

Loss of appetite that accompanies active nephrosis creates a perplexing problem for nurses. During this time the combined efforts of the nurse, dietitian, parents, and child are needed to formulate a nutritionally adequate and attractive diet. Salt and fluids are restricted during the edema phase. Every effort should be made to serve attractive meals with a minimum of fuss, but it usually requires a considerable amount of ingenuity and enticement to get the child to eat. Games, rewards, and special treats often help, but each child is unique, and it may require considerable trial and error to arrive at a successful strategy. Also, the same strategy may not work consistently. (See Feeding the Sick Child, Chapter 27.)

As the edema subsides, children are allowed increased salt and water. Suitable recreational and diversional activities are also an important part of their care. Once the edema fluid has been lost, children resume their usual activities without problems. Irritability and mood swings accompanying the disease process and steroid therapy are not unusual manifestations in these children and create an additional challenge to the nurse and the family.

**Family Support and Home Care.** Many children are treated at home during exacerbations. Parents are taught to detect signs of relapse and to bring the child for treatment at the earliest indications. Home care is preferred unless the edema and proteinuria are severe or the parents for some reason are unable to care for the ill child. Parents are instructed in urine testing for albumin, administration of medications, and general care. Urine testing is usually daily while the child is receiving medicine for nephrotic syndrome, twice a week during remission and when off medication, and when the youngster has any type of childhood illness. Salt is restricted to no additional salt during relapse and steroid therapy, but a regular diet is suitable for the child in remission. Parents are instructed regarding avoiding contact with infected playmates, but the child is permitted to attend school. It is important for parents of children on corticosteroid therapy to be aware of the common side effects of steroid therapy (e.g., rounding of the face, increased appetite, abdominal distention, and hirsutism) and to distinguish some of these from the edema formation of the disease. They should be reassured that the symptoms will disappear gradually after discontinuation of the drug. The child should receive close medical or nursing observation to detect unusual but more serious side effects. (See Critical Thinking Exercise box.)

The prolonged course of the relapsing form of nephrotic syndrome is taxing to both the child and the family. In the worst cases of frequent remissions and exacerbations with periodic disruption of family life by hospitalization a severe strain is placed on the child and the family, both psychologically and financially. Parents of children with frequent relapses poorly responsive to medications need reassurance regarding this characteristic of the course of the disease so they do not become discouraged. At the same time, it is important to impress on them the importance of long-term care to gain their cooperation. A satisfactory response is more likely when relapses are detected and therapy is instituted early, and remissions are prolonged when instructions are carried out faithfully. For example, one child had an exacerbation when his mother reduced the dosage of his drug because it was so expensive.

Social isolation is a concomitant problem for these children. Isolation is related to frequent hospitalization or confinement during relapse, the risk of infection that may precipitate an exacerbation, lack of energy, and the child's reluctance to face friends at home or school because of the changes in appearance resulting from the disease or the medication. Both parents and child need someone to listen to their complaints, to assist them in coping with both short-term and long-term problems associated with the disease, and to find solutions to their problems. Continuous support of the child and family is one of the major nursing considerations. (See Nursing Care Plan: The Child with Nephrotic Syndrome.*)

## RENAL TUBULAR DISORDERS

Disorders of renal tubular function include a variety of conditions in which there are one or more abnormalities in specific mechanisms of tubular transport or reabsorption, whereas initially glomerular function is normal or comparatively less impaired. Eventually there may be more widespread kidney destruction with renal failure. In some cases the dysfunction has little, if any, effect on renal function. These disorders may be permanent or transient and may originate as primary defects or arise as a secondary effect of

metabolic disease or exogenous toxins. Renal tubular disorders may be congenital (usually displaying characteristic patterns of genetic transmission), appear without evidence of hereditary transmission, or be acquired as a result of known or unknown causes.

Unlike the classic manifestations of glomerular diseases, edema and hypertension are absent and the blood urea nitrogen level and routine urinalysis are usually normal. Tubular proteinuria may be demonstrated. Manifestations of tubular disorders are primarily metabolic disturbances or deficiencies, such as failure to thrive, metabolic bone disease, or persistent acidosis. The variety of these disorders is extensive, and the incidence is rare.

### Tubular Function

The function of the proximal tubules is the reabsorption of substances from the glomerular filtrate, including sodium, potassium, chloride, bicarbonate, glucose, phosphate, and amino acids. A number of disorders feature impairment of reabsorption of one or more filtrate constituents, and most involve defects in the transport mechanisms for these substances. Impaired tubular reabsorption of any specific substance causes that substance to appear in the urine, sometimes with reduced levels in the blood. Examples include bicarbonate and phosphate.

The primary functions of the distal renal tubules are acidification of urine, potassium secretion, and the selective and differential reabsorption of sodium, chloride, and water, which determines the final urinary concentration. Because the contribution of the distal tubule to urine composition depends in part on the volume and composition of the filtrate from the proximal tubule, the net contribution of the distal tubule is related to proximal tubular function and glomerular filtration.

### Renal Tubular Acidosis

Renal tubular acidosis is a syndrome of sustained metabolic acidosis in which there is impaired reabsorption of bicarbonate or excretion of net hydrogen ion but in which glomerular function is normal or comparatively less impaired. On the basis of underlying pathophysiology, renal tubular acidosis is divided into *proximal renal tubular acidosis,* which results from a defect in bicarbonate absorption, and *distal renal tubular acidosis,* which results from inability to establish an adequate gradient of pH between blood and tubular fluid.

#### Proximal Tubular Acidosis (Type II)

Proximal tubular acidosis is caused by impaired bicarbonate reabsorption in the proximal tubule. It may occur as an isolated defect (primary); however, more often it appears in association with other proximal tubular disorders (secondary). As a result of a depressed renal threshold, bicarbonate reabsorption in the proximal tubule is incomplete, causing the plasma concentration of bicarbonate to stabilize at a lower level than normal. This results in a hyperchloremic metabolic acidosis. There is no impairment of

*In Wong DL, Hess CS: *Wong and Whaley's clinical manual of pediatric nursing,* ed 5, St Louis, 2000, Mosby.

distal tubular integrity or, in most cases, of the distal acidifying mechanism.

A more complex abnormality in the proximal tubules is the *Fanconi syndrome,* in which transport mechanisms are damaged by the accumulation of toxic metabolites or the tubular epithelium is damaged by heavy metals such as lead, cadmium, or platinum.

Fanconi syndrome can be part of a number of hereditary diseases, be acquired, or be idiopathic, in which the cause is not identifiable. The major clinical manifestation and presenting symptom of Fanconi syndrome is growth failure. Tachypnea from hyperchloremic metabolic acidosis is also evident. Dehydration, vomiting, episodic fever, nephrolithiasis secondary to hypercalciuria, muscle weakness or paralysis as a result of hypokalemia, and episodes of severe, life-threatening acidemia (sometimes triggered by a concurrent infection) may also be seen. Complications are rare. The disorder appears to be transient and resolves spontaneously in time.

## Distal Tubular Acidosis (Type I)

Distal tubular acidosis is caused by the inability of the kidney to establish a normal pH gradient between tubular cells and tubular contents. Its most characteristic feature is the inability to produce a urinary pH below 6.0 despite the presence of severe metabolic acidosis.

Distal renal tubular acidosis may occur as a primary, isolated defect or in association with other diseases or disorders. Most secondary causes are rare. The primary disorder is usually considered to be a hereditary defect with a variable degree of expression and a greater penetrance in females. After the age of 2 years the child usually has growth failure, although there is often a history of vomiting, polyuria, dehydration, anorexia, and failure to thrive. Evidence of bone demineralization may be present, along with the occasional formation of urinary calculi (urolithiasis) in older children.

The inability to secrete hydrogen ions causes an accumulation of the ion in the body, which soon depletes the available hydrogen buffer and produces a sustained acidosis. Acidosis slows normal somatic growth, and demineralization of bone occurs as bone salts are mobilized to buffer the excessive hydrogen ions. Increased serum levels of both calcium and phosphorus contribute to the development of stones within the renal system. Both sodium and potassium are secreted in larger amounts. Serum potassium levels are depleted as the distal tubules excrete large amounts of potassium ions in an attempt to conserve sodium because hydrogen ions are unable to participate in the exchange. Hyponatremia stimulates increased aldosterone secretion, which further aggravates the hypokalemia. With the depletion of bicarbonate ions, more chloride is reabsorbed in the proximal tubule to create a hyperchloremia.

**Prognosis.** The primary disorder is usually permanent. However, secondary effects on growth and stone formation can be avoided with early diagnosis and therapy. When the disorder occurs as a secondary complication and renal damage is prevented, the prognosis is good.

## Therapeutic Management

Treatment of both proximal and distal disorders consists of the administration of sufficient bicarbonate or citrate to balance metabolically produced hydrogen ions, to maintain the plasma bicarbonate level within normal range, and to correct associated electrolyte disorders, especially hypokalemia. Proximal disorders require large volumes of bicarbonate to compensate for urinary losses; in distal disorders the alkali required to maintain a normal plasma concentration is low. Most authorities favor a mixture of sodium and potassium bicarbonate (or citrate) in order to prevent deficiencies of either cation. The citrate solutions (Bicitra, Polycitra, or Shohl solution) are usually more easily tolerated than bicarbonate solutions. Shohl solution is very effective but has the disadvantage of requiring preparation by a pharmacist.

## Nursing Considerations

Nursing goals include recognizing the possibility of renal tubular acidosis in children who fail to thrive or who display other symptoms suggestive of the disorders and referring these children for medical evaluation. Helping parents understand the importance of adhering to the medication plan as a long-term goal is essential. (See Compliance, Chapter 27, and Administration of Medication, Chapter 27.) Children who must continue the medication indefinitely are taught the importance of taking the medications as soon as they are old enough to assume responsibility for their own care.

# Nephrogenic Diabetes Insipidus (NDI)

NDI is the major disorder associated with a defect in the ability to concentrate urine. In this disorder the distal tubules and collecting ducts are insensitive to the action of antidiuretic hormone or its exogenous counterpart, vasopressin. The nature of the defect is unknown but occurs primarily in males, which supports X-linked recessive inheritance. The disease is more variable in female carriers of the defective gene, who may exhibit only a mild defect in urine-concentrating ability. The differential diagnosis for NDI should include chronic obstructive renal disorders, sickle cell disease, renal tuberculosis, and other renal disorders, which may cause high urinary output with failure of the kidney to respond to vasopressin.

## Clinical Manifestations

NDI is manifested in the newborn period by vomiting, unexplained fever, failure to thrive, and severe recurrent dehydration with hypernatremia. The passage of copious amounts of dilute urine, which produces severe dehydration and hypoelectrolytemia, is a serious threat to life during this period and may be responsible for the high incidence of mental and motor retardation found in affected persons. Growth retardation is probably related to diminished food intake and poor general health because of uncontrolled polydipsia. Diagnosis is suspected on the basis of the patient and family history and confirmed by a urine osmolality value consistently below that of plasma. Lack of response to vasopressin administration rules out other causes.

## Therapeutic Management

Therapy involves provision of adequate volumes of water to compensate for urinary losses. As a result of an insatiable thirst, most of the child's time is spent drinking and voiding, with little time for activity and stimulation. These children may go to great lengths to satisfy their thirst. A low-sodium/low-solute diet and the use of chlorothiazide or ethacrynic acid diuretics to increase the reabsorption of sodium and water in the proximal tubule help to reduce the amount of tubular fluid delivered to the distal tubules and to diminish the volume of water excreted. Urinary output has been reported to be reduced when nonsteroidal antiinflammatory drugs are administered in conjunction with chlorothiazide (Behrman, Kliegman, and Jenson, 2000). Supplemental potassium may be required to prevent hypokalemia as a result of thiazide therapy. Normal growth can be expected and a normal life span anticipated if the disease is recognized early and treatment is instituted and maintained.

## Nursing Considerations

Nursing goals for children and families with NDI are to recognize signs of the disorder early and assist them in coping with the long-term inconvenience of the continual thirst and elimination problems. Families need to be taught to administer medications and help with diet planning for those on sodium restriction and needing supplemental potassium. The problem of ensuring adequate hydration is lifelong, and families need to adapt to away-from-home fluid needs and avoid activities that contribute to dehydration when fluids may not be available. Genetic counseling is recommended.

# MISCELLANEOUS RENAL DISORDERS
## Hemolytic Uremic Syndrome (HUS)

HUS is an acute renal disease characterized by a triad of manifestations: acute renal failure, hemolytic anemia, and thrombocytopenia. HUS occurs primarily in infants and small children between the ages of 6 months and 3 years. It has been recognized predominantly in whites and, although it occurs worldwide, is more prevalent in South Africa, Argentina, and the west coasts of North and South America. HUS represents one of the main causes of acute renal failure in early childhood (Berhman, Kliegman, and Jenson, 2000).

## Etiology

In the majority of cases of HUS no causative agents have been identified, although recent theories implicate genetic factors, prostacyclin deficiency, neuraminidase and agglutination, endotoxins (especially *Shigella* endotoxin), antithrombin-III deficiency, deficiency of antioxidants, and reduced platelet aggregation. The appearance of the disease

has been associated with *Rickettsia;* viruses such as coxsackievirus, echovirus, and adenovirus; *E. coli;* pneumococci; *Shigella;* and *Salmonella* and may represent an unusual response to these infections. Multiple cases of HUS caused by enteric infection of the *E. coli* O157:H7 serotype have been traced to undercooked meat, especially ground beef, unpasteurized apple juice, alfalfa sprouts, and public pools (Centers for Disease Control and Prevention, 1997; Cieslak and others, 1997).

The disease usually follows an acute gastrointestinal or upper respiratory tract infection and tends to occur in scattered outbreaks in small geographic areas. HUS is clinically and pathologically similar to thrombocytopenic purpura, except for the hypertension associated with HUS. Some authorities have speculated that thrombocytopenic purpura may be the adult version of the HUS of infancy and early childhood.

## Pathophysiology

The primary site of injury appears to be the endothelial lining of the small glomerular arterioles, but other organs and tissues may be involved (e.g., the liver, brain, heart, pancreatic islet cells, and muscles). The endothelium becomes swollen and occluded with the deposition of platelets and fibrin clots (intravascular coagulation). Red blood cells are damaged as they move through the partially occluded blood vessels. These fragmented red blood cells are removed by the spleen, causing acute hemolytic anemia. Fibrinolytic action on the precipitated fibrin causes these fibrin-split products to appear in the serum and urine. The characteristic thrombocytopenia is produced by the platelet aggregation within damaged blood vessels or the damage and removal of platelets.

## Clinical Manifestations

The disease is preceded by a prodromal period during which there is an episode of diarrhea and vomiting. Less often the illness is an upper respiratory tract infection or, occasionally, varicella, measles, or a urinary tract infection.

The hemolytic process persists for several days to 2 weeks. During this time the child is anorectic, irritable, and lethargic. There is marked and rapid onset of pallor accompanied by hemorrhagic manifestations such as bruising, purpura, or rectal bleeding. Severely affected patients are anuric and often hypertensive. Seizures and stupor suggest central nervous system involvement, and there may be signs of acute heart failure. Mild cases demonstrate anemia, thrombocytopenia, and azotemia; urinary output may be reduced or increased.

In children infected with *E. coli* O157:H7, risk factors for developing HUS include the use of antimotility drugs, an age under 5 years, vomiting, and an elevated white blood cell count (Bell and others, 1997).

## Diagnostic Evaluation

The triad of anemia, thrombocytopenia, and renal failure is sufficient for diagnosis. Renal involvement is evidenced by proteinuria, hematuria, and the presence of urinary casts;

blood urea nitrogen and serum creatinine levels are elevated. A low hemoglobin and hematocrit and a high reticulocyte count confirm the hemolytic nature of the anemia.

### Therapeutic Management

In general, treatment is directed toward control of the complications and hematologic manifestations of renal failure. The initial supportive measures for most children are those used in managing renal failure—fluid replacement (calculated with great care), treatment of hypertension, and correction of acidosis and electrolyte disorders. The most consistently effective treatment is early hemodialysis, peritoneal dialysis, or continuous hemofiltration, which is instituted in any child who has been anuric for 24 hours or who demonstrates oliguria with uremia or hypertension and seizures. Blood transfusions with fresh, washed packed cells are administered for severe anemia but are used with caution to prevent circulatory overload from added volume.

Once vomiting and diarrhea have resolved, the child is restarted on enteral nutrition. Sometimes parenteral nutrition is required for children with severe, persistent colitis and for those in whom tissue catabolism is marked. There is no substantial evidence that heparin, corticosteroids, or fibrinolytic agents are beneficial, and in some instances they may aggravate the condition. The usefulness of plasma infusion for treatment of HUS is currently being studied; it may be useful in selected cases.

**Prognosis.** With prompt treatment the recovery rate is approximately 95%, but residual renal impairment ranges from 10% to 50% in various areas. Death is usually caused by residual renal impairment or central nervous system injury.

### Nursing Considerations

Nursing care is the same as that provided in acute renal failure and, for children with continued impairment, includes management of chronic disease. Because of the sudden and life-threatening nature of the disorder in a previously well child, parents are often ill prepared for the impact of hospitalization and treatment. Therefore support and understanding are especially important aspects of care.

> **NURSING ALERT**
>
> To prevent infection from contaminated meat, the internal temperature of the food, such as hamburger, should be at least 165° F. Cooking the ground beef until no pink color is seen may not be sufficient to kill the bacteria. Therefore a meat thermometer is needed to ensure a safe product. Discourage parents from giving children unpasteurized apple juice and unwashed raw vegetables. Also discourage the use of antimotility drugs for diarrhea.

## Familial Nephritis (Alport Syndrome)

The syndrome of chronic hereditary glomerulopathy consists of hematuria, high-frequency sensorineural deafness, ocular disorders, and chronic renal failure. The disease appears to be inherited as an autosomal-dominant trait, which suggests a possible X-linked dominant trait, although rare male-to-male transmission does occur. Alport syndrome is uncommon but not rare and accounts for a significant percentage of persistent glomerular disease in childhood.

The clinical manifestations are indistinguishable from mild acute nephritis. Initial symptoms include hematuria, proteinuria, malaise, and mild edema. Onset of gross hematuria may be associated with an acute respiratory infection. The average age of onset is 6 years, but the condition may be noted in infancy. It begins slowly and progresses until uncontrollable renal failure develops in adolescence or early adulthood. There is usually a positive family history. Most untreated boys develop severe symptoms, whereas affected girls generally have a milder disease and a normal life expectancy.

Treatment is symptomatic and supportive. Dialysis and renal transplantation are ultimate therapeutic measures for end-stage renal disease. Hearing loss and ocular disorders should receive appropriate attention, and families should be counseled regarding the genetic implications of the disease.

## Unexplained Proteinuria

Often apparently healthy children with no suggestion of renal disease demonstrate proteinuria on routine urinalysis. The percentage of children with unexplained proteinuria ranges from 1% at 6 years of age to 11% at puberty, reaching a maximum prevalence at age 13 in girls and age 16 in boys.

Unexplained proteinuria can be categorized as (1) transient (inconstant), (2) persistent, or (3) orthostatic, or postural. *Transient proteinuria* is a common finding with no known cause but sometimes increases with febrile illness, exercise, cold, or emotions.

*Persistent proteinuria* usually signifies renal disease. *Orthostatic proteinuria* is seen in 3% to 5% of adolescents and young adults and, although proteinuria is evident in both the recumbent and the erect position, it is quantitatively and qualitatively greater in the erect position. The cause is unknown, but minor glomerular changes occur in many instances. The condition is benign and generally resolves over a period of time.

In cases of unexplained proteinuria, it is important to confirm or exclude renal disease with appropriate diagnostic tests. Repeated examination for proteinuria, an orthostatic test, urine culture, and (if proteinuria is persistent) more definitive tests—including 24-hour protein excretion, renal ultrasound, and renal scan—are indicated.

## Renal Trauma

Serious injuries of the genitourinary tract are not uncommon in the pediatric age-group, with a peak incidence between ages 10 and 20 years. The kidneys are among the organs most often injured in children despite their relatively protected location. However, the kidneys in children are more mobile than they are in adults, and the outer borders are less well protected. They are separated from the skin surface by only 2 to 3 cm (¾ to 1¼ inches) in young children. Most injuries are of the nonpenetrating or "blunt" type and usually involve falls, athletic injuries, and motor vehicle accidents. Penetrating trauma (e.g., gunshot or stab wound) is much less common in children. In many children are found preexisting renal abnormalities, particularly congenital anomalies associated with mild to moderate hydronephrosis, which were unrecognized before the injury.

Renal injury can be suspected in children who complain of flank pain, and often there are abrasions or contusions on the overlying skin. Hematuria is consistently present, but the amount of blood in the urine is not a reliable indicator of the seriousness of the injury. Many relatively insignificant injuries are associated with grossly bloody urine, whereas some of the most severe injuries are found in children with only microscopic hematuria (Box 30-5).

Renal rupture involves the actual splitting open of the kidney capsule, causing extravasation of blood or a mixture of blood and urine into the surrounding retroperitoneal space. Renal vascular injury, although unusual, requires immediate recognition and surgical intervention. Because the volume-per-minute blood flow through the kidney is greater (25% of cardiac output) than to any other abdominal organ, *injury to the kidney may result in a rapid loss of blood.*

In active children there may or may not be a history of unusual trauma. Abdominal or flank pain and tenderness are caused by bleeding around the kidney and may or may not be associated with fever. Clots passing down the ureter may cause pain similar to that of renal colic, and dysuria is common. Patients with more severe injuries may complain of nausea or abdominal pain. There may be a palpable abdominal mass caused by loss of blood or urine into the retroperitoneum. The fibrous capsule enclosing the kidney prevents expansion of a hematoma; therefore exsanguination and shock are seldom observed, even in severe renal trauma.

Diagnosis is made on the basis of intravenous pyelography, angiography, or retrograde pyelography. Unsuspected hydronephrosis often is first detected as a result of traumatic injury.

### Therapeutic Management

Severe injury requires close observation in the hospital intensive care unit, as well as blood replacement if there is severe internal or external bleeding. In most cases bleeding subsides spontaneously. Surgical exploration is indicated if there are multiple injuries, extravasation of blood around the kidneys, or disruption of the major vessels or the collecting system. Children with less severe injuries, such as contusions only, are placed on bed rest. They should remain on bed rest for 3 days after cessation of gross bleeding, because the substance released from injured renal tissue (urinary urokinase) has strongly fibrinolytic properties that may precipitate serious bleeding. The prognosis depends on the nature and extent of the injury.

### Nursing Considerations

Nursing management is directed toward recognizing and assisting in the diagnosis of renal injury. Care of both the child and the family is primarily supportive. All the concepts related to emergency hospitalization and care are implemented. (See Chapter 26.) Postsurgical care, if indicated, is the same as for any other surgical patient.

## RENAL FAILURE

Renal failure is the inability of the kidneys to excrete waste material, concentrate urine, and conserve electrolytes. The disorder can be acute or chronic and affects most of the systems in the body. Two terms that are often used in relation to renal failure need some clarification: *azotemia* is the accumulation of nitrogenous waste within the blood, whereas *uremia* is a more advanced condition in which retention of nitrogenous products produces toxic symptoms. Azotemia is not life-threatening, whereas uremia is a serious condition that often involves other body systems.

### Acute Renal Failure (ARF)

ARF is said to exist when the kidneys suddenly are unable to regulate the volume and composition of urine appropriately in response to food and fluid intake and the needs of the organism. The principal feature is oligoanuria* associated with azotemia, acidosis, and diverse electrolyte disturbances. ARF is not common in childhood, but the outcome depends on the cause, associated findings, and prompt recognition and treatment.

### Etiology

ARF can develop as a result of a large number of related or unrelated clinical conditions—poor renal perfusion, acute renal injury, or the final expression of chronic, irreversible renal disease. The most common cause in children is transient renal failure resulting from dehydration or other causes of poor perfusion that respond to restoration of fluid volume. Causes of ARF are usually classified as prerenal, intrinsic renal, and postrenal causes. Severe or long-standing prerenal or postrenal etiologies can produce severe secondary renal damage.

**Prerenal Causes.** Prerenal causes of ARF are most common in children and are always related to the reduction of

---

> **Box 30-5** ■ ■ ▫
> ### Classification According to Extent of Renal Injury
>
> **Type I:** A relatively mild renal contusion in which the capsule, parenchyma, and collecting system are usually intact but subcapsular bleeding commonly occurs into the parenchyma and appears in the urine. Renal contusion is an important cause of gross hematuria in active children.
> **Type II:** Laceration of the kidney, injury to a major renal vessel, or injury to the collecting system with intracapsular extravasation of urine.
> **Type III:** Multiple renal lacerations or injury to the main renal artery.

---

*The definition of oligoanuria varies extensively in the literature—from 1.8 to 4 dl/m²/24 hours.

renal perfusion in an anatomically and physiologically normal kidney and collecting system. Dehydration secondary to diarrheal disease or persistent vomiting is the most common cause of prerenal failure in infants and children. Surgical shock and trauma (including burns) are also common causes. Hypovolemia and decreased renal perfusion cause a decreased glomerular filtration rate and stimulate the secretion of renin, aldosterone, and antidiuretic hormone, which further diminish urine flow. Extended and severe hypoperfusion (secondary to procedures such as cardiac surgery) can produce cortical or tubular necrosis; however, when medical care is available, this is seldom allowed to occur. In general, the azotemia that accompanies this type of renal failure is rapidly reversible with prompt attention to expansion of the extracellular fluid volume. Prerenal failure is often difficult to distinguish from tubular or cortical necrosis. Renal artery stenosis, altered peripheral vascular resistance related to sepsis, and hepatorenal syndrome are less common causes.

**Intrinsic Renal Causes.** Intrinsic renal causes of ARF constitute the largest group that requires extended management. These include diseases and nephrotoxic agents that damage the glomeruli, tubules, or renal vasculature. Glomerular disease is the most common cause of glomerular damage, whereas tubular destruction is more often caused by ischemia or nephrotoxins. Vascular damage is an uncommon cause of renal failure in childhood. The type and extent of damage determine the degree and duration of renal insufficiency, and it is difficult to predict in any given case whether or not acute necrosis will develop.

**Postrenal Causes.** ARF resulting from obstructive uropathy is uncommon in children except during the first year of life. Renal function can be restored by relief of the obstruction. The degree of recovery depends on the duration of the renal failure.

## Pathophysiology

ARF is usually reversible, but the deviations of physiologic function can be extreme, and mortality in the pediatric age-group is still high. There is severe reduction in the glomerular filtration rate, an elevated blood urea nitrogen level, and decreased tubular reabsorption of sodium from the proximal tubule. Consequently, there is increased concentration of sodium in the distal tubule, which causes stimulation of the renin mechanism. The local action of angiotensin causes vasoconstriction of the afferent arteriole, which further reduces glomerular filtration and prevents urinary losses of sodium. There is a significant reduction in renal blood flow.

The pathologic conditions that produce acute renal failure caused by glomerulonephritis, hemolytic uremic syndrome, and other renal disorders have been discussed in relation to those disease processes. The necrotic processes within the nephron can be cortical, tubular, or both.

**Cortical Necrosis.** Complete cortical necrosis usually results from severe ischemia, infection, or intravascular coagulation and represents a severe, irreversible cause of acute renal failure. In the pediatric age-group this occurs as a fatal event, most commonly during the neonatal period as a result of hypoxia and shock. When cortical destruction is incomplete, some recovery of renal function may occur. Intravascular coagulation is believed to play a significant role as an intermediate factor in the development of ARF, especially in cases related to sepsis.

**Tubular Necrosis.** Damage to the renal tubules can be broadly classified as (1) secondary to renal ischemia and (2) associated with the ingestion or inhalation of substances toxic to the kidneys. Renal tubules are particularly vulnerable to a wide variety of toxic agents that produce vasoconstriction and to focal patches of ischemia that cause a uniform necrosis of the tubular epithelium down to, but not including, the basement membrane. A lesion produced by sustained reduction in renal blood flow also involves the basement membrane, which may become fragmented and ruptured to the extent that the continuity of tubular structure is disrupted. The lesions may affect any segment of the tubules, appearing at irregular intervals along with normal segments throughout the kidney.

Healing of tubular lesions is accomplished by reepithelialization in the areas with intact basement membrane. Such healing is unable to take place in areas in which the basement membrane has been disrupted; connective tissue grows through the ruptured membrane, thus preventing reestablishment of tubular integrity. Individual cells within the nephron, but not the entire nephron, are capable of regeneration.

**Clinical Course.** The clinical course of the child with ARF is variable and depends on the cause. In reversible ARF there is a period of severe oliguria, or a low-output phase, followed by an abrupt onset of diuresis, or a high-output phase; this phase is followed by a gradual return to, or toward, normal urine volumes. The length of the oliguric phase in older children and adolescents is 10 to 14 days but is highly variable at all ages. It tends to be shorter (3 to 5 days) in infants, children, and milder cases. The onset of the diuretic phase appears unexpectedly, and over several days it proceeds in stepwise fashion from very low to above-normal urine volumes. During the oliguric phase, manifestations of uremia are present but may also be accompanied by other clinical disorders that make assessment difficult, such as infection, anoxia, and shock.

## Clinical Manifestations

In many instances of ARF the infant or child is already critically ill with the precipitating disorder, and the explanation for development of oliguria may or may not be readily apparent. The underlying illness often overshadows the renal failure and often assumes the priority of care (e.g., the patient who is in shock from endotoxemia, the infant who is severely dehydrated from gastroenteritis, or a child who is subject to seizures as a result of hypertensive encephalopathy associated with acute glomerulonephritis).

The prime manifestation of ARF is oliguria, generally a urinary output of less than 1 ml/kg/hr or 300 ml/m². Anuria (no urinary output in 24 hours) is uncommon except in obstructive disorders. Other symptoms related to ARF include edema, drowsiness, circulatory congestion, and cardiac arrhythmia from hyperkalemia. Seizures may be caused by hyponatremia or hypocalcemia and tachypnea from metabolic acidosis. With continued oliguria, biochemical abnormalities can develop rapidly, and circulatory and central nervous system manifestations appear.

## Diagnostic Evaluation

When a previously well child develops ARF without obvious cause, a careful history is obtained to reveal symptoms that may be related to glomerulonephritis, obstructive uropathy, or exposure to nephrotoxic chemicals, such as ingestion of heavy metals or inhalation of carbon tetrachloride or other organic solvents or drugs (e.g., methicillin, sulfonamides, neomycin, polymyxin, and kanamycin). Laboratory data reflect the kidney dysfunction—hyperkalemia, hyponatremia, metabolic acidosis, hypocalcemia, anemia, or azotemia (Table 30-7).

## Therapeutic Management

The most effective management of ARF is prevention. The development of ARF is a known risk in certain situations. This should be anticipated and recognized, and adequate therapy should be implemented (e.g., fluid therapy for children with hypovolemia in conditions such as dehydration, burns, and hemorrhage). Nephrotoxic drugs should be used with caution or avoided in children with renal disease, and all personnel should be knowledgeable about precautions related to their administration. For example, a generous fluid intake is needed for children receiving antimetabolite drugs and after radiotherapy.

The treatment of ARF is directed toward (1) treatment of the underlying cause, (2) management of the complications of renal failure, and (3) provision of supportive therapy within the constraints imposed by the renal failure. Treatment of poor perfusion resulting from dehydration consists of volume restoration as described in the treatment of dehydration. (See Chapter 28.) If oliguria persists after restoration of fluid volume or if the renal failure is caused by intrinsic renal damage, the physiologic and biochemical abnormalities that have resulted from kidney dysfunction must be corrected or controlled. Central venous pressure monitoring is usually implemented.

Initially a Foley catheter is inserted to rule out urine retention, to collect available urine for electrolytes and analysis, and to monitor the results of diuretic administration. The catheter may or may not be removed. Many authorities who believe that it serves little purpose during the oliguric phase and predisposes to bladder infection prefer collection bags for measuring urine output. Others maintain a catheter for hourly urine measurements.

**Oliguria.** When there is persistent oliguria in the presence of adequate hydration and no lower tract obstruction, mannitol, furosemide, or both may be administered rapidly as a test to provoke a flow of urine. When glomerular function is intact, the administration of these substances will behave as nonreabsorbable solute in the tubular fluid to evoke an osmotic diuresis. The presence of mannitol in tubular fluid and the obligatory water that follows it also serve to dilute the concentration of any nephrotoxin that may be present in the tubules to below toxic levels. The furosemide blocks reabsorption of tubular filtrate. If urine flow is generated to the extent of 6 to 10 ml/kg of body weight in 1 to 3 hours, the initial dosage is reduced and continued, if needed, to sustain the flow. If no urine is produced within 2 hours after the single dose, the drugs are not repeated, and an oliguric regimen is instituted to control water balance and other abnormalities.

**Fluid and Calories.** The amount of exogenous water provided should not exceed the amount needed to maintain zero water balance. It is calculated on the basis of estimated endogenous water formation and losses from sensible (primarily gastrointestinal) and insensible sources. No allotment is calculated for urine as long as oliguria persists.

The child with ARF has a tendency to develop water intoxication and hyponatremia, both of which make it diffi-

**TABLE 30-7**   Laboratory findings associated with acute renal failure

| Clinical Problem | Mechanism | Clinical Considerations |
|---|---|---|
| **Azotemia**<br>   **Elevated BUN levels** | Ongoing protein catabolism<br>Significantly decreased excretion | Lower rate of production in neonates and persons with depleted protein stores<br>Increased in situations involving large amounts of necrotic tissue or extravasated blood |
| **Elevated plasma**<br>   **creatinine levels** | Continued production<br>Significantly decreased excretion | Production less affected by other factors<br>More sensitive measure of intensity of azotemia<br>Low in neonate because of small muscle mass relative to size |
| **Metabolic acidosis** | Continued endogenous acid production<br>Significantly decreased excretion<br>Depletion of extracellular and intracellular fluid buffers | Compensatory hyperventilation<br>Opisthotonos<br>Major threat to life |
| **Hyponatremia** | Dilution of extracellular fluid<br>Decreased excretion of water | May develop cerebral signs |
| **Hyperkalemia** | Ongoing protein catabolism<br>Decreased excretion compounded by metabolic acidosis | Most important electrolyte to be considered in acute renal failure<br>May contribute to cardiac arrhythmia<br>With electrocardiogram (ECG) changes, major threat to life<br>May be lost from gastrointestinal tract |
| **Hypocalcemia** | Associated with metabolic acidosis and hyperphosphatemia | During alkali therapy, may cause tetany |

cult to provide calories in sufficient amounts to meet the needs of the child and reduce the tissue catabolism, metabolic acidosis, hyperkalemia, and uremia. If the child is able to tolerate oral foods, concentrated food sources high in carbohydrates and fat but low in protein, potassium, and sodium may be provided. However, many children have functional disturbances of the gastrointestinal tract, such as nausea and vomiting; therefore the IV route is generally preferred, and nourishment usually consists of essential amino acids or a combination of essential and nonessential amino acids administered by the central venous route.

Control of water balance in these patients requires careful monitoring of feedback information, such as accurate intake and output, body weight, and electrolyte measurements. In general, during the oliguric phase no sodium, chloride, or potassium is given unless there are other large, ongoing losses. Regular measurement of plasma electrolytes, pH, blood urea nitrogen, and creatinine levels is required to assess the adequacy of fluid therapy and to anticipate complications that require specific treatment.

**Hyperkalemia.** An elevated serum potassium level is the most immediate threat to the life of the child with ARF. Potassium ions are not being excreted, whereas at the same time the release of potassium from cells is accelerated by acidosis, stress, and tissue breakdown in cases associated with internal bleeding or trauma. Because cardiac arrhythmia and cardiac arrest may result, electrocardiograms (ECGs) and serum potassium ion levels are monitored regularly. Hyperkalemia can be minimized and sometimes avoided by eliminating potassium from all food and fluids, by reducing tissue catabolism, and by correcting acidosis.

> **NURSING ALERT**
> Any of the following signs of hyperkalemia constitute an emergency situation and should be reported immediately:
> Serum potassium concentrations in excess of 7 mEq/L
> Presence of ECG abnormalities, such as loss of P wave, prolonged RS complex, depressed ST segment, tall and tented T waves, bradycardia, or heart block

Several measures are available to reduce the serum potassium concentration, and the priority of implementation is usually based on the rapidity with which the measures are effective. Temporary measures that produce a rapid but transient effect are as follows:

- Calcium gluconate, 0.5 ml/kg, administered intravenously over 2 to 4 minutes, with continuous ECG monitoring, exerts a protective effect on cardiac conduction.
- Sodium bicarbonate, 2 to 3 mEq/kg, administered intravenously over 30 to 60 minutes, elevates the serum pH to cause a transient shift of extracellular fluid potassium into the intracellular fluid. However, there is risk of hypocalcemia, tetany, and fluid overload.
- Glucose, 50%, and insulin, 1 U/kg, administered intravenously, accelerate glycogen synthesis, causing glucose and potassium to move into the cells. Insulin facilitates the entry of glucose into cells.

These effects produce only transient protection by redistributing existing potassium stores; they do not remove potassium from the body. However, they provide relief while more definitive but slower-acting measures are being implemented. Potassium can be removed by the following:

- Administration of a cation exchange resin such as sodium polystyrene sulfonate (Kayexalate), 1 g/kg, administered orally or rectally, to bind potassium and remove it from the body. This requires time to be effective, and a sodium ion is exchanged for each potassium ion. This increased sodium concentration adds to the body fluids, which may contribute to fluid overload, hypertension, and cardiac failure.
- Dialysis or continuous hemofiltration (see p. 1293). Hemodialysis is efficient but requires specialized facilities. Peritoneal dialysis is simpler and can be carried out in almost any hospital setting. Indications for dialysis in ARF are continued oliguria associated with any of the following:
  Severe, persistent acidosis
  Inability to reduce serum potassium levels to a safe range with other methods
  Clinical uremic syndrome consisting of nausea and vomiting, drowsiness, and progression to coma
  Circulatory overload, hypertension, and evidence of cardiac failure

A popular philosophy is to institute renal replacement therapy (see p. 1293) after 24 to 48 hours of oliguria, regardless of other symptoms. Supporters of this approach believe that early intervention is associated with reduced morbidity and mortality and permits improved nutrition with relaxed diet restrictions. The combination of renal replacement therapy and nutrition tends to reduce the complications of ARF.

**Hypertension.** Hypertension is a common and serious complication of ARF, and blood pressure determinations are taken every 4 to 6 hours to detect it early. The most common cause of hypertension in ARF is overexpansion of the extracellular fluid and plasma volume together with activation of the renin-angiotensin system. The goal of therapy is to prevent hypertensive encephalopathy and avoid overtaxing the cardiovascular system.

When there is a threat of encephalopathy, labetalol (a beta and alpha blocker) may be administered intravenously as bolus infusions or a continuous drip. Sodium nitroprusside may be given but requires close monitoring. For less urgent situations, hydralazine, clonidine, or verapamil may be given intravenously. Oral drugs used for acute hypertension include nifedipine, captopril, minoxidil, hydralazine, propranolol, or furosemide (Lasix).

**Other Complications.** Other complications that may occur with ARF are anemia, seizures and coma, cardiac failure, and pulmonary edema. *Anemia* is commonly associated with ARF, but transfusion is not recommended unless the hemoglobin level drops below 6 g/dl. Transfusions consist of fresh, packed red blood cells given slowly to reduce the likelihood of increasing blood volume, hypertension, and hyperkalemia.

*Seizures* occur rather often when renal failure progresses to uremia and are also related to hypertension, hyponatremia, and hypocalcemia. Treatment is directed toward the specific cause when known. More obscure etiologies are managed with antiepileptic drugs.

*Cardiac failure* with pulmonary edema is almost always associated with hypervolemia. Treatment is directed toward reduction of fluid volume, with water and sodium restriction and administration of diuretics. Digitalis is ineffective and can be hazardous.

**Diuretic, or High-Output, Phase.** When the output begins to increase, either spontaneously or in response to diuretic therapy, the intake of fluid, potassium, and sodium must be monitored, and adequate replacement must be provided to prevent depletion and its consequences. In some cases the high-output phase is mild and lasts only a few days; in others enormous amounts of electrolyte-rich urine are passed.

**Prognosis.** The prognosis of ARF depends largely on the nature and severity of the causative factor or precipitating event and the promptness and competence of management. The mortality rate is less than 20%. The outcome is least favorable in children with rapidly progressive nephritis and cortical necrosis. Children in whom ARF is a result of hemolytic uremic syndrome or acute glomerulitis may recover completely, but residual renal impairment or hypertension is more often the rule. Complete recovery is usually expected in children whose renal failure is a result of dehydration, nephrotoxins, or ischemia. ARF following cardiac surgery is less favorable. It is often impossible to assess the extent of recovery for several months.

### Nursing Considerations

Nursing care of the infant or child with ARF involves care of the underlying cause plus careful observation and management of the renal status. The major goal is reestablishment of renal function (with emphasis on providing an adequate caloric intake to minimize reduction of protein stores), prevention of complications, and monitoring of fluid balance, laboratory data, and physical manifestations. The probability of dialysis or continuous hemofiltration must be considered and the necessary equipment made available in anticipation of such an eventuality. Because the child requires intensive observation and often specialized equipment, the usual disposition is admission to an intensive care unit where equipment and personnel trained in its use are available.

The major nursing task in the care of the infant or child with ARF is monitoring and assessing fluid and electrolyte balance. Limiting fluid intake requires ingenuity on the part of caregivers to cope with the child who is thirsty. One strategy involves rationing the daily intake with small amounts of fluid served in containers that give the impression of larger volumes. Older children who understand the rationale of fluid limits can help determine how their daily ration should be distributed.

Meeting nutritional needs is sometimes a problem because the child may be nauseated and because getting the child to eat concentrated foods without fluids may be difficult. When nourishment is provided by the IV route, careful monitoring is essential to prevent fluid overload. IV fluid management related to fluid overload can become a major challenge in the face of nutritional requirements and administration of IV medications. The IV drugs being used may be nephrotoxic, which can require a specified volume of solution for delivery. In some instances blood products must also be delivered. Collaborating to prevent fluid overload while delivering medications and calories requires a concerted effort. In addition, nursing measures such as maintaining an optimum thermal environment, reducing any elevation of body temperature, and reducing restlessness and anxiety are used to decrease the rate of tissue catabolism.

The nurse must be continually alert for behavior changes that indicate the onset of complications. Infection from reduced resistance, anemia, and general morbidity is a constant threat. Fluid overload and electrolyte disturbances can precipitate cardiovascular complications such as hypertension and cardiac failure. Fluid and electrolyte imbalances, acidosis, and accumulation of nitrogenous waste products can produce neurologic involvement manifested by coma, seizures, or alterations in sensorium.

Although children with ARF are usually quite ill and voluntarily diminish their activity, infants may become restless and irritable, and children are often anxious and frightened. Frequent, painful, and stress-producing treatments and tests must be performed. The presence of a supportive, empathetic nurse can provide comfort and stability in a threatening and unnatural environment.

**Family Support.** Providing support and reassurance to parents is among the major nursing responsibilities. The seriousness and emergency nature of ARF are stressful to parents, and most feel some degree of guilt regarding the child's condition, especially when the illness is the result of ingestion of a toxic substance, dehydration, or a genetic disease. They need reassurance and an empathetic listener. They also need to be kept informed of the child's progress and provided explanations regarding the therapeutic regimen. The equipment and the child's behavior are sometimes frightening and anxiety-provoking. Nurses can do much to help parents comprehend and deal with the stresses of the situation. (See Nursing Care Plan: The Child with Acute Renal Failure.*)

## Chronic Renal Failure (CRF)

The kidneys are able to maintain the chemical composition of fluids within normal limits until more than 50% of functional renal capacity is destroyed by disease or injury. Chronic renal failure or insufficiency begins when the diseased kidneys can no longer maintain the normal chemical structure of body fluids under normal conditions. Progressive deterioration over months or years produces a variety of clinical and biochemical disturbances that eventually culminate in the clinical syndrome known as *uremia.* The final stage of chronic renal failure, *end-stage renal disease (ESRD),* is irreversible. Treatment with dialysis or transplantation is required when the glomerular filtration rate (GFR) decreases below 10% to 15% of normal. The pattern of renal dysfunction is remarkably uniform no matter what disease process initiates the advanced disease.

*In Wong DL, Hess CS: *Wong and Whaley's clinical manual of pediatric nursing,* ed 5, St. Louis, 2000, Mosby.

## Etiology

A variety of diseases and disorders can result in CRF (Fig. 30-5). The most common causes of CRF before age 5 years are congenital renal and urinary tract malformations (particularly renal hypoplasia and dysplasia and obstructive uropathy) and vesicoureteral reflux. Glomerular and hereditary renal disease predominate in children 5 to 15 years of age. The glomerular diseases that most commonly lead to CRF are chronic pyelonephritis, chronic glomerulonephritis, and glomerulonephropathy associated with systemic diseases such as anaphylactoid purpura and lupus erythematosus. Hereditary nephritis, congenital nephrotic syndrome, Alport syndrome, polycystic kidney, and several other hereditary disorders result in renal failure in childhood. Renal vascular disorders such as hemolytic uremic syndrome, vascular thrombosis, or cortical necrosis are less common causes.

## Pathophysiology

Early in the course of progressive nephron destruction, the child remains asymptomatic with only minimal biochemical abnormalities. Unless its presence is detected in the process of routine assessment, signs and symptoms that indicate advanced renal damage often emerge only late in the course of the disease. Midway in the disease process, as increasing numbers of nephrons are totally destroyed and most others are damaged to varying degrees, the few that remain intact are hypertrophied but functional. These few normal nephrons are able to make sufficient adjustments to stresses to maintain reasonable degrees of fluid and electrolyte balance. Definitive biochemical examination at this time will reveal restricted tolerance to excesses or restrictions. As the disease progresses to the end stage because of severe reduction in the number of functioning nephrons, the kidneys are no longer able to maintain fluid and electrolyte balance, and the features of the uremic syndrome appear.

The pathophysiology of specific biochemical abnormalities is briefly summarized in the following sections.

**Retention of Waste Products.** A moderate decrease in renal function is not associated with a rise in fasting blood urea nitrogen concentration. With progressive nephron destruction and diminished function, the serum level of these end products of protein metabolism increases. However, the blood urea nitrogen level is affected by protein intake, whereas the creatinine concentration depends on muscle mass; therefore creatinine is a more reliable index of renal failure.

**Water and Sodium Retention.** The damaged kidneys are able to maintain sodium and water balance under normal circumstances, although the few remaining functional nephrons are required to increase their rate of filtration and reabsorption in proportion to their numbers. The limitations of this capacity become apparent under stress. The nature of abnormalities in adjustment depends on the underlying renal disease: infants and small children with kidney dysplasia or urinary obstructive disease tend to excrete large volumes of dilute urine low in sodium content; children with glomerular disease tend to retain both sodium and water as a result of a greater reduction of glomerular filtration than of tubular reabsorption; and children with defective sodium reabsorption from tubular disease tend to lose sodium with a corresponding osmotic water loss. Consequently, sodium excesses may cause edema and hypertension, whereas sodium deprivation can result in hypovolemia and circulatory failure. Only in ESRD is markedly reduced glomerular filtration inadequate to handle normal amounts of sodium and water. Retention of these substances leads to edema and vascular congestion.

**Hyperkalemia.** Dangerous hyperkalemia is an uncommon occurrence in CRF until the end stage. However, the

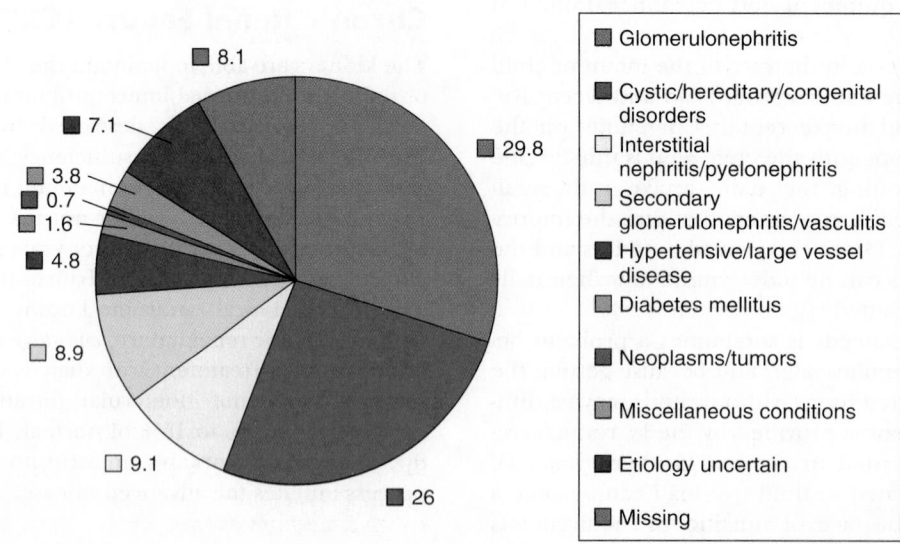

**Fig. 30-5** Primary disease incidence in pediatric ESRD patients, ages birth to 19 years (1993-1997 data).

kidneys are unable to adjust readily to increased ingestion of potassium, and they require a longer period of time to rid the body of this excess.

**Acidosis.** A sustained metabolic acidosis is characteristic of CRF; it results from the inability of the damaged kidney to excrete a normal load of metabolic acids generated by normal metabolic processes. There is reduced capacity of the distal tubules to produce ammonia and impaired reabsorption of bicarbonate. Although there is continual hydrogen ion retention and bicarbonate loss, the plasma pH is maintained at a level compatible with life by other buffering mechanisms, particularly the bone salt (see the following sections).

**Calcium and Phosphorus Disturbances.** One of the distressing features of CRF is its effect on calcium and phosphorus homeostasis. Profound and complex disturbances in the metabolism of these substances result in significant bone demineralization and impaired growth. This appears to be related to several factors (Box 30-6). The result of these complex disturbances in calcium, phosphorus, and bone metabolism produces growth arrest or delay, bone pain, and deformities known as *renal osteodystrophy,* sometimes called *renal rickets,* because the disorganization of bone growth and demineralization are similar to that caused by vitamin D–resistant rickets.

**Anemia.** A consistent feature of chronic renal insufficiency is anemia, which appears to result from several factors (Box 30-7).

**Growth Disturbance.** One of the most striking effects of CRF in childhood, and one that can have profound psychologic and social consequences for the developing child, is delayed growth. The cause is poorly understood but may be related to nutritional and biochemical factors (Box 30-8).

Sexual maturation may be delayed or may not occur in children with CRF, and secondary amenorrhea commonly develops in girls past puberty. CRF can also cause sexual dysfunction by creating imbalances in gonadal hormone levels. Decreased testosterone levels impair spermatogenesis in males; decreased estrogen, luteinizing hormone, and progesterone cause anovulation and menstrual irregularities (usually amenorrhea) in females. Autonomic neuropathy and anemia are also factors that can alter sexual function.

**Other Disturbances.** Children with CRF are more susceptible to infection, especially pneumonia, urinary tract infection, and septicemia, although the reason for this is not entirely clear. Hyperventilation, a manifestation of the respiratory compensatory mechanism for metabolic acidosis, and pulmonary edema may contribute to upper respiratory tract infection. These children become extraordinarily sensitive to changes in vascular volume that may cause, in addition to pulmonary overload, cerebral symptoms and circulatory manifestations such as hypertension and cardiac failure.

Numerous neurologic manifestations appear with advanced renal failure, although no specific toxin or biochemical defect has been identified. However, disturbances in enzyme function, disturbances in water and electrolyte balance, altered calcium ion concentration, hypertension, and accumulation of various "uremic toxins" have been implicated.

### Clinical Manifestations

The first evidence of difficulty is usually loss of normal energy and increased fatigue on exertion. For example, the

---

**Box 30-6**

**Factors Related to Bone Demineralization in Chronic Renal Failure**

1. In a state of acidosis there is dissolution of the alkaline salts of bone, which serve as buffers, and the release of phosphorus and calcium into the bloodstream.
2. Reduced glomerular filtration and excretion of inorganic phosphate lead to an elevation of plasma phosphate with a concomitant decrease in serum calcium.
3. Decreased serum calcium concentration stimulates the secretion of parathyroid hormone (PTH), which results in resorption of calcium from bones. Under normal circumstances parathyroid hormone inhibits the tubular reabsorption of phosphates.
4. Diseased kidneys are unable to complete the synthesis of vitamin D to its most active form, 1,25-dihydroxycholecalciferol, which is necessary for the absorption of calcium from the gastrointestinal tract and deposition of calcium in bone. This acquired resistance to vitamin D decreases calcium absorption, permits retention of phosphorus, and contributes to secondary hyperparathyroidism.

---

**Box 30-7**

**Causes of Anemia in Chronic Renal Failure**

1. Shortened life span of red blood cells caused by some extracorpuscular factor associated with the uremic state
2. Impaired red blood cell production resulting from decreased production of erythropoietin
3. Blood loss related to increased tendency to bleed, associated with a prolonged bleeding time, probably related to impaired platelet function and laboratory blood samples
4. Hyperparathyroidism
5. Hypersplenism, which may be related to silicone deposition (from dialysis blood lines) and granuloma formation in the spleen
6. Diseases related to hemolytic anemia, such as systemic lupus erythematosus and sickle cell disease

---

**Box 30-8**

**Probable Causes of Growth Failure in Chronic Renal Failure**

1. Renal osteodystrophy
2. Poor nutrition associated with dietary restrictions (especially protein) and loss of appetite
3. Biochemical abnormalities associated with renal failure, such as sustained acidosis renal sodium wasting
4. Hypertension
5. Corticosteroid treatment
6. Tissue resistance to growth hormone
7. Trace mineral and vitamin deficiencies

child may prefer quiet, passive activities rather than participation in more active games and outdoor play. The child is usually somewhat pale, but the change is often so inconspicuous that it may not be evident to parents or others. Blood pressure is sometimes elevated. Growth is affected early in the development of chronic renal failure, and falling behind on the growth chart is often the first measurable sign.

Other manifestations may appear as the disease progresses. The child does not eat as well (especially breakfast), shows less interest in normal activities such as schoolwork or play, and has a decreased or increased urinary output and a compensatory intake of fluid. For example, a child who has achieved bladder control may wet the bed at night. Pallor becomes more evident as the skin develops a characteristic sallow, muddy appearance as a result of anemia and deposition of urochrome pigment in the skin. The child may complain of headache, muscle cramps, and nausea. Other signs and symptoms include weight loss, facial puffiness, malaise, bone or joint pain, growth retardation, dryness or itching of the skin, bruised skin, and sometimes sensory or motor loss. Amenorrhea is common in adolescent girls.

Therapy is generally initiated before the appearance of the *uremic syndrome,* although there are occasions in which the symptoms may be observed. Manifestations of untreated uremia reflect the progressive nature of the homeostatic disturbances as well as general toxicity. Gastrointestinal symptoms include loss of appetite and nausea and vomiting. Bleeding tendencies are apparent in bruises, bloody diarrheal stools, stomatitis, and bleeding from the lips and mouth. There is intractable itching, probably related to hyperparathyroidism. Deposits of urea crystals may appear on the skin as "uremic frost" but are seldom seen because of the availability of dialysis and transplantation (Gilman and Frauman, 1998). There may be an unpleasant "uremic" odor to the breath. Respirations become deeper as a result of metabolic acidosis, and circulatory overload is manifested by hypertension, congestive heart failure, and pulmonary edema. Neurologic involvement is reflected by progressive confusion, dulling of the sensorium and ultimately coma. Other signs may include tremors, muscular twitching, and seizures.

### Diagnostic Evaluation

The diagnosis of CRF is usually suspected on the basis of any of a number of clinical manifestations, a history of prior renal disease, or biochemical findings. The onset is usually gradual, and the initial signs and symptoms are vague and nonspecific. Laboratory and other diagnostic tools and tests are of value in assessing the extent of renal damage, biochemical disturbances, and related physical dysfunction. Often they can help establish the nature of the underlying disease and differentiate between other disease processes and the pathologic consequences of renal dysfunction.

### Therapeutic Management

In irreversible renal failure the goals of medical management are to promote effective renal function, maintain body fluid and electrolyte balance within acceptable limits, treat systemic complications, and promote as active and nor-mal a life as possible for the child for as long as possible. This becomes increasingly difficult as the disease progresses toward its inevitable end. Even therapeutic measures designed to relieve one manifestation may prove detrimental to another. For example, antihypertensive agents may further impair renal function.

**Activity.** Children are allowed unrestricted activity and to set their own limits regarding rest and extent of exertion. They are encouraged to attend school. When the effort is too great, home tutoring is arranged.

**Diet.** Regulation of diet has been seen as the most effective means, short of dialysis, for reducing the quantity of materials that require renal excretion. The goal of the diet in renal failure is to provide sufficient calories and protein for growth while minimizing the excretory demands made on the kidney, to limit metabolic bone disease (osteodystrophy), and to minimize fluid and electrolyte disturbances. Dietary protein intake is limited only to the recommended daily allowance (RDA) for the child's age. Restriction of protein intake below the RDA is believed to negatively impact growth and neurodevelopment. Dietary phosphorus may need to be restricted. It should be remembered that any attempt to restrict dietary intake in children potentially restricts caloric intake and can impact growth.

Protein in the diet should include foods of high biologic value. When given with meals, substances that bind phosphorus in the intestines prevent its absorption and allow a more liberal intake of phosphorus-containing protein. Sodium and water are not usually limited unless there is evidence of edema or hypertension.

Potassium is not restricted as long as creatinine clearance remains at acceptable limits ((30 to 35 ml/min). However, restrictions are instituted for patients with oliguria or anuria. Restrictions of any or all these minerals may be imposed in later stages or at any time in which factors cause abnormal serum concentrations.

Because of modified dietary intake, altered metabolism, and poor appetite, some dietary supplementation is usually needed. Because fat-soluble vitamins can accumulate in patients with CRF, vitamins A, E, and K are not supplemented beyond normal dietary intake. An active form of vitamin D is prescribed, and water-soluble vitamin supplementation may be required if the diet is inadequate. Other dietary needs are discussed in relation to osteodystrophy and anemia. Dietary management of the child with renal failure is a difficult and complex problem that necessitates collaboration with a registered dietitian who is knowledgeable about pediatric nutrition and the impact of renal failure.

**Osteodystrophy.** Measures directed at prevention or correction of the calcium/phosphorus imbalance are reduction of dietary phosphorus, administration of a phosphorus-binding agent, provision of supplemental calcium, control of acidosis, and administration of an active form of vitamin D.

Dietary phosphorus can be controlled by the reduction of protein and milk intake. Phosphorus levels can be further reduced by the oral administration of phosphorus-binding agents that combine with the phosphorus to decrease gastrointestinal absorption and thus the serum levels of phosphate.

Calcium carbonate preparations can be used as phosphorus binders. These medications act as (1) phosphate binders, (2) calcium supplements, and (3) alkalizing agents. Calcium carbonate preparations can be given with meals to bind phosphorus if the child is hyperphosphatemic or mildly hypocalcemic. If given 1 to 2 hours after meals, they act as calcium supplements for children with stable phosphorus but low calcium levels. Calcium acetate can also be used.

Aluminum hydroxide gels are effective phosphorus binders but have been shown to cause aluminum loading when used in children with renal failure. Aluminum intoxication leads to altered sensorium, an inability to talk, ataxia, seizures, and severe bone disease.

When serum phosphate levels are within a normal range, appropriate therapy with an active form of vitamin D is instituted. These drugs are administered to increase the absorption of calcium through the gastrointestinal tract and include dihydrotachysterol (Hytakerol) or calcitriol (Rocaltrol). The serum calcium level is monitored weekly during periods when the drugs are being changed or regulated. Parathyroid hormone levels are measured every 2 to 3 months.

Osseous deformities that result from renal osteodystrophy, especially those related to ambulation, are troublesome and require correction if they occur. Careful attention to the management of osteodystrophy and bone growth can prevent deformities from occurring in some children.

**Acidosis.** Pharmacologic treatment of acidosis is initiated early in children who have chronic renal insufficiency. In addition to reducing the formation of metabolic acids by decreasing the dietary intake of protein, acidosis is alleviated by alkalizing agents such as sodium bicarbonate or a combination of sodium and potassium citrate (Bicitra, Polycitra, or Shohl solution*). Correction of acidosis is best attempted after calcium levels are elevated, because rapid correction may precipitate tetany in a hypocalcemic child.

**Anemia.** Because the anemia associated with renal failure is related to decreased production of erythropoietin, it usually cannot be successfully managed with hematinic agents. Sufficient sources of folic acid and iron should be provided in the diet, although this is difficult when protein sources are restricted. Inadequate intake and iron losses that may occur are managed by supplemental iron, usually ferrous sulfate. Providing adequate sources of ascorbic acid at the same time that iron-rich foods or supplements are given enhances the absorption.

The medication **recombinant human erythropoietin (r-HuEPO)** corrects anemia (improving energy level and general well-being) and eliminates the need for frequent blood transfusions in patients with CRF (Jabs and others, 1994). To support the formation of new RBCs before rHuEPO therapy, iron stores must be adequate. Iron supplements are required in conjunction with rHuEPO.

**Hypertension.** Hypertension of advanced renal disease may be managed initially by cautious use of a low-sodium diet, fluid restriction, and perhaps diuretics such as thiazides or furosemide. Strict restriction of sodium intake may be necessary in patients with oliguria. Severe hypertension may require the combination of a beta blocker and a vasodilator (propranolol and hydralazine). Other drugs that may be used include nifedipine, atenolol, minoxidil, prazosin, captopril, or labetalol, either singly or in combinations.

**Growth Retardation.** One major consequence of CRF is growth retardation. Children with onset of renal failure earlier in life have more severe growth impairment than those diagnosed later (Fine and others, 1996). These children grow poorly both before and after initiation of dialysis. In addition to a number of metabolic abnormalities, depletion of body protein is characteristic of children with CRF. The use of recombinant human growth hormone has shown marked acceleration in growth velocity in children with growth retardation secondary to CRF (Burg and others, 1996).

**Miscellaneous Complications.** Intercurrent infections are treated with appropriate antimicrobials at the first sign of infection. Most of these drugs are excreted through the kidneys; therefore the dosage is usually reduced in proportion to the decrease in renal function, and the interval between doses is extended in these children to avoid possible toxic effects from accumulation. Any drug eliminated through the kidneys is administered with caution. Serum levels of ototoxic or nephrotoxic drugs (e.g., aminoglycosides or vancomycin) are assessed regularly to ensure a safe, nontoxic level.

Dental defects are common in children with chronic kidney disease; the earlier the onset of the disease, the more severe the dental manifestations. These defects include hypoplasia, hypomineralization, tooth discoloration, alteration in the size and shape of teeth, malocclusion (secondary to deficient skeletal growth), ulcerative stomatitis, occasional oral hematomas, and an increase in calcific deposits around the teeth. Regular dental care is especially important in these children. Other nondental complications are treated symptomatically (e.g., chlorpromazine [Thorazine] or prochlorperazine [Compazine] is given for nausea, antiepileptics are given for seizures, and diphenhydramine [Benadryl] is given for pruritus). Once evidence of ESRD appears in a child, the disease runs its relentless course and terminates in death in a few weeks unless waste products and toxins are removed from body fluids by dialysis or kidney transplantation. Since the adaptation of these techniques for infants and small children, the outlook for these patients has improved remarkably. In cases in which the patient has other serious illnesses or organ system failures and aggressive care is considered futile, the appropriate end-of-life recommendation may be for palliative care and comfort measures only (Currier, 1994).

### Nursing Considerations

### ■ Assessment

Assessment of the child with CRF is primarily one of observation for signs of complications and evidence of improvement through therapy. Some of the first changes observed

---

*Each milliliter of Shohl solution contains 1 mEq of citrate ion, which metabolizes to yield 1 mEq of bicarbonate. Citric acid exerts no effect on acid-base balance but enhances the palatability of the mixture.

are growth failure, developmental delay, bone disease, and hypertension.

## ◾ Nursing Diagnoses

A number of nursing diagnoses become evident on assessment of the child. Those most relevant in the majority of cases are outlined in the Nursing Care Plan on pp. 1294-1295. Others may be appropriate for individual children and their families.

## ◾ Planning

The goals of care for the child with CRF, especially one in ESRD, and family are as follows:

1. The child will receive encouragement in his or her normal growth and development, minimizing the impact of the disease process.
2. The child will remain free of complications.
3. The child and family will receive appropriate support, guidance, and education.

The child with CRF has a life maintained by drugs and artificial means, and the multiple stresses placed on these children and their families are often overwhelming. The unrelenting course of the disease process is one of progressive deterioration. There is no means by which to prevent the irreversible progress of renal insufficiency, nor is there any known cure. As the affected child progresses from renal insufficiency to uremia and then to dialysis and transplantation with a need for intensity of therapy, the need for supportive nursing care is also intensified. Team effort is more important than ever and involves coordination of personnel from medicine, nursing, social services, child life, physical/occupational therapy, dietetics, and psychologic or psychiatric specialties.

Progressive disease places a number of stresses on the child and family. There is a continuing need for repeated examinations that often entail painful procedures, side effects, and frequent hospitalizations. Diet therapy can become progressively more restrictive and intense, and parents may need help in learning to select appropriate foods, read labels carefully for sodium and potassium content, and modify meals to accommodate the special needs of the child. The child is required to take a variety of medications. Compliance is difficult when long-term therapies are involved. Ever present in all aspects of the treatment regimen is the agonizing realization that, without treatment, death is the inevitable outcome.

ESRD presents the same nonspecific stresses on child and family as any other chronic (Chapter 22) or life-threatening (Chapter 23) illness. The reactions and adaptation of the child and family depend on the age and developmental stage of the child, the cultural and socioeconomic background of the family, the quality of the interpersonal relationships of family members, and the communication patterns within the family. In general the problems observed and the emotional responses to the stress of the illness are influenced less by the nature of the illness than by the family relationships and personalities of its members. (See Family Focus box.)

One of the first and most noticeable changes is the alteration in physical appearance—fluctuations in weight, anemia, and failure to grow. Children must adjust to the fact that they will always be different from their peers in some ways. They will be shorter, often more tired, and unable to participate in all the activities that are attractive to young people. Children who have had diversion procedures, dialysis, and other surgeries or who urinate into a bag need to learn positive coping strategies for the alterations in their body image and for the questions and potential teasing of peers. It is not difficult or unusual for children with chronic conditions to exhibit behavioral regression. This is particularly so for children with renal failure because their appearance is often of a child much younger than their chronologic age.

School is often difficult for these children. Frequent absences for illnesses, evaluations, or treatments disrupt the educational process and socialization. Teachers and school systems are not always sympathetic to the rights and needs of a child with a chronic illness (e.g., the right to equal education and the need for flexibility and special help at times), which places an additional burden on the parents. Sometimes a teacher will pass a failing child because of pity.

In some families illness and stressful experiences act as a unifying force; in other families stress aggravates preexisting problems and contributes to family disharmony. The relentless nature of the disease and its therapies not only places physical and emotional stresses on the family but is also a chronic drain on the family finances. Insurance rarely covers the full cost of the multiple hospitalizations and outpatient expenses. ESRD care is funded by the federal Medicare program, for which most children qualify. However, hidden costs abound, such as transportation to special treatment centers, meals and, sometimes, lodging away from home. Some temporary assistance may be provided by private foundations, churches, and community groups, and nurses should become familiar with those in the area of their practice that can be of financial and educational service to these families. For example, the **National Kidney**

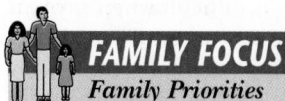

## FAMILY FOCUS
### *Family Priorities*

Families who have children with long-term chronic illnesses, such as end-stage renal disease, spend much time in hospitals, outpatient clinics, and primary health care facilities. When they miss appointments or respond less quickly than anticipated, sometimes they are quickly labeled "noncompliant." It is important to remember that families have to develop priorities for the unit as a whole. Sometimes the family may decide that it is more important for the parent to go to work or to attend a sibling's school performance than to attend an appointment scheduled for them by health care personnel. The chronically ill child cannot and should not always be the number-one priority for the family. The professional staff who works with the family can help the parents prioritize the needs of the ill child within the needs of the family constellation.

Teresa Hall, MS, RN
Hathaway Children's Services
Sylmar, CA

Foundation* and numerous other agencies provide services and information for families, including pamphlets and descriptive literature. Particularly useful are booklets written for children with renal disease.†

Certain specific stresses related to ESRD and its treatment are predictable. When it first becomes apparent that kidney failure is inevitable, both the child and the parents experience great depression and anxiety. Acceptance is particularly difficult if renal failure progresses rapidly after the diagnosis. Denial and disbelief are usually pronounced, especially among parents. Denial can also develop when progression to ESRD has been prolonged and both the child and the parents develop a denial pattern of believing it will never occur.

Once the kidney failure is established and the symptoms become progressively more distressing, the initiation of hemodialysis is usually perceived as a positive experience. After the initial concerns of implementing the treatment, the child begins to feel better, and parental anxiety is relieved for a time.

## ▓ Evaluation

The effectiveness of nursing interventions is determined by continual reassessment and evaluation of care based on the following observational guidelines:

1. Observe and interview the family regarding their adherence to the medical and dietary regimen.
2. Monitor vital signs, growth measurements, laboratory reports, behavior, and appearance.
3. Observe and interview child and family regarding their feelings, concerns, and fears; observe reactions to therapies and prognosis.

The *expected outcomes* are described in the Nursing Care Plan on pp. 1294-1295.

## RENAL REPLACEMENT THERAPY

Technologic advances in the care of children with acute and chronic renal failure provide several renal replacement therapies for maintaining excretory function in acute disease and for prolonging life in those with ESRD. The primary modalities are hemodialysis, peritoneal dialysis, hemofiltration, and transplantation.

*Dialysis* is the process of separating colloids and crystalline substances in solution by the difference in their rate of diffusion through a semipermeable membrane. This movement across the membrane is accomplished by three processes: osmosis, diffusion, and ultrafiltration (Box 30-9).

Methods of dialysis currently available for clinical management of renal failure are:

Hemodialysis, in which blood is circulated outside the body through artificial cellophane membranes that permit a similar passage of water and solutes

Peritoneal dialysis, wherein the abdominal cavity acts as a semipermeable membrane through which water and solutes of small molecular size move by osmosis and diffusion according to their respective concentrations on either side of the membrane

Hemofiltration, in which blood filtrate is circulated outside the body by hydrostatic pressure exerted across a semipermeable membrane and replaced (simultaneously) by electrolyte solution

The choice of whether to use hemodialysis, peritoneal dialysis, or hemofiltration is determined by the nature of the renal failure (acute vs chronic) and the cause of the renal failure. For chronic dialysis, family lifestyles and preferences are considered in choice of treatment. Hemodialysis is more efficient than peritoneal dialysis but is technically more difficult in infants and very young children. In these children hemofiltration may be a viable substitute for dialysis. As a rule, dialysis is reserved for children who are in end-stage renal failure, because it requires creation of an access and special equipment. It may be used acutely for conditions such as severe metabolic acidosis, accidental poisoning, chronic heart failure with fluid overload, hyperkalemia, severe hypernatremia, severe hyperphosphatemia, and tumor lysis syndrome.

The absolute indications for dialysis are life-threatening electrolyte abnormalities, severe volume overload, and children with bilateral neoplastic disease or bilateral nephrectomies performed for various reasons, including intractable hypertension. Although each child is assessed on an individual basis, indications for instituting dialysis in CRF are biochemical abnormalities, including elevated blood urea nitrogen, acidosis, severe hyperphosphatemia, and elevated potassium. Other indications include deteriorating central nervous system function or congestive heart failure that is unresponsive to other therapy. Growth failure, severe osteodystrophy, insufficient caloric intake, and an inability to carry out normal activities are sometimes criteria for dialysis.

Most children show rapid clinical improvement with the implementation of dialysis, although it is directly related to the duration of uremia before dialysis and the extent to which dietary regulations are followed. Growth rate and skeletal maturation improve, but recovery of normal growth is uncommon. In many cases sexual development, although delayed, has progressed to completion.

## Hemodialysis

Hemodialysis is the preferred dialytic method for children with acute conditions such as life-threatening hyperkalemia

---

*30 E 33rd St, New York, NY 10016, (212) 889-2210 or (800) 622-9010; www.kidney.org.
†A recommended resource for children and parents is *Understanding Kidney Failure: A Handbook for Parents* by F. Orrbine and N.N. Wolfish, available from Children's Hospital of Eastern Ontario Foundation, 385 Smyth Rd, Ottawa, Ontario, Canada K1H 8L2.

---

### Box 30-9 ▪ ▪ ▪
### Processes of Fluid and Electrolyte Movement

**Osmosis**—Passive movement of water from a solution of lower concentration to a solution of higher concentration of particles
**Diffusion**—Random movement of particles from an area of greater concentration to an area of lower concentration
**Ultrafiltration**—Process by which plasma water is removed because of a pressure gradient between the blood and dialysate compartments

## Nursing Care Plan
### The Child with Chronic Renal Failure (CRF)

> NURSING DIAGNOSIS: Risk for injury related to accumulated electrolytes and waste products

**PATIENT GOAL 1:** Will maintain near-normal electrolyte levels

- **NURSING INTERVENTIONS/*RATIONALES***

*Assist with dialysis *to maintain excretory function*

*Administer cation exchange resins as prescribed *to reduce serum potassium levels*

Provide diet low in protein, potassium, sodium, and phosphorus, if prescribed, *to reduce excretory demand on kidneys*

Observe for evidence of accumulated waste products (hyperkalemia, hyperphosphatemia, uremia) *to ensure prompt treatment*

- **EXPECTED OUTCOME**

Child exhibits no evidence of waste product accumulation

> NURSING DIAGNOSIS: Fluid volume excess related to failure of renal regulatory mechanisms

**PATIENT GOAL 1:** Will maintain appropriate fluid volume

- **NURSING INTERVENTIONS/*RATIONALES***

*Assist with dialysis *to maintain excretory function*

Monitor progress *to assess adequacy of therapy and detect possible complications*

- **EXPECTED OUTCOME**

Child exhibits no evidence or complications of accumulated fluid between dialysis sessions

*Dependent nursing action.

**PATIENT GOAL 2:** Will maintain appropriate fluid volume through regulation of fluid intake

- **NURSING INTERVENTIONS/*RATIONALES***

*Administer oral fluids as prescribed

Use strategies to prevent undesirable intake

Review daily fluid restrictions with parents and child *to encourage cooperation*

Suggest ways to divide total volume of fluid into small quantities to be spread over entire day

Keep mouth moist by other means, such as hard candy, ice chips, fine mist spray of cool water *to prevent feeling of dryness*

- **EXPECTED OUTCOME**

Child exhibits no evidence of fluid gain

> NURSING DIAGNOSIS: Imbalanced nutrition: less than body requirements related to restricted diet

**PATIENT GOAL 1:** Will consume appropriate diet

- **NURSING INTERVENTIONS/*RATIONALES***

Provide dietary instructions for foods *that reduce excretory demands on kidney and provide sufficient calories and protein for growth*

*Limit phosphorus, salt, and potassium as prescribed

Encourage intake of carbohydrates *to provide calories for growth* and foods high in calcium *to prevent bone demineralization*

Arrange for renal dietitian to meet with family to review allowable foods and assist in dietary planning *so that family understands dietary needs of child*

Help hemodialysis patients to fill out menu requests for meals

Administer water-soluble vitamins as prescribed

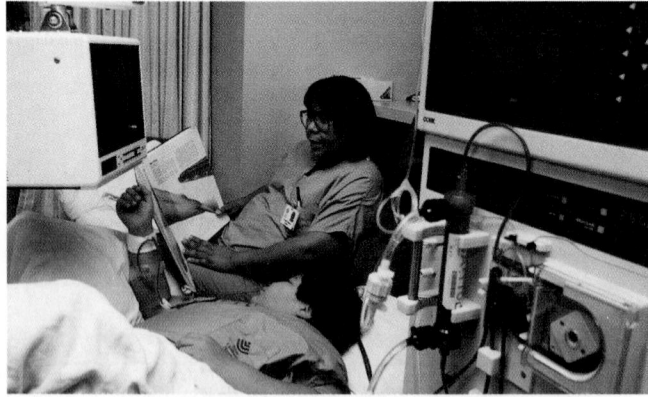

**Fig. 30-6** Fifteen-year-old receiving hemodialysis treatment.

or poisoning with dialyzable compounds. Protein loss is less extensive than with peritoneal dialysis. However, hemodialysis is technically difficult in small children less than 20 kg because their delicately balanced cardiovascular dynamics may be upset by the rapid changes in blood volume and systemic blood pressure that may occur with this method. In addition, it may be difficult to place vascular access for hemodialysis in small children.

Hemodialysis is the preferred form of dialysis for certain family situations in which any one person is unable to take the time and responsibility to perform the procedures at home. It is best suited to children who live close to the dialysis center, because they must come to the center as often as three or more times a week for treatments. Children who are not good candidates for peritoneal dialysis because of family noncompliance, recurrent peritoneal infections, or unstable living conditions must elect to have hemodialysis.

### Procedure

Hemodialysis requires the use of special dialysis equipment—the hemodialyzer, or so-called artificial kidney (Fig. 30-6). Hemodialyzers are available in two forms: parallel flow (plate) and hollow fiber. Hollow fiber dialyzers are preferable for children because their blood compartment is rigid and available in relatively small volumes (Evans and Greenbaum,

# Nursing Care Plan
## The Child with Chronic Renal Failure (CRF)—cont'd

- **EXPECTED OUTCOMES**

Child consumes an adequate amount of appropriate foods

Child shows no evidence of deficiencies or weight loss

> NURSING DIAGNOSIS: Disturbed body image related to chronic illness, impaired growth, and perception of being "different"

**PATIENT GOAL 1:** Will develop positive self-esteem and understanding of disease

- **NURSING INTERVENTIONS/*RATIONALES***

Provide education about CRF, including management, treatment, and long-term outcome

Encourage child's independence with care and management of CRF, *because independence helps child develop positive self-esteem*

　Allow child to participate in dialysis procedures

　Allow child to participate in making decisions when appropriate

Promote self-esteem in child with CRF

　Organize patient support group or suggest counseling as needed

　Provide positive reinforcement during dialysis procedures and follow-up visits

- **EXPECTED OUTCOMES**

Child demonstrates an understanding of CRF and complies with therapies

Child exhibits signs of positive self-esteem

> NURSING DIAGNOSIS: Interrupted family processes related to a child with a chronic disease

**PATIENT (FAMILY) GOAL 1:** Will exhibit positive coping behaviors

- **NURSING INTERVENTIONS/*RATIONALES***

Assist parents in diet planning and support their efforts to adjust diet to meet needs of all family members

Provide anticipatory guidance regarding probable and expected events, such as symptoms, diet, and effects of medications

Assist parents in decision making regarding dialysis and transplantation *because these are the alternatives once palliative care is no longer effective*

Prepare child and family for hemodialysis or kidney transplantation *because preparation is essential for positive coping*

Prepare child and family for home hemodialysis or continuous home peritoneal dialysis

Maintain periodic contact with family *for ongoing support*

Refer family to special agencies and support groups *for long-term support*

- **EXPECTED OUTCOME**

Child and family demonstrate ability to cope with stresses of illness (specify)

See also:

Nursing Care Plan: The Child with a Chronic Illness or Disability, Chapter 22

Nursing Care Plan: The Child in the Hospital, Chapter 26

Nursing Care Plan: The Family of the Child Who Is Ill or Hospitalized, Chapter 26

Nursing Care Plan: The Child Who Is Terminally Ill or Dying, Chapter 23

---

1995). Pediatric dialysis can be safely carried out when the total dialysis circuit volume does not exceed 10% of the child's estimated blood volume.

Hemodialysis also requires three means of blood access: grafts, fistulas, or external access devices. An ***arteriovenous fistula*** is an access in which a vein and artery are connected surgically. The preferred site is the radial artery and a forearm vein. The creation of a subcutaneous (internal) arteriovenous fistula by anastomosing a segment of the radial artery and brachiocephalic vein produces dilation and thickening of the superficial vessels of the forearm to provide easy access for repeated venipuncture. Fewer complications and less restriction of activity are observed with this approach. If vessels are inadequate for an autogenous fistula, a ***synthetic graft*** may be placed in the arm or thigh with either a loop or straight configuration. Both the graft and the fistula require needle insertion at each dialysis. For short-term external vascular access, percutaneous catheters are inserted in the femoral or internal jugular veins, even in very small children. Subclavian access should be avoided because of the potential complication of stenosis. For long-

term external vascular access, cuffed, dual-lumen (single-lumen for infants) catheters can be surgically placed similarly to other central venous access devices. They are ready to be used immediately, and no needles are required.

Various hemodialysis schedules are used, but most centers recommend dialysis three times a week for 3 to 5 hours, depending on the size of the child. The length of a hemodialysis treatment, the blood flow rate, and dialyzer characteristics contribute to adequacy of treatment. Current target levels for adequacy are a urea reduction ratio (URR) of 65% or higher or a Kt/V (clearance/time/volume) of 1.4 or higher. For a complete description of the highly specialized process of hemodialysis, the reader is directed to the numerous references available on this topic.

Dietary limitations are necessary in chronic dialysis to avoid biochemical complications. Fluid and sodium are restricted to prevent fluid overload and its associated symptoms of hypertension, cerebral manifestations, and congestive heart failure. Potassium is restricted to prevent complications related to hyperkalemia; phosphorus restriction helps to prevent parathyroid hyperactivity and its attendant risk of abnormal calcification in soft tissues. Adequate protein intake is necessary to maximize growth potential. Fluid limitations are determined by residual urine output and the need to limit intradialytic weight gain.

Seizures during or after hemodialysis are now uncommon. With the current practice of hemodialysis, cerebral edema caused by alterations in osmolality in the brain when the blood urea nitrogen level is lowered rapidly (associated with dialysis disequilibrium syndrome) is rare.

### Home Hemodialysis

With appropriate cannulization and proper training and education of both the child and the parents, hemodialysis can be performed at home. Time spent in transportation is eliminated, the environment is more pleasant and secure, and the child is able to assume a more active role in the treatment program. Home dialysis is especially advantageous for children waiting for a transplant who live a great distance from the dialysis center or for children who have had one or more kidney transplant failures.

Home hemodialysis units are available to some children, and the preparation and management are similar to that required for hemodialysis in the hospital. The patient is equipped with a dialysis unit that is used with the vascular access established for outpatient dialysis. Parents of children on home hemodialysis must know how to operate the equipment, connect the unit to the vascular access, and assess the status of the child. Home hemodialysis is more prevalent in sparsely populated regions of the country.

### Nursing Considerations

Initiating a hemodialysis regimen is a traumatic and anxiety-provoking experience for most children. After surgery for implantation of the graft, fistula, or long-term external access device, the initial experience with the hemodialysis machine and its implication is frightening to most children. They need reassurance about the nature of the preparations for dialysis and the conduct of the treatment. They are anxious about repeated venipunctures (with implanted shunts and for blood chemistries) and about the sight of their blood leaving their body and entering the machine. (See Atraumatic Care box.) Anxiety can also be caused by the child's physiologic response to the treatment (e.g., nausea and vomiting, cramps, or seizures). These are usually individual responses related to the child's overall well-being and degree of compliance with the total medical regimen. Once the initial fear of the machine has been resolved, children can be helped to develop strategies for dealing with restricted activity and movement for the duration of each treatment (Fig. 30-7).

With their increased need for independence and their urge for rebellion, adolescents may adapt less well. They resent the control and enforced dependence imposed by the rigorous and unrelenting therapy program. They resent dependency on a machine, parents, and professional staff. Depression, hostility, or both are common in adolescents undergoing hemodialysis. The adverse consequences of the disease include the need for diet restrictions, limitations in physical activity (resulting from lack of energy, frequent illnesses, and specific restrictions related to access), and the sense of being different from other children. Withdrawal from peers and social isolation are the rule, and noncompliance with the therapeutic regimen is not uncommon.

Body changes related to the disease process, such as growth retardation, skin color, and lack of sexual maturation, are stress provoking. Dietary restrictions are particularly burdensome for both children and parents. Children feel deprived when unable to eat foods previously enjoyed and unrestricted for other family members. Consequently, failure to cooperate is not uncommon. Diet restrictions are interpreted as punishment, because they may not be able to fully understand the purpose of the restrictions, some will sneak forbidden food items at every opportunity. Allowing children, especially adolescents, maximum participation in and responsibility for their own treatment program is helpful. The extent of adherence and adjustment depends on the personalities of the involved persons, the quality of their relationships, and their coping mechanisms.

After weeks, months, or years of hemodialysis, the parents and the child feel anxiety associated with the prognosis and continued pressures of the treatment. The relentless need for treatment interferes with family plans and activities, including school. Graft and fistula problems are not uncommon and present a common source of aggravation. Most families and children on hemodialysis look to renal transplantation as a desirable alternative to long-term treatment.

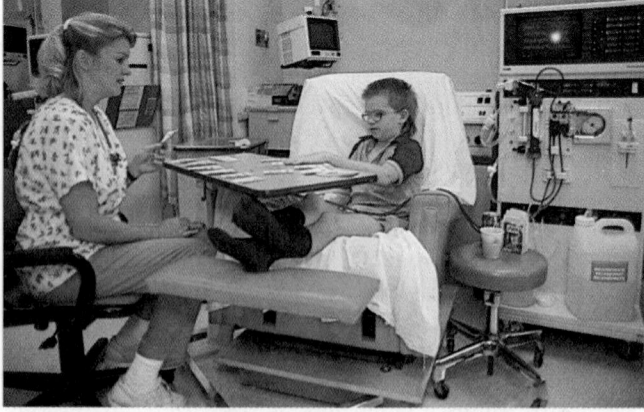

**Fig. 30-7** Diversional activities help lessen the boredom children can experience during hemodialysis.

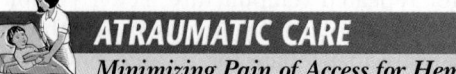

### ATRAUMATIC CARE
*Minimizing Pain of Access for Hemodialysis*

Use buffered lidocaine or one of the more rapid-onset novacaines (e.g., procaine) with a small-gauge needle (30 gauge) to anesthetize the area before venipuncture of the graft/fistula. Or apply an anesthetizing topical preparation such as EMLA (eutectic mixture of local anesthetics [lidocaine and prilocaine]) 1 hour before venipuncture. (See Pain Management, Chapter 26.)

## Peritoneal Dialysis (PD)

For acute conditions, *PD* is quick, relatively easy to learn and safe to perform, and requires a minimal amount of equipment and specially trained nurses. PD is a slow, gentle process, which decreases the stress on body organs that can occur with the rapid chemical and volume changes of hemodialysis. The procedure is indicated for neonates, children with severe cardiovascular disease, or those who are poor risks for vascular access.

*Chronic PD* is the preferred form of dialysis for children/parents who are independent, families who live a long distance from the medical center, infants, school-age children, and adolescents, who prefer fewer dietary restrictions and a gentler form of dialysis. Chronic peritoneal dialysis is most often performed at home.

Contraindications for the use of PD include recent abdominal surgery or peritoneal adhesions and scarring. A higher rate of infection (peritonitis) is observed with this modality.

### Procedure

In acute situations PD catheter insertion may be accomplished at the bedside; catheters for long-term use are placed surgically in the operating room with the patient under anesthesia. A catheter is inserted through the anterior abdominal wall, and the catheter cuff is sutured into place. Chronic PD catheters are tunneled through a subcutaneous tract before exiting the skin in a manner similar to implantation of central venous access devices. At the time of dialysis a commercially prepared dialysis solution is allowed to flow by gravity through the catheter and into the peritoneal cavity, where it remains while equilibrium between plasma and dialysis fluid takes place. Approximately 30 to 50 ml/kg, or 1100 ml/m$^2$, of dialysis solution is instilled at each cycle. The fluid is then allowed to flow by gravity drainage into a receptacle, and fresh dialysis solution is again instilled.

In PD each pass or cycle is characterized by inflow time, dwell time, and drain time. The length of each portion of the cycle is part of the dialysis prescription. The dwell time varies according to the goals of the treatment (i.e., removal of water, solute, electrolyte, or all of these). The procedure is usually continued until renal function is restored, waste products are reduced, or (in prolonged need) the patient is switched to a form of chronic PD—*continuous ambulatory peritoneal dialysis (CAPD)* or *continuous cycling peritoneal dialysis (CCPD)*. An acute PD catheter may remain in place for several weeks provided that aseptic technique is adhered to by all who enter the system.

### Home Dialysis

The development of satisfactory methods for CAPD and its alternative, CCPD, has provided additional means for managing ESRD at home. In both methods commercially available sterile dialysis solution is instilled into the peritoneal cavity through the surgically implanted indwelling catheter. The warmed solution is allowed to enter the peritoneal cavity by gravity and remains a variable length of time according to the procedure used. Dialysis solution is infused and dialysate drained through a single catheter.

In CAPD the dialysis solution is instilled, the line is clamped off, and worn attached to the abdomen or thigh or even placed in a pocket. Manufacturers offer a variety of disconnect devices (e.g., "Y" set), all of which minimize the connectivity and amount of tubing the patient carries between exchanges. The solution is allowed to remain in the peritoneum for 4 to 6 hours. The dialysate is then drained via gravity into a bag. Another warmed bag is infused, and the process is repeated so that there is fluid in the abdomen continuously. The procedure is performed at a minimum of three times during the day and once at night. For an active child CAPD has proved to be a satisfactory alternative to hemodialysis.

CCPD is a modification of CAPD and intermittent peritoneal dialysis. The dialysis exchange is usually performed at night using a peritoneal dialysis machine that warms the dialysis fluid and automates the cycles of inflow of dialysis fluid and outflow of dialysate. As with CAPD, the CCPD system is opened twice as opposed to multiple times per day. Nighttime dialysis allows the child more freedom during the day and relieves parents of needing to perform multiple exchanges (Evans and Greenbaum, 1995).

The care and management of the procedure are the responsibility of the parents of young children. Older children and adolescents are able to carry out the procedure themselves, thus providing them with some control and less dependency. This is especially important for adolescents.

**Complications.**   CAPD and CCPD are presently considered to be the methods of choice for most children who require dialysis because they are easier to initiate and maintain than hemodialysis. Peritonitis is the major complication of home peritoneal dialysis. The patients are treated intraperitoneally with antibiotics, and some may require catheter replacement. Although the risk of infection is continuously present, most practitioners believe it is not great enough to discourage the use of these methods.

However, other complications have been noted in patients on home peritoneal dialysis. Tunnel infections are evidenced by swelling, warmth, and tenderness along the subcutaneous catheter tract; however, they can be managed with administration of antibiotics or catheter replacement. Peritoneal leaks and ventral hernias caused by the sustained intraabdominal pressure that develops within the peritoneum have also been found in a significant number of children. Few of these patients respond to a reduction in dialysis solution volume, and many require surgical intervention.

**NURSING ALERT**   Observe for changes in the color of the dialysis solution draining from the child. The solution should be straw-colored and clear. If the color is pink, bright yellow, or brown, or, if the solution is cloudy, notify the practitioner immediately.

### Nursing Considerations

The availability of home dialysis has offered a greater degree of freedom for persons undergoing long-term dialysis. The need for a residence convenient to a dialysis unit and the necessity for frequent trips to the unit are eliminated, except for monthly evaluations. The nurse is responsible for teaching the family. Education focuses on (1) the disease, its implications, and the therapeutic plan; (2) the possible psychologic effects of the disease and the treatment; and (3) the technical aspects of the procedure.

The family must learn how to take vital signs before and after the dialysis and how to interpret the significance of blood pressure and temperature variations. They need to know how to vary the composition of the dialysis solution to compensate for variations in the vital signs and to maintain an accurate record of all aspects of the treatment.

Parents of the young child using CAPD are taught how to exchange bags and manage the procedure at home. Even newborn infants are able to benefit from peritoneal dialysis. Older children can be taught to take responsibility for their own treatments as much as possible. The family is encouraged to ask questions throughout the preparation time, including those that clarify anatomy and physiology, mechanical functioning, and side effects of the disease and the treatment. The peritoneal dialysis schedule is outlined to meet the individual needs of the patient and family. Most schedules are arranged for uninterrupted sleep at night and coordination of the dialysis with school and other activities. The diet, medication, and activity are discussed, and feelings about the entire therapeutic program are explored with the child and family.

Infection is the greatest hazard of peritoneal dialysis; therefore the family is instructed to contact the appropriate persons at the earliest evidence of peritonitis. In most instances of peritonitis the infection can be controlled with administration of antibiotics. Unfortunately, there is a high incidence of peritonitis, and repeated infections may necessitate replacement of the catheter or its removal and abandonment of the peritoneum as an access route.

The importance of emotional, as well as material, support cannot be overemphasized. The National Kidney Foundation, mentioned previously, provides a number of services and information for families of children with renal disease. A relatively new organization, the **American Association of Kidney Patients (AAKP),*** has been organized to promote the interest and welfare of kidney patients. It provides education and support for patients and public education regarding all areas of kidney disease. (See Critical Thinking Exercise box.)

## Continuous Venovenous Hemofiltration (CVVH)

A third type of "dialysis" or renal replacement therapy used primarily in acute care settings is CVVH. This type of therapy uses specialized equipment (hemofilter, blood pump, tubing connected to a vascular access) to ultrafiltrate blood continuously at a very slow rate. With this procedure, fluid balance may be achieved within 24 to 48 hours after initiation. CVVH(D) is used to remove excess fluid from patients with severe oliguric fluid overload.

CVVH(D) is an ideal form of renal replacement therapy for children with fluid overload from surgical procedures (e.g., cardiovascular surgery) who do not have severe biochemical abnormalities. It is commonly used for critically ill children who require volume-expanding fluids such as hyperalimentation solution, albumin, or packed red cells. It creates space for the infusion of these replacement solutions in fluid-sensitive patients. CVVH(D) has proved to be a highly successful alternative form of dialysis for critically ill children who might not survive the rapid volume changes that occur with hemodialysis and peritoneal dialysis.

## Transplantation

Renal transplantation is the preferred means of renal replacement therapy in the pediatric age-group. Although peritoneal dialysis and hemodialysis are life preserving and

## Critical Thinking Exercise

### End-Stage Renal Disease

Jamie is a 20-month-old boy with end-stage renal disease secondary to obstructive uropathy. He is currently in the hospital for replacement of his peritoneal dialysis catheter. In reviewing his admission data base, you identify that he has not had the measles-mumps-rubella (MMR) vaccine. Of the following actions, which is the most critical given that you would interview his primary caretaker to verify that the immunization status is correct?

FIRST, THINK ABOUT IT . . .
- What precise question are you trying to answer?
- What information are you using?

1. Include instructions on the need for completing Jamie's infant immunizations and the locations of local immunization clinics in your discharge teaching with Jamie's parents.
2. Bring the immunization status to the attention of Jamie's primary health care practitioner as soon as possible.
3. Recognize that Jamie's chronic condition has contributed to his incomplete immunization status and that his immunizations will be completed before he receives a renal transplant.
4. Recommend that Jamie receive the MMR vaccine in 4 to 6 weeks, when he has recovered from his surgery.

*The best response at this time is two. The primary health care practitioner can potentially order the immunizations to be given before discharge from this hospitalization. Jamie's immunization status is most likely related to his chronic illness. Precisely, he must receive the immunizations before becoming eligible for renal transplantation because the MMR vaccine contains live viruses that the immunosuppressive medications required after renal transplantation would preclude. Jamie's recent surgery is not a contraindication to vaccination at this time, and waiting simply delays his transplant eligibility. Educating his parents is also appropriate; however, the objective at this time is immediate immunization.*

---

*100 South Ashley Dr, Suite 280, Tampa, FL 33602 (800) 749-2257; www.aakp.org.

are able to be carried out in the home in a large number of cases, neither method is compatible with a normal lifestyle. Transplantation, on the other hand, offers the opportunity for a relatively normal life.

Kidneys for transplant are available from either of two sources: (1) *a living related donor (LRD),* usually a parent, grandparent, or sibling; or (2) *a cadaver donor (CD),* wherein the family of a dead or brain-dead patient consents to donation of a healthy kidney. The criteria for selection of kidney recipients are quite liberal, but uniform criteria have not been established among the various centers that specialize in the procedure. In general there is no limit to age. In some cases a person's mental status (e.g., severe mental retardation, emotional instability, or nonadherance to drug therapy) may be reason to defer transplantation until the recipient's psychoemotional status improves and it is reasonable to assume that the posttransplant regimen will be carried out. (See Family Focus box.)

Children who have ESRD secondary to uncontrolled malignancy must be cancer-free for a specified period of time before transplantation (in remission for 2 years with patient off chemotherapy). Generalized infection must be eradicated before attempted transplantation, and the recipient should have adequate bladder capacity. Some children may have bladder augmentation or other genitourinary surgery as preparation for transplantation. Children with abnormal urinary tracts may be subject to more posttransplant urologic complications and infection than they would otherwise be.

## Procedure

The kidney graft is placed in the extraperitoneal space, usually the anterior iliac fossa; the renal artery is anastomosed to the internal iliac or hypogastric artery; the renal vein is anastomosed to the hypogastric vein; and the ureter is implanted into the bladder or anastomosed to the recipient's ureter. Small children receiving a large donor kidney may require placement within the abdomen with vessel anastomoses to the aorta and inferior vena cava. Unless there is medical contraindication, the recipient's failed kidneys are left in place. Severe hypertension, neoplasm, large and continuous protein losses, and persistent severe vesicoureteral reflux are the usual reasons for nephrectomy.

The primary goal in transplantation is the long-term survival of the grafted tissue. The means by which this is attempted include (1) securing tissues that are antigenically similar to that of the recipient and (2) suppressing the recipient's immune mechanism.

### Selection of Donor Tissue

The source of a donor kidney is either a live person or a cadaver soon after death. The closer the genetic relationship between the donor and recipient, the better the possibility of long-term survival. The only truly compatible tissue match is that between identical twin siblings. The next best possible match is a sibling, then a parent or grandparent. In some states the use of siblings is impossible until the possible donor is of age to give consent for removal of a kidney. Unrelated donors are least likely to be compatible. Careful immunologic studies are carried out to determine the donor whose kidney is least likely to be rejected by the recipient.

### Suppression of the Immune Response

After the best possible tissue match is obtained for a transplant, the survival time can be significantly lengthened by suppressing the immune response of the recipient. The immunosuppressant therapy of choice in kidney transplantation is corticosteroids (prednisone) in conjunction with cyclosporine and azathioprine. Other therapies include antilymphocyte globulin or monoclonal antibodies, administered intravenously for 14 days either for induction or rescue from rejection.

The administration of these drugs is not without hazard. The major problem encountered with nonspecific immunosuppression is that it not only suppresses the immune response to the grafted tissue but also suppresses the body's capacity to respond to other antigenic stimuli. Consequently, the child is vulnerable to overwhelming infections.

Prednisone is an immunosuppressant and antiinflammatory agent that acts to stabilize cell walls, reduce migration of white blood cells into the inflamed area, and inhibit deposition of fibrin and collagen. It also depresses T-cells, B-cells, and phagocytes. A number of complications from corticosteroid therapy are cause for concern. Interference with linear growth has led many centers to use alternate-day administration in an effort to improve growth rates and to decrease other long-term side effects such as cataracts, fluid and sodium retention, hypertension, gastric ulcer, and obesity.

Cyclosporine is a powerful immunosuppressant that acts to decrease the production of T-cells. The side effects of this

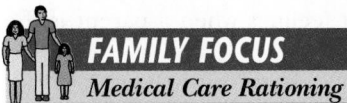

## FAMILY FOCUS
### Medical Care Rationing

The criteria for selection of renal transplant recipients sometimes create dilemmas for professionals. In most cases the decision is simply a matter for the transplant team and the family to resolve for the benefit of the child involved. However, in some situations the solution is less clear, especially in view of the scarcity of donor kidneys and the expense of the procedure. The matter creates more questions than answers.

For example, should a child without a severe mental or physical disability take priority over one with these disabilities? Should financial responsibility be a consideration? Some youngsters with renal transplants have discontinued taking their medications, thereby either causing damage to their kidney or losing the graft. Should these youngsters receive a second transplant? Should very young children whose families have proved to be too unreliable in adhering to a therapeutic regimen be given a transplant when the success of the graft depends on following a prescribed therapeutic plan? Are very young, single adolescent mothers likely to be less adherent in following the prescribed medical regimen? Can persons on limited incomes manage to acquire the costly medications? If not, should the government subsidize payment?

What solutions to these dilemmas are available, and how are decisions justified? Who should make the decisions?

drug are hypertension, which may appear within several days of transplant; hirsutism; and nephrotoxicity. Maintenance doses of cyclosporine are determined by serum blood levels. After the initial IV therapy immediately following the transplant, the drug is administered orally. When the liquid form is used, each center has specific instructions for administering cyclosporine. The concerns are that the complete dose will be taken and absorption of the medication will be maximized.

Azathioprine, another immunosuppressant, interferes with cellular protein synthesis. The problem related to the toxic effect of azathioprine is mainly neutropenia, which is usually managed by reduced dosage. (See Chapter 36 for a discussion of immunosuppressant therapy and related nursing care.)

## Rejection

Rejection of a transplanted kidney is the most common cause of transplant failure. Rejection can be one of three types—hyperacute, acute, or chronic. *Hyperacute rejection* is irreversible, develops immediately or within a few hours after revascularization, and is related to circulating antibodies preformed in the recipient against the donor tissue antigens.

*Acute rejection* usually occurs between the first few days and months after transplantation but may occur years later, especially if the patient becomes poorly compliant with immunosuppressant medications. Rejection is evidenced by both biochemical and clinical abnormalities. The most common finding is fever, which is usually accompanied by swelling and tenderness over the graft, hypertension, and diminished urinary output. A severe reaction may cause oliguria. Increases in serum blood urea nitrogen and creatinine levels are laboratory evidence of decreased transplant function. Most acute rejection episodes respond to IV administration of methylprednisolone sodium succinate (Solu-Medrol), antilymphocyte globulin, or monoclonal antibodies.

> **NURSING ALERT**
>
> The child with a recent kidney transplant (a few days) or one who was grafted approximately 6 months previously who exhibits any of the following should be evaluated immediately for possible rejection:
> Fever
> Swelling and tenderness over graft area
> Diminished urinary output
> Elevated blood pressure

*Chronic rejection* is characterized by slow, gradual deterioration of renal function that typically begins 6 months or more after transplantation. Evidence of rejection may be heralded by proteinuria or hematuria, and the rejection may have symptomatology indistinguishable from the original kidney disease. No present therapy can halt the progressive process, which inevitably leads to loss of the implanted kidney.

## Prognosis

The overall primary graft survival rate for kidneys at 1 year is 81%; at 3 years, 72%; and at 5 years, 64% (Elshihabi and others, 2000). One-year survival rates for cadaver kidney grafts increased from 72% in 1987 to 88% in 1995, and living-donor kidney grafts improved from 88% in 1987 to 93% in 1995. Predictors of graft survival for children include age at transplantation, pretransplantation dialysis, early rejection, and race. Over time, adolescents and African-Americans appeared to have the lowest graft survival (Ishitani and others, 2000). Long-term graft survival is not guaranteed, and many children require a second or third transplant. Successful renal transplantation does improve rehabilitation of children with CRF, both educationally and psychologically.

## Nursing Considerations

The possibility of renal transplantation often comes as a hope for relief from the rigors of dialysis or the restriction of a conservative management regimen. Most children and families respond well to a kidney transplant. Children with successful renal transplants are usually able to resume life activities similar to those of their unaffected age-mates within 1 year after the transplant. The rehabilitation of children with renal transplants is influenced primarily by their pattern of functioning before becoming ill. It is important to remember that transplantation is a treatment that makes a much less negative impact on the normal life activities of a child. However, stresses remain for the child and family in relation to the uncertainty of the future, the child's health and well-being, social isolation, and financial burdens (Fedewa and Oberst, 1996).

A variety of serious emotional and psychologic conflicts may arise as a consequence of donor selection, including ambivalence of donors faced with surgery and relinquishing a kidney, feelings of guilt if one should prove to be unacceptable as a donor, and the emotional impact of having a live relative–donated kidney rejected by the recipient. This especially can result in guilt feelings when a parent is the donor.

The child recipient responds in various ways to a kidney transplant. The concept of having a foreign body, especially a cadaver kidney, inside their own body is sometimes disturbing to children. They often speculate about the age, sex, personality, and physical characteristics of the donor. They may fear that the kidney will wear out if it came from an older person. Some children are distressed to find that their donor kidney came from a person of the opposite sex. Corticosteroid therapy, necessary in kidney transplants, creates undesirable side effects (e.g., growth failure, obesity, characteristics of Cushing syndrome [see Fig. 38-4], acne, and hirsutism) that are often a source of emotional and social problems for older children. Gum hyperplasia, brittle fingernails, and hair breaking can also occur (Olin and others, 1998).

The most common reason for poor adherence in childhood renal transplant recipients is dislike of undesirable side effects. The cosmetic implications of the side effects can be overwhelming, especially to adolescent girls. Deliberate discontinuation of the drugs is most commonly observed in teenage girls. Problems with adherence are also commonly seen in children from poorly communicating families who are not very supportive. (See Compliance, Chapter 27.)

Working with children and their families during the various stages of renal failure, dialysis, and transplantation is a difficult and challenging experience. Nurses must become familiar with the family; assess family strengths, weaknesses, and coping mechanisms; and be prepared to provide intensive support and guidance during the prolonged experience. The child and family need help in accepting what is happening to them, in learning anticipatory guidance regarding predictable stresses, and in dealing constructively with the physical, emotional, and financial burdens that are an ongoing part of this prolonged disability.

## KEY POINTS

- The main function of the kidney is to maintain the composition and volume of body fluids in equilibrium.
- Common inflammatory disorders of the genitourinary tract include urinary tract infection, nephrotic syndrome, and acute glomerulonephritis.
- Management of urinary tract infections is directed at eliminating infection, detecting and correcting functional or anatomic abnormalities, preventing recurrences, and preserving renal function.
- Vesicoureteral reflux is the retrograde flow of bladder urine into the ureters.
- Common features of acute glomerulonephritis are oliguria, edema, hypertension, circulatory congestion, hematuria, and proteinuria.
- Therapeutic management of acute glomerulonephritis is maintenance of fluid balance and treatment of hypertension.
- Nephrotic syndrome is characterized by increased glomerular permeability to protein.
- Management of nephrotic syndrome is aimed at reducing excretion of protein, reducing or preventing fluid retention by tissues, and preventing infection and other complications. These are accomplished through dietary control, use of diuretics, corticosteroid therapy, and immunosuppressant therapy.

- Primary functions of the renal tubules are acidification of urine, potassium secretion, and selective and differential reabsorption of sodium, chloride, water, and other substances.
- The most common renal tubular disorders are renal tubular acidosis and nephrogenic diabetes insipidus.
- Management of hemolytic-uremic syndrome is aimed at control of hematologic manifestations and complications of renal failure.
- In acute renal failure, management is directed at determining treatment of the underlying cause, managing the complications of renal failure, and providing supportive therapy.
- Abnormalities in chronic renal failure are waste product retention, water and sodium retention, hyperkalemia, acidosis, calcium and phosphorus disturbance, anemia, hypertension, and growth disturbances.
- When the child will need home dialysis, the nurse educates the family about the disease, its implications, the therapeutic plan, possible psychologic effects of the disease, and the treatment and technical aspects of the procedure.
- The major concerns in renal transplantation are tissue matching and prevention of rejection, as well as psychologic concerns involving self-image as related to possible body changes resulting from the effects of corticosteriod therapy.

## REFERENCES

AAP Committee on Quality Improvement, Subcommittee on Urinary Tract Infections: Practice parameters: the diagnosis, treatment and evaluation of the initial urinary tract infection in febrile infants and young children, *Pediatrics* 103(4):843-853, 1999.

Bell BP and others: Predictors of hemolytic uremic syndrome in children during a large outbreak of *Escherichia coli* O157-H7 infections, *Pediatrics* 100(1):127, 1997; *www.pediatrics.org/cgi/content/full/100/1/e12*.

Berhman RE, Kliegman RM, Jenson, HB: *Nelson textbook of pediatrics*, ed 16th, Philadelphia, 2000, WB Saunders.

Burg FD and others: *Gellis and Kagan's current pediatric therapy*, Philadelphia, 1996, WB Saunders.

Centers for Disease Control and Prevention: Outbreaks of *Escherichia coli* O157:H7 infection associated with eating alfalfa sprouts—Michigan and Virginia, June-July 1997, *MMWR* 46(32):741-744, 1997.

Cieslak PR and others: Hamburger-associated *Escherichia coli* O157:H7 infection in Las Vegas: a hidden epidemic, *Am J Public Health* 87(2):176-180, 1997.

Colodner R, Keness Y: Evaluation of Dip-Streak containing CNA-MacConkey agar: a new bedside urine culture device, *Isr Med Assoc J* 2(7):563-565, 2000.

Connolly LP and others: Vesicoureteral reflux in children: incidence and severity in siblings, *J Urol* 157(6):2287-2290, 1997.

Currier H: Ethical issues in the neonatal patient with end stage renal disease, *J Perinat Neonatal Nurs* 8(11):74-78, 1994.

Elshihabi I and others: Continuing improvement in cadaver donor graft survival in North American children: the 1998 annual report of the North American Pediatric Renal Transplant Cooperative Study, *Pediatr Transplant* 4:221-234, 2000.

Evans ED, Greenbaum LA: Principles of renal replacement therapy in children, *Pediatr Nephrol* 42(6):1579-1602, 1995.

Fedewa MM, Oberst MT: Family caregiving in a pediatric renal transplant population, *Pediatr Nurs* 22(5):402-407, 1996.

Fine RN and others: Long-term treatment of growth-retarded children with chronic renal insufficiency, with recombinant human growth hormone, *Kidney Int* 49(3):781-785, 1996.

Froom P and others: Stability of common analytes in urine refrigerated for 24 hours before automated analysis by test strips, *Clin Chem* 46(9):1384-1386, 2000.

Gilman C, Frauman AC: The pediatric patient. In Parker J: *Contemporary nephrology nursing*, Pitman, NJ, 1998, Jannetti.

Goldman M and others: Imaging after urinary tract infection in male neonates, *Pediatrics* 105(6):1232-1235, 2000.

Gray ML: *Genitourinary disorders,* St Louis, 1992, Mosby.

Greenfield SP, Wan J: The relationship between dysfunctional voiding and congenital vesicoureteral reflux, *Curr Opin Urol* 10(6):607-610, 2000.

Ishitani M and others: Predictors of graft survival in pediatric living related kidney transplant recipients, *Transplantation* 70(2):288-292, 2000.

Jabs K and others: Primary results from the US Multicenter Pediatric Recombinant Erythropoietin Study (abstract), *J Am Soc Nephrol* 5:456, 1994.

Koff SA: Non-neuropathic vesicourethral dysfunction in children. In O'Donnel B, Koff SA, editors: *Pediatric urology,* Oxford, 1997, Butterworth-Heinemann.

Kunin C: Urinary tract infections in children. In O'Donnell B, Koff SA, editors: *Pediatric urology,* Oxford, 1997, Butterworth-Heinemann.

Lama G and others: Primary vesicoureteric reflux and renal damage in the first year of life, *Pediatr Nephrol* 15(3-4):205-210, 2000.

Milford DV: Glomerulonephritis in children, *Br J Hosp Med* 54(2/3):87-91, 1995.

Miller KL: Urinary tract infections: children are not little adults, *Pediatr Nurs* 22(6):473-480, 544, 1996.

Olin BR and others: *Drug facts and comparisons,* St Louis, 1998, Facts and Comparisons.

Plachter NB, Schulman SL, Canning DA: Identification and management of urinary tract infection in the preschool child, *J Pediatr Health Care* 13(6 Pt 1):268-272, 1999.

Raymond J, Sauvestre C: Microbiological diagnosis of urinary tract infections in the child: importance of rapid tests, *Arch Pediatr* 5(suppl 3):260S-265S, 1998.

Rushton HG: Urinary tract infections in children: epidemiology, evaluation, and management, *Urol Clin North Am* 44(5):1133-1169, 1997.

Schlager TA and others: Effect of cranberry juice on bacteriuria in children with neurogenic bladder receiving intermittent catheterization, *J Pediatr* 135(6):698-702, 1999.

Schoen EJ, Colby CJ, Ray GT: Newborn circumcision decreases incidence and costs of urinary infections during the first year of life, *Pediatrics* 105(4 Pt 1):789-793, 2000.

Soygur T and others: Relationship among pediatric voiding dysfunction and vesicoureteral reflux and renal scars, *Urology* 54(5):905-908, 1999.

Sugarman RA: Structure and function of the neurologic system. In Huether SE, McCance KL: *Understanding pathophysiology,* ed 2, St Louis, 2000, Mosby.

Walsh PC and others: *Campbell's urology,* ed 2, Philadelphia, 1998, WB Saunders.

Warshaw B: Nephrotic syndrome, *Pediatr Ann* 23(9):495-497, 1994.

Wiswell TE: The prepuce, urinary tract infections, and the consequences, *Pediatrics* 105(4 Pt 1):860-861, 2000.

Chapter **31**

# The Child with Disturbance of Oxygen and Carbon Dioxide Exchange

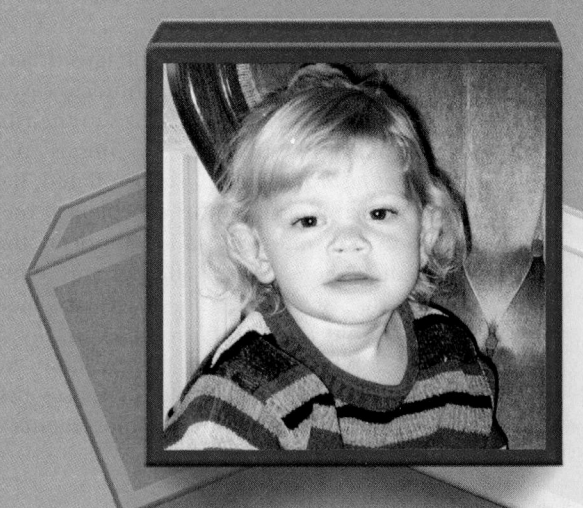

## Chapter Outline

**RESPIRATORY TRACT STRUCTURE AND FUNCTION, 1303**
**Structure, 1303**
  Chest, 1304
  Airways, 1305
  Respiratory Units, 1306
**Function, 1306**
  Gas Exchange, 1308
  Defenses of the Respiratory Tract, 1310
**ASSESSMENT OF RESPIRATORY FUNCTION, 1310**
**Physical Assessment, 1310**
  Respiration, 1310
  Associated Observations, 1310
**Diagnostic Procedures, 1312**
  Pulmonary Function Tests, 1312

Radiology and Other Diagnostic
  Procedures, 1312
Blood Gas Determination, 1313
**RESPIRATORY THERAPY, 1317**
**Oxygen Therapy, 1317**
  Oxygen Administration, 1317
  Oxygen Toxicity, 1319
**Aerosol Therapy, 1319**
**Bronchial (Postural) Drainage, 1320**
**Chest Physiotherapy (CPT), 1320**
**Artificial Ventilation, 1323**
  Care of the Patient, 1324
  Endotracheal Airways, 1324
**Tracheostomy, 1325**
  Tracheostomy Care, 1326
  Decannulation, 1329

Home Care of the Child with a
  Tracheostomy, 1329
**RESPIRATORY EMERGENCY, 1331**
**Respiratory Failure, 1331**
  Conditions That Predispose to Respiratory
    Failure, 1331
  Recognition of Respiratory Failure, 1332
**Management and Related Nursing
  Considerations, 1332**
  Observation and Monitoring, 1332
  Family Support, 1333
**Cardiopulmonary Resuscitation (CPR), 1333**
  Resuscitation Procedure, 1334
**Airway Obstruction, 1338**
  Infants, 1338
  Children, 1341

## Related Topics

The Child with Respiratory Dysfunction,
  Ch. 32
Discharge Planning and Home Care, Ch. 26

Family-Centered Home Care, Ch. 25
High Risk Related to Disturbed Respiratory
  Function, Ch. 10

Physical Examination: Chest, Lungs, Ch. 7
Preparation for Procedures, Ch. 27
Shock, Ch. 29

## RESPIRATORY TRACT STRUCTURE AND FUNCTION

Disorders of the respiratory tract occur frequently in infancy and childhood. Anatomically, several factors influence the manner in which children, particularly infants, respond to respiratory disturbances.

The ***respiratory tract*** consists of many complex structures. The primary responsibility of these structures is to distribute air and exchange gases so that cells are supplied with oxygen ($O_2$) for body metabolism while carbon dioxide ($CO_2$), the volatile product of metabolism, is removed. The structures of the respiratory system—nose, pharynx, larynx, tra-

chea, bronchi, and lungs—provide the means whereby gases enter the body. The circulatory system distributes gases to and from the millions of cells throughout the body. All of the structures of the respiratory system except the minute air sacs (alveoli) of the lung tissue function in air distribution. It is within the alveoli that gas exchange takes place.

## Structure

The ***thoracic cavity***, which is encased in the bony framework provided by the ribs, vertebrae, and sternum, consists of three major partitions: the ***three-lobed lung*** on the right, the ***two-lobed lung*** on the left, and the space between them—the

■ Marilyn L. Winkelstein, PhD, RN, revised this chapter.

*mediastinum*—which contains the esophagus, trachea, large blood vessels, and heart. The entire thoracic cavity is lined by smooth *parietal pleura,* which adheres to the ribs and superior surface of the diaphragm. Each lung is encased in a separate *visceral pleural sac* that, when inflated, lies against the parietal pleura. Normally the two pleural membranes are separated by only enough fluid to lubricate the surface for painless movement during filling and emptying of the lungs. In disease states, this space may contain air *(pneumothorax),* fluid *(pleural effusion),* serum *(hydrothorax),* blood *(hemothorax),* or pus *(pyothorax,* also known as *empyema).* Inflammation of the pleura causes the painful friction of pleurisy during respiratory movements.

## Chest

The chest has a relatively round configuration at birth but changes gradually to one that is more or less flattened in the anteroposterior (front-to-back) diameter in adulthood. In some lung diseases chronic overinflation causes changes in these measurements. For example, in severe obstructive lung disease (e.g., asthma, cystic fibrosis) the anteroposterior measurement approaches the transverse (side-to-side) measurement to produce the so-called *barrel chest.* Periodic measurements provide clues to the course of the lung disease or the efficacy of therapy. Increased size indicates progressive obstructive lung disease.

The elliptic shape of the ribs and the angle at which they are attached to the spine allow the thorax to change size during respiration. Contraction of the intercostal muscles lifts the ribs from a downward angle to a more horizontal angle, which increases both the anteroposterior and the lateral dimensions of the chest (Fig. 31-1, *A*). This also changes the diameter of the bronchi; the diameter increases during inspiration and decreases during expiration,

an important factor when the bronchi are narrowed as a result of obstruction or inflammation. Contraction and relaxation of the diaphragm cause the chest cavity to lengthen and shorten, which also increases the volume of the chest cavity during inspiration. Normal expiration is passive, although contraction of the internal intercostal muscles pulls the rib cage downward, and contraction of the abdominal muscles forces the diaphragm upward to decrease the chest size actively. (See Fig. 7-34.)

An adult's ribs articulate with the vertebrae and sternum from a downward and lateral angle. During inspiration the respiratory muscles contract and the thorax enlarges. In the newborn infant, however, the ribs articulate with the spine at a horizontal rather than a downward slope; consequently, during inspiration the diameter of the chest is decreased (Fig. 31-1, *B*). The infant relies almost entirely on diaphragmatic-abdominal breathing. During inspiration the diaphragm is forced downward, increasing the available space for lung expansion; the intercostal muscles serve primarily as stabilizing forces. The processes of *compliance,* the elastic property of lung tissue that allows it to expand and recoil, and *resistance,* which affects the amount of flow through the airways, facilitate respiration (see p. 1307).

Variations occur in lung volume relative to posture. In the upright position the evenly distributed weight of the abdominal contents contributes to uniform application of negative intrathoracic pressure. However, in the supine position the abdominal contents apply weight caudally to create a nonuniform distribution of positive pressure to the diaphragm. Consequently, lung volume is increased in the upright position and decreased in the supine position. In addition, the mechanical attachment of the diaphragm to the rib cage is such that contraction will elevate the rib cage in the upright position but in the supine position tends to pull in the rib cage (Fig. 31-2).

In the newborn the diaphragm is attached higher in front. Therefore this already-stretched diaphragm is unable to contract as far or as forcefully as that of the older infant or child. Young infants are also less able to withstand diaphragmatic fatigue because of fewer energy-producing components. Abdominal distention from gas or fluid can impede diaphragmatic excursion significantly.

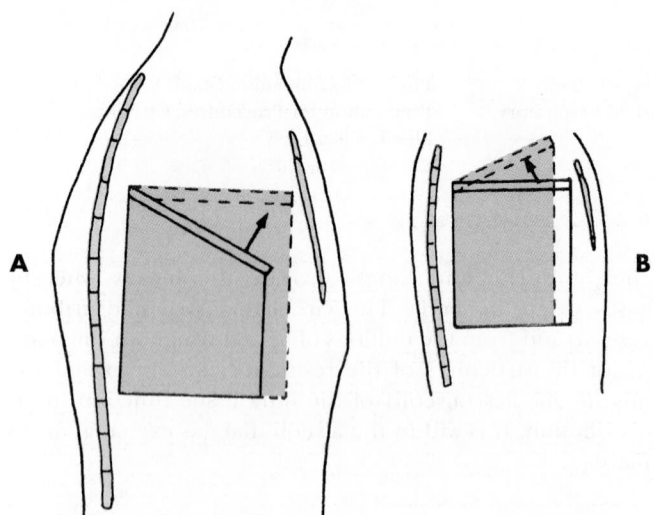

**Fig. 31-1** Mechanisms of respiratory excursion. **A,** Downward and lateral position of rib in adult and expansion of lung capacity on thoracic inspiration. **B,** More horizontal position of rib in infant and decreased expansion of lung capacity on thoracic inspiration.

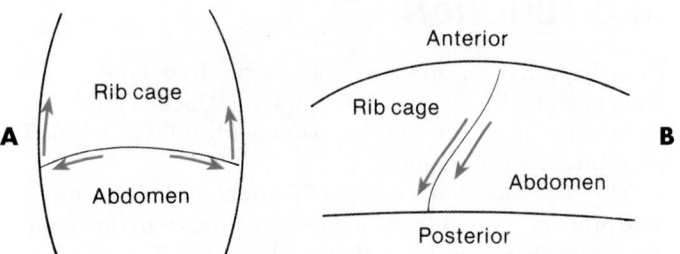

**Fig. 31-2** Relationship of diaphragm and abdominal contents in **A,** upright, and **B,** supine positions.

## Airways

The rigid *nasal structures,* which are lined with ciliated mucous membranes, serve as passageways for air, warming and moistening air, filtering it of impurities, and destroying microorganisms that come in contact with immune defenses in the mucosa. In infancy the nasal passages are narrow, and infants are primarily nose breathers. Any factor that decreases the size of the nasal passages and increases airway resistance, such as nasal mucosal swelling and mucus accumulation, hampers breathing and feeding.

The *upper airway* (oronasopharynx, pharynx, larynx, and upper part of the trachea) is shared by both the respiratory and the alimentary tracts, and many of the muscles in this area participate in several complex acts. However, the sequence of airway muscle activation is different in breathing and swallowing. The upper airway dilates during inspiration and constricts during exhalation. During some activities these dimensions are modified; for example, inspiration is short during crying, coughing, and sneezing, but with crying the larynx and pharynx dilate. The net result of swallowing is closure of the upper airway with interruption of airflow. Consequently, the timing and magnitude of muscle activation have important implications for airway size and patency.

The *pharynx* is a passageway for the entry and exit of air, and it plays a role in phonation by helping to produce vowel sounds. The pharynx contains the palatine and lingual tonsils, which are involved in infection control.

The *larynx,* situated at the upper end of the trachea, is constructed of a rigid circular framework of cartilage and contains the epiglottis and the glottis (vocal cords). These structures prevent solids or liquids from entering the airway during swallowing, and the vibrations of the vocal cords produce voice sounds. In infancy the *glottis* is located more cephalad (toward the head) than in later childhood, and

the laryngeal reflexes are very active. The *epiglottis* is longer and projects further posteriorly in infants. The narrowest portion of the larynx is at the level of the *cricoid cartilage.* In the infant and young child the ciliated columnar epithelium below the vocal cords is loosely bound with areolar tissue and is therefore more susceptible to edema formation. Swelling of the glottis and epiglottis produces hoarseness and often life-threatening obstruction of this portion of the airway.

The *lower airway* is made up of the lower trachea, mainstem bronchi, segmental bronchi, subsegmental bronchioles, terminal bronchioles, and alveoli. The *trachea,* which is composed of smooth muscle supported by C-shaped rings of cartilage, ensures an open airway to the bronchi and lungs. The trachea divides at the *carina* into two primary *bronchi.* The right one is situated slightly more vertical than the left, which causes aspirated objects to lodge more frequently in the right bronchus. Each bronchus enters the lung on its respective side, where it divides into secondary bronchi that continue to branch and divide into progressively smaller *bronchioles.* The entire bronchial tree is lined with mucous membrane and is composed of spiral smooth muscle supported by rings of cartilage. As the bronchioles become smaller, the cartilaginous rings become increasingly irregular and then disappear completely in the smallest bronchioles, the walls of which consist of only a single layer of cells (Fig. 31-3). There is a range of 23 to 26 levels of branches divided into two categories: the *conducting airways* and the *terminal respiratory units.* These branch levels are called *generations* (Thompson and others, 1997).

All of the structures are subject to obstruction from edema or foreign objects, but the degree of obstruction from constriction of smooth muscle differs. The diameter of the relatively rigid upper airway is less subject to constriction than the lower airway structures, which contain very lit-

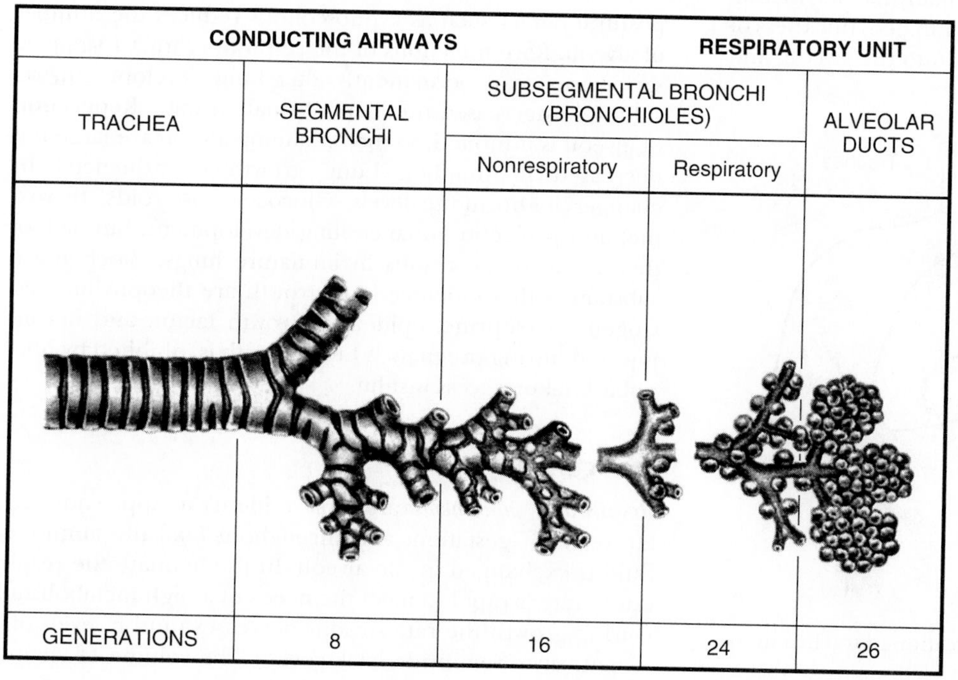

| CONDUCTING AIRWAYS | | | | RESPIRATORY UNIT |
|---|---|---|---|---|
| TRACHEA | SEGMENTAL BRONCHI | SUBSEGMENTAL BRONCHI (BRONCHIOLES) | | ALVEOLAR DUCTS |
| | | Nonrespiratory | Respiratory | |
| GENERATIONS | 8 | 16 | 24 | 26 |

**Fig. 31-3** Structures of the lower airway. (From Thompson JM and others: *Mosby's clinical nursing,* ed 4, St Louis, 1997, Mosby.)

tle cartilaginous support. The highly reactive bronchiolar smooth muscle of the lower airway structures can cause life-threatening obstruction during bronchoconstriction. The airway cartilage in young infants is very soft and compressible; therefore the intrathoracic airways are highly reactive to stimuli, such as vagal nerve stimulation.

The airways of the newborn have very little smooth muscle, but in children 4 to 5 months of age they contain sufficient muscle to cause narrowing in response to irritating stimuli. By 1 year of age, smooth muscle development and reactivity are comparable to that in the adult. Growth of the respiratory system follows the general growth curve during the early weeks of life, but the airways grow faster than the thoracic and cervical portions of the vertebral column. Consequently, the larynx and trachea descend in relation to the upper spine. For example, the bifurcation of the trachea that lies opposite the third thoracic vertebra in the infant descends to a position opposite the fourth in adulthood (Fig. 31-4). Likewise, the cricoid cartilage descends from a position opposite the fourth cervical vertebra in the infant to opposite the sixth cervical vertebra in the adult. These anatomic changes produce differences in the angle of access to the trachea at various ages and must be considered when the infant or child is positioned for resuscitation and airway clearance.

The function of the tracheobronchial tree is to distribute air to the alveoli of the lung. A variety of diseases and conditions, such as mucosal swelling, muscular contraction, and mechanical obstruction by mucus or a foreign body, can cause localized or generalized airway occlusion.

## Respiratory Units

The two cone-shaped lungs consist of the bronchi, bronchioles, and innumerable small **air sacs,** or **alveoli.** Through these thin-walled sacs, gas exchange occurs by simple diffusion between the inspired air and the bloodstream. The amount of gas exchanged depends on many factors, including the amount and composition of air inhaled, thickness of the alveolar wall, adequacy of circulation to the alveoli, and

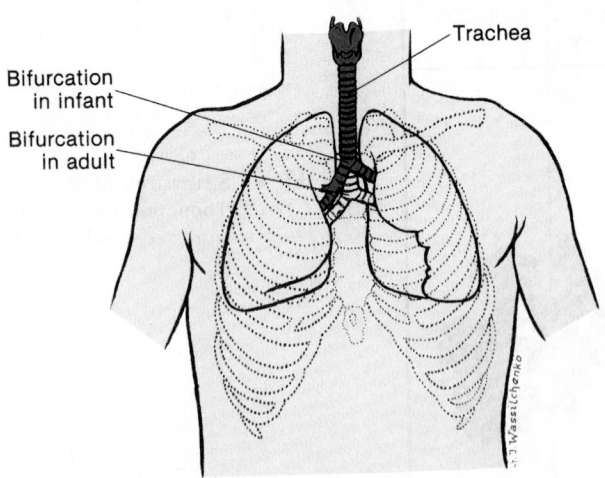

**Fig. 31-4** Difference in level of bifurcation of trachea in the infant and adult.

substances within the alveoli that either prevent their inflation (e.g., surface-active substance surfactant) or prevent gas exchange (e.g., fluids).

With age, changes take place in the air passages that increase the respiratory surface area. The major changes are in the number and size of alveoli and in the increased branching of terminal bronchioles. Although the number of conducting airways is complete early in fetal life, the air sacs are shallow with wide necks and have few shared walls, or *septa,* at birth. This promotes patency but limits surface area for gas exchange. The alveoli are large with thick septa that have little elastic recoil (not unlike the emphysemic lung). During the first year, bronchioles continue to branch, and the globular alveoli formed earlier in the terminal units rapidly increase in number with each generation. These alveoli partition and divide existing alveoli to form smaller lobular units separated by thinner septa, thus enlarging the area available for gas exchange.

Alveoli increase steadily in number, but it is unclear when septal division ceases and an increase in size begins. It appears to occur sometime during middle childhood, although evidence indicates that an increase in the number of alveoli for each terminal airway takes place at puberty. Approximately nine times as many alveoli are present at age 12 years than at birth. In later stages of growth the structures lengthen and enlarge. In addition, collateral pathways of ventilation develop, including pores through alveolar walls and possibly pathways between bronchioles.

All of these factors have significant implications for respiratory disorders in children. Infants and young children have less alveolar surface area for gas exchange, the narrowly branching peripheral airways become easily obstructed, and lack of collateral pathways inhibits ventilation beyond obstructed units. Consequently, young children are subject to obstruction and atelectasis, especially as a result of repeated infection.

A variety of pathologic conditions affect **lung growth.** A postural defect such as kyphoscoliosis reduces the number of alveoli. Rare infections of the respiratory tract (e.g., coxsackievirus) can permanently alter lung development, resulting in decreased numbers of small airways. Replication of alveoli is inhibited, so the remaining alveoli are large but decreased in number. Lung growth is influenced by changes in hormone levels. Glucocorticosteroids, thyroxine, and prolactin enhance lung development, but lack of thyroid hormone results in immature lungs. Biochemical substances that enhance lung growth are theophylline, estrogen, isoxsuprine, epidermal growth factor, and heroin injected during pregnancy. Lung growth is inhibited by phenobarbital or excess insulin.

## Function

**Respiratory movements** are first evident at approximately 20 weeks of gestation, and throughout fetal life amniotic fluid is exchanged in the alveoli. In the neonate the respiratory rate is rapid to meet the needs of a high metabolism. During growth the rate steadily decreases until it levels off at maturity. (See inside back cover.) The volume of air inhaled increases with the growth of the lungs and is closely related to body size. In addition, a qualitative difference exists in expired air at different ages. During growth the amount of $O_2$ in the expired air gradually decreases and the amount of $CO_2$ increases.

*Ventilation,* the passage of air in and out of the lungs, results from changes in pressure gradients created by changes in the size of the thoracic cavity. Contraction of the diaphragm and external intercostal muscles increases the size of the thorax and decreases the intrathoracic pressure. As a result, air moves from the atmosphere, which has a higher pressure, into the lungs, which have a lower pressure. The principles of *artificial ventilation* are based on this concept. Artificial respiratory devices increase the pressure entering the air passages *(positive-pressure breathing devices)* or lower the pressure around the body *(negative-pressure ventilator).*

The two primary forces that affect the mechanics of breathing are compliance and resistance; conditions that either increase or decrease these two forces are listed in Box 31-1. Compliance is a measure of chest wall and lung distensibility. It represents the relative ease with which the chest and lungs expand with increasing volume and then collapse away from the pleural wall with decreasing volume (elastic recoil). The two major factors determining compliance are (1) *alveolar surface tension,* which is lowered by **surfactant,** a lipoprotein at the air-fluid interface that allows alveolar expansion and prevents alveolar collapse, and (2) *elastic recoil,* the tendency of the lungs to return to the resting state after inspiration (a passive process that requires no muscular effort). Other factors influencing compliance include the degree of tissue hydration, lung blood volume, surface forces at the air-fluid interface, and chest or lung tissue pathology (i.e., fibers of elastin or collagen). Factors that interfere with compliance and recoil increase the work of breathing.

Compliance is normally very high in the newborn and infant because of a more pliant (flexible) rib cage. This greater compliance causes the rib cage to be easily distorted with increased negative pressure in the pleural cavity or when factors inhibit the stabilizing action of the intercostal muscles. As the child grows, chest wall compliance decreases and elastic recoil increases; therefore ventilation be-

comes progressively more efficient. In pathologic states an increase in compliance indicates that the lungs or chest wall are abnormally easy to inflate and have lost some elastic recoil, such as in asthma. A decrease in compliance indicates that the lungs or chest wall are abnormally stiff or difficult to inflate, such as in respiratory distress syndrome (McCance and Huether, 1998).

*Resistance* is determined primarily by airway size. Three sources of resistance must be overcome during breathing: tissue resistance in the chest wall (about 20% resistance), tissue resistance in the lungs (about 15% resistance), and, most important, flow resistance in the airways (which often increases with respiratory disease). The four factors determining resistance are flow rate velocity, gas viscosity, length of airway, and airway diameter. If any of the first three variables increases, resistance to airflow will also increase. If airway diameter decreases, resistance increases exponentially.

The small diameter of children's airways increases the potential risk of any condition that reduces airway size. (See Critical Thinking Exercise on p. 1308.) Fig. 31-5 illustrates the difference that airway size plays in older children's and infants' responses to airway compromise.

**NURSING ALERT**   Any condition that decreases or increases compliance or increases airway resistance results in increased work of breathing (increased respiratory rate, retractions, nasal flaring). If respiratory muscle fatigue develops, respiratory failure can occur.

The diameter of the airways and thus the airflow are determined by the balance of forces that tend to widen or narrow the airways. One of these is neural regulation of bronchial smooth muscles mediated through autonomic nerves. Sympathetic impulses relax the airways; parasympathetic impulses constrict them. Reflex constriction occurs in response to irritating inhalants such as dust, smoke, or sulfur dioxide; arterial hypoxemia and hypercapnia; cold air; and some drugs, such as acetylcholine and histamine. Other factors that alter airway size are peribronchial pressure, which tends to narrow the airways, and intraluminal pressure, which tends to keep the airways open. For example, forced expiration causes increased peribronchial pressure

---

**Box 31-1**

**Conditions and Diseases Affecting Lung Compliance and Resistance**

| COMPLIANCE | | RESISTANCE | |
|---|---|---|---|
| **DECREASED** | **INCREASED** | **INCREASED** | **DECREASED** |
| Pulmonary edema | Lobar emphysema | Asthma | Normal lung fields |
| Pneumothorax | Asthma | Cystic fibrosis | |
| Atelectasis | | Bronchopulmonary dysplasia (BPD) | |
| Pulmonary fibrosis | | Bronchiolitis | |
| Absence of muscles of breathing | | Tracheostenosis | |
| Neuromuscular conditions | | Conditions with high amount of secretions | |
| Surfactant deficiency | | | |
| Distended fluid spaces | | | |
| Engorged blood vessels | | | |

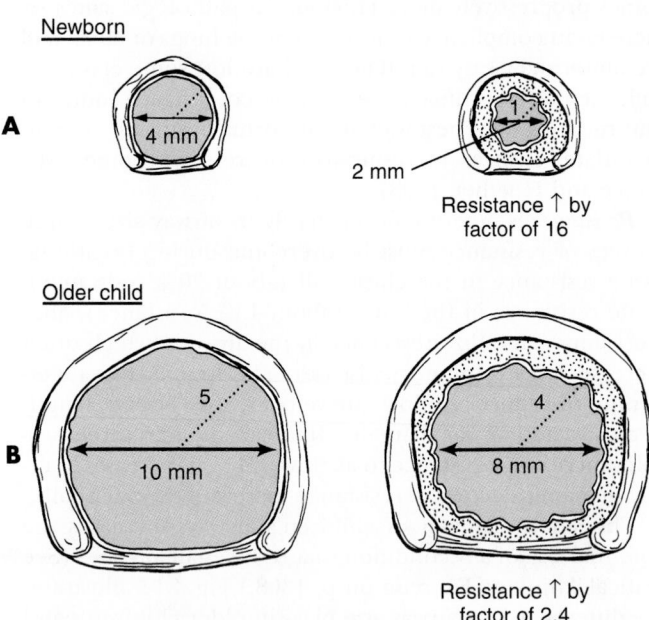

Newborn

A

4 mm

2 mm

Resistance ↑ by
factor of 16

Older child

B

5

10 mm

4

8 mm

Resistance ↑ by
factor of 2.4

**Fig. 31-5** Effects of 1 mm of circumferential edema in small neonate and an older child. **A,** The neonate possesses a larynx approximately 4 mm in diameter and 2 mm in radius. If 1 mm of circumferential edema develops, it will halve the airway radius and increase resistance to air flow by a factor of 16. **B,** The older child possesses a larynx approximately 10 mm in diameter and 5 mm in radius. The 1 mm of circumferential edema will reduce the radius by 20% (from 5 mm to 4 mm) and increase resistance to air flow by a factor of 2.4 (From Hazinski MF, editor: *Nursing care of the critically ill child,* ed 2, St Louis, 1992, Mosby.)

## Critical Thinking Exercise

### Anatomic Differences in Respiratory Structures

Susie is 4 months old and is hospitalized because of respiratory problems. Susie's nurse, Mary, has only been working in pediatrics for 1 month although she has been a nurse for 5 years and previously cared for many adults with respiratory disorders. In providing nursing care for Susie, Mary will need to remember that infants are more vulnerable to respiratory alterations than adults for which of the following reasons?

FIRST, THINK ABOUT IT . . .
• What is the purpose of your thinking?
• What conclusions are you coming to?

1. Oxygen consumption in infants is lower in proportion to body surface area.
2. The cilia lining an infant's airways are nonfunctional.
3. Infants have fewer accessory muscles to use for respiration.
4. The smaller diameter of infants' airways places them at risk for conditions that further reduce their airway size.

*The best response is four. The diameter of the infant's airways is anatomically smaller than those of an adult. Thus the correct conclusion is that conditions that further reduce the diameter, such as irritants, edema, or infection, significantly increase airway resistance and the work of breathing for the infant. The first answer is incorrect because both the respiratory rate and oxygen consumption are high in proportion to body surface area in the infant. However, the cilia and accessory muscles are adequately developed in infants.*

and hence narrowing of the airways; a positive-pressure breathing apparatus increases intraluminal pressure, keeping the airways open.

### Gas Exchange

Gases in the blood are measured by the *partial pressures (tensions)* of the individual gases and are expressed in millimeters of mercury. With $O_2$ therapy it is important to understand the relationship between the concentration of the inspired gas and the partial pressure of that gas in the arteries ($PaO_2$). Inspired $O_2$ is expressed as the *fraction of inspired $O_2$ ($FIO_2$),* with 1.0 indicating 100% $O_2$, 0.5 indicating 50% $O_2$, and so on. Patients breathing room air have an $FIO_2$ of 0.21 because ambient air contains 21% $O_2$.

Ambient air is composed of 21% $O_2$, trace amounts of $CO_2$, and 79% nitrogen (N). Water vapor ($H_2O$) also exerts a pressure. The water vapor does not change with the barometric pressure ($PB$) but exerts a constant pressure of 47 mm Hg when the gas is fully saturated at body temperature. Each gas contributes to the total $PB$ as follows:

$$PB = PO_2 + PCO_2 + PN_2 + PH_2O$$

At sea level, the total pressure of gases in the atmosphere and the blood ($PB$) is always equal to 760 mm Hg.

The significance of inspired gases lies in the $FIO_2$ and the pressure it exerts ($PIO_2$). At sea level this can be calculated as follows:

$$PIO_2 = FIO_2 \times (PB - PH_2O)$$
$$PIO_2 = 0.21 \times (760 - 47)$$
$$PIO_2 = 0.21 \times 713$$
$$PIO_2 = 150 \text{ mm Hg}$$

When the $FIO_2$ is increased (for example to 50%), the pressure exerted also increases:

$$PIO_2 = 0.50 \times (760 - 47)$$
$$PIO_2 = 0.50 \times 713$$
$$PIO_2 = 356.5 \text{ mm Hg}$$

As the inspired gas travels down the airway and reaches the alveoli, the pressure drops as $CO_2$ is added to the mixture. Ambient air contains only traces of $CO_2$. As the gas diffuses from the capillary blood to the alveoli, however, the amount and pressure of $CO_2$ in the alveoli increase to the $CO_2$ levels in the venous blood (approximately 40 mm Hg). By subtracting the $PCO_2$ from the $PIO_2$, the alveolar $O_2$ pressure ($PAO_2$) can be determined. The $PACO_2$ is first divided by 0.8. This correlation factor, or respiratory quotient (RQ), is used to calculate the ratio of $O_2$ absorbed to

$CO_2$ eliminated. The alveolar pressure can then be expressed as:

$$PAo_2 = PIo_2 - (PAco_2 \div 0.8)$$
$$PAo_2 = 150 - (40 \div 0.8)$$
$$PAo_2 = 150 - 50$$
$$PAo_2 = 100 \text{ mm Hg}$$

Because normal venous $Po_2$ is approximately 40 mm Hg, a gradient is created when the $PAo_2$ is 100 mm Hg and diffusion occurs between the alveoli and capillary blood. When the patient's $Pao_2$ decreases, the $FIo_2$ can be raised to increase the $PAo_2$, thereby increasing the gradient for diffusion.

Because $CO_2$ is more soluble than $O_2$, it diffuses 21 times faster; therefore diffusion of $CO_2$ from the blood to the alveoli is not impaired. The amount of $O_2$ that diffuses into the blood and the amount of $CO_2$ removed by the lungs depend on several factors (Box 31-2).

**Oxygen/Carbon Dioxide Transport.** Once $O_2$ has diffused from the alveolus to the pulmonary capillary, it is transported throughout the body in two ways. A small amount ($Pao_2$) is transported as a solute dissolved in the plasma and the water of red blood cells. A larger portion (40 to 70 times as much) is carried by hemoglobin as *oxyhemoglobin.* Because each gram of hemoglobin can combine with 1.34 ml of $O_2$, the transport capacity is largely determined by the amount of hemoglobin present. Thus children with severe anemia tend to be fatigued and breathe more rapidly. In addition, increasing the amount of $O_2$ delivered to the alveoli can increase the amount carried by the blood only in relation to the amount of hemoglobin present. For example, at a $Pao_2$ of 100 mm Hg, hemoglobin is 97.5% saturated. Hemoglobin saturation is commonly termed *arterial oxygen saturation ($Sao_2$)* or *oxyhemoglobin saturation.* The *nonlinear* relationship between the $Pao_2$ and the $Sao_2$ is described by the oxyhemoglobin dissociation curve (see Fig. 31-10).

$CO_2$ is carried in the blood in a number of ways. A small amount ($Paco_2$) is transported dissolved in the plasma and the water of red blood cells. A large amount (more than half) hydrates to form carbonic acid, which dissociates and is carried as bicarbonate and hydrogen ions. The remaining $CO_2$ combines with certain plasma proteins and hemoglobin. The association of $CO_2$ with hemoglobin is accelerated by an increasing $Paco_2$ and a decreasing $Pao_2$ and is decreased by the opposite conditions. The diffusion of $CO_2$ into the alveoli is very rapid. Thus the equilibrium between the $Paco_2$ of the pulmonary capillaries and the alveoli is achieved promptly. Transport between blood and tissue cells is accomplished down a diffusion gradient, just as it is between the blood and the alveoli.

**Regulation of Respiration.** The mechanisms that control respiration are divided into two categories: (1) a *neural system* that maintains a coordinated, rhythmic respiratory cycle and regulates the depth of respiration and (2) a *chemical* system that regulates alveolar ventilation and maintains normal blood gas pressures.

*Neural control* in the respiratory center is located in three areas: a *pneumotaxic center,* which modulates the respiratory frequency and depth; an *apneustic center,* which produces an inspiratory spasm and is modulated by the pneumotaxic and medullary centers and by vagal afferent impulses; and the *medullary respiratory centers,* both inspiratory and expiratory, which regulate the rhythmicity of respirations. Impulses from other areas also affect the respiratory centers. *Proprioceptive vagal impulses* in the lung parenchyma are sensitive to stretching. When lungs become stretched, impulses are transmitted by the vagus nerve to the respiratory center, which inhibits further inflation and prevents overdistention—the *Hering-Breuer reflex.* The cerebral cortex also helps to control respirations by voluntary inhibition or acceleration of the rate and depth of respirations. Reflex apnea can result from sudden painful stimulation, sudden cold stimulation, and stimulation to the larynx or pharynx (the choking reflex, which serves to prevent aspiration).

*Chemical control* is mediated by specialized structures that respond to changes in pH, $Pco_2$, and $Po_2$—*central chemoreceptors,* located in the medulla, and *peripheral chemoreceptors,* located in the great vessels. Peripheral chemoreceptors of greatest physiologic importance are the carotid bodies, located at the division of the common carotid artery into its external and internal branches, and the aortic bodies that lie between the ascending aorta and the pulmonary artery. $CO_2$ and hydrogen ions control respiration by acting directly on the respiratory center; the peripheral chemoreceptors respond to changes in $Po_2$. Thus an increase in ventilation can result from either (1) stimulation of the respiratory center by an increased $Paco_2$ or pH or (2) a decreased $Pao_2$, which stimulates the carotid and aortic bodies. These bodies then transmit signals to the brain to excite the respiratory center.

The lungs also have an important role in *acid-base balance.* Less rapid than the chemical buffers, the respiratory mechanism begins to act within 1 to 3 minutes to make adjustments in pH by eliminating or retaining $CO_2$. When the levels of $CO_2$ are altered sufficiently, the respiratory centers in the brain respond by either increasing or decreasing the rate and depth of respirations. For example, when the pH of the blood drops, as from increased exercise, a compensatory increase in respirations rids the body of the $CO_2$ derived from carbonic acid, which is formed from buffered acid metabolites. $CO_2$ buildup from breath holding produces the same response, again increasing the carbonic acid and reducing the serum pH. Therefore the lungs serve as compensatory organs in metabolic disturbances and respond quite rapidly.

### Defenses of the Respiratory Tract

The respiratory tract has several anatomic and biochemical characteristics that provide natural defenses against the many biologic and inanimate agents that can damage respiratory tissues. Intact defenses help to repel and resist the impact of injurious agents; factors that reduce the integrity of these mechanisms increase the vulnerability of these tissues to invasion and disease. Respiratory tract defenses include:

**Lymphoid tissues**—Faucial, lingual, and pharyngeal tonsils (adenoids) and other pharyngeal lymphoid tissues form a protective circle around the entrance to the respiratory tract. These help to localize and contain invading organisms so that they can be destroyed by the body's humoral defense mechanisms.

**Mucous blanket**—The epithelium of the respiratory tract secretes a sticky mucus to which airborne organisms adhere.

**Ciliary action**—The mucus secreted by the columnar epithelium of the respiratory tract is kept flowing, carrying microorganisms and other foreign agents away from the lungs to be coughed or swallowed.

**Epiglottis**—The epiglottis and the epiglottis reflex protect the respiratory tract from invading material, including infectious exudate from the upper tract, and prevent such material from being aspirated into the lower tract.

**Cough**—The expulsive force of the cough reflex propels foreign material out of the lower tract.

**Tracheobronchial dynamics**—The tracheobronchial tree elongates and dilates on inspiration and shortens and narrows on expiration.

**Position changes**—Changes in body position encourage drainage of tracheobronchial passages.

**Lymphatics**—Lymphatics draining the terminal bronchi and bronchioles remove invading organisms, which are filtered and destroyed in the regional lymph nodes.

**Humoral defenses**—Organisms and other foreign material are removed or destroyed by phagocytes, enzymes, and immunoglobulins, especially immunoglobulin A (IgA), secreted by the bronchial epithelium.

Some children have conditions that predispose them to infection as a result of interference with the efficiency of these mechanisms (e.g., chronic asthma, cystic fibrosis, and the various immunodeficiency disorders). Frequent, intense exposure to organisms that accompany conditions of crowding or continual exposure to irritating substances in the air results in breakdown of healthy defenses. Concurrent illness, malnutrition, or fatigue reduces the efficiency of natural defenses. Drying of the mucous membranes also inhibits the activity of humoral defenses, such as immunoglobulins.

## ASSESSMENT OF RESPIRATORY FUNCTION

### Physical Assessment

Information about the child's respiratory status is obtained from observations of physical signs and behavior. However, to make a useful assessment, the nurse must know what to look for and how to interpret findings. (See Physical Examination: Chest, Chapter 7.) *Auscultation* of the lung fields is helpful in identifying specific pathologies and in assessing the child's responses to treatment. Auscultation is essential when determining airway patency. *Palpation* and *percussion* provide information regarding areas of pain and tissue density. Breath sounds and their terminology are described in Chapter 7.

### Respiration

The configuration of the chest and the pattern of respiratory movement, including rate, regularity, symmetry of movements, depth, effort expended in respiration, and use of accessory muscles of respiration, should be assessed. To determine deviations, the nurse must know the normal type and rate of respiration in relation to the child's size and age. (See inside back cover.) Respirations (ventilations) are best determined when the child is sleeping or quietly awake.

*Tachypnea* (rapid respirations) is observed with anxiety, elevated temperature, severe anemia, and metabolic acidosis. It may also be associated with respiratory alkalosis caused by psychoneurosis and with central nervous system disturbances. The progress of disorders that contribute to low compliance, such as the pneumonias, pulmonary edema, and pleural effusion, can be followed and evaluated by observing changes in respiratory rate.

Alterations in the depth of respirations—too deep *(hyperpnea)* or too shallow *(hypopnea)*—are recognized as abnormal only in the extremes. Hyperpnea is noted with fever, severe anemia, respiratory alkalosis associated with psychosis, central nervous system disturbances, and respiratory acidosis that accompanies disorders such as diabetes mellitus or diarrhea. Hypoventilation is less easily detected and occurs with metabolic alkalosis in conditions such as pyloric stenosis and respiratory acidosis that accompanies diaphragmatic paralysis or central nervous system depression.

### Associated Observations

*Retractions,* or a sinking in of soft tissues relative to the cartilaginous and bony thorax, may be noted in some pulmonary disorders. In disease states (particularly in severe airway obstruction), retraction becomes extreme. Subcostal retraction, observed anteriorly at the lower costal margins, indicates a flattened diaphragm because it not only lowers the floor of the thorax, but also pulls on the rib cage in response to a greater than normal decrease in intrathoracic pressure. In severe obstruction, retractions extend to the supraclavicular areas and the suprasternal notch. See Fig. 31-6 for location of retractions.

*Nasal flaring* is a sign of respiratory distress and a very significant finding in an infant. The enlargement of the nos-

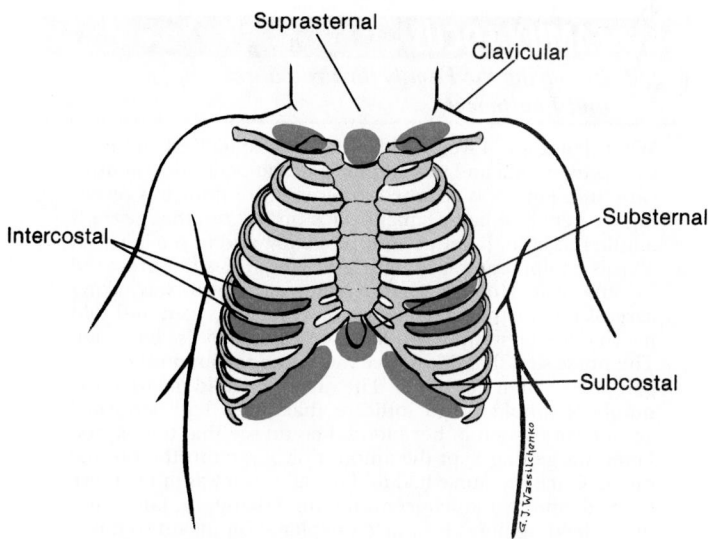

**Fig. 31-6**   Location of retractions.

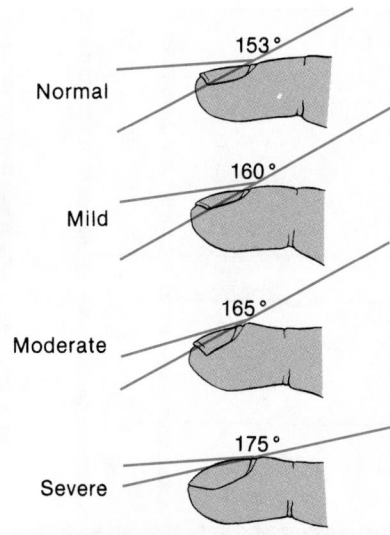

**Fig. 31-7**   Stages of clubbing. Degree of angle formed above finger at skin-nail junction indicates extent of clubbing. Angle greater than 160 degrees and decided curvature of nail are good criteria for presence of clubbing. (Modified from Waring WW: The history and physical examination. In Chernick V, editor: *Kendig's disorders of the respiratory tract in children*, ed 6, Philadelphia, 1998, WB Saunders.)

trils helps reduce nasal resistance and maintains airway patency. Nasal flaring may be intermittent or continuous and should be described as minimal or marked.

*Head bobbing* in a sleeping or exhausted infant is a sign of dyspnea. The head, supported on the caregiver's arm only at the suboccipital area, will bob forward with each inspiration. This is caused by neck flexion resulting from contraction of the scalene and sternocleidomastoid muscles. *Noisy breathing* such as "snoring" is frequently associated with hypertrophied adenoidal tissue, choanal obstruction, polyps, or a foreign body in the nasal passages.

*Grunting* is frequently a sign of chest pain, suggesting acute pneumonia or pleural involvement. It is also observed in pulmonary edema and is a characteristic of respiratory distress syndrome. It serves to increase end-respiratory pressure and thus prolong the period of $O_2$ and $CO_2$ exchange across the alveolocapillary membrane.

*Color changes* of the skin, especially mottling, pallor, and cyanosis, are important. Except for the peripheral bluish discoloration resulting from circulatory stasis in the newborn or the mottling or peripheral cyanosis resulting from a cool environment, mottling and cyanosis are significant and usually indicate cardiopulmonary disease.

*Chest pain* may be a complaint of older children and may have a variety of causes, both pulmonary and nonpulmonary. It may be caused by disease of any of the chest structures—esophagus, pericardium, diaphragm, pleura, or chest wall. *Parietal pleural pain* is usually localized over the affected area and is aggravated by respiratory movements. The pain of *diaphragmatic pleural irritation* may be referred to the base of the neck posteriorly and anteriorly or to the abdomen. Most pleural pain is related to respiration; therefore respiratory movements are shallow and rapid.

*Clubbing*, or proliferation of tissue about the terminal phalanges, accompanies a variety of conditions, frequently those associated with chronic hypoxia, primarily cardiac defects and chronic pulmonary disease. Although club-

---

**Box 31-3**
**Causes of Cough**

Inflammatory disorders
   Asthma, infections
Lung disease
   Cystic fibrosis, bronchiolitis, retained foreign body, congenital malformations
Focal or anatomic lesions
Psychogenic or habit cough
Postnasal drip or sinusitis

---

bing often worsens with lung disease, it does not reflect disease progression accurately. The degree of clubbing is determined by the extent to which the nail base is lifted on the dorsal surface of the phalanx by the tissue proliferation. The greater the angle formed above the finger or toe at the skin-nail junction, the more pronounced the clubbing, especially when there is a decided curvature to the nail (Fig. 31-7).

*Cough* is often associated with respiratory disease, although it may suggest other disorders (Box 31-3). It serves as a protective mechanism as well as an indicator of irritation. A cough can be initiated voluntarily but is usually a result of a complex reflex consisting of three components: afferent nerve fibers, the cough center, and efferent nerve fibers. The respiratory epithelium contains afferent receptors that are sensitive to mechanical or chemical stimuli. These receptors are concentrated in the areas of the larynx, the carina, and the bifurcations of the large and medium-sized bronchi. When a stimulus is applied to these areas, impulses are transmitted via the vagus nerve to the cough cen-

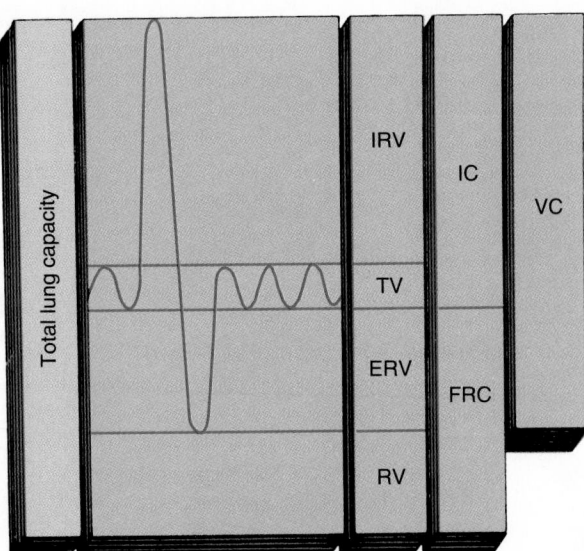

**Fig. 31-8**   Divisions of total lung capacity. Total lung capacity *(TLC)* is the maximum amount of air contained in the lungs. The total lung capacity is divided into four primary volumes: *IRV,* inspiratory reserve volume; *TV,* tidal volume; *ERV,* expiratory reserve volume; and *RV,* residual volume. **Capacities** are combinations of two or more lung volumes. These include inspiratory capacity *(IC),* functional residual capacity *(FRC),* and vital capacity *(VC).* (From Shapiro BA, Harrison RA, Walton R: *Clinical application of blood gases,* ed 3, St Louis, 1982, Mosby.)

---

**Box 31-4 ■ ■ ▫**
**Cough Assessment**

**Onset and duration**
**Type**—Dry, hacking, moist, barking, brassy, paroxysmal (a sudden attack, outburst, or intensification of symptoms)
**Progress**—Better, worse, unchanged, persistent
**Pattern**—Daytime, nighttime, both, different intensity with time or activity
**Associated symptoms**—Sore throat, dyspnea, pain and its location
**Secretions**—Sputum presence, consistency, color, frequency, evidence of swallowing sputum, postnasal drip

---

ter in the brainstem. Efferent impulses travel via the vagus, phrenic, and spinal motor nerves to the larynx, intercostal muscles, diaphragm, abdominal muscles, and pelvic floor. An inspiratory gasp and closure of the glottis are followed by contraction of muscles in the chest wall, diaphragm, abdomen, and pelvic floor. The resulting compression and increase in pleural, alveolar, and subglottic pressure cause a sudden opening of the glottis and immediate release of trapped air at extremely rapid expiratory flow rates, which forces undesirable material from the respiratory tract.

Inflammation or infection in the upper or lower respiratory tract may produce coughing. Some types of cough are characteristic of specific diseases. For example, a severe cough is associated with measles and cystic fibrosis, and the paroxysmal cough accompanied by an inspiratory "whoop" is typical of pertussis. A brassy cough is part of the sympto-

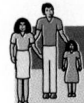
matology of croup and foreign body aspiration. Because there are no cough receptors in the alveoli, a cough may be absent in a child with pneumonia in the early stages of the disease but is a common feature during active pneumonia and recovery. Cough is assessed according to the features listed in Box 31-4.

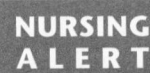

**NURSING ALERT**   Coughing is not normal and should be investigated further.

## Diagnostic Procedures

Several procedures are available for assessing respiratory function and diagnosing respiratory disease. All of these procedures require preparation and support of the child and the family to ensure cooperation and accurate results. (See Family Focus box.) These procedures not only are useful in diagnosis, but also provide information that guides nursing interventions, such as positioning, use of supplemental $O_2$, and assistance with coughing or deep breathing.

### Pulmonary Function Tests

Noninvasive pulmonary mechanics are often measured at the bedside of infants and children with the use of pneumotachography or spirometry. However, information obtained limits diagnosis because the same functional abnormality may occur in different diseases. These tests are useful to evaluate the severity and course of a disease and to study the effects of treatment. A listing of the measured parameters is provided in Table 31-1 and Fig. 31-8.

### Radiology and Other Diagnostic Procedures

Radiography is used frequently in diagnostic evaluation of children. Although no definitive information exists on the

**TABLE 31-1    Pulmonary function and blood gas tests used in children**

| Test | Measurement | Significance |
|------|-------------|--------------|
| Forced vital capacity (FVC) (peak flow) | Maximum amount of air that can be expired after maximum inspiration | Reduced in obesity<br>Reduced in obstructive airway disease<br>Normal in restrictive disease |
| Forced expiratory volume in 1 ($FEV_1$) or 3 ($FEV_3$) seconds | Amount of air that can be forced from lungs after maximum inspiration in 1 and 3 seconds | Normally 80% of FVC in 1 second<br>Reduced in obstructive disease<br>Is the single best measure of airway function |
| Tidal volume (TV or $V_T$) | Amount of air inhaled and exhaled during any respiratory cycle | Multiplied by respiratory rate to provide minute volume<br>Information needed to determine rate and depth of artificial ventilation<br>Allows for aeration of alveoli |
| Functional residual volume (FRV); functional residual capacity (FRC) | Volume of air remaining in lungs after passive expiration | Increased in hyperinflated lungs of obstructive lung disease |
| Dynamic compliance | Relationship between change in volume and pressure difference | Reflects elastic recoil of lung<br>Normal volume but decreased airflow in obstructive disease (e.g., asthma)<br>Normal flow but decreased volume in restrictive disease (e.g., pulmonary fibrosis) |
| Pulmonary resistance | Changes in pressure with changes in flow on inspiration and expiration | |
| Work of breathing | Total work expended moving lung and chest | |
| Respiratory time constancy | Time for proximal and alveolar airway pressure to equilibrate | |
| Blood oxygenation | | |
| Transcutaneous $O_2/CO_2$ monitoring (TCM) | Skin surface electrodes heated and applied to well-perfused areas of trunk; measurements in mm Hg | Provides continuous and reliable trends of arterial $O_2$ and $CO_2$<br>Noninvasive |
| Oximetry | Photometric measurement of $O_2$ saturation ($SaO_2$) Measurements in percentages | Provides continuous noninvasive measurements of hemoglobin saturation |
| Capnography | Measures $CO_2$ during inhalation and exhalation cycle and produces a graph of $CO_2$ concentration over time | Provides end-tidal $CO_2$ levels to determine trends and identify shunts |
| Arterial puncture | Arterial blood obtained from temporal (neonates), brachial, radial, posterior tibial, and femoral arteries | Obtains blood for gas analysis ($PO_2$, $PCO_2$, pH) |
| $FEV_1$ or $FEV_3$/FVC | Percentage of maximum inspiration that is expired in 1 or 3 seconds | Normally 95% of FVC in 3 seconds<br>Reduced in obstructive disease |

effects of low-dose radiation, measures are carried out to protect vulnerable areas from possible damage. When possible, technicians and others try to prevent unnecessary exposure of the child (and personnel), and the more radiosensitive areas are protected. Careful protection of the immature gonads of the infant or child with lead shields is essential. Other sensitive areas are the thyroid gland, ocular lens, and bone marrow.

Although nurses have limited control over the length, frequency, and correct application of the x-ray beam, they can make certain that the infant or child receives proper protection from possible hazards. Lead shields, correctly placed and consistently applied to areas not needed for diagnostic purposes, are essential. Play and modification of methodology can be used effectively to reduce the trauma sometimes associated with the procedure and to gain the child's cooperation. Special radiologic examinations used in respiratory diagnosis are outlined in Table 31-2.

Several other procedures are used to diagnose lung disorders (Table 31-3). Most require specialized equipment and skills. All require preparation of the child.

## Blood Gas Determination

Blood gas measurements are sensitive indicators of change in respiratory status in acutely ill patients (see Table 31-4). They provide valuable information regarding lung function, lung adequacy, and tissue perfusion and are essential for monitoring conditions involving hypoxemia, $CO_2$ retention, and pH. For the acutely ill patient, this information also guides decisions regarding therapeutic interventions, such as adjusting the ventilator, increasing chest physiotherapy, administering $O_2$, or positioning the child for maximum ventilation. Both invasive and noninvasive methods are available. (See Atraumatic Care box on p. 1314.)

*Pulse oximetry* provides a continuous or intermittent noninvasive method of determining $O_2$ saturation ($SaO_2$). A sensor comprising a light-emitting diode (LED) and a photodetector is placed in opposition around a foot, hand, finger, toe, or earlobe, with the LED placed on top of the nail when digits are used (Fig. 31-9). The diode emits red and infrared lights that pass through the skin to the photodetector. The photodetector measures the amount of each type of light absorbed by *functional hemoglobins* (those

**TABLE 31-2**    Radiologic examinations

| Test | Description | Purpose | Comment |
|---|---|---|---|
| Radiography | Pictures obtained by passing x-rays through body and recording them on sensitized film | Produces images of internal structures of chest, including air-filled lungs, airways, vascular markings, heart, and great vessels | Requires preparation, cooperation, and immobilization of child |
| Fluoroscopy | Projection of electronically intensified image on viewing screen | Used primarily to study diaphragmatic excursion and respiratory motion of lungs<br>Examination of barium-filled esophagus to outline mediastinal abnormalities | Requires preparation and immobilization of child |
| Bronchography | Contrast medium is instilled directly into bronchial tree through opaque catheter inserted via orotracheal tube | Valuable to demonstrate and inspect bronchiectasis<br>Detects distal bronchial obstruction<br>Detects malformations | Carried out with child under general anesthesia or sedation<br>Used less frequently than other examinations<br>Prepare child for anesthesia |
| Barium swallow | Esophagus is outlined when barium solution or colloid is swallowed | Esophageal displacement defines mediastinal masses<br>Detects swallowing disorders and malformations (e.g., tracheoesophageal fistula) | Valuable adjunct for diagnosis<br>Performed under fluoroscope<br>Prepare child for procedure |
| Angiography | Injection of dye to produce image of pulmonary vasculature | Investigation of pulmonary vascular anomalies and pulmonary hypertension | Performed with child under general anesthesia<br>Prepare child for anesthesia |
| Computed tomography (CT) | Sequence of x-rays, each representing a cross section or "cut" through lung tissue at different depth | Useful in identifying presence of calcium or a cavity within a lesion, hilar adenopathy, mediastinal masses, or abnormalities | Usually reserved for children old enough to suspend respiration voluntarily<br>Prepare child for procedure |
| Magnetic resonance imaging (MRI) | Use of large magnet and radio waves to produce two- or three-dimensional image | Clearly identifies soft tissues | Requires cooperation or sedation of child<br>Prepare child for procedure or anesthesia |
| Radioisotope scanning | Intravenous injection of albumin labeled with radioisotopes or inhalation of radioactive aerosols or xenon gas followed by radiation scanning | Delineates defects in pulmonary arterial perfusion and diseased areas of lung<br>Detects location of aspirated foreign body | Requires cooperation or sedation of child<br>Prepare child for procedure |
| Ultrasonography | Transmission of sound waves through chest | Identifies opacification | Limited use in diagnosis of respiratory disorders<br>Prepare child for procedure |

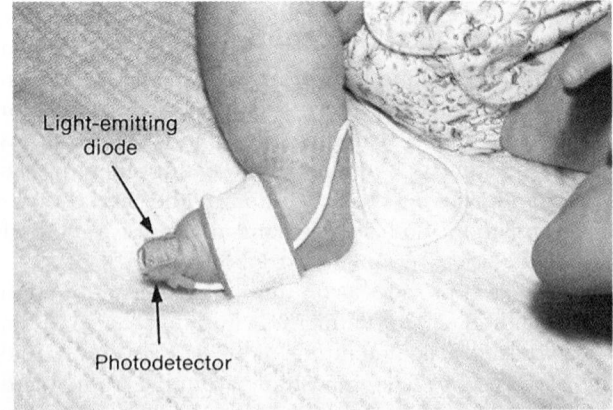

**Fig. 31-9**    Oximeter sensor on great toe. Note that sensor is positioned with light-emitting diode opposite photodetector. Cord is secured to foot with self-adhering band (not tape) to minimize movement of sensor.

**ATRAUMATIC CARE**
*Blood Gas Monitoring*

For continuous monitoring of blood gases, noninvasive measurements are used whenever possible. Oximetry should be used before arterial punctures are performed when information about $O_2$ saturation is sufficient to evaluate the child's condition.

capable of carrying $O_2$). Hemoglobin saturated with $O_2$ *(oxyhemoglobin)* absorbs more infrared light than does hemoglobin not saturated with $O_2$ *(deoxyhemoglobin).* A microprocessor determines the difference between absorption of the red and infrared light. The percentage of the total normal hemoglobin that is oxygenated is displayed on a monitor. Pulsatile blood flow is the primary physiologic factor that influences accuracy of the pulse oximeter.

Another noninvasive method is *transcutaneous monitoring (TCM),* which provides continuous monitoring of transcu-

**TABLE 31-3    Diagnostic procedures used in respiratory disorders**

| Procedure | Description | Purpose |
|---|---|---|
| Tracheal aspiration | Sputum obtained by direct aspiration from trachea | Obtains secretions for examination, culture |
| Bronchoscopy | Direct observation of tracheobronchial tree via bronchoscope | Localizes abnormalities in major airways<br>Provides access to (1) remove aspirated foreign bodies from major airways, (2) remove obstructive mucous plugs, and (3) perform bronchial lavage |
| Lung puncture | Needle aspiration of lung fluid via syringe and needle through intercostal space | Obtains lung aspirate for histologic study or culture |
| Lung biopsy | Removal of lung tissue via open thoracotomy or closed-needle procedures | Used for diagnosis of protracted pulmonary disease unexplained by other means |
| Brush biopsy | Material for biopsy obtained with nylon brush on end of wire passed through tube placed via nose, pharynx, trachea, and airways (via fluoroscope) to involved lung segment | Obtains material for culture and histologic examination |
| Percutaneous transtracheal aspiration | Needle and catheter aspiration of tracheal secretions through thyroid cartilage | Obtains secretions for laboratory examination and culture |

taneous partial pressure of $O_2$ in arterial blood (tcPa$O_2$) and, with some devices, of $CO_2$ in arterial blood (tcPa$CO_2$). An electrode is attached to the warmed skin to facilitate arterialization of cutaneous capillaries. The site of the electrode must be changed every 3 to 4 hours to prevent burning the skin, and the machine must be calibrated with every site change. This monitoring is used frequently in neonatal intensive care units, but it may not reflect Pa$O_2$ in infants with impaired local circulation or in older infants whose skin is thicker.

The Pa$O_2$ can be correlated with the Sa$O_2$ by means of the *oxyhemoglobin dissociation curve* (Fig. 31-10), although changes in Pa$O_2$ do not cause identical (linear) changes in Sa$O_2$. The curve represents the relationship between Pa$O_2$ (measured in the blood) and Sa$O_2$ (measured by the pulse oximeter). As seen on the graph, when the Pa$O_2$ is 60 mm Hg, the Sa$O_2$ is 90%. Increasing the Pa$O_2$ above this point does not significantly increase Sa$O_2$ or greatly improve oxygen delivery to the tissues. At this point, further increases in the Pa$O_2$ will only increase the dissolved $O_2$ in the blood and will not, under normal conditions, contribute significantly to the arterial $O_2$ content. On the lower part of the curve, however, even small changes in the Pa$O_2$ produce large changes in saturation. This is an advantage at the tissue level, especially in low oxygen states (hypoxia) because a small decrease in Pa$O_2$ will cause a relatively large unloading of oxygen to the tissues.

**NURSING TIP** A quick formula for calculating correlation of Pa$O_2$ with Sa$O_2$ is the 30-60, 60-90 rule. Assuming a normal pH, Pa$CO_2$, and body temperature, this rule can apply: when Pa$O_2$ = 30, Sa$O_2$ = 60; when Pa$O_2$ = 60, Sa$O_2$ = 90.

Oximetry is insensitive to hyperoxia because hemoglobin approaches 100% saturation for all Pa$O_2$ readings above approximately 100 mm Hg, which is a dangerous situation for the preterm infant at risk for developing retinopathy of prematurity. (See Chapter 10.) Therefore the preterm infant being monitored with oximetry should have upper limits identified, such as 90% to 95%, and a protocol should be established for decreasing $O_2$ when saturations are high.

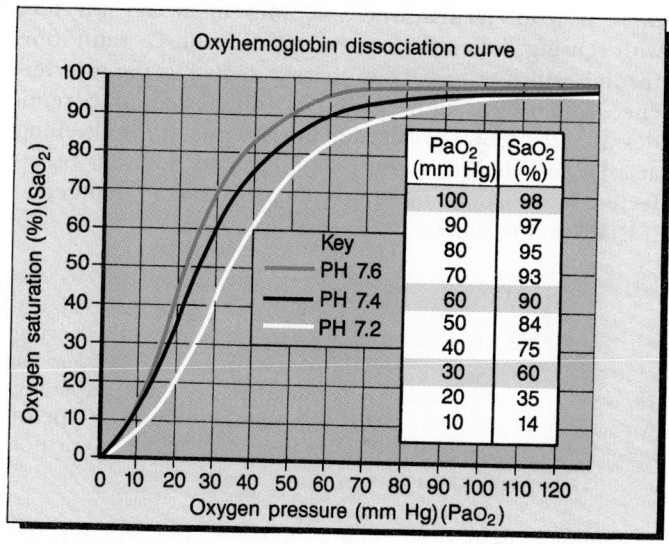

**Fig. 31-10**  Oxyhemoglobin dissociation curve. Changes in the affinity of hemoglobin for oxygen shift the position of the oxyhemoglobin dissociation curve. *Standard curve* (black): Assumes normal pH (7.4), temperature, and Pco$_2$ levels. *Shift to left* (blue): Increased $O_2$ affinity of hemoglobin: increased pH, decreased temperature and Pco$_2$. *Shift to right* (white): Decreasesd $O_2$ affinity of hemoglobin: decreased pH, increased temperature and Pco$_2$.

The degree to which $O_2$ combines with hemoglobin is affected by several factors. A *shift of the curve to the left* causes an increased affinity of hemoglobin for $O_2$, but the $O_2$ is not easily released to the tissues. This represents an increase in the Sa$O_2$ if it is measured against the same Pa$O_2$ of the normal oxyhemoglobin dissociation curve. This left shift can be caused by an increase in blood pH or a decrease in arterial $CO_2$ pressure (Pa$CO_2$) or body temperature.

A *shift of the curve to the right* causes a decreased affinity of hemoglobin for $O_2$ but improved $O_2$ release to the tissues. This represents a lower Sa$O_2$ if measured against the same Pa$O_2$ of the normal oxyhemoglobin dissociation curve. This rightward shift can be caused by a decrease in blood pH or an increase in PaCO₂ or body temperature.

Oximetry offers several advantages over TCM. Oximetry (1) does not require heating the skin, thus reducing the risk of burns, (2) eliminates a delay period for transducer equilibration, and (3) maintains an accurate measurement regardless of the patient's age or skin characteristics or the presence of lung disease.

> **NURSING ALERT**   It is important to make certain that sensory connectors and oximeters are compatible. Wiring that is incompatible can generate considerable heat at the tip of the sensor, causing second- and third-degree burns under the sensors. Pressure necrosis can also occur from sensors attached too tightly. Therefore inspect the skin under the sensor frequently.

Applying the sensor correctly is essential for accurate SaO₂ measurements. Because the sensor must identify every pulse beat to calculate the SaO₂, movement can interfere with sensing. Some devices synchronize the O₂ saturation reading with the heartbeat, thereby reducing the interference caused by motion. Sensors are not placed on extremities used for blood pressure monitoring or with indwelling arterial catheters, because pulsatile blood flow can be affected. It is recommended that the probe site be changed at least every 4 to 8 hours in preterm infants.

> **NURSING TIP**   *For the infant:* Secure the sensor to the great toe and tape the wire to the sole of the foot (or use a commercial holder that fastens with a self-adhering closure). Place a snugly fitting sock over the foot. *For the child:* Secure the sensor to the index finger and tape the wire to the back of the hand. Use self-adhering Ace type of wrap (e.g., Coban) around the finger or hand to further secure the sensor and wire.

Ambient light from ceiling lights and phototherapy, as well as high-intensity heat and light from radiant warmers, can interfere with readings. Therefore the sensor should be covered to block these light sources. Intravenous dyes; green, purple, or black nail polish; nonopaque synthetic nails; and possibly ink used for footprinting can also cause inaccurate SaO₂ measurements. The dyes should be removed or, in the case of porcelain nails, a different area used for the sensor. Skin color, thickness, and edema do not affect the readings. Elevated levels of carboxyhemoglobin, methemoglobin, and fetal hemoglobin affect the accuracy of the device because it can only distinguish between oxyhemoglobin and deoxyhemoglobin.

*Arterial blood gas (ABG) sampling* may be performed on blood from an artery or a capillary. Some controversy surrounds the collection of "arterialized" capillary blood for blood gas measurements. However, many believe it to be a safe, convenient, and relatively accurate method. The blood samples are obtained by taking a deep heelstick after dilation of the vascular bed by warming. (See Fig. 27-19.) The first drop of blood is discarded, and subsequent blood is collected directly into heparinized capillary tubes held in a horizontal position. The tubes are delivered to the laboratory as soon as possible.

> **ATRAUMATIC CARE**
> *Arterial Blood Punctures*
>
> Arterial blood punctures are painful. Buffered lidocaine, a local anesthetic, may be administered intradermally immediately over the artery to minimize discomfort during the blood-drawing procedure. However, small volumes of anesthetic should be used because large volumes can produce arterial spasm (Zander and Hazinski, 1992). EMLA, a topical anesthetic, can be applied under an occlusive dressing 1 hour before the procedure.

ABG samples may also be obtained through an indwelling catheter (e.g., arterial line, multilumen catheter, or Swan-Ganz catheter) or by arteriopuncture. The sites most commonly used for arterial puncture include the radial, dorsalis pedis, posterior tibial, and femoral arteries. The femoral artery is the last choice because hemorrhage and hematomas are difficult to control in this area and the risk for limb ischemia is high if the femoral artery is damaged (Curley and Moloney-Harmon, 2001). (See Atraumatic Care box.) Before a radial artery puncture, the ***Allen test*** is performed to assess adequacy of the collateral circulation. To perform the test, the extremity distal to the puncture site is elevated and blanched by squeezing gently (such as making a fist). The two arteries supplying blood flow to the extremity (such as the radial and ulnar arteries in the wrist) are then occluded. The extremity is lowered, and pressure is removed from *one* artery (such as the ulnar). Color return to the blanched extremity in less than 5 seconds indicates collateral circulation.

> **NURSING ALERT**   Nurses should perform the Allen test as a precautionary measure regardless of whether or not they perform the arterial puncture.

Unclotted whole or capillary blood is required; therefore a heparinized syringe or capillary tube is used to draw blood samples. No air bubbles should enter the sample to alter the blood gas concentration. Many institutions use prepackaged ABG sampling kits. These kits allow air-free samples to be drawn without the need for heparin dilutions. The amount collected depends on the child's size. Depending on the laboratory facilities, as little as 0.1 ml may be sufficient in small infants. After the blood sample is obtained, it is packed in ice to reduce blood cell metabolism and taken to the laboratory immediately for analysis. Table 31-4 lists normal ABG and pH measurements on room air at sea level for adults and children 7 to 19 years of age.

Although ABG values are similar for children and adults, neonates can have slightly lower values and still be considered normal. For example, normal pH values for a newborn range from 7.26 to 7.29; the average PaO₂ is 70 mm Hg; the average PaCO₂ is 33 mm Hg; and the average HCO₃ is 20 mEq/L (Johns Hopkins Hospital Department of Pediatrics, 2000).

ABG values also depend on the concentration of O₂ the child is breathing. The arterial PO₂ should rise in proportion to the O₂ concentration being inhaled. Therefore, when ABG values are evaluated, the following are consid-

**TABLE 31-4**   Blood gas analysis

| Component | Definition | Normal Value | Acidosis | Alkalosis |
|---|---|---|---|---|
| pH | Indicates acid-base status of body | 7.35-7.45 (adult) 7.39 (child 7-19 years) | Less than 7.35 indicates an excess of acid | Greater than 7.45 indicates an excess of base |
| $PCO_2$ | Pressure exerted by dissolved $CO_2$ in blood Under control of lungs Respiratory component | 35-45 mm Hg (adult) 37 mm Hg (child 7-19 years) | Greater than 45 mm Hg Causes: obstructive lung disease, hypoventilation of any cause | Less than 35 mm Hg Causes: hypoxia, pulmonary embolism, hyperventilation of any cause |
| $HCO_3$ | Buffers effect of acid in blood Under control of kidneys Metabolic component | 22-26 mEq/L (adult) 22 mEq/L (child 7-19 years) | Less than 22 mEq/L Causes: diarrhea, lactic acidosis, renal failure, shock, therapy with acetazolamide, diabetic ketoacidosis, drainage of pancreatic juice | Greater than 26 mEq/L Causes: fluid loss from upper gastrointestinal tract, diuretics, corticosteroid therapy |
| Base excess (BE) | Reflects status of all bases in blood | ±2 (adult) ±3 (child 7-19 years) | More negative | More positive |
| $PO_2$ | Pressure exerted by dissolved $O_2$ in blood Indicates effectiveness of oxygenation by lungs | 90-110 mm Hg (adult) 96 mm Hg (child 7-19 years) | Less than 80 mm Hg: hypoxia Causes: obstructive lung disease, high $CO_2$ levels, low $FIO_2$, hypoventilation | Greater than 100 mm Hg; hyperoxygenation Causes: high $FIO_2$, hyperventilation |

Modified from Siberry GK, Iannone R, editors, Johns Hopkins Hospital Department of Pediatrics: *The Harriet Lane handbook*, ed 15, St Louis, 2000, Mosby.
NOTE: The $SaO_2$ printed with blood gas reports cannot be used as a standard to confirm oximetry readings. Blood gas analyzers provide only approximate blood $O_2$ saturations based on calculations using measured blood gases, pH, and $PaO_2$.

ered: the percentage of $O_2$ administered (if any); the child's body temperature (as little as 1° F can alter the blood gas values 5% to 8%); and the presence of anxiety (if children hyperventilate, $CO_2$ is exhaled) or crying (can cause breath holding and apnea, resulting in decreased $PaO_2$).

The significance of ABG determination is related primarily to the relationships among three parameters: pH, $PO_2$, and $PCO_2$. (See Acid-Base Imbalance, Chapter 28.) Any change in a blood gas value must be compared with the other values and with previous readings, as well as with the child's clinical appearance and behavior, medical history, and associated physiologic factors.

Clinical indications for blood gas analysis include changes in color (e.g., mottling, pallor, cyanosis, or duskiness), depth or rate of respirations (e.g., shallow and rapid), behavior or sensorium, and vital signs. The nurse may or may not obtain the blood sample by arteriopuncture, depending on the institution's policies. Regardless of whether the nurse does or does not obtain the blood sample, nurses must understand the results of blood gas analyses because these results provide essential information to guide nursing interventions (e.g., changing the position, performing suction, administering prescribed drugs, or notifying the practitioners).

## RESPIRATORY THERAPY

### Oxygen Therapy

The indication for administration of $O_2$ is *hypoxemia* (reduced blood oxygenation). $O_2$ is delivered by mask, nasal cannula, tent, hood, face tent, or ventilator (Table 31-5). The mode of delivery is selected on the basis of the concentration needed and the child's ability to cooperate in its use. The concentration of $O_2$ delivered should be regulated according to the individual child's needs. There are hazards related to its use; therefore $O_2$ should be continued only as long as needed. Because medical-grade $O_2$ from piped systems or tanks is anhydrous, humidification of the gas before administration to the patient is essential.

$O_2$ therapy is frequently administered in the hospital, although increasing numbers of children are receiving $O_2$ in the home. It is the responsibility of the nurse or respiratory care practitioner to ensure uninterrupted delivery of the appropriate $O_2$ concentration and to monitor the child's response to the therapy.

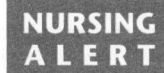 **NURSING ALERT**   Oxygen is a drug and is only administered as prescribed by dose, typically in liters per minute.

### Oxygen Administration

$O_2$ delivered to infants is best tolerated by using a ***plastic hood*** (Fig. 31-11). Low and high concentrations of $O_2$ can be easily maintained in this head hood, and most nursing procedures can be continued without interrupting the $O_2$ delivery. This is not possible when delivering $O_2$ directly into the incubator. At least 4 to 5 L/min of flow is needed to maintain $O_2$ concentrations and remove the exhaled $CO_2$.

The humidified $O_2$ should not be blown directly into the face of an infant in a hood. Cold fluid or air applied to the face stimulates receptors that trigger the diving reflex, which causes bradycardia and shunting of blood from peripheral to central circulation. The $O_2$ hood should not rub against the infant's neck, chin, or shoulder. Older infants and children can use a ***nasal cannula*** or ***prongs. Masks*** are not well tolerated by children.

For children beyond early infancy, the ***oxygen tent*** may be a satisfactory means for $O_2$ administration (Fig. 31-12). A

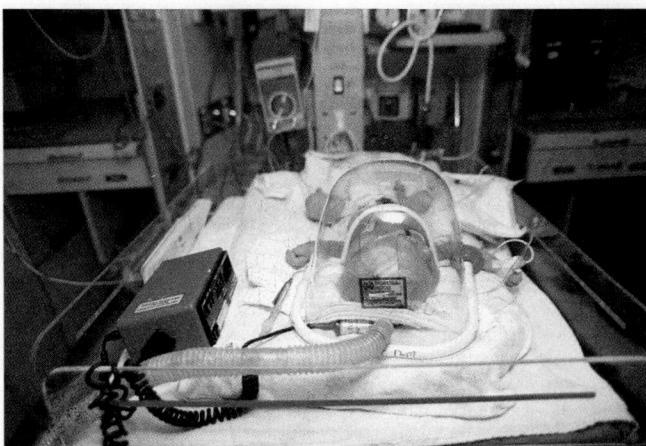

**Fig. 31-11**   Oxygen administered to infant by means of a plastic hood. Note oxygen analyzer (blue machine).

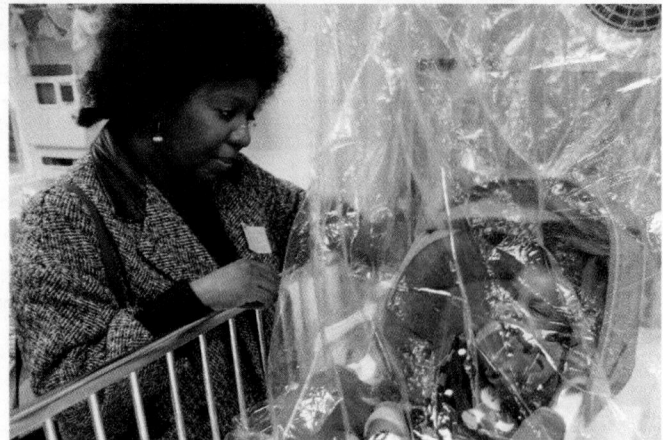

**Fig. 31-12**   The tent provides a comfortable method for oxygen administration.

| TABLE 31-5 | Advantages and disadvantages of various oxygen-delivery systems | |
| --- | --- | --- |
| **Systems** | **Advantages** | **Disadvantages** |
| **Oxygen mask** | Various sizes available; delivers higher oxygen conception than cannula | Skin irritation |
| | Ability to provide a predictable concentration of oxygen (with Venturi mask) whether child breathes through nose or mouth | Fear of suffocation |
| | | Accumulation of moisture on face |
| | | Possibility of aspiration of vomitus |
| | | Difficulty in controlling $O_2$ concentrations |
| **Nasal cannula** | Provides low-moderate oxygen concentration (22%-40%) | Must have patent nasal passages |
| | Child can eat and talk while getting oxygen | Possibility of causing abdominal distention and discomfort or vomiting |
| | Possibility of more complete observation of child because nose and mouth remain unobstructed | Difficulty of controlling $O_2$ concentrations if child breathes through mouth |
| | | Inability to provide mist if desired |
| **Oxygen tent** | Achievement of lower $O_2$ concentrations ($FIO_2$ of 0.3-0.5) | Necessity for right fit around bed to prevent leakage of gas |
| | Child receives increased inspired $O_2$ concentration even while eating. | Cool and wet tent environment |
| | | Poor access to patient—inspired $O_2$ levels will fall whenever tent is entered |
| **Oxygen hood, face tent** | Achievement of high $O_2$ concentrations ($FIO_2$ up to 1.00) | High humidity environment |
| | Free access to patient's chest for assessment | Need to remove patient for feeding and care |

Modified from Hazinski MF, editor: *Nursing care of the critically ill child,* ed 2, St Louis, 1992, Mosby.

tent does not require any device to come into direct contact with the face, but the concentration of $O_2$ within the tent is difficult to control and to maintain above 30% to 50%. A major difficulty with the use of the tent is keeping the tent closed so that $O_2$ concentration is maintained.

To reduce $O_2$ loss, nursing care is planned carefully so that the tent is opened as little as possible. Because $O_2$ is heavier than air, loss will be greater at the bottom of the tent; therefore the tent is tucked in snugly without open edges. The bottom of the tent should be examined more often when the child is restless, fussy, or likely to pull the covers loose. Some tents are even open at the top. Because of the rapid diffusing qualities of $CO_2$, the levels of the gas do not build up within these enclosures.

After the tent has been opened for an extended period of time, it is flushed with $O_2$ by increasing the flow meter for a few minutes to quickly raise the $O_2$ and mist concentration. The flow meter is then reset to the prescribed number of liters.

The enclosed tent becomes very warm; therefore some type of cooling mechanism is provided. Although the cool environment can reduce fever and airway inflammation, it can also produce hypothermia and cold stress. Because $O_2$ is drying to the tissues, the gas is humidified, which causes moisture to condense on the tent walls.

**NURSING ALERT**   Keep the child warm and dry by checking the temperature inside the tent and the child's bedding and clothing frequently. Adjust the temperature and change clothing as often as needed.

The reactions of children to the oxygen tent are variable. Some, especially older children, feel comfortable in the tent and like the cozy, close privacy it affords. Others, more often younger children, may be frightened by the forced enclosure. The plastic walls distort their view of the world and constitute a barrier between them and their parent. Their distress can be minimized if they are able to see someone

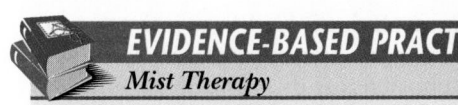

## EVIDENCE-BASED PRACTICE
### Mist Therapy

Continuous administration of mist, or aerosolized water, often viewed as a traditional and helpful remedy, is not a treatment of choice for most inflammatory conditions of the airways. The exception is the child with mild viral croup, who might be helped by cool-mist therapy, including a walk outside in the cool, humid, night air. The beneficial effect of cool mist may include moistening of airway secretions, a reflex reaction to the cool air that slows rapid respiration, and a feeling of reassurance from holding the child near the mist that may help lessen the anxiety for both the child and the parent (Kaditis and Wald, 1999). Mist therapy may not help the child with reactive airway disease and croup because humidity may worsen the bronchospasm.

The notion that inhaled mist can influence the viscosity of mucus in dehydrated children is erroneous. If dehydration is evident, oral or parenteral rehydration will normalize the water content of respiratory mucus.

nearby and are reassured that they will not be left alone. A favorite toy or object can be placed inside the tent. Other familiar items can be placed at the foot of the bed or in view.

> **NURSING ALERT**
> Inspect all toys for safety and suitability (e.g., vinyl or plastic—not stuffed items that absorb moisture and are difficult to keep dry). The high $O_2$ environment makes any source of sparks (such as mechanical or electrical toys) a potential fire hazard.

In some instances the child can be removed from the oxygen tent for activities such as feeding and bathing, whereas in other cases the child is placed in the tent only during periods of rest. Some children may require $O_2$ continuously and can be removed from the tent or incubator only if an $O_2$ source is held close to the child's face. Any change in color, increased respiratory effort, or restlessness is an indication to return the child to the oxygen tent.

### Oxygen Toxicity

$O_2$ is essential to life and a valuable therapeutic aid. Prolonged exposure to high $O_2$ tensions, however, can be damaging to lung tissue. Although the exact pathogenesis of the pulmonary changes is unclear, evidence indicates damage to lung capillaries, which causes diffuse microhemorrhagic changes, diminished mucus flow, inactivation of surfactant, and altered ciliary function. The result of these changes is a gradual impairment of alveolar ventilation.

*Atelectasis* may occur as a result of the "washing out" of nitrogen from the alveoli by the high concentrations of $O_2$. This is more likely to occur in persons with low tidal volume and retention of mucus or other secretions.

*$O_2$-induced $CO_2$ narcosis* is a physiologic hazard of $O_2$ therapy that may occur in persons with chronic pulmonary disease. It is seldom encountered in children except those with cystic fibrosis. These children have chronic alveolar hypoventilation with a concomitant chronic $CO_2$ retention and hypoxemia. In these patients the respiratory center has adapted to the continuously higher $PaCO_2$ levels, and therefore hypoxia becomes the more powerful stimulus to respiration. When the $PaO_2$ is elevated during $O_2$ administration, the hypoxic drive is removed, causing progressive hypoven-

tilation and increased $PaCO_2$ levels, and the child rapidly becomes unconscious. $CO_2$ narcosis can also be induced by the administration of sedation in these patients.

Other suspected toxic effects of $O_2$ include changes in the renal tubules, sympathoadrenal medullary stimulation precipitating neurogenic seizures, and an increased rate of destruction of red blood cells. In preterm infants the risk of retinopathy of prematurity is a major concern in $O_2$ administration. (See Chapter 10.)

## Aerosol Therapy

Aerosol therapy can be effective in depositing medication directly into the airway. However, the value of aerosolized water or "mist therapy" is controversial. (See Evidence-Based Practice box.) This route of administration can be useful in avoiding the systemic side effects of certain drugs and in reducing the amount of drug necessary to achieve the desired effect. Bronchodilators, steroids, and antibiotics, suspended in particulate form, can be inhaled so that the medication reaches the small airways. Aerosol therapy is particularly challenging in children who are too young to cooperate with controlling the rate and depth of breathing. Administration of this therapy requires skill, patience, and creativity.

Medications can be aerosolized or nebulized with air or with $O_2$-enriched gas. *Hand-held nebulizers* are frequently used. The medicated "mist" is discharged into a small plastic mask, which the child holds over the nose and mouth.* To avoid particle deposition in the nose and pharynx, the child is instructed to take slow, deep breaths through an open mouth during treatment. For home or school use an air compressor–driven nebulizer is necessary to force air through the liquid medication to form the aerosol. Compact, portable units can be obtained or rented from health equipment companies.

The *metered dose inhaler (MDI)* is a self-contained, hand-held device that allows for intermittent delivery of a specified amount of medication. Many bronchodilators are available in this form and are used successfully by children with asthma or cystic fibrosis. (See Chapter 32.) For children less than 5 or 6 years of age or children who have difficulty learning to use an MDI, a *spacer device* or holding chamber attached to the MDI can help coordinate breathing and aerosol delivery. The spacer allows the aerosolized particles to remain in suspension for a longer time. Dry powder inhalers such as the Rotahaler and Turbuhalers are also commonly used for inhaled medications.

A major nursing responsibility during aerosol therapy is to assess the effectiveness of the treatment, the patient's tolerance of the procedure and the patient's ability to perform the procedure and use equipment correctly. Assessment of breath sounds and work of breathing should be performed before and after treatments. Young children who become upset with a mask held close to the face may become fatigued from fighting the procedure and may appear worse during and immediately after the therapy. It may be neces-

---

*An aerosolized medication device is available for infants—PediNeb, Westmed, Inc, 5580 S. Nogales Hwy, Unit 170, Tucson, Arizona (800) 975-7987; fax (520) 294-6061; www.westmedinc.com.

sary to spend a few minutes calming the child after the therapy and allowing vital signs to return to baseline levels to accurately assess changes in breath sounds and work of breathing.

## Bronchial (Postural) Drainage

Bronchial drainage is indicated whenever excessive fluid or mucus in the bronchi is not removed by normal ciliary activity and cough. Positioning the child to take maximum advantage of gravity facilitates removal of secretions. Postural drainage can be very effective in children with chronic lung disease characterized by thick mucus secretions, such as cystic fibrosis.

Postural drainage is carried out three to four times daily and is more effective when it follows other respiratory therapy, such as bronchodilator or nebulization medication. Bronchial drainage is generally performed before meals (or 1 to 1½ hours after meals) to minimize the chance of vomiting and is repeated at bedtime. The duration of treatment depends on the child's condition and tolerance—usually 20 to 30 minutes. There are several positions to facilitate drainage from all major lung segments (Fig. 31-13); all positions are not used at each session. Children will usually cooperate for four to six positions, but more than six tends to exceed their limits of tolerance. Older children can tolerate longer periods.

In the hospital an older child can be positioned over an elevated knee rest. Small children and infants can be positioned with pillows or on the therapist's lap and legs (Fig. 31-14). Infants should not be placed in the Trendelenburg position, because they do not have an autonomic regulation of blood flow to the head. Special modifications of the techniques are required in children whose conditions contraindicate the standard positioning, such as head injuries, some types of surgical incisions or burns, and casts or traction. At home small children can be positioned on a padded ironing board.* Children who require postural drainage over a period of months or years may benefit from specially constructed tables padded and adjusted to their individual needs. The position used and the frequency and duration of treatment are individualized.

## Chest Physiotherapy (CPT)

CPT usually refers to the use of postural drainage in combination with adjunctive techniques that are thought to enhance the clearance of mucus from the airway. These techniques include manual percussion, vibration, and squeezing of the chest; cough; forceful expiration; and breathing exercises. Special mechanical devices are also currently used to perform CPT (e.g., the ThAIRapy Vest) (see p. 1408).

Postural drainage in combination with forced expiration has been shown to be beneficial. In addition, noninvasive inspiratory nasal pressure support ventilation (PSV) used in combination with CPT has demonstrated a significant improvement in respiratory muscle performance and a reduction in oxygen desaturation (Fauroux and others, 1999).

The most common technique used in association with postural drainage is manual *percussion* of the chest wall. Nurses are often responsible for this procedure, and they should become skilled in the technique. The patient is dressed in a light shirt and placed in a postural drainage position. The practitioner then gently but firmly strikes the chest wall with a cupped hand (Fig. 31-15, *A*). For infants, special devices are available for percussing small areas (Fig. 31-15, *B*). A "popping," hollow sound should be the result, not a slapping sound. The procedure should be done over the rib cage only and should be painless. Percussion can be performed with a soft, circular mask (adapted to maintain air trapping) or a percussion cup marketed especially for the purpose of aiding the loosening of secretions (Fig. 31-15, *B*).

*Vibration* can be used to help move secretions cephalad during exhalations. Hand-held vibrators should be approved for use in an $O_2$-enriched environment (tent, head hood). Larger children may benefit from a more powerful vibrator. This therapy is subject to patient tolerance, and oximetry is an excellent monitoring tool for therapy tolerance.

CPT is contraindicated when patients have pulmonary hemorrhage, pulmonary embolism, end-stage renal disease, increased intracranial pressure, osteogenesis imperfecta, or minimum cardiac reserves. Guidelines for performing CPT are included in the Guidelines box.

*Squeezing* is sometimes useful while the child is in the drainage position. The child is directed to take a deep breath and then exhale through the mouth rapidly and as completely as possible. The depth of the expiratory effort is increased by brief, firm pressure from the practitioner's hands compressing the sides of the chest. This decreases the volume of the tracheobronchial tree and facilitates the expression of secretions. Inspiration after the activity often stimulates a deep, productive cough.

*Deep breathing* is encouraged when the child is relaxed and in the desired position for drainage. The child is directed to take several deep breaths using diaphragmatic breathing. The use of deep breathing enlarges the tracheobronchial tree, enabling air to circulate around and through secretions that are not affected by usual tidal volumes. Expirations after these deep breaths often carry secretions and may stimulate a cough. Other methods that can be employed to stimulate deep breathing are the use of incentive spirometers, and incorporation of play that extends the expiratory time and increases expiratory pressure. For example, play may include blowing pinwheel toys, mov-

---

*Home care instructions are available in Wong DL, Hess CS: *Wong and Whaley's clinical manual of pediatric nursing*, ed 5, St Louis, 2000, Mosby.

---

### GUIDELINES
#### Performing Chest Physiotherapy

Chest physiotherapy should be used for patients who have increased sputum production. It is probably of no value to the uncomplicated postoperative patient or the patient with pneumonia.

Forced expiration combined with postural drainage is more effective than cough alone.

Appropriate use of bronchodilators before chest physiotherapy will enhance mucus clearance.

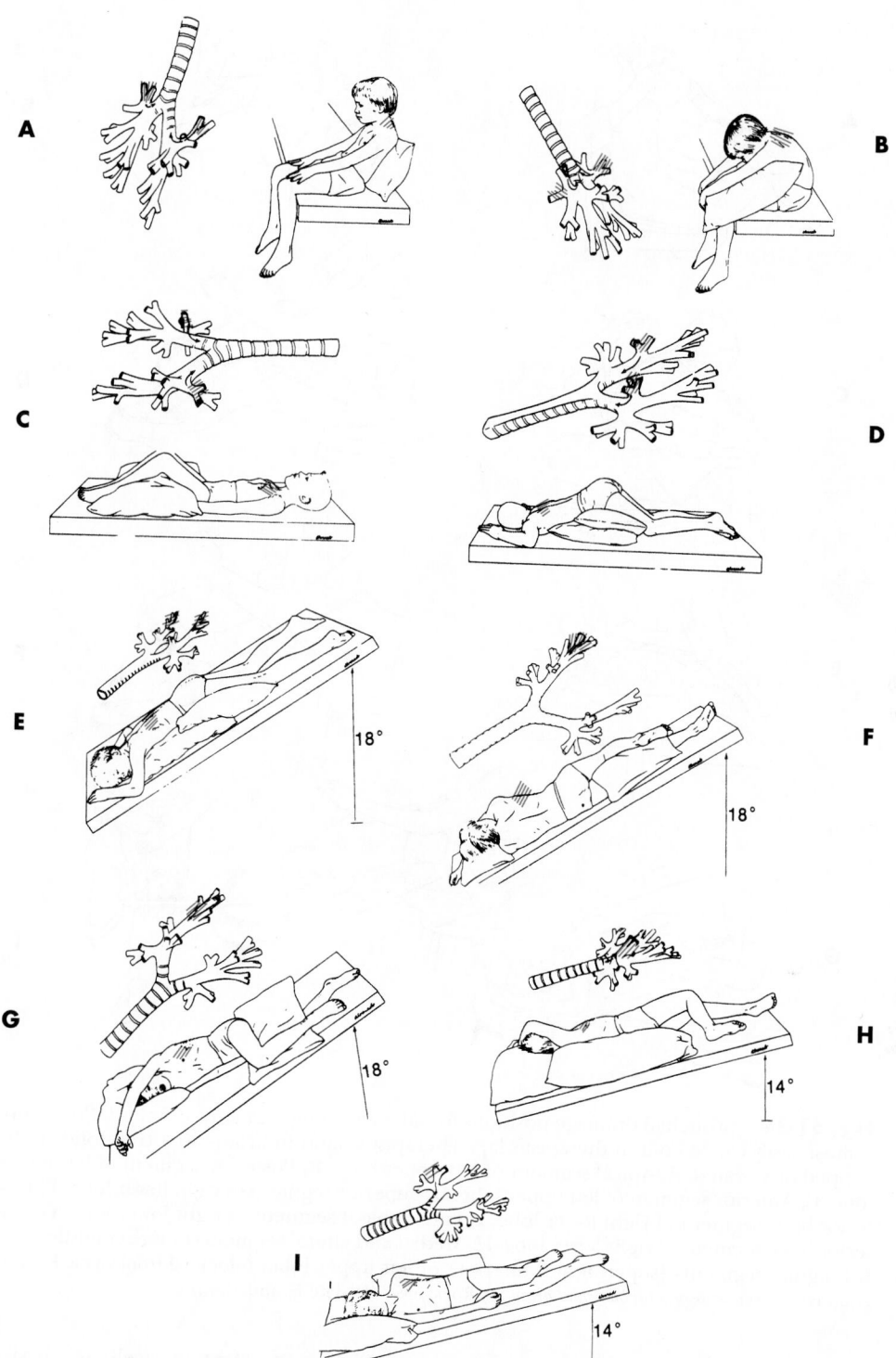

**Fig. 31-13**   Bronchial drainage positions for all major lung segments of child. For each position, model of tracheobronchial tree is projected beside child to show segmental bronchus *(striped)* being drained and pathway of secretions out of bronchus. Drainage platform is horizontal unless otherwise noted. Striped area on child's chest indicates area to be cupped or vibrated by therapist. **A,** Apical segment of right upper lobe and apical subsegment of apical-posterior segment of left upper lobe. **B,** Posterior segment of right upper lobe and posterior subsegment of apical-posterior segment of left upper lobe. **C,** Anterior segments of both upper lobes; child should be rotated slightly away from side being drained. **D,** Superior segments of both lower lobes. **E,** Posterior basal segments of both lower lobes. **F,** Lateral basal segments of right lower lobe; left lateral basal segment would be drained by mirror image of this position (right side down). **G,** Anterior basal segment of left lower lobe; right anterior basal segment would be drained by mirror image of this position (left side down). **H,** Medial and lateral segments of right middle lobe. **I,** Lingular segments (superior and inferior) of left upper lobe (homologue of right middle lobe). (From Chernick V, editor: *Kendig's disorders of the respiratory tract of children,* ed 6, Philadelphia, 1998, WB Saunders.)

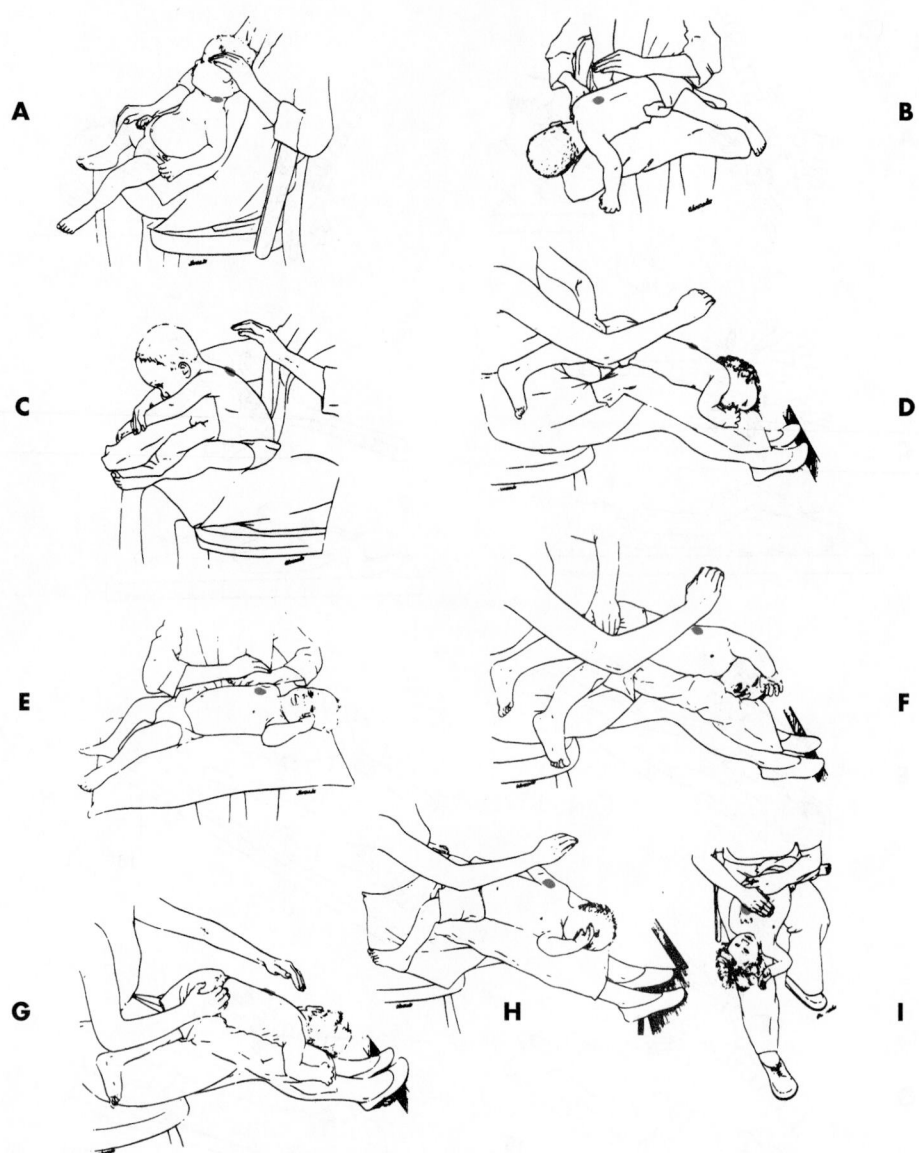

**Fig. 31-14** Bronchial drainage positions for all major lung segments of infant. Procedure is most easily carried out in therapist's lap. Therapist's hand indicates area (red solid) to be cupped or vibrated. **A,** Apical segment of left upper lobe. **B,** Posterior segment of left upper lobe. **C,** Anterior segment of left upper lobe. **D,** Superior segment of right lower lobe. **E,** Posterior basal segment of right lower lobe. **F,** Lateral basal segment of right lower lobe. **G,** Anterior basal segment of right lower lobe. **H,** Medial and lateral segments of right middle lobe. **I,** Lingular segments (superior and inferior) of left upper lobe. (Modified from Cystic Fibrosis Foundation: *Infant segmental bronchial drainage,* Rockville, MD, The Foundation.)

ing small items by blowing through a straw, blowing cotton balls or a Ping-Pong ball on a table, preventing a tissue from falling by blowing it against a wall, blowing up balloons (under supervision), singing loudly (especially songs with a lot of words between breaths), or blowing soap bubbles.

With or without stimulation, children are encouraged to *cough,* not to suppress a cough, and not to waste strength and energy with repeated weak and ineffective coughs. One or two hard coughs after a deep breath are more efficient. Because many children have difficulty coughing when in a dependent position, they are encouraged to sit up while they cough. Having the child hug a stuffed toy or a small pil-

low offers comfort, as well as physical support, during coughing. As an alternative, the practitioner can reinforce the child's efforts by encircling the chest with the practitioner's hands and compressing the sides of the lower chest in synchrony with the cough. This is less fatiguing and increases the effectiveness of the cough efforts.

*Breathing* and *postural exercises* are useful techniques with motivated children and children with kyphoscoliosis, cystic fibrosis, asthma, and bronchiectasis. Breathing exercises are employed as part of a total therapy program and are more convenient when performed in association with bronchial drainage.

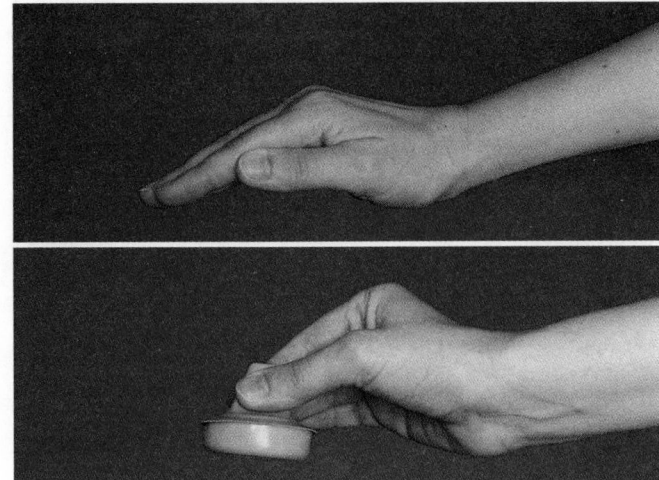

**Fig. 31-15  A,** Cupped hand position for percussion. **B,** Device for infant percussion.

---

**Box 31-5** ■ ■ ■
**Indications for Mechanical Ventilation**

Progressive hypoxia, despite $O_2$ therapy, measured by decreasing $O_2$ saturations or blood gas analysis (high $PaCO_2$ and low pH)
Inadequate ventilation due to:
  Apnea
  Central nervous system injury or infection
  Alveolar hypoventilation
  Respiratory muscle weakness
  Medication toxicity
  Infectious pathology
  Foreign body obstruction
Excessive work of breathing, manifested by retractions, tachypnea, decreasing $O_2$ saturation, abnormal respiratory patterns
Inadequate respiratory effort
Hyperventilation for treatment of increased intracranial pressure (ICP)

---

The goals of breathing exercises are to (1) develop more effective diaphragmatic and lower intercostal breathing; (2) relax all muscles, especially those of the upper chest, shoulder girdle, and neck; and (3) attain correct posture. The number and type of exercises depend on the child's age, motivation, and strength, as well as the type and extent of the physiologic disturbance. Breathing exercises are selected to meet the specific child's needs. The most important exercises are diaphragmatic breathing and side bending, with emphasis on abdominal expansion and lateral expansion.

## Artificial Ventilation

If a child's respiratory status is deteriorating and the respiratory effort is excessive or inadequate, mechanically assisted ventilation may become necessary (Box 31-5).

A variety of methods are available for controlling or assisting ventilation. Temporary assistance can be provided by a hand-operated self-inflating ventilation bag with a mask and a nonreturnable valve to prevent rebreathing, commonly referred to as a *bag-valve-mask (BVM).* With the mask placed on the nose and mouth, the bag is rhythmically compressed, forcing gas from the bag into the patient's airways. The self-inflating bag is equipped with a reservoir so that a high percentage of $O_2$ can be delivered. To avoid barotrauma, self-inflating bags should be equipped with a preset (or adjustable) pop-off valve that allows maximum peak inspiratory pressure of 30 to 35 cm $H_2O$ (Curley and Moloney-Harmon, 2001).

Another type of bag used for manual ventilation is the uninflated "anesthesia bag." This type of bag reinflates only if a continuous source of $O_2$ is available. The bag is commonly used in intensive care units and requires skill and training of the personnel who use it. Regardless of the type of manual ventilation bag used, an open airway is established by correct positioning with the patient's chin directed forward and the neck extended to the "sniffing" position. It is important not to hyperextend an infant's neck, because this can occlude the airway.

Recently several types of noninvasive positive-pressure ventilation (NPPV) have been used to support pediatric patients who have respiratory difficulties in acute, chronic, and home settings (O'Neill, 1998). NPPV does not require endotracheal intubation or a tracheotomy and is delivered via a nasal or oral mask attached to a ventilation system. Three types of NPVV can be delivered: (1) continuous positive airway pressure (CPAP), (2) intermittent positive-pressure breathing (IPPB), and (3) bilevel positive airway pressure (BiPAP). CPAP provides a constant flow of positive pressure to prevent collapse of the alveoli. IPPB is a type of CPAP used intermittently to deliver aerosol medications. BiPAP provides constant positive pressure at two different pressure settings—one for inspiration and one for expiration. BiPAP has been used for pediatric patients with obstructive sleep apnea, tracheomalacia, diaphragm paralysis, progressive neuromuscular disorders, cystic fibrosis, and asthma (Curley and Moloney-Harmon, 2001).

For more prolonged assistance, mechanical ventilation is used to replace the function of the diaphragm and thoracic chest wall muscles. Ventilators are attached to the patient by endotracheal (ET) tube or tracheostomy. The lungs are inflated by application of either positive or negative pressure. A *positive-pressure* machine inflates the lungs by creating a pressure at the airway opening that is greater than intraalveolar pressure, which then forces pressurized gas into the lungs. Application of positive pressure by mechanical means usually improves gas distribution within the lung and often reinflates partially collapsed lung segments. The overall effect is improvement of gas exchange. *Negative-pressure ventilators* create a subatmospheric pressure around the chest wall and inside the chest, thus allowing air to move into the chest. This form of ventilation is occasionally used for patients with neuromuscular disease.

Ventilators are usually classified according to the factors that regulate cycling. The method by which inspiration is terminated can be categorized as pressure cycled, volume cycled, or time cycled (Box 31-6). *High-frequency ventilation* is a generic term for several types of mechanical ventilation.

---

**Box 31-6**
**Types of Ventilators**

**Pressure-cycled ventilator**—Terminates the respiratory cycle when a preset inspiratory pressure is reached. Volume will differ greatly, depending on the flow rate of the delivery of gas. The compliance of the lung will affect the tidal volume even though the pressure will remain constant.

**Volume-cycled ventilator**—Terminates respiration when a preset volume (tidal volume) is delivered. The compliance and resistance of the lung will change the pressure needed to deliver the preset volume.

**Time-cycled ventilator**—Terminates inspiration when a preset time is reached. Tidal volume is greatly affected by the compliance of the ventilator tubing, compliance and resistance of the lung, and flow rate of the delivered gas. The duration of the inspiratory pressure will be affected by the preset inspiratory time and the flow rate of the delivered gas.

---

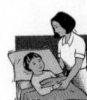

**ATRAUMATIC CARE**
*Extubation and the Use of Opioids*

If opioids are being given for pain, it is not necessary to withhold them (Furdon and others, 1998). If respiratory depression occurs following extubation, a small dose of naloxone (Narcan) (0.5 µg/kg) can be given to determine the cause of the respiratory effect. No change in respiratory rate indicates that the opioids are not the cause.

---

Some specific types of high-frequency ventilation include high-frequency jet, high-frequency flow interrupter, and high-frequency positive-pressure ventilation, and high-frequency oscillation ventilation. All of these devices use a rapid cycling rate and deliver small tidal volumes with each cycle. During high-frequency ventilation, lung volume is held relatively constant, the cycle of inflation and deflation associated with conventional ventilation is reduced, and gas exchange is maintained with less lung injury (Curley and Moloney-Harmon, 2001). Although high-frequency ventilation has improved ventilation in critically ill neonates in whom conventional ventilation has failed, more research is needed to determine the role of high-frequency ventilation in improving outcomes (Donn and Sinha, 2001). *Extracorporeal membrane oxygenation (ECMO)* is a form of cardiopulmonary bypass, which provides both pulmonary and cardiac support using an external oxygenation device and a pump.

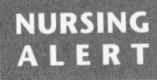

**NURSING ALERT** Patients requiring mechanical ventilation should always have a self-inflating ventilation bag with a reservoir at the bedside. When the patient's condition or the ventilator's operation is in doubt, the ventilation bag is used.

### Care of the Patient

The regulation and maintenance of mechanical ventilators is the responsibility of respiratory care practitioners. However, nurses should understand the function of the ventilator and how to detect signs of malfunction and deviations from the desired settings. The nurse also promotes the effectiveness of ventilation by suctioning, positioning, ensuring that adequate humidification is provided, and providing support and reassurance to the child and the family. (See Chapter 10 for assisted and controlled ventilation in the neonate.)

**NURSING ALERT** The use of a mechanical ventilator does not guarantee that the child is actually being ventilated. Nursing assessment of ventilatory status therefore is essential.

Nursing assessment of the child requiring mechanical ventilation focuses on physical examination, vital signs, pulmonary status, oxygenation, and airway patency (e.g., obstruction or dislodgment), as well as laboratory analysis and pulse oximetry. All infants and children who are intubated and on mechanical ventilation should be placed on a cardiorespiratory monitor.

Other important criteria to assess include nutritional status, intake and output (urinary output should be at least 2 ml/kg/hr for the younger child and 1 ml/kg/hr for the older child), and skin integrity (especially around the face and lips for the child with an ET tube, and around the neck and stoma for the child with a tracheostomy).

Weaning the patient from a ventilator involves gradual physical and psychologic withdrawal from dependence on the mechanical device. Criteria for beginning the weaning process vary with the primary disease.

The child who is to be extubated is allowed nothing by mouth to avoid the risk of aspiration. Steroids may be administered before the extubation to control laryngeal edema. Sedation or other respiratory depressants may be withheld before the procedure so that the child can be observed for respiratory activity. (See Atraumatic Care box.) The child should remain on a cardiorespiratory monitor, and resuscitation and reintubation equipment must be available at the bedside.

CPT and suctioning are ordinarily performed just before tube removal, and cool mist is begun immediately after extubation. The child is monitored for respiratory distress, and ABG measurements are observed. The most common complications are airway edema, fatigue, and atelectasis. Airway edema often responds to nebulized racemic epinephrine, which can be given several times to prevent reintubation.

### Endotracheal Airways

An artificial airway is usually used in association with artificial ventilation and in children with upper airway obstruction (Box 31-7). ET intubation can be accomplished by the *nasal (nasotracheal), oral (orotracheal),* or *direct tracheal (tracheostomy)* routes. Oral intubation is usually the method of choice for emergency situations, but for prolonged intubation a nasotracheal tube is used. Nasotracheal intubation facilitates oral hygiene and provides more stable fixation, which reduces the complication of tracheal erosion and the danger of accidental extubation.

Only uncuffed ET tubes should be used in children less than 8 years of age (Curley and Moloney-Harmon, 2001). Although newborn infants have been successfully maintained on ET tubes for longer periods, tracheostomy is usually considered in older children who require intubation for an extended period of time.

**NURSING TIP**   The size of an ET tube can be determined in three ways:

Using patient length and the Broselow resuscitation tape*

$$\text{ET tube size} = \frac{\text{Age (years)} + 16}{4}$$

"Pinky" rule: the diameter of a child's pinky is approximately the size of the trachea.

The decision to change from an ET tube to a tracheostomy is made on an individual basis. The tracheostomy allows the child to speak (by temporarily occluding the opening with a clean fingertip or with a special device) and eat and also facilitates clearing of secretions. Suctioning an ET tube is carried out with the same care as suctioning a tracheostomy.

**Complications.**   The most severe complication related to immediate intubation is hypoxia with accompanying bradycardia. Patients must be closely monitored during intubation attempts, and if hypoxia occurs, the procedure is discontinued until vital signs are stable. Ventilation with bag-valve-mask and $O_2$ is reinstituted. Other complications include trauma to the mouth and teeth, epistaxis, creation of air leaks, and vagal-mediated changes in vital signs. The most common sequela of intubation is a sore throat, which disappears within 48 to 72 hours without therapy, although a humidified atmosphere is beneficial. Other complications include traumatic laryngitis, infection, glottic edema, and mucosal lesions of the larynx secondary to pressure exerted by the rigid ET tube. The most severe sequela of intubation is subglottic stenosis secondary to fibrosis.

## Tracheostomy

Tracheostomy is a surgical opening in the trachea between the second and fourth tracheal rings (Fig. 31-16). Congenital or acquired structural defects, such as subglottic stenosis, tracheomalacia, and vocal cord paralysis, account for many long-term tracheostomies. A tracheostomy may be required in an emergency situation for epiglottitis, croup, or foreign

*Vital Signs, 20 Campus Rd, Totowa, NJ 07512, (800) 932-0760; www. vital-signs.com.

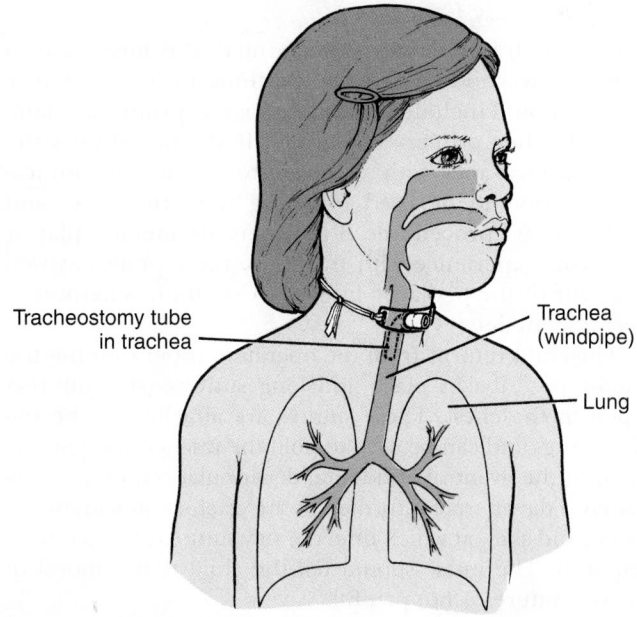

**Fig. 31-16**   Tracheostomy tube in trachea and securely tied with cloth tape.

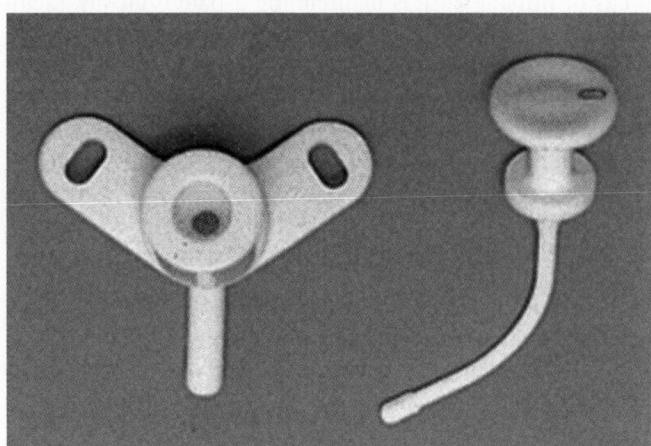

**Fig. 31-17**   Silastic pediatric tracheostomy tube and oburator.

body aspiration. These tracheostomies remain in place for a short time. An infant or child requiring long-term ventilatory support may also have a tracheostomy.

Pediatric tracheostomy tubes are usually made of plastic or Silastic (Fig. 31-17). The most common types are the Hollinger, Jackson, Aberdeen, and Shiley tubes. These tubes are constructed with a more acute angle than adult tubes, and they soften at body temperature, conforming to the contours of the trachea. Because these materials resist the formation of crusted respiratory secretions, they are made without an inner cannula. Some children require a metal tracheostomy tube (usually made of sterling silver or stainless steel), which contains an inner cannula. The principal advantage of metal tubes is their nonreactivity and decreased chance for an allergic reaction.

## Tracheostomy Care

Before the tracheostomy is performed, it is important to prepare the child and family. Teaching prior to the procedure should include the child (if age-appropriate), family, and other primary caregivers. It should address the child's appearance with a tracheostomy, the communication method to be used following the procedure, and postoperative procedures. If time permits, medical play or hands-on experience with tracheostomy supplies, as well as a tour of the pediatric intensive care unit, is helpful to decrease anxiety.

The child returns from the operating room with the tracheostomy tube in place and long sutures (stay sutures) taped to the chest. These sutures are attached to the tracheal rings and can be used to hold the tracheostomy stoma open in the event of accidental decannulation. In approximately 5 days a tract is formed in the trachea, subcutaneous tissue, and skin, at which time the stay sutures are no longer required. The nurse should tell the child that removal of the stay sutures is not painful.

Children who have undergone a tracheostomy must be closely monitored for complications such as hemorrhage, edema, aspiration, accidental decannulation, tube obstruction, and the entrance of free air into the pleural cavity. The focus of nursing care is maintaining a patent airway, facilitating the removal of pulmonary secretions, providing humidified air or $O_2$, cleansing the stoma, monitoring the child's ability to swallow, and teaching while simultaneously preventing complications.

Because the child may be unable to signal for help, direct observation of the child, as well as the use of respiratory and cardiac monitors, is essential. Respiratory assessments (including breath sounds and work of breathing, vital signs, tightness of the tracheostomy ties, and the type and amount of secretions) are performed every 15 minutes until the patient is stable and then every 1 to 2 hours for the first 24 hours. Assessments thereafter are performed every 2 to 4 hours or more frequently if needed.

> **NURSING ALERT**　Large amounts of bloody secretions are uncommon and should be considered a sign of hemorrhage. The practitioner should be notified immediately if this occurs.

The child is positioned with the head of the bed raised, or in the position most comfortable to the child, with the call light easily available. Suction catheters, the suction source, gloves, sterile saline, sterile gauze for wiping away secretions, scissors, an extra tracheostomy tube of the same size with ties already attached, another tracheostomy tube one size smaller, and the obturator are kept at the bedside. A source of humidification is provided, because the normal humidification and filtering functions of the airway have been bypassed. Intravenous fluids ensure adequate hydration until the child is able to swallow sufficient amounts of fluids.

**Suctioning.** The airway must remain patent and requires frequent suctioning during the first few hours after a tracheostomy to remove mucous plugs and excessive secretions. Hyperoxygenation should be provided before suctioning. Proper vacuum pressure and suction catheter size are important to prevent atelectasis and decrease hypoxia from the suctioning procedure. Vacuum pressure should range from 60 to 100 mm Hg for infants and children and from 40 to 60 mm Hg for preterm infants. Unless secretions are thick and tenacious, the lower range of negative pressure is recommended. Tracheal suction catheters are available in a variety of sizes. The catheter selected should have a diameter one half the diameter of the tracheostomy tube. If the catheter is too large, it can block the airway. The catheter is constructed with a side port so that the catheter is introduced without suction and removed while simultaneously intermittent suction is applied by covering the port with the thumb (Fig. 31-18). The catheter is inserted to 0.5 cm beyond or just to the end of the tracheostomy tube.

The practice of instilling sterile saline in the tracheostomy tube before suctioning is not supported by research and is no longer recommended by many institutions. (See Evidence-Based Practice box.)

> **NURSING ALERT**　Suctioning should require no more than 5 seconds.

Counting 1—one thousand, 2—one thousand, 3—one thousand, and so on while suctioning is a simple means for monitoring the time. Without a safeguard, the airway may

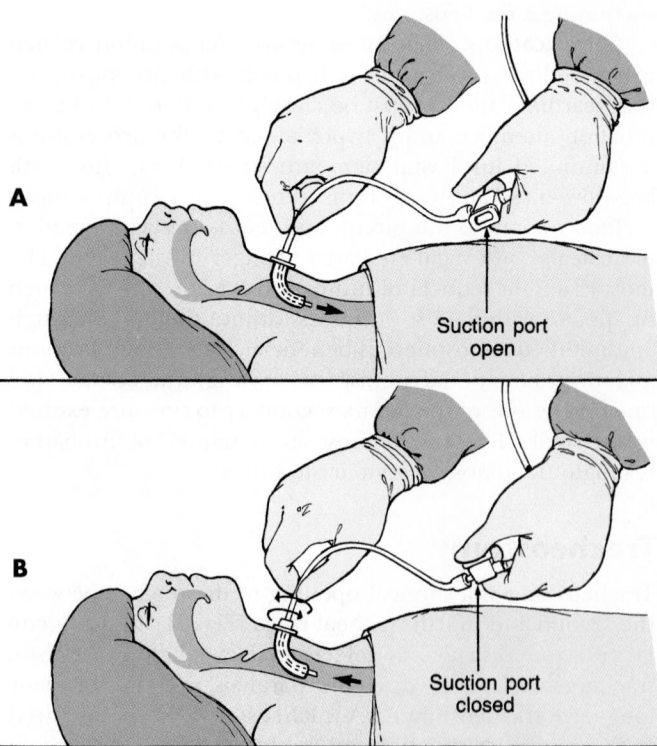

**Fig. 31-18** Tracheostomy suctioning. **A,** Insertion, port open. **B,** Withdrawal, port occluded. Note that catheter is inserted just slightly beyond end of tracheostomy tube.

be obstructed for too long. Hyperventilating the child with 100% $O_2$ before and after suctioning (using a bag-valve-mask or increasing the $FIO_2$ ventilator setting) is also performed to prevent hypoxia. Closed tracheal suctioning systems that allow for uninterrupted $O_2$ delivery may also be used. In a closed suction system a suction catheter is directly attached to the ventilator tubing. This system has several advantages. First, there is no need to disconnect the patient from the ventilator, which allows for better oxygenation. Second, the suction catheter is enclosed in a plastic sheath, which reduces the risk of exposure to the patient's secretions (Carroll, 1998).

The child is allowed to rest for 30 to 60 seconds after each aspiration to allow $O_2$ saturation to return to normal; then the process is repeated until the trachea is clear. Suctioning should be limited to about three aspirations in one period. Oximetry is an effective feedback tool to monitor suctioning and prevent hypoxia.

**NURSING ALERT** Suctioning is carried out *only* as often as *needed* to keep the tube patent. Signs of mucus partially occluding the airway include an increased heart rate, a rise in respiratory effort, a drop in $O_2$ saturation, cyanosis, or an increase in the positive inspiratory pressure (PIP) on the ventilator.

In the acute care setting, aseptic technique is used during care of the tracheostomy. Secondary infection is a major concern because the air entering the lower airway bypasses the natural defenses of the upper airway. Gloves are worn

## EVIDENCE-BASED PRACTICE
### Suctioning, Catheter Length, and Saline

Traditional technique for suctioning endotracheal (ET) or tracheostomy tubes recommends advancing a suction catheter into the tube until it meets resistance, then withdrawing it slightly and applying suction. However, studies indicate that this approach causes trauma to the tracheobronchial wall. This trauma can be avoided by inserting the catheter and advancing it to the premeasured depth of just to the tip (especially in infants) or no more than 0.5 cm beyond the tube (Kleiber, Krutzfield, and Rose, 1988).

Calibrated catheters are easier to use for premeasured suctioning technique, but unmarked catheters can also be used. To measure the length for catheter insertion, place the catheter near a sample ET or tracheostomy tube (same size as child's tube), with the end of the catheter at the correct position. Grasp the catheter with a sterile-gloved hand to mark the length, and insert the catheter until the hand reaches the stoma.

It has been common practice to instill a bolus of normal saline into the tube before suctioning. However, this technique may contribute to lower airway colonization and nosocomial pneumonia through repeated washing of organisms from the tube's surface into the lower airway (Haglar and Traver, 1994). The use of saline has been shown to have an adverse effect on $SaO_2$ and should not be used routinely in patients receiving mechanical ventilation who have a pulmonary infection (Ackerman, 1998). Although the pediatric research is scarce, routine use of normal saline with ET tube suctioning should be avoided (Curley and Moloney-Harmon, 2001).

during the aspiration procedure, although a sterile glove is needed only on the hand touching the catheter. A new sterile suction catheter and sterile gloves are used each time. (See Critical Thinking Exercise box.)

**Routine Care.** The tracheostomy stoma requires daily care. Assessments of the stoma area include observations for signs of infection and breakdown of the skin. The skin is kept clean and dry, and secretions around the stoma may be gently removed with half-strength hydrogen peroxide. Hydrogen peroxide should not be used with sterling silver tracheostomy tubes because it tends to pit and stain the silver surface. The nurse should be aware of wet tracheostomy dressings, which

## Critical Thinking Exercise
### Planning for Home Tracheostomy Care

Jose Munoz, 18 months old, has been ventilator-dependent since birth. He is presently hospitalized with pneumonia that has responded well to antibiotic therapy. You are discussing plans for discharge and home care with the family. Jose lives with his mother and her parents. Home nursing support is available only during the day. The family does not want to take Jose home because he is frequently suctioned at night. What should your initial intervention be?

FIRST, THINK ABOUT IT . . .

• What conclusions are you reaching?
• If you accept the conclusions, what are the implications?

1. Talk with the night nurses about their suctioning program.
2. Design a plan for the family that allows them to each assume responsibility for night care with scheduled suctioning times.
3. Arrange with social services to request additional financial support for the family.
4. Suggest that Jose stay in the hospital until he needs less frequent suctioning.

*The best response is one. If the family managed with daytime nursing assistance before this hospitalization and the pneumonia has resolved, the child should not require intensive suctioning. In talking with the night staff, you find that the nurses suction anytime they walk past the room and hear Jose "gurgling." Also, if you accept the conclusion that they do not use premeasured suctioning technique, the implications are that you need to discuss with them a program of premeasured suctioning only as needed to reduce the production of secretion that may be from tracheal irritation.*

*The other three responses assume that the frequent suctioning is needed and are not appropriate initial interventions. Suctioning should be performed not on a set schedule, but only as needed. Requesting additional financial support does not contain costs and does not allow the family to return to their prehospitalization status. Jose should be discharged as soon as possible to avoid nosocomial infection, promote normalization for a toddler, and contain health care costs. In this case, changing the suctioning regimen decreased the frequency to a minimum of once or twice a night—a level of care the family was able to manage.*

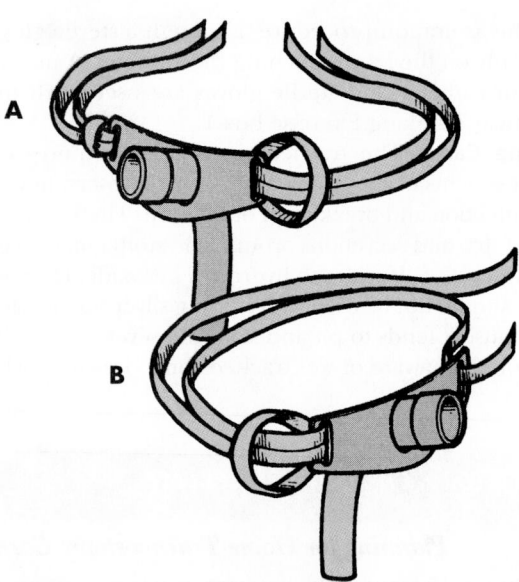

**Fig. 31-19** Pediatric tracheostomy tube. **A,** Cloth tape secured at both sides to be tied in back. **B,** Cloth tape secured on one side and looped through other side to be tied at side.

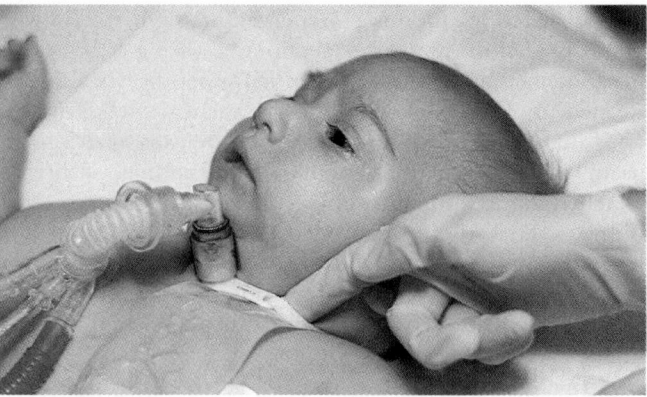

**Fig. 31-20** Tracheostomy ties are snug but allow one finger to be inserted.

can predispose the peristomal area to skin breakdown. Several products are available to prevent or treat excoriation. The Allevyn tracheostomy dressing is a hydrophilic sponge with a polyurethane back that is highly absorptive. Other possible barriers to help maintain skin integrity include the use of hydrocolloid wafers (e.g., Duoderm CGF, Hollister Restore) under the tracheostomy flanges, as well as the use of extrathin hydrocolloid wafers under the chin.

The tracheostomy tube is held in place with tracheostomy ties made of a durable, nonfraying material. The ties are changed daily and when soiled. New ties are looped through the flanges (Fig. 31-19) and tied snugly in a triple knot at the side of the neck *before* the soiled ties are cut and removed. Some nurses have found that threading the ties through a piece of ¼-inch surgical tubing cushions the ties; others have found the tubing to be irritating to the skin. The ties should be tight enough to allow just a fingertip to be inserted between the ties and the neck (Fig. 31-20). It is easier to ensure a snug fit if the child's head is flexed rather than extended while the ties are being secured. Ties fastened with self-adhering closures are also available. These devices, such as the Dale tracheostomy tube holder, are made of a soft, cushioning, and slightly stretchy material that is very comfortable. They are becoming increasingly popular because of their ease of use and ability to maintain better skin integrity. However, nurses and family members must consider the safety factor and use them only on children who will not pull and undo the fastener.

Routine tracheostomy tube changes are usually carried out weekly after a tract has been formed to minimize formation of granulation tissue. The first change is usually performed by the surgeon; subsequent changes are performed by the nurse and, if the child is discharged home with the tracheostomy, by either a parent or a visiting nurse. Ideally, two caregivers participate in the procedure to assist with positioning the child.

Changing the tracheostomy tube is accomplished using sterile technique. Tube changes should occur before meals or 2 hours after the last meal. Continuous feedings should be turned off at least an hour before a tube change. The new, sterile tube is prepared by inserting the obturator and attaching new ties. The child is suctioned before the procedure to minimize secretions, then restrained and positioned with the neck slightly extended. One caregiver cuts the old ties and removes the tube from the stoma. The new tube is inserted gently into the stoma (using a downward and forward motion that follows the curve of the trachea), the obturator is removed, and the ties are secured. The adequacy of ventilation must be assessed after a tube change because the tube can be inserted into the soft tissue surrounding the trachea; therefore breath sounds and respiratory effort are carefully monitored.

Supplemental $O_2$ is always delivered with a humidification system to prevent drying of the respiratory mucosa (Fig. 31-21). Humidification of room air for an established tracheostomy can be intermittent if secretions remain thin enough to be coughed or suctioned from the tracheostomy. Direct humidification via tracheostomy mask can be provided during naps and at night so that the child is able to be up and around unencumbered during much of the day. Room humidifiers are also used successfully.

The inner cannula, if used, should be removed with each suctioning, cleaned with sterile saline and pipe cleaners to remove crusted material, dried thoroughly, and reinserted.

**Emergency Care: Tube Occlusion and Accidental Decannulation.** Occlusion of the tracheostomy tube is life-threatening. Infants and children are at greater risk than adults because of the smaller diameter of the tube. Maintaining patency of the tube is accomplished with suctioning and routine tube changes to prevent formation of crusts that can occlude the tube.

**NURSING ALERT** Life-threatening occlusion is apparent when the child displays signs of respiratory distress and a suction catheter cannot be passed to the end of the tube despite several attempts and instillation of saline. This situation requires an immediate tube change.

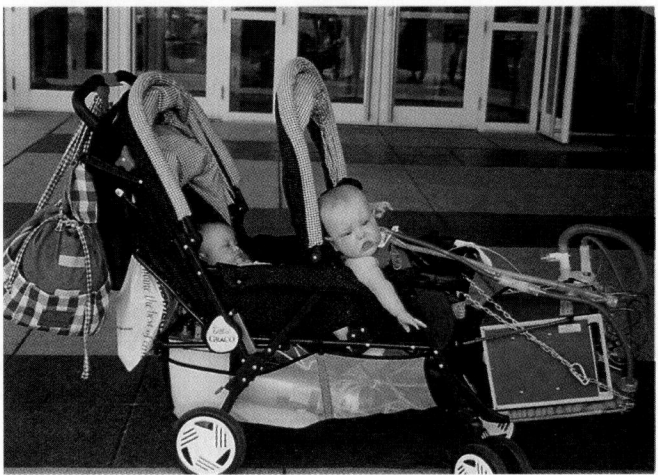

**Fig. 31-21**   Child with a tracheostomy.

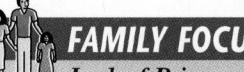

**FAMILY FOCUS**
*Lack of Privacy: Children with*
*Respiratory Problems in Home Care*

Currently, many children with chronic respiratory problems are discharged home on apnea monitors, on oxygen, or with a tracheostomy or ventilator assistance. When a child is on an apnea monitor, the family may need to make only a few adjustments in their routines to accommodate this need. However, when a child has a tracheostomy or requires ventilator assistance, many family routines may need to be changed. In particular, the family will need to give up some of their privacy to accommodate many different people coming into the home. Nurses, equipment vendors, respiratory therapists, rehabilitation therapists, and social workers may all need to visit frequently. One mother of a child in home care counted a total of 25 different health-related professionals who came to her home in a single day. All of these intrusions seriously limit privacy and tax the family's coping strategies. Many mothers of children in home care state that no one prepared them for the constant interruptions in daily routines, the continuous demands on their time, the loss of family leisure time, and the need to interact with so many different people. Nurses who work with families of children in home care because of respiratory problems need to provide information concerning the changes the family can anticipate in their everyday routines, the stress these changes can produce, the need for respite care, and the benefits of support groups in providing emotional support.

Accidental decannulation also requires immediate tube replacement. Some children have a fairly rigid trachea, so that the airway remains partially open when the tube is removed. However, others have malformed or flexible tracheal cartilage, which causes the airway to collapse when the tube is removed or dislodged. Because many infants and children with upper airway problems have little airway reserve, if replacement of the dislodged tube is impossible, a smaller-sized tube should be inserted. Ventilation with a bag-valve-mask should be provided to the stoma if the child is apneic. If the stoma cannot be cannulated with another tracheostomy tube, oral intubation should be performed.

### Decannulation

The tracheostomy tube is removed as soon as it is no longer needed. Diseases of short duration (e.g., croup) usually allow early removal, but some conditions (e.g., tracheomalacia, tracheostenosis, paralysis) may require that the tube remain in place indefinitely. Opinions differ regarding the best means for removing the tube, especially after lengthy intubation. The usual procedure is to wean the child to the smallest possible tracheostomy tube. Once this has been accomplished and the child's respiratory status is unimpaired for 24 hours, the tube is occluded, with removal within the next 24 hours. A small bandage is usually placed over the open stoma, which will close within a short period of time. The procedure is carried out in a clinical setting where continuous observation is available and emergency reintubation can be accomplished without delay, if necessary. Following successful decannulation, the child remains under close observation for an additional period of time.

### Home Care of the Child with a Tracheostomy

The early return of the infant or child with a tracheostomy to a home setting can reduce the amount of developmental delay or social handicap related to prolonged hospitalization. Placement in the home also allows for reestablishment of routines and a regular schedule of normal activities. Physical or occupational therapy, as well as speech therapy, is continued in the home setting. Nursing care may also be continued in the home through private-duty care or by routine, frequent nursing visits.

Preparing the family to care for the child with a tracheostomy at home is multifaceted. (See Family Focus box.) Teaching sessions should be short, and written material must accompany instructions to reinforce what is taught.* The family must be able to demonstrate tracheostomy care before the child is discharged from the hospital. Home-based care of a tracheostomy includes suctioning the tracheostomy, cleaning the stoma, changing the tracheostomy ties, changing the tracheostomy tube, adjusting or adapting the home environment, and recognizing warning signs of obstruction, infection, or a worsening condition.

To prepare for any emergency, the family must be taught infant or child cardiopulmonary resuscitation (CPR). The local utilities company and local emergency medical service (EMS) should be notified of the child's condition and the equipment used in the home. Prior notification allows for a quick response if help is needed.

The home should have all the necessary equipment before the child arrives. Supplies include sterile saline, a portable, battery-operated suction machine (as well as a DeLee suction trap), connecting tubing for suction, suction catheters, hydrogen peroxide, tracheostomy dressings, twill tape or self-adhering tracheostomy ties, pipe cleaners or a tracheostomy brush, sterile jars, an extra tracheostomy tube, a ventilator bag, and a cool mist humidifier. Many children receive $O_2$ at home; so this too must be in place. Finally, an apnea monitor or oximeter may be needed.

---

*Home care instructions for tracheostomy care and postural drainage are available in Wong DL, Hess CS: *Wong and Whaley's clinical manual of pediatric nursing*, ed 5, St Louis, 2000, Mosby.

The family should be encouraged to take the child out of the home for routine outings. Two people should always be present when traveling because the child may need attention while riding in the car or at the destination. In addition to routine child care supplies, the family should always bring the portable suction machine, sterile suction catheters, an extra tracheostomy tube, and a complete sterile tracheostomy care kit.

**Management of the Tracheostomy.** Clean technique and thorough, strict handwashing is taught for suctioning, cleaning the tracheostomy site, and changing the tracheostomy tube. One sterile suction catheter per day is usually sufficient. After initial use, the catheter is rinsed with sterile water and then stored between uses in a sterile cup or jar.

Skin at the tracheostomy site is assessed for areas of breakdown or drainage. The area can be cleansed with an antibacterial soap and water.

The family is encouraged not to oversuction the child because this causes increased mucus production and irritation to the mucosal lining. The care provider should be alert to changes in the child's secretions regarding the amount, color, or viscosity. Awareness of these changes can prompt early medical interventions if necessary.

When dealing with the child's secretions, the family must be able to take care of a plugged, clogged, or obstructed tracheostomy tube. This situation can result in life-threatening circumstances. The family must be able to remove the plugged tube and replace it with a clean one.

Older children and adolescents should be taught to care for their tracheostomies. The child should be encouraged to assume as much of his or her care as is developmentally appropriate. Independence is enhanced as the child takes responsibility for tracheostomy care.

**Home Environment.** Changes in the home environment may be necessary before bringing the child home. Toys, blankets, clothing, and pets that shed fine hair or lint, as well as aerosols, powders, dust, and smoke, should be avoided. Fine particles from any of these items can accumulate in the tracheostomy tube and obstruct the airway. Toys that have small removable parts (that could become foreign bodies if placed in the tracheostomy tube) should also be eliminated.

Clothing should have a loose-fitting collar that does not cover the tracheostomy tube opening. When the child is outside, the artificial nose or a thin cloth such as a bandanna can be placed loosely over the tracheostomy tube to prevent cold air, dust, dirt, or sand from entering the tube. The latter also camouflages the tracheostomy and allows a sense of normalcy to occur.

Bathing can be performed in a tub filled with shallow water, although it is important to ensure that no water or soap enters the tracheostomy tube. If this does occur, the tracheostomy should be suctioned immediately. Older children may shower if they are able to tolerate plugging the tube while under the shower spray.

**Vocalization.** The life of a child with a tracheostomy should be normalized. After the child returns home, routines should be established that allow the child to renew skills and enhance childhood development. Verbalization and speaking are major tasks that are often overlooked. Vocalization for the child with a tracheostomy has recently become a reality. Several tracheostomy speaking valves have been created to aid in the development of uninterrupted speech without the necessity of finger occlusion. When the speaking valve is used, air enters through the tracheostomy but is expelled over the vocal cords and through the mouth and nose. This creates a more normal passage of air through the upper airway.

Many benefits are afforded to the child with a speaking valve. An improved self-image is developed, because the tracheostomy can be disguised and finger occlusion for speech is not needed. The ability to swallow improves, because pressure can now accumulate as a result of the decreased amount of air released from the tracheostomy. This also allows for the creation of back pressure into the lungs. The lungs then remain open for improved gas exchange. Other advantages of this redirection of air by a speaking valve into the upper airway include improved senses of smell and taste. Secretion production is decreased because of normal evaporation, and secretions can now be coughed into the mouth, decreasing the amount of suctioning required.

Several speaking valves are available. The *Passy-Muir* valve* is a one-way valve that attaches to the hub of all types and sizes of tracheostomies. The Passy-Muir valve will not function properly without an air leak around the tracheostomy tube and is contraindicated if there is a lack of air leak around the tube or there is an upper airway obstruction (Kaut, Turcott, and Lavery, 1996). Therefore a cuffed tracheostomy tube must be fully deflated when using the Passy-Muir valve. If the cuff is not deflated, and the Passy Muir valve is attached, the patient will lose his or her airway. This valve can be used in infants and in children who are ventilator assisted (Engleman and Turnage-Carrier, 1997).

The Pilling Company† makes two types of speaking valves for adolescents and adults. The first, the *Kistner valve*—a part of all Kistner tracheostomy tubes—is made of thin, soft plastic and does not protrude into the trachea. (Jackson metal tracheostomy tubes can also be used with a Kistner valve.) The second type is the *Tucker valve,* which is built into the inner cannula as a one-way leaflet. The leaflet opens on inspiration to allow air in and closes on expiration to force air into the upper airway. The Tucker valve inner cannula can be used with Tucker tracheostomy tubes sizes 4 to 9 and with Jackson tracheostomy tubes sizes 4 to 8. Tucker valves can only be used with sterling silver tracheostomy tubes.

Tracheostomy speaking valves are inappropriate for use in children who require an inflated cuff tracheostomy; who have a laryngectomy, severe tracheostenosis, or copious or excessive secretions; and in unconscious or seriously ill children.

**Socialization.** School-age children can be placed in a regular classroom environment and participate in school ac-

---

*Further information can be obtained from Passy & Passy, Inc, 4521 Campus Dr, Suite 273, Irvine, CA 92612, (800) 634-5397, fax (949) 833-8299, e-mail: info@passy.muir.com; www.passy-muir.com.
†Further information can be obtained from The Pilling Company, 420 Delaware Dr, Fort Washington, PA 19034, (800) 523-6507.

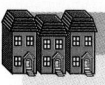

tivities as their physical abilities will allow it. (See Community Focus box.) They should be encouraged to interact with their peers to facilitate socialization. Participation in ability-appropriate extracurricular activities should also be advocated.

Many children with tracheostomies benefit from attending summer camps for children with tracheostomies who may or may not be ventilator dependent. Camping environments provide the child with independent living and a normal camping experience. Some camping sites allow the family to vacation together yet provide special care and assistance for the child with a tracheostomy.

## RESPIRATORY EMERGENCY

### Respiratory Failure

An inadequate supply of $O_2$ results in blood *hypoxemia* and tissue *hypoxia;* inadequate $CO_2$ removal causes *hypercapnia.* Often both gases may be insufficiently exchanged. In general, the term *respiratory insufficiency* is applied to two conditions: (1) when there is increased work of breathing but gas exchange function remains near normal and (2) when normal blood gas tensions cannot be maintained and hypoxemia and acidosis develop secondary to $CO_2$ retention.

*Respiratory failure* is defined as the inability of the respiratory apparatus to maintain adequate oxygenation of the blood, with or without $CO_2$ retention. This process involves pulmonary dysfunction that generally results in impaired alveolar gas exchange, which can lead to hypoxemia or hypercarbia.

*Respiratory arrest* is the cessation of respiration.

*Apnea* is generally defined as cessation of breathing for more than 20 seconds or for a shorter period when associated with hypoxemia or bradycardia (Curley and Moloney-Harmon, 2001). Apnea can be (1) *central,* in which respiratory efforts are absent; (2) *obstructive,* in which respiratory efforts are present; and (3) *mixed,* in which both central and obstructive components are present.

Effective pulmonary gas exchange requires clear airways, normal lungs and chest wall, and adequate pulmonary circulation. Anything that affects these functions or their relationships can compromise respiration.

Respiratory dysfunction may have an abrupt or an insidious onset. Respiratory failure can occur as an emergency situation or may be preceded by gradual and progressive deterioration of respiratory function. Most clinical manifestations are nonspecific and are affected by variations among individual patients and differences in the severity and duration of inadequate gas exchange.

The diagnosis of respiratory failure is determined by the combined application of three sources of information:

1. Presence or history of a condition that might predispose to respiratory failure
2. Observation of respiratory failure
3. Measurement of arterial blood gases (ABGs) and pH

### Conditions That Predispose to Respiratory Failure

Respiratory disorders are classified according to three dominant functional abnormalities, although all three types may be present in the disease. In *obstructive lung disease* there is increased resistance to airflow in either the upper or the lower respiratory tract. Obstruction can result from anomalies (e.g., tracheomalacia, choanal atresia, vocal paralysis), aspiration (e.g., meconium, mucus, vomitus, foreign body), infection (e.g., epiglottitis, pneumonia, pertussis, severe tonsillitis), tumors (e.g., hemangioma), anaphylaxis, and laryngospasm from local irritation (e.g., intubation, drowning, aspiration).

In *restrictive lung disease* there is impaired lung expansion resulting from loss of lung volume, decreased distensibility, or chest wall disturbance. Causes of pulmonary restriction include respiratory distress syndrome, pneumonia, cystic fibrosis, pneumothorax, pulmonary edema, plural effusion, near-drowning, diaphragmatic hernia, abdominal distention, muscular dystrophy, and paralytic conditions (e.g., polio, botulism).

In *primary inefficient gas transfer* there is insufficient alveolar ventilation for $CO_2$ removal or impaired oxygenation of pulmonary capillary blood as a result of dysfunction of the respiratory control mechanism or a diffusion defect. Causes of *respiratory center depression* include cerebral trauma (birth injuries); intracranial tumors; central nervous system infection (meningitis, encephalitis, sepsis); overdose with barbiturates, opioids, benzodiazepines (diazepam [Valium] or midazolam [Versed]); severe asphyxia (hypercapnia, hypoxemia); and tetanus. *Pulmonary diffusion defects* include pulmonary edema, fibrosis, embolism, or hypertension; collagen disorders; *Pneumocystis carinii* infection; anemia; and hemorrhage.

## Recognition of Respiratory Failure

Respiratory failure that occurs as a result of acute obstruction of a major airway or cardiac arrest is sudden and readily apparent. Gradual and more covert development of signs and symptoms is less easily recognized. Insufficient alveolar ventilation from any cause ultimately leads to hypoxemia and hypercapnia. However, situations occur in which severe respiratory distress may be present without significant $CO_2$ retention, and hypoxemia may occur without clinically detectable cyanosis. Therefore evaluation of respiratory adequacy is based on both clinical assessment and laboratory studies. Nursing observation and judgment are vital to successful management of respiratory failure. Nurses must be able to assess a situation and initiate appropriate action within moments.

Unless respiratory arrest occurs suddenly, signs of hypoxemia and hypercapnia are usually subtle in their development and become more obvious as respiratory failure progresses. The unknowing observer may attribute early signs such as mood changes and restlessness to other causes, and some signs can be altered by other factors. Clinical manifestations of respiratory failure are outlined in Box 31-8.

In clinical situations in which impaired ventilation can be anticipated or clinical manifestations indicate impending hypoxemia, serial measurements of blood gases should be obtained and monitored to detect impending respiratory failure, and therapy should be implemented before respiratory acidosis becomes extreme.

---

### Box 31-8 ■ ■ ■
### Clinical Manifestations of Respiratory Failure

**CARDINAL SIGNS**

Restlessness
Tachypnea
Tachycardia
Diaphoresis

**EARLY BUT LESS OBVIOUS SIGNS**

Mood changes, such as euphoria or depression
Headache
Altered depth and pattern of respirations
Hypertension
Exertional dyspnea
Anorexia
Increased cardiac output and renal output
Central nervous system symptoms (decreased efficiency, impaired judgment, anxiety, confusion, restlessness, irritability, depressed level of consciousness)
Flaring nares
Chest wall retractions
Expiratory grunt
Wheezing or prolonged expiration

**SIGNS OF MORE SEVERE HYPOXIA**

| | |
|---|---|
| Hypotension or hypertension | Depressed respirations |
| Dimness of vision | Bradycardia |
| Somnolence | Cyanosis, peripheral or |
| Stupor |   central |
| Coma | |
| Dyspnea | |

---

## Management and Related Nursing Considerations

The interventions used in the management of respiratory failure are often dramatic, requiring special skills, and are frequently emergency procedures. If respiratory arrest occurs, the primary objectives are to recognize the situation and immediately initiate resuscitative measures, such as suctioning, CPR, or intubation. When the situation is not an arrest, the suspicion of respiratory failure is confirmed by assessment and the severity is defined by ABG analysis. Interventions such as supplemental $O_2$, positioning, stimulation, suctioning, and early intubation may avert an arrest. When severity is established, an attempt is made to determine the underlying cause by thorough evaluation.

Treatment of respiratory dysfunction involves both specific and nonspecific therapy. Specific therapies are directed toward reversal of the causative factors. However, nonspecific measures are needed to maintain oxygenation and enhance $CO_2$ removal until specific methods take effect. The major reasons for implementing nonspecific treatments are (1) unknown etiology, (2) lack of specific treatment for a known cause, (3) lack of time for a specific treatment to take effect, and (4) need for specialized personnel or equipment for specific treatment.

The principles of management are to (1) treat the underlying cause, (2) correct hypoxemia/hypercapnia, (3) maintain ventilation and maximize $O_2$ delivery, (4) minimize extrapulmonary organ failure, (5) apply specific and nonspecific therapy to control $O_2$ demands, and (6) anticipate complications. Monitoring the patient's condition is critical.

### Observation and Monitoring

The child is monitored to evaluate the cause of the failure, determine a course of action, and assess the patient's response to treatment. If close, continuous monitoring is required, the child is transferred to an intensive care unit. The child is kept as comfortable as possible, and observation is geared toward general appearance, responsiveness, pulse oximetry, and vital signs. The child is positioned to allow maximum lung expansion and comfort, such as sitting upright or leaning forward.

Recently, prone positioning has been used to improve oxygenation and lung mechanics in adult patients with acute lung injury and acute respiratory distress syndrome. A preliminary study of pediatric patients indicated that these patients may also experience improved oxygenation without serious iatrogenic injury after prone positioning (Curley, Thompson, and Arnold, 2000). Future randomized clinical trials should indicate the safety and effectiveness of this type of positioning on clinical outcomes in pediatric patients (Curley and Moloney-Harmon, 2001).

The child's cardiac and respiratory status are monitored by observation and by electronic means. However, no monitoring equipment can replace conscientious nursing observations (Box 31-9), which should focus primarily on the child's airway, oxygenation, ventilation, and skin perfusion.

Because one goal of therapy is to control the $O_2$ demands of the body, assessments of fever and pain should be frequent. Both conditions (as well as cold stress) can dramatically increase $O_2$ requirements, especially in younger children, and therefore increase respiratory effort. Oxygenation is measured by the use of pulse oximetry or blood gases.

## Family Support

Children who are fatigued and in distress before a procedure, such as a tracheostomy, often relax after establishment of an airway. However, unless they remain unconscious or semiconscious, they will be anxious and frightened when they are unable to communicate. Children who are old enough to write and not too fatigued can use a pad of paper and a pencil or spelling board to express their needs and concerns. Other alternative means for communication are pictures illustrating various items and activities. Simple sign language is an effective and easily learned communication method.

It is a terrifying experience for young children to discover that they are unable to make vocal sounds, including crying. It is also stressful to parents to watch their children plead with frightened eyes and cry noiselessly. It is important to talk to children and reassure them that their voices will return when the tube is removed. Children can also be taught to occlude the opening with a clean finger so that they can use the vocal cords to communicate.

Parents have many concerns relative to tracheostomies, ET tubes, and ventilators. Before intubation or a tracheostomy, the reasons for the decision to implement the therapy, the expected results, and the approximate length of time it will remain in place should be discussed with them. Parental concern is centered around the (often) life-threatening implications generated by the need for the procedure and the possible long-term effects on the child, both physiologic and psychologic. Parents are concerned about the visible wound and the scar. Parents who must face the possibility of caring for the child with a tracheostomy or a ventilator at home have additional worries regarding their ability to assume this responsibility (see p. 1329 and Fig. 31-22.)

For those families whose child has a respiratory arrest, support focuses on keeping the family informed of the child's status and helping them cope with a near-death experience or an actual death. (See Chapter 23.) Knowing that their child requires CPR is a frightening and often overwhelming experience for parents. Uncertainty regarding outcome—both mortality and morbidity—is a primary concern. Traditionally family members have not been allowed to be present during resuscitation efforts. (See Evidence-Based Practice box on p. 1334.) Nurses can serve as the family's advocate by either being present with them or making sure a support person, such as the clergy, is present. After the child's recovery or death, the family needs continued support and thorough medical information regarding life-saving measures, the prognosis if the child survives, and the cause of death if the child dies.

## Cardiopulmonary Resuscitation (CPR)*

Cardiac arrest in the pediatric population is less often of cardiac origin than from prolonged hypoxemia secondary to inadequate oxygenation, ventilation, and circulation (shock). Some causes include injuries, suffocation (e.g., foreign body aspiration), smoke inhalation, sudden infant death syndrome (SIDS), and infection. Respiratory arrest is associated with a better survival than cardiac arrest. Once cardiac arrest occurs, the outcome of resuscitative efforts is poor. There is a 25% mortality rate for children who experience a respiratory arrest, and an 87% mortality rate when cardiac arrest occurs (Young and Seidel, 1999).

Complete apnea signals the need for rapid and vigorous action to prevent cardiac arrest. In such situations nurses must be prepared to initiate action immediately. In the hospital, emergency equipment should be readily available in areas in which respiratory arrest might take place, and the status of this resuscitation equipment should be checked at least once daily. Regardless of the cause of the arrest, basic procedures are carried out and modified somewhat according to the child's size.

---

*Home care instructions for CPR are available in Wong DL, Hess CS: *Wong and Whaley's clinical manual of pediatric nursing*, ed 5, St Louis, 2000, Mosby.

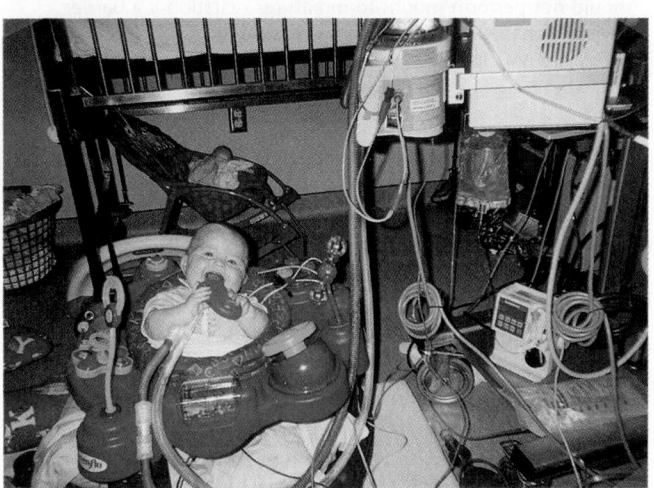

**Fig. 31-22** Child with a tracheostomy being managed at home.

---

**Box 31-9** ■ ■ ■
### Nursing Observations for the Child with Respiratory Failure

Visual inspection of skin color to estimate level of arterial $O_2$ saturation
Observation of respiratory effort or distress—nasal flaring, grunting, gasping, retraction, agonal respirations
Observation of diaphragmatic movement, lung expansion, and use of accessory muscles—depth, symmetry, inspiration/expiration ratio
Auscultation of thorax to assess:
  Breath sounds—presence, intensity, quality, symmetry
  Abnormal sounds—stridor, wheezes, crackles, rubs, crepitation, increase or decrease in sounds
  Tube placement and need for endotracheal suction when child is intubated

In the past, few acute care facilities have allowed parents to remain during CPR or a "code." The traditional thinking was that this experience would be upsetting to parents and that family members would require care that would interfere with resuscitation efforts. However, recent studies indicate that family presence during emergencies alleviates the family's anger about being separated from the patient during a crisis, reduces their anxiety, eliminates doubts about what was done to help the patient, and facilitates the grieving process (Anderson and others, 1994; Powers and Rubenstein, 1999; Sacchetti and others, 1996).

Currently many nurses foster efforts to permit parental presence during resuscitation (Eichhorn and others, 1996). The Emergency Nurses Association (1995) not only supports but has developed national guidelines for family presence during invasive procedures and CPR. These guidelines include recommendations for assessing family members to determine if family presence is appropriate and the use of a family facilitator (e.g., a nurse, child-life specialist, or chaplain) who remains with the family during resuscitation to answer questions, clarify information, and offer comfort. Recently the Parkland Health and Hospital System conducted an investigation of these guidelines. The study included interviews with 39 family members and 96 health care providers who were present in the emergency department during invasive procedures or CPR (Meyers and others, 2000). Thirty-one percent of the invasive procedures or CPR efforts in this study involved pediatric patients. All family members who participated believed their presence at the procedure was helpful and stated they would do it again. Ninety-six percent of the nurses and 79% of the attending physicians supported family presence and felt it should be continued at the hospital. As a result of this study a hospital-wide protocol for family presence was approved.

Results of these empirical studies indicate that flexible programs to facilitate parental presence during CPR can be implemented in acute care settings. Not all parents will want to take advantage of such programs, but family presence represents an effort to preserve the wholeness, integrity, and dignity of the family unit (Eichhorn and others, 1996).

---

> **NURSING ALERT**
>
> Rescuers who have infections that may be transmitted by blood or saliva or who believe they have been exposed to such an infection should not perform mouth-to-mouth resuscitation if a barrier device or mask with a one-way valve is not available. If CPR efforts are anticipated in the workplace or other out-of-hospital settings, rescuers should have access to these devices (American Heart Association, 2000).

Outside the hospital the first action in an emergency is to quickly assess the extent of any injury and determine whether the child is unconscious. A child who is struggling to breathe but conscious should be transported immediately to an advanced life support (ALS) facility, allowing the child to maintain whatever position affords the most comfort. Attempting to transport a child by automobile wastes valuable time in obtaining help. Transport by EMS is recommended. Services in larger communities can institute ALS immediately or en route to a medical facility.

An unconscious child is managed with care to prevent additional trauma if a head or spinal cord injury has been sustained. The circumstances in which the child is found of-fer clues to a possible injury. For example, a child who has been thrown from a bicycle or has fallen from a tree is more likely to have sustained trauma than a child who is discovered in bed. The child should be turned as a unit with firm support to the head and neck to prevent rolling, twisting, or tilting backward or forward.

### Resuscitation Procedure

The American Heart Association (2000) implemented several changes in CPR guidelines in July 2001. The new guidelines incorporate the use of the automated external defibrillator as a part of the treatment of cardiorespiratory arrest in adults and children older than 8 years of age. Health care providers are advised to give adults and children older than 8 years a defibrillatory shock within 5 minutes of collapse outside the hospital and within 3 minutes in the hospital. Other changes in the guidelines focus on the lay rescuer. Changes for the lay rescuer are discussed in the text. The sequence of CPR steps for the health care provider are discussed in both the text and in Figs. 31-23 and 31-24.

For effective CPR the victim is placed on the back on a firm, flat surface, employing appropriate precautions. **Unlike rescuers of adults, who initiate EMS first, pediatric rescuers provide 1 minute of basic life support (BLS) before activating EMS.** Because pediatric arrests are most commonly due to respiratory arrest, maintaining ventilation is primary.

With loss of consciousness, the tongue, which is attached to the lower jaw, relaxes and falls back, obstructing the airway. To open the airway, the head is positioned with either a head tilt/chin lift or a jaw thrust. Health professionals should be able to use both maneuvers. A **head tilt** is accomplished by placing one hand on the victim's forehead and applying firm, backward pressure with the palm to tilt the head back. The fingers of the free hand are placed under the bony portion of the lower jaw near the chin to lift and bring the chin forward *(chin lift)*. This supports the jaw and helps tilt the head back (Fig. 31-25, *A*).

The *jaw thrust* is accomplished by grasping the angles of the victim's lower jaw and lifting with both hands, one on each side, displacing the mandible upward and outward (Fig. 31-25, *B*). In suspected neck injuries the jaw thrust method should be used while the cervical spine is completely immobilized. After restoration of a patent airway by removal of foreign material and secretions (if indicated) and if the child is not breathing, continuation of the airway is maintained and rescue breathing is initiated. To ventilate the lungs in the infant (from birth to 1 year of age), the bag-valve-mask or operator's mouth is placed in such a way that both the mouth and the nostrils are included (Fig. 31-25, *C*). Children (over 1 year of age) are ventilated through the mouth while the nostrils are firmly pinched for airtight contact (Fig. 31-25, *D*).

> **NURSING ALERT**
>
> The volume of air in an infant's lungs is small, and the air passages are considerably smaller, with resistance to flow potentially higher than in adults. Small puffs of air should be delivered, and the rise of the chest should be assessed.

| | Objectives | ACTIONS | | |
|---|---|---|---|---|
| | | Adult (over 8 yr) | Child (1 to 8 yr) | Infant (under 1 yr) |
| **A. AIRWAY** | 1. Assessment: Determine unresponsiveness. | Tap or gently shake shoulder. | | |
| | | Say, "Are you okay?" | | Speak loudly. |
| | 2. Get help. | Activate EMS. | Shout for help. If second rescuer available, have person activate EMS. | |
| | 3. Position the victim. | Turn on back as a unit, supporting head and neck if necessary (4-10 sec). | | |
| | 4. Open the airway. | Head tilt/chin lift. | | |
| **B. BREATHING** | 5. Assessment: Determine breathlessness. | Maintain open airway. Place ear over mouth, observing chest. Look, listen, feel for normal breathing (no more than 10 sec).* | | |
| | 6. Give 2 rescue breaths. | Maintain open airway. | | |
| | | Pinch nose, seal mouth to mouth. | | Mouth to nose and mouth. |
| | | Give 2 slow effective breaths. Observe chest rise. Allow lung deflation between breaths. | | |
| | | 2 sec each | 1 to 1½ sec each | |
| | 7. Option for obstructed airway. | a. Reposition victim's head. Try again to give rescue breaths. | | |
| | | | b. Activate EMS. | |
| | | c. Give 5 subdiaphragmatic abdominal thrusts (the Heimlich maneuver). | | c. Give 5 back blows. |
| | | | | c. Give 5 chest thrusts. |
| | | d. Tongue-jaw lift and finger sweep. | d. Tongue-jaw lift, but finger sweep only if you see a foreign object. | |
| | | If unsuccessful, repeat a, c, and d until successful. | | |
| **C. CIRCULATION** | 8. Assessment: Determine pulselessness. | Feel for carotid pulse with one hand; maintain head-tilt with other hand (no more than 10 sec). | | Feel for brachial pulse: keep head tilt. |
| **CPR** | Pulse absent: Begin chest compressions: 9. Landmark check. | Use 2-3 fingers to locate lower margin of rib cage. Follow rib margin to base of sternum (xiphoid process). | | Imagine a line drawn between the nipples. |
| | 10. Hand position. | Place one hand above fingers of first hand on lower half of sternum. | | Place 2 fingers on sternum 1 finger's width below line. Depress ½-1 in.† |
| | | Place other hand on top of hand on sternum. Depress 1½-2 in. | Use heel of one hand. Depress 1-1½ in. | |
| | 11. Compression rate. | 80-100 per min | 100 per min | At least 100 per min |
| | 12. Compressions to breaths. | 2 breaths to every 15 compressions | 1 breath to every 5 compressions | |
| | 13. Number of cycles. | 4 | 20 (approximately 1 min) | |
| | 14. Reassessment. | Feel for carotid pulse. | | Feel for brachial pulse. |
| | | If no pulse, resume CPR, starting with compressions. | If alone, activate EMS. If no pulse, resume CPR, starting with compressions. | |
| | Pulse present; not breathing: Begin rescue breathing. | 1 breath every 5 sec (12 per min) | 1 breath every 3 sec (20 per min) | |

* If victim is breathing or resumes breathing, place in recovery position: (1) move head, shoulders, and torso simultaneously; (2) turn onto side; (3) leg not in contact with ground may be bent and knee moved forward to stabilize victim; (4) victim should not be moved in any way if trauma is suspected and should not be placed in recovery position if rescue breathing or CPR is required.
† Use the 2 thumb–encircling hands technique if two rescuers are available for infant CPR.

**Fig. 31-23**  One-rescuer CPR. (Modified from Stapleton ER and others: *BLS for healthcare providers*, Dallas, 2001, American Heart Association.)

The correct volume for each breath is the volume that causes the chest to rise. If air enters freely and the chest rises, the airway is assumed to be clear. Breaths should be given slowly with sufficient volume to make the chest rise. Volume must be provided without causing abdominal distention. Gastric distention, which interferes with di-aphragmatic excursion, occurs when more volume than necessary is delivered and the breaths are delivered too rapidly.

After an initial two breaths, the pulse is palpated by the health care provider to ascertain the presence of a heartbeat. The carotid is the most central and accessible artery

| Step | Objective | Actions |
|------|-----------|---------|
| **1. AIRWAY** | **One rescuer (ventilator):** Assessment: Determine unresponsiveness. | Tap or gently shake shoulder. |
| | | Shout, "Are you okay?" |
| | Call for help. | Activate EMS. |
| | Position the victim. | Turn on back if necessary (4-10 sec). |
| | Open the airway. | Use a proper technique to open airway. |
| **2. BREATHING** | Assessment: Determine breathlessness. | Look, listen, and feel (3-5 sec). |
| | Ventilate twice (2 slow breaths). | Observe chest rise: 2 sec/inspiration. |
| **3. CIRCULATION** | Assessment: Determine pulselessness. | Feel for carotid pulse (5-10 sec). |
| | State assessment results. | Say "No pulse." |
| | **Other rescuer (compressor):** Get into position for compressions. | Hand, shoulders in correct position. |
| | Locate position on sternum. | Check hand position. |
| **4. COMPRESSION/ VENTILATION CYCLES** | **Compressor:** Begin chest compressions. | Correct ratio compressions/ventilations: 15:2 |
| | | Compression rate: 100/min (2 compressions per sec). |
| | | Say any helpful mnemonic (such as "1 and 2 and 3"). |
| | | Stop compressing for each ventilation. |
| | **Ventilator:** Ventilate twice after 15 compressions and check compression effectiveness. (Minimum of 10 cycles.) | Ventilate 1 time (2 sec/inspiration). |
| | | Check pulse occasionally to assess compressions. |
| **5. CALL FOR SWITCH** | **Compressor:** Call for switch when fatigued. | Give clear signal to change. |
| | | Compressor completes 15th compression. |
| | | Ventilator completes ventilation after 15th compression. |
| **6. SWITCH** | Simultaneously switch: | |
| | **Ventilator:** Move to chest. | Become compressor. |
| | | Get into position for compressions. |
| | | Locate position on sternum and hand position. |
| | **Compressor:** Move to head. | Become ventilator. |
| | | Check carotid pulse (5 sec). |
| | | Say "No pulse." |
| | | Ventilate once (2 sec/inspiration). |
| **7. CONTINUE CPR** | Resume compression/ventilation cycles. | Resume Step 4. |

**Fig. 31-24** Two-rescuer CPR. (NOTE: Two-rescuer CPR for children 1 to 8 years of age can be performed similarly to that for adults with appropriate changes in chest compressions and ventilations.) (Modified from Stapleton ER and others: *BLS for healthcare providers*, Dallas, 2001, American Heart Association.)

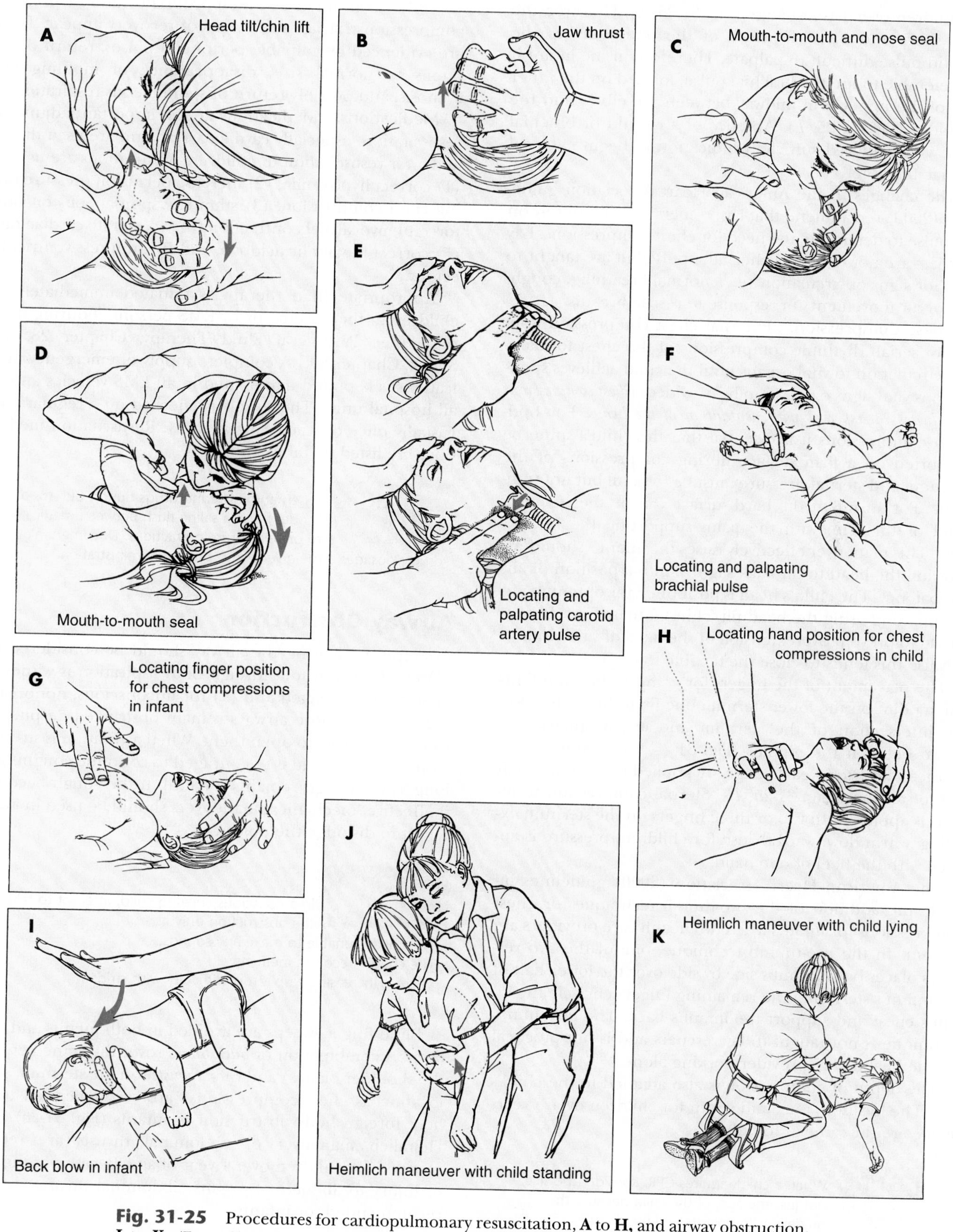

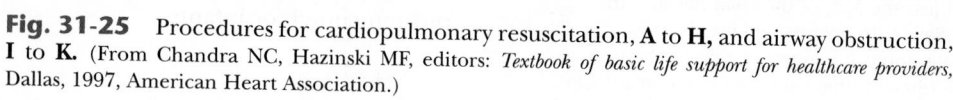

**Fig. 31-25**   Procedures for cardiopulmonary resuscitation, **A** to **H,** and airway obstruction, **I** to **K.** (From Chandra NC, Hazinski MF, editors: *Textbook of basic life support for healthcare providers,* Dallas, 1997, American Heart Association.)

in children over 1 year of age (Fig. 31-25, *E*). However, the very short and often fat neck of the infant makes the carotid pulse difficult to palpate. Therefore in the infant it is preferable to use the brachial pulse, located on the inner side of the upper arm midway between the elbow and the shoulder (Fig. 31-25, *F*). Absence of a carotid or brachial pulse is considered sufficient indication to begin external cardiac massage.

The changes in the American Heart Association guidelines (2000) recommend that lay rescuers should not rely on the pulse to determine the need for chest compressions. Lay rescuers are not taught to check the pulse but are taught to look for signs of circulation (e.g., normal breathing, coughing, or air movement) in response to rescue breaths.

**Chest Compression.** External chest compression consists of serial, rhythmic compressions of the chest to maintain circulation to vital organs until the child achieves spontaneous vital signs or ALS can be provided. *Chest compressions are always interspersed with ventilation of the lungs.* For optimum compressions it is essential that the child's spine be supported on a firm surface during compressions of the sternum, and sternal pressure must be forceful but not traumatic. For an infant the hard surface can be the rescuer's hand or forearm, with the palm supporting the infant's back. This maneuver effectively raises the infant's shoulders, allowing the head to tilt back slightly, into a position of airway patency. The child's head is positioned for optimum airway opening using the head tilt/chin lift maneuver. It is essential to prevent overextension of the head of small infants because this tends to close the flexible trachea.

The placement of the fingers for compression in infants is at a point on the lower sternum one fingerbreadth below the intersection of the sternum and an imaginary line drawn between the nipples (Fig. 31-25, *G*). Compressions on the child 1 to 8 years of age are applied to the lower half of the sternum (Fig. 31-25, *H*). Sternal compression to infants is applied with two or three fingers on the sternum exerting a firm downward thrust; for children, pressure is applied with the heel of one hand.

The American Heart Association (2000) guidelines include the addition of the two-thumb technique for chest compressions for infants when two health care providers are present. In the two-thumb technique, one of the two rescuers places both thumbs side by side over the lower half of the infant's sternum. The remaining fingers encircle the infant's chest and support the infant's back. The two-thumb technique is not taught to lay rescuers and is not practical for the health care provider working alone.

The depth of compression is also adapted to the child's size. The location, rate, and depth for children over 8 years of age are the same as for adults.

> **NURSING ALERT**
>
> When a child requires CPR, consider the size, not just the age, of the child because the guidelines for infants and for children ages 1 to 8 years may not always apply. For example, young children who can be placed on the rescuer's thigh should receive infant CPR. Because many older children with severe chronic illness or disability remain small in size, pediatric, not adult CPR, may be appropriate.

CPR is continued at the appropriate ratio of breaths/compressions for age until signs of recovery appear. These are evidenced by palpable peripheral pulses, return of the pupils to normal size, disappearance of mottling and cyanosis, and possibly return of spontaneous respiration.

**Medications.** Medications are an important adjunct to resuscitation, especially cardiac arrest, and are used during and after resuscitation in children. Medications are used to (1) correct hypoxemia, (2) increase perfusion pressure during chest compression, (3) stimulate spontaneous or more forceful myocardial contraction, (4) accelerate cardiac rate, (5) correct metabolic acidosis, and (6) suppress ventricular ectopy.

Appropriate fluid therapy is initiated immediately for children in the hospital or by EMS personnel during transport. (See Parenteral Fluid Therapy, Chapter 28, and Shock, Chapter 29.) A complete supply of emergency medications is kept and maintained in all EMS vehicles and on all hospital units. The supply is checked on a regular basis (usually once on each 8-hour shift). Resuscitation medications are listed in Table 31-6.

> **NURSING ALERT**
>
> When administering drugs during CPR (or a "code"), use a saline flush between medications to prevent drug interactions. Document all drugs, dosages, time given, and route of administration.

## Airway Obstruction

Attempts at clearing the airway should be considered for (1) children in whom foreign body aspiration is witnessed or strongly suspected and (2) for unconscious, nonbreathing children whose airways remain obstructed despite the usual maneuvers to open them. When aspiration is strongly suspected, the child is encouraged to continue coughing as long as the cough remains forceful. If the cough becomes ineffective, mechanical maneuvers should be used in an attempt to dislodge the object.

> **NURSING ALERT**
>
> In a conscious choking child, attempt to relieve the obstruction only if:
> The child is unable to make any sounds.
> The cough becomes ineffective.
> There is increasing respiratory difficulty with stridor.

Blind finger sweeps are avoided in both infants and children. A combination of **back blows** (over the spine between the shoulder blades) and **chest thrusts** (on the sternum, same location as chest compressions) are recommended to relieve foreign body obstruction in infants (Fig. 31-26). The Heimlich maneuver or abdominal thrusts are recommended for children over 1 year of age. Because of the risk of injury to abdominal organs, abdominal thrusts are not recommended for infants.

### Infants

A choking infant is placed face down over the rescuer's arm with the head lower than the trunk and the head supported (Fig. 31-25, *I*, and Fig. 31-26). For additional support, the

**TABLE 31-6**   Drugs for pediatric cardiopulmonary resuscitation

| Drug/Dose | Action | Implications |
|---|---|---|
| **Epinephrine HCl\*** <br> IV/IO: 0.01 mg/kg (1:10,000) <br> ET: 0.1 mg/kg (1:1000) <br> Repeat doses = 0.1 ml/kg (1:1000) | Adrenergic <br> Acts on both alpha and beta receptor sites, especially heart and vascular and other smooth muscle | Most useful drug in cardiac arrest <br> Disappears rapidly from bloodstream after injection; instill 2-3 ml saline following ET administration <br> May produce renal vessel constriction and decreased urine formation |
| **Sodium bicarbonate** <br> IV/IO: 1 mEq/kg <br> Newborn: 0.5 mEq/ml <br> 2 mg/kg | Alkalinizer <br> Buffers pH | Infuse slowly and only when ventilation is adequate; flush with saline before and after administration <br> Do not mix with catecholamines or calcium <br> Incompatible with epinephrine |
| **Atropine sulfate\*** <br> 0.02 mg/kg/dose <br> Minimum dose: 0.1 mg <br> Maximum single dose: infants and children, 0.5 mg; adolescents, 1.0 mg | Anticholinergic-parasympatholytic <br> Increases cardiac output, heart rate by blocking vagal stimulation in heart | Used to treat bradycardia after ventilatory assessment; always provide adequate ventilation and monitor $O_2$ saturation <br> Produces pupil dilation, which constricts with light |
| **Calcium chloride 10%** <br> 20 mg/kg IV <br> 0.2 mg/kg/dose q 10 min | Electrolyte replacement <br> Needed for maintenance of normal cardiac contractility | Used only for hypocalcemia, calcium blocker overdose, hyperkalemia, or hypermagnesemia <br> Administer slowly, very sclerosing, administer in central vein <br> Incompatible with phosphate solutions |
| **Lidocaine HCl\*** <br> 1 mg/kg/dose | Antiarrhythmic <br> Inhibits nerve impulses from sensory nerves | Used for ventricular arrhythmias only |
| **Amiodarone** <br> IV (limited data): 5 mg/kg over 30 min followed by continuous infusion starting at 5 μg/kg/min <br> May increase to maximum 10 μg/kg/min | Antiarrhythmic agent <br> Inhibits adrenergic stimulation; prolongs action potential and refractory period in myocardial tissues; decreased atrioventricular (AV) conduction and sinus node function | Recommended as first choice for shock-refractory ventricular tachycardia <br> Contraindicated in severe sinus node dysfunction, marked sinus bradycardia, second- and third-degree AV block <br> Monitor for hypotension |
| **Adenosine** <br> 0.1 to 0.2 mg/kg <br> Maximum single dose: 12 mg <br> Follow with 2-3 ml normal saline flush | Antiarrhythmic, for supraventricular tachycardia (SVT) <br> Causes a temporary block through the AV node and interrupts the reentry circuits | Administer by rapid IV push followed by saline flush <br> May cause transient bradycardia |
| **Naloxone (Narcan)\*** <br> 0.1 mg/kg/dose† <br> May repeat q 2 to 3 min | Reverses respiratory arrest due to excessive opiate administration | Evaluate level of pain following administration because analgesic effects of opioids are reversed with large dose of naloxone |
| **Magnesium** <br> 25-50 mg/kg <br> Maximum: 2 g | Inhibits calcium channels and causes smooth muscle relaxation | Given by rapid IV infusion for suspected hypomagnesemia <br> Have calcium gluconate (IV) available as antidote |
| **Infusions** | | |
| **Epinephrine HCl infusion** <br> 0.1-1.0 μg/kg/min | Adrenergic <br> See above | Titrated to desired hemodynamic effect |
| **Dopamine HCl infusion** <br> 2-20 μg/kg/min | Agonist <br> Acts on alpha receptors, causing vasoconstriction <br> Increases cardiac output | Titrated to desired hemodynamic response |
| **Dobutamine HCl infusion** <br> 2.5-15 μg/kg/min | Adrenergic direct-acting β₁-agonist <br> Increases contractility and heart rate | Titrated to desired hemodynamic response <br> Little vasoconstriction, even at high rates |
| **Lidocaine HCl infusion** <br> 20-50 μg/kg/min | Antiarrhythmic <br> Increases electrical stimulation threshold of ventricle | See above <br> Lower infusion dose used in shock <br> Used for ventricular tachycardia |

*These drugs may be administered via the ET tube if an IV is not available.
†Dose of naloxone to reverse respiratory depression without reversing analgesia from opioids is 0.5 μg/kg in children <40 kg (American Pain Society, 1992).

| Signs of life-threatening obstruction: truly choking child *cannot speak*, *becomes cyanotic*, and *collapses* | | | | |
|---|---|---|---|---|
| | Objectives | Actions | | |
| | | Adult (over 8 yr) | Child (1 to 8 yr) | Infant (under 1 yr) |
| **CONSCIOUS VICTIM** | 1. Assessment: Determine airway obstruction. | Ask, "Are you choking?" Determine if victim can cough or speak. | | Observe breathing difficulty, ineffective cough, no strong cry. |
| | 2. Act to relieve obstruction. | Perform up to 5 subdiaphragmatic abdominal thrusts (Heimlich maneuver). | | Give 5 back blows. |
| | | | | Give 5 chest thrusts. |
| | Be persistent. | Repeat Step 2 until obstruction is relieved or victim becomes unconscious. | | |
| **VICTIM WHO BECOMES UNCONSCIOUS** | 3. Position the victim: call for help. | Turn on back as a unit, supporting head and neck, face up, arms by sides. Call out, "Help!" Activate EMS. If second rescuer available, have person activate EMS. | | |
| | 4. Check for foreign body. | Perform tongue-jaw lift and finger sweep. | Perform tongue-jaw lift. Remove foreign object only if you actually see it. | |
| | 5. Give rescue breaths. | Open the airway with head tilt/chin lift. Try to give rescue breaths. If airway is obstructed, reposition head and try to ventilate again. | | |
| | 6. Act to relieve obstruction. | Perform up to 5 subdiaphragmatic abdominal thrusts (Heimlich maneuver). | | Give 5 back blows. |
| | | | | Give 5 chest thrusts. |
| | 7. Be persistent. | Repeat steps 4-6 until obstruction is relieved. | | |
| **UNCONSCIOUS VICTIM** | 1. Assessment: Determine unresponsiveness. | Tap or gently shake shoulder. Shout, "Are you okay?" | Tap or gently shake shoulder. | |
| | | If unresponsive, activate EMS. | | |
| | 2. Call for help: position the victim. | Turn on back as a unit, supporting head and neck, face up, arms by sides. | | |
| | | | Call out for help. | |
| | 3. Open the airway. | Head-tilt/chin-lift. | | Head tilt/chin lift, but do not tilt too far. |
| | 4. Assessment: Determine breathlessness. | Maintain an open airway. Ear over mouth; observe chest. Look, listen, feel for breathing (no more than 10 sec). | | |
| | 5. Give rescue breaths. | Make mouth-to-mouth seal. | | Make mouth-to-mouth-and-nose seal. |
| | | Try to give rescue breaths. | | |
| | 6. If chest not rising, try again to give rescue breaths. | Reposition head. Try rescue breaths again. | | |
| | 7. Activate the EMS system. | | If airway obstruction not relieved after about 1 min, activate EMS as rapidly as possible. | |
| | 8. Act to relieve obstruction. | Perform up to 5 subdiaphragmatic abdominal thrusts (Heimlich maneuver). | | Give 5 back blows. |
| | | | | Give 5 chest thrusts. |
| | 9. Check for foreign body. | Perform tongue-jaw lift and finger sweep. | Perform tongue-jaw lift. Remove foreign object only if you actually see it. | |
| | 10. Rescue breaths. | Open the airway with head tilt/chin lift. Try again to give rescue breaths. If airway is obstructed, reposition head and try to ventilate again. | | |
| | 11. Be persistent. | Repeat steps 8-10 until obstruction is relieved. | | |

**Fig. 31-26** Foreign body airway obstruction management. (Modified from Stapleton ER and others: *BLS for healthcare providers,* Dallas, 2001, American Heart Association.)

rescuer should support the arm firmly against the thigh. Up to five quick, sharp back blows are delivered between the infant's shoulder blades with the heel of the rescuer's hand. Less force is required than would be applied to an adult. After delivery of the back blows, the rescuer's free hand is placed flat on the infant's back so that the infant is "sandwiched" between the two arms, making certain the neck and chin are well supported. While the rescuer maintains support with the infant's head lower than the trunk, the infant is turned and placed supine, supported on the rescuer's thigh, where up to five quick downward chest thrusts are applied in rapid succession in the same location

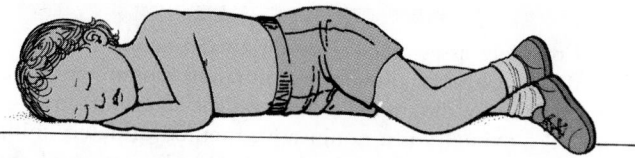

**Fig. 31-27** Recovery position for child after respiratory emergency.

## Critical Thinking Exercise

### Airway Obstruction

John, an experienced pediatric nurse, is attending a family reunion. A family member asks John to come quickly to help an infant who appears to be choking. As John approaches the infant, he notices that the infant is conscious but not coughing or crying. Which actions should John perform next?

FIRST, THINK ABOUT IT . . .
• What information are you using?
• How are you interpreting that information?

1. Open the infant's mouth and perform a blind finger sweep.
2. Position the infant in a face-down, prone position over his (John's) arm and administer five quick blows between the infant's shoulder blades.
3. Place the infant flat on his or her back and administer abdominal thrusts until the obstruction is removed.
4. Begin to perform the Heimlich maneuver on the infant.

*The best response is two. Important information reveals that John has determined that the infant is conscious and unable to make vocalizations. The next step is to relieve the obstruction. In an infant the procedure involves placing the infant in a prone position and delivering five sharp back blows between the infant's shoulder blades. The back blows are followed by five chest thrusts. Blind finger sweeps are avoided in both infants and children; abdominal thrusts and the Heimlich maneuver are also avoided in infants.*

as the external chest compressions described for CPR. Back blows and chest thrusts are continued until the object is removed or the infant becomes unconscious. (See Critical Thinking Exercise box.)

### Children

The *Heimlich maneuver*, a series of *subdiaphragmatic abdominal thrusts*, is recommended for children over 1 year of age. The maneuver creates an artificial cough that forces air, and with it the foreign body, out of the airway. The procedure is

carried out with the child in a standing, sitting, or lying position (Fig. 31-25, *J* and *K*). In the conscious choking child, upward thrusts are delivered to the upper abdomen with the fisted hand at a point just below the rib cage (Fig. 31-25, *J*, and Fig. 31-26). To prevent damage to the internal organs, the rescuer's hands should not touch the xiphoid process of the sternum or the lower margins of the ribs. Up to five thrusts are repeated in rapid succession until the foreign body is expelled.

It is neither necessary nor desirable to squeeze or compress the arms during the procedure. It is not a punch or a bear hug. The child may vomit after relief of the obstruction and should be positioned to prevent aspiration. After breathing is restored, the child should receive medical attention and be assessed for complications.

The success of the technique is primarily a result of the obstruction occurring at the end of a maximum respiration. The victim is most likely to choke on food during inspiration; therefore the tidal volume plus expiratory reserve volume is present in the lungs. When pressure is exerted on the diaphragm by the maneuver, the food bolus is ejected with considerable force by this trapped air.

**NURSING ALERT** If the victim is breathing or resumes effective breathing after emergency interventions, place in the recovery position: move the head, shoulders, and torso simultaneously and turn onto the side. The leg not in contact with the ground may be bent and the knee moved forward to stabilize the victim (Fig. 31-27). The victim should not be moved in any way if trauma is suspected and should not be placed in the recovery position if rescue breathing or CPR is required.

## KEY POINTS

■ The major functions of the respiratory tract are to distribute air and exchange gases to supply cells with oxygen ($O_2$) and to remove carbon dioxide ($CO_2$).

■ Several anatomic features predispose infants and young children to airway obstruction and atelectasis: there is less alveolar surface for gas exchange; narrowly branching peripheral airways become easily obstructed; and lack of collateral pathways inhibits ventilation beyond obstructed units.

■ Gas exchange depends on the amount and composition of gases inhaled, thickness of the alveolar wall, adequacy of circulation to the alveoli, and substances

within the alveoli that prevent their inflation or gas exchange.

■ The amount of $O_2$ that diffuses into the blood depends on a pressure gradient between alveolar air and capillary blood, the total functional surface area of the alveolocapillary membrane, minute volume, and alveolar ventilation.

■ Defense mechanisms of the respiratory tract include the lymphatic system, mucus secretions, ciliary action, epiglottis, cough reflex, tracheobronchial dynamics, body position changes, and humoral defenses.

- Complete assessment of respiratory function involves a detailed history, physical examination, pulmonary function tests, radiography, and blood gas determination.
- Pulse oximetry is a noninvasive method of determining the $O_2$ saturation in the blood. One limitation of the technology is that it does not identify dangerously high $O_2$ levels.
- Improvement in respiratory function may be accomplished with measures such as $O_2$ therapy, positioning, humidification, aerosol therapy, and artificial ventilation.
- $O_2$ for administration must always be humidified.
- Chest physiotherapy is useful for patients with increased sputum production but is contraindicated for some.
- Implications for possible intubation include airway obstruction, respiratory arrest, pulmonary toilet, neuromuscular compromise or paralysis, and hypoxemia.
- Respiratory failure is defined as the inability of the respiratory system to maintain adequate oxygenation of the blood, with or without $CO_2$ retention.

- Management of respiratory failure is to provide $O_2$, maintain ventilation, apply appropriate therapy, and anticipate complications.
- Endotracheal and tracheostomy suctioning involves premeasured insertion of the catheter, application of suction for 3 to 4 seconds when withdrawing the catheter, and supplemental $O_2$ before and after suctioning.
- Occlusion of the endotracheal and tracheostomy tube is life-threatening; therefore equipment for replacing a tube must always be available.
- Pediatric cardiopulmonary resuscitation (CPR) includes 1 minute of ventilations and compressions before summoning emergency help.
- Two essentials of CPR are to support the patient's spine and to apply forceful, but not traumatic, sternal pressure.
- The Heimlich maneuver is reserved for children for whom aspiration is witnessed or strongly suspected. A combination of back blows and chest thrusts is used for infants with obstructed airways.

# REFERENCES

Ackerman MH: Instillation of normal saline before suctioning in patients with pulmonary infections: a prospective randomized controlled trial, *Am J Crit Care* 7(4): 261-266, 1998.

American Heart Association: Part 9: pediatric basic life support, *Resuscitation* 46:301-341, 2000.

American Pain Society: *Principles of analgesic use in the treatment of acute pain and chronic cancer pain*, ed 3, Glenview, IL, 1992, The Society.

Anderson B and others: A review of children's dying in a paediatric intensive care unit, *N Z Med J* 107(985):345-347, 1994.

Blackwood B: Normal saline instillation with endotracheal suctioning: primum non nocere (first do no harm), *J Adv Nurs* 29(4):928-934, 1999.

Carroll P: Closing in on safer suctioning, *RN* 61(5):22-27, 1998.

Chandra NC, Hazinski MF, editors: *Textbook of basic life support for healthcare providers*, Dallas, 1997, American Heart Association.

Curley MAQ, Moloney-Harmon PA: *Critical care nursing of infants and children*, ed 2, Philadelphia, 2001, WB Saunders.

Curley MA, Thompson JE, Arnold JH: The effects of early and repeated prone positioning in pediatric with acute lung injury, *Chest* 118:156-163, 2000.

Donn S, Sinha S: Newer modes of mechanical ventilation for the neonate, *Curr Opin Pediatr* 13(2):93-103, 2001.

Eichhorn DJ and others: Opening the doors: family presence during resuscitation, *J Cardiovasc Nurs* 10:59-70, 1996.

Emergency Nurses Association: *Presenting the option for family presence*, (program educational booklet), Park Ridge, IL, 1995, The Association.

Engleman SG, Turnage-Carrier C: Tolerance of the Passy-Muir speaking valve™ in infants and children less than 2 years of age, *Pediatr Nurs* 23:571-573, 1997.

Fauroux B and others: Chest physiotherapy in cystic fibrosis: improved tolerance with nasal pressure support ventilation, *Pediatrics* 103(3):e32, 1999.

Furdon S and others: Outcome measures after standardized pain management strategies in postoperative patients in the NICU, *J Perinatal Neonatal Nurs* 12(1):58-69, 1998.

Johns Hopkins Hospital Department of Pediatrics: Siberry GK, Iannone R, editors: *The Harriet Lane handbook*, ed 15, St Louis, 2000, Mosby.

Hagler DA, Traver GA: Endotracheal saline and suction catheters: sources of lower airway contamination, *Am J Crit Care* 3(6):444-447, 1994.

Kaditis AG, Wald ER: Viral croup: current diagnosis and treatment, *Contemp Pediatr* 16(2):139-153, 1999.

Kaut K, Turcott JC, Lavery M: Passy-Muir speaking valve, *Dimens Crit Care Nurs* 15:298-306, 1996.

Kleiber C, Krutzfield N, Rose EF: Acute histologic changes in tracheobronchial tree associated with different suction catheter insertion techniques, *Heart Lung* 17:10-14, 1988.

Krier JJ: Involvement of educational staff in the health care of medically fragile children, *Pediatr Nurs* 19(3):251-254, 1993.

McCance KL, Huether SE: *Pathophysiology: the biological basis for disease in adults and children*, ed 3, St Louis, 1998, Mosby.

Meyers TA and others: Family presence during invasive procedures and resuscitation, *Am J Nurs* 100(2):32-42, 2000.

O'Neill N: Improving ventilation in children using bilevel positive airway pressure, *Pediatr Nurs* 24(4):377-381, 1998.

Powers KS, Rubenstein JS: Family presence during invasive procedures in the pediatric intensive care unit: a prospective study, *Arch Pediatr Adolesc Med* 153(9):955-958, 1999.

Sacchetti A and others: Family member presence during pediatric emergency department procedures, *Pediatr Emerg Care* 12(4): 268-271, 1996.

Stapleton ER and others: *BLS for healthcare providers*, Dallas, 2001, American Heart Association.

Thompson JM and others: *Mosby's clinical nursing*, ed 4, St. Louis, 1997, Mosby.

Young KD, Seidel JS: Pediatric cardiopulmonary resuscitation: a collective review, *Ann Emerg Med* 33:195-204, 1999.

Zander J, Hazinski MF: Pulmonary disorders. In Hazinski MF, editor: *Nursing care of the critically ill child*, ed 2, St Louis, 1992, Mosby.

# Chapter 32

# The Child with Respiratory Dysfunction

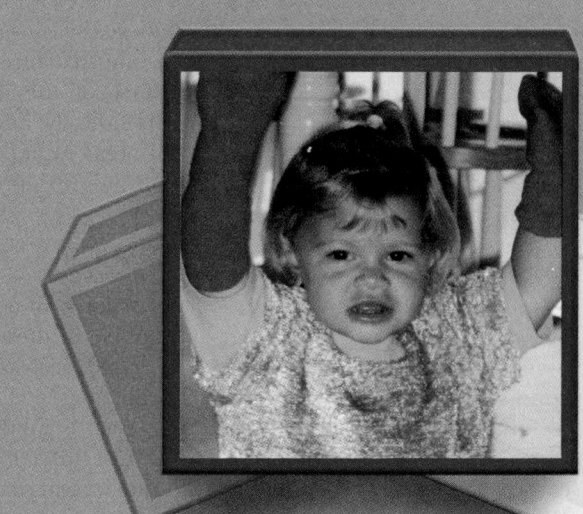

## Chapter Outline

**RESPIRATORY INFECTION, 1343**
**General Aspects of Respiratory Infections, 1343**
*Nursing Care Plan: The Child with Acute Respiratory Infection, 1347*
**UPPER RESPIRATORY TRACT INFECTIONS (URIs), 1350**
**Acute Viral Nasopharyngitis, 1350**
**Acute Streptococcal Pharyngitis, 1351**
**Tonsillitis, 1352**
**Infectious Mononucleosis, 1354**
**Influenza, 1356**
**Otitis Media (OM), 1356**
**Otitis Externa, 1361**
**CROUP SYNDROMES, 1361**
**Acute Epiglottitis, 1362**
**Acute Laryngitis, 1363**
**Acute Laryngotracheobronchitis (LTB), 1363**
**Acute Spasmodic Laryngitis, 1365**

Bacterial Tracheitis, 1365
**INFECTIONS OF THE LOWER AIRWAYS, 1365**
**Bronchitis, 1366**
**Respiratory Syncytial Virus (RSV)/Bronchiolitis, 1366**
**PNEUMONIA, 1368**
**Viral Pneumonia, 1369**
**Primary Atypical Pneumonia, 1369**
**Bacterial Pneumonia, 1369**
**Chlamydial Pneumonia, 1371**
**OTHER INFECTIONS OF THE RESPIRATORY TRACT, 1371**
**Pertussis (Whooping Cough), 1371**
**Tuberculosis (TB), 1372**
**PULMONARY DISTURBANCE CAUSED BY NONINFECTIOUS IRRITANTS, 1376**

**Foreign Body (FB) Aspiration, 1376**
**Foreign Body (FB) in the Nose, 1378**
**Aspiration Pneumonia, 1378**
   Hydrocarbon Pneumonia, 1378
   Lipoid Pneumonia, 1379
   Powder, 1379
**Acute (Adult) Respiratory Distress Syndrome (ARDS), 1379**
**Smoke Inhalation Injury, 1380**
**Passive Smoking, 1382**
**LONG-TERM RESPIRATORY DYSFUNCTION, 1383**
**Allergic Rhinitis, 1383**
**Asthma, 1385**
*Nursing Care Plan: The Child with Asthma, 1402*
**Cystic Fibrosis (CF), 1401**

## Related Topics

Administration of Medication, Ch. 27
The Child with Disturbance of Oxygen and Carbon Dioxide Exchange, Ch. 31
Compliance, Ch. 27
Controlling Elevated Temperatures, Ch. 27
Family-Centered Care of the Child with Chronic Illness or Disability, Ch. 22

Family-Centered Home Care, Ch. 25
High Risk Related to Disturbed Respiratory Function, Ch. 10
Immunizations, Ch. 12
Infection Control, Ch. 27
Ingestion of Injurious Agents, Ch. 16

Maintaining Healthy Skin, Ch. 27
Pain Assessment; Pain Management, Ch. 26
Physical Examination: Ears, Nose, Mouth and Throat, Chest, Lungs, Ch. 7
Surgical Procedures, Ch. 27
Tobacco (Use), Ch. 21

# RESPIRATORY INFECTION

## General Aspects of Respiratory Infections

Infections of the respiratory tract are described according to the areas of involvement. The *upper respiratory tract,* or *upper airway,* consists primarily of the nose and pharynx.

The *lower respiratory tract* consists of the bronchi and bronchioles (the reactive portion of the airway because of their smooth muscle content and ability to constrict) and the alveoli. Authorities disagree about the designation for the structurally stable portion of the airway (including the epiglottis, larynx, and trachea). For this discussion the trachea is considered with lower tract disorders, and infections of the epiglottis and larynx are categorized as croup syndromes.

■ Marilyn L. Winkelstein, PhD, RN, revised this chapter.

Respiratory infections spread from one structure to another because of the contiguous nature of the mucous membrane lining the entire tract. Consequently, infections of the respiratory tract involve several areas rather than a single structure, although the effect on one may predominate in any given illness.

## Etiology and Characteristics

Respiratory infections account for the majority of acute illnesses in children. The etiology and course of these infections are influenced by the age of the child, season, living conditions, and preexisting medical problems.

**Infectious Agents.** The respiratory tract is subject to a wide variety of infective organisms. Most infections are caused by viruses, particularly respiratory syncytial virus (RSV). Other agents involved in primary or secondary invasion include group A β-hemolytic streptococci, staphylococci, *Haemophilus influenzae*, *Chlamydia trachomatis*, *Mycoplasma*, and pneumococci.

**Age.** Infants under age 3 months have a lower infection rate, presumably because of the protective function of maternal antibodies. The infection rate increases from age 3 to 6 months, the time between the disappearance of maternal antibodies and the infant's own antibody production. The viral infection rate continues to remain high during the toddler and preschool years. By the time the child reaches 5 years of age, viral respiratory infections are less frequent, but the incidence of *Mycoplasma pneumoniae* and group A β-hemolytic streptococcus infections increases. The amount of lymphoid tissue increases throughout middle childhood, and repeated exposure to organisms confers increasing immunity as children grow older.

Some viral agents produce a mild illness in older children but cause severe lower respiratory tract illness or croup in infants. For example, whooping cough is a relatively harmless tracheobronchitis in childhood but a serious disease in infancy.

**Size.** Anatomic differences influence the response to respiratory tract infections. The diameter of the airways is smaller in young children and subject to considerable narrowing from edematous mucous membranes and increased production of secretions. In addition, the distance between

---

### Box 32-1 ■ ■ ■
### Signs and Symptoms Associated with Respiratory Infections in Infants and Small Children

**FEVER**

May be absent in newborn infants
Greatest at ages 6 months to 3 years
  Temperature may reach 39.5° to 40.5° C (103° to 105° F) even
    with mild infections
Often appears as first sign of infection
May be listless and irritable or somewhat euphoric and more
    active than normal, temporarily; some children talk with unac-
    customed rapidity
Tendency to develop high temperatures with infection in certain
    families
    May precipitate febrile seizures (see Chapter 37)
    Febrile seizures uncommon after 3 or 4 years of age

**MENINGISMUS**

Meningeal signs without infection of the meninges
Occurs with abrupt onset of fever
Accompanied by:
    Headache
    Pain and stiffness in the back and neck
    Presence of Kernig and Brudzinski signs
Subsides as the temperature drops

**ANOREXIA**

Common with most childhood illnesses
Frequently the initial evidence of illness
Persists to a greater or lesser degree throughout febrile stage of
    illness; often extends into convalescence

**VOMITING**

Small children vomit readily with illness
A clue to the onset of infection
May precede other signs by several hours
Usually short-lived but may persist during the illness

**DIARRHEA**

Usually mild, transient diarrhea but may become severe
Often accompanies viral respiratory infections
Is frequent cause of dehydration

**ABDOMINAL PAIN**

Common complaint
Sometimes indistinguishable from pain of appendicitis
Mesenteric lymphadenitis may be cause
Muscle spasms from vomiting may be a factor, especially in
    nervous, tense children

**NASAL BLOCKAGE**

Small nasal passages of infants easily blocked by mucosal swelling
    and exudation
Can interfere with respiration and feeding in infants
May contribute to the development of otitis media and sinusitis

**NASAL DISCHARGE**

Frequent occurrence
May be thin and watery (rhinorrhea) or thick and purulent
    Depends on the type and/or stage of infection
Associated with itching
May irritate upper lip and skin surrounding the nose

**COUGH**

Common feature
May be evident only during the acute phase
May persist several months after a disease

**RESPIRATORY SOUNDS**

Sounds associated with respiratory disease:
    Cough
    Hoarseness
    Grunting
    Stridor
    Wheezing
Auscultation:
    Wheezing
    Crackles
    Absence of sound

**SORE THROAT**

Frequent complaint of older children
Young children (unable to describe symptoms) may not complain
    even when highly inflamed
Often child will refuse to take oral fluids or solids

structures within the tract is shorter in the young child; therefore organisms move more rapidly down the respiratory tract for more extensive involvement. The relatively short and open eustachian tube in infants and young children allows pathogens easy access to the middle ear.

**Resistance.** The ability to resist invading organisms depends on several factors. Deficiencies of the immune system place the child at risk for infection. Other conditions that decrease resistance are malnutrition, anemia, fatigue, and chilling of the body. Conditions that weaken defenses of the respiratory tract and predispose to infection include allergies (e.g., allergic rhinitis), asthma, cardiac anomalies that cause pulmonary congestion, and cystic fibrosis. Daycare attendance, especially if the caregivers smoke, also increases the likelihood of infection (Blumer, 1998).

**Seasonal Variations.** The most common respiratory tract pathogens appear in epidemics during the winter and spring months, but mycoplasmal infections occur more often in autumn and early winter. Infection-related asthma (e.g., asthmatic bronchitis) occurs more frequently during cold weather. Winter and spring are typically the "RSV seasons."

## Clinical Manifestations

Infants and young children, especially those between 6 months and 3 years of age, react more severely to acute respiratory tract infection than older children. Young children display a number of generalized signs and symptoms, as well as local manifestations, that differ from those seen in older children and adults. Signs and symptoms associated with respiratory illnesses are listed in Box 32-1.

## Nursing Considerations

### ⬛ Assessment

Assessment of the respiratory system follows the guidelines described in Chapter 7 (for nose, mouth and throat, chest, and lungs). In addition, special attention is given to the observations outlined in Box 32-1 and the components in Box 32-2.

### ⬛ Nursing Diagnoses

After a thorough assessment, several nursing diagnoses may be identified. Others may be apparent in individual cases. (See Nursing Care Plan on pp. 1347-1350.)

### ⬛ Planning

The goals for the child with an acute respiratory infection and the family are as follows:

1. Child will exhibit normal respiratory efforts.
2. Child will receive adequate rest.
3. Child will remain comfortable.
4. Child will not spread primary infection to others.
5. Child's temperature will remain within normal limits.
6. Child will maintain normal hydration and adequate nutrition.
7. Child will experience no complications.
8. Child and family will receive information, especially for home care, and support.

### ⬛ Implementation

**Ease Respiratory Efforts.** Many acute respiratory infections are mild and cause few symptoms. Although children may feel uncomfortable and have a "stuffy" nose and some mucosal swelling, respiratory distress occurs infrequently. The interventions described in the following discussion are usually sufficient to relieve minor discomfort and ease respiratory efforts. However, children with croup or epiglottitis may develop sufficient swelling to obstruct the airway. These children may require hospitalization for observation and therapy.

Warm or cool mist is a common therapeutic measure for symptomatic relief of respiratory discomfort. The moisture soothes inflamed membranes and is beneficial when there is hoarseness or laryngeal involvement. Mist tents are fre-

---

**Box 32-2** ⬛ ⬛ ⬛

## Components for Assessing Respiratory Function

### RESPIRATIONS

The pattern of respirations is observed for rate, depth, ease, and rhythm of breathing:

**Rate**—Rapid (tachypnea), normal, or slow for the particular child

**Depth**—Normal depth, too shallow (hypopnea), too deep (hyperpnea); usually estimated from the amplitude of thoracic and abdominal excursion

**Ease**—Effortless, labored (dyspnea), orthopnea, associated with intercostal or substernal retractions (inspiratory "sinking in" of soft tissues in relation to the cartilaginous and bony thorax), pulsus paradoxus (blood pressure falls with inspiration and rises with expiration), flaring nares, head bobbing (head of sleeping child with suboccipital area supported on caregiver's forearm bobs forward in synchrony with each inspiration), grunting, or wheezing

**Labored breathing**—Continuous, intermittent, becoming steadily worse, sudden onset, at rest or on exertion, associated with wheezing, grunting, associated with pain

**Rhythm**—Variation in rate and depth of respirations

### OTHER OBSERVATIONS

In addition to respirations, particular attention is addressed to the following:

**Evidence of infection**—Check for elevated temperature, enlarged cervical lymph nodes, inflamed mucous membranes, and purulent discharges from the nose, ears, or lungs (sputum)

**Cough**—Observe the characteristics of the cough (if present); under what circumstances the cough is heard (e.g., night only, on arising), the nature of the cough (paroxysmal with or without wheeze, "croupy" or "brassy"), frequency of the cough, associated with swallowing or other activity, character of the cough (moist or dry), productivity

**Wheeze**—Expiratory or inspiratory, high-pitched or musical, prolonged, slowly progressive or sudden, associated with labored breathing

**Cyanosis**—Note distribution (peripheral, perioral, facial, trunk as well as face), degree, duration, associated with activity

**Chest pain**—May be a complaint of older children. Note location and circumstances: localized or generalized, referred to base of neck or abdomen, dull or sharp, deep or superficial, associated with rapid, shallow respirations or grunting

**Sputum**—Older children may provide sputum sample by coughing, whereas young children may need use of bulb suction to provide a sample. Note volume, color, viscosity, and odor

**Bad breath**—May be associated with some lung infections

quently used in the hospital for humidifying the air and relieving discomfort. However, the use of steam vaporizers in the home should be discouraged because of the hazards related to their use and limited evidence to support their efficacy. Shallow pans with wide surface areas for evaporation increase humidity, but they should be placed where they do not pose a safety hazard.

A time-honored method of producing steam is the shower. Running a shower of hot water into the empty bathtub or open shower stall with the bathroom door closed produces a quick source of steam. Keeping a child in this environment for 10 to 15 minutes offers the same advantages as the mist tent without the fear and restraint often associated with the confines of a tent. A small child can be held on the lap of a parent or other adult. Older children can sit in the bathroom under the supervision of an adult.

**Promote Rest.** Children who have an acute febrile illness should be placed on bed rest. This is usually not difficult while the temperature is elevated but may become difficult when children begin to feel better. Often children are more apt to comply with bed rest if they are allowed to lie quietly on a couch where they can watch television or participate in a quiet activity. If children protest, allowing them to play quietly serves the purpose of rest better than allowing them to cry excessively in bed.

**Promote Comfort.** Older children are usually able to manage nasal secretions with little difficulty. Parents are instructed in the correct administration of nose drops and throat irrigations, if ordered. For very young infants, who normally breathe through their noses, an infant nasal aspirator or a rubber ear syringe is helpful in removing nasal secretions before feeding. This practice, followed by instillation of saline nose drops, may clear nasal passages and promote feeding. Saline nose drops can be prepared at home by dissolving 1 teaspoon of salt in 1 pint of warm water.*

For older infants and children who can tolerate decongestants, vasoconstrictive nose drops may be administered 15 to 20 minutes before feeding and at bedtime. Two drops are instilled, and, because this shrinks only the anterior mucous membranes, two more drops are instilled 5 to 10 minutes later. Phenylephrine (Neo-Synephrine) 0.25% and ephedrine 1% are frequently prescribed. Older cooperative children often prefer nasal sprays. They are taught to compress the plastic container at the moment of inspiration. Spray bottles and bottles of nose drops should be used for one child only and only for one illness, because they become easily contaminated with bacteria. To avoid rebound congestion, nose drops or sprays should not be administered for more than 3 days.

Hot or cold applications sometimes provide relief for children with painful cervical adenitis. An ice bag or heating pad applied to the neck decreases the discomfort, but safety precautions must be observed to prevent burns. The ice bag or heating device must be covered, and the heating pad should not be set at high ranges.

**Prevent Spread of Infection.** Careful handwashing is carried out when caring for children with respiratory infections. Children and families are taught to use a tissue or their hand to cover their nose and mouth when they cough or sneeze and to dispose of the tissues properly, as well as to wash their hands. Used tissues should be immediately thrown into the wastebasket, and tissues should not be allowed to accumulate in a pile. Children with respiratory infections should not share drinking cups, washcloths, or towels.

**NURSING ALERT**  To avoid contamination with respiratory viruses, wash hands and do not touch your eyes or nose.

Every endeavor should be made to remove affected children from contact with other children. Parents are encouraged to keep affected children out of school or daycare settings to prevent the spread of infection. Ideally, ill children should be isolated in a separate bedroom at the first sign of illness. This may be a problem when living arrangements are crowded and there are several children in the family. An effort should be made to teach well children to stay away from ill children.

**Reduce Temperature.** If the child has a significantly elevated temperature, controlling the fever is important. The parent should know how to take a child's temperature and read the thermometer accurately. Nurses should not assume that all parents can read a thermometer; those who cannot require instruction.

If the practitioner has prescribed an antipyretic such as ibuprofen or acetaminophen, parents may need help administering the drug. Most parents can read the label and calculate the desired dose, but some may require careful instruction.* It is important to emphasize accuracy in both the amount of drug given and the time intervals at which the drug is administered to avoid accumulative effects. To reduce the temperature and minimize the chances of dehydration, cool liquids are encouraged. (See Controlling Elevated Temperatures, Chapter 27.)

**Promote Hydration.** Dehydration is always a hazard when children are febrile or anorexic, especially when vomiting or diarrhea is also present. Adequate fluid intake is encouraged by offering small amounts of favorite fluids at frequent intervals. High-calorie liquids, such as colas, fruit juices, water flavored and sweetened with corn syrup, or similar drinks, help prevent catabolism and dehydration but should be avoided if diarrhea is present. Oral rehydration solutions, such as Infalyte or Pedialyte, should be considered for infants, and sports drinks, such as Gatorade or Exceed, should be considered for older children. Fluids should not be forced, and children should not be awakened to take fluids. Forcing fluids may create the same difficulties as urging unwanted food. Gentle persuasion with preferred beverages is usually successful.

---

*Home care instructions for administration of nose drops and nasal aspiration are available in Wong DL, Hess CS: *Wong and Whaley's clinical manual of pediatric nursing,* ed 5, St Louis, 2000, Mosby.

*Home care instructions for measuring temperature and administration of medication are available in Wong DL, Hess CS: *Wong and Whaley's clinical manual of pediatric nursing,* ed 5, St Louis, 2000, Mosby.

To assess their child's level of hydration (see Chapter 28), parents are advised to observe the frequency of voiding and to notify the nurse or practitioner if there is insufficient voiding.

> **NURSING TIP** Counting the number of wet diapers in a 24-hour period is a satisfactory method of assessing output in infants and toddlers.

**Provide Nutrition.** Loss of appetite is characteristic of children with acute infections, and in most cases, children can be permitted to determine their own need for food. Urging foods on anorexic children may precipitate nausea and vomiting and cause an aversion to feeding that can extend into the convalescent period and beyond. Many children show no decrease in appetite, and others respond well to foods such as gelatin, soup, and puddings. (See Feeding the Sick Child, Chapter 27.)

**Family Support and Home Care.** Young children with respiratory infections are irritable and difficult to comfort. Therefore the family needs support, encouragement, and practical suggestions concerning comfort measures and administration of medication.

In addition to antipyretics and nose drops, the child may require antibiotic therapy. Parents of children receiving oral antibiotics need to understand the importance of regular administration and continuing the drug for the prescribed length of time, regardless of whether the child appears to be ill.

Parents are also cautioned against giving the child any medications that are not approved by the health practitioner. Adverse effects have been noted in children who have received preparations intended for adults (e.g., some long-acting nose drops [Neo-Synephrine II] and dextromethorphan cough squares [mistaken for candy]). They are also cautioned about giving the child unprescribed antibiotics left over from a previous illness. Self-medication with unprescribed antibiotics can produce serious side effects, and the likelihood of adverse reactions is increased when medications are administered to children without consultation with the practitioner. (See Chapter 27 for administration of medications and teaching parents.)

## ⚒ Evaluation

The effectiveness of nursing interventions is determined by continual reassessment and evaluation of care based on the following observational guidelines:

1. Observe child's respiratory effort and movement.
2. Observe signs and symptoms for progress toward status before illness.
3. Observe child's behavior and activity.
4. Observe other family members and contacts for evidence of infection.
5. Take temperature.
6. Observe for signs of adequate hydration.
7. Observe eating behavior.
8. Assess complications, such as dehydration, weight loss, or spread of infection to other areas of the body.
9. Observe family's behavior and interview members regarding their feelings and concerns.

The *expected outcomes* are described in the Nursing Care Plan on pp. 1347-1350.

## *Nursing Care Plan*
## The Child with Acute Respiratory Infection

> **NURSING DIAGNOSIS:** Ineffective breathing pattern related to inflammatory process

**PATIENT GOAL 1:** Will exhibit normal respiratory function

• **NURSING INTERVENTIONS/RATIONALES**

Position for maximum ventilation (i.e., open airway and permit maximum lung expansion)

Allow position of comfort (e.g., tripod position of child with epiglottitis or maintain head elevation of at least 30 degrees)

Check child's position frequently to ensure child does not slide down *to avoid compressing the diaphragm*

Avoid constricting clothing or bedding

Use pillows and padding *to maintain open airway (e.g., in infant or child with hypotonia)*

*Provide increased humidity and supplemental oxygen by placing child in small tent or hood (infant) or administer via nasal cannula or mask (preferred methods for children older than infancy because of safety issues)

Promote rest and sleep by scheduling appropriate activity and rest periods

Encourage relaxation techniques

Teach child and family measures *to ease respiratory efforts (i.e., appropriate positioning)*

For most respiratory illnesses use cool-mist humidifier in child's room

For spasmodic croup create warm mist by running hot water in a closed bathroom (warm mist, often used for children with spasmodic croup, may be helpful because of its relaxing effect, but mostly because child is being held upright in the shower)

• **EXPECTED OUTCOMES**

Respirations remain within normal limits (See inside back cover for normal variations)

Respirations are unlabored

Child rests and sleeps quietly

---

*Dependent nursing action.

*Continued*

# Nursing Care Plan
## The Child with Acute Respiratory Infection—cont'd

**PATIENT GOAL 2:** Will receive optimum oxygen supply

• **NURSING INTERVENTIONS/RATIONALES**
Position for maximum ventilatory efficiency (See Goal 1)
Use pulse oximetry *to monitor oxygen saturations*
Place in cool, humidified environment, using appropriate oxygen delivery system
*Provide oxygen as prescribed or needed

• **EXPECTED OUTCOMES**
Child breathes easily
Respirations remain within normal limits (see inside back cover for normal variations)
Oxygen saturation is ≥95%

---

**NURSING DIAGNOSIS:** Fear/anxiety related to difficulty breathing, unfamiliar procedures, and possibly environment (hospital)

---

**PATIENT GOAL 1:** Will experience reduction of fear/anxiety

• **NURSING INTERVENTIONS/RATIONALES**
Explain unfamiliar procedures and equipment to child in developmentally appropriate terms
Establish rapport with child and parents
Remain with child and parent during procedures
Use calm, reassuring manner
Provide frequent attendance during acute phase of illness
Provide comfort measures child prefers (e.g., rocking, stroking, music)
Provide attachment objects (e.g., familiar toy, blanket)
Encourage family-centered care with increased parental attendance and, when possible, involvement
Do nothing to make child more anxious or fearful
Instill confidence in both parents and child
Try to avoid any intrusive or painful procedures
Be aware of child's rest/sleep cycle or pattern in planning nursing activities
Assess and implement appropriate pain management therapy (i.e., sedatives or analgesics) (see Pain Assessment; Pain Management, Chapter 26)
Provide diversional activities appropriate to child's cognitive ability and condition
*Administer medications that promote improved ventilation (e.g., bronchodilators, expectorants) as prescribed

• **EXPECTED OUTCOMES**
Child exhibits no signs of respiratory distress or physical discomfort
Parents remain with child and provide comfort
Child engages in quiet activities appropriate for age, interest, condition, and cognitive level

---

**NURSING DIAGNOSIS:** Ineffective airway clearance related to mechanical obstruction, inflammation, increased secretions, pain

---

**PATIENT GOAL 1:** Will maintain patent airway

• **NURSING INTERVENTIONS/RATIONALES**
Position child in proper body alignment *to allow better lung expansion and improved gas exchange, as well as to prevent aspiration of secretions* (prone, semiprone, side lying; for infants not at risk for aspiration, use supine or side-lying position for sleeping)
Suction secretions from airway as needed
　　Limit each suction attempt to 5 seconds with sufficient time between attempts to allow reoxygenation
Position supine with head in "sniffing" position with neck slightly extended and nose pointed to ceiling
　　Avoid neck hyperextension
Assist child in expectorating sputum
*Administer expectorants if prescribed
Perform chest physiotherapy
Give nothing by mouth *to prevent aspiration of fluids* (e.g., child with severe tachypnea)
*Administer appropriate pain management
Have emergency equipment available *to avoid delay in treatment if needed*
Avoid throat examination and culture with suspected epiglottitis, *because it could cause airway obstruction*
Assist child in splinting any incisional/injured area *to maximize effects of coughing and chest physiotherapy*

• **EXPECTED OUTCOMES**
Airways remain clear
Child breathes easily; respirations are within normal limits (see inside back cover)

**PATIENT GOAL 2:** Will expectorate secretions adequately

• **NURSING INTERVENTIONS/RATIONALES**
Ensure adequate fluid intake *to liquefy secretions*
Provide humidified atmosphere *to prevent crusting of nasal secretions and drying of mucous membranes*
Explain importance of expectoration to child and family
Assist child in coughing effectively; provide tissues
Remove accumulated mucus; suction if needed
*Administer pain medications as indicated before attempt to clear airway
Provide nebulization with appropriate solution and equipment as prescribed
Assist with splinting *so child will experience minimal discomfort*
*Perform percussion, vibration, and postural drainage *to facilitate drainage of secretions*

• **EXPECTED OUTCOME**
Older child expectorates secretions without undue stress and fatigue; younger child will be able to have a productive cough

---

*Dependent nursing action.

# Nursing Care Plan
## The Child with Acute Respiratory Infection—cont'd

---

**NURSING DIAGNOSIS:** Risk for infection related to presence of infective organisms

**PATIENT GOAL 1:** Will exhibit no signs of secondary infection

• **NURSING INTERVENTIONS/RATIONALES**
Maintain aseptic environment, using sterile suction catheters and good handwashing
Isolate child as indicated *to prevent nosocomial spread of infection*
Administer antibiotics as prescribed *to prevent or treat infection*
Provide nutritious diet according to child's preferences and ability to consume nourishment *to support body's natural defenses*
Encourage good chest physiotherapy
Teach child and family manifestations of illness

• **EXPECTED OUTCOME**
Child exhibits evidence of diminishing symptoms of infection

**PATIENT GOAL 2:** Will not spread infection to others

• **NURSING INTERVENTIONS/RATIONALES**
Use standard precautions (see Infection Control, Chapter 27)
Instruct others (parents, members of staff) in appropriate precautions
Teach affected children protective methods to prevent spread of infection (e.g., handwashing, disposal of soiled tissues)
Limit the number of visitors/family members/siblings and screen for any recent illness in visitors
Try to keep infants and small children from placing hands and objects in contaminated areas
Assess home situation and implement protective measures as feasible in individual circumstances
*Administer antimicrobial medications if prescribed

• **EXPECTED OUTCOME**
Others remain free from infection

---

**NURSING DIAGNOSIS:** Activity intolerance related to inflammatory process, imbalance between oxygen supply and demand

**PATIENT GOAL 1:** Will maintain adequate energy levels

• **NURSING INTERVENTIONS/RATIONALES**
Assess child's level of physical tolerance
Assist child in those activities of daily living that may be beyond tolerance

Provide diversional activities appropriate to child's age, condition, capabilities, and interest
Provide diversional play activities that promote rest and quiet but prevent boredom and withdrawal
Provide rest and sleep periods appropriate to age and condition
Instruct child to rest when feeling tired
Balance rest and activity when ambulatory

• **EXPECTED OUTCOMES**
Child plays and rests quietly and engages in activities appropriate to age and capabilities (specify)
Child exhibits no evidence of increased respiratory distress
Child tolerates increasingly more activity

**PATIENT GOAL 2:** Will receive optimum rest

• **NURSING INTERVENTIONS/RATIONALES**
Provide quiet environment
Organize activities for maximum sleep time
Do not perform nonessential treatments or procedures *to maximize rest*
Schedule visiting to allow for sufficient rest
Encourage parents to remain with child
Schedule treatments or other activities around the needs of the child *so that fatigue will be minimized*
*Administer sedatives and analgesics as indicated if ordered for restlessness and pain
Encourage frequent rest periods and regular sleep times
Follow child's usual routine for bedtime and nap time
Implement measures to ensure sleep, such as quiet, darkened room

• **EXPECTED OUTCOMES**
Child remains calm, quiet, and relaxed
Child rests a sufficient amount (specify)

---

**NURSING DIAGNOSIS:** Acute pain related to inflammatory process, surgical incision

**PATIENT GOAL 1:** Will experience no pain or reduction of pain/discomfort to level acceptable to child

• **NURSING INTERVENTIONS/RATIONALES**
Use local measures (gargles, troches, warmth or cold) *to reduce throat pain*
Apply heat or cold as appropriate to affected area
*Administer analgesic as prescribed (see Pain Management, Chapter 26)
Assess response to pain control measures (see Pain Assessment, Chapter 26)
Encourage diversional activities appropriate to age, condition, capabilities

• **EXPECTED OUTCOME**
Child has no pain or acceptable level of pain

---

*Dependent nursing action.

*Continued*

*Nursing Care Plan*
## The Child with Acute Respiratory Infection—cont'd

> **NURSING DIAGNOSIS:** Interrupted family processes related to illness or hospitalization of a child

**PATIENT (FAMILY) GOAL 1:** Will experience reduction of anxiety and increased ability to cope

- **NURSING INTERVENTIONS/*RATIONALES***

Recognize parental concern and need for information and support

Explore family's feelings and "problems" surrounding hospitalization and child's illness

Explain therapy and child's behavior

Provide support as needed

Encourage family-centered care and encourage family to become involved in their child's care

- **EXPECTED OUTCOME**

Parents ask appropriate questions, discuss child's condition and care calmly, and become involved positively in child's care

See also:

Nursing Care Plan: The Family of the Child Who Is Ill or Hospitalized, Chapter 26

Nursing Care Plan: The Child in the Hospital, Chapter 26

# UPPER RESPIRATORY TRACT INFECTIONS (URIs)

## Acute Viral Nasopharyngitis

Acute nasopharyngitis (the equivalent of the "common cold") is caused by a number of viruses, usually rhinoviruses, RSV, adenovirus, influenza virus, or parainfluenza virus.

### Clinical Manifestations

Symptoms of nasopharyngitis are more severe in infants and children than in adults. Fever is common, especially in young children. Older children have low-grade fevers, which appear early in the illness. In children 3 months to 3 years, fevers occur suddenly and are associated with irritability, restlessness, decreased appetite, and decreased activity. Nasal inflammation may lead to obstruction of passages, producing open-mouth breathing. Vomiting and diarrhea may also be evident.

The initial symptoms in older children are dryness and irritation of nasal passages and the pharynx, followed by sneezing, chilly sensations, muscular aches, an irritating nasal discharge, and sometimes cough. Nasal inflammation may lead to obstruction. Continual wiping away of secretions causes skin irritation to nares.

The disease is self-limited and usually resolves within 4 to 10 days without complications. Occasionally fever recurs and a child might experience otitis media (particularly infants); this usually occurs early or after the initial phase of nasopharyngitis is past. Pneumonia is less frequent but may be observed in infants.

### Therapeutic Management

Children with nasopharyngitis are managed at home. There is no specific treatment, and effective vaccines are not available. Antipyretics are prescribed for mild fever and discomfort. (See Chapter 27 for management of fever.) Rest is recommended until the child is free of fever for at least 1 day. Decongestants may be prescribed for children and infants over 6 months of age to shrink swollen nasal passages. The decongestants that exert their effect by vasoconstriction are usually less effective when taken orally than when applied topically as nose drops. Because these drugs affect *all* vascular beds, they should be given with caution to children with diabetes.

Cough suppressants containing dextromethorphan may be prescribed for a dry, hacking cough. Some preparations contain up to 22% alcohol; they should not be administered to young children continuously and must be stored securely away from children.

Antihistamines are largely ineffective in treatment of nasopharyngitis. These drugs have a weak atropine-like effect that dries secretions, but they can cause drowsiness or, paradoxically, have a stimulatory effect on children. There is no support for the usefulness of expectorants, and antibiotics are usually not indicated.

**Prevention.** Nasopharyngitis is so widespread in the general population that it is impossible to prevent. Children are more susceptible to colds because they have not yet developed resistance to many types of viruses. Very young infants are subject to relatively serious complications; therefore attempts should be made to protect them from exposure.

### Nursing Considerations

A cold is often the parents' first introduction to an illness in their infants. Most discomfort of nasopharyngitis is related to the nasal obstruction, especially in small infants. Elevating the head of the bed or crib mattress assists with drainage of secretions; suctioning and vaporization may also help provide relief. Saline nose drops and gentle suction with a bulb syringe, particularly before feeding, are useful.

Maintaining adequate fluid intake is essential during any infectious process. Although a child's appetite for solid foods is usually diminished for several days, it is important to offer favorite fluids to prevent dehydration. Fluids can be cool or warm, depending on individual preference.

Because nasopharyngitis is spread from secretions, the best means for prevention is avoiding contact with affected

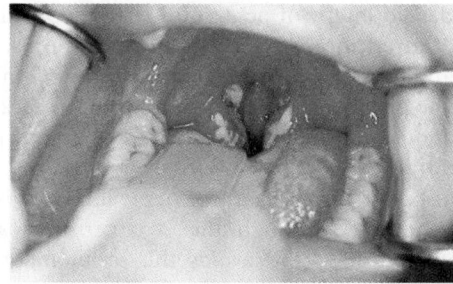

**Fig. 32-1**  Tonsillitis and pharyngitis. (Courtesy Dr. Edward L. Applebaum, Head, Department of Otolaryngology, University of Illinois Medical Center, Chicago, Illinois.)

persons. This goal is difficult when large numbers of people are confined in a small area for a long time, such as daycare centers and classrooms. Family members with a cold should try to "keep it to themselves" by carefully disposing of tissues; not sharing towels, glasses, or eating utensils; covering the mouth and nose with tissues when coughing or sneezing; and washing the hands thoroughly after nose blowing or sneezing. The most frequent carriers of infection are the human hands, which deposit viruses on doorknobs, faucets, and other everyday objects. Children should be taught to wash their hands thoroughly before putting them near their nose, mouth, or eyes.

**Family Support.**  Support and reassurance are important elements of care for families of young children with recurrent URIs. Because URIs are so frequent in children less than 3 years of age, families may feel they are on an endless roller coaster of illness. They can be reassured that frequent colds are a normal part of childhood and that by 5 years of age, most children will have developed immunity to many viruses. Parents who work outside the home should expect to take time off to care for ill children during the fall and winter months. If the children are cared for routinely in daycare centers, the infection rate will be higher than if they were cared for in the home. Parents should know the signs of respiratory complications and should notify a health professional if any signs of complications appear or if the child does not improve within 2 or 3 days (Box 32-3).

## Acute Streptococcal Pharyngitis

Group A β-hemolytic streptococcus (GABHS) infection of the upper airway *(strep throat)* is not in itself a serious disease, but affected children are at risk for serious sequelae: *acute rheumatic fever (ARF),* an inflammatory disease of the heart, joints, and central nervous system (see Chapter 34); and *acute glomerulonephritis,* an acute kidney infection (see Chapter 30). Permanent damage can result from these sequelae, especially ARF.

### Clinical Manifestations

GABHS is generally a relatively brief illness that varies in severity from subclinical (no symptoms) to severe toxicity. The onset is often abrupt and characterized by pharyngitis, headache, fever, and (especially in small children) abdominal pain. The tonsils and pharynx may be inflamed and covered with exudate (50% to 80% of cases) (Fig. 32-1), which usually appears by the second day of illness. However, streptococcal infections should be suspected in children over the age of 2 years who have pharyngitis even if no exudate is present (Thuma, 1997).

Anterior cervical lymphadenopathy (30% to 50% of cases) usually occurs early, and the nodes are often tender. Pain can be relatively mild to severe enough to make swallowing difficult. Clinical manifestations usually subside in 3 to 5 days unless complicated by sinusitis or parapharyngeal, peritonsillar, or retropharyngeal abscess. Nonsuppurative complications may appear after the onset of GABHS—acute nephritis in about 10 days and rheumatic fever in an average of 18 days.

### Diagnostic Evaluation

Although 80% to 90% of all cases of acute pharyngitis are viral, a throat culture should be performed to rule out GABHS. Because some children normally harbor streptococci in their throats, a positive culture is not always conclusive evidence of active disease. Most streptococcal infections are short-term illnesses, and antibody (antistreptolysin O) responses appear later than symptoms and are useful only for retrospective diagnosis.

Rapid identification of GABHS with diagnostic test kits is possible in the office or clinic setting. However, because these kits have questionable sensitivity, they are not yet considered to be a substitute for culture, and a confirmatory throat culture is recommended in patients who have a negative test result with a rapid diagnostic test kit (American Academy of Pediatrics, 2000).

### Therapeutic Management

If streptococcal sore throat infection is present, oral penicillin is prescribed in a dose sufficient to control the acute local manifestations and to maintain an adequate level for at least 10 days to eliminate organisms that might remain to initiate rheumatic fever symptoms. Penicillin does not prevent the development of acute glomerulonephritis in susceptible children; however, it may prevent the spread of a nephrogenic strain of GABHS to others in the family. Penicillin usually produces a prompt response within 24 hours. Some patients require retreatment if the organism is not eradicated.

Intramuscular (IM) benzathine penicillin G is also an appropriate therapy. Although this drug ensures adequate blood concentrations and avoids the problem of compliance, it is very painful and not the first choice for children. Orally administered erythromycin is indicated for children allergic to penicillin. Other drugs that have been used to treat GABHS pharyngitis include clarithromycin, azithromycin and clindamycin, oral cephalosporins, amoxicillin, and amoxicillin with clavulanic acid (McMillan and Feigin, 1999). A combination of penicillin and rifampin is more effective in eradicating GABHS than penicillin alone and is recommended for carriers.

### Nursing Considerations

The nurse often obtains a throat swab for culture and instructs the parents about administering penicillin and analgesics as prescribed. Most children prefer to remain in bed during the acute phase of the illness. Cold or warm compresses to the neck may provide relief. In children old enough to cooperate, warm saline gargles offer some relief of throat discomfort. Pain may interfere with oral intake, and the child should not be forced to eat. Cool liquids or ice chips are usually more acceptable than solids and are encouraged.

Special emphasis is placed on correct administration of oral medication and completing the course of antibiotic therapy. (See Administration of Medication, Chapter 27, and Compliance, Chapter 27.) If injections are required, they must be administered deep into a large muscle mass

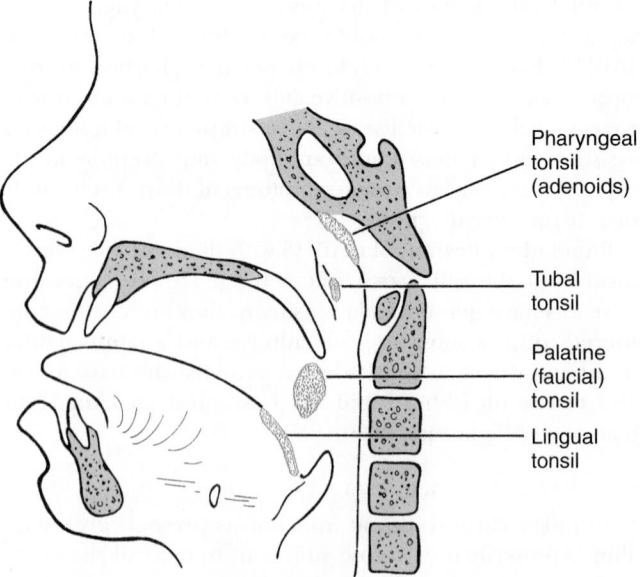

**Fig. 32-2** Location of various tonsillar masses.

(e.g., the vastus lateralis or ventrogluteal muscle). Parents need to be aware of the residual tenderness, which may cause the child to limp for a day or two. Local applications of heat are helpful in relieving discomfort. (For other atraumatic strategies to reduce injection pain, such as application of EMLA over the site for 2½ hours, see Administration of Medication: Intramuscular Administration, Chapter 27.)

**Prevention.** No immunization is available for prevention of streptococcal disease. The organism is spread by close contact with affected persons—direct projection of large droplets or physical transfer of respiratory secretions containing the organism. Spread of infection is common in families, classrooms, and daycare centers. Children with streptococcal infection are noninfectious to others 24 hours after initiation of antibiotic therapy. It is generally recommended that children not return to school or daycare until they have been taking antibiotics for a full 24-hour period.

> **NURSING ALERT** When nurses become aware that children have positive throat cultures for streptococcal infection, they should remind the children to discard their toothbrush and replace it with a new one after they have been taking antibiotics for 24 hours.

It is important to know when the organism is epidemic in the community so that families can be alert for symptoms. Directors of daycare centers and school officials should share infectious disease information with parents. Obtaining throat cultures from children who are close family contacts of patients with streptococcal infection is advised.

## Tonsillitis

The tonsils are masses of lymphoid tissue located in the pharyngeal cavity. The tonsils filter and protect the respiratory and alimentary tracts from invasion by pathogenic organisms. They also play a role in antibody formation. Although the size of tonsils varies, children generally have larger tonsils than adolescents or adults. This difference is thought to be a protective mechanism because young children are especially susceptible to URIs.

### Pathophysiology

Several pairs of tonsils are part of a mass of lymphoid tissue encircling the nasal and oral pharynx, known as the *Waldeyer tonsillar ring* (Fig. 32-2). The *palatine*, or *faucial*, *tonsils* are located on either side of the oropharynx, behind and below the pillars of the fauces (opening from the mouth). A surface of the palatine tonsils is usually visible during oral examination. The palatine tonsils are those removed during tonsillectomy. The *pharyngeal tonsils*, also known as the *adenoids*, are located above the palatine tonsils on the posterior wall of the nasopharynx. Their proximity to the nares and eustachian tubes causes difficulties in instances of inflammation. The *lingual tonsils* are located at the base of the tongue. The *tubal tonsils*, found near the posterior nasopharyngeal opening of the eustachian tubes, are not part of the Waldeyer tonsillar ring.

## Etiology

Tonsillitis often occurs with pharyngitis. Because of the abundant lymphoid tissue and the frequency of URIs, tonsillitis is a common cause of morbidity in young children. The causative agent may be viral or bacterial.

## Clinical Manifestations

The manifestations of tonsillitis are caused by inflammation. As the palatine tonsils enlarge from edema, they may meet in the midline (kissing tonsils), obstructing the passage of air or food. The child has difficulty swallowing and breathing. When enlargement of the adenoids occurs, the space behind the posterior nares may become blocked, making it difficult or impossible for air to pass from the nose to the throat. As a result, the child breathes through the mouth.

If mouth breathing is continuous, the mucous membranes of the oropharynx become dry and irritated. There may be an offensive mouth odor and impaired senses of taste and smell. Because air cannot be trapped for proper speech sounds, the voice has a nasal and muffled quality. A persistent cough is also common. Because of the proximity of the adenoids to the eustachian tubes, this passageway is frequently blocked by swollen adenoids, interfering with normal drainage and frequently resulting in otitis media or difficulty hearing.

## Therapeutic Management

**Medical Treatment.**  Because the illness is self-limiting, treatment of viral pharyngitis is symptomatic. Throat cultures positive for GABHS infection warrant antibiotic treatment. It is important to differentiate between viral and streptococcal infection in febrile exudative tonsillitis. Because the majority of infections are of viral origin, early rapid tests can eliminate unnecessary antibiotic administration.

**Surgical Treatment.**  Surgical treatment of chronic tonsillitis is controversial. Except in documented cases of recurrent, frequent streptococcal infection or a history of development of a peritonsillar abscess, tonsillectomy is not indicated in the child who has recurrent pharyngitis (Thuma, 1997).

*Tonsillectomy* (removal of the palatine tonsils) may be indicated for massive hypertrophy that results in difficulty breathing or eating (Derkay, Darrow, and LeFebvre, 1995). Absolute indications are malignancy and obstruction of the airway that result in cor pulmonale. *Adenoidectomy* (removal of the adenoids) is recommended for those children in whom hypertrophied adenoids obstruct nasal breathing. Their removal may be warranted in the child under 3 years of age and should be performed without a tonsillectomy. Follow-up after adenoidectomy should include assessment of hearing, smell, and taste for expected improvement. Contraindications to either tonsillectomy or adenoidectomy are (1) cleft palate because both tonsils help minimize escape of air during speech; (2) acute infections at the time of surgery because the locally inflamed tissues increase the risk of bleeding; and (3) uncontrolled systemic diseases or blood dyscrasias.

Generally removal of the tonsils should not occur until after 3 or 4 years of age because of the problem of excessive blood loss in young children and the possibility of regrowth or hypertrophy of lymphoid tissue. The tubal and lingual tonsils often enlarge to compensate for the lost lymphoid tissue, resulting in continued pharyngeal and eustachian tube obstruction.

## Nursing Considerations

Nursing care of the child with tonsillitis involves providing comfort and minimizing activities or interventions that precipitate bleeding. A soft to liquid diet is generally preferred. A cool-mist vaporizer keeps the mucous membranes moist during periods of mouth breathing. Warm saltwater gargles, throat lozenges, and analgesic/antipyretic drugs such as acetaminophen (Tylenol) are useful to promote comfort. Often opioids are needed to reduce the pain in order for the child to drink. Combination nonopioid and opioid elixirs or tablets such as Tylenol with Codeine or Lortab (acetaminophen and hydrocodone) relieve pain and should be given routinely every 4 hours.

If surgery is needed, the child requires the same psychologic preparation and physical care as for any procedure. (See Chapters 26 and 27.) The following discussion focuses on specific nursing care for tonsillectomy and adenoidectomy (T & A), although both procedures may not be performed.

A complete history is taken, with special notation of any bleeding tendencies because the operative site is highly vascular. Baseline vital signs are important for postoperative monitoring and observation. Signs of any URI are noted and reported, and bleeding and clotting times are included in the usual laboratory work requests. During physical assessment the presence of any loose teeth is noted. (See Surgical Procedures, Chapter 27.)

Until they are fully awake, children are placed on the abdomen or side to facilitate drainage of secretions. Suctioning is performed carefully to avoid trauma to the oropharynx. When alert, children may prefer sitting up, although they should remain in bed for the remainder of the day. They are discouraged from coughing frequently, clearing their throat, blowing their nose, or any activities that may aggravate the operative site.

Some secretions are common, particularly dried blood from surgery. All secretions and vomitus are inspected for evidence of fresh bleeding (some blood-tinged mucus is expected). Dark brown (old) blood is usually present in the emesis, as well as in the nose and between the teeth. If parents are not prepared for this, they may be frightened at a time when they need to be calm and reassuring.

The throat is very sore after surgery. An ice collar may provide relief, but many children find it bothersome and refuse to use it. Most children experience moderate pain after a T & A and need pain medication for at least the first 24 hours. Analgesics may need to be given rectally or intravenously to avoid the oral route. Because pain is continuous, analgesics should be administered at regular intervals. Local anesthetics, such as tetracaine lollipops or ice pops, and transdermal antiemetics, such as promethazine (Phenergan), can be compounded by some pharmacists. (See Pain Management, Chapter 26.)

Food and fluid are restricted until children are fully alert and there are no signs of hemorrhage. Cool water, crushed ice, flavored ice pops, or dilute fruit juice are given, and fluids with a red or brown color are avoided to distinguish fresh or old blood in emesis from the ingested liquid. Citrus juice may cause discomfort and is usually poorly tolerated.

Milk, ice cream, or pudding are not usually offered until clear fluids are retained because milk products coat the mouth and throat, causing the child to clear the throat, which may initiate bleeding. However, in a study in which children were offered milk or apple juice, more youngsters chose the juice, but over a third also drank the milk. The researchers concluded that children should be given an unrestricted diet postoperatively to increase their food and liquid consumption (Thomas, Moore, and Reilly, 1995).

Soft foods, particularly gelatin, cooked fruits, sherbet, soup, and mashed potatoes, are started on the first or second postoperative day or as the child tolerates feeding. The pain from surgery often inhibits intake, reinforcing the need for adequate pain control.

Postoperative hemorrhage is unusual but can occur. The nurse observes the throat directly for evidence of bleeding, using a good source of light and, if necessary, carefully inserting a tongue depressor. Other signs of hemorrhage are increased pulse (greater than 120 beats/min), pallor, frequent clearing of the throat or swallowing by a younger child, and vomiting of bright red blood. Restlessness, an indication of hemorrhage, may be difficult to differentiate from general discomfort after surgery. Decreasing blood pressure is a much later sign of shock.

> **NURSING ALERT** The most obvious early sign of bleeding is the child's continuous swallowing of the trickling blood. While the child is sleeping, note the frequency of swallowing. If continuous bleeding is suspected, notify the surgeon immediately.

Surgery may be required to ligate a bleeding vessel. Airway obstruction may also occur as a result of edema or accumulated secretions and is indicated by signs of respiratory distress, such as stridor, drooling, restlessness, agitation, increasing respiratory rate, and progressive cyanosis. Suction equipment and oxygen should be available after tonsillectomy.

**Family Support and Home Care.** Discharge instructions include (1) avoiding foods that are irritating or highly seasoned, (2) avoiding the use of gargles or vigorous toothbrushing, (3) discouraging the child from coughing or clearing the throat or putting objects in the mouth, (4) using analgesics or an ice collar for pain, and (5) limiting activity to decrease the potential for bleeding. Hemorrhage may occur up to 10 days after surgery as a result of tissue sloughing from the healing process. Any sign of bleeding warrants immediate medical attention. Objectionable mouth odor and slight ear pain with a low-grade fever are common for a few days postoperatively. However, persistent

severe earache, fever, or cough requires medical evaluation. Most children are ready to resume normal activity within 1 to 2 weeks after the operation.

A T & A often represents the first hospitalization experience for the child and family. Because the surgery is usually an elective procedure, there is ample opportunity to prepare both children and parents for this event. Both need reassurance about what to expect at the time of admission, before and after surgery, and at discharge. Most children are admitted to "same-day surgery units" and discharged home after a recovery period. If the child is hospitalized, parents are encouraged to room-in if possible and participate in their child's care. Children are honestly informed about postoperative discomfort and reassured that they will be able to talk. Some children believe that the procedure will immediately "make the throat all better" and are dismayed to find that it still hurts after the surgery. Ideally, children should have an opportunity to discuss the experiences to gain a feeling of mastery and to overcome any fears or misconceptions. (See Nursing Care Plan: The Child with a Tonsillectomy.*)

## Infectious Mononucleosis

Infectious mononucleosis is an acute, self-limiting infectious disease that is common among young people under 25 years of age. The disease is characterized by an increase in the mononuclear elements of the blood and by symptoms of an infectious process. The course is usually mild but occasionally can be severe or, rarely, accompanied by serious complications.

### Etiology/Pathophysiology

The herpes-like *Epstein-Barr (EB) virus* is the principal cause of infectious mononucleosis. It appears in both sporadic and epidemic forms, but the sporadic cases are more common. The mechanism of spread has not been proved, although it is believed to be transmitted by direct intimate contact with oral secretions. It is mildly contagious, and the period of communicability is unknown. The incubation period following exposure is 4 to 6 weeks.

### Clinical Manifestations

Symptoms of infectious mononucleosis appear anywhere from 10 days to 6 weeks after exposure and may be acute or insidious. The common presenting symptoms vary greatly in type, severity, and duration. The characteristics of the disease are malaise, sore throat, and fever with generalized lymphadenopathy and splenomegaly that may persist for several months. Often the symptoms appear insidiously with fatigue, lack of energy, and sore throat. The youngster's chief complaint is difficulty in maintaining the usual level of activity. This is often attributed to lack of sleep or a URI. In many instances the manifestations never arouse enough concern to bring the affected individual to medical atten-

---

*In Wong DL, Hess CS: *Wong and Whaley's clinical manual of pediatric nursing,* ed 5, St Louis, 2000, Mosby.

tion. The clinical manifestations of infectious mononucleosis are usually less severe (often subclinical or unapparent) and the convalescent phase is shorter in younger children than in older children and young adults. Many young children do not develop all of the expected clinical and laboratory findings; often a complication is the only or presenting symptom.

A skin rash that involves a discrete macular eruption (most prominent over the trunk) is present in some cases. More young children have rashes, and older children have abdominal pain. Other symptoms include headache, epistaxis, and a severe sore throat. The tonsils may be enlarged, reddened, and sometimes covered with a diphtheria-like membrane. In about half of the cases, the spleen is enlarged and may present a risk of possible rupture. Hepatic involvement is almost always present, often in association with jaundice, which may cause the disease to be confused with infectious hepatitis. The extensive mononuclear infiltration produces symptoms related to any body tissue, and the clinical picture can resemble that of many conditions, including neurologic manifestations and cardiac involvement.

### Diagnostic Evaluation

The diagnosis is established on the basis of clinical manifestations, absolute increase in atypical leukocytes in a peripheral blood smear, and a positive heterophil agglutination test. Differential diagnosis depends on the clinical symptoms present. For example, the pharyngitis may simulate symptoms of diphtheria and streptococcal pharyngitis. Lymphadenopathy, fever, malaise, jaundice, nervous system manifestations, and skin eruptions may be similar to symptoms seen in a variety of conditions. The leukocyte count may be normal or low, but usually lymphocyte leukocytosis develops.

The *heterophil antibody test* determines the extent to which the patient's serum will agglutinate sheep red blood cells. In infectious mononucleosis a titer of 1:160 is considered diagnostic, although a rising titer during the earlier stages is the best indicator. Because young children have a lower rate of heterophil antibody responses, the diagnosis may be overlooked in this group.

The *spot test (Monospot)* is a slide test of high specificity for the diagnosis of infectious mononucleosis. It is rapid, sensitive, inexpensive, and easy to perform, and it has the advantage that it can detect significant agglutinins at lower levels, thus permitting earlier diagnosis. Blood is usually obtained for the test by finger puncture and is placed on special paper. If the blood agglutinates, forming fragments or clumps, the test is positive for the infection.

### Therapeutic Management

No specific treatment exists for infectious mononucleosis. Common symptoms are ordinarily relieved by simple remedies. A mild analgesic is usually sufficient to relieve the bothersome symptoms of headache, fever, and malaise. Bed rest is encouraged for fatigue but is not imposed for any specified time. Affected youngsters are instructed to regulate activities according to their own tolerance unless complicating factors are present. If the spleen is enlarged, activities in which children might receive a blow to the abdomen or chest are avoided.

A short course of oral penicillin is sometimes prescribed for sore throat, especially if β-hemolytic streptococci are present. Administration of ampicillin frequently precipitates a maculopapular rash in affected persons; therefore its use is contraindicated. Sore throat, which can be severe, can be relieved by gargles, hot drinks, analgesic or anesthetic troches, or analgesics, including opioids. Although corticosteroids have been used to treat respiratory distress from tonsillar hypertrophy, hemolytic anemia, thrombocytopenia, and neurologic complications, the routine use of steroids is not recommended (Barone and Krilov, 2001).

**Prognosis.** The course of infectious mononucleosis is self-limiting and usually uncomplicated. Contrary to popular belief, mononucleosis is not necessarily a difficult, prolonged, or disabling disease, and the prognosis is generally good. Acute symptoms usually disappear within 7 to 10 days, and the persistent fatigue subsides within 2 to 4 weeks. A number of affected youngsters may need to restrict activities for 2 to 3 months; the disease rarely extends for longer periods.

Complications are uncommon but can be serious and require appropriate management. Liver involvement is present to some degree in almost all cases and may become chronic. Neurologic complications are seen in some outbreaks and vary in severity and outcome. Other complications include pneumonitis, myocarditis, hemolytic anemia, thrombocytopenia, and ruptured spleen. Some evidence indicates a depressed cellular immune reactivity during the course of the disease and for some time afterward; thus live vaccines are best avoided until several months after recovery.

> **NURSING ALERT**   Advise family to seek medical evaluation of the youngster if:
> Breathing becomes difficult.
> Abdominal pain develops.
> Sore throat pain is so severe that the child is unable to eat or drink.

### Nursing Considerations

Nursing responsibilities are directed toward providing comfort measures to relieve the symptoms and toward helping affected youngsters and their families determine appropriate activities for the stage of the disease and their interests. They may need diet counseling to select foods that contain sufficient calories to meet growth and energy needs but are easy to swallow. Every effort should be made to prevent a secondary infection; therefore the adolescent is counseled to limit exposure to persons outside the family, especially during the acute phase of illness.

The protracted nature of the illness and its associated weakness and fatigue can cause depression and resentment in vigorous, active teenagers. It is important to spend time with youngsters to listen to their concerns and to allow them to express their feelings and vent their anger. Adolescents need reassurance that the limitations are temporary, that social activities—so essential at this stage of development—

can be resumed after the acute phase, and that they will have sufficient autonomy to determine the extent of their capabilities and the rate of resumption of activities.

## Influenza

Influenza, or "flu," is caused by three of the orthomyxoviruses, which are antigenically distinct: types A and B, which cause epidemic disease, and type C, which is unimportant epidemiologically. The viruses undergo significant changes from time to time. Major changes that occur at intervals of usually 5 to 10 years are called *antigenic shift;* minor variations within the same subtypes, *antigenic drift,* occur almost annually. Consequently, antigenic drift can alter the virus sufficiently to result in susceptibility of individuals to a type for which they were previously immunized or infected.

The disease is spread from one individual to another by direct contact (large-droplet infection) or by articles recently contaminated by nasopharyngeal secretions. There is no predilection for a specific age-group, but attack rates are highest in young children who have not had previous contact with a strain. It is frequently most severe in infants and the elderly. During epidemics, infection among school-age children is believed to be a major source of transmission in a community. Influenza is more common during the winter months.

The disease has a 1- to 3-day incubation period, and affected persons are most infectious for 24 hours before and after the onset of symptoms. The virus has a peculiar affinity for epithelial cells of the respiratory tract mucosa, where it destroys ciliated epithelium with metaplastic hyperplasia of the tracheal and bronchial epithelium with associated edema. The alveoli may also become distended with a hyaline-like material. The viruses can be isolated from nasopharyngeal secretions early after the onset of infection, and serologic tests identify the type by complement fixation or the subgroups by hemagglutination inhibition.

### Clinical Manifestations

The manifestations of influenza may be subclinical, mild, moderate, or severe. In most cases the throat and nasal mucosa are dry, and there is a dry cough and a tendency toward hoarseness. A sudden onset of fever and chills is accompanied by flushed face, photophobia, myalgia, hyperesthesia, and sometimes prostration. Subglottal croup is common, especially in infants. The symptoms last for 4 to 5 days. Complications include severe viral pneumonia (often hemorrhagic), encephalitis, and secondary bacterial infections, such as otitis media, sinusitis, or pneumonia.

### Therapeutic Management

Uncomplicated influenza in children usually requires only symptomatic treatment: acetaminophen or ibuprofen for fever and sufficient fluids to maintain hydration. Amantadine hydrochloride (Symmetrel) has been effective in reducing symptoms associated with type A disease if administered within 24 to 48 hours after their onset. It is ineffective against type B or C influenza or other viral diseases. It

should not be given to children under 1 year of age but is recommended for unvaccinated high-risk children.

Zanamivir and rimantadine are two other medications that have been approved for the treatment of flu symptoms in children under 18 years of age. Both these medications must also be started within 48 hours of symptom onset. Zanamivir is an inhaled medication effective for viruses Types A and B influenza. The drug is taken twice daily for 5 days and is administered by a specially designed oral inhaler (Diskhaler). Zanamivir cannot be used for children less than 7 years of age. Bronchospasm and a decline in lung function can occur when zanamivir is used in patients with underlying airway disease such as asthma or chronic obstructive pulmonary disease. Rimantadine is effective only for Type A virus; this drug is taken orally in tablet or syrup twice daily for 7 days. Rimantadine cannot be used for children less than 1 year of age (Palencia, 2000). Children with influenza (or other similar viruses) should not receive aspirin because of its possible link with Reye syndrome.

**Prevention.**    Inactivated influenza viral vaccines are safe and effective for prevention of influenza provided that the antigens in the vaccine correlate with circulating influenza viruses. (See Immunizations, Chapter 12.)

### Nursing Considerations

Nursing care is the same as for any child with a URI, including helping the family to implement measures to relieve symptoms. The greatest danger to affected children is development of a secondary infection.

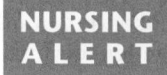 **NURSING ALERT**    Prolonged fever or appearance of fever during early convalescence is a sign of secondary bacterial infection and should be reported to the practitioner for antibiotic therapy.

## Otitis Media (OM)

Otitis media (OM) is one of the most prevalent diseases of early childhood. Approximately 80% of children have had at least one episode, and nearly 50% have had three or more episodes by 3 years of age (Kline, 1999). The incidence is highest in children ages 6 months to 2 years; it then gradually decreases with age, except for a small increase at age 5 or 6 years, the time of school entry. OM occurs infrequently in children over 7 years of age. Preschool-age boys are affected more frequently than preschool-age girls. The incidence of acute otitis media (AOM) is highest in the winter months. Children living in households with many members (especially smokers) are more likely to have OM than those living with fewer persons, and children who have siblings or parents with a history of chronic OM have a higher incidence than those who do not.

Passive smoking has been established as a significant factor in the development of OM. Tobacco smoke inhalation may increase the risk of a blocked eustachian tube by impairing mucociliary function, causing congestion of soft nasopharyngeal tissues, or predisposing patients to URI. Daycare attendance and living with a smoker are also risk factors for OM (Adair-Bischoff and Sauve, 1998; Nafstad and others, 1999).

OM has been defined in a variety of ways. The standard terminology to describe OM is outlined in Box 32-4.

## Etiology

AOM is frequently caused by *Streptococcus pneumoniae, H. influenzae,* and *Moraxella catarrhalis.* The etiology of the non-infectious type is unknown, although it is frequently the result of blocked eustachian tubes from the edema of URIs, allergic rhinitis, or hypertrophic adenoids. Chronic OM is frequently an extension of an acute episode.

A relationship has been observed between the incidence of OM and infant feeding methods. Infants fed breast milk have a lower incidence of OM compared with formula-fed infants. Breast-feeding may protect infants against respiratory viruses and allergy because it contains secretory immunoglobulin A (IgA), which limits the exposure of the eustachian tube and middle ear mucosa to microbial pathogens and foreign proteins. Reflux of milk up the eustachian tubes is less likely in breast-fed infants because of the semivertical positioning during breast-feeding compared with bottle-feeding.

## Pathophysiology

OM is primarily a result of a dysfunctioning eustachian tube. The eustachian tube is part of a contiguous system composed of the nares, nasopharynx, eustachian tube, middle ear, and mastoid antrum and air cells. (See Fig. 7-26.) Eustachian tubes have three functions relative to the middle ear: (1) protection of the middle ear from nasopharyngeal secretions, (2) drainage of secretions produced in the middle ear into the nasopharynx, and (3) ventilation of the middle ear to equalize air pressure within the middle ear with atmospheric pressure in the external ear canal and replenishment of oxygen that has been absorbed.

Mechanical or functional obstruction of the eustachian tube causes accumulation of secretions in the middle ear. Intrinsic obstruction can be caused by infection or allergy; extrinsic obstruction is usually a result of enlarged adenoids or nasopharyngeal tumors. Persistent collapse of the tube during swallowing can cause functional obstruction associated with decreased stiffness or an inefficient opening mechanism. Eustachian tube obstruction results in negative middle ear pressure and, if persistent, produces a transudative middle ear effusion. Drainage is inhibited by sustained negative pressure and impaired ciliary transport within the tube. When the passage is not totally obstructed, contamination of the middle ear can take place by reflux, aspiration, or insufflation during crying, sneezing, nose blowing, and swallowing when the nose is obstructed.

Several factors predispose infants and young children to development of OM (Box 32-5).

**Complications.**   The consequences of prolonged middle ear disorders can be either functional or structural. The principal functional consequence is **hearing loss,** although loss in most children is conductive in nature and mild in severity. The causes of hearing loss are negative middle ear pressure, the presence of effusion in the middle ear, or structural damage to the tympanic membrane. However, the most feared consequence of hearing loss is its adverse effect on development of speech, language, and cognition. Children who have prolonged periods of middle ear effusion perform less well on speech and language tests than those who have few if any middle ear diseases.

Structural complications or sequelae involve primarily the tympanic membrane. *Tympanic membrane retraction* or *retraction pocket* occurs when continued negative middle ear pressure draws the tympanic membrane inward, and in areas of low tensile strength or atrophic segments of the drum head, retraction pockets appear. This retraction may result in impaired sound transmission, perforation of the thinned-out areas, or infection in the pockets and, later, cholesteatoma.

---

**Box 32-5** ■ ■ ▫
### Factors Predisposing to Development of Otitis Media in Children

The eustachian tubes are short, wide, and straight and lie in a relatively horizontal plane (Fig. 32-3).

The cartilage lining is undeveloped, making the tubes more distensible and therefore more likely to open inappropriately.

The normally abundant pharyngeal lymphoid tissue readily obstructs the eustachian tube openings in the nasopharynx.

Immature humoral defense mechanisms increase the risk of infection.

The usual lying-down position of infants favors the pooling of fluid, such as formula, in the pharyngeal cavity.

---

**Box 32-4** ■ ■ ▫
### Standard Terminology for Otitis Media

**Otitis media**—An inflammation of the middle ear without reference to etiology or pathogenesis

**Acute otitis media (AOM)**—A rapid and short onset of signs and symptoms lasting approximately 3 weeks

**Otitis media with effusion (OME)**—An inflammation of the middle ear in which a collection of fluid is present in the middle ear space

**Chronic otitis media with effusion**—Middle ear effusion that persists beyond 3 months

---

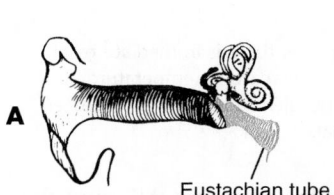
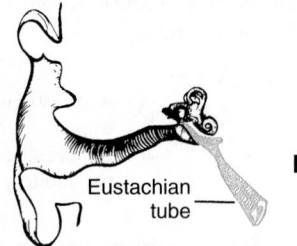

**Fig. 32-3**   Comparison of anatomic position of eustachian tube in, **A,** child and, **B,** adult. The eustachian tube is shorter, wider, straighter, and more horizontal in the child than in the adult.

*Tympanosclerosis* (eardrum scarring) is the deposition of hyaline material into the fibrous layer of the tympanic membrane. It is often seen in children with inflammatory middle ear disease or those with repeated tympanoplasty tube placement. Eardrum *perforation* is a common complication in AOM and often accompanies chronic disease. Persistent perforation is a complication of tympanostomy tube placement. Surgery is required to close some perforations.

*Adhesive otitis media* (glue ear) is a thickening of the mucous membrane by proliferation of fibrous tissue that can cause fixation of the ossicles with a resultant hearing loss. *Chronic suppurative otitis media,* an inflammation of the middle ear and mastoid, is evidenced by perforation and discharge (otorrhea) for up to 6 weeks' duration. *Labyrinthitis,* infection of the inner ear, and *mastoiditis,* infection of the mastoid sinus, are rare since the advent of antibiotic therapy. *Meningitis* and other suppurative intracranial complications are possible complications of extension of infection from the middle ear or mastoid. However, these complications occur infrequently when adequate antibiotic therapy is implemented.

*Cholesteatoma* is the least common but most potentially dangerous sequela of otitis media with effusion (OME). A cholesteatoma is formed when the keratinizing, stratified, squamous epithelial cell lining desquamates to form scales that accumulate within the middle ear space. As it enlarges, the cholesteatoma erodes all of the structures it encounters, especially bone, destroying the ossicles and gaining entry to the inner ear and meninges. Clinical signs are a foul-smelling, grayish yellow discharge, sometimes pain, and permanent, progressive hearing loss. Treatment is surgical excision of the entire cholesteatoma.

## Clinical Manifestations

As purulent fluid accumulates in the small space of the middle ear chamber, pain results from the pressure on surrounding structures. Infants become irritable and indicate their discomfort by holding or pulling at their ears and rolling their head from side to side. Young children usually verbally complain of the pain. A temperature as high as 40° C (104° F) is common, and postauricular and cervical lymph glands may be enlarged. Rhinorrhea, vomiting, and diarrhea, as well as signs of concurrent respiratory or pharyngeal infection, may also be present. Loss of appetite typically occurs, and sucking or chewing tends to aggravate the pain. In children with OME, exudate will accumulate and pressure will increase, with the potential for tympanic membrane rupture.

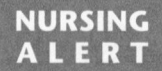 **NURSING ALERT** As a result of rupture, there is immediate relief of pain, a gradual decrease in temperature, and the presence of purulent discharge in the external auditory canal.

Severe pain or fever is usually absent in OME, and the child may not appear ill. Instead there is a feeling of "fullness" in the ear, a popping sensation during swallowing, and a feeling of "motion" in the ear if air is present above the level of fluid. Because chronic serous OM is the most fre-

quent cause of conductive hearing loss in young children, audiometry may reveal deficient hearing.

## Diagnostic Evaluation

In AOM, otoscopy reveals an intact membrane that appears bright red and bulging, with no visible landmarks or light reflex. The usual landmarks of the bony prominence from the long and the short process of the malleus are obscured by the outwardly bulging membrane. In OME, otoscopic findings may include a slightly injected, dull gray membrane, obscured landmarks, and a visible fluid level or meniscus behind the eardrum if air is present above the fluid.

Several tests provide an assessment of mobility of the tympanic membrane. *Pneumatic otoscopy* and *tympanometry* are discussed under Auditory Testing in Chapter 7. Acoustic reflectometry measures the level of sound transmitted and reflected from the middle ear to a microphone located in a probe tip placed against the ear canal opening and directed toward the tympanic membrane. The information provides a measure of canal length and presence of effusion. The greater the cancellation of transmitted sound by reflected sound, the greater the probability of middle ear effusion.

Diagnosis is usually based on clinical manifestations, but if purulent discharge is present, it should be cultured and a specific antibiotic chosen for that organism.

## Therapeutic Management: Acute Otitis Media (AOM)

Because of concerns about penicillin resistance, infectious disease authorities recommend judicious use of antibiotics. Some experts advise that AOM be treated only in children who meet one of the following criteria: more than three ear infections in the past year; a positive respiratory culture; and a high risk for bacterial infections because of immunosuppression, a splenectomy, cystic fibrosis, sickle cell disease, attendance at a daycare center, or living with a smoker (Armitage, Gross, and Yamauchi, 1999). When antibiotics are warranted, a variety can be used. Oral amoxicillin is a reasonable first choice for older infants and children because of its ease of use, relatively inexpensive cost, and availability. An important consideration for deciding which drug to prescribe is compliance by the parent in giving the antibiotic. Another consideration is the organism causing the OM. Eleven serotypes of *S. pneumoniae* account for approximately 85% of the cases of OM caused by that organism. These serotypes are susceptible to penicillin. However, many strains of *H. influenzae* and most strains of *M. catarrhalis* produce β-lactamase and are resistant to amoxicillin and penicillin (Kline, 1999).

In addition to amoxicillin, other oral antibiotics prescribed include sulfonamides, trimethoprim-sulfamethoxazole (Bactrim, Septra), erythromycin-sulfisoxazole (Pediazole), azithromycin, and the cephalosporins, which are often selected because of their broad-spectrum activity, dosage schedule, decreased side effects, and bactericidal activity against β-lactamase–producing pathogens (Montville and White, 1998).

Single-dose parenteral drugs have been used to treat AOM. These drugs provide an advantage to children who might have poor absorption of an oral drug due to vomiting or diarrhea, who refuse to take oral medications, or who have decreased compliance due to family circumstances. A single IM dose of ceftriaxone was found to be comparable in clinical efficacy to 10 days' dosage of oral trimethoprim-sulfamethoxazole (TMP-SMZ) for treatment of AOM (Barnett and others, 1997).

An important consideration with the use of single-dose IM injections is the pain involved in this therapy. One strategy to minimize pain at the injection site is to mix the cephalosporin with lidocaine. (See Atraumatic Care box.)

For fever or discomfort associated with OM, analgesic/antipyretic drugs such as acetaminophen or ibuprofen may be given. Antihistamines and decongestants are not recommended. Antibiotic eardrops have no value in treating AOM.

Children with AOM should be seen after antibiotic therapy is complete to evaluate the effectiveness of the treatment and to identify potential complications, such as effusion or hearing impairment. It is often difficult for parents to determine hearing loss; therefore audiometric testing should be done. (Screening tests for hearing are discussed in Chapter 7.)

### Therapeutic Management: Recurrent Otitis Media

Therapy for recurrent AOM has included chemoprophylaxis with long-term antibiotic therapy, immunotherapy, and surgery. Children receiving long-term antibiotic therapy should be evaluated once a month to detect any evidence of effusion. Any acute infection during prophylaxis is treated with an alternate antibiotic regimen. According to guidelines published by the **Agency for Healthcare Research and Quality (AHRQ)*** (formerly AHCPR), steroids are not recommended for treatment of OME in children of any age.

Polyvalent pneumococcal polysaccharide vaccines have reduced the incidence of pneumococcal OM by 50% in children older than 2 years, but these vaccines are not effective in infants, who do not normally develop antibodies to polysaccharide vaccines (Andrews, 2001). In some high-risk infants an immune globulin containing antibodies against bacterial polysaccharides (BPIG) has resulted in significantly fewer cases of AOM caused by *S. pneumoniae.*

Although there is controversy over the efficacy of this procedure, a myringotomy with surgical placement of tubes may be performed if there is severe pain, significant conductive hearing loss secondary to the presence of recurrent and chronic OM, or failure of medical management with prophylactic antibiotics (Andrews, 2001). Tubes are usually placed in the anteroinferior quadrant of the membrane. If, however, a eustachian tube remains blocked, fluid will return after a fairly rapid spontaneous healing of the myringotomy. Adenoidectomy may be successful in treating OM if a blocked eustachian tube secondary to hypertrophy of ade-

---

*A parent guide (94-0624) and more detailed *Clinical Practice Guidelines* (94-0620) are available in English and Spanish from AHCPR Publications Clearinghouse, OME/AAP, PO Box 8547, Silver Spring, MD 20907, (800) 358-9295.

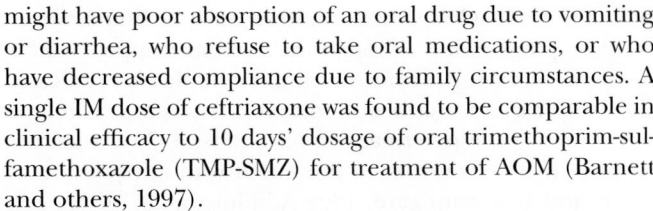

**ATRAUMATIC CARE**

*Intramuscular Ceftriaxone (Rocephin)*

To reduce the pain from IM administration of ceftriaxone, use lidocaine 1% as the diluent (Barnett and others, 1997). The lidocaine can be buffered at the time of use to further reduce stinging or burning. If time permits, apply EMLA cream to the IM site 2½ hours before the injection.

noids is the cause. Mastoidectomy may be performed when antibiotic therapy has failed and the child's life is threatened by infection, with tympanoplasty (middle ear reconstructive surgery) possibly being done after surgery.

### Therapeutic Management: Otitis Media with Effusion (OME)

Some children have fluid that persists in the middle ear for weeks or months. OME is frequently associated with mild to moderate impairment of hearing. The major goal of therapy is to establish and maintain an aerated middle ear that is free of fluid with a normal mucosa and ultimately to achieve normal hearing.

A child who has had fluid in both middle ears for a total of 3 months should have a hearing evaluation. A course of antibiotics is not indicated for the initial treatment of OME but may be indicated for children who have had persistent effusion for more than 3 months (Dowell and others, 1998). If bilateral effusion has persisted and the child has hearing loss, surgical myringotomy is an option. Placement of tympanostomy tubes is recommended after a total of 4 to 6 months of bilateral effusion with a bilateral hearing deficit (Andrews, 2001). This therapy allows for mechanical drainage of the fluid, which promotes healing of the membrane and prevents scar formation and loss of elasticity. The tubes (or ventilatory pressure-equalizer [PE] tubes or grommets) facilitate continued drainage of fluid and allow ventilation of the middle ear. The primary objective is to allow the eustachian tube a period of recovery while the surgically placed tube performs its functions. The surgery is relatively benign; however, sometimes the tubes may become plugged and often require reinsertion. Complications of repeated or long-term tube placement are tympanosclerosis, localized or diffuse atrophy of the membrane, persistent perforation, or, rarely, cholesteatoma. Tonsillectomy is not beneficial for OME (Kline, 1999).

**Prognosis.**   Most cases of OM resolve eventually. However, hearing loss, typically conductive, is a common complication of OM. The degree of hearing loss can vary from none to severe. Although conductive hearing loss is most often associated with OM, sensorineural hearing loss may also be present, especially in severe forms of chronic or recurrent OM, because of the passage of toxic products from fluids into the cochlea through the tympanic membrane. The longer the fluid is present, the greater the sensorineural hearing loss. Children who are prone to OM should be referred to a pediatric otolaryngologist and possibly a pediatric allergist for identification and treatment of the etiology of their eustachian tube dysfunction. They should also be referred to a speech/language pathologist for primary prevention counseling. In addition, the child should ideally be followed by an audiologist to evaluate the adequacy of hearing.

## Nursing Considerations

Nursing objectives for the child with AOM include (1) relieving pain, (2) facilitating drainage when possible, (3) preventing complications or recurrence, (4) educating the family in care of the child, and (5) providing emotional support to the child and family.

Analgesics are helpful to reduce severe earache. High fever, particularly in infants, should be reduced with antipyretic drugs. An advantage of using ibuprofen rather than acetaminophen is its longer duration of action (about 6 hours), especially for nighttime comfort. The application of heat may reduce pain in some children but may aggravate discomfort in others. Local heat should be placed over the ear while the child lies on the affected side. This position also facilitates drainage of the exudate if the eardrum has ruptured or if myringotomy was performed. An ice compress placed over the affected ear may also provide comfort, because it reduces edema. If the child is cooperative, either procedure can be tried to determine which offers maximum relief.

If the ear is draining, the external canal may be cleansed with sterile cotton swabs or pledgets soaked in hydrogen peroxide. If ear wicks or lightly rolled sterile gauze packs are placed in the ear after surgical treatment, they should be loose enough to allow accumulated drainage to flow out of the ear; otherwise the infection may be transferred to the mastoid process. Parents should be told to keep these wicks dry during shampoos or baths. Occasionally drainage is so profuse that the pinna and surrounding skin become excoriated from exudate. This is prevented by frequent cleansing and application of various moisture barriers (e.g., Aloe Vesta, Proshield Plus) or petrolatum jelly (e.g., Vaseline).

Parents require anticipatory guidance regarding temporary hearing loss that accompanies OM. For example, they may need to speak louder, at closer proximity, and while facing the child. They are reminded that the child is not ignoring them.

The child may not be able to localize where a sound is coming from because awareness and understanding of speech are reduced either unilaterally or bilaterally, depending on the degree of hearing deficit. The family should also be aware of possible behavioral changes with hearing loss, including inattentiveness to or lack of awareness of environmental sounds; requests for repetition in conversation or mishearing of content; softer or louder voice than usual; poor attention span and fidgety behavior when in a group (e.g., classroom) listening situation; aggressiveness and low frustration tolerance because of the frustration of frequent communication breakdown; and impaired speech and language skills. Persistent difficulty in hearing beyond the acute stage should be evaluated.

Preventing recurrence requires adequate parent education regarding antibiotic therapy. Because the symptoms of pain and fever usually subside within 24 to 48 hours, nurses must emphasize that although the child may appear well in a couple of days, the infection is not completely eradicated until all of the prescribed medication is taken. It is important to stress the potential complications of OM, especially hearing loss, which can be prevented with adequate treatment and follow-up care. (See Administration of Medication, Chapter 27, and Compliance, Chapter 27.*)

Tympanostomy tubes may allow water to enter the middle ear. Several studies indicate that small amounts of water pose little hazard and that even swimming without earplugs or occlusive bathing caps carries no increased risk of infection. However, diving, jumping, and submerging is forbidden by some practitioners. Bathwater and shampoo water should be kept out of the ear, if possible, because soap reduces the surface tension of water, facilitating entry through the tube. Lake water, as well as bathwater, is contaminated; therefore wearing earplugs, although not watertight earplugs, prevents total flooding of the external canal and provides sufficient protection. Parents should be aware of the appearance of a grommet (usually a tiny, white plastic, spool-shaped tube) so that they can recognize it if it falls out. They are reassured that this is normal and requires no immediate intervention, although they should notify the practitioner.

Parents sometimes ask about preventing ear discomfort in their infants during ascent or descent of an airplane. During ascent, air in the middle ear expands, but decompression takes place through a normal eustachian tube. If the tissues are congested with a URI, the passage of air may be blocked. A nasal mucosa–shrinking spray or oral decongestant before the trip may be helpful. During descent, the air within the middle ear decreases as atmospheric pressure increases. Swallowing is the simplest and most effective method for inflating the middle ear on descent; therefore feeding or offering a pacifier to infants during descent is beneficial.

Reducing the chances of OM is possible with simple measures, such as sitting or holding an infant upright for feedings. Propping bottles is discouraged to avoid the supine position and to encourage human contact during feeding. Eliminating tobacco smoke and known allergens is also recommended. Forceful nose blowing during a URI is discouraged to avoid forcing organisms to ascend through the eustachian tube. Early detection of middle ear effusion is essential in prevention of complications. Infants and preschool children should be screened for effusion, and all schoolchildren, especially those with learning disabilities, should be tested for middle ear effusion. Frequent audiologic evaluations, medical consultation, and education of parents and children are advised when middle ear effusion is detected. (See Nursing Care Plan: The Child with Acute Otitis Media.†)

---

*Home care instructions for administration of medications are available in Wong DL, Hess CS: *Wong and Whaley's clinical manual of pediatric nursing,* ed 5, St Louis, 2000, Mosby.

†In Wong DL, Hess CS: *Wong and Whaley's clinical manual of pediatric nursing,* ed 5, St Louis, 2000, Mosby.

## Otitis Externa

Infections of the external ear result from normal ear flora (*Staphylococcus epidermidis* and *Corynebacterium*) that assume pathogenic characteristics under conditions of excessive wetness or dryness. Ordinarily the external ear canal is protected by a waxy, water-repellent coating composed of highly viscid secretions of the sebaceous glands and the watery, pigmented secretions of apocrine glands in combination with exfoliated surface cells. Inflammation occurs when this environment is altered by swimming, bathing, or increased environmental humidity *(swimmer's ear);* by infection, dermatoses, or insufficient cerumen; or by trauma from a foreign body or a finger.

Secondary invasion of foreign pathogens also occurs. In addition to the resident flora, the offending agents can be *Pseudomonas aeruginosa* (most common), *Enterobacter aerogenes, Proteus mirabilis, Klebsiella pneumoniae,* streptococci, and fungi such as *Candida* and *Aspergillus* organisms. The ear canal becomes irritated, and maceration takes place.

The predominant symptom of external ear infection is ear pain accentuated by manipulation of the pinna, especially pressure on the tragus. The pain often appears to be out of proportion to the degree of inflammation. Conductive hearing loss may be present as a result of the edema, secretions, and accumulation of debris within the canal. Edema, erythema, and a cheesy green-blue-gray discharge and tenderness appear as the infection progresses. The external canal may be so tender and swollen that visualization is difficult. There may be fever. In advanced cases the pain is intense, constant, and aggravated by jaw motion or ear manipulation.

Therapeutic objectives include relief of pain, edema, and itching and restoration of normal flora, cerumen, and canal epithelium. Analgesics are prescribed for pain. Debris is removed with gentle suction and wisps of cotton on metal cotton carriers. Otic preparations containing neomycin with either colistin or polymyxin and corticosteroids are instilled in the canal. A gauze wick is usually inserted to facilitate the medication reaching the site of inflammation. The wick is removed after swelling and pain have subsided, but the drops are continued for at least 3 days after relief of pain. The best management for external ear inflammation is prevention.

### Nursing Considerations

Nurses can teach parents or patients to apply simple measures to prevent recurrent infections. Children are advised to limit their stay in the water to less than an hour, if possible, and ears should dry completely (1 to 2 hours) before children enter the water again. Shaking the head and judicious use of the corner of a towel can remove most excess water. The ear canal can also be dried with a small tuft of cotton (not a swab). Placing a combination of white vinegar and rubbing alcohol (50:50) in both ear canals on arising, at bedtime, and at the end of each swim is effective in preventing recurrence. The solution could remain in the canal for 5 minutes. Youngsters are cautioned not to pick at the ears with a pencil, cotton swab, bobby pin, or other object, which can injure or infect the ear canal.

**NURSING TIP**   To keep the ear dry, pull the auricle up and out to straighten the canal, then use a conventional hair dryer, set on *low* or *no heat,* held at a distance of 18 to 24 inches for 30 seconds, three times a day.

## CROUP SYNDROMES

*Croup* is a general term applied to a symptom complex characterized by hoarseness, a resonant cough described as "barking" or "brassy" (croupy), varying degrees of inspiratory stridor, and varying degrees of respiratory distress resulting from swelling or obstruction in the region of the larynx. Acute infections of the larynx are of greater importance in infants and small children than they are in older children, because of the increased incidence in children in this age-group and the smaller diameter of the airway, which renders it subject to significantly greater narrowing with the same degree of inflammation (Fig. 32-4).

Croup is a common respiratory disease of childhood and occurs more often in boys than in girls. The number of croup cases increases in the late autumn through early

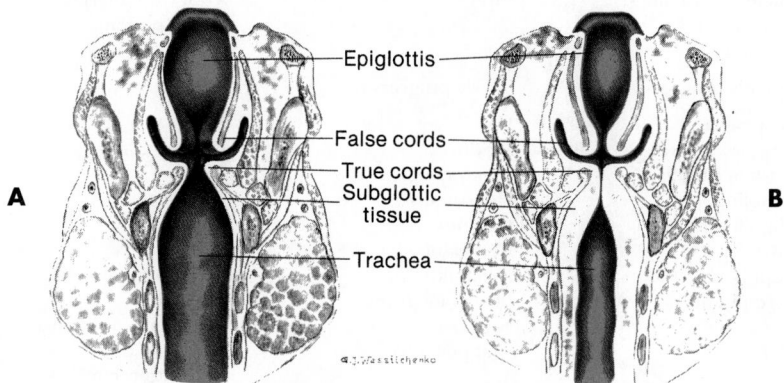

**Fig. 32-4   A,** Normal larynx. **B,** Obstruction and narrowing resulting from edema of croup.

winter months and occurs primarily in children 6 months to 3 years of age. Hospitalization may be necessary for some children with croup, and intubation is required for a small percentage of hospitalized children.

*Croup syndromes* affect to varying degrees the larynx, trachea, and bronchi. However, laryngeal involvement often dominates the clinical picture because of the severe effects on the voice and breathing. Croup syndromes are usually described according to the primary anatomic area affected (i.e., epiglottitis [or supraglottitis], laryngitis, laryngotracheobronchitis [LTB], and tracheitis). In general, LTB tends to occur in very young children, whereas epiglottitis is more characteristic of older children. A comparison of croup syndromes is given in Table 32-1.

Because croup is one of the most benign conditions causing upper airway obstruction, it is vitally important to identify correctly and distinguish what type of croup syndrome or condition is actually occurring (i.e., spasmodic croup or LTB as opposed to a potentially life-threatening condition such as epiglottitis, bacterial tracheitis, foreign body aspiration, or a peritonsillar abscess). The key differences between LTB and epiglottitis are the absence of cough, the presence of dysphagia, and the high degree of toxicity in children with epiglottitis. *Children with epiglottitis usually look worse than they sound, in contrast to children with LTB, who sound worse than they look.*

# Acute Epiglottitis

Acute epiglottitis, or acute supraglottitis, is a serious obstructive inflammatory process that occurs principally in children between 2 and 5 years of age but can occur from infancy to adulthood. The disorder requires *immediate* attention. The obstruction is supraglottic, as opposed to the subglottic obstruction of laryngitis. The responsible organism is usually *H. influenzae;* LTB and epiglottitis do not occur together.

## Clinical Manifestations

The onset of epiglottitis is abrupt, less often preceded by cold symptoms and more often by a sore throat. It can rapidly progress to severe respiratory distress. The child usually goes to bed asymptomatic to awaken later, complaining of sore throat and pain on swallowing. The child has a fever and appears sicker than clinical findings suggest. The child insists on sitting upright and leaning forward, with the chin thrust out, mouth open, and tongue protruding (tripod position). Drooling of saliva is common because of the difficulty or pain on swallowing and excessive secretions.

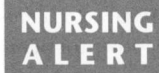 **NURSING ALERT** Three clinical observations that have been found to be predictive of epiglottitis are absence of spontaneous cough, presence of drooling, and agitation.

The child is irritable and extremely restless and has an anxious, apprehensive, and frightened expression. The voice is thick and muffled, with a froglike croaking sound on inspiration. The child is not hoarse. Suprasternal and substernal retractions may be visible. The child seldom struggles to breathe, and slow, quiet breathing provides better air exchange. The sallow color of mild hypoxia may progress to frank cyanosis. The throat is red and inflamed, and a distinctive, large, cherry red, edematous epiglottis is visible on careful throat inspection. *Throat inspection should be attempted only when immediate intubation can be performed if needed.*

## Therapeutic Management

The course of epiglottitis may be fulminant, with respiratory obstruction appearing suddenly. Progressive obstruction

| **TABLE 32-1** Comparison of croup syndromes | | | | |
|---|---|---|---|---|
| | **Acute Epiglottitis (Supraglottitis)** | **Acute Laryngotracheobronchitis** | **Acute Spasmodic Laryngitis (Spasmodic Croup)** | **Acute Tracheitis** |
| **Age-group affected** | 1-8 years | 3 months-8 years | 3 months-3 years | 1 month-6 years |
| **Etiologic agent** | Bacterial, usually *H. influenzae* | Viral | Viral with allergic component | Bacterial, usually *Staphylococcus aureus* |
| **Onset** | Rapidly progressive | Slowly progressive | Sudden; at night | Moderately progressive |
| **Major symptoms** | Dysphagia<br>Stridor aggravated when supine<br>Drooling<br>High fever<br>Toxic<br>Rapid pulse and respirations | URI<br>Stridor<br>Brassy cough<br>Hoarseness<br>Dyspnea<br>Restlessness<br>Irritability<br>Low-grade fever<br>Nontoxic appearance | URI<br>Croupy cough<br>Stridor<br>Hoarseness<br>Dyspnea<br>Restlessness<br>Symptoms awaken child<br>Symptoms disappear during day<br>Tends to recur | URI<br>Croupy cough<br>Stridor<br>Purulent secretions<br>High fever<br>No response to LTB therapy |
| **Treatment** | Antibiotics<br>Airway protection | Humidity<br>Racemic epinephrine | Humidity | Antibiotics |

leads to hypoxia, hypercapnia, and acidosis followed by decreased muscular tone, reduced level of consciousness and, when obstruction becomes more or less complete, a rather sudden death. A presumptive diagnosis of epiglottitis constitutes an emergency.

The child suspected of epiglottitis should be examined where facilities are available for coping with this type of emergency. The child is best transported while sitting in a parent's lap to reduce distress. Examination of the throat with a tongue depressor is contraindicated until properly experienced personnel and equipment are at hand to proceed with immediate intubation or tracheostomy in the event that the examination precipitates further or complete obstruction.

If a lateral neck film is indicated, the same experienced personnel should accompany the child to the radiology department. However, most practitioners prefer that the child not be transported but remain on the parent's lap in the examination area during portable radiology.

Endotracheal intubation or tracheostomy is usually considered for the child with *H. influenzae* epiglottitis with severe respiratory distress. It is recommended that the intubation or tracheostomy and any invasive procedure, such as starting an intravenous (IV) infusion, be performed in the operating room. Whether or not there is an artificial airway, the child requires intensive observation by experienced personnel. The epiglottal swelling usually decreases after 24 hours of antibiotic therapy, and the epiglottis is near normal by the third day. Intubated children are generally extubated at this time.

Children with suspected bacterial epiglottitis are given antibiotics intravenously, followed by oral administration to complete a 7- to 10-day course. The use of corticosteroids for reducing edema may be beneficial during the early hours of treatment; most intubated children will have had a course of corticosteroids for 24 hours before extubation.

**Prevention.** The American Academy of Pediatrics (2000) recommends that all children, beginning at 2 months of age, receive the *H. influenzae* type B conjugate vaccine. Since administration of the vaccine has become a routine part of the regular immunization schedule, a decline in the incidence of epiglottitis has occurred. Patients now tend to be older and have disease caused by other organisms. (See Immunizations, Chapter 12.)

## Nursing Considerations

Epiglottitis is a serious and frightening disease for the child, family, and health professionals. It is important to act quickly but calmly and provide support without unduly increasing anxiety. The child is allowed to remain in the position that provides the most comfort and security, and parents are reassured that everything possible is being done to obtain relief for their child.

**NURSING ALERT** Nurses who suspect epiglottitis should not attempt to visualize the epiglottis directly with a tongue depressor or take a throat culture but should refer the child to a physician immediately. (See Critical Thinking Exercise box.)

Acute care of the child is the same as that described for the child with acute respiratory distress and artificial airways in Chapter 31. Continuous monitoring of respiratory status, including blood gases, is part of nursing observations, and the IV infusion is maintained. (See Chapter 28.)

## Acute Laryngitis

Acute infectious laryngitis is a common illness in older children and adolescents. Infants and smaller children experience more generalized involvement. (See following section on LTB.) Viruses are the usual causative agents, and the principal complaint is hoarseness, which may be accompanied by other upper respiratory symptoms (e.g., coryza, sore throat, nasal congestion) and systemic manifestations (e.g., fever, headache, myalgia, malaise). Other complaints vary with the infecting virus. For example, adenoviruses and influenza viruses are responsible for more systemic involvement; parainfluenza viruses, rhinoviruses, and RSV cause more mild illness.

### Therapeutic Management and Nursing Considerations

The disease is almost always self-limited without long-term sequelae. Treatment is symptomatic with fluids and humidified air. (See Nursing Care Plan on pp. 1347-1350.)

## Acute Laryngotracheobronchitis (LTB)

LTB is the most common type of croup experienced by children admitted for hospitalization and primarily affects chil-

### Critical Thinking Exercise

#### Epiglottitis

Kim Lee, 4 years old, is admitted to the emergency department with a sore throat, pain on swallowing, drooling, and a fever of 39° C (102.2° F). She looks ill, is agitated, and prefers to sit up and lean over. Which of the following medical orders should you question?

FIRST, THINK ABOUT IT. . .

• How are you interpreting the information?
• What would the consequences be if you put your thoughts into action?

1. Obtain a complete blood count (CBC) and throat culture immediately.
2. Place child on oxygen saturation monitor.
3. Start an IV line of 5% dextrose in normal saline to run at 30 ml/hr.
4. Have pediatric-size tracheostomy tray available.

*The best response is one. Interpreting the information correctly, the nurse should question the order for a throat culture because the child's symptoms suggest epiglottitis. Negative consequences may result if inappropriate nursing actions are taken because the action can precipitate obstruction of the airway. The CBC and other interventions are appropriate.*

dren less than 5 years of age. Organisms responsible for LTB are the parainfluenza virus type 1, followed by virus types 3 and 2, RSV, influenza A and B, and *M. pneumoniae.* The disease is usually preceded by a URI, which gradually descends to adjacent structures. It is characterized by the gradual onset of low-grade fever.

Inflammation of the mucosa lining the larynx and trachea causes a narrowing of the airway. When the airway is significantly narrowed, the child struggles to inhale air past the obstruction and into the lungs, producing the characteristic inspiratory stridor and suprasternal retractions; other classic manifestations include cough and hoarseness. The typical child with LTB is a toddler who develops the classic barking or seallike cough and acute stridor after several days of coryza. The child may be in slight to moderate respiratory distress, with mild wheezing and a low-grade fever. When the child is unable to inhale a sufficient volume of air, symptoms of hypoxia become evident. As the work of forcing air past the obstruction increases, negative pressure generated in the thoracic cavity also increases, leading to leakage of pulmonary vascular fluid into interstitial spaces and causing uneven ventilation and hypoxia. Obstruction severe enough to prevent adequate exhalation of carbon dioxide causes respiratory acidosis, and, eventually, the child experiences respiratory failure (see progression of symptoms outlined in Box 32-6).

### Therapeutic Management

The major objective in medical management of infectious LTB is maintaining an airway and providing for adequate respiratory exchange. Children with mild croup (no stridor at rest) are managed at home. Parents are taught the signs of respiratory distress so that professional help can be summoned if needed. Children whose symptoms progress to stage II should receive medical attention.

High humidity with cool mist provides relief for most children. A cool-air vaporizer can be used at home. In the hospital, hoods for infants or mist tents for toddlers may be used to provide increased humidity and supplemental oxygen.

The cool-temperature therapy modalities assist by constricting edematous blood vessels. In the home environment, suggestions to provide cool air include taking the child outside to breathe in cool night air, use of a cold-water vaporizer or humidifier, standing in front of the open freezer, and taking the child to a cool basement or garage.

Controversy surrounds the use of mist therapy to treat croup. Studies have failed to demonstrate any improvement in subglottic edema with mist therapy. Any apparent effectiveness of mist therapy is probably due to the calming effect of the caregiver's or parent's presence. Despite this, mist therapy continues to be used in the home and emergency department for mildly distressed children (Wald, 1999).

It is essential to allow children with mild croup to continue to drink beverages they like and to encourage parents to use comforting measures with their child (e.g., being held, rocked, walked, sung to). If the child is unable to take oral fluids, IV fluid therapy may be indicated.

---

**NURSING ALERT**   Children with severe respiratory distress (traditionally, a respiratory rate >60 breaths/min for infants) should not be given anything by mouth to prevent aspiration and increase in the work of breathing.

---

Nebulized epinephrine *(racemic epinephrine)* is often used in children with more severe disease, stridor at rest, retractions, or difficulty breathing. The α-adrenergic effects cause mucosal vasoconstriction and subsequent decreased subglottic edema. The onset of action is rapid. Peak effect is observed in 2 hours. Additional doses may be administered every 20 to 30 minutes in the intensive care unit or 3 to 4 hours in a regular hospital unit (Wald, 1999). In a significant number of children, however, improvement persists and additional treatments are not necessary.

The use of corticosteroids is beneficial because the antiinflammatory effects decrease subglottic edema. The onset of action is clinically detectable as early as 6 hours after administration, with continued improvement over a period of 12 to 24 hours. Children receiving corticosteroids also have shortened stays in the emergency department and reduced admission rates (Wald, 1999).

### Nursing Considerations

The most important nursing function in the care of children with LTB is continuous, vigilant observation and accurate assessment of respiratory status. Cardiac, respiratory, and noninvasive blood gas monitoring equipment supplement visual observations. Changes in therapy are frequently based on nurses' observations and assessment of a child's

---

**Box 32-6** ▪ ▪ ▫
**Progression of Symptoms in Laryngotracheobronchitis**

**STAGE 1**
Fear
Hoarseness
Croupy cough
Inspiratory stridor when disturbed

**STAGE II**
Continuous respiratory stridor
Lower rib retraction
Retraction of soft tissue of neck
Use of accessory muscles of respiration
Labored respiration

**STAGE III**
Signs of anoxia and carbon dioxide retention
Restlessness
Anxiety
Pallor
Sweating
Rapid respiration

**STAGE IV**
Intermittent cyanosis
Permanent cyanosis
Cessation of breathing

From Walter EB, Shurin PA: Acute respiratory infections. In Krugman S and others: *Infectious diseases of children,* ed 9, St Louis, 1992, Mosby.

status, response to therapy, and tolerance of procedures. The trend away from early intubation of children with LTB emphasizes the importance of nursing observation and the ability to recognize impending respiratory failure so that intubation can be implemented without delay. Intubation equipment should be readily accessible and taken with the child during transport to other areas (e.g., radiology, operating room).

> **NURSING ALERT**   Early signs of impending airway obstruction include increased pulse and respiratory rate; substernal, suprasternal, and intercostal retractions; flaring nares; and increased restlessness.

To conserve energy, children are given every opportunity to rest. Infants or small children find that being enclosed within a mist tent, coughing, having laryngeal spasms, and needing IV therapy are additional sources of distress. Infants and small children prefer sitting upright, and most want to be held. Children need the security of the parent's presence. Because crying increases respiratory distress and hypoxia, a child's individual tolerance for these therapies must be assessed. An extremely fussy child may do better when held in the parent's lap with cool mist directed toward the child's face.

The rapid progression of croup, the alarming sound of the cough and stridor, and the child's apprehensive behavior and ill appearance combine to create a very frightening experience for the parents. They need reassurance regarding the child's progress and an explanation of treatments. They may feel guilty for not having suspected the seriousness of the condition sooner. The family should be allowed to remain with their child as much as possible, especially when this decreases the child's distress.

The nurse can provide the parents with an opportunity to express their feelings, thus minimizing any blame or guilt. They need frequent reassurance provided in a calm, quiet manner and education regarding what they can do to make their child more comfortable. Fortunately, as the crisis subsides and the child responds to therapy, breathing becomes easier and recovery is generally prompt. Home care after discharge includes continued humidity, adequate hydration, and nourishment. Parents are encouraged to ask questions about home care and preparation for discharge. Referral to a public health agency for follow-up care may be advisable.

## Acute Spasmodic Laryngitis

Acute spasmodic laryngitis (spasmodic croup, "midnight croup," or "twilight croup") is distinct from laryngitis and LTB and characterized by paroxysmal attacks of laryngeal obstruction that occur chiefly at night. Signs of inflammation are absent or mild, and there is often a history of previous attacks lasting for 2 to 5 days followed by uneventful recovery. It usually affects children ages 1 to 3 years. Some children appear to be predisposed to the condition; allergy and psychogenic factors are implicated in some cases.

The child goes to bed well or with some very mild respiratory symptoms but awakes suddenly with characteristic barking, metallic cough, hoarseness, noisy inspirations, and restlessness. The child appears anxious, frightened, and prostrated. Dyspnea is aggravated by excitement. However, there is no fever, the attack subsides in a few hours, and the child appears well the next day.

### Therapeutic Management and Nursing Considerations

Children with spasmodic croup are managed at home. Cool mist is recommended for the child's room. Warm mist provided by steam from hot running water in a closed bathroom may be helpful. Humidification may help, but warm temperatures will not relieve the constriction. Sometimes the spasm is relieved by sudden exposure to cold air (as when the child is taken out into the night air to see the practitioner). Parents are usually advised to have the child sleep in humidified air until the cough has subsided so that subsequent episodes may be prevented. Children with moderately severe symptoms may be hospitalized for observation and therapy with cool mist and racemic epinephrine, as for LTB. Patients may respond to corticosteroid therapy. The disease is usually self-limited.

## Bacterial Tracheitis

Bacterial tracheitis, an infection of the mucosa of the upper trachea, is a distinct entity with features of both croup and epiglottitis. The disease is seen in children ages 1 month to 6 years and may be a serious cause of airway obstruction—severe enough to cause respiratory arrest. It is believed to be a complication of LTB, and although *Staphylococcus aureus* is the most frequent organism responsible, group A β-hemolytic streptococci and *H. influenzae* have also been implicated.

Many of the manifestations of bacterial tracheitis are similar to those of LTB but are unresponsive to LTB therapy. There is a history of previous URI with croupy cough, stridor unaffected by position, toxicity, and high fever. A prominent manifestation is the production of thick, purulent tracheal secretions. Respiratory difficulties are secondary to these copious secretions.

### Therapeutic Management and Nursing Considerations

Bacterial tracheitis requires vigorous management. Humidified oxygen, antipyretics, and antibiotics are prescribed. Most children require endotracheal intubation and frequent tracheal suctioning to prevent airway obstruction. The emphasis in this disorder is early recognition in order to prevent catastrophic airway obstruction.

# INFECTIONS OF THE LOWER AIRWAYS

The *reactive portion* of the lower respiratory tract includes the bronchi and bronchioles in children. Cartilaginous support of the large airways is not fully developed until adolescence. Consequently, the smooth muscle in these structures represents a major factor in the constriction of the airway, particularly in the bronchioles, that portion that extends from the bronchi to the alveoli.

Table 32-2 compares some of the major features of bronchial and bronchiolar infections.

## Bronchitis

Bronchitis (sometimes referred to as *tracheobronchitis*) is inflammation of the large airways (trachea and bronchi), which is frequently associated with a URI. Viral agents are the primary cause of the disease, although *M. pneumoniae* is a common cause in children older than 6 years of age. The condition is characterized by a dry, hacking, and nonproductive cough that is worse at night and becomes productive in 2 to 3 days.

Bronchitis is a mild, self-limiting disease that requires only symptomatic treatment, including analgesics, antipyretics, and humidity. Cough suppressants may be useful to allow rest but can interfere with clearance of secretions. Most patients recover uneventfully in 5 to 10 days.

## Respiratory Syncytial Virus (RSV)/Bronchiolitis

Bronchiolitis is an acute viral infection with maximum effect at the bronchiolar level. The infection occurs primarily in winter and spring and is rare in children over 2 years of age. Although few children with bronchiolitis require hospitalization, it can be a serious disease.

Although adenoviruses and parainfluenza viruses can cause acute bronchiolitis, *respiratory syncytial virus (RSV)* is responsible for 80% or more of cases of bronchiolitis during epidemic periods (Long, 1999). It is considered the single most important respiratory pathogen in infancy and early childhood.

### Etiology

RSV is a paramyxovirus containing a single strand of ribonucleic acid (RNA) and related to parainfluenza virus. There are two major subgroups of RSV strains: A (the more virulent) and B. More children develop bronchiolitis and pneumonia from RSV subgroup A infections than from subgroup B infections during major outbreaks.

The disease usually begins in the fall, reaches a peak during the winter, and then decreases during the spring. In tropical regions, peaks of activity are less pronounced, and outbreaks tend to occur in rainy seasons.

### Pathophysiology

RSV affects the epithelial cells of the respiratory tract. The ciliated cells swell, protrude into the lumen, and lose their cilia. RSV produces a fusion of the infected cell membrane with cell membranes of adjacent epithelial cells, thus forming a giant cell with multiple nuclei. At the cellular level this fusion results in multinucleated masses of protoplasm, or "syncytia," being created.

The bronchiole mucosa swell, and lumina are subsequently filled with mucus and exudate. The walls of the bronchi and bronchioles are infiltrated with inflammatory cells, and peribronchiolar interstitial pneumonitis is usually present. Because luminal epithelial cells are shed into the bronchioles when they die, the lumina are frequently obstructed, particularly on expiration. The varying degrees of obstruction produced in small air passages lead to hyperinflation, obstructive emphysema resulting from partial obstruction, and patchy areas of atelectasis. Dilation of bronchial passages on inspiration allows sufficient space for intake of air, but narrowing of the passages on expiration

| **TABLE 32-2** | **Comparison of conditions affecting the bronchi** | | |
|---|---|---|---|
| | **Viral-Induced Asthma*** | **Bronchitis** | **Bronchiolitis** |
| **Description** | Exaggerated response of bronchi to infection<br>Bronchospasm, exudation, and edema of bronchi | Usually occurs in association with URI<br>Seldom an isolated entity | More common infectious disease of lower airways<br>Maximum obstructive impact at bronchiolar level |
| **Age-group affected** | Late infancy and early childhood | Affects children in first 4 years of life | Usually children 2-12 months; rare after age 2<br>Peak incidence approximately age 6 months |
| **Etiologic agents** | Most often viruses but may be any of a variety of URI pathogens | Usually viral<br>Other agents (e.g., bacteria, fungi, allergic disorders, airborne irritants) can trigger symptoms | Viruses, predominantly respiratory syncytial viruses; also adenoviruses, parainfluenza viruses, and *M. pneumoniae* |
| **Predominant characteristics** | Wheezing, productive cough | Persistent dry, hacking cough (worse at night) becoming productive in 2-3 days | Dyspnea, paroxysmal nonproductive cough, tachypnea with retractions and flaring nares, emphysema, may be wheezing |
| **Treatment** | Bronchodilators | Cough suppressants if needed | Oxygen mist<br>Ribavirin may be used for high-risk populations |

*See Asthma, p. 1385.

prevents air from leaving the lungs. Thus air is trapped distal to the obstruction and causes progressive overinflation *(emphysema)*.

## Transmission

The transmission of RSV is predominantly through direct contact with respiratory secretions, mainly as a result of inoculation from hand to eye, nose, or other mucous membranes; by direct inoculation by large-particle aerosols; or by self-inoculation from contaminated fomites (Long, 1999).

RSV in secretions can survive for hours on countertops, gloves, paper tissues, and cloth, and for half an hour on skin; it remains infectious when transferred from hands or objects. Distant spread of RSV by small-particle aerosols (airborne transmission) has not been documented.

## Clinical Manifestations

The younger the infant, the greater the likelihood that severe lower respiratory tract disease requiring hospitalization will occur. The peak incidence for RSV is 2 to 5 months of age, but reinfection with RSV is very common at all ages, with the highest rates being reported from daycare centers. The severity of RSV tends to diminish with age and repeated infections.

The illness usually begins with a URI after an incubation of about 5 to 8 days. Symptoms such as rhinorrhea and low-grade fever often appear first. Otitis media and conjunctivitis may also be present. In time a cough may develop. If the disease progresses, it becomes a lower respiratory tract infection and manifests typical symptoms (Box 32-7). With infants there may be several days of URI symptoms or no symptoms except slight lethargy, poor feeding, or irritability.

Once the lower airway is involved, classic manifestations include signs of altered air exchange, such as wheezing, re-

---

> ### Box 32-7 ■ ■ □
> ### Signs and Symptoms of Respiratory Syncytial Virus
>
> **INITIAL**
> Rhinorrhea
> Pharyngitis
> Coughing/sneezing
> Wheezing
> Possible ear or eye infection
> Intermittent fever
>
> **WITH PROGRESSION OF ILLNESS**
> Increased coughing and wheezing
> Air hunger
> Tachypnea and retractions
> Cyanosis
>
> **SEVERE ILLNESS**
> Tachypnea >70 breaths/min
> Listlessness
> Apneic spells
> Poor air exchange; poor breath sounds

---

tractions, crackles, dyspnea, tachypnea, and diminished breath sounds.

## Diagnostic Evaluation

Because RSV infection may be manifested as a URI, it is often difficult to identify the specific etiologic agent by clinical criteria alone. The most difficult distinction is between RSV and asthma, because both conditions involve the lower airway and have similar symptoms.

Identification has been simplified by the development of tests done on nasal or nasopharyngeal secretions, using either rapid immunofluorescent antibody (IFA) or enzyme-linked immunosorbent assay (ELISA) techniques for RSV antigen detection. Both tests have sensitivities and specificities of about 85% (Long, 1999). The more traditional viral culture is becoming obsolete, because it takes several days to get a result.

## Therapeutic Management

Bronchiolitis is treated symptomatically with high humidity, adequate fluid intake, rest, and medications. Most children with bronchiolitis can be managed at home. Hospitalization is usually recommended for children with complicating conditions, such as underlying lung or heart disease or associated debilitated states, or if the adequacy of the caregiver is questionable. The child who is tachypneic, has marked retractions, seems listless, or has a history of poor fluid intake should also be admitted. Mist therapy is generally combined with oxygen by hood or tent in concentrations sufficient to alleviate dyspnea and hypoxia, after which mist alone is continued for mild dyspnea. Fluids by mouth may be contraindicated because of tachypnea, weakness, and fatigue; therefore IV fluids are preferred until the acute stage of the disease has passed.

Clinical assessments, noninvasive oxygen monitoring, and blood gas values guide therapy. Medical therapy for bronchiolitis is controversial. Bronchodilators, corticosteroids, antihistamines, and antibiotics have not been shown to be effective in controlled studies and are not recommended for routine use. *Ribavirin,* an antiviral agent (synthetic nucleoside analog), is the only specific therapy approved for children hospitalized with RSV (Long, 1999). This drug is aerosolized and delivered via a small-particle aerosol generator (SPAG). It may be administered by hood, tent, or mask, or through ventilator tubing for 12 to 20 hours daily; average duration of therapy is 3 days (Long, 1999).

The use of ribavirin aerosol treatment for RSV is highly controversial. The high cost, aerosol route of administration, concern about potential toxic effects among exposed health care personnel, and conflicting results of efficacy trials have all contributed to this controversy (American Academy of Pediatrics, 1996). Therefore decisions about the use of ribavirin should be made on a case-by-case basis.

Currently, *respiratory syncytial virus immune globulin (RSV-IGIV* or *RespiGam)* is used prophylactically to prevent RSV infection in high-risk infants. RespiGam is an IV preparation of immunoglobulin G that provides neutralizing antibodies against subtype A and B strains of RSV. The drug is given on an inpatient or outpatient basis before or during the RSV epidemic season (November through April). Subsequent doses are given every month to maintain protection. A clinical trial of RSV-IGIV prophylaxis indicated that monthly administration of RespiGam was safe, well tolerated, and effective in reducing the incidence and total days of both hospitalization for RSV and overall hospitalization for respiratory conditions in infants with a history of prematurity or bronchopulmonary dysplasia (PREVENT Study Group, 1997). Another study of RespiGam indicated that monthly infusions may have the additional benefit of preventing acute otitis media in high-risk populations (Simoes and others, 1996). RespiGam is not approved by the Food and Drug Administration for patients with congenital heart disease (CHD) and should not be used in patients with cyanotic CHD (American Academy of Pediatrics, 2000).

In 1998 a genetically engineered RSV monoclonal antibody, palivizumab (Synagis), was approved for prophylactic treatment of RSV. A multicenter trial indicated that monthly IM injections of palivizumab were associated with 55% overall reduction in RSV-related hospitalizations. For most high-risk children, palivizumab is favored over RSV-IGIV because it can be given monthly in an IM injection, it has none of the risks of complications associated with IV administration of human immune globulin products, and it does not interfere with the measles-mumps-rubella and varicella vaccines (American Academy of Pediatrics, 1998b; Driver and Oertel, 1999).

Recommendations for the use of palivizumab or RSV-IVIG (American Academy of Pediatrics, 2000) are as follows:

1. Infants and children younger than 2 years of age with chronic lung disease (CLD) who have received medical therapy for CLD within 6 months before the anticipated RSV season. Patients with more severe CLD may benefit from prophylaxis for two RSV seasons.
2. Infants born at 32 weeks of gestation or earlier without CLD also may benefit from RSV prophylaxis.
3. Children with severe immunodeficiencies (e.g., severe combined immunodeficiency or acquired immunodeficiency syndrome) may benefit from prophylaxis.
4. Prophylaxis for RSV should be initiated at the onset of the RSV season and terminated at the end of the season.
5. In hospitalized infants the major means to prevent RSV disease is strict observance of infection control practice and segregation of RSV-infected infants.

### Nursing Considerations

Children admitted to the hospital with suspected RSV infection may be assigned separate rooms or grouped with other RSV-infected children. A variety of infection control procedures have been employed over the years, the most important of which is consistent handwashing, not touching the nasal mucosa or conjunctiva, and use of gloves and gowns when entering the patient's room. Other isolation procedures of potential benefit are those aimed at diminishing the number of hospital personnel, visitors, and uninfected patients in contact with the child. Another measure includes making patient assignments so that nurses assigned

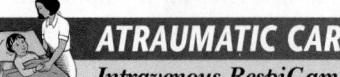

**ATRAUMATIC CARE**

*Intravenous RespiGam and Intramuscular Palivizumab*

To reduce the pain of the monthly IV infusion and intramuscular (IM) injections, apply EMLA cream to at least two possible venous sites (for IV insertion) 60 minutes or to the IM site 2½ hours before the procedure.

to children with RSV are not caring for other patients who are considered high risk.

If patient care warrants opening the tent while the SPAG is running and ribavirin is administered, the nurse should shut the machine off and wait a few moments before opening the tent. Gloves and gowns are not essential, because dermal absorption appears to be negligible. Scavenger devices are commercially available to help decrease the escape of aerosolized ribavirin.

**NURSING ALERT** Pregnant health care providers should not care for a child receiving ribavirin.

Nursing care of infants and children receiving RespiGam is the same as that involved in caring for any individual receiving an IV immunoglobulin product. RespiGam is made from human plasma and carries the possibility for transmission of blood-borne pathogens. Children with underlying pulmonary problems should be monitored for symptoms of fluid volume overload during administration. However, complications related to fluid volume are uncommon and are generally managed with modifications in the infusion rate (PREVENT Group, 1997). Frequent monitoring of vital signs, careful observations of any signs of discomfort at the needle insertion or IM injection site, or symptoms of an anaphylactic reaction are also important. (See Atraumatic Care box.) Antibodies present in the IV immune globulin preparation may interfere with the immune response to live virus vaccines, such as measles-mumps-rubella and chickenpox. Therefore these vaccines should be deferred for 9 months after RespiGam infusion (American Academy of Pediatrics, 2000). Palivizumab does not interfere with the response to vaccines.

## PNEUMONIA

Pneumonia, an inflammation of the pulmonary parenchyma, is common in childhood but occurs more frequently in infancy and early childhood. Clinically, pneumonia may occur either as a primary disease or as a complication of another illness.

Pneumonia can be classified according to morphology, etiologic agent, or clinical form. Although morphologic classification is typically used (Box 32-8), the most useful classification is based on the etiologic agent (i.e., viral, bacterial, mycoplasmal, or aspiration of foreign substances).

**Box 32-8** ■ ■ ■
**Types of Pneumonia**

**Lobar pneumonia**—All or a large segment of one or more pulmonary lobes is involved. When both lungs are affected, it is known as *bilateral* or *double pneumonia*.
**Bronchopneumonia**—Begins in the terminal bronchioles, which become clogged with mucopurulent exudate to form consolidated patches in nearby lobules; also called *lobular pneumonia*.
**Interstitial pneumonia**—The inflammatory process is more or less confined within the alveolar walls (interstitium) and the peribronchial and interlobular tissues.

The causative agent is usually introduced into the lungs through inhalation or from the bloodstream. Pneumonia may be caused by histomycosis, coccidioidomycosis, and other fungi. Other terms that describe pneumonias are hemorrhagic, fibrinous, and necrotizing. *Pneumonitis* is a localized acute inflammation of the lung without the toxemia associated with lobar pneumonia.

The clinical manifestations of pneumonia vary depending on the etiologic agent, the age of the child, the child's systemic reaction to the infection, the extent of the lesions, and the degree of bronchial and bronchiolar obstruction. The etiologic agent is identified largely from the clinical history, the child's age, the general health history, the physical examination, radiography, and the laboratory examination.

## Viral Pneumonia

Viral pneumonias occur more frequently than bacterial pneumonias and are seen in children of all age-groups. They are often associated with viral URIs, and the pathologic changes involve interstitial pneumonitis with inflammation of the mucosa and the walls of bronchi and bronchioles. Viruses that cause pneumonia in children include RSV in infants and parainfluenza, influenza, and adenovirus in older children. There are few clinical symptoms to distinguish between the responsible organisms, and differentiations between viruses can be made only by laboratory examination.

### Clinical Manifestations

The onset may be acute or insidious, and symptoms vary from mild fever, slight cough, and malaise to high fever, severe cough, and prostration. Early in the illness, the cough is likely to be unproductive or productive of small amounts of whitish sputum. Breath sounds may include a few wheezes or fine crackles. Radiography reveals diffuse or patchy infiltration with a peribronchial distribution.

### Therapeutic Management and Nursing Considerations

The prognosis is generally good, although viral infections of the respiratory tract render the affected child more susceptible to secondary bacterial invasion. Treatment is usually symptomatic and includes measures to promote oxygena-

tion and comfort, such as oxygen administration with cool mist, chest physiotherapy and postural drainage, antipyretics for fever management, fluid intake, and family support. Although some authorities recommend antimicrobial therapy in the hope of reducing or preventing secondary bacterial infection, it is usually reserved for children in whom the presence of such infection is demonstrated by appropriate cultures.

## Primary Atypical Pneumonia

*M. pneumoniae* is the most common cause of pneumonia in children between ages 5 and 12 years. It occurs principally in the fall and winter months and is more prevalent in crowded living conditions.

### Clinical Manifestations

The onset may be sudden or insidious and is usually accompanied by general systemic symptoms, including fever, chills (in older children), headache, malaise, anorexia, and muscle pain (myalgia). These symptoms are followed by rhinitis, sore throat, and a dry, hacking cough. The cough, initially nonproductive, produces seromucoid sputum that later becomes mucopurulent or blood streaked. The duration and degree of fever vary widely, and the fever may last from several days to 2 weeks. Dyspnea occurs infrequently.

Radiographic examination reveals evidence of pneumonia before physical signs are apparent. There may be fine crepitant crackles over various areas of the lung fields, but consolidation is usually not demonstrated. The pathologic process consists of interstitial round cell infiltration and edema of alveolar septa and varying distribution of areas of inflammation, necrosis, and ulceration of the mucosal lining of bronchi and bronchioles. Areas of consolidation and emphysema are present.

### Therapeutic Management and Nursing Considerations

Most affected persons recover from acute illness in 7 to 10 days with symptomatic treatment, followed by a week of convalescence. Hospitalization is rarely necessary.

## Bacterial Pneumonia

Bacterial pneumonia is often a serious infection. The pathogenetic mechanisms involved are often aspiration or hematogenous dissemination. The cause varies depending on the age and underlying illness of the child and the degree of immunosuppression or competency.

### Etiology and Epidemiology

Etiology of bacterial pneumonia varies with the age of the child. *S. pneumoniae* (pneumococcus), group A streptococcus, staphylococcus, or enteric bacilli are the most likely agents in infants under 3 months of age. Chlamydial infection is also a cause of pneumonia in this age-group. In the 3-month to 5-year age-group, *S. pneumoniae*, *M. catarrhalis*, and group A streptococci are common causes. *H. influenzae* type b (Hib) is causing fewer infections because of the Hib vaccine. *S. aureus* pneumonia is also now rarely seen in infants and toddlers. *M. pneumoniae* and *S. pneumoniae* are the dominant organisms in children over 5 years of age (Modlin, 1999).

## Clinical Manifestations

Clinical manifestations of bacterial pneumonia in normal children (Box 32-9) include an acute onset, fever, and toxic appearance; infants and young children develop more severe symptoms than older children. The older child may complain of headache, chills, abdominal pain, chest pain, or meningeal symptoms *(meningism)*. Respiratory distress may or may not be present. In some cases the only finding may be an increased respiratory rate.

Initially, the cough is usually hacking and nonproductive, and breath sounds are diminished or heard as scattered crackles. When consolidation is present, breath sounds may be tubular in quality with no adventitious noises. As the infection resolves, coarse crackles and wheezing are heard and the cough becomes productive with purulent sputum.

Lack of specific signs indicating infection makes diagnosis in infancy particularly difficult. An early sign of infection is often irritability or lethargy and poor feeding. Abrupt fever may be accompanied by seizures. Respiratory distress is evident with air hunger, tachypnea, and circumoral cyanosis. Because pneumonia in newborns carries a high morbidity and mortality, bacterial infection should be suspected in all neonates with respiratory symptoms.

Staphylococcal pneumonia is rare but particularly progressive and must be treated aggressively. The onset is rapid, with rapid deterioration. Conjunctivitis and furuncles are signs of a probable staphylococcal infection.

## Diagnostic Evaluation

The key to a preliminary diagnosis is finding pulmonary infiltrates on radiographic examination, usually revealing lobar consolidation and, in some severe cases, pleural effusion. Laboratory studies include Gram stain and culture of sputum, nasopharyngeal specimens, blood cultures, and lung aspiration and biopsy. The white blood cell count may be elevated, but it may be normal for infants with staphylococcal disease. Children with streptococcal disease usually have an elevated antistreptolysin O (ASO) titer. The infant or child with recurrent pneumonia should be further evaluated for cystic fibrosis or an immune deficiency disease.

## Therapeutic Management

Antimicrobial therapy has significantly reduced the morbidity and mortality from bacterial pneumonia.

Oral amoxicillin is used widely for outpatient management of infants and children younger than 5 years of age. Amoxicillin clavulanate (Augmentin) or a second-generation cephalosporin (cefuroxime, cefadroxil) should be given to patients incompletely immunized against *H. influenzae.* Erythromycin is the drug of choice for older children and adolescents because of its activity against *M. pneumonia.* In the hospital, medications are given parenterally for rapid action and maximum effect. A variety of drugs, including ampicillin-sulbactam (Unasyn) and cefuroxime, are given parenterally. IV or oral erythromycin should be added for children older than 5 years of age until *M. pneumoniae* is ruled out. Penicillin G is no longer considered reliable therapy because of β-lactamase production by many anaerobes (Modlin, 1999).

Most older children with pneumonia can be treated at home, especially if the condition is recognized and treatment initiated early. Antibiotic therapy, bed rest, liberal oral intake of fluid, and administration of antipyretics for fever are the principal therapeutic measures. Hospitalization is indicated when pleural effusion or empyema accompanies the disease and is mandatory for children with staphylococcal pneumonia. Pneumonia in the infant or young child may also require hospitalization because the course of illness is variable and complications are more common in very young patients. In addition, IV fluid administration is frequently necessary, and oxygen may be required if the child is in respiratory distress.

**Prognosis.** The prognosis for pneumonia is generally good, with rapid recovery when it is recognized and treated early. The course of staphylococcal pneumonia is generally prolonged. The prognosis varies with the length of the illness before treatment, although early recognition and treatment are usually beneficial.

The use of pneumococcal polysaccharide vaccine is recommended in selected individuals, such as children over age 2 years who are at risk of acquiring pneumococcal infection or are at risk of serious disease. (See Immunizations, Chapter 12.)

**Complications.** At present the classic features and clinical course of pneumonia are rarely seen because of early and vigorous antibiotic and supportive therapy. However, some children, especially infants, with staphylococcal pneumonia develop empyema, pyopneumothorax, or tension pneumothorax. Acute otitis media and pleural effusion are common in children with pneumococcal pneumonia. A diagnostic needle aspiration or thoracentesis is performed if fluid is suspected in the pleural cavity. Nonpurulent effusions do not require surgical drainage.

Continuous closed chest drainage is instituted when purulent fluid is aspirated. If a large amount of purulent drainage is obtained, an appropriate antibiotic is instilled into the cavity and the suction is discontinued for approxi-

---

**Box 32-9** ■ ■ ■
### General Signs of Pneumonia

Fever: usually quite high
Respiratory
    Cough: unproductive to productive with whitish sputum
    Tachypnea
    Breath sounds: rhonchi or fine crackles
    Dullness with percussion
    Chest pain
    Retractions
    Nasal flaring
    Pallor to cyanosis (depends on severity)
Chest x-ray film: diffuse or patchy infiltration, with peribronchial distribution
Behavior: irritable, restless, lethargic
Gastrointestinal: anorexia, vomiting, diarrhea, abdominal pain

mately 1 hour after the installation. Closed drainage is continued until drainage fluid is free of pathogens, which rarely requires more than 5 to 7 days. Sometimes, repeated pleural taps are sufficient to remove fluid; however, if the purulent drainage accumulates rapidly and is highly viscous, continuous drainage is preferred. In addition, continuous drainage is less traumatic to the child than repeated thoracentesis.

**Thoracentesis.** Dyspnea resulting from pressure from fluid accumulation in the pleural cavity requires removal by thoracentesis. Thoracentesis is also performed to obtain fluid for culture or to instill antibiotics directly into the pleural cavity. Nursing responsibilities include obtaining and setting up equipment, preparing the child physically and psychologically, and assisting with the procedure. If continuous closed chest drainage is anticipated, this equipment should also be available. Thoracentesis is performed with the child in a sitting position, preferably with the arms and trunk bent forward over pillows or over an overbed table with a pillow. Infants are positioned in a semirecumbent position on the unaffected side. (See Atraumatic Care box.) The nurse provides explanation, offers emotional support during the procedure, and observes the child for any changes in color, respiration, or pulse and for any alterations in behavior (e.g., coughing) or sensorium.

After the procedure the child is made comfortable, and observations and recording of physical and emotional responses, the amount and description of the fluid obtained, and any medication instilled are recorded. Specimens are sent to the laboratory for culture. Continuous closed chest drainage is managed according to the same protocol as for the child with a thoracotomy. (See Chapter 34.)

### Nursing Considerations

Nursing care of the child with pneumonia is primarily supportive and symptomatic but necessitates thorough respiratory assessment and administration of oxygen and antibiotics. The child's respiratory rate and status, as well as general disposition and level of activity, are frequently assessed. Isolation procedures are instituted according to hospital policy; rest and conservation of energy are encouraged by the relief of physical and psychologic stress. The child is disturbed as little as possible by clustering care to encourage the child's regular sleep cycle. If the cough is disturbing, the use of antitussives, especially before rest times and meals, is often helpful. To prevent dehydration, fluids are frequently administered intravenously during the acute phase. Oral fluids, if allowed, are given cautiously to avoid aspiration and to decrease the possibility of aggravating a fatiguing cough.

Children may be placed in a mist tent. Cool humidification moistens the airways and provides an atmosphere that assists in temperature reduction. Children often require frequent clothing and linen changes to prevent chilling in the damp atmosphere. They are usually more comfortable in a semierect position but should be allowed to determine the position of comfort. Lying on the affected side (if pneumonia is unilateral) splints the chest on that side and reduces the pleural rubbing that often causes discomfort. If needed, oxygen is delivered into the hood or mist tent or administered via a nasal cannula. Fever is controlled by the cool environment and administration of antipyretic drugs as prescribed. Temperature is monitored regularly to detect a rise that might trigger a febrile seizure.

Vital signs and chest sounds are monitored to assess the progress of the disease and to detect early signs of complications. Children with ineffectual cough or those with difficulty handling secretions, especially infants, require suctioning to maintain a patent airway. A simple bulb suction syringe is usually sufficient for clearing the nares and nasopharynx of infants, but mechanical suction should be readily available if needed. Older children can usually handle secretions without assistance. Postural drainage and chest physiotherapy are generally prescribed every 4 hours or more often, depending on the child's condition.

The hospitalized child is apprehensive, and the treatments and tests are frightening and stress producing. It is important to involve the entire family in the care as appropriate and to encourage questions and facilitate effective communication. Reducing anxiety and apprehension reduces psychologic distress in the child, and when the child is more relaxed, the respiratory efforts are lessened. Easing respiratory efforts makes the child less apprehensive, and encouraging the presence of the caregiver provides the child with a source of comfort and support.

## Chlamydial Pneumonia

*C. trachomatis*, an intracellular microorganism similar to gram-negative bacteria, is responsible for one of the most common sexually transmitted diseases. Newborn infants acquire pulmonary infection from their mothers via ascending infection just before or in the process of birth.

Chlamydial pneumonia is a severe, diffuse disease. It occurs in children between 1 and 3 months of age. It is characterized by a persistent cough, tachypnea, and minimal or absent fever. Radiographs show nonspecific abnormalities. Erythromycin given for 2 to 3 weeks is the treatment of choice (Hammerschlag, 1999). Nursing care is the same as for any infant with pneumonia.

# OTHER INFECTIONS OF THE RESPIRATORY TRACT

## Pertussis (Whooping Cough)

Pertussis, or whooping cough, is an acute respiratory infection caused by *Bordetella pertussis* that occurs primarily in children younger than 4 years of age who have not been

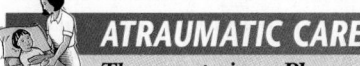

### ATRAUMATIC CARE
*Thoracentesis or Placement of Chest Tube*

To reduce the pain of the needle or incision, local anesthesia should be administered with buffered lidocaine and EMLA cream. Appropriate conscious sedation should *also* be provided.

immunized. It is highly contagious and is particularly threatening in young infants, who have a higher morbidity and mortality rate. (See Table 16-1 for signs, symptoms, and management of pertussis.) The incidence is highest in the spring and summer months, and a single attack confers lifetime immunity. Pertussis vaccine is effective, but the immunity diminishes with time after the initial infection or immunization.

## Tuberculosis (TB)

TB remains the most important chronic infectious disease in the world in terms of morbidity, mortality, and cost (Starke, 1999). Cases of TB for all ages are highest in urban, low-income areas and among nonwhite racial and ethnic groups; the highest rates of infection and disease are among first-generation immigrants from endemic countries, Native Americans, the homeless, and residents of correctional facilities (American Academy of Pediatrics, 2000). The incidence of TB is increasing in the United States. From 1985 through 1997 more than 80,000 additional cases of TB were reported in the United States than would have been expected if the previous decline had continued (Starke,

---

**Box 32-10** ◼ ◼ ◻
**Factors Affecting Resistance to Tuberculosis**

**HEREDITY**
No positive evidence to indicate hereditary tendency
Evidence that resistance to infection may be genetically
  transmitted

**SEX**
Early years: no sex differences in incidence
Later childhood and adolescence: morbidity and mortality
  higher in girls than in boys

**AGE**
Diminished resistance to infection in infancy
  Delay in development of acquired immunity
  Diminished capacity to resist extension of infective process
Increased tendency to develop disease during puberty and
  adolescence
  New infection superimposed on a previous one
  Increased contacts
  Indigenous reinfection stimulated by metabolic changes or
    suboptimum diets during a period of rapid growth

**STRESS STATES**
Temporary stressful circumstances (e.g., injury or illness,
  undernutrition, emotional distress, chronic fatigue) may
  increase susceptibility to infection
Increased secretion of adrenal steroids suppresses protective
  inflammatory response and permits infection to spread
Therapeutic administration of corticosteroids (similar effect)

**NUTRITION**
Active disease inversely proportional to state of nutrition
Excellent nutrition is essential to young children's recovery
  from disease

**INTERCURRENT INFECTION**
Infectious diseases (especially human immunodeficiency virus
  [HIV], measles, pertussis) may activate latent tuberculosis
Noncompliance with therapy

---

1999). The increases are attributed in part to the many foreign-born persons immigrating to the United States, the increase in homelessness, and the human immunodeficiency virus (HIV) epidemic (Hoffman, Kelly, and Futterman, 1996).

### Etiology

TB is caused by *Mycobacterium tuberculosis,* an acid-fast bacillus not readily decolorized by acids after staining. Children are susceptible to the human *(M. tuberculosis)* and the bovine *(Mycobacterium bovis)* organisms. In parts of the world where TB in cattle is not controlled or pasteurization of milk is not practiced, the bovine type is a common source of infection.

Although the causative agent is the tubercle bacillus, other factors influence the degree to which the organism is able to produce an altered state in the host. Multidrug-resistant strains of *M. tuberculosis* have caused outbreaks in hospitals. Resistance to the TB bacillus can be modified by many factors (Box 32-10).

### Pathophysiology

The source of infection in children is usually an infected member of the household or any frequent visitor to the household, such as a baby-sitter or domestic worker. Transmission of *M. tuberculosis* occurs when the child inhales microdroplets (usually 1 to 5 mm in size) into the respiratory tract after someone has coughed or sneezed. Although the lung is the most frequent portal of entry in humans, the organism *M. bovis* can be ingested via infected milk. When the *M. tuberculosis* droplet is inhaled, it passes down the bronchial tree, implants in either a bronchiole or alveolus, and starts to multiply.

Epithelial cells surround and encapsulate the multiplying bacilli in an attempt to wall off the invading organisms, thus forming the typical **tubercle.** During the inflammatory process, some bacilli leave the focal area and are carried to the regional lymph nodes that drain the anatomic area of the organism; as a result, the child develops a fever. Radiographic examinations may be positive if such tests are performed when the child is known to have been exposed. The tuberculin test is positive.

Extension of the primary lesion at the original site causes progressive tissue destruction as it spreads within the lung, discharges material from foci to other areas of the lungs (e.g., bronchi or pleura), or produces pneumonia. Erosion of blood vessels by the primary lesion can cause widespread dissemination of the tubercle bacillus to near and distant sites *(miliary TB).* Organisms deposited in the upper lung zones, bones, kidneys, and brain may find favorable environments for growth, but organs and tissue such as bone marrow, liver, and spleen appear to inhibit multiplication of the bacilli.

For children not immunosuppressed or compromised, a strong cell-mediated immune response provides specific immunity that usually limits further multiplication of the bacilli. These children remain asymptomatic, and the lesions will usually heal. *TB infection* is manifested by a positive skin test only. In a small percentage of persons with newly acquired TB, replication of the organism continues and *TB disease* occurs, as evidenced by a positive chest radiograph, positive sputum culture, and signs of disease.

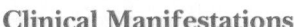

## Clinical Manifestations

Clinical manifestations of TB in children are extremely variable. The disease may be asymptomatic or produce a broad range of symptoms, including general responses such as fever, malaise, anorexia, and weight loss or more specific symptoms related to the site of infection (e.g., lungs, bone, brain, kidneys). Lung disease may or may not include cough (which progresses slowly over weeks to months), aching pain and tightness in the chest, and (rarely) hemoptysis.

As increasing amounts of lung tissue become involved, the respiratory rate increases, the lung on the affected side does not expand as well as the other, auscultation reveals diminished breath sounds and crackles, and there is dullness to percussion. In children (usually infants) who are unable to contain the spread of infection, the fever persists; the generalized symptoms are manifest; and children develop pallor, anemia, weakness, and weight loss.

## Diagnostic Evaluation

Diagnosis is based on information derived from physical examination, history, reaction to a tuberculin test, organism cultures, and radiographic examinations. In addition, it must be determined if the lesion is in the active, quiescent, or healed stage.

**History.**   Symptoms generally do not contribute significantly to a diagnosis. A history of possible contact with a person known to be infected or subsequently found to be in-

fected is helpful. All contacts of an affected child are examined for the disease.

**Tuberculin Test.**   The *tuberculin test* is the single most important test to determine whether a child has been infected with the tubercle bacillus. A primary infection initiates a hypersensitivity reaction to the protein fraction of the tubercle bacillus, which can be detected 2 to 10 weeks after the infection. The standard dose of *purified protein derivative (PPD)* is 5 tuberculin units (TU) in 0.1 ml of solution, injected intradermally *(Mantoux test)* (American Academy of Pediatrics, 2000). In the past, multiple puncture tests (MPTs) such as the tine test were used, but these tests have significant problems and are no longer recommended (Starke, 1999). Recommendations for TB skin testing of children are listed in Box 32-11.

A *positive reaction* indicates that the person has been infected and has developed a sensitivity to the protein of the tubercle bacillus; it does not confirm the presence of active disease. Once individuals react positively, they will always react positively. A positive reaction in a previously negative reactor indicates that the person has been infected since the last test. Guidelines for interpreting the Mantoux skin test are listed in Box 32-12.

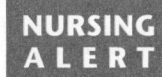 The American Academy of Pediatrics (2000) recommends that Mantoux skin test results be read by health care professionals.

---

### Box 32-11
### Revised Tuberculin Skin Test Recommendations*

**CHILDREN FOR WHOM IMMEDIATE SKIN TESTING IS INDICATED**

Contacts of persons with confirmed or suspected infectious tuberculosis (TB) (contact investigation). This includes children identified as contacts of family members or associates in jail or prison in the last 5 years.
Children with radiographic or clinical findings suggesting TB.
Children emigrating from endemic regions (e.g., Asia, Middle East, Africa, Latin America).
Children with travel histories to endemic countries or significant contact with indigenous persons from such countries.

**CHILDREN WHO SHOULD BE TESTED ANNUALLY FOR TB†**

Children infected with human immunodeficiency virus (HIV) or living in household with HIV-infected persons.
Incarcerated adolescents.

**CHILDREN WHO SHOULD BE TESTED EVERY 2 TO 3 YEARS†**

Children exposed to the following individuals: HIV-infected, homeless, residents of nursing homes, institutionalized adolescents or adults, users of illicit drugs, incarcerated adolescents or adults, ar.d migrant farm workers; foster children with exposure to adults in the preceding high-risk groups are included.

**CHILDREN WHO SHOULD BE CONSIDERED FOR TB SKIN TESTING AT AGES 4 TO 6 AND 11 TO 16 YEARS**

Children whose parents emigrated (with unknown tuberculin skin test status) from regions of the world with a high prevalence of

TB. Continued potential exposure by travel to the endemic areas or household contact with persons from the endemic areas (with unknown tuberculin skin test status) should be an indication for repeat tuberculin skin testing.
Children without specific risk factors who reside in high-prevalence areas. In general a high-risk neighborhood or community does not mean an entire city is at high risk; rates in any area of the city may vary by neighborhood, or even from block to block. Physicians should be aware of these patterns in determining the likelihood of exposure. Public health officials or local TB experts should help clinicians identify areas with appreciable TB rates.

**RISK FOR PROGRESSION TO DISEASE**

Children with other medical risk factors, including diabetes mellitus, chronic renal failure, malnutrition, and congenital or acquired immunodeficiencies deserve special consideration; without recent exposure, these persons are not at increased risk of acquiring TB infection. Underlying immune deficiencies associated with these conditions theoretically would enhance the possibility for progression to severe disease. Initial histories of potential exposure to TB should be included for all of these patients. If these histories or local epidemiologic factors suggest a possibility of exposure, immediate and periodic TB skin testing should be considered. An initial TB skin test should be performed before initiation of immunosuppressive therapy in any child with an underlying condition that necessitates immunosuppressive therapy.

Modified from American Academy of Pediatrics, Committee on Infectious Diseases, Pickering L, editor: *2000 Red book: report of the Committee on Infectious Diseases*, ed 25, Elk Grove Village, IL, 2000, The Academy.
*Bacille Calmette-Guérin (BCG) immunization is not a contraindication to tuberculin skin testing.
†Initial tuberculin skin testing at the time of diagnosis or circumstance, beginning at 3 months of age.

## Box 32-12 ▣ ▣ ▢
### Definition of Positive Mantoux Skin Test (5 TU-PPD) in Children*

Tuberculin skin test should be read at 48 to 72 hours after placement

**INDURATION ≥5 mm**

Children in close contact with persons who have known or suspected contagious cases of tuberculosis:
  Households with active or previously active cases if (1) treatment cannot be verified as adequate before exposure, (2) treatment was initiated after the child's contact, or (3) reactivation is suspected
Children suspected to have tuberculous disease:
  Chest roentgenogram consistent with active or previously active tuberculosis
  Clinical evidence of tuberculosis
Children receiving immunosuppressive therapy or with immunosuppressive conditions, including HIV infection

**INDURATION ≥10 mm**

Children at increased risk of disseminated disease:
  Young age: less than 4 years of age
  Other medical risk factors, including Hodgkin disease, lymphoma, diabetes mellitus, chronic renal failure, or malnutrition
Children with increased exposure to tuberculosis disease:
  Born, or whose parents were born, in regions of the world where tuberculosis is highly prevalent
  Frequently exposed to adults who are HIV infected, homeless, users of illicit drugs, residents of nursing homes, incarcerated or institutionalized persons or migrant farm workers
  Travel and exposure to high-prevalence regions of the world

**INDURATION ≥15 mm**

Children 4 years of age or older without any risk factors

From American Academy of Pediatrics, Committee on Infectious Diseases: *2000 Red book: report of the Committee on Infectious Diseases,* ed 25, Elk Grove Village, IL, 2000, The Academy.
*These recommendations apply regardless of previous BCG immunization.

## Box 32-13 ▣ ▣ ▢
### Circumstances Producing False-Negative Reactions to Tuberculin Tests

**Tuberculin reaction suppressed** by:
  Intercurrent diseases (e.g., viral diseases such as measles, rubella, influenza, mumps, varicella, and probably others [about 4 weeks])
  Viral vaccines (e.g., measles, mumps, and rubella vaccines [about 4 weeks])
  Corticosteroids and other immunosuppressive agents
**Cellular immunodeficiency disease**
**Severe malnutrition**
**Too early testing** before the body develops a sensitivity to the protein fraction of the tubercle bacillus
**Use of outdated testing material**—Mixture that has been prepared for too long or has been exposed to sunlight
**Faulty technique** (e.g., deep injection, no wheal formed, improper measurement of solution, or leaking of solution from a defective or loosely fitting syringe)
**Overwhelming tuberculosis infections**—End-stage and terminal miliary disease

---

A *negative reaction* usually means that the child has never been infected with the organism. Several factors can produce false-negative results (Box 32-13). Tuberculin testing should not be carried out at the same time as measles immunization. Viral interference from the measles vaccine may cause a false-negative reaction.

**Bacteriologic Examination.** A definitive diagnosis is made by demonstrating the presence of mycobacteria in culture. The organism is identified from microscopic examination of properly prepared and stained smears from early-morning gastric washings or from sputum, pleural fluid, urine, spinal fluid, draining lymph nodes, and other body fluids.

**Radiographic Studies.** Radiographic examinations may be done, but the lesions of numerous chronic intrathoracic diseases resemble tuberculous lesions. Therefore x-ray examinations are used to supplement other diagnostic methods.

### Therapeutic Management

Medical management of tuberculous lesions in children consists of adequate nutrition, chemotherapy, general supportive measures, prevention of unnecessary exposure to other infections that further compromise the body's defenses, prevention of reinfection, and sometimes surgical procedures.

First-line drugs for treating tuberculosis include isoniazid (INH), rifampin, pyrazinamide (PZA), ethambutol, and streptomycin. Second-line drugs such as paraaminosalicylic acid, ethionamide, capreomycin, kanamycin, fluoroquinolones, and cycloserine, are used when drug resistance or intolerance is encountered (Starke, 1999). A multidrug regimen (i.e., giving two or more drugs simultaneously) is helpful in preventing the development of bacterial resistance to a single drug (Stevenson, 1997b).

Preventive therapy is intended to keep latent infection from progressing to clinically active TB and to prevent initial infection in persons in high-risk situations. The most commonly used drug for this is isoniazid (INH) for 9 months and up to 12 months for the HIV-infected child. This is given daily in a single dose, usually 10 mg/kg orally, with a maximum dose of 300 mg. The drug has no effect on the child's reaction to tuberculin; therefore, the test continues to be useful in detecting acquired infection.

For the child with clinically active tuberculosis, the goal is to achieve sterilization of the tuberculous lesion. A 6-month regimen consisting of INH, rifampin, and PZA given daily for the first 2 months is recommended. After this 2-month period, a regimen of INH and rifampin given twice weekly is acceptable if administration of the drugs is observed directly for the remaining 4 months. Additional medications such as streptomycin (IM injection only) or ethambutol are added if the child is suspected to have multidrug-resistant TB (American Academy of Pediatrics, 2000; Starke, 1999).

**NURSING ALERT** Direct observation means that a health care worker or other responsible, mutually agreed-on individual is present when medications are administered to the patient. If the reliability of self-administration of medications is in doubt, directly observed, twice-weekly therapy administered by a health care professional must be provided.

*Surgical procedures* may be required to remove the source of infection in tissues that are inaccessible to chemotherapy or that are destroyed by the disease. Orthopaedic procedures for correction of bone deformities, bronchoscopy for removal of a tuberculous granulomatous polyp, or resection of a portion of a diseased lung may also be performed.

**Prognosis.**   Most children recover from primary TB infection and may be unaware of its presence. However, very young children have a higher incidence of disseminated disease. It is a serious disease during the first 2 years of life, during adolescence, and in children infected with HIV. Except in cases of tuberculous meningitis, death seldom occurs in treated children. Antibiotic therapy has decreased mortality and hematogenous spread from primary lesions.

**Prevention.**   The only certain means to prevent TB is to avoid contact with the tubercle bacillus. Maintaining an optimum state of health with adequate nutrition and avoiding fatigue and debilitating infections promote natural resistance but do not prevent infection.

Pasteurization of milk and routine testing and elimination of diseased cattle have helped reduce the incidence of bovine tuberculosis. Infants and children should be given only pasteurized milk from TB-free cattle.

A source of concern is that the infected child and/or family members may spread the disease when visiting in the hospital. Most children with TB need not be isolated and can be hospitalized on an open ward if they are receiving chemotherapy. Children and adolescents with infectious pulmonary TB (i.e., those whose sputum smears show acid-fast bacillus), should be on isolation precautions until effective chemotherapy has been initiated, their sputum smears show a diminishing number of organisms, and their cough is improving. Masks are indicated only when the child is coughing and does not reliably cover his or her mouth. Gowns are indicated only if needed to prevent gross contamination of clothing. Family members should be managed with airborne precautions when visiting until they are demonstrated not to have infectious TB.

Limited immunity can be produced by administration of **BCG (bacille Calmette-Guérin)** vaccine containing bovine bacilli with reduced virulence. The freshly prepared vaccine, injected intradermally, produces definite although incomplete protection (ranging from 0% to 80%) against TB (Starke, 1999). In most instances, positive tuberculin reactions develop after inoculation. The distribution of BCG vaccine is controlled by local or state health departments, and the vaccine is not used extensively, even in areas with a high prevalence of disease. BCG vaccination is not generally recommended for use in the United States. However, it may be recommended for long-term protection of infants and children with negative tuberculin skin tests who (1) are at high risk for continuing exposure to persons with infectious TB, (2) are continuously exposed to persons with tuberculosis who have bacilli resistant to both isoniazid and rifampin, or (3) are at high risk for noncompliance (Starke, 1999).

### Nursing Considerations

Hospitalization is seldom necessary. Only those children with the more serious forms of the disease are placed in the hospital. The major nursing care of children with TB involves nurses in ambulatory settings: outpatient departments, schools, and public health agencies.

Asymptomatic children can lead an essentially unrestricted life. They can and should attend school (or daycare), but older children are restricted from vigorous activities such as competitive games and contact sports during the active stage of primary TB. They should be protected from stresses, including parental anxieties, overprotection, and pressures regarding nutritional intake. The regular immunization schedule should be continued. Care should be exerted to maintain optimum health with proper diet, adequate rest, and avoidance of infection.

Nurses assume several roles in management of the disease, including helping the family to understand the rationale for diagnostic procedures, assisting with radiographic examinations, performing skin tests, and obtaining specimens for laboratory examination. Skin tests must be carried out correctly to obtain accurate results. The tuberculin is injected intradermally with the bevel of the needle pointing upward. A wheal 6 to 10 mm in diameter should form between the layers of the skin when the solution is injected properly. If the wheal is not formed, the procedure is repeated. The volar or dorsal surface of the forearm is the usual injection site (Macquire, 1997). The reaction to the skin test is determined in 48 to 72 hours. The size of the transverse diameter of induration, not the erythema, is measured. The diameter transverse to the long axis of the forearm is the only one standardized for measurement purposes (Starke, 1999).

Sputum specimens are difficult or impossible to obtain from an infant or young child because they swallow any mucus coughed from the lower respiratory tract. The best means for obtaining material for smears or culture is by *gastric washing* (i.e., aspiration of lavaged contents from the fasting stomach). The procedure is carried out and the specimen obtained early in the morning before the customary breakfast time.

**Ambulatory Care.**   Nursing supervision of the child at home involves teaching the parents and child about the disease and its ramifications. Because children usually acquire the disease from an adult in the home, parents often feel guilty. Historically the disease has been regarded with fear, and numerous misconceptions need to be clarified. Reducing parental anxieties helps them to deal with the illness more constructively and to collaborate more effectively in planning the child's continued care. Because the success of therapy depends on compliance with drug therapy, parents are instructed regarding the importance of giving the medication as often and as long as it is ordered. (See Compliance, Chapter 27.) Promoting optimum general health and preventing intercurrent infections and reinfections with the tubercle bacillus are very important. Excellent patient education materials can be obtained from the **American Lung Association.***

**Case Finding.**   Case finding and follow-up of known contacts are important nursing responsibilities. Every case of tuberculosis identified in the community involves nurses

---

*1740 Broadway, New York, NY 10019-4374, (212) 315-8700; www. lungusa.org.

in follow-up of known contacts—individuals from whom the affected person may have acquired the disease and persons who may have been exposed to the diseased individual. Early diagnosis affords a means for early protection or treatment and prevents further spread of the disease.

# PULMONARY DISTURBANCE CAUSED BY NONINFECTIOUS IRRITANTS
## Foreign Body (FB) Aspiration

Small children characteristically explore objects with their mouth and are prone to aspirate foreign bodies into the air passages. Aspiration of an FB can occur at any age but is most common in older infants and children ages 1 to 3 years. Severity is determined by the location, type of object aspirated, and extent of obstruction. For example, dry vegetable matter, such as a seed, nut, or piece of carrot or popcorn, that does not dissolve and that may swell when wet creates a particularly difficult problem. The high fat content of potato chips and peanuts may cause the added risk of lipoid pneumonia. "Fun foods" of any kind are among the worst offenders. Offending foods in the order of frequency of aspiration are hot dog, round candy, peanut or other nut, grape, cookie or biscuit, other meat, carrot, apple, and peanut butter. Round foods are the most frequent offenders. The first four items together make up more than 40% of all aspirated food items.

A sharp or irritating object produces irritation and edema. A round, pliable object that does not readily break apart is more likely to occlude an airway than an object with a different shape. Latex balloons (uninflated, inflated, or in broken pieces) are especially hazardous. It takes only a small piece of the pliable, impermeable latex to totally occlude the airway. A small object may cause little if any pathologic change, whereas an object of sufficient size to obstruct a passage can produce various changes, including atelectasis, emphysema, inflammation, and abscess.

### Pathophysiology

Most inhaled FBs lodge in a mainstem or lobar bronchus, a few find their way into more distal portions of the lung field, and the remaining FBs lodge in the trachea. The site is determined by the size, weight, and configuration of the object. For example, heavy objects such as bullets, coins, and nails are more likely to drop into the dependent portions of the tracheobronchial tree. The object may remain in the same location or move in the airway. It can be coughed from a smaller to a larger airway and reaspirated in a different passage—or it might be ejected forcefully into the mouth and subsequently swallowed.

Signs of obstruction caused by an FB in a bronchus are explained by the same mechanisms that control the flow of fluids in pipes (Fig. 32-5). During normal respiration the caliber of bronchi and bronchioles becomes larger during inspiration and smaller during expiration. When a small object partially obstructs a passage, air passes around the obstruction during both inspiration and expiration (bypass valve). In this type of obstruction a wheeze is heard. A somewhat larger obstruction will allow air to enter the distal portion when bronchioles enlarge during inspiration, but when they diminish in caliber during expiration, the lumen becomes occluded and air becomes trapped distal to the obstruction (check valve). This type of obstruction produces obstructive emphysema. When there is complete blockage of the bronchus by an FB or by the FB and swollen mucosa, air is unable to move in either direction (stop valve), and the air distal to the obstruction is absorbed, leaving an area of obstruction atelectasis. The right bronchus, with its shorter length and straighter angle, is the usual site of bronchial obstruction.

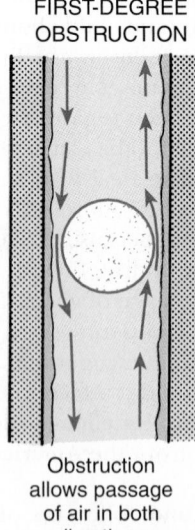

**FIRST-DEGREE OBSTRUCTION**

Obstruction allows passage of air in both directions

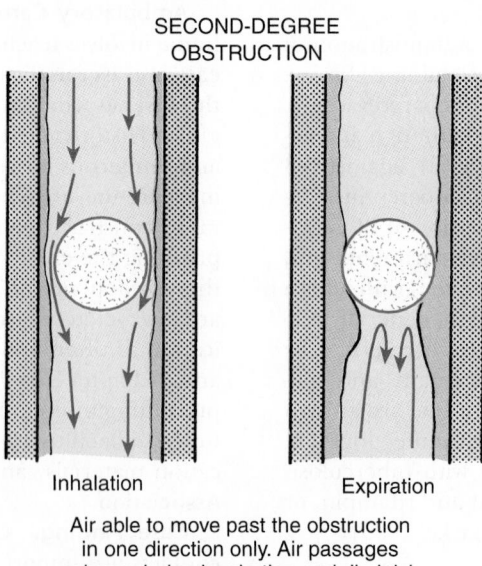

**SECOND-DEGREE OBSTRUCTION**

Inhalation

Air able to move past the obstruction in one direction only. Air passages enlarge during inspiration and diminish during expiration.

Expiration

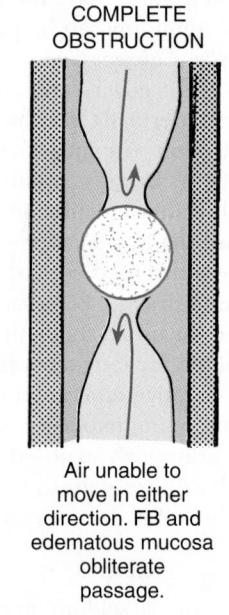

**COMPLETE OBSTRUCTION**

Air unable to move in either direction. FB and edematous mucosa obliterate passage.

**Fig. 32-5** Mechanisms of airway obstruction by foreign body (FB).

## Clinical Manifestations

Initially, an FB in the air passages produces choking, gagging, or coughing, but symptoms depend on the site of obstruction and on the interval between aspiration and presentation. Laryngotracheal obstruction most commonly causes dyspnea, cough, stridor, and hoarseness because of a decreased air entry. Cyanosis may also occur if the obstruction becomes worse. Bronchial obstruction usually produces cough (frequently paroxysmal), wheezing, asymmetric breath sounds, decreased airway entry, and dyspnea.

If the obstruction progresses, the child's face may become livid, and sometimes the child becomes unconscious and dies of asphyxiation if the object is not removed. If obstruction is partial, hours, days, or even weeks may pass without symptoms after the initial period. Secondary symptoms are related to the anatomic area in which the FB is lodged and are usually caused by a persistent respiratory infection located distally to the obstruction. A history of recurrent intractable pneumonia is reason to consider an FB in an airway. Often, by the time secondary symptoms appear, the parents have forgotten the initial episode of coughing and gagging. The most common symptoms observed in children brought to medical attention are stridor, wheezing, sternal retraction, and cough. When an object is lodged in the larynx, there is inability to speak or breathe.

## Diagnostic Evaluation

The diagnosis of FB is usually suspected on the basis of the history and physical signs. Radiographic examination reveals opaque FBs but is of limited value in localizing vegetable matter. Bronchoscopy is required for a definitive diagnosis of objects in the larynx and trachea. Fluoroscopic examination is valuable in detecting FBs in the bronchi.

On fluoroscopy a check-valve–obstructed lung will remain expanded, the diaphragm will remain low and fixed on the obstructed side, and the heart and mediastinum will shift to the unobstructed side during expiration. In a stop-valve obstruction the heart and mediastinum are drawn to the obstructed side and remain there during both inspiration and expiration. The diaphragm on the obstructed side remains high, whereas that on the unobstructed side moves normally.

The mainstay of diagnosis and management of foreign bodies is endoscopy. If there is doubt about the presence of an FB, endoscopy can be diagnostic as well as therapeutic (Lorin, 1999). When endoscopy is used to remove an FB, the procedure should be performed by an endoscopist who is experienced and comfortable caring for children. The endoscopist should also have access to state-of-the art endoscopy equipment, and the procedure should be performed in a setting that can accommodate any complication or emergency.

## Therapeutic Management

FB aspiration may result in life-threatening airway obstruction, especially in infants because of the small diameters of their airways. Current recommendations for the emergency treatment of the choking child include the use of abdominal thrusts for children over 1 year of age and back blows and chest thrusts for children less than 1 year of age. (See Cardiopulmonary Resuscitation, Chapter 31.) An FB is rarely coughed up spontaneously; therefore it must be removed by endoscopy.

Removal of the FB must be done as quickly as possible, because the progressive local inflammatory process triggered by the foreign material hampers removal, a chemical pneumonia soon develops, and vegetable matter begins to macerate within a few days, causing it to be even more difficult to remove. After removal of the FB, the child is placed in a high-humidity atmosphere, and observed for signs of airway edema. Any secondary infection is treated with appropriate antibiotics.

## Nursing Considerations

A major role of nurses caring for a child who has aspirated an FB is to recognize the signs of FB aspiration and implement immediate measures to relieve the obstruction.

All persons working with children should be prepared to deal effectively with aspiration of an FB. Choking on food or other material should not be fatal. Two simple procedures—back blows and the Heimlich maneuver, which can be used by both health professionals and lay persons—can save lives. It is the obligation of nurses to learn these techniques and teach them to parents and other groups. (See Figs. 31-25 and 31-26.)

To aid a child who is choking, nurses need to recognize the signs of distress. Not every child who gags or coughs while eating is truly choking.

> **NURSING ALERT**
>
> The child in distress (1) *cannot speak,* (2) *becomes cyanotic,* and (3) *collapses.* These three signs indicate that the child is truly choking and requires immediate and quick action. The child can die within 4 minutes. Follow-up care after the foreign body is removed include monitoring for respiratory distress and education of the parents.

**Prevention.** Small children should not be allowed access to small objects that they might place in their mouth. Rubber balloons are high-risk items for children; Mylar balloons are the only safe variety. Aluminum tabs from soft drink containers, adhesive bandages applied to fingers of infants or very small children, plastic tabs from protective coverings on containers and price tags from clothing can become FBs. Peanut butter, a staple in the diet of children, should never be given to a child unless it is spread thinly on bread or a cracker. A spoonful of peanut butter can obstruct the airway and stick to mucous membranes, becoming difficult or impossible for the child to dislodge.

Nurses are in a position to teach prevention in a variety of settings. (See Community Focus box on p. 1378.) They can educate parents singly or in groups about hazards of aspiration in relation to the developmental level of their children and encourage them to teach their children safety. Parents should be cautioned about behaviors that their children might imitate (e.g., holding foreign objects, such as pins, nails, and toothpicks, in their lips or mouth). (Prevention based on the child's age is discussed in Chapters 12 and 14.)

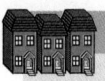

## Foreign Body (FB) in the Nose

Children sometimes place foreign objects, such as food, crayons, small toys, pieces of plastic, beans, beads, erasers, wads of paper, and small stones, into their nose. An FB is suspected when there is unilateral nasal discharge that is foul smelling, local obstruction with sneezing, mild discomfort, and (rarely) pain. The irritation produces local mucosal swelling if the items increase in size as they absorb moisture (hygroscopic). Signs of obstruction and discomfort may increase with time. Infection usually follows, as evidenced by foul breath and a purulent or bloody discharge from one nostril.

Although the object is usually situated anteriorly, unskilled attempts at removal may move it further posteriorly. Removal should be carried out as soon as possible to prevent the risk of aspiration and local tissue necrosis. Removal is easily accomplished with conscious sedation, general anesthesia, or topical anesthesia and either forceps or suction. Sometimes phenylephrine added to the topical anesthesia helps shrink swollen membranes. Inflammation and irritation usually disappear after removal.

## Aspiration Pneumonia

*Aspiration pneumonia* occurs when food, secretions, inert materials, volatile compounds, or liquids enter the lung and cause inflammation and a chemical pneumonitis. Many conditions increase the risk of aspiration (Box 32-14). Aspiration of fluid or food substances is particularly hazardous in the child who has difficulty with swallowing or is unable to swallow because of paralysis, weakness, debility, congenital anomalies such as cleft palate or tracheoesophageal fistula, or absent cough reflex (unconscious) or who is force-fed, especially while crying or breathing rapidly.

Clinical signs of the aspiration of oral secretions may not be distinguishable from other forms of acute bacterial pneumonia. For example, if vegetable matter has been aspirated, manifestations may not appear for several weeks after the event. Classic symptoms include an increasing cough or fever with foul-smelling sputum, deteriorating chest radiographs, and other signs of lower airway involvement.

---

**Box 32-14** ▪ ▪ ▪
**Conditions That Increase Risk of Aspiration**

**ALTERED LEVEL OF CONSCIOUSNESS**
Central nervous system injury or disease (e.g., meningitis, seizures, paralysis, trauma, poisoning, toxic ingestion)
Sedation
General anesthesia
Cardiopulmonary resuscitation

**DYSPHAGIA**
Esophageal dysmotility
Neurologic deficit
Gastroesophageal reflux

**MECHANICAL DISRUPTION OF DEFENSIVE BARRIERS**
Endotracheal tube
Tracheostomy
Cleft lip/palate

**PERSISTENT VOMITING**
Gastrointestinal infection
Chemotherapy
Emetic (e.g., ipecac)
Postanesthesia

---

Modified from Hazinski MF, editor: *Nursing care of the critically ill child,* ed 2, St Louis, 1992, Mosby.

---

These deviations may persist for weeks, however, while the child starts to feel better.

The newborn may develop a severe pneumonia from aspirating amniotic fluid and debris during birth. Rarely, aspiration causes immediate death from asphyxia; more often the irritated mucous membrane becomes a site for secondary bacterial infection. In addition to fluids, food, vomitus, and nasopharyngeal secretions, other substances that may cause pneumonia are hydrocarbons, lipids, powder, and barium.

### Hydrocarbon Pneumonia

Children frequently develop pneumonia secondary to the ingestion of various forms of hydrocarbons, such as kerosene, gasoline, solvents, lighter fluid, furniture polish, and mineral oil. Petroleum distillates are generally impure substances contaminated with heavy metals or other toxic chemicals that cause systemic, as well as local, effects. Many hydrocarbons are made from petroleum and are found in the home or garage.

Hydrocarbons are usually packaged in attractive containers and have a pleasant aroma; consequently, they are frequently ingested accidentally by young children. On the average, children will swallow less than 30 ml (often about 3 to 4 ml). They begin coughing severely and swallow no more. Although central nervous system abnormalities, gastrointestinal irritation, myocardiopathy, and renal toxicity can occur, the most serious complication is pneumonitis.

Distillates that have high volatility (evaporate quickly), decreased viscosity (thinner solution), and low surface tension are more likely to be aspirated and produce respiratory complications. Decreased viscosity enhances penetration into distal airways; lower surface tension facilitates spread over a larger area of lung surface. Consequently, ingestion of lighter fluid, kerosene, or gasoline is more likely to cause a pathologic condition than substances that have high viscosity (e.g., petroleum jelly, tar, or lubricating oil).

**Pathogenesis.**   The severity of the lung injury depends on the pH of the aspirated material, the presence of bacteria, and the volatility/viscosity of the substance. Pulmonary involvement may also be caused by irritation from aspiration during swallowing, vomiting, or gastric lavage. Pathologic changes include signs of inflammation (edema, hyperemia, infiltration of polymorphonuclear cells), vascular thrombosis and hemorrhage, and necrosis of bronchial, bronchiolar, and alveolar tissues. Other reactions are bronchospasm, atelectasis, emphysema, pulmonary hemorrhage, necrosis, surfactant impairment, and pulmonary edema. Even in small amounts, hydrocarbons spread over the surface of tissues and the lungs and interfere with gas exchange. Aspiration of inert fluids may not produce a chemical or bacterial pneumonia, but these fluids can decrease lung compliance and cause hypoxemia.

**Clinical Manifestations.**   Acid aspiration may produce immediate pulmonary symptoms that worsen over the first 24 hours. Coughing and vomiting, which occur almost immediately after ingestion, contribute to the aspiration. Central nervous system symptoms include agitation, restlessness, confusion, drowsiness, and coma. The temperature is elevated (37.8° to 40° C [100° to 104° F]). (See Ingestion of Injurious Agents, Chapter 16.)

After swallowing, coughing, and choking, the child becomes short of breath, and older children complain of dyspnea. There are varying degrees of cyanosis, tachycardia, tachypnea, nasal flaring, and retractions. Intercostal retractions, grunting, cough, and fever may appear within 30 minutes or be delayed for a few hours. Localized areas of dullness are felt on percussion, and moderately intense wheezes and crackles are heard. Severe injury causes hemoptysis, pulmonary edema, severe cyanosis, and death within 24 hours of aspiration.

**Therapeutic Management.**   Inducing the child to vomit is contraindicated because of the renewed danger of aspiration. Hydrocarbons are readily absorbed by the gastrointestinal tract and excreted by the lungs. Bronchitis or pneumonia usually develops early (within the first 24 hours) but may be delayed. Recovery from pulmonary involvement occurs in most instances despite a severe clinical course. Death is generally the result of hepatic failure complicated by pulmonary factors. Treatment is the same as for any lower respiratory tract inflammation and consists of high humidity, oxygen, hydration, and treatment of any secondary infection. Further treatment modalities include support of the respiratory system using supplemental oxygen to maintain oxygen saturations greater than 95%, as well as preparing for possible endotracheal intubation.

### Lipoid Pneumonia

Oily substances aspirated into the respiratory passages initially cause an interstitial proliferative inflammation that may include an exudative pneumonia. The next stage involves a diffuse, chronic, proliferative fibrosis that is often complicated by acute bronchopneumonia. The final stage features multiple localized nodules or tumorlike paraffinomas. There are no characteristic manifestations. Cough is usually present, and dyspnea is seen in severe cases. Secondary bronchopneumonia is common. The outcome depends on the extent of pulmonary damage, the general condition of the infant or child, and discontinuing the oily inhalation. No specific treatment exists.

### Powder

A significant number of infants suffer talcum powder aspiration. Commercial talcum powder is predominantly a mixture of talc (hydrous magnesium silicate) and other silicates. Severe respiratory distress occurs immediately as a result of an inflammatory reaction in small bronchioles initiated by deep inhalation of the extremely light powder. (See Chapter 12 for further discussion of powder inhalation.)

### Nursing Considerations

Care of the child with aspiration pneumonia is the same as that described for the child with pneumonia from other causes. However, the major thrust of nursing care is aimed at prevention of aspiration. Proper feeding techniques should be carried out for weak, debilitated, and uncooperative children, and preventive measures are used to prevent aspiration of any material that might enter the nasopharynx.

Oily nose drops and oil-based vitamin preparations are not appropriate for infants and small children. Solvents, lighter fluid, and other hydrocarbon substances should be kept away from older infants and small children who are apt to put anything in their mouth and who may be attracted by the slightly sweet smell.

Talcum powder should not be used. If used, careful application (placing it on the caregiver's hand and then on the child's skin) and proper storage are essential.

Infants and debilitated children should be positioned on the right side after feedings to minimize the possibility of aspirating vomitus or regurgitated feeding.

## Acute (Adult) Respiratory Distress Syndrome (ARDS)

ARDS is recognized in children, as well as adults, and has been associated with clinical conditions and injuries such as sepsis, viral pneumonia, smoke inhalation, and near-drowning (Mariscalco, 1999). It is characterized by respiratory distress and hypoxemia that occur within 72 hours of a serious injury or surgery in a person with previously normal lungs.

The hallmark of ARDS is increased permeability of the alveolocapillary membrane that results in pulmonary edema. During the acute phase of ARDS, the alveolocapillary membrane is damaged, with an increasing pulmonary capillary permeability and resulting interstitial edema. Later stages are characterized by pneumocyte and fibrin infiltration of the alveoli, with the start of either the healing process or fibrosis. When fibrosis occurs, the child may demonstrate respiratory distress and the need for mechanical ventilation.

In ARDS the lungs become stiff, gas diffusion is impaired, and eventually there is bronchiolar mucosal swelling and congestive atelectasis. The net effect is decreased functional residual capacity and increased intrapulmonary right-to-left shunting of pulmonary circulation. Surfactant secretion is reduced, and the atelectasis and fluid-filled alveoli provide an excellent medium for bacterial growth.

The criteria for diagnosis of ARDS in children are an acute antecedent illness or injury, acute respiratory distress or failure, no evidence of prior cardiopulmonary disease, and diffuse bilateral infiltrates evidenced on chest radiography. The child with ARDS may first demonstrate only symptoms caused by an injury or infection but, as the condition deteriorates, hyperventilation, tachypnea, increasing respiratory effort, cyanosis, and decreasing oxygen saturation occur. At times the developing hypoxemia is not responsive to oxygen administration.

### Therapeutic Management

Treatment involves the supportive approaches listed in the Guidelines box. When delivering oxygen, it is extremely important to monitor saturations and the amount being delivered because increased levels can promote atelectasis by reabsorption. The use of endotracheal intubation and positive end-expiratory pressure (PEEP) may be required to ensure maximum oxygen delivery by increasing functional residual capacity, reducing intrapulmonary shunting, and shifting pulmonary fluids to secondary areas of the lungs.

Current advances in the treatment of ARDS in children include the use of lung-protective ventilator strategies, permissive hypercapnia, inhaled nitric oxide, high-frequency ventilation, and extracorporeal life support (Redding 2001). Recently a study of 25 pediatric patients with acute lung injury demonstrated improvements in oxygenation without serious iatrogenic injury after prone positioning (Curley, Thompson, and Arnold, 2000).

**Prognosis.** In spite of advances in understanding and treating ARDS, mortality in children ranges from 40% to 75% (Mariscalco, 1999). The precipitating disorder influences the outcome; the worst prognosis is associated with uncontrolled sepsis, bone marrow transplantation, cancer, and multisystem involvement with hepatic failure. Children who recover may have persistent cough and exertional dyspnea.

### Nursing Considerations

Nursing care involves careful monitoring of pulse, heart rate, perfusion, capillary filling, and urinary output, as well as assessment of respiratory status. Blood gas analysis and pulse oximetry are important evaluation tools. Respiratory distress is a frightening situation for both the child and the parents, and attention to their psychologic needs is a major element in the care of these children. Because the mortality rate of ARDS is high, the family is kept informed of the child's progress and made aware of the possibility of death. (See Family-Centered End-of-Life Care, Chapter 23.)

## Smoke Inhalation Injury

A number of noxious substances that may be inhaled are toxic to humans. They are primarily products of incomplete combustion and cause more deaths from fires than flame injuries. The severity of the injury depends on the nature of the substances generated by the material being burned, whether the victim is confined in a closed space, and the duration of contact with the smoke.

### General Aspects

Possible inhalation injury is suspected when there is a history of flames in a closed space whether or not burns are present. Sooty material around the nose or in the sputum, singed nasal hairs, or mucosal burns of the nose, lips, mouth, or throat are all signs that the affected person demands observation for possible pulmonary injury from inhalants. A hoarse voice and cough are further evidence of airway involvement, and increased inspiratory and expiratory stridor indicates severe damage to the upper passages. Signs of respiratory distress are also indicated by tachypnea, tachycardia, and diminished or abnormal breath sounds, including crackles and wheezes.

Three distinct stages occur in the child suffering from inhalation injury: (1) pulmonary insufficiency, usually during the initial 12 hours; (2) pulmonary edema, usually after 6 to 72 hours, with an increase in the lung fluid and interstitial edema; and (3) bronchopneumonia, usually after 72 hours with a resulting airway obstruction or atelectasis. Strangulation may also occur from the cervical eschar secondary to a severe burn (Sockrider, 1999).

Smoke inhalation causes three different types of injury: heat, local chemical, and systemic.

**Heat Injury.** Heat causes thermal injury to the upper airway, but because air has low specific heat, the injury goes no further than the upper airway. Reflex closure of the glottis prevents injury to the lower airway. Heat may reach the middle airway occasionally, but it rarely penetrates to the lungs.

**Chemical Injury.** A wide variety of gases may be generated during the combustion of materials such as clothing,

---

### GUIDELINES

*Management of the Child with Acute (Adult) Respiratory Distress Syndrome (ARDS)*

1. Maintain diligent surveillance for secondary infection.
2. Maintain intravascular volume and hydration status.
3. Monitor urinary output.
4. Treat fever.
5. Establish and maintain neutral thermal environment.
6. Maintain tissue oxygenation:
   a. Oxygen administration
   b. Correct and appropriate position to improve functional residual capacity
   c. Mechanical ventilation when needed, with positive end-expiratory pressure (PEEP) therapy
   d. Suctioning
7. Employ comfort measures, and treat pain.
8. Provide psychologic and emotional support.
9. Provide nutritional support, with appropriate calories given via tube feeding for child unable to tolerate oral intake or parenteral nutrition.
10. Provide meticulous fluid and blood-product management.

furniture, and floor coverings. Acids, alkalis, and their precursors in smoke can produce chemical burns. These substances can be carried deep into the respiratory tract, including the lower respiratory tract, in the form of insoluble gases. Soluble gases tend to dissolve in the upper respiratory tract.

Synthetic materials are especially toxic, producing gases such as oxides of sulfur and nitrogen, acetaldehyde, formaldehyde, hydrocyanic acid, and chlorine. Heated plastics are the source of extremely toxic vapors, including chlorine and hydrochloric acid from polyvinylchloride and hydrocarbons, aldehydes, ketones, and acids from polyethylene. Irritant gases such as nitrous oxide or carbon dioxide combine with water in the lungs to form corrosive acids; aldehydes cause denaturation of proteins, cellular damage, and edema of pulmonary tissues. Chemical burns to the airways are similar to burns on the skin, except they are painless because the tracheobronchial tree is relatively insensitive to pain.

Inhalation of small amounts of noxious irritants produces alveolar and bronchiolar damage that can lead to obstructive bronchiolitis. Severe exposure causes further injury, including alveolocapillary damage with hemorrhage, necrotizing bronchiolitis, inhibited secretion of surfactant, and formation of hyaline membranes—manifestations of ARDS.

**Systemic Injury.**   Gases that are nontoxic to the airways (e.g., carbon monoxide, hydrogen cyanide) can cause injury and death by interfering with or inhibiting cellular respiration. *Carbon monoxide (CO)* is a colorless, odorless gas with an affinity for hemoglobin 200 to 250 times greater than that of oxygen. When CO enters the bloodstream, it readily binds with hemoglobin to form *carboxyhemoglobin (COHb)*. Because CO combines more readily and is released less readily, very low levels of tissue oxygen must be reached before appreciable amounts of oxygen are released from the hemoglobin. Therefore tissue hypoxia reaches dangerous levels before oxygen is available to meet tissue needs.

> **NURSING ALERT**
>
> The oxygen saturation ($SaO_2$) obtained by pulse oximetry will be normal because the device measures only oxygenated and deoxygenated hemoglobin; it does not measure dysfunctional hemoglobin, such as COHb.

Accidental CO poisoning is most often a result of exposure to fumes from heaters or smoke from structural fires, although poorly ventilated recreational vehicles with improperly operated or maintained gas lamps or stoves and cooking in underventilated areas with charcoal grills or hibachis are also frequent causes. CO is produced by incomplete combustion of carbon or carbonaceous material, such as wood or charcoal.

The signs and symptoms of CO poisoning are secondary to tissue hypoxia and vary with the level of COHb. Mild manifestations include headache, visual disturbances, irritability, and nausea, whereas more severe intoxication causes confusion, hallucinations, ataxia, and coma (Box 32-15). CO may increase cerebral blood flow, increase cerebral capillary permeability, and increase cerebrospinal fluid pressure, all of which

contribute to the central nervous system signs observed. The bright, cherry red lips and skin often described are less often observed; more frequently, pallor and cyanosis are seen.

### Therapeutic Management

The treatment of children with smoke toxicity is largely symptomatic. The most widely accepted treatment is placing the child on humidified 100% oxygen as quickly as possible and monitoring for signs of respiratory distress and impending failure. Blood gases are drawn to determine baseline arterial blood gases and COHb levels. Surprisingly, arterial oxygen partial pressure may be within normal limits unless there is marked respiratory depression. If CO poisoning is confirmed, 100% oxygen is continued until COHb levels fall to the nontoxic range of about 10%.

Respiratory distress may occur early in the course of smoke inhalation as a result of hypoxia, or patients who are breathing well on admission may suddenly develop respiratory distress. Therefore intubation and tracheostomy equipment should be readily available. Early endotracheal intubation is recommended in many cases because upper airway edema frequently occurs and makes later intubation very difficult. Indications for intubation include full-thickness burns of the face or neck; children with altered sensorium with inability to protect the airway, such as an absent gag reflex; visible edema on bronchoscopy; and clinical signs indicating obstruction, such as stridor, wheezing, or grunting.

Tracheostomy is usually reserved for situations in which acute respiratory distress occurs in a child who cannot undergo endotracheal intubation or fails to tolerate extubation. Pulmonary toilet may be facilitated by bronchodilators, humidification, and chest physical therapy to enhance the removal of necrotic material, minimize bronchocon-

---

**Box 32-15**

**Inhalation Injury Related to Carboxyhemoglobin Concentration**

| Signs and Symptoms | Percent of COHb Concentration |
|---|---|
| Usually none (often questioned) | 0-5 |
| Tightness across forehead, may or may not be headache, cutaneous blood vessel dilation | 5-15 |
| Throbbing headache plus above | 15-30 |
| Severe headache, weakness, dizziness, dimmed vision, nausea, vomiting, cardiovascular collapse (especially infants, anemic children, and those with pulmonary disease) | 30-40 |
| Same as above but worse, with greater possibility of cardiovascular collapse, syncope, coma, and lactic acidemia | 40-50 |
| Syncope, tachycardia, poor cardiac output, seizures, Cheyne-Stokes respirations, death* | 50-60 |
| Coma, seizures, decreased cardiac output, respiratory depression and failure, death if not treated* | 60-80 |

*Death can occur with lower concentrations in infants and in children with pulmonary disease or anemia.

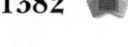

striction, and avoid atelectasis. Bronchoscopy may be needed to clear inspissated secretions.

Carbon monoxide is excreted primarily through the lungs. Treatment of CO intoxication with 100% oxygen reduces the COHb level by one half in 40 to 60 minutes. The role of *hyperbaric oxygen* remains controversial. Although hyperbaric oxygen lowers COHb levels more rapidly, it is questionable whether it provides an advantage over the administration of an inspired concentration of oxygen of 1.0 and whether hyperbaric oxygen affects delayed neurologic complications in patients whose COHb levels are already less than 30% on arrival at the hospital (Sockrider, 1999).

Corticosteroids have no established benefit and may increase the risk of infection. Prophylactic antibiotics offer no benefit and may lead to the development of resistant organisms (Sockrider, 1999).

### Nursing Considerations

Nursing care of the child with inhalation injury is the same as that for any child with respiratory distress. Vital signs and other respiratory assessments are performed frequently, and the pulmonary status is carefully observed and maintained. Pulmonary physiotherapy is usually part of the therapeutic program, as well as mechanical ventilation if needed. Fluid requirements for children experiencing inhalation injury are greater than those with surface burns alone. However, one concern is the development of pulmonary edema; therefore accurate monitoring of intake and output is essential.

In addition to the observation and management of the physical aspects of inhalation injury, the nurse also deals with the psychologic needs of a frightened child and distraught parents. As with any accidental injury, the parents feel overwhelming guilt, even when the injury occurred through no fault of their own. Parents need support and reassurance, as well as information about their child's condition, treatment, and progress.

## Passive Smoking

Numerous investigations indicate that parental smoking is an important cause of morbidity and mortality in children. Involuntary tobacco exposure contributes to millions of cases of disease and disability among children. Pediatric passive smoking also produces significant direct medical costs and economic costs in terms of lives lost. A recent study indicated that parental smoking resulted in an annual direct medical expenditure in the United States of $4.6 billion and annual loss-of-life costs of $8.2 billion (Aligne and Stoddard, 1997).

Children exposed to parental tobacco smoke have an increased incidence of respiratory illnesses, such as bronchiolitis and asthma, and reduced pulmonary function tests. Acute otitis media and otitis media with effusion are also increased in children who have smoking parents (Aligne and Stoddard, 1997). Among children with asthma, exposure to parental cigarette smoking increases asthma symptoms, trips to the emergency department, and medication use and impairs recovery after hospitalization for acute asthma (Abulhosn and others, 1997).

Exposure to cigarette smoking by the mother is particularly dangerous to infants and children. Maternal passive smoke exposure has been associated with increased respiratory symptoms and illnesses in infants and children; decreased fetal growth; increased deliveries of low–birth-weight, preterm, and stillborn infants; and a greater incidence of sudden infant death syndrome (SIDS).

The amount of passive smoke exposure in infants and children is directly related to the presence of smoking parents and the number of smokers in a household. Past studies that have measured passive smoke exposure have analyzed the amount of urinary cotinine in a child's urine. *Cotinine,* a by-product of nicotine, is considered a valid biochemical marker for environmental smoke exposure. Recent studies have indicated that urinary cotinine levels are increased in children who live in homes with smokers and that these levels increase proportionally with the number of smokers in the home (Winkelstein, Tarzian, and Wood, 1997). Cotinine levels have also been used to document exposure to passive smoke in the fetus and newborn. Nonsmoking pregnant women exposed to cigarette smoke had significant amounts of cotinine in the hair of their developing fetus (Eliopoulos and others, 1994). Cotinine has also been found in the meconium of infants born to mothers exposed to passive smoke (Ostrea and others, 1994).

The American Academy of Pediatrics has renewed its statement on the hazards of passive smoking (American Academy of Pediatrics, 1994). The report states: "The dangers to children of both active and passive tobacco exposure, including smokeless forms, are so well established that pediatricians should make the elimination of this threat a major issue as they pursue the goal of a tobacco-free generation by the year 2000."

### Nursing Considerations

Passive smoke exposure during childhood may also contribute to the development of chronic lung disease in adulthood. Nurses and other health care professionals need to include assessments of passive smoke exposure in all children, especially those with respiratory illnesses. In families where smokers refuse to quit, house rules should be established for reducing smoke in the child's environment. (See Family Home Care box.) Nurses should also inform caregivers of the health hazards of children's exposure to tobacco smoke,* set an example for children and families, and become advocates for "no smoking" ordinances in pub-

---

*For a copy of the EPA report *Respiratory Health Effects of Passive Smoking,* write to CERI, US EPA, 26 W Martin Luther King Dr, Cincinnati, OH 45268, (513) 569-7562.

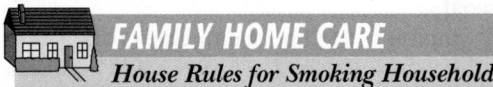

### FAMILY HOME CARE
*House Rules for Smoking Households*

Maintain a smoke-free home.
Do not smoke around children.
Restrict smoking to an isolated, outdoor area.
Do not smoke in motor vehicles with children.
Do not smoke in rooms children use.
Do not allow visitors to smoke in the home.

lic places, prohibition of advertising tobacco products in the media, and inclusion of health warnings of sidestream smoke on tobacco products.

# LONG-TERM RESPIRATORY DYSFUNCTION

## Allergic Rhinitis

Allergic rhinitis affects up to 20% of the pediatric population and is associated with numerous airway disorders, including asthma, otitis media with effusion, and chronic sinusitis. *Seasonal allergic rhinitis* (also known as "hay fever") usually follows a spring-fall pattern and is caused by tree, grass, and weed pollens. Seasonal allergic rhinitis usually does not develop until the individual has been sensitized by two or more pollen seasons. Year-round or perennial allergic rhinitis is more common and is triggered by household inhaled allergens such as feathers, household dust, animal dander, air pollutants, and molds. Peak incidence for allergic rhinitis is in the adolescent and postadolescent age-groups, but younger children are also affected.

### Pathophysiology

Allergic rhinitis requires two conditions: a familial predisposition to develop allergy and exposure of a sensitized person to the allergen. Inhalants in the form of microscopic airborne particles (i.e., pollens, mold, animal danders, and environmental dusts) enter the upper respiratory tract with inhalation and bind to submucosal mast cells in the respiratory tract epithelium.

In the allergic child, symptoms are mediated by immunoglobulin E (IgE), which is produced by the child's B-lymphocytes. The IgE molecules on the cell surfaces trigger the rapid release of mast cell mediators (e.g., histamine, prostaglandins, and leukotrienes), as well as the slower synthesis of cell interactive compounds called cytokines (Simons, 1999). Histamine, a potent vasodilator, acts directly on local receptors to produce vasodilation, mucosal edema, and increased production of mucus. The cytokines summon cells to the area and are responsible for the slower "late-phase allergic" reaction of inflammation and destruction of the mucosal surface that progresses to chronic nasal obstruction (Wood, 2001). Repeated exposure of these sensitized membranes to specific aeroallergens results in clinical allergic disease.

### Clinical Manifestations

Children who have allergic rhinitis have a history of watery rhinorrhea, nasal obstruction, sneezing, or nasal pruritus. Symptoms may be chronic, recurrent, or acute and include itching of the nose, eyes, palate, pharynx, and conjunctiva. The nasal stuffiness sometimes progresses to partial or total obstruction of airflow, and mucus secretion with postnasal drainage can occur. Nasal itching is troublesome, and the affected child attempts to alleviate the symptoms by rubbing the nose—the "allergic salute" (Fig. 32-6). Other symptoms include snoring during sleep, fatigue, malaise, and poor school performance. Frequently children have an associated upper respiratory tract infection.

On physical examination, children may display dark circles or "allergic shiners" beneath their eyes secondary to obstruction of normal outflow from regional lymphatics and veins. If the nasal obstruction is severe, the child will become an obligate mouth breather and present with an open mouth or "allergic gape." Facial findings include a horizontal nasal crease across the lower third of the nose due to frequent rubbing induced by the nasal pruritus, and Dennie lines, or extra wrinkles below the lower eyelids. The child may develop facial tics and mannerisms in an attempt to avoid scratching the nose. Examination of the child's nose often reveals a pale, boggy nasal mucosa with enlarged nasal turbinates.

Symptoms that appear during peak symptom periods include tearing and soreness of the eyes and gelatinous conjunctival discharge in the morning, irritability, fatigue, depression, and loss of appetite.

When allergic rhinitis is suspected, it is important to obtain information regarding clinical signs of related disorders, including middle ear disease, ear pain, delayed speech or language development, chronic cough, wheezing, exercise intolerance, eczema, or urticaria. It is also important to ask about any family history of allergies and to obtain information about specific triggers or environmental changes that may have precipitated an episode of rhinitis, such as seasonal pollens, pets, cigarette smoking, or the use of a woodburning stove for cooking or as a heat source. Chronic rhinitis with significant nasal obstruction can lead to various abnormalities in growth and development and in psychosocial and intellectual development.

### Diagnostic Evaluation

Diagnosis of allergic rhinitis is based on a thorough history and physical examination. Because allergic rhinitis is often associated with atopic dermatitis or asthma, examination of the skin and chest is indicated. Diagnostic tests include a

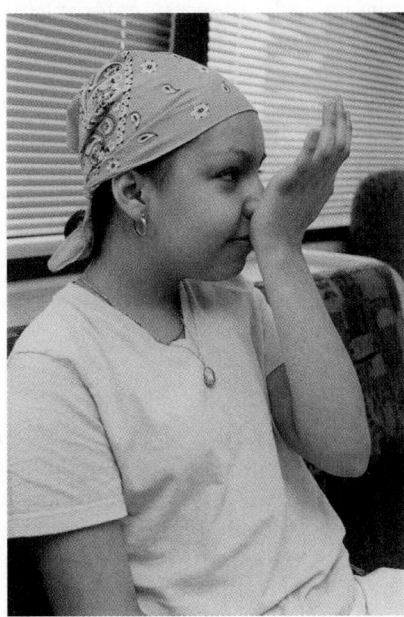

**Fig. 32-6** "Allergic salute." (Courtesy Paul Vincent Kuntz, Texas Children's Hospital.)

nasal smear to determine the number of eosinophils in the nasal secretions, blood examination for total IgE and elevated eosinophils, skin tests, radioallergosorbent tests (RASTs), and various challenge tests. RAST testing is used to determine the level of specific IgE antibodies to specific allergens. This test is generally used as a supplemental test rather than a screening test and requires a blood sample.

A recent screening test designed to detect allergy is the Phadiatope. This test requires a specimen of blood from a vein or finger stick. The test measures IgE antibodies to a group of common allergens. Results of this test are interpreted as positive or negative for a general diagnosis of allergy (Wood, 1995).

*Skin testing* is the most commonly used diagnostic test for allergy. Skin testing involves the injection of specific allergens and should be performed by a practitioner trained in allergy who has access to reliable reagents, experience in the interpretation of results, and adequate facilities to treat adverse reactions to the procedure (Pearlman and others, 1997). The allergenic extract is introduced into the epidermis by (1) scratch, prick, or puncture; (2) a single intradermal injection of a dilute concentration of specific allergen; or (3) serial dilution (threefold or tenfold) injections to determine the end point of reactivity. After a suitable time period (10 to 30 seconds), the size of the resultant wheal and flare reaction is measured to assess the patient's sensitivity. The magnitude of the wheal and flare response correlates roughly with the severity of symptoms produced by natural exposure to the same allergen; however, a positive skin test does not always indicate the presence of clinical reactivity (Wood, 1995).

Skin testing and immunotherapy are generally safe procedures, but they are not without risk. Severe and even fatal reactions can occur within a short time, depending on the type of extract used and the sensitivity of the individual. To minimize the risk of severe reactions, the American Academy of Allergy and Immunology (1990) recommends that the patient remain under observation for at least 20 minutes after injection and longer for high-risk patients. In other countries (e.g., United Kingdom), in which extracts unapproved in the United States are used, the recommended waiting period is 2 hours.

> **NURSING ALERT**
>
> The onset of a reaction is often insidious. Mild initial symptoms may include local pruritus, pallor, flushing, cyanosis, shortness of breath, dyspnea, cough, malaise, or abdominal pain. Later developments include hypotension, airway obstruction, chest pain, ventricular fibrillation, and loss of consciousness.

## Therapeutic Management

Therapy is directed toward avoidance of offending allergens, and use of medication and immunotherapy (hyposensitization or desensitization). Avoidance measures involve removing allergens from the environment and are usually effective for allergy to foods, drugs, and animals. (See Family Home Care box on p. 1398.)

If a patient is unable to avoid allergens, symptoms can be controlled with medication, but treatment should be individualized. Antihistamines and nasal corticosteroids are the first-line drugs used for allergic rhinitis. When used in combination, these medications nearly always relieve symptoms (Kaliner, Spector, and Wenzel, 1999).

Antihistamines are effective in treating sneezing, rhinorrhea, and nasal itching. Antihistamines act by inhibiting the effects of histamine by binding to $H_1$ receptors. Classic antihistamines such as diphenhydramine (Benadryl) and chlorpheniramine (Chlor-Trimeton) are effective but may produce undesirable side effects such as sedation, restlessness, dry mouth, urinary retention, constipation, and impaired school performance. Newer antihistamines such as astemizole (Hismanal), loratadine (Claritin), and cetirizine hydrochloride (Zyrtec) are approved for use in children 6 years of age and older (Pearlman and others, 1997); fexofenadine hydrochloride (Allegra) has been approved for children 12 years of age and older. These drugs are nonsedating and have few cardiovascular adverse effects (Simons, 1999).

If nasal obstruction is a prominent feature, α-adrenergic decongestants, such as pseudoephedrine, phenylephrine, and phenytpropanolamine may be given. Nasal or oral administration often provides symptomatic relief. Caution should be taken, however, with long-term use because of "rebound effects" (return of symptoms) and habituation (lessened effectiveness). Other side effects of these drugs include nervousness and tachycardia (Wood, 2001).

Cromolyn sodium is used prophylactically on a regular basis and is effective in preventing both the early and the late responses to antigen. Its usefulness is limited by the fact that it must be taken four to six times a day, a schedule that is very difficult to maintain in children.

Topical nasal corticosteroids (beclomethasone [Vancenase and Beconase], flunisolide [Nasalide], fluticasone (Flovent) triamcinolone [Nasacort], and budesonide [Rhinocort or Plumicort]) are safe, effective alternatives to the use of cromolyn sodium and can be used effectively on a short-term basis during periods of exacerbation (Simons, 1999). Side effects are minimal, with occasional nasal irritation and epistaxis.

*Immunotherapy* may be necessary if drug therapy and avoidance of allergens are ineffective in controlling symptoms or if drugs evoke undesirable side effects. Before immunotherapy is begun, a positive skin test reaction to the allergen should be confirmed. Immunotherapy involves a series of injections with extracts of the specific allergens that cause symptoms for the child. Initially treatment is given weekly with dilute exposures, and the tolerated dosage is then gradually increased. This process takes about 4 to 8 months to complete, and once this level is reached, maintenance treatment is continued every 3 to 4 weeks for 3 to 5 years. Immunotherapy is most effective in reducing symptoms caused by seasonal pollen-related allergy.

## Nursing Considerations

Nurses can help by recognizing the existence of rhinitis and referring children for diagnosis and therapy.

An important aspect of caring for the child with allergic rhinitis is preparation for skin tests and immunotherapy injections. These procedures are a source of stress for many children. Young children, in particular, cannot understand how uncomfortable injections that must be given regularly over a long period of time will make them feel better. All children who receive skin tests need an explanation of the procedure, and many children benefit from strategies that minimize trauma. (See Atraumatic Care box.)

**NURSING TIP** To distinguish allergies from colds, be aware that:
Allergies occur repeatedly and are often seasonal.
Allergies are seldom accompanied by fever.
Allergies often involve itching in the eyes and nose.
Allergies usually trigger constant and consistent bouts of sneezing.
Allergies are often accompanied by ear and eye problems.

Children with allergic rhinitis and their family members also need specific and detailed information relating to their medications. In the case of seasonal rhinitis, antihistamines or topical antiinflammatory medications are often started approximately 2 weeks before the "allergy season" begins (Pearlman and others, 1997). Phone or mailed reminders to families to start their medications are very helpful in preventing lower respiratory complications of allergic rhinitis. In addition, some nasal sprays may not reach their maximum effect or improve symptoms until a week after they are started. Antihistamines that have sedation as a side effect should not be given to teenagers who are driving, and children should be cautioned to avoid hazardous activities such as bicycling or skating if drowsiness occurs. School nurses, teachers, and parents should monitor children receiving sedating antihistamines for any changes in learning or intellectual functioning in school. Follow-up is essential to be sure that children or their parents do not exceed the correct dosage and that correct administration procedures are followed, especially with the use of inhaled medications (see pp. 1391 and 1399).

**NURSING ALERT** Parents should be aware of the possibility of drug interactions with antihistamines. For example, astemizole (Hismanal) should not be given with erythromycin or antifungal agents such as ketoconazole; giving these drugs together can result in life-threatening cardiac arrhythmias (Pearlman and others, 1997).

**ATRAUMATIC CARE**
*Reducing Pain of Allergy Skin Tests and "Allergy Shots"*

To help allay children's fears of skin tests, give them a careful and thorough explanation of what is to be done and how many "pricks" are involved (usually a series of 8 on each site, for a total of 30 tests). Very young anxious patients may benefit from one prick on the arm to demonstrate how it feels. The skin is pierced with a stylet rather than a regular needle and syringe, then a drop of allergen is placed on the site. Another helpful strategy is to have the child count off the number of pricks with the nurse as a distraction. For intradermal skin injections, EMLA, a topical anesthetic, reduces or eliminates pain without altering test results.

## Asthma

Asthma is defined as a chronic inflammatory disorder of the airways in which many cells play a role, in particular, mast cells, eosinophils, and T-lymphocytes. In susceptible children, inflammation causes recurrent episodes of wheezing, breathlessness, chest tightness, and cough, particularly at night or in the early morning. These episodes are usually associated with variable airflow limitation or obstruction that is reversible either spontaneously or with treatment. The inflammation that occurs in asthma also causes an associated increase in bronchial hyperresponsiveness to a variety of stimuli (National Asthma Education and Prevention Program, 1997). Recognition of the importance of inflammation has made the use of antiinflammatory agents, especially inhaled steroids, a key component in the treatment of asthma.

Asthma prevalence, morbidity, and mortality are increasing in the United States and other nations (Burt and Knapp, 1996). These increases may result from increasing air pollution, poor access to medical care, or underdiagnosis and undertreatment. Asthma is the most common chronic disease of childhood, the primary cause of school absences, and responsible for a major proportion of pediatric admissions to emergency departments and hospitals. Although the onset of asthma may occur at any age, 80% to 90% of children have their first symptoms before 4 or 5 years of age. Boys are affected more frequently than girls until adolescence, when the trend reverses. The severity of the disease varies among children and is not influenced by sex.

In 1995 the National Heart, Lung, and Blood Institute developed a classification of asthma based on clinical or symptom indexes of disease severity (National Heart, Lung, and Blood Institute, 1995). The National Asthma Education and Prevention Program accepted this classification in 1997 and placed the classification in the revision of the *Guidelines for the Diagnosis and Management of Asthma*. This classification includes four categories of asthma: mild intermittent, mild persistent, moderate persistent, and severe persistent (Box 32-16 on p. 1386). Clinical features used to determine these categories include the frequency of daytime and nighttime symptoms, the frequency and severity of exacerbations, and lung function. These four categories are listed as steps because they also provide a stepwise approach to pharmacologic therapy and management. For example, if control of asthma is not maintained at one level or step, pharmacologic therapy for the next step up should be considered. If control is adequate at one step, a gradual stepwise reduction in therapy may be possible. The stepwise approach is presented as a guide to assist clinical decision making. The stepwise approach is not a specific prescription. Therapy and management should be reviewed every 1 to 6 months and should be individualized to the patient. In addition to pharmacologic management, environmental control and educational interventions are essential at each step (National Asthma Education and Prevention Program, 1997).

Studies of children with asthma indicate that allergy influences both the persistence and the severity of the disease. In fact, atopy, or the genetic predisposition for the development of an IgE-mediated response to common

### Box 32-16 ■ ■ □
### Asthma Severity Classification in Children Five Years of Age and Older: Clinical Features*

**STEP 4: SEVERE PERSISTENT ASTHMA**

Continual symptoms
Frequent exacerbations
Frequent nighttime symptoms
Limited physical activity
Peak expiratory flow (PEF) or forced expiratory volume in
   1 second (FEV$_1$) ≤60% of predicted value
PEF variability >30%

**STEP 3: MODERATE PERSISTENT ASTHMA**

Daily symptoms
Daily use of inhaled short-acting $\beta_2$-agonists
Exacerbations affect activity
Exacerbations ≥2 times a week
Exacerbations may last days
Nighttime symptoms >1 time a week
PEF/FEV$_1$ >60% to <80% of predicted value
PEF variability >30%

**STEP 2: MILD PERSISTENT ASTHMA**

Symptoms >2 times/week, but <1 time a day
Exacerbations may affect activity
Nighttime symptoms >2 times a month
PEF/FEV$_1$ ≥80% of predicted value
PEF variability 20% to 30%

**STEP 1: MILD INTERMITTENT ASTHMA**

Symptoms ≤2 times a week
Exacerbations brief (from a few hours to a few days); intensity
   may vary
Nighttime symptoms ≤2 times a month
Asymtomatic and normal PEF between exacerbations
PEF or FEV$_1$ ≥80% of predicted value
PEF variability <20%

From National Asthma Education and Prevention Program: *Expert Panel report II: guidelines for the diagnosis and management of asthma,* Bethesda, MD, 1997, National Heart, Lung, and Blood Institute, National Institutes of Health.
*The presence of one clinical feature of severity is sufficient to place a patient in that category. An individual should be assigned to the most severe grade in which any feature occurs. The characteristics in this table are general and may overlap because asthma is highly variable. An individual's classification may change over time.

### Box 32-17 ■ ■ □
### Triggers Tending to Precipitate or Aggravate Asthmatic Exacerbations

Allergens
   **Outdoor:** Trees, shrubs, weeds, grasses, molds, pollens, air
      pollution, spores
   **Indoor:** Dust or dust mites, mold, cockroach antigen
Irritants: tobacco smoke, wood smoke, odors, sprays
Exposure to occupational chemicals
Exercise
Cold air
Changes in weather or temperature
Environmental change: moving to new home, starting new
   school, etc.
Colds and infections
Animals: cats, dogs, rodents, horses
Medications: aspirin, nonsteroidal antiinflammatory drugs
   (NSAIDs), antibiotics, beta blockers
Strong emotions: fear, anger, laughing, crying
Conditions: gastroesophageal reflux, tracheoesophageal fistula
Food additives: sulfite preservatives
Foods: nuts, milk/dairy products
Endocrine factors: menses, pregnancy, thyroid disease

der involving biochemical, immunologic, infectious, endocrine, and psychologic factors.

### NURSING ALERT

Risk factors for asthma include:

Age
Heredity
Gender
Children of young mothers under age 20
Smoking
Ethnicity: African-Americans at greatest risk
Previous life-threatening attacks
Lack of access to medical care
Psychologic and psychosocial problems

## Pathophysiology

There is general agreement that inflammation contributes to heightened airway reactivity in asthma. The mechanisms contributing to airway inflammation are multiple and involve a number of different pathways. It is unlikely that asthma is caused by either a single cell or a single inflammatory mediator; rather, it appears that asthma results from complex interactions among inflammatory cells, mediators, and the cells and tissues present in the airways (National Asthma Education and Prevention Program, 1997). The sequence for the initial trigger in an asthmatic episode may occur as follows (Fig. 32-7):

1. An initial release of inflammatory mediators from bronchial mast cells, macrophages, and epithelial cells
2. Migration and activation of other inflammatory cells
3. Alterations in epithelial integrity and autonomic neural control of airway tone
4. Increase in the airway smooth muscle responsiveness, which then results in several physiologic manifestations, such as wheezing and dyspnea with eventual obstruction

aeroallergens, is the strongest identifiable predisposing factor for developing asthma (National Asthma Education and Prevention Program, 1997). In addition to allergens, other substances and conditions can serve as triggers that may induce exacerbations of asthma (Box 32-17).

The allergic reaction in the airways is significant for two reasons: (1) it can cause an immediate reaction, with obstruction occurring, and (2) it can precipitate a late bronchial obstructive reaction several hours after the initial exposure. This delayed bronchial response is associated with an increase in the airway hyperresponsiveness to nonimmunologic stimuli and can persist for several weeks or more after a single allergen exposure (National Heart, Lung, and Blood Institute, 1995).

Although allergens play an important role in asthma, 20% to 40% of children with asthma have no evidence of allergic disease (Eggleston, 1999). Asthma is a complex disor-

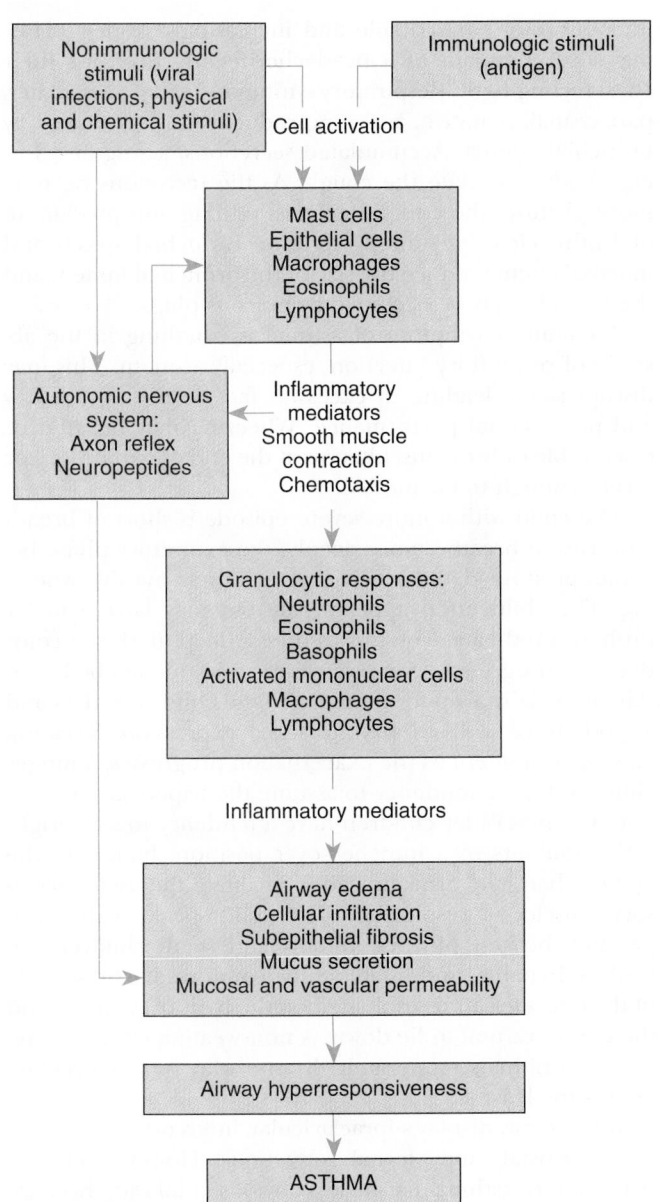

**Fig. 32-7**   Proposed pathways in pathogenesis of bronchial inflammation and airway hyperresponsiveness. (From National Heart, Lung, and Blood Institute, National Institutes of Health: *Guidelines for the diagnosis and management of asthma*, Pub No 91-3042, Bethesda, MD, Aug, 1991.)

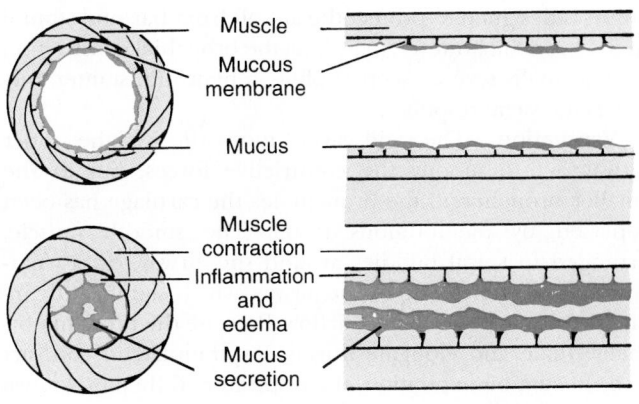

**Fig. 32-8**   Mechanisms of obstruction in asthma.

The role that each of these mechanisms plays varies from child to child as well as during the course of the disease.

Another important component of asthma is bronchospasm and obstruction. The mechanisms responsible for the obstructive symptoms in asthma include (Fig. 32-8):

- Inflammation and edema of the mucous membranes
- Accumulation of tenacious secretions from mucous glands
- Spasm of the smooth muscle of the bronchi and bronchioles, which decreases the caliber of the bronchioles

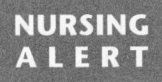 **NURSING ALERT**   Airflow is determined by the size of the airway lumen, degree of bronchial wall edema, mucus production, smooth muscle contraction, and muscle hypertrophy.

**Exacerbations.**   Exacerbations are episodes of progressively worsening shortness of breath, cough, wheezing, chest tightness, or some combination of these changes. They also are characterized by decreases in expiratory airflow. Airways narrow because of bronchospasm, mucosal edema, and mucous plugging, with air being trapped behind occluded or narrowed airways. Functional residual capacity rises because the child is breathing close to total lung capacity; hyperinflation enables the child to keep the airways open and permits gas exchange to occur. Hypoxemia can occur during episodes because of the mismatching of ventilation and perfusion. This is seen as increasing carbon dioxide tension and decreasing oxygen tension levels.

**Immunologic Factors.**   Many children with asthma exhibit an allergic component. Allergy is the strongest epidemiologic risk factor for chronic asthma morbidity and mortality. Many substances in the environment can induce an asthmatic response, but the most significant are those that are antigenic (i.e., that evoke the immune response). The antigen (or foreign substance) is deposited on the respiratory mucosa, where lysozymes immediately digest its outer coating, releasing fragments of foreign protein that initiate the immune sequence. The antibody (immunoglobulin) most active in allergic disorders, including asthma, is IgE, located primarily in skin and mucous membranes.

IgE mediates the immediate hypersensitive reaction in the bronchial mucosa that leads to *specific tissue binding.* IgE attaches to surfaces of mast cells and basophils, where it reacts with the specific antigen to which they have developed a bonding capacity. Antigenic substances trigger an immediate hypersensitivity reaction with subsequent release of chemical mediators from mast cells and basophils: histamine, leukotrienes, platelet-activating factor, and other substances, including prostaglandins, serotonin, and various kinins. The major effects of the mediators in the airways are increased permeability of the blood vessels, contraction of smooth muscle, and stimulation of mucus secretion.

**Vagal Stimulation.**   Normally the balance of vagal and sympathetic nerve influences maintains the tone of bronchial smooth muscle. Irritant receptors on the bronchial mucosa stimulated by various antigenic (pollens, dust) or nonantigenic (smoke, fumes, cold) stimuli trigger a reflex bronchospasm that narrows the airway. This normal reflex mechanism is designed to protect the alveoli from harmful stimuli in the bronchi; however, in asthma the bronchial constriction is abnormally severe. Acetylcholine, a neurotransmitter, mediates the vagal response.

**Ventilation.** The rigid cartilaginous rings of the upper airway act to modify the constrictive forces, but in the smaller bronchi and the bronchioles the cartilage has been replaced by membranous tissue. The smooth muscle, arranged in spiral bundles around the airway, causes narrowing and shortening of the airway, which significantly increases airway resistance to airflow. Because the bronchi normally dilate and elongate during inspiration and contract and shorten on expiration, the respiratory difficulty is more pronounced during the expiratory phase of respiration.

Increased resistance in the airway causes forced expiration through the narrowed lumen. The volume of air trapped in the lungs increases as airways are functionally closed at a point between the alveoli and the lobar bronchi. As the severity of the asthma increases, the airways close at higher residual volume. This gas trapping is the central physiologic feature in the clinical manifestations of asthma. Because gas trapping forces the individual to breathe at a higher and higher lung volume, the work of breathing increases. Consequently, the person with asthma fights to inspire sufficient air. Hyperinflation of alveoli increases the diameter of the airways by exerting lateral traction on bronchiolar walls. Gas exchange is facilitated, but more energy is required during inspiration to overcome the tension of already-stretched elastic lung tissues. The expenditure of effort for breathing causes fatigue, decreased respiratory effectiveness, and increased oxygen consumption and cardiac output at a time when gas exchange and cardiac output are also compromised. In addition, the inspiration occurring at higher lung volumes reduces the effectiveness of the cough. The child becomes progressively dyspneic, cyanotic, and tachypneic.

**Gas Exchange.** The degree to which impaired respiration interferes with gas exchange depends on the ratio of poorly ventilated and hyperextended alveoli to well-ventilated alveoli. When the number of poorly ventilated alveoli increases, the degree of arterial hypoxemia also increases. If there are a sufficient number of well-ventilated alveolocapillary units, perfusion remains adequate and carbon dioxide elimination is not impaired. As the severity of obstruction increases, there is a reduced alveolar ventilation with carbon dioxide retention, hypoxemia, respiratory acidosis, and eventually respiratory failure.

## Clinical Manifestations

The classic manifestations of asthma are dyspnea, wheezing, and coughing. However, the timing of these symptoms varies among children. Bronchoconstriction in response to an allergen can have an immediate, histamine type of pattern or a late response with airway hypersensitivity lasting for days, weeks, or months. A second wave of symptoms can occur 6 to 8 hours after the initial antigen exposure.

Children may experience a prodromal itching localized at the front of the neck or over the upper part of the back. An asthmatic episode usually begins with children feeling uncomfortable or irritable and increasingly restless. They may also complain of a headache, feeling tired, or their chest feeling tight. Respiratory symptoms include a hacking, paroxysmal, irritative, and nonproductive cough caused by bronchial edema. Accumulated secretions, acting as a foreign body, stimulate the cough. As the secretions become more profuse, the cough becomes rattling and productive of frothy, clear, gelatinous sputum. Bronchial spasm and mucosal edema reduce the size of the bronchial lumen, and the bronchi may be occluded by mucous plugs.

A common symptom of asthma is coughing in the absence of respiratory infection, especially at night. This may disrupt sleep, leading to excessive fatigue during the day and poor school performance. Wheezing may be mild or discernible only on auscultation at the end of expiration, or severe enough to be audible.

The child with a more severe episode is short of breath and tries to breathe more deeply; the expiratory phase becomes prolonged and is accompanied by an audible wheezing. The child often appears pale but may have a malar flush and red ears. The lips assume a deep, dark red color that may progress to cyanosis observed in the nail beds and skin, especially around the mouth. The child is restless and apprehensive with an anxious facial expression. Sweating may be prominent as the exacerbation progresses. Younger children have a tendency to assume the tripod sitting position, whereas older children have a tendency to sit upright with shoulders in a hunched-over position, hands on the bed or chair, and arms braced to facilitate the use of accessory muscles of respiration. The child speaks with short, panting, broken phrases. Infants and small children are restless, irritable, and unable to be comforted. The severity of the episode can be evaluated on the basis of sweating and the child's refusal to lie down. A nonsweating child who remains upright is moderately ill; one who remains recumbent is the least ill.

Infants may display supraclavicular, intercostal, suprasternal, subcostal, and sternal retractions. However, clinical symptoms of asthma may be less obvious in infancy. Because infants have a more pliant (flexible) chest, a prolonged expiratory phase may not be easily observed. In addition, wheezing (a characteristic symptom of asthma) can occur in infants with respiratory infections, cardiac defects, cystic fibrosis, and aspiration. The difficulty of differentiating asthma from other conditions in infancy has caused some practitioners to delay or avoid making a diagnosis of asthma. In addition, health care providers are often reluctant to label an infant as "asthmatic" because of a fear that this diagnosis will increase parental anxiety needlessly (Ladebauche, 1997) and may jeopardize health care coverage if the diagnosis is not correct.

Examination of the chest reveals hyperresonance on percussion. Breath sounds are coarse and loud, with sonorous crackles throughout the lung fields. Expiration is prolonged. Coarse rhonchi can be heard, as well as generalized inspiratory and expiratory wheezing that becomes more high pitched as obstruction progresses. With minimal obstruction, wheezing may be mild (discernible only on auscultation at the end of expiration) or even absent.

With severe spasm or obstruction, breath sounds and crackles may become inaudible. Cough is ineffective despite repeated hacking maneuvers. This represents a lack of air movement and may be misinterpreted as improvement by unknowing examiners.

> **NURSING ALERT**
> Shortness of breath with air movement in the chest restricted to the point of absent breath sounds accompanied by a sudden rise in respiratory rate is an ominous sign indicating ventilatory failure and imminent asphyxia.

Children with chronic asthma develop generalized vascularization, mucosal thickening, and hypertrophy of the mucous glands and fibers of the bronchial musculature. With repeated episodes the thoracic cavity becomes fixed in a hyperaerated state (barrel chest), with a depressed diaphragm, elevated shoulders, and increased use of accessory muscles of respiration.

## Diagnostic Evaluation

The diagnosis of asthma is determined on the basis of clinical manifestations, history, physical examination, and laboratory tests. Radiographic examinations are used primarily to rule out other diseases and to evaluate coexisting disease.

Generally, chronic cough in the absence of infection or diffuse wheezing during the expiratory phase of respiration is sufficient to establish a diagnosis. Several conditions may mimic asthma (Box 32-18). For example, localized, monophonic wheezing may indicate the obstruction of a single bronchus, caused by foreign body aspiration, bronchial stenosis, or intrathoracic tumor. Stridor, heard primarily on inspiration, usually indicates an extrathoracic obstruction such as laryngotracheomalacia, croup, or epiglottitis.

*Pulmonary function tests (PFTs)* provide an objective method of evaluating the presence and degree of lung disease, as well as the response to therapy. Spirometry can generally be performed reliably on children by the age of 5 or 6 years and includes either the traditional and simple mechanical spirometer often used in clinics, offices, and the home or the new computerized versions. The Expert Panel recommends that spirometry testing be done at the time of initial assessment of asthma, after treatment is initiated and symptoms have stabilized, and at least every 1 to 2 years to assess the maintenance of airway function (National Asthma Education and Prevention Program, 1997).

Another tool or instrument used to monitor pulmonary function is the *peak expiratory flow rate (PEFR)*. PEFR measures the maximum flow of air that can be forcefully exhaled in 1 second. PEFR is measured in liters per minute. PEFR can be measured with inexpensive and portable peak flow meters. However, because measurement of PEFR depends on effort and technique, children need instructions, demonstrations, and frequent reviews of technique. (See Family Home Care box on p. 1399.) PEFR monitoring can be used for short-term monitoring, managing exacerbations, and daily long-term monitoring. Three zones of measurement are typically used to interpret PEFR. The zone system is patterned after a traffic light so that the categories are easier to use and remember. (See Guidelines box.)

Each individual child's PEFR varies according to age, height, sex, and race. The child's value may be consistently higher or lower than average predicted norms. Each child needs to establish his or her *personal best value.* A personal best value can be established during a 2- to 3-week period during which the child records PEFR at least twice a day. The personal best value is usually achieved in the early afternoon after maximal therapy has stabilized the asthma. A course of oral corticosteroids may be needed to establish the personal best PEFR. Once the personal best value has been established, the child's current PEFR on any given occasion can be compared with the personal best value.

The Expert Panel recommends that peak flow monitoring be used in children with moderate to severe persistent asthma to determine the severity of an exacerbation and to guide therapeutic decisions in the home, school, clinician's

---

> **Box 32-18 ■ ■ ■**
> **Conditions That May Mimic Asthma**
>
> **OBSTRUCTION INVOLVING LARGE AIRWAYS**
> Foreign body in trachea, bronchus, or esophagus
> Vascular rings
> Laryngotracheomalacia
> Enlarged lymph nodes
> Tumor laryngeal webs
> Tracheostenosis or bronchostenosis
> Vocal cord paralysis
>
> **OBSTRUCTION INVOLVING BOTH LARGE AND SMALL AIRWAYS**
> Bronchiolitis: viral or obliterative
> Cystic fibrosis
> Bronchopulmonary dysplasia
> Aspiration from swallowing dysfunction; gastroesophageal reflux; tracheoesophageal fistula
> Pulmonary edema
> Acute inflammation of the airways

---

> **GUIDELINES**
> *Interpreting Peak Expiratory Flow Rates\**
>
> ● *Green (80% to 100% of personal best)* signals all clear. Asthma is under reasonably good control. No symptoms are present, and the routine treatment plan for maintaining control can be followed.
> ● *Yellow (50% to 79% of personal best)* signals caution. Asthma is not well controlled. An acute exacerbation may be present. Maintenance therapy may need to be increased. Call the practitioner if the child stays in this zone.
> ● *Red (below 50% of personal best)* signals a medical alert. Severe airway narrowing may be occurring. A short-acting bronchodilator should be administered. Notify the practitioner if the PEFR measure does not return immediately and stay in yellow or green zones.
>
> ---
> \*These zones are guidelines only. Specific zones and management should be individualized for each child.

office, or emergency department. Long-term daily peak flow monitoring in children with moderate to severe persistent asthma can also be used to detect early changes in disease status that require treatment, to evaluate responses to changes in therapy, to provide assessment of severity for children who are unable to perceive airflow obstruction, and to provide a quantitative measure of impairment (National Asthma Education and Prevention Program, 1977). Although children with mild intermittent or mild persistent asthma may not require long-term daily peak flow monitoring, such monitoring may be useful in guiding therapeutic decisions and when these children develop severe exacerbations.

Bronchial challenges using methacholine, histamine, or exercise may be performed to assess airway responsiveness. Although these tests are highly specific and sensitive, they place the child at risk for an asthmatic episode and should be done under close observation in a qualified laboratory or clinic.

Skin testing is useful in identifying specific allergens, and those obtained by the puncture technique correlate better than intracutaneous tests with symptoms and measurements of specific IgE antibody. Provocative testing, direct exposure of the mucous membranes to a suspected antigen in increasing concentrations, helps to identify inhaled allergens. The RAST test helps identify antigens against various foods and is often useful in determining appropriate therapy. The 1997 revised guidelines for the treatment of asthma recommend that all patients with persistent asthma be tested with skin tests or laboratory analysis of the patient's blood to determine sensitization to perennial allergens (i.e., house dust mite, cat, dog, cockroach, and fungus) (National Asthma Education and Prevention Program, 1997).

In addition to these tests, other important tests include laboratory tests (complete blood count with differential) and chest x-ray films. The complete blood count may show a slight elevation in the white blood cell count during acute asthma, but elevations to more than 12,000/mm$^3$ or an increased percentage of band cells may indicate respiratory infection. The presence of eosinophilia of greater than 500/mm$^3$, however, tends to suggest an allergic or inflammatory disorder. Frontal and lateral x-ray films show infiltrates and hyperexpansion of the airways, with the anteroposterior diameter on physical examination indicating an increased diameter (suggestive of barrel chest).

## Therapeutic Management: General

The overall goal of asthma management is to prevent disability, to minimize physical and psychologic morbidity, and to assist the child in living as normal and happy a life as possible. This includes facilitating the child's social adjustments in the family, school, and community and normal participation in recreational activities and sports. To accomplish these goals, several treatment principles need to be followed (National Asthma Education and Prevention Program, 1997):

- A continuous care approach with regular visits (at least every 6 months) to the health care provider are necessary to control symptoms and prevent exacerbations.

- Prevention of exacerbations includes avoidance of triggers, avoidance of allergens, and the use of medications as needed.
- Therapy includes efforts to reduce underlying inflammation and to relieve or prevent symptomatic airway narrowing.
- Therapy includes patient education, environmental control, and pharmacologic management, as well as the use of objective measures to monitor the severity of disease and course of therapy.

**Allergen Control.** The goal of nonpharmacologic therapy is prevention and reduction of the child's exposure to airborne allergens and irritants. Basic to any therapeutic plan is an evaluation of the child's general health and an assessment of the specific allergenic factors that precipitate symptoms. *House dust mites* and other components of house dust are the agents identified most often in children allergic to inhalants. The most important method to eliminate dust mites is to keep the humidity in the house under 50%, the level below which dust mites do not survive (Kaliner, Spector, and Wenzel, 1999).

The *cockroach,* another common household inhabitant, has also been identified as an important allergen in children with asthma (Kuster, 1996). In some locations (i.e., inner-city environments) and among some ethnic groups, the cockroach is a more common allergen than the house dust mite (Rosenstreich and others, 1997). In addition, sensitivity to the cockroach allergen has been shown to be an important risk factor for frequent episodes of asthma among patients in emergency departments. Effective environmental control of cockroaches requires repeated, vigorous extermination of not only the affected house or apartment but also neighboring houses or apartments. In addition to exterminating living cockroaches, carefully cleaning kitchen floors and cabinets, putting food away quickly after eating, and taking trash out in the evening are necessary measures to eliminate the residue left by cockroaches (Kuster, 1996).

Recently two studies identified mouse allergen as a significant allergen, second only to the cockroach, in the homes of inner-city children with asthma. Researchers in these studies recommended aggressive extermination of not only cockroaches but also mice from inner city homes (Phipatankul and others, 2000a; Phipatanakul and others, 2000b).

Specific allergens are identified by skin testing, and steps are taken to eliminate or avoid the offending allergens. (See Family Home Care box on p. 1398.) Often, simply removing the offending environmental factors will decrease the frequency of asthmatic episodes (e.g., removal of a dog or cat from the bedroom or home of a child sensitive to animal dander). Nonspecific factors that may trigger an episode, such as extremes of temperature, are sometimes controlled by dehumidifiers or air conditioners.

**Drug Therapy.** Pharmacologic therapy is used to prevent and control asthma symptoms, reduce the frequency and severity of asthma exacerbations, and reverse airflow obstruction. A stepwise approach to pharmacologic therapy is recommended, with the type and amount of medication dictated by the severity of the asthma. For example, children with mild intermittent asthma usually require medication only when they have an acute exacerbation. Children with persistent asthma (mild, moderate, and severe) may, however, require daily long-term medications in addition to medications to treat acute exacerbations. Because inflammation is considered an early and persistent feature of asthma, therapy for persistent asthma is directed toward long-term suppression of the inflammation. Thus the most effective medications for long-term control are those with antiinflammatory effects.

Medications used to treat asthma are categorized into two general classes: *long-term control medications* (also called *preventor medications*) to achieve and maintain control of inflammation and *quick-relief medications* (also referred to as *rescue medications*) to treat acute symptoms and exacerbations (National Asthma and Education Program, 1997). Quick-relief and long-term medications are often used in combination. Corticosteroids, cromolyn sodium and nedocromil, long-acting $\beta_2$-agonists, methylxanthines, and leukotriene modifiers are used as long-term control medications. Short-acting $\beta_2$-agonists, anticholinergics, and systemic corticosteroids are used as quick-relief medications. $\beta_2$-agonists can be used as both quick-relief and long-term medications.

Many medications used to treat asthma are given by inhalation with a nebulizer or metered-dose inhaler (MDI). An MDI is a small, handheld device with a mouthpiece. When the MDI is activated, a precise dose of medication is delivered through the mouth to the lungs. Some MDIs use chlorofluorocarbons (CFCs) as the propellant, and they may have a spacing unit or reservoir attached to make it easier for young children to use (Fig. 32-9). Because CFCs have been linked to damage and depletion of the earth's ozone layer, the manufacturing of CFCs is now banned in the United States by an international agreement known as the Montreal Protocol. Although MDIs were granted a temporary exemption, pharmaceutical companies are striving to produce safe and effective CFC-free alternatives. Hydrofluorocarbons (HFCs) will eventually replace CFCs. At the present time, Proventil HFC is the only CFC-free aerosol MDI available in the United States. It contains the propellant hydrofluoroalkane (HFA).

Other CFC-free MDIs, such as the Diskus inhaler and the *Turbuhaler*, deliver inhaled powder. The Turbuhaler is easier for children to use because it eliminates the coordination of the actuation of the device with inhalation and holding the breath. It delivers a tasteless and odorless fine particulate powder to the lungs that is approximately twice the dose of the drug when compared with the same drug delivered via an aerosol inhaler. The favorable ratio of lung deposition to systemic absorption suggests that the same degree of asthma control can be achieved with a lower dose of the steroid budesonide (Pulmicort) (National Asthma Education and Prevention Program, 1997). Persons accustomed to using the propellant devices, which leave an unpleasant taste, may think that no medication was inhaled with the Turbuhaler. Patients are cautioned not to repeat the inhalation.

All children and families using an MDI need careful instructions and assistance to learn how to use the MDI correctly. (See Family Home Care box on p. 1399.) Many children do not use their MDI correctly. A recent study of school-age urban children with asthma indicated that only 7% of these children had effective MDI skills (Winkelstein and others, 2000). Adolescents also use MDIs incorrectly and have been noted to overuse their MDIs to administer $\beta_2$-agonists (Beausoleil, Weldon, and McGeady, 1997). Overuse can worsen the severity of the asthma and may contribute to fatal or near-fatal asthma. Infants and very young children who have difficulty using the MDI can obtain effective relief with **nebulization.** The medication is mixed with saline and then nebulized with compressed air by a machine. When using the nebulizer, children are instructed to breathe normally with the mouth open to provide a direct route to the trachea for the medicine.

*Corticosteroids.* Corticosteroids are antiinflammatory drugs used to treat reversible airflow obstruction and to control symptoms and reduce bronchial hyperreactivity in chronic asthma (Eggleston, 1999). Clinical studies of corticosteroids have indicated significant improvement of all asthma parameters, including decreasing symptoms, emergency visits, and medication requirements.

Corticosteroids can be administered parenterally, orally, or by inhalation. Oral medications are metabolized slowly, with an onset of action up to 3 hours after administration and peak effectiveness occurring within 6 to 12 hours. Oral systemic steroids may be given for a short period of time (i.e., a 3- to 10-day "burst") to gain prompt control of inadequately controlled persistent asthma. Oral steroids may also be used to manage severe persistent asthma. These drugs should be given in the lowest effective dose. For long-term use, morning dosing every other day produces the least toxicity. Long-term use also poses the risk of significant adverse effects, such as osteoporosis, hypertension, Cushing syndrome, impaired immune mechanisms, cataracts, diabetes, and hypothalamic-pituitary-adrenal suppression (National Asthma Education and Prevention Program, 1997).

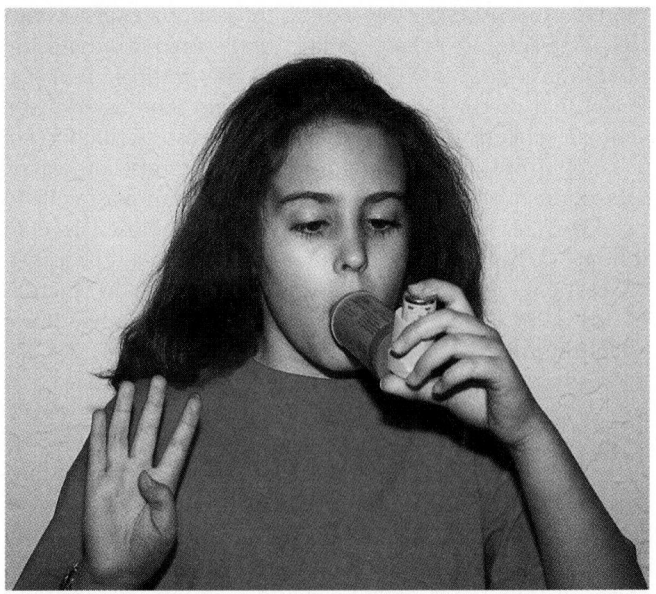

**Fig. 32-9** Child using metered-dose inhaler with spacer. Fingers are used for counting to 10 seconds.

Consideration should also be given to coexisting conditions that could be worsened by systemic steroids, such as herpes virus infections, varicella, and tuberculosis.

Inhaled corticosteroids are used for long-term prevention of symptoms as well as suppression, control, and reversal of inflammation. In addition to MDI preparations of corticosteroids, an inhalation suspension of budesonide was recently approved by the U.S. Food and Drug Administration (FDA) for use in children as young as 12 months (Kemp and others, 1999). Inhaled steroids have few side effects (cough, dysphonia, and oral thrush), and their use has reduced the need for long-term use of oral steroids (National Asthma Education and Prevention Program, 1997).

*Cromolyn and nedocromil sodium.* Cromolyn sodium is a nonsteroidal antiinflammatory drug. This drug blocks both the early and late reaction to allergens. Cromolyn also stabilizes mast cell membranes, inhibits activation and release of mediators from eosinophils and epithelial cells, and inhibits the acute airway narrowing after exposure to exercise, cold dry air, and sulfur dioxide. However, there is no way to reliably predict whether a child will respond to the drug. Cromolyn sodium has minimal side effects, but recent research questioning its efficacy in the preschool child with mild to moderate asthma has led to the recommendation against its use as first-line preventive therapy (Skoner, 2002).

Nedocromil sodium has both antiallergic and antiinflammatory properties. This drug inhibits the bronchoconstrictor response to inhaled antigens and inhibits the activity of and release of histamine, leukotrienes, and prostaglandins from inflammatory cells associated with asthma. The drug is used for maintenance therapy in asthma and is not effective for reversal of acute exacerbations. This drug has few side effects, but some patients complain of the drug's unpleasant taste.

*β-adrenergic agents.* β-Adrenergic agonists (primarily albuterol, metaproterenol, and terbutaline) are used for quick relief of acute exacerbations and for the prevention of exercise-induced bronchospasm. These drugs bind with the beta receptors on the smooth muscle of airways, where they activate adenylate cyclase and convert adenosine monophosphate (AMP) to cyclic AMP (cAMP). It is believed that the increased cAMP enhances binding of intracellular calcium (Ca) to the cell membrane, reducing the availability of Ca and thus allowing smooth muscle to relax. Other effects of the drug help stabilization of mast cells to prevent release of mediators. Most β-adrenergics used in asthma therapy affect predominantly the beta$_2$ receptors, which help eliminate bronchospasm. Beta$_1$ effects, such as increased heart rate and gastrointestinal disturbances, have been minimized.

β-Adrenergic agonists can be given via inhalation or as oral or parenteral preparations. The inhaled drug, administered by an MDI or nebulizer, has a more rapid onset of action than the oral form. Inhalation also reduces troublesome systemic side effects: irritability, tremor, nervousness, and insomnia.

Inhaled β-adrenergics should not be taken more than three to four times daily for acute symptoms (Meng and Martorell, 1997). Regularly scheduled, daily use of short-acting β$_2$-agonists is generally not recommended. If a child is requiring increasing use of short-acting β$_2$-agonists each day or is using more than one canister of this medication in 1 month, this indicates inadequate control of asthma and the need to seek medical care and ask about initiating or intensifying antiinflammatory therapy (National Asthma Education and Prevention Program, 1997). Children with exercise-induced bronchospasm are advised to use their β$_2$-agonist prophylactically 10 to 15 minutes before exercise.

*Salmeterol (Serevent)* is a long-acting bronchodilator that is used twice a day. This drug is added to antiinflammatory therapy and is used for long-term prevention of symptoms, especially nocturnal symptoms. Salmeterol is not used in children less than 12 years of age, and it is not to be used to treat acute symptoms or exacerbations. If a child requires increasing doses of a rescue β$_2$-agonist to control acute symptoms while also taking salmeterol, the physician should be consulted, because this may indicate that the asthma is not under control and that the child is at risk for a severe exacerbation.

*Methylxanthines.* The methylxanthines, principally theophylline, have been used for decades to relieve symptoms and prevent asthma attacks. Theophylline, however, is now considered a third-line agent and perhaps even unnecessary for treating asthma exacerbations. It is a weaker bronchodilator than the β-adrenergics, and because inflammation contributes to asthma, other drugs are of increased benefit (Eggleston, 1999).

Theophylline may be administered intravenously, intramuscularly, orally, or rectally (seldom used). The drug is also available in sustained-release tablets and capsules. In addition to its bronchodilator effect, theophylline is a central respiratory stimulant and increases respiratory muscle contractility. Theophylline is also losing popularity to β-adrenergics because it is associated with toxicity and complex pharmacokinetics (Eggleston, 1999).

Several factors affect the metabolism of theophylline (Box 32-19). For example, children under 12 months of age metabolize the drug faster than older children and adults. In general, theophylline is used when a child is not responsive to other inhaled medications or for long-term

---

**Box 32-19** ■ ■ ■
**Factors Affecting Theophylline Clearance**

**SUBSTANCES THAT ACCELERATE CLEARANCE**
Phenytoin
Rifampin
Phenobarbital
Valproic acid
Cigarette and marijuana smoking

**FACTORS THAT DELAY CLEARANCE**
**Medication:** Antibiotics (especially erythromycin), cimetidine (Tagamet), carbamazepine (Tegretol), quinoline, oral contraceptives, propranolol (Inderal), furosemide, allopurinol
**Illnesses:** Liver or heart dysfunction, congestive heart failure, fever for more than 24 hours, acute viral illness
**Other:** Obesity

control and prevention of symptoms, especially nocturnal symptoms.

When theophylline is used, serum concentrations of the drug must be monitored. Both therapeutic and toxic effects are related directly to plasma levels with a therapeutic range of 5 to 15 $\mu$g/ml suggested. Maximum levels of 15 $\mu$g/ml are recommended for outpatient care (Eggleston, 1999).

**NURSING ALERT**   Theophylline toxicity can occur with serum levels 20 $\mu$g/ml or greater. Side effects from theophylline include nausea, vomiting, headache, irritability, and insomnia. Early signs of toxicity are distractibility, poor school performance, nausea, tachycardia, and irritability; seizures and arrhythmias occur at blood theophylline levels greater than 30 $\mu$g/ml.

The signs and symptoms of theophylline intoxication involve several organ systems. Nausea and vomiting are the most common early symptoms. Cardiopulmonary effects include tachycardia, arrhythmias, and stimulation of the respiratory center (tachypnea), with the possibility of diuresis, irritability, and even seizures.

*Anticholinergics.*   Anticholinergic therapy, the oldest form of bronchodilator therapy for asthma, reduces intrinsic vagal tone to the airways and blocks reflex bronchoconstriction caused by inhaled irritants. Anticholinergics are used for relief of acute bronchospasm. However, these drugs have adverse side effects that include drying of respiratory secretions, blurred vision, and cardiac and central nervous system stimulation. The primary drugs used are atropine or its derivative, ipratropium, which does not cross the blood-brain barrier and therefore elicits no central nervous system effects. Ipratropium has been shown to be effective during status asthmaticus when used in nebulized form in combination with $\beta$-adrenergic agents (Schuh and others, 1995).

*Leukotriene modifiers.*   Leukotrienes are potent inflammatory mediators released from mast cells, eosinophils, and basophils. These substances cause transient increases in airway hyperresponsiveness, triggering airway spasms. By blocking the leukotriene receptors, leukotriene receptor antagonists or modifiers block pathogenic effects such as bronchospasm and inflammatory cell infiltration. The leukotriene receptor antagonists montelukast (Singulair), zafirlukast (Accolate), and zileuton (Zyflo) are given orally (tablets). Current guidelines indicate that leukotrine modifiers can be a suitable alternative to low-dose inhaled corticosteroids (ICS) in mild persistent asthma and an effective addition to ICS in moderate persistent asthma (Skoner, 2002). These drugs are not to be used to treat acute episodes of asthma. Montelukast is administered once a day and can be taken by children as young as 6 years. Zafirlukast and zileuton are indicated for children older than 12 years of age. Only zafirlukast may be taken during pregnancy, and neither zafirlukast or zileuton is recommended for use by breast-feeding women (Stevenson, 1997a).

*Heliox and magnesium.*   For children manifesting bronchospasm or difficulty in ventilation, heliox (helium/oxygen mixture) has been used. Helium is nonreactive

with biologic membranes and is virtually insoluble in lung tissue. Carbon dioxide diffuses more readily through a mixture of helium/oxygen than through air because of the decreased density, resulting in less turbulent airflow.

Helium can be delivered via a nonrebreathing face mask from premixed tanks, which may be blended in a stand-alone unit or within a ventilator. An oxygen analyzer must be placed in line after mixing the gases to measure the concentration of oxygen that the patient is actually receiving. The usual ratio of helium to oxygen is either 60:40 or 70:30. Although limited studies have suggested that heliox may be an effective and exciting addition to the traditional treatment of status asthmaticus (Browne-Heitschmidt and Cassidy, 1997), more careful studies of its long-term or repeated use are necessary (Manthous and others, 1995).

In the past, IV infusions of magnesium have been found to produce improvement in pulmonary function and peak flow rate among pediatric patients treated in the emergency department (ED) with moderate to severe asthma (Ciarallo, Sauer, and Shannon, 1996). Another, more recent study indicated that children with moderate to severe asthma who were treated with doses of 40 mg/kg of IV magnesium sulfate showed remarkable short-term improvement in predicted PEFR, forced expiratory volume in 1 second, and forced vital capacity (Ciarallo, Brousseau, and Reinert, 2000). In the last 2 years several questions have been raised about the treatment of acute asthma with magnesium sulfate. A randomized trial of children with moderate to severe asthma who came to the ED indicated that routine administration of high-dose magnesium in addition to albuterol and corticosteroids was not efficacious (Scarfone and others, 2000). In addition, a meta-analysis of seven randomized trials of IV magnesium failed to demonstrate statistically significant evidence of a beneficial effect for all patients who came to the ED with acute asthma. However, a beneficial effect was obvious in patients who presented with severe acute asthma (Rowe and others, 2000). Clearly, additional research is needed to determine exactly which patients with asthma benefit from magnesium and the optimal dose that is beneficial for pediatric patients.

**Chest Physiotherapy (CPT).**   CPT includes breathing exercises and physical training. These therapies help produce physical and mental relaxation, improve posture, strengthen respiratory musculature, and develop more efficient patterns of breathing. For the motivated child, breathing exercises and controlled breathing are of value in preventing overinflation and improving efficiency of the cough. Although pursed-lip and other forms of controlled breathing may help to maintain calm during respiratory distress, these techniques are not recommended during acute exacerbations of asthma (National Asthma Education and Prevention Program, 1997).

**Hyposensitization.**   The role of immunotherapy or hyposensitization for childhood asthma has become controversial. In the past, immunotherapy was widely used for treatment of seasonal allergy and when single substances were identified as the offending allergen. Immunotherapy has not been recommended for allergens that can be eliminated effectively, such as foods, drugs, and animal dander.

Injection therapy is usually limited to clinically significant allergens. The initial dose of the offending allergen(s), based on the size of the skin reaction, is injected subcutaneously. The amount is increased at weekly intervals until a maximum tolerance is reached, after which a maintenance dose is given at 4-week intervals. This may be extended to 5- or 6-week intervals during the off-season for seasonal allergens. Successful treatment is continued for a minimum of 3 years and then stopped. If no symptoms appear, acquired immunity is said to be retained; if symptoms recur, treatment is reinstituted.

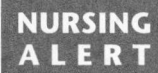 Hyposensitization injections should be administered only with emergency equipment and medications readily available in the event of an anaphylactic reaction.

Previous studies of children with allergic asthma who are sensitive to single allergens, such as house dust, pollens, and molds, have indicated that immunotherapy reduces airway sensitivity to allergens, decreases signs and symptoms provoked by natural exposure, and improves basal airway function (Abramson, Puy, and Weiner, 1995). However, a double-blind placebo-controlled experimental trial of multiple-allergen immunotherapy of 121 allergic children with moderate to severe perennial asthma indicated no significant differences in medication use between children who received immunotherapy and children who received the placebo (Adkinson and others, 1997). Parents of children with asthma should consult their physician before making any decisions and if they have any questions about immunotherapy as a treatment for asthma.

**Exercise.** *Exercise-induced bronchospasm (EIB)* is caused by a loss of heat and/or water from the lungs during exercise because of hyperventilation of air that is cooler and dryer than that of the respiratory tract. If untreated, EIB can limit and disrupt normal activities of childhood. Although EIB should be anticipated in all patients with asthma, in some patients EIB may be a marker for inadequate asthma management. These patients should be monitored regularly to be sure that they have no symptoms of asthma in the absence of exercise. EIB typically occurs during or minutes after vigorous activity, reaches its peak 5 to 10 minutes after stopping the activity, and usually resolves in another 20 to 30 minutes. Cough, shortness of breath, chest pain or tightness, wheezing, and endurance problems during exercise are characteristic symptoms of EIB, but an exercise challenge test in a laboratory setting is used to establish the diagnosis (National Asthma Education and Prevention, 1997).

EIB should not limit either participation or success in vigorous activities. One goal of management is to enable children to participate in any activity they choose without experiencing asthma symptoms. The use of $\beta_2$-agonists will usually prevent EIB in more than 80% of patients (National Asthma Education and Prevention, 1997). The use of short-acting inhaled $\beta_2$-agonists immediately before exercise is often effective for 2 to 3 hours. Cromolyn and nedocromil may also be used. In children over 12 years of age, salmeterol has been shown to prevent EIB for 10 to 12 hours. A

**TABLE 32-3** **Estimating severity of asthma exacerbations**

| Sign/Symptom/ Assessment | Mild | Moderate | Severe | Respiratory Arrest Imminent |
|---|---|---|---|---|
| Breathless | While walking<br>Can lie down | While talking (infant—softer, shorter cry; difficulty feeding)<br>Prefers sitting | While at rest (infant—stops feeding)<br>Sits upright | |
| Talks in | Sentences | Phrases | Words | |
| Alertness | May be agitated | Usually agitated | Usually agitated | Drowsy or confused |
| Respiratory rate | Increased | Increased | Often >30/min | |
| Accessory muscle use; retractions | Usually not present | Commonly present | Usually present | Abnormal thoracoabdominal movement |
| Wheeze | Moderate, often only end expiratory | Loud, throughout exhalation | Usually loud throughout inhalation and exhalation | Absence of wheeze |
| Peak expiratory flow rate | 80% of predicted or personal best | 50% to 80% of predicted or personal best | <50% of predicted or personal best | |
| Oxygen saturation ($SaO_2$), (on air) at sea level | >95% | 91% to 95% | <91% | |
| $PaO_2$ (on air) | Normal | >60 mm Hg | <60 mm Hg; possible cyanosis | |
| $PaCO_2$ | <42 mm Hg | <42 mm Hg | ≥42 mm Hg; possible respiratory failure | |

From National Asthma Education and Prevention Program: *Expert Panel Report II: guidelines for diagnosis and management of asthma,* Bethesda, MD, 1997, National Heart, Lung, and Blood Institute, National Institutes of Health.

lengthy warm-up period before exercise may also benefit some children. Teachers and coaches need to be notified when children have EIB and told that the children can participate in physical activities but will need time to take their inhaled medication before the activity.

Children with EIB and asthma are often excluded from exercise by parents, teachers, and physicians as well as by the children themselves because they are fearful that activity will provoke an episode. This can seriously hamper peer interaction and physical health. Exercise is advantageous for children with asthma, and the majority of these children can participate in activities at school and in sports with minimal difficulty, provided that the asthma is under control. Participation is encouraged but should be evaluated on an individual basis in terms of tolerance for duration and intensity of effort.

## Therapeutic Management: Specific

Children with asthma have exacerbations at varying intervals, with severity ranging from wheezing to life-threatening status asthmaticus (Table 32-3).

Protocols have been developed for treating the child experiencing an asthmatic episode at home, in the emergency department, or in the hospital (National Asthma Education and Prevention Program, 1997) (Table 32-4).

Successful home management of acute asthma begins before symptoms develop. All patients and family members should be taught how to monitor symptoms to recognize early signs of deterioration. Children with moderate to severe persistent asthma and those with a history of severe exacerbations should be taught how to monitor their peak

flow rate to assess the severity of the exacerbation and the response to therapy. All children should be given a *written action plan* to be followed in the event of symptoms or an exacerbation. This plan should include information on how to adjust medications in response to signs, symptoms, and peak flow measurements and when to seek medical help. School-age children should have a written action plan that is appropriate for the school setting.

**Status Asthmaticus.** Children who continue to display respiratory distress despite vigorous therapeutic measures, especially the use of sympathomimetics (i.e., albuterol, epinephrine), are considered to be in *status asthmaticus.* The condition may develop gradually or rapidly, often coincident with complicating conditions, such as pneumonia, that can influence the duration and treatment of the exacerbation. Status asthmaticus is a medical emergency that can result in respiratory failure and death if untreated.

Persistent hypoventilation leads to an accumulation of carbon dioxide, with a decrease in arterial pH and respiratory acidosis. Compensatory buffering mechanisms become overtaxed, and the pH may drop to dangerous levels. Vomiting and dehydration cause further reduction of arterial pH. Therapy for status asthmaticus is directed toward correction of dehydration and acidosis, improvement of ventilation, and treatment of any concurrent infection.

A child suspected of having status asthmaticus is usually seen in the emergency department and is often admitted to a pediatric intensive care unit for close observation and continuous cardiorespiratory monitoring.

Oxygen is recommended and should be given to maintain an oxygen saturation greater than 90%. Frequent

---

**TABLE 32-4** Initial assessment and emergency treatment of acute exacerbations of asthma in a child who is capable of using a peak flow meter*

| Assessment | Recommended Actions |
|---|---|
| Does the patient have:<br>Altered level of consciousness<br>Marked dyspnea, speaks only in single words or short phrases<br>Severe intercostal or sternocleidomastoid retractions<br>Cyanosis, pallor, or diaphoresis<br>Inaudible breath sounds<br>Subcutaneous or other extrapulmonary air<br>Oxygen saturation <90% if oximeter available<br>Peak expiratory flow rate <50% of predicted norm or baseline<br>$P_{CO_2}$ >40 mm Hg if arterial blood gases are available | If any of these conditions exist:<br>Give oxygen by ventimask or nasal cannula. If unable to generate PEFR, give epinephrine subcutaneously (SC), 0.01 ml/kg/dose of 1:1000 epinephrine with a maximum dose of 0.3 ml or SC terbutaline 0.01 mg/kg/dose. If able to generate PEFR, give nebulized albuterol 0.15 mg/kg/dose with 6-8 L/min of $O_2$ flow. Give systemic steroids at a prednisone equivalent of 2 mg/kg. Consider transfer to an appropriate emergency setting at an $FIO_2$ of 0.40 or greater and intermittent albuterol treatments every 20 min or continuous albuterol treatments at 0.5 mg/kg/hr if initial response is inadequate. If patient responds well to initial albuterol treatment, repeat twice every 20 minutes and provide *follow-up treatment.* |
| Does the patient have a history of:<br>Steroid-dependent asthma<br>Panic attacks with acute exacerbations<br>Duration of asthma >12 hours<br>History of respiratory failure<br>Premonitions of death<br>≥2 visits to office or ED in 24 hours<br>>3 visits in 48 hours<br>Paroxysmal attacks, especially at night | THIS IS A HIGH-RISK PATIENT. Begin therapy immediately as outlined above for moderate or severe exacerbation, regardless of the severity of the current episode. These are high-risk factors that should be considered in the decision to urgently transfer the patient to an appropriate emergency setting. If there is not a prompt clinical response to therapy, consider transfer and give systemic steroids (oral or parenteral) at a prednisone equivalent of 1-2 mg/kg before transfer. |

From American Academy of Pediatrics, Provisional Committee on Quality Improvement: Practice parameter: the office management of acute exacerbations of asthma in children, *Pediatrics* 93(1):119-126, 1994c; and National Asthma Education and Prevention Program: *Practical guide for the diagnosis and management of asthma,* NIH Pub No 97-4053, Bethesda, MD, October 1997, The Program.

*NOTE: This table presents only *one part* of the treatment of acute asthmatic episodes.

pulse oximetry measurements and observations of color, respiratory effort, and level of consciousness are essential. Humidified oxygen is administered by nasal prongs, hood, or face mask to maintain an arterial oxygen tension greater than 65 mm Hg but less than 100 mm Hg to avoid the danger of oxygen narcosis. Mist tents do not allow for the close observation needed for the severely affected child. Because oxygen is a stimulus for respiration, high levels may significantly depress respirations. Controlled ventilation with endotracheal intubation may be needed if the condition progresses to respiratory failure.

Inhaled aerosolized short-acting $\beta_2$-agonists are recommended for all patients. In the emergency department three treatments of $\beta_2$-agonists spaced 20 to 30 minutes apart are usually given as initial therapy. Systemic prednisone is also given. An anticholinergic such as ipratropium bromide may be added to the aerosolized solution of the $\beta_2$-agonist. Anticholinergics have been shown to result in additional bronchodilation in patients with severe airflow obstruction (Schuh and others, 1995). An IV infusion is often begun to provide a means for hydration and administering medications. Correction of dehydration, acidosis, hypoxia, and electrolyte disturbance is guided by frequent determination of arterial pH, blood gases, and serum electrolytes. If the pH is lower than 7.25, sodium bicarbonate may be administered to correct acidosis, because values this low tend to impair systemic, pulmonary, and coronary blood flow; normal pH enhances the response of bronchial smooth muscle to bronchodilator therapy.

IV fluids are infused at maintenance rates; rates higher than maintenance can cause pulmonary edema (Meng and Martorell, 1997). Aggressive hydration is not recommended for older children and adults but may be indicated for infants and young children. Infants and young children can become dehydrated as a result of increased respiratory rate and decreased oral intake. In caring for infants and young children, assessments of urine output, urine specific gravity, mucous membrane moisture, and electrolytes provide important data for decisions related to hydration (National Asthma Education and Prevention Program, 1997).

> **NURSING ALERT**
> Dehydration should be corrected slowly; overhydration can increase the accumulation of interstitial pulmonary fluid to exacerbate small airway obstruction.

Theophylline/aminophylline is not recommended in the emergency department because it usually provides no additional benefit to inhaled $\beta_2$-agonists and may increase adverse effects (Eggleston, 1999). If the child is currently taking a theophylline-containing preparation, however, a serum theophylline concentration should be obtained to rule out toxicity (National Asthma Education and Prevention Program, 1997). Antibiotics are given if pneumonia, otitis media, or sinusitis is present. As the attack subsides, fluids and medication are given orally (adrenergic agonists may be administered by MDI), and plans for discharge and follow-up care are made.

**Prognosis.** The outlook for children with asthma varies widely. Some children become asymptomatic at puberty, but up to two thirds of children with asthma continue to suffer from the disorder through puberty and adulthood.

The prognosis for control or disappearance of symptoms varies in children from those who have rare and infrequent episodes to those who are constantly wheezing or are subject to status asthmaticus. In general, when the symptoms are severe and numerous, when the symptoms have been present for a long time, and when there is a family history of allergy, there is a greater likelihood of a poor prognosis. Many children who "outgrow" their exacerbations continue to have airway hyperresponsiveness and cough as adults, and airway hyperresponsiveness in adults appears to be associated with an increase in the rate of decline of lung function (National Heart, Lung, and Blood Institute, 1995).

Although deaths from asthma have been relatively uncommon, especially in the young age-groups, since the 1970s the rate of death from asthma has increased steadily in the United States and other countries (Sherman and Capen, 1997). The adolescent age-group appears to be the most vulnerable, with the greatest increase occurring in children 10 to 14 years of age. No reliable data exist to explain this increase. Factors that have been postulated include exposure of atopic persons to more allergens, change in the severity of the disease, abuse of drug therapy (toxicity), failure of families and practitioners to recognize the severity of the asthma, and psychologic factors, such as denial or refusal to accept the disease. Risk factors for asthma deaths appear to be an onset at an early age, frequent attacks, difficult-to-manage disease, adolescence, history of respiratory failure, psychologic problems (refusal to take medications), dependency on or misuse of drugs (high use), presence of physical stigmata (barrel chest, intercostal retractions), and abnormal pulmonary function tests.

### Nursing Considerations: Acute Care

Children who are admitted to the hospital with acute asthma are ill, anxious, and uncomfortable. In many instances children are admitted from the emergency department in status asthmaticus and acute distress. The importance of continual observation and assessment cannot be overemphasized.

> **NURSING ALERT**
> The child who sweats profusely and remains sitting upright and refuses to lie down is in severe distress. Also, the child who suddenly becomes agitated, or the agitated child who suddenly becomes quiet, may be seriously hypoxic and requires immediate intervention.

When $\beta_2$-agonists and corticosteroids are given, the child is monitored closely and continuously for relief of respiratory distress and signs of side effects or toxicity. Vital signs are checked frequently.

Older children usually prefer the high-Fowler position, although they may be more comfortable sitting upright or leaning slightly forward. When possible, the nurse communicates in such a way that a child can reply in a few words to avoid fatigue. Shortness of breath makes talking difficult.

Children in status asthmaticus are apprehensive, anxious, and usually tired from respiratory efforts and loss of sleep. The calm, efficient presence of a nurse helps to reassure them that they are safe and will be cared for during this stressful period. It is important to assure children that they will not be left alone and that their parents will be allowed to remain with them.

Parents need reassurance and information about their child's condition and therapies. They are upset and apprehensive and may feel that they have in some way contributed to the child's condition or could have prevented the episode. They may be concerned about the appearance of symptoms despite their efforts to prevent or control the exacerbation. Reassurance about their efforts and their parenting capabilities helps to alleviate their stress. Efforts to reduce parental apprehension will also reduce the child's distress. Anxiety is easily communicated to the child from parents and members of the staff.

### Nursing Considerations: General Care

Nursing care of children with asthma involves both acute and long-term care. Nurses who are involved with children in the home, clinic, or practitioner's office play an important role in helping children and their families learn to live with the condition. The disease can be managed so that it does not require hospitalization or interfere with family life, physical activity, or school attendance.

## ⊞ Assessment

Physical assessment of asthma involves the same observations and techniques described in Chapters 7 and 31. In addition, physical characteristics of chronic respiratory involvement are noted and evaluated, including chest configuration (e.g., barrel chest), posturing, and type of breathing. A history of the current and previous episodes and precipitating factors or events provides important information.

Nurses assist with diagnostic tests, pulmonary function tests, and skin testing, as well as a general health assessment. Nurses also obtain assessments of how asthma impacts the child's everyday activities and self-concept, as well as the child and family's adherence to the prescribed therapy and their personal treatment goals. Every effort is made to build a partnership between the child and the family and the health care team. Communication is an essential part of this partnership, and health care providers should routinely assess the effectiveness of patient-provider communication. In particular, the child and family's satisfaction with asthma control and satisfaction with the quality of care should be assessed. The nurse should also assess the child and family's perception of the severity level of the disease, the family's level of social support, and any cultural or ethnic beliefs or practices that may influence self-management activities and necessitate modifications in the educational approaches to meet the needs of the family.

## ⊞ Nursing Diagnoses

Based on a thorough assessment, several nursing diagnoses are identified. The more common diagnoses for the child with asthma are included in the Nursing Care Plan on pp. 1402-1404. Others may apply in specific situations.

## ⊞ Planning

The goals for a child with asthma and the family include the following:

1. Child will not experience an asthmatic episode.
2. Child will exhibit improved ventilatory capacity.
3. Child will maintain optimum health.
4. Child will not develop complications.
5. Child will engage in normal activities for age.
6. Child and family will receive appropriate support and education regarding the disease and its management.

## ⊞ Implementation

The major emphasis of nursing care is directed toward outpatient management by the family. Parents are taught how to avoid allergens, to recognize and respond to symptoms of bronchospasm, to maintain health and prevent complications, and to promote normal activities. In some situations a case management approach by the nurse can be very successful in empowering patients and their families to manage their child's asthma (Kropfelder and Winkelstein, 1996).

**Avoid Allergens.** One goal of asthma management is avoidance of an exacerbation. Parents need to know how to avoid allergens and relieve asthmatic episodes. The nurse assists the parent in modifying the environment to reduce contact with the offending allergen(s). (See Family Home Care box on p. 1398.) The parents are cautioned to avoid exposing a sensitive child to excessive cold, wind, or other extremes of weather.

Foods known to provoke symptoms should be eliminated from the diet. Food additives, especially monosodium glutamate (MSG); sulfites, such as sulfur dioxide; sodium and potassium salts of sulfite, bisulfite, and metabisulfite; and dyes have been reported to produce allergic responses in sensitive persons. Families are taught to read labels carefully for the presence of these substances.

Approximately 2% to 6% of children with asthma are sensitive to aspirin; therefore nurses should caution parents to use other analgesic/antipyretic drugs for discomfort or fever and to read package labeling. Although aspirin is rarely given to children in the United States, salicylate compounds are in other common medications, such as Pepto-Bismol. Acetaminophen is safe for these children and is recommended as the analgesic of choice. Children with aspirin-induced asthma may also be sensitive to nonsteroidal antiinflammatory drugs and tartrazine (yellow dye number 5, a common food coloring). Other drugs to avoid are antihistamines (dry airway secretions, making expectoration difficult), cough suppressants (impair clearance of secretions), and sedatives (depress respirations and aggravate hypoventilation).

**Relieve Bronchospasm.** Parents and older children are taught to recognize early signs and symptoms of an im-

## FAMILY HOME CARE
### "Allergy-Proofing" the Home and Community

Keep humidity between 30% and 50%; use dehumidifier or air conditioner if available; keep air conditioners clean and free of mold; do not use vaporizers or humidifiers.

Encase pillows in zippered allergen-impermeable covers or wash pillows in hot water (at least 54.4° C [130° F]) every week.

Encase mattress and box springs in zippered allergen-impermeable cover.

Use foam rubber mattress and pillows or Dacron pillows and synthetic blankets.

Wash bed linens every 7 to 10 days in hot water (at least 54.4° C).

Encase polyester comforters in allergen-impermeable covers or wash in hot water (at least 54.4° C) every week; if possible, do not use comforters and use cotton blankets.

Do not use a canopy above the bed; children should not sleep on the bottom bunk of a bunk bed.

Store nothing under the bed; keep clothing in a closet with the door shut.

Use washable window shades; avoid heavy curtains; if curtains are used, launder them frequently.

Remove all carpeting if possible; if not possible, vacuum carpet once or twice a week while the child wears a mask; have child remain out of the room while vacuuming occurs and for 30 minutes after vacuuming.

If possible, use a central vacuum cleaner with a collecting bag outside of the home or use cleaner filters (e.g., high-efficiency particulate air [HEPA] filters).

Have air and heating ducts cleaned annually; change or clean filters monthly; cover heating vents with filter material (e.g., cheesecloth) to prevent circulation of dust, especially when heat is turned on after summer.

Remove unnecessary furniture, rugs, stuffed or real animals, toys, books, upholstered furniture, plants, aquariums, and wall hangings from child's room.

Use wipeable furniture (wood, plastic, vinyl, or leather) in place of upholstered furniture; avoid rattan or wicker furniture.

Cover walls with washable paint or wallpaper.

Limit child's exposure to animals, rabbits, gerbils, hamsters at school; teach child to stay away from zoos, petting farms, and neighbor's pets.

Change child's clothes after playing outdoors; wash child's hair nightly if child is outside and pollen count is high.

Keep child indoors while lawn is being mowed, bushes/trees are being trimmed, or pollen count is high.

Keep windows and doors closed during pollen season; use air conditioner if possible or go to places that are air conditioned, such as libraries and shopping malls, when the weather is hot.

Wet-mop bare floors weekly; wet-dust and clean child's room weekly; child should not be present during cleaning activities.

Wash showers and shower curtains with bleach or Lysol at least once a month.

Limit or avoid child's exposure to tobacco and wood smoke; do not allow cigarette smoking in the house or car; select daycare centers, play areas, and shopping malls that are smoke-free.

Avoid odors or sprays (e.g., perfumes, talcum powder, room deodorizers, chalk dust at school, fresh paint, or cleaning solutions).

Avoid cellar (basement) as a play area if it is damp and use a dehumidifier in damp basement.

Cover all food, including pet food, and put food away in cabinets.

Store garbage in closed containers.

Use pesticide sprays, roach bait traps, and boric acid powder to kill cockroaches; if living in an apartment or adjacent housing, encourage neighbors to work together to get rid of cockroaches and mice.

Repair leaking or dripping faucets; seal cracks and crevices in cabinets and pantry areas.

---

pending attack so that it can be controlled before symptoms become distressing. Many children can recognize prodromal symptoms well before an attack (about 6 hours), and preventive therapy can be implemented. Objective signs that parents may observe include rhinorrhea, cough, low-grade fever, irritability, itching (especially in front of the neck and chest), apathy, anxiety, sleep disturbance, abdominal discomfort, and loss of appetite. A variety of easy-to-use, inexpensive *peak expiratory flow meters (PEFMs)* are available for use in the home and at school to assess changes in pulmonary function. (See Family Home Care box.)

In general, children 5 years of age and older are able to use a peak flow meter successfully. However, young children need to be supervised while they are learning to use their peak flow meter, and their technique should be checked frequently to be sure it is correct. Children should use the same peak flow meter over time, and they should bring their peak flow meter for use at every follow-up visit. Using the same brand of meter is recommended because different brands can give significantly different values. Measurements from the same brand are fairly consistent, and once children establish their personal best on their own meter, they can obtain reliable and clinically meaningful readings each time a peak flow measurement is obtained. Specific peak flow values for the child's individual red, yellow, and green

zones should be noted on the child's written asthma action plan. This plan should be kept in a convenient place both at home and in school. When the child's peak flow meter is replaced, the child needs to reestablish the personal best value with the new meter.

Children who use a *metered dose inhaler (MDI)* (see Fig. 32-9) need to learn how to use the device correctly. The MDI delivers medication directly to the airways; therefore the child needs to learn to breathe slowly and deeply for better airway distribution. (See Family Home Care box.)

*Spacers or holding chambers* are devices that attach to an MDI and hold the medication in the chamber long enough for the patient to inhale the medicine during one or two slow, deep breaths. (See Critical Thinking Exercise box.) Spacers provide proper dosing and delivery of medications to the small airway and can be beneficial to children of all ages, especially those who have difficulty using proper inhalation technique (Togger and Brenner, 2001). Spacers or holding chambers may be used with all inhaled medications, but they are recommended for use with inhaled steroids to prevent yeast infections in the mouth.

The child and parents also need to be cautioned about the adverse effects of prescribed drugs and the dangers of overuse of $\beta_2$-agonists. They should know that it is important to use them when needed but not indiscriminately or as a

## FAMILY HOME CARE
### Use of a Peak Expiratory Flow Meter

1. Before each use, make sure the sliding marker or arrow on the PEFM is at the bottom of the numbered scale.
2. Stand up straight.
3. Remove gum or any food from the mouth.
4. Close your lips tightly around the mouthpiece. Be sure to keep your tongue away from the mouthpiece.
5. Blow out as hard and as quickly as you can, a "fast hard puff."
6. Note the number by the marker on the numbered scale.
7. Repeat entire routine three times; but wait at least 30 seconds between each routine.
8. Record the *highest* of the three readings, not the average.
9. Measure your peak expiratory flow rate (PEFR) close to the same time and same way each day (i.e., morning and evening; before and 15 minutes after taking medication).
10. Keep a chart of your PEFRs.

## Critical Thinking Exercise

### Asthma

Traditional thinking about the pathophysiology of asthma has changed in recent years. Which one of the following treatments reflects this better understanding of the mechanisms involved in an asthmatic episode?

FIRST, THINK ABOUT IT . . .

• What precise question are you trying to answer?
• What conclusions are you reaching?

1. Peak expiratory flow meter (PEFM)
2. Metered-dose inhaler (MDI)
3. Allergy hyposensitization
4. Chest physiotherapy

*The best response is two. Inflammation of the bronchial airways is now recognized as a critical component in the pathophysiology of asthma. The conclusion that MDIs are used to deliver corticosteroids to decrease the inflammation is correct. The PEFM is an assessment device; the other two choices have been used traditionally.*

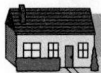

## FAMILY HOME CARE
### Use of a Metered-Dose Inhaler*

**STEPS FOR CHECKING HOW MUCH MEDICINE IS IN THE CANISTER**

1. If the canister is new, it is full.
2. If the canister has been used repeatedly, it might be empty. (Check product label to see how many inhalations should be in each canister.)
3. The most accurate way to determine how many doses remain in an MDI is to count and record each actuation as it is used.
4. Many dry powder inhalers have a dose-counting device or dose indicator on the canister to let you know when the canister is empty.
5. Placing dry powder inhalers or MDIs with hydrofluoroalkanes in water will destroy these inhalers.

**STEPS FOR USING THE INHALER**

1. Remove the cap and hold inhaler upright.
2. Shake the inhaler.
3. Tilt the head back slightly and breathe out slowly.
4. With the inhaler in an upright position, insert the mouthpiece:
   a. About 3 to 4 cm from the mouth *or*
   b. Into an aerochamber *or* spacer
   c. Into the mouth, forming an airtight seal between the lips and the mouthpiece
5. At the end of a normal expiration, depress the top of the inhaler canister firmly to release the medication (into either the aerochamber or the mouth), and breathe in slowly (about 3 to 5 seconds). Relax the pressure on the top of the canister.
6. Hold the breath for at least 5 to 10 seconds to allow the aerosol medication to reach deeply into the lungs.
7. Remove the inhaler and breathe out slowly through the nose.
8. Wait 1 minute between puffs (if an additional puff is needed).

Modified from Nurses' Asthma Education Working Group: *Nurses: partners in asthma care*, NIH Pub No 95-3308, Bethesda, MD, 1995, National Heart Lung and Blood Institute, National Institutes of Health.
*NOTE: Inhaled dry powder such as Pulmicort requires a different inhalation technique. To use a dry powder inhaler, the base of the device is turned until a click is heard. It is important to close the mouth tightly around the mouthpiece of the inhaler and inhale rapidly.

---

substitute for avoiding the symptom-provoking allergen. Parents and children are taught to report any changing reaction to a drug or if the drug appears to be losing its effectiveness, as evidenced by a more frequent need for the drug. Parents are also cautioned against purchasing over-the-counter preparations because these medications can place the child at risk for increased dosage of a drug and toxicity.

**Maintain Health and Prevent Complications.** The child should be protected from a respiratory infection that can trigger an attack or aggravate the asthmatic state, especially in young children, whose airways are mechanically smaller and more reactive. It is well established that viral respiratory infections (in particular, infections with the respiratory syn-

cytial virus [RSV], rhinovirus, and influenza virus) can exacerbate asthma. Annual influenza vaccinations are recommended for patients with persistent asthma (American Academy of Pediatrics, 1998a). (See Immunizations, Chapter 12.)

The equipment used for the child, such as nebulizers, must be kept absolutely clean to decrease the chance of contamination with bacteria and fungi. Oral candidiasis is a major complication of aerosolized steroids; therefore children with severe asthma who are taking steroids by this route are taught to use a spacer and to rinse the mouth thoroughly with water after each treatment to minimize the risk of infection.

Breathing exercises and controlled breathing are taught and encouraged for the motivated youngster. The nurse can provide information concerning activities that promote diaphragmatic breathing, side expansion, and improved mobility of the chest wall.

**NURSING TIP** Play techniques that can be used as breathing exercises for younger children to extend their expiratory time and increase expiratory pressure include blowing cotton balls or a Ping-Pong ball on a table, blowing a pinwheel, or preventing a tissue from falling by blowing it against the wall.

**NURSING TIP** To reduce the probability of an asthmatic episode triggered by cold air, teach the child to breathe through the nose (not the mouth). Also, a reservoir of warm air can be created by having the child wear a mask or swaddling the nose and mouth in a scarf when in cold air.

Asthma camps have become popular in recent years as a means of encouraging physical activity in a more homogeneous, controlled, and less competitive environment. Children who attend asthma camps have improved attitudes toward asthma, increased participation in sports activities, improved self-management skills, and reduced school absences and hospital visits (Meng, 1997).

**Promote Normal Activities.** Self-care is the hallmark of effective asthma management, and self-management programs are important in helping the child and family to learn as much as possible about the factors that precipitate an asthmatic episode and the most effective means of bringing the disease under control.

However, self-care does not mean self-treatment. For young children, co-management concepts are important: the child, family, and health care provider must all work together as a team. (See Family Focus box.)

Effective management programs focus on building skills and confidence, not just providing information. When appropriate, nurses should use the following six Rs in their interactions with children and their family members (Nurses' Asthma Education Working Group, 1995):

1. Respect the child and the parents and show them that they are important and valued.
2. Recognize the family's belief system and remember that beliefs provide the basis for the development of a treatment plan and can aid in the success of the plan.
3. Reach agreement on goals and what is expected in the asthma treatment plan.
4. Rehearse important skills such as how to use the MDI, nebulizer, and peak flow meter, as well as what to do when an exacerbation occurs.
5. Repeat key points three times during a session; have more than one person repeat key information during office visits.
6. Reinforce in the form of praise in subsequent sessions; ask school personnel, including teachers and sports coaches, to reinforce the same messages.

Most self-management programs convey several principles to the child and family. First, asthma is a common disease, and to have asthma is annoying but not disgraceful. Even though emotions have been implicated in asthma, psychologic aspects are primarily a response to it rather than a cause. Emotions and stress can be major triggers, but the disease, not the individual, is responsible for the symptoms.

Second, persons with asthma can live full and active lives. Learning about others who have accomplished their goals (e.g., Theodore Roosevelt) and meeting children of the

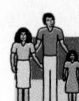

**FAMILY FOCUS**
*Asthma: The Relief of Knowing*

Today we have very different feelings about our son's asthma than we did when he had his first attack. My husband and I were terrified then; we didn't know what was going on. We only knew that our child, John, could not breathe. We felt so helpless and were afraid that he might die. After rushing John to the emergency department and spending the night there, we were referred to an allergist. After performing several tests, this doctor told us that John definitely had asthma and that he would work with us to help us manage John's condition. He placed John on several daily asthma medications and told us the purpose for all the medications. He gave us specific written instructions and a plan to follow that we put on the refrigerator at home and also gave to the school nurse. Before we left the allergy clinic, we also spoke with the nurse, who gave us several pamphlets and books about asthma. She showed us how to use John's inhaler and his flow meter, and told us she would call us to see how we were doing in the next week. When we left the office, we felt such a sense of relief. For us, just knowing what our child had was so helpful. Although it has not always been easy, and despite the fact that John still has some asthmatic episodes, we now feel more confident that we know what to look for, how to read the cues to impending danger, and how to cope with this condition that was once so terrifying.

Mother of John (10), who has had asthma for 5 years

same age who are dealing effectively with their disease, including engaging in age-related activities (e.g., sports), provide positive examples of what is possible.

Third, it is much easier to prevent than to treat an asthmatic episode. Compliance with a therapeutic program and learning the activities or factors that trigger an episode are important. Appropriate drug therapy, environmental control, education, and self-management skills can prevent exacerbations.

Many approaches are used to facilitate self-management. Self-contained programs and brochures for patient education are available from the **Asthma and Allergy Foundation of America (AAFA)*** and the **American Lung Association.†** The **National Heart, Lung, and Blood Institute‡** provides educational materials for asthma education in the school setting and also copies of the *Expert Panel Report II: Guidelines for the Diagnosis and Management of Asthma* for the practitioner. Another publication designed for health care practitioners is entitled *Pediatric Asthma: Promoting Best Practice.* This publication can be obtained from the **American Academy of Allergy, Asthma and Immunology.§**

Asthma education and awareness are an important aspect of asthma management. Although the principles of self-management and the educational programs designed for children with asthma are fairly generic, specific content and intervention strategies must be personalized to the con-

---

*1125 15th St, Washington, DC 20005, (202) 466-7643 or (800) 7-ASTHMA; www.aafa.org.
†National office: 1740 Broadway, New York, NY 10019, (212) 315-8700 or (800) LUNG-USA; www.lungusa.org.
‡National Heart, Lung, and Blood Institute Information Center, Code AS-ASHA, PO Box 30105, Bethesda, MD 20824-0105, fax: (301) 251-1223; www.nhlbi.nih.gov/nhlbi.htm.
§611 E Wells St, Milwaukee, WI 53202, (414) 272-6071; fax: (414) 272-6070.

cerns and agendas of individual children and their families (Yoos and McMullen, 1996).

**Child and Family Support.** The nurse working with children with asthma can provide support in several ways. Many asthmatic children voice frustration because asthmatic episodes interfere with their daily activities and social lives. Children need reassurance from the health team and reinforcement of their coping mechanisms.

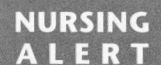 Be aware of children, especially adolescents, who are depressed and may not comply with therapy as a means of passive suicide. Refer these youngsters for psychologic support.

Both short- and long-term adaptation of affected children depends on the family's acceptance of the disorder. The task of living day to day with affected children involves the family continually. There are periodic crises and the ever-present threat of a crisis, requiring parental vigilance, sleepless nights, frequent trips to the physician's office or hospital, and often overwhelming medical expenses. Throughout these stresses, parents are encouraged to promote as normal a life as possible for their children.

## ⁝⁝ Evaluation

The effectiveness of nursing interventions is determined by continual reassessment and evaluation of care based on the following observational guidelines:

1. Interview family about removal or avoidance of known allergens.
2. Observe child for evidence of respiratory symptoms.
3. Assess child's general health.
4. Observe child and interview family about any infections or other complications.
5. Interview child about daily activities.
6. Determine the degree to which the family and child understand the child's condition and the extent to which the therapies are carried out.

The **expected outcomes** are described in the Nursing Care Plan on pp. 1402-1404.

## Cystic Fibrosis (CF)

CF, a condition characterized by exocrine (or mucus-producing) gland dysfunction that produces multisystem involvement, is the most common lethal genetic illness among white children, adolescents, and young adults.

It is estimated that 1 in 29 Caucasians in the United States are symptom-free carriers. Although more than 95% of the documented cases of CF occur in Caucasians (1 in 3300 live births), the incidence in African-Americans is 1 in 16,300 births and in Asians 1 in 32,100 births (Rosenstein, 1999).

In 1966 the median life expectancy for individuals with CF was 7.5 years; by 1996, the median life expectancy had increased to 31 years (Rosenstein, 1999). Recent advances in new therapies, the impact of protein and gene therapy, continued aggressive chest physiotherapy, aerosolized antibiotic therapy, and nutritional education make the outlook more hopeful.

### Etiology

CF is inherited as an autosomal recessive trait; the affected child inherits the defective gene from both parents, with an overall incidence of 1:4. (See Chapter 5.) The mutated gene responsible for CF is located on the long arm of chromosome 7. This gene codes a protein of 1,480 amino acids called the *cystic fibrosis transmembrane regulator (CFTR)*. The CFTR protein is related to a family of membrane-bound glycoproteins. The glycoproteins constitute a cAMP-activated chloride channel and also regulate other chloride and sodium channels at the surfaces of the epithelial cells. Functional expression of the CF defect reduces the ability of the epithelial cells in the airways and pancreas to transport chloride. Abnormal transport of sodium and chloride across the epithelium is thought to lead to increased viscosity of airway mucus, abnormal mucociliary clearance, and lung disease.

The F508 gene mutation is the most common alteration found in CF. It occurs in 70% of all known CF chromosomes and is closely related to pancreatic insufficiency. Most of the remaining cases of CF are explained by more than 700 other mutations. However, approximately 2% of the cases of CF cannot be explained genetically (Rosenstein, 1999).

### Pathophysiology

With the discovery of the CFTR gene, research is continuing to determine its multisystem effects on the body. CF is characterized by several unrelated clinical features: increased viscosity of mucous gland secretions, a striking elevation of sweat electrolytes, an increase in several organic and enzymatic constituents of saliva, and abnormalities in autonomic nervous system function. Although both sodium and chloride are affected, the defect appears to be primarily a result of abnormal chloride movement.

Children with CF demonstrate decreased pancreatic secretion of bicarbonate and chloride and an increase in sodium and chloride in both saliva and sweat. This last characteristic is the basis for the sweat chloride diagnostic test.

The sweat electrolyte abnormality is present from birth, continues throughout life, and is unrelated to the severity of the disease or the extent to which other organs are involved. The sodium and chloride content of sweat in children with CF is two to five times greater than that of the controls in 98% to 99% of affected children.

The primary factor, and the one responsible for many of the clinical manifestations of the disease, is mechanical obstruction caused by the increased viscosity of mucous gland secretions (Fig. 32-10 on p. 1405). Instead of forming a thin, freely flowing secretion, the mucous glands produce a thick, inspissated mucoprotein that accumulates and dilates them. Small passages in organs such as the pancreas and bronchioles become obstructed as secretions precipitate or coagulate to form concretions in glands and ducts.

**Respiratory Tract.** Because of the increased viscosity of bronchial mucus, there is greater resistance to ciliary action (probably secondary to infection and ciliary destruction), a slower flow rate of mucus, and incomplete expectoration, which also contributes to the mucous obstruction. This retained mucus serves as an excellent medium for bacterial

# Nursing Care Plan
## The Child with Asthma

---

**NURSING DIAGNOSIS:** Risk for suffocation related to interaction between individual and allergen(s)

---

**PATIENT GOAL 1:** Will experience no asthmatic episode

- **NURSING INTERVENTIONS/*RATIONALES***

Teach child and family how to avoid conditions or circumstances that precipitate asthmatic episode

Assist parents in eliminating allergens or other stimuli that trigger exacerbation (see Box 32-17 for complete listing), such as:

Meal planning to eliminate allergenic foods

Removal of pets

Modification of environment: "allergy-proof" home, especially no smoking in home

Avoid extremes of environmental temperature

When child is exposed to cold air, recommend breathing through nose (not mouth) and wearing a mask or scarf, or cupping hand over nose and mouth *to create a reservoir of warm air to breathe*

Assist parents in obtaining and installing device to control environment (dehumidifier, air conditioner, electronic air filter)

Teach child and family to recognize early signs and symptoms *so that an impending episode can be controlled before it becomes distressful*

Teach child and family correct use of bronchodilators and antiinflammatory drugs (e.g., corticosteroids, cromolyn sodium), adverse effects, and dangers of overuse or underuse of drugs

Teach child to understand how equipment works

Teach child correct use of inhalers, nebulizers, and peak expiratory flow meters (PEFMs)

Teach child and family prophylactic treatment when appropriate (e.g., prevent exercise-induced bronchospasm by using medication before exercise)

Explain to child and family possible benefits of hyposensitization therapy when allergen(s) can be defined and cannot be avoided (e.g., pollen, mold) or controlled satisfactorally by drugs

*Administer hyposensitization therapy if prescribed

- **EXPECTED OUTCOMES**

Family makes every effort to remove or avoid possible allergens or precipitating events

Child/family are able to detect signs of an impending episode early and implement appropriate actions

Child/family are able to administer medications and use inhalers and other equipment

---

**PATIENT GOAL 2:** Will experience optimum health

- **NURSING INTERVENTIONS/*RATIONALES***

Encourage sound health practices *to support body's natural defenses:*

Balanced, nutritious diet

Adequate rest

Good hygiene

Appropriate exercise

Follow-up care

Prevent respiratory infection *because it can trigger an attack or aggravate the asthmatic state*

Avoid exposure to infection

Take meticulous care of equipment *to avoid bacterial or fungal growth*

Use good handwashing

- **EXPECTED OUTCOMES**

Child and parents practice sound health practices

Child exhibits no evidence of infection

---

**NURSING DIAGNOSIS:** Ineffective airway clearance related to allergenic response and inflammation in the bronchial tree

---

**PATIENT GOAL 1:** Will exhibit evidence of improved ventilatory capacity

- **NURSING INTERVENTIONS/*RATIONALES***

Instruct in or supervise breathing exercises and controlled breathing *to promote proper diaphragmatic breathing, side expansion, and improved chest wall mobility*

Use play techniques for breathing exercises with young children (e.g., blow a pinwheel or blow cotton balls on table *to extend expiratory time and increase expiratory pressure*)

Teach correct use of prescribed medications

Teach correct use of PEFM, nebulizer, and metered-dose inhaler (MDI) if indicated

Teach family to perform percussion and postural drainage and to encourage coughing if indicated

Encourage physical exercise

Recommend activities requiring short bursts of energy (e.g., baseball, sprints, skiing) *because they may be better tolerated than those requiring endurance exercise* (e.g., soccer, distance running)

Recommend swimming *because child breathes air saturated with moisture, and exhaling underwater prolongs expiration and increases end-expiratory pressure*

Restrict physical activity only when child's condition makes it necessary

Encourage good posture *for maximum lung expansion*

Assist child and family in selecting activities appropriate to child's capabilities and preferences

- **EXPECTED OUTCOMES**

Child breathes easily and without dyspnea

Child exhibits improved ventilatory capacity (specify)

Child engages in activities according to abilities and interest (specify)

---

**NURSING DIAGNOSIS:** Activity intolerance related to imbalance between oxygen supply and demand

---

**PATIENT GOAL 1:** Will receive optimum rest

- **NURSING INTERVENTIONS/*RATIONALES***

Encourage activities appropriate to child's condition and capabilities (specify)

---

*Dependent nursing action.

# Nursing Care Plan
## The Child with Asthma—cont'd

Provide ample opportunities for sleep, rest, and quiet activities to conserve oxygen supply

- **EXPECTED OUTCOMES**

Child engages in appropriate activities (specify)
Child appears rested

> **NURSING DIAGNOSIS:** Interrupted family processes related to having a child with a chronic illness

**PATIENT/FAMILY GOAL 1:** Will exhibit positive adaptation to the condition

- **NURSING INTERVENTIONS/***RATIONALES*

Foster positive family relationships
Reinforce positive coping mechanisms of child and family
Use every opportunity to increase parents' and child's understanding of the disease and its therapies, *because adequate knowledge is related to family's timely use of preventive and emergency intervention*
Reinforce the need for responding to early signs of impending asthma episode using prescribed medications as needed *to decrease potential for a severe exacerbation*
Intervene appropriately if there is evidence of maladaptation
Be alert to signs of parental rejection or overprotection
Be alert to signs that child is depressed and make appropriate referral for psychologic support, *because depressed children, especially adolescents, may not comply with therapies as a means of passive suicide*
Teach child and family how to give respiratory treatments *to eliminate any confusion* regarding medication or inhalers/nebulizers
Encourage family to contact school personnel (e.g., nurse, teachers, coaches, principal) to develop a consistent plan of care for school setting
Refer family to appropriate support groups and community agencies

- **EXPECTED OUTCOMES**

Family copes with symptoms and effects of the disease and provides a normal environment for the child
See Nursing Care Plan: The Child with Chronic Illness or Disability, Chapter 22

## STATUS ASTHMATICUS (SPECIAL NEEDS)

> **NURSING DIAGNOSIS:** Risk for suffocation related to bronchospasm, mucus secretions, edema

**PATIENT GOAL 1:** Will experience cessation of bronchospasm

- **NURSING INTERVENTIONS/***RATIONALES*

Establish IV infusion *for administration of medication and hydration*
*Administer aerosolized bronchodilators and either oral or IV corticosteroids with or without epinephrine as prescribed *to relieve bronchospasm*
Carefully monitor IV aminophylline infusion or oral theophylline *for maximum efficacy and minimum side effects*

*Dependent nursing action.

Closely monitor vital signs before, during, and after administration for maximum efficacy and minimum side effects
Interview parents to determine medications given before admission to avoid possible overdose
Have emergency equipment and medications readily available *to prevent delay in treatment*

- **EXPECTED OUTCOMES**

Child breathes more easily
Child does not suffocate

**PATIENT GOAL 2:** Will exhibit normal respiratory function

- **NURSING INTERVENTIONS/***RATIONALES*

Administer humidified oxygen by tent, face mask, or cannula *to maintain satisfactory oxygenation*
Closely monitor oxygen saturations and blood gases via pulse oximetry *to detect early or impending hypoxia*
Closely monitor percentage of oxygen delivered, *because high levels may depress respirations*
Position *for optimum lung expansion*
  High-Fowler position
  Provide overbed table with pillow on which to lean if more comfortable for child
Implement measures to reduce fear/anxiety *to decrease respiratory efforts and oxygen consumption*
Encourage relaxation techniques *to decrease anxiety and promote lung expansion*
*Administer sedatives and tranquilizing agents, if prescribed, with extreme caution and when agitation is not caused by anoxia, *because these drugs can depress respirations and mask signs of anoxia*
Organize activities to allow for rest, sleep, and minimum expenditure of energy

- **EXPECTED OUTCOMES**

Child's respirations are unlabored and within normal limits (see inside back cover)
Child rests and sleeps comfortably
Child does not experience decreased oxygen saturations

**PATIENT GOAL 3:** Will successfully expel bronchial secretions

- **NURSING INTERVENTIONS/***RATIONALES*

Provide adequate hydration, oral or IV, *to liquefy secretions for easier removal*
Maintain nothing by mouth (NPO), if necessary, *to prevent aspiration of fluids and food*
Provide humidified atmosphere *to prevent drying of mucous membranes*
Encourage child to cough effectively
  Provide tissues
  Explain need to remove secretions
Suction, using correct technique, only when necessary
Do not use chest physiotherapy (CPT) during an acute episode, *because it will only agitate an already-anxious, dyspneic child and aggravate the episode*
Position, if necessary, *to prevent aspiration of secretions*
  Semiprone
  Side-lying

*Continued*

# Nursing Care Plan
## The Child with Asthma—cont'd

- **EXPECTED OUTCOMES**

Secretions are adequately and easily expelled

Child coughs effectively

Child does not aspirate secretions, food, or fluids

> **NURSING DIAGNOSIS:** Risk for deficient fluid volume related to difficulty taking fluids, insensible fluid losses from hyperventilation, and diaphoresis

**PATIENT GOAL 1:** Will exhibit adequate hydration

- **NURSING INTERVENTIONS/*RATIONALES***

Maintain IV infusion at appropriate rate, *because fluid therapy will enhance liquifaction of secretions* (IV usually run two-thirds to three-quarters maintenance [unless dehydration present] in order to minimize the risk of pulmonary edema because of high inspiratory pressures)

Encourage oral fluids

Offer fluids when acute respiratory distress subsides *to decrease risk of aspiration*

Avoid cold liquids *because they can trigger reflex bronchospasm*

Give fluids (and food) in small, frequent feedings *to avoid abdominal distention that might interfere with diaphragmatic excursion*

Use play techniques appropriate to child's age *to encourage fluid intake*

Measure intake and output

Correct dehydration slowly, *because overhydration can increase the accumulation of interstitial pulmonary fluid, leading to increased airway obstruction*

- **EXPECTED OUTCOME**

Child exhibits adequate hydration

> **NURSING DIAGNOSIS:** Risk for injury (respiratory acidosis, electrolyte imbalance) related to hypoventilation, dehydration

**PATIENT GOAL 1:** Will not experience acidosis

- **NURSING INTERVENTIONS/*RATIONALES***

Closely monitor blood pH, *because pH less than 7.25 impairs systemic, pulmonary, and coronary blood flow, and normal pH enhances effect of bronchodilators*

*Administer sodium bicarbonate as ordered *to prevent or correct acidosis*

---

*Dependent nursing action.

Maintain IV infusion *for administration of emergency medications and to prevent dehydration*

Prevent vomiting and subsequent dehydration; initially child will experience alkalosis, but if vomiting becomes severe or uncontrolled, can lead to acidosis

Implement measures to improve ventilation; *hypoventilation may cause an accumulation of carbon dioxide, which will decrease pH*

- **EXPECTED OUTCOME**

Child exhibits no evidence of respiratory acidosis

**PATIENT GOAL 2:** Will exhibit normal serum electrolytes

- **NURSING INTERVENTIONS/*RATIONALES***

Closely monitor serum electrolytes, *because dehydration, as well as medications, can alter normal serum electrolytes*

Maintain IV infusion at appropriate rate

Prevent dehydration and vomiting, *because they cause electrolyte imbalances*

- **EXPECTED OUTCOME**

Child exhibits normal serum electrolytes

> **NURSING DIAGNOSIS:** Interrupted family processes related to emergency hospitalization of child

**PATIENT/FAMILY GOAL 1:** Will experience reduction of anxiety

- **NURSING INTERVENTIONS/*RATIONALES***

Keep parents informed of child's condition

Encourage expression of feelings, especially severity of condition and prognosis

Allow parents to be with child as much as possible by encouraging family-centered care concepts

Point out any evidence of improvement *to encourage positive coping behaviors*

If/when possible, schedule treatments and care to child's routines

Reduce sensory stimuli by maintaining quiet, relaxed environment

- **EXPECTED OUTCOMES**

Family verbalizes concerns and spends time with child

Family exhibits no signs of distress

See also:

Nursing Care Plan: The Family of the Child Who Is Ill or Hospitalized, Chapter 26

Nursing Care Plan: The Child in the Hospital, Chapter 26

---

growth. Reduced oxygen–carbon dioxide exchange causes variable degrees of hypoxia, hypercapnia, and acidosis. In severe, progressive lung involvement, compression of pulmonary blood vessels and progressive lung dysfunction frequently lead to pulmonary hypertension, cor pulmonale, respiratory failure, and death.

Pulmonary complications are present in almost all children with CF, but the onset and extent of involvement are variable. Symptoms are produced by stagnation of mucus in the airways, with eventual bacterial colonization leading to destruction of lung tissue. The abnormally viscous and tenacious secretions are difficult to expectorate and gradually obstruct the bronchi and bronchioles, causing scattered areas of bronchietasis, atelectasis, and emphysema. The stagnant mucus offers a favorable environment for bacterial growth.

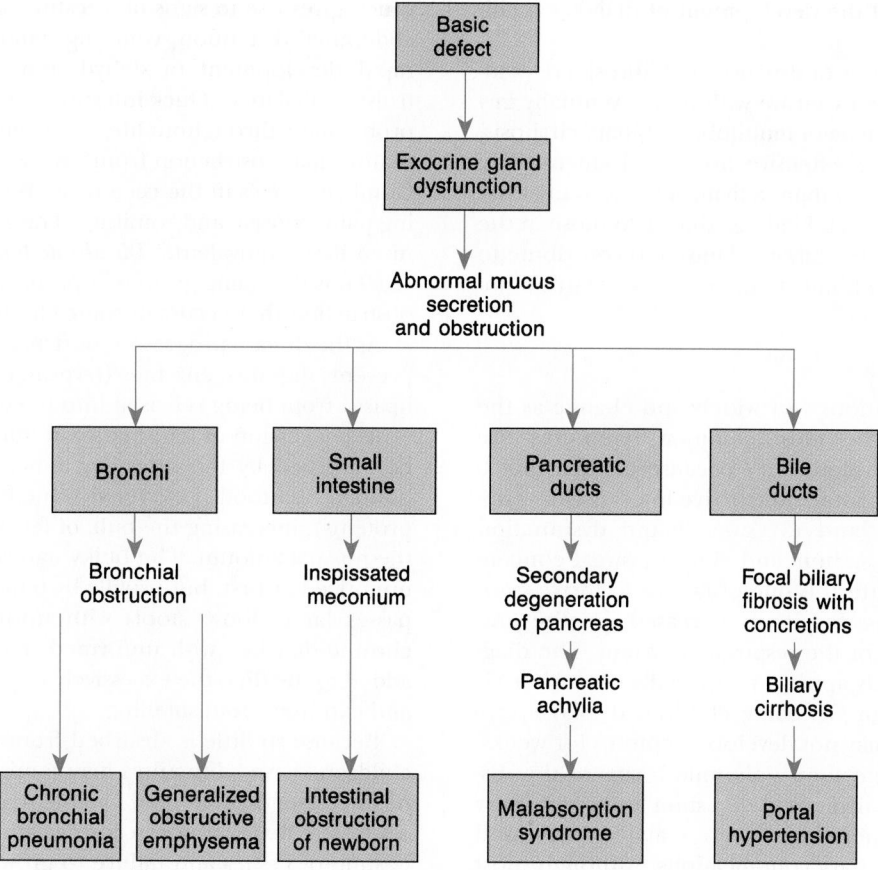

**Fig. 32-10**   Various effects of exocrine gland dysfunction in cystic fibrosis.

The most common pathogens are *Pseudomonas aeruginosa, Burkholderia cepacia, S. aureus, H. influenzae, Escherichia coli,* and *Klebsiella pneumoniae* (Hagemann, 1996). The pseudomonal strains are particularly pathogenic for children with CF because in most patients the alveolar macrophages cannot destroy *Pseudomonas* organisms. The pseudomonal strains also quickly develop resistance to most medications by developing mucoid strains, and once a person with CF is colonized with these organisms, they are difficult to eradicate. *B. cepacia* is especially worrisome, because this organism is extremely virulent, produces a bacteremia, and has been associated with rapid pulmonary function deterioration and death in approximately 20% of patients with mild or moderate CF (Rosenstein, 1999).

*P. aeruginosa* infection is not specific for CF but occurs much more frequently in CF than in other diseases characterized by chronic airway obstruction. Multiple antibodies developed by the patient to the bacteria are ineffective in controlling infection, and the host is able to tolerate large concentrations of bacteria without overt evidence of worsening.

Gradual progression of pulmonary disease follows chronic infection; bronchial epithelium is destroyed; and infection spreads to peribronchial tissues, resulting in weakening of bronchial walls and peribronchial fibrosis. The pattern is chronic, progressive fibrosis with decreased oxygen–carbon dioxide exchange and a concurrent alteration in pulmonary vasculature. Chronic hypoxemia causes contraction and hypertrophy of medial muscle fibers in pulmonary arteries and arterioles, leading to pulmonary hypertension and eventual cor pulmonale. Pneumothorax may occur when peripheral bullae rupture; hemoptysis can occur with the erosion of bronchial arteries into a bronchus.

**Gastrointestinal Tract.**   The extent of gastrointestinal involvement varies. In the pancreas of many patients, the thick secretions block the ducts, leading to cystic dilations of the acini (small lobes of the gland), which then undergo degeneration and progressive diffuse fibrosis. This event prevents essential pancreatic enzymes from reaching the duodenum, which causes marked impairment in the digestion and absorption of nutrients, particularly fats, proteins, and, to a lesser degree, carbohydrates. Disturbed absorption is reflected in excessive stool fat *(steatorrhea)* and protein *(azotorrhea).*

The endocrine function of the pancreas often remains unchanged, because the islets of Langerhans are normal but may decrease in number as pancreatic fibrosis progresses. The incidence of diabetes mellitus is greater in CF children than in the general population, which may be caused by changes in pancreatic architecture and diminished blood supply over time. Consequently, with increased survival, type 1 diabetes is becoming a more frequent finding. There is no relationship between the progression of pulmonary disease and the development of diabetes mellitus in CF.

In the liver, focal biliary obstruction and fibrosis are common and become more extensive with time, eventually giving rise to a distinctive type of multilobular biliary cirrhosis. A few children develop extensive liver involvement. The gallbladder is small and contains a firm, gelatinous material that also fills the cystic duct. Findings similar to those in the pancreas are found in the salivary glands and contribute to a dry mouth and susceptibility to infection as a result of interference with salivation.

## Clinical Manifestations

The clinical manifestations vary widely and change as the disease progresses. The most common symptoms are (1) pancreatic enzyme deficiency because of duct blockage, (2) progressive chronic obstructive lung disease associated with infection, and (3) sweat gland dysfunction resulting in increased sodium and chloride sweat concentrations. The usual pattern is one of failure to thrive, with an increased weight loss despite an increased appetite, and gradual deterioration of the respiratory system. The diagnosis may not be readily apparent, especially when there is no familial evidence of CF. Some children display symptoms at birth; others may not develop symptoms for weeks, months, or years. Some show only mild forms of the disease, with limited impairment of digestion and respiratory problems, whereas others have severe malabsorption and life-threatening pulmonary complications. Although most affected children display both pulmonary and gastrointestinal symptoms, a few have only enzyme deficiency without pulmonary disease, and a few have only pulmonary disease without pancreatic insufficiency.

**Respiratory Tract.** Initial pulmonary manifestations are often wheezing respirations and a dry, nonproductive cough. Eventually diffuse bronchial and bronchiolar obstruction leads to irregular aeration with progressive pulmonary disturbance and secondary infection. The most prominent and constant feature of pulmonary involvement is chronic cough. Dyspnea increases, the cough often becomes paroxysmal, and the mucoid impactions within the small air passages cause a generalized obstructive emphysema and patchy areas of atelectasis.

Progressive pulmonary involvement with hyperaeration of functioning alveoli produces the overinflated, barrel-shaped chest in which the anteroposterior diameter approaches the lateral diameter. When ventilation and subsequent diffusion and gas exchange are significantly impaired, cyanosis and clubbing of the fingers and toes may occur. The child has repeated episodes of bronchitis and bronchopneumonia and is subject to chronic nasal congestion, rhinitis, chronic sinusitis, and nasal polyps. The incidence of ear, nose, and throat surgeries is higher in this group of children when compared with the general population.

**Gastrointestinal Tract.** The earliest postnatal manifestation of CF is *meconium ileus,* which occurs in 7% to 10% of newborns with the disease (McMullen, 2000). Thick, putty-like, tenacious, mucilaginous meconium blocks the lumen of the small intestine usually at or near the ileocecal valve,

which gives rise to signs of intestinal obstruction, including abdominal distention, vomiting, failure to pass stools, and rapid development of dehydration with associated electrolyte imbalance. Thick intestinal secretions continue to be problematic throughout life. Children of all ages are subject to intestinal obstruction from inspissated or impacted feces. Gumlike masses in the cecum can obstruct the bowel, causing pain, nausea, and vomiting. This is referred to as "meconium ileus equivalent." *Distal intestinal obstruction syndrome (DIOS)* is the name given to a partial or complete intestinal obstruction that occurs in some children with CF.

As the disease progresses, obstruction of pancreatic ducts prevents digestive enzymes (trypsin, chymotrypsin, amylase, lipase) from being released into the duodenum, which prevents conversion of ingested food into compounds that can be absorbed by the intestinal mucosa. Consequently, the nondigested food is excreted (chiefly unabsorbed fats and proteins), increasing the bulk of feces to two or three times the normal amount. The bulky nature of the stools may go unnoticed at first, but usually by 6 months of age the child passes large, loose stools with normal frequency or has chronic diarrhea with unformed stools. As solid foods are added to the diet, the excessively large stools become frothy and extremely foul smelling.

Because so little is absorbed from the intestine, affected children have difficulty maintaining weight despite a healthy appetite and diet. Unable to compensate for the fecal losses, many children lose weight and exhibit marked wasting of tissues and failure to grow. The abdomen is distended, the extremities are thin, and the sallow skin droops from wasted buttocks. The impaired ability to absorb fats results in a deficiency of the fat-soluble vitamins A, D, E, and K, which causes easy bruising. Anemia is a common complication. Failure to thrive is also a frequent initial diagnosis in young children with CF. Many patients with CF have an increased prevalence of gastroesophageal reflux, and a high incidence of peptic ulcer disease has been reported in African-American adolescents with CF (Rosenstein, 1999). Another common gastrointestinal complication associated with CF is *prolapse of the rectum,* which occurs in infancy and early childhood and is related to large, bulky stools, malnutrition, and increased intraabdominal pressure secondary to paroxysmal cough. Every patient with rectal prolapse should be evaluated for CF (Rosenstein, 1999).

**Reproductive System.** Delayed puberty in females with CF is common even when their nutritional and clinical status is good (Johannesson, Gottlieb, and Hjelte, 1997). The reproductive systems of both males and females with CF are affected. Females with CF have normal fallopian tubes and ovaries. Fertility can be inhibited by highly viscous cervical secretions, which act as a plug, blocking sperm entry. Women with CF who become pregnant have an increased incidence of premature labor and delivery and low birth weight in the infant. Favorable nutritional status and pulmonary function are positively correlated with favorable pregnancy outcomes (Rosenstein, 1999). Most adult males (98%) with CF are sterile, which may be caused by blockage of the vas deferens with abnormal secretions or by failure of normal development of the wolffian duct structures (vas deferens, epididymis, and seminal vesicles), resulting in decreased or absent sperm production.

**Integumentary System.** The consistent finding of abnormally high sodium and chloride concentrations in the sweat is a unique characteristic of CF. Parents frequently observe that their infants taste "salty" when they kiss them. The chloride channel defect in sweat glands prevents reabsorption of sodium and chloride, which leaves the affected person at risk for abnormal salt loss, dehydration, and hypochloremic and hyponatremic alkalosis during hyperthermic conditions. This is especially important to the infant because of limited fluid stores and the potential for inadequate sodium intake with most commercially prepared infant formulas.

The disease is sometimes expressed in other ways (e.g., hypoelectrolytemia caused by massive losses through sweat, especially in high environmental temperatures or febrile episodes). Infants with CF who fail to thrive frequently demonstrate hypoalbuminemia resulting from diminished absorption of protein, which in severe cases causes generalized edema.

## Diagnostic Evaluation

An initial evaluation is conducted with overall appraisal in the areas of general activity, physical findings, nutritional status, and findings on chest radiographs. The diagnosis of CF is suspected in the child who fails to thrive or has frequent upper respiratory tract infections and is established on the basis of duplicate sweat chloride tests. Diagnosis of CF requires a positive sweat test result in the presence of either clinical symptoms consistent with CF or a family history of CF.

The *quantitative sweat chloride test (pilocarpine iontophoresis)* involves stimulating the production of sweat with a special device, collecting the sweat, and measuring the sweat electrolytes. The quantitative analysis requires a sufficient volume of sweat (>75 mg). Two separate samples are collected to ensure the reliability of the test for any individual. Because newborns do not have active sweat glands, it is often difficult to obtain an adequate sample for analysis. Therefore, if results are questionable, the test is repeated at a later date. The test should be performed only by personnel skilled in the procedure.

Normally sweat chloride content is less than 40 mEq/L, with a mean of 18 mEq/L. A chloride concentration greater than 60 mEq/L is diagnostic of CF; in infants less than 3 months, a sweat chloride concentration greater than 40 mMol/L is highly suggestive of CF. Children with questionable results are followed for any evidence of pulmonary system symptoms.

Detection of CF mutations and the measurement of nasal electrical potential difference (PD) can also be used for diagnosis. The active transport of ions across epithelial surfaces generates a PD that can be measured. CF patients have abnormalities in ion transport in their respiratory epithelia, and their pattern of nasal PD differs from that of individuals without CF.

Chest radiography reveals characteristic patchy atelectasis and obstructive emphysema. Pulmonary function tests are sensitive indexes of lung function, providing evidence of abnormal small airway function in CF. Other diagnostic tools that may aid in diagnosis include stool fat or enzyme analysis. Stool analysis requires a 72-hour sample with accurate recording of food intake during that time. Radiographs, including barium enema, are used for diagnosis of meconium ileus.

## Screening

Newborn screening for CF has been possible since 1979. The standard methods of diagnosis include detection of abnormal chloride secretion in sweat. In some situations DNA testing may be substituted for the sweat test. The presence of a mutation known to cause CF on each CFTR gene predicts with a high degree of certainty that the individual has CF. In newborns an immunoreactive trypsinogen (IRT) analysis is commonly performed and is generally followed by direct analysis of DNA for the presence of the F508 mutation or other mutations. An in utero diagnosis of CF is also possible, based on detection of two CF mutations in the fetus.

Carrier screening is available and reliable for siblings and family members of a child with CF. DNA probes can detect the major gene defect (F508) for CF, which is located in about 70% of Caucasian patients and 30% of African-American patients. Although the technology is available to conduct carrier screening for the general population, this issue remains controversial and widespread implementation of screening programs is not recommended.

## Therapeutic Management

Improved survival among patients with CF during the past two decades is attributable largely to antibiotic therapy and improved nutritional management. Goals of therapy therefore include (1) to prevent or minimize pulmonary complications, (2) to ensure adequate nutrition for growth, (3) to encourage appropriate physical activity, and (4) to promote a reasonable quality of life for the child and family. To attain these goals a multisystem approach to treatment is used. Current research and modern technologies are exploring methods to attack the defect itself. For example, a number of clinical trials are underway to examine the feasibility of correcting the underlying genetic defect using gene therapy.

**Management of Pulmonary Problems.** Management of pulmonary problems is directed toward prevention and treatment of pulmonary infection by improving aeration, removing mucopurulent secretions, and administering antimicrobial agents. The large amounts and viscosity of respiratory secretions in children with CF contribute to the likelihood of infection. Once infection becomes established, it is difficult to eradicate.

Prevention of infection involves a daily routine of *chest physiotherapy (CPT)* to maintain pulmonary hygiene. (See Chapter 31.) Postural drainage and percussion of the lungs loosen and move secretions toward the glottis to facilitate expectoration. Exercise, deep breathing, and coughing are also effective in clearing secretions. Patients with CF have been found to regress when conventional CPT is discontinued. Therefore, although it is time-consuming for the child and family, CPT remains the cornerstone of pulmonary therapy.

CPT is usually performed twice daily (on rising and in the evening) and more frequently if needed, especially during pulmonary infection. Bronchodilator medications (such as albuterol, metaproterenol, and terbutaline) delivered via a MDI or nebulizer open bronchi for easier expectoration and are administered before CPT to improve pulmonary function and lessen wheezing.

The **Flutter mucus clearance device*** is a small, handheld plastic pipe with a stainless-steel ball on the inside that facilitates removal of mucus (Fig. 32-11). The Flutter has the advantage of increasing sputum expectoration and can be used without an assistant. Most children are able to clear the airway in 5 to 15 minutes.

**NURSING ALERT** The Flutter should be stored away from young children because, if the device separates, the steel ball can pose a choking hazard.

Another device that may be used in children and adolescents with CF is the **ThAIRapy vest.** This device provides high-frequency chest wall oscillation, which helps to loosen secretions.†

Forced expiration, or "huffing," with the glottis partially closed helps move secretions from the small airways so that subsequent coughing can move secretions forcefully from the large airways. Several studies indicate that this maneuver enhances the pulmonary function of patients with CF.

A regular daily physical exercise program is an important adjunct to daily CPT. Exercise not only stimulates mucus secretion, it also provides a sense of well-being and increased self-esteem. Any aerobic exercise that is enjoyed by the patient should be encouraged. The ultimate aim of exercise is to establish a good habitual breathing pattern.

---

*Manufactured by Scandipharm, Inc, 22 Inverness Center Parkway, Birmingham, AL 35242, (205) 991-8085 or (800) 950-8085; www.scandipharm.com.
†For information about the ThAIRapy vest, contact American Biosystems, 20 Yorkton Ct, St Paul, MN 55117, (800) 426-4224.

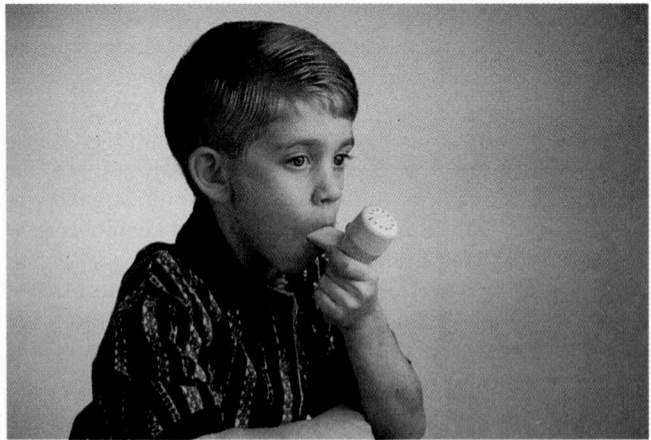

**Fig. 32-11** Child using Flutter mucus clearance device. (Courtesy Scandipharm, Inc.)

Another aerosolized medication used in CF is **recombinant human deoxyribonuclease (DNase),** known generically as **dornase alfa (Pulmozyme).** This medicine is given daily via nebulization. It decreases the viscosity of mucus, is well tolerated, and has no major adverse effects (minor reactions are voice alterations and laryngitis). This medication has resulted in improvements in spirometry, pulmonary function tests, dyspnea scores, and perceptions of well-being as well as producing a reduction in the viscosity of sputum.

Pulmonary infections are treated as soon as they are recognized. Some practitioners prefer to prescribe oral antibiotics prophylactically at the time of diagnosis; others begin therapy when pulmonary symptoms arise. Sputum culture and sensitivity guide the choice of antibiotic. The trend is toward aggressive therapy even for milder disease.

Colonization with *P. aeruginosa* and *B. cepacia* signal progressive involvement. Although the bacteria are impossible to eradicate, they can be successfully controlled. Inhaled antibiotics are administered as a prophylactic measure in some centers, but once the organisms have become established, antibiotic therapy is most effective when given intravenously. Patients with CF metabolize antibiotics more rapidly than normal; therefore drug dosage is often higher than would be expected. Depending on the sensitivity of the organism, *P. aeruginosa* is usually treated with aminoglycosides in combination with antipseudomonal β-lactam antibiotics (ticarcillin, piperacillin, ceftazidime). Antibiotic treatment of *B. cepacia* should be based on susceptibility and synergy testing (Rosenstein, 1999). The duration of therapy depends on the patient's response, measured with clinical indicators including cough, fatigue, and exercise intolerance in addition to tests such as pulmonary function tests, chest radiography, and oxygen and carbon dioxide measurements.

IV antibiotics are usually administered at home as an alternative to hospitalization as long as the family agrees and regular monitoring for toxicity can be accomplished. Most children have central venous access devices for home administration of IV medications. When pulmonary function does not improve with outpatient management, hospitalization is necessary for continued antibiotic therapy and vigorous CPT.

Aerosolized antibiotics have been used in children with CF. These medications are usually administered by jet or ultrasonic nebulizers after CPT is performed. This type of delivery system allows for direct antimicrobial application with little systemic absorption. Agents that have been used include tobramycin, ticarcillin, and gentamicin. Studies of the use of these agents indicate that aerosolized antibiotics may be beneficial in patients with frequent exacerbations and may slow the development of the exacerbations or slow the colonization with *P. aeruginosa* (Hagemann, 1996).

Oxygen administration is usually recommended for children with acute episodes, but, because many of these children have chronic carbon dioxide retention, the unsupervised use of oxygen can be harmful. (See Oxygen Toxicity, Chapter 31.)

Pneumothorax is most often caused by rupture of subpleural blebs through the visceral pleura and usually occurs in patients with more advanced disease.

**NURSING ALERT**    Signs of a pneumothorax are usually nonspecific and include tachypnea, tachycardia, dyspnea, pallor, and cyanosis.

Some pneumothoraces resolve spontaneously; others require more aggressive therapy, such as chest tube insertion. For those patients unresponsive to such therapy, other options include partial pleurectomy, limited surgical pleurodesis, chemical pleurodesis, and oversewing or stapling of the subpleural blebs (Rosenstein, 1999). To prevent pneumothorax, patients with CF should avoid activities such as power weight lifting, intensive isometric exercise, and scuba diving, which lead to marked fluctuations in intrapleural pressure.

Blood streaking of the sputum is usually associated with increased pulmonary infection and often requires no specific treatment. Hemoptysis greater than 240 ml in 24 hours for the older child (less for a younger child) indicates a potentially life-threatening event and needs to be treated immediately. Sometimes bleeding can be controlled with bed rest, IV antibiotics, replacement of acute blood loss, IV conjugated estrogens (Premarin) or pitressin, and correction of any coagulation defects with vitamin K or fresh frozen plasma. If hemoptysis persists, the site of bleeding should be localized via bronchoscopy and cauterized or embolized (Rosenstein, 1999).

Treatment of nasal polyps includes intranasal glucosteroids, oral antihistamines, and decongestants. If these measures are ineffective, surgical interventions may be necessary.

Because pulmonary damage in patients with CF is believed to be caused by the inflammatory process that occurs with frequent infections, the use of corticosteroids has been studied. A 4-year multicenter study of 284 pediatric patients with CF indicated that patients who received prednisone every other day had better pulmonary function than patients who received a placebo every other day (Eiger and others, 1995).

However, treatment with corticosteroids for longer than 24 months has been associated with linear growth retardation, glucose abnormalities, and cataract formation (Rosenstein, 1999). Antiinflammatory medications such as ibuprofen are becoming more important in the treatment of CF. Long-term daily ibuprofen given in a dose sufficient to achieve a peak plasma concentration between 50 and 100 $\mu$g/ml has been shown to slow the rate of decline in pulmonary function and to decrease the need for IV antibiotics in young patients with mild pulmonary involvement (Rosenstein, 1999). Although this therapy is generally well tolerated, careful monitoring for adverse effects is essential.

***Lung transplantation*** is a final therapeutic option for some patients. Heart-lung and double-lung procedures have been successfully performed in children with advanced pulmonary vascular disease and hypoxia. The obstacles surrounding this technique are availability of donated organs and complications from surgery.

**Management of Gastrointestinal Problems.**    The principal treatment for pancreatic insufficiency is replacement of pancreatic enzymes, which are administered with meals and snacks to ensure that digestive enzymes are mixed with food in the duodenum. Enteric-coated products prevent the neutralization of enzymes by gastric acids, thus allowing activation to occur in the alkaline environment of the small bowel. The amount of enzymes depends on the severity of the insufficiency, the response of the child to enzyme replacement, and the frequency and character of the patient's stools. Usually one to five capsules are administered with a meal, and a smaller amount is taken with snacks. Capsules can be swallowed whole or taken apart and the contents sprinkled on a small amount of food to be taken at the beginning of the meal. The amount of enzyme is adjusted to achieve normal growth and a decrease in the number of stools to two or three per day. (See Critical Thinking Exercise box.)

 *Critical Thinking Exercise*

### Cystic Fibrosis

Sam, an 8-year-old boy with cystic fibrosis, comes to the outpatient clinic for a routine checkup following the completion of a course of IV antibiotics at home. Since his last clinic visit, he has gained 2 pounds and his mother states that his appetite has improved. Sam tells the nurse that he has been having more large, foul-smelling stools than usual in the past week. When discussing Sam's diet and care, which of the following teaching points should the nurse emphasize?

FIRST, THINK ABOUT IT . . .

- What information are you using?
- How are you interpreting that information?

1. To reduce the number of stools, Sam should take his pancreatic enzymes between meals and just before bedtime.
2. Sam should always remember to stop taking his pancreatic enzymes when he is receiving antibiotics.
3. Sam needs to remember to take his pancreatic enzymes each time he eats a meal and with all snacks; when he increases his intake, he will need to increase his enzymes.
4. Sam should decrease his pancreatic enzymes when he notices an increase in his stools.

The best response is three. Pancreatic enzymes should be taken within 30 minutes of each meal and with every snack to make sure that the digestive enzymes are mixed with food in the duodenum. If Sam's appetite has increased and he is eating more, he needs to increase, not decrease, the number of enzymes he takes, which is important information. Taking pancreatic enzymes between meals will not provide the enzymes when they are needed. The enzymes need to be present when food is in the duodenum, and taking the enzymes at the correct time should improve digestion and decrease the number of stools. Finally, children with cystic fibrosis receive antibiotic therapy frequently for pulmonary exacerbations, and they should continue to take their pancreatic enzymes throughout their antibiotic treatment.

Children with CF require a well-balanced, high-protein, high-calorie diet. The diet should be high in calories because of the impaired intestinal absorption. In fact, these children often require up to 150% of the recommended daily allowances to meet their needs for growth. Breastfeeding with enzyme supplementation should be continued whenever possible for parents who prefer this method and, when necessary, supplemented with a higher-calorie-per-ounce formula. For formula-fed infants, commercial cow's milk formulas are usually adequate, although frequently a hydrolysate formula with medium-chain triglycerides (e.g., Pregestimil or Alimentum) may be recommended. Enzymes are mixed into cereal or fruit, such as applesauce. Because the uptake of fat-soluble vitamins is decreased, water-miscible forms of these vitamins (A, D, E, K) are given, along with multivitamins and the enzymes. Although fat restriction is not necessary, one concern is that other nutrients might not be provided from a diet with increased fats. When high-fat foods are eaten, the child is encouraged to add extra enzymes. Pancreatic enzymes should be taken within 30 minutes of eating, and the beads should not be chewed or crushed; by destroying the enteric coating, inactivation of the enzymes and excoriation of oral mucosa can occur.

Children with CF should thrive with adequate replacement therapy and caloric intake. Failure to thrive despite adequate nutritional support usually indicates deterioration of pulmonary status. Occasionally patients will be placed on supplemental tube feedings or parenteral alimentation in an effort to build up nutritional reserves if there has been a history of inability to maintain weight.

Meconium ileus and meconium ileus equivalent, or total or partial intestinal obstruction, can occur at any age. Constipation is often the result of a combination of malabsorption (either from inadequate pancreatic enzyme dosage or a failure to take the enzymes), decreased intestinal motility, and abnormally viscous intestinal secretions. These problems usually do not require surgical interventions and may be treated with GoLYTELY or Colyte (osmotic solutions given orally or by nasogastric tubes), other laxatives, stool softeners, or rectal administration of meglumine diatrizoate (Gastrografin). Once the obstruction has been relieved, a low-fat diet and long-term use of some combination of stool softener, mild stimulant, bulk laxative, and added bulk to the diet may be recommended (McMullen, 2000).

Rectal prolapse occurs in about 25% of children, usually in the first 3 years of life (McMullen, 2000). The first episode of rectal prolapse is frightening to both parents and child. Its reduction usually requires immediate guidance and intervention, which is managed by simply guiding the rectum back into place with a gloved, lubricated finger. Further management usually involves attempting to decrease the bulk of daily stools through enzyme replacement.

Salt depletion through sweating can be a problem during hot weather or physical exertion. Most children are able to adjust salt to their needs, and older children often exhibit a preference for salty foods. Salt supplementation is often needed during hot weather or febrile periods and should include use of fluids such as Gatorade or Exceed, which provide an adequate supply of electrolytes.

**Prognosis.** Despite considerable progress and a recent surge in new treatment modalities, CF remains a progressive and incurable disease. The pulmonary involvement ultimately determines the patient's outcome because pancreatic enzyme deficiency is less of a problem if adequate nutrition is ensured. With advances in technology, parents and adolescents are challenged to set future goals that may include college, careers, social relationships, and marriage. Concurrently they are faced with increasing morbidity and higher rates of CF complications as they grow older.

## Nursing Considerations

Assessment of the child with CF involves both pulmonary and gastrointestinal observations. Pulmonary assessment is the same as that described for asthma (see p. 1388), with special attention to lung sounds, observation of cough, and evidence or degree of finger clubbing. Gastrointestinal assessment primarily involves observing the frequency and nature of the stools and abdominal distention. The observer is also alert to evidence of failure to thrive (e.g., weight loss, wasting, pallor, fatigue). Family members are interviewed to determine the child's eating and eliminating habits, to determine salty perspiration, and to confirm a history of frequent respiratory infections or bowel obstruction in infancy.

On initial contact, frequently in the hospital setting, nurses are involved in performing or assisting with diagnostic tests, primarily sweat for laboratory analysis of chloride content and, less often, stool specimens for trypsin and fat. The child, usually an infant, needs comfort during the procedures; young children need distraction while they are confined during iontophoresis. Even short periods of inactivity seem long to an active child. Children beyond very early childhood need an explanation of the strange, and sometimes painful, procedures and the equipment used for tests and treatments.

The respiratory equipment is also frightening, especially for infants and very young children. The child needs support and guidance in using the equipment. Accepting uncharacteristic behavior and explaining this normal stress response to parents are important nursing functions.

Parents are anxious and puzzled. Few of them have any understanding of the disease process and the long-term implications it has for their family. They need careful explanations of the disease, how it might affect their family, and what they can do to provide the best possible care for their child.

The shock associated with the diagnosis is overwhelming to parents. They must face the impact of the chronic, life-threatening nature of the disease and the prospect of intensive treatment, for which they must assume a major part of the responsibility and for which they are ill prepared. They often fear that they will be unable to provide the care the child needs. One of the most difficult aspects of the diagnosis is the implications inherent in its etiology (i.e., the recognition that each parent contributed the gene responsible for the defect in their child).

**Hospital Care.** When the child is hospitalized for confirmation of the diagnosis or for pulmonary complications, aerosol therapy is instituted or continued. Respiratory therapy is usually initiated and supervised by a trained respiratory therapist or physiotherapist. In institutions with large support staffs, support personnel may provide all treatments. Otherwise, it becomes the responsibility of the nurse to perform the prescribed aerosol therapy and CPT and to teach supervised breathing exercises. CPT should not be performed before or immediately after meals. Planning the activity so that it does not coincide with meals is difficult in the hospital situation. However, it is very important and is often overlooked by nursing personnel.

Oxygen is cautiously administered to children in respiratory distress, and the child requires frequent assessment. The hazard of oxygen narcosis is a constant threat in children with long-standing disease who receive oxygen. (See Chapter 31.) The child requires close observation to assist with cough and expectoration.

The diet is implemented for the newly diagnosed child or continued for the child who is hospitalized for pulmonary disease. Children in the early stages of the disease maintain a good appetite, and some will eat excessively. With infection and increased lung involvement, however, the appetite diminishes. Eventually, it becomes a challenge to tempt failing appetites. (See Feeding the Sick Child, Chapter 27.) Some younger children may object to the extra fluids that are encouraged to prevent dehydration. Food is considered therapy for these patients. The caloric intake should be increased significantly. Pancreatic enzymes are supplied for each meal or snack, and adequate salt is provided, especially for febrile children.

Frequent skin care is carried out to prevent irritation and skin breakdown over bony prominences. Particular attention is necessary after use of the bedpan or when the diaper is changed. Careful cleansing helps to reduce irritation and odor from offensive stools, and the use of moisture barriers is designed to protect the skin. (See Diaper Dermatitis, Chapter 13, and Maintaining Healthy Skin, Chapter 27.)

The child will need support for the many treatments and tests that are a necessary part of the hospital therapy. IV fluids and blood tests are almost always a part of the treatment, and the child soon associates hospitalization with these stress-provoking procedures. Because these children are usually quite thin with little muscle mass, careful selection of injection sites is required.

Because of the high risk of transmission of *B. cepacia* in the hospital environment, many hospitals now place children who have a positive culture for *B. cepacia* on room isolation and separate patients with *B. cepacia* from other patients with CF (Henskens, 2000). In the past, children with CF were allowed to interact with each other when they were hospitalized. Changes in policy or hospital procedures may cause some children with CF to view these changes as punitive and unusually restrictive. Children and their family members need careful explanations of all hospital procedures designed to reduce the spread of *B. cepacia* among pa-

tients with CF.* Careful handwashing by everyone who interacts with CF patients (family members, visitors, and especially all hospital personnel) is essential.

Giving support to both the child and the family is a vital part of nursing care. The progressive nature of the disease makes each illness requiring hospitalization a potentially life-threatening event. Skilled nursing care and sympathetic attention to the emotional needs of the child and family help them cope with the stresses associated with repeated respiratory infections and hospitalization.

When discussing the nature of the illness and the genetic etiology, families should be informed of genetic counseling services in the community. It is important that the family understands the 1:4 likelihood of an affected child with each pregnancy. (See Chapter 5.)

**Home Care.** After the diagnosis is confirmed and a treatment program determined, preparation for home care is implemented. The plan of care should be flexible enough so that family activities are disrupted as infrequently as possible. Parents need help in finding inhalation equipment available for home use that best meets their needs. They need opportunities to learn how to use the equipment and become familiar with the problems they may encounter.

Parents also need to learn how to provide a diet of nutritious meals with tolerated fat, increased protein and carbohydrate, and the administration of pancreatic enzymes. For infants and young children the enzymes can be mixed with pureed fruit, such as applesauce, and fed with a spoon. Capsules are suitable for older children. It is important to stress to parents that the enzymes, in the amount regulated to the child's needs, should be administered about 30 minutes before all meals and snacks. They are cautioned about not restricting salt, especially during hot weather, and ensuring an adequate fluid intake, because dehydration aggravates the thick mucus secretions. Oral hygiene is important because of interference with salivation and the increased susceptibility to oral infections.

One of the most important aspects of educating parents for home care is teaching chest physiotherapy and breathing exercises. The success of a therapy program depends on conscientious performance of these treatments regularly as prescribed. The number of times these therapies are performed each day is determined on an individual basis, and often parents readily learn to adjust the number and intensity of the treatments to the child's needs. Although it is usually the physiotherapist who instructs the parents, nurses frequently follow up the care in the home and assist the family with innovative approaches to therapy. For example, using games and normal childhood activities to achieve the desired end reduces the likelihood that treatment will meet with resistance from the child. When additional respiratory exercises are introduced to estab-

---

*Information for families is available from **Home Infusion and Pharmacy Services,** a subsidiary of the **Cystic Fibrosis Foundation,** 6931 Arlington Rd, Suite T-200, Bethesda MD 20814-9650, (800) 541-4959, fax: (800) 233-3504; www.CFF.org. A suggested article is "*Burkholderia cepacia*—The Facts," by L Saiman in a special (August 1996) edition of *Homeline*.

lished routines, the family will need to be reeducated in new techniques, such as "huffing."

Postural drainage can be achieved with simple activities that are fun, such as hanging by the knees from a bar or low-hanging trapeze that can be easily built in the backyard (or indoors), turning somersaults, or playing "wheelbarrow" with the child suspended head down and propelling with the hands while the adult holds on to the feet. Parents soon learn to respond to cues from their children and incorporate spontaneous activities into the treatment regimen.

For pulmonary infection, home IV antibiotics are typically prescribed. Home IV care is preferred for willing and competent families, because it reduces tension and usually brings a sense of belonging to the family members. With use of the venous access devices, such as percutaneously inserted central catheters (or PICC lines), the parents and child are taught the technique of direct administration into the IV line.* (See Venous Access Devices, Chapter 28.) Unfortunately, around-the-clock administration may be difficult for families because it may require waking at least once during the night to give the drug.

Families also need information about medications and possible side effects. If a child is receiving ibuprofen, serum drug levels need to be monitored closely to establish therapeutic doses, and observations for side effects such as gastrointestinal irritation are essential.

Children with CF should receive routine primary care with special attention to diet, growth and development, and immunizations. Primary care providers should be alert to any weight loss or flattening in the growth curve associated with loss of appetite, which could indicate a pulmonary exacerbation in children with CF (McMullen, 2000). In addition to all the recommended routine immunizations, CF patients should be immunized against influenza starting at age 6 months and followed by a yearly booster (American Academy of Pediatrics, 2000). Anticipatory guidance concerning issues of discipline, how to incorporate aspects of the treatment regimen into the school environment, and delayed pubertal development are also important considerations for the primary care provider.

The nurse can assist the family in contacting resources that provide help to families with affected children. Various special child health services, many local clinics, private agencies, service clubs, and other community groups often offer equipment and medications either free or at reduced rates. The **Cystic Fibrosis Foundation†** has chapters throughout the United States to provide education and services to families and professionals.

**Family Support.** One of the most important and difficult aspects of providing care for the family of a child with CF is coping with the emotional needs of the child and family. The diagnosis, treatment, and prognosis are fraught with many problems, frustrations, and feelings. The diagnosis, with all its implications, evokes feelings of guilt and self-recrimination in parents. These feelings may be particularly marked if the newly diagnosed child is the second affected child in the family and the parents had been counseled about the 1:4 risk of such an event occurring.

The long-range problems are those encountered in the care of a child with a chronic illness. (See Chapter 22.) Both the child and the family must make many adjustments, the success of which depends on their ability to cope and also on the quality and quantity of support they receive from outside sources. Combined efforts of a variety of health professionals offer the most comprehensive services to families. It is often the responsibility of the nurse to organize and coordinate these services, to assess the home situation, and to collect the data needed to evaluate the effectiveness of the services in meeting the family's needs.

For the family, the illness means modification of numerous family activities. Meals require planning in order not to place too many restrictions on the affected child or deprive the other members of the family. Limits on mobility restrict family recreational activities, especially when the child's therapy includes respiratory equipment that is not transportable. CPT must be continued wherever the child may be, and some families may hesitate to take the child too far from familiar and trusted medical care. The illness even determines the family's place of residence and employment because the child's condition dictates that the family live near medical care facilities that offer the specialized care the child needs.

The persistent need for treatment several times daily also places a strain on the family. Someone must perform the procedures, such as postural drainage, even on older children who are able to assume responsibility for their own exercises and respiratory therapy. Children often balk at the treatments, and the parents are placed in the position of insisting on compliance. Sometimes the stress and anxiety related to this continual routine generate feelings of resentment, which are frequently focused on one aspect of the regimen, such as the diet or equipment. When possible, occasional trusted respite care should be made available to the parent or parents to allow them the opportunity to leave the situation for short periods without undue anxiety about the child's welfare.

The affected child also may become resentful about the disease, its relentless routine of therapy, and the necessary curtailment it places on activities and relationships. The child's activities are interrupted or built around treatment, medications, and diet that impose hardships (such as carrying medication to school and other places where the child may eat away from home), and the growth retardation associated with most chronic illnesses may be trying. Any of these aspects of the disease may be the cause of ridicule from other children. However, the child should be encouraged to attend school, participate in physical exercise, and

---

*Home care instructions for giving medications to children are available in Wong DL, Hess CS: *Wong and Whaley's clinical manual of pediatric nursing*, ed 5, St Louis, 2000, Mosby.

†6931 Arlington Rd, Bethesda, MD 20814-3205, (301) 951-4422 or (800) FIGHT CF; www.cff.org. In Canada: **Canadian Cystic Fibrosis Foundation,** 586 Eglinton Ave E, Suite 204, Toronto, Ontario M4P 1P2. Two excellent publications available from the Cystic Fibrosis Foundation are *What Everyone Should Know About Cystic Fibrosis* and *Cystic Fibrosis: A Summary of Symptoms, Diagnosis, and Treatment.* For information about specialized medications, especially Pulmozyme, and equipment for CF and other pulmonary diseases, contact **Cystic Fibrosis Pharmacy, Inc,** HHCS Pharmacy Services, 633 E Colonial Dr, Orlando, FL 32803, (800) 741-4427.

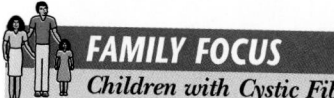

join age-appropriate groups to foster a life that is as normal and productive as possible.

Families afflicted with CF have psychologic hurdles similar to those of all families coping with a child with a chronic illness. (See Chapter 22.) Another constant source of anxiety for both parents and child is the fear of death. Despite the prognosis of a shortened life span, numerous hospitalizations, and unpleasant complications, children with CF have been found to be well-adjusted. Patients and their siblings also have generally healthy self-esteem, and family functioning is normal.

As the disease progresses, however, family stress should be expected, and the patient may become angry and noncompliant. It is important for the nurse to recognize the changing needs of the family and the grief they may experience as the CF worsens. (See Family Focus box.) Families should be made aware of sources for counseling. Patients need to be guided into activities that enable them to express anger, sorrow, and fear without guilt.

As life expectancy continues to rise for children with CF, issues related to marriage, childbearing, and career choice become more pressing. Men must be informed at some point that they will be unable to produce offspring. It is important that the distinction be made between sterility and impotence. Normal sexual relationships can be expected. Female patients may be able to bear children but must be made aware that their children will be carriers of the CF gene. Adolescent females may need counseling concerning the use of oral contraceptives and other contraceptive options (McMullen, 2000).

Life as an independent adult should be encouraged for children with CF. From the time that children can take par-

> ### FAMILY FOCUS
> *Children with Cystic Fibrosis*
>
> When I walk by Jeff's room, I still look in to see him, even though I know he will not be there. I took care of Jeff for 3 years, and during that time we became very close. He died of CF at 19 years of age. During his short life he did not have a normal childhood and he had no future, but he was very sensitive to people and their feelings. In addition to having CF, Jeff also had growth hormone deficiency: he had the body of a child and the mind of a young man. I miss Jeff, but I know that he can now breathe easier and is free of his disease.
>
> Children with CF come from all walks of life. As nurses, we must recognize this fact and treat them as normally as the situation allows, never imposing our values on them. Let them know they are loved; their bodies may be affected, but their minds are not.
>
> *Imogene Smith, RN*
> *The Children's Hospital at Saint Francis*
> *Tulsa, OK*

tial responsibility for their own care (e.g., CPT and taking enzymes), independence and accountability should be fostered. Although the prognosis for these children has improved, many will need continued support as they cope with the demands of surviving with CF.

Anticipatory grieving and other aspects related to care of a child with a terminal illness are also part of nursing care. (See Chapter 23.) (See Nursing Care Plan: The Child with Cystic Fibrosis.*)

---

*In Wong DL, Hess CS: *Wong and Whaley's clinical manual of pediatric nursing*, ed 5, St Louis, 2000, Mosby.

## KEY POINTS

- Acute infection of the respiratory tract is the most common cause of illness in infancy and childhood.
- The incidence and severity of respiratory tract infections are influenced by the infectious agent involved, the child's age, and the child's natural defenses.
- Symptoms of respiratory tract infections include fever, anorexia, vomiting, diarrhea, abdominal pain, nasal blockage and discharge, wheezing, cough, adventitious respiratory sounds, and sore throat.
- Common respiratory tract infections of childhood include acute nasopharyngitis, acute pharyngitis, influenza, tonsillitis, and otitis media.
- Severe bleeding from the tonsil site can occur within 6 hours to 5 to 10 days after tonsillectomy.
- Factors that predispose children to otitis media are the shape and position of eustachian tubes, undeveloped cartilage lining, abundant pharyngeal lymphoid tissue, immature humoral defense mechanisms, and the recumbent position (in infants).
- The most common upper respiratory tract infections are categorized as croup syndromes, which include acute laryngotracheobronchitis, acute spasmodic laryngitis, and acute epiglottitis.
- Epiglottitis is a medical emergency and is characterized by high fever, toxic appearance, and difficulty swallowing.
- The primary nursing function in the care of children with croup is observation for signs of respiratory embarrassment and relief of laryngeal obstruction.
- Lower airway conditions constitute the majority of respiratory problems in children and are usually viral in nature (excluding foreign body aspiration).
- Common infections of the lower airway include bacterial tracheitis, asthmatic bronchitis, bronchitis, bronchiolitis, and pneumonia.
- Pneumonias are generally classified either by site (lobar, bronchial, or interstitial) or by etiologic agent (viral, bacterial, mycoplasmal, or associated with foreign bodies).
- Management of uncomplicated bronchiolitis and viral pneumonia is symptomatic in otherwise healthy infants.
- In tuberculosis, resistance to the bacillus can be altered by heredity, sex, age, stress states, poor nutrition, intercurrent infection, and noncompliance with therapy.

- Signs of choking include inability to speak, color change, and decreased level of activity.
- Inhaled objects are rarely coughed up spontaneously; therefore they must be removed by direct laryngoscopy or bronchoscopy.
- Inducing a child to vomit is contraindicated in the event of hydrocarbon ingestion because of the danger of hydrocarbon aspiration.
- Asthma is the leading cause of chronic illness in children.
- General therapeutic management of asthma includes allergen control, drug therapy, controlled exercise, and sometimes hyposensitization.

- Support for the family of the child with asthma includes education about the disease and its therapy and facilitation of self-management.
- Cystic fibrosis is the most frequently occurring inherited disease of white children and is transmitted by an autosomal recessive gene located on chromosome 7.
- Diagnosis of cystic fibrosis is based on family history, absence of pancreatic enzymes, chronic pulmonary involvement, and an abnormally high sweat chloride concentration, with the pilocarpine test (or sweat test) being the most commonly used diagnostic test.

# REFERENCES

Abramson MJ, Puy RM, Weiner JM: Is allergen immunotherapy effective in asthma? A meta-analysis of randomized controlled trials, *Am J Respir Crit Care Med* 151(4):969-974, 1995.

Abulhosn RS and others: Passive smoke exposure impairs recovery after hospitalization for acute asthma, *Arch Pediatr Adolesc Med* 151(2):135-139,1997.

Adair-Bischoff CE, Sauve RS: Environmental tobacco smoke and middle ear disease in preschool-age children, *Arch Pediatr Adolesc Med* 152(2):127-133, 1998.

Adkinson NF and others: A controlled trial of immunotherapy for asthma in allergic children, *N Engl J Med* 336(5):324-331, 1997.

Aligne CA, Stoddard JJ: Tobacco and children: an economic evaluation of the medical effects of parental smoking, *Arch Pediatr Adolesc Med* 151(7):648-653, 1997.

American Academy of Allergy and Immunology, Executive Committee: The waiting period after allergen skin testing and immunotherapy, *Pediatrics* 85(2):526-527, 1990.

American Academy of Pediatrics: *Influenza: guidelines for parents,* Elk Grove Village, IL, 1998a, The Academy.

American Academy of Pediatrics, Committee on Infectious Diseases and Committee on Fetus and Newborn: Prevention of respiratory syncytial virus infections: indications for the use of palivizumab and update on the use of RSV-IVIG, *Pediatrics* 102(5):1211-1216, 1998b.

American Academy of Pediatrics, Committee on Infectious Diseases: Reassessment of the indications for ribavirin therapy in respiratory syncytial virus infections, *Pediatrics* 97(1):137-140, 1996.

American Academy of Pediatrics, Committee on Infectious Diseases, Pickering L, editor: *2000 Red book: report of the Committee on Infectious Diseases,* ed 25, Elk Grove Village, IL, 2000, The Academy.

American Academy of Pediatrics, Committee on Substance Abuse: Tobacco-free environment: an imperative for the health of children and adolescents, *Pediatrics* 93(5):866-868, 1994.

Andrews JS: Otitis media and otitis externa. In Hoekelman RA and others, editors: *Primary pediatric care,* ed 4, St Louis, 2001, Mosby.

Armitage KB, Gross P, Yamauchi T: Respiratory infections: which antibiotics for empiric therapy? *Patient Care N P,* pp 30-46, Jan 1999.

Barnett ED and others: Comparison of ceftriaxone and trimethoprim-sulfamethoxazole for acute otitis media, *Pediatrics* 99(1):23-28, 1997.

Barone SR, Krilov LR: Infectious mononucleosis and other Epstein-Barr virus infections. In Hoekelman RA and others, editors: *Primary pediatric care,* ed 4, St Louis, 2001, Mosby.

Beausoleil JL, Weldon DP, McGeady SJ: Beta 2-agonist metered dose inhaler overuse: psychological and demographic profiles, *Pediatrics* 99(1):40-43, 1997.

Blumer JL: Traditional management of acute otitis media. In Klein JO, editor: *Otitis media management strategies for the 21st century,* Bala Cynwyd, PA, 1998, Meniscus Educational Institute.

Browne-Heitschmidt MG, Cassidy JB: Heliox: a new treatment for life-threatening asthma, *Pediatr Nurs* 23(5):479-482, 1997.

Burt CW, Knapp DE: Ambulatory care visits for asthma: United States, 1993-1994, *Advance Data from Vital and Health Statistics,* No 277, Hyattsville, MD, 1996, National Center for Health Statistics.

Ciarallo L, Brousseau D, Reinert S: Higher-dose intravenous magnesium therapy for children with moderate to severe acute asthma, *Arch Pediatr Adolesc Med* 154(10):979-983, 2000.

Ciarallo L, Sauer AH, Shannon MW: Intravenous magnesium therapy for moderate to severe pediatric asthma: results of a randomized placebo-controlled trial, *J Pediatr* 129(6):809-814, 1996.

Curley MA, Thompson JE, Arnold JH: The effects of early and repeated prone positioning in pediatric patients with acute lung injury, *Chest* 118(1):156-163, 2000.

Derkay CS, Darrow D, LeFebvre S: Pediatric tonsillectomy and adenoidectomy procedures, *AORN J* 62(6):887-904, 1995.

Dowell SF and others: Otitis media: principles of judicious use of antimicrobial agents, *Pediatrics* 101(1, suppl, pt 2 of 2):165-171, 1998.

Driver LC, Oertel MD: Synagis: an anti-RSV monoclonal antibody, *Pediatr Nurs* 25(5):527-530, 1999.

Eggleston PA: Asthma. In McMillan J and others, editors: *Oski's pediatrics: principles and practice,* ed 3, Philadelphia, 1999, Lippincott Williams & Wilkins.

Eiger H and others: A multicenter study of alternate-day prednisone therapy in patients with cystic fibrosis, *J Pediatr* 126(4):515-523, 1995.

Eliopoulos C and others: Hair concentrations of nicotine and cotinine in women and their newborn infants, *JAMA* 271(8):621-623, 1994.

Hagemann T: Cystic fibrosis—drug therapy, *J Pediatr Health Care* 10(3):127-134, 1996.

Hammerschlag MR: Chlamydial infections. In McMillan J and others, editors: *Oski's pediatrics: principles and practice,* ed 3, Philadelphia, 1999, Lippincott Williams & Wilkins.

Henskens JE, VonNessen SK: *Burkholderia cepacia* in cystic fibrosis: implications for nursing practice, *Pediatr Nurs* 26(3):325-328, 2000.

Hoffman N, Kelley C, Futterman D: Tuberculosis infection in human immunodeficiency virus-positive adolescents and young adults: a New York City cohort, *Pediatrics* 97(2):198-203, 1996.

Johannesson M, Gottlieb C, Hjelte L: Delayed puberty in girls with cystic fibrosis despite good clinical status, *Pediatrics* 99(1):29-34, 1997.

Kaliner MA, Spector SL, Wenzel SE: Treating allergic rhinitis for better asthma control, *Patient Care N P,* pp. 2-7, May 1999.

Kemp JP and others: Once-daily budesonide inhalation suspension for the treatment of persistent asthma in infants and young children, *Ann Allergy Asthma Immunol* 83(3):231-239, 1999.

Kline MW: Otitis media. In McMillan J and others, editors: *Oski's pediatrics: principles and practice,* ed 3, Philadelphia, 1999, Lippincott Williams & Wilkins.

Kropfelder L, Winkelstein M: A case management approach to pediatric asthma, *Pediatr Nurs* 22(4):291-295, 1996.

Kuster PA: Reducing risk of house dust mite and cockroach allergen exposure in inner-city children with asthma, *Pediatr Nurs* 22(4):297-303, 1996.

Ladebauche PL: Managing asthma: a growth and development approach, *Pediatr Nurs* 23(1):37-44, 1997.

Long SS: Respiratory syncytial virus. In McMillan J and others, editors: *Oski's pediatrics: principles and practice*, ed 3, Philadelphia, 1999, Lippincott Williams & Wilkins.

Lorin MI: Foreign bodies. In McMillan J and others, editors: *Oski's pediatrics: principles and practice*, ed 3, Philadelphia, 1999, Lippincott Williams & Wilkins.

Macquire MC: Tuberculosis skin testing at the end of a century, *Pediatr Nurs* 23(2):209-211, 1997.

Manthous CA and others: Heliox improves pulsus paradoxus and peak expiratory flow in nonintubated patients with severe asthma, *Am J Respir Crit Care Med* 151(2 Pt 1):310-314, 1995.

Mariscalco MM: Acute respiratory distress syndrome. In McMillan J and others, editors: *Oski's pediatrics: principles and practice*, ed 3, Philadelphia, 1999, Lippincott Williams & Wilkins.

McMillan JA, Feigin RD: Group A streptococcal infections. In McMillan J and others, editors: *Oski's pediatrics: principles and practice*, ed 3, Philadelphia, 1999, Lippincott Williams & Wilkins.

McMullen A: Cystic fibrosis. In Jackson PL, Vessey JA, editors: *Primary care of the child with a chronic condition*, ed 3, St Louis, 2000, Mosby.

Meng A: An asthma day camp, *MCN Am J Matern Child Nurs* 22(3):135-141, 1997.

Meng A, Martorell N: The hospitalized child with asthma, *MCN Am J Matern Child Nurs* 22(3):128-134, 1997.

Modlin JF: Bacterial pneumonia. In McMillan J and others, editors: *Oski's pediatrics: principles and practice*, ed 3, Philadelphia, 1999, Lippincott Williams & Wilkins.

Montville NH, White MA: Diagnosis and pharmacological management of acute otitis media, *Pediatr Nurs* 23(5):423-429, 1998.

Nafstad P and others: Day care centers and respiratory health, *Pediatrics* 103(4):753-758, 1999.

National Asthma Education and Prevention Program: *Expert Panel Report II: guidelines for the diagnosis and management of asthma*, Bethesda, MD, 1997, National Heart Lung and Blood Institute, National Institutes of Health.

National Heart Lung and Blood Institute, National Institutes of Health: *Global initiative for asthma*, Pub No 95-3659, Bethesda, MD, 1995.

Nurses' Asthma Education Working Group: *Nurses: partners in asthma care*, NIH Pub No 95-3308, Bethesda, MD, 1995, National Heart, Lung, and Blood Institute, National Institutes of Health.

Ostrea EM and others: Meconium analysis to assess fetal exposure to nicotine by active and passive maternal smoking, *J Pediatr* 124(3):471-476, 1994.

Palencia S: Treating the flu: available medications, *Allergy Asthma Health*, pp 30-32, Fall 2000.

Pearlman DS and others: Allergy and the pediatric population, *Dialog Redefin Allergy* 1:1-16, 1997.

Phipatanakul W and others: Mouse allergen. I. The prevalence of mouse allergen in inner-city homes. The National Cooperative Inner-City Asthma Study, *J Allergy Clin Immunol* 106(6):1070-1074, 2000a.

Phipatanakul W and others: Mouse allergen. II. The relationship of mouse allergen exposure to mouse sensitization and asthma morbidity in inner-city children with asthma, *J Allergy Clin Immunol* 106(6):1075-1080, 2000b.

The PREVENT Study Group: Reduction of respiratory syncytial virus hospitalization among premature infants and infants with bronchopulmonary dysplasia using respiratory syncytial virus immune globulin prophylaxis, *Pediatrics* 99(1):93-99, 1997.

Redding GJ: Current concepts in adult respiratory distress syndrome in children, *Curr Opin Pediatr* 13(3):261-266, 2001.

Rosenstein BJ: Cystic fibrosis. In McMillan J and others: editors: *Oski's pediatrics: principles and practice*, ed 3, Philadelphia, 1999, Lippincott Williams & Wilkins.

Rosenstreich DL and others: The role of cockroach allergy and exposure to cockroach allergen in causing morbidity among inner-city children with asthma, *N Engl J Med* 336(19):1356-1363, 1997.

Rowe BH and others: Intravenous magnesium sulfate treatment for acute asthma in the emergency department: a systematic review of the literature, *Ann Emerg Med* 36(3):181-190, 2000.

Scarfone RJ and others: A randomized trial of magnesium in the emergency department treatment of children with asthma, *Ann Emerg Med* 36(6):572-578, 2000.

Schuh S and others: Efficacy of frequent nebulized ipratropium bromide added to frequent high-dose albuterol therapy in severe childhood asthma, *J Pediatr* 126(4):639-645, 1995.

Sherman JM, Capen CL: The red alert program for life-threatening asthma, *Pediatrics* 100(2):187-191, 1997.

Simoes EAF and others: Respiratory syncytial virus–enriched globulin for the prevention of acute otitis media in high-risk children, *J Pediatr* 129(2):214-219, 1996.

Simons FER: Allergic rhinitis and associated disorders. In McMillan J and others, editors: *Oski's pediatrics: principles and practice*, ed 3, Philadelphia, 1999, Lippincott Williams & Wilkins.

Skoner, DP: Balancing safety and efficacy in pediatric asthma management, *Pediatrics* 109(2) (suppl):381-392, 2002.

Sockrider MM: Respiratory complications of burns and smoke inhalation (respiratory burns). In McMillan J and others, editors: *Oski's pediatrics: principles and practice*, ed 3, Philadelphia, 1999, Lippincott Williams & Wilkins.

Starke JR: Tuberculosis. In McMillan J and others, editors: *Oski's pediatrics: principles and practice*, ed 3, Philadelphia, 1999, Lippincott Williams & Wilkins.

Stevenson AM: Leukotriene receptor antagonists: the newest in asthma drugs, *MCN Am J Matern Child Nurs* 22(3):170, 169, 1997a.

Stevenson AM: Tuberculosis treatment of women and children, *MCN Am J Matern Child Nurs* 22(5):282, 1997b.

Thomas PC, Moore P, Reilly JS: Child preferences for post tonsillectomy diet, *Intern J Pediatr Otorhinolaryngol* 31(1):29-33, 1995.

Thuma PE: Pharyngitis and tonsillitis. In Hoekelman RA and others, editors: *Primary pediatric care*, ed 3, St Louis, 1997, Mosby.

Togger DA, Brenner PS: Metered dose inhalers, *AJN* 101(10):26-32, 2001.

Wald ER: Croup. In McMillan J and others, editors: *Oski's pediatrics: principles and practice*, ed 3, Philadelphia, 1999, Lippincott Williams & Wilkins.

Winkelstein ML, Tarzian A, Wood RA: Parental smoking behavior and passive smoke exposure in children with asthma, *Ann Allergy Asthma Immunol* 78(4):419-423, 1997.

Winkelstein ML and others: Factors associated with medication self-administration in children with asthma, *Clin Pediatr* 39(6):337-345, 2000.

Wood RA: Allergic rhinitis. In Hoekelman RA and others, editors: *Primary pediatric care*, ed 4, St Louis, 2001, Mosby.

Wood RA: *Taming asthma and allergy by controlling your environment: a guide for patients*, Baltimore, 1995, Asthma and Allergy Foundation.

Yoos HL, McMullen A: Illness narratives of children with asthma, *Pediatr Nurs* 22(4):285-290, 1996.

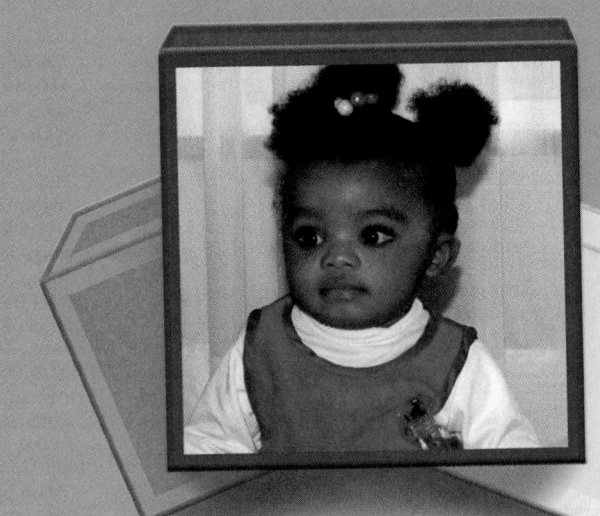

Chapter

# 33

# The Child with Gastrointestinal Dysfunction

## Chapter Outline

**GASTROINTESTINAL (GI) STRUCTURE AND FUNCTION, 1416**

**Development of the Gastrointestinal Tract, 1416**
Digestion, 1417
Absorption, 1418
Assessment of Gastrointestinal Function, 1419

**INGESTION OF FOREIGN SUBSTANCES, 1419**
Pica, 1422
Foreign Bodies, 1423

**DISORDERS OF MOTILITY, 1424**
Constipation, 1424

Hirschsprung Disease (Congenital Aganglionic Megacolon), 1426
Gastroesophageal Reflux (GER), 1429
Irritable Bowel Syndrome (IBS), 1432
**INFLAMMATORY CONDITIONS, 1432**
Acute Appendicitis, 1432
*Nursing Care Plan: The Child with Appendicitis, 1436*
Meckel Diverticulum, 1435
Inflammatory Bowel Disease (IBD), 1437
  Ulcerative Colitis (UC), 1438
  Crohn Disease (CD), 1438
Peptic Ulcer Disease (PUD), 1443

**OBSTRUCTIVE DISORDERS, 1446**
Hypertrophic Pyloric Stenosis (HPS), 1446
Intussusception, 1448
Malrotation and Volvulus, 1449
**MALABSORPTION SYNDROMES, 1450**
Celiac Disease (Gluten-Sensitive Enteropathy), 1450
Short Bowel Syndrome (SBS), 1451
**GASTROINTESTINAL BLEEDING, 1454**
Upper and Lower Gastrointestinal Bleeding, 1454
**HEPATIC DISORDERS, 1456**
Acute Hepatitis, 1456
Cirrhosis, 1460

## Related Topics

Central Venous Access Devices, Ch. 28
Cystic Fibrosis, Ch. 32
Disorders of the Gastrointestinal Tract, Ch. 11
Encopresis, Ch. 18
Feeding Resistance, Ch. 10

Gastric Feeding Techniques, Ch. 27
Gastrointestinal Disorders, Ch. 29
Intestinal Parasitic Diseases, Ch. 16
Nursing Care of High-Risk Newborns, Ch. 10
Ostomies, Ch. 27

Pain Assessment; Pain Management, Ch. 26
Preparation for Procedures, Ch. 27
Procedures Related to Elimination, Ch. 27
Sudden Infant Death Syndrome, Ch. 13
Surgical Procedures, Ch. 27

## GASTROINTESTINAL (GI) STRUCTURE AND FUNCTION

The primary function of the GI tract is the digestion and absorption of nutrients. The GI tract also has secretory, barrier, endocrine, and immunologic functions (Box 33-1). The extensive surface area of the GI tract and its digestive function represent the major means of exchange between the human organism and the environment. Thus any dysfunction of the GI tract can cause significant problems with the exchange of fluids, electrolytes, and nutrients.

■ Carolyn V. Daigneau, MS, RN-CS, PNP, revised this chapter.

## Development of the Gastrointestinal Tract

The development of the GI tract (from mouth to anus) occurs in several stages from conception through birth. The GI tract may be divided into three parts in intrauterine life: *foregut* (esophagus, stomach, and proximal duodenum), *midgut* (distal duodenum, jejunum, ileum, cecum, and proximal colon), and *hindgut* (distal colon and rectum). The *salivary glands, liver, gallbladder,* and *pancreas* are outgrowths of the foregut and midgut.

The *esophagus* develops from the foregut and can be identified by 4 weeks of gestation. It elongates rapidly after the fourth week to a length of approximately 10 cm at term. The stomach also develops from the primitive foregut and

**Box 33-1** ■ ■ ☐
**Functions of the Gastrointestinal Tract**

Process and absorb nutrients necessary to maintain metabolic processes and to support growth and development

Perform an excretory function for both digestive residue and other waste products that pour into the intestine from the blood or are excreted in the bile

Provide detoxification while other routes of elimination (kidneys, liver, skin) are still immature

Participate in maintaining fluid and electrolyte balance in infancy

Serve a lymphoid function by providing a barrier to bacteria, viruses, parasites; the liver also processes antigens and produces immunoglobulins

can be identified by the fourth week of gestation. It continues to develop in the second trimester. From the fifth week of gestation until term, the intestine lengthens a thousandfold.

The third trimester is the period of most extensive and rapid growth of the gut. At full term, the **small intestine** is approximately 250 to 300 cms and will grow to approximately 2 to 4 meters in the adult. The **large intestine** develops from the midgut and the hindgut and is approximately 30 to 50 cm at term.

During pregnancy the fetus receives nutrients via the placenta. At birth the full-term infant is capable of adaptation to extrauterine nutrition. This adaptation process includes coordinated sucking and swallowing, efficient gastric emptying and intestinal motility, regulation of digestive secretions and enzymes, efficient digestion and absorption, and excretion of waste products. The capacity of the infant to adapt to enteral nutrition depends on the gestational age at birth and the type of nutrients to which the GI tract is exposed.

Movement of nutrients through the GI tract occurs as a result of contraction of the intestinal smooth muscles. Gastrointestinal movement is regulated by a combination of myogenic, neural, and neuroendocrine input during fasting and digestion. By 26 weeks of gestation, uncoordinated contractions occur, but gastric emptying is slow. By 36 weeks of gestation, motility is similar to the full-term infant, and coordinated sucking and swallowing allow preterm infants to feed orally (Blank, 1999). Intestinal motility improves with gestational age, but it is not known if the introduction of enteral feeding initiates coordinated motor activity. *Meconium,* a thick greenish black material consisting of epithelial cells, digestive tract secretions, and residue of swallowed amniotic fluid, is normally expelled from the intestine shortly after birth and provides evidence of patency of the GI tract.

At term the mechanical functions of digestion are relatively immature. *Swallowing* is an automatic reflex action for the first 3 months, and the infant has no voluntary control of swallowing until the striated muscles in the throat establish their cerebral connections. This begins at approximately 6 weeks of age. By 6 months the infant is capable of swallowing, holding food in the mouth, or spitting it out at will. The mechanism of *sucking* is also a reflexive activity in the newborn, and the muscular action of the tongue has a

typical forward thrust. With neural and muscular development, the infant gradually acquires the ability to perform the coordinated muscular action typical of the adult type of swallowing. (See Chapter 12.) The *chewing* function is facilitated by eruption of the primary teeth. The timing of dietary changes closely parallels these progressive developmental capabilities. First foods are those that require merely swallowing, then those that need no mastication, and finally those that require biting and chewing.

The *stomach,* which lies horizontally, is round until the child is approximately 2 years of age. It then gradually elongates until approximately 7 years of age, when it assumes the shape and anatomic position of the adult stomach. This anatomic placement of the stomach in infancy influences positioning practices during and after feeding. (See Chapter 8.) At birth the stomach capacity is small, but it increases rapidly with age.

The frequency and character of stools are affected by the rate of peristalsis and the nature of ingested food. The frequent, yellow stools of the neonate gradually assume a more adult regularity and character in the infant. When compared with the older child, the capacity of the infant's stomach is decreased, but the emptying time is faster. Both the stomach capacity and the emptying time have implications for the amount and frequency of feedings during infancy.

The *secretory cells* of the GI tract are believed to be functional at birth. However, because most of the digestive enzymes depend on a specific pH, their efficiency may be impaired. The newborn produces only small amounts of saliva, which contain the starch-splitting enzyme amylase; therefore its primary purpose at this time is to moisten the mouth and throat. By the end of the second year, the salivary glands have increased in size about five times to reach their full size and function.

## Digestion

Three processes—digestion, absorption, and metabolism—are necessary for the body to convert nutrients into forms it can use. *Nutrients* are composed of six major substances: carbohydrates, proteins, fats, vitamins, minerals, and water. *Digestion* is the initial preparation of food for use by the body. Two basic activities are involved: mechanical or muscular activity producing GI motility (movement) and chemical or enzymatic activity resulting from GI secretions.

*Mechanical digestion* occurs through a series of neuromuscular actions that move and mix food along the GI tract at a rate suitable for digestion and absorption. Three types of muscles in the stomach and intestines contribute to this motility: (1) *circular muscles* churn and mix food particles; (2) *longitudinal muscles* propel the food mass; and (3) *sphincter muscles* (the lower esophageal, pyloric, ileocecal, and anal sphincters) control passage of the food mass to the next segment. The nervous system regulates these muscular actions. The *intramural plexus* forms the complex network of nerves within the GI wall that control smooth muscle contractions.

*Chemical digestion* involves five types of GI secretions: (1) *enzymes* (specific actions on degradation of nutrients),

(2) *hormones* (stimulate or inhibit GI secretions), (3) *hydrochloric acid* (produces the pH necessary for the activity of specific enzymes), (4) *mucus* (lubricates and protects the GI tract), and (5) *water and electrolytes* (transport nutrients for digestion and absorption). Numerous cells and glands produce these secretions. The cells that secrete mucus and GI hormones are found primarily in the *mucosa* of the stomach and small intestine. The *salivary glands* secrete enzymes, and the *gastric glands* secrete enzymes and hydrochloric acid. The *pancreas* also secretes enzymes, and the liver secretes bile.

Mechanical and chemical digestion begins in the mouth. *Biting* and *chewing* mix food with saliva and reduce the food into a *bolus.* The saliva moistens the food to aid in swallowing. Salivary *amylase* begins the process of digestion of complex carbohydrates or starches.

The next phase of digestion is *swallowing,* or *deglutition.* Safe swallowing requires coordination of the oral and pharyngeal phases of swallowing to prevent food material from entering the airway. The coordination of swallowing is controlled by the interaction of the cranial nerves and the muscles of the mouth, pharynx, and esophagus. The *oral phase* of swallowing is voluntary. The *pharyngeal phase* is involuntary and consists of elevation of the palate, uvula, and larynx, followed by a peristaltic wave. The *upper esophageal sphincter (UES)* then relaxes to allow passage of the bolus into the esophagus. *Peristalsis* (wavelike movements that squeeze food along the entire length of the alimentary tract) moves the food through the esophagus, and the *lower esophageal sphincter (LES)* relaxes to allow the food to enter the stomach.

Once a bolus of food has entered the stomach, the LES contracts to prevent food from refluxing (returning) into the esophagus. The stomach stores, mixes, and empties the food during digestion. The gastric glands secrete enzymes, hydrochloric acid, and mucus, which mix with the food to continue the process of digestion. The enzyme *pepsin,* formed from pepsinogen, begins the breakdown of whole proteins into polypeptides. Hydrochloric acid, secreted by the parietal cells, aids in the digestion of proteins. The hormone *gastrin* is released in the stomach in response to food. Gastrin stimulates the parietal cells to produce more hydrochloric acid. When the pH is very low, a feedback mechanism stops secretion of gastrin to prevent excessive acid formation. The mucus serves primarily to form a protective barrier between the acid and the gastric mucosa.

Partially digested food and watery secretions *(chyme)* are delivered to the small intestine. Up to this time, most of the digestion has been mechanical. The major part of chemical digestion, as well as several types of movement that aid in mechanical digestion, occurs in the small intestine. The small intestine secretes a large number of enzymes, each of which is specific for one of the fundamental types of nutrients. The mucosa of the small intestine secretes *disaccharidases (maltase, lactase,* and *sucrase)* that convert maltose, lactose, and sucrose to monosaccharides (glucose, fructose, and galactose). *Aminopeptidase* and *dipeptidase* convert polypeptides to smaller peptides and amino acids.

Secretions from the liver and pancreas complete the process of chemical digestion. The pancreas produces insulin, a hormone necessary for the metabolism of carbohydrates, fats, and proteins, and several enzymes that digest nutrients. Amylase converts starch to disaccharides. *Trypsin* and *chymotrypsin* convert proteins and polypeptides to smaller polypeptides. *Lipase* converts fats to glycerides and fatty acids. These pancreatic enzymes become active only after the inactive forms are secreted into the small intestine. For example, the enzyme *enterokinase,* secreted by the intestinal mucosal glands, is necessary for trypsinogen to be converted into trypsin. Otherwise, activated enzymes would digest the pancreas and pancreatic duct.

Another important aid in digestion and absorption in the small intestine is *bile.* Bile is produced in the liver and stored by the gallbladder. When fat enters the small intestine, the hormone *cholecystokinin,* which stimulates the gallbladder to release bile, is secreted by the intestinal mucosal glands. Bile, an emulsifying agent for fats that facilitates the digestion of fats by lipase, is necessary for the absorption of the fat-soluble vitamins A, D, E, and K. Absence of bile causes increased amounts of ingested fat to appear in the feces *(steatorrhea),* as well as a deficiency of these vitamins.

## Absorption

After digestion of the food is complete, the simplified nutrient end products—monosaccharides (glucose, fructose, and galactose) from carbohydrates, fatty acids and glycerides from fats, and small peptides and amino acids from proteins—are ready for absorption. Vitamins and minerals are also released as a result of digestion. Water and electrolytes contribute to the fluid food mass that is finally absorbed.

The principal site for absorption of nutrients in the GI tract is the *small intestine.* The inner mucosa of the small intestine consists of folds and projections that are progressively smaller in size. These mucosal folds, villi, and microvilli increase the inner surface area approximately 600 times over the outer serosa, yielding an extremely large surface for absorption.

The *mucosal folds* are elevated folds along the mucosa. The *villi* can be seen by light microscope and are small, fingerlike projections covering the mucosal folds. The villi increase the surface area further. Each villus has a vascular supply, including *venous* and *arterial capillaries* and *lacteals* (lymphatic vessels in the small intestine that contain the substance chyle). The *microvilli,* numerous minute projections on the surface of each villus (visible by electron microscope), form the *brush border* (Fig. 33-1).

There are several mechanisms of absorption by the small intestine, including passive diffusion, carrier-mediated diffusion, active energy-driven transport, and engulfment. *Passive diffusion (osmosis)* occurs across the epithelial membrane in the direction from higher concentration to lower concentration. *Carrier-mediated diffusion* occurs as molecules are carried across the epithelial cells of microvilli by a molecule that serves as a vehicle. Large molecules must be combined with a smaller molecule to pass from a greater pressure gradient to a lesser one. For example, vitamin $B_{12}$ requires intrinsic factor to be carried into the intestinal circulation.

In *active energy-driven transport,* nutrients require energy to be absorbed and to cross the intestinal epithelial membrane. This mechanism is referred to as a *pump.* The pump transports molecules across the membrane by means of energy supplied by the cell's metabolism. The sodium pump, which transports glucose, is an example of this mechanism.

*Engulfment,* or *pinocytosis,* is the process that allows large macromolecules to be absorbed by the epithelial cells of the villi. The epithelial cell engulfs the macromolecule and opens to allow the particle to enter the interior of the cell. The particle then enters the capillary blood. Some whole proteins and fat droplets are transported by this mechanism.

Following absorption by these mechanisms, the end products of carbohydrates and proteins are absorbed into the intestinal capillaries and enter the portal blood circulation of the liver, where further metabolic conversion occurs. The transfer of the end products of fat digestion is unique in that the fat molecules pass between the cells of the intestinal mucosa and into the lacteals of the villi. From there, they enter the larger lymph vessels and then the portal blood flow at the thoracic duct. Exceptions include the medium- and short-chain fatty acids, which can be absorbed directly into the blood circulation of the villi. Most of the fats commonly consumed are long-chain fatty acids, however, which are transported by way of the lacteals.

Fat-soluble vitamins are absorbed with digested fats in the presence of bile. Water-soluble vitamins, vitamin B complex, and vitamin C are absorbed in the small intestine. Absorption of vitamin $B_{12}$ takes place only in the ileum. The majority of water and electrolyte absorption also takes place in the small intestine.

The *large intestine* completes the process of absorption and functions primarily to absorb sodium and additional water. The remainder of the products of digestion pass into the large intestine through the ileocecal valve. The muscular activity of the large intestine propels the mass forward. Most of the water and sodium is absorbed into the bloodstream in the proximal half of the colon. The colonic bacteria synthesize vitamin K, vitamin $B_{12}$, and some of the vitamin B complex. Bacteria also affect the color and odor of the stool and gas formation. The odor is primarily caused by products of bacterial action and depends on the type of colonic flora and ingested food. (Defects in digestion or absorption notably alter the odor, as well as the appearance, of feces.) Color is the result of bilirubin end products converted by bacteria to urobilinogen and then oxidized to urobilin (stercobilin). The *feces* that are excreted consist of undigested residue, water, bacteria, and mucus. Defecation occurs when the internal and external anal sphincters relax following distention of the rectum by feces.

## Assessment of Gastrointestinal Function

The most common consequences of GI disease in children include malabsorption, fluid and electrolyte disturbances, malnutrition, and poor growth. (See Dehydration, Chap-

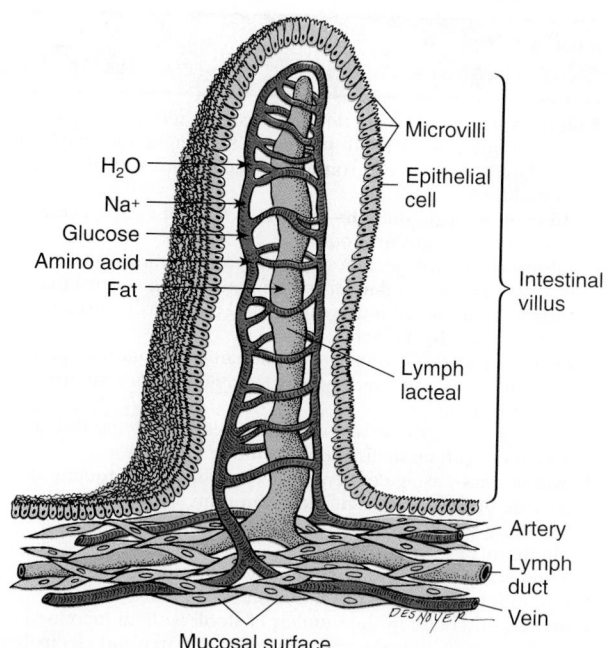

**Fig. 33-1**  Intestinal villus. Presence of intestinal villi and microvilli increases absorptive surface area of the intestinal mucosa. Most absorbed substances enter the blood in intestinal capillaries, with the exception of fat, which enters lymph by way of the intestinal lacteals. (From Thibodeau GA, Patton KT: *Anatomy and physiology,* ed 3, St Louis, 1996, Mosby.)

ter 28, and Acute Diarrheal Disease, Chapter 29.) A thorough GI assessment includes history questions, general observations, clinical examination, and specific tests and procedures. The most important basic nursing assessments include measurement of intake and output, heights and weights, abdominal examination, and simple stool and urine tests.

Numerous clinical manifestations provide clues to specific GI problems (Box 33-2). Some cases involve only one manifestation, whereas others may involve several signs and symptoms as part of the disease complex or syndrome.

A number of tests assess GI function (Table 33-1). Nurses are often responsible for collecting specimens. (See Collection of Specimens, Chapter 27.) Because children may refuse to drink contrast media, generally dislike enemas, and are frightened of unfamiliar equipment, they need preparation for procedures and collection of specimens. (See Preparation for Procedures, Chapter 27.)

## INGESTION OF FOREIGN SUBSTANCES

Children are prone to ingesting foreign substances, because they may put their hands or other objects or substances in their mouth. Infants and small children in particular explore items with the mouth instinctively. Older children often place items in their mouth and accidentally swallow them. Rarely, a child deliberately swallows unusual objects or substances. Hands come into contact with dirt and cont-

## Box 33-2 ■ ■ ■
## Clinical Manifestations of Gastrointestinal Dysfunction in Children

**Failure to thrive**—Deceleration from established growth pattern or consistently below the 5th percentile for height and weight on standard growth charts; sometimes accompanied by developmental delays

**Spitting up or regurgitation**—Passive transfer of gastric contents into the esophagus or mouth

**Vomiting**—Forceful ejection of gastric contents; involves a complex process under central nervous system control that causes salivation, pallor, sweating, and tachycardia; usually accompanied by nausea

*Projectile vomiting*—Vomiting accompanied by vigorous peristaltic waves and typically associated with pyloric stenosis or pylorospasm

**Nausea**—Unpleasant sensation vaguely referred to the throat or abdomen with an inclination to vomit

**Constipation**—Passage of firm or hard stools or infrequent passage of stool with associated symptoms such as difficulty expelling the stools, blood-streaked stools, and abdominal discomfort

**Encopresis**—Overflow of incontinent stool causing soiling; often due to fecal retention or impaction

**Diarrhea**—Increase in the number of stools with an increased water content as a result of alterations of water and electrolyte transport by the GI tract; may be acute or chronic

**Hypoactive, hyperactive, or absent bowel sounds**—Evidence of intestinal motility problems that may be caused by inflammation or obstruction

**Abdominal distention**—Protuberant contour of the abdomen that may be caused by delayed gastric emptying, accumulation of gas or stool, inflammation, or obstruction

**Abdominal pain**—Pain associated with the abdomen that may be localized or diffuse, acute or chronic; often caused by inflammation, obstruction, or hemorrhage

**Gastrointestinal bleeding**—Bleeding from an upper or lower GI source; may be acute or chronic

*Hematemesis*—Vomiting of bright red blood or denatured blood that results from bleeding in the upper GI tract or from swallowed blood from the nose or oropharynx

*Hematochezia*—Passage of bright red blood per rectum, usually indicating lower GI tract bleeding

*Melena*—Passage of dark-colored, "tarry" stools due to denatured blood, suggesting upper GI tract bleeding or bleeding from the right colon

**Jaundice**—Yellow coloration of the skin and sclerae associated with liver dysfunction

**Dysphagia**—Difficulty swallowing caused by abnormalities in the neuromuscular function of the pharynx or upper esophageal sphincter or by disorders of the esophagus

**Dysfunctional swallowing**—Impaired swallowing due to central nervous system defects or structural defects of the oral cavity, pharynx, or esophagus; can cause feeding problems or aspiration

**Fever**—Common manifestation of illness in children with GI disorders; usually associated with dehydration, infection, or inflammation

## TABLE 33-1  Gastrointestinal diagnostic procedures

| Test | Description | Purpose | Comments |
|---|---|---|---|
| Stool examination | Gross, microscopic, and chemical examination of stool specimen | To detect presence of normal and abnormal constituents | Explanation of process for collecting samples should be given<br>Fresh specimen is optimal |
| Ova and parasites (O&P) | Microscopic examination of stool contents for presence of parasites or their eggs | To aid in diagnosis of parasitic infections | Requires several fresh specimens placed in special preservative<br>Obtaining three samples improves probability of detection of organism |
| Bacterial culture | Sample contents are grown on culture medium | To detect presence of bacterial pathogens in stool | Fresh specimen important to improve probability of detection of organism<br>Serologic tests will determine presence of bacterial toxins |
| Stool assay for viral pathogens | ELISA (enzyme-linked immunosorbent assay) | To detect presence of viral pathogens in stool | Standard ELISA test available for detection of rotavirus and adenovirus |
| *Giardia* antigen | ELISA | To detect presence of *Giardia* | More sensitive than a single stool for O&P |
| Quantitative fat | Determination of presence of abnormal quantities of fat in stool | To aid in diagnosis of pancreatic insufficiency or malabsorption by measuring stool-reducing substances | Requires 72-hour collection of stool and a simultaneous food intake record.<br>Patient is instructed to consume more than 50 g of fat |
| Reducing substances | Unabsorbed sugars can be measured in the stool (glucose, fructose, lactose, galactose, and pentose) | Elevated levels of reducing substances in stool is abnormal and suggests carbohydrate malabsorption | Requires random fresh stool specimen delivered immediately to the laboratory. Fermentation by bacteria can give false low if stool not tested immediately |
| pH | Stool pH <5 suggests carbohydrate malabsorption; colonic bacterial fermentation produces short-chain fatty acids, which lower stool pH | To detect carbohydrate malabsorption | Requires random fresh stool<br>Refrigerate<br>Avoid barium procedures and laxatives prior to study. These can alter test results |
| Occult blood guaiac test | Stool is smeared on guaiac-impregnated paper, and 2 drops of developing solution are added to reverse side; blue color indicates hemoglobin | To detect presence of blood in stool | Easily and quickly measured screening test<br>Small amounts of blood (e.g., from bleeding mouth, gums, nose) may give positive results |

**TABLE 33-1** Gastrointestinal diagnostic procedures—cont'd

| Test | Description | Purpose | Comments |
|------|-------------|---------|----------|
| ***Helicobacter pylori* testing** | | | |
| Serology test | Blood test for antibody to *H. pylori* (Anti-HpIgG) | To assess for exposure to *H. pylori* | Does not determine if infection is acute or chronic |
| C-urea breath test | Collection of breath after ingestion of isotopic urea with either carbon-14 or carbon-13; measures labeled carbon dioxide in expired air | To determine if there is active infection with *H. pylori* in the stomach | One of the most accurate methods to determine *H. pylori* infection in children aged 2 or older, carbon-13 nonradioactive (preferred) and carbon-14 very low level radioactive |
| Urease test | Biopsy of stomach, which is stained and placed in Christensen urea medium, which turns color in presence of *H. pylori* | To determine presence of *H. pylori* in the stomach | Must be obtained during endoscopy |
| **Pancreatic function** | Pancreatic secretions are collected via duodenal tube under stimulated conditions and analyzed for water, ions, and enzymes<br>Serial samples are collected | To determine functional secretory capacity of the pancreas | Nothing by mouth (NPO) prior to procedure<br>Family and child preparation for study<br>Invasive and expensive test |
| **Radiography** | | | |
| Plain films | Anteroposterior and lateral radiographs of abdomen and pelvis | To detect foreign body or mass, reveal bowel gas patterns, and detect obstruction or perforation in GI tract | Family and child preparation for study<br>No special physical preparation required |
| Contrast studies—upper GI and lower GI series | Radiopaque media (barium or water-soluble contrast) or air is swallowed or administered as an enema. | To assess structure and function of GI tract and to detect luminal abnormalities, mucosal defects, or masses | Barium enema sometimes requires cleansing enemas and oral cathartics before procedure<br>Contrast material may be given by nasogastric (NG) or gastrostomy tube<br>Contrast enemas may reduce intussusception<br>Family and child preparation for swallowing contrast media, NG tube insertion, or enema<br>Encourage fluids following procedure |
| **Ultrasonography (sonography)** | Measures and records reflection of pulsed or continuous high-frequency sound waves | To locate, measure, and delineate abdominal organs | Family and child preparation for study<br>Noninvasive techniques<br>No radiation involved<br>Doppler studies demonstrate presence and direction of blood flow; often requires intravenous (IV) contrast material |
| **Computed tomography (CT)** | Pinpoint x-ray is directed on horizontal or vertical plane to provide series of "cuts" or "slices" that are fed into computer and assembled in image displays on video screen and transferred to permanent record | To visualize horizontal and vertical cross section of abdomen at any axis<br>To distinguish density of various tissue structure of organs<br>To detect blunt trauma to internal organs and masses | Family and child preparation for study<br>Usually noninvasive, but may require oral or IV contrast material<br>May require sedation |
| **Magnetic resonance imaging (MRI)** | Images are formed by reemission of radio signals by atomic nuclei stimulated in a magnetic field | Permits visualization of internal body structures in any plane<br>Permits soft tissue discrimination unavailable with many techniques | Requires family and child preparation<br>Usually noninvasive, but may require oral or IV contrast material<br>May require sedation for lengthy procedure NPO 3-4 hours prior to study; immobilization; time of test is long<br>No exposure to ionizing radiation<br>No magnetic material can be present in scanner |
| **Manometry** | | | |
| Esophagus | A multilumen catheter is inserted into esophagus, and water perfusion or solid state is sensed by a transducer and recorded | Evaluate dysphagia, esophageal spasm, achalasia, dysmotility | Teaching and preparation before procedure<br>NPO 6-8 hrs before procedure<br>Need patient cooperation |
| Rectal | Records reflex responses of anal sphincter to transient distention of rectal balloon | Measures and sphincter function especially to screen for constipation and Hirschsprung disease | Teaching and preparation before procedure<br>Enema to clear rectum before procedure |

*Continued*

**TABLE 33-1** Gastrointestinal diagnostic procedures—cont'd

| Test | Description | Purpose | Comments |
|---|---|---|---|
| **Biopsy** | | | |
| Liver | Removal of small piece of living tissue for microscopic examination by needle or surgically. General sedation or local anesthesia | Evaluate for biliary obstruction, hepatitis, metabolic disease. Assess response to treatment interventions | Teaching and preparation before procedure. Preliminary laboratory studies needed. Contraindicated with prolonged bleeding or clotting times, anemia, infection, or obstructive jaundice |
| Esophagus, stomach, intestine | Small sample of mucosal tissue taken for microscopic evaluation | To evaluate for infection, inflammation, mucosal abnormalities | Teaching and preparation before procedure<br>Requires conscious or general sedation<br>Usually obtained with endoscopy |
| **Endoscopy** | | | |
| Upper GI, colonoscopy, flexible sigmoidoscopy, anoscopy | Endoscope is introduced into the area to be examined<br>Endoscope has flexible-tip light source and aspiration and instrument channel | Allows direct visualization of GI tract to evaluate abnormalities, detect lesions, obtain biopsies. Perform therapeutic procedures—polypectomies, remove foreign bodies, sclerotherapy of esophageal varices, placement of feeding tubes, percutaneous catheters | Teaching and preparation before procedure.<br>NPO 4-8 hours before procedure<br>Lower GI requires bowel cleansing<br>Requires conscious or general sedation |
| **Esophageal pH monitoring** | A probe that measures pH is placed through the nose into the distal esophagus and records pH over time | To determine frequency and duration of gastric acid refluxed into the esophagus (GER)<br>To establish an association between patient symptoms (pain, apnea, failure to thrive, asthma, wheezing, hoarseness) and acid reflux | Teaching and preparation before procedure<br>Usually done over 24-hour period<br>Usually done with an events diary to determine association/relation to acid/GER<br>NPO 4 hours before tube passed; discontinue antacids and other medications 24 hours to 7 days (omeprazole) before study |
| **Breath hydrogen test** | Noninvasive study to assess for carbohydrate intolerance<br>Hydrogen is generated in colon by bacterial fermentation of undigested carbohydrates and is then absorbed into blood, where it diffuses into expired air via lungs | Evaluate for bacterial overgrowth, lactase or sucrase-isomaltase deficiency<br>A rise in expired hydrogen after oral loading with a specific carbohydrate indicates its malabsorption or bacterial overgrowth | Teaching and preparation before procedure<br>NPO 12 hours before test<br>Previous nights' dinner should consist of meat, rice, and water; avoid starches<br>Antibiotics may reduce hydrogen levels |
| **D-Xylose absorption test** | D-xylose solution is administered orally; serum levels of D-xylose are measured at 30, 60, 90, and 120 minutes. Urine is collected for total of 5 hours to measure D-xylose excretion | To evaluate absorptive capacity of small intestinal mucosa. Diagnosis of small bowel malabsorption caused by celiac disease | Teaching and preparation before procedure<br>NPO 4-8 hours before test<br>Test used less often, largely replaced by endoscopic biopsies to evaluate for villous atrophy |
| **Hepatobiliary scintigraphy** | Nuclear medicine study<br>Radiopharmaceutical is administered intravenously<br>Sequential images of the liver, biliary system, and bowel are obtained | To evaluate conditions of the liver and biliary tract abnormalities and gallbladder disease. Helpful in diagnosis and monitoring of these conditions, such as biliary atresia | Need to prepare family and child for study<br>Images may be obtained for up to 24 hours if excretion is delayed |

aminated objects that may contain lead, bacteria, or parasites. (See Chapter 16.)

## Pica

Pica is an eating disorder characterized by the compulsive and excessive ingestion of both food and nonfood substances. *Food picas* include the excessive eating of ordinary foods or unprepared food substances, such as coffee grounds or uncooked cereals. *Nonfood picas* include the ingestion of substances such as clay, soil, stones, laundry starch, paint chips, ice, hair, paper, rubber, and feces. Pica is more common in children, women (especially during pregnancy), individuals who are autistic or mentally retarded, and those with anemia or chronic renal failure. In some cultures pica is an accepted practice based on the presumed nutritional or therapeutic properties or on religious or superstitious beliefs.

There are several theories regarding the cause of pica, including psychologic theories (compulsive neurosis) and nutritional theories (craving caused by a nutrient deficiency). Pica has been found to be clearly associated with both iron and zinc deficiencies, although controversy exists regarding whether pica is the cause or the result of the deficiency. Pica has also been reported to be the presenting symptom in children with celiac disease thought to be caused by iron deficiency. Pica for dirt (geophagia) is the principal risk factor for visceral larva migrans (a common parasite in children and adults).

In some instances pica is relatively harmless. However, when the ingested substance contains a toxic ingredient (e.g., lead in paint), the consequences can cause serious complications. Surgical complications, such as intestinal obstruction, perforation, inflammation, or hemorrhage, can result.

Pica may be detected by the history, physical examination, and radiologic studies. However, it is often unrecognized, and children may deny any unusual eating behaviors. Pica should be considered when children known to be at risk for this condition develop abdominal pain, other GI symptoms, or anemia. Children exhibiting signs of this disorder should be evaluated, and if a potentially harmful substance is involved, it should be removed from the environment of the child. Nursing education regarding the dangers of pica, especially lead, and assistance in helping families remove the substance are important. (See Chapter 16.)

## Foreign Bodies

Foreign body ingestions are most common in infants and children between the ages of 6 months and 3 years. Coins, buttons, batteries, and toys are the items most frequently swallowed, at these ages. Older children and adolescents with mental retardation or psychiatric illness may swallow anything. Adults tend to have more problems with bones and meats (Byrne, 1999). Foreign bodies tend to become impacted at normally narrow sites of the GI tract or at areas of pathologic narrowing. Foreign bodies, including food boluses, are more likely to become impacted in the esophagus of children with motility disorders or other esophageal abnormalities. Pathologic narrowing of the intestine or intestinal stomas can also be a cause of foreign body obstruction.

Foreign bodies are generally classified as sharp or dull, pointed or blunt, and toxic or nontoxic. Impaction by toxic foreign bodies can lead to local damage from pressure necrosis and corrosive action or burns from the alkaline contents of a battery.

Important variables in the application of treatment guidelines include the type of foreign object, its location in the GI tract, and whether the patient is symptomatic. Of all foreign bodies that reach the stomach, 80% to 90% pass spontaneously, 10% to 20% require endoscopic removal, and 1% require surgery (Byrne, 1999). The progress of a foreign body may be followed radiographically. All stools should be examined to detect the passage of the object. The child should be fed the usual diet. Sharp objects such as long pins or chicken or fish bones should be removed endoscopically rather than risk perforation by allowing them to pass spontaneously (Byrne, 1999). Interventions such as magnetic or Foley catheter removal are not recommended.

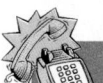

**EMERGENCY TREATMENT**
*Foreign Body Ingestion*

1. Seek medical treatment immediately if:
   a. Any sharp or large object or a battery was ingested.
   b. There are signs that the object may have been aspirated (i.e., coughing, choking, inability to speak, or difficulty breathing). (See Chapter 31 for emergency treatment of acute airway obstruction.)
   c. There are signs of GI perforation (i.e., chest or abdominal pain, evidence of bleeding in vomitus, stool, hematocrit, or vital signs).
   d. There are signs that the object may be lodged in the esophagus (i.e., increased salivation, drooling, gagging, or difficulty swallowing).
   e. There are signs that the object may be lodged in the pharynx (i.e., discomfort in the throat or chest—more likely with a fish or chicken bone or large piece of meat).
2. Seek medical advice even if the object is smooth and small (usually less than the size of a nickel).
3. If no treatment is advised, check the stool for passage of the object; do not give laxatives.

These methods offer no control of the object and increase the risk that the object will be dropped during removal, causing a potential pulmonary aspiration.

### Nursing Considerations

The primary nursing intervention is prevention of foreign body ingestion through family teaching. All children who are old enough to understand are taught not to put anything in their mouth except food. Infants and young children who cannot follow such advice must have their environment protected.

Prevention includes supervision, as well as ongoing education as the child matures. Any small items, diaper pins, or sharp objects are placed out of the area where an infant is usually cared for, plays, or sleeps. As the infant becomes more mobile, the environment is inspected carefully for hazardous objects. Any potentially dangerous items are placed out of reach of a young child or discarded where they cannot be retrieved easily. Toys are carefully examined for small or removable parts that could be accidentally ingested. If infants and small children wear earrings, the earrings should have screwbacks to prevent them from falling off. Infants and small children who wear other jewelry should be carefully supervised. Infants or young children should not be allowed to play with marbles, coins, or objects with small batteries.

Once an object is swallowed, parents need guidelines on seeking treatment. (See Emergency Treatment box.) When no treatment is advised and the object is left to pass spontaneously, parents should examine all stools for verification that the object has passed safely through the GI tract, usually within 3 to 4 days. For children in diapers, this is easily accomplished by squeezing the stool between the diaper to locate the object. In toilet-trained children, a piece of plastic wrap placed across the toilet bowl to collect the stool makes it easier to examine the feces. A tongue blade or similar disposable object may be needed to break up the stool for inspection.

# DISORDERS OF MOTILITY
## Constipation

*Constipation* is an alteration in the frequency, consistency, or ease of passing stool. In children, constipation is defined as 3 or more days without the passage of stool, painful bowel movements that are often blood streaked, or the retention of stool with or without soiling, even with a stool frequency of more than 3 stools per week (Loening-Bauke, 1995). The frequency of bowel movements is not the only diagnostic criterion because frequency varies widely among children. Normal frequency is daily to every other day. Having extremely long intervals between defecation is termed *obstipation*. *Encopresis* is the term used for constipation with fecal soiling.

Constipation may arise secondary to a variety of organic disorders of the GI tract or in association with systemic disorders. Structural disorders of the intestine, such as strictures, ectopic anus, and Hirschsprung disease, may be associated with constipation. Systemic disorders include hypothyroidism, hypercalcemia due to hyperparathyroidism or vitamin D excess, and chronic lead poisoning. Constipation is also a side effect of drugs such as antacids, diuretics, antiepileptics, antihistamines, opioids, and iron supplements. Spinal cord lesions may be associated with loss of rectal tone and sensation; affected children are prone to chronic fecal retention and overflow incontinence.

The majority of children have *idiopathic* or *functional constipation*, because no underlying organic cause can be clearly identified. Chronic constipation may be initiated by environmental, psychosocial factors, or a combination of both. Transient illness, travel, dietary changes, personality, and emotional factors may play a role in the etiology of constipation. The experience of passing a painful stool may trigger stool-withholding behavior in an effort to avoid pain. During toilet training many children also withhold stool either because they do not wish to interrupt play or in response to overzealous toilet training. Repeated stool withholding leads to stretching or dilating of the rectum and decreases the sensation or "urge" to defecate. Some children with chronic constipation and encopresis have abnormal defecation dynamics; the external anal sphincter contracts rather than relaxing during attempts to defecate.

Normally the *newborn* passes a first meconium stool within 24 to 36 hours of birth. Any infant who does not do so should be assessed for evidence of intestinal atresia or stenosis, Hirschsprung disease (congenital aganglionic megacolon), hypothyroidism, meconium plugs, or meconium ileus. *Meconium plugs* are caused by meconium that has reduced water content and are usually evacuated following digital examination but may require irrigation with a hypertonic solution or contrast medium.

*Meconium ileus,* often the initial manifestation of cystic fibrosis, is the luminal obstruction of the distal small intestine by abnormal meconium. Treatment is the same as for a meconium plug. Early surgical intervention may be necessary to evacuate the small intestine.

Frequently the onset of constipation occurs in infancy and may be related to diet. It is important to differentiate constipation resulting from organic causes such as Hirschsprung disease, hypothyroidism, and strictures from functional constipation. The history should always include the age of onset, duration of symptoms, frequency and consistency of bowel movements, current diet, and any history of pain, bleeding, or withholding behaviors.

Constipation is less common in breast-fed infants who tend to have softer stools than formula-fed infants. Occasionally, breast-fed infants have infrequent stools, but this is a normal phenomena because of the digestability of breast milk and the lack of residue forming stool. Often problems occur with the transition from breast-feeding to formula feeding and the transition from infant formula to whole cow's milk. Simple measures such as adding or increasing the amount of cereal, vegetables, and fruit in the diet may correct this problem. Often when an infant passes a hard stool that results in an anal fissure, stool-withholding behaviors may begin in response to pain on defecation. (See Critical Thinking Exercise box.)

Constipation in early childhood may result from environmental changes or normal development when a child begins to attain control over bodily functions. A child who has experienced discomofrt during bowel movements may deliberately withhold stool. Over time the rectum accommodates to the stool accumulation by dilating, and the urge to defecate passes. When the bowel contents are ultimately evacuated, the accumulated feces are passed with pain, thus reinforcing the desire to withhold stool.

Constipation in the school-age child may represent an ongoing chronic problem or a first-time event. The onset of constipation at this age is often the result of environmental changes, stresses, and changes in toileting patterns. A common cause of new-onset constipation at school entry is fear of using school bathrooms, which are noted for their lack of privacy. Early and hurried departure for school immediately after breakfast may also impede bathroom use.

### Therapeutic Management

Treatment of constipation depends on the cause and duration of symptoms. A complete history and physical examination are essential to determine appropriate management. Meconium plugs are often evacuated following digital examination.

It may be necessary to facilitate passage of the obstruction by irrigation with a hypertonic solution or water-soluble enema such as Gastrografin or Hypaque. If the constipation is due to Hirschsprung disease, surgical treatment may include resection of the intestine and saline irrigations.

Management of the infant should include education of the parents concerning normal bowel habits. Short, transient periods of constipation usually require no intervention. Mild constipation usually resolves as solid food is introduced in the diet.

Stool softeners such as malt extract or lactulose may be used for hard stools or anal fissures. The persistent use of rectal stimulation with thermometers or cotton-tipped applicators is discouraged because these methods often result in anal fissures and increased pain that may trigger stool withholding.

The management of simple constipation consists of a plan to keep the bowel relatively empty of stool and dietary management to prevent further constipation.

Management of chronic constipation requires an organized approach. The goals for management include restoring regular evacuation of stool, shrinking the distended rectum to its normal size, and promoting a regular toileting routine. This requires a combination of therapies and should include bowel cleansing, maintenance therapy to prevent stool retention, modification of diet, bowel habit training, and behavioral modification.

There is not total agreement as to the most effective way to treat chronic constipation. It is important to remove hard, impacted stool. This may be accomplished with suppositories, enemas, and occasionally the use of polyethylene glycol electrolyte solution (GoLYTELY) administered orally or by nasogastric tube. A severe impaction may require a combination of mineral oil to soften the mass and enemas. Suppositories are not usually effective for severe impactions. Sometimes surgical removal may be required.

> **NURSING ALERT**
>
> Mineral oil must be given carefully to avoid the risk of aspiration.

After the impaction is removed, maintenance therapy is necessary to promote easy passage of stool and to prevent stool retention. Maintenance therapy includes mineral oil, stool softeners, and laxatives. Stool softeners are often not effective for severe constipation; laxative therapy may be necessary to return the rectum to its normal size. Milk of magnesia and polyethylene glycol (Miralax) are the safest laxatives to use because they act to increase fluid in the colon. The additional volume of fluid stimulates the urge to defecate.

Changes in the diet may be helpful but are usually not effective alone. Encouraging the intake of fiber will ultimately help to maintain regular elimination once the rectum returns to normal size and the child is tapered off laxatives. Effective counseling is an essential element of the treatment plan for children with chronic constipation. Normal bowel function, the purpose of interventions, and the need for persistence should be explained to the child and family. Erroneous concepts concerning this condition should be corrected.

Retraining therapy involves habit training, reinforcement for sitting on the toilet and defecation, and emotional support. A regular toilet time should be established once or twice a day, preferably after a meal. A reasonable amount of time (5 to 10 minutes) should be spent attempting to defecate completely. Biofeedback may be indicated as a form of behavior modification and as a means to teach children to relax the anal sphincter during defecation.

### Nursing Considerations

Unfortunately, constipation tends to be self-perpetuating. A child who has difficulty or discomfort when attempting to evacuate the bowels has a tendency to retain the bowel contents, and thus constipation becomes a chronic problem.

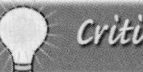

## Critical Thinking Exercise

### Constipation

An 8-month-old infant is seen by the pediatric nurse practitioner. The infant's mother states that the infant usually has one hard stool every 4 to 5 days, which causes discomfort when the stool is passed. Once the infant had an episode of diarrhea and twice has had ribbonlike stools. Abdominal distention and vomiting have not accompanied the constipation, and the infant's growth has been normal. The infant's diet consists of cow's milk formula only. The infant's mother reports that the infrequent passage of hard stools began approximately 6 weeks ago when she stopped breast-feeding. Which of the following interventions should the nurse practitioner include in the initial management of this infant's problem?

FIRST, THINK ABOUT IT . . .

- What are you taking for granted?
- What would the consequences be if you put your thoughts into action?

---

1. Prescribe several medications to be given daily to maintain a loose consistency of stools.
2. Tell the infant's mother that she stopped breast-feeding too soon and that if she resumes breast-feeding, the constipation will resolve.
3. Reassure the mother that constipation may occur with a change in diet and recommend that the mother slowly introduce cereal and prune juice into the infant's diet.
4. Refer the mother to a pediatric gastroenterologist for further evaluation.

---

*The best responses are three and four. Although functional constipation often occurs in infancy with a change in diet, the episode of diarrhea and the passage of ribbonlike stools may be manifestations of a medical cause. The referral is needed to rule out conditions such as Hirschsprung disease, which should not be taken for granted. If this infant is determined to have functional constipation, simple measures such as dietary modifications may help to remedy the problem. Often, functional constipation resolves as solid food is introduced into the diet. One or two offerings of fruit juice each day may also help to prevent further constipation. Although breast-fed infants may have constipation less frequently than bottle-fed infants, telling the mother to resume breast-feeding may make her feel responsible for her infant's constipation and instill guilt. Medications may be needed if dietary measures fail or if the child is found to have a medical cause for the constipation. However, pharmacologic intervention is not the intervention of choice at this time.*

Nursing assessment begins with a history of bowel habits, diet, events that may be associated with the onset of constipation, drugs or other substances that the child may be taking, and the consistency, color, frequency, and other characteristics of the stool. If there is no evidence of a pathologic condition that requires further investigation, the major task of the nurse is to educate the parents regarding normal stool patterns and to participate in the education and treatment of the child.

Dietary modifications are helpful in preventing constipation. Fiber is an important part of the diet. Parents benefit from guidance about foods high in fiber (Box 33-3) and ways to promote healthy food choices in children. If bran is added to the diet, creative ways to disguise the consistency, such as adding it to cereal, peanut butter, mashed potatoes, fruit shakes, and baked goods, are helpful. Beans are often found in Mexican dishes children enjoy and can be added to soups, salads, and stews. Beyond the age when foreign body aspiration is a hazard, a good source of fiber is corn and popcorn.

Parents need reassurance concerning the prognosis for establishing normal bowel habits. Many parents are very concerned about constipation and view the condition as dangerous. Families need thorough instructions about the treatment plan. If the child needs enemas or medication, the family is given appropriate instructions.* It is important to discuss attitudes and expectations regarding toilet habits and the treatment plan.

## Hirschsprung Disease (Congenital Aganglionic Megacolon)

Hirschsprung disease is a congenital anomaly that results in mechanical obstruction from inadequate motility of part of the intestine. It accounts for about one fourth of all cases of neonatal intestinal obstruction. The incidence is 1 in 5000 live births. It is four times more common in males than in females and follows a familial pattern in a small number of cases. It has been estimated that 80% of the cases of Hirschsprung disease are due to autosomal domi-

---

*Home care instructions for administering oral medications and enemas are available in Wong DL, Hess CS: *Wong and Whaley's clinical manual of pediatric nursing*, ed 5, St Louis, 2000, Mosby.

nant genetic mutations with incomplete penetrance (Klein and Burd, 1999). Hirschsprung disease is associated with other anomalies, such as Down syndrome. Depending on its presentation, it may be an acute, life-threatening condition or a chronic disorder.

### Pathophysiology

The pathology of Hirschsprung disease relates to the absence of ganglion cells in the affected areas of the intestine, resulting in a loss of the rectosphincteric reflex and an abnormal microenvironment of the cells of the affected intestine. The term *congenital aganglionic megacolon* describes the primary defect, which is the absence of ganglion cells in the myenteric plexus of Auerbach and the submucosal plexus of Meissner (Fig. 33-2). These ganglion cells were formerly known as intramural ganglia of the parasympathetic nervous system and are now classified as elements of an independent enteric nervous system (ENS). The absence of ganglion cells in the affected bowel results in a lack of ENS stimulation, which decreases the ability of the internal sphincter to relax. Unopposed sympathetic stimulation of the intestine results in increased intestinal tone. In addition to the contraction of the abnormal bowel and the resulting lack of peristalsis, there is a loss of the rectosphincteric reflex. Normally when a stool bolus enters the rectum, the internal sphincter relaxes and the stool is evacuated. In Hirschsprung disease, the internal sphincter does not relax. The disease appears to result from a failure of neural crest cells to migrate along the GI tract during the fifth and twelfth weeks of gestation. The earlier this arrest in migration occurs, the longer the aganglionic segment (Klein and Burd, 1999). In most cases the aganglionic segment includes the rectum and some portion of the distal colon. However, the entire colon or part of the small intestine may be involved. Occasionally, skip segments or total intestinal aganglionosis may occur.

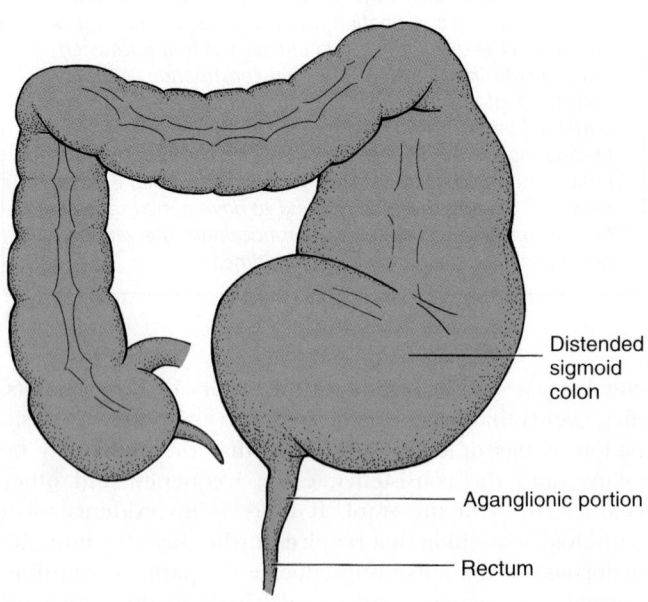

**Fig. 33-2**  Hirschsprung disease.

Distended sigmoid colon

Aganglionic portion

Rectum

---

**Box 33-3** ■ ■ ■
**High-Fiber Foods**

**BREAD, GRAINS**
Whole-grain bread or rolls
Whole-grain cereals
Bran
Pancakes, waffles, and muffins with fruit or bran
Unrefined (brown) rice

**VEGETABLES**
Raw vegetables, especially broccoli, cabbage, carrots, cauliflower, celery, lettuce, and spinach
Cooked vegetables, such as those listed above, and asparagus, beans, brussels sprouts, corn, potatoes, rhubarb, squash, string beans, and turnips

**FRUITS**
Prunes, raisins, or other dried fruits
Raw fruits, especially those with skins or seeds, other than ripe banana or avocado

**MISCELLANEOUS**
Legumes (beans), popcorn, nuts, seeds
High-fiber snack bars

## Clinical Manifestations

Clinical manifestations vary according to the age when symptoms are recognized, the length of the affected bowel, and the occurrence of complications such as enterocolitis. In the newborn period, abdominal distention, vomiting, constipation, and failure to pass meconium within the first 48 hours of life are likely to occur. Neonates may also have signs of acute intestinal obstruction, including abdominal distention and bilious vomiting. Some infants have abdominal distention that is relieved by rectal simulation or enemas. In older infants and children the presenting clinical features are constipation, abdominal distention, vomiting, and a history of delayed meconium passage. Chronic constipation with passage of ribbonlike, foul-smelling stools and abdominal distention are the most common features. Older children often have evidence of previous gastrointestinal dysfunction, failure to thrive, or chronic constipation (Klein and Burd, 1999).

## Diagnostic Evaluation

In the neonate the diagnosis is suspected on the basis of clinical signs of intestinal obstruction or failure to pass meconium. In infants and children the history is an important part of diagnosis and typically includes a chronic pattern of constipation. On examination the rectum is empty of feces, the internal sphincter is tight, and leakage of liquid stool and accumulated gas may occur if the aganglionic segment is short. A barium enema often demonstrates the transition zone between the dilated proximal colon (megacolon) and the aganglionic distal segment. However, this typical megacolon and narrow distal segment may not develop until the age of 2 months or later.

To confirm the diagnosis, rectal biopsy is performed either surgically to obtain a full-thickness biopsy specimen or by suction biopsy for histologic evidence of the absence of ganglion cells. A noninvasive procedure that may be used is *anorectal manometry,* in which a catheter with a balloon attached is inserted into the rectum. The test records the reflex pressure response of the internal anal sphincter to distention of the balloon. A normal response is relaxation of the internal sphincter followed by a contraction of the external sphincter. In Hirschsprung disease the external sphincter contracts normally but the internal sphincter fails to relax.

## Therapeutic Management

The majority of children with Hirschsprung disease require surgery rather than medical therapy with frequent enemas. Once the child is stabilized with fluid and electrolyte replacement, if needed, surgery is performed with a high rate of success. Surgical management consists primarily of the removal of the aganglionic portion of the bowel to relieve obstruction, restore normal motility, and preserve the function of the external anal sphincter. In most cases this is accomplished in two stages. First, a temporary ostomy is created proximal to the aganglionic segment, to relieve obstruction and allow the normally innervated dilated bowel to return to normal size.

Following this initial surgery a second complete, corrective surgery is performed, usually when the child weighs approximately 9 kg (20 pounds). There are several operations that can be performed, including the Swenson, Duhamel, Boley, and Soave procedures. The *Soave endorectal pull-through procedure* is often performed and consists of pulling the end of the normal bowel through the muscular sleeve of the rectum, from which the aganglionic mucosa has been removed. The ostomy is usually closed at the time of the final, definitive surgery.

With earlier diagnosis the proximal bowel may not be extremely distended, thus allowing for a primary pull-through or one-stage procedure and eliminating the need for a temporary colostomy. Simpler operations, such as an anorectal myomectomy, may be indicated in very-short-segment disease. Recently, minimally invasive laparoscopic techniques have been used. These approaches may improve morbidity, and although they are more expensive, they have shortened the duration of hospitalization (Klein and Burd, 1999).

Following the pull-through procedure, anal stricture and incontinence may occur and require further therapy, including dilations or bowel-retraining therapy.

## Nursing Considerations

The nursing concerns depend on the child's age and the type of treatment. Observation of passage of meconium and bowel patterns in the neonatal period is an important factor in early diagnosis. If the disorder is diagnosed during the neonatal period, the main objectives are helping the parents adjust to the congenital disorder, fostering infant-parent bonding, preparing the parents for the medical/surgical intervention, and assisting them in caring for the colostomy after discharge.

When the disorder is not discovered during infancy, the nurse can facilitate establishing a diagnosis by carefully listening to the history, with a special emphasis on bowel habits. In Hirschsprung disease, several areas must be investigated: (1) frequency of bowel movements; (2) character of stools, particularly ribbonlike and foul-smelling stools; and (3) onset of constipation, especially if present since birth. Other clues in the history and physical examination include poor feeding habits, fussiness and irritability, distended abdomen, and signs of undernutrition, such as thin extremities, pallor, muscle weakness, and fatigue.

In unusual cases when the child is managed with occasional enemas, the nurse needs to teach the parents the correct procedure, as well as inform them of the dangers associated with using tap water, concentrated salt solutions, soap solutions, or phosphate preparations. Normal saline solution can be purchased without a prescription from a pharmacy or can be prepared at home by adding 1 level measuring teaspoon of noniodized salt to 1 pint of tap water. Because the instructions for preparing the solution and administering the enema require several steps, all of the directions should be written down, as well as verbally explained.* (See Chapter 27 for suggested amounts of solution according to the child's age.)

---

*Home care instructions for giving an enema are available in Wong DL, Hess CS: *Wong and Whaley's clinical manual of pediatric nursing,* ed 5, St Louis, 2000, Mosby.

**Preoperative Care.** The child's preoperative care depends on the age and clinical condition. A child who is malnourished may not be able to withstand surgery until the physical status improves. Often this involves symptomatic treatment with enemas; a low-fiber, high-calorie, and high-protein diet; and in severe situations, the use of *total parenteral nutrition (TPN)*.

Physical preoperative preparation entails the same procedures that are common to any surgery. (See Chapter 27.) In the newborn, bowel is sterile; no additional preparation is required. In older children, preoperative preparation for the pull-through procedure should include a complete bowel preparation with nasogastric (NG) tube administration of GoLYTELY to empty the bowel and the administration of systemic antibiotics and rectal irrigations.

In children with enterocolitis, emergency preoperative care includes frequent monitoring of vital signs and blood pressure for signs of shock; monitoring fluid and electrolyte replacements, plasma, or other blood derivatives; and observing for symptoms of bowel perforation, such as fever, increasing abdominal distention, vomiting, increased tenderness, irritability, dyspnea, and cyanosis.

Because progressive distention of the abdomen is a serious sign, abdominal circumference is measured with a paper tape measure at the largest diameter, usually at the level of the umbilicus. The point of measurement is marked with a pen to ensure reliability. It is best to record the measurement in serial order so that a change will be readily apparent. (See Atraumatic Care box.)

The child's age dictates the type and extent of psychologic preparation necessary for the child and the parents. Older children need to be emotionally prepared and educated for an ostomy. (See Ostomies, Chapter 27.) Because a colostomy represents a change in body function, the nurse should investigate the caregiver's previous knowledge of this procedure. Family members may have misconceptions regarding an ostomy or may have concerns regarding the appearance or care of the stoma. Education and emotional support are the most helpful nursing interventions at this time.

Teaching children and family members about an ostomy is best done by a verbal explanation, as well as through the use of a drawing or a teaching doll. It is important to stress to parents and older children that the colostomy for Hirschsprung disease is temporary, unless so much bowel is involved that a permanent ileostomy must be performed. In most instances the extent of bowel resection is known before surgery, although the nurse should be aware of those instances when doubt exists concerning repair. The nurse

should also keep in mind that although a temporary colostomy is favorable in terms of future help and adjustment, it also necessitates additional surgery, which may be very stressful to parents and children.

**Postoperative Care.** Postoperative care following a colostomy or pull-through procedure is similar to that following any abdominal surgery. The infant or child should have nothing by mouth and will often have an NG tube to suction. Intake and output, including NG tube losses and stool from the ostomy, are measured. To prevent contamination of the abdominal wound with urine in the infant, the diaper should be pinned below the dressing. Sometimes a Foley catheter is used in the immediate postoperative period to divert the flow of urine away from the abdomen. Intravenous (IV) fluids are monitored to maintain adequate hydration and electrolyte balance. An abdominal assessment, including monitoring of return of bowel sounds and passage of stool, will indicate when oral feeding can be initiated. Following a colostomy procedure, ostomy care is an important nursing responsibility. Ongoing education of the older child and caregivers regarding ostomy care will begin with preparation for their discharge home.

When family members initially visit their child postoperatively, they are often anxious about the numerous tubes and IV lines attached to various body parts. The nurse should explain the function of each piece of equipment, stressing features that permit the child to be safely moved and handled, such as length of tubing, use of arm boards and IV sites, and tape to secure the NG tube to the nose. Parents are encouraged and assisted in holding and comforting their child.

**Home Care.** Postoperatively parents need instruction concerning colostomy care at home, including skin care, emptying and changing the ostomy appliance, and monitoring for problems.* (See Ostomies, Chapter 27.) During the early postoperative period, including parents and the older child in dressing changes can enhance teaching of colostomy care when an appliance is fitted and promote gradual acceptance of the body change. Even a preschooler can be included in the care by handing articles to the parent, rolling up the colostomy bag after it has been emptied, or applying cream to the surrounding skin. Because these children may have had difficulties with bowel training before surgery because of constipation and erratic stool patterns, the period during the temporary ostomy can relieve the pressures previously associated with bowel control. Although Hirschsprung disease occurs less frequently in school-age children or adolescents, if it is discovered in older children, they should be involved in colostomy care to the point of total responsibility.

In some institutions an enterostomal therapist is available to provide additional expert assistance in planning for home care, such as preparation of the skin, application of the collecting appliance, care of the appliance, control of odor, and signs of complications, such as ribbonlike stools,

---

### ATRAUMATIC CARE
*Abdominal Circumference Measurements*

To reduce any stress to the acutely ill child when frequent measurements of abdominal circumference are needed, leave the tape measure in place beneath the child. Measure the abdomen at the same time that vital signs are taken to avoid frequently disturbing the child.

---

*Home care instructions for caring for the child with a colostomy are available in Wong DL, Hess CS: *Wong and Whaley's clinical manual of pediatric nursing,* ed 5, St Louis, 2000, Mosby.

excessive diarrhea, bleeding, prolapse, or failure to pass flatus or stool.

Sometimes families require financial assistance and additional psychologic support, and referral to a social worker or other service agency may be necessary. Additional supervision of care, reinforcement of child and family education, and support are often required in the home setting to maintain continuity of care. A referral to a home health care agency for home nursing visits can meet this need. (See Nursing Care Plan: The Child with Hirschsprung Disease [Megacolon].*)

## Gastroesophageal Reflux (GER)

GER is defined as the transfer of gastric contents into the esophagus. Although GER occurs occasionally in everyone, it is the frequency, persistency, and complications of occurrence that make it abnormal. Approximately 1 in 300 to 1 in 1000 children have GER. It is important to differentiate GER from gastroesophageal reflux disease (GERD). GERD includes symptoms of tissue damage that result from GER. However, GER may occur without GERD. GER becomes the disease (GERD) when complications such as failure to thrive, bleeding, or dysphagia develop. GERD has also been associated with respiratory conditions such as apnea, bronchospasm, laryngospasm, and pneumonia (Zeiter and Hyams, 1999).

The causes of GER are related to dysfunction of the lower esophageal sphincter (LES), delay in gastric emptying, poor clearance of esophageal acid, and the susceptibility of the esophageal mucosa to acid injury (Zeiter and Hyams, 1999). In the past, GER was thought to result from decreased LES tone; however, it now appears that transient relaxation of the lower esophageal sphincter is the most common cause. Factors that may cause LES pressure to vary include gastric distention, increased abdominal pressure caused by coughing, central nervous system disease, delayed gastric emptying, hiatal hernia, and gastrostomy placement. Medications can also increase GER by relaxing the LES or increasing gastric acid production and secretion.

Infants and children who are prone to develop GER include premature infants, infants with bronchopulmonary dysplasia, and children who have had tracheoesophageal or esophageal atresia repairs, neurologic disorders, scoliosis, asthma, cystic fibrosis, and cerebral palsy.

### Clinical Manifestations

The most common clinical manifestation of GER is passive regurgitation or emesis. Other, less common symptoms that may appear in children with a significant problem include poor weight gain, heme-positive emesis or stools, anemia, irritability or heartburn, gagging or choking after a feeding, apnea, or recurrent pneumonias.

Recurrent reflux of acidic gastric contents can lead to *esophagitis*, which can cause bleeding from the esophageal

mucosa. Blood loss produces anemia and is seen as hematemesis or melena (blood in stools). Heartburn is a frequent symptom in older children who are able to describe it, but it may be unrecognized in preverbal infants. Esophagitis can also cause discomfort in the chest area, which may be manifested as unusual irritability or poor intake of nutrients. Poor weight gain and poor growth may occur in a child with an insufficient intake of nutrients or with a very large amount of regurgitation.

Multiple respiratory abnormalities have been linked to GER, but it is difficult to distinguish whether respiratory problems are a result or a contributing cause of reflux. In newborns, particularly premature infants, a few symptoms, such as apnea and bradycardia, have been attributed to GER. In addition, microaspiration may occur in some infants and children. The cause may include a swallowing disorder leading to aspiration of refluxed gastric contents or an esophagovagal reflex rather than GER. GER may also serve as a trigger for asthma in some children.

### Diagnostic Evaluation

The history and physical examination is an important part of the diagnostic evaluation for GER. The history should include questions regarding feeding habits, frequency and characteristics of emesis, behavior, and respiratory symptoms, including the time at which they occur and any associated events. The physical examination should include a stool guaiac test and assessment of growth and nutritional status.

Diagnostic studies to further evaluate GER include a barium swallow and an upper GI series. The barium swallow is performed to observe for reflux following swallowing. The upper GI series is important to exclude other anatomic obstructions, such as an esophageal, gastric, or duodenal web; pyloric mass; or malrotation.

Another study to aid in the evaluation of GER is *esophageal pH monitoring*. A probe is placed through the nose down to the distal esophagus and connected to a pH monitoring device. A 24-hour pH probe study provides information regarding the frequency of acid reflux, the amount of time there is acid in the distal esophagus, and the time it takes for the acid to be cleared from the esophagus. The effects of feeding, positioning, sleep, and other events on GER can be determined. Occasionally a pH probe study can be done simultaneously with a cardiorespiratory recording monitor to address the relationship of GER and respiratory symptoms such as apnea.

Endoscopy may be performed when GER is suspected to assess whether esophagitis is present. The esophagus is examined visually for evidence of inflammation or ulceration. Mucosal biopsies are obtained to assess microscopic changes consistent with GER and to determine the severity of reflux.

Scintigraphy and manometry are also used in the diagnosis of GER. During *scintigraphic studies* a radionuclide is added to the infant's formula, and a gamma counter detects the presence of formula refluxed to the esophagus or lungs. Scintigraphy is a useful tool for assessing delayed gastric emptying, which may contribute to GER.

---

*Home care instructions for caring for the child with a colostomy are available in Wong DL, Hess CS: *Wong and Whaley's clinical manual of pediatric nursing,* ed 5, St Louis, 2000, Mosby.

## Therapeutic Management

Therapeutic management of GER depends on its severity and on whether complications such as poor growth, esophagitis, or respiratory problems are present. For the majority of infants with reflux, only conservative management is indicated to minimize the symptoms until the problem resolves. Small, frequent feedings are often beneficial to decrease the amount of regurgitation. Occasionally, continuous NG tube feedings are indicated if severe regurgitation and poor growth are present.

Controversies surround both thickened feedings and positioning therapy as treatment for GER. Small, frequent feedings of thickened formula and frequent burping are generally accepted as reasonable strategies to minimize reflux.

Thickening is usually accomplished by adding enough rice cereal to the formula to achieve a concentration that necessitates enlarging the nipple to allow adequate flow. Evaluation of this therapy using pH probe and scintigraphy has not shown a decrease in reflux but has shown a decrease in the number and total volume of emesis. Thickening feedings decreases crying and increases the caloric density of the formula, which may help infants with nutritional deficits due to regurgitation with reflux. Whether thickened feedings are helpful for infants with nonregurgitant reflux is not yet resolved (Orenstein, 1999). Increased frequency of feedings may also result in increasing the postprandial time when most reflux occurs. Recommending smaller, more frequent feedings may be a reasonable approach for infants who were previously fed large-volume feedings infrequently (Orenstein, 1999).

Positioning therapy has been a topic of much controversy and research. The prone position decreases reflux, improves gastric emptying, decreases aspiration, energy expenditure, and crying time. Prone positioning also has beneficial effects on respiratory disease. The American Academy of Pediatrics (1996) recommends that infants be placed supine (or side-lying) for sleep to minimize the risk of sudden infant death syndrome (SIDS). However, infants with GERD are exempt. Any additional risk of SIDS may be eliminated by avoiding puffy, potentially suffocating bedding (Orenstein, 1999).

Pharmacologic therapy is sometimes used to treat infants and children with GER when reflux is causing complications such as esophagitis, respiratory symptoms, or failure to thrive. The medications used are prokinetic agents that act to increase sphincter pressure and promote gastric emptying and acid suppressors. Antacids or histamine receptor antagonists ($H_2$ blockers), such as cimetidine (Tagamet), ranitidine (Zantac), or famotidine (Pepcid), reduce the amount of acid present in gastric contents and may prevent esophagitis. Omeprazole (Prilosec) and lansoprazole (Prevacid) are proton pump inhibitors that act to block the proton pump in the parietal cells of the gastric mucosa. These drugs bind to the hydrogen-potassium ATPase enzyme. This enzyme, also known as the proton pump, is necessary for the last step in the gastric acid secretion process (Hochwald and Farrington, 1996). Side effects of proton pump inhibitors include nausea, vomiting, diarrhea, constipation, abdominal pain, headache, and dizziness.

Prokinetic medications are often prescribed as a treatment for GER. Bethanecol (Urecholine) and metoclopramide (Reglan) have both been used to decrease reflux. Bethanecol is a cholinergic drug that acts to increase LES pressure, esophageal peristaltic amplitude and duration, and salivary flow (Orenstein, 1999). However, this drug has not been shown to decrease reflux by pH probe studies (Hillemeier, 1999), and it may exacerbate respiratory symptoms such as wheezing and bronchospasm. Metoclopramide increases LES pressure and improves gastric emtpying and esophageal peristalsis. However, metoclopromide should be used with caution because there is a narrow therapeutic margin between the effectiveness of this drug and its side effects, which include restlessness, drowsiness, and extrapyramidal reaction (Orenstein, 1999).

Cisapride (Propulsid) was very effective in promoting gastric emptying, but this drug was discontinued because of the risk of serious cardiac arrhythmias and death associated with its use. This drug is available only through an investigational limited-access program.

Surgical management of GER is selected for infants and children who have failed to respond to medical therapy or who have an anatomic abnormality that is contributing to the symptoms. Several antireflux procedures are available, but the **Nissen fundoplication** is the most frequently performed procedure. The principle behind this procedure is to establish an intraabdominal portion of the esophagus and to develop a lower esophageal sphincter that resists the passage of gastric contents from the stomach to the esophagus. The surgeon creates an antireflux valve around the portion of the intraabdominal esophagus by bringing a portion of the fundus of the stomach around the esophagus (Foglia, 1999) (Fig. 33-3). The purpose of the surgery is to create a high-pressure zone in this portion of the esophagus by de-

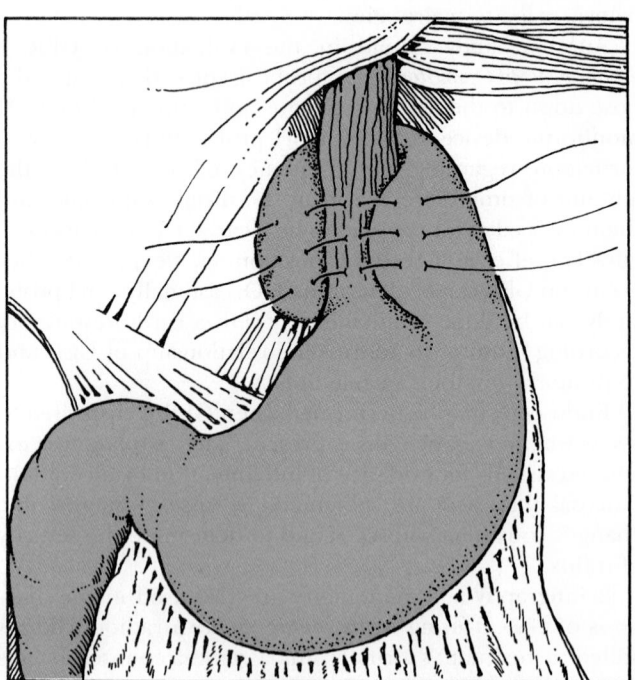

**Fig. 33-3** Nissen fundoplication sutures passing through esophageal musculature. (Redrawn from Campbell A, Ferrara B: Toupet partial fundoplication, *AORN J* 57:671-679, 1993.)

creasing the diameter of the distal esophagus, thereby increasing the opening pressure necessary to initiate reflux while preserving the angle of His. Patients with delayed gastric emptying may also have a pyloroplasty performed (Foglia, 1999). Unfortunately, complications can occur following fundoplication; therefore the decision to perform this procedure should be carefully considered. Postoperative problems include small-bowel obstruction, failure with continued GER, wrap hernia, retching, gas-bloat syndrome, and dumping syndrome. For children with neurologic impairment who are continuously tube fed, an alternative to fundoplication with gastrostomy tube placement is a nonsurgical percutaneous gastrojejunostomy and placement of a jejunostomy tube (Fonkalsrud and others, 1998).

**Prognosis.** The majority of infants with GER have a mild problem that generally improves by 12 to 18 months of age and requires only conservative lifestyle changes or medical therapy. If GER is severe and remains unsuccessfully treated, multiple complications can occur. Esophageal strictures caused by persistent esophagitis with scarring is one of the most significant complications. Recurrent respiratory distress with aspiration pneumonia, another serious complication, is an indication for surgery. Failure to thrive caused by GER can often be managed with medical therapy and nutritional support.

## Nursing Considerations

Nursing care is directed at (1) identifying children with symptoms suggestive of GER; (2) educating parents regarding home care, including feeding, positioning, and medications when indicated; and (3) if appropriate, caring for the child undergoing surgical intervention. For the majority of infants, parental reassurance of the benign nature of the condition and its relationship to physiologic maturity is the most important intervention. To help parents cope with the inconvenience of dealing with a child who spits up or regurgitates frequently, simple measures such as using bibs and protective clothes during feeding and prone positioning after feeding are beneficial.

It is important to educate and reassure parents about positioning. In the past, recommendations encouraged upright positioning for both infants and older children. Further studies indicated that poor truncal tone of infants may make the seated position detrimental. The prone position is desirable when the infant is not being held strictly vertical by the caretaker. Elevation of the head of the bed has long been recommended for infants in the prone position, but a large controlled study failed to show significant benefit of head elevation compared to the simple flat prone position (Orenstein, 1990). For older children, the recommendation is standing or sitting upright while awake and sleeping in the prone position. Parents will need reassurance about the prone position for infants because most parents are aware of the recommendation to position infants in the supine position to prevent SIDS.

Feeding modification may require some rescheduling of the family's routine to accommodate more frequent feeding times. If formula is thickened with cereal, the nipple opening may need to be enlarged for easier sucking. Usually breast-feeding may continue, and the mother may provide more frequent feeding times or express the milk for thickening with rice cereal. Parents should avoid feeding the child fatty foods, chocolate, tomato products, and carbonated liquids, which decrease LES pressure, and fruit juices, citrus products, and spicy foods, which increase secretion of gastric acid. Other practical advice relating to feedings includes advising the parents to avoid vigorous play following feedings and to avoid feeding just before bedtime.

When regurgitation is severe and growth is a problem, continuous NG tube feedings may decrease the amount of emesis and provide constant buffering of gastric acid. Special preparation of caregivers is required when this type of nutritional therapy is indicated.

The nurse can support the family by providing information about all aspects of treatment. Parents often require specific information about the medications given for GER. For example, omeprazole and lansoprazole are available in capsules. Usually the capsule is swallowed whole without chewing. However, this is often not possible for infants and young children. In these situations the capsule may be opened and added to a weakly acidic vehicle such as apple juice, applesauce, or yogurt. The granules should not be mixed with water or saline. If a dose is smaller than the capsule size, the granules should be divided before mixing. The remaining granules can then be stored in a tightly closed container and retained for the next scheduled dose (Woods and McClintock, 1993). Many pharmacies will compound the medication in a liquid form for administration. However, the liquid form needs to be dispensed in smaller amounts, thus necessitating more frequent trips to the pharmacy, because the potency of the medication expires quickly. Currently many pharmaceutical companies are working to develop new formulations that will be easier to administer to infants and children.

If a child is receiving medications through a jejunostomy feeding tube, the granules should be mixed with sodium bicarbonate to dissolve the enteric coating and facilitate absorption in the normally alkaline environment of the intestines and should be given immediately.

Postoperative nursing care following the Nissen fundoplication is similar to that for other types of abdominal surgery. (See Chapter 27.) Gastric decompression by an NG tube or gastrostomy must be maintained to avoid distention in the immediate postoperative period. Usually the NG tube should not be replaced by the nurse if it is accidentally removed, because of the risk of injury to the operative site. When postoperative ileus resolves, the NG tube is removed or the gastrostomy tube is elevated in preparation for feeding. If bolus feedings are initiated through the gastrostomy, the tube may need to remain vented for several days or longer to avoid gastric distention from swallowed air. Edema surrounding the surgical site and a tight gastric wrap may prohibit the infant from expelling air through the esophagus. Some infants benefit from clamping of the tube for increasingly longer intervals until they are able to tolerate continuous clamping between feedings. During this time, if the infant displays increasing irritability and evidence of cramping, some relief may be provided by venting the tube.

**Preparation for Home Care.** If medical management is prescribed or surgery is performed, nursing responsibilities include educating caregivers about administering drugs at home,* special feeding regimens or formula preparation, gastrostomy care, and postoperative care. (See Chapter 27.) After surgery, reflux is completely controlled in most cases, with these children attaining normal health and growth. If a gastrostomy tube is inserted during surgery, it may be removed after several months unless nutritional supplementation is needed. In severe cases of bloating or dumping syndrome, continuous tube feedings may be better tolerated. Caregivers should be aware of potential postoperative problems, such as difficulty vomiting, bloating symptoms, or discomfort with large solid-food meals, and seek guidance from their health care provider as needed.

## Irritable Bowel Syndrome (IBS)

IBS is one of the most common problems treated by adult gastroenterologists. Recently IBS has been identified as a cause of recurrent abdominal pain in children. (See Recurrent Abdominal Pain, Chapter 18.) A recent study indicated that 14% of high school students and 6% of middle school students had recurrent abdominal pain symptoms (Hyams and others, 1996). Unlike the adult population in which women are more frequently affected, boys and girls are equally affected in the pediatric population.

IBS is classified as a functional gastrointestinal disorder. As with other forms of recurrent abdominal pain, the symptoms should be present either recurrently or constantly over a 3-month period (Mahajan and Wyllie, 1999).

Children with IBS often have alternating diarrhea and constipation, flatulence, bloating or a feeling of abdominal distention, lower abdominal pain, a feeling of urgency when needing to defecate, and a feeling of incomplete evacuation of the bowel. IBS also has psychosocial effects. Children with symptoms of IBS report that they feel different from other children, are embarrassed about their health problems, and feel that their health problems prevent them from going out with their friends (Thomson and Dancey, 1996). In addition, among adolescents symptoms of IBS are associated with higher anxiety and depression scores on standardized tests (Hyams and others, 1996).

The cause of IBS is not clear, but it is believed to involve a combination of motor, autonomic, and psychologic factors. Children with IBS are evaluated to rule out organic causes for their symptoms such as inflammatory bowel disease, lactose intolerance, and parasitic infections. Many children with symptoms appear active and healthy and have normal growth. Their physical examination and laboratory studies are also generally normal (Mahajan and Wyllie, 1999).

### Therapeutic Management

The long-range goal of treatment is development of regular bowel habits and relief of symptoms. As with other variants of functional abdominal pain, environmental modifications, stress management, and psychosocial intervention may re-

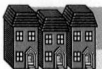
**COMMUNITY FOCUS**
*Irritable Bowel Syndrome*

Parents, school nurses, and teachers frequently interact with children and adolescents who complain of abdominal pain. Complaints of abdominal pain can lead to interruption of activities and absence from school. In addition, children and adolescents who complain of abdominal pain may have accompanying symptoms of irritable bowel syndrome, as well as anxiety and depression (Hyams and others, 1996). Parents, school nurses, and teachers should be aware of this symptom complex and become skilled in the identification of its manifestations. If the student has other worrisome features, such as weight loss, rectal bleeding, or significant fatigue, further diagnostic evaluation may be necessary. However, many students with uncomplicated abdominal pain and irritable bowel syndrome benefit from reassurance, diet counseling, and stress management. Parents, school nurses, and teachers should also remember that helping adolescents to learn to cope with life events may also influence their anxiety and depression and ultimately reduce the symptoms of abdominal pain and irritable bowel syndrome.

lieve stress and GI symptoms. A high-fiber diet with psyllium supplements (i.e., Metamucil, Fiberall) is often beneficial for the treatment of IBS. Antispasmodics, antidiarrheal drugs, and simethicone may benefit some children.

### Nursing Considerations

The primary nursing goal is family support and education. The disorder is very stressful to children and parents. Providing support and reassurance that although the symptoms of the disorder are difficult to deal with, the disorder is not generally a threat to the child's health is helpful. Nurses can help the child and family to identify and implement strategies that decrease symptoms, including eating slowly, avoiding carbonated beverages, adding fiber to the diet, and relieving environmental stressors. (See Community Focus box.)

## INFLAMMATORY CONDITIONS
### Acute Appendicitis

Appendicitis, inflammation of the vermiform appendix (the blind sac at the end of the cecum) is the most common abdominal surgical emergency in childhood. Approximately 1% of children younger than 15 years of age develop appendicitis each year with the peak incidence between 10 to 12 years of age (Pegoli, 1999). More than 80,000 children undergo appendectomies each year (Mattei, Stevenson, and Ziegler, 1999). Although many normal appendices are found at the time of surgery, at least one third of all cases of acute appendicitis in children are diagnosed after the appendix has perforated (Mattei, Stevenson, and Ziegler, 1999). Although uncommon in children younger than 2 years of age, it is associated with increased complications and mortality in this age-group. Primarily an acute disorder, appendicitis rapidly progresses to perforation and peritonitis if it remains undiagnosed. It is a significant pediatric problem; early diagnosis is frequently delayed because children are unable to verbalize symptoms and because the signs of acute appendicitis may be mistaken for other illnesses. Because there is no single diagnostic study to confirm or exclude acute appendicitis in a reliable and cost-effective way, it remains a significant cause of illness and serious morbidity in the pediatric population (Mattei, Stevenson, and Ziegler, 1999).

## Etiology

The exact cause of appendicitis is poorly understood, but it is almost always a result of obstruction of the lumen of the appendix by hardened fecal material (*fecalith*), foreign bodies, microorganisms, or parasites. Sometimes a fold of peritoneum causes the appendix to adhere to the cecum, resulting in an obstructive kink. Other causes include lymphoid hyperplasia, fibrous stenosis from an earlier inflammation, and tumors.

The risk of developing appendicitis for individuals living in the United States is estimated to be approximately 6% to 20% (Pegoli, 1999). Dietary habits may play a role with diets high in sugars and low in fibers. Fiber increases the bulk and softness of the stool—a factor that minimizes the chance of obstruction and promotes evacuation. Pinworms have not been shown to be a cause of appendicitis.

## Pathophysiology

With acute obstruction, the outflow of mucus secretions is blocked, and pressure builds within the lumen, resulting in compression of blood vessels. The luminal bacteria proliferate and invade the wall of the appendix, causing progressive local inflammatory changes and potential bacteremia. The infectious process is typically polymicrobial (both aerobes and anaerobes). The most common organisms isolated are *Escherichia coli* and *Klebsiella* with occasional *Streptococcus, Pseudomonas, Enterobacter, Bacteroides,* and *Clostridium* species (Mattei, Stevenson, and Ziegler, 1999).

The pathophysiology of acute appendicitis is determined by the stage at which the symptoms are recognized and when surgical intervention occurs. *Early simple appendicitis* may have minimal findings. *Suppurative appendicitis* often manifests with congestion and marked edema of the appendix. *Gangrenous appendicitis* is characterized by focal areas and circumferential necrosis of the wall of the appendix and possibly purulent ascites with areas of near perforation. A *perforated or ruptured appendix* presents with frank peritonitis or a walled-off appendix (Mattei, Stevenson, and Ziegler, 1999). Progressive peritoneal inflammation results in functional intestinal obstruction of the small bowel (*ileus*). Because the peritoneum represents a major portion of total body surface, the loss of extracellular fluid to the peritoneal cavity leads to electrolyte imbalance and hypovolemic shock.

## Clinical Manifestations

The first symptom of appendicitis is usually colicky, cramping, abdominal pain located around the umbilicus. *Referred pain* is the term used for this vague periumbilical localization. The midgut shares the same T10 dermatome, so pain is often perceived to be coming from this area. Generally this pain progresses and becomes constant.

The most important physical finding is focal abdominal tenderness. As the inflammation progresses to involve the

serosa of the appendix and the peritoneum of the abdominal wall, the pain may shift to the right lower quadrant. *McBurney's point,* located two thirds the distance along a line between the umbilicus and the anterior superior iliac spine, is the most common point of tenderness. Localized peritoneal signs may be found with gentle percussion or maneuvers such as heel strike or shaking the bed. Another helpful finding is Rovsing sign, a tenderness in the right lower quadrant that is elicited by palpation or percussion of other abdominal quadrants (Pearl and others, 1998). *Rebound tenderness,* deep palpation with sudden release, is often present, but may be of little use. Eliciting rebound tenderness can be extremely painful to the child and is not necessarily a finding specific only to appendicitis (Mattei, Stevenson, and Ziegler, 1999). Nausea, vomiting, and anorexia typically occur after the pain starts. Diarrhea, as well as other common signs of childhood illness such as upper respiratory tract congestion, poor feeding, lethargy, or irritability may accompany appendicitis. The child may not be able to walk well and may complain of pain in the right hip due to inflammation in the psoas or iliopsoas muscles. Low grade fever (greater than 100.5° F) may be present but occurs in only about 55% of all patients. The absence of fever does not exclude appendicitis. Temperature elevations of 102° to 103° F can occur after perforation; however, very high fevers (greater than 103° F) are uncommon (Pearl and others, 1998). **Because of the great variability in the presentation and location of appendicitis, any child with focal tenderness, regardless of the location, should be considered to potentially have acute appendicitis.** (See Community Focus box.)

**NURSING ALERT** Signs of peritonitis in addition to fever usually include sudden relief from pain after perforation; subsequent increase in pain, which is usually diffuse and accompanied by rigid guarding of the abdomen; progressive abdominal distention; tachycardia; rapid, shallow breathing as the child refrains from using abdominal muscles; pallor; chills; irritability; and restlessness.

## Diagnostic Evaluation

Diagnosis is not always straightforward. Numerous infectious and inflammatory processes have similar features. For example, fever, vomiting, abdominal pain, and an elevated blood count are associated with inflammatory bowel disease, acute infectious diarrhea, pelvic inflammatory disease, urinary tract infection, gastroenteritis, right lower lobe pneumonia, mesenteric adenitis, Meckel diverticulum, and intussusception. In adolescent females the symptoms may be caused by an ectopic pregnancy.

The diagnosis is based primarily on the history and physical examination. The only laboratory studies indicated are a complete blood count, urinalysis, and in adolescent females, a serum human chorionic gonadotropin (β-HCG). A white blood count (WBC) greater than 10,000/mm is common, but not necessarily specific for appendicitis. However, a normal white blood count and a temperature less than 100.5° F may be helpful to exclude appendicitis. An elevated percentage of bands (often called a "shift to the left") may indicate an inflammatory process. Urinalysis results are used to rule out a urinary tract infection, and the serum β-HCG in adolescents is helpful to rule out an ectopic pregnancy.

Ultrasonography and a computed tomography (CT) scan may be helpful in the differentiation of pediatric abdominal pain from other causes. Findings such as visualization of the appendix and the presence of fluid around the appendix are important sonographic signs (Borowski, 1994).

### Therapeutic Management

The treatment for appendicitis before perforation is surgical removal of the appendix (appendectomy). Usually antibiotics are administered preoperatively. IV fluids and electrolytes are often required before surgery, especially if the child is dehydrated as a result of the marked anorexia characteristic of appendicitis.

The operation is usually performed through a right lower quadrant incision *(open appendectomy)*. *Laparoscopic surgery* has been used to treat nonperforated acute appendicitis in selected pediatric patients. Three cannulas are inserted in the abdomen: one in the umbilicus, one in the left lower abdominal quadrant, and one in the suprapubic area. A small telescope is inserted through the left lower quadrant cannula, and an endoscopic stapler is inserted through the umbilical cannula. The appendix is ligated with the stapler and removed through the umbilical cannula. Advantages of laparoscopic appendectomy include reduced time in surgery and under anesthesia and also reduced risk of postoperative wound infection (Holcomb, 2001).

**Ruptured Appendix.** Management of the child diagnosed with peritonitis caused by a ruptured appendix begins with IV administration of fluid and electrolytes, systemic antibiotics, and decompression of the GI tract with an NG tube preoperatively. Postoperative management includes IV fluids and electrolytes, continued administration of antibiotics, and NG tube suction for abdominal decompression until intestinal motility returns. The child with peritonitis is given antibiotics, including ampicillin, gentamicin, and clindamycin, for 7 to 10 days.

In some instances the wound is closed following irrigation of the peritoneal cavity. Many surgeons, however, leave the wound open *(delayed closure)* to prevent wound infection and abscess formation. A Penrose drain may be used to permit transperitoneal drainage. Wound irrigations and wet-to-dry dressings may be ordered.

The treatment of a localized perforation with an appendiceal abscess is controversial. Some surgeons prefer to treat these children with antibiotics and IV fluids and allow the abscess to drain spontaneously. An elective appendectomy is then performed 2 to 3 months later.

**Prognosis.** Complications are uncommon following a simple appendectomy, and recovery is usually rapid and complete. The mortality rate from perforating appendicitis has improved from nearly certain death a century ago to 1% or less at the present time (Strahlman, 2001). Complications, however, including wound infection and intraabdominal abscess, are not uncommon. Early recognition of the illness is important to prevent complications.

## Nursing Considerations

### ✦ Assessment

Because successful treatment of appendicitis is based on prompt recognition of the disorder, a primary nursing objective is to assist in establishing a diagnosis. Because abdominal pain is a common childhood complaint, the nurse needs to make some preliminary assessment of the severity of the pain. (See Chapter 26.) One of the most reliable estimates is the degree of change in behavior. A child who stays home from school and voluntarily lies down or refuses to play is much more likely to have considerable pain than a child who is absent from school but plays contentedly at home. The younger, nonverbal child may assume a rigid, side-lying position with the knees flexed and have decreased range of motion of the right hip. For those nurses involved in primary ambulatory care, the responsibility of recognizing a possible case of appendicitis and prompt medical or surgical referral is particularly important. (See Community Focus box.) A detailed history and thorough abdominal examination cannot be overemphasized. Palpating the abdomen should be delayed until all other assessments have been made. The child is instructed to point with one finger to the site of the abdominal pain. Rebound tenderness may be present but is not always a sufficiently reliable test in children. Light palpation will satisfactorily elicit pain without causing excessive trauma. (See Atraumatic Care box.)

### ATRAUMATIC CARE
*Palpating the Abdomen for Abdominal Pain*

Because children associate the stethoscope with "listening," use the bell piece for initial palpation of the abdomen for tenderness. Children usually endure pressure from the stethoscope that they would not tolerate from a probing hand. Follow with manual palpation, using a gentle touch without lifting the hand from the abdomen while observing the child's face for signs of discomfort, such as a grimace and watchful eyes on the examination of the abdomen.

Ask the child with mild pain to lift the heels and drop them to the floor two or three times, to hop on one foot, or to "puff out" or "pull in" the abdomen to check for tenderness without more painful probing.

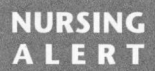

Other techniques for assessment of the abdomen are discussed in Chapter 7.

> **NURSING ALERT**
> In any instance in which severe abdominal pain is observed, the nurse must be aware of the danger of administering laxatives or enemas. Such measures stimulate bowel motility and increase the risk of perforation.

## Nursing Diagnoses

Based on a thorough assessment, several nursing diagnoses are identified. The more common diagnoses for the child with acute appendicitis are included in the Nursing Care Plan on p. 1436. Others may apply in specific situations.

## Planning

The goals for the child with acute appendicitis and the family include the following:

1. Child and family will be prepared for surgical intervention.
2. Child will receive postoperative care as described for the child undergoing surgery in Chapter 27.
3. Child with peritonitis will not experience postoperative complications, such as spread of infection.
4. Child and family will receive support and education.

## Implementation

Physical preparation of the child with appendicitis is similar to that for any child undergoing surgery. (See Chapter 27.) In situations in which medical treatment is required to correct problems associated with peritonitis, the nurse must anticipate procedures and set up equipment as quickly as possible to prevent any delay in preparing the child for surgery. Psychologic preparation of the child and parents is similar to that used in other emergency situations. (See Chapter 27.)

**Postoperative Care.** Postoperative care for the nonperforated appendix is the same as for most abdominal operations. Care of the child with a ruptured appendix and peritonitis involves more complex care. The child may need to remain in the hospital for several days or may be discharged with home care services to provide IV antibiotics and dressing changes.

Postoperatively the child is maintained on IV fluids and antibiotics, is allowed nothing by mouth (NPO), and remains on low, intermittent gastric decompression until there is evidence of return of intestinal motility. Listening for bowel sounds and observing for other signs of bowel activity (such as passage of stool) are part of the routine assessment.

A drain is often placed in the wound during surgery, and frequent dressing changes with meticulous skin care are essential to prevent excoriation of the surgery area. If the wound is left open, moist dressings (usually saline-soaked gauze), as well as wound irrigations with antibacterial solution, are used to provide an optimum healing environment.

Pain management is an essential part of the child's care. Not only is the incision painful, but the repeated dressing changes and irrigations also cause considerable distress. Because pain is continuous during the first few postoperative days, analgesics, especially opioids, are given around the clock. Procedures are performed when the analgesics are at peak effect. (See Pain Assessment; Pain Management, Chapter 26.)

Psychosocial care after surgery is also important. Sudden, acute illnesses cause unique stress, because there is little time for preparation or planning. Parents and older children need an opportunity to express their feelings and concerns regarding the events surrounding the illness and hospitalization. The nurse can provide important education and psychosocial support to promote adequate coping, with alleviation of anxiety for both the child and the family.

## Evaluation

The effectiveness of nursing interventions is determined by continual reassessment and evaluation of care based on the following observational guidelines:

1. Observe child preoperatively for reaction to the situation and compliance with care.
2. Observe for documentation regarding child's emotional and physical needs, especially assessment of pain and administration of analgesics.
3. Monitor child for evidence of infection.
4. Interview and observe child and family for evidence of their understanding of the condition, especially its sudden onset and the need for surgery.

The *expected outcomes* are described in the Nursing Care Plan on p. 1436.

# Meckel Diverticulum

Meckel diverticulum is a remnant of the fetal omphalomesenteric duct that connects the yolk sac with the primitive midgut during fetal life. Normally the structure is obliterated by the seventh to eighth week of gestation, when the placenta replaces the yolk sac as the source of nutrition for the fetus. Failure of obliteration may result in an *omphalomesenteric fistula* (a fibrous band connecting the small intestine to the umbilicus), known as Meckel diverticulum.

Meckel diverticulum is a true diverticulum because it arises from the antimesenteric border of the small intestine and includes all layers of the intestinal wall. The position of the diverticulum is variable, but it is usually found within 40 to 50 cm of the ileocecal valve. The diverticulum may develop in a variety of shapes and lengths, but most typically it is approximately 3 to 6 cm in length and smaller than the diameter of the intestine (Schwartz, 1999).

Meckel diverticulum is the most common congenital malformation of the GI tract and is present in 1% to 4% of the population, with more frequent occurrence in males than females (Schwartz, 1999). Often it exists without ever causing symptoms. Most symptomatic cases are seen in childhood. A survey of patients requiring surgery indicated that most were less than 10 years of age and about 50% were less than 2 years of age (Schwartz, 1999).

### Pathophysiology

The symptomatic complications of Meckel diverticulum are caused by bleeding, obstruction, or inflammation. Gastric

# Nursing Care Plan
## The Child with Appendicitis

### PREOPERATIVE CARE

> **NURSING DIAGNOSIS:** Acute pain related to inflamed appendix

**PATIENT GOAL 1:** Will experience no pain or reduction of pain to level acceptable to child

- **NURSING INTERVENTIONS/***RATIONALES*
See Pain Assessment; Pain Management, Chapter 26
Allow position of comfort (usually with legs flexed) *because it may vary among children*
Provide small pillow *for splinting of abdomen*
*Administer analgesia *to provide pain relief*

- **EXPECTED OUTCOME**
Child rests quietly, reports or exhibits no evidence of discomfort

> **NURSING DIAGNOSIS:** Risk for deficient fluid volume related to decreased intake and losses secondary to loss of appetite, vomiting

**PATIENT GOAL 1:** Will receive fluids for adequate hydration

- **NURSING INTERVENTIONS/***RATIONALES*
Maintain NPO *to minimize losses through vomiting and minimize abdominal distention*
Maintain integrity of infusion site *for IV fluids and electrolytes*
*Administer IV fluids and electrolytes as prescribed
Monitor intake and output *to assess hydration*

- **EXPECTED OUTCOMES**
Child receives sufficient fluids to replace losses
Child exhibits signs of adequate hydration (specify)

> **NURSING DIAGNOSIS:** Risk for infection related to possibility of rupture

**PATIENT GOAL 1:** Will experience minimized risk of infection

- **NURSING INTERVENTIONS/***RATIONALES*
Closely monitor vital signs, especially for increased heart rate and temperature and rapid, shallow breathing, *to detect ruptured appendix*
Observe for other signs of peritonitis (e.g., sudden relief of pain [sometimes] at time of perforation, followed by increased, diffuse pain and rigid guarding of the abdomen, abdominal distention, bloating, belching [from accumulation of air], pallor, chills, and irritability) *for appropriate treatment to be initiated*
Avoid administering laxatives or enemas, *because these measures stimulate bowel motility and increase risk of perforation*
Monitor WBC count *as indicator of infection*

- **EXPECTED OUTCOMES**
Child remains free of symptoms of peritonitis
Signs of peritonitis are recognized early (specify)

### POSTOPERATIVE CARE

See Postoperative Care in Nursing Care Plan: The Child Undergoing Surgery, Chapter 27

### RUPTURED APPENDIX

> **NURSING DIAGNOSIS:** Risk for infection related to presence of infective organisms in abdomen

**PATIENT GOAL 1:** Will experience minimized risk of spread of infection

- **NURSING INTERVENTIONS/***RATIONALES*
Provide wound care and dressing changes as prescribed *to prevent infection*
Monitor vital signs and WBC count *to assess presence of infection*
*Administer antibiotics as prescribed

- **EXPECTED OUTCOME**
Child demonstrates resolution of peritonitis as evidenced by lack of fever, clean wound, normal WBC

> **NURSING DIAGNOSIS:** Risk for injury related to absence of bowel motility

**PATIENT GOAL 1:** Will not experience abdominal distention, vomiting

- **NURSING INTERVENTIONS/***RATIONALES*
Maintain NPO in early postoperative period *to prevent abdominal distention and vomiting*
Maintain NG tube decompression *until bowel motility returns*
Assess abdomen for distention, tenderness, presence of bowel sounds *to assess presence of peristalsis*
Monitor passage of flatus and stool *as indicator of bowel motility*

- **EXPECTED OUTCOME**
Child does not exhibit signs of discomfort; abdomen remains soft and nondistended; child does not vomit

> **NURSING DIAGNOSIS:** Interrupted family processes related to illness and hospitalization of child

**PATIENT (FAMILY) GOAL 1:** Will receive adequate support

- **NURSING INTERVENTIONS/***RATIONALES*
Encourage expression of feelings and concerns *to enhance coping*
Encourage child to discuss hospital admission and treatments *in order to clarify misconceptions*
See Nursing Care Plan: The Child in the Hospital, Chapter 26
See Nursing Care Plan: The Family of the Child Who Is Ill or Hospitalized, Chapter 26

- **EXPECTED OUTCOMES**
Child and family express feelings and concerns
Child and family demonstrate understanding of hospitalization and treatments

*Dependent nursing action.

mucosa is the most common ectopic tissue found in a Meckel diverticulum. Bleeding, which is the most common problem in children, is caused by peptic ulceration or perforation because of the unbuffered acidic secretion. Several mechanisms may cause obstruction. Intussusception may be led by Meckel diverticulum. Obstruction may also be caused by entanglement of the small intestine around a fibrous cord, by trapping of a loop of intestine under the band, by incarceration within a hernia sac, or by volvulus of the intestinal segment containing the diverticulum. Diverticulitis occurs when peptic ulceration or obstruction leads to inflammation.

### Clinical Manifestations

Signs and symptoms are based on the specific pathologic process, such as inflammation, bleeding, or intestinal obstruction. The most common clinical presentation is rectal bleeding caused by ulceration at the junction of the ectopic gastric mucosa and normal ileal mucosa. The bleeding is usually painless and may be dramatic and occur as bright red or currant jelly–like stools, or it may occur intermittently and appear as tarry stools (Schwartz, 1999). The bleeding may be significant enough to cause hypotension. Obstruction occurs more often in adults, but volvulus and intussusception are common obstructive symptoms in children with Meckel diverticulum.

### Diagnostic Evaluation

Diagnosis is usually based on the history, physical examination, and radiographic studies. Radionucleotide scintigraphy (Meckel scan) confirms the diagnosis in 90% of cases. It consists of IV injection of an isotope, which is taken up by functional gastric mucosa, including ectopic locations. Laboratory studies are usually part of the general workup to rule out any bleeding disorder and to evaluate the severity of the anemia. Abdominal radiographs, barium enema, and arteriography have generally been unsuccessful as aids in diagnosis.

### Therapeutic Management

The standard treatment for symptomatic Meckel diverticulum is surgical removal. In instances in which severe hemorrhage increases the surgical risk, medical intervention to correct hypovolemic shock (e.g., blood replacement, IV fluids, and oxygen) may be necessary. In diverticulitis, antibiotics may be used preoperatively to control infection. If intestinal obstruction has occurred, appropriate preoperative measures are used to correct fluid and electrolyte imbalances and prevent abdominal distention.

**Prognosis.** If Meckel diverticulum is diagnosed and treated early, full recovery is likely. The mortality rate of untreated Meckel diverticulum has been reported to range from 2.5% to 15%. The serious complications of untreated Meckel diverticulum include GI hemorrhage and bowel obstruction.

### Nursing Considerations

Nursing objectives are the same as for any child undergoing surgery. (See Chapter 27.) When intestinal bleeding is present, specific preoperative considerations include (1) frequent monitoring of vital signs and blood pressure, (2) keeping the child on bed rest, and (3) recording the approximate amount of blood lost in stools.

Postoperatively the child will require IV fluids and an NG tube for decompression and evacuation of gastric secretions. Because the onset of illness is usually rapid, psychologic support is important, as in other acute conditions, such as appendicitis. It is important to remember that massive rectal bleeding is most often traumatic to both the child and the parents and may significantly affect their emotional reaction to hospitalization and surgery.

## Inflammatory Bowel Disease (IBD)

Inflammatory bowel disease, IBD, should not be confused with irritable bowel syndrome. IBD is a term that has been used to refer to two major forms of chronic intestinal inflammation—Crohn disease (CD) and ulcerative colitis (UC). CD and UC have similar epidemiologic, immunologic, and clinical features, but they are distinct disorders.

In addition to GI symptoms, both CD and UC are characterized by extraintestinal and systemic inflammatory responses. Exacerbations and remissions without complete resolution are also characteristics of IBD. Growth failure, particularly common in CD, is an important problem unique to the pediatric population. CD is also more disabling, has more serious complications, and medical and surgical treatment is often less effective for CD. Because UC is confined to the colon, theoretically it may be cured by a colectomy.

Study of the epidemiology of IBD has been complicated by the insidious onset of the disease, the lack of universal diagnostic criteria, and the occasional misclassification of patients (Hyams, 1999). Over the past 30 years, the incidence of CD has risen while the incidence of UC in children has remained stable. Although sources differ, the incidence of UC in children has been estimated as 3.5 new cases per 100,000 per year (Jackson and Grand, 1999). The incidence of CD has been reported as 3.11 per 100,000 (Hyams, 1999).

### Etiology

The exact cause of IBD is unknown, although there is evidence for a multifactorial etiology. It is proposed that IBD results from one or more influences, including the infectious organisms, dietary habits, and environmental toxins, that promote disease in genetically susceptible individuals. Current research focuses on theories of defective immunoregulation of the inflammatory response to bacteria or viruses in the GI tract in individuals with a genetic predisposition. There is a familial tendency in approximately 20% to 25% of cases. Individuals from higher socioeconomic levels and more whites are affected. The incidence is also greater among Jews living in Europe and North America and among individuals living in urban settings. Males and females are affected equally (Leichtner, Jackson, and Grand, 1999, Hyams, 1999). A primary role for psychologic factors has not been supported by evidence, although psychologic problems may occur secondary to IBD and may intensify symptoms and influence the course of the disease.

## Ulcerative Colitis (UC)

**Pathophysiology and Clinical Manifestations.** The inflammation is limited to the colon and rectum, with the distal colon and rectum often the most severely affected. Inflammation usually is limited to the mucosa and submucosa and involves continuous segments along the length of the bowel with varying degrees of ulceration, bleeding, and edema. Water and electrolytes are poorly absorbed by the inflamed mucosa of the colon, resulting in loose stools. Thickening of the bowel wall and fibrosis are unusual, but long-standing disease can result in shortening of the colon and strictures.

The presentation of UC may be mild, moderate, or severe, based on the extent of mucosal inflammation and systemic symptoms. Most include bloody diarrhea or occult fecal blood, abdominal pain, and varying degrees of systemic manifestations and growth abnormalities (Leichtner, Jackson, and Grand, 1999).

One of the earliest signs of UC may be growth failure with decreased linear growth velocity (Leichtner, Jackson, and Grand, 1999). Growth failure is most likely due to chronic poor dietary intake caused by anorexia due to GI symptoms. UC often presents with the insidious onset of diarrhea, possibly with hematochezia, and usually without fever or weight loss. The course of the disease may remain mild with intermittent exacerbations. Some children and adolescents present with grossly bloody diarrhea, cramps, urgency with defecation, mild anemia, fever, anorexia, weight loss, and moderate signs of systemic illness. Severe UC is characterized by very frequent bloody stools, abdominal pain, significant anemia, fever, and weight loss. *Extraintestinal manifestations* are less common in UC than in CD and may precede colitis. The erythrocyte sedimentation rate may be elevated, indicating the presence of a systemic response to an inflammatory process. Enlarged lymph nodes (lymphadenopathy), arthritis, and the skin lesions of erythema nodosum may be present.

## Crohn Disease (CD)

**Pathophysiology and Clinical Manifestations.** The chronic inflammatory process of CD may involve any part of the GI tract from the mouth to the anus but most commonly

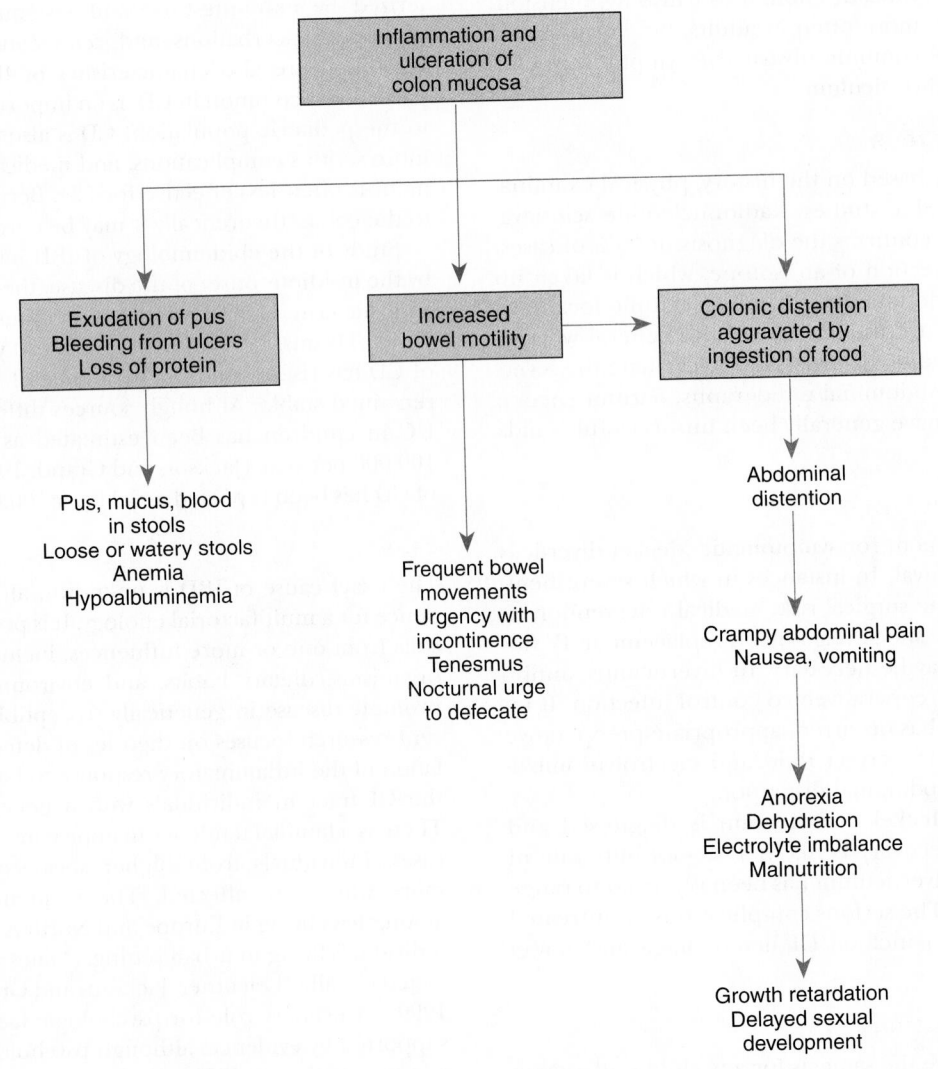

**Fig. 33-4** Effects of ulcerative colitis or Crohn disease.

affects the terminal ileum. CD involves all layers of the bowel wall (transmural) in a discontinuous fashion, meaning there are areas of affected mucosa between areas of intact mucosa (skip lesions). As with UC, the extent of the disease involvement correlates with the clinical manifestations. The inflammation may result in ulcerations, fibrosis, adhesions, stiffening of the bowel wall, stricture formation, and fistulas to other loops of bowel, bladder, vagina, or skin. The effects of UC and CD are listed in Fig. 33-4.

Common presenting manifestations of CD include diarrhea, abdominal pain with cramps, fever, and weight loss. Mild GI symptoms, poor growth, and extraintestinal manifestations may be present for several years before overt GI symptoms are present.

Nonspecific GI symptoms such as satiety, nausea, and burning epigastric pain may be present. Gastroduodenal abnormalities and symptoms are usually due to the CD rather than peptic ulcer disease, although the symptoms of each are similar. With small intestinal involvement, diarrhea with malabsorption is present as a result of mucosal inflammation, partial bowel obstruction with stasis and bacterial overgrowth, or fistulas. Both malabsorption and anorexia are factors that contribute to the growth problems that are prevalent in CD.

The disease process can also involve the colon, causing diarrhea, cramps, and urgency with defecation. Signs of colitis, such as gross rectal bleeding or stool with occult blood, are similar to those seen in UC. Perianal disease, including skin tags, abscesses, fissures, and fistulas, is a feature of CD.

*Extraintestinal manifestations,* including erythema nodosum, large joint arthritis, uveitis, mouth ulcers, liver disease, and renal calculi, are common in CD. Children with CD often have anemia and an elevated white blood cell count and erythrocyte sedimentation rate during exacerbations of the disease. Various forms of arthritis and skin lesions of erythema nodosum or erythema multiforme may be present. The symptoms of arthritis and the skin lesions appear to correspond to the clinical activity in the bowel and often improve when the intestinal inflammation is controlled. In a small number of children, serum aminotransferase levels may be elevated during disease flares. When elevations are prolonged, sclerosing cholangitis or chronic hepatitis can develop with significant liver dysfunction (Hyams, 1999). Uveitis (inflammation of the uveal tract of the eye, including the iris, ciliary body, and choroid) occurs in only a small number of children. Decreased growth velocity may precede GI symptoms in about 20% of children with CD, and an absolute height deficiency is present in approximately 30% of children at the time of diagnosis. Permanent growth failure has also been reported (Hyams, 1999). Table 33-2 provides a comparison of UC and CD.

## Diagnostic Evaluation

The diagnosis of UC and CD is usually suspected based on findings from the history, physical examination, and laboratory evaluation. However, the diagnosis is confirmed by radiologic, endoscopic, and histologic findings. Laboratory tests include a complete blood count to evaluate anemia and an erythrocyte sedimentation rate to assess the systemic reaction to the inflammatory process. Levels of total protein, albumin, iron, zinc, magnesium, vitamin $B_{12}$, and fat-soluble vitamins are measured, because they may be low in children with CD. Stool is examined for the presence of blood, leukocytes, and infectious organisms. Another specific diagnostic laboratory study used to differentiate UC from other forms of colitis is a serologic test for the detec-

**TABLE 33-2** Comparison of inflammatory bowel diseases—ulcerative colitis and Crohn disease

| Characteristics | Ulcerative Colitis | Crohn Disease |
|---|---|---|
| **Pathologic changes** | | |
| Extent of involvement | Diffuse, mucosal | Focal, transmural (entire wall) |
| Ulceration | Superficial, extensive | Deep |
| Distribution of lesions | Contiguous, symmetric | Segmental, asymmetric with "skip" areas |
| Lymph nodes | Normal | Affected |
| **Areas of involvement** | Colon, rectum | May include any part of alimentary tract from mouth to anus; terminal ileum often involved |
| **Clinical features** | | |
| Intestinal bleeding | Common, mild to severe | Uncommon, mild to severe |
| Diarrhea | Often severe | Mild to severe |
| Abdominal pain | Less frequent | Common |
| Anorexia | Mild to moderate | May be severe |
| Weight loss | Mild to moderate | May be severe |
| Growth retardation | Usually mild | May be severe |
| Anal and perianal lesions | Rare | Common |
| Fistulas and strictures | Rare | Common |
| **Surgical resection of affected bowel** | Curative | May be indicated if strictures or fistulas are present |
| | | Long-term outcome may be unsatisfactory because of frequent recurrence of disease |
| **Risk of carcinoma** | Related to duration of disease | Occurs less frequently |
| | Prevented by colectomy | Not prevented by surgery |

tion of circulating perinuclear antineutrophil cytoplasmic antibody. Circulating pANCA is found in about 70% of adults with UC and only in about 6% of CD patients. A pediatric study of this serologic test indicated a detection sensitivity of 67% for pANCA, with a specificity of 97%, a negative predictive value of 67%, and a 97% positive predictive value for identifying UC in children (Hyams, 1999).

An upper GI series with small bowel follow-through is necessary to evaluate small bowel disease in children suspected of having CD; the terminal ileum may be rigid and narrowed with partial obstruction. A CT scan may be indicated to evaluate abscesses or bowel wall thickening. A barium or air contrast enema is usually performed in children with suspected colitis unless the colitis is severe.

Diagnosis of IBD is usually confirmed following endoscopy of the lower and upper GI tracts. Endoscopy with direct visualization and biopsy of the affected segments permits an accurate determination of the extent and distribution of the colitis. The bowel is examined grossly for ulcerations or strictures. Multiple mucosal biopsies are obtained during endoscopy, and the tissue is examined for microscopic changes consistent with inflammation caused by IBD. Diffuse inflammation beginning at the anal verge and progressing proximally is consistent with UC on endoscopy. Rectal sparing is common in CD, but may be present in early cases of UC. Endoscopic findings consistent with CD include patchiness of inflammation with interspersing of areas of abnormal-appearing tissue and areas of normal tissue. Deep fissuring ulcers and pseudopolyps may be present, and the ileocecal valve may appear granular, friable, and edematous with the terminal ileum revealing marked nodularity, inflammation, and ulceration.

### Therapeutic Management

The goals of current medical, surgical, and nutritional therapies for IBD are (1) to control the inflammatory process in order to reduce or eliminate the symptoms, (2) to obtain long-term remission, (3) to promote normal growth and development, and (4) to allow as normal a lifestyle as possible. Treatment must be individualized and focused on management of current symptoms. A pediatric CD activity index may be used to standardize assessment of disease activity.

**Medical Treatment.** Symptomatic improvement is often accomplished with antiinflammatory drugs. Corticosteroids have been the most effective drugs for treating moderate to severe IBD. High doses of IV steroids are administered for acute exacerbations and are then transitioned to oral forms and tapered according to the clinical response. Steroid enemas may be used for relief of symptoms caused by sigmoid and rectal inflammation. Generally the steroid dose is decreased or discontinued as soon as possible to minimize side effects, such as adrenal suppression, hypertension, osteoporosis, glaucoma, cataracts, hirsutism, diabetes, altered body composition, and growth retardation.

Compliance problems and steroid dependence may also occur. Many children and adolescents find side effects such as mood swings, acne, weight gain, and a moon face intol-

erable. Although many patients have symptomatic improvement with steroids, attempts to taper the dose can result in a return of symptoms. Budesonide, a new synthetic steroid with potent antiinflammatory activity, is expected to be available soon in the United States. Although this drug has fewer side effects, its effectiveness in the management of inflammatory symptoms has not been evaluated.

Aminosalicylates such as sulfasalazine (Azulfidine) and mesalamine (Asacol and Pentasa) are useful in the treatment of IBD because of their antiinflammatory effects. Asacol is active in the terminal ileum; Pentasa acts from the proximal jejunum to the colon. The only controlled clinical trials for these medications have been done in adults. The aminosalicylates have been shown to be effective in maintaining remission in mild to moderate UC. Although mesalamine is usually well tolerated, side effects may include worsening diarrhea, rectal bleeding, nephritis, pancreatitis, hair loss, hepatitis, and pericarditis. Sulfasalzine is effective for mild to moderate CD but has no documented benefit in small bowel disease. Side effects of sulfasalazine include nausea, abdominal pain, headache, and rash. Because this drug interferes with the absorption of folic acid, daily supplements of folic acid are often prescribed.

Immunomodulators such as 6-mercaptopurine, azathioprine, methotrexate, and cyclosporine, are frequently used to treat CD. Azathioprine and 6-mercaptopurine are effective when initiated during corticosteroid therapy. These drugs facilitate remission, the tapering of steroids, and decrease the likelihood of recurrence of disease in patients in remission. However, it takes 3 to 6 months to determine whether these drugs are effective. A potential side effect of both 6-mercaptopurine and azathioprine is myelosuppression. Bone marrow toxicity may be seen shortly after therapy begins, and regular blood testing is mandatory to monitor for side effects. Bone marrow suppression can cause leukopenia and opportunistic infections. Other side effects include pancreatitis, hepatitis, fever, rash, and arthralgias. There may be a slight risk for the development of malignancies with long-term therapy. Potential side effects for methotrexate therapy include hepatitis, nausea, and rash. There is also a low risk for hepatic fibrosis in patients treated with methotrexate. IV cyclosporine has been effective in improving symptoms in a small group of children with refractory colitis. Side effects of cyclosporine include renal disease, abnormal hair growth, gingival hyperplasia, tremor, and the risk of opportunistic infections and malignancy.

New agents currently being evaluated for the treatment of CD include a chimeric human-mouse IgG1 monoclonal antibody to tumor necrosis factor alpha (anti-TNFα, infliximab [Remicade]). This drug has resulted in clinical improvement in perirectal disease. Similar results have been found with a nonchimeric anti-TNFα antibody. Interleukin-10, a cytokine with antiinflammatory activity, is also being studied (Hyams, 1999).

Antibiotics have not been extremely helpful in the treatment of UC. Metronidazole may be used as an adjunctive therapy in children with CD or with complications such as perianal disease or small bowel bacterial overgrowth. Ciprofloxacin may be given with metronidazole. Potential side effects of metronidazole include nausea, a metallic taste, and rarely peripheral neuropathy.

**Nutritional Support.**   Nutritional support is an important component of therapeutic management of IBD. There is some evidence to support the importance of nutritional support as an adjunctive therapy, and possibly as a primary therapy in lieu of corticosteroids, in children with CD. Nutritional support is not effective as a therapy for UC; however, it may be useful to correct growth retardation or to improve nutritional status before surgery.

Growth failure is a common serious complication of IBD, especially in CD. Growth failure is characterized by weight loss, alteration in body composition, retarded height, and delayed sexual maturation. Malnutrition is the cause of growth failure in IBD. The etiology of the malnutrition is multifactorial and includes inadequate dietary intake, excessive GI losses, malabsorption, drug-nutrient interactions, and increased nutritional requirements. Inadequate dietary intake occurs as a result of anorexia associated with chronic disease and episodes of increased disease activity. Excessive losses of nutrients occur secondary to intestinal mucosal inflammation and diarrhea. Stool losses include protein, blood, electrolytes, and minerals. Malabsorption due to mucosal injury and bacterial overgrowth is common in CD. Carbohydrate, lactose, fat, vitamin, and mineral malabsorption can occur in small bowel disease. Vitamin $B_{12}$ and folic acid deficiencies are common in children with disease or resection of the terminal ileum. Nutritional requirements are increased with increased inflammatory activity, fever, fistulas, and periods of rapid growth, such as adolescence.

The goals of nutritional support include (1) correction of specific nutrient deficits and replacement of ongoing losses, (2) provision of adequate energy and protein for healing, and (3) provision of adequate nutrients to promote normal growth. Nutritional support may include both enteral and parenteral nutrition. A well-balanced, high-protein, high-calorie diet is recommended for children whose symptoms do not prohibit an adequate oral intake. There is little evidence that avoiding specific foods influences the severity of the disease. Foods containing fiber (which is mechanically difficult to digest), such as seeds, popcorn, and corn, may produce symptoms and obstruction in children with intestinal strictures. Supplementation with multivitamins, iron, and folic acid is generally recommended. A recent study of adult patients with CD indicated that patients who received an enteric-coated fish oil preparation were significantly less likely to have relapses than patients who received a placebo (Belluzzi and others, 1996). Fish oil has an antiinflammatory action and may increase enteral absorption of nutrients, resulting in improvement of nutrition.

Enteral formulas, given by mouth or by continuous NG tube infusion (often at night), may be required to correct nutritional deficiencies and growth retardation. Both polymeric and elemental formulas may correct malnutrition and promote catch-up growth. Elemental formulas have been used successfully to improve nutritional status, as well as to induce remission, in children and adolescents with CD. Elemental formulas are completely absorbed in the small intestine with almost no residue. Several studies have demonstrated that a diet consisting only of elemental formula not only improved nutritional status, but also induced remission either without steroids or with a diminished dosage of steroids. An elemental diet is a safe and potentially effective primary therapy for patients with CD.

Total parenteral nutrition (TPN) has been shown to improve nutritional status in children with IBD. Short-term remission of symptoms has been achieved following TPN, although complete "bowel rest" has not been proved to reduce inflammation or to add to the benefits of improved nutrition achieved by TPN (Leichtner, Jackson, and Grand, 1999). Nutritional support in patients with UC is less likely to induce a remission than in patients with CD. Improvement of nutritional status is important, however, in preventing deterioration of the patient's health status and in preparing the patient for surgery.

**Surgical Treatment.**   Surgery is indicated for UC when medical and nutritional therapies fail to prevent significant complications. Surgical options include a **subtotal colectomy** and **ileostomy** that leaves a rectal stump as a blind pouch. A **J pouch** or **Kock pouch,** consisting of terminal ileum, may be created to aid in continence. An **ileoanal pull-through** preserves the normal pathway for defecation. In many cases UC can be cured with a total colectomy.

Surgery may be required in children with CD when complications cannot be controlled by medical and nutritional therapy. Segmental intestinal resections are performed for small-bowel obstructions or fistulas. Partial colonic resection is not curative, however, because the disease often recurs. Surgical intervention is often necessary for toxic megacolon, a complication of inflammatory bowel disease. In toxic megacolon an acute dilation of the colon occurs secondary to severe inflammation of the bowel mucosa. The marked dilation of the inflamed bowel causes the colon to lose its tone, and subsequent ileus or microperforations can occur. In some cases the colon thins out and shreds, leading to hemorrhage, peritonitis, and death. Signs and symptoms of toxic megacolon include spiking fever, acute abdominal pain, and distention. If toxic megacolon does not resolve with supportive medical therapy or if bowel perforation occurs, emergency surgery (a total colectomy with ileostomy) is necessary.

**Prognosis.**   IBD is a chronic disease, often with exacerbations followed by relatively long periods of remission. The outcome of the disease process is influenced by the severity of GI involvement and the regions of bowel affected, as well as by appropriate therapeutic management. Malnutrition, growth failure, intestinal strictures, fistulas, GI bleeding, and toxic megacolon are serious complications. The overall prognosis for UC is good; surgery to remove the diseased colon often provides a cure. There is no cure for CD.

Carcinoma of the colon is a long-term complication of UC and less often of CD. In UC (not CD), removal of the diseased bowel alleviates symptoms and reduces the risk of cancer (Martin, 1997).

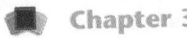
## Nursing Considerations

Many nursing considerations relate directly to the therapeutic management of IBD. However, the scope of nursing responsibilities includes (1) continued guidance of families in terms of dietary management and drug compliance; (2) coping with factors that increase stress and emotional lability; (3) adjusting to remissions and exacerbations, and (4) when indicated, preparing the child and parents for the possibility of diversionary bowel surgery.

Because nutritional support is an important component of therapy, encouraging the anorectic child to consume sufficient quantities of food is often a challenge. An approach that is more likely to meet with success involves including the child in meal planning; encouraging small, frequent meals or snacks rather than three large meals a day; serving meals around medication schedules, when diarrhea, mouth pain, and intestinal spasm are controlled; and encouraging high-protein, high-calorie foods, such as milk shakes, cream soups, puddings, and custard (if lactose is tolerated). (See Feeding the Sick Child, Chapter 27.)

Foods that are known to aggravate the condition are avoided. The routine practice of using bran or a high-fiber diet for IBD is not advised. Bran, even in small amounts, has been shown to worsen the patient's condition. Occasionally the occurrence of aphthous stomatitis complicates adherence to dietary management. (See Stomatitis, Chapter 16.) The mouth ulcers generally resolve with control of the disease process, but they contribute to poor oral intake. Gentle mouth care before eating, the selection of bland foods, and the avoidance of hot liquids or foods usually relieve the discomfort of mouth sores. A nutritionist may also be consulted to provide dietary counseling for the child and the family.

Nurses have an important role in preparing children and families to administer NG tube feedings or TPN when indicated. The purpose and the expected outcomes of these therapies should be explained, anxieties should be acknowledged, and the child and family members should be given adequate time to demonstrate the skills necessary to continue the therapy at home if needed.* (See Critical Thinking Exercise box.) A referral to a home health agency to ensure continuity of care is beneficial for the child receiving home nutritional support. (See Family-Centered Home Care, Chapter 25.)

The importance of continued drug therapy despite remission of symptoms must be stressed to the child and caregivers. Failure to adhere to the pharmacologic regimen can result in exacerbation of the disease. (See Compliance, Chapter 27.)

Attending to the emotional aspects of a chronic condition requires a thorough assessment of disease-related stress factors. Frequently the nurse can help these children to adjust to the problems of growth retardation, delayed sexual maturation, dietary restrictions, feelings of being different or sickly, inability to compete with peers, and necessary absence from school during the exacerbations of the illness. (See Chapter 22.) Complications of IBD, especially growth failure, can negatively affect self-esteem, school performance, and social interactions. Nurses can promote positive coping skills by educating the child regarding the disease and the rationale for all therapies. Many children benefit from peer support provided by other children with IBD. (See Chapter 22.)

If a permanent colectomy/ileostomy is required, the nurse can assist the child and family in accepting and ad-

---

 *Critical Thinking Exercise*

### Inflammatory Bowel Disease (IBD)

A 13-year-old girl is admitted to the hospital because of bloody diarrhea, abdominal pain, and weight loss. After a thorough evaluation, including laboratory tests, radiographic studies, and GI endoscopy procedures, the diagnosis of Crohn disease (CD) is made. Medical treatment, including corticosteroid drugs and nutritional support, is initiated in the hospital. Enteral formula administered by continuous nighttime nasogastric (NG) tube infusion and vitamin and mineral supplements will need to be continued at home after the hospitalization. Which of the following interventions would *not* be included as part of important preparations for successful home care?

FIRST, THINK ABOUT IT . . .

- What information are you using?
- How are you interpreting that information?

---

1. Educate the adolescent and family regarding the disease process.
2. Educate the adolescent and family regarding medication therapy and administration of NG tube feedings.
3. Provide psychosocial support to aid in the adjustment to a chronic disease of remissions and exacerbations.
4. Restrict school attendance and extracurricular activities for the duration of home therapy.

---

*The best response is four. The information provided in the first sentence indicates the age of the girl, which is a very important factor. School absences or inability to compete with peers in some activities may occur during exacerbations of the disease, but self-esteem, positive school performance, and social interactions are enhanced through support and guidance by family members and interactions with peers. Once the acute disease exacerbation is under control, the adolescent should resume school attendance and participate with peers in activities of interest. Important nursing responsibilities include educating the adolescent and her family regarding the disease process and therapeutic management and promoting adjustment to the chronic nature of the disease. The importance of continued drug therapy as prescribed despite remission of symptoms should be emphasized. The purpose and expected outcomes of nutrition support therapy should be explained, and the adolescent and her family members should be given adequate time to demonstrate skills relating to NG tube feedings in the hospital environment under supervision before the girl is discharged.*

---

*Home care instructions on gastrostomy feedings and caring for a central venous catheter (for TPN) are available in Wong DL, Hess CS: *Wong and Whaley's clinical manual of pediatric nursing*, ed 5, St Louis, 2000, Mosby.

justing to the change by teaching them how to care for the ileostomy, emphasizing the positive aspects of surgery (particularly, accelerated growth and sexual development, permanent recovery, and eliminated risk of colonic cancer) and stressing the normality of life despite bowel diversion. Introducing the child and parents to other ostomy patients, especially those of the child's age, can be helpful. Whenever possible, the newer continent ostomies should be offered as options to the child, although they are not performed in all centers throughout the United States.

Because of the chronic and often lifelong nature of the disease, families benefit from many of the services provided by organizations such as the **Crohn's and Colitis Foundation of America, Inc. (CCFA),*** which has branches in many major communities and provides education regarding the management of IBD. If diversionary bowel surgery is indicated, the **United Ostomy Association†** and the **Wound Ostomy and Continence Nurses Society‡** are available to assist with ileostomy care and provide important psychologic support through their self-help group. Adolescents often benefit by participating in peer-support groups, which are sponsored in some areas by the CCFA. (See Nursing Care Plan: The Child with Inflammatory Bowel Disease.§)

# Peptic Ulcer Disease (PUD)

PUD is an ulcerative condition causing a circumscribed loss of tissue of the mucosal, submucosal, and sometimes muscular layer in parts of the GI tract exposed to acid-pepsin gastric secretions. Ulcers are described as gastric or duodenal and as primary or secondary. A *gastric ulcer* involves the mucosa of the stomach, and a *duodenal ulcer* involves the pylorus or duodenum. Most *primary ulcers* are chronic, occurring in the absence of a predisposing factor, and are frequently located in the duodenum. *Secondary ulcers,* or *stress ulcers,* are generally acute and tend to occur as a result of the stress of a severe underlying disease or injury (e.g., severe burns, sepsis, intracranial disease, severe trauma, multisystem organ failure), or ingestion of an ulcerogenic drug (e.g., salicylates, nonsteroidal antiinflammatory agents, ferrous sulfate). They are most often located in the stomach.

Stress ulcers occur in all pediatric age-groups, including high-risk newborns. Critically ill patients are at the highest risk. Typically, stress ulcers occur as multiple lesions involving the gastric mucosa. Less commonly, lesions may occur in the duodenum or involve the gastric mucosa more diffusely (as in acute hemorrhagic gastritis). The proposed pathophysiology of stress ulceration may be related to acid hyper-

secretion, prostaglandin deficiency, mucus deficiency, and hypoxia (Motil, 1999).

In older children and adolescents the majority of ulcers are primary. The incidence of ulcers in boys is two to three times greater than the incidence in girls although this difference is less in very young children.

## Etiology

The exact cause of PUD in children is unknown, although infectious, genetic, and environmental factors are important. There is an increased familial incidence and an increased incidence in persons with blood group O.

Current evidence indicates that some children less than 18 years of age who present with duodenal and gastric ulcers with no identified cause may have a family history of peptic ulcer disease. Many of these children and adolescents, however, are found to have *Helicobacter pylori.* Recent investigations indicate that *H. pylori* is associated with a significant proportion of the duodenal ulcers and a lesser number of gastric ulcers in children (Gold and Blecker, 1999).

In addition to ulcerogenic drugs, both alcohol and smoking are known to contribute to ulcer formation. There is no conclusive evidence to implicate particular foods, such as caffeine-containing beverages or spicy foods, as a cause of PUD. Polyunsaturated fats and fiber may play a role in ulcer prevention.

Psychologic factors may play a role in the development of PUD. Stressful life events and dependency, passiveness, and hostility have all been implicated as contributing factors in PUD. Many psychologic studies, however, are uncontrolled, which makes it difficult to determine the pathogenesis of emotional factors in PUD.

## Pathophysiology

Most likely, the pathogenesis of PUD is due to an imbalance between destructive factors that promote the formation of peptic ulcers and protective factors that guard against ulcer formation. The gastric duodenal epithelium secretes a layer of water-insoluble mucus that serves as a protective barrier against hydrogen ions, which are neutralized by the bicarbonate within the mucosa. Prostaglandins appear to play a role in mucosal defense, because they stimulate both mucus and alkali secretions. Abnormalities of the mucus-bicarbonate barrier, such as infection with *H. pylori,* contribute to ulcer formation.

The most important endogenous destructive factors include gastric acid and pepsin production. When abnormalities in the protective barrier exist, the mucosa is vulnerable to damage by acid and pepsin. Exogenous factors, such as aspirin and nonsteroidal antiinflammatory drugs, have been shown to cause gastric ulcers by inhibition of prostaglandin synthesis. Zollinger-Ellison syndrome may occur in children who have multiple, large, or recurrent ulcers. This syndrome is characterized by hypersecretion of gastric acid, intractable ulcer disease, and intestinal malabsorption caused by a gastrin-secreting tumor of the pancreas (Motil, 1999). The pathogenesis, manifestations, and complications of PUD are outlined in Fig. 33-5.

---

*386 Park Ave S, 17th Floor, New York, NY 10016, (800) 932-2423; www.ccfa.org.

†19772 MacArthur Blvd, Suite 200, Irvine, CA 92612-2405, (714) 660-8624; www.uoa.org.

‡1550 South Coast Highway, Suite 201, Laguna Beach, CA 92651, (888) 224-9626; www.wocn.org. In Canada: **Crohn's and Colitis Foundation of Canada;** www.ccfc.ca; and **United Ostomy Association, Canada,** PO Box 46057, College Park Post Office, 444 Yonge St, Toronto, Ontario M5B2L8, (416) 595-5452, fax: (416) 595-9924.

§In Wong DL, Hess CS: *Wong and Whaley's clinical manual of pediatric nursing,* ed 5, St Louis, 2000, Mosby.

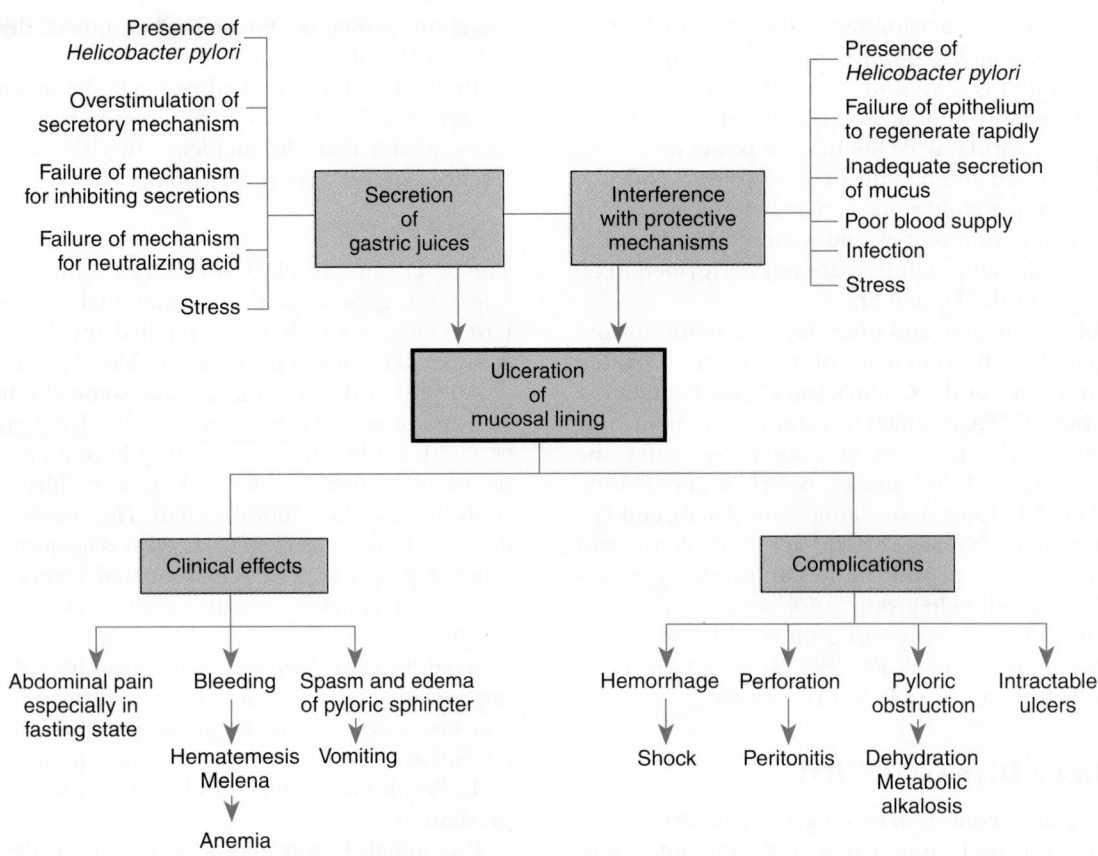

**Fig. 33-5**  Possible causes and effects of peptic ulcer.

## Clinical Manifestations

The clinical manifestations of PUD vary according to the age of the child and the location of the ulcer (Table 33-3). Common clinical manifestations include chronic abdominal pain, especially when the stomach is empty, such as during the night or early morning; recurrent vomiting; hematemesis; melena; chronic anemia; and abdominal tenderness.

## Diagnostic Evaluation

Diagnosis is based on the history (pattern of pain) and physical examination.

Frequently a history of epigastric and periumbilical pain accompanies PUD. However, children often find it difficult to describe the location of their pain and frequently indicate the location by moving their hand in a circular movement all around the stomach area. Asking the child to take one finger and point to the area where it hurts the most often helps to identify the location of the pain. Pain may also be elicited during the examination with palpation. Routine laboratory studies to diagnosis PUD include a complete blood count with differential, erythrocyte sedimentation rate, blood chemistry studies, a urinalysis, and stool analysis to identify anemia or inflammation and to rule out infection. A 13 C-urea breath test is often performed to determine the presence of antibodies to *H. pylori*. An upper GI series is rarely helpful in identifying ulcers in children; a fiberoptic endoscopy is the most reliable way to detect PUD in children. Direct visualization of the gastric and duodenal mucosa with biopsy to determine the presence of *H. pylori* is the most commonly used and effective way to determine the diagnosis.

## Therapeutic Management

The major goals of therapy for children with PUD are to relieve discomfort, promote healing, and prevent complications and recurrence. Management is primarily medical and consists of administration of medications to treat the infection or reduce or neutralize gastric acid secretion. Whenever possible, known stressors are reduced.

***Antacids*** have been beneficial medications that neutralize gastric acid. However, in terms of healing the ulcer or in the eradication of *H. pylori,* antacids are not as effective as the medications that inhibit acid secretion.

Mucosal protective agents, such as sucralfate and bismuth-containing preparations, may be prescribed. ***Sucralfate*** is an aluminum-containing agent that forms a protective barrier for ulcerated mucosa against acid and pepsin. Sucralfate also comes in liquid form. It is given four times a day and binds to the erosive surface of the ulcer and protects the mucosa from further damage. It is important to instruct the family not to give this medication at the same time as other medications because it may interfere with their absorption and decrease their effectiveness. Bismuth compounds have been used in combination with antibiotics in the treatment of *H. pylori*.

**TABLE 33-3   Characteristics of peptic ulcers**

| Type of Ulcer | Clinical Manifestations | Comments |
|---|---|---|
| **Neonates** | | |
| Usually gastric and secondary | Perforation may be first sign that massive bleeding may occur | Commonly has history of prematurity respiratory distress, sepsis, hypoglycemia, or an intraventricular hemorrhage |
| **Infants to 3-year-old children** | | |
| Most likely to have secondary ulcer located equally in the stomach or duodenum. Primary ulcers less common and usually located in the stomach | Hematemesis, melena, or perforation | Likely to present in relation to illness, surgery, or trauma |
| **3- to 6-year-old children** | | |
| Primary or secondary ulcers Located equally in stomach and duodenum | Periumbilical pain, poor eating, vomiting, irritability, nighttime waking, hematemesis, melena | Diagnosis often made based on history. Perforation more likely in secondary ulcers |
| **Children 6 years and older** | | |
| Usually primary and most often duodenal | Epigastric pain or vague abdominal pain Nighttime waking, hematemesis, melena, and anemia may occur | More typical of adult type Chance of recurrence greater Often associated with *H. pylori* |

Currently the recommended therapy for treatment of *H. pylori* is triple-drug therapy. Several combinations of drugs are used. One combines bismuth, amoxicillin, and metronidazole for 2 weeks. Another combines ranitidine or famotidine with amoxicillin and clarithromycin for 2 weeks. The combination of a proton pump inhibitor (e.g., omeprazole, lansoprazole) and amoxicillin and clarithromycin is currently the most effective therapy in children. Combination therapy has demonstrated 90% effectiveness in eradication of *H. pylori* when compared with antibiotic monotherapy (Motil, 1999). Concern has been raised about the use of bismuth. Excessive use may result in encephalopathy and acute renal failure. To date no adverse effects with the use of this drug have been reported in children. Concern has also been raised about the presence of salicylate in bismuth subsalicylate and the risk of Reye syndrome when this drug is used in children. Salicylates must always be used with caution when treating children. However, to date Reye syndrome has never been reported in association with bismuth subsalicylate therapy for the treatment of ulcer.

*Antisecretory agents* may be prescribed for children with PUD. These agents include the histamine ($H_2$) receptor antagonists cimetidine (Tagamet), ranitidine (Zantac), and famotidine (Pepcid). These drugs suppress gastric acid production and have few side effects.

Proton pump inhibitors such as omeprazole and lansoprazole act to inhibit the hydrogen ion pump in the parietal cells, thus blocking the final pathway in the production of acid. Although these drugs have not been well studied in children, they are used in clinical practice to treat ulcers, as well as gastroesophageal reflux, esophagitis, and gastritis. They appear to be well tolerated and have infrequent side effects.

The child is provided with a nutritious diet but is advised to avoid caffeine. Adolescents are warned about gastric irritation that occurs as a result of alcohol use and smoking cigarettes.

A child with an acute ulcer who has developed complications such as massive hemorrhage requires emergency care.

Administration of IV fluids, blood, or plasma depends on the amount of blood loss. Replacement with whole blood or packed cells may be necessary for significant blood loss.

*Surgical intervention* may be required in the management of complications of PUD, such as hemorrhage, perforation, or gastric outlet obstruction. Ligation of the source of bleeding or closure of a perforation may be performed. A vagotomy and pyloroplasty may be indicated in children with recurring ulcers despite aggressive medical treatment.

**Prognosis.** The long-term prognosis for PUD is variable. Many ulcers can be successfully treated with medical therapy; however, primary duodenal peptic ulcers frequently recur. Complications, such as GI bleeding, can occur and extend into adulthood. The effect of maintenance drug therapy on long-term morbidity remains to be established with further studies.

## Nursing Considerations

The main nursing objective is to promote healing of the inflamed mucosa through compliance with the medication regimen. If an analgesic/antipyretic is needed during the course of therapy, acetaminophen, not aspirin, is used. Drug compliance is essential and can be a problem with the need for frequent administration of antacids. Strategies to improve compliance are instituted early in the course of therapy. (See Chapter 27.) For traveling and during school, the use of antacid tablets rather than liquid is more convenient. The child and caregiver should be educated about the disease process and the rationale for drug therapy.

Although the exact role that stress plays in the pathogenesis of PUD in children is unclear, the nurse should be aware of environmental conditions that contribute to stress. Critically ill neonates, infants, and children in intensive care units should receive antacids and $H_2$ blockers to prevent stress ulcers. All critically ill patients and patients receiving IV $H_2$ blockers should have their gastric pH values checked at frequent intervals and buffered with antacid if necessary.

The role of stress in ulcer formation should also be considered for nonhospitalized children with chronic illnesses.

Many ulcers in children occur secondary to other conditions, and nurses should be aware of family and environmental conditions that may precipitate or aggravate the condition. Children may benefit from psychologic counseling and from learning how to cope more constructively with stresses in their lives. (See Nursing Care Plan: The Child with Peptic Ulcer Disease.*)

## OBSTRUCTIVE DISORDERS

Obstruction in the GI tract occurs when the passage of nutrients and secretions is impeded by a constricted or occluded lumen, or when there is impaired motility *(paralytic ileus)*. Obstructions may be congenital or acquired (Box 33-4). Congenital obstructions, such as esophageal or intestinal atresias and malrotation, usually appear in the neonatal period. (See Chapter 11.) Obstruction in the GI tract from many causes is characterized by similar signs and symptoms, although the progression may vary greatly.

Usually, acute intestinal obstruction is characterized by abdominal pain, nausea, vomiting, abdominal distention, and a change in stooling patterns. *Pain* is caused by intermittent muscular contractions proximal to the obstruction as the bowel attempts to move luminal contents along the normal path and may be due to severe abdominal distention. *Abdominal distention* is a result of accumulation of gas and fluid above the level of the obstruction. As abdominal distention progresses, the abdomen may become extremely tender, rigid, and firm.

When abdominal contents continue to accumulate, nausea and vomiting occur. *Vomiting of gastric contents* is often the first sign of a high obstruction, such as obstruction of the pylorus, and *vomiting of bile-stained material* is a sign of obstruction of the small intestine. Persistent vomiting can lead to dehydration and electrolyte disturbances. *Constipation* and *obstipation* (prolonged absence of defecation) are early signs of low obstructions and later signs of higher obstructions. In acute conditions such as intussusception, the clinical manifestations are apparent within a few hours of the onset of the disorder. In other conditions such as pyloric

*In Wong DL, Hess CS: *Wong and Whaley's clinical manual of pediatric nursing,* ed 5, St Louis, 2000, Mosby.

---

**Box 33-4** ■ ■ ▫
**Causes of Intestinal Obstruction in Children**

| CONGENITAL | ACQUIRED |
|---|---|
| Atresia | Pyloric stenosis |
| Incarcerated hernia | Intussusception |
| Imperforate anus | Postoperative adhesions or |
| Meckel diverticulum | strictures |
| Hirschsprung disease | Tumor |
| Stricture | Foreign body |
| Malrotation | |
| Volvulus | |
| Meconium plug | |
| Meconium ileus | |
| Annular pancreas | |

---

stenosis, the signs and symptoms may have a more gradual onset. *Bowel sounds* may initially be hyperactive, then diminish or cease. *Respiratory distress* may occur when the diaphragm is pushed up into the pleural cavity as a result of severe abdominal distention.

## Hypertrophic Pyloric Stenosis (HPS)

HPS occurs when the circumferential muscle of the pyloric sphincter becomes thickened, resulting in elongation and narrowing of the pyloric channel. This produces an outlet obstruction and compensatory dilation, hypertrophy, and hyperperistalsis of the stomach. This condition usually develops in the first few weeks of life, causing projectile vomiting, dehydration, metabolic alkalosis, and failure to thrive. The precise etiology of HPS is not known. Firstborn children and males are affected four to six times more frequently than females. HPS is seen less frequently in black and Asian infants than in white infants. It is more likely to affect a full-term infant than a premature one. Inheritance is polygenic, with an increased risk in siblings and the offspring of affected persons. The greatest risk of recurrence (20%) is in the first-born male offspring of a mother who was affected (Milla, 1999).

### Pathophysiology

The circular muscle of the pylorus thickens as a result of hypertrophy. This produces severe narrowing of the pyloric canal between the stomach and the duodenum. Consequently, the lumen at this point is partially obstructed. Over time the size of the opening is reduced, and the partial obstruction may progress to complete obstruction. The hypertrophied pylorus may be palpable as an olivelike mass in the upper abdomen.

Pyloric stenosis is not a congenital disorder. Evidence suggests that local innervation may be involved in the pathogenesis. In most cases this is an isolated lesion; however, it may be associated with intestinal malrotation, esophageal and duodenal atresia, and anorectal anomalies (Fig. 33-6).

### Clinical Manifestations

Infants with HPS have nonbilious vomiting in the early stages. The vomiting may be projectile and progressive, becoming brown in color in later stages if gastritis develops. Vomiting usually begins at 3 weeks of age but can start as early as 1 week and as late as 5 months. Initially the infant is hungry and irritable, but prolonged vomiting may lead to dehydration, weight loss, and failure to thrive. Gastric peristalsis may be visible on examination, and the olive-shaped mass in the epigastrium just to the right of the umbilicus may be palpated (Fig. 33-6, *A*).

### Diagnostic Evaluation

The diagnosis of HPS is often made following the history and physical examination. The olivelike mass is most easily palpated when the stomach is empty, the infant is quiet, and the abdominal muscles are relaxed. If the diagnosis is inconclusive from the history and physical examination, ultrasonography will demonstrate an elongated mass surrounding a long pyloric channel. If ultrasonography does not demonstrate a hypertrophied pylorus, upper GI radiography should be done to rule out other causes of vomiting.

Laboratory findings reflect the metabolic alterations created by severe depletion of both water and electrolytes from extensive and prolonged vomiting. There are decreased serum levels of both sodium and potassium, although these may be masked by the hemoconcentration from extracellular fluid depletion. Of greater diagnostic value are a decrease in serum chloride levels and increases in pH and bicarbonate (carbon dioxide content), indicative of metabolic alkalosis. The blood urea nitrogen will be elevated as evidence of dehydration.

### Therapeutic Management

Surgical relief of the pyloric obstruction by pyloromyotomy is the standard therapy for this disorder. Preoperatively the infant must be rehydrated, and metabolic alkalosis is corrected with parenteral fluid and electrolyte administration. Replacement fluid therapy usually delays surgery for 24 to 48 hours. The stomach is decompressed with an NG tube. In infants with no evidence of fluid and electrolyte imbalance, surgery is performed without delay.

The surgical procedure is performed through a right upper quadrant incision and consists of a longitudinal incision through the circular muscle fibers of the pylorus down to, but not including, the submucosa (*pyloromyotomy,* sometimes called *Fredet-Ramstedt procedure*) (Fig. 33-6, *B*). The procedure has a very high success rate. *Laparoscopy* has been found to be safe and successful for infants with HPS (Najmaldin and Tan, 1995). The use of a small incision for the laparoscope may result in a shorter surgical time, more rapid postoperative feeding, and shorter hospital stay.

Feedings are usually begun 4 to 6 hours postoperatively, beginning with small, frequent feedings of glucose, water, or electrolyte solution. If clear fluids are retained, about 24 hours after surgery formula is started in the same small increments. The amount and the interval between feedings are gradually increased until a full feeding schedule is reinstated, which usually takes about 48 hours.

**Prognosis.**  The prognosis is excellent, and the mortality is low. Postoperative complications include persistent pyloric obstruction and wound dehiscence. Approximately 15% of infants with HPS also have gastroesophageal reflux (Milla, 1999).

### Nursing Considerations

Nursing care involves primarily observation for clinical features that help establish the diagnosis, careful regulation of fluid therapy, and reestablishment of normal feeding patterns. Nurses must be alert to signs of HPS in infants and refer them for medical evaluation. The possibility of HPS should be considered in the very young infant who appears alert but fails to gain weight and has a history of vomiting after meals. Assessment is based on observation of eating behaviors, evidence of characteristic clinical manifestations, hydration, and nutritional status.

Preoperatively the emphasis is on restoring hydration and electrolyte balance. The infant is allowed nothing by mouth and given IV fluids of glucose and electrolytes based on serum electrolyte values—usually sodium chloride solution with added potassium (when there is adequate urinary output). Careful monitoring of the IV fluids and strict monitoring of intake, output, and urine specific gravity are important. Accurate description of any vomiting, as well as the number and character of stools, is recorded.

Observations include assessment of vital signs, particularly those that indicate fluid or electrolyte imbalances. These infants are especially prone to metabolic alkalosis from loss of hydrogen ions and depletion of potassium, sodium, and chloride, all of which are contained in gastric secretions. The skin and mucous membranes are assessed for alterations in hydration status, and daily weights provide added clues to water gain or loss. (See Chapter 28 for manifestations of fluid and electrolyte disturbances.)

When stomach decompression and gastric lavage are part of preoperative management, the nurse is responsible for ensuring that the NG tube is patent and functioning properly and that the type and amount of NG drainage is recorded. General hygienic care, with particular attention to the skin and mouth in dehydrated infants, is important. Protection from infection is essential because infants with impaired nutritional status are more susceptible to infection than normal newborns.

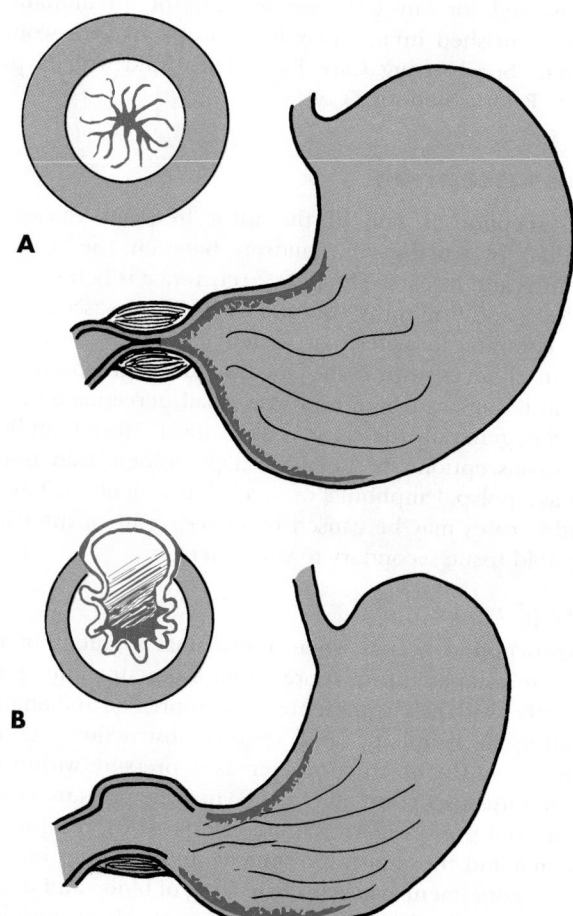

**Fig. 33-6**  Hypertrophic pyloric stenosis. **A,** Enlarged muscular tumor nearly obliterates pyloric channel. **B,** Longitudinal surgical division of muscle down to submucosa establishes adequate passageway.

Parents are encouraged to visit and become involved in the child's care. Most parents need support and reassurance that the condition is caused by a structural problem and is not a reflection of their parenting skills and capacities.

**Postoperative Care.** Postoperative vomiting is not uncommon, and most infants, even with successful surgery, exhibit some vomiting during the first 24 to 48 hours. IV fluids are administered until the infant is taking and retaining adequate amounts by mouth. Much of the same care that was instituted before surgery is continued postoperatively, including observation of vital signs, monitoring of IV fluids, and careful monitoring of intake and output. In addition, the infant is observed for responses to the stress of surgery and for evidence of pain. Appropriate analgesics should be given around the clock, because pain is continuous.

The NG tube may be maintained after surgery for a short time. Feedings are usually instituted within 24 hours postoperatively, beginning with clear liquids containing glucose and electrolytes. They are offered in small quantities at frequent intervals. If the infant has been breast-fed, breast milk, expressed by the mother, may be given by bottle when the infant is able to tolerate feedings, or the mother is instructed to limit nursing time and gradually increase the time to previous patterns. Supervision of feedings is an important part of postoperative care. The operative site should be observed for any drainage or signs of inflammation. Poorly nourished infants may have problems with wound healing. (See Nursing Care Plan: The Child with Hypertrophic Pyloric Stenosis.*)

## Intussusception

Intussusception is one of the most frequent causes of intestinal obstruction in children between the ages of 3 months and 3 years. The peak occurrence is between the ages of 5 and 9 months (Brandt, 1999). Intussusception is more common in males than in females and is more common in children with cystic fibrosis. Although specific intestinal lesions can be found in a small percentage of the children, generally the cause is not known. More than 90% of intussusceptions do not have a pathologic lead point, such as a polyp, lymphoma, or Meckel diverticulum. The idiopathic cases may be caused by hypertrophy of intestinal lymphoid tissue secondary to viral infection.

### Pathophysiology

Intussusception occurs when a proximal segment of the bowel telescopes into a more distal segment, pulling the mesentery with it. The mesentery is compressed and angled, resulting in lymphatic and venous obstruction. As the edema from the obstruction increases, pressure within the area of intussusception increases. When the pressure equals the arterial pressure, arterial blood flow stops, resulting in ischemia and the pouring of mucus into the intestine. Venous engorgement also leads to leaking of blood and mucus into the intestinal lumen, forming the classic currant-jelly

*In Wong DL, Hess CS: *Wong and Whaley's clinical manual of pediatric nursing,* ed 5, St Louis, 2000, Mosby.

stools (Brandt, 1999). The most common site is the *ileocecal valve (ileocolic),* where the ileum invaginates into the cecum and then further into the colon (Fig. 33-7). Other forms include *ileoileal* (one part of the ileum invaginates into another section of the ileum) and *colocolic* (one part of the colon invaginates into another area of the colon) intussusceptions, usually in the area of the hepatic or splenic flexure or at some point along the transverse colon.

### Clinical Manifestations

Intussusception usually presents with the sudden onset of crampy abdominal pain, inconsolable crying, and a drawing up of the knees to the chest in an otherwise healthy child. Between episodes the child appears normal. As the obstruction progresses, bilious vomiting may occur and lethargy increases. The classic triad of pain, a palpable sausage-shaped abdominal mass, and currant-jelly stools occurs in only 15% to 20% of children when they are seen initially. In one series of 209 patients the most frequent symptoms included emesis, abdominal pain, rectal bleeding or Hematest-positive stools, a palpable abdominal mass, lethargy, or sepsis (West and Grosfeld, 1999). With atypical cases, lethargy may be the primary symptom. If the distal bowel remains distended, necrosis and perforation are possible.

> **NURSING ALERT**
>
> The classic signs and symptoms of intussusception may not be present; a more chronic picture may occur, characterized by diarrhea, anorexia, weight loss, occasional vomiting, and periodic pain. The older child may have pain without other signs or symptoms. Because this condition is potentially life threatening, be aware of such signs and closely observe and refer these children for further medical investigation.

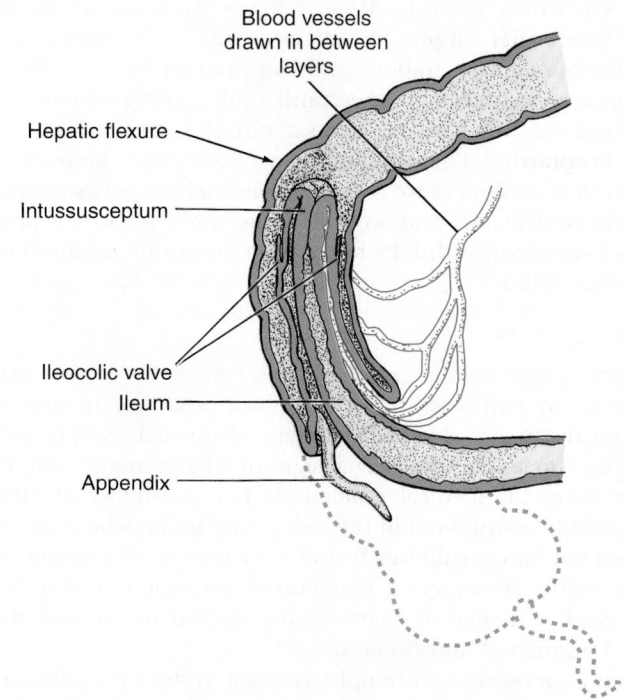

**Fig. 33-7** Ileocolic intussusception.

## Diagnostic Evaluation

Frequently the diagnosis can be made on subjective findings alone. However, definitive diagnosis is based on a barium enema, which clearly demonstrates the obstruction to the flow of barium. Initially an abdominal radiograph is obtained to detect intraperitoneal air from a bowel perforation, which would contraindicate a barium enema. A rectal examination reveals mucus, blood, and occasionally a low intussusception itself.

## Therapeutic Management

In many cases the initial treatment of choice is nonsurgical hydrostatic reduction, traditionally by barium enema. In this procedure correction of the invagination is carried out at the same time as the diagnostic testing. The force exerted by the flowing barium is usually sufficient to push the invaginated portion of the bowel into its original position, similar to pushing an inverted "finger" out of a glove. This procedure is not recommended if there are clinical signs of shock or perforation.

The use of barium as the contrast agent is becoming less routine. A high percentage of radiologists use water-soluble contrast and air pressure to reduce intussusceptions. The increased use of water-soluble contrast reflects concern regarding the risk of barium peritonitis. The administration of air pressure to reduce intussusception is as successful as and more rapid than barium, without the risk of peritonitis. IV fluids, NG decompression, and antibiotic therapy may be given before attempts at hydrostatic reduction are made.

Because these procedures are not always successful, the child may require surgical intervention. Surgery involves manually reducing the invagination and, where indicated, resecting any nonviable intestine.

**Prognosis.** Nonoperative reduction is successful in more than 75% of cases. Surgery is required for those patients in whom the contrast enema was unsuccessful. If untreated, approximately 10% of children will have spontaneous reduction or chronic intussusception. The other 90% of untreated children will suffer from complications such as perforation, peritonitis, and sepsis. With early diagnosis and treatment, serious complications and death are very uncommon.

## Nursing Considerations

The nurse helps establish a diagnosis by obtaining the parent's description of the child's physical and behavioral symptoms. Although parents may not know the medical problem, they can detect a change in the child's behavior.

**NURSING ALERT** A report of severe, colicky abdominal pain in a child with vomiting and currant jelly–like stools is a significant clue to intussusception.

As soon as intussusception is suspected, the nurse should prepare the parents for the usual nonsurgical techniques and the possibility of surgery. It is important to explain the basic defect of intussusception and how an intussusception is corrected with contrast enemas.

**NURSING TIP** Intussusception is easily demonstrated by pushing the end of a "finger" on a rubber glove back into itself or using the example of a telescoping rod. The principle of reduction by hydrostatic pressure can be simulated by filling the glove with water, which pushes the finger into a fully extended position.

Even though nonsurgical intervention is often successful, preoperative procedures may be performed. For the child with signs of electrolyte imbalance, hemorrhage, or peritonitis, additional medical preparations such as replacement fluids, antibiotics, and NG suctioning may be indicated. All stools are examined before hydrostatic reduction or surgery.

**NURSING ALERT** Passage of a normal brown stool usually indicates that the intussusception has reduced itself. This is immediately reported to the physician, who may choose to alter the diagnostic/therapeutic plan of care.

Following hydrostatic reduction, the nurse observes for passage of barium or water-soluble contrast material with stools. The child should be admitted to the hospital for 12 to 24 hours for observation. The parents should be educated about the risk of recurrence. If intussusception recurs, hydrostatic reduction is usually attempted. A laparotomy is considered for multiple recurrences. If surgical reduction or bowel resection is performed, postoperative care is similar to that following any abdominal surgery. (See Chapter 27.)

**Family Support.** Because hospitalization to correct intussusception may be the child's first separation from the parents, it is important to preserve the parent-child relationship by encouraging rooming-in or extended visiting. Parents should also be prepared for procedures such as IV therapy, frequent vital sign and blood pressure monitoring, and special orders, such as nothing by mouth. Because of the rapidity of the onset, diagnosis, and treatment, parents may be left with the feeling of stunned numbness. They may ask few questions, or they may constantly make inquiries, sometimes the same ones several times. (See Nursing Care Plan: The Child with Intussusception.*)

## Malrotation and Volvulus

Malrotation of the intestine is caused by abnormal rotation of the intestine around the superior mesenteric artery during embryologic development. Malrotation may present in utero or may be asymptomatic throughout life. Infants with malrotation have intermittent vomiting, recurrent abdominal pain, distention, or lower GI bleeding. Malrotation is the most serious type of intestinal obstruction because, if the intestine undergoes complete volvulus (the intestine twisting around itself), compromise of the blood supply will result in intestinal necrosis, peritonitis, perforation, and death.

*In Wong DL, Hess CS: *Wong and Whaley's clinical manual of pediatric nursing,* ed 5, St Louis, 2000, Mosby.

### Diagnostic Evaluation

It is imperative that malrotation and volvulus be diagnosed promptly and surgical treatment be instituted quickly. Any infant with bilious vomiting should be evaluated for malrotation, volvulus, and obstruction. An upper GI series is the definitive procedure to diagnose this condition.

### Therapeutic Management

Surgery is performed to remove the affected area. However, if the lesion is extensive, short-gut syndrome can occur postoperatively.

### Nursing Considerations

Preoperative nursing care is the same as that provided to any infant or child with intestinal obstruction. Postoperative nursing care is similar to that provided to an infant or child who has undergone abdominal surgery.

## MALABSORPTION SYNDROMES

Malabsorption syndromes are characterized by chronic diarrhea and malabsorption of fluid and nutrients. An important complication of malabsorption syndromes in children is failure to thrive. Cases of malabsorption are classified according to the location of the anatomic or biochemical defect. The term *celiac disease* is often used to describe a symptom complex that has four characteristics in common: (1) steatorrhea (fatty, foul, frothy, bulky stools), (2) general malnutrition, (3) abdominal distention, and (4) secondary vitamin deficiencies.

Malabsorption may be caused by *digestive defects* in which the enzymes necessary for digestion are diminished or absent, as in (1) cystic fibrosis or chronic pancreatitis, in which pancreatic enzymes are absent; (2) biliary or liver disease, in which bile flow is affected; or (3) lactase deficiency, in which there is congenital or secondary lactose intolerance.

Malabsorption is also caused by *absorptive defects,* in which the intestinal mucosa transport system is impaired. Absorptive defects may occur as primary defects (e.g., celiac disease or food allergies) or primary enzyme deficiencies (sucrase-isomaltase deficiency), or secondary to infection or inflammatory disease of the bowel that results in impaired absorption (e.g., ulcerative colitis). Obstructive disorders (e.g., Hirschsprung disease) can also cause secondary malabsorption from enterocolitis.

*Anatomic defects,* such as extensive resection of the bowel or "short bowel syndrome," affect digestion by decreasing the transit time of substances and compromising the absorptive surface.

## Celiac Disease (Gluten-Sensitive Enteropathy)

Celiac disease, also known as *gluten-induced enteropathy, gluten-sensitive eneropathy (GSE),* and *celiac sprue,* is a permanent intestinal intolerance to dietary wheat gliadin and related proteins that produces mucosal lesions in genetically susceptible individuals. It is second only to cystic fibrosis as a cause of malabsorption in children.

The incidence is variable and has been reported as 1 in 3000 and 1 in 4000. The disease is seen more frequently in Europe than in the United States. It is more prevalent in women than men and is rarely reported in Asians or African-Americans. Although the exact cause is unknown, it is now generally accepted that celiac disease is an immunologically mediated small intestine enteropathy. The mucosal lesions contain features that suggest both humoral and cell-mediated immunologic overstimulation.

### Pathophysiology

Celiac disease is characterized by villous atrophy in the small bowel in response to the protein *gluten.* Gluten is found in wheat, barley, rye, and oat grains. When individuals are unable to digest the gliadin component of gluten, an accumulation of a toxic substance that is damaging to the mucosal cells occurs. Damage to the mucosa of the small intestine leads to villous atrophy, hyperplasia of the crypts, and infiltration of the epithelial cells with lymphocytes. Villous atrophy leads to malabsorption due to the reduced absorptive surface area (see Fig. 33-1 and the discussion of absorption on p. 1418).

### Clinical Manifestations

Symptoms of celiac disease appear when solid foods such as beans and pasta are introduced in the child's diet between the ages of 1 and 5 years. There is usually an interval of several months between the introduction of gluten into the diet and the onset of symptoms. Intestinal symptoms are common in children diagnosed within the first 2 years of life. Other symptoms include failure to thrive, chronic diarrhea, abdominal distention, muscle wasting, anorexia, and irritability.

### Diagnostic Evaluation

The definitive diagnosis of celiac disease is based on (1) the finding of villous atrophy with hyperplasia of the crypts and abnormal epithelium in a child who is eating a diet with gluten and (2) a full remission of symptoms after the withdrawal of gluten from the diet. The presence of antigliadin and antiendomysial IgG and IgA antibodies and their disappearance when gluten is removed from the diet are important findings that aid in the diagnosis (Lifschitz, 1999).

### Therapeutic Management

Treatment of celiac disease consists primarily of dietary management. Although a gluten-free diet is prescribed, it is difficult to remove every source of this protein. Some patients are able to tolerate restricted amounts of gluten. Because gluten is found mainly in the grains of wheat and rye, but also in smaller quantities in barley and oats, these four foods are eliminated. Corn, rice, and millet are substitute grain foods.

Children with untreated celiac disease may have lactose intolerance, especially if their mucosal lesions are extensive. Lactose intolerance usually improves as the mucosa heals with gluten withdrawal. Specific nutritional deficiencies, such as iron, folic acid, and fat-soluble vitamin deficiencies, are treated with appropriate supplements.

**Prognosis.** Celiac disease is generally regarded as a chronic disease; its severity varies greatly among children.

The most severe symptoms usually occur in early childhood and again in adult life. Most children who comply with dietary management are healthy and remain free of symptoms and complications. Strict dietary avoidance of gluten may minimize the risk of developing lymphoma, especially of the small intestine, one of the most serious complications of the disease.

### Nursing Considerations

The main nursing consideration is helping the child adhere to dietary management. Considerable time is involved in explaining the disease process to the child and the parents, the specific role of gluten in aggravating the disorder, and those foods that must be restricted. It is difficult to maintain a diet indefinitely when the child has no symptoms and temporary transgressions result in no difficulties. However, evidence indicates that the majority of individuals who relax their diet will experience a relapse of their disease and possibly exhibit growth retardation, anemia, or osteomalacia. There is also the risk of developing malignant lymphoma of the small intestine or other GI malignancies.

Although the chief source of gluten is cereal and baked goods, grains are frequently added to processed foods as thickeners or fillers. To compound the difficulty, gluten is added to many foods as hydrolyzed vegetable protein, which is derived from cereal grains. The nurse must advise parents of the necessity of reading all label ingredients carefully to avoid hidden sources of gluten.

Many of children's favorite foods contain gluten, including bread, cake, cookies, crackers, donuts, pies, spaghetti, pizza, prepared soups, some processed ice cream, many types of chocolate candy, milk preparations such as malts, hot dogs, luncheon meats, meat gravy, and some prepared hamburgers. Many of these products can be eliminated from the infant's or young child's diet fairly easily, but monitoring the diet of the school-age child or adolescent is more difficult. Luncheon preparation away from home is particularly difficult, because bread, luncheon meats, and instant soups are not allowed. For families on restricted food budgets, the diet adds an additional financial burden because many inexpensive or convenient foods cannot be used.

In addition to restricting gluten, other dietary alterations may be necessary. For example, in some children who have more severe mucosal damage, the digestion of disaccharides is impaired, especially in relation to lactose. Therefore, these children often need a temporarily lactose-free diet, which necessitates eliminating all milk products. In general, dietary management includes a diet high in calories and proteins, with simple carbohydrates such as fruits and vegetables, but low in fats. Because the bowel is usually inflamed as a result of the pathologic processes in absorption, high-fiber foods, such as nuts, raisins, raw vegetables, and raw fruits with skin, are avoided until inflammation has subsided.

It is important to stress long-range complications, as well as to remind parents of the child's physical status before dietary treatment and the dramatic improvement following treatment. The nurse can be instrumental in allowing the child to express concerns and frustration while focusing on ways in which the child can still feel normal. The child and parents can be encouraged to find new recipes using suit-able ingredients, such as Mexican or Chinese dishes that use corn or rice. A nutritionist should be consulted to provide children and their families with detailed dietary instructions and education.

Several resources are available to assist children and parents in all aspects of coping with celiac disease. The **Celiac Sprue Association/United States of America*** is an organization that provides support and guidance to families and supplies educational materials concerning a gluten-free diet, food sources, recipes, and travel information.† (See Nursing Care Plan: The Child with Celiac Disease.‡)

## Short Bowel Syndrome (SBS)

SBS is a malabsorptive disorder that occurs as a result of decreased mucosal surface area, usually due to extensive resection of the small intestine. Malabsorption may be exacerbated by other factors, such as bacterial overgrowth and dysmotility. The most common causes of SBS in children are necrotizing enterocolitis, volvulus, jejunal atresias, and gastroschisis. Other causes include midgut volvulus and diffuse small bowel Crohn disease in older children. Less frequent causes include trauma to the GI tract and total colonic aganglionosis with extension into the small bowel. Two primary problems occurs with SBS: (1) decreased intestinal surface area for absorption of fluid, electrolytes, and nutrients and (2) increased and disorganized transit time for intestinal contents (Treem, 1999). The prognosis for infants with SBS has improved dramatically in the past 20 to 30 years as a result of advances in parental nutrition and enteral feeding.

### Therapeutic Management

The goals of therapy for infants and children with SBS include the following: (1) preserve as much length of bowel as possible during surgery; (2) maintain optimum nutritional status, growth, and development while intestinal adaptation occurs; (3) stimulate intestinal adaptation with enteral feeding; and (4) minimize complications related to the disease process and therapy.

**Nutritional Support.** Nutritional support is the long-term focus of care for children with SBS. The *initial phase* includes *total parenteral nutrition (TPN)* as the primary source of nutrients. Occasionally, additional parenteral fluids are required to manage fluid and electrolyte losses.

Numerous complications are associated with SBS and long-term TPN. *Central venous catheter infections* can occur from contamination of the parenteral nutrition solutions, administration sets, or the catheter itself. The GI tract can also be a source of microbial seeding of the catheter. Small intestine *bacterial overgrowth* and bowel atrophy, which may foster increased intestinal permeability of bacteria, may con-

---

*PO Box 31700, Omaha, NE 68131-0700, (402) 558-0600, e-mail: celia-cusa@aol.com. In Canada: **Canadian Celiac Association, Inc,** 190 Britannia Rd E, Unit 11, Mississauga, Ontario, (905) 507-6208.

†A booklet, *Pointers for Parents: Coping with Celiac Sprue,* which provides information on shopping, cooking, and living with an affected child, is available from the Clinical Dietetics Department, Children's Memorial Hospital, 2300 Children's Plaza, Chicago, IL 60614, (773) 880-4793.

‡In Wong DL, Hess CS: *Wong and Whaley's clinical manual of pediatric nursing,* ed 5, St Louis, 2000, Mosby.

tribute to bacterial translocation and increase the risk of central line infections.

*Metabolic complications* of parenteral nutrition can occur secondary to the composition of the parenteral nutrition solution or to impaired metabolic function. These complications include electrolyte disturbances, hyperglycemia, hypoglycemia, and hyperlipidemia.

*Technical complications* include catheter occlusion, catheter migration, venous thrombosis, and pulmonary embolus. The catheter may also become damaged or perforated, resulting in leakage of the TPN solution and increasing the risk of microbial contamination. When the major blood vessels become thrombosed following multiple central venous catheterizations, a lack of adequate central venous access becomes a significant problem for the child in need of long-term parenteral nutrition.

*Cholestasis* and *liver dysfunction,* as evidenced by abnormal liver function tests, may occur as a complication of parenteral nutrition. In some cases cholestasis may be severe enough to progress to cirrhosis and liver failure. The incidence and severity of the cholestasis is multifactorial. However, prolonged TPN, and a lack of enteral feeding play independent and significant roles.

The introduction of *enteral feeding* constitutes the *second phase* of nutritional support and is instituted as soon as possible following surgery. Generally a continuous infusion of a partially elemental formula via an NG or gastrostomy tube is recommended. These special formulas contain glucose, sucrose and glucose polymers, hydrolyzed proteins, and medium-chain triglycerides, which are more readily absorbed. Continuous feedings are advantageous over bolus feedings because of enhanced absorption and tolerance. Enteral feedings are gradually advanced as tolerated. Stool volume, pH, and reducing substances are monitored closely for signs of severe malabsorption. Severe malabsorption may indicate fluid and electrolyte imbalance and a need to be cautious when increasing enteral feedings. Advances in feedings should be made slowly, and TPN must be adjusted so total protein and caloric intake is not compromised and normal growth is promoted. Dehydration and severe metabolic acidosis are contraindications to increasing the enteral feeding concentration or rate. Oral feedings of partially elemental formula, electrolyte solutions, water, and small amounts of solids may be offered in addition to tube feedings so that the child can learn to suck and swallow. Oral feedings help to minimize problems with oral hypersensitivity and food aversion when the bowel can tolerate more complex foods.

A *final phase* of nutritional support occurs when exclusively enteral feedings can sustain adequate growth and development. During this phase the continuous feedings of partially elemental formula may be decreased as tolerance and acceptance of oral foods increases. The risk of developing specific nutritional deficiencies increases once TPN is discontinued. Malabsorption of fat-soluble vitamins (A, D, E, and K) and trace minerals (iron, selenium, zinc) is common in children with SBS. Vitamin $B_{12}$ deficiency often occurs following resection of the ileum. Serum vitamin and mineral levels should be monitored, and enteral supplementation of vitamins and minerals may be required.

**Adaptation Process.**   Long-term survival without TPN depends on the ability of the small intestine to increase its absorptive capacity so that nutritional needs may be provided through the enteral route. Many children develop the ability to live without TPN because of the adaptation response of the small intestine following massive resection. The compensatory increase in the mucosal surface area occurs primarily by villus hyperplasia. The small intestine length and diameter increase a small amount in children as well. This *adaptation response* is characterized by an increase in cell number and cell mass per villus column. The increased villus length and increased number of enterocytes available for absorption per centimeter of bowel allows for a gradual increase in absorption of nutrients. The capacity for adaptation is greater after proximal small bowel resection than after distal resection.

Stimulation of the adaptation process is an important goal of therapy; the primary stimulus is enteral feeding. Atrophy of the mucosa of the intestine occurs when no intraluminal nutrition is provided, even though nutrients are given parenterally. Intraluminal nutrients stimulate the mucosal adaptation through several mechanisms: (1) direct contact of nutrients with the mucosal surface appears to stimulate intestinal hyperplasia; (2) trophic hormones are secreted in response to intraluminal nutrients, which stimulate production of enterocytes; and (3) trophic upper GI secretions are released by stimulation from the presence of intraluminal nutrients (Vanderhoof and others, 1992).

**Medical and Surgical Therapy.**   Common problems associated with SBS are treated medically. *Bacterial overgrowth* is likely to occur when the ileocecal valve is absent or when stasis exists as a result of a partial obstruction or a dilated segment of bowel with poor motility. Alternating cycles of broad-spectrum antibiotics may be used to reduce bacterial overgrowth; treatment may decrease the risk of bacterial translocation and subsequent central venous catheter infections.

Another complication of bacterial overgrowth and carbohydrate malabsorption is *metabolic acidosis.* Malabsorbed carbohydrates are fermented by bacteria in the intestine, and short-chain fatty acids are produced that accumulate in the bloodstream, causing acidosis. The treatment for metabolic acidosis may include antibiotic therapy, low-carbohydrate formulas, and supplemental administration of citrate or bicarbonate.

*Gastric acid hypersecretion* is caused by a disruption of normal feedback mechanisms from the small intestine to the stomach following bowel resection. Histamine receptor antagonist drugs are administered to treat this problem.

Although nutritional and medical therapy are the primary forms of treatment for SBS, additional surgery may be indicated. If severe dilation of the small bowel occurs with subsequent complications, an *intestinal tapering procedure* may be beneficial. Other surgical interventions, including intestinal valves, antiperistaltic segments, recirculating loops, and intestinal lengthening procedures, have been attempted in order to delay the intestinal transit time or increase the absorptive surface area. However, these surgical procedures are not yet used routinely. *Intestinal transplantation* has been performed successfully in some children, but developments in this area have been delayed because of problems related to immunosuppression and graft-versus-host disease (GVHD). Transplantation may be seriously considered for children with SBS if they also have end-stage liver disease, less than 15 cm of remaining jejunum (especially if the ileocecal valve is removed), microvillus inclusion disease, generalized polyposis syndrome, potentially fatal complications (esophageal and small bowel variceal bleeding, pulmonary embolism, permanent intestinal dysfunction), or congenital transport defects.

**Prognosis.** Although the prognosis for infants with SBS has improved with advances in parenteral nutrition and enteral nutrition, prognosis depends in part on the length of the residual small intestine and on whether the ileocecal valve was preserved. An intact ileocecal valve improves the prognosis. Up to 50% of the intestine can be lost without affecting the child's health, unless the loss includes the distal ileum. A loss of greater than 70% of the small bowel results in severe malabsorption. However, the remaining intestine and stomach may adapt to the loss through compensatory growth, provided the child is kept alive with special nutritional support. Small bowel transplantation or liver and small bowel transplantation may further improve the prognosis.

Infants and children with SBS usually die of TPN-related problems, such as fulminant sepsis or severe TPN cholestasis.

## Nursing Considerations

The most important components of nursing care for children with SBS include administration and monitoring of nutritional therapy. During TPN therapy, care must be taken to minimize the risk of complications related to the central venous access device, such as catheter infections, occlusions, dislodgment, or accidental removal. For example, the catheter is secured away from the diaper area to prevent contamination of the line from stool or gastrostomy tube drainage. All connections are taped, and the tubing is secured to and covered by the child's clothing. (See Chapter 28 regarding care of central venous access devices.)

Care of enteral feeding tubes and monitoring of enteral feeding tolerance are important nursing responsibilities. The NG tube needs to be changed periodically, and proper tube placement needs to be checked frequently (possibly every 8 hours) to identify problems early. The gastrostomy tube requires frequent site care and monitoring for signs of tube migration or local infection. Assessing enteral feeding tolerance includes daily measuring of intake and output, urine specific gravity, frequent weights; daily stool testing for occult blood, reducing substances, and pH; and monitoring for vomiting, abdominal distention, and increased frequency and volume of stools. (See Critical Thinking Exercise box.)

**Home Care.** When long-term TPN is required, preparation of the family for home care of the child is a major nursing responsibility. Preparation for home nutritional support is initiated as early as possible to prevent lengthy hospitalizations with subsequent problems such as developmental delays and family stresses.

Many infants and children can be successfully cared for at home with enteral and parenteral nutrition if the family is thoroughly prepared and provided with adequate support

services. Most families benefit from home nursing care to assist with and supervise therapy. Nurses can advocate, on behalf of patients and families, for necessary services and supplies for home care. Careful follow-up care by a multidisciplinary nutritional support service is essential. Most home health agencies now provide portable enteral and parenteral equipment, which enables the child and family to maintain a more normal and active lifestyle.

In addition to TPN, central venous catheter care, and tube feedings,* nursing care of infants with SBS should include nonnutritive sucking, oral stimulation, and provision of small amounts of oral feeding as prescribed to prevent later food aversion. Inadequate oral stimulation during a

---

*See Chapters 27 and 28 for additional nursing care related to these procedures. Home care instructions for caring for a central venous catheter, giving NG tube feedings, giving gastrostomy feedings, and caring for the child with a colostomy are available in Wong DL, Hess CS: *Wong and Whaley's clinical manual of pediatric nursing*, ed 5, St Louis, 2000, Mosby.

---

 ## Critical Thinking Exercise

### Short Bowel Syndrome

The parents of a 2-year-old boy with short bowel syndrome call their health care professional to report that their child has passed many more stools than usual with an increased watery consistency in the past 24 hours. He also has a fever of 39° C (102.2° F) and has vomited several times. The boy is admitted to the hospital. During the initial period of nursing assessment, which of the following would you monitor?

FIRST, THINK ABOUT IT . . .

• What precise question are you trying to answer?
• How are you interpreting the information?

1. Stool pH, urine pH, vital signs
2. Vital signs, weight, urine specific gravity, measurement of intake and output
3. Vital signs, stool-reducing substances, stool culture
4. Urine specific gravity, stool for blood, electrolytes

*The best response is two.* Precisely, dehydration and electrolyte disturbances are common with diarrhea. Important initial nursing interventions include assessment of the child's hydration status, including vital signs, weight, urine specific gravity, and measurement of intake and output. Children with chronic malabsorption may have severe diarrhea and are particularly susceptible to dehydration and electrolyte imbalance with an acute episode of illness such as infectious gastroenteritis. Additional factors contributing to dehydration include vomiting and fever.

*Laboratory analyses, including serum electrolytes, blood urea nitrogen, and creatinine, will also be necessary in order to guide the fluid and electrolyte therapy. Stool samples may need to be obtained to detect bacterial or viral pathogens. However, obtaining these tests is not an independent nursing function. Ongoing assessment may include testing of stool-reducing substances and pH (to detect carbohydrate malabsorption) and stool Hematest (to detect bleeding from intestinal mucosal inflammation or ischemia).*

critical period of 6 to 12 months of age may result in difficulty establishing successful oral feeding at a later date. Food aversion may require treatment by a multidisciplinary feeding team using behavioral therapy, as well as the expertise of speech-language and occupational therapists. (See Feeding Resistance, Chapter 10.)

Many infants with SBS have an intestinal ostomy performed at the time of the initial bowel resection. Routine ostomy care is another important nursing responsibility.* Since infants and children with SBS have chronic diarrhea, perineal skin irritation is often a problem following ostomy closure. Frequent diaper changes, gentle perineal cleansing, and protective skin ointments help prevent skin breakdown. (See Diaper Dermatitis, Chapter 13.)

When hospitalization is prolonged, the child's developmental and emotional needs must be part of the plan of care. This often requires special efforts to promote normal family adaptation to hospital routines. It may be months to years before the child no longer requires specialized nutritional support. Family members require psychosocial support and education to cope successfully with SBS.

# GASTROINTESTINAL BLEEDING

GI bleeding in infants and children is common but rarely life threatening. Most actual or apparent instances of GI bleeding cause great anxiety in the parents or caregivers. Blood may be vomited or passed per rectum, but the origin of the blood may not be the GI tract. In the newborn, swallowed maternal blood at the time of delivery may account for some episodes of apparent GI bleeding. A bleeding site on the nipple of a nursing mother may lead to heme-positive stools in the breast-fed infant. Finally, blood can be swallowed during epistaxis and then be passed as hematemesis or melena.

## Upper and Lower Gastrointestinal Bleeding

Once it has been established that the cause of bleeding is from a source in the GI tract, further investigation for the source and cause is done. *Upper GI bleeding* comes from above the ligament of Treitz, which is attached to the duodenum at its junction with the jejunum. *Lower GI bleeding* comes from a source distal to the ligament of Treitz. Diagnostic studies such as endoscopy, scintigraphy, and angiography have improved the ability to localize the site of bleeding (Brown, 1999).

### Etiology

The esophagus is a common site of upper GI bleeding. Esophagitis due to gastroesophageal reflux may lead to chronic and often occult blood loss. Esophageal varices secondary to portal hypertension may cause massive bleeding.

Peptic inflammation (gastritis and duodenitis) or ulceration is the most common cause of upper GI bleeding in children. Hemorrhagic gastritis may occur in the newborn infant following a difficult delivery or asphyxia. In this circumstance gastric perforation is a serious complication that requires emergent treatment. Less common causes of upper GI bleeding include bleeding disorders, vascular malformations, GI duplications, Mallory-Weiss syndrome (an esophageal tear caused by protracted vomiting), and hematobilia (bleeding into biliary passages).

In lower GI bleeding, small amounts of bright red blood in the stool of a healthy child may be due to an anal fissure. Colonic polyps are another cause of passage of bright red blood per rectum in toddlers and older children. Bleeding associated with diarrhea may indicate a serious problem. Enteric infections remain the leading cause, but necrotizing enterocolitis, hemolytic-uremic syndrome, inflammatory bowel disease, and food allergy should be considered. Other causes are intussusception with the passage of blood per rectum (see p. 1448) or Meckel diverticulum with the painless passage of currant jelly–like stools (see p. 1435).

### Pathophysiology

The GI tract has an extensive surface area and a rich vascular supply. Bleeding can occur anywhere along the GI tract from a vein, artery, or vascular malformation. Children with coagulopathies, including hemophilia A or B, have an incidence of GI bleeding of 10% to 25% (Perrault and Berry, 1999). Many of these children have peptic ulcer disease. Children with liver disease may also have deficient coagulation factors because of poor synthesis and malabsorption of vitamin K, which is a risk factor for GI bleeding.

Portal hypertension may lead to GI bleeding, because the formation of portosystemic shunts can result in dilated venous channels in vulnerable locations such as the esophagus and stomach. These dilated venous channels (*varices*) may bleed, causing severe GI hemorrhage.

### Diagnostic Evaluation

The diagnosis of GI bleeding is often made on the basis of the history and physical examination. *Hematemesis* is the vomiting of bright red blood or denatured blood that looks like "coffee grounds," usually representing an upper GI source of bleeding. *Hematochezia* is the passage of bright red blood per rectum, indicating lower GI bleeding. This blood may precede or follow a bowel movement or be mixed with or coat the stool. Bright red blood that coats the stool may be due to a hard bowel movement, hemorrhoids, or anal fissures. Blood mixed with stool indicates a bleeding source proximal to the rectum. Blood passed alone following a bowel movement is most likely due to bleeding in the perianal or rectal area, possibly caused by a polyp. Blood with mucus in the stool indicates an inflammatory or infectious condition, and currant jelly–like stools indicate vascular compromise, such as intussusception. *Melena* is the passage of black, tarry stools that contain denatured (digested) blood and suggests an upper GI source of bleeding. Occasionally, bright red blood may be passed per rectum from an upper GI source of bleeding when the bleeding is massive.

---

*See Chapters 27 and 28 for additional nursing care related to these procedures. Home care instructions for caring for a central venous catheter, giving NG tube feedings, giving gastrostomy feedings, and caring for the child with a colostomy are available in Wong DL, Hess CS: *Wong and Whaley's clinical manual of pediatric nursing*, ed 5, St Louis, 2000, Mosby.

It is important to test emesis or stool for the presence of occult blood to differentiate true bleeding from the ingestion of food containing food coloring. In older children, false-positive stool tests for occult blood can also occur with the ingestion of red meats and iron preparations.

Laboratory studies are determined on the basis of the history and physical examination. In many instances, a complete blood count with platelet quantification, prothrombin, partial thromboplastin, and coagulation studies will be done. Children who have acute illness, fever, and joint pain in addition to GI bleeding will need an erythrocyte sedimentation rate and stool studies with culture to evaluate for enteric pathogens, ova and parasites, and *Clostridium difficile*. When inflammatory bowel disease is suspected, a metabolic panel to determine total protein and albumin may be added to a complete blood count, erythrocyte sedimentation rate, and liver function tests. The child with massive painless rectal bleeding may require a nuclear medicine scan to rule out Meckel diverticulum. If there is evidence of portal hypertension or chronic liver disease, liver function tests, liver imaging studies, and a liver biopsy may be necessary. A barium enema is performed if intussusception is suspected.

Imaging studies help to differentiate among several suspected diagnoses. CT of the sinuses helps to localize bleeding that is coming from the nasopharynx or sinuses. A chest radiograph may distinguish hemoptysis related to cystic fibrosis, bronchiectasis, or other chronic lung conditions from hematemesis. Angiography can be used to identify the source of bleeding and to allow embolization or vasopressin infusion for treatment. Endoscopy is the diagnostic method chosen when the source of bleeding is thought to be secondary to gastritis, esophagitis, PUD, colitis, or polyps. Endoscopic examinations also permit visualization of the intestinal mucosa and collection of biopsy specimens and cultures (Heitlinger and McClung, 1999).

### Therapeutic Management

Treatment of GI bleeding in children depends on its severity and cause. The first step in management of acute GI bleeding is to assess the magnitude of blood loss and restore the child's hemodynamic stability. Severe bleeding necessitates hospitalization. IV fluids (normal saline or lactated Ringer's solution) are administered rapidly. Oxygen therapy is indicated if the bleeding is severe. Transfusion of blood products may be required if the blood loss is significant, and any existing coagulopathy should be corrected.

Upper GI mucosal lesions are usually treated with $H_2$ receptor antagonists (cimetidine [Tagamet], ranitidine [Zantac], or famotidine [Pepcid]) or proton pump inhibitors (omeprazole [Prilosec] or lansoprazole [Prevacid]) and antacids to reduce acidity and promote mucosal healing. Variceal hemorrhage can be treated with peripheral vasopressin infusion and endoscopic sclerotherapy to hasten tissue fibrosis. Balloon tamponade to place pressure on the bleeding area may be performed as a temporary measure until endoscopic sclerotherapy can be done.

Therapy for lower GI bleeding is directed toward the primary underlying condition. The treatment may include medical or surgical management. Surgery may be required if the bleeding is severe despite aggressive medical intervention.

### Nursing Considerations

The infant or child with acute and severe GI bleeding requires emergency care. Initial management includes assessment of the magnitude of bleeding and hemodynamic status and assistance with resuscitation efforts. (See Critical Thinking Exercise box.)

**NURSING ALERT**

Monitor closely for signs of shock: restlessness; increased respiratory and heart rate; poor capillary refill; pallor; cool, clammy extremities; and decreased blood pressure (a late sign). Call for assistance immediately if these signs are observed.

---

 *Critical Thinking Exercise*

### Hematemesis

A 6-month-old infant is seen in the emergency room. The parents brought the infant to the hospital because he spit up formula with blood streaks. In the emergency room the infant is tachypneic, has tachycardia, and is febrile with a temperature of 39° C (102.2° F). A chest x-ray film shows pneumonia. The infant is admitted to the hospital to receive antibiotics and for observation. Several hours after admission to the inpatient unit, the mother calls the nurse when the infant vomits a large amount of bright red blood. The infant is pale and lethargic. Which of the following should *not* be included in the initial nursing actions?

FIRST, THINK ABOUT IT . . .

- What precise question are you trying to answer?
- What conclusions are you coming to?

1. Call for assistance and estimate the amount of blood loss.
2. Obtain vital signs and monitor capillary refill, skin color, and behavior.
3. Prepare to pass a nasogastric tube, obtain blood for laboratory analyses, and start an IV line.
4. Test stool for blood (Hematest or Hemoccult).

*The best response is four. Because this infant has acute severe GI bleeding, initial nursing actions include an assessment of hemodynamic status for possible shock (option 2). The infant should not be left unattended, and the nurse should call for assistance because further vomiting and potential aspiration may occur. The nurse should also anticipate that a nasogastric tube will be inserted to lavage the stomach and monitor for further bleeding. A correct conclusion is that blood will need to be drawn, including a hemoglobin, hematocrit, platelet count, white blood cell count, and a type and crossmatch for potential transfusion. An IV line will need to be inserted to administer fluids and possibly blood products.*

*Once the patient is stabilized, additional information and evaluation will be necessary in order to identify the cause of the bleeding. In this case a potential cause of bleeding is stress-induced gastritis or peptic ulceration because of infection. Hematest of the stool will add no useful information at this point.*

Oxygen should be administered, and suction equipment should be available. An IV catheter should be inserted, and preparation should be made for the administration of IV fluids, usually normal saline or lactated Ringer's solution. Blood should be drawn for laboratory analysis, including a hemoglobin, hematocrit, blood urea nitrogen, creatinine, coagulation studies, and type and crossmatch. The nurse should be prepared to insert an NG tube to help locate the site of bleeding and to lavage the stomach with normal saline at room temperature if upper GI bleeding is suspected. Rectal temperatures are avoided to prevent further irritation or damage to the rectal mucosa of a child suspected of having rectal bleeding or fissures. After the child is stabilized, ongoing monitoring in an intensive care setting may be indicated.

In cases of mild or chronic bleeding, there is more time for a thorough history and diagnostic evaluation, and this type of evaluation is often performed in an outpatient setting. Important nursing responsibilities include assisting with the history and physical examination, diagnostic procedures, and education regarding the therapeutic plan.

The parents or caregivers of a child with GI bleeding may be extremely anxious and panic-stricken. They need reassurance that most instances of bleeding are self-limited and can be treated successfully. In life-threatening situations, special emotional support is required. The family is kept informed about the source, cause, and treatment of the bleeding.

# HEPATIC DISORDERS

The liver is an active, vital organ whose functions can be divided into several groups: (1) vascular functions of storing and filtering blood; (2) secretory function of producing bile; (3) metabolism of carbohydrate, protein, and fat; (4) synthesis of blood-clotting components and storage of iron and vitamins (A, D, B$_{12}$, and K); and (5) detoxification and excretion of certain drugs and metabolic substances. Many disorders can cause liver dysfunction in children, including biliary atresia, hepatitis, and cirrhosis. (See Chapter 11).

## Acute Hepatitis

Hepatitis is an acute or chronic inflammation of the liver that can result from several different causes. One cause is infection. Many types of hepatitis are caused by viruses such as the hepatitis viruses, Epstein-Barr virus (EBV), the cytomegalovirus (CMV), and the human immunodeficiency virus (HIV). Other causes of hepatitis are nonviral (abscess, amebiasis), autoimmune, metabolic, chemical, neoplastic, anatomic (choledochal duct cyst and biliary atresia), hemodynamic (shock, congestive heart failure), and idiopathic (sclerosing cholangitis and Reye syndrome) (Evans, 1999).

## Etiology

The majority (90%) of cases of viral hepatitis are caused by six viruses:

1. Hepatitis A virus (HAV)
2. Hepatitis B virus (HBV)
3. Hepatitis C virus (HCV)
4. Hepatitis D virus (HDV)
5. Hepatitis E virus (HEV)
6. Hepatitis G virus (HGV)

In the United States, most non-A, non-B hepatitis is caused by HCV (Castiglia, 1996). In addition, CMV, EBV, and herpes simplex virus (HSV) may occasionally cause hepatitis. The clinical symptoms of these viruses are similar. Epidemiologic features and serologic testing are used to differentiate the causes. Table 33-4 compares the features of HAV, HBV, and HCV.

*Hepatitis A* is widespread, affecting approximately 25,000 people in the United States each year. There is no chronic or carrier state. The virus is spread directly or indirectly by the fecal-oral route either by ingestion of contaminated foods, direct exposure to infected fecal material, or close contact with an infected person. The virus is particularly prevalent in developing countries with poor living conditions, inadequate sanitation, crowding, and poor personal hygiene practices. The spread of HAV has been associated with improper food handling and high-risk areas such as households with infected persons, residential centers for the disabled, and daycare centers. The average incubation period is about 4 weeks, with a range of 15 to 50 days. Fecal shedding of the virus can occur for 2 to 3 weeks before and for a week after the onset of jaundice. During this time, although the individual is asymptomatic, the virus is most likely to be transmitted. Infants with HAV infection are likely to be asymptomatic (anicteric hepatitis). Children often have diarrhea, and their symptoms are frequently attributed to gastroenteritis. Only 1 in 12 young children will develop jaundice. Most adults develop clinical signs with icteric hepatitis. The prognosis of HAV infection is usually good, and complications are rare. The fatality rate from fulminant hepatitis in children less than 14 years of age is 0.1% (Evans, 1999).

*Hepatitis B* can be an acute or chronic infection, ranging from an asymptomatic, limited infection to fatal, fulminant (rapid and severe) hepatitis. There are no environmental or animal reservoirs for the HBV. Humans are the main source of infections. HBV may be transmitted parentally, percutaneously, or transmucosally. Hepatitis B surface antigen (HBsAg) has been found in all body fluids, including feces, bile, breast milk, sweat, tears, vaginal secretions, and urine, but only blood, semen, and saliva have been found to contain infectious HBV particles. HBV infection from human bites has been documented, but transmission from feces has not. Hepatitis B has been acquired following blood transfusion, but this likelihood has been reduced as a result of blood product–screening procedures. Adults whose occupations are associated with considerable exposure to blood or blood products, such as health care workers, are at an increased risk of contracting HBV.

**TABLE 33-4**    Comparison of types A, B, and C hepatitis

| Characteristics | Type A | Type B | Type C |
|---|---|---|---|
| Incubation period | 15-50 days, average 25-30 days | 45-160 days, average 90 days | 2 weeks-6 months, average 6-7 weeks |
| Period of communicability | Unknown<br>Virus in blood and feces 2-3 weeks before onset of jaundice and for about 1 week after onset of jaundice | Variable<br>Virus in blood or other body fluids during late incubation period and acute stage of disease; may persist in carrier state for years to lifetime | Begins before onset of symptoms<br>May persist in carrier state for years |
| Mode of transmission | Principal route—fecal-oral<br>Rarely—parenteral | Principal route—parenteral<br>Less frequent route—oral, sexual, any body fluid<br>Perinatal transfer—transplacental blood (last trimester), at delivery, or during breast-feeding, especially if mother has cracked nipples | Principal route—parenteral<br>Nonparenteral spread possible |
| **Clinical features** | | | |
| Onset | Usually rapid, acute | More insidious | Usually insidious |
| Fever | Common and early | Less frequent | Less frequent |
| Anorexia | Common | Mild to moderate | Mild to moderate |
| Nausea and vomiting | Common | Sometimes present | Mild to moderate |
| Rash | Rare | Common | Sometimes present |
| Arthralgia | Rare | Common | Rare |
| Pruritus | Rare | Sometimes present | Sometimes present |
| Jaundice | Present (many cases anicteric) | Present | Present |
| Immunity | Present after one attack; no crossover to type B or C | Present after one attack; no crossover to type A or C | Present after one attack; no crossover to type A or B |
| Carrier state | No | Yes | Yes |
| Chronic infection | No | Yes | Yes |
| **Prophylaxis** | | | |
| Immune globulin (IgG) | Passive immunity<br>Successful, especially in early incubation period and preexposure prophylaxis | Passive immunity<br>Inconsistent benefits; probably of no use | Not currently recommended by Centers for Disease Control and Prevention |
| HAV vaccine | Two inactivated vaccines are approved for children ages 2-18 years: Havrix and Vaqta; Havrix is given in either a 3-dose schedule (1 month between first and second doses with third dose in 6-12 months) or a 2-dose schedule (6-12 months between doses); Vaqta is given in a 2-dose schedule (6-12 months between doses) | | |
| HBV immune globulin (HBIG) | No benefit | Postexposure protection possible if given immediately after definite exposure | No benefit |
| HBV vaccine (see Table 12-1) | | Provides active immunity<br>Universal vaccination recommended for all newborns | |
| Mortality | 0.1% to 0.2% | 0.5% to 2.0% in uncomplicated cases; may be higher in complicated cases | 1% to 2% in uncomplicated cases; may be higher in complicated cases |

Most HBV infection in children is acquired perinatally. Transmission from mother to infant during the perinatal period (i.e., transmission from HBsAg-positive mothers) results in chronic infection in 70% to 90% of infants if the mother is hepatitis Be antigen (HBeAg)–positive (American Academy of Pediatrics, 2000). Perinatal infection is thought to occur during the birthing process when the infant comes in contact with maternal body fluids, most likely blood. It is still not known if the virus enters the infant via mucosal membranes, intestinal tract, or skin abrasions. HBsAg has been detected in breast milk, but it is not clear whether HBV infection is transmitted through ingested breast milk or from swallowed maternal blood from injured nipples (Evans, 1999). Infants and children who are not infected during the perinatal period remain at high risk for acquiring person-to-person transmission from their mother during the first 5 years of life.

HBV infection occurs in children and adolescents in specific high-risk groups: (1) individuals with hemophilia or other disorders who have received multiple transfusions, (2) children and adolescents involved in IV drug abuse, (3) institutionalized children, (4) preschool children in endemic areas, and (5) individuals engaged in heterosexual activity or sexual activity with homosexual males. The incubation period for HBV infection ranges from 45 to 160 days with an average of 90 days (American Academy of Pediatrics, 2000). HBV infection can cause a carrier state and lead to chronic hepatitis with eventual cirrhosis or hepatocellular carcinoma in adulthood.

*Hepatitis C* was previously "non-A, non-B hepatitis" because of the absence of HAV and HBV serologic markers of infection. HCV is transmitted parenterally through exposure to blood and blood products from HCV-infected persons. Recent improvements in donor screening and inactivation procedures for blood products such as the factor concentrates used for hemophilia patients have significantly reduced the risk of transmission through blood products. The mechanism of nonparenteral or nonpercutaneous transmission of HCV is uncertain. Sexual transmission among monogamous couples and among family contacts is uncommon. Maternal coinfection with HIV has been associated with increased risk of perinatal transmission of HCV and may depend on the HCV genotype and the serum titer of maternal HCV-RNA. All persons with HCV antibody or HCV-RNA in their blood are considered to be infectious (American Academy of Pediatrics, 2000). The clinical course is variable. The incubation period for HCV ranges from 2 weeks to 6 months with an average of 6 to 7 weeks. The natural history of the disease in children is not well defined. Some children may be asymptomatic, but hepatitis C can become a chronic condition and can cause cirrhosis and hepatocellular carcinoma. About 60% to 70% of individuals infected with HCV develop chronic disease. Infection with HCV is the leading reason for liver transplantation in the United States (America Academy of Pediatrics, 2000).

*Hepatitis D* occurs in children already infected with HBV. HDV is a defective RNA virus that requires the helper function of HBV. The incubation period is from 2 to 8 weeks. Both acute and chronic forms of hepatitis D tend to be more severe than hepatitis B and can lead to cirrhosis. HDV infection occurs mostly in drug abusers, individuals with hemophilia, and persons immigrating from endemic areas.

*Hepatitis E* is enterically transmitted non-A, non-B hepatitis. Transmission may occur through the fecal-oral route or from contaminated water. The incubation period is 2 to 9 weeks. This illness is uncommon in children, does not cause chronic liver disease, is not a chronic condition, and has no carrier state. However, it can be a devastating disease among pregnant women with an unusually high case-fatality rate.

*Hepatitis G* virus is blood-borne but can also be transmitted by organ transplantation. High-risk groups include transfusion recipients, IV drug users, and individuals infected with HCV. Individuals with the virus are often asymptomatic, and most infections are chronic. The incubation period is unknown.

## Pathophysiology

Pathologic changes occur primarily in the parenchymal cells of the liver and result in variable degrees of swelling, infiltration of liver cells by mononuclear cells, and subsequent degeneration, necrosis, and fibrosis. Structural changes within the hepatocyte are thought to account for altered liver functions, such as impaired bile excretion, elevated transaminase levels, and decreased albumin synthesis. The disorder may be self-limiting, with regeneration of liver cells without scarring, leading to a complete recovery. There are, however, forms of hepatitis that do not result in complete return of liver function. These include *fulminant hepatitis,* which is characterized by a severe, acute course with massive destruction of the liver tissue causing liver failure and high mortality within 1 to 2 weeks, and *subacute* or *chronic active hepatitis,* which is characterized by progressive liver destruction, uncertain regeneration, scarring, and potential cirrhosis.

## Clinical Manifestations

The clinical manifestations and course of uncomplicated acute viral hepatitis are similar for most of the hepatitis viruses. Usually the prodromal or *anicteric phase* (absence of jaundice) lasts 5 to 7 days. Anorexia, malaise, lethargy, and easy fatigability are the most common symptoms. Fever may be present, especially in adolescents. Nausea, vomiting, and epigastric or right upper quadrant abdominal pain or tenderness may occur. Arthralgia and skin rashes may occur and are more likely in children with hepatitis B than those with hepatitis A. The transaminases, rather than the bilirubin, will often be elevated in acute hepatitis, and hepatomegaly may be present. Some mild cases of acute viral hepatitis do not cause symptoms or can be mistaken for influenza.

In young children most of the prodromal symptoms disappear with the onset of jaundice, or the *icteric phase.* Many children with acute viral hepatitis, however, never develop jaundice. If jaundice occurs, it is often accompanied by dark urine and pale stools. Pruritis may accompany jaundice and can be bothersome for children.

Children with chronic active hepatitis may be asymptomatic but more commonly have nonspecific symptoms of malaise, fatigue, lethargy, weight loss, or vague abdominal pain. Hepatomegaly may be present, and the transaminases are often very high, with mild to severe hyperbilirubinemia.

Fulminant hepatitis is due primarily to hepatitis B or hepatitis C. Many children with fulminant hepatitis develop characteristic clinical symptoms and rapidly develop manifestations of liver failure, including encephalopathy, coagulation defects, ascites, deepening jaundice, and an increasing white blood cell count. Changes in mental status or personality indicate impending liver failure. Although children with acute hepatitis may have hepatomegaly, a rapid decrease in the size of the liver (indicating loss of tissue due to necrosis) is a serious sign of fulminant hepatitis. Complications of fulminant hepatitis include GI bleeding, sepsis, renal failure, and disseminated coagulopathy.

### Diagnostic Evaluation

Diagnosis is based on the history, physical examination, and serologic markers for hepatitis A, B, and C. No liver function test is specific for hepatitis, but serum aspartate and serum aminotransferase levels are markedly elevated. Serum bilirubin levels peak 5 to 10 days after clinical jaundice appears. Histologic evidence from liver biopsy may be required to establish of the diagnosis and to assess the severity of the liver disease. Serologic markers indicate the antibodies or antigens formed in response to the specific virus and confirm the diagnosis. Serum immunologic tests are not available to detect HAV antigen, but there are two HAV antibody tests, anti-HAV IgG and IgM. Anti-HAV antibodies are present at the onset of the disease and persist for life. A positive anti-HAV antibody test indicates the following: acute infection, immunity from past infection, passive antibody acquisition (e.g., transfusion, serum immune globulin infusion), or immunization. To diagnose an acute or recent HAV infection, a positive anti-HAV IgM test that is present with the onset of the disease and that persists for only 2 to 3 days is required.

Diagnosis of hepatitis B is confirmed by the detection of various hepatitis virus antigens and the antibodies that are produced in response to the infection. A listing of these antibodies and antigens and their significance includes:

**HBsAg**—Hepatitis B surface antigen (found on the surface of the virus) indicates ongoing infection or carrier state

**anti-HBs**—Antibody to surface antigen HBsAg indicates resolving or past infection

**HBcAg**—Hepatitis B core antigen (found on the inner core of the virus) can be detected only in the liver

**anti-HBc**—Antibody to core antigen HBcAg indicates ongoing or past infection

**HBeAg**—Hepatitis Be antigen (another component of the HBV core) indicates active infection

**anti-HBe**—Antibody to HBeAg indicates resolving or past infection

**IgM anti-HBc**—IgM antibody to core antigen

Tests are available for detection of all of the HBV antigens and antibodies except HBcAg. HBsAg is detectable during acute infection. Presence of the HBsAg antigen indicates that the individual has been infected with the hepatitis virus. If the infection is self-limited, HBsAg disappears in most patients before serum anti-HBs can be detected (termed the window phase of infection). IgM anti-HBc is highly specific in establishing the diagnosis of acute infection, as well as during the window phase in older children and adults. However, IgM anti-HBc usually is not present in perinatal HBV infection (American Academy of Pediatrics, 2000). Neonatal infection is most likely to occur in infants born to mothers who are HBeAg-positive. In contrast, hepatitis B is much less likely to occur in infants whose mothers are HBsAg-positive but HBeAg-negative and who have antibodies to HBeAg (Jonas, 1999).

Clinical improvement is usually associated with a decrease in or disappearance of these antigens, followed by the appearance of their antibodies. For example, anti-HBc of the IgM class is seen early in the disease, followed by a rise in anti-HBc of the IgG class. Because the antibodies persist indefinitely, they are used to identify the *carrier state* (individuals with HBV who have no clinical disease but are able to transmit the organism). Persons with chronic HBV infection have circulating HBsAg and anti-HBc, and on rare occasions anti-HBsAg is present. Both anti-HBs and anti-HBc are detected in persons with resolved infection, but anti-HBs alone are present in individuals who have been immunized with the HBV vaccine.

HCV-RNA is the earliest serologic marker for HCV. HCV-RNA can be detected during the incubation period before symptoms of HCV disease are expressed. A positive HCV-RNA indicates active infection, and persistence of HCV-RNA indicates chronic infection. A negative test correlates with resolution of the disease. HCV-RNA is also used to determine patient response to antiviral therapy for HCV.

The history of all patients should include questions to seek evidence of (1) contact with a person known to have hepatitis, especially a family member; (2) unsafe sanitation practices, such as contaminated drinking water; (3) eating certain foods, such as clams or oysters (especially from polluted water); (4) multiple blood transfusions; (5) ingestion of hepatotoxic drugs, such as salicylates, sulfonamides, antineoplastic agents, acetaminophen, anticonvulsants, and many other medications; and (6) parenteral administration of illicit drugs or sexual contact with a person who uses these drugs.

### Therapeutic Management

Treatment options for viral hepatitis are limited. The goals of management include early detection, support and monitoring of the disease, recognition of chronic liver disease, and prevention of spread of the disease. No specific effective therapy for either acute or chronic hepatitis B or hepatitis C exists. Special high-protein, high-carbohydrate, low-fat diets are generally not of value. The use of corticosteroids alone or with immunosuppressive drugs is not advocated in the treatment of chronic viral hepatitis; however, steroids have been used to treat chronic autoimmune hepatitis. Hospitalization is required in the event of coagulopathy or fulminant hepatitis. Human interferon-a has been used in the treatment of chronic hepatitis B and C in adults but is not approved by the U.S. Food and Drug Administration (FDA) for children (American Academy of Pediatrics, 2000). Therapy for hepatitis depends on the severity of inflammation and the cause of the disorder.

**Prevention.** Proper handwashing and standard precautions prevent the spread of viral hepatitis. Prophylactic use of standard immune globulin (IG) is effective in preventing hepatitis A in situations of preexposure (such as anticipated travel to areas where HAV is prevalent) or within 2 weeks of exposure.

Hepatitis B immune globulin (HBIG) is effective in preventing HBV infection following one-time exposures such as accidental needle punctures or other contact of contaminated material with mucous membranes and should be given to newborns whose mothers are HBsAg-positive. HBIG is prepared from plasma that contains high titers of antibodies against HBV. HBIG should be given within 72 hours of exposure.

Vaccines have been developed to prevent HAV and HBV infection (see Table 33-4). HBV vaccination is recommended for all newborns and for high-risk groups; only selected individuals should receive HAV vaccine. (See Immunizations, Chapter 12.) In addition, the American Academy of Pediatrics (2000) recommends universal immunization of all adolescents with the HBV vaccine. Because HDV cannot be transmitted in the absence of HBV infection it is possible to prevent HDV infection by preventing HBV infection. The U.S. Public Health Service recommends that individuals who received an IV immune globulin preparation called Gammagard between April 1, 1993, and February 23, 1994, be screened for HCV infection and tested for aminotransferase concentrations and for the anti-HCV globulin. Routine serologic testing for anti-HCV of children born to women previously identified as being infected with HCV is also recommended (American Academy of Pediatrics, 2000).

**Prognosis.** The prognosis for children with hepatitis is variable and depends on the type of virus, the child's age, and immunocompetency. Hepatitis A and E are usually mild, brief illnesses with no carrier state. Hepatitis B can cause a wide spectrum of acute and chronic illness. Infants are more likely than older children to develop chronic hepatitis. Hepatocellular carcinoma during adulthood is a potentially fatal complication of chronic HBV infection. Hepatitis C frequently becomes chronic, and cirrhosis may develop in these children. Limited data concerning hepatitis G suggests that the rate of progression to cirrhosis with this virus may be very low. The highest mortality occurs in hepatitis D. Approximately 50% of the cases of fulminant hepatic failure are caused by viral hepatitis. The mechanism by which fulminant hepatic failure occurs is not well understood, and survival varies (Novak, Suchy and Balistreri, 1999).

### Nursing Considerations

Nursing objectives depend largely on the severity of the hepatitis, the medical treatment, and factors influencing the control and transmission of the disease. Because children with mild viral hepatitis are frequently cared for at home, explaining any medical therapies and infection control measures is frequently left to the clinic or office nurse. When further assistance is needed for parents to comply with instructions, a public health nursing referral is necessary.

A well-balanced diet and a schedule of rest and activity adjusted to the child's condition are encouraged. Because the child with HAV is not infectious within a week after the onset of jaundice, the child may feel well enough to resume school shortly thereafter. Parents are cautioned about administering any medication to the child, because normal doses of many drugs may become dangerous because of the liver's inability to detoxify and excrete them.

Standard precautions are followed when children are hospitalized. However, these children are not usually isolated in a separate room unless they are fecally incontinent or their toys and other personal items are likely to become contaminated with feces. Children are discouraged from sharing their toys. (See Infection Control, Chapter 27.)

Handwashing is the single most effective measure in prevention and control of hepatitis in any setting. (For a discussion of preventive measures in the daycare center, see Chapter 15; see also Infection Control, Chapter 27.) Parents and children need an explanation of the usual ways in which HAV (fecal-oral route) and HBV (parenteral route) are spread.* Parents should also be aware of the recommendation for universal vaccination against HBV for newborns and adolescents. (See Chapter 12.)

In young people with HBV infection who have a known or suspected history of illicit drug use, the nurse has the responsibility of helping them realize the associated dangers of drug abuse, stressing the parenteral mode of transmission of hepatitis and encouraging them to seek counseling through a drug program. (See Nursing Care Plan: The Child with Acute Hepatitis.†)

## Cirrhosis

Cirrhosis occurs as an end stage of many chronic liver diseases, including biliary atresia and chronic hepatitis. Severe liver damage can be caused by infectious, autoimmune, or toxic factors and by chronic diseases such as hemophilia and cystic fibrosis. A cirrhotic liver is irreversibly damaged.

### Pathophysiology

Cirrhosis occurs as a result of hepatocyte injury with necrosis, fibrosis, regeneration, and eventual degeneration. The diminished parenchymal cell mass causes regeneration of tissue with nodular areas of proliferating hepatocytes that stretch the surrounding connective tissue. Hepatocytes respond to injury with deposition of collagen that forms fibrous connective tissue. This scar tissue and nodular areas of regeneration impair the intrahepatic blood flow. Ongoing necrosis and self-perpetuation of this pathologic process are the result of cirrhosis.

Failure of hepatocellular function and portal hypertension occur and often lead to complications, including ascites, severe cholestasis, encephalopathy (hepatic coma), and GI bleeding.

### Clinical Manifestations

Clinical manifestations of cirrhosis include jaundice, poor growth, anorexia, muscle weakness, and lethargy. Ascites,

---

*Home care instructions for preventing AIDS and hepatitis infection are available in Wong DL, Hess CS: *Wong and Whaley's clinical manual of pediatric nursing,* ed 5, St Louis, 2000, Mosby.
†In Wong DL, Hess CS: *Wong and Whaley's clinical manual of pediatric nursing,* ed 5, St Louis, 2000, Mosby.

edema, GI bleeding, anemia, and abdominal pain may be present in children with impaired intrahepatic blood flow. Pulmonary function may be impaired because of pressure against the diaphragm due to hepatosplenomegaly and ascites. Dyspnea and cyanosis may occur, especially on exertion. Intrapulmonary arteriovenous shunts may develop, which can also cause hypoxemia. Spider angiomas and prominent blood vessels on the upper torso are often present.

## Diagnostic Evaluation

The diagnosis of cirrhosis is based on (1) the history, especially in regard to prior liver disease, such as hepatitis; (2) physical examination, particularly hepatosplenomegaly or a sudden decrease in liver size; (3) laboratory evaluation, especially liver function tests, such as bilirubin and aminotransferases, ammonia, albumin, cholesterol, and prothrombin time; and (4) liver biopsy for characteristic changes. Doppler ultrasonography of the liver and spleen is useful to confirm ascites, to evaluate the blood flow through the liver and spleen, and to determine the patency and size of the portal vein if liver transplantation is considered.

**NURSING ALERT**   The most common complication from percutaneous liver biopsy is internal bleeding. Monitor vital signs and laboratory values, especially hematocrit, for evidence of hemorrhage and shock.

## Therapeutic Management

Unfortunately, there is no successful treatment to arrest the progression of cirrhosis. The goals of management include monitoring liver function and managing specific complications such as esophageal varices and malnutrition. Assessment of the child's degree of liver dysfunction is important so that the child may be evaluated for transplantation at the appropriate time.

*Liver transplantation* has improved the prognosis substantially for many children with cirrhosis. The combination of new immunosuppressive medications and new surgical techniques have resulted in 90% 1-year survival rates in many large hospital centers. Recent changes in the policy governing the allocation of livers for transplantation by the United Network for Organ Sharing (UNOS) will allow patients with acute fulminant liver failure plus those with failed liver grafts and the sickest pediatric patients to be placed at the top of the UNOS transplantation lists (Ott, 1997). Although this change will benefit many pediatric patients, the shortage of available donors for children will continue to dictate transplantation decisions, and many children will continue to die while waiting for a suitable donor. (See Biliary Atresia, Chapter 11.)

Nutritional support is an important therapy for children with cirrhosis and malnutrition. Supplements of fat-soluble vitamins are often required, and mineral supplements may be indicated. In some instances aggressive nutritional support in the form of continuous tube feedings or parenteral nutrition may be necessary.

Esophageal and gastric varices are a life-threatening complication of portal hypertension. Acute hemorrhage is man-

### FAMILY FOCUS
#### End-Stage Liver Disease

In many cases the child with liver disease and the family must cope with an uncertain progression of the disease. The only hope for long-term survival may be liver transplantation. Transplantation can be very successful, but the waiting period may be long, because there are many more children in need of organs than there are donors. The procedure is very expensive and is only performed at designated medical centers, which are often far from the family's home. The nurse should recognize the unique stresses of coping with end-stage liver disease and waiting for transplantation, and should offer support and assistance to the family in coping with these stressors. The assistance of social workers and support from other parents can also be very beneficial.

aged with IV fluids, blood products, vasopressin, and gastric lavage. Balloon tamponade with a Sengstaken-Blakemore tube may be indicated. Endoscopic sclerotherapy or endoscopic banding ligation are also effective therapies for esophageal and gastric varices.

Ascites may be managed by sodium restriction and diuretics. Severe ascites with respiratory compromise may be managed with administration of albumin or by paracentesis.

Although the full mechanism of hepatic encephalopathy is unknown, failure of the damaged liver to remove endogenous toxins, such as ammonia, plays a role. Treatment is directed at limiting the ammonia formation and absorption that occur in the bowel, especially with the drugs neomycin and lactulose. Because ammonia is formed in the bowel by the action of bacteria on ingested protein, neomycin reduces the number of intestinal bacteria so less ammonia is produced. The fermentation of lactulose by colonic bacteria produces short-chain fatty acids, which lower the colonic pH, thereby inhibiting bacterial metabolism. This decreases the formation of ammonia from bacterial metabolism of protein.

**Prognosis.**   The success of liver transplantation has revolutionized the approach to liver cirrhosis. Liver failure and cirrhosis are indications for transplantation. Careful monitoring of the child's condition and quality of life are necessary to evaluate the need for and timing of transplantation.

## Nursing Considerations

Nursing care of the child with cirrhosis is influenced by several factors, including the cause of the cirrhosis, the severity of complications, and the prognosis. The prognosis is often poor unless successful liver transplantation occurs. Therefore nursing care of this child is similar to that for any child with a life-threatening illness. (See Chapter 23.) Hospitalization is required when complications such as hemorrhage, severe malnutrition, or hepatic failure occur. Nursing assessments are directed at monitoring the child's condition, and interventions are aimed at treatment of specific complications. If liver transplantation is an option, the family needs support and assistance to cope. (See Family Focus box.)

# KEY POINTS

- The essential functions of the gastrointestinal (GI) system are to process and absorb nutrients necessary to maintain metabolic processes and support growth and development, to perform excretory functions, to provide detoxification, to maintain fluid and electrolyte balance, and to serve a lymphoid function.
- Digestion is the catabolism of foodstuffs (water, vitamins, minerals, carbohydrates, proteins, and fats) from their original complex form to simple, assimilable nutrients.
- The small intestine is the principal absorptive site in the GI system.
- Most ingested foreign bodies pass through the alimentary tract without difficulty. Those lodged in the esophagus or objects with sharp edges require further evaluation.
- Constipation is managed with diet changes and laxative therapy in an organized program to promote regular bowel habits.
- Hirschsprung disease requires surgical removal of aganglionic segments of bowel.
- Nursing care of gastroesophageal reflux is aimed primarily at instructing caregivers regarding home care feeding and positioning, and caring for the child undergoing surgical intervention.
- Although the cause of appendicitis is poorly understood, it is typically a result of obstruction of the lumen, usually by a fecalith. Common signs and symptoms are colicky abdominal pain, guarding of the abdomen, and fever.
- Meckel diverticulum is a congenital malformation of the GI tract characterized by bloody stools.
- Inflammatory bowel disease refers to ulcerative colitis and Crohn disease. Chronic diarrhea and growth abnormalities are common features.
- Management of inflammatory bowel disease includes nutritional support, sulfasalazine, corticosteroids or other immunosuppressive drugs, antibiotics, and general supportive therapy. Current research is focused on drugs that block the inflammatory response. Surgical removal of inflamed bowel may be necessary.
- Peptic ulcers are poorly understood, but contributing factors include interference with the normal protective mechanisms of the mucosal lining and the presence of *Helicobacter pylori*.
- General signs of GI obstruction include abdominal pain, nausea and vomiting, abdominal distention, and a decline in the amount of stool excreted.
- Hypertrophic pyloric stenosis is characterized by projectile vomiting without loss of appetite, dehydration, and metabolic alkalosis. Therapy is surgical pyloromyotomy.
- Intussusception is a common cause of intestinal obstruction during infancy. Treatment is either nonsurgical hydrostatic reduction or surgical reduction.
- Malabsorption syndromes are disorders associated with some degree of impaired digestion or absorption. They include digestive defects, absorptive defects, and anatomic defects.
- The prognosis for children with short bowel syndrome improved dramatically as a result of advances in parenteral and enteral nutritional support, which is the primary therapy for this condition. Home care is an important component of these children's quality of life.
- Celiac disease is characterized by an intolerance for gluten. The major role of the nurse is to help the parents and child adhere to diet therapy.
- GI bleeding may be upper or lower GI tract bleeding. Initial management should include assessment of the magnitude of bleeding and restoration of hemodynamic stability.
- Viral hepatitis is caused by six types of virus—hepatitis A virus, hepatitis B virus, hepatitis C virus, hepatitis D virus, hepatitis E virus, and hepatitis G virus.
- Hepatitis A virus is spread by a fecal-oral route, whereas hepatitis B and C viruses are transmitted primarily by the parenteral route. The single most effective measure in prevention and control of hepatitis in any setting is handwashing.
- Universal immunization against hepatitis B virus is recommended for all newborns.
- Liver transplantation offers hope to children with end-stage liver disease.

# REFERENCES

American Academy of Pediatrics, Committee on Infectious Diseases, Pickering L, editor: *2000 Red book: report of the Committee on Infectious Diseases*, Elk Grove Village, IL, 2000, The Academy.

American Academy of Pediatrics Task Force on Infant Positioning and SIDS: Positioning and sudden infant death syndrome (SIDS): update, *Pediatrics* 98(6):1216-1218, 1996.

Belluzzi A and others: Effect of an enteric-coated fish-oil preparation on relapses in Crohn's disease, *N Engl J Med* 334(24):1557-1560, 1996.

Blank E: Motility disorders. In McMillan JA and others, editors: *Oski's pediatrics: principles and practice*, ed 3, Philadelphia, 1999, Lippincott Williams & Wilkins.

Borowski S: Common pediatric surgical problems, *Nurs Clin North Am* 29(4):551-562, 1994.

Brandt ML: Intussusception. In McMillan JA and others, editors: *Oski's pediatrics: principles and practice*, ed 3, Philadelphia, 1999, Lippincott Williams & Wilkins.

Brown MR: Gastrointestinal bleeding. In McMillan JA and others, editors: *Oski's pediatrics: principles and practice*, ed 3, Philadelphia, 1999, Lippincott Williams & Wilkins.

Byrne WJ: Foreign bodies. In Wyllie R, Hyams JS, editors: *Pediatric gastrointestinal disease: physiology, diagnosis, management*, ed 2, Philadelphia, 1999, WB Saunders.

Castiglia PT: Hepatitis in children, *J Pediatr Health Care* 10(6):286-288, 1996.

Evans JS: Acute and chronic hepatitis. In Wyllie R, Hyams JS, editors: *Pediatric gastrointestinal disease: physiology, diagnosis, management*, ed 2, Philadelphia, 1999, WB Saunders.

Foglia RP: Gastroesophageal reflux. In Oldham KT, Colombani PM, Foglia RP, editors: *Surgery of infants and children: scientific principles and practice*, ed 2, Philadelphia, 1999, WB Saunders.

Fonkalsrud EW and others: Surgical treatment of gastroesophageal reflux in children: a combined hospital study of 7467 patients, *Pediatrics* 101(3):419-422, 1998.

Gold BD, Blecker U: Peptic ulcer disease. In Wyllie R, Hyams JS, editors: *Pediatric gastrointestinal disease: physiology, diagnosis, management*, ed 2, Philadelphia, 1999, WB Saunders.

Heitlinger LA, McClung HJ: Gastrointestinal hemorrhage. In Wyllie R, Hyams JS, editors: *Pediatric gastrointestinal disease: physiology, diagnosis, management*, ed 2, Philadelphia, 1999, WB Saunders.

Hillemeier A: Reflux and esophagitis. In Walker WA and others, editors: *Pediatric gastrointestinal disease: pathophysiology, diagnosis, management*, ed 3, St Louis, 1999, Mosby.

Hochwald C, Farrington E: Omeprazole (Prilosec), *Pediatr Nurs* 22(5):453-454, 442, 1996.

Holcomb GW: Minimally invasive surgery. In Hoekelman RA and others, editors: *Primary pediatric care*, ed 4, St Louis, 2001, Mosby.

Hyams JS: Inflammatory bowel disease. In Wyllie R, Hyams JS, editors: *Pediatric gastrointestinal disease: physiology, diagnosis, management*, ed 2, Philadelphia, 1999, WB Saunders.

Hyams JS and others: Abdominal pain and irritable bowel syndrome in adolescents: a community-based study, *J Pediatr* 129(2):220-226, 1996.

Jackson WD, Grand RJ: Crohn's disease. In McMillan JA and others, editors: *Oski's pediatrics: principles and practice*, ed 3, Philadelphia, 1999, Lippincott Williams & Wilkins.

Jonas MM: Postnatal infections of the liver. In Walker WA and others, editors: *Pediatric gastrointestinal disease: pathophysiology, diagnosis management*, ed 3, St Louis, 1999, Mosby.

Klein MD, Burd RS: Hirschsprung's disease. In Wyllie R, Hyams JS, editors: *Pediatric gastrointestinal disease: physiology, diagnosis, management*, ed 2, Philadelphia, 1999, WB Saunders.

Leichtner AM, Jackson WD, Grand RJ: Crohn's disease. In Walker WA and others, editors: *Pediatric gastrointestinal disease: pathophysiology, diagnosis, management*, ed 3, St Louis, 1999, Mosby.

Lifschitz CH: Celiac disease. In McMillan JA and others, editors: *Oski's pediatrics: principles and practice*, ed 3, Philadelphia, 1999, Lippincott Williams & Wilkins.

Loening-Baucke V: Functional constipation, *Semin Pediatr Surg* 4(10):26-34, 1995.

Mahajan L, Wyllie R: Chronic abdominal pain of childhood and adolescence. In Wyllie R, Hyams JS, editors: *Pediatric gastrointestinal disease: physiology, diagnosis, management*, ed 2, Philadelphia, 1999, WB Saunders.

Martin FL: Ulcerative colitis, *Am J Nurs* 97(8):38-39, 1997.

Mattei PA, Stevenson RJ, Ziegler MM: Appendicitis. In Wyllie R, Hyams JS, editors: *Pediatric gastrointestinal disease: physiology, diagnosis, management*, ed 2, Philadelphia, 1999, WB Saunders.

Milla P: Motor disorders including pyloric stenosis. In Walker WA and others, editors: *Pediatric gastrointestinal disease: pathophysiology, diagnosis, management*, ed 3, St Louis, 1999, Mosby.

Motil K: Peptic ulcer disease. In McMillan JA and others, editors: *Oski's pediatrics: principles and practice*, ed 3, Philadelphia, 1999, Lippincott Williams & Wilkins.

Najmaldin A, Tan HL: Early experience with laparoscopic pyloromyotomy for infantile hypertrophic pyloric stenosis, *J Pediatr Surg* 30(1):37-38, 1995.

Novak DA, Suchy FJ, Balistreri WF: Disorders of the liver and biliary system relevant to clinical practice. In McMillan JA and others, editors: *Oski's pediatrics: principles and practice*, ed 3, Philadelphia, 1999, Lippincott Williams & Wilkins.

Orenstein SR: Prone positioning in infant gastroesophageal reflux: is elevation of the head worth the trouble? *J Pediatr* 117(2):184-187, 1990.

Orenstein SR: Gastroesophageal reflux. In Wyllie R, Hyams JS, editors: *Pediatric gastrointestinal disease: physiology, diagnosis, management*, ed 2, Philadelphia, 1999, WB Saunders.

Ott BB: Changes in liver transplantation policy, *Pediatr Nurs* 23(2):167-168, 1997.

Pearl RH and others: The approach to common abdominal diagnoses in infants and children, *Pediatr Clin North Am* 45(6):1287-1326, 1998.

Pegoli W: Appendicitis. In McMillan JA and others, editors: *Oski's pediatrics: principles and practice*, ed 3, Philadelphia, 1999, Lippincott Williams & Wilkins.

Perrault J, Berry R: Gastrointestinal bleeding. In Walker WA and others, editors: *Pediatric gastrointestinal disease: pathophysiology, diagnosis, management*, ed 3, St Louis, 1999, Mosby.

Schwartz MZ: Meckel diverticulum. In Wyllie R, Hyams JS, editors: *Pediatric gastrointestinal disease: physiology, diagnosis, management*, ed 2, Philadelphia, 1999, WB Saunders.

Strahlman RS: Appendicitis. In Hoekelman RA and others, editors: *Primary pediatric care*, ed 4, St Louis, 2001, Mosby.

Thomson S, Dancey CP: Symptoms of irritable bowel in school children: prevalence and psychosocial effects, *J Pediatr Health Care* 10(6):280-285, 1996.

Treem WR: Short bowel syndrome. In Wyllie R, Hyams JS, editors: *Pediatric gastrointestinal disease: physiology, diagnosis, management*, ed 2, Philadelphia, 1999, WB Saunders.

Vanderhoof J and others: Short bowel syndrome, *J Pediatr Gastroenterol Nutr* 14(4):359-370, 1992.

West KW, Grosfeld JL: Intussusception in infants and children. In Wyllie R, Hyams JS, editors: *Pediatric gastrointestinal disease: physiology, diagnosis, management*, ed 2, Philadelphia, 1999, WB Saunders.

Woods DJ, McClintock AD: Omeprazole administration, *Ann Pharmacother* 27(5):651, 1993.

Zeiter DK, Hyams JS: Gastroesophageal reflux: pathogenesis, diagnosis and treatment, *Allergy Asthma Proc* 20(1):45-49, 1999.

# Chapter 34

# The Child with Cardiovascular Dysfunction

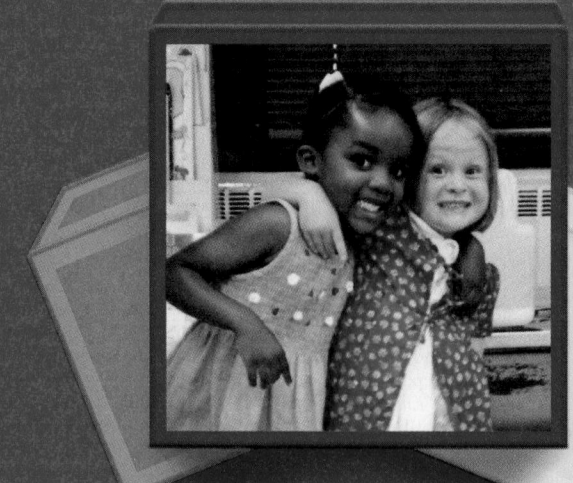

## Chapter Outline

**CARDIAC STRUCTURE AND FUNCTION, 1465**
**Cardiac Development and Function, 1465**
Embryologic Development, 1465
Postnatal Development, 1466
Basic Cardiac Physiology, 1468
**Assessment of Cardiac Function, 1468**
History, 1468
Physical Examination, 1469
**Tests of Cardiac Function, 1469**
Radiography, 1469
Electrocardiography, 1469
Echocardiography, 1471
Cardiac Catheterization, 1471
**CONGENITAL HEART DISEASE (CHD), 1474**
**Altered Hemodynamics, 1474**
**Classification and Clinical Consequences, 1475**
**Congestive Heart Failure (CHF), 1476**
*Nursing Care Plan: The Child with Congestive Heart Failure, 1485*
**Hypoxemia, 1484**
Altered Hemodynamics, 1484

Pulmonary Artery Hypertension, 1490
**Defects with Increased Pulmonary Blood Flow, 1491**
Atrial Septal Defect (ASD), 1492
Ventricular Septal Defect (VSD), 1493
Atrioventricular Canal (AVC) Defect, 1493
Patent Ductus Arteriosus (PDA), 1494
**Obstructive Defects, 1491**
Coarctation of the Aorta (COA), 1494
Aortic Stenosis (AS), 1495
Pulmonic Stenosis (PS), 1496
**Defects with Decreased Pulmonary Blood Flow, 1496**
Tetralogy of Fallot (TOF), 1497
Tricuspid Atresia, 1497
**Mixed Defects, 1498**
Transposition of the Great Arteries (TGA) or Transposition of the Great Vessels (TGV), 1499
Total Anomalous Pulmonary Venous Connection (TAPVC), 1499
Truncus Arteriosus (TA), 1500
Hypoplastic Left Heart Syndrome (HLHS), 1501

**Nursing Care of the Family and Child with Congenital Heart Disease, 1498**
Help Family Adjust to the Disorder, 1498
Educate Family About the Disorder, 1502
Help Family Cope with Effects of the Disorder, 1502
Prepare Child and Family for Surgery, 1503
Provide Postoperative Care, 1504
Provide Emotional Support, 1508
Plan for Discharge and Home Care, 1509
**ACQUIRED CARDIOVASCULAR DISORDERS, 1509**
**Bacterial (Infective) Endocarditis (BE), 1509**
**Rheumatic Fever (RF), 1511**
**Kawasaki Disease (KD) (Mucocutaneous Lymph Node Syndrome), 1514**
**Systemic Hypertension, 1516**
**Hyperlipidemia (Hypercholesterolemia), 1519**
**Cardiomyopathy, 1522**
**Cardiac Dysrhythmias, 1523**
**HEART TRANSPLANTATION, 1526**

## Related Topics

Birth of a Child with a Physical Defect, Ch. 11
Compliance, Ch. 27
Controlling Elevated Temperatures, Ch. 27
Family-Centered Care of the Child with Chronic Illness or Disability, Ch. 22
Family-Centered Care of the Child with Life-Threatening Illness/Unexpected Death, Ch. 23

Heart (Physical Assessment), Ch. 7
High Risk Related to Cardiovascular/Hematologic Complications, Ch. 10
Neonatal Loss, Ch. 10
Neonatal Pain, Ch. 10
Nursing Care of the Surgical Neonate, Ch. 11
Pain Assessment; Pain Management, Ch. 26

Physiologic Measurements, Ch. 7
Preparation for Procedures, Ch. 27
Skin (Physical Assessment), Ch. 7
Surgical Procedures, Ch. 27
Tissue Donation/Autopsy, Ch. 23
Transplantation, Ch. 30
Vulnerable Child Syndrome, p. 424

# CARDIAC STRUCTURE AND FUNCTION

Cardiovascular disorders in children are divided into two major groups: congenital cardiac defects and acquired heart disorders. ***Congenital heart defects*** are anatomic abnormalities present at birth that result in abnormal cardiac function. The clinical consequences of congenital heart defects fall into two broad categories: congestive heart failure and hypoxemia. ***Acquired cardiac disorders*** refer to disease processes or abnormalities that occur after birth and can be seen in the normal heart or in the presence of congenital heart defects. They result from various factors, including infection, autoimmune responses, environmental factors, and familial tendencies.

Understanding the effects of congenital and acquired heart defects requires knowledge of the normal heart's structure and function, including embryologic development, fetal circulation, and the changes that occur with postnatal growth. Basic cardiac physiology is presented in this section; altered hemodynamics are discussed on p. 1474.

## Cardiac Development and Function

The heart is a muscular four-chambered organ whose primary purpose is to pump blood throughout the body. It is located slightly to the left of the sternum in the space between the two pleural cavities, called the ***mediastinum.*** The main mass of the heart is formed by the muscular tissue, the ***myocardium.*** Lining the inner surface of the myocardium is the ***endocardium,*** a thin layer of endothelial tissue. The heart also has its own special covering, a double-walled membrane called the ***pericardium.*** Between the two layers is a slight space ***(pericardial space),*** which is filled with a few drops of serous fluid ***(pericardial fluid).*** These layers provide for frictionless movement of the heart muscle.

The interior of the heart is divided into four chambers. The two upper chambers are called ***atria;*** the two bottom chambers are ***ventricles.*** The atria are divided into the right atrium (RA) and the left atrium (LA) by the atrial septum. The ventricles are divided into the right ventricle (RV) and the left ventricle (LV) by the ventricular septum. Located within the heart are four ***valves,*** whose main function is to prevent the backflow of blood. The ***tricuspid valve,*** so named because it has three leaflets, or cusps, of endocardial tissue projecting into the ventricles, is located between the RA and the RV. The ***mitral valve*** has two leaflets and is located between the LA and the LV. Together these two valves are often termed ***atrioventricular (AV) valves.*** The valve leaflets are attached to the heart muscle by several cordlike structures called ***chordae tendineae.*** The ***semilunar valves*** are located in the pulmonary artery ***(pulmonic valve)*** and the aorta ***(aortic valve).*** Heart sounds ($S_1$ and $S_2$) are related to the vibrations that result during closing of these valves. (See Chapter 7.)

### Embryologic Development

The heart and other components of the circulatory system (blood, blood vessels, lymph) begin to develop from the mesoderm during the fourth week of gestation and are completed by the eighth week. Cardiac development parallels the embryo's increasing nutritional needs.

During the third week, two endocardial tubes fuse to become the heart tube. As the tube elongates, it begins to coil to the right (dextro or D-looping). This looping occurs by approximately the twenty-eighth day, when the heart begins to beat. Concentrations of mesenchymal cells enlarge and cause their lining (endocardium) to bulge into the heart lumen. These internal bulges are called ***endocardial cushions*** and eventually merge to divide the heart chambers.

The developing heart tube bulges until it finally lies in the pericardial cavity. The tube remains attached to the pericardium at its cephalic and caudal ends but is free at the midsection. During the fifth week the midcardiac tube grows rapidly and assumes a characteristic convoluted shape with identifiable structures. These structures ultimately give rise to the heart chambers and great vessels and include (1) a ***common atrium;*** (2) a ***common ventricle;*** (3) the ***bulbus cordis,*** which eventually helps form the outflow tracts of the ventricles; (4) the ***sinus venosus,*** which develops into the ***inferior*** and ***superior vena cava*** and ***coronary sinus;*** and (5) the ***truncus arteriosus,*** which divides into the pulmonary artery and aorta and also gives rise to the aortic arch.

The formation of the heart's internal structures, particularly the cardiac septa (partitions), takes place almost simultaneously. The ***atrial septum*** is formed by the growth of both the ***septum primum*** and the ***septum secundum*** at about the fourth week of fetal growth. Overlapping of the septum primum and septum secundum before fusion results in a temporary flap opening known as the ***foramen ovale.***

The ***ventricular septum*** develops from the joining of the muscular and membranous ventricular septa during the fourth to eighth weeks of growth. The ***muscular septum*** develops when the right and left ventricular chambers fuse, whereas the ***membranous septum*** develops out of an intricate growth of the endocardial cushions, conal cushions, and conotruncal septum (Fig. 34-1). During this partitioning

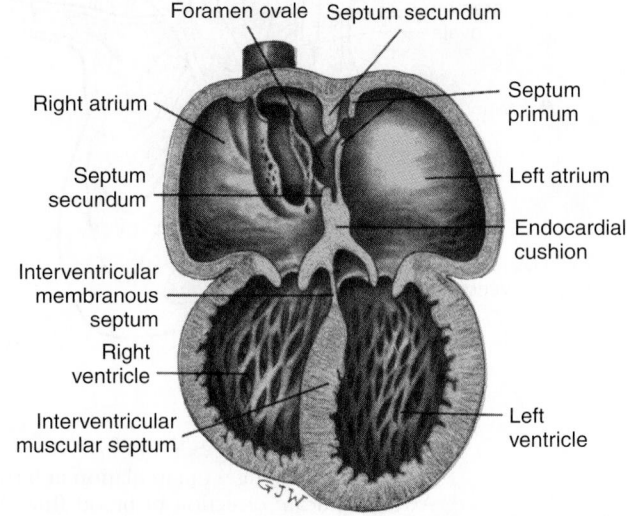

Foramen ovale   Septum secundum

Right atrium

Septum secundum

Interventricular membranous septum

Right ventricle

Interventricular muscular septum

Septum primum

Left atrium

Endocardial cushion

Left ventricle

**Fig. 34-1** Septal development of the heart.

■ Patricia O'Brien, MSN, RN, PNP, and Annette L. Baker, MSN, RN, revised this chapter.

process, congenital defects may result if the formation of various structures is disturbed.

**Fetal Circulation.** The characteristics of fetal circulation ensure that the most vital organs and tissues receive the maximum concentration of oxygenated blood. The fetal brain requires the highest oxygen concentration. The lungs are essentially nonfunctional, and the liver is only partially functional; therefore less blood is needed in these organs in fetal life.

Blood carrying oxygen and nutritive materials from the placenta enters the fetal system through the umbilicus via the large umbilical vein (Fig. 34-2, *A*). The blood then travels to the liver, where it divides; part of the blood enters the portal and hepatic circulation of the liver, and the remainder travels directly to the inferior vena cava (IVC) by way of the *ductus venosus.* Because of the higher pressure of blood entering the RA from the IVC, it is directed posteriorly in a straight pathway across the RA and through the foramen ovale to the LA. In this way the better-oxygenated blood enters the LA and LV to be pumped through the aorta to the head and upper extremities. Blood from the head and upper extremities entering the RA from the superior vena cava (SVC) is directed downward through the tricuspid valve into the RV. From there it is pumped through the pulmonary artery, where the major portion is shunted to the descending aorta via the *ductus arteriosus.* A small amount flows to and from the nonfunctioning fetal lungs. Blood is returned to the placenta from the descending aorta through the two umbilical arteries.

Before birth, the high pulmonary vascular resistance created by the collapsed fetal lung causes greater pressures in the right side of the heart and the pulmonary artery. At the same time, the free-flowing placental circulation and the ductus arteriosus produce a low systemic vascular resistance in the remainder of the fetal vascular system. With the clamping of the umbilical cord and the expansion of the lungs at birth, the hemodynamics of the fetal vascular system undergo pronounced and abrupt changes. These changes are the direct result of cessation of the placental blood flow and the beginning of lung respiration. The changes occurring at birth are discussed in Chapter 8, and the circulatory changes in the heart are shown in Fig. 34-2, *B.*

## Postnatal Development

In infancy the size of the heart in relation to total body size is larger, and the heart occupies a larger space within the mediastinum. The ventricle walls are more or less equal in thickness at birth. With a postnatal rise in systemic vascular resistance, the LV walls become thicker than the walls of the RV and the pressures on the left side of the heart rise.

Right-sided pressures decrease because the RV is pumping blood to the low-pressure pulmonary bed. An increase in heart size accompanies the adolescent growth spurt, with a resulting increase in blood pressure (BP) and decrease in heart rate. The heart rate at any age shows an inverse relationship to body size. (See inside back cover.)

The arteries and veins elongate to keep pace with expanding body dimensions, and the vessel walls thicken to cope with the increased pressure. The systolic BP after birth is low, reflecting the weaker LV of the neonate. With the developing strength and power of the left side of the heart, the

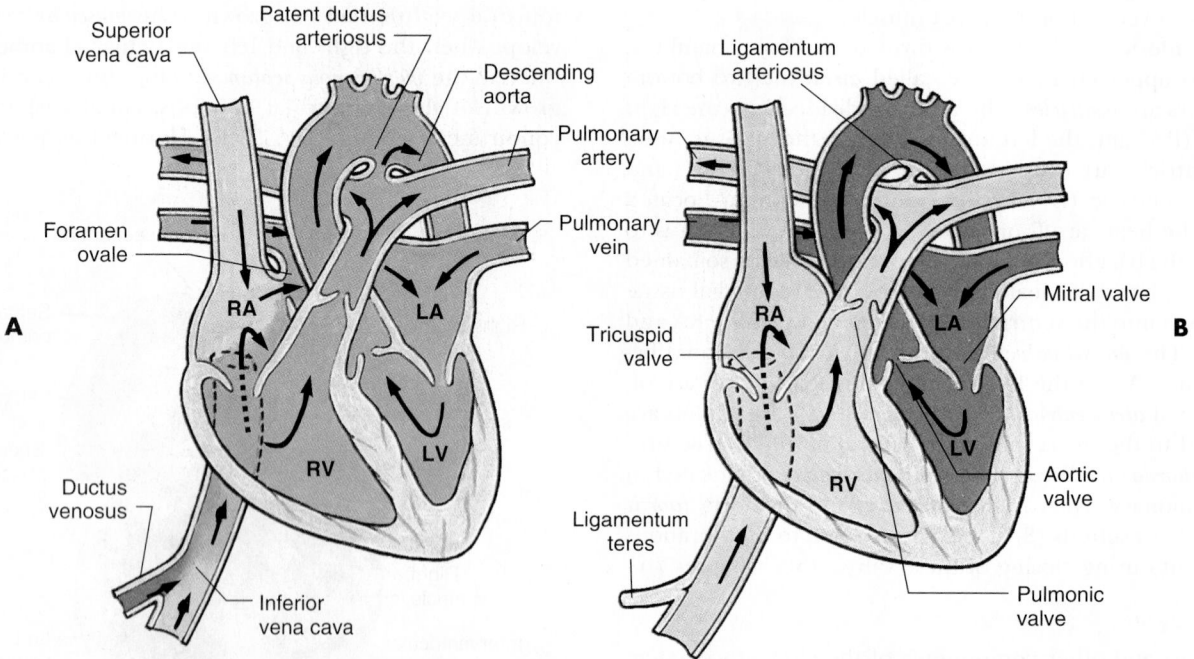

**Fig. 34-2** Changes in circulation at birth. **A,** Prenatal circulation. **B,** Postnatal circulation. Arrows indicate direction of blood flow. Although four pulmonary veins enter the LA, for simplicity this diagram shows only two. *RA,* Right atrium; *LA,* left atrium; *RV,* right ventricle; *LV,* left ventricle.

systolic pressure rises rather sharply during the first 6 weeks and continues to rise but at a much slower rate until shortly before puberty, at which point it rises rapidly to adult levels. (See inside back cover.)

**Postnatal Circulation.** Once the cardiorespiratory system adjusts to the changes necessary to support extrauterine life, the circulation through the heart assumes a pathway that allows for oxygenation of blood by the lungs and delivery of oxygenated blood to the systemic circulation. Blood returning from the body via the SVC and IVC is received in the RA. It flows to the RV through the tricuspid valve. The RV pumps the blood through the pulmonic valve into the pulmonary artery and then to the lungs, where the blood becomes saturated with oxygen. The blood is then returned from the lungs via the pulmonary veins into the LA, where it flows through the mitral valve to the LV, and finally through the aortic valve to the aorta and into the systemic circulation (see Fig. 34-2, *B*).

Arteries are thicker-walled blood vessels with thin muscular layers that carry highly oxygenated blood away from the heart to the capillary bed, which supplies oxygen and nutrients to the tissues. Veins are thin-walled blood vessels that return desaturated blood to the heart. The arterial system provides resistance to blood flow to maintain BP and circulation. The venous system acts as a collecting system and a reservoir to accommodate changes in circulating blood volume. Both work together to provide equilibrium and maintain BP.

The heart muscle receives its blood supply through the coronary circulation. The right and left *coronary arteries,* which arise above the aortic valve, supply all of the myocardium. The heart is the first organ to receive blood with each heartbeat; the brain is next. These two organs depend most on adequate oxygen levels for normal function. *Coronary veins* collect the blood and return it directly to the RA or through the coronary sinus, which drains into the RA.

**Conduction System.** To maintain an orderly and effective pumping action, the heart has a specialized electrical conduction system—electrical impulses generated within the heart initiate the mechanical contraction leading to the circulation of blood. Although all myocardial cells are capable of developing an action potential and depolarizing without external stimulation, certain specialized cells make up the heart's normal conduction system. These structures include the following (Fig. 34-3):

> **Sinoatrial (SA) node,** located within the RA wall near the opening of the SVC
>
> **Atrioventricular (AV) node,** also located within the RA but near the lower end of the septum
>
> **Atrioventricular bundle (bundle of His),** which extends from the AV node along each side of the interventricular septum and then divides into right and left bundle branches
>
> **Purkinje fibers,** which extend from the AV bundle into the walls of the ventricles

The SA node is normally the heart's pacemaker and initiates an impulse. The impulse spreads from the SA node throughout the atria to cause depolarization. As the atria depolarize, impulses spread to the AV node to conduct to the ventricles. The AV node is the major pathway by which the impulses from the atria can be transmitted to the ventricles. The impulses then spread to the AV bundle and Purkinje fibers to cause simultaneous depolarization of the ventricles.

A *cardiac cycle* is composed of sequential contraction *(systole)* and relaxation *(diastole)* of both the atria and the ventricles. First the atria contract, ejecting blood into the relaxed ventricles. Then, as the atria relax, the ventricles contract to eject blood into the pulmonary artery and aorta. During diastole, blood enters the atria from the systemic and pulmonary veins, thus completing one cardiac cycle.

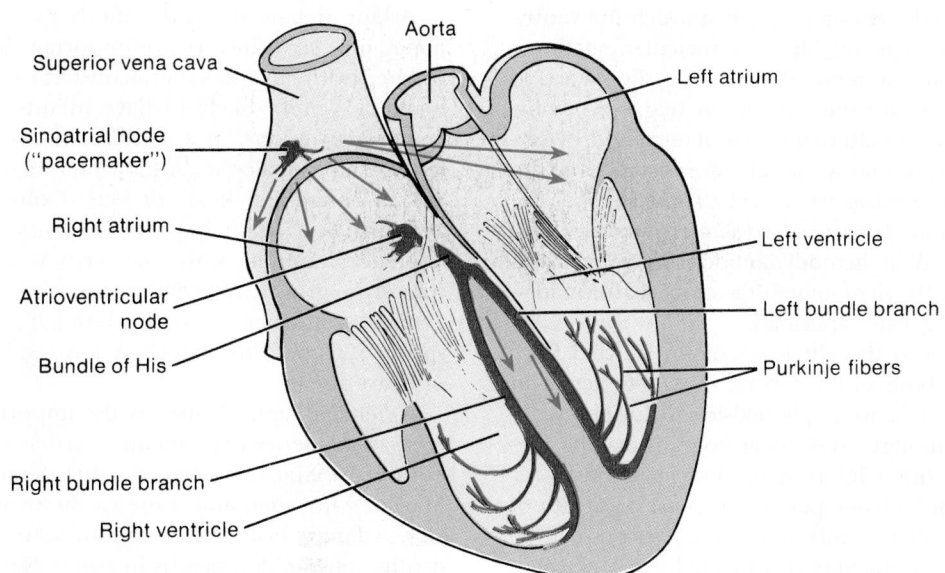

**Fig. 34-3** Conduction system of the heart.

## Basic Cardiac Physiology

The heart is basically a complex pump, ejecting blood throughout the body. The heart and lungs function together to deliver oxygen to the tissues and remove waste products such as carbon dioxide. The primary function of the cardiopulmonary system is to provide effective oxygen transport to meet the body's metabolic needs. To perform this function, the heart must maintain an adequate cardiac output. By definition, *cardiac output* is the volume of blood ejected by the heart in 1 minute. It is derived by multiplying the heart rate (HR) (number of beats per minute) by the stroke volume. *Stroke volume* is the amount of blood ejected by the heart in any one contraction. Stroke volume is influenced by three factors: preload, afterload, and contractility.

$$\text{Cardiac output} = \text{HR} \times \text{Stroke volume}$$
$$\uparrow$$
$$\text{Preload}$$
$$\text{Afterload}$$
$$\text{Contractility}$$

HR is influenced by the autonomic nervous system. The sympathetic fibers increase HR, and the parasympathetic fibers, acting through the vagus nerve, decrease HR. Levels of circulating catecholamines and other hormones also influence HR. Generally an increase in HR will increase cardiac output, and a decrease or irregularity in HR (bradycardia, dysrhythmia) will impair cardiac output. However, a very fast HR shortens diastole and impairs coronary artery perfusion, causing eventual impairment of cardiac muscle function.

In simple terms, *preload* is the volume of blood returning to the heart, or the circulating blood volume. In physiologic terms, preload refers to myocardial fiber length. If the amount of blood delivered to the heart increases, then the myocardial fibers lengthen, and a greater amount of blood is pumped out of the heart. The circulating blood volume is most easily assessed clinically using the central venous pressure.

*Afterload* refers to the resistance against which the ventricles must pump when ejecting blood (ventricular ejection). Conditions that make it more difficult for the heart to pump blood forward into the circulation (e.g., severe hypertension) increase the afterload. It is determined by several complex factors, primarily the relative resistances of the systemic circulation *(systemic vascular resistance)* and the pulmonary circulation *(pulmonary vascular resistance)*. Clinically, without the aid of hemodynamic monitoring, measurement of arterial BP gives some indication of afterload—higher BP indicates greater afterload.

*Contractility* refers to the efficiency of myocardial fiber shortening, or the ability of the cardiac muscle to act as an efficient pump. There is no simple bedside technique to assess contractility, although an echocardiogram may be useful. Contractility is often inferred in clinical practice. Assessments of peripheral tissue perfusion (pulses, warmth of extremities, and capillary refill) and urinary output can be helpful. Decreased contractility is suspected if the extremities are cool with thready pulses and urinary output is diminished. Certain states are known to depress contractility

(e.g., hypoxia, acidosis). It is often decreased following cardiac surgery in the early postoperative period.

Adequate systemic perfusion depends on an appropriate HR, adequate circulating blood volume, efficient pump function, appropriate systemic and pulmonary vascular resistances, capillary permeability, and tissue utilization of oxygen. The body makes frequent adjustments in the various determinants of cardiac output to maintain a steady state.

Several clinical examples are useful to illustrate these principles. The **Starling law (Frank-Starling curve)** demonstrates that an increase in ventricular end-diastolic volume (caused by an increased preload) somewhat increases stroke volume. Because the myocardial fibers can stretch only to a certain point and still function effectively, any increase in volume beyond this point impairs cardiac output. When decreased cardiac output results from decreased preload (e.g., in hypovolemia due to blood loss), treatment involves providing volume, either with intravenous (IV) fluids or blood products. If decreased cardiac output results from a dramatic increase in afterload (e.g., severe hypertension) that increases the myocardial workload, treatment involves reducing afterload with vasodilating drugs. Contractility can be enhanced by medications such as digoxin or IV inotropic medications such as dopamine or dobutamine. Adjustments in HR are the most common response to changes in cardiac output; HR is slowest during sleep and can more than double with strenuous physical exercise.

## Assessment of Cardiac Function

### History

Taking an accurate health history is an important first step in assessing an infant or child for possible heart disease. Parents may have specific concerns such as poor feeding or fast breathing in their infant or that their 7-year-old can no longer keep up with his friends on the soccer field. Others may not realize that their child has a medical problem; their child has always been pale and a fussy baby.

Asking details about the mother's health history, pregnancy, and birth history are important in assessing infants. Mothers with chronic health conditions, such as diabetes or lupus, are more likely to have infants with heart disease. Some medications, such as dilantin, are teratogenic to the fetus. Maternal alcohol use or illicit drug use increases the risk of congenital heart defects. Exposures to infections, such as rubella, early in pregnancy may result in congenital anomalies. Infants with low birth weight because of intrauterine growth retardation are more likely to have congenital anomalies. High–birth-weight infants, often offspring of diabetic mothers, also have an increased incidence of heart disease.

A detailed family history is also important. There is an increased incidence of congenital cardiac defects if either parent or a sibling has a heart defect. Some diseases, such as Marfan syndrome, and some cardiomyopathies are hereditary. A family history of frequent fetal loss, sudden infant deaths, and sudden deaths in adults may indicate heart disease. Congenital heart defects are seen in many syndromes such as Down syndrome and Turner syndrome.

The health history of an infant should elicit details about feeding patterns, weight gain, and development. Feeding difficulties with fatigue, rapid breathing, and sweating with feeds and poor weight gain are common in infants with heart disease. The incidence of respiratory infections and breathing problems should be discussed. The onset and frequency of color changes, particularly cyanosis, should be reported.

With older children and adolescents a history should include questions about exercise tolerance and activities, presence of edema and respiratory problems, chest pain, palpitations, and neurologic problems such as fainting or headaches. Recent infections or toxic exposures may precede heart diseases, such as cardiomyopathy or rheumatic fever.

In all patients a review of all other health problems and the presence of other congenital anomalies is important. All medications, including over-the-counter medications and herbal supplements, should be reviewed because prolonged or incorrect use of many medications can cause cardiac symptoms.

## Physical Examination

Assessment of vital signs is helpful in screening patients for diseases of the cardiovascular system. An abnormally fast heart rate *(tachycardia)* or slow heart rate *(bradycardia)* may indicate cardiac disease. A fast respiratory rate *(tachypnea)* may indicate congestive heart failure. Hypertension is diagnosed by serial BP measurements. Differences in BP between the upper and lower extremities may indicate coarctation of the aorta (see Box 34-3).

> **NURSING ALERT**
>
> A systolic blood pressure value 8 to 10 mm Hg higher in the arm than in the leg should be considered a significant finding in terms of coarctation of the aorta (Park, Lee, and Johnson, 1993).

Several aspects of physical examination may yield evidence of heart disease. (See Chapter 7 for a general discussion of physical assessment of the heart.) During inspection a general examination of skin color (particularly the presence of cyanosis), position of comfort, and overall nutritional status is performed. During palpation the point of maximum intensity and the apical impulse should be established, because they may offer clues to the position of the heart. The presence of a thrill, a soft vibration over the heart that reflects the transmitted sound of a heart murmur, should be noted. The quality of chest activity ("active precordium"), quality and symmetry of all pulses, warmth of extremities, and presence or absence of edema are assessed. Locating the hepatic and splenic borders for evidence of organ enlargement is also important.

Auscultation of heart sounds begins with assessment of heart rate and rhythm. The normal heart sounds $S_1$ and $S_2$ are auscultated, and the normal physiologic splitting of $S_2$ is noted. The presence of additional heart sounds, such as a gallop or a murmur, is noted. Auscultation of lung sounds, in particular noting the presence of crackles, wheezing, grunting, or decreased or absent breath sounds

in some areas, is also important in the assessment of cardiovascular disease.

Murmurs are heart sounds that reflect the flow of blood within the heart. They may occur in systole or diastole or occur in both (a continuous murmur). They may reflect blood flow through a normal heart (particularly in periods of increased cardiac output such as fever, anemia, or rapid growth) or reflect abnormalities within the heart or the great arteries. (See Chapter 7 for a more detailed discussion of heart murmurs.) About 50% of children have an innocent murmur at some point (Allen and others, 1994). Innocent murmurs are present in infants and children with normal cardiac anatomy and heart function.

## Tests of Cardiac Function

A variety of invasive and noninvasive tests may be employed in the diagnosis of heart disease. Table 34-1 briefly outlines cardiac diagnostic procedures. The more frequently conducted tests are described here.

### Radiography

A chest x-ray examination is the most frequently ordered radiographic test for children with suspected cardiac problems. A chest film provides a permanent record of (1) the heart's size and configuration, its chambers, and the great vessels; and (2) the pattern of blood flow, especially in the pulmonary vessels. Fluoroscopy is used mainly in conjunction with cardiac catheterization.

### Electrocardiography

An electrocardiogram (ECG) measures the electrical activity of the heart and records it on graph paper. This allows the evaluation of the sequence and magnitude of the electrical impulses generated by the heart (Fig. 34-4). The normal ECG consists of the P wave, P-R interval, QRS complex, T wave, Q-T interval, and ST segment:

**P wave**—Represents the spread of the impulse over the atria (atrial depolarization). The sinus node's electrical activity is not represented in the ECG.

**P-R interval**—Represents the time that elapses from the beginning of atrial depolarization to the beginning of ventricular depolarization. It is termed P-R instead of P-Q because the Q wave is frequently absent.

**QRS complex**—Represents ventricular depolarization. It is actually composed of three separate waves—the Q, the R, and the S—that result from the currents generated when the ventricles depolarize before their contraction.

**T wave**—Represents ventricular repolarization.

**Q-T interval**—Represents ventricular depolarization and repolarization. This interval varies with heart rate—the faster the rate, the shorter the Q-T interval. Therefore in children this interval is normally shorter than in adults.

**ST segment**—Represents the time that the ventricles are in absolute refractory period, the period between ventricular depolarization and repolarization.

Information supplied by an ECG includes heart rate and rhythm, abnormalities of conduction, muscular damage (ischemia), hypertrophy, effects of electrolyte imbalance, the influence of various drugs, and pericardial disease. The

ECG gives no direct information about the mechanical performance of the heart as a pump.

Special uses of the ECG include (1) continuous ambulatory monitoring, which employs a *Holter monitor,* a transistorized tape recorder attached to chest leads, and (2) an *exercise stress test,* in which the ECG is monitored during controlled exercise, usually on a treadmill.

An ECG is taken by placing leads or electrodes on the skin to transmit electrical impulses back to a recording machine. Usually the electrodes are attached to the extremities

| TABLE 34-1 | Procedures for cardiac diagnosis |
|---|---|
| **Procedure** | **Description** |
| **Chest radiograph (x-ray)** | Provides information on heart size and pulmonary blood flow patterns |
| **Electrocardiography (ECG)** | Graphic measure of the electrical activity of the heart |
| Holter monitor | 24-hour continuous ECG recording used to assess dysrhythmias |
| **Echocardiography** | Use of high-frequency sound waves obtained by a transducer to produce an image of cardiac structures |
| Transthoracic | Done with transducer on chest |
| M-mode | One-dimensional graphic view used to estimate ventricular size and function |
| Two-dimensional (2-D) | Real-time, cross-sectional views of heart used to identify cardiac structures and cardiac anatomy |
| Doppler | Identifies blood flow patterns and pressure gradients across structures |
| Fetal | Imaging fetal heart in utero |
| Transesophageal (TEE) | Transducer placed in esophagus behind the heart to obtain images of posterior heart structures or in patients with poor images from chest approach |
| **Cardiac catheterization** | Imaging study using radiopaque catheters placed in a peripheral blood vessel and advanced into heart to measure pressures and oxygen levels in heart chambers and visualize heart structures and blood flow patterns |
| Hemodynamics | Measures pressures and oxygen saturations in heart chambers |
| Angiography | Use of contrast material to illuminate heart structures and blood flow patterns |
| Biopsy | Use of special catheter to remove tiny samples of heart muscle for microscopic evaluation; used in assessing infection, inflammation, or muscle dysfunction disorders; also to evaluate for rejection after heart transplant |
| Electrophysiology (EPS) | Speical catheters with electrodes employed to record electrical activity from within heart; used to diagnose rhythm disturbances |
| **Exercise stress test** | Monitoring of heart rate, blood pressure, electrocardiogram (ECG), and oxygen consumption at rest and during progressive exercise on a treadmill or bicycle |
| **Cardiac magnetic resonance imaging (MRI)** | Newest noninvasive imaging technique; used in evaluation of vascular anatomy outside of heart (i.e., coarctation of the aorta, vascular rings), estimates of ventricular mass and volume; uses for MRI are expanding |

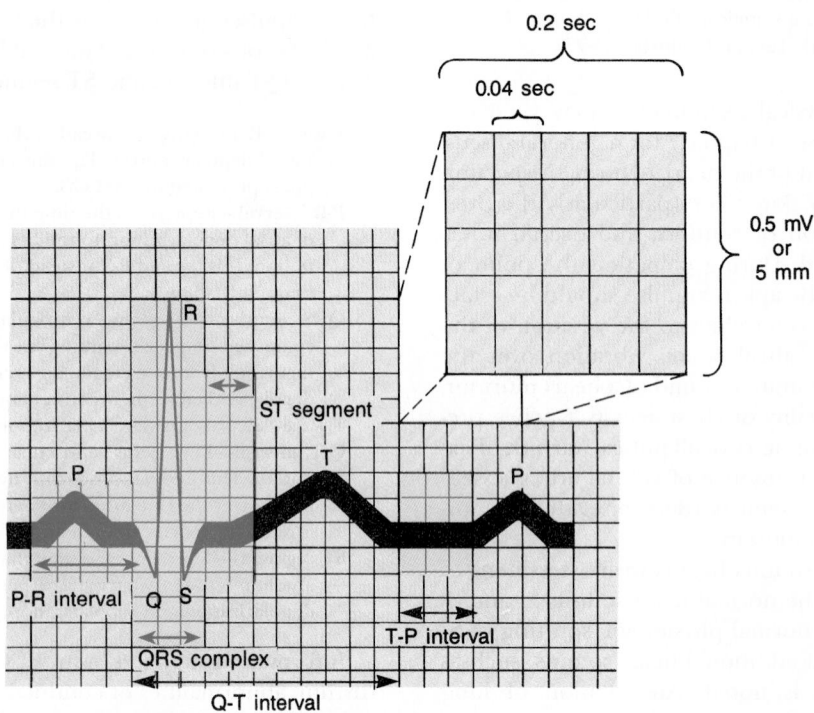

**Fig. 34-4** Normal electrocardiogram pattern. Inset (*upper right*) shows conventional time and voltage or amplitude (height) calibrations.

and chest with adhesive, such as hydrogel, or with a suction bulb. An electrolyte lubricant is placed between the skin and the lead to increase conductivity. Chest leads must be positioned correctly because even minor misplacement can cause considerable inaccuracy in the recording. The standard adult ECG has 12 leads (6 limb leads and 6 chest leads). The standard pediatric ECG has actually 15 leads with the addition of leads on the right side of the chest and on the left lateral chest area. Although all of these tests are painless, the leads can be frightening. Children old enough to understand can benefit from an explanation of the procedure. The child must remain still for the standard ECG; infants and young children may be more cooperative if they are held in the parent's lap during the procedure.

Bedside cardiac monitoring with the ECG is commonly used in pediatrics, especially in the care of children with heart disease. The bedside monitor provides valuable information about heart rate and rhythm through a graphic display of the ECG tracing and a digital display. An alarm can be set with parameters for individual patient requirements and will sound if the heart rate is above or below the set parameters. Gelfoam electrodes are commonly used and placed on the right side of the chest (above the level of the heart) and on the left side of the chest, and a ground electrode is placed on the abdomen (Fig. 34-5). Electrodes should be changed every 1 to 2 days because they are irritating to the skin. Bedside monitors are an adjunct to patient care and should never be substituted for direct assessment and auscultation of heart sounds. The nurse should assess the patient, not the monitor.

**NURSING TIP**  Electrodes for cardiac monitoring are often color coded: white for right, green (or red) for ground, and black for left. Always check to ensure that these colors are placed correctly.

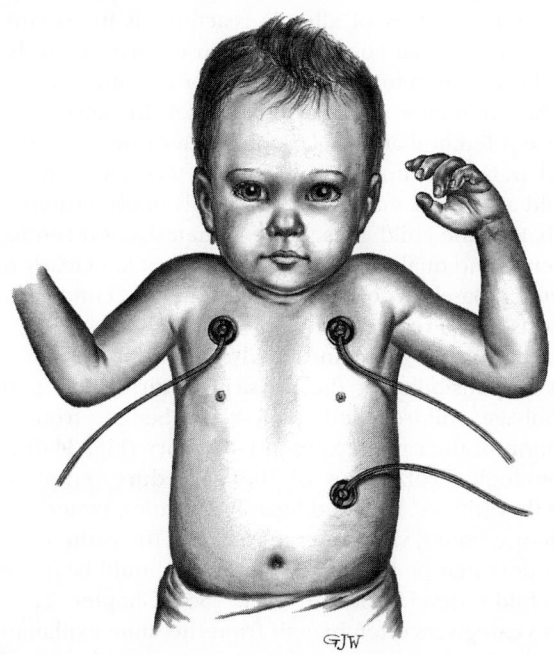

**Fig. 34-5**  Electrode placement for standard chest lead II in cardiac monitoring.

## Echocardiography

Echocardiography is one of the most frequently used tests for detecting cardiac dysfunction in children. Recent improvements in echocardiographic techniques have made it increasingly possible to confirm the diagnosis without resorting to cardiac catheterization. In increasing instances a prenatal diagnosis of congenital heart disease can be made by fetal echocardiography.

Echocardiography involves the use of ultra-high-frequency sound waves to produce an image of the heart's structure. A transducer placed directly on the chest wall delivers repetitive pulses of ultrasound and processes the returned signals (echoes).

There are two types of transthoracic echocardiograms. *Motion mode (M-mode)* provides a one-dimensional view of the heart and is useful in determining its size, the presence or absence of structures, and their relationship to one another. A *two-dimensional (2-D)*, or *cross-sectional*, echocardiogram provides information about spatial relationships between structures. A *pulse*, or *continuous Doppler*, echocardiogram is primarily a velocity-sensing system and is generally used with 2-D "echo" to provide information about volume flow rate. Depending on the type of test, information can be obtained regarding the integrity of septa; chamber size; position and contractility; presence, position, size, and function of the valves; velocity of blood flow; and relationship between, and size of, the great vessels.

Although the test is noninvasive, painless, and associated with no known side effects, it can be stressful for children. The child must lie quietly in the standard echocardiographic positions; crying, nursing, or sitting up often leads to diagnostic errors or omissions. Therefore infants and young children may need a mild sedative (see Preoperative Sedation, p. 1112); older children benefit from psychologic preparation for the test. The distraction of a videotape is often helpful.

*Transesophageal echocardiograms (TEEs)* can provide information in cases where it is difficult to obtain information using the transthoracic approach. A transducer is passed into the esophagus to an area behind the atria. This procedure is more complicated and may require intubation to protect the airway of smaller children. Patients require IV sedation before this test. TEE is frequently used in the operating room to assess for residual problems before coming off cardiopulmonary bypass. Underleider and others (1995) reported that less than 10% of patients underwent revision of the surgical repair based on TEE findings and a decrease in length of stay and hospital costs were seen using intraoperative TEE.

## Cardiac Catheterization

The most invasive diagnostic procedure is cardiac catheterization, in which a radiopaque catheter is inserted through a peripheral blood vessel into the heart. It is usually combined with angiography (angiocardiography), in which a radiopaque contrast material is injected through the catheter and into the circulation. Cardiac catheterization provides information regarding:

- *Oxygen saturation* of blood within the chambers and great vessels
- *Pressure changes* within these structures

- *Cardiac output* or *stroke volume* (the amount of blood pumped out of the LV into the aorta with each contraction)
- *Anatomic abnormalities,* such as septal defects or obstruction to flow

Cardiac catheterization may be for diagnostic, interventional, or electrophysiologic purposes. The two main types of *diagnostic cardiac catheterizations* are (1) *right-sided,* or *venous, catheterization,* in which the catheter is introduced from a vein into the RA, and (2) *left-sided,* or *arterial, catheterization,* in which the catheter is threaded by way of a systemic artery retrograde into the aorta and LV, or from a right-sided approach to the LA by means of a septal puncture or through an existing abnormal septal opening. In children the most common method is a right-sided catheterization, because septal defects permit entry into the left side of the heart.

The catheter is usually introduced through a percutaneous puncture into the femoral vein (the catheter is threaded over a guide wire inserted through a large-bore needle). Rarely, a cutdown procedure is needed to gain access to the vein, but this approach is associated with an increased risk of infection, hemorrhage, and obstruction. Once the vessel is entered, the catheter is guided through the heart with the aid of fluoroscopy. As the tubing is advanced, the child may feel pressure at the insertion site and vasospasm (fluttering) of the small vessels. Once the catheter is within the heart, blood samples and pressure readings are taken for analysis. Then the contrast material may be injected, and films are taken of the dilution and circulation of the material. As the contrast medium is administered, the child may experience warmth, nausea, vomiting, restlessness, or headache.

*Interventional cardiac catheterization* has become an alternative to surgery in some congenital heart defects, such as isolated valvular pulmonic stenosis and patent ductus arteriosus (Table 34-2).

Electrophysiologic studies are increasingly being used to evaluate and treat dysrhythmias. *Diagnostic electrophysiologic catheterizations* employ catheters with tiny electrodes that record the heart's electrical impulses directly from the conduction system. *Interventional electrophysiologic catheterizations* use radiofrequency ablation to destroy accessory pathways, which cause some tachydysrhythmias.

**Nursing Considerations.** Cardiac catheterization has become a routine diagnostic procedure and may be done on an outpatient basis. Catheterization is not, however, without risks, especially in neonates and seriously ill infants and children. Typical reactions include acute hemorrhage from the entry site (more likely with interventional procedures because larger catheters are used), low-grade fever, nausea, vomiting, loss of a pulse in the catheterized extremity (usually transient, resulting from a clot, hematoma, or intimal tear), and transient dysrhythmias (generally catheter induced). In a large review of pediatric cardiac catheterizations, the incidence of vascular complications was 3.5% and mortality related to the procedure was 0.12% (Vitiello and others, 1998). Therefore it is essential that the nurse employ good nursing judgment and physical assessment before and after the procedure.

**TABLE 34-2** Current interventional cardiac catheterization procedures in children

| Intervention | Diagnosis |
|---|---|
| Balloon atriaseptostomy (BAS)<br>  Well-established in newborns<br>  May also be done under echo guidance | Transposition of the great arteries<br><br>Some complex single-ventricle defects |
| Balloon dilation<br>  Treatment of choice | Valvular pulmonic stenosis<br>Branch pulmonary artery stenosis<br>Congenital valvular aortic stenosis<br>Rheumatic mitral stenosis<br>Recurrent coarctation of the aorta<br>Further follow-up required in:<br>  Native coarctation of the aorta in patients >7 months<br>  Congenital mitral stenosis |
| Coil occlusion<br>  Accepted alternative to surgery | Patent ductus arteriosus (<4 mm) |
| Transcatheter device closure<br>  Several devices in clinical trials | Atrial septal defect |
| Stent placement | Pulmonary artery stenosis<br>Other lesions investigational |
| Radiofrequency ablation | Some tachydysrhythmias |

Data from Allen HD and others: Pediatric therapeutic cardiac catheterization, AHA scientific statement, *Circulation* 97:609-625, 1998.

**Preprocedural Care.** A complete nursing assessment is necessary to ensure a safe procedure with a minimum of complications. This assessment should include an accurate height (essential to correct catheter selection) and weight. Obtaining a history of allergic reactions is important, because some of the contrast agents used are iodine based. Specific attention to signs and symptoms of infection is crucial. Severe diaper rash may be a reason to cancel the procedure if femoral access is required. Because assessment of pedal pulses is important after catheterization, the nurse should assess and mark pulses (dorsalis pedis, posterior tibial) before the child goes to the catheterization room. The presence and quality of pulses in both feet are clearly documented. Baseline oxygen saturation in children with cyanosis is also recorded.

Preparing the child and family for the procedure is the joint responsibility of the physician, nurse, and parents. School-age children and adolescents benefit from a description of the catheterization laboratory (Fig. 34-6) and a chronologic explanation of the procedure, emphasizing what they will see, feel, and hear. Preparation materials such as picture books, videotapes, or tours of the catheterization laboratory may be helpful. Preparation should be geared to the child's developmental level. (See Chapter 27.) The child's caregivers often benefit from the same explanations. Additional information, such as the expected length of the catheterization, description of the child's appearance after

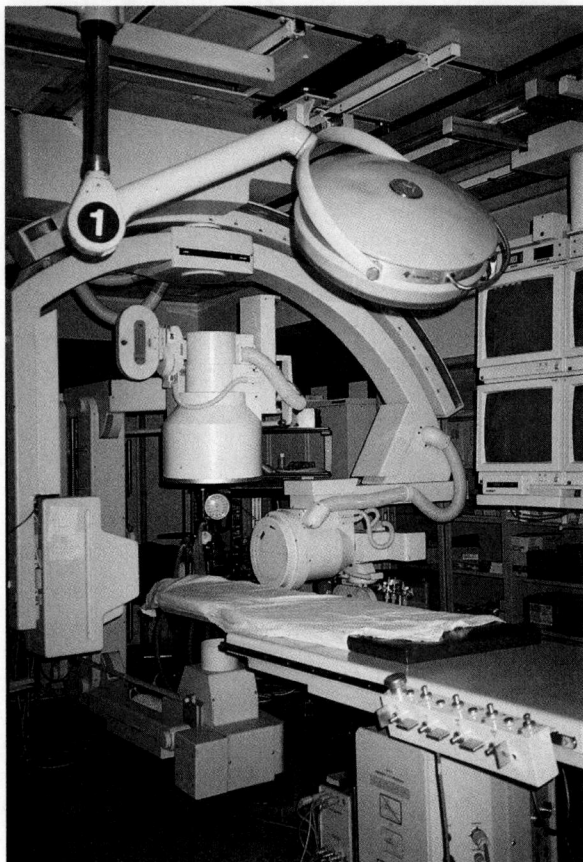

**Fig. 34-6** Cardiac catheterization laboratory.

## Critical Thinking Exercise

### Cardiac Catheterization

Tommy, a 4-year-old with tetralogy of Fallot, has just returned from the catheterization laboratory. He has vomited, and his mother calls you to the bedside to tell you that he is bleeding. You arrive to find Tommy crying and sitting up in a puddle of blood. What is the first thing you should do?

FIRST, THINK ABOUT IT . . .
- What concepts are central to your thinking?
- What are the implications?

1. Increase the rate of his IV fluids.
2. Give an antiemetic and keep Tommy NPO (nothing by mouth).
3. Call the cardiologist.
4. Lie Tommy down, remove the dressing, and apply direct pressure above the catheterization site.

*The best response is four. This may be an arterial bleed, and the implications are that Tommy is at risk for losing a large amount of blood in a short time. Your first priority should be to control the bleeding. Pressure is applied above the visible catheterization site where the vessel was entered. Placing the child flat decreases the effect of gravity on the rate of bleeding and is the appropriate position in case of shock. When this is done, you can notify the practitioner and replace fluids and control emesis as ordered.*

catheterization, and usual postprocedure care, should be outlined.

Methods of sedation vary among institutions and may include oral or intravenous medications. (See Preoperative Sedation, p. 1112.) General anesthesia is usually unnecessary except in selected interventional procedures. Unconscious sedation may be induced with ketamine or propofol (Diprivan). Typically the child is allowed nothing by mouth before catheterization, although polycythemic infants and children may require IV fluids to prevent dehydration, and neonates may need dextrose solution for up to 2 hours before the procedure to prevent hypoglycemia. Usually the morning dose of all oral medications is withheld, although this is clarified beforehand with the practitioner.

**Postprocedural Care.** Patients may recover from the catheterization procedure in a recovery unit or in their hospital room. Some may require care in the intensive care unit (ICU). Patients are usually placed on a cardiac monitor and a pulse oximeter for the first few hours following catheterization.

The most important nursing responsibility is observation of the following for signs of complications. (See Critical Thinking Exercise box.):

- Pulses, especially below the catheterization site, for equality and symmetry (pulse distal to the site may be weaker for the first few hours after catheterization but should gradually increase in strength)

- Temperature and color of the affected extremity, since coolness or blanching may indicate arterial obstruction
- Vital signs, which may be taken as frequently as every 15 minutes, with special emphasis on the heart rate, which is counted for 1 full minute for evidence of dysrhythmias or bradycardia
- BP, especially for hypotension, which may indicate hemorrhage from cardiac perforation or bleeding at the site of initial catheterization
- Dressing, for evidence of bleeding or hematoma formation in the femoral or antecubital area
- Fluid intake, both IV and oral, to ensure adequate hydration (Blood loss in the catheterization laboratory, the child's status of nothing by mouth [NPO], and diuretic actions of contrast material used during the procedure put children at risk for hypovolemia and dehydration.)

Infants are particularly at risk for hypoglycemia. They should receive dextrose-containing IV fluids, and blood glucose levels should be checked.

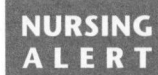

**NURSING ALERT** If bleeding occurs, direct continuous pressure is applied 2.5 cm (1 inch) *above* the percutaneous skin site to localize pressure over the vessel puncture.

Depending on hospital policy, the child may be kept in bed with the affected extremity maintained straight for 4 to 6 hours after venous catheterization and 6 to 8 hours after arterial catheterization to facilitate healing of the cannu-

## FAMILY HOME CARE
### Following Cardiac Catheterization

Remove pressure dressing the day after catheterization. Cover site with an adhesive bandage strip for several days.

Keep site clean and dry. Avoid tub baths for several days; may shower.

Observe site for redness, swelling, drainage, and bleeding. Monitor for fever. Notify practitioner if these occur.

Avoid strenuous exercise for several days. May attend school.

Resume regular diet without restrictions.

Use acetaminophen or ibuprofen for pain.

Keep follow-up appointments per practitioner's instruction.

Modified from Children's Hospital (Boston) Cardiovascular Program, 1994.

**TABLE 34-3** Prevalence of the most common congenital heart defects: data from the Baltimore-Washington Infant Heart Study, 1981-1989

| Defect | Prevalence per 10,000 live births |
|---|---|
| Ventricular septal defect | 15.6 |
| Pulmonary valve atresia/stenosis | 9 |
| Tricuspid atresia | 3.6 |
| AV septal defects | 3.3 |
| Transposition of the great arteries | 2.6 |
| Tetralogy of Fallot | 2.6 |
| Atrial septal defects | 2.3 |
| Hypoplastic left heart syndrome | 1.8 |
| Coarctation of the aorta | 1.4 |
| Patent ductus arteriosus | 0.8 |

Modified from Ferencz C and others, editors: *Epidemiology of congenital heart defects: the Baltimore-Washington Infant Heart Study 1981-1989*, Mt Kisco, NY, 1993, Futura.

lated vessel. If younger children have difficulty complying, they can be held in the parent's lap with the leg maintained in the correct position. The child's usual diet can be resumed as soon as tolerated, beginning with sips of clear liquids and advancing as the condition allows it. The child is encouraged to void to clear the contrast material from the blood. Generally there is only slight discomfort at the percutaneous site. Acetaminophen with or without codeine or ibuprophen can be given for pain. The catheterization site is covered with an occlusive waterproof pressure dressing (usually a foam tape dressing tightly applied) to prevent bleeding and contamination that could cause infection. The dressing is left on until the next day. Home care instructions are outlined in the Family Home Care box.

## CONGENITAL HEART DISEASE (CHD)

The incidence of congenital heart disease in children is approximately 5 to 8 per 1000 live births (Behrman, Kliegman, and Jenson, 2000). About 2 to 3 in 1000 infants will be symptomatic during the first year of life. CHD is the major cause of death (other than prematurity) in the first year of life. Although there are more than 35 well-recognized defects, the most common heart anomaly is ventricular septal defect (VSD) (Table 34-3).

The exact etiology of 90% of the congenital cardiac defects is unknown. Most are thought to be a result of multifactorial inheritance: a complex interaction of genetic and environmental factors. The tremendous amount of information being discovered in molecular biology and the human genome project will likely increase our understanding of the genetic etiologies of congenital heart defects.

Some risk factors are known to increase the incidence of congenital heart defects. Maternal factors include chronic illnesses such as diabetics or poorly controlled phenylketonuria (PKU), alcohol consumption, and exposure to environmental toxins and infections. Family history of a cardiac defect in a parent or sibling increases the likelihood of a cardiac anomaly. The risk of congenital heart disease increases if a first-degree relative (parent or sibling) is affected (Behrman, Kliegman, and Jenson, 2000). The familial risk is higher with left-sided obstructive lesions.

Congenital heart anomalies are often associated with chromosomal abnormalities, syndromes, or congenital defects in other body systems. In a large population-based epidemiologic study, 28% of children with cardiac defects had another anomaly (Ferencz and others, 1997). Down syndrome (trisomy 21) and trisomy 13 and 18 are highly correlated with congenital heart defects. Syndromes associated with heart defects include Noonan syndrome (pulmonary valve anomalies and cardiomyopathy), Williams syndrome (aortic and pulmonic stenosis), and Holt-Oram syndrome (upper limb anomalies and atrial septal defect [ASD]). Extracardiac defects such as tracheoesophageal fistula, renal abnormalities, and diaphragmatic hernia are seen.

Recent research in gene mapping has identified deletion of part of the 22 chromosome (22q11), which is present in the majority of patients with DiGeorge syndrome, velocardiofacial syndrome (VCFS), and conotruncal anomaly face syndrome. The features of these syndromes include congenital cardiac defects, soft palate abnormalities, dysmorphic facial features, and speech and developmental delays. Mild immunologic abnormalities of T-cells, absence or hypoplasia of the thymus, and parathyroid abnormalities resulting in hypocalcemia are seen with DiGeorge syndrome. Commonly associated cardiac defects are interrupted aortic arch, truncus arteriosus, tetralogy of Fallot, and posterior malaligned ventricular septal defects (Goldmuntz and others, 1998). There is a very variable clinical expression of this syndrome with some patients minimally affected and others having all characteristics.

## Altered Hemodynamics

To understand the physiology of heart defects, it is necessary to review the role of pressure gradients, flow, and resistance within the circulation. Blood flows because of pressure gradients in different parts of the body and because of the heart's pumping action. As with any fluid, blood flows from an area of high pressure to one of low pressure and takes the path of least resistance. The rate of flow is directly proportional to the pressure gradient (i.e., the higher the pressure gradient, the greater the rate of flow) and inversely proportional to the resistance (i.e., the higher the resistance, the less the rate of flow). However, increased resistance does not always decrease flow. If the proximal cardiac chamber can increase the driving pressure proportionately, flow can remain unchanged.

Normally the pressure on the right side of the heart is lower than that on the left side, and the resistance in the pulmonary circulation is less than that in the systemic circulation. Likewise, vessels entering or exiting from these chambers have corresponding pressures (e.g., lower pressure in the pulmonary artery and higher pressure in the aorta). Therefore, if an abnormal connection exists between the heart chambers, such as a septal defect, blood flows from an area of higher pressure (left side) to one of lower pressure (right side). This directional flow of blood is termed a *left-to-right shunt*. If the opening is small, the amount of blood shunted to the atrium or ventricle may be minimal.

An understanding of saturations within the heart is also helpful in understanding CHD. The blood returning to the heart via the great veins, the SVC and the IVC, should have the lowest oxygen saturation because the tissues should have extracted oxygen, leaving the venous blood desaturated. Saturations in the RA, RV, and pulmonary artery should be equal. Blood returning from the lungs to the heart through the pulmonary veins should be fully saturated, the most oxygen-rich blood in the body. Saturations on the left side of the heart should all be equal, with fully saturated blood entering the aorta and first supplying the heart muscle through the coronary arteries and then supplying the brain (Fig. 34-7). Normally, saturated blood circulates separately from desaturated blood. Depending on the type of defect, mixing of saturated and desaturated blood may occur. The amount of mixed blood that reaches the systemic circulation is a significant feature of several cardiac anomalies and results in varying degrees of hypoxemia and cyanosis.

## Classification and Clinical Consequences

Congenital heart defects have been classified into several categories. Traditionally a physical characteristic, cyanosis, has been used as the distinguishing feature, dividing the anomalies into *acyanotic* and *cyanotic defects.* In clinical practice this system is problematic because children with acyanotic defects may develop cyanosis. Also, more often, those with cyanotic defects may be pink and have more clinical signs of congestive heart failure (CHF). Because of the complexity of many defects and the variability of their clinical manifestations, the cyanotic-acyanotic classification system has proved to be inadequate and misleading.

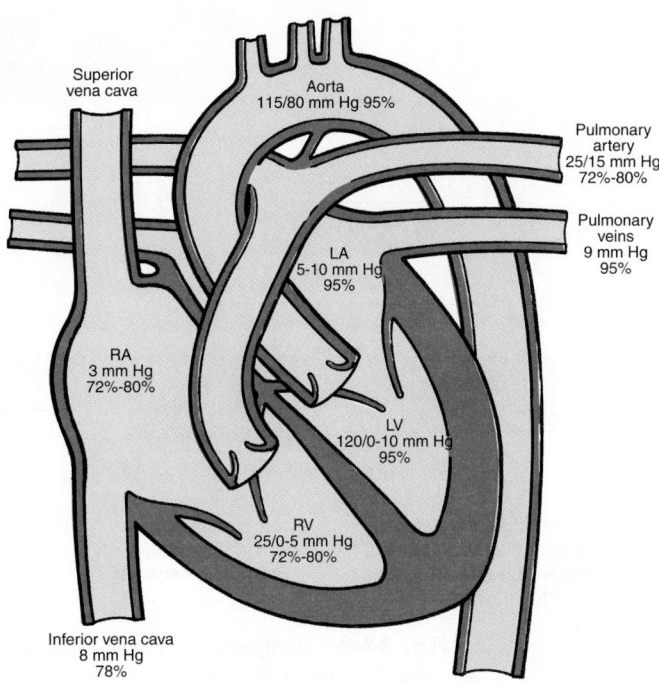

**Fig. 34-7**   Normal chamber pressures (mm Hg) and oxygen saturations (SaO₂) in cardiac chambers and great arteries. For simplicity, only two of the four pulmonary veins are shown. See Fig. 34-2 for abbreviations.

A more useful classification system is based on *hemodynamic characteristics,* or movements involved in circulation of blood. The defining characteristic is blood flow patterns: (1) increased pulmonary blood flow, (2) decreased pulmonary blood flow, (3) obstruction to blood flow out of the heart, and (4) mixed blood flow, in which saturated and desaturated blood mix within the heart or great arteries. Both classification systems are outlined in Fig. 34-8.

With the hemodynamic classification system, the clinical manifestations of each group are more uniform and predictable. Defects that allow blood flow from the high-pressure left side of the heart to the lower-pressure right side (left-to-right shunt) result in increased pulmonary blood flow and cause CHF. Obstructive defects impede blood flow out of the ventricles; obstruction on the left side of the heart results in CHF, whereas severe obstruction on the right side causes cyanosis. Defects that cause decreased pulmonary blood flow result in cyanosis. Mixed lesions present a variable clinical picture based on the degree of mixing and amount of pulmonary blood flow; hypoxemia (with or without cyanosis) and CHF usually occur together. (For more detailed explanations, see specific defects later in this chapter.)

Depending on the severity of the cardiac defect and the altered hemodynamics, two principal clinical consequences can occur: CHF and hypoxemia. The conditions can occur alone or together. Nursing care plays a critical role in the early identification and supportive management of these conditions.

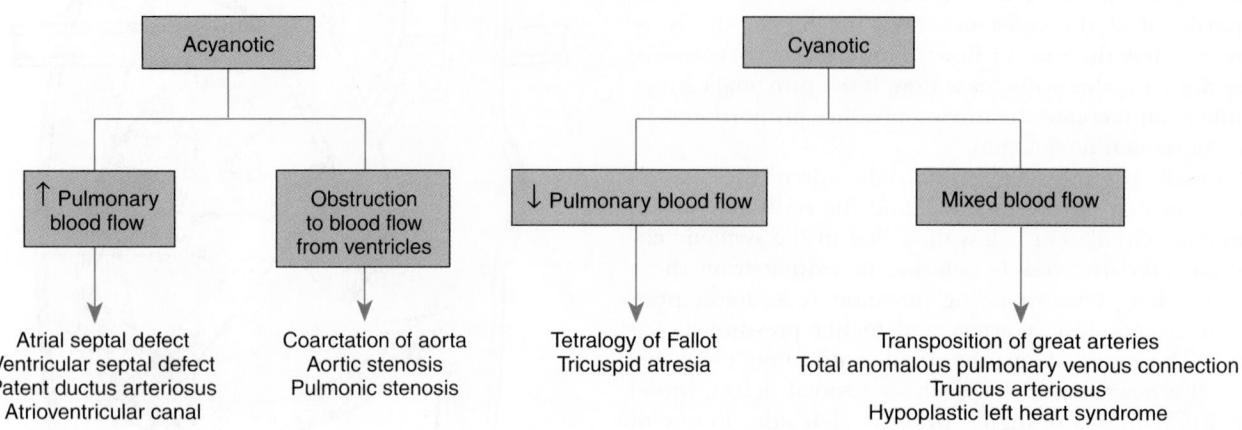

**Fig. 34-8** Comparison of acyanotic-cyanotic and hemodynamic classification systems of congenital heart disease.

# Congestive Heart Failure (CHF)

CHF is inability of the heart to pump an adequate amount of blood to the systemic circulation at normal filling pressures to meet the body's metabolic demands. Causes of CHF can be classified according to the following changes:

> **Volume overload,** especially with left-to-right shunts that may cause the RV to hypertrophy in order to compensate for the additional blood volume
>
> **Pressure overload,** primarily resulting from obstructive lesions, such as valvular stenosis or coarctation of the aorta
>
> **Decreased contractility,** primarily factors that affect the contractility of the myocardium, such as cardiomyopathy or myocardial ischemia from severe anemia or asphyxia, heart block, acidemia, and low levels of potassium, glucose, calcium, or magnesium
>
> **High cardiac output demands,** in which the body's need for oxygenated blood exceeds the heart's cardiac output (even though the volume may be normal), such as in sepsis, hyperthyroidism, and severe anemia

In children CHF occurs most frequently secondary to congenital heart defects in which structural abnormalities result in an increased volume load or increased pressure load on the ventricles. For example, septal defects can cause large left-to-right shunts, resulting in a volume load on the RV. Obstruction to flow out of the LV, such as narrowing of the aorta (coarctation of the aorta), can cause increased pressure inside the ventricle. CHF can also be a result of an excessive workload on a normal myocardium. Myocardial failure, in which the contractility of the heart muscle is impaired, can result from cardiomyopathy, drugs, electrolyte imbalances, dysrhythmias, and other causes. Diseases in other organ systems, particularly the lungs, also can cause CHF. Obstructive changes in the lungs result in increased pulmonary vascular resistance, which increases the RV workload. In time, the right side of the heart has difficulty pump-

ing blood forward to the lungs, becomes dilated, and hypertrophies; then signs and symptoms of right-sided heart failure are seen. **Cor pulmonale** is the term for CHF resulting from obstructive lung diseases such as cystic fibrosis or bronchopulmonary dysplasia.

## Pathophysiology

Theoretically heart failure may be divided into two classifications: right-sided failure and left-sided failure. In **right-sided failure,** RV function is suboptimal. RV end-diastolic pressure rises, causing increased central venous pressure and systemic venous engorgement. Systemic venous hypertension causes hepatomegaly and may cause edema in the extremities. In **left-sided failure,** LV dysfunction occurs and LV end-diastolic pressure rises, resulting in increased pressure in the LA and also in the pulmonary veins. The lungs become congested with blood, causing elevated pulmonary pressures and pulmonary edema.

Although each type of heart failure produces different signs and symptoms, clinically it is unusual to observe solely right- or left-sided failure in children. Because both sides of the heart depend on adequate function of the other side, failure of one chamber causes a reciprocal change in the opposite chamber.

**Compensatory Mechanisms.** The heart initially tries to meet the body's demand for increased cardiac output through several compensatory mechanisms called the **cardiac reserve.** These include hypertrophy and dilation of the cardiac muscle and stimulation of the sympathetic nervous system (Fig. 34-9).

**Hypertrophy and dilation of the cardiac muscle.** In response to the need to increase cardiac output, the cardiac muscle hypertrophies, developing greater tension. It is able to generate increased pressure within the ventricle, pump-

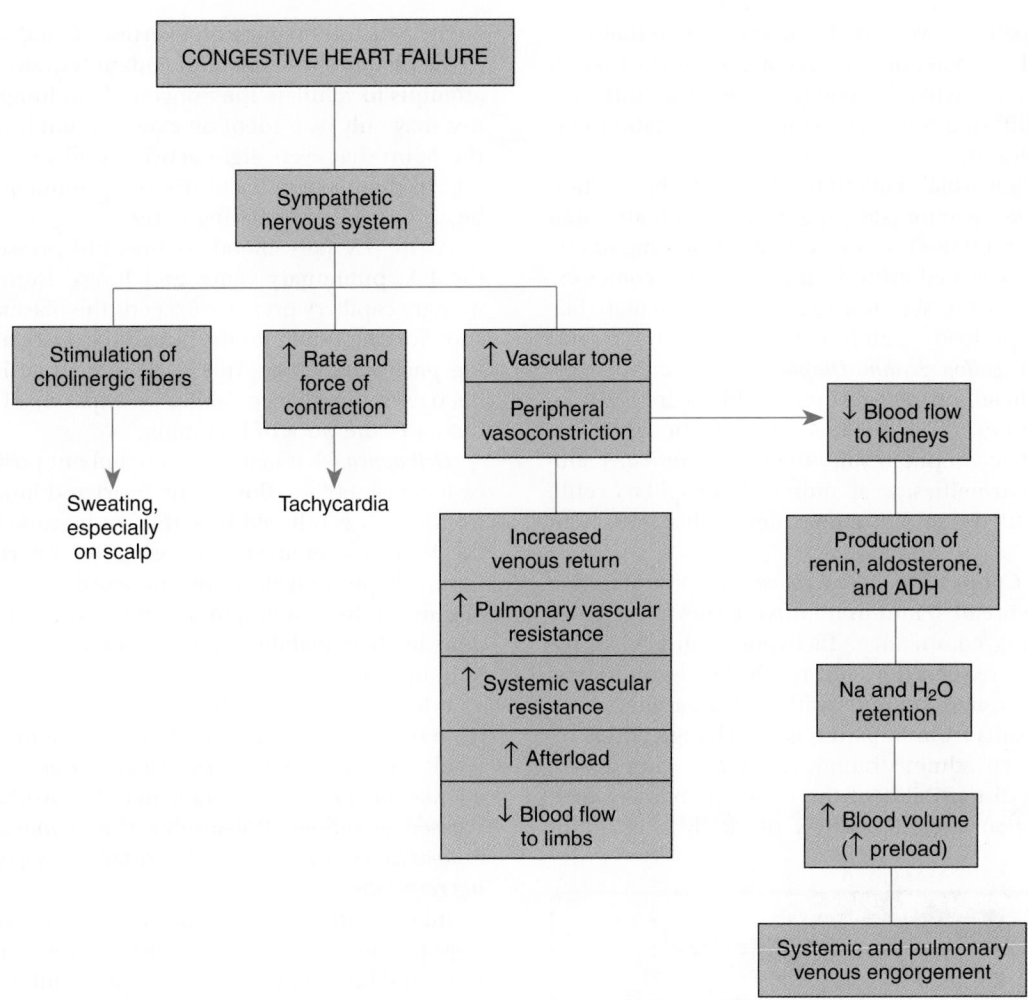

**Fig. 34-9** Pathophysiology of congestive heart failure.

ing blood out of the heart at a higher pressure. Also the cardiac muscle can dilate and increase the stretch of its fibers, which increases the force of contraction. However, both hypertrophy and dilation have potentially negative effects. Hypertrophy may result in decreased ventricular compliance over time. Decreased compliance requires a higher filling pressure to produce the same stroke volume. The increased muscle mass impairs oxygenation to the heart muscle. Beyond a certain amount of dilation, the force of contraction decreases and the heart fails. (See discussion of Starling law, p. 1468.)

*Stimulation of the sympathetic nervous system.* When the cardiac output begins to fall, stretch receptors and baroreceptors in the blood vessels stimulate the sympathetic nervous system, releasing catecholamines. Catecholamines increase the force and rate of myocardial contraction, as manifested by tachycardia. They cause peripheral vasoconstriction, resulting in increased systemic vascular resistance, increased venous return, and reduced blood flow to the limbs, viscera, and kidneys. Sympathetic cholinergic fibers cause sweating.

Although initially successful in increasing cardiac output, prolonged sympathetic stimulation also has negative

effects. By shortening the diastolic period, tachycardia increases oxygen consumption by the heart muscle, eliminates the heart's resting phase, and impairs coronary artery perfusion. A continued increase in systemic vascular resistance increases the afterload on the heart muscle, which requires extra work by the heart muscle and reduces systemic blood flow.

The renal system is particularly sensitive to reductions in blood flow and renal perfusion, activating the renin-angiotensin-aldosterone mechanism. Renin-angiotensin secretion causes vasoconstriction and leads to an increase in aldosterone secretion, which causes retention of salt and water. Retention of salt and water causes an increase in preload. Although at first helpful to the failing heart, the sodium and water retention becomes excessive, resulting in signs of systemic venous congestion and fluid overload.

### Clinical Manifestations

As the compensatory mechanisms are exceeded, the child will exhibit signs of CHF because of decreased myocardial contraction, increased preload, and increased afterload. The signs and symptoms of CHF can be divided into three groups: (1) impaired myocardial function, (2) pulmonary congestion, and (3) systemic venous congestion (Box 34-1). Because these hemodynamic changes occur from different causes and at differing times, the clinical presentation may vary among children.

**Impaired Myocardial Function.** One of the earliest signs of CHF is *tachycardia* (sleeping heart rate greater than 160 beats/min in infants) as a direct result of sympathetic stimulation. It is elevated even during rest but becomes extremely rapid with the slightest exertion. Ventricular dilation and excess preload result in extra heart sounds $S_3$ and $S_4$, referred to as *gallop rhythm. Diaphoresis* is often seen, especially on the head during exertion. Children are easily fatigued, have poor exercise tolerance, and are often irritable. Decreased cardiac output results in *poor perfusion,* manifested by cold extremities, weak pulses, slow capillary refill, low BP, and mottled skin. Extreme pallor or duskiness is an ominous sign.

**Pulmonary Congestion.** *Tachypnea* (respiratory rate greater than 60 breaths/min in infants) occurs in response to decreased lung compliance. Tachypnea can lead to hypoxemia because oxygen does not reach the alveoli for gas exchange in adequate amounts with fast breathing rates. *Mild cyanosis* results from impaired gas exchange and is relieved with oxygen administration. *Dyspnea* is caused by a decrease in the distensibility of the lungs. Inability to feed with resultant poor weight gain is primarily a result of tachypnea and dyspnea on exertion. *Costal retractions* occur as the pliable chest wall in the infant is drawn inward during attempts to ventilate the noncompliant lungs. Initially dyspnea may only be evident on exertion, but it may progress to the point that even slight activity results in labored breathing. In infants dyspnea at rest is a prominent sign and may be accompanied by flaring nares.

As the LV fails, blood volume and pressure increase in the LA, pulmonary veins, and lungs. Eventually the pulmonary capillary pressure exceeds the plasma osmotic pressure, forcing fluid into the interstitial space and finally causing *pulmonary edema.* Increased interstitial lung water also decreases compliance (ability to expand) of the lungs and increases the work of breathing.

*Orthopnea* (dyspnea in the recumbent position) is caused by increased blood flow to the heart and lungs from the extremities. It is relieved by sitting up because blood pools in the lower extremities, decreasing venous return. In addition, this position decreases pressure from the abdominal organs on the diaphragm. In infants orthopnea may be evident in their inability to lie supine and their desire to be held upright.

Edema of the bronchial mucosa may produce *wheezing* from obstruction to airflow. Mucosal swelling and irritation result in a persistent, dry, hacking *cough.* As pulmonary edema increases, the cough may be productive from increased secretions. Pressure on the laryngeal nerve results in *hoarseness.* A late sign of heart failure is *gasping* and *grunting respirations.*

Infants with CHF have an increased metabolic rate and require additional caloric intake to grow. The work of the heart and breathing demands all of the infant's energy, leaving little for normal activity. As a result of poor weight gain and activity intolerance, infants with CHF demonstrate *developmental delays.* Because of the physical energy and strength needed to sit up, pull to stand, and walk, these infants are delayed most in gross motor activities. The fine motor, social, and cognitive aspects of development seem less impaired. Following surgical correction, most children will catch up to their peers with time. Older children with severe CHF will have decreased exercise tolerance and persistent developmental delays.

**Systemic Venous Congestion.** Systemic venous congestion from right-sided failure results in increased pressure and pooling of blood in the venous circulation. *Hepatomegaly* occurs from pooling of blood in the portal circulation and transudation of fluid into the hepatic tissues. The liver may be tender on palpation, and its size is an indication of the course of heart failure.

*Edema* forms as the sodium and water retention causes systemic vascular pressure to rise. The earliest sign is *weight gain.* However, as additional fluid accumulates, it leads to swelling of soft tissue that is dependent and favors the flow of gravity, such as the sacrum and scrotum (when recumbent) and loose periorbital tissues. In infants edema is usually generalized and difficult to detect. Gross fluid accumulation may produce *ascites* and *pleural effusions.*

*Distended neck* and *peripheral veins* result from a consistently elevated central venous pressure. Normally neck and

---

**Box 34-1** ■ ■ ■
**Clinical Manifestations of Congestive Heart Failure**

**IMPAIRED MYOCARDIAL FUNCTION**
Tachycardia
Sweating (inappropriate)
Decreased urinary output
Fatigue
Weakness
Restlessness
Anorexia
Pale, cool extremities
Weak peripheral pulses
Decreased blood pressure
Gallop rhythm
Cardiomegaly

**PULMONARY CONGESTION**
Tachypnea
Dyspnea
Retractions (infants)
Flaring nares
Exercise intolerance
Orthopnea
Cough, hoarseness
Cyanosis
Wheezing
Grunting

**SYSTEMIC VENOUS CONGESTION**
Weight gain
Hepatomegaly
Peripheral edema, especially periorbital
Ascites
Neck vein distention (children)

hand veins collapse when the head or hands are raised above the level of the heart, because the blood drains by gravity back to the heart. However, when the venous pressure is high, it slows venous return, causing the veins to remain distended. Distended neck veins are difficult to detect in the short, fat neck of infants and are usually observed only in older children.

## Diagnostic Evaluation

Diagnosis is made on the basis of clinical symptoms such as tachypnea and tachycardia at rest, dyspnea, retractions, activity intolerance (especially during feeding in infants), weight gain caused by fluid retention, and hepatomegaly. A chest x-ray film demonstrates cardiomegaly and increased pulmonary vascular markings due to increased pulmonary blood flow. Ventricular hypertrophy appears on the ECG. An echocardiogram is done to determine the cause of CHF such as a congenital heart defect or poor ventricular function.

## Therapeutic Management

The goals of treatment are to (1) improve cardiac function (increase contractility and decrease afterload), (2) remove accumulated fluid and sodium (decrease preload), (3) decrease cardiac demands, and (4) improve tissue oxygenation and decrease oxygen consumption. For most infants diagnosed with CHF the cause is a CHD. Infants are stabilized on medical therapy and then referred for surgical repair. For children newly diagnosed with CHF, the cause may be worsening ventricular function following a previous cardiac repair, cardiomyopathy, arrhythmia, or other causes. In addition to management of CHF, the underlying cause is treated if possible.

**Improve Cardiac Function.**    Two groups of drugs are used to enhance myocardial performance in CHF: (1) digitalis glycosides, which improve contractility and (2) angiotensin-converting enzyme inhibitors, which reduce the afterload on the heart, making it easier for the heart to pump.

Digitalis has three major actions. It (1) increases the force of contraction (positive inotropic), (2) decreases the heart rate (negative chronotropic) and slows the conduction of impulses through the AV node (negative dromotropic), and (3) indirectly enhances diuresis by increased renal perfusion. The beneficial effects are increased cardiac output, decreased heart size, decreased venous pressure, and relief of edema.

In pediatrics, *digoxin (Lanoxin)* is used because of its rapid onset and decreased risk of toxicity as a result of a relatively short half-life (1½ days) compared with other digitalis preparations. It is available as an elixir (50 $\mu g$/ml) for oral administration or in a parenteral preparation (0.1 mg/ml). For infants the dose is often calculated in micrograms (1000 $\mu g$ = 1 mg). Because digoxin has a very narrow margin of safety, the dosage must be calculated exactly. Premature infants are more sensitive to digoxin and require smaller doses because the drug accumulates in the blood faster than in full-term infants and children because of impaired renal excretion (Park, 1996).

Treatment is based on a digitalizing dose, given intravenously or orally, in divided doses over 24 hours to bring the child's serum digoxin level into the therapeutic range. A maintenance dose, usually one eighth of the digitalizing dose, is given orally twice a day to maintain blood levels (Table 34-4). During digitalization the child is monitored with an ECG to observe for the desired effects (prolonged P-R interval and reduced ventricular rate) and to detect side effects, especially dysrhythmias.

Digoxin is the only oral inotropic agent generally available for infants and children, although other oral inotropic agents are being used in clinical trials in adults. For patients with severe CHF, IV inotropic agents such as dopamine, dobutamine, or milrinone are used to improve contractility. They are generally given in ICU settings.

Another group of drugs used in the treatment of CHF, the *angiotensin-converting enzyme (ACE) inhibitors,* inhibit the normal function of the renin-angiotensin system in the kidney. The production of renin triggers the production of angiotensin I and angiotensin II, which cause vasoconstriction and aldosterone secretion. The ACE inhibitors block the conversion of angiotensin I to angiotensin II so that instead of vasoconstriction, vasodilation occurs. Vasodilation results in decreased pulmonary and systemic vascular resistance, decreased BP, a reduction in afterload, and decreased right and left atrial pressures. It also reduces the secretion of aldosterone, which reduces preload by preventing volume expansion from fluid retention and decreases the risk of hypokalemia. Renal blood flow is improved, which enhances diuresis.

ACE inhibitors are frequently used in pediatrics: *captopril (Capoten),* given three times a day, *enalapril (Vasotec),* given twice a day, and *lisinopril, (Zestil),* given once daily, are most common. Captopril is used in infants and young children because it can be given in smaller doses; its principal side effects are hypotension, renal dysfunction, and cough. Captopril may also have some immune-based side effects, including fever and allergic reactions. Because enalapril has the same principal side effects but fewer immune-based side effects, patients may be switched from one preparation to the other (see Box 34-11). (Phillips and Somers, 2000).

> **NURSING ALERT**    Because ACE inhibitors also block the action of aldosterone, the addition of potassium supplements or spironolactone (Aldactone) to the drug regimen of patients taking diuretics is usually not needed and may cause hyperkalemia.

**TABLE 34-4    Oral digoxin dosage in infants and children***

| Age | Total Digitalizing Dose† | Daily Maintenance Dose‡ |
|---|---|---|
| Premature infant | 20 | 5 |
| Full-term infant | 30 | 8-10 |
| <2 years | 40-50 | 10-12 |
| >2 years | 30 | 8-10 |

*Dosage in $\mu g$/kg of body weight.
†Total dose given in several divided doses over 12 to 24 hours.
‡Maintenance dose given in two divided doses.

Carvedilol, a beta blocker, is the newest medication to be added to the treatment of some children with chronic CHF. It blocks the α- and β-adrenergic receptors, causing decreased heart rate, decreased blood pressure, and vasodilation. It has been shown to decrease morbidity and mortality in some adults with heart failure and is being used selectively in children. The efficacy of carvedilol in the management of children with heart failure is being studied.

**Remove Accumulated Fluid and Sodium.** Treatment consists of diuretics, possible fluid restriction, and possible sodium restriction. Diuretics are the mainstay of therapy to eliminate excess water and salt to prevent reaccumulation. The most commonly used agents are listed in Table 34-5. Because furosemide and the thiazides cause loss of potassium, potassium supplements and rich dietary sources of the electrolyte are given.

> **NURSING ALERT**
>
> A fall in the serum potassium level enhances the effects of digoxin, increasing the risk of digoxin toxicity. Increased serum potassium diminishes digoxin's effect. Therefore serum potassium levels (normal range 3.5 to 5.5 mmol/L) must be carefully monitored.

Fluid restriction may be required in the acute stages of CHF and must be carefully calculated to avoid dehydrating the child, especially if cyanotic CHD and significant polycythemia are present. Infants rarely need fluid restrictions because CHF makes feeding so difficult that they struggle to take maintenance fluids.

Sodium-restricted diets are used less often in children than in adults to control CHF because of their potential negative effects on the child's appetite and ultimate growth. If salt intake is restricted, the diet usually consists of avoiding additional table salt and highly salted foods. Low-salt formulas are available but used infrequently because infants need a normal sodium source to offset the sodium depletion of chronic diuretic therapy. Most infant formulas have slightly more sodium than does breast milk.

**Decrease Cardiac Demands.** To lessen the workload on the heart, metabolic needs are minimized by (1) providing a neutral thermal environment to prevent cold stress in infants, (2) treating any existing infections, (3) reducing the effort of breathing (semi-Fowler position), (4) using medication to sedate an irritable child, and (5) providing rest and decreasing environmental stimuli.

**TABLE 34-5** Diuretics used in congestive heart failure

| Drug | Action | Comments | Nursing Considerations |
|---|---|---|---|
| Furosemide (Lasix) | Blocks reabsorption of sodium and water in proximal renal tubule and interferes with reabsorption of sodium in loop of Henle and in most proximal portion of distal tubule | Drug of choice in severe CHF Causes excretion of chloride and potassium (hypokalemia may precipitate digitalis toxicity) | Begin to record output as soon as drug is given Observe for dehydration caused by profound diuresis Observe for side effects (nausea and vomiting, diarrhea, ototoxicity, hypokalemia, dermatitis, postural hypotension) Encourage foods high in potassium and give potassium supplements Monitor chloride and acid-base balance with long-term therapy |
| Chlorothiazide (Diuril) | Acts directly on distal tubules and possibly proximal tubules to decrease sodium, water, potassium, chloride, and bicarbonate absorption Decreases urinary diluting capacity | Less frequently used drug Causes hypokalemia, acidosis from large doses May be given on alternate days or for 4 or 5 days and stopped for 2 days to allow for reabsorption of potassium | Observe for side effects (nausea, weakness, dizziness, paresthesia, muscle cramps, skin eruptions, hypokalemia, acidosis) Encourage foods high in potassium and give potassium supplements |
| Spironolactone (Aldactone) | Blocks action of aldosterone, allows retention of potassium | Weak diuretic Has potassium-sparing effect; frequently used with thiazides, furosemide Poorly absorbed from gastrointestinal tract Takes several days to achieve maximum actions | Observe for side effects (skin rash, drowsiness, ataxia, hyperkalemia) Do not administer potassium supplements |
| Bumetanide (Bumex) | Loop diuretic similar to furosemide Much more potent than furosemide (1 mg = 40 mg furosemide) | May be used for severe CHF when furosemide is less effective Use cautiously because of profound diuresis and electrolyte imbalances | Monitor for dehydration and electrolyte imbalances Observe for side effects (similar to those for furosemide) Observe for renal toxicity and electrolyte disturbances |
| Metolazone (Zaroxolyn) | Unique thiazide diuretic Appears effective in patients with reduced renal function | Chronic diuretic; useful in long-term therapy, not for acute diuresis Duration of action: 24 hours Use cautiously (once a day or several times weekly) because of profound diuresis and electrolyte imbalances | Observe for side effects, especially dehydration, nausea, vomiting, electrolyte imbalances Provide foods high in potassium and administer potassium supplements |

**Improve Tissue Oxygenation.** All of the preceding measures serve to increase tissue oxygenation either by improving myocardial function or by lessening tissue oxygen demands. In addition, supplemental cool humidified oxygen may be administered to increase the amount of available oxygen during inspiration. Oxygen administration is especially helpful in patients with pulmonary edema, intercurrent respiratory infections, and increased pulmonary vascular resistance (oxygen is a vasodilator that decreases pulmonary vascular resistance).

**NURSING ALERT** Oxygen is a drug and is only administered with an appropriate order. There are some uncommon circumstances in patients with complex hemodynamics when oxygen can be detrimental.

An oxygen hood is preferred with young infants to provide increased concentration of the gas. A nasal cannula or face tent may be useful with older infants and children. Nasal cannulas are ideal for long-term oxygen administration because the child can be ambulatory and can easily eat and drink. Cool humidification is necessary to counteract the drying effect of oxygen. The amount of cool humidity is carefully regulated to prevent chilling.

### Nursing Considerations

The infant or child with CHF is usually quite ill and may be admitted to an ICU. Expert nursing care is essential to reduce the cardiac demands that strain the failing heart muscle. During this time the child and family require emotional support; for some children severe CHF represents end-stage cardiac disease.

### ⚏ Assessment

Nurses need to be alert to signs of CHF in children with CHD and in infants with suspected CHD (see Box 34-1).

### ⚏ Nursing Diagnoses

Following a thorough assessment, several nursing diagnoses are evident (see Nursing Care Plan, p. 1485-1486). Others may become apparent in special circumstances and with children in different age-groups.

### ⚏ Planning

The goals for the infant or child with CHF and the family are as follows:

1. Child will exhibit improved cardiac output.
2. Child will experience decreased cardiac demands.
3. Child will exhibit improved respiratory function.
4. Child will maintain adequate nutritional status.
5. Child will exhibit no evidence of fluid excess.
6. Child and family will receive adequate support and education.

### ⚏ Implementation

Although the objectives of nursing care are the same, the interventions differ depending on the child's age. Interventions for infants are quite different from those for older children.

**Assist in Measures to Improve Cardiac Function.** The nurse's responsibility in administering digoxin includes observing for signs of toxicity, calculating and administering the correct dosage, and instituting parental teaching regarding drug administration at home. The child's apical pulse is always checked before administering digoxin. As a general rule, the drug is not given if the pulse is below 90 to 110 beats/min in infants and young children or below 70 beats/min in older children (the cutoff point for adults is 60). However, because the pulse rate varies in children in different age-groups, the written drug order should specify at what heart rate the drug is withheld. The nurse should also use judgment in evaluating the pulse rate. If it is significantly lower than the previous recording, the dose should be withheld until the practitioner is notified.

The apical rate is taken because a pulse deficit (radial pulse rate lower than apical) may be present with decreased cardiac output. It is auscultated for 1 full minute to evaluate alterations in rhythm. If the child is monitored by means of an ECG, a rhythm strip is obtained and attached to the chart for rate and rhythm analysis, such as abnormal lengthening of the P-R interval (more than a 50% increase over predigitalization interval) and dysrhythmias.

Digoxin is a potentially dangerous drug because the margin of safety of therapeutic, toxic, and lethal doses is very narrow. Many toxic responses are extensions of its therapeutic effects. Therefore the nurse must maintain a high index of suspicion for signs of toxicity when administering digoxin. The most common signs of digoxin toxicity in infants and children are bradycardia (although other dysrhythmias may occur), anorexia, nausea, and vomiting. Although vomiting should alert the nurse to observe for other evidence of cardiac toxicity, one episode of vomiting does not warrant cessation of the drug, because vomiting from other causes frequently occurs, especially in infants. Vomiting associated with digoxin toxicity is often unrelated to feedings, and infants are usually less interested in feeding, with a recent decrease in oral intake. When in doubt regarding the cause of the vomiting and if another dose of digoxin should be given, the nurse should seek the practitioner's advice before administering the next dose. When there is concern about possible digoxin toxicity, the digoxin drug level is checked.

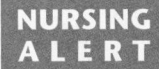 **NURSING ALERT** Therapeutic serum digoxin levels range from 0.8 to 2 µg/L. Observe for signs of toxicity, especially bradycardia and vomiting.

Other extracardiac signs of toxicity are neurologic or visual disturbances, which are extremely difficult to identify in children and consequently are of little value in assessing toxicity in infants.

Because digoxin toxicity can occur from accidental overdose, great care must be taken in properly calculating and measuring the dosage. When converting milligrams to micrograms to milliliters, the nurse carefully checks the placement of the decimal point, because an error causes a significant change in dosage. For example, 0.1 mg is 10 times the dosage of 0.01 mg.

Infants rarely receive more than 1 ml (50 μg, or 0.05 mg) in one dose; a higher dose is an immediate warning of a dosage error. To ensure safety, compare the calculation with another staff member before giving digoxin.

If digoxin toxicity occurs, especially as a result of a drug overdose, all subsequent doses are withheld. The child is closely monitored for dysrhythmias, which are treated appropriately if they occur. Digoxin immune Fab fragments are used as an antidote to digoxin in cases of severe digitalis toxicity (Phillips and Somers, 2000). Because of the long half-life of digoxin (32 to 48 hours in patients with normal renal function; longer in those with renal impairment), it may be several days before the blood level returns to normal (Frishman, 1995).

These same principles are taught to parents in preparation for discharge, although the correct dose in milliliters is usually specified on the container, thus reducing potential errors in calculation. The nurse observes the parent measuring the elixir in the dropper and stresses the level mark as the meniscus of the fluid that is observed at eye level. Other instructions for administering digoxin are listed in the Family Home Care box.

Parents are also advised of the signs of toxicity. According to the practitioner's preference, they may be taught to take the pulse before giving the drug. A return demonstration of the procedure from both parents or principal caregivers is included as part of the teaching plan. Their level of anxiety in counting the pulse is assessed because overconcern about the heart rate may result in excessive withholding of the drug.

**Reduce Afterload.**  For patients receiving ACE inhibitors for afterload reduction, the nurse should carefully monitor BP before and after dose administration, observe for symptoms of hypotension, and notify the practitioner if BP is low. Serum electrolyte levels should be monitored. Because ACE inhibitors also block the action of aldosterone, they act as potassium-sparing agents. Most patients do not need potassium supplements or spironolactone (Aldactone) while receiving these medications. Numerous medications affecting the kidney can potentiate renal dysfunction, so children taking multiple diuretics along with an ACE inhibitor require careful assessment.

**Decrease Cardiac Demands.**  The infant requires rest and conservation of energy for feeding. Every effort is made to organize nursing activities to allow for uninterrupted periods of sleep. Whenever possible, parents are encouraged to stay with their infant to provide the holding, rocking, and cuddling that help children sleep more soundly. To minimize disturbing the infant, changing bed linen and complete bathing are done only when necessary. Feeding is planned to accommodate the infant's sleep and wake patterns. The child is fed when hungry, such as when sucking on fists rather than when crying for a bottle because the stress of crying exhausts the limited energy supply. Because infants with CHF tire easily and may sleep through feedings, smaller feedings every 3 hours may be helpful. Gavage feedings may be instituted to provide adequate nutrition and allow the infant to rest.

Every effort is made to minimize unnecessary stress. With infants this primarily involves preserving the parent-child relationship and meeting their needs to reduce frustration. Older children need an explanation of what is happening to them to decrease anxiety about their illness and necessary treatments, such as cardiac monitoring, oxygen administration, and medications. Outlining a plan for the day, preparing the child for tests and procedures, providing quiet activities, and providing adequate rest periods are all helpful interventions with older children. Some infants and children require sedation during the acute phase of illness to allow them to rest.

Temperature is carefully monitored for hyperthermia (a sign of infection) or hypothermia (loss of heat to ambient air). Fever is reported because infection must be promptly treated. Fever increases oxygen demands and is poorly tolerated. If body temperature is low, the child is kept warm with additional blankets or the use of a radiant heater. Maintaining body temperature is very important for the child who is receiving cool, humidified oxygen and for one who tends to be diaphoretic, losing heat via evaporation.

Skin breakdown from edema is prevented with frequent change of position and use of pressure-relieving or pressure-reducing mattresses or beds. The skin, especially over the sacrum, is checked for evidence of redness from pressure. Respiratory infections can exacerbate CHF and

## FAMILY HOME CARE
### Administering Digoxin

Give digoxin at regular intervals, usually every 12 hours, such as 8 AM and 8 PM.

Plan the times so that the drug is given *1 hour before or 2 hours after* feedings.

Use a calendar to mark off each dose that is given or post a reminder, such as a sign on the refrigerator.

Have the prescription refilled *before* the medication is completely used.

Administer the drug carefully by slowly directing it on the side and back of the mouth.

Do not mix it with other foods or fluids, because refusal to consume these results in inaccurate intake of the drug.

If the child has teeth, give water after administering the drug; whenever possible, brush the teeth to prevent tooth decay from the sweetened liquid.

If a dose is missed and more than 4 hours has elapsed, withhold the dose and give the next dose at the regular time; if less than 4 hours has elapsed, give the missed dose.

If the child vomits, do not give a second dose.

If more than two consecutive doses have been missed, notify the physician or other designated practitioner.

Do not increase or double the dose for missed doses.

If the child becomes ill, notify the physician or other designated practitioner immediately.

Keep digoxin in a safe place, preferably a locked cabinet.

In case of accidental overdose of digoxin, call the nearest poison control center immediately; the number is usually listed in the front of the telephone directory.

Modified from Jackson PL: Digoxin therapy at home: keeping the child safe, *MCN* 4(2):105-109, 1979.

should be appropriately treated and prevented if possible. The child is protected from persons with respiratory infections and has a noninfectious roommate. With an older child, it is advantageous to choose a roommate who is also confined to bed and relatively quiet in order to promote a restful environment. Good handwashing technique is practiced before and after caring for any hospitalized child. Antibiotics may be given to combat respiratory infection. The nurse ensures that the drug is given at equally divided times over a 24-hour schedule to maintain high blood levels of the antibiotic.

**Reduce Respiratory Distress.** Careful assessment, positioning, and oxygen administration can reduce respiratory distress. Respirations are counted for 1 full minute during a resting state. Any evidence of increased respiratory distress is reported, because this may indicate worsening heart failure.

Infants should be positioned to encourage maximum chest expansion, with the head of the bed elevated; they should sit up in an infant seat or be held at a 45-degree angle. Children prefer to sleep on several pillows and remain in a semi-Fowler or high Fowler position during waking hours. Shirts and diapers are pinned loosely to allow maximum chest expansion. Safety restraints, such as those used with the infant seats, are applied low on the abdomen and loosely enough to provide safety and maximum expansion.

The infant or child is often given humidified supplemental oxygen via an oxygen hood or tent, nasal cannula, or mask. The child's response to oxygen therapy is carefully evaluated by noting the respiratory rate, ease of respiration, color, and especially oxygen saturations, as measured by oximetry.

**Maintain Nutritional Status.** Meeting the nutritional needs of infants with CHF or serious cardiac defects is a nursing challenge. The metabolic rate of these infants is greater because of poor cardiac function and increased heart and respiratory rates. Their caloric needs are greater than those of the average infant because of their increased metabolic rate, yet their ability to take in adequate calories is hampered by their fatigue. Feeding for a fragile infant with serious CHD is similar to exercise in an adult, and they often do not have the energy or cardiac reserve to do extra work. The nurse seeks measures to enable the infant to feed easily without excess fatigue and to increase the caloric density of the formula.

The infant should be well rested before feeding and fed soon after awakening so as not to expend energy on crying. A 3-hour feeding schedule works well for many infants. (Feeding every 2 hours does not provide enough rest between feedings, and a 4-hour schedule requires an increased volume of feeding, which many infants are unable to take.) The feeding schedule should be individualized to the infant's needs. A soft preemie nipple or a slit in a regular nipple to enlarge the opening decreases the energy expenditure of the infant while sucking. Infants should be well supported and fed in a semiupright position. The infant may need to rest frequently and may need to have the jaw and cheeks stroked to encourage sucking. Generally, giving an infant about a half hour to complete a feeding is reason-

able. Prolonging the feeding time can exhaust the infant and decrease the rest period between feedings.

Infants with feeding difficulties are often gavage fed using a nasogastric tube to supplement oral intake and ensure adequate calories. If they are very stressed and fatigued, in respiratory distress, or tachypneic to 80 to 100 breaths/min, oral feedings may be withheld and all nutrition given by gavage feedings. Gavage feedings are usually a temporary measure until the infant's medical status improves and nutritional needs can be met through oral feedings. Some infants with severe CHF, neurologic deficits, or significant gastroesophageal reflux may need placement of a gastrostomy tube to allow adequate nutrition. (See Critical Thinking Exercise box.)

Increasing the caloric density of formulas by concentration and then adding corn or MCT oil or Polycose is frequently done. Infant formulas provide 20 kcal per ounce, and the use of additives can increase the calories to 30 kcal or more per ounce. This allows the infant to obtain more calories despite a smaller-volume intake of formula. The caloric density of the formula needs to be increased slowly (by 2 kcal per ounce per day) to prevent diarrhea or formula intolerance. Breast-feeding mothers may be encouraged to provide the infant with alternating feedings of breast milk and high-calorie formulas. Some lactating mothers will prefer to feed the child expressed breast milk that has been for-

---

 *Critical Thinking Exercise*

### Congestive Heart Failure

A 6-week-old infant is admitted from the clinic in congestive heart failure following diagnosis of a ventricular septal defect. On admission, HR is 170, RR is 84, BP is 76/40, and $O_2$ saturation is 96%. He is very tired and irritable and has mild retractions but no edema. He has been feeding poorly for several days. He is started on digoxin and Lasix. In planning fluid and nutrition for the next 12 hours, you would expect which of the following interventions to be ordered?

FIRST, THINK ABOUT IT . . .
- What is the purpose of your thinking?
- What information are you using?

1. Push bottle feedings every 3 hours.
2. Make him NPO and run IV fluids at one-half maintenance.
3. Place a nasogastric feeding tube and institute gavage feedings to meet maintenance fluid requirements.
4. Begin infant on high-calorie formula and bottle-feed every 4 to 5 hours.

*The best response is three, begin gavage feedings. The infant is in mild respiratory distress with tachypnea and is very tired, which is important information. Bottle-feedings would be too tiring, and he would not receive adequate fluids or nutrition. Gavage feedings will allow the infant to rest and supply needed nutrition. Enteral feedings are always preferred over IV hydration because more calories can be given. Fluid restriction is not needed, because the infant is behind on fluid intake, and Lasix therapy has begun, so further fluid restriction would risk dehydration.*

tified with Similac or Enfamil powder, Polycose, or corn oil to increase caloric intake. A supplemental nurser may also be helpful. A diet plan specific to the individual infant's needs is calculated and prescribed by the nutritionist in collaboration with the other health personnel. The nurse needs to reinforce this information with the parents as necessary.

**Assist in Measures to Promote Fluid Loss.**  When diuretics are given, the nurse records fluid intake and output and monitors body weight at the same time each day to evaluate benefit from the drug. Because profound diuresis may cause dehydration and electrolyte imbalance (loss of sodium, potassium, chloride, bicarbonate), the nurse observes for signs indicating either complication, as well as signs and symptoms suggesting reactions to the drugs. Diuretics should be given early in the day to children who are toilet trained to avoid the need to urinate at night. If potassium-losing diuretics are given, the nurse encourages foods high in potassium, such as bananas, oranges, whole grains, legumes, and leafy vegetables, and administers prescribed supplements.

**NURSING TIP**   Mix the potassium supplement elixir with fruit juice (red punch or grape juice works well) to disguise the bitter taste and to prevent intestinal irritation from a concentrated solution.

**NURSING ALERT**   Observe for signs of hypokalemia (muscle weakness, hypotension, dysrhythmias, tachycardia or bradycardia, irritability, drowsiness) or hyperkalemia (muscle weakness, twitching, bradycardia, ventricular fibrillation, oliguria, apnea) from supplement overdose.

Fluid restriction is rarely necessary in infants because of their difficulty in feeding. However, if fluids are restricted, the nurse plans fluid intake schedules for a 24-hour period, allowing for most fluids during waking hours. With toddlers and preschoolers it is psychologically advantageous to give small amounts of liquid in small cups so that the containers appear full. Suitable utensils are decorated medicine cups, small paper cups, doll-sized teacups, or measuring cups. It is also important to avoid leaving extra fluids at the bedside because older children may help themselves to additional servings. Older children's cooperation is gained by placing them in charge of recording fluid intake.

If salt is limited, the nurse discusses food sources of sodium with the family and discourages their bringing salt-containing treats to the child. At mealtime the child's tray is checked to make sure the appropriate diet is given.

**Support Child and Family.**  CHF is a serious complication of heart disease. Parents and older children are usually acutely aware of the critical nature of the condition. Because stress places additional demands on cardiac function, the nurse should focus on reducing anxiety through anticipatory preparation, frequent communication with the parent regarding the child's progress, and constant reassurance that everything possible is being done.

Home care involves many of the same interventions discussed under Plan for Discharge and Home Care (see p. 1509). The nurse teaches the family about the medications that need to be administered and alerts them to the signs of worsening CHF that require medical attention, such as increased sweating, decreased urinary output (noted in fewer wet diapers or infrequent use of the toilet), or poor feeding. Compliance is a major issue, and every effort is extended to improve the family's adherence to the medication schedule. (See Chapter 27.) Written instructions regarding correct administration of digitalis (digoxin) are essential (see Family Home Care box on p. 1482), including an explanation regarding signs of toxicity.

If CHF is the end stage of a severe heart defect, the nurse cares for this child the same as for any child who is terminally ill, using the principles discussed in Chapter 23.

## ■■ Evaluation

The effectiveness of nursing interventions for the family and the child with CHF is determined by continual reassessment and evaluation of care based on the following observational guidelines:

1. Monitor heart rate and quality, respiratory rate and efforts, and color, and observe behaviors that provide clues to expended effort.
2. Observe nutritional intake, feeding behaviors, and weight.
3. Monitor intake, output, and weight.
4. Interview and observe behaviors of family.

The *expected outcomes* are described in the Nursing Care Plan on pp. 1485-1486.

## Hypoxemia

*Hypoxemia* refers to an arterial oxygen tension (or pressure, $PaO_2$) that is less than normal and can be identified by a decreased arterial oxygen saturation ($SaO_2$) or a decreased $PaO_2$. *Hypoxia* is a reduction in tissue oxygenation that results from low $SaO_2$ and $PaO_2$ and results in impaired cellular processes. *Cyanosis* is a blue discoloration in the mucous membranes, skin, and nail beds of the child with reduced oxygen saturation. It results from the presence of deoxygenated hemoglobin (hemoglobin not bound to oxygen) in a concentration of 5 g/dl of blood or more. Cyanosis is usually apparent when $SaO_2$ is 85% or lower. Determination of cyanosis is subjective. It can vary depending on skin pigment, quality of light, color of the room, or clothing worn by the child. The presence of cyanosis may not accurately reflect arterial hypoxemia, because both $SaO_2$ and the amount of circulating hemoglobin are involved. Children with severe anemia may not be cyanotic despite severe hypoxemia, because the hemoglobin level may be too low to produce the characteristic blue color. Conversely, patients with polycythemia may appear cyanotic despite a near-normal $PaO_2$.

### Altered Hemodynamics

Heart defects that cause hypoxemia and cyanosis result from desaturated venous blood (blue blood) entering the systemic circulation without passing through the lungs. Three types of defects cause cyanosis in the infant. The first results from severe obstruction to pulmonary blood flow and blood shunting from the right side to the left side of the heart, or *right-to-left shunting*. Tetralogy of Fallot is the most

# *Nursing Care Plan*
## The Child with Congestive Heart Failure

---

**NURSING DIAGNOSIS:** Decreased cardiac output related to structural defect, myocardial dysfunction

**PATIENT GOAL 1:** Will exhibit improved cardiac output

- **NURSING INTERVENTIONS/***RATIONALES*
*Administer digoxin (Lanoxin) as ordered, using established precautions *to prevent toxicity*
Make certain dosage is within safe limits
Infants rarely receive more than 1 ml (50 µg or 0.05 mg) in one dose; *a higher dose is an immediate warning of a dosage error*
Ascertain correct preparation for route
Check dosage with another nurse *to ensure safety*
Count apical pulse for 1 full minute before giving drug
Withhold medication and notify practitioner if pulse rate is less than 90 to 110 beats/min (infants) or 70 to 85 beats/min (older children), depending on previous pulse readings
Recognize signs of digoxin toxicity (nausea, vomiting, anorexia, bradycardia, dysrhythmias)
Often an ECG rhythm strip is taken *to assess cardiac status before administration*
Ensure adequate intake of potassium
Observe for signs of hypokalemia (muscle weakness, hypotension, dysrhythmias, tachycardia or bradycardia, irritability, drowsiness) or hyperkalemia (muscle weakness, twitching, bradycardia, ventricular fibrillation, oliguria, apnea)
Monitor serum potassium levels *because decrease enhances digoxin toxicity*
*Administer medications to decrease afterload, as ordered
Check blood pressure
Observe for signs of hypotension
Monitor electrolyte levels
Attach cardiac monitor if ordered

- **EXPECTED OUTCOMES**
Heartbeat is strong, regular, and within normal limits for age (see inside back cover)
Peripheral perfusion is adequate

---

**NURSING DIAGNOSIS:** Ineffective breathing pattern related to pulmonary congestion

**PATIENT GOAL 1:** Will exhibit improved respiratory function

- **NURSING INTERVENTIONS/***RATIONALES*
Place in inclined posture of 30 to 45 degrees *to encourage maximum chest expansion;* tilt mattress support of incubator: place older infant in infant seat
Avoid any constricting clothing or restraints around abdomen and chest
*Administer humidified oxygen as prescribed
Assess respiratory rate, ease of respiration, color, and oxygen saturations as measured by oximetry

---

*Dependent nursing action.

- **EXPECTED OUTCOME**
Respirations remain within normal limits, color is good, and child rests quietly (see inside back cover for normal variations in respirations)

**PATIENT GOAL 2:** Will experience reduction of anxiety

- **NURSING INTERVENTIONS/***RATIONALES*
Employ flexible feeding schedule *that reduces fretfulness associated with hunger*
Handle child gently
Hold and comfort infant
Employ comfort measures found effective for individual child
Encourage family to provide comfort and solace
Explain equipment and procedures to child *to decrease anxiety*

- **EXPECTED OUTCOME**
Child rests quietly and breathes easily

---

**NURSING DIAGNOSIS:** Fluid volume excess related to fluid accumulation (edema)

**PATIENT GOAL 1:** Will exhibit no evidence of fluid excess

- **NURSING INTERVENTIONS/***RATIONALES*
*Administer diuretics as prescribed
Maintain accurate intake and output
Weigh daily at same time and on same scale *to assess fluid gain or loss*
Assess for evidence of increased or decreased edema
Maintain fluid restriction, if ordered
Provide skin care for children with edema
Change position frequently *to prevent skin breakdown associated with edema*
Use alternating-pressure mattress

- **EXPECTED OUTCOME**
Infant exhibits evidence of fluid loss (frequent urination, weight loss)

---

**NURSING DIAGNOSIS:** Activity intolerance related to imbalance between oxygen supply and demand

**PATIENT GOAL 1:** Will exhibit no additional respiratory or cardiac stress

- **NURSING INTERVENTIONS/***RATIONALES*
Maintain neutral thermal environment *because hypothermia or hyperthermia increases need for oxygen*
Place newborn in incubator or under warmer
Keep infant warm
Treat fever promptly
Feed small volumes at frequent intervals (every 2 to 3 hours) using soft nipple with moderately large opening, *because infants with CHF tire easily*
Implement gavage feeding if infant becomes fatigued before taking an adequate amount

*Continued*

## Nursing Care Plan
### The Child with Congestive Heart Failure—cont'd

**PATIENT GOAL 1—cont'd**

• **NURSING INTERVENTIONS/*RATIONALES*—cont'd**
Time nursing activities to disturb child as little as possible
Implement measures to reduce anxiety
Respond promptly to crying or other expressions of distress

• **EXPECTED OUTCOME**
Child rests quietly

> **NURSING DIAGNOSIS:** Risk for infection related to reduced body defenses, pulmonary congestion

See Infection Control, Chapter 27
See Nursing Care Plan: The Child with Congenital Heart Disease†

> **NURSING DIAGNOSIS:** Interruptd family processes related to a child with a life-threatening illness

**PATIENT (FAMILY) GOAL 1:** Will receive adequate support

• **NURSING INTERVENTIONS/*RATIONALES* AND EXPECTED OUTCOMES**
See Nursing Care Plan: The Family of the Child Who Is Ill or Hospitalized, Chapter 26

---

†In Wong DL, Hess CS: *Wong and Whaley's clinical manual of pediatric nursing,* ed 5, St Louis, 2000, Mosby.

**PATIENT (FAMILY) GOAL 2:** Will be prepared for home care

• **NURSING INTERVENTIONS/*RATIONALES***
Teach family:
Medication administration and side/toxic effects
Signs and symptoms of CHF and to report them to designated practitioner
Feeding techniques and nutritional requirements
Positioning
Need for rest
Growth and developmental considerations
Growth is slowed
Gross motor skills may be delayed more than fine motor skills
Refer to outpatient services and community resources as needed *for ongoing support*

• **EXPECTED OUTCOMES**
Family demonstrates an understanding of the condition and required care at home
Family uses appropriate community resources

---

common example. The second is mixing of arterial and venous blood within the chambers of the heart itself; a single ventricle is an example. The third defect, transposition of the great arteries, presents a unique situation in which the pulmonary and systemic circulations are parallel rather than in sequence. Fully oxygenated blood returns to the lungs, and desaturated blood returns to the body. Newborns with transposition of the great arteries depend on intracardiac mixing from a patent foramen ovale, septal defect, or ductus arteriosus to allow oxygenation.

Infants and children with some complex cardiac anomalies can be both hypoxemic and cyanotic and have symptoms of CHF. Defects resulting in one functional ventricle, hypoplastic left heart syndrome (HLHS), and transposition of the great arteries with a ventricular septal defect are examples.

Adolescents and young adults may become cyanotic because of unrepaired septal defects in which the increased pulmonary blood flow over many years results in pulmonary vascular changes. *Eisenmenger complex (syndrome)* refers to the clinical situation in which a left-to-right shunt becomes a right-to-left shunt because of a progressive increase in pulmonary vascular resistance. With increasing pulmonary vascular thickening, the resistance in the pulmonary circula-

tion can exceed or equal that in the systemic circulation, causing a reversal of blood flow from the right to the left ventricle.

### Clinical Manifestations

Over time, two physiologic changes occur in the body in response to chronic hypoxemia: polycythemia and clubbing. Persistent hypoxemia stimulates erythropoiesis, resulting in *polycythemia,* an increased number of red blood cells. Theoretically a greater number of red blood cells increases the oxygen-carrying capacity of the blood. However, this increased red blood cell formation may result in anemia if iron is not readily available for the formation of hemoglobin. In addition, polycythemia increases the viscosity of the blood and tends to crowd out platelets and other coagulation factors. *Clubbing,* a thickening and flattening of the tips of the fingers and toes, is thought to occur because of chronic tissue hypoxemia and polycythemia (Fig. 34-10).

Infants with mild hypoxemia may be asymptomatic except for cyanosis and exhibit near-normal growth and development. Those with more severe hypoxemia may exhibit fatigue with feeding, poor weight gain, tachypnea, and dyspnea. Flaccidity is usually a sign of severe cardiovascular compromise.

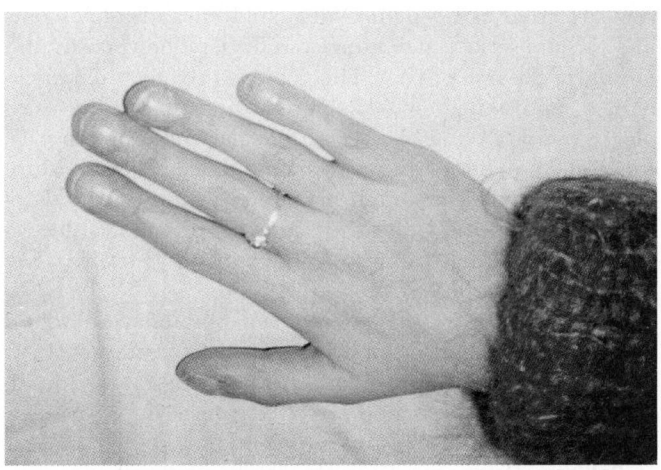

**Fig. 34-10**   Clubbing of the fingers.

*Squatting* is rarely seen today because of early surgical repair in the first year of life. It has similar benefits to the knee-chest position during a hypercyanotic spell.

Severe hypoxemia resulting in tissue hypoxia is manifested by clinical deterioration and signs of poor perfusion. The infant is pale and dusky with increased cyanosis, cool to touch with diminished pulses, and lethargic with signs of respiratory distress, including hyperpnea and gasping respirations. Tissue hypoxia causes metabolic acidosis, leading to hyperventilation and a rapidly worsening clinical course unless prompt treatment is instituted.

*Hypercyanotic spells,* also referred to as blue spells or "tet" spells because they are often seen in infants with tetralogy of Fallot, may occur in any child whose heart defect includes obstruction to pulmonary blood flow and communication between the ventricles (see Fig. 34-8). The infant becomes acutely cyanotic and hyperpneic because sudden infundibular spasm decreases pulmonary blood flow and increases right-to-left shunting (the proposed mechanism in tetralogy of Fallot). With other anomalies an increase in oxygen requirements, which the infant is unable to meet, may cause a spell. Hypoxia causes acidosis, which further increases pulmonary vascular resistance, which further decreases pulmonary blood flow; thus a vicious circle ensues. Spells, rarely seen before 2 months of age, occur most frequently in the first year of life and more often in the morning, and they may be preceded by feeding, crying, or defecation. Because profound hypoxemia causes cerebral hypoxia, hypercyanotic spells require prompt assessment and treatment to prevent brain damage or possibly death.

Persistent cyanosis as a result of cyanotic cardiac defects places the child at risk for significant neurologic complications. Polycythemia and the resultant increased viscosity of the blood increase the risk of thromboembolic events. *Cerebrovascular accidents (CVAs),* or strokes, may occur; infants with severe cyanosis and iron deficiency anemia are at greatest risk (O'Brien and Smith, 1994). They may occur spontaneously but often follow an acute febrile illness, a hypoxic spell, cardiac catheterization, or cardiac surgery, or following the Fontan procedure with an open fenestra-

tion (see Box 34-4, p. 1498). Signs and symptoms of CVA include sudden paralysis, altered speech, extreme irritability or fatigue, and seizures. The incidence of brain abcess is very low. Rarely seen in children under age 2 years, it should be suspected in older children with fever, headaches, focal neurologic signs, or seizures. Prompt treatment with antibiotics and surgical drainage is critical because death or significant neurologic impairment may result. Also, children who are cyanotic, especially those with systemic-to-pulmonary shunts, are at increased risk of *bacterial endocarditis* (see p. 1509).

Negative developmental consequences, particularly in the area of motor and cognitive development, may result from chronic hypoxemia. Fifty percent of postnatal brain growth occurs in the first year of life, so chronic hypoxemia, poor growth, and nutrition during this period can have significant adverse effects. If the risks of CVA, periods of profound cyanosis and hypoxia during hypercyanotic spells, and multiple surgeries, hospitalizations, and cardiac catheterizations are added, the possibility of neurologic insult resulting in developmental delays becomes significant and increases with each year of life. Minimizing these risks is an important factor in the trend toward early corrective surgical repair of cyanotic defects in infancy.

Children who are cyanotic from birth are generally smaller than their peers, exhibit poor weight gain, have dyspnea on exertion, fatigue easily, and have poor exercise tolerance. Hematologic abnormalities are also seen, such as thrombocytopenia, abnormal platelet function, fewer coagulation factors, and prolonged clotting time. These hematologic changes increase the likelihood of postoperative bleeding.

### Diagnostic Evaluation

Cyanosis in the newborn can be a result of cardiac, pulmonary, metabolic, or hematologic disease, although cardiac and pulmonary causes occur most often. To distinguish between the two, a hyperoxia test may be helpful. The infant is placed in a 100% oxygen environment, and blood gases are monitored. A $PaO_2$ of 150 mm Hg or more suggests lung disease, and a $PaO_2$ less than 100 mm Hg suggests cardiac disease (the problem is related to inadequate perfusion of the pulmonary bed) (Park, 1996). An accurate history, a chest radiograph (demonstrating reduced pulmonary blood flow), and especially an echocardiogram contribute to the diagnosis of cyanotic heart disease.

### Therapeutic Management

Newborns generally exhibit cyanosis within the first few days of life as the ductus arteriosus, which provided pulmonary blood flow, begins to close. Prostaglandin $E_1$, which causes vasodilation and smooth muscle relaxation, thus increasing dilation and patency of the ductus arteriosus, is administered intravenously to reestablish pulmonary blood flow. The use of prostaglandins has been lifesaving for infants with ductus-dependent cardiac defects. The increase in oxygenation allows the infant to be stabilized and for a complete diagnostic evaluation to be performed before further treatment is needed.

Hypercyanotic spells occur suddenly, and prompt recognition and treatment are essential. In the hospital setting, spells are often seen during blood drawing or IV line insertion, when the child is highly agitated, or following cardiac catheterization. Treatment of a hypercyanotic spell is outlined in the Guidelines box. Placing an infant in the knee-chest position reduces the venous return from the legs (which is desaturated) and increases systemic vascular resistance, which diverts more blood flow into the pulmonary artery. Morphine, administered subcutaneously or through an existing IV line, is helpful in reducing infundibular spasm. A spell indicates the need for prompt surgical treatment (Beekman, 2001). Rarely, propranolol (Inderal) may be given in the interim to prevent infundibular spasm.

The cyanotic infant and child are well hydrated to keep the hematocrit and blood viscosity within acceptable limits to reduce the risk of CVA. Fevers are carefully evaluated because bacteremia can result in bacterial endocarditis. The infant is monitored closely for anemia because of the risk of CVAs and the reduced arterial oxygen-carrying capacity that occurs. Iron supplementation and possibly blood transfusion are used as needed. Older children and adolescents may require serial phlebotomy to reduce blood viscosity and minimize the risk of CVA. The goal is to reduce the hematocrit to approximately 60% by removing small aliquots of blood and replacing blood with normal saline or other IV solutions to maintain intravascular volume. This procedure is a temporary measure but may relieve symptoms of dyspnea, headache, and malaise for short periods and can be repeated every 1 or 2 months if polycythemia is severe. (See Critical Thinking Exercise box.)

Respiratory infections or reduced pulmonary function from any cause can worsen hypoxemia in the cyanotic child. Aggressive pulmonary hygiene, chest physiotherapy, administration of antibiotics, and use of oxygen to improve arterial saturations are important interventions.

**Palliative Surgery.** Severely hypoxemic newborns with cardiac defects not amenable to corrective repair may have a palliative surgical procedure called a *shunt.* The shunt serves the same purpose as the ductus arteriosus: to increase blood flow to the lungs through a systemic artery-to-pulmonary artery connection. Currently a *modified Blalock-Taussig shunt* using a Gore-Tex or Impra tube graft to create a communication between the right or left subclavian

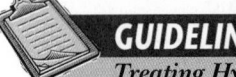

## GUIDELINES
### Treating Hypercyanotic Spells

Place infant in knee-chest position (Fig. 34-11).
Employ calm, comforting approach.
Administer 100% oxygen by face mask.
Give morphine subcutaneously or through existing IV line.
Begin IV fluid replacement and volume expansion, if needed.
Repeat morphine administration.

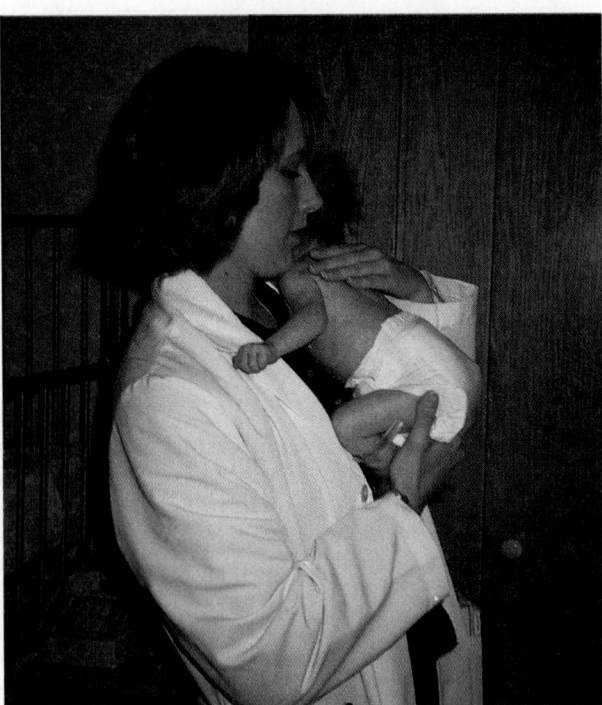

**Fig. 34-11** Infant held in knee-chest position.

### Critical Thinking Exercise

#### Hypercyanotic Spell

A 4-month-old infant known to have tetralogy of Fallot is seen in the emergency department because of a 2-day history of diarrhea, low-grade fever, and poor oral intake. When blood tests are done, he becomes acutely cyanotic with rapid shallow respirations. What should you do?

FIRST, THINK ABOUT IT . . .
• What precise questions are you trying to answer?
• If you accept the conclusions, what are the implications?

1. Begin cardiopulmonary resuscitation (CPR).
2. Calm the infant, place in the knee-chest position and administer blow-by oxygen, and call for assistance.
3. Continue the procedure; this is expected for an infant with tetralogy of Fallot.
4. Stop the procedure and wait for color to improve before completing the blood test.

*The best response is two. Precisely, the questions are focused on what symptoms is the infant experiencing, and what is the priority nursing action. The infant is having a hypercyanotic or "tet" spell, and the first actions should be to calm the infant, place in the knee-chest position, and give supplemental oxygen. A hypercyanotic spell will likely worsen without intervention, so prompt action is needed. CPR is inappropriate at this time because the infant has an adequate heart rate and effective respirations. If you fail to accept the conclusions, negative implications may result, because a severe hypercyanotic spell may require IV medications, hydration, and resuscitative measures to stabilize the infant.*

artery and the pulmonary artery on the same side is the preferred procedure. Because of the higher resistance in the systemic circulation, blood flows from the subclavian artery to the pulmonary artery and to the lungs for oxygenation. The small diameter of the subclavian artery (as opposed to the aorta) automatically restricts the volume of blood flow to the pulmonary artery. This procedure sacrifices the brachial and radial pulse on the affected side, and the hand initially may be slightly cooler and paler until collateral circulation develops. Table 34-6 outlines the different shunt procedures (Fig. 34-12). Corrective surgical repair is always preferred to a palliative shunt procedure if it can be performed at low risk. Corrective techniques are described with the cardiac defect.

Following a shunt procedure, the infant must be assessed for signs of increased or decreased pulmonary blood flow. If the shunt is too small or narrowed, the newborn may remain severely hypoxemic, with oxygen saturations below 70%. Surgically revising the shunt or placement of an additional shunt may be needed. More often the shunt is too large and the pulmonary blood flow may be excessive, resulting in signs and symptoms of CHF and oxygen saturations above 85%. The infant may require digoxin and diuretic therapy (see discussion of CHF). Some surgeons place infants on low-dose aspirin therapy for several months to prevent platelet aggregation and subsequent narrowing of the shunt. Acute cyanosis and signs of tissue hypoxia may occur if the shunt is occluded and pulmonary blood flow is severely limited; shunt occlusion is a medical emergency.

## Nursing Considerations

The general appearance of infants and children with significant cyanosis poses unique concerns. Blue lips and fingernails are obvious signs of their hidden cardiac defect. Clubbing and small, thin stature in older children further indicate severe heart disease. Body image concerns are important; these children are often teased about their appearance and singled out as different. Adolescents are especially concerned about their body image, and cyanosis can become a particular issue for them. Many children, when asked what surgery will do, reply, "Make me pink." Their joy

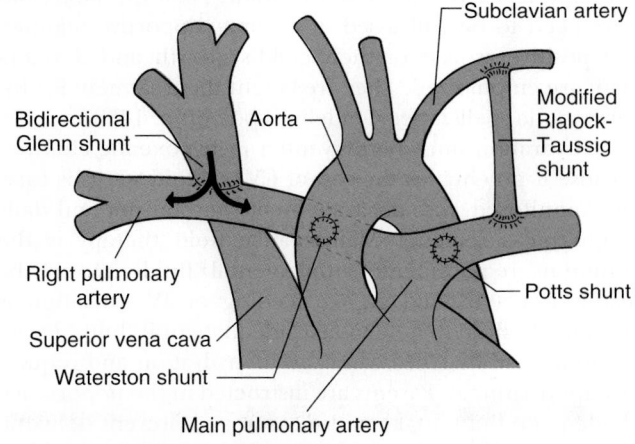

**Fig. 34-12** Schematic diagram of cardiac shunts.

| TABLE 34-6 Shunt procedures for children with cardiac defects | |
| --- | --- |
| **Type of Shunt/Location** | **Comments** |
| **Blalock-Taussig (BT)**<br>Subclavian artery to pulmonary artery | Replaced by modified version<br>More difficult to perform in small infants because of small subclavian artery<br>Ligation of subclavian artery may cause growth retardation in affected arm |
| **Modified Blalock-Taussig**<br>Subclavian artery or pulmonary artery using Gore-Tex or Impra tube graft | Shunt flow sometimes excessive, requiring use of diuretics<br>Possibility of thrombosis; antiplatelet therapy may be used postoperatively<br>Easy to ligate at time of definitive correction<br>Shunt size fixed and may become too small as child grows |
| **Central**<br>Ascending aorta to main pulmonary aorta using Gore-Tex graft | Length of shunt acts to restrict blood flow, limiting symptoms of CHF; may require diuretics<br>Uncommon; used when BT shunt or modified BT shunt cannot be done<br>Easy to perform and remove at time of repair |
| **Classic Glenn**<br>Superior vena cava to side of right pulmonary artery, which is ligated from main pulmonary artery<br>Blood flow to right lung only | Used as a second shunt procedure if complete repair not possible<br>High mortality in infants under age 6 months<br>Superior vena cava syndrome may occur<br>Pulmonary arteriovenous fistulas may occur many years later<br>Difficult to take down at time of definitive repair |
| **Bidirectional Glenn (cavopulmonary anastomosis)**<br>Superior vena cava to side of right pulmonary artery<br>Blood flow to both lungs | Done as a second shunt; often as a staging step to a Fontan procedure<br>Can be incorporated into eventual modified Fontan procedure<br>Relieves cyanosis and decreases volume overload on ventricle |

NOTE: Two early shunt procedures—Waterston shunt (ascending aorta to right pulmonary artery) and Potts shunt (descending aorta to left pulmonary artery)—are no longer performed because of problems with excessive pulmonary blood flow and distortion of the pulmonary arteries. Adult patients may have had these shunts done as their initial repair.

and excitement following surgery are evident when they see their pink fingers. Accentuating the normal and positive and being careful not to call attention to their cyanosis are helpful interventions. Meeting other children who are cyanotic in the clinic or hospital reassures them that they are not the only ones who are blue.

Parents are often fearful of their child's bluish color because cyanosis is usually associated with lack of oxygen and severe illness. They also must deal with comments from relatives, friends, and strangers in the community about their child's abnormal color. They need a simple explanation of hypoxemia and cyanosis and reassurance that cyanosis does not imply a lack of oxygen to the brain. Their questions and fears need to be addressed in a calm, supportive manner, and positive aspects of their child's growth and development are emphasized. They are taught the treatment for hypercyanotic spells. (See Guidelines box on p. 1488.)

Dehydration must be prevented in hypoxemic children because it potentiates the risk of CVAs. Fluid status is carefully monitored, with accurate intake and output and daily weight measurements. Maintenance fluid therapy is the minimum requirement; supplemental fluids should be readily available, and gavage feeding or IV hydration is given to children unable to take adequate oral fluids. Fever, vomiting, and diarrhea can cause dehydration and require prompt treatment. Parents are instructed in the importance of adequate fluid intake and measures to prevent dehydration. An oral electrolyte solution such as Pedialyte should be available at home in the event that the infant is unable to tolerate the usual formula. The practitioner should be notified of fever, vomiting, diarrhea, or other problems.

Preventive measures and accurate assessment of respiratory infection are important nursing considerations. Any compromise in pulmonary function will increase the infant's hypoxemia. Good handwashing and protection from individuals with an obvious respiratory infection are important. Aggressive pulmonary hygiene, treatment with antibiotics or antiviral agents as indicated, and supplemental oxygen to decrease hypoxemia are necessary measures. Infants may need to be gavage fed or given parenteral hydration if respiratory distress prevents oral feeding.

> **NURSING ALERT** Intracardiac shunting of blood from the right side (desaturated) to the left side of the heart allows air in the venous system to go directly to the brain, resulting in an air embolism. Therefore all IV lines should have filters in place to prevent air from entering the system, and the entire tubing and any syringes used for flushing or administering medication are checked for air. Any air is removed, and all connections are taped securely.

## Pulmonary Artery Hypertension

Pulmonary artery hypertension (PAH) describes a group of rare disorders that result in an elevation of pulmonary artery pressure above 25 mm Hg at rest after the neonatal period (Barst, 1999). These disorders are poorly understood, and until recently there was no treatment beyond supportive care. PAH is a progressive, eventually fatal disease for which there is no known cure. It can be difficult to diagnose in the early stages. Often when patients become symptomatic and a diagnosis is made, their disease is rapidly progressing, treatment is unsuccessful, and death occurs within several years. Recent therapeutic advances, including anticoagulation and vasodilator therapy with nitric oxide and prostacyclin, have improved the outlook for this group of patients. Improvements in quality of life, exercise capacity, pulmonary hemodynamics, and long-term survival have been seen (Barst, 1999).

PAH can be caused by increased pulmonary blood flow or increased pulmonary vascular resistance. Why some children develop the disease and others do not is unclear. There are many possible causes of PAH. Cardiac causes occur primarily in patients with a large left-to-right shunt (such as in ventricular septal defect [VSD], patent ductus arteriosis [PDA], or complete atrioventricular canal [CAVC]) producing increased pulmonary blood flow. If these defects are not repaired early, the high pulmonary flow will cause changes in the pulmonary artery vessels and the vessels will lose their elasticity. This causes increased resistance in the pulmonary bed and results in eventual right heart failure because the heart cannot pump against the greater resistance. The flow of blood becomes right to left, and cyanosis is seen. This is known as Eisenmenger's syndrome. Other causes of PAH include hypoxic lung diseases, thromboembolic diseases causing pulmonary vascular obstruction, collagen vascular diseases, and exposure to toxic substances. Many of the patients have no identifiable cause for PAH and have primary or idiopathic PAH.

The diagnostic workup is extensive and includes evaluation of cardiac and pulmonary function, coagulation studies, collagen vascular evaluation, and other studies. An evaluation for possible transplantation may also be indicated. A cardiac catheterization is done to evaluate the degree of pulmonary hypertension and the response to vasodilator therapy. Oxygen, nitric oxide, and prostacyclin may all be used during the catheterization to assess the ability of various therapies to reduce pulmonary artery pressure.

The mechanisms that cause PAH are poorly understood. It is likely that injury to the vascular endothelium in the pulmonary arteries or imbalances in the production or metabolism of vasoactive mediators leads to the release of vasoconstrictive substances, which causes changes in the vessel wall, muscular proliferation, progressive vascular obstruction, and eventual obliteration of the vessel (Barst, 1999). Another hypothesis maintains that primary pulmonary hypertension is a disease of individuals with overly reactive lung vessels and exposure to various stimuli causes vasoconstriction and eventual obstruction (Wagenvoort and Wagenvoort, 1977).

### Clinical Manifestations

The clinical manifestations include dyspnea with exercise, chest pain, and syncope. Dyspnea is the most common symptom and is caused by impaired oxygen delivery. Chest pain is the result of coronary ischemia in the right ventricle from severe hypertrophy. Syncope reflects a limited cardiac output leading to decreased cerebral blood flow. Right heart dysfunction is steadily progressive as the pulmonary vessels become obstructed and the pulmonary artery pressure increases. The right ventricle hypertrophies to attempt to maintain a normal cardiac output. With time and continued increases in pulmonary vascular resistance, the cardiac output decreases. When signs of right heart failure with systemic venous congestion and edema are evident, the prognosis is poor.

### Therapeutic Management

Although no cure is known, several therapies have shown promise in slowing the progression of the disease and improving quality of life. In general, situations that may exacerbate the disease and cause hypoxia are avoided. Exercise should be limited if symptoms are increased. High altitudes should be avoided because of the relative hypoxia, and some patients have moved to sea level to slow the progress of the disease. Supplemental oxygen, especially at night while sleeping, is commonly used to relieve hypoxia. Patients with PAH are at risk for thromboembolic events. Anticoagulation has been shown to increase survival in adults. Many patients are treated with warfarin (Coumadin) to prevent pulmonary emboli, which can be a fatal event. Digoxin and diuretics are often used to treat right heart failure.

Vasodilator therapy has improved the survival of patients with PAH. Vasodilators reduce pulmonary artery pressure by relaxing vascular smooth muscle and increasing cardiac output. The limiting factor is systemic hypotension. Oral calcium channel blockers have been successful in about 40% of children. Younger patients and those who had a favorable response to vasodilator therapy during cardiac catheterization are most likely to do well on calcium channel blockers. Five-year survival was 97% in this group compared to 35% in the children who did not respond to vasodilator therapy (Barst, 1999).

Continuous IV prostacyclin or chronic inhaled nitric oxide have been used with some success in the 60% of children who did not respond to a trial of vasodilation during catheterization. Prostacyclin imitates a natural prostacyclin that dilates smooth muscle. It also prevents thrombus formation. It is given by a continuous IV infusion through an indwelling catheter with a portable battery-operated pump. Improved 5-year survival (92%) has been shown with this treatment compared with only 29% in untreated patients (Barst, 1999). Side effects include hypotension, pulmonary edema, headaches, facial flushing, and jaw pain. Nitric oxide is an endothelium-derived relaxing factor. When inhaled, it can relax pulmonary vascular smooth muscle. It is short-acting and is inactivated by contact with hemoglobin in the capillary bed. It is a selective pulmonary vasodilator with minimal hemodynamic side effects. Nitric oxide has been used most often in the ICU to manage acute pulmonary hypertensive crisis following congenital cardiac surgery or for diagnostic purposes in the cardiac catheterization laboratory. The experience with chronic use in the outpatient setting is limited (Channick and others, 1996).

Lung transplantation may be another treatment option for children, especially for those with primary pulmonary hypertension who tend to have rapid progression of their disease. The use of vasodilator therapy may be a bridge to transplantation.

### Nursing Considerations

The diagnosis of pulmonary artery hypertension is devastating for the child and family. There is no known cure, and the treatments require significant lifestyle changes and commitment on the part of patient and family to make them successful. Anxiety, depression, and fear of the future are common. Patients and families require extensive education about the disease and its management. They need emotional support to cope with a poor prognosis and make decisions about treatment options.

The medical treatment is complex and involves different medications and therapies. Families are often referred to a specialized center that has experience in the management of PAH. This involves travel far from home and the accompanying emotional and financial hardships. The patient and family must cope with the symptoms of the disease and the side effects of the treatment. Dealing with a continuous IV infusion or continuous oxygen or nitric oxide requires a major adjustment in lifestyle to accommodate the therapy. The prostacyclin infusion cannot be interrupted at any time because symptoms can worsen and cause acute pulmonary hypertensive crisis, which can be fatal. Back-up systems need to be in place at all times. The patient and family must make a commitment to adhere to a complex regimen of preparing the infusion, maintaining the equipment, and maintaining sterility of the central line. Nitric oxide is short acting, and the delivery of the gas must be continuous to prevent symptoms from worsening. Both these therapies are very expensive, so insurance coverage and financial issues must be considered. Nurses have an important role in preparing families to perform these complex therapies. Discharge planning involves many team members and outside agencies. The nurse has a pivotal role in coordinating the child's care in the hospital and the transition to home.

## Defects with Increased Pulmonary Blood Flow

In this group of cardiac defects, intracardiac communications along the septum or an abnormal connection between the great arteries allows blood to flow from the high-pressure left side of the heart to the lower-pressure right side of the heart (Fig. 34-13). Increased blood volume on the right side of the heart increases pulmonary blood flow at the expense of systemic blood flow. Clinically patients demonstrate signs and symptoms of CHF. Atrial and ventricular septal defects and patent ductus arteriosus are typical anomalies in this group (Box 34-2).

## Obstructive Defects

Obstructive defects are those in which blood exiting the heart meets an area of anatomic narrowing (stenosis), causing obstruction to blood flow. The pressure in the ventricle and in the great artery before the obstruction is increased, and the pressure in the area beyond the obstruction is decreased. The location of the narrowing is usually near the valve (Fig. 34-14):

**Valvular**—At the site of the valve itself
**Subvalvular**—Narrowing in the ventricle below the valve (also referred to as the *ventricular outflow tract*)
**Supravalvular**—Narrowing in the great artery above the valve

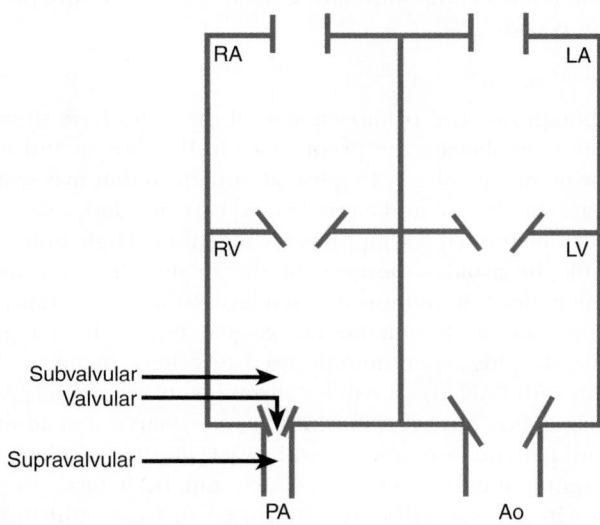

**Fig. 34-13** Hemodynamics in defects with increased pulmonary blood flow. See Fig. 34-2 for abbreviations.

Coarctation of the aorta (narrowing of the aortic arch), aortic stenosis, and pulmonic stenosis are typical defects in this group (Box 34-3). Hemodynamically there is a pressure load on the ventricle and decreased cardiac output. Clini-

*Text continued on p. 1496*

**Fig. 34-14** Obstruction to ventricular ejection can occur at the valvular level (shown), below the valve (subvalvular), or above the valve (supravalvular). Pulmonary stenosis is shown here. See Fig. 34-2 for abbreviations.

---

## Box 34-2 ■ ■ ■
### Defects with Increased Pulmonary Blood Flow

**ATRIAL SEPTAL DEFECT (ASD)**

**Description:** Abnormal opening between the atria, allowing blood from the higher-pressure left atrium to flow into the lower-pressure right atrium. There are three types:

*Ostium primum (ASD 1)*—Opening at lower end of septum; may be associated with mitral valve abnormalities
*Ostium secundum (ASD 2)*—Opening near center of septum
*Sinus venosus defect*—Opening near junction of superior vena cava and right atrium; may be associated with partial anomalous pulmonary venous connection

**Pathophysiology:** Because left atrial pressure slightly exceeds right atrial pressure, blood flows from the left to the right atrium, causing an increased flow of oxygenated blood into the right side of the heart. Despite the low pressure difference, a high rate of flow can still occur because of low pulmonary vascular resistance and the greater distensibility of the right atrium, which further reduces flow resistance. This volume is well tolerated by the right ventricle because it is delivered under much lower pressure than in a ventricular septal defect. Although there is right atrial and ventricular enlargement, cardiac failure is unusual in an uncomplicated ASD. Pulmonary vascular changes usually occur only after several decades if the defect is unrepaired.

**Clinical manifestations:** Patients may be asymptomatic. They may develop congestive heart failure (CHF). There is a characteristic murmur. Patients are at risk for atrial dysrhythmias (probably caused by atrial enlargement and stretching of conduction fibers) and pulmonary vascular obstructive disease and emboli formation later in life from chronic increased pulmonary blood flow.

**Surgical treatment:** Surgical patch closure (pericardial patch or Dacron patch) of moderate to large defects similar to closure of ventricular septal defects. Open repair with cardiopulmonary

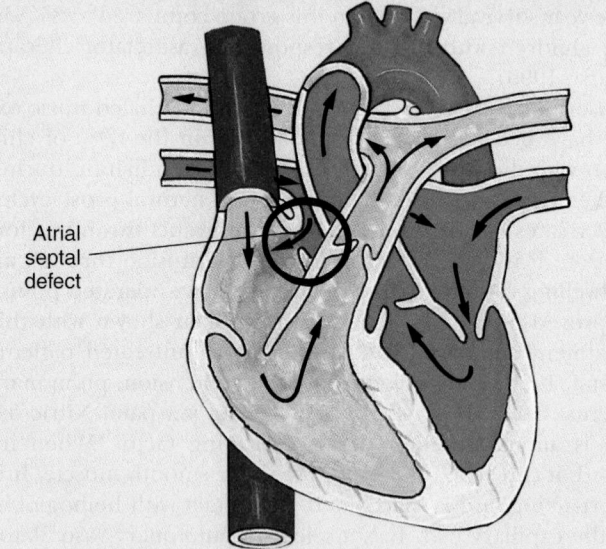

Atrial septal defect

bypass is usually performed before school age. In addition, the sinus venosus defect requires patch placement, so the anomalous right pulmonary venous return is directed to the left atrium with a baffle. The ASD 1 may require mitral valve repair or, rarely, replacement of the mitral valve.

**Nonsurgical treatment:** ASD 2 may also be closed using devices during cardiac catheterization. This technique is in clinical trials in some centers.

**Prognosis:** Very low operative mortality, less than 1%.

**Box 34-2** ■ ■ ■
**Defects with Increased Pulmonary Blood Flow—cont'd**

### VENTRICULAR SEPTAL DEFECT (VSD)

**Description:** Abnormal opening between the right and left ventricles. May be classified according to location: membranous (accounting for 80%) or muscular. May vary in size from a small pinhole to absence of the septum, resulting in a common ventricle. Frequently associated with other defects, such as pulmonary stenosis, transposition of the great vessels, patent ductus arteriosus, atrial defects, and coarctation of the aorta. Many VSDs (20% to 60%) are thought to close spontaneously. Spontaneous closure is most likely to occur during the first year of life in children having small or moderate defects. A left-to-right shunt is caused by the flow of blood from the higher-pressure left ventricle to the lower-pressure right ventricle.

**Pathophysiology:** Because of the higher pressure within the left ventricle and because the systemic arterial circulation offers more resistance than the pulmonary circulation, blood flows through the defect into the pulmonary artery. The increased blood volume is pumped into the lungs, which may eventually result in increased pulmonary vascular resistance. Increased pressure in the right ventricle as a result of left-to-right shunting and pulmonary resistance causes the muscle to hypertrophy. If the right ventricle is unable to accommodate the increased workload, the right atrium may also enlarge as it attempts to overcome the resistance offered by incomplete right ventricular emptying. In severe defects, Eisenmenger syndrome may develop (see p. 1486).

**Clinical manifestations:** CHF is common. There is a characteristic murmur. Patients are at risk for bacterial endocarditis and pulmonary vascular obstructive disease. In severe defects, Eisenmenger syndrome may develop.

**Surgical treatment:**
*Palliative:* Pulmonary artery banding (placing a band around the main pulmonary artery to decrease pulmonary blood flow) in infants may be done with multiple muscular VSDs or complex anatomy. Improvements in surgical techniques and postoperative care make complete repair in infancy the preferred approach.
*Complete repair (procedure of choice):* Small defects are repaired with a pursestring approach. Large defects usually require a

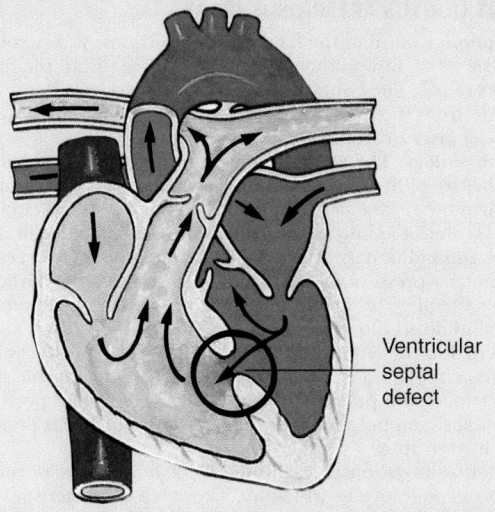

Ventricular septal defect

knitted Dacron patch sewn over the opening. Both procedures are performed via cardiopulmonary bypass. The repair is generally approached through the right atrium and the tricuspid valve. Postoperative complications include residual VSD and conduction disturbances.

**Nonsurgical treatment:** Device closure during cardiac catheterization is under clinical trials in some centers for closure of muscular defects that carry a high operative risk.

**Prognosis:** Risks depend on the location of the defect, number of defects, and other associated cardiac defects. Single membranous defects have a low mortality (less than 5%); multiple muscular defects can have a risk of more than 20%.

### ATRIOVENTRICULAR CANAL (AVC) DEFECT

**Description:** Incomplete fusion of endocardial cushions. Consists of a low atrial septal defect that is continuous with a high ventricular septal defect and clefts of the mitral and tricuspid valves, creating a large central atrioventricular (AV) valve that allows blood to flow between all four chambers of the heart. The directions and pathways of flow are determined by pulmonary and systemic resistance, left and right ventricular pressures, and the compliance of each chamber, although flow is generally from left to right. It is the most common cardiac defect in children with Down syndrome.

**Pathophysiology:** The alterations in the hemodynamics depend on the defect's severity and the child's pulmonary vascular resistance. Immediately after birth, while the newborn's pulmonary vascular resistance is high, there is minimum shunting of blood through the defect. Once this resistance falls, left-to-right shunting occurs and pulmonary blood flow increases. The resultant pulmonary vascular engorgement predisposes to development of CHF.

**Clinical manifestations:** Patients usually have moderate to severe CHF. There is a characteristic murmur. There may be mild cyanosis that increases with crying. Patients are at high risk for developing pulmonary vascular obstructive disease.

**Surgical treatment:**
*Palliative:* Pulmonary artery banding for infants less than 5 kg with severe symptoms may be done. Complete repair in infancy is recommended.
*Complete repair:* Surgical repair consists of patch closure of the septal defects and reconstruction of the AV valve tissue (either repair of the mitral valve cleft or fashioning two AV valves). If the mitral valve defect is severe, a valve replacement

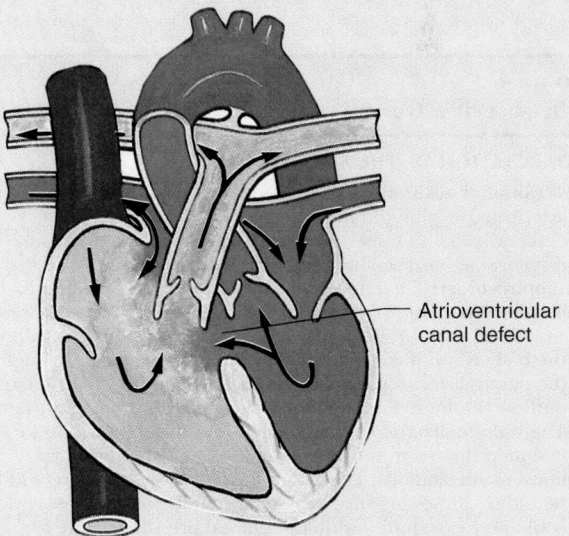

Atrioventricular canal defect

may be needed. Postoperative complications include heart block, CHF, mitral regurgitation, dysrhythmias, and pulmonary hypertension.

**Prognosis:** Operative mortality is less than 10%. Potential later problem is mitral regurgitation, which may require valve replacement.

*Continued*

## Box 34-2 ■ ■ ■
### Defects with Increased Pulmonary Blood Flow—cont'd

### PATENT DUCTUS ARTERIOSUS (PDA)

**Description:** Failure of the fetal ductus arteriosus (artery connecting the aorta and pulmonary artery) to close within the first weeks of life. The continued patency of this vessel allows blood to flow from the higher-pressure aorta to the lower-pressure pulmonary artery, causing a left-to-right shunt.

**Pathophysiology:** The hemodynamic consequences of PDA depend on the size of the ductus and the pulmonary vascular resistance. At birth the resistance in the pulmonary and systemic circulations is almost identical, thus equalizing the resistance in the aorta and pulmonary artery. As the systemic pressure exceeds the pulmonary pressure, blood begins to shunt from the aorta, across the duct, to the pulmonary artery (left-to-right shunt). The additional blood is recirculated through the lungs and returned to the left atrium and left ventricle. The effect of this altered circulation is increased workload on the left side of the heart, increased pulmonary vascular congestion and possibly resistance, and potentially increased right ventricular pressure and hypertrophy.

**Clinical manifestations:** Patients may be asymptomatic or show signs of congestive heart failure. There is a characteristic machinery-like murmur. A widened pulse pressure and bounding pulses result from runoff of blood from the aorta to the pulmonary artery. Patients are at risk for bacterial endocarditis and pulmonary vascular obstructive disease in later life from chronic excessive pulmonary blood flow.

**Medical management:** Administration of indomethacin (prostaglandin inhibitor) has proved successful in closing a patent ductus in premature infants and some newborns.

**Surgical treatment:** Surgical division or ligation of the patent vessel via a left thoracotomy. A newer technique, visual assisted thoracoscopic surgery (VATS), uses a thoracoscope and instruments placed through three small incisions on the left side of the chest

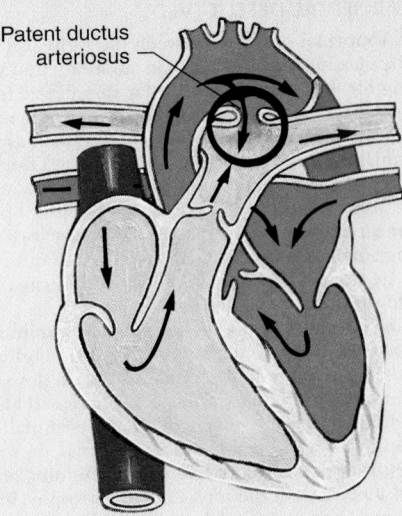

Patent ductus arteriosus

to place a clip on the ductus. It is used in some centers and eliminates the need for a thoracotomy, thereby speeding postoperative recovery.

**Nonsurgical treatment:** Use of coils to occlude the PDA in the catheterization laboratory is done in many centers. Small infants (with small-diameter femoral arteries) and those patients with large or unusual PDAs may require surgery.

**Prognosis:** Both procedures can be done at low risk with less than 1% mortality.

## Box 34-3 ■ ■ ■
### Obstructive Defects

### COARCTATION OF THE AORTA (COA)

**Description:** Localized narrowing near the insertion of the ductus arteriosus, resulting in increased pressure proximal to the defect (head and upper extremities) and decreased pressure distal to the obstruction (body and lower extremities).

**Pathophysiology:** The effect of a narrowing within the aorta is increased pressure proximal to the defect and decreased pressure distal to it. In the preductal type of COA the lower half of the body is supplied with blood by the right ventricle through the ductus arteriosus. In the postductal type, right ventricular outflow cannot maintain blood flow to the descending aorta. Therefore collateral circulation develops during fetal life to maintain flow from the ascending to the descending aorta.

**Clinical manifestations:** There may be high blood pressure and bounding pulses in arms, weak or absent femoral pulses, and cool lower extremities with lower blood pressure. There are signs of congestive heart failure (CHF) in infants. Often these patients' hemodynamic condition deteriorates rapidly, and they are admitted to the intensive care unit near death, usually severely acidotic and hypotensive. Mechanical ventilation and inotropic support are often necessary before surgery. Older children may experience dizziness, headaches, fainting, and epistaxis resulting from hypertension. Patients are at risk for hypertension, ruptured aorta, aortic aneurysm, or stroke.

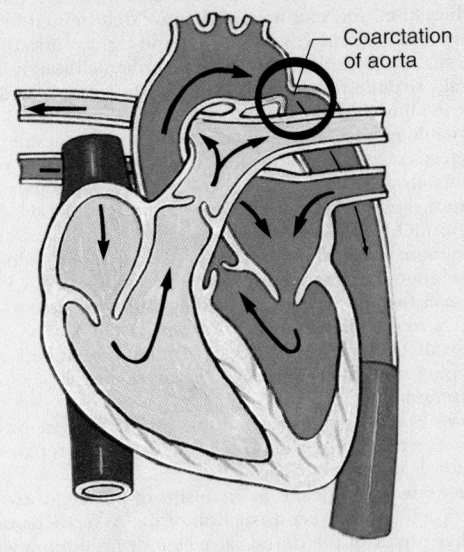

Coarctation of aorta

## Box 34-3 ■ ■ ■
## Obstructive Defects—cont'd

### COARCTATION OF THE AORTA (COA)—cont'd

**Surgical treatment:** Either resection of the coarcted portion with an end-to-end anastomosis of the aorta or enlargement of the constricted section using a graft of prosthetic material or a portion of the left subclavian artery. Because this defect is outside the heart and pericardium, cardiopulmonary bypass is not required and a thoracotomy incision is used. Postoperative hypertension (greater than 160 mm Hg) is treated with intravenous sodium nitroprusside or amrinone, followed by oral medications, such as captopril, hydralazine, or propranolol. Residual permanent hypertension after repair of COA seems to be related to age and time of repair. To prevent both hypertension at rest and exercise-provoked systemic hypertension after repair, elective surgery for COA is advised within the first 2 years of life. There is a 15% to 30% risk of recurrence in patients who underwent surgical repair as infants (Beekman, 2001). Percutaneous balloon angioplasty techniques have proved to be very effective in relieving residual postoperative coarctation gradients.

**Nonsurgical treatment:** Balloon angioplasty as a primary intervention for COA is being performed in some centers. Recent studies have demonstrated that balloon angioplasty is effective in children and that aneurysm formation is rare. The high restenosis rate in infants less than 7 months of age limits its application in this group (Allen and others, 1998).

**Prognosis:** Less than 5% mortality in patients with isolated coarctation; increased risk in infants with other complex cardiac defects.

### AORTIC STENOSIS (AS)

**Description:** Narrowing or stricture of the aortic valve, causing resistance to blood flow in the left ventricle, decreased cardiac output, left ventricular hypertrophy, and pulmonary vascular congestion. The prominent anatomic consequence of AS is the hypertrophy of the left ventricular wall, which eventually will lead to increased end-diastolic pressure, resulting in pulmonary venous and pulmonary arterial hypertension. Left ventricular hypertrophy also interferes with coronary artery perfusion and may result in myocardial infarction or scarring of the papillary muscles of the left ventricle, causing mitral insufficiency. *Valvular stenosis,* the most common type, is usually caused by malformed cusps resulting in a bicuspid rather than tricuspid valve or fusion of the cusps. *Subvalvular stenosis* is a stricture caused by a fibrous ring below a normal valve; *supravalvular stenosis* occurs infrequently. Valvular AS is a serious defect for the following reasons: (1) the obstruction tends to be progressive; (2) sudden episodes of myocardial ischemia, or low cardiac output, can result in sudden death; and (3) surgical repair rarely results in a normal valve. This is one of the rare instances in which strenuous physical activity may be curtailed because of the cardiac condition.

**Pathophysiology:** A stricture in the aortic outfow tract causes resistance to ejection of blood from the left ventricle. The extra workload on the left ventricle causes hypertrophy. If left ventricular failure develops, left atrial pressure will increase; this causes increased pressure in the pulmonary veins, resulting in pulmonary vascular congestion (pulmonary edema).

**Clinical manifestations:** Infants with severe defects demonstrate signs of decreased cardiac output with faint pulses, hypotension, tachycardia, and poor feeding. Children show signs of exercise intolerance, chest pain, and dizziness when standing for a long period. There is a characteristic murmur. Patients are at risk for bacterial endocarditis, coronary insufficiency, and ventricular dysfunction.

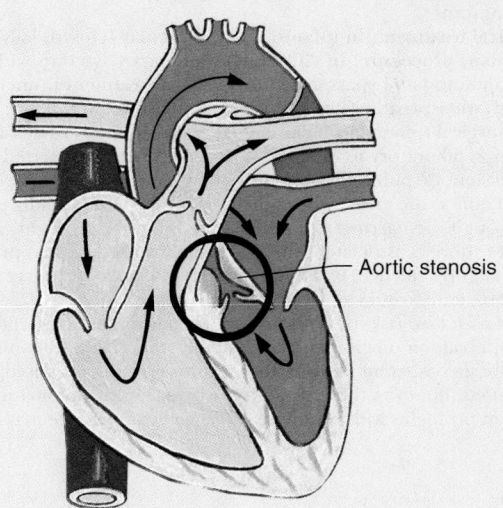

Aortic stenosis

#### Valvular Aortic Stenosis

**Surgical treatment:** Aortic valvotomy under inflow occlusion.

**Prognosis:** Aortic valvotomy in critically ill neonates and infants still carries a mortality of 10% to 20% in major medical centers (Hawkins and others, 1998). Results of aortic valvotomy in older children are very good, with mortality close to 0%. However, aortic valvotomy remains a palliative procedure, and approximately 25% of patients require additional surgery within 10 years for recurrent stenosis. A valve replacement may be required at the second procedure. An aortic homograft with a valve may also be used *(extended aortic root replacement),* or the pulmonary valve may be moved to the aortic position and replaced with a homograft valve *(Ross procedure).*

**Nonsurgical treatment:** Dilating narrowed valve with balloon angioplasty in the catheterization laboratory.

**Prognosis:** Complications include aortic insufficiency or valvular regurgitation, tearing of the valve leaflets, and loss of pulse in the catheterized limb. Relief of obstruction is similar to that for surgical valvotomy (Allen and others, 1998).

#### Subvalvular Aortic Stenosis

**Surgical treatment:** May involve incising a membrane if one exists or cutting the fibromuscular ring. If the obstruction results from narrowing of the left ventricular outflow tract and a small aortic valve annulus, a patch may be required to enlarge the entire left ventricular outflow tract and annulus and replace the aortic valve, an approach known as the *Konno* procedure.

**Prognosis:** Mortality from surgical repairs of subvalvular AS is less than 5% in major centers; however, about 20% of these patients develop recurrent subaortic stenosis and require additional surgery (Freed, 2001).

*Continued*

**Box 34-3** ■ ■ □
## Obstructive Defects—cont'd

### PULMONIC STENOSIS (PS)

**Description:** Narrowing at the entrance to the pulmonary artery. Resistance to blood flow causes right ventricular hypertrophy and decreased pulmonary blood flow. *Pulmonary atresia* is the extreme form of PS in that there is total fusion of the commissures and no blood flows to the lungs. The right ventricle may be hypoplastic.

**Pathophysiology:** When PS is present, resistance to blood flow causes right ventricular hypertrophy. If right ventricular failure develops, right atrial pressure will increase, and this may result in reopening of the foramen ovale, shunting of unoxygenated blood into the left atrium, and systemic cyanosis. If PS is severe, CHF occurs, and systemic venous engorgement will be noted. An associated defect such as a patent ductus arteriosus (PDA) partially compensates for the obstruction by shunting blood from the aorta to the pulmonary artery and into the lungs.

**Clinical manifestations:** Patients may be asymptomatic; some have mild cyanosis or CHF. Newborns with severe narrowing will be cyanotic. There is a characteristic murmur. Cardiomegaly is evident on chest x-ray film. Patients are at risk for bacterial endocarditis, with progressive narrowing causing increased symptoms.

**Surgical treatment:** In infants, transventricular (closed) valvotomy (*Brock*) procedure. In children, pulmonary valvotomy with cardiopulmonary bypass. Need for surgical treatment is uncommon with widespread use of balloon angioplasty techniques.

**Nonsurgical treatment:** Balloon angioplasty in the cardiac catheterization laboratory to dilate the valve. A catheter is inserted across the stenotic pulmonic valve into the pulmonary artery, and a balloon at the end of the catheter is inflated and rapidly passed through the narrowed opening. (See figure below, right.) The procedure is associated with few complications and has proved to be highly effective. It is the treatment of choice for discrete PS in most centers and can be done safely in neonates.

**Prognosis:** Low risk for both procedures; less than 2% mortality. Both balloon dilation and surgical valvotomy leave the pulmonic valve incompetent because they involve opening the fused valve leaflets; however, these patients are clinically asymptomatic. Long-term problems with restenosis or valve incompetence may occur.

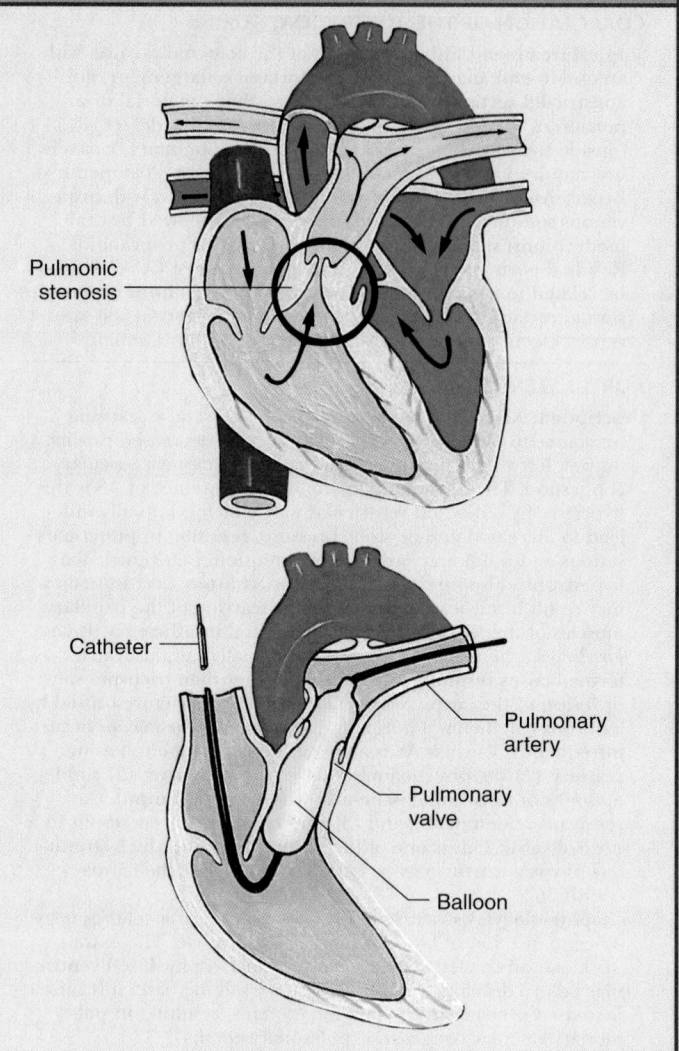

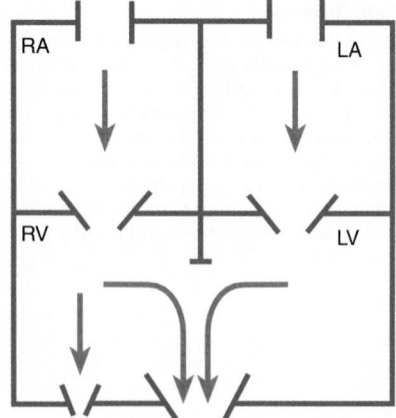

**Fig. 34-15** Hemodynamic defects with decreased pulmonary blood flow. See Fig. 34-2 for abbreviations.

cally infants and children exhibit signs of CHF. Children with mild obstruction may be asymptomatic. Rarely, as in severe pulmonic stenosis, hypoxemia may be seen.

## Defects with Decreased Pulmonary Blood Flow

In this group of defects, there is obstruction of pulmonary blood flow and an anatomic defect (atrial septal defect [ASD] or ventricular septal defect [VSD]) between the right and left sides of the heart (Fig. 34-15). Because blood has difficulty exiting the right side of the heart via the pulmonary artery, pressure on the right side increases, exceeding left-sided pressure. This allows desaturated blood to shunt right to left, causing desaturation in the left side of the heart and in the systemic circulation. Clinically these patients are hypoxemic and usually appear cyanotic. Tetralogy of Fallot and tricuspid atresia are the more common defects in this group (Box 34-4).

## Box 34-4 ■ ■ ■
## Defects with Decreased Pulmonary Blood Flow

### TETRALOGY OF FALLOT (TOF)

**Description:** The classic form includes four defects: (1) ventricular septal defect, (2) pulmonic stenosis, (3) overriding aorta, and (4) right ventricular hypertrophy.

**Pathophysiology:** The altered hemodynamics vary widely, depending primarily on the degree of pulmonary stenosis, but also on the size of the ventricular septal defect (VSD) and the pulmonary and systemic resistance to flow. Because the VSD is usually large, pressures may be equal in the right and left ventricles. Therefore the shunt direction depends on the difference between pulmonary and systemic vascular resistance. If pulmonary vascular resistance is higher than systemic resistance, the shunt is from right to left. If systemic resistance is higher than pulmonary resistance, the shunt is from left to right. Pulmonic stenosis decreases blood flow to the lungs and consequently the amount of oxygenated blood that returns to the left side of the heart. Depending on the position of the aorta, blood from both ventricles may be distributed systemically.

**Clinical manifestations:**

*Infants:* Some infants may be acutely cyanotic at birth; others have mild cyanosis that progresses over the first year of life as the pulmonic stenosis worsens. There is a characteristic murmur. There are acute episodes of cyanosis and hypoxia, called blue spells or tet spells (see p. 1488). Anoxic spells occur when the infant's oxygen requirements exceed the blood supply, usually during crying or after feeding. Patients are at risk for emboli, seizures, and loss of consciousness or sudden death following an anoxic spell.

**Surgical treatment:**

*Palliative shunt:* In infants who cannot undergo primary repair, a palliative procedure to increase pulmonary blood flow and increase oxygen saturation may be performed. The preferred procedure is the ***Blalock-Taussig*** or *modified Blalock-Taussig shunt,* which provides blood flow to the pulmonary arteries from the left or right subclavian artery. (See Table 34-6.) In general, however, shunts are avoided because they may result in pulmonary artery distortion.

*Complete repair:* Elective repair is usually performed in the first year of life. Indications for repair include increasing cyanosis and the development of hypercyanotic spells. Complete repair involves closure of the VSD and resection of the infundibular stenosis, with a pericardial patch to enlarge the right ventricular outflow tract. The procedure requires a median sternotomy and the use of cardiopulmonary bypass.

**Prognosis:** The operative mortality for total correction of TOF is less than 5%. With improved surgical techniques there is a lower incidence of dysrhythmias and sudden death; surgical heart block is rare. CHF may occur postoperatively.

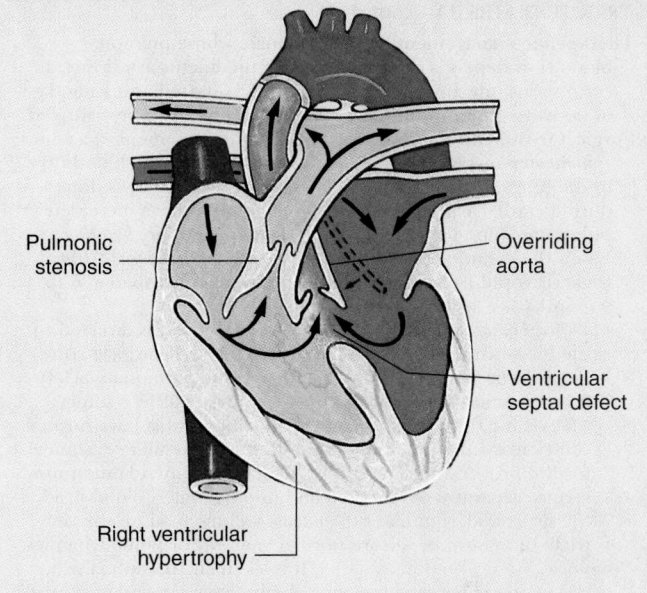

Pulmonic stenosis

Overriding aorta

Ventricular septal defect

Right ventricular hypertrophy

### TRICUSPID ATRESIA

**Description:** Failure of the tricuspid valve to develop; consequently there is no communication from the right atrium to the right ventricle. Blood flows through an atrial septal defect (ASD) or a patent foramen ovale to the left side of the heart and through a VSD to the right ventricle and out to the lungs. It is often associated with pulmonic stenosis and transposition of the great arteries. There is complete mixing of unoxygenated and oxygenated blood in the left side of the heart, resulting in systemic desaturation and varying amounts of pulmonary obstruction, causing decreased pulmonary blood flow.

**Pathophysiology:** At birth the presence of a patent foramen ovale (or other atrial septal opening) is required to permit blood flow across the septum into the left atrium; the patent ductus arteriosus allows blood flow to the pulmonary artery into the lungs for oxygenation. A VSD allows a modest amount of blood to enter the right ventricle and pulmonary artery for oxygenation. Pulmonary blood flow usually is diminished.

**Clinical manifestations:** Cyanosis is usually seen in the newborn period. There may be tachycardia and dyspnea. Older children have signs of chronic hypoxemia with clubbing. Patients are at risk for bacterial endocarditis, brain abscess, and stroke.

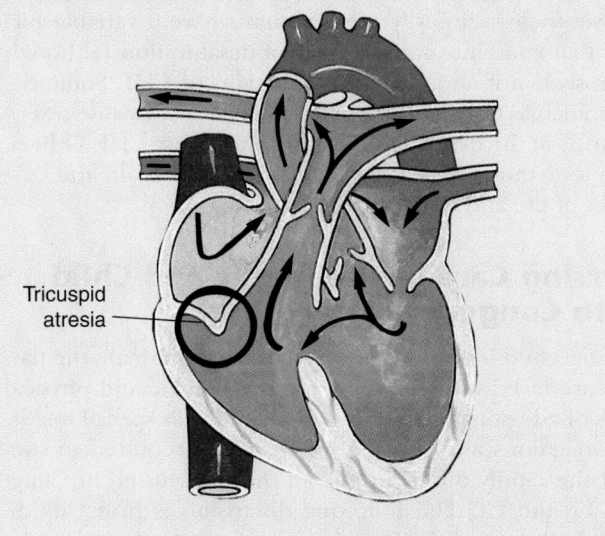

Tricuspid atresia

*Continued*

## Box 34-4 ■ ■ ■
## Defects with Decreased Pulmonary Blood Flow—cont'd

### TRICUSPID ATRESIA—cont'd

**Therapeutic management:** For the neonate whose pulmonary blood flow depends on the patency of the ductus arteriosus, a continuous infusion of prostaglandin $E_1$ is started at 0.1 mg/kg of body weight/min until surgical intervention can be arranged.

**Surgical treatment:** *Palliative* treatment is the placement of a shunt *(pulmonary–to–systemic artery anastomosis)* to increase blood flow to the lungs. If the ASD is small, an atrial septostomy is done during cardiac catheterization. Some children have increased pulmonary blood flow and require *pulmonary artery banding* to lessen the volume of blood to the lungs. A *bidirectional Glenn shunt* (cavopulmonary anastomosis) may be performed at 6 to 9 months as a second stage.

*Modified Fontan procedure:* Systemic venous return is directed to the lungs without a ventricular pump through surgical connections between the right atrium and the pulmonary artery. A fenestration (opening) in the right atrial baffle is sometimes done to relieve pressure. The patient must have normal ventricular function and a low pulmonary vascular resistance for the procedure to be successful. The modified Fontan procedure separates oxygenated and unoxygenated blood inside the heart and eliminates the excess volume load on the ventricle but does not restore normal anatomy or hemodynamics.

**Prognosis:** Surgical mortality varies. It is less than 10% in many centers and increases with more complex anatomy and other risk factors. Postoperative complications include dysrhythmias, systemic venous hypertension, pleural and pericardial effusions, and ventricular dysfunction. Long-term concerns are the development of protein-losing enteropathy, atrial dysrhythmias, late ventricular dysfunction, and developmental delays.

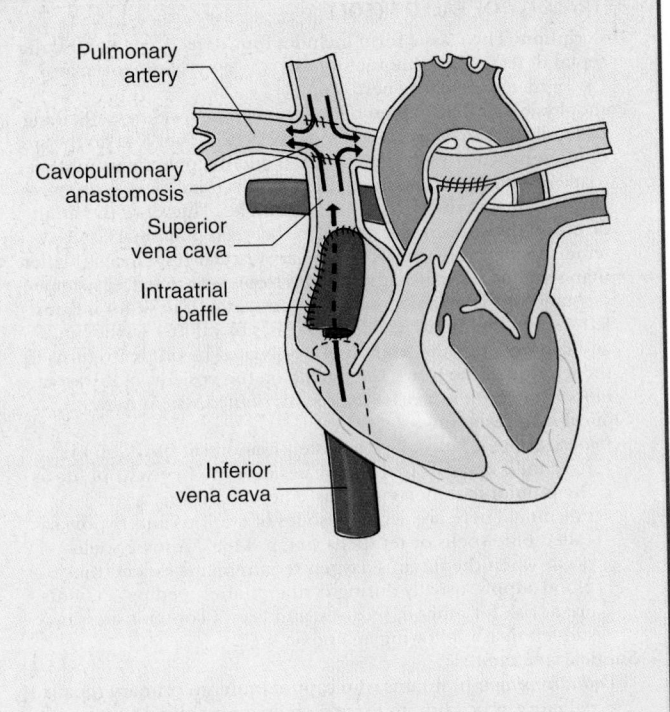

## Mixed Defects

Many complex cardiac anomalies are classified together in the *mixed* category (Box 34-5) because survival in the postnatal period depends on mixing of blood from the pulmonary and systemic circulations within the heart chambers. Hemodynamically, fully saturated systemic blood flow mixes with the desaturated pulmonary blood flow, causing a relative desaturation of the systemic blood flow. Pulmonary congestion occurs because the differences in pulmonary artery pressure and aortic pressure favor pulmonary blood flow. Cardiac output decreases because of a volume load on the ventricle. Clinically these patients have a variable picture that combines some degree of desaturation (although cyanosis is not always visible) and signs of CHF. Some defects, such as transposition of the great arteries, cause severe cyanosis in the first days of life and later cause CHF. Others, such as truncus arteriosus, cause severe CHF in the first weeks of life and mild desaturation.

## Nursing Care of the Family and Child with Congenital Heart Disease

When a child is born with a severe cardiac anomaly, the parents are faced with the immense psychologic and physical tasks of adjusting to the birth of a child with special needs. The reactions and nursing interventions required to support the family differ little from those discussed in Chapters 11 and 22. The following discussion is primarily directed (1) toward the family of an infant who has a serious heart defect and requires home care before definitive repair and (2) toward preparation and care of the child and family when heart surgery is performed. For nursing care related to the child with hypoxemia and CHF, the reader should refer to earlier discussions of these topics.

Nursing care of the child with a congenital heart defect begins as soon as the diagnosis is suspected. Prenatal diagnosis of congenital heart defects is becoming increasingly frequent. New demands are being placed on nurses to counsel and support families, as well as assess the fetus with known heart defects as families prepare for the birth of these infants.

### Help Family Adjust to the Disorder

Once parents learn of the heart defect, they are initially in a period of shock, followed by high anxiety, especially fear of the child's death. This reaction may occur soon after the child's birth or at a later period in life. Whatever its timing, the family needs a period of grief before assimilating the meaning of the defect. Unfortunately, the demands for medical treatment may not allow this, necessitating that the parents be informed of the condition in order to give informed consent for diagnostic/therapeutic procedures. The nurse can be instrumental in supporting parents in their loss, assessing their level of understanding, supplying information as needed, and helping other members of the health team to understand the parents' reactions.

Severely distressed newborns usually remain in the hospital. This can seriously affect parent-infant attachment unless parents are encouraged to hold, touch, and look at

*Text continued on p. 1501*

## Box 34-5 ■ ■ ■
## Mixed Defects

### TRANSPOSITION OF THE GREAT ARTERIES (TGA) OR TRANSPOSITION OF THE GREAT VESSELS (TGV)

**Description:** The pulmonary artery leaves the left ventricle, and the aorta exits from the right ventricle, with no communication between the systemic and pulmonary circulations.

**Pathophysiology:** Associated defects such as septal defects or patent ductus arteriosus must be present to permit blood to enter the systemic circulation or the pulmonary circulation for mixing of saturated and desaturated blood. The most common defect associated with TGA is a patent foramen ovale. At birth there is also a patent ductus arteriosus (PDA), although in most instances this closes after the neonatal period. Another associated anomaly may be a ventricular septal defect (VSD). The presence of these defects increases the risk of congestive heart failure (CHF), because they often produce high pulmonary blood flow under high pressure. For example, a large VSD permits blood to flow from the right to the left ventricle, into the pulmonary artery, and finally to the lungs. However, it also produces high pulmonary blood flow under high pressure, which can result in pulmonary vascular resistance. The same series of events occurs with a large PDA, because blood directly from the aorta flows under high pressure into the pulmonary artery and lungs.

**Clinical manifestations:** Depend on the type and size of the associated defects. Children with minimum communication are severely cyanotic and depressed at birth. Those with large septal defects or a patent ductus arteriosus may be less severely cyanotic but may have symptoms of congestive heart failure (CHF). Heart sounds vary according to the type of defect present. Cardiomegaly is usually evident a few weeks after birth.

**Therapeutic management:**

*To provide intracardiac mixing:* The administration of intravenous prostaglandin $E_1$ may be initiated to temporarily increase blood mixing if systemic and pulmonary mixing is inadequate to provide an oxygen saturation of 75% or to maintain cardiac output. During cardiac catheterization a balloon atrial septostomy *(Rashkind procedure)* may also be performed to increase mixing and maintain cardiac output over a longer period.

**Surgical treatment:**

*Arterial switch procedure:* Procedure of choice performed in first weeks of life. Involves transecting the great arteries and anastomosing the main pulmonary artery to the proximal aorta (just above the aortic valve) and anastomosing the ascending aorta to the proximal pulmonary artery. The coronary arteries are switched from the proximal aorta to the proximal pulmonary artery, creating a new aorta. Reimplantation of the coronary arteries is critical to the infant's survival, and they must be reattached without torsion or kinking to provide the heart with its supply of oxygen. The advantage of the arterial switch procedure is the reestablishment of normal circulation, with the left ventricle acting as the systemic pump. Potential complications of the arterial switch include narrowing at the great artery anastomoses or coronary artery insufficiency.

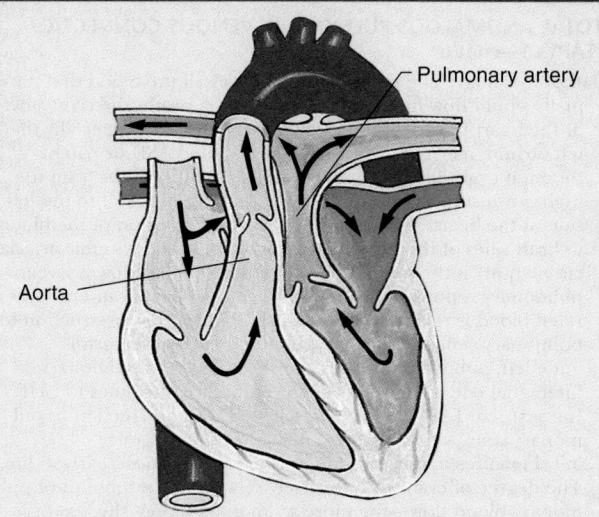

Pulmonary artery

Aorta

**Prognosis:** Operative mortality is less than 5% in most centers (Wernovsky and Jonas, 1998). Long-term problems include suprapulmonic stenosis (5% to 30%) and neoaorta dilation and regurgitation. Long-term outcomes are excellent with more than 90% survival with excellent cardiac function (Wernovsky, 2001).

*Intraatrial baffle repairs:* Intraatrial baffle repairs are rarely performed, although many adolescents and adults survive today with repairs that were done 10 to 25 years ago. An intraatrial baffle is created to divert venous blood to the mitral valve and pulmonary venous blood to the tricuspid valve using the patient's atrial septum *(Senning procedure)* or a prosthetic material *(Mustard procedure)*. Performed in first year of life. A disadvantage is the continuing role of the right ventricle as the systemic pump and the late development of right ventricular failure and rhythm disturbances. Other potential postoperative complications include loss of normal sinus rhythm, baffle leaks, and ventricular dysfunction.

*Rastelli procedure:* Operative choice in infants with TGA, VSD, and severe pulmonic stenosis (PS). It involves closure of the VSD with a baffle, directing left ventricular blood through the VSD into the aorta. The pulmonic valve is then closed, and a conduit is placed from the right ventricle to the pulmonary artery, creating a physiologically normal circulation. Unfortunately, this procedure requires multiple conduit replacements as the child grows.

**Prognosis:** Operative mortality is about 5% to 10% with atrial procedures. There is a later risk of dysrhythmias (loss of sinus rhythm in 50% of patients at 10 years), right ventricular dysfunction, baffle obstruction, and sudden death (2% to 10%). Ten-year survival is about 85% (Wernovsky, 2001). Operative mortality for the Rastelli repair is 5% with 40% intermediate survival (Vouhe and others, 1992).

### TOTAL ANOMALOUS PULMONARY VENOUS CONNECTION (TAPVC)

**Description:** Rare defect characterized by failure of the pulmonary veins to join the left atrium. Instead, the pulmonary veins are abnormally connected to the systemic venous circuit via the right atrium or various veins draining toward the right atrium, such as the superior vena cava. The abnormal attachment results in mixed blood being returned to the right atrium and shunted from the right to the left through an atrial septal defect (ASD). The type of TAPVC is classified according to the pulmonary venous point of attachment as:

*Supracardiac*—Attachment above the diaphragm, such as to the superior vena cava (most common form) (see Fig. 34-12)
*Cardiac*—Direct attachment to the heart, such as to the right atrium or coronary sinus
*Infracardiac*—Attachment below the diaphragm, such as to the inferior vena cava (most severe form)
TAPVC is also called total anomalous pulmonary venous return (TAPVR) or total anomalous pulmonary venous drainage (TAPVD).

*Continued*

## Box 34-5 ■ ■ □
## Mixed Defects—cont'd

### TOTAL ANOMALOUS PULMONARY VENOUS CONNECTION (TAPVC)—cont'd

**Pathophysiology:** The right atrium receives all the blood that normally would flow into the left atrium. As a result, the right side of the heart hypertrophies, whereas the left side, especially the left atrium, may remain small. An associated ASD or patent foramen ovale allows systemic venous blood to shunt from the higher-pressure right atrium to the left atrium and into the left side of the heart. As a result, the oxygen saturation of the blood in both sides of the heart (and ultimately in the systemic arterial circulation) is the same. If the pulmonary blood flow is large, pulmonary venous return is also large and the amount of saturated blood is relatively high. However, if there is obstruction to pulmonary venous drainage, pulmonary venous return is impeded, pulmonary venous pressure rises, and pulmonary interstitial edema develops and eventually contributes to CHF. Infracardiac TAPVC is often associated with obstruction to pulmonary venous drainage and is a surgical emergency.

**Clinical manifestations:** Most infants develop cyanosis early in life. The degree of cyanosis is inversely related to the amount of pulmonary blood flow—the more pulmonary blood, the less cyanosis. Children with unobstructed TAPVC may be asymptomatic until pulmonary vascular resistance decreases during infancy, increasing pulmonary blood flow, with resulting signs of CHF. Cyanosis becomes worse with pulmonary vein obstruction; once obstruction occurs, the infant's condition usually deteriorates rapidly. Without intervention, cardiac failure will progress to death.

**Surgical treatment:** Corrective repair in early infancy. The surgical approach varies with the anatomic defect. In general, however, the common pulmonary vein is anastomosed to the left atrium, the ASD is closed, and the anomalous pulmonary venous connection is ligated. The cardiac type is most easily repaired; the infracardiac type has the highest morbidity and mortality

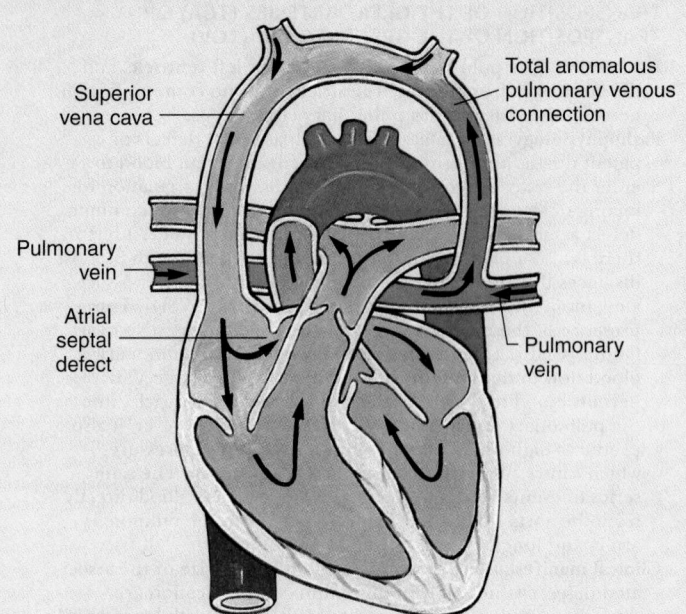

Superior vena cava

Total anomalous pulmonary venous connection

Pulmonary vein

Atrial septal defect

Pulmonary vein

because of the higher incidence of pulmonary vein obstruction. Potential postoperative complications include reobstruction; bleeding; dysrhythmias, particularly heart block; pulmonary artery hypertension; and persistent heart failure.

**Prognosis:** The cardiac type has a surgical mortality of less than 5%; the incidence of morbidity is greater with the other types and increases with the presence of pulmonary vein obstruction.

### TRUNCUS ARTERIOSUS (TA)

**Description:** Failure of normal septation and division of the embryonic bulbar trunk into the pulmonary artery and the aorta, resulting in a single vessel that overrides both ventricles. Blood from both ventricles mixes in the common great artery, causing desaturation and hypoxemia. Blood ejected from the heart flows preferentially to the lower-pressure pulmonary arteries, causing increased pulmonary blood flow and reduced systemic blood flow. There are three types:

*Type I*—A single pulmonary trunk arises near the base of the truncus and divides into the left and right pulmonary arteries.

*Type II*—The left and right pulmonary arteries arise separately but in close proximity and at the same level from the back of the truncus.

*Type III*—The pulmonary arteries arise independently from the sides of the truncus.

**Pathophysiology:** Blood ejected from the left and right ventricles enters the common trunk, mixing pulmonary and systemic circulations. Blood flow is distributed to the pulmonary and systemic circulations according to the relative resistances of each system. The amount of pulmonary blood flow depends on the size of the pulmonary arteries and the pulmonary vascular resistance. Generally resistance to pulmonary blood flow is less than systemic vascular resistance, resulting in preferential blood flow to the lungs. Pulmonary vascular disease develops at an early age in patients with truncus arteriosus.

**Clinical manifestations:** Most infants are symptomatic with moderate to severe CHF and variable cyanosis, poor growth, and activity intolerance. There is a characteristic murmur. Thirty-five percent of patients have 22q11 deletions (Goldmuntz and others, 1998).

**Surgical treatment:** Early repair in the first few months of life. It involves closing the VSD so that the truncus arteriosus receives the outflow from the left ventricle, excising the pulmonary arteries from the aorta, and attaching them to the right ventri-

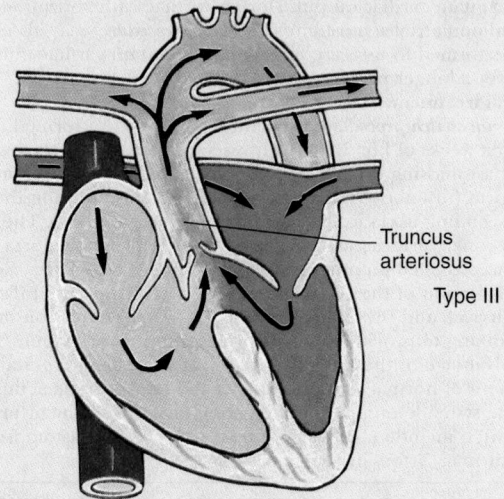

Truncus arteriosus

Type III

cle by means of a homograft. Currently homografts (segments of cadaver aorta and pulmonary artery that are treated with antibiotics and cryopreserved) are preferred over synthetic conduits to establish continuity between the right ventricle and pulmonary artery. Homografts are more flexible and easier to use during the procedure and appear less prone to obstruction. Postoperative complications include persistent heart failure, bleeding, pulmonary artery hypertension, dysrhythmias, and residual VSD. These children require additional procedures to replace the conduit as its size becomes inadequate in relation to the children's growth.

**Prognosis:** Mortality is greater than 10%; future operations are required to replace the conduits.

## Box 34-5 ■ ■ ■
## Mixed Defects—cont'd

### HYPOPLASTIC LEFT HEART SYNDROME (HLHS)

**Description:** Underdevelopment of the left side of the heart, resulting in a hypoplastic left ventricle and aortic atresia. Most blood from the left atrium flows across the patent foramen ovale to the right atrium, to the right ventricle, and out the pulmonary artery. The descending aorta receives blood from the patent ductus arteriosus supplying systemic blood flow.

**Pathophysiology:** An ASD or patent foramen ovale allows saturated blood from the left atrium to mix with desaturated blood from the right atrium, and to flow through the right ventricle and out into the pulmonary artery. From the pulmonary artery the blood flows to the lungs, then through the ductus arteriosus into the aorta and out to the body. The amount of blood flow to the pulmonary and systemic circulations depends on the relationship between the pulmonary and systemic vascular resistances. The coronary and cerebral vessels receive blood by retrograde flow through the hypoplastic ascending aorta.

**Clinical manifestations:** There is mild cyanosis and signs of congestive failure until the patent ductus arteriosus closes, then progressive deterioration with cyanosis and decreased cardiac output, leading to cardiovascular collapse. It is usually fatal in the first months of life without intervention.

**Therapeutic management:** Neonates require stabilization with mechanical ventilation and inotropic support preoperatively. A prostaglandin $E_1$ infusion is needed to maintain ductal patency, ensuring adequate systemic blood flow.

**Surgical treatment:** Several-staged approach: First stage is *Norwood procedure* or anastomosis of the main pulmonary artery to the aorta to create a new aorta, shunting to provide pulmonary blood flow, and creation of a large atrial septal defect. Postoperative complications include imbalance of systemic and pulmonary blood flow, bleeding, low cardiac output, and persistent heart failure. The second stage is often a *bidirectional Glenn shunt* done at 6 to 9 months of age to relieve cyanosis and reduce the volume load on the right ventricle. The final repair is a *modified Fontan procedure*. (See Tricuspid Atresia in Box 34-4.)

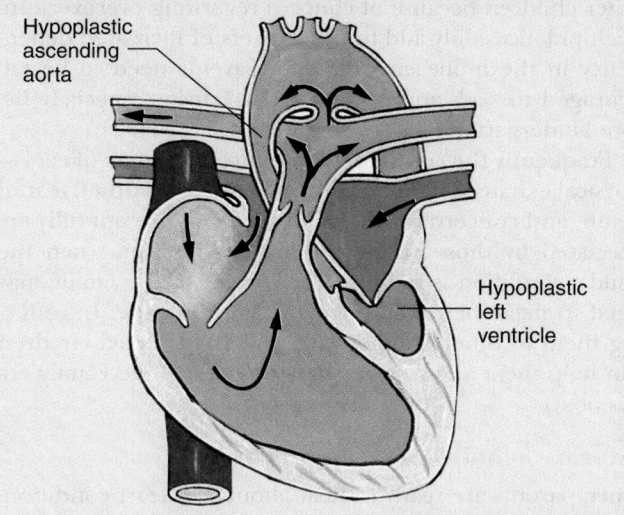

Hypoplastic ascending aorta

Hypoplastic left ventricle

**Transplantation:** Some programs believe that heart transplantation in the newborn period is the best option for these infants. Problems include the shortage of newborn organ donors, risk of rejection, long-term problems with chronic immunosuppression, and infection. (See Heart Transplantation, p. 1526.)

**Prognosis:** Mortality rates are high, with 1-month survival of 67% to 77% and 3-year survival of 50% to 60% reported in a multiinstitutional study including both stage 1 repairs and transplantation (Jacobs, Blackstone, and Bailey, 1998). Survival rates vary widely in different centers. Long-term problems with repair include worsening ventricular function, dysrhythmias, and developmental delays.

---

their child. Every effort must be made by health personnel to foster attachment. (See Chapter 10 for suggestions for promoting attachment between parents and their hospitalized newborn.)

The effect of a child with a serious heart defect on the family is complex. No member, regardless of the degree of positive adjustment, is unaffected. Mothers frequently feel inadequate in their mothering ability because they gave birth to a child with a defect and are unable to keep their child well. Mothers often feel constantly exhausted from the pressures of caring for this child and the other family members. Likewise, fathers and siblings may feel neglected and resentful, a reaction similar to the feelings of family members toward other chronic conditions. (See Chapter 22.) Often parents do not feel confident leaving the child in another's care because they believe that the child will be upset by a change in routine and that the baby-sitter will be unable to cope with the child's symptoms. This often sets up a trap for parents, especially mothers, who become locked into the child's care with no relief. Although the parents' fears are justified, they can be minimized by gradually teaching someone else (a reliable relative or neighbor) how to care for the child.

The need to maintain discipline and set consistent limits cannot be overemphasized. Using behavior-modification techniques, either concrete awards (e.g., a favorite food) or social reinforcement (e.g., approval), can be effective. However, these techniques are most beneficial if employed *before* the child learns to control the family. Therefore guiding parents toward the need for discipline while the child is in infancy is necessary to prevent later problems. It also teaches these children how to tolerate frustration and delayed gratification, which often are lacking because of immediate satisfaction of all of their needs.

Another problem that may develop within family relationships is the child's overdependency. This is often a result of parental fear that the child may die and overcompensation through what has been termed the benevolent overreaction. (See Chapter 22.) The best approach to dealing with this dilemma is prevention. Parents need guidance to recognize the eventual hazards of continuing dependency and protectiveness as the child grows older, and the nurse can assist parents in learning ways to foster optimum development. Unless parents are helped to see what activities the child can do, they may focus on physical limitations and encourage dependency.

The child also needs opportunities for social development. These children do not need to be isolated from known sources of infection or prevented from playing with other children because of concern regarding overexertion. Such practices only add to the dangers of increased dependency in the home environment. Parents need to be encouraged to seek appropriate social activity, especially before kindergarten.

Frequently the continuing unremitting stresses of care—physical exhaustion, financial costs, emotional upset, fear of death, and concern for the child's future—are not fully appreciated by those caring for the family. Even when the child's condition is stabilized or corrected, the family may need to make new adjustments in their lifestyle. Introducing them to other families with similarly affected children can help them adjust to the daily stresses.* (See Family Focus box.)

### Educate Family About the Disorder

Once parents are ready to hear about the heart condition, it is essential that they be given a clear explanation based on their level of understanding. A review of normal cardiac anatomy is helpful before explaining the anatomic defect. A simple diagram, pictures, or a model of the heart can be most helpful in visualizing the heart and the congenital defect. Parents appreciate receiving written information about the specific condition.† Health care professionals should take advantage of subsequent encounters with the family to assess parental understanding of the condition and clarify information as needed.

Different health personnel may convey the same information using different diagrams and medical terms. To pre-

vent this from becoming a problem, the same type of diagram should be used, and the parents should write down any unclear terms or ask for clarification. Sometimes it is helpful to provide the family with a glossary of frequently used words for reference.

Increasingly families are using the Internet as a source of information about heart disease in children.* They are also finding support through contacts with other parents and parent groups. Several Internet sites with pertinent information are listed below. It is important for parents to realize that not all Web sites offer medically accurate information and information from other parents may not be applicable to their own situation. Some children with rare, complex heart defects require individualized treatment plans, and general information on the Internet or in books may not apply to their child. Parents should use their health care team, in particular their cardiologist, to discuss information they have received from other sources.

Parents are primarily interested in information concerning two areas: prognosis and surgery. They are frequently upset by indefinite answers to either. The family should be assured that the health care team will be honest in keeping them informed of the child's condition and of decisions regarding future procedures and treatments. The nurse needs to be aware of alterations in the plan of therapy in order to convey similar messages to the family.

Children of various ages have different ideas about their heart. Children between ages 4 and 6 years have heard about the heart, know its approximate anatomic location in the chest or back, illustrate it as being shaped like a valentine, characterize it by the sounds *tick-tock* or *thump,* and visualize blood as flowing freely (not in vessels). Children ages 7 to 10 have a clearer concept of the heart, realizing that it is not shaped like a valentine and that it has vital functions, such as, "It makes you live." However, their knowledge of its integrated functions to pump blood through a system of vessels to all parts of the body is still hazy. By age 10 or 11, children have a much more involved concept of the heart, with knowledge of veins, valves, pumping action, and circulation. They are beginning to appreciate why death occurs when the heart stops.

Information given to the child must be tailored to the child's developmental age. As the child matures, the level of information is revised to meet the child's new cognitive level. Preschoolers need basic information about what they will experience more than what is actually occurring physiologically. School-age children benefit from a concrete explanation of the defect. Preadolescents and adolescents often appreciate a more detailed description of how the defect affects their heart. Children of all ages need to express their feelings concerning the diagnosis.

### Help Family Cope with Effects of the Disorder

Parents should be aware of the symptoms of their child's cardiac condition (if the child is symptomatic). Parents of children who may develop CHF should be familiar with the

---

*Some local American Heart Associations have organized parent groups.
†**American Heart Association,** 7272 Greenville Ave, Dallas, TX 75231, (800) AHA USA1, www.americanheart.org; **Kids with Heart National Association for Children's Heart Disorders,** 1578 Careful Dr, Green Bay, WI 54304, www.execpc.com/~kdswhrt/.

---

### FAMILY FOCUS
#### The Diagnosis of Heart Disease

Remember, we don't have your experience. We don't see children everyday who have heart disease. We would have been upset finding out our child had to have his tonsils out. How could we ever be prepared for this? Please remember, we only know people who have trivial heart murmurs. How could we ever expect this to happen? And to us, this is the worst problem we've ever heard of.

We still fear most what we don't know and understand. Be honest with us. If you don't know either, tell us. But at least don't leave us wondering about what you know and we don't. Not knowing anything really can be worse than knowing something bad. Be honest, but don't strip us of hope. . . .

Please, remember we are trying to learn complex information in a moment of time. And trying to learn it in a context of great pain and emotional investment. This is our lives you're talking about. Please be thorough, but keep it simple. Tell us again, maybe even again and again, when we can hear better.

From Schrey C, Schrey M: A parent's perspective: our needs and our message, *Crit Care Nurs Clin North Am* 6(1):113-119, 1994.

---

*The Children's Health Information Network, www.tchin.org; PediHeart, www.pediheart.org/parents/index.html; NASPE (information on arrhythmias), www.naspe.org.

symptoms (see p. 1479) and know when to contact the practitioner. Parents of children with cyanosis should be informed about fluid management and hypercyanotic spells (see p. 1488). Parents should know how to contact their child's cardiologist at all times and know what to do in an emergency.

Another area of parental concern is the child's level of physical activity. Children do not need to restrict activity, and the best approach is to treat the child normally and allow self-limited activity. Exceptions to self-determined activity primarily involve strenuous recreational and competitive sports in children with specific cardiac problems. Activities and exercise restrictions should be discussed with the child's cardiologist. Deliberately attempting to prevent crying should be avoided because it can establish a maladaptive parental pattern of relating to the infant.

Infants and children with CHD require good nutrition. Providing infants with adequate nutrition is especially difficult because of their high caloric requirements and inability to suck effectively because of fatigue and tachypnea. Instructing parents in feeding methods that decrease the work of the infant and giving high-calorie formula are important interventions (see p. 1483 for a discussion on feeding the infant with CHF).

Children with severe cardiac defects are often anorexic. Encouraging them to eat can be a tremendous challenge. Because of the parents' concern over eating, children learn early to manipulate parents through eating, such as making unrealistic demands for foods that are not available. The nurse advises parents of this potential problem, because prevention yields greater success than intervention. For example, the child should be given a choice of available high-nutrient foods. Suggestions for encouraging sick children to eat are discussed in Chapter 27.

The family also needs to be knowledgeable regarding the therapeutic management of the disorder, especially in terms of the medications that the child is receiving. Parents are taught the correct procedure for giving medications* and cautioned to keep them in a safe area to prevent accidental ingestion. (See Family Home Care box on p. 1482.)

## Prepare Child and Family for Surgery

Few surgical procedures demand as much planning for preoperative preparation and postoperative care as does heart surgery. The general principles for preparing children for procedures, such as surgery, are discussed in Chapter 27, and the reader is urged to review them. This discussion focuses on those measures specific to the cardiovascular procedure. Technical differences exist between closed- and open-heart surgery because the latter involves the use of cardiopulmonary bypass (extracorporeal circulation). Consequently there are some additions to physical care postoperatively in open-heart surgery. However, in general the term *heart surgery* is used regardless of the actual procedure, and the same nursing interventions apply.

Outpatient preoperative workups for heart surgery are becoming common for most elective procedures. Children are then admitted on the morning of surgery. Preoperative teaching is often done in the clinic setting and may include a tour of the ICU and the in-patient facilities. No well-documented research exists on how extensive the preoperative preparation should be, and the nurse must use considerable judgment in planning the aspects of teaching. Preparation can be divided into three categories: environment, equipment, and procedures. It is assumed that the child and parent understand the defect and planned surgical repair; otherwise this information is also included.

**Introduce Child and Family to the Environment.** If a visit to the recovery room and ICU is planned, it should take place when there is minimum activity in the area, when the parents can accompany the child, and when the child is well rested. Usually the day before surgery is ample time to allow the child to ask questions and to prevent undue fantasizing about the experience. If a visit is not included in the teaching plan, the nurse can use a book, preferably with pictures or photographs of the actual rooms, to explain the environment to the child.

During the visit to the ICU, the child and parents should experience everything that directly affects the child's care, such as the sounds of ECG monitors, oxygen tents, and placement of the bed. All positive, nonfrightening aspects of the environment are emphasized, such as the play area, visitors' section, pictures or mobiles in the room, or television. If it is a pediatric ICU, the nurse can introduce the family to other children who may be recovering from surgery. The child should be protected from the frightening sights in the unit, and equipment not in view postoperatively, such as equipment located behind or below the bed, needs less attention. The child and parents are encouraged to ask questions or to explore further any equipment in the room, but they should not be pushed to assimilate more information than they appear to be tolerating.

**Familiarize Child and Family with Equipment and Procedures.** Some of the equipment, such as stethoscopes, sphygmomanometers, and thermometers, will already be familiar to the child and parents. However, the nurse emphasizes that procedures involving such equipment will be done more frequently. The child is told about the placement of an oximeter sensor on the skin, usually the finger.

Types of equipment new to many families are oxygen masks, suction equipment, chest tubes, endotracheal (ET) tubes, incentive spirometers, nasogastric tubes, and IV tubing. These are shown and demonstrated either on a doll or on the child, if he or she appears ready. With a younger child, miniaturized equipment suitable for use with a doll or puppet often produce less anxiety than the actual samples. If other children in the unit have an IV infusion or an oxygen mask, the older child may benefit from seeing them, but this must be planned carefully to avoid frightening the child.

Several IV lines are inserted perioperatively: (1) a peripheral line for infusion of fluids; (2) a venous pressure line, inserted into the right subclavian or jugular vein; and (3) an arterial line for direct measurement of arterial pressure and to obtain blood samples. Younger children need

---

*Home care instructions on giving medications to children are available in Wong DL, Hess CS: *Wong and Whaley's clinical manual of pediatric nursing,* ed 5, St Louis, 2000, Mosby.

only know the location of the tubing and that both arms may be restrained to prevent dislodging the tubing. Older children may appreciate knowing the reason for each infusion, especially when venous and arterial measurements are taken. Because the lines are inserted during surgery, they are not painful, only uncomfortable because of the restricted movement.

The type and size of dressing the child will have after surgery are discussed and can be shown on a doll. Usually one of two types of incisions is made: a *median sternotomy,* which splits the sternum, or a *lateral thoracotomy,* which extends from the midaxillary line to the scapula. Increasingly a ministernotomy, in which only the lower half of the sternum is opened, is being done for simple repairs. Frequently no sutures are visible because subcuticular, absorbable sutures may be used. If this is done, it should be pointed out to the child and parents, who may fear that the incision will open. Sometimes a butterfly incision is used for cosmetic reasons in girls instead of the regular median sternotomy.

The child may be told about chest tubes and their purpose in draining fluid from around the heart and lungs. A picture of the equipment used for drainage can be shown to the child, or the setup can be simulated by attaching one end of the tubes to a doll with a chest dressing and the other end to small bottles (e.g., empty medicine vials). The nurse stresses that the child must move even though the tubes are in place. It can be demonstrated on the doll that the tubing is long enough to permit turning. Since this information may cause anxiety in the child, it is best left to the end of the teaching session or may be eliminated if the child appears too anxious.

An ET tube is inserted during surgery and may be left in place for ventilatory assistance and tracheobronchial suctioning. However, it may be best to prepare older children for the ET tube only if *prolonged* ventilatory support is planned. The ET tube can be presented as a "breathing tube" that is placed in the nose or mouth. The nurse explains that while the tube is in, the child will feel it in the throat and will not be able to talk, but nothing is wrong. The child can express desires by pointing or using a picture communication board. The nurse stresses that the tube will be removed as soon as possible, often during the first postoperative day.

Preoperative physical care differs little, if any, from that for any other surgery and is discussed in Chapter 27. The child should be assured that the parents will be there when the child wakes up; they should be allowed to accompany their child as far as possible to the operating suite. (See Evidence-Based Practice box on p. 1107.) After all of the equipment and procedures have been explained, it is important to talk about "getting well" and going home. If a doll was used during the preparatory session, the tubes can be removed and the doll can be dressed in regular clothes in anticipation of discharge.

## Provide Postoperative Care

Immediate postoperative care is usually provided by specially trained nurses in the ICU. Many of the procedures, such as arterial pressure and central venous pressure monitoring and the observations related to vital functions, require advanced educational training (the reader should refer to critical care texts for further information). However, nurses caring for the child before surgery and during the convalescent period need to be familiar with the major principles of care.

**Observe Vital Signs and Arterial/Venous Pressures.** Vital signs, including BP, are recorded frequently until the child is stable. The heart rate and respirations are counted for 1 full minute, compared with the ECG monitor, and recorded with activity. The heart rate is normally increased after surgery. The nurse observes cardiac rhythm and notifies the practitioner of any changes in regularity. Dysrhythmias may occur postoperatively secondary to administration of anesthetics, acid-base and electrolyte imbalance, hypoxia, surgical intervention, or trauma to conduction pathways.

At least hourly, the lungs are auscultated for breath sounds. Diminished or absent breath sounds may indicate an area of atelectasis, pleural effusion, or pneumothorax. All necessitate further assessment. Auscultation guides the nurse's selective use of postural drainage and percussion to those pulmonary lobes most in need. It also allows a more objective evaluation of effective ventilation.

Temperature changes are typical during the early postoperative period. Hypothermia is expected immediately after surgery from hypothermia procedures, effects of anesthesia, and loss of body heat to the cool environment. During this period the child is kept warm to prevent additional heat loss. Infants may be placed under radiant heat warmers. During the next 24 to 48 hours the body temperature may rise to 37.8° C (100° F) or slightly higher as part of the inflammatory response to tissue trauma. After this period an elevated temperature is most likely a sign of infection and warrants immediate investigation for probable cause.

*Intraarterial monitoring* of BP is almost always done following open-heart surgery. Residual vasoconstriction after cardiopulmonary bypass makes indirect BP readings less reliable, and intraarterial monitoring permits continuous rather than intermittent observation. A catheter is passed into the radial artery or the dorsalis pedis or posterior tibial artery, and the other end is attached to an electronic monitoring system, which provides a continuous recording of the BP. Continuous BP readings are compared with those taken indirectly with a sphygmomanometer or oscillometry (Dinamap). A discrepancy between the two may indicate a change in peripheral vascular resistance, a malfunction in the electronic device, or human error in using the wrong-size BP cuff. The nurse also observes for potential complications of intraarterial monitoring, such as arterial thrombosis, infection, air emboli, or blood loss through the catheter. Prevention of each of these hazards is similar to care for any other type of infusion.

The intraarterial line is maintained with a low-rate, constant infusion of heparinized saline to prevent clotting. The amount of irrigant is recorded as intake fluid. The dressing at the site is changed daily.

*Intracardiac monitoring* lines, placed intraoperatively, provide data on cardiac function and output. A central venous pressure (CVP) line is usually inserted in the superior vena cava in the neck. Monitoring lines allow assessment of pressures inside the cardiac chambers, which gives vital information on blood volume, cardiac output, ventricular function, pulmonary artery pressures, and responses to drug therapy in the immediate postoperative period. The RA and CVP lines may also be used to infuse fluids and medications. Left atrial lines and pulmonary artery lines are used with more complex repairs. Intracardiac lines are used only in the ICU, although CVP lines may remain for use as a central IV line outside the ICU. All lines must be treated with strict aseptic technique to prevent infection. Patients must be carefully assessed for bleeding at the time of line removal. See critical care texts for a more complete discussion of intracardiac lines.

**Maintain Respiratory Status.** Infants usually require mechanical ventilation in the immediate postoperative period. Children may be extubated in the operating room or in the first few postoperative hours, especially children who did not require cardiopulmonary bypass. When weaning and extubation are completed, humidified oxygen is delivered by mask, hood, or nasal cannula to prevent drying of mucosa. The child is encouraged to turn and deep breathe at least hourly. Every measure is employed to enhance ventilation and decrease pain, such as splinting of the operative site and use of analgesics.

Suctioning is performed only as needed and is performed carefully to avoid vagal stimulation (which can trigger cardiac dysrhythmias) and laryngospasm, especially in infants. Suctioning is intermittent and maintained for no more than 5 seconds to prevent depleting the oxygen supply. Supplemental oxygen is administered with a manual resuscitation bag before and after the procedure to prevent hypoxia. The heart rate is monitored after suctioning to detect changes in rhythm or rate, especially bradycardia. The child should always be positioned facing the nurse to permit assessment of the child's color and tolerance to the procedure.

> **NURSING ALERT**
>
> During suctioning, observe for signs and symptoms of respiratory distress, such as tachypnea, use of accessory muscles for breathing, and restlessness.

Chest tubes are inserted into the pleural or mediastinal space during surgery or in the immediate postoperative period to remove secretions and air in order to allow reexpansion of the lung. The chest tube is attached to a disposable water-seal drainage system. The purpose of the underwater drainage is to prevent air from traveling up the tube into the pleural space, causing a pneumothorax. The nursing considerations include the following: (1) do not interrupt water-seal drainage unless the chest tube is clamped, (2) check for tube patency (fluctuation in the water-seal chamber), and (3) maintain sterility.

Drainage is checked hourly for color and quantity. Immediately postoperatively the drainage may be bright red, but afterward it should be serous. The largest volume of drainage occurs in the first 12 to 24 hours, and drainage is greater in extensive heart surgery.

> **NURSING ALERT**
>
> Chest tube drainage greater than 3 ml/kg/hr for more than 3 consecutive hours or 5 to 10 ml/kg in any 1 hour is excessive and may indicate postoperative hemorrhage. The surgeon is notified immediately because cardiac tamponade can develop rapidly and is life-threatening.

Chest radiographs are taken when the tubes are inserted to check their location and after they are removed to evaluate the inflation of the lungs. Chest tubes are usually removed on the second to third postoperative day. Lung expansion is evidenced by decreased fluctuation in the tube and absence of drainage.

Removal of chest tubes can be a painful, frightening experience. (See Atraumatic Care box.) Children are forewarned that they will feel a sharp, momentary pain. After the suture is cut, the tubes are quickly pulled out at the end of full inspiration to prevent intake of air into the pleural cavity. A purse-string suture (placed when the tubes were inserted) is pulled tight to close the opening. A petrolatum-covered gauze dressing is immediately applied over the wound and securely taped on all four sides to the skin so that an airtight seal is formed. The dressing is checked for signs of drainage and any evidence of infection. Breath sounds are auscultated because pneumothorax is a possible complication of chest tube removal.

**Provide Maximum Rest.** After heart surgery maximum rest should be provided to decrease the workload of the heart and promote healing. Nursing care is planned according to the child's usual activity and sleep patterns. The simplest way to ensure individualized, efficient, high-quality care is to plan at the beginning of the shift the nursing procedures to be done. Periods of rest are identified. The schedule should be shared with parents to allow them to visit at the most advantageous times, such as after a rest period when no special treatments are anticipated.

**Provide Comfort.** Heart surgery is both painful and frightening for children, and providing comfort is a primary nursing concern. In the past, children often poorly medicated for pain after surgery, especially were children who are unable to verbally communicate discomfort. (See Pain Assessment, Chapter 26.) However, studies show that adequate analgesia and anesthesia decrease the body's stress response to surgery and improve postoperative morbidity and mortality (Anand and Hickey, 1992; Wessel, 1993). (See also Neonatal Pain, Chapter 10.) Increased awareness of the importance of pain control has increased the use of postoperative analgesia in children (McRae and others, 1997).

Continuous IV opioid infusions, particularly morphine and fentanyl, are safe and effective methods of pain con-

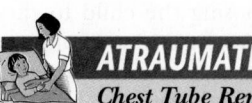

**ATRAUMATIC CARE**
*Chest Tube Removal*

Analgesics given intravenously such as morphine sulfate (0.1 mg/kg), often in combination with midazolam (Versed), may be given before the procedure. Oral analgesics and sedatives have also been used.

trol. Patient-controlled analgesia may be used with children old enough to understand the concept (Macfadyen and Buckmaster, 1999). Epidural morphine is another option. Paralyzing agents such as pancuronium (Pavulon) or metocurine (Metubine) may also be used with the analgesics for children who are very agitated or hemodynamically unstable. Children receiving opioid infusions for a prolonged period are weaned slowly from the medication to prevent withdrawal symptoms.

Most patients need IV analgesics for pain control during the 24- to 48-hour postoperative period. Following removal of lines and tubes, pain may be controlled with oral medications such as codeine with acetaminophen (Tylenol) or oxycodone and acetaminophen (Tylox). Nonsteroidal antiinflammatory agents such as IV ketorolac (Toradol) or oral ibuprofen may be used to provide relief of moderate postoperative pain. Thoracotomy incisions are usually painful because the incision is through muscle. Higgins and others (1999) have found round-the-clock use of Tylenol or ibuprofen to augment narcotics is advantageous in providing pain relief after heart surgery. Tylenol or ibuprofen alone is usually adequate pain control after discharge (See Pain Management, Chapter 26.)

In addition to pharmacologic pain control, every effort is made to minimize the discomfort of procedures, such as using a firm pillow or favorite stuffed animal placed against the chest incision during coughing, and performing treatments *after* pain medication is given, preferably at a time that coincides with the drug's peak effect. Nonpharmacologic measures are employed to lessen the perception of pain, and parents are encouraged to comfort their child as much as possible. (See Pain Management, Chapter 26.)

**Monitor Fluids.** Intake and output of all fluids must be accurately calculated. Intake is primarily IV fluids; however, a record of fluid used to flush the arterial and CVP lines or to dilute medications is also kept. Output includes hourly recordings of urine (usually a Foley catheter is inserted and attached to a closed collecting device), drainage from chest and nasogastric tubes, and blood drawn for analysis. Urine is analyzed for specific gravity to assess the kidneys' concentrating ability and to assess approximately the body's degree of hydration. Renal failure is a potential risk from a transient period of low cardiac output.

> **NURSING ALERT**
> The signs of renal failure are decreased urinary output (less than 1 ml/kg/hr) and elevated levels of blood urea nitrogen and serum creatinine.

Fluids are restricted during the immediate postoperative period to prevent hypervolemia, which places additional demands on the myocardium, predisposing the child to cardiac failure. Two factors influence increased blood volume. In open-heart surgery the cardiopulmonary pump is primed with a large volume of fluid (usually electrolyte solution), which may greatly dilute the patient's blood. The large fluid volume also diffuses into the interstitial spaces, causing total-body edema and pulmonary edema. Postoperatively the increased interstitial fluid diffuses back into the systemic circulation, where it can be excreted by the kidney. Diuretics help accelerate this process.

In addition, the physiologic changes of open- or closed-heart surgery stimulate the adrenal cortex to secrete aldosterone, which increases renal reabsorption of sodium. This results in water retention but increased excretion of potassium. Concurrently the hypothalamus secretes additional antidiuretic hormone (ADH), which causes the distal and collecting tubules to reabsorb more water. Not only can this process result in hypervolemia, but it also may cause electrolyte imbalances, principally hypokalemia. Decreased potassium affects myocardial function and may increase the risk of dysrhythmias. The nurse assesses electrolyte imbalances by observing for signs of hypokalemia (see Table 34-5) and checking all blood electrolyte reports.

Fluid requirements are based on the child's weight and body surface area. The child is weighed daily, preferably in the morning, using the same scale and similar clothing. The child is usually given nothing by mouth for the first 24 hours. If an ET tube is inserted, oral fluids are usually withheld until the child is extubated. Fluid restrictions are unusual. The nurse calculates the distribution over a 24-hour period based on the child's preoperative weight and drinking habits. The distribution should allow for the majority of fluid to be given during the child's most wakeful and active periods.

**Plan for Progressive Activity.** Fatigue and weakness are common after heart surgery, as a result of both the surgical trauma to the heart and sleep deprivation during the immediate postoperative period. However, moderate activity is essential to prevent pulmonary and vascular complications. Initially, turning, coughing, and deep breathing are sufficient to promote respiratory expansion. However, passive range-of-motion exercises, especially to the lower extremities, are instituted to prevent venous stasis. All infusion sites are inspected for evidence of thrombophlebitis and emboli. The areas are passively exercised to promote circulation.

A progressive schedule of ambulation and activity is planned, based on the child's preoperative activity patterns and postoperative cardiovascular and pulmonary function. Toys that were enjoyed before surgery are provided to encourage movement. It is important to plan the activity at times when the child is well rested, is comfortable (usually has had analgesic medication), and is not scheduled for any strenuous procedure or treatment immediately afterward.

Ambulation is initiated early, usually by the second postoperative day, when chest tubes, arterial lines, and assisted ventilatory equipment may be removed. The nurse begins ambulation for this child the same as for a child who had any other postsurgical procedure, progressing from sitting on the edge of the bed and dangling the legs to standing up and to sitting in a chair. The heart rate and respirations are carefully monitored to assess the degree of cardiac demand imposed by each activity. Tachycardia, dyspnea, cyanosis, desaturation, progressive fatigue, or dysrhythmias indicate the need to limit further energy expenditure. Even if the child is able to ambulate to a chair with a moderate increase in heart rate, the effort required to return to bed must be considered. After ambulation a rest period is scheduled.

**Observe for Complications of Heart Surgery.** Several complications can occur after heart surgery, most of which are related to open-heart surgery and use of cardiopulmonary bypass. Many of the procedures discussed in the preceding paragraphs are aimed at preventing these problems. Only those that have not already been discussed are included here. A serious complication, bacterial endocarditis, is discussed on p. 1509.

*Cardiac changes.* Preoperatively the workload of the heart is increased because of the abnormal hemodynamics caused by the congenital defect. In the initial postoperative period the heart is under increased stress because of the effect of surgery and the use of the heart-lung machine. In some cases cardiac function can actually be worse in the early postoperative period despite repair of the congenital defect. CHF, hypoxia, low cardiac output, dysrhythmias, and tamponade are all potential postoperative problems.

*CHF* may occur postoperatively because of excessive pulmonary blood flow or fluid overload (see p. 1481 for assessment and management of CHF). *Hypoxia* may occur because of inadequate pulmonary blood flow or because of respiratory problems. Rapid assessment of the causes of hypoxia and appropriate interventions to improve ventilation and perfusion are vital because hypoxia can rapidly lead to acidosis, which can impair ventricular function.

*Low cardiac output syndrome* and *decreased peripheral perfusion* can occur from hypothermia or inability of the LV to maintain systemic circulation. The most important signs of adequate peripheral perfusion are rapid capillary refill, good skin color, warm extremities, and strong pulses. Evidence of low cardiac output is similar to signs of shock (i.e., decreased BP, decreased pulse pressure, cool extremities, metabolic acidosis, and oliguria). Low cardiac output states are aggressively treated with IV inotropic medications such as dopamine, dobutamine, and milrinone. If maximum medical therapy is failing, cardiac assist devices such as, extracorporeal membrane oxygenation (ECMO) or a ventricular assist device may be used in some centers under certain circumstances. Assist devices may be used as a bridge to transplantation. Mortality is greater than 50% for patients who require mechanical support. Patients who have recovery of ventricular function within 2 to 3 days and have a short period of support have the best outcomes (Craig, Smith, and Fineman, 2001).

*Dysrhythmias* can result from electrolyte imbalance, especially hypokalemia and surgical intervention to the septum or myocardium. The heart rate and rhythm are carefully monitored by observing the ECG pattern and by counting the apical pulse for 1 full minute. Dysrhythmias that impair cardiac performance are bradycardia, tachycardia, extrasystole, or heart block. When assessing dysrhythmias, nurses need to be aware of normal rates for age to determine abnormally fast and slow rhythms. The child is assessed for signs of decreased cardiac output, because in some children a faster than normal rate may be required to maintain an adequate cardiac output in the postoperative period. Epicardial pacing wires may be inserted during surgery for managing cardiac dysrhythmias postoperatively.

*Cardiac tamponade* is compression of the heart by blood and other effusion (clots) in the pericardial sac, which severely restricts the normal heart movement. Another sign is *paradoxical pulse pressure,* in which the systolic pressure drops during inspiration because accumulated blood compresses the heart, resulting in a drop in cardiac output. Signs include rising and equalizing right and left atrial filling pressures, narrowing pulse pressure, tachycardia, dyspnea, apprehension, and an abrupt stop to chest tube drainage from mediastinal tubes.

Any evidence of this potentially fatal complication is immediately reported. An echocardiogram will confirm the diagnosis. Treatment consists of prompt pericardiocentesis to remove the blood or fluid. If active hemorrhage and coagulopathy are present, steps are taken to enhance blood clotting.

*Pulmonary changes.* Areas of atelectasis are common immediately after surgery as a result of deflation of the lung during cardiopulmonary bypass. Other pulmonary complications include pneumothorax, especially caused by faulty chest tubes; pulmonary edema from increased pulmonary blood flow or heart failure; and pleural effusion caused by persistent venous congestion. Signs of pneumothorax are persistent decreased breath sounds, sudden dyspnea, tachycardia, rapid shallow respirations, cyanosis, and sometimes sharp chest pain. Signs of pulmonary edema are tachypnea, rales, wheezing, moist dyspneic respirations, tachycardia, cyanosis, and restlessness. Signs and symptoms of pleural effusions include increased respiratory rate, vomiting, decreased breath sounds, fatigue, irritability, and decreased oxygen saturation. (See Critical Thinking Exercise box on p. 1508.)

*Neurologic changes.* *Cerebral edema* and *brain damage* may occur during open-heart surgery. Although the exact cause is unknown, it is thought to be a result of tissue ischemia or emboli. The nurse checks the equality of strength and reflexes in both extremities for evidence of paralysis; assesses the pupil size, equality, and reaction to light and accommodation; and assesses the child's orientation to the environment. Any evidence of cerebral damage is immediately reported. The nurse also observes for focal or generalized *seizure* activity. Seizures identified by electroencephalogram (EEG) have been seen in up to 20% of infants who undergo repair of congenital cardiac defects (Helmers and others, 1997).

*Infection.* All patients are at risk for infections postoperatively, especially infants, those with poor cardiac function, and those who require multiple invasive lines and procedures for a prolonged period. Prophylactic antibiotics are given for the first 1 or 2 days. All dressings are done with aseptic technique. Patients are monitored closely for fever and signs of infection. Appropriate treatment is instituted if an infection is identified.

*Hematologic changes.* While passing through the heart-lung machine, blood is exposed to substantial trauma by direct contact with oxygen, mechanical action, foreign substances, and massive doses of anticoagulants. The result of mechanical trauma is red blood cell hemolysis and potential renal tubular necrosis. Heparinization of the blood during extracorporeal circulation can result in clotting abnormalities from decreased thrombin and prothrombin, decreased platelets, and altered platelet aggregation.

Hemolysis of red blood cells results in blood loss and anemia, which may require packed red blood cell transfusion. The nurse monitors results of complete blood counts to identify the severity of the hemolysis. All urine is tested for the presence of blood. If transfusions are required, the child is closely observed for signs of reaction and fluid overload. (See Table 35-2.) The necessity of measuring urinary output hourly has already been discussed.

Because blood clotting mechanisms are affected, signs of hemorrhage, especially bleeding from the chest tubes and a fall in arterial/venous pressures, are important observations. Hemorrhage is more likely to occur in patients who have repair of cyanotic heart defects because of the associated physiologic thrombocytopenia.

Normally the filter and bubble trap on the heart-lung machine remove air emboli, tiny clots, fat debris, and organisms from the arterialized (oxygenated) blood before its return to the body. However, impure blood entering the systemic circulation can cause fat emboli, thromboemboli, and infection anywhere in the body, but most importantly in the brain.

***Postpericardiotomy syndrome.*** This syndrome of fever, leukocytosis, pericardial friction rub, or pericardial and pleural effusion can occur anytime the pericardium is opened, either in the immediate postoperative period or after surgery, typically around day 7 to 21. The cause is unknown, although etiologic theories include a viral infection, autoimmune response to myocardial tissue, or a reaction to blood in the pericardium. It is self-limited and is treated with rest, salicylates, nonsteroidal antiinflammatory drugs (NSAIDs) and sometimes steroids. Pericardiocentesis or pleurocentesis may be needed to treat large effusions.

### Provide Emotional Support

Children may become depressed after surgery. This is thought to be caused by preoperative anxiety, postoperative psychologic and physiologic stress, and sensory overstimulation. Typically the child's disposition improves on leaving the ICU. (See Chapter 26.)

Children may also be angry and uncooperative after surgery as a response to the physical pain and to the loss of control imposed by the surgery and treatments. They need an opportunity to express feelings, either verbally or through activity. The nurse can be supportive by reassuring children that the procedures that require cooperation, such as coughing and deep breathing, are difficult to perform. Nurses can praise children for their efforts to cooperate and should refrain from expecting too much courage or bravery. Children often regress in their behavior during the stress of surgery and hospitalization. This approach allows children to express feelings with the nurse's acceptance, regardless of their emotional response. Children also may express feelings of anger or rejection toward parents. The nurse must reassure parents that this is normal and that with continued support the anger will subside.

The nurse can support the parents by being available for information and explaining all the procedures to them. The first few postoperative days are particularly difficult because parents see their child in pain and realize the potential risks from surgery. They often are overwhelmed by the physical environment of the ICU and feel useless because they can do so little for their child. The nurse can minimize such feelings by including parents in caregiving activities and comfort and play activities; by providing information about the child's condition; and by being sensitive to their emotional and physical needs. The importance of their presence in making the child feel more secure is stressed, even if they do not provide physical care.

## Critical Thinking Exercise

### Postoperative Cardiac Care

Four-year-old Amy is 2 days postoperative following repair of coarctation of the aorta. She has a left thoracotomy and a chest tube in place. During your assessment you note an absence of breath sounds in the left upper lobe, a mildly elevated respiratory rate of 32 breaths/min, and a decreased $O_2$ saturation of 90%. She is not in any respiratory distress but is complaining of left shoulder pain. The chest tube has drained 30 ml of serous fluid in the past 12 hours. Which of the following is the best course of action?

FIRST, THINK ABOUT IT . . .

• What are you taking for granted?
• What would the consequences be if you put your thoughts into action?

1. You should consider a possible pneumothorax, carefully check the chest tube placement and connections, and notify the practitioner.
2. You should reassure her that decreased or absent breath sounds on the affected side are typical of patients with thoracotomy incisions.
3. You should administer codeine and acetaminophen as ordered because her respiratory findings are likely the result of pain.
4. You should consider a pleural effusion, check amount of chest tube drainage, and change her position frequently to promote drainage of the pleural space.

*The best response is one. A pneumothorax is a common complication in patients with chest tubes, and Amy is experiencing typical symptoms of absent breath sounds, increased respiratory rate, decreased $O_2$ saturation, and pain. The chest tube is carefully assessed to make sure it is properly in place, all connections are tight and there is no air leak, and the drainage system is functioning correctly. The practitioner is notified and will likely take action and request a chest x-ray film, which will distinguish between a pneumothorax, a pleural effusion, or atelectasis. A pneumothorax due to a leak in the chest drainage system will continue to worsen and may lead to significant respiratory distress. Therefore it needs to be promptly assessed and treated. If her symptoms are related to atelectasis, then chest physical therapy, pain management to decrease splinting, frequent position changes and ambulation are all indicated.*

## Plan for Discharge and Home Care

Ideally discharge planning begins on admission for cardiac surgery and includes an assessment of the parents' adjustment to the child's altered state of health. As mentioned earlier, one of the most common parental reactions is overprotection, and the nurse needs to be aware of times when the family may need help in recognizing the child's improved health status. With surgical correction of heart anomalies occurring during infancy, there is less likelihood of this pattern of overdependency developing.

The family will need verbal as well as written instructions on medication, nutrition, activity restrictions, subacute bacterial endocarditis, return to school, wound care, and signs and symptoms of infection or complications. Referrals to community agencies may be warranted to assist parents in the transition from hospital to home and to reinforce the teaching. (See Family Home Care box.)

The parents will also need clear instructions on when to seek medical care, such as for a change in the child's behavior or an unexplained fever. Follow-up with the cardiologist is also arranged before discharge. Appropriate medical identification, such as a Medic-Alert bracelet, is indicated for children with a pacemaker or a heart transplant and for those receiving anticoagulation therapy or antidysrhythmic medication.

The nurse also discusses common behavior disturbances that may occur after discharge, such as nightmares, sleep disturbances, separation anxiety, and overdependence. A supportive, consistent response is essential to allow the child to overcome the surgical experience. The child may work out feelings and fears through therapeutic play, and this should be encouraged.

Although surgical correction of heart defects has improved dramatically, it is still not possible to totally repair many of the complex anomalies. For many children, repeat procedures are required to replace conduits or grafts or to manage complications, such as restenosis. Consequently the long-term prognosis is uncertain, and full recovery is not always possible. For these families medical follow-up and continued emotional support are essential. The nurse can often serve as an important primary health care professional and as a resource for referrals when needed.

# ACQUIRED CARDIOVASCULAR DISORDERS

Acquired cardiac disorders refer to disease processes or abnormalities that occur after birth and can be seen in the normal heart or in the presence of congenital heart defects. They occur for a variety of reasons, including infection, autoimmune responses, environmental factors, and familial tendencies. Nursing care often plays a critical role in the identification and supportive management of these cardiovascular disorders.

## Bacterial (Infective) Endocarditis (BE)

BE, or infective endocarditis (IE), or subacute bacterial endocarditis (SBE), is an infection of the valves and inner lining of the heart. Although it can occur without underlying heart disease, it most often is a sequela of bacteremia in the child with acquired or congenital anomalies of the heart or great vessels. It especially affects children with valvular abnormalities, prosthetic valves, ventricular septal defects, patent ductus arteriosus, tetralogy of Fallot, or rheumatic heart disease with valve involvement. Children with indwelling catheters are also at risk. Endocarditis can occur without any known risk factors, usually affecting the mitral or aortic valves. The incidence of BE appears to have increased in the pediatric and neonatal population, most likely due to improved survival among children at risk for BE (those with congenital heart defects and hospitalized infants) (Ferrieri and others, 2001).

The most common causative agent is *Streptococcus viridans;* other causative agents are *Staphylococcus aureus,* gram-negative bacteria, and fungi, such as *Candida albicans.* (Gutschik, 1999).

### Pathophysiology

The microorganisms usually grow on a section of the endocardium that has been subjected to abnormal blood streaming and turbulence, such as occurs when the flow of blood is restricted by an anatomic narrowing or forced through an abnormal opening. Growth may also begin where the abnormal jet of blood strikes the opposing endocardium, causing a thickening of the lining. Changes in the endocardium predispose it to the growth of invading organisms.

Organisms may enter the bloodstream from any site of localized infection. The most common portals of entry are oral from dental work *(S. viridans);* the urinary tract, such as from urinary tract infection after catheterization (gram-negative bacilli); the heart from cardiac surgery, especially if synthetic material is used (valves, patches, conduits); and the bloodstream from long-term indwelling catheters. The microorganisms grow on the endocardium, forming vegetations (verrucae), deposits of fibrin, and platelet thrombi.

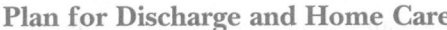

**FAMILY HOME CARE**

*Topics to Include in Discharge Teaching
Following Cardiac Surgery*

Medication teaching (for digoxin, see p. 1482)
Activity restrictions
Diet and nutrition
Wound care (include dressings if any, suture removal, bathing)
Bacterial endocarditis prophylaxis (see p. 1482)
Follow-up appointments (cardiologist, primary care provider)
   Community agencies as needed (visiting nurse service, early developmental intervention)
When to call practitioner; signs and symptoms of postoperative problems
Review of cardiac defect and surgical repair

The lesion may grow to invade adjacent tissues, such as aortic and mitral valves and myocardium, and may break off and embolize elsewhere, especially in the spleen, kidney, central nervous system, lung, skin, and mucous membranes.

## Clinical Manifestations

The onset of symptoms is usually insidious, with unexplained low-grade, intermittent fever. Other common nonspecific symptoms are malaise, myalgias, arthralgias, headache, diaphoresis, and weight loss. A new murmur or a change in a previously existing one is frequently found as a result of damage to valves or perforation of the myocardium. Another finding, especially in those with prolonged illness, is splenomegaly. Other signs that result from emboli formation elsewhere in the body include splinter hemorrhages (thin black lines) under the nails, Osler nodes (red, painful intradermal nodes with white centers found on the pads of the phalanges), Janeway spots (painless hemorrhagic areas on the palms and soles), and petechiae on the oral mucous membranes. Neonates may have feeding difficulties, respiratory distress, tachycardia, CHF, or symptoms of septicemia (Ferrieri and others, 2001).

## Diagnostic Evaluation

Several laboratory findings may indicate BE, such as ECG changes (prolonged P-R interval), radiographic evidence of

---

### Box 34-6 ■ ■ ■
### Endocarditis Prophylaxis Recommendations

**DENTAL PROCEDURES**

Dental extractions
Periodontal procedures, including surgery, scaling and root planing, probing, and recall maintenance
Dental implant placement and reimplantation of avulsed teeth
Endodontic (root canal) instrumentation or surgery only beyond the apex
Subgingival placement of antibiotic fibers/strips
Initial placement of orthodontic bands but not brackets
Intraligamentary local anesthetic injections
Prophylactic cleaning of teeth or implants where bleeding is anticipated

**OTHER PROCEDURES**
*Respiratory Tract*

Surgical operations that involve respiratory mucosa
Bronchoscopy with a rigid bronchoscope
Tonsillectomy and/or adenoidectomy

*Gastrointestinal Tract*

Sclerotherapy for esophageal varices
Esophageal stricture dilation
Endoscopic retrograde cholangiography with biliary obstruction
Biliary tract surgery
Surgical operations that involve intestinal mucosa

*Genitourinary Tract*

Prostatic surgery
Cystoscopy
Urethral dilation

From Dajani AS and others: Prevention of bacterial endocarditis: recommendations by the American Heart Association, *JAMA* 277:1794-1801, 1997.

---

cardiomegaly, anemia, an elevated erythrocyte sedimentation rate, leukocytosis, and microscopic hematuria. Definitive diagnosis can be made after growth of the organism and identification of the causative agent in the blood. Usually several blood specimens are drawn for culturing to rule out contamination during venipuncture and dilution technique. Strict sterile technique is practiced in obtaining cultures to avoid contamination. Three separate blood cultures are recommended. As soon as an organism is isolated, sensitivity studies are done to determine appropriate antibiotic therapy. Vegetation formation and myocardial abscess may be visualized on 2-D echocardiography. A diagnosis of culture-negative endocarditis is made when the patient has echo or clinical evidence of BE but no organism can be cultured (Ferrieri and others, 2001).

## Therapeutic Management

Treatment is administration of high-dose antibiotics (usually penicillin, ampicillin, methicillin, cloxacillin, streptomycin, or gentamicin for specific bacteria or amphotericin B or flucytosine for fungi) given intravenously for between 2 to 8 weeks. Blood cultures are taken periodically to evaluate the response to antibiotic therapy. In instances when antibiotic therapy is unsuccessful, CHF develops, valvular obstruction occurs, or recurrent systemic emboli are present, surgical intervention is warranted. This may include replacing damaged valves with prostheses, debriding and draining myocardial abscesses, excising areas of infection, and removing vegetations (Dajani and Taubert, 2001).

Successful early medical treatment, especially with BE, occurs in approximately 80% of affected patients. However, cases diagnosed late, those caused by antibiotic-resistant organisms or fungi, or those occurring in infants or patients without preexisting heart disease carry a higher mortality and may necessitate surgical intervention. Death is most often caused by CHF, myocardial infarction from coronary emboli, or cardiac perforation. Nonfatal complications result from embolism to other organs, especially to the central nervous system (causing hemiplegia, aphasia, meningitis, convulsions), kidney (resulting in hematuria, proteinuria), spleen, and bowel.

Prevention of BE in susceptible children is of utmost importance and includes all children with CHD except those with (1) isolated ASD secundum or (2) surgical repair of ASD secundum, VSD, or PDA without residual effects after 6 months. In addition, patients with mitral valve prolapse without mitral regurgitation do not require prophylaxis (Dajani and others, 1997).

Prevention involves administration of prophylactic antibiotic therapy 1 hour before procedures known to increase the risk of entry of organisms (Box 34-6). Drugs of choice include amoxicillin, ampicillin, clindamycin, cephalexin, cefadroxil, azithromycin, and clarithromycin. The drugs may be given orally or parenterally, depending on the procedure to be performed. The newest recommendations for BE prophylaxis divide patients with cardiac conditions into high-, moderate-, and low-risk categories based on the potential for morbidity and mortality. Prophylaxis is recommended for those patients who fall into the high- and moderate-risk categories. Published recommendations provide guidelines for antibiotic prophylaxis, but they are complex and must be individualized for the child (Dajani and others, 1997).

### Nursing Considerations

Ideally, the objective of nursing care is to counsel parents of high-risk children concerning the need for prophylactic antibiotic therapy before procedures such as dental work. The family's regular dentist should be advised of existing cardiac problems in the child as an added precaution to ensure preventive treatment. These children should also maintain the highest level of oral health to reduce the chance of bacteremia from oral infections. (See also discussion on dental care in Chapter 14.)

Parents should also have a high index of suspicion regarding potential infections. Without unduly alarming them, the nurse stresses that any unexplained fever, weight loss, or change in behavior (lethargy, malaise, anorexia) must be brought to the practitioner's attention. Such symptoms should not be self-diagnosed as a cold or flu. Early treatment is important in preventing further cardiac damage, embolic complications, and growth of resistant organisms.

Treatment of endocarditis requires long-term hospitalization for the duration of parenteral drug therapy. In some cases IV antibiotics may be administered at home with nursing supervision for part of the treatment course. Nursing goals during this period are (1) preparation of the child for IV infusion, usually with an intermittent-infusion device, and several venipunctures for blood cultures; (2) observation for side effects of antibiotics, especially inflammation along venipuncture sites; (3) observation for complications, including embolism and CHF; and (4) education regarding the importance of follow-up visits for cardiac evaluation, echocardiographic monitoring, and blood cultures.

## Rheumatic Fever (RF)

RF is a poorly understood inflammatory disease that occurs after infection with group A β-hemolytic streptococcal pharyngitis. It is a self-limited illness that involves the joints, skin, brain, serous surfaces, and heart. Cardiac valve damage (referred to as *rheumatic heart disease*), is the most significant complication of RF (Vasan and others, 1996; Bitar and others, 2000). In developed countries RF and rheumatic heart disease have become uncommon, probably as a result of antibacterial control of streptococcal infection, successful treatment of rheumatic heart disease, and a change in the organism itself. However, RF remains a devastating problem in developing (third world) countries and has reappeared in some parts of the United States (Gentles and others, 2001).

### Etiology

Strong evidence supports a relationship between upper respiratory tract infection with group A β-hemolytic streptococci and subsequent development of RF (usually within 2 to 6 weeks). In almost all cases of RF a previous infection with group A β-hemolytic streptococci can be documented by laboratory evidence of rising antibody titers. Diagnosis and treatment of group A β-hemolytic streptococcal infection prevents RF.

### Pathophysiology/Clinical Manifestations

The principal manifestations of RF are observed in the heart, joints, skin, and central nervous system. Inflammatory hemorrhagic bullous lesions, called *Aschoff bodies,* are formed, which cause swelling, fragmentation, and alterations in the connective tissue. Aschoff bodies are found in virtually all patients with clinical rheumatic activity. These lesions are found in the heart, blood vessels, brain, and serous surfaces of the joints and pleura.

The major cardiac manifestation of RF is *carditis* involving the endocardium, pericardium, and myocardium. In the acute illness, clinical signs and symptoms reflect valvulitis, myocarditis, and pericarditis. Clinically, rheumatic carditis is most commonly associated with the mitral valve (Vasan and others, 1996). The presence of an apical systolic murmur reflecting mitral regurgitation is a common clinical finding in acute rheumatic carditis. This murmur is a long, high-pitched, blowing murmur that begins with the first heart sound ($S_1$) and continues throughout systole. Other murmurs in the acute phase may reflect aortic regurgitation. In addition, myocarditis produces tachycardia that is out of proportion to the degree of fever, especially during rest or sleep. Signs and symptoms of CHF may result, and cardiomegaly may be demonstrated by chest x-ray examination. Signs and symptoms of pericarditis include muffled heart sounds because of pericardial effusion. In addition, the patient may demonstrate a pericardial friction rub and complain of chest pain. Pericardial effusions can be documented by echocardiography. Patients with mitral or aortic valve involvement may experience progressive valvar damage as time goes on. Carditis is the only manifestation that can lead to permanent damage (Narula and others, 1999).

The second major manifestation is *polyarthritis* caused by edema, inflammation, and effusions in joint tissue. The arthritis is reversible and migratory, favoring large joints such as the knees, elbows, hips, shoulders, and wrists. The affected joint is swollen, hot, red, and exquisitely painful for 1 to 2 days, after which a different joint is affected. Joint manifestations usually accompany the acute febrile period, most often in the first 1 to 2 weeks; however, they can persist for 4 weeks in untreated patients.

The third major manifestation is *erythema marginatum.* This is a distinct, erythematous macule with a clear center and wavy, well-demarcated border. This transitory, nonpruritic rash is most often found on the trunk and proximal portion of extremities.

The fourth major manifestation is the development of *subcutaneous nodules,* which are small (0.5 to 1 cm), nontender swellings that persist indefinitely after onset of the disease and gradually resolve with no resulting damage. They are rare but may be found in crops over bony prominences, such as feet, hands, elbows, scalp, scapulae, and vertebrae.

The last major manifestation reflects central nervous system involvement characterized by *chorea,* which is referred to as *St. Vitus dance* or *Sydenham chorea.* Chorea is characterized by sudden, aimless, irregular movements of the extremities, involuntary facial grimaces, speech disturbances, emotional lability, and muscle weakness that can be profound. It is usually exaggerated by anxiety and attempts at deliberate fine motor activity and is relieved by rest, especially sleep.

In addition to these major manifestations, minor manifestations that may support the diagnosis include arthralgia and fever, which may be low grade and which often spikes in the late afternoon. Laboratory findings reflect an inflammatory process. Other vague signs and symptoms include unexplained epistaxis, abdominal pain that may be severe enough to simulate appendicitis, weakness, fatigue, pallor, anorexia, and weight loss.

## Diagnostic Evaluation

There is no single symptom or laboratory test that can definitely diagnose RF. Rather, the diagnosis is based on a set of guidelines recommended by the American Heart Association. These guidelines were revised so that they are designed to aid only in the diagnosis of the initial episode of RF (Box 34-7). Clinical and laboratory findings are divided into major and minor manifestations and are accompanied by evidence of recent streptococcal infection in the majority of instances.

Although the majority of patients with RF meet criteria, there are three circumstances where exceptions are allowed. In patients who have chorea as the only symptom and in patients who present late with continued carditis, the late diagnosis may preclude supporting manifestations and laboratory findings. Finally, a recurrence of RF in a patient with a previous history may not fulfill the standard Jones criteria. However, if there is a single major or several minor

manifestations in a patient with a history of prior disease along with evidence of recent group A streptococcal infection, the diagnosis may be made without classic adherence to the criteria.

Streptolysin-O (O because it is oxygen labile) is a streptococcal extracellular product that produces lysis of the red blood cell. *Antistreptolysin-O (ASLO) titers* measure the concentration of antibodies formed in the blood against this product. Normally the titers begin to rise about 7 days after onset of the infection and reach maximum levels in 4 to 6 weeks. Therefore a rising titer demonstrated by at least two ASLO tests is the most reliable evidence of recent streptococcal infection. Normal values are between 0 and 120 Todd units. Elevations over 333 Todd units indicate recent streptococcal infection in children.

## Therapeutic Management

The goals of management include (1) eradication of group A β-hemolytic streptococci *(primary prevention)*, (2) prevention of permanent cardiac damage, (3) palliation of the other symptoms, and (4) prevention of recurrences *(secondary prevention)* (Dajani and others, 1995).

Penicillin remains the drug of choice (oral or intramuscular injections), with macrolides or cephalosporins as a substitute in penicillin-sensitive children. Initial therapy includes a full 10-day course of penicillin or an alternative antibiotic (Table 34-7).

Children who have had acute RF are susceptible to recurrent RF for the rest of their lives, and therefore prophylactic treatment against recurrence of RF is started immediately after the initial course of antibiotics is complete. Secondary prevention involves monthly intramuscular injections of benzathine penicillin G, two daily oral doses of penicillin V, or one daily dose of sufadiazine/sufisoxazole or erythromycin (see Table 34-7). The duration of long-term prophylaxis varies and depends on whether the child has had cardiac involvement (Box 34-8).

---

**Box 34-7 ■ ■ □**

### Guidelines for the Diagnosis of Initial Attack of Rheumatic Fever (RF) (Jones Criteria, 1992 Update)*

| MAJOR MANIFESTATIONS | MINOR MANIFESTATIONS |
|---|---|
| Carditis | Clinical findings |
| Polyarthritis | Arthralgia |
| Chorea | Fever |
| Erythema marginatum | Laboratory findings |
| Subcutaneous nodules | Elevated acute-phase reactants |
| | Erythrocyte |
| | sedimentation rate |
| | C-reactive protein |

#### SUPPORTING EVIDENCE OF ANTECEDENT GROUP A STREPTOCOCCAL INFECTION

Positive throat culture or rapid streptococcal antigen test
Elevated or rising streptococcal antibody titer

---

From Guidelines for the diagnosis of rheumatic fever. Jones criteria, 1992 update, *JAMA* 268(15):2070, 1992.
*If supported by evidence of preceding group A streptococcal infection, the presence of two major manifestations or of one major and two minor manifestations indicates a high probability of acute RF.

---

**Box 34-8 ■ ■ □**

### Duration of Secondary Rheumatic Fever Prophylaxis

| CATEGORY | DURATION |
|---|---|
| Rheumatic fever with carditis and residual heart disease (persistent valvar disease*) | At least 10 years since last episode and at least until age 40 years, sometimes lifelong prophylaxis |
| Rheumatic fever with carditis but no residual heart disease (no valvar disease*) | 10 years or well into adulthood, whichever is longer |
| Rheumatic fever without carditis | 5 years or until age 21 years, whichever is longer |

---

From Dajani AS and others: Treatment of acute streptococcal pharyngitis and prevention of rheumatic fever: a statement for health professionals, *Pediatrics* 96:758-764, 1995.
*Clinical or echocardiographic evidence.

The antibiotic regimens used to prevent recurrences of RF are inadequate for the prevention of BE, and therefore other antibiotics need to be used in situations where these children require SBE prophylaxis (e.g., dental work, invasive procedures).

Salicylates are used to control the inflammatory process, especially in the joints, and to reduce fever and discomfort. Patients with arthritis from RF are generally very responsive to salicylate therapy; however, salicylates should not be instituted before diagnosis, because their use may mask the polyarthritis. Prednisone may be indicated in some patients with pancarditis and valvular involvement (Behrman, Kliegman, and Jenson, 2000). Neither salicylcates nor predisone has been shown to affect cardiac sequelae. Traditionally bed rest or at least limited activity has been recommended during the acute illness.

## Nursing Considerations

The objectives of nursing care for the child with RF are to (1) encourage compliance with drug regimens, (2) facilitate recovery from the illness, (3) provide emotional support, and (4) prevent recurrence of the disease. Because compliance is a major concern in long-term drug therapy, every effort is made to encourage adherence to the therapeutic plan. (See Compliance, Chapter 27.) When compliance is poor, monthly injections may be substituted for daily oral administration of antibiotics, and children need preparation for this often dreaded procedure.

Interventions during home care are primarily concerned with providing rest and adequate nutrition. Usually, once the febrile stage is over, children can resume moderate activity and their appetite improves. If carditis is present, the family must be aware of any activity restrictions and may need help in choosing less strenuous activities for the child.

One of the most disturbing and frustrating manifestations of the disease is chorea. The onset is gradual and may occur weeks to months after the illness, sometimes even occurring in children who have not been diagnosed with RF. It may be mistaken for nervousness, clumsiness, behavioral changes, inattentiveness, and learning disability. It is usually a source of great frustration to the child because the movements, incoordination, and weakness severely limit physical ability. The child needs an opportunity to verbalize feelings. Of utmost importance is stressing to parents and schoolteachers the involuntary, sudden nature of the movements, that the chorea is transitory, and that all manifestations eventually disappear.

Nurses also have a role in prevention, primarily in screening school-age children for sore throats that may be caused by group A streptococci. This may involve actively participating in throat culture screening programs or referring children with a possible streptococcal infection for testing. (See Nursing Care Plan: The Child with Rheumatic Fever.*)

*In Wong DL, Hess CS: *Wong and Whaley's clinical manual of pediatric nursing,* ed 5, St Louis, 2000, Mosby.

---

**TABLE 34-7　Prevention of rheumatic fever (treatment of streptococcal tonsillopharyngitis)**

| Agent | Dose | Mode | Duration |
|---|---|---|---|
| **Primary Prevention** | | | |
| Benzathine penicillin G | 600 000 U for patients ≤27 kg (60 lb)<br>1 200 000 U for patients >27 kg (60 lb)<br>or | Intramuscular | Once |
| Penicillin V (phenoxymethyl penicillin) | Children: 250 mg 2-3 times daily<br>Adolescents and adults: 500 mg 2-3 times daily | Oral | 10 d |
| *For Individuals Allergic to Penicillin*<br>Erythromycin: | | | |
|   Estolate | 20-40 mg/kg/d 2-4 times daily (maximum 1 g/d)<br>or | Oral | 10 d |
|   Ethylsuccinate | 40 mg/kg/d 2-4 times daily (maximum 1 g/d) | Oral | 10 d |

| Prevention of Recurrent Attacks of Rheumatic Fever | | |
|---|---|---|

| Agent | Dose | Mode |
|---|---|---|
| Benzathine penicillin G | 1 200 000 U every 4 weeks*<br>or | Intramuscular |
| Penicillin V | 250 mg twice daily<br>or | Oral |
| Sulfadiazine | 0.5 g once daily for patients ≤27 kg (60 lb)<br>1.0 g once daily for patients >27 kg (60 lb) | Oral |
| *For Individuals Allergic to Penicillin and Sulfadiazine*<br>Erythromycin | 250 mg twice daily | Oral |

Modified from Dajani AS and others: Treatment of acute streptococcal pharyngitis and prevention of rheumatic fever: a statement for health professionals, *Pediatrics* 96:758-764, 1995.
*In high-risk situations, administration every 3 weeks is justified and recommended.

# Kawasaki Disease (KD) (Mucocutaneous Lymph Node Syndrome)

KD is an acute systemic vasculitis of unknown cause. Approximately 80% of cases occur in children under the age of 5 years, with peak incidence in the toddler age-group. The acute disease is self-limited. Without treatment, however, approximately 20% to 25% of children develop cardiac sequelae. Damage to the blood vessels that supply the heart muscle (the coronary arteries) and damage to the heart muscle itself can occur. The most common sequela is dilation of the coronary arteries, resulting in *ectasia* (dilation) or *aneurysm* formation. Infants less than 1 year of age are at the greatest risk for heart involvement. Recent data have suggested that children more than 5 years old are also at increased risk of developing coronary sequelae, perhaps because KD is often not suspected in older children, leading to delayed diagnosis and treatment. KD has become a leading cause of acquired heart disease in children in the United States.

KD is seen in children of most racial and ethnic groups and is the leading cause of heart disease in children in the United States and Japan. The incidence rates are between 120 and 150 cases per 100,000 children under 5 years of age. KD occurs 1.5 times more frequently in males than females, and 85% of the children are under 5 years of age (Burns and others, 2000).

The etiology of KD remains unconfirmed. Although KD is not spread by person-to-person contact, several factors support an infectious etiology. It is often seen in geographic and seasonal outbreaks, with most cases reported in the late winter and early spring. KD is also a pediatric illness, suggesting the development of passive immunity. Because an etiologic agent has not been found, some experts believe that the illness may represent a "final common pathway" to more than one potential agent.

## Pathophysiology

KD involves widespread inflammation of the small and medium-sized blood vessels (Conner and McCance, 2000), with the coronary arteries being the most susceptible to damage. During the acute stage of the illness there is progressive inflammation of the small vessels (capillaries, venules, arterioles) along with pancarditis. This inflammation is reflected in the clinical signs and symptoms as well as in laboratory markers of inflammation, which are elevated in the acute illness. This vasculitis progresses to the medium-sized muscular arteries, potentially damaging the walls of the vessels and leading to the formation of coronary artery aneurysms in some children. Enlargement of the coronary arteries can be detected as early as day 7 of illness. Affected vessels continue to enlarge for several weeks and generally reach their largest diameter approximately 4 to 6 weeks from the onset of fever. Longer duration of fever (most likely reflecting the severity of inflammation) is strongly associated with the development of aneurysms. Aneurysms of the peripheral vessels (axillary, brachial, iliac, cervical, and renal arteries) can occur, although this is very rare and usually occurs only in children who also have large coronary aneurysms. In the acute phase myocarditis (inflammation of the myocardium) is usually present. Decreased left ventricular function may be seen on echocardiogram, but children do not often have clinical signs of heart failure. The systemic inflammation gradually subsides and eventually ceases in 6 to 8 weeks.

Over time, affected vessels may attempt to heal whereby cells in the vessels multiply in an attempt to restore a "normal" lumen diameter. However, even if the lumen size is restored, the vessel is never completely normal again. The affected vessel walls are thicker and are subject to scarring and calcification, especially at the distal ends of the aneurysm.

Almost all of the morbidity and morality resulting from KD is caused by cardiac complications. Coronary thrombosis may result from sluggish blood flow in a dilated/aneurysmal vessel. Over years, stenosis and scarring may also lead to impeded blood flow, predisposing the patient to myocardial ischemia or infarction.

## Clinical Manifestations

KD manifests in three phases: acute, subacute, and convalescent. The *acute phase* begins with an abrupt onset of high fever that is unresponsive to antibiotics and antipyretics. Over the next week or so, the diagnostic symptoms become evident. The bulbar conjunctiva of the eyes become reddened, with clearing around the iris (limbal sparing). The eyes are generally dry, without drainage. Inflammation of the pharynx and the oral mucosa develops, with red, cracked lips and the characteristic "strawberry tongue" (the normal coating of the tongue sloughs off, leaving the large papillae exposed, resembling a strawberry). The rash of KD differs from child to child but is never vesicular. It is most often accentuated in the perineum. Often the area affected by the rash may desquamate. In addition, the child's hands and feet become edematous, and the palms and soles become erythematous. The child may have cervical lymphadenopathy (at least a single node 1.5 cm or larger). During this stage the child is typically *very* irritable and inconsolable. Complications during this period include myocarditis with resultant ECG changes, decreased LV function, and occasional symptoms of CHF. Coronary arteries may begin to show enlargement during this phase. Approximately one third of patients will develop a temporary arthritis beginning in the small joints.

The *subacute phase* begins with resolution of the fever and lasts until all outward clinical signs of KD have disappeared. If changes in the coronary arteries occur, they generally become evident by echocardiography during the second week of illness. Damaged vessels continue to stretch and will reach their maximum diameter approximately 4 weeks from the onset of illness. Thrombocytosis and hypercoagulability in children with expanding aneurysms and disrupted blood flow place the child at risk for coronary thrombosis. During this period the child often has the characteristic periungual desquamation (peeling that begins under the fingertips and toes) of the hands and feet. Arthritis may be evident during this phase and usually affects the larger weight-bearing joints. Irritability persists during this phase.

In the *convalescent phase* all of the clinical signs of KD have resolved. The laboratory values, however, have not yet returned to normal. The erythrocyte sedimentation rate may remain elevated, reflecting lingering inflammation. Thrombocytosis may still be present. Arthritis may continue into this stage, and coronary complications may remain a concern. This phase is complete when all blood values return to normal (6 to 8 weeks after onset). At the end of this stage, parents report that the child appears to have returned to normal in terms of temperament, energy, and appetite.

**Cardiac Involvement.**    The most serious complication of KD is the potential for myocardial infarction, which generally results from thrombotic occlusion or stenotic occlusion of a coronary aneurysm. The group at highest risk for thrombus formation are children with "giant" aneurysms (greater than 8 mm in diameter). The main symptoms of acute myocardial infarction in children are abdominal pain, vomiting, restlessness, inconsolable crying, pallor, and shock. Complaints of chest pain are more typical in older children (Kato, Ichinose, and Kawasaki, 1986).

## Diagnostic Evaluation

Currently no specific diagnostic test exists for KD. Therefore the diagnosis is established on the basis of clinical findings and associated laboratory results (Box 34-9).

These criteria should be used as guidelines. Many children with KD do not fulfill standard diagnostic criteria, and infants often have an atypical presentation. It is therefore important to consider KD as a possible diagnosis in any infant or child with prolonged elevated temperature that is unresponsive to antibiotics and is not attributable to another cause.

Several associated laboratory findings, when combined with clinical data, can be helpful in making the diagnosis. The typical child with KD is anemic and has a leukocytosis with a "shift to the left" (increased immature white blood cells) during the acute phase. An elevated erythrocyte sedimentation rate reflects ongoing inflammation and generally persists for 6 to 8 weeks. Microscopic urinalysis reveals a

sterile pyuria with mononuclear cells. This will not be evident with a regular dipstick test, because the white blood cells are not polymorphonuclear neutrophils. A transient elevation of liver enzymes typically occurs. Thrombocytosis with hypercoagulability becomes evident in the subacute phase and peaks 3 to 4 weeks after the onset of fever.

Echocardiograms are used to monitor myocardial and coronary artery status. A baseline echocardiogram should be obtained at the time of diagnosis for comparison with future studies. In addition, follow-up echocardiograms should be performed at approximately 2 weeks after onset and again at 4 to 6 weeks from the onset of fever to determine the diameter of the coronary arteries, as well as LV contractility and valvular function. If cardiac involvement is evident, more frequent studies may be necessary.

## Therapeutic Management

The current treatment of KD includes high-dose IV immune globulin (IVIG) along with salicylate therapy. IVIG reduces the duration of fever and the incidence of coronary artery abnormalities when given within the first 10 days of the illness. A single large infusion of 2 g/kg over 10 to 12 hours is recommended (American Academy of Pediatrics, 2000).

Aspirin is given initially in an antiinflammatory dose (80 to 100 mg/kg/day in divided doses every 6 hours) to control fever and symptoms of inflammation. Once fever has subsided, aspirin is continued at an antiplatelet dose (3 to 5 mg/kg/day). Low-dose aspirin is continued in patients without echocardiographic evidence of coronary abnormalities until the platelet count has returned to normal (6 to 8 weeks). If the child develops coronary abnormalities, salicylate therapy is continued indefinitely. Additional anticoagulatory therapy, such as warfarin (Coumadin), may be indicated in those children with giant aneurysms (>8 mm), who are at the greatest risk for morbidity and mortality (O'Brien and others, 2000).

**Prognosis.**    Most children with KD recover fully following treatment. However, when cardiovascular complications occur, serious morbidity may result. Death occurs rarely (0.3%) and almost always results from ischemia caused by coronary thrombosis or stenosis. Children with coronary abnormalities are followed with periodic ECGs, echocardiograms, and myocardial perfusion scans based on their individual risk. Although echocardiography is very sensitive in visualizing coronary dilation, it does not detect stenoses of the coronary arteries. Cardiac catheterization of the coronary arteries remains the gold standard and may be performed in children who still have significant abnormalities at 1 year and in situations where myocardial ischemia is suspected by noninvasive testing.

Children without coronary artery aneurysms have been followed for over 30 years in Japan and the United States and do not show an increased incidence of premature heart disease. However, some research studies have suggested that both coronary and peripheral arteries may be stiffer than normal, even in children who did not suffer obvious coronary artery dilation. For this reason it is especially important that children who have had KD have as few other risk factors

---

**Box 34-9** ■ ■ ■
### Diagnostic Criteria for Kawasaki Disease

The child must exhibit five of the following six criteria, including fever:
1. Fever for 5 or more days (often diagnosed with shorter duration of fever if other symptoms are present)
2. Bilateral conjunctival injection (inflammation) without exudation
3. Changes in the oral mucous membranes, such as erythema, dryness, and fissuring of the lips; oropharyngeal reddening; or "strawberry tongue" (large papillae are exposed)
4. Changes in the extremities, such as peripheral edema, erythema of the palms and soles, and periungual desquamation (peeling) of the hands and feet
5. Polymorphous rash
6. Cervical lymphadenopathy (one lymph node >1.5 cm)

for coronary disease as possible. Cholesterol levels and BP should be monitored, and these children should be encouraged to have a heart-healthy lifestyle in terms of diet, exercise, and avoidance of smoking.

### Nursing Considerations

The nursing care of children with KD is challenging. Inpatient care focuses on symptomatic relief, emotional support, diagnostic assistance, medication administration, and education of the child and family.

In the initial phase the nurse must monitor the child's cardiac status carefully. Intake and output and daily weight measurements are recorded. Although the child may be reluctant to eat and therefore may be partially dehydrated, fluids need to be administered with care because of the usual finding of myocarditis. The child should be assessed frequently for signs of CHF, including decreased urinary output, gallop rhythm, tachycardia, and respiratory distress. Cardiac monitoring is suggested in the following cases: before the initial ECG and echocardiogram are completed and shown to be normal, during the infusion of IV gamma globulin (because of the large fluid load), for children less than 1 year of age, and for any child with cardiac symptoms. Sedation is generally required before echocardiography in children under 2½ to 3 years of age, because the child needs to remain still for up to an hour.

Nursing care primarily focuses on symptomatic relief. To minimize skin discomfort, cool cloths, unscented lotions, and soft, loose clothing are helpful. During the acute phase, mouth care, including applying lubricating ointment to the lips, is important for the mucosal inflammation. Clear liquids and soft foods can be offered. Elevated temperatures need to be carefully monitored. Acetaminophen can be given for fever. (See Controlling Elevated Temperatures, Chapter 27.) If arthritis develops, passive range-of-motion exercise may be indicated and can be done most easily during the child's bath.

The administration of gamma globulin should follow the same guidelines as for any blood product, with frequent monitoring of vital signs. Patients must be watched for allergic reactions. (See Table 35-2.) Cardiac status needs monitoring because of the large volume being administered to patients who may have myocarditis or diminished LV function. Patency of the IV line is checked because extravasation can result in tissue damage. Hypercoagulability and venous fragility often make it difficult to maintain IV access in children with KD (Conner and McCance, 2000).

Patient irritability is perhaps the most challenging problem. These children need to be placed in a quiet environment that promotes adequate rest. Their parents need to be supported in their efforts to comfort an often inconsolable child. They may need time away from their child, and nurses can often provide respite care for the family. Parents need to understand that irritability is a hallmark of KD and that they need not feel guilty or embarrassed about their child's behavior.

**Discharge Teaching.** Parents need accurate information about the usual course of KD, including the importance of follow-up monitoring and when they should contact their practitioner. Irritability is likely to persist for up to 2 months after the onset of symptoms. Peeling of the hands and feet is painless and occurs primarily in the second and third weeks. Arthritis, especially of the larger weight-bearing joints, may persist for several weeks. Children are typically most stiff in the mornings, during cold weather, and after naps. Passive range-of-motion exercises in the bathtub are often helpful in increasing flexibility. Although the arthritis in KD is always temporary, it can be severe enough that some children require treatment with antiarthritic agents once they are no longer on high-dose aspirin. (NOTE: high-dose non-steroidal antiinflammatory agents should not be given with high-dose salicylates).

Despite treatment with IVIG, some children develop recurrent fever and symptoms, necessitating retreatment with IVIG (2 g/kg) in approximately 10% of children. Temperature should be recorded after discharge until the child has been afebrile for several days. Parents should be educated about the signs and symptoms of KD; if any occur together with a temperature of 38.4° C (101° F) or above, they are instructed to notify their practitioner.

Parents also need to be instructed about the administration of salicylates and, if the child is receiving high doses, made aware of the signs of aspirin toxicity—ringing in the ears (tinnitus), headache, dizziness, and confusion. The only side effect of low-dose aspirin is easy bruising. In addition, the aspirin should be stopped and the practitioner notified if the child is exposed to chickenpox or influenza because of the drug's possible association with Reye syndrome.

All parents should understand the unlikely but real possibility of myocardial infarction, as well as the signs and symptoms of cardiac ischemia in a child. At discharge the ultimate cardiac sequela is generally not known, because changes occur up to a month after the onset of KD. In addition, the parents of children with known severe coronary artery sequelae should be taught cardiopulmonary resuscitation.* Finally, children with coronary abnormalities may require indefinite antiplatelet therapy with low-dose aspirin or additional anticoagulants. In this situation contact sports should be avoided and yearly administration of influenza vaccine is indicated. The administration of measles-mumps-rubella (MMR) vaccine should be delayed for 11 months after the administration of IVIG, because the body might not produce the appropriate amount of antibodies. In addition, the varicella vaccine should not be given for at least 11 months after IVIG therapy (American Academy of Pediatrics, 2000).

## Systemic Hypertension

*Hypertension* is the consistent elevation of BP beyond values considered the upper limits of normal. The two major cate-

---

*Home care instructions for measuring a child's temperature, for administering oral medication, and for infant and child cardiopulmonary resuscitation are available in Wong DL: *Wong and Whaley's clinical manual of pediatric nursing,* ed 5, St Louis, 2000, Mosby.

gories of hypertension are *essential,* or *primary* (no identifiable cause), and *secondary* (subsequent to an identifiable cause) hypertension. Traditionally, primary hypertension has been considered a disease of older adults and is a major health problem. Hypertension is the most common cause of a CVA and is a major risk factor in myocardial infarction. However, in recent years there has been increasing interest in this disorder in children and in whether early detection may decrease later morbidity and mortality. Some evidence suggests that primary hypertension of adulthood may begin in childhood. However, findings reveal that many adults with high BP had normal BP as children and that children with high BP have normal BP as adults (Gillman and others, 1993). These findings emphasize the importance of BP evaluation for all individuals at each health visit.

## Etiology

Most instances of hypertension observed in young children occur secondary to a structural abnormality or an underlying pathologic process, although this observation is being challenged by screening programs of relatively healthy children. The most common cause of secondary hypertension is renal disease (90%), followed by cardiovascular, endocrine, and some neurologic disorders. Miscellaneous conditions such as lead poisoning and ingestion of excessive amounts of licorice are causes unique to children. As a rule, the younger the child and the more severe the hypertension, the more likely it is to be secondary. The conditions associated with secondary hypertension in children and adolescents are listed in Box 34-10.

The causes of primary hypertension are undetermined. There is evidence that both genetic and environmental factors play a role. In younger children hypertension is most commonly due to secondary causes; however, in adolescents primary hypertension is seen more often than the secondary forms. The incidence of hypertension is greater in children with a family history of hypertension. African-Americans have a higher incidence of hypertension than whites. In the African-American population hypertension develops earlier and is frequently more severe, resulting in mortality at an earlier age. Environmental factors that contribute to the risk of developing hypertension include obesity, salt ingestion, smoking, and stress.

## Clinical Manifestations

Although clinical manifestations associated with hypertension depend largely on the underlying cause, some observations can provide clues to the practitioner that an elevated BP may be a factor. Adolescents and older children with hypertension may complain of frequent headaches, dizziness, or changes in vision. In infants or young children who cannot communicate symptoms, observation of behavior provides clues, although gross behavioral changes may not be apparent until complications are present. Parents of infants and small children who have been treated for hypertension report that their child had previously been irritable, often indulged in an abnormal degree of head banging or rubbing, and may have wakened screaming in the night (when BP tends to be highest).

## Diagnostic Evaluation

It is clear from the increasing numbers of hypertensive or potentially hypertensive children and adolescents being identified that a BP determination should be a routine part of annual assessment in children. In addition, any child who is ill should have BP measurements taken, because the signs and symptoms of hypertension in children are often vague. The BP of children at any age should be measured if they are diagnosed as having or are suspected of having coarctation of the aorta, unexplained heart failure, unexplained heart murmurs, unexplained seizures or other

---

**Box 34-10** ■ ■ ■
### Conditions Associated with Secondary Hypertension in Children

**RENAL DISORDERS**
Congenital defects
    Polycystic kidney, ectopic kidney, horseshoe kidney
    Obstructive anomalies
    Hydronephrosis
Renal tumor
    Wilms tumor
    Renovascular
Abnormalities of renal arteries
Renal vein thrombosis
Acquired disorders
    Glomerulonephritis—acute or chronic
    Pyelonephritis
    Nephritis associated with collagen disease

**CARDIOVASCULAR DISEASE**
Coarctation of aorta
Arteriovenous fistulas
Patent ductus arteriosus
Aortic or mitral insufficiency

**METABOLIC AND ENDOCRINE DISEASES**
Adrenal tumors
    Adenoma
    Pheochromocytoma
    Neuroblastoma
    Cushing syndrome
    Adrenogenital syndrome
    Hyperthyroidism
    Aldosteronism
    Hypercalcemia
    Diabetes mellitus

**NEUROLOGIC DISORDERS**
Space-occupying lesions of cranium (increased intracranial pressure)
    Tumors, cysts, hematoma
    Cerebral edema
    Encephalitis (including Guillain-Barré and Reye syndromes)

**MISCELLANEOUS CAUSES**
Drugs (corticosteroids, oral contraceptives, pressor agents, amphetamines)
Burns
Genitourinary surgery
Trauma (e.g., stretching of femoral nerve with leg traction)
Insect bites (e.g., scorpion)
Intravascular overload (blood, fluid)
Hypernatremia
Toxemia of pregnancy
Heavy metal poisoning

neurologic signs, an abdominal mass or masses, edema, ascites, or evidence of renal failure, hypernatremia, failure to thrive, respiratory distress, hyperlipidemia, or unexplained headaches.

No definitive cutoff values are used in the diagnosis of hypertension in the pediatric patient. The National Institutes of Health (1996) has suggested the classification found on the inside back cover. *Significant hypertension* is considered a BP persistently between the 95th and 99th percentiles for age, sex, and height. *Severe hypertension* is a BP persistently at or above the 99th percentile for age, sex, and height. These newer guidelines take into account the differences in body size. It is important to note that a child who is large for age may normally have a higher BP than a child who is of average size.

Before a diagnosis is made, BP should be measured on at least three separate occasions. To obtain an accurate reading, care is taken to quiet the child or relax the adolescent while the measurement is recorded to avoid false readings caused by excitement. The chief cause of falsely elevated BP readings is the use of improperly fitting, narrow cuffs. Therefore attention to correct measurement technique is essential. (See Blood Pressure, Chapter 7.) Twenty-four-hour BP monitoring devices detect changes in pressure throughout the day, thus giving a more realistic picture. These devices are best used with older children who are able to tolerate being attached to an ambulatory monitor.

A careful family history should be obtained to screen for other relatives with hypertension or other cardiovascular risk factors. In children with suspected primary hypertension, initial laboratory data are also obtained. This generally includes a urinalysis, renal function studies such as a creatinine and blood urea nitrogen, a lipid profile, complete blood count, and electrolytes. Additional laboratory data may include urine and blood catecholemines and aldosterone. In children who have significant hypertension, secondary causes should be investigated thoroughly. A renal ultrasound scan provides a first-line screen of renovascular hypertension. In addition, it is often useful to assess left ventricular mass by echocardiography. If the LV mass is higher than normal, it indicates chronically elevated blood pressure because heart muscle thickens in response to chronic hypertension.

## Therapeutic Management

Therapy for secondary hypertension involves diagnosis and treatment of the underlying cause. In those cases amenable to surgical repair, the nature of the condition, the type of surgery, and the age of the child are all important considerations. Children or adolescents with consistently elevated BP readings from no known cause or those with secondary hypertension not amenable to surgical correction may be treated with a combination of nonpharmacologic and pharmacologic interventions. Dietary practices and lifestyle changes are important in the control of hypertension both for children and for adults. Nonpharmacologic measures, such as limitation of dietary salt, weight control, increased exercise, and avoidance of stress and smoking, carry no risk and should be instituted first,

except in severe cases. Because the long-term effects of antihypertensive agents on children are not known, drug treatment of asymptomatic children with mild or borderline hypertension is not recommended.

Because obesity and hypertension are closely related, a weight reduction program is recommended for overweight youngsters. In salt-sensitive children, high salt intake increases the risk of hypertension for those genetically predisposed and aggravates existing hypertension unless salt intake is limited. Modifying salt intake in children is difficult and takes time and support. Regular exercise augments weight reduction and alone has been shown to normalize BP. The exercise regimen is tailored to the child's interest. Aerobic exercise, such as swimming, running, or cycling, is highly recommended. Stress reduction strategies may be beneficial and include biofeedback and relaxation. Smoking is discouraged. If the adolescent is taking oral contraceptives, these may need to be discontinued and other contraceptive options provided.

Drug therapy in children is instituted with caution. Indications for antihypertensive drug therapy include significant elevations of BP resistant to nonpharmacologic intervention. The National Institutes of Health (NIH) Second Task Force on Blood Pressure Control in Children (1996) recommends beginning with one drug and adding other agents only if control is not obtained. Compliance with antihypertensive drug regimens is often difficult.

The oral antihypertensive drugs used most often in children include the ACE inhibitors (lisinopril, captopril, and enalapril), beta blockers (propranolol), diuretics, and occasionally a vasodilator (hydralazine). Calcium channel blockers remain controversial for the pediatric population. The practitioner should keep in mind that beta blockers can cause lipid abnormalities or mood disturbances such as depression in some children. Pharmacologic intervention is tailored to meet the needs of individual children and is determined by the hypotensive effect produced and the appearance of any side effects. The goal is to achieve a normotensive state throughout the day without accompanying side effects. With many antihypertensive drugs, minimal data are available regarding their side effects in children. Therefore any behavioral or physical changes that occur after institution of therapy should be considered a possible effect, and therapy may need to be revised.

## Nursing Considerations

The nurse is a valuable link in the health care delivery system in relation to hypertension in the pediatric age-group. Active in detection, diagnosis, and therapy in any setting—hospital, school, clinic, private office, public health services, and private practice—nurses are frequently the persons who operate well-child care and follow-up units and are usually the primary contact between health services and the child and family.

A BP measurement should always be a part of the routine assessment of infants and children. In carrying out the procedure, it is important to use the correct cuff size. Any questionable reading is repeated. When an elevated pressure is detected, the procedure should be carried out in the supine, sitting, and standing positions as feasible. In addition, initial comparisons should be made between the upper and lower extremities.

Nursing counseling and guidance of affected children is a challenge. Education aimed at the understanding of hypertension and its implication over the life span is essential in promoting patient and family compliance with both nonpharmacologic and pharmacologic therapies. (See Compliance, Chapter 27.)

Home BP measurements can facilitate surveillance in youngsters with chronic hypertension and can document effectiveness of therapy. A family member can be instructed in how to take and record accurate BP measurements, thus decreasing the number of trips to a health care facility. This individual needs to understand when to contact the practitioner regarding elevated values. When this option is not feasible, the school nurse can often be a valuable resource in monitoring BP.

The nurse plays an important role in assessing individual families and providing targeted information regarding nonpharmacologic modes of intervention, such as diet, weight loss, smoking, and exercise programs. If extensive dietary counseling is required, the child should be referred to a registered dietitian with expertise in working with children and adolescents. Exercise regimens should be individualized. Schoolchildren and young adolescents generally prefer team sports rather than individual training, which they may view as a burden rather than an enjoyable activity. If peers and family members can be encouraged to participate in any of the management strategies, the child's compliance is likely to be greater.

If drug therapy is prescribed, the nurse needs to provide information to the family regarding the reasons for drug therapy, how the drug works, and possible side effects (Box 34-11). It is important to explain that the drug needs to be taken consistently to achieve any prolonged control of BP. The need for follow-up is stressed, especially because antihypertensive therapy can sometimes be safely discontinued if BP remains under control over time.

Learning needs vary greatly depending on developmental levels and individual differences. Some children and families require a great deal of support, education, and guidance, whereas others need only education and periodic follow-up. A positive approach is essential; negative feedback will serve only to alienate the family. Exploring the reasons for difficulty in compliance can often provide realistic alternatives. Continued education, support, and reinforcement for positive behavior is a major nursing responsibility.

## Hyperlipidemia (Hypercholesterolemia)

*Hyperlipidemia* is a general term for excessive lipids (fat and fatlike substances); *hypercholesterolemia* refers to excessive cholesterol in the blood. High lipid or cholesterol levels are believed to play an important role in producing *atherosclerosis* (fatty plaques on the arteries), which eventually can lead to *coronary artery disease (CAD)*, a primary cause of morbidity and mortality in the adult population. The risk of premature CAD has been shown to increase directly with

---

### Box 34-11
### Antihypertensive Drugs Commonly Used in the Treatment of Pediatric Hypertension, with Nursing Interventions*

**ACE INHIBITORS**

*Action:* Acts primarily by interfering with the production of angiotensin II, a potent vasoconstrictor

**Captopril (Capoten)**
Monitor blood pressure and pulse.
Instruct to take 1 hour before meals to increase absorption.
Instruct patient to report any evidence of infection.
Advise to avoid rapid position changes (can initially cause dizziness).

**Enalapril (Vasotec)**
Monitor blood pressure and pulse (may cause hypotension).
Instruct to report any swelling of face or lips and difficulty breathing (may rarely cause laryngeal edema).
Instruct to report any evidence of infection.
Advise not to use potassium supplements (can increase serum levels).

**Lisinopril (Zestril, Prinivil)**
Longer half-life; able to administer in a single daily dose.
May cause hypotension, dizziness.
Monitor electrolytes/blood urea nitrogen/creatinine (can increase serum levels).

**BETA BLOCKERS**

*Actions:* Blocks response to beta stimulation Depresses renin output

**Propranolol (Inderal)**
Monitor pulse and blood pressures (can cause bradycardia and hypotension).
Instruct to take with meals.
Advise that drug may cause fatigue, a decrease in exercise tolerance, weakness, and cold extremities.
Warn males of possible impotence.

**Atenolol (Tenormin)**
Monitor pulse and blood pressures (can cause bradycardia and hypotension).
Advise that drug can be given once a day.
Instruct patients not to discontinue abruptly (needs to be withdrawn over a 2-week period).

**VASODILATORS**

*Actions:* Acts on vascular smooth muscle Thought to produce its effect by direct action on blood vessels to cause arterial vasodilation

**Hydralazine (Apresoline)**
Instruct to take with meals.
Advise that drug may cause drowsiness and to use caution operating machinery or doing other hazardous activity.
Instruct to report if sore throat, fever, muscle and joint aches, or skin rash develops.

**DIURETICS**
(See Table 34-5.)

---

*For the use of all drugs, instruct child or adolescent (and family) to:
Rise slowly from a horizontal position and avoid sudden position changes.
Take drug as prescribed.
Notify practitioner if unpleasant side effects occur but do not discontinue drug.
Avoid alcohol and stay on prescribed diet.

---

plasma concentrations of total cholesterol and certain types of lipids. Interventions that decrease low-density lipoproteins (LDLs) and increase high-density lipoproteins (HDLs) have been shown to lower the risk for CAD (American Academy of Pediatrics [AAP], 1998). Current research indicates that a presymptomatic phase of atherosclerosis begins in childhood. As a result, preventive cardiology is focusing on the screening and management of lipid levels in childhood. The goal is to identify those children at high risk and intervene early.

The rationale for lipid screening and management in children is evolving as lipid levels have been followed from childhood into adulthood. Children who demonstrate cholesterol levels in the upper percentiles seem to have an increased risk of remaining in the upper percentiles into adulthood. The more severely affected children are generally the ones targeted for dietary and possibly pharmacologic intervention. On the other hand, children in the lower percentiles are unlikely to have high cholesterol levels as adults. Cholesterol in childhood appears to be a major population predictor for adult cholesterol levels (AAP, 1998). From known data on lipid levels and their relationship to cardiovascular disease in adults, some experts believe that children with hypercholesterolemia may suffer an increased risk of cardiovascular disease in adulthood.

To date no definitive studies can predict the long-term risk of heart disease for children with hyperlipidemia. Research in this area is logistically difficult to complete because of the long period of clinical follow-up extending over 40 to 60 years. As a result, pediatric guidelines are inferred from adult data. Lifestyle habits, including diet, exercise patterns, and smoking, all known to be potential risk factors for cardiovascular disease, are normally established at a young age.

*Cholesterol,* a fatlike steroid alcohol, is part of the lipoprotein complex in plasma that is essential for cellular metabolism. *Triglycerides,* natural fats synthesized from carbohydrates, are used for energy. Both are major lipids transported on lipoproteins, a combination of lipids and proteins, which include:

**Chylomicrons**—Produced in the intestine in response to the intake of dietary fat. These are the principal transporters of dietary fat (triglycerides) from the intestine to the blood and ultimately to the fatty tissue. Chylomicrons are usually not present in the blood after a 12- to 14-hour fast.

**Very-low-density lipoproteins (VLDLs)**—Contain high concentrations of triglycerides, moderate concentrations of cholesterol, and little protein.

**Low-density lipoproteins (LDLs)**—Contain low concentrations of triglycerides, high levels of cholesterol, and moderate levels of protein. The end product of VLDL synthesis, LDLs are the major carriers of cholesterol to the cells. Cells use cholesterol for synthesis of membranes and steroid production. Elevated levels of circulating LDL are a strong risk factor in cardiovascular disease.

**High-density lipoproteins (HDLs)**—Contain very low concentrations of triglycerides, relatively little cholesterol, and high levels of protein. HDLs transport free cholesterol to the liver for secretion in the bile. High levels of HDL are thought to protect against cardiovascular disease.

The formula used for a standard fasting lipid profile that reflects total cholesterol (TC) is:

$$TC = LDL + HDL + \frac{Triglycerides}{5}$$

LDL concentration can be calculated from this formula. It is considered accurate as long as the fasting triglyceride level is below 450 mg/dl.

$$LDL = TC - \left(HDL + \frac{Triglycerides}{5}\right)$$

## Diagnostic Evaluation

Diagnosis of hyperlipidemia is based on analysis of blood for a full lipid profile. Two samples drawn in the fasting state (12 hours) should be analyzed, and the average of the values used for diagnosis. Blood samples should be collected after having the child sit for 5 minutes, and the tourniquet should be applied immediately before the needle puncture, because posture and vascular stasis may affect results. Diagnostic values for acceptable, borderline, and high total cholesterol and LDL cholesterol levels are listed in Table 34-8.

Screening children for hypercholesterolemia is a controversial issue, with some authorities advocating universal screening and others proposing selective screening. Current guidelines recommended by the American Academy of Pediatrics, Committee on Nutrition (1998) recommend a strategy that combines two complementary approaches: (1) a *population approach* that aims to lower the average levels of blood cholesterol among all American children through population-wide changes in nutrient intake and eating patterns, and (2) an *individualized approach* based on selective screening. (See Evidence-Based Practice box.)

## Therapeutic Management

Treatment of high cholesterol is primarily dietary. The American Academy of Pediatrics guidelines recommend a two-step dietary approach that restricts the intake of cholesterol and fat. Children with borderline LDL cholesterol are advised to follow the *step one diet.* It recommends the same nutrient intake as for the general population (i.e., less than 10% of total calories from saturated fatty acids, no more than 30% of calories from total fat, less than 300 mg/day of cholesterol, and adequate calories to support growth and development and to reach or maintain desirable body weight). Children with high LDL cholesterol levels initially are also placed on this diet. If these dietary modifications fail to achieve satisfactory levels of LDL after 3 months of therapy, the *step two diet* is initiated. These dietary restric-

**TABLE 34-8** Classification of total and low-density lipoprotein (LDL) cholesterol levels in children and adolescents from families with hypercholesterolemia or premature cardiovascular disease

| Category | Total Cholesterol (mg/dl) | LDL-Cholesterol (mg/dl) |
|---|---|---|
| Acceptable | <170 | <110 |
| Borderline | 170-199 | 110-129 |
| High | ≥200 | ≥130 |

From National Cholesterol Education Program: Report of the Expert Panel on Blood Cholesterol Levels in Children and Adolescents, *Pediatrics* 89(3, pt 2): 527, 1992.

tions include a further reduction of saturated fatty acid intake to 7% of calories and of cholesterol intake to less than 200 mg/day.

New research continues to support the benefit of diets low in saturated fats. However, current debate among experts revolves around the optimum amount of total fat for lipid-lowering diets. In overly fat-restricted diets, HDL values (good cholesterol) tend to drop along with LDL values, thus decreasing the potential benefits of this approach. Further concern arises when patients replace fat calories with foods high in simple sugars, which can raise triglyceride values, decreasing the effectiveness of nutritional interventions.

Current thinking favors a "Mediterranean"-type diet. Whole grains, fruits, and vegetables form the foundation of this diet. In addition, this diet allows the use of monounsaturated fats, such as olive oil and canola oil, which have beneficial effects on HDL-cholesterol values. The use of these fats also makes the diet more realistic. Dietary recommendations can be confusing, and individualized guidelines should be made by a certified dietitian with expertise in lipid management.

For children with severe hypercholesterolemia who fail to respond to dietary modifications, drug therapy may be necessary. Two drugs recommended for treatment are the bile acid–binding resins or sequestrants *cholestyramine* and *colestipol*. These drugs act by binding bile acids in the intestinal lumen. Because they are not absorbed by the intestine, they do not produce systemic toxicity and are safe for children. Cholestyramine (Questran) and colestipol (Colestid) are both powders that are mixed with water or juice just before ingestion. Some patients cannot tolerate the medication because of the taste and the side effects, the most significant being constipation, abdominal pain, gastrointestinal bloating, flatulence, and nausea. Patients often complain of the "gritty" consistency of the medication. The average dose for a child is 4 g three times daily or 6 g twice daily. Colestid is now available in pill form (1 g/tablet); however, the pills are very large, and 5 pills equal 1 packet of powder. An older child or adolescent may still prefer to take the pills. However, the pills should be taken with adult supervision and plenty of water because of their size.

> **NURSING ALERT**
>
> The Report of the Expert Panel on Blood Cholesterol Levels in Children and Adolescents regarding recommendations for fat intake is not intended for infants from birth to 2 years of age, whose fast growth requires a higher percentage of calories from fat. Toddlers 2 to 3 years of age may safely make the transition to the recommended eating pattern as they begin to eat with the family. No treatment recommendations are made for any child younger than 2 years of age.

Patients should be instructed to take one multivitamin supplement with iron daily because cholestyramine may interfere with the absorption of fat-soluble vitamins. It may also interfere with absorption of other medications, which should be given at least 1 hour before or 6 hours after the bile acid–binding agent is ingested. The results of a complete blood count, chloride and folate levels, and serum concentrations of vitamins A, D, and E should be evaluated yearly.

### Nursing Considerations

Nurses play an important role in the screening, education, and support of children with hyperlipidemia and their families. When a child is referred to a lipid clinic, it is essential that the family be adequately prepared for the first visit. Generally the parents will be asked to keep a dietary history of the child before this visit. Sometimes they will need to complete a questionnaire regarding the child's normal dietary habits over the preceding year. Families are instructed to keep their child fasting for at least 12 hours before screening. Therefore it is important to schedule the blood test early in the morning and to arrange for nourishment immediately thereafter. At the visit a complete family history is taken, including the health of both parents and all first-degree relatives, including questions about early heart disease, hypertension, CVAs, sudden death, hyperlipidemia, diabetes, and endocrine abnormalities. Nurses may also uncover risk factors when obtaining a health history for other purposes. It is therefore important that nurses be familiar with current screening practices and the availability of resources for children with positive family histories.

---

## EVIDENCE-BASED PRACTICE
### Cholesterol Screening for Children

Practitioners' opinions differ regarding lipid screening in childhood. In 1992 the National Cholesterol Education Program (NCEP) issued a consensus statement that provides guidelines for cholesterol screening in the pediatric population. Currently, selective screening is recommended for children who have a family history of premature cardiovascular disease (<55 years old) or children who have at least one parent with a high blood cholesterol level (>240 mg/dl). In addition, if a child's complete family history is not available, practitioners may consider screening. Finally, cholesterol values should be obtained in children who have any individual risk factors, such as a history of diabetes, Kawasaki disease, hypertension, or obesity.

Selective screening is favored by many experts because high blood cholesterol levels aggregate in families as a result of shared genetic and environmental factors (American Academy of Pediatrics, 1998). In addition, the most severely affected children generally come from families where there is a high incidence of early heart disease.

Advocates of selective screening oppose universal screening for various reasons. Screening is costly, and the laboratory data may vary significantly from center to center, resulting in inappropriate diagnosis.

Those favoring universal screening believe that selective screening is too limited and overlooks many children with hyperlipidemia. With varying family constellations a common situation today, family history may be incomplete. In addition, a negative history from a parent may be inaccurate, since approximately half of well-educated adults do not know their own cholesterol levels.

In your practice, how many adult family members know their "numbers"? Also, observe how often pediatric practitioners ask about parents' cholesterol levels and heart disease as part of the child's health assessment. From your observations do you believe that selective screening is being implemented?

Parents and extended families are informed about cholesterol and hyperlipidemia. This education should include a brief introduction to the different lipoprotein categories, including cholesterol, HDL, LDL, and triglycerides. Also, behavioral risk factors for heart disease, such as smoking and exercise, are reviewed. For management to be effective, parents need to understand the rationale for dietary and pharmacologic intervention. The key is prevention of future cardiovascular disease.

Stringent dietary guidelines may become an issue of control and a source of great stress for many families. Children are not viewed as having a disease. Rather, the positive aspects of healthy eating, regular exercise, and avoiding smoking are emphasized. Basic dietary changes are encouraged for the whole family so that the affected child is not singled out. The focus is positive, with emphasis on what can be eaten, such as substituting chicken and fish for hot dogs and hamburgers and substituting frozen yogurt for ice cream (Table 34-9). Cultural differences must be considered and recommendations individualized. For example, it is more realistic to suggest frying food in a monounsaturated oil such as canola oil than to forbid frying food altogether in

families where this is common practice. Substitution rather than elimination needs to be emphasized. Visual aids are often helpful, especially for children (e.g., test tubes depicting the amount of fat in a hot dog). Diets should be flexible and individually tailored by a nutritionist experienced in combining recommendations that meet both the nutritional demands of the growing child and lipid modifications. Parents are encouraged to participate in dietary and educational sessions, ask questions, and share ideas and experiences.

Parents often feel guilty about the hereditary component of hyperlipidemia. Many of these same parents believe they have failed if the diet alone is not making a significant difference in their child's lipid profile. They are reassured that a dietary approach alone is often not sufficient, especially for children with values greater than the 95th percentile.

Parents of children who require pharmacologic therapy need to understand the purpose, dosage, and possible side effects of the various drugs. Medication schedules should remain flexible and should not interfere with the child's daily activities. As an example, children of elementary school age may have better compliance if they take a resin-binding agent (e.g., cholestyramine, colestipol) twice a day (i.e., before school and at night) rather than the standard three times a day. Follow-up phone calls by the nurse between visits allow parents to discuss their concerns and ask any questions that have arisen.

## Cardiomyopathy

Cardiomyopathy refers to abnormalities of the myocardium in which the cardiac muscles' ability to contract is impaired. Cardiomyopathies are relatively rare in children. Possible etiologic factors include familial or genetic causes, infection, deficiency states, metabolic abnormalities, and collagen vascular diseases. Most cardiomyopathies in children are considered primary or idiopathic, in which the cause is unknown and the cardiac dysfunction is not associated with systemic disease. Recent research in metabolic and genetic causes of cardiomyopathies suggest that many may be a result of abnormalities of the cell function of the cardiac myocyte (Canter and Strauss, 1995). Some of the known causes of **secondary** cardiomyopathy are anthracycline toxicity (the antineoplastic agents doxorubicin [Adriamycin] and daunomycin), hemochromatosis (from excessive iron storage), Duchenne muscular dystrophy, Kawasaki disease, collagen diseases, and thyroid dysfunction.

Cardiomyopathies can be divided into three broad clinical categories according to the type of abnormal structure and dysfunction present: dilated cardiomyopathy, hypertrophic cardiomyopathy, and restrictive cardiomyopathy. **Dilated cardiomyopathy** is characterized by ventricular dilation and greatly decreased contractility resulting in symptoms of CHF. This is the most common type of cardiomyopathy in children. Its cause is often unknown, although carnitine and selenium deficiency, metabolic diseases, drug toxicities, dysrhythmias, and infection causing myocarditis should be considered. Familial inheritance may be the etiology of nearly 25% of these cardiomyopathies (Grunig and others, 1998). The clinical findings are of CHF with tachycardia, dyspnea,

**TABLE 34-9** Low-cholesterol substitutes for common foods

| Foods High in Cholesterol and Saturated Fats | Substitutions Low in Cholesterol and Saturated Fats |
|---|---|
| Red meat | Skinless chicken, broiled or baked |
| | Turkey |
| | Tofu |
| | Meatless main dishes (e.g., vegetarian chili or lasagna) |
| | Fish |
| Hot dogs | Low-fat hot dogs |
| Processed luncheon meats and fast foods | Turkey |
| | Low-fat ham |
| | Tuna fish |
| | Grilled, skinless chicken or salads |
| Regular milk (4% fat) | Skim milk |
| Ice cream | Nonfat frozen yogurt |
| | Sherbet without cream |
| | Frozen fruit juice bars |
| Butter, shortening, lard | Olive oil, canola oil |
| | Fat-free margarine |
| | Fat-free mayonnaise |
| Cheddar/American cheese | Part-skim mozzarella sticks |
| | Fat-free yogurt |
| | Fat-free cottage cheese |
| | Fat-free American cheese |
| Egg noodles | Yolkless noodles |
| | Other grains (rice and pasta) |
| Potato chips | Pretzels |
| | Plain popcorn |
| | Vegetable sticks |
| Chocolate | Cocoa-containing foods |
| Cookies/crackers | Low-fat cookies/crackers (graham, animal, saltines) |

Modified from American Academy of Pediatrics National Cholesterol Education Program: Report of the Expert Panel on Blood Cholesterol Levels in Children and Adolescents, *Pediatrics* 89(suppl):525-584, 1992.

hepatosplenomegaly, fatigue, and poor growth. Dysrhythmias may be present and may be more difficult to control with worsening heart failure. Chest radiography demonstrates cardiomegaly and congested lung fields. The echocardiogram demonstrates poor ventricular contractility, dilated LV, and reduced shortening and ejection fraction. Cardiac catheterization with endomyocardial biopsy is usually done for diagnosis and to identify a possible infectious cause.

*Hypertrophic cardiomyopathy* is characterized by an increase in heart muscle mass without an increase in cavity size, usually occurring in the LV and associated with abnormal diastolic filling. Half of these patients have a familial autosomal dominant genetic abnormality (Burch and Blair, 1999). Infants of diabetic mothers may have a hypertrophic cardiomyopathy that resolves with time. Clinical symptoms usually present in school-age period or adolescence and may include anginal chest pain, dysrhythmias, and syncope. Sudden death is possible. Presentation in infancy includes signs of CHF and has a poor prognosis. Chest radiography shows a mildly enlarged heart; the ECG demonstrates LV hypertrophy, often with ST-T changes. The echocardiogram is most helpful and demonstrates asymmetric septal hypertrophy and an increase in LV wall thickness, with a small LV cavity.

*Restrictive cardiomyopathy,* rare in children, describes a restriction to ventricular filling caused by endocardial or myocardial disease or both. Thrombus formation and embolic events are common, and elevation of pulmonary vascular resistance may occur (Denfield and others, 1997). Symptoms are of CHF (see p. 1477).

### Therapeutic Management

Treatment is directed toward correcting the underlying cause whenever feasible. However, in most affected children this is not possible, and treatment is aimed at managing CHF (see p. 1479) and dysrhythmias. Digoxin, diuretics, and aggressive use of afterload reduction agents have been found to be helpful in managing symptoms in those with dilated cardiomyopathy. Digoxin and inotropic agents are usually not helpful in the other forms of cardiomyopathy because increasing the force of contraction may exacerbate the muscular obstruction and actually impair ventricular ejection. Beta blockers such as propranolol (Inderal) or calcium channel blockers such as verapamil (Calan) have been used to reduce LV outflow obstruction and improve diastolic filling in those with hypertrophic cardiomyopathy.

Careful monitoring and treatment of dysrhythmias is essential. Anticoagulants may be given to reduce the risk of thromboemboli, a complication of the sluggish circulation through the heart. For worsening heart failure and signs of poor perfusion, IV inotropic support with dobutamine for several days has been successfully used in children, with symptomatic improvement lasting beyond the infusion. Severely ill children may benefit from mechanical ventilation, oxygen administration, and IV afterload reduction agents such as nitroprusside or amrinone. Heart transplantation may be a treatment option for patients who have worsening symptoms despite maximum medical therapy (see p. 1526).

### Nursing Considerations

Because of the poor prognosis in many children with cardiomyopathy, nursing care is consistent with that for any child with a life-threatening disorder. (See Chapter 23.) One of the most difficult adjustments for the child may be the realization of failing health and the need for restricted activity, especially the normally active youngster with hypertrophic cardiomyopathy. The child should be included in decisions regarding activity and allowed to discuss feelings, particularly if the disease follows a progressively fatal course. Once symptoms of CHF or dysrhythmias develop, the same nursing interventions are implemented as discussed on pp. 1481-1484. If cardiac transplantation is considered, the needs of the child and family are great in terms of psychologic preparation and postoperative care. The nurse plays an important role in assessing the family's understanding of the procedure and long-term consequences. Children of school age and older should be fully informed to give their assent to the procedure. (See Informed Consent, Chapter 27.)

## Cardiac Dysrhythmias

Dysrhythmias, or abnormal heart rhythms, can occur in children with structurally normal hearts, as features of some congenital heart defects, and in patients following surgical repair of congenital heart defects. They are also seen in patients with cardiomyopathy and with cardiac tumors. They can occur secondary to metabolic and electrolyte imbalances. Recently some dysrhythmias have been found to have a genetic of familial etiology (Fish and Benson, 2001). They can be classified in several ways, such as by heart rate characteristics (bradycardia and tachycardia) or by the origin of the dysrhythmia in the atria or ventricles. Most are due to abnormalities in impulse generation in the right atria or to abnormalities in the conduction pathways.

Some dysrhythmias are well tolerated and self-limiting. Others may cause decreased cardiac output with associated symptoms. Some dysrhythmias can cause sudden death. Treatment depends on the cause of the dysrhythmia and its severity. Underlying causes are treated if possible (such as electrolyte imbalances). Some (such as congenital heart block causing bradycardia) are well tolerated and may not require treatment for many years. Others may require medications, radiofrequency ablation, or pacemaker placement. Some can be difficult to treat and involve multiple therapies.

Many advances have been made in the diagnosis and treatment of pediatric dysrhythmias in the past decade. Improvements in technology have allowed better diagnosis, the development of ablation techniques and the expansion of pacemaker capabilities. New antidysrhythmic medications have proven safe and effective in children. Radiofrequency ablation has offered a cure for some dysrhythmias. Pediatric electrophysiology has become a highly specialized field, and the student is referred to more detailed sources for an in-depth discussion. The following sections will address diagnostic studies and a general discussion of the most common tachycardia (supraventricular tachycardia [SVT]) and the most common bradycardia (complete heart block) that require treatment in the pediatric population.

## Diagnostic Evaluation

Before diagnosing an infant or child with an abnormal rate, nurses must be familiar with the standards of normal heart rate for the particular age-group. (See inside back cover.) Heart rate variations considered normal for a particular child can vary tremendously. An initial nursing responsibility is recognition of an abnormal heartbeat, either in rate or rhythm. When a dysrhythmia is suspected, the apical rate is counted for 1 full minute and compared with the radial rate, which may be lower because not all of the apical beats are felt. Consistently high or low heart rates should be regarded as suspicious. Accurate nursing assessment is essential. The patient should be placed on a cardiac monitor with recording capabilities. A 12-lead ECG yields more information than the monitor recording and should be done as soon as possible. Recent advances in bedside telemetry allow storage of ECG tracings for later analysis.

Several advances in the diagnosis of cardiac dysrhythmias have greatly improved the understanding and treatment of these conditions in children. The basic diagnostic procedure is the ECG, including 24-hour Holter monitoring. However, more definitive procedures include both noninvassive and invasive techniques.

*Electrophysiologic cardiac catheterization* allows for identification of the conduction disturbance and immediate investigation of drugs that may control the dysrhythmia. Electrode catheters are introduced intravenously and directed toward the right side of the heart. The heart is then selectively stimulated to induce dysrhythmias. Once a dysrhythmia occurs, different antidysrhythmic drugs are administered intravenously to monitor which pharmacologic agent is most successful in terminating the dysrhythmia. Preparation for the procedure is similar to a cardiac catheterization (see p. 1471). These studies can be lengthy, lasting more than 4 hours. Sedation or general anesthesia is required.

Another procedure that may be employed is *transesophageal recording*. An electrode catheter is passed to the lower esophagus and, when in position at a point proximal to the heart, is used to stimulate and record dysrhythmias.

The onset and diagnosis of a cardiac dysrhythmia are frightening experiences for parents and the older child. Sometimes the dysrhythmia rapidly leads to heart failure and a medical crisis. In this situation parents need much support to express their feelings and to understand the diagnosis and its treatment. Often an unspoken fear of potential death exists even if the dysrhythmia is benign. and repeated explanations are needed to allay anxiety.

**Bradydysrhythmias.** *Sinus bradycardia* in children can be due to the influence of the autonomic nervous system, as with hypervagal tone, or in response to hypoxia and hypotension. Once the infant receives adequate oxygenation and any acidosis is eliminated, the heart rate will often return to baseline. Sinus bradycardias are also known to develop after atrial repairs involving extensive atrial suture lines such as atrial baffle procedures (Mustard and Senning repairs for transposition of the great arteries) and the Fontan procedure.

Complete atrioventricular block (AV block) is also referred to as complete heart block (Fig. 34-16). This can be either congenital (occurring in children with structurally normal hearts) or acquired following surgery to repair cardiac defects. *AV blocks* are most often related to edema around the conduction system and resolve without treatment. Temporary epicardial wires are placed in most patients at surgery; if a rhythm disturbance occurs, temporary pacing can be employed. Just before discharge the health practitioner removes the wires by pulling slowly and deliberately down on them from the site of insertion. In some cases permanent pacemaker implantation may be necessary to treat complete AV blocks that do not resolve by the eight to tenth postoperative day (Fish and Benson, 2001).

A permanent pacemaker may be needed in some children, such as those with postsurgical AV block or, less frequently, congenital AV block. The pacemaker takes over or assists in the conduction function of the heart. The surgical implantation of a pacemaker is usually a low-risk procedure. Once the wire has been introduced, a small incision is made and a pocket is formed under the muscle to house and prottect the generator. Continuous ECG monitoring is necessary during the recovery phase to assess pacemaker function. The nurse should be aware of the programmed rate and expected individual generator variations. A baseline ECG and chest x-ray film are obtained for future comparison. The pacemaker insertion site is monitored for signs of infection. Analgesics are given for pain.

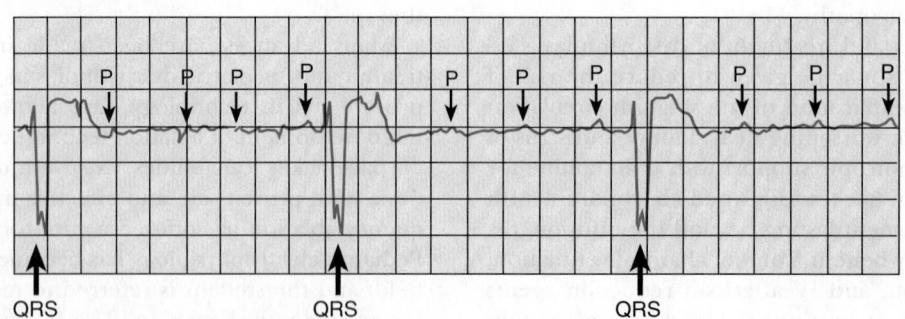

**Fig. 34-16** Complete heart block. Note slow rhythm and several P waves not followed by a QRS complex.

Pacemaker functions have become dramatically more sophisticated; they can control heart rate according to activity, cardiac output, and respirations. In addition, some models can be programmed for overdrive pacing or cardioversion when the generator detects accelerated rates beyond established normal values.

When a *pacemaker* is implanted, the education of the parents and child includes an explanation of the device, a description of the component parts, the surgical procedure, and discharge teaching. The pacemaker is made up of two basic parts: the pulse generator and the lead. The *pulse generator* is composed of the battery and the electronic circuitry. The function is to produce the electrical impulse sent to the heart and to receive and respond to signals produced by the heart. The *lead* is an insulated, flexible wire that conducts the electrical impulse from the pulse generator to the heart. Two types of leads ar available: transvenous and epicardial. The child's size and the heart's structure determine which lead is more appropriate. *Transvenous leads* are inserted into a large vein, often the subclavian, and advanced into the right side of the heart. Placement is secured by engaging a small corkscrew or fishhook attachment at the end of the lead into the endocardium. *Epicardial leads* are directly attached to the epicardial layer of the heart. Parents should be aware of which type of lead their child has in place.

Discharge teaching includes information about the signs and symptoms of infection, general wound care, and activity restrictions. Parents, and patients if they are old enough, should be taught to take a pulse and know the settings of the pacemaker. If the patient's low rate is set at 80 beats/min and the heart rate is only 68 beats/min, there is a possible problem with the pacemaker that needs to be investigated. Instructions for telephone transmission of ECG readings are also given. Telephone transmission can be used to transmit ECG strips and also to monitor battery life and pacemaker function. The pacemaker generator will have to replaced periodically because of battery depletion. Children with pacemakers should wear a medical alert device, and their parents should have a paper identification card with specific pacer data in case of an emergency. CPR instruction is suggested for parents.

**Tachydysrhythmias.** *Sinus tachycardia* (abnormally fast heart rate) secondary to fever, anxiety, pain, anemia, dehydration, or any other etiologic factor requiring increased cardiac output should be ruled out first before diagnosing an increased heart rate as pathologic. *Supraventricular tachycardia (SVT),* the most common tachydysrhythmia found in children, refers to a rapid regular heart rate of 200 to 300 beats/min (Fig. 34-17). The rapid rhythm originates in the atria. The onset and termination of SVT are abrupt. The QRS complex is usually narrow (in contrast with ventricular tachycardia, in which the QRS complexes are typically wide), and the P waves are often absent. Infants and young children with SVT may be unable to compensate for the rapid heart rate, and the clinical course can progress to CHF. Important signs in the infant and young child are poor feeding, extreme irritability, and pallor. Children may experience palpitations, dizziness, chest pain, and diaphoresis.

Ventricular tachycardias are rare in children and will not be discussed here.

The treatment of SVT depends on the degree of compromise imposed by the dysrhythmia. In some instances, *vagal maneuvers,* such as applying ice to the face, massaging the carotid artery (on *one* side of the neck only), or having an older child perform a Valsalva maneuver (e.g., exhaling against a closed glottis, blowing on the thumb as if it were a trumpet for 30 to 60 seconds), have reversed the SVT. When vagal maneuvers fail, adenosine may be used to end the episode of SVT by impairing AV node conduction. Adenosine must be given by rapid IV push with a saline bolus immediately following the drug. Incrementally increasing doses given about 2 minutes apart may be needed. The desired effect usually occurs in 10 to 20 seconds. The very short half-life (less than 10 seconds) of adenosine minimizes side effects such as flushing, headache, and dizziness (Phillips and Somers, 2000).

If the infant or child is minimally symptomatic, digitalization should be undertaken, with careful monitoring of vital signs and patient response to the intervention. More aggressive pharmacologic treatment with medications such as propranolol (Inderal) or amiodarone may be needed for those with more severe symptoms or recurrence of SVT while on digoxin. If cardiac output is significantly compromised or signs of CHF exist, esophageal overdrive pacing or synchronized cardioversion can be employed in the intensive care setting.

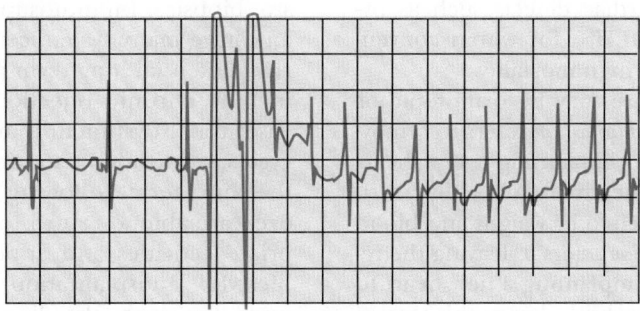

**Fig. 34-17**   Supraventricular tachycardia (SVT). Note normal sinus rhythm (three PQRST complexes) on the left and abrupt onset of a very fast rhythm (SVT) on the right.

*Transesophageal atrial overdrive pacing* is accomplished through placement of a protected lead into the esophagus, behind the left atrium of the heart. The lead is then attached to a stimulator capable of pacing at very rapid rates to interrupt the tachydysrhythmia. *Synchronized cardioversion* is the timed delivery of a preset amount of energy through the chest wall in an attempt to reestablish an organized rhythm. Sedation is needed for both procedures. Cardioversion should never be done in a conscious patient.

Radiofrequency (RF) ablation has become first-line therapy for some types of SVT. The procedure is done in the cardiac catheterization laboratory and begins with mapping of the conduction system to identify the dysrhythmia focus. A catheter delivering radiofrequency current is directed at the site, and the identified area is heated to destroy the tissue in the area. Complications include complete heart block and vascular and endothelial damage (Saul, 2001). Success rates vary between 60% and 90% depending on the type of SVT (Le Roy, 2001). A successful ablation is curative and antidysrhythmic medications can be discontinued.

Preparation is similar to that for cardiac catheterization and other electrophysiology studies. The risks and benefits of ablation need to reviewed. These are lengthy procedures, often 6 to 8 hours, and sedation or general anesthesia is required. Postprocedure care is similar to that for cardiac catheterization (see p. 1473) with the addition of careful dysrhythmia monitoring. Patients and their families often have great hope for a cure and are disappointed if the ablation is unsuccessful.

A primary focus of nursing care is education of the family regarding the symptoms of SVT and the treatment. SVT may occur again despite therapy. Following the first episode of SVT, parents should be taught to take a radial pulse for 1 full minute. If medication is prescribed, instructions regarding accurate dosage and the importance of administering the correct dose at specified intervals are stressed.

## HEART TRANSPLANTATION

Heart transplantation has become a treatment option for infants and children with worsening heart failure and a limited life expectancy despite maximum medical and surgical management. Indications for cardiac transplantation in children are cardiomyopathy and end-stage congenital heart disease. It is also an option for patients with some forms of complex congenital cardiac defects such as hypoplastic left heart syndrome (HLHS) for whom conventional surgical approaches have a high mortality.

The heart transplant procedure may be orthotopic or heterotopic. *Orthotopic heart transplantation* refers to removing the recipient's own heart and implanting a new heart from a donor who has had brain death but a healthy heart. The donor and recipient are matched by weight and blood type. *Heterotopic heart transplantation* refers to leaving the recipient's own heart in place and implanting a new heart to act as an additional pump or "piggyback" heart; this type of transplant is rarely done in children.

Before transplantation, potential recipients undergo a careful cardiac evaluation to determine if there are any other medical or surgical options to improve the patient's cardiac status. Other organ systems are assessed to identify problems that might preclude or increase the risk of transplantation. A psychosocial evaluation of the patient and family is done to assess family function, support systems, and the family's ability to comply with the complex medical regimen after the transplant. Support services to help the family successfully care for their child are provided when possible. Parents and older adolescents need extensive education about the risks and benefits of transplantation so that they can make an informed decision. In a study of factors that influenced parent decision making about heart transplantation, family beliefs and values were found to be most important (Higgins and Kayser-Jones, 1996).

Patients are listed on a national computer network organized by the **United Network for Organ Sharing (UNOS)** to match donors and recipients. (See Tissue Donation/Autopsy, Chapter 23.)

The number of heart transplants in pediatric patients has been constant for the last decade, between 340 and 400 transplants per year (Boucek and others, 2001). This likely reflects a limit in the number of available donors. Waiting times have more than doubled in all age groups in the last decade (UNOS Scientific Registry, 2000). A multicenter study evaluating waiting times found that 31% of infants died while awaiting transplantation (Morrow and others, 1997). Infants are the largest group of pediatric transplant recipients. The International Society for Heart and Lung Transplantation Registry data for all pediatric heart transplant recipients from 1982 to 1999 demonstrated a 1-year actuarial survival rate of 78% and a 9-year actuarial survival rate of 59%. Data for the most recent era (1996 to 1999) showed an improved 1-year actuarial survival rate of 86% and a 4-year actuarial survival rate of 79% (Boucek and others, 2001). In all eras the largest mortality is in the early posttransplant period.

The posttransplant course is complex. Although heart function is greatly improved or normal following transplantation, the risk of rejection is serious. The leading cause of death after heart transplantation is rejection (Fortuna, Chinnock, and Bailey, 1999). Rejection of the heart is diagnosed primarily by endomyocardial biopsy in older children. Serial echocardiograms are often used in infants and young children to reduce the need for invasive biopsies. Immunosuppressants must be taken for life and have many systemic side effects. Infection is always a risk. Potential long-term problems that may limit survival include chronic rejection, causing coronary artery disease; renal dysfunction and hypertension resulting from cyclosporine administration; lymphoma; and infection. In the short term, following successful transplantation, children are able to return to full participation in age-appropriate activities and appear to adapt well to their new lifestyle. Transplantation is not a cure, because patients must live with the lifetime consequences of chronic immunosuppression.

## Nursing Considerations

Nursing care following transplantation is demanding and complex, with careful attention to both the physical needs of the child and the emotional needs of the child and family. Successfully caring for a child following a heart transplant requires the expertise and dedication of many members of the health care team. Nurses play vital roles in assessment, coordination of care, psychosocial support, and patient and family education. The heart transplant recipient must be carefully monitored for signs of rejection, infection, and the side effects of the immunosuppressant medications. The patient and family's psychosocial well-being also needs to be assessed to identify issues such as increased family stress, depression, substance abuse, and school problems. Noncompliance with an intense medication regimen, especially during adolescence, can lead to serious medical problems and can be fatal. Immunosuppressants and nursing implications are discussed in Chapter 30 in relation to renal transplantation. Care of the immunosuppressed child is reviewed in Chapter 36. Psychosocial concerns and appropriate interventions for the child with a life-threatening disorder are presented in Chapter 23.

The first 6 months to 1 year following the transplant are most intense, because the risk of complications is greatest and the patient and family are adjusting to a new lifestyle. Patients are monitored closely by the health care team, with frequent visits and laboratory tests. Care is usually shared between local health care providers and the transplant center. Many patients are able to return to school and other age-appropriate activities within 2 to 3 months after the transplant.

## KEY POINTS

- Congenital heart disease is the most common form of cardiac disease in children.
- Major categories to investigate in the cardiac history are poor weight gain, poor feeding habits, and fatigue during feeding; frequent respiratory infections and difficulties; and evidence of exercise intolerance.
- The most common tests used in assessing cardiac function are radiography, electrocardiography, echocardiography, and cardiac catheterization.
- Cardiac catheterization procedures can be divided into three groups: (1) diagnostic procedures, including angiography that measure pressures and saturations to establish cardiac diagnosis; (2) interventional procedures, in which catheters or balloon devices are used to correct cardiac defects; and (3) electrophysiologic procedures for diagnosis and treatment of dysrhythmias.
- Cardiac catheterization provides important information about oxygen saturation of blood within the chambers and great vessels, pressure changes, changes in cardiac output or stroke volume, and anatomic abnormalities.
- Several prenatal factors may predispose children to congenital heart disease: maternal rubella during pregnancy, maternal alcoholism, and maternal type 1 diabetes.
- Congenital heart defects can be divided into four main groups, as determined by hemodynamic patterns: (1) defects that result in increased pulmonary blood flow, (2) obstructive defects, (3) defects that result in decreased pulmonary blood flow, and (4) mixed defects.
- Cardiac output is determined by the interaction of several factors: preload, afterload, contractility, and heart rate.
- Clinical consequences of congenital heart defects include congestive heart failure (CHF) and hypoxemia. A child can have both hypoxemia and CHF, although usually they occur independently.
- Clinical manifestations of CHF are impaired myocardial function (tachycardia, cardiomegaly), pulmonary congestion (dyspnea, tachypnea, orthopnea, cyanosis), and systemic congestion (hepatosplenomegaly, edema, distended veins).
- Nursing measures in the care of a child with CHF are to assist in improving cardiac function, decrease cardiac demands, reduce respiratory distress, maintain nutritional status, promote fluid loss, and provide family support.
- Clinical manifestations of hypoxemia are cyanosis, polycythemia, clubbing, and delayed growth and development. The child is at increased risk for hypercyanotic spells, cerebrovascular accidents, brain abscess, and bacterial endocarditis.
- Caring for the child with congenital heart disease (CHD) and the family requires helping them adjust to the disorder and cope with the effects of the defect and fostering growth-promoting family relationships.
- Preoperative care of the child with a congenital defect involves introducing the child and family to the hospital and preparing them for preoperative and postoperative procedures.
- Providing postoperative care includes observing vital signs and arterial/venous pressures, maintaining respiratory status, allowing maximum rest, providing comfort, monitoring fluids, planning for progressive activities, giving emotional support, observing for complications of surgery, and planning for discharge and home care.
- Acquired cardiovascular disorders include bacterial endocarditis, rheumatic fever, Kawasaki disease, systemic hypertension, hyperlipidemia, cardiomyopathy, and cardiac dysrhythmias.
- Prevention of bacterial endocarditis in certain children with CHD involves administration of prophylactic antibiotics when specific procedures are performed.
- Acute rheumatic fever is a systemic inflammatory disease that can damage the cardiac valves and is associated with previous group A β-hemolytic streptococcal infection. Its incidence has increased in some areas of the United States.
- Kawasaki disease is an extensive inflammation of small vessels and capillaries that may progress to involve the

coronary arteries, causing aneurysm formation. The administration of gamma globulin is an important aspect of treatment.

■ Education of the child and family with hypertension focuses on drug therapy, diet control, and appropriate exercise.

■ Cholesterol screening in children is controversial; currently children with known risk factors for hyperlipidemia are screened and treated as needed. The influence of childhood cholesterol levels on later development of coronary artery disease is under investigation.

■ Cardiomyopathy, or abnormality of the myocardium, is a serious, often fatal, disorder. Heart transplantation may offer more favorable options for some children than drug or other regimens.

■ Common dysrhythmias in children include slow rhythms (bradycardias, heart block) and fast rhythms (sinus tachycardia, supraventricular tachycardia).

■ Heart transplantation may benefit infants and children with cardiomyopathy and complex congenital heart defects resulting in severe ventricular dysfunction.

# REFERENCES

Allen H and others: Heart murmurs in children: when is a workup needed? *Contemp Pediatr* 2:29-52, 1994.

Allen HD and others: Pediatric therapeutic cardiac catheterization: AHA scientific statement, *Circulation* 97(6):609-625, 1998.

American Academy of Pediatrics: Cholesterol in childhood, *Pediatrics* 101(1, part 1):141-147, 1998.

American Academy of Pediatrics, Committee on Infectious Diseases, Pickering LK, editor: *2000 Red book: report of the Committee on Infectious Diseases,* ed 25, Elk Grove Village, IL, 2000, The Academy.

Anand KJS, Hickey PR: Halothane-morphine compared with high dose sufentanil for anesthesia and postoperative analgesia in neonatal cardiac surgery, *N Engl J Med* 326(1):1-9, 1992.

Barst RJ: Recent advances in the treatment of pediatric pulmonary artery hypertension, *Pediatr Clin North Am* 46(2):333-345, 1999.

Beekman RH: Coarctation of the aorta. In Allen HD and others, editors: *Moss and Adams' heart disease in infants, children and adolescents,* ed 6, Philadelphia, 2001, Lippincott Williams & Wilkins.

Behrman RE, Kliegman RM, Jenson, HA: *Nelson textbook of pediatrics,* ed 16, Philadelphia, 2000, WB Saunders.

Boucek MM and others: The Registry of the International Society for Heart and Lung Transplantation: fourth official pediatric report—2000, *J Heart Lung Transplant* 20:39-52, 2001.

Brashers V and others: Alterations of cardiovascular function. In Huether S, McCance K, editors: *Understanding pathophysiology,* ed 2, St Louis, 2000, Mosby.

Burch M, Blair E: The inheritance of hypertrophic cardiomyopathy, *Pediatr Cardiol* 20(5):313-316, 1999.

Burns J and others: Kawasaki disease: a brief history, *Pediatrics* 106(2):e27, 2000.

Canter CE, Struss A: Cardiomyopathies: when to think of congenital causes, *Contemp Pediatr* 12(4):25-38, 1995.

Channick RN and others: Pulsed delivery of inhaled nitric oxide to patients with primary pulmonary hypertension: an ambulatory delivery system and initial clinical tests, *Chest* 109(6):1545-1549, 1996.

Connor J, McCance K: Alterations of cardiovascular function. Huether S, McCance K, editors: *Understanding pathophysiology,* ed 2, St Louis, 2000, Mosby.

Craig J, Smith JB, Fineman LD: Tissue perfusion. In Curley MAQ, Moloney-Harmon P, editors: *Critical care nursing of infants and children,* ed 2, Philadelphia, 2001, WB Saunders.

Dajani AS, Taubert KA: Infective endocarditis. In Allen HD and others, editors: *Moss and Adams' heart disease in infants, children, and adolescents,* ed 6, Philadelphia, 2001, Lippincott Williams & Wilkins.

Dajani AS and others: Treatment of acute streptococcal pharyngitis and prevention of rheumatic fever: a statement for health professionals, *Pediatrics* 96:758-764, 1995.

Dajani AS and others: Prevention of bacterial endocarditis: recommendations by the American Heart Association, *JAMA* 277:1794-1801, 1997.

Denfield S and others: Restrictive cardiomyopathies in childhood, *Tex Heart Inst J* 24:38-44, 1997.

Ferencz C and others, editors: *Epidemiology of congenital heart disease: the Baltimore-Washington Infant Heart Study 1981-1989,* Mt Kisco, NY, 1997, Futura.

Ferencz C and others, editors: *Genetic and environmental risk factors of major cardiovascular malformations: the Baltimore-Washington Infant Heart Study 1981-1989,* Armonk, NY, 1997, Futura.

Ferrieri P and others: *Unique features of infective endocarditis in childhood,* From the Committee on Rheumatic Fever, Endocarditis and Kawasaki Disease, Council on Cardiovascular Disease in the Young, American Heart Association, 2001 (in press).

Fish FA and Benson WD: Disorders of rhythm and conduction. In Allen HD and others, editors: *Moss and Adams' heart disease in infants, children and adolescents,* ed 6, Philadelphia, 2001, Lippincott Williams & Wilkins.

Fortuna RS, Chinnock RE, Bailey LL: Heart transplantation among 233 infants during the first six months of life: the Loma Linda experience, *Clin Transpl* 1999:263-272, 1999.

Freed MD: Aortic stenosis. In Allen HD and others: *Moss and Adams' heart disease in infants, children and adolescents,* ed 6,

Philadelphia, 2001, Lippincott Williams and Wilkins.

Frishman WH, editor: *Current cardiovascular drugs,* ed 2, Philadelphia, 1995, Current Medicine.

Gentles T and others: Left ventricular mechanics during and after acute rheumatic fever: contractile dysfunction is closely related to valve regurgitation, *J Am Coll Cardiol* 37(1):201-207, 2001.

Gillman MW and others: Identifying children at high risk for the development of essential hypertension, *J Pediatr* 122:837-846, 1993.

Goldmuntz E and others: Frequency of 22q11 deletion in patients with conotruncal defects, *J Am Coll Cardiol* 32:492-498, 1998.

Grunig E and others: Frequency and phenotypes of familial dilated cardiomyopathy, *J Am Coll Cardiol* 31:186-194, 1998.

Gutschik E: New developments in the treatment of infective endocarditis, *Int J Antimicrob Agents* 13:79-92, 1999.

Hawkins JA and others: Late results and reintervention after aortic valvotomy for critical aortic stenosis, *Ann Thorac Surg* 65:1758-1762, 1998.

Helmers S and others: Perioperative electroencephalographic seizures in infants undergoing repair of complex congenital cardiac defects, *Electroencephalogr Clin Neuro Physiol* 102:27-36, 1997.

Higgins SS, Kayser-Jones J: Factors influencing parent decision making about pediatric cardiac transplantation, *J Pediatr Nurs* 11(3):152-160, 1996.

Higgins SS and others: Prescription and administration of around the clock analgesics in postoperative pediatric cardiovascular surgery patients, *Progr Cardiovasc Nurs* 14:19-24, 1999.

Jacobs ML, Blackstone EH, Bailey LL: Intermediate survival in neonates with aortic atresia: a multi-institutional study, *J Thorac Cardiovasc Surg* 116:417-431, 1998.

Kato H, Ichinose E, Kawasaki T: Myocardial infarction in Kawasaki disease: clinical analyses in 195 cases, *J Pediatr* 108(6):923-927, 1986.

LeRoy SS: Clinical dysrhythmias after surgical repair of congenital heart disease, *AACN Clin Issues* 12:87-99, 2001.

Macfayden AJ, Buckmaster MA: Pain management in the PICU, *Crit Care Clin* 15:185-200, 1999.

McRae ME and others: Development of a research-based standard for assessment, intervention, and evaluation of pain after neonatal and pediatric cardiac surgery, *Pediatr Nurs* 23(3):263-271, 1997.

Morrow WR and others: Outcome of listing for heart transplantation in infants younger than six months: predictors of death and interval to transplantation, *J Heart Lung Transplant* 16:1255-1266, 1997.

Narula J and others: Diagnosis of acute rheumatic carditis, *Circulation* 100: 1576-1581, 1999.

National Institutes of Health, National Heart, Lung, and Blood Institute: *Update on the Task Force Report (1987) on High Blood Pressure in Children and Adolescents,* Bethesda, MD, 1996, The Institutes.

O'Brien P, Smith P: Chronic hypoxemia in children with cyanotic heart disease, *Crit Care Nurs Clin North Am* 9(2):215-226, 1994.

O'Brien M and others: Ticlopidine plus aspirin for coronary thrombosis in Kawasaki disease, *Pediatrics* 105(5):e64, 2000.

Park MK: *Pediatric cardiology for practitioners,* ed 3, St Louis, 1996, Mosby.

Park MK, Lee DH, Johnson GA: Oscillometric blood pressures in the arm, thigh and calf in healthy children and those with aortic coarctation, *Pediatrics* 91(4):761-765, 1993.

Phillips BG, Somers VK: *Drug information handbook for cardiology 2000-2001,* Cleveland, 2000, Lexi-Comp.

Saul JP: Electrophysiologic therapeutic catheterization. In Allen HD and others, editors: *Moss and Adams' heart disease in infants, children, and adolescents,* ed 6, Philadelphia, 2001, Lippincott Williams & Wilkins.

Siwik ES, Patel C, Zahka KG: Tetralogy of Fallot. In Allen HD and others, editors: *Moss and Adams' heart disease in infants, children, and adolescents,* ed 6, Philadelphia, 2001, Lippincott Williams & Wilkins.

Underleider RM and others: Intraoperative echocardiograms during congenital heart operation: experiences with 1000 cases, *Ann Thorac Surg* 60:S539-542, 1995.

United Network for Organ Sharing: *UNOS Scientific Registry Annual Report,* Richmond, VA, 2000, UNOS.

Vasan R and others: Echocardiographic evaluation of patients with acute rheumatic fever and rheumatic carditis, *Circulation* 94(1):73-82, 1996.

Vitiello R and others: Complications associated with pediatric cardiac catheterization, *J Am Coll Cardiol* 32:1433-1440, 1998.

Vouhe PR and others: Transposition of the great arteries, ventricular septal defect, pulmonic stenosis, *J Thorac Cardiovasc Surg* 102:428-436, 1992.

Wagenvoort CA, Wagenvoort N: *Pathology of pulmonary hypertension,* New York, 1977, Wiley.

Wernovsky G: Transposition of the great arteries. In Allen HD and others, editors: *Moss and Adams' heart disease in infants, children and adolescents,* ed 6, Philadelphia, 2001, Lippincott Williams & Wilkins.

Wernovsky G, Jonas RA: Transposition of the great arteries. In Hanley FL, Wernovsky AC, Chang AC, editors: *Pediatric cardiac intensive care,* Philadelphia, 1998, Lippincott Williams & Wilkins.

Wessel DL: Hemodynamic responses to perioperative pain and stress in infants, *Crit Care Med* 21(9, suppl):S361-S362, 1993.

# Chapter 35

# The Child with Hematologic or Immunologic Dysfunction

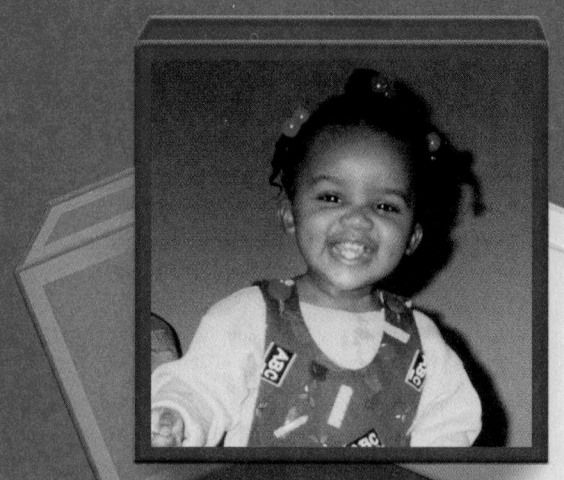

## Chapter Outline

**THE HEMATOLOGIC SYSTEM AND ITS FUNCTION, 1530**
**Origin of Formed Elements, 1530**
    Red Blood Cells (RBCs, Erythrocytes), 1532
    Hemoglobin (Hgb), 1532
    White Blood Cells (WBCs, Leukocytes), 1534
    Platelets, 1535
**Assessment of Hematologic Function, 1535**
**RED BLOOD CELL DISORDERS, 1535**
**Anemia, 1535**
**Blood Transfusion Therapy, 1540**
**ANEMIA CAUSED BY NUTRITIONAL DEFICIENCIES, 1542**
**Iron Deficiency Anemia, 1542**
**ANEMIAS CAUSED BY INCREASED DESTRUCTION OF RED BLOOD CELLS, 1546**

Hereditary Spherocytosis (HS), 1546
Sickle Cell Anemia (SCA), 1547
*Nursing Care Plan: The Child with Sickle Cell Anemia, 1555*
β-Thalassemia, 1555
**ANEMIAS CAUSED BY IMPAIRED OR DECREASED PRODUCTION OF RED BLOOD CELLS, 1559**
**Aplastic Anemia, 1559**
**DEFECTS IN HEMOSTASIS, 1561**
**Mechanisms Involved in Normal Hemostasis, 1561**
    Vascular Influence, 1561
    Platelet Role, 1561
    Clotting Factors, 1561
**Hemophilia, 1561**
**von Willebrand Disease (vWD), 1566**
**Idiopathic Thrombocytopenic Purpura (ITP), 1566**

Disseminated Intravascular Coagulation (DIC), 1567
**OTHER HEMATOLOGIC DISORDERS, 1568**
**Neutropenia, 1568**
**Henoch-Schönlein Purpura (HSP), 1569**
**IMMUNOLOGIC DEFICIENCY DISORDERS, 1570**
**Mechanisms Involved in Immunity, 1571**
    Specific Immune Mechanisms, 1572
**Human Immunodeficiency Virus (HIV) Infection and Acquired Immunodeficiency Syndrome (AIDS), 1572**
*Nursing Care Plan: The Child and Adolescent with HIV Infection, 1577*
**Wiskott-Aldrich Syndrome, 1577**
**Severe Combined Immunodeficiency Disease (SCID), 1579**

## Related Topics

Administration of Medication, Ch. 27
Bone Marrow Aspiration/Biopsy, Ch. 27
Bone Marrow Transplantation, Ch. 36
Collection of Specimens, Ch. 27
Compliance, Ch. 27
Family-Centered Care of the Child with Chronic Illness or Disability, Ch. 22
Family-Centered Care of the Child During Illness and Hospitalization, Ch. 26

Family-Centered End-of-Life Care, Ch. 23
Hemolytic Disease of the Newborn, Ch. 9
Human Immunodeficiency Virus Encephalopathy, Ch. 37
Human Immunodeficiency Virus Infection and Acquired Immunodeficiency Syndrome, Ch. 20

Immunizations, Ch. 12
Infection Control, Ch. 27
Leukemias, Ch. 36
Lymphomas, Ch. 36
Pain Assessment; Pain Management, Ch. 26
Physical Examination: Skin, Ch. 7
Preparation for Procedures, Ch. 27

## THE HEMATOLOGIC SYSTEM AND ITS FUNCTION

### Origin of Formed Elements

Blood is composed of a fluid portion called plasma and a cellular portion known as the formed elements of the

■ Rosalind Bryant, MN, RN-CS, PNP, revised this chapter.

blood. The two components are approximately equal in volume. *Plasma* is about 90% water and 10% solutes. The principal solutes are albumin, electrolytes, and proteins. Among the proteins are clotting factors, globulins, circulating antibodies, and fibrinogen. The *cellular elements* sequentially develop into mature red blood cells (RBCs, erythrocytes), white blood cells (WBCs, leukocytes), and platelets (thrombocytes) (Fig. 35-1).

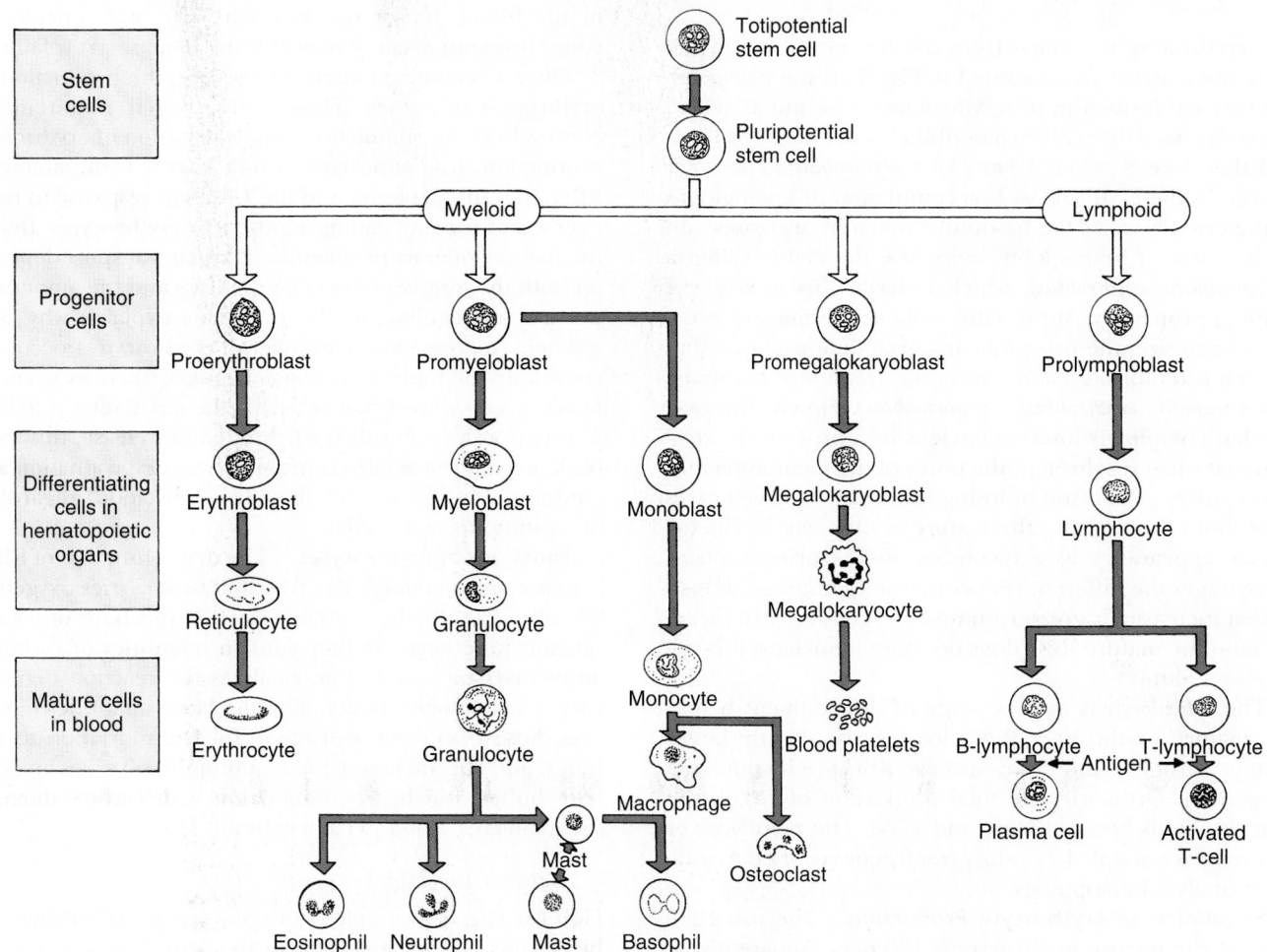

**Fig. 35-1**   Bone marrow and stem cell systems. (Modified from McCance KL, Huether SE: *Pathophysiology: the biologic basis for disease in adults and children,* ed 3, St Louis, 1998, Mosby.)

The major *hemopoietic organs* (blood-forming organs) of the body are the *red bone marrow (myeloid tissue)* and the *lymphatic system,* which consists of lymph (fluid), lymphatic vessels, and lymphoid structures—the lymph nodes, spleen, thymus, and tonsils. Although the lymphatic system plays an important role in regulating blood cells, the lymph vessels and fluids do not produce cells. The *lymph nodes* regulate the manufacture of WBCs. The *spleen* and *liver* are the primary organs for hematopoiesis in the young fetus and cell removal in postnatal life. *Macrophages* (formerly called reticular cells) are cells of mesodermal origin that are widely dispersed in the lining of the vascular and lymph channels. Macrophages form a network and are capable of phagocytosis (ingestion and digestion of foreign substances), formation of immune bodies, and differentiation into other cells, such as hemocytoblasts, myeloblasts, or lymphoblasts.

All of the formed elements of the blood, except to some extent the agranulocytes, are believed to be formed in myeloid tissue during postnatal life. During embryonic development the mesenchyme, spleen, liver, thymus, and yolk sac serve as additional sites of blood cell formation. In certain blood disorders these sites, particularly the spleen, can be stimulated to produce blood cells and constitute *ex-*

*tramedullary hemopoiesis.* In infants and young children all of the bone contains red marrow (so called because of its color from the formation of erythrocytes), but as bone growth ceases near the end of adolescence, only the ribs, sternum, vertebrae, and pelvis continue to produce blood cells. The remainder of the bone marrow becomes yellow from deposition of fat. However, in conditions of increased demand for blood cells, the yellow marrow can revert to red marrow as another hemopoietic source.

Although the progressive development of each blood cell is fairly well delineated, there is considerable controversy regarding the origin of the blood cell. One of the most widely held theories (monophyletic) is that each blood cell originates from a primordial (primitive) cell called a *blast,* or *totipotential stem cell,* which has the ability to self-replicate and transform into all the blood components.

The second-generation stem cell called a pluripotential stem cell is committed to produce erythroblast, myeloblast, monoblast, lymphoblast, and megakaryoblast (see Fig. 35-1). The blast cells sequentially develop into mature red blood cells (RBCs, erythrocytes), white blood cells (WBCs, leukocytes), platelets (thrombocytes), and other cells (such as mast cells and macrophages) (see Fig. 35-1).

## Red Blood Cells (RBCs, Erythrocytes)

The erythrocyte is formed from the hemocytoblast in the red bone marrow. As illustrated in Fig. 35-1, the *pluripotential stem cell* forms the proerythroblast. The initial cell of this series has a deep blue (basophilic)—staining cytoplasm and therefore is called a *basophilic erythroblast.* The chief change in the erythroblast is accumulation of hemoglobin in the cytoplasm. As the basophilic material decreases and the amount of hemoglobin increases, the cell is called a *polychromatic erythroblast,* which describes its mixture of staining properties. At the same time as the nucleus is decreasing in size, the basophilic material disappears, so that the cell is uniformly stained by eosin dye, hence the name *orthochromatic erythroblast,* or *normoblast.* Finally, the normoblast completely loses its nucleus by a process of extrusion as it squeezes through the pores of the membrane into the capillary. As a result of losing its nucleus, the cell caves in on both sides, giving the mature erythrocyte its characteristic appearance as a biconcave disk. During each of these stages the different cells continue to undergo mitosis so that increasingly greater numbers of cells are produced. Because the mature RBC does not have a nucleus, it is unable to multiply.

The *reticulocyte* is the last stage of development before the mature erythrocyte. Reticulocytes are slightly larger than erythrocytes and indicate active RBC production (*erythropoiesis*). Ordinarily the total proportion of circulating reticulocytes is between 0.5% and 1.5%. The *reticulocyte* or *retic count* is a simple laboratory test frequently used to indirectly analyze hemopoiesis.

### Regulation of Erythrocyte Production.

The usual life span of the mature erythrocyte is 120 days. Apparently, as RBCs grow old, their membranes become fragile and eventually rupture. The contents of the cell fragment as they circulate through the blood vessels and are phagocytized by the macrophages in the spleen, liver, and bone marrow. The hemoglobin is broken down into the iron-containing pigment hemosiderin and the bile pigments biliverdin and bilirubin. Most of the iron is reused by the bone marrow for production of new RBCs or stored in the liver and other tissues for future use. The bile pigments are excreted by the liver in bile.

Normally there is a homeostatic balance between the regulation of RBC production and destruction. This balance ensures adequate tissue oxygenation and a blood viscosity that allows the blood to flow freely through the vessels. The basic regulator of erythrocyte production is believed to be tissue oxygenation and renal production of *erythropoietin* (also called *erythropoietic-stimulating factor*). In states of tissue hypoxia, erythropoietin is released by the kidneys into the bloodstream. As a result the bone marrow is stimulated to produce new RBCs. The major activity seems to be an increase in both the maturation rate and mitosis of all stages of erythrocyte production, but primarily at the stem cell level.

During this rapid increase in RBC production, the circulating erythrocytes may not be totally mature. Consequently the number of reticulocytes may increase dramatically (as high as 30% or more of the total RBC count). Even normoblasts or nucleated red blood cells (NRBCs) may appear in the blood. If this rise in erythrocyte and reticulocyte count does not occur, it may indicate bone marrow failure.

Once tissue oxygenation is adequate, the production of erythropoietin ceases. Thus tissue oxygen requirements control both the stimulation and termination of erythrocyte production. It is important to note that it is the ability of RBCs to transport oxygen to the tissues in response to their needs, not the circulating numbers of erythrocytes, that is the basic regulatory mechanism. Oxygen transport depends on both the number of circulating RBCs and the amount of normal hemoglobin in the cell. This explains why *polycythemia* (increase in the number of erythrocytes) occurs in conditions of prolonged tissue hypoxia, such as cyanotic heart defects. (See Chapter 34.) If the circulating numbers of erythrocytes controlled erythropoietin release, this feedback mechanism would control erythrocyte production at a constant level (4.5 to 5.5 million/mm$^3$ of blood) regardless of existing tissue hypoxia.

### Functions of Erythrocytes.

The major function of RBCs is to transport hemoglobin, which in turn carries oxygen to all cells of the body. However, erythrocytes have other significant functions: (1) they contain quantities of carbonic anhydrase, an enzyme that catalyzes the reaction between carbon dioxide and water, allowing large quantities of carbon dioxide to react with blood for transportation to the lungs, and (2) the hemoglobin, a protein, serves as an acid-base buffer, which, in combination with carbon dioxide, maintains the blood pH at a constant level.

## Hemoglobin (Hgb)

Hgb (or Hb) is a complex molecule composed of four globin chains. The type of Hgb in the cells depends on both the stage of life and any abnormalities in the genes that regulate the production of Hgb. *Fetal Hgb,* composed of two alpha ($\alpha$)- and two gamma ($\gamma$)-chains, has a greater affinity for oxygen and is best suited to the fetal environment. During the latter part of pregnancy, the fetus begins developing *adult Hgb* (two $\alpha$- and two beta ($\beta$)-chains). When a defect in Hgb synthesis is present (e.g., sickle cell disease or thalassemia), fetal Hgb may be produced into adulthood. Research is currently under-way to develop cell-free Hgb that can be used for oxygen and carbon dioxide transport. Hgb values vary according to the child's age. (See Appendix D.)

Several tests offer important information about Hgb. The *hematocrit (Hct),* which is approximately three times the concentration of Hgb (in grams per deciliter), indicates the percentage volume of circulating packed RBCs of the total blood. Under normal conditions, Hgb and Hct are in a fixed relationship with each other and vary according to the child's age (Dixon, 1997).

*Red blood cell indexes* are based on ratios of packed RBC volume, Hgb concentration, and RBC count, and they are a useful way of designating different types of anemias. Values for mean corpuscular volume (MCV) and mean corpuscular Hgb (MCH) do not stay constant during infancy and childhood. However, MCH concentration (MCHC) values are more constant (Dixon, 1997).

*Mean corpuscular volume (MCV)* indicates the average (mean) volume or size of a single RBC. Normal RBCs (normocytes), small cells (microcytes), and large cells (macrocytes) have the normal ranges listed in Table 35-1 on p. 1536.

***Mean corpuscular hemoglobin (MCH)*** indicates the average weight of Hgb in each RBC. The normal MCH ranges are listed in Table 35-1. Normochromic cells are those with a normal Hgb content or normal MCH. Those cells with below-normal MCH are called hypochromic, and those with above-normal MCH are hyperchromic (Dixon, 1997).

***Mean corpuscular hemoglobin concentration (MCHC)*** indicates the average concentration of Hgb in the RBC. The MCHC is calculated from the amount of Hgb in 100 ml of RBCs rather than the amount of Hgb in whole blood. At 6 months of age, the normal MCHC value of 33 g/dl is reached (Brugnara and Platt, 1998).

Fig. 35-2 reveals the use of RBC indexes as indicators of different types of anemias.

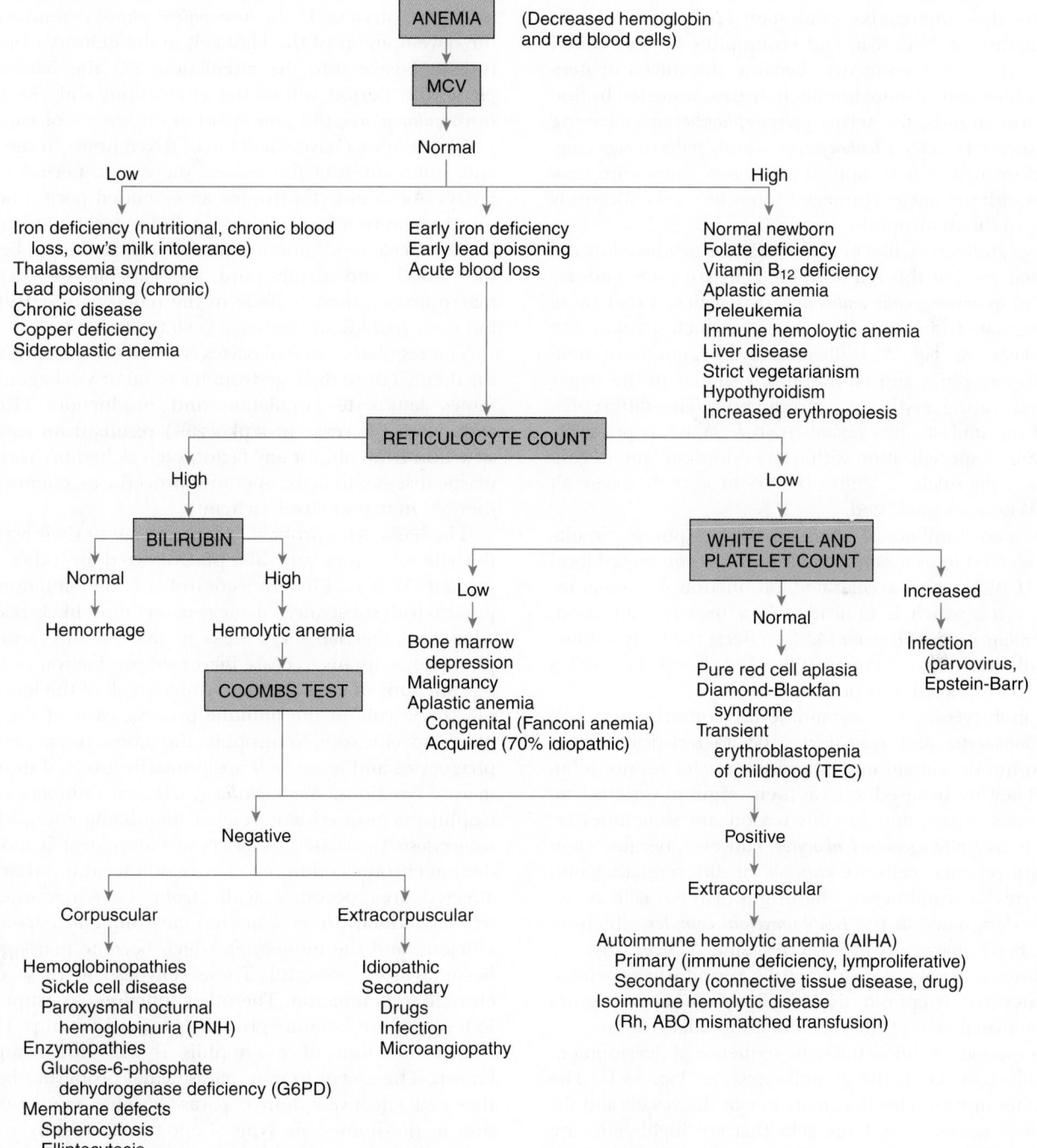

**Fig. 35-2**  Approach to the diagnosis of anemia by MCV and reticulocyte count. (Modified from Lanzkowsky P: *Manual of pediatric hematology and oncology*, New York, 2000, Churchill Livingstone; Scott JP: Hematology. In Behrman RE, Kliegman RM, editors: *Nelson essentials of pediatrics*, Philadelphia, 1998, WB Saunders.)

## White Blood Cells (WBCs, Leukocytes)

The leukocytes refer to a number of cells with similar yet distinct functions. They are divided into two major classifications—granulocytes and agranulocytes—based on the presence or absence, respectively, of granules within the cytoplasm of the cells.

**Granulocytes.** There are three types of granulocytes: *neutrophils, basophils,* and *eosinophils.* The name of each of these refers to the characteristic staining property of the granule during laboratory analysis. Neutrophils stain neutral to the dyes, whereas basophils stain a purple color to the basic methylene blue dye, and eosinophils take on a red color to the acidic eosin dye. Because the nuclei of neutrophils have two or more lobules that are connected by fine chromatin strands, the terms *polymorphonuclear* (meaning "many-formed nuclei") *leukocytes* or simply *polys* or *segs* (segmented or mature neutrophils) and *bands* (immature neutrophils with the nuclei connected) may be used collectively to refer to the neutrophils.

The granulocytes, like erythrocytes, are produced in the bone marrow. For this reason these cells are sometimes referred to as *myelogenous leukocytes.* It is believed that these cells originate from primitive stem cells, which develop into myeloblasts. As Fig. 35-1 illustrates, the genesis of neutrophils, basophils, and eosinophils is similar to the stages observed during erythrocyte production. The differentiation of myeloblasts into various mature WBCs is primarily the result of specialization within the cytoplasm and degeneration of the nucleus. Unlike the erythrocyte, however, all of the WBCs are nucleated.

Increased numbers of bands in the peripheral circulation (referred to as a *shift to the left* on the complete blood count [CBC]) is an accelerated production of immature granulocytes, which is indicative of a bacterial infection. The *absolute neutrophil count (ANC)* reflects the body's ability to handle bacterial infections. If the ANC is less than 500, a severe risk of infection is present.

**Agranulocytes.** The agranulocytes comprise two cell types: *monocytes* and *lymphocytes.* Characteristically these cells do not develop granules, and the nuclei are not lobulated. They are believed to have their origin in various lymphogenous organs and for this reason are sometimes referred to as *lymphogenous leukocytes.* However, because stem cells and reticular cells are capable of differentiating into monocytes or lymphocytes, the origin of these cells is frequently designated as the *lymphomyeloid complex,* which includes bone marrow, lymph nodes, spleen, liver, thymus, subepithelial lymphoid tissue (tonsils, vermiform appendix, and intestinal lymphoid tissues), and connective tissues (mesenchymal cells of the reticuloendothelial system).

The monocytes follow the same sequence of development from the stem cell as the granulocytes (see Fig. 35-1). The monocytes in turn have the ability to exit the vessels and develop into *macrophages,* large cells that are highly effective phagocytes. *Kupffer cells* are macrophages located in the liver. *Histiocytes* are macrophages in the connective tissue. These names are remnants of the old reticular endothelial system.

*Lymphocytopoiesis* (lymphocyte formation) is believed to take place anywhere in the lymphomyeloid complex. Lymphocytes develop from blast (stem) cells (see Fig. 35-1). The lymphocyte has the potential to develop into other cells. For example, lymphocytes may become T-cells or B-cells (see p. 1531).

**Regulation of Leukocyte Production.** The exact life span of the leukocytes is not as clearly defined as that of the erythrocytes, because their existence in the circulation is primarily for transportation to extravascular areas, where they reside in reservoirs or where they are needed to resist infection. Therefore their survival rate has been divided into three phases: (1) the *hemopoietic phase,* extending from the development of the blast cell to the delivery of the mature leukocyte into the circulation; (2) the *intravascular phase,* the period within the circulation; and (3) the *extravascular phase,* the time spent in the viscera or tissues.

Granulocytes have a half-life of 6 to 8 hours in the blood and, after entering the tissues, die over a period of 4 to 5 days. Agranulocytes live for an extended period because they remain in inflamed tissue areas longer than the granulocytes. Because monocytes wander back and forth between the blood and tissues and are capable of becoming macrophages, their half-life in the blood is 8 to 10 hours, but their half-life in the tissue is 60 to 90 days.

The regulation of leukocytes is based on the body's need for them. Tissue damage from bacterial or viral agents promotes leukocyte circulation and production. However, *leukocytosis* (increase in leukocytes) results from tissue destruction from almost any factor, such as hemorrhage, neoplastic disease, toxicity, operative procedures, chemical and thermal injury, or tissue ischemia.

The leukocytes probably die as a result of their activity at the site of injury and are phagocytized by other newly formed WBCs. Effective control of the inflammatory process with subsequent tissue recovery most likely results in a feedback mechanism to the bone marrow and causes lymphogenous organs to cease increased production of WBCs.

**Functions of Leukocytes.** Although all of the leukocytes play some role in the immune process, each of the WBCs plays a specific role. Neutrophils and monocytes are effective phagocytes and as a result are primarily involved in inflammatory reactions. *Neutrophilia* (increased numbers of neutrophils) is most evident in an acute inflammation, whereas *monocytosis* (increased numbers of monocytes) is more evident in chronic conditions. The reason for this is that as the affected area becomes acidic from tissue necrosis, neutrophils, which prefer a neutral environment, become less efficient, and the monocytes, which become macrophages, become more powerful. These cells also increase during chronic inflammation. The other functions of lymphocytes in terms of the immune process are discussed on p. 1572.

The function of eosinophils is still not completely known. They seem to have parasiticidal properties because they can selectively destroy parasites. They may also function in the immediate type of allergic or anaphylactic hypersensitivity reactions because *eosinophilia* (increased numbers of eosinophils) is well documented in such conditions. Eosinophils also are thought to release a substance called *profibrinolysin,* which, when activated to form fibrinolysin, digests *fibrin,* thereby helping dissolve a clot.

The function of basophils is also not completely understood, although *basophilia* (increased numbers of basophils) occurs during the healing phase of inflammation and during prolonged inflammation. Basophils in the blood exit the vessels and become mast cells in the tissue. They are responsible for histamine release, resulting in increased permeability of the vessels to allow WBCs to exit the vessels at the site of injury.

### Platelets

Platelets are actually small fragments of megakaryocytes. They are smaller than blood cells, do not possess a cellular structure, and consist of a clear substance containing granules. The origin of platelets is part of the myelogenous group of WBCs (see Fig. 35-1). Platelets are formed when the megakaryocytic membrane invaginates, fuses within the cell to separate the cytoplasm, and then fragments.

**Regulation of Platelet Production.** The life span of platelets has been estimated as 8 to 10 days. Apparently the body regulates platelets to maintain a fairly constant level (between 150,000 and 400,000/mm³). Platelet production is probably regulated by a hormone, thrombopoietin, but the source and mode of action of this substance are unknown. Old platelets are most likely removed by the liver and spleen.

**Function of Platelets.** The term *thrombocyte* means "clot" (*thrombo*) and "cell" (*cyte*) and accurately describes the main function of platelets. When there is a break in the continuity of a blood vessel, the platelets, which are normally round or oval disks, come in contact with the wet vessel surface and dramatically change their shape to become swollen spheres with long, irregular projections called *pseudopodia* (false feet). As a result the platelets begin to adhere to the wet endothelium and to each other. The initial platelets at the site of injury release substances that attract other thrombocytes to the area. This causes a layering of platelets, which eventually forms a *plug*. This plug is large enough to partially or totally occlude the opening in the vessel wall but small enough to allow blood flow to continue unimpaired through the vessel.

In small vessel tears, the platelet plug is sufficient to produce hemostasis, and additional blood coagulation is not necessary. However, when platelet counts are low, these numerous small ruptures, which occur continually in the body as a result of general functioning, are not repaired. Consequently, small hemorrhagic areas called *petechiae* form under the skin. Their appearance is similar to reddish freckles or tiny spiderwebs.

Platelets also influence hemostasis by releasing a substance called *serotonin* at the site of injury. Serotonin is a vasoconstrictor that produces vascular spasm to decrease the amount of blood flow to the injured area.

## Assessment of Hematologic Function

Several tests can be performed to assess hematologic function, including additional procedures to identify the cause of the dysfunction. The following discussion is limited to a description of the most common and one of the most valuable tests, the *complete blood count (CBC)*. Other procedures, such as those related to iron, coagulation, and immune status, are discussed throughout the chapter as appropriate.

The CBC consists of the following determinations: RBC count, WBC count, hematocrit, hemoglobin, differential WBC, RBC indexes (MCV, MCH, and MCHC), and peripheral smear. Additional tests may be included, such as the reticulocyte count, RBC volume distribution width (RDW), and platelet count. Each of these is summarized in Table 35-1. Most of the determinations can be performed on a small quantity of blood (micromethod) and are automatically computed. The nurse should be familiar with the significance of the findings from the CBC (see Table 35-1) and be aware of normal values for age, which are listed in Appendix D.

The history and physical examination are essential to identification of hematologic dysfunction, and the nurse is often the first person to suspect a problem based on information from these sources. Comments by the parent regarding the child's lack of energy, food diary with decreased sources of iron, frequent infections, and bleeding that is difficult to control offer clues to the more common disorders affecting the blood. A careful physical appraisal can reveal findings such as persistent fatigue, pallor, petechiae, or bruising that may indicate minor or serious hematologic conditions. Nurses need to be aware of the clinical manifestations of blood diseases in order to assist in recognizing symptoms and establishing a diagnosis.

# RED BLOOD CELL DISORDERS

## Anemia

Anemia is defined as reduction of RBCs and/or hemoglobin concentration compared with age-matched normal values (Kline, 1996; Worrall, Tompkins and Rust, 1999). The anemias are the most common hematologic disorders of infancy and childhood and are not disease but a manifestation of an underlying pathologic process (see Fig. 35-2).

### Classification

Anemias can be classified using two basic approaches: (1) *etiology* manifested by erythrocyte or hemoglobin depletion and (2) *morphology*, the characteristic changes in RBC size, shape, and color (Box 35-1).

Although the morphologic classification is useful in the laboratory evaluation of anemia, the etiology provides direction for planning nursing care. For example, anemia with reduced hemoglobin concentration may be caused by a dietary depletion of iron, and the principal intervention is replenishing iron stores.

The main causes of anemia are (1) inadequate production of RBCs or RBC components, (2) increased destruction of RBCs and (3) excessive loss of RBCs through hemorrhage. Each of these causes affects the amount of hemoglobin that is available to carry oxygen to the cells (see Box 35-1). Therefore the etiology is based on the various conditions that can result from any of these physiologic changes.

**TABLE 35-1** Tests performed as part of the complete blood count

| Test (Average Value)* | Description | Comments |
|---|---|---|
| Red blood cell (RBC) count (4.5-5.5 million/mm³) | Number of RBCs/mm³ of blood | Indirectly estimates Hgb content of blood<br>Reflects function of bone marrow |
| Hemoglobin (Hgb) determination (11.5-15.5 g/dl) | Amount of Hgb/dl of whole blood | Total blood Hgb primarily depends on number of circulating RBCs, but also on amount of Hgb in each cell |
| Hematocrit (Hct) (35%-45%) | Percentage or volume of packed RBCs to whole blood | Indirectly measures Hgb content<br>Is approximately three times Hgb content |
| **RBC indexes** | | |
| Mean corpuscular volume (MCV) (77-95 μm³) | Average of mean volume (size) of a single RBC $$MCV = \frac{Hct\ (\%) \times 10}{RBC\ count\ (millions/mm^3)}$$ | MCV and MCH depend on accurate counts of RBCs, whereas MCHC does not; therefore MCHC is often more reliable<br>All indexes depend on *average* cell measurements and do not show individual RBC (anisocytosis) variations<br>MCV values expressed as cubic microns (μm³) or femtoliters (fl) |
| Mean corpuscular hemoglobin (MCH) (25-33 pg/cell) | Average or mean quantity (weight) of Hgb of a single RBC $$MCH = \frac{Hgb\ (g)/dl \times 10}{RBC\ count\ (millions/mm^3)}$$ | MCH values expressed as picograms (pg) or micromicrograms (μμg) |
| Mean corpuscular hemoglobin concentration (MCHC) (31%-37% Hgb [g]/dl RBC) | Average concentration of Hgb in a single RBC $$MCHC = \frac{Hgb\ (g)/dl \times 100}{Hct\ (\%)}$$ | MCHC values expressed as % Hgb (g)/cell or Hgb (g)/dl RBC |
| RBC volume distribution width (RDW) (13.4% ± 1.2%) | Average size of RBCs | Differentiates some types of anemia |
| Reticulocyte count (0.5%-1.5% erythrocytes) | % Reticulocytes to RBCs | Index of production of mature RBCs by bone marrow<br>Decreased count indicates depressed bone marrow function<br>Increased count indicates erythrogenesis in response to some stimulus<br>When reticulocyte count is extremely high, other forms of immature RBCs (normoblasts, even erythroblasts) may be present<br>Indirectly estimates hypochromic anemia |
| White blood cell (WBC) count (4.5-13.5 × 10³ cells/mm³) | Number of WBCs/mm³ of blood | Total number of WBCs is less important than differential count |
| Differential WBC count | Inspection and quantification of WBC types present in peripheral blood | Values are expressed as percentages; to obtain absolute number of any type of WBCs, multiply its respective percentage by total number of WBCs |
| Neutrophils (polys) (54%-62%) (3.0-5.8 × 10³ cells/mm³) | | Primary defense in bacterial infection; capable of phagocytizing and killing bacteria |
| Bands (3%-5%) (0.15-0.4 × 10³ cells/mm³) | Immature neutrophil | Increased numbers in bacterial infection<br>Also capable of phagocytosis and killing bacteria |
| Eosinophils (1%-3%) (0.05-0.25 × 10³ cells/mm³) | Named for their staining characteristics with eosin dye | Increased in allergic disorders, parasitic diseases, certain neoplasms, and other diseases |
| Basophils (0.075%) (0.015-0.030 cells/mm³) | Named for their characteristic basophilic stippling | Contain histamine, but their function is unknown |
| Lymphocytes (25%-33%; 1.5-3.0 × 10³ cells/mm³) | | Involved in development of antibody and delayed hypersensitivity |
| Monocytes (3%-7%) | | Large phagocytic cells that are involved in early stage of inflammatory reaction |
| Absolute neutrophil count (ANC) (>1000) | % Neutrophils and bands × WBC count | Indicates body's capability to handle bacterial infections |
| Platelet count (150-400 × 10³/mm³) | Number of platelets/mm³ of blood | Cellular fragments that are necessary for clotting to occur |
| Stained peripheral blood smear | Visual estimation of amount of Hgb in RBCs and overall size, shape, and structure of RBCs | Various staining properties of RBC structures may be evidence of immature forms of erythrocyte<br>Shows variation in size and shape of RBCs—microcytic, macrocytic, poikilocytic (variable sizes) |

*See Appendix D for normal values according to ages and for explanation of units of measurement.

## Pathophysiology and Clinical Manifestations

The basic physiologic defect caused by anemia is a decrease in the oxygen-carrying capacity of blood and consequently a reduction in the amount of oxygen available to the cells. When the anemia has developed slowly, the child usually adapts to the declining hemoglobin level. Most children seem to have a remarkable ability to function quite well despite low levels of hemoglobin. Also, compensatory mechanisms such as a shift in the oxyhemoglobin dissociation curve may delay the development of any obvious signs. (See p. 1315.)

When the hemoglobin level falls sufficiently to produce clinical manifestations, the signs and symptoms are due to tissue *hypoxia* (e.g., weakness, fatigue, and a waxy pallor in severe anemia) (Box 35-2). Cyanosis, the result of the quantity of deoxygenated hemoglobin in arterial blood, is typically not evident. Hemoglobin levels generally must *exceed* 5 g/dl before cyanosis is evident. Anemia is caused by decreased hemoglobin or RBCs, not inadequate oxygen saturation of existing hemoglobin.

Central nervous system manifestations include headache, dizziness, light-headedness, irritability, slowed thought processes, decreased attention span, apathy, and depression.

Growth retardation resulting from decreased cellular metabolism and coexisting anorexia is a common finding in chronic severe anemia. It is frequently accompanied by delayed sexual maturation in the older child.

The effects of anemia on the circulatory system can be profound. A reduction in hemoglobin concentration that results in decreased oxygen-carrying capacity of the blood is associated with a compensatory increase in heart rate and cardiac output (see Box 35-2). Initially this greater cardiac output compensates for the lower oxygen-carrying capacity of the blood, because blood replenished with oxygen returns to the tissues at a faster than normal rate. The increased circulation and turbulence within the heart may produce a heart murmur. Because the cardiac workload is increased during exercise, infection, or emotional stress, cardiac failure may ensue.

*Acute or chronic hemorrhage* results in loss of plasma and all formed elements of the blood. After acute hemorrhage the body replaces plasma within 1 to 3 days, maintaining blood volume. However, this results in a low concentration of RBCs, which are gradually replaced within 3 to 4 weeks. During this period there is usually a normocytic, normochromic anemia, provided that there are sufficient iron stores for hemoglobin synthesis.

In chronic blood loss the actual number of RBCs may be normal because of continual replacement. However, insufficient iron is available to form hemoglobin as quickly as it is lost. As a result erythrocytes are usually microcytic and hypochromic.

**Routine Screening.**   The "Put Prevention into Practice Program" developed for the U.S. Public Health Service identifies the following recommendations of major authorities:

**American Academy of Family Physicians** and **U.S. Preventive Services Task Force**—All children should be screened for anemia once during infancy.

**American Academy of Pediatrics**—Hemoglobin or hematocrit should be measured once during infancy (between 6 and 9 months), early childhood (between 1 and 5 years), late childhood (between 5 and 12 years), and adolescence (between 14 and 20 years).

**Canadian Task Force on the Periodic Health Examination**—Hemoglobin concentration screening should be performed on children at high risk for iron deficiency anemia: preterm infants; infants born of a multiple pregnancy or an iron-deficient woman; and children in low socioeconomic conditions.

---

**Box 35-1 ■ ■ ■**
**Red Blood Cell (RBC) Morphology**

| DESCRIPTION OF RED BLOOD CELL | CHARACTERISTICS OF RED BLOOD CELL |
|---|---|
| Size (cell size) | Variation in RBC sizes (anisocytocytes) |
| | Normocytes (normal cell size) |
| | Microcytes (smaller than normal cell size) |
| | Macrocytes (larger than normal cell size) |
| Shape (irregular shape) | Variation in RBC shapes (poikiolocytes) |
| | Spherocytes (globular cells) |
| | Drepanocytes (sickle-shaped cells) |
| | Numerous other irregular-shaped cells |
| Color (staining characteristics) | Variation in hemoglobin concentration in the RBC |
| | Normochromic (sufficient or normal amount of hemoglobin per RBC) |
| | Hypochromic (reduced amount of hemoglobin per RBC) |
| | Hyperchromic (increased amount of hemoglobin per RBC) |

---

**Box 35-2 ■ ■ ■**
**Signs and Symptoms of Anemia**

| DECREASED RED BLOOD CELL PRODUCTION | INCREASED RED BLOOD DESTRUCTION | INCREASED RED BLOOD CELL LOSS |
|---|---|---|
| Pallor | Icteric sclera | Pallor |
| Tachycardia | Jaundice | Fatigue |
| Fatigue (shortness of breath and frequent resting) | Tachycardia | Muscle weakness |
| Muscle weakness | Dark urine | Cool skin |
| Systolic heart murmur | Splenomegaly | Tachycardia |
| | Hepatomegaly | Decreased peripheral pulses |
| | Frontal bossing | Low blood pressure (late sign of shock) |

## Diagnostic Evaluation

In general, anemia may be suspected from findings on the history and physical examination, such as lack of energy, easy fatigability, and pallor, but unless the anemia is severe, the first clue to the disorder may be alterations in the CBC, such as decreased RBCs, and decreased hemoglobin and hematocrit levels. Although anemia is sometimes defined as a hemoglobin level below 10 or 11 g/dl, this arbitrary cutoff is inappropriate for all children, because hemoglobin levels normally vary with age (see Table 35-1 and Appendix D).

Various findings on the CBC are also significant, such as increased reticulocytes, which indicate the body's response to an increased demand for RBCs. A peripheral smear may demonstrate significant changes in the shape of RBCs, such as sickled cells. Tests to measure the amount of hemoglobin in a single cell are helpful in determining the cause of the anemia (see Table 35-1 and p. 1544). Sometimes a bone marrow aspiration may be necessary to evaluate the body's ability to produce normal cells. For example, in leukemia the bone marrow is *hyperplastic* (producing increased numbers of cells), whereas in aplastic anemia the bone marrow is **hypoplastic** (producing decreased numbers of cells) or **aplastic** (producing no cells).

Tests for hematologic function do not always reflect the *immediate* changes occurring in the blood. For example, in acute massive hemorrhage the hemoglobin and hematocrit values may not be reliable, because the plasma volume may not increase for several hours. Without the hemodilution caused by the reexpansion of the vascular space, the hemoglobin and hematocrit may be close to normal, and the RBC loss may not be apparent. Consequently, assessing the quantity of blood loss in a seriously ill child may be difficult. The estimated volume of blood loss must be analyzed in conjunction with the total blood volume of the child to determine the percent of blood loss. Blood specimens obtained from central lines may more accurately reflect the patient's status than specimens obtained from an extremity, because of the vasoconstriction of the peripheral vasculature. Decreased blood pressure changes are a late sign because of the compensatory mechanisms.

## Therapeutic Management

The objective of medical management is to reverse the anemia by treating the underlying cause. In nutritional anemias the specific deficiency is replaced. In blood loss from acute hemorrhage, RBC transfusion may be given. In patients with severe anemia, supportive medical care may include oxygen therapy, bed rest, and replacement of intravascular volume with intravenous (IV) fluids. In addition to these general measures, more specific interventions may be implemented depending on the cause, and these are discussed in the next sections.

## Nursing Considerations

The physical examination yields valuable evidence regarding the severity of the anemia and some indication of its possible etiology (see Fig. 35-2 and Box 35-2). In interviewing the family, the nurse stresses the following areas: (1) nutrition, especially if lactose intolerant or inadequate intake of iron; (2) past history of chronic, recurrent infection; (3) eating habits, particularly pica (eating non-food items such as dirt, starch, lead-based paint chips, paper); (4) bowel habits and presence of frank blood in stools or black, tarry stools as a result of chronic blood loss; and (5) familial history of hereditary diseases, such as sickle cell disease or thalassemia.

The nurse should also be aware of the significance of a thorough history to obtain pertinent information that may aide in identifying the cause of the anemia. For example, such statements as "the baby drinks too much milk" or "my teenager is on a liquid or vegetarian diet" are clues related to iron deficiency.

**Prepare Child and Family for Laboratory Tests.** Several blood tests may be sequentially ordered, therefore the child may experience multiple finger/heel sticks or venipunctures. These invasive procedures need not be painful with the application of a topical anesthetic called EMLA.

The nurse is responsible for preparing the child for the tests by (1) explaining the significance of each test, particularly why the tests are not done at one time; (2) physically being with the child during the procedure whenever possible; and (3) allowing the child to play with the equipment on a doll or participate in the actual procedure (e.g., by holding the Band-Aid).

Older children may appreciate the opportunity to observe the blood cells under a microscope or in photographs. This is especially important if a serious blood disorder, such as leukemia, is suspected, because it serves as a foundation for explaining the pathophysiology of the disorder.

---

**NURSING TIP** Suggested explanations for teaching children about blood components are:

**Red blood cells**—Carry the oxygen you breathe from your lungs to all parts of your body.

**White blood cells**—Help keep germs from causing infection.

**Platelets**—Small parts of cells that help make bleeding stop; platelets help your body stop bleeding by forming a clot (scab) over the hurt area.

**Plasma**—The liquid portion of blood; has clotting factors that help make bleeding stop.

---

Bone marrow is not a routine hematologic test but is essential for definitive diagnosis of the leukemias, lymphomas, and certain anemias. (Information for preparing the child is presented in Chapter 27.)

**Decrease Tissue Oxygen Needs.** Because the basic pathology in anemia is a decrease in oxygen-carrying capacity of the RBCs, an important nursing responsibility is to minimize tissue oxygen needs by continual assessment of the child's energy level. In most instances of anemia this is not necessary, but when it is, several important interventions are implemented. These same interventions apply to any child with a nursing diagnosis of fatigue or activity intolerance.

The child's level of tolerance for activities of daily living and play is assessed, and adjustments are made to allow as much self-care as possible without undue exertion. During periods of rest the nurse takes vital signs and observes behavior to establish a baseline of nonexertion energy expenditure. During periods of activity the nurse repeats these measurements and observations to compare them with resting values.

> **NURSING ALERT**
> Signs of exertion include tachycardia, palpitations, tachypnea, dyspnea, shortness of breath, hyperpnea, breathlessness, dizziness, light-headedness, diaphoresis, and change in skin color. The child looks fatigued (sagging, limp posture; slow, strained movements; inability to tolerate additional activity; difficulty sucking in infants).

Once a baseline of physical tolerance has been established, the nurse anticipates those activities that are physically taxing, such as dressing, feeding, or getting out of bed, and allows for conservation of energy by assisting the child as needed. However, because dependency can be threatening, the child is allowed as much control in the environment as possible. For example, a child with severe anemia may be unable to walk to the bathroom but may be able to use a bedside commode or be transported in a wheelchair to the lavatory rather than having to use a bedpan. Scheduling activities throughout the day with planned rest periods in between maximizes the child's energy potential without causing undue exertion. Safety measures are anticipated and implemented, (e.g., staying with the child when out of bed and raising siderails when in the bed to prevent falls).

Diversional activities are planned that promote rest but prevent boredom and withdrawal. Because short attention span, irritability, and restlessness are common in anemia and increase stress demands on the body, appropriate activities are planned, such as listening to music; using a tape recorder; watching television; playing video games; reading or listening to stories or comics; continuing a favorite hobby, such as stamp collecting; coloring or drawing; playing board and card games; or being wheeled in a carriage or chair. Choosing the appropriate roommate, such as a child of similar age with a diagnosis that also requires restricted activity, is another helpful intervention.

If infants or young children are hospitalized, the importance of preventing separation from parents must be considered. Crying and fretfulness place increased stress demands on the body, which increases oxygen needs. Parents may need help in understanding the importance of their presence and the basis for their child's mood changes.

**Prevent Complications.** Children with anemia are prone to infection because tissue hypoxia causes cellular dysfunction and the disturbed metabolic processes weaken the host's defenses against foreign agents. Infection also worsens the anemia by increasing metabolic needs and in instances of chronic infection also interferes with erythropoiesis and shortens the survival time of RBCs. All of the usual precautions are taken to prevent infection, such as practicing thorough handwashing, appropriate room selection in a noninfectious area, restricting visitors or hospital personnel with active infection, and maintaining adequate nutrition. The nurse also observes for signs of infection, particularly temperature elevation and leukocytosis. How-

ever, an elevated WBC count sometimes occurs in anemia without the presence of systemic or local infection.

Multiple blood samples may present a problem with cumulative blood loss, necessitating blood replacement. This situation occurs most often in infants with severe anemia. To prevent this, blood may be withdrawn through a continuous IV line and replaced after the exact amount needed has been tested and discarded. As a precaution, a record is kept of the volume of blood being withdrawn. Using micromethods of testing whenever possible minimizes the amount of blood required for the test. The nurse needs to observe for cumulative effects of blood loss, particularly signs of shock and increased hypoxia, and to explain to parents the necessity of multiple blood samples and the reason for blood replacement. (See Cultural Awareness box and Critical Thinking Exercise box on p. 1540.)

The main complication of anemia is cardiac decompensation, which can result from excessive demands on the heart by increased metabolic needs or cardiac overload. The nurses need to observe for signs and symptoms of heart failure such as tachycardia, dyspnea, rales, moist respirations, cough, shortness of breath, and sweating. Obviously,

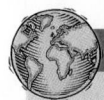

## CULTURAL AWARENESS
### Jehovah's Witnesses and Blood Transfusions

Jehovah's Witnesses are members of a worldwide religious group that strongly opposes the use of blood products, especially blood transfusions, for themselves and their children. They believe that the Old Testament (Leviticus 17:10) forbids eating the blood of any flesh, and they consider blood transfusions to be equivalent to oral ingestion of blood. Among the members there are differing interpretations of the prohibition of blood, from loss of salvation to a forgivable sin.

Transfusions of whole blood, packed RBCs, WBCs, platelets, and plasma (fresh or frozen) are forbidden. Banking of the person's own blood or salvage from suction during surgery is also forbidden because Witnesses believe that blood that has left the body should be discarded.

The use of albumin, immune globulin, and factor concentrates, as in hemophilia, is an individual decision. Nonblood plasma expanders, such as saline solution, Ringer's lactate, and hetastarch, are acceptable, and Witnesses may give blood for a sample.

The consequences of parents giving consent for a blood transfusion require them to leave the church, family, friends, and the Jehovah's Witness community. Refusal of blood is a basic component of the Jehovah's Witness faith, and if this covenant is broken, the individual may lose eternal salvation. Families are often shunned by the community (Catlin, 1997; McNeil, 1997).

For children from the Jehovah's Witness faith, every attempt should be made to treat with nonblood products. With advances in health care, more products are being developed, such as recombinant factor VIII concentrate, that are considered nonblood products. When this is not possible, consultation with experts in treating individuals who are of this faith is important. For the parents' sake, it is better to obtain a court order for lifesaving transfusion than to ask for their permission (Catlin, 1997). This removes the decision from the parents and prevents the parents and child from being ostracized, because the matter was taken out of their control. The nurse's role is to be an advocate for the family and a consultant to other members of the health team regarding the family's beliefs.

preventing heart failure through minimizing hypoxia and closely monitoring IV infusions is of first priority. Packed RBCs are usually administered to prevent circulatory hypervolemia. When blood transfusions are required in severe anemia to increase the hemoglobin level, all of the usual precautions for administering blood and observing for signs of transfusion reactions are instituted (Table 35-2).

## Blood Transfusion Therapy

Technologic advances in blood banking and transfusion medicine enable the administration of only the blood component needed by the child such as packed RBCs in anemia or platelets for bleeding disorders (Table 35-3 on p. 1543). Regardless of the blood component administered, the nurse must be aware of the possibility of transfusion reactions.

Although hemolytic reactions are rare, ABO incompatibility remains the most common cause of death from blood transfusion, and human error is usually responsible (administration of wrong type to patient or mislabeling of blood product) (Labovich, 1997; Lubin, 1995). Blood is usually matched between the donor and recipient for blood groups (A, B, AB, or O) and Rh factors (positive or negative). However, AB-type RBCs can be transfused to individuals with blood types A, B, and AB, and Rh-negative RBCs can be used for Rh-positive individuals. (See Chapter 9 for a discussion of blood groups and ABO and Rh incompatibility.)

When blood is mismatched, the A or B antiagglutinin is mixed with RBCs containing A or B agglutinogens, respectively, and agglutination (clumping) of the RBCs occurs. The agglutinins, which are bivalent, attach themselves to two different erythrocytes at the same time, causing the cells to clump together and clog small blood vessels. Over a few hours to days, the entrapped cells degenerate and hemolyze, liberating excessive quantities of hemoglobin into the circulation. The eventual hemolysis of large numbers of RBCs decreases the blood volume, causing circulatory failure and *shock*. Treatment is aimed at replacing lost blood and using plasma volume expanders.

Acute kidney shutdown and eventual *renal failure* are the result of renal vasoconstriction from antigen-antibody complexes derived from the RBC surface. The greatly reduced blood flow causes complete renal failure and death within 7 to 12 days. Treatment involves promoting diuresis with rapid, dilute IV fluids and diuretics, such as furosemide and mannitol, and alkalinizing body fluids, which render hemoglobin more soluble.

Another consequence of hemolysis is the release of large quantities of phospholipids, which are capable of stimulating *disseminated intravascular coagulation (DIC)* (see p. 1567). As a result the plasma is depleted of the coagulation factors needed to prevent hemorrhage. Without treatment with heparin to prevent the coagulation and blood components to initiate clotting, death from generalized hemorrhage can occur.

In addition to the nursing precautions and responsibilities outlined in Table 35-2, some general guidelines that apply to all transfusions include:

■ Take vital signs, including blood pressure, *before* administering blood to establish baseline data for intratransfusion and posttransfusion comparison, then every 15 minutes for 1 hour while blood is infusing.

■ Check the identification of the recipient with the donor's blood group and type, regardless of the blood product used.

■ Administer the first 50 ml of blood or initial 20% volume (whichever is smaller) *slowly* and stay with the child.

■ Administer with normal saline on a piggyback setup, or have normal saline available.

■ Administer blood through an appropriate filter to eliminate particles in the blood and prevent the precipitation of formed elements—gently shake the container frequently.

■ Use blood within 30 minutes of its arrival from the blood bank; if it is not used, return to the blood bank—do not store in a regular unit refrigerator.

■ Infuse a unit of blood (or the specified amount) within 4 hours. If the infusion will exceed this time, the blood should be divided into appropriate-size quantities by the blood bank, with the unused portion refrigerated under controlled conditions.

**TABLE 35-2**  Nursing care of the child receiving blood transfusions

| Complication | Signs/Symptoms | Precautions/Nursing Responsibilities |
|---|---|---|
| **Immediate Reactions** | | |
| *Hemolytic Reactions* | | |
| Most severe type, but rare Incompatible blood Incompatibility in multiple transfusions | Chills Shaking Fever Pain at needle site and along venous tract Nausea/vomiting Sensation of tightness in chest Red or black urine Headache Flank pain Progressive signs of shock and/or renal failure | Verify patient identification Identify donor and recipient blood types and groups before transfusion is begun; verify with another nurse or other practitioner Transfuse blood slowly for first 15 to 20 minutes or initial 20% volume of blood; remain with patient Stop transfusion immediately in event of signs or symptoms, maintain patent intravenous (IV) line, and notify practitioner Save donor blood to recrossmatch with patient's blood Monitor for evidence of shock Insert urinary catheter and monitor hourly outputs Send samples of patient's blood and urine to laboratory for presence of hemoglobin (indicates intravascular hemolysis) Observe for signs of hemorrhage resulting from disseminated intravascular coagulation (DIC) Support medical therapies to reverse shock |
| *Febrile Reactions* | | |
| Leukocyte or platelet antibodies Plasma protein antibodies | Fever Chills | May give acetaminophen for prophylaxis Leukocyte-poor RBCs are less likely to cause reaction Stop transfusion immediately; report to practitioner for evaluation |
| *Allergic Reactions* | | |
| Recipient reacts to allergens in donor's blood | Urticaria Flushing Pruritus Asthmatic wheezing Laryngeal edema | Give antihistamines for prophylaxis to children with tendency toward allergic reactions Stop transfusion immediately Administer epinephrine for wheezing or anaphylactic reaction |
| *Circulatory Overload* | | |
| Too rapid transfusion (even a small quantity) Excessive quantity of blood transfused (even slowly) | Sudden severe headache Precordial pain Tachycardia Dyspnea Rales Cyanosis Dry cough Distended neck veins Hypertension | Transfuse blood slowly Prevent overload by using packed RBCs or administering divided amounts of blood Use infusion pump to regulate and maintain flow rate Stop transfusion immediately if signs of overload Place child upright with feet in dependent position to increase venous resistance |
| *Air Emboli* | | |
| May occur when blood is transfused under pressure | Sudden difficulty in breathing Sharp pain in chest Apprehension | Normalize pressure before container is empty when infusing blood under pressure Clear tubing of air by aspirating air with syringe at nearest Y-connector if air is observed in tubing; disconnect tubing and allow blood to flow until air has escaped only if a Y-connector is not available |
| *Hypothermia* | Chills Low temperature Irregular heart rate Possible cardiac arrest | Allow blood to warm at room temperatures (less than 1 hour) Use approved mechanical blood warmer or electric warming coil to rapidly warm blood; never use microwave oven Take temperature if patient complains of chills; if subnormal, stop transfusion |
| *Electrolyte Disturbances* | | |
| Hyperkalemia (in massive transfusions or in patients with renal problems) | Nausea, diarrhea Muscular weakness Flaccid paralysis Paresthesia of extremities Bradycardia Apprehension Cardiac arrest | Use washed RBCs or fresh blood if patient is at risk |

*Continued*

**TABLE 35-2**   Nursing care of the child receiving blood transfusions—cont'd

| Complication | Signs/Symptoms | Precautions/Nursing Responsibilities |
|---|---|---|
| **Delayed Reactions** | | |
| *Transmission of Infection* | | |
| Hepatitis<br>Human immunodeficiency virus (HIV)<br>Malaria<br>Syphilis<br>Bacteria or viruses | Signs of infection (e.g., jaundice)<br>Toxic reaction: high fever, severe headache or substernal pain, hypotension, intense flushing, vomiting/diarrhea | Blood is tested for antibodies to human immunodeficiency virus (HIV), hepatitis C virus, and hepatitis B core antigen; in addition, blood is tested for hepatitis B surface antigen (HBsAg) and alanine aminotransferase (ALT), and a serology test is performed for syphilis; positive units are destroyed; individuals at risk for carrying certain viruses are deferred from donation<br>Report any sign of infection and, if occurring during transfusion, stop transfusion immediately, send sample for culture and sensitivity tests, and notify physician |
| *Alloimmunization* | | |
| (Antibody formation)<br>Occurs in patients receiving multiple transfusions | Increased risk of hemolytic, febrile, and allergic reactions | Use limited number of donors<br>Observe carefully for signs of reactions |
| *Delayed Hemolytic Reaction* | Destruction of RBCs and fever 5 to 10 days after transfusion (anemia, jaundice, dark urine) | Observe for posttransfusion anemia and decreasing benefit from successive transfusions |

■ If a reaction of any type is suspected, take vital signs, stop the transfusion, maintain a patent IV line with normal saline and new tubing, notify the practitioner, and do not restart the transfusion until the child's condition has been medically evaluated.

Blood is usually administered to children by infusion pump; therefore the usual precautions and management related to pumps apply. When the blood is started with a standard transfusion set, the filter chamber is filled to allow the total filter to be used. The drip chamber is partially filled with blood to permit counting of the drops. In adjusting the flow rate, it is important to remember that blood administration sets do not use microdrops (60 drops/ml) but regular drops (usually 10 or 15 drops/ml). Therefore this must be considered when calculating the flow rate.

Oxygen may be administered to provide optimum environmental conditions for hemoglobin saturation. However, oxygen is of limited value because each gram of hemoglobin is able to carry a limited amount of the gas. In addition, prolonged supplemental oxygen can decrease erythropoiesis. Therefore the child is monitored closely for evidence of decreasing benefit from oxygen. One of the first signs of hypoxia is restlessness. (See the Nursing Care Plan: The Child with Anemia.*)

# ANEMIA CAUSED BY NUTRITIONAL DEFICIENCIES

## Iron Deficiency Anemia

Anemia caused by an inadequate supply or loss of iron is the most prevalent nutritional disorder in the United States and the most preventable mineral disturbance. Without iron-fortified formula and cereals, 20% of lower-income

inner-city children 6 to 24 months of age will become anemic (Andrews and Bridges 1998; Felt and Lozoff, 1996). Female adolescents are also at risk for iron deficiency because of their rapid growth rate, menses, and poor eating habits (Pappas and Cheng, 1998). Over the past three decades, a decline in the prevalence of iron deficiency anemia in the United States may be primarily attributed to the initiation of the Women, Infants, and Children (WIC) program (Kwaitkowski and others, 1999). The promotion of breast-feeding, introduction of iron-fortified infant formula and cereal, weaning the bottle by 1 year of age, and delayed introduction of cow's milk into the diet have all contributed to the decreased incidence of iron deficiency anemia in infants and young children (Bogen and others, 2000). However, iron deficiency still occurs in infants and children of all races and ethnic groups (Buchanan, 1999) and continues to be a significant health problem.

### Etiology

Iron deficiency anemia can be caused by any number of factors that decrease the supply of iron, impair its absorption, increase the body's need for iron, or affect the synthesis of hemoglobin (Box 35-3). Although the clinical manifestations and diagnostic evaluation are quite similar regardless of the cause, the therapeutic and nursing considerations depend on the specific reason for the iron deficiency. The following discussion is limited to iron deficiency anemia resulting from inadequate iron in the diet.

At birth the full term infant's supply of iron is approximately 300 mg, or 75 mg/kg of body weight. During the last trimester of pregnancy, iron is transferred from the mother to the fetus at the rate of 4 mg/day. Most of the iron is stored in the circulating hemoglobin of the erythrocytes, and the remainder is deposited in the liver, spleen, and bone marrow. Maternal iron stores are adequate for the first 5 to 6 months in the full-term infant but only for about 2 to

*In Wong DL, Hess CS: *Wong and Whaley's clinical manual of pediatric nursing,* ed 5, St Louis, 2000, Mosby.

**TABLE 35-3**  Blood components and nursing administration

| Components/Indications | Dose | Nursing Administration |
|---|---|---|
| **Packed red blood cells (PRBCs)**<br>Symptomatic anemia<br>Renal/liver disease<br>Hemolysis<br>Decreased erythropoiesis<br>Thalassemia major<br>Splenic/liver sequestration | Volume packed RBC = weight<br>(kg) × change in hematocrit<br>(Hct) desired | 1. Regulate infusion rate using microaggregate filter via infusion pump at 5 ml/kg/hr over 2-4 hours (usual rate). Do not use the tubing to infuse more than 1 unit of blood.<br>2. Monitor vital signs before transfusion, 15 minutes after initiation, and at the end of transfusion.<br>3. Do not refrigerate blood in the nursing unit. Only the blood bank refrigerator may be used. |
| **Whole blood** (rarely used)<br>Acute massive blood loss | Volume of whole blood = weight<br>(kg) × change in Hct desired × 2 | 4. Ensure that each unit is infused in 4 hours or less. If a longer infusion time is needed, the unit must be divided in the blood bank.<br>5. Do not infuse solutions other than normal saline in the line with RBCs. |
| **Fresh frozen plasma (FFP)**<br>Deficiencies of plasma clotting factors in bleeding patients (e.g., disseminated intravascular coagulopathy [DIC]), liver failure, vitamin K deficiency with bleeding, or replacement of antithrombin III (ATIII), protein C, or protein S | 10-15 ml/kg (use within 6-24 hours of thawing) | 1. Use microaggregate filter over 1-2 hours every 12-24 hours until hemorrhage stops at a rate of 20 ml/min.<br>2. Monitor prothrombin time (PT) and partial thromboplastin time (PTT) before and after FFP.<br>3. Monitor other coagulation factors (e.g., fibrinogen, fibrin split products, D-Dimer, ATIII, protein C, and protein S). |
| **Platelets (plt)**<br>Active hemorrhage, DIC<br>Thrombocytopenia with bleeding or if indicated by clinical status | 1 unit/10 kg or 6 units/m² intravenously (IV) | 1. Regulate infusion rate using 170 $\mu$m microaggregate filter at 10 cc/kg/hr, IV push or over an hour or as fast as patient can tolerate.<br>2. Monitor vital signs before transfusion, 15 minutes after initiation, and at the end of infusion.<br>3. Obtain postplatelet count 60 minutes to 24 hours after infusion. |
| **Granulocytes** (rarely used)<br>As an adjunct with other measures in treatment of severe infections in the septic neonate or high-risk patient (e.g., proven bacterial infection in severe neutropenic patient nonresponsive to antibiotic therapy) | 10-15 ml/kg IV usually daily × 4 days | 1. Monitor vital signs before transfusion, 15 minutes after initiation, and at the end of transfusion.<br>2. Premedicate 1 hour before transfusion, usually antihistamines, acetaminophen, or steroids.<br>3. Infuse at slow rate (2-4 hours) using 170 $\mu$m blood filter within a 24-hour period.<br>4. Recommend minimal 4-6 hours between amphotericin B and granulocyte infusion. |
| **Factor VIII** (plasma-derived or recombinant)<br>Hemophilia A<br>Acquired factor VIII deficiency | 1 unit/kg IV of factor VIII = 2% of factor activity<br>35-50 units/kg IV of factor VIII every 12-24 hours | 1. Use reconstituted factor within 3 hours of mixing.<br>2. Inject reconstituted factor intravenously over 2-5 minutes.<br>3. Assess for signs of an adverse reaction such as hives, itchy wheals with redness, tightness in chest, wheezing, low blood pressure, or trouble breathing. Notify health care provider immediately if symptoms are present. |
| **Factor IX** (plasma-derived or recombinant)<br>Hemophilia B | 1 unit/kg IV of factor IX = 1% of factor activity<br>30-50 units/kg IV every 24 hours | |
| **FEIBA (Factor eight inhibitor by-pass activity)** plasma-derived<br>Hemophilia A or B with inhibitors (antibodies) | 75-100 units/kg IV every 8-24 hours (maximum dose 200 units/kg/day) | |
| **Factor VII a** (recombinant)<br>Hemophilia A or B with inhibitors | 90 $\mu$g/kg IV every 2 hours (35-120 $\mu$g/kg) dosage range | |
| **Cryoprecipitate (CRYO)** (rarely used)<br>Control bleeding in patients with DIC<br>Hypofibrinogenemia | 4 bags CRYO/10 kg IV | 1. Monitor closely PT/PTT, fibrinogen, fibrinogen split products, D-Dimer.<br>2. Use a filter needle to draw up and administer within 15-30 minutes. |

3 months in premature infants or infants of multiple births. If dietary sources of iron are not supplied to meet the infant's growth demands following depletion of fetal iron stores, iron deficiency anemia results. Physiologic anemia should not be confused with iron deficiency anemia resulting from nutritional causes. (See Chapter 12.)

Vegetarian diets, popular among teenage girls, have been associated with nutritional deficiencies. Infants and toddlers who have been fed inappropriate vegetarian diets have been reported to have severe protein-energy malnutrition, as well as deficiencies of iron, vitamin $B_{12}$, and vitamin D. Unrefined cereals contain substances that modify the absorption of minerals such as zinc, calcium, and iron. Individuals with vegetarian diets that include a large amount of unrefined cereals could be at a greater risk of rickets and iron deficiency anemia (Sanders, 1995).

## Pathophysiology

Iron is required for the production of hemoglobin. One molecule consists of *protein (globin)* combined with four molecules of a *pigmented compound (heme)*. Each molecule of heme contains one atom of iron. When iron stores are deficient, the production of hemoglobin is reduced. Consequently, the main effect of iron deficiency is decreased hemoglobin and reduced oxygen-carrying capacity of the blood.

## Clinical Manifestations

The clinical manifestations are directly attributed to the reduction in the amount of oxygen available to tissues and resemble those seen in any type of anemia. Usually the signs are insidious and obscure, and the severity is directly related to the duration of the dietary deficiency.

Although the majority of infants with iron deficiency anemia are underweight, many are overweight because of excessive milk ingestion (known as *milk baby*). These children become anemic for two reasons: milk, a poor source of iron, is given almost to the exclusion of solid foods, and 50% of iron-deficient infants fed cow's milk have an increased fecal loss of blood. This asymptomatic loss of hemoglobin has been thought to cause iron deficiency (Kwaitkowski and others, 1999). Although chubby, these infants are pale, usually demonstrate poor muscle development, and are prone to infection. The skin color may be described as porcelain-like.

Although the mechanism is unknown, iron deficiency anemia enhances the leakage of plasma proteins in infants, causing edema, retarded growth, and decreased serum concentration of the proteins albumin, gamma globulin, and

transferrin (a protein that binds iron and transports it through the plasma). Other manifestations of iron deficiency include irritability, tachycardia, fatigue, glossitis, angular stomatitis, and koilonychia (concave or "spoon" fingernails). The precise relationship of iron deficiency anemia to behavioral and intellectual functioning is not clear, but increasing evidence suggests that chronic severe iron deficiency during infancy results in impaired cognitive skills, social and behavioral problems. (Halterman and others, 2001; Lozoff and others, 2000).

## Diagnostic Evaluation

Laboratory tests that measure or describe hemoglobin, the morphologic changes in the RBC, and iron concentration are usually performed (see Table 35-1). The RBC count may be normal, borderline, or moderately reduced in the child with iron deficiency anemia. Typically the nearly normal number of erythrocytes is strikingly out of proportion to the low hemoglobin concentration. RBCs are typically small in size (microcytic), which have a decreased mean corpuscular volume (MCV) (see Box 35-1). For infants 1 year of age, an MCV below 70 $\mu m^3$ is considered diagnostic. In the child from 1 to 10 years of age an MCV of 70 $\mu m^3$ plus the child's age in years is a quick calculation of the lower limit of normal.

The reticulocyte count is usually normal or slightly reduced because of decreased stores of iron (see Table 35-1). However, in severe anemia, when tissue hypoxia exerts an erthyropoietic response, the reticulocyte count may be elevated to 3% or 4%. The level of erythrocyte protoporphyrin (EP), the immediate precursor of heme, becomes elevated in RBCs whenever heme synthesis is disturbed.

In terms of differential diagnosis, a stool analysis for occult blood (guaiac test) is commonly performed to confirm or rule out the possibility of chronic fecal blood loss, especially from milk intolerance or structural anomalies such as diverticulitis.

**Iron Studies.** In addition to those tests that indirectly indicate the level of iron by the effects of iron deficiency on the RBC, several other tests are usually performed that more directly measure the amount of circulating iron. The *serum-iron concentration (SIC)* measures the amount of circulating iron and normally is about 70 $\mu g/dl$ in infants and slightly higher in older children. Lower limits of serum iron vary not only with age but also with the time of day; they are highest in the morning, when the test should be performed.

The *total iron-binding capacity (TIBC)* measures the amount of *transferrin,* or iron-binding globulin, which is necessary for the transport of iron in the bloodstream. When combined with transferrin, the iron is loosely bound to the globulin molecule so that it can be released easily to tissue cells anywhere in the body. In iron deficiency anemia the TIBC is elevated above the normal range of 350 $\mu g/dl$ (6 months to 2 years) or 450 $\mu g/dl$ (children older than 2 years and adults). The elevated TIBC represents the body's compensatory mechanisms to absorb more exogenous sources of iron during states of deficiency than normally. The combination of a reduced SIC and an elevated

TIBC is of significant diagnostic value because it is not found in any other condition except hypochromic, microcytic anemia caused by inadequate intake or absorption of iron. The *transferrin saturation* is calculated by dividing the SIC by the TIBC and multiplying the result by 100 to express the value as a percentage. A transferrin saturation of 10% suggests anemia.

## Therapeutic Management

Prevention is the primary goal and is achieved through optimum nutrition and appropriate iron supplementation. In infants the American Academy of Pediatrics (AAP) (1999a) recommends the following guidelines to prevent iron deficiency:

- Use only breast milk or iron-fortified formula (containing between 4.0 to 12 mg/l of iron) for the first 12 months.
- Begin iron supplementation (preferably iron-fortified commercial formula or, in breast-fed infants, iron-fortified infant cereal) to provide 1 mg/kg/day of iron by 4 to 6 months of age in fullterm infants and by 2 months of age in preterm infants.
- Administer iron (ferrous sulfate) drops at a dose of 2 to 3 mg/kg/day to a maximum of 15 mg/day to breast-fed preterm infants after 2 months of age and give iron-fortified infant cereal when solid foods are introduced.
- Limit the amount of formula to no more than 1 L/day to encourage intake of iron-rich solid foods.

Once the diagnosis of iron deficiency anemia is made, therapeutic management focuses on increasing the amount of supplemental iron the child receives. This is usually done through dietary counseling and the administration of oral iron supplements. In formula-fed infants the most convenient and best sources of supplemental iron are iron-fortified commercial formula and iron-fortified infant cereal (Buchanan, 1999). Iron-fortified formula provides a relatively constant and predictable amount of iron and is not associated with an increased incidence of gastrointestinal symptoms, such as colic, diarrhea, or constipation. Infants under 12 months of age should not be given fresh cow's milk to decrease the possibility of gastrointestinal blood loss occurring from allergy to the milk protein.

Dietary addition of iron-rich foods may not provide sufficient supplemental quantities of the mineral. Oral supplements of ferrous iron are given because this form is more readily absorbed than ferric iron, resulting in higher hemoglobin levels. Ingested iron is absorbed largely from the duodenum, and absorption is facilitated by an acid environment. Children absorb an average of 10% to 20% of oral iron supplements, but during periods of iron deficiency they absorb an additional 5% to 10%. Oral iron supplementation is prescribed as 3 to 6 mg of elemental iron/kg/day. Lower doses of iron are associated with fewer side effects. Ideally the daily dose of iron should be given in two or three divided doses between meals. Side effects of oral iron therapy include nausea, gastric irritation, diarrhea or constipation, and anorexia, but these occur infrequently, especially in infants. If the iron produces vomiting and diarrhea, it should be administered with meals and in gradually increasing doses.

The response to oral iron therapy is reflected in a peak increase in the reticulocyte count by the fifth to the tenth day of administration. Following the reticulocyte rise, the hemoglobin and hematocrit levels and RBC count increase. The hemoglobin level rises an average of 0.17 to 0.25 g/dl/day; therefore a substantial increase should occur by the end of 1 month.

If the hemoglobin is very low or if levels fail to rise after 1 month of oral therapy, it is important to assess whether or not the iron is being administered correctly. Parenteral iron administration is painful, expensive, and occasionally associated with regional lymphadenopathy or serious allergic reaction (Frewin, Henson, and Provan, 1997; Miller, 1995). Therefore parenteral iron is reserved for children who have iron malabsorption or chronic hemoglobinuria. The Z-track method of intramuscular injection must be used to minimize staining of the skin, and careful observation is required because of the risk of anaphylaxis. Transfusions are indicated for the most severe anemia and in cases of serious infection, cardiac dysfunction, or surgical emergency when anesthesia is required. Packed RBCs (2 to 3 ml/kg), not whole blood, are used to minimize the chance of circulatory overload. Supplemental oxygen is administered when tissue hypoxia is severe.

*Vitamin B$_{12}$ deficiency* develops when the gastric mucosa fails to secrete sufficient amounts of intrinsic factor, which is essential for absorption of vitamin B$_{12}$. Deprived of vitamin B$_{12}$, the bone marrow produces fewer but larger (macrocytic) RBCs. The erythrocytes are usually immature and, because of their extremely fragile cell membranes, are rapidly destroyed during circulation. Treatment initially involves the administration of 25 to 100 $\mu$g intramuscularly for several days, followed by injections of 500 or 1000 $\mu$g of vitamin B$_{12}$ every 1 to 2 months.

**Prognosis.** Prognosis for a child with this condition is very good. However, there is evidence that if the iron deficiency anemia is severe and long-standing, then diminished cognitive function, behavior changes, delayed infant growth and development, decreased exercise tolerance, and impaired immune function may develop (Bogen and others, 2000).

## Nursing Considerations

A primary nursing objective is to prevent nutritional anemia through family education. Nurses need to be aware of recommendations regarding iron supplementation during infancy and appropriate sources of dietary iron. One of the difficulties in terms of infant feeding is encouraging parents to limit the quantity of milk, use iron-fortified infant formulas, and introduce solid foods when they believe milk is best for the infant and equate the resultant weight gain with a "healthy child." Although milk is an excellent food, it is deficient in iron, vitamin C, zinc, and fluoride. Sources of each of these nutrients and the role they play in preventing deficiencies need to be discussed with the family, especially the person who is responsible for feeding the infant. For example, the mother may have less decision-making power regarding feeding than the grandmother who cares for the child.

It is also stressed that overweight is not synonymous with good health. If the infant has obvious signs of anemia, such as pallor, listlessness, frequent infections, and muscular weakness, they are pointed out as evidence of suboptimum health. In some instances it is helpful to chart the hemoglobin or hematocrit values to visually impress on parents the change in iron levels. Often, increased blood values correspond to improved physical status and reinforce the benefit of dietary or oral iron supplementation.

Instructing parents regarding proper administration of oral iron supplements is an essential nursing responsibility. Several factors affect the absorption of iron, such as stomach acidity. (See Table 13-2.) Ideally iron supplements are administered in two divided doses between meals, when the presence of free hydrochloric acid is greatest, and are accompanied by a citrus fruit or juice, which helps reduce iron to its most soluble state. An inadequate dietary intake of calcium helps bind and remove agents, such as phosphates and phytates, that react with iron to render it insoluble. In cultures in which tea is drunk as a common beverage, iron should be administered with some other liquid, because the tannins in tea form an insoluble complex with iron from foods other than meat. In addition, some substances in herbal teas may adversely affect the uptake of iron (Beard and Tobin, 2000). Adequate dosage of oral iron turns the stools a tarry green or black color. The nurse advises parents of this normally expected change and inquires about its occurrence on follow-up visits. Absence of the greenish black stool may be a clue to poor compliance. If compliance is an issue, every effort should be made to institute strategies to improve adherence to the medication regimen, such as administering the drug once a day at the most convenient time. (See Compliance, Chapter 27.)

Oral iron supplements are available in liquid or tablet form. Liquid preparations may temporarily stain the teeth. If possible, the medication should be taken through a straw or given through a syringe or medicine dropper placed toward the back of the mouth. Brushing the teeth after administration of the drug lessens the discoloration.

> **NURSING ALERT**
>
> Because iron ingested in excessive quantities is toxic, even fatal, parents should keep no more than a 1-month supply in the home and store it safely away from the reach of children.

Counseling families whose children are anemic is often a difficult and challenging task. Meal planning must be based on their budget, cultural pattern, and food preferences. Often this requires more than a brief discussion with the mother or usual caregiver about foods high in iron. (See Table 13-2.) For teaching to be effective, the nurse may need to offer recipes, assist in planning a shopping list, and investigate food prices for economy. Because the physical effects of anemia are insidious, parents may not consider their child ill and consequently may view the medication and diet changes as unnecessary. Stressing what the physical and behavioral improvements will be and what effect the improved diet will have on all family members may encourage parents to adhere to the treatment plan.

Diet education of teenagers is difficult, especially because teenage girls are particularly prone to following weight-reduction diets. Emphasizing the effect of anemia on appearance (pallor) and energy level (difficulty maintaining popular activities) may be useful. (See Table 13-2 and Mineral Disturbances, Chapter 13, for sources of iron-rich foods.)

# ANEMIAS CAUSED BY INCREASED DESTRUCTION OF RED BLOOD CELLS

*Excessive destruction* or *hemolysis* of erythrocytes can occur from a defect within the RBC (intracorpuscular) that shortens the life span of the cell, preventing production from keeping pace with destruction. Sickle cell anemia and thalassemia have decreased erythrocyte life spans because of a hemoglobin defect, whereas spherocytosis has a decreased erythrocyte life span due to a defective red cell membrane. Extracorpuscular factors are those conditions that cause hemolysis in otherwise normal RBCs. A classic example is blood group incompatibility, such as hemolytic disease of the newborn or incompatibility secondary to mismatched blood transfusion. Damage to a normal red cell may be caused by toxic drugs, burns, poisonings (such as from lead), infections such as malaria, and splenic sequestration (hypersplenism).

## Hereditary Spherocytosis (HS)

HS, the most common of the hemolytic disorders, is caused by a defect in the proteins that form the RBC membrane (Delhommeau and others, 2000). It is primarily prevalent in persons of Northern European heritage with reported incidence of 1 in 5000 (Bader-Meunier and others, 2001; Sackey, 1999).

It is transmitted as an autosomal dominant condition. However, 25% of the cases are thought to represent new mutations, autosomal recessive or autosomal dominant with reduced penetrance (Sackey, 1999). The affected cells have a smaller surface area relative to their volume than normal RBCs, which results in an inflexible sphere known as a *spherocyte*. Inflexibility of these cells makes it difficult for them to circulate through the spleen and leads to their early destruction.

Clinical manifestations vary widely and include anemia (usually mild), splenomegaly (usually modest and does not correlate with severity of disease), and jaundice (most often scleral-icterus). HS frequently presents in the first 24 hours of the newborn's life as severe hyperbilirubinemia. Folic acid supplementation should be given to these children to prevent deficiency due to the rapid cell turnover. Laboratory findings include the following: hemoglobin level between 7 to 10 g/dl, reticulocyte count of 3% to 15% (inversely correlated with the hemoglobin), and an increase in osmotic fragility.

Aplastic crisis, which results in a sudden cessation of RBC production by the bone marrow, is a serious complication. Hemoglobin and hematocrit values drop rapidly, resulting in severe anemia. Transfusion support may be needed, and close monitoring of the child's cardiovascular status is necessary.

Splenectomy, a treatment for HS, is generally reserved for children more than 5 years of age with symptomatic anemia. The splenectomy corrects the hemolysis but not the RBC defect. Occasionally splenectomy is performed in children less than 5 years of age who are severely anemic and are showing signs of failure to thrive. Children who are scheduled to undergo a splenectomy should be evaluated for the presence of gallstones before surgery. If gallstones are present, a cholecystectomy is performed at the time of splenectomy. Because of the risk of life-threatening bacterial infection after splenectomy, these children are immunized with the pneumococcal, meningococcal, and *Haemophilus influenzae* type b (Hib) vaccines before surgery and receive prophylactic penicillin for several years after splenectomy. Parents must be instructed in the importance of seeking immediate medical attention if their child develops fever over 38.3° C (101° F) (Kline and Mooney, 1998; Lanzkowsky, 2000).

## Sickle Cell Anemia (SCA)

SCA is a part of a group of diseases collectively termed *hemoglobinopathies,* in which normal adult hemoglobin (*hemoglobin A [HgbA]*) is partly or completely replaced by abnormal *sickle hemoglobin (HgbS). Sickle cell disease (SCD)* refers to a group of hereditary disorders, all of which are related to the presence of HgbS. Even though SCD is sometimes used to refer to SCA, this use is incorrect. Correct terms for SCA are *HgbSS* and *homozygous sickle cell disease.* In the United States the most common forms of SCD are:

Sickle cell anemia (SCA)—The homozygous form of the disease (HgbSS), in which valine, an amino acid, is substituted for glutamic acid at the sixth position of the β-chain.

Sickle cell–C disease—A heterozygous variant of SCD, including both HgbS and hemoglobin C (HgbSC), in which lysine is substituted for glutamic acid at the sixth position of the β-chain.

Sickle thalassemia disease—A combination of sickle cell trait and β-thalassemia trait. $\beta^+$ (beta plus) refers to the ability to still produce some normal adult hemoglobin. $\beta^0$ (beta zero) indicates that there is no ability to produce normal adult hemoglobin.

Of the SCDs, SCA is the most common form in African-Americans in the United States, followed by sickle cell–C disease and sickle β-thalassemia. Numerous other sickle syndromes exist that have paired with rare mutant globins.

SCD is the most common genetic disease in the United States with an incidence of 1 in 375 births and approximately 70,000 cases among African-Americans. However, SCD affects other nationalities, including Africans, Hispanics, Arabs, Italians, Native Americans, Caribbeans, Iranians, Turks, and infrequently American whites (primarily of Mediterranean descent). The incidence of the disease varies in different geographic locations. Among African-Americans, the incidence of sickle cell trait is about 8%, whereas the frequency of sickle cell trait is reported to be as high as 40% among inhabitants of West Africa. The high incidence of sickle cell trait in these individuals is believed by some to be a result of selective protection of trait carriers against malaria caused by *Plasmodium falciparum.*

### Mode of Transmission

The gene that determines the production of HgbS is situated on an autosome. The expected pattern of transmission from two parents who carry the heterozygous gene HgbAS is illustrated in Fig. 5-6. Therefore, when both parents have sickle cell trait, there is a 25% chance with each pregnancy of producing an offspring with SCA. In the United States it is estimated that 1 in 12 African-Americans carries the trait; therefore the risk of two African-American parents having a child with the disease is 0.7%. The occurrence of other forms of SCD is a result of the union between two individuals who carry the heterozygous form of hemoglobin variants.

### Basic Defect

The basic defect responsible for the sickling effect of erythrocytes is in the globin fraction of hemoglobin, which is composed of 574 amino acids. Under conditions of dehydration, acidosis, hypoxia, and temperature elevations, the relatively insoluble HgbS changes its molecular structure to form long, slender crystals. These filamentous crystals cause distortion of the cell membrane from a pliable disk to a crescent- or sickle-shaped RBC. The filamentous forms are associated with much greater viscosity than the normal holly leaf structure of HgbA.

In most instances the sickling response is reversible under conditions of adequate oxygenation and hydration. During this time the RBCs are indistinguishable from normal erythrocytes on peripheral examination. RBCs with HgbS can sickle and unsickle under adverse conditions. After repeated cycles of sickling and unsickling, the RBC becomes irreversibly sickled.

Although the defect is inherited, the sickling phenomenon is usually not apparent until later in infancy because of the presence of fetal hemoglobin (HgbF). HgbF is composed of two α- and two γ-polypeptide chains. At 32 weeks of gestation, the production of β- and δ-chains begins. These combine with α-chains to form the major adult hemoglobins: HgbA (two α and two β-chains) and HgbA₂ (two α- and two δ-chains). As long as the newborn has predominately HgbF, sickling does not occur in these cells because there are no β-chains carrying the defect. The newborn has from 60% to 80% fetal hemoglobin, but this rapidly decreases during the first year, so that the child is at risk for sickle cell–related complications (Yaster, Kost-Byerly and Maxwell, 2000; AAP, 2002).

**Sickle Cell Trait.**  Persons with sickle cell trait have the same basic defect, but only about 35% to 45% of the total hemoglobin is HgbS. The remainder is HgbA. Normally these individuals are asymptomatic. Although rare, complications have been described in individuals with sickle cell trait. Nonpainful, gross hematuria is the major complication, seen primarily in the teenage and adult years. Under conditions of extreme or prolonged deoxygenation, such as riding in an unpressurized aircraft or military training, splenic sequestration with profound anemia can occur, resulting in death.

### Pathophysiology and Clinical Manifestations

The clinical manifestations of SCA are primarily the result of (1) *obstruction* caused by the sickled RBCs and (2) increased RBC *destruction.* The entanglement and enmeshing of rigid sickle-shaped cells with one another intermittently block the microcirculation, causing vaso-occlusion. The resultant absence of blood flow to adjacent tissues causes local hypoxia, leading to tissue ischemia and infarction (cellular death) (Box 35-4). Most of the complications seen in SCA can be traced to this process and its impact on various organs of the body (Fig. 35-3).

Initially the *spleen* may become enlarged from congestion and engorgement with sickled cells. This repeated insult to the splenic sinuses results in infarction. The functioning cells are gradually replaced with fibrotic tissue until by the age of 5 years the spleen is decreased in size and totally replaced by a fibrous mass (*functional asplenia*). Without the spleen to filter bacteria and to promote the release of large numbers of phagocytic cells, these individuals are highly susceptible to infection.

The *liver* is also altered in form and function. Liver failure and necrosis are the result of severe impairment of hepatic blood flow from anemia and capillary obstruction. Moderate hepatomegaly is common by age 1 and usually persists throughout childhood and early adulthood. The

rapid destruction of RBCs often results in the development of pigmented gallstones. Obstruction of the common bile duct by gallstones is uncommon; therefore cholecystectomy for asymptomatic patients is generally not recommended. If recurrent episodes of right upper abdominal pain occur, cholecystectomy may be indicated.

*Kidney* abnormalities are probably the result of the same cycle of congestion of glomerular capillaries and tubular arterioles with sickle cells and hemosiderin, tissue necrosis, and eventual scarring. The principal results of kidney ischemia are hematuria, inability to concentrate urine, enuresis, and occasionally nephrotic syndrome.

*Bone* changes include hyperplasia and congestion of the bone marrow, resulting in osteoporosis, widening of the medullary spaces, and thinning of the cortices. As a result of the weakening of bone, especially in the lumbar and thoracic regions, skeletal deformities, particularly lordosis and kyphosis, may occur. From chronic hypoxia, the bone becomes susceptible to osteomyelitis, frequently from *Salmonella* organisms. Aseptic necrosis of the femoral head from chronic ischemia is an occasional problem.

Changes in the *central nervous system* are primarily vascular from the same cyclic reaction of occlusion, ischemia, and infarction. Stroke, or cerebrovascular accident, is a major complication that occurs in approximately 10% of children with SCD (peak incidence between 4 and 6 years) and can result in permanent paralysis or death (Gribbons, Zahr and Opas, 1995; Wethers, 2000). Any number of neurologic symptoms can herald a minor cerebral insult, such as headache, aphasia, weakness, convulsions, visual disturbances, or unilateral hemiplegia. Loss of vision is usually the result of progressive retinopathy and retinal detachment. Cognitive impairment from SCA without any signs of neurologic injury, known as "silent" infarct or stroke, is being investigated (Wethers, 2000).

*Heart* problems are mainly attributable to the stress of chronic anemia, which can eventually result in decompensation and failure. Cardiomegaly is visualized on chest x-ray examination, and a systolic flow murmur is frequently present as a consequence of the anemia. An echocardiogram shows cardiomegaly, septal hypertrophy, and contractility (Covitz and others, 1995; Lanzkowsky, 2000).

With the formation of sickled erythrocytes, mechanical fragility is increased, thereby decreasing the life span of the RBC. Hemolysis occurs both during intravascular circulation and as a result of stagnation of sickled cells in the congested spleen (see Fig. 35-3). Although the body attempts to compensate through stimulated erythropoietic activity, as evidenced by a hyperplastic bone marrow, the rate of destruction exceeds the rate of production. A normocytic, normochromic anemia results. With increased hemolysis, hemosiderosis (increased storage of iron) is present in the liver, spleen, bone marrow, kidneys, and lymph nodes (see Box 35-4).

**Other Signs and Symptoms.** In addition to the effects of sickling on various organ structures, the child with SCA may have a variety of complaints, such as exercise intolerance, anorexia, jaundiced sclera, and gallstones. Chronic leg ulcers are common in adolescents and adults and are

---

**Box 35-4** ■ ■ ■
## Clinical Manifestations of Sickle Cell Anemia

**GENERAL**
Possible growth retardation
Chronic anemia (Hgb 6 to 9 g/dl)
Possible delayed sexual maturation
Marked susceptibility to sepsis

**VASO-OCCLUSIVE (CRISIS)**
Pain in area(s) of involvement
Manifestations related to ischemia of involved areas:
  Extremities—painful swelling of hands and feet (sickle cell dactylitis, or hand-foot syndrome), painful joints
  Abdomen—severe pain resembling acute surgical condition
  Cerebrum—stroke, visual disturbances
  Chest—symptoms resembling pneumonia, protracted episodes of pulmonary disease
  Liver—obstructive jaundice, hepatic coma
  Kidney—hematuria
  Genital—priapism (painful constant penile erection)

**SEQUESTRATION CRISIS**
Pooling of large amounts of blood:
  Hepatomegaly
  Splenomegaly
  Circulatory collapse

**EFFECTS OF CHRONIC VASO-OCCLUSIVE PHENOMENA**
Heart—cardiomegaly, systolic murmurs
Lungs—altered pulmonary function, susceptibility to infections, pulmonary insufficiency
Kidneys—inability to concentrate urine, progressive renal failure, enuresis
Liver—hepatomegaly, cirrhosis, intrahepatic cholestasis
Spleen—splenomegaly, susceptibility to infection, functional reduction in splenic activity progressing to autosplenectomy
Eyes—intraocular abnormalities with visual disturbances, sometimes progressive retinal detachment and blindness
Extremities—avascular necrosis of hip/shoulder, skeletal deformities, especially lordosis and kyphosis, chronic leg ulcers, susceptibility to osteomyelitis
Central nervous system—hemiparesis, seizures

thought to be a result of decreased circulation due to vaso-occlusion and tissue ischemia. Other generalized effects include growth retardation in both height and weight, delayed sexual maturation, and decreased fertility. When the child reaches adulthood, sexual development and adult height are usually achieved.

**Sickle Cell Crises.** The clinical manifestations of SCA vary markedly in severity and frequency. The most acute symptoms of the disease occur during periods of exacerbation called *crises.* There are several types of episodic crises: vaso-occlusive, acute splenic sequestration, aplastic, hyperhemolytic, stroke, chest syndrome, and infection. The crises may occur individually or concomitantly with one or more other crises.

*Vaso-occlusive crises (VOCs)* are the most common non–life-threatening crises, preferably called "painful episodes or events." They are characterized by ischemia causing mild to severe pain that may last from minutes to days. A child with a VOC alone may have localized or generalized pain, acute abdominal pain from visceral hypoxia or gallstones, priapism (an unwanted, prolonged penile erection), and arthralgia. The pain is often migratory, with presence of a low-grade fever but without an exacerbation of anemia.

VOCs can result in a variety of skeletal problems. One of the more frequent is the *hand-foot syndrome (dactylitis),* which occurs primarily in young children ages 6 months to 2 years. It is caused by infarction of short tubular bones and is characterized by pain and swelling of the soft tissue over the hands and feet. It usually resolves spontaneously within a couple of days to weeks. Localized swelling over joints with arthralgia can occur from erythrostasis with sickle cells.

*Sequestration crises* are caused by the pooling of large quantities of blood, usually in the spleen and infrequently in the liver, causing a decrease in blood volume and ultimately shock. The splenic crisis may be acute or chronic. The chronic manifestation is termed *hypersplenism.* The acute form occurs most commonly in children between 2 months and 5 years of age and may result in death from profound anemia and cardiovascular collapse. Splenic sequestration has been reported in older children and adolescents with sickle cell–C disease or sickle β-thalassemia.

*Aplastic crisis* is diminished RBC production, usually triggered by a viral (especially the human parvovirus) or other infection. When it is superimposed on the existing rapid destruction of RBCs, a profound anemia results. Packed RBC transfusion is occasionally required in children exhibiting signs and symptoms of congestive heart failure.

*Megaloblastic anemia* is attributed to an excessive nutritional need for folic acid and/or vitamin $B_{12}$ during periods of pronounced erythropoiesis. Because infection is not always antecedent to aplastic or hypoplastic crises, it is possible that folic acid deficiency is a causative agent.

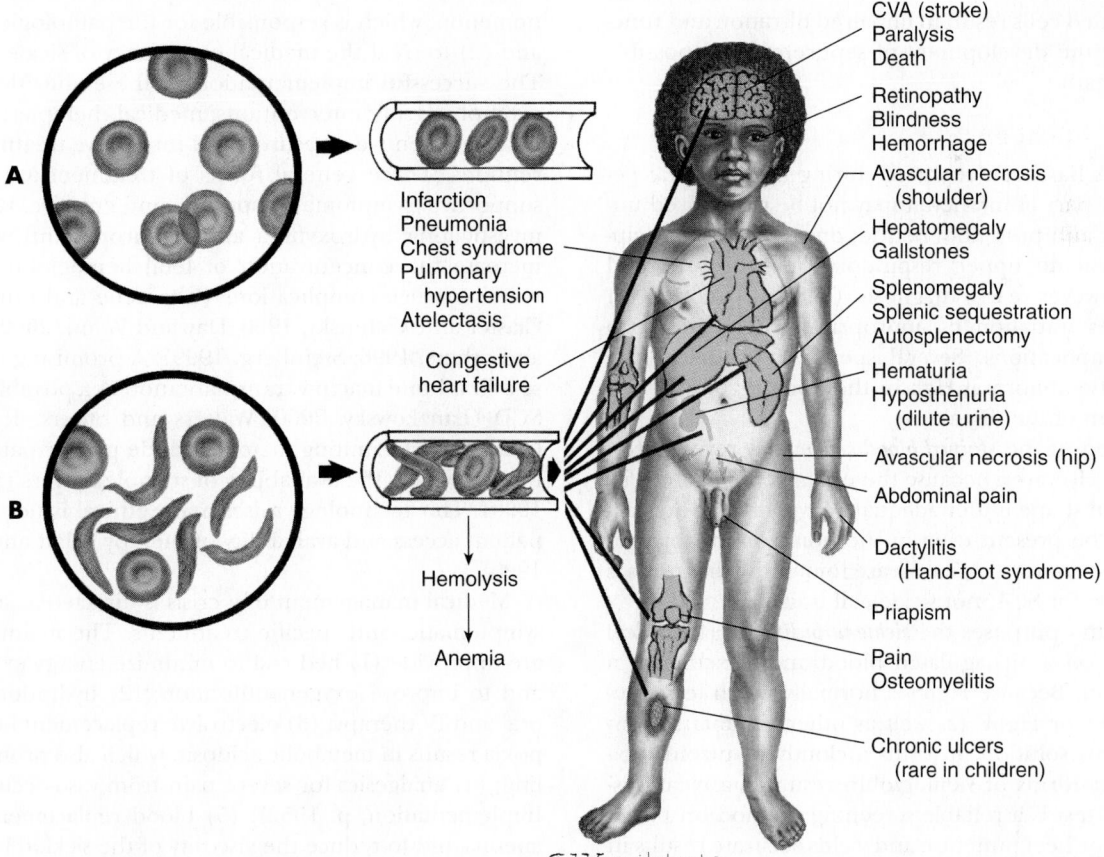

**Fig. 35-3** Differences between **A,** normal RBCs, and **B,** sickled RBCs in circulation with related complications.

*Hyperhemolytic crisis* is an accelerated rate of RBC destruction characterized by anemia, jaundice, and reticulocytosis. This complication frequently suggests other coexisting conditions, such as viral illness, transfusion reactions to alloantibodies, or glucose-6-phosphate dehydrogenase (G6PD) deficiency, which is also common in African-Americans.

A *cerebrovascular accident (CVA, stroke)* is a sudden and severe complication, often with no related illnesses. Sickled cells block the major blood vessels in the brain, resulting in cerebral infarction, which causes variable degrees of neurologic impairment. Repeat strokes causing progressively greater brain damage occur in approximately 50% of children who have already experienced one stroke and do not receive monthly transfusions (Steinberg, 1999).

Another serious complication is *chest syndrome,* which is clinically similar to pneumonia. It is the presence of a new pulmonary infiltrate associated with chest pain, fever, cough, tachypnea, wheezing, and hypoxia (Platt, 2000; Vichinsky and others, 2000). It is believed that a VOC or infection results in sickling in the small blood vessels of the lungs, with ensuing occlusion, stasis, and anemia. Repeated episodes of chest syndrome may cause restrictive lung disease and pulmonary hypertension.

*Overwhelming infection,* especially with *Streptococcus pneumoniae* and *H. influenzae* type b as a result of defective splenic function, is the major cause of death in children under the age of 5 with SCD. Repeated insults on the splenic sinuses by sickled cells result in impaired filtration and function, allowing the development of septicemia and possibly subsequent death.

### Diagnostic Evaluation

Although SCA has been reported during the neonatal period and early part of infancy, it may not be recognized until the toddler and preschool period, during a crisis precipitated by an acute upper respiratory or gastrointestinal infection. However, early diagnosis (before 3 months of age) facilitates initiation of appropriate interventions to minimize complications. Several specific tests detect the presence of the abnormal Hgb in the homozygous or heterozygous form of the disease.

Examination of the *stained blood smear* may reveal a few sickled RBCs. However, because the erythrocyte assumes its normal discoid shape under adequate oxygenation, no sickled cells may be present even in the homozygous form of the disease. Whenever sickle cells are found, the diagnosis is usually positive for SCA, not sickle cell trait.

For screening purposes the *sickle-turbidity test (Sickledex)* is performed on anticoagulated blood and mixed with a special solution. Because HgbS is normally much less soluble than HgbA or HgbF (as well as other variants), when mixed with this solution, it forms a cloudy or turbid mixture. All other forms of hemoglobin result in a clear suspension. This test is a reliable screening method on blood from a finger or heel puncture and yields accurate results in 3 minutes. However, if the test is positive, hemoglobin electrophoresis is necessary to distinguish between those children with the trait and those with the disease.

*In hemoglobin electrophoresis,* the blood is specially prepared and separated into various hemoglobins by high-voltage electrophoresis. The resulting pattern of the separated peptides as it appears on paper is referred to as *fingerprinting* of the protein. This test is accurate, rapid, and specific for detecting the homozygous and heterozygous forms of the disease as well as the percentages of the various hemoglobins.

**Newborn Screening.** Screening for SCA in the newborn period can identify children with hemoglobinopathies. Newborn screening for SCA is performed in 41 states and the District of Columbia (Panepinto, and others, 2000). It provides early identification of these children before complications develop. Early diagnosis facilitates parental education regarding the importance of immunizations, penicillin prophylaxis, detection of splenomegaly, and the dangers of fever and increasing pallor, which all may be lifesaving (Steinberg, 1999).

There has been a decrease in the death rate from splenic sequestration and septicemia. Parents are taught to palpate the child's abdomen and seek medical attention at the first sign of complications (Dover and Platt, 1998). Penicillin prophylaxis is started by 2 months of age, and parents are instructed to seek medical attention if their child develops a fever of 38.3° C (101° F) or higher.

### Therapeutic Management

The aims of therapy are (1) to prevent the sickling phenomenon, which is responsible for the pathologic sequelae, and (2) to treat the medical emergency of sickle cell crisis. The successful implementation of these aims depends on prompt nursing interventions, medical therapies, child and family preventive measures, and innovative treatment interventions. Three general forms of treatment are available: supportive/symptomatic, specific, and curative. Research is investigating hydroxyurea and erythropoietin, which may increase the concentration of fetal hemoglobin and ultimately reduce complications (Charache and others, 1996; Claster and Vichinsky, 1996; Day and Wynn, 2000; Jayabose and others, 1996; Steinberg, 1999). A promising area of research is bone marrow transplantation as a possible cure for SCD (Lanzkowsky, 2000; Walters and others, 1996). (See Chapter 36.) Limiting factors include proper patient selection, as well as the availability of suitable donors (Steinberg, 1999). This technology raises many ethical issues regarding patient access and availability of therapy (Platt and Guinan, 1996).

Medical management of a crisis is directed at supportive, symptomatic, and specific treatments. The main objectives are to provide (1) bed rest to minimize energy expenditure and to improve oxygen utilization; (2) hydration through oral and IV therapy; (3) electrolyte replacement because hypoxia results in metabolic acidosis, which also promotes sickling; (4) analgesics for severe pain from vaso-occlusion (see Implementation, p. 1552); (5) blood replacement to treat anemia and to reduce the viscosity of the sickled blood; and (6) antibiotics to treat any existing infection. Administration of pneumococcal, Hib, and meningococcal vaccines is recommended for these children because of their susceptibility to infection from functional asplenia. (See Immunizations, Chapter 12.) Oral penicillin prophylaxis is recommended by 2 months of age to reduce the chance of pneumococcal sepsis. The nurse assumes an important role in helping the family to comply with a medication regimen as well as seeking medical attention immediately when the child has a fever 38.3° C (101° F) or higher, increase in spleen size, or severe pallor (Hendricks-Fenguson and Nelson 1999).

Short-term oxygen therapy may be helpful if a child has symptoms of respiratory difficulty. Although oxygen may prevent more sickling, it usually is not effective in reversing sickling or in pain reduction because, with the vessels clogged with cells, the oxygen is not able to reach the enmeshed sickled RBCs (Chiocca, 1996). In addition, prolonged administration of oxygen can depress bone marrow activity, further aggravating the anemia (Dover and Platt, 1998; Khoury and Grimsley, 1995).

The use of blood transfusions is another important component of care. An RBC transfusion is used in aplastic, hyperhemolytic, and splenic sequestration crises. Exchange transfusion is a successful, rapid method of reducing the number of circulating sickle cells and therefore slowing down the vicious circle of hypoxia, tissue ischemia, and injury. It is used in chest syndrome and after a stroke to prevent recurrence and further cerebral damage. Routine transfusions to maintain the hemoglobin value between 9 and 10 g/dl in children with central nervous system disease can minimize the chances of further neurologic problems. In the event of major surgery, exchange or partial exchange transfusions are given preoperatively to prevent anoxia and suppress the formation of new sickle cells and postoperatively to replace lost blood. For minor surgeries a simple packed RBC transfusion to raise the hemoglobin value to 10 g/dl, as well as vigorous hydration preoperatively and postoperatively, is sufficient to prevent sickling complications secondary to anesthesia (Dover and Platt, 1998; Koshy and others, 1995; Vichinsky and others, 1995).

However, multiple transfusions carry the risk of transmission of viral infection, hyperviscosity, transfusion reactions, alloimmunization, and hemosiderosis (Lane, 1996; Lanzkowsky, 2000). To reduce iron overload, home subcutaneous chelation therapy may be started (see p. 1558). Although the appropriate time for beginning treatment is controversial, chelation is often initiated when the ferritin level is greater than 1000 ng/ml, which is increasingly recognized as an ineffective test to determine iron overload (Olivieri, 1999). The liver biopsy is an accurate measurement of iron concentration yet is not without risk of hemorrhage, infection, or discomfort (Olivieri, 1999). A new noninvasive approach being developed on the basis of magnetic susceptibility is known as magnetic susceptometry, which is an accurate measurement of hepatic iron (Angelucci and others, 2000).

In children with recurrent life-threatening splenic sequestration, splenectomy may be a lifesaving measure. However, the spleen usually atrophies on its own through progressive fibrotic changes (functional asplenia) by 6 years of age in the child with SCA. However, surgical or autosplenec-

tomy has several advantages because the spleen is the major site of sickling, sequestration, and destruction of RBCs.

**Prognosis.**   The prognosis varies, yet most patients live into their fifth decade. The greatest risk is usually in children under 5 years of age, and the majority of deaths in these children are caused by overwhelming infection. However, as the child grows older, the crises usually become less severe and less frequent, although death in early adulthood is not uncommon. Consequently SCA is a chronic illness with a potentially terminal outcome. Physical and sexual maturation are delayed in adolescents with SCA. Although adults achieve normal height, weight, and sexual function, the delay may present problems to the adolescent (Gribbons, Zahr, and Opas, 1995; Lemanek, Steiner and Grossman, 1999). In some young people chronic pain becomes a significant problem. Bone marrow transplantation offers the hope of a cure for about 1% of children with SCA, although the mortality related to the procedure is significant (Platt and Guinan, 1996; Steinberg, 1999; Walters and others, 1996).

Children and adolescents younger than 16 years of age who have severe complications (stroke, recurrent acute chest syndrome, or refractory pain) and have an HLA-matched donor available are the best candidates for transplantation (Steinberg, 1999).

## Nursing Considerations

### ▓ Assessment

Many nurses are involved in screening programs for SCA to identify persons with the abnormal hemoglobin in order to implement therapy for homozygotes and provide genetic counseling for heterozygotes. Young children from families of at-risk racial or geographic origin who exhibit any of the signs previously described are advised to seek medical attention immediately.

Assessment of the child in sickle cell crisis involves all areas and systems that can be affected by circulatory obstruction, including vital signs, neurologic signs, vision, and hearing, as well as the respiratory, gastrointestinal, renal, and musculoskeletal systems. It is also important to assess the location and intensity of pain.

### ▓ Nursing Diagnoses

Nursing diagnoses are derived from observation and assessment of children at risk or who demonstrate evidence of SCD. Some of the general aspects of nursing management are included in the Nursing Care Plan on pp. 1555-1556. Others will become apparent, depending on the state of the child's health, the organs involved, and the individual needs of the child and family.

### ▓ Planning

The primary goals for the child with SCD and the family are as follows:

1. Child will experience minimal effects of sickling.
2. Family and child (when appropriate) will receive adequate education regarding the sickling phenomenon, possible consequences, and genetic counseling.

3. Child and family will adjust to a lifelong, potentially fatal hereditary disease.

## ■ Implementation

**Minimize Tissue Deoxygenation.** Anything that increases cellular metabolism also results in tissue hypoxia. For the child this includes (1) frequent rest periods during physical activities; (2) avoiding contact sports if the spleen is enlarged, because rupture will cause massive internal hemorrhage; (3) avoiding environments of low oxygen concentration, such as high altitudes or nonpressurized airplane flights; and (4) avoiding known sources of infection. If the child has even a mild infection, the parents must seek medical attention at once.

**Promote Hydration.** The nurse emphasizes the importance of adequate hydration to prevent sickling and delay the vaso-occlusion and hypoxia–ischemia cycle. The nurse calculates the child's fluid requirements (approximately 1600 ml/m²/day), which is the minimum daily fluid intake. The nurse also assesses the child's usual fluid consumption to evaluate its adequacy and makes adjustments based on this knowledge. It is not sufficient to advise parents to "force fluids" or "encourage drinking." They need specific instructions on how many glasses or bottles of fluid are required. Many foods are also a source of fluid, particularly soups, popsicles, yogurt, ice cream, sherbet, gelatin, and puddings.

Children can be encouraged to drink by giving them a "special" cup, thermos, or water bottle with a straw to drink from throughout the day. The nurse advises parents to take advantage of thirsty times, such as on awakening or after playing; serving frequent, small portions; and leaving the cup in easy reach for self-service. Flavored ice pops and crushed ice "slurpies" are sources of fluid commonly accepted by children.

Because the kidneys' ability to concentrate urine is impaired, the child is especially prone to dehydration. Dilute urine or low specific gravity is no longer a valid sign of adequate hydration. Parents are taught to observe for other indications of fluid loss, such as dry mucous membranes, dry diapers, weight loss, and a sunken fontanel in infants. In addition, without the ability to conserve water by concentrating urine, the child is prone to dehydration from environmental factors, particularly overheating. The nurse alerts parents to the need for wearing proper indoor and outdoor clothing and avoiding excess exposure to the sun.

### FAMILY FOCUS
*Fear of Addiction*

Although the pain is usually severe and opioids are needed, many families fear that their child will become addicted to the narcotic. Unfortunately, misinformed health professionals may foster this unfounded fear, resulting in needless suffering. Extremely few children who receive opioids for severe pain become behaviorally addicted to the drug (Gribbons, Zahr, and Opas, 1995). Families and older children, especially adolescents, need to be reassured that opioids are medically indicated, high doses may be needed, and children rarely become addicted.

Increased fluids combined with impaired kidney function result in the problem of enuresis. Parents who are unaware of this fact frequently employ the usual measures to discourage bed-wetting, such as limiting fluids at night, and may resort to punishment and shame to force bladder control. The nurse discusses this problem with parents, stressing the child's ability to concentrate urine is impaired. Reminding the child to urinate frequently is helpful during the day, and waking him or her during the night may prove beneficial if the child's sleep patterns are not disturbed. Parents who are toilet training their toddlers should be aware of the more frequent pattern of urination and increased difficulty in learning control. Enuresis is treated as a complication of the disease to alleviate parental pressure on the child and to prevent any fluid restriction.

**Minimize Crises.** Because infection is the major cause of death due to the body's inability to resist infection, the nurse stresses to parents the importance of adequate nutrition, frequent medical supervision, proper handwashing, and isolation from known sources of infection. The last measure must be tempered with an awareness of the child's need for living a normal life. Overprotection can be as devastating emotionally as an infection is physically. Parents need to be aware of the necessity of seeking prompt medical care at the first sign of any infection.

The family should be taught the signs and symptoms of crises and advised to seek medical attention immediately. Teaching parents spleen palpation for earlier detection of splenic sequestration can reduce mortality from this serious complication.

**Promote Supportive Therapies.** The success of many of the medical therapies relies heavily on nursing implementation. Management of pain is an especially difficult problem and often involves experimenting with various analgesics, including opioids, and schedules before relief is achieved. Unfortunately, these children tend to be undermedicated, resulting in "clock watching" and demands for additional doses sooner than might be expected. Often this incorrectly raises suspicions of drug addiction, when in fact the problem is one of inadequate pain control. (See Family Focus box.) In choosing and scheduling analgesics, *the goal is prevention of pain.*

The most frequent problem for patients with SCD is pain from VOCs (Fig. 35-4). In one study with a group of 17 children with SCD, 3- to 12-year-olds reported less severe pain than 13- to 18-year-olds (Sporrer and others, 1995). The severity of pain was not related to the number of painful sites, but the duration of pain was longer when more sites were involved. Patients with pain scores greater than 2 out of 5 had longer hospitalizations. Beyer (2000) found that 15 of 21 children with sickle cell disease who were receiving IV pain medication for a painful crisis continued to report moderate to severe pain. Recommendations for continuous adjustment of analgesics were emphasized in this study. The chronic nature of this pain can greatly affect the child's development. A multidisciplinary approach is best for its management. When mild to moderate pain is reported, acetaminophen or ibuprofen is initially used. If acetaminophen or ibuprofen is not effective alone, codeine can be added. The dosages of the drugs are titrated (adjusted) to a therapeutic level. Opioids such as immediate- and sustained-release morphine, oxycodone, hydromorphone, and methadone are administered parenterally or orally for severe pain and are given around the clock. Patient-controlled analgesia (PCA) has been used successfully for sickle cell–related pain. The PCA reinforces the patient's role and responsibility in managing the pain and provides flexibility for pain, which may vary in severity over time. If PCA devices are not available, and if the pain is not readily controlled with IV boluses administered around the clock, a low-dose infusion with rescue boluses administered every 2 hours on a flexible dosing basis can provide a safe and effective alternative. Continuous IV infusion of opioids, particularly morphine, provides better pain control than intermittent opioid therapy (Doven and Platt, 1998; Gribbons, Zahr, and Opas 1995).

**NURSING ALERT** Meperidine (pethidine [Demerol]) is not recommended. Normeperidine, a metabolite of meperidine, is a central nervous system stimulant that produces anxiety, tremors, myoclonus, and generalized seizures when it accumulates with repetitive dosing. Patients with SCD are particularly at risk for normeperidine-induced seizures (Dover and Platt, 1998; Simon, Lobo and Jackson, 1999).

Medication given by mouth can be as effective as by the IV route when equianalgesic dosages are prescribed. (See Chapter 26.)

Any pain program should be combined with psychologic support to help the child deal with the depression, anxiety, and fear that accompany the disease. This includes regular visits with the child to discuss his or her concerns during the hospitalization and positive reinforcement of adaptive coping skills, such as successful methods of dealing with the pain and compliance with treatment prescriptions. To reduce the negative connotation associated with the term "crisis," it is best to say "pain episode."

Frequently heat to the affected area is soothing. Cold compresses are not applied to the area because doing so enhances vasoconstriction and occlusion. Bed rest is usually well tolerated during a crisis, although actual rest depends a great deal on pain alleviation and organized schedules of nursing care. Although the objective of bed rest is to minimize oxygen consumption, some activity, particularly passive range-of-motion exercises, is beneficial to promote circulation. Usually the best course of action is to let children dictate their activity tolerance.

If blood transfusions or exchange transfusions are given, the nurse has the responsibility of observing for signs of transfusion reaction (see Table 35-2). Because hypervolemia from too rapid transfusion can increase the workload of the heart, the nurse also is alert to signs of cardiac failure.

In splenic sequestration the size of the spleen is gently measured because increasing splenomegaly is an ominous sign. A spleen that is decreasing in size denotes response to therapy. Vital signs and blood pressure are also closely monitored for impending shock. Anemia is typically not a

presenting complication in VOCs but is a critical problem in other types of crises. The nurse monitors for evidence of increasing anemia and institutes appropriate nursing intervention.

Oxygen is not beneficial in vaso-occlusive episodes unless hypoxemia is present (Chiocca, 1996). It does not reverse sickled RBCs, and if used in the nonhypoxic patient, it will decrease erythropoiesis (Vichinsky and Styles, 1996). (See Critical Thinking Exercise box on p. 1554.) Because prolonged oxygen can aggravate the anemia, signs of lack of therapeutic benefit, such as restlessness, increased pallor, and continued pain, are reported.

Intake, especially of IV fluids, and output are recorded. The child's weight should be taken on admission, because it serves as a baseline for evaluating hydration. Because diuresis can result in electrolyte loss, the nurse observes for signs of hypokalemia and should be familiar with normal serum electrolyte values to report changes. Nurses also need to be aware of the signs of chest syndrome and stroke, both potentially fatal complications. (See Nursing Alert on p. 1555.)

**Decrease Surgical Risks.**   The main surgical risk is hypoxia from anesthesia. However, emotional stress, the demands of wound healing, and the possibility of infection potentially increase the sickling phenomenon, both in children with the disease and in those with the trait. The primary nursing objectives are aimed at minimizing each of these threats preoperatively and postoperatively by keeping

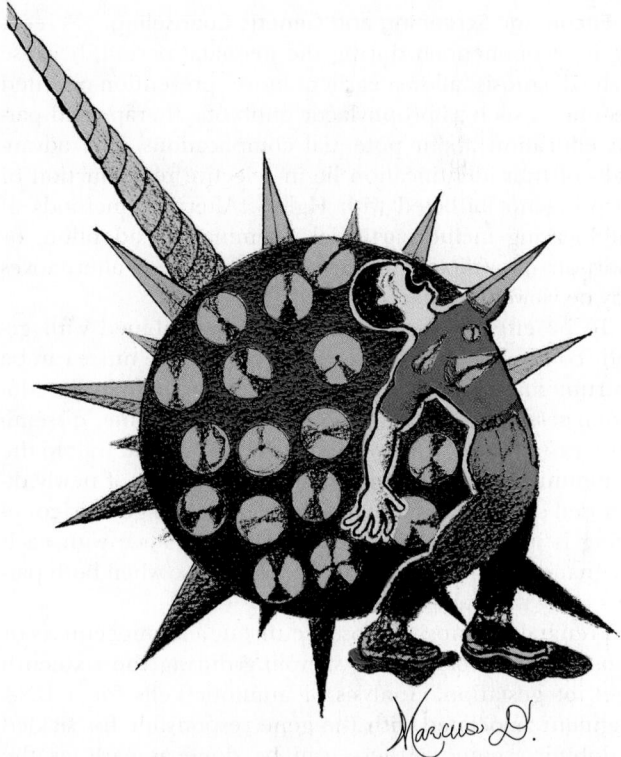

**Fig. 35-4**  Drawing of sickle cell pain by Marcus D., a 17-year-old boy. When asked what message he would like to give health care professionals about treating pain, he stated, "Tell them to listen to the patient and family. They know about the pain."

## Critical Thinking Exercise

### Sickle Cell Anemia

Samantha Lipe, 7 years old, is brought to the emergency department experiencing a vaso-occlusive sickle cell crisis. She is treated with IV fluids for hydration and analgesics for pain management. Mr. Lipe tells you that for all previous crises, oxygen was used and Samantha seemed to recover quicker. What should be your initial response to Mr. Lipe?

FIRST, THINK ABOUT IT . . .

• What precise question are you trying to answer?
• What information are you using?

1. Suggest that he discuss this with the practitioner.
2. Set up the oxygen and nasal cannula.
3. Ask him how he thinks oxygen helps.
4. Help him understand vaso-occlusive crises.

*The best response is three. Before offering an explanation regarding oxygen's lack of effect when cells are sickled, you want to know what the father understands and has been told. Based on this information, you can clarify any misconceptions or suggest that he talk with the attending practitioner. Oxygen is a drug and is administered only as ordered.*

the child well hydrated, preparing the child psychologically, and preventing infection.

**Encourage Screening and Genetic Counseling.** Screening is recommended during the neonatal period, because early diagnosis allows earlier, more prevention-oriented treatment, such as prophylactic antibiotic therapy and parent education about potential complications. The advantages of trait identification lie in selective reproduction of offspring not afflicted with Hgb S. Alternate methods of childbearing include artificial insemination, adoption, or abortion of afflicted fetuses. However, these alternatives may be viewed as unacceptable.

To be effective, screening must be combined with genetic counseling and long-term follow-up. The nurse can be instrumental in such programs by conducting parent education sessions, following the family in the home, disseminating correct information about the disease and trait to the community, and rendering support to parents of newly diagnosed children. A primary consideration in genetic counseling is informing parents of the 25% chance with each pregnancy of having a child with the disease when both parents carry the trait. (See Chapter 5.)

Prenatal diagnosis is possible through amniocentesis or fetoscopy and fetal blood sampling during the sixteenth week of gestation. Analysis of amniotic cells for a DNA fragment associated with the gene responsible for sickled β-globulin chain synthesis can be done as early as the twelfth week with chorionic sampling. In the event of an affected fetus, the decision regarding termination of the pregnancy should be left to the couple.

**Explain the Disease.** Because SCA may be recognized when the child is a toddler, most of the nurse's counseling is with parents. The nurse explains to parents the basic effect of tissue hypoxia on RBCs and the effect of sickling on the circulation (see Fig. 35-3). Taking time to establish a sound basis of understanding why certain measures are beneficial to the child encourages parents to practice them.*†

**NURSING TIP** One simple yet graphic way of illustrating the difference between normal discoid RBCs and sickle cells is to roll round or oval objects, such as marbles, through a tube to demonstrate normal blood cell circulation and then roll pointed objects such as screws or jacks through the tube. The effect of sickling and clumping of the pointed objects is especially noticeable at a bend or slight narrowing of the tube. This same idea can be expanded to discuss the importance of increased fluid in keeping the pointed objects suspended away from each other to prevent concentration.

The nurse advises the parents to inform all treating practitioners of the child's condition. The use of a medical identification bracelet is another way of ensuring awareness of the disease. Some people view such identification as "negative labeling." The nurse can stress the benefits of displaying this information, especially in emergencies when the use of anesthesia may be required.

**Support Family.** Families need the opportunity to discuss their feelings regarding transmitting a potentially fatal, chronic illness to their child. Some parents are able to cope with this fact; some feel great guilt and remorse for giving their child the disease, whereas others regret not knowing that they carried the trait. For many parents the decision regarding subsequent pregnancies is viewed with doubt and ambivalence.

Because of the widely publicized prognosis for children with SCA, many parents express their fear of death. The prognosis varies; with early diagnosis and treatment these

---

*National Association for Sickle Cell Disease, Inc, 3345 Wilshire Blvd, Suite 1106, Los Angeles, CA 90010-1880 (213) 736-5455 or (800) 421-8453; www.sicklecelldisease.org; Center for Sickle Cell Disease, Howard University, 2121 Georgia Ave NW, Washington, DC 20059, (202) 806-7930; and National Heart, Lung, and Blood Institute, 9000 Rockville Pike, Building 31, Room 4A-21, Bethesda, MD 20892, (301) 496-4236; www.nhlbi.nih.gov/nhlbi/nhlbi.htm. The Agency for Healthcare Research and Quality (AHRQ) (formerly AHCPR) has published three booklets on sickle cell disease: Sickle Cell Disease: Comprehensive Screening, Diagnosis, Management, and Counseling in Newborns and Infants, Clinical Practice Guideline No 6, Pub No AHCPR-0562; Sickle Cell Disease: Comprehensive Screening and Management in Newborns and Infants, Quick Reference Guide for Clinicians No 6, Pub No AHCPR-0563; and Sickle Cell Disease in Newborns and Infants: A Guide for Parents, Pub No AHCPR 93-0564. They are available from the AHCPR Publications Clearinghouse, PO Box 8547, Silver Spring, MD 20907, (800) 358-9295; www.ahcpr.gov/. Also available is Guideline for the Management of Acute and Chronic Pain in Sickle-Cell Disease from American Pain Society, 4700 W Lake Ave, Glenview, IL 60025-1485, (847) 375-4715, fax: (847) 375-6315, email: info@ampainsoc.org; www.ampainsoc.org; and Clinical Reference Guide for Health Care Providers; Sickle Cell Related Pain: Assessment And Management—a Guide for Patients and Parents from the New England Regional Genetics Groups (NERGG), No 28 Clarendon St, Newton, MA 02460, (617) 243-3033, email: maryaten@mediaone.net; www.acadia.net/NERGG.

†A video, Sickle Cell Disease Is More Than Pain Management, is available from Maxishare, PO Box 2041, Milwaukee, WI 53201, (800) 444-7747. Information is also available from the Sickle Cell Disease Association of America, Inc, 200 Cooperate Pointe, Suite 495, Culver City, CA 90230-7633.

children are living longer. However, because there is no way to predict which child's condition will follow a favorable course, the nurse should care for the family as she or he would for any family with a child who has a chronic and life-threatening illness, with particular emphasis on the siblings' reactions, the stress on the marital relationship, and the childrearing attitudes displayed toward the child. (See Chapters 22 and 23.) (See Nursing Care Plan: The Child with Sickle Cell Disease.*)

**NURSING ALERT**

Report signs of the following immediately:

Chest syndrome:
  Severe chest pain, back or abdominal pain
  Fever of 38.3° C (101° F) or higher
  Cough
  Dyspnea, tachypnea
  Retractions
  Declining oxygen saturation (oximetry)
Stroke:
  Jerking or twitching of the face, legs, or arms
  Convulsions or seizures
  Strange, abnormal behavior
  Inability to move an arm or a leg
  Stagger or an unsteady walk
  Stutter or slurred speech
  Weakness in the hands, feet, or legs
  Changes in vision
  Severe, unrelieved headaches
  Severe vomiting

*In Wong DL, Hess CS: *Wong and Whaley's clinical manual of pediatric nursing,* ed 5, St Louis, 2000, Mosby.

## Evaluation

The effectiveness of nursing interventions is determined by continual reassessment and evaluation of care based on the following observational guidelines:

1. Observe child for any evidence of sickling; monitor preventive strategies and therapies.
2. Interview family regarding genetic counseling.
3. Interview family regarding their understanding of the disease, the sickling phenomenon, and its consequences.
4. Interview and observe child and family regarding the way in which the disease has affected their lives.

The *expected outcomes* are described in the Nursing Care Plan on pp.1555-1556.

## β-Thalassemia

The term *thalassemia* comes from the Greek word *thalassa,* meaning "sea," and is applied to a variety of inherited blood disorders characterized by deficiencies in the rate of production of specific globin chains in hemoglobin. The name appropriately refers to people or their descendants living near the Mediterranean Sea, namely, Italians, Greeks, and Syrians. Evidence suggests that the high incidence of the disorder among these groups is a result of selective advantage of the trait in protection against malaria as is postulated in sickle cell disease. However, the disorder has a wide geographic distribution, probably as a result of genetic migration through intermarriages or possibly as a result of spontaneous mutation.

The thalassemias are classified according to the hemoglobin chain affected and by the amount of the globin chain that is synthesized; for example, if α-chains are affected, the thalassemia is classified as α-thalassemia. Each

---

# *Nursing Care Plan*
## The Child with Sickle Cell Anemia

**NURSING DIAGNOSIS:** Risk for injury related to abnormal hemoglobin, decreased ambient oxygen, dehydration

**PATIENT GOAL 1:** Will maintain adequate tissue oxygenation

• **NURSING INTERVENTIONS/*RATIONALES***
Explain measures to minimize complications related to physical exertion and emotional stress *to avoid additional tissue oxygen needs*
  Prevent infection
  Avoid low-oxygen environment

• **EXPECTED OUTCOME**
Child avoids situations that reduce tissue oxygenation

**PATIENT GOAL 2:** Will maintain adequate hydration

• **NURSING INTERVENTIONS/*RATIONALES***
Calculate recommended daily fluid intake (1600 ml/m²/day) and base child's fluid requirements on this *minimum* amount (specify) *to ensure adequate hydration*
Increase fluid intake above minimum requirements during physical exercise/emotional stress and during a crisis *to compensate for additional fluid needs*
Give parents written instructions regarding specific quantity of fluid required *to encourage compliance*
Encourage child to drink *to encourage compliance*
Teach family signs of dehydration *to avoid delay in rehydration therapy* (see Chapter 28)
Stress importance of avoiding overheating *as source of fluid loss*

• **EXPECTED OUTCOME**
Child drinks an adequate amount of fluid and shows no signs of dehydration

*Continued*

# Nursing Care Plan
## The Child with Sickle Cell Anemia—cont'd

**PATIENT GOAL 3:** Will remain free of infection

- **NURSING INTERVENTIONS/**_RATIONALES_

Stress importance of adequate nutrition; routine immunization, including pneumococcal and meningococcal vaccines; protection from known sources of infection; and frequent health supervision

Report any sign of infection to practitioner immediately _to avoid delay in treatment_

Promote compliance with antibiotic therapy both _to prevent and to treat infection_

- **EXPECTED OUTCOME**

Child remains free of infection

**PATIENT GOAL 4:** Will experience decreased risks associated with a surgical procedure

- **NURSING INTERVENTIONS/**_RATIONALES_

Explain reason for preoperative blood transfusion (_given to increase concentration of HgbA_)

Keep child well hydrated _to prevent sickling_

Decrease fear through appropriate preparation, _because anxiety increases oxygen needs_

*Administer pain medications _to keep child comfortable and reduce stress response_

Avoid unnecessary exertion _to avoid additional oxygen needs_

Promote pulmonary hygiene postoperatively _to prevent infection_

Use passive range-of-motion exercises _to promote circulation_

*Administer oxygen, if prescribed, _to saturate hemoglobin_

Monitor for evidence of infection _to avoid delay in treatment_

- **EXPECTED OUTCOME**

Child undergoes a surgical procedure without crisis

> **NURSING DIAGNOSIS:** Acute pain related to tissue anoxia (vaso-occlusive crisis)

**PATIENT GOAL 1:** Will have no pain or pain relieved to level acceptable to child

- **NURSING INTERVENTIONS/**_RATIONALES_

Plan preventive schedule of medication around the clock, not as needed, _to prevent pain_

Recognize that various analgesics, including opioids, and medication schedules may need to be tried _to achieve satisfactory pain relief_

Avoid administration of meperidine (Demerol) _because of increased risk of normeperidine-induced seizures_

Reassure child and family that analgesics, including opioids, are medically indicated, high doses may be needed, and children rarely become addicted, _because needless suffering may result from their unfounded fears_

Apply heat to affected area _because it may be soothing_

Avoid applying cold compresses _because this enhances sickling and vasoconstriction_

- **EXPECTED OUTCOME**

Child will experience no or minimal pain

> **NURSING DIAGNOSIS:** Interrupted family processes related to a child with potentially life-threatening disease

**PATIENT/FAMILY/TEACHER GOAL 1:** Will receive education regarding disease.

- **NURSING INTERVENTIONS/**_RATIONALES_

Teach family and older children characteristics of basic defect and measures _to minimize complications of sickling_

Stress importance of informing significant health personnel of child's disease _to ensure prompt and appropriate treatment (e.g., for pain)_

Explain signs of developing crisis, especially fever, pallor, respiratory distress, and pain, _to avoid delay in treatment_

Reinforce basics of trait transmission and refer to genetic counseling services _for family to make informed reproductive decisions_

Teach parents to be an advocate for their child _to secure the best care_

Educate the teacher/students regarding etiology of SCD and measures to avoid complications (e.g., allow fluids throughout school day, allow frequent bathroom privileges)

Educate the teacher regarding SCD complications such as fever, severe headache, weakness, severe vaso-occlusive episodes and importance of reporting them immediately to medical personnel

Stress to educators the need to provide tutorials and to allow time to make up schoolwork during medical-related absences

- **EXPECTED OUTCOME**

Child, family, and teacher demonstrate an understanding of the disease, its etiology, and its therapies

**PATIENT/FAMILY GOAL 2:** Will receive adequate support

- **NURSING INTERVENTIONS/**_RATIONALES_

Refer to special organizations and agencies _for ongoing support_

Refer child to comprehensive sickle cell clinic _for ongoing care_

Be especially alert to family's needs when two or more members are affected

See Nursing Care Plan: The Child with a Chronic Illness or Disability, Ch. 22

- **EXPECTED OUTCOMES**

Family takes advantage of community services (specify); child receives ongoing care from appropriate facility

See also:
   Nursing Care Plan: The Child in the Hospital, Ch. 26
   Nursing Care Plan: The Family of the Child Who Is Ill or Hospitalized, Ch. 26

---

*Dependent nursing action.

of the abnormal genes that cause thalassemia is seen in particular populations (e.g., β-thalassemia: Greeks, Italians, and Syrians; α-thalassemia: Chinese, Thai, African, and Mediterranean peoples).

*β-thalassemia* is the most common of the thalassemias and occurs in four forms: two heterozygous forms, *thalassemia minor,* generally an asymptomatic silent carrier state, and *thalassemia trait,* which produces a mild microcytic anemia; *thalassemia intermedia,* which is manifested as splenomegaly and moderate to severe anemia. Lastly, there is a homozygous form, *thalassemia major* (also known as *Cooley anemia*), which results in a severe anemia that is not compatible with life without transfusion support.

### Mode of Transmission

Thalassemia is an autosomal-recessive disorder with varying expressivity. Both parents must be carriers to produce a child with β-thalassemia major (Drake, 1997). The exact mode of transmission between parents who are heterozygous for thalassemia is illustrated in Fig. 5-6.

### Pathophysiology and Clinical Manifestations

Normal postnatal hemoglobin A (HgbA) is composed of two α-and two β-polypeptide chains. In β-thalassemia there is a partial or complete deficiency in the synthesis of the β chain of the Hgb molecule. Consequently there is a compensatory increase in the synthesis of α-chains, and γ-chain production remains activated, resulting in defective Hgb formation. This unbalanced polypeptide unit is very unstable; when it disintegrates, it damages the RBCs, causing severe anemia. To compensate for the hemolytic process, an overabundance of erythrocytes is formed unless the bone marrow is suppressed by transfusion therapy. Excess iron from packed RBC transfusions and from the rapid destruction of defective cells is stored in various organs (hemosiderosis).

The onset of clinical manifestations in thalassemia major may be insidious and not recognized until late infancy or early toddlerhood (Box 35-5). The clinical effects of thalassemia major are primarily attributable to (1) defective synthesis of hemoglobin A, (2) structurally impaired RBCs, and (3) the shortened life span of the erythrocyte. The major consequences of thalassemia are caused by the pathologic condition, resultant chronic hypoxia, and iron overload from the supportive treatment of multiple blood supplements (Fig. 35-5 and Box 35-5).

*Anemia* results from the body's inability to maintain a level of erythropoiesis commensurate with hemolysis. The bone marrow compensates by increasing production of large numbers of immature cells, such as normoblasts and erythroblasts, large cells that are extremely thin and form bizarre shapes, and *target cells,* which have abnormal staining properties. As a result of the excessive production of abnormal RBCs, their life span is severely shortened.

Anemia also is exaggerated by aplastic crises after infection, folic acid deficiencies from demands of bone marrow hyperplasia, and progressive hemolysis from repeated blood transfusions. The spleen becomes greatly enlarged as a result of extramedullary hemopoiesis, rapid destruction of the defective erythrocytes and, rarely, progressive fibrosis from hemochromatosis. Splenomegaly may progress until the organ's very size interferes with the function of other abdominal organs and respiratory expansion.

With progressive anemia, signs of chronic hypoxia, namely, headache, irritability, precordial and bone pain, de-

---

**Box 35-5**

**Clinical Manifestations of β-Thalassemia**

**ANEMIA (BEFORE DIAGNOSIS)**
Pallor
Unexplained fever
Poor feeding
Enlarged spleen/liver

**WITH PROGRESSIVE ANEMIA**
Signs of chronic hypoxia
  Headache
  Precordial and bone pain
  Decreased exercise tolerance
Listlessness
Anorexia

**OTHER FEATURES**
Small stature
Delayed sexual maturation
Bronzed, freckled complexion (if not chelated)

**BONE CHANGES (OLDER CHILDREN IF UNTREATED)**
Enlarged head
Prominent frontal and parietal bosses
Prominent malar eminences
Flat or depressed bridge of the nose
Enlarged maxilla
Protrusion of the lip and upper central incisors and eventual malocclusion
Oriental appearance of eyes

---

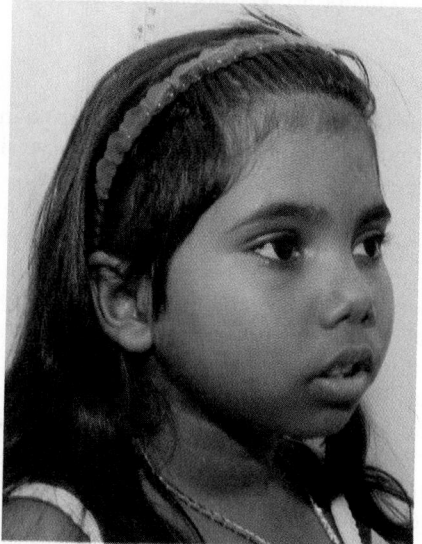

**Fig. 35-5**  A young girl with β-thalassemia demonstrating mild frontal bossing of the right forehead and mild maxillary prominence. (Courtesy James DeLeon, Texas Children's Hospital.)

creased exercise tolerance, listlessness, and anorexia, may develop. Another common symptom in these children is frequent epistaxis, although the exact reason is unknown. Hyperuricemia and gout from rapid cellular catabolism are also seen.

*Hemosiderosis* refers to excess iron storage in various tissues of the body, especially the spleen, liver, lymph glands, heart, and pancreas, but without associated tissue injury. *Hemochromatosis* refers to excess iron storage with resultant cellular damage. The mechanism for tissue destruction resulting from iron storage is not known. Chronic hypoxia is believed to be an important contributing factor.

In thalassemia, excess *hemosiderin,* the iron-containing pigment from the breakdown of hemoglobin, results from decreased hemoglobin synthesis and increased hemolysis of transfused erythrocytes. Decreased production of hemoglobin results in an excess supply of available iron. In addition, the body probably responds to the anemia by increasing the rate of gastrointestinal absorption of dietary iron, because ineffective erythropoiesis is a potent controlling factor in regard to exogenous iron use. However, the primary source of additional iron is from the hemolysis of supplemental erythrocytes and rapid destruction of defective RBCs. With the prophylactic use of deferoxamine to minimize excess iron storage, the characteristic changes in body structures from hemochromatosis have been greatly reduced.

*Retarded growth* and, especially, *delayed sexual maturation* are common findings. There is evidence that both may also be caused by pituitary failure, although the exact reasons for this are unclear, but the impaired growth is probably related to hemochromatosis. It is possible that the endocrine glands are extremely sensitive to iron toxicity and that even small amounts of deposited iron can produce organ dysfunction. Children with severe disease usually achieve normal growth rates until puberty, when height becomes markedly retarded. Secondary sexual characteristics are delayed or absent in many adolescents (Tolis, Viachopapadopoulou, and Karydis, 1996).

## Diagnostic Evaluation

Hematologic studies reveal the characteristic changes in the RBC (i.e., microcytosis, hypochromia, anisocytosis, poikilocytosis, target cells, and basophilic stippling of various stages). Low hemoglobin and hematocrit levels are seen in severe anemia, although they are typically lower than the reduction in the RBC count because of the proliferation of immature erythrocytes.

*Hemoglobin electrophoresis* confirms the diagnosis and is helpful in distinguishing the type and severity of the various thalassemias because it analyzes the quantity and specific hemoglobin variants found in blood. In β-thalassemia, hemoglobin F (HgbF) and hemoglobin $A_2$ (HgbA$_2$; a type of normal adult hemoglobin) are elevated because neither depends on β-chain polypeptides for synthesis.

## Therapeutic Management

The objective of supportive therapy is to maintain sufficient hemoglobin levels to prevent bone marrow expansion and bony deformities and to provide sufficient RBCs to support growth and normal physical activity. Transfusions are the foundation of medical management. Recent studies have evaluated the benefits of maintaining the hemoglobin level above 9.5 g/dl, a goal that may require transfusions as often as every 3 weeks. The advantages of this therapy include (1) improved physical and psychologic well-being because of the ability to participate in normal activities, (2) decreased cardiomegaly and hepatosplenomegaly, (3) fewer bone changes, (4) normal or near-normal growth and development until puberty, and (5) fewer infections.

One of the potential complications of frequent blood transfusions is iron overload (hemosiderosis). Because the body has no effective means of eliminating the excess iron, the mineral is deposited in body tissues. To minimize the development of hemosiderosis and hemochromatosis, *deferoxamine (Desferal),* an iron-chelating agent, is given with oral supplements of vitamin C. Vitamin C should only be used in patients who are ascorbate depleted and only while deferoxamine is being administered. Administration of vitamin C significantly augments iron excretion by delaying the conversion of ferritin to hemosiderosis, which allows more iron to remain in chelatable form (Orkin and Nathan, 1998).

Deferoxamine adminstration regimen is given intravenously or subcutaneously at home via portable infusion pump over a period of 8 to 10 hours (usually during sleep) for 5 to 7 days a week. It is also given intravenously over a period of 4 hours at the time of blood transfusion in many centers. Significant liver fibrosis and growth impairment may be prevented if chelation therapy is initiated as early as 2 to 4 years of age (Benz and Giardinia, 1995). However, in addition to the intensive schedule required for chelation therapy, deferoxamine use has been linked with decreased height and other bony changes (Levin and others, 1995). Creative strategies such as behavioral contracting have been used to assist the child in complying with the deferoxamine regimen. The availability of an oral chelator would be a major advance in the care of the chronically transfused patient. Deferiprone, an oral chelator being investigated, has been noted to have several adverse side effects and seems to be considerably less effective as a chelator than previously thought (Olivieri and Brittenham, 1997). However, clinical trials continue to further investigate Deferiprone as a possible oral chelator.

In some children with severe splenomegaly who require repeated transfusions, a splenectomy may be necessary to decrease the disabling effects of abdominal pressure and to increase the life span of supplemental RBCs. Over time the spleen may accelerate the rate of RBC destruction and therefore increase transfusion requirements. After a splenectomy children generally require fewer transfusions, although the basic defect in hemoglobin synthesis remains unaffected. A major postsplenectomy complication is severe and overwhelming infection. Therefore these children are kept on prophylactic antibiotics with close medical supervision for many years and should receive the pneumococcal and meningococcal vaccines in addition to the regularly scheduled immunizations. (See Immunizations, Chapter 12.)

**Prognosis.** Most children treated with blood transfusion and early chelation therapy survive well into adulthood (Orkin and Nathan, 1998). This intensive therapy allows them to lead a nearly normal life (Olivieri, 1999). The most common cause of death is heart disease, followed by infection, liver disease, and malignancy secondary to hemochromatosis (Benz and Giardinia, 1995). A promising treatment for some children is bone marrow transplantation. (See Bone Marrow Transplantation, Chapter 36.) In one study, children under 16 years of age who underwent allogenic bone marrow transplantation had a high rate of complication-free survival. Children with thalassemia who undergo allogenic bone marrow transplantation currently have a 60% to 90% chance of cure (Olivieri, 1999).

### Nursing Considerations

The objectives of nursing care are to (1) promote compliance with transfusion and chelation therapy, (2) assist the child in coping with the anxiety-provoking treatments and the effects of the illness, (3) foster the child's and family's adjustment to a chronic illness, and (4) observe for complications of multiple blood transfusions. Basic to each of these goals is explaining to parents and older children the defect responsible for the disorder, its effect on RBCs, and potential effects of untreated hemosiderosis (such as delayed growth and maturation and heart disease). Because the prevalence of this condition is high among families of Mediterranean descent, the nurse also inquires about the family's previous knowledge about thalassemia. All families with a child with thalassemia should be tested for the trait and referred for genetic counseling.

**Support Family.** As with any chronic illness, the needs of the family must be met for optimum adjustment to the stresses imposed by the disorder. (See Chapter 22.) Sources of information for the family are the **Cooley's Anemia Foundation**\* and the **Thalassemia Action Group**.† Genetic counseling for the parents and fertile offspring is mandatory, and both prenatal diagnosis using amniocentesis or fetal blood sampling and screening for thalassemia trait are available. There has been a marked decrease in the number of new cases of thalassemia in the United States and Canada. This is thought to be a result of education and testing of parents (Olivieri, 1999).

**Assist in Coping with Effects of the Disorder.** Body image alterations, decreased growth, and sexual immaturity are frequently difficult adjustment problems for older children. These children feel different from their peers, and the delayed sexual development is a major issue for the maturing adolescent with an improved life expectancy. Adolescents need an opportunity to express their thoughts and feelings about these complex issues. They can learn grooming aids that make them appear more sexually mature, such as up-to-date clothing, new hairstyles, and well-applied makeup. Children with the characteristic bone changes may benefit from surgery or orthodontic appliances to improve facial structure.

With frequent transfusion therapy there is less restriction imposed on physical activity because of severe anemia, and these children should be encouraged to pursue activities commensurate with their exercise tolerance. However, the frequency of treatment can interfere with a normal lifestyle. To minimize disruptions, the nurse can be instrumental in arranging for blood transfusions and medical supervision at times that interfere least with the child's regular activities, especially school. In addition, children are more likely to cooperate with medical treatments that do not interfere significantly with their routine.

## ANEMIAS CAUSED BY IMPAIRED OR DECREASED PRODUCTION OF RED BLOOD CELLS

Impaired or decreased production of red blood cells can occur as a result of either bone marrow failure or deficiency of essential nutrients. *Bone marrow failure* may be caused by (1) replacement of bone marrow by fibrosis or by neoplastic cells, such as in leukemia; (2) depression of marrow activity from irradiation, chemicals, or drugs; or (3) interference with bone marrow activity from other systemic diseases, such as severe infection, chronic renal disease, widespread malignancy (without marrow infiltration), collagen diseases, or hypothyroidism. When depression of the hematologic system is extensive, aplastic anemia develops.

The reason for various systemic disorders affecting erythrocyte production varies according to the condition. For example, in *severe chronic infection* there is evidence that depression of erythropoiesis is caused by a defect in the conversion of protoporphyrin into hemoglobin. In addition, there is some degree of hemolysis, although the exact mechanism is not known.

### Aplastic Anemia

*Aplastic anemia* refers to a condition in which all formed elements of the blood are simultaneously depressed. The peripheral blood smear demonstrates pancytopenia or the triad of profound anemia, leukopenia, and thrombocytopenia. *Hypoplastic anemia* is characterized by a profound depression of RBCs but normal or slightly decreased WBCs and platelets. A type of hypoplastic anemia is *pure RBC aplasia,* which can be congenital or acquired. The acquired defect in erythropoiesis is an autoimmune condition that is seen mostly in adults (Miller, 1995). The congenital condition (*Diamond-Blackfan syndrome*) is marked by complete or almost complete absence of all cells of the erythroid series with normal production of the other myeloid cells. Its treatment, which consists of transfusions, splenectomy, and administration of corticosteroids, is similar to that of other diseases, such as the thalassemias, that result in profound anemia. The prognosis varies, although long-term survival is possible. The principal causes of death are cardiac failure, hepatitis from transfusion therapy, and sepsis. Hemosiderosis and hemochromatosis (p. 1558) also affect vital tissues necessary for survival.

---

\*129-09 26th Ave, Flushing, NY 11354, (718) 321-2873 or (800) 522-7222, fax: (718) 321-3340; www.thalassemia.org.
†129-09 26th Ave, Flushing, NY 11354, (718) 321-2873 or (800) 522-7222, fax: (718) 321-3340; www.geocities.com/hotsprings/8730/.

Aplastic anemia can be *primary* (*congenital,* or present at birth) or *secondary* (*acquired*). The best-known congenital disorder of which aplastic anemia is an outstanding feature is *Fanconi syndrome,* a rare hereditary disorder charac-terized by pancytopenia, hypoplasia of the bone marrow, and patchy brown discoloration of the skin due to the de-position of melanin and associated with multiple congeni-tal anomalies of the musculoskeletal and genitourinary sys-tems. The syndrome appears to be inherited as an autosomal recessive trait with varying penetrance; there-fore affected siblings may demonstrate several different combinations of defects.

Several factors contribute to the development of ac-quired hypoplastic anemia, including suppressed erythro-poiesis from multiple transfusion therapy; hemolytic syn-dromes (such as sickle cell anemia); and autoimmune or allergic states. The most common causes of acquired aplas-tic anemia are listed in Box 35-6. These include infection with human parvovirus (HPV), hepatitis, or overwhelming infection; irradiation; drugs such as the chemotherapeutic agents and several antibiotics, especially chloramphenicol; industrial and household chemicals, including benzene and its derivatives, which are found in petroleum products, dyes, paint remover, shellac, and lacquers; infiltration and re-placement of myeloid elements, such as in leukemia or the lymphomas; and idiopathic factors, in which no identifiable precipitating cause can be found. The following discussion focuses on acquired severe aplastic anemia, which carries a poorer prognosis and follows a more rapidly fatal course than the primary types.

### Diagnostic Evaluation

The onset of clinical manifestations, which include anemia, leukopenia, and decreased platelet count, is usually insidi-ous, not unlike that seen in leukemia. Definitive diagnosis is determined from bone marrow aspiration, which demon-strates the conversion of red bone marrow to yellow, fatty bone marrow.

### Therapeutic Management

The objectives of treatment are based on the recognition that the underlying disease process is failure of the bone marrow to carry out its hematopoietic functions. Therefore therapy is directed at restoring function to the marrow and involves two main approaches: (1) immunosuppressive ther-apy to remove the presumed immunologic functions that prolong aplasia or (2) replacement of the bone marrow through transplantation. Bone marrow transplantation is the treatment of choice for severe aplastic anemia when a suitable donor exists.

However, in the last 15 years new treatment strategies have been developed to improve the prognosis for children with acquired aplastic anemia who do not have a matched sibling donor. *Antilymphocyte globulin (ALG)* or *antithymocyte globulin (ATG)* are similar products; therefore the terms are used interchangeably.

The use of immunosuppressive therapy, including cy-closporin A (CSA) and ATG, with the addition of human recombinant granulocyte- or granulocyte-macrophage–colony-stimulating factor (G-CSF or GM-CSF) and methyl-prednisolone (to prevent ATG serum sickness) has greatly improved the prognosis for patients with aplastic anemia.

The rationale for using ATG is based on the theory that aplastic anemia may be a result of autoimmunity. ATG and CSA suppress T-cell–dependent autoimmune responses but do not cause bone marrow suppression. The optimum schedule for ATG administration is still under investiga-tion. It is usually given intravenously over 12 to 16 hours daily for 4 days, after a test dose to check for hypersensitiv-ity. A course may be repeated, depending on the reduction in circulating lymphocytes and the patient's response (see Nursing Considerations on p. 1561). Cyclosporine is ad-ministered orally for a duration of several weeks to months. G-CSF or GM-CSF, given parenterally, is used to enhance bone marrow production.

In children who fail to respond to ATG, CSA, and growth factors, success has been achieved using high-dose cyclophosphamide as an effective immunosuppressive agent. Androgens may be used with ATG to stimulate eryth-ropoiesis if the aplastic anemia is nonresponsive to initial therapies.

*Bone marrow transplantation* should be considered *early* in the course of the disease if a compatible donor can be found. Transplantation is more successful when performed before multiple transfusions have sensitized the child to leukocyte and HLA antigens. Children who are eligible for transplantation should be transferred to one of the medical centers that specialize in this procedure. Many different preparative regimens are available, and all aim to decrease the rate of graft-vs-host disease. All regimens include im-munosuppressive therapy. Some regimens include im-munosuppressive therapy and irradiation (either total body or thoracoabdominal). Patients who have received a large number of transfusions before bone marrow transplanta-tion have a higher rejection and shorter survival rate (Miller, 1995).

With effective use of immunosuppressive therapy or a bone marrow transplant, the prognosis for patients with aplastic anemia has improved in recent years to over 80% of the children being long-term survivors (Pitcher and others, 1999).

## Nursing Considerations

The care of the child with aplastic anemia is similar to that of the child with leukemia (i.e., preparing the family for the diagnostic and therapeutic procedures, preventing complications from the severe pancytopenia, and emotionally supporting them in terms of a potentially fatal outcome.)* (See Chapters 23 and 36.) Because each of these nursing considerations has been discussed, only the exceptions will be presented. (Bone marrow transplantation is discussed in Chapter 36.)

During administration of ATG, whether using a central venous catheter or peripheral vein, vigilant attention must be directed to the infusion to prevent extravasation. Meticulous care of the venous access catheter is essential because of the child's susceptibility to infection. Although anaphylactic reactions to ATG are rare, emergency preparations should be planned in advance, with epinephrine and oxygen readily available. The nurse should observe for immediate reactions to ATG, which include fever and skin rash. Delayed reactions (serum sickness) may also occur within 7 to 14 days of a course of ATG, and the manifestations are similar to immediate reactions. The symptoms are reversed and in the case of serum sickness may be prevented with corticosteroids. Because growth factors are usually given subcutaneously over several days, an anesthetic cream, EMLA, may be used to minimize pain at the injection site.

Because chemotherapeutic agents may be used, many of the reactions, such as nausea and vomiting, alopecia, and mucosal ulceration, may be encountered. In addition, extensive ecchymotic areas of the oral mucosa from thrombocytopenia require meticulous mouth care to prevent breakdown, bleeding, and infection. Fortunately, these lesions, which look painful, cause little or no discomfort. Local anesthetics are not necessary, but anorexia is still a consequence because of the edematous nature of the lesions. Liquid, bland, and soft diets are usually tolerated best. (See Feeding the Sick Child, Chapter 27.)

# DEFECTS IN HEMOSTASIS

*Hemostasis* is the process that stops bleeding when a blood vessel is injured. Vascular and plasma clotting factors, as well as platelets, are required. A complex system of clotting, anticlotting, and clot breakdown (fibrinolysis) mechanisms exists in equilibrium to ensure clot formation only in the presence of blood vessel injury and to limit the clotting process to the site of vessel wall injury. Dysfunction in these systems will lead to bleeding or abnormal clotting.

## Mechanisms Involved in Normal Hemostasis

To understand the role that factor deficiencies play in promoting bleeding tendencies, it is necessary to review the nor-

*Additional information is available from the **Aplastic Anemia and MDS International Foundation, Inc,** PO Box 613, Annapolis, MD 21404, (800) 747-2820; www.aamds/international.org.

mal coagulation process of the blood. Although the coagulation process is complex, clotting depends on three main factors: vascular influence, platelet role, and clotting factors.

### Vascular Influence

At the time and site of injury, several events occur to initiate hemostasis: local vasoconstriction, compression of the blood vessels by extravasated blood, release of von Willebrand factor (VWF) by endothelial walls, and the presence of collagen in exposed subendothelial cells that acts as a site for platelet adhesion.

### Platelet Role

Normally the platelets do not adhere to each other or to normal endothelium. However, at the time a blood vessel is injured, the following occur. Platelet adhesion occurs at the site of the injury, providing a plug. The platelets change shape, develop pseudopods, and release a variety of chemicals to stimulate vasoconstriction and vessel repair and to activate and recruit more platelets to the injury site. Receptor sites are located on the platelets for fibrinogen and other adhesive proteins, causing the platelets to stick together (aggregation). As the membrane of the platelet changes, the phospholipids necessary for blood coagulation are exposed, resulting in fibrin production, which secures the platelet plugs to the site. Finally, the clot compresses and is secured to the injury.

Defects in platelets and clotting factors are the most common causes of bleeding during childhood. The following discussion focuses on the major conditions that require nursing intervention.

### Clotting Factors

The clotting factors (Table 35-4) are activated in sequence to develop a fibrin clot. Two mechanisms exist that can generate prothrombin to produce thrombin:

1. *Intrinsic pathway.* Factor XII, high-molecular-weight kininogen (HMK, Fitzgerald factor), and prekallikrein (KAL, Fletcher factor) react on a negative-charged surface (contact activation reaction) to activate factor XI (PTA, plasma thromboplastin antecedent). The partial thromboplastin time (PTT) measures abnormalities in the intrinsic pathway (abnormalities in factors I, II, V, VIII, IX, X, XII, HMK, and KAL).
2. *Extrinsic pathway.* A lipoprotein tissue factor stimulates activation of factor VII. The prothrombin time (PT) measures abnormalities of the extrinsic pathway (abnormalities in factors I, II, V, VII, and X).

Laboratory tests to assess hemostasis are presented in Table 35-5.

## Hemophilia

The term *hemophilia* refers to a group of bleeding disorders resulting from a congenital deficiency of specific coagulation proteins (DiMichele and Neufeld, 1998). Although the symptomatology is similar regardless of which clotting factor is deficient, the identification of specific factor deficiencies has allowed definitive treatment with replacement agents.

In about 80% of all cases of hemophilia, the inheritance pattern is demonstrated as X-linked recessive. (See Chapter 5.) The two most common forms of the disorder are *factor VIII deficiency* (*hemophilia A* or *classic hemophilia*) and *factor IX deficiency* (*hemophilia B* or *Christmas disease*). The following discussion is primarily concerned with factor VIII deficiency, which accounts for about 75% of all cases.

| TABLE 35-4 | Blood-clotting factors |
|---|---|
| **Factor Number** | **Synonyms** |
| I | Fibrinogen |
| II | Prothrombin |
| III | Platelet factor 3, thromboplastin |
| IV | Calcium |
| V | Labile factor, proaccelerin, Ac globulin |
| VII | Serum prothrombin conversion accelerator (SPCA), proconvertin, stable factor |
| VIII | Antihemophilic factor (AHF), |
| IX | Plasma thromboplastin component (PTC), Christmas factor |
| X | Stuart-Prower factor |
| XI | Plasma thromboplastin antecedent (PTA) |
| XII | Hageman factor |
| XIII | Fibrin-stabilizing factor (FSF) |
| KAL | Prekallikrein, Fletcher factor |
| HMK | High-molecular-weight kininogen, Fitzgerald factor |

## Modes of Transmission

Hemophilia is transmitted as an X-linked recessive disorder; however, only about 60% of affected children have a positive family history for the disease. As many as one third of the cases of hemophilia may be caused by gene mutation. The most frequent pattern of transmission is through the mating of an unaffected male with a trait-carrier female. (See Fig. 5-8.) With improved treatment for persons with hemophilia, it is important to consider the results of mating between an affected male and a normal female or a carrier female. For example, the mating of an affected male with a carrier female results in a 1 in 4 chance of producing either an affected son or daughter, a carrier daughter, or a normal son. This is one of the few ways in which a female inherits the disorder. Female carriers may have low levels of factor VIII and be symptomatic.

## Pathophysiology and Clinical Manifestations

The basic defect of hemophilia A is a deficiency of factor VIII (antihemophilic factor [AHF]). AHF is produced by the liver and is necessary for the formation of thromboplastin in phase I of blood coagulation. The less AHF found in the blood, the more severe the disease.

A major feature of hemophilia is that its expression varies markedly in the degree of bleeding severity. Hemophilia is generally classified into three groups according to the severity of the factor deficiency; approximately 60% to 70% of

| TABLE 35-5 | Laboratory tests for hemostasis* | |
|---|---|---|
| **Test** | **Description** | **Comments** |
| **Platelet Function** | | |
| **Bleeding time** | Measures time it takes for bleeding from small superficial wound to cease | Function depends on platelet aggregation and vasoconstriction; two common methods used: Ivy (incision made on forearm) and Duke (incision made on earlobe) |
| **Tourniquet test** | Measures platelet function and capillary fragility; apply pressure to forearm with tourniquet for 5 to 10 minutes | Normal response is absence of petechiae or fewer than 10 Abnormal in platelet and connective tissue disorders |
| **Clot retraction test** | Measures degree to which clot shrinks and expresses serum | Depends on platelet function |
| **Blood-Clotting Mechanisms** | | |
| **Whole blood–clotting time** | Measures time it takes for clot to form *within* blood | Prolonged clotting time indicates problem in thrombin-to-fibrin phase or in any factor in intrinsic clotting mechanism; difficult test to standardize; therefore often unreliable results |
| **Prothrombin time (PT)** | Measures activity of prothrombin, as well as factors necessary for its conversion to thrombin and fibrinogen | Actually does not measure prothrombin levels, but activity; because it bypasses intrinsic-extrinsic mechanism, detects deficiencies of factors V, VII, X, and fibrinogen as well as prothrombin |
| **Partial thromboplastin time (PTT) test** | Similar to PT but measures activity of thromboplastin, which depends on intrinsic clotting factors | Specific for factor deficiencies, except factor VII, which results in a normal PTT but prolonged PT |
| **Thromboplastin generation test (TGT)** | Measures blood's ability to generate thromboplastin | Allows for determination of specific factor deficiencies, especially distinguishing between factors VIII and IX |
| **Prothrombin consumption test** | Indirectly measures thromboplastin generation and prothrombin response | Normally, as blood clots, prothrombin is converted to thrombin so that serum is depleted of prothrombin; if thromboplastin is decreased (as a result of extrinsic factor deficiencies), not all prothrombin will be converted and removed from serum |
| **Fibrinogen level** | Directly measures fibrinogen levels in blood | Not dependent on phase I or II deficiencies |

*Normal values are listed in Appendix D.

children with hemophilia demonstrate the severe form of the disorder:

| Clinical Severity | Factor VIII Activity | Bleeding Tendency |
|---|---|---|
| Severe | 1% | Spontaneous bleeding without trauma |
| Moderate | 1%-5% | Bleeding with trauma |
| Mild | 5%-50% | Bleeding with severe trauma or surgery |

The effect of hemophilia is prolonged bleeding anywhere from or in the body. With severe factor deficiencies, hemorrhage can occur as a result of minor trauma, such as after circumcision, during loss of deciduous teeth, or as a result of a slight fall or bruise. However, in children with less severe deficiencies the bleeding tendency may not be noted until the onset of walking.

Subcutaneous and intramuscular hemorrhages are common. *Hemarthrosis,* which refers to bleeding into the joint cavities, especially the knees, elbows, and ankles, is the most frequent form of internal bleeding. Bony changes and crippling deformities occur after repeated bleeding episodes over several years. Early signs of hemarthrosis are a feeling of stiffness, tingling, or ache in the affected joint, followed by a decrease in the ability to move the joint. Obvious signs and symptoms are warmth, redness, swelling, and severe pain with considerable loss of movement. Spontaneous hematuria is not uncommon. Epistaxis may occur but is not as frequent as other kinds of hemorrhage. Petechiae are uncommon in persons with hemophilia because repair of small hemorrhages depends on platelet function, not on blood-clotting mechanisms.

Bleeding into the tissue can occur anywhere but is serious if it occurs in the neck, mouth, or thorax, because the airway can become obstructed. Intracranial hemorrhage can have fatal consequences and is one of the major causes of death. Hemorrhage anywhere along the gastrointestinal tract can lead to anemia, and bleeding into the retroperitoneal cavity is especially hazardous because of the large space for blood to accumulate. Hematomas in the spinal cord can cause paralysis.

## Diagnostic Evaluation

The diagnosis is usually made on a history of bleeding episodes, evidence of X-linked inheritance (only one third of the cases are new mutations), and laboratory findings. To understand the significance of various tests of hemostasis, it is helpful to recall the usual mechanisms to control bleeding (i.e., the function of platelets and of clotting factors). Tests that measure platelet function, such as the bleeding time, are all normal in persons with hemophilia, whereas tests that assess clotting factor function may be abnormal (see Table 35-5). The tests specific for hemophilia include factor VIII and IX assays, procedures normally done by specialized laboratories. Other tests are those that depend on specific factors for a reaction to occur, especially the partial thromboplastin time (PTT) test. Carrier detection is possible in classic hemophilia using DNA testing and is an important consideration in families in which female offspring may have inherited the trait.

## Therapeutic Management

The primary therapy for hemophilia is replacement of the missing clotting factor. The products currently available are *factor VIII concentrate,* from genetically engineered recombinant or from pooled plasma to be reconstituted with sterile water immediately before use. *DDAVP (1-deamino-8-D-arginine vasopressin),* a synthetic form of vasopressin, is the treatment of choice in mild hemophilia and von Willebrand disease (in type I and IIA only) if the child shows an appropriate response. After DDAVP administration a threefold to fourfold rise in factor VIII activity should occur. Because the goal is to raise the factor VIII level at least 30%, patients with moderate factor VIII deficiency do not benefit. In addition, various therapies are employed when bleeding occurs or is anticipated (Table 35-6).

*Cryoprecipitate* is no longer recommended for use in treating factor VIII deficiency. Since 1988, with the advent of highly purified factor VIII concentrate (monoclonal), and since the licensing of recombinant factor VIII concentrate in 1992 (not marketed as a blood product but as a drug), practitioners have been advised by the National Hemophilia Foundation to use only these products. Cryoprecipitate cannot be treated to safely eliminate hepatitis or human immunodeficiency virus (HIV) infection.

Aggressive factor concentrate replacement therapy is initiated to prevent chronic crippling effects from joint bleeding. If replacement therapy is begun immediately, local measures such as ice applications and splinting are seldom needed.

Other drugs may be included in the therapy plan, depending on the source of the hemorrhage. Corticosteroids are given for hematuria, acute hemarthrosis, and chronic synovitis. Nonsteroidal antiinflammatory drugs (NSAIDs), such as ibuprofen, are effective in relieving pain caused by synovitis; however, they must be used with caution because they inhibit platelet function (Dragone and Karp, 1996; Hilgartner and Corrigan, 1995). Oral use of epsilon

| TABLE 35-6 | Adjunct therapies for hemophilia A |
|---|---|
| **Site of Bleed** | **Treatment** |
| Joint | Rest |
| | Ice |
| | Elevation |
| | Splint/Ace wrap/crutches |
| | Physical therapy |
| Soft tissue (substraneous) | Ice |
| | Elevation |
| | Splint/Ace wrap |
| Muscle | Rest |
| | Ice |
| | Elevation |
| | Splint/Ace wrap/crutches |
| | Physical therapy |
| | Complete bed rest for iliopsoas muscle bleed |
| Mucous membrane (e.g., nose, mouth) | Pressure to nares (for nosebleed) |
| | Topical antifibrinolytic agent (epsilon amino-caproic acid) |
| | Nasal pack (sometimes necessary) |

aminocaproic acid (EACA, Amicar) prevents clot destruction. Its use is limited to mouth, trauma, or surgery; and a dose of factor concentrate must be given first. The child may rinse the mouth with this medicine and then swallow it.

A regular program of exercise and physical therapy is an important aspect of management. If started early and continued throughout adulthood, planned, individualized physical activity strengthens muscles around joints and may decrease the number of spontaneous bleeding episodes.

> **NURSING ALERT**   Passive range-of-motion exercises should never be part of an exercise regimen after an acute episode because the joint capsule could easily be stretched and bleeding could recur. Active range-of-motion exercises are best so that the patient can control his or her own pain tolerance.

Treatment without delay results in more rapid recovery and a decreased likelihood of complications; therefore most children are treated at home. The family is taught the technique of venipuncture and how to administer the AHF to children over 2 to 3 years of age. The child learns the procedure for self-administration at 8 to 12 years of age. Home treatment is highly successful, and the rewards, in addition to the immediacy, are less disruption of family life, fewer school or work days missed, and enhancement of the child's self-esteem and independence.

Primary prophylaxis in hemophilia patients has been practiced for many years in European countries and has proved to be effective in preventing arthropathy. Primary prophylaxis involves the infusion of factor VIII concentrate on a regular basis before the onset of joint damage. A recent study using primary prophylaxis supported decreased joint damage but at prohibitative cost (Smith and others, 1996). Secondary prophylaxis involves the infusion of factor VIII concentrate on a regular basis after the child experiences his or her first joint bleed. The infusions are given three times a week. Aggressive factor replacement may be a cost-effective alternative to primary prophylaxis, yet showed no decrease in the development of joint disease (Smith and others, 1996). This involves the infusion of a high dose of factor VIII concentrate when a joint bleed occurs, followed by 2 days of more standard doses of factor VIII concentrate, which stops the bleeding (Cross and Koerper, 1997) but does not prevent long-term joint damage.

**Prognosis.**   The progress made in hemophilia care over the past two decades has been striking. The advent of home infusion therapy coupled with recent advances in producing safer and more effective factor concentrates has revolutionized the treatment and management of hemophilia (DiMichele and Neufeld, 1998). Home infusion therapy enables early recognition of joint and muscle bleeds, as well as immediate adequate treatment with clotting factor. Early treatment has significantly reduced the morbidity formerly associated with hemophilia. The concept of comprehensive hemophilia treatment centers offers the child with hemophilia and the family a coordinated multidisciplinary approach to meeting their needs and improving the child's health and well-being.

Although there is no cure for hemophilia, its symptoms can be controlled and its potentially crippling deformities markedly reduced or even avoided. Today many children with hemophilia function with minimal or no joint damage. They are normal with an average life expectancy in every aspect but one: they have a tendency to bleed, which is a significant inconvenience but not necessarily a life-threatening event.

Unfortunately, those individuals with hemophilia who were treated before current purification techniques for factor VIII concentrate (between 1979 and 1985) may have been exposed to HIV. It is estimated that over 50% of these patients have seroconverted to HIV-positive status, and 30% have acquired immunodeficiency syndrome (AIDS) (Hilgartner and Corrigan, 1995). As these individuals become sexually active, the issue of sexual transmission of HIV becomes increasingly important. The adolescent must be knowledgeable regarding safe sexual behavior. Individuals with hemophilia diagnosed and treated with factor concentrates since 1985 are at virtually no risk for developing HIV infection from treatment.

Gene therapy may prove to be a treatment option in the future. This therapy involves introducing a working copy of the factor VIII gene into a patient who has a flawed copy of the gene (Cross and Koerper, 1997). The scientific community remains undaunted in its attempt to make gene-addition therapy a twenty-first century reality for patients with hemophilia A and B. Therapeutically the retroviruses that ravaged one generation of hemophiliac patients are the most used vectors for gene transfer and may now participate in the cure for the next generation of patients with hemophilia (DiMichele and Neufeld, 1998).

### Nursing Considerations

The earlier a bleeding episode is recognized, the more effectively it can be treated. Signs that indicate internal bleeding are especially important to recognize. Children are aware of internal bleeding and are very reliable in telling the examiner the location of an internal bleed. In addition, the nurse maintains a high level of suspicion when a child with hemophilia demonstrates signs, such as headache, slurred speech, loss of consciousness (from cerebral bleeding), and black, tarry stools (from gastrointestinal bleeding).

**Prevent Bleeding.**   The goal of prevention of bleeding episodes is directed toward decreasing the risk of injury. Prevention of bleeding episodes is geared mostly toward appropriate exercises to strengthen muscles and joints and to allow age-appropriate activity. During infancy and toddlerhood the normal acquisition of motor skills creates innumerable opportunities for falls, bruises, and minor wounds. Restraining the child from mastering motor development can herald more serious long-term problems than allowing the behavior. However, the environment should be made as safe as possible, with close supervision maintained during playtime, to minimize incidental injuries.

For older children the family usually needs assistance in preparing for school. A nurse who knows the family can be instrumental in discussing the situation with the school nurse and in jointly planning an appropriate schedule of activity. Because almost all persons with hemophilia are boys, the physical limitations in regard to active sports may be a difficult adjustment and activity restrictions must be tempered with sensitivity to the child's emotional, as well as physical, needs. Appropriate safety equipment should always be used. Children and adolescents with severe hemophilia are encouraged to participate in noncontact sports such as swimming and golf. Football, boxing, hockey, soccer, and rugby are strongly discouraged because the risk of injury outweighs the physical and psychosocial benefits of participating in these sports (Buzzard, 1996; Dragone and Karp, 1996; National Hemophilia Foundation and American Red Cross, 1996).

To prevent oral bleeding, some readjustment in dental hygiene may be needed to minimize trauma to the gums, such as use of a water irrigating device, softening the toothbrush in warm water before brushing, or using a sponge-tipped disposable toothbrush. A regular toothbrush should be soft bristled and small in size. Adolescents also need to be advised of the dangers of using safety razors with blades and be encouraged to use an electric shaver.

Because any trauma can lead to a bleeding episode, all persons caring for these children must be aware of their disorder. These children should wear medical identification, and older children are encouraged to recognize situations in which disclosing their condition is important, such as during dental extractions or injections. Health personnel need to take special precautions to prevent the use of procedures such as intramuscular injections. The subcutaneous route is substituted for intramuscular injections whenever possible. Venipunctures for blood samples are usually preferred by these children. There is usually less bleeding after the venipuncture than after finger or heel punctures. Neither aspirin nor any aspirin-containing compound should be used. Acetaminophen (Tylenol) is a suitable aspirin substitute, especially for use during control of pain at home.

**Recognize and Control Bleeding.** The earlier a bleeding episode is recognized, the more effectively it can be treated. Factor replacement therapy should be instituted according to established medical protocol, and supportive measures may be implemented, such as *RICE*, which is (1) **r**est, (2) **i**ce, (3) **c**ompression, and (4) **e**levation. When parents and older children are taught such measures beforehand, they can be prepared to initiate immediate treatment before blood loss is excessive. Plastic bags of ice or cold packs should be kept in the freezer for such emergencies. However, such measures should not take the place of factor replacement.

**Prevent Crippling Effects of Bleeding.** As a result of repeated episodes of hemarthrosis, incompletely absorbed blood in the joints, and limitation of motion, bone and muscle changes occur that may result in flexion contractures and joint fixation. Obviously prevention of bleeding is the ideal goal. However, because spontaneous bleeding is not uncommon in persons with severe hemophilia, definitive measures, including replacement therapy and physical therapy, are necessary to limit joint damage.

During bleeding episodes the joint is elevated and immobilized. Active range-of-motion exercises are usually in-

stituted after the acute phase. This allows the child to control the degree of exercise according to the level of discomfort. Physical therapy is beneficial to promote maximum function of the joint and unaffected body parts. Success of a physical therapy plan involves control of pain by administering analgesics before therapy and adjusting the dose to provide maximum benefit.

If an exercise program is instituted in the home, a physical therapist or public health nurse may need to supervise compliance with the regimen. Rarely, orthopaedic intervention, such as casting, application of traction, or aspiration of blood, may be necessary to preserve joint function. Diet is also an important consideration, because excessive body weight can increase the strain on affected joints, especially the knees, and predispose the child to hemarthrosis. Consequently calories need to be supplied in accordance with energy requirements.

**Support Family and Prepare for Home Care.** The discovery of factor concentrates has greatly changed the outlook for these children. Bleeding can be minimized, and the child can live a much more normal, unrestricted life. Children are taught to take responsibility for their disease at an early age. They learn their limitations and other preventive measures as well as self-administration of the factor replacement.

The needs of families who have children with hemophilia are best met through a comprehensive team approach of physicians (pediatrician, hematologist, orthopaedist), nurse practitioner, nurse, social worker, and physical therapist. Parent-group discussions are beneficial in meeting those needs often best met by similarly affected families. For example, with the improved prognosis for these children, parents and adolescents with hemophilia are faced with vocational and financial problems in addition to concern over future childbearing. Once children reach 21 years of age, many insurance companies will no longer insure them. This can be disastrous in terms of the cost of treatment, which can exceed $10,000 per year. The **National Hemophilia Foundation*** and the **Canadian Hemophilia Society†** provide numerous services/publications for both health care providers and families.

Children who have become infected with HIV through transfusions and factor replacement products are faced with the consequences of this dreaded disease. Consequently they need the support of health professionals, especially in the area of safe sexual practices to avoid disease transmission and public education regarding AIDS and ways to deal with public reactions to persons who have AIDS (see p. 1572 for a discussion of AIDS). (See Nursing Care Plan: The Child with Hemophilia.‡)

**Identify Persons at Risk.** Genetic counseling is essential as soon as possible after diagnosis. Unlike many other disorders in which both parents carry the trait, the feeling of responsibility for this condition usually rests with the

---

*116 W 32ⁿᵈ St, 11ᵗʰ floor, New York, NY 10001, (212) 431-8541 or (800) 42HANDI, fax: (212) 431-0906; www.hemophilia.org
†625 President Kennedy, Suite 1210, Montreal, Quebec, Canada H3A 1K2, (514) 848-0503, e-mail: chs@odysee.net.
‡In Wong DL, Hess CS: *Wong and Whaley's clinical manual of pediatric nursing*, ed 5, St Louis, 2000, Mosby.

mother. Without an opportunity to discuss her feelings, the couple's relationship may suffer. Prenatal DNA testing can identify affected fetuses and identify carriers in most cases.

## von Willebrand Disease (vWD)

vWD is a hereditary bleeding disorder characterized by a deficiency or defective protein called von Willebrand factor (vWF) with usually a deficiency of factor VIII (Cordoni, 2000; Mannucci and others, 2002). This results in prolonged bleeding time because platelets fail to adhere to the walls of the ruptured vessel to form a platelet plug. vWD can cause mild, moderate, or severe bleeding. Most cases are mild and require intervention only for dental and surgical procedures.

The most characteristic clinical feature of vWD is an increased tendency toward bleeding from mucous membranes. The most common symptom is frequent nosebleeds, followed by gingival bleeding, easy bruising, and excessive menstrual bleeding (menorrhagia) in females. Unlike hemophilia, vWD affects both males and females because its inheritance is autosomal dominant. However, the treatment and final outcome are similar in both disorders. Treatment of bleeding is with DDAVP and/or a specially concentrated clotting factor called Humate-P.

### Nursing Considerations

The nursing goals are similar to those for hemophilia, with special considerations related to epistaxis. Nosebleeds are often a frightening experience for the child and parents. A calm, reassuring manner can alleviate anxiety and promote the child's cooperation. Because most of the nosebleeding originates in the anterior part of the nasal septum, bleeding can be controlled by applying pressure to the nose with the thumb and forefinger. (See Emergency Treatment box.) During this time the child breathes through the mouth. If local measures are not successful at stopping the bleeding, a single dose of DDAVP is usually effective.

For menorrhagia, factor replacement therapy or the administration of DDAVP may be beneficial on the first day of the menstrual cycle to lessen the flow. Teaching the adolescent methods to prevent embarrassing accidents during menstruation, such as wearing plastic-lined underpants and using double sanitary pads, helps her adjust to the inconvenience. Interestingly, these females frequently do not experience excessive bleeding at the time of delivery (Pavlovich-Danis, 2001). This is thought to be because of increased levels of factor VIII during pregnancy. Decisions regarding childbearing are difficult because of the dominant pattern of inheritance.

## Idiopathic Thrombocytopenic Purpura (ITP)

ITP is an acquired hemorrhagic disorder that is characterized by (1) excessive destruction of platelets (*thrombocytopenia*), (2) *purpura* (a discoloration caused by petechiae beneath the skin), and (3) normal bone marrow with a usual increase in large, young platelets. Although the cause is unknown, it is believed to be an autoimmune response to disease-related antigens. It is the most frequently occurring thrombocytopenia of childhood, with 80% presenting between 2 and 10 years of age and recovering completely within 6 months (Murphy, Nepo and Sills, 1999).

The disease occurs in one of two forms: an acute, self-limiting course or a chronic condition (greater than 6 months' duration). The acute form is most commonly seen after upper respiratory tract infections; after the childhood diseases of measles, rubella, mumps, and chickenpox; or after infection with human parvovirus.

Clinical symptoms include petechiae, bruising, bleeding from mucous membranes, or prolonged bleeding from abrasions. Symptomatic bleeding is not usually seen until the platelet count is less than 20,000/mm³. Fatal hemorrhages have been reported in less than 1% of all patients.

### Diagnostic Evaluation

In ITP the platelet count is reduced to below 20,000 mm³/dl; therefore tests that depend on platelet function, such as the tourniquet test, bleeding time, and clot retraction, are abnormal. Although there is no definitive test on which to establish a diagnosis of ITP, several tests are usually performed to rule out other disorders in which thrombocytopenia is a manifestation, such as systemic lupus erythematosus, lymphoma, or leukemia.

### Therapeutic Management

Management of ITP is primarily supportive because the course of the disease is self-limited in the majority of cases. Activity is restricted at the onset while the platelet count is low and while active bleeding or progression of lesions is occurring. Treatment for acute presentation is symptomatic and has included prednisone, IV immune globulin (IVIG), and anti-D antibody. These are not curative therapies. Some experts suggest that no therapy is necessary for the asymptomatic patient because there is no difference in the recovery time of platelet counts. *Anti-D antibody* is a relatively new therapy for ITP. Infusion of anti-D antibody causes a transient hemolytic anemia in the patient. Along with the clearance of antibody-coated RBCs, there is prolonged survival of platelets due to the blockade of the Fc receptors of the reticuloendothelial cells. The platelet count does not increase until 48 hours after an infusion of anti-D antibody; therefore it is not appropriate therapy for patients who are actively bleeding. The benefits of choosing anti-D antibody therapy over prednisone or IVIG is that anti-D antibody can be given in one dose over a period of 5 to 10 minutes and is significantly less expensive than IVIG. Historically patients who are treated with prednisone first undergo a bone marrow examination to rule out leukemia, which is now controversial because leukemia rarely presents with a low platelet count alone (Bolton-Magap, 2000). Therefore the use of anti-D antibody and IVIG alleviates the need for a bone marrow examination. Before the initial administration of anti-D antibody, patients must meet certain criteria (Box 35-7). Premedication with acetaminophen (such as Tylenol) 5 to 10 minutes before infusion is recommended.

Box 35-7 ■ ■ ■
**ITP Patients Eligible for Anti-D Antibody Therapy**

Children >1 year and <19 years of age
Rh(D)-positive blood type
Normal WBC and hemoglobin for age; platelets <30,000/μl
No active mucosal bleeding
No prior history of reaction to plasma products
No patient known to be IgA deficient
No concurrent infection
No patient with Evans syndrome (characterized by the combination of idiopathic thrombocytopenia purpura and autoimmune hemolytic anemia)
No patient with suspected lupus or other collagen/vascular disorder
No patient with splenectomy

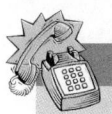
**EMERGENCY TREATMENT**
*Epistaxis*

Have child sit up and lean forward (not lying down).
Apply continuous pressure to nose with thumb and forefinger for at least 10 minutes.
Insert cotton or wadded tissue into each nostril and apply ice or cold cloth to bridge of nose if bleeding persists.
Keep child calm and quiet.

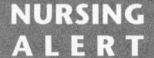
**NURSING ALERT**   After administration of anti-D antibody, observe the child for a minimum of 1 hour and maintain a patent IV line. Obtain baseline vital signs before the infusion and again 5, 20, and 60 minutes after beginning the infusion. Fever, chills, and headache may occur during or shortly after the infusion. If fever, chills, or headache occurs, diphenhydramine (Benadryl) and Solu-Cortef should be given and the patient should be observed for an additional hour.

Splenectomy is reserved for chronic severe ITP patients who are not responsive to pharmacologic management. It is the only treatment associated with long-term remission for 60% to 90% of children, therefore removing the risk of hemorrhage (Chu, Korb, and Sakamoto, 2000). Before considering splenectomy, it is generally recommended to wait until the child is more than 5 years of age because of the increased risk of bacterial infection. Pneumococcal, meningococcal, and *H. influenzae* vaccines are recommended before splenectomy (if not previously administered). The child also receives penicillin prophylaxis after splenectomy. The length of prophylactic-therapy is controversial, but in general, a minimum of 3 years is recommended.

**Prognosis.** The majority of children have a self-limited course without major complications. Some children will develop chronic ITP and require ongoing therapy. A splenectomy may modify the disease process, and the child will be asymptomatic.

### Nursing Considerations

Nursing care is largely supportive and should include teaching regarding possible side effects of therapy and limitation in activities while the child's platelet count is <50,000 to 100,000/mm³. Children with ITP should not participate in *any* contact sports, bike riding, skateboarding, in-line skating, gymnastics, climbing, or running. Parents are encouraged to engage their children in quiet activities and to prevent any injuries to the child's head (e.g., by using protective head gear and lining crib with protective padding). The parents are instructed to obtain prompt medical evaluation if the child sustains head or abdominal trauma.

The harmful effects of using aspirin and NSAIDs to control pain are critical for these children; therefore substitutes (such as acetaminophen) are always used. As in any condition with an uncertain outcome, the family needs emotional support.

## Disseminated Intravascular Coagulation (DIC)

DIC, also known as *consumption coagulopathy* is not a primary disease but a secondary disorder of coagulation that complicates a number of pathologic processes (such as hypoxia, acidosis, shock, and endothelial damage [burns]) and many severe systemic disease states (such as congenital heart disease, necrotizing enterocolitis, gram-negative bacterial sepsis, rickettsial infections, and some severe viral infections). The disease is characterized by bleeding and clotting, which occur simultaneously and are the hallmarks of this disorder.

### Pathophysiology

DIC occurs when the first stage of the coagulation process is abnormally stimulated. Although there is no well-defined sequence of events, two distinct phases can be identified. First, when the clotting mechanism is triggered in the circulation, thrombin is generated in greater amounts than can be neutralized by the body. Consequently there is rapid conversion of fibrinogen to fibrin with aggregation and destruction of platelets. Local and widespread fibrin deposition occurs in blood vessels. Obstruction is caused by the thrombi impeding the blood flow with eventual necrosis of tissues. Concurrently, the fibrinolytic mechanism is activated, causing extensive destruction of clotting factors. With a deficiency of clotting factors the child is vulnerable to uncontrollable hemorrhage into vital organs. An additional complication is damage and hemolysis of RBCs (Fig. 35-6).

### Clinical Manifestations

Signs and symptoms of DIC are those of many other diseases, which often confuses the diagnosis. There is evidence of bleeding—petechiae, purpura, bleeding from openings in the skin (e.g., a venipuncture site or surgical incision), hypotension, and dysfunction of organs from infarction and ischemia.

### Diagnostic Evaluation

DIC is suspected when there is an increased tendency to bleed (Box 35-8). Hematologic findings include prolonged prothrombin (PT), partial thromboplastin (PTT), and

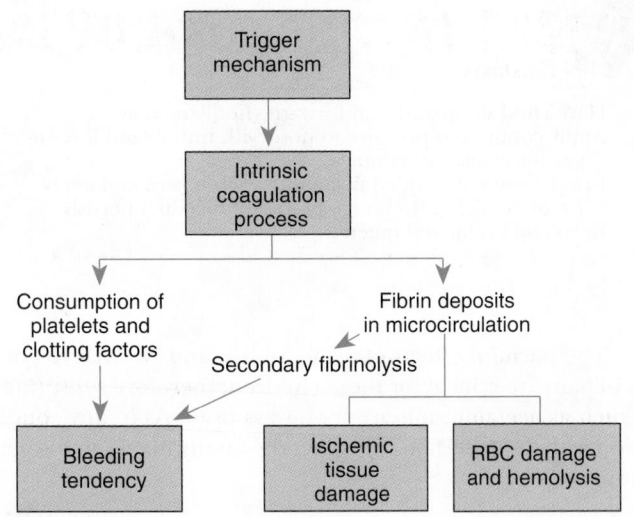

**Fig. 35-6** Effects of disseminated intravascular coagulation.

thrombin time (TT). There is a profoundly depressed platelet count, fragmented RBCs, and depleted fibrinogen.

### Therapeutic Management

Treatment is directed toward control of the underlying or initiating cause, which in most instances stops the coagulation problem spontaneously. Platelets and fresh frozen plasma may be needed to replace lost plasma components, especially in the child whose underlying disease remains uncontrolled. The extremely ill newborn infant may require exchange transfusion with fresh blood. The administration of IV heparin to inhibit thrombin formation is most often restricted to cases that have not responded to treatment of the underlying disease or replacement of coagulation factors and platelets.

### Nursing Considerations

The goals of nursing care are to be aware of the possibility of DIC in the severely ill child and to recognize signs that might indicate its presence. The skills needed to monitor IV infusion and blood transfusions and to administer heparin are the same as for any child receiving these therapies. Because the child is usually cared for in an intensive care unit, the special needs of the family must be considered. (See Chapter 26.)

## OTHER HEMATOLOGIC DISORDERS

### Neutropenia

Neutropenia is a reduction in circulating *neutrophils* and is usually defined as an *absolute neutrophil count (ANC)* of less than 1000/mm³ (in infants 2 weeks to 1 year of age) or less than 1500/mm³ (in children more than 1 year of age). African-Americans have ANCs that are 100 to 200/mm³ lower than whites (Lanzkowsky, 2000). The ANC is calculated by multiplying the total WBC count by the percentage of neutrophils and bands in the differential (see Table 35-1). When the ANC is less than 500/mm³, the risk for infec-

tion is high (Baehner and Miller, 1995a; Boxer, 2000; Lanzkowsky, 2000). Several different types of neutropenia occur in children (Table 35-7). This discussion focuses on the most common type, *chronic benign neutropenia.*

### Diagnostic Evaluation

Chronic benign neutropenia presents at 8 to 11 months of age, with 90% of children being diagnosed before 14 months of age. The median duration is usually 6 to 54 months (Dinaver, 1998). Neutropenia is often found as an incidental finding during the evaluation of a child with fever. The ANC is usually below 500/mm³, and the only physical findings (if any) are those related to infection. Oral ulcerations and skin infections are the most common manifestation of chronic benign neutropenia. However, most children have no infections despite the markedly reduced ANC. Bone marrow aspiration shows normal cellularity with absence of mature neutrophils. Antineutrophil antibodies are usually present, but their absence does not exclude the diagnosis.

To determine a child's neutrophil response during times of infection, a steroid stimulation test may be performed. The child is given a dose of IV steroid, and the neutrophil count is measured at hourly intervals for 4 to 5 hours. If the ANC increases to greater than 1000/mm³ after the dose of steroid, the child will have the same response during times of infection. If the ANC does not increase, it is an indication for increased vigilance and medical attention if the child develops fever of 38.3°C (101°F) or higher. These children may require hospitalization and aggressive treatment with broad-spectrum IV antibiotics, depending on the severity of illness.

### Therapeutic Management

Therapy to increase the ANC is rarely required. Children who have recurrent or severe infections, however, may benefit from the use of G-CSF.

*Colony-stimulating factors (CSFs)* are a naturally occurring group of glycoproteins. They were first discovered and characterized from their effect on growth and differentiation of marrow cells. Recombinant DNA technology has enabled the production of large quantities of highly purified CSFs that are nearly identical to the naturally occurring substances and have successfully increased the neutrophil count in a wide variety of neutropenic conditions (Dinauer, 1998). Children with chronic benign neutropenia have nor-

**TABLE 35-7**    Clinical and hematologic features of some congenital neutropenias

| Feature | Severe Congenital Neutropenia (Kostmann's Disease) | Familial Benign Neutropenia | Chronic Benign Neutropenia; Idiopathic Autoimmune Neutropenia | Reticular Dysgenesis |
|---|---|---|---|---|
| Etiology | Autosomal-recessive (ocassionally autosomal dominant) | Dominant | Antineutrophil antibodies detected in almost all cases | Failure of stem cells to produce myeloid and lymphoid cells |
| Severity | Severe illness Life-threatening pyogenic infections in first months of life | Variable; benign to severe infections | Benign | Severe, fatal thymic dysplasia; lymphoid hypoplasia |
| Clinical findings | Skin infection Aphthous ulcers Septicemia Meningitis Peritonitis Lung abscess Lymphadenopathy Splenomegaly (20%) | Less troublesome infection to severe infection | Paronychia Gingivitis Impetigo: mild infections, localized | Severe bacterial and viral infection Neonatal death |
| Hematologic findings | Anemia Neutropenia, <200/mm³ Monocytosis Eosinophilia Risk of leukemia | Neutropenia, usually <300/mm³ Monocytosis | No anemia Absent mature PMN Some band forms Monocytosis | Neutropenia Lymphopenia |
| Marrow findings | ↑Promyelocytes Absent MM, B, PMN ↑Monocytes ↑Eosinophils ↑Plasma cells | ↓MM, B, PMN "Maturation arrest" | Absent PMN Normal myeloid cells to band stage; lymphocytes increased | Absent myeloid and absent lymphoid cells Normal thrombopoiesis and erythropoiesis |
| Treatment | Antibiotics Supportive measures G-CSF Bone marrow transplantation | No therapy G-CSF if indicated | Antibiotics, as indicated G-CSF, if indicated | Bone marrow transplantation |

Modified from Lanzkowsky P: *Manual of pediatric hematology and oncology*, San Diego, 2000, Academic Press.
Notes: *B*, bands; *MM*, metamyelocytes; *PMN*, polymorphonuclear leukocytes; *G-CSF*, granulocyte colony-stimulating factor.

mal cellular immunity; therefore they should be given their routine childhood immunizations.

### Nursing Considerations

The care of the child with neutropenia primarily focuses on educating the parents. Parents should be instructed to keep their child away from large indoor crowds (e.g., grocery store on Saturday morning, movie theaters, daycare centers, church nursery) and individuals who are ill. Parents also need to be instructed to seek medical attention if their child has a fever of 38.3°C (101°F) or higher, or if skin lesions develop. Because G-CSF is administered parenterally only, parents must be instructed regarding administration of subcutaneous injections.

**Support Family.**    Neutropenia can have many effects on family life. Some parents must quit their jobs to avoid use of daycare. Financial counseling should be provided as indicated. Parents of children with neutropenia need a listening ear for their frustrations and continued encouragement that these children usually recover by the age of 4½ years.*

---

*Information is available from **Severe Chronic Neutropenia Inc**, 600 Steward St, Suite 1503, Seattle, WA 98101, (800) 726-4463; www.dpts. washington.edu/registry/.

## Henoch-Schönlein Purpura (HSP)

HSP, also referred to as allergic vasculitis, allergic purpura, or anaphylactoid purpura, is a relatively common acquired disorder in children characterized by a nonthrombocytopenic purpura, arthritis, nephritis, and abdominal pain.

The etiology is unknown, but the disease often follows an upper respiratory tract infection, and allergy or drug sensitivity plays a role in some instances. The disease occurs in children ages 6 months to 16 years but more frequently in children ages 2 to 11 years. It is observed more often in white children than in other races and in boys almost twice as often as in girls.

### Pathophysiology

The disease is characterized by inflammation of small blood vessels, and the manifestations observed are influenced by the size and distribution of the affected vessels. A generalized vasculitis of dermal capillaries (and to a lesser extent small arterioles and veins), causing extravasation of RBCs, produces the petechial skin lesions. Inflammation and hemorrhage may also occur in the gastrointestinal tract, synovium, glomeruli, and central nervous system.

## Clinical Manifestations

The onset of the disease may be abrupt, with the simultaneous appearance of several manifestations, or gradual, with the sequential appearance of different manifestations. The primary feature, however, is a symmetric purpura that involves the buttocks and lower extremities but may extend to include the extensor surfaces of the upper extremities and, less commonly, the upper trunk and face (Fig. 35-7). The rash may be associated with maculopapular lesions, urticaria, and erythema. There is often marked edema of the scalp, eyelids, lips, ears, and dorsal surfaces of the hands and feet—especially in infants and younger children. In severe cases, the skin may slough, leaving denuded areas that are similar in appearance and treatment to partial-thickness burns.

Arthritic effects are evident in two thirds of affected children and range from asymptomatic swelling around a single joint to painful, tender swelling of several joints, most often the knees and ankles. The involvement is periarticular and resolves in a few days without permanent damage or deformity.

Two thirds of the children have gastrointestinal involvement manifested by recurrent colicky midabdominal pain, often associated with nausea and vomiting. The stools contain gross or occult blood and mucus.

Renal involvement occurs in up to 50% of affected children and is potentially the most serious long-term complication. Initially the nephritis is manifested as hematuria, casts, and proteinuria. Although the majority of children with renal involvement recover completely, some develop chronic renal disease with eventual renal failure.

## Diagnostic Evaluation

Diagnosis is usually established on the basis of the history and clinical manifestations. Laboratory tests are used to assess gastrointestinal and renal involvement and to determine adequacy of hemostatic function. Tests for occult blood in the stool are performed. Increased levels of immunoglobulin A are a frequent finding.

## Therapeutic Management

Management is primarily supportive, with close observation for signs of renal or gastrointestinal manifestations. Edema, rash, malaise, and arthralgia are usually managed with ap-

propriate analgesics, such as NSAIDs, and mild sedation if necessary. Corticosteroids may be prescribed for relief of more severe edema, arthralgia, and colicky abdominal pain. The nephropathy requires careful monitoring of fluid and electrolyte balance, salt intake, and blood pressure. Antihypertensive agents may be needed.

The majority of children recover without the need for hospitalization, and in most instances a single acute episode clears spontaneously within a month. Others may have periodic recurrences for as long as 2 to 3 years before attaining permanent remission from symptoms. Rarely, death occurs from severe gastrointestinal complications, acute renal failure, or central nervous system involvement. Children with HSP nephritis should receive long-term follow-up (Jonides, 1996; Tizard, 1999).

## Nursing Considerations

Nursing care of the child hospitalized with HSP is primarily supportive, with vigilant observation for signs of complications. Vital signs are taken and recorded at regular intervals, specimens are obtained for laboratory examination, and medication is administered as prescribed. Urine and stools are carefully observed for fresh and occult blood.

If the child suffers from joint pain, positioning, careful movement, and administration of analgesics, including opioids, help reduce discomfort. More severe involvement, such as gastrointestinal symptoms and nephritis, is managed as for any such disorder.

Concern about the unsightly appearance of the rash is common. The child and parents can be reassured that it is only a temporary phenomenon, and the child can be encouraged to wear clothing that helps hide the rash, such as long sleeves, pants, and a robe. Emphasizing good grooming and attractive apparel helps promote a more positive self-image. If the skin surface is denuded, treatment may involve debridement and dressing changes similar to care of burns. (See Chapter 29.)

# IMMUNOLOGIC DEFICIENCY DISORDERS

A number of disorders can cause profound, often life-threatening alterations within the body's immune system. The most serious are those conditions that completely depress immunity, such as severe combined immunodeficiency disease. However, the one disorder that generates the most anxiety within both the family and the community is *human immunodeficiency virus (HIV) infection* and the subsequent development of *acquired immunodeficiency syndrome (AIDS).*

Several classifications of immune dysfunction exist. For example, in AIDS; severe combined immunodeficiency syndrome (SCIDS), and Wiskott-Aldrich syndrome are syndromes wherein the body is unable to mount an immune response. The immune response can also be misdirected. In autoimmune disorders, antibodies, macrophages, and lymphocytes attack healthy cells. Some disorders and their target organs include myasthenia gravis, muscle cells; Graves disease, thyroid cells; and type 1 diabetes, B-cells in the pancreas. With the exception of AIDS, SCIDS, and Wiskott-

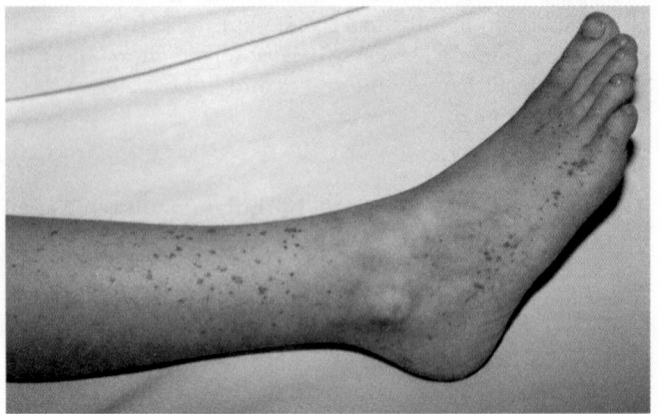

**Fig. 35-7** Henoch-Schönlein purpura.

Aldrich syndrome, the other disorders are discussed elsewhere in the book.

## Mechanisms Involved in Immunity

The function of the immune system is to recognize "self" from "nonself" and to initiate response to eliminate the "nonself" or the foreign substance known as *antigen.* All cells in the body have specific cell surface markers unique to the individual. These cell surface markers are known as the *major histocompatibility complex (MHC).* Because the markers were first identified on human leukocytes, they are commonly referred to as *human leukocyte antigens (HLAs).*

The protective mechanisms of the body consist of complex, overlapping defense systems. Intact skin serves as the first line of protection for the body. Body secretions such as saliva, sweat, and tears contain chemicals that can kill many organisms. The stomach contains acids that can destroy swallowed pathogens. Organisms trapped in the mucus of the nose and mouth, are expelled by sneezing or coughing. If the foreign substance has penetrated these barriers, cellular elements are mobilized.

The immune system is composed of the *primary lymphoid organs* (thymus, bone marrow, and probably liver) and the *secondary lymphoid organs* (lymph nodes, spleen, and gut-associated lymphoid tissue [GALT]). There are two types of functions of the immune system: nonspecific and specific (Fig. 35-8). *Nonspecific immune defenses* are activated on exposure to any foreign substance but react similarly regardless of the type of antigen; they are unable to identify the

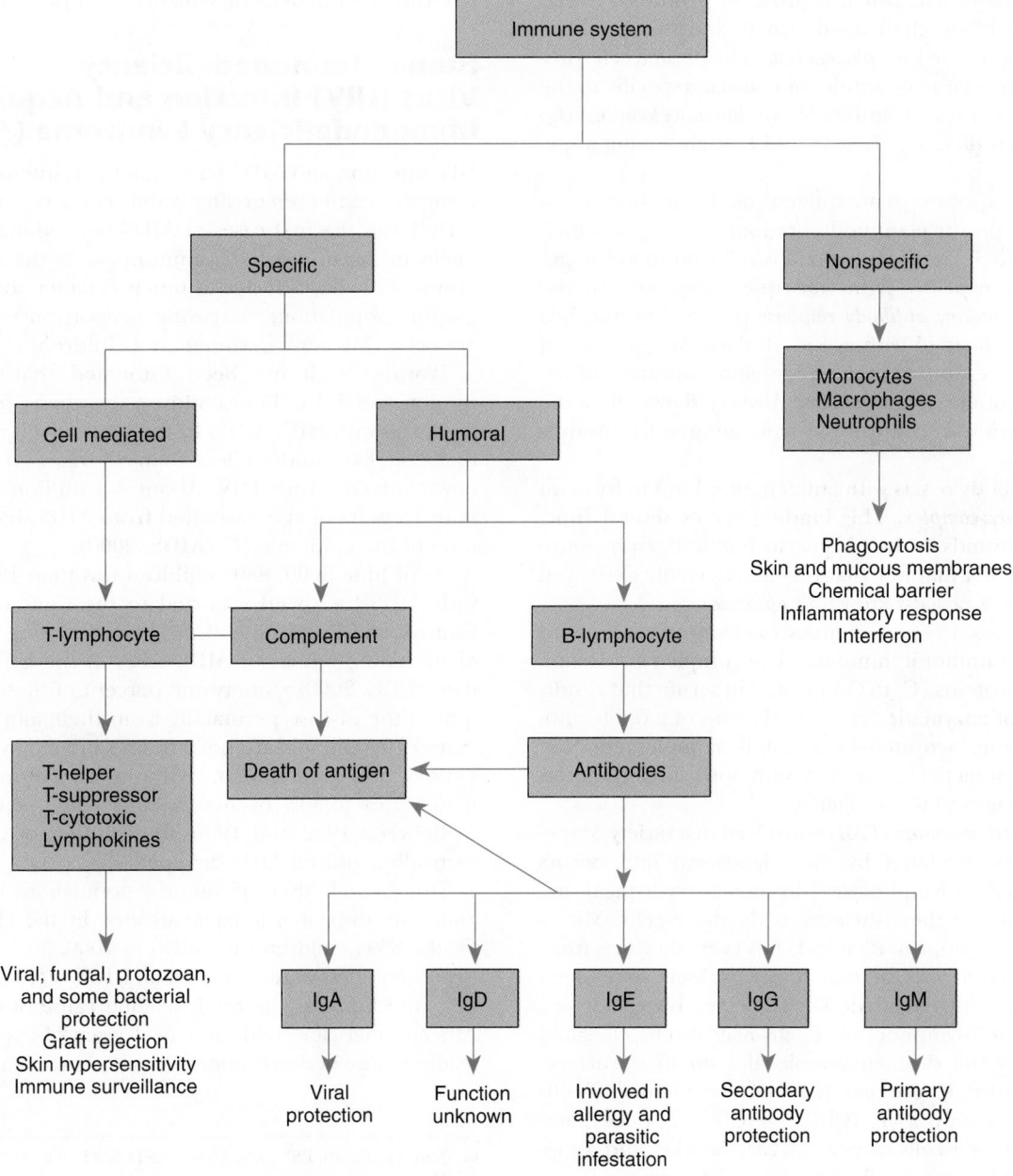

**Fig. 35-8**   Components of immune system.

antigen, except to know that it is "nonself." The principal activity of this system is *phagocytosis,* the process of ingesting and digesting foreign substances. Phagocytic cells include neutrophils and monocytes (see p. 1534). Specific defenses are discussed in the following section.

### Specific Immune Mechanisms

*Specific (adaptive) defenses* are those that have the ability to recognize the antigen and respond selectively. The components of adaptive immunity are humoral immunity and cell-mediated immunity. The cells responsible for these two forms of immunity are the lymphocytes, specifically B-lymphocytes and T-lymphocytes.

*Humoral immunity* is involved with antibody production and complement and is concerned with immune processes occurring *outside* the cells, such as on cell surfaces or in body fluids. The principal cell involved in antibody production is the *B-lymphocyte* which is probably produced in the bone marrow. When challenged with an antigen, B-cells divide and differentiate into *plasma cells.* The plasma cells produce and secrete large quantities of *antibodies* specific to the antigen. Five classes of antibodies of *immunoglobulins (Ig)* have been identified: G, M, A, D, and E, each serving a specific function.

On initial exposure to an antigen, the B-lymphocyte system begins to produce antibody, predominantly IgM, which appears in 2 to 3 days. This process is referred to as the *primary antibody response.* With subsequent exposure to the antigen, a *secondary antibody response* occurs. Specific IgG antibodies are formed within 4 to 10 days. An example of the secondary response is subsequent administration of immunizations, often called *boosters.* *Memory B-cells* allow the immune system to recognize the same antigen for months or years.

When antibody reacts with antigen, they bind to form an *antigen-antibody complex.* This binding serves several functions. Antibody aids in the phagocytosis of antigen by sensitizing it in such a manner that it is more readily destroyed by phagocytes, a process known as *opsonization.*

Antibody also activates or fixes *complement,* the second component of humoral immunity. The complement system is a series of proteins ($C_1$ to $C_9$) present in serum that results in a cascade of enzymatic actions and death of a viable antigen. After being activated by antibody, complement produces a chemotactic factor that summons T-lymphocytes and macrophages to the antigen site.

*Cell-mediated immunity (CMI)* is involved in a variety of specific functions mediated by the *T-lymphocyte* and occurs *within* the cell. T-lymphocytes do not carry typical immunoglobulins on their surfaces as do the B-cells. Microscopically T-cells appear identical; however, they are functionally heterogeneous in that several subsets have been identified, including cytotoxic T-cells, helper T-lymphocytes, and suppressor T-lymphocytes. T-cells may also be classified structurally by the distinctive molecules on their surface, known as *cluster designations (CDs).* Once mature, T-cells carry markers known as $T_2$ ($CD_2$), $T_3$ ($CD_3$), $T_5$ ($CD_5$), and $T_7$ ($CD_7$). Helper T-cells carry a $T_4$ ($CD_4$) marker and a suppressor, and cytotoxic T-cells carry a $T_8$ ($CD_8$) marker.

Specific functions of CMI include (1) protection against most viral, fungal, and protozoan infections and slow-growing bacterial infections, such as tuberculosis; (2) rejection of histoincompatible grafts; (3) mediation of cutaneous delayed hypersensitivity reactions, such as in tuberculin testing; and (4) probably immune surveillance for malignant cells. In addition, they also have regulatory functions within the immune system. For example, helper T-lymphocytes assist B-lymphocytes and other types of T-cells to mount an optimum immune response.

The cellular immune response is initiated when a T-lymphocyte is sensitized by antigen. In response to this contact, the T-cell releases numerous humoral factors called *lymphokines,* which eventually bring about death of the antigen. *Interferons* are a group of proteins secreted by leukocytes and infected host cells that nonspecifically inhibit viral replication, promote phagocytosis, and stimulate the killer activity of sensitized lymphocytes.

## Human Immunodeficiency Virus (HIV) Infection and Acquired Immunodeficiency Syndrome (AIDS)*

HIV infection and AIDS have generated intense medical investigation and even greater public concern and fear. In the early 1980s the first cases of AIDS were identified in adult males in urban coastal communities. As the epidemic has grown, HIV has affected a much broader social and geographic population; increasing proportions of AIDS cases are occurring among women and children.

Worldwide, it has been estimated that 16.4 million women and 1.4 million children less than 15 years of age are living with HIV/AIDS. In the year 2000 it was estimated that 600,000 children less than 15 years of age became newly infected with HIV. About 4.3 million children less than 15 years of age have died from AIDS since the beginning of the epidemic (UNAIDS, 2000).

As of June 2000, 8804 children less than 13 years of age with AIDS had been reported to the Centers for Disease Control and Prevention (CDC), representing less than 2% of the total number of AIDS cases in the United States to date (CDC, 2000). Ninety-one percent of these children acquired the disease perinatally from their mothers. An estimated 7000 infants are born to HIV-infected women in the United States each year. Without intervention, approximately 15% to 30% of these infants would be infected.

Between 1992 and 1996, the number of children with vertically acquired AIDS dropped 43% (CDC, 1998c).

However, children of minority populations in the United States are disproportionately affected by the HIV epidemic. Of the 8804 children with AIDS in 2000, 59% were African-American, 23% were Hispanic, and 18% were white. In 1998 HIV infection was the tenth leading cause of death among African-American children 1 to 4 years of age, the seventh leading cause of death among African-American children 5 to

■ *Nancy R. Calles, BSN, RN, ACRN, and Cara L. Simon, MSN, RN, CPNP, ACRN, revised this section.

14 years of age, and the sixth leading cause of death for African-Americans 15 to 24 years of age (National Vital Statistics Report, 2000).

Sexual contact and IV drug use are the major sources of HIV infection in adolescents. As of June 2000, 3865 adolescents 13 to 19 years of age and 26,518 young people from 20 to 24 years of age had been diagnosed with AIDS. Although this accounts for only 4% of the cumulative total of AIDS cases in the United States, HIV infection is the ninth leading cause of death in the United States for all races 15 to 24 years of age and the sixth leading cause of death for African-Americans 15 to 24 years of age (National Vital Statistics Report, 2000).

## Etiology

HIV is the primary cause of AIDS. There are different strains of HIV. HIV-2 is prevalent in Africa, whereas HIV-1 is the more common form in the United States and elsewhere. *Horizontal transmission* of HIV occurs through intimate sexual contact or parenteral exposure to blood or body fluids containing visible blood. *Vertical (perinatal) transmission* occurs when an HIV-infected pregnant woman passes the infection to her infant. There is no evidence that *casual* contact between infected and uninfected individuals can spread the virus.

The majority of children with HIV infection are less than 7 years of age. Children with HIV fall into three subpopulations: infants born to HIV-infected women, children who received infected blood products before the initiation of HIV screening in 1985, and adolescents infected as a result of high-risk behaviors.

Perinatal transmission accounts for 91% of the AIDS cases to date in children (CDC, 1999a). This is a direct consequence of the increasingly large number of infected women. The transmission of HIV can occur in utero, intrapartum, or after delivery through breast-feeding. Maternal risk factors (e.g., viral load, stage of disease) influence the rate of perinatal transmission, which can range from 15% to 30%. In 1994 results of clinical trials demonstrated a two-thirds decrease in perinatal transmission with zidovudine therapy for HIV-infected pregnant women and their newborns (Connor and others, 1994). Nevirapine, a nonnucleoside reverse transcriptase inhibitor, may be a particularly attractive option for preventing perinatal transmission of HIV in the developing world because of its ease of administration and low cost. The clinical trial, HIVNET 012, conducted in Kampala, Uganda, proved its effectiveness in reducing HIV transmission compared with zidovudine therapy (Owor and others, 2000). The Public Health Service issued recommendations in 1994 for zidovudine treatment to reduce perinatal HIV transmission (CDC, 1994), and the American Academy of Pediatrics (1995) recommended routine HIV counseling and voluntary testing for all pregnant women in the United States.

Transfusion of infected blood or blood products has accounted for 7% of pediatric AIDS cases to date (CDC, 1999a). Before donor blood was routinely tested for HIV in 1985, children with hemophilia were especially at risk because factor concentrates were prepared from pooled plasma. Since the initiation of donor blood screening, transfusion-associated HIV infection has become virtually nonexistent.

Sexual contact is the leading cause of exposure to HIV in the United States. In the pediatric population this is an infrequent route of transmission; a small number of children have been infected through sexual abuse. In contrast, sexual activity is a major cause of HIV infection in adolescents. Through June 2000, 3865 adolescents 13 to 19 years of age infected with HIV have been reported to the CDC (CDC, 1999a). This number represents only a fraction of those in this age-group who become infected with HIV. Given that the average period of time from HIV infection to the development of AIDS in adults is 10 years, most people in their twenties with AIDS were likely infected in their teen years. Adolescents commonly take risks and experiment; participation in high-risk behaviors, including IV drug use and unsafe sexual practices, increases their risk of becoming infected with HIV.

## Pathophysiology

HIV primarily infects a specific subset of T-lymphocytes, the $CD_4^+$ T-cells, but it can also invade cells of the monocyte-macrophage lineage. The virus takes over the machinery of the $CD_4^+$ lymphocyte, using it to replicate itself, rendering the $CD_4^+$ cell dysfunctional. Such suppression of cell-mediated immunity places a person at risk for opportunistic infections. HIV also causes dysfunction of B-cells and antigen-presenting cells, resulting in suppression of humoral immunity.

Although the course of HIV infection varies among individuals, a common progression of events has been recognized. Immediately after primary infection, there is dissemination of virus and seeding of lymphoid organs, along with a transient decrease in the number of $CD_4^+$ lymphocytes in peripheral blood. An immune response follows, and the resulting level of plasma virus is generally maintained for years. A period of clinical latency ensues that may be longer than 10 years in adults. The $CD_4^+$ lymphocyte count gradually decreases over time; at some point, physical symptoms appear. The count eventually reaches a critical level below which there is substantial risk of opportunistic illnesses followed by death.

A more rapid progression of disease is seen in perinatally infected children. This is primarily due to the naivete and immaturity of the developing immune system. Two general patterns of illness in children with perinatally acquired HIV infection have been observed. About 20% have an accelerated disease course, developing manifestations of AIDS in the first year of life; most of these children die by age 4 years. The remaining 80% have a slower rate of disease progression, many not developing manifestations of AIDS until school entry or even adolescence; these children survive to age 5 years and beyond (Katz, 1998).

## Clinical Manifestations

The majority of infants with perinatally acquired HIV infection are clinically normal during infancy, developing symptoms by 18 to 24 months of age. Clinical manifestations (Box 35-9) are varied. Diarrhea may be a result of pathogens or HIV itself. Malabsorption of carbohydrate, protein, and fat has been documented in both symptomatic and asymptomatic HIV-infected children (Castaldo and others, 1996). HIV-infected children often do not grow normally; they may be proportionally smaller in both length and weight for age.

The diagnosis of AIDS in children is based on the occurrence of certain illnesses or conditions (CDC, 1994). The most common AIDS-defining conditions observed among American children are listed in Box 35-10. Recurrent bacterial infections, parotitis, lymphoid interstitial pneumonitis (LIP), and early onset of progressive neurologic deterioration are characteristic of children with HIV infection but rarely seen in affected adults. Kaposi's sarcoma, one of the hallmarks of adult disease, is found in less than 1% of affected children. *Pneumocystis carinii* pneumonia (PCP), a frequent cause of death, is common in both age-groups.

Central nervous system abnormalities attributed to direct effects of HIV infection are seen in most children with AIDS. Secondary infections with opportunistic and common pathogens are infrequent in this population. Either global or specific neuropsychologic deficits may occur at random intervals. Many affected children display evidence of a developmental disability. Deficits in motor skills, communication, and behavioral functioning are common. Expressive language (use of language) is more frequently impaired than receptive language (understanding of language).

## Diagnostic Evaluation

For children 18 months of age and older, the HIV enzyme-linked immunosorbent assay (ELISA) and Western blot immunoassay are performed to determine HIV infection. In infants born to HIV-infected mothers, these assays will be positive because of the presence of maternal antibodies derived transplacentally. Maternal antibodies may persist in the infant up to 18 months of age. Therefore other diagnostic tests are employed: virus culture, polymerase chain reaction (PCR) for detection of proviral DNA, and p24 antigen detection, which is HIV-specific. With these techniques more than 95% of infected infants can be diagnosed by 1 to 3 months of age. Positive results on two separate tests performed on separate blood specimens are required for the diagnosis of HIV infection. Infants born to HIV-infected women are also considered HIV infected if they meet the CDC surveillance case definition for AIDS. Before testing, counseling should be provided to the parent or guardian, including an explanation of HIV infection, the reason for the test, implications of positive test results, confidentiality issues, risk reduction behaviors, and beneficial effects of early intervention.

The CDC (1994) has developed a classification system to describe the spectrum of HIV disease in children (Table 35-8). The system indicates the severity of clinical signs/symptoms and the degree of immunosuppression. Mild signs/symptoms include lymphadenopathy, parotitis, hepatosplenomegaly, and recurrent or persistent sinusitis or otitis media. Moderate signs/symptoms include lymphoid interstitial pneumonitis

---

**Box 35-9** ◼ ■ ▫
**Common Clinical Manifestations of HIV Infection in Children**

Lymphadenopathy
Hepatosplenomegaly
Oral candidiasis
Chronic or recurrent diarrhea
Failure to thrive
Developmental delay
Parotitis

---

**Box 35-10** ◼ ■ ▫
**Common AIDS-Defining Conditions in Children**

*Pneumocystis carinii* pneumonia
Lymphoid interstitial pneumonitis
Recurrent bacterial infections
Wasting syndrome
Candidal esophagitis
HIV encephalopathy
Cytomegalovirus disease
*Mycobacterium avium-intracellulare* complex infection
Pulmonary candidiasis
Herpes simplex disease
Cryptosporidiosis

---

**TABLE 35-8** Pediatric human immunodeficiency virus (HIV) classification*

| Immunologic Categories | Clinical Categories | | | |
| --- | --- | --- | --- | --- |
| | N: No Signs/Symptoms | A: Mild Signs/Symptoms | B: Moderate Signs/Symptoms† | C: Severe Signs/Symptoms† |
| No evidence of suppression | N1 | A1 | B1 | C1 |
| Evidence of moderate suppression | N2 | A2 | B2 | C2 |
| Severe suppression | N3 | A3 | B3 | C3 |

From Centers for Disease Control and Prevention: 1994 revised classification system for human immunodeficiency virus infection in children less than 13 years of age, *MMWR* 43(RR-12):1-10, 1994.
*Children whose HIV infection status is not confirmed are classified by using the above table with a letter E (for perinatally exposed) placed before the appropriate classification code (e.g., EN2).
†Both category C and lymphoid interstitial pneumonitis in category B are reportable to state and local health departments as aquired immunodeficiency syndrome.

(LIP) and a variety of organ-specific dysfunctions or infections. Severe signs/symptoms include AIDS-defining illnesses with the exception of LIP. Children with LIP have a better prognosis than those with other AIDS-defining illnesses.

The clinical and immunologic classification categories are mutually exclusive. Once classified, an infant or child may not be reclassified in a less severe category even if improvement in clinical or immunologic status occurs in response to antiretroviral therapy or other factors. In children whose HIV infection is not yet confirmed, the letter *E* (vertically exposed) is placed in front of the classification. The immune categories are based on $CD_4^+$ lymphocyte counts and percentages. Age adjustment of these numbers is necessary because normal counts, which are relatively high in infants, decline steadily until 6 years of age, when they reach adult norms (Table 35-9).

## Therapeutic Management

The goals of therapy for HIV infection include slowing the growth of HIV, promoting or restoring normal growth and development, preventing complicating infections and cancers, improving quality of life, and prolonging survival. ***Antiretroviral drugs*** work at various stages of the HIV life cycle to prevent reproduction of functional new virus particles. Antiretroviral therapy regimens are continually evolving. Classes of antiretroviral agents include nucleoside reverse transcriptase inhibitors (e.g., zidovudine, didanosine, stavudine, lamivudine, abacavir); nonnucleoside reverse transcriptase inhibitors (e.g., nevirapine, delavirdine, efavirenz); and protease inhibitors (e.g., indinavir, saquinavir, ritonavir, nelfinavir, amprenavir, lopinavir/ritonavir). Combinations of these drugs are being used more frequently to forestall the emergence of drug resistance, which has been observed in some children receiving a single drug. In addition, investigational drugs are available through pediatric clinical trials. Although not a cure, antiretroviral drugs can delay progression of the disease (MMWR, 2002).

Strict scheduling guidelines, side effects, and multiple medications, which at times are not very palatable, make it difficult for children and adolescents to take their medications at the right time and in proper coordination with their meals. Yet, adhering to the medication schedule is critical to preventing the development of resistant forms of HIV (CDC, 1998a; MMWR, 2002). Clinical improvements include weight gain in children with previous growth retardation, decreased hepatosplenomegaly, improvement in symptoms of HIV-associated encephalopathy, and improvement in immune system function.

PCP is the most common opportunistic infection of children infected with HIV. It occurs most frequently between 3 and 6 months of age, when HIV status may be indeterminate. Therefore, all infants born to HIV-infected women should receive prophylaxis during the first year of life according to guidelines set by the CDC. After 1 year of age, the need for prophylaxis is determined by the presence of severe immunosuppression or a history of PCP. Trimethoprim-sulfamethoxazole (TMP-SMZ) is the agent of choice. If adverse effects are experienced with this medication, dapsone or pentamidine may be used.

Prophylaxis is often employed for other opportunistic infections, such as disseminated *Mycobacterium avium-intracellulare* complex (MAC), candidiasis, and herpes simplex. IV immunoglobulin has been helpful in preventing recurrent or serious bacterial infections in some HIV-infected children; however, HIV-infected children who are already receiving PCP prophylaxis with TMP-SMX seem to derive little additional benefit from IV immunoglobulin (Spector and others, 1994).

Immunization against common childhood illnesses is recommended for all children exposed to and infected with HIV, including the pneumococcal and influenza vaccines. The varicella and measles-mumps-rubella (MMR vaccine) can be administered if there is no evidence of the presence of severe immunocompromise (CDC 1999b; CDC 1998b). Because antibody production to vaccines may be poor or decrease over time, immediate prophylaxis after exposure to several vaccine-preventable diseases (e.g., measles, varicella) is warranted. It should be recognized that children receiving IV gamma globulin prophylaxis may not respond to the MMR vaccine (American Academy of Pediatrics, 2000).

HIV infection often leads to marked failure to thrive and multiple nutritional deficiencies. Nutritional management may be difficult because of recurrent illness, diarrhea, and other physical problems. Intensive nutritional interventions should be instituted when the child's growth begins to slow or weight begins to decrease.

**Prognosis.**   Early recognition and improved medical care have changed HIV disease from a rapidly fatal to a chronic disease. Children diagnosed with AIDS, particularly as a result of PCP, in the first year of life are more likely to have a shorter life expectancy. Progressive encephalopathy

---

**TABLE 35-9**   Immunologic categories based on age-specific $CD_4^+$ T-lymphocyte counts, and percent of total lymphocytes

| | Age of Child | | | | | |
|---|---|---|---|---|---|---|
| | **<12 Months** | | **1-5 Years** | | **6-12 Years** | |
| **Immunologic Category** | $\mu l$ | **(%)** | $\mu l$ | **(%)** | $\mu l$ | **(%)** |
| No evidence of suppression | ≥1500 | (≥25) | ≥1000 | (≥25) | ≥500 | (≥25) |
| Evidence of moderate suppression | 750-1499 | (15-24) | 500-999 | (15-24) | 200-499 | (15-24) |
| Severe suppression | <750 | (<15) | <500 | (<15) | <200 | (<15) |

From Centers for Disease Control and Prevention: 1994 revised classification system for human immunodeficiency virus infection in children less than 13 years of age, *MMWR* 43(RR-12):1-10, 1994.

also carries a poor prognosis. In contrast, LIP is associated with a later onset of symptoms and prolonged survival.

## Nursing Considerations

Education concerning transmission and control of infectious diseases, including HIV infection, is essential for children with HIV infection and anyone involved in their care. The basic tenets of standard precautions should be presented in an age-appropriate manner, with careful consideration of the educational levels of the individuals. (See Infection Control, Chapter 27.) Safety issues, including appropriate storage of special medications and equipment (e.g., needles and syringes), are emphasized. Unfortunately, relatives, friends, and others in the general public are very fearful of contracting HIV infection, and criticism and ostracism of the child and family are common. In an effort to protect the child and deal with the community's fear, the family may limit the child's activities outside the home. Although certain precautions are justified in limiting exposure to sources of infections, they must be tempered with concern for the child's normal developmental needs. Both the family and the community need ongoing education about HIV to dispel many of the myths that have been perpetuated by uninformed persons.

Prevention is a key component of HIV education. Educating adolescents about HIV is essential in preventing HIV infection in this age-group. Education should include the routes of transmission, the hazards of IV and other recreational drug use, and the value of sexual abstinence and safe sex practices (AAP, 2001). Such education should be a part of anticipatory guidance provided to all adolescent patients. Nurses can also encourage adolescents at risk to undergo HIV counseling and testing. In addition to identifying infected teenagers and getting them into care, such counseling affords adolescents an opportunity to learn about, and possibly change, their risk behaviors. (See Human Immunodeficiency Virus Infection and Acquired Immunodeficiency Syndrome, Chapter 20.)

The nurse's role in the care of the child with HIV is multifaceted. (See Nursing Care Plan on pp. 1577-1578.) The nurse serves as educator, direct care provider, case manager, and advocate. As with all chronic illnesses, these children will have much involvement with the health care system. Clinic visits and hospitalizations may become frequent as the disease progresses. The physiologic care of the child is directed at minimum exposure to infections; delaying the development of viral resistance; nutritional support; comfort measures, including pain management; and assessment and recognition of changes in status that may indicate new complications. The scope of nursing care will change with new symptoms, changes in treatment, and disease progression. Psychologic interventions will vary with the unique circumstances of each child and family.

Common psychosocial concerns include disclosure of the diagnosis to the child, making custody plans when the parent is infected, and anticipating the loss of a family member. Other stressors may include financial difficulties, HIV-associated stigma, striving to keep the diagnosis a secret, other infected family members, and the multiple losses associated with HIV. Most mothers of these children are single mothers who are also HIV infected. As primary caretakers, they often attend to the needs of their child first, neglecting their own health in the process. The nurse can encourage the mother to receive regular health care. Family members are often involved in the care of the child, particularly if the mother has symptomatic illness. After the death of the mother, a grandparent or other relative typically assumes responsibility for the care of the child. Nursing can provide support and encouragement for the new surrogate parent, particularly during the transition phase. If no family member is available, the child may be placed in a foster or group home. Nursing is an integral part of the multidisciplinary team necessary for the successful management of the complex medical and social problems of these families.

The multiple complications associated with HIV disease are potentially painful. Hirschfeld and others (1996) documented a high prevalence of pain in children with HIV infection. Aggressive pain management is essential in order for these children to have an acceptable quality of life. Their pain may be due to infections (e.g., otitis media, dental abscess), encephalopathy (e.g., spasticity), adverse effects of medications (e.g., peripheral neuropathy), or an unknown source (e.g., deep musculoskeletal pain). Sources of pain are related not only to disease processes, but also to various treatments these children often undergo, including venipunctures, lumbar punctures, biopsies, and endoscopies. Ongoing assessment of pain is crucial and is most easily accomplished in older children who are able to communicate. Nonverbal and developmentally delayed children are more difficult to assess. Be alert for other signs of pain: emotional detachment, lack of interactive play, irritability, and depression. Effective pain management depends on the appropriate use of pharmacologic agents, including EMLA (eutectic mixture of local anesthetics) cream, acetaminophen, NSAIDs, muscle relaxants, and opioids. Tolerance to opioids may indicate increased dosing; monitored use ensures safety. Nonpharmacologic interventions (guided imagery, hypnosis, relaxation and distraction techniques) are useful adjuncts.

A major concern for both the family and the community has been school and daycare attendance for children with HIV infection. The American Academy of Pediatrics has published a policy statement (1999b) regarding issues related to HIV transmission in schools, child care settings, medical settings, the home, and the community. HIV-infected children should be admitted to health care settings and schools without restrictions and allowed to participate in all activities, including sports, to the extent that their health permits (American Academy of Pediatrics, 1999b). It is well established that the risk of HIV transmission in school settings is minimal. The CDC and World Health Organization's (WHO's) standard precautions guidelines should be followed in all child care settings and schools regardless of the incidence of HIV infection in the community (CDC, 1989). School nurses play a vital role in educating the public and in monitoring the needs of the affected child.

Confidentiality is another major issue in daycare or school attendance. Parents and legal guardians have the right to decide whether they inform a school or daycare agency of a child's HIV diagnosis.*

Nursing care of the child with *AIDS* is summarized in the Nursing Care Plan on pp. 1577-1578.

---

*Additional information is available from the **National Pediatric & Family HIV Resource Center,** 30 Bergen St, ADMC #4, Newark, NJ 07103, (973) 972-0410 or (800) 362-0071; www.pedihivaids.org; and from the **Baylor Pediatric AIDS Initiative,** Baylor College of Medicine, 6621 Fannin, Houston, TX 77030, (832) 824-1038, (877) 498-6497; www.bayloraids.org.

## Wiskott-Aldrich Syndrome

The Wiskott-Aldrich syndrome is a congenital X-linked recessive disorder characterized by a triad of abnormalities: (1) thrombocytopenia with small platelets, (2) eczema, and (3) immunodeficiency.

### Pathophysiology

The exact defect is unknown. A variety of pathologic findings are evident. The platelets are abnormally small in size and have a shortened life span, possibly because of a metabolic defect in their synthesis. The primary immunologic defect consists of the inability of phagocytes (macro-

---

# Nursing Care Plan
## The Child and Adolescent with HIV Infection

**NURSING DIAGNOSIS:** Risk for infection related to impaired body defenses, presence of infective organisms

**PATIENT GOAL 1:** Will experience minimized risk of infection

- **NURSING INTERVENTIONS/***RATIONALES*

Use thorough handwashing technique *to minimize exposure to infective organisms*

Advise visitors to use good handwashing technique *to minimize exposure to infective organisms*

Place child in room with noninfectious children or in private room

Restrict contact with persons who have infections, including family, other children, friends, and members of staff; explain that child is highly susceptible to infection *to encourage cooperation and understanding*

Observe medical asepsis as appropriate *to decrease risk of infection*

Encourage good nutrition and adequate rest *to promote body's remaining natural defenses*

Explain to family and older child importance of contacting health professional if exposed to childhood illnesses (e.g., chickenpox, measles) *so that appropriate immunizations can be given*

*Administer appropriate immunizations as prescribed *to prevent specific infections*

*Administer antibiotics as prescribed

- **EXPECTED OUTCOMES**

Child does not come in contact with infected persons or contaminated articles

Child and family apply good health practices

Child exhibits no evidence of infection

**PATIENT GOAL 2:** Will not spread disease to others

- **NURSING INTERVENTIONS/***RATIONALES*

Implement and carry out standard precautions *to prevent spread of virus* (see Infection Control, Chapter 27)

---

*Dependent nursing action.

Instruct others (e.g., family, members of staff) in appropriate precautions; clarify any misconceptions about communicability of virus, *since this is a frequent problem and may interfere with use of appropriate precautions*

Teach affected children protective methods *to prevent spread of infection,* (e.g., handwashing, handling genital area, care after using bedpan or toilet)

Endeavor to keep infants and small children from placing hands and objects in contaminated areas

Place restrictions on behaviors and contacts for affected children who bite or who do not have control of their bodily secretions

Assess home situation and implement protective measures as feasible in individual circumstances

- **EXPECTED OUTCOME**

Others do not acquire the disease

**NURSING DIAGNOSIS:** Imbalanced nutrition: less than body requirements related to recurrent illness, diarrheal losses, loss of appetite, oral candidiasis

**PATIENT GOAL 1:** Will receive optimum nourishment

- **NURSING INTERVENTIONS/***RATIONALES*

Provide high-calorie, high-protein meals and snacks *to meet body requirements for metabolism and growth*

Provide foods child prefers *to encourage eating*

Fortify foods with nutritional supplements (e.g., powdered milk or commercial supplements) *to maximize quality of intake*

Provide meals when child is most likely to eat well

Use creativity to encourage child to eat (see Feeding the Sick Child, Chapter 27)

Monitor child's weight and growth *so that additional nutritional interventions can be implemented if growth begins to slow or weight drops*

*Administer antifungal medication as ordered *to treat oral candidiasis*

*Administer appetite stimulants as ordered.

- **EXPECTED OUTCOME**

Child consumes a sufficient amount of nutrients (specify)

*Continued*

## Nursing Care Plan
### The Child and Adolescent with HIV Infection—cont'd

**NURSING DIAGNOSIS:** Impaired social interaction related to physical limitations, hospitalizations, social stigma toward HIV

**PATIENT GOAL 1:** Will participate in peer-group and family activities

- **NURSING INTERVENTIONS/*RATIONALES***

Assist child in identifying personal strengths *to facilitate coping*

Educate school personnel and classmates about HIV *so that child is not unnecessarily isolated*

Encourage child to participate in activities with other children and family

Encourage child to maintain phone contact with friends during hospitalization *to lessen isolation*

- **EXPECTED OUTCOME**

Child participates in activities with peer group and family

**NURSING DIAGNOSIS:** Ineffective sexuality patterns related to risk of disease transmission

**PATIENT GOAL 1:** Will exhibit healthy sexual behavior

- **NURSING INTERVENTIONS/*RATIONALES***

Educate adolescent about the following *so that adolescent has adequate information to identify safe, healthy expressions of sexuality*

Sexual transmission

Risks of perinatal infection

Dangers of promiscuity

Abstinence, use of condoms

Avoidance of high-risk behaviors

Encourage adolescent to talk about feelings and concerns related to sexuality *to facilitate coping*

- **EXPECTED OUTCOMES**

Adolescent exhibits a positive sexual identity

Adolescent does not infect other individuals

**NURSING DIAGNOSIS:** Chronic pain related to disease process (i.e., encephalopathy, treatments)

**PATIENT GOAL 1:** Will exhibit minimal or no evidence of pain or irritability

- **NURSING INTERVENTIONS/*RATIONALES***

Assess pain (see Pain Assessment, Chapter 26)

Use nonpharmacologic strategies *to help child manage pain*

For infants, may try general comfort measures (i.e., rocking, holding, swaddling, reducing environmental stimuli [may or may not be effective because of encephalopathy])

Use pharmacologic strategies (see Pain Management, Chapter 26)

Plan preventive schedule if analgesics are effective in relieving continuous pain

Encourage use of premedication for painful procedures *to minimize discomfort* (i.e., use of EMLA)

Child may benefit from use of adjunctive analgesics (e.g., antidepressants) that are effective against neuropathic pain

Use pain assessment record *to evaluate effectiveness of pharmacologic and nonpharmacologic interventions*

- **EXPECTED OUTCOME**

Child exhibits absence of or minimal evidence of pain or irritability

**NURSING DIAGNOSIS:** Interrupted family processes related to having a child with a dreaded and life-threatening disease

**PATIENT (FAMILY) GOAL 1:** Will receive adequate support and will be able to meet needs of child

- **NURSING INTERVENTIONS/*RATIONALES* AND EXPECTED OUTCOMES**

See Nursing Care Plan: The Family of the Child Who Is Ill or Hospitalized, Chapter 26

**NURSING DIAGNOSIS:** Anticipatory grieving related to having a child with a potentially fatal illness

See Nursing Care Plan: The Child Who Is Terminally Ill or Dying, Chapter 23

---

phages) to process foreign antigens, particularly polysaccharides such as pneumococci. As a result, immunologically competent cells fail to produce normal immunoglobulin patterns. Early in life the immunoglobulin levels may be normal, but later, reduced levels of IgM are observed, and elevated levels of IgG, IgA, and IgE (Baehner and Miller, 1995b; Bonilla, Rosen, and Geha, 1998). Typically isohemagglutinins (anti-A and anti-B agglutinins in the blood) are decreased or absent. Eczema is a result of a decrease in $CD_3$- and $CD_8$-positive T-suppressor lymphocytes (Baehner and Miller, 1995b).

The thymus and lymph nodes are normal at birth but become progressively dysfunctional with age until a profound cellular immunodeficiency results. Consequently these children are highly susceptible to infection and malignancy, especially lymphoma and leukemia.

## Clinical Manifestations

At birth the major effect of the disorder is bleeding because of the thrombocytopenia, especially bloody diarrhea, which may be the presenting feature (Bonilla, Rosen, and Geha, 1998). As the child grows older, recurrent infection and eczema become more severe, and the bleeding becomes less frequent.

Eczema is typical of the allergic type and readily becomes superinfected. Chronic infection with herpes simplex is a frequent problem and may lead to chronic keratitis with loss of vision. From infection, chronic pulmonary disease, sinusitis, and otitis media result. In those children who survive the bleeding episodes and overwhelming infections, malignancy presents an additional threat to survival.

## Diagnostic Evaluation

The diagnosis can usually be made during the neonatal period because of the thrombocytopenia. Specific tests for immunologic function confirm the diagnosis. Carrier detection is also possible.

## Therapeutic Management

Medical treatment primarily involves (1) counteracting the bleeding tendencies with platelet transfusions; (2) using IV immunoglobulin to provide passive immunity (Baehner and Miller, 1995b) (but it is ineffective in preventing platelet destruction [Beardsley and Nathan, 1998]); (3) administering prophylactic antibiotics to prevent and control infection; and (4) using aggressive local therapy for the eczema. Splenectomy may improve the platelet count, although the risk of asplenic sepsis in these infants is extremely high. These children require the same prophylactic antibiotic and appropriate immunizations as any child with asplenia. Despite their immune deficiency, they are able to mount an adequate immunologic response to the inactivated vaccines. When an HLA-matched donor exists, bone marrow transplantation is the treatment of choice.

## Nursing Considerations

Because of the poor prognosis for these children, the main nursing consideration is supporting the family in the care of a child with a life-threatening illness. (See Chapter 23.) Physical care is directed at controlling the problems imposed by the disorder. The measures used to control bleeding are similar to those used for hemophilia and von Willebrand disease (see earlier discussions). Another major goal is to prevent or control infection. Because eczema is a troublesome problem, nursing measures specific to this condition are especially important.

The genetic implications of this X-linked recessive disorder differ little from any other X-linked disorder. However, the multiplicity of defects tends to affect emotional adjustment and physical care to a greater degree than other X-linked disorders. The nurse can be especially supportive by providing short-term goals during periods of hospitalization and by focusing on long-range needs through coordinated efforts with a public health nurse.

# Severe Combined Immunodeficiency Disease (SCID)

SCID is a defect characterized by absence of both humoral and cell-mediated immunity (Champi, 2002). The terms *Swiss-type lymphopenic agammaglobulinemia*, an autosomal-recessive form of the disease, and *X-linked lymphopenic agammaglobulinemia* have been used to describe this disorder, which, as the names imply, can follow either mode of inheritance.

## Pathophysiology

The exact cause of SCID is unknown. The theories include (1) a defective stem cell that is incapable of differentiating into B- or T-cells; (2) defective organs responsible for the differentiating process, primarily the thymus and lymphoid complex; or (3) an enzymatic defect that suppresses lymphocytic cell function.

The consequence of the immunodeficiency is an overwhelming susceptibility to infection and to the *graft-vs-host reaction,* which can occur when any histoincompatible (unmatched) tissue from an immunocompetent donor is infused into the immunodeficient recipient. Because of its immunodeficiency, the body is unable to reject the foreign, incompatible tissue. Therefore the antigenic donor cells attack the host's tissues. The graft-vs-host reaction is a serious complication in the only known treatment for SCID, bone marrow transplantation.

## Clinical Manifestations

The most common manifestation is susceptibility to infection early in life, most often in the first month of life. Specifically, the disorder in children is characterized by chronic infection, failure to completely recover from an infection, frequent reinfection, and infection with unusual agents. In addition, the history reveals no logical source of infection. Failure to thrive is a consequence of the persistent illness.

If the child should receive a foreign tissue (e.g., blood supplements), signs of graft-vs-host reaction, such as fever, skin rash, alopecia, hepatosplenomegaly, and diarrhea, are expected. Because the reaction requires 7 to 20 days for tissue damage to become evident, the symptoms may be mistaken for an infection. However, the presence of a graft-vs-host reaction increases the child's susceptibility to overwhelming infection and therefore is a grave complication.

## Diagnostic Evaluation

Diagnosis is usually based on a history of recurrent, severe infections from early infancy, a familial history of the disorder, and specific laboratory findings, which include lymphopenia, lack of lymphocyte response to antigens, and absence of plasma cells in the bone marrow. Documentation of immunoglobulin deficiency is difficult during infancy because of the normally delayed response of infants to produce their own immunoglobulins and maternal transfer of immunoglobulin G.

## Therapeutic Management

The only definitive treatment is a histocompatible bone marrow transplant. The most suitable donor is a sibling with a matched HLA bone marrow. Because SCID is inherited, an identical twin, who usually is a perfect donor, is not a candidate because that offspring would also display the disorder. Mild to severe graft-vs-host reaction is seen in the majority of patients who undergo an HLA-matched bone marrow transplant (Champi, 2002).

Other approaches to SCID include providing passive immunity with IV immunoglobulin and maintaining the child in a sterile environment. The latter is effective only if it is instituted before the existence of any infectious process in the infant, and it represents an extreme effort to prevent life-threatening infections. Other investigational transplant procedures include nonidentical HLA bone marrow grafts and fetal liver or thymus transplants. However, the results are still uncertain, although they provide potential hope for future children born with the disorder.

## Nursing Considerations

Nursing care depends on the type of therapy used. If bone marrow transplantation is attempted, the care is consistent with that needed for bone marrow transplantation for any condition. (See Chapter 36.) To prevent infection, all interventions aimed at protecting the immunocompromised child are implemented (see Nursing Care Plan: The Child with HIV Infection, pp. 1577-1578). However, even with exacting environmental control, these children are prone to opportunistic infection. Chronic fungal infections of the mouth and nails with *Candida albicans* are frequent problems despite vigorous efforts at prevention or treatment. A hoarse voice may result from repeated esophageal and vocal cord erosions from the fungus. It is important to stress to parents that such conditions are not a result of laxity on their part in preventing them but are a result of the severe immunologic disorder. Parents should be encouraged to immediately notify a physician regarding any evidence of a worsening infection.

Because the prognosis for SCID is very poor if a compatible bone marrow donor is not available, nursing care is directed at supporting the family in caring for a child with a life-threatening illness. (See Chapter 23.) Genetic counseling is essential because of the modes of transmission in either form of the disorder.

## KEY POINTS

- Major functions of the hematologic system include production of cells, oxygenation, nutrient distribution to the cells, immune protection, and waste collection from the cells heat regulation.
- The major blood-forming organs of the body are red bone marrow, the lymphatic system, and the reticuloendothelial system.
- Anemia is defined as reduction of the RBCs and/or hemoglobin concentration compared with age-matched normal values. The disorders are classified either by etiology or by morphology.
- The nurse's role in treatment of anemia is to assist in establishing a diagnosis, prepare the child for laboratory tests, decrease tissue oxygen needs, implement safety precautions, and observe for complications.
- The main nursing goal in prevention of nutritional anemia is parent education regarding well-balanced meals.
- Four types of sickle cell crises are vaso-occlusive, splenic sequestration, aplastic, and hyperhemolytic.
- Nursing care of the child with sickle cell disease is aimed at family recognition and prevention of the sickling phenomena, managing pain during splenic crises, and helping the child and parents adjust to a lifelong, chronic disease.
- Nursing care of the child with thalassemia entails observing for complications of multiple blood transfusions, helping the child cope with the effects of illness, and fostering parent-child adjustment to long-term illness.
- Common causes of aplastic anemia are irradiation, drugs, industrial and household chemicals, infections, infiltration and replacement of myeloid elements, and idiopathic conditions.
- Nursing care of the child with hemophilia involves preventing bleeding by decreasing the risk of injury, recognizing and managing bleeding, preventing the crippling effects of joint degeneration, and preparing and supporting the child and family for home care.
- Henoch-Schönlein purpura is characterized by a nonthrombocytic purpura and variable joint and visceral abnormalities. Nursing care is primarily supportive, with observation for complications and provision of comfort being key nursing goals.
- Pediatric clinical manifestations of AIDS include failure to thrive, interstitial pneumonitis, and hepatosplenomegaly.

# REFERENCES

American Academy of Pediatrics: Perinatal human immunodeficiency virus testing, *Pediatrics* 95(2):303-307, 1995.

American Academy of Pediatrics: Pickering LK, editor: *2000 Red book: report of the Committee on Infectious Diseases*, ed 25, Elk Grove Village, IL, 2000, The Academy.

American Academy of Pediatrics, Committee on Nutrition: Iron fortification of infant formulas, *Pediatrics* 104(1):119-123, 1999a.

American Academy of Pediatrics, Committee on Pediatric AIDS and Committee on Adolescence: Adolescents and human immunodeficiency virus infection: the role of the pediatrician in prevention and intervention, *Pediatrics* 107(1):188-190, 2001.

American Academy of Pediatrics, Committee on Pediatric AIDS and Committee on Infectious Diseases: Issues related to human immunodeficiency virus transmission in school, child care, medical settings, the home, and community, *Pediatrics* 104(2):318-324, 1999b.

American Academy of Pediatrics, Section on Hematology/Oncology, Committee on Genetics: Health supervision for children with sickle cell disease, *Pediatrics* 109(3):526-535, 2002.

Andrews NC, Bridges KR: Disorders of iron metabolism and sideroblastic anemia. In Nathan DG, Orkin SH, editors: *Hematology of infancy and childhood*, ed 5, Philadelphia, 1998, WB Saunders.

Angelucci E and others: Hepatic iron concentration and total body iron stores in thalassemia major, *N Engl J Med* 343(5):327-331, 2000.

Bader-Meunier B and others: Long-term evaluation of the beneficial effect of subtotal splenectomy for management of hereditary spherocytosis, *Blood* 97(2):399-403, 2001.

Baehner RL, Miller DR: Disorders of granulopoiesis. In Miller DR, Baehner RL, editors: *Blood diseases of infancy and childhood*, ed 7, St Louis, 1995a, Mosby.

Baehner RL, Miller DR: Lymphocytes. In Miller DR, Baehner RL, editors; *Blood diseases of infancy and childhood*, ed 7, St Louis, 1995b, Mosby.

Beard J, Tobin B: Iron status and exercise, *Am J Clin Nutr* 72(suppl): 594S-597S, 2000.

Beardsley DS, Nathan DG: Platelet abnormalities in infancy and childhood. In Nathan DG, Orkin SH, editors: *Nathan and Oski's hematology of infancy and childhood*, ed 5, Philadelphia, 1998, WB Saunders.

Benz EJ, Giardinia PJV: Thalassemia syndromes. In Miller DR, Baehner RI, editors: *Blood diseases of infancy and childhood*, ed 7, St Louis, 1995, Mosby.

Beyer JE: Judging the effectiveness of analgesia for children and alolescents during vaso-occlusive events of sickle cell disease, *J Pain Symptom Manage* 19(1):63-72, 2000.

Bogen DL and others: Screening for iron deficiency anemia by dietary history in a high-risk population, *Pediatrics* 105(6):1254-1259, 2000.

Bolton-Maggs PHB: Idiopathic thrombocytopenic purpura, *Arch Dis Child* 83:220-222, 2000.

Bonilla FA, Rosen FS, Geha RS: Primary immunodeficiency diseases. In Nathan DG, Orkin SH, editors: *Nathan and Oski's hematology of infancy and childhood*, ed 5, Philadelphia, 1998, WB Saunders.

Boxer LA: Neutropenia. In Behrman RE, Kliegman RM, Jenson HB, editors: *Nelson textbook of pediatrics*, ed 16, Philadelphia, 2000, WB Saunders.

Brugnara C: Reference values in infancy and childhood. In Nathan DG, Orkin SH, editors: *Nathan and Oski's hematology of infancy and childhood*, ed 5, Philadelphia, 1998, WB Saunders.

Buchanan GR: The tragedy of iron deficiency during infancy and early childhood, *J Pediatr* 135(4):413-415, 1999.

Buzzard BM: Sports and hemophilia, *Clin Orthop* 328:25-30, 1996.

Castaldo A and others: Iron deficiency and intestinal malabsorption in HIV disease, *J Pediatr Gastroenterol Nutr* 22(4):359-363, 1996.

Catlin AJ: Commentary on Johnny's story: transfusing a Jehovah's Witness, *Pediatr Nurs* 23(3):289-290, 1997.

Centers for Disease Control and Prevention: Guidelines for the prevention of transmission of human immunodeficiency virus and hepatitis B virus to health-care workers and public-safety workers, *MMWR* 38(S-6), 1989.

Centers for Disease Control and Prevention: Guidelines for the use of anti-retroviral agents in HIV-infected adults and adolescents, *MMWR* 47(RR-5):42-82, 1998a.

Centers for Disease Control and Prevention: *HIV/AIDS surveillance report* 11(1):1999a.

Centers for Disease Control and Prevention: *HIV/AIDS surveillance report* 12(1):2000.

Centers for Disease Control and Prevention: Guidelines for using anti-retroviral agents among HIV-infected adults and adolescents, *MMWR* 51(RR-7):1-55, 2002.

Centers for Disease Control and Prevention: Measles, mumps, and rubella vaccine use and strategies for elimination of measles, rubella, and congenital rubella syndrome and control of mumps: recommendations of the Advisory Committee on Immunization Practices (ACIP), *MMWR* 47(RR-8):21, 1998b.

Centers for Disease Control and Prevention: 1994 revised classification system for human immunodeficiency virus infection in children less than 13 years of age, *MMWR* 43(RR-12):1-10, 1994.

Centers for Disease Control and Prevention: *Trends in the HIV/AIDS epidemic*, Atlanta, GA, 1998c, Department of Health and Human Services.

Centers for Disease Control and Prevention: Prevention of varicella: updated recommendations of the Advisory Committee on Immunization Practices (ACIP), *MMWR* (RR-6):1-5, 1999b.

Champi, C: Primary immunodeficiency disorders in children: prompt diagnosis can lead to lifesaving treatment, *J Pediatr Health Care* 16(1):16-21, 2002.

Charache S and others: Hydroxyurea and sickle cell anemia: clinical utility of a myelosuppresive switching agent, *Medicine* 75(6):300-326, 1996.

Chiocca EM: Sickle cell crisis: severe pain and potential tissue necrosis are the major concerns, *Am J Nurs* 96(9):49, 1996.

Chu Y-W, Korb J, Sakamoto KM: Idiopathic thrombocytopenic purpura, *Pediatr Rev* 21(3):95-104, 2000.

Claster S, Vichinsky E: First report of reversal of organ dysfunction in sickle cell anemia by the use of hydroxyurea: splenic regeneration, *Blood* 88(6):1951-1953, 1996.

Conner EM and others: Reduction of maternal-infant transmission of human immunodeficiency virus type 1 with zidovudine treatment, *N Engl J Med* 331(18):1173-1180, 1994.

Cordoni A: von Willebrand's disease: diagnosis and treatment, *Am J Nurse Pract* 9-16, 2000.

Covitz W and others: The heart in sickle cell anemia: the cooperative study of sickle cell disease (CSSCD), *Chest* 108(5):1214-1219, 1995.

Cross S, Koerper M: Symposium report: prophylaxis in hemophilia—primary, secondary, and beyond, *Hemaware* 2(2):7-12, 34, 1997.

Day SW, Wynn LW: Sickle cell pain and hydroxyurea, *Am J Nurs* 100(11):34-39, 2000.

Delhommeau F and others: Natural history of hereditary spherocytosis during the first year of life, *Blood* 95(2):393-397, 2000.

DiMichele D, Neufeld EJ: Hemophilia, a new approach to an old disease, *Hematol Oncol Clin North Am* 12(6):1315-1344, 1998.

Dinauer MC: The phagocyte system and disorders of granulopoiesis and granulocyte function. In Nathan DG, Orkin SH, editors: *Nathan and Oski's hematology of infancy and childhood,* ed 5, Philadelphia, 1998, WB Saunders.

Dixon LR: The complete blood count: physiologic basis and clinical usage, *J Perinatal Neonatal Nurs* 11(3):1-18, 1997.

Dover GJ, Platt OS: Sickle cell disease. In Nathan DG, Orkin SH, editors: *Nathan and Oski's hematology of infancy and childhood,* ed 5, Philadelphia, 1998, WB Saunders.

Dragone MA, Karp S: Bleeding disorders. In Jackson PL, Vessey JA, editors: *Primary care of the child with a chronic condition,* St Louis, 1996, Mosby.

Drake EE: Anemia. In Fox JA, editor: *Primary health care of children,* St Louis, 1997, Mosby.

Felt BT, Lozoff B: Brain iron and behavior of rats are not normalized by treatment of iron deficiency anemia during early development, *J Nutr* 126(3):693-701, 1996.

Frewin R, Henson A, Provan D: ABC of clinical haematology: iron deficiency anaemia, *Br Med J* 314(7090):1333-1336, 1997.

Gribbons D, Zahr LK, Opas SR: Nursing management of children with sickle cell disease: an update, *J Pediatr Nurs* 10(4):232-242, 1995.

Halterman JS and others: Iron deficiency and cognitive achievement among school-aged children and adolescents in the United States, *J Pediatr* 107(6):1381-1386, 2001.

Hendricks-Ferguson VL, Nelson M: Update of the health care management needs of infants with sickle cell disease, *J Pediatr Health Care* 13(5):217-222, 1999.

Hilgartner MW, Corrigan JJ: Coagulation disorders. In Miller DR, Baehner RL, editors: *Blood diseases of infancy and childhood,* ed 7, St Louis, 1995, Mosby.

Hirschfield and others: Pain in pediatric human immunodeficiency virus infection: incidence and characteristics in a single-institution pilot study, *Pediatrics* 98(3):449-452, 1996.

Jayabose S and others: Clinical and hematologic effects of hydroxyurea in children with sickle cell anemia, *J Pediatr* 129(4):559-565, 1996.

Jonides LK: Infant with a purpuric rash, *J Pediatr Health Care* 10(3):139, 147-148, 1996.

Katz LS: Immunizations for HIV-infected children. In Pizzo PA, Wilfert CM, editors: *Pediatric AIDS: the challenge of HIV in infants, children, and adolescents,* Baltimore, Maryland, 1998 Lippincott.

Khoury H, Grimsley E: Oxygen inhalation in nonhypoxic sickle cell patients during vasoocclusive crisis, *Blood* 86(10):3998, 1995.

Kline NE: A practical approach to the child with anemia, *J Pediatr Health Care* 10(3):99-105, 1996.

Kline NE, Mooney KH: Alterations in hematologic function in children. In McCance KL, Huether SE, editors: *Pathology: the biological basis for disease in adults and children,* ed 2, St Louis, 1998, Mosby.

Koshy M and others: Surgery and anesthesia in sickle cell disease, *Blood* 86(10):3676-3684, 1995.

Kwiatkowski JL and others: Severe iron deficiency anemia in young children, *J Pediatr* 135(4):514-516, 1999.

Labovich TM: Transfusion therapy: nursing implications, *Clin J Oncol Nurs* 1(3):61-72, 1997.

Lane PA: Sickle cell disease, *Pediatr Hematol* 43(3):639-664, 1996.

Lanzkowsky P: *Manual of pediatric hematology and oncology,* ed 3, San Diego, 2000, Academic Press.

Lemanek KL, Steiner SM, Grossman NJ: Too little, too late: primary vs. secondary interventions for adolescents with sickle cell disease, *Adolesc Med* 10(3):385-400, 1999.

Levin TL and others: MRI marrow observations in thalassemia: the effects of the primary disease, transfusional therapy, and chelation, *Pediatr Radiol* 25(8):607-613, 1995.

Lozoff B and others: Poorer behavioral and developmental outcome more than 10 years after treatment for iron deficiency in infancy, *Pediatrics* 105(4):1-11, 2000.

Lubin NLC: Blood groups and blood component transfusion. In Miller DR, Baehner RL, editors: *Blood diseases of infancy and childhood,* ed 7, St Louis, 1995, Mosby.

Manucci and others: Treatment of von Willebrand disease with a high-purity factor VIII/von Willebrand factor concentrate: a prospective, multicenter study, *Blood* 99(2):450-456, 2002.

McNeil SB: Johnny's story: transfusing a Jehovah's Witness, *Pediatr Nurs* 23(3):287-288, 1997.

Miller DR: Erythropoiesis, hypoplastic anemias, and disorders of heme synthesis. In Miller DR, Baehner RL, editors: *Blood diseases of infancy and childhood,* ed 7, St Louis, 1995, Mosby.

Murphy S, Nepo A, Sills R: Thrombocytopenia, *Pediatr Rev* 20(2):64-68, 1999.

National Hemophilia Foundation and American Red Cross: *Hemophilia sports and exercise,* New York, 1996, National Hemophilia Foundation.

National Vital Statistics Report: Deaths: final data for 1998, *Natl Vital Stat Rep* 48(11):2000.

Olivieri NF: The B-thalassemias, *N Engl J Med* 341(2):99-109, 1999.

Olivieri NF, Brittenham GM: Iron-chelating therapy and the treatment of thalassemia, *Blood* 89(3):739-761, 1997.

Olivieri NF, Vichinsky EP: Hydroxyurea in children with sickle cell disease: impact on splenic function and compliance with therapy, *J Pediatr Hematol Oncol* 20(1):26-31, 1998.

Orkin SH, Nathan DG: The thalassemias. In Nathan DG, Orkin SH, editors: *Nathan and*

*Oski's hematology of infancy and childhood,* ed 5, Philadelphia, 1998, WB Saunders.

Owor M and others: *The one-year safety and efficacy data of the HIVNET 012 trial.* Program and Abstracts for the XIII International AIDS Conference, Durban, South Africa, July 2000. Abstract LbOrl.

Panepinto JA and others: Universal versus targeted screening of infants for sickle cell disease: a cost-effectiveness analysis, *J Pediatr* 136(2):201-208, 2000.

Pappas DE, Cheng TL: Iron deficiency anemia, *Pediatr Rev* 19(9):321-322, 1998.

Pavlovich-Danis S: Update on von Willebrand's disease, *Clin Advisor* Nov-Dec:28-32, 37-39, 2001.

Pitcher LA and others: Improved prognosis for acquired aplastic anaemia, *Arch Dis Child* 80(2):158-162, 1999.

Platt OS, Guinan EC: Bone marrow transplantations in sickle cell anemia: the dilemma of choice, *N Engl J Med* 335(6):426-427, 1996.

Platt OS: The acute chest syndrome of sickle cell disease, *N Engl J Med* 342(25):1904-1907, 2000.

Sackey K: Hemolytic anemia, part I, *Pediatr Rev* 20(5):152-208, 1999.

Sanders TAB: Vegetarian diets and children, *Pediatr Clin North Am* 42(4):955-965, 1995.

Simon K, Lobo ML, Jackson S: Current knowledge in the management of children and adolescents with sickle cell disease. I. Physiological issues, *J Pediatr Nurs* 14(5):281-295, 1999.

Smith PS and others: Episodic versus prophylactic infusions for hemophilia A: a cost-effectiveness analysis, *J Pediatr* 129(3):424-431, 1996.

Spector SA and others: A controlled study of the intravenous immunoglobulin for the prevention of serious bacterial infections in children receiving zidovudine for advanced human immunodeficiency virus infection, *N Engl J Med* 331(18):1181, 1994.

Sporrer KA and others: Pain in children and adolescents with sickle cell anemia: a prospective study utilizing self-reporting, *Pain Med J Club J* 191:31-33, 1995.

Steinberg MH: Management of sickle cell disease, *N Engl J Med* 340(13):1021-1030, 1999.

Tizard EJ: Henoch-Schonlein purpura, *Arch Dis Child* 80(4):380-383, 1999.

Tolis GJ, Viachopapadopoulou E, Karydis I: Reproductive health in patients with beta thalassemia, *Curr Opin Pediatr* 8(4):406-410, 1996.

United Nations Programme on HIV/AIDS (UNAIDS)/World Health Organization (WHO): *AIDS epidemic update: 2000,* Geneva, 2000, UNAIDS/WHO.

Vichinsky E, Styles L: Sickle cell disease: pulmonary complications, *Hematol Oncol Clin North Am* 10(6):1275-1287, 1996.

Vichinsky EP and others: A comparison of conservative and aggressive transfusion regimens in the perioperative management of sickle cell disease, *N Engl J Med* 332(4):206-213, 1995.

Vichinsky EP and others: Causes and outcomes of the acute chest syndrome in sickle cell disease, *N Engl J Med* 342(25): 1855-1866, 2000.

Walters MC and others: Bone marrow transplantation for sickle cell disease, *N Engl J Med* 335(6):369-376, 1996.

Wethers DL: Sickle cell disease in childhood. II. Diagnosis and treatment of major complications and recent advances in treatment, *Am Fam Physician* 62(6):1309-1314, 2000.

Worrall LM, Tompkins CA, Rust DM: Recognizing and managing anemia, *Clin J Oncol Nurs* 3(4):153-160, 1999.

Yaster M, Kost-Byerly S, Maxwell LG: The management of pain in sickle cell disease, *Pediatr Clin North Am* 47(3):699-710, 2000.

# Chapter 36

## The Child with Cancer

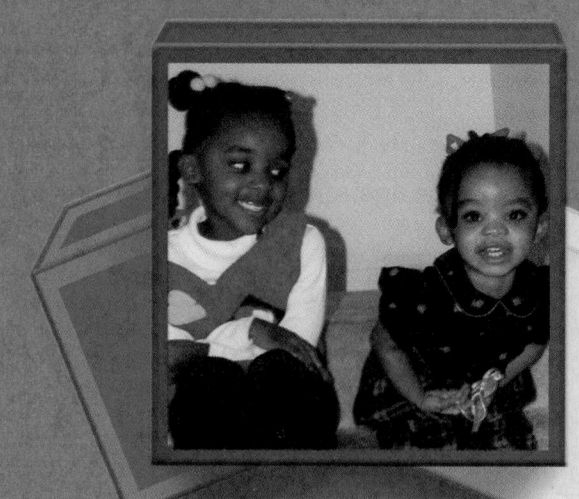

## Chapter Outline

**CANCER IN CHILDREN, 1584**
**Etiologic Factors, 1585**
  Prevention, 1586
**Diagnostic Evaluation, 1587**
  Complete History, 1587
  Review of Symptoms, 1587
  Physical Examination, 1587
  Laboratory Tests, 1587
  Imaging Studies, 1587
  Biopsy, 1587
**Modes of Therapy, 1588**
  Surgery, 1588
  Chemotherapy, 1588
  Radiation Therapy, 1594
  Biologic Response Modifiers (BRMs), 1594
  Bone Marrow Transplantation (BMT), 1595
**Complications of Therapy, 1596**
  Pediatric Oncologic Emergencies, 1596

**NURSING CARE OF THE CHILD WITH CANCER, 1597**

Assessment, 1597
  Signs and Symptoms of Cancer in
    Children, 1597
**Nursing Diagnoses, 1597**
**Planning, 1598**
**Implementation, 1598**
  Managing Side Effects of Treatment, 1598
  Nursing Care During Bone Marrow
    Transplantation (BMT), 1602
  Preparation for Procedures, 1603
  Pain Management, 1604
  Health Promotion, 1604
  Family Education, 1605
  Cessation of Therapy, 1606
**Evaluation, 1606**
*Nursing Care Plan: The Child with Cancer, 1606*

**CANCERS OF THE BLOOD AND LYMPH SYSTEMS, 1610**
**Leukemias, 1610**
**Lymphomas, 1616**

**Hodgkin Disease, 1616**
**Non-Hodgkin Lymphoma (NHL), 1618**

**NERVOUS SYSTEM TUMORS, 1619**
**Brain Tumors, 1619**
**Neuroblastoma, 1625**

**BONE TUMORS, 1626**
**General Considerations, 1626**
**Osteogenic Sarcoma, 1627**
**Ewing Sarcoma (Primitive Neuroectodermal
  Tumor [PNET] of the Bone), 1628**

**OTHER SOLID TUMORS, 1629**
**Wilms Tumor, 1629**
**Rhabdomyosarcoma, 1631**
**Retinoblastoma, 1632**
**Testicular Tumors, 1635**

**THE CHILDHOOD CANCER SURVIVOR, 1635**
**Long-Term Sequelae of Treatment, 1635**

## Related Topics

Administration of Medication, Ch. 27
Anaphylaxis, Ch. 29
Anemia, Ch. 35
Biologic Development (Adolescence), Ch. 19
Bone Marrow Aspiration/Biopsy, Ch. 27
The Child with Cerebral Dysfunction, Ch. 37
Dental Health, Ch. 14
Drug Reactions, Ch. 18

Epistaxis (Nosebleeding), Ch. 35
Family-Centered Care of the Child During
  Illness and Hospitalization, Ch. 26
Family-Centered Care of the Child with
  Chronic Illness or Disability, Ch. 22
Family-Centered End-of-Life Care, Ch. 23
Immunizations, Ch. 12
Infection Control, Ch. 27

Lumbar Puncture, Ch. 27
Pain Assessment; Pain Management, Ch. 26
Physical Examination, Ch. 7
Preparation for Procedures, Ch. 27
Stomatitis, Ch. 16
Sunburn, Ch. 18
Surgical Procedures, Ch. 27
Venous Access Devices, Ch. 28

## CANCER IN CHILDREN

There are few situations in nursing that exceed the challenges of caring for a child with cancer. Despite the dramatic improvements in survival rates for these children, the needs of the family are tremendous as they cope with

a serious physical illness, as well as the fear that the child will not be cured. Support of the patients and their families should be based on the premise that communication promotes understanding and clarity; with understanding, fear diminishes; in the absence of fear, hope emerges; and in the presence of hope, anything is possible (Stovall, 1995).

■ Rosalind Bryant, MN, RN-CS, PNP, revised this chapter.

**TABLE 36-1**   Most common forms of childhood malignancy with incidence in the United States and peak age at diagnosis

| Malignancy | Peak Age (y) | Rate (million/y) |
|---|---|---|
| Leukemia | | |
|   Acute lymphocytic | 2-5 | 24.7 |
|   Acute nonlymphocytic | Constant | 5.0 |
| Lymphomas | | |
|   Non-Hodgkin | 6-16 | 9.3 |
|   Hodgkin | >10 | 7.5 |
| CNS tumors | | |
|   Gliomas | Constant | 13.4 |
|   Medulloblastomas | 5-10 | 4.9 |
|   Ependymoma | <5 | 2.1 |
| Solid tumors | | |
|   Neuroblastoma | <3 | 8.0 |
|   Wilms tumor | <5 | 6.9 |
|   Retinoblastoma | <3 | 3.0 |
|   Rhabdomyosarcoma | 2-6 and 14-18 | 3.7 |
|   Ewing sarcoma/PNET | 10-18 | 2.1 |
|   Osteosarcoma | 10-18 | 3.1 |
|   Hepatoblastoma | <2 | 1.6 |
|   Germ cell tumors | <2 and >14 | 0.4 |

From Herrera JM and others: Childhood tumors, *Surg Clin North Am* 80(2):748, 2000.

This chapter is concerned primarily with the physical problems associated with several types of childhood cancer. The general psychologic needs of these children and their families are discussed in Chapter 22 in terms of chronic illness and in Chapter 23 for situations when the outcome becomes life-threatening and death is a possibility.

Childhood cancer is the second leading cause of death in children ages 1 to 14 years (Greenlee and others, 2000; Parker and others, 1997). The incidence of cancer in this age-group is approximately 129 per million children (Gurney and Bondy, 2002). The projected number of new cases is an estimated 8200 per year in the United States, with an estimated 1600 deaths per year (Parker and others, 1997). A 15% increased incidence in cancer among infants, consisting of central nervous system (CNS) tumors, neuroblastoma, retinoblastoma, and teratomas, was identified in a study by Kenney and others (1998), which may account for the rise in new cases.

During childhood there are changing incidences for various types of cancer. For children in all pediatric age-groups, leukemia is the most frequent type of cancer, followed by brain tumors and lymphomas (Table 36-1). Tumors of the kidney and soft tissue are more common in African-Americans, whereas tumors of the bone are more common in whites. Males are affected more often by cancer than females (ratio of 1.2:1), although this varies with the type of cancer. This is accounted for by an increased risk among young males for acute lymphoid leukemia, lymphoma, and medulloblastoma (Gurney and Bondy, 2002).

Probably the most significant aspect of childhood cancer is the improved prognosis during the last 3 decades. Mor-

tality among children with cancer has declined from 8.8 per 100,000 in 1950 to 2.9 per 100,000 in 1993 (Parker and others, 1997). Currently, more than 75% of all children with malignant neoplasms treated at major cancer centers will now survive more than 5 years (Greenlee and others, 2000; Lanzkowsky, 2000; Parker and others, 1997). The cancers demonstrating the greatest improvement in survival rates are acute leukemia, lymphomas, Wilms tumor, rhabdomyosarcoma, osteosarcoma, and Ewing sarcoma. However, African-American children with cancer do more poorly than white children (Parker and others, 1997).

Although survival is discussed in terms of "cure," the term *biologic cure* is not absolute because it is not possible to demonstrate definitively complete eradication of all cancer cells, and late recurrences do occur. The definition of cure includes the criteria of (1) cessation of therapy, (2) continuous freedom from clinical and laboratory evidence of cancer, and (3) minimum or no risk of relapse, as determined by previous experience with the disease. The time that must elapse before a child clinically free of cancer is considered cured varies with each type of cancer but typically ranges from 2 to 5 years.

## Etiologic Factors

The cause of cancer is not known. Although there are numerous hypotheses concerning its origin, the most enduring theory is that some genetic alteration results in the unregulated proliferation of cells. Recent studies have demonstrated the existence of genes activated in human tumors that are capable of causing uncontrolled proliferation of cells when transmitted to normal cells.

The retinoblastoma (RB) gene is an example of the role genes can play in the development of cancer. Like most genes, the RB gene is present in two copies on each cell and is responsible for controlling cell growth. When just one of these copies is lost, the cell remains normal. However, when the second copy is lost, abnormal cell proliferation occurs and retinoblastoma develops (Lanzkowsky, 2000; MacDonald and Lessick, 2000).

Some childhood cancers, in particular retinoblastoma, Wilms tumor, and neuroblastoma, may demonstrate patterns of inheritance that suggest a genetic basis for the disorder. The Philadelphia chromosome was the first chromosome abnormality to be found in a malignancy. It occurs as a result of a translocation between chromosomes 9 and 22 and is observed in almost all individuals with chronic myelogenous leukemia (Altman, 2002; Grier and Civin, 1998). Chromosome abnormalities have also been found in children with acute leukemia and lymphoma as well as numerous pediatric solid tumors (Look and Kirsch, 2002). Bilateral Wilms tumor is associated with an increased incidence of congenital anomalies, which include aniridia, hemihypertrophy, and urogenital anomalies (Green and others, 1996; Lanzkowsky, 2000). In addition, children with certain types of chromosome abnormalities, especially those syndromes caused by abnormal numbers of chromosomes, have an increased incidence of cancer. For example, in children with Down syndrome the probability of developing leukemia is about 20 times greater than in the general population (Plon and Malkin, 2002; Taub, 2001). Other chromosome syndromes associated with a predisposition to cancer are Fanconi syndrome (a deficiency of all cellular elements of the blood), Bloom syndrome (dwarfism and skin changes), ataxia-telangiectasia (progressive cerebellar ataxia and oculocutaneous vascular lesions), Klinefelter syndrome, and nevoid basal cell sarcoma syndrome.

Children with immune deficiencies, such as Wiskott-Aldrich syndrome or acquired immunodeficiency syndrome (AIDS), or children whose immune system has been suppressed, such as following transplant procedures, are at a greater risk for developing various cancers. Of major concern is the increased risk of secondary cancers in some children successfully treated for their primary malignancy.

Population studies of siblings and offspring of children with cancer suggest that there is not, in general, a strong constitutional genetic component for childhood cancers other than retinoblastoma (Buckley and others, 1996; MacDonald, and Lessick, 2000).

Genes having the potential to transform normal cells into malignant ones are called *oncogenes.* What causes the induction of cell transformation is speculative, but RNA tumor viruses (also called *retroviruses* because they have the ability to translate RNA back to DNA) may play a role in the transfer of DNA from a malignant cell to a normal cell (Kennedy and others, 1996). The Epstein-Barr virus (EBV) has been found to be involved in the pathogenesis of a significant number of cases of childhood Hodgkin disease (Flavell and Murray, 2000; Lanzkowsky, 2000).

Despite the lack of knowledge about the origin of cancer, there is considerable information on risk factors that increase the likelihood of children developing specific types of cancer. The following is a brief overview of some of the etiologic factors implicated in childhood cancer.

Several environmental agents that are *carcinogenic* (capable of producing cancer) in adults have been described, but only one of these—ionizing radiation—has been implicated in children. Low doses of radiation have been known to cause thyroid cancer and leukemia. There is some evidence that exposing pregnant women to diagnostic radiographic procedures increases the occurrence of leukemia and other forms of cancer among their children (Wakeford, 1995).

The overall percentage of childhood cancers that are clearly inherited disorders or caused by significant environmental exposure is low. Genetic alterations that have been passed on to the child from the parents have been seen in families of children with cancer. Optic glioma and retinoblastoma have the highest inherited rates (MacDonald and Lessick, 2000).

Exposure to power lines as a causative factor in the development of childhood leukemia has been a subject of controversy in the past few years. Recent studies have found marginally significant relationships between cancer and electromagnetic exposure (Schuz and others, 2001; Thomas and others, 1999). However, future studies are necessary to further identify the seriousness of the risk.

Although drugs, particularly those containing radioisotopes and immunosuppressive agents, can increase the risk of developing childhood cancer, the one drug most notably recognized for its carcinogenic effect is diethylstilbestrol. Large doses of this hormone given to pregnant women to prevent abortion cause adenocarcinoma of the vagina in a significant proportion of the female offspring when they reach adolescence and early adulthood (Zahm and Devesa, 1995).

Other factors associated with increased risk of cancer are parental occupational exposures to chemicals, solvents, paints, and pesticides; maternal alcohol use; cigarette smoking during pregnancy; and maternal history of prior fetal loss (Bhatia and others, 2001; Freedman and others, 2001; Schneider and Freeman, 2001).

There is much interest in discovering if certain foods or nutrients provide protection against cancer in children. Some studies have suggested that breast-feeding longer than 6 months provides protection against certain leukemias and lymphomas (Bener, Denic and Galadari, 2001; Shu and others, 1999). Some aspects of the maternal diet, especially early prenatal multivitamin use, may have a role in preventing primitive neuroectodermal tumors, such as medulloblastoma, in young children (Thorne and others, 1994). This finding is especially intriguing in light of the association between supplemental doses of folic acid and the reduced risk of neural tube defects. (See Spina Bifida/Myelodysplasia, Chapter 11.) The neural tube is lined with neuroepithelial cells, which are the precursor cells of primitive neuroectodermal tumors.

## Prevention

Knowledge of the risk factors that increase the likelihood of cancer holds the promise of prevention. Unfortunately, in children the known carcinogens are limited to radiation and a few drugs given to the mother during pregnancy. Therefore at present there is really no known prevention.

Health professionals do have two roles, however. One is aimed at preventing adult type of cancers by educating parents and children about the hazards of known carcinogens, particularly the effects of cigarette smoking and excessive exposure to sunlight. Lung cancer is the leading cause of death from cancer in adults, and malignant melanoma is the leading cause of death from diseases of the skin. Children at higher risk for skin cancer are those with light-colored eyes, complexion, and hair; those who sunburn easily; and those who live near the equator (Loescher and others, 1995). Not only these children but all children should be protected from overexposure to the sun. (See Chapter 18.) In addition, to provide early detection of other types of cancer, males should be taught testicular self-examination; female adolescents should be taught breast self-examination and be encouraged to seek periodic health examinations, including a Papanicolaou (Pap) smear.*

---

*Information on self-instructional materials on testicular and breast self-examination is available from the local chapters of the **American Cancer Society, Inc,** or the national office, 1599 Clifton NE Rd, Atlanta, GA 30329, (404) 320-3333 (headquarters), (800) ACS-2345 (for general cancer information); www.cancer.org.

Second, health care professionals need to be aware of the cardinal symptoms of childhood cancer (see Box 36-1). Unfortunately, fever and pain are manifestations of common childhood disorders, and without a high index of suspicion, they may be attributed to minor ailments. The other signs are subtle and easily missed. If parents suspect an abnormality, their concerns must be taken seriously. The greatest weapons against all forms of cancer are early detection and treatment.

## Diagnostic Evaluation

The evaluation of a child suspected of having cancer may take several days to complete. Signs and symptoms depend on the type of cancer and its location. The following are essential components of a comprehensive evaluation for childhood cancer.

### Complete History

**History of present illness**—Onset of symptoms, severity and duration, alleviating or potentiating factors

**History of previous illnesses**—Communicable diseases, infections, previous hospitalizations or surgeries, exposure to blood products, immunization status

**Family history**—Previous family members with cancer: type, treatment, and outcome

**Present health status of family members**—History of illness or disease in other family members

**Developmental**—Milestones obtained, recent regression in any milestones

**Psychosocial**—Include family concerns or problems

### Review of Symptoms

**Skin**—History of bruising or bleeding, lesions or sores (leukemia)

**Head, eyes, ears, nose, and throat (HEENT)**—History of infection, proptosis, pupil discoloration, eye muscle weakness (neuroblastoma, retinoblastoma)

**Heart**—History of murmur or thrill

**Lungs**—History of infection, cough, wheezing, shortness of breath (lung metastasis, lymphoma), dyspnea

**Abdomen**—History of abdominal swelling, pain, mass, change in bowel or bladder patterns (Wilms tumor, neuroblastoma, lymphoma)

**Musculoskeletal**—History of weakness in extremities, limited range of motion, tenderness or swelling, joint pain (osteogenic sarcoma, primitive neuroectodermal tumor [PNET] of the bone, rhabdomyosarcoma)

**Neurologic**—Altered consciousness, decreased sensations, abnormal reflexes, abnormal cerebellar functions (brain tumors)

**Lymphatic**—History of enlarged lymph nodes, frequent infections (leukemia, lymphoma)

**Hematologic**—History of bruising, nosebleeds or gum bleeding, paleness, fatigue, bloody or tarry-colored stools (leukemia)

### Physical Examination

See Physical Assessment, Chapter 7.

**General**—Orientation, state of health

**Skin**—Petechiae or ecchymosis, lesions or sores, presence of blood from gum or nose, color of skin (leukemia)

**HEENT**—Evidence of infection, proptosis, pupil discoloration, extraocular movements not intact, limited peripheral vision, nystagmus (retinoblastoma, brain tumor)

**Heart**—Murmur or thrill, peripheral pulses

**Lungs**—Evidence of infection, rales or rhonchi, decreased breath sounds (lymphoma)

**Abdomen**—Hepatosplenomegaly (leukemia, lymphoma), mass, decreased bowel sounds, striae (Wilms tumor, neuroblastoma, rhabdomyosarcoma)

**Neurologic**—Altered consciousness, decreased sensations, abnormal reflexes, abnormal cerebellar functions, unstable gait (brain tumor)

**Lymphatic**—Enlarged lymph nodes (lymphoma, leukemia)

### Laboratory Tests

Any number of laboratory tests may be performed, but most often a complete blood count and chemistry, and urinalysis will be done. Malignancies of the blood-forming organs manifest signs early, and these frequently cause decreased elements of the blood, increased production of immature cells, or overproduction of some cells, such as leukocytosis. Because many of the chemotherapeutic agents depress bone marrow function, repeated blood counts are a constant feature of follow-up care.

Blood chemistry yields important information concerning renal and liver function and electrolyte balance. Evaluation of renal and liver function is important not only for detection of cancer or metastasis to these organs, but also for monitoring during treatment because of the extra burden placed on these systems to metabolize and excrete the chemotherapeutic drugs. Consequently, regular blood chemistries and urinalysis are standard procedures through the course of the disease.

A lumbar puncture (LP) is a routine test employed in leukemia, brain tumors, and other cancers that may metastasize to the spinal cord and brain. An LP is also performed to administer intrathecal drugs, such as methotrexate and cytosine arabinoside, when this mode of administration is part of the treatment protocol.

### Imaging Studies

Advances in imaging procedures have greatly aided in the diagnosis of solid tumors and have minimized the need for invasive techniques. Depending on the suspected site of the malignancy, initial preliminary radiologic studies include conventional films of the chest, abdomen, bone, and skull and more specialized tests such as the intravenous (IV) pyelogram for kidney involvement. However, these radiographs are generally followed by much more sophisticated imaging procedures, including computed tomography (CT), ultrasound, nuclear scan, and magnetic resonance imaging (MRI). (See Table 37-2.)

### Biopsy

As part of the diagnostic evaluation, biopsies are essential to determine the classification and stage of the disease. *Classification* refers to the biologic characteristics of the tumor, and *staging* refers to the extent of the disease at the time of diagnosis. Although the classification of the tumor may not change, the stage often does and is usually directly related to prognosis (the higher the stage, the poorer the prognosis).

Biopsies may be performed during surgical removal of the tumor, or in the case of lymphomas, surgery may be performed specifically to obtain tissue samples of the spleen and involved lymph nodes. Easily accessed nodes, such as those in the cervical, inguinal, or axillary region, may be removed for biopsy. Whenever there is concern for metastasis to the hematologic system or when the primary site is the blood-forming organs, bone marrow studies are performed.

A **bone marrow test** may be accomplished by (1) **aspiration,** obtaining marrow through a large- or fine-bore needle, or (2) **biopsy,** obtaining a piece of bone through a special type of needle. Examination of bone marrow is used to determine the extent of involvement by malignant cells. In leukemia, involvement is classified by the percentage of leukemia cells present in bone marrow, where $M_1$ is less than 5%, $M_2$ is greater than 5% but less than 25%, and $M_3$ is greater than 25% (Margolin, Steuber, and Poplack, 2002).

# Modes of Therapy

Several advances in the understanding of cancer and improvements in technical procedures have greatly influenced present modes of therapy, including (1) surgery, (2) chemotherapy, (3) radiotherapy, (4) immunotherapy, and (5) bone marrow transplantation. Although there have been significant developments in new modes of treatment, one of the major reasons for more effective treatment regimens has been the use of clinical trials and protocols. Because of the relatively small number of children with cancer, the **National Cancer Institute (NCI)** set up cooperative groups of pediatric oncologists (physicians specializing in the care of children with cancer) from different regions of the United States to systematically combine data regarding treatment and other aspects of cancer care. Based on the evaluation of success from different types of treatment, these experts plan and initiate comparative **clinical trials.** * Although clinical trials may involve any aspect of cancer care (prevention, treatment, or long-term effects), they are frequently concerned with evaluating investigational drugs. For example, one group of patients (control group) typically receives the best possible treatment presently known. The experimental group(s) receives treatment that is thought to be even better. The formalized outline of the clinical study, which among other details includes the treatment plan (administration and evaluation), is called a **protocol.**

Over the past 3 decades the use of clinical trials and protocols has been responsible for major changes in the approaches to cancer treatment. Some of the recent strategies include reduction of toxicity with prolonged and continuous rather than intermittent IV infusion, shortening of duration of maintenance therapy, the use of intensive combination therapy, and the administration of as many effective agents as possible in the highest doses possible during the initiation of therapy. The following is an overview of the major modes of therapy. In addition, specific aspects of therapy

---

*A suggested reference for families is *What Are Clinical Trials All About?* NIH Publication No 92-2706, available from the **National Cancer Institute,** NCI Public Inquiries Office, Building 31, Room 10A03, 31 Center Dr, MSC 2580, Bethesda, MD 20892-2580, (800) 4 Cancer, fax: (800) 624-2511; cancermail@cips.nci.nih.gov.

are discussed later in the chapter when applicable to the individual type of cancer.

## Surgery

The main goal of surgery, besides obtaining biopsies, is to remove all traces of tumor and restore normal body functioning. Surgery is most successful when the tumor is encapsulated and localized (confined to the site of origin). It may only be palliative when the cancer is regional (metastasized to an area adjacent to the original site) or advanced (widespread throughout the body). Obviously the best prognosis is directly related to early detection of the tumor.

The recent trend is toward more conservative surgical excision. For example, in some types of bone cancer, such as osteosarcoma, patients are successfully treated with resection of the diseased portion of the bone rather than amputation. There is an increasing emphasis on the use of combination drug therapy and radiotherapy after limited surgical intervention.

## Chemotherapy

Chemotherapy may be the primary form of treatment, or it may be used as an adjunct to surgery or radiotherapy. Although several drugs with antineoplastic capabilities have been found effective in treating different forms of cancer, the remarkable survival rates have been the result of improved combination-drug regimens. Combining drugs allows for optimum cell cycle destruction with minimum toxic effects and decreased resistance by the cancer cells to the agent. For example, VAC (vincristine [Oncovin], doxorubicin [Adriamycin], and cyclophosphamide [Cytoxan]) combines complementary cytotoxic effects with nonsimilar side effects. Doxorubicin and cyclophosphamide are myelosuppressive, whereas vincristine is neurotoxic.

In addition to more effective combinations of drugs, several advances in the administration of chemotherapy have permitted continuous or intermittent IV administration without multiple venipunctures. The use of venous access devices (catheters and implantable infusion ports) has greatly facilitated safe and effective drug administration with minimum discomfort for the child. (See Chapter 28.) Continuous infusions over an extended period using syringe pumps have made possible the administration of certain drugs, such as cytosine arabinoside, in higher doses with less toxicity than when the drug is administered intermittently.

Chemotherapeutic agents are classified according to their cytotoxic action. **Alkylating agents** replace a hydrogen atom of a molecule by an alkyl group. The irreversible combination of alkyl groups with nucleotide chains, particularly DNA, causes unbalanced growth of unaffected cell constituents so that the cell eventually dies. They are radiomimetic in that their action is similar to irradiation. **Antimetabolites** resemble essential metabolic elements needed for cell growth but are sufficiently altered in molecular structure to inhibit further synthesis of DNA or RNA. **Plant alkaloids** arrest cells in metaphase (a phase of mitosis) by binding to microtubular protein needed for spindle formation. **Antitumor antibiotics** are natural products that interfere with cell division by reacting with DNA in such a way as to prevent further replication of DNA and transcription of RNA.

Both adrenal and gonadal *hormones* have antineoplastic properties. The precise mechanism of action is still unclear. Adrenocorticosteroids are thought to bind with DNA and alter the transcription process. Although there are a number of cortisone preparations, prednisone or dexamethasone is most frequently used.

A number of agents are not categorized according to the preceding classifications. For example, L-asparaginase is an enzyme isolated from extracts of bacterial cultures of *Escherichia coli* or *Erwinia carotovora*. It hydrolyzes L-asparagine, an amino acid, to L-aspartic acid, which prevents the cell from synthesizing protein needed for DNA and RNA synthesis. Because L-asparagine is synthesized by normal cells but must be exogenously supplied to certain leukemic and lymphoma cells, administration of the enzyme destroys the essential exogenous supply while sparing normal cells of untoward effects.

An understanding of drugs' actions and side effects is essential to nursing care of children with cancer (Table 36-2). Unfortunately, almost all drugs are not selectively cytotoxic for malignant cells, and other cells with a high rate of proliferation, such as the bone marrow elements, hair, skin, and epithelial cells of the gastrointestinal tract, are also affected. Frequently the problems related to the destruction of these normal cells require more nursing care than the disease itself.

**Precautions in Administering and Handling Chemotherapeutic Agents.** Many chemotherapeutic agents are *vesicants (sclerosing agents)* that can cause severe cellular damage if even minute amounts of the drug infiltrate surrounding tissue. Only nurses experienced with chemotherapeutic agents should administer vesicants. Guidelines are available* and must be followed meticulously to prevent tissue damage to patients. Interventions for extravasation vary, but each nurse should be aware of the institution's policies and implement them at once.

> **NURSING ALERT**
> Chemotherapeutic drugs must be given through a free-flowing IV line. The infusion is stopped *immediately* if any sign of infiltration (pain, stinging, swelling, or redness at needle site) occurs.

*Giving Cancer Drugs Intravenously: Some Guidelines* is available from the **American Cancer Society,** 1599 Clifton NE Rd, Atlanta, GA 30329, (404) 320-3333 (headquarters), (800) ACS-2345 (for general cancer info) www.cancer.org.

**TABLE 36-2** Summary of chemotherapeutic agents used in the treatment of childhood cancers*

| Agent/Administration | Side Effects and Toxicity | Comments and Specific Nursing Considerations |
|---|---|---|
| **Alkylating Agents** | | |
| **Mechlorethamine (nitrogen mustard, Mustargen)** IV† | N/V‡ (½-8 hours later) (severe)<br>BMD§ (2-3 weeks later)<br>Alopecia<br>Local phlebitis | Vesicant‖<br>May cause phlebitis and discoloration of vein<br>Use within 15 minutes after reconstitution |
| **Cyclophosphamide (Cytoxan, CTX, Neosar)** PO, IV, IM | N/V (3-4 hours later) (severe at high doses)<br>BMD (10-14 days later)<br>Alopecia<br>Hemorrhagic cystitis<br>Severe immunosuppression<br>Stomatitis (rare)<br>Syndrome of inappropriate antidiuretic hormone (SIADH) with seizures<br>Hyperpigmentation<br>Transverse ridging of nails<br>Infertility<br>Cardiac toxicity | BMD has platelet-sparing effect<br>Give dose early in day to allow adequate fluids afterward<br>Mesna is given to prevent hemorrhagic cystitis<br>Force fluids before administering drug and for 2 days after to prevent chemical cystitis; encourage frequent voiding even during night<br>Warn parents to report signs of burning on urination or hematuria to practitioner |
| **Ifosfamide (Ifos, IFF)** IV | Hemorrhagic cystitis<br>BMD (10-14 days later)<br>Alopecia<br>Neurotoxicity—lethargy, disorientation, somnolence, seizures (rare) | Mesna is given to prevent hemorrhagic cystitis<br>Hydrate as with CTX<br>Myelosuppression less severe than with CTX |

*Table includes principal drugs used in the treatment of childhood cancers. Several other conventional and investigational chemotherapeutic agents may be employed in the treatment regimen.
†*IV,* Intravenous; *PO,* by mouth; *IM,* intramuscular; *SC,* subcutaneous; *IT,* intrathecal. For parenteral injections, apply EMLA 60 minutes before IV and 2½ hours before IM administration.
‡*N/V,* Nausea and vomiting. Mild = <20% incidence; moderate = 20% to 70% incidence; severe = >75% incidence.
§*BMD,* Bone marrow depression.
‖Vesicants (sclerosing agents) can cause severe cellular damage if even minute amounts of the drug infiltrate surrounding tissue. Only nurses experienced with chemotherapeutic agents should administer vesicants. These drugs must be given through a free-flowing IV line. The infusion is stopped *immediately* if any sign of infiltration (pain, stinging, swelling, or redness at needle site) occurs. Interventions for extravasation vary, but each nurse should be aware of the institution's policies and implement them at once.

*Continued*

**TABLE 36-2** Summary of chemotherapeutic agents used in the treatment of childhood cancers—cont'd

| Agent/Administration | Side Effects and Toxicity | Comments and Specific Nursing Considerations |
|---|---|---|
| **Alkylating Agents—cont'd** | | |
| **Melphalan (L-phenylalanine mustard, Alkeran, L-Pam)** PO, IV | N/V (severe)<br>BMD (2-3 weeks later)<br>Diarrhea<br>Alopecia | Potent irritant<br>Give over 30 minutes to 1 hour<br>Administer within 60 minutes of reconstitution |
| **Procarbazine (Matulane)** PO | N/V (moderate)<br>BMD (3-4 weeks later)<br>Lethargy<br>Dermatitis<br>Myalgia<br>Arthralgia<br>Less commonly:<br>  Stomatitis<br>  Neuropathy<br>  Alopecia<br>  Diarrhea<br>Azoospermia<br>Cessation of menses | Central nervous system depressants (phenothiazines, barbiturates) enhance central nervous system symptoms<br>Monoamine oxidase (MAO) inhibition sometimes occurs, causing increased norepinephrine; foods containing high levels of tyramine may elevate norepinephrine to toxic levels; foods to avoid are over-ripe or aged products (e.g., cheese; avocados, bananas; tea, coffee; broad beans, fava beans; red wines; yogurt, chocolate) (Baquiran and Gallagher, 1998); to avoid drug interactions, all other drugs are avoided unless medically approved |
| **Dacarbazine (DTIC-Dome)** IV | N/V (severe)<br>BMD (7-14 days later)<br>Alopecia<br>Flulike syndrome<br>Burning sensation in vein during infusion (not extravasation) | Vesicant (less sclerosive)<br>Must be given cautiously in patients with renal dysfunction<br>Decrease IV rate or use cold pack along vein to decrease burning |
| **Cisplatin (Platinol)** IV | Renal toxicity (severe)<br>N/V (1-4 hours later) (severe)<br>BMD (mild, 2-3 weeks later)<br>Ototoxicity<br>Neurotoxicity (similar to that for vincristine)<br>Electrolyte disturbances, especially hypomagnesemia, hypocalcemia, hypokalemia, and hypophosphatemia<br>Anaphylactic reactions may occur | Renal function (creatinine clearance) must be assessed before giving drug<br>Must maintain hydration before and during therapy (specific gravity of urine is used to assess hydration)<br>Mannitol may be given IV to promote osmotic diuresis and drug clearance<br>Monitor intake and output<br>Monitor for signs of ototoxicity (e.g., ringing in ears) and neurotoxicity; report signs immediately; ensure that routine audiogram is done before treatment for baseline and routinely during treatment<br>Do not use aluminum needle; reaction with aluminum decreases potency of drug<br>Monitor for signs of electrolyte loss (i.e., hypomagnesemia—tremors, spasm, muscle weakness, lower extremity cramps, irregular heartbeat, convulsions, delirium)<br>Have emergency drugs at bedside¶ |
| **Carboplatin (CBDCA)** IV | BMD (14 days later)<br>N/V (mild)<br>Mild hepatotoxicity<br>Alopecia | Do not use saline dilution<br>Less nephrotoxic and ototoxic than cisplatin<br>Do not use aluminum needle |
| **Thiotepa (triethylene thiophosphoramide, TESPA)** IV, IT, IM, SQ intracavity, intratumor | N/V (mild)<br>BMD (7-14 days later)<br>Headache, dizziness<br>Stomatitis<br>Dermatitis<br>Alopecia | Use 0.22-μm filter when preparing to eliminate haze<br>Do not use with succinylcholine |
| **Antimetabolites** | | |
| **5-Azacytidine (5-AzaC)** IV | N/V (moderate)<br>BMD (7-14 days later)<br>Diarrhea | Infuse slowly via IV drip to decrease severity of N/V |

¶Emergency drugs include oxygen and parenteral preparations of epinephrine 1:1000, diphenhydramine or similar antihistamine, aminophylline, corticosteroids, and vasopressors.

**TABLE 36-2**   Summary of chemotherapeutic agents used in the treatment of childhood cancers—cont'd

| Agent/Administration | Side Effects and Toxicity | Comments and Specific Nursing Considerations |
|---|---|---|
| **Antimetabolites—cont'd** | | |
| **Cytosine arabinoside (Ara-C, Cytosar, Cytarabine, arabinosyl cytosine)** IV, IM, SC, IT | Alopecia<br>N/V (mild but severe at high doses)<br>BMD (7-14 days later)<br>Ara-C syndrome (fever, conjunctivitis, maculopapular rash)<br>Mucosal ulceration<br>Immunosuppression<br>Hepatitis (usually subclinical) | Crosses blood-brain barrier<br>Use with caution in patients with hepatic dysfunction<br>Conjunctivitis with high doses<br>Administer steroid eye drops to prevent conjunctivitis |
| **5-Fluorouracil (5-FU, Adrucil, fluorouracil)** IV | N/V (moderate)<br>Stomatitis<br>BMD (7-14 days later)<br>Alopecia<br>Diarrhea<br>Dermatitis | Infuse slowly via IV |
| **Mercaptopurine (6-MP, Purinethol)** PO, IV | N/V (mild)<br>Diarrhea<br>Anorexia<br>Stomatitis<br>BMD (4-6 weeks later)<br>Immunosuppression<br>Dermatitis<br>Less commonly may be hepatotoxic | 6-MP is an analog of xanthine; therefore allopurinol (Zyloprim) delays its metabolism and increases its potency, necessitating a lower dose ($\frac{1}{3}$ to $\frac{1}{4}$) of 6-MP |
| **Methotrexate (MTX, Amethopterin)** PO, IV, IM, IT<br>May be given in conventional doses (mg/m²) or high doses (g/m²) | N/V (severe at high doses)<br>Diarrhea<br>Mucosal ulceration (2-5 days later)<br>BMD (10 days later)<br>Immunosuppression<br>Dermatitis<br>Photosensitivity<br>Alopecia (uncommon)<br>Toxic effects include:<br>  Hepatitis (fibrosis)<br>  Osteoporosis<br>  Nephropathy<br>  Pneumonitis (fibrosis)<br>Neurologic toxicity with IT use—pain at injection site, meningismus (signs of meningitis without actual inflammation, especially fever and headache); potential sequelae—transient or permanent hemiparesis, convulsions, dementia, death | Side effects and toxicity are dose related<br>Potency and toxicity increased by reduced renal function, salicylates, sulfonamides, and aminobenzoic acid; avoid use of these substances, such as aspirin<br>Use sunblock<br>High-dose therapy:<br>  Citrovorum factor (folinic acid or leucovorin) decreases cytotoxic action of MTX; used as an antidote for overdose and to enhance normal cell recovery following high-dose therapy; avoid use of vitamins containing folic acid during MTX therapy unless prescribed by physician<br>IT therapy:<br>  Drug *must* be mixed with preservative-free diluent<br>  Report signs of neurotoxicity immediately |
| **6-Thioguanine (6-TG, Thioguan)** PO | N/V (mild)<br>BMD (7-14 days later)<br>Stomatitis<br>Rarely:<br>  Dermatitis<br>  Photosensitivity<br>  Liver dysfunction | Side effects are unusual<br>Take oral dose once daily on an emtpy stomach |
| **Plant Alkaloids** | | |
| **Vincristine (Oncovin)** IV | Neurotoxicity—paresthesia (numbness); ataxia; weakness; footdrop; hyporeflexia; constipation (adynamic ileus); hoarseness (vocal cord paralysis); ptosis; abdominal, chest, and jaw pain; mental depression<br>Fever<br>N/V (mild)<br>BMD (minimal; 7-14 days later)<br>Alopecia<br>SIADH | Vesicant<br>Report signs of neurotoxicity because may necessitate cessation of drug<br>Individuals with underlying neurologic problems may be more prone to neurotoxicity<br>Monitor stool patterns closely; administer stool softener<br>Excreted primarily by liver into biliary system; administer cautiously to anyone with biliary disease<br>Maximum dose is 2 mg |

*Continued*

**TABLE 36-2   Summary of chemotherapeutic agents used in the treatment of childhood cancers—cont'd**

| Agent/Administration | Side Effects and Toxicity | Comments and Specific Nursing Considerations |
|---|---|---|
| **Plant Alkaloids—cont'd** | | |
| **Vinblastine (Velban)** IV | Neurotoxicity (same as for vincristine but less severe)<br>N/V (mild)<br>BMD (especially neutropenia; 7-14 days later)<br>Alopecia | Same as for vincristine |
| **VP-16 (etoposide, VePesid)** IV, PO | N/V (mild to moderate)<br>BMD (7-14 days later)<br>Alopecia<br>Hypotension with rapid infusion<br>Bradycardia<br>Diarrhea (infrequent)<br>Stomatitis (rare)<br>May reactivate erythema of irradiated skin (rare)<br>Allergic reaction with anaphylaxis possible<br>Neurotoxicity | Give slowly via IV drip with child recumbent<br>Have emergency drugs available at bedside¶ |
| **VM-26 (teniposide)** IV | Same as for VP-16 | Same as for VP-16 |
| **Antibiotics** | | |
| **Actinomycin D (dactinomycin, Cosmegen, ACT-D)** IV | N/V (2-5 hours later) (moderate)<br>BMD (especially platelets; 7-14 days later)<br>Immunosuppression<br>Mucosal ulceration<br>Abdominal cramps<br>Diarrhea<br>Anorexia (may last a few weeks)<br>Alopecia<br>Acne<br>Erythema or hyperpigmentation of previously irradiated skin<br>Fever<br>Malaise | Vesicant<br>Enhances cytotoxic effects of radiation therapy but increases toxic effect<br>May cause serious desquamation of irradiated tissue |
| **Doxorubicin (Adriamycin)** IV | N/V (moderate)<br>Stomatitis<br>BMD (7-14 days later)<br>Fever, chills<br>Local phlebitis | Vesicant (extravasation may *not* cause pain)<br>Observe for any changes in heart rate or rhythm and signs of failure<br>Cumulative dose must not exceed 375 mg/m², less with radiation |
| **Doxorubicin (Adriamycin)** IV | Alopecia<br>Cumulative-dose toxicity includes:<br>    Cardiac abnormalities<br>    ECG changes<br>    Heart failure | Warn parents that drug causes urine to turn red (for up to 12 days after administration); this is normal, not hematuria |
| **Daunorubicin (daunomycin, rubidomycin)** IV | Similar to doxorubicin | Similar to doxorubicin |
| **Bleomycin (Blenoxane)** IV, IM, SC | Allergic reaction—fever, chills, hypotension, anaphylaxis<br>Fever (nonallergic)<br>N/V (mild)<br>Stomatitis<br>Cumulative dose effects include:<br>    Skin—rash, hyperpigmentation, thickening, ulceration, peeling, nail changes, alopecia<br>    Lungs—pneumonitis with infiltrate that can progress to fatal fibrosis | Should give test dose (SC) before therapeutic dose administered<br>Have emergency drugs at bedside¶<br>Hypersensitivity occurs with first one to two doses<br>May give acetaminophen before drug to reduce likelihood of fever<br>Concentration of drug in skin and lungs accounts for toxic effects<br>Follow pulmonary function tests: baseline, before therapy, and after therapy |

¶Emergency drugs include oxygen and parenteral preparations of epinephrine 1:1000, diphenhydramine or similar antihistamine, aminophylline, corticosteroids, and vasopressors.

**TABLE 36-2**   Summary of chemotherapeutic agents used in the treatment of childhood cancers—cont'd

| Agent/Administration | Side Effects and Toxicity | Comments and Specific Nursing Considerations |
|---|---|---|
| **Hormones/Corticosteroids** | | |
| **Prednisone (Meticorten, Deltasone, Paracort)** PO; IV<br>**Dexamethasone (Decadron)** PO, IV<br>**Hydrocortisone (Solu-Cortef)** IV, IT<br>**Methylprednisolone (Solu-Medrol)** PO, IV | For short-term use, no acute toxicity<br>Usual side effects are mild; moon face, fluid retention, weight gain, mood changes, increased appetite, gastric irritation, insomnia, susceptibility to infection<br>Hyperglycemia<br>Long-term effects of chronic steroid administration are mood changes, hirsutism, trunk obesity (buffalo hump), thin extremities, muscle wasting and weakness, osteoporosis, poor wound healing, bruising, potassium loss, gastric bleeding, hypertension, diabetes mellitus, growth retardation, immuno-suppression, and avascular necrosis of bone | Explain expected effects, especially in terms of body image, increased appetite, and personality changes<br>Monitor weight gain<br>Recommend moderate salt restriction<br>Administer with antacid and early in morning (sometimes given every other day to minimize side effects)<br>May need to disguise bitter taste (crush tablet and mix with syrup, jam, ice cream, or other highly flavored substance; use ice to numb tongue before administration; place tablet in gelatin capsule if child can swallow it)<br>Observe for potential infection sites; usual inflammatory response and fever are absent<br>Encourage foods high in potassium (bananas, raisins, prunes, coffee, chocolate)<br>Test stools for occult blood<br>Monitor blood pressure<br>Test blood for sugar and urine for acetone<br>Observe for signs of abrupt steroid withdrawal; flulike symptoms, hypotension, hypoglycemia, shock |
| **Enzymes** | | |
| **l-Asparaginase (Elspar)** IV, IM, SQ<br>**Erwinia L-Asparaginase**<br>**PEG-L-Asparaginase (long-acting form)** | Allergic reactions (including anaphylactic shock)<br>Fever<br>N/V (mild)<br>Anorexia<br>Weight loss<br>Arthralgia<br>Toxicity:<br>  Liver dysfunction<br>  Hyperglycemia<br>  Renal failure<br>  Pancreatitis<br>Coagulation abnormalities | Observe patient 1 hour after dose for signs of allergic reaction<br>Have emergency drugs at bedside¶<br>Record signs of allergic reaction, such as urticaria, facial edema, hypotension, or abdominal cramps<br>Check weight daily<br>Normally, blood urea nitrogen (BUN) and ammonia levels rise as a result of drug; not evidence of liver damage<br>Check urine for sugar and blood amylase |
| **Nitrosoureas** | | |
| **Carmustine (BCNU)** IV<br>**Lomustine (CCNU)** PO | N/V (2-6 hours later) (severe)<br>BMD (3-4 weeks later)<br>Burning pain along IV infusion (usually due to alcohol diluent)<br>BCNU—flushing and facial burning on infusion<br>Alopecia | Prevent extravasation; contact with skin causes brown spots<br>Oral form—give 4 hours after meals when stomach is empty<br>Reduce IV burning by diluting drug and infusing slowly via IV drip<br>Crosses blood-brain barrier |
| **Other Agents** | | |
| **Hydroxyurea (Hydrea)** PO | N/V (mild)<br>Anorexia<br>Less commonly:<br>  Diarrhea<br>  BMD<br>  Mucosal ulceration<br>  Alopecia<br>  Dermatitis | Must be given cautiously in patients with renal dysfunction |

In addition to extravasation, a potentially fatal complication is anaphylaxis, especially from L-asparaginase, bleomycin, cisplatin, and etoposide. (See Chapter 29.) Hypersensitivity reactions to these chemotherapeutic agents are characterized by the presence of urticaria, angioedema, flushing, rashes, or hypotension. Nursing responsibilities include prevention of, recognition of, and preparation for serious reactions. Prevention begins with a careful history of known allergy. (See Chapter 6.)

> **NURSING ALERT**
>
> When chemotherapeutic and immunologic agents are given, the child must be observed for 1 hour after the infusion for signs of anaphylaxis (cyanosis, hypotension, wheezing, severe urticaria). Emergency equipment (especially blood pressure monitor and bag-valve-mask) and emergency drugs (especially oxygen, epinephrine, antihistamine, aminophylline, corticosteroids, and vasopressors) must be available.

If a reaction is suspected, the drug is discontinued, the IV line is flushed and maintained with saline, and the child's vital signs and subsequent responses are monitored.

In addition to the many responsibilities nurses must have in regard to the child and family, they must also use safeguards to protect themselves. Handling chemotherapeutic agents may present risks to handlers and to their offspring, although the exact degree of risk is not known.

The **Oncology Nursing Society** has published comprehensive guidelines for safe practice issues related to administration of chemotherapy.* Safe management procedures for chemotherapy administered in the home have also been established (Close and others, 1995; Directorate of Technical Support, 1995). Basic nursing guidelines are listed in the Guidelines box.

---

*Cancer Chemotherapy Guidelines* can be obtained from the **Oncology Nursing Society**, 501 Holiday Dr, Pittsburgh, PA 15220-2749, (412) 921-7373, www.ons.org.

> **GUIDELINES**
> *Handling Chemotherapeutic Agents*
>
> Use utmost care and strict aseptic technique in handling chemotherapeutic agents to prevent any physical contact with the substance.
> Prepare drugs in a properly ventilated room or biologic safety cabinet (incorporates protective front panel and vertical laminar airflow to reduce potential for inhalation during preparation).
> Wear disposable gloves and protective clothing and discard in special container after each use.
> Use a sterile gauze pad when priming IV tubing, connecting and disconnecting tubing, inserting syringes into vials, breaking glass ampules, or any other procedure in which antineoplastic drugs may be inadvertently discharged.
> Dispose of all contaminated needles, syringes, IV tubing, and other contaminated equipment in a leakproof and puncture-resistant container; do not recap or break needles.

## Radiation Therapy

Radiation therapy is frequently used in the treatment of childhood cancer, usually in conjunction with chemotherapy or surgery. It can be used for curative purposes and is often employed for palliation to relieve symptoms by shrinking the size of the tumor. Recent advances in radiation therapy have optimized its beneficial effects and minimized many of the undesirable side effects, although high-dose irradiation is associated with many serious late effects.

Ionizing radiation is cytotoxic in at least three different ways: (1) damaging the pyrimidine bases cytosine, thymine, and uracil, needed for the synthesis of nucleic acids; (2) causing single-strand breaks in the DNA or RNA molecule; or (3) causing double helical–strand breaks in these molecules. The effect of disturbing cellular metabolic and reproductive functions is either sublethal or lethal damage.

*Lethal damage* refers to the death of the cell. *Sublethal damage* refers to injured cells that may subsequently be repaired. Many of the acute side effects are the result of lethal damage to radiosensitive tissue, particularly proliferating cells such as those of the bone marrow, gastrointestinal tract, and hair follicles. Late effects are usually the result of cell death.

The acute untoward reactions from radiation therapy depend primarily on the area to be irradiated. *Total-body irradiation (TBI)* is associated with the most severe reactions and is employed to prepare the immune system for bone marrow transplantation. Table 36-3 summarizes the acute effects of radiation therapy and nursing interventions that may be helpful in lessening or preventing them.

## Biologic Response Modifiers (BRMs)

BRMs modify the relationship between tumor and host by therapeutically changing the host's biologic response to tumor cells. These agents or interventions may affect the host's immunologic mechanisms (immunotherapy), have direct antitumor activity, or stimulate cell growth, reducing the hematologic toxicity associated with chemotherapy (Calabresi and Gamucci, 1995; Wakeling, 1999). A new immunotherapy being investigated is known as adoptive immunotherapy because it adopts the patient's T-cells (the cells most responsible for the immune response). The patient's T-cells are sensitized to the antigen expressed by the tumor, cloned in a laboratory, and then administered as an infusion. The hope is that the T-cells will zero in on and destroy the cancer cells (Wakeling, 1999).

Much of the current work in biotherapy is directed toward the use of monoclonal antibodies in the diagnosis and treatment of cancers. Through a complex process, special cells are fused to form a hybrid clone or hybridoma that produces antibodies that recognize a single specific antigen, hence the term *monoclonal antibody* (*mono* meaning *one* and *clone* meaning *exact duplicate*). These clones are then frozen, maintained in culture, or grown as tumors in mice to produce large quantities of the antibody in ascites fluid (Roselli and others, 1996). Although there are many prospective uses for monoclonal antibodies, their current role has been in diagnosing subclasses of leukemia cells to enhance understanding of which types of leukemia respond to different treatments and to determine if the subclass is related to the prognosis. Monoclonal antibodies have also been used to deplete allogeneic bone marrow of T-cells to reduce graft-vs-host disease and to selectively eliminate malignant cells from autologous marrow for transplanting back into the patient (Naparstek and others, 1995). Results from these studies have been encouraging, but further work is needed to define the role monoclonal antibodies and other BRMs will have in cancer care.

## Bone Marrow Transplantation (BMT)

Another approach to the treatment of childhood cancer is BMT. Candidates for transplantation are children who have malignancies that are unlikely to be cured by other means. (See Family Focus box.) BMT allows for lethal doses of chemotherapy, often combined with radiation therapy, to

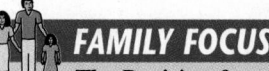

**FAMILY FOCUS**
*The Decision for a Bone Marrow Transplant*

A family's decision for a child to undergo a bone marrow transplant may be fraught with challenges. Often the child is facing certain death from the malignancy. The preparation of the child for the transplant also places the patient at great medical risk.

Once the preparatory regimen is begun and the child's immune system is destroyed, there is no turning back. Unlike kidney transplantation, BMT does not have a "rescue" procedure, such as dialysis, for supportive therapy. If the donor is a sibling, the issue of his or her marrow "saving" the brother or sister can be a concern, especially if the transplant fails. Parents often must leave the home to stay at the transplant center and encounter additional stressors such as arranging child care, taking a leave from work, and managing finances. The patient faces the greatest stress—fear of BMT failure or life-threatening complications.

| TABLE 36-3   Early side effects of radiation therapy | |
|---|---|
| **Site/Effects** | **Nursing Interventions** |
| **Gastrointestinal Tract** | |
| Nausea/vomiting | Give antiemetic around the clock |
| | Measure amount of emesis to assess for dehydration |
| Anorexia | Encourage fluids and foods best tolerated, usually light, soft diet and small, frequent meals |
| | Monitor weight loss |
| Mucosal ulceration | Use frequent mouthrinses and oral hygiene to prevent mucositis |
| Diarrhea | Can be controlled with antispasmodics and kaolin pectin preparations |
| | Observe for signs of dehydration |
| **Skin** | |
| Alopecia (within 2 weeks; may regrow by 3-6 months) | Introduce idea of wig |
| | Stress necessity of scalp hygiene and need for head covering in cold weather |
| Dry or moist desquamation | Do not refer to skin change as a "burn" (implies use of too much radiation) |
| | Keep skin clean |
| | Wash daily, using soap (e.g., Tone, Dove) sparingly |
| | Do not remove skin marking for radiation fields |
| | Avoid exposure to sun |
| | For dryness, apply lubricant |
| | For desquamation, consult practitioner for skin hygiene and care |
| **Head** | |
| Nausea/vomiting (from stimulation of vomiting center in brain) | Same as for gastrointestinal tract |
| Alopecia | Same as for skin |
| Mucositis | Encourage regular dental care, fluoride treatments |
| Potential effects | May need analgesics to relieve discomfort |
|  Parotitis | |
|  Sore throat | |
|  Loss of taste | |
|  Xerostomia (dry mouth) | Combat severe dryness of mouth with oral hygiene and liquid diet |
| **Urinary Bladder** | |
| Rarely cystitis | More likely to occur with concomitant use of cyclophosphamide |
| | Encourage liberal fluid intake and frequent voiding |
| | Evaluate for hematuria |
| **Bone Marrow** | |
| Myelosuppression | Observe for fever (temperature above 38.3° C [101° F]) |
| | Initiate workup for sepsis as ordered |
| | Administer antibiotics as prescribed |
| | Avoid use of suppositories, rectal temperatures |
| | Institute bleeding precautions |
| | Observe for signs of anemia |

be given in order to rid the body of all cancer cells (Abramovitz and Senner, 1995). Once the body is free of malignant cells and the immune system is suppressed to prevent rejection of the transplanted marrow, the donor marrow or stem cells or the cells previously stored from the patient are given to the patient by IV transfusion. The newly transfused marrow or stem cells will begin to produce functioning nonmalignant blood cells. In essence, a new blood-forming organ will be accepted by the recipient.

The selection process of a suitable donor and the potential complications in transplantation are related to the *human leukocyte antigen (HLA) system complex.* Some of the major HLA antigens are A, B, C, D, and DR. There is a wide diversity for each of these HLA loci. There are more than 20 different HLA-A antigens that can be inherited and more than 40 different HLA-B antigens.

The genes are inherited as a single unit or *haplotype.* A child inherits one unit from each parent; thus a child and each parent have one identical and one nonidentical haplotype. Because the possible haplotype combinations among siblings follow the laws of mendelian genetics, there is a 1 in 4 chance that two siblings have two identical haplotypes and are perfectly matched at the HLA loci.

The importance of HLA matching is to prevent the serious complication known as *graft-vs-host disease (GVHD).* Because the child's immune system is essentially rendered nonfunctional, there is little difficulty with bone marrow rejection by the recipient. However, the donor's marrow may contain antigens not matched to the recipient's antigens, which begin attacking body cells. The more closely the HLA systems match, the less likely GVHD is to develop. However, it can occur even with a perfect HLA match because there are as yet unidentified and thus unmatched histocompatibility antigens (Guinan, Krance, and Lehman, 2002).

Different types of BMT are now performed in children with cancer. *Allogeneic BMT* involves the matching of a histocompatible donor with the recipient. However, allogeneic BMT is limited by the presence of a suitable marrow donor.

Because of the limited numbers of patients having HLA-identical siblings, other types of allogeneic transplants have evolved. *Umbilical cord blood stem cell transplantation* is a new source of hematopoietic stem cells for use in children with cancer (Rocha and others, 2000; Wagner and others, 1995). Because stem cells can be found with high frequency in the circulation of newborns, cord blood transplantation has become an alternative for some children (Amos and Gordon, 1995; Rocha and others, 2000). The benefit of using umbilical cord blood is the blood's relative immunodeficiency at birth, allowing for partially matched unrelated cord blood transplants to be successful, with a lower risk of GVHD-related problems (Varadi and others, 1995).

*Autologous BMTs* use the patient's own marrow that was collected from disease-free tissue, frozen, and sometimes treated to remove malignant cells. Children with solid tumors such as neuroblastoma, Hodgkin disease, non-Hodgkin lymphoma, rhabdomyosarcoma, Ewing sarcoma, and Wilms tumor have been treated with autologous BMTs.

*Peripheral stem cell transplants (PSCTs)* are also used in children with cancer. PSCT, a type of autologous transplant, differs in the way stem cells are collected from the patient. Colony-stimulating factor (CSF) is first given to stimulate the production of many stem cells (Lanzkowsky, 2000; Matsubara and others, 2001). Once the white blood cell count is high enough, the stem cells are collected by an "apheresis" machine. This machine filters out peripheral stem cells from whole blood, returning the remainder of the blood cells and plasma to the child. Stem cells have been collected in very small children weighing 20 kg or less, without problems (Takaue and others, 1995). The peripheral stem cells are then frozen until the patient is ready for the PSCT.

## Complications of Therapy

Although tremendous advances have been achieved through current modes of cancer therapy, the successes are not without consequences. Numerous side effects are expected with chemotherapy and radiotherapy, and these are discussed in the Nursing Care Plan on pp. 1606-1611. However, other complications that are less frequently seen but generally more serious are described here.

### Pediatric Oncologic Emergencies

Life-threatening conditions may develop in children with cancer as a result of aggressive treatment modalities or from the malignancy itself. *Acute tumor lysis syndrome* is caused by the rapid release of intracellular metabolites during the initial treatment of malignancies such as Burkitt and T-cell lymphomas and acute leukemia. Rapid tumor lysis leads to hyperuricemia, hypocalcemia, hyperphosphatemia, and hyperkalemia (Lanzkowsky, 2000).

Children develop flank pain, lethargy, nausea and vomiting, oliguria, pruritus, tetany, and altered level of consciousness. Renal failure can occur, which may necessitate the use of renal dialysis. Management consists of hydration and alkalinization, and the use of allopurinol to reduce uric acid formation and promote excretion of by-products of purine metabolism. Exchange transfusions are sometimes necessary to reduce the metabolic consequences of massive tumor lysis, especially in children with a high tumor burden.

*Hyperleukocytosis,* defined as a peripheral white blood cell count greater than $100,000/mm^3$, can lead to capillary obstruction, microinfarction, and organ dysfunction. Children experience respiratory distress and cyanosis; neurologic changes include altered level of consciousness, visual disturbances, agitation, confusion, ataxia, and delirium. Management consists of rapid cytoreduction by chemotherapy, with hydration, urinary alkalinization, and allopurinol. Leukophoresis or exchange transfusion may be necessary.

*Obstruction* may create an oncologic emergency for a child with cancer. Space-occupying lesions, especially from Hodgkin disease and non-Hodgkin lymphoma (NHL), located in the chest, may cause *superior vena cava syndrome (SVCS)* (compression of mediastinal structures), leading to airway compromise and potentially to respiratory failure.

SVCS has also been reported with central venous catheters from the formation of a thrombus or a fibrotic reaction (Mayo, Pearson, and Horne, 1997).

Children present with cyanosis of the face, neck, and upper chest; upper extremity edema; and distended neck veins. They may have dyspnea from airway obstruction. Management consists of airway protection and alleviation of respiratory distress. Rapid cytoreduction is instituted.

Children may have a mass obstructing the spinal cord, as manifested by symptoms ranging from tingling to paresthesias and loss of bowel and bladder control. Children with brain tumors may develop symptoms ranging from increased intracranial pressure to respiratory compromise and herniation, depending on the location and size of the tumor.

Presentation depends on the tumor location and age of the child. Motor impairment from muscle weakness or paralysis can occur. Sensory impairment with numbness, tingling, sensation of cold, and pain on light touch can be assessed. Back pain and urinary or bowel incontinence or retention can occur. Early intervention is critical in preventing permanent damage. Rapid cytoreduction is essential and may include radiation therapy, chemotherapy, steroids, and possible surgery.

***Overwhelming infections*** in the immunocompromised child constitute an emergency situation. Gram-negative sepsis can result in numerous complications, including disseminated intravascular coagulation (DIC), created by bacteria or fungus causing damage to the endothelial system. Life-threatening hemorrhage can occur from DIC in combination with thrombocytopenia (platelet count 20,000/mm³), and leukocytosis (leukocyte count 100,000/mm³). Leukocytosis may cause intracranial bleeding from increased viscosity of the blood. The resulting leukocytosis leads to vascular damage and subsequent hemorrhage.

# NURSING CARE OF THE CHILD WITH CANCER

This section presents an overview of general nursing concepts that apply to most childhood cancers. Specific nursing care for the child with a particular type of cancer is discussed under each disease section later in this chapter. The focus of this discussion is on the physical aspects of care. Emotional aspects are presented in Chapter 22 (chronic illness) and in Chapter 23 (terminal illness).

## ✷ Assessment

### Signs and Symptoms of Cancer in Children

Early detection is critical to early treatment and eventual cure. Cancers in children are often difficult to recognize. Therefore being alert to the persistence of unusual symptoms is essential (Box 36-1). Some of the more significant clues to pediatric cancer are discussed here.

***Pain*** may be an early or late initial sign of cancer and requires a careful history of its onset, characteristics, location, intensity, and alleviating factors. Pain may be generalized or present at a specific location. For example, bone pain occurs in approximately 20% of children with leukemia. Pain, swelling, and tenderness at the tumor site may be the initial sign in bone tumors.

***Fever*** is a frequent occurrence during childhood and is caused by numerous illnesses, including cancer. Fever is most often caused by infection secondary to the malignant process.

A careful ***skin*** assessment will reveal signs and symptoms of a low platelet count. Ecchymosis and petechiae are most commonly found on the child's extremities, and nosebleeding may occur when the platelet count falls below 20,000/mm³.

The child with malignant invasion of the bone marrow often appears pale, with symptoms of lethargy, weight loss, and generalized malaise. These symptoms may be attributed to the development of ***anemia*** caused by the replacement of normal cells with malignant cells in the bone marrow. The nurse should assess for signs and symptoms of anemia. (See Chapter 35.)

An ***abdominal mass*** is a typical finding in children with Wilms tumor and neuroblastoma. The presence of an abdominal mass in a child must be evaluated for a malignancy.

***Swollen lymph glands*** are another common finding in children. However, enlarged, firm, lymph nodes in a child with fever for more than 1 week, a recent history of weight loss, or an abnormal chest x-ray film may indicate a serious disease and should be evaluated further.

The presence of a ***white reflection*** as opposed to the normal red pupillary reflex in the pupil of a child's eye is the classic sign of retinoblastoma. The presence of squinting, strabismus, or swelling can indicate other solid tumors of the eye.

The child with a brain tumor will develop signs and symptoms according to the exact area of the brain involved. The nurse must perform a thorough assessment to identify the specific area of tumor involvement (see Table 36-5).

## ✷ Nursing Diagnoses

A number of nursing diagnoses become apparent following an assessment of the child with cancer and the family. Some are considered in the Nursing Care Plan on pp. 1606-1611. Others are identified here in specific situations.

---

**Box 36-1 ■ ■ □**
**Cardinal Symptoms of Cancer in Children**

Unusual mass or swelling
Unexplained paleness and loss of energy
Sudden tendency to bruise
Persistent, localized pain or limping
Prolonged, unexplained fever or illness
Frequent headaches, often with vomiting
Sudden eye or vision changes
Excessive, rapid weight loss

---

Data from Hockenberry M, Kline NE: Nursing support of the child with cancer. In Pizzo PA, Poplack DP, editors: *Principles and practices of pediatric oncology,* ed 4, Philadelphia, 2002, JB Lippincott.

## ■ Planning

The goals for the child with cancer and the family include the following:

1. Child will receive appropriate primary health care.
2. Child and family will be prepared for diagnostic and therapeutic procedures.
3. Child will experience minimal complications from treatment.
4. Problems of irradiation and drug toxicity will be managed.
5. Child and family will receive adequate support and education.

## ■ Implementation

### Managing Side Effects of Treatment

Cancer care encompasses more than treatments aimed at eliminating the malignant cells. Because of the delicate balance between killing malignant cells and preserving functional cells, supportive therapy is frequently needed during those times that serious damage occurs to normal body tissues.

**Infection.** A major concern for the child receiving treatment for cancer is the risk for the development of complications secondary to the treatment. Major complications include fever, bleeding, and anemia.

The nurse caring for the child with fever must be aware of the signs and symptoms of septic shock, as discussed in Chapter 29. The child with fever who has an **absolute neutrophil count (ANC)** lower than 500/mm³ is at risk for the following (see Guidelines box):

- Overwhelming infection
- General malaise
- Dehydration
- Seizures (young infants and children)
- Invasion of organisms producing secondary infections

The child with fever is evaluated for potential sites of infection, such as from a needle puncture, mucosal ulceration, minor abrasion, or skin tears (e.g., a hangnail). Although the body may not be able to produce an adequate inflammatory response to the infection and the usual clinical signs of infection may be partially expressed or absent, fever will occur. Therefore temperature is monitored closely. To identify the source of infection, blood, stool, urine, and nasopharyngeal cultures and chest x-ray films are taken.

Once infection is suspected, broad-spectrum IV antibiotic therapy is begun before the organism is identified and may be continued for 7 to 10 days. If the child does not have

### GUIDELINES

#### Calculating the Absolute Neutrophil Count (ANC)

1. Determine the total percent of neutrophils ("polys or segs" and "bands").
2. Multiply white blood cell (WBC) count by percent of neutrophils.
   *Example:* WBC = 1000, neutrophils = 7%, nonsegmented neutrophils (bands) = 7%
   Step 1: 7% + 7% = 14%
   Step 2: 0.14 × 1000 = 140 ANC

a venous access device, a heparin lock should be inserted to prevent the inconvenience of multiple venipunctures in maintaining a patent IV line and to prevent limited activity imposed by an immobilized body part.

The organisms most lethal to these children are (1) viruses, particularly varicella (chickenpox), herpes zoster, herpes simplex, measles, rubella, mumps, and poliomyelitis; (2) *Pneumocystis carinii* (a protozoan); (3) fungi, especially *Candida albicans;* (4) gram-negative bacteria, such as *Pseudomonas aeruginosa, E. coli, Proteus,* and *Klebsiella;* and (5) gram-positive bacteria, especially *Staphylococcus aureus, Staphylococcus epidermidis,* and group A β-hemolytic streptococcus (Quadri and Brown, 2000). As prophylaxis against these various organisms, broad-spectrum antibiotics are usually prescribed. Ensuring compliance with this long-term regimen is an important nursing responsibility.

Prophylaxis against *P. carinii* is routinely given to most children during treatment for cancer (American Academy of Pediatrics, 2000). Trimethoprim/sulfamethoxazole (Bactrim, Septra) is usually given three times a week during treatment.

*Colony-stimulating factors (CSFs),* a family of glycoprotein hormones that regulate the reproduction, maturation, and function of blood cells, are now routinely used as supportive measures to prevent the side effects caused by low blood counts. CSFs promote stem cell proliferation and stimulate a more rapid maturation of the cells, allowing them to enter the bloodstream earlier. *G-CSF (granulocyte colony-stimulating factor)* (filgrastim [Neupogen]) directs granulocyte development and can decrease the duration of neutropenia following immunosuppressive therapy. This reduces the incidence and duration of infection in children receiving treatment for cancer. G-CSF is also being used to decrease the bone marrow recovery time following BMT (Freifeld and Pizzo, 1996; Matsubara and others, 2001). G-CSF is usually administered intravenously or subcutaneously 24 hours after chemotherapy is discontinued and is given for 10 to 14 days. G-CSF is discontinued when the ANC surpasses 10,000/mm³. During G-CSF therapy, children may experience bone pain, fever, rash, malaise, and headaches.

Prevention of infection continues as a priority after discharge from the hospital. Some institutions allow the child to return to school when the ANC is above 500/mm³. Other institutions place no restrictions on the child, regardless of the blood count. If the level falls below this value, cautious isolation from crowded areas, such as shopping centers or subways, is advisable. At all times family members are encouraged to practice good handwashing to prevent introducing pathogens into the home.

**Hemorrhage.** Before the use of transfused platelets, hemorrhage was a leading cause of death in children with some types of cancer. Now most bleeding episodes can be prevented or controlled with judicious administration of platelet concentrates or platelet-rich plasma. Severe spontaneous internal hemorrhage varies, but usually does not occur until the platelet count is 10,000/mm³ or less (Hockenberry and Kline, 2002; Rossetto and McMahon, 2000).

Because infection increases the tendency toward hemorrhage, and because bleeding sites become more easily infected, special care is taken to avoid performing skin punctures whenever possible. When finger sticks, venipunctures, intramuscular injections, and bone marrow tests are performed, aseptic technique must be employed with continued observation for bleeding. Meticulous mouth care is essential, because gingival bleeding with resultant mucositis is a frequent problem. Because the rectal area is prone to ulceration from various drugs, hygiene is essential. To prevent additional trauma, rectal temperatures and suppositories are avoided. Frequent turning and the use of a pressure-reducing mattress under bony prominences prevent development of pressure areas and decubital ulcers.

Platelet transfusions are generally reserved for active bleeding episodes that do not respond to local treatment and that may occur during induction or relapse therapy. Epistaxis and gingival bleeding are the most common. The nurse teaches parents and other children measures to control nosebleeding (see p. 1567). Applying pressure at the site without disturbing clot formation is the general rule. (See Critical Thinking Exercise box.)

Two of the problems with multiple platelet transfusions are the risk of febrile reactions and decreased life span of the platelets. Platelet concentrates normally do not have to be crossmatched for blood group or type. However, because platelets contain specific antigen components similar to blood group factors, children who receive multiple transfusions may become sensitized to a platelet group other than their own. Therefore platelets are crossmatched with the donor's blood components whenever possible.

Transfused platelets generally survive in the body for 1 to 3 days. The peak effect is reached in about 2 hours and decreased by half in 24 hours. Therefore after a transfusion the nurse observes and records the approximate time when hemostasis of bleeding sites occurs. Delayed hemostasis is evidence of platelet destruction. For long-term patients, multiple transfusion therapy becomes progressively less effective.

During bleeding episodes the parents and child need much emotional support. The sight of oozing blood is very upsetting. Often parents will request a platelet transfusion, unaware of the necessity of trying local measures first. The nurse can be instrumental in allaying anxiety by explaining the reason for delaying a platelet transfusion until absolutely necessary. Because compatible donors decrease the risk of antigen formation in the recipient, the nurse should encourage parents to locate suitable donors for eventual blood use.

Children at home who have low platelet counts (usually below 100,000/mm³) are advised to avoid activities that might cause injury or bleeding, such as riding bicycles or skateboards, roller skating or in-line skating, climbing trees or playground equipment, and contact sports such as football or soccer. These restrictions can be terminated once the platelet count rises. In addition, aspirin and aspirin-containing products are not used; for mild pain or significantly elevated temperature, acetaminophen is substituted.

**Anemia.** Initially anemia may be profound from complete replacement of the bone marrow by cancer cells. During induction therapy, blood transfusions with packed red blood cells may be necessary to raise the hemoglobin to levels approaching 10 g. The usual precautions in caring for the child are instituted. (See Chapter 35.)

Anemia is also a consequence of drug-induced myelosuppression. Although not as severely affected as the white blood cells, erythrocyte production may be delayed. Because children have an amazing capacity to withstand low hemoglobin levels, the best approach is to allow the child to regulate activity with reasonable adult supervision. It may be necessary for the parents to alert the schoolteacher to the child's physical limitations, particularly in terms of strenuous activity.

**Nausea and Vomiting.** The nausea and vomiting that occur shortly after administration of several of the drugs and as a result of cranial or abdominal irradiation can be profound. 5-HT$_3$ receptor antagonists are the antiemetics of choice used to manage nausea and vomiting caused by chemotherapy and radiation therapy (Engstrom and others, 1999). The advantage of these agents over conventional drugs is that they produce no extrapyramidal side effects, such as difficulty in speaking or swallowing, shuffle walk, slow movements, trembling, stiffness of the arms and legs, or loss of balance. Multiple studies have shown ondansetron (Zofran) to be effective for patients receiving cisplatin, cyclophosphamide, ifosfamide, and anthracyclines (Anastasia, 2000; Kurylak and others, 1995). Ondansetron in combination with dexamethasone has been more effective than ondansetron alone (Roila, Aapro, and Stewart, 1998) and has been superior to meto-

---

### Critical Thinking Exercise

#### Bleeding

Paul Jones, 14 years old, is undergoing chemotherapy for leukemia but has recently been hospitalized because of pneumonia. His platelet count is 50,000/mm³. After morning report, you visit him and note the following. Which one requires further assessment because it potentially increases his risk of bleeding?

FIRST, THINK ABOUT IT . . .
• What is the purpose of your thinking?
• What information are you using?

1. A sign over his bed reads "no needle punctures."
2. He is receiving 6 L of oxygen via nasal cannula.
3. He has an intermittent infusion device in his hand.
4. A tympanic membrane sensor is in the room.

*The best response is two. You should assess if the oxygen is being humidified. The nose is vascular and can bleed easily if the mucosa is dried by the oxygen, which is important information. Also, inspect the placement of the nasal prongs for any sign of irritation and ask Paul if the prongs are comfortable.*

*The other aspects of care—the sign to remind staff to avoid any skin punctures, the infusion device to maintain access to the vein if needed, and the temperature measurement device using the ear and thus avoiding the rectal route and possible mucosal damage—are aimed at preventing bleeding.*

clopramide (Reglan) for cisplatin-induced emesis (ASHP, 1999; Rhodes and others, 1995). Most institutions use a three-dose IV regimen of 0.15 mg/kg/dose with or without further oral doses of 4 to 8 mg three times daily. A single IV dose of 5 mg/m² followed by oral doses of 2 to 4 mg every 8 hours has also been used.

For mild to moderate vomiting, phenothiazine type of drugs remain the mainstay of therapy. Promethazine (Phenergan), chlorpromazine (Thorazine), prochlorperazine (Compazine), or trimethobenzamide (Tigan) may be effective agents. Metoclopramide is a more effective antiemetic for severe vomiting. Unfortunately, the drug causes a number of side effects in children, particularly extrapyramidal reactions, such as muscle tremors or twitching, agitation, grimacing, dysarthria, and oculogyric crisis (fixation of eyes in one position for minutes or hours). Metoclopramide should be administered with dexamethasone or diphenhydramine (Berde, Billett, and Collins, 2002).

Another drug that has yielded promising results is THC (δ-9-tetrahydrocannabinol), the active component of marijuana. Synthetic cannabinoids are now being used in children undergoing chemotherapy. Nabilone was developed to overcome the problems associated with the naturally occurring cannabinoids.

The most beneficial regimen for antiemetic control has been the administration of the antiemetic *before* the chemotherapy begins (30 minutes to 1 hour before) and regular (not as-needed [PRN]) administration every 2, 4, or 6 hours for at least 24 hours after chemotherapy. There is some evidence that beginning antiemetic therapy up to 24 hours before the chemotherapy adds to its effectiveness (Rhodes and others, 1995; Roila, Aapro, and Stewart, 1998). The goal is to prevent the child from ever experiencing nausea or vomiting, because this can prevent the development of anticipatory symptoms (the conditioned response of developing nausea and vomiting before receiving the drug). Other nonpharmacologic interventions (similar to those discussed for pain management in Chapter 26) can be useful in controlling posttherapy and anticipatory nausea and vomiting. Giving the antineoplastic drug with a mild sedative at bedtime is also helpful for some children, and there is evidence that nighttime administration of drugs such as methotrexate and 6-mercaptopurine may be more effective cytotoxically than morning administration.

**Altered Nutrition.** Altered nutrition is a common side effect of treatment. Continued assessment of the child's nutritional status must occur throughout treatment. Regular evaluation of the child's intake should be recorded. The child's height, weight, and head circumference (for children under 3 years of age) must be measured routinely during visits to the hospital or clinic. When appropriate, energy reserves, evaluated by skinfold measurements, should be followed. Biochemical assays may be helpful in some children and include serum prealbumin, transferrin, and albumin (Han-Markey, 2000; Nitenberg and Raynard, 2000). Criteria for nutrition intervention in children with cancer are found in Box 36-2.

Nutritional status is important to maintain because it can contribute to reduced tolerance to treatment, altered metabolism of chemotherapy drugs, prolonged episodes of neutropenia, and increased risk for infection.

Supportive nutrition measures include oral supplements with high-protein and high-calorie foods. Ways to increase calories include substituting cream for milk, adding tofu (high in protein) to most meals, eating full-fat yogurt and ice cream instead on nonfat or low-fat items, cooking with butter, putting sugar on cereal, and making high-calorie snacks such as trail mix, peanut butter, or dried fruit readily available for the child. Enteral feeding may be necessary when children are unable to maintain the necessary calories to prevent weight loss. The use of parental hyperalimentation is used most frequently for children who have digestive problems or are postsurgery or BMT patients. These interventions are discussed in more detail in Chapter 27.

> **NURSING ALERT** It is important to remember that some children develop aversions to certain foods if they are eaten during chemotherapy. It is best to refrain from offering the child's favorite foods when the child is receiving chemotherapy.

Some children still do not eat despite such approaches. The following theories have been postulated to explain persistent anorexia. It is (1) a physical effect related to the cancer that is nonspecific; (2) a conditioned aversion to food from nausea and vomiting during treatment; (3) a response to stress in the environment, related to eating or to the child's condition; (4) a result of depression; (5) a control mechanism when so much else has been imposed on the child; and (6) an opportunity to express anger at parents and punish them for "allowing" the child to become sick. When loss of appetite and weight persists, the nurse should investigate the family situation to determine if any of these variables are contributing to the problem.

**Mucosal Ulceration.** One of the most distressing side effects of several drugs is gastrointestinal mucosal cell damage, which results in ulcers anywhere along the alimentary tract. Oral ulcers (stomatitis) are red, eroded, painful areas in the mouth or pharynx. (See Stomatitis, Chapter 16.) Similar lesions may extend along the esophagus and in the rectal area. They greatly compound anorexia because eating is ex-

---

**Box 36-2** ◼ ◼ ◼
**Criteria for Nutrition Intervention in Children with Malignancies**

Interval or total weight loss >5% of the pre-illness body weight
Relative weight-for-height of ≤90% or weight-for-height ≤10th percentile (determined from the NCHS growth chart)
Serum albumin level <3.2 mg/dl
Arm fat area or subscapular skinfolds <5th percentile for age and sex
Current percentile for weight or height that is 2 percentile channels <pre-illness percentile

Modified from Kumar S and others: Protein energy malnutrition and skeletal muscle wasting in childhood acute lymphoblastic leukemia, *Indian Pediatr* 37:722, 2000.

tremely uncomfortable. When oral ulcers develop, the following interventions are helpful: (1) a bland, moist, soft diet; (2) use of a soft sponge toothbrush (Toothette)* or cotton-tipped applicator; (3) frequent mouthrinses with normal saline (using a solution of 1 teaspoon of table salt and 1 pint of water) or sodium bicarbonate and salt mouthrinses (using a solution of 1 teaspoon of baking soda and 1/2 teaspoon of table salt in 1 quart of water); and (4) local anesthetics without alcohol, such as a Benadryl/Maalox solution or Ulcerease (Kennedy and Diamond, 1997; Larson and others, 1998). Although local anesthetics are effective in temporarily relieving the pain, many children dislike the taste and numb feeling they produce.

**NURSING ALERT**

Viscous lidocaine is not recommended for young children; if applied to the pharynx, it may depress the gag reflex, increasing the risk of aspiration. Seizures have also been associated with the use of oral viscous lidocaine, most likely as result of the rapid absorption into the bloodstream via the oral lesions (Cho, Cheng, and Cheng, 2000).

Oral preparations used to prevent or treat mucositis include Ulcerease, which is used to soothe mucositis and gum irritations; chlorhexidine gluconate (Peridex) is effective against candidal and bacterial infections (Kennedy and Diamond, 1997). Antifungal troches (lozenges) or mouthrinse is typically used prophylactically in patients with myelosuppression, especially for children who have undergone BMT.

**NURSING ALERT**

Agents such as lemon glycerin swabs, hydrogen peroxide, and milk of magnesia are avoided because of the drying effects on the mucosa. In addition, lemon may be irritating to eroded tissue and can decay the teeth (Kennedy and Diamond, 1997).

A strategy that may be helpful in reducing oral pain is massaging the area on the backs of both hands between the thumb and index finger with an ice cube for 5 to 7 minutes until the area becomes numb.

Administering mouth care is particularly difficult in infants and toddlers. A satisfactory method of cleaning the gums is to wrap a piece of gauze around a finger, soak it in saline or plain water, and swab the gums, palate, and inner cheek surfaces with the finger. Mouthrinses are best accomplished with plain water or saline because the child cannot gargle or spit out excess fluid. Mouth care is done routinely before and after any feeding and as often as every 2 to 4 hours to rid mucosal surfaces of debris, which becomes an excellent medium for bacterial and fungal growth.

Dental hygiene can become a serious problem if the child wears an orthodontic appliance. The accumulated debris on braces is difficult to remove without vigorous brushing, and the appliance itself traumatizes the gums. Sometimes braces are removed during chemotherapy.

*Manufactured by Halbrand, Inc, Willoughby, OH.

Difficulty in eating is a major problem with stomatitis and may warrant hospitalization if the child refuses fluids. The child will usually choose the foods that are best tolerated. Surprisingly, some children prefer salty foods to more bland ones. Drinking can usually be encouraged if a straw is used to bypass the ulcerated oral mucosa. The nurse should encourage parents to relax any eating pressures because the anorexia accompanying stomatitis is well justified. In addition, because it is a temporary condition, once the ulcers heal, the child can resume good food habits. Ordinarily, severe mucosal ulceration indicates a need for decreased chemotherapy until complete healing takes place, usually within a week. Analgesics, including opioids, may be needed when treatment cannot be altered, such as during BMT.

If rectal ulcers develop, meticulous toilet hygiene, warm sitz baths after each bowel movement, and an occlusive ointment applied to the ulcerated area promote healing; the use of stool softeners is necessary to prevent further discomfort. Parents are advised to record bowel movements because the child may voluntarily avoid defecation to prevent discomfort. Rectal temperatures and suppositories are avoided because they may further traumatize the affected area.

**Neurologic Problems.**   Vincristine, and to a lesser extent vinblastine, can cause various neurotoxic effects, one of the more common of which is severe constipation from decreased bowel innervation. Constipation is further aggravated by opioids. The nurse advises parents to record bowel movements and to notify the practitioner of a change in stool habits. Physical activity and stool softeners are helpful in preventing the problem, but laxatives, such as Peri-Colace, or enemas are often necessary to stimulate evacuation. Dietary changes such as increased fiber may not be effective, because the increased bulk tends to increase fecal distention and discomfort without producing the necessary mechanical stimulation.

Footdrop, weakness, and numbness of the extremities may cause difficulty in walking or fine hand movement. The nurse should look for these problems and warn parents of these side effects, which are reversible once the drug is stopped. If the child is on bed rest, a footboard is used to preserve proper alignment. If weakness occurs while the child is attending school, a temporary alteration of activity may be necessary. The teacher should be apprised of the situation so that unrealistic expectations of the child's abilities are not made.

Another side effect that can be severe is jaw pain. Analgesics may be necessary to relieve the discomfort. Avoiding movement by not talking or chewing is usually self-imposed, although continuous chewing, such as with gum, may actually reduce the pain. Because the pain is temporary, usually lasting for a day or two, the child can be given fluids through a straw.

A neurologic syndrome (*postirradiation somnolence*) may develop 5 to 8 weeks after central nervous system irradiation and may last for 4 to 15 days. It is characterized by somnolence with or without fever, anorexia, and nausea and vomiting. Parents should be warned of the possibility of such symptoms and encouraged to seek medical evaluation because somnolence may be an early indicator of long-term neurologic sequelae after cranial irradiation.

**Hemorrhagic Cystitis.** Sterile hemorrhagic cystitis is a side effect of chemical irritation to the bladder from chemotherapy or radiation therapy. It can be prevented by (1) a liberal oral or parenteral fluid intake (at least one and one-half times the recommended daily fluid requirement [2 L/m²/day]); (2) frequent voiding immediately after feeling the urge, including immediately before bed and after arising (may include one nighttime void); (3) administration of the drug early in the day to allow for sufficient fluids and frequent voiding; and (4) administration of mesna, a drug that inhibits the urotoxicity of cyclophosphamide and ifosfamide (Lanzkowsky, 2000).

> **NURSING ALERT** If signs of cystitis such as burning on urination occur, prompt medical evaluation is needed. Hemorrhagic cystitis warrants cessation of the drug.

In some cases IV fluids are given before, during, and after the drug to ensure adequate hydration, thereby eliminating the need for the child's drinking large amounts of fluid. If oral home administration is prescribed, the family needs *specific* instructions on exactly how much fluid the child must have.

**Alopecia.** Hair loss is a side effect of several chemotherapeutic drugs and cranial irradiation. Not all children lose their hair during drug therapy; however, retaining hair is the exception rather than the rule. It is better to warn children and parents of this side effect than to allow them to think that it is only a remote possibility.

The family should know that the hair falls out in clumps, causing patchy baldness. To lessen the trauma of seeing large amounts of hair on bed linen or clothing, the child can wear a disposable surgical cap to collect the shed hair during the period of greatest hair loss or the hair can be cut short. Families should also be aware that wigs are tax deductible and that hair regrows in 3 to 6 months (at a rate of about ½ inch a month). The hair frequently is darker, thicker, and curlier than before.

> **NURSING TIP** Encouraging children to choose a wig similar to their own hairstyle and color *before* the hair falls out is helpful in fostering later adjustment to hair loss.

If the child chooses not to wear a wig, attention to some type of head covering is important, especially in cold or sunny climates. Scalp hygiene is also important. The scalp should be washed regularly as with any other body part.

Many children demonstrate increased tolerance to hair loss on reinduction therapy. Rather than complete baldness, the child may experience thinning of the hair. If the hair is cut short, kept clean, and blow-dried with an electric hair drier, it usually can look full enough to make a wig unnecessary. This can be a tremendous psychologic boost to the child who is already depressed about learning of a relapse and the need for additional chemotherapy.

**Steroid Effects.** Short-term steroid therapy produces no acute toxicities and often results in two beneficial reactions—

increased appetite and a sense of well-being. However, it does produce alterations in body image, which, although not clinically significant, can be extremely distressing to older children. One of these is **moon face.** The child's face becomes rounded and puffy. (See Fig. 38-5.) Unlike hair loss, little can be done to camouflage this obvious change, although careful avoidance of salt and salt-containing foods can help reduce fluid accumulation. It is not unusual for other children to make fun of the child, with such remarks as "Porky Pig" or "fat face." It is helpful to reassure the child that after cessation of the drug the facial contours will return to normal. If the child resumes activity early in the course of treatment, the change may be less noticeable to peers than after a long absence. Also, the use of loose-fitting clothes, such as warm-up outfits, can help camouflage the change in weight.

In contrast, parents may appreciate the full-rounded appearance because it simulates the look of a well-nourished, healthy child. Because of their own needs, they may be less able to understand the child's misery over altered body image. The nurse can foster a better understanding between the parents and child if both parties are encouraged to openly discuss their feelings.

Children receiving steroid therapy do look healthy. The moon face, red cheeks, supraclavicular fat pads, protuberant abdomen, and fluid retention indicate weight gain. However, the actual weight gain resulting from increased muscle mass and subcutaneous tissue may be small. Therefore the nurse should evaluate weight gain by observing the extremities and measuring skinfold thickness and arm circumference during steroid therapy to determine if the weight gain is a result of increased dietary intake.

Shortly after beginning steroid therapy, children may experience a number of **mood changes,** which range from feelings of well-being and euphoria to depression and irritability. If parents are unaware of these drug-induced changes, they may become unduly concerned. Therefore the nurse should warn them of the reactions and encourage them to discuss the behavioral changes with each other and the child.

### Nursing Care During Bone Marrow Transplantation (BMT)

Many of the side effects previously discussed occur in the child undergoing BMT. However, because of the aggressive preconditioning programs used to ablate the marrow and the use of growth factors to promote engraftment of transplanted stem cells, these children are usually hospitalized for several weeks after BMT. Because of the risk of infection, the unit may employ such measures as strict handwashing, screening visitors, laminar airflow rooms, and institutional isolation policies.

BMT patients must have numerous procedures performed, such as the insertion of a venous access device, administration of intensive chemotherapy and irradiation, and continued meticulous personal hygiene. In addition, side effects and complications may occur after the preoperative cytotoxic regimen, which include development of infection, severe mucositis, parotitis, nausea, vomiting, diarrhea, syndrome of inappropriate antidiuretic hormone (SIADH), nephropathy, and heart failure (Poliquin, 1997).

During the period after transplantation and before the new marrow begins adequately replacing granulocytes, the child is extremely susceptible to infection. Interstitial or nonbacterial pneumonia is another serious complication with a high mortality rate. However, the most common complication in allogeneic transplants is GVHD, which can affect the skin, gastrointestinal tract, liver, heart, lungs, lymphoid tissue, and marrow. GVHD is characterized by a hardening of the tissues and drying of the mucous membranes. The severity of the manifestations varies, but once vital organs are affected, death can ensue. Treatment involves the use of steroids or azathioprine (Imuran). However, these immunosuppressive drugs further increase the risk of infection. All blood products should be irradiated to minimize the introduction of additional antigens. Another unfortunate post-transplant possibility is recurrence of the malignancy after engraftment. Emphasis is now placed on the prevention of GVHD, using various agents such as cyclosporine, methotrexate, and steroids (Guinan, Krance, and Lehman, 2002).

Skin breakdown and delayed wound healing occur frequently in the patient undergoing BMT. Preventive interventions to minimize pressure on dependent areas of the skin include the use of pressure-relieving or pressure-reducing beds or mattresses and frequent turning. Measures to promote healing when breakdown occurs include frequent sitz baths for the perianal area; transparent dressings, such as Tegaderm, over bony prominences; and protective skin barriers, such as hydrocolloid dressings or occlusive ointments. Throughout this long ordeal there is the family's concern for successful engraftment and fear of fatal complications. Consequently nurses involved with the child and family need to provide sensitive care and maintain a supportive attitude during the many crises that may arise. If the procedure is not successful, the care needed by these families is consistent with that required by the family of any child with a life-threatening disorder. (See Chapter 23.)

## Preparation for Procedures

Children in particular need psychologic preparation for the various treatment modalities, which often involve surgery, IV injections, bone marrow aspiration, and lumbar punctures. The diagnostic procedures initially employed to confirm the diagnosis and those that are repeated to monitor treatment are often a source of discomfort and stress to the child and family. Even noninvasive procedures such as imaging and radiologic tests are frightening to a young child. Many of these tests require the child to lie absolutely motionless for a prolonged time in a confined space with little or no communication with a supportive adult. Consequently infants and young children are usually sedated, and older children need an explanation of what to expect and reminders during the test of how much longer they must remain still. The same principles for preparing children for procedures that are discussed in Chapter 27 apply here, including the option of having parents stay with the child whenever possible. (See Evidence-Based Practice box on p. 1107.) Children who undergo repeated tests need additional preparation and emotional support to experience decreasing levels of stress (Kazak and others, 1998).

Two procedures, bone marrow studies and lumbar punctures, are so commonly performed in many types of childhood cancer that they deserve special consideration in preparing children (Fig. 36-1). Both tests can be frightening to children because they are done behind the child's field of vision. Consensus among professionals caring for children with cancer recommend the use of sedation for the initial procedures and subsequent developmentally appropriate support using both pharmacologic and nonpharmacologic approaches. Most sedation protocols combine an opioid analgesic with a benzodiazepine for anxiolysis and sedation (Kazak and others, 1998; Macpherson and Lundblad, 1997). (See Critical Thinking Exercise box on p. 1604.) Sedation is induced with agents such as ketamine, propofol (Diprivan), and methohexital (Brevital) (Freyer and others, 1997).

EMLA cream, a topical anesthetic preparation that adequately penetrates intact skin, is used as a local anesthetic before intrusive procedures, including venipunctures, implanted port access, lumbar punctures, and subcutaneous or intramuscular injections of growth factors or other drugs (Hockenberry-Eaton and others, 1999; Lloyd-Thomas, 1999). (See Fig. 27-16.) Local intradermal anesthesia is frequently used for lumbar puncture and bone marrow examination. To reduce the stinging sensation from lidocaine, sodium bicarbonate should be added. (See Pain Management, Chapter 26.) Deeper infiltration of the muscle and periosteum of the bone with buffered lidocaine further reduces the pain from the large-bore aspiration/biopsy needle entering the bone.

For bone marrow studies and lumbar punctures, as well as other procedures, children of preschool age and beyond should be prepared beforehand. If this is not possible, the nurse should explain each step of the procedure as it occurs, stressing what will be done and what it will feel like. If each step is explained beforehand, having the child recall the next step during the procedure can be a distraction mechanism.

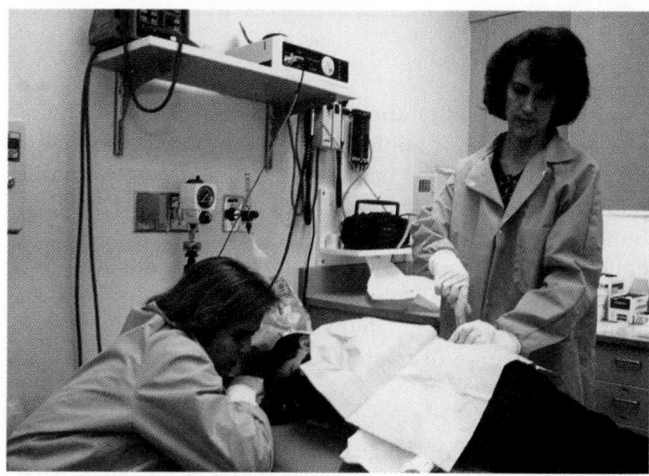

**Fig. 36-1**   Child with leukemia undergoing a bone marrow aspiration.

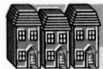

## Critical Thinking Exercise

### Bone Marrow Test

Suzy Long, 5 years old, is admitted to the hospital for diagnosis of possible leukemia. During your nursing admission history regarding Suzy's pain experience, Mrs. Long tells you that her daughter is very cooperative when she receives injections. Suzy agrees and adds that they hurt, but just for a second. With this information you discuss with the nurse practitioner who will perform the bone marrow test the type of preparation that is appropriate for Suzy. You both believe that the best option would be which of the following?

FIRST, THINK ABOUT IT . . .

• What assumptions are you making?
• If you accept the assumptions, what are the implications?

1. Tell Suzy what the test will be like and teach her a simple breathing exercise to help her relax.
2. Use a local anesthetic at the bone marrow site to lessen the painful entry of the needle.
3. Administer midazolam and fentanyl intravenously just before the procedure to produce sedation.
4. Offer Suzy the above choices and let her select one.

*All of the options are potentially acceptable, but for Suzy the best response is three, considering her age, the type of painful procedures she has experienced, the pain intensity of the bone marrow test, and the possibility of future invasive procedures.*

*Suzy is too young to compare the first three choices critically. Injections are typically less painful than a bone marrow test, which Suzy has never had. Relaxation works well in some children for procedures that produce mild to moderate pain, such as venipunctures, but there is no way to predict its success. A local anesthetic lessens the pain, but not the sensation of pushing to insert the needle or the aspiration of the marrow. Also, the bone marrow test for diagnosis takes longer to perform than most other bone marrow tests because a larger amount of marrow is needed. Sometimes two punctures may be done. Using fentanyl and midazolam will reduce the pain and produce amnesia, making the procedure less stressful and preventing fear and anxiety for future tests.*

Physical care after the procedures is minimal. A small pressure bandage is applied to the bone marrow puncture site, and an adhesive bandage is applied to the lumbar puncture site. No activity restriction is necessary after the bone marrow test, although the site is usually sore and the child may prefer to remain quiet. Recommendations after the lumbar puncture vary. If medication was instilled, the child may be placed in a slight Trendelenburg position to facilitate circulation of the medicated spinal fluid.

## Pain Management

Nurses must be knowledgeable about the basic pathophysiology of cancer pain and treatment-related side effects. The World Health Organization's (WHO's) three-step analgesic

pain ladder should be incorporated into the approach to pain management for every child with cancer* (Hellsten, 2000; McGrath, 1996; WHO, 1998). Nurses must acquire extensive knowledge of nonopioid and opioid analgesics used in pediatric pain management. (See Chapter 26.) Interdisciplinary pain management teams are used in many pediatric cancer centers. These teams serve as consultants and provide expertise in the assessment and management of pain. The nurse often serves as the coordinator of care, playing a key role in cancer pain management.

Pharmacologic management of disease-related pain involves a variety of methods that are discussed in detail in Chapter 26. It is important to consider that it may take more than a trial of one type of medication to find the appropriate agent to manage a patient's pain. The route of administration must be considered as well. Providing "pain relief" by administering painful intramuscular injections, as an alternative to the IV route, is not appropriate therapy because many oral preparations are now available with comparable efficacy. Nonsteroidal antiinflammatory drugs (NSAIDs), acetaminophen with codeine, oxycodone, and morphine are commonly used agents in the management of disease-related pain (Kumar, Rajagopal, and Naseema, 2000; Lloyd-Thomas, 1999; McGrath, 1996). All are available in the oral form, and morphine and the NSAID ketorolac (Toradol) are available as IV preparations. Appropriate dosing is imperative. Doses are titrated to increase the amount of analgesia and minimize side effects.

### Health Promotion

Children with cancer require the same basic health supervision as any child. Sometimes the overwhelming needs and demands placed on the family coupled with the singular concern focused on the cancer by both family and practitioners result in a lack of attention to normal health care needs. Nurses should monitor the type of primary care the child receives, using as a guideline recommendations for health supervision. (See Chapter 7 and Commu-

 *For additional information, please view "Pain Assessment and Management" in *Whaley and Wong's Pediatric Nursing Video Series,* St Louis, 1996, Mosby, (800) 426-4545, www.mosby.com.

nity Focus box.) As discussed under the Assessment section, areas of particular concern are growth, physical and cognitive development, and neurologic status. Two other areas are also important: (1) dental care, because of potential side effects from treatment; and (2) immunizations, because of concern with live virus vaccines and immunosuppression.

**Dental Care.** Irradiation to the head and neck can cause a number of late complications (Dreyer, Blatt, and Bleyer, 2002). Some are irreversible, such as facial asymmetry, but those affecting the teeth and gums (caries, periodontal disease) benefit from excellent oral hygiene, including regular use of systemic and topical fluoride. (See Dental Health, Chapter 14.) There is also evidence of delayed or absent development of the permanent teeth (Dreyer, Blatt, and Bleyer, 2002; Oeffinger and others, 2000). Depending on the child's age, this can be a source of acute psychologic distress, especially during early school-age years, when "losing a tooth" is a status symbol. Children need to be aware of this possibility and need help to explain the delay to peers.

Daily toothbrushing and flossing is encouraged in children with granulocyte counts in excess of $500/mm^3$ and platelet counts above $40,000/mm^3$. Fluoride rinses are used as discussed in Chapter 14. Oral hygiene for children whose counts are below these parameters is limited to wiping the teeth with moistened gauze sponges or Toothettes.

**Immunizations.** Viral replication following the administration of live vaccine for polio, measles, rubella, and mumps can cause serious disease in immunocompromised children who receive these vaccines.

The child receiving chemotherapy for cancer should not receive live, attenuated vaccines. Inactivated vaccines can be given to immunosuppressed children, but the immune response is likely to be suboptimal, so delaying vaccinations is usually recommended (American Academy of Pediatrics, 2000; McFarland, 1999). Siblings and household contacts may receive the live measles, mumps, and rubella (MMR) vaccine without risk to the child with cancer. Children who are immunosuppressed should not receive the varicella vaccine (McFarland, 1999). Siblings and other family members can receive the varicella vaccine without risk to the child who is immunosuppressed.

> **NURSING ALERT**
>
> Children vaccinated 2 weeks before or during chemotherapy should be considered unimmunized and should be revaccinated or receive live virus vaccines 3 months after chemotherapy has stopped (American Academy of Pediatrics, 2000).

A very important indication for isolation is an outbreak of childhood disease, especially chickenpox. Ideally the school nurse should work with the treating practitioner to decide the optimum time for school reattendance. If the child has been exposed to the varicella virus, varicella-zoster immune globulin (VZIG) given within 72 hours may favorably alter the course of the disease, or antiviral agents, such as acyclovir, may be given if the child develops varicella. These antiviral agents are very effective in preventing serious disease if given during the first 3 days of the appearance of symptoms (American Academy of Pediatrics, 2000). Without treatment, death from disseminated varicella (about 7%) is usually caused by pneumonia; other serious although nonfatal complications include hepatitis, pancreatitis, meningitis, and bacterial skin infections. (See also Immunizations, Chapter 12.)

## Family Education

Nurses working with children who have cancer have a significant supportive role in helping the family understand the various therapies, preventing or managing expected side effects or toxicities, and observing for late effects of treatment. Education is a constant feature of the nursing role, especially in terms of new treatments, clinical trials, and home care. Because of the anxiety generated by the diagnosis of cancer, some families may resort to unproven methods of treatment that are frequently referred to as "cancer quackery." These unorthodox approaches may produce unnecessary harm by themselves or, if benign, render injury because other proven modes of therapy are avoided. In many instances this causes financial burden and emotional strife among family members.

Nurses can be instrumental in working against cancer quackery by being aware of factors that increase a family's likelihood of seeking unproven remedies, such as social pressure to "leave no stone unturned" and feelings of depression, helplessness, and hopelessness. Communicating effectively with families about the diagnosis and forms of therapy and providing all possible support and reassurance during treatment are also important interventions to counteract the factors that lead to dissatisfaction with conventional care. Nurses must be fortified with knowledge to substantiate present treatment protocols and to discredit unauthorized methods. The American Cancer Society and local and state medical societies are reliable sources of information concerning research on investigational vs quack methods of cancer therapy. The **National Association of Pediatric Oncology Nurses**[*] has developed numerous educational materials for family and child teaching. The **Candlelighters Childhood Cancer Foundation**[†] is an international organization providing support, education, and advocacy programs for children with cancer and their families.

Instruction regarding home care frequently involves teaching about medication schedules, observation for side effects or toxicities that require further evaluation, measures to prevent or manage these problems, and care of special devices such as central venous catheters.[‡] Compliance

---

[*]4700 W Lake Ave, Glenview, IL 60025-1485, (847) 375-4724, fax: (847) 375-6325; www.apon.org.

[†]3910 Warner St, Kensington, MD 20895, (800) 366-2223 or (301) 962-3520, fax: (301) 962-3521; www.candlelighters.org.

[‡]Home care instructions for giving medications to children and caring for a central venous catheter are available in Wong DL, Hess CS: *Wong and Whaley's clinical manual of pediatric nursing*, ed 5, St Louis, 2000, Mosby.

is a very important issue, because poor adherence to drug regimens can result in a relapse. Every effort must be made to ensure that the family understands the importance of adhering to the prescribed treatment schedule and measures to improve compliance. (See Chapter 27.)

### Cessation of Therapy

Care does not end when the child completes therapy. With the increasing awareness of late effects, nurses play an important role in the assessment of the child for problems such as delayed growth, secondary malignancies, and disturbances in any body system. These children require regular follow-up, and the family needs to be aware of the importance of continued medical supervision. Other health care professionals caring for the child, such as school nurses, family physicians, and dentists, should be informed of the child's previous diagnosis of cancer. As children reach adulthood, they may benefit from genetic counseling regarding cancers that are likely to be inherited. If the possibility of sterility exists, pretreatment sperm banking may be offered to adolescent boys, which allows additional options regarding family planning in adulthood.

### ❖ Evaluation

The effectiveness of nursing interventions is determined by continual reassessment and evaluation of care based on the following observational guidelines:

1. Compare number of visits for primary health with recommended schedule of health supervision.
2. Monitor growth, development, and other aspects of regular health assessment; check mouth for adequacy of dental hygiene; review immunization record for age-appropriate vaccines and the use of non–live virus preparations.
3. Interview child and family regarding their understanding of treatments and diagnostic tests.
4. Employ pain assessment techniques for procedural pain.
5. Make careful observations of physical status:
   Take vital signs regularly.
   Observe for evidence of bleeding, infection, neuropathy, cystitis, and mucosal ulceration.
   Observe and record intake and output.
6. Interview child and family and observe behaviors as a result of complications of therapies.
7. Interview child and family and observe behaviors that provide clues to their response to the disease, its therapy, and nursing interventions.

The *expected outcomes* are described in the Nursing Care Plan on pp. 1606-1611.

---

## Nursing Care Plan
### The Child with Cancer

**NURSING DIAGNOSIS:** Risk for injury related to malignant process, treatment

**PATIENT GOAL 1:** Will experience partial or complete remission from disease

- **NURSING INTERVENTIONS/RATIONALES**

*Administer chemotherapeutic agents as prescribed
Assist with radiotherapy as ordered
Assist with procedures for administration of chemotherapeutic agents (e.g., lumbar puncture for intrathecal administration)
†Prepare child and family for surgical procedure if appropriate

- **EXPECTED OUTCOME**

Child achieves a partial or complete remission from disease

**PATIENT GOAL 2:** Will not experience complications of chemotherapy

- **NURSING INTERVENTIONS/RATIONALES**

Follow guidelines for administration of chemotherapeutic agents
Observe for signs of infiltration at intravenous site: pain, stinging, swelling, redness
Immediately stop infusion if any sign of infiltration occurs *to prevent severe tissue damage*
Implement policies of institution *to treat infiltration*

Obtain careful history for known allergies *to prevent anaphylaxis*
Observe child for 20 minutes after infusion for *signs of anaphylaxis* (cyanosis, hypotension, wheezing, severe urticaria)
Stop infusion of drug and flush intravenous line with normal saline if reaction is suspected
Have emergency equipment (especially blood pressure monitor and manual resuscitation bag and mask) and emergency drugs (especially oxygen, epinephrine, antihistamine, aminophylline, corticosteroids, and vasopressors) readily available *to prevent delay in treatment*

- **EXPECTED OUTCOMES**

Child will not experience complications of chemotherapy
Child will receive prompt, appropriate treatment of complications

**NURSING DIAGNOSIS:** Risk for infection related to depressed body defenses

**PATIENT GOAL 1:** Will experience minimized risk of infection

- **NURSING INTERVENTIONS/RATIONALES**

Place child in private room *to minimize exposure to infective organisms*
Advise all visitors and staff to use good handwashing technique *to minimize exposure to infective organisms*
Screen all visitors and staff for signs of infection *to minimize exposure to infective organisms*
Use scrupulous aseptic technique for all invasive procedures
Monitor temperature *to detect possible infection*

---

*Dependent nursing action.
†Indicates content that is specific to a particular malignancy.

# Nursing Care Plan
## The Child with Cancer—cont'd

Evaluate child for any potential sites of infection (e.g., needle punctures, mucosal ulceration, minor abrasions, dental problems)

Provide nutritionally complete diet for age *to support body's natural defenses*

Avoid giving live attenuated virus vaccines (e.g., measles, varicella, mumps, rubella) to child with depressed immune system *because these vaccines can result in overwhelming infection*

*Give inactivated virus vaccines (e.g., Salk polio, influenza) as prescribed and indicated *to prevent specific infections*

*Administer antibiotics as prescribed

*Administer granulocyte colony-stimulating factor (G-CSF) as prescribed

- **EXPECTED OUTCOMES**

Child does not come in contact with infected persons or contaminated articles

Child consumes diet appropriate for age (specify)

Child does not exhibit signs of infection

> **NURSING DIAGNOSIS:** Risk for injury (hemorrhage, hemorrhagic cystitis) related to interference with cell proliferation

**PATIENT GOAL 1:** Will exhibit no evidence of bleeding

- **NURSING INTERVENTIONS/***RATIONALES***

Use all measures to prevent infection, especially in ecchymotic areas, *because infection increases tendency toward bleeding*

Use local measures (e.g., apply pressure, ice) to stop bleeding

Restrict strenuous activity *that could result in accidental injury*

Involve child in responsibility for limiting activity when platelet count drops *to encourage compliance*

Avoid skin punctures when possible *to prevent bleeding*

Observe for bleeding after procedures such as venipuncture, bone marrow aspiration

Turn frequently and use pressure-reducing or pressure-relieving mattress *to prevent decubitus ulcers*

Teach parents and older child measures to control nosebleeding

Prevent oral and rectal ulceration *because ulcerated skin is prone to bleeding*

Avoid aspirin-containing medications *because aspirin interferes with platelet function*

*Administer platelets as prescribed *to raise platelet count*

- **EXPECTED OUTCOME**

Child exhibits no evidence of bleeding

**PATIENT GOAL 2:** Will exhibit no evidence of hemorrhagic cystitis

- **NURSING INTERVENTIONS/***RATIONALES***

Observe for signs of cystitis (e.g., burning and pain on urination)

Report signs of cystitis to practitioner *because prompt medical evaluation is needed*

Give liberal (3000 ml/m²/day) fluid intake (meters squared is calculated from West Nomogram, p. 1150)

Encourage frequent voiding, including during nighttime, *to minimize metabolites' contact with bladder mucosa*

*Administer drugs irritating to bladder early in the day *to allow for sufficient fluid intake and voiding*

- **EXPECTED OUTCOMES**

Child voids without discomfort

No hematuria is present

**PATIENT GOAL 3:** Will experience minimal effects of anemia

- **NURSING INTERVENTIONS/***RATIONALES* **AND EXPECTED OUTCOMES**

See Nursing Care Plan: The Child with Anemia‡

> **NURSING DIAGNOSIS:** Risk for deficient fluid volume related to nausea and vomiting

**PATIENT GOAL 1:** Will experience no nausea or vomiting

- **NURSING INTERVENTIONS/***RATIONALES***

*Administer initial dose of antiemetic before chemotherapy begins *to prevent child from ever experiencing nausea and vomiting, thus preventing an anticipatory response*

*Administer antiemetic around the clock for as long as nausea and vomiting typically last *to prevent any episodes from occurring*

Assess child's response to antiemetic, *because no antiemetic drug is uniformly successful*

Avoid foods with strong odors *that may induce nausea and vomiting*

Uncover hospital food tray outside of child's room *to reduce food odors that may induce nausea*

Encourage frequent intake of fluids in small amounts, *because small portions are usually better tolerated*

*Administer intravenous fluid, as prescribed, *to maintain hydration*

- **EXPECTED OUTCOMES**

Child retains food and fluid

Child does not experience nausea or vomiting

> **NURSING DIAGNOSIS:** Impaired oral mucous membrane related to administration of chemotherapeutic agents

**PATIENT GOAL 1:** Will not develop oral mucositis

- **NURSING INTERVENTIONS/***RATIONALES***

Inspect mouth daily for oral ulcers; report evidence of ulcers to practitioner *for early treatment*

Avoid oral temperatures *to prevent trauma*

Institute meticulous oral hygiene as soon as a drug is used that causes oral ulcers

    Use soft-sponge toothbrush, cotton-tipped applicator, or gauze-wrapped finger *to avoid trauma*

    Administer frequent (at least every 4 hours and after meals) mouthrinses (normal saline with or without sodium bicarbonate solution) *to promote healing*

---

*Dependent nursing action.

‡In Wong DL, Hess CS: *Wong and Whaley's clinical manual of pediatric nursing,* ed 5, St. Louis, 2000, Mosby.

*Continued*

# Nursing Care Plan
## The Child with Cancer—cont'd

### PATIENT GOAL 1—cont'd

• **NURSING INTERVENTIONS/*RATIONALES*—cont'd**

Apply local anesthetics to ulcerated areas before meals and as needed *to relieve pain*

Avoid using viscous lidocaine for young children *because if applied to pharynx, it may depress gag reflex, increasing risk of aspiration, and may cause seizures*

Apply lip balm *to keep lips moist and prevent cracking or fissuring*

Serve bland, moist, soft diet; offer food best tolerated by child

Encourage fluids; use a straw *to help bypass painful areas*

Encourage parents to relax any eating pressures, *because stomatitis is a temporary condition*

Avoid juices containing ascorbic acid and hot or cold or spicy foods if they cause further discomfort

Avoid using lemon glycerin swabs *(irritate eroded tissue and can decay teeth)*, hydrogen peroxide *(delays healing by breaking down protein)*, and milk of magnesia *(dries mucosa)*

Explain to parents that child may require hospitalization for hydration, parenteral nutrition, and pain control (often with intravenous morphine) *if stomatitis interferes with food and fluid intake*

*Administer antiinfective medication *to prevent or treat mucositis*

*Administer analgesics, including opioids, *to control pain*

• **EXPECTED OUTCOMES**

Mucous membranes remain intact

Ulcers show evidence of healing

Child reports and exhibits no evidence of discomfort

### PATIENT GOAL 2: Will not develop rectal ulceration

• **NURSING INTERVENTIONS/*RATIONALES***

Wash perianal area after each bowel movement *to lessen irritation*

Use warm sitz baths or tub baths *to promote healing*

Expose reddened but not ulcerated areas to air *to keep skin dry*

Apply protective skin barriers (transparent film dressings, occlusive ointment) to perineal area *to protect skin from direct contact with urine or feces and to promote healing*

Observe for constipation *resulting from child's voluntary refusal to defecate or from chemotherapy or opioids*

Record bowel movements; use stool softener *to prevent constipation*; may need stimulants *for evacuation*

Avoid rectal temperatures and suppositories *to prevent trauma*

• **EXPECTED OUTCOMES**

Rectal mucosa remains clean and intact

Ulcerated areas heal without complications

Child has regular bowel movements

---

**NURSING DIAGNOSIS:** Imbalanced nutrition: less than body requirements related to loss of appetite

---

### PATIENT GOAL 1: Will receive adequate nutrition

• **NURSING INTERVENTIONS/*RATIONALES***

Encourage parents to relax pressures placed on eating; explain that loss of appetite *is a direct consequence of nausea and vomiting caused by chemotherapy*

Allow child *any* food tolerated; plan to improve quality of food selections when appetite increases

Explain expected increase in appetite from steroids *to prepare child and parents for this change*

Take advantage of any hungry period: serve small "snacks" *because small portions are usually better tolerated*

Fortify foods with nutritious supplements, such as powdered milk or commercial supplements, *to maximize quality of intake*

Allow child to be involved in food preparation and selection *to encourage eating*

Make food appealing

Remember usual food practices of children in each age-group, such as food jags in toddlers or normal occurrence of physiologic anorexia, *to distinguish these expected changes from actual refusal to eat*

Assess family for additional problems (e.g., use of food by child as a control mechanism) if appetite does not improve despite improved physical status *to identify areas that require intervention*

• **EXPECTED OUTCOME**

Nutritional intake is adequate

---

**NURSING DIAGNOSIS:** Impaired skin integrity related to administration of chemotherapeutic agents, radiotherapy, immobility

---

### PATIENT GOAL 1: Will maintain skin integrity

• **NURSING INTERVENTIONS/*RATIONALES***

Provide meticulous skin care, especially in mouth and perianal regions, *because they are prone to ulceration*

Change position frequently *to stimulate circulation and relieve pressure*

Encourage adequate caloric-protein intake *to prevent negative nitrogen balance*

• **EXPECTED OUTCOME**

Skin remains clean and intact

### PATIENT GOAL 2: Will experience minimal negative effects of therapy

• **NURSING INTERVENTIONS/*RATIONALES***

Select loose-fitting clothing over irradiated area *to minimize additional irritation*

Protect area from sunlight and sudden changes in temperature (avoid ice packs, heating pads) during radiotherapy or administration of methotrexate

• **EXPECTED OUTCOME**

Child and family comply with suggestions (specify)

---

**NURSING DIAGNOSIS:** Impaired physical mobility related to neuromuscular impairment (neuropathy)

---

### PATIENT GOAL 1: Will experience minimal negative effects of peripheral neuropathy

• **NURSING INTERVENTIONS/*RATIONALES***

Encourage ambulation when child is able

Alter activity, including school attendance, *to prevent injuries if weakness occurs*

Use footboard or high-top shoes *to prevent footdrop*

---

*Dependent nursing action.

## Nursing Care Plan
### The Child with Cancer—cont'd

Provide fluids and soft foods *to lessen chewing movements with jaw pain*

- **EXPECTED OUTCOME**

Child ambulates without incident or difficulty

> **NURSING DIAGNOSIS:** Disturbed body image related to loss of hair, moon face, debilitation

**PATIENT/FAMILY GOAL 1:** Will exhibit positive coping behaviors

- **NURSING INTERVENTIONS/***RATIONALES*

Introduce idea of wig before hair loss
  Encourage child to select a wig similar to child's own hairstyle and color before hair falls out *to foster later adjustment to hair loss*
Provide adequate covering during exposure to sunlight, wind, or cold, *because natural protection is lost*
Suggest keeping thin hair clean, short, and fluffy *to camouflage partial baldness*
Explain that hair begins to regrow in 3 to 6 months and may be a slightly different color or texture *to prepare child and family for changes in appearance of new hair*
Explain that alopecia during a second treatment with same drug may be less severe
Encourage good hygiene, grooming, and sex-appropriate items (e.g., wig, scarves, hats, makeup, attractive sex-appropriate clothing) *to enhance appearance*

- **EXPECTED OUTCOMES**

Child verbalizes concern regarding hair loss
Child helps determine methods to reduce effects of hair loss and applies these methods
Child appears clean, well-groomed, and attractively dressed

**PATIENT GOAL 2:** Will exhibit adjustment to altered facial appearance

- **NURSING INTERVENTIONS/***RATIONALES*

Encourage rapid reintegration with peers *to lessen contrast of changed facial appearance*
Stress that this reaction is temporary *to provide reassurance that usual appearance will return*
Evaluate weight gain carefully (*in weight gain resulting from administration of steroids, extremities remain thin*)
Encourage visits from friends before discharge *to prepare child for reactions and questions*

- **EXPECTED OUTCOMES**

Family demonstrates understanding of consequences of therapies
Child resumes former activities and relationships within capabilities

**PATIENT GOAL 3:** Will express feelings

- **NURSING INTERVENTIONS/***RATIONALES*

Provide opportunities for child to discuss feelings and concerns

---

*Dependent nursing action.

Provide materials for nonverbal expression (e.g., play, art)

- **EXPECTED OUTCOME**

Child expresses feelings regarding altered body in words, play, art (specify)

> **NURSING DIAGNOSIS:** Acute pain related to diagnosis, treatment, physiologic effects of neoplasia

**PATIENT GOAL 1:** Will experience no pain or reduction of pain to level acceptable to child

- **NURSING INTERVENTIONS/***RATIONALES*

Whenever possible, make use of procedures (e.g., noninvasive temperature monitoring, venous access device) to minimize discomfort
Assess need for pain management (See Chapter 26.)
Evaluate effectiveness of pain relief with degree of alertness vs sedation *to determine need for change in dosage, time of administration, or drug*
Implement appropriate nonpharmacologic pain reduction techniques *as adjunct to analgesics*
*Administer analgesics as prescribed
  Avoid aspirin or any of its compounds (e.g., other nonsteroidal antiinflammatory agents) *because aspirin increases bleeding tendency*
*Administer drugs on preventive schedule (around the clock) *to prevent pain from recurring*
Monitor effectiveness of therapy on pain assessment record

- **EXPECTED OUTCOME**

Child rests quietly, reports and exhibits no evidence of discomfort, verbalizes no complaints of discomfort

> **NURSING DIAGNOSIS:** Fear related to diagnostic tests, procedures, treatments

**PATIENT GOAL 1:** Will exhibit reduced fear related to diagnostic procedures and tests

- **NURSING INTERVENTIONS/***RATIONALES*

Explain procedure carefully at child's level of understanding *to reduce fear of the unknown*
Explain what will take place and what child will feel, see, and hear *to increase sense of control*
Use recall of each step *as method of distraction*
Explain special requests of child (e.g., need to remain motionless during test or radiotherapy) *to encourage cooperation*
Provide child with some means for involvement with procedure (e.g., holding a piece of equipment, such as bandage or tape, counting with the operator, answering questions) *to promote sense of control, encourage cooperation, and support child's coping skills*
Implement distracting techniques and pain reduction techniques as indicated
(See Guidelines box, Preparing Children for Procedures, on pp. 1104-1105)

- **EXPECTED OUTCOMES**

Child readily responds to verbal directives
Child repeats information accurately

*Continued*

# Nursing Care Plan
## The Child with Cancer—cont'd

**NURSING DIAGNOSIS:** Fear related to diagnosis, prognosis

See Nursing Care Plan: The Child Who Is Terminally Ill or Dying, Chapter 23

**NURSING DIAGNOSIS:** Deficient diversional activity related to restricted environment (private room)

**PATIENT GOAL 1:** Will have opportunity to participate in diversional activities

• **NURSING INTERVENTIONS/RATIONALES**
Provide age-appropriate toys that can be properly cleaned *to provide diversion without risk of infection*
Involve child-life specialist or other supportive services in planning diversional activities

• **EXPECTED OUTCOMES**
Child engages in activities appropriate for age and interests
Suitable toys are provided

**NURSING DIAGNOSIS:** Interrupted family processes related to having a child with a life-threatening disease

**PATIENT (FAMILY) GOAL 1:** Will demonstrate knowledge about diagnostic/therapeutic procedures

• **NURSING INTERVENTIONS/RATIONALES**
Explain reason for each test and procedure
Explain reason for radiotherapy, chemotherapy
Explain operative procedure honestly (if appropriate)
Avoid overemphasis on benefits, which may not be immediately evident (applies primarily to brain tumors) *to avoid unrealistic expectations*
(See Guidelines box, Preparing Children for Procedures, on pp. 1104-1105)

• **EXPECTED OUTCOME**
Child and family demonstrate understanding of procedures (specify learning and manner of demonstration)

**PATIENT (FAMILY) GOAL 2:** Will receive adequate support

• **NURSING INTERVENTIONS/RATIONALES**
Teach parents about disease process
Explain all procedures that will be done to child
Schedule time for family to be together, without interruptions from staff, *to encourage communication and expression of feelings*
Help family plan for future, especially for helping child live a normal life, *to promote child's optimum development*
Encourage family to discuss feelings regarding child's course before diagnosis and child's prognosis
Discuss with family how they will tell child about outcome of treatment and need for additional treatment (if appropriate) *to maintain open and honest communication*
Refer to local chapter of American Cancer Society or other organizations

• **EXPECTED OUTCOMES**
Family demonstrates knowledge of child's disease and treatments (specify methods of learning and evaluation)
Family expresses feelings and concerns and spends time with child
See also:
Nursing Care Plan: The Child in the Hospital, Chapter 26
Nursing Care Plan: The Family of the Child Who Is Ill or Hospitalized, Chapter 26

**NURSING DIAGNOSIS:** Interrupted family processes related to a child undergoing therapy

**PATIENT (FAMILY) GOAL 1:** Will demonstrate understanding of side effects and complications of treatment

• **NURSING INTERVENTIONS/RATIONALES**
Advise family of expected side effects vs toxicities; clarify which demand medical evaluation (mucosal ulceration, hemorrhagic cystitis, peripheral neuropathy, evidence of infection or dehydration) *to prevent delay in treatment*
Reassure family that such reactions are not caused by return of cancer cells *to minimize undue concern*

# CANCERS OF THE BLOOD AND LYMPH SYSTEMS

## Leukemias

Leukemia, cancer of the blood-forming tissues, is the most common form of childhood cancer. The annual incidence is 3 to 4 cases per 100,000 white children (Margolin, Steuber, and Poplack, 2002). It occurs more frequently in males than in females after age 1 year, and the peak onset is between 2 and 6 years of age. It is one of the forms of cancer that have demonstrated dramatic improvements in survival rates. Before the use of antileukemic agents in 1948, a child with acute lymphocytic leukemia (ALL) lived 2 to 3 months. Current long-term disease-free survival rates for children with ALL approach 80% in major research centers.

### Classification

*Leukemia* is a broad term given to a group of malignant diseases of the bone marrow and lymphatic system. It is a complex disease of varying heterogeneity. Consequently classification has become increasingly complex, sophisticated, and essential because identification of the subtype of leukemia has therapeutic and prognostic implications. The following is an overview of the major classification systems currently being used.

## Nursing Care Plan
### The Child with Cancer—cont'd

Interpret prognostic statistics carefully, realizing family's temporary need to interpret them as they see necessary, *to present a realistic, but hopeful, future*

Prepare family for expected mood changes from steroids

Interpret mood changes based on drugs or reactions to disease/treatment *to prevent any unwarranted negative reaction to child (e.g., punishment)*

• **EXPECTED OUTCOMES**

Family demonstrates knowledge of instructions (specify method of learning and evaluation)

Family demonstrates understanding of behavior changes

**PATIENT GOAL 2:** Will receive adequate support during treatment

• **NURSING INTERVENTIONS/***RATIONALES*

Explain reason for antibiotics or transfusions, particularly why platelets are reserved for acute, uncontrolled bleeding episodes

Observe for signs of transfusion reaction (see Table 35-2)

Record appropriate time for hemostasis to occur after administration of platelets *to determine if transfusions are becoming less effective*

• **EXPECTED OUTCOME**

Child demonstrates understanding of procedures and tests (specify method and learnings)

**PATIENT (FAMILY) GOAL 3:** Will be prepared for home care

• **NURSING INTERVENTIONS/***RATIONALES*

Teach preventive measures at discharge (e.g., handwashing and isolation from crowds) *to prevent infection*

Stress importance of isolating child from any known cases of chickenpox or other childhood diseases; work with school nurse and physician to determine optimum time for school reattendance *to prevent unnecessary absences or risk of infection*

Teach home care instructions specific to child's needs

• **EXPECTED OUTCOME**

Family demonstrates ability to provide home care for child (specify)

---

**NURSING DIAGNOSIS:** Anticipatory grieving related to perceived potential loss of a child

---

**PATIENT (FAMILY) GOAL 1:** Will acknowledge and cope with possibility of child's death

• **NURSING INTERVENTIONS/***RATIONALES*

Provide consistent contact with family *to establish a trusting relationship that encourages communication*

Clarify, refocus, and supply information as needed

Help family plan care of child, especially at terminal stage (e.g., extent of extraordinary lifesaving measures) *to ensure their wishes are implemented*

Provide or arrange for hospice care if family desires it

Arrange for spiritual support in accordance with family's beliefs or affiliations

• **EXPECTED OUTCOMES**

Family remains open to counseling and nursing contact

Family and child discuss their fears, concerns, needs, and desires at terminal stage

Family investigates hospice care

Appropriate religious representative is contacted (specify)

**PATIENT (FAMILY) GOAL 2:** Will receive adequate support

• **NURSING INTERVENTIONS/***RATIONALES* **AND EXPECTED OUTCOMES**

See also:

Nursing Care Plan: The Child Who Is Terminally Ill or Dying, Chapter 23

---

**Morphology.** In children, two forms are generally recognized: *acute lymphoid leukemia (ALL)* and *acute myelogenous leukemia (AML).* Synonyms for ALL include lymphatic, lymphocytic, lymphoblastic, and lymphoblastoid leukemia. Usually the terms *stem* or *blast cell leukemia* also refer to the lymphoid type of leukemia.

Because of the confusion and inconsistency in classifying the leukemias, acute lymphoblastic and acute nonlymphoblastic leukemias are further subdivided according to another system known as the *French-American-British (FAB) system.* In the FAB system the subtypes are determined after a thorough study of the morphology (structure) and cytochemical reactivity of the leukemic cells. Accordingly, ALL

is divided into three subtypes: $L_1$, $L_2$, and $L_3$. $L_1$ morphology is the most common subtype, accounts for 84% of children with ALL and has the best prognosis (Landier, 2001; Margolin, Steuber, and Poplack, 2002). AML is classified into eight subtypes that constitute 20% of leukemias in children. The subtypes of AML are not clearly related to prognosis as is the case with ALL.

**Cytochemical Markers.** Leukemic cells demonstrate different reactions when they are exposed to certain chemicals. For example, terminal deoxynucleotidyl transferase is able to provide excellent differentiation between ALL and ANLL. Several other chemicals are available to further differentiate various cell types.

**Chromosome Studies.** Chromosome analysis of leukemic cells has become an important tool in the diagnosis of ALL. For example, children with trisomy 21 have 20 times the risk of other children for developing ALL (Plon and Milkin, 2002). Children with more than 50 chromosomes (DNA index >1.16) have a better prognosis.

Children with trisomies 4 and 10 have a good prognosis with a low risk of treatment failure (Margolin, Steuber, and Poplack, 2002). Translocations of chromosomes are also found in leukemic cells. The t(1:19)(q23;p13) translocation is one of the most common chromosome abnormalities in children with leukemia and is associated with a poor prognosis. However, intensive chemotherapy has improved survival for this group to nearly 80% (Landier, 2001). The t(9;22)(q34;p11) translocation, known as the Philadelphia chromosome, is found in approximately 5% of children with ALL and is associated with a poor outlook.

**Cell-Surface Immunologic Markers.** Most childhood leukemias are of B-cell lineage. Early pre–B-cell (common) ALL is the most frequent type of cancer found in children. Most (>80%) of these children have the common acute lymphocytic leukemia antigen (CALLA) on their cell surface (Margolin, Steuber, and Poplack, 2002). Children with ALL who are CALLA-positive have better survival rates.

Other subtypes of ALL include pre–B-cell ALL, characterized by the presence of cytoplasmic immunoglobulins (CIg), B-cell ALL that secretes immunoglobulin on the cell surface, and T-cell ALL (revealed by the presence of T-cell surface antigens and heat-stable rosette formation in the presence of sheep red blood cells). A small group of patients ( <5%) who lack T- or B-cell elements and the CALLA antigen have null-cell ALL (Margolin, Steuber, and Poplack, 2002).

At present, cell-surface markers for AML are still rudimentary. However, current research with monoclonal antibodies may provide significant information about the nonlymphoid cells.

## Pathologic and Related Clinical Manifestations

Leukemia is an unrestricted proliferation of immature white blood cells in the blood-forming tissues of the body. Although not a "tumor" as such, the leukemic cells demonstrate the neoplastic properties of solid cancers. Therefore the resultant pathologic and clinical manifestations of the disease are caused by infiltration and replacement of any tissue of the body with nonfunctional leukemic cells. Highly vascular organs, such as the spleen and liver, are most severely affected.

To understand the pathophysiology of the leukemic process, it is important to clarify two common misconceptions. First, although leukemia is an overproduction of white blood cells, most often in the acute form the leukocyte count is low. Instead, the peripheral blood smear and, more definitively, the bone marrow examination reveal greatly elevated counts of immature cells or "blasts." Second, these immature cells do not deliberately attack and destroy the normal blood cells or vascular tissues. Cellular destruction is by the process of infiltration and subsequent competition for metabolic elements. The following discussion elaborates on the pathologic process and related clinical manifestations in the most susceptible organs of the body (Fig. 36-2).

**Bone Marrow Dysfunction.** In all types of leukemia the proliferating cells depress bone marrow production of the formed elements of the blood by competing for and depriving the normal cells of the essential nutrients for metabolism. The three main consequences are (1) *anemia* from decreased erythrocytes, (2) *infection* from neutropenia, and (3) *bleeding* from decreased platelet production.

The invasion of the bone marrow with leukemic cells gradually causes a weakening of the bone and a tendency toward fractures. As leukemic cells invade the periosteum, increasing pressure causes severe pain.

The most frequent presenting signs and symptoms of leukemia are a result of infiltration of the bone marrow. These include fever, pallor, fatigue, anorexia, hemorrhage (usually petechiae), and bone and joint pain. In the presence of neutropenia the body's normal bacterial flora can become aggressive pathogens. Any break in the skin is a potential site of infection. Frequently, vague abdominal pain is caused by areas of inflammation from normal flora within the intestinal tract.

**Disturbance of Involved Organs.** The spleen, liver, and lymph glands demonstrate marked infiltration, enlargement, and eventually fibrosis. Hepatosplenomegaly is typically more common than lymphadenopathy.

The next most important site of involvement is the central nervous system. Initially, leukemic cells do not tend to invade this area because of the protective blood-brain barrier. However, this normal protective mechanism also prevents the antileukemic drugs, with the exception of a few agents, from entering the brain in sufficient therapeutic doses to be effective. Before prophylactic use of cranial irradiation or intrathecal methotrexate, central nervous system involvement was frequent in children who survived 6 months or more. However, newer modes of therapy have significantly changed the course of the disease, although central nervous system complications still occur, even during bone marrow remission.

The usual effect of leukemic infiltration of the meninges is increased intracranial pressure. The pathogenesis is presumably attributable to invasion of the arachnoid by proliferating cells, which then interfere with the flow of cerebrospinal fluid in the subarachnoid space and at the base of the brain. The increased fluid pressure causes dilation of all four ventricles and consequently the signs and symptoms normally associated with this condition, such as severe headache, vomiting, papilledema, irritability, lethargy, and eventually coma. Irritation of the meninges also causes pain and stiffness in the neck and back.

Additional sites of involvement may be the cranial nerves, most often cranial nerve VII, or the facial nerve, and spinal nerves, particularly of the lumbosacral plexus, hypothalamus, and cerebellum. Clinical manifestations for these sites are directly related to the area involved. For example, with lumbosacral invasion, there is weakness in the lower extremities, pain radiating down the legs to the feet, and difficulty in voiding. Although such signs may suggest a brain

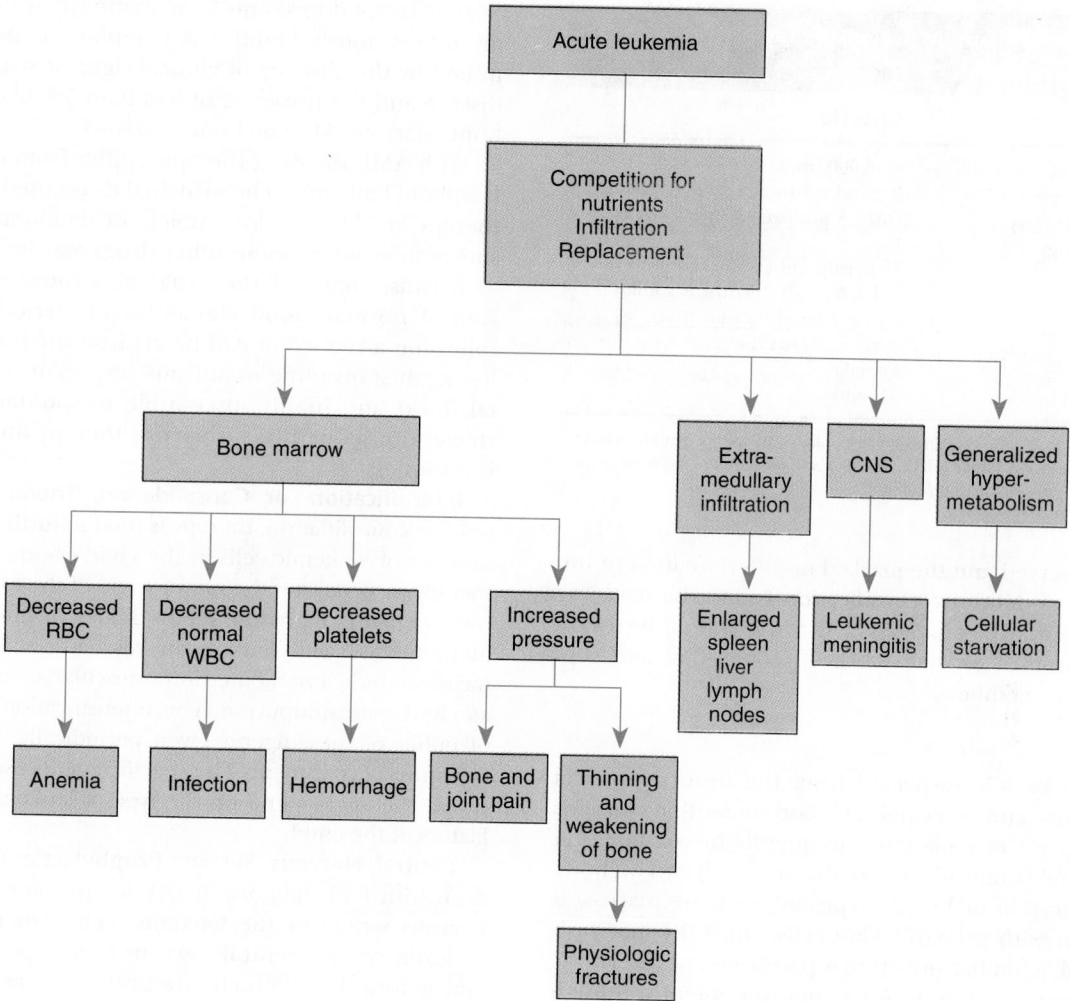

**Fig. 36-2** Principal sites of tissue involvement in leukemia.

tumor, the absence of localized signs often leads to the discovery of central nervous system involvement in leukemia.

Other sites that may become invaded with leukemic cells include the kidneys, testes, prostate, ovaries, gastrointestinal tract, and lungs. With long-term survivors becoming increasingly common, such extramedullary sites of leukemic invasion, especially the testes, are becoming more important clinically.

### Onset

The onset of leukemia varies from acute to insidious. In most instances the child displays remarkably few symptoms. For example, leukemia may be diagnosed when a minor infection, such as a cold, fails to completely disappear. The child continues to be pale, listless, irritable, febrile, and anorexic. Parents often suspect some underlying problem when they observe the weight loss, petechiae, bruising without cause, and continued complaints of bone and joint pain.

At other times leukemia is diagnosed after an extended history of signs and symptoms mimicking such conditions as rheumatoid arthritis or mononucleosis. There are also occasions when the diagnosis of leukemia accompanies some

totally unrelated event, such as a routine physical examination or injury.

The history not only yields valuable medical information regarding the subsequent course of the illness, but also bears heavily on the parents' emotional reaction to the diagnosis. In most instances the diagnosis is an unexpected revelation of catastrophic proportion.

### Staging and Prognostic Factors

The most important prognostic factors in determining long-term survival for children with ALL are the initial white blood cell count, the patient's age at diagnosis, cytogenetics, the immunologic subtype, and the child's sex (Table 36-4).

For children with AML, prognostic factors associated with a poorer prognosis include certain chromosome abnormalities (monosomy 7), a high white blood cell count ($>100,000/mm^3$), and AML developing after a myelodysplastic syndrome. The absence of Auer rods in the $M_1$ subtype of AML has also been correlated with a low remission rate (Golub and Arceci, 2002).

From the time of establishment of the diagnosis, the nurse has some idea of the expected course the child will follow. However, in some instances, because of the variety of

**TABLE 36-4** Favorable prognostic factors for acute lymphocytic leukemia

| Factor | Criteria |
| --- | --- |
| Leukocyte count | <50,000/mm³ |
| Age | >2 and <10 years |
| Immunologic subtype | CALLA-positive, early pre–B-cell |
| FAB morphology | L₁ |
| Cytogenetics | Hyperdiploid (>50 chromosomes, DNA index >1.16); trisomies 4 and 10 and translocations t(12; 21)(p12; q22) |
| Sex | Female |
| Leukemia cell burden | Minimal |

Modified from Margolin JP, Steuber CP, Poplack DG: Acute lymphoblastic leukemia. In Pizzo PA, Poplack DG: *Principles and practice of pediatric oncology,* ed 4, Philadelphia, 2002, JB Lippincott.

cell types observed and the marked undifferentiation of immature cells, a definitive classification cannot be made or the diagnosis may be changed. The nurse should be aware of the importance of such events in counseling and supporting family members.

## Diagnostic Evaluation

Leukemia is usually suspected from the history, physical manifestations, and a peripheral blood smear that contains immature forms of leukocytes, frequently in combination with low blood counts. Definitive diagnosis is based on bone marrow aspiration or biopsy. Typically the bone marrow is hypercellular with primarily blast cells. Once the diagnosis is confirmed, a lumbar puncture is performed to determine if there is any central nervous system involvement, although a very small number of children have central nervous system involvement and most are asymptomatic.

## Therapeutic Management

Treatment of leukemia involves the use of chemotherapeutic agents with or without cranial irradiation in four phases: (1) *induction,* which achieves a complete remission or disappearance of leukemic cells; (2) *intensification, or consolidation, therapy,* which further decreases the tumor burden; (3) *central nervous system prophylactic therapy,* which prevents leukemic cells from invading the central nervous system; and (4) *maintenance,* which serves to maintain the remission phase. Although the combination of drugs and possibility of irradiation may vary according to the institution, the prognostic or risk characteristics of the patient, and the type of leukemia being treated, the following general principles for each phase are consistently employed.

**Remission Induction.** Almost immediately after confirmation of the diagnosis, induction therapy is begun and lasts for 4 to 6 weeks (Margolin, Steuber, and Poplack, 2002). The principal drugs used for induction in ALL are the corticosteroids (prednisone or dexamethasone), vincristine, and L-asparaginase, with or without doxorubicin (see Table 36-2). Oral steroids are administered daily in divided doses to maintain consistently high blood levels. Vincristine is given by IV infusion once a week for a total

of four to six doses, and L-asparaginase or doxorubicin is given at various schedules. A complete remission is determined by the absence of clinical signs or symptoms of the disease and the presence of less than 5% blast cells in the bone marrow (M₁-type bone marrow).

With AML the drug therapies differ from those used for lymphoid leukemia. The principal drugs used for induction therapy in AML are doxorubicin or daunomycin and cytosine arabinoside; various other drugs may be added.

Because many of the drugs also cause myelosuppression of normal blood elements, the period immediately following a remission can be critical; the body is defenseless against invading organisms (especially normal bacterial flora) and highly susceptible to spontaneous hemorrhage. Consequently, supportive therapy during this time is essential.

**Intensification, or Consolidation, Therapy.** Intensification, or consolidation, therapy is used to further decrease the number of leukemic cells in the child's body. Intensification therapy incorporates the use of some of the following agents: L-asparaginase, high-dose methotrexate or intermediate-dose methotrexate with leukovorin rescue, vincristine, doxorubicin, steroids, cytarabine, intramuscular or oral methotrexate, and mercaptopurine. The intensification phase consists of pulses of these agents given periodically during the first 6 months of treatment. The specific agents used for intensification therapy depend on the type of leukemia and the risk factors of the child.

**Central Nervous System Prophylactic Therapy.** Children with leukemia are at risk for invasion of the central nervous system by the leukemic cells. For this reason, all children receive central nervous system prophylactic therapy. Before the 1980s children with ALL received cranial/spinal irradiation. Because of the concern regarding late effects of cranial irradiation, this mode of therapy is now generally reserved for high-risk patients or those with central nervous system disease. Depending upon protocol, intrathecal methotrexate or triple intrathecal chemotherapy (consisting of methotrexate, cytarabine, and hydrocortisone) is used during induction and intensification (consolidation) and maintenance therapy to prevent central nervous system disease.

**Maintenance.** The goal of maintenance therapy is to preserve remission and further reduce the number of leukemic cells. Combined drug regimens have been more successful in maintaining remissions and preventing drug resistance. A variety of agents are used during maintenance therapy including a daily dose of oral 6-mercaptopurine, weekly doses of methotrexate, with intermittent pulses of steroids and vincristine, which are standard in most treatment regimens.

During maintenance therapy, weekly or monthly complete blood counts are taken to evaluate the marrow's response to the drugs. If myelosuppression becomes severe (usually indicated by an absolute neutrophil count below 1000/mm³), or if toxic side effects occur, therapy is temporarily stopped or the dose decreased.

Duration of therapy has been based on clinical experience comparing survival rates for various time intervals and is concerned with preventing deleterious effects of excessive treatment. Although the optimum time for discontinuing therapy is not known, current practice is to continue treatment for 2½ to 3 years. All children after cessation of therapy require regular medical evaluation for surveillance of relapse and long-term sequelae of treatment. Most relapses (16%) occur during the first year off therapy, about 2% to 3% of the relapses occur during each of the next 3 years, and very few relapses occur after 6 years (Margolin, Steuber, and Poplack, 2002).

**Reinduction Following Relapse.**   For many children, additional therapy becomes necessary when a relapse occurs, as evidenced by the presence of leukemic cells within the bone marrow. Usually reinduction for ALL includes the use of prednisone and vincristine with a combination of other drugs not previously used. Although remissions may be achieved after more than one relapse, each relapse heralds an increasingly poor prognosis. However, more long-term second and subsequent remissions are occurring, and these may have better outlooks than previously thought.

A site that is resistant to chemotherapy and is responsible for leukemic relapse is the testes. A minority of males experience relapse during maintenance therapy or have occult disease after cessation of therapy. Treatment for testicular disease includes bilateral testicular irradiation, intensive systemic chemotherapy, and central nervous system prophylactic therapy (Landier, 2001).

**Bone Marrow Transplantation (BMT).**   BMT has been used successfully in treating some children with ALL and AML. In general, BMT is not recommended for children with ALL during the first remission because of the excellent results possible with chemotherapy. The group with the best results have been those with ALL who received the graft during the second remission (Guinan, Krance, and Lehman, 2002). Because of the poorer prognosis in children with AML, transplantation may be considered during the first remission when a suitable donor is available (Guinan, Krance, and Lehman, 2002).

**Prognosis.**   The majority of children with newly diagnosed leukemia who receive effective multiagent chemotherapy will survive. One long-term comprehensive study reported that the rates of complete remission ranged from 90% to 95%. Almost 80% of the children achieved long-term disease-free survival, and the majority of these children developed no obvious health problems from the leukemia or its treatment. It appears that the risk of relapse is rare after 3 to 4 years of complete remission following cessation of therapy.

Prognosis after transplantation varies with the timing of the procedure and the type of leukemia; reported ranges for long-term survival are between 25% and 50% (Guinan, Krance, and Lehman, 2002). However, because many of these children faced almost certain death without transplantation, even these low figures represent a major advance in eliciting a cure. Still, the use of BMT remains controversial.

## Nursing Considerations

Nursing care of the child with leukemia is directly related to the regimen of therapy. Secondary complications that necessitate supportive physical care are caused by myelo-suppression, drug toxicity, and leukemic infiltration. This discussion focuses on supportive interventions for the child with leukemia and the family. General aspects of care appropriate for the child with leukemia are discussed earlier under Nursing Care of the Child with Cancer. (Psychologic interventions appropriate for children with leukemia during significant phases of therapy are discussed in Chapter 23.)

**Prepare Family for Diagnostic/Therapeutic Procedures.** From the time before diagnosis to cessation of therapy, children must undergo several tests, the most traumatic of which are bone marrow aspiration or biopsy and lumbar punctures. Multiple finger sticks and venipunctures for blood analysis and drug infusion are common occurrences for several years after the diagnosis. Therefore the child needs an explanation of why each procedure is done and what can be expected. (See Preparation for Procedures, Chapter 27.)

Depending on the age of the child, one way of beginning diagnostic preparation is to explain the tests, procedures, and treatment plan.* Using a drawing or letting the child look at a drop of blood under a microscope not only teaches, but also encourages trust between the nurse and the child. It also allows the nurse to assess the child's level of understanding. An error many health professionals make is to overestimate children's knowledge about their bodies. For example, a bone marrow aspiration makes sense only when it is clarified that the center of a bone is hollow and contains the cells that later become "working" blood cells or leukemic cells.

**Provide Continued Emotional Support.**   Nursing care of the child with leukemia is based on typical problems with which the family is confronted during the treatment phases. It is not unusual for a child who discontinues therapy after 2 or 3 years and maintains a permanent remission to experience many of these side effects. Therefore the nurse's role is continually one of support, guidance, clarification, and judgment. Parents need to know how to recognize symptoms that demand medical attention. Although some of the reactions discussed are expected, parents should still report them to their practitioner. Warning parents of their possible occurrence beforehand also allows parents an opportunity to prepare for them. At the same time, it reassures them that these reactions are not caused by a return of leukemic cells.

The nurse must also use judgment in recognizing which side effects are normal reactions and which indicate toxicity. Frequently it is the office or clinic nurse who screens such telephone calls and gives advice when appropriate. Usually nausea and vomiting are not indications for drug cessation. However, severe vomiting may require immediate intervention to prevent dehydration. Signs of infection, mucosal ulceration, hemorrhagic cystitis, peripheral neuropathy, and obstipation require medical evaluation.

---

*Especially recommended is the book *The C-Word: Teenagers and Their Families Living with Cancer* by E. Dorfman (1994, New Sage Press, Troutdale, OR).

Another aspect of continued emotional support involves prognosis. Although leukemia is not invariably fatal, present statistics must also be correctly interpreted. While more than 95% of children with ALL will achieve an initial remission and almost 80% of them will live 5 years or longer, it must be remembered that these are *average* estimates and apply to those children treated with the most successful protocols since diagnosis (Shusterman and Meadows, 2000). For the low-risk child the chances may be better, but for the high-risk child they may be significantly poorer. Of those who do survive after discontinuing therapy, a portion will relapse. At present only the passage of time is positive confirmation of the child who is "cured" of the disease.

The nurse must be familiar with these statistics in order to interpret them correctly to parents. At the same time, the nurse must realize that a realistic understanding of the chances for survival requires an adjustment period. For example, it is not unusual for parents to interpret the "95% remission" as the probability for a cure. When a relapse occurs, parents may for the first time be able to "hear" the correct facts.

Statistics are numbers. Sometimes they bring hope, and at other times they bring despair. Although they are very important in terms of research, better treatment, and identification of high- or low-risk populations, they present a general picture of what to expect. The nurse who is working with family members must individualize the "numbers" to relate to the people. An understanding of each member's emotional needs, as well as competent care of physical ones, is essential to the positive, growth-promoting support of the family. Comprehensive emotional support for the family through all phases of the illness is discussed in Chapter 23.

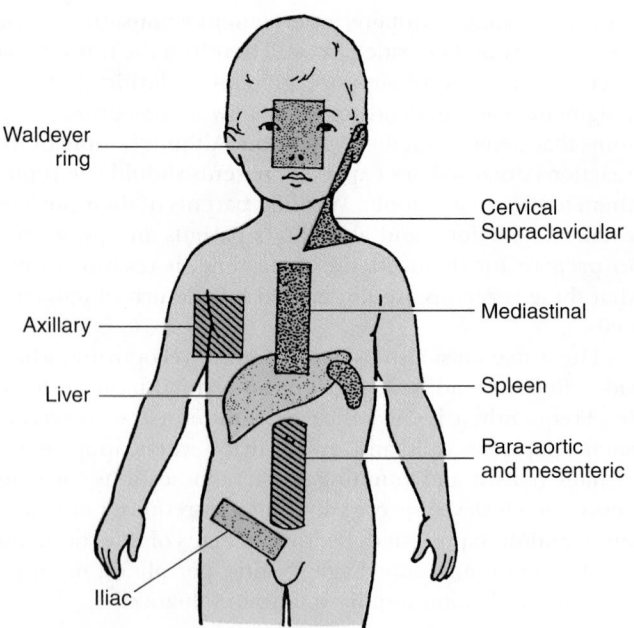

**Fig. 36-3** Main areas of lymphadenopathy and organ involvement in Hodgkin disease.

## Lymphomas

The lymphomas, a group of neoplastic diseases that arise from the lymphoid and hemopoietic systems, are divided into Hodgkin disease and non-Hodgkin lymphoma (NHL). These diseases are further subdivided according to tissue type and extent of disease (staging). In children NHL is more common than Hodgkin disease. Although Hodgkin disease is extremely rare before 5 years of age, there is a striking increase in children ages 15 to 19 years, when it occurs with almost the same frequency as leukemia.

## Hodgkin Disease

Hodgkin disease affects about 5 in 1 million children, mostly adolescents. The malignancy originates in the lymphoid system and primarily involves the lymph nodes. It predictably metastasizes to nonnodal or extralymphatic sites, especially the spleen, liver, bone marrow, lungs, and mediastinum (mass of tissues and organs separating the lungs; includes the heart and its vessels, trachea, esophagus, thymus, and lymph nodes), although no tissue is exempt from involvement (Fig. 36-3). It is classified according to four histologic types: (1) lymphocytic predominance, (2) nodular sclerosis, (3) mixed cellularity, and (4) lymphocytic depletion. With present treatment protocols, the histologic stage of the disease has less prognostic significance.

### Clinical Staging and Prognosis

Accurate staging of the extent of disease is the basis for treatment protocols and expected prognosis. More than one staging system exists; the one in Box 36-3 is known as the *Ann Arbor Staging Classification.*

Each stage is further subdivided into A or B. *A* denotes absence of associated general symptoms. *B* indicates presence of symptoms such as night sweats, fever (>38° C [100.4° F]), or weight loss of 10% or more during the preceding 6 months. In stages II and III, subtype B has a significantly poorer prognosis than subtype A.

The prognosis for patients with Hodgkin disease has improved dramatically in the past few years, largely as a result of the systematic staging procedure and improved treatment protocols. The prognosis is excellent in children with

---

**Box 36-3 ■ ■ □**
### Stages of Hodgkin Disease

**Stage I:** Lesions are limited to one lymph node area or only one additional extralymphatic site (IE), such as the liver, lungs, kidney, or intestines.
**Stage II:** Two or more lymph node regions on the same side of the diaphragm or one additional extralymphatic site or organ (IIE) on the same side of the diaphragm is involved.
**Stage III:** Lymph node regions on both sides of the diaphragm are involved, or one extralymphatic site (IIIE), spleen (IIIS), or both (IIISE).
**Stage IV:** Cancer has metastasized diffusely throughout the body to one or more extralymphatic sites with or without involvement of associated lymph nodes.

localized disease. The overall 10-year survival rate is as high as 90%. For relapses, complete remission may occur in 20% to 40% of patients; BMT may represent hope for a cure (Lanzkowsky, 2000). Even in those with disseminated disease, long-term remissions are possible in more than half of the patients. Unfortunately, a number of children may have late recurrences of the original disease or develop a second malignancy, especially osteosarcoma, breast cancer, thyroid carcinoma, or leukemia. The risk is higher in females than in males (Mueller and Grufferman, 1999). The most common complication of irradiation to the neck area is hypothyroidism (Vose, Constine, and Sutcliffe, 1999).

### Clinical Manifestations

Hodgkin disease is characterized by painless enlargement of lymph nodes. The most common finding is enlarged, firm, nontender, movable nodes in the supraclavicular or cervical area. In children the "sentinel" node located near the left clavicle may be the first enlarged node. Enlargement of axillary and inguinal lymph nodes is less frequent (see Fig. 36-3).

Other signs and symptoms depend on the extent and location of involvement. Mediastinal lymphadenopathy may cause a persistent nonproductive cough. Enlarged retroperitoneal nodes may produce unexplained abdominal pain. Systemic symptoms include low-grade or intermittent fever (Pel-Ebstein disease), anorexia, nausea, weight loss, night sweats, and pruritus. Generally such symptoms indicate advanced lymph node and extralymphatic involvement.

### Diagnostic Evaluation

The history and physical examination often yield important clues to the disease, such as fevers, night sweats, weight loss, and enlarged lymph nodes, spleen, or liver. Because of the multiple organs that can become involved, diagnosis consists of several tests to confirm the presence of Hodgkin disease and to assess the extent of involvement for accurate staging. Tests include complete blood count, uric acid levels, liver function tests, erythrocyte sedimentation rate, serum copper, ferritin level, fibrinogen, immunoglobulins, T-cell function studies, and urinalysis. Radiographic tests include CT scans of the neck, chest, abdomen, and pelvis; a gallium scan (identifies metastatic/recurrent disease); a chest x-ray film; and if clinically indicated, a bone scan to detect metastasis.

A special procedure, lymphangiography (LAG) involves the intradermal injection of a contrast material (usually alphazurine) in the first interdigital space of each foot for visualization of the lymphatic vessels to determine the presence of disease in various lymph node regions (Mendenhall, Holland, and Sombeck, 1994). However, most centers have replaced lymphangiography with the CT and the gallium scan even though the LAG is more accurate.

A lymph node biopsy is essential to establish histologic diagnosis and staging. The presence of **Sternberg-Reed cell,** is considered diagnostic of Hodgkin disease because it is ab-

sent in the other lymphomas; however, it may occur in infectious mononucleosis. A bone marrow aspiration or biopsy is also usually performed. With the advent of the CT and gallium scans to identify metastatic disease and multiagent chemotherapy and radiation therapy to eradicate metastatic disease, a laparotomy is avoided except in a few selected cases.

### Therapeutic Management

The primary modalities of therapy are irradiation and chemotherapy. Each may be used alone or in combination based on the clinical staging. The goal of treatment is obviously a cure; however, aggressive therapy increases the chances of complications in the disease-free state and can seriously compromise the quality of life. Consequently, numerous research studies are presently investigating treatment options to minimize long-term sequelae. Because of the diversity of approaches to treatment, the following is an overview of general principles that may or may not apply to all children. One of the major concerns with combined radiation and antineoplastic drug therapy is the serious late effects in children with an excellent prognosis.

Radiation may involve *involved field (IF)*, *extended field (EF) radiation* (involved areas plus adjacent nodes), or *total nodal irradiation (TNI)* (the entire axial lymph node system), depending on the extent of involvement. In stage IV disease, chemotherapy is the primary form of treatment, although limited irradiation may be given to areas of bulky disease. The most effective combination of chemotherapy widely used in the past has been MOPP (mechlorethamine [Mustargen], vincristine [Oncovin], prednisone, and procarbazine) alternating with, adriamycin, bleomycin, vinblastine, and dacarbazine (ABVD) (Behrendt, Brinkhuis, and Van Leeuwen, 1996; Hough and Hancock, 1999).

However, this therapy combination caused severe late effects, including secondary malignancies. For this reason other drug combinations such as BEACOPP (doxorubicin, cyclophosphamide, etoposide, procarbazine, prednisone, vincristine, bleomycin) or ABVD are being used (Mauch and others, 1999; Hough and Hancock, 1999).

Follow-up care of children no longer receiving therapy is essential to identify relapse and second malignancies. In children with splenectomy because of laparotomy, prophylactic antibiotics are administered for an indefinite period. Also, immunizations against pneumococci and meningococci are recommended before the splenectomy. (See Chapter 12.)

### Nursing Considerations

Nursing care involves (1) preparation for diagnostic and operative procedures, (2) explanation of treatment side effects, and (3) child and family support. (See Nursing Care Plan: The Child with Cancer.*) Once the child is hospitalized for suspected Hodgkin disease, a battery of diagnostic tests is ordered. The family needs an explanation of why

---

*In Wong DL, Hess CS: *Wong and Whaley's clinical manual of pediatric nursing,* ed 5, St Louis, 2000, Mosby.

each test is performed because many of them, such as bone marrow aspiration and lymph node biopsy, are invasive procedures. (See Chapter 27.)

Explanations of chemotherapeutic reactions vary with the specific drug regimen. Drugs commonly used are outlined in Table 36-2, and the most common side effects, such as nausea and vomiting, body image changes, neuropathy, and mucosal ulceration, are discussed under Nursing Care of the Child with Cancer. If radiation results in few side effects, sometimes consisting only of a mild skin reaction. With EF radiation to the chest and abdomen, nausea and vomiting, weight loss, and mucosal ulceration (esophagitis, gastric ulcers) are common. The usual measures for providing relief are discussed on pp. 1598-1602 and are outlined in Table 36-3.

The most common side effect of extensive irradiation is malaise, which may result from damage to the thyroid gland, causing hypothyroidism. Lack of energy is particularly difficult for adolescents because it prevents them from keeping up with their peers. Sometimes adolescents will push themselves to the point of physical exhaustion rather than admit fatigue and succumb to the decreased activity tolerance. Parents are advised to observe for such behavior, such as extreme fatigue at the end of the day, falling asleep at the dinner table, inability to concentrate on homework, or an increased susceptibility to infection. Regular bedtimes and periodic rest times are important for these children, especially during chemotherapy, when myelosuppression increases the risk of infection and debilitation. Before discharge, the nurse should discuss a feasible school schedule with the parents and child. If alterations are necessary, such as elimination of strenuous physical education, they are discussed with the teacher, nurse, and principal. Follow-up care is essential to diagnose hypothyroidism early and institute thyroid replacement.

An area of concern for adolescents is the high risk of sterility from irradiation and chemotherapy. Both irradiation to the gonads and drugs, particularly procarbazine and alkylating agents, may lead to infertility. Younger patients with a greater complement of oocytes are more likely to retain ovarian function.

Although sexual function is not altered, the appearance of secondary sexual characteristics and menstruation may be delayed in the pubescent child. Adolescents should be informed of these side effects early in the course of the diagnosis and treatment. Delayed sexual maturation may be an extremely sensitive and painful area for children. (See Chapter 20.)

## Non-Hodgkin Lymphoma (NHL)

Approximately 60% of pediatric lymphomas are classified as NHL with an incidence of 7 to 8 children per million under age 15 (Magrath, 2002). Histologic classification of childhood NHL is strikingly different from that of Hodgkin disease and adult NHL in several respects (Reiter and others, 1995):

- The disease is usually diffuse rather than nodular.
- The cell type is either undifferentiated or poorly differentiated.

- Dissemination occurs earlier, more often, and more rapidly.
- Mediastinal involvement and invasion of meninges typically occur.

### Staging and Prognosis

NHL is heterogeneous, exhibiting a variety of morphologic, cytochemical, and immunologic features, not unlike the diversity seen in leukemia. Classification is based on the pattern of histologic presentation: (1) lymphoblastic, (2) Burkitt or non-Burkitt, or (3) large cell (Reiter and others, 1995). Immunologically these cells are also classified as T-cells, B-cells (an example of which is Burkitt lymphoma), or non-T–non-B–cells, which lack specific immunologic properties.

The clinical staging system used in Hodgkin disease is of little value in NHL, although that system has been modified for NHL and other systems have been developed. A favorable prognosis is defined by (1) lymph node involvement only and limited to one or two adjacent lymphatic regions (excluding the mediastinum); (2) an extranodal site in the nasopharynx, oropharynx, or other isolated extranodal site, with or without regional lymphadenopathy; or (3) gastrointestinal involvement, with or without regional lymphadenopathy, limited to the mesentery (Magrath, 2002). The most commonly used staging system is presented in Box 36-4.

The use of aggressive combination chemotherapy has had a major impact on the survival rates of children with NHL. The most effective treatment regimens result in cure in almost all children with limited disease involvement; 75% to 90% of children with extensive disease are cured (Magrath, 2002; Reiter and others, 1995).

### Clinical Manifestations

Clinical manifestations depend on the anatomic site and extent of involvement. Many of those seen in Hodgkin disease may be present in NHL, although rarely does a single symptom give rise to the diagnosis. Rather, metastasis to the bone marrow or central nervous system may produce signs and symptoms typical of leukemia. Lymphoid tumors compressing various organs may cause intestinal or airway obstruction, cranial nerve palsies, or spinal paralysis.

The exception to the usual presentation of NHL is **Burkitt lymphoma,** a type of cancer that is rare in the United States but endemic in parts of Africa. It is a rapidly growing neoplasm that is most commonly seen as a mass in the jaw, abdomen, or orbit. However, no anatomic site appears ex-

---

**Box 36-4** ▪ ▪ ▫
**Staging System for Non-Hodgkin Lymphoma**

**Stage I:** Single tumor at a single site
**Stage II:** Single tumor with regional involvement on same side of diaphragm
**Stage III:** Tumor on both sides of abdomen; also, all primary thoracic, intraabdominal, and paraspinal or epidural tumors
**Stage IV:** Any of the involvement in stages I and II, with central nervous system or bone marrow involvement

empt from involvement. Peripheral lymphadenopathy, hepatosplenomegaly, or signs of conversion to leukemia are rarely seen.

### Diagnostic Evaluation

Because widespread disease exists in most children with NHL at diagnosis, thorough pathologic staging is unnecessary. Current recommendations for staging include a surgical biopsy for histopathologic confirmation of disease with immunophenotyping and cytogenetic evaluation; bone marrow aspiration; radiologic studies, especially CT scans of the lungs and gastrointestinal organs; and lumbar puncture.

### Therapeutic Management

The present treatment protocols for NHL include an aggressive approach using irradiation and chemotherapy. Similar to leukemic therapy, the protocols include induction, consolidation, and maintenance phases, some with intrathecal chemotherapy. At present the differentiation between lymphoblastic lymphoma and all other lymphomas is widely used as a way to categorize patients for specific treatment regimens (Magrath, 2002). Children with lymphoblastic lymphoma are treated with several drug protocols, most containing several chemotherapeutic agents. One of the most commonly used regimens includes cyclophosphamide or ifosfamide, vincristine, intrathecal chemotherapy, prednisone, daunomycin, 6-thioguanine, cytosine arabinoside, BCNU, and L-asparaginase.

Children with nonlymphoblastic lymphoma are treated with cyclic drug combinations, including cyclophosphamide and intermediate-dose or high-dose methotrexate (Magrath, 2002). Most protocols also include an anthracycline. These children receive central nervous system prophylaxis with combination intrathecal chemotherapy. These multiagent regimens are administered for 6 to 24 months.

### Nursing Considerations

Nursing care of the child with NHL is very similar to the care discussed under Nursing Care of the Child with Cancer. Because of the intensive chemotherapy protocol, nursing care is primarily directed toward managing the side effects of these agents.

## NERVOUS SYSTEM TUMORS

Two major forms of childhood cancer are derived from neural tissue. **Brain tumors** are the most common solid tumors that occur in children and are second only to leukemia as a form of cancer. **Neuroblastomas** are the most common malignant tumors of infancy and are second only to brain tumors as the type of solid malignancy seen during the first 10 years (Lanzkowsky, 2000; Matthay, 1995). Both of these tumors have presented difficulties in identifying successful modes of treatment and have not demonstrated the dramatic improvements in survival seen in many other forms of cancer.

## Brain Tumors

Tumors of the central nervous system account for about 20% of all childhood cancers and have an annual incidence of 2.4 per 100,000 children under 15 years of age. About 60% of the tumors are **infratentorial** (below the tentorium cerebelli), which means that they occur in the posterior third of the brain, primarily in the cerebellum or brainstem. This anatomic distribution accounts for the frequency of symptoms resulting from increased intracranial pressure (ICP). The other tumors are **supratentorial**, or within the anterior two thirds of the brain, mainly the cerebrum. Major brain tumors of childhood are outlined in Box 36-5.

Because the neoplasms can arise from any cell within the cranium, it is possible to have tumors originating from the glial cells, nerve cells, neuroepithelium, cranial nerves, blood vessels, pineal gland, and hypophysis. Within each of these structures, specific cells may be involved to provide a histologic classification of the major tumors found in children. **Astrocytes,** cells that form most of the supportive tissue for the neurons, may form **astrocytomas,** the most common glial tumor (Armstrong and Gilbert, 1996; Strickler and Phillips, 2000). Brain tumors may be benign or malignant.

### Clinical Manifestations

The signs and symptoms of brain tumors are directly related to their anatomic location and size and to some extent the age of the child. In infants, whose sutures are still open, virtually no early detectable symptoms develop. It is not until spinal fluid obstruction causes markedly increased head size that a lesion may be suspected. Head circumference allows for detection of increased head size. Even in older children, clinical manifestations are nonspecific. However, the most common symptoms are headache, especially on awakening, and vomiting that is not related to feeding. The headache occurs from traction on pain-sensitive areas, such as large blood vessels and cranial nerves, and possibly from dural stretching. The headache is worse in the morning from the compression of these structures during sleep. It typically subsides or improves during the day. Vomiting occurs from increased ICP that compresses the brainstem, directly stimulating the vomiting center in the medulla (Armstrong and Gilbert, 1996; Strother and others, 2002; Strickler and Phillips, 2000). The common presenting symptoms of brain tumors are presented in Table 36-5.

### Diagnostic Evaluation

Diagnosis of a brain tumor is based subjectively on presenting clinical signs and objectively on neurologic tests. Because the signs and symptoms are vague and easily overlooked, early diagnosis necessitates a high index of suspicion during history taking. A number of tests may be employed in the neurologic evaluation (see Table 37-2), but the gold standard diagnostic procedure is MRI, which permits early diagnosis of brain tumors as well as assessment of tumor growth during or following treatment. Magnetic resonance (MR) angiography can be performed during the same session as MRI to determine the vascularity of the tumor (Brunelle, 2000). Another test is CT, which permits direct visualization of the brain parenchyma, ventricles, and

## Box 36-5 ◼ ◼ ◻
## Major Brain Tumors of Childhood

### LOW-GRADE OR HIGH-GRADE ASTROCYTOMAS

Most common pediatric brain tumor; about 23% are low grade and 11% are high grade.

Usually infiltrates brain parenchyma without distinct boundaries.

Low-grade tumors have more highly differentiated cells and are less malignant than high-grade tumors.

Characteristic presenting signs include headache, nausea, seizures, and sometimes bizarre behavior (staring spells and automatic movements).

Extensive surgical excision is attempted and may require repeated operations; chemotherapy and irradiation are used after incomplete resection.

Five-year survival rate is 75% to 85% for low-grade astrocytomas, less for high-grade tumors.

### MEDULLOBLASTOMA (PRIMITIVE NEUROECTODERMAL TUMOR)

Accounts for 20% to 25% of pediatric brain tumors.

Fast growing, highly malignant.

Characteristic presenting signs include headache, vomiting, and ataxia.

Improved survival rates with excision of most or all of tumor plus chemotherapy with or without irradiation.

Overall 5-year survival rate is greater than 70%.

Period for risk of recurrence is age at diagnosis plus 9 months.

### CEREBELLAR ASTROCYTOMA

Accounts for about 15% of pediatric brain tumors.

Slow growing if low grade.

Characteristic presenting signs include headache, clumsiness (usually one hand), awkward gait (stumbling to one side), and vomiting.

With no postoperative residual tumor, likelihood of cure is 70% to 90%.

### BRAINSTEM GLIOMA

Accounts for about 15% of pediatric brain tumors.

Often grows to a very large size before causing symptoms.

Characteristic presenting signs include diplopia, facial weakness, and difficulty walking (headache and vomiting are uncommon).

Surgical excision is very difficult because of tumor location in vital brain centers; removal is attempted whenever possible, followed by irradiation.

Palliative therapy with irradiation shrinks tumor to prolong survival, which depends on size, cell type, and location of tumor.

Prognosis is poor, because most tumors are highly resistant to therapy.

### EPENDYMOMA

Accounts for about 4% of brain tumors.

Demonstrates varying rates of growth.

Most invade ventricles, obstructing flow of cerebrospinal fluid.

Characteristic presenting signs include vomiting, headache, ataxia, hemiparesis, papilledema, and, in infants, hydrocephalus.

Goal of surgery is total resection; risks associated with total resection are greater with brainstem infiltration, which occurs in about 50% of patients.

Overall 5-year survival rate is about 45% and improves to about 80% if no postoperative residual tumor.

Modified from Shiminiski-Maher T: Central nervous system tumors. In Hockenberry-Eaton MJ and others, editors: *Essentials of pediatric oncology nursing: a core curriculum*, Glenview, IL, 1998, Association of Pediatric Oncology Nurses.

---

surrounding subarachnoid space. Through the IV injection of radiographic contrast agents, intracranial blood vasculature can be demonstrated (Strother and others, 2002). MR spectroscopy is a new radiographic technique under investigation that is able to differentiate between malignant tumors and areas of necrosis (Brunelle, 2000; Lanzkowsky, 2000).

When a positive CT scan is obtained, angiography may be done to provide information about the tumor's blood supply and degree of vascularity, which may assist the surgeon in planning the operative approach. Other tests (e.g., electroencephalography, tomographies, lumbar puncture, or ventriculography) may be performed. Lumbar puncture is dangerous in the presence of increased ICP because of possible brainstem herniation following sudden release of pressure.

Definitive diagnosis is based on tissue specimens obtained during surgery. Occasionally, special techniques are required for determining the cell type. This period of waiting is one of anxiety for family members, who are aware of the relevance of cell type to prognosis.

### Therapeutic Management

Treatment may involve the use of surgery, radiotherapy, and chemotherapy. All three may or may not be used, depending on the type of tumor. The treatment of choice is total re-

moval of the tumor without residual neurologic damage. Patients with the most complete tumor removal have the greatest chance of survival. Several surgical advances have allowed the biopsy and removal of tumors in areas previously considered too dangerous for traditional operative techniques. *Stereotactic surgery* involves the use of CT and MRI in conjunction with other special computer techniques to reconstruct the tumor in three dimensions. With computer-assisted instruments, removal is sometimes possible. Stereotactic biopsy is performed with CT or MRI computer guidance for inserting the biopsy needle. This procedure has the benefit of a short hospital stay and a lower morbidity and mortality rate in comparison with an open craniotomy (Armstrong and Gilbert, 1996; Strother and others, 2002). Other procedures include the use of *lasers* to vaporize tumor tissue and *brain mapping* to determine the precise location of critical brain areas that are avoided during surgery.

Radiotherapy is used to treat most tumors and to shrink the size of the tumor before attempting surgical removal. The use of chemotherapy has emerged in the past decades with an increasingly important role, either in combination with irradiation or alone. The drugs most commonly used are carmustine (BCNU), lomustine (CCNU), vincristine (Oncovin), cisplatin (Platinol), carboplatin (CBDCA), etoposide (VP-16), thiotepa (TSPA), and cyclophosphamide

**TABLE 36-5  Clinical manifestations and assessment of brain tumors**

| Signs and Symptoms | Assessment |
|---|---|
| **Headache**<br>Recurrent and progressive<br>In frontal or occipital areas<br>Usually dull and throbbing<br>Worse on arising, less during day<br>Intensified by lowering head and straining, such as during bowel movement, coughing, sneezing | Record description of pain, location, severity, and duration<br>Use pain rating scale to assess severity of pain (see Chapter 26)<br>Note changes in relation to time of day and activity<br>Observe changes in behavior in infants (persistent irritability, crying, head rolling) |
| **Vomiting**<br>With or without nausea or feeding<br>Progressively more projectile<br>More severe in morning<br>Relieved by moving about and changing position | Record time, amount, and relationship to feeding, nausea, and activity |
| **Neuromuscular Changes**<br>Incoordination or clumsiness<br>Loss of balance (use of wide-based stance, falling, tripping, banging into objects)<br>Poor fine motor control<br>Weakness<br>Hyporeflexia or hyperreflexia<br>Positive Babinski sign<br>Spasticity<br>Paralysis | Test muscle strength, gait, coordination, and reflexes (see Chapter 7) |
| **Behavioral Changes**<br>Irritability<br>Decreased appetite<br>Failure to thrive<br>Fatigue (frequent naps)<br>Lethargy<br>Coma<br>Bizarre behavior (staring, automatic movements) | Observe behavior regularly<br>Compare observations with parental reports of normal behavioral patterns<br>Monitor growth and food intake<br>Monitor activity and sleep |
| **Cranial Nerve Neuropathy**<br>Cranial nerve involvement varies according to tumor location<br>Most common signs<br>  Head tilt<br>  Visual defects (nystagmus, diplopia, strabismus, episodic "graying out" of vision, visual field defects) | Assess cranial nerves, especially VII (facial), IX (glossopharyngeal), X (vagus), V (trigeminal, sensory roots), and VI (abducens) (see Chapter 7)<br>Assess visual acuity, binocularity, and peripheral vision (see Chapter 7) |
| **Vital Sign Disturbances**<br>Decreased pulse and respiration<br>Increased blood pressure<br>Decreased pulse pressure<br>Hypothermia or hyperthermia | Measure vital signs frequently<br>Monitor pulse and respirations for 1 full minute<br>Record pulse pressure (difference between systolic and diastolic blood pressure) |
| **Other Signs**<br>Seizures<br>Cranial enlargement*<br>Tense, bulging fontanel at rest*<br>Nuchal ridigity<br>Papilledema (edema of optic nerve) | Record seizure activity (see Chapter 37)<br>Measure head circumference daily (infant and young child)<br>Perform funduscopic examination if skilled in procedure |

*Present only in infants and young children.

(Cytoxan) (Shiminski-Maher, 1998; Strickler and Phillips, 2000). In addition, other drugs, such as corticosteroids, may be needed to manage complications, such as brain edema.

The problems of treatment are compounded by the serious late effects of all three modes of therapy. Surgery may cause injury to important areas of the brain, especially when the surgeon is attempting to remove invasive tumors. Irradiation has serious long-term consequences, including radiation somnolence syndrome (see p. 1601), brain necrosis, endocrine dysfunction, and behavioral/intellectual deficits. For these reasons, the use of irradiation is deferred for as long as possible in young children, although there is limited information regarding a "safe age," which is considered over age 3 for most centers (Mainprize, Taylor, and Rutka, 2000). Chemotherapy is also not without effects (see Table 36-2).

## Nursing Considerations

Nursing care of the child with a brain tumor is similar regardless of the type of intracranial lesion. Because a brain tumor is potentially fatal, the reader is urged to incorporate the psychologic interventions discussed in Chapter 23 with those elaborated on in this section.

**Assess for Signs and Symptoms.** A child admitted to the hospital with neurologic dysfunction is often suspected of having a brain tumor, although the actual diagnosis is as yet unconfirmed. Establishing a baseline of data on which to compare preoperative and postoperative changes is an essential step toward planning physical care and preventing complications. It also allows the nurse to assess the degree of physical incapacity and the family's emotional reaction to the diagnosis. For example, children with cerebellar astrocytoma may have displayed vague cerebellar symptoms for several years before a tumor is suspected. For these parents the revelation of a neoplasm may be more of a shock than for those who have witnessed a rapid deterioration in their child's abilities. Common presenting signs and assessment procedures to document significant changes in the child's condition are summarized in Table 36-5.

**Prepare Family for Diagnostic/Operative Procedures.** The suspected diagnosis of a brain tumor is always a crisis event. Despite the fact that some tumors are removed with excellent results, the physician can rarely give definitive answers regarding the prognosis until after surgery. Therefore parents and older children require much emotional support to face the diagnostic procedures and a craniotomy.

How the child is prepared for the diagnostic tests depends on the child's age and previous experience. Because most of the tests involve x-ray equipment, the child may be familiar with the procedure. Preparing children for an MRI or a CT scan is discussed in Chapter 37. Once surgery is scheduled, the child needs an explanation of what to expect. By the time most children are late preschoolers, they know that the head and brain are important parts of their body. It may be helpful to have children draw their concept of the brain in order to clarify misconceptions and base the explanation on their level of understanding.

Although the temptation is to justify the need for surgery by stating that removing the tumor will take away various symptoms, the nurse should refrain from emphasizing this point too strenuously. Postsurgical headaches and cerebellar symptoms, such as ataxia, may be aggravated rather than improved. Surgery may not improve vision. With optic gliomas the child will be blind in one eye. Finally, surgical removal of the mass may be impossible, and after surgery there may be temporary deterioration of functioning. Being honest before surgery most often makes honesty after the procedure easier because no false hopes were created.

It is best to deliver information in small amounts to let the child pursue additional answers. For example, some children will ask about what happens when part of the tu-

mor is left in. An honest reply is that after surgery the practitioner will try to shrink the tumor with a special radiation machine or drugs. A further explanation of irradiation or chemotherapy should be delayed until a decision regarding these treatments is made.

The hair is usually shaved in the operating room just before surgery, or sometimes in the child's room, usually the night before surgery. When shaving is done with the child awake, the procedure is approached in a sensitive, positive way. If the child's hair is long, it should be braided so that the long swatch can be saved. Showing children how they look at different stages of the process helps them prepare for the final appearance.

Once the hair is clipped very short or shaved, the child can be given a cap or scarf to wear in order to camouflage the baldness. Every precaution is taken to provide privacy during the procedure and to protect the child from teasing or ridicule by other children before surgery. It is also emphasized that the hair will regrow shortly after surgery. Depending on the child's immediate adjustment to the hair loss, the nurse may introduce the idea of wearing a wig until the hair is grown in, particularly if additional irradiation or chemotherapy is anticipated.

Children are also told about the size of the dressing. Usually the entire scalp is covered to maintain a tight wound closure, even if a small incision is made. Infratentorial head dressings may be attached to the upper back and extend forward to the neck in order to maintain slight extension and alignment as a precaution against wound rupture. Applying a similar dressing or "special hat" to a doll is often a less traumatic way of demonstrating the physical appearance.

Children also need a brief explanation of how they will feel after surgery and where they will be. Ordinarily they will return to a special intensive care unit, which they may visit beforehand depending on hospital policy. They should be aware that they may be sleepy for some time after surgery and that a headache is likely, although it should last only a few days.

Parents need similar explanations before surgery, especially in terms of special equipment used in the intensive care unit, dressings, and their child's behavior. For example, they should know that it is not unusual for the child to be comatose or lethargic for a few days after surgery. The nurse may wish to encourage less frequent visiting during this period so that parents can rest and be able to support their child when the child is awake.

The nurse should participate in preoperative conferences with the physician and parents. The nurse needs to know what information the parents have been given in order to be able to give further explanations or emotional support when necessary.

**Prevent Postoperative Complications.** Usually the surgeon will prescribe specific orders for vital signs, positioning, fluid regulation, and medication. These vary somewhat, depending on the location of the craniotomy. The following are general principles of care for infratentorial or supratentorial surgery. Additional aspects of care are discussed in Chapter 37, such as care of the child with seizures and care of the unconscious child in terms of respiratory status and neurologic assessment.

**Assessment.**   Vital signs are taken as frequently as every 15 to 30 minutes until stable. Temperature measurement is particularly important because of hyperthermia resulting from surgical intervention in the hypothalamus or brainstem and from some types of general anesthesia. To prepare for this reaction, a cooling blanket may be placed on the bed *before* the child returns to the unit, or it may be used when needed. Because the temperature control centers are affected, the nurse monitors body temperature often when any cooling measures are employed, because hypothermia can occur suddenly.

> **NURSING ALERT**
>
> When temperature is elevated, an infectious process must always be suspected, particularly if the febrile state occurs 1 to 2 days after surgery.

The most likely types of infection are meningitis and respiratory tract infection. The probable cause of meningitis is wound contamination. Signs of meningitis, such as opisthotonos, Kernig and Brudzinski signs (see Chapter 7), and nuchal rigidity (see Chapter 37), are very similar to those of increased ICP and must be carefully evaluated to determine whether they indicate an infection.

The risk of respiratory infections is high because of the imposed immobility, danger of aspiration, and possible depression from the brainstem. The usual precautions of deep breathing and turning as allowed are instituted. Regular pulmonary assessments are performed to identify adventitious sounds or any areas of diminished or absent breath sounds. Blood pressure is also taken at frequent intervals. The deflated cuff is left on the arm between readings to allow for the least movement and disturbance of the child. Ocular signs are recorded at least every hour.

> **NURSING ALERT**
>
> Sluggish, dilated, or unequal pupils are reported immediately because they may indicate increased ICP and potential brainstem herniation—a medical emergency.

Observations for function are not instituted until the child regains consciousness. However, as soon as possible the nurse should begin testing reflexes, handgrip, and functioning of the cranial nerves. Muscle strength is usually less after surgery because of general weakness but should improve daily. Ataxia may be significantly worse with cerebellar intervention, but it will slowly improve. Edema near the cranial nerves may depress important functions such as the gag, blink, or swallowing reflex.

Neurologic checks are an essential aspect of care and include pupillary reaction to light, level of consciousness (LOC), sleep patterns, and response to stimuli. Although children may be comatose for a few days, once they regain consciousness, there should be a steady increase in alertness. Regression to a lethargic, irritable state indicates increasing pressure, possibly caused by meningitis, hemorrhage, or edema.

Dressings are observed for evidence of drainage. If soiled, the dressing is not removed but reinforced with dry sterile gauze. The approximate amount of drainage is estimated and recorded.

> **NURSING ALERT**
>
> To keep an accurate account of drainage, the soiled area is circled with a pen every hour or so to identify continuous bleeding. The presence of colorless drainage is reported immediately because it most likely is cerebrospinal fluid from the incisional area. A foul odor from the dressing may indicate an infection. Such a finding is reported, and a culture is taken.

Once the younger child is alert, the arms may need to be restrained to preserve the dressing. Even a child who has been cooperative before surgery must be closely supervised during the initial stages of regaining consciousness, when disorientation and restlessness are common. Elbow restraints are satisfactory to prevent the hands from reaching the head, although additional restraint may be necessary to preserve an infusion line and maintain a specific position.

**Positioning.**   Correct positioning after surgery is critical to prevent pressure against the operative site, reduce intracranial pressure, and avoid the danger of aspiration. If a large tumor was removed, the child is not placed on the operative side, because the brain may suddenly shift to that cavity, causing trauma to the blood vessels, linings, and the brain itself. The nurse confers with the surgeon to be certain of the correct position, including the degree of neck flexion. The first 24 to 48 hours after brain surgery are critical. If positioning is restricted, notice of this is posted above the head of the bed. When the child is turned, every precaution is used to prevent jarring or malalignment in order to prevent undue strain on the sutures. Two nurses, one supporting the head and the other the body, are needed. The use of a turning sheet may facilitate turning a heavy child.

The child with an infratentorial procedure is usually positioned flat and on either side. Pillows should be placed against the child's back, not head, to maintain the desired position. Ordinarily the head and neck are kept in midline with the body and slightly extended. In a supratentorial craniotomy the head is usually elevated above the heart to facilitate cerebrospinal fluid drainage and decrease excessive blood flow to the brain to prevent hemorrhage.

> **NURSING ALERT**
>
> The Trendelenburg position is contraindicated in both infratentorial and supratentorial surgeries because it increases intracranial pressure and the risk of hemorrhage. If shock is impending, the practitioner is notified immediately, before the head is lowered.

**Fluid regulation.**   With an infratentorial craniotomy the child is allowed nothing by mouth for at least 24 hours and longer if the gag and swallowing reflexes are depressed or the child is comatose. With a supratentorial procedure, feeding may be resumed soon after the child is alert, sometimes within 24 hours. Clear water is always started first because of the danger of aspiration. If the child vomits, oral liquids are stopped. Vomiting not only predisposes the child to aspiration, but also increases ICP and the risk for incisional rupture.

IV fluids are continued until fluids are well tolerated. Because of the cerebral edema postoperatively and the danger of increased ICP, fluids are carefully monitored and usually infused at one half the maintenance rate. If drugs, such as prophylactic antibiotics, are given intravenously, the medication amount is calculated as part of the IV fluid. For example, if the child is to receive 20 ml/hr and the diluted drug is 5 ml, the IV solution is reduced to 15 ml for that hour.

A hypertonic solution such as mannitol or dextrose may be necessary to remove excess fluid. These drugs cause rapid diuresis. After surgery the child may have a Foley catheter in place. Urinary output is monitored after administration of these drugs to evaluate their effectiveness.

When able to take fluids, the child should be fed to conserve strength and minimize movement. If there is any sign of facial paralysis, the child is fed slowly to prevent choking or aspiration. Scrupulous mouth care is essential to prevent oral infection. Sometimes gavage feeding is necessary when bodily functions are too depressed to permit safe oral feedings or the child refuses to eat or drink. In the latter instance the nurse should employ every measure to encourage acceptance of fluids or solids. (See Chapter 27 for nursing interventions.)

*Comfort measures.* Headache may be severe and is largely the result of cerebral edema. Measures to relieve some of the discomfort include providing a quiet, dimly lit environment, restricting visitors to a minimum, preventing any sudden jarring movement, such as banging into the bed, and preventing an increase in ICP. The last is most effectively achieved by proper positioning and prevention of straining, such as during coughing, vomiting, or defecating. The use of opioids, such as morphine, to relieve pain is controversial because it is thought that they may mask signs of altered consciousness or depress respirations. However, they can be given safely because naloxone can be used to reverse opioid effects, such as sedation or respiratory depression. Acetaminophen and codeine are also effective analgesics. Regardless of the drugs used, adequate dosage and regular administration are essential to providing optimum pain relief. (See Pain Assessment; Pain Management, Chapter 26.)

Bowel movements are monitored to prevent constipation. Stool softeners may be given as soon as liquids are tolerated to facilitate easy passage of stool. Placing an ice bag on the forehead may also provide some headache relief, especially if facial edema is severe.

Brain edema may severely depress the gag reflex, necessitating suctioning of oral secretions. Facial edema may also be present, necessitating eye care if the lids remain partially open. Ice compresses applied to the eyes for short periods help in relieving the edema. A depressed blink reflex also predisposes the corneas to ulceration. Irrigating the eyes with saline drops and covering them with eye dressings are important steps in preventing this complication.

**Support Family.** The emotional needs of the family are great when the diagnosis is a brain tumor, and feelings are influenced by the extent of surgery, any neurologic deficits, the expected prognosis, and additional therapy. Because few definitive answers can be given before surgery, the sur-

geon's report is a significant finding that can vary from a completely benign, resected neoplasm to a highly malignant, invasive, and only partially removed tumor. Although parents try to prepare themselves for a potentially fatal diagnosis, it is a shock for them.

Ideally, a nurse should be with the family when the physician discusses with parents the expected prognosis and plan of therapy. Although parents may hear only a fraction of what they are told, they can begin to put the future into perspective. Although some children will be cured, those with residual tumor may die within a relatively short time or live for several years. Regardless of the future prospects, the parents' thinking must be directed toward helping the child recover and resume a normal life to his or her fullest potential. Providing the opportunity for the family to share their concerns and questions with other families who have a child with a brain tumor helps the family cope with the ongoing situation.*

It is also a time to encourage parents to verbalize their feelings about the diagnosis. Often they express guilt for attributing the insidious onset of symptoms, such as ataxia, visual difficulty, or headache, to minor "complaints" by the child. Parents may have punished their child for clumsiness, mistaking it for carelessness. The nurse listens to such statements, emphasizing the normalcy of the parents' reactions. Sometimes it may be helpful to precipitate such a discussion with a statement such as "It is difficult to know when a child's complaints are significant because so often they are caused by minor ailments." Any comments that insinuate that the parents should have sought medical advice sooner are avoided because such remarks only add to the parents' guilt feelings.

During this period the nurse should also discuss with parents what they plan to tell the child. If the child was prepared honestly as described previously, the diagnosis can be expressed in a similar manner, such as "The surgeon removed most of the tumor, and the rest will be treated with special drugs and x-ray treatments." During recovery the child will need additional explanation about the treatment, as well as the reason for residual neurologic effects, such as ataxia or blindness. Because the hair was shaved before surgery, hair loss from treatment is less of a concern, although its regrowth will be delayed by 3 to 6 months, depending on the length of therapy. At this point it is advisable to reinforce the idea of a wig.

**Promote Return to Optimum Functioning.** The ultimate goal is a cured child who has maximum functioning. As soon as possible, the child should resume usual activities within tolerable limits, especially returning to school.† Until the skull is completely healed, the child may need to wear a helmet when engaging in any active sport. The school nurse and teacher should confer with the parents to discuss

---

*Information about support groups is available from the **National Brain Tumor Foundation,** 414 13th St, Suite 700, Oakland, CA 94612, (800) 934-CURE, fax: (510) 839-9779, e-mail: mdts@braintumor.org; www.braintumor.org.
†Excellent publications, including the pamphlet, *When Your Child Is Ready to Return to School,* are available from the **American Brain Tumor Association,** 2720 Red Rd, Suite 146, Des Plaines, IL 60018, (847) 827-9910, fax: (847) 827-9918, e-mail: info@abta.org; www.abta.org.

activity restrictions, such as physical education, and the reactions of schoolmates to the child's appearance. Since children often equate brain surgery with "going crazy," it is important to prepare the child for possible remarks to this effect. As one child told a classmate, "It's *your* head they should have fixed, because you're crazy. Can't you see that I'm all better?"

After discharge the family needs continuing medical and emotional support from health personnel. Even with children who are long-term survivors after treatment for a brain tumor, residual disabilities, such as growth retardation, cranial nerve palsies, sensory defects, motor abnormalities (especially ataxia), intellectual deficits, dysphagia, dysgraphia, and behavioral problems, may occur (Strother and others, 2002; Loring and Meador, 2000; Riva and Giorgi, 2000). It is difficult to assess the exact cause of the nonphysical disabilities, because numerous variables influence the total rehabilitation of the child. However, the high frequency of late effects attests to the tremendous need for follow-up care despite successful treatment of the tumor.

The realm of possible consequences following the diagnosis of a brain tumor is vast. They are not discussed here. Rather, the reader is urged to refer to other sections of the text that deal with possible outcomes, such as the paralyzed, visually impaired, or unconscious child or the child with a ventricular shunt, seizure disorder, or meningitis. Numerous physical problems can occur with progression of the tumor that may necessitate additional procedures. For example, frequent vomiting, anorexia, and nausea may require nonoral routes of feeding, such as gastrostomy or parenteral alimentation. Trials with chemotherapy may necessitate the use of central venous access devices. Whenever these procedures are instituted, the nurse may be responsible for teaching the family appropriate home care to allow the child the highest quality of life for the longest period of time. (See discussion of discharge planning and home care in Chapter 26 and Nursing Care Plan: The Child with a Brain Tumor.*)

## Neuroblastoma

Neuroblastoma occurs in about 1 in 10,000 live births, with a slightly higher incidence in males. About half the cases occur in children under 2 years of age, and another fourth occur in children under age 4. These tumors originate from embryonic neural crest cells that normally give rise to the adrenal medulla and the sympathetic nervous system. Consequently the majority of the tumors arise from the adrenal gland or from the retroperitoneal sympathetic chain. Therefore the primary site is within the abdomen. Other sites may be within the head, neck, chest, or pelvis.

### Clinical Manifestations

The signs and symptoms of neuroblastoma depend on the location and stage of the disease. Most presenting signs are caused by compression of adjacent structures. With abdominal tumors the most common presenting sign is a firm, nontender, irregular mass in the abdomen that crosses the midline (in contrast to Wilms tumor, which is usually confined to one side). Compression of the kidney, ureter, or bladder may cause urinary frequency or retention.

Distant metastasis frequently causes supraorbital ecchymosis, periorbital edema, and proptosis (exophthalmos) from invasion of retrobulbar soft tissue. Lymphadenopathy, especially in the cervical and supraclavicular areas, may also be an early presenting sign. Bone pain may or may not be present with skeletal involvement. Vague symptoms of widespread metastasis include pallor, weakness, irritability, anorexia, and weight loss.

Other primary tumors may cause significant clinical effects, such as neurologic impairment from an intracranial lesion, respiratory obstruction from a thoracic mass, or varying degrees of paralysis from compression of the spinal cord. Infrequently a child may have symptoms of increased catecholamine excretion, such as flushing, hypertension, tachycardia, and diaphoresis (Grosfeld, 1998; Matthay, 1995).

### Diagnostic Evaluation

Diagnostic evaluation is aimed at locating the primary site and areas of metastasis. A skeletal survey; skull, neck, chest, abdominal, bone scan; CT scans; and bilateral bone marrow aspirate and biopsies are used to locate a tumor mass or metastasis. Metaiodobenzylguanidine (MIBG) scans are used to determine bone/tissue involvement; however, they are only available at certain centers. Neuroblastomas, particularly those arising on the adrenal glands or from a sympathetic chain, excrete the catecholamines epinephrine and norepinephrine. Urinary excretion of catecholamines is detected in approximately 95% of children with adrenal or sympathetic tumors. Analyzing the breakdown products that are normally excreted in the urine, namely, vanillylmandelic acid (VMA), homovanillic acid (HVA), dopamine, and norepinephrine, permits detection of a suspected tumor both before and after medical/surgical intervention. Amplification of the N-myc gene and abnormalities in chromosomes have been associated with a poorer prognosis (Grosfeld, 2000; Matthay, 1995). Increased ferritin, neuron-specific enolase (NSE), and ganglioside ($GD_2$) are associated with neuroblastoma.

### Staging and Prognosis

Neuroblastoma is a "silent" tumor. In more than 70% of cases, diagnosis is made after metastasis occurs, with the first signs caused by involvement in the nonprimary site, usually the lymph nodes, bone marrow, skeletal system, skin, or liver. Because of the frequency of invasiveness, the prognosis for neuroblastoma is poor.

The age of the child and the stage of the disease (Box 36-6) at diagnosis are important prognostic factors. Survival is inversely correlated with age. If all stages are grouped together, the survival rates are 75% for children under 1 year of age and less than 50% for children over 1 year of age. This marked difference in survival rates by age is partly accounted for by the larger proportion of

---

*In Wong DL, Hess CS: *Wong and Whaley's clinical manual of pediatric nursing,* ed 5, St Louis, 2000, Mosby.

very young children with stage I, II, or IV-S disease and the absence of the N-myc gene amplification (Grosfeld, 1998; Schor, 1999).

Infants who remain free of disease for 1 year after treatment are usually cured, but older children have experienced relapses several years after cessation of treatment. Surgical resection of the tumor in stage I infants diagnosed by ultrasonography done for other reasons appears to be near 90% curative (Grosfeld, 2000).

Neuroblastoma is one of the few tumors that demonstrate spontaneous regression (especially stage IV-S), possibly as a result of maturity of the embryonic cell or development of an active immune system.

### Therapeutic Management

Accurate clinical staging is important for establishing initial treatment. Therefore surgery is employed both to remove as much of the tumor as possible and to obtain biopsies. In stages I and II, complete surgical removal of the tumor is the treatment of choice. If the tumors are large, partial resection is attempted, with a course of irradiation postoperatively to shrink the tumor in the hope of complete removal at a later date. Surgery is usually limited to biopsy in stages III and IV because of the extensive metastasis, although the use of additional surgery to assess tumor regression or remove a regressed tumor is not unlikely.

The precise role of radiotherapy is unclear. It does not appear to be of any benefit in children with stage I and II disease; it is commonly used with stage III disease, although it may not improve survival expectancy; and it may make a large tumor operable. Radiotherapy provides emergency management of a massive neuroblastoma causing spinal cord compression (Nguyen and others, 2000). It also offers palliation for metastatic lesions in bones, lungs, liver, or brain.

Chemotherapy is the mainstay of therapy for extensive local or disseminated disease. The drugs of choice are vincristine, doxorubicin, cyclophosphamide, cisplatin, teniposide, etoposide, ifosfamide, and carboplatin. They are administered in a variety of combinations, but none has proved to be superior. There is a 10% to 20% survival rate for children over 2 years of age with recurrent disease, using

retinoic acid and high-dose chemotherapy with BMT or peripheral stem cell rescue.

### Nursing Considerations

Nursing considerations are similar to those discussed previously under Nursing Care of the Child with Cancer, including psychologic and physical preparation for diagnostic and operative procedures; prevention of postoperative complications for abdominal, thoracic, or cranial surgery; and explanation of chemotherapy and radiotherapy and their side effects (see Tables 36-2 and 36-3).

Because this tumor carries a poor prognosis for many children, every consideration must be given to the family in terms of coping with a life-threatening illness. (See Chapter 23.) Because of the high degree of metastasis at the time of diagnosis, many parents suffer much guilt for not having recognized signs earlier. Often the guilt is expressed as anger toward professionals for not diagnosing it sooner. Parents need much support in dealing with these feelings and expressing them to the appropriate people.

## BONE TUMORS

Malignant bone tumors represent less than 5% of all malignant neoplasms, but 85% of all primary malignant bone tumors in children are either osteogenic sarcoma and Ewing sarcoma. The peak ages during childhood are 15 to 19 years. The sexes are affected equally until puberty, at which time the ratio approaches 2:1 in favor of males. This propensity for males with a peak incidence during adolescence is thought to result from the accelerated growth rate of osseous tissue.

## General Considerations

Neoplastic disease can arise from any tissues involved in bone growth, such as osteoid matrix, bone marrow elements, fat, blood and lymph vessels, nerve sheath, and cartilage. They have several characteristics in common, which are discussed in the following sections. Specific information about each tumor is then presented.

### Clinical Manifestations

Most malignant bone tumors produce localized pain in the affected site, which may be severe or dull and may be attributed to trauma or the vague complaint of "growing pains." The pain is often relieved by a flexed position, which relaxes the muscles overlying the stretched periosteum. Frequently it draws attention when the child limps, curtails physical activity, or is unable to hold heavy objects.

### Diagnostic Evaluation

Diagnosis begins with a thorough history and physical examination. A primary objective is to rule out causes such as trauma or infection. Careful questioning regarding pain is essential in attempting to determine the duration and rate of tumor growth. Physical assessment focuses on functional status of the affected area, signs of inflammation, size of the mass, involvement of regional lymph nodes, and any systemic indication of generalized malignancy, such as anemia, weight loss, and frequent infection.

Definitive diagnosis is based on radiologic studies, such as CT to determine the extent of the lesion; MRI to assess soft tissue, tumor boundaries, nerve and vessel involvement; radioisotope bone scans to evaluate metastasis; and either needle or surgical bone biopsy to determine the histologic pattern. Radiologic findings are characteristic for each type of tumor. In osteogenic sarcoma, needlelike new bone formation growing at right angles to the diaphysis (shaft) produces a "sunburst" appearance. In Ewing sarcoma the deposits of new bone in layers under the periosteum produce an "onionskin" appearance. In both types of bone tumors, soft tissue infiltration may be apparent.

At present there is no reliable biochemical test for bone cancers. Elevated alkaline phosphatase levels may occur in osteoid tumors. Several tests may be done for differential diagnosis in terms of secondary bone metastasis from Wilms tumor, neuroblastoma, retinoblastoma, rhabdomyosarcoma, lymphoma, or leukemia. Lung tomography is usually a standard procedure, because pulmonary metastasis is the most common complication of primary bone tumors. Bone marrow aspiration is helpful in diagnosing Ewing sarcoma in the rare event that the child has bone marrow metastasis.

### Prognosis

A better understanding of the biology of neoplastic growth has resulted in more aggressive treatment and an improved prognosis. The natural history of osteogenic sarcoma and Ewing sarcoma suggests that multiple submicroscopic foci of metastatic disease are present at the time of diagnosis despite clinical evidence of localized involvement. Before the use of aggressive multimodal therapy, pulmonary metastasis invariably appeared in 6 to 24 months in patients with osteogenic sarcoma who were treated with surgical excision of the tumor. Now, with surgery for osteosarcoma or intensive radiotherapy for Ewing sarcoma combined with chemotherapy, survival statistics are improving for both types of bone cancer. Survival rates differ according to the specific treatment protocols and are influenced by a number of factors, such as the site of the primary tumor, especially in Ewing sarcoma, and the presence or absence of metastatic disease at diagnosis.

## Osteogenic Sarcoma

Osteogenic sarcoma (osteosarcoma) is the most common bone cancer in children. Its peak incidence is between 10 and 25 years of age. It presumably arises from bone-forming mesenchyme, which gives rise to malignant osteoid tissue. Most primary tumor sites are in the metaphysis (wider part of the shaft, adjacent to the epiphyseal growth plate) of long bones, especially in the lower extremities. More than half occur in the femur, particularly the distal portion, with the rest involving the humerus, tibia, pelvis, jaw, and phalanges.

### Therapeutic Management

Optimum treatment of osteosarcoma is surgery and chemotherapy. The surgical approach consists of surgical biopsy followed by either limb salvage or amputation. Depending on the tumor site, surgery includes amputation of the affected extremity at least 7.5 cm (3 inches) above the proximal tumor margin or above the joint proximal to the involved bone. With tumors of the distal femur, preservation of the hip joint may be possible. Other procedures include an above-the-knee amputation for tumors of the tibia or fibula, a hemipelvectomy for tumors of the innominate (hip) bone, and a forequarter amputation (removal of arm, scapula, and portion of the clavicle on the affected side) for tumors of the upper humerus. The other surgical approach for selected patients is the limb salvage procedure, which involves en bloc resection of the primary tumor with prosthetic replacement of the involved bone. For example, with osteosarcoma of the distal femur, a total femur and joint replacement is performed. Frequently children undergoing a limb salvage procedure will receive preoperative chemotherapy in an attempt to decrease the tumor size and make surgery more manageable (Lanzkowsky, 2000; Link, Gebhardt, and Myers, 2002).

Chemotherapy plays a vital role in treatment of osteosarcoma. Antineoplastic drugs, such as high-dose methotrexate with citrovorum factor rescue, doxorubicin, bleomycin, actinomycin D, cyclophosphamide, ifosfamide, and cisplatin, may be administered singly or in combination and may be employed both before and after surgery. When pulmonary metastasis is found, thoracotomy and chemotherapy have resulted in prolonged survival and potential cure. These combined-modality approaches have significantly improved the prognosis in osteosarcoma to approximately 85% in nonmetastatic patients (Lanzkowsky, 2000). New trials have recently been completed using muramyl tripeptide phosphatidylethanolamine (MTP-PE) to eradicate micrometastases by stimulating macrophages to kill tumor cells not eliminated by chemotherapy (Lanzkowsky, 2000).

### Nursing Considerations

Nursing care depends on the type of surgical approach. Obviously the family may have more difficulty adjusting to an amputation than a limb salvage procedure. In either instance, preparation of the child and family is critical. Straightforward honesty is essential in gaining the cooperation and trust of the child. The diagnosis of cancer should not be disguised with falsehoods such as "infection." To accept the need for radical surgery, the child must be aware of the lack of alternatives for treatment. Although the responsibility of telling the child is generally left to the physician, the nurse should be present at the discussion or be aware of exactly what is said to the child. The child should be told a few days before surgery to allow the child time to think about the diagnosis and consequent treatment and to ask questions. (See Nursing Care Plan: The Child with a Bone Tumor.*)

---

*In Wong DL, Hess CS: *Wong and Whaley's clinical manual of pediatric nursing,* ed 5, St Louis, 2000, Mosby.

Sometimes children have many questions about the prosthesis, limitations on physical ability, and prognosis in terms of cure. At other times they react with silence or with a calm manner that belies their concern and fear. Either response must be accepted, because it is part of the grieving process of a loss. For those who wish information, it may be helpful to introduce them to another amputee before surgery or to show them pictures of the prosthesis.* However, the nurse must be careful not to overwhelm children with information. A sound approach is to answer their questions without offering additional information. For those who do not pursue additional information, the nurse expresses a willingness to talk.

The child is also informed of the need for chemotherapy and its side effects before surgery. Caution must be exercised in offering too much information at one time. It is wise to discuss hair loss with an emphasis on positive aspects, such as wearing a wig. Because bone tumors affect adolescents and young adults, it is not unusual for them to become angry over all the radical body alterations.

If an amputation is performed, the child is usually fitted with a temporary prosthesis immediately after surgery, which permits early functioning and fosters psychologic adjustment. If this is not done, the child requires stump care, which is the same as for any amputee. A permanent prosthesis is usually fitted within 6 to 8 weeks. During hospitalization the child begins physical therapy to become proficient in the use and care of the device.

***Phantom limb pain*** may develop following amputation. This symptom is characterized by sensations such as tingling, itching and, more frequently, pain felt in the amputated limb. The child and family need to know that the sensations are real, not imagined. Amitriptyline (Elavil), has been used successfully in children to decrease the pain (Olsson, 1999).

Discharge planning must begin early during the postoperative period. Once the child has begun physical therapy, the nurse should consult with the therapist and practitioner to evaluate the child's physical and emotional readiness to reenter school. It is an opportune time to involve a community nurse in the home care of the child. Every effort is made to promote normalcy and gradual resumption of realistic preamputation activities.† Role-playing in anticipation of such experiences is very beneficial in preparing the child for the inevitable confrontation by others. Environmental barriers, such as stairs, are assessed in terms of the accessibility in the school and home, especially because the child may need to use crutches or a wheelchair before complete healing and prosthetic competency are achieved.

The nurse encourages the child to select clothing that best camouflages the prosthesis, such as pants or long-sleeved shirts. Well-fitted prostheses are so natural looking that girls can usually wear sheer stockings without revealing the device. Emphasizing feminine or masculine apparel helps the child regain a feeling of self-identity. Even during the postoperative period, encouraging the child to wear blue jeans and a shirt may distract attention from the deformity and focus it on familiar aspects of appearance.

The family and child need much support in adjusting not only to a life-threatening diagnosis but also to alteration in body form and function. Because loss of a limb constitutes a grieving process, those caring for the child need to recognize that the reactions of anger and depression are normal and necessary. Often parents view the anger as a direct affront to them for allowing the amputation to occur, or they see the depression as rejection. These are not interpersonal attacks but the child's attempts to cope with a loss.

## Ewing Sarcoma (Primitive Neuroectodermal Tumor [PNET] of the Bone)

Ewing sarcoma, classified as a PNET, is the second most common malignant bone tumor (after osteosarcoma) in childhood (Lanzkowsky, 2000). Ewing sarcoma arises in the marrow spaces of the bone rather than from osseous tissue. The tumor originates in the shaft of long and trunk bones, most often affecting the femur, tibia, fibula, humerus, ulna, vertebra, scapula, ribs, pelvic bones, and skull. It occurs almost exclusively in individuals under age 30, with the majority being between 4 and 25 years of age.

### Therapeutic Management

Surgical amputation is not routinely recommended but may be considered when the results of radiotherapy render the extremity useless or deformed (e.g., from retarded growth in young children) or the tumor appears resectable. The treatment of choice is intensive irradiation of the involved bone combined with chemotherapy. A widely used drug regimen includes vincristine, actinomycin D, cyclophosphamide or ifosfamide, VP-16, and doxorubicin. The addition of Ifosfamide and etoposide has increased the 3-year survival to 80% (Lanzkowsky, 2000).

### Nursing Considerations

The psychologic adjustment to Ewing sarcoma is typically less traumatic than it is to osteogenic sarcoma because of the preservation of the affected limb. Many families accept the diagnosis with a sense of relief in knowing that this type of bone cancer does not necessitate amputation, and initially they may not be aware of the damaging effects on the irradiated site. Consequently they need preparation for the various diagnostic tests, including bone marrow aspiration and surgical biopsy, and adequate explanation of the treatment regimen. High-dose radiotherapy often causes a skin reaction of dry or moist desquamation followed by hyperpigmentation. The child should wear loose-fitting clothes over the irradiated area to minimize additional skin irritation. Because of increased sensitivity, the area is protected from sunlight and sudden changes in temperature, such as from heating pads or ice packs. The child is encouraged to

---

*Information about protheses can be obtained from the **National Amputation Foundation, Inc,** 3840 Church St, Malverne, NY 11565, (516) 887-3600.
†Information about special programs for children with amputations is available from the **Candlelighters Childhood Cancer Foundation,** 3910 Warner St, Kensington, MD 20895, (800) 366-2223 or (301) 962-3520, fax: (301) 962-3521, www.candlelighters.org.

use the extremity as tolerated. Occasionally an active exercise program may be planned by the physical therapist to preserve maximum function.

The child needs the same considerations for adjusting to the effects of chemotherapy as any other patient with cancer. The drug regimen usually results in hair loss, severe nausea and vomiting, peripheral neuropathy, and possibly cardiotoxicity. Every effort should be made to outline a treatment plan that allows the child maximum resumption of a normal lifestyle and activities. (See Nursing Care Plan: The Child with a Bone Tumor.*)

## OTHER SOLID TUMORS

In addition to the cancers already discussed, several other types of solid tumors may occur in children. Wilms tumor, rhabdomyosarcoma, and retinoblastoma are unique in that they tend to be diagnosed early, typically before 5 years of age. Wilms tumor and retinoblastoma are also unusual in that they are among the few types of cancer that may occur in both hereditary and nonhereditary forms.

### Wilms Tumor

Wilms tumor, or nephroblastoma, is the most common intraabdominal and kidney tumor of childhood (Skoldenberg and others, 2001). Its frequency is estimated to be 9 cases per million in white children less than 15 years of age (Lanzkowsky, 2000). Eighty percent of patients with Wilm's tumor are diagnosed under 5 years of age, and it has a peak incidence between 3 and 4 years of age (Lanzkowsky, 2000; Pertruzzi and Green, 1997). Wilms tumor is one of the childhood cancers that show an increased incidence among siblings and identical twins, reflecting evidence of genetic inheritance. The mode of inheritance in familial cases, which account for less than 2% of all Wilms tumors, is autosomal dominant with variable penetrance and expressivity (Green and others, 2002). Wilms tumor is heritable in about 15% to 20% of all cases, including some unilateral sporadic cases (Green and others, 2002). Unfortunately, there is no method of identification of gene carriers.

Wilms tumor is also associated with several congenital anomalies; the most common are aniridia, hemihypertrophy, genitourinary anomalies (such as hypospadias, cryptorchidism, ambiguous genitalia), and Beckwith-Wiedemann syndrome (Green and others, 1996; Lanzkowsky, 2000). Other, less common anomalies are microcephaly, pigmented and vascular nevi, pinna deformities, and mental and growth retardation.

#### Clinical Manifestations

The most common presenting sign is a swelling or mass within the abdomen. The mass is characteristically firm, nontender, confined to one side, and deep within the flank. If it is on the right side, it may be difficult to distinguish from the liver, although, unlike that organ, it does not move with respiration. Parents usually discover the mass during routine bathing or dressing of the child.

Other clinical manifestations are the result of compression from the tumor mass, metabolic alterations secondary to the tumor, or metastasis. Hematuria occurs in less than one fourth of children with Wilms tumor. Anemia, usually secondary to hemorrhage within the tumor, results in pallor, anorexia, and lethargy. Hypertension, probably caused by secretion of excess amounts of renin by the tumor, occurs occasionally. Other effects of malignancy include weight loss and fever. If metastasis has occurred, symptoms of lung involvement, such as dyspnea, cough, shortness of breath, and pain in the chest, may be evident.

#### Diagnostic Evaluation

In a child suspected of having Wilms tumor, special emphasis is placed on the history and physical examination for the presence of congenital anomalies, a family history of cancer, and signs of malignancy, such as weight loss, size of the liver and spleen, indications of anemia, and lymphadenopathy. Specific tests include radiographic studies, including abdominal ultrasound, CT, MRI, hematologic studies (polycythemia is sometimes present if the tumor secretes excess erythropoietin), biochemical studies, and urinalysis. Studies to demonstrate the relationship of the tumor to the ipsilateral kidney and the presence of a normally functioning kidney on the contralateral side are essential. If a large tumor is present, an inferior venacavogram is necessary to demonstrate possible tumor involvement adjacent to the vena cava. A bone marrow aspiration is electively performed to rule out metastasis, which is rare in children with Wilms tumor.

#### Staging and Prognosis

Wilms tumor probably arises from a malignant, undifferentiated metanephrogenic blastoma (a cluster of primordial cells capable of initiating the regeneration of an abnormal structure). Its occurrence slightly favors the left kidney, which is advantageous because surgically this kidney is easier to manipulate and remove. Although the tumor may become quite large, it remains encapsulated for an extended period. During surgery the tumor is staged to maximize the effectiveness of treatment protocols (Box 36-7).

The histology of the tumor cells is also identified and classified according to two groups: favorable histology (FH) and unfavorable histology (UH). Only about 12% of Wilms tumors demonstrate UH, which is associated with a poorer

---

| Box 36-7 ■ ■ ■ |
| --- |
| **Staging of Wilms Tumor** |

**Stage I:** Tumor is limited to kidney and completely resected.
**Stage II:** Tumor extends beyond kidney but is completely resected.
**Stage III:** Residual nonhematogenous tumor is confined to abdomen.
**Stage IV:** Hematogenous metastases; deposits are beyond stage III, namely, to lung, liver, bone, and brain.
**Stage V:** Bilateral renal involvement is present at diagnosis.

---

*In Wong DL, Hess CS: *Wong and Whaley's clinical manual of pediatric nursing,* ed 5, St Louis, 2000, Mosby.

prognosis and demands a more aggressive treatment protocol, regardless of the clinical stage.

Survival rates for Wilms tumor are one of the highest among all childhood cancers. Children with localized tumor (stages I and II) have a 90% chance of cure with multimodal therapy. FH of the tumor, a first complete remission of more than 12 months' duration before relapse, and nonabdominal relapse sites are each associated with a significantly better survival expectancy (Green and others, 1996).

### Therapeutic Management

Combined treatment of surgery and chemotherapy with or without irradiation is based on the clinical stage and histologic pattern. In unilateral disease a large transabdominal incision is performed for optimum visualization of the abdominal cavity; the tumor, affected kidney, and adjacent adrenal gland are removed. Great care is taken to keep the encapsulated tumor intact because rupture can seed cancer cells throughout the abdomen, lymph channel, and bloodstream. The contralateral kidney is carefully inspected for evidence of disease or dysfunction. Regional lymph nodes are inspected, and a biopsy is performed when indicated. Any involved structures, such as part of the colon, diaphragm, or vena cava, are removed. Metal clips are placed around the tumor site for exact marking during radiotherapy.

If both kidneys are involved, the child may be treated with radiotherapy or chemotherapy preoperatively to shrink the tumor, allowing more conservative therapy (Graf, Tournade, and deKraker, 2000; Lanzkowsky, 2000). In some cases a partial nephrectomy is performed on the less affected kidney, with a total nephrectomy performed on the opposite side. When a transplant is feasible, such as from a twin, sibling, or parent, bilateral nephrectomy is considered as a last resort.

Postoperative radiotherapy is indicated for children with large tumors, metastasis, residual disease at the primary tumor site, UH, or recurrence. Chemotherapy is indicated for all stages. The most effective agents for treating Wilms tumor are actinomycin D and vincristine; doxorubicin and cyclophosphamide may be used for UH or advanced-stage disease (Green and others, 2002; Lanzkowsky, 2000). The duration of therapy varies, ranging from 6 to 15 months.

### Nursing Considerations

The nursing care of the child with Wilms tumor is similar to that of other cancers treated with surgery, irradiation, and chemotherapy. However, some significant differences are discussed for each phase of nursing intervention.

**Preoperative Care.** As with many of the other cancers, the diagnosis of Wilms tumor is a shock. Frequently the child has no physical indication of the seriousness of the disorder other than a palpable abdominal mass. Because it is the parents who usually discover the mass, the nurse needs to take into account their feelings regarding the diagnosis. Whereas some parents are grateful for their detection of the tumor, others feel guilty for not finding it sooner or anger toward the practitioner for missing it on earlier examinations.

The preoperative period is one of swift diagnosis. Typically, surgery is scheduled within 24 to 48 hours of admission. The nurse is faced with the challenge of preparing the child and parents for all laboratory and operative procedures. Because of the little time available, explanations should be kept simple and repeated often with attention to what the child will experience. Besides usual preoperative observations, blood pressure is monitored, because hypertension from excess renin production is a possibility.

There are several special preoperative concerns, the most important of which is that the tumor is not palpated unless absolutely necessary because manipulation of the mass may cause dissemination of cancer cells to adjacent and distant sites.

> **NURSING ALERT** To reinforce the need for caution, it may be necessary to post a sign on the bed that reads "DO NOT PALPATE ABDOMEN." Careful bathing and handling are also important in preventing trauma to the tumor site.

Because radiotherapy and chemotherapy are usually begun immediately after surgery, parents need an explanation of what to expect, such as major benefits and side effects, although the timing of the information should be considered to avoid overwhelming the family. Ideally the nurse should be present during physician-parent conferences to answer questions as they arise. It is usually better to postpone telling the child about these side effects until after surgery. Alopecia, usually of most concern to older children, does not occur until 2 weeks after the initial treatment regimen. Therefore the child can be prepared for the hair loss postoperatively.

**Postoperative Care.** Despite the extensive surgical intervention necessary in many children with Wilms tumor, the recovery period is usually rapid. The major nursing responsibilities are those following any abdominal surgery. (See Nursing Care Plan: The Child Undergoing Surgery, Chapter 27.) Because these children are at risk for intestinal obstruction from vincristine-induced adynamic ileus, radiation-induced edema, and postsurgical adhesion formation, gastrointestinal activity, such as bowel movements, bowel sounds, distention, and vomiting, is monitored. Other considerations are frequent evaluation of blood pressure and observation for signs of infection, especially during chemotherapy. Because of the myelosuppression from the drugs, pulmonary hygiene measures are instituted in the immediate postoperative period to prevent complications.

**Family Support.** The postoperative period is frequently difficult for parents. The shock of seeing their child immediately after surgery may be the first realization of the seriousness of the diagnosis. It also marks the confirmation of the stage of the tumor. During this period the nurse should again be with parents to assure them of the child's recovery after surgery and to assess their understanding of the pathology report.

Older children need an opportunity to deal with their feelings concerning the many procedures to which they have been subjected in rapid succession. Play therapy with dolls, puppets, or drawing can be extremely beneficial in helping them adjust to the surgery and hair loss. It is not unusual for children to feel betrayed because they were not adequately prepared for the extent of surgery, the need for additional therapy, or the seriousness of the disorder.

Because the child is left with only one kidney, certain precautions, such as avoiding contact sports or any other activity that has a high risk potential, are recommended to prevent injury to the organ. Urinary tract infections should be prevented with good hygiene, especially in girls. Prompt detection and treatment of any genitourinary signs or symptoms is mandatory.

## Rhabdomyosarcoma

Soft tissue sarcomas are the fourth most common type of solid tumors in children. These malignant neoplasms originate from undifferentiated mesenchymal cells in muscles, tendons, bursae, and fascia, or in fibrous, connective, lymphatic, or vascular tissue. They derive their name from the specific tissue(s) of origin, such as myosarcoma (*myo*—muscle). Rhabdomyosarcoma (*rhabdo*—striated) is the most common soft tissue sarcoma in children. Because striated (skeletal) muscle is found almost anywhere in the body, these tumors occur in many sites, the most common of which are the head and neck, especially the orbit. The disease occurs in children in all age-groups but is most common in children younger than 5 years of age. Its incidence is approximately 8.5 per million for white children but only 4.0 per million for African-American children in the age-group from 2 to 19 years (Lanzkowsky, 2000).

Rhabdomyosarcoma arises from embryonic mesenchyme. Three subtypes are recognized and described in Box 36-8.

### Clinical Manifestations

The initial signs and symptoms are related to the site of the tumor and compression of adjacent organs (Table 36-6). Some tumor locations, particularly the orbit, produce symptoms early in the course of the illness and contribute to rapid diagnosis and an improved prognosis. Other tumors, such as those of the retroperitoneal area, produce no symptoms until they are large, invasive, and widely metastasized. Unfortunately, many of the signs and symptoms attributable to rhabdomyosarcoma are vague and frequently suggest a common childhood illness, such as "earache" or "runny nose." In some instances a primary tumor site is never identified.

---

**Box 36-8** ■ ■ □
**Subtypes of Rhabdomyosarcoma**

**Embryonal**—Most common type; most frequently found in the head, neck, abdomen, and genitourinary tract
**Alveolar**—Second most common type; most often seen in deep tissues of the extremities and trunk
**Pleomorphic**—Rare in children (adult form); most often occurs in soft parts of extremities and trunk

---

## Diagnostic Evaluation

Diagnosis begins with a careful examination of the head and neck area, particularly palpation of a nontender, firm, hard mass. The nasopharynx and oropharynx are inspected for any evidence of a visible mass.

Radiographic studies to isolate a tumor site are performed, accompanied by chest x-ray examinations, CT, MRI, bone surveys, and bone marrow aspiration to rule out metastasis. A lumbar puncture is indicated for head and neck tumors to examine the cerebrospinal fluid for malignant cells. An excisional biopsy is done to confirm the histologic type.

## Staging and Prognosis

Careful staging is extremely important for planning treatment and determining the prognosis. The Intergroup Rhabdomyosarcoma Study has established clinical staging (Lanzkowsky, 2000; Wexler, Crist, and Helman, 2002) (Box 36-9).

With the change in treatment from radical surgery or radiotherapy to a multimodal approach, survival rates for all stages have increased considerably. Five-year survival rates are approximately 65% (Lanzkowsky, 2000; Wexler, Crist, and Helman, 2002). Data suggest that children who remain disease-free for 2 years are probably cured; however, if relapse occurs, the prognosis for long-term survival is extremely poor.

---

**TABLE 36-6** Clinical manifestations of rhabdomyosarcoma according to tumor site

| Location | Signs and Symptoms |
|---|---|
| **Orbit** | Rapidly developing unilateral proptosis<br>Ecchymosis of conjunctiva<br>Loss of extraocular movements (strabismus) |
| **Nasopharynx** | Stuffy nose (earliest sign)<br>Nasal obstruction—dysphagia, nasal voice (obstruction of posterior nasal conchae), serous otitis media (obstruction of eustachian tube)<br>Pain (sore throat and ear)<br>Epistaxis<br>Palpable neck nodes<br>Visible mass in oropharynx (late sign) |
| **Paranasal sinuses** | Nasal obstruction<br>Local pain<br>Discharge<br>Sinusitis<br>Swelling |
| **Middle ear** | Signs of chronic serous otitis media<br>Pain<br>Sanguinopurulent drainage<br>Facial nerve palsy |
| **Retroperitoneal area** (usually a "silent" tumor) | Abdominal mass<br>Pain<br>Signs of intestinal or genitourinary obstruction |
| **Perineum** | Visible superficial mass<br>Bowel or bladder dysfunction (from tumor compression) |

---

**Box 36-9** ▪ ■ ◾
**Staging of Rhabdomyosarcoma**

**Group I:** Localized disease; tumor completely resected and regional nodes not involved
**Group II:** Localized disease with microscopic residual, or regional disease with no residual or with microscopic residual
**Group III:** Incomplete resection or biopsy with gross residual disease
**Group IV:** Metastatic disease present at diagnosis

---

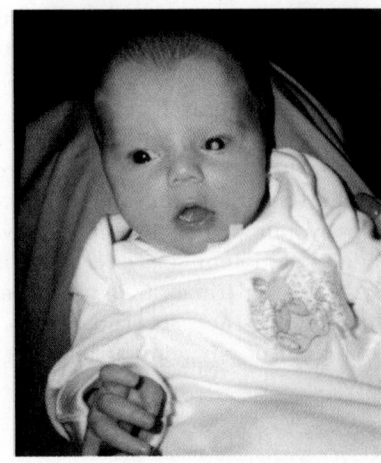

**Fig. 36-4** Cat's eye reflex. Whitish appearance of lens is produced as light falls on tumor mass in left eye.

### Therapeutic Management

Because this tumor is highly malignant, with metastasis frequently occurring at the time of diagnosis, aggressive multimodal therapy is recommended. In the past, radical surgical removal of the tumor was the treatment of choice, but with improved survival from combined chemotherapy and irradiation, surgery plays a lesser role. Complete removal of the primary tumor is advocated whenever possible. However, only biopsy is required in certain tumor locations, such as those of the orbit, when followed by irradiation and chemotherapy. This is a fortunate change, because it avoids the devastating effects of enucleation, amputation, or pelvic exenteration.

High-dose irradiation to the primary tumor is recommended, except in group I tumors. Chemotherapy plays a major role in treatment of all groups. Drugs that are cytotoxic for rhabdomyosarcoma are vincristine, actinomycin D, ifosfamide, cisplatin, VP-16, carboplatin, etoposide, and cyclophosphamide, topotecan, melphalan, and Adriamycin, for 1 to 2 years, depending on the stage of the disease (Lanzkowsky, 2000; Lyos and others, 1996).

### Nursing Considerations

The nursing responsibilities are similar to those for other types of cancer, especially the solid tumors when surgery is employed. Specific objectives include (1) careful assessment for signs of the tumor, especially during well-child examinations; (2) preparation of the child and family for the multiple diagnostic tests (see p. 1603); and (3) supportive care during each stage of multimodal therapy. The reader is urged to review the Nursing Considerations section for cancer and Chapter 23 for emotional support of the family in the event of a poor prognosis.

## Retinoblastoma

Retinoblastoma, which arises from the retina, is the most common intraocular malignancy of childhood (Tsinopoulos and others, 2001). Approximately 11 cases per million occur annually, primarily in children under 5 years of age. The average age of the child at the time of diagnosis is 17 months; it is usually diagnosed earlier in hereditary cases and later in nonhereditary types. Of all cases, 60% are nonhereditary and unilateral, 15% are hereditary and unilateral, and 25% are hereditary and bilateral.

Retinoblastoma may be caused by (1) a somatic mutation, (2) a germinal mutation, or (3) a chromosome aberration. *Somatic mutations* (those occurring in the general body cells, as opposed to the germ cells or gametes) are a sporadic, nonhereditary event. They result in unilateral tumors. *Germinal mutations* are passed to future generations. Almost all bilateral retinoblastomas are considered hereditary, and 15% of individuals with unilateral disease have the hereditary form (Hurwitz and others, 2002; Tsinopoulos and others, 2001). Hereditary retinoblastomas are transmitted as an autosomal dominant trait, with a 90% penetrance (Lanzkowsky, 2000). Consequently 10% of gene carriers remain unaffected.

Retinoblastoma has also been associated with partial deletion of the long arm of a group D chromosome 13 (Lanzkowsky, 2000; Tsinopoulos and others, 2001) and polyploidy (excessive number of chromosomes), such as trisomy 21. In children who have chromosome aberrations and retinoblastoma, there is often an increased incidence of mental retardation and congenital malformations although the vast majority of children with retinoblastomas apparently have normal chromosomes and intelligence.

### Clinical Manifestations

Retinoblastoma has few grossly obvious signs. Typically it is the parent who first observes a whitish "glow" in the pupil, known as the *cat's eye reflex* or *leukokoria* (Fig. 36-4). The reflex represents visualization of the tumor as the light momentarily falls on the mass. When a tumor arises in the macular region (area directly at the back of the retina when the eye is focused straight ahead), a white reflex may be seen when the tumor is quite small. It is best observed when a bright light is shining toward the child as the child looks forward. It is sometimes accidentally discovered by parents when taking a photograph of their child using a flash attachment.

When the tumor arises in the periphery of the retina, it must grow to a considerably large size before light can strike it sufficiently to produce the cat's eye reflex. In this situation it is seen only when the child looks in certain directions (sideways) or if the observer stands at an oblique angle to the child's face as the child looks straight ahead. The fleet-

---

**Box 36-10 ■ ■ ■**
**Staging of Retinoblastoma**

**Group I:** Very favorable
   Solitary tumor, less than 4 DD, at or behind the equator
   Multiple tumors, none greater than 4 DD, all at or behind
      the equator
**Group II:** Favorable
   Solitary tumors, 4 to 10 DD, at or behind the equator
   Multiple tumors, 4 to 10 DD, behind the equator
**Group III:** Doubtful
   Any lesion anterior to the equator
   Solitary tumors larger than 10 DD behind the equator
**Group IV:** Unfavorable
   Multiple tumors, some larger than 10 DD
   Any lesion extending anteriorly to the ora serrata
**Group V:** Very unfavorable
   Massive tumors involving more than half the retina
   Vitreous seeding

---

ing nature of the reflex often results in a delayed diagnosis because health care professionals fail to appreciate the ominous significance of the parents' findings.

The next most common sign is strabismus resulting from poor fixation of the visually impaired eye, particularly if the tumor develops in the macula, the area of sharpest visual acuity. Blindness is usually a late sign, but it frequently is not obvious unless the parent consciously observes for behaviors indicating loss of sight, such as bumping into objects, slowed motor development, or turning of the head to see objects lateral to the affected eye.

Another common presenting sign is a red, painful eye, often accompanied by glaucoma. Other common clinical manifestations include orbital cellulitis, unilateral mydriasis, a change in the color of the iris, hyphema, white spots on the iris, nystagmus, and complaints indicating systemic metastasis, such as weight loss, poor appetite, or fatigue.

### Diagnostic Evaluation

The first step in diagnosis is carefully listening to and recognizing the significance of reports from family members regarding suspected abnormalities within the eye. *Parental remarks that in any way suggest the presence of such findings must be taken seriously and investigated further.* For example, if the parent indicates that the child has a strange expression or an unusual glow in the eye, every attempt is made to duplicate the circumstances necessary to observe these changes. Children suspected of having this disorder are referred to an ophthalmologist. Definitive diagnosis is usually based on indirect ophthalmoscopy employing scleral indentation, which is done with the patient under general anesthesia and with maximum dilation of the pupils.

Metastatic disease at time of retinoblastoma diagnosis is rare (Singh, Shields, and Shields, 2000). Therefore staging procedures such as bone marrow aspiration, bone survey, and lumbar puncture are not performed.

### Staging and Prognosis

Staging of retinoblastomas is done under indirect ophthalmoscopy before surgery to determine accurately the tumor size (measured in disc diameters [DD]) and location (ac-

cording to an imaginary line called the equator drawn on the midplane of the eye) (Hurwitz and others, 2002; Lanzkowsky, 2000). The classification by Reese-Ellsworth is commonly used (Box 36-10).

The classification system has been used to define cure in terms of numbers of years free of disease and in terms of preservation of useful vision in the affected eye (favorable, doubtful, or unfavorable). Cure rates for survival are much better than for retention of useful vision. The overall 10-year survival rate is nearly 90% for unilateral and bilateral tumors; most of the deaths occur in children with group V disease (Hurwitz and others, 2002; Singh, Shields, and Shields, 2000). Retinoblastoma is one of the tumors that may spontaneously regress.

Of major concern in long-term survivors is the development of secondary tumors, especially osteogenic sarcoma. Children with bilateral disease (hereditary form) are more likely to develop secondary cancers than are children with unilateral disease. It is thought that these individuals are predisposed to developing cancer, and radiation increases their risk.

### Therapeutic Management

Treatment of retinoblastoma depends chiefly on the stage of the tumor at diagnosis. In general, unilateral retinoblastomas in stages I, II, and III are treated with irradiation. The aim of radiotherapy is to preserve useful vision in the affected eye and eradicate the tumor.

Other approaches toward treating small, localized tumors involve (1) *plaque brachytherapy* (surgical implantation of an iodine-125 applicator on the sclera until the maximum radiation dose has been delivered to the tumor), (2) *photocoagulation* (use of a laser beam to destroy retinal blood vessels that supply nutrition to the tumor), and (3) *cryotherapy* (freezing of the tumor, which destroys the microcirculation to the tumor and the cells themselves through microcrystal formation). One of the reasons for investigating treatments other than radiotherapy is to minimize the risk of radiation-induced malignancies later in life.

With advanced tumor growth, especially optic nerve involvement, enucleation of the affected eye is the treatment of choice. The use of chemotherapy in advanced disease, even in group V, is controversial and has not shown improved survival. Drugs that may be used in the treatment of metastatic disease include vincristine, cyclophosphamide, Adriamycin, cisplatin, carboplatin, and etoposide. In the case of central nervous system disease, intrathecal chemotherapy may be administered (Hurwitz and others, 2002; Lanzkowsky, 2000).

With bilateral disease, every attempt is made to preserve useful vision in the less affected eye with enucleation of the severely diseased eye. When bilateral tumors are found very early, enucleation may be prevented with the use of radiotherapy to both eyes.

### Nursing Considerations

**Prepare Family for Diagnostic/Therapeutic Procedures and Home Care.** Because the tumor is usually diagnosed in infants or very young children, most of the preparation for diagnostic tests and treatment involves parents. After indirect ophthalmoscopy the child may not see very clearly, or the eyes may be sensitive to light because of pupillary dilation. Parents are made aware of these normal reactions before the procedure.

Once the disease is staged, the physician confers with the parents regarding treatment. Unless the diagnosis is made very early, an enucleation is performed. Parents are told about the procedure, as well as about the benefits of a prosthesis. Parents often believe the procedure is bloody and mutilating, envisioning that the eye is "ripped out of its socket." Actually, the surgery is very similar to scooping a nut out of its shell. All of the adnexal structures of the eye, such as the lids, lashes, and tear glands, are left undisturbed.

Showing parents pictures of another child with an artificial eye may be very helpful in their adjustment to the thought of disfigurement (Fig. 36-5). Although the idea of loss of vision is a very distressing one, most parents seem to realize that there is no alternative. The facts that the unaffected eye retains normal vision and that the affected eye is probably already blind are particularly helpful in promoting acceptance of the imposed impairment and should be emphasized.

After surgery the parents need to be prepared for the child's facial appearance. An eye patch is in place, and the child's face may be edematous or ecchymotic. Parents often fear seeing the surgical site because they imagine a cavity in the skull. On the contrary, the lids are usually closed, and the area does not appear sunken because a surgically implanted sphere maintains the shape of the eyeball. The implant is covered with conjunctiva, and when the lids are open, the exposed area resembles the mucosal lining of the mouth. Once the child is fitted for a prosthesis, usually within 3 weeks, the facial appearance returns to normal.

After an uneventful recovery from enucleation, plans can be made for discharge from the hospital, usually within 3 to 4 days postoperatively. Parents need instruction regarding care of the surgical site and preparation for any additional therapy. They should be given the opportunity to see the socket as soon after surgery as possible. A good time to do this without unduly pressuring them is during dressing changes. They should then be encouraged to participate in the dressing changes.

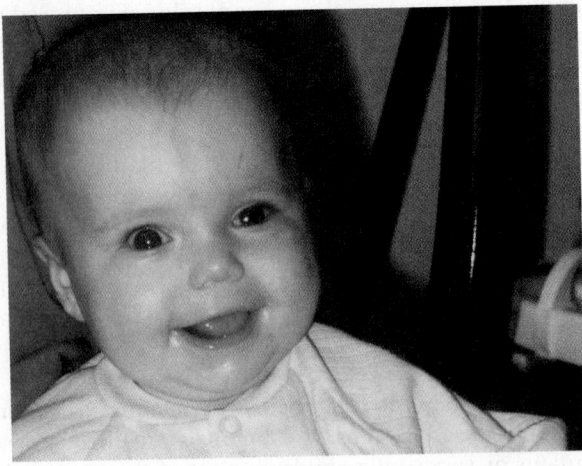

**Fig. 36-5** Infant with left prosthetic eye.

Care of the socket is minimal and easily accomplished. The wound itself is clean and has little or no drainage. If an antibiotic ointment is prescribed, it is applied in a thin line on the surface of the tissues of the socket. To cleanse the site, an irrigating solution may be ordered and is instilled daily or more frequently if necessary, *before* application of the antibiotic ointment. The dressing consists of an eye pad changed daily. Self-adhesive eye pads can also be used as dressings. Once the socket has healed completely, a dressing is no longer necessary, although there are several reasons for having the child continue to wear an eye patch. Infants and toddlers explore their environment with their hands, and without an eye patch in place, the socket is available to exploring fingers. Although there is little danger of the child injuring the socket, parents may feel more secure with the socket covered. This also helps prevent infection.

Initial instructions for care of the prosthesis are given by the ocularist, who fits and manufactures the device. Once in place, the prosthesis need not be removed unless cleaning is necessary, in which case it is taken out by gently pulling down on the lower lid, which frees the lower edge of the prosthesis, and applying pressure to the upper lid. If the child resists by forcing the lids shut, a small rubber instrument resembling a plunger can be used to facilitate removal and reinsertion. The end of the plunger is moistened and placed on top of the prosthetic iris. The lower eyelid is retracted, and the prosthesis is pulled out with a downward motion.

The prosthesis is cleaned by placing it in hot water and soaking it for several minutes. Reinsertion is easier if the prosthesis remains wet. To reinsert the prosthesis, the lids are separated, and with the prosthesis held in the correct position (it should be marked to indicate the nasal side), it is pushed up under the upper lid, allowing the lower lid to cover its lower edge.

Because the prosthesis is easily removed, the child may accidentally cause it to dislodge. Reactions of children vary from fear that they have "lost" their eye to matter-of-fact acceptance. The first time can be disturbing to both parents and child, but it is just one part of the child's adjusted lifestyle. If children are old enough to understand, parents can explain that they have a "special" eye that can accidentally fall out but that can also be quickly put back in place.

Safety is a major concern to prevent damage to the unaffected eye. Safety measures should be practiced at all times, and rough contact sports should be avoided or protective eye wear worn during such activity.

**Support Family.** The diagnosis of retinoblastoma presents some special concerns in addition to those created by any type of cancer. Families with a history of the disorder may feel great guilt for transmitting the defect to their offspring, especially if they knowingly "played the odds" and parented an affected child. Conversely, when parents are aware of the probability and have an affected child, early treatment results in such favorable outcomes that parental adjustment may be rapid. In families with no history of retinoblastoma, the discovery of the diagnosis is a shock, frequently complicated by guilt for not having discovered it sooner. Because parents frequently are the first to observe the cat's eye reflex, they may feel angry at themselves or others, especially professionals, for delaying a more thorough examination. Each of these variables needs to be considered in offering supportive care to the family.

Other concerns are also related to the hereditary aspects of the disease. Of great importance to parents is the recurrence risk of retinoblastoma in their subsequent offspring and in the offspring of the surviving affected child. With improving prognoses for these children, the necessity of genetic counseling to prevent transmission of the disease is assuming greater importance. (See Chapter 5 for a discussion of the nurse's role in genetic counseling.) Determining the risk of transmission is possible through DNA/RNA studies of the tumor cells. If a germinal mutation is found, blood samples from family members can be analyzed to see if they carry the mutation (Hurwitz and others, 2002; Smith and others, 2000).

These families are also encouraged to seek regular follow-up care for the affected child to detect secondary tumors, and all subsequent offspring of unaffected parents and survivors should undergo regular ophthalmoscopy to detect retinoblastoma at its earliest stage (Shields and Shields, 2001). (See Nursing Care Plan: The Child with Cancer.*)

## Testicular Tumors

Tumors of the testes are not a common condition, but when manifested in adolescence they are generally malignant. Testicular cancer is the most common form of cancer in males ages 15 to 44 years (Braga and others, 2001). Approximately 80% of pediatric testicular tumors remain localized to the testis, compared with 39% in adults (Kusumakumary and others, 2000). The usual presenting symptom is a heavy, painless testicular swelling, which described the presentation of boys with testicular tumors in a study by Kusumakumary and others (2000). The tumor may be smooth or nodular and does not transilluminate unless it is accompanied by a hydrocele. The involved testicle hangs lower and is therefore more susceptible to trauma. Although not all scrotal masses are malignant, any firm swelling of the testis demands immediate evaluation. If swelling is noted, the youth should be subjected to a minimum of preoperative palpation and referred immediately for surgical exploration. There is seldom delay in seeking medical advice if the mass is painful, but in the absence of pain the condition may go unattended for some time.

Treatment for testicular cancer consists of surgical removal of the affected testicle (orchiectomy) and the adjacent lymph nodes, if affected. If metastases are evident in more distant nodes or organs, chemotherapy (such as cisplatin, etoposide, bleomycin, vinblastine) and radiation therapy are implemented.

### Nursing Considerations

To supplement routine health assessment, every adolescent male should be taught to perform frequent testicular self-examination (TSE) to familiarize himself with his own

anatomy and to ensure early detection of any abnormality. Ideally self-examination should be performed once a month beginning when physical development reaches Tanner stage 3, usually about age 13 or 14 years. (See Fig. 19-6.) Each testicle is examined individually, preferably after a warm bath or shower (when scrotal skin is more relaxed), using the thumbs and fingers of both hands and applying a small amount of firm, gentle pressure. The normal testicle is a firm organ with a smooth egg-shaped contour. The epididymis can be palpated as a raised swelling on the superior aspect of the testicle and should not be confused with an abnormality. The efficacy of teaching TSE to adolescent males has been tested and found to be successful (Han and Peschel, 2000; Turner, 1995).

## THE CHILDHOOD CANCER SURVIVOR

It is estimated that by the year 2000, one individual in 900 will have survived childhood cancer (Fig. 36-6). These young adults are at risk for the development of numerous late effects caused by the cancer or its treatment. These complications are defined as posttherapeutic disabilities, ranging from impaired cognitive development to the onset of second malignancies.

Psychosocial, cognitive, emotional, and physical development may be affected by treatment as well as by the disease. Table 36-7 describes the systemic late effects caused by cancer treatment that require careful nursing assessment.

### Long-Term Sequelae of Treatment

Vigorous treatment of childhood cancers has resulted in dramatically improved survival rates. However, treatment programs combining surgery, irradiation, and chemotherapy are not without their complications. Some may occur immediately, such as loss of a limb from surgical amputation or asplenia from splenectomy in Hodgkin disease. However, current concern is with late effects—adverse changes related to treatment modalities, interactions between modes of treatment, individual characteristics of the child, and the disease process that may appear months to years after lifesaving treatment. Because of the greater number of children who are cured and survive into adulthood, increasing documentation of late effects is emerging (see Table 36-7). Almost no organ is exempt, and almost every antineoplastic agent (including and especially irradiation) is responsible for some adverse effect. Although many factors influence the development of late effects from irradiation, some of the more important ones include the total cumulative dose given, the age of the child (the younger the child, the more radiosensitive the body organs are), and the location of the tumor.

Radiation therapy to growing bones or reproductive glands responsible for growth-related hormones can delay or stunt growth. Nurses must document growth by assessing height and weight at each visit. Any decrease in growth velocity should be further evaluated. Further assessment includes documenting parental heights, obtaining a wrist x-

*In Wong DL, Hess CS: *Wong and Whaley's clinical manual of pediatric nursing,* ed 5, St Louis, 2000, Mosby.

## TABLE 36-7 Late effects of cancer treatment

| Systemic Effects/Clinical Manifestations | Associated Mode of Treatment |
| --- | --- |
| **Central Nervous System (CNS)** | |
| Leukoencephalopathy (syndrome ranging from lethargy, dementia, and seizures to quadriplegia and death) | Methotrexate or CNS irradiation |
| Mineralizing microangiopathy (headaches, focal seizures, incoordination, gait abnormalities) | Methotrexate or CNS irradiation |
| Peripheral neuropathy (footdrop, incoordination) | Vincristine |
| Cognitive deficits (intelligence, nonlanguage skills) | Intrathecal chemotherapy or cranial irradiation (especially before age 3 years) |
| **Cardiovascular** | |
| Cardiomyopathy (tachycardia, tachypnea, dyspnea, shortness of breath, edema, palpitations) | Anthracyclines (doxorubicin and daunorubicin) or irradiation to heart<br>High-dose cyclophosphamide |
| Pericardial damage (pleural effusion, cardiomegaly) | Mediastinal irradiation |
| **Respiratory** | |
| Pneumonitis (dyspnea, nonproductive cough, fever) | Lung irradiation, alkylating agents, possibly bleomycin, vinblastine, cisplatin |
| Pulmonary fibrosis (dyspnea, restrictive ventilation, decreased exercise tolerance) | |
| **Gastrointestinal** | |
| Chronic enteritis (colic, abdominal pain, vomiting, diarrhea, obstipation, bleeding) | Abdominal irradiation, methotrexate, cytosine arabinoside |
| Hepatic fibrosis (jaundice, hepatomegaly) | Methotrexate, 6-mercaptopurine |
| **Urinary** | |
| Hemorrhagic cystitis (chronic microscopic hematuria to gross hemorrhage) | Cyclophosphamide, ifosfamide, irradiation, especially with radiomimetic chemotherapeutic agents (i.e., doxorubicin and daunorubicin) |
| Bladder fibrosis (decreased bladder capacity, ureteral reflux) | Cisplatin |
| Tubular necrosis (decreased creatinine clearance) | |
| **Endocrine** | |
| Growth retardation (abnormal growth velocity) | Irradiation to the thyroid, pituitary gland, testes, ovaries |
| Thyroid dysfunction (see Chapter 38) | |
| Gonadal dysfunction (see Reproductive) | |
| **Reproductive** | |
| Possible gonadal damage—both sexes (amenorrhea, decreased sperm counts, increased follicle-stimulating and luteinizing hormones [FSH, LH], decreased testosterone/estrogen) | Alkylating agents<br>Irradiation to the pituitary gland, testes, ovaries |
| **Skeletal** | |
| Linear growth retardation (short stature) | Irradiation, long-term steroids |
| Spinal deformities, scoliosis, kyphosis, asymmetric growth, pathologic fractures | Irradiation |
| **Immune** | |
| Asplenia (overwhelming infection, fever) | Splenectomy (Hodgkin disease) |
| **Sensory Organs** | |
| Cataracts (opacity over pupil) | Cranial irradiation, high-dose steroids |
| Hearing (decreased hearing associated with high-frequency loss) | Cisplatin |
| **Additional Effects** | |
| *Dental Problems* | |
| Increased caries, periodontal disease, hypoplastic teeth, hypodontia (delayed or absent tooth development) | Irradiation to maxilla and mandible |
| *Second Malignancies* | |
| Bone and soft tissue tumors | Irradiation, alkylating agents |
| Leukemia | |
| Nonlymphocytic leukemia | |

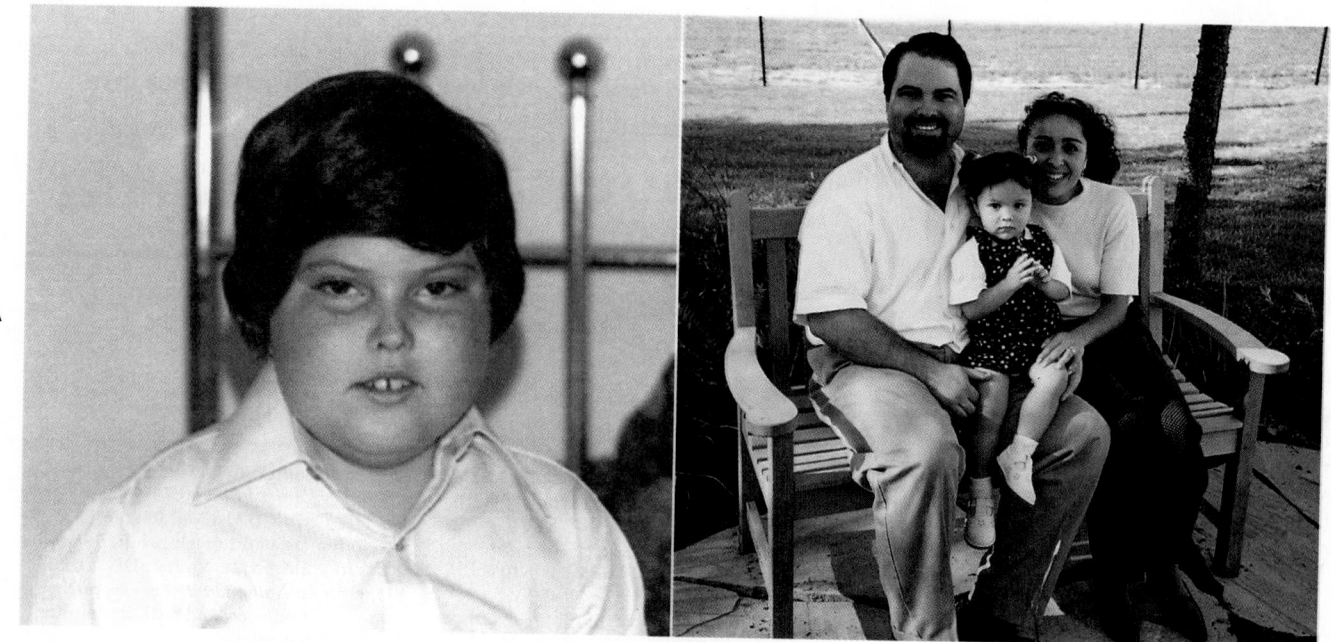

**Fig. 36-6** T-cell leukemia patient. **A,** At age 10 (wearing wig because of hair loss during treatment). **B,** 20 years later with wife and daughter.

ray film to predict further growth potential, and assessing gonadal development and pituitary function.

Radiation therapy and the alkylating agents can cause hormonal dysfunction, decreased fertility, and sterility. The potential for gonadal dysfunction depends on the child's age, sex, type of treatment, and the duration and total doses of treatment. Nursing assessment must begin with careful documentation of the child's sexual development using the Tanner staging scale. (See Pubertal Sexual Maturation, Chapter 19.)

Irradiation to developing bone and cartilage may cause numerous abnormalities. Assessment includes close observation of the irradiated bone for defects, such as spinal kyphoscoliosis, leg length discrepancy, and skull and facial disfigurement.

Irradiated bones are more fragile and may fracture easily, have functional limitations, and heal slowly in the presence of infection. Osteoporosis may develop. Children who have received irradiation to the mandibular area are at risk for dental caries, arrested tooth development, and incomplete dental calcification. A careful assessment of the oral cavity in children who have received irradiation to the mandible is performed at each clinic visit.

## KEY POINTS

- Criteria used to determine cure of cancer include cessation of therapy, continuous freedom from clinical and laboratory evidence of cancer, and minimum or no risk of relapse, as determined by previous experience with the disease.
- Although the cure rate for most types of childhood cancer has improved, the late effects of treatment are of increasing concern.
- Determination of malignancy and metastasis is made by history and physical examination, laboratory tests, imaging techniques, and biopsy.
- The major modes of cancer therapy are surgery, chemotherapy, radiotherapy, immunotherapy, and bone marrow transplantation.
- Chemotherapeutic agents are classified according to their cytotoxic action: alkylating agents, antimetabolites, plant alkaloids, antitumor antibiotics, and hormones.

- Types of bone marrow transplants are allogeneic and autologous.
- Nursing goals in the care of the child with cancer are to prepare the family for diagnostic and therapeutic procedures, prevent complications of myelosuppression (infection, hemorrhage, anemia), manage problems of irradiation and drug toxicity (nausea and vomiting, anorexia, mucosal ulceration, neuropathy, hemorrhagic cystitis, alopecia, moon face, mood changes), and provide continued emotional support.
- Leukemia is the most common form of childhood cancer. Current 5-year survival rates exceed 80% in major research centers, and the majority of these children will be cured.
- The lymphomas include Hodgkin disease and non-Hodgkin lymphoma; Hodgkin disease affects primarily adolescents.

- Nursing care of the child with a brain tumor includes observing for signs and symptoms related to the tumor, preparing the child and family for diagnostic tests and operative procedures, preventing postoperative complications, planning for discharge, and promoting a return to optimum health.
- The treatment of osteosarcoma is limb salvage or amputation followed by chemotherapy.

- Wilms tumor shows an increased incidence among siblings and identical twins, demonstrating a hereditary predisposition.
- Rhabdomyosarcoma may occur almost anywhere in the body, but the most common sites are the head and neck.
- Common presenting signs in retinoblastoma are cat's eye reflex, strabismus, and red, painful eye.
- Male adolescents should be taught to perform monthly testicular self-examination to detect testicular tumors.

# REFERENCES

Abramovitz LZ, Senner AM: Pediatric bone marrow transplantation update, *Oncol Nurs Forum* 22(1):107-115, 1995.

Altman AJ: Chronic leukemias of childhood. In Pizzo PA, Poplack DG, editors: *Principles and practices of pediatric oncology*, ed 4, Philadelphia, 2002, JB Lippincott.

American Academy of Pediatrics: Pickering LK, editor: *2000 Red book: report of the Committee on Infectious Diseases*, ed 25, Elk Grove Village, IL, 2000, The Academy.

Amos TA, Gordon MY: Sources of human hematopoietic stem cells for transplantation: a review, *Cell Transplant* 4(6):547-569, 1995.

Anastasia PJ: Effectiveness of oral 5-HT$_3$ receptor antagonists for emetogenic chemotherapy, *Oncol Nurs Forum* 27(3): 483-493, 2000.

Armstrong TS, Gilbert MR: Glial neoplasms: classification, treatment and pathways for the future, *Oncol Nurs Forum* 23(4):615-625, 1996.

ASHP Commission of Therapeutics and Approved by the ASHP Board of Directors: ASHP therapeutic guidelines on the pharmacologic management of nausea and vomiting in adult and pediatric patients receiving chemotherapy or radiation therapy or undergoing surgery, *Am J Health Syst Pharm* 56:729-764, 1999.

Baquiran DC, Gallagher J: *Lippincott's cancer chemotherapy handbook*, Philadelphia, 1998, Lippincott-Raven.

Behrendt H, Brinkhuis M, Van Leeuwen EF: Treatment of childhood Hodgkin's disease with ABVD without radiotherapy, *Med Pediatr Oncol* 26(4):244-248, 1996.

Bener A, Denic S, Galadari S: Longer breast-feeding and protection against childhood leukaemia and lymphomas, *Eur J Cancer* 37(2):234-238, 2001.

Berde CB, Billett AL, Collins JJ: Symptom management in supportive care. In Pizzo PA, Poplack DG, editors: *Principles and practices of pediatric oncology*, ed 4, Philadelphia, 2002, JB Lippincott.

Bhatia S and others: Solid cancers after bone marrow transplantation, *J Clin Oncol* 19(2): 464-471, 2001.

Braga FJHN and others: Bone scintigraphy in testicular tumors, *Clin Nucl Med* 26(2): 117-118, 2001.

Brunelle F: Noninvasive diagnosis of brain tumours in children, *Childs Nerv Syst* 16(10-11):731-734, 2000.

Buckley JD and others: Concordance for childhood cancer in twins, *Med Pediatr Oncol* 26(4):223-229, 1996.

Calabresi F, Gamucci T: Biological response modifiers, *Lung Cancer* 12(suppl 1):S193-S198, 1995.

Cho S, Cheng AC, Cheng MCK: Oral care for children with leukaemia, *Hong Kong Med J* 6(2):203-208, 2000.

Close P and others: A prospective, controlled evaluation of home chemotherapy for children with cancer, *Pediatrics* 95(6):896-900, 1995.

Directorate of Technical Support: Controlling occupational exposure to hazardous, *OSHA Instruction* CPL 2-2.20B CH-4:21-34, 1995.

Dreyer ZE, Blatt J, Bleyer WA: Late effects of childhood cancer and its treatment. In Pizzo PA, Poplack DG, editors: *Principles and practices of pediatric oncology*, ed 4, Philadelphia, 2002, JB Lippincott.

Engstrom C and others: The efficacy and cost effectiveness of new antiemetic guidelines, *Oncol Nurs Forum* 26(9):1453-1458, 1999.

Flavell KJ, Murray PG: Hodgkin's disease and the Epstein-Barr virus, *Mol Pathol* 53(5): 262-269, 2000.

Freedman DM and others: Household solvent exposures and childhood acute lymphoblastic leukemia, *Am J Public Health* 91(4):564-567, 2001.

Freifeld AG, Pizzo PA: The outpatient management of febrile neutropenia in cancer patients, *Oncology* 10(4):599-6161, 1996.

Freyer DR and others: IV methohexital for brief sedation of pediatric oncology outpatients: physiologic and behavioral responses (electronic abstract), *Pediatrics* 99(5):725, 1997, www.pediatric.org/cgi/content/full/99/5/e8.

Golub TR, Arceci RJ: Acute myelogenous leukemia. In Pizzo PA, Poplack DG, editors: *Principles and practices of pediatric oncology*, ed 4, Philadelphia, 2002, JB Lippincott.

Graf N, Tournade MF, deKraker JD: The role of preoperative chemotherapy in the management of Wilms' tumor, *Urol Clin North Am* 27(3):443-454, 2000.

Green DM and others: Wilms tumor, *CA Cancer J Clin* 46(1):46-63, 1996.

Green DM and others: Wilms tumor. In Pizzo PA, Poplack DG, editors: *Principles and practices of pediatric oncology*, ed 4, Philadelphia, 2002, JB Lippincott.

Greenlee RT and others: Cancer statistics, 2000, *CA Cancer J Clin* 50:7-33, 2000.

Grier HE, Civin CI: Myeloid leukemias, myelodysplasia and myeloproliferative diseases in children. In Nathan DG, Orkin SH, editors: *Nathan and Oski's hematology of infancy and childhood*, ed 5, Philadelphia, 1998, WB Saunders.

Grosfeld JL: Neuroblastoma. In Grossfeld JL and others, editors: *Pediatric surgery*, ed 5, St Louis, 1998, Mosby.

Grosfeld JL: Risk-based management of solid tumors in children, *Am J Surg* 180(5):322-327, 2000.

Guinan EC, Krance RA, Lehman LE: Stem cell transplantation in pediatric oncology. In Pizzo PA, Poplack DG, editors: *Principles and practices of pediatric oncology*, ed 4, Philadelphia, 2002, JB Lippincott.

Gurney JG, Bondy MG: Epidemiologic research methods and childhood cancer. In Pizzo PA, Poplack DG, editors: *Principles and practices of pediatric oncology*, ed 4, Philadelphia, 2002, JB Lippincott.

Han S, Peschel RE: Father-son testicular tumors: evidence for genetic anticipation? *Cancer* 88(10):2319-2325, 2000.

Han-Markey T: Nutritional considerations in pediatric oncology, *Semin Oncol Nurs* 16(2):146-151, 2000.

Hellsten MB: All the king's horses and all the king's men: pain management from hospital to home, *J Pediatr Oncol Nurs* 17(3):149-159, 2000.

Hockenberry M, Kline NE: Nursing support of the child with cancer. In Pizzo PA, Poplack DG, editors: *Principles and practices of pediatric oncology*, ed 4, Philadelphia, 2002, JB Lippincott.

Hockenberry-Eaton M and others: *Pain management in children with cancer*, Austin, 1999, Texas Cancer Council.

Hough RE, Hancock BW: Principles of chemotherapy in Hodgkin's disease. In Mauch PM and others, editors: *Hodgkin's disease*, Philadelphia, 1999, Lippincott, Williams & Wilkins.

Hurwitz RL and others: Retinoblastoma. In Pizzo PA, Poplack DG, editors: *Principles and practices of pediatric oncology*, ed 4, Philadelphia, 2002, JB Lippincott.

Kazak AE and others: Pharmacologic and psychologic interventions for procedural pain, *Pediatrics* 102(1):59-66, 1998.

Kennedy L, Diamond J: Assessment and management of chemotherapy-induced mucositis in children, *J Pediatr Oncol Nurs* 14(3):164-174, 1997.

Kennedy D and others: An RNA recognition motif in Wilms' tumor protein (WT1) revealed by structural modeling, *Nat Genet* 12(3):329-331, 1996.

Kenney LB and others: Increased incidence of cancer in infants in the US: 1980-1990, *Cancer* 82(7):1396-1400, 1998.

Kumar KS, Rajagopal MR, Naseema AM: Intravenous morphine for emergency treatment of cancer pain, *Palliat Med* 14:183-188, 2000.

Kurylak A and others: Estimation of effectiveness of antiemetic treatment with Zofran given in one dose to children with neoplasms, *Pediatr Pol* 70(11):925-928, 1995.

Kusumakumary P and others: Testicular germ cell tumors in prepubertal children, *Pediatr Hematol Oncol* 17:105-111, 2000.

Landier W: Childhood acute lymphoblastic leukemia: current perspectives, *Oncol Nurs Forum* 28(5):823-833, 2001.

Lanzkowsky P: *Manual of pediatric hematology and oncology*, San Diego, 2000, Academic Press.

Larson PJ and others: The PRO-Self© mouth aware program: an effective approach for reducing chemotherapy-induced mucositis, *Cancer Nurs* 21(4):263-268, 1998.

Link MP, Gebhardt MC, Myers PA: Osteosarcoma. In Pizzo PA, Poplack DG, editors: *Principles and practices of pediatric oncology*, ed 4, Philadelphia, 2002, JB Lippincott.

Lloyd-Thomas AR: Modern concepts of paediatric analgesia, *Pharmacol Ther* 83(1):1-20, 1999.

Loescher LJ and others: Public education projects in skin cancer: the evolution of skin cancer prevention education for children at a comprehensive cancer center, *Cancer* 75(suppl 2):651-656, 1995.

Look AT, Kirsch I: Molecular basis of childhood cancer. In Pizzo PA, Poplack DG, editors: *Principles and practices of pediatric oncology*, ed 4, Philadelphia, 2002, JB Lippincott.

Loring DW, Meador KJ: Corticosteroids and cognitive function in humans: methodological considerations, *J Pediatr Hematol Oncol* 22(3):193-196, 2000.

Lyos AT and others: Soft tissue sarcoma of the head and neck in children and adolescents, *Cancer* 77(1):193-200, 1996.

MacDonald DJ, Lessick M: Hereditary cancers in children and ethical and psychosocial implications, *J Pediatr Nurs* 15(4):217-225, 2000.

Macpherson CF, Lundblad LA: Conscious sedation of pediatric oncology patients for painful procedures: development and implementation of a clinical practice protocol, *J Pediatr Oncol Nurs* 14(1):33-42, 1997.

Magrath IT: Malignant non-Hodgkin's lymphomas in children. In Pizzo PA, Poplack DG, editors: *Principles and practices of pediatric oncology*, ed 4, Philadelphia, 2002, JB Lippincott.

Mainprize TG, Taylor MD, Rutka JT: Pediatric brain tumors: a contemporary prospectus, *Clin Neurosurg* 47:259-302, 2000.

Margolin JF, Steuber CP, Poplack DG: Acute lymphoblastic leukemia. In Pizzo PA, Poplack DG, editors: *Principles and practices of pediatric oncology*, ed 4, Philadelphia, 2002, JB Lippincott.

Matsubara H and others: Possible clinical benefits of the use of peripheral blood stem cells over bone marrow in the allogeneic transplantation setting for the treatment of childhood leukemia, *Jpn J Clin Oncol* 31(1):30-34, 2001.

Matthay KK: Neuroblastoma: a clinical challenge and biologic puzzle, *CA Cancer J Clin* 45(3):179-192, 1995.

Mauch PM and others: Treatment of favorable prognosis stage I-II Hodgkin's disease. In Mauch PM and others, editors: *Hodgkin's disease*, Philadelphia, 1999, Lippincott, Williams & Wilkins.

Mayo DJ, Pearson DC, Horne MK: Superior vena cava thrombosis associated with a central venous access device: a case report, *Clin J Oncol Nurs* 1(1):5-10, 1997.

McFarland E: Immunizations for the immunocompromised child, *Pediatr Ann* 28(8):487-496, 1999.

McGrath PA: Development of the World Health Organization Guidelines on Cancer Pain Relief and Palliative Care in Children, *J Pain Symptom Manage* 12(2):87-92, 1996.

Mendenhall NP, Holland KW, Sombeck MD: The role of lymphangiography in designing fields for elective pelvic node irradiation on Hodgkin's disease, *Int J Radiat Oncol Biol Phys* 30(4):993-995, 1994.

Mueller NE, Grufferman S: The epidemiology of Hodgkin's disease. In Mauch PM and others, editors: *Hodgkin's disease*, Philadelphia, 1999, Lippincott, Williams & Wilkins.

Naparstek E and others: T-cell depleted allogenic bone marrow transplantation for acute leukaemia using Campath-1 antibodies and post-transplant administration of donor's peripheral blood lymphocytes for prevention of relapse, *Br J Haematol* 89(3):506-515, 1995.

Nguyen NP and others: Neuroblastoma producing spinal cord compression: rapid relief with low dose of radiation, *Anticancer Res* 20(6c):4687-4690, 2000.

Nitenberg G, Raynard B: Nutritional support of the cancer patient: issues and dilemmas, *Crit Rev Oncol/Hematol* 34(3):137-168, 2000.

Oeffinger KC and others: Providing primary care for long-term survivors of childhood acute lymphoblastic leukemia, *J Fam Prac* 49(12):1133-1146, 2000.

Olsson GL: Neuropathic pain in children. In McGrath PJ, Finley GA, editors: *Chronic and recurrent pain in children and adolescents*, Seattle, 1999, IASP Press.

Parker SL and others: Cancer statistics, 1997, *CA Cancer J Clin* 47(1):5-27, 1997.

Pertruzzi MJ, Green DM: Wilm's tumor, *Pediatr Clin North Am* 40(4):939-949, 1997.

Plon SE, Milkin D: Childhood cancer and heredity. In Pizzo PA, Poplack DG, editors: *Principles and practices of pediatric oncology*, ed 4, Philadelphia, 2002, JB Lippincott.

Poliquin CM: Overview of bone marrow and peripheral blood stem cell transplantation, *Clin J Oncol Nurs* 1(1):11-17, 1997.

Quadri TL, Brown AE: Infectious complications in the critically ill patient with cancer, *Semin Oncol* 27(3):335-346, 2000.

Reiter A and others: Non-Hodgkin's lymphomas of childhood and adolescence: results of a treatment stratified for biologic subtypes and stage—a report of the Berlin-Frankfurt-Munster Group, *J Clin Oncol* 13(2):359-372, 1995.

Rhodes VA and others: Nurses' perceptions of antiemetic effectiveness, *Oncol Nurs Forum* 22(8):1243-1252, 1995.

Riva D, Giorgi C: The neurodevelopmental price of survival in children with malignant brain tumors, *Childs Nerv Syst* 16(10-11):751-754, 2000.

Rocha V and others: Graft-versus-host disease in children who have received a cord-blood or bone marrow transplant from an HLA-identical sibling, *N Engl J Med* 342(25):1846-1854, 2000.

Roila F, Aapro M, Stewart A: Optimal selection of antiemetics in children receiving cancer chemotherapy, *Support Care Cancer* 6(3):215-220, 1998.

Roselli M and others: Tumor markers as targets for selective diagnostic and therapeutic procedures, *Anticancer Res* 16(4B):2187-2192, 1996.

Rossetto CL, McMahon JE: Current and future trends in transfusion therapy, *J Pediatr Oncol Nurs* 17(3):160-173, 2000.

Ruble K, Kelly KP: Radiation therapy in childhood cancer, *Semin Oncol Nurs* 15(4):292-302, 1999.

Schneider D, Freeman N: Children's environmental health risks: a state-of-the-art conference, *Arch Environ Health* 56(2):103-110, 2001.

Schor NF: Neuroblastoma as a neurobiological disease, *J Neurooncol* 41(2):159-166, 1999.

Schuz J and others: Residential magnetic fields as a risk factor for childhood acute leukaemia: results from a German population-based case-control study, *Int J Cancer* 91(5):728-735, 2001.

Shields JA, Shields CL: Pediatric ocular and periocular tumors, *Pediatr Ann* 30(8):491-501, 2001.

Shiminski-Maher T: Central nervous system tumors. In Hockenberry-Eaton MJ and others, editors: *Essentials of pediatric oncology nursing: a core curriculum*, Glenview, IL, 1998, Association of Pediatric Oncology Nurses.

Shu XO and others: Breast-feeding and risk of childhood acute leukemia, *J Nat Cancer Inst* 91(20):1765-1772, 1999.

Shusterman S, Meadows AT: Long term survivors of childhood leukemia, *Curr Opin Hematol* 7(4):217-222, 2000.

Singh AD, Shields CL, Shields JA: Prognostic factors in retinoblastoma, *J Pediatr Ophthalmol Strabismus* 37(3):134-141, 2000.

Skoldenberg EG and others: Angiogenesis and angiogenic growth factors in Wilms tumor, *J Urol* 165(6, Part 2 of 2) Suppl:2274-2279, 2001.

Smith JH and others: Siblings of retinoblastoma patients: are we underestimating their risk? *Am J Ophthalmol* 129(3):396-398, 2000.

Stovall E: Self-advocacy and cancer survivorship, *Illness Crisis Loss* 5(1):199-203, 1995.

Strickler R, Phillips ML: Astrocytomas: the clinical picture, *Clin J Oncol Nurs* 4(4):153-158, 2000.

Strother DR and others: Tumors of the central nervous system. In Pizzo PA, Poplack DG, editors: *Principles and practices of pediatric oncology,* ed 4, Philadelphia, 2002, JB Lippincott.

Takaue Y and others: Collection and transplantation of peripheral blood stem cells in very small children weighing 20 kg or less, *Blood* 86(1):372-380, 1995.

Taub JW: Relationship of chromosome 21 and acute leukemia in children with down syndrome, *J Pediatr Hematol Oncol* 23(3):175-178, 2001.

Thomas DC and others: Residential magnetic fields predicted from wiring configurations. II. Relationships to childhood leukemia, *Bioelectromagnetics* 20(7):414-422, 1999.

Thorne RN and others: Decline in incidence of medulloblastoma in children, *Cancer* 74(12):3240-3244, 1994.

Tsinopoulos I and others: Retinoblastoma with an unusual presentation in a child with polydactyly: clinical associations and genetic implications, *Acta Ophthalmol Scand* 79(1):79-80, 2001.

Turner D: Testicular cancer and the value of self-examination, *Nurs Times* 91(1):30-31, 1995.

Varadi G and others: Human umbilical cord blood for hematopoietic progenitor cells transplantation, *Leuk Lymphoma* 20(1-2):51-58, 1995.

Vose JM, Constine LS, Sutcliffe SB: Other complications of the treatment of Hodgkin's disease. In Mauch PM and others, editors: *Hodgkin's disease,* Philadelphia, 1999, Lippincott, Williams & Wilkins.

Wagner JE and others: Allogeneic sibling umbilical-cord-blood transplantation in children with malignant and non-malignant disease, *Lancet* 346(8969):214-219, 1995.

Wakeford R: The risk of childhood cancer from intrauterine and preconceptional exposure to ionizing radiation, *Environ Health Perspect* 103(11):1018-1025, 1995.

Wakeling KS: The latest weapon in the war against cancer, *RN* 62(7):58-60, 1999.

Wexler LH, Crist WM, Helman LJ: Rhabdomyosarcoma and the undifferentiated sarcomas. In Pizzo PA, Poplack DG, editors: *Principles and practices of pediatric oncology,* ed 4, Philadelphia, 2002, JB Lippincott.

World Health Organization in conjunction with IASP: *Cancer pain relief and palliative care in children,* (Order No 1150459), WHO Publications Center USA, 1998, WHO.

Zahm SH, Devesa SS: Childhood cancer: overview of incidence trends and environmental carcinogens, *Environ Health Perspect* 103(suppl 6):177-184, 1995.

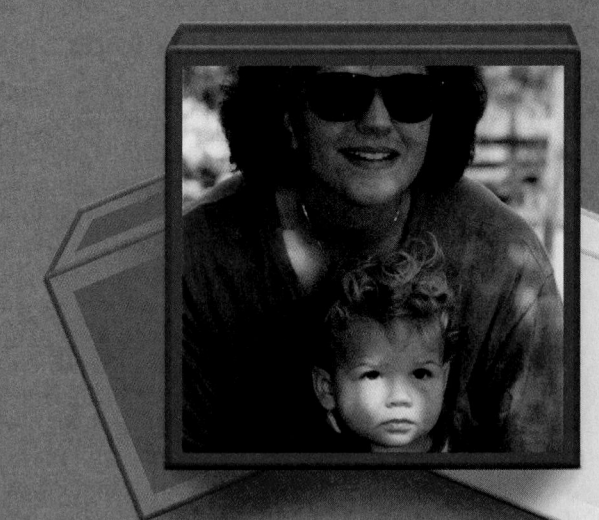

# Chapter 37

# The Child with Cerebral Dysfunction

## Chapter Outline

**CEREBRAL STRUCTURE AND FUNCTION, 1641**
**Development of the Neurologic System, 1642**
**Central Nervous System (CNS), 1642**
   Brain Coverings, 1642
   The Brain, 1643
**Increased Intracranial Pressure (ICP), 1645**
**EVALUATION OF NEUROLOGIC STATUS, 1646**
**Assessment: General Aspects, 1646**
   History, 1646
   Physical Examination, 1646
**Altered States of Consciousness, 1647**
   Level of Consciousness (LOC), 1647
   Coma Assessment, 1647
**Neurologic Examination, 1649**
   Vital Signs, 1649
   Skin, 1650
   Eyes, 1650

Motor Function, 1651
Posturing, 1651
Reflexes, 1651
**Special Diagnostic Procedures, 1652**
**THE CHILD WITH CEREBRAL COMPROMISE, 1654**
**Nursing Care of the Unconscious Child, 1654**
   Respiratory Management, 1656
   Intracranial Pressure Monitoring, 1656
   Nutrition and Hydration, 1658
   Medications, 1658
   Thermoregulation, 1659
   Elimination, 1659
   Hygienic Care, 1659
   Positioning and Exercise, 1659
   Stimulation, 1659
   Family Support, 1660
*Nursing Care Plan: The Unconscious Child, 1662*
**Head Injury, 1661**

**Near-Drowning, 1674**
**INTRACRANIAL INFECTIONS, 1676**
**Bacterial Meningitis, 1677**
**Nonbacterial (Aseptic) Meningitis, 1680**
**Tuberculous (TB) Meningitis, 1681**
**Brain Abscess, 1681**
**Encephalitis, 1681**
**Rabies, 1682**
**Reye Syndrome (RS), 1683**
**Human Immunodeficiency Virus (HIV) Encephalopathy, 1684**
**SEIZURE DISORDERS, 1684**
**Epilepsy, 1684**
*Nursing Care Plan: The Child with Epilepsy, 1697*
**Febrile Seizures, 1696**
**HEADACHE, 1698**
**Assessment, 1698**
**Migraine Headache, 1699**

## Related Topics

Administration of Medication, Ch. 27
Anencephaly, Ch. 11
Brain Tumors, Ch. 36
Controlling Elevated Temperatures, Ch. 27
Cranial Deformities, Ch. 11
Family-Centered Home Care, Ch. 25

High Risk Related to Neurologic Disturbance, Ch. 10
Human Immunodeficiency Virus Infection and Acquired Immunodeficiency Syndrome, Chs. 20 and 35
Hydrocephalus, Ch. 11

Infection Control, Ch. 27
Injuries—The Leading Killer, Ch. 1
Maintaining Healthy Skin, Ch. 27
Neurologic Assessment, Chs. 7 and 8
Pain Assessment; Pain Management, Ch. 26
Preparation for Procedures, Ch. 27

## CEREBRAL STRUCTURE AND FUNCTION

The nervous system comprises three intimately connected and functioning parts: (1) the *central nervous system (CNS)*, composed of two cerebral hemispheres, the brainstem, the cerebellum, and the spinal cord; (2) the *peripheral nervous system*, composed of the cranial nerves that arise from or travel to the brainstem and the spinal nerves that travel to or from the spinal cord and which may be motor (efferent) or sensory (afferent); and (3) the *autonomic nervous system (ANS)*, composed of the sympathetic and parasympathetic systems, which provide automatic control of vital functions.

This chapter is concerned primarily with disturbances of the brain. The structure and function of the spinal cord and ANS are discussed in more detail in Chapter 40.

■ Nancy E. Kline, PhD, RN, CPNP, and Jill Brace O'Neill, MS, RN-CS, PNP, revised this chapter.

## Development of the Neurologic System

In contrast to other body tissues, which grow rapidly after birth, the nervous system grows proportionately more rapidly before birth. Two periods of rapid brain cell growth occur during fetal life. At 15 to 20 weeks of gestation there is a dramatic increase in the number of neurons; another increase in rate begins at 30 weeks of gestation and extends to 1 year of age. This rapid growth during infancy continues during early childhood and slows to a more gradual rate during later childhood and adolescence. Brain volume is readily reflected in head circumference, which increases six times as much during the first year as during the second year of life. One half of the postnatal brain growth is achieved by age 1 year, 75% by age 3, and 90% by age 6. Cerebral blood flow and oxygen consumption in childhood (up to age 6 years) is almost twice that of adults, which reflects an increased metabolic requirement consistent with growth and development.

The growth and final form of the brain depend on the development and multiplication of neurons. Creation of new cells is believed to occur only during the first 100 days of gestation. During the remainder of gestation, cells divide and multiply at the astonishing rate of 250,000 per minute. It is believed that no new nerve cells appear after the sixth month of fetal life. Postnatal growth consists of increasing the amount of cytoplasm around the nuclei of the 10 billion existing cells, increasing the number and intricacy of communications with other cells, and advancing their peripheral axons to keep pace with expanding body dimensions.

The brain constitutes 12% of the body weight at birth. It doubles its weight in the first year, and by age 5 or 6 years its weight at birth has tripled. Thereafter growth slows until in adulthood the brain is only about 2% of the total body weight. The surface configuration of the brain also changes with development. The early embryonic brain surface is smooth, but the sulci deepen with advancing development. This process continues throughout childhood. At birth the cortex is only about one half of its adult thickness, although all the major surface features are present. There is little cortical control over body movements at birth, with movements guided principally by primitive reflexes. (See Chapter 8.) With advancing development and maturation, the brain, through association pathways, exercises increasing control over much of the reflex activity. This allows the growing child to perform progressively complex tasks that require coordinated movements. Persistence of primitive reflexes may suggest defective cortical development.

Cortical control is closely associated with the acquisition of a myelin coating on the nerves. Although nerve fibers are able to conduct impulses without this myelin sheath, the impulses travel at a slower rate and with more likelihood of diffusion. Myelinization of the various nerve tracts in the CNS, which allows progressive neuromotor function, follows the cephalocaudal (head-to-toe) and proximodistal (near-to-far) sequence. It appears first with the fibers of the spinal cord and cranial nerves, then in the brainstem and corticospinal tracts.

Development of the nervous system proceeds on a continuum. The brain and spinal cord are among the first of the major organ systems to be recognized in the embryo and one of the last to finish significant development after birth. The rate of myelogenesis accelerates rapidly after birth. In general the pathways concerned with sensation are myelinated early, before the motor pathways. The acquisition of motor skills depends on the maturation and myelination of the nervous system, and no amount of special training or practice will hasten the process. Most of the advancing performance in an infant is a direct result of brain development indirectly influenced by environmental stimuli.

## Central Nervous System (CNS)

The bony skull forms the strongest covering and provides the primary protection to the brain. It is an expansible structure in the infant and young child but becomes rigid in the older child and adolescent. Blood is supplied to the dura mater by the middle meningeal artery, a branch of the external carotid artery. It enters the skull at a point inferior to the temporal bone, then branches over the surface of the dura, usually encased in a groove in the temporal and parietal bones after 2 years of age. Damage to this artery or to its branches is a common cause of an epidural hematoma.

### Brain Coverings

Within the skull the brain is covered and protected further by three membranes, the *meninges*—the dura mater, arachnoid membrane, and pia mater (Fig. 37-1). The tough outer membrane, the *dura mater,* is a double layer that serves as the outer meningeal layer and the inner periosteum of the cranial bones; these two layers are separated by the *epidural space.* The dura is closely attached to the skull in infancy, causing slower spread of blood in epidural hemorrhage. Because of this adherence, epidural hemorrhages are uncommon in the first 2 years of life.

Between these layers of dura inside the skull lie large venous sinuses. Sheets of the dura mater also extend downward and inward to form partitions within the cranium. Projecting downward into the longitudinal fissure is a sheet of dura called the *falx cerebri,* which separates the cerebral hemispheres, and the *falx cerebelli,* which separates the cerebellar hemispheres. Another segment is a tentlike structure, the *tentorium,* which separates the cerebellum from the occipital lobe of the cerebrum. The large gap through which the brainstem passes is the *tentorial hiatus,* the site of herniation in untreated intracranial pressure.

The middle meningeal layer, the *arachnoid membrane,* is a delicate, avascular, weblike structure that loosely surrounds the brain. Between the arachnoid and the dura mater lies the *subdural area,* a potential space that normally contains only enough fluid to prevent adhesion between the two membranes. During cerebral trauma, the fine blood vessels that bridge the subdural space are stretched and ruptured, causing venous blood to escape and spread freely and forming a subdural hemorrhage. The subdural space is small in children; therefore small amounts of blood can increase intracranial hemorrhage significantly.

The innermost covering layer, the *pia mater,* is a delicate transparent membrane that, unlike the other coverings, adheres closely to the outer surface of the brain, conforming to the folds (gyri) and furrows (sulci). Within the pial layer

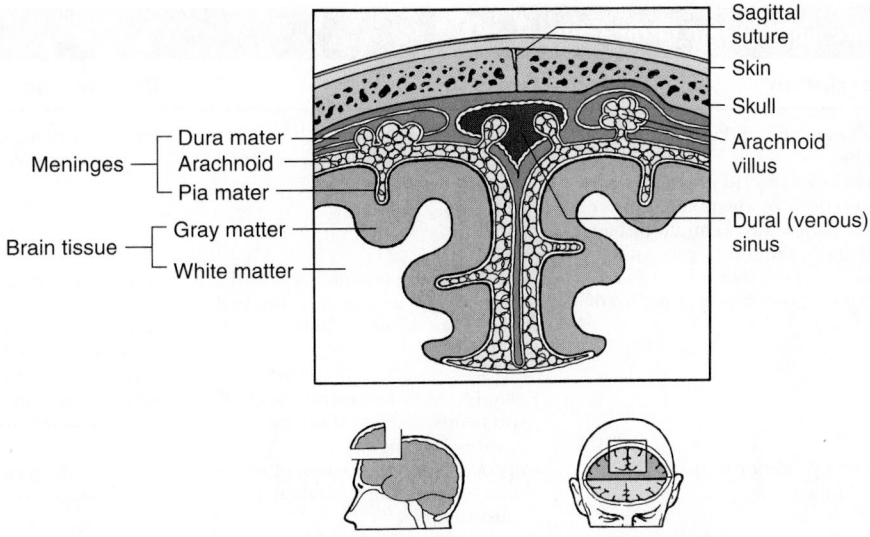

**Fig. 37-1**   Coronal section of the top of the head showing meningeal layers. (Redrawn from Cohen BJ: *Memmler's structure and function of the human body,* ed 7, Philadelphia, 2000, Lippincott Williams & Wilkins.)

lie the arteries and veins of the brain. Between the pia mater and the arachnoid membrane is the *subarachnoid space.* Cerebrospinal fluid (CSF) fills the entire subarachnoid space surrounding the brain and spinal cord and acts as a protective cushion for the brain tissue. Further protection is provided by fibrous filaments known as *arachnoid trabeculae,* which help anchor the brain. When the head receives a blow, these attachments allow the arachnoid to slide on the dura, preventing excessive movement.

## The Brain

Each section of the brain plays a vital role in regulation and control of body function. Each hemisphere is artificially divided into lobes. Pressure on or damage to these lobes produces observable signs or symptoms directly related to the area of pathology; these signs provide clues to the location of the damage. The major structures of the brain and their functions are briefly outlined in Table 37-1.

The two large cerebral hemispheres that occupy the anterior and medial fossae of the skull are separated in the upper part by the *longitudinal fissure.* This separation is complete anteriorly and posteriorly, but centrally the hemispheres are joined by the block of fibers known as the *corpus callosum,* the largest fiber bundle in the brain. These fibers interconnect cortical areas of the right and left hemispheres. Destruction of the corpus callosum causes hemispheric independence, or "split brain."

Situated deeply within each hemisphere and on each side of the midline are the *basal ganglia* (or cerebral nuclei), which serve as vital sorting areas for messages passing to and from the hemispheres. Connected to the hemispheres by thick bunches of nerve fibers is the *brainstem,* through which all nerve fibers traverse as they pass from the hemispheres to the cerebellum and spinal cord. The brainstem extends from the base of the hemispheres through the foramen magnum, where it is continuous with the spinal cord. Within the cranium and behind the brainstem is the cerebellum. Any pressure exerted on the intracranial structures can cause compression of the brainstem and prolapse of the cerebellum through the foramen magnum.

**Cerebral Blood Flow (CBF).**   The blood supply to the brain tissue is carried by the internal carotid arteries, which branch to supply the various brain segments. The volume of blood to the brain, which constitutes only 17% of the cardiac output, supplies the brain with 20% of the body oxygen. The brain, an "inactive" organ, uses 10 times the oxygen used by the body as a whole. Only the heart uses more oxygen per gram of tissue.

CBF is the result of two opposing forces—cerebral blood pressure (the difference between systemic arterial pressure and cerebral venous pressure) and cerebral vascular resistance. CBF remains constant at a cerebral blood pressure between 50 and 150 mm Hg. Because cerebral venous pressure is usually very low and relatively constant, cerebral blood pressure is determined mainly by systemic arterial pressure.

**Autoregulation.**   One of the most important factors in the control of CBF is *autoregulation,* the unique ability of cerebral arterial vessels to change their diameter in response to fluctuating cerebral perfusion pressure (CPP). The CPP is the mean arterial pressure (MAP) minus the intracranial pressure (ICP):

$$CPP = MAP - ICP$$

As a result, cerebral vessels maintain a constant blood flow during alterations in blood pressure and perfusion caused by body posture, increased ICP, decreased cardiac output, or narrowing or occlusion in the major blood vessels of the neck. Autoregulation fails when the limits of cerebrovascular dilation are reached; at this point CBF decreases, causing clinical symptoms of ischemia (nausea, fainting, dizziness, dim vision). Conversely, increased MAP leads to "breakthrough of autoregulation," with increased CBF leading to microhemorrhages and cerebral edema. Autoregulation may be impaired locally or globally as a result of trauma or ischemia.

| **TABLE 37-1** | Structure and function of the brain | | |
|---|---|---|---|
| **Structure** | **Description** | **Function** | **Dysfunction** |
| **Cerebrum** | Two hemispheres divided into lobes<br>Upper parts divided anteriorly and posteriorly by longitudinal fissure<br>Lower parts joined centrally by block of fibers, the corpus callosum | Center for consciousness, thought, memory, sensory input, motor activity | Pressure or damage produces signs and symptoms specific to involved areas |
| Frontal lobes | Most anteriorly located of all lobes that end posteriorly at fissure of Rolando | Posterior portion contains cells that control motor activity in the body<br>Basis for social interaction<br><br>Recognition of cause-and-effect relationships, abstract thinking, expressive language | Impaired movement of body part directly related to motor center for that part<br>Injury or damage to anterior portion may cause personality changes, altered intellectual functioning<br>Memory deficits<br>Language deficits, dysfunction |
| Parietal lobes | Situated posterior to fissure of Rolando | Important for appreciation of sensation, somatic interpretation and integration | Aphasia, apraxia, motor and sensory loss to lower extremities, atopognosia |
| Occipital lobe | At posterior base of skull<br>Most posteriorly placed lobe | Receives stimuli for vision<br>Spatial orientation<br>Visual recognition | Injury produces impaired vision, functional blindness |
| Temporal lobes | Situated anterior to occipital lobe and inferior to parietal lobes | Receives and interprets stimuli for taste, vision, sound, smell<br>Converts crude visual impressions into recognizable images | Injury or destruction causes inability to interpret meanings of sensory experiences |
| | Point where temporal, parietal, and occipital lobes converge | Primary interpretive area | Impairment causes inability to interpret sensory stimuli, difficulty in understanding higher levels of meaning of body sensory experiences |
| | Point where temporal, parietal, and frontal lobes converge | Center for speech, hearing, receptive language | Impairment produces aphasia<br>Hearing dysfunction |
| **Cerebellum** | Located just below posterior part of cerebrum and separated from it by tentorium<br>Contains two lateral lobes joined by midline portion, the vermis | Necessary for refinement and coordination of all muscle movements, including walking, talking, control of muscle tone and balance | Dysmetria, ataxia, dysarthria, hypotonia, nystagmus, dystonia<br>Rest tremor |
| **Basal ganglia** | Situated deeply within cerebral hemispheres on either side of midline | Unconscious or automatic control of lower motor centers<br>Excitation causes inhibition of muscle tone throughout body | Chorea, athetosis<br>Dystonia<br>Rest tremor |
| **Diencephalon** | Situated between cerebrum and mesencephalon | Contains diffuse fibers that compose reticular activating system | Stupor |
| Thalamus | Rounded mass forms most of lateral wall of third ventricle and part of floor of lateral ventricles | Major relay station for sensory impulses to cerebral cortex<br>Activates cerebral cortex | Impaired consciousness |
| Hypothalamus | Lies beneath thalamus<br>Forms floor of third ventricle | Vital control center for involuntary functions (e.g., blood pressure, satiety, hunger, rage, feeding, water conservation, temperature, sleep regulation, libido)<br>Controls secretion of tropic hormones | Impairment causes alterations in vegetative functions<br>Somnolence, coma<br>Anorexia, loss of weight, fever, diabetes insipidus, loss of libido<br>Endocrine disorders |
| **Brainstem** | Extends from cerebral hemisphere to spinal cord | All cranial nerves (except I) arise from brainstem | Stupor, coma |
| Mesencephalon (midbrain) | Lies below inferior surface of cerebellum and above pons | Main connection between forebrain and hindbrain<br>Contains nuclei for cranial nerves III, IV, part of V | Impaired consciousness<br>No independent movement or verbal response<br>Decerebrate posturing<br>Neurologic hyperventilation |
| | Ventral portion composed of cerebral peduncles | Control of eye movement | Impaired function of muscles supplied by these nerves |
| Pons | Located just above medulla oblongata | Contains pneumotaxic center—control of respiration<br>Cranial nerves V through VIII | Deep, rapid, or periodic breathing<br><br>Impaired function of muscles supplied by these nerves |
| Medulla | Forms attachment of brain to spinal cord<br>Separated from pons by horizontal groove | Contains vital centers, including respiratory and vasomotor cranial nerves IX, X, XI, XII | Impaired vital functions<br>No response to any stimuli<br>Ataxic (Biot) breathing<br>Flaccid muscle tone<br>Deep tendon, gag, corneal reflexes absent |

Changes in arterial oxygen pressure ($PaO_2$) or arterial carbon dioxide pressure ($PaCO_2$) have a profound effect on autoregulation. Hypercapnia ($PaCO_2$ >40 mm Hg) or increased levels of lactic acid have a pronounced dilating effect on cerebral arterioles, which increases CBF and thus cerebral volume. Hypocapnia ($PaCO_2$ 25 to 30 mm Hg) constricts cerebral arterioles and decreases CBF. $PaO_2$ values between 70 and 100 mm Hg have little effect on the cerebrovascular system. Profound hypoxia ($PaO_2$ <50 mm Hg) dramatically increases CBF. Consequently maintenance of the airway and effective hyperventilation are of primary importance in the initial management of the neurologically impaired patient. CPP is the most important physiologic determinant because the brain relies on the delivery of oxygen and nutrients to function.

**Oxygen.** Metabolic requirements for oxygen by the brain are not affected by rest or sleep, but they are reduced by narcosis and coma and are altered by changes in temperature. CBF is not altered when body temperature is maintained between 35° and 40° C (95° and 104° F). Oxygen consumption by the brain is increased by hyperthermia and decreased by hypothermia. The brain depends on a constant supply of oxygen-rich blood and, because the oxygen need of the brain is great in relation to the volume of blood supplied, it extracts more oxygen from each unit of circulating blood.

Oxygen supply to the brain is compromised when the supply is inadequate as a result of impaired respiration, hypotension, increased ICP or vascular damage, spasm, or compression. Neurons are highly susceptible to elevated $PaCO_2$ (a potent vasodilator), and the metabolic damage to brain tissue caused by an inadequate supply of well-oxygenated blood can often exceed the effects of trauma. Respiratory acidosis resulting from increased $PaCO_2$ levels can produce symptoms indistinguishable from those of head injury.

**Blood-Brain Barrier.** The blood-brain barrier (BBB) is an anatomic-physiologic feature of the brain that separates the brain parenchyma from the blood. Unlike capillaries in other parts of the body, cerebral capillaries have no fenestrations or pores. The tight junctions of the vascular endothelium are thought to be responsible for the selective nature of the BBB. The mature BBB allows facilitated diffusion of glucose and passive diffusion of water and carbon dioxide but is impermeable to protein and does not permit passage of many active substances. However, the BBB of the fetus and newborn is normally indiscriminately permeable, allowing protein and other large and small molecules to pass freely between the cerebral vessels and the brain. Conditions that cause cerebrovascular dilation (hypertension, hypercapnia, hypoxia, acidosis) disrupt the BBB. Hyperosmotic fluids, which cause shrinkage of vascular endothelium and widen the vascular junctions, also disrupt the BBB.

## Increased Intracranial Pressure (ICP)

The brain, tightly enclosed in the solid bony cranium, is well protected but highly vulnerable to pressure that may accumulate within the enclosure. Its total volume—brain (80%),

CSF (10%), and blood (10%)—must remain approximately the same at all times. A change in the proportional volume of one of these components (e.g., increase or decrease in intracranial blood) must be accompanied by a compensatory change in another (e.g., decrease or increase in CSF). In this way the volume and pressure normally remain constant. Examples of compensatory changes are reduction in blood volume, decrease in production of CSF, increase in CSF absorption, or shrinkage of brain mass by displacement of intracellular and extracellular fluid.

Children with open fontanels compensate by skull expansion and widened sutures. However, at any age the capacity for spatial compensation is limited. An increase in ICP may be caused by tumors or other space-occupying lesions, accumulation of fluid within the ventricular system, bleeding, or edema of cerebral tissues. Once compensation is exhausted, any further increase in volume results in a rapid rise in ICP.

The early signs and symptoms of increased ICP are often subtle (e.g., headache, vomiting), involving personality changes, irritability, and fatigue (Box 37-1). In older children

---

**Box 37-1**

**Clinical Manifestations of Increased Intracranial Pressure in Infants and Children**

**INFANTS**

Tense, bulging fontanel
Separated cranial sutures
Macewen (cracked-pot) sign
Irritability
High-pitched cry
Increased frontaloccipital circumference
Distended scalp veins
Poor feeding
Crying when disturbed
Setting-sun sign

**CHILDREN**

Headache
Nausea
Forceful vomiting
Diplopia, blurred vision
Seizures

**PERSONALITY AND BEHAVIOR SIGNS**

Irritability, restlessness
Indifference, drowsiness
Decline in school performance
Diminished physical activity and motor performance
Increased sleeping
Inability to follow simple commands
Lethargy
Drowsiness

**LATE SIGNS**

Bradycardia
Decreased motor response to command
Decreased sensory response to painful stimuli
Alterations in pupil size and reactivity
Decerebrate or decorticate posturing
Cheyne-Stokes respirations
Papilledema
Decreased consciousness
Coma

subjective symptoms are headache, especially when lying flat (e.g., on awakening in the morning) or when coughing, sneezing, or bending over, and nausea and vomiting. The child may complain of double vision or blurred vision with movement of the head. Seizures may occur. In children whose cranial sutures have not closed, there is an increase in the head circumference and bulging fontanels. Cranial sutures may become diastatic or may split; head circumference can enlarge until the child is 5 years of age if the condition progresses slowly. As pressure increases, the pupils become progressively sluggish in reaction and eventually become fixed and dilated. The level of consciousness progressively deteriorates from drowsiness to eventual coma. Problems related to increased ICP are discussed later in this chapter in relation to head injury. (See Brain Tumors, Chapter 36, and Hydrocephalus, Chapter 11.)

Physiologic and biochemical changes within the cerebral vasculature serve to complicate the primary causes of increased ICP. Especially in cases of trauma, there is often an initial increase in blood flow as a result of venous congestion or vasomotor paralysis. If cerebral hypoxia is associated with the cerebral dysfunction, the compensatory vasodilation caused by oxygen deficiency will tend to increase the cerebral flow. However, blood flow is reduced as ICP progressively increases, with diminished blood supply to the brain tissues. The classic responses observed in adults (widening pulse pressure, increased blood pressure) are rarely seen in children and, if so, are very late signs. Periodic or irregular breathing is an ominous sign of brainstem (especially medullary) dysfunction that often precedes apnea.

# EVALUATION OF NEUROLOGIC STATUS

Earlier chapters discuss methods used to evaluate neurologic function in relation to numerous aspects of child care. The neurologic examination is an integral part of the health assessment (see Chapter 7) and newborn assessment (see Chapter 8). Some of the tests used to differentiate neuromuscular disorders are discussed in Chapter 40. The assessment tools and examinations in this chapter are primarily those used to assess intracranial integrity.

## Assessment: General Aspects

Children younger than 2 years of age require special evaluation because they are unable to respond to directions designed to elicit specific neurologic responses. Early neurologic responses in infants are primarily reflexive; these responses are gradually replaced by meaningful movement in the characteristic cephalocaudal direction of development. This evidence of progressive maturation reflects more extensive myelinization and changes in neurochemical and electrophysiologic properties.

Most information about infants and small children is gained through observation of their spontaneous and elicited reflex responses, by their development of increasingly complex locomotor and fine motor skills, and by elic-

iting progressively sophisticated communicative and adaptive behaviors. Delay or deviation from expected milestones helps to identify high-risk children. Persistence or reappearance of reflexes that normally disappear indicates pathology. In evaluating the infant or young child, it is important to obtain the history of the pregnancy, delivery, respiratory status at birth, and neonatal health in order to determine the possible effect of intrauterine and extrauterine environmental influences on the orderly maturation of the CNS. These influences include maternal infections, chemicals, trauma, and metabolic insults.

## History

A family history can sometimes offer clues regarding possible genetic disorders with neurologic manifestations. A review of family members often identifies conditions that might otherwise be overlooked, especially in siblings who have died or in relatives whose conditions have been hidden from memory. Questions regarding specific neurologic problems are asked, such as mental retardation, deafness, epilepsy, blindness, unusual movements, weakness, ataxia, stroke, and progressive mental deterioration.

A history is very important because it provides valuable clues regarding the cause of neurologic deficit or change in consciousness. There may have been an injury or short febrile illness, or the child may have diabetes or sickle cell disease. A history of any event that led to the health care assessment is probed, especially when it involves injury, an encounter with an animal or insect, ingestion of neurotoxic substances, inhalation of chemicals, or past illness. Sudden or progressive alterations in movement or mental abilities may provide clues for investigation.

## Physical Examination

Physical examination includes observation of the size and shape of the **head,** spontaneous **activity** and postural **reflex activity,** and **sensory responses.** Note whether the patient is lethargic, drowsy, stuporous, alert, active, or irritable. The attitude is observed. It is noted whether the infant assumes a normal flexed posture or one of extreme extension, opisthotonos, or hypotonia. The extremities are observed for symmetry of **movement.** Seizure activity is suspected if holding the extremity snugly does not stop the activity.

Facial features may suggest a specific syndrome, and a high-pitched, piercing cry is associated with CNS disorders. An abnormal respiratory cycle, such as prolonged apnea, ataxic breathing, paradoxic chest movement, and hyperventilation, may be the result of a neurologic problem.

Older children can be evaluated by the usual methods used in a neurologic examination. In addition, an estimation of the **level of development** provides essential information about neurologic function. This assessment is discussed throughout the book in relation to evaluation for specific disorders such as mental retardation, failure to thrive, attention deficit disorder, cerebral palsy, cerebral tumors, and other physical or behavioral problems. Developmental screening tests can be used to assess developmental progress in the young child. (See Appendix B.)

**Muscular Activity.** Muscular activity and coordination, including ocular movements and gait, are valuable sources of information. Ocular movements, pupillary response, facial movements, and mouth functions provide clues regarding CNS involvement or impingement. (See Chapter 7 for CNS and reflex testing.) Testing reflexes, strength, and coordination and for the presence and location of tremors, twitching, tics, or other unusual movements (Box 37-2) are also aspects of the neurologic assessment. Abnormalities of gait that indicate cerebral dysfunction are described in Box 37-3.

## Altered States of Consciousness

*Consciousness* implies awareness—the ability to respond to sensory stimuli and have subjective experiences. There are two aspects of consciousness: *alertness,* an arousal-waking state that includes the ability to respond to stimuli, and *cognitive power,* which includes the ability to process stimuli and produce verbal and motor responses.

An altered state of consciousness usually refers to varying states of unconsciousness that may be momentary or may last for hours, days, or indefinitely. *Unconsciousness* is depressed cerebral function—the inability to respond to sensory stimuli and have subjective experiences. *Coma* is defined as a state of unconsciousness from which the patient cannot be aroused, even with powerful stimuli.

> **NURSING ALERT**
>
> Lack of response to painful stimuli is abnormal and must be reported immediately.

The seat of consciousness, or "alerting area," of the brain is in the reticular formation—the central core of the brainstem. The reticular formation extends from the midbrain to the medulla. The reticular activating system (RAS) receives collaterals from and is stimulated by *every* major somatic and special sensory pathway in the brain. Disturbances of consciousness may occur when any part of the reticular, thalamic, hypothalamic, and cortical circuits is sufficiently impaired. However, the effects may vary according to the areas involved. For example, small lesions of the reticular or hypothalamic regions produce a profound effect, whereas extensive impairment of the cortex is required to produce quantitatively similar results.

### Etiology

An altered state of consciousness may be the outcome of several processes that affect the CNS. Impaired neurologic function can result from a direct or indirect cause. Some altered states, such as the diffuse changes observed in encephalitis, are directly related to cerebral insult; others are the result of dysfunction in other organs or processes. For example, biochemical changes can impair neurologic function without morphologic findings, as in hypoglycemia.

### Level of Consciousness (LOC)

Assessment of LOC remains the earliest indicator of improvement or deterioration in neurologic status. LOC is determined by observations of the child's responses to the environment. Other diagnostic tests, such as motor activity, reflexes, and vital signs, are more variable and do not necessarily directly parallel the depth of the comatose state. The most consistently used terms are described in Box 37-4.

### Coma Assessment

Diminished alertness as a result of pathologic conditions occurs as a continuum and is designated as the *comatose state,* which extends from somnolence at one end to deep coma at the other. To produce coma, one of the following must

---

### Box 37-2 ■ ■ ■
### Description of Abnormal Involuntary Muscular Movements

**Ataxia**—Gross incoordination that may become worse with the eyes closed
**Spasm**—Involuntary contraction of a muscle
**Spasticity**—Prolonged and steady contraction of a muscle characterized by clonus (alternating relaxation and contraction of the muscle) and exaggerated reflexes
**Rigidity**—Inability to flex or extend a joint
**Tremors**—Constant small involuntary movements
**Twitching**—Spasmodic movements of short duration
**Tic**—Involuntary, compulsive, stereotyped movement of an associated group of muscles
**Choreiform movements**—Quick, jerky, grossly uncoordinated, irregular movements that may disappear on relaxation
**Athetosis**—Slow, writhing, wormlike, constant, grossly uncoordinated movements that increase on voluntary activity and decrease on relaxation
**Dystonia**—Slow twisting movements of limbs or trunk
**Associated movements**—Voluntary movement of one muscle accompanied by involuntary movement of another muscle
**Mirroring movements**—Same as associated movements except with symmetric muscle groups

---

### Box 37-3 ■ ■ ■
### Abnormalities of Gait That Indicate Cerebral Dysfunction

**Ataxia**—Impaired ability to coordinate movements; staggering gait and postural imbalance.
**Spastic paraplegic gait**—Narrow-based gait with a tendency to walk on toes, along with flexion at knees and hips, and shuffling. Hips are adducted, and knees may strike each other with each step; in younger children a "scissoring" position results when lower limbs cross because of increased adductor tone. Patients walk stiffly and take slow, deliberate steps. Difficulty when attempting to walk on heels or run.
**Spastic hemiplegic gait**—Involved leg extended, circumducted, plantar flexion. The affected arm is flexed, adducted, and does not swing.
**Cerebellar gait**—Staggering, unsteadiness, wide-based. Tendency to veer in one lateral direction. Often accompanied by swaying of the trunk.
**Extrapyramidal gait**—Rigidity, few automatic movements, and bradykinesia (slowness of all movements) with associated bending of trunk and head, arms adducted at shoulders and flexed at elbows and wrists, fingers extended; festination (upper body moves forward in advance of lower part), causing rapid steps and risk of falling.

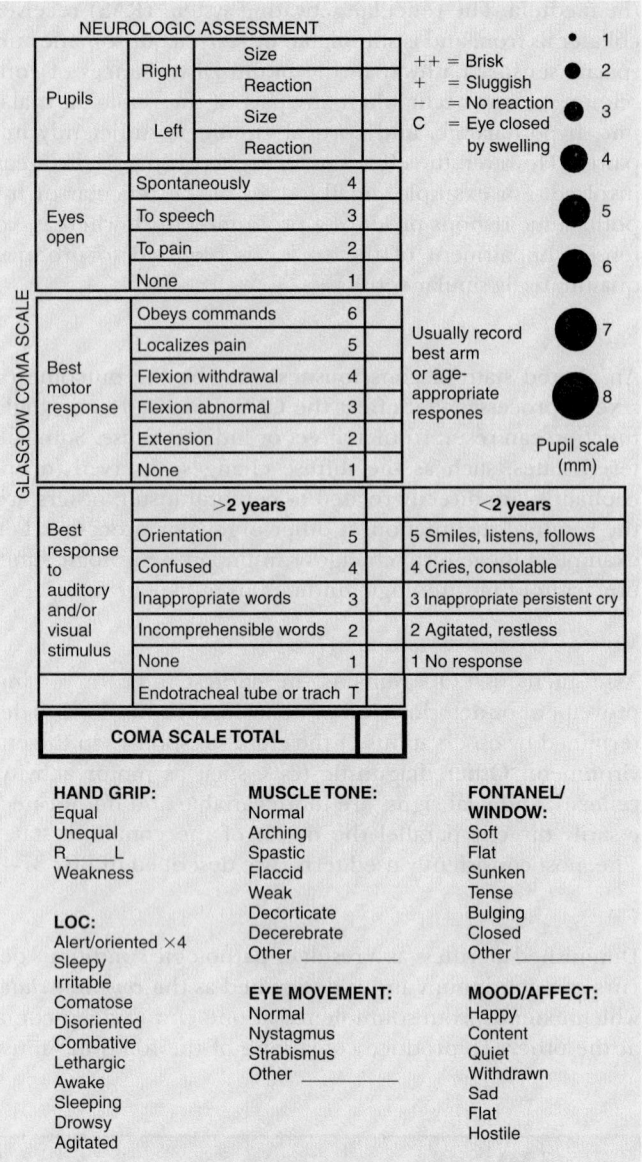

**Fig. 37-2** Pediatric coma scale.

**Box 37-4**
## Levels of Consciousness

**Full consciousness**—Awake and alert, orientated to time, place and person; behavior appropriate for age

**Confusion**—Impaired decision making

**Disorientation**—Confusion regarding time, place; decreased level of consciousness

**Lethargy**—Limited spontaneous movement, sluggish speech, drowsy, falls asleep quickly

**Obtundation**—Arousable with stimulation

**Stupor**—Remains in a deep sleep, responsive only to vigorous and repeated stimulation, simple motor or moaning responses to stimuli, responses slow

**Coma**—No motor or verbal response or decerebrate posturing to noxious (painful) stimuli

**Persistent vegetative state (PVS)**—Permanently lost function of the cerebral cortex; eyes follow objects only by reflex or when attracted to the direction of loud sounds; all four limbs are spastic but can withdraw from painful stimuli; hands show reflexive grasping and groping; the face can grimace, some food may be swallowed, and the child may groan or cry but utter no words

Modified from Seidel HM and others, editors: *Mosby's guide to physical examination,* ed 4, St Louis, 1999, Mosby.

age. The pediatric coma scale does not assess verbal responses as such but records smiling, crying, and interaction; it uses a 6-point motor scale that is inappropriate for children below the age of 6 months. In children under 5 years of age, speech is understood to be any sound at all, even crying. Young children will demonstrate orientation by identifying their parents correctly or giving their own names. The scale with variations adapted to the young patient is provided in Fig. 37-2. When assessing LOC in young children, it is often useful to have a parent present to help elicit a desired response. An infant or child may not respond in an unfamiliar environment or to unfamiliar voices.

Numeric values of 1 to 5 are assigned to the levels of response in each category. The sum of these numeric values provides an objective measurement of the patient's LOC. The lower the score, the deeper the coma. A person with an unaltered LOC would score the highest, 15; a score of 8 or below is generally accepted as a definition of coma; the lowest score, 3, indicates deep coma or death.

The GCS in itself is not sufficient to determine the responses of all children. For example, because a child with quadriplegia cannot respond to commands physically, the child can score very low but be cerebrally intact. Nevertheless, the GCS provides a more objective method for evaluating the state of consciousness in most cases. Severely injured children (GCS of 8 or less) may have a consistent grading of motor response, verbal response, and eye opening.

The GCS at admission is predictive of abnormal neurologic findings at discharge only when profoundly depressed (6 or less); otherwise the GCS is not useful as a prognostic tool when used alone (White and others, 2001). GCS scores less than 8 in combination with other abnormal findings (e.g., hypoxia on admission and abnormal computerized tomography [CT] results) were associated with poor outcome (Ong and others, 1996).

occur: (1) extensive, diffuse, bilateral cerebral hemispheric destruction (the brainstem may be intact); (2) a lesion in the diencephalon; or (3) destruction of the brainstem down to the level of the lower pons.

Several scales have been devised in an attempt to standardize the description and interpretation of the degree of depressed consciousness. The most popular of these is the **Glasgow Coma Scale (GCS),** which consists of a three-part assessment: eye opening, verbal response, and motor response. The GCS was created to meet a clinical need: the desire of experienced nurses for objective criteria for the conscious level. For clinical purposes, the primary role of observation of the LOC is to detect a life-threatening complication such as cerebral edema. The GCS requires observational skills and is readily reproducible between observers.

A pediatric version of the GCS recognizes that expected verbal and motor responses must be related to the child's

## GUIDELINES
### Establishing Brain Death in Children

1. Coma and apnea must coexist. Child must exhibit complete loss of consciousness, vocalization, and volitional activity.
2. Brainstem function must be absent, as defined by:
   a. Midposition or fully dilated pupils that do not respond to light. Drugs may influence and invalidate pupillary assessment.
   b. Absence of spontaneous eye movements and those induced by oculocephalic and caloric (oculovestibular) testing.
   c. Absence of movement of bulbar musculature, including facial and oropharyngeal muscles. The corneal, gag, cough, sucking, and rooting reflexes are absent.
   d. Respiratory movements are absent when child is removed from respirator. Apnea testing using standardized methods can be performed but is done after other criteria are met.
3. Child must not be significantly hypothermic or hypotensive for age.
4. Flaccid tone and absence of spontaneous or induced movements, including spinal cord events such as reflex withdrawal or spinal myoclonus, should exist.
5. Examination should remain consistent with brain death throughout the observation and testing period.
6. Observation periods according to age:

| | |
|---|---|
| 7 days to 2 months | Two examinations and two EEGs, separated by at least 48 hours |
| 2 months to 1 year | Two examinations and two EEGs, separated by at least 24 hours |
| Over 1 year | Observation period of at least 12 hours |
| | If irreversible cause exists, no laboratory testing needed |
| | If difficult to assess extent of reversibility of brain damage, observation indicated for at least 24 hours |

Modified from Task Force for the Determination of Brain Death in Children: Guidelines for the determination of brain death in children, *Ann Neurol* 21:616, 1987; Janakiraman N: Brain death, *Indian J Pediatr* 65:525-527, 1998.

**Irreversible Coma.** There is no precise diagnosis for clinical death. Different tissues undergo permanent damage after varying periods of exposure to an ongoing insult; therefore the brain (especially the cerebrum) has become the tissue of most importance in determining the time of death. The current concept of dying is a process that takes place over a finite interval of time rather than an event that occurs spontaneously. *Brain death* is the total cessation of brainstem and cortical brain function that may result from irreversible traumatic, anoxic, or metabolic conditions. The pronouncement of brain death requires two conditions: (1) complete cessation of clinical evidence of brain function (as evidenced by lack of activity on flow study) and (2) irreversibility of the condition. The child who meets the criteria for brain death will eventually suffer cardiovascular collapse (usually within hours). Brain death cannot be determined if certain CNS medications have been given (e.g., phenobarbital).

Organ transplantation has created a need to subdivide the process of death in order to obtain viable tissues at a time when the brain is already dead. The clinical criteria for brain death must be constituted so that there is *no error*. Although the legal status of the concept of death varies among individual states and communities in the United States, the Task Force for the Determination of Brain Death in Children has established Guidelines for the Determination of Brain Death in Children. (See Guidelines box.) (See Tissue Donation/Autopsy, Chapter 23.)

Substantial variability exists in the criteria used by clinicians for the diagnosis of brain death (e.g., number of coma examinations, number and duration of apnea tests, $PCO_2$ measurements at the end of the apnea test, ancillary tests used to confirm brain death, organ procurement, and reasons for nonprocurement) (DeVita, 2001).

## Neurologic Examination

The purpose of the neurologic examination is to establish an accurate, objective baseline of neurologic function. Therefore it is essential that the neurologic examination be documented in a fashion that is *reproducible*. In this way a comparison of baseline, previous, and current findings allows the observer to detect subtle changes in the neurologic status that might not otherwise be evident. Descriptions of behaviors should be simple, objective, and easily interpreted: "Drowsy but awake and conversationally rational/oriented," "Sleepy but arousable with vigorous physical stimuli. Pressure to nail base of right hand results in upper extremity flexion/lower extremity extension."

Vital signs, observation of posture and movement (both spontaneous and elicited), eye examination, cranial nerve (CN) testing, and reflex testing all provide valuable clues regarding the LOC, the site of involvement, and the probable cause, but they do not necessarily parallel the depth of a comatose state.

### Vital Signs

*Pulse, respiration,* and *blood pressure* provide information regarding the adequacy of circulation and the possible underlying cause of altered consciousness. *Autonomic activity* is most intensively disturbed in deep coma and in brainstem lesions. *Body temperature* is often elevated; sometimes the elevation is extreme and unresponsive to therapeutic measures. High temperature is most often a sign of an acute infectious process or heatstroke but may be caused by ingestion of some drugs (especially salicylates, alcohol, and barbiturates) or intracranial bleeding. Hypothalamic involvement may cause elevated or decreased temperature. Serious infection may produce hypothermia.

The pulse is variable and may be rapid, slow and bounding, or feeble. Blood pressure may be normal, elevated, or very low. The Cushing reflex, or pressor response that causes a slowing of the pulse and an increase in blood pressure, is uncommon in children; when it does occur, it is a very late sign. Vital signs are also affected by medications. For assessment purposes, *changes* in pulse and blood pressure are more important than the direction.

Respirations are more often slow, deep, and irregular. Slow and deep breathing is often seen in the heavy sleep caused by sedatives, after seizures, or in cerebral infections. Slow, shallow breathing may result from sedatives or narcotics. Hyperventilation (deep and rapid respirations) is usually the result of metabolic acidosis or abnormal stimulation of the respiratory center in the medulla caused by salicylate poisoning, hepatic coma, or Reye syndrome.

Breathing patterns have been described with a number of terms (e.g., apneustic, cluster, ataxic, Cheyne-Stokes). However, it is better to describe what is being observed rather than placing a label on it. The terms are often used and interpreted incorrectly. Periodic and irregular breathing are signs of brainstem (especially medullary) dysfunction. This is an ominous sign that often precedes complete apnea. The odor of the breath may provide additional clues (e.g., the fruity and acetone odor of ketosis, the foul odor of uremia, the fetid odor of hepatic failure, or the odor of alcohol).

## Skin

The skin may offer clues to the cause of unconsciousness. The body surface should be examined for the presence of injury, needle marks, petechiae, bites, and ticks. Evidence of toxic substances may be found on the hands, face, mouth, and clothing—especially in small children.

## Eyes

Pupil size and reactivity are assessed (Fig. 37-3). Pupils either react or do not react to light. Pinpoint pupils are commonly observed in poisoning (e.g., opiate or barbiturate poisoning) or in brainstem dysfunction. Widely dilated and reactive pupils are often seen after seizures and may involve only one side. Widely dilated and fixed pupils suggest paralysis of CN III secondary to pressure from herniation of the brain through the tentorium. A unilateral fixed pupil usually suggests a lesion on the same side. Bilateral fixed pupils usually imply brainstem damage if present for more than 5 minutes. Dilated and nonreactive pupils are also seen in hypothermia, anoxia, ischemia, poisoning with atropine-like substances, or prior instillation of mydriatic drugs. Some of the therapies used (e.g., barbiturates) can alter pupil size and reaction.

**NURSING ALERT** The sudden appearance of a fixed and dilated pupil is a neurosurgical emergency.

The description of eye movements should indicate whether one or both eyes are involved and how the reaction was elicited. The parents should be asked if the child has a strabismus, which will cause the eyes to appear normal under compromise.

Blinking observed at rest or in response to a sudden loud noise or bright light implies that the pontine reticular formation is intact. The *corneal reflex,* blinking of the eyelids when the cornea is touched with a wisp of cotton or a camel hair pencil, is used to test the integrity of the ophthalmic division of CN V. A posttraumatic strabismus indicates CN VI damage.

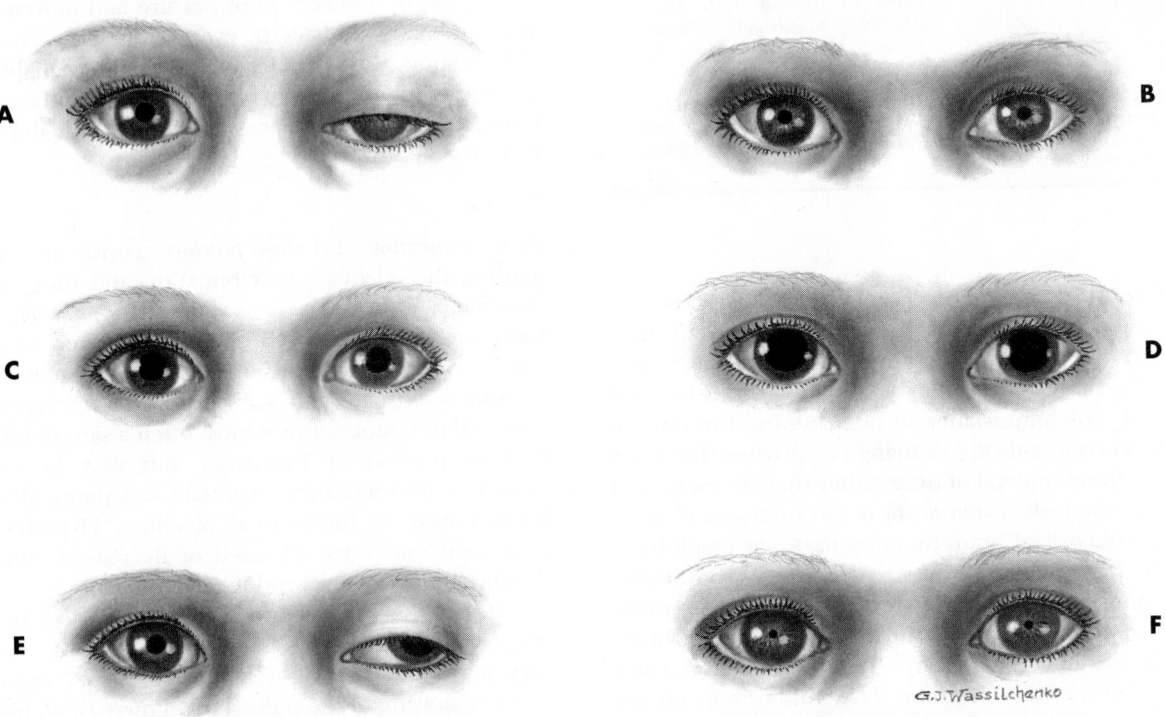

**Fig. 37-3** Variations in pupil size with altered states of consciousness. **A,** Ipsilateral pupillary constriction with slight ptosis. **B,** Bilateral small pupils. **C,** Midposition, light fixed to all stimuli. **D,** Bilateral dilated and fixed pupils. **E,** Dilated pupils, left eye abducted with ptosis. **F,** Pinpoint pupils.

Eye movements are assessed by the *doll's head maneuver*, in which the child's head is rotated quickly to one side and then to the other. When the brainstem centers for eye movement are intact, there is conjugate (paired or working together) movement of the eyes in the direction opposite the head rotation. Absence of this response suggests dysfunction of the brainstem or oculomotor nerve (CN III). Downward or lateral deviation is often observed in association with pupillary dilation in dysfunction of CN III.

> **NURSING ALERT**   Any tests that require head movement are not attempted until after cervical spine injury has been ruled out.

The *caloric test,* or *oculovestibular response,* is elicited by irrigating the external auditory canal with 10 ml of ice water over a period of approximately 20 seconds (head of bed elevated at a 30-degree angle). This test normally causes movement of the eyes toward the side of stimulation. This response is lost when the pontine centers are impaired and thus provides important information in assessment of the comatose patient.

> **NURSING ALERT**   The ice water caloric test is painful and is never performed on the awake child or if the tympanic membranes are ruptured.

Funduscopic examination reveals additional clues. Because it takes 24 to 48 hours to develop, *papilledema* (optic disc swelling, indistinct margins, hemorrhages, tortuosity of vessels, absence of venous pulsations), if it develops at all, will not be evident early in the course of unconsciousness. The presence of preretinal hemorrhages in children is usually the result of acute trauma with intracranial bleeding, usually subarachnoid or subdural hemorrhage.

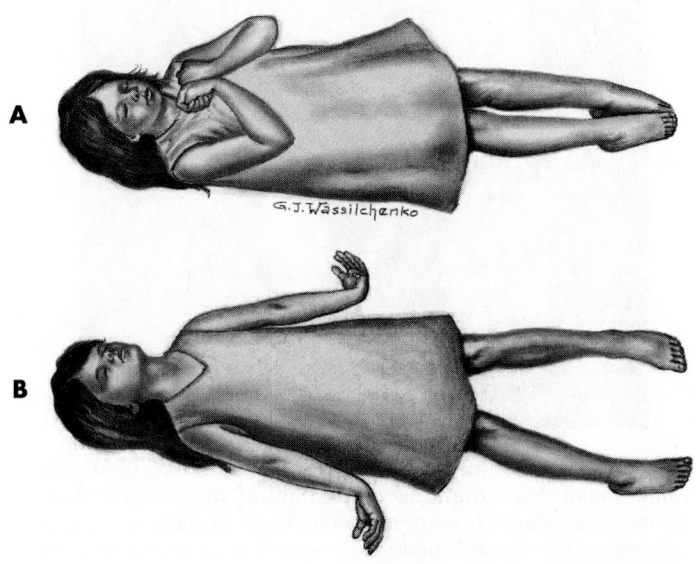

**Fig. 37-4**   **A,** Decorticate posturing. **B,** Decerebrate posturing.

## Motor Function

Observation of spontaneous activity, posture, and response to painful stimuli provides clues to the location and extent of cerebral dysfunction. Even subtle movements (e.g., the out-turning of a hip) should be noted and the child observed for other signs. Asymmetric movements of the limbs or the absence of movement suggests paralysis. In hemiplegia the affected limb lies in external rotation and will fall uncontrollably when lifted and allowed to drop.

In the deeper comatose states there is little or no spontaneous movement, and the musculature tends to be flaccid. There is considerable variability in motor behavior in lesser degrees of coma. For example, the child may be relatively immobile or restless and hyperkinetic; muscle tone may be increased or decreased. Tremors, twitching, and spasms of muscles are common observations. The patient may display purposeless plucking or tossing movements. Combative or negativistic behavior is not uncommon. Hyperactivity is more common in acute febrile and toxic states than in cases of increased ICP. Seizures are common in children and may be present in coma as a result of any cause. Any repetitive or seizure movements are described.

## Posturing

Primitive postural reflexes emerge as cortical control over motor function is lost in brain dysfunction. These reflexes are evident in posturing and motor movements directly related to the area of the brain involved. Posturing reflects a balance between the lower exciting and the higher inhibiting influences, and strong muscles overcome weaker ones. *Decorticate posturing* (Fig. 37-4, *A*) is seen with severe dysfunction of the cerebral cortex or with lesions to corticospinal tracts above the brainstem. Typical decorticate posturing includes rigid flexion, with arms held tightly to the body, flexed elbows, wrists, and fingers, plantar flexed feet, legs extended and internally rotated, and possibly presence of fine tremors or intense stiffness. *Decerebrate posturing* (Fig. 37-4, *B*), is a sign of dysfunction at the level of the midbrain or lesions to the brainstem. It is characterized by rigid extension and pronation of the arms and legs, flexed wrists and fingers, clenched jaw, extended neck, and possibly an arched back. Unilateral decerebrate posturing is often caused by tentorial herniation.

Posturing may not be evident when the child is quiet but can usually be elicited by applying painful stimuli, such as a blunt object pressed on the base of the nail. Nurses should avoid applying thumb pressure to the supraorbital region of the frontal bone (risk of orbital damage). Noxious stimuli (e.g., suctioning) will elicit a response, as may turning or touching. When describing posturing, the stimulus needed to provoke the response is as important as the reaction.

## Reflexes

Testing of certain reflexes, such as those present in an intact spinal cord, may be of limited value. (See Chapter 7.) In general, the corneal, pupillary, muscle-stretch, superficial, and plantar reflexes tend to be absent in deep coma. The state of reflexes is variable in lighter grades of unconsciousness and depends on the underlying pathologic process and the location of the lesion. The doll's eye reflex maneuver, described previously, reflects paralysis of CN III. The absence of corneal reflexes (CN V) and the presence of a tonic neck reflex are associated with severe brain damage. The Babinski reflex, in which the lateral portion of the foot is stroked, may be of value if it is found to be present consistently in children older than 1 year. A positive Babinski reflex is significant in the assessment of pyramidal tract lesions when it is unilateral and associated with other pyramidal signs. A fluctuating Babinski reflex is often observed after seizures. (See Fig. 8-9, *B*.)

> **NURSING ALERT**
> Three key reflexes that demonstrate neurologic health in young infants are the Moro, tonic neck, and withdrawal reflexes.

## Special Diagnostic Procedures

Numerous diagnostic procedures are used for assessment of cerebral function. Laboratory tests that may help to delineate the cause of unconsciousness include blood glucose, urea nitrogen, and electrolyte (pH, sodium, potassium, chloride, calcium, and bicarbonate) tests; clotting studies, hematocrit, and a complete blood count; liver function tests; blood cultures if there is fever; and sometimes studies to detect lead or other toxic substances, such as drugs.

An electroencephalogram (EEG) may provide important information. For example, generalized random slow activity suggests suppressed cortical function, and localized slow activity suggests a space-occupying lesion. A flat tracing is one of the criteria used as evidence of brain death. Examination of spinal fluid is carried out when toxic encephalopathy or infection is suspected. Lumbar puncture is ordinarily delayed if intracranial hemorrhage is suspected and is contraindicated in the presence of ICP because of the potential for tentorial herniation.

Auditory and visual evoked potentials are sometimes used in neurologic evaluation of very young children. Brainstem auditory evoked potentials are useful for evaluating the continuity of brainstem auditory tracts and are particularly useful for detecting demyelinating disease and neoplasms of the brainstem and distinguishing between brainstem and cortical lesions. For example, a normal evoked potential in a comatose patient suggests involvement of the cerebral hemispheres.

Highly sophisticated tests are carried out with specialized equipment. Two imaging techniques, CT and magnetic resonance imaging (MRI) (Fig. 37-5), assist in diagnosis by scanning both soft tissues and solid matter. Most of these tests are outlined in Table 37-2. Because such tests can be threatening to children, a child will need preparation for these tests, with support and reassurance during them. (See Preparation for Procedures, Chapter 27.)

Children who are old enough to understand require careful explanation of the procedure, why it is being done, what they will experience, and how they can help. School-age children usually appreciate a more detailed description of why contrast material is injected. The importance of lying

still for tests, particularly CT, needs to be stressed. Children unfamiliar with the machines can be shown a picture beforehand. Although radiographic examinations are not painful, the machinery is often so frightening in appearance that the child protests because of anxiety.

This is especially true of CT and MRI, both of which require that the child's head be placed within a special immobilizing device. Chin and cheek pads are sometimes used to prevent the slightest head movement, and straps are applied to the body to prevent a slight change in body position. The nurse can explain these events to a frightened child by comparing them to an astronaut's preparation for a space flight. It is very important to emphasize to the child that at no time is the procedure painful.

It is helpful for nurses to become acquainted with the equipment and the general environment in which the test will take place so they can better explain the procedure to children at their level of understanding. Written material describing the procedure should be available for parents and may be appropriate to share with children. Equipment is often strange and ominous to children and may be perceived as a frightening monster. They need constant reassurance from a trusted companion. Because children are particularly frightened of needles, they need to be informed of any medication or contrast media that will be administered intravenously.

The nurse should not expect cooperation from a young child. Sedation may be required. Many different agents are currently used for sedation of children undergoing neurologic diagnostic procedures. Chloral hydrate (CH) has been used for decades as a short-term sedative agent and remains a safe method of pediatric outpatient sedation (Kao and

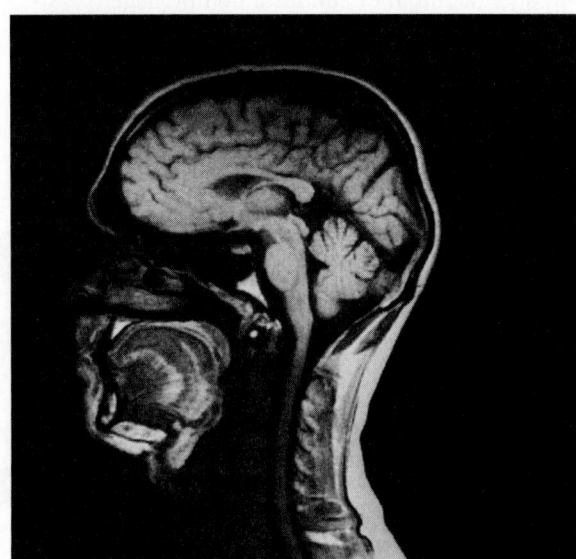

**Fig. 37-5** MRI. Midsagittal image produces excellent anatomic detail. Note the clear delineation of structures such as the pituitary gland, brainstem, spinal cord, cerebellum, corpus callosum, and sylvian aqueduct. (Courtesy Philips Medical Systems. From Nolte J: *The human brain: an introduction to its functional anatomy*, ed 3, St Louis, 1993, Mosby.)

others, 1999). CH is used alone for sedating children for procedures such as MRI.

In recent years other sedative agents have been used safely, alone and in combination, for children in the outpatient setting. These include intravenous (IV) sodium pento-barbital (Nembutal), IV midazolam (Rosen and Rosen, 1998), and intranasal midazolam (Ljungman and others, 2000; Lloyd, Alredy and Lloyd, 2000).

As a result of an increase in the use of sedatives, analgesics, and general anesthetic agents in the outpatient set-

**TABLE 37-2** Neurologic diagnostic procedures

| Test | Description | Purpose | Comments |
|---|---|---|---|
| **Lumbar puncture (LP)** | Spinal needle is inserted between L3 and L4 or L4 and L5 vertebral spaces into subarachnoid space; cerebrospinal fluid (CSF) pressure is measured, and sample is collected for examination | Diagnostic—measures spinal fluid pressure, obtains CSF for laboratory analysis<br>Therapeutic—injection of medication | Contraindicated in patients with increased intracranial pressure (ICP) or infected skin over puncture site |
| **Subdural tap** | Needle is inserted into anterior fontanel or coronal suture (midline to pupil) | Helps rule out subdural effusions<br>Removes CSF to relieve pressure | Infant is placed in semierect position after subdural tap to minimize leakage from site; prevent child from crying if possible<br>Check site frequently for evidence of leakage |
| **Ventricular puncture** | Needle is inserted into lateral ventricle via coronal suture (midline to pupil) | Removes CSF to relieve pressure | Risk of intracerebral or ventricular hemorrhage |
| **Electroencephalography (EEG)** | Records changes in electric potential of brain<br>Electrodes are placed at various points to assess electrical function in a particular area<br>Impulses are recorded by electromagnetic pen or digitally | Detects spikes, or bursts of electrical activity that indicate the potential for seizures<br>Used to determine brain death | Patient should remain quiet during procedure<br>May require sedation<br>Reduce external stimuli to a minimum during procedure |
| **Nuclear brain scan** | Intravenous (IV) injection of radioisotope that is counted and recorded after fixed time intervals | Radioisotope accumulates in areas where blood-brain barrier is defective<br>Identifies focal brain lesions (e.g., tumors, abscesses)<br>Positive uptake of material with encephalitis and subdural hematoma<br>Visualizes CSF pathways | Requires IV access; may require sedation<br>In normal children or noncommunicating hydrocephalus there is no retrograde filling of ventricles<br>Areas of concentrated uptake of material are termed "hot spots" |
| **Echoencephalography** | Pulses of ultrasonic waves are beamed through head; echoes from reflecting surfaces are recorded graphically | Identifies shifts in midline structures from their normal positions as a result of intracranial lesions<br>May show ventricular dilation | Simple, safe, rapid procedure<br>Fontanel must be patent |
| **Real-time ultrasonography (RTUS)** | Similar to CT but uses ultrasound instead of ionizing radiation | Allows high-resolution anatomic visualization in variety of imaging planes | Produces images similar to CT scan<br>Especially useful in neonatal CNS problems<br>Anterior fontanel must be patent |
| **Radiography** | Skull films are taken from different views—lateral, posterolateral, axial (submentoventricular), half-axial | Shows fractures, dislocations, spreading suture lines, craniostenosis<br>Shows degenerative changes, bone erosion, calcifications | Simple, noninvasive procedure |
| **Computed tomography (CT) scan** | Pinpoint x-ray beam is directed on horizontal or vertical plane to provide series of "images" that are fed into computer and assembled in image displayed on video screen<br>Uses ionizing radiation | Visualizes horizontal and vertical cross section of brain in three planes (axial, coronal, sagittal)<br>Distinguishes density of various intracranial tissues and structures—congenital abnormalities, hemorrhage, tumors, demyelinating and inflammatory processes, calcification | Requires IV access if contrast agent is used<br>May require sedation<br>Rapid |

*Continued*

**TABLE 37-2**   Neurologic diagnostic procedures—cont'd

| Test | Description | Purpose | Comments |
|---|---|---|---|
| Magnetic resonance imaging (MRI) | Produces radiofrequency emissions from elements (e.g., hydrogen, phosphorus), which are converted to visual images by computer | Permits visualization of morphologic features of target structures<br>Permits tissue discrimination unavailable with many techniques | Noninvasive procedure except when IV contrast agent is used<br>No exposure to radiation<br>May require sedation<br>Parent or attendant can remain in room with child<br>Does not visualize bone detail or calcifications<br>No metal can be present in the scanner |
| Positron emission tomography (PET) | IV injection of positron-emitting radionucleotide; local concentrations are detected and transformed into a visual display by computer | Detects and measures blood volume and flow in brain, metabolic activity, biochemical changes within tissues | Requires lengthy period of immobility<br>Minimal exposure to radiation<br>May require sedation |
| Digital subtraction angiography (DSA) | Contrast dye injected IV; computer "subtracts" all tissues without contrast medium, leaving clear image of contrast medium in vessels studied | Visualizes vasculature of target tissue<br>Visualizes finite vascular abnormalities | Safe alternative to angiography<br>Patient must remain still during procedure<br>May require sedation |
| Single-photon emission computed tomography (SPECT) | IV injection of photon-emitting radionuclide; radionuclides are absorbed by healthy tissue at a different rate than diseased or necrotic tissue; the data are transferred to a computer that converts the image to film | Provides information regarding blood flow to tissues; analyzing blood flow to an organ may help determine how well it is functioning | Requires lengthy period of immobility<br>Minimal exposure to radiation<br>May require sedation |

ting, the American Academy of Pediatrics (1992) developed Guidelines for Monitoring and Management of Pediatric Patients During and After Sedation for Diagnostic and Therapeutic Procedures. These guidelines were reaffirmed in 1998. Nurses involved in caring for children receiving sedation should be familiar with these guidelines. (See Pain Management, Chapter 26.)

Physical preparation for the diagnostic test may involve administration of a sedative. If so, children should be helped through the preparation and administration and assured that someone will remain with them (if this is possible) (Kociela, 1998). Children need continual support and reinforcement during procedures in which they will remain conscious. Vital signs and physiologic responses to the procedure are monitored throughout. Many diagnostic procedures performed on an outpatient basis require sedation, and children need recovery time and observation. Written instructions should be reviewed with parents if the child is discharged following a procedure. (See Critical Thinking Exercise box.)

Children who have undergone a procedure with a general anesthetic require postanesthesia care, including positioning to prevent aspiration of secretions and frequent assessment of the vital signs and LOC. In addition, other neurologic functions such as pupillary responses, motor strength, and movement are tested at regular intervals. Any surgical wound resulting from the test is checked for bleeding, CSF leakage, and other complications. Children who undergo repeated subdural taps should have their

hematocrit monitored to detect excessive blood loss from the procedure.

The emotional reaction of children to the procedure should be considered. They should be allowed and encouraged to express their feelings about the experience through verbal expression and the use of therapeutic play. Parents also seek and are entitled to an explanation of the results of tests and procedures performed on their children. Nurses are in a unique position to provide support and education to parents regarding procedures.

# THE CHILD WITH CEREBRAL COMPROMISE

## Nursing Care of the Unconscious Child

The unconscious child requires continuous nursing attendance with observation, recording, and evaluation of changes in objective signs. These observations provide valuable information regarding the patient's progress and often serve as a guide to diagnosis and treatment. Therefore careful and detailed observations are essential for the child's welfare. In addition, vital functions must be maintained and complications prevented through conscientious and meticulous nursing care. The outcome of unconsciousness may be early and complete recovery, death within a few hours or days, persistent and permanent unconsciousness, or recovery with varying degrees of residual mental or physical disability. The outcome and recov-

## Critical Thinking Exercise

### Sedation

Brian, 4 weeks old, is returned to his room after a CT scan to evaluate a seizure episode. Upon examination you find a sleepy infant who is arousable with vigorous stimulation and has pale, dusky colored skin and mucous membranes. The vital signs are temperature of 35.8° C, pulse of 110, respiratory rate of 30, and blood pressure of 82/40; the oxygen saturation is 89% to 92%. His weight is 5 kg, and he received 500 mg of chloral hydrate (<10 kg: 75-100 mg/kg dosage) as ordered before leaving for the CT. During the report the CT nurse reviews the sedation record, and you note it does not include the infant's temperature. An additional dosage of 250 mg of chloral hydrate was administered in CT to achieve sleep for Brian. What is the best intervention?

FIRST, THINK ABOUT IT . . .

- What information are you using?
- What conclusions are you reaching?

1. Monitor the vital signs and cover the infant.
2. Administer oxygen, place a radiant warmer over the infant, and notify the physician.
3. Fill out a medication error report.
4. Allow the infant to sleep.

*The best response is two. The information provided indicates that Brian is experiencing thermoregulation problems compounded by the administration of too much chloral hydrate for sedation. You may appropriately conclude that the maximum dosage of sedation was exceeded for this infant. Sedation flow sheets to record vital signs often do not include temperature measurement, which is an essential observation in infants because of their inability to maintain body temperature.*

ery of the unconscious child may depend on the level of nursing care and observational skills.

Emergency measures are directed toward ensuring patent airway, breathing, and circulation (ABC's); stabilizing the spine when indicated; treating shock; and reducing ICP (if present). Delayed treatment often leads to increased damage. Therapies for specific causes of unconsciousness are begun as soon as emergency measures have been implemented—in many cases concurrently. Because nursing care is closely related to the medical management, both are considered here.

## ⠿ Assessment

Continual observation of the LOC, pupillary reaction, and vital signs is essential to management of CNS disorders. Regular assessment of neurologic and vital signs is an integral part of the nursing care of comatose children. The frequency depends on the cause of coma, the status, and the progression of cerebral involvement. Intervals between observation may be as short as every 15 minutes or as long as every 2 hours. Significant alterations are reported immediately. The temperature is measured every 2 to 4 hours, depending on the child's condition.

An elevated temperature may occur in children with CNS dysfunction; therefore a light covering may be sufficient. Vigorous efforts, such as tepid sponge baths or application of a hypothermia blanket, are needed to prevent brain damage if temperature exceeds 40° C (104° F).

The LOC is assessed periodically, including pupillary size, equality, and reaction to light, as well as signs of meningeal irritation, such as nuchal rigidity. This also includes response to vocal commands, spontaneous behavior, resistance to care, and response to painful stimuli. Motions of any type, changes in muscle tone or strength, and body position are noted. Seizure activity is described according to type and length of seizure and the body areas involved (see Box 37-11).

Pain management for the comatose child requires astute nursing observation and management. Signs of pain include changes in behavior (e.g., increased agitation and rigidity, alteration in vital signs and perfusion); usually, an increased heart rate, respiratory rate, and blood pressure; and decreased oxygen saturation. Because these findings are not specific for pain, the nurse should be alert for their appearance during times of induced or suspected pain and for their disappearance following the inciting procedure or the administration of analgesia. A pain assessment record is used to document indications of pain and the effectiveness of interventions. (See Pain Assessment, Chapter 26.)

The use of opioids, such as morphine, to relieve pain is controversial because they can mask signs of altered consciousness or depress respirations. However, unrelieved pain can elevate ICP. To block the stress response, some authorities advocate the use of analgesics, sedatives and, in some cases such as head injury, paralyzing agents via continuous IV infusion. A commonly used combination is fentanyl, midazolam (Versed), and vecuronium. If there are concerns about assessing the LOC or respiratory depression, naloxone can be used to reverse the opioid effects. Acetaminophen and codeine may also be effective analgesics for mild to moderate pain. Regardless of the drugs used, adequate dosage and regular administration are essential to providing optimum pain relief.

Other measures to relieve discomfort include providing a quiet, dimly lit environment, restricting visitors to a minimum, preventing any sudden jarring movement, such as banging into the bed, and preventing an increase in ICP. The latter is most effectively achieved by proper positioning and prevention of straining, such as during coughing, vomiting, or passing stool. (See Pain Management, Chapter 26.)

**NURSING ALERT**   When opioids are used, bowel elimination must be closely monitored because of the potential constipating effect. A stool softener should be given regularly with laxatives as needed to prevent constipation.

Antiepileptic drugs, such as phenytoin (Dilantin) or phenobarbital, may be ordered for control of seizure activity.

## ⠿ Nursing Diagnoses

Based on a thorough assessment, several nursing diagnoses are identified. The more common diagnoses for the unconscious child are included in the Nursing Care Plan on pp. 1662-1664. Others may apply in specific situations.

## ▓ Planning

The goals for the unconscious child and the family include the following:

1. Child will maintain respiratory integrity.
2. Child will not experience increasing ICP.
3. Child will have basic needs (hygiene, nutrition, hydration, elimination) met.
4. Child will not experience complications of immobility.
5. Family will receive adequate support and education.

## ▓ Implementation

### Respiratory Management

Respiratory effectiveness is the primary concern in the care of the unconscious child, and establishment of an adequate airway is *always* the first priority. Carbon dioxide has a potent vasodilating effect and will increase cerebral blood flow and ICP. Cerebral hypoxia at normal body temperature that lasts longer than 4 minutes nearly always causes irreversible brain damage.

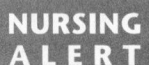 **NURSING ALERT**   Respiratory obstruction and subsequent compromise leads to cardiac arrest. Always maintain an adequate, patent airway.

Children in lighter stages of coma may be able to cough and swallow, but those in deeper states of coma are unable to manage secretions, which tend to pool in the throat and pharynx. Dysfunction of CN IX and X places the child at risk of aspiration and cardiac arrest; therefore the child is positioned with the head and body to the side to prevent aspiration of secretions, and the stomach is emptied to reduce the likelihood of vomiting. In infants the blockage of air passages from secretions can happen in seconds. In addition, upper airway obstruction from laryngospasm is a common complication in comatose children.

An oral airway can be used for the child who is suffering a temporary loss of consciousness, such as after a seizure or anesthesia. For children who remain unconscious for a time, a nasotracheal or orotracheal tube is inserted to maintain the open airway and facilitate removal of secretions. A tracheostomy is performed in cases in which laryngoscopy for introduction of an endotracheal tube would be difficult or dangerous or for a child who needs long-term ventilatory support. Suctioning is used only as needed to clear the airway, exerting care to prevent increasing ICP. Respiratory status is observed and evaluated regularly. Signs of respiratory distress may indicate a need for ventilatory assistance.

Mechanical ventilation is usually indicated when the respiratory center is involved. (See Chapter 31.) Blood gas analysis is performed regularly, and oxygen is administered when indicated. Moderately severe hypoxia and respiratory acidosis are often present but not always evident from clinical manifestations. Hyperventilation often accompanies unconsciousness and may lead to respiratory alkalosis, or it may represent the body's attempt to compensate for metabolic acidosis. Therefore blood gas and pH determinations

are essential guides for electrolyte therapy. Chest physiotherapy is carried out on a regular basis, and the child's position is changed at least every 2 hours to prevent pulmonary complications.

### Intracranial Pressure Monitoring

Continuous ICP monitoring was first introduced 30 years ago.

Prompt intervention can be lifesaving in the comatose patient who has evidence of a marked increase in ICP. When increased ICP is the result of accumulation of CSF from obstruction of CSF flow, a ventricular tap will provide relief quickly and effectively. This group includes children with obstruction due to infection, acute hemorrhages, or neoplasms. Evacuation of a hematoma reduces pressure from this source. The selection of the type of ICP monitor should be guided by the clinical presentation and the therapeutic strategy that is chosen for each child. Indications for inserting an ICP monitor are (1) Glasgow Coma Scale evaluation of less than 7, (2) Glasgow Coma Scale evaluation of less than 8 with respiratory assistance, (3) deterioration of condition, and (4) subjective judgment regarding clinical appearance and response.

Four major types of ICP monitors are (1) intraventricular catheter with or without fibroscopic sensors attached to a monitoring system, (2) subarachnoid bolt (Richmond screw), (3) epidural sensor, and (4) anterior fontanel pressure monitor. Transducers for both ventricular and subarachnoid monitoring should be set up without the use of a flush device. Direct ventricular pressure measurement remains the gold standard of ICP monitoring.

The ventricular catheter method involves introduction of a catheter into the lateral ventricle on the nondominant side, if known, or placement in the subdural space. The catheter has the advantage of providing a means of therapeutic drainage of CSF to reduce pressure. A drainage bag attached to the system is kept at the level of the ventricles and can be lowered to decrease ICP. (See Critical Thinking Exercise box.) This device requires full penetration of the brain, skill and experience with placement, and carries the risk of infection (Luerssen, 1997).

**NURSING ALERT**   If the external ventricular drain (EVD) is unclamped for CSF drainage, carefully monitor the level of the collection container. If the container is positioned too low, improper CSF decompression could lower ICP too rapidly, causing bleeding and pain.

With the bolt method the end of the bolt is placed into the subarachnoid space. The bolt cannot be adequately secured in a small child's pliant skull, although special modifications have been developed for children under 6 years of age. The placement of the bolt is not adjusted by anyone except the neurosurgeon who placed the device. The neurosurgeon is notified if a satisfactory wave form is not observed.

**NURSING ALERT**   The bolt is stabilized with dressings, but these are not changed or disturbed, not even to check the site.

An epidural sensor can be placed between the dura and the skull through a burr hole and connected to a stopcock assembly and a transducer, which provides a readout of the pressure. Although less invasive, correlation of pressure readings may be inconsistent. In infants a fontanel transducer can be used to detect impulses from a pressure sensor and convert them to electrical energy. The electrical energy is then converted to visible waves or numeric readings on an oscilloscope. ICP measurement from the anterior fontanel, although noninvasive, may prove to be inaccurate if the equipment is poorly placed or inconsistently recalibrated.

ICP can be increased by direct instillation of solutions; therefore antibiotics are administered systemically if a positive CSF culture is obtained. However, ICP monitoring rarely causes infection. Because CSF is a body fluid, standard precautions should be implemented according to hospital policy. (See Infection Control, Chapter 27.)

Nurses caring for patients with intracranial monitoring devices must be acquainted with the system, assist with insertion, interpret the monitor readings, and be able to distinguish between danger signals and mechanical dysfunction. Because systemic blood pressure, ICP, and therefore cerebral perfusion pressure are normally lower in children, the age of the child must be taken into account when deciding what constitutes abnormally high ICP or abnormally low cerebral perfusion pressure.

## Critical Thinking Exercise

### Hydrocephalus

Three-year-old Emma underwent surgery 5 days ago for removal of a posterior fossa tumor. Although an external ventricular drain (EVD) was placed to treat her hydrocephalus, she continues to demonstrate signs of increased ICP, including holding the back of her head, anorexia, crying when moved or when strangers enter room, and lethargy. On examination, fluid drainage is noted on the mother's clothes, and Emma is experiencing repetitive, rapid eyelid blinking. What is the best intervention?

FIRST, THINK ABOUT IT . . .

- What precise question are you trying to answer?
- What conclusions are you reaching?

1. Lower the EVD drain.
2. Check the EVD dressing site, perform a neurologic examination, and notify the practitioner.
3. Change the dressing to a transparent adhesive.
4. Request a CT scan.

*The best response is two. Precisely, the question is whether the EVD is draining correctly. Your conclusion should be that it is not draining properly but is taking the path of least resistance through the insertion site. Lowering the EVD may cause rapid drainage of the CSF, resulting in subdural complications. The dressing may need to be changed to a clear adhesive so that the site can be observed. A CT may be required, but the priority is to stabilize Emma, who is demonstrating signs of increased ICP and cranial neuropathy.*

Several medical measures are available to treat increased ICP resulting from cerebral edema. Osmotic diuretics are reserved to control intracranial hypertension that does not respond to sedation and CSF drainage. Although their effect is transient and lasts only about 6 hours, they can be lifesaving in emergencies. These substances are rapidly excreted by the kidneys and carry with them large quantities of sodium and water. Mannitol (or sometimes urea) administered intravenously is the drug most commonly used for rapid reduction of ICP. The infusion is generally given slowly but may be pushed rapidly if there is herniation or impending herniation. Because of the profound diuretic effect of the drug, an indwelling catheter is inserted to ensure bladder emptying. $PaCO_2$ should be maintained at 25 to 30 mm Hg to produce vasoconstriction, which reduces CBF, thereby decreasing ICP. Recording and analyzing the child's volume state, plasma sodium concentration, and serum osmolarity can avert potential fluid and electrolyte problems. Administration of adrenocorticosteroids is not recommended for cerebral edema secondary to head trauma.

**Nursing Activities.** In cases of high levels of increased ICP, nursing procedures tend to trigger reactive pressure waves in many children. For example, increased intrathoracic or abdominal pressure will be transmitted to the cranium. The goals of monitoring a child who is neurologically compromised include maintaining central perfusion pressure; controlling ICP, cerebral edema, and factors that increase cerebral metabolism (fever, seizures); and maintaining hemodynamic stability. Particular care should be taken in positioning these patients to avoid neck vein compression, which may further increase ICP by interfering with venous return.

**NURSING ALERT** The head of the bed is elevated 15 to 30 degrees, and the child is positioned so that the head is maintained in midline to facilitate venous drainage and avoid jugular compression. Turning side to side is contraindicated because of the risk of jugular compression.

Sandbags or other support devices may be needed to maintain correct head position. The child can be propped to one side or the other, and the use of a pressure-relieving or pressure-decreasing mattress decreases the chance of prolonged pressure to vulnerable skin areas. Frequent clinical assessment of the child cannot be replaced by an ICP monitoring device.

It is important to avoid activities that might trigger a seizure or those that that may cause pain, emotional stress, or crying and thus increase ICP. Gentle range-of-motion exercises can be carried out but should not be performed vigorously. Nontherapeutic touch can cause an increase in ICP. Any disturbing procedures to be performed should be scheduled to take advantage of therapies that reduce ICP, such as osmotherapy and sedation. Efforts are made to minimize or eliminate environmental noise. Assessment and intervention to relieve pain are important nursing functions to decrease ICP.

Although controversies remain, nurses have studied intracranial responses to environmental stimuli in an effort to minimize unnecessary elevations and decrease secondary brain damage. The data support the theory that touch may help to stabilize ICP and that a child in a coma may still receive and process verbal and tactile stimuli at some level. Individualizing nursing activities and minimizing environmental stimuli by decreasing noxious procedures help to control ICP (Vernon-Levett, 1998).

**Suctioning.** Suctioning and percussion are poorly tolerated and are therefore contraindicated unless there are concurrent respiratory problems. Hypoxia and the Valsalva maneuver associated with cough both acutely elevate ICP. Vibration, which does not increase ICP, accomplishes excellent results and should be tried first if treatment is needed. If suctioning is necessary, it should be used judiciously and preceded by hyperventilation with 100% oxygen, which can be monitored during suctioning with a pulse oxygen sensor reading to determine oxygen saturation.

## Nutrition and Hydration

In the comatose child fluids and calories are supplied initially by the IV route. (See Chapter 28.) An IV infusion is started early, and the type of fluid administered is determined by the general condition of the patient. Fluid therapy requires careful monitoring and adjustment based on neurologic signs and electrolyte determinations. Comatose children often cannot tolerate the same amounts of fluid as when they are healthy, and overhydration must be avoided to prevent fatal cerebral edema.

Long-term nutrition is provided in a balanced formula given by nasogastric or gastrostomy tube. The nasogastric tube is usually taped in place, with care taken to prevent pressure on the nares. Most children have continuous feedings, but if bolus feedings are used, the tube is rinsed with water after each feeding. Tubes are replaced according to institutional policy. Irritation of the nasal mucosa is prevented by alternating nares each time the nasogastric tube is replaced.

Overfeeding is avoided to prevent vomiting and the associated risk of aspiration. Stomach contents are aspirated with a syringe and measured before feeding to ascertain the amount remaining in the stomach. The removed contents are refed. If the residual volume is excessive (depending on the size of the child), the dietitian and physician should be consulted regarding the composition and amount of formula and whether changes are required to provide the needed calories and nutrients in a smaller volume.

Hydration is maintained in the same manner. When cerebral edema is a threat, fluids may be restricted to reduce the chance of fluid overload. Skin and mucous membranes are examined for signs of dehydration. Adjustments to fluid administration are based on urine output, serum electrolytes and osmolarity, blood pressure, and arterial filling pressure. Observation for signs of altered fluid balance related to abnormal pituitary secretions is a part of nursing care.

**Altered Pituitary Secretion.** An altered ability to handle fluid loads is attributed in part to the syndrome of inappro-

priate antidiuretic hormone (SIADH) and diabetes insipidus (DI) resulting from hypothalamic dysfunction. (See Chapter 38.) SIADH often accompanies CNS diseases such as head injury, meningitis, encephalitis, brain abscess, brain tumor, and subarachnoid hemorrhage. In the child with SIADH, scant quantities of urine are excreted, electrolyte analysis reveals hyponatremia and hyposmolality, and manifestations of overhydration are evident. It is important to evaluate all parameters because the reduced urinary output might be erroneously interpreted as a sign of dehydration.

The treatment of SIADH consists of restriction of fluids until serum electrolytes and osmolality return to normal levels. Because SIADH often occurs with meningitis in children, fluid restriction is often prescribed until serum electrolytes and osmolality return to normal levels. Likewise, DI may occur following intracranial trauma. There is increased urinary volume and the accompanying danger of dehydration. See Table 37-3 for comparison of fluid changes in SIADH and DI. Adequate replacement of fluids is essential, and observation of electrolyte balance is necessary to detect signs of hypernatremia and hyperosmolality. Exogenous vasopressin may be administered.

## Medications

The cause of unconsciousness determines specific drug therapies. Children with infectious processes are given antibiotics to treat the infecting organism. Corticosteroids are prescribed for inflammatory conditions and edema. Cerebral edema is an indication for osmotic diuretics. Sedatives or antiepileptics are prescribed for seizure activity. Sedation in the combative child provides amnesic and anxiolytic properties in conjunction with a paralytic agent. The combination decreases ICP and allows treatment of cerebral edema. Usual drugs include morphine, midazolam (Versed), and pancuronium. Midazolam is attractive because of its short half-life.

Deep coma induced by the administration of barbiturates is controversial in the management of ICP. Barbiturates are currently reserved for the reduction of increased ICP when all else has failed. Barbiturates decrease the cerebral metabolic rate for oxygen and protect the brain during times of reduced central perfusion pressure. Barbiturate coma requires extensive monitoring, cardiovascular and respiratory support, and ICP monitoring to assess response to therapy. Paralyzing agents such as pancuronium (Pavulon) also may be needed to aid in performing diagnostic tests, improving effectiveness of therapy, and reducing the risks of

**TABLE 37-3** Effects of altered pituitary secretion

| Measurement | Diabetes Insipidus | Syndrome of Inappropriate Antidiuretic Hormone |
|---|---|---|
| Urinary output | Increased | Decreased |
| Specific gravity | Decreased | Increased |
| Serum sodium | Increased (hypernatremia) | Decreased (hyponatremia) |

secondary complications. Elevation of ICP or heart rate in patients who are being given paralyzing agents or are under sedation may indicate the need for another dose of either or both medications.

## Thermoregulation

Hyperthermia often accompanies cerebral dysfunction; if present, measures are implemented to reduce the temperature to prevent brain damage from hyperthermia and to reduce metabolic demands generated by the increased body temperature. Antipyretics are the method of choice for fever reduction; cooling devices are used for hyperthermia. (See Controlling Elevated Temperatures, Chapter 27.) Laboratory tests and other methods are used in an attempt to determine the cause, if any, of the hyperthermia. Treatment with hypothermia and barbiturates increases the risk of iatrogenic complications.

## Elimination

A urinary catheter is usually inserted in the unconscious child, although diapers may be used and weighed to record urinary output. The child who previously had bowel and bladder control is generally incontinent. If the child remains comatose for a long period, the indwelling catheter may be removed and periodic bladder emptying accomplished by intermittent catheterization. Stool softeners are usually sufficient to maintain bowel function, but suppositories or enemas may be needed occasionally for adequate elimination and to prevent fecal impaction. The passage of liquid stool after a period of no bowel activity is usually a sign of impaction. To avoid this preventable problem, daily recording of bowel activity is essential.

## Hygienic Care

Routine measures for cleansing and maintaining skin integrity are an integral part of nursing care of the unconscious child. Skin folds require special attention to prevent excoriation. The child who is unable to move is prone to develop tissue breakdown and necrosis; therefore the child is placed on a resilient appliance (e.g., alternating-pressure or water-filled mattress) to prevent pressure on prominent areas of the body. The goal is prevention by regular change of position and inspection of vulnerable areas (e.g., the ankle, heels, trochanter, sacrum, and shoulder). Unconscious children undergo numerous invasive procedures, and the skin sites used for these procedures require special assessment and intervention to promote healing and to prevent infection. Bed linen and any clothing are kept dry and free of wrinkles. Rubbing the back and extremities with lotion stimulates circulation and helps prevent drying of the skin. However, to prevent further tissue damage, reddened and nonblanching skin is not massaged. (See Maintaining Healthy Skin, Chapter 27.) If the child requires surgery or radiography, the nurse checks all dressings, bony sites, catheters, and IV access lines before and after the procedure.

Mouth care is performed at least twice daily because the mouth tends to become dry or coated with mucus. The teeth are carefully brushed with a soft toothbrush or cleaned with gauze saturated with saline. Commercially prepared cleansing devices, such as Toothettes, are convenient for cleansing the mouth and teeth. Lips are coated with ointment (e.g., A & D ointment, or wax-based lipstick-style balm) to protect them from drying, cracking, or blistering.

The deeply comatose child is also prone to eye irritation. The corneal reflexes are absent; therefore the eyes are easily irritated or damaged by linen, dust, or other substances that may come in contact with them. There is excessive dryness as a result of decreased secretions, especially if there is incomplete closure of the lids or if the child is undergoing osmotherapy to reduce or prevent brain edema.

> **NURSING ALERT**
> The eyes are examined regularly and carefully for early signs of irritation or inflammation. Artificial tears (methylcellulose) are placed in the eyes every 1 to 2 hours. Eye patches may be required to protect the eyes from possible damage.

The child's hair should be kept combed and secured to prevent tangling. The scalp is kept clean with dry or wet shampoos as needed. The child's head may be shaved for tests or surgical procedures. If so, the hair should be saved if possible and given to the family.

## Positioning and Exercise

The unconscious child is positioned to minimize ICP and to prevent aspiration of saliva, nasogastric secretions, and vomitus. The head of the bed is elevated, and the child is placed in a side-lying or semiprone position. A small, firm pillow is placed under the head, and the uppermost limbs are flexed and supported with pillows. The weight of the body should not rest on the dependent arm. In the semiprone position the child lies with the dependent arm at the side behind the body; the opposite side is supported on pillows, and the uppermost arm and leg are flexed and resting on the pillows. This position prevents undue pressure on the dependent extremities. The dependent position of the face encourages drainage of secretions and prevents the flaccid tongue from obstructing the airway.

Normal range-of-motion exercises help to maintain function and prevent contractures of joints. Exercises should be performed gently and with full range of motion. A small rolled pad can be placed in the palms to help maintain proper positioning of fingers; footboards or high-top shoes (e.g., running or tennis shoes) can be used to help prevent footdrop; splinting may be needed to prevent severe contractures of the wrist, knee, or ankle in decerebrate children.

## Stimulation

Sensory stimulation is as important in the care of the unconscious child as it is in the care of the alert child. For the temporarily unconscious or semiconscious child, sensory stimulation helps to arouse the child to the conscious state and orient the child in terms of time and place. Auditory and tactile stimulation is especially valuable. Tactile stimulation is not appropriate for a child in whom it may elicit an undesirable response. However, for other children tactile contact often has a relaxing and calming effect. When the child's condition permits, holding or rocking the child has a soothing effect and provides the body contact needed by young children.

The auditory sense is often intact in a state of coma. Hearing is the last sense to be lost and the first one to be regained; therefore the child should be spoken to as if he or she can hear. Conversation around the child should not include thoughtless or derogatory remarks. Soft music is often used to provide auditory stimulation. Singing the child's favorite songs or reading a favorite story is a tactic used to maintain the child's contact with a familiar world. Having parents tape songs or stories provides a continuous source of familiar voices.

## Family Support

Dealing with the parents of an unconscious child is especially difficult. They may demonstrate all the guilt, fear, hos-

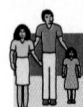

### FAMILY FOCUS
#### *Understanding the Child's Recovery from a Comatose State*

Recovering from coma is a complex process and may be confusing for parents and family members, who are already anxious and overwhelmed. Understanding the stages of recovery may assist parents in coping with the situation. It is important to remember that comatose children may not complete all stages of the recovery process and that they may manifest characteristics of more than one stage at a time.

**Level 1:** No response—child does not respond to stimuli but may be able to hear what is said in the room.
**Level 2:** Generalized response—child responds to painful or unpleasant stimuli; responses may not be consistent and may be delayed.
**Level 3:** Localized response—child responds purposefully to painful or unpleasant stimuli by trying to pull away; turns toward sounds; responds to simple commands.
**Level 4:** Confused, agitated—child becomes restless, aggressive, frustrated; exhibits abnormal behavior; forgets answers to frequently asked questions.
**Level 5:** Confused, inappropriate, nonagitated—child behaves more calmly; behavior starts to normalize but may become frustrated; voice and face lack expression; follows simple commands; performs simple tasks.
**Level 6:** Confused, appropriate—child is less frustrated and is able to concentrate for longer periods of time (up to 30 minutes); short-term memory is improving; responses to questions are more appropriate but may not be correct.
**Level 7:** Automatic, appropriate—child's memory continues to improve, although details may not be clear; continues to have difficulty concentrating; preexisting behavioral or learning problems may be worse than before the comatose state.
**Level 8:** Purposeful—child's basic thinking skills will have recovered to the maximum extent; incidental changes in social skills, memory, and concentration may continue for months; will fully understand what happened and may grieve over how things have changed.

Modified from *A Booklet for Parents: Recovering from Brain Injury*, Toronto, 1996, The Hospital for Sick Children. Stages for recovery are based on the Rancho Los Amigos Scale, copyright Rancho Los Amigos, 1989; revised by CJ Wright, MSN, RNC, Children's Hospital Trauma Center.

tility, and anxiety of any parent of a seriously ill child. (See Chapter 23.) In addition, these parents are faced with the uncertain outcome of the cerebral dysfunction. The fear of death, mental retardation, or other permanent disability is present. Nursing intervention with parents depends on the nature of the pathologic condition, the personality of the parents, and the parent-child relationship before injury or illness. (See Family Focus box.)

The child may regain consciousness within a short time. If there is little or no residual effect, the child will be discharged or transferred to home care fairly soon. The parents need the most intensive nursing intervention during the period of crisis and uncertainty. During the recovery phase they are given information, which is clarified as needed, and are encouraged to become involved in the child's care. Often the child's hospitalization is brief; however, some children require extended hospitalization for intensive therapy and rehabilitation.

The parents of children who die require support and guidance in order to cope with the reality of the death and resolving their grief. (See Chapter 23.)

Probably the most difficult situations are those that involve children who never regain consciousness. Unlike losing a child through death, finality is lacking for these parents, which often leaves them in a state of suspended grief. Like parents of dying children, parents of the comatose child search for any signs of hope. Well-meaning friends and relatives relate instances of miraculous recoveries. The parents seek confirmation and support for such possibilities and assign erroneous meanings to any sign in the child that might be interpreted as evidence of recovery (e.g., reflexive muscle contractions).

At these times nurses need to respond with compassion and honesty. They can acknowledge that miraculous recoveries do occur but are rare. The important message is to maintain open communication with the family.

Like parents who lose a child through death, the parents of a child who is comatose attempt to construct a representation of the child. They bring items that belong to the child, such as favorite toys, music, and other objects. This is interpreted as an attempt to provide stimulation for the child in the hope of eliciting a response, to let the hospital staff know the child as the unique individual he or she was, and to reconstitute an image of the child "lost" to them and for whom they mourn. An awareness of these behaviors and coping mechanisms provides nurses with an understanding that helps them support the parents throughout the grief process.

In addition to the process of grieving for the "lost" child are the difficult decisions the parents may face. When the child is so neurologically impaired that vital functions must be maintained by artificial means, the parents must make the final decision to remove the life-support systems. Because this decision is so difficult for parents, the practitioner is often placed in a position of making the decision indirectly. After providing the parents with all the information, the practitioner may suggest that the child be removed from life support to "see if the child can make it without help." The approach relieves the parents of the decision and can be effective, but it is based on an evaluation of the parents' intellectual level and emotional state. Sometimes parents may even choose to refuse treatment if they believe doing so is best for the child and the family (informed dissent). At other times parents request that "everything possible" be done for the child.

The nurse can be instrumental in providing guidance and clarifying information—a valued but demanding undertaking. It is not unusual for the family to ask the same questions and to compare responses elicited from different staff members. A child's death is an intensely personal issue that deserves direct involvement by the nurse and auxiliary support systems.

When the child has survived the illness or injury that produced the brain damage but is left permanently unconscious, the parents must decide whether to place the child in a chronic care facility or to care for the child at home. The nurse can listen to the parents' discussions regarding alternatives, provide information where appropriate, and support the family in their decision. The nurse can help the family to prepare for the transfer of the child and make referrals to persons or agencies that can provide additional assistance.

When the child has survived the cerebral insult and is not comatose but has limited physical or mental capacity (either minimal or severe), families must cope with the long and tedious rehabilitation process and uncertain outcome. The drain on financial, emotional, and social resources can be enormous.

For parents who choose to care for their child at home, planning for home care begins early in the process of recovery. Family members should become involved with the care of the child as soon as they indicate an interest and ability to do so. They need education and support in learning to care for the child, regular follow-up observation and assessment of the home management, and planning for respite care. Parents need to understand that it is important to plan for periodic relief from the continual care of the child. (See Discharge Planning and Home Care, Chapter 26, and Family-Centered Home Care, Chapter 25.)

## ■■ Evaluation

The effectiveness of nursing interventions for the unconscious child is determined by continual reassessment and evaluation of care based on the following observational guidelines:

1. Monitor child's neurologic signs, vital signs, and behavior. Compare neurologic status and behavior with preillness/trauma state.
2. Observe child's response to nursing activities, therapies, and diagnostic procedures; monitor ICP.
3. Observe child's color, position, and motor activity; measure fluid and nutritional intake and output.
4. Monitor status of child's respiratory, renal, and gastrointestinal systems and skin.
5. Observe family behaviors and interview members regarding their understandings, feelings, and concerns.

The *expected outcomes* are described in the Nursing Care Plan on pp. 1662-1664.

## Head Injury

Head injury is a pathologic process that involves the scalp, skull, meninges, or brain as a result of mechanical force. According to national statistics and the Safe Kids Campaign,* injuries are the number one health risk for children and the leading cause of death in children older than 1 year of age. Each year, one child in four in the United States will suffer an injury serious enough to require medical attention. Tragically, 8000 children are killed every year by injuries, and nearly 120,000 are permanently disabled. It has been estimated that, each year, 300 per 100,000 children have a traumatic brain injury, with 10 per 100,000 children dying as a result of the brain injury. Studies indicate that as many as three fourths of the childhood deaths caused by mechanical trauma are the direct result of a brain injury.

### Etiology

The three major causes of brain damage in childhood, in order of importance, are falls, motor vehicle injuries, and bicycle injuries (Fig. 37-6). Neurologic injury accounts for the highest mortality, with boys usually affected twice as often as girls. Falls account for 35% of all head injuries in children (Fisher, 1997). Motor vehicle accidents account for approximately 80% of children with severe head injury. Children less than 2 years of age are almost exclusively injured as passengers, whereas older children may also be injured as pedestrians or cyclists. The majority of deaths from brain trauma caused by bicycle injuries occur between the ages of 5 and 15 years. With the advent of bike helmet laws, this should be a decreasing trend.

Many of the physical characteristics of children predispose them to craniocerebral trauma. For example, infants are often left unattended on beds, in high chairs, and in other places from which they can fall. Because the head of

*SAFE KIDS, 1301 Pennsylvania Ave NW, Suite 1000, Washington, DC 20004-1707, (202) 662-0600, fax: (202) 393-2072; www.safekids.org.

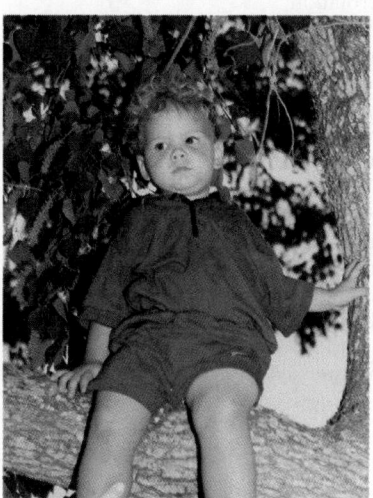

**Fig. 37-6** Children possess a sense of adventure and wonder; however, falls remain the leading cause of head injury in children under 5 years of age.

# Nursing Care Plan
## The Unconscious Child

**NURSING DIAGNOSIS:** Risk for suffocation (aspiration): ineffective airway clearance related to depressed sensorium, impaired motor function

**PATIENT GOAL 1:** Will maintain patent airway

- **NURSING INTERVENTIONS/*RATIONALES***

Position for optimum ventilation
   Insert oral airway if indicated
   Position with neck slightly extended and nose in "sniffing" position *to open trachea fully*
   Avoid neck hyperextension, *which can block airway*
   Place in semiprone or side-lying position *to prevent aspiration*
Remove accumulated secretions promptly *to prevent aspiration*
Provide routine care of endotracheal tube or tracheostomy if appropriate; have equipment available for emergency insertion for respiratory distress *to prevent delay in treatment*
Monitor artificial ventilation

- **EXPECTED OUTCOME**

Airway remains patent

**NURSING DIAGNOSIS:** Risk for injury related to physical immobility, depressed sensorium, intracranial pathology

**PATIENT GOAL 1:** Will maintain stable intracranial pressure (ICP)

- **NURSING INTERVENTIONS/*RATIONALES***

Elevate head of bed 15 to 30 degrees with child's head in midline position *to facilitate venous drainage and avoid jugular compression*
Avoid positions or activities that increase ICP
   Pressure on neck veins
      Turning side-to-side *(risk of jugular compression)*
   Flexion or hyperextension of neck
   Head rotation
   Valsalva maneuver
   Painful stimuli
   Respiratory procedures (especially suctioning, percussion)
Prevent constipation *(Valsalva maneuver increases ICP)*
   *Administer stool softener as prescribed
   Closely monitor bowel elimination when child is receiving codeine *(constipating effect)*
Minimize emotional stress and crying *(increased ICP)*
   Provide quiet, subdued environment
   Use therapeutic touch
   Avoid emotionally stressful conversation (e.g., about pain, condition, prognosis)
   *Administer sedation, if ordered, for extreme agitation or restlessness

Prevent or relieve pain, *(increased ICP)*
   Closely observe child for signs of pain, especially changes in behavior (e.g., agitation); increased heart rate, respiratory rate, and blood pressure *(usually increase with pain);* decreased oxygen saturation
   Observe child's response during times of induced or suspected pain
   Observe child's response following a painful procedure or the administration of analgesia
   Use pain assessment record (see Chapter 26)
   *Administer paralyzing and analgesic agents if prescribed
Schedule disturbing procedures to take advantage of therapies that reduce ICP (e.g., bathe child after sedation or osmotherapy)
Monitor ICP monitoring device

- **EXPECTED OUTCOMES**

ICP remains within safe limits
Child shows no evidence of sustained increased ICP

**PATIENT GOAL 2:** Will exhibit no signs of cerebral hypoxia

- **NURSING INTERVENTIONS/*RATIONALES***

Maintain patent airway *(respiratory obstruction leads to cardiac arrest)*
Provide oxygen as indicated by objective signs or as ordered
*Hyperventilate at prescribed intervals if ordered
Monitor blood gases and pH
If child is on mechanical ventilation:
   Monitor for correct settings, proper functioning
   Prepare to provide artificial ventilation in case of ventilatory failure; have manual resuscitation bag at bedside
*Administer medications as ordered *to prevent cerebral edema and improve cerebral circulation*

- **EXPECTED OUTCOME**

Child breathes easily; respirations are within normal limits (see inside back cover)

**PATIENT GOAL 3:** Will exhibit no evidence of cerebral edema

- **NURSING INTERVENTIONS/*RATIONALES***

Elevate head of bed to 15 to 30 degrees *to facilitate venous drainage*
Maintain IV fluids as prescribed
   Avoid overhydration *to prevent cerebral edema*
Monitor intake and output
Monitor electrolyte balance and specific gravity *to detect signs of hypernatremia and hyperosmolality; diabetes insipidus and the syndrome of inappropriate antidiuretic hormone commonly occur with CNS diseases and trauma*
*Administer hyperosmolar fluids as prescribed
*Administer corticosteroids as ordered

- **EXPECTED OUTCOME**

Child exhibits no signs of sustained increased ICP

*Dependent nursing action.

# Nursing Care Plan
## The Unconscious Child–cont'd

**PATIENT GOAL 4:** Will experience no seizures

- **NURSING INTERVENTIONS/***RATIONALES***

Avoid stimulation that precipitates undesirable responses
Cluster nursing activities for minimum disturbance
*Administer antiepileptic drugs as prescribed
    IV fosphenytoin (Cerebyx) is often used to treat seizures
       instead of IV phenytoin because of possible complica-
       tions associated with IV phenytoin
    If IV phenytoin is ordered, administer carefully and
       observe the following precautions:
       Administer via slow IV push (not to exceed 50 mg/min)
          *(rapid administration may cause cardiac dysrhythmias)*
       Infuse completely in 1 hour *(drug tends to precipitate)*
       Never mix phenytoin with 5% dextrose *(drug will*
          *precipitate)*
       Dilute phenytoin with normal saline *to decrease vein*
          *irritation and pain*

- **EXPECTED OUTCOME**

Child exhibits no seizure activity or undue restlessness and
    agitation

**PATIENT GOAL 5:** Will exhibit stable body
temperature

- **NURSING INTERVENTIONS/***RATIONALES***

Closely monitor child's temperature *(hypothermia, hyperthermia*
    *often occur with CNS dysfunction)*
Remove excess coverings
*Administer antipyretics if prescribed for fever
Give tepid sponge bath if indicated, only for hyperthermia,
    not for fever, *(it may induce shivering)*
Apply and monitor hypothermia blanket if indicated and
    ordered

- **EXPECTED OUTCOME**

Body temperature remains within safe limits (See inside back
    cover.)

**PATIENT GOAL 6:** Will exhibit no evidence of
respiratory tract infection

- **NURSING INTERVENTIONS/***RATIONALES***

Turn frequently—at least every 2 hours, as tolerated, unless
    contraindicated by increased ICP
Keep persons with upper respiratory tract infection away
    from child
Use good handwashing technique
Keep all equipment in contact with child clean or sterile
Provide good oral hygiene *to decrease risk of infection*
Perform chest physiotherapy if prescribed and as tolerated;
    avoid percussion

- **EXPECTED OUTCOME**

Child exhibits no evidence of pulmonary dysfunction

**PATIENT GOAL 7:** Will experience no corneal
irritation

- **NURSING INTERVENTIONS/***RATIONALES***

Patch eye, if indicated
Keep lids completely closed *to protect corneas when corneal*
    *reflexes are absent*
Instill "artificial tears" *to lubricate eyes*
Assess eyes carefully for early signs of irritation or
    inflammation

- **EXPECTED OUTCOME**

Corneas remain clear and moist

**PATIENT GOAL 8:** Will exhibit no breakdown in
mucous membrane integrity

- **NURSING INTERVENTIONS/***RATIONALES***

Provide meticulous mouth care, *because mouth tends to become*
    *dry or coated with mucus*
Avoid drying products (e.g., lemon glycerin and alcohol)

- **EXPECTED OUTCOME**

Mucous membranes remain moist and free of irritation

**PATIENT GOAL 9:** Will experience no physical injury

- **NURSING INTERVENTIONS/***RATIONALES***

Keep siderails up *to prevent falls*
Pad hard surfaces *that may injure extremities during spontaneous*
    *or involuntary movements*

- **EXPECTED OUTCOME**

Child remains free of physical injury

**PATIENT GOAL 10:** Will maintain limb flexibility and
full range of motion

- **NURSING INTERVENTIONS/***RATIONALES***

Perform passive range-of-motion exercises *to prevent contractures*
Position *to reduce contractures*
    Place small, rolled pad in palms to *maintain proper position*
       *of fingers*
    Use footboard or ankle-high shoes *to prevent footdrop*
    Splint joints, if needed, *to prevent severe contractures of*
       *wrists, knees, and ankles*

- **EXPECTED OUTCOME**

Joints remain flexible and retain full range of motion

> **NURSING DIAGNOSIS:** Risk for impaired skin
> integrity related to immobility, bodily secretions, inva-
> sive procedures

**PATIENT GOAL 1:** Will maintain skin integrity

- **NURSING INTERVENTIONS/***RATIONALES***

Place child on pressure-reducing surface *to prevent tissue*
    *breakdown and pressure necrosis*
Change position frequently unless contraindicated by
    increased ICP
Protect pressure points (e.g., trochanter, sacrum, ankle,
    heels, shoulder, occiput)

---

*Dependent nursing action.

*Continued*

## Nursing Care Plan
### The Unconscious Child–cont'd

Inspect skin surfaces regularly for signs of irritation, redness, excoriation

Cleanse skin regularly, at least once daily

Protect skinfold and surfaces that rub together *to prevent excoriation*

Keep clothing and linen clean, dry, and free of wrinkles

Provide out good perineal care

Gently massage skin with lotion or other lubricating substance, unless on existing reddened pressure areas, *to stimulate circulation and prevent drying*

Protect lips with cream or ointment *to prevent drying and cracking*

• **EXPECTED OUTCOME**

Skin remains clean, intact, and free of irritation

---

**NURSING DIAGNOSIS:** Feeding, bathing/hygiene, toileting self-care deficits related to physical immobility, perceptual and cognitive impairment

---

**PATIENT GOAL 1:** Will receive optimum nutrition

• **NURSING INTERVENTIONS/***RATIONALES*

Provide nourishment in manner suitable to child's condition

Monitor IV feedings when ordered

Record intake and output

Weigh daily or as ordered

• **EXPECTED OUTCOME**

Child obtains sufficient nourishment

**PATIENT GOAL 2:** Will receive proper hygienic care

• **NURSING INTERVENTIONS/***RATIONALES*

Bathe daily or more often if indicated

Dress appropriately

Keep hair clean

• **EXPECTED OUTCOME**

Child appears clean and as well groomed as possible within limitations of condition

**PATIENT GOAL 3:** Will void and defecate adequately

• **NURSING INTERVENTIONS/***RATIONALES*

Provide sufficient liquid intake, unless contraindicated by cerebral edema or if overhydration is a threat

Apply urine-collecting device or insert indwelling catheter (if ordered)

Provide proper care of catheter

Clean skin well after elimination *to prevent skin irritation*

Diaper as needed *to contain stool and urine*

Check abdomen for evidence of distention

  Measure abdominal girth *to detect enlargement*

*Administer stool softener *to prevent constipation*

*Administer suppositories or enema as indicated *to promote evacuation*

• **EXPECTED OUTCOMES**

Child eliminates sufficient urine (in accordance with intake)

Bowel is evacuated daily

Child's diaper area remains clean and free of irritation

---

**NURSING DIAGNOSIS:** Disturbed sensory perception (visual, auditory, kinesthetic, gustatory, tactile, olfactory) related to central nervous system impairment, bed rest

---

**PATIENT GOAL 1:** Will receive appropriate sensory stimulation

• **NURSING INTERVENTIONS/***RATIONALES*

Provide tactile stimulation as tolerated

Provide auditory stimulation (e.g., by voice, radio, music box)

Provide visual stimuli appropriate for age

Provide proprioceptive stimulation (e.g., by rocking, cuddling) suitable for the child's condition

Encourage family to participate in stimulation program

• **EXPECTED OUTCOMES**

Child receives sensory stimulation appropriate to age and condition

Child appears relaxed and rests quietly

Stimulation does not induce seizures or increase ICP

**PATIENT GOAL 2:** Will exhibit no evidence of pain

• **NURSING INTERVENTIONS/***RATIONALES*

Assess for evidence of pain

Use pain assessment record *to document effectiveness of interventions*

*Administer pain medication as needed

• **EXPECTED OUTCOME**

Child exhibits no evidence of pain

---

**NURSING DIAGNOSIS:** Interrupted family processes related to a child hospitalized with a potentially fatal condition or permanent disability

---

**PATIENT (FAMILY) GOAL 1:** Will receive adequate support

• **NURSING INTERVENTIONS/***RATIONALES* **AND EXPECTED OUTCOMES**

See Nursing Care Plan: The Family of the Child Who Is Ill or Hospitalized, Chapter 26.

**PATIENT (FAMILY) GOAL 2:** Will express feelings and concerns

• **NURSING INTERVENTIONS/***RATIONALES*

Provide needed information

Answer family's questions; encourage expression of feelings

Refer to persons or agencies for further information and clarification

Support parents' decisions

• **EXPECTED OUTCOME**

Family verbalizes feelings and concerns

---

*Dependent nursing action.

an infant or toddler is proportionally large and heavy in relation to other body parts, it is the most likely to be injured. Incomplete motor development contributes to falls at young ages, and the natural curiosity and exuberance of children increase their risk for injury.

## Pathophysiology

The pathology of brain injury is directly related to the force of impact. Intracranial contents (brain, blood, CSF) are damaged because the force is too great to be absorbed by the skull and musculoligamentous support of the head. The elastic, pliable skulls of infants and young children absorb much of the direct energy of physical impact to the head and afford some protection to intracranial structures. Although nervous tissue is delicate, it usually requires a severe blow to cause significant damage.

A child's response to head injury is different from that of adults. The larger head size and insufficient musculoskeletal support render the very young child particularly vulnerable to acceleration-deceleration injuries. The surface area of the child's scalp is large and has remarkable vascularity; therefore a child can bleed to death from a severe scalp laceration.

Primary head injuries are those that occur at the time of trauma and include skull fractures, contusions, intracranial hematomas, and diffuse injuries. Secondary injury includes hypoxic brain damage, increased ICP, infection, and cerebral edema. The predominant feature of a child's brain injury is the diffuse amount of swelling that occurs. Hypoxia and hypercapnia threaten the energy requirements of the brain and increase CBF. The added volume across the blood-brain barrier plus the loss of autoregulation exacerbates cerebral edema. Pressure inside the skull that is greater than arterial pressure results in inadequate perfusion.

Cerebral edema results from an increase in the fluid content of brain tissue and causes an increase in ICP (Vernon-Levett, 1998). Because the cranium of very young children has the ability to expand and the thin skull is more compliant, they may tolerate increases in ICP better than older children and adults.

Physical forces act on the head through *acceleration, deceleration,* or *deformation.* Acceleration or deceleration is more descriptive of the circumstances responsible for most head injuries. When the stationary head receives a blow, the sudden acceleration causes deformation of the skull and mass movement of the brain. Continued movement of the intracranial contents allows the brain to strike parts of the skull (e.g., the sharp edges of the sphenoid or the irregular surface of the anterior fossa) or the edges of the tentorium.

Although the brain volume remains unchanged, significant distortion and cavitation occur as the brain changes shape in response to the force transmitted from the impact to the skull. This deformation can cause bruising at the point of impact *(coup)* or at a distance as the brain collides with the unyielding surfaces opposite or far removed from the point of impact *(contrecoup)* (Fig. 37-7). Children with an acceleration/deceleration injury demonstrate diffuse generalized cerebral swelling produced by increased blood volume or by a redistribution of cerebral blood volume

(cerebral hyperemia) rather than by the increased water content (edema) seen in adults. Thus a blow to the occipital region can cause severe injury to the frontal and temporal areas of the brain. Sudden deceleration, as takes place during a fall, causes the greatest cerebral injury at the point of impact.

Another effect of brain movement is *shearing forces,* which are caused by unequal movement or different rates of acceleration at various levels of the brain. A shearing force may tear small arteries that travel from the cerebral surfaces through the meninges to the dural sinuses to cause subdural hemorrhages. Shearing or stretching effects can also be transmitted to nerve fibers. Maximum stress from the shearing force occurs at the interface between structures of different density so that the gray matter (cell body) rapidly accelerates while the white matter (axons) tends to lag behind. Although shearing forces are maximum at the cerebral surface and extend toward the center of rotation within the brain, the most serious effects are often in the area of the brainstem.

Another source of damage occurs when severe compression of the skull causes the brain to be forced through the tentorial opening. This can produce irreparable damage to the brainstem (Fig. 37-8). Because the uncus of the temporal lobe is the presenting part, this complication is usually referred to as uncal herniation.

As a whole, head injuries can be regarded as localized or generalized. In *localized injuries* the force is spent on a local area of both the skull and underlying tissues; in *gen-*

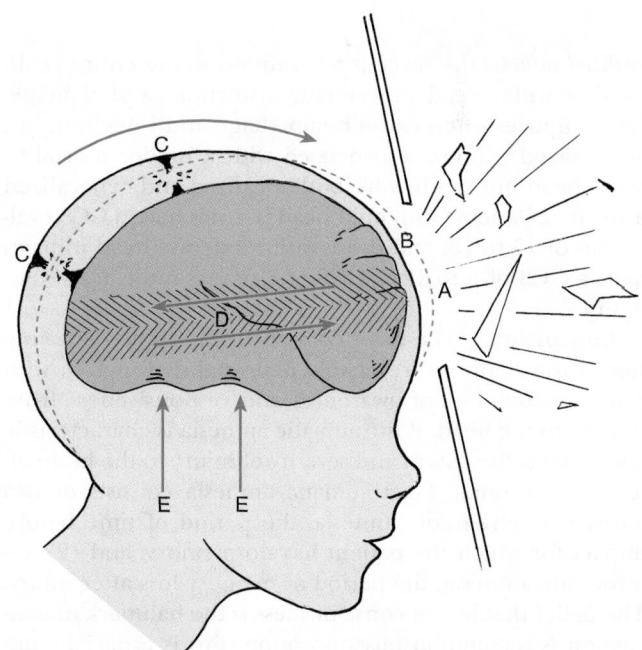

**Fig. 37-7** Mechanical distortion of cranium during closed head injury. **A,** Preinjury contour of skull. **B,** Immediate postinjury contour of skull. **C,** Torn subdural vessels. **D,** Shearing forces. **E,** Trauma from contact with floor of cranium. (Redrawn from Grubb RL, Coxe WS: Central nervous system trauma: cranial. In Eliasson SG, Presky AL, Hardin WB Jr, editors: *Neurological pathophysiology,* New York, 1974, Oxford University Press.)

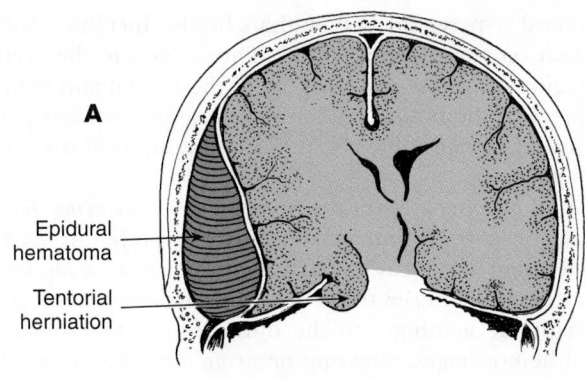

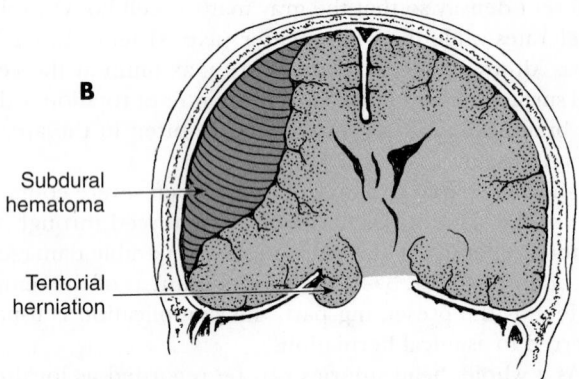

**Fig. 37-8** **A,** Epidural (extradural) hematoma and compression of temporal lobe through tentorial hiatus. **B,** Subdural hematoma.

*eralized injuries* the force is transmitted to the entire skull, causing widespread movement, distortion, and damage. Local injuries often cause hemorrhage and infection, but generalized trauma is associated with a higher mortality. Many head injuries involve both localized and generalized disorders. Patients with mild head injuries have a GCS evaluation of 13 to 15, and those with moderate head injuries have a GCS of 9 to 12; a GCS of 8 or less indicates severe injury.

**Concussion.**   The most common head injury is *concussion,* a transient and reversible neuronal dysfunction with instantaneous loss of awareness and responsiveness from trauma to the head. Posttraumatic amnesia is characteristic and reflects the extent and severity of injury to the brain after blunt trauma. Posttraumatic amnesia consists of two parts: (1) retrograde amnesia, the period of time before impact for which the patient has no memory, and (2) anterograde amnesia, the period of memory loss after injury. The belief that loss of consciousness is the hallmark of concussion is a common misconception; this is especially untrue for children. Concussion is correctly defined as "a traumatically induced alteration in mental status." Confusion and amnesia following head impact are the hallmarks of concussion.

The pathogenesis of concussion is still unclear but may be a result of shearing forces that cause stretching, com-

pression, and tearing of nerve fibers, particularly in the area of the central brainstem, the seat of the reticular activating system. It has also been suggested that the anatomic alterations of nerve fibers cause the release of large quantities of acetylcholine into the CSF and a reduction in oxygen consumption with increased lactate production.

**Contusion and Laceration.**   The terms *contusion* and *laceration* are used to describe actual bruising and tearing of cerebral tissue. Contusions represent petechial hemorrhages or localized bruising along the superficial aspects of the brain at the site of impact (coup injury) or a lesion remote from the site of direct trauma (contrecoup injury). In serious accidents there may be multiple sites of injury.

The major areas of the brain susceptible to contusion or laceration are the occipital, frontal, and temporal lobes. Also, the irregular surfaces of the anterior and middle fossae at the base of the skull are capable of producing bruises or lacerations on forceful impact. Contusions may cause focal disturbances in strength, sensation, or visual awareness. The degree of brain damage in the contused areas varies according to the extent of vascular injury. Signs vary from mild, transient weakness of a limb to prolonged unconsciousness and paralysis. However, the signs and symptoms may be clinically indistinguishable from concussion.

The lower incidence of cerebral contusion in infancy has been attributed to the infant's pliable skull, with less convolutional markings of the inner space between brain tissue and bone. The infant's brain tissue has a softer consistency, which also reduces surface injury. However, infants who are roughly shaken (shaken baby syndrome) can sustain profound neurologic impairment, seizures, retinal hemorrhages (usually bilateral), and intracranial subarachnoid or subdural hemorrhages (McCabe and Donahue, 2000). In addition to these classic injuries other skeletal fractures and injury may occur (Castiglia, 2001).

Cerebral lacerations are generally associated with penetrating or depressed skull fractures. However, they may occur without fracture in small children. When brain tissue is actually torn, with bleeding into and around the tear, more severe and prolonged unconsciousness and paralysis usually occur, leaving permanent scarring and some degree of disability.

**Fractures.**   Because of its flexibility, the immature skull is able to sustain a greater degree of deformation than the adult skull before incurring a fracture. It requires a great deal of force to produce a fracture in the skull of an infant. A fracture may occur with little or no brain damage, or severe and fatal brain injury can take place without fracture. The undersurface of the skull contains grooves in which the meningeal arteries lie. A fracture that runs through one of these grooves may tear the artery and produce severe and damaging hemorrhage. Hypovolemic hypotension can occur in infants with skull fractures.

The types of fractures that occur are linear, depressed, compound, basilar, and diastatic. As a rule, the faster the blow, the greater the likelihood of a depressed fracture; a low-velocity impact tends to produce a linear fracture. *Linear fractures* are uncommon before 2 to 3 years of age but constitute the majority of childhood skull fractures.

The lines of the fracture are predetermined by the site and velocity of the impact, as well as the strength of the bone. Linear fractures are often asymptomatic in older children and heal in 3 to 4 months without special treatment unless they involve a blood vessel, enter the paranasal sinuses, or impinge on the brainstem or cranial nerves. The location of the fracture often provides clues to the possibility of such complications. For example, a fracture that extends through the squamous portion of the temporal bone is more apt to be associated with laceration of the middle meningeal artery, and fractures extending through the base of the skull may cause leakage of CSF or blood into either the auditory or the nasal passages. In infants the uneven ossification and the absence of buttresses cause fracture lines to be irregular and follow no predictable pattern.

*Depressed fractures* are those in which the bone is locally broken, usually into several irregular fragments that are pushed inward, causing pressure on the brain. This pressure constitutes a neurosurgical emergency that requires surgical intervention to elevate the fracture. The inner portion of the bone is more extensively fragmented than the outer portion, which almost invariably produces tears in the dura. Depressed skull fractures may be associated with direct underlying parenchymal damage and should be suspected when a child's head appears misshapen. Both linear and comminuted (fracture consisting of several breaks in the bone) depressed fractures are uncommon before 2 to 3 years of age. In infants and very young children the soft, malleable bone may become dented in a peculiar rounded or "Ping-Pong ball" depression without laceration of either skin or dura. This effect is encountered occasionally in difficult deliveries, resulting from either pressure of the head against the pelvis, incorrect application of forceps or use of vacuum extraction.

*Compound fractures* consist of a skin laceration that extends to the site of the bony fracture, which can be linear, depressed, or comminuted. Prompt surgical debridement is needed (unless contraindicated by the child's clinical condition), as is reduction of the fracture either by elevating or removing fragmented bone. Antibiotic therapy is implemented.

*Basilar fractures* involve the basilar portion of the frontal, ethmoid, sphenoid, temporal, or occipital bones and usually result in a dural tear. The diagnosis of basilar fractures is difficult to make from radiographs because of the complex structure of the base of the skull. Because of the proximity of the fracture line to structures surrounding the brainstem, a basal skull fracture is a serious head injury. Clinical features include hemorrhage into the nose, nasopharynx, or middle ear (hemotympanum if it occurs behind the eardrum). Effusion of blood is seen on the posterior neck and under and posterior to the ear (Battle sign). Anterior basal fracture produces the characteristic hemorrhage about the eyes ("raccoon eyes"). CN palsies may occur and primarily involve CN I, VIII, and VII (in order of decreasing frequency). Leakage of CSF can occur between the brain floor and the nose, ears, or both. Meningitis, although rare, is always a potential risk with CSF leakage. The use of prophylactic antibiotics is controversial, and the trend has been to treat only documented cases of meningitis.

*Diastatic fractures* are traumatic separations of cranial sutures. These most commonly affect the lambdoid suture and are rarely seen beyond the first 4 years of life. They require no specific treatment but should be observed for "growing fractures." The syndrome of growing skull fracture occurs exclusively in infants and young children. For this entity to occur, the child must sustain a skull fracture (usually parietal) and a dural tear. The ongoing normal growth of a child's brain is an underlying aggravating factor. The development of a pulsatile mass or enlarging skull defect can be detected by physical examination.

## Complications

The major complications of trauma to the head are hemorrhage, infection, edema, and herniation through the tentorium. Infection is always a hazard in open injuries, and edema is related to tissue trauma. Vascular rupture may occur even in minor head injuries, causing hemorrhage between the skull and cerebral surfaces. Compression of the underlying brain produces effects that can be rapidly fatal or insidiously progressive.

**NURSING ALERT**   Posttraumatic meningitis should be suspected in children with increasing drowsiness and fever who also have basilar skull fractures.

**Epidural Hemorrhage.** Epidural (extradural) hemorrhage is usually arterial in origin, most often as a result of a skull fracture that penetrates the groove in the skull occupied by the middle meningeal artery. The lower incidence of epidural hematoma in childhood has been attributed to the fact that the middle meningeal artery is not embedded in the bone surface of the skull until approximately 2 years of age. Therefore a fracture of the temporal bone is less likely to lacerate the artery. Second, the dura closely adheres to the inner table of the skull, especially at the level of the sutures, making separation from bleeding less likely. However, a child's skull can be indented with sufficient force to tear the middle meningeal artery without causing a fracture. Hemorrhage can also originate from dural veins or the dural sinuses, especially in infants and small children, in whom fracture is less likely to occur. In 20% to 40% of children a skull fracture is not detectable.

The blood accumulates between the dura and the skull to form a hematoma. Because of the difficulty with which dura is stripped from bone, this accumulation forces the underlying brain contents downward and inward as it expands (see Fig. 37-8, *A*). Because bleeding is generally arterial, brain compression occurs rapidly. Most often the expanding hematoma is located in the parietotemporal region, which forces the medial portion of the temporal lobe under the edge of the tentorium, where it causes pressure on nerves and blood vessels. Pressure on the arterial supply and venous return to the reticular formation causes loss of consciousness; pressure on CN III (oculomotor nerve) produces dilation and (later) fixation of the ipsilateral pupil. Pressure on the fibers of the pyramidal tract is evidenced by contralateral weakness or paralysis and increased deep tendon reflexes. Extreme pressure may extend to the brainstem to cause decerebrate signs and disturbances in the respiratory and other vegetative centers.

The classic clinical picture of epidural hemorrhage (momentary unconsciousness followed by a normal period, then lethargy or coma) is seldom evident in children. The period of impaired consciousness is often lacking, and the symptom-free period is atypical because of nonspecific complaints such as irritability, headache, and vomiting. The symptom-free period often lasts longer than 48 hours. Clinically significant epidural hematomas are uncommon in children younger than 4 years of age. These differences may be caused by the decreased tendency of the resilient skull to fracture; the ability of blood to escape through widened sutures, an open fontanel, or a fracture; bleeding from smaller vessels with less rapid and massive bleeding; lower systolic blood pressure in children; and possibly the brain being less susceptible to pressure changes in children. An epidural hematoma can be detected by an initial CT scan. If the severity of the child's symptoms is not recognized, herniation and death will result. See Table 37-4 for a comparison of epidural and subdural hematomas.

**Subdural Hemorrhage.**   A subdural hemorrhage is bleeding between the dura and the cerebrum, usually venous in origin secondary to the rupture of the cortical veins

**TABLE 37-4**   Features of acute epidural and subdural hematomas

|  | Epidural | Subdural |
|---|---|---|
| **Supratentorial** | | |
| Frequency | Less | 5 to 10 times greater |
| Skull fracture | 70% | 30% |
| Source of hemorrhage | Arterial or venous | Almost always venous |
| Age | Usually older than 2 years | Usually younger than 1 year |
| Location | Usually temporoparietal | Usually frontoparietal |
| Laterality | Usually unilateral | 75% bilateral |
| Seizures | Less than 25% | 75% |
| (Pre-)retinal hemorrhages | Uncommon | Very frequent |
| Increased ICP | Present | Present |
| CT configuration | Usually lenticular | Curvilinear or crescentic |
| Mortality | Relatively high | Usually lower |
| Morbidity | Low | High |
| **Infratentorial** | | |
| Frequency | 2 to 3 times greater | Less |
| Skull fracture | Almost always | Frequent |
| Source of hemorrhage | Venous | Venous |
| Impaired consciousness | Frequent | Frequent |
| Acute hydrocephalus/ medullary compression | Variable | Variable |
| Other posterior fossa signs | Variable | Variable |

From Swaiman KF: *Pediatric neurology: principles and practice,* ed 3, St Louis, 1999, Mosby.

that bridge the subdural space (see Fig. 37-8, *B*). Subdural hematomas are 10 times more common than epidural hematomas and occur most often in infancy, with a peak incidence at 6 months.

Unlike epidural hemorrhage, which develops inwardly against the less resistant brain tissue, subdural hemorrhage tends to develop more slowly and spreads thinly and widely until it is limited by the dural barriers—the falx and tentorium. Subdural hematoma is fairly common in infants, often as a result of birth trauma, falls, assaults, or violent shaking. The small subdural space and the dura, which is firmly attached to the skull in this area, are highly vulnerable to increased ICP.

Subdural hemorrhage can cause either acute or chronic subdural hematoma. *Acute subdural hematoma* may be associated with contusions or lacerations and develops within minutes or hours of injury. *Chronic subdural hematoma* is more common. The clinical course and manifestations vary, depending on the damage sustained by the brain and the age of the child. Delayed symptoms are common in children with open fontanels and sutures. The usual presenting manifestations in children are seizures, vomiting, drowsiness, increased head circumference, and irritability or other personality changes. Older children may complain of headache.

Presenting signs of acute hematoma include evidence of increased ICP, such as increased head size and bulging fontanels (in the infant), retinal hemorrhages, extraocular palsies (especially CN VI), hemiparesis, quadriplegia and, sometimes, elevated temperature. An infant who has an altered LOC and in whom the CT scan shows subarachnoid hemorrhage or a subdural hematoma may have been physically abused.

**NURSING ALERT**   Children with a subdural hematoma and retinal hemorrhages should be evaluated for the possibility of child abuse, especially shaken baby syndrome (SBS).

Older children may display an unsteady gait, and papilledema is usually present. Because papilledema is a late sign of increased ICP, it constitutes an emergency. In infants the bleeding may be extensive enough to lower the hematocrit significantly and may be observed before any change in LOC in fast-expanding lesions. The mortality of subdural hematoma of infancy is high, probably because of severe diffuse brain injury.

Repeated subdural taps often provide relief in the infant as revealed by follow-up CT scans, improved neurologic status, and a flat anterior fontanel. Surgical evacuation of the hematoma is the treatment of choice in the older child and is often required in infants.

**Other Hemorrhagic Lesions.**   Subarachnoid and intracerebral hemorrhages may occur as a result of head injury. Seizures, nuchal rigidity, and altered consciousness are features of subarachnoid hemorrhage. Manifestations of intracranial bleeding depend on the size and location of the resulting hematoma.

**Cerebral Edema.**   Some degree of brain edema is expected after craniocerebral trauma and often accompanies any of the previously mentioned disorders. Cerebral edema peaks at 24 to 72 hours following injury and may account for changes in a child's neurologic status. Cerebral edema caused by direct cellular injury or vascular injury induces vascular stasis, anoxia, and further vasodilation. Increased tissue pressure within the skull causes venules to collapse, which leads to venous stasis and tissue anoxia. This results in loss of selective permeability of tissue membranes with increased loss of fluid from the vascular compartment to the cerebral tissues, thereby increasing cerebral edema.

There is considerable evidence indicating that cerebral autoregulatory function and $CO_2$ reactivity are impaired or absent in traumatized areas of the brain. Thus a self-perpetuating sequence of events is repeated. If this progression continues unchecked, ICP exceeds arterial pressure, fatal anoxia ensues, or the pressure causes herniation of a portion of the brain over the edge of the tentorium, compressing the brainstem and occluding the posterior cerebral arteries. Children at risk for deterioration can be identified by abnormalities seen on admitting CT scans (Ong and others, 1996).

## Diagnostic Evaluation

A detailed health history, both past and present, is essential in evaluating the child with craniocerebral trauma. Certain disorders such as drug allergies, hemophilia, diabetes mellitus, or epilepsy may produce similar symptoms. Events surrounding the injury often supply significant data. For example, if a child stumbles and falls while running and strikes the head on the sidewalk, it is usually safe to assume that the neurologic manifestations are a direct result of the injury. However, if a child collapses and in doing so strikes the head, there may be other causes that contributed to the injury. Sometimes a traumatic injury, even a minor one, will aggravate a preexisting disease process, thereby producing neurologic signs out of proportion to the injury.

Whether or not the infant or child exhibited alterations in consciousness must be determined. Usually this information is easily elicited from older children, but in young children it may be difficult to differentiate between a breath-holding spell and a seizure. The parents are asked if the infant cried immediately after the injury. After a minor injury, initial unconsciousness (if present) is brief and the child will ordinarily exhibit a transient period of confusion, somnolence, and listlessness, with this period most often accompanied by irritability, pallor, and one or more episodes of vomiting.

A severe head injury, such as one sustained in a fall from a significant height (greater than the height of the child) or a motor vehicle accident, requires immediate evaluation and treatment. Because head injuries are often accompanied by injuries in other areas (spine, viscera, extremities), the examination is performed with care to avoid further damage. Manifestations of head injury are listed in Box 37-5.

> **NURSING ALERT**
> Stabilize the spine after head injury until spinal cord injury is ruled out.

**Initial Assessment.**   Priorities in the initial phase in the care of a child with a head injury include assessment of the ABCs (airway, breathing, circulation); assessment for spinal cord injury; evaluation for shock; a neurologic examination, especially LOC; pupillary symmetry and response to light; and seizures. The assessment is carried out quickly in relation to vital signs. (See Emergency Treatment box on p. 1671.)

> **NURSING ALERT**
> Deep, rapid, periodic, or intermittent and gasping respirations; wide fluctuations or noticeable slowing of the pulse; and widening pulse pressure or extreme fluctuations in blood pressure are signs of brainstem involvement. Marked hypotension may represent internal injuries.

Ocular signs such as fixed, dilated, and unequal pupils; fixed and constricted pupils; and pupils that are poorly reactive or unreactive to light and accommodation indicate increased ICP or brainstem involvement. It is important to remain with the patient who demonstrates fixed and dilated pupils, because these are ominous signs with the probability of respiratory arrest. Dilated, nonpulsating blood vessels indicate increased ICP before the appearance of papilledema. Retinal hemorrhages are seen with acute head injuries, specifically with shaken baby syndrome.

> **NURSING ALERT**
> Observation of asymmetric pupils or one dilated, unreactive pupil in a comatose child is a neurosurgical emergency that may require evacuation of an epidural hematoma.

---

**Box 37-5** ■ ■ ■
**Clinical Manifestations of Acute Head Injury**

**MINOR INJURY**
May or may not lose consciousness
Transient period of confusion
Somnolence
Listlessness
Irritability
Pallor
Vomiting (one or more episodes)

**SIGNS OF PROGRESSION**
Altered mental status (e.g., difficulty rousing child)
Mounting agitation
Development of focal lateral neurologic signs
Marked changes in vital signs

**SEVERE INJURY**
Signs of increased ICP (see Box 37-1)
   Bulging fontanel (infant)
Retinal hemorrhages
Extraocular palsies (especially CN VI)
Hemiparesis
Quadriplegia
Elevated temperature
Unsteady gait
Papilledema

**ASSOCIATED SIGNS**
Scalp trauma
Other injuries (e.g., to extremities)

---

**Box 37-6** ◼ ◼ ◻
**Clinical Manifestations of Posttraumatic Syndromes**

**POSTCONCUSSION SYNDROME**

*Infants*
Pallor
Sweating
Irritability
Sleepiness
Possible vomiting

*Children*
Behavioral disturbances
  Aggressiveness
  Disobedience
  Withdrawal
  Regression
  Anxiety
Sleep disturbances
Phobias
Emotional lability
Irritability
Altered school performance
Seizures

*Adolescents*
Headache
Dizziness
Impaired concentration

**STRUCTURAL COMPLICATIONS**
Hydrocephalus
Focal deficits
  Optic atrophy
  Cranial nerve palsies
  Motor deficits
  Diabetes insipidus
  Aphasia
  Seizures

---

## *Critical Thinking Exercise*

### *Postconcussion Syndrome*

Two weeks ago 4-year-old Thomas attempted to climb the shelves of a storage cabinet in the garage of his home. The shelves and Thomas fell to the concrete floor. Thomas cried immediately. Because of the large occipital hematoma and a vomiting episode, the parents took their son to an emergency department within 1 hour of the incident. He was released after a negative CT scan, suturing of his occipital scalp laceration, and a GCS of 15.

At his 2-week follow-up visit, his mother reports changes in Thomas's behavior that include enuresis, crying episodes, vomiting in the morning, a poor appetite, and an increase in wanting to be held. What is your initial intervention?

FIRST, THINK ABOUT IT . . .
- What precise question are you trying to answer?
- What are the implications?

1. Review the signs and symptoms of postconcussion syndrome with the mother.
2. Advise the mother to give the child extra attention at home.
3. Report the symptoms to the physician.
4. Reassure the mother that these symptoms can occur during the first month following injury.

*The correct answer is three. The worsening postconcussion symptoms and signs of increased ICP, especially early-morning vomiting, require urgent consultation. The behavioral signs should not be dismissed as "attempts for attention."*

*The other two interventions are not appropriate as the initial action, although you would want to inform parents that children can exhibit postconcussion syndrome for up to 1 month following the injury, the time required for the bruised brain to heal. Because subsequent falls involving a head injury can compound the original injury, protecting the child during this period is especially important.*

---

Fundoscopic examination should be performed routinely to detect retinal hemorrhages in a child with CNS trauma. Cortical blindness, defined as a complete bilateral visual loss associated with normal pupillary responses to light, can be a brief or transient consequence of head trauma. Theories of possible etiologies are vasospasm or localized cerebral edema. Transient blindness following mild head trauma may not be obvious in children unless this diagnosis is considered and evaluated.

Less urgent but important additional assessments include examination of the scalp for lacerations and palpation for depressed skull fractures, widely separated sutures, and the size and tension of fontanels, which indicate intracranial hemorrhage or rapidly developing cerebral edema. However, a significant amount of blood loss can occur from scalp lacerations. An underlying skull fracture should be ruled out by palpation and radiography.

**NURSING ALERT** Bleeding from the nose or ears needs further evaluation, and a watery discharge from the nose (rhinorrhea) that is positive for glucose (as tested with reagent strips [e.g., Dextrostix]) suggests leaking of CSF from a skull fracture.

**Posttraumatic Syndromes.** *Postconcussion syndrome* is a common sequela to brain injury, and the manifestations vary with the age of the child. Most often there are behavioral disturbances (e.g., aggressiveness, withdrawal, regression), sleep disturbances, phobias, emotional lability, irritability, and alterations in school performance. The younger the child with severe head trauma, the higher the risk of late behavioral and emotional sequelae.

Postconcussion syndrome is very common in children under 1 year of age. Within minutes to an hour after a minimum head injury, the child sweats; becomes pale, irritable,

and sleepy; and may vomit. In children beyond 1 year of age a severe degree of concussion causes acute brain swelling, which may progress to coma with pupillary changes, apnea, and even death. Death from concussion is preventable unless overwhelming secondary brain injury has occurred (Durkin and others, 1998) (Box 37-6). (See Critical Thinking Exercise box.)

**NURSING ALERT** If a child loses consciousness or vomits more than three times, medical attention should be sought.

*Posttraumatic seizures* occur in a number of children who survive a head injury and are more common in children than in adults. Seizures are more likely to occur in children with severe head injury and usually occur within the first few days (Chiretti and others, 2000). Seizure activity may mimic brainstem herniation signs in children following head injuries.

*Structural complications* may occur as a result of head injuries. Hydrocephalus is seen when there has been subarachnoid hemorrhage or infection. Normal-pressure hy-

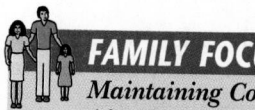

## FAMILY FOCUS
*Maintaining Contact with Parents After Head Injury*

Maintaining contact with parents for continued observation and reevaluation of the child, when indicated, facilitates early diagnosis and treatment of possible complications from head injury, such as hematoma, hydrocephalus, cysts, and posttraumatic seizures. Children are generally hospitalized for 24 and 48 hours' observation if their family lives far from medical facilities or lacks transportation or a telephone, which would provide access to immediate help. Other circumstances, such as language or other communication barriers or even emotional trauma, may hinder learning and make it difficult for families to feel confident in caring for their child at home.

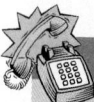

## EMERGENCY TREATMENT
*Head Injury*

1. Assess child:
   A—Airway
   B—Breathing
   C—Circulation
   Neurologic and thermoregulatory status
2. Stabilize neck and spine immediately. Use jaw thrust to open airway, not chin lift.
3. Clean any abrasions with soap and water.
   Apply clean dressing.
   If bleeding, apply ice to relieve pain and swelling.
4. Keep NPO until instructed otherwise.
5. Give no analgesics or sedatives.
6. Check pupil reaction every 4 hours (including twice during night) for 48 hours.
7. Awaken two times during night to check level of consciousness.
8. Seek medical attention if there is any of the following:
   Injury sustained
   - At high speed (e.g., auto)
   - Fall from a significant distance (height greater than that of the child)
   - From great force (e.g., baseball bat)
   - Under suspicious circumstances
   Loss of consciousness
   Discomfort (crying) more than 10 minutes after injury
   Headache that is severe, worsening, interferes with sleep, or lasts more than 24 hours
   Vomiting three or more times
   Swelling in front of or above earlobe or swelling that increases in size
   Blackened eyes
   Confused or not behaving normally
   Difficult to rouse from sleep
   Difficulty with speaking
   Blurring of vision or seeing double
   Unsteady gait
   Difficulty using extremities
   Neck pain or stiffness
   Pupils dilated, fixed or unequal
   Infant with bulging fontanel
   Seizures

drocephalus is a complication of traumatic brain injury. The clinical signs and symptoms include cognitive deterioration, gait changes, and incontinence. These signs are also seen during posttraumatic amnesia, making early recognition of this syndrome difficult. Focal deficits, including optic atrophy, CN palsies, motor deficits, diabetes insipidus, or aphasia, may be seen. The type of residual effect depends on the location and nature of the trauma. True mental retardation occurs only after severe injuries.

Evaluation of reflexes provides information about cerebral and pyramidal involvement, although transient abnormalities of the abdominal reflexes and Babinski sign may be present in children with mild head trauma. Conscious, cooperative children are examined for cerebellar signs such as ataxia. Children may display unsteadiness, clumsiness, or tremor with intentional movement after head injury.

Temperature may be moderately elevated for 1 or 2 days following an initial mild hypothermia after injury. A persistent fever may indicate subarachnoid hemorrhage or infection.

An accurate assessment of these various clinical signs provides baseline information. Serial evaluations, preferably by a single observer, help to detect changes in the neurologic status. Alterations in mental status, evidenced by increased difficulty in rousing the child, mounting agitation, development of focal lateral neurologic signs, or marked changes in vital signs, usually indicate extension or progression of the basic pathologic process.

**Special Tests.** After a thorough clinical examination, a variety of diagnostic tests are helpful in providing a more definitive diagnosis of the type and extent of the trauma. The severity of a head injury may not be apparent on clinical examination of the child but will be detectable on a CT scan. Whenever the child has a history consistent with a serious head injury (as with an unrestrained occupant in a severe motor vehicle accident or a fall), it is important that a scan be performed even if the child initially appears alert and oriented. All children with head injuries who have any alteration of consciousness, headache, vomiting, skull fracture, or seizure should undergo CT scanning.

MRI and neurobehavioral assessment following early head injury may be useful in documenting cognitive impairment in relation to structural alterations in the young brain. MRI provides details of soft tissues and cerebral

edema better than any other noninvasive device. Scanning with MRI is reserved for stable or recovering children because the metal devices used when treating a trauma, such as a ventilator, may not be placed in proximity to the magnetic field.

Skull x-ray films and other radiographic tests may be indicated. Electroencephalography is not helpful for early diagnosis but is useful for defining sites of potential seizure activity after the acute phase of illness. Lumbar puncture is rarely used for craniocerebral trauma and is contraindicated in the presence of increased ICP because of the possibility of herniation.

### Therapeutic Management

The majority of children with mild to moderate concussion who have not lost consciousness can be cared for and observed at home after careful examination reveals no serious intracranial injury. Parents are advised to bring the child in for examination in 1 or 2 days. The manifestations of epidural hematoma in children do not generally appear until 24 hours or more after injury. (See Family Focus box and Emergency Treatment box.)

Children with severe injuries, those who have lost consciousness for more than a few minutes, and those with prolonged and continued seizures or other focal or diffuse neurologic signs must be hospitalized until their condition is stable and their neurologic signs have diminished. The child is maintained on NPO status (nothing by mouth) or restricted to clear liquids (if able to take fluids by mouth) until it is determined that vomiting will not occur. IV fluids are indicated for the child who is comatose or displays dulled sensorium and for the child with persistent vomiting.

The volume of IV fluid is carefully monitored to minimize the possibility of overhydration in case of SIADH and cerebral edema. However, damage to the hypothalamus or pituitary gland may produce diabetes insipidus with its accompanying hypertonicity and dehydration. Fluid balance is closely monitored by daily weight, strict intake and output measurement, and serum osmolality (detect early signs of water retention). Observe for excessive dehydration and states of hypertonicity or hypotonicity.

Sedating drugs are usually withheld in the acute phase. Headache is usually controlled with acetaminophen, although opioids may be needed (see p. 1655). Antiepileptics are used for seizure control and often in cases of suspected contusion or laceration. Antibiotics are administered if there are lacerations or penetrating injuries. Prophylactic tetanus toxoid is given as appropriate. (See Chapter 12.) Cerebral edema is managed as described for the unconscious child. Hyperthermia is controlled with a hypothermia blanket.

**Surgical Therapy.**   Scalp lacerations are sutured after careful examination of underlying bone. Torn dura is also sutured. (See Atraumatic Care box.) Depressed fractures require surgical reduction and removal of bone fragments. A skull fracture depressed more than the thickness of the skull or an intracranial hematoma that causes more than 5 mm midline shift is an indication for surgery. Direct pressure should not be applied to a depressed skull fracture. "Ping-Pong ball" skull fractures in very young infants can correct themselves within a few weeks or may require surgical elevation.

**Prognosis.**   The outcome of craniocerebral trauma depends on the extent of injury and complications. However, the outlook is generally more favorable for children than for adults. More than 90% of children with concussions or simple linear fractures recover without symptoms after the initial period. Children have a significantly higher percentage of good outcomes and a lower mortality rate, as well as

a lower incidence of surgical mass lesions after severe head trauma. However, their thinner, softer brain may sustain greater long-term damage than previously suggested.

The concern regarding outcome is increasingly focused on cognitive, emotional, or mental problems. Recent studies indicate that children experience a higher frequency of psychologic disturbances following head injury, whereas adults are more prone to complaints of a physical nature. Children may be more vulnerable than adults to long-term cognitive and behavioral dysfunction after diffuse brain injury.

True coma (not obeying commands, eyes closed, and not speaking) usually does not last more than 2 weeks. A child's eventual outcome can range from brain death to a persistent vegetative state to complete recovery. However, even the best recovery may be associated with personality changes, including mood lability and loss of confidence, impaired short-term memory, headaches, and subtle cognitive impairments. Many children are left with significant disabilities after head injury that appear months later as learning difficulties, behavioral changes, or emotional disturbances (Cattelani and others, 1998). In general, 90% of the long-term neurologic outcome has been achieved within 6 months to 1 year after the injury.

### Nursing Considerations

The hospitalized child requires careful neurologic assessment and evaluation (see p. 1646). Frequent nursing assessments can provide information needed to establish a correct diagnosis, identify signs and symptoms of increased ICP, determine clinical management, and prevent many complications. The goals of nursing management of the child with a head injury are to maintain adequate ventilation, oxygenation, and circulation; to monitor and treat increased ICP; to minimize cerebral oxygen requirements; and to provide support to the child and family during the recovery phases.

The child is placed on bed rest, usually with the head of the bed elevated slightly. Appropriate safety measures, such as siderails kept up and seizure precautions, are implemented. The extremely restless child may require that hard surfaces be padded and restraints used to prevent the possibility of further injury. Care is individualized according to the specific needs of the child.

A key nursing role is to provide sedation and analgesia for the child. The conflict between the need to promote comfort and relieve anxiety in the child versus the need to be able to assess for neurologic changes presents a dilemma. Both goals can be achieved with close observation of the child's LOC and response to analgesics (using a pain assessment record) and effective communication with the practitioner. Decreasing restlessness after administration of an analgesic most likely reflects pain control rather than a decreasing LOC. (See Pain Assessment; Pain Management, Chapter 26.)

Children may be restless and irritable, but more often their reaction is to fall asleep when left undisturbed. A quiet environment helps reduce the restlessness and irritability. Bright lights are irritating. This often makes checking the

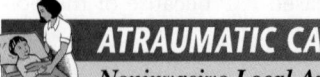

**ATRAUMATIC CARE**

*Noninvasive Local Anesthesia*

The use of topical lidocaine, epinephrine, and tetracaine (LET) solution (Adler, Dubinsky, and Eisen 1998) or lidocaine, adrenaline, and tetracaine (LAT) gel provides noninvasive anesthesia for suturing (Ernst and others, 1997). Both of these preparations provide an acceptable alternative to tetracaine, adrenaline, and cocaine (TAC), which is more expensive, is a restricted narcotic, and carries a higher potential for toxicity (Keyes, Tallon, and Rizos, 1998).

ocular responses more difficult to perform and more aggravating to the child.

Frequent examinations of vital signs, neurologic signs, and LOC are extremely important nursing observations. When possible, they should be performed by a single observer in order to better detect subtle changes that may indicate worsening of neurologic status. Pupils are checked for size, equality, reaction to light, and accommodation. After the initial elevations usually seen after injury, the vital signs generally return to normal unless there is brainstem involvement.

The most important nursing observation is assessment of the child's LOC. In the progression of an injury, alterations in consciousness appear earlier than alterations of vital signs or focal neurologic signs (see p. 1647 for evaluation of responsiveness). Certain expected responses may be misinterpreted as deviations from the normal. Frequent examinations of alertness are fatiguing to the child; therefore the child often desires to fall asleep, which may be confused with depressed consciousness. When left alone, the child promptly dozes. It is not uncommon to observe ocular divergence through the partially closed eyelids.

Observations of position and movement provide additional information. Any abnormal posturing is noted, as well as whether it occurs continuously or intermittently. Questions nurses might ask themselves include:

- Are the child's hand grips strong and equal in strength?
- Are there any signs of decerebrate or decorticate posturing?
- What is the child's response to stimulation?
- Is movement purposeful, random, or absent?
- Are movement and sensation equal on both sides or restricted to one side only?

The child may complain of headache or other discomfort. The child who is too young to describe a headache will be fussy and resist being handled. The child who suffers from vertigo will often vigorously resist being moved from a position of comfort. Forcible movement causes the child to vomit and display spontaneous nystagmus. Seizures are relatively common in children at the time of head injury and may be of any type. Any seizure activity should be carefully observed and described in detail (see Box 37-11). Children in postictal states are more lethargic, with sluggish pupils.

Drainage from any orifice should be documented. Bleeding from the ear suggests the possibility of a basal skull fracture. The amount and characteristics of the drainage are observed.

**NURSING ALERT**  Suctioning through the nares is contraindicated because there is a risk the catheter entering the brain through a fracture in the skull.

Head trauma is often accompanied by other undetected injuries; therefore any bruises, lacerations, or evidence of internal injuries or fractures of the extremities are noted and reported. Associated injuries are evaluated and treated appropriately.

The child with a normal LOC is usually allowed clear liquids unless fluid is restricted. If the child has an IV infusion, it is maintained as prescribed. The diet is advanced to that appropriate for the child's age as soon as the condition permits. Intake and output are measured and recorded, and any incontinence of bowel or bladder is noted in the child who has been toilet trained.

The child is observed for any unusual behavior, but interpretation of behavior is made in relation to the child's normal behavior. For example, urinary incontinence during sleep would be of no consequence in a child who routinely wets the bed but would be highly significant for one who is always dry. Parents are invaluable resources in evaluating objective behaviors of their children. Information obtained from parents at or shortly after admission is essential in evaluating the child's behavior (e.g., the ease with which the child is roused normally, the usual sleeping position, how much the child sleeps during the day, motor activities of the child [rolling over, sitting up, climbing], hearing and visual acuity, appetite, and manner of eating [spoon, bottle, cup]). There would be less concern about a child who falls asleep several times during the day if this particular pattern of sleeping is consistent with the child's usual behavior.

When the child is discharged, the parents are advised of probable posttraumatic symptoms that may be expected, such as behavioral changes, sleep disturbances, phobias, and seizures. They should understand observations that should be made and how to contact the practitioner or health facility in case the child develops any unusual signs or symptoms. (See Critical Thinking Exercise box on p. 1670.) The importance of follow-up evaluation is emphasized.

**Family Support.**   The emotional and educational support of the family presents a challenge. Witnessing the parents' grief and helplessness on seeing their child in an intensive care unit connected to monitoring equipment and in an altered state evokes empathy. The nurse can encourage the family to be involved in the child's care, to bring in familiar belongings, or to make a tape recording of familiar voices and sounds. Parents may need a demonstration on how to touch or cuddle their child and may want to talk about their grief. The nurse can listen attentively, reinforce what is being done to assist the child, and direct parents toward signs and symptoms of recovery to instill hope without promises. Honesty and kindness, along with consistent and competent care, can help families through this difficult time.

**Rehabilitation.**   Rehabilitation and management of the child with permanent brain injury are essential aspects of care. Rehabilitation of children with brain injury is begun as soon as feasible and usually involves the family and a rehabilitation team. Careful assessment of the child's capabilities, limitations, and probable potential is made as early as possible, and appropriate interventions are implemented to maximize the residual capacities. **The Brain Injury Association*** provides information and listings of rehabilitation services and support groups throughout the country.

Pediatric trauma rehabilitation is a national concern. Twenty million children are injured by accidents each year; 50,000 children are permanently disabled, and 2 million

---

*105 North Alfred St, Alexandria, VA 22314, (703) 236-6000, fax: (703) 236-6001; www.biausa.org.

children have temporary disabilities (Spivak, 1999). Coordinating care and services for early rehabilitation involves identifying the child and family's response to the traumatic injury and disability, securing available resources, and recognizing the parents' role in the process.

The child with a disability resulting from head trauma requires assessment on a physical, cognitive, emotional, and social level. The child has experienced separation, pain, sensory deprivation and overload, changes in circadian cycle, and fear of the unknown. Recovery and transition require new coping strategies at the same time that regressive and acting-out behaviors may start. Parents and children need honest communication for decision making. Rehabilitation is recommended when the child is making progress beyond what can be provided in a hospital setting. The Rancho Los Amigos Scale provides a systematic assessment of the progress that a child with a severe head injury may achieve. (See Family Focus box on p. 1660.)

Pediatric rehabilitation focuses on the strengths and needs of the child. The rehabilitation team should include physical medicine, rehabilitation nursing, nutritional counseling, physical therapy, special education, occupational therapy, speech therapy, and psychologic, neuropsychologic, child-life, and social services. Families need to know what to look for when visiting a pediatric rehabilitation center. Before the child's transfer, the hospital team should provide a detailed care plan of the child's needs and abilities, especially communication skills; a description of the child's usual schedule; nursing care interventions; and the concerns and needs of the family. To augment the care plan, a videotape introducing the child and family and showing any unique aspects of their care can be sent to the rehabilitation center.

**Prevention.** Preventive strategies are underused in almost all cases of accidental childhood injury. Head injuries occur in the most serious accidental injuries—especially motor vehicle accidents, sports, and falls.

Tremendous strides have been taken in the prevention of cerebral damage after head injury in children. New developments are directed towards the prevention of cellular injury or the primary insult. The roles of calcium, oxyradicals, and prostaglandins, are being investigated. However, the greatest benefit lies in prevention of head injuries. Nurses can exert a valuable influence on behalf of children through education. Accidents remain preventable because unnecessary risks go unchecked. Inadequate supervision combined with a child's natural sense of curiosity and exploration can lead to lethal results. Nurses are in the unique position of influencing caregivers in terms of growth and development. Banning the use of infant walkers is an example. This equipment does not help develop motor skills but places infants at risk for head and neck injuries from falls, especially down steps. Public education coupled with legislative support can prevent childhood injuries.

For extensive discussions of childhood injuries, see the information on injury prevention in Chapters 12, 14, 15, 17, and 19 as well as Injuries—The Leading Killer, Chapter 1. (See Nursing Care Plan: The Child with a Head Injury.*)

---

*In Wong DL, Hess CS: *Wong and Whaley's clinical manual of pediatric nursing,* ed 5, St Louis, 2000, Mosby.

## Near-Drowning

Drowning ranks second as a cause of accidental death in children. Most cases of drowning are accidental, usually involving children who are helpless in water, such as inadequately attended children in or near swimming pools or infants in bathtubs; small children who fall into ponds, streams, and flooded excavations, usually near home; occupants of pleasure boats who fail to wear life preservers; children who have diving accidents; and children who are able to swim but overestimate their endurance. Accidental drowning occurs five times more often in boys than in girls; 50% of children are under the age of 4, and 90% of cases occur in private swimming pools (National Center for Injury Prevention and Control, 1999) (Fig. 37-9).

Accidental drowning occurs more often in males than in females; in almost all cases, supervision is absent. Most of the drownings are related to the characteristics of specific age-groups. For example, infants drown in bathtubs, preschool children in swimming pools, and teenagers in lakes and rivers. The largest proportion of drownings for all children occurs in private swimming pools, with the highest rate among children 2 to 3 years of age. Drowning as a form of fatal child abuse also occurs. Homicidal drownings are unwitnessed, usually occur in the home, and the victims are either infants or toddlers.

Drowning can take place in any body of water, including such unlikely places as a pail of water or a toilet bowl. Top-heavy toddlers fall headfirst into a pail of water, their arms become trapped, and they are unable to free themselves. Hot tubs and whirlpool spas have been implicated in childhood drowning injury. The suction created at the outlet is strong enough to trap even larger children underwater.

### Pathophysiology

Near-drowning occurs when a victim of a submersion incident survives at least 24 hours after rescue, regardless of the

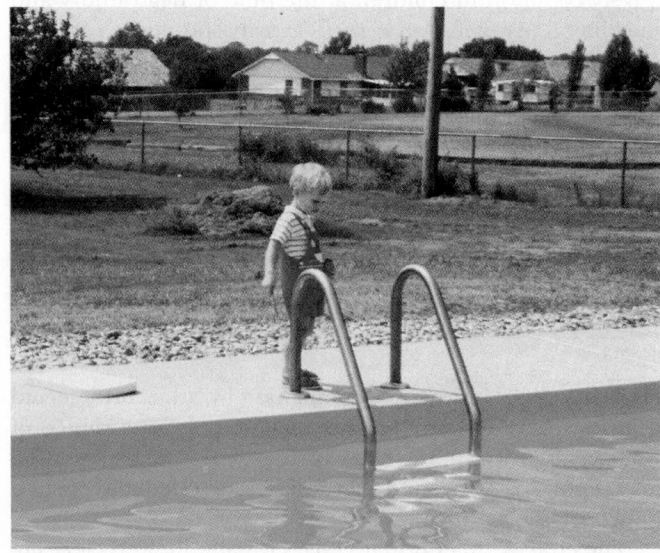

**Fig. 37-9** Water is fascinating for children; however, drowning is the second leading cause of accidental death in unsupervised situations.

final outcome (Box 37-7). Physiologically most organ systems will be affected, especially the pulmonary, cardiovascular, and neurologic systems. The major pulmonary changes that occur in drowning are directly related to the length of submersion (regardless of the type and amount of fluid aspirated), the physiologic response of the victim, and the development and degree of immersion hypothermia. In addition, cerebral recovery may depend on the effectiveness of initial resuscitation and subsequent critical care measures to support cerebral salvage.

Physiologic factors that influence the extent of damage from immersion include resistance to asphyxia and anoxia, which shows some individual variation. There is greater resistance with diminishing age; young children can withstand longer periods of submersion. More important is the drowning, or diving, reflex. This neurologic response is triggered by immersion of the face in cold water. Blood is shunted away from the periphery, and the flow is predominantly concentrated to the brain and heart. There is profound bradycardia, but the diminishing supply of oxygen is delivered to these essential organs.

Submerged children struggle initially. There is laryngospasm, and they swallow water and often vomit. This is followed by gasping and aspiration. Cardiopulmonary arrest is secondary to asphyxia after approximately 4 to 6 minutes of complete submersion. The problems created by near-drowning are (1) hypoxia and asphyxiation, (2) aspiration, and (3) hypothermia (except near-drowning in hot tubs).

Hypoxia is the primary problem because it results in global cell damage, with different cells tolerating variable lengths of anoxia. Neurons, especially cerebral cells, sustain irreversible damage after 4 to 6 minutes of submersion. The heart and lungs can survive up to 30 minutes. Regardless of the amount of water aspirated, there is arterial hypoxemia (resulting from atelectasis with shunting of blood through the nonventilated alveoli), combined respiratory acidosis (resulting from retained carbon dioxide), and metabolic acidosis (caused by buildup of acid metabolites due to anaerobic metabolism). Although electrolyte imbalances are contributing factors, they are not the major causes of morbidity and mortality. The pathologic events are directly related to the duration of submersion. The major difficulty is acute ventilatory insufficiency. Approximately 10% of drowning victims die without aspirating fluid but succumb from acute asphyxia as a result of prolonged reflex laryngospasm.

Aspiration of fluid occurs in the majority of drownings. The aspirated fluid results in pulmonary edema, atelectasis, airway spasm, and pneumonitis, which aggravates hypoxia. It was previously thought that the physiologic response to near-drowning differed between submersion in salt water and fresh water. However, there is no clinically significant difference in human survivors, and the type of water does not alter the therapy or outcome.

Hypothermia occurs rapidly in infants and children, partly because of their large surface area relative to size and partly as a result of the cold water itself. Profound hypothermia is usually evidence of lengthy submersion. Although small children may tolerate submersion in *very* cold water, severe neurologic damage results from hypoxia within 3 to 6 minutes.

## Clinical Manifestations

Clinical manifestations are directly related to the degree of consciousness following rescue and resuscitation. The manifestations and management are categorized in Table 37-5.

## Therapeutic Management

With rapid treatment some children can and are being saved. Resuscitative measures should begin at the scene, and the victim should be transported to the hospital with maximum ventilatory and circulatory support. Many victims need care for some time after aspiration of fluid. In the hospital intensive pulmonary care is implemented and continued according to the needs of the patient.

In general, management of the near-drowning victim is based on the degree of cerebral insult. The first priority is to restore oxygen delivery to the cells and prevent further hypoxic damage. A spontaneously breathing child will do well in an oxygen-enriched atmosphere; the more severely affected child will require endotracheal intubation and mechanical ventilation. Blood gases and pH are monitored at frequent intervals as a guide to oxygen, fluid, and electrolyte therapies.

> **NURSING ALERT**
> All children who have a near-drowning experience should be admitted to the hospital for observation. Although many patients do not appear to have suffered adverse effects from the event, complications (e.g., respiratory compromise, cerebral edema) may occur 24 hours after the incident.

Because of the frequency of complications after near-drowning, patients should be hospitalized for 12 to 48 hours for observation. Potential causes for altered neurologic function in the pediatric near-drowning victim (e.g., head injury, drug intoxication, or hypothermia) require evaluation. Aspiration pneumonia is a common complication that occurs approximately 48 to 72 hours after the episode.

---

**Box 37-7**
### Terms Describing Drowning Injury

**Drowning**—Death from asphyxia while submerged, regardless of whether fluid has entered the lungs
**Near-drowning**—Survival at least 24 hours after submersion in a fluid medium
These terms can be further described as:
**Drowning without aspiration**—Death from respiratory obstruction and asphyxia while submerged, usually as a result of prolonged laryngospasm; also called "dry drowning" (approximately 10% of drownings)
**Drowning with aspiration**—Death from the combined effects of asphyxia and changes secondary to fluid aspiration while submerged
**Near-drowning without aspiration**—Survival, at least temporarily, following asphyxia after submersion in a fluid medium
**Near-drowning with aspiration**—Survival, at least temporarily, following aspiration of fluid while submerged
**Delayed death caused by drowning**—Death as a result of complications subsequent to successful resuscitation following submersion

**TABLE 37-5** Clinical manifestations and management of near-drowning related to degree of consciousness

| Category | Characteristics | Management |
|---|---|---|
| A | Awake, minimum injury<br>Fully conscious; may have mild hypothermia, mild chest radiograph changes, mild arterial blood gas abnormalities | Symptomatic treatment with oxygen administration and warming<br>Laboratory assessment of electrolytes<br>Usually well enough to be discharged in 12 to 24 hours |
| B | Blunted sensorium, moderate injury<br>Obtund, stuporous, purposeful response to painful stimuli, mild to moderate hypothermia, frequent respiratory distress, abnormal chest radiographs, arterial blood gas abnormalities | Symptomatic, as for category A<br>Regular monitoring of neurologic and respiratory status<br>Correction of acidosis<br>Furosemide to stimulate diuresis |
| C | Comatose, severe anoxia<br>Patient unarousable, abnormal response to pain, abnormal respiratory pattern, seizures, shock, marked arterial blood gas abnormalities, abnormal chest radiographs, arhythmias, metabolic acidosis, hyperkalemia, hyperglycemia, disseminated intravascular coagulation | Invasive life-support measures<br>Mechanical ventilation for at least 12 to 24 hours (to reduce energy expenditure)<br>More severely affected children managed as any unconscious child<br>Increased ICP usually not a problem in children who do well, but when present (even with treatment), associated with death or significant neurologic damage<br>Symptomatic management |
| C1 | Decorticate, Cheyne-Stokes respirations | |
| C2 | Decerebrate, central hyperventilation | |
| C3 | Flaccid, apneustic or cluster breathing | |
| C4 | Flaccid, apneic, no detectable circulation | |

Bronchospasm, alveolar-capillary membrane damage, atelectasis, abscess formation, and hyaline membrane disease are other complications that occur after aspiration of fluid.

**Prognosis.** In one study the best predictors of a good outcome were length of submersion in nonicy water (>5° C [41° F]) of less than 5 minutes and the presence of sinus rhythm, reactive pupils, and neurologic responsiveness at the scene. The worst prognoses—death or severe neurologic impairment—were for children submerged for more than 10 minutes and not responding to advanced life support within 25 minutes. All children without spontaneous purposeful movement and normal brainstem function 24 hours after near-drowning suffered severe neurologic deficits or death (Sachdeva, 1999).

### Nursing Considerations

Nursing care depends on the condition of the child. A child who survives may need intensive respiratory nursing care with attention to vital signs, mechanical ventilation or tracheostomy, blood gas determination, chest therapy, and IV infusion. Often the child has sustained a hypoxic insult and requires the same care as an unconscious child.

Probably the most difficult aspect in the care of the child victim of near-drowning is dealing with the parents, whose guilt reactions are severe. The magnitude of the event is so great that efforts to provide comfort and support are of only limited success. Parents need to hear that everything possible is being done to treat the child, and this message needs to be repeated often.

Most drownings, particularly of infants or small children, could have been prevented with adequate supervision. If the child dies, the sudden, unexpected nature of the death and the particular circumstances of the accident, especially in terms of guilt for not preventing it, compound the grief. (See Chapter 23.) The parents of the child who is saved from death are faced with the anxiety of not knowing what the outcome will be and sometimes wish for the death of the child, or they continue to hope the child will "wake up" in the face of cerebral hypoxia. Because their situation generates such intense feelings of loneliness, it is important for families to know they are not alone. Additional sources of support that can be recommended are psychiatric and social work consultants, community services, and religious support. Self-help groups are excellent if available in the community.

Nurses often have difficulty relating to the parents if obvious neglect has precipitated the accident and subsequent problems; therefore, it is important for those who care for these children and their families to assess their own feelings about the situation, as well as the coping abilities and resources of the family. Caring for near-drowning victims and their families requires the nurse to be sensitive to the needs of the child and the family and to recognize his or her own reactions and emotions.

**Prevention.** Water safety and survival training should be required for all school-age children, and nurses can be active advocates in their communities. Nurses are also in a position to emphasize the importance of adequate adult supervision when children are in or near the water (Nieves and others, 1996). Young children should never be left unattended. Parents with pools should know cardiopulmonary resuscitation (CPR) techniques. (See Injury Prevention, Chapters 12, 14, 15, 17, and 19.)

## INTRACRANIAL INFECTIONS

The nervous system is subject to infection by the same organisms that affect other organs of the body. However, the nervous system is limited in the ways in which it responds to injury. Laboratory studies are needed to identify the causative agent. The inflammatory process can affect the meninges (*meningitis*) or brain (*encephalitis*).

Meningitis can be caused by a variety of organisms, but the three main types are (1) *bacterial*, or pyogenic, caused by pus-forming bacteria, especially the meningococcus, pneumococcus, and haemophilus organisms; (2) *viral*, or aseptic, caused by a wide variety of viral agents; and (3) *tuberculous*, caused by the tuberculin bacillus. The majority of children with acute febrile encephalopathy have either bacterial meningitis or viral meningitis as the underlying cause.

# Bacterial Meningitis

Bacterial meningitis is an acute inflammation of the meninges and CSF. The advent of antimicrobial therapy has had a marked effect on the course and prognosis, although the use of conjugate vaccines against *Haemophilus influenzae* type b in 1990 has led to the most dramatic change in the epidemiology of bacterial meningitis (Feigin and Perlman, 1998). In 1993 the incidence of *H. influenzae* was 2 cases per 100,000 children younger than 5 years, whereas the incidence was 41 per 100,000 in 1987 (Anderson and others, 1994). By 1996, cases of invasive *H. influenzae* disease (among children age >5 years) were at or near the lowest numbers ever recorded and near elimination target levels (Centers for Disease Control and Prevention [CDC], 1999b). Practitioners are optimistic that the use of the new pneumoccal conjugate vaccine will produce a rapid and adequate antibody response in young children. If so, bacterial meningitis from *Streptococcus pneumoniae* will soon be on the decline (Eskola, 2000). Bacterial meningitis remains a significant cause of illness in the pediatric age-groups. Its importance lies primarily in the residual damage caused by undiagnosed and untreated or inadequately treated cases. Ninety percent of reported cases occur between 1 month and 5 years of age (Feigin and Perlman, 1998).

## Etiology

Bacterial meningitis can be caused by any of a variety of bacterial agents. Currently *H. influenzae* (type B), *S. pneumoniae*, and *Neisseria meningitidis* (meningococcus) organisms are responsible for bacterial meningitis in 95% of children older than 2 months.

Other organisms are β-hemolytic streptococcus, *Staphylococcus aureus*, and *Escherichia coli*. The leading causes of neonatal meningitis are group B streptococci, *E. coli*, and *Listeria monocytogenes*. *E. coli* infection is seldom seen beyond infancy. Meningococcal meningitis occurs in epidemic form and is the only type readily transmitted by droplet infection from nasopharyngeal secretions. Although this condition may develop at any age, the risk of meningococcal infection increases with the number of contacts; therefore it occurs predominantly in school-age children and adolescents.

There appear to be some seasonal variations. Meningitis caused by *H. influenzae* primarily occurs in autumn or early winter. Pneumococcal and meningococcal infections can occur at any time but are more common in later winter or early spring.

Several factors may predispose the child to the development of bacterial meningitis. Males are affected more often than females, and this is somewhat more pronounced in the neonatal period. The greatest morbidity after meningitis appears to involve children who were afflicted between birth and 4 years of age. Maternal factors, such as premature rupture of fetal membranes and maternal infection during the last week of pregnancy, are major causes of neonatal meningitis.

Deficiencies in the immune mechanisms and decreased leukocyte activity may influence the incidence in newborns, children with immunoglobulin deficiencies, and children receiving immunosuppressant drugs. Meningitis appears to occur as an extension of a variety of bacterial infections, probably as a result of the lack of acquired resistance to the various etiologic organisms. Preexisting CNS anomalies, neurosurgical procedures or injuries, chronic diseases such as sickle cell, cystic fibrosis, diabetes, or immunesuppression, and primary infections elsewhere in the body are factors related to increased susceptibility.

## Pathophysiology

The most common route of infection is vascular dissemination from a focus of infection elsewhere. For example, organisms from the nasopharynx invade the underlying blood vessels and enter the cerebral blood supply or form local thromboemboli that release septic emboli into the bloodstream. Invasion by direct extension from infections in the paranasal and mastoid sinuses is less common. Organisms also gain entry by direct implantation after penetrating wounds, skull fractures that provide an opening into the skin or sinuses, lumbar puncture or surgical procedures, anatomic abnormalities such as spina bifida, or foreign bodies such as an internal ventricular shunt or an external ventricular device. Once implanted, the organisms spread into the CSF, by which the infection spreads throughout the subarachnoid space.

Altered permeability of the BBB can be produced by bacterial products; the release of tumor necrosis factor (TNF) appears to initiate meningeal inflammation (Feigin and Perlman, 1998).

The infective process is like that seen in any bacterial infection—inflammation, exudation, white blood cell accumulation, and varying degrees of tissue damage. The brain becomes hyperemic and edematous, and the entire surface of the brain is covered with a layer of purulent exudate that varies with the type of organism. For example, meningococcal exudate is most marked over the parietal, occipital, and cerebellar regions; the thick, fibrinous exudate of pneumococcal infection is confined chiefly to the surface of the brain, particularly the anterior lobes; and the exudate of streptococcal infections is similar to that of pneumococcal infections, but thinner.

As infection extends to the ventricles, thick pus, fibrin, or adhesions may occlude the narrow passages and obstruct the flow of CSF.

## Clinical Manifestations

The clinical manifestations of acute bacterial meningitis depend to a large extent on the age of the child. The picture is also influenced to some degree by the type of organism, the effectiveness of therapy for antecedent illness, and whether it occurs as an isolated entity or as a complication of another illness or injury.

**Children and Adolescents.** The onset of illness is likely to be abrupt, with fever, chills, headache, and vomiting that are associated with or quickly followed by alterations in sensorium. Often the initial sign is a seizure, which may recur as the disease progresses. The child is extremely irritable and agitated and may develop photophobia, confusion, hallucinations, aggressive behavior, drowsiness, stupor, and coma. Sometimes the onset is slower and is often preceded by several days of respiratory or gastrointestinal symptoms. Occasionally a prior infection treated with antibiotics masks or delays the signs of meningitis.

The child resists flexion of the neck; as the disease progresses, the neck stiffness (nuchal rigidity) becomes marked until the head is drawn into extreme overextension (opisthotonos). Kernig and Brudzinski signs are positive. Reflex responses are variable, although they show hyperactivity. (See Reflexes, Chapter 7.) The skin may be cold and cyanotic with poor peripheral perfusion.

Other signs and symptoms may appear that are specific to individual organisms. Petechial or purpuric rashes occur in 50% of cases and indicate a meningococcal infection (meningococcemia), especially when the eruption is associated with a septic shock–like state. Joint involvement is seen in meningococcal and *H. influenzae* infection. A chronically draining ear commonly accompanies pneumococcal meningitis. *E. coli* infection may be associated with a congenital dermal sinus that communicates with the subarachnoid space.

**Infants and Young Children.** Between 3 months and 2 years of age the illness is characterized by fever, poor feeding, vomiting, marked irritability, restlessness, and seizures, which are often accompanied by a high-pitched cry. A bulging fontanel is the most significant finding, and nuchal rigidity and Brudzinski and Kernig signs may occur late in the young child (Feigin and Perlman, 1998).

**Neonates.** Meningitis in newborn and premature infants is extremely difficult to diagnose. The vague and nonspecific manifestations, which are characteristic of all neonatal sepsis, bear little resemblance to the findings in older children. These infants are usually well at birth but within a few days begin to appear ill. They refuse feedings, have poor sucking ability, and may vomit or have diarrhea. They display poor muscle tone and lack of movement and have a poor cry. Other nonspecific signs that may be present include hypothermia or fever (depending on the maturity of the infant), jaundice, irritability, drowsiness, seizures, respiratory irregularities or apnea, cyanosis, and weight loss. The full, tense, and bulging fontanel may or may not be present until late in the course of the illness, and the neck is usually supple. Untreated, the child's condition will decline to cardiovascular collapse, seizures, and apnea.

**Complications.** The incidence of complications from acute bacterial meningitis has been significantly reduced with early diagnosis and vigorous antimicrobial therapy. If infection extends to the ventricles, thick pus, fibrin, or adhesions may occlude the narrow passages, thereby obstructing the flow of CSF and causing obstructive hydrocephalus.

Subdural effusions often occur, and thrombosis may occur in meningeal veins or venous sinuses. Destructive changes may take place in the cerebral cortex, and brain abscesses may form by direct extension of the infection or by vascular dissemination. Extension of the infection to the areas of the cranial nerves or compression necrosis from increased pressure may cause deafness, blindness, or weakness or paralysis of facial or other muscles of the head and neck.

One of the most dramatic and serious complications usually associated with meningococcal infections is *meningococcal sepsis,* or *meningococcemia.* When the onset is severe, sudden, and rapid (fulminate), it is known as the *Waterhouse-Friderichsen syndrome.* The syndrome is characterized by overwhelming septic shock, disseminated intravascular coagulation (DIC), massive bilateral adrenal hemorrhage, and purpura (Fig. 37-10). Meningococcemia requires immediate emergency treatment, hospitalization, and intensive care. The mortality is as high as 90% (Feigin and Perlman, 1998).

> **NURSING ALERT** Any child who is ill and develops a purpuric or petechial rash may have (overwhelming) meningococcemia and must receive medical attention immediately (see Fig. 37-10).

Other acute complications of meningitis include SIADH (see Chapter 38), subdural effusions, seizures, cerebral edema and herniation, and hydrocephalus. Obstruction to the flow of CSF occurs during the acute phase of illness by clumping of purulent material in the drainage channels and during the chronic phase by adhesive arachnoiditis or fibrotic obstruction through any of the ventricular foramina. Postmeningitic complications in neonates include ventriculitis, which results in cystic, walled-off areas of the brain with fluid accumulation and pressure.

Extension of the inflammation to cranial nerves or compression and destruction of the nerves from ICP can produce permanent impairment of vision or hearing and other nerve palsies. Auditory nerve damage is usually followed by permanent deafness. Other long-term complications include cerebral palsy, mental handicap, learning disorder, attention deficit hyperactivity disorder, and seizures.

Hemiparesis and quadriparesis may result from damage caused by arteritis or thrombosis or other mechanisms. Be-

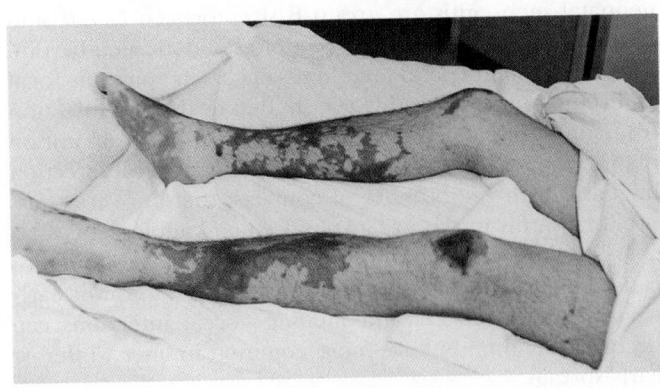

**Fig. 37-10** Purpura of the lower extremities of child suffering from meningococcemia.

havioral changes are noted in some children. Also, evidence indicates that psychometric and behavioral defects may be a significant concomitant sign of meningitis in childhood, although it is difficult to determine the degree to which meningitis affects the intelligence of young children. Meningitis in the neonatal period is more likely to cause developmental problems (Monzo, 2002).

## Diagnostic Evaluation

A lumbar puncture (LP) is the definitive diagnostic test. The fluid pressure is measured, and samples are obtained for culture, Gram stain, blood cell count, and determination of glucose and protein content. The findings are usually diagnostic. Culture and sensitivity are needed to identify the causative organism. Spinal fluid pressure is usually elevated, but interpretation is often difficult when the child is crying. Sedation with fentanyl and midazolam (Versed) can alleviate the child's pain and fear associated with this procedure. (See Atraumatic Care box.) If there is evidence or suspicion of increased ICP (papilledema, focal neurologic deficits, bulging fontanelle), a CT scan of the head may be warranted before the procedure.

There is generally an elevated white blood cell count, often predominantly polymorphonuclear leukocytes. The glucose level is reduced, generally in proportion to the duration and severity of the infection. The relationship between the CSF glucose and serum glucose levels is important in evaluating the glucose content of CSF; therefore a serum glucose sample is drawn approximately ½ hour before the LP. Protein concentration is usually increased.

A blood culture is advisable for all children suspected of meningitis and occasionally will be positive when CSF culture is negative. Nose and throat cultures may provide helpful information in some cases.

## Therapeutic Management

Acute bacterial meningitis is a medical emergency that requires early recognition and immediate institution of therapy to prevent death and avoid residual disabilities. The initial therapeutic management includes:

- Isolation precautions
- Initiation of antimicrobial therapy
- Maintenance of hydration
- Maintenance of ventilation
- Reduction of increased ICP
- Management of systemic shock
- Control of seizures
- Control of temperature
- Treatment of complications

The child is isolated from other children, usually in an intensive care unit for close observation. An IV infusion is started in order to facilitate the administration of antimicrobial agents, fluids, antiepileptic drugs, and blood if needed. The child is placed on a cardiac monitor and respiratory isolation.

**Drugs.**   Until the causative organism is identified, the choice of antibiotic is based on the known sensitivity of the organism most likely to be the infective agent. Following identification of the organism, antimicrobial agents are adjusted accordingly.

Dexamethasone may play a role in the initial management of increased ICP and cerebral herniation, but the ability of dexamethasone to reduce long-term complications of bacterial meningitis remains controversial. There is evidence that dexamethasone therapy prevents bilateral deafness in children with *H. influenzae* type b meningitis (Wald and others, 1995). Dexamethasone is currently recommended for the treatment of *H. influenzae* type b meningitis and should be considered for use in other bacterial types of meningitis (American Academy of Pediatrics, 2000a). It should not be used if aseptic or nonbacterial meningitis is suspected (Feigin and Perlman, 1998).

Signs of gastrointestinal hemorrhage or secondary infection may complicate steroid administration. Antibiotic treatment with cephalosporins demonstrates superiority for promptly sterilizing the CSF and reducing the incidence of severe hearing impairment.

**Nonspecific Measures.**   Maintaining hydration is a prime concern, and IV fluids and the type and amount of fluid are determined by the patient's condition. The optimum hydration involves correction of any fluid deficits followed by fluid restriction as ordered to prevent cerebral edema. Cerebral edema and electrolyte disturbances are associated with poor neurologic outcome following bacterial meningitis (Feigin and Perlman, 1998). Children with bacterial meningitis must be monitored for signs of increased ICP. If needed, measures to decrease ICP are implemented (see p. 1656).

Complications are treated appropriately, such as aspiration of subdural effusion in infants and treatment for disseminated intravascular coagulation syndrome. Shock is managed by restoration of circulating blood volume and maintenance of electrolyte balance. Seizures can occur during the first few days of treatment. These are controlled with the appropriate antiepileptic drug. Hearing loss is not uncommon. The patient should undergo auditory evaluation 6 months after the illness has resolved.

Lumbar puncture is carried out as needed to determine the effectiveness of therapy. The patient is evaluated neurologically during the convalescent period.

**Prognosis.**   Ten percent to 15% of cases of bacterial meningitis are fatal (CDC, 2000b). The age of the child, the duration of illness before antibiotic therapy, the rapidity of diagnosis after onset, the type of organism, and the adequacy of therapy are important in the prognosis of bacterial meningitis. Bacterial meningitis can result in brain damage, hearing loss, or learning disability (CDC, 2000b).

Neonatal meningitis carries the highest mortality. However, with the development of new antibiotics and the advent of aggressive supportive care measures, the mortality

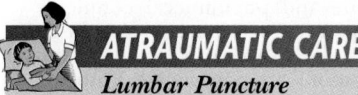

## ATRAUMATIC CARE
### Lumbar Puncture

EMLA cream, a topical anesthetic, may be applied to the skin overlying L3 to L5 to reduce pain. For maximum effect, the cream should be applied at least 1 hour before the procedure.

rate for bacterial meningitis in children caused by *H. influenzae* type b, *S. pneumoniae*, and *N. meningitidis* (meningococcal meningitis) is less than 10% in most studies (Kaplan, 1997).

The sequelae of bacterial meningitis are seen most often when the disease occurs in the first 2 months of life and least often in children with meningococcal meningitis. The residual deficits in infants are primarily a result of communicating hydrocephalus and the greater effects of cerebritis on the immature brain. In older children the residual effects are related to the inflammatory process itself or result from vasculitis associated with the disease. Bacterial meningitis continues to cause substantial morbidity in infants and children. The mortality rate and incidence of poor neurologic outcome is highest in patients with pneumococcal meningitis (Kaplan, 1997).

Hearing impairment is the most common sequela of this disease. Evaluation of CN VIII is needed for at least a 6-month follow-up period to assess for possible hearing loss.

**Prevention.** Vaccines are available for types A, C, Y, and W-135 meningococci and *H. influenzae* type b. Routine meningococcal vaccination of children is not recommended. However, routine vaccinations for *H. influenzae* type b are recommended for all children beginning at 2 months of age. (See Immunizations, Chapter 12.) Pneumococcal conjugate vaccine is now recommended for all children beginning at 2 months of age (American Academy of Pediatrics, 2000a, b).

### Nursing Considerations

Nurses should take the necessary precautions to protect themselves and others from possible infection. Parents are taught the proper procedures and supervised in their application.

> **NURSING ALERT**
>
> A major priority of nursing care of a child suspected of having meningitis is to administer antibiotics as soon as they are ordered. The child is placed on respiratory isolation for at least 24 hours after implementation of antimicrobial therapy.

The room is kept as quiet as possible, and environmental stimuli are kept at a minimum because most children with meningitis are sensitive to noise, bright lights, and other external stimuli. Most children are more comfortable without a pillow and with the head of the bed slightly elevated. A side-lying position is more often assumed because of nuchal rigidity. The nurse should avoid actions that cause pain or increase discomfort, such as lifting the child's head. Evaluating the child for pain and implementing appropriate relief measures are important during the initial 24 to 72 hours. Acetaminophen with codeine is often used. Measures are used to ensure safety because the child is often restless and subject to seizures.

The nursing care of the child with meningitis is determined by the child's symptoms and treatment. Observation of vital signs, neurologic signs, LOC, urinary output, and other pertinent data is carried out at frequent intervals. The child who is unconscious is managed as described previously (see p. 1654), and all children are observed carefully for signs of the complications just described, especially for

signs of increased ICP, shock, or respiratory distress. Frequent assessment of the open fontanel(s) is needed in the infant because subdural effusions and obstructive hydrocephalus can develop as a complication of meningitis.

Fluids and nourishment are determined by the child's status. The child with dulled sensorium is usually given nothing by mouth. Other children are allowed clear liquids initially and, if tolerated, progress to a diet suitable for their age. Careful monitoring and recording of intake and output are needed to determine deviations that might indicate impending shock or increasing fluid accumulation, such as cerebral edema or subdural effusion.

One of the most difficult problems in the nursing care of children with meningitis is maintaining IV infusion for the length of time needed to provide adequate antimicrobial therapy (usually 10 days). Because continuous IV fluids are usually not necessary, an intermittent infusion device is used. In some cases children who are recovering uneventfully are sent home with the device, and the parents are taught IV drug administration. (See Nursing Care Plan: The Child with Acute Bacterial Meningitis.*)

**Family Support.** The sudden nature of the illness makes emotional support of the child and parents extremely important. (See Family Focus box.) Parents are very upset and concerned about their child's condition and often feel guilty for not having suspected the seriousness of the illness sooner. They need much reassurance that the natural onset of meningitis is sudden and that they acted responsibly in seeking medical assistance when they did. The nurse encourages the parents to openly discuss their feelings to minimize blame and guilt. They also are kept informed of the child's progress and of all procedures, results and treatments. In the event that the child's condition worsens, they need the same psychologic care as parents who face the possible death of their child. (See Chapter 23.)

## Nonbacterial (Aseptic) Meningitis

Aseptic meningitis is caused by many different viruses. The onset may be abrupt or gradual. The initial manifestations are headache, fever, malaise, and gastrointestinal symptoms.

---

*Home care instructions for caring for an intermittent infusion device and nursing care plan are available in Wong DL, Hess CS: *Wong and Whaley's clinical manual of pediatric nursing*, ed 5, St Louis, 2000, Mosby.

> **FAMILY FOCUS**
> *Preventing Bacterial Meningitis*
>
> With the change in immunization schedules calling for administration of Hib vaccine and pneumoccal conjugate vaccine to infants at 2 months of age, parents should be encouraged to bring their child to a health facility so that the full series of immunizations are completed. With the high mortality associated with bacterial meningitis, early immunization can prevent families from experiencing the tragic death of a child. Nurses play a significant role in educating families regarding preventive measures, such as early vaccination.

Signs of meningeal irritation develop 1 or 2 days after the onset of illness. Onset is more insidious in infants and toddlers. Signs and symptoms are vague and are often thought to be associated with a minor illness.

Diagnosis is based on clinical features and CSF findings. Variations in CSF values in bacterial and viral meningitis are listed in Table 37-6. It is important to differentiate this self-limited disorder from the more serious forms of meningitis.

Treatment is primarily symptomatic, such as acetaminophen for headache and muscle pain, maintenance of hydration, and positioning for comfort. Until a definitive diagnosis is made, antimicrobial agents may be administered and isolation enforced as a precaution against the possibility that the disease might be of bacterial origin. Nursing care is similar to the care of the child with bacterial meningitis.

## Tuberculous (TB) Meningitis

TB meningitis must be considered, especially in persons traveling or living in, and in immigrants from, developing countries. The advent of drug-resistant TB may predispose an increasing number of children to this organism. Tuberculous meningitis is more likely to be disseminated (including CNS involvement) in very young or immunosuppressed children.

Ischemic infarction can occur with TB meningitis. The most common clinical findings are meningeal signs, fever, alteration of consciousness, CN involvement, seizures, and focal neurologic deficit.

Early diagnosis of TB meningitis in the child can significantly reduce the disability caused by hydrocephalus, a common complication of this type of meningitis. Nursing care is similar to the care of the child with bacterial meningitis and involves administration of medications, support of the child, control of pain, and neurologic monitoring.

## Brain Abscess

Intracerebral abscesses form when pyogenic organisms gain access to neural tissue by way of the bloodstream from foci of infection or from direct inoculation of organisms from meningitis, penetrating trauma, or surgical procedures. Chronic ear infection, mastoiditis, and cyanotic congenital heart disease are the most common predisposing factors for children with brain abscesses. Meningitis and ventriculitis

are dominant etiologies in infants. It is important to note that the incidence of a concomitant brain abscess is very high when an infant is diagnosed with *Citrobacter diversus* meningitis (Kline, 1988). The most common pyogenic organisms include staphylococci, streptococci, and *Proteus*. However, a large number of children with brain abscesses have no discernible source of infection.

The most common sites of intracerebral abscesses are the temporal and frontal lobes between the gray and white matter. Early signs of the disease are vague, and the insidious onset often includes vomiting, lethargy, fever, seizures, and progression to coma. Specific neurologic signs are related to the area invaded by the infectious process and, as this area enlarges, resemble those produced by an intracranial tumor. Cerebellar abscesses produce signs and symptoms associated with any posterior fossa mass. (See Brain Tumors, Chapter 36.) Because mortality rates from brain abscesses may exceed 20%, a prompt diagnosis is critical. Successful management consists of surgical drainage and antibiotic therapy. Surgical drainage is necessary if medical therapy does not resolve the abscess. Where possible, the source of the infection is eradicated. Children may experience seizure disorders as a long-term complication.

## Encephalitis

Encephalitis is an inflammatory process of the CNS that is caused by a variety of organisms, including bacteria, spirochetes, fungi, protozoa, helminths, and viruses. Most infections are associated with viruses, and this discussion is limited to these agents.

### Etiology

Encephalitis can occur as a result of (1) direct invasion of the CNS by a virus or (2) postinfectious involvement of the CNS after a viral disease. Often the specific type of encephalitis may not be identified. The cause of more than half the cases reported in the United States is unknown. The majority of cases of known etiology are associated with the childhood diseases of measles, mumps, varicella, and rubella and, less often, with the enteroviruses, herpes viruses, and West Nile virus.

Herpes simplex encephalitis is an uncommon disease, but 30% of cases involve children. The initial clinical findings are nonspecific (fever, altered mental status), but

**TABLE 37-6**   Variation in CSF analysis in bacterial and viral meningitis

| Type of Meningitis | WBC Count | Protein Content | Glucose Content | Gram Stain; Bacterial Culture | Color |
|---|---|---|---|---|---|
| Bacterial* | Elevated; increased polys | Elevated | Decreased | Positive | Turbid or cloudy |
| Viral | Slightly elevated; increased lymphs | Normal or slightly increased | Normal | Negative | Clear or slightly cloudy |

*Results may vary in the neonate.

most cases evolve to demonstrate focal neurologic signs and symptoms. Children may experience focal seizures. The CSF is abnormal in most cases. Because of a rise in the number of children with herpes simplex virus encephalitis, suspected cases require prompt attention, especially because the diagnosis can be difficult. The clinical diagnosis can be confirmed by the rapid appearance of IgM antibody to herpes simplex virus type 1 in CSF and serum. The early use of IV acyclovir reduces mortality and morbidity. Empiric therapy with acyclovir is given before precise virologic diagnosis has been established. CSF should be sent for viral titers.

The multiplicity of causes of viral encephalitis makes diagnosis difficult. Most are those involved with arthropod vectors (togaviruses and bunyaviruses) and those associated with hemorrhagic fevers (arenaviruses, filoviruses, and hantaviruses). In the United States, the vector reservoir for most agents pathogenic for humans is the mosquito (St. Louis encephalitis; West Nile); therefore most cases of encephalitis appear during the hot summer months and subside during the autumn.

### Clinical Manifestations

The clinical features of encephalitis are similar regardless of the agent involved. Manifestations can range from a mild benign form that resembles aseptic meningitis, lasts a few days, and is followed by rapid and complete recovery, to a fulminating encephalitis with severe CNS involvement. The onset may be sudden or may be gradual with malaise, fever, headache, dizziness, apathy, stiffness of the neck, nausea and vomiting, ataxia, tremors, hyperactivity, and speech difficulties. In severe cases there is high fever, stupor, seizures, disorientation, spasticity, and coma that may proceed to death. Ocular palsies and paralysis also may occur.

### Diagnostic Evaluation

The diagnosis is made on the basis of clinical findings and, where possible, identification of the specific virus. Early in the course of encephalitis, CT scan results may be normal. Later, hemorrhagic areas in the frontotemporal region may be seen. Togaviruses (some of which were formerly labeled arboviruses) are rarely detected in the blood or spinal fluid, but viruses of herpes, mumps, measles, and enteroviruses may be found in the CSF. Serologic testing may be required. The first blood sample should be drawn as soon as possible after onset, with the second sample drawn 2 or 3 weeks later.

### Therapeutic Management

Patients suspected of having encephalitis are hospitalized promptly for observation. Treatment is primarily supportive and includes conscientious nursing care, control of cerebral manifestations, and adequate nutrition and hydration, with observations and management as for other cerebral disorders. Viral encephalitis can cause devastating neurologic injury. Cerebral hyperemia occurs in severe viral encephalitis, and ICP monitoring to reduce the pressure may be needed (Willoughby, 1997). Follow-up care with periodic reevaluation and rehabilitation is important for patients who develop residual effects of the disease.

The prognosis for the child with encephalitis depends on the child's age, the type of organism, and residual neurologic damage. Very young children (younger than 2 years of age) may exhibit increased neurologic disability, including learning difficulties and seizure disorders.

### Nursing Considerations

Nursing care of the child with encephalitis is the same as for any unconscious child and for the child with meningitis. Additional nursing interventions include observation for deterioration in consciousness. Isolation of the child is not necessary; however, good handwashing technique must be followed. A main focus of nursing management is the control of rapidly rising ICP. Neurologic monitoring, administration of medications, and support of the child and parents are the major aspects of care.

## Rabies

Rabies is an acute infection of the nervous system caused by a virus that is almost invariably fatal if left untreated. It is transmitted to humans by the saliva of an infected mammal and is introduced through a bite or skin abrasion. After entry into a new host, the virus multiplies in muscle cells and is spread through neural pathways without stimulating a protective host immune response.

Approximately greater than 85% of rabies cases come from wild animals. Carnivorous wild animals (skunks, raccoons, and bats) are the animals most often infected with rabies and the cause of most indigenous cases of human rabies in the United States (CDC, 2001). The likelihood of human exposure to a rabid domestic animal has decreased greatly.

The circumstances of a biting incident are important. An unprovoked attack is more likely than a provoked attack to indicate a rabid animal. Bites inflicted on a child attempting to feed or handle an apparently healthy animal can generally be regarded as provoked. Any child bitten by a wild animal is assumed to be exposed to rabies.

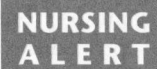 **NURSING ALERT** Unusual behavior in an animal is cause for suspicion; children should be warned to beware of wild animals that appear to be friendly.

Although rabies is common among wildlife species, human rabies is rarely acquired. Modern-day prophylaxis is nearly 100% successful. The highest incidence occurs in children under age 15 years. The incubation period usually ranges from 1 to 3 months but may be as short as 10 days or as long as 8 months. Only 10% to 15% of persons bitten develop the disease, but once symptoms are present, rabies progresses to a fatal outcome. In the United States, human fatalities associated with rabies occur in people who fail to seek medical attention, usually because they are unaware of their exposure.

The disease is characterized by a period of general malaise, fever, and sore throat followed by a phase of excitement that features hypersensitivity and increased reaction to external stimuli, convulsions, maniacal behavior, and choking. Attempts at swallowing may cause such severe spasm of respiratory muscles that apnea, cyanosis, and anoxia are produced—the characteristics from which the term *hydrophobia* was derived.

Diagnosis is made on the basis of history and clinical features. Treatment is of little avail once symptoms appear, but the long incubation period allows time for the induction of active and passive immunity before the onset of illness.

### Therapeutic Management

Two types of immunizing products are available for use in humans: (1) the inactivated rabies vaccines, which induce an active immune response; and (2) the globulins, which contain preformed antibodies. The two types of products should be used concurrently for rabies postexposure treatment when prophylaxis is indicated.

The current therapy for a rabid animal bite consists of thorough cleansing of the wound and passive immunization with *human rabies immune globulin (HRIG)* as soon as possible after exposure to provide rapid, short-term passive immunity (CDC, 1999a).

Of the 21 cases of human rabies reported since 1980 that were caused by bat-associated rabies virus, only one patient had a definite history of a bat bite. Therefore, unless the bat is available for testing and is determined to be negative for rabies, postexposure prophylaxis is recommended for all persons who have had a bat bite, scratch, or mucous membrane exposure (CDC, 1999a).

Postexposure active immunity is conferred by administration of the *human diploid cell rabies vaccine (HDCV)*. The first intramuscular injection of the vaccine is given at the same time as the immune globulin (day 0) and is followed by injections at 3, 7, 14, and 28 days after the first dose (CDC, 1999a). An additional dose in 90 days is recommended by the World Health Organization. Before antirabies prophylaxis is initiated, the local or state health department should be consulted.

### Nursing Considerations

Parents, as well as children, are frightened by the urgency and seriousness of the situation. They need anticipatory guidance for the therapy as well as support and reassurance regarding the efficacy of the preventive measures for this dreaded disease. The vaccine is well tolerated by children, although they need preparation for the series of injections. Mass immunization is unnecessary and unlikely to be implemented. In areas in which rabies is rare, the schedule given is sufficient. However, certain circumstances may warrant preexposure vaccination, such as when a child is being taken to an area of the world where rabies in stray dogs is still a problem.

## Reye Syndrome (RS)

RS is a disorder defined as toxic encephalopathy associated with other characteristic organ involvement. It is characterized by fever, profoundly impaired consciousness, and disordered hepatic function.

The etiology of RS is not well understood, but most cases follow a common viral illness, most commonly influenza or varicella. RS is a condition characterized pathologically by cerebral edema and fatty changes of the liver. The onset of RS is notable for profuse vomiting and varying degrees of neurologic impairment, including personality changes and deterioration in consciousness (Belay and others, 1999). The pathology of RS is a mitochondrial insult induced by different viruses, drugs, exogenous toxins, and genetic factors. Elevated serum ammonia levels tend to correlate with the clinical manifestations and prognosis.

Definitive diagnosis is established by liver biopsy. The staging criteria for RS are based on liver dysfunction and on neurologic signs that range from lethargy to coma (Box 37-8). Children who in the past would have been diagnosed with RS are now diagnosed with other illnesses as a result of improved diagnostic techniques. Many children are now correctly diagnosed as having viral or metabolic diseases. Cases of unrecognized, drug-induced encephalopathy by antiemetics given to children during viral illnesses have symptoms similar to those of RS.

The potential association between aspirin therapy for the treatment of fever in children with varicella or influenza and the development of RS precludes its use in these patients. However, by the time aspirin product labeling was required by the Food and Drug Administration (FDA) in 1986, most of the decline in RS incidence had already occurred. However, many experts maintain that adequate labeling to alert the public to potential hazards from administration of aspirin has been a factor in the virtual disappearance of RS.

### Nursing Considerations

The most important aspect of successful management of the child with RS is early diagnosis and aggressive therapy. Cerebral edema with increased ICP represents the most immediate threat to life. Recovery from RS is rapid and usually

---

**Box 37-8**
**Staging Criteria for Reye Syndrome**

**STAGE I**
Vomiting, lethargy, and drowsiness; liver dysfunction; type I EEG, follows commands, pupillary reaction brisk

**STAGE II**
Disorientation, combativeness, delirium, hyperventilation, hyperactive reflexes, appropriate responses to painful stimuli; evidence of liver dysfunction; type I EEG, pupillary reaction sluggish

**STAGE III**
Obtunded, coma, hyperventilation, decorticate rigidity, preservation of pupillary reaction and oculovestibular reflexes (although sluggish); type II EEG

**STAGE IV**
Deepening coma, decerebrate rigidity, loss of oculocephalic reflexes, large and fixed pupils, loss of doll's eye reflex, loss of corneal reflexes; minimum liver dysfunction; type III or IV EEG, evidence of brainstem dysfunction

**STAGE V**
Seizures, loss of deep tendon reflexes, respiratory arrest, flaccidity; type IV EEG; usually no evidence of liver dysfunction

without sequelae if there has been early diagnosis and implementation of therapy. In about one third of patients RS causes death or long-term neurologic sequelae (Belay and others, 1999).

Care and observations are implemented as for any child with an altered state of consciousness (see p. 1656) and increasing ICP. Accurate and frequent monitoring of intake and output is essential for adjusting fluid volumes to prevent both dehydration and cerebral edema. Because of related liver dysfunction, laboratory studies to determine impaired coagulation, such as prolonged bleeding time, should be monitored.

Parents of children with RS need to be kept informed regarding the child's progress, to have diagnostic procedures and therapeutic management explained, and to be given concerned and sympathetic support.* Families need to be aware that salicylate, the alleged offending ingredient in aspirin, is contained in other products (e.g., Pepto-Bismol). They should refrain from administering any product for influenza-like symptoms without first checking the label for "hidden" salicylates.

## Human Immunodeficiency Virus (HIV) Encephalopathy

Documented routine HIV testing and counseling for all pregnant women in the United States is recommended (American Academy of Pediatrics, 1995). Consent is obtained before testing. The use of zidovudine (AZT) by HIV-infected pregnant women significantly reduces the chance that the mother will pass the virus on to her infant.

---

*National Reye's Syndrome Foundation, Inc, (800) 233-7393 (United States only) or (419) 636-2679, fax: 419-636-9897, e-mail: nrsf@reyessyndrome.org.

### EVIDENCE-BASED PRACTICE
#### *Terminology for Epilepsy*

Many words are used synonymously with the term *epilepsy*, *seizure disorder*, or *seizure*. Epilepsy used to belong to the medical discipline of psychiatry, and therefore words such as "attacks" and "fits" are sometimes used to describe seizure events. These words, however, still create images of medieval superstitions, evil spirits, and the horrors of mental institutions. For these reasons, parents are often hesitant to inform caregivers and the school that their child has a seizure disorder for fear of prejudice and misunderstandings.

The words "convulsion," "convulsive disorder," and "anticonvulsive drugs" are often used to cover all seizure types and antiepileptic drugs. However, the word "convulsion" conjures up images of a raving, wild person who is out of control and possibly dangerous. Therefore the wisdom of referring to all seizures as convulsions is questionable, because most seizures are not convulsive in nature. Therefore in this chapter the words "event," "episode," or "experience" are used to describe a seizure; likewise, medications are referred to as antiepileptic drugs. In working with families, health professionals should consider the words they use to discuss epilepsy and seizures. Correct terminology can help lessen the stigma and fear often associated with words such as "convulsions" or "fits."

HIV infection is acquired through direct exposure to blood, semen, or vaginal fluid or via breast milk. The majority of pediatric HIV cases worldwide are acquired vertically from an infected mother. HIV DNA polymerase chain reaction (PCR) can identify HIF infection in over 90% of newborns 1 month of age. In the United States, antiretroviral therapy is recommended for all HIV-infected infants less than 1 year of age.

Children with HIV infection can develop neurologic manifestations, including progressive multifocal encephalopathy, myelopathy, peripheral neuropathy, and developmental delay or arrest. Changes on CT examination, including generalized brain atrophy and bilateral calcifications of the basal ganglia, may be seen. The advent of highly active antiretroviral therapy (HAART) has reversed, stopped, or delayed the onset of neurologic changes in many children with HIV (Kline, 2001).

HIV-infected children with an IQ of less than 70 at baseline have the highest risk for disease progression (56%) compared with borderline low (IQ 70 to 89, 26%) or average or above (IQ greater than 90, 18%) functioning. Motor dysfunction at study entry is also a predictor of early disease progression (Pearson and others, 2000).

## SEIZURE DISORDERS

Seizures are caused by malfunctions of the brain's electrical system that result from cortical neuronal discharge. Seizures are determined by the site of origin, and signs and symptoms may include unconsciousness or altered consciousness, involuntary movements, and changes in perception, behaviors, sensations, and posture. Seizures are the most commonly observed neurologic dysfunction in children and can occur with a wide variety of CNS conditions.

### Epilepsy

Once it is determined that the child has had a seizure, it is important to distinguish whether the episode was an epileptic or a nonepileptic seizure. Seizures are the indispensable characteristic of epilepsy; however, not every seizure is epileptic. (See Evidence-Based Practice box.) Epilepsy is a condition characterized by two or more unprovoked seizures. The careful diagnosis of epilepsy should be made and substantiated with clinical evidence because of the important prognostic and therapeutic implications, which also involve the identification and treatment of the etiology.

A simple seizure event should not be classified as epilepsy and is generally not treated with long-term antiepileptic drugs. Some seizures may result from an acute medical or neurologic illness and cease once the illness is treated. In other cases children may have a single seizure without the cause ever being known.

#### Etiology

Seizures in children have many different causes. Most seizures are *idiopathic*. Although the cause of idiopathic epilepsy is unknown, it may indicate genetic factors that in some way alter the seizure threshold to influence neuronal discharge. Infant and children with congenital defects and some genetic disorders (e.g., tuberous sclerosis) may have seizures. Febrile seizures are related to a lowered seizure threshold. Hereditary EEG abnormalities have been detected in some families, and there is a higher incidence of seizures among relatives of children with idiopathic seizure disorders.

A seizure disorder also can be *acquired* as a result of brain injury during prenatal, perinatal, or postnatal periods. This injury may be caused by trauma, hypoxia, infections, exogenous or endogenous toxins, and a variety of other factors. Biochemical events (e.g., hypoglycemia, hypocalcemia, certain nutritional deficiencies) produce seizure activity. A partial list of causative factors is presented in Box 37-9.

Epilepsy and seizures affect about 2.3 million Americans. People of all ages are affected, but particularly the very young and the elderly. The incidence of causative factors associated with childhood seizures is often related to the age of the child. Seizures are more common during the first 2 years of life than during any other period of childhood. In very young infants the most common causes are birth injuries (e.g., intracranial trauma, hemorrhage, or anoxia and congenital defects of the brain). Acute infections are a common cause of seizures in late infancy and early childhood but become an uncommon cause in middle childhood. In children older than 3 years, the most common cause is idiopathic epilepsy.

Excessive fluid intake or fluid retention, such as occurs during the premenstrual period, produces alterations in the serum (and brain) concentrations of sodium, potassium, and water, which may precipitate seizures. There appear to be periods of functional instability of the brain, normally when falling asleep or awakening from sleep. At these times seizures are more likely to occur. The hormonal and metabolic changes associated with adolescence can alter the seizure threshold. In some instances photogenic stimulation by such commonplace things as television, video games, rays of the sun, or certain types of music have been implicated in precipitating seizures. For further information contact the local Epilepsy Foundation.

## Pathophysiology

Regardless of the etiologic factor or type of seizure, the basic mechanism is the same. The electric discharges (1) may arise from central areas in the brain that affect consciousness; (2) may be restricted to one area of the cerebral cortex, producing manifestations characteristic of that particular anatomic focus; or (3) may begin in a localized area of the cortex and spread to other portions of the brain which, if sufficiently extensive, produce generalized seizure activity.

Seizure activity is believed to be caused by spontaneous electric discharge initiated by a group of hyperexcitable cells referred to as the *epileptogenic focus.* As evidenced on EEG tracings, these cells display increased electric excitability but may remain quiescent over time while discharging intermittently. Normally these discharges are restrained from spreading beyond the focal area by normal inhibitory mechanisms.

In response to physiologic stimuli, such as cellular dehydration, abnormal blood sugar levels, electrolyte imbalance, fatigue, emotional stress, and endocrine changes, these hyperexcitable cells activate normal cells in surrounding areas and in distant, synaptically related cells. A generalized seizure develops when the neuronal excitation from the epileptogenic focus spreads to the brainstem, particularly the midbrain and reticular formation. These centers within the brainstem, known as the centrencephalic system, are responsible for the spread of the epileptic potentials. The discharges can originate spontaneously in the centrencephalic system or be triggered by a focal area in the cortex. On the basis of these characteristic neuronal discharges (as recorded by the EEG), seizures are designated as partial, generalized, and unclassified epileptic seizures (Menkes and Sankar, 2000). In a large proportion of children focal seizures spread to other areas, ultimately becoming generalized with loss of consciousness.

### Seizure Classification and Clinical Manifestations

Seizures are classified into three major categories: (1) *partial seizures,* formerly called focal seizures, which are limited to a particular local area of the brain; (2) *generalized seizures,* which involve both hemispheres of the brain; and (3) *unclassified epileptic seizures* (Box 37-10). In addition to the seizures classified by the international system, several types of epileptic syndromes display a group of signs and symptoms that collectively characterize or indicate a particular condition (Commission on Classification and Terminology of the International League Against Epilepsy, 1985). Several syndromes associated with epilepsy occur in infants and

---

**Box 37-9** ■ ■ ▫
### Etiology of Seizures in Children

| NONRECURRENT (ACUTE) | RECURRENT (CHRONIC) |
|---|---|
| Febrile episodes | Idiopathic epilepsy |
| Intracranial infection | Epilepsy secondary to: |
| Intracranial hemorrhage | Trauma |
| Space-occupying lesions | Hemorrhage |
| (cyst, tumor) | Anoxia |
| Acute cerebral edema | Infections |
| Anoxia | Toxins |
| Toxins | Degenerative phenomena |
| Drugs | Congenital defects |
| Tetanus | Parasitic brain disease |
| Lead encephalopathy | Hypoglycemia injury |
| *Shigella, Salmonella* | Epilepsy—sensory stimulus |
| Metabolic alterations | Epilepsy-stimulating states |
| Hypocalcemia | Narcolepsy and catalepsy |
| Hypoglycemia | Psychogenic |
| Hyponatremia or | Tetany from hypocalcemia, |
| hypernatremia | alkalosis |
| Hypomagnesemia | Hypoglycemic states |
| Alkalosis | Hyperinsulinism |
| Disorders of amino | Hypopituitarism |
| acid metabolism | Adrenocortical insufficiency |
| Deficiency states | Hepatic disorders |
| Hyperbilirubinemia | Uremia |
| | Allergy |
| | Cardiovascular dysfunction or |
| | syncopal episodes |
| | Migraine |

children. The two syndromes that occur most often are infantile spasms and Lennox-Gastaut syndrome.

**Partial Seizures.** Partial seizures may arise from any area of the cerebral cortex, but the frontal, temporal, and parietal lobes are most often affected and are characterized by localized motor symptoms; somatosensory, psychic, or autonomic symptoms; or a combination of these. The abnormal EEG discharges remain unilateral and are evident as focal spikes or sharp waves. Partial seizures are subdivided into three types:

1. **Simple partial seizures**—Elementary or simple symptoms and no alteration of consciousness (also called an aura; see discussion under Complex Partial Seizures)
2. **Complex partial seizures**—Complex symptoms and impairment of consciousness
3. **Simple or complex seizures secondarily generalized**—Simple or complex seizures that evolve into generalized seizures, usually a tonic-clonic event

Partial seizures exhibit manifestations related to where they occur in the brain. A clear description of the seizure *(ictal state)* by an eyewitness is a valuable aid in localizing the brain area involved. The initial event may provide the best clue for assessing the type of seizure and its localization. Correctly localizing the area of the brain involved during a seizure event is of crucial importance for diagnostic/therapeutic reasons. Many antiepileptic drugs exist and are specific for each type of seizure. Therefore assigning the appropriate classification is crucial for treatment.

---

**Box 37-10** ◼ ◼ ◻

## Classification of Seizures and Epilepsy Syndromes

**PRIMARY GENERALIZED**
*Seizure Types*
Tonic-clonic
Absence
Atonic
Myoclonic

*Epilepsy Syndromes*
Infantile spasms (West syndrome)
Lennox-Gastaut syndrome
Childhood absence epilepsy
Juvenile myoclonic epilepsy

**PARTIAL**
*Seizure Types*
Simple partial
Complex partial
Partial seizures that generalize

*Epilepsy Syndromes*
Benign partial epilepsy of childhood
Epilepsia partialis continua

*Unclassified*
Neonatal seizures
Febrile seizures
Pseudoseizures

Adapted from Commission on Classification and Terminology of the International League Against Epilepsy: Proposal for classification of epilepsies and epileptic syndromes, *Epilepsia* 26(3):268-278, 1985.

---

In addition to the initial event, the circumstances that precipitated the episode are important. Identifying and eliminating triggering factors may be the only treatment needed (see p. 1695). The *postictal state* (the period following a seizure) may be varied. The child may be drowsy, be uncoordinated, have transient aphasia or confusion, and display some sensory or motor impairment. Neurologic changes should be documented. Weakness, hypotonia, or inactivity of a body part may indicate an epileptogenic focus in the corresponding contralateral cortical region.

*Simple partial seizures.* **Simple partial seizures with motor signs** arise from the area of the brain that controls muscle movement. A common motor seizure in children occurs when the eye or eyes and head turn away from the side of the focus. In some children the upper extremity toward which the head turns is abducted and extended and the fingers are clenched, giving the impression that the child is looking at the closed fist. The child may be aware of the movement.

A common form is the *rolandic (sylvian) seizure,* in which there are tonic-clonic movements involving the face, salivation, and arrested speech (Holmes and Stafstrom, 1998). These are most common during sleep. On rare occasions children may have another type of simple motor seizure that displays the *jacksonian march.* The march consists of orderly, sequential progression of clonic movements that begin in a foot, hand, or face and, as electric impulses spread from the irritable focus to contiguous regions of the cortex, affect body parts activated by these cerebral regions. Motor seizures are particularly common in hemiplegic children. The movements, which are usually clonic, begin in the hemiplegic hand, spread to the entire affected side and, in many cases, become generalized seizures (typically of the tonic-clonic type).

Eye movements provide clues to the focus or origin of the seizure. Discharge in the cortex of one hemisphere tends to cause the eyes to deviate to the opposite side. Bilateral discharges tend to cause the eyes to move upward or straight ahead. When the child's eyes are closed during the seizure episode, a gentle attempt to open them may provide valuable information.

*Simple partial seizures with sensory signs* are characterized by various sensations, including numbness, tingling, paresthesia, or pain that originates in one area (e.g., face or extremities) and spreads to other parts of the body. Visual sensations, hallucinations, light flashes, tastes, smells, or sounds may be experienced. For example, the child may run into the living room because he or she hears a favorite program on television, only to discover that the television is not on. Autonomic activity may include pallor, sweating, flushing, and pupillary dilation.

*Complex partial seizures.* Partial seizures with complex symptoms are the most difficult to diagnose and control. Because they involve more organized and high-level cerebral function, as well as sensory and motor function, they have also been termed *psychomotor seizures.* These are the most common type of seizures. Complex partial seizures are observed more often in children from 3 years of age through adolescence. These seizures may begin with an *aura*—a simple partial seizure that is usually a sensation or sensory phenomenon that reflects the complicated connections and integrative functions of that area of the brain. The most common sensation is a strange feeling at the bottom of the stomach that rises toward the throat. This feeling may be accompanied by odd or unpleasant odors or taste, complex auditory or visual hallucinations, or ill-defined feelings of elevation or strangeness (e.g., *deja vu*, a feeling of familiarity in a strange environment). Small children may emit a cry as a manifestation of an aura. Strong feelings of fear and anxiety, as well as a disturbed sense of time, can be associated with an aura. The aura is part of the seizure event and is associated with EEG changes (Shafer, 1999).

*Impaired consciousness* is another characteristic of the complex partial seizure. The child may appear dazed and confused and be unable to respond when spoken to or to follow instructions.

Another feature of this seizure is *automatisms* (repeated activities without purpose and carried out in a dreamy state). The predominant observations may be oropharyngeal activities such as smacking, chewing, drooling, or swallowing; ambulatory activities such as wandering or running; and verbal manifestations such as repeating words ("please, please," "help, help," or "oh, oh"). These automatisms may be exhibited by antisocial behaviors, such as removing clothes in public or attempting to open the door of a moving car. The child may begin walking or racing around the room, knocking over chairs and lamps. It is important to realize that the child's consciousness is impaired and that these actions are not deliberate.

It is sometimes difficult to determine whether such behavior is related to the seizure activity or to a behavioral deviation. If the behavior results from seizure activity, all attempts to control such behavior with counseling or behavior plans are ineffective. The child may suddenly cease activity, appear dazed, stare into space, become confused or apathetic, become limp or stiff, or display some form of posturing.

If the seizure involves areas of the brain that control motor function, the child will exhibit movements such as jerking of the hands, arms, and so on. This seizure generally lasts for a few minutes but can last for hours and days.

Following the seizure, the postictal period occurs with signs of confusion and lack of recollection of the ictal period. Depending on the brain area involved during the episode, the child may sleep for a period of time. (See Table 37-7 for a comparison of simple partial, complex partial, and absence seizures.)

*Partial seizures that generalize.*   Simple or complex partial seizures may spread and become generalized, usually into a tonic-clonic seizure. In such a case the partial seizure is considered the primary seizure event, and the generalized seizure is considered the secondary one. In such a case it would be stated that the tonic-clonic seizure was not generalized at the onset but was a partial seizure that secondarily generalized.

**Generalized Seizures.**   Generalized seizures without a focal onset appear to arise in the reticular formation, and the clinical observations indicate that the initial involvement is from both hemispheres. Loss of consciousness occurs and is the initial clinical manifestation. Unlike partial seizures that become generalized, there is no aura. Seizures occur at any time, day or night, and the interval between events may be minutes, hours, weeks, or even years. Most affected persons first experience seizures in childhood, and children whose seizures begin before age 4 years have mental retardation and behavioral and learning problems more often than those whose seizures begin after age 4.

*Tonic-clonic seizures.*   The generalized tonic-clonic seizure, formerly known as "grand mal," is the most dramatic of all seizure manifestations of childhood (Wiederholt, 2000). The seizure usually occurs without warning and consists of two distinct phases: tonic and clonic.

In the *tonic phase,* there is a rolling of the eyes upward and immediate loss of consciousness. If standing, the child falls to the ground. The musculature stiffens in a generalized and symmetric tonic contraction of the entire body. The arms usually flex, and the legs, head, and neck extend. This tonic phase lasts approximately 10 to 20 seconds, during which the child is apneic and may become cyanotic. Autonomic stimulation causes increased salivation.

In the *clonic phase,* the tonic rigidity is replaced by intense jerking movements as the trunk and extremities undergo rhythmic contraction and relaxation. During this time the child cannot control oral secretions and may be

**TABLE 37-7**   Comparison of simple partial, complex partial, and absence seizures

| Clinical Manifestations | Simple Partial | Complex Partial | Absence |
| --- | --- | --- | --- |
| Age of onset | Any age | Uncommon before age 3 years | Uncommon before age 3 years |
| Frequency (per day) | Variable | Rarely over 1-2 times | Multiple |
| Duration | Usually less than 30 seconds | Usually over 60 seconds, rarely less than 10 seconds | Usually less than 10 seconds, rarely more than 30 seconds |
| Aura | May be sole manifestation of seizure | Frequently | Never |
| Impaired consciousness | Never | Always | Always, brief loss of consciousness |
| Automatisms | No | Frequently | Frequently |
| Clonic movements | Frequently | Occasionally | Occasionally |
| Postictal impairment | Rare | Frequently | Never |
| Mental disorientation | Rare | Common | Unusual |

incontinent of urine and feces. As the seizure ends, the movements become less intense and occur at less frequent intervals until they cease entirely. The clonic phase can last from only a few seconds to a half hour or longer.

In the postictal state children appear to relax but may remain semiconscious and difficult to rouse. They may awaken in a few minutes but remain confused for several hours. They have mild impairment of fine motor movements. Children may have visual and speech difficulties and may vomit or complain of headache. When left alone, they usually sleep for several hours. On awakening, they are fully conscious but usually feel tired and complain of sore muscles and headache, and they have no recollection of the event.

*Absence seizures.*    Absence seizures, formerly called "petit mal" or "lapses," are characterized by a brief loss of consciousness with minimal or no alteration in muscle tone and may go unrecognized because the child's behavior changes very little. These seizures almost always first appear during childhood. In most instances the onset occurs between 4 and 12 years of age. Absence seizures may persist into adulthood.

The onset of absence seizures is abrupt, with the child suddenly experiencing 20 or more events daily. Characteristically the brief loss of consciousness appears without warning and usually lasts approximately 5 to 10 seconds. Slight loss of muscle tone may cause the child to drop objects, but the child seldom falls. There may be minor movements such as lip smacking, twitching of the eyelids or face, or slight hand movements. The sudden arrest of activity and consciousness is not accompanied by incontinence, and the child will not remember the episode.

If the child is involved in a group activity, such as classroom reading or discussion, he or she may need help to catch up with the group after the seizure. An episode is often mistaken for inattentiveness or daydreaming. Frequent episodes can result in slowed intellectual processes and deterioration in schoolwork and behavior, which is sometimes the first indication of the problem. Seizures can be precipitated by hyperventilation, hypoglycemia, stress (emotional and physiologic), fatigue, or sleeplessness.

During these brief seizure episodes, there is a lapse of consciousness, and the child appears to be inattentive or daydreaming. The child's schoolwork may deteriorate, and the child may become very frustrated and develop behavior problems. It is important that the absence seizure be distinguished from daydreaming and attention deficit hyperactivity disorder (ADHD), which are also exhibited by inattentiveness or short attention span.

*Atonic seizures.*    Atonic seizures are manifested as a sudden, momentary loss of muscle tone. The onset is usually between 2 and 5 years of age. Depending on the severity of the seizure, the child may or may not lose consciousness. During a mild seizure the child may simply experience several sudden brief head drops. During a more severe episode, the child will suddenly fall to the ground (generally face down), will lose consciousness briefly, and after a few seconds will get up as if nothing happened. If a child is known to have frequent atonic seizures, he or she should

wear a helmet with a face guard because falls can result in an injury to the face.

*Myoclonic seizures.*    Myoclonic seizures include a variety of convulsive episodes characterized by sudden, brief contractures of a muscle or group of muscles. These seizures occur singly or repetitively without loss of consciousness or postictal state. The seizure may or may not be symmetric and may be isolated as benign essential myoclonus or may occur in association with other seizure forms. Myoclonus often appears normally in the course of falling asleep or is observed as a nonspecific symptom in many diseases of the nervous system, such as viral encephalitis, uremic encephalopathy, and degenerative diseases of the cerebrum.

The myoclonic seizure can be confused with the exaggerated startle reflex but may be distinguished by placing one's palm against the back of the child's head. If it is possible to push the child's head forward, this indicates an exaggerated startle reflex. In the case of a myoclonic seizure, the child's head resists attempts to bring the head forward.

**Unclassified Epileptic Seizures.**    *Infantile spasms* refer to a rare disorder that has an onset within the first 6 to 8 months of life. Nearly all children with infantile spasms will have some degree of mental retardation (Shields, 2000). The pathophysiology is unknown, but recent evidence suggests the involvement of certain regions in the brainstem associated with sleep cycling. The underlying cause may be a disturbance of the central neurotransmitter regulation at a specific phase of brain development.

This disorder (a specific spike in the EEG) is also known as infantile myoclonus, massive spasm, hypsarrhythmia, or infantile myoclonic spasms. It is twice as common in males as in females. In infants who are able to sit but not stand, the seizure is observed as a sudden dropping forward of the head and neck with trunk flexed forward and knees drawn up—the *salaam* or *jackknife seizure.* The episode may consist of a series of sudden, brief, symmetric, muscular contractions by which the head is flexed, the arms extended, and the legs drawn up. The eyes may roll upward or inward, and the seizure may be preceded or followed by a cry or giggling. There may or may not be loss of consciousness, and the infant will sometimes flush, turn pale, or become cyanotic. The child may have numerous seizures during the day without postictal drowsiness or sleep.

Less often, alternate clinical forms of infantile spasms are observed and include extensor spasms rather than head nodding and flexion of arms, legs, and trunk. Lightning attacks, which involve a single, momentary, shocklike contraction of the entire body, are another variant.

Infantile spasms are often associated with cerebral abnormalities, such as structural malformations, severe anoxic brain damage, phenylketonuria, and degenerative changes. Microcephaly, choreoathetoid or tonic posture, and abnormal movements are often present. There may be a history of maternal infection, prematurity, or birth injury, and development is delayed before the onset of the seizures. Children with infantile spasms are also at risk for cortical visual impairment (Castano and others, 2000). The long-term prognosis is poor, both mentally and developmentally.

Adrenocorticotropic hormone (ACTH) is used to treat infantile spasms, but it is associated with significant adverse effects (e.g., immunosuppression, hypertension) (Ito and others, 2000; Koo, 1999). Still, many providers advocate its use (Wong and Travathan, 2001). Vigabatrin (Sabril) is also used in many countries (Cossette, Riviello, and Carmant, 1999; Granstrom, Gaily, and Liukkonen, 1999; Riikonen, 2000) to treat infantile spasms but has been associated with irreversible visual field deficits (Riikonen, 2000; Wong and Travathan, 2001). Vigabatrin acts to increase levels of the neurotransmitter γ-aminobutyric acid (GABA) in order to decrease seizure activity.

Many children who have infantile spasms eventually develop **Lennox-Gastaut syndrome (LGS).** LGS is diagnosed on the evidence of mixed seizure types (atonic, tonic-clonic, tonic, and atypical absence), slow mental development, poor response to treatment, and typical EEG changes (diffuse slow spike waves at <3 Hz while awake or burst of fast rhythms [10 Hz] while asleep) (Swaiman, 1999). Onset of LGS is between 1 and 10 years of age, after which it is far less common. When the onset of LGS occurs before 1 year of age, it is important that it not be confused with infantile spasm seizure. The cause of LGS remains unknown. LGS is classified as idiopathic or symptomatic.

*Idiopathic LGS,* also called *cryptogenic LGS,* appears in children with normal psychomotor development and no history of epilepsy or evidence of brain damage. Seizures may occur after infectious illness, vaccination, or febrile seizure. In school-age children behavioral disturbances and changes in personality are common.

*Symptomatic LGS* reveals a history of encephalopathy and mental retardation or epilepsy. The prognosis is poorer than in the cryptogenic type. The evolution of LGS is severe. Seizure episodes continue with high frequency and with episodes of status epilepticus. Intellectual impairment is progressive.

Treatment is very difficult, and most cases do not respond to therapy. Drugs are chosen according to the types of seizures. Valproate continues to be the drug of choice for LGS. Other drugs include benzodiazepines, especially clonazepam, nitrazepam, and clobazam. Felbamate has been shown to be an effective treatment for LGS, but it is associated with a considerable risk of aplastic anemia and hepatotoxicity (Yoon and Jagoda, 2000).

High doses of immunoglobulins and a ketogenic diet have been used, but the results have been poor. The prognosis varies but can be poor. Additional family support is often required to maintain the child at home.

### Diagnostic Evaluation

Establishing a diagnosis is critical. The process of diagnosis in a child with a seizure disorder has two major foci: (1) to ascertain the type of seizure the child has experienced, and (2) to attempt to understand the cause of the event. The assessment and diagnosis rely heavily on a thorough history, skilled observation, and the use of several diagnostic tests.

It is especially important to differentiate epilepsy from other brief alterations in consciousness or behavior. Clinical entities that mimic seizures include migraine headaches, toxic effects of drugs, syncope (fainting), hyperventilation, transient ischemic attacks, breath-holding spells in infants and young children, and brainstem herniation. Cocaine intoxication should be considered in the differential diagnosis of new-onset seizure activity in newborn infants.

Because it is unusual to observe the child during a seizure, a complete, accurate, and detailed history should be obtained from a reliable and knowledgeable informant. The history involves prenatal, perinatal, and neonatal periods, including any episodes of infection, apnea, colic, or poor feeding, and information regarding any previous accidents or serious illnesses. If the diagnosis is clear, the seizure can be identified as an isolated event that is unlikely to recur (e.g., a febrile seizure) or as a symptom of an underlying disease (e.g., a brain tumor).

The history of the seizure(s) should be equally detailed, including the type of seizure or description of the child's behavior during the event(s), the age at onset, and the time at which the seizure occurs (i.e., early morning, before meals, while awake, or during sleep). Any factors that may have precipitated the seizure are important, including fever, infection, head trauma, anxiety, fatigue, and activity (e.g., hyperventilation or exposure to strong stimuli such as bright flashing lights or loud noises). If the child can describe any sensory phenomena, these are recorded. The duration and progression of the seizure (if any) and the postictal feelings and behavior (e.g., confusion, inability to speak, amnesia, headache, and sleep) are recorded. The ability to identify seizure types accurately has resulted from the technologic advances in video recording and long-term EEG monitoring that may last hours or days.

A complete physical and neurologic examination, including developmental assessment of language, learning, behavior, and motor abilities, often provides clues to neurologic disturbances. A family history can offer clues to paroxysmal disorders such as migraines, breath-holding spells, febrile seizures, or neurologic diseases.

Laboratory studies that may prove to be of value include a venous lead level if the history warrants or white blood cell count (for signs of infection). Blood glucose may give evidence of hypoglycemic episodes, and serum electrolytes, blood urea nitrogen, calcium, and other blood studies may indicate metabolic disturbances. Lumbar puncture can confirm a suspected diagnosis of meningitis. MRI can identify brain lesions.

The EEG is obtained for all children with seizures and is the most useful tool for evaluating seizure disorders. The EEG is carried out under varying conditions—with the child asleep, awake, awake with provocative stimulation (flashing lights, noise), and hyperventilating. Stimulation elicits abnormal electrical activity, which is recorded on the EEG. Various seizure types produce characteristic EEG patterns—high-voltage spike discharges are seen in tonic-clonic seizures, with abnormal patterns in the intervals between seizures; a three-per-second spike and wave pattern is observed in an absence seizure; and absence of electrical activity in an area suggests a large lesion, such as an abscess or subdural collection of fluid. A normal EEG does not rule out seizures because the EEG is only a surface recording and may represent normal interictal activity.

A variation of the EEG is long-term video-EEG recordings of the patient during waking or sleeping. The full body image may be recorded on video, with selected EEG channels displayed on the same screen for simultaneous recording and viewing. EEG monitoring is also available in digital EEG and digital video imaging, which allows for greater selection of EEG channels and is available in both routine and long-term EEGs.

Polygraph equipment may also be used to monitor physiologic data such as respiratory effort, eye movements, heart rate, and systemic blood pressure. These techniques can be used concurrently and are especially valuable in differentiating epileptic activity from paroxysmal behavior or nonepileptic motor events.

## Therapeutic Management

The goal of treatment of seizure disorders is to control the seizures or to reduce their frequency and severity, discover and correct the cause when possible, and help the child to live as normal a life as possible. If the seizure activity is a manifestation of an infectious, traumatic, or metabolic process, the seizure therapy is instituted as part of the general therapeutic regimen.

**Drug Therapy.** It is known that persons predisposed to epilepsy have seizures when their basal level of neuronal excitability exceeds a critical point; no event occurs if the excitability is maintained below this threshold. The administration of antiepileptic drugs serves to raise this threshold and prevent seizures. Consequently the primary therapy for seizure disorders is the administration of the appropriate antiepileptic drug or combination of drugs in a dosage that provides the desired effect without causing undesirable side effects or toxic reactions. Antiepileptic drugs are believed to exert their effect primarily by reducing the responsiveness of normal neurons to the sudden, high-frequency nerve impulses that arise in the epileptogenic focus. Thus the seizure is effectively suppressed; the abnormal brain waves may or may not be altered. Complete control can be achieved in 75% of children with epilepsy; good control can be achieved in another 15% (Shafer, 1999). The drugs used for control of seizures are outlined in Table 37-8.

Therapy is begun with a single drug known to be effective for the child's particular type of seizure; the dosage is gradually increased until the seizures are controlled or the child develops signs of toxicity. If the drug is effective but does not sufficiently control the seizures, a second drug is added in gradually increasing doses. Once seizures are controlled, the drug or drugs are continued for a prolonged time. Monotherapy remains the treatment method of choice for new-onset epilepsy, but, due to the availability of many new antiepileptic drugs, polypharmacy may be a viable alternative for children who cannot attain seizure control with only one agent (Leppik, 2000).

Periodic measurement of blood levels of the drug is important to assess the continued effectiveness and to alter the dose if needed. The dosage will need to be increased as the child grows. Blood cell counts, urinalysis, and liver function tests are obtained at frequent intervals in children receiving particular antiepileptic medications due to known side effects.

Discontinuation of antiepileptic therapy follows a predesigned protocol, which is usually begun when the child has been seizure-free for at least 2 years and has a normal EEG. Recurrence is most likely within the first year after discontinuance of the medication. When a medication is discontinued, the dosage should be reduced gradually over several weeks. Sudden withdrawal of a drug can cause an increase in the number and severity of seizures, often precipitating status epilepticus. If the time for reducing the medication coincides with puberty or, in younger children, occurs during periods when the child is subject to frequent infections, the drug is continued for a longer period.

**Complications of Drug Therapy.** The side effects of continued use of antiepileptic medications are sometimes distressing to the child and the family. Most side effects are transient and dose related but warrant immediate attention. Drug reactions require clinical evaluation and serum drug levels. Combination therapy, such as with barbiturates and carbamazepine, can potentiate drug levels. Careful monitoring is necessary to avoid toxicity. To avoid possible complications of tissue damage and difficulties with administration of IV phenytoin, fosphenytoin should be used.

> **NURSING ALERT**
>
> Fosphenytoin (Cerebyx) is often used to treat seizures instead of IV phenytoin because of possible complications and drug interactions associated with IV phenytoin. If IV phenytoin is used, it should be administered via slow IV push and at a rate that does not exceed 50 mg/min. Because phenytoin precipitates when mixed with glucose, only normal saline is used to flush the tubing or catheter. Fosphenytoin may be given in saline or glucose solutions at a rate of up to 150 mg PE (phenytoin equivalent)/min, and it may be given intramuscularly if necessary.

Chronic treatment with phenytoin may cause lymphoid hyperplasia that is most noticeable in the gums. Surgical removal of the excess tissue may be needed in severe cases. Enlargement of the tonsillar and adenoidal tissue can cause partial airway obstruction, which produces snoring during sleep.

Common side effects, such as ataxia and rashes, often disappear when drug dosages are reduced. Depression, which has been reported in children with epilepsy who are taking barbiturate antiepileptics, can be relieved by changing drugs.

**Surgical Therapy.** When seizures are determined to be caused by a hematoma, tumor, or other cerebral lesion, surgical removal is the treatment. In children with epilepsy, surgery is reserved for those who suffer from incapacitating, refractory seizures. The epileptogenic area should be in a surgically removable and functionally silent region of the brain. Early removal of the symptomatic area is associated with seizure control and decreased use of antiepileptic drugs (Mathern and others, 1999). Because a very extensive

**TABLE 37-8    Common antiepileptic medications**

| Drug | Indications | Half-life (hours) | Usual Dose (mg/kg/day) | Therapeutic Levels (μg/ml) | Adverse Effects |
|------|-------------|-------------------|------------------------|----------------------------|-----------------|
| Carbamazepine | Partial, secondary generalized | 3-23 (18-55 initially) | 5-25 5-10 (monotherapy) | 4-12 | Allergic rashes, nausea, diplopia, blurry vision, dizziness, hypersensitivity hepatitis, aplastic anemia |
| Phenytoin | Partial, secondary generalized, primary generalized | 7-42 (nonlinear kinetics) | 5-7 | 10-20 (occasionally lower) | Rashes, hirsutism, gingival hyperplasia, coarse features, psychomotor slowing, neuropathy, folate deficiency, myelosuppression, drug-induced lupus |
| Valproic acid | Primary generalized, absence, myoclonic, akinetic, febrile, infantile spasms, some partial | 6-16 | 10-30 20-50 (infants and in polytherapy) | 50-100 (150 if tolerated) | Nausea, tremor, weight gain, hair loss, thrombocytopenia, hepatic failure, pancreatitis |
| Phenobarbital | Neonatal, febrile, partial, secondary generalized, primary generalized, akinetic | 36-120 | 3-5 (<25 kg) 2-3 (25-50 kg) 1-2 (>50 kg) | 10-40 | Sedation, inattention, hyperactivity, irritability, cognitive impairment, rare hypersensitivity reactions |
| Ethosuximide | Absence, myoclonic, akinetic | 15-68 | 15-40 | 40-100 | Nausea, abdominal discomfort, hiccups, drowsiness, behavioral problems, dystonias, myelosuppression, drug-induced lupus |
| Primidone | Partial, secondary generalized, primary generalized | 3-20 | 5-10 (1-2 initially) | 5-12 | Sedation, irritability, psychomotor slowing, rare hematological and hypersensitivity reactions |
| Clonazepam | Absence, primary generalized, infantile spasms | 20-36 | 0.01-0.2 | 0.01-0.07 | Sedation, hyperactivity, inattention, aggressiveness, tolerance, ataxia, withdrawal seizures |
| Acetazolamide | Absence, myoclonic, akinetic, partial | 10-12 | 10-20 | 10-14 | Diuresis, paresthesias, sedation, $CO_2$ retention, rashes |
| Felbamate | Partial (in patients >12 years), Lennox-Gastaut syndrome | 20 (in monotherapy) | 15-45 (maximum of 3600 mg) | — | Anorexia, weight loss, nausea, insomnia, headache, fatigue, aplastic anemia |
| Gabapentin | Partial, with or without secondary generalized seizures in patients >12 years | 5-7 | Total daily dose 900-1800 mg | — | Somnolence, dizziness, ataxia, fatigue |
| Lamotrigine | Partial, primary generalized, absence, atypical absence, atonic, and myoclonic | 7 to 45 | 5-15 without valproic acid, 1-5 with valproic acid | — | Somnolence, rash, vomiting |
| Topiramate | Partial, primary generalized, tonic, atonic, atypical absence | 20-30 | 1-9 | — | Somnolence, anorexia, fatigue, difficulty with concentration, nervousness |
| Tigabine | Partial | 3-9 | 0.25-1.5 (maximum of 56 mg) | | Dizziness, somnolence, headache, depression |

From Hoekelman RA and others: *Primary pediatric care,* St Louis, 2001, Mosby.

medical (e.g., invasive EEG monitoring), psychosocial, and psychometric evaluation is required, prospective candidates should be able to cooperate and tolerate the testing.

There are three types of surgical interventions. In *resective surgery* the focal area of the seizure activity is excised with the expectation that serious deficits will not be produced and that existing deficits will not be increased. Surgical excision of the epileptogenic focus does not eliminate the need for continuation of drug therapy. Drug administration is restarted as soon as the patient regains consciousness and is continued until the patient is free of seizures. *Callosotomy* involves the separation of the connections between the two hemispheres of the brain and is used in some generalized seizures. In *multiple subpial transection*, horizontal fibers of the motor cortex are divided to reduce seizures, whereas the vertical fibers are spared to allow for function (Mathern and others, 1999).

Another treatment for refractory seizures is the use of the *ketogenic diet*, which severely restricts carbohydrate and protein intake and uses fat as the primary fuel to produce ketosis. A recent review of the effects of the diet support that some children have reduced seizures during treatment, but the long-term effects, such as increased blood lipids, are not known (Lefevre and Aronson, 2000).

**Vagus Nerve Stimulation.** Vagus nerve stimulation uses an implantable device that reduces seizures in individuals who have not had effective control with drug therapy. It is currently indicated for use in patients 12 years and older whose epileptic disorder is dominated by partial seizures (with or without secondary generalization). An implanted, programmable signal generator delivers a precise pattern of stimulation to the vagus nerve and can be activated by the patient if needed.

**Status Epilepticus.** Status epilepticus is a continuous seizure that lasts more than 30 minutes or a series of seizures from which the child does not regain a premorbid level of consciousness. The initial treatment is directed toward support and maintenance of vital functions—including maintenance of an adequate airway, administration of oxygen, and hydration—followed by IV administration of antiepileptic agents.

Rectal diazepam is a simple, effective, and safe treatment for home or prehospital management (Mitchell and others, 1999). It is available in a prefilled rectal gel syringe (Diastat) for easier administration. Valproic acid has also been reported to be effective in status epilepticus when given rectally or intravenously (Yamamoto and Yim, 2000). Lorazepam (Ativan) may be replacing IV diazepam as the drug of choice. It has a longer duration of action and causes less respiratory distress in children over 2 years of age. Concurrent IV loading with phenytoin is usually necessary for sustained control of seizures. Midazolam (Versed) has been given successfully by intranasal route for treatment of acute epileptic seizures (Fisin and others, 2000; Kutler and others, 2000; Scheepers and others, 2000).

| NURSING ALERT | Diazepam is incompatible with many drugs. To give intravenously, inject slowly and directly into the vein or through tubing as close as possible to the vein insertion site. |

The child must be closely monitored during administration to detect early alterations in vital signs that may indicate impending respiratory depression. When diazepam is ineffective, phenytoin or phenobarbital is given intravenously as the initial medication, often in extremely high levels that may require respiratory support. Patients who do not respond to drug therapy may require the use of IV lidocaine, a general anesthetic, or a potent paralyzing agent. Although paralyzing agents resolve the physical manifestations of the seizure, they have no effect on the EEG. The child may continue to seize and may require continuous EEG monitoring and treatment for electrographic seizures.

Status epilepticus is a medical emergency that requires immediate intervention to prevent possible brain injury or death. Equally imperative to halting the tonic-clonic movement is correct diagnosis of the underlying problem. The outcome is related to the etiology and duration of the status epilepticus.

### Prognosis

Most children who experience a second seizure will experience additional seizures. Therefore a history of two seizures is sufficient to diagnose epilepsy (Shinner and others, 2000). Onset of seizures before 1 year of age, a symptomatic etiology, and a high frequency of seizures before treatment are thought to be early predictors of intractability (Cassetta and others, 1999) although others have identified the etiology of the seizure as the single most important factor (Ramos-Lizana, 2000).

Children who had only two seizures in the 6 months following diagnosis were more likely to have remission of seizures for 1 year when compared with children who had more than two seizures during this period (95% vs 75%). In the 5-year period after diagnosis, 47% of the children in low-risk group remained seizure-free in contrast to 24% in the high-risk group (MacDonald and others, 2000).

Convulsive status epilepticus is convincingly related to serious morbidity and mortality and is often associated with a severe neurologic abnormality, uncontrolled seizure disorder, or concurrent serious illness or infection. In one study, 79% of children who suffered status epilepticus had neurologic abnormalities. The highest morbidity was in patients with a nonidiopathic, nonfebrile cause, whereas children with idiopathic or febrile status epilepticus had a more favorable outcome (Barnard and Wirrell, 1999).

### Nursing Considerations

### ◼ Assessment

An important nursing responsibility includes observing the seizure episode and accurately documenting the events. Any alterations in behavior preceding the seizure and the characteristics of the episode, such as sensory-hallucinatory phenomena (e.g., an aura), motor effects (e.g., eye movements, muscular contractions), alterations in consciousness, and postictal state, are noted and recorded (Box 37-11). Describe only what is observed, rather than trying to label a seizure type.

Generalized seizures and other types with dramatic manifestations are easily detected, but absence seizures present more difficulties. They are easily misinterpreted as inattention. Any unusual behavior, even seemingly inconsequential, such as a momentary interruption of activity, staring, or mental blankness, should be described. The more detailed these descriptions, the more valuable they are for assessment. The nurse notes the time that the seizure began and times the length of the seizure. This is especially important if the child becomes cyanotic.

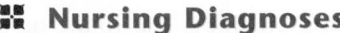

## 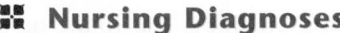 Nursing Diagnoses

Based on a thorough assessment, several nursing diagnoses are identified. The more common diagnoses for the child with a seizure disorder are included in the Nursing Care Plan on p. 1697-1698. Others may apply in specific situations.

## 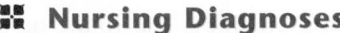 Planning

The goals for the child with a seizure disorder and the family include the following:

1. Child will be protected during a seizure.
2. Influencing or triggering factors will be determined, and adjustments will be made to lessen seizure events.
3. Child will experience as few seizures as possible.
4. Child and family will cope with the challenges associated with the disorder.
5. Child will develop a positive self-image.

## 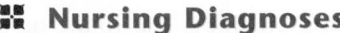 Implementation

The child must be protected from injury during the seizure; nursing observations made during the event provide valuable information for diagnosis and management of the disorder. (See Emergency Treatment box on p. 1695.)

It is impossible to halt a seizure once it has begun, and no attempt should be made to do so. The nurse must remain calm, stay with the child, and prevent the child from sustaining any harm during the seizure. If possible, the child should be isolated from the view of others by closing a door or pulling screens. A seizure can be very upsetting to the child, other visitors, and their families. If other persons are present, they should be assured that everything is being done for the child. After the seizure, they can be given a simple explanation about the event as needed.

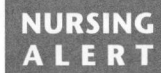 Do not move or forcefully restrain the child during a tonic-clonic seizure, and do not place a solid object between the teeth.

If the nurse is able to reach the child in time, he or she is eased to the floor immediately. During (and sometimes after) the tonic-clonic seizure, the swallowing reflex is lost, salivation increases, and the tongue is hypotonic. Therefore the child is at risk for aspiration and airway occlusion. Placing the child on the side facilitates drainage and helps to maintain a patent airway. Suctioning of the oral cavity and posterior oropharynx may be necessary. Vital signs should be taken. The child is allowed to rest if at school or away from home. When feasible, the child is integrated into the environment as soon as possible. Sending a child with a chronic seizure disorder home from school is not necessary unless requested by the parents.

---

### Box 37-11 ■ ■ ■
### General Observations: The Child During a Seizure

**OBSERVE SEIZURE**

**Describe**

Order of events (before, during, and after)
Duration of seizure
   Tonic-clonic—from first signs of event until jerking stops
   Absence—from loss of consciousness until regains consciousness
   Complex partial—from first sign of unresponsiveness, motor activity, automatisms until there are signs of responsiveness to environment

**Onset**

Time of onset
Significant preseizure precipitating events—bright lights, noise, excitement, stress
Behavior
   Change in facial expression
   Cry or other sound
   Stereotypic or automatous movements
   Random activity (wandering)
Position of eyes, head, body, extremities
   Unilateral or bilateral posturing of one or more extremities

**Movement**

Change of position, if any
Site of commencement—hand, thumb, mouth, generalized
Tonic phase—length, parts of body involved
Clonic phase—twitching or jerking movements, parts of body involved, sequence of parts involved, generalized, change in character of movements
Lack of movement or muscle tone of body part or entire body

**Face**

Color change—pallor, cyanosis, flushing
Perspiration
Mouth—position, deviating to one side, teeth clenched, tongue bitten, frothing at mouth, flecks of blood or bleeding
Lack of expression
Assymetric expression

**Eyes**

Position—straight ahead, deviation upward or outward, conjugate or divergent gaze
Pupils—change in size, equality, reaction to light and accommodation

**Respiratory Effort**

Presence and length of apnea

**Other**

Incontinence

**OBSERVE POSTICTALLY**

Duration of postictal period
State of consciousness
Orientation
Arouseable
Motor ability
   Any change in motor function
   Ability to move all extremities
   Paresis or weakness
Speech
Sensations
   Complaint of discomfort or pain
   Any sensory impairment
   Recollection of preseizure sensations aura

---

**Box 37-12** ■ ■ ■
**Seizure Precautions**

Extent of precautions depends on type, severity, and frequency of seizures.
May include:
  Siderails raised when child is sleeping or resting
  Siderails and other hard objects padded
  Waterproof mattress/pad on bed/crib
  Appropriate precautions during potentially hazardous activities:
    Swimming with a companion
    Use of protective helmet and padding during bicycle riding, skateboarding, in-line skating
    Supervision during use of hazardous machinery or equipment
Have child carry or wear medical identification.
Alert other caregivers to need for any special precautions.

---

Seizure precautions are required for children who are known to have seizures or who are under observation for seizures. The extent of these measures depends on the type and frequency of the seizure (Box 37-12).

**Long-Term Care.** Care of the child with a recurrent seizure disorder involves physical care and instruction regarding the importance of the drug therapy and, probably more significant, the problems related to the emotional aspects of the disorder. Few diseases generate as much anxiety among relatives as epilepsy. Fears and misconceptions about the disease and its treatment abound in the layperson's mind. For many it represents the archetype of severe hereditary affliction. Nurses can assist the child and family in dealing with the psychologic and sociologic problems related to the disorder.

**Physical Aspects.** Children with known seizure disorders are prescribed antiepileptic therapy. These medications are dosed at regular intervals to maintain adequate levels in the blood.

**NURSING ALERT** Children taking phenobarbital or phenytoin should receive adequate vitamin D and folic acid, because deficiencies of both have been associated with these drugs. Phenytoin should not be taken with milk.

It is important to impress on the family the necessity of continuing the medication regularly without interruption for as long as required. This is usually 2 to 3 years after the last seizure, at which point the drug is discontinued slowly over a period of weeks to avoid the possibility of precipitating a seizure. It is sometimes easy to skip doses or omit them for a variety of reasons, especially when the child is free of seizures most of the time. This is particularly so when the child is older and assumes responsibility for the medication. Parents should notify the health professional if the child has an illness, including vomiting, diarrhea, or fever. Vomiting and diarrhea can interfere with drug absorption; fever may increase metabolic requirements. Both can precipitate seizure activity.

Rectal preparations of some antiepileptic medications are highly effective when a child is unable to take oral medications because of repeated vomiting, gastrointestinal surgery, or status epilepticus. Administration of rectal antiepileptic medication can be learned by parents for home treatment.* Rectal diazepam is a useful adjunctive home treatment for children at risk for prolonged cluster seizures. Hospitalization is minimized, and parental confidence is enhanced. However, knowledge of CPR is indicated for caregivers who are responsible for administering rectal diazepam.

Nurses need to educate the child and parents about the possible adverse reactions to the medications used to treat seizure disorders in children. They should understand the common side effects so they can report any unusual observations that might indicate unfavorable reactions. Parents should understand that the child needs periodic physical assessment and laboratory studies. Possible adverse effects on the hematopoietic system, liver, and kidneys may be reflected in symptoms such as fever, sore throat, enlarged lymph nodes, jaundice, and bleeding (e.g., easy bruising, petechiae, ecchymoses, epistaxis). A common factor in status epilepticus is inadequate blood levels of antiepileptic drugs.

Parents need to be warned of possible behavioral changes as the seizures are controlled in children taking primidone, phenobarbital, or phenytoin. Changes in personality, indifference to school activities and family, hyperactivity, or even psychotic behavior may sometimes be observed. The potential effects of epileptic drugs on learning and behavior should be considered. Progressive intellectual deterioration in a child with epilepsy requires investigation of the present medication plus the role of the underlying cerebral pathology.

The degree to which activities are restricted is individualized for each child and depends on the type, frequency, and severity of the seizures; the child's response to therapy; and the length of time the seizures have been controlled. Most normal activities are encouraged for children, and participation in competitive sports is determined on an individual basis. With encouragement, most older children can accept the restrictions placed on activities. To reduce the likelihood of needlessly accentuating differences, only the essential restrictions are placed on children regarding sports and peer activity; these restrictions are approached in a positive way in terms of what the child can do rather than what the child cannot do. Parents sometimes curtail the child's activities more than necessary.

To prevent head injuries, children should wear appropriate safety devices, such as helmets. Activities involving heights should be avoided. To prevent submersion injury, they should never swim alone. Showers are recommended for older children, and close supervision is required when children are in a bathtub.

Because the child is encouraged to attend school, camp, and other normal activities, the school nurse and the teacher should be made aware of the child's condition and therapy. They can help to ensure regularity of medication

---

*Home care instructions for administration of medications and CPR instructions are available in Wong DL, Hess, CS: *Wong and Whaley's clinical manual of pediatric nursing,* ed 5, St Louis, 2000, Mosby.

## Critical Thinking Exercise

### Seizures

Since age 2 years, Jane has had epilepsy that is well controlled with medication. However, now that she has begun elementary school, her seizures have returned. On the way home Jane usually has a seizure on the bus; however, on weekends and holidays she is seizure-free. As the school nurse, what should you advise Jane's parents to do?

FIRST, THINK ABOUT IT . . .

• What information are you using?
• How are you interpreting that information?

1. Take her for medical reevaluation.
2. Increase her antiepileptic medication.
3. Drive her home from school.
4. Ride with her on the school bus.

*The best response is four. Your first priority is to help the family identify triggering events, which would yield pertinent and necessary information. At your suggestion, the mother rode the school bus home with Jane. As the child began to have a seizure, the mother noted that they had just passed a white picket fence, the triggering factor. Once the child was seated on the other side of the bus, the seizure episodes stopped.*

*With the consistent pattern and abrupt onset of the seizures, seeking medical reevaluation should be advised only if no triggering event is identified. An accurate interpretation of the information is that it is not within the scope of nursing practice for you to change the dosage of the medication. Even if the child rides home in a car, the seizures may occur if Jane sits in the same position as on the school bus.*

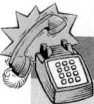

## EMERGENCY TREATMENT
### Seizures

### TONIC-CLONIC SEIZURE

#### During the Seizure

Remain calm.
Time seizure episode.
If child is standing or seated, ease child down to the floor.
Place pillow or folded blanket under child's head.
Loosen restrictive clothing.
Remove eyeglasses.
Clear area of any hazards or hard objects.
Allow seizure to end without interference.
If vomiting occurs, turn child to one side.
Do not:
    Attempt to restrain child or use force
    Put anything in child's mouth
    Give any food or liquids

#### After the Seizure

Time postictal period.
Check for breathing. Check position of head and tongue.
    Reposition if head is hyperextended. If breathing is not present, give rescue breathing and call emergency medical services (EMS).
Keep child on side.
Remain with child.
Do not give food or liquids until fully alert and swallowing reflex has returned.
Call EMS when necessary.
Look for medical identification, and determine what factors occurred before onset of seizure that may have been triggering factors.
Check head and body for possible injuries.
Check inside of mouth to see if tongue or lips have been bitten.

### COMPLEX PARTIAL SEIZURE

#### During the Seizure

Do not restrain.
Remove harmful objects from area.
Redirect to safe area.
Do not agitate; instead, talk in calm, reassuring manner.
Do not expect child to follow instructions.
Watch to see if seizure generalizes.

#### After the Seizure

Stay with child and reassure until fully conscious.

### CALL EMERGENCY MEDICAL SERVICE IF:

Child stops breathing.
There is evidence of injury or child is diabetic or pregnant.
Seizure lasts for more than 5 minutes (unless duration of seizure is typically longer than 5 minutes) and written medical order is present.
Status epilepticus occurs.
Pupils are not equal after seizure.
Child vomits continuously 30 minutes after seizure has ended (sign of possible acute problem).
Child cannot be awakened and is unresponsive to pain after seizure has ended.
Seizure occurs in water.
This is child's first seizure.

Modified from *Seizure recognition and first aid*, 2001, Epilepsy Foundation, *www.efa.org*.

---

administration and provision of any special care the child might need. Teachers, child care providers, camp counselors, youth organization leaders, coaches, and other adults who assume responsibility for children should be instructed regarding care of the child during a seizure so that they can act in a calm manner for the welfare of the child and influence the attitude of the child's peers.*

**Triggering Factors.** Careful and detailed documentation of seizures over time may indicate a pattern. When this occurs, the nurse or responsible adult may intervene to identify the triggering factors and make changes in the environment that may prevent or decrease seizure frequency. Often the necessary changes are very simple but can make an enormous difference in the lives of the child and family. (See Critical Thinking Exercise box.)

Factors that may trigger seizures in children include changes in dark-light patterns, such as those that occur with a flash on a camera, automobile headlights, reflections of light on snow or water, or rotating blades on a fan; sudden loud noises; startling or sudden movements; extreme or drastic changes in temperature; dehydration; fatigue; hy-

perventilation; hypoglycemia; caffeine; and insufficient protein in the diet (protein is needed to metabolize some antiepileptic drugs). There are children who have seizures while playing video games. These children are sensitive to

---

*An excellent resource is *Students with Seizures: A Manual for School Nurses* by N. Santilli, W.E. Dodson, and A.V. Walton (1991, Epilepsy Foundation) and *The Brainstorms Family: Epilepsy on Our Terms—Stories by Children with Seizures and Their Parents* by S.C. Schachter, G.D. Montouris, and J.M. Pellock (1996, Lippincott Williams & Wilkins).

intermittent photic stimulation that can trigger an epileptic episode (Fylan and others, 1999; Ricci and Vigevano, 1999). However, the overwhelming majority of children with epilepsy can play video games without the risk of seizures.

Factors that trigger seizure episodes should be considered in activities of daily living. If a child is photosensitive, it may be necessary to avoid such things as video games. A pattern of early-morning seizures could indicate hypoglycemia; a snack at bedtime and a glass of juice before arising may prevent this. Other dietary modifications, such as the use of caffeine-free sodas, coffee, and tea, as well as adequate protein and fluids, especially in hot weather, may prevent seizure episodes.

**Family Support.** Parental attitudes and management of a child with a seizure disorder are varied. Whether the seizures result from illness, injury, or unknown etiology, the parents may feel guilt, anxiety and, often, humiliation. They want to know if the seizures will affect the child's mental capacities. Many persons erroneously associate epilepsy with mental deficiency. Seizures do commonly accompany other manifestations of severe brain damage from disease or injury, but most children with seizures, as in any population of healthy children, display a wide range of intelligence.

Parents also wonder how the illness will affect the child's future. They need reassurance that the illness will not shorten the life of the child and that the child can attend school, marry, and elect to have children. The child may need vocational guidance, and the parents will need to become familiar with the laws in their state regarding any limitations that might be imposed on the child because of the disorder. It should be emphasized that the seizures can be controlled or greatly reduced in the large majority of affected children. Parents need reassurance that there is less stigma attached to the condition than in the past.

It is important to encourage a healthy attitude toward the child and the condition and to help the parents feel competent in their ability to meet their responsibilities to the child. The child should be reared in the same manner as any normal child, with natural concern tempered by the understanding of the need not to overprotect. Many parents refrain from correcting or punishing the child, especially if they have had the experience of such an emotional stress precipitating a seizure. The child must not be made to feel different in any way. Parents should be encouraged to be honest and open about the disorder with the child and with others. Some parents are tempted to try to conceal the nature of the child's illness because of their belief that the disorder is shameful or a disgrace to the family.

Educational materials and support groups may prove beneficial for families. The **Epilepsy Foundation**\* is a national organization that works for the welfare of persons with epilepsy and their families, helps with employment and legal problems, and provides education to patients, families, and communities.

**The Child with Epilepsy.** The child who is provided the security of a loving family, rewards and punishments no dif-

ferent from those of other children, and support in acquiring self-esteem is more apt to have a positive attitude toward the condition. Children derive their self-concept and self-esteem from observations of others' reactions to them and from their own perceptions of their capabilities. The suddenness and unpredictability of the seizures and the reactions of others further influence their feelings. When others consider children to be different, inferior, or objects of ridicule, they come to view themselves as different, inferior, and incapable.

Children with epilepsy need to learn about their condition and the role that the medication plays in contributing to their prolonged well-being. As soon as they are old enough, children should assume responsibility for taking their own medication and should be advised to carry medical identification with pertinent information about their condition. Planning activities with children and emphasizing those in which they can engage rather than those in which they cannot participate helps them to succeed and to gain satisfaction in their achievements. They should be offered opportunities and encouraged to exercise judgment in their daily lives.

The adolescent period may prove to be a trying time for the child with epilepsy. Limits imposed on the young person's activities at a time when freedom and independence are desired may bring the disability into sharp focus. For example, all U.S. states have a defined seizure-free period before a driver's license can be obtained.

Epilepsy should not be a severe impairment to most youngsters. The nurse can help to provide positive outcomes for the child and family by assuming the role of patient advocate, helping to educate the public regarding the condition, working toward making opportunities available to persons with the disorder, and lobbying for legislation that recognizes the needs of the individual with a seizure disorder.

## ■■ Evaluation

The effectiveness of nursing interventions for the child with epilepsy is determined by continual reassessment and evaluation of care based on the following observational guidelines:

1. Observe child's behavior for evidence of seizure activity and assess the environment for situations that could cause injury to child in the event of a seizure; interview family regarding management of child during a seizure.
2. Interview child and family regarding compliance with the medication regimen and identification of triggering factors.
3. Observe and interview family regarding their feelings and concerns and their understanding of child's condition.
4. Observe child's interactions with others, and interview child about any feelings or concerns regarding health.

The *expected outcomes* are described in the Nursing Care Plan on pp. 1697-1698.

## Febrile Seizures

Febrile seizures are transient disorders of children that occur in association with a fever. They are one of the most common neurologic disorders of childhood, affecting ap-

\*4351 Garden City Dr, Landover, MD 20785-7223, (301) 459-3700 or (800) EFA-1000; www.efa.org. In Canada: **Epilepsy Canada,** 1470 Peel St, Suite 745, Montreal, Quebec H3A 1TI, (514) 845-7855.

## Nursing Care Plan
## The Child with Epilepsy

---

**NURSING DIAGNOSIS:** Risk for injury related to type of seizure

**PATIENT GOAL 1:** Will not experience seizure activity

- **NURSING INTERVENTIONS/*RATIONALES***

*Administer antiepileptic medication

Teach family and child, when appropriate, the administration of medications

Stress importance of compliance

Avoid situations that are known to precipitate a seizure (e.g., blinking lights, fatigue)

- **EXPECTED OUTCOME**

Child remains free of seizure activity

**PATIENT GOAL 2:** Will not experience complications from medication

- **NURSING INTERVENTIONS/*RATIONALES***

Be aware of and teach family to recognize unfavorable reactions to medications

Encourage periodic physical and laboratory assessment *to determine possible deviations from normal findings*

Encourage good dental care during phenytoin therapy *to reduce gingival hyperplasia from phenytoin*

Encourage adequate vitamin D and folic acid with phenytoin and phenobarbital therapy *to prevent deficiency*

- **EXPECTED OUTCOME**

Child and family demonstrate an understanding of possible unfavorable responses to medications and the appropriate intervention (specify)

**PATIENT GOAL 3:** Will not experience injury

- **NURSING INTERVENTIONS/*RATIONALES***

Educate parents and child regarding appropriate activities for child (depends on type, frequency, and severity of seizures)

Explore appropriate modifications or adaptations to situations *that pose a danger during a seizure* (climbing trees, swimming)

Provide companionship during permissible activities, such as swimming, biking

Recommend showering, or close supervision during bathing

Educate teachers and other persons who are associated with child regarding correct assistance during and after seizure

- **EXPECTED OUTCOMES**

Child and family agree on appropriate activities or modifications of activities for child

Individuals in contact with child intervene appropriately during and after seizure

---

**NURSING DIAGNOSIS:** Risk for injury, hypoxia, and aspiration related to motor activity and loss of consciousness (tonic-clonic seizure)

**PATIENT GOAL 1:** Will not experience injury, respiratory distress, or aspiration

- **NURSING INTERVENTIONS/*RATIONALES***

Time seizure *to determine possible hypoxia and need for emergency care*

Protect child during seizure

Do not attempt to restrain child or use force *to prevent inflicting injury to child or self*

If child is standing or sitting in wheelchair at beginning of episode, ease child to floor *to prevent falls*

Place small cushion or blanket under child's head *to prevent injury*

Do not put anything in child's mouth (e.g., tongue blades, food, or fluids) *that can cause injury, obstruct breathing, or be aspirated*

Remove eyeglasses *to protect eyes from trauma*

Loosen clothing *that may restrict movement or breathing*

Prevent child from hitting head on objects *that might cause injury*

Remove hazards (furniture)

Pad objects such as crib, siderails, or wheelchair *to lessen injury*

Keep siderails raised when child is sleeping, resting, or having a seizure *to avoid falls*

Allow seizure to end without interference

Position child with head in midline, not hyperextended, *to promote adequate ventilation*

If child begins to vomit, turn to side *to prevent aspiration*

Protect child after seizure (postictal period)

Time postictal period

Maintain child in side position

Call emergency medical service (EMS) (see Emergency Treatment box, p. 1695)

- **EXPECTED OUTCOME**

Child exhibits no sign of physical or mental injury or aspiration

---

**NURSING DIAGNOSIS:** Risk for injury related to impaired consciousness and automatisms (complex partial seizure)

**PATIENT GOAL 1:** Will not experience injury and will remain calm

- **NURSING INTERVENTIONS/*RATIONALES***

Time seizure *to establish duration and possible need for emergency care*

Protect child during seizure

Do not restrain, unless child is in danger, *to prevent injury to child or self*

Remove hazards in immediate environment

Redirect child to safe area, especially away from windows, stairs, heating elements, or sources of water, *to prevent falls, burns, and drowning*

---

*Dependent nursing action.

*Continued*

## Nursing Care Plan
### The Child with Epilepsy—cont'd

**PATIENT GOAL 1—cont'd**

- **NURSING INTERVENTIONS/**_RATIONALES_**—cont'd**

  Do not agitate; rather, talk in calm voice and reassuring manner

  Do not expect child to follow instructions _because of impaired consciousness_

  Watch to see if seizure generalizes into a tonic-clonic seizure

  Protect child after seizure (postictal)

  Time postictal period

  Stay and reassure child until fully alert _because child may be confused and frightened_

  Call EMS (see Emergency Treatment box, p. 1695)

- **EXPECTED OUTCOME**

  Child exhibits no sign of physical injury and remains calm

---

> **NURSING DIAGNOSIS:** Interrupted family processes related to a child with a chronic illness

---

**PATIENT (FAMILY) GOAL 1:** Will receive adequate support

- **NURSING INTERVENTIONS/**_RATIONALES_

  See Nursing diagnosis: Interrupted family processes in Nursing Care Plan: The Child with Chronic Illness or Disability, Chapter 22

  Refer to special support groups and agencies (e.g., Epilepsy Foundation)

- **EXPECTED OUTCOME**

  Family becomes involved with support group

  See also:

  Nursing Care Plan: The Child with Chronic Illness or Disability, Chapter 22

  Nursing Care Plan: The Unconscious Child, pp. 1662-1663

---

proximately 3% of children. Most febrile seizures occur after 6 months of age and usually before age 3 years, with increased frequency in children younger than 18 months. They are unusual after 5 years of age. Boys are affected about twice as often as girls, and there appears to be an increased family susceptibility

The cause of febrile seizures is still uncertain. In most children the height, but not the rapidity, of the temperature elevation seems to be a factor. The temperature usually exceeds 38.8° C (101.8° F), and the seizure occurs _during_ the temperature rise rather than after a prolonged elevation. Sometimes it constitutes the dramatic beginning of an illness, often an upper respiratory or gastrointestinal infection.

Most febrile seizures have stopped by the time the child is taken to a medical facility. However, if the seizure continues, treatment consists of controlling the seizure with IV or rectal diazepam (Valium) and reducing the temperature with administration of acetaminophen. Antiepileptic prophylaxis may be considered for a child (1) who experiences focal or prolonged seizures, (2) who has neurologic abnormalities, (3) who has a first-degree relative with febrile seizures, (4) who is younger than age 1 year, and (5) in whom multiple seizures occur within a 24-hour period. In children with simple febrile seizures prophylactic antiepileptic therapy is not recommended.

Parental education and emotional support are important interventions (American Academy of Pediatrics, 1999). Parents need reassurance regarding the benign nature of febrile seizures (almost 95% to 98% of children with febrile seizures will not develop epilepsy or any neurologic damage). They also need education regarding protecting the child from harm and observing exactly what happens to the child during the event. Attempts to lower the temperature

will not prevent a seizure. Tepid sponge baths are not recommended for several reasons: they are ineffective in significantly lowering the temperature, the shivering effect further increases metabolic output, and cooling causes discomfort in the child.

Long-term antiepileptic therapy is usually not required for children with simple febrile seizures. Vigorous antipyretic therapy during febrile illness may prevent a seizure.

> **NURSING ALERT**   If a febrile seizure lasts more than 5 minutes, parents should seek medical attention right away. Instruct them to call for emergency assistance (911) and not to place the child who is actively having a seizure in the car.

## HEADACHE

Headaches are a common complaint of children and are associated with different pathologies, including extracranial disease, intracranial disease, vascular abnormalities, psychogenic disorders, or a combination of the above (Table 37-9).

### Assessment

It is important to determine the pattern of the headache—single acute episode, paroxysmal, acute and recurrent, chronic and progressive, chronic nonprogressive, or mixed. Other assessment information includes the presence of seizures, ataxia, lethargy, weakness, nausea or vomiting, or any personality changes. Factors related to early development and past illnesses and a family history of headaches

**TABLE 37-9** Characteristics of headaches

| Type of Headache | Characteristics |
|---|---|
| **Extracranial** | |
| Acute sinusitis (may also be classified as inflammatory) | Usually accompanied by fever and tenderness over involved sinuses: *Ethmoid sinuses:* Referred pain to orbital and temporal areas *Frontal sinuses:* Pain above the eyes |
| Ocular abnormalities | Headaches usually occur late in the day, precipitated by schoolwork, driving, or television viewing |
| Dental disorders (may be classified as inflammatory) | Frontal or temporal headaches caused by malocclusion, caries, abscess, temporomandibular joint (TMJ) dysfunction TMJ headaches may be exacerbated by chewing or stress Pain localized to affected structures |
| Respiratory infections (pharyngitis, otitis media) | |
| Viral infections/febrile illnesses (may also be classified as vascular) | Viral infections such as influenza or bacterial infections such as streptococcus pharyngitis may cause headache |
| Inflammatory illnesses (meningitis, encephalitis) | Global headache usually accompanied by nuchal rigidity, fever, mental status changes |
| Trauma | Localized to area of trauma; related to nerve and tissue injury Postconcussion syndrome (See Posttraumatic Syndromes, Box 37-6, p. 1670) |
| **Acute Recurrent** | |
| Vascular: migraine syndrome (see migraine classification in Box 37-14) | Intermittent attacks of vasoconstriction Paroxysmal Nausea, vomiting, fatigue, pallor Positive family history May be triggered by stress, fatigue, trauma, exercise, menses, medications, diet, sleep deprivation, environmental factors |
| **Chronic Progressive** | |
| Intracranial abnormalities | Symptoms of increased ICP |
| Tumors | Early morning headaches primarily |
| Hydrocephalus | Bulging fontanel, suture splitting in infants and young children, symptoms of increased ICP |
| Subdural hematoma | Usually results from trauma Seizures and focal neurologic deficits more common than headaches |
| Brain abscess | Rare but may be associated with chronic otitis media or sinusitis, cyanotic heart disease, and immunosuppression |
| Pseudotumor cerebri | Increased ICP without obstruction of CSF |
| **Chronic Nonprogressive** | |
| Muscle contraction and psychogenic | Common in children Adjustment reaction, anxiety related Conversion reaction (anxiety converted to somatic symptoms) |

may also be pertinent. A "headache diary," which includes time of onset and termination of headaches, intensity, associated events, and actions taken and their effects, can be very helpful for the patient and practitioner.

The family history may provide clues to etiology, including information about the home or social situation (e.g., divorce, separation, alcoholism, school avoidance). Specific questions that often elicit needed information are listed in Box 37-13. Thorough physical and neurologic examinations are performed, and further diagnostic tests (e.g., a CT, an MRI, or an EEG) are ordered if indicated.

Tension headaches are the most common form of headache in children. Simple analgesics, including acetaminophen and ibuprofen, are usually the most effective pharmacologic intervention. Biofeedback and relaxation techniques may be useful nonpharmacologic interventions in children with recurrent tension headaches (Diamond, 1999).

## Migraine Headache

Migraine, an autosomal dominant disorder, occurs in children, as well as adults. The cause is unknown, but attacks may be precipitated by stress, hypoglycemia, sleep deprivation, environmental factors, sympathetic stimulation, nervous system, fatigue, exercise, menses, conflict, anxiety, or certain foods such as chocolate. It is characterized by a chronic and recurrent headache, is often preceded by an aura, and is accompanied by nausea and vomiting. Pediatric migraine headaches can be a challenging problem to diagnose because younger children often have difficulty describing their symptoms.

The exact pathophysiology of migraines and all of their components continues to be researched. It is believed that migraine headaches are the result of vascular and neural dysfunction, which causes paroxysmal vasoconstriction and vasodilation of the cerebral vasculature. Altered serotonin neurotransmission and platelet activity is also believed to play a part in the onset of migraine headaches. Several pat-

---

**Box 37-13 ■ ■ □**
## Questions for Evaluating Headaches

1. Do you have more than one type of headache?
2. How did the headache begin? Trauma? Infection?
3. How long has it been present?
4. Are the symptoms getting worse or staying the same?
5. How often do they occur?
6. How long do they last?
7. Do they occur at any special time or when certain things happen?
8. Do you have warning signs?
9. Where does it hurt?
10. How does the pain feel? Pounding? Sharp?
11. Do you feel sick in other ways during the headache? Abdominal pain? Nausea, vomiting?
12. Do you stop what you are doing during the headache?
13. Do you have any other health problems?
14. Are you taking any medicines regularly?
15. Are there some things you do that make the headache worse or better?
16. Does any one medicine make the headache better?
17. Does anyone else in your family have headaches?
18. What do you think is causing your headaches?

Modified from Rothner AD: Management of headaches in children and adolescents, *J Pain Symptom Manage* 8(2):81-86, 1993.

---

**Box 37-14 ■ ■ ■**
## Migraine Patterns

**CLASSIC MIGRAINE**

Preceded by visual aura
Fatigue, malaise, pallor, irritability
Followed by throbbing, usually unilateral headache coupled with nausea, vomiting, photophobia, and phonophobia with a desire to sleep
On awakening the child is usually well

**COMMON MIGRAINE**

Aura less pronounced and usually consists of malaise, pallor, and irritability
Headache coupled with nausea and vomiting, photophobia, and phonophobia with a desire to sleep

**HEMIPLEGIC MIGRAINE**

Associated with recurrent paralysis
Hemiplegia may precede or follow headache
Hemiplegia resolves, lasting from a few minutes up to a day
May be familial

**BASILAR MIGRAINE**

Recurrent attacks
Symptoms and signs referable to brainstem and cerebellum
Paroxysmal acute ataxia, vertigo, occipital headache, occasional loss of consciousness

**PAROXYSMAL VERTIGO**

Episodes of vertigo in young child (ages 2 to 4 years)
Inability to maintain posture; nystagmus
Headaches, nausea, and vomiting are absent

**CYCLIC VOMITING**

Unexplained recurrent episodes of vomiting
Abdominal pain usually present
Headache absent

**CONFUSIONAL MIGRAINE**

Disturbed sensorium, agitation
Receptive or expressive aphasia
(Rule out encephalopathy and drug use)

**OPHTHALMOPLEGIC MIGRAINE**

Ptosis, mydriasis, and outward deviation of eyes (has been associated with stroke and seizures)

---

terns of migraines have been identified and are described in Box 37-14. Common migraine is one of the types most often experienced by children. The duration and localization of migraines are different in adults and children. Many children have migraine headaches of shorter duration than those of adults (deGrauw, 1999).

Symptoms may include pallor, malaise, irritability, and fatigue. Nausea and vomiting often follow a throbbing bilateral headache, although it may be unilateral. Depending on the type of migraine, the patient may experience a visual aura before the symptoms. The child often experiences photophobia and seeks out a quiet, dark room. Sleep will often terminate a migraine episode.

A family history of migraine is elicited in 70% of children; 5% of all children who have migraines will experience a headache before age 15 years. Before the onset of puberty, migraines are more common in males; this trend reverses after puberty.

**NURSING ALERT** During the health history and neurologic assessment, the following abnormal signs require immediate follow-up for children:
The headache progresses in frequency and severity over a brief period of time (2 to 3 weeks); awakens the child from sleep (may also be migraine); occurs in early morning; is worse on arising; is characterized by persistent, occipital, or frontal pain; is accompanied by unexplained vomiting; is associated with change in gait, personality, or behavior; or is exacerbated by Valsalva maneuver (intensified by lowering head and straining, such as during a bowel movement, coughing, or sneezing).

Symptomatic pain relief with oral, rectal, or IV analgesics is the basis for headache management regardless of cause. Intervention should be multifaceted. If triggers are identi-

fied, the child can learn to avoid them to assist in controlling a potential attack.

Migraine therapy, if administered early in the course of the headache, may provide rapid relief. For children who experience frequent or refractory migraines, prophylactic medications such as cyproheptadine, propranolol, or amitriptyline may be used. In adolescents who experience infrequent migraine episodes, serotonin agonists (sumatriptan, Imitrex), Excedrin, Midrin, or ergotamine may be used (Annequin, Tourniaire, and Massiou, 2000).

Although ergotamine preparations are used in the treatment of adult vascular headaches, they are not typically used in children because of side effects. Opioids also are not often used because they rarely act on the mechanism of pain.

The outlook for a child with migraine is good, but the child and parents should be informed that predisposition to the headaches may be lifelong. Severe headaches can adversely affect the child's routine activities of daily living, including family relations and school performance.

## KEY POINTS

- The central nervous system (CNS) is composed of the brain and spinal cord.
- Gait abnormalities that may indicate cerebral dysfunction include ataxia, spastic paraplegic gait, hemiplegic gait, cerebellar gait, and extrapyramidal gait.
- Level of consciousness (LOC) is the most important indicator of neurologic health; altered levels include sleep, confusion, delirium, and comatose states.
- Complete neurologic examination includes LOC; gait, motor, sensory, cranial nerve (CN), and reflex testing; and vital signs.
- Nursing care of the unconscious child focuses on respiratory management, neurologic assessment, increased intracranial pressure (ICP) monitoring, supplying adequate nutrition and hydration, drug therapy, promoting elimination, maintenance of hygiene positioning and exercise, stimulation, and family support.
- Primary head injury involves events that occur at the time of trauma, including fractured skull, contusions, intracranial hematoma, and diffuse injury. Secondary complications include hypoxic brain damage, increased ICP, infection, cerebral edema, and posttraumatic syndromes.
- The young child's response to head injury is different because of the following features: larger head size in proportion to body, larger blood volume to the brain, small subdural spaces, and thinner, softer brain tissue.
- Fractures resulting from head injuries may be classified as linear, depressed, compound, basilar, and diastatic.
- Problems resulting from near-drowning are caused by hypoxia and include asphyxiation, aspiration, and hypothermia.
- Nursing care of the child with meningitis includes administration of antibiotics, vital signs monitoring, intravenous therapy, and promotion of fluid, nutritional status, and family support
- Routine immunization of infants against H. influenzae type b infection has reduced the incidence of bacterial meningitis.
- Encephalitis may result from direct invasion of the CNS by a virus or from postinfectious involvement of the CNS after viral illness.
- A seizure is a symptom of underlying pathology and may be manifested by sensory-hallucinatory phenomena, motor effects, sensorimotor effects, or impaired or loss of consciousness.
- Partial seizures are categorized as simple (without associated impairment of consciousness) or complex primary generalized; both types may become generalized.
- Generalized seizures are categorized as tonic-clonic, absence, atonic, akinetic, or myoclonic.
- Long-term care of the child involves teaching caregivers appropriate interventions during a seizure, emphasizing the importance of antiepileptic therapy, giving practical advice regarding drug administration and scheduling, and fostering the child's and family's coping with diagnosis.
- Febrile seizures are the most common type of childhood seizure. The most important nursing intervention is to reassure parents of their benign nature and educate parents regarding protection of their child and meaningful observation during the event.
- A child's complaint of headache requires a thorough history and physical with a neurologic assessment to rule out increased ICP. Stress the most common cause of recurrent headache in children.

## REFERENCES

Adler AJ, Dubinsky I, Eisen J: Does the use of topical lidocaine, epinephrine and tetracaine solution provide sufficient anesthesia for laceration repair? *Acad Emerg Med* 5:108-112, 1998.

American Academy of Pediatrics, Committee on Drugs: Guidelines for monitoring and management of pediatric patients during and after sedation for diagnostic and therapeutic procedures, *Pediatrics* 89(6): 1110-1115, 1992.

American Academy of Pediatrics, Committee on Quality Improvement, Subcommittee on Febrile Seizures: Practice parameter: long-term treatment of the child with simple febrile seizures, *Pediatrics* 103(6): 1307-1309, 1999.

American Academy of Pediatrics: Dexamethasone therapy for bacterial meningitis in infants and children. In Peter G, editor: *2000 Red book: report of the Committee on Infectious Diseases*, ed 25, Elk Grove Village, IL, 2000a, The Academy.

American Academy of Pediatrics: Perinatal human immunodeficiency virus testing, *Pediatrics* 95(2):303-307, 1995.

American Academy of Pediatrics: Recommendations for the prevention of pneumococcal infections, including the use of pneumococcal conjugant vaccine, pneumococcal polysaccharide vaccine and antibiotic prophylaxis, *Pediatrics* 106(2): 362-366, 2000b.

Anderson G and others: Progress toward elimination of *Haemophilus influenzae* type b disease among infants and children: United States, 1987-1993, *MMWR* 43:144-148, 1994.

Annequin D, Tourniaire B, Massiou H: Migraine and headache in childhood and adolescence, *Pediatr Clin North Am* 47(3):617-631, 2000.

Barnard C, Wirrell E: Does status epilepticus cause developmental deterioration and development of epilepsy? *J Child Neurol* 14(12):787-794, 1999.

Belay ED and others: Reye's syndrome in the United States from 1981 through 1997, *N Engl J Med* 340(18):1377-1382, 1999.

Cassetta I and others: Early predictors of intractability in childhood epilepsy: a community based case-control study, *Acta Neurol Scand* 99:329-333, 1999.

Castano G and others: Cortical visual impairment in children with infantile spasms, *J AAPOS* 4(7):175-178, 2000.

Castiglia PT: Shaken baby syndrome, *J Pediatr Health Care* 15:78-80, 2001.

Cattelani R and others: Traumatic brain injury in childhood: intellectual, behavioral and social outcome into adulthood, *Brain Inj* 12:283-296, 1998.

Centers for Disease Control and Prevention: Compendium of animal rabies prevention and control, 2001, National Association of State Public Health Veterinarians, Inc, *MMWR* 50(RR-8):1-9, 2001.

Centers for Disease Control and Prevention: Human rabies prevention: United States, 1999, *MMWR* 48(RR-1):1-21, 1999a.

Centers for Disease Control and Prevention: Meningococcal disease, 2000, *www.cdc.gov/ ncidod/dbmd/diseaseinfo/meningococcal_t. htm.*

Centers for Disease Control and Prevention: Progress toward eliminating *Haemophilus influenzae* type-b disease among infants and children: United States 1987-1997, *JAMA* 281(5):409-410, 1999b.

Chiretti A and others: Early post-traumatic seizures in children with head injury, *Childs Nerv Syst* 16:862-866, 2000.

Commission on Classification and Terminology of the International League Against Epilepsy: Proposal for classification of epilepsies and epileptic syndromes, *Epilepsia* 26(3):268-278, 1985.

Cossette P, Riviello TT, Carmant L: ACTH versus vigabatrin therapy in infantile spasms: a retrospective study, *Neurology* 52:1691-1694, 1999.

de Grauw TJ and others: Diagnosis of migraine in children attending a pediatric headache clinic, *Headache* 39(7):481-485, 1999.

DeVita MA: The death watch: certifying death using cardiac criteria, *Prog Transplant* 11(1):58-66, 2001.

Diamond S: Tension-type headache, *Clin Cornerstone* 1(6):33-44, 1999.

Durkin MS and others: The epidemiology of urban pediatric neurological trauma: evaluation of, and implications for, injury prevention programs, *Neurosurgery* 42(2):300-310, 1998.

Ernst AA and others: Topical lidocaine adrenaline tetracaine (LAT gel) versus injectable buffered lidocaine for local anesthesia in laceration repair, *West J Med* 167(2):79-81, 1997.

Eskola T: Immunogenicity of pneumococcal conjugate vaccines, *Pediatr Infect Dis J* 19(4):388-393, 2000.

Feigin RD, Perlman E: Bacterial meningitis beyond the neonatal period. In Feigin RD, Cherry JD, editors: *Textbook of pediatric infectious diseases*, ed 4, Philadelphia, 1998, WB Saunders.

Fisher MD: Pediatric traumatic brain injury, *Crit Care Nurs Q* 20(1):36-51, 1997.

Fisin T and others: Nasal midazolam effects on childhood acute seizures, *J Child Neurol* 15(12):833-835, 2000.

Fylan F and others: Mechanisms of video game epilepsy, *Epilepsia* 40(Suppl 4):28-30, 1999.

Granstrom ML, Gaily E, Liukkonen E: Treatment of infantile spasms: results of a population-based study with vigabatrin as the first drug for spasms, *Epilepsia* 40(7):950-957, 1999.

Holmes GL, Stafstrom CE: The epilepsies. In David RB: *Child and Adolescent Neurology*, St Louis, 1998, Mosby.

Ito M and others: Subdural hematoma during low-dose ACTH therapy in patients with West syndrome, *Neurology* 54(12):2346-2347, 2000.

Kao SC and others: A survey of post-discharge side-effects of conscious sedation using chloral hydrate in pediatric CT or MR imaging, *Pediatr Radiol* 29(4):287-290, 1999.

Kaplan SL: Acute bacterial meningitis beyond the neonatal period. In Long SS, Pickering IK, Prober CG, editors: *Principles and practice of pediatric infectious diseases*, New York, 1997, Churchill Livingstone.

Keyes PD, Tallon JM, Rizos J: Topical anesthesia, *Can Fam Physician* 44:2152-2156, 1998.

Kline MW: *Citrobacter* meningitis and brain abscess in infancy: epidemiology, pathogenesis, and treatment, *J Pediatr* 113(3):430-434, 1988.

Kline N: *Neurologic manifestations of HIV-infection*, HIV Nursing Curriculum, Houston, 2001, Baylor College of Medicine.

Kociela VL: Pediatric flexible bronchoscopy under conscious sedation: nursing considerations for preparation and monitoring, *J Pediatr Nurs* 13(6):343-348, 1998.

Koo B: Vigabatrin in the treatment of infantile spasms, *Pediatr Neurol* 20:106-110, 1999.

Kutler NO and others: Intranasal midazolam for prolonged convulsive seizures, *Brain Dev* 22(6):359-361, 2000.

Lefevre F, Aronson N: Ketogenic diet for the treatment of refractory epilepsy in children: a systematic review of efficacy, *Pediatrics* 105(4):e46, 2000, *www.pediatrics.org/cgi/content/full/105/4/c46*.

Leppik IE: Monotherapy and polypharmacy, *Neurology* 55(suppl 3):525-529, 2000.

Ljungman G and others: Midazolam nasal spray reduces procedural anxiety in children, *Pediatrics* 105(1 Pt 1):73-78, 2000.

Lloyd CJ, Alredy T, Lloyd JC: Intranasal midazolam as an alternative to general anaesthesia in the management of children with oral and maxillofacial trauma, *Br J Oral Maxillofac Surg* 38(6):593-595, 2000.

Luerssen TJ: Intracranial pressure: Current status in monitoring and management, *Semin Pediatr Neurol*, 4(3):146-155, 1997.

MacDonald BK and others: Factors predicting prognosis of epilepsy after presentation with seizures, *Ann Neurol* 48(6):833-841, 2000.

Mathern GW and others: Postoperative seizure control and antiepileptic drug use in pediatric epilepsy surgery patients: the UCLA experience, 1986-1997, *Epilepsia* 40(12):1740-1749, 1999.

McCabe CF, Donahue SP: Prognostic indicators for vision and mortality in shaken baby syndrome, *Arch Ophthalmol* 118(3):373-377, 2000.

Menkes JH, Sankar R: Paroxysmal disorders. In Menkes JH, Sarnat HB: *Child neurology*, Philadelphia, 2000, Lippincott Williams and Wilkins.

Mitchell WG and others: An open-label study of repeated use of diazepam rectal gel (Diastat) for episodes of acute breakthrough seizures and clusters: safety, efficacy, and tolerance, North American Diastat Group, *Epilepsia* 40(11):1610-1617, 1999.

Monzo J: Meningitis in infancy increases risk of long-term disabilities, *Infect Dis Child* 15(1):14, 2002.

National Center for Injury Prevention and Control: *Unintentional injury: drowning fact sheet*, 1999, *www.cdc.gov/ncipc/duip/drown.htm*.

Nieves JA and others: Childhood drowning: review of the literature and clinical implications, *Pediatr Nurs* 22(3):206-210, 1996.

Ong I and others: The prognostic value of the Glasgow Coma Scale: hypoxia and computerized tomography in outcome prediction of pediatric head injury, *Pediatr Neurosurg* 24(6):285-291, 1996.

Pearson DA and others: Predicting HIV disease progression in children using measures of neuropsychological and neurological functioning, Pediatric AIDS Clinical Trials 152 Study Team, *Pediatrics* 106(6):E76, 2000.

Ramos-Lizana J and others: Seizure recurrence after a first unprovoked seizure in childhood: a prospective study, *Epilepsia* 1(8):1005-1013, 2000.

Ricci S, Vigevano F: The effect of video-game software in video-game epilepsy, *Epilepsia* 40(suppl 4):31-37, 1999.

Riikonen RS: Steroids or vigabatrin in the treatment of infantile spasms? *Pediatr Neurol* 23(5):403-408, 2000.

Rosen DA, Rosen KR: Intravenous conscious sedation with midazolam in paediatric patients, *Int J Clin Pract* 52(1):46-50, 1998.

Sachdeva RC: Near drowning, *Crit Care Clin* 15(2):281-296, 1999.

Scheepers M and others: Is intranasal midazolam an effective rescue medication in adolescents and adults with severe epilepsy? *Seizure* 9(6):417-422, 2000.

Shafer PO: Epilepsy and seizures: advances in seizure assessment, treatment, and self-management, *Nurs Clin North Am* 34(3):743-759, 1999.

Shields WD: Catastropic epilepsy in childhood, *Epilepsia* 41(suppl 2):52-56, 2000.

Shinner S and others: Predictors of multiple seizures in a cohort of children prospectively followed from the time of their first unprovoked seizure, *Ann Neurol* 48(2):140-147, 2000.

Spivak M: Keeping kids safe: injury prevention programs, *Emerg Med Serv* 28(5):45, 47, 49-51, 1999.

Swaiman KF: *Pediatric neurology: principles and practice*, ed 3, St Louis, 1999, Mosby.

Vernon-Levett P: Neurologic system. In Slota MC, editor: *Core curriculum for pediatric critical care nursing*, Philadelphia, 1998, WB Saunders.

Wald ER and others: Desamethasone therapy for children with bacterial meningitis, *Pediatrics* 95(1):21-28, 1995.

White JR and others: Predictors of outcome in severely head-injured children, *Crit Care Med* 29(7):534-540, 2001.

Wiederholt WC: Neurology for non-neurologists, ed 4, Philadelphia, 2000, WB Saunders.

Willoughby RE: Encephalitis, meningoencephalitis, and postinfactious encephalomyelitis. In Long SS, Pickering LK, Prober CG, editors: *Principles and practice of pediatric infectious diseases*, New York, 1997, Churchill Livingstone.

Wong M, Travathan E: Infantile spasms, *Pediatr Neurol* 24(2):89-98, 2001.

Yamamoto LG, Yim GK: The role of intravenous valproic acid in status epilepticus, *Pediatr Emerg Care* 16(4):296-298, 2000.

Yoon U, Jagoda A: New antiepileptic drugs and preparations, *Emerg Med Clin North Am* 18(4):755-765, 2000.

# Chapter 38

# The Child with Endocrine Dysfunction

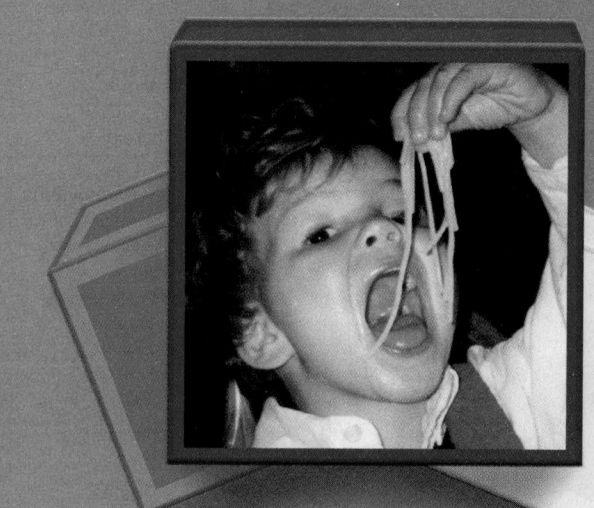

## Chapter Outline

**THE ENDOCRINE SYSTEM, 1703**
**Hormones, 1703**
  Control of Hormone Secretion, 1704
**Neuroendocrine Interrelationships, 1705**
**DISORDERS OF PITUITARY FUNCTION, 1706**
**Hypopituitarism, 1706**
**Pituitary Hyperfunction, 1713**
**Precocious Puberty, 1714**
**Diabetes Insipidus (DI), 1715**
**Syndrome of Inappropriate Antidiuretic Hormone (SIADH), 1716**

**DISORDERS OF THYROID FUNCTION, 1717**
**Juvenile Hypothyroidism, 1717**
**Goiter, 1718**
**Lymphocytic Thyroiditis, 1718**
**Hyperthyroidism, 1719**
**DISORDERS OF PARATHYROID FUNCTION, 1721**
**Hypoparathyroidism, 1722**
**Hyperparathyroidism, 1722**
**DISORDERS OF ADRENAL FUNCTION, 1723**
**Adrenal Hormones, 1723**

  Adrenal Cortex, 1723
  Adrenal Medulla, 1724
**Acute Adrenocortical Insufficiency, 1725**
**Chronic Adrenocortical Insufficiency (Addison Disease), 1726**
**Cushing Syndrome, 1727**
**Congenital Adrenal Hyperplasia (CAH), 1729**
**Hyperaldosteronism, 1731**
**Pheochromocytoma, 1731**
**DISORDERS OF PANCREATIC HORMONE SECRETION, 1732**
**Diabetes Mellitus (DM), 1732**
*Nursing Care Plan: The Child with Diabetes Mellitus, 1752*

## Related Topics

Abnormal Sexual Development, Ch. 11
Administration of Medication, Ch. 27
Family-Centered Home Care, Ch. 25

Genetic Evaluation and Counseling, Ch. 5
Hypocalcemia, Ch. 9

Hypoglycemia, Ch. 9
Single-Gene (Monogenic) Disorders, Ch. 5

## THE ENDOCRINE SYSTEM

The endocrine system consists of three components: (1) the *cell,* which sends a chemical message by means of a hormone; (2) the *target cells,* or *end organs,* which receive the chemical message; and (3) the *environment* through which the chemical is transported (blood, lymph, extracellular fluids) from the site of synthesis to the sites of cellular action. The endocrine system controls or regulates metabolic processes governing energy production, growth, fluid and electrolyte balance, response to stress, and sexual reproduction (Baxter and Ribeiro, 2001).

The endocrine glands, which are distributed throughout the body, are listed in Box 38-1; also listed are several additional structures sometimes considered endocrine glands, although they are not usually included.

## Hormones

A hormone is a complex chemical substance produced and secreted into body fluids by a cell or group of cells that exerts a physiologic controlling effect on other cells (Behrman, Kliegman, and Jenson, 2000). Some are *local hormones,* creating their effect near the point of secretion. For example, acetylcholine, released at the parasympathetic and skeletal nerve endings, mediates the synaptic activity of the nervous system; secretin, a digestive hormone secreted by certain cells lining the duodenum, stimulates the pancreas to release a watery secretion; and the prostaglandins, or tissue hormones, secreted by a wide variety of organs (including the seminal vesicles, kidneys, lungs, iris, brain, and thymus), usually diffuse only a short distance to integrate activities of neighboring cells.

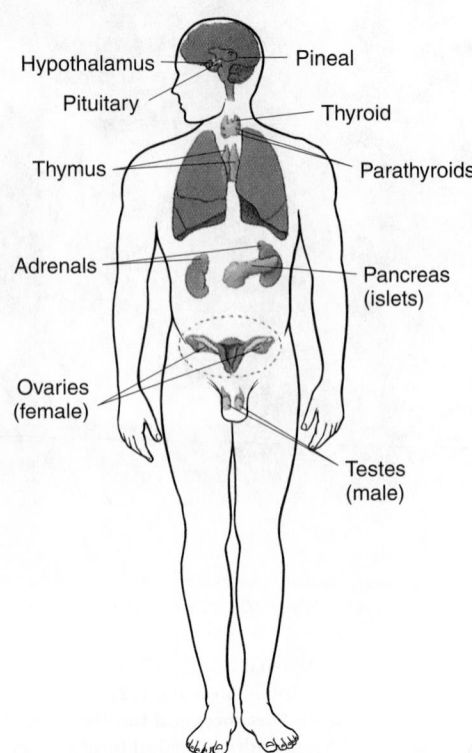

**Fig. 38-1** Location of the endocrine glands. (From Thibodeau GA, Patton KT: *Structure and function of the body*, ed 10, St Louis, 1997, Mosby.)

*General hormones* are produced in one organ or part of the body and are carried through the bloodstream to a distant part, or parts, of the body where they initiate or regulate physiologic activity of an organ or group of cells. Some of these hormones (such as thyroid hormone and growth hormone) affect most cells of the body, whereas others (such as the tropic hormones) produce their effects on specific tissues, called *target tissues.* For example, the pituitary hormones stimulate the adrenal glands and the thyroid gland to secrete adrenocorticotropin and thyrotropic hormone, respectively.

### Control of Hormone Secretion

Hormones are released by endocrine glands into the bloodstream, where they are carried to responsive tissues (Fig. 38-1). These responsive, or target, tissues may be another endocrine gland, an organ, or tissue (Baxter and Ribeiro, 2001). Regulation of hormonal secretion is based on negative feedback. As a general rule, endocrine glands have a tendency to oversecrete their particular hormones. However, once the physiologic effect of the hormone has been achieved, this information is transmitted to the producing gland, either directly or indirectly, to inhibit further secretion. If the gland undersecretes, the inhibition is relieved, and the gland increases production of the hormone. As a result, the hormone is secreted according to the amount needed. This is the primary function of the tropic hormones.

The endocrine gland primarily responsible for stimulation and inhibition of target glandular secretions is the *anterior pituitary,* or "master gland." *Tropic* (which literally means "turning") hormones secreted by the anterior pituitary regulate the secretion of hormones from various target organs (Fig. 38-2). As blood concentrations of the target hormones reach normal levels, a negative message is sent to the anterior pituitary to inhibit release of the tropic hormone. For example, thyroid-stimulating hormone (TSH) responds to low levels of circulating thyroid hormone (TH). As blood levels of thyroid hormone reach normal concentrations, a negative feedback message is sent to the anterior pituitary, resulting in diminished release of TSH.

The pituitary gland is, in turn, controlled by either hormonal or neuronal signals from the hypothalamus. Two types of substances are secreted from the hypothalamus: (1) *releasing hormones* and (2) *inhibitory hormones,* which are secreted within the hypothalamus and transported by way of the pituitary portal system to the anterior pituitary, where they stimulate the secretion of tropic hormones. An example of this is the secretion of corticotropin-releasing factor (CRF) by the hypothalamus, which stimulates the pituitary to secrete adrenocorticotropic hormone (ACTH). In this instance the anterior pituitary is

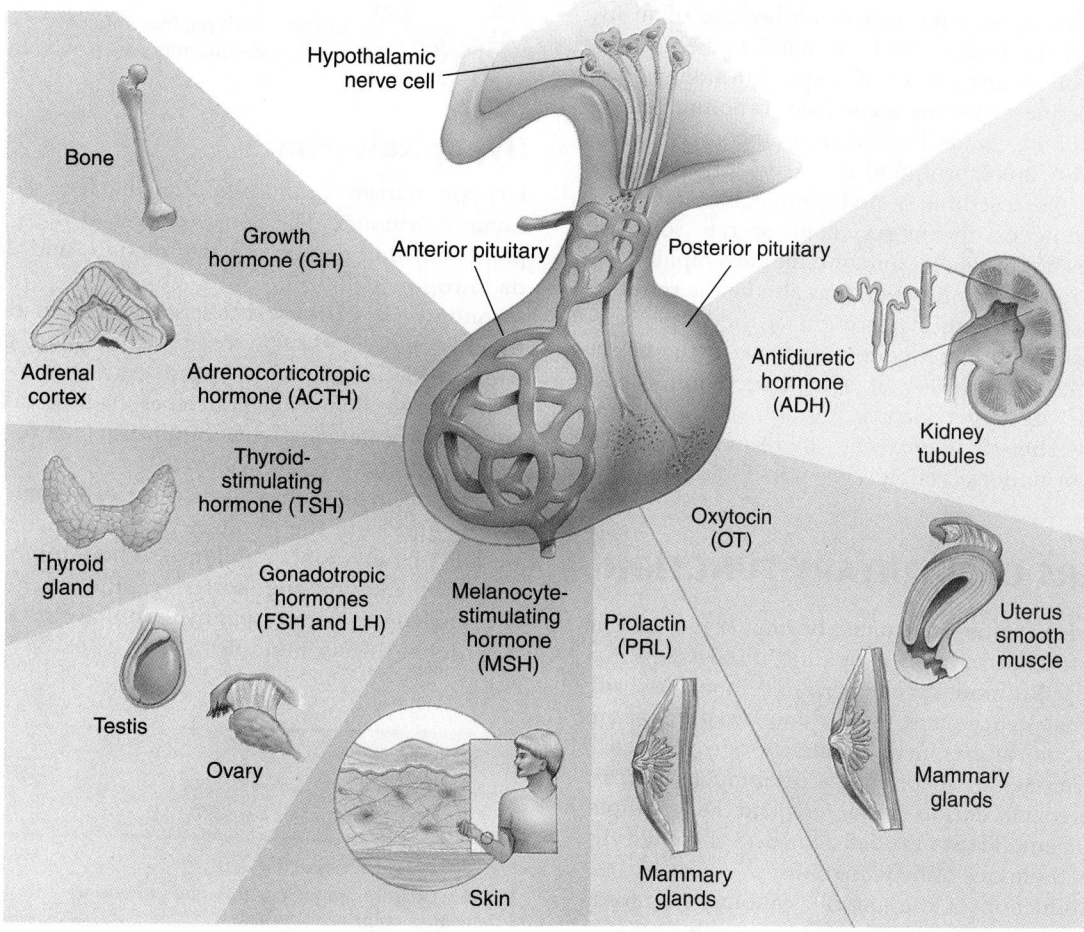

**Fig. 38-2**   Principal anterior and posterior pituitary hormones and their target organs. (From Thibodeau GA, Patton KT: *Structure and function of the body,* ed 10, St Louis, 1997, Mosby.)

the target of the hypothalamus and secondarily effects a response from another target gland, the adrenals. The adrenals in turn secrete glucocorticoids, which have multiple target sites throughout the body. Pituitary hormones that lack feedback control from the product of a target tissue (growth hormone, prolactin, and melanocyte-stimulating hormone) require hypothalamic inhibitors and stimulators for their control.

Not all hormones depend on other hormones for their release. For example, insulin is secreted in response to blood glucose concentrations. Other glandular hormones that are not under the control of the pituitary gland are glucagon, parathyroid hormone (parathormone, PTH), antidiuretic hormone (ADH), and aldosterone.

## Neuroendocrine Interrelationships

Homeostasis is maintained by two regulatory systems: the endocrine and the autonomic nervous systems (collectively known as the ***neuroendocrine system***) (Baxter and Ribeiro, 2001). The *autonomic nervous system* consists of the sympathetic and parasympathetic systems, which control nonvoluntary functions, specifically of smooth muscle, myocardium, and glands. The *parasympathetic system,* in particular, is primarily involved in regulating digestive processes, whereas the *sympathetic system* functions to maintain homeostasis during stress.

The higher autonomic centers, located in the hypothalamus and limbic system, help control the functioning of both autonomic systems. Both sympathetic and parasympathetic nerve fibers secrete ***neurotransmitting substances***— acetylcholine, released by cholinergic fibers, and norepinephrine, released by adrenergic fibers. Release of norepinephrine into the plasma produces the same effects as secretion of this substance by the adrenal medulla. Thus the interrelatedness between the two systems is demonstrated.

The neuroendocrine system acts by synthesizing and releasing various chemical substances that regulate body functions. Information is carried by means of neural impulses in the autonomic system and by the blood in the endocrine system. In general, neural responses are more rapid and localized; endocrine responses are more lasting and widespread. The two systems function synergistically because neural impulses transmitted to the central nervous system stimulate the hypothalamus to manufacture and release several ***releasing*** or ***inhibiting factors.***

Because of the interdependent relationship of these glands, a malfunction in one gland produces effects elsewhere. Endocrine dysfunction may result because of an intrinsic defect in the target gland (primary) or because of a diminished or elevated level of tropic hormones (secondary). Endocrine problems occur from hypofunction or hyperfunction of the glands. Primary hypofunction is usually associated with a more profound deficiency of the target gland hormone because little or no hormone is secreted. In secondary dysfunction the target glands secrete some of their hormones but in smaller amounts and less rapidly.

Hyperfunction or hypofunction may also be the result of an increase or a decrease in secretion of the tropic hormones (primary) with a consequent increase in the target gland hormones (secondary) or a hypersecretion or hyposecretion of the target glands. A summary of the endocrine glands, their functions, and the primary effects of oversecretion or undersecretion is given in Table 38-1.

## DISORDERS OF PITUITARY FUNCTION

Deficiencies of the anterior pituitary hormones may be due to organic defects or have an idiopathic etiology and may occur as a single hormonal problem or in combination with other hormonal deficiencies. The clinical manifestations depend on the hormones involved and the age of onset. If the tropic hormones are involved, the resulting disorder reflects the altered stimulus to the target gland. For example, if TSH is deficient, TH is also deficient, and the child displays the manifestations of hypothyroidism.

An overproduction of the anterior pituitary hormones can result in gigantism (caused by excess growth hormone [GH] production during childhood), hyperthyroidism, hypercortisolism (Cushing syndrome), and precocious puberty from excessive gonadotropins. Overproduction is thought to be caused by hyperplasia of the pituitary cells—which may eventually progress to a tumor (adenoma)—or a primary hypothalamic defect that results in excess of the hormone's respective releasing factor. Although the initial clinical manifestations are a result of pituitary hypersecretion, eventually pituitary insufficiency occurs, and the signs of panhypopituitarism become evident.

## Hypopituitarism

Hypopituitarism is diminished or deficient secretion of pituitary hormones. The consequences of the condition depend on the degree of dysfunction and lead to gonadotropin deficiency with absence or regression of secondary sex characteristics; somatotropin deficiency, in which children display retarded somatic growth; thyrotropin deficiency, which produces hypothyroidism; and corticotropin deficiency, which results in manifestations of adrenal hypofunction. Hypopituitarism can result from any of the conditions listed in Box 38-2.

The most common organic cause of pituitary hyposecretion is tumors in the pituitary or hypothalamic region, especially the craniopharyngiomas. These tumors usually invade the anterior and posterior pituitary lobes and the hypothalamus, causing panhypopituitarism, a generalized disorder involving multiple systems (Box 38-3). The child

---

**Box 38-2 ■ ■ ■**
**Etiology of Hypopituitarism**

Aplasia or hypoplasia
  Developmental defects
  Idiopathic—sporadic; genetic
Destructive lesions
  Trauma—perinatal; child abuse; basal skull fracture
  Infiltrative lesions—tumors; tuberculosis; toxoplasmosis; hemochromatosis; sarcoidosis
Irradiation—central nervous system (CNS); eye; middle ear
Autoimmune hypophysitis
Surgery—removal of pharyngeal pituitary; ablation of craniopharyngioma or other tumor
  Vascular—aneurysm; infarct
Functional deficiency
  Psychosocial dwarfism
  Anorexia nervosa

---

**Box 38-3 ■ ■ ■**
**Clinical Manifestations of Panhypopituitarism**

**GROWTH HORMONE (GH)**
Short stature but proportional height and weight
Delayed epiphyseal closure
Retarded bone age proportional to height
Premature aging common in later life
Increased insulin sensitivity

**THYROID-STIMULATING HORMONE (TSH)**
Short stature with infantile proportions
Dry, coarse skin, yellow discoloration, pallor
Cold intolerance
Constipation
Somnolence
Bradycardia
Dyspnea on exertion
Delayed dentition, loss of teeth

**GONADOTROPINS**
Absence of sexual maturation or loss of secondary sex characteristics
Atrophy of genitalia, prostate gland, breasts
Amenorrhea without menopausal symptoms
Decreased spermatogenesis

**ADRENOCORTICOTROPIC HORMONE (ACTH)**
Severe anorexia, weight loss
Hypoglycemia
Hypotension
Hyponatremia, hyperkalemia
Adrenal apoplexy, especially in response to stress
Circulatory collapse

**ANTIDIURETIC HORMONE (ADH)**
Polyuria
Polydipsia
Dehydration

**MELANOCYTE-STIMULATING HORMONE (MSH)**
Decreased pigmentation

## TABLE 38-1   Summary of the endocrine system

| Gland/Hormone | Effect | Hypofunction | Hyperfunction |
|---|---|---|---|
| **Adenohypophysis (Anterior Pituitary)*** | | | |
| Somatotropic hormone (STH) or growth hormone (GH) (somatotropin) Target tissue: bones | Promotes growth of bone and soft tissues Has main effect on linear growth Maintains a normal rate of protein synthesis Conserves carbohydrate utilization and promotes fat mobilization Is essential for proliferation of cartilage cells at epiphyseal plate Is ineffective for linear growth after epiphyseal closure Has hyperglycemic effect (antiinsulin action) | Epiphyseal fusion with cessation of growth Prepubertal dwarfism Pituitary cachexia (Simonds disease) Generalized growth retardation Hypoglycemia | Prepubertal gigantism Acromegaly (after full growth is attained) Diabetes mellitus Postpubertal hypoproteinemia |
| Thyrotropin (thyroid-stimulating hormone [TSH]) Target tissue: thyroid gland | Promotes and maintains growth and development of thyroid gland Stimulates thyroid hormone secretion | Hypothyroidism Marked delay of puberty Juvenile myxedema | Hyperthyroidism Thyrotoxicosis Graves disease |
| Adrenocorticotropic hormone (ACTH) Target tissue: adrenal cortex | Promotes and maintains growth and development of adrenal cortex Stimulates adrenal cortex to secrete glucocorticoids and androgens | Acute adrenocortical insufficiency (Addison disease) Hypoglycemia Increased skin pigmentation | Cushing syndrome |
| Gonadotropins Target tissue: gonads | Stimulate gonads to mature and produce sex hormones and germ cells | Absent or incomplete spontaneous puberty | Precocious puberty Early epiphyseal closure |
| Follicle-stimulating hormone (FSH) Target tissue: ovaries, testes | Male: Stimulates development of seminiferous tubules Initiates spermatogenesis Female: Stimulates graafian follicles to mature and secrete estrogen | Hypogonadism Sterility Absence or loss of secondary sex characteristics Amenorrhea | Precocious puberty Primary gonadal failure Hirsutism Polycystic ovary Early epiphyseal closure |
| Luteinizing hormone (LH)† Target tissue: ovaries, testes | Male: Stimulates differentiation of Leydig cells, which secrete androgens, principally testosterone Female: Produces rupture of follicle with discharge of mature ovum Stimulates secretion of progesterone by corpus luteum | Hypogonadism Sterility Impotence Absence or loss of secondary sex characteristics Ovarian failure Eunuchism | Precocious puberty Primary gonadal failure Hirsutism Polycystic ovary Early epiphyseal closure |
| Prolactin (luteotropic hormone) Target tissue: ovaries, breasts | Stimulates milk secretion Maintains corpus luteum and progesterone secretion during pregnancy | Inability to lactate Amenorrhea | Galactorrhea Functional hypogonadism |
| Melanocyte-stimulating hormone (MSH) Target tissue: skin | Promotes pigmentation of skin | Diminished or absent skin pigmentation | Increased skin pigmentation |
| **Neurohypophysis (Posterior Pituitary)** | | | |
| Antidiuretic hormone (ADH) (vasopressin) Target tissue: renal tubules | Acts on distal and collecting tubules, making them more permeable to water, thus increasing reabsorption and decreasing excretion of urine | Diabetes insipidus | Syndrome of inappropriate secretion of ADH Fluid retention Hyponatremia |
| Oxytocin Target tissue: uterus, breasts | Stimulates powerful contractions of uterus Causes ejection of milk from alveoli into breast ducts (letdown reflex) | | |
| **Thyroid** | | | |
| Thyroxine ($T_4$) and triiodothyronine ($T_3$) | Regulates metabolic rate; controls rate of growth of body cells Especially important for growth of bones, teeth, and brain Promotes mobilization of fats and gluconeogenesis | Hypothyroidism Myxedema Hashimoto thyroiditis General growth is greatly reduced; extent depends on age at which deficiency occurs Mental retardation in infant | Exophthalmic goiter (Graves disease) Accelerated linear growth Early epiphyseal closure |
| Thyrocalcitonin | Regulates calcium and phosphorus metabolism Influences ossification and development of bone | | |

*For each anterior pituitary hormone there is a corresponding hypothalamic-releasing factor. A deficiency in these factors caused by inhibiting anterior pituitary hormone synthesis produces the same effects. (See text for more detailed infomation.)
†In the male, LH is sometimes known as interstitial cell–stimulating hormone (ICSH).

*Continued*

**TABLE 38-1** Summary of the endocrine system—cont'd

| Gland/Hormone | Effect | Hypofunction | Hyperfunction |
|---|---|---|---|
| **Parathyroid Glands** | | | |
| Parathyroid hormone (PTH) | Promotes calcium reabsorption from blood, bone, and intestines<br>Promotes excretion of phosphorus in kidney tubules | Hypocalcemia (tetany) | Hypercalcemia (bone demineralization)<br>Hypophosphatemia |
| **Adrenal Cortex** | | | |
| Mineralocorticoids<br>Aldosterone | Stimulate renal tubules to reabsorb sodium, thus promoting water retention but potassium loss | Adrenocortical insufficiency | Electrolyte imbalance<br>Hyperaldosteronism |
| Sex hormones (androgens, estrogens, progesterone) | Influence development of bone, reproductive organs, and secondary sexual characteristics | Male feminization | Adrenogenital syndrome |
| Glucocorticoids<br>Cortisol (hydrocortisone and compound F)<br>Corticosterone (compound B) | Promote normal fat, protein, and carbohydrate metabolism<br>In excess, tend to accelerate gluconeogenesis and protein and fat catabolism<br>Mobilize body defenses during period of stress<br>Suppress inflammatory reaction | Addison disease<br>Acute adrenocortical insufficiency<br>Impaired growth and sexual function | Cushing syndrome<br>Severe impairment of growth with slowing in skeletal maturation |
| **Adrenal Medulla** | | | |
| Epinephrine (adrenaline), norepinephrine (noradrenaline) | Produces vasoconstriction of heart and smooth muscles (raises blood pressure)<br>Increases blood sugar via glycolysis<br>Inhibits gastrointestinal activity<br>Activates sweat glands | | Hyperfunction caused by:<br>Pheochromocytoma<br>Neuroblastoma<br>Ganglioneuroma |
| **Islets of Langerhans of Pancreas** | | | |
| Insulin (beta cells) | Promotes glucose transport into the cells<br>Increases glucose utilization, glycogenesis, and glycolysis<br>Promotes fatty acid transport into cells and lipogenesis<br>Promotes amino acid transport into cells and protein synthesis | Diabetes mellitus | Hyperinsulinism |
| Glucagon (alpha cells) | Acts as antagonist to insulin, thereby increasing blood glucose concentration by accelerating glycogenolysis<br>Able to inhibit secretion of both insulin and glycogen | | Hyperglycemia<br>May be instrumental in genesis of diabetic ketoacidosis (DKA) in diabetes mellitus |
| Somatostatin (delta cells) | Able to inhibit secretion of both insulin and glycogen | | |
| **Ovaries** | | | |
| Estrogen | Accelerates growth of epithelial cells, especially in uterus following menses<br>Promotes protein anabolism<br>Promotes epiphyseal closure of bones<br>Promotes breast development during puberty and pregnancy<br>Plays role in sexual function<br>Stimulates water and sodium reabsorption in renal tubules<br>Stimulates ripening of ova | Lack of or repression of sexual development | Precocious puberty, early epiphyseal closure |
| Progesterone | Prepares uterus for nidation of fertilized ovum and aids in maintenance of pregnancy<br>Aids in development of alveolar system of breasts during pregnancy<br>Inhibits myometrial contractions<br>Has effect on protein catabolism<br>Promotes salt and water retention, especially in endometrium | | |
| **Testes** | | | |
| Testosterone | Accelerates protein anabolism for growth<br>Promotes epiphyseal closure<br>Promotes development of secondary sex characteristics<br>Plays role in sexual function<br>Stimulates testes to produce spermatozoa | Delayed sexual development or eunuchoidism | Precocious puberty, early epiphyseal closure |

may experience growth retardation for quite some time before developing any symptoms or signs of increased intracranial pressure, local compression, or the destructive effects of the tumor. Other causes of panhypopituitarism sometimes include encephalitis, head trauma (rarely), and congenital hypoplasia of the hypothalamic area.

*Idiopathic hypopituitarism,* or *idiopathic pituitary growth failure,* is usually related to *growth hormone (GH) deficiency,* which inhibits somatic growth in all cells of the body (Allen, Johanson, and Blizzard, 1996). Growth failure is defined as an absolute height <−2 SD for age, or a linear growth velocity consistently <−1 SD for age. When this occurs without the presence of hypothyroidism, systemic disease, or malnutrition, then an abnormality of the GH/IGF axis should be considered (Hochberg, 1999). Although children with hypopituitarism are normal at birth, they show growth patterns that progressively deviate from the normal growth rate, often beginning in infancy. The chief complaint in most instances is short stature. Of those who seek help, boys outnumber girls 3 to 1. The extent of idiopathic GH deficiency may be complete or partial, but the cause is unknown. It is frequently associated with other pituitary hormone deficiencies, such as deficiencies of TSH and ACTH; thus it is theorized that the disorder is probably secondary to hypothalamic deficiency. It has also been observed that there is a higher than average frequency in some families, which indicates a possible genetic etiology in a number of instances.

Not all children with short stature have GH deficiency. In most instances the cause of short stature is either familial short stature or a simple constitutional growth delay. *Familial short stature* refers to otherwise healthy children who have ancestors with adult height in the lower percentiles, and whose height during childhood is appropriate for genetic background. Fig. 38-3 provides an overview of the possible causes of short stature in children.

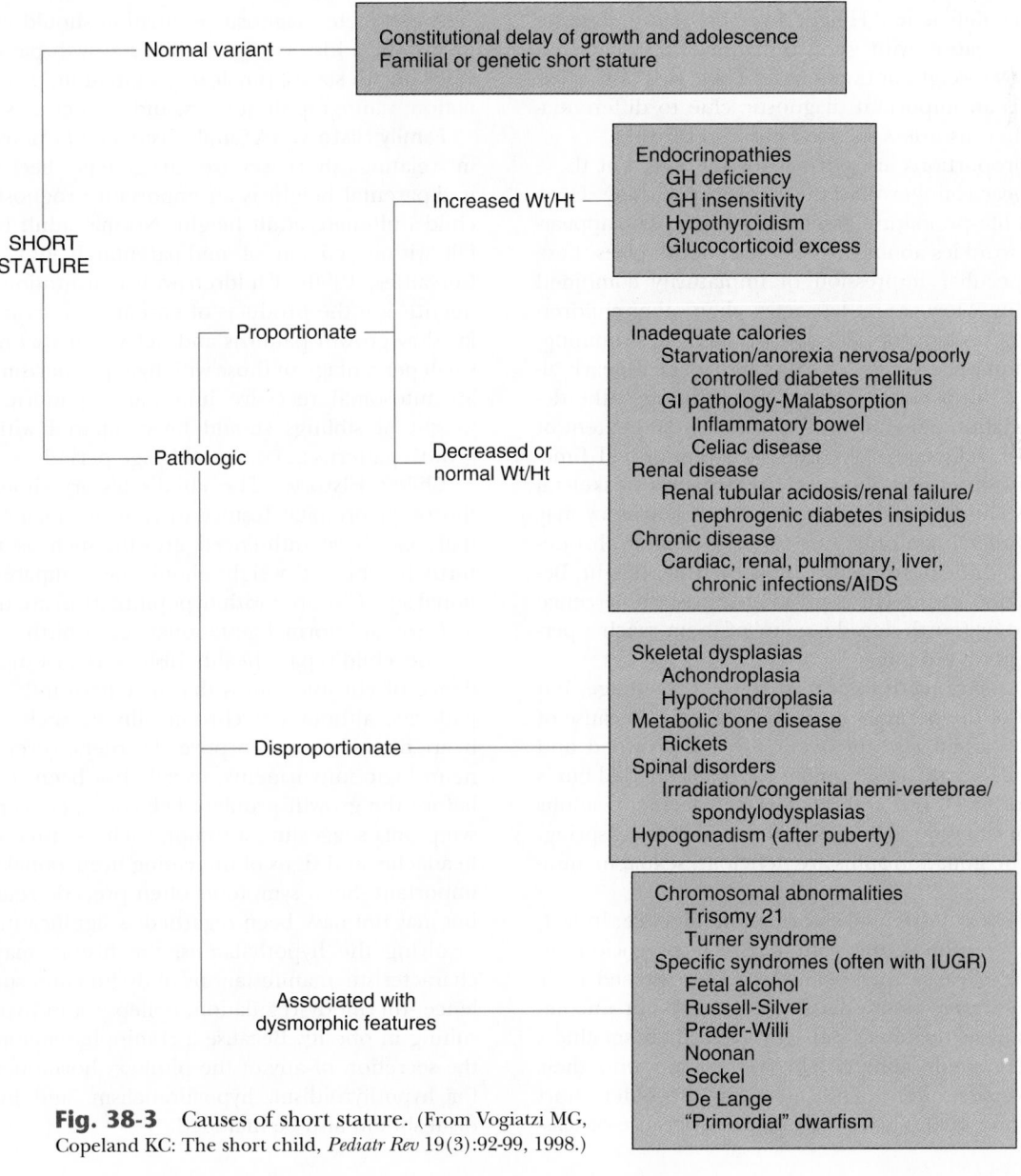

**Fig. 38-3**   Causes of short stature. (From Vogiatzi MG, Copeland KC: The short child, *Pediatr Rev* 19(3):92-99, 1998.)

*Constitutional growth delay* refers to individuals (usually boys) with delayed linear growth and skeletal and sexual maturation that is behind that of age-mates (Lifshitz and Cervantes, 1996). Typically these children will reach normal adult height. Often there is a history of a similar pattern of growth in one of the parents or other family members of children with constitutional growth delay. The untreated child will proceed through normal changes as expected on the basis of bone age. These changes, although occurring later than in the average child, will appear in normal sequence and manner, and treatment with GH is not usually indicated. However, its use has become a controversial issue, especially in relation to parental and child requests for treatment to accelerate growth.

## Clinical Manifestations

These children generally grow normally during the first year and then follow a slowed growth curve that is below the third percentile. In children with a partial GH deficiency, the growth retardation is less marked than in children with complete GH deficiency. Height may be retarded more than weight because, with good nutrition, these children can become overweight or even obese. Their well-nourished appearance is an important diagnostic clue to differentiation from other disorders such as failure to thrive.

Skeletal proportions are normal for the age, but these children appear younger than their chronologic age. However, later in life premature aging is common. The appearance of fine wrinkles about the eyes and mouth gives these children a peculiar impression of immaturity combined with presenility. They are no less active than other children if directed to size-appropriate sports, such as swimming, wrestling, gymnastics, soccer, or ballet. Bone age is nearly always retarded but is closely related to height age—the degree of retardation depends on the duration and extent of the hormonal deficiency. Children with diminished function of recent onset may show little retardation in skeletal age, whereas children with a long-standing deficiency may evidence a skeletal age only 40% to 50% of their chronologic age. It is difficult to predict their eventual height. Because the period of growth is prolonged past adolescence into the third or fourth decade, many of them reach a permanent height of 4 to 5 feet.

Usually, primary teeth appear at the expected age, but the eruption of the permanent teeth is delayed. Because of the underdeveloped jaw, the teeth are overcrowded and malpositioned. Sexual development is usually delayed but is otherwise normal. Even without GH replacement, adults with GH deficiency are able to reproduce normal offspring. However, if the gonadotropins are deficient, sexual maturation is absent.

Most of these children have normal intelligence. In fact, during early childhood they often appear precocious in their learning because their ability seems to exceed their small size. However, emotional problems are not uncommon, especially as they near puberty, when their smallness becomes increasingly apparent in comparison with their peers. Anecdotal evidence indicates that the older short child has poorer-quality social interactions because of teasing and ridicule about his or her size. Height discrepancy has been significantly correlated with emotional adjustment problems and may be a valuable predictor of the extent to which GH-delayed children will experience difficulty with anxiety, social skills, and positive self-esteem (Stabler and others, 1996). Also, academic problems are not uncommon. A history will often reveal repeated classes or enrollment in classes for children with learning disabilities. These children are usually not pushed to perform at their chronologic age but at their height age.

## Diagnostic Evaluation

Only a small number of children with delayed growth or short stature have hypopituitary dwarfism. In the majority of instances the cause is constitutional delay. Diagnostic evaluation is aimed at isolating organic causes, which, in addition to GH deficiency, may include hypothyroidism, hypersecretion of cortisol, gonadal aplasia, chronic illness, or nutritional inadequacy as well as Russell-Silver dwarfism or hypochondroplasia.

A complete diagnostic evaluation should include a family history, a history of the child's growth patterns and previous health status, physical examination, psychosocial evaluation, radiographic surveys, and endocrine studies.

**Family History.** A family history is of utmost importance in relating short stature to genetic background. The mid-parental height is an important prognosticator of the child's ultimate adult height. Normal adult height should fall within ±5 cm of mid-parental height (Lifshitz and Cervantes, 1996). Children with constitutional delays frequently are the products of parents who experienced similar slow growth patterns and delayed sexual maturation. A small percentage of those with hypopituitarism demonstrate an autosomal recessive inheritance pattern. Height and weight of siblings should be compared with the child's growth patterns at comparable age periods.

**Child's History.** The child's history should include a thorough prenatal history to rule out maternal disorders that may have influenced growth, such as malnutrition. Birth height and weight should be compared with gestational age. Children with hypopituitarism are usually of normal size and normal gestational age at birth.

The child's past health history is investigated for evidence of chronic illness that may have influenced growth patterns, although a chronic illness, such as congenital heart disease, malabsorptive disorders, severe anemia, or neurologic impairments, usually has been identified long before the growth problem becomes a concern. Signs and symptoms suggesting a tumor, such as visual disturbances, headache, and signs of increasing intracranial pressure, are important. Such symptoms often precede retarded growth but may not have been regarded as significant. With lesions involving the hypothalamus, the history may also reveal characteristic manifestations of dysfunction such as somnolence, thermodysregulation, epilepsy, and hyperphagia, resulting in obesity. Because a craniopharyngioma can affect the secretion of any of the pituitary hormones, assessment for hypothyroidism, hypoadrenalism, and hypoaldosteronism should also be included.

Whenever possible, the child's growth patterns since birth should be evaluated, especially growth velocity, and compared with standard measurements. The age of onset of short stature provides a significant diagnostic clue. When the clinician evaluates the results of plotting height and weight, upward or downward changes in height velocity in children older than 3 years may indicate a growth abnormality (Vogiatzi and Copeland, 1998). Progressive retardation in height and weight since early childhood suggests idiopathic hypopituitary dwarfism, whereas a recent change from normal growth is more characteristic of a tumor. In addition, these children are usually well nourished, ruling out other causes of growth failure.

**Physical Examination.**    Accurate measurement of height (using a calibrated stadiometer) and weight and comparison with standard growth charts are essential (Box 38-4). Multiple height measures reflect a more accurate assessment of abnormal growth patterns (Hall, 2000). Other measurements may include crown-to-pubis and pubis-to-heel length to compare body proportions, and sexual development should be assessed and compared with age-appropriate development. Observation of general appearance yields valuable clues, especially signs of premature aging and infantile facial features. A funduscopic examination and testing for visual acuity should be performed to detect evidence of ocular damage from a tumor.

**Radiographic Surveys.**    A skeletal survey in children less than 3 years of age and radiographic examination of the hand/wrist for centers of ossification (bone age) (Box 38-5)

in older children are important in evaluating growth. Epiphyseal maturation is retarded in hypopituitarism but consistent with retardation in height. This is in contrast to hypothyroidism, in which bone maturation is greatly retarded, or gonadal dysplasia, such as Turner syndrome, in which bone age is near normal. Radiographic studies should also include a skull series, which helps in identifying abnormalities such as an abnormally small sella turcica or evidence of a space-occupying lesion such as craniopharyngioma. Computed tomography (CT) radionuclear scans, or carotid angiograms may be needed to establish diagnosis and localization of lesions.

**Endocrine Studies.**    Definitive diagnosis is based on absent or subnormal reserves of pituitary GH. Because GH levels are normally so low in children that differentiation from abnormal concentrations is unreliable, GH secretion should be stimulated, followed by measurement of blood levels. Exercise is a natural and benign stimulus for GH release, and elevated levels can be detected after 20 minutes of strenuous exercise in normal children. Also, GH levels are elevated 45 to 90 minutes following the onset of sleep.

Initial assessment of the serum insulin-like growth factor (IGF-I) and GF-binding protein (IGFBP-3) indicates a need for further evaluation of GH dysfunction if levels are lower than $-1$ SD below the mean for age. It is recommended that GH stimulation tests be reserved for children with low serum IGF-I and IGFBP-3 levels and poor growth (Hochberg, 1999).

Many of the traditional pharmacologic tests involve the use of neuromodulators such as levodopa or agents such as arginine, insulin, propranolol, or glucagon, which are known to stimulate the release of GH directly or indirectly (American Academy of Pediatrics [AAP], 1997; Guyda, 2000). Recent studies have shown that traditional GH stimulation test results can be substantially lower than previously accepted (Guyda, 2000; Mauras and others, 2000). GH-dependent growth factors may be more sensitive indicators of GH defficiency than GH stimulation tests. Increasingly sensitive radioimmunoassays for GH levels have been developed.

---

**Box 38-4 ■ ■ ■**
**Evaluating the Growth Curve**

1. **Ensure reliability of measurements.**
   Accurately obtain and plot height and weight measurements.
2. **Determine absolute height.**
   The absolute height of a child bears some relationship to the likelihood of a pathologic condition. However, the majority of children who have a height below the lowest percentile (either 3rd or 5th percentile on the height curve) do not have a pathologic growth problem.
3. **Assess height velocity.**
   The most important aspect of a growth evaluation is the observation of a child's height over time or height velocity. Accurate determination of height velocity requires at least 4 and preferably 6 months of observation. A substantial deceleration in height velocity (crossing several percentiles) between 3 and 12 or 13 years of age indicates pathology until proven otherwise.
4. **Determine weight-to-height relationship.**
   Determination of the weight-to-height ratio has some diagnostic value in ascertaining the cause of growth retardation in a short child.
5. **Project target height.**
   The height of a child can be judged inappropriately short only in the context of his or her genetic potential. Determine the target height of the child with the formula: [father's height (cm) + mother's height (cm) + 13]/2 for boys or [father's height (cm) + mother's height (cm) − 13]/2 for girls. Most children achieve an adult stature within approximately 10 cm of the target height.

Modified from Vogiatzi MG, Copeland KC: The short child, *Pediatr Rev* 19(3):92-99, 1998.

---

**Box 38-5 ■ ■ ■**
**Bone Age for Evaluating Growth Disorders**

1. Bone age refers to a method of assessing skeletal maturity by comparing the appearance of repesentative epiphyseal centers obtained on x-ray with age-appropriate published standards.
2. Most conditions that cause poor linear growth also cause a delay in skeletal maturation and a retarded bone age. Observation of even a profoundly delayed bone age is never diagnostic or even indicative of a specific diagnosis. A delayed bone age merely indicates that the associated short stature is to some extent "partially reversible" because linear growth will continue until epiphyseal fusion is complete. In comparison, a bone age that is not delayed in a short child is of much greater concern and may in fact, be of some diagnostic value under certain circumstances.

Modified from Vogiatzi MG, Copeland KC: The short child, *Pediatr Rev* 19(3):92-99, 1998.

## Therapeutic Management

Treatment of GH deficiency caused by organic lesions is directed toward correction of the underlying disease process (e.g., surgical removal or irradiation of a tumor). The definitive treatment of GH deficiency is replacement of GH and is successful in 80% of affected children. For more than 20 years cadaver-derived human growth hormone (HGH) was used successfully to enhance linear growth in short children. In 1985 the Food and Drug Administration (FDA) stopped use of the hormone in response to reported deaths due to *Creutzfeldt-Jakob disease (CJD)* in three former HGH recipients. To date, more than 20 patients have been identified who both received and became infected with CJD, a rare and fatal neurodegenerative condition iatrogenically transmitted through human tissue (Wetterau and Cohen, 2000). Donation of organs or tissues from HGH recipients for transplantation should be prohibited because of the inability to test for infection with CJD. Blood banks do not accept donations from former HGH recipients. *Biosynthetic GH* prepared by recombinant DNA technology (and without the risk of CJD) is now available and is the therapy of choice (Wetterau and Cohen, 2000).

The daily administration of GH at a dose of 25 to 50 μg/kg to short, prepubertal children has resulted in an increased growth velocity (Wetterau and Cohen, 2000). Many children who respond to therapy have maintained this accelerated rate until achievement of height that is more appropriate to family height. Typically growth velocity improves from a pretreatment rate of less than 5 cm/yr to 10 to 12 cm in the first year, and then to 7 to 9 cm/yr during the next several years (Anhalt and Chin, 2000). For children to achieve their genetic growth potential, early diagnosis of and intervention for growth disorders is essential.

The decision to stop GH therapy is made jointly by the child, family, and health care team. Radiologic evidence of epiphyseal closure is a criterion for ending therapy. Dosage is increased as the time of epiphyseal closure nears in order to gain the best advantage of the GH. Children with other hormone deficiencies require replacement therapy to correct the specific disorders. This may involve administration of thyroid extract, cortisone, testosterone, or estrogens and progesterone. The sex hormones are usually begun during adolescence to promote normal sexual maturation.

## Nursing Considerations

The principal nursing consideration is identifying children with growth problems. Despite the fact that the majority of growth problems are not a result of organic causes, any delay in normal growth and sexual development poses special emotional adjustments for these children.

The nurse may be a key person in helping to establish a diagnosis. For example, if serial height and weight records are not available, the nurse can question parents about the child's growth in comparison with that of siblings, peers, or relatives. Investigating clothing sizes is often helpful in determining growth at different ages. Parents of these children frequently comment that the child wears out clothes before growing out of them or that, if the clothing fits the body, it often is too long in the sleeves or legs.

Because the behavioral or physical changes that suggest a tumor are insidious, they are frequently overlooked. It is important to correlate the onset of any positive findings with the initial evidence of growth retardation. For example, visual problems and headache are not uncommon in school-age children and can coincidentally occur after a growth problem is recognized. In fact, headache may represent the emotional trauma caused by short stature rather than be a symptom of a tumor. This line of questioning should be pursued cautiously to avoid alarming parents unduly about the possibility of a brain tumor.

Part of a nurse's role in helping establish a diagnosis is assisting with diagnostic tests. Preparation of the child and family is especially important if a number of tests are being performed, and the child will require particular attention during provocative testing. Blood samples are usually taken every 30 minutes for a 3-hour period. (See Atraumatic Care box.) Children also have difficulty overcoming hypoglycemia generated by tests with insulin, so they must be observed carefully for signs of hypoglycemia, whereas those receiving glucagon are at risk of nausea and vomiting.

**Child and Family Support.** Once a diagnosis is made confirming an organic cause of the problem, the parents and child need an opportunity to express their thoughts and feelings. Not infrequently, a growth problem that was present since birth is missed until adolescence, at which time the child's difference in body development becomes dramatically evident in comparisons with peers. Family members may feel anger and resentment toward members of the health staff for not detecting the problem sooner. Parents may experience guilt for not seeking medical attention earlier, especially if the child has been miserable from experiencing ridicule and criticism from associates. Appropriate emotional support from the nurse can include an affirmation of each person's justified feelings, such as anger or guilt, and emphasis on the treatment plan and prospects for improvement in the future.

Children undergoing hormone replacement require additional support. Education for patient self-management during the school-age years should be provided.* Nursing functions include family education concerning medication preparation and storage, injection sites, injection technique, and syringe disposal. (See Chapter 27.) Administration of GH is facilitated by family routines that include a specific time of day for the injection. Younger children may enjoy using a calendar and colorful stickers to designate received injections.

### ATRAUMATIC CARE
*Avoiding Pain of Venipuncture*

To avoid the pain of repeated venipunctures, apply EMLA to the site at least 60 minutes before the first blood sample. Use an intermittent infusion device and flush with saline to keep patent.

---

*Home care instructions on giving subcutaneous injections are available in Wong DL, Hess, CS: *Wong and Whaley's clinical manual of pediatric nursing*, ed 5, St Louis, 2000, Mosby.

**NURSING ALERT** Optimum dosing is often achieved when GH is administered at bedtime. Physiologic release is more normally simulated as a result of pituitary release of GH during the first 45 to 90 minutes after the onset of sleep.

Even when hormone replacement is successful, these children attain their eventual adult height at a slower rate than their peers; therefore they need assistance in setting realistic expectations regarding improvement. Both sexes need guidance toward appropriate vocational goals. For example, children with aspirations for athletic sports such as basketball would be better advised to explore other activities not so dependent on excessive height.

Because these children appear younger than their chronologic age, others frequently relate to them in infantile or childish ways. Children having school problems will need special counseling. Parents and teachers benefit from guidance directed toward setting realistic expectations for the child based on age and abilities. (See Critical Thinking Exercise box.) For example, in the home such children should have the same age-appropriate responsibilities as their siblings. As they approach adolescence, they should be encouraged to participate in group activities with their peers. They should wear styles that accentuate their actual age, not their size. If abilities and strengths are emphasized rather than physical size, such children are more likely to develop a positive self-image.

Professionals and families may find education and support from the **Human Growth Foundation.*** The treatment is expensive—up to $10,000 to $50,000 per year, depending on the dosage (AAP, 1997). Usually the cost is partially covered by insurance if the child has a *documented* deficiency. Children with panhypopituitarism should be advised to wear medical identification at all times.

## Pituitary Hyperfunction

Excess GH before closure of the epiphyseal shafts results in proportional overgrowth of the long bones until the individual reaches a height of 8 feet or more. Vertical growth is accompanied by rapid and increased development of muscles and viscera. Weight is increased but is usually in proportion to height. Proportional enlargement of head circumference also occurs and may result in delayed closure of the fontanels in young children. Children with a pituitary-secreting tumor may also demonstrate signs of increasing intracranial pressure, especially headache.

If hypersecretion of GH occurs after epiphyseal closure, growth is in the transverse direction, producing a condition known as *acromegaly*. Typical facial features include overgrowth of the head, lips, nose, tongue, jaw, and paranasal and mastoid sinuses; separation and malocclusion of the teeth in the enlarged jaw; disproportion of the face to the cerebral division of the skull; increased facial hair; thick-

ened, deeply creased skin; and increased tendency toward hyperglycemia and diabetes mellitus.

### Diagnostic Evaluation

Diagnosis is based on a history of excessive growth during childhood and evidence of increased levels of GH. Radiographic studies may reveal a tumor in an enlarged sella turcica, normal bone age, enlargement of bones (such as the paranasal sinuses), and evidence of joint changes. Endocrine studies to confirm excess of other hormones, specifically thyroid, cortisol, and sex hormones, should also be included in the differential diagnosis.

### Therapeutic Management

If a lesion is present, surgical treatment by cryosurgery or hypophysectomy is performed to remove the tumor when feasible. Other therapies aimed at destroying pituitary tissue include external irradiation and radioactive implants. Depending on the extent of surgical extirpation and degree of

 *Critical Thinking Exercise*

#### Growth Hormone Deficiency

Kevin, an 11-year-old boy, is being treated for GH deficiency. A work-up was initiated after Kevin's mother noticed that his pants size had not changed in 2 years and that his 8-year-old brother was rapidly becoming taller than Kevin. Kevin has become increasingly hostile to his brother and is refusing to attend school on a regular basis. Kevin's mother is administering the daily injections of GH. Which of the following interventions should be initiated first to allow Kevin to regain feelings of mastery and control over his environment?

FIRST, THINK ABOUT IT . . .
- What concepts or ideas are central to your thinking?
- What conclusions are you coming to?

1. Preparation for home schooling.
2. Family counseling related to sibling rivalry.
3. Education and support related to self-administration of GH.
4. Encouragement and assurance that the therapy is temporary and will maximize his adult height.

*The best response is three. The idea that children with GH deficiency may develop behaviors related to feelings of inadequacy and loss of control is developmentally sound. Often families, teachers, and peers relate to the child relative to his short height rather than his chronologic age. A child of 11 years is competent to draw up and administer daily injections of GH, which will allow the child increased control over his environment and a feeling that he is responsible for treatment of his growth deficit.*

*Option one is incorrect; these children must remain in regular school. At this point option two is probably not necessary, because increasing Kevin's control may reduce his hostility. Although option four is always appropriate, it does not address the principal issue—the conclusion that Kevin should be independently responsible for his therapy.*

*7777 Leesburg Pike, Suite 202—South, Falls Church, VA 22043, (800) 451-6434, e-mail: hgfound@erols.com.

pituitary insufficiency, hormone replacement with thyroid extract, cortisone, and sex hormones may be necessary.

## Nursing Considerations

The primary nursing consideration is early identification of children with excessive growth rates. Although medical management is unable to reduce growth already attained, further growth can be retarded, and the earlier the treatment, the more control there is in predetermining a normal adult height. Nurses in ambulatory settings who are frequently involved in growth screening should refer children who demonstrate excessive linear growth for a medical evaluation. They should also observe for signs of a tumor, especially headache, and evidence of concurrent hormonal excesses, particularly the gonadotropins, which cause sexual precocity.

Children with excessive growth rates require as much emotional support as those with short stature. However, girls may suffer from the effects of excessive height much more than boys. In fact, males may find the tallness an asset when pursuing sports such as basketball. Children and their parents need an opportunity to express their thoughts. A compassionate nurse can be very supportive to these children, especially before adolescence when they are larger than their peers. The nurse can emphasize to a tall girl that as boys grow older they become taller and that she will not always be looking down at them. Because early adolescence is a time of idol worship, the nurse can point out marriages

of celebrities in which the woman is taller than the man to help the girl gain a perspective that not all heterosexual relationships must follow stereotypic models.

## Precocious Puberty

Manifestations of sexual development before age 9 years in boys or age 8 years in girls have traditionally been considered precocious development, and these chhildren were recommended for further evaluation (Klein, 1999). Recent examination of the age limit for defining when puberty is precocious reveals that the onset of puberty in girls is occurring earlier than previous studies have documented (Kaplowitz and Oberfield, 1999; Klein, 1999; Palmert, Malin, and Boepple, 1999). Breast and pubic hair development appeared on average 1 year earlier in Caucasian girls and 2 years earlier in African-American girls. Based on recent findings, precocious puberty evaluation for a pathologic etiology should be performed for Caucasian girls younger than 7 years of age or for African-American girls younger than 6 years of age (Kaplowitz and Oberfield, 1999). No change in the guidelines for evaluation of precocious puberty in boys is recommended.

Normally the hypothalamic-releasing factors stimulate secretion of the gonadotropic hormones from the anterior pituitary at the time of puberty. In the male, interstitial cell-stimulating hormone stimulates Leydig cells of the testes to secrete testosterone; in the female, follicle-stimulating hormone and luteinizing hormone stimulate the ovarian follicles to secrete estrogens. This sequence of events is known as the *hypothalamic-pituitary-gonadal axis.* If for some reason there is premature activation of this cycle, the child will display evidence of advanced or precocious puberty. Causes of precocious puberty are found in Box 38-6.

Isosexual precocious puberty is more common among girls than boys. Approximately 50% of children will have *central precocious puberty (CPP),* in which pubertal development is activated by the hypothalamic *gonadotropin-releasing hormone (Gn-RH).* This produces early maturation and development of the gonads with secretion of sex hormones, development of secondary sex characteristics, and sometimes production of mature sperm and ova (Lee, 1999; Root, 2000). CPP may be the result of congenital anomalies; infectious, neoplastic, or traumatic insults to the central nervous system (CNS) or treatment of long-standing sex hormone exposure (Box 38-6). CPP occurs more frequently in girls and is usually idiopathic with 95% demonstrating no causative factor (Root, 2000). A CNS insult or structural abnormality is found in more than 90% of boys with CPP (Root, 2000).

*Peripheral precocious puberty (PPP)* includes early puberty resulting from hormone stimulation other than the hypothalamic Gn-RH–stimulated pituitary gonadotropin release.

Isolated manifestations that are usually associated with puberty may be seen as variations in normal sexual development. They appear without other signs of pubescence and are probably caused by unusual end-organ sensitivity to prepubertal levels of estrogen or androgen. Included are *premature thelarche*—development of breasts in prepubertal females; *premature pubarche (premature adrenarche)*—early develop-

---

**Box 38-6** ▪ ▪ ▫
**Causes of Precocious Puberty**

**CENTRAL PRECOCIOUS PUBERTY**
☐ Idiopathic: With/without hypothalamic hamartoma
☐ Secondary
    Congenital anomalies
    Postinflammatory: encephalitis, meningitis, abscess, granulomatous disease
    Radiation therapy
    Trauma
    Neoplasms
☐ Following effective treatment of long-standing pseudoisosexual precocity

**PERIPHERAL PRECOCIOUS PUBERTY**
☐ Familial male-limited precocious puberty
☐ McCune-Albright syndrome
☐ Gonadal/extragonadal tumors
☐ Adrenal
    Congenital adrenal hyperplasia:
    Adenoma, carcinoma
    Glucocorticoid resistance
☐ Exogenous sex hormones
☐ Primary hypothyroidism

**INCOMPLETE PRECOCIOUS PUBERTY**
☐ Premature thelarche
☐ Premature menarche
☐ Premature pubarche/adrenarche

Modified from Root AW: Precocious puberty, *Pediatr Rev* 21(1):10-19, 2000.

ment of sexual hair; and *premature menarche*—isolated menses without other evidence of sexual development.

## Therapeutic Management

Treatment of precocious pseudopuberty is directed toward the specific cause when known. Precocious puberty of central (hypothalamic-pituitary) origin is managed with monthly injections of a synthetic analog of *luteinizing hormone–releasing hormone (LH-RH),* which regulates pituitary secretions. (Carel and Chaussain, 1999; Lee, 1999). The available preparation, leuprolide acetate (Lupron Depot), is given in a dose of 0.2 to 0.3 mg/kg intramuscularly once every 4 weeks. Breast development regresses or does not advance, and growth returns to normal rates, enhancing predicted height. Recent studies suggest that not all patients attain adult targeted heights and the addition of growth hormone therapy may be warranted (Walvoord and Pescovitz, 1999). Treatment is discontinued at a chronologically appropriate time, allowing pubertal changes to resume. Psychologic management of the patient and family is an important aspect of care. Both parents and the affected child should be taught the injection procedure.

## Nursing Considerations

Psychologic support and guidance of the child and family are the most important aspects of management. Parents need anticipatory guidance, support and information resources, and reassurance of the benign nature of the condition (Williams, 1995). Dress and activities for the physically precocious child should be appropriate to the chronologic age. Heterosexual interest is not usually advanced beyond the child's chronologic age, and parents need to understand that the child's mental age is congruent with the chronologic age and that the child's normal, overt manifestations of affection are age-appropriate and do not represent sexual advances.

Despite the early sexual development, maturation of the gonads and the appearance of secondary sexual characteristics proceed in the usual order. The most difficult time for the child is usually the school years before adolescence. After puberty, physical differences from peers are no longer present.

Although the child's heterosexual behavior is appropriate for the chronologic age, the nurse should emphasize to parents that the child is fertile. Usually no form of contraception is necessary unless the child is sexually active. In this situation proper counseling is important because hormonal forms of birth control, such as estrogen pills, will prematurely initiate epiphyseal closure, resulting in stunted linear growth.

## Diabetes Insipidus (DI)

The principal disorder of posterior pituitary hypofunction is DI, also known as *neurogenic DI,* resulting from hyposecretion of *antidiuretic hormone (ADH),* or *vasopressin,* and producing a state of uncontrolled diuresis. (Bode, Crawford, and Danon, 1996). This disorder is not to be confused with nephrogenic DI, a rare hereditary disorder affecting primar-

ily males and caused by unresponsiveness of the renal tubules to the hormone. (See Chapter 30.)

Neurogenic DI may result from a number of different causes. Primary causes are familial or idiopathic; of the total groups, approximately 45% to 50% are idiopathic. Secondary causes include trauma (accidental or surgical), tumors, granulomatous disease, infections (meningitis or encephalitis), and vascular anomalies (aneurysm). Certain drugs, such as alcohol or phenytoin (diphenylhydantoin), can cause a transient polyuria.

## Clinical Manifestations

The cardinal signs of DI are polyuria and polydipsia. In the older child, signs such as excessive urination accompanied by a compensatory insatiable thirst may be so intense that the child does little more than go to the toilet and drink fluids. Not infrequently, the first sign is enuresis. In the infant the initial symptom is irritability that is relieved with feedings of water but not milk. The infant is also prone to dehydration, electrolyte imbalance, hyperthermia, azotemia, and potential circulatory collapse.

Dehydration is usually not a serious problem in older children, who are able to drink larger quantities of water. However, any period of unconsciousness, such as after trauma or anesthesia, may be life-threatening because the voluntary demand for fluid is absent. During such instances careful monitoring of urine volumes, blood concentration, and intravenous (IV) fluid replacement is essential to prevent dehydration.

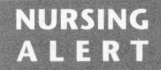 **NURSING ALERT**    The child with DI complicated by congenital absence of the thirst center must be encouraged to drink sufficient quantities of liquid to prevent electrolyte imbalance.

## Diagnostic Evaluation

The simplest test used to diagnose this condition is restriction of oral fluids and observation of consequent changes in urine volume and concentration. Normally, reducing fluids results in concentrated urine and diminished volume. In DI, fluid restriction has little or no effect on urine formation but causes weight loss from dehydration. Accurate results from this procedure require strict monitoring of fluid intake, urinary output, measurement of urine concentration (specific gravity or osmolality), and frequent weight checks. A weight loss between 3% and 5% indicates significant dehydration and requires termination of the fluid restriction.

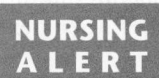 **NURSING ALERT**    Small children require close observation during fluid deprivation to prevent them from drinking, even from toilet bowls, plants, or other unlikely sources of fluid.

If this test is positive, the child should be given a test dose of injected *aqueous vasopressin (Pitressin),* which should alleviate the polyuria and polydipsia. Unresponsiveness to exogenous vasopressin usually indicates nephrogenic DI.

An important diagnostic consideration is to differentiate DI from other causes of polyuria and polydipsia, especially diabetes mellitus. Other tests used in the diagnostic evaluation include CT of the brain or magnetic resonance imaging (MRI) to detect a tumor, kidney function tests and blood electrolyte levels to assess renal failure, and specific endocrine studies to isolate associated problems. In rare instances a psychologic consultation may be warranted to confirm the possibility of compulsive water drinking related to psychogenic causes.

## Therapeutic Management

The usual treatment is hormone replacement, either with an intramuscular or subcutaneous injection of *vasopressin tannate* in peanut oil or with a nasal spray of *aqueous lysine vasopressin* (Bode, Crawford, and Danon, 1996). The injectable form has the advantage of lasting for 48 to 72 hours, which affords the child a full night's sleep. However, it has the disadvantage of requiring frequent injections as well as proper preparation of the drug.

> **NURSING ALERT**
>
> To be effective, vasopressin must be thoroughly resuspended in the oil by being held under warm running water for 10 to 15 minutes and shaken vigorously before being drawn into the syringe. If this is not done, the oil may be injected minus the ADH. Small brown particles, which indicate drug dispersion, must be seen in the suspension.

The nasal spray has the benefit of being a simple, painless route of administration. However, applications must be repeated every 8 to 12 hours to prevent recurrence of symptoms. To provide longer relief during the night, a cotton pledget moistened with the spray can be inserted into the nostril. However, mucous membrane irritation caused by a cold or allergy renders this route unreliable. Although the vaginal and buccal mucosae are substitute routes for the spray, they can be inconvenient. *Desmopressin acetate (DDAVP)*, a long-acting analog of arginine vasopressin, which has fewer side effects, is available and administered intranasally by way of a flexible tube to achieve adequate control. The response pattern of the child is variable, with duration ranging from 6 to 24 hours (Bode, Crawford, and Danon, 1996). It is usually administered twice daily—at bedtime to allow the child to sleep through the night and in the morning to allow fewer interruptions in the school day. Some "breakthrough" urination is allowed during the evening hours as a precaution against overmedication. The signs of overmedication are similar to manifestations associated with inappropriate secretion of ADH. (See next section.)

## Nursing Considerations

The initial objective is identification of the disorder. Because an early sign may be sudden enuresis in a child who is toilet trained, excessive thirst with bed-wetting is an indication for further investigation. Another clue is persistent irritability and crying in an infant that is relieved only by bottle-feedings of water. Following head trauma or cer-tain neurosurgical procedures, the development of DI can be anticipated; therefore these patients must be closely monitored.

Assessment includes measurement of body weight, serum electrolytes, blood urea nitrogen, hematocrit, and urine specific gravity taken before surgery and every other day following the procedure. Fluid intake and output should be carefully measured and recorded. Alert patients are able to adjust intake to urine losses, but unconscious or very young patients will require closer fluid observation. In children who are not toilet trained, collection of urine specimens may require application of a urine-collecting device.

After confirmation of the diagnosis, parents need a thorough explanation regarding the condition with specific clarification that DI is a different condition from diabetes mellitus. They must realize that treatment is lifelong. If children are to receive the injectable vasopressin (Pitressin), ideally two caregivers should be taught the correct procedure for preparation and administration of the drug. Once children are old enough, they should be encouraged to assume full responsibility for their care.*

For emergency purposes, these children should wear medical alert identification. Older children should carry the nasal spray with them for temporary relief of symptoms. School personnel need to be aware of the problem so that they can grant children unrestricted use of the lavatory. Failure to permit this may result in embarrassing accidents that often result in a child's unwillingness to attend school.

## Syndrome of Inappropriate Antidiuretic Hormone (SIADH)

The disorder that results from hypersecretion of the posterior pituitary hormone, or ADH (vasopressin), is known as SIADH. It is observed with increased frequency in a variety of conditions, especially those involving infections, tumors, or other CNS disease or trauma.

The manifestations are directly related to fluid retention and hypotonicity. Excess ADH causes most of the filtered water to be reabsorbed from the kidneys back into central circulation. Serum osmolality is low, and urine osmolality is inappropriately elevated. When serum sodium levels are diminished to 120 mEq/L, affected children display anorexia, nausea (and sometimes vomiting), stomach cramps, irritability, and personality changes. With progressive reduction in sodium, other neurologic signs, stupor, and convulsions may be evident. The symptoms usually disappear when the underlying disorder is corrected.

The immediate management consists of restricting fluids. Subsequent management depends on the cause and severity. Fluids continue to be restricted to one-fourth to one-half maintenance. When there are no fluid abnormalities but SIADH can be anticipated, fluids are often restricted expectantly at two-thirds to three-fourths maintenance.

---

*Home care instructions on giving subcutaneous injections are available in Wong DL, Hess CS: *Wong and Whaley's clinical manual of pediatric nursing,* ed 5, St Louis, 2000, Mosby.

## Nursing Considerations

The first goal of nursing management is recognizing the presence of SIADH from symptoms described in patients at risk, especially those in the pediatric intensive care unit (PICU).

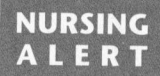

**NURSING ALERT** Nausea, vomiting, and malaise may precede the onset of more severe stages such as disorientation, confusion, coma, and seizures (Bode, Crawford, and Danon, 1996).

Accurately measuring intake and output, noting daily weight, and observing for signs of fluid overload are primary nursing functions, especially in the child receiving IV fluids. Seizure precautions are implemented, and the child and family need education regarding the rationale for fluid restrictions. The rare child with chronic SIADH will be placed on long-term ADH-antagonizing medication, and the child and family will require instructions for its administration.

## DISORDERS OF THYROID FUNCTION

The thyroid gland secretes two types of hormones: *thyroid hormone (TH),* which consists of the hormones *thyroxine (T$_4$)* and *triiodothyronine (T$_3$),* and *thyrocalcitonin.* The secretion of thyroid hormones is controlled by *thyroid-stimulating hormone (TSH)* from the anterior pituitary, which in turn is regulated by thyrotropin-releasing factor (TRF) from the hypothalamus as a negative feedback response. Consequently, hypothyroidism or hyperthyroidism may result from a defect in the target gland or from a disturbance in the secretion of TSH or TRF. Because the functions of T$_3$ and T$_4$ are qualitatively the same, the term *thyroid hormone (TH)* is used throughout the discussion (Box 38-7).

The synthesis of TH depends on available sources of dietary iodine and tyrosine. The thyroid is the only endocrine gland capable of storing excess amounts of hormones for release as needed. During circulation in the bloodstream, T$_4$ and T$_3$ are bound to carrier proteins (thyroxine-binding globulin [TBG]). They must be unbound before they are able to exert their metabolic effect.

The main physiologic action of TH is to regulate the basal metabolic rate and thereby control the processes of growth and tissue differentiation, as outlined in Box 38-7. Unlike GH, TH is involved in many more diverse activities that influence the growth and development of body tissues. Therefore a deficiency of TH exerts a more profound effect on growth than that seen in hypopituitarism.

Thyrocalcitonin helps maintain blood calcium levels by decreasing the calcium concentration. Its effect is the opposite of parathormone in that it inhibits skeletal demineralization and promotes calcium deposition in the bone.

## Juvenile Hypothyroidism

Hypothyroidism is one of the most common endocrine problems of childhood. It may be either congenital (see

---

**Box 38-7**
### Physiologic Effects of Thyroid Hormone

Regulates metabolic rate of all cells; protein, fat, and carbohydrate catabolism; and nitrogen excretion

Regulates body heat production and heat-dissipating mechanisms

Regulates protein synthesis and catabolism, amino acid incorporation into protein, and transcription of messenger RNA

Increases gluconeogenesis and peripheral utilization of glucose

Maintains appetite and secretion of gastrointestinal substances

Maintains calcium mobilization

Stimulates cholesterol synthesis and hepatic mechanisms that remove cholesterol from the circulation; stimulates lipid turnover and free fatty acid release

Regulates hepatic conversion of carotene to vitamin A

Maintains growth hormone secretion, skeletal maturation, and tissue differentiation

Is necessary for muscle tone and vigor and normal skin constituents

Maintains cardiac rate, force, and output

Affects respiratory rate, depth of oxygen utilization, and carbon dioxide formation

Affects central nervous system development and cerebration during first 2 to 3 years

Affects milk production during lactation and menstrual cycle fertility

Maintains sensitivity to insulin and insulin degradation

Affects red cell production

Affects cortisol secretion, probably caused by direct effect on adrenal glands and by increasing ACTH secretion

---

Chapter 9) or acquired and represents a deficiency in secretion of TH (Foley, 2001). Hypothyroidism from dietary insufficiency of iodine is now rare in the United States because iodized salt is a readily available source of the nutrient.

Beyond infancy, primary hypothyroidism may be caused by a number of defects. For example, a congenital hypoplastic thyroid gland may provide sufficient amounts of TH during the first year or two but be inadequate when rapid body growth increases demands on the gland. A partial or complete thyroidectomy for cancer or thyrotoxicosis can leave insufficient thyroid tissue to furnish hormones for body requirements. Radiation therapy for Hodgkin disease or other malignancies may be a cause of hypothyroidism (Hockenberry-Eaton and others, 1998). Infectious processes may be a cause of hypothyroidism. It can also occur when dietary iodine is deficient.

Clinical manifestations depend on the extent of dysfunction and the age of the child at the onset. Primary congenital hypothyroidism is characterized by low levels of circulating thyroid hormones and raised levels of thyrotropin at birth (Macchia, 2000). The presenting symptoms are decelerated growth from chronic deprivation of TH or thyromegaly. Impaired growth and development are less when hypothyroidism is acquired at a later age, and, because brain growth is nearly complete by 2 to 3 years of age, mental retardation and neurologic sequelae are not associated with juvenile hypothyroidism. Other manifestations are myxedematous skin changes (dry skin, puffiness around the eyes, sparse hair), constipation, sleepiness, and mental decline.

Therapy is TH replacement, the same as for hypothyroidism in the infant, although the prompt treatment needed in the infant is not required in the child. In children with severe symptoms, the restoration of euthyroidism is achieved more gradually with administration of increasing amounts of L-thyroxine over a period of 4 to 8 weeks to avoid symptoms of hyperthyroidism, which can occur with treatment of chronic hypothyroidism. Researchers have found that children treated early continue to have mild delays in reading, comprehension, and arithmetic with catchup by grade 6 (Rovet and Ehrlich, 2000). However, adolescents may demonstrate problems with memory, attention, and visuospatial processing.

### Nursing Considerations

The importance of early recognition in the infant has already been discussed in Chapter 9. Growth cessation or retardation in a child whose growth has previously been normal should alert the observer to the possibility of hypothyroidism. Following diagnosis and implementation of thyroxine therapy, the importance of compliance and periodic monitoring of response to therapy should be stressed to parents. Children should learn to take responsibility for their own health as soon as they are old enough, at about 9 to 10 years of age.

## Goiter

A goiter is an enlargement or hypertrophy of the thyroid gland. It may occur with deficient (hypothyroid), excessive (hyperthyroid), or normal (euthyroid) TH secretion. It can be congenital or acquired. Congenital disease usually occurs as a result of maternal administration of antithyroid drugs or iodides during pregnancy. Acquired disease can result from increased secretion of pituitary TSH in response to decreased circulating levels of TH or from infiltrative neoplastic or inflammatory processes. In areas where dietary iodine (essential for TH production) is deficient, goiter can be endemic.

Enlargement of the thyroid gland may be mild and noticeable only when there is an increased demand for TH (e.g., during periods of rapid growth). Where iodine deficiency is severe, a large percentage of the population display goiters. Enlargement of the thyroid at birth can be sufficient to cause severe respiratory distress. Sporadic goiter is usually caused by lymphocytic thyroiditis, and intrinsic biochemical defects in synthesis of the hormones are associated with goiters. TH replacement is necessary to treat the hypothyroidism and reverse the TSH effect on the gland.

### Nursing Considerations

Large goiters are identified by their obvious appearance. Smaller nodules may be evident only on palpation. Nurses in ambulatory settings need to be aware of the possibility of goiters and report such findings. Benign enlargement of the thyroid gland may occur during adolescence and should not be confused with pathologic states. Nodules rarely are caused by a cancerous tumor but always require evaluation.

Questions regarding exposure to radiation should be included in the assessment.

> **NURSING ALERT** If an infant is born with a goiter, immediate precautions are instituted for emergency ventilation, such as supplemental oxygen and a tracheostomy set. Hyperextension of the neck often facilitates breathing.

Immediate surgery to remove part of the gland may be lifesaving in infants born with a goiter. When thyroid replacement is necessary, parents have the same needs regarding its administration as discussed for the parents of children who have hypothyroidism. (See Chapter 9.)

## Lymphocytic Thyroiditis

Lymphocytic thyroiditis (*Hashimoto disease, juvenile autoimmune thyroiditis*) is the most common cause of thyroid disease in children and adolescents and accounts for the largest percentage of juvenile hypothyroidism (Szymborska and Staroszczyk, 2000). It accounts for many of the enlarged thyroid glands formerly designated as thyroid hyperplasia of adolescence or "adolescent goiter." Although it can occur during the first 3 years of life, it occurs more frequently after age 6. It reaches a peak incidence during adolescence, and there is evidence that the disease is self-limited.

### Pathophysiology

There is a strong genetic predisposition to the development of autoimmune thyroiditis, although no mode of inheritance has been delineated and the basic stimulus or autoimmune defect is unknown. There is a close relationship between this disease and other thyroid disorders (Graves disease, idiopathic hypothyroidism, idiopathic myxedema) and autoimmune disorders (pernicious anemia, Addison disease, type 1 diabetes mellitus, and hypoparathyroidism) in families. An increased incidence of the histocompatibility antigens HLA-DR3 and HLA-DR5 has been observed in patients with autoimmune thyroiditis (Huang and others, 1996).

The disease is characterized by lymphocytic infiltration of the gland, germinal center inflammation, and, in many patients, replacement with fibrous tissue. In the early stages there may be only hyperplasia. A defect in autoregulation allows the persistence of a T-cell clone, which induces a cell-mediated immune response. Several antithyroid antibodies have been recognized in patients with thyroiditis.

### Clinical Manifestations

The presence of the enlarged thyroid gland is usually detected by the practitioner during a routine examination, although it may be noted by parents when the youngster swallows. In most children the entire gland is enlarged symmetrically (but may be asymmetric) and is firm, freely movable, and nontender. There may be manifestations of moderate tracheal compression (sense of fullness, hoarseness, and dysphagia), but it is extremely rare for a nontoxic diffuse goiter to enlarge to the extent that its size causes mechanical obstruction. Most children are euthyroid, but some display symptoms of hypothyroidism. Others have signs suggestive of hyperthyroidism, such as nervousness, irritability, tachycardia, increased sweating, or hyperactivity.

### Diagnostic Evaluation

Thyroid function tests are usually normal, although TSH levels may be slightly or moderately elevated. With progressive disease the $T_4$ decreases, followed by a decrease in $T_3$ levels and an increase in TSH. A variety of abnormalities in radioactive iodine uptake may be noted. The majority of children have serum antibody titers to thyroid antigens, but fewer children have a positive red blood cell hemagglutination test result. When both tests are used, almost all children with thyroid autoimmunity are detected. However, levels in children are lower than in adults; therefore repeated measurements may be needed in doubtful cases because titers may increase later in the disease.

### Therapeutic Management

In many cases the goiter is transient and asymptomatic and regresses spontaneously within a year or two. Therapy of a nontoxic diffuse goiter is usually simple, uncomplicated, and effective. Oral administration of TH will decrease the size of the gland significantly. It provides the feedback needed to suppress TSH stimulation, and the hyperplastic thyroid gland gradually regresses in size. Surgery is contraindicated in this disorder. Untreated patients should be evaluated periodically.

### Nursing Considerations

Nursing care consists of identifying the youngster with thyroid enlargement, reassuring the child that the condition is probably only temporary, and reinforcing instructions for thyroid therapy.

## Hyperthyroidism

The largest percentage of hyperthyroidism in childhood is caused by Graves disease, which is usually associated with an enlarged thyroid gland and exophthalmos. (Zimmerman and Lteif, 1998). Most cases of Graves disease occur in children ages 6 to 15, with a peak incidence at 12 to 14 years of age, but the disease may be present at birth in children of thyrotoxic mothers. The incidence is five times higher in girls than in boys.

The hyperthyroidism of Graves disease is apparently caused by an autoimmune response to TSH receptors, but no specific etiology has been identified. There is definitive evidence for familial association, with a high concordance incidence in twins. Patients with Graves disease possess the histocompatibility antigen, $A^1$, $B_8$, and $DR_3$ (Dallas and Foley, 1996.)

### Clinical Manifestations

The development of manifestations is highly variable. Signs and symptoms develop gradually, with an interval between onset and diagnosis of approximately 6 to 12 months. The principal clinical features are excessive motion—irritability, hyperactivity, short attention span, tremors, insomnia, and emotional lability. Gradual weight loss despite a voracious appetite is observed in half of the cases. Linear growth and bone age are usually accelerated. Muscle weakness often occurs. Hyperactivity of the gastrointestinal tract may cause vomiting and frequent stooling. Cardiac manifestations include a rapid, pounding pulse even during sleep, widened pulse pressure, systolic murmurs, and cardiomegaly. Dyspnea occurs during slight exertion, such as climbing stairs. The skin is warm, flushed, and moist. Heat intolerance may be severe and is accompanied by diaphoresis. The hair is unusually fine and unable to hold a wave.

*Exophthalmos* (protruding eyeballs), observed in many children, is accompanied by a wide-eyed staring expression, increased blinking, lid lag, lack of convergence, and absence of wrinkling of the forehead when looking upward. As protrusion of the eyeball increases, the child may not be able to completely cover the cornea with the lid. Visual disturbances may include blurred vision and loss of visual acuity. Ophthalmopathy can develop long before or after the onset of hyperthyroidism. A consistent pathogenic link between them has not been identified, and the cause of Graves ophthalmopathy is not known (Bartley and others, 1996).

### Diagnostic Evaluation

The presence of a thyroid mass in a child requires a thorough history, including inquiry into prior irradiation to the head and neck and exposure to a goitrogen. The diagnosis is established on the basis of increased levels of $T_4$ and $T_3$. TSH is suppressed to unmeasurable levels. Other tests are rarely indicated.

### Therapeutic Management

Therapy for hyperthyroidism is controversial, but all methods are directed toward retarding the rate of hormone secretion. The three acceptable modes available are the antithyroid drugs, which interfere with the biosynthesis of TH, including propylthiouracil (PTU) and methimazole (MTZ, Tapazole); subtotal thyroidectomy; and ablation with radioiodine ($^{131}$I-iodide). (Zimmerman and Lteif, 1998). Each is effective, but each has advantages and disadvantages.

When affected children exhibit signs and symptoms of hyperthyroidism (i.e., increased weight loss, pulse, pulse pressure, and blood pressure), their activity should be limited to class work only. Vigorous exercise is restricted until thyroid levels are decreased to normal or near-normal values.

**Drug Therapy.** Most centers favor drugs as an initial therapy. An effective response to these drugs occurs after a latent period because they inhibit production of additional TH but do not retard secretion of stored supplies. Generally, some improvement is noted within the first 2 weeks, with evidence of decreased nervousness, less fatigue, increased strength, a lowered pulse, and weight gain. In many children an initial treatment course of 1 to 2 years will be followed by a complete remission of the disorder. Those who relapse may benefit from a second course of therapy but may also be candidates for surgical intervention.

Disadvantages include toxic drug reactions requiring alternate therapy, chronic dependency on the drug, and failure to produce remission in a large number of patients. The most serious side effect of these antithyroid drugs is agranulocytosis (severe leukopenia), which generally occurs within the initial weeks or months of therapy. It is usually accompanied by a sore throat and fever. Treatment involves immediate discontinuation of the drug, social isolation of the child, and administration of antibiotics and glucocorticoids until symptoms resolve. (See Critical Thinking Exercise box.)

**Thyroidectomy.** Surgical treatment involves surgical ablation of the thyroid (thyroidectomy). Although this approach has the advantage of being a long-lasting form of therapy without the need for multiple-dose drug therapy, it has a number of serious disadvantages, including an increased incidence of hypothyroidism and the need for thyroxine therapy, infrequent recurrent laryngeal nerve palsy and permanent hypoparathyroidism, keloid formation of the anterior cervical scar, and (rarely) surgical mortality. Therefore surgery in most centers is reserved for children who do not respond to or comply with the use of antithyroid drugs or who are prone to recurrences.

**Radioiodine Therapy.** Radioiodine may be a therapy of choice in young patients with Graves disease who relapse after medical treatment (Cheetham and others, 1998). Radioiodine therapy has become an even more acceptable option since it has become apparent that lifelong thyroxine replacement is required after either surgery or radioiodine therapy. **The Thyroid Society for Education and Research*** has an extensive web site with information relation to prevention, treatment, and cure of thyroid disease.

**Thyrotoxicosis.** Thyrotoxicosis (thyroid "crisis" or thyroid "storm") may occur from sudden release of the hormone. Although thyrotoxicosis is unusual in children, a crisis can be life-threatening. These "storms" are evidenced by the acute onset of severe irritability and restlessness, vomiting, diarrhea, hyperthermia, hypertension, severe tachycardia, and prostration. There may be rapid progression to delirium, coma, and even death. A crisis may be precipitated by acute infection, surgical emergencies, or discontinuation of antithyroid therapy. Treatment in addition to antithyroid drugs is administration of β-adrenergic blocking agents (propranolol), which provide relief from the adrenergic hyperresponsiveness that produces the disturbing side effects of the reaction. Therapy is usually required for 2 to 3 weeks.

## Nursing Considerations

The initial nursing objective is identification of children with hyperthyroidism. Because the clinical manifestations often appear gradually, the goiter and ophthalmic changes may not be noticed, and the excessive activity may be attributed to behavioral problems. Nurses in ambulatory settings, particularly those caring for children in school, need to be alert to signs that suggest this disorder, especially weight loss despite an excellent appetite, academic difficulties resulting from a short attention span and inability to sit still, unexplained fatigue and sleeplessness, and difficulty with fine motor skills, such as writing. Exophthalmos may develop, but is less common in adults than children (Jospe, 2001).

Much of these children's care is related to treating physical symptoms before a response to drug therapy is achieved. These children need a quiet, unstimulating environment that is conducive to rest. Sometimes hospitalization is necessary during the immediate treatment phase to remove a child from a troubled home. A regular routine is beneficial in providing frequent rest periods, minimizing the stress of coping with unexpected demands, and meeting the children's needs promptly. Physical activity is restricted. For example, school physical education classes are discontinued.

Because the manifestations often interfere with schoolwork, a consultation with the child's teachers is important in advising them of the medical reason for the problem and

## Critical Thinking Exercise

### Graves Disease

Susie, 15 years old, has noticed a racing pulse, ravenous appetite with continued weight loss, heat intolerance, sensitivity, and eyes that appear to be bulging from their sockets. After a diagnosis of Graves disease Susie is started on a therapeutic dose of propylthiouracil. Because of tachycardia, Susie is advised to participate in sedentary activities only and to discontinue school physical education classes. Environmental temperature and appropriate dress related to heat sensitivity, as well as dietary adjustments to meet increased metabolic needs, are addressed by the nurse. Susie is shown that exopthalmus can be minimized with artful application of cosmetics. Episodic emotional lability is discussed with Susie and her family. The drug regimen is explained with special emphasis on its side effects. After 6 weeks of treatment Susie presents with a sore throat and fever. Which of the following interventions is most appropriate?

FIRST, THINK ABOUT IT . . .

- What precise question are you trying to answer?
- What conclusions are you coming to?

1. Immediate follow-up by the practitioner.
2. Further instruction related to heat sensitivity.
3. Instruction related to symptomatic relief of the common cold.
4. Psychosocial interventions related to somatization of emotional lability.

*The best response is one. Precisely, the question is focused on the complications of propylthiouracil. Therapeutic levels of propylthiouracil can be accompanied by the grave complication of leukocytopenia. Any indication of infection must be promptly evaluated and appropriate therapy instituted. An accurate conclusion is that none of the other options addresses the immediate problem.*

*7515 S Main St, Suite 545, Houston, TX 77030, (800) 849-7643, e-mail: help@the-thyroid-society.org. A 200-page book on thyroid problems and answers called *Could It Be My Thyroid* can be purchased through the Society.

suggesting ways of helping the child adjust. For example, the child may benefit from a shortened school day or at least study periods in a quiet area. Limiting demands on the child, such as reciting in class or participating in extracurricular activities, may help conserve strength for academic studies. Despite the excessive activity of these children, they tire easily, experience muscle weakness, and are unable to relax to recover their strength.

Emotional lability is often manifested by sudden episodes of crying or elation. Such behavior, coupled with irritability, disrupts interpersonal relationships, creating difficulties within and outside the home. Parents need help in understanding the uncontrollable nature of these outbursts and ways of minimizing them through decreased environmental stimulation, stress, and frustration. The child should be encouraged to express feelings about behavior and the effect that it has on others. The nurse can encourage the child to concentrate on friendship with one special peer rather than a group until such time as the condition is stabilized.

Heat intolerance may produce considerable family conflict. Preferring a cooler environment than others, the child is likely to open windows, complain about the heat, wear minimal clothing, and remove blankets while sleeping. Although the child should dress in accordance with climatic conditions, the use of light cotton clothing in the home, good ventilation, air conditioning or fans, frequent baths, and adequate hydration is helpful in providing comfort. Hygiene should be stressed because of excessive sweating.

Dietary requirements should be adjusted to meet the child's increased metabolic rate. Although the need for calories is increased, these should be provided in wholesome foods rather than "junk" foods. The child may require vitamin supplements to meet the daily requirement. Rather than three large meals, the child's appetite may be better satisfied by five or six moderate meals throughout the day. Family members should refrain from making remarks about the child's appetite because the child may voluntarily restrict his or her eating to avoid such attention.

Once therapy is instituted, the nurse explains the drug regimen, emphasizing the importance of observing for side effects of antithyroid drugs. Untoward effects of propylthiouracil and related compounds include urticarial rash, fever, arthritis, or arthralgia. There may be enlargement of the salivary and cervical lymph glands, a diminished sense of taste, hepatitis, and edema of the lower extremities.

**NURSING ALERT**

Children being treated with propylthiouracil or methimazole must be carefully monitored for side effects of the drug. Because sore throat and fever accompany the grave complication of leukopenia, these children should be seen by a practitioner if such symptoms occur. Parents and children should be taught to recognize and report symptoms immediately.

Parents should also be aware of the signs of hypothyroidism, which can occur from overdose of the drugs. The most common indications are lethargy and somnolence.

**Surgical Care.** If surgery is anticipated, iodine is usually administered for a few weeks before the procedure. Because oral iodine preparations are unpalatable, they should be mixed with a strong-tasting fruit juice, such as grape or punch flavors, and be given through a straw. Compliance with iodine therapy is essential to avoid the danger of thyroid crisis after sudden discontinuation.

Psychologic preparation of children for thyroidectomy is similar to that for any other surgical procedure. (See Chapter 27). However, of special consideration is the site of the incision. The fear of having the throat cut is very real and in older children is associated with death. The nurse should explain that the throat is not cut, only the skin, to remove the gland. Showing children a picture of the anatomic location of the thyroid around the trachea is often helpful. Children should be prepared for the dressing around the neck and the possibility of an endotracheal or "breathing" tube after surgery.

Postoperative care involves positioning with the neck slightly flexed to avoid strain on the sutures and observation for bleeding and complications. The children are taught to support the neck in this position when they sit up. Damage to the recurrent laryngeal nerve is evidenced by severe stridor or hoarseness, although some hoarseness is expected. Laryngospasm, a spasmodic contraction of the larynx, can be a life-threatening complication of thyroidectomy. Signs of laryngospasm are stridor, hoarseness, and a feeling of tightness in the throat. A tracheostomy set should be placed near the bed for emergency use. Observation for signs of hypoparathyroidism, which causes hypocalcemia, should be implemented in the immediate postoperative period.

**NURSING ALERT**

The earliest indication of hypoparathyroidism may be anxiety and mental depression, followed by paresthesia and evidence of heightened neuromuscular excitability, such as:

**Chvostek sign**—Facial muscle spasm elicited by tapping the facial nerve in the region of the parotid gland
**Trousseau sign**—Carpal spasm elicited by pressure applied to nerves of the upper arm
**Tetany**—Carpopedal spasm (sharp flexion of wrist and ankle joints), muscle twitching, cramps, seizures and stridor

## DISORDERS OF PARATHYROID FUNCTION

The parathyroid glands secrete *parathormone (PTH)*, the main function of which, along with vitamin D and calcitonin, is homeostasis of serum calcium concentration. (Perheentupa, 1996). The effect of PTH on calcium is opposite that of thyrocalcitonin. The principal effects of PTH on its target sites are listed in Box 38-8.

The net result of the integrated action of PTH and vitamin D is maintenance of serum calcium levels within a narrow normal range and the mineralization of bone. Secretion of PTH is controlled by a negative feedback system involving the serum calcium ion concentration. Low ionized calcium levels stimulate PTH secretion, causing absorption of calcium by the target tissues; high ionized calcium concentrations suppress PTH.

> **Box 38-8** ■ ■ ☐
> **Physiologic Effects of Parathyroid Hormone**
>
> **Bones**—Increases osteoclastic activity, causing phosphate-producing bone demineralization
> **Kidneys**—Increases absorption of calcium and excretion of phosphate
> **Gastrointestinal tract**—Promotes calcium absorption

## Hypoparathyroidism

Hypoparathyroidism (HP) is a spectrum of disorders with a deficient parathyroid hormone effect. Congenital HP may be caused by a specific defect in the synthesis or cellular processing of the parathyroid hormone or from aplasia or hypoplasia of the gland (Perheentupa, 1996).

Hypoparathyroidism can also occur secondary to other causes. Postoperative hypoparathyroidism may follow thyroidectomy with acute or gradual onset and be transient or permanent. Two forms of transient hypoparathyroidism may be present in the newborn, both of which are the result of a relative PTH deficiency. One type is caused by maternal hyperparathyroidism or maternal diabetes mellitus. A more common, later form appears almost exclusively in infants fed a milk formula with a high phosphate-to-calcium ratio.

### Clinical Manifestations

Symptoms vary from none to significant morbidity if treatment is not initiated. Mild deficiency may be identified through laboratory studies. Muscle cramps is an early symptom, progressing to numbness, stiffness, and tingling in the hands and feet. A positive Chvostek or Trousseau sign or laryngeal spasms may be present. Convulsions with loss of consciousness may occur. These episodes may be preceded by abdominal discomfort, tonic rigidity, head retraction, and cyanosis. Headaches and vomiting with increased intracranial pressure and papilledema may occur and may suggest a brain tumor (Behrman, Kliegman, and Jenson, 2000).

Children with long-standing deficiency may have dry, scaly, course skin with eruptions often caused by *Candida* (Behrman, Kliegman, and Jenson, 2000). Dental and enamel hypoplasia often occurs. Cataracts develop in patients with untreated disease. Because hypoparathyroidism results in decreased bone resorption and inactive osteoclastic activity, skeletal growth is retarded.

### Diagnostic Evaluation

The diagnosis of hypoparathyroidism is made on the basis of clinical manifestations associated with *decreased serum calcium* and *increased serum phosphorus*. Levels of plasma PTH are low in idiopathic hypoparathyroidism but high in pseudohypoparathyroidism. End-organ responsiveness is tested by the administration of PTH with measurement of urinary cyclic adenosine monophosphate (cAMP). Kidney function tests are included in the differential diagnosis to rule out renal insufficiency. Although bone radiographs are usually normal, they may demonstrate increased bone density and suppressed growth.

### Therapeutic Management

The objective of treatment is to maintain normal serum calcium and phosphate levels with minimum complications. Acute or severe tetany is corrected immediately by IV and oral administration of calcium gluconate and follow-up daily doses to achieve normal levels. Twice-daily serum calcium measurements are taken to monitor the efficacy of therapy and prevent hypercalcemia. When diagnosis is confirmed, *vitamin D therapy* is begun. Vitamin D therapy is somewhat difficult to regulate because the drug has a prolonged onset and a long half-life. Some authorities advocate beginning with a lower dose with stepwise increases and careful monitoring of serum calcium until stable levels are achieved. Others prefer rapid induction with higher doses and rapid reduction to lower maintenance levels.

Long-term management consists of administration of massive doses of vitamin D, and oral calcium supplementation may be useful in maintaining adequate serum calcium levels, although it is not essential. Blood calcium and phosphorus are monitored frequently until the levels have stabilized; they are then monitored monthly and less often until the child is seen at 6-month intervals. Renal function, blood pressure, and serum vitamin D levels are measured every 6 months. Serum magnesium levels are measured every 3 to 6 months to permit detection of hypomagnesemia, which may raise the requirement for vitamin D.

### Nursing Considerations

The initial objective is recognition of hypocalcemia. Unexplained convulsions, irritability (especially to external stimuli), gastrointestinal symptoms (diarrhea, vomiting, cramping), and positive signs of tetany should lead the nurse to suspect this disorder. Much of the initial nursing care is related to the physical manifestations and includes institution of seizure and safety precautions, reduction of environmental stimuli (e.g., avoiding sudden or loud noise, bright lights, stimulating activities), and observation for signs of laryngospasm, such as stridor, hoarseness, and a feeling of tightness in the throat. A tracheostomy set and injectable calcium gluconate should be located near the bedside for emergency use. The administration of calcium gluconate requires precautions against extravasation of the drug and tissue destruction.

After initiation of treatment, the nurse discusses with the parents the need for continuous daily administration of calcium salts and vitamin D. Because vitamin D toxicity can be a serious consequence of therapy, parents are advised to watch for signs that include weakness, fatigue, lassitude, headache, nausea, vomiting, and diarrhea. Early renal impairment is manifested by polyuria, polydipsia, and nocturia.

## Hyperparathyroidism

Hyperparathyroidism is rare in childhood but can be primary or secondary. The most common cause of primary hyperparathyroidism is adenoma of the gland (Behrman, Kliegman, and Jenson, 2000). The most common causes of secondary hyperparathyroidism are chronic renal disease, renal osteodystrophy, and congenital anomalies of the urinary tract. The common factor is *hypercalcemia.* The manifestations of hyperparathyroidism are listed in Box 38-9.

## Diagnostic Evaluation

Blood studies to identify *elevated calcium* and *decreased phosphorus levels* are routinely performed. Measurement of PTH, as well as several tests to isolate the cause of the hypercalcemia, such as renal function studies, should be included. Other procedures used to substantiate the physiologic consequences of the disorder include electrocardiography and radiographic bone surveys.

## Therapeutic Management

Treatment depends on the cause of hyperparathyroidism. The treatment of primary hyperparathyroidism is surgical removal of the tumor or hyperplastic tissue. Treatment of secondary hyperparathyroidism is directed at the underlying contributing cause, which subsequently restores the serum calcium balance. However, in some instances the underlying disorder is irreversible, such as in chronic renal failure. In this instance treatment is aimed at raising serum calcium levels in order to inhibit the stimulatory effect of low levels on the parathyroids. This includes oral administration of calcium salts, high doses of vitamin D to enhance calcium absorption, a low-phosphorus diet, and administration of a phosphorus-mobilizing aluminum hydroxide to reduce phosphate absorption.

## Nursing Considerations

The initial nursing objective is recognition of the disorder. Because secondary hyperparathyroidism is a consequence of chronic renal failure, the nurse is always alert to signs that suggest this complication, especially bone pain and fractures. Because urinary symptoms are the earliest indication, assessment of other body systems for evidence of high calcium levels is indicated when polyuria and polydipsia coexist. Change in behavior, especially inactivity, unexplained gastrointestinal symptoms, and cardiac irregularities provide clues to the possibility of hyperparathyroidism.

Much of the initial nursing care is related to the physical symptoms and prevention of complications. To minimize renal calculi formation, hydration is essential. Fruit juices that maintain a low urinary pH, such as cranberry or apple juice, are encouraged, since acidity of body fluids promotes calcium absorption. All urine should be strained for evidence of renal casts.

Safety precautions, such as siderails in place at all times and assistance with ambulation, are instituted because of the tendency toward fractures and muscular weakness. Children with renal rickets (osteodystrophy) may wear braces to minimize skeletal deformities. These should be worn as prescribed. If the child is confined to bed, the nurse should consult with the physical therapist regarding proper use of orthopaedic appliances.

Vital signs should be taken frequently, and the pulse should be counted for 1 full minute to detect irregularities. A decrease in pulse rate should be reported, since it may signal severe bradycardia and cardiac arrest. The diet needs supervision to ensure compliance with low-phosphate foods,

---

> ### Box 38-9 ■ ■ □
> ### Clinical Manifestations of Hyperparathyroidism
>
> **Gastrointestinal**—Nausea, vomiting, abdominal discomfort, and constipation
> **Central nervous system**—Delusions, confusion, hallucinations, impaired memory, lack of interest and initiative, depression, and varying levels of consciousness
> **Neuromuscular**—Weakness, easy fatigability, muscle atrophy (especially proximal muscles of the lower limbs), twitching of the tongue, and paresthesias in extremities
> **Skeletal**—Vague bone pain, subperiosteal resorption of phalanges, spontaneous fractures, and absence of lamina dura around the teeth
> **Renal**—Polyuria and polydipsia, renal colic, and hypertension

particularly dairy products. The nurse should instruct parents regarding foods that need to be avoided and the necessity of administering calcium and vitamin D.

If surgery is anticipated, care is similar to that discussed for the child with hyperthyroidism. Because hypocalcemia is a potential complication, observation for signs of tetany, institution of seizure precautions, and having calcium gluconate available for emergency use are part of the nursing care.

# DISORDERS OF ADRENAL FUNCTION
## Adrenal Hormones

The adrenal glands consist of two distinct portions: the cortex, or outer section, and the medulla, or inner core. The *adrenal cortex* secretes the hormones, collectively called *steroids,* which are essential to life. The adrenal medulla produces the *catecholamines (epinephrine)* and *norepinephrine.* Because these chemicals are also produced by the sympathetic nervous system, absence of the adrenal supply is not incompatible with life.

### Adrenal Cortex

The cortex secretes three groups of hormones that are classified according to their biologic activity: (1) *glucocorticoids* (cortisol, corticosterone), (2) *mineralocorticoids* (aldosterone), and (3) *sex steroids* (androgens, estrogens, and progestins). The glucocorticoids and mineralocorticoids influence metabolic regulation and stress adaptation. The sex steroids influence sexual development but are not essential because the gonads secrete the major supply of these hormones.

**Glucocorticoids.**   The most important glucocorticoids in humans are *cortisol* and *corticosterone,* the principal effects of which are outlined in Box 38-10. Normally the hypothalamus secretes *corticotropin-releasing factor (CRF),* which causes the pituitary gland to produce *adrenocorticotropic hormone (ACTH),* which stimulates the adrenal glands to synthesize glucocorticoids (primarily cortisol). The switch that controls this feedback is cortisol. When blood levels of cortisol are low, the system turns on. When blood levels of cortisol rise, the system turns off.

In times of stress, the anterior pituitary is stimulated by CRF from the hypothalamus, which causes the release of in-

---

**Box 38-10** ■ ■ ■
**Physiologic Effects of Glucocorticoids**

Stimulation of gluconeogenesis by the liver (a hyperglycemic effect)
Increased protein catabolism with resulting reduction in protein stores (except in the liver)
Increased mobilization and utilization of fatty acids for energy
Increased storage of adipose tissue in certain sites
Decreased inflammatory and allergic actions
Regulation of fluid and electrolytes by promoting sodium retention and potassium excretion by the kidneys and by water diuresis through direct antagonistic action against antidiuretic hormone
Increased gastric acid and pepsin production
Suppression of lymphocytes, eosinophils, and basophils, but elevation of neutrophils, erythrocytes, and thrombocytes

---

**Box 38-11** ■ ■ ■
**Physiologic Effects of Catecholamine Secretion**

Increased cardiac activity
Vasoconstriction of blood vessels (elevation of blood pressure)
Increased rate and depth of respirations
Bronchial dilation
Inhibition of gastrointestinal activity
Increased muscular contraction
Pupillary dilation
Increased metabolic rate
Heightened sensory awareness
Diaphoresis

---

creased amounts of ACTH. Stressful stimuli capable of provoking this response include trauma, anesthesia, surgical intervention, sepsis, acute anoxia, hypothermia, hypoglycemia, and emotional states, especially panic, anxiety, or anger.

Secretion of the glucocorticoids is also regulated by body rhythms. Blood levels of cortisol demonstrate a typical diurnal or circadian pattern. In individuals who follow a regular routine of nighttime sleeping, cortisol levels are highest in the early morning hours after arising and lowest in the evening hours before bedtime.

**Mineralocorticoids.** The most important mineralocorticoid is *aldosterone.* Like cortisol, it promotes sodium retention and potassium excretion in the renal tubules. The effect of aldosterone is many times more potent than that of the glucocorticoids in maintaining extracellular fluid volume, acid-base balance, and normal potassium levels.

Aldosterone synthesis is regulated primarily by the renin-angiotensin system of the kidney. A block in aldosterone synthesis will cause very high plasma *renin* activity levels (Huether, 2000). The juxtaglomerular cells of the kidney respond to decreased arterial pressure or blood volume and to decreased sodium concentrations by secreting the enzyme renin into the blood. Renin in turn converts *angiotensinogen* to *angiotensin* I and then to angiotensin II. Increased levels of angiotensin stimulate the adrenal cortex to secrete aldosterone, which preserves sodium, thereby retaining water. The renin-angiotensin mechanism also results in increased blood pressure.

**Sex Steroids.** Except for the first few days of life, the sex hormones are normally secreted in only minimal amounts until adolescence, at which time they play a role in pubertal changes. Their actions are the same as those of the gonadal hormones on internal and external sexual structures and skeletal growth.

### Adrenal Medulla

The adrenal medulla secretes the catecholamines epinephrine and norepinephrine. Both hormones have essentially the same effects on different organs as those caused by direct sympathetic stimulation, except that the hormonal effects last several times longer. Their major actions are outlined in Box 38-11.

Although the catecholamines evoke similar responses from target sites, there are some important differences. Epinephrine has a greater effect on cardiac activity than norepinephrine, but it causes only weak constriction of the blood vessels of muscles in comparison with the effect of norepinephrine. As a result, norepinephrine elevates blood pressure, whereas epinephrine increases cardiac output. Another important difference is their effect on metabolism. Epinephrine increases the metabolic rate to a much greater extent than norepinephrine. These differences in action have been attributed to the catecholamines' effects on α- or β-adrenergic receptors. Supposedly norepinephrine can only affect those effector cells that contain alpha receptors, which are mostly excitatory (constriction and contraction). Epinephrine, however, can affect both alpha and beta receptors, and beta receptors are mostly inhibitory (dilation and relaxation).

Control of secretion of catecholamines, primarily in response to physiologic or emotional stress, is through the hypothalamus. Also, stimulation of the sympathetic nervous system results in the release of epinephrine and norepinephrine from the sympathetic nerves and adrenal medulla. Both systems support each other, and one can be substituted for the other. For this reason there is no condition attributable to hypofunction of the adrenal medulla. Even in bilateral adrenalectomy, catecholamine replacement is not necessary, because the sympathetic release of these chemicals is sufficient to meet all of the physiologic functions required to cope with stressful events.

Catecholamine-secreting tumors are the primary cause of adrenal medullary hyperfunction. In children the most common neoplasms of this type are pheochromocytoma (see p. 1731), neuroblastoma, and ganglioneuroma. Ganglioneuromas are thought to be neuroblastomas that have undergone maturation into a benign tumor composed of ganglion cells. These tumors are associated with less abnormal catecholamine secretion than the other two types, but persons with ganglioneuromas may have a clinical picture of chronic diarrhea, failure to thrive, skin rash, hypokalemia, persistent cough, and abdominal distention. The exact reason for these symptoms is unknown, although they are attributable to the tumor because they disappear after surgical removal of the mass.

# Acute Adrenocortical Insufficiency

The acute form of adrenocortical insufficiency (*adrenal crisis*) may result from a number of causes during childhood. Although a rare disorder, some of the more common etiologic factors include hemorrhage into the gland from trauma, which may be caused by a prolonged, difficult labor; fulminating infections, such as meningococcemia, which result in hemorrhage and necrosis (Waterhouse-Friderichsen syndrome); abrupt withdrawal of exogenous sources of cortisone or failure to increase exogenous supplies during stress; or as a result of congenital adrenogenital hyperplasia of the salt-losing type.

## Clinical Manifestations

Early symptoms of adrenocortical insufficiency include increased irritability, headache, diffuse abdominal pain, weakness, nausea and vomiting, and diarrhea. Generalized hemorrhagic manifestations are present in the *Waterhouse-Friderichsen syndrome.* Fever increases as the condition worsens and is accompanied by signs of CNS involvement, such as nuchal rigidity, convulsions, stupor, and coma. The child is in a shocklike state with a weak, rapid pulse, decreased blood pressure, shallow respirations, cold clammy skin, and cyanosis. Circulatory collapse is the terminal event.

In the newborn, adrenal crisis is accompanied by extreme hyperpyrexia (high temperature), tachypnea, cyanosis, and seizures. Usually there is no evidence of infection or purpura. However, hemorrhage into the adrenal gland may be evident as a palpable retroperitoneal mass.

## Diagnostic Evaluation

There is no rapid, definitive test for confirmation of acute adrenocortical insufficiency. Routine procedures such as measurement of plasma cortisol levels are too time-consuming to be practical. Therefore diagnosis is usually made based on clinical presentation, especially when a fulminating sepsis is accompanied by hemorrhagic manifestations and signs of circulatory collapse despite adequate antibiotic therapy. Because there is no real danger in administering a cortisol preparation for a short period, treatment should be instituted immediately. Improvement with cortisol therapy confirms the diagnosis.

## Therapeutic Management

Treatment involves replacement of cortisol, replacement of body fluids to combat dehydration and hypovolemia, administration of glucose solutions to correct hypoglycemia, and specific antibiotic therapy in the presence of infection. Initially IV hydrocortisone (Solu-Cortef) is administered. Normal saline containing 5% glucose is given parenterally to replace lost fluid, electrolytes, and glucose. If hemorrhage has been severe, whole blood may be replaced. In the event that these measures do not reverse the circulatory collapse, vasopressors are used for immediate vasoconstriction and elevation of blood pressure.

Once the child's condition is stabilized, oral doses of cortisone, fluids, and salt are given, similar to the regimen used for chronic adrenal insufficiency. To maintain sodium retention, aldosterone is replaced by synthetic salt-retaining steroids.

## Nursing Considerations

Because of the abrupt onset and potentially fatal outcome of this condition, prompt recognition is essential. Vital signs and blood pressure are taken every 15 minutes to monitor the hyperpyrexia and shocklike state. Seizure precautions are instituted, because convulsions from the elevated temperature are not uncommon. As soon as therapy is instituted, the nurse should monitor the child's response to fluid and cortisol replacement. Too rapid administration of fluids can precipitate cardiac failure, whereas overdosage with cortisol produces hypotension and a sudden fall in temperature.

An ascending flaccid paralysis may occur on the second to third day of treatment because of an abnormally low serum potassium level that results from overtreatment with cortisol and sodium chloride. The nurse should regulate IV infusions carefully to guard against too rapid administration of drugs. Intake and urinary output are recorded.

Once the acute phase is over and the hypovolemia is corrected, the child is given oral fluids, such as small quantities of ginger ale, fruit juice, or salted broth. Too rapid ingestion of oral fluids may induce vomiting, which increases dehydration. Therefore the nurse should plan a gradual schedule for reintroducing liquids. For children who refuse to drink, the prospect of having the IV infusion removed once oral fluids are increased is often a motivating factor.

> **NURSING ALERT**   Monitor serum electrolyte levels and observe for signs of hypokalemia or hyperkalemia (e.g., weakness, poor muscle control, paralysis, cardiac dysrhythmias, and apnea). The condition is rapidly corrected with IV or oral potassium replacement.

> **NURSING TIP**   When an oral potassium preparation is given, it should be mixed with a small amount of strongly flavored fruit juice to disguise its bitter taste.

The sudden, severe nature of this disorder necessitates a great deal of emotional support for the child and family. The child may be placed in an intensive care unit where the surroundings are strange and frightening. Despite the need for emergency intervention, the nurse must be sensitive to the family's psychologic needs and prepare them for each procedure, even if this is as brief as a statement such as "The intravenous infusion is necessary to replace fluid that the child is losing." Because recovery within 24 hours is often dramatic, the nurse should keep the parents apprised of the child's condition, emphasizing signs of improvement, such as a lowered temperature and elevated blood pressure. If paralysis occurs, the nurse should assure them that this condition is temporary and quickly reversed.

If treatment needs to be continued past the acute stage, parents require the same preparation as in the case of children with chronic adrenal insufficiency. Preparation for discharge should begin as soon as possible after the child's condition has stabilized.

# Chronic Adrenocortical Insufficiency (Addison Disease)

Chronic adrenocortical insufficiency is rare in children. When it does occur, it is usually caused by a destructive lesion of the adrenal gland or neoplasms, or the cause is idiopathic. At one time, generalized tuberculosis was the leading cause of adrenal gland destruction.

Evidence of this disorder is usually gradual in onset, because 90% of adrenal tissue must be nonfunctional before signs of insufficiency are manifested. However, during periods of stress, when demands for additional cortisol are increased, symptoms of acute insufficiency may appear in a previously well child (Table 38-2).

Definitive diagnosis is based on measurements of functional cortisol reserve. The cortisol and urinary 17-hydroxy-corticosteroid levels are low and fail to rise while plasma ACTH levels are elevated with corticotropin (ACTH) stimulation, the definitive test for the disease.

## Therapeutic Management

Treatment involves replacement of glucocorticoids (cortisol) and mineralocorticoids (aldosterone). Some children are able to be maintained solely on oral supplements of cortisol (cortisone or hydrocortisone preparations) with a liberal intake of salt. During stressful situations, such as fever, infection, emotional upset, or surgery, the dosage must be tripled to accommodate the body's increased need for glu-

cocorticoids. Failure to meet this requirement will precipitate an acute crisis. Overdosage produces appearance of cushingoid signs (Fig. 38-4).

Children with more severe states of chronic adrenal insufficiency require mineralocorticoid replacement to maintain fluid and electrolyte balance. Other forms of therapy include monthly injections of desoxycorticosterone acetate or implantation of desoxycorticosterone acetate pellets subcutaneously every 9 to 12 months.

## Nursing Considerations

Once the disorder is diagnosed, parents need guidance concerning drug therapy. They must be aware of the continuous need for cortisol replacement. Sudden termination of the drug because of inadequate supplies or inability to ingest the oral form because of vomiting places the child in danger of an acute adrenal crisis. Therefore parents should always have a spare supply of the medication in the home. Ideally they will have a prefilled syringe of hydrocortisone in the home and be instructed in proper technique for intramuscular administration of the drug in case of crisis.* As mentioned earlier, unnecessary administration of cortisone will not harm the child but, if needed, may be lifesaving. Any evidence of acute insufficiency should be reported to the practitioner immediately.

Parents also need to be aware of side effects of the drugs. Undesirable side effects of cortisone include gastric irritation, which is minimized by ingestion with food or the use of an antacid; increased excitability and sleeplessness; weight gain that may require dietary management to prevent obesity; and, rarely, behavioral changes, including depression or euphoria. Parents should be aware of signs of overdose and report these to the practitioner. In addition, the drug has a very bitter taste, which creates a challenge for nurses and parents in its administration.

**NURSING TIP** Taste a drop of the different preparations of cortisone because some are less bitter than others. Although using the concentrated form means a smaller volume of liquid to ingest, this form is also the most bitter.

The side effects of mineralocorticoids are primarily caused by overdosage and include generalized edema, which is first noticed around the eyes; hypertension, which may cause headaches; cardiac arrhythmias; and signs of hypokalemia. The child should be evaluated periodically for evidence of excessive medication. Emphasizing the importance of routine follow-up care is a significant nursing responsibility.

Because the body cannot supply endogenous sources of cortical hormones during times of stress, the home environment should be stable and relatively unstressful. Parents need to be aware that during periods of emotional or physical crisis the child requires additional hormone replacement. The child should wear medical identification, such as a bracelet, to permit medical personnel to adjust requirements during emergency care.

| TABLE 38-2 | Clinical manifestations of adrenocortical insufficiency |
|---|---|
| **Signs and Symptoms** | **Clinical Manifestations** |
| **Glucocorticoid** | |
| Fasting hypoglycemia | Headache, diaphoresis, weakness, trembling, hunger, seizures (rare) |
| Decreased gastric acidity | Anorexia, nausea, vomiting |
| Fatigue | Increased sleeping, listlessness |
| Psychologic symptoms | Irritability, apathy, negativism |
| **Mineralocorticoid** | |
| Muscle weakness | Generalized weakness that is aggravated by slight additional exertion or minor illness |
| Weight loss | Dehydration and anorexia |
| Fatigue | Increased sleeping, listlessness |
| Gastrointestinal symptoms | Nausea, vomiting, anorexia |
| Nutritional symptoms | Salt craving |
| Circulatory | Hypotension, small heart size, syncope (fainting), dizziness |
| Electrolyte imbalances | Hyperkalemia, hyponatremia, acidosis |
| Psychologic symptoms | Irritability, apathy, negativism |
| **Androgen Deficiency (Older Children and Adults)** | |
| Integumentary changes | Decreased pubic and axillary hair |
| Psychologic symptoms | Decreased libido |
| **Increased ACTH and β-Lipotropin** | |
| Dermatologic changes | Hyperpigmentation (elbow, knees, waist), pigmentary changes of previous scars, palmar creases |

---

*Home care instructions on giving subcutaneous injections are available in Wong DL, Hess CS: *Wong and Whaley's clinical manual of pediatric nursing*, ed 5, St Louis, 2000, Mosby.

# Cushing Syndrome

Cushing syndrome is a characteristic group of manifestations caused by excessive circulating free cortisol. It can result from a variety of etiologies, which generally fall into one of five categories (Box 38-12).

Cushing syndrome is uncommon in children. When seen, it is often caused by excessive or prolonged steroid therapy that produces a cushingoid appearance (Fig. 38-4). This condition is reversible once the steroids are gradually discontinued. Abrupt withdrawal will precipitate acute adrenal insufficiency. Gradual withdrawal of exogenous supplies is necessary to allow the anterior pituitary an opportunity to secrete increasing amounts of ACTH to stimulate the adrenals to produce cortisol.

## Clinical Manifestations

Because the actions of cortisol are widespread, clinical manifestations are equally profound and diverse (Table 38-3). Those symptoms that produce changes in physical appearance occur early in the disorder and are of considerable concern to school-age and older children (Fig. 38-5). The physiologic disturbances, such as hyperglycemia, susceptibility to infection, hypertension, and hypokalemia, may have life-threatening consequences unless recognized early and treated successfully. Children with short stature may be responding to increased cortisol levels, resulting in Cushing syndrome. Cortisol inhibits the action of GH.

---

**Box 38-12 ■ ■ □**
**Etiology of Cushing Syndrome**

**Pituitary**—Cushing syndrome with adrenal hyperplasia, usually attributed to an excess of ACTH
**Adrenal**—Cushing syndrome with hypersecretion of glucocorticoids, generally the result of adrenocortical neoplasms
**Ectopic**—Cushing syndrome with autonomous secretion of ACTH, most often caused by extrapituitary neoplasms
**Iatrogenic**—Cushing syndrome, frequently the result of administration of large amounts of exogenous corticosteroids
**Food dependent**—Inappropriate sensitivity of adrenal glands to normal postprandial increases in secretion of gastric inhibitory polypeptide.

---

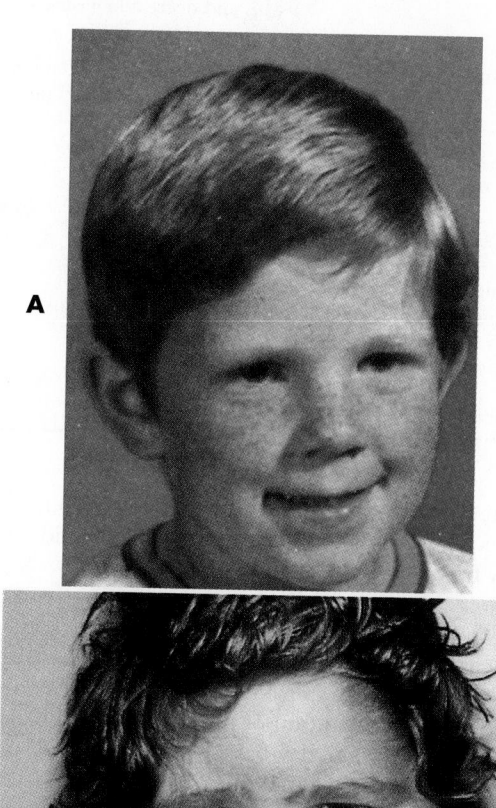
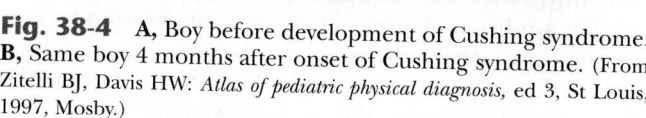

**Fig. 38-4    A,** Boy before development of Cushing syndrome. **B,** Same boy 4 months after onset of Cushing syndrome. (From Zitelli BJ, Davis HW: *Atlas of pediatric physical diagnosis,* ed 3, St Louis, 1997, Mosby.)

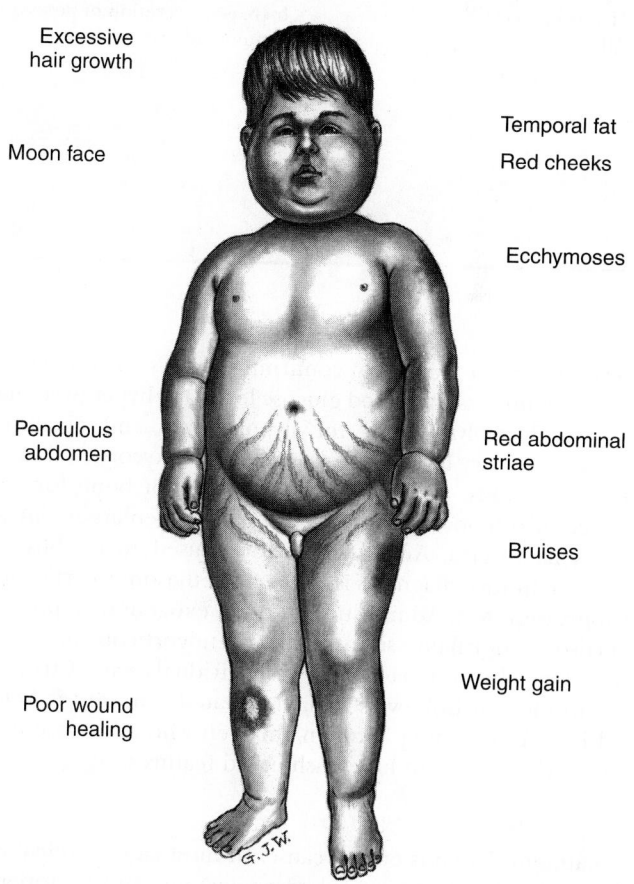

Excessive hair growth
Moon face
Temporal fat
Red cheeks
Ecchymoses
Pendulous abdomen
Red abdominal striae
Bruises
Poor wound healing
Weight gain

**Fig. 38-5    Characteristics of Cushing syndrome.**

**TABLE 38-3** Clinical manifestations of Cushing syndrome

| Signs/Symptoms | Physiologic Cause | Signs/Symptoms | Physiologic Cause |
|---|---|---|---|
| Centripetal fat distribution<br>  Truncal obesity<br>  Supraclavicular fat pads<br>  Fat pads on neck and back ("Buffalo hump")<br>Rounded or "moon" face | Increased appetite and deposition of fat | Osteoporosis<br>  Compression fractures of vertebrae<br>  Kyphosis<br>  Backache<br>  Retarded linear growth (short stature)<br>  Delayed bone age | Increased glomerular filtration rate and excretion of calcium and decreased absorption of calcium from intestinal tract<br>Increased levels of cortisol interfere with the action of GH |
| Muscular wasting<br>  Thin extremities<br>  Pendulous abdomen<br>  Muscle weakness<br>Thin skin and subcutaneous tissue<br>Poor wound healing | Increased protein catabolism resulting in negative nitrogen balance | Hypercalciuria—renal calculi | Excessive amount of calcium in urine |
| | | Psychoses<br>  Irritability<br>  Insomnia<br>  Euphoria<br>  Depression<br>  Frank psychoses | Cause unknown |
| Increased frequency of infection<br>Decreased inflammatory response | Decreased production and circulating levels of antibodies by lysis of fixed plasma cells and lymphocytes | | |
| Excessive bruising<br>Petechial hemorrhages | Capillary weakness resulting from loss of protein | Peptic ulcer | Increased production of hydrochloric acid and pepsin and decreased gastric mucus production |
| Facial plethora ("red cheeks")<br>Reddish purple abdominal striae | Thin skin that allows capillary blood to be visible, increased color from polycythemia | Hyperglycemia<br>  Glycosuria | Increased gluconeogenesis by liver and decreased rate of glucose utilization by cells |
| Hypertension—arteriosclerosis | Increased salt and water retention (hypervolemia) | Latent or overt diabetes | Overstimulation of islets of Langerhans |
| Hypokalemia<br>Alkalosis | Increased excretion of potassium and hydrogen ions | Virilization<br>  Hirsutism (excessive body hair)<br>  Acne<br>  Deepening of voice<br>  Clitoral enlargement<br>  Tendency toward male physique in female<br>  Amenorrhea<br>  Impotence | Excess production of androgens |

## Diagnostic Evaluation

Several tests are helpful in confirming excess cortisol levels. They include fasting blood glucose levels for hyperglycemia, serum electrolyte levels for hypokalemia and alkalosis, 24-hour urinary levels of elevated 17-hydroxycorticoids and 17-ketosteroids, and radiographic studies of bone for evidence of osteoporosis and of the skull for enlargement of the sella turcica. Another procedure used to establish a more definitive diagnosis is the dexamethasone (cortisone) suppression test. Administration of an exogenous supply of cortisone normally suppresses adrenocorticotropic hormone production. However, in individuals with Cushing syndrome, cortisol levels remain elevated. This test is helpful in differentiating between children who are obese and those who appear to have cushingoid features.

## Therapeutic Management

Treatment depends on the cause. In most cases surgical intervention involves bilateral adrenalectomy and postoperative replacement of the cortical hormones (the therapy for this is the same as that outlined for chronic adrenal insufficiency). If a pituitary tumor is found, surgical extirpation or irradiation may be chosen. In either of these instances, treatment of panhypopituitarism with replacement of GH, thyroid extract, ADH, gonadotropins, and steroids may be necessary for an indefinite period.

## Nursing Considerations

Nursing care also depends on the cause. When cushingoid features are caused by steroid therapy, the effects may be lessened with administration of the drug early in the morning and on an alternate-day basis. Giving the drug early in the day maintains the normal diurnal pattern of cortisol secretion. If given during the evening, it is more likely to produce symptoms because endogenous cortisol levels are already low and the additional supply exerts more pronounced effects. An alternate-day schedule allows the anterior pituitary an opportunity to maintain more normal hypothalamic-pituitary-adrenal control mechanisms.

If an organic cause is found, nursing care is related to the treatment regimen. Although a bilateral adrenalectomy permanently solves one condition, it reciprocally produces another syndrome. Before surgery, parents need to be adequately informed of the operative benefits and disadvantages. Postoperative teaching regarding drug replacement is the same as discussed in the previous section.

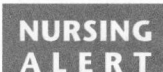 **NURSING ALERT** Postoperative complications of adrenalectomy are related to the sudden withdrawal of cortisol. Observe for shocklike symptoms (e.g., hypotension, hyperpyrexia).

Anorexia and nausea and vomiting are very common and may be improved with the use of nasogastric decompression. Muscle and joint pain may be severe, requiring use of analgesics. The psychologic depression can be profound and may not improve for months. Parents should be aware of the physiologic reasons behind these symptoms in order to be supportive of the child.

## Congenital Adrenal Hyperplasia (CAH)

CAH is a family of disorders caused by decreased enzyme activity required for cortisol production in the adrenal cortex. The most common defect is 21-hydroxylase deficiency, which constitutes more than 90% of all cases of CAH (AAP, 2000; Levine, 2000). This deficiency occurs in approximately 1 per 12,000 to 1 per 15,000 births and causes overproduction of the adrenal androgens, resulting in virilization of the female fetus.

### Pathophysiology

Interference in the biosynthesis of cortisol during fetal life results in an increased production of ACTH, which stimulates hyperplasia of the adrenal gland. Depending on the enzymatic defect, increased quantities of cortisol precursors and androgens are secreted. There are six major types of biochemical defects. The most common is partial or complete *21-hydroxylase deficiency*. With partial deficiency, enough aldosterone is produced to preserve sodium, and adequate cortisol is produced to prevent signs of adrenocortical insufficiency.

In the complete or salt-losing form, insufficient amounts of aldosterone and cortisol are produced. If salt-losing CAH is not diagnosed and treated at birth, infants will exhibit symptoms of failure to thrive, weakness, vomiting, and dehydration, and a salt-losing crisis will ensue (Behrman, Kliegman, and Jenson, 2000). In *11-hydroxylase deficiency* there is an increase in the mineralocorticoid 11-desoxycorticosterone, which leads to hypertension. In each of these types there is excess production of androgens, which causes ambiguous female genitalia in females and precocious genital development in males. Other forms of CAH do not result in excess production of androgens but cause various degrees of hypoaldosteronism or hyperaldosteronism.

### Clinical Manifestations

Excessive androgens cause masculinization of the urogenital system at approximately the tenth week of fetal development. The most pronounced abnormalities occur in the female, who is born with varying degrees of ambiguous genitalia. Masculinization of external genitalia causes the clitoris to enlarge so that it appears as a small phallus. Fusion of the labia produces a saclike structure resembling the scrotum without testes. However, no abnormal changes occur in the internal sexual organs, although the vaginal orifice is usually closed by the fused labia. (See also Abnormal Sexual Development, Chapter 11.) The label *ambiguous genitalia* should be applied to any infant with hypospadias or micropenis and no palpable gonads, and a diagnostic evaluation for CAH should be contemplated. Males do not display genital abnormalities at birth (New, Ghizzoni, and Speiser, 1996).

Increased pigmentation of skin creases and genitalia caused by increased ACTH may be a subtle sign of adrenal insufficiency. A salt-wasting crisis frequently occurs, usually within the first few weeks of life (Behrman, Kliegman, and Jenson, 2000). Infants fail to gain weight, and hyponatremia and hyperkalemia may be significant. Cardiac arrest can occur.

Untreated CAH results in early sexual maturation, with enlargement of the external sexual organs; development of axillary, pubic, and facial hair; deepening of the voice; acne; and marked increase in musculature with changes toward an adult male physique. However, in contrast to precocious puberty, breasts do not develop in the female, and she remains amenorrheic and infertile. In the male the testes remain small, and spermatogenesis does not occur. In both sexes linear growth is accelerated, and epiphyseal closure is premature, resulting in short stature by the end of puberty.

### Diagnostic Evaluation

Clinical diagnosis is initially based on congenital abnormalities that lead to difficulty in assigning sex to the newborn and on signs and symptoms of adrenal insufficiency or hypertension. Definitive diagnosis is confirmed by evidence of increased 17-ketosteroid levels in most types of CAH (Levine, 2000). Usually the level of 17-hydroxycorticoids is low or near normal. In complete 21-hydroxylase deficiency, blood electrolytes demonstrate loss of sodium and chloride and elevation of potassium. In older children bone age is advanced, and linear growth is increased. Chromosome typing for positive sex determination and to rule out any other genetic abnormality (e.g., Turner syndrome) is always done in any case of ambiguous genitalia.

Another test that can be used to visualize the presence of pelvic structures is ultrasonography, a noninvasive, painless imaging technique that does not require anesthesia or sedation. It is especially useful in CAH because it readily identifies the absence or presence of female reproductive organs in a newborn or child with ambiguous genitalia. Because ultrasonography yields immediate results, it has the advantage of determining the child's gender long before the more complex laboratory results for chromosome analysis or steroid levels are available.

### Therapeutic Management

The initial medical objective is to confirm the diagnosis and assign a sex to the child, usually according to the genotype. In both sexes cortisone is administered to suppress the abnormally high secretions of ACTH. If cortisone is begun early enough, it is very effective. Cortisone depresses the secretion of ACTH by the adenohypophysis, which in turn inhibits the secretion of adrenocorticosteroids, which stems the progressive virilization. The signs and symptoms of masculinization in the female gradually disappear, and excessive early linear growth is slowed. Puberty occurs normally at the appropriate age.

The recommended oral dosage is divided to simulate the normal diurnal pattern of ACTH secretion. Because these children are unable to produce cortisol in response to stress, it is necessary to increase the dosage during episodes of infection, fever, or other stresses. Acute emergencies require immediate IV or intramuscular administration. Emergency situations include bacterial and viral infections, vomiting, surgery, fractures, major injuries, and sometimes insect stings.

Children with the salt-losing type of CAH require aldosterone replacement, as outlined under chronic adrenal insufficiency, and supplementary dietary salt. Frequent laboratory tests are conducted to assess the effects on electrolytes, hormonal profiles, and renin levels. The frequency of testing is individualized to the child.

Depending on the degree of masculinization in the female, reconstructive surgery may be required to reduce the size of the clitoris, separate the labia, and create a vaginal orifice. Surgery is performed when the infant is physically able to withstand the procedure but before she is old enough to be aware of the abnormal genitalia. Plastic surgery is generally done in stages and yields excellent cosmetic results. Reports concerning sexual satisfaction after partial clitoridectomy indicate that the capacity for orgasm and sexual gratification is not necessarily impaired.

Unfortunately, not all children with CAH are diagnosed at birth and raised in accordance with their genetic sex. Particularly in the case of affected females, masculinization of the external genitalia may have led to sex assignment as a male. In males, diagnosis is usually delayed until early childhood, when signs of virilism appear. In these situations it is advisable to continue rearing the child as a male in accordance with assigned sex and phenotype. Hormonal replacement may be required to permit linear growth and to initiate male pubertal changes. Surgery is usually indicated to remove the female organs and reconstruct the phallus for satisfactory sexual relations. These individuals are not fertile.

## Nursing Considerations

Of major importance is recognition of ambiguous genitalia in newborns. If there is any question regarding assignment of sex, the parents need to be told immediately to prevent the embarrassing situation of informing family members of the child's sex and then having to change the announcement. As with any congenital defect, the parents require an adequate explanation of the condition and a period of time to grieve for the loss of perfection. In this instance they may also need to grieve for the loss of the desired-sex child. For example, the birth of a phenotypically male infant may fulfill their wish for a son. Knowledge of the child's actual sex may leave them disappointed. Such situations may also lead them to discuss the possibility of raising the child as a male despite the actual sex. This is a difficult question that requires thoughtful discussion among the parents and members of the health team.

In general, rearing the genetically female child as a female is preferred because of the success of surgical intervention and the satisfactory results with hormones in reversing virilism and providing a prospect of normal puberty and the ability to conceive. This is in contrast to the choice of rearing the child as a male, in which case the child is sterile and may never be able to function satisfactorily in heterosexual relationships. If the parents persist in their decision to assign a male sex to a genetically female child, a psychologic consultation should be requested to explore their motivations and ensure their understanding of the future consequences for the child.

Parents need an explanation regarding this disorder that facilitates their explaining it to others. Before confirmation of the diagnosis and sex of the child, the nurse should refer to the infant as "child" or "baby" rather than "he" or "she" and definitely not "it." When referring to the external genitalia, it is preferable to refer to them as sex organs and to emphasize the similarity between the penis/clitoris and scrotum/labia during fetal development. It can be explained that the sex organs were overdeveloped because of too much male hormone secretion. Using a correct vocabulary allows parents to explain the abnormalities to others in a straightforward manner, just as if the defect involved the heart or an extremity.

Parents often fear that the infant will retain "male behavioral characteristics" because of prenatal masculinization and will not be able to develop female characteristics. It is also important to stress that sex assignment and rearing depend on psychosocial influences, not on genetic sex hormone influences during fetal life. Because the prognosis for normal sexual development is excellent after early treatment, the nurse should foster identification with the child as one sex only. Ambiguous genitalia have no relationship with sexual preference for partners later in life.

As soon as the sex is determined, parents should be informed of the findings and encouraged to choose an appropriate name, and the child should be identified as a male or female, with no reference to ambiguous sex. If the appearance of the enlarged genitalia in a female child concerns the parents, they should be encouraged to discuss their feelings. Suggesting ways to avoid questioning remarks from visitors, such as diapering the child in a separate room, is also helpful. If surgery is anticipated, showing parents before-and-after photographs of reconstruction helps to reinforce the expected cosmetic benefits.

Nursing considerations regarding cortisol and aldosterone replacement are the same as those discussed for chronic adrenocortical insufficiency. However, because parents may be overwhelmed with the diagnosis and obvious abnormalities at the time of birth, they may not hear all of the discharge instructions regarding the medication schedule. A follow-up visit by a public health nurse may be desirable to ensure that parents understand and comply with the treatment regimen. Likewise, nurses in well-child facilities should assume responsibility for guidance and supervision regarding this aspect of care during each visit.

Because infants are especially prone to dehydration and salt-losing crises, parents need to be aware of signs of dehydration and the urgency of immediate medical intervention to stabilize the child's condition. Parents should have injectable hydrocortisone available and know how to prepare and administer the intramuscular injection. Parents, and later the child, need to understand that the medical regimen must be a lifelong commitment; therefore, they should be provided with the education and counseling that is most likely to ensure informed and willing compliance. They also need to know that growth retardation that may have occurred before therapy cannot be overcome and that normal stature is not a realistic expectation, even though growth velocity may improve with medication. The parents are also taught to give necessary injections.* (See Chapter 27.)

In the unfortunate situation in which the sex is erroneously assigned and the correct sex determined later, parents need a great deal of help in understanding the reason for the incorrect sex identification and the options for sex reassignment or medical/surgical intervention. Because children become aware of their sexual identity by 18 months to 2 years of age, it is believed that any reassignment after this period can cause tremendous psychologic conflicts in the child. Therefore sex rearing should be continued as previously established with medical/surgical intervention as required.

> **NURSING ALERT**
>
> The parents should be advised that there is no physical harm in treating for suspected adrenal insufficiency that is not present, whereas the consequence of not treating acute adrenal insufficiency can be fatal (Ruble, 1996).

A dilemma often arises, however, regarding what these children should know about their condition, especially gender identification. Because the knowledge that one has been reared opposite to the genetic gender can initiate profound psychologic problems, it is recommended that children not be told this fact but rather be given an explanation regarding their physical disabilities, such as infertility, and the need for hormone replacement and plastic surgery. Parents, in turn, must believe that these children have been raised according to their "true sex," which is absolutely honest, because sex is not solely a biologic entity but an expression of multiple environmental influences.

Because the hereditary form of adrenal hyperplasia is an autosomal recessive disorder, parents should be referred for genetic counseling before conceiving another child. The nurse's role is to ensure that parents understand the probability of transmitting the trait or disorder with each pregnancy. Affected offspring also require genetic counseling because both sexes are generally able to reproduce. (See Chapter 5 for recurrence risks and genetic counseling.)

## Hyperaldosteronism

Excessive secretion of aldosterone may be caused by an adrenal tumor or, in some types of adrenal-genital syndromes, may be a result of enzymatic deficiency. The signs and symptoms are caused by increased sodium levels, water retention, and potassium loss. Hypervolemia causes hypertension and resultant headaches. Paradoxically, funduscopic changes resulting from increased blood pressure and edema from water retention are minimal. Hypokalemia results in muscular weakness, paresthesia, episodes of paralysis, and tetany and may be responsible for polyuria and consequent polydipsia.

The clinical diagnosis is suspected when there are findings of hypertension, hypokalemia, and polyuria that fail to respond to ADH administration. Renin and angiotensin titers are abnormally low. Urinary levels of 17-hydroxycorticosteroids and 17-ketosteroids are normal in primary hyperaldosteronism caused by an aldosterone-secreting tumor but are usually abnormal in adrenogenital syndrome.

### Therapeutic Management

Temporary treatment of the disorder involves replacement of potassium and administration of spironolactone (Aldactone), a diuretic that blocks the effects of aldosterone, thereby promoting excretion of sodium and water while preserving potassium. Definitive treatment is similar to that for chronic adrenocortical insufficiency.

### Nursing Considerations

An important nursing consideration is recognition of the syndrome, particularly in children who demonstrate high blood pressure. Other clues include bed-wetting, excessive thirst, and unexplained weakness. After the diagnosis, nursing care should be related to the treatment regimen. If diuretics are used, they should be administered in the morning to avoid accidents during the night. Children need unrestricted restroom privileges at school. Potassium supplements should be mixed with fruit juice such as grape juice to increase their acceptability, and potassium-rich foods should be encouraged. Parents need to be aware of the signs of hypokalemia and hyperkalemia.

After an adrenalectomy, nursing care is similar to that for chronic adrenocortical insufficiency.

## Pheochromocytoma

Pheochromocytoma is a rare tumor characterized by secretion of catecholamines. The tumor most commonly arises from the chromaffin cells of the adrenal medulla but may occur wherever these cells are found, such as along the paraganglia of the aorta or thoracolumbar sympathetic chain. Approximately 10% of these tumors are located in extraadrenal sites. In children they are frequently bilateral or multiple and are generally benign. Often there is a familial transmission of the condition as an autosomal dominant trait (Behrman, Kliegman, and Jenson, 2000).

### Clinical Manifestations

The clinical manifestations of pheochromocytoma are caused by an increased production of catecholamines, producing hypertension, tachycardia, headache, decreased gastrointestinal activity with resultant constipation, increased metabolism with anorexia, weight loss, hyperglycemia, polyuria, polydipsia, hyperventilation, nervousness, heat in-

---

*Home care instructions are available in Wong DL, Hess CS: *Wong and Whaley's clinical manual of pediatric nursing*, ed 5, St Louis, 2000, Mosby.

tolerance, and diaphoresis. In severe cases, signs of congestive heart failure are evident.

### Diagnostic Evaluation

The clinical manifestations mimic those of other disorders, such as hyperthyroidism or diabetes mellitus. Tests specific to these conditions may be performed as part of the differential diagnosis. In a small number of instances a palpable tumor suggests the diagnosis. Usually the tumor is identified by a CT scan or MRI. Definitive tests include 24-hour measurement of urinary levels of the catecholamine metabolites; histamine stimulation, which will provoke a hypertensive attack from sudden release of large amounts of catecholamines; and alpha-blocking agents, which will produce a hypotensive episode by inhibiting the action of circulating catecholamines.

### Therapeutic Management

Definitive treatment consists of surgical removal of the tumor. In children the tumors may be bilateral, requiring a bilateral adrenalectomy and lifelong glucocorticoid and mineralocorticoid therapy. The major complications that can occur during surgery are severe hypertension, tachyarrhythmias, and hypotension. The first two are caused by excessive release of catecholamines during manipulation of the tumor, and the latter results from catecholamine withdrawal and hypovolemic shock.

Preoperative medication to inhibit the effects of catecholamines is begun 1 to 3 weeks before surgery to prevent these complications. The major group of drugs used is the α-adrenergic blocking agents with or without β-adrenergic blocking agents. The most commonly used α-adrenergic blocker is phenoxybenzamine (Dibenzyline), a longer-acting medication given orally every 12 hours. The shorter-acting phentolamine (Regitine) is equally effective but less satisfactory for long-term use, although it is useful for acute hypertension. To control catecholamine release when α-adrenergic blocking agents are inadequate, the child is given β-adrenergic blocking agents.

Success of therapy is judged by lowering of blood pressure to normal, absence of hypertensive attacks (flushing or blanching, fainting, headache, palpitations, tachycardia, nausea and vomiting, profuse sweating), heat tolerance, decrease in perspiration, and disappearance of hyperglycemia. A disadvantage of these drugs is their inability to block the effects of catecholamines on beta receptors.

### Nursing Considerations

An initial nursing objective is identification of children with this disorder. Outstanding clues are hypertension and hypertensive attacks. Because of behavioral changes (nervousness, excitability, overactivity, even psychosis), increased cardiac and respiratory activity may appear to be related to an acute anxiety attack. Therefore a careful history of the onset of symptoms and association with stressful events is helpful in distinguishing between an organic and a psychologic cause for the symptoms.

Preoperative nursing care involves frequent monitoring of vital signs and observing for evidence of hypertensive attacks and congestive heart failure. Therapeutic effects are evidenced by normal vital signs and absence of glycosuria. Daily blood glucose levels, urine acetone, and any signs of hyperglycemia are noted and reported immediately.

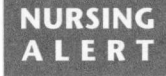 **NURSING ALERT** Do not palpate the mass. Preoperative palpation of the mass releases catecholamines, which can stimulate severe hypertension and tachyarrhythmias.

The environment is made conducive to rest and free of emotional stress. This requires adequate preparation during hospital admission and before surgery. Parents are encouraged to room-in with their child and to participate in the care. Play activities need to be tailored to the child's energy level but not be overly strenuous or challenging because these can increase metabolic rate and promote frustration and anxiety.

After surgery the child is observed for signs of shock from removal of excess catecholamines. If a bilateral adrenalectomy was performed, the nursing interventions are those discussed for chronic adrenocortical insufficiency.

## DISORDERS OF PANCREATIC HORMONE SECRETION*
### Diabetes Mellitus (DM)

DM is a chronic disorder of metabolism characterized by a partial or complete deficiency of the hormone *insulin.* It is the most common metabolic disease, resulting in metabolic adjustment or physiologic change in almost all areas of the body. DM affects approximately 15.7 million persons in the United States, and, although estimates of prevalence in the United States vary, most sources estimate a rate of 20 per 100,000 children and adolescents (LaPorte, Matsushima, and Chang, 1995). DM in children can occur at any age but has a peak incidence between ages 10 and 15 years, with 75% diagnosed before 18 years of age. The incidence in boys is slightly higher than in girls (1:1 to 1.2:1).

Type 1 DM is more prominent in whites, with an incidence of 20 per 100,000; the incidence in African-Americans is 11 per 100,000; the incidence in Hispanics is 15.2 per 100,000; and the incidence in Cubans is 2.6 per 100,000. Native Americans tend to develop type 2 DM rather than type 1 DM even when diagnosed in childhood. The Pima Tribe reports a 55+% incidence of type 2 DM.

### Classification

Traditionally DM had been classified according to the type of treatment needed. The old categories were insulin-dependent diabetes mellitus (IDDM), or type I; and non–insulin-dependent diabetes mellitus (NIDDM), or type II. In 1997 these terms were eliminated because treatment can vary (some people with NIDDM require insulin) and because the terms do not indicate the underlying problem. The new terms are type 1 and type 2, using Arabic symbols to avoid confusion (e.g., type II could be read as type eleven) (American Diabetes Association, 2001). The characteristics of type 1 DM and type 2 DM are outlined in Table 38-4.

---

■ *Barbara Schreiner, RN, MN, CDE, BC-ADM, revised this section.

**TABLE 38-4**  Comparison of characteristics of types 1 and 2 diabetes mellitus

| Characteristic | Type 1 | Type 2 |
|---|---|---|
| Age at onset | Less than 20 years | Over 30 years; although increasingly occurring in adolescents |
| Type of onset | Abrupt | Gradual |
| Sex ratio | Males slightly more than females | Females outnumber males |
| Percentage of diabetic population | 5%-8% | 85%-90% |
| Heredity: | | |
|    Family history | Sometimes | Frequently |
|    Human leukocyte antigen (HLA) | Associations | No associations |
|    Twin concordance | 25%-50% | 90%-100% |
|    Ethnic distribution | Primarily whites | Increased incidence in Native Americans/Hispanics/African-Americans |
| Presenting symptoms | Three Ps* common | May be related to long-term complications |
| Nutritional status | Underweight | Overweight |
| Insulin (natural): | | |
|    Pancreatic content | Usually none | Over 50% normal |
|    Serum insulin | Low to absent | High or low |
|    Primary resistance | Minimum | Marked |
| Islet cell antibodies | 80%-85% | Less than 5% |
| Therapy: | | |
|    Insulin | Always | 20%-30% of patients |
|    Oral agents | Ineffective | Often effective |
|    Diet only | Ineffective | Often effective |
| Chronic complications | Greater than 80% | Variable |
| Ketoacidosis | Common | Infrequent |

*Polyuria, polydipsia, and polyphagia.

*Type 1 diabetes* is characterized by destruction of the pancreatic beta cells, which produce insulin; this usually leads to absolute insulin deficiency. Type 1 diabetes has two forms. *Immune-mediated diabetes mellitus* results from an autoimmune destruction of the beta cells; it typically starts in children or young adults who are slim, but it can arise in adults of any age. *Idiopathic type 1* refers to rare forms of the disease that have no known cause.

*Type 2 diabetes* usually arises because of insulin resistance, in which the body fails to use insulin properly, combined with relative (rather than absolute) insulin deficiency. People with type 2 can range from predominantly insulin resistant with relative insulin deficiency to predominantly deficient in insulin secretion with some insulin resistance. It typically occurs in those who are over 45, are overweight and sedentary, and have a family history of diabetes.

Several other specific types of DM have been defined, such as those resulting from genetic defects of beta-cell function, pancreatic diseases (e.g., cystic fibrosis), and defects in insulin action. *Maturity-onset diabetes of the young (MODY)* is associated with monogenetic defects in beta-cell function that are characterized by impaired insulin secretion with minimal or no defects in insulin action. The disease is inherited as an autosomal dominant pattern, and the onset of hyperglycemia occurs at an early age (generally before age 25 years).

## Etiology

The clinical syndrome of DM results from a large variety of etiologic and pathogenic mechanisms. Type 1 DM is an autoimmune disease that arises when a person with a genetic predisposition is exposed to a precipitating event, such as a viral infection. Type 2 DM is more likely to be influenced by stronger, but as yet unknown, genetic factors. Thus its origin is considered to be polygenic.

**Genetic Factors.**  Type 1 DM is not inherited, but heredity is a prominent factor in the etiology. There are more than 40 rare genetic syndromes of which diabetes is a major feature (Harris, 2000). No simple mendelian pattern is found for DM. Children born to fathers with type 1 DM are about three times more likely to develop type 1 DM (approximately 7% frequency) than children born to mothers with type 1 DM (approximately 2% frequency).

At least 60% of the genetic susceptibility to type 1 diabetes is conferred by human leukocyte antigen (HLA) on chromosome 6. Several alleles have been implicated, including DR3, DR4, and DQ8. The highest-risk alleles (DR3 and DR4) are found in 95% of patients with diabetes. Only 50% of nondiabetic persons have these alleles. Certain alleles, such as DR2, may actually protect the individual from diabetes (Yongsoo and Eisenbarth, 2000).

Studies of type 2 DM in identical twins demonstrate a 100% concordance throughout the life span, whereas studies of type 1 DM in identical twins demonstrate a 30% to 50% concordance rate, suggesting that both environmental and gentic factors are important in the development of type 1 DM (Redondo, Fain, and Eisenbarth, 2001).

**Autoimmune Mechanisms.**  Pancreatic islet cell antibodies (ICAs) are found in about 70% to 85% of patients newly diagnosed with type 1 DM. The antibodies disappear by 1 year after diagnosis in most persons, but in some they may persist for years. The current theory is that the presence of the HLA genes causes a defect in the immune system that renders the possessor susceptible to a trigger event, which can be a dietary source, a virus, bacteria, or a chemical irritant. The predisposing factor initiates an autoimmune process that gradually destroys beta cells. Without beta cells no insulin can be produced. It is unclear whether the ICAs are a result of the inflammatory process or a significant aspect of the beta-cell destruction. Controversy exists regarding whether the autoimmune response is primarily mediated by the lymphocyte response or the humoral (antibody) response or is a result of the two.

There is a strong association between type 1 DM and other autoimmune endocrine disorders. An increased incidence of other autoimmune endocrine disorders, such as thyroiditis and Addison disease, has been found in families of children with DR3-associated type 1 DM.

It has also been found that anti–islet cell antibodies are detected in a number of unaffected first-degree relatives of children with type 1 DM (Gardner, and others, 1999). These findings offer hope of identifying persons at risk for diabetes with the eventual possibility of screening and implementation of therapy.

Research continues to identify genetic risk and environmental triggers with the hope of developing prevention strategies such as immunizations.

Treatment with cyclosporine or other forms of immunosuppression has been tested as an early intervention in the newly diagnosed person with type 1 DM. The effects of lifelong immunosuppression must be carefully weighed against the lifelong effects of diabetes.

**Diet.**  Cow's milk has been implicated as a possible trigger of the autoimmune response that destroys pancreatic beta cells in genetically susceptible hosts, thus causing DM (Kimpimaki and others, 2001). Further research is needed.

**Viruses.**  A variety of viruses, including mumps, Coxsackie B, and congenital rubella, have been implicated as the prime environmental factor in the etiology of DM. Islet cells appear to be particularly susceptible to either direct viral damage or chemical insult. The body reacts to this damaged or changed tissue in an autoimmune phenomenon. Therefore the virus serves as a precipitating factor or "trigger." A viral etiology also helps explain the seasonal variation in the onset of DM. Although this seasonal variation is not evident in children under 5 years of age, the marked increase in older children during the winter months strongly suggests an infectious disease relationship in either etiology or expression of diabetes in children.

**Type 2 Diabetes.**  Type 1 DM is the predominant form of diabetes in the pediatric age-group, and type 2 diabetes is more rare. The disturbed carbohydrate metabolism of type 2 DM may be a result of a sluggish or insensitive secretory response in the pancreas or a defect in body tissues that requires unusual amounts of insulin, or it may be that the insulin secreted is rapidly destroyed, inhibited, or inactivated in affected persons. Children with type 2 diabetes often have other features of insulin resistance syndrome: polycystic ovary syndrome and acanthosis nigricans (AN). AN may be found in as many as 90% of children with type 2 diabetes

and is characterized by velvety hyperpigmented areas in skin folds. Risk factors include non-European ancestry, family history of type 2 diabetes, obesity, insulin resistance, and age (Brosnan, Upchurch, and Schreiner, 2001).

While performing routine scoliosis screenings, school nurses will often identify AN on the child's neck. Such children should be referred to their primary care provider for further metabolic evaluation.

### Pathophysiology

Insulin is needed to support the metabolism of carbohydrates, fats, and proteins, primarily by facilitating the entry of these substances into the cell. Insulin is needed for the entry of glucose into the muscle and fat cells, prevention of mobilization of fats from fat cells, and storage of glucose as glycogen in the cells of liver and muscle. Insulin is not needed for the entry of glucose into nerve cells or vascular tissue. The chemical composition and molecular structure of insulin are such that it fits into receptor sites on the cell membrane. Here it initiates a sequence of poorly defined chemical reactions that alter the cell membrane to facilitate the entry of glucose into the cell and stimulate enzymatic systems outside the cell that metabolize the glucose for energy production.

With a deficiency of insulin, glucose is unable to enter the cell, and its concentration in the bloodstream increases. The increased concentration of glucose (*hyperglycemia*) produces an osmotic gradient that causes the movement of body fluid from the intracellular space to the interstitial space, then to the extracellular space and into the glomerular filtrate in order to "dilute" the hyperosmolar filtrate. Normally the renal tubular capacity to transport glucose is adequate to reabsorb all of the glucose in the glomerular filtrate. When the glucose concentration in the glomerular filtrate exceeds the renal threshold (±180 mg/dl), glucose "spills" into the urine (*glycosuria*) along with an osmotic diversion of water (*polyuria*), a cardinal sign of diabetes. The urinary fluid losses cause the excessive thirst (*polydipsia*) observed in diabetes. This water "washout" results in a depletion of other essential chemicals, especially potassium.

Protein is also wasted during insulin deficiency. Because glucose is unable to enter the cells, protein is broken down and converted to glucose by the liver (*glucogenesis*); this glucose then contributes to the hyperglycemia. These mechanisms are similar to those seen in starvation when substrate (glucose) is absent. The body is actually in a state of starvation during insulin deficiency. Without the use of carbohydrates for energy, fat and protein stores are depleted as the body attempts to meet its energy needs. The hunger mechanism is triggered, but increased food intake (*polyphagia*) enhances the problem by further elevating blood glucose (Fig. 38-6).

**Ketoacidosis.**  When insulin is absent or there is an altered insulin sensitivity, glucose is unavailable for cellular metabolism, and the body chooses alternate sources of energy, principally fat. Consequently fats break down into fatty acids, and glycerol in the fat cells is converted by the liver to ketone bodies (β-hydroxybutyric acid, acetoacetic acid, acetone). Any excess is eliminated in the urine (*ketonuria*) or the lungs *(acetone breath)*. The ketone bodies in the blood *(ketonemia)* are strong acids that lower serum pH, producing **ketoacidosis.**

**Ketones** are organic acids that readily produce excessive quantities of free hydrogen ions, causing a fall in plasma pH. Then chemical buffers in the plasma, principally bicarbonate, combine with the hydrogen ions to form carbonic acid, which readily dissociates into water and carbon dioxide. The respiratory system attempts to eliminate the excess carbon dioxide by increased depth and rate—**Kussmaul respirations,** or the hyperventilation characteristic of metabolic acidosis. The ketones are buffered by sodium and potassium in the plasma. The kidney attempts to compensate for the increased pH by increasing tubular secretion of hydrogen and ammonium ions in exchange for fixed base, thus depleting the base buffer concentration.

With cellular death, potassium is released from the cell (intracellular fluid [ICF]) into the bloodstream (extracellular fluid [ECF]) and excreted by the kidney, where the loss is accelerated by osmotic diuresis. The total body potassium is then decreased, even though the serum potassium level may be elevated as a result of the decreased fluid volume in which it circulates. Alteration in serum and tissue potassium can make cardiac arrest a potential problem.

If these conditions are not reversed by insulin therapy in combination with correction of the fluid deficiency and electrolyte imbalance, progressive deterioration occurs with dehydration, electrolyte imbalance, acidosis, coma, and death. Diabetic ketoacidosis (DKA) should be diagnosed promptly in a seriously ill patient, and therapy instituted in an intensive care unit.

**Long-Term Complications.**    Long-term complications of diabetes involve both the microvasculature and the macrosvasculature. The principal microvascular complications are **nephropathy, retinopathy,** and **neuropathy.** Microvascular disease develops during the first 30 years of diabetes, beginning in the first 10 to 15 years after puberty, with renal involvement evidenced by proteinuria and clinically apparent retinopathy.

With poor diabetic control, vascular changes can appear as early as 2½ to 3 years after diagnosis; however, with good to excellent control, changes have been postponed for 20 or more years. Intensive insulin therapy appears to delay the onset and slow the progression of clinically important retinopathy, including vision-threatening lesions, nephropathy, and neuropathy, by 35% to more than 70%, according to studies on treatment and complications of type 1 DM (Diabetes Control and Complications Trial Research Group, 1993.)

The postpubertal duration, not the total duration, of type 1 DM is implicated as a risk factor for the development of microvascular disease (Schultz and others, 1999). The process appears to be one of **glycosylation,** wherein proteins from the blood become deposited in the walls of small vessels (e.g., glomeruli), where they become trapped by "sticky" glucose compounds (glycosyl radicals). The buildup of these substances over time causes narrowing of the vessels, with subsequent interference with microcirculation to the affected areas (Beisswenger, Szwergold, and Yeo, 2001). Macrovascular disease develops after 25 years of diabetes and creates the predominant problems in patients with type 2 DM.

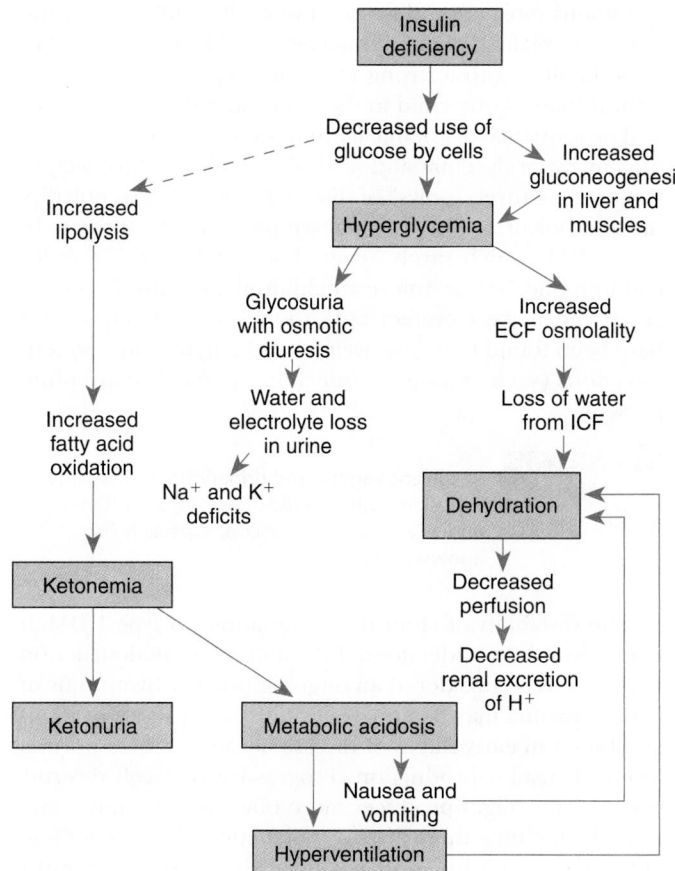

**Fig. 38-6**    Pathophysiology of acidosis in diabetes mellitus.

Other complications have been observed in children with type 1 DM. Hyperglycemia appears to influence thyroid function, and altered function is frequently observed at the time of diagnosis, as well as in poorly controlled diabetes. Limited mobility of small joints of the hand occurs in 30% of 7- to 18-year-old children with type 1 DM and appears to be related to changes in the skin and soft tissues surrounding the joint as a result of glycosylation.

**Mild Diabetes.**    Although most cases of childhood diabetes are recognized during the rapid initial deterioration in carbohydrate metabolism, other cases with more benign disease are being identified with increasing frequency. A few are detected accidentally by urinalysis before overt symptoms occur. MODY, for instance, is a rare genetic type of diabetes resulting from mutations at one of five genes and transmission by an autosomal dominant inheritance (Fajans and Bell, 2000). Children with this type of diabetes phenotypically resemble type 2 DM but are usually not obese. MODY is characterized by beta-cell dysfunction and is often treated similarly to type 2 DM.

## Clinical Manifestations

The symptomatology of diabetes is more readily recognizable in children than in adults, so it is surprising that the diagnosis may sometimes be missed or delayed. Diabetes is a great imitator; influenza, gastroenteritis, and appendicitis are the conditions most often diagnosed when it turns out that the disease is really diabetes. Diabetes should be suspected in those families with a strong family history of diabetes, especially if there is one child in the family with diabetes.

The sequence of chemical events described previously results in hyperglycemia and acidosis, which produce weight loss and the three "polys" of diabetes—polyphagia, polydipsia, and polyuria—the cardinal symptoms of the disease. In type 2 DM (which rarely occurs but may be seen in older children and Native American children), the insulin values are found to be elevated; 80% to 90% of this population have been found to be overweight, and fatigue and frequent infections (such as monilial infections in females) are often present.

**NURSING ALERT** Recurrent vaginal and urinary tract infections, especially with *Candida albicans,* are often an early sign of type 2 DM, especially in adolescents.

The variability of clinical manifestations in type 1 DM at diagnosis is best understood if the autoimmune destruction of islet cells is considered an ongoing process. Symptoms of hyperglycemia may be apparent only during stress (such as an illness) in early stages of disease because of near-normal levels of insulin production. Progressive islet cell destruction of later stages produces more obvious signs and symptoms. By the time there are overt diabetic symptoms, 80% to 90% of islet cell function has been destroyed. Frequently identified symptoms of overt diabetes include enuresis, irritability, and unusual fatigue.

Abdominal discomfort is common. Weight loss, though quite observable on the charts, may be a less frequent presenting complaint because the family might not have noticed the change over time. Another outstanding feature of diabetes is thirst. One couple reported that their child, during a trip from California to Kansas, drank the contents of a gallon jug of water between each gas station stop. As abdominal discomfort and nausea increase, the child may actually refuse fluid and food, adding to the increasing state of dehydration and malnutrition. Other symptoms include dry skin, blurred vision, and sores that are slow to heal. More commonly in children, fatigue and bed-wetting are the chief complaints that prompt parents to take their child for evaluation.

At diagnosis, the child may be *hyperglycemic,* with elevated blood glucose levels and glucose in the urine; *ketotic,* with ketones measurable in the blood and urine, with or without dehydration; or suffering from *diabetic ketoacidosis (DKA),* with dehydration, electrolyte imbalance, and acidosis.

## Diagnostic Evaluation

Three groups of children who should be considered as candidates for diabetes are (1) children who have glycosuria, polyuria, and a history of weight loss or failure to gain despite a voracious appetite; (2) those with transient or persistent glycosuria; and (3) those who display manifestations of metabolic acidosis, with or without stupor or coma. In every case diabetes must be considered if there is glycosuria, with or without ketonuria, and unexplained hyperglycemia.

Glycosuria by itself is not diagnostic of diabetes. Other sugars, such as galactose, can produce a positive result with certain test strips, and other conditions may cause a mild degree of glycosuria. These are infection, trauma, emotional or physical stress, hyperalimentation, and some renal or endocrine diseases.

An 8-hour fasting blood glucose level ≥126 mg/dl, a random blood glucose value of ≥200 accompanied by classic signs of diabetes, or an oral glucose tolerance test (OGTT) finding ≥200 mg/dl in the 2-hour sample is almost certain to indicate diabetes (American Diabetes Association, 2001). Postprandial blood glucose determinations and the traditional OGTTs have yielded low detection rates in children and are not usually necessary for establishing a diagnosis. Serum insulin levels may be normal or moderately elevated at the onset of diabetes; delayed insulin response to glucose indicates the presence of impaired glucose tolerance.

Ketoacidosis must be differentiated from other causes of acidosis or coma, including hypoglycemia, uremia, gastroenteritis with metabolic acidosis, salicylate intoxication encephalitis, and other intracranial lesions. DKA is a state of relative insulin insufficiency and may include the presence of hyperglycemia (blood glucose level ≥330 mg/dl), ketonemia (strongly positive), acidosis (pH <7.30 and bicarbonate <15 mmol/L), glycosuria, and ketonuria (Magee and Bhatt, 2001). Tests used to determine glycosuria and ketonuria are the glucose oxidase tapes (Keto-Diastix).

## Therapeutic Management

The management of the child with type 1 DM consists of a multidisciplinary approach involving the family, the child (when appropriate), and professionals, including a pediatric endocrinologist, diabetes nurse educator, and nutritionist, as well as an exercise physiologist. Often psychologic support from a mental health professional is also needed. Communication among the team members is essential and extends to other individuals in the child's life, such as teachers, the school nurse, school guidance counselor, and coach. (See Community Focus box.)

The definitive treatment is replacement of insulin that the child is unable to produce. However, insulin needs are also affected by emotions, nutritional intake, activity, and other life events, such as illnesses and puberty. The complexity of the disease and its management requires that the child and family incorporate diabetes needs into their lifestyle. Medical and nutritional guidance are primary, but management also includes continuing diabetes education, family guidance, and emotional support.

**Insulin Therapy.** Insulin replacement is the cornerstone of management of type 1 DM. Insulin dosage is tailored to each child based on home blood glucose monitoring (HBGM). The goal of insulin therapy is maintaining near-normal blood glucose values while avoiding too frequent episodes of hypoglycemia. Insulin is administered as two or more injections per day or as continuous subcutaneous infusion using a portable insulin pump.

Healthy pancreatic cells secrete insulin at a low but steady basal rate with superimposed bursts of increased secretion that coincide with intake of nutriments. Consequently insulin levels in the blood increase and decrease coincidentally with rises and falls in blood glucose levels. In addition, insulin is secreted directly into the portal circulation; therefore the liver, which is the major site of glucose disposal, receives the largest concentration of insulin. No matter which method of insulin replacement is used, this normal pattern cannot be duplicated. Subcutaneous injection results in absorption of the drug into the general circulation, thus reducing the concentrations of insulin to which the liver is exposed.

*Insulin preparations.*  Insulin is available in highly purified pork preparations; and in human insulin biosynthesized by and extracted from bacterial or yeast cultures. Human and pork varieties are less allergenic, and the animal insulins are less expensive than the synthetic human insulins. Insulin is available in rapid-, intermediate-, and long-acting preparations, and all are packaged in the strength of 100 U/ml. Some insulins are available as premixed insulins, such as 70/30 and 50/50 ratios, the first indicating percentage of intermediate and the second number identifying the percentage of rapid-acting insulin.

Lispro-H (Humalog)* and insulin as part (NovoLog)† (Eli Lilly, 2000) are human insulin analogs. One unit of the analog has the same glucose-lowering effect as 1 unit of human rapid-acting insulin, but the effect is even more rapid and of shorter duration. One benefit is less risk for hypoglycemia, because the peak effect is reached in 1½ to 2 hours. Because of its rapid onset, each of the analogs must be injected within 15 minutes before eating.

> **NURSING ALERT**  The human insulins from various manufacturers may be interchangeable, but human insulin and pork insulin or pure pork insulin should *never* be substituted for one another.

*Dosage.*  Conventional management has consisted of a twice-daily insulin regimen consisting of a combination of *rapid-acting (regular)* and *intermediate-acting (NPH or Lente)* insulin drawn up into the same syringe and injected before breakfast and before the evening meal. The amount of morning regular insulin is determined by patterns in the late morning and lunchtime blood glucose values. The morning intermediate-acting dosage is determined by patterns in the late afternoon and supper blood glucose values. Fasting blood glucose patterns at breakfast help determine the evening dose of intermediate insulin, and the blood glucose patterns at bedtime help determine the evening dose of rapid-acting (regular) insulin. For some children, better morning glucose control is achieved by a later (bedtime) injection of intermediate-acting insulin.

Regular insulin is best administered at least 30 minutes before meals. This allows sufficient time for absorption and results in a significantly more reduced postprandial rise in blood glucose than if the meal were eaten immediately following the insulin injection. Some children require more frequent administration of insulin. This includes children with difficult-to-control diabetes and children during the adolescent growth spurt. Intensive therapy consists of mul-

tiple injections throughout the day with a once- or twice-daily dose of long-acting (Ultralente) insulin to simulate the basal insulin secretion and injections of rapid-acting insulin before each meal. A *multiple daily injection (MDI)* program has been shown to reduce microvascular complications of diabetes in young, healthy patients who have type 1 DM (Diabetes Control and Complications Trial Research Group, 1993).

The precise dose of insulin needed cannot be predicted. Therefore the total dosage and percentage of regular- to intermediate-acting insulin should be determined empirically for each child. Usually 60% to 75% of the total daily

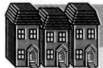

## COMMUNITY FOCUS
### The Adolescent with Type 1 DM

As a nurse caring for adolescents with type 1 DM, I am constantly aware of the wide range of adolescent behaviors that affect the course of this disease. Education of the child and the parents can often make the difference between a disease in control of the teen and a teen in control of the disease.

I have cared for many adolescent females who have episodes of hyperglycemia at the time of menstruation that can result in DKA. I have found that education regarding sick-day protocol with sliding-scale regular insulin instituted at the first sign of hyperglycemia, which may occur 1 to 2 days before onset of menses, can keep the adolescent girl out of the ICU and in control of her diabetes.

Eating disorders, such as bulimia or anorexia nervosa, in the teenager with type 1 DM pose a serious health hazard. (Jones and others, 2000). Also, insulin manipulation or omission has been identified as a weight loss method used by some female adolescents (Hoffman, 2001). Nurses working with these adolescents, especially females, must be aware of the hazards and openly discuss the risks with the young person. A referral for specialized intervention may be needed.

Another group of adolescents with diabetes who are at risk are those who drink alcohol. I have found that confusion about the effects of alcohol on blood glucose is common. Teens may believe that alcohol will increase blood glucose levels, when in fact the opposite occurs. Ingestion of alcohol inhibits the release of glycogen from the liver, therefore resulting in hypoglycemia. Teens with diabetes who drink alcohol may become hypoglycemic but be treated as if they were inebriated (drunk). Behaviors may be similar, such as shakiness, combativeness, slurred speech, and loss of consciousness.

Education regarding the effects of alcohol is important and must be included in a teaching plan. If teens insist on drinking alcohol, they can be cautioned to use sweetened mixers or eat snacks when consuming alcoholic beverages.

Episodes of hyperglycemia or hypoglycemia may become a serious issue for adolescents who are leaving home for the first time. One teenager confided that her mother always recognized her combative, antisocial behavior as impending hypoglycemia and treated her with the appropriate intervention. The teen feared that a college roommate might be offended by the behavior and leave her alone with impending hypoglycemia.

One young man realized he could not live alone when he "took a nap because of feeling tired" and woke up 4 days later in the hospital. Fortunately, his family realized he was in a coma and summoned emergency medical service. The fatigue signaled the beginning of a viral infection, which led to a blood glucose level of 410 mg/dl. Nurses need to address these fears openly and facilitate ways in which the teen can enlist the aid of significant peers who may be available during hyperglycemic or hypoglycemic episodes.

Susan Zekauskas, RN, MSN, PNP

*Eli Lilly & Co, Indianapolis, IN 46285.
†NovoNordisk, Princeton, NJ 08540.

dose is given before breakfast, and the remainder before the evening meal. Furthermore, insulin requirements do not remain constant but change continuously during growth and development; the need varies according to the child's activity level and pubertal status. For example, less insulin is required during spring and summer months, when the child is more active. Illness also alters insulin requirements. Some children require more frequent insulin administration. This includes children with difficult-to-control diabetes and children during the adolescent growth spurt.

*Methods of administration.* Daily insulin is administered subcutaneously by twice-daily injections, by multiple-dose injections, or by means of an insulin infusion pump. The *insulin pump* is an electromechanical device designed to deliver fixed amounts of regular or lispro insulin continuously (basal rate), thereby more closely imitating the release of the hormone by the islet cells. Although the pump delivers a programmed amount of basal insulin, the child or parent must program a dose for the pump to deliver before each meal.

The system consists of a syringe to hold the insulin, a plunger, and a mechanism to drive the plunger. The insulin flows from the syringe through a catheter to a needle inserted into subcutaneous tissue (the abdomen or thigh), and the lightweight device is worn on a belt or a shoulder holster. The needle and catheter are changed every 48 to 72 hours by the child or parent, using aseptic technique, and taped in place.

Although the pump provides more consistent insulin delivery, it has certain disadvantages. Pump therapy is expensive and requires commitment from the parent and child. A certain level of math skills is required to calculate infusion rates. Like any other mechanical device, it may malfunction. However, the pumps are equipped with alarms that signal problems that may arise, such as a low battery reserve, an occluded needle or tubing, or an uncontrolled insulin delivery rate.

Various routes for insulin administration are being studied. Inhaled insulin, for instance, has been found to be an effective and safe means to control postprandial glucose levels (Skyler and others, 2001). Although not commercially available, inhaled insulin is still being studied in both adults and children.

**Future Therapies.** *Islet cell* or *whole pancreas transplantation* may offer hope to patients in the future. Viable insulin-producing cells have been injected into the portal vein, where they are transported via the circulation to the liver and eventually produce up to two thirds of the required insulin. The major use of transplants has been in persons who have serious complications, particularly those whose deteriorating kidneys have required renal transplantation and who are receiving immunosuppressive therapy. However, islet cell and pancreatic transplants tend not to be sustainable over time despite continuation of therapy. The use of nonhuman islet cells encapsulated in immunoprotective, semipermeable membranes may have a future in the treatment of type 1 DM (Robertson, and others, 2000).

**Monitoring.** Daily monitoring of blood glucose levels is an essential aspect of appropriate DM management.

*Blood glucose.* *Self-monitoring of blood glucose (SMBG)* has improved diabetes management and is used successfully by children from the onset of their diabetes. By testing their own blood, children are able to change their insulin regimen to maintain their glucose level in the euglycemic (normal) range of 80 to 120 mg/dl. Diabetes management depends to a great extent on SMBG. In general, children tolerate the testing well.

*Glycosylated hemoglobin.* The measurement of glycosylated hemoglobin (hemoglobin $A_{1c}$) levels is a satisfactory method for assessing the control of the diabetic patient. As red blood cells circulate in the bloodstream, glucose molecules gradually attach to the hemoglobin A molecules and remain there for the lifetime of the red blood cell, approximately 120 days. The attachment is not reversible; therefore, this glycosylated hemoglobin reflects the average blood glucose levels that have taken place during the previous 2 to 3 months. The test is a satisfactory method for assessing control, detecting incorrect testing, monitoring effectiveness of changes in treatment, defining patients' goals, and detecting nonadherence.

*Urine.* Urine testing for glucose is no longer used for diabetic management; there is poor correlation between simultaneous glycosuria and blood glucose concentrations. However, urine testing can be carried out to detect evidence of ketonuria.

**NURSING ALERT** It is recommended that urine be tested for ketones every 3 hours during an illness and whenever the blood glucose level is ≥240 mg/dl when illness is not present.

**Nutrition.** Essentially the nutritional needs of children with diabetes are no different from those of healthy children. Children with diabetes need no special foods or supplements. They need sufficient calories to balance daily expenditure for energy and to satisfy the requirement for growth and development. Unlike the child without diabetes, whose insulin is secreted in response to food intake, insulin injected subcutaneously has a relatively predictable time of onset, peak effect, duration of action, and absorption rate depending on the type of insulin used. Consequently the timing of food consumption must be regulated to correspond to the time and action of the insulin prescribed.

Meals and snacks must be eaten according to peak insulin action, and the total number of calories and proportions of basic nutrients must be consistent from day to day. The constant release of insulin into the circulation makes the child prone to hypoglycemia between the three daily meals unless a snack is provided between meals and at bedtime. The distribution of calories should be calculated to fit the activity pattern of each child. For example, a child who is more active in the afternoon will need the larger snack at that time. This larger snack might also be split to allow some food at school and some food after school. Alterations in food intake should be made so that food, insulin, and exercise are balanced. Extra food is needed for increased activity.

The food intake may be planned in a variety of ways but is based on a balanced diet that incorporates six basic food groups: milk, meat, vegetables, fat, fruit, and starch. There are several meal-planning approaches, including the exchange system and carbohydrate counting. The exchange system from the American Diabetes Association (ADA) groups foods by nutrient content. Within each group, portion sizes of foods are calculated to give an equivalent amount of the nutrient. In the fruit list, for instance, one small apple has the equivalent amount of carbohydrate as a half banana. In the exchange system, food groups are important: fruits exchanged with fruits, starches exchange with starches.

Carbohydrate counting became popular with the Diabetes Control and Complications Trial. Portion sizes are still important, but all carbohydrates are considered equivalent. In this system, food groups are not as important as carbohydrate content. For example, one small apple and one slice of bread have the same carbohydrate amount (15 g) and may be used interchangeably.

Concentrated sweets are discouraged, and because of the increased risk for atherosclerosis in persons with DM, fat is reduced to 30% or less of the total caloric requirement. Dietary fiber has become increasingly important in dietary planning because of its influence on digestion, absorption, and metabolism of many nutrients. It has been found to diminish the rise in blood glucose after meals.

Correctly used, the diet allows for flexibility and the incorporation of preferred foods in most instances. For the growing child, food restriction should never be used for diabetic control, although caloric restrictions may be imposed for weight control if the child is overweight. In general the child's appetite should be the guide for the amount of calories needed, with the total caloric intake adjusted to appetite and activity. Basic principles of diet management are outlined in Box 38-13.

**Exercise.**   Exercise is encouraged and never restricted unless indicated by other health conditions. Exercise lowers blood glucose levels, depending on the intensity and duration of the activity. Consequently exercise should be included as part of diabetic management, and the type and amount of exercise should be planned around the child's interests and capabilities. However, in most instances children's activities are unplanned, and the resulting decrease in blood glucose can be compensated for by providing extra snacks before (and, if the exercise is prolonged, during) the activity. In addition to a feeling of well-being, regular exercise aids in utilization of food and often results in a reduction of insulin requirements.

Physical training tends to increase tissue sensitivity to insulin, even in the resting state. Consequently it is especially important to understand the relationship between the activity and the diabetic regimen. Vigorous muscular contraction increases regional blood flow and accelerates the absorption and circulation of insulin that is injected into the area, which can contribute to development of hypoglycemia. If exercise involving leg muscles is planned, it is recommended that nonexercised sites (arm or abdomen) be used for insulin injection. This practice may replace the need for further increased carbohydrate intake or a reduced insulin dose (or both) to avoid exercise-induced hypoglycemia.

Children with poorly controlled diabetes are particularly at risk for hyperglycemia with exercise, or exercise may actually stimulate ketoacid production. Therefore the child who has marked hyperglycemia (blood glucose level ≥240 mg/dl) and ketonuria should be discouraged from strenuous physical activity until satisfactory control of the diabetes is achieved by appropriate adjustments of insulin and diet.

Athletes and those youngsters who regularly participate in organized sports are advised to adjust their insulin dosage in anticipation of sustained physical activity during the part of the day devoted to strenuous exercise. Team sports may encourage overexertion and subsequent hypoglycemia. Insulin dosage decreases are used for participation in organized sports or prolonged activities, such as swimming for several hours. It is important that the patient consult with the practitioner for advice on insulin dose adjustment.

**Hypoglycemia.**   Occasional episodes of hypoglycemia are an integral part of insulin therapy, and an objective of diabetic management is to achieve the best possible glycemic control while minimizing the frequency and severity of hypoglycemia. Even with good control, a child may frequently experience mild symptoms of hypoglycemia. If the signs and symptoms are recognized early and promptly relieved by appropriate therapy, the child's activity should be interrupted for no more than a few minutes.

**NURSING ALERT**   Hypoglycemic episodes most commonly occur before meals, or when the insulin effect is peaking.

The most common causes of hypoglycemia are bursts of physical activity without additional food, or delayed, omitted, or incompletely consumed meals. Reglycosylation of muscles may occur over the ensuing 24 hours. Particular vigilance related to hypoglycemia may be necessary during the night after vigorous exertion. Occasionally, hypoglycemic reactions occur unexpectedly and without apparent cause. They may be the result of an inadvertent or deliberate error in insulin administration.

---

**Box 38-13** ■ ■ ■
**Nutritional Management in Type 1 DM**

**GOAL**
Attain metabolic control of glucose and lipid levels

**OBJECTIVES**
1. Appropriate meal and snack planning:
   ☐ Achieve a dietary balance of carbohydrates, fats, and proteins.
   ☐ Provide extra food during periods of exercise.
   ☐ Time meals consistently to prevent hypoglycemia.
   ☐ Avoid high-sugar foods to prevent hyperglycemia.
2. Develop an appropriate insulin regimen and physical activity program:
   ☐ Administer insulin as directed before eating.
   ☐ Increase insulin dose or activity level when extra food is eaten.
   ☐ Decrease insulin dose during periods of strenuous activity.

Gastroenteritis, in which there is gastric stasis, may impede the absorption of food, even though the child is eating reasonably well. It can also occur when the blood glucose level is so low that it causes stasis. Then the child may eat a meal or snack and still have an insulin reaction. Continued feeding does not seem to alter the blood glucose level, because the simple glucose or sugar remains in the stomach.

The signs and symptoms of hypoglycemia are caused by both increased adrenergic activity and impaired brain function. The increased adrenergic nervous system activity plus increased secretion of catecholamines produces nervousness, pallor, tremulousness, palpitations, sweating, and hunger. Weakness, dizziness, headache, drowsiness, irritability, loss of coordination, seizures, and coma are more severe responses and reflect CNS glucose deprivation and the body's attempts to elevate the serum glucose levels (Fig. 38-7).

It is often difficult to distinguish between hyperglycemia and a hypoglycemic reaction (Table 38-5). Because the symptoms are similar and usually begin with changes in behavior, the simplest way to differentiate between the two is to test the blood glucose level. The blood glucose level is low in hypoglycemia, whereas in hyperglycemia the glucose level will be significantly elevated. Urinary ketones may be present following hypoglycemia as a result of starvation ketone production. In doubtful situations it is safer to give the child some simple carbohydrate. This will help alleviate the symptoms in the case of hypoglycemia but will do little harm if the child is hyperglycemic.

Children are usually able to detect the onset of hypoglycemia, but some are too young to implement treatment. Parents should become adept at recognizing the onset of symptoms—for example, a change in a child's behavior, such as tearfulness or euphoria. In the majority of cases, 10 to 15 g of simple carbohydrate, such as 1 tablespoon of table sugar, will elevate the blood glucose level and alleviate the symptoms. The simpler the carbohydrate, the more rapidly it will be absorbed (8 ounces of milk equals 15 g of carbohydrate). The rapid-releasing sugar is followed by a complex carbohydrate such as a slice of bread or a cracker and by a protein such as peanut butter or milk.

For a mild reaction, milk or fruit juice is a good food to use in children. Milk supplies them with lactose or milk sugar, as well as a more prolonged action from the protein and fat (aids in decreased absorption). Other glucose sources include Insta-Glucose (cherry-flavored glucose), carbonated drinks (not sugarless), sherbet, gelatin, or cake icing. All children with diabetes should carry with them glucose tabs, Insta-Glucose, sugar cubes, or sugar-containing candy, such as Life Savers or Charms. A difficulty with candies or icing is that the child may learn to fake a reaction to get the sweets; therefore commercial treatment products such as Insta-glucose or glucose tabs may be the preferred treatment.

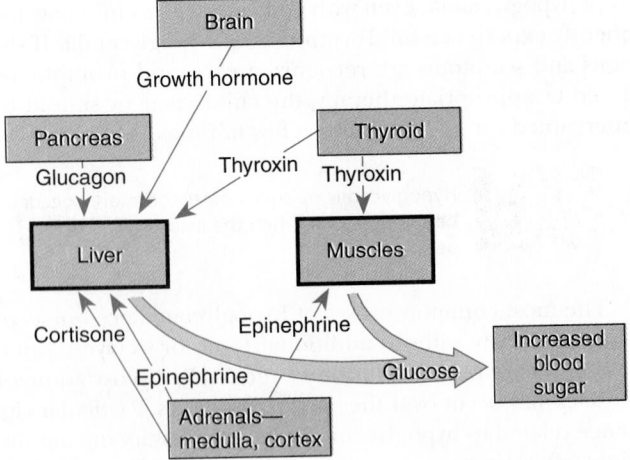

**Fig. 38-7** Body systems respond to hypoglycemia in various ways to increase blood glucose level.

| **TABLE 38-5** | Comparison of manifestations of hypoglycemia and hyperglycemia | |
|---|---|---|
| **Variable** | **Hypoglycemia** | **Hyperglycemia** |
| Onset | Rapid (minutes) | Gradual (days) |
| Mood | Labile, irritable, nervous, weepy, combative | Lethargic |
| Mental status | Difficulty concentrating, speaking, focusing, coordinating | Dulled sensorium Confused |
| Inward feeling | Shaky feeling, hunger Headache Dizziness | Thirst Weakness Nausea/vomiting Abdominal pain |
| Skin | Pallor Sweating | Flushed Signs of dehydration |
| Mucous membranes | Normal | Dry, crusty |
| Respirations | Shallow | Deep, rapid (Kussmaul) |
| Pulse | Tachycardia | Less rapid, weak |
| Breath odor | Normal | Fruity, acetone |
| Neurologic | Tremors Late: hyperreflexia, dilated pupils, convulsion | Diminished reflexes Paresthesia |
| Ominous signs | Shock, coma | Acidosis, coma |
| Blood: | | |
|   Glucose | Low: below 60 mg/dl | High: 240 mg/dl or more |
|   Ketones | Negative/trace | High/large |
|   Osmolarity | Normal | High |
|   pH | Normal | Low (7.25 or less) |
|   Hematocrit | Normal | High |
|   HCO$_3$ | Normal | Less than 15 mEq/L |
| Urine: | | |
|   Output | Normal | Polyuria (early) to oliguria (late) |
|   Sugar | Negative | High |
|   Acetone | Negative/trace | High |

When in doubt, it is best to assume hypoglycemia and treat, but overtreatment could result in hyperglycemia. The treatment may be repeated in 10 to 15 minutes if the initial response is not satisfactory. Rest and the addition of food should be part of the plan.

An *insulin reaction* is often the most feared aspect of diabetes because severe brain symptoms may develop. In a severe reaction the various areas of the brain respond in sequence: the forebrain with increased drowsiness and perspiration, the hypothalamus and thalamus with tachycardia and loss of consciousness, the midbrain with seizure activity that may be started from stimulation initially from the hypothalamus, and finally the hindbrain with responses of deeper coma and decreasing reflexes. The treatment of choice for severe hypoglycemia is 50% glucose administered intravenously.

*Glucagon* is sometimes prescribed for home treatment of hypoglycemia. It is available as an emergency kit that must be mixed at the time of use and is administered intramuscularly or subcutaneously. Glucagon functions by releasing stored glycogen from the liver and requires about 15 to 20 minutes to elevate the blood glucose level.

> **NURSING ALERT**
>
> Vomiting may occur after administration of glucagon; therefore precautions against aspiration must be taken (e.g., placing the child on the side), because the child will be unconscious.

Once the child is responsive, the lost glycogen stores are replaced by small amounts of sugar-containing fluid administered frequently until the child feels comfortable about trying solid foods.

**Morning Hyperglycemia.**    The management of elevated morning blood glucose levels depends on whether the increase is a true dawn phenomenon, insulin waning, or a rebound hyperglycemia (the *Somogyi effect*). Insulin waning is a progressive rise in blood glucose levels from bedtime to morning. It is treated by increasing the nocturnal insulin dose. The true dawn phenomenon shows a relatively normal blood glucose level until about 3 AM, when the level begins to rise. The Somogyi effect may occur at any time but often shows an elevated blood glucose level at bedtime and a drop at 2 AM with a rebound rise following. The treatment for this phenomenon is adjusting (down) the nocturnal insulin dose to prevent the 2 AM hypoglycemia from occurring. The rebound rise in the blood glucose level is a result of counter-regulatory hormones (epinephrine, GH, and corticosteroids), which are stimulated by hypoglycemia. More frequent blood monitoring (especially at times of anticipated peak insulin action) will usually identify these conditions. Trace amounts of urinary ketones aid in identifying undetected hypoglycemia.

**Illness Management.**    Illness alters diabetes management, and maintaining control is usually related to the seriousness of the illness. In the well-controlled child an illness will run its course as it does in the unaffected child. The goals during an illness are to restore euglycemia, treat urinary ketones, and maintain hydration. Blood glucose levels and urinary ketones should be monitored every 3 hours.

Some hyperglycemia and ketonuria are expected in most illnesses, even with diminished food intake, and are an indication for increased insulin. Insulin should never be omitted during an illness, although dosage requirements may increase, decrease, or remain unchanged, depending on the severity of the illness and the child's appetite. Often the child will need supplemental insulin between usual dose times. If the child vomits more than one time, if blood glucose levels remain above 240 mg/dl, or if urinary ketones remain high, the health care practitioner should be notified. Simple carbohydrates may be substituted for carbohydrate-containing exchanges in the meal plan. Although insulin and diet are important tools in sick-day care, fluids are the most important intervention. Fluids must be encouraged to prevent dehydration and to flush out ketones.

**Surgery.**    The physiologic and emotional stresses related to surgery require careful adjustment of insulin. Because the child receives IV glucose during surgery and the stress of the surgery itself will also raise the blood glucose level, the risk of an insulin reaction is very slight. Short-acting insulins should be continued until the child is able to tolerate oral feedings and a return to the routine pattern of insulin administration.

**Prevention.**    Major advances have been made in the ability to detect susceptibility to type 1 DM, and animal studies indicate that the disease can be prevented by various immunologic interventions (Skyler and Marks, 2000). Recent sources also indicate that early immunosuppression may preserve long-term endogenous insulin secretion in individuals with type 1 DM.

It has been shown previously that immunosuppressive drugs can be used to induce metabolic remissions in newly diagnosed patients. However, more recent studies have shown that the metabolic remission is temporary despite continuation of therapy. Cyclosporine, mycophenolic acid, and nicotinamide have shown promise in delaying beta-cell destruction or lowering the incidence of type 1 DM in relatives of children afflicted with the disease. Much progress has been made in respect to the identification of islet cell antigens targeted by the immune response. Many potential treatments to prevent type 1 DM have appeared, and human trials have begun.

## Therapeutic Management: Diabetic Ketoacidosis (DKA)

DKA, the most complete state of insulin deficiency, is a life-threatening situation. Management consists of rapid assessment, adequate insulin to reduce the elevated blood glucose level, fluids to overcome dehydration, and electrolyte replacement (especially potassium).

DKA constitutes an emergency situation; therefore the child should be admitted to an intensive care facility for management. The priority is to obtain a venous access for administration of fluids, electrolytes, and insulin. The child should be weighed, measured, and placed on a cardiac monitor. Blood glucose and ketone levels are determined at the bedside, and samples are obtained for laboratory measurements of glucose, electrolytes, blood urea nitrogen, arterial pH, $Po_2$, $Pco_2$, hemoglobin, hematocrit, white blood cell count and differential, and calcium and phosphorus.

Oxygen may be administered to patients who are cyanotic and in whom arterial oxygen is less than 80%. Gastric suction is applied to unconscious children to avoid the possibility of pulmonary aspiration. Antibiotics may be administered to febrile children after appropriate specimens are obtained for culture. A Foley catheter may or may not be inserted for urine samples and measurement. Unless the child is unconscious, a collection bag is usually sufficient for accurate assessments.

**Fluid and Electrolyte Therapy.** All patients with DKA suffer from dehydration (10% of total body weight in severe ketoacidosis) due to the osmotic diuresis, accompanied by depletion of electrolytes, sodium, potassium, chloride, phosphate, and magnesium. Serum pH and bicarbonate reflect the degree of acidosis. Prompt and adequate fluid therapy restores tissue perfusion and suppresses the elevated levels of stress hormones.

The initial hydrating solution is 0.9% saline solution. Traditionally deficits have been replaced at a rate of 50% over the first 8 to 12 hours and the remaining 50% over the next 16 to 24 hours. Current trends suggest more cautious fluid management to reduce the risk of cerebral edema. The fluid deficit is replaced evenly over a period of 24 to 48 hours.

> **NURSING ALERT** Potassium must never be given until the serum potassium level is known to be normal or low, and urinary voiding is observed. All maintenance IV fluids should include 20 to 40 mEq/L of potassium. Never give potassium as a rapid IV bolus or cardiac arrest may result.

Serum potassium levels may be normal on admission, but following fluid and insulin administration, the rapid return of potassium to the cells can seriously deplete serum levels, with the attendant risk of cardiac arrhythmias. As soon as the child has established renal function (is voiding at least 25 ml/hr) and insulin has been given, vigorous potassium replacement is implemented. The cardiac monitor is used as a guide to therapy, and configuration of T waves should be followed every 30 to 60 minutes to determine changes that might indicate alterations in potassium concentration (widening of the Q-T interval and the appearance of a U wave following a flattened T wave indicate hypokalemia; an elevated and spreading T wave and shortening of the Q-T interval indicate hyperkalemia).

Insulin should not be given until urine ketones and a blood glucose level have been obtained. Continuous IV regular insulin is given at a dose of 0.1 U/kg/hr. Insulin therapy should be started after the initial rehydration bolus, because serum glucose levels fall rapidly after volume expansion. Blood glucose levels should decrease by 50 to 100 mg/dl/hr. When blood glucose levels fall to 250 to 300 mg/dl, dextrose is added to the IV solution. The goal is to maintain blood glucose levels between 120 and 240 mg/dl by adding 5% to 10% dextrose. Sodium bicarbonate is used conservatively; it is used for pH <7.0, severe hyperkalemia, or cardiac instability. Because sodium bicar-

bonate has been associated with increased risk for cerebral edema, children receiving this substance must be carefully monitored for changes in level of consciousness (Glaser and others, 2001).

When the critical period is over, the task of regulating insulin dosage to diet and activity is started. Children should be actively involved in their own care and are given responsibility according to their ability and the guidance of the nurse.

> **NURSING ALERT** Because insulin can chemically bind to plastic tubing and in-line filters, thereby reducing the amount of the medication reaching the systemic circulation, an insulin mixture is run through the tubing to saturate the insulin-binding sites before the infusion is started.

## Nursing Considerations: Acute Care

Children with DM may be admitted to the hospital at the time of their initial diagnosis, during illness or surgery, or for episodes of ketoacidosis, which may be precipitated by any of a variety of factors. Many children are able to keep the disease under control with periodic assessment and adjustment of insulin, diet, and activity as needed under the supervision of a practitioner. Under most circumstances these children can be managed very well at home and require hospitalization only for a serious illness or upset.

However, a small number of children with diabetes exhibit a degree of metabolic lability and have repeated episodes of DKA that require hospitalization, which interferes with education and social development. These children appear to display a characteristic personality structure. They tend to be unusually passive and nonassertive and to come from families that are inclined to smooth over conflicts without resolution. Children in this type of setting experience emotional arousal with little, if any, opportunity or ability to bring about its resolution. Other children from psychosocially dysfunctional families display behavioral and personality problems. This emotional stress causes an increased production of endogenous catecholamines, which stimulates fat breakdown, leading to ketonemia and ketonuria.

Loving discipline is a supportive measure for any child; however, children with poorer diabetic control come from predominantly disruptive family units with little or no discipline as part of the family lifestyle. Lack of control is psychologically harmful. Because many of the psychosocial problems are not immediately apparent, psychosocial assessment by professionals is required, together with ongoing emotional support and counseling to reverse the patterns of ketoacidosis (Kaufman and Halvorson, 1999).

**Hospital Management.** The child with DKA requires intensive nursing care. Vital signs should be observed and recorded frequently. Hypotension caused by the contracted blood volume of the dehydrated state may cause decreased peripheral blood flow, which can be particularly hazardous to the heart, lungs, and kidneys. An elevated temperature may indicate the presence of infection and should be reported so that treatment can be implemented immediately.

Careful and accurate records should be maintained, including vital signs (pulse, respiration, temperature, blood pressure), weight, IV fluids, electrolytes, insulin, blood glucose level, and intake and output. A urine collection device or retention catheter is used to obtain the urine measurements, which include volume, specific gravity, and glucose and ketone values. The volume relative to the glucose content is important because 5% glucose in a 300-ml sample is a significantly greater amount than a similar reading from a 75-ml sample. A diabetic flow sheet maintained at the bedside provides an ongoing record of the vital signs, urine and blood tests, amount of insulin given, and intake and output of the patient. The level of consciousness is assessed and recorded at frequent intervals. The comatose child generally regains consciousness fairly soon after initiation of therapy but is managed as any unconscious child during that time.

When the critical period is over, the task of regulating insulin dosage to diet and activity is begun. The same meticulous records of intake and output, urine glucose and acetone levels, and insulin administration are maintained. Capable children should be actively involved in their own care and are given responsibility for keeping the intake and output record, testing the blood and urine, and, when appropriate, administering their own insulin—all under the supervision and guidance of the nurse.

### Nursing Considerations: General Care

#### ⁙ Assessment

Diabetic management involves a constant state of assessment. Daily monitoring of blood glucose levels, periodic urinalysis for ketones, and observation for signs of hypoglycemia, hyperglycemia, or other complications is part of the daily life of children with diabetes and their families. Diabetes can be suspected in any child who exhibits the manifestations of hypoglycemia or hyperglycemia (see Table 38-5), and the child should be referred for further assessment and appropriate testing.

The nurse should be alert to evidence of complications, although these are usually not manifested until adulthood. Assessment of skin for evidence of breakdown is important in order that appropriate care can be implemented to facilitate healing and prevent infection. Because illnesses, such as respiratory infections or gastrointestinal upsets, complicate the diabetes management, they should be detected early.

#### ⁙ Nursing Diagnoses

Based on a thorough assessment, several nursing diagnoses are identified. The more common diagnoses for the child with DM are included in the Nursing Care Plan on pp. 1752-1755. Others may apply in specific situations.

#### ⁙ Planning

The goals for the child with DM and the family include the following:

1. Child and family will be educated about the disease, assessment techniques, and therapy.

2. Child will experience a minimum of ill effects from complications of diabetes.
3. Child will develop a positive self-image.
4. Child and family will receive adequate support.

#### ⁙ Implementation

Education is the cornerstone of diabetes management and the major responsibility in diabetes nursing care. This includes education and reinforcement of information for the family and for children who are old enough to participate in self-management of the disease. With younger children, parents must supervise and manage their therapeutic program, but children should assume some responsibility for self-management as soon as they are capable. Children can assist with blood glucose testing at a relatively young age, and most should be able to administer their own insulin at about 9 years of age. In situations in which the parents are inconsistent or unreliable, the child should be taught self-care at an earlier age. It must be understood, however, that education programs cannot be conducted as one-time activities with the expectation that they will achieve permanent behavior changes. Education is an ongoing nursing activity as family and patient needs change and new findings are applied.

**Concepts of Child and Family Education.** Children and their families vary in educational background and the capacity to learn and understand the various aspects of the therapeutic program. Some families respond best to very simple explanations and directions, whereas others expect thorough, in-depth information about the physiologic processes and responses associated with the disease and its therapy. All of the principles of teaching and learning are applied in the educational process; therefore, before beginning, the nurse must determine the optimum time, place, method, and content to be taught. Self-management, the ultimate goal for children with diabetes, is more likely to occur when children understand the disease and the care it requires. Properly educated and motivated, most families should be able to follow a program of regulated control satisfactorily.

When to teach a family is best judged by the psychologic state and emotional readiness of the family and the child. When a child is newly diagnosed, the psychologic adjustment to the disease can block the learning process completely. For example, members of the family may in a follow-up visit state that it is the first time that they have heard a certain bit of information when in reality the specific material had been covered several times in the course of teaching.

Certainly the first 3 or 4 days after diagnosis is not an optimum time for complex learning. In fact, the later the more complex material is presented, the better. For example, one successful program teaches only essential, or survival, information first and intense information a month later. Another program advocates, as a choice of time for teaching, 1 week after diagnosis followed by a review of survival techniques 2 weeks after discharge. Probably a most inopportune and ineffective time for teaching is the day or so after diagnosis, when the education must be compressed into a few hours or days so that the child can be discharged early. Regardless of the teaching plan, the ability of the individuals involved to learn must be accurately assessed. This includes assessment of the educational background and emotional stability of the individual(s) involved and the use of appropriate measurement tools, such as a pretest or an objective assessment of the learner's educational level. The stepped approach to patient education employs the method of simple to complex. The stepped approach involves three phases: (1) use good interpersonal skills; (2) teach about the illness and regimen; and (3) overcome obstacles to behavior change.

The setting for the educational process can facilitate the learning process. An environment that is too hot or too cold or one in which there is too much noise will distract the learner. Outpatient education for the newly diagnosed but well child has been found to be as effective as hospitalizing all new-onset patients for education (Siminerio and others, 1999). If hospitalized, bedside education may be necessary in some cases, but the coming and going of a number of people is distracting. There are times in the educational process when individual instruction is needed, but contact with other children or parents can assist in adjustment to the reality of the disease and the implications of having a chronic condition. Supplementary material such as audiovisual aids enhances the learning process and promotes retention of information.

A child learns best when sessions are kept short, no more than 15 to 20 minutes. The parents do best with periods of 45 to 60 minutes, or longer if they are inquisitive. Education should involve all of the senses, and although visual aids are valuable tools, participation is the most effective method for learning. For example, to teach blood glucose testing, the technique is explained, the procedure is demonstrated, and the learner is allowed to perform the procedure; this is followed by a review of the material by visual aids, with learning validated by some testing method that includes feedback. A variety of teaching methods and teaching aids can be used. Some visual aids may be beautifully illustrated but miss a major point; therefore materials should be previewed for accuracy and appropriateness. Varying the presentation with a variety of audiovisual materials, including films, slide-tape programs, and books, stimulates the senses and helps the individual to learn.

Several organizations are prepared to assist with education and dissemination of knowledge about diabetes. The **American Diabetes Association (ADA)**,* **Canadian Diabetes Association,**† **Juvenile Diabetes Research Foundation International,**‡ and **American Association of Diabetes Educators**§ are valuable resources for a wide variety of educational materials. The **National Diabetes Information Clearinghouse**‖ publishes a number of comprehensive annotated bibliogra-

phies, including *Educational Materials for and About Young People with Diabetes,* a compilation of resource materials for children, siblings, parents, teachers, and health professionals, and *Sports and Exercise for People with Diabetes.*

The content of the educational course must include all aspects of the disease as they specifically relate to the individual child. There are many aspects of the disease that may not be covered in an initial educational course but can be postponed until subsequent office or clinic visits or can be done through referral sources such as the American Diabetes Association. The minimum information needed is that which will help the family manage from one day to the next; expanded information helps the individual with the biopsychosocial adjustment that is basic to in-depth knowledge about the disease. The more the family understands about the disease in relation to body needs, the better it is able to maintain a high degree of control. Important content needed for minimum management is discussed briefly in the following sections.

**Identification.**   One of the first things that should be called to the attention of the parents is the need for the child to wear some means of medical identification. Usually recommended is the Medic-Alert identification, a stainless steel, silver, or gold-plated identification bracelet that is visible and immediately recognizable. It contains a collect telephone number that medical personnel can call around the clock for medical records and personal information.

**Nature of Diabetes.**   The better the parents understand the pathophysiology of diabetes and the function and action of insulin and glucagon in relation to caloric intake and exercise, the better will be their understanding of the disease and its effects on the child. Parents need answers to a number of questions (voiced or unvoiced) because those answers can provide them an increased feeling of security in coping with the disease. For example, they may want to know about the various procedures performed on their child and treatment rationale, such as what is being put in the IV bottle and the expected effect.

**Meal Planning.**   Normal nutrition is a major aspect of the family education program. Diet instruction is usually conducted by the nutritionist, with reinforcement and guidance from the nurse (Fig. 38-8). The emphasis is on adequate intake for age, consistent menus, complex carbohydrates, and consistent eating times. The family is taught how the meal plan relates to the requirements of growth and development, the disease process, and the insulin regimen. Meals and snacks are modified around the child and the present food menu, preserving cultural patterns and preferences as much as possible. Extensive exchange lists are available that include foods that are compatible with most lifestyles.

Learning about foods within specific food groups helps in making choices. Weights and measures of foods are used as eye-training devices for defining serving sizes and should be practiced for about 3 months, with gradual progression to estimation of food portions. Even when the child and family become competent in estimating portion sizes, reassessment should take place weekly or monthly and when there is any change of brands. Members of the family

---

*1701 N Beauregard St, Alexandria, VA 22311, (800) 342-2383; www. diabetes.org.
†15 Toronto St, Suite 800, Toronto, ON M5C 2E3, (800)-BANTING; www. diabetes.ca.
‡120 Wall St, New York, NY 10005, (800)JDF-CURE; www.jdf.org.
§100 W Monroe St, Suite 400, Chicago, IL 60603-1901, (800)338-3633; www.aadenet.org.
‖ Information Way, Bethesda, MD 20892-3560, (800) 860-8747; www. niddk.nih.gov.

should also be guided in reading labels for the nutritional value of foods and food content.

Family members should also become familiar with the carbohydrate content of food groups. Substitution with foods of equal carbohydrate content is the skill needed for successful carbohydrate counting. Substitution might be necessary if a food is not available in sufficient quantity or for the teenager who wishes to eat fast food with peers. The use of MDI lends flexibility to the timing of meals.

Educating children or teenagers to make healthy food choices is an ongoing task. Younger children might be taught to choose from a special treat box stocked with sugar-free items when high-sugar treats are brought to the classroom by others. Discussions with school-age children might include situations encountered at school or parties, such as choosing food in the cafeteria or bringing substitute treats to parties. Role-playing and discussion help teenagers deal with food choices when on dates, with friends, or on a food break after school.

Lists of popular fast-food items and items served at the major fast-food chains can be obtained from the restaurants to help guide food selections. It is important that the child know the nutritional value of these items (the major chains are remarkably uniform), but the child should be cautioned to avoid high-fat and high-sugar items; for example, the child could choose a plain hamburger instead of a double cheeseburger. See Table 38-6 for a small sample of some popular fast-food items.

Children should use sugar substitutes with moderation in items such as soft drinks. Artificial sweeteners have been shown to be safe, but if there is any question about amounts, the physician, dietitian, or nurse specialist can provide guidelines based on body weight. "Sugar-free" chewing gum and candies made with sorbitol may be used in moderation by children with DM. Although sorbitol is less cariogenic than other varieties of sugar substitutes, it is an alcohol sugar that is metabolized to fructose and then to glucose. Furthermore, large amounts can cause osmotic diarrhea. Most dietetic foods contain sorbitol. They are more expensive than regular foods. Also, while a product may be "sugar free," it is not necessarily carbohydrate free.

**Traveling.** Traveling requires advance planning, especially when a trip involves crossing time zones. A number of tips are included in pamphlets available free of charge.* Suggestions for traveling include what will be needed from the practitioner before leaving, what and how much to take along, needs in transit, what to consider at the destination, and planning for when the child returns home. Planning is needed no

*Vacations, Travel, and Diabetes, available from Becton, Dickson & Co, Rochelle Park, NJ 07662.

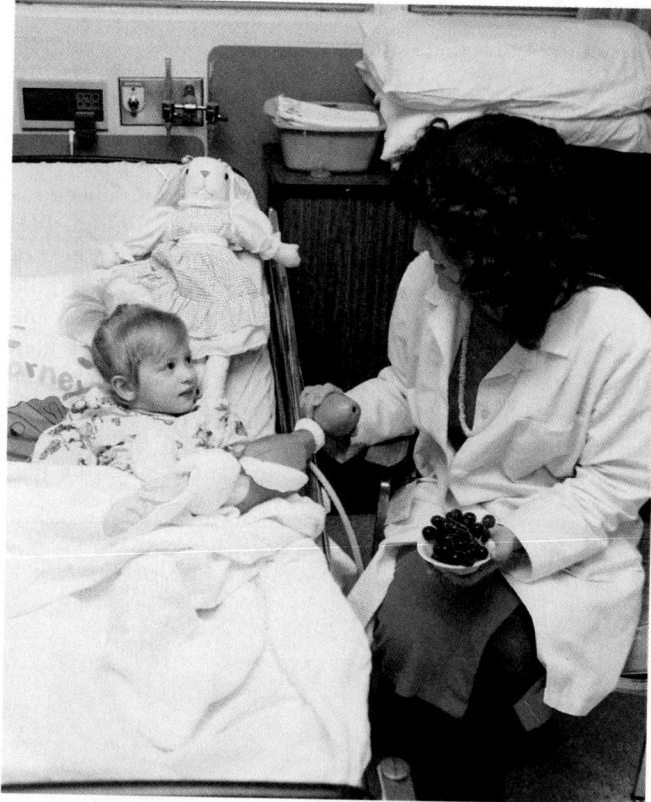

**Fig. 38-8** Nutritionist instructs child, using food to explain food exchanges.

**TABLE 38-6**  Exchange equivalents and carbohydrate content for selected fast food items

| Food | Carbohydrate Counting | | | | Exchange System | | | |
|---|---|---|---|---|---|---|---|---|
| | CHO choices | CHO (g) | Protein (g) | Fat (g) | Medium fat | Starch/ Bread | Fat | Vegetable |
| Arby's roast beef sandwich (regular) | 2½ | 36 | 23 | 20 | 2 (lean) | 2½ | 3 | — |
| Burger King Whopper ® | 3 | 47 | 29 | 40 | 3 | 3 | 5 | 1 |
| KFC Original (two pieces chicken, potatoes, gravy, cole slaw, roll) | 4 | 71 | 33 | 48 | 4 | 3½ | 4½ | 1 |
| McDonald's Big Mac® | 3 | 45 | 26 | 32 | 2 | 3 | 4 | 2 |
| Pizza Hut cheese pizza (three slices) | 9 | 129 | 42 | 27 | 3 | 9 | 3 | — |
| Taco Bell | | | | | | | | |
|   Taco | 1 | 12 | 9 | 10 | 1 | 1 | 1 | — |
|   Beef burrito | 4 | 54 | 24 | 23 | 2 | 4 | 3 | 2 |
| Wendy's cheeseburger (single) | 2 | 37 | 25 | 20 | 3 | 2 | 1 | — |

Modified from *Nutrition in the fast lane,* Indianapolis, IN, 2000, Eli Lilly.

matter what type of travel is considered—automobile, plane, bus, or train. Diabetic supplies should not be left in a hot environment.

**Insulin.** Families need to understand the treatment method and the insulin prescribed, including the effective duration, onset, and peak action. They also need to know the characteristics of the various types of insulins, the proper mixing and dilution of insulins, and how to substitute another type when their usual brand is not available (insulin is a nonprescription drug). Insulin need not be refrigerated but should be maintained at a temperature between 15° C (59° F) and 29.4° C (85° F). Freezing renders insulin inactive.

Insulin bottles that have been "opened" (i.e., the stopper has been punctured) should be stored at room temperature or refrigerated for up to 28 to 30 days. After one month these vials should be discarded. Unopened vials should be refrigerated and are good until the expiration date on the label.

**Injection Procedure.**   Learning to give insulin injections is a source of anxiety for both parents and children. It is helpful for the learner to know that this important aspect of care will become as routine as brushing the teeth. First, the basic injection technique is taught, using an orange or similar item and sterile normal saline for practice.* To gain children's confidence, the nurse can demonstrate the technique by giving a skillful injection to the parent and then having the parent return the demonstration by giving the nurse an injection. With practice and confidence, the par-

---

*Home care instructions on giving subcutaneous injections are available in Wong DL, Hess CS: *Wong and Whaley's clinical manual of pediatric nursing,* ed 5, St Louis, 2000, Mosby.

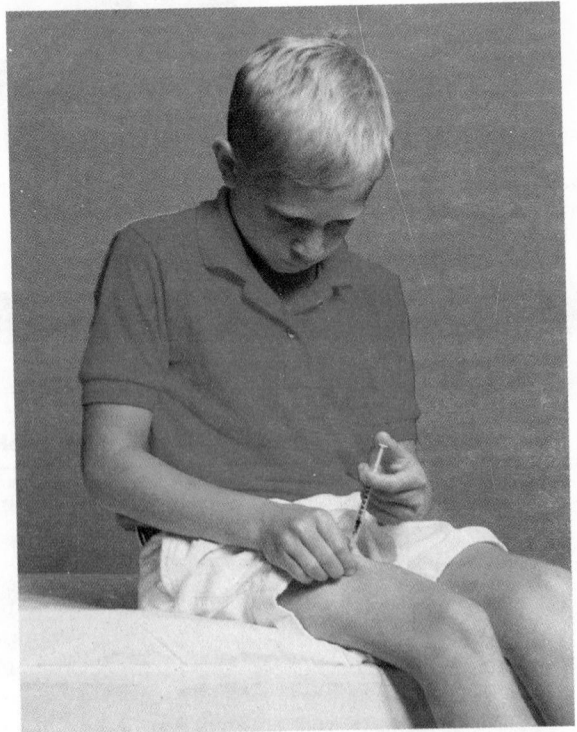

**Fig. 38-9**   School-age children are able to administer their own insulin.

ents will soon be able to give the insulin injection to their children, and their children will trust them. Another effective strategy is to instruct the children and then have them teach the technique to the parents while the nurse observes. Both parents should participate, and as little time as possible should elapse between instruction and the actual injection, especially with parents and teenage learners.

Insulin can be injected into any area in which there is adipose (fat) tissue over muscle; the drug is injected at a 90-degree angle. Newly diagnosed children may have lost adipose tissue, and care should be exerted not to inject intramuscularly. The pinch technique is the most effective method for obtaining tenting of the skin to allow easy entrance of the needle to subcutaneous tissues in children. The site selected will sometimes depend on whether children or parents administer the insulin. The arms, thighs, hips, and abdomen are usual injection sites for insulin. The children can reach the thighs, abdomen, and part of the hip and arm easily but may require help to inject other sites. For example, a parent can pinch a loose fold of skin of the arm while the child injects the insulin.

The parents and child are helped to work out a rotation pattern to various areas of the body to enhance absorption because insulin absorption is slowed by the fat pads that develop in overused injection areas. The most efficient rotation plan involves giving about four to six injections in one area (each injection about 1 inch [2.5 cm] apart, or the diameter of the insulin vial from the previous injection) and then moving to another area.

It is important to remember that the absorption rate varies in different parts of the body (Table 38-7). The methodical use of one anatomic area and then moving to another (as described in the previous paragraph) minimizes variation in absorption rates. However, absorption is also altered by vigorous exercise, which enhances absorption from exercised muscles; therefore it is recommended that a site be chosen other than the exercising extremity (e.g., avoiding legs and arms when playing in a tennis tournament).

Injection sites for an entire month can be determined in advance on a simple chart. For example, the "paper doll" (body outline) described on p. 172 can be constructed and insulin sites marked by the child. After injection, the child places the date on the appropriate site. To keep in practice, it is a good idea for the parent to give two or three injections a week in the areas that are difficult for the child to reach.

The same basic methodology is used when teaching children to give their own insulin injections (Fig. 38-9). They should practice first on an orange or a doll, building

**TABLE 38-7**   Onset and duration of action related to injection site

| | Site of Injection | | | |
|---|---|---|---|---|
| | **Abdomen** | **Arm** | **Leg** | **Buttock** |
| Rate | Very fast | Fast | Slow | Very slow |
| Duration | Very short | Short | Long | Very long |

From Albisser AM, Sperlich M: Adjusting insulins, *Diabetes Educ* 18(3):211-218, 1992.

courage gradually. The first attempt will undoubtedly be awkward because children tend to slowly push the needle through the skin rather than using a quick approach. It is best not to pressure them into assuming this responsibility until they are ready. When children participate in a group learning situation or have an opportunity to observe their peers giving their own injections, they may become more strongly motivated. Parents should be warned that at some time children will give themselves an uncomfortable injection at home and that they will need parental support and encouragement. Otherwise children may not wish to give themselves injections for some time.

Other devices are available for insulin injection and may offer advantages to some children. Children who do not wish to give themselves injections can be taught to use a syringe-loaded injector *(Injectease)*. With the device, puncture is always automatic. Adolescents respond well to a self-contained and compact device resembling a fountain pen *(NovoPen\*),* which eliminates conventional vials and syringes. Preloaded pens may also cause less pain, because the needle is not blunted by piercing the rubber top of the insulin vial (Lteif and Schwenk, 1999).

Teaching includes the proper way to equalize pressure in the bottle by injecting an amount of air equal to the amount of solution withdrawn and how to remove air bubbles from the syringe. When insulin dosages are small, an air bubble in the syringe can displace a significant amount of medication. Since the introduction of the 0.5-ml and 0.3-ml syringes, the risk of incorrect dosage has diminished. Patients who have small doses of mixed insulins should be advised and instructed to use one of these syringes. Insulin syringes should be compared for accuracy, comfort, and strength. The family and child should be able to choose both "their" insulin and "their" syringe from a variety of samples. The needle length and gauge are also factors to consider from the point of view of comfort (e.g., use the shortest and smallest-gauge needle available). Some brands of syringes may be more comfortable than others. When currently available syringes are used, insulin injections of less than 2 units of U100 may have an unacceptably large error. Diluted insulin is sometimes used if the prescribed dose is less than 2 units. Special diluent is needed and is available from the insulin manufacturers (Eli Lilly, 2000).

When the child's dosage requires the injection of both short- and intermediate-acting insulin at the same time, most families prefer to mix the two and use a single injection. Insulin can be premixed and stored in the refrigerator for later use. Commercially prepared insulin mixtures are also available (i.e., 70/30 and 50/50).

To obtain maximum benefit from mixing insulins, the recommended practice is to (1) inject the measured amount of air (equivalent to the dosage) into the long-acting insulin, (2) inject the measured amount of air into the rapid-acting (clear) insulin, and without removing the needle, (3) withdraw the clear insulin and (4) insert the needle (already containing the clear insulin) into the long-acting (cloudy) insulin and then withdraw the desired amount.

**NURSING ALERT**

When mixing types of insulin, always withdraw the clear, rapid-acting insulin into the syringe first, then the long-acting insulin. This avoids contaminating the short-acting insulin with the longer-acting insulin.

The mixture should be injected in less than 5 minutes after mixing (before the zinc content of the long-acting insulin affects the action time of the short-acting insulin) or not until 15 or more minutes after mixing (to allow the insulins to resume long-acting and short-acting properties).

**NURSING ALERT**

Inject insulin within 5 minutes if mixing rapid-acting insulin with an intermediate- or long-acting insulin.

It is acceptable practice to reuse disposable needles and syringes for 1 to 3 days. Bacterial counts are unaffected, and there is a considerable cost saving. It is essential to stress the importance of vigorous handwashing before handling any equipment, as well as capping the syringe immediately after use and storing it in the refrigerator to reduce the growth of organisms. Nurses should also teach proper disposal of equipment after use in the home. Although not standard practice in the hospital, the use of a needle clipper is recommended to safely remove and house the used needle. The syringe plunger can be broken before disposal. An excellent means for syringe disposal is in an opaque, puncture-resistant container, such as an empty coffee can, bleach bottle, or milk carton. The container is labeled "biohazardous waste" and is discarded with similar material only, not with household refuse and consistent with local regulations.

***Continuous subcutaneous insulin infusion.*** Some children are considered candidates for use of a portable insulin pump, and even some young children with unsatisfactory metabolic control can benefit from its use. The child and the parents are taught to operate the device, including the mechanics of the pump, battery changes, and alarm systems. A number of devices are available on the market that vary in the basal rates they are able to deliver and in the cost of the equipment. Families can investigate the various devices and select the model that best suits their needs. Product information is available from pump manufacturers and distributors.\*

Parents and children learn (1) the technical aspects of the pump and self-monitoring of blood glucose; (2) how to prevent and treat hyperglycemia, sick-day management, and meal planning; (3) the effects of exercise, stress, and diet on blood glucose levels; and (4) decision-making strategies to evaluate blood glucose patterns and how to make adjustments in all aspects of the regimen.

Numerous blood glucose measurements (at least four times per day) are an essential part of infusion pump use. Intensive education and supervision are critical to obtaining maximum efficiency and control. This is particularly important if the family has been accustomed to a conventional insulin regimen. They must realize that simply wearing the

---

\*NovoNordisk, Princeton, NJ 08540.

\*Minimed Technologies, Inc, www.minimed.com; Disetronic, www.disetronic-usa.com; Animas, www.animascorp.com.

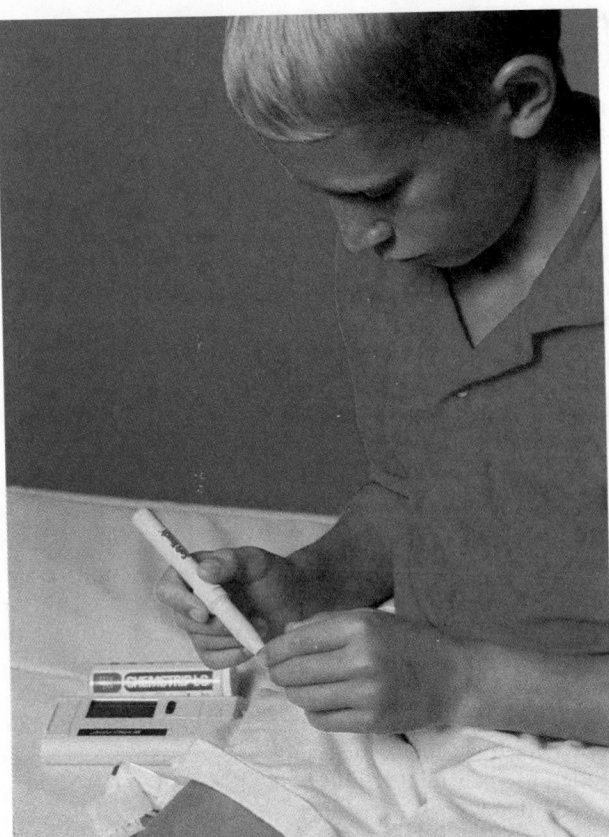

**Fig. 38-10** Child using finger-stick device to obtain blood sample. Blood glucose monitor and reagent strips are nearby.

### ATRAUMATIC CARE
*Minimizing Pain of Blood Glucose Monitoring*

To enhance blood flow to the finger, hold it under warm water for a few seconds before the puncture.

When obtaining blood samples, use the ring finger or thumb (blood flows more easily to these areas), and puncture the finger just to the side of the finger pad (more blood vessels and fewer nerve endings).

To prevent a deep puncture, press the platform of the lancet device lightly against the skin and avoid steadying the finger against a hard surface.

Use lancet devices with adjustable-depth tips. Begin with the most shallow setting.

Use glucose monitors that require very small blood samples to avoid repunctures (e.g., Glucometer Elite).

---

the child and family should learn to use both methods in the event of mechanical failure. Several lancet devices are available from which to choose, and each provides a means for obtaining a large drop of blood for testing (Fig. 38-10).

**NURSING ALERT** Caution children not to allow anyone else to use their lancet because of the risk of contracting hepatitis B virus or human immunodeficiency virus (HIV) infection.

The blood sample may be obtained from either fingertips or alternate sites such as the forearm. Alternate site testing requires a meter that can test small volume of blood. Not all meters are capable of this.

Signs of redness and soreness at the site of finger puncture should be examined by the practitioner. It may be evidence of poor technique, poor hygiene, or poor skin healing relative to poor control. (See Atraumatic Care box.)

Many types of blood-testing meters are available for home use. Newer technology has brought about improvements in meter size and ease of use. The family should be shown features of several meters, including advantages and disadvantages, and allowed to choose equipment that best meets their needs. Availability of acceptable noninvasive technology is still several years away.

The least expensive testing method uses a reagent strip to which blood is applied. After blotting, the color change is compared against a color scale for an estimation of the blood glucose level. The strips can be cut in half (although this is not recommended by all professionals) to obtain two readings per strip. This method is not accepted practice but may be necessary for some families or situations.

*Urine testing.* Testing for urinary ketones is recommended during times of illness or when blood glucose values are elevated. Information on a specific ketone testing product should include correct procedure, storage, and product expiration. Families need a clear understanding of home management of ketones: fluids and additional insulin as directed by the health care team.

*Shopping.* Diabetic maintenance is not an inexpensive necessity. Families are advised to investigate all sources of obtaining supplies for managing the disease. Prices are of-

pump will not normalize blood glucose. The pump is merely an insulin delivery device, and frequent, routine blood glucose determinations are necessary to adjust the insulin delivery rate.

The major problem with use of the insulin pump is inflammation from irritation or infection at the insertion site. The site should be cleaned thoroughly before the needle is inserted and then covered with a transparent dressing. The site is changed and rotated every 48 to 72 hours (this may vary) or at the first sign of inflammation. Nurses working where the pumps are part of the therapeutic regimen should become familiar with the operation of the specific device being used and the protocol of disease management. Others should be aware of this management technique and be prepared to assist patients who have this method in operation.

**Monitoring.** Nurses should also be prepared to teach and supervise blood glucose monitoring. SMBG is associated with very few complications, and although it does not necessarily lead to improved metabolic control, it provides a more accurate assessment of blood glucose levels than can be obtained with the historical urine testing. Blood glucose monitoring has the added advantage that it can be performed anywhere.

Blood for testing can be obtained by two different methods: manually or with a mechanical bloodletting device. A mechanical device is recommended for children, although

ten lower when supplies are purchased in volume; however, it is not advisable to buy bulk items that are unfamiliar or untried, because the new items may not be satisfactory for the individual child or may become outdated before they are used. Costs vary considerably among pharmacies and other suppliers, including the numerous discount mail-order establishments. When buying by mail, it is important to find a supplier that responds to the family's satisfaction and to allow ample time for delivery to avoid running out of supplies. Parents are also cautioned not to substitute insulins or the type of insulin syringe (e.g., a 1-ml syringe for the low-dose type) simply to save money. Parent groups and the local ADA can offer some suggestions for investigation. Most states have legislation mandating that insurance companies cover the cost of diabetes supplies and education.

**Hyperglycemia.** Severe hyperglycemia is most often caused by illness, growth, emotional upset, or missed insulin doses. Emotional stress from school finals or examinations or physical response to immunizations are examples of causes of hyperglycemia. With careful glucose monitoring, any elevation can be managed by adjustment of insulin or food intake. Parents should understand how to adjust food, activity, and insulin at the time of illness or when the child is treated for an illness with a medication known to raise the blood glucose level (e.g., steroids). The hyperglycemia is managed by increasing insulin soon after the increased glucose level is noted. Health care professionals should be aware that adolescent girls often become hyperglycemic around the time of their menses and should be advised to increase insulin dosages if necessary.

**Hypoglycemia.** Hypoglycemia is caused by imbalances of food intake, insulin, and activity. Ideally hypoglycemia should be prevented, and parents need to be prepared to prevent, recognize, and treat the problem. They should be familiar with the signs of hypoglycemia and instructed in treatment, including care of the child with seizures. (See Chapter 37.) Early signs are *adrenergic,* including sweating and trembling, which help raise the blood glucose level, much like the reaction when an individual is startled or anxious. The second set of symptoms that follow an untreated adrenergic reaction are *neuroglycopenic* (also called brain hypoglycemia). These symptoms typically include difficulty with balance, memory, attention, or concentration; dizziness or light-headedness; and slurred speech. Severe and prolonged hypoglycemia leads to seizures, coma, and possible death (Cryer, 2000). Hypoglycemia can be managed effectively as outlined in the Emergency Treatment box.

It is advisable for parents to plan for anticipated excitement or exercise. In addition, gastroenteritis may decrease insulin needs slightly as a result of poor appetite, vomiting, or diarrhea. If the blood glucose level is low but urinary ketones are present, the family should be aware of the increased need for simple carbohydrates and liquids.

**Hygiene.** All aspects of personal hygiene should be emphasized for the child with diabetes. The child should be cautioned against wearing shoes without socks, wearing sandals, or walking barefoot. Correct nail and extremity care tailored to the individual child (with the guidance of a po-

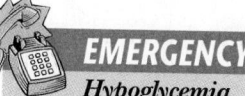

## EMERGENCY TREATMENT
### Hypoglycemia

**MILD REACTION: ADRENERGIC SYMPTOMS**

Give child 10 to 15 g of simple, high carbohydrate (preferably liquid, e.g., 3 to 6 ounces of orange juice).
Follow with starch-protein snack.

**MODERATE REACTION: NEUROGLYCOPENIC SYMPTOMS**

Give child 10 to 15 g of simple carbohydrate as above.
Repeat in 10 to 15 minutes if symptoms persist.
Follow with larger snack.
Watch child closely.

**SEVERE REACTION: UNRESPONSIVE, UNCONSCIOUS, OR SEIZURES**

Administer glucagon as prescribed.
Follow with planned meal or snack when child is able to eat, or add a snack of 10% of daily calories.

**NOCTURNAL REACTION**

Give child 10 to 15 g of simple carbohydrate.
Follow with snack of 10% of daily calories.

diatrist) can begin health practices that last a lifetime. Eyes should be checked once a year unless the child wears glasses, and then as directed by the ophthalmologist. Regular dental care is emphasized, and cuts and scratches should be treated with plain soap and water unless otherwise indicated. Diaper rash in infants and candidal infections in teens may indicate poor diabetes control.

**Exercise.** Exercise is an important component of the treatment plan. If the child is more active at one time of the day than at another time, food or insulin can be altered to meet the activity pattern of the individual child. Food should be increased in the summer, when children tend to be more active. Decreased activity on return to school may require a decrease in food intake or increase in insulin dosage. The child who is active in team sports will need additional food intake in the form of a snack about ½ hour before the anticipated activity. Races or other competition may call for a slightly higher food intake than practice times.

Food intake will usually need to be repeated for prolonged activity periods, often as frequently as every 45 minutes to 1 hour. Families should be informed that if increased food is not tolerated, decreased insulin is the next course of action. If the timing of the exercise is changed so that the supper meal is delayed, the insulin in the second or third dose of the day may be moved back to precede the mealtime. Sugar may sometimes be needed during exercise periods for quick response. Elevated blood glucose levels following extreme activity may represent the body's adrenergic response to exercise. If the blood glucose level is elevated (≥240 mg/dl) before planned exercise, urine ketones should be checked and the activity may need be postponed until the blood glucose is controlled.

Without adequate insulin levels the cells are unable to receive glucose, the preferred fuel, despite the high level of blood glucose. The low insulin level allows glucagon to act, uninhibited, to increase hepatic glucose production, further raising the blood glucose level with no means to use sugar at the muscle site. Breakdown of fat (lipolysis) is the alternative, and the end product of lipolysis is ketone body production (White, 2000).

> **NURSING ALERT**
> Ketonuria in the presence of hyperglycemia is an early sign of ketoacidosis and a contraindication to exercise.

**Record Keeping.** Home records are an invaluable aid to diabetes self-management. The nurse and family devise a method to chart insulins administered, blood glucose values, urine ketone results, and other factors and events that affect diabetes control. The child and family are encouraged to observe for patterns of blood glucose responses to events such as exercise. If lapses in management occur (such as eating a candy bar), the child should be encouraged to note this and not be criticized for the transgression.

**Complications.** The implications of the disease should be presented in a tactful, clear, and nonfearful manner. Knowledge of the complications of diabetes and their relationship to control provides a basis for knowledgeable decision making. Eye and kidney disease are the greatest threats, with neurologic complications close behind. Clear explanations of these problems clarify false information often given by well-meaning friends. The information should include discussion of research so that the family is left with the positive impression that others are concerned about finding answers and preventing complications. It also gives them hope that somehow, some way, a prevention or cure will be possible.

**Self-Management.** Self-management is the key to close control. Being able to make changes at the time they are needed rather than waiting until the next contact with health care professionals is important for self-management and gives the individual and family the feeling that they have control over the disease. Psychologically this helps the family members feel that they are useful and participating members of the team. Learning to look at records objectively gives the child support. As children grow and assume more responsibility for self-management, they develop confidence in their ability to manage their disease and confidence in themselves as persons. They learn to respond to the disease and to make more accurate interpretations and changes in self-management when they become adults.

Self-management techniques to be mastered are the testing and adjustment of insulin and diet with alterations in day-to-day activities and anticipation of unusual occurrences. However, guidelines should be provided regarding when to consult with the health care professionals. For instance, the degree of metabolic control before an illness is a determining factor in seeking medical help during the illness. In an individual with poor control, it takes only a few hours before the trouble is severe, whereas if control is good before the illness, several days may elapse before help is needed. Patients and families should be cautioned to seek assistance if glucose levels are elevated and urine is not clear of ketones after 24 hours of self-management.

**Child and Family Support.** Just as the physiologic responses affect the child, the parents and other family members of the child with newly diagnosed DM experience various emotional responses to the crisis. Care in the acute setting is short but may create fears and frustrations. The prospect of a chronic illness in their child engenders all of the feelings and concerns that are faced by parents of children with other chronic illnesses. (See Chapter 22.) The threat of complications and death is always present, as well as the continuing drain on emotional and financial resources.

Certain fears may develop as a result of past experiences with the disease. A severe insulin reaction with seizures is certainly one experience that contributes to fear of repetition. Once parents observe a seizure or the adolescent has one in a public place, the desire to maintain better control is reinforced. They must understand how to prevent problems and how to handle problems calmly and coolly if they occur, and they must understand the complexities of the body, the disease, and its complications. Young children usually adjust well to problems related to the disease. With toddlers and preschoolers, insulin injections and glucose testing may be difficult at first. However, they usually accept the procedures when the parents use a matter-of-fact approach without calling attention to a "hurt" and treat the procedure like any other routine part of the child's life. Following the injection, time with some special and positive attention, such as reading, talking, or another pleasant activity, is one way to convert children who initially refuse injections to those who accept them.

Children in the years before adolescence probably accept their condition most easily. They are able to understand the basic concepts related to their disease and its treatment. They are able to test blood glucose and urine, recognize food groups, give injections, keep records, and distinguish between feelings of fear, excitement, and hypoglycemia. They understand how to recognize, prevent, and treat hypoglycemia. However, they still need considerable parental involvement.

> **NURSING TIP** Ongoing motivation to adhere to a regimen is difficult. An older child and parent (or another caregiver) may enjoy negotiating a day off when the responsibility for testing and recording blood glucose is delegated from the child to the caregiver (or vice versa).

Adolescents appear to have the most difficulty in adjusting. Adolescence is a time when there is much stress toward being perfect and being like one's peers, and no matter what others say, having diabetes is being different. Some adolescents are more upset about not being able to have a candy bar than about injections, diet, and other aspects of management. If children can accept the difference as a part of life, in other words, that each person is different in some way, then with adequate parental support they should be able to adjust well.

Problems of adjustment to diabetes are especially difficult for the young person whose disease is diagnosed in adolescence. Denial is sometimes expressed by omitting insulin, not performing tests, and eating incorrectly, although denial of the disease usually diminishes during this period as the adolescent with DM begins to feel competent and worthy. Diabetes makes the teenager different when conformity and sameness are desired; having the disease emphasizes vulnerability and imperfection when the search for identity is the foremost developmental task of adolescence. It is often difficult for the adolescent to know what to tell friends.

Camping and other special groups are very useful. At diabetes camp, children learn that they are not alone. As a result, they become more independent and resourceful in the nondiabetes camp setting, especially if they have had experience in a diabetes camp. Useful information about such camps and organizations can be obtained from the ADA. A list of accredited camps specifically for children and teenagers with diabetes is also available from the **American Camping Association.**\*

Puberty is associated with decreased sensitivity to insulin that normally would be compensated for by an increased insulin secretion. Health care professionals should anticipate that pubertal patients will have more difficulty maintaining glycemic control. Insulin doses commonly need to be increased, often dramatically (McConnell and others, 2001). Patients should be taught to give themselves additional doses of rapid-acting insulin (5% to 10% of their daily dose) when their blood glucose levels are increased. The use of supplemental rapid-acting insulin is preferred to withholding food in the adolescent.

Eating disorders, such as bulimia or anorexia nervosa, in the teenager with type 1 DM (see Chapter 21) pose a serious health hazard (Jones and others, 2000). The nurse should be alert to a history of preoccupation with weight, food faddism, excessive caloric restriction, or unexplained hypoglycemia. Moreover, insulin manipulation or omission has been identified as a weight loss tool used by some female adolescents (Bryden and others, 1999).

Inaccurate doses of insulin may occur inadvertently or, if they occur frequently, may be an attention-seeking device; in a number of cases they may demonstrate adolescent depression and, more seriously, a subconscious but socially accepted method of suicide. Excessive intake of food leads to obesity and may also be symptomatic of depression. Psychiatric counseling may be needed if suicidal tendencies are amplified by the diabetes.

Rehospitalizations are most often related to poor control of the disease, although it is also possible that they are indirectly related to noncoping and are a method of avoiding the pressures caused by family and peers. The hospital may represent an environment that is peaceful and free of stress. The goal for this problem is to determine the cause of the hospitalization. It may be related to poor control,

poor self-management, or the need for better supportive management at home. Evaluation should be based on the physiologic and psychologic adjustment of the child and the family.

***Parents.*** Parents develop guilt feelings when they have a child with any chronic disease, especially one with a hereditary component. They cope with these feelings in a number of ways. For example, they may be overprotective or neglectful. Guilt-ridden parents may blame themselves for the disease, consciously or subconsciously. Nevertheless, they must come to realize through education and counseling that there was nothing they could have done to prevent the disease and that it was not their fault, because environmental, as well as hereditary, factors may be involved in the development of the disease.

Parents who are overprotective of the child suffer from feelings of guilt, as well as fear of the unknown. Overprotection is a mechanism that alters the guilt responses to justify the parents' own needs—for example, "If the child is in my sight, nothing worse will happen than has already happened by the child getting diabetes. Therefore I am going to watch this child every single minute so that nothing further can happen to him." The overprotective parent becomes the smothering parent, one who hampers the growth, development, and maturation of the affected child.

The neglectful parent, on the other hand, has a different problem. This response is a mechanism developed to block feelings that give pain and provide relief from feelings of guilt—"This is your disease, and I have no responsibilities related to your disease; therefore, if anything bad happens to you as a result of your having this disease, it is not my fault." The neglectful parent assigns responsibilities to the child before the child is mature enough to accept a more adult role.

Threatened parents look at the disease as a way to keep the child tied to them. If the child learns to be independent, as is expected of the child in a camping experience, the parent may feel threatened and place obstacles in the child's path to independent development. Problems in the parental response provide a challenge for the nurse to assist by counseling or, if severe enough, by appropriately referring the parents to resources designed to help them alter their behavior. (See Critical Thinking Exercise box on p. 1752.)

Children who are sufficiently mature may be seen alone by the health care professional, although the parents should not be made to feel that they are being left out. Time should be set aside during the child's health visit or afterward to meet the needs of the parents. They should also be included in special sessions to keep them abreast of the child's management, to help them continue to participate in the child's care, and to provide them with an opportunity to express their own feelings concerning their own or their child's adjustment to the disease. The amount of information that they offer at this time can give clues to their level of support of the child and help assist in decisions concerning the therapeutic management of the child. This helps guide the

---

\*American Camping Association, 5000 State Rd 67 N, Martinsville, IN 46151, (765) 342-8456; www.acacamps.org.

## Critical Thinking Exercise

### Type 1 Diabetes Mellitus

Rebecca, 15 years old, has a 3-year history of DM and has been admitted to the pediatric intensive care unit for treatment of diabetic ketoacidosis (DKA). This is her fifth hospital admission for DKA in the past year. Rebecca's parents are divorced, and she has four younger siblings, none of whom have diabetes. Rebecca's mother has maintained two jobs for the past 5 years and frequently leaves Rebecca in charge of the household. In anticipation of her discharge, you plan a patient education program for Rebecca and her mother. Areas of diabetes management that must be emphasized are (1) careful dietary management, (2) an appropriate exercise program, (3) conscientious self-testing of blood glucose and appropriate administration of daily insulin, (4) adherence to sliding scale insulin therapy as prescribed, (5) urine ketone testing when blood glucose levels are elevated, and (6) effective methods of handling emotional stressors. Of the following issues that might be influencing the recurrent episodes of DKA, which one should you address initially?

FIRST, THINK ABOUT IT . . .

- What concepts or ideas are central to your thinking?
- What would the consequence be if you put your thoughts into action?

1. The responsibility Rebecca feels for the care of her four younger siblings
2. Fluctuation of blood glucose levels around the time of menses with inadequate insulin dosage
3. Stress related to the absence of Rebecca's mother and the loss of the close relationship Rebecca shared with her father
4. Adolescent issues, such as seeking independence, feeling different from her peers, and alcohol use

*The best response is two. The nurse should concentrate first on situations directly related to hyperglycemia. The concept that adolescent females with diabetes tend to have frequent fluctuation of blood glucose levels, especially increased blood glucose immediately before, during, or after their menses, is correct. Emotional stress related to increased responsibilities, normal developmental tasks of adolescence, and personal loss from divorce can also precipitate a stress response and elevate blood glucose levels. The nurse should address these issues if there is time during teaching or make a referral for special support services, because negative consequences could result if no action is taken.*

child through the most disruptive time of life—the teenage years.

Health care professionals must be aware of parents who voice support and appear to be supporting the child to the optimum level but who, with more in-depth interviewing, are found to be supporting the child in word but not by action. These parents seldom see the need for following through from verbalizing to fulfilling the real needs of the child, and they unknowingly place obstacles in the child's path. They may be helping the child grow up too fast and therefore insecurely. Counseling is urgently needed for these parents, who need to realize how their behavior affects the child. The classroom experience, group therapy, or parenting programs can help guide the parents' relationships with their children. All parents should be guided to recognize that as children grow and develop, they are children first and children with diabetes second. The ultimate goal for these parents is to be supportive of their children, to communicate more effectively with them, and to help their children develop in a more acceptable manner (Wysocki, 1997).

### ▓ Evaluation

The effectiveness of nursing interventions is determined by continual reassessment and evaluation of care based on the following observational guidelines:

1. Interview the family to determine their understanding of the disease; have the child and family demonstrate and discuss the needed assessment and the therapeutic techniques involved.
2. Interview the family regarding their understanding of tight control; analyze and evaluate management records.
3. Discuss the disease with child.
4. Interview the family and child regarding their feelings and concerns about the disease.

The *expected outcomes* are described in the Nursing Care Plan on pp. 1752-1755.

## Nursing Care Plan
### The Child with Diabetes Mellitus

### HOSPITAL CARE

> **NURSING DIAGNOSIS:** Risk for injury related to insulin deficiency

**PATIENT GOAL 1:** Will exhibit normal blood glucose levels

- **NURSING INTERVENTIONS/*RATIONALES***

Obtain blood glucose level *to determine most appropriate dose of insulin*

\*Administer insulin as prescribed *to maintain normal blood glucose level*

Understand the action of insulin

    Understand the differences in composition, time of onset, and duration of action for the various insulin preparations *to ensure accurate insulin administration*

Employ insulin techniques when preparing and administering insulin

Subcutaneous injection; depth according to thickness of subcutaneous tissue

Rotation of sites *to enhance absorption of insulin*

- **EXPECTED OUTCOME**

Child demonstrates normal blood glucose levels

---

\*Dependent nursing action.

# Nursing Care Plan
## The Child with Diabetes Mellitus—cont'd

---

**NURSING DIAGNOSIS:** Risk for injury related to hypoglycemia

**PATIENT GOAL 1:** Will exhibit no evidence of hypoglycemia

- **NURSING INTERVENTIONS/*RATIONALES***

Recognize signs of hypoglycemia early
    Be particularly alert at times when blood glucose levels are lowest (11:00 AM and 2:30 AM) (e.g., bursts of physical activity without additional food, or delayed, omitted, or incompletely consumed meal or snack)
    Test blood glucose
Offer 10 to 15 g of readily absorbed carbohydrates, such as orange juice, hard candy, or milk, *to elevate blood glucose level and alleviate symptoms of hypoglycemia*
Follow with complex carbohydrate and protein, such as bread or cracker spread with peanut butter or cheese *to maintain blood glucose level*
\*Administer glucagon to unconscious child *to elevate blood glucose level;* position child *to minimize risk of aspiration, because vomiting may occur*

- **EXPECTED OUTCOMES**

Child ingests an appropriate carbohydrate
Child displays no evidence of hypoglycemia

## PREPARATION FOR HOME CARE

---

**NURSING DIAGNOSIS:** Deficient knowledge (diabetes management) related to care of a child with newly diagnosed diabetes mellitus

**PATIENT/FAMILY GOAL 1:** Will accept teaching provided

- **NURSING INTERVENTIONS/*RATIONALES***

Select methods, vocabulary, and content appropriate to the level of the learner *to maximize learning*
Allow 3 or 4 days for family and child to begin to adjust to the initial impact of the diagnosis
Select an environment conducive to learning
Allow ample time for the education process
Restrict length of teaching sessions *because this is how people learn best*
    Child—15-20 minutes
    Parents—45-60 minutes
Involve all senses and employ a variety of teaching strategies, especially participation *because it is usually the most effective method for learning*
Provide pamphlets or other supplementary materials *for future referral*

- **EXPECTED OUTCOME**

Child and/or family display attitudes conducive to learning

**PATIENT/FAMILY GOAL 2:** Will demonstrate understanding of the disease and its therapy

- **NURSING INTERVENTIONS/*RATIONALES***

Provide information regarding the pathophysiology of diabetes and the function and actions of insulin and glucagon in relation to caloric intake and exercise
Answer questions and clarify misconceptions *to ensure optimum learning*
Explain function and expected effects of procedures and tests *because these are a necessary part of diabetes management*

- **EXPECTED OUTCOME**

Child and family demonstrate an understanding of the disease and its therapy (specify indicators)

**PATIENT/FAMILY GOAL 3:** Will demonstrate understanding of meal planning

- **NURSING INTERVENTIONS/*RATIONALES***

Enlist the services of a dietitian *to teach meal planning*
Emphasize the relationship between normal nutritional needs and the disease *to encourage a sense of normalcy*
Become familiar with family's culture and food preferences *so that these are included in meal planning*
Teach or reinforce learners' understanding of the basic food groups and the meal plan prescribed (e.g., carbohydrate counting, exchange diet)
Help child and family estimate portion sizes *because this is more practical than weighing food*
Suggest low-carbohydrate snack items
Guide family in assessing the labels of food products for carbohydrate content *because concentrated sugars are minimized in the diet*
Teach or reinforce an understanding of the concept of exchanges or carbohydrate choices *because these systems ensure day-to-day consistency in total intake while allowing a choice of foods*
Relate constant carbohydrate equivalents to familiar foods
Retain cultural patterns and family preferences as much as possible *so that child and family are more likely to adhere to diet requirements*

- **EXPECTED OUTCOME**

Child and family demonstrate an understanding of meal planning and food selection (specify indicators)

**PATIENT/FAMILY GOAL 4:** Will demonstrate knowledge of and ability to administer insulin

- **NURSING INTERVENTIONS/*RATIONALES***

Teach child and family the characteristics of the insulins prescribed for child, *because there are several insulin preparations*
Teach proper mixing of insulins
Teach injection procedure
    Impress on learners that the procedure will be a routine part of child's life *in order to decrease anxiety and increase cooperation*
    Involve caregivers and child, if old enough, *so that more than one person learns procedure*
    Teach basic techniques using an orange or similar item *so that learner can gain confidence before injecting a person*

---

\*Dependent nursing action.

*Continued*

# Nursing Care Plan
## The Child with Diabetes Mellitus—cont'd

### PATIENT/FAMILY GOAL 4—cont'd

- **NURSING INTERVENTIONS/*RATIONALES*—cont'd**

Teach injection procedure—cont'd

Use demonstration and return demonstration techniques on another before injecting child *because this is usually less stressful*

Help families and child work out a set rotational pattern *because this is important for maximum absorption of insulin*

Teach proper care of insulin and equipment

Teach management of continuous infusion pump (if used)

- **EXPECTED OUTCOMES**

Child and family demonstrate an understanding of insulin, its various forms, and action (specify indicators)

Child and family demonstrate injection technique correctly

Child and family develop an injection site rotation plan

Child and family demonstrate correct use of pump and care of injection site

### PATIENT/FAMILY GOAL 5: Will demonstrate ability to test blood glucose level

- **NURSING INTERVENTIONS/*RATIONALES***

Teach family and child, if old enough:

Blood glucose monitoring or use of equipment selected for use

Interpretation of results *so that they learn how to adjust insulin based on blood glucose level*

Care and maintenance of equipment

- **EXPECTED OUTCOME**

Child and family demonstrate correct use of the glucose monitoring equipment

### PATIENT/FAMILY GOAL 6: Will demonstrate ability to test urine

- **NURSING INTERVENTIONS/*RATIONALES***

Teach family and child, if old enough:

Urine ketone testing and interpretation of results

Proper care of test strips

- **EXPECTED OUTCOME**

Child and family demonstrate urine testing and interpretation

### PATIENT/FAMILY GOAL 7: Will demonstrate understanding of proper hygiene

- **NURSING INTERVENTIONS/*RATIONALES***

Emphasize the importance of personal hygiene *so that child establishes health practices that last a lifetime*

Encourage regular dental care and yearly ophthalmologic examinations *because these are important for child's general health*

Teach proper care of cuts and scratches *to minimize risk of infection*

Teach proper foot care *because this will become a high priority during adulthood*

- **EXPECTED OUTCOME**

Child and family demonstrate an understanding of the importance of proper hygiene

### PATIENT/FAMILY GOAL 8: Will demonstrate understanding of importance of exercise regimen

- **NURSING INTERVENTIONS/*RATIONALES***

Arrange for occupational therapy program that includes physical activity, *because this is an important part of diabetic management*

Work with child, family, and others (e.g., coaches) to help plan a home exercise program

Reiterate practitioner's instructions regarding adjustment of food or insulin to meet child's activity pattern; reinforce with examples *so that child and family are adequately prepared*

- **EXPECTED OUTCOME**

Child and family help child outline and carry out a regular exercise program

### PATIENT/FAMILY GOAL 9: Will demonstrate understanding and management of hyperglycemia and hypoglycemia

- **NURSING INTERVENTIONS/*RATIONALES***

Instruct learners in how to recognize signs of hyperglycemia and hypoglycemia (especially hypoglycemia) *to prevent delay in treatment*

Explain the relationship of insulin needs to illness, activity, and intense emotion (either positive or negative)

Teach how to adjust food, activity, and insulin at times of illness and during other situations that alter blood glucose levels

Suggest carrying source of carbohydrate, such as sugar cubes or hard candy, in pocket or handbag *so that it is readily available to treat hypoglycemia*

Instruct parents and child in how to treat hypoglycemia with food, simple sugars, or glucagon

- **EXPECTED OUTCOME**

Child and family demonstrate an understanding of the signs and management of a hypoglycemic reaction (specify)

### PATIENT GOAL 10: Will wear medical identification

- **NURSING INTERVENTIONS/*RATIONALES***

Encourage acquisition of a means of identification, such as an identification bracelet, that explains child's condition *in case of emergency*

Explain to child why identification is important *so that child is more likely to comply*

- **EXPECTED OUTCOME**

Family acquires and child wears identification bracelet

### PATIENT/FAMILY GOAL 11: Will keep proper records of insulin administration and testing procedures

- **NURSING INTERVENTIONS/*RATIONALES***

Help child and family to design a form for keeping records of the following *because this information is useful to both practitioner and family in managing diabetes:*

Insulin administered

Blood and urine tests

Food intake

Marked variation in exercise

Illness

# Nursing Care Plan
## The Child with Diabetes Mellitus—cont'd

- **EXPECTED OUTCOME**

Family and child keep accurate record of insulin administration, glucose testing, and so on

- **PATIENT/FAMILY GOAL 12:** Will engage in self-management

- **NURSING INTERVENTIONS/RATIONALES**

Encourage honesty in recording, such as eating a forbidden candy bar, *so that recording is accurate and useful*

Encourage independence in applying the concepts learned in teaching sessions *because diabetes management is a lifelong endeavor*

Instruct when to seek assistance from medical personnel *to prevent delay in treatment*

- **EXPECTED OUTCOME**

Child takes responsibility for management of disease commensurate with age and capabilities

> **NURSING DIAGNOSIS:** Interrupted family processes related to situational crisis (child with a chronic disorder)

See also Nursing Care Plan: The Child with Chronic Illness or Disability, Chapter 22

## KEY POINTS

- The endocrine system has three components: the cell, which sends a chemical message via a hormone; target cells, which receive the message; and the environment through which the chemical is transported from the site of synthesis to the sites of cellular action.
- Pituitary dysfunction is manifested primarily by growth disturbance.
- The main physiologic action of the thyroid hormone is to regulate the basal metabolic rate and control the processes of growth and tissue differentiation.
- Disorders of thyroid function include hypothyroidism, autoimmune thyroiditis, goiter, and hyperthyroidism.
- Therapy for hyperthyroidism is directed at retarding the rate of hormone secretion and may include drug therapy, thyroidectomy, or radioiodine therapy.
- Classic forms of hypoparathyroidism in childhood are idiopathic—deficient production of parathormone (PTH)—and pseudohypoparathyroidism—increased PTH production with end-organ unresponsiveness to PTH.

- The adrenal cortex secretes three important groups of hormones: glucocorticoids, mineralocorticoids, and sex steroids.
- Disorders of adrenal function include acute adrenocortical insufficiency, chronic adrenocortical insufficiency, Cushing syndrome, congenital adrenal hyperplasia, and hyperaldosteronism.
- Five categories of Cushing syndrome are pituitary, adrenal, ectopic, iatrogenic, and food dependent.
- Management of congenital adrenal hyperplasia includes assignment of a sex according to genotype, administration of cortisone, and, possibly, reconstructive surgery.
- Diabetes mellitus is categorized as type 1 diabetes, type 2 diabetes, and maturity-onset diabetes of youth.
- The focus of type 1 diabetes management is insulin replacement, diet, and exercise.
- Education of families includes explanation of diabetes, meal planning, administering insulin injections, monitoring general hygienic practices, promoting exercise, record keeping, and observing for complications.

## REFERENCES

Allen DB, Johanson AJ, Blizzard RM: Growth hormone treatment. In Lifshitz F, editor: *Pediatric endocrinology*, ed 3, New York, 1996, Marcel Dekker, Inc.

American Academy of Pediatrics, Committee on Drugs and Committee on Bioethics: Considerations related to the use of recombinant human growth hormone in children, *Pediatrics* 99(1):122-129, 1997.

American Academy of Pediatrics, Section on Endocrinology and Committee on Genetics: Technical report: congenital adrenal hyperplasia, *Pediatrics* 106(6):1511-1518, 2000.

American Diabetes Association: Type 2 diabetes in children and adolescents, *Pediatrics* 105(3):671-680, 2000a.

American Diabetes Association: Type 2 diabetes in children and adolescents, *Diabetes Care* 22(12):381-389, 2000b.

American Diabetes Association: Report of the Expert Committee on the Diagnosis and Classification of Diabetes Mellitus, *Diabetes Care* 24(suppl 1):S5-S20, 2001.

Anhalt H, Chin D: Endocrine treatment for short stature, *Pediatr Ann* 29(9):576-581, 2000.

Bartley GB and others: Chronology of Graves' ophthalmopathy in an incidence cohort, *Am J Ophthalmol* 121(4):426-434, 1996.

Baxter JD, Ribeiro RCJ: Introduction to endocrinology. In Greenspan FS, Gardner DG, editors: *Basic and clinical endocrinology*, ed 6, New York, 2001, Lange Medical Books/McGraw-Hill.

Behrman RE, Kliegman RM, Jenson HB: *Nelson textbook of pediatrics*, ed 16, Philadelphia, 2000, WB Saunders.

Beisswenger P, Szwergold B, Yeo K: Glycated proteins in diabetes, *Clin Lab Med* 21(10):53-78, 2001.

Blondell RD, Foster MB, Dave KC: Disorders of puberty, *Am Fam Physician* 60(1):209-218, 1999.

Bode HH, Crawford JD, Danon M: Disorders of antidiuretic hormone homeostasis: diabetes insipidus and SIADH. In Lifshitz F, editor: *Pediatric endocrinology*, ed 3, New York, 1996, Marcel Dekker.

Brosnan C, Upchurch S, Schreiner B: Type 2 diabetes in children and adolescents: an emerging disease, *J Pediatr Health Care* 15(4):187-193, 2001.

Bryden K and others: Eating habits, body weight, and insulin misuse: a longitudinal study of teenagers and young adults with type 1 diabetes, *Diabetes Care* 22(12): 1956-1960, 1999.

Carel J-C, Chaussain J-L: Gonadotropin releasing hormone against treatment for central precocious puberty, *Horm Res* 51(suppl 3):64-69, 1999.

Cheetham TD and others: Treatment of hyperthyroidism in young people, *Arch Dis Child* 78(3):207-209: 1998.

Cryer P: Glucose counterregulatory hormones: physiology, pathophysiology, and relevance to clinical hypoglycemia. In Le Roith D, Taylor S, Olefsky J, editors: *Diabetes mellitus: a fundamental and clinical text*, ed 5, Philadelphia, 2000, Lippincott, Williams & Wilkins.

Dallas JS, Foley TP: Hyperthyroidism. In Lifshitz F, editor: *Pediatric endocrinology*, ed 3, New York, 1996, Marcel Dekker.

Diabetes Control and Complications Trial Research Group: The effect of intensive treatment of diabetes on the development and progression of long-term complications in insulin-dependent diabetes mellitus, *N Eng J Med* 329(14):977-986, 1993.

Eli Lilly: *Humalog package insert*, Indianapolis, May 1, 2000, Eli Lilly.

Fagot-Campagna A: Emergence of type 2 diabetes mellitus in children: epidemiological evidence, *J Pediatr Endocrinol Metab* 13(suppl 6):1395-1402, 2000.

Fajans S, Bell G: Maturity-onset diabetes of the young: a model for genetic studies of diabetes mellitus. In Le Roith D, Taylor S, Olefsky J, editors: *Diabetes mellitus: a fundamental and clinical text*, ed 2, Philadelphia, 2000, Lippincott, Williams & Wilkins.

Foley TP: Hypothyroidism. In Hoekelman RA and others, editors: *Primary pediatric care*, ed 4, St Louis, 2001, Mosby.

Gardner SG and others: Progression to diabetes in relatives with islet autoantibodies, *Diabetes Care* 22(12):2049-2054, 1999.

Glaser N and others: Risk factors for cerebral edema in children with diabetic ketoacidosis. *N Engl J Med* 344(4):302-303, 2001.

Guyda HJ: Growth hormone testing and the short child, *Pediatr Res* 48(5):579-580, 2000.

Hall DMB: Growth monitoring, *Arch Dis Child* 82(1):10-15, 2000.

Harris M: Definition and classification of diabetes mellitus and the new criteria for diagnosis. In Le Roith D, Taylor S, Olefsky J, editors: *Diabetes mellitus: a fundamental and clinical text*, ed 5, Philadelphia, 2000, Lippincott, Williams & Wilkins.

Hochberg Z: *Practical algorithms in pediatric endocrinology*, Basel, Switzerland, 1999, S Karger AG.

Hockenberry-Eaton M and others: *Essentials of pediatric oncology nursing: a core curriculum*, Glenview, Ill, 1998, Association of Pediatric Oncology Nurses.

Hoffman RP: Eating disorders in adolescents with Type 1 diabetes: a closer look at a complicated condition, *Postgrad Med* 109(4):67-69, 73-74, 2001.

Huang W and others: Although DR3-DQBI*0201 may be associated with multiple component disease of the autoimmune polyglandular syndromes, the human leukocyte antigen DR4-DQBI*0302 haplotype is implicated only in beta-cell autoimmunity, *J Clin Endocrinol Metab* 81(7):2559-2563, 1996.

Huether SE: Fluids and electrolytes, acids and bases. In Huether SE, McCance KL, editors: *Understanding pathophysiology*, ed 2, St Louis, 2000, Mosby.

Jones J and others: Eating disorders in adolescent females with and without type 1 diabetes: cross sectional study, *Br Med J* 320(7249):1563-1566, 2000.

Jospe N: Hyperthyroidism. In Hoekelman RA and others, editors: *Primary pediatric care*, ed 4, St. Louis, 2001, Mosby.

Kaplowitz PB, Oberfield SE and the Drug and Therapeutics and Executive Committees of the Lawson Wilkins Pediatric Endocrine Society: Reexamination of the age limit for defining when puberty is precocious in girls in the United States: implications for evaluation and treatment, *Pediatrics* 104(4):936-941, 1999.

Kaufman FR, Halvorson M: The treatment and prevention of diabetic ketoacidosis in children and adolescents with type 1 diabetes mellitus, *Pediatr Ann* 28(9):576-582, 1999.

Kimpimaki T and others: Short term exclusive breastfeeding predisposes young children to increased genetic risk of Type 1 diabetes to progressive beta-cell autoimmunity, *Diabetolgia* 44(1):63-69, 2001.

Klein KO: Precocious puberty: who has it? Who should be treated? *J Clin Endocrinol Metab* 84(2):411-414, 1999.

LaPorte R, Matsushima M, Chang Y: Prevalence and incidence of insulin dependent diabetes. In National Diabetes Data Group, NIH: *Diabetes in America*, ed 2, NIH Pub No 95-1468, Bethesda, Md, 1995, NIH.

Lee PA: Central precocious puberty: an overview of diagnosis, treatment, and outcome, *Endocrinol Metab Clin North Am* 28(4):901-918, 1999.

Levine LS: Congenital adrenal hyperplasia, *Pediatr Rev* 21(5):159-170, 2000.

Lifshitz F, Cervantes CD: Short stature. In Lifshitz F, editor: *Pediatric endocrinology*, ed 3, New York, 1996, Marcel Dekker.

Lteif AN, Schwenk WF: Accuracy of pen injectors versus insulin syringes in children with type 1 diabetes, *Diabetes Care* 22(10): 137-140, 1999.

Macchia PE: Recent advances in understanding the molecular basis of primary congenital hypothyroidism, *Mol Med Today* 6(1): 36-42, 2000.

Magee MF, Bhatt BA: Management of decompensated diabetes: diabetic ketoacidosis and hyperglycemic hyperosmolar syndrome, *Crit Care Clin* 17(1):75-106, 2001.

Mauras N and others: Growth hormone stimulation testing in both short and normal statured children: use of an immunofunctional assay, *Pediatr Res* 48(5):614-618, 2000.

McConnell EM and others: Achieving optimal diabetic control in adolescence: the continuing enigma, *Diabetes Metab Res Rev* 17(10):67-74, 2001.

New MI, Ghizzoni L, Speiser PW: Update on congenital adrenal hyperplasia. In Lifshitz F, editor: *Pediatric endocrinology*, ed 3, New York, 1996, Marcel Dekker.

Palmert MR, Malin HV, Boepple PA: Unsustained or slowly progressive puberty in young girls: initial presentation and long-term follow-up of 20 untreated patients, *J Clin Endocrinol Metab* 84(2):415-423, 1999.

Perheentupa J: Hypoparathyroidism and mineral homeostasis. In Lifshitz F, editor: *Pediatric endocrinology*, ed 3, New York, 1996, Marcel Dekker.

Redondo M, Fain P, Eisenbarth G: Genetics of type 1A diabetes, *Recent Prog Horm Res* 56:69-89, 2001.

Robertson RP and others: Pancreas and islet transplantation for patients with diabetes (technical review), *Diabetes Care* 23:112-116, 2000.

Root AW: Precocious puberty, *Pediatr Rev* 21(1):10-19, 2000.

Rovet JF, Ehrlich R: Psychoeducational outcome in children with early-treated congenital hypothyroidism, *Pediatrics* 105(3):515-522, 2000.

Ruble JA: Congenital adrenal hyperplasia. In Jackson PL, Vessey JA, editors: *Primary care of the child with a chronic condition*, ed 2, St Louis, 1996, Mosby.

Schultz CJ and others: Microalbuminuria prevalence varies with age, sex, and puberty in children with type 1 diabetes followed from diagnosis in a longitudinal study, *Diabetes Care* 22(3):495-502, 1999.

Siminerio LM, and others: Comparing outpatient and inpatient diabetes education for newly diagnosed pediatric patients, *Diabetes Educ* 25(6):895-906, 1999.

Skyler J and others: Efficacy of inhaled human insulin in type 1 diabetes mellitus: a randomised proof-of-concept study, *Lancet* 357(9253):324-325, 2001.

Skyler J, Marks J: Immune intervention. In Le Roith D, Taylor S, Olefsky J, editors: *Diabetes mellitus: a fundamental and clinical text*, ed 2, Philadelphia, 2000, Lippincott, Williams & Wilkins.

Stabler, B and others: Evidence of social phobia and other psychiatric disorders in adults who were growth hormone deficient during childhood, *Anxiety* 2(2):86-89, 1996.

Szymborska M, Staroszczyk B: Thyroiditis in children, *Med Wieku Rozwoj* IV(4):383-391, 2000.

Vogiatzi MG, Copeland KC: The short child, *Pediatr Rev* 19(3):92-99, 1998.

Walvoord EC, Pescovitz OH: Combined use of growth hormone and gonadotropin-releasing hormone analogues in precocious puberty: theoretic and practical considerations, *Pediatrics* 104(4):1010-1020, 1999.

Wetterau L, Cohen P: New paradigms for growth hormone therapy in children, *Horm Res* 53(suppl 3):31-36, 2000.

White NH: Diabetic ketoacidosis in children, *Endocrinol Metab Clin North Am* 29(4): 657-682, 2000.

Williams JA: Parenting a daughter with precocious puberty or Turner syndrome, *J Pediatr Health Care* 9(3):109-114, 1995.

Wysocki T: *The ten keys to helping your child grow up with diabetes*, Alexandria, Va, 1997, American Diabetes Association.

Yongsoo P, Eisenbarth G: The natural history of autoimmunity in type 1A diabetes mellitus. In Le Roith D, Taylor S, Olefsky J, editors: *Diabetes mellitus: a fundamental and clinical text*, ed 2, Philadelphia, 2000, Lippincott, Williams & Wilkins.

Zimmerman D, Lteif AN: Thyrotoxicosis: thyrotoxicosis in children, *Endocrinol Metab Clin North Am* 27(1):109-126, 1998.

# Chapter 39

# The Child with Musculoskeletal or Articular Dysfunction

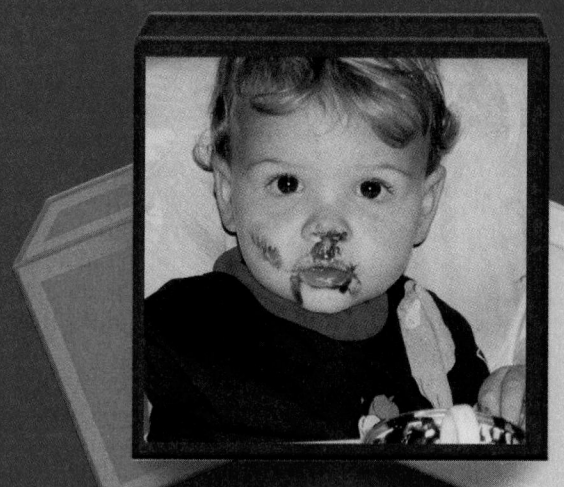

## Chapter Outline

**THE CHILD AND TRAUMA, 1758**
**Trauma Management, 1758**
  Epidemiology of Trauma, 1758
  Prevention of Injury, 1759
**Assessment of Trauma, 1760**
  Emergency Management, 1760
  Systematic Assessment, 1761

**THE IMMOBILIZED CHILD, 1761**
**Immobilization, 1761**
  Physiologic Effects of Immobilization, 1762
  Psychologic Effects of Immobilization, 1766
  Effect on Families, 1767
*Nursing Care Plan: The Child Who Is Immobilized, 1772*
**Mobilization Devices, 1773**
  Orthotics and Prosthetics, 1773
  Crutches and Canes, 1775
  Wheelchairs, 1776

**THE CHILD WITH A FRACTURE, 1776**
**Fractures, 1776**
  Bone Healing and Remodeling, 1781
**The Child in a Cast, 1784**
  The Cast, 1784
**The Child in Traction, 1787**
  Purposes of Traction, 1788
  Types of Traction (General), 1788
  Upper Extremity Traction, 1789
  Lower Extremity Traction, 1789

  Cervical Traction, 1790
**Distraction, 1792**
**External Fixation, 1792**
**Internal Fixation, 1793**
**Fracture Complications, 1793**
  Circulatory Impairment, 1793
  Nerve Compression Syndromes, 1793
  Compartment Syndromes, 1793
  Epiphyseal Damage, 1794
  Nonunion, 1794
  Malunion, 1794
  Infection, 1794
  Kidney Stones, 1794
  Pulmonary Emboli, 1795
**Amputation, 1795**

**INJURIES AND HEALTH PROBLEMS RELATED TO SPORTS PARTICIPATION, 1796**
**Preparation for Sports, 1796**
**Types of Injury, 1797**
**Contusions, 1798**
**Dislocations, 1798**
**Sprains and Strains, 1799**
**Overuse Syndrome, 1800**
  Stress Fractures, 1801
**Heat Injury/Illness, 1801**
**Underwater Sports–Related Injuries, 1802**
  Sports and Accidental Drowning, 1802

**Health Concerns Associated with Sports, 1802**
  Nutrition, 1802
  Considerations for the Female Athlete, 1804
  Drug Misuse by Athletes, 1804
  Sudden Death, 1805
**Nurse's Role in Children's Sports, 1805**

**MUSCULOSKELETAL DYSFUNCTION, 1807**
**Torticollis, 1807**
**Legg-Calvé-Perthes Disease, 1807**
**Slipped Femoral Capital Epiphysis, 1808**
**Kyphosis and Lordosis, 1809**
**Scoliosis, 1810**
*Nursing Care Plan: The Child with Structural Scoliosis, 1815*

**ORTHOPAEDIC INFECTIONS, 1817**
**Osteomyelitis, 1817**
**Septic Arthritis, 1818**
**Tuberculosis, 1818**
  Skeletal Tuberculosis, 1818

**SKELETAL AND ARTICULAR DYSFUNCTION, 1819**
**Osteogenesis Imperfecta (OI), 1819**
**Juvenile Rheumatoid Arthritis, (Juvenile Idiopathic Arthritis), 1820**
*Nursing Care Plan: The Child with Juvenile Rheumatoid Arthritis, 1826*
**Systemic Lupus Erythematosus (SLE), 1825**

## Related Topics

Back and Extremities, Ch. 7
Birth Injuries, Ch. 9
Care of the Family Experiencing Unexpected Childhood Death, Ch. 23
Compliance, Ch. 27
Congenital Clubfoot, Ch. 11
Developmental Dysplasia of the Hip, Ch. 11

Family-Centered Care of the Child with Chronic Illness or Disability, Ch. 22
Family-Centered Home Care, Ch. 25
Head Injury, Ch. 37
Injuries—The Leading Killer, Ch. 1

Injury Prevention: Infant, Ch. 12; Toddler, Ch. 14; Preschooler, Ch. 15; School-Age Child, Ch. 17; Adolescent, Ch. 19
Maintaining Healthy Skin, Ch. 27
Pain Assessment; Pain Management, Ch. 26
Physical Abuse, Ch. 16
Physical Activity, Ch. 17

# THE CHILD AND TRAUMA

## Trauma Management

### Epidemiology of Trauma

Trauma is a leading cause of death in children over age 1 year (see Chapter 1) and an important cause of disability during childhood and adolescence. In many ways, childhood trauma differs little from trauma in adults. However, many aspects of injury are affected by the developmental stage of the child in both the type of injury that is incurred and the physiologic response to injury.

**Nonintentional Injury.** Among the leading causes of morbidity in children are medical problems resulting from traumatic injury at home, at school, in an automobile, or associated with recreational activities. Children's everyday activities include vigorous play, such as climbing, falling, running into immovable objects, and receiving blows to any part of their body. All of these activities make them prone to injury. School-age children and adolescents are vulnerable to multiple and severe trauma because they are mobile on bikes and motorcycles and in automobiles; they are also active in sports. Speed and congested surroundings often intensify the chance of injury.

Young children and teenagers usually do not calculate risks as they learn to manipulate their environment and achieve developmental goals. Therefore accidents are a part of many childhood experiences. Fortunately, when children fall or are hit, their body's resilience protects them from incurring serious damage to soft tissue, the musculoskeletal system, or other body organs. Their bones are more flexible

---

■ Jean Brown, MS, RNC, and David Wilson, MS, RNC, revised this chapter.

---

and therefore do not offer the rigid resistance to external forces that are likely to cause fractures (as occurs in more mature bones).

**Child Abuse Injury.** Unfortunately, careless handling of an infant or child (in some instances intentional physical abuse) is not uncommon. A multitude of different types of bone and soft tissue injuries are inflicted on children by adults, and smaller children who are unable to protect themselves are most vulnerable. It is estimated that perhaps 25% of fractures in children under 3 years of age are the result of child abuse. Emergency department and pediatric of-

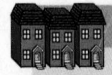

## COMMUNITY FOCUS
### General Injury Prevention Guidelines

**MOTOR VEHICLE ACCIDENTS**

For infants, use a rear-facing infant seat in the middle of the backseat. After 20 pounds, use front-facing infant/toddler seat until child is approximately 4 years/40 pounds, then use a booster seat. Avoid front seat if air bags are present. Provide supervision while playing near and crossing streets. For teenagers, provide driver's education and education regarding hazards of drinking and driving. Encourage helmets while riding motorcycles and all-terrain vehicles.

**FIRES/BURNS**

Set hot water tanks to a maximum safe temperature. Temperatures warmer than 48.9° C (120° F) are considered "too hot for tots." Install smoke detectors. Cover electric outlets. Turn pot handles in on stove. With school-age child, practice stop-drop-roll and escape routes. Keep away from matches, cigarette lighters, and other instant lighters.

**DROWNING**

Never leave child alone in tub. Fence in pools, fish tanks, ground-level garden ponds; provide supervision while swimming; and encourage swimming lessons. Warn teenagers about risks of drinking and swimming/boating.

**FALLS**

Never leave infant unattended on changing table or other raised surface. Avoid walkers and place gates at top and bottom of stairs. Install window guards.

**BICYCLE INJURIES**

Use approved and properly fitting helmets. Teach bike safety.

**FIREARM INJURIES**

Remove guns from home or use secure storage practices. Teach children not to touch a gun if found. Teach older children proper use of a firearm for hunting purposes.

**SPORTS INJURIES**

Encourage proper training, conditioning, and warm-up. Deemphasize competition and emphasize "fun" aspect of sports activities (see Community Focus box, on p. 1806).

**POISONINGS**

Choose childproof lids on medications and vitamins. Store medications and household cleaning products out of child's reach or in locked area. Inspect motor vehicle exhaust system and adequately ventilate heating systems.

---

Data from Crawley T: Childhood injury: significance and prevention strategies, *J Pediatr Nurs* 11(4):225-232, 1996; and Rivara FP, Grossman DC: Prevention of traumatic deaths to children in the United States: how far have we come and where do we need to go? *Pediatrics* 97(6):791-797, 1996.

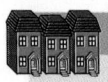

## COMMUNITY FOCUS
### Distinguishing Nonintentional from Intentional Fractures

Distinguishing abusive from nonintentional fractures can be challenging. The history, location of the injury, x-ray data, and associated injuries must be carefully considered. Details of the history to consider include delay in seeking medical care and an inappropriate clinical history or the report of a change in the child but no report of injury.

Although not diagnostic of an intentional injury, the location of a fracture can raise suspicions about the actual cause. In an infant, midshaft or metaphyseal humerus fractures and radius/ulna, tibia/fibula, or femur fractures are not common and raise suspicion about the likelihood of abusive behavior. Rib fractures, scapular fractures, bilateral fractures, complex skull fractures, and vertebral fractures or subluxations are also suspicious (Della-Giustina and Della-Guistina, 1999). In contrast, in children over 1 year of age, supracondylar humerus fractures and fractures of the clavicle, distal extremity, and femur are most frequently related to a nonintentional injury. In children of all ages, x-ray evidence of previous fractures at different stages of healing may be indicative of repeated trauma and raise concern about intentional injuries. The presence of bruising, burns, and additional soft tissue injuries in children may also prompt further evaluation to see if the child has been subjected to intentional harm. One mnemonic used for awareness to consider the possibility of abuse is "B-5: *bumps, bruises, breaks, burns,* and anything that happens in the *bathroom.*"

fice personnel should be alert to situations in which the child's injuries are not congruent with the parent's description of the incident; in which the child's behaviors, such as fearful mannerisms or lack of crying, are not the expected ones; or in which x-ray films show multiple healed fractures. Accounts of injury inconsistent with developmental abilities can alert the provider to possible abuse. For example, a 6-month-old infant can not "climb out of the crib and break her or his leg." Reporting these incidents will aid in securing help for the child and family. A traumatic incident that produces physical injury to an infant or child may be the outcome of an accident that was no one's fault, or it may be associated with child abuse. A well-documented history and a careful examination are essential to determine the cause of the injury. (See Community Focus box; see Physical Abuse, Chapter 16.)

**Childhood Characteristics.** Certain developmental characteristics of children at various ages render them more susceptible to injury. For example, the large head of infants and toddlers predisposes them to head injury, especially in falls or motor vehicle injuries. Also, the relatively large spleen and liver and the broad costal arch make these organs prone to direct trauma. Because of their light weight and small size, infants and small children are easily thrown around in a moving vehicle. Their natural curiosity and their propensity for using large muscles lure them to attempt potentially hazardous activities.

Later, in school-age children and adolescents, whose bone growth outstrips muscle growth, difficulty controlling movement can contribute to physical injury. It is also a time when many of these youngsters are attempting to engage in activities beyond their capabilities to keep up with more agile companions. They are also vulnerable to a "dare." Risk-taking compounded by a feeling of invulnerability is also characteristic of adolescence.

### Prevention of Injury

Increasingly, health care providers are recognizing the importance of injury prevention efforts in preserving the health and well-being of children. Nurses have an important role to play in these efforts. (See Community Focus box and Evidence-Based Practice box.)

## EVIDENCE-BASED PRACTICE
### Injury Prevention

Leading causes of injury to children include violence (assault), motor vehicle accidents, fires and burns, bicycle accidents, pedestrian injuries, falls, drowning, and firearms (Crawley, 1996). A recent survey of childhood injuries found that violence, motor vehicle trauma, and burns accounted for a major portion of injuries to children over 1 year of age. Injuries in adolescents accounted for 49% of all injuries (Scheidt and others, 2000). Vital statistics show that 43.9% of deaths in children over 1 year of age in 1998 occurred as a result of unintentional injuries; homicide accounted for 9.5% of all childhood deaths (1 to 19 years of age), and firearms were involved in 7% of all injury deaths in the same age group (Guyer and others, 2000).

Poisonings also occur in the young child, and sports injuries occur in school-age children and adolescents. Unintentional preventable injury is the primary cause of pediatric mortality and a significant contributor to morbidity, including permanent disability. Both morbidity and mortality could be reduced dramatically by improved efforts at injury prevention (Cramer, 1995; Patterson, 1999). Studies have shown that there is a general lack of public awareness regarding risks, causes, and prevention of injury to children. Studies indicate that injury prevention counseling is effective both in reducing hazards in the home and in increasing car seat use (Bass and others, 1993). One literature review cites the effectiveness of building fences around pools to prevent drownings in preschool children (Thompson and Rivara, 2000). Nurses can be active in legislative efforts, public awareness campaigns, group classes on injury prevention, and individual prevention counseling with children and families.

Rivara (1992) suggests the following guidelines for parental prevention education: suggest passive one-time strategies (such as placing a car seat in the automobile), provide specific advice related to the age of the child, and concentrate efforts on problems that are frequent and severe and for which prevention strategies exist (such as seat belts, motorcycle and bicycle helmets, and protective gear for sports).

In one study, practitioners questioned about pediatric injury prevention reported a greater emphasis on passive environmental strategies, such as car seats, smoke detectors, lowering the temperature of the hot water heater, and fencing in home pools, and a lesser emphasis on active, educational strategies (Cohen and others, 1997). Because of both time constraints and a concern to not overwhelm parents, most practitioners in the study limited prevention counseling to four or fewer strategies in a single visit, introducing some new messages and reinforcing others. Counseling was thought to be best directed to developmentally relevant issues. (See example of prevention guidelines in the Community Focus box on p. 1758 and in health promotion sections of individual chapters of this text.)

Another strategy to increase accident awareness and prevent childhood injuries has been to implement home visits by school-based home visitors to families of low-income children attending preschool. Home visitors identified potential sources of danger in the home and distributed items such as smoke detectors and ipecac. Follow-up visits were favorable for the continued implementation of injury prevention by families involved (Johnston and others, 2000).

Crawley (1996) suggests many strategies for nurses. Nursing history or hospital admission forms can include screening questions about safety issues. Discharge planning or primary care visits might be a time to provide a family with information on safety practices. Films/videos on auto, firearm, and bike safety can be shown in waiting rooms. Home health care nurses can easily assist a family in a safety assessment. School nurses can develop safety education programs for different ages. Nurses in emergency department and outpatient clinic settings can provide instructions related to injury prevention on an individual basis as developmentally appropriate.

Accident prevention among teenagers presents a unique challenge to all health care workers. In order for accident prevention to be effective, adolescents must perceive the specific interventions as having an impact on their lives. Adolescents are very much concerned with body image and often feel indestructable unless their own lives or the life of a close friend is touched by the tragedy of a catastrophic debilitating injury or death. With increased emphasis in society on having fun and enjoying life to its fullest (today) regardless of the consequences (tomorrow), it is difficult for adolescents to understand the necessity to abide by the rules of persons who are authority figures. At the time of this writing there is increased concern about injuries to teens by all-terrain motor vehicles (in which there is no law for age limit), snowmobiles, in-line skating, trampolines, and motor vehicles.

What efforts are you making in your practice or institution to incorporate injury prevention education into the care of children and families? What additional efforts could you make?

## Assessment of Trauma

The site of the injury usually influences the order of priority of interventions when emergency care is being instituted. The safety of both the victim and the "Good Samaritan" rescuers must be considered to prevent further injury.

For example, removing a child from a burning building or the bottom of a swimming pool is the obvious action to the logically thinking person, but anxious rescuers may not consider their own safety to be of prime importance. The major reason for thinking through steps to be taken in an emergency before the actual incident occurs is to have a mental repertoire of preplanned actions available at a stimulus-response level.

> **NURSING ALERT**    Always consider personal safety a top priority because the victim cannot be helped if the rescuer is injured.

### Emergency Management

Guidelines for care of the child at the scene of an injury are outlined in the Emergency Treatment box. Following assessment of level of consciousness, the concerns are for *airway, breathing,* and *circulation (ABCs),* after which other injuries are managed as indicated by the assessment. The *airway* is opened using the *modified jaw-thrust maneuver,* which is accomplished by grasping the angles of the victim's lower jaw and lifting with both hands, one on each side, displacing the mandible upward and outward and without head-tilt or chin-lift.

*Spinal cord injury* cannot be adequately assessed in the prehospital setting. It requires radiographs, a computed tomography (CT) scan, or magnetic resonance imaging (MRI) for diagnosis. Spinal cord injury is always suspected in the patient with head, trunk, or multisystem trauma. Only in a fully equipped trauma center with radiographs and other diagnostic tests can spinal cord injury be ruled out. Therefore the patient is treated as if injury is present. The cervical spine is immobilized by holding the head in a neutral position and not allowing movement of the head or body in any direction.

> **NURSING ALERT**    Improper movement of the injured child with undetected spinal injury may lead to serious, permanent injury or death. It is virtually impossible to rule out spinal injury outside of the hospital; therefore, all victims with *any possibility* of spinal injury are treated as if injury is present.

*Breathing* is assessed after the airway is opened. If the child is not breathing, rescue breaths are given at a rate of 20 per minute. Oxygen should be provided when possible. Circulation is assessed only after the airway has been maintained and breathing is established. In children under 1 year of age, a brachial pulse is assessed. After 1 year of age, a carotid pulse is palpated. Chest compressions should be initiated if necessary. (See Cardiopulmonary Resuscitation, Chapter 31.)

*Bleeding* is first controlled by direct pressure with a *gloved* hand. If this does not work, a pressure dressing is applied.

The next step is to elevate the body part and then attempt to control hemorrhage with arterial pressure points. A tourniquet is a *last resort.* Once applied, it is not removed or loosened. Below the tourniquet site, skin and tissue necrosis begins. If the tourniquet is loosened or removed, it allows release of the toxins into the circulation in high concentrations and may induce a systemic, deadly, tourniquet shock. With the tourniquet in place, the patient has a better chance of survival, even though it may mean the loss of a limb.

Assessment of the child involves observation from head to toe because infants and young children are unable to communicate except by crying and other behaviors. Therefore pinpointing areas of pain is very difficult. To check for any motor or sensory dysfunction in extremities, the nurse should note any spontaneous movement, which provides the best clue in infants and young children. Older children are able to follow directions for wiggling toes or fingers demonstrating a grasp, "pushing down on the gas pedal," or lifting legs off the bed. The child is identified as soon as feasible by anyone who knows the child. It is important to determine if the child has any existing health problems that might have implications for the circumstances of the injury and for therapeutic management. Any witnesses are asked for details about the incident to aid in assessment of the child's emotional responses.

In the prehospital setting the role of the nurse consists of activating the *Emergency Medical Service (EMS)* and providing basic life support until EMS personnel arrive on the scene. The role of the nurse is limited to basic life support because the nurse has no standing orders or protocols to work under in the prehospital setting. (See Emergency Treatment box.) Emergency services are called as soon as possible so that the patient can receive advanced life support before and during transport. A pediatric trauma triage system with personnel designated to the care of an injured child is essential in order to provide excellent trauma patient care. Nuss, Dietrich, and Smith (2001) discussed the use of a two-tier trauma assessment system that triages patients into level 1 and level 2 trauma alert categories. This triage system more effectively predicted which patients were more likely to have serious injury. Some trauma centers use the Injury Severity Score, a tool that predicts the degree of trauma experienced by an individual (Grisoni and others, 2001).

A paramedic-level ambulance provides at least one *paramedic* with skills in advanced cardiac life support (ACLS), pediatric advanced life support (PALS), and neonatal resuscitation (NRP). A paramedic's skills include electrocardiogram (ECG) interpretation and defibrillation, advanced airway management (including endotracheal intubation, as well as intravenous [IV] and pharmacologic therapy), placement of a pneumatic antishock garment (PASG), pleural decompression (chest tube), and placement of a nasogastric tube and Foley catheter. Other advanced life support skills include expertise in spinal immobilization, extrication, management of fractures and bleeding, and emergency scene management. The paramedic remains in constant contact with the emergency department physician by means of a radio or cellular telephone for situations requiring medical control.

An *emergency medical technician (EMT)* has training in basic life support (BLS) measures, including basic airway management, hemorrhage control, fracture management, and spinal immobilization. In some areas EMTs may have additional training that allows them to perform some advanced airway procedures, IV therapy, and automated defibrillation, as well as to use the PASG.

> **NURSING ALERT**  Emergency medical services with paramedics or EMTs are used to manage all out-of-hospital emergencies and have specialized equipment to manage such emergencies. It is imperative that EMS be called to respond as soon as possible. Family, friends, or strangers should not transport the trauma victim.

## Systematic Assessment

There are several factors that can affect a child's response to trauma. An undetected congenital anomaly can contribute to a complicated injury. Acute gastric distention is a frequent occurrence in children because of the crying and screaming that accompany an injury. The temperature of young children is unstable because of their large surface area related to body mass, and temperature maintenance is critical in trauma management. Children also experience rapid metabolic changes. When they are ill, children are really ill; but as they recover, they change very rapidly. In addition, children have a small amount of blood volume in the absolute sense. Whereas blood volume is 60% of total body weight in the adult, it is 70% to 85% in the child.

The first priority on admission to an emergency facility is *rapid assessment of the ABC status.* Because the overwhelming majority of childhood injuries are the result of blunt-impact trauma, multiple organ involvement is a common finding; therefore it is essential to perform a systematic assessment of the trauma victim.

The secondary survey is a comprehensive assessment that is a *systematic "head-to-toe" search* for the remaining injuries not originally addressed in the primary survey. However, children are often an exception to the "head-to-toe" approach. It may be necessary to complete the secondary survey on the injured child in the "toe-to-head" manner. This approach may allow the rescuer to gain the child's confidence as the survey progresses. With this approach, the rescuer gradually moves into the child's "personal space" while gaining the child's trust. An example of a complete secondary survey is given in the Guidelines box on p. 1762. Throughout the assessment, the nurse observes for areas of deformity, edema, ecchymosis, bleeding, hematoma, paralysis, or pain.

# THE IMMOBILIZED CHILD
## Immobilization

One of the most difficult aspects of illness is the immobility it often imposes on a child. Children's natural tendency to be mobile influences all elements of growth and development—physical, social, psychologic, and emotional. Impaired physical mobility related to disability or imposed activity restrictions presents a definite challenge to the child, staff, and parents providing care.

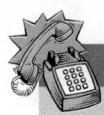

## EMERGENCY TREATMENT
### Trauma

*Before* entering trauma area, observe for dangers to rescuers and bystanders. Be aware of potential for further injuries to child.

Observe scene for signs and mechanism of injury (e.g., head-on motor vehicle injury) (helps to determine proper course of action for treating child's injuries).

Do not move child before arrival of emergency medical services (EMS) unless child is in danger of further injury. If it is necessary to move child, follow appropriate steps to prevent further injury (e.g., exacerbating spinal injury by failing to maintain cervical spine stabilization during movement).

### PRIMARY ASSESSMENT AND INTERVENTION

Assess *level of consciousness.* Use the AVPU method:
  **A** Child is *alert*
  **V** Child responds to *verbal* stimulus
  **P** Child responds to *painful* stimulus
  **U** Child is *unresponsive* to any stimulus
Open *airway,* using appropriate method.
  In child with head, trunk, or multisystem trauma, modified jaw-thrust is preferred method (see p. 1760). At this point, cervical spine should be manually immobilized and held in alignment with rest of spinal column and should not be released until EMS personnel have immobilized child with appropriate equipment.
Assess for *breathing.* If necessary, begin rescue breathing.
Assess for *circulation.* If necessary, begin chest compressions.
  Palpate carotid artery in children 1 year or older.
  Palpate brachial artery in infants less than 1 year old.
Observe for hemorrhage. Control bleeding with a *gloved or protected hand:*
  1. Apply direct pressure to wound site.
  2. Elevate wound site.
  3. Apply pressure to appropriate arterial pressure point.
  4. Apply tourniquet only as a last resort. Once a tourniquet is applied, it should *not* be loosened.
Assess for further injury.
Do not remove objects protruding from child's body.
Check for evidence of decreased motor or sensory function in extremities:
  Infant and young child—observe spontaneous movement in extremities.
  Older child—ask if able to wiggle extremities.
Evaluate pain—present, absent; severe, mild.
  Attempt to alleviate with nonpharmacologic techniques.
  Encourage use of analgesics when EMS arrive.
Assess pulses in extremity distal to injury.
  Check color and temperature of extremities.
Manage any injuries appropriately (e.g., splint fractures) (see Emergency Treatment box, p. 1781)
Maintain body heat.
Identify child.
Obtain information regarding the injury from witnesses, if any.
Call EMS or other transport team to take child to nearest facility, preferably a pediatric trauma center.

## Etiology of Immobilization

The usual reason for immobilizing or restricting the activity of a child without disabilities is illness or injury. Bed rest or mechanical restraining devices are frequently prescribed to aid in the healing and restorative processes. When children are ill, they are content to remain quiet, and most of them instinctively reduce their activity. It is children who are forced to remain inactive because of physical limitations or therapy who display the multiple effects of restricted movement. The most frequent reasons for immobility are con-

## GUIDELINES
### Assessing Trauma

**Primary assessment**
   *Blood pressure* (if available)
   *Respirations*—Assess rate and quality, auscultate lung sounds.
   *Pulse*—Assess rate and quality.
   *Skin*—Assess color, temperature, and condition. Treat for shock if mechanism of injury and vital signs indicate possible need. Administer high-flow oxygen if available. Elevate lower extremities (if no possibility of spinal injury). Maintain body heat.
**Systematic head-to-toe (or toe-to-head) assessment**
   *Neck and cervical spine*—Palpate for point tenderness, observe for stoma, distended neck veins, tracheal shift, medical alert tags.
   Immobilize neck with cervical collar and towel rolls/foam head blocks (to prevent lateral neck movement) if available. (Manual cervical spine immobilization should still be in effect from emergency assessment and intervention.)
   *Scalp and skull*—Palpate for indentions, deformity, etc. Observe for cerebrospinal fluid in ears, Battle sign (bruising behind ears, indicating possible skull fracture).
   *Face*—Observe for deformity, cerebrospinal fluid in nose.
   *Eyes*—Observe for pupillary response, equality.
   *Mouth*—Observe for possible obstructions, breath odor, loose teeth.
   *Chest and ribs*—Palpate for possible fractures, deformity; observe and feel for equal expansion, asymmetry.
   *Abdomen*—Auscultate, then palpate all quadrants for deformity, rigidity (indicating possible intraabdominal bleed).
   *Lumbar spine*—Palpate for deformity, tenderness.
**Reassessment of level of consciousness, airway patency**
   *Pelvis and hips*—Perform three-way compression test for possible fracture without rocking the hip (contraindicated if known pelvic fracture).
   *Groin*—Observe for bleeding, priapism (indicating possible severe spinal injury).
   *Extremities*—Palpate and observe all extremities for deformity, crepitus, bleeding, sensory, motor and circulatory function, medical alert tags.
**Reevaluate** treatment for shock, level of consciousness, airway, breathing, circulation, bleeding control, and vital signs.

genital defects (e.g., spina bifida), degenerative disorders (e.g., muscular dystrophy), and infections or injuries that impair the integumentary system (severe burns), the musculoskeletal system (fractures or osteomyelitis), or the neurologic system (spinal cord injury, polyneuritis, or head injury). Sometimes therapies, such as traction and spinal fusion, are responsible for prolonged immobilization, although the trend is toward early mobilization, early discharge, and outpatient care.

## Physiologic Effects of Immobilization

Many clinical studies, including space program research, have documented predictable consequences that occur following immobilization and the absence of gravitational force. Functional and metabolic responses to restricted movement can be noted in most of the body systems. Each has a direct influence on the child's growth and development because homeostatic mechanisms thrive on normal use and need feedback to maintain dynamic equilibrium. Inactivity leads to

a decrease in the functional capabilities of the whole body as dramatically as the lack of physical exercise leads to muscle weakness. Although children usually become mobile once they feel well, the effects of immobility may be offset by a process termed *prehabilitation*, a process whereby one's functional capacity is enhanced before prolonged immobility to withstand the stress of such a condition on the body's vital function. Prehabilitation has been proposed for ICU adult patients who require prolonged immobilization (Topp and others, 2002) and could be used for children anticipating immobility. Prehabilitation is used by athletes to decrease the incidence of injuries and increase vital function of cardiorespiratory, muscle, and metabolic functions.

Most of the pathologic changes that take place during immobilization arise from decreased muscle strength and mass, decreased metabolism, and bone demineralization, which are closely interrelated, with one change leading to or affecting another. Some results of immobilization are primary and produce a direct effect; other pathophysiologic consquences occur frequently but seem to be more indirect and are therefore secondary effects. Many pathophysiologic changes affect more than one body system, with the primary or secondary effect being demonstrated in both systems.

Children who are confined to bed during an illness or traumatic injury are usually restricted in movement for a relatively short time or are sufficiently active to avoid the physical consequences of immobility. Most physical and biologic effects of immobilization are the result of complete immobility, usually as a result of paralysis caused by nervous system infection (e.g., poliomyelitis, encephalitis, or polyneuritis) or trauma to the brain or spinal cord. Partial paralysis or weakness may be caused by birth defects (e.g., myelomeningocele), trauma, infection, or degenerative disease, such as muscular dystrophy or muscular atrophy.

The major effects of immobilization (Fig. 39-1) are related directly or indirectly to decreased muscle activity, which produces numerous primary changes in both muscular and bone structures with secondary alterations in the cardiovascular, respiratory, metabolic, and renal systems. The major consequences are:

- Significant loss of muscle strength, endurance, and muscle mass (atrophy)
- Bone demineralization leading to osteoporosis
- Loss of joint mobility and contractures

The larger the portion of the body immobilized and the longer the immobilization, the greater the hazards of immobility.

**Muscular System.**   Inactive muscle loses strength at the rate of 3% per day and, in instances without primary neuromuscular deficit, sometimes requires several weeks or months to regain function. A stretching can occur as muscle loses its tone or as excessive strain is put on weakened muscle (e.g., stretching by tight bed covers or poor body position that produces wristdrop or footdrop experienced by some children with a disability). The disuse leads to tissue breakdown and loss of muscle mass *(atrophy)*. The chief intracellular muscle enzyme, creatine, is released into the serum as the muscle atrophies; therefore serum levels provide an indication of the

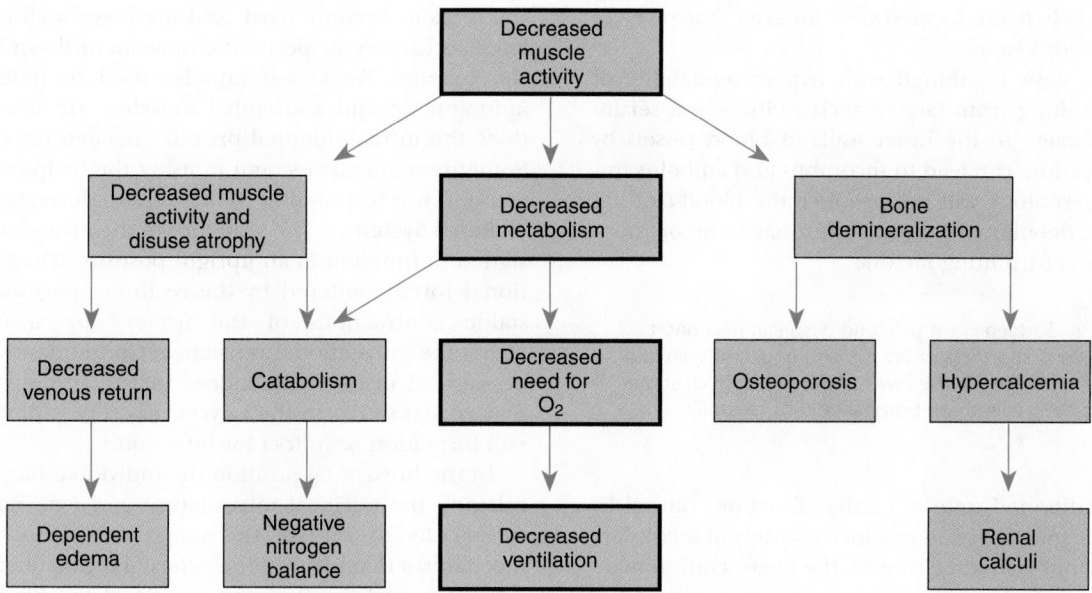

**Fig. 39-1**   Physiologic effects of immobilization.

amount of muscle mass undergoing degeneration. Inactive muscle also affects the cardiovascular system by decreasing venous return and cardiac output. In general, muscle atrophy causes decreased strength and endurance. Stiffness of joints, as well as joint and intraarticular dysfunction, may be prevented, by passive or active range of motion and proper positioning.

**Skeletal System.**   The daily stresses on bone created by motion and weight bearing maintain the balance between bone formation *(osteoblastic activity)* and bone resorption *(osteoclastic activity)*. When these stresses are diminished, bone formation ceases, whereas the bone destruction continues, thus disrupting the state of equilibrium. Bone calcium becomes severely depleted, and there is increased secretion of phosphorus and nitrogen. This demineralization of the bone *(osteopenia)* makes the skeletal structures prone to pathologic fractures and increases calcium ion concentration in the blood *(hypercalcemia).*

In children who have limited mobility, such as the child who is unconscious or paralyzed or the child with rheumatoid arthritis, joint mobility becomes restricted. In the absence of normal structural stretching, collagen fibers generated within the joint become fibrotic and further limit movement. This *tissue fibrosis* creates a shortening of the muscles and a contracture of the joint. Any decrease in circulation to the joint by edema, inflammation, or restrictive positioning will contribute to further fibrotic changes. The problem rapidly becomes cyclic as the contracture leads to muscle fatigue and pain, which causes the child to protect the site, thus leading to more fibrosis. This process is further exaggerated because body flexor muscles are stronger than the extensor muscles, and unless range of motion is instituted within 3 to 7 days, *contractures* will develop. Frequent disabling contractures are hip flexion, knee flexion, shoulder stiffness, and plantar flexion of the feet.

**Cardiovascular System.**   There are three major cardiovascular consequences of immobility: *orthostatic intolerance, increased workload of the heart,* and *thrombus formation.* During movement, muscle contraction causes pressure on peripheral veins, which in turn causes the venous valves to close, thus assisting return of the blood to the heart when the individual is in an upright position. In the absence of this assistance, blood tends to pool in the dependent areas, reducing the blood supply to the trunk and brain. In addition, direct reflex stimulation to the splanchnic and peripheral vessels causes them to constrict when a person is upright. Impairment of this neurovascular orthostatic reflex activity from lack of motion causes further interference with venous return. The individual displays signs of excessive autonomic activity (i.e., pallor, sweating, and restlessness, which are frequently followed by fainting). The child with a spinal cord injury has unique problems with orthostatic intolerance, which is discussed in Chapter 40.

Changes in vascular resistance caused by the horizontal position and immobility alter the distribution of blood within the body. The reduction in gravity pressure to the extremities causes much of the total blood volume to be redistributed from lower extremities to other parts of the body. Consequently there is an increase in the venous return and the volume of blood to be handled by the heart, which is reflected in an elevated blood pressure. Therefore cardiac output and stroke volume are increased, and a progressive increase in heart rate occurs. When immobilization extends over a period of time, there is a compensatory decrease in blood volume and a decrease in heart rate and blood pressure.

Without muscle contraction venous stasis and increased intravascular pressure in the extremities lead to dependent edema. If undue pressure is exerted on the major veins by positioning or mechanical devices, the likelihood of interstitial edema is increased. Most frequently this situation is seen when a child is placed on the side with one leg resting on the other or when the youngster is permitted to sit for a long time with pressure on the large veins behind the knee and in the groin. Edematous tissue is prone to infection and trauma, especially tissue located over an area that receives much of the body's weight.

Circulatory stasis combined with hypercoagulability of the blood, resulting from factors such as increased serum calcium or damage to the inner walls of blood vessels by trauma or infection, can lead to thrombus and embolus formation. Bed rest alone will not produce the blood-clotting problems, but debilitated persons often have one or more of these other contributing factors.

> **NURSING ALERT**
> Sudden chest pain and dyspnea, new onset of shortness of breath, air hunger, or pain and swelling in the lower extremities, which sometimes indicates deep vein thrombosis, should be carefully evaluated.

The deconditioned state of cardiac function, caused by skeletal muscle inactivity, can produce a variety of secondary problems in other systems. However, the major clinical manifestation is increased pulse and heart rate in response to an active exercise program. After prolonged immobility the child should build up activity tolerance slowly to allow the heart to regain optimum capabilities.

**Respiratory System.** Initially the effects of immobilization are compensatory or adaptive. The basal metabolic rate is decreased because with reduced expenditure of energy the cells require less oxygen and produce less carbon dioxide. Lessened demand for oxygen–carbon dioxide exchange causes the respirations to become slower and more shallow. Chest expansion may be limited by the supine posture; by abdominal distention caused by accumulation of feces, gas, or fluid; and by mechanical restriction such as a body cast, brace, or tight binders. Reduced muscle power and coordination secondary to altered innervation can also hinder respiratory movement. More effort is required to expand the lungs in the supine position.

Prolonged immobility also reduces the normal movement of secretions from the tracheobronchial tree, particularly in the presence of impaired muscle function and positional changes that normally facilitate removal of secretions. A weak and ineffectual cough reflex contributes to stasis of secretions and the possibility of airway obstruction. Shallow respirations and obstruction of the airway with thick mucus contribute to the development of secondary complications such as atelectasis, hypostatic pneumonia, and respiratory acidosis.

**Gastrointestinal System.** Prolonged immobility produces a state of negative nitrogen balance resulting from the increased catabolic activity related to muscle atrophy. This and the reduced energy requirements contribute to a diminished appetite and a resulting decrease in ingestion of nutrients. The mechanisms of eating and feeding become more difficult with immobility, and the risk of aspiration is increased. Intake is further influenced by associated psychologic factors.

The process of elimination depends on the integration of smooth and skeletal muscle activity and on visceral reflex patterns. Immobility may interfere with these mechanisms, as well as with the gravitational effect on stool passing through the intestines. Slowing of stool in the colon causes the feces to become hard, and the bowel wall is not stimulated to further its peristaltic movement down the tract to the rectum. Weakened muscles used in defecation (diaphragmatic and abdominal muscles) are unable to produce the intraabdominal pressure needed for elimination. Sometimes embarrassment in using the bedpan may be the cause of not responding to the urge to defecate.

**Renal System.** The structure of the urinary system is designed to function in an upright posture. When the gravitational force is altered by the reclining position, the peristaltic contractions of the ureters are insufficient to overcome gravitational resistance. Consequently there may be stasis of urine in the kidney pelves, and any particulate matter that settles in the calyces may serve as nuclei for calculi formation or as foci for infection.

In the horizontal position the individual has difficulty in relaxing the perineal musculature and external sphincter sufficiently to initiate the integrated reflex micturition mechanism that involves the external sphincter, the internal sphincter, and the detrusor muscle of the bladder wall. If adequate intraabdominal pressure is exerted, voiding can occur, but if the individual does not respond to the sensation to void, bladder distention leads to stasis and its complications add to overflow incontinence, a source of embarrassment. In time, reflux and back pressure may impair renal function, and urinary tract infection is always a hazard with urine retention.

Normally the kidney is able to handle the increased metabolites from protein breakdown and bone demineralization. However, the increased level of calcium excreted may predispose to the formation of calculi. *Calculi formation* ("kidney stones") is further favored by urinary stasis, infection, and an alkaline urine caused by the decreased production of the acid by-products of metabolism. Hematuria may be the only clue to diagnosis.

**Metabolism.** Immobility or severe restriction of activity is often accompanied by decreased or inappropriate nutritional intake, which frequently leads to a decreased basal metabolic rate, a negative nitrogen balance associated with catabolism, and a high serum calcium level.

All body systems are influenced by a decrease in metabolism. The altered energy level leads to further fatigue and lack of motivation for moving. Although less of a problem in children, immobilized persons often feel sluggish and have a poor appetite, particularly for protein foods. The protein breakdown in the body related to a loss of muscle and other tissues is more apt to be severe after injury or surgery. Protein breakdown produces nitrogenous wastes, and on the fifth or sixth day of catabolic protein metabolism, an increase in urinary nitrogen develops that contributes to anemia and delayed healing.

Another metabolic problem is hypercalcemia associated with bone catabolism. Completely immobilized youngsters are especially prone to hypercalcemia. Symptoms that include nausea and vomiting, polydipsia, polyuria, and lethargy usually appear 4 to 8 weeks after immobilization. In quadriplegia, symptoms may occur within 10 days and last for as long as 6 months. The accelerated rate of bone metabolism in youngsters makes the bone demineralization a greater hazard. Larger amounts of calcium are released into the blood than the kidney can excrete, and calcium continues to accumulate in serum. High levels of serum calcium decrease neuronal permeability, which can lead to a depression of central and peripheral nervous systems. Symptoms that include smooth and skeletal muscle fatigue, diminished reflexes, and atony of the gastrointestinal tract are a result of the depressed nervous system.

Medical treatment for hypercalcemia consists of restricting dietary calcium, increasing weight bearing when this is possible and, most important, vigorous hydration (e.g., 3000 to 4000 ml/day of fluid for a teenager). Electrolyte imbalances are corrected, and diuretics are administered to promote removal of calcium. Sometimes pharmacologic agents, such as corticosteroids, oral phosphates, and thyrocalcitonin, may be used to lower serum calcium levels. Any urinary tract infection is treated.

A child with bone demineralization may not develop hypercalcemia, but the excess amount of calcium that the kidneys are required to excrete may produce a negative calcium balance, with more calcium than citric acid lost in the urine. This imbalance causes the urine to become alkaline, with the potential danger of renal calculi, especially if there is an accompanying retention of urine.

**Integumentary System.** Circulation to the skin is reduced during inactivity and may be further impeded by dependent edema. Circulation is especially compromised in places where the bone surface is near the skin, such as areas over the sacrum, occiput, trochanter, and ankle, and continued impairment causes rapid necrosis with ulcer formation. Mechanical irritation from appliances, such as straps, rods, and ropes, and the friction of bedclothes during turning or other movement can produce skin breakdown. Healing capacity is also impaired by poor circulation, negative nitrogen balance, and anemia. Immobilization often makes

it difficult to carry out adequate cleansing and hygienic measures, which may also contribute to tissue breakdown in areas that are difficult to reach. Children with neurologic deficit should be guarded against extremes of heat and cold in direct contact with the skin.

Cellular breakdown caused by prolonged pressure can be identified by several characteristics. Normally when pressure is applied to the skin, the skin appears pale but becomes very red, or hyperemic, after the pressure is removed. This reactive hyperemia should disappear within 5 to 15 minutes. Prolonged redness (over 30 minutes) indicates that a pressure area is developing and treatment should be instituted. Other manifestations of tissue ischemia include an increase in temperature in the area, blistering, swelling, or dark purple or black areas. The pressure area may be limited to the skin and subcutaneous layers or may be deeper and more extensive. The skin changes observed may represent the top of a cone-shaped area with widespread tissue destruction, beneath which tissue rapidly ulcerates and creates a large hole that sometimes extends to the bone. The skin may be broken, and there may even be a purulent drainage. Fig. 39-2 illustrates the sequence of events in tissue breakdown.

**Neurosensory System.** Studies indicate that immobilization does not produce neurosensory consequences directly; however, two occurrences—loss of innervation and sensory and perceptual deprivation—are common.

Peripheral nerves, in contrast to skeletal muscles, do not degenerate with disuse, but loss of innervation takes place if nerves are damaged by pressure or if their blood supply is disrupted. Improper body positioning or poorly applied casts or restraints can place excessive pressure on nerves and blood vessels that can lead to ischemia and nerve degeneration. Frequent sites of this compression phenome-

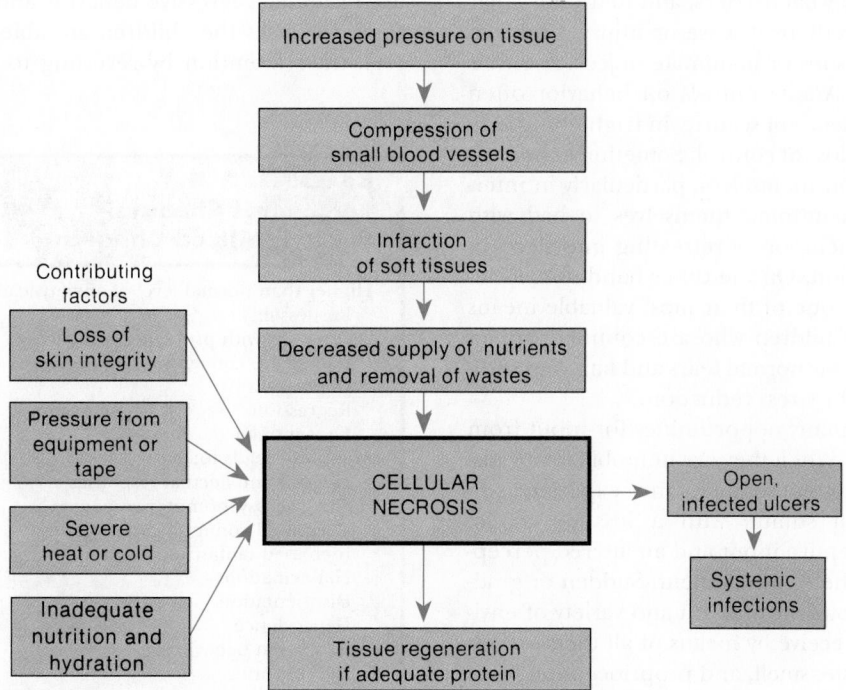

**Fig. 39-2**   Sequence of events in tissue breakdown.

non are on the peroneal nerve, where pressure results in footdrop, and on the radial nerve, where pressure leads to wristdrop. These complications significantly interfere with attempts to regain functional use of extremities, but they can be prevented by conscientious nursing assessment and intervention. Preventing pressure on vulnerable areas and avoiding unnatural positions of flexion and extension that apply inappropriate pressure on nerves and blood vessels reduce the likelihood of compression injury. Periodic plantar flexion and dorsiflexion of the feet and hands will stimulate circulation and keep nerves from becoming pinched.

| **NURSING ALERT** | Numbness, tingling, change in sensation, and loss of motion are symptoms of neurologic impairment and should be evaluated immediately. |
|---|---|

### Psychologic Effects of Immobilization

For children, one of the most difficult aspects of illness is immobilization. Throughout childhood, physical activity is an integral part of daily life and is essential for physical growth and development. It also serves children as an instrument for communication and expression and as a means for learning about and understanding their world. Activity helps them deal with a variety of feelings and impulses and provides a mechanism by which they can exert control over inner tensions. Children respond to anxiety with increased activity. Removal of this power deprives them of necessary input and a natural outlet for their feelings and fantasies. Through movement children also gain sensory input, which provides an essential element for developing and maintaining a body image.

In daily life, children's activity is restricted in many ways: limits are set on behavior and expression, activity is restricted by physical and verbal barriers, and neuromuscular function is affected directly by disease or injury. Children perceive restraint by persons or inanimate objects as either comforting or stressful. Adult controls on behavior often provide children with a sense of security in frightening situations or when they fear loss of control. Sometimes children will impose restrictions on themselves, particularly in interaction with others, by confining themselves to bed with blankets pulled about them, or by retreating into sleep in the presence of stimulation. On the other hand, forced inactivity deprives them of one of their most valuable means for dealing with stress. Children who are confined to bed may become victims of their normal fears and fantasies without the physical means for stress reduction.

Active children have many opportunities for input from a wide variety of settings. When they are immobilized by disease or as a part of a treatment regimen, they experience diminished environmental stimuli with a loss of tactile, vestibular, and proprioceptive input and an altered perception of themselves and their environment. Sudden or gradual immobilization narrows the amount and variety of environmental stimuli they receive by means of all their senses: touch, sight, hearing, taste, smell, and proprioception. This *sensory deprivation* frequently leads to a feeling of isolation,

boredom, and being forgotten, especially by peers. Nursing interventions involving the use of diversional activities, schoolwork, structured television, computer games, or video programs can assist the child with maintaining usual activities. (See Chapter 26.)

Sensorimotor activity is a predominant mode of activity in infants; even newborns respond with protest when they are physically restrained. Physical interference with the activity of infants and young children gives them a feeling of helplessness. It has also been found that speech and language skills require sensorimotor activity/experience. There appears to be a significant relationship between physical restraint and the incidence of language problems. Children who are restrained by casts, splints, or straps during the first 3 years of life have more difficulty with language than children whose activities were unrestricted. Language delay is even more marked in children with neurologic impairment.

The struggle for independence is thwarted by imposed immobility. For toddlers, exploration and imitative behaviors are essential to developing a sense of autonomy; preschoolers' expression of initiative is evidenced by their penchant for vigorous physical activity; school-age children's development is strongly influenced by physical achievement and competition; and adolescents rely on mobility to achieve independence. The quest for mastery at every stage of development is related to mobility. To children, the inability to move is threatening to self-preservation and reactivates the struggle between activity and passivity, and between dependence and independence.

Behavioral changes are noted when children experience prolonged sensory deprivation. Some of these behaviors are demonstrated by a higher than normal level of anxiety (Box 39-1). (See Family Focus box.) Children are likely to become depressed over their loss of ability to function or the marked changes in body image. Significant others are apt to notice regressive behavior and a greater reliance on them for tasks the children are able to perform. Children seek their attention by reverting to earlier developmental

| **Box 39-1** ▨ ▪ ▫<br>**Behavioral Changes<br>in Immobilized Children** |
|---|
| Higher than normal level of anxiety leads to:<br>   Restlessness<br>   Difficulty with problem solving<br>   Inability to concentrate on activities<br>   Depression<br>   Regression<br>   Egocentrism<br>Monotony leads to:<br>   Sluggish intellectual responses<br>   Sluggish psychomotor responses<br>   Decreased communication skills<br>   Increased fantasizing<br>   Hallucinations<br>   Disorientation<br>   Dependence<br>   Acting-out behavior<br>   Depression |

behaviors, such as wanting to be fed, bed-wetting, and baby talk. In many ways immobilized children are realistically dependent on others; therefore intelligent and sensitive care is required to prevent major developmental regressions during the period of immobility.

Limbs in casts or traction transmit less than normal sensory data. The presence of sensory impairment may be a concomitant problem of the involved part. Numbness or loss of feeling markedly alters proprioception. Children who have limited ability to feel others touching them not only experience less tactile stimuli in a physical sense but are also deprived of warm, loving feelings that arise from being touched. The loss of feeling derived from touch can further add to their sense of being isolated and unwanted.

The type and extent of immobilization influence the emotional response. When children are able to see the reason for their restraint (e.g., a cast), they are less likely to be resistant. The child whose activity is restricted because of an invisible disorder finds it difficult to understand the reason for adult restrictions on activity, imagines the worst, and may react with noncompliance and overactivity when unobserved. Children may react to immobility by active protest, anger, and aggressive behavior, or they may become quiet, passive, and submissive. Often children believe that the immobilization is a justified punishment for misbehavior. Children should be allowed to express their anger, but it should be within the limits of safety to their self-esteem and not damaging to the integrity of others. For example, providing an object to attack rather than a person or a valued possession is safe and therapeutic.

Unfortunately, adults may be confused by, resent, and find it difficult to deal with the acting-out behavior of children. Too often this behavior is considered "bad" even when it is a release of tension. In some cases, such as with the paralyzed child, parents and nurses may feel inadequate to cope with the child's profound distress and feelings of hopelessness, and the professional help of a mental health specialist is needed.

The most difficult situations are those involving major injuries and diseases that produce a disfigurement or a severe loss of function that directly affects children's self-image,

such as burns, amputation, or the sudden, catastrophic effects of an accident that leaves healthy, active children paralyzed for life. Feelings of anger and hostility are difficult for children to express when they are at the mercy of the environment. They dare not speak out against or defy the authorities on whom they depend so completely. Consequently their aggression may be masked by cheerfulness or rigidity. When they are unable to express their anger, the aggression is often displayed inappropriately through regressive behavior and outbursts of crying or temper tantrums over insignificant irritations. Adolescents and older school-age children should be allowed to vary their daily routine to fit their needs for independence; allowing this age-group to stay up late at night and sleep in during the daytime (within reasonable limits of treatment needs) may help decrease struggles over other inconsequential matters and at the same time allow a daily pattern of life. Parents are encouraged to continue setting limits and not abandon disciplinary measures with children who are confined to bed due to trauma or illness.

### Effect on Families

Brief periods of immobilization have few effects on the family; however, catastrophic illness or disability may severely tax their resources. The needs for instruction concerning medical and nursing care, community resources to contact, and emotional support are paramount. Many families are already plagued by unmet needs, operate from crisis to crisis, and are often unable to use outside help appropriately. For these families the new situation can be quite disruptive; therefore the rehabilitation team must help the family members identify unmet needs and actively help in the family's problem-solving process. The following are commonly occurring problems:

- Financial strains may decrease or totally eliminate the family's resources.
- The focus of attention is placed, at least temporarily, on the affected member; therefore other members of the family, especially siblings, may feel neglected or their needs may not be met.
- The family may have difficulty in accepting the child's altered body image.
- Individual family members may be unable to express their feelings and may have difficulty coping in the face of the crisis.
- Parents often experience guilt over their child's condition and need for immobilization. Their perception of failing to protect the child forms the basis for their difficulty coping.

The family's needs often must be met by the services of a multidisciplinary team, and nurses play a key role in anticipating the services they will need and in coordinating conferences to plan care. In preparation for discharge, home visits are advisable, and home management is frequently planned weeks in advance of the actual discharge, including special considerations for cultural, economic, physical, and psychologic needs. A child with a severe disability is very dependent, and caregivers need rest periods to revitalize themselves. Individual and group counseling is beneficial for preproblem-solving situations and provides an emotional support system. Parent groups are also helpful and often allow nonthreatening social contact. The families of

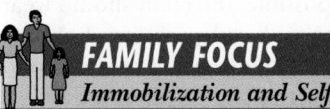

### FAMILY FOCUS
#### Immobilization and Self-Esteem

Immobilization, as with any illness or disorder that is debilitating in some way, may restrict children from participating in age-appropriate activities. These children may be labeled as "different," and over time this may result in a child feeling unaccepted. In young children, acceptance by their peers is an important component in the formulation of their self-esteem. The assessment of self-esteem in young children is a critical attribute to their well-being. It is important to educate children about their illness and encourage them to engage in activities. Children who have a strong sense of self-worth and confidence are able to initiate activities and explore their environment. They approach tasks and relationships with the expectation that they will be well received and successful.

children with permanent disabilities need long-term resources because some of the most difficult problems arise as they try to sustain high-quality care for many years. (See Chapter 22.)

## Nursing Considerations

### ▓ Assessment

Physical assessment of the child who is immobilized as a result of an injury or a degenerative disease includes a focus on not only the injured part (e.g., fracture or damaged joint), but also the functioning of other systems that may be affected secondarily—the circulatory, renal, respiratory, muscular, and gastrointestinal systems. With long-term immobilization there may also be neurologic impairment and changes in electrolytes (especially calcium), nitrogen balance, and the general metabolic rate. The psychologic impact of immobilization should also be assessed.

### ▓ Nursing Diagnoses

Based on a thorough assessment, several nursing diagnoses may be identified. The more common diagnoses for the immobilized child are included in the Nursing Care Plan on p. 1772. Others may apply in specific situations.

### ▓ Planning

The goals for the immobilized child should be developed with the family and may include the following:

1. Child will have opportunity for mobilization within capabilities.
2. Child will maintain skin integrity.
3. Child will experience no physical injury.
4. Child will engage in diversional activity.
5. Child and family will receive adequate support.

### ▓ Implementation

Frequent position changes and the use of antiembolism stockings or Ace wraps may minimize or prevent dependent edema and fluid movement to third spaces and help to stimulate circulation, respiratory function, gastrointestinal motility, and neurologic sensations. When the condition allows it, the child can periodically assume the upright position on a tilt table or similar device to stimulate gastrointestinal and renal function and increase the stress on bones.

Each metabolic disturbance is treated specifically. Metabolism is increased by activity within the limitations of the disability and the capabilities of the child. High-protein, high-calorie foods are encouraged for correction of negative nitrogen balance. This may be difficult to correct by diet, especially if there is loss of appetite. It is desirable to determine the child's favorite foods and to allow the family to bring special foods from home or a favorite fast-food restaurant, as appropriate. This is especially helpful for children from varied cultural backgrounds. Stimulating the appetite with small servings of attractively arranged, preferred foods may be sufficient. Sometimes supplementary nasogastric feedings or hyperalimentation may be needed.

Diet modification for the child with increased serum calcium presents problems because the dairy foods that children often desire are high in this mineral. Acid ash foods, such as cereals, meats, poultry, fish, and cranberry or apple juice, are encouraged. Lying in a prone position may precipitate problems with swallowing or self-feeding. Therefore offering small bites, controlling swallowing with semisolid food, and using a straw for fluids are nursing interventions that will prevent choking. A suction machine should be in the vicinity for emergencies if the child has difficulty with secretions or food. The primary nursing measure for hypercalcemia is conscientious hydration and active remobilization as soon as possible.

Adequate hydration promotes bowel and kidney function and helps prevent complications in these systems. A knowledge of previous bowel habits and of a method to get the child to a toilet helps promote elimination and will be valuable data if needed for a bowel program. It is important to determine the words the child uses for elimination. Embarrassment can be avoided by a mutually satisfactory communication system. Whenever possible, the child should be helped into an upright position to use a fracture urinal or a bedpan. Providing privacy for toileting and encouraging the child to participate in solving toileting problems will increase the chances of a successful program.

Children are encouraged to be as active as their condition and restrictive devices allow. This usually poses few problems for children, whose innate ingenuity and natural inclination toward mobility provide them with the impetus for physical activity. They need the opportunity, the materials or objects to stimulate activity, and the encouragement and participation of others. Those who are unable to move will need passive exercise and movement, perhaps in consultation with a physical therapist (PT). An occupational therapist (OTR) and child-life specialist may also be involved to assist in planning activities to decrease the boredom of inactivity and to help regain lost skills such as self-feeding. A child psychologist may be consulted to discuss issues with the child and family such as depression, anger management, or the effects of the illness on family function.

Whenever possible, transporting the child by stretcher, stroller, or wagon outside the confines of the room will increase environmental stimuli and provide social contact with others. While hospitalized, the child will benefit from frequent visitors, clocks and calendars, and a program of diversional therapy, which will help the child to function in a more normal way. As soon as possible, the child should wear "street clothes" and resume school and preinjury hobbies. Play is the most useful tool of nursing (see Chapter 26), and activities, which are selected on the basis of interest, ability, and limitations, should include some form of physical activity that encourages the use of uninvolved muscles and joints. Any activity that is tolerated (e.g., turning in bed or changing the position of the bed in the room) helps to alter the monotony of immobilization and dissipates tension and frustration (Fig. 39-3). (See Critical Thinking Exercise box.)

Using dolls or a stuffed animal such as a bear to illustrate and explain the restraining method is a valuable tool for small children. Placing a cast, tubing, or other restraining equipment on the doll or stuffed animal offers the child a nonthreatening opportunity to express, through the doll, feelings concerning the restrictions and feelings toward the

## Critical Thinking Exercise

### The Child Who Is Immobilized

Jimmy, 5 years old, has been immobilized for 3 days because of a fracture of the femur. One parent has been with him since he was admitted. This morning he is yelling at his mother. You suspect which of the following reasons for his behavior?

FIRST, THINK ABOUT IT . . .

• What concepts or ideas are central to your thinking?
• What assumptions are you making?

1. The mother has been with him too long and should leave him to be cared for by the nurses.
2. He has no appropriate outlet for tensions.
3. He may be in pain.
4. All of the above.

*The correct answers are two and three. Jimmy is 5 years old. Central to your thinking are several concepts. First, at this age, children are usually physically active and often manage stress in physical ways. Jimmy should be provided with appropriate diversional and physical activities (e.g., playing with clay, coloring materials, punching bag). Also, both traction and a fracture can be painful. Pain assessment and management are key nursing responsibilities. Most children will be more comfortable lashing out at parents than at hospital personnel. Nonetheless, it is appropriate for a parent to stay with a 5-year-old while the child is hospitalized. Some parents may need help understanding the source of the child's anger so that they do not personalize it.*

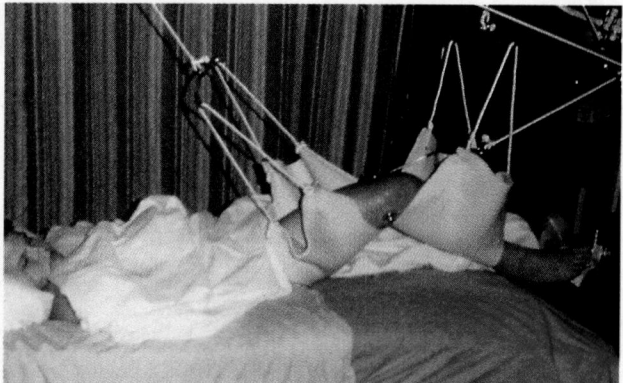

**Fig. 39-3**   Immobilized child. (Courtesy Paul Vincent Kuntz, Texas Children's Hospital.)

Visits from significant persons, such as family members and friends, offer occasions for emotional support and also provide opportunities for learning how to care for the child. Some privacy is needed, particularly by the adolescent, and most long-term health care facilities recognize that rooms shared by two to four youngsters are better environments for habilitation or rehabilitation. When roommates are selected according to age and companionship, a chance is available to test out thoughts and feelings safely with others. If a traumatic incident caused the child's disability, guilt feelings may be displayed overtly or masked behind regressive or aggressive behavior. The feeling that "I must have been bad to receive this fate" is common, and honest feed-back stating, "It just happened—it was an accident," needs repeating many times. Additional aspects of grieving are involved if there was a loss of another person or if permanent disability occurred as a result of the accident. All of these feelings need to be brought out and dealt with. In addition, professional persons working with these children must not "baby" or overprotect them but must help them to cope with their altered body image and reestablish their self-esteem.

For a child with greatly restricted movement (e.g., a child with quadriplegia or a child with a large bilateral hip spica cast), nursing care is a challenge. These situations require long-term care either in the hospital or, increasingly, at home. Wherever the care occurs, consistent planning and coordination of activities with professionals and significant others is vital. Nursing assessment includes psychosocial data, as well as physical manifestations, because long-term immobilization has a profound effect on the child and the family. Nursing approaches are evaluated frequently and continued, discontinued, or modified to meet the changing problems and goals. Physical effects of immobilization and appropriate nursing considerations are summarized in Table 39-1.

## ✖ Evaluation

The effectiveness of nursing interventions is determined by continual reassessment and evaluation of care based on the following observational guidelines:

1. Observe vital signs, neurologic signs, and respiratory, gastrointestinal, and renal functioning; inspect skin; observe effects of

nurse and other health care providers. It also provides a means for anticipatory teaching and explanation of needed restraining devices.

One of the most useful interventions to help children cope with immobility is participation in their own care. Self-care to the maximum extent is usually well received by children. They can help plan their daily routine, select their diet (when possible), and choose the clothes they are to wear, including innovative adornment, such as a baseball cap, brightly colored stockings, or other items of apparel that express each child's autonomy and individuality. They should be encouraged to do as much for themselves as they are able in order to keep muscles active and their interest alive. If feasible, they should be placed where they can benefit from the company of other children which assures them that they are not being singled out for this treatment.

It is important for children to understand behavioral limitations or rules. Their questions should be answered. For example, children need to know the reasons for medical, nursing, occupational, and physical therapy and to know that some schedules are necessary. In some areas they have a choice; in others they do not. They may or may not be permitted to sleep late, but they can choose their own clothing. Most of children's activity of daily living is play; therefore therapies that incorporate this concept are more apt to gain their cooperation.

**TABLE 39-1** Summary of physical effects of immobilization with nursing interventions*

| Primary Effects | Secondary Effects | Nursing Considerations |
|---|---|---|
| **Muscular System** | | |
| Decreased muscle strength, tone, and endurance | Decreased venous return and decreased cardiac output | Use antiembolism stockings or wrap legs with Ace bandages to promote venous return (monitor circulatory and neurovascular status of extremities when such devices are used) |
| | Decreased metabolism and need for oxygen | Plan play activities to use uninvolved extremities |
| | Decreased exercise tolerance | Place in upright posture when possible |
| | Bone demineralization | |
| Disuse atrophy and loss of muscle mass | Catabolism | Perform range-of-motion, active, passive, and stretching exercises |
| | Loss of strength | |
| Loss of joint mobility | Contractures, ankylosis of joints | Maintain correct body alignment |
| | | Use joint splints as indicated to prevent further deformity |
| | | Maintain range of motion |
| Weak back muscles | Secondary spinal deformities | Maintain body alignment |
| Weak abdominal muscles | Impaired respiration | See nursing considerations for respiratory system |
| **Skeletal System** | | |
| Bone demineralization—osteoporosis, hypercalcemia | Negative bone calcium uptake | With paralysis, use upright posture on tilt table |
| | Pathologic fractures | Handle extremities carefully when turning and positioning |
| | Calcium deposits | Administer calcium-mobilizing drugs (diphosphonates) and normal saline infusions if ordered |
| | Extraosseous bone formation, especially at hip, knee, elbow, and shoulder | Ensure adequate intake of fluid; monitor output |
| | Renal calculi | Acidify urine |
| | | Promptly treat urinary tract infections |
| Negative bone calcium uptake | Life-threatening electrolyte imbalance | Monitor serum levels of calcium |
| | | Provide electrolyte replacement as indicated |
| **Metabolism** | | |
| Decreased metabolic rate | Slowing of all systems | Mobilize as soon as possible |
| | Decreased food intake | Perform active and passive resistance and deep-breathing exercises |
| | | Ensure adequate food intake |
| | | Provide a high-protein diet |
| Negative nitrogen balance | Decline in nutritional state | Encourage small, frequent feedings with protein and preferred foods |
| | Impaired healing | Prevent pressure areas |
| Hypercalcemia | Electrolyte imbalance | See nursing considerations for skeletal system |
| Decreased production of stress hormones | Decreased physical and emotional coping capacity | Identify etiologies of stress |
| | | Implement appropriate interventions to lower physical and psychosocial stresses |
| **Cardiovascular System** | | |
| Decreased efficiency of orthostatic neurovascular reflexes | Inability to adapt readily to upright position | Monitor peripheral pulses and skin temperature changes |
| | Pooling of blood in extremities in upright posture | Use antiembolism stockings to decrease pooling when upright |
| Diminished vasopressor mechanism | Orthostatic intolerance with syncope, hypotension, decreased cerebral blood flow, tachycardia | Provide abdominal support |
| | | In severe cases, use antigravitational pants |
| | | Administer peripheral sympathetic stimulating agents such as ephedrine if ordered |
| | | Position horizontally |
| Altered distribution of blood volume | Increased cardiac workload | Monitor hydration, blood pressure, and urine output |
| | Decreased exercise tolerance | |
| Venous stasis | Pulmonary emboli or thrombi | Encourage and assist with frequent position changes |
| | | Elevate extremities without knee flexion |
| | | Ensure adequate fluid intake |
| | | Perform active or passive exercises or movement, as needed |
| | | Prescribe routine wearing of antiembolic stockings |
| | | Monitor for signs of pulmonary embolism: sudden dyspnea, chest pain, respiratory arrest |

*Individualize care according to child's needs—interventions may vary in each institution.

**TABLE 39-1** Summary of physical effects of immobilization with nursing interventions—cont'd

| Primary Effects | Secondary Effects | Nursing Considerations |
|---|---|---|
| **Cardiovascular System—cont'd** | | |
| Venous stasis—cont'd | | Promptly intervene to maintain adequate oxygen if signs and symptoms of pulmonary emboli are noted |
| | | Measure circumference of extremities periodically |
| | | Give anticoagulant drugs as ordered |
| Dependent edema | Tissue breakdown and susceptibility to infection | Administer skin care |
| | | Turn every 2 hours |
| | | Monitor skin color, temperature, and integrity |
| | | Use pressure-relief mattress as necessary to prevent skin breakdown (see Chapter 27) |
| **Respiratory System** | | |
| Decreased need for oxygen | Altered oxygen–carbon dioxide exchange and metabolism | Exercise as tolerated |
| | | Use position for optimum chest expansion |
| Decreased chest expansion and diminished vital capacity | Diminished oxygen intake | Use prone positioning without pressure on abdomen to allow gravity to aid in diaphragmatic excursion |
| | Dyspnea and inadequate arterial oxygen saturation; acidosis | When sitting, maintain proper alignment to prevent pressure on respiratory mechanism |
| Poor abdominal tone and distention | Interference with diaphragmatic excursion | Avoid restriction of chest and abdominal musculature |
| | | Supply torso support to promote chest expansion |
| Mechanical or biochemical secretion retention | Hypostatic pneumonia | Change position frequently |
| | Bacterial and viral pneumonia | Carry out percussion, vibration, and drainage (or suctioning) as necessary |
| | Atelectasis | Monitor breath sounds |
| Loss of respiratory muscle strength | Poor cough | Encourage coughing and deep breathing |
| | | Support chest wall when coughing |
| | | Use special devices such as a rocking bed, breathing bag, incentive spirometers |
| | | Observe for signs of acute respiratory distress with pulse oximetry or blood gases as necessary |
| | Upper respiratory infection | Avoid contact with infected persons |
| | | Provide adequate hydration |
| | | Administer immunizations as necessary (pneumococcal, meningococcal) |
| **Gastrointestinal System** | | |
| Distention caused by poor abdominal muscle tone | Interference with respiratory movements | Monitor bowel sounds |
| | | Encourage small, frequent feedings |
| | Difficulty in feeding in prone position | Sit in upright position if possible |
| No specific primary effect | Gravitation effect on feces through ascending colon or weakened smooth muscle tone may cause constipation | Carry out bowel-training program with hydration, stool softeners, increased fiber intake, and mild laxatives if necessary |
| | Anorexia | Stimulate appetite with favored foods |
| **Urinary System** | | |
| Alteration of gravitational force | Difficulty in voiding in prone position | Position as upright as possible to void |
| Impaired ureteral peristalsis | Urinary retention in calyces and bladder | Hydrate to ensure adequate urinary output for age |
| | Infection | Collect specimens as needed |
| | Renal calculi | Stimulate bladder emptying with warm running water, water, as necessary |
| | | Catheterize only for severe retention |
| | | Administer antibiotics as indicated |
| **Integumentary System** | | |
| Altered tissue integrity | Decreased circulation and pressure leading to tissue injury | Turn and position at least every 2 hours |
| | Difficulty with personal hygiene | Frequently inspect total skin surface |
| | | Eliminate mechanical factors causing pressure, friction, or irritation |
| | | Assess ability to perform hygienic care and assist with bathing, grooming, and toileting as needed |
| | | Ensure adequate intake of protein, vitamins, and minerals |

correct functioning of equipment and appliances (restraints, traction, cast, braces).

2. Observe child's behavior; engage in dialogue to elicit feelings, concerns, and interests.

3. Observe child's activities and interests.

4. Interview child and family regarding their feelings and concerns.

The *expected outcomes* are described in the Nursing Care Plan on p. 1772.

# Nursing Care Plan
## The Child Who Is Immobilized

---

**NURSING DIAGNOSIS:** Impaired physical mobility related to mechanical restrictions, physical disability (specify level)

**PATIENT GOAL 1:** Will have opportunity for mobilization

- **NURSING INTERVENTIONS/*RATIONALES***

Transport child by stretcher, stroller, wagon, bed, wheelchair or other conveyance from confines of room *to provide for mobilization despite restrictions*

Change position of bed in room *to alter monotony of immobilization*

Change position in bed when possible *to decrease feelings of being immobilized*

- **EXPECTED OUTCOMES**

Child moves from confines of room or within room

Child's position is changed when possible

**PATIENT GOAL 2:** Will maintain optimum autonomy

- **NURSING INTERVENTIONS/*RATIONALES***

Instruct child in use of orthoses, crutches, wheelchair *to facilitate independent mobility*

Provide mobilizing devices (orthoses, crutches, wheelchair)

Assist with acquisition of specialized equipment *to encourage independence*

Instruct in use of equipment *to ensure safety*

Encourage activities that require mobilization

Allow as much freedom of movement as possible and encourage normal activities *to maintain a sense of autonomy*

Encourage child to participate in own care as much as possible *to encourage sense of autonomy and independence*

Allow child to make choices (e.g., daily routine, food, clothes) *to encourage sense of autonomy despite limitations*

- **EXPECTED OUTCOMES**

Child moves about without assistance

Child engages in activities appropriate to limitations and developmental level

---

**NURSING DIAGNOSIS:** Risk for impaired skin integrity related to immobility, therapeutic appliances

**PATIENT GOAL 1:** Will maintain skin integrity

- **NURSING INTERVENTIONS/*RATIONALES***

Place child on pressure-reducing surface (mattress overlay or special bed) *to prevent tissue breakdown and pressure necrosis*

Change position frequently, unless contraindicated, *to prevent dependent edema and stimulate circulation*

Protect pressure points (e.g., trochanter, sacrum, ankle, shoulder, occiput)

Inspect skin surfaces regularly for signs of irritation, redness, evidence of pressure

Eliminate mechanical factors causing pressure, friction, or irritation (e.g., keep linen and clothing free of wrinkles)

Maintain meticulous skin cleanliness

Gently massage only *healthy* skin with lubricating substance *to stimulate circulation*

See also Maintaining Healthy Skin, Chapter 27

- **EXPECTED OUTCOME**

Skin remains clean and intact with no evidence of irritation

---

**NURSING DIAGNOSIS:** Risk for injury related to impaired mobility

**PATIENT GOAL 1:** Will experience no physical injury

- **NURSING INTERVENTIONS/*RATIONALES***

Teach correct use of mobilizing devices or apparatus *to ensure safety*

Assist with moving and ambulating as needed *to ensure safety*

Remove hazards from environment (specify)

Modify environment as needed (specify)

Keep call button within reach

Keep siderails up at all times *to prevent falls*

Help child to use bathroom or commode if possible

Implement safety measures appropriate to child's developmental age (specify)

- **EXPECTED OUTCOME**

Child remains free of injury

---

**NURSING DIAGNOSIS:** Deficient diversional activity related to impaired mobility, musculoskeletal impairment, confinement to hospital or home

**PATIENT GOAL 1:** Will engage in diversional activity

- **NURSING INTERVENTIONS/*RATIONALES* AND EXPECTED OUTCOMES**

See also Nursing Care Plan: The Child in the Hospital, Chapter 26

---

**NURSING DIAGNOSIS:** Risk for interrupted family processes related to a child with disability, illness

**PATIENT (FAMILY) GOAL 1:** Will receive support as desired

- **NURSING INTERVENTIONS/*RATIONALES* AND EXPECTED OUTCOMES**

See also Nursing Care Plan: The Family of the Child Who Is Ill or Hospitalized, Chapter 26

# Mobilization Devices

## Orthotics and Prosthetics

Developments in the disciplines of *orthotics* (fabrication and fitting of braces) and *prosthetics* (fabrication and fitting of artificial limbs) have resulted in lighter and better-fitting devices and thus greater patient compliance. *Orthoses* are often used to prevent deformity, increase energy efficiency of gait, and control alignment. Paralyzed or markedly weakened extremities can sometimes be stabilized by braces that facilitate walking. Some are designed to stabilize the extremities and offer support during ambulation. Special joint hinges permit the hip, knee, and ankle to flex during sitting, whereas the leg is held rigid during ambulation. Well-fitted orthoses promote ambulation, whereas ill-fitting braces are dangerous to the balance of the child and frequently cause muscle stress and tissue breakdown. Braces for the growing child will need frequent adjusting and replacement by the orthotist if long-term use is necessary.

A standing frame or a parapodium (a standing frame on a circular base) is used to get small children in an upright position and begin mobilization. Children learn to use their arms and shift their weight to swivel the base of the parapodium to mobilize. Four common types of orthoses are used in older children and are described based on the joints controlled by the orthosis. The *ankle-foot orthosis (AFO)* is used to prevent footdrop due to bed rest, trauma to the foot, or paralysis of muscles that flex the foot; to prevent heel cord tightening following heel cord–lengthening surgery; or to support the foot in proper position for standing and walking (Fig. 39-4). AFOs are now available in patterns and colors.

The *knee-ankle-foot orthosis (KAFO)* is used to prevent buckling of the knee, to support the extremity when there is paralysis or marked weakness of the knee extension or quadriceps muscle, or to protect the limb when the bone structure is weak (Fig. 39-5). The *hip-knee-ankle-foot orthosis (HKAFO)* is used to provide various types of control for the knee and ankle joints (as described above), as well as the hip (e.g., flail lower limb and paralysis). The *reciprocal gait orthosis (RGO)* is a type of HKAFO that has a mechanism allowing children with significant paraplegia to walk in a reciprocal fashion on a flat surface. RGOs are used in children with spinal cord injury, sacral agenesis, and spina bifida.

The *thoracolumbosacral orthosis (TLSO)* is custom molded and fits snugly around the trunk of the body to exert pressure on the ribs and back, to support the spine in a straight position (Fig. 39-6). The *Boston brace* is an underarm orthosis customized from prefabricated plastic shells, with cor-

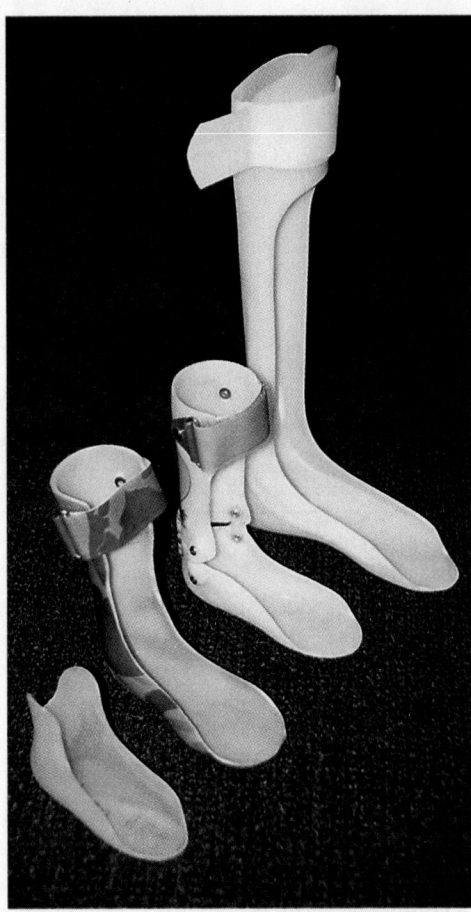

**Fig. 39-4** *Left to right:* Supramalleolar ankle-foot orthosis (AFO), solid ankle AFO, articulating ankle AFO, floor reaction AFO.

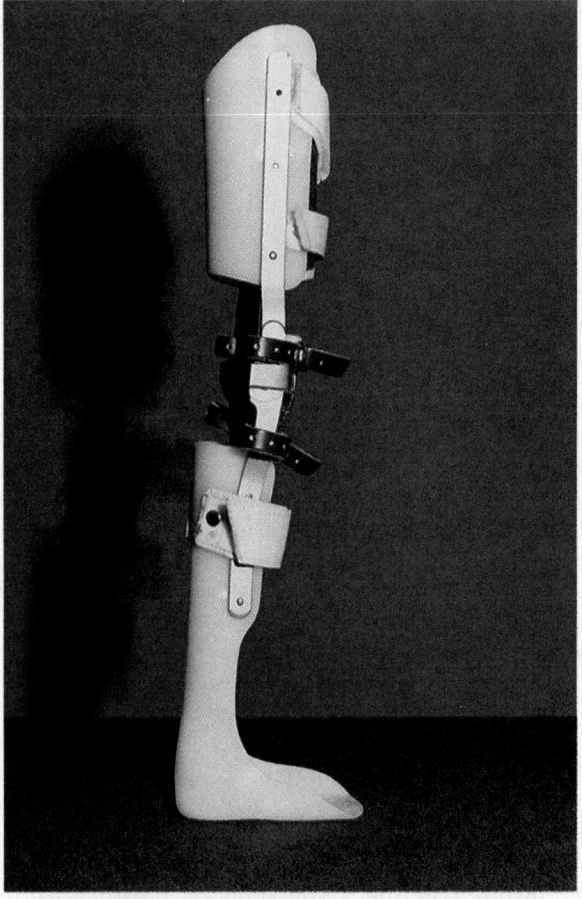

**Fig. 39-5** Knee-ankle-foot orthosis (KAFO).

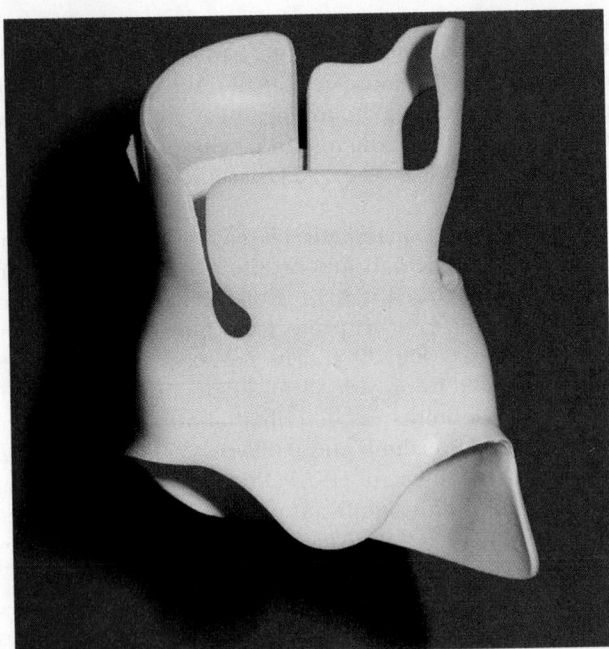

**Fig. 39-6** Thoracolumbosacral orthosis (TLSO).

---

**Box 39-2** ■ ■ ■
**Types of Amputations**

**Syme**—Ankle disarticulation
**BK**—Below knee
**KD**—Knee disarticulation
**AK**—Above knee
**HD**—Hip disarticulation
**WD**—Wrist disarticulation
**BE**—Below elbow
**ED**—Elbow disarticulation
**AE**—Above elbow
**SD**—Shoulder disarticulation

---

rective forces for each patient supplied by lateral pads. These braces may prevent the progression of curves in the spine, such as scoliosis, or provide needed torso support in a child with paraplegia. The *Jewett-Taylor brace* is sometimes used to support the spine and trunk during ambulation to prevent compression after fracture of the spinal column.

An orthosis must fit each body curvature to avoid undue pressure on tissues and imbalance between muscle groups. Bony prominences where a brace has contact, such as along the spine, chin, and iliac crests, are observed closely for pressure or irritation and are padded as necessary.

When *prostheses* are prescribed, many factors are considered—level of amputation, age, weight, activity, agility, and skin condition. Each prosthesis is custom-made or fabricated of various plastic and foam materials. The style of the prosthesis depends on the most distal joint involved in the amputation or prosthetic fitting. Common abbreviations used to describe types of amputations are listed in Box 39-2.

Prosthetic advances and developments are constantly evolving in both fabrication and fitting. Myoelectric devices,

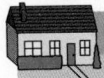

cosmetic materials used in terminal gloves and feet, and CAD-CAM (computer-aided design—computer-aided manufacturing) socket construction are but a few of the recent changes that have positively affected patients who require prostheses.

## Nursing Considerations

Meticulous skin care under a brace is necessary. At times, protective clothing should be worn under braces to protect the skin from friction and pressure. Assessment of all areas that make contact with the brace, every 2 to 4 hours for the first few days following application, is recommended. If any area is reddened, the brace is removed for ½ to 1 hour. If redness does not disappear, the nurse should notify the practitioner or orthotist. (See Family Home Care box.)

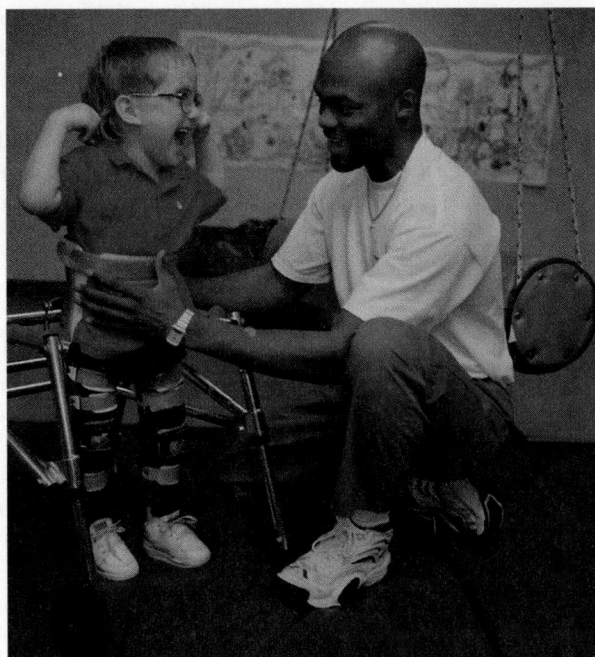

**Fig. 39-7**   Young child with a rear-rolling walker. (Courtesy Paul Vincent Kuntz, Texas Children's Hospital.)

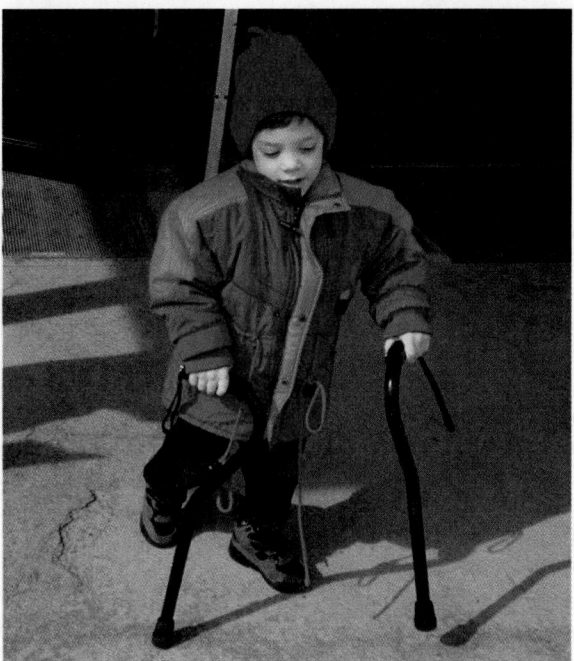

**Fig. 39-8**   Child learning to walk with canes.

It is important to assess the condition of the skin, especially noting areas of redness or breaks in the integrity of the skin, before application of a prosthesis. Prevention of skin breakdown is best accomplished through good hygiene of the residual limb, proper fitting of the artificial limb, and prosthetic training. (See Family Home Care box.)

Safety is another important consideration. Parallel bars provide secure handrails on both sides of children as they learn to walk again with or without braces or a prosthesis. As they become more proficient, a walker with or without wheels is substituted for the bars and children are no longer confined to a limited territory. Children then progress to crutches if their age and condition permit it.

## Crutches and Canes

Crutches are used when children are not allowed to bear weight, need support for balance while walking in braces, or can only place part of their body weight on an extremity, such as with most lower leg injuries. A variety of crutches can be employed, and the selection is determined by the individual needs of the child. *Axillary crutches* are used most frequently as temporary assistance. *Forearm crutches* are the usual selection for children who anticipate permanent use, such as paraplegic children who are able to use braces. For children with limited hand and arm strength or function, *trough crutches* allow the weight to be assumed by the elbow. For habilitating small children who have not yet learned to walk or who are unsteady, front- or rear-rolling walkers are typically used until the children can progress to crutches (Fig. 39-7).

Children must be properly fitted for a crutch or cane to prevent both poor posture and crutch pressure on the axilla during ambulation. Measuring for crutches and teaching crutch and cane use are usually assumed by a physical ther-

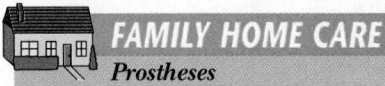

**FAMILY HOME CARE**
*Prostheses*

**CARE OF RESIDUAL LIMB**

Wash with mild, nonperfumed soap, rinse, and dry thoroughly daily.
A small amount of powder may be used on the skin, but no alcohol.
Check skin for redness, sensitive areas, or signs of infection.

**CARE OF PROSTHESIS**

The socket should be routinely washed with water and mild soap, rinsed, and dried thoroughly.
Straps and rubber bands should be checked with each application.
Check joints to ensure that they operate smoothly.
Replace worn or broken parts (heels, soles, straps) as needed.
Wear stump socks to absorb perspiration, prevent skin friction, and provide comfort.
Change socks daily and wash and dry following instructions provided by prosthetist.

apist; however, nurses in some areas such as the emergency department do teach children crutch walking. Nurses are also the persons who supervise the use of crutches and canes in pediatric units and in the home (Fig. 39-8). The type of crutch gait taught to children depends on their degree of stability, whether or not the knees can be flexed, the amount of weight bearing allowed, and the specific goal established for each child.

Bed exercises for strengthening arms and shoulders are important before crutch use if immobilization has been prolonged. The youngster gains confidence in ambulating by wearing a safety belt held by the therapist. The types of gaits used and instructions to children are similar to those given to adults. They are conveyed in language children understand and with a demonstration. Most children grasp the techniques readily.

### Wheelchairs

Wheelchairs are used temporarily or permanently as a means of transportation. For temporary use, a wheelchair should fit the child and contain any adaptations needed, such as an elevating leg rest or reclining back. The child is taught how to transfer in and out of the chair and how to propel it safely. Prescribing a wheelchair for permanent use is the joint responsibility of the physician and therapist after an assessment of home and surroundings. A wheelchair should be neither too small nor too large and preferably should be one that can be adapted to the child's growth needs (Fig. 39-9). Detachable or rotating armrests, which permit easy transfer in and out, are needed for children with spinal cord injuries.

Other desirable features are detachable and swing-away footrests and detachable desk arms. Elevating leg rests are required for children who are prone to contractures, and a reclining back rest is needed for those who may have poor trunk balance (Fig. 39-10). A pressure-relief cushion should be provided for the child who has decreased sensation. Hand rim and brake lever projections are helpful for the child with upper extremity weakness. For children who have the use of only one arm, a special "one-arm drive" wheelchair is available. Children with paraplegia will require upper arm strengthening exercises and instruction on transfer techniques before wheelchair mobilization. Often a tilt table must be used to overcome the problems of orthostatic hypotension before wheelchair sitting can be tolerated.

Various motorized chairs are available for marked upper extremity weakness, and mouth- or cheek-operated models are available for children who do not have the use of upper extremities so that they can operate them independently. Very small children who have permanent paralysis of the lower extremities are provided with specially designed units that allow independent mobility. A detachable handle on these units permits their conversion to strollers.

## THE CHILD WITH A FRACTURE

The process of *ossification,* the gradual conversion of precursor substances (namely cartilage) to bony structures, begins in the embryo and continues until the child is 18 to 21 years of age. In long bones this process progresses outwardly from the *diaphysis,* the hard shaftlike portion that constitutes the major portion of the bone. Within this hard, compact shaft is the hollow medullary canal composed of the bone marrow.

The *epiphysis,* located at the ends of long bones, consists of layers of cartilage, subchondral bone, and spongelike cancellous bone. Situated between the diaphysis and epiphysis is the *epiphyseal plate,* which plays a major role in the longitudinal growth of the developing child (Fig. 39-11). The *periosteum,* the thin, tough membrane covering all bones, contains blood vessels that nourish the living bone. Damage to this thin membrane can be a major problem in bone growth and healing.

### Fractures

Bones fracture when the resistance of the bone against the stress being exerted yields to the stress force. Fractures are a common injury at any age but are more likely to occur in children and elderly persons. The natural tendency toward

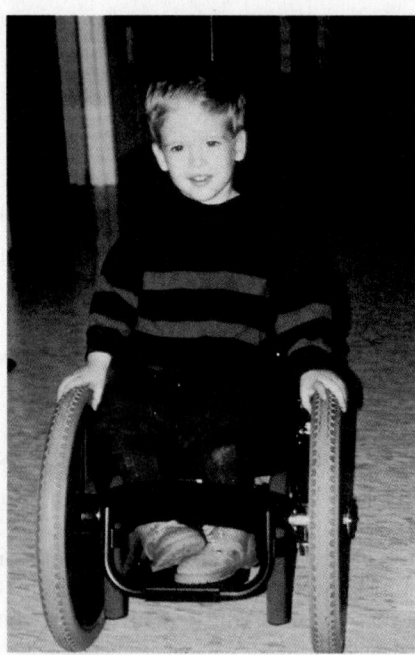

**Fig. 39-9** Wheelchair should be sized appropriately to the child.

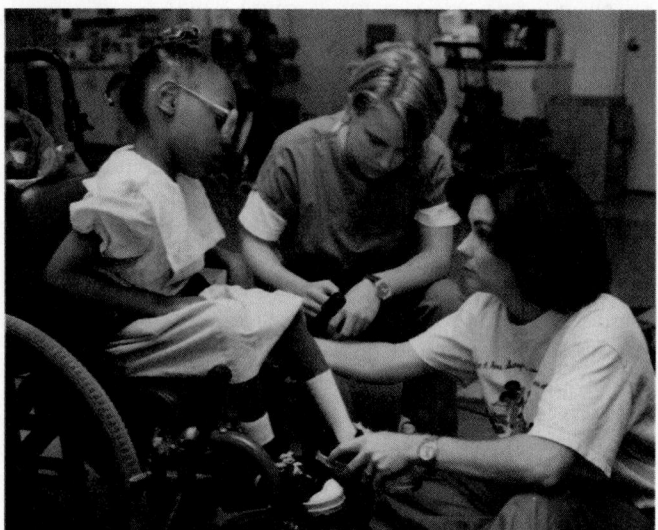

**Fig. 39-10** Child in wheelchair with elevating leg rests and reclining back rest. (Courtesy Paul Vincent Kuntz, Texas Children's Hospital.)

active mobility and their limited gross motor coordination make children susceptible to physical injury.

## Etiology

The causes of fracture injuries in children are those described for general traumatic injuries in childhood. Fractures in infancy are more often the result of birth trauma, injury, or child abuse. Aside from motor vehicle injuries, true accidents rarely occur in infancy; therefore injuries in children in that age-group warrant further investigation. (See Critical Thinking Exercise box.) Most often, early bone trauma in infants consists of periosteal bleeding in the long bones of the arms and legs, usually caused by rough handling, twisting, and pulling, which is not evident on radiographic examination until 3 to 6 weeks after the injury. Any investigation of fractures in infants, particularly multiple fractures, should include the suspicion of osteogenesis imperfecta (see p. 1819). In any small child, radiographic evidence of fractures at various stages of healing, with few exceptions, indicates physical abuse. (See Community Focus box on p. 1758.)

Fractures of the forearm are common bone injuries in childhood and are usually caused when the child extends the palm of the hand to break a fall. The force resulting from a fall on the outstretched hand progresses up the length of the extremity with the possibility of injury to the finger, wrist, elbow, shoulder, or clavicle (Fig. 39-12). The clavicle is probably the bone most frequently broken in children; approximately half of clavicle fractures occur in children under 10 years of age. Many occur at birth. Hip fractures are rare in children and require a great deal of force to produce. A femoral neck fracture may be sustained in children 6 or 7 years of age as a result of pedestrian-automobile accidents because their hip height is on the same level as an automobile bumper. In older children the femur is the most likely target; in adolescents knee injuries are common.

Children fall from heights (e.g., trees, roofs) as their insatiable curiosity and immature judgment lure them to places of danger. Fractures in school-age children are often the result of bicycle-automobile collision, skateboard or scooter injury. Sports, organized or not, are a frequent cause of injury in the school-age child and adolescent.

At all ages motor vehicle mishaps are a frequent cause of bone injury. Most children who are hit by an automobile are between 4 and 7 years of age and sustain a triad of injuries, which must be kept in mind when making an assessment: (1) the child's femur, which is at the level of the bumper, is fractured; (2) the hood of the automobile produces injuries to the child's trunk; and (3) a contralateral head injury is usually sustained when the child is thrown to the ground by the impact (Fig. 39-13). Therefore a child with any of these injuries who was struck by an automobile should be examined for evidence of the other two.

## Pathophysiology

The anatomic, biomechanical, and physiologic nature of children's skeletons causes differences in the pattern

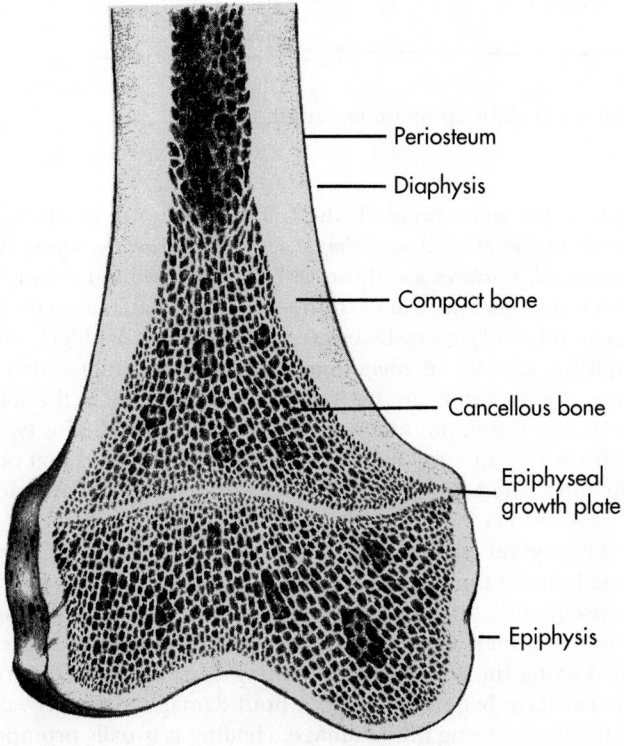

**Fig. 39-11** Bone showing relationships of compact and cancellous bone, epiphysis, epiphyseal plate, and diaphysis. (From Thompson JM and others: *Mosby's clinical nursing,* ed 4, St Louis, 1997, Mosby.)

Labels on figure:
- Periosteum
- Diaphysis
- Compact bone
- Cancellous bone
- Epiphyseal growth plate
- Epiphysis

---

### Critical Thinking Exercise

#### Femur Fracture in an Infant

A family arrives at the emergency department with an 8-month-old infant who has a fractured right femur. They say they are not sure how it happened. Your initial action should be which of the following?

**FIRST, THINK ABOUT IT . . .**

- What information are you using?
- What are you taking for granted, what assumptions are you making?

1. Call social services, because child abuse is likely.
2. Consider the possibility of osteogenesis imperfecta.
3. Assess the child.
4. Apply a temporary splint to the affected limb.

*The correct answer is three. A thorough nursing assessment of any injury is the first step in triage and is important to the provision of proper care. At the same time, astute practitioners will be aware that a fractured femur in an infant is unusual and should raise suspicions of posssible child abuse, especially when parents can provide no explanation. Osteogenesis imperfecta is another important consideration in unexplained fractures (see p. 1819). Option number four should not be carried out until the child's injury has been thoroughly evaluated by a specialist.*

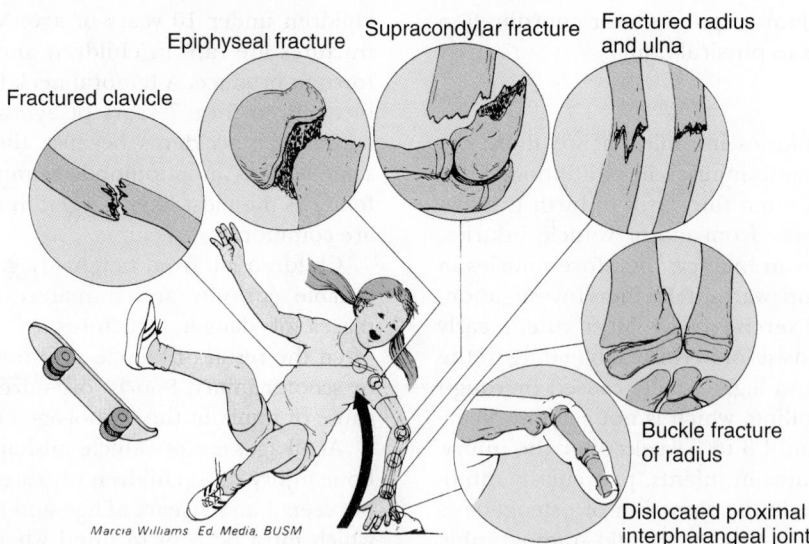

**Fig. 39-12** Trauma resulting from progression of force in fall on outstretched hand. (From Segal D: Pediatric orthopedic emergencies, *Pediatr Clin North Am* 26(4):793-802, 1979.)

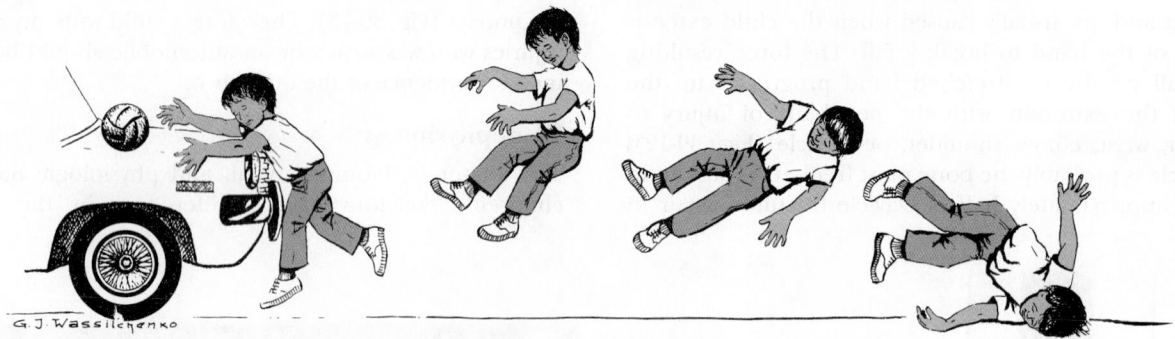

**Fig. 39-13** Triad of injuries sustained when child is struck by automobile: femur, trunk, and contralateral head injury.

of fractures, the problems of diagnosis, and the methods of treatment. The bones of the adult are strong and require a violent traumatic force to fracture, which is accompanied by massive injury to surrounding soft tissues. In children the bones are more easily injured, and fractures may result from minor falls or twists and are less likely to be accompanied by soft tissue damage. Features of children's fractures not observed in the adult are outlined in Box 39-3.

**Types of Fractures.** A fractured bone consists of fragments—the fragment closest to the midline, or the proximal fragment, and the fragment farthest from the midline, or the distal fragment. When fracture fragments are separated, the fracture is *complete;* when fragments remain attached, it is said to be *incomplete.* The fracture line can be:

Transverse—Crosswise, at right angles to the long axis of the bone
Oblique—Slanting but straight, between a horizontal and a perpendicular direction
Spiral—Slanting and circular, twisting around the bone shaft

All fractures affect the entire cross-section of the bone. The twisting of an extremity while the bone is breaking re-

sults in the spiral break. If the fracture does not produce a break in the skin, it is a *simple,* or *closed, fracture. Open,* or *compound, fractures* are those with an open wound through which the bone protrudes. If the bone fragments cause damage to other organs or tissues (e.g., the lung or bladder), the injury is said to be *complicated.* When small fragments of bone are broken from the fractured shaft and lie in the surrounding tissue, the fracture is called *comminuted.* This type of fracture is rare in children. The types of fractures that occur most often in children are shown in Fig. 39-14 and described in Box 39-4.

**Epiphyseal (or Physeal) Injuries.** The weakest point of long bones is the cartilage growth plate, or epiphyseal plate. Consequently this is a frequent site of damage during trauma. Under most conditions, fractures in this area proceed along the zone of degenerating cartilage cells, before the cartilage begins to ossify, without damage to the growth plate, thus causing little damage. Healing is usually prompt. When fracture lines deviate from a transverse direction through the degenerating cells, more serious damage to the epiphysis and the plate may occur. Fig. 39-15 illustrates the types of epiphyseal injuries in order of increasing risk of

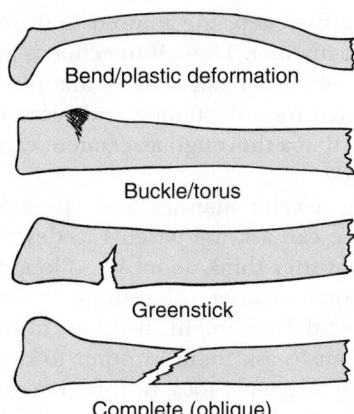

**Fig. 39-14** Common types of fractures in children. Note that there are subclassifications of complete fractures based on a description of the fracture line.

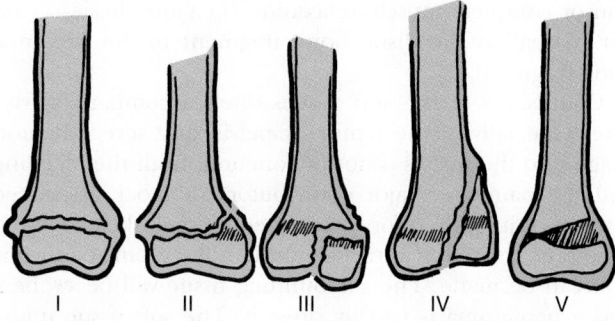

**Fig. 39-15** Types of epiphyseal injuries in order of increasing risk. The injuries are classified as follows: *type I,* separation or slip of growth plate without fracture of the bone; *type II,* separation of growth plate *and* breaking off of a section of metaphysis; *type III,* fracture of the epiphysis extending through the joint surface; *type IV,* fracture of the growth plate, epiphysis, *and* metaphysis; *type V,* crushing injury of epiphysis (can only be diagnosed in retrospect). This classification of epiphyseal injuries was developed by orthopedists RB Salter and WR Harris. (First published in Salter RB, Harris WR: Injuries involving the physeal plate, *J Bone Joint Surg Am* 45[3]:587-622, 1963.)

---

**Box 39-3** ▪ ■ ▫
**Features of Fractures in Children**

1. The growth plate, a thick, elastic portion of bone where growth takes place, serves to absorb shock and protect joint surfaces from injury and is the means by which the limb is able to grow and to straighten itself. Growth is stimulated by a fracture in the diaphysis, whereas damage to the growth plate can cause shortening and often a progressive angular deformity.
2. The periosteum of a child's bone is thicker, stronger, and has more active osteogenic potential as compared with the adult.
3. The pliable bones of growing children are more porous than those of the adult, which allows them to bend, buckle, and break in a "greenstick" manner. The greater porosity increases the flexibility of the bone and dissipates and absorbs a significant amount of the force on impact.
4. Healing is more rapid in children, and the rapidity is inversely related to the age of the child. The younger the child, the more rapid the healing process. Nonunion of bone fragments is almost unknown in children.
5. Stiffness is unusual and, unlike in adults, an uninjured joint in a child can be immobilized for a long period without producing stiffness that lasts longer than a few minutes. Injured joints do become stiff, however, and the current trend is toward early mobilization and active range-of-motion exercises as preventive measures.
6. Children only complain when something is wrong. Unreasonable crying, restlessness, and calling for the parents are usually indications that something is amiss and requires investigation.

---

**Box 39-4** ▪ ■ ▫
**Types of Fractures in Children**

**Bends**—A child's flexible bone can be bent 45 degrees or more before breaking. However, if bent, the bone will straighten slowly, but not completely, to produce some deformity but without the angulation that exists when the bone breaks. Bends occur more commonly in the ulna and fibula, often in association with fractures of the radius and tibia.

**Buckle fracture**—Compression of the porous bone produces a buckle, or torus, fracture. This appears as a raised or bulging projection at the fracture site. Torus fractures occur in the most porous portion of the bone near the metaphysis (the portion of the bone shaft adjacent to the epiphysis) and are more common in young children.

**Greenstick fracture**—Occurs when a bone is angulated beyond the limits of bending. The compressed side bends and the tension side fails, causing an incomplete fracture similar to the break observed when a green stick is broken.

**Complete fracture**—Divides the bone fragments. They often remain attached by a periosteal hinge, which can aid or hinder reduction. Complete fractures are subclassified by a description of the fracture line as transverse, spiral, oblique, comminuted (multiple fractures at the site), or butterfly (a large, central fragment at the site).

---

permanent epiphyseal damage and possible growth disturbance. The Salter-Harris classification is typically used to describe epiphyseal injuries, as indicated in Fig. 39-15.

Detection of epiphyseal injuries is sometimes difficult, and they may be mistaken for dislocations or ligamentous injuries. Fractures involving the epiphysis or epiphyseal plate present special problems in determining whether or not bone growth will be affected. Early and correct assessment is essential to minimize the incidence of longitudinal growth problems and angular deformities. The medical/surgical management of these injuries is different than that

for other fractures because open reduction and internal fixation are often employed to prevent complications. If the affected limb is shorter, epiphyseal surgery is performed either to stimulate the involved epiphysis or to retard growth in the unaffected leg.

**Associated Problems.** Immediately after a fracture occurs, the muscles contract and physiologically splint the injured area. This phenomenon accounts for the muscle tightness observed over a fracture site and the deformity that is produced as the muscles pull the bone ends out of alignment. This muscle response must be overcome by traction or complete muscle relaxation (i.e., anesthesia) in order to realign the distal bone fragment to the proximal bone fragment.

Contusions of the soft tissues often accompany a fracture, especially of the femur or pelvis, and severe hemorrhage into the tissues is not uncommon. Both the bleeding and the pain are major contributors to shock associated with this injury; therefore, suspected musculoskeletal injury should be treated as a fracture until radiographic confirmation can be made. The surrounding tissue will be swollen, and a hematoma is usually present. The soft tissue injury must be treated as any other contusion. Because the injury may cause damage to essential structures, the circulatory and neurologic status of tissues distal to the fracture is carefully assessed, especially for fractures of the femur and supracondylar fractures of the elbow.

## Clinical Manifestations

Children demonstrate the usual signs of injury—generalized swelling, pain or tenderness, and diminished functional use of the affected part. There may be bruising, severe muscular rigidity, and sometimes crepitus (a grating sensation at the fracture site), which are also frequent signs in adults. More often the fracture is remarkably stable because of the usually intact periosteum. The child may even be able to use an affected arm or walk on a fractured leg.

> **NURSING ALERT**   A fracture should be strongly suspected in a small child who refuses to walk or crawl.

Although neurologic and vascular damage is much less frequent in children than in adult patients, the integrity of these structures must be thoroughly assessed. This is often difficult in infants and young children who are unable to cooperate. Vascular injury is most likely to occur with supracondylar fractures of the humerus and femur. Femoral and popliteal vessels and the sciatic nerve are prone to trauma in femoral fractures; humeral fractures may cause damage to the medial, ulnar, or radial nerves and to the brachial artery.

> **NURSING ALERT**   The five "Ps" of ischemia from a vascular injury—*pain, pallor, pulselessness, paresthesia,* and *paralysis*—should be included in an assessment.

**NURSING TIP**   A radial head dislocation, or "nursemaid's elbow," is often seen in children 1 to 3 years of age and is commonly mistaken for a fracture because the child refuses to use the affected arm and holds it against the body (see p. 1799).

## Nursing Assessment

Nurses often make the initial assessment of a child with a suspected fracture. (See Emergency Treatment box.) The child and the parents are frightened and upset, the child is in pain, and, because some fractures are obvious, the parents and frequently the child are already convinced of the diagnosis. As a first step, the injured limb should be supported in some manner. Then, if the child is alert and there is no evidence of hemorrhage, the initial nursing interventions are directed toward calming and reassuring the child and parents so that a thorough assessment can be more easily accomplished.

Maintaining a calm manner and speaking in a quiet voice, the nurse can ask the parents to describe what happened and what they think about it. As long as the limb is supported in some manner, this minute or two does not delay or endanger the treatment. It is best not to touch children initially but to ask them to point to the painful area and wiggle their fingers or toes. By this time they usually feel relatively safe and will allow someone to touch them gently to feel the pulse and test for sensation. A child's anxiety is greatly influenced by previous experiences with injury and health care personnel. However, children need to be told what will happen and what they can do to help. The affected limb need not be palpated and should not be moved unless properly splinted. Some type of splint should be applied carefully if the child must be transported to a hospital or to the radiology department and cast room.

## Diagnostic Evaluation

A history of the injury or events leading up to the injury may be lacking for childhood injuries. Infants and toddlers are unable to clearly communicate the details of what occurred. Older children may not be reliable informants or volunteer information (even under direct questioning) if the injury occurred during forbidden activities. In cases of child abuse, parents or caregivers may give false information deliberately in order to protect themselves. Whenever possible, it is helpful to get information from someone who witnessed the injury.

**Radiography.**   Radiographic examination is the most useful diagnostic tool for assessing skeletal trauma. The calcium deposits in mature bone make the entire structure radiopaque. However, in normal growth and development, much of the skeleton of infants and young children is composed of radiolucent growth cartilage that does not appear on radiographs. In addition, the epiphyseal cartilage and undisplaced separations of the epiphysis, which often occur, are not easily detected on x-ray films. Radiographs are sometimes less reliable in predicting extremity fractures than are gross deformity and point tenderness.

Many practitioners obtain a film of the uninjured limb for a direct comparison to help identify minor alterations in alignment and configuration of the epiphysis and associated injuries that might be missed. Radiographic films are also taken after fracture reduction and in some situations may be taken during the healing process to determine satisfactory progress.

**Laboratory Evaluation Studies.**   Severe soft tissue, muscle, and bone injury often results in the destruction of red blood cells with a rise in bilirubin and a fall in the hemoglobin or hematocrit reading. The child's homeostatic mechanisms are activated to correct the problem, and generally only supportive therapy with a high-protein diet and iron replacement is needed. When muscle integrity is disrupted, enzymes nor-

---

**Box 39-5** ■ ■ ■
**Criteria for Determining Use
of Reduction Method for Fractures**

Age of child
Degree of displacement
Amount of overriding
Degree of edema
Condition of skin and soft tissue
Sensation and circulation distal to fracture

---

**Box 39-6** ■ ■ ■
**Medical Interventions Associated
with Fracture Injury**

Control of pain, hemorrhage, and edema
Relief of muscle spasms
Realignment of fracture fragments
Promotion of bone healing
Immobilization of fracture until adequate healing has begun
Prevention of secondary complications
Limitation of disuse syndrome
Restoration of function

---

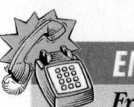

## EMERGENCY TREATMENT
### Fracture

Assess extent of injury—5 "Ps":
  Pain and point of tenderness
  Pulselessness—distal to the fracture site (late and
    ominous sign)
  Pallor
  Paresthesia—sensation distal to the fracture site
  Paralysis—movement distal to the fracture site
Determine the mechanism of injury.
Move injured part as little as possible.
Cover open wounds with sterile or clean dressing.
Immobilize the limb, including joints above and below frac-
  ture site; do not attempt to reduce fracture or push pro-
  truding bone under the skin.
  Soft splint (pillow or folded towel)
  Rigid splint (rolled newspaper or magazine)
  Uninjured leg can serve as splint for leg fracture if no
    splint is available
Reassess neurovascular status.
Apply traction if circulatory compromise is present.
Elevate the injured limb if possible.
Apply cold to the injured area (no longer than 20 minutes
  with each application).
Call EMS or transport to medical facility.

---

mally contained within muscles are released into the bloodstream. Serum levels of creatine phosphokinase (CPK), alkaline phosphatase, serum glutamic-oxaloacetic transaminase (SGOT), and lactate dehydrogenase (LDH) may increase in proportion to the amount of muscle damage.

A normal physiologic response to tissue injury is the inflammatory process with a slight elevation of white blood cells, especially neutrophils. When infection occurs, a rise in leukocytes is anticipated and the accompanying symptoms of fever and lethargy develop.

### Therapeutic Management

The goals of fracture management are:

1. To regain alignment and length of the bony fragments (reduction)
2. To retain alignment and length (immobilization)
3. To restore function to the injured parts
4. To prevent further injury

In children the bone fragments are usually realigned and immobilized by traction or by closed manipulation and casting until adequate callus is formed. Internal and external fixation is also used. Weight bearing and active movement for the purpose of regaining function can begin after the fracture site is stable. The child's natural tendency to be active is usually sufficient to restore normal mobility, and physical therapy is rarely needed. Open reduction is seldom required and is limited to fractures that cannot be maintained by conservative methods and when there is interposed tissue or injury to arteries or nerves. However, surgical reductions are more apt to delay normal healing and often predispose to nonunion. In the majority of cases children's fractures can be managed by closed reduction and plaster immobilization, which is often provided on an outpatient basis with

reevaluation in 7 to 10 days. The use of local and regional blocks and conscious sedation, as well as dissociative anesthesia, enables the child to be treated in the outpatient setting comfortably and safely (McCarty and others, 1999).

Children are most frequently hospitalized for fractures of the femur and the supracondylar area of the distal humerus. If simple reductions cannot be achieved or a neurovascular problem is detected after injury, observation in a hospital unit is indicated. Severe contusions with profound swelling cannot be treated with a cast, which would act as a tourniquet on the extremity, and badly malaligned fractures require traction for a time before a cast is applied. The method of fracture reduction is determined by several criteria (Box 39-5).

Medical interventions associated with fracture injury involve both the physician and the nurse, as well as the family, in their management (Box 39-6). Specific interventions and nursing responsibilities associated with the care of a child with a fracture are discussed later in the chapter.

### Bone Healing and Remodeling

Bone healing follows a patterned sequence. Fig. 39-16 shows three broad overlapping phases: inflammatory, restorative, and remodeling. Bone healing is described more definitively in five stages (Table 39-2). When the bone breaks, the envelope of subcutaneous tissue, muscle, and periosteal tissue surrounding the site is torn, blood vessels rupture, and a hematoma forms. The ends of the fractured bone segments, deprived of circulation, die as far back as the nearest collateral circulation. Necrotic tissue accumulates, and an inflammatory response takes place at the site, with its characteristic vasodilation, plasma exudation, and edema. The organization and resorption of the hematoma proceeds, and the restorative phase begins with the reestablishment of

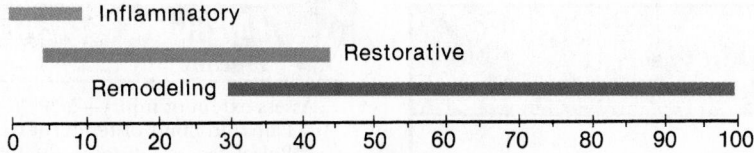

**Fig. 39-16** Approximate time devoted to inflammatory, restorative, and remodeling phases of bone healing. Scale indicates percentage of healing time.

| **TABLE 39-2** | Stages of bone healing | | | |
|---|---|---|---|---|
| **Time*** | **Physiologic Events** | | **Time** | **Physiologic Events** |
| **Stage 1: Hematoma Formation** | | | **Stage 3: Callus Formation** | |
| Impact | Fracture<br>Injury to soft tissue envelops site<br>Periosteal tissue torn<br>Vessels rupture | | 6-10 days | Fibroblasts form in granulation tissue; form bone in areas adjacent to surface of bone shaft; form cartilage at surfaces more distal to blood supply<br>*Provisional callus* develops, bridging fracture ends; holds bone together but will not support body weight |
| 3-5 minutes | Bleeding from bone and tissues into area between and around bone fragments | | | |
| First 24 hours | Hematoma forms and clots; fibrin assists in clotting periosteal membrane to aid in repair<br>Clot provides fibrin network for cellular invasion<br>Granulation tissue forms by fibroblasts and new capillaries<br>Osteoblastic activity stimulated | | 14-21 days | *True callus* develops, seen on radiographs; forms more than needed, but with remodeling, excess callus absorbs<br>Cartilage differentiates to bone tissue |
| | | | **Stage 4: Ossification** | |
| | | | 3-10 weeks | Callus forms into bone, which grows beneath periosteum of fragments; fuses fracture defect (knits together)<br>Also called the *union stage* |
| **Stage 2: Cellular Proliferation** | | | | |
| After 24 hours | Blood supply increases, bringing available calcium, phosphate, and fibroblasts<br>Cells proliferate at ends of bone fragments and differentiate into cartilage and connective tissue | | **Stage 5: Consolidation and Remodeling** | |
| | | | After 9 months | Bone marrow cavity restored<br>Compact bone formed according to stress patterns<br>Remodeling according to Wolff's law<br>Fracture line always visible on radiographs |
| Next few days | Hematoma becomes granulation tissue, which forms into a framework for bone-forming substances<br>Fibroblasts convert to osteoblasts (bone-forming cells) | | | |
| 2-3 days | *Halisteresis* (softening of bone ends) $\frac{1}{8}$ to $\frac{1}{4}$-inch; absorption of bone cells | | | |

*Healing time more rapid in infants and in cancellous (spongy) bone; may be delayed with complications.

local circulation. Repair requires an adequate blood supply and immobilization of the fracture fragments.

When there is a break in the continuity of bone, the periosteal and intraosseous osteoblasts are in some way stimulated to maximum activity. New osteoblasts are formed in immense numbers almost immediately after the injury and begin building a bridge, as evidenced by a bulging growth of osteoblastic tissue and new bone matrix between the fractured bone fragments. This is followed by deposition of calcium salts to form *callus,* which provides stability (Fig. 39-17, *B*).

Bone healing is characteristically rapid in children because of the thickened periosteum and generous blood supply. In the young child, for example, there is frequently a solid union of the femoral shaft in 3 to 4 weeks, whereas in the adult, callus sufficient to avoid deformities from constant muscle contraction associated with movement may not

take place in less than 10 to 16 weeks. The approximate healing times for a femoral shaft are:

- Neonatal period—2 to 3 weeks
- Early childhood—4 weeks
- Later childhood—6 to 8 weeks
- Adolescence—8 to 12 weeks

*Remodeling* is a unique process that occurs in the healing of long bone fractures before epiphyseal closure. When a bone remodels, the irregularities produced by the fracture become indistinct because hollows are filled in and angles are rounded off in the healing process, which gives the bone a straighter appearance. It does not alter the alignment of the bone. The buildup of new bone or callus will restore a portion of the normal bone structure in most cases despite observable malalignment. The younger the child and the

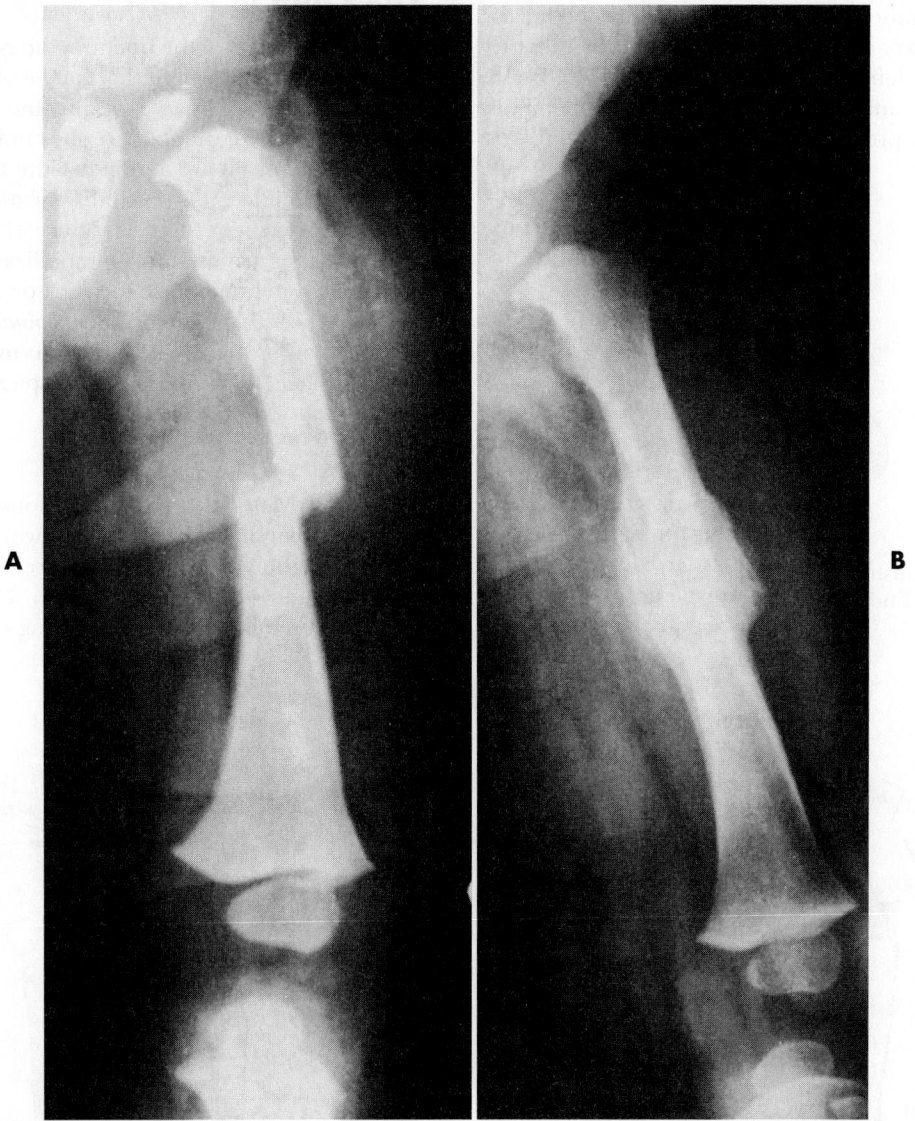

**Fig. 39-17**   Fractured femur. Most fractured femurs in childhood are of spiral type shown here. Note comparison of **A,** original x-ray film with **B,** 6-month postfracture film showing callus formation. (Courtesy Henrietta Egleston Hospital for Children, Atlanta, GA. From Hilt NE, Schmitt EW: *Pediatric orthopedic nursing*, St Louis, 1975, Mosby.)

closer the proximity of the fracture to the growth plate, the more likely it is that spontaneous correction will take place. In some instances a 90-degree angle will straighten in a year, but rotational deformities do not correct themselves. Various factors such as the type and location of the fracture, the age of the child, and the amount of fragment angulation or rotation will influence the degree of correction in alignment that can be obtained by remodeling.

The position of the bone fragments in relation to one another influences the rapidity of healing and the residual deformity. For example, a gap between fragments delays (or prevents) healing (Fig. 39-18, *A*). Healing is prompt and complete with end-to-end apposition (Fig. 39-18, *B*), but the fracture stimulates accelerated growth of the neighboring epiphysis, which causes bony overgrowth and increased length of the extremity. Angulation deformity caused by an

incomplete fracture (Fig. 39-18, *C*) may remodel in the young child, but the degree of residual deformity depends on the relationship of the angulation of the bone fragments to the angle of the joint. This requires careful evaluation and reduction to prevent permanent deformity.

Wolff's law is applied to treating children with orthopaedic problems. Paraphrased, it states that bone will grow in the direction in which stress is placed on it. Examples of the use of this law are the hip spica cast with an abduction bar for treating developmental hip dysplasias and application of casts or traction at a selected angle to influence the direction of bone healing.

Bone healing in persons of any age-group is greatly influenced by the general health of the traumatized person. The child with a fracture requires adequate nutrition for optimum bone healing. When nutritional intake is insufficient, vitamin and mineral supplementation may be necessary. No special dietary changes need to be made except to correct nutritional deficiencies. Monitoring of fluid and electrolyte balance, renal function, and possible anemia is equally important to promote wellness of the child.

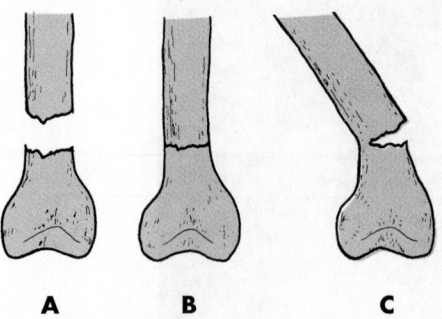

**Fig. 39-18** Relationships of fracture fragments. **A,** Gap between fragments. **B,** End-to-end apposition. **C,** Angulation of incomplete fracture.

## The Child in a Cast

The completeness of the fracture, the type of bone involved, and the amount of weight that can be placed on the limb influence how much of an extremity must be included in the cast to immobilize the fracture site completely. In most situations the joints above and below the fracture are immobilized to eliminate the possibility of movement that might cause displacement at the fracture site. Four major categories of casts are used for immobilization of fractures: *upper extremity* to immobilize the wrist or elbow, *lower extremity* to immobilize the ankle or knee, *spinal* and *cervical* for immobilization of the spine, and *spica casts* to immobilize the hip and knee (Fig. 39-19). A full spica cast with a hip abductor is shown in Fig. 39-20.

### The Cast

**Casting Materials.** Casts are constructed from gauze strips and bandages impregnated with plaster of paris or synthetic lighter-weight and water-resistant materials (e.g., fiberglass and polyurethane resin). The lightweight casts are being used more often for casting of children. They are

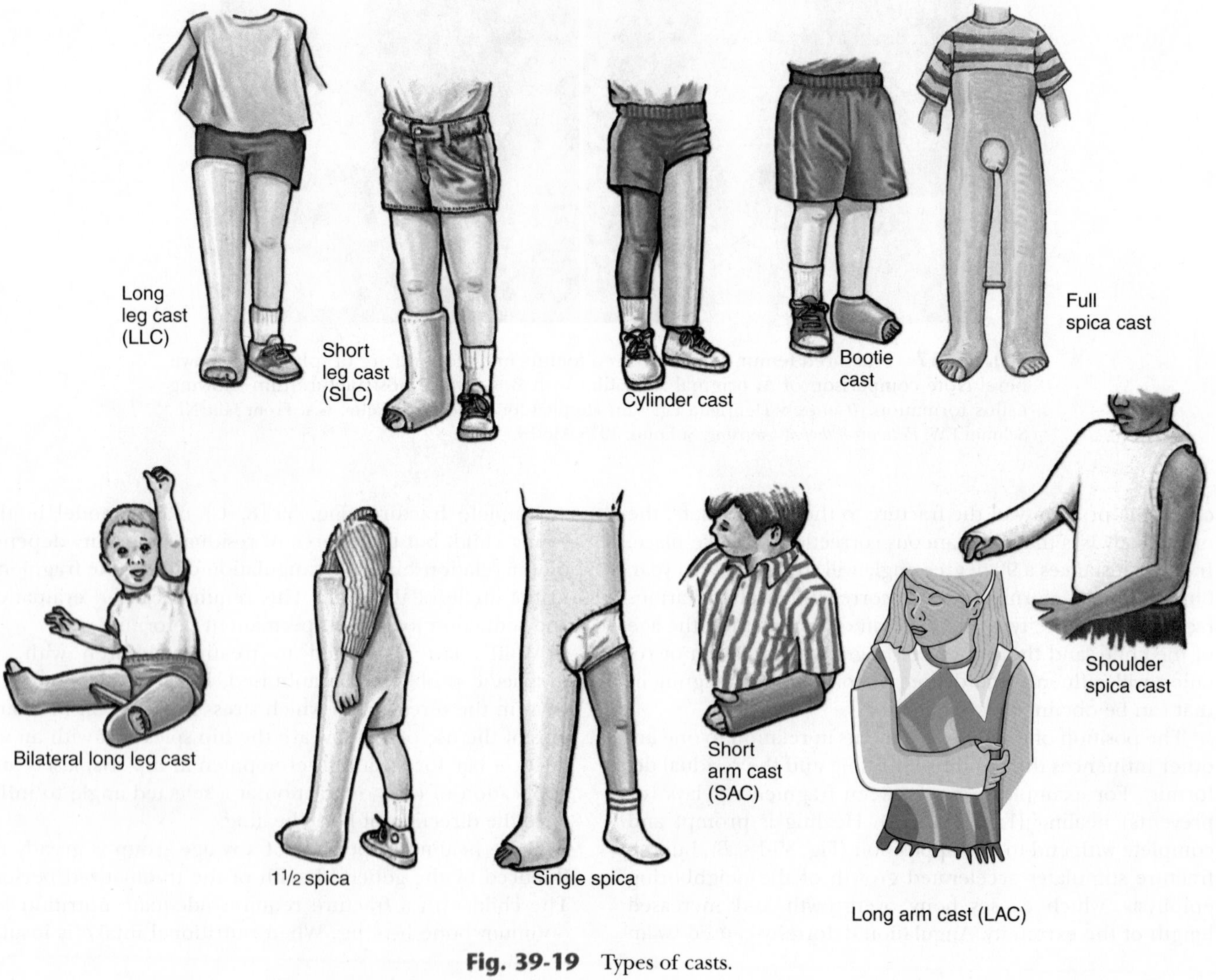

Long leg cast (LLC)

Short leg cast (SLC)

Cylinder cast

Bootie cast

Full spica cast

Bilateral long leg cast

1½ spica

Single spica

Short arm cast (SAC)

Long arm cast (LAC)

Shoulder spica cast

**Fig. 39-19** Types of casts.

available in colors and prints. Plaster casts are usually reserved for situations that require close conformity such as "total contact" casting for wounds or small irregularly shaped areas such as the hand. Table 39-3 compares the relative merits of plaster and synthetic casts.

**Cast Application.**  A nurse may assist in cast application by holding the extremity in alignment. Special cast tables that hold the child's body are used for applying large hip spica casts. If possible, children should be allowed to play with a small doll that has a cast so that they understand what will be done. Before the cast is applied, the extremities are checked for any abrasions, cuts, or other alterations in the skin surface and for the presence of rings or other items that might cause constriction from swelling; such objects are removed. Identification bands are placed on a noninjured extremity if hospitalization is required.

A tube of stockinette is stretched over the area to be casted, and bony prominences are padded with soft cotton sheeting. Some practitioners use a special plastic material or Gore-Tex under a spica cast to prevent skin breakdown (Killian, Wilkinson, and Dulaney, 1995). Dry rolls of gauze impregnated with plaster of Paris are immersed in a pail of tepid water with the open end of the roll angled downward to allow soaking of the bandage. The wet plaster rolls are put on in a bandage fashion and molded to the extremity. A heat-producing chemical reaction occurs between the plaster and water as the plaster becomes a crystalline gypsum. During application of the cast, the underlying stockinette is

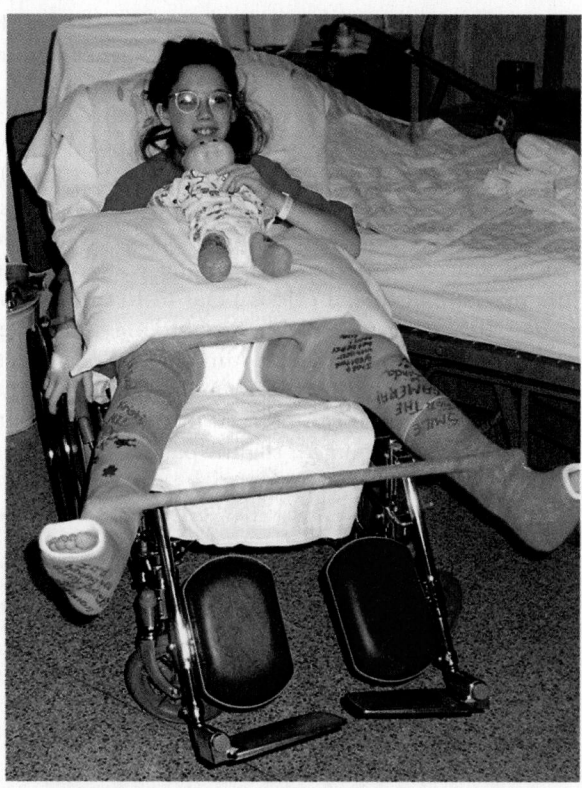

**Fig. 39-20**  Spica cast with hip abductor. Note casts on doll as well.

| TABLE 39-3 | Comparison of plaster of Paris and synthetic cast | |
|---|---|---|
| | **Plaster of Paris** | **Synthetic** |
| Composition and preparation | Cotton tape permeated with calcium sulfate crystals that interlock as tape dries (tepid water activated) | 1. Polyester/cotton tape permeated with polyurethane resin (cool water activated) 2. Knitted fiberglass tape with polyurethane resin (tepid water activated or photoactivated) 3. Knitted thermoplastic polyester fabric (hot water activated) |
| Setting time | 3 to 8 minutes | 3 to 15 minutes |
| Drying time | 10 to 72 hours (varies with cast size) | 5 to 30 minutes (varies with type of cast) |
| Indentations | Slow drying time increases possibility | Rapid drying time reduces likelihood of indentations; allows rapid use |
| Weight | Relatively heavy; bulky; difficulty wearing regular clothing | Lightweight; less bulky; can wear with regular clothing; allows for greater range of activity |
| Conformity | Molds readily to body part | Does not mold easily to body parts; unsuitable for small children or severely displaced fractures |
| Surface | Smooth exterior; does not scratch clothing or furniture | Rough exterior; can snag clothing or furniture; abrasive to skin |
| Cost | Relatively inexpensive; an advantage if cast changes anticipated | Expensive; cost three to seven times that of plaster casts |
| Stability | Relatively stable; must keep cast dry | May get cast wet or immerse in water with permission from practitioner (with use of nonabsorbent synthetic lining); clean with small amount of mild soap and water; dry with towel followed by blow dryer on cool or warm setting |
| Miscellaneous | Child may feel uncomfortable warming or burning sensation under cast while drying (chemical reaction) Skin under cast may become irritated Cast must be protected when around water (bathing) | Child may feel uncomfortable warming or burning sensation under cast while drying (chemical reaction) Special aids may be required for application or removal of some types Increased activity may displace fracture Skin under cast may become macerated from inadequate drying after water immersion |

pulled over the raw edges of the cast and secured with a layer of wet plaster $\frac{1}{2}$ to 1 inch below the rim to form a smooth, padded edge to protect the skin.

If the operator does not form such a protective edge with stockinette, the raw edges of the cast can be protected by a "petaled" edge. Small pieces approximately 2 to 3 inches long are cut from 1- or 1½-inch-wide moleskin or adhesive tape. The edges are rounded with scissors, and each of these "petals" is placed over the edge of the cast, each petal slightly overlapping the previous petal to form a smooth, neat edge. It is easier to apply the petal to the underside of the cast first and then bring the unadhered edge to the front, pressing firmly so the edges remain securely attached. Adhesive strip bandages can be used instead of tape petals for quicker preparation and a slightly padded cast edge.

### FAMILY HOME CARE
#### Cast Care

Expose the plaster cast to air until dry.
Keep the casted part of the body elevated on pillows or similar support for the first day, or as directed by the health care professional.
Lift and support the wet cast with the palms of the hands only, to avoid indenting with the fingers.
Observe the fingers or toes for any evidence of swelling or discoloration (darker or lighter than a comparable extremity) and contact the health care professional immediately if noted.
Check movement and sensation of the visible fingers and toes frequently and contact the health care professional regarding any changes noted.
Follow health professional's orders regarding any restriction of activities.
Restrict strenuous activities for the first few days.
  Engage in quiet activities but encourage use of muscles.
  Move the joints above and below the cast on the affected extremity.
  Specific exercises for the child should be demonstrated by hospital staff, and a written copy should be provided to the parents.
Encourage frequent rest for a few days, keeping the injured arm or leg elevated while resting.
Avoid allowing the affected limb to hang down for more than 30 minutes.
  Keep an injured arm or hand elevated (e.g., in a sling) most of the time; supporting it on pillows at chest level is helpful.
  Elevate a leg when sitting and avoid standing for more than 30 minutes.
Do not allow the child to put anything inside the cast.
  Keep small items that might be placed inside the cast away from young children.
Visualize skin at cast edges to check for irritation or breakdown and pad cast accordingly.
Itching may be relieved by an ice pack and administering medication as recommended by the physician.
Keep a clear path for ambulation.
  Remove toys, hazardous floor rugs, pets, or other items over which the child might stumble.
Use crutches appropriately if lower limb fracture.
  The crutches should fit properly, have a soft rubber tip to prevent slipping, and be well padded at the axilla. The axilla should not rest on the crutches.
Instruct child and parents to avoid placing the cast in water (e.g., tub, shower, swimming pool).
If patient is incontinent, protect the cast with waterproof tape and plastic. Use diapers, pull-ups, or other guards.

## Nursing Considerations

The complete evaporation of the water from a hip spica cast can take 24 to 48 hours when plaster materials are used. Drying occurs within minutes with fiberglass materials. The cast must remain uncovered to allow it to dry from the inside out. Turning the child in a plaster cast at least every 2 hours will help to dry a body cast evenly and prevent complications related to immobility. A regular fan or cool-air hair dryer used to circulate air may be helpful when the humidity is high.

> **NURSING ALERT** Heated fans or dryers are not used because they cause the cast to dry on the outside and remain wet beneath, thus becoming moldy. They also cause burns from heat conduction by way of the cast to the underlying tissue.

A wet cast should be handled by the palms of the hands to prevent indenting the cast and creating pressure areas and supported by a pillow covered with plastic. A dry plaster-of-paris cast produces a hollow sound when tapped with the finger.

During the first few hours after a cast is applied, the chief concern is that the extremity may continue to swell to the extent that the cast becomes a tourniquet, shutting off circulation and producing neurovascular complications. A measure for reducing the likelihood of this potential problem is to elevate the body part, thereby increasing venous return. If edema is excessive, casts are bivalved (i.e., cut to make anterior and posterior halves that are held together with an elastic bandage). The cast and the involved extremity are observed frequently for neurovascular integrity and any signs of compromise. Permanent muscle and tissue damage can occur within 6 to 8 hours, for which nurses can be held liable. Once the cast has dried, "hot spots" felt on the cast surface or foul-smelling areas of the cast may indicate infection underneath and should be reported. Often the cast is windowed over the area of suspicion to directly observe and treat the area if necessary.

> **NURSING ALERT** Observations including the five "Ps" of ischemia should be reported immediately: *pain,* especially with passive range of motion; *pallor; pulselessness* (a dismal and late sign); *paresthesia;* and *paralysis.*

When casting an extremity that has sustained an open fracture, a window is often left over the wound area to allow for observation and for dressing of the wound. A surgical reduction is usually casted as for a closed fracture.

Usually the child is discharged to home care after a cast is applied in the emergency department or clinic. Parents need instructions on drying and caring for the cast and checking for signs and symptoms that indicate the cast is too tight. (See Family Home Care box.) They should also be told to take the child to the health care professional for attention if the cast becomes too loose, because a loose cast no longer serves its purpose. A cast may represent a badge of honor for the child and serves as visible evidence of an otherwise invisible injury.

**Cast Removal.**   Cutting the cast to remove it or to relieve tightness is frequently a frightening experience for children. They fear the sound of the cast cutter and are terrified that their flesh, as well as the cast, will be cut. Because it works by vibration, a cast cutter cuts only the hard surface of the cast. This can be demonstrated by the person removing the cast. The oscillating blade vibrates very rapidly back and forth and will not cut when placed lightly on the skin. Children have described it as producing a "tickly" sensation. The vibration also generates heat that may be felt by the child. Both of these sensations should be explained.

Preparation for the procedure will help reduce anxiety, especially if a trusting relationship has been established between the child and the nurse. Many young children come to regard the cast as part of themselves, which intensifies their fear of removal (Fig. 39-21). Using the analogy of having fingernails or hair cut sometimes helps reduce their anxiety. They need continual reassurance that all is going well and that their behavior is accepted.

Home care for children in casts creates problems of various magnitude, especially with large casts (e.g., a hip spica). Commonplace situations become problematic (e.g., returning the child home safely and comfortably). Standard seat belts and car seats are not readily adapted for use by children in casts. (See Developmental Dysplasia of the Hip, Chapter 11.) Sitting can be impossible in a spica cast, and leg casts require extra space in a small room, under a table, or in a bathroom. Children in spica casts usually find the prone position easier for self-feeding from a small table placed next to the dining table or on the floor. The conventional toilet is almost impossible for a child in a spica cast. Small bedpans or other containers offer alternatives for elimination. The use of a Gore-Tex pantaloon, a protective skin barrier, and adult underguards has been described as a way of reducing urine burns and heat rash and increasing hygiene with a hip spica cast. (Killian, Wilkinson, and Dulaney, 1995).

Nurses can help families adapt the child's environment to meet the temporary encumbrance of a cast (e.g., devising plastic wraps for waterproofing casts for a shower). Baths are possible only if the plaster cast is kept out of the water and covered to prevent it from becoming wet from splashes. Some synthetic casts are waterproof, but skin can become irritated from water that collects beneath the cast.

After the cast is removed, the skin surface will be caked with desquamated skin and sebaceous secretions. Simple soaking in a bathtub is usually sufficient for their removal, but it may require several days to eliminate the accumulation completely. Application of olive oil or lotion may provide comfort. The parents and child should be instructed not to pull or forcibly remove this material with vigorous scrubbing because it may cause excoriation and bleeding.* When cast care will be long-term, the nurse can help the family train a baby-sitter to provide care; the nurse can also help the family network with other parents in a similar situation. (See Nursing Care Plan: The Child with a Fracture and Nursing Care Plan: The Child in a Cast.†)

## The Child in Traction

Bone fragments that cannot be reduced with simple traction and stabilization with a cast may require the extended pulling force obtained with continuous traction. Traction is also used for other purposes (Box 39-7). Muscle relaxants may be administered for muscle spasms.

With the increased emphasis on outpatient treatment of acute and chronic illnesses to cut healthcare costs, developmental and social considerations, immobilization problems, and newer surgical techniques, traction is used with decreasing frequency. The appeal of skeletal fixation (internal or external) and early ambulation of the child replaces the use of traction in many instances.

---

*Home care instructions for the child in a cast and nursing care plan are available in Wong DL, Hess CS: *Wong and Whaley's clinical manual of pediatric nursing*, ed 5, St Louis, 2000, Mosby.
†In Wong DL, Hess CS: *Wong and Whaley's clinical manual of pediatric nursing*, ed 5, St Louis, 2000, Mosby.

---

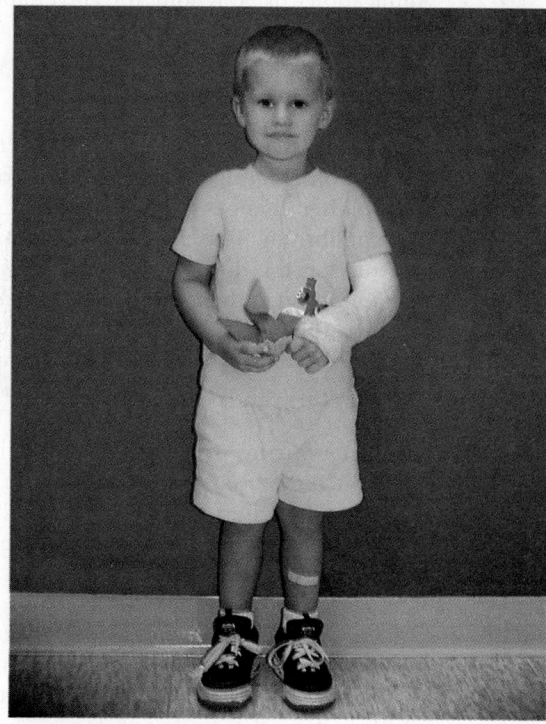

**Fig. 39-21**   Young children come to regard a cast as part of their body. They usually adapt well but may fear its removal.

---

**Box 39-7** ■ ■ ◻
**Purposes of Traction**

To realign bone fragments
To provide rest for an extremity
To help prevent or improve contracture deformity
To correct a deformity
To treat a dislocation
To allow preoperative or postoperative positioning and alignment
To provide immobilization of specific areas of the body
To reduce muscle spasms (rare in children)

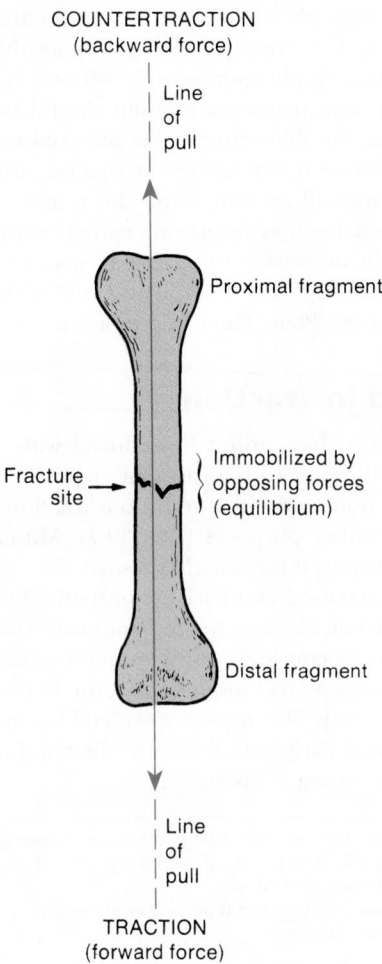

**Fig. 39-22** Application of traction for maintaining equilibrium.

## Purposes of Traction

When forces having both direction and magnitude act on an object at the same point simultaneously from opposite directions, the object either changes its state of rest or motion or remains in equilibrium. The use of traction in the management of fractures is the direct application of these forces to produce equilibrium at the fracture site. A *forward force (traction)* is produced by attaching weight to the distal bone fragment, which is balanced by the *backward force* of the muscle pull (*countertraction*) and the *frictional force* between the patient and the bed (Fig. 39-22).

To reduce or realign a fracture site, traction is provided by weights applied to the distal bone fragment; body weight provides countertraction. By adjusting the line of pull upward or downward or by adducting or abducting the extremity, the operator uses these forces to align the distal and proximal bone fragments. To attain equilibrium, the amount of forward force is adjusted by adding weight to or subtracting weight from the traction, or countertraction can be increased by elevating the foot of the bed to create a greater gravitational pull to the backward force. A bed board placed under the mattress of heavy children prevents sagging, which might otherwise change the direction of the forces applied to the fracture.

**Manual traction**—Traction applied to the body part by the hand placed distally to the fracture site. Nurses frequently provide manual traction during cast application to realign bone fragments. It is used in uncomplicated arm or leg fractures in which there is little overriding of the bones and minimum muscle pull to overcome.

**Skin traction**—Pull applied directly to the skin surface and indirectly to the skeletal structures. The pulling mechanism is attached to the skin with adhesive material or an elastic bandage. Both types are applied over soft foam-backed traction straps to distribute the traction pull. It is applied when there is minimum displacement and little muscle spasticity but is contraindicated when there is associated skin damage. Skin traction has specific limits of weight that it can pull without causing tissue breakdown.

**Skeletal traction**—Pull applied directly to the skeletal structure by a pin, wire, or tongs inserted into or through the diameter of the bone distal to the fracture. It is employed when significant traction pull must be applied in order to achieve realignment and immobilization. By inserting a pin or wire into the bone, the stress is placed on the bone and not on the surrounding tissue.

The three primary purposes of traction for reduction of fractures are:

1. To fatigue the involved muscle and reduce muscle spasm so that bones can be realigned
2. To position the distal and proximal bone ends in desired realignment to promote satisfactory bone healing
3. To immobilize the fracture site until realignment has been achieved and sufficient healing has taken place to permit casting or splinting

Fatiguing of a muscle is accomplished by applying constant stress to the muscle so that the buildup of lactic acid will produce muscle relaxation. The all-or-none law, characteristic of muscle contractility, influences the complete relaxation. When muscle is stretched, muscle spasm ceases and permits the realignment of the bone ends. The continuous maintenance of traction is important during this phase because releasing the traction allows the muscle's normal contracting ability to again cause a malpositioning of the bone ends.

The realignment of the fragments is a gradual process that is achieved more rapidly in infants, who have limited muscle tone, than in muscular teenagers. The desired line of pull and callus formation are checked periodically by radiographic examination. The traction pull to some degree immobilizes the fracture site; however, adjunctive immobilizing devices such as splints or casts are sometimes used with skeletal traction. In injuries in which there is severe soft tissue swelling or vascular and nerve damage, it is customary to use traction until these complications have been resolved and it is safe to apply a cast. Immobilization with traction will be maintained until the bone ends are in satisfactory realignment, after which a less-confining type of immobilization, usually a cast, will be applied.

### Types of Traction (General)

The pull needed for traction can be applied to the distal bone fragment in several ways (Box 39-8). The type of traction applied is determined primarily by the age of the child,

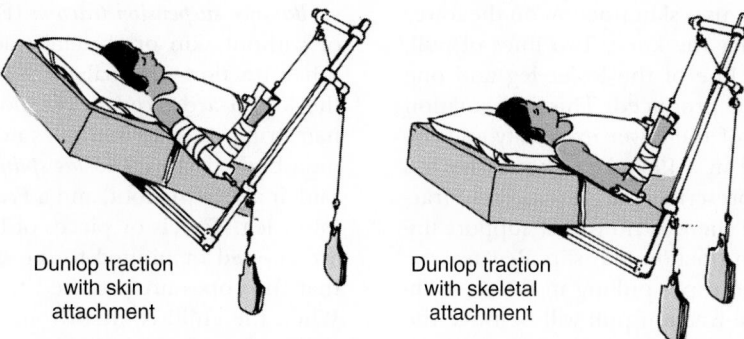

Dunlop traction
with skin
attachment

Dunlop traction
with skeletal
attachment

**Fig. 39-23**   Dunlop traction. (Figs. 39-23 to 39-28 redrawn from Hilt NE, Schmitt EW: *Pediatric orthopedic nursing,* St Louis, 1975, Mosby.)

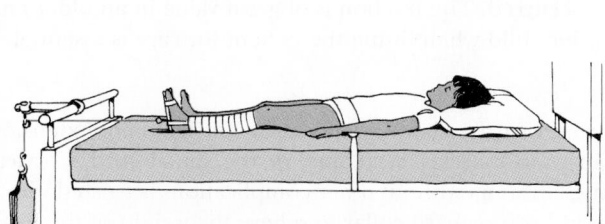

**Fig. 39-24**   Buck extension traction.

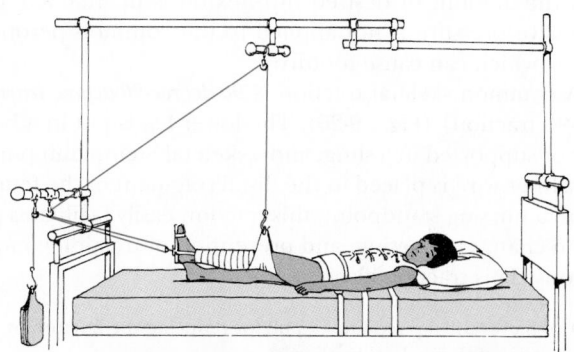

**Fig. 39-25**   Russell traction.

the condition of the soft tissues, and the type and degree of displacement of the fracture. Fractures most commonly treated by application of traction are those involving the humerus, femur, and vertebrae. The major types of traction for specific fractures are discussed in the following sections.

### Upper Extremity Traction

Treatment of fractures of the humerus by traction is accomplished either (1) by *overhead suspension,* in which the arm, bent at the elbow, is suspended vertically by skin or skeletal attachment and traction is applied to the distal end of the humerus, or (2) by *Dunlop traction.* With Dunlop traction (Fig. 39-23) the arm is suspended horizontally, using either skin or skeletal attachment.

When skin traction is used, straps are placed on the lower and upper arm with the arm flexed to accomplish pull in two directions: one along the longitudinal direction of the upper arm and one to maintain alignment of the lower arm. In instances such as supracondylar fractures, the amount of traction pull needed to align the site more critically requires a skeletal wire placed in the upper arm to allow the additional weight.

Fractures of the humerus, which are usually the result of a fall with the arm in extension, frequently involve the supracondylar portion. There are three major complications associated with this injury: Volkmann contractures (p. 1793); traumatic injury to the median, ulnar, or radial nerves; and angulation deformities. The fracture must be carefully reduced, sometimes with the child under anesthesia, and because of the danger of complications, children with closed reduction of supracondylar fractures are often

hospitalized for observation. In severely malaligned fractures, closed reduction with the child under anesthesia is followed by application of skeletal traction for 2 to 3 weeks, after which a long arm cast is applied for an additional 2 to 3 weeks.

### Lower Extremity Traction

The frequent site for a femoral fracture is in the middle one third of the shaft (see Fig. 39-17, *A*). With this fracture there is significant overriding but minimal displacement. In a fracture in the lower one third of the shaft, the pull of the gastrocnemius muscle causes the distal fragment to become downwardly displaced. The severity of the fracturing force and the ability of the muscles to hold the fracture out of alignment will determine the fracture type and the amount of overriding of the fragments. The periosteum may remain intact, which helps maintain alignment.

When traction is required, several types may be employed, based on the initial assessment. *Bryant traction,* a type of running traction in which the pull is only in one direction, is not recommended because of the gravitational vascular draining of the elevated extremities, the possible tourniquet effect of the bandages, and the effect of the traction, which can trigger vasospasms and avascular necrosis.

*Buck extension traction* (Fig. 39-24) is a type of skin traction with the legs in an extended position. Buck extension is used primarily for short-term immobilization, such as preoperative management of a child with a dislocated hip, or for correcting contractures or bone deformities, such as in Legg-Calvé-Perthes disease. A side-lying position may be permissible if the leg is stable.

***Russell traction*** (Fig. 39-25) uses skin traction on the lower leg and a padded sling under the knee. Two lines of pull, one along the longitudinal line of the lower leg and one perpendicular to the leg, are produced. This combination of pulls allows realignment of the lower extremity and immobilizes the hip and knee in a flexed position. The hip flexion must be kept at the prescribed angle to prevent fracture malalignment, because there is no direct support under the fracture and the skin traction may slip. Because the traction is set up to have two ropes pulling in the same direction at the foot plate, the traction pull will be twice the amount of weight at the end of the bed. For example, 5 pounds of weight produces 10 pounds of pull. Special nursing measures include carefully checking the position so that the amount of desired hip flexion is maintained and excessive pressure is not applied to the common peroneal nerve, which can cause footdrop.

A common skeletal traction is ***90-degree-90-degree traction*** (90-90 traction) (Fig. 39-26). The lower leg is put in a boot cast or supported in a sling, and a skeletal Steinmann pin or Kirschner wire is placed in the distal fragment of the femur. From a nursing standpoint, this traction easily facilitates position changes, toileting, and prevention of traction complications. This traction also:

- Achieves the desired line of pull for reducing the fracture by means of the skeletal traction
- Allows a 90-degree flexion of both the hip and the knee
- Supports the lower extremity in a desired position with good venous return
- Provides adequate immobilization of the fracture site

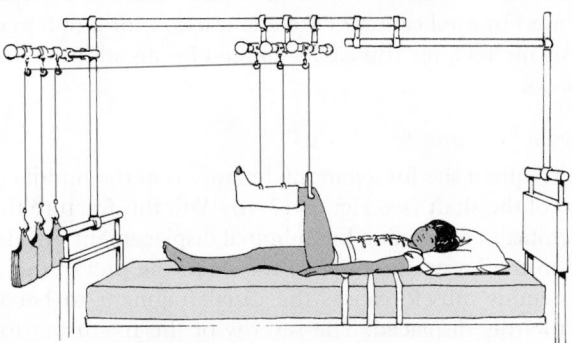

**Fig. 39-26**   "90-90" traction.

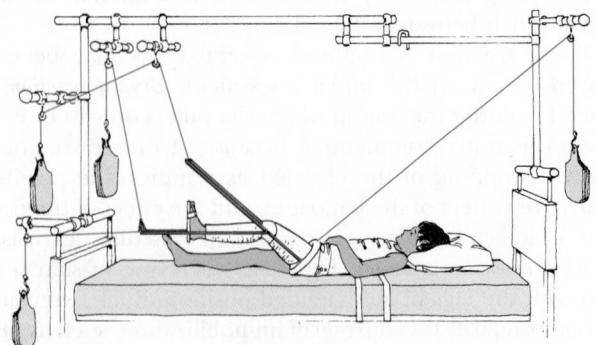

**Fig. 39-27**   Balance suspension with Thomas ring splint and Pearson attachment.

***Balance suspension traction*** (Fig. 39-27) may be used with or without skin or skeletal traction. Unless used with another traction, the balanced suspension merely suspends the leg in a desired flexed position to relax the hip and hamstring muscles and does not exert any traction directly on a body part. A ***Thomas splint*** extends from the groin to midair above the foot, and a ***Pearson attachment*** supports the lower leg. Towels or pieces of felt covered with stockinette are clipped or pinned to the splints for leg support. Note that the ropes are attached to create a balanced traction. When the child is lifted from the bed, the traction lifts as well, with no loss of alignment.

The Pearson attachment will stay wherever positioned. Many times the practitioner will put a rope between the end of the Pearson attachment and the end of the Thomas splint to prevent any knee flexion alteration while the child is moved. This traction requires very careful checking of splints and ropes to make certain that no slippage or fraying has occurred. The traction is of great value in an older and heavier child when lifting the patient for care is essential.

## Cervical Traction

The cervical area is a vulnerable site for flexion or extension injuries to muscles, vertebrae, or the spinal cord. Cervical muscle trauma without other complications is treated with a cervical soft or hard collar to relieve the weight of the head from the fracture site. Intermittent cervical skin traction might be employed with a head halter and weight to decrease muscle spasms (Fig. 39-28). Injuries limited to cervical muscles can be very uncomfortable but, with prompt medical care, usually resolve with conservative treatment.

When a child displaces or fractures a cervical vertebra, it is necessary to reduce and immobilize the site with cervical skeletal traction. The spinal cord runs through the intravertebral canal, and dislocation or fracture of the vertebrae can also cause spinal cord trauma.

Physical examination, especially a neurologic assessment, and radiographic studies are essential diagnostic aids to determine:

- The presence of a vertebral fracture
- The degree of vertebral dislocation
- Displacement of an intervertebral disk

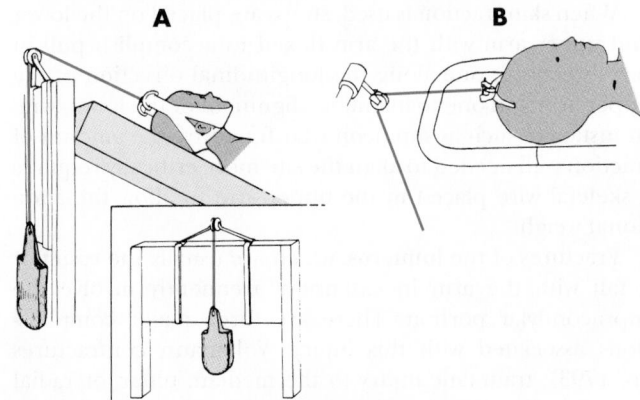

**Fig. 39-28**   **A,** Cervical traction. **B,** Crutchfield tong traction.

- Compression of the spinal cord and other neurologic structures
- Sensory, motor, and autonomic nerve deficits

Cervical traction is usually accomplished by insertion of Crutchfield, Barton, or Gardner-Wells tongs through burr holes in the skull. The head is placed in a hyperextended position, and, as the neck muscles fatigue with constant traction pull, the vertebral bodies gradually are pulled apart and the cord is no longer pinched between the vertebrae. Immobilization until fracture healing can occur is an essential goal of cervical traction. If the injury has been limited to a vertebral fracture without neurologic deficit, a halo vest can be applied to permit earlier ambulation. Halos are also used preoperatively and postoperatively to stabilize the cervical spine in children undergoing surgery.

## Nursing Considerations

To assess the child in traction, it is essential to know the purpose for which the traction is applied. Regular assessment of both the child and the traction apparatus is required, as outlined in the Guidelines box. The child is also assessed for evidence of adverse effects of immobilization (see p. 1762).

Evaluating the therapeutic effects and possible negative consequences of traction is essential to good patient care. Many of the nursing problems associated with a child in traction are related to immobility. However, there are a number of physical needs that require attention and vigilance.

**NURSING ALERT** Skeletal traction is never released by the nurse (unless under direct supervision of practitioner). This precaution includes not lifting weights (e.g., for moving the child in bed, for repositioning) that are applying traction.

However, when indicated by the attending practitioner, the nurse may remove nonadhesive skin traction. In these

---

## GUIDELINES
### Traction Care

**UNDERSTAND THERAPY**

Understand purpose of traction.
Understand function of traction in each specific situation.

**MAINTAIN TRACTION**

Check desired line of pull and relationship of distal fragment to proximal fragment.
    Check whether fragment is being directed upward, adducted, or abducted.
Check function of each component:
    Position of bandages, frames, splints
    Ropes: in center track of pulley, taut, no fraying, knots tied securely
    Pulleys:
        In original position on attachment bar; have not slid from original site
        Wheels freely movable
    Weights:
        Correct amount of weight
        Hanging freely
        In safe location
Check bed position—head or foot elevated as directed for desired amount of pull and countertraction.
Do not remove skeletal traction or adhesive traction straps on skin traction.
Assess for pain or discomfort from traction.

**MAINTAIN ALIGNMENT**

Observe for correct body alignment with emphasis on alignment of shoulder, hip, and leg.
Check after child has moved.
Apply restraints only if ordered.
Maintain correct angles at joints.

**CARE FOR SKIN TRACTION**

Replace nonadhesive straps or elastic bandage on skin traction *when permitted* or absolutely necessary, but make certain that traction on limb is maintained by someone during procedure.
Assess bandages to ascertain if they are correctly applied (diagonal or spiral), not too loose or too tight, which could cause slippage and malalignment of traction.

**CARE FOR SKELETAL TRACTION**

Check pin sites frequently for signs of bleeding, inflammation, or infection.
Cleanse and dress pin sites as ordered.
Apply topical antiseptic or antibiotic daily if ordered.
Cover ends of pins with protective or padding to prevent child's being scratched by pin.
Note pull of traction on pin; pull should be even.
Check pin screws to be certain that screws are tight in metal clamp that attaches traction apparatus to pin.

**PREVENT SKIN BREAKDOWN**

Provide pressure-reducing mattress.
Make total body skin checks for redness or breakdown, especially over areas that receive greatest pressure (see Nursing Tip on p. 1792)
Wash and dry skin at least daily.
Stimulate circulation with gentle massage only over healthy skin.
Change position at least every 2 hours to relieve pressure (see Maintaining Healthy Skin, Chapter 27).

**PREVENT COMPLICATIONS**

Check pulse in affected areas.
Assess circular dressings for excessive tightness.
Assess restraining devices:
    Make certain that they are not too loose or too tight.
    Remove periodically and check for pressure areas.
Encourage deep breathing, coughing, incentive spirometry.
Note any neurovascular changes, such as:
    Color in skin and nail beds
    Capillary refill
    Alterations in sensation, increased pain
    Alterations in motor ability
    Skin temperature
Take immediate action to correct problem or report to practitioner if neurovascular changes are found.
Record findings of neurovascular changes.
Carry out passive, active, or active-with-resistance exercises of uninvolved joints.
Note if any tightness, weakness, or contractures are developing in uninvolved joints and muscles.
Take measures to correct or prevent further development of weakness, such as applying foot board to prevent footdrop.
Check beneath child for small objects (e.g., food, toys, candy).

cases intermittent traction is periodically released and reapplied as ordered. When skin traction must be constantly maintained, such as in fractures, nurses may occasionally remove and reapply the Ace bandage if this is approved by the attending practitioner, provided that *someone manually maintains the traction during the rewrapping process.* A child may have several types of traction at one time, and each traction must be assessed separately to avoid problems.

In addition to routine skin observation and care (see The Immobilized Child, p. 1761), children in skeletal traction will need special skin care at the pin site according to hospital policy or practitioner preference. In a recent review of pin-site care in children and adults, it was concluded that pin sites should be frequently assessed and cleaned to prevent infection. However, the best choice for cleansing agent, frequency, crust removal, and dressing application is as yet unknown (Bernardo, 2001). A pressure reduction device, such as a foam overlay or an alternating-pressure mattress placed beneath the hips and back, reduces the chance of skin breakdown in these vulnerable areas.

**NURSING TIP**  A small hand mirror facilitates visualization of inaccessible skin areas.

When the child is first placed in traction, an increase in discomfort is common as a result of the traction pull fatiguing the muscle. It has been determined that orthopaedic conditions are associated with a higher-than-average number of painful events and a higher percentage of bodily symptoms than other common conditions (Wong and Baker, 1988). Analgesics, including opioids, and muscle relaxants help during this phase of care and should be administered liberally.

Helping children cope with the confinement and new experience requires more than medications. An explanation should be given according to each child's level of development about what is happening and why the child must remain in the device. Children should be reassured that someone will always be available to aid them in adjusting to the traction and to cope with the problems of immobilization.

Some devices assist children in performing activities independently. An overhead trapeze, which they can use to help lift themselves, facilitates hygiene and repositioning and provides exercise for uninvolved muscles.

Later, when traction is released, muscle spasms can be quite severe. Pain assessment and pain management should be part of care at this phase. (See Chapter 26.) (See Nursing Care Plan: The Child in Traction.*)

## Distraction

Unlike traction, which helps bones realign and fuse properly, *distraction* is the process of separating opposing bone to encourage regeneration of new bone in the created space. Distraction can also be used when limbs are of unequal lengths and new bone is needed to elongate the shorter limb.

---

*In Wong DL, Hess CS: *Wong and Whaley's clinical manual of pediatric nursing,* ed 5, St Louis, 2000, Mosby.

## External Fixation

The *Ilizarov external fixator (IEF)* is the most common external fixation device. It uses a system of wires, rings, and telescoping rods that permits limb lengthening to occur by manual distraction. In addition to lengthening bones, the device can be used to correct angular or rotational defects or to immobilize fractures. It allows earlier mobilization and earlier hospital discharge, and it obviates the need for traction. The device is attached surgically by securing a series of external full or half rings to the bone with wires. External telescoping rods connect the rings to each other. Manual distraction is accomplished by manipulating the rods to increase the distance between the rings. A percutaneous osteotomy is performed when the device is applied to create a "false" growth plate. A special osteotomy or corticotomy involves cutting only the cortex of the bone while preserving its blood supply, bone marrow, endosteum, and periosteum. Capillary blood flow to the transected area is essential for proper bone growth. Cut bone ends typically grow at a rate of 1 cm/month. IEF can result in up to a 15-cm gain in length.

Other types of external fixation are used in the management of certain types of fractures—for example, fracture of a distal radius or a tibia in an adolescent.

### Nursing Considerations

Success of the IEF depends on the child's and family's cooperation; therefore before surgery they must be fully informed of the appearance of the device, how it accomplishes bone growth, alterations in activities, and home and follow-up care. Children are involved in learning to adjust the device to accomplish distraction. Children who participate actively in their care report less discomfort. Because the device is external (Fig. 39-29), the child and family need to be prepared for the reactions of others and assisted in camouflaging the device with appropriate apparel, such as wide-legged pants that close with self-adhering fasteners around the device. Partial weight bearing is allowed, and the child needs to learn to walk with crutches. Alterations in activity include modifications at school and in physical edu-

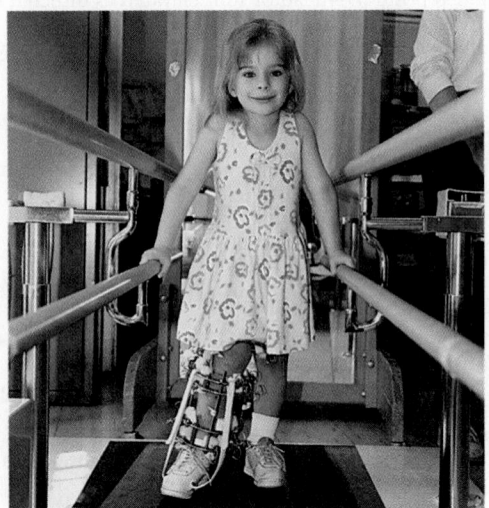

**Fig. 39-29**  Children with the Ilizarov external fixator must learn to walk and cope with the visible nature of the device.

cation. Full weight bearing is not allowed until the distraction is completed and bone consolidation has occurred. Parents should be instructed in pin care, including observation for infection and loosening of pins. Pin care varies among practitioners but usually includes using normal saline, removing crusts, avoiding ointments, and using clean technique for home care (McKenzie, 1999). Follow-up care is essential to maintain appropriate distraction until the desired leg length is achieved. The child may need to use crutches or have a cast for 4 to 6 weeks following removal of the device.

## Internal Fixation

Internal fixation methods require surgery and include screw and plate fixation and intramedullary fixation. When surgical intervention is necessary to realign a fracture, the child needs physical and psychologic preparation. The preoperative teaching is the same as for any other surgical procedure, except that orthopaedic surgery uses a variety of rods, screws, staples, and plates, and the child needs to know about these unfamiliar objects and how they will appear when he or she returns from the procedure. The fixating devices are made of substances that do not act as proteins foreign to the body and therefore are not rejected. Usually the rods are driven down the shaft of the long bones, whereas screws and plates are attached to the side of the bone shaft. Postoperatively the bone healing takes place with callus formation, as it does in a new fracture. Generally the child with an internal fixation device sits in a chair and walks with a walker or crutches within a few hours or days. The most common postoperative complication is infection. The nurse's responsibility includes close monitoring of neurovascular changes in the involved extremity and the prevention of postanesthesia problems. The family should be alerted to signs of infection and instructed in appropriate weight-bearing and activity plans. Occasionally, supplemental casting or bracing is needed.

## Fracture Complications

### Circulatory Impairment

If the trauma or immobilizing device restricts veins or arteries in the affected extremity, bone healing will be seriously impaired. Careful assessment of the pulses, capillary refill, skin color, and temperature is an important nursing responsibility. After injury, swelling of tissues occurs more rapidly in the child than in the adult. In the upper extremity, brachial, radial, ulnar, and digital pulses are felt. In the leg, femoral, popliteal, posterior tibial, and dorsalis pedis pulses are checked.

**NURSING ALERT**  When circulatory impairment is evident (absence of pulse, discoloration, swelling, pain), the nurse takes quick action to relieve the problem by reporting the situation immediately. If the practitioner is unable to come and release the pressure, the nurse or orthopaedic technician must be able to cut the cast in half to form a bivalve cast or make a large window in it to decrease the pressure.

Closely associated with an inadequate blood supply is a low hematocrit value, which can result from the initial blood loss or surgically induced anemia. Although the blood flow may be adequate, a lowered amount of hemoglobin will not provide a sufficient supply of oxygen for tissue repair.

### Nerve Compression Syndromes

Nerve damage can take place at the time of injury, develop in the process of realignment, or be a complication of an immobilizing apparatus. The syndromes are classified according to the anatomic area affected and can involve the median (carpal tunnel syndrome), ulnar (at wrist or elbow), radial, posterior tibial (tarsal tunnel syndrome), common peroneal, or sciatic nerves. Peroneal nerve damage can result in footdrop, and radial nerve impairment produces wristdrop. Both of these disabilities can significantly interfere with activities of daily living.

Sensory testing with touch and pinprick and evaluating motor strength by asking the child to move the unaffected joint distal to the injury are common means of determining neurologic involvement. Subjective symptoms are pain or discomfort, muscular weakness, a burning sensation, limitation of motion, and altered sensation. Because the fear of pain limits the child's cooperation, play can be the nurse's most valuable tool.

Treatment is alleviation of pressure on the nerve. The practitioner determines whether correcting the alignment will alleviate pressure on the nerve or if surgical intervention is necessary. At times sensory or motor changes indicate ischemia, and the treatment is correction of the vascular disturbance.

### Compartment Syndromes

A **compartment** is a group of muscles surrounded by tough, inelastic fascial tissue. The compartment syndrome occurs when increased pressure within this closed space rises and compromises circulation to the muscles and nerves within the space. Muscles and nerves of both upper and lower extremities are enclosed within such compartments. The most frequent causes of compartment syndrome are tight dressings or casts, hemorrhage, trauma, burns, and surgery. Other causes include an increase in compartment content (hemorrhage, venous obstruction, infiltrated IV infusion, exudate) and externally applied pressure, such as lying on the affected limb (Harvey, 2001).

Signs and symptoms of compartment syndrome reflect a deficit or deterioration of neuromuscular status in the anatomic area surrounding the involved structures. These include motor weakness and pain out of proportion to the injury and requiring opioids for pain control (Horn and others, 1997). Compartment syndrome clinical manifestations may occur as early as 30 minutes after the ischemia develops (Harvey, 2001). Tenseness may be noted on palpation of the area. Because early detection is important in preventing permanent damage to tissues, in certain high-risk situations specialists may recommend continuous monitoring of compartment pressures by way of a small, slit-tip catheter inserted into the compartment. Treatment of compartment syndrome is immediate relief of pressure, which sometimes requires fasciotomy.

*Volkmann contracture* (ischemic muscular atrophy) is a serious, persistent flexion contraction of the forearm and hand caused by massive infarction of muscle. Pressure from a cast or tight bandage or from swelling from the injury in the area of the elbow begins with arterial occlusion and then progresses to muscle anoxia and reflex vasospasms. Finally, the lack of blood supply leads to muscle necrosis and replacement with fibrous tissue, which produces paralysis and a clawlike hand contracture. Any fracture that requires excessive traction can be complicated by Volkmann contracture; however, it occurs most often in the elbow.

The neuromuscular symptoms are severe pain (although pain is not always a manifestation), pallor or cyanosis, edema, absence of pulses in the extremity, and loss of sensitivity. Unrelieved, the occlusive hypoxic process can cause some contracture if ischemia lasts as little as 6 hours. A great deal of muscle damage occurs after 12 to 24 hours; 48 hours of ischemia produces severe deformity, with muscle fibrosis and contractures in 5 to 10 days. If not treated, the contracture leads to severe deformity and paralysis.

The immediate treatment is to remove any mechanically obstructive materials, such as tight bandages, and extend the joint to free blood vessels. If the symptoms do not improve within a few hours, arteriography is done in anticipation that surgery may be needed to decrease arterial spasms and to improve the blood supply by separation of the fascial sheaths of the involved muscles.

### Epiphyseal Damage

Growth of bone originates from the epiphyseal plate, and damage to this structure can result in an unequal extremity length. Surgical intervention to the epiphysis on the affected extremity or to the epiphyseal line on the opposite extremity is the usual treatment.

### Nonunion

Bone healing and callus formation can span and repair only a limited space between fragments. When inadequate reduction, poor immobilization, or a damaged or softened cast cannot maintain the bone fragments in correct align-

---

**Box 39-9** ■ ■ □
**Factors That Interfere with Bone Healing**

Separation of bone fragments at fracture site
Loss of hematoma
Interposition of tissue between bone fragments
Loss of bone tissue, especially from necrosis
Infection
Poor nutrition
Interruption of blood supply
Diseases that influence calcium metabolism (e.g., thyroid disorder)
Bone cancer
Administration of steroids

---

ment for repair, bone healing is impaired. Based on the physiologic needs for bone healing, the factors most likely to interfere with bone healing and cause delayed union or nonunion are listed in Box 39-9.

The hematoma, which becomes the matrix for bone deposition in the break, must be free of infection or bits of adipose or connective tissue. The constant supply of nutrients and bone-forming cells brought to the area by way of the bloodstream provides the vital ingredients for repair.

Sometimes artificial means are employed to facilitate bone healing. Bone grafting becomes necessary when bone nonunion occurs. The donor site is usually the tibia or the iliac crest. Bleeding of bone ends may need to be artificially stimulated, and at times holes are drilled near the bone ends in an attempt to increase circulation. Postsurgical immobilization of the recipient area is crucial to a successful graft. The Ilizarov procedure and protocol for care are frequently used to assist bone healing in patients with this type of fracture (see p. 1792).

### Malunion

Malunion is fracture union with increased angulation or deformity at the fracture site. It can be detected at any stage in the healing process or after complete healing. Unsatisfactory reduction is the usual reason for malunion. A cast or splint that allows fracture movement will also likely result in malunion. Periodic radiographic examinations will help detect this complication and avoid its becoming a major problem over a long period.

Excessive deformity can be corrected during the healing process through realignment and reimmobilization. However, attempts at correction may cause delayed union or nonunion; therefore the degree of deformity is carefully evaluated in light of these complications. The probability of sufficient spontaneous alignment that occurs with growth and continuation of the healing process also is considered. Correction of the malunion when healing is near completion requires surgical intervention.

### Infection

Osteomyelitis, infection of the bone, is often secondary to a bloodstream infection but is a potential problem in open fractures, from pressure ulcers, or when bone surgery has been performed. Any bacterial organism can cause this infectious process; however, *Staphylococcus aureus* is the most frequent pathogen (see p. 1817 for a discussion of osteomyelitis).

### Kidney Stones

Although uncommon in children, renal calculi are a potential risk whenever the child has a limb that is non–weight bearing for a long time, especially if the circumstances also produce urinary stasis. Preventive measures for renal calculi are to maintain good hydration, to mobilize the child as much as possible, and to check closely the amount and characteristics of urinary output. Any urinary tract infection should be treated promptly with appropriate antimicrobials and urine acidification because the nucleus of the calculi is often composed of bacterial debris or calcium and the buildup of stone is precipitated by alkaline urine. An associated problem, hypercalcemia, is reviewed under problems of the immobilized child.

## Pulmonary Emboli

Blood, air, or fat emboli can be a hazard to the child with a fracture. As postinjury bleeding and clotting occur, a small piece of the clot can travel to vital organs, such as the lung, heart, or brain, and produce a life-threatening vascular obstruction and ischemia. Generally the pulmonary system is the most frequent site for emboli deposition, but it may not occur until 6 to 8 weeks after the injury.

Fat emboli are the greatest threat to an individual with multiple fractures, particularly in fractures of the long bones such as the femur. Fat droplets from the marrow are transferred to the general circulation by means of the venous-arterial route, where they can be transported to the lung or brain. This type of emboli phenomenon occurs within the first 24 hours, generally in the second 12 hours after the injury occurs. Adolescents are the usual victims in the pediatric age-groups.

Emboli in the vital organs produce the classic symptoms of shock. Petechial hemorrhages of the chest and shoulders are the outstanding signs that differentiate this condition from other kinds of shock. Deep breathing, coughing, and mechanical respiratory assistance are important to maintain adequate alveolar gas exchange. An IV infusion is established to treat shock and administer medications such as an anticoagulant and corticosteroids.

Sequential pneumatic compression devices may also be used to prevent venous pooling in lower extremities when prolonged immobilization is required. These devices are inflatable sleeves that allow cyclic emptying and filling of leg veins; the devices are used in children with spinal cord injury once mobilization is initiated to decrease the effects of orthostatic intolerance.

> **NURSING ALERT**
> Pulmonary embolism should be suspected in the child with recent surgery, major trauma, or prolonged immobilization who suddenly develops chest pain and dyspnea. The severe dyspnea must be treated immediately by elevating the head when possible and administering oxygen by means of a mask or nasal cannula. This is a medical emergency.

## Amputation

A child may be born with the congenital absence of a body part, have a traumatic loss of an extremity, or need a surgical amputation for a pathologic condition such as osteogenic sarcoma. With today's surgical technology and the quick thinking of bystanders who save a traumatically amputated body part, some children have had fingers and arms sewn back on with variable degrees of functional use regained. A severed part should be rinsed in saline, wrapped gently but completely in sterile gauze and placed in a watertight bag labeled with the child's name, the date, and the time. The bag is then placed in ice water to keep the limb chilled but not frozen. The part should not be packed in ice because damage to the tissue may make reimplantation impossible.

Surgical amputation or the surgical repair of a permanently severed limb focuses on constructing an adequately nourished stump. A smooth, healthy, padded stump, free of nerve endings, is important in prosthesis fitting and subsequent ambulation. In some situations in which there is no vascular or neurologic deficit, a cast is applied to the stump immediately after the procedure, and a pylon, metal extension, and artificial foot are attached so that the patient can walk on the temporary prosthesis within a few hours.

### Nursing Considerations

Stump shaping is done postoperatively with special elastic bandaging using a figure-8 bandage, which applies pressure in a cone-shaped fashion. This technique decreases stump edema, controls hemorrhage, and aids in developing desired contours so that the child will bear weight on the posterior aspect of the skin flap rather than on the end of the stump. When appropriate, the use of a stump shrinker, in addition to an Ace wrap, may be used. Stump elevation may be used during the first 24 hours, but after this time the extremity should not be left in this position because contractures in the proximal joint will develop and seriously hamper ambulation. Monitoring proper body alignment will further decrease the risk of flexion contractures. Postoperatively, children who undergo amputation of the lower extremity should not only be turned from side to side but also from front to back. As the child progresses he or she should be encouraged to lie prone at least three times a day, increasing the time prone to tolerance of an hour at a time.

For older children and adolescents, arm exercises and bed push-ups, as well as exercises with parallel bars, which are used in prosthesis training programs, help to build up the arm muscles necessary for walking with crutches. Full range-of-motion exercises of joints above the amputation must be performed several times daily, using active and isotonic exercises. Young children are spontaneously active and require little encouragement.

Depending on the age, children or their parents will need to learn stump care, including careful washing with soap and water every day and checking for skin irritation, breakdown, or infection. A tube of stockinette or talcum powder is used to slide the prosthesis on more easily. A careful skin check must be done every time the prosthesis is removed, and prosthesis tolerance time must be adjusted to prevent skin breakdown.

Limb pain, especially pain that increases with ambulation, should be evaluated for the possibility of a neuroma at the free nerve endings in the stump and for a poorly fitting prosthesis. Chronic pain may also relate to weakness or joint instability, injury to the nerve, or fibrosis of soft tissues. Pain in the contralateral extremity may result from asymmetric weight bearing.

> **NURSING ALERT**
> For an amputated limb or body part do the following:
> Rinse limb in saline
> Loosely wrap limb in sterile gauze
> Place in a watertight bag
> Chill, without freezing, bag in ice water
> Transport patient and limb by EMS to trauma center

For children who have had an amputation, *phantom limb pain* is an expected experience because the nerve-brain connections are still present. Phantom pain is "real" pain and should be treated appropriately with analgesics and other pain-relieving measures. Gradually these sensations fade, although in many amputees they persist for years. Preoperative discussion of this phenomenon will help a child to understand these feelings and not hide the experience from others.

## INJURIES AND HEALTH PROBLEMS RELATED TO SPORTS PARTICIPATION

Adolescents probably spend more time and energy practicing and participating in sports activities than members of any other age-group. The practice of sports and games contributes significantly to growth and development, to the education process, and to better health. It provides exercise for growing muscles, interactions with peers, and a socially acceptable means of enjoying stimulation and conflict. In addition, competitive activities help the teenager in the process of self-appraisal, development of self-respect, and concern for others.

Every sport has some potential for injury to the participant—whether the young person engages in serious competition or participates for pure enjoyment. Serious injury is not limited to the athlete who competes in rough contact sports; a large number of severe or fatal injuries occur to persons engaging in less rough physical activity who are not physically prepared for the activity. For example, a body build may not be suited to the sport, muscles and support systems (respiratory and cardiovascular) may not have been sufficiently conditioned to withstand the rigors of the physical stress, or youngsters may not possess insight and judgment to recognize when an activity is beyond their capabilities. Rapidly growing bones, muscles, joints, and tendons are especially vulnerable to unusual strain.

The awkward and inexperienced youngster may suffer more injury than the more skilled and experienced one; strong muscles are less easily damaged than weak ones and will provide better protection to the joints they cross; and fatigue significantly impairs muscle function and judgment. More injuries occur during recreational sports participation than in organized athletic competition. Likewise, most injuries occur in practices rather than in games. And although team sports have frequent injuries (25% to 75%), serious injuries resulting from recreational and individual sports are generally more common (Saperstein and Nicholas, 1996). The increase in strength and vigor in adolescence may tempt youngsters to overextend themselves, especially boys who are egged on by teammates or are stimulated by the admiration of female observers.

Not only does the activity itself pose a hazard of greater or lesser degree, but the environment and the sports or recreational equipment present additional risks. Adolescents participate in physical activity in a variety of environments, both indoors and outdoors, on floors, on the ground, on snow, on or beneath water surfaces, and some-times in free air space. These activities frequently involve equipment that intensifies the risk factor.

## Preparation for Sports

The degree of physical maturation varies greatly among adolescents of the same age, and many of the physical characteristics important in sports are related to hormone production. Consequently, physical strength, coordination, endurance, and size vary considerably among youngsters who wish to compete against each other. Sports competition between young people who differ markedly in strength and agility is unfair and hazardous. Matching of candidates for sports should be made relative to physical maturity, height, weight, and physical fitness and skills, particularly in a sport involving rigorous body contact. Age is a less important consideration.

---

**Box 39-10 ◼ ◼ ◻**
**Classification of Sports**

| CONTACT SPORTS | NONCONTACT SPORTS |
|---|---|
| *Contact/Collision* | *Strenuous* |
| Basketball | Aerobic dancing |
| Boxing* | Canoeing/kayaking (flat |
| Diving | water) |
| Field hockey | Crew or rowing |
| Football (tackle) | Dancing (ballet, modern, |
| Hockey (ice)† | jazz) |
| Lacrosse | Field (discus, javelin, |
| Martial arts | shot put) |
| Rodeo | Rope jumping |
| Rugby | Running |
| Ski jumping | Scuba diving |
| Soccer | Swimming |
| Team handball | Tennis |
| Wrestling | Track |
| Water polo | Weight lifting |
| | |
| *Limited Contact/Collision* | *Moderately Strenuous* |
| Baseball | Badminton |
| Bicycling | Body building |
| Canoeing or kayaking | Curling |
| Cheerleading | Orienteering |
| Fencing | Sailing |
| Field (high jump, pole vault) | Table tennis |
| Flag football | Walking |
| Gymnastics | |
| Handball | *Nonstrenuous* |
| Horseback riding | Archery |
| Skating (ice, roller, in-line) | Bowling |
| Skiing (cross-country, | Golf |
| downhill, water) | Hunting |
| Skateboarding | Riflery |
| Snowboarding | |
| Softball | |
| Squash | |
| Ultimate frisbee | |
| Volleyball | |
| White water canoeing/kayaking | |
| Windsurfing or surfing | |

*Participation not recommended by AAP.
†AAP recommends limiting amount of body checking allowed in players <15 years.
Modified from American Academy of Pediatrics, Committee on Sports Medicine and Fitness: Medical conditions affecting sports participation, *Pediatrics* 107(5):1205-1209, 2001.
NOTE: This categorization does not reflect the relative risk of injury.

The American Academy of Pediatrics (2001) has developed a classification that divides sports according to strenuousness and probability of collision (Box 39-10). Collision sports such as tackle football, basketball, hockey, and soccer have the highest injury rate, followed by other contact sports (Figs. 39-30 and 39-31). The American Academy of Pediatrics (2001) has also prepared a table that provides criteria for determining inclusion or exclusion of the young athlete relative to common medical and surgical conditions and relative risks in various-sports categories. This serves as a useful guideline for the health professional in counseling youth for activities.

A recent child sports injury survey in the District of Columbia found that injury rates were higher for males and falls accounted for the most injuries, followed by being struck by or against an object. Of injuries requiring hospitalization, 51% involved other persons, 12% were equipment related, and 8% were attributed to a poor field surface. Examples of injuries in specific sports were as follows: baseball, 55% involved being hit by a ball or bat; football, 7% involved being hit by an opponent's helmet, and 9% involved falls on or against glass, concrete, or other fixed objects. The authors emphasize the need for improved head protection gear, increased supervision by officials, and enforcement of safety rules (Cheng and others, 2000). The American Academy of Pediatrics (2000a) encourages sports participation by young persons and encourages adults close to sports activities to be aware of early warning signs of fatigue, dehydration, and injury. Athletes are encouraged to seek assistance when an injury is suspected and not "work through" injuries caused by overuse (shin splints, stress fractures, tendinitis, and apophysitis).

The role of health care professionals in relation to sports injuries is directed toward prevention, treatment, and rehabilitation. Of these, the area of *prevention* is perhaps the most important. However, it is difficult to "sell" prevention, especially to children. Anticipatory guidance is an important aspect of preventive counseling for sports injuries because many injuries occur when the child is tired and not concentrating on his or her activity; injuries are also more common when the participant is distracted by events off the field of play, such as not really wanting to play or personal problems. Everyone wants to play the game, not practice. Often, if an 8- to 15-minute warm-up is suggested, youngsters will warm up for 30 seconds and say they are ready to go. To this end, those youth who are actively involved in athletic programs need medical evaluation as a prerequisite to participation; education in sports skills with correct training and conditioning methods; omission of those tactics that are dangerous beyond the ordinary risk associated with the specific sport; use of appropriate protective equipment, properly maintained and suited to the individual; and an environment with maximum provision for safety and availability of first-aid and medical services.

The same protective principles apply to noncompetitive sports enthusiasts. They need the same education in basic safety precautions, encouragement to acquire proper instruction in the skills required for performance of the activity (instruction in water safety, skiing techniques, and so on), and proper maintenance of equipment.

## Types of Injury

The injuries sustained in sports or recreational activities can involve any part of the body and extend from relatively minor cuts, bruises, and abrasions to totally incapacitating central nervous system injuries or death. Some of these injuries are discussed in chapters devoted to the major topic (e.g., spinal cord injuries [Chapter 40] and head injuries [Chapter 37]). Fractures are discussed earlier in this chapter.

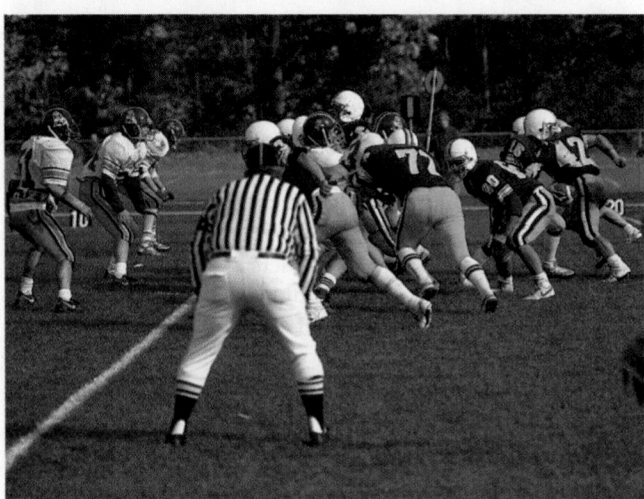

**Fig. 39-30** Football is an example of a strenuous collision sport with a high risk of serious injury.

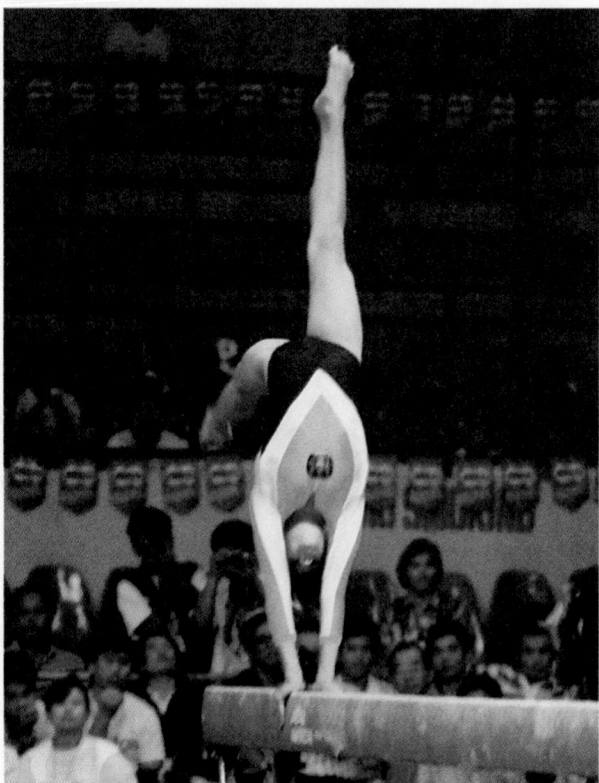

**Fig. 39-31** Gymnastics is an example of a strenuous limited-contact/collision sport with a high risk of serious injury.

Some sports are particularly dangerous for children. Snowmobiles, all-terrain motor vehicles, in-line skates, scooters, bicycles, wave runners, and trampolines are examples of sports and recreation activities that have significant injuries as a result of inappropriate use, not wearing protective equipment, or participation of children who are under age (American Academy of Pediatrics, 1999; Bercher and others, 2001; Brown and Lee, 2000; Helmkamp, 2000; Rice, Alvanos, and Kenney, 2000).

A variety of injuries can result when an external force is exerted with severe stress on tissue, muscle, and skeletal structures (Fig. 39-32). The body structures attempt to accommodate the force, but when they are unable to do so, injuries occur. Two general types of injury are recognized. The first is *acute* trauma, which is defined as a sudden, acute injury from a major force. The injuries incurred include fractures of long bones and the axial skeleton; sprains of joint ligaments; strains of muscle tendon units; and contusions, including those of muscle tendon units and overlying soft tissue. The second is repetitive overuse, or *microtrauma,* which results from repetitive injury to tissue over a long period of time. Overuse injuries include stress fractures, bursitis, tendonitis, apophysitis of tendon insertions, and at times injuries of the joint surface. More than 95% of sports injuries involve the soft tissues, not the bony skeleton. About two thirds of these consist of strains and sprains, and most injuries involve the extremities. Acute overload injuries are those that occur suddenly during an activity and produce immediate symptoms. They can be caused by a blow or over-stretching, twisting, or otherwise causing a sudden stress to tissues.

## Contusions

Contusions are probably the most common of sports injuries and are often considered to be "part of the game." A contusion is damage to the soft tissue, subcutaneous structures, and muscle. The tearing of these tissues and small blood vessels and the inflammatory response lead to hemorrhage, edema, and associated pain when the youngster attempts to move the injured part. The escape of blood into the tissues will be observed as *ecchymosis,* a black-and-blue discoloration.

The most serious contusions are those involving the quadriceps and are common in strenuous, collision-type sports, usually as a result of getting kicked or "kneed" in the thigh. Large contusions cause gross swelling, pain, and disability and usually receive immediate attention from health care personnel. The less spectacular smaller injuries may go unnoticed, allowing continued participation. However, they can become disabling after rest because of pain and muscle spasm. The young athlete is frequently instructed to work it out or disregard the pain. Unfortunately, this can result in myositis ossificans, which requires a lengthy recovery.

Immediate treatment of a contusion consists of cold application for no more than 20 to 30 minutes, as in the treatment of sprains described on p. 1799. Return to participation is allowed when the strength and range of motion of the affected extremity are equal to those of the opposite extremity.

Although not always directly related to sports, crush injuries occur in children when they slam their fingers (in doors, folding chairs, or equipment) or hit their fingers (as when hammering a nail). A severe crush injury involves the bone, with swelling and bleeding beneath the nail (subungual) and sometimes laceration of the pulp of the distal phalanx. The subungual hematoma can be released by a special cautery device that "burns" a hole at the proximal end of the nail.

## Dislocations

Long bones are held in approximation to one another at the joint by ligaments. Joints can be tight or loose, and loose joints are more likely to be dislocated. For certain sports the joints need to be limber (e.g., gymnastics and acrobatic dancing); a tight joint is needed for sports such as football. One of the most vulnerable joints is the shoulder, which is structurally insecure, having only a rotator cuff to maintain the shoulder in place. The joint is shallow with relatively little muscle protection; therefore the capsule becomes stretched and the joint dislocates easily. There is a high incidence of shoulder injuries in male gymnasts and an even greater incidence of shoulder injuries in players of contact sports, such as football.

Dislocations are less common in children than in older persons, but some types are peculiar to the younger age-groups. Before final closure of the epiphyses, injuries to the joints are more likely to cause epiphyseal separation than

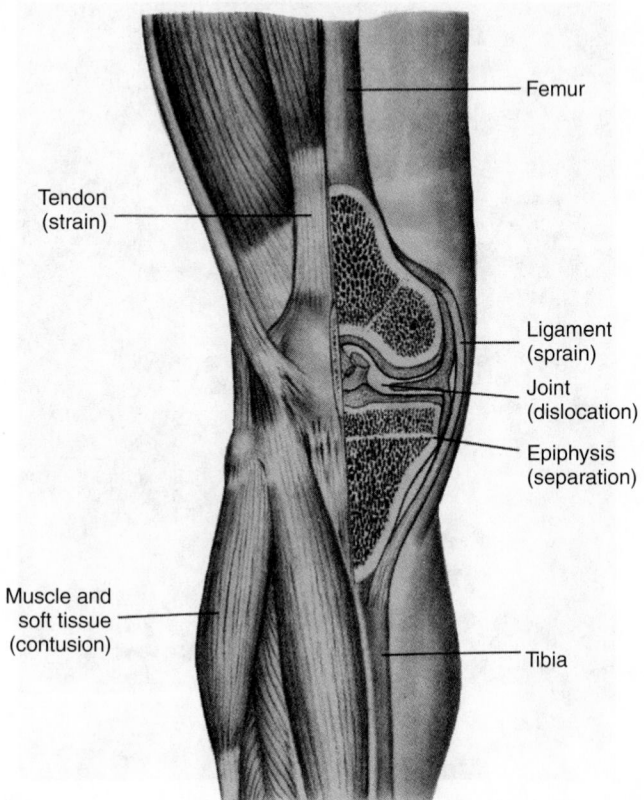

**Fig. 39-32** Sites of injuries to bones, joints, and soft tissues.

Femur

Tendon (strain)

Ligament (sprain)

Joint (dislocation)

Epiphysis (separation)

Muscle and soft tissue (contusion)

Tibia

dislocation. For example, shoulder dislocation occurs most often in older adolescents, and dislocation unaccompanied by fracture is rare. Dislocation of the phalanges is the most common type seen in children, followed by elbow dislocations. Injury to the hip causes dislocation more frequently than femoral neck fracture (often experienced by persons in the older age-groups).

In children younger than 5 years of age, the hip can be dislocated by a fall. The greatest risk following this injury is the potential loss of blood supply to the head of the femur. Children with naturally lax joints, such as children with Down syndrome, are more prone to recurrent dislocation of the hip.

A dislocation occurs when the force of stress on the ligament is so great as to displace the normal position of the opposing bone ends or the bone end to its socket. The predominant symptom is pain that increases with attempted passive or active movement of the extremity. In dislocations there may be an obvious deformity and inability to move the joint. Temporary restriction of the joint, with a sling or bandage that secures the arm to the chest in a shoulder dislocation, provides sufficient comfort and immobilization until the youngster can receive medical help.

The best chance for prevention of damage to the head of the femur is to relocate the hip within 60 minutes after the injury occurs. As the length of time between injury and hip relocation increases, the risk of irreparable damage increases. Simple dislocations should be reduced with the child under conscious sedation and often local anesthesia. Use of sedative/analgesic agents such as midazolam, ketamine, propofol, and fentanyl can produce partial or complete analgesia (Baltes-Messner and others, 1999). (See Surgical Procedures, Chapter 27.) An unreduced dislocation will be complicated by increased swelling, making reduction difficult and increasing the risk of neurovascular problems. Treatment depends on the severity of the injury.

Dislocation of the *patella* is a recurrent experience in some children; in others it is a result of injury. It is common among adolescent girls. The patella is always dislocated laterally. Most dislocations are reduced either spontaneously or by a companion before the child is seen by a practitioner. Therapy is immobilization for 3 to 4 weeks. Surgery may be needed for recurrent dislocations.

The most common dislocation injury is subluxation or partial dislocation of the *radial head* in the elbow, also called "pulled elbow" or "nursemaid's elbow." In the vast majority of cases the injury occurs in a child between ages 1 and 3 years who receives a sudden longitudinal pull or traction at the wrist while the arm is fully extended and the forearm pronated. It usually occurs when an adult who is holding the child by the hand or wrist gives a sudden jerk to prevent a fall, attempts to lift the child by pulling the wrist, or the child suddenly pulls away by dropping to the floor (or ground). The child has an anxious expression, whines, complains of pain in the elbow and wrist, refuses to move the arm, and holds it with the opposite hand and in a slightly flexed and pronated position against his or her body.

The practitioner manipulates the arm by applying firm finger pressure to the head of the radius and then supinates and flexes the forearm to return the bone structures to normal alignment. A click is heard, and functional use of the arm returns within 20 to 30 minutes. However, the longer the subluxation is present, the longer it takes for the child to recover mobility after treatment. A radiograph may be needed if attempts to reduce the dislocation are not successful (Della-Giustina and Della-Giustina, 1999).

## Sprains and Strains

A *sprain* occurs when trauma to a joint is so severe that a ligament is either stretched or partially or completely torn by the force created as a joint is twisted or wrenched. This is often accompanied by damage to associated blood vessels, muscles, tendons, and nerves. As a guideline for management and prognosis, sprains are classified according to the degree of injury (Box 39-11). Because of all of the ligaments required to maintain knee stability, the knee is the most commonly injured joint relative to sports injuries. It is also the largest joint and consequently more prone to injury.

The presence of joint laxity is the most valid indicator of the severity of a sprain. In a severe injury the athlete complains of the joint "feeling loose" or as if "something is coming apart" and may describe hearing a "snap," "pop," or "tearing." Pain is seldom the principal subjective symptom. There is a rapid onset with swelling, often diffuse, accompanied by immediate disability and appreciable reluctance to use the injured joint.

A *strain* is a microscopic tear to the musculotendinous unit and has features in common with sprains. The area is painful to touch and is swollen. The severity is evaluated in grades I, II, and III, except that the degree of laxity does not apply. Even with severe grade III injuries, complaints of laxity are rare. Most strains are incurred over time rather than suddenly, and the rapidity of the appearance provides clues regarding severity. In general the more rapidly the strain occurs, the more severe the injury. When the strain involves the muscular portion, there is more bleeding, often palpable soon after injury and before edema obscures the hematoma.

### Therapeutic Management

The first 6 to 12 hours is the most critical period for virtually all soft tissue injuries. Basic principles of managing

---

**Box 39-11** ■ ■ □
**Classification of Sprains**

**Grade I:** Mild injury; involves overstretching or microscopic tearing but without hemorrhage or increased instability of the involved joint. Swelling may develop later.

**Grade II:** Moderate injury; involves partial, overt tearing of the ligament with at least some ligamentous continuity remaining; usually immediate pain and swelling with decreased function.

**Grade III:** Severe injury; total loss of ligamentous continuity (i.e., disruption of one or more ligaments or the musculotendinous unit). Pain is immediate but subsides because none of the pain fibers is being stretched. Swelling may be minimal because hemorrhage extravasates outside of the area into soft tissues.

sprains and other soft tissue injuries are summarized in the acronyms RICE and ICES:

**R**—Rest              **I**—Ice
**I**—Ice               **C**—Compression
**C**—Compression       **E**—Elevation
**E**—Elevation         **S**—Support

Soft tissue injuries should be iced immediately. This is best accomplished with crushed ice wrapped in a towel or encased in a screw-top ice bag or plastic bag (e.g., a resealable storage bag). A wet elastic wrap is applied to provide compression and to keep the ice pack in place. A single layer of the wrap or cloth is placed over the injured area to protect the skin under the ice pack, and the remainder of the bandage secures the pack in place. The wet wrap transfers the cold better than a dry wrap. Some athletic trainers keep wet elastic wraps refrigerated for ready use.

**NURSING TIP**   A plastic bag of frozen vegetables, such as peas, serves as a convenient ice pack for soft tissue injuries occurring at home. It is clean, watertight, and easily molded to the injured part. Snow placed in a plastic bag works well also.

There is still controversy regarding the use of heat or ice during the rehabilitative phase of management. Regardless of the method used, it is accompanied by appropriate exercise, depending on the severity of the injury, and carried out under the direction of a competent professional experienced in care of sports injuries.

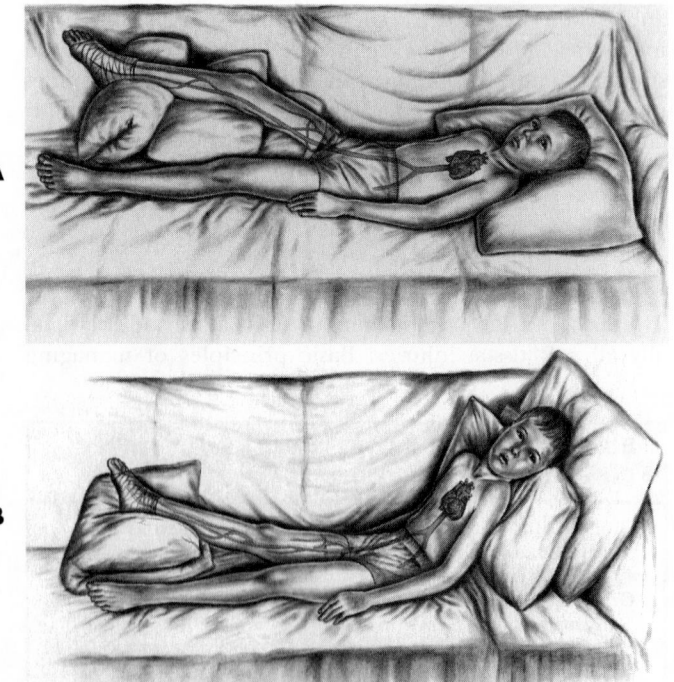

**Fig. 39-33**   Correct and incorrect methods for elevating a lower extremity. **A,** Correct method: lower leg elevated on pillows; ankle above heart level. **B,** Incorrect positioning: ankle below level of heart.

Ice has a rapid cooling effect on tissues that reduces pain and the magnitude of the stretch reflex by decreasing muscle spindle response, afferent nerve discharge, and the afferent loop response (monosynaptic reflex). Secondary effects are achieved by vasoconstriction, slowing muscle nerve velocity, and increasing muscle viscosity. Also, the decreased temperature slows metabolism, thus reducing tissue oxygen requirements. Edema formation is reduced when fewer histamine-like substances are released. Nine to 15 minutes of ice exposure produces a deep-tissue vasodilation without increased metabolism. However, the effects last up to 7 hours. Ice therapy should never be applied for more than 30 minutes.

Elevating the extremity uses gravity to facilitate venous return and reduce edema formation in the damaged area. The point of injury should be kept several inches above the level of the heart for therapy to be effective (Fig. 39-33). Several pillows can be used effectively for elevation. Allowing the extremity to be dependent causes excessive fluid accumulation in the area of injury, delaying healing and causing painful swelling.

Major sprains or tears to the ligamentous tissue rarely occur in growing children. Ligaments are stronger than bone, and the epiphysis and growth plate are the weakest areas of the bone; therefore the more usual sites of injury are at the growth plate. (See Fractures, p. 1776). Torn ligaments, especially those in the knee, are now commonly treated with arthroscopy and ligament repair as necessary. These injuries are particularly common in adolescents who participate in contact sports, such as football and soccer or skiing. Postoperative mobilization of the affected joint is implemented with a continuous passive motion (CPM) device immediately. The CPM device provides passive range of motion to the injured extremity and decreases postoperative complications related to restricted mobility. The patient is often ambulatory within hours on crutches and discharged late on the day of surgery or the following day.

## Overuse Syndrome

To excel in sports, the young athlete is forced to train longer, harder, and earlier in life than previously. The rewards are an increased level of fitness, better performance, faster times, and the satisfaction of attaining a personal goal. However, the risk of overuse injury is always present and can be related to several factors: training errors, muscle-tendon imbalance, anatomic malalignment (i.e., femoral anteversion, excessive lumbar lordosis, or tibial torsion), incorrect footwear or playing surface, an associated disease state, and growth (growth cartilage is less resistant to microtrauma). Athletes who run extensively frequently experience shin splints. The ligaments tear away from the shaft (tibial), and this creates the pain. Ice, rest, and nonsteroidal antiinflammatory drugs, such as ibuprofen or naproxen, are the usual treatment. Shin splints are rarely serious.

Chronic pain in athletes is often associated with overuse injuries, which can occur at any level of athletic participation. The common feature in overuse injuries is the *repetitive microtrauma* that occurs to a particular anatomic structure. Performing the same movements time and again sometimes causes several types of injury: (1) *frictional*, rubbing of one structure against another; (2) *tractional*, repeated pull on a ligament or tendon; or (3) *cyclic loading* of impact forces (stress fractures). The end result is inflammation of the involved structure with complaints of pain, tenderness, swelling, and disability.

Bursae, tendons, muscles, ligaments, joints, and bones are all subject to overuse. Some of the common overuse syndromes are briefly outlined in Table 39-4. Plantar fasciitis is very common in athletes, and Osgood-Schlatter disease is seen in children who do a lot of jumping. The overuse type of injuries, such as sore shoulders and strained elbows, may indicate that too much is being requested of the child in too short a period of time.

## Stress Fractures

With intensity and duration of training, many young athletes suffer stress fractures, especially after a recent increase in training regimens. These fractures occur as a result of repeated muscle contraction and are seen most often in repetitive weight-bearing sports such as running, gymnastics, and basketball. They occur less often in swimmers (upper extremity). Tibial fractures are most common.

The most common symptoms of stress fracture are a sharp, persistent, progressive pain or a deep, persistent dull ache located over the bone. Sometimes there is pain on impact (heel strike), but the most important clinical sign is pain over the involved bony surface. Diagnosis is established on the basis of clinical observation. Plain radiographs are rarely diagnostic of stress fractures during the initial few weeks, because callus formation is not yet evident. Occasionally a bone scan may be needed, which will indicate a "hot spot."

## Therapeutic Management

Development of inflammation is common to all overuse syndromes; therefore the management is directed toward rest or alteration of activities, physical therapies, and medication. Rest is the primary therapy, usually interpreted as reduced activity and use of alternative exercise—*not* bed rest or immobilization with casting. The primary purpose is to alleviate the repetitive stress that initiated the symptoms. It is important to keep the youngster mobile, and training can be continued. Alternative exercise is selected that maintains conditioning without aggravating the injury. For example, pool running (treading water in the deep end of a pool) can use the same movements as running but without the weight bearing; bicycling, swimming, and rowing are viable alternatives.

Other modalities include cryotherapy and cold whirlpools, and sometimes taping, bracing, splinting, and other orthoses are employed, according to the injury. Medications, such as nonsteroidal antiinflammatory drugs (see Table 26-4), are sometimes prescribed to reduce inflammation and pain. Topical medications are of questionable value.

## Heat Injury/Illness

Infants, children, and adolescents are at high risk for heat-related illness. Several characteristics of infants and children render them more vulnerable to heat injury. The

| TABLE 39-4 | Selected overuse injuries | |
|---|---|---|
| **Disorder** | **Cause** | **Manifestations** |
| Plantar fasciitis | Repetitive stretching of the plantar fascia (calcaneus to metatarsal heads) | Pain in arch or heel |
| Achilles tendinitis | Repeated forcible traction on short tendon | Pain on palpation; pain with plantar flexion against resistance |
| Sever disease | Epiphysitis of the calcaneus | Pain over insertion of Achilles tendon into tip of calcaneus |
| Anterior leg pain ("shin splints") | Irritation of posterior tibial muscle in unconditioned athlete or one not conditioned to a new sport | Pain in leg along anterior or medial edge of midshaft or distal third of tibia |
| Osgood-Schlatter disease | Traction apophysitis of tibial tubercle | Pain and tenderness; overprominence of involved tubercle |
| Sinding-Larsen syndrome ("jumper's knee") | A variant of Osgood-Schlatter disease; traction apophysitis on inferior pole of patella | Same as above; pain slightly lower than Osgood-Schlatter |
| Patellofemoral syndromes | Malalignment of extensors, increased patellar compression, and increased training intensity | Chronic knee pain, especially following forced leg extension from flexion or after running |
| "Tennis elbow" | Lateral epicondylitis from repetitive strain on elbow | Pain in elbow, aggravated by use |
| "Little League elbow" | Osteochondritis of the capitellum; tendinitis of flexor-origin medial epicondyle from repetitive valgus strain to elbow from throwing | Pain in elbow that increases with activity |
| "Little League shoulder" | Microfracture of proximal humeral growth plate from repetitive throwing | Pain and characteristic contracture; loss of internal rotation and increased external rotation |
| "Swimmer's shoulder" | Supraspinatus tendinitis from repetitive shoulder movement | Pain in shoulder that increases with activity |

greater ratio of surface area to body mass in infants and young children leads to increased transfer of heat between the body and the environment. Children produce more metabolic heat for body mass during exercise and have a reduced capacity to convey heat from the body core to the skin. Also, children do not have the sweating capacity of adults and take longer to become acclimated to hot conditions. Young children may also not feel the need to drink a sufficient amount of fluid during extended exercise.

*Heat cramps* are caused by sodium depletion, which in turn potentiates the effects of calcium on skeletal muscle. It most often occurs as a result of strenuous exercise in a hot environment. Cramps most often involve the leg muscles. Vital signs are usually normal, but the core temperature may be elevated. The child sweats profusely, but mentation is normal. Treatment is rest and replacement of fluid and electrolytes. Dilute sports drinks or electrolyte replacement liquids are helpful. Electrolyte replacement liquids are now available as popsicles and are well tolerated with less vomiting.

*Heat exhaustion,* or heat collapse, is a common condition that usually occurs during vigorous exercise in a hot environment. It results from excessive loss of fluids, especially in poorly acclimated and dehydrated children. The onset may be gradual, with initial complaints that include thirst, headache, fatigue, dizziness, anxiety, or nausea and vomiting. The child usually has a clear sensorium but may be somewhat disoriented. The temperature can be normal or mildly elevated; sweating is profuse. Tachycardia, hypotension (usually postural), and syncope may be observed secondary to intravascular volume depletion. Treatment is to move the child to a cool environment, provide rest, and replace fluid volume. The child with a clear sensorium can be given oral replacement fluids but often IV fluids are required due to vomiting. External cooling methods are not necessary.

*Heatstroke* represents a failure of normal thermoregulatory mechanisms. Heatstroke usually occurs during or immediately following physical activity, especially in the unacclimated adolescent who is exercising vigorously. The onset is rapid with initial symptoms of headache, weakness, and disorientation. Central nervous system manifestations may be agitation, confusion, and lethargy; loss of consciousness may occur without warning and may be accompanied by nuchal rigidity, posturing, and convulsions. Sweating may not be present. The temperature is typically greater than 40° C (104° F), and there is severe volume depletion. Immediate care is relocation to a cool environment, removal of clothing, application of cool water (wet towels or immersion), and use of fans. The child is transported to the hospital for intensive care.

Hospital care includes rapid cooling until core temperature reaches 102° F to prevent "overcooling." Antipyretics are not used because they are metabolized by the liver, which is already not functioning properly. Renal and liver failure are common sequelae to heatstroke. Treatment includes careful monitoring of temperature and other vital signs, supportive care such as supplemental oxygen, and fluid and electrolyte replacement. *Prevention* remains the best treatment for hyperthermia. If the temperature is elevated, time in the sun should be decreased. Activity should be stopped if the humidity is elevated as well. The athlete should drink plenty of fluids, preferably with low sugar content.

Nonexertional, or classic, heatstroke has a slow onset with insidious development of anorexia, nausea, vomiting, headache, development of mental manifestations, and loss of intravascular volume. Classic heatstroke occurs primarily in children with abnormal thermoregulation (e.g., children with cystic fibrosis) and infants subjected to prolonged neglect in a hot environment.

## Underwater Sports–Related Injuries

Children who venture into water at least waist deep generally start to play underwater. It is not unusual for children to be able to swim underwater before they are able to swim on the surface. The injuries that are sustained from diving or swimming underwater are serious and deserve brief mention. Near-drowning is primarily a respiratory and neurologic problem and is discussed in Chapters 32 and 37; the major injury from diving or surfing is damage to the cervical spine. (See Spinal Cord Injuries, Chapter 40.)

Other underwater sports injuries include ear squeeze, which occurs when middle ear pressures are not equalized during diving; decompression sickness (the bends) and air emboli from too rapid decompression after deep dives; and nitrogen narcosis.

### Sports and Accidental Drowning

Young people ages 15 to 24 years have the highest drowning rates. At highest risk are males between ages 15 and 19 years, with concurrent alcohol use present in approximately 40% of drowning incidents. Alcohol not only impairs judgment but also increases the likelihood of water aspiration. Jet skiing is a popular but hazardous activity. Preventive measures to decrease the number of deaths have been unsuccessful. Suggested methods of intervention have been to (1) reduce the amount of alcohol consumed by adolescents, (2) increase the proportion of the population who are able to swim, and (3) encourage routine use of protective devices, such as life vests, when boating or fishing. Because most drownings are witnessed but resuscitation methods are often not quickly or appropriately initiated, public education programs have been suggested as a potential remedy for this problem (American Academy of Pediatrics, 1993a).

## Health Concerns Associated with Sports
### Nutrition

Most athletes are motivated to enhance their performance by any and all means available. They are eager to learn about nutrition, and many become subject to misconceptions, fads, and superstitions regarding certain foods. Physical performance is affected by energy and body composition. The young athlete must maintain a diet that provides sufficient nutrients and energy to meet metabolic needs for optimum functioning. Physical training increases the need for energy, as well for more nutrients that convert food energy into chemical energy for physical performance.

There is no evidence to indicate that food supplements, extra vitamins, sports bars, or high-protein diets are needed to meet the demands of heavy physical exercise or improve physical performance. In addition, there is no scientific data supporting the benefits of such supplements to improve physical performance other than anecdotal incidents (Steen, 1996). However, young athletes need considerably more calories than the recommended daily allowance. When the basic requirements for growth and activity are met by a balanced diet of protein, grains and cereals, fruits and vegetables, and dairy products, the additional calories needed for the extra exertion can be selected as desired. These extra caloric needs can be supplied by eating additional helpings from any of the basic four food groups, but many of the additional calories are provided by complex carbohydrates found in such foods as vegetables, pastas, and bread. The recommended dietary energy intake for adolescents involved in sports is as follows: 55% to 60% of total energy from carbohydrate, 12% to 15% from protein, and 25% to 30% from fat (Steen, 1996). It should be noted however that energy requirements will vary depending on the sport, age, and body build of the child. The use of laxatives, diuretics, salt tablets, and especially fluid restriction is not recommended for enhancing performance (Steen, 1996). Adolescent athletes need additional iron and calcium intake from appropriate food sources to meet growth and developmental needs as well as to replace those lost in competition (Steen, 1996). A summary of nutrition pointers for young athletes is presented in Box 39-12.

**Water and Electrolytes.**    Considerable water is lost from the body through perspiration, urination, and evaporation from the respiratory tract. Water losses, especially from the skin, increase with the duration and intensity of exercise and in higher environmental temperatures. Although the thirst mechanism is experienced early in dehydration, it is unreliable as an indicator of fluid deficit. Athletes participating in multiple daily exercise sessions in warm environments are at risk for dehydration and should receive all the water they desire.

Very little water is exchanged in the stomach and must reach the intestines for absorption. The best fluids for rapid gastric emptying are cold, of low osmolality, and have a large volume. Those containing simple sugars or glucose polymers with few or no electrolytes are better than plain water. Gatorade and other "sports" drinks contain excess carbohydrate (6% to 8%) and should be diluted with one or two parts water to one part drink.

Small amounts of electrolytes are lost during exercise, especially sodium and chloride. Because sweat is quite dilute relative to plasma concentrations, excessive perspiration can result in excessive loss of water and an increase in plasma concentrations of sodium chloride. Therefore it is more important to **replace water** than sodium and chloride. Children should be well hydrated before beginning strenuous exercise/sports, especially in warm climates or environments. Periodic drinking breaks are encouraged, and adults or other team members should be alerted to the child who has complaints such as headache, cramping, nausea, and vertigo. One suggestion is to take a break each 15 to 20 minutes of strenuous play/exercise and hydrate with 5 to 9 ounces of water or a flavored salted beverage (add 1 g salt

---

### Box 39-12  ■ ■ □
### Fifteen Steps to Good Sports Nutrition

1. A well-balanced diet consists of elements from the Food Guide Pyramid. The recommended percentages of major nutrients are 55% to 75% carbohydrates, 25% to 30% fat, and 15% to 20% protein.*
2. Athletes should take water at regular intervals during exercise.
3. For each pound of fluid lost through exercise, the athlete should consume 16 ounces of water.
4. Any athlete who loses more than 3% of body weight in an exercise session should not return to activity until the fluid is restored. Monitoring body weight can prevent chronic dehydration.
5. Beverages with small amounts of simple sugars or glucose polymers with little or no electrolytes are better sources of hydration than plain water.
6. Salt tablets are rarely needed and may actually do harm by increasing dehydration.
7. Glycogen loading is of value only for endurance exercises that take more than 1 hour, such as marathons and cross-country ski races. It is not recommended for children.
8. Protein and amino acid supplementation are potentially harmful and should be discouraged.
9. Vitamin supplements are usually unnecessary and a waste of money; excessive doses may be harmful. One daily multivitamin is not harmful for youngsters who do not consume well-balanced meals.
10. Mineral supplements are usually not needed, except for young athletes, especially menstruating females, who develop a specific deficiency such as iron.
11. Any weight loss program should be designed to lose body fat primarily and not lean body tissue or water. The goal should be to achieve a certain percentage of body weight as fat.
12. Athletes should not lose more than 1 to 2 pounds per week. They should not reduce daily caloric intake to less than 1200 calories for girls and 1500 calories for boys.
13. Athletes who wish to gain weight can do so by combining increased caloric intake with muscle work (i.e., weight training). Nutritional supplements are not usually needed.
14. Athletes should gain weight no more rapidly than 1 to 2 pounds per week. They should be monitored for percentage of body fat.
15. The pregame meal should be eaten at least 2½ hours before competition. It should consist primarily of carbohydrates and not foods that are slowly digested (fats) or that have excessive concentrated sugars (desserts).

Modified from Primos WA, Landry GL: Fighting the fads in sports nutrition, *Contemp Pediatr* 6(9):14-50, 1989.
*Note that percentages may vary among authorities and should take into consideration the energy expended, body build, and age of the athlete.

to 2 pints of the flavored drink) (American Academy of Pediatrics, 2000a). Salt tablets are unnecessary and may actually be harmful. Athletes usually derive sufficient salt replacement from their diet.

**Minerals.** The basic diet will not satisfy the iron requirement of 10% to 15% of female athletes. The largest group are those teenage girls who may become iron depleted after menarche. Young boys who are experiencing rapid adolescent growth and who have irregular and inadequate diets also are at risk of iron depletion. These youngsters will need iron supplements.

Adequate calcium intake during puberty is essential to promote mineralization of the growing skeleton. In addition, calcium plays a vital role in nerve transmission, muscle contraction, and blood coagulation. Female athletes who engage in intensive training and subsequently develop amenorrhea may require additional calcium intake to prevent osteoporosis. The best sources of calcium for athletes are nonfat dairy products.

**Glycogen.** Energy is derived primarily from glycogen previously stored in muscles and the liver. Energy for prolonged exercise is derived from high-carbohydrate food (e.g., bread, cereals, pancakes, potatoes, rice, spaghetti) consumed 24 to 48 hours before the activity, not from a meal eaten just before the activity. The meal before a physical contest should be eaten at least 2 to 4 hours before the exertion and consist mainly of carbohydrates. Carbohydrate (glycogen) loading is a technique reserved for competition in prolonged aerobic endurance events and requires dietary changes a week before the competitive event. For more information regarding carbohydrate loading and other techniques for improving athletic performance, the reader is directed to texts on sports medicine and sports training.

**Weight.** Control of body weight by restriction of water intake, food restriction, or encouragement of sweat loss is dangerous; these are highly undesirable means for meeting a minimum weight classification. Young athletes need to learn something about nutrition to dispel the allure of prevalent fads and fallacies about diet and performance. The optimum diet for an athlete is one that contains the essential food groups and that is adjusted to the energy requirements of the sport in which the youngster is engaged. Such a dietary plan should provide adequate nutrition for top physical efficiency and performance, maintenance of physical fitness and desirable body weight, and optimum function of all organ systems.

The "bottom line" for athletes to build stronger bodies and enhance performance is to consume well-balanced meals including the four major food groups from the Food Guide Pyramid with additional carbohydrate servings and to use high-protein drinks or sports bars sparingly. Sports bars and high-protein drinks should not become substitutes for a meal (Ryan-Krause, 1998).

## Considerations for the Female Athlete

The female athlete triad consists of amenorrhea, osteoporosis, and disoriented eating. The triad was originally described in athletes in whom thinness was desired (gymnasts, ballet dancers, figure skaters, and long distance runners),

yet is now recognized in virtually all sports (American Academy of Pediatrics, 2000b; Callahan, 2000). The phenomenon has been attributed to a complex interplay of physical, genetic, hormonal, nutritional, psychologic, and environmental factors that include the stress of competition, decreased protein consumption, and altered lean-to-fat body ratio.

Amenorrhea has been reported for girls who engage in strenuous exercise. Except for swimmers, menarche is attained later in athletes than in nonathletes. Gymnasts, figure skaters, and ballet dancers have the latest mean ages of menarche; track athletes have less of a delayed maturity than gymnasts and ballet dancers, who also tend to be smaller, lighter, and leaner than other female athletes. Swimmers, who tend to be larger, have a mean age of menarche that approximates that for nonathletes. Also, there appears to be an association between delayed menarche and more advanced competitive levels; that is, athletes at the more advanced levels have a greater delay than those at lower competitive levels.

An area for counseling the female athlete with delayed menarche regards pregnancy. Sexually active teenagers, regardless of menstruation, need to be reminded to take contraceptive precautions. Most teenage girls erroneously believe that because they do not menstruate, they cannot become pregnant.

Osteoporosis from decreased levels of estrogen in these athletes, complicated by poor nutritional intake, leads to loss of bone resorption and stress fractures. The peak of bone density is reached in late adolescence and is related to circulating estrogen levels. Girls with diminished estrogen secretion in delayed menarche will reach late adolescence with low bone density and will be subject to osteoporosis. Hypoestrogenic bone loss greatly increases the risk of injury.

Disordered eating is less severe and more subtle than eating disorders such as anorexia and bulimia. Disordered eating includes food restrictions, rigid food patterns, fasting, vomiting, and the use of diet pills and laxatives. The goal is to achieve a specific body image that is seen as desirable for the sport and is influenced by others such as a coach, teammates, or peers. Disordered eating results in poor protein intake, low fat intake, and inadequate caloric intake. Teenage girls need to be counseled to increase calcium intake to four to six servings per day (1500 mg of calcium is recommended daily intake for amenorrheic athletes), which should be supplied by low-fat dairy products. In addition, they should be encouraged to have adequate protein and caloric intake to meet the energy and metabolic needs related to exercise. Trainers and coaches also need to be aware of the potentially long-term results of intensive, prolonged exercise in pubertal girls.

## Drug Misuse by Athletes

Young athletes have used various substances in an attempt to augment their athletic performance. These substances, known as *ergogenic aids*, are believed by athletes to increase strength and endurance, delay the onset of fatigue, increase the ability to concentrate, and decrease sensitivity to pain. Although use of these substances is prohibited in international Olympic competition, there are no means at present to enforce a prohibition on their use in other sports participation.

The principal drugs misused by athletes are the psychomotor stimulants (e.g., amphetamines) and the anabolic steroids. Amphetamines and related drugs, such as methylphenidate (Ritalin) and phenmetrazine (Preludin), as well as caffeine, are taken to provide a sense of increased alertness and relief of fatigue; however, obscuring fatigue may permit participants to exceed their limits and precipitate a sudden collapse. These drugs can also make the users more aggressive, which can contribute to injuries to themselves and others.

Anabolic steroids, such as nandrolone phenpropionate (Durabolin) and methandrostenolone (Dianabol), are a source of concern to health professionals. The majority of these drugs are no longer manufactured in the United States by legitimate companies. Black market supplies of anabolic steroids are of poor quality and potency. In an attempt to enhance muscle strength, these drugs are administered to athletes by coaches, managers, athletic trainers, and even physicians. The user develops larger-appearing muscles and increased body weight and body water, but reports on the effectiveness in improving performance have been conflicting. Although the psychologic effect may be beneficial, many valid studies have failed to demonstrate any improvement in performance.

The precise incidence of use of anabolic steroids by adolescent athletes remains debatable but may range from 5% to 11% of high school athletes. Coaches and health professionals who work with youth report a trend toward increased use of these agents. Teenagers rely on poor sources of information about the potential hazards of steroids (friends, television, muscle magazines) and are generally poorly informed of their potential negative side effects. Health care professionals need to be aware of the clinical manifestations of steroid use. Clinical signs such as severe acne, a sudden increase in strength and muscle, a sudden decrease in body fat, a male pattern of baldness, and water retention are common. In females a male pattern of hair growth and a deepening voice are significant observations.

The dangers of continued use are well-known and include hypertension; virilization in females; oligospermia, testicular atrophy, infertility, and gynecomastia in males; and premature closure of the epiphyses, acne, increased blood cholesterol levels, and hepatocellular carcinoma in both genders. Mood changes have been observed, including aggressiveness, changes in libido, and mood swings, which are often dramatic, such as "roid rage." Health hazards outweigh any potential gain that might be induced.

Other drugs that are often misused include nutritional aids, local anesthetic agents, narcotic analgesics such as Nubain, beta blockers (to reduce circulating catecholamines and thus reduce anxiety related to somatic type of stress), and antiinflammatory drugs, such as dimethyl sulfoxide (DSMO) (which is not approved for use and is available only as a veterinary or an industrial preparation), and corticosteroids. The possibility of their use by the adolescent athlete should be considered when performing a health assessment.

### Sudden Death

A death associated with sports produces renewed anxiety in both parents and health care professionals. The term *sudden,* or *instantaneous death* is applied to death that occurs within minutes of the onset of the cause of death or within 24 hours of the episode. Causes of sudden death are related to three main risk factors: (1) sports with a high inherent risk for sport-related sudden death; (2) children with recognized or unknown underlying medical problems; and (3) the sport environment (i.e., the rules, equipment, practice fields or areas of sport participation, and the ambient temperature of the geographic area). (Chapter 23 discusses the impact of sudden death on the family and relevant nursing interventions.)

**Sports.**  Sports that create the greatest risk of sudden death are those involving collision and frequent body contact. Examples of collision sports include football, ice hockey, rugby, and boxing. There is a high potential for serious injury or fatality in sports such as mountain or rock climbing and hang gliding. Sports that involve high-velocity objects, such as baseball and ice hockey, may cause death as a result of serious head or chest injuries. Riding vehicles such as snowmobiles, mopeds, water ski jets, all-terrain vehicles, minibikes, and motorcycles can also be considered high-risk sports.

**Medical Conditions.**  The most frequent medical causes of sudden death during sports activity are cardiac abnormalities, especially *idiopathic hypertrophic subaortic stenosis (hypertrophic cardiomyopathy).* Manifestations suggestive of hypertrophic cardiomyopathy include a typical triad of severe chest pain with dizziness, prominent pulses, and a murmur at the left lower sternal border. A history of sudden death of a relative, or relatives, in the second and third decade often offers a clue to recognition.

Well-trained athletes often display evidence of hypertrophic cardiomyopathy, the so-called athlete's heart, but the condition is not pathologic. Congenital heart problems are infrequent causes of sudden death in sports involving children and adolescents. Children with systemic hypertension, some types of cardiac arrhythmias, and some forms of heart block will require restrictions in the type and amount of exercise they can tolerate safely.

**Environmental Causes.**  Environmental factors that are potential causes of death include playing conditions, clothing, equipment, rules used by officials governing a sport, and outdoor temperature. Heatstroke and hypothermia (see Chapter 18) are probably the most serious uncontrollable environmental causes of death in athletes.

## Nurse's Role in Children's Sports

Nurses may become involved in sports activities in the areas of preparation and evaluation for activities, prevention of injury, treatment of injuries, and rehabilitation after injury. Selecting an appropriate sport for both recreation and competition is a joint effort of the youngster, parents, and health professionals. Children are introduced to sports as part of family activities, neighborhood games, and school physical education programs, and both parents and children are influenced by media exposure to a variety of sports. Children are highly influenced by the popularity and exposure afforded athletics in the school setting, especially in high school.

The best approach to counseling children and parents regarding sports participation is to encourage activities that are most likely to provide pleasure and physical benefits throughout childhood and into adulthood. Exposure to a variety of sports activities is probably better for young children than limiting them to only one sport. Parents should be cautioned against overprogramming children so the children have ample time for other activities and associations.

Nurses are sometimes members of a sports medicine team. Although the training and rehabilitation are usually managed by certified sports trainers and other specialists in sports medicine, the nurse should have input regarding injury prevention. Nurses should be able to provide emergency treatment for any type of injury and know when to refer the injured child for evaluation and care. Sports injuries can occur in free play as well as in organized athletic programs, and a school nurse is often the first person who attends an injured child.

When children sustain athletic injuries, nurses are often responsible for instructing the children and their parents regarding care. Instructions, such as follow-up appointments, application of ice, and any restrictions in activity, should be made clear and preferably be accompanied by written directions. The importance of taking medications as prescribed is emphasized because they may be needed for an extended period of time and compliance may be difficult. For children continuing with activities, medication administration an hour before practice or competition is advantageous.

Prevention of sports injuries is probably the most important aspect of any athletic program. The children should be suited to the activity; the environment and equipment should be made safe for physical activity; and the children should be adequately prepared for the sport, especially if it is one that requires strenuous or continuous physical exertion. Nurses collaborate with coaches and athletic trainers to ensure that safety measures are carried out. Stretching exercises, warming-up and cooling-down activities, and an appropriate training program are only some of the requisites for safe participation. Protective measures, such as pads, taping, wrapping, or other devices, are employed for areas at risk. Nurses are also on the alert for environmental safety risks.

Participation of youth in sports programs has grown significantly in the past several decades. This trend toward greater participation by both genders has been encouraged because of its demonstrated effect on reducing obesity and lowering blood pressure, and its beneficial impact on lowering cholesterol and lipid levels.

For some athletes, the whole of life revolves around sports participation. When a serious injury occurs, the athlete's self-esteem and self-image may suffer a devastating blow. Nursing assessment may reveal an athlete who appears to have difficulty dealing with the event and actually rejects any positive reinforcement. The nurse may help the child and family in establishing a support system. The athlete may need to learn new coping skills and explore other avenues to foster feelings of increased self-worth and a sense of accomplishment.

Attrition and exercise aversion are sometimes the aftermath of declining interest in sports after participation during the school years and adolescence. Motivation can be al-

---

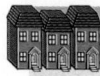

## COMMUNITY FOCUS

### Parental Pressure and Youth Sports

There is often great peer and parental pressure to participate in sports, and the stress felt by the adolescent who performs in competitive situations may be great. There is much fear of failure related to the pressure to be like friends or parents.

Although positive aspects are important and inherent in sports activities, nurses should be alert to some parental behaviors and motivations that interfere with a youngster's enjoyment of the activities.

First, some parents are unwilling to allow the activity to remain child oriented and place unrealistic demands on the child. Both the youngster's physical and emotional age must be considered. Second, some parents are unable to maintain the appropriate emotional distance from the activity and make the youngster's involvement in sports an extension of their own ego. These youngsters may recognize that they are being exploited and exhibit extreme forms of rebellion. Third, in some cases, parents' manipulative behaviors can have a profound negative effect on their youngsters. Guilt-producing verbal manipulation (e.g., pointing out what they and others have sacrificed for the child) is a powerful weapon that creates a form of emotional bondage. Fourth, there are parents who lose sight of the meaning of the sport because they become entrapped in dreams and fantasies that their youngsters' athletic ability can become a passport to status and economic freedom.

The pressures that some parents impose on their children negate most of the psychologic values of sports, such as fun, emotional release, and learning to relate effectively with peers. Winning becomes more important than playing. Overemphasis on sports has the potential for interfering with the emotional and social growth of a child, especially when ego integration is tied to recognition and reward through such a narrow range of personal characteristics. Ego vulnerability is great in youngsters whose identity, self-esteem, and feelings of self-worth depend entirely on the psychologic and social rewards of athletic achievement.

When children need medical attention because of repeated injuries, disinterest should be suspected and investigated. Obtaining separate histories from the youth and the parents may illuminate possible psychologic complications as a cause of injury. Alternative sports or other means for gaining self-esteem and regard from parents and peers can be explored and encouraged for children not interested in or suited for athletic competition.

Children may wish to remain in the sport but want less parental pressure. To minimize parents' becoming "sideline coaches," nurses can suggest other options for participation, such as organizing fund-raising, acting as social director to boost team morale, or operating concession stands at games.

The **National Youth Sports Safety Foundation** has information for parents, children, and coaches regarding sports activities and child participation aimed at reducing sports injuries and encouraging sports participation at 333 Longwood Ave, Suite 202, Boston, MA 02115, (617) 277-1171, e-mail: NYSSF@aol.com, web site: *www.nyssf.org*.

tered or permanently destroyed by failure to appreciate youngsters' needs related to sports activities. Ridicule or derogation during acquisition of motor skills can shatter a youngster's self-esteem, producing anxiety and self-doubt that may result in a lifelong aversion to sports. Every child should have the opportunity to develop a strong sense of personal worth through the process of motor learning and acquisition of skills. *All* participants should have the opportunity to participate and be rewarded with positive encouragement for their contribution, no matter how small; all participants should be rewarded for what they do right. (See Community Focus box.)

# MUSCULOSKELETAL DYSFUNCTION
## Torticollis

Torticollis (wry neck) is a congenital or acquired condition of limited neck motion in which the neck is flexed and turned to the affected side. It may be associated with a variety of conditions, some quite serious (Ballock and Song, 1996). In early infancy a firm, nontender mass may be felt in the midportion of the muscle. The mass regresses and is replaced by fibrous tissue. If the condition remains untreated, there is permanent limitation of neck movement, and the head and face become asymmetric, probably as a result of impaired blood supply to the depressed side of the head.

Treatment of simple torticollis consists of gentle stretching exercises. The face is turned toward the affected muscle while the head is tilted in the opposite direction with the neck extended. A physical therapist will typically establish the treatment regimen to be followed by the nurse and family. The exercises are best performed by two persons—one to control the torso and one to manipulate the head. If stretching exercises are unsuccessful, surgical release of the sternocleidomastoid muscle may be needed. Increasingly, surgical correction by age 12 to 18 months is recommended to prevent muscle contractures.

### Nursing Considerations

Nurses are alert to the possibility of torticollis in infants with limited head movement. After diagnosis it is frequently a nursing responsibility to teach and supervise the family in performing the exercises. The exercises require very explicit instructions to the family, and compliance is mandatory. The nurse should also suggest that the child be placed in the crib or playpen in a way that encourages turning the head away from the deformity in order to observe activities and interesting items. Feeding and play with the child can be used to encourage turning the head in the direction desired for correction.

## Legg-Calvé-Perthes Disease

Legg-Calvé-Perthes disease (LCPD) sometimes called *coxa plana* or *osteochondritis deformans juvenilis,* is a self-limited disorder in which there is aseptic necrosis of the femoral head. The disease affects children ages 3 to 12 years, but most cases occur in boys between 4 and 8 years of age as an isolated event. In approximately 10% to 15% of cases the involvement is bilateral; most of the affected children have a skeletal age significantly below their chronologic age. The male/female ratio is 4:1 or 5:1; white children are affected 10 times more frequently than African-American children.

### Pathophysiology

The cause of the disease is unknown, but there is a disturbance of circulation to the femoral capital epiphysis that produces an ischemic aseptic necrosis of the femoral head. During middle childhood, circulation to the femoral epiphysis is more tenuous than at other ages, being supplied almost entirely by lateral retinacular vessels. These can become obstructed by trauma, inflammation, coagulation defects, and a variety of other causes (Burg and others, 1998). This circulatory impairment appears to extend to the epiphysis and acetabulum as well. The pathologic events seem to take place in four stages (Box 39-13), although there is controversy regarding prognostic classification. The entire disease process may encompass as little as 18 months or continue for several years. The reformed femoral head may be severely altered or appear entirely normal.

### Clinical Manifestations

The onset is insidious, and the history may reveal only intermittent appearance of a limp on the affected side or a symptom complex including hip soreness, ache, or stiffness that can be constant or intermittent. The pain may be experienced in the hip, along the entire thigh, or in the vicinity of the knee joint. The pain and limp are usually most evident on arising and at the end of a long day of activities. The pain is usually accompanied by joint dysfunction and limited range of motion. There may be a vague history of trauma. The diagnosis is established by radiographic examination.

### Therapeutic Management

Because deformity occurs early in the disease process, the aim of treatment is to keep the head of the femur contained in the acetabulum, which serves as a mold to preserve the spherical shape of the head and to maintain a full range of

---

**Box 39-13**
**Stages of Legg-Calvé-Perthes Disease**

**Stage I:** Aseptic necrosis or infarction of the femoral capital epiphysis with degenerative changes producing flattening of the upper surface of the femoral head—the *avascular stage.*
**Stage II:** Capital bone absorption and revascularization with fragmentation (vascular resorption of the epiphysis) that gives a mottled appearance on radiographs—the *fragmentation,* or *revascularization stage.*
**Stage III:** New bone formation, which is represented on radiographs as calcification and ossification or increased density in the areas of radiolucency; this filling-in process appears to take place from the periphery of the head centrally—the *reparative stage.*
**Stage IV:** Gradual reformation of the head of the femur without radiolucency and, it is hoped, to a spherical form—the *regenerative stage.*

motion. However, there is no agreement regarding the best treatment in terms of conservative vs surgical approaches (Poussa and others, 1993). Surgical intervention appears to provide the best outcome with respect to a round femoral head in severe cases (Herring, 1994). LCPD is a biologic process, however, and a mechanical intervention may not prove to be successful (Roy, 1999). Often treatment approaches vary with the severity of presentation (Rang, 1996). Activity causes microfractures of the soft, ischemic epiphysis, which tend to induce synovitis, stiffness, and adductor contracture. The initial therapy is rest and non–weight bearing, which helps reduce inflammation and restore motion. Later, active motion is encouraged. In some cases traction is applied to stretch tight adductor muscles.

Containment can be accomplished in several ways. One is the use of non–weight-bearing devices, such as an abduction brace, leg casts, or a leather harness sling, that prevent weight bearing on the affected limb. Another includes the use of various weight-bearing appliances, such as abduction-ambulation braces or casts after a period of bed rest and traction. A third consists of surgical reconstruction and containment procedures. Conservative therapy must be continued for 2 to 4 years, although braces constructed from lightweight materials allow the child to maintain a nearly normal activity level. Surgical correction, although subjecting the child to additional risks (e.g., from anesthesia, infection, blood transfusion), returns the child to normal activities in 3 to 4 months. The use of home traction has been explored (Stevens and others, 1995).

The disease is self-limited, but the ultimate outcome of therapy depends on early and efficient treatment and the age of the child at onset of the disorder. Younger children, whose epiphyses are more cartilaginous, have the best prognosis for complete recovery. The later the diagnosis is made, the more femoral damage has occurred before treatment is

implemented. In most cases, with good patient compliance the prognosis is excellent.

### Nursing Considerations

Nurses are often the first health care professionals to identify affected children and to refer them for medical evaluation. They are also persons on whom the child and family can rely to help them understand and adjust to the therapeutic measures. Because most care of these children is conducted on an outpatient basis, the major emphasis of nursing care is on teaching the family the care. The family needs to learn the purpose, function, application, and care of the corrective device and the importance of compliance in order to achieve the desired outcome.

One of the most difficult aspects associated with the disorder is coping with normally active children who feel well but must remain relatively inactive. It is important to emphasize that children continue to attend school and engage in former activities that can be adapted to the therapeutic appliance. School adaptation may need to be arranged with school personnel.

Suitable activities must be devised to meet the needs of the child in the process of developing a sense of initiative or industry. Activities that meet the creative urges are well received. This is also an opportune time to encourage the child to begin a hobby such as collections, model building, or crafts. (See Family Focus box.)

## Slipped Femoral Capital Epiphysis

Slipped femoral capital epiphysis (SFCE), or *coxa vara*, refers to the spontaneous displacement of the proximal femoral epiphysis in a posterior and inferior direction. It develops most frequently shortly before or during accelerated growth and the onset of puberty (children between the ages of 10 and 16 years—median age, 13 for boys, 11 for girls) and is most frequently observed in obese children. Bilateral involvement has been reported in up to 40% of cases (Loder, 1998).

### Pathophysiology

Most cases of SFCE are idiopathic, although it can be associated with endocrine disorders, growth hormone therapy, renal osteodystrophy, and radiation therapy. The cause of idiopathic SFCE is multifactorial and includes obesity, physeal architecture and orientation, and puberty hormone changes that affect physeal strength. Although obesity stresses the physeal plate, SFCE can also occur in children who are not obese (Loder, 1998). Radiographs show medial displacement of the epiphysis and uncovered upper portion of the femoral neck adjacent to the physis. There is a widened growth plate and irregular metaphysis. The capital femoral epiphysis remains in the acetabulum, but the femoral neck slips, deforming the femoral head and stretching blood vessels to the epiphysis.

### Clinical Manifestations

The following different varieties of clinical behavior have been observed: (1) an episode of trauma in which the epi-

---

**FAMILY FOCUS**
*Legg-Calvé-Perthes Disease*

A family gifted with five healthy children were one day startled to learn that their 2-year-old son could no longer walk. He was diagnosed with Legg-Calvé-Perthes disease. Through several years of prosthetic devices and numerous physician visits, hospitalizations and surgeries, this family turned a potentially devastating experience into one with cherished memories.

Today the parents reflect on how their family coped with the reality of a debilitating disease. It was difficult for the parents to observe an eager, energetic child watch other children riding bicycles, running, or playing outdoor games. Also, they are warmed by memories of watching their other children make the difference for their sibling. They all developed a strong bond through caring and sharing with one another. Coping as a family was an easy adjustment and, most of all, therapeutic. Today, over 20 years later, the parents feel that each family member has grown with feelings of faith and trust. The experience proved to them that life will go on, and that life is what you make it!

Shona Swenson Lenss, BSN, RN
Cheyenne Children's Clinic
Cheyenne, WY

physis is acutely displaced in a previously functional joint; (2) gradual displacement without definite injury, with progressively increased hip disability; (3) intermittent bouts of displacement alternating with periods of well-being, with gradual appearance of symptoms associated with ambulation (e.g., external rotation); and (4) a combined gradual and traumatic displacement in which there is gradual slippage, with further displacement caused by injury.

Slipped femoral epiphysis is suspected when an adolescent or preadolescent youngster, especially one who is obese or tall and lanky, begins to limp and complains of pain in the hip continuously or intermittently. The pain is frequently referred to the groin, anteromedial aspect of the thigh, or knee. Physical examination reveals early restriction of internal rotation on adduction and external rotation deformity with loss of abduction and internal rotation as the severity increases. The diagnosis is confirmed by radiographic examination.

### Therapeutic Management/Nursing Considerations

Treatment goals include avoiding avascular necrosis, avoiding chondrolysis, preventing further slip, and correcting the deformity (Aronsson and Loder, 1996). Surgical treatment varies with the degree of displacement; methods include presurgury bed rest/traction followed by a single pin, multiple pins and screws, or osteotomy for deformity correction

if needed. Postsurgery care includes non–weight bearing with crutch ambulation until acceptable, painless range of motion is achieved (Aronsson and Loder, 1996). SFCE is an emergency and requires early diagnosis and treatment to increase the likelihood of a satisfactory cure. Nursing care is the same as that for a child in a cast or a child in traction, as discussed earlier in this chapter.

## Kyphosis and Lordosis

The spine, consisting of numerous segments, can acquire deformation curves of three types: kyphosis, lordosis, and scoliosis (Fig. 39-34).

*Kyphosis* is an abnormally increased convex angulation in the curvature of the thoracic spine (Fig. 39-34, *B*). It can occur secondary to disease processes such as tuberculosis, chronic arthritis, osteodystrophy, or compression fractures of the thoracic spine. The most common form of kyphosis is "postural." Children, especially during the time when skeletal growth outpaces growth of muscle, are prone to exaggeration of a tendency toward kyphosis. This is particularly common in self-conscious adolescent girls who assume a round-shouldered slouching posture in an attempt to hide their developing breasts and increasing height. *Scheuermann kyphosis* is defined as a thoracic curve of greater than 45 degrees with wedging of more than 5 degrees of at least three adjacent vertebral bodies and vertebral irregularity. Postural

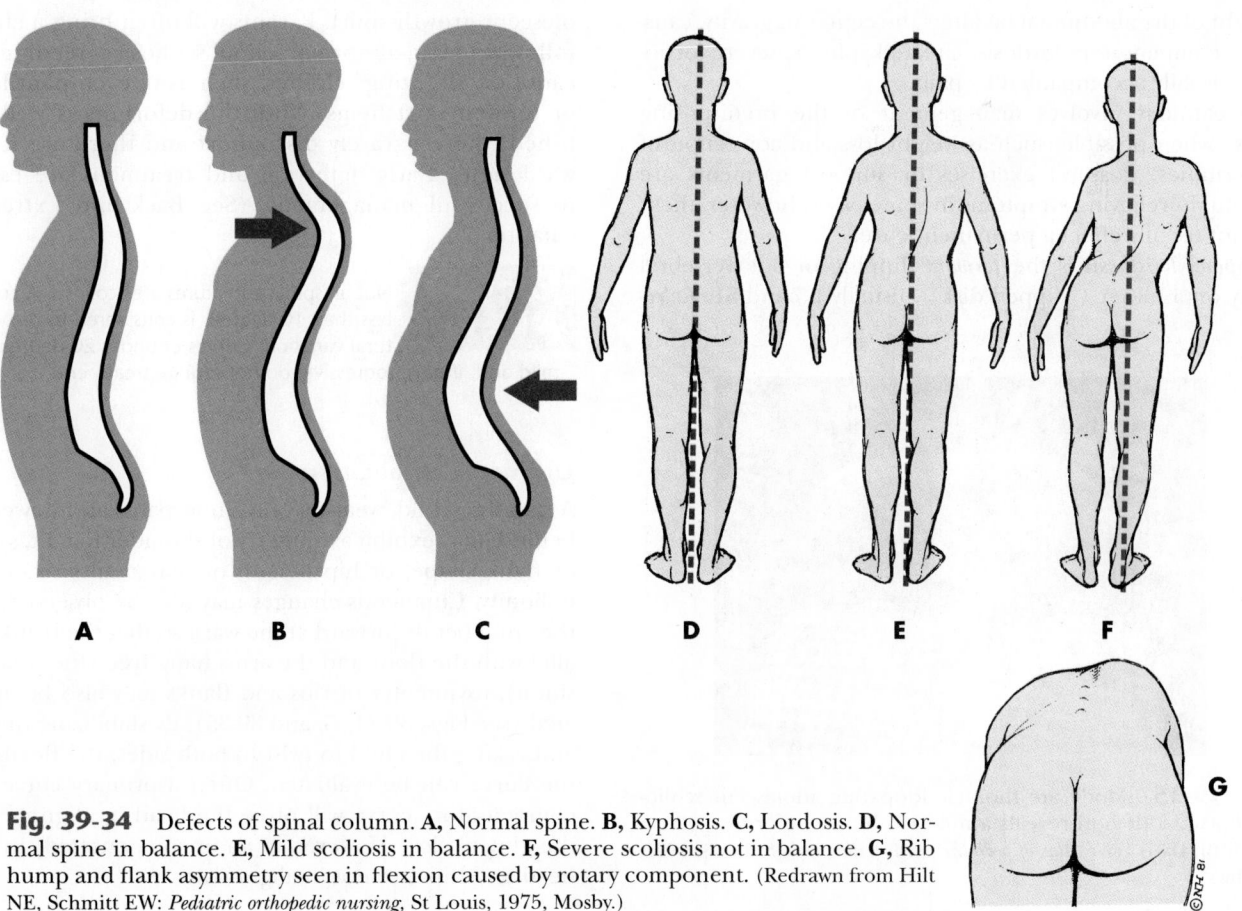

**Fig. 39-34**   Defects of spinal column. **A,** Normal spine. **B,** Kyphosis. **C,** Lordosis. **D,** Normal spine in balance. **E,** Mild scoliosis in balance. **F,** Severe scoliosis not in balance. **G,** Rib hump and flank asymmetry seen in flexion caused by rotary component. (Redrawn from Hilt NE, Schmitt EW: *Pediatric orthopedic nursing,* St Louis, 1975, Mosby.)

kyphosis is almost always accompanied by a compensatory postural lordosis, an abnormally exaggerated concave lumbar curvature.

Treatment of kyphosis consists of postural exercises to strengthen shoulder and abdominal muscles and bracing for more marked deformity. Unfortunately, treatment is difficult because of the nature of the adolescent personality. The best approach is to emphasize the cosmetic value of corrective therapy and to place the responsibility on the adolescent for carrying out an exercise program at home with regular visits to and assessments by a therapist.

Most adolescents respond well to selected sports as a supplement to regular exercise, such as weight lifting (preferably performed from a prone or supine position on a bench), track sports, and dance classes (ballet or modern). Swimming is excellent and has the added advantages of exercising all muscles, eliminating gravity, and teaching breath control. Treatment with a brace may be indicated until skeletal maturity, and surgical fusion may be considered for severe, painful, or progressive kyphotic curves.

*Lordosis* is an accentuation of the lumbar curvature beyond physiologic limits (Fig. 39-34, *C*). It may be a secondary complication of a disease process, the result of trauma, or idiopathic. Lordosis is a normal observation in toddlers and, in older children, is often seen in association with flexion contractures of the hip, obesity, congenital dislocated hip, and slipped femoral capital epiphysis. During the pubertal growth spurt, lordosis of varying degrees is observed in teenagers, especially girls. In obese children the weight of the abdominal fat alters the center of gravity, causing a compensatory lordosis. Unlike kyphosis, severe lordosis is usually accompanied by pain.

Treatment involves management of the predisposing cause when possible, such as weight loss and correction of deformities. Postural exercises or support garments are helpful in relieving symptoms in some cases; however, these do not usually effect a permanent cure.

*Spondylolisthesis* is the *forward* slipping of one vertebral body on another ("slipped disk"), usually L5 and S1. *Retro-*

*spondylolisthesis* or *retrolisthesis* is the *posterior* slipping or displacement of one vertebral body on another. Either condition can have multiple causes, including congenital deficiency or fracture of part of the vertebra. This condition may be asymptomatic, or it may cause low back pain or neurologic compromise. Spondylolisthesis can usually be treated nonsurgically, although spinal fusion may be indicated in severe, progressive slips.

## Scoliosis

Scoliosis is a complex spinal deformity in three planes, usually involving lateral curvature, spinal rotation causing rib asymmetry, and thoracic hypokyphosis (Fig. 39-35). It is the most common spinal deformity. It can be congenital, or it can develop during infancy or childhood, but it is most common during the growth spurt of early adolescence. Scoliosis can be caused by a number of conditions and may occur alone or in association with other diseases, particularly neuromuscular conditions. In most cases, however, there is no apparent cause, and it is called **idiopathic scoliosis.** There is evidence that it may be genetic and transmitted as an autosomal dominant trait with incomplete penetrance, or it may be multifactorial. The various causes of scoliosis are outlined in Box 39-14.

### Clinical Manifestations

Idiopathic scoliosis is seldom apparent before 10 years of age and is most noticeable at the beginning of the preadolescent growth spurt. Parents will often bring a child for follow-up of an abnormal school scoliosis screening or because of "ill-fitting" clothes, such as uneven pant lengths or uneven skirt hems. Until the deformity is well established, there is rarely discomfort and there are few outward signs. Early detection and treatment are essential to successful management. (See Back and Extremities, Chapter 7.)

> **NURSING ALERT**
>
> Not all spinal curvatures are scoliosis. A curve of less than 10 degrees is considered to be a postural variation. Curves of under 20 degrees are mild and, if nonprogressive, do not require treatment.

### Diagnostic Evaluation

A standing child, wearing only underpants and viewed from behind, may exhibit asymmetry of shoulder height, scapular or flank shape, or hip height, or may demonstrate pelvic obliquity. Cutaneous changes may also be observed. When the child bends forward at the waist so that the trunk is parallel with the floor and the arms hang free (the Adams position), asymmetry of ribs and flanks may also be appreciated (see Figs. 39-34, *G*, and 39-35). By stabilizing the pelvis and asking the child to twist to both sides, the flexibility of the curve can be evaluated. Often a primary curve and a compensatory curve will place the head in alignment with the gluteal cleft. However, in an uncompensated curve, the head and hips are not in alignment.

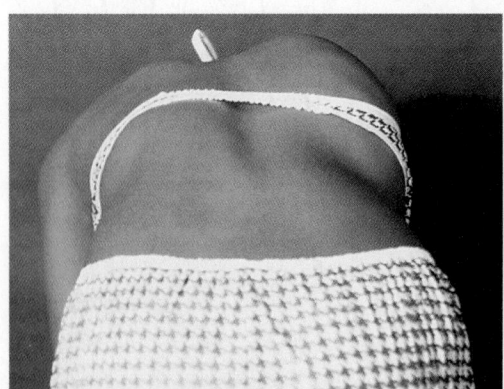

**Fig. 39-35** Moderate thoracic idiopathic adolescent scoliosis. Forward flexion reveals a mild rib hump deformity. (From Zitelli BJ, Davis HW: *Atlas of pediatric physical diagnosis*, St Louis, 1997, Mosby.)

Radiographs taken with the child in the standing position are measured using the Cobb technique for curve magnitude. In addition, the Risser sign, determined by evaluating the extent of excursion of the iliac apophysis, helps to establish the skeletal maturity of the individual.

Intraspinal pathology or other disease processes that can cause scoliosis must be ruled out. The presence of pain, sacral dimpling or hairy patches, cutaneous vascular changes, absent or abnormal reflexes, bowel or bladder incontinence, or a left thoracic curve may indicate an intraspinal abnormality such as *syringomyelia, diastematomyelia,* or *tethered cord syndrome.* An MRI should be obtained for evaluation.

**Screening.** Screening for scoliosis remains controversial. Some groups support screening, believing that early detection permits use of bracing rather than surgery to prevent further curvative formation. However, some researchers question the value of school-based scoliosis screening based upon the large number of children who were referred but did not require treatment (Yawn and others, 1999; Greiner, 2002). The American Academy of Pediatrics recommends scoliosis screening at the time of primary practitioner visits.

### Therapeutic Management: Bracing and Exercise

Current management options include observation with regular clinical and radiographic evaluation, orthotic intervention (bracing), and spinal fusion surgery (Fig. 39-36). Treatment decisions are based on the magnitude, location, and type of curve; the age and skeletal maturity of the child; and any underlying or contributing disease process.

For many curves in the growing child and adolescent, bracing—although not curative—may be the treatment of choice. The application of a properly constructed and well-fitted external spinal orthosis, used with close supervision, is successful in halting or slowing the progression of most curvatures while the child reaches skeletal maturity. The two most commonly used braces are (1) the *Boston brace,* or underarm orthosis, customized from prefabricated plastic shells, with corrective forces for each patient, using lateral pads and decreasing lumbar lordosis, and (2) the *TLSO* (see p. 1773), which is an underarm custom-molded plastic jacket that is shaped to correct or hold the deformity (Fig. 39-37). The *Milwaukee brace,* an individually adapted plastic and metal brace that includes a neck ring, is used for kyphosis but only rarely for scoliosis. The type of brace and wearing schedule (usually between 16 and 23 hours a day) are based on the nature of the curve, age of the child, and any underlying condition associated with the curve.

Exercises alone are rarely of value with scoliosis. However, supplemental exercises are employed daily in and out of the brace to prevent atrophy of spinal and abdominal muscles. External electrical stimulation of spinal muscles transmitted by pads on the back during sleep have not been effective alternatives to orthotic treatment.

---

### Box 39-14  ■ ■ ■
### Causes of Scoliosis

**IDIOPATHIC SCOLIOSIS**

Infantile
  Age of onset—birth to 3 years of age
  More common in males
  Usually left thoracic curve
  Poor prognosis
Juvenile
  Age of onset—4 to 10 years of age
  More equal distribution between sexes
  Usually right thoracic curve
  Severity increases with growth
Adolescent (most common)
  Age of onset—10 years of age to skeletal maturity
  Predominant in females, about 7:1
  Right thoracic and thoracolumbar curves more common

**CONGENITAL SCOLIOSIS**

May be associated with meningomyelocele or other dysrhaphism
Hemivertebrae or failure of segmentation

**NEUROMUSCULAR SCOLIOSIS**

Caused by muscular imbalance or weakness
Neurogenic
  Lower motor neuron disease such as poliomyelitis, spinal muscular atrophy
  Upper motor neuron disease such as cerebral palsy
Myogenic
  Progressive disease such as muscular dystrophy
  Static disease such as amyotonia congenita
Mixed—weakness and overpull by stronger trunk muscles, such as in Friedreich ataxia

**NEUROFIBROMATOSIS**

Short, sharp thoracic curve often associated with kyphosis

**TRAUMATIC**

Thoracogenic—result of thoracotomy and thoracoplasty with rib resection
Spinal trauma
  Irradiation such as tumor therapy
  Fractures

**MISCELLANEOUS**

Secondary to irritation
  Tumor
  Inflammation
Nutritional—rickets
Metabolic—renal osteodystrophy
Intraspinal, cord tether, syringomyelia

**MESENCHYMAL DISEASE**

Congenital disorders
  Dwarfism
  Disease of connective tissue such as arachnodactyly, arthrogryposis multiplex congenita
  Disease of bone such as osteogenesis imperfecta
Acquired disorders—rheumatoid arthritis

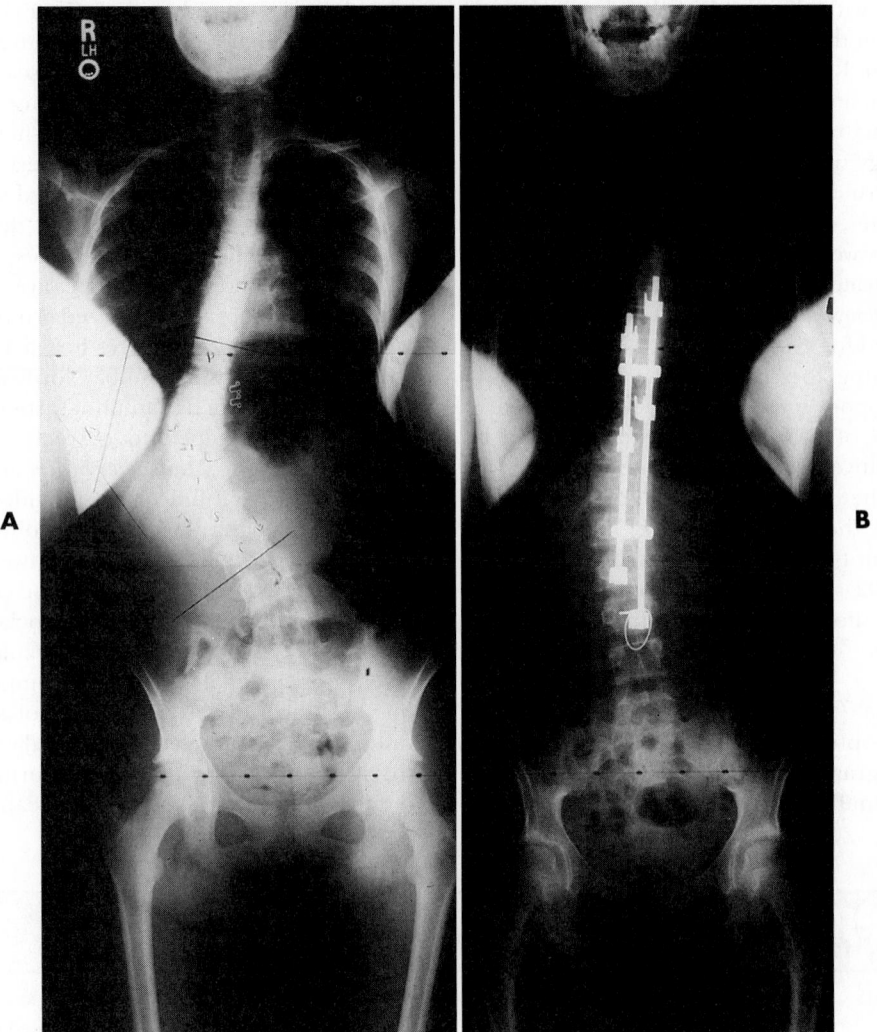

**Fig. 39-36**  Radiographs showing severe scoliosis before surgical correction (**A**) and surgical correction of scoliosis including internal fixation (**B**).

## Therapeutic Management: Operative

Surgical intervention may be required for correction of severe curves (see Fig. 39-36). The degree of curvature and the cause determine the decision for surgery. Bracing and exercise have been universally disappointing in curves greater than 40 degrees, and paralytic and congenital curves, which will eventually progress, are best treated with early surgical stabilization if the health status of the child will allow major surgery. The age of the child and location of the curvature influence the decision for surgery, and any progressive or severe curve that does not respond to more conservative orthotic measures requires surgical correction. Difficulties with balance or seating, respiratory excursion, or pain are also considered.

The surgical technique consists of realignment and straightening with internal fixation and instrumentation combined with bony fusion (*arthrodesis*) of the realigned spine. The goals of surgical intervention are to correct the curvatures on the sagittal and coronal planes and to have a solid, pain-free fusion in a well-balanced torso, with maximum mobility of the remaining spinal segments.

The preoperative workup usually involves radiographic series, including bending and traction films, pulmonary function studies, and laboratory studies, including prothrombin, partial thromboplastin, bleeding time, blood count, electrolytes, urinalysis and urine culture, and levels of any medications. Autologous blood donations are routinely obtained from the youngster before the surgery to replace blood loss during the operation.

There are many instrumentation systems available, including Harrington, Dwyer, Zielke, Luque, Cotrel-Dubousset, Isola, TSRH (Texas Scottish Rite Hospital), and Moss-Miami. Posterior or anterior approaches can be used. The **Harrington system,** the first internal spinal instrumentation device, consists of distraction and compression rods, hooks, and nuts. The posterior spinal elements are decorticated, and chips and strips of bone from the iliac crest are placed across the vertebra to provide fusion. Following instrumentation, the child is logrolled to prevent spinal motion. A molded plastic jacket is used to provide external stabilization of the spine while the child resumes activities.

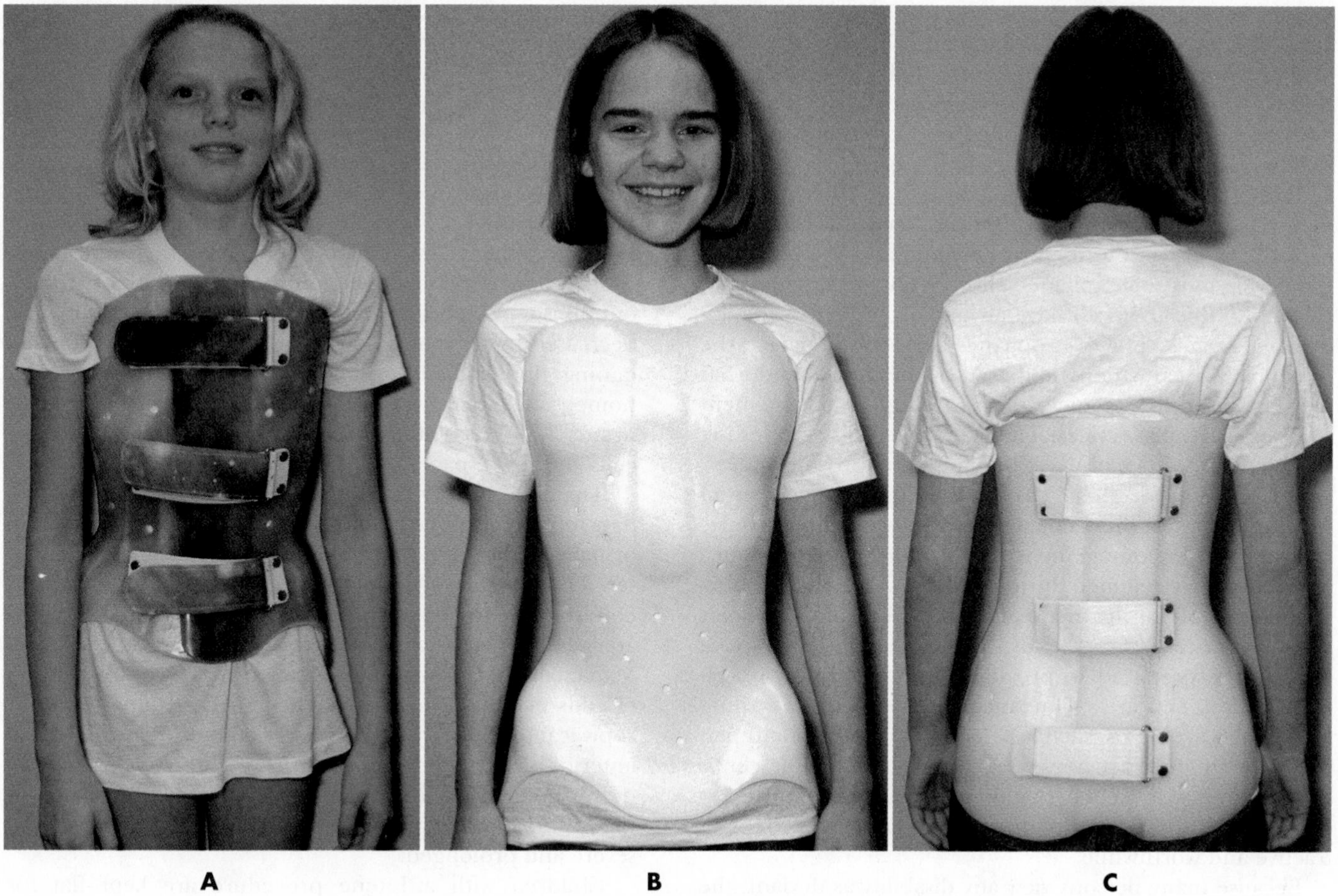

**Fig. 39-37** **A,** Standard TLSO brace for idiopathic scoliosis. Note the color and design incorporated into the brace to make it more acceptable to children and adolescents. **B,** Variation of a standard TLSO brace that fastens in the back, **C,** to provide needed support for the spine curvature.

The ***Luque segmental spinal instrumentation*** provides segmental stability by the use of wires and flexible L-shaped rods. By way of a posterior approach, wires are threaded beneath the laminae of each vertebra and tightened around the rods resting along the transverse processes so that the spinal column is stabilized by transverse traction on each vertebra. The spine is fused with a bone graft taken from the iliac crest. The advantages of this procedure are that the patient can be mobile within a few days and that no postoperative immobilization is required. The disadvantage is the risk of spinal nerve damage.

The ***Cotrel-Dubousset (CD)*** approach combines the Harrington and Luque systems. Anterior approaches using ***Dwyer*** or ***Zielke instrumentation*** involve screws into the vertebral bodies connected by a cable or rod. These systems require postoperative immobilization with a custom-fitted plastic jacket.

## Nursing Considerations

Nursing care and management of the child with scoliosis involves the same care as that of any child with a partial immobilization and a potential alteration in carrying out the routines of daily living. The child's needs are assessed on an individual basis, however, and care is planned according to the child's physical, growth, and developmental needs.

### Assessment

One of the major functions of nurses is to learn to detect the presence of scoliosis. School nurses routinely evaluate children in their care, and most are a part of scoliosis screening programs. The methods of assessment are those described in Chapter 7 and in relation to Diagnostic Evaluation, p. 1810.

### Nursing Diagnoses

Based on a thorough assessment, several nursing diagnoses are identified. The more common diagnoses for the child with scoliosis are included in the Nursing Care Plan on pp. 1815-1816. Others may apply in specific situations.

### Planning

The goals for the child with scoliosis and the family include the following:

1. Child will adjust to the method of therapeutic management.
2. Child will experience an acceptable level of pain relief.
3. Child will experience no complications.
4. Child and family will receive appropriate support, encouragement, and education.

### Implementation

Treatment for scoliosis extends over a significant portion of the child's period of growth. In adolescents this period is the one in which their physical and psychologic identity is formed. Treatment may mean a modified lifestyle and being "different" from their peers, even though they are usually able to engage in most activities enjoyed by other youngsters. Pen pals and support groups may be of value, particularly for adolescents, in helping them to feel less isolated and different because of their scoliosis.

When the child first faces the prospect of a prolonged period in a brace, the therapy program and the nature of the device must be explained thoroughly to the child and parents so that they will have an understanding of the anticipated results, how the appliance corrects the defect, the freedoms and constraints imposed by the device, and what they can do to help achieve the desired goal. Management involves skills and services of a team of specialists, including orthopaedist, nurse, physical therapist, and prosthetist.

It is difficult for a child to be restricted at any phase of development, but the teenager needs continual positive reinforcement, encouragement, and as much independence as can be safely assumed during this time. Although adolescents cope well for the first year or two of bracing, problems may arise as the time extends. Nurses need to be aware of this and be prepared to provide support and encouragement if problems arise. Guidance and assistance regarding anticipated problems, such as selection of clothing and participation in social activities, are appreciated by adolescents. Socialization with peers should be encouraged, and every effort should be expended to help the adolescent feel attractive and worthwhile.

Because many persons view any disability as deviant, the child needs help in learning how to deal with reactions of others to the appliance. Preparation for such responses places the child at an advantage. The best approach is usually for the child to initiate the interaction by mentioning the device and its purpose. This alleviates the ambiguity surrounding the appliance and its purpose and reduces anxiety on the part of the child and other persons. Most important, the child should be helped to view the condition and appliance in a positive way and avoid seeing them as a stigma. Some youngsters who receive patient teaching, peer counseling, and support find positive aspects to wearing a brace.

**Preoperative Care.** Surgery for spinal fusion is quite complex and often adolescents who require the procedure because of idiopathic scoliosis are not familiar with medical terms and have not had experience with medical procedures. Detailed preoperative teaching is critical for the adolescent to be able to cooperate and participate in his or her treatment and recovery and to maintain some sense of control during this time.

**Postoperative Care.** Postoperatively patients are usually monitored closely in an acute care facility and logrolled when changing position to prevent damage to the fusion and instrumentation. Skin care is very important, and pressure-relieving beds may be needed to prevent pressure wounds. (See Maintaining Healthy Skin, Chapter 27.)

In addition to the usual postoperative assessment—of wound, circulation, and vital signs—the neurologic status of the patient, especially that of the extremities, requires special attention. Prompt recognition of any neurologic impairment is imperative because delayed paralysis may develop that requires surgical intervention. The patient is encouraged to exercise by contracting and relaxing the thigh and calf muscles periodically.

There may be some degree of paralytic ileus following the procedure; therefore, nursing intervention includes care of the nasogastric tube (if used) and assessment for returning bowel function. Urinary retention is common—an indwelling catheter is often used for the first 24 to 48 hours. Because of the extensive blood loss during the surgical procedure and renal hypoperfusion, observation of urinary output is especially important. Initially urine output may be decreased because of blood loss during surgery, and maintaining fluid balance is important. As the body regains homeostasis, there will be a period of diuresis that usually occurs 3 to 4 days after surgery as the fluid shifts from the cells and third spaces.

The child usually has considerable pain for the first few days following surgery and requires frequent administration of pain medication, preferably the use of opioids administered on a regular schedule, as opposed to "as needed." For children able to understand the concept, patient-controlled analgesia (PCA) is a recommended alternative. (See Pain Management, Chapter 26.) Pain can also be controlled with opioids or long-acting anesthetics, such as bupivacaine or ropivacaine through an epidural catheter. Because of the anterior approach, patients with Dwyer instrumentation require thoracotomy care in addition to the care related to the fusion and realignment procedures. Their pain is more severe and prolonged.

Children with a Luque procedure are kept flat for 12 hours before logrolling is begun. The head of the bed can be elevated on the second day, and range-of-motion exercises begun. Activity is initiated by instructing the patient to roll from a side-lying position to a sitting position. Next, walking slowly with the aid of a safety belt and walker is allowed and, finally, unassisted ambulation, which is usually achieved before discharge. Most patients are ambulatory by the second or third postoperative day and are discharged home by 1 week (Rodts, 1998).

All patients are started on physiotherapy as soon as they are able, beginning with range-of-motion exercises and many of the activities of daily living. Self-care, such as washing and eating, is always encouraged. Throughout hospitalization, diversional activities and contact with family and friends are an important part of nursing care and planning.

The family is encouraged to become involved with the patient's care to facilitate the transition from hospital to home management. Family members learn to apply and care for the brace or learn cast care, with special attention given to jagged edges on the cast, padding of the appliance, and daily skin checks for reddened areas, especially in areas such as under the arms or over the hips. The family may need assistance in modifying the environment for limited ambulation and acquiring needed home care items, such as a raised toilet seat or overhead trapeze bar. The child and family need to learn efficient ways to move and carry out various activities of daily living. The diet may require modification. Overeating and constipation can be problems related to limited activity. Arrangements for homebound schooling initially and then partial-day school attendance should be made with the child's school.

Several organizations provide education and services to both families and professionals. The **National Scoliosis Foundation, Inc.*** is devoted to awareness and action for early detection and prevention of spinal deformity. This organization offers educational support materials for parents, schools, and health care providers. A list of books, pamphlets, and other materials is available on request. The **American Academy of Orthopaedic Surgeons** and **Scoliosis Research Society (SRS)†** have published a booklet called *Scoliosis;* SRS also has educational information available on its web site.

---

*5 Cabot Pl, Stoughton, MA 02072, (617) 341-6333 or (800) 673-6922, fax: (617) 341-8333, e-mail: scoliosis@aol.com.
†6300 N River Rd, Rosemont, IL 60018-4262; (847) 698-1627; www.srs.org.

## ▓ Evaluation

The effectiveness of nursing interventions is determined by continual reassessment and evaluation of care based on the following observational guidelines:

1. Observe and interview child regarding problems and solutions experienced.
2. Observe and interview child regarding pain level experience and adequacy of pain management.
3. Observe child for untoward effects related to the management of scoliosis (i.e., prevention of complications such as skin breakdown).
4. Discuss with child and family their feelings and concerns about scoliosis, management, and effects on family and child.

The **expected outcomes** are described in the Nursing Care Plan on pp. 1815-1816.

# Nursing Care Plan
## The Child with Structural Scoliosis

---

> **NURSING DIAGNOSIS:** Risk for injury related to unaccustomed brace

**PATIENT GOAL 1:** Will not experience injury related to wearing brace

- **NURSING INTERVENTIONS/***RATIONALES*
Assess environment for hazards *to prevent injuries*
Teach safety precautions such as using handrail on stairways and avoiding slippery surfaces *to prevent falls*
Help develop safe methods of mobilization

- **EXPECTED OUTCOME**
Child remains free of injury related to wearing brace

**PATIENT GOAL 2:** Will adjust to restricted movement

- **NURSING INTERVENTIONS/***RATIONALES*
Demonstrate alternative modes of accomplishing tasks such as getting in and out of bed, dressing
Help devise alternatives for restricted activities and coping with awkwardness

- **EXPECTED OUTCOME**
Child demonstrates appropriate adaptation to corrective device (specify)

> **NURSING DIAGNOSIS:** Risk for impaired skin integrity related to corrective device

**PATIENT GOAL 1:** Will not experience skin irritation or breakdown

- **NURSING INTERVENTIONS/***RATIONALES*
Examine skin surfaces in contact with brace for signs of irritation *so that appropriate treatment is instituted*
Implement corrective action to treat or prevent skin breakdown
Suggest nonirritating fabrics and clothing such as cotton T-shirts that can be worn under brace *to minimize risk of skin irritation*
Recommend daily bath or shower followed by thorough drying *to maintain cleanliness and minimize risk of skin irritation*

- **EXPECTED OUTCOME**
Skin remains clean with no evidence of irritation

> **NURSING DIAGNOSIS:** Disturbed body image related to perception of defect in body structure

**PATIENT GOAL 1:** Will exhibit signs of physical adjustment to appliance

- **NURSING INTERVENTIONS/***RATIONALES*
Plan *with* the child *to encourage compliance and adjustment*
Attempt to determine source of any discomfort *so that appropriate care is instituted*
Refer to orthotist for needed adjustment and service
Assist with plan for personal hygiene
Help in selection of appropriate and attractive apparel to wear over brace
Advise regarding selection of appropriate footwear *to maintain proper balance*
Reinforce teaching regarding removal and reapplication of appliance *so that child receives maximum benefit of appliance*

- **EXPECTED OUTCOMES**
Brace fits well and produces no discomfort
Child complies with directions for wear and care of brace
Child is well-groomed and wears attractive attire and proper footwear

**PATIENT GOAL 2:** Will exhibit positive coping behaviors

- **NURSING INTERVENTIONS/***RATIONALES*
Encourage child to discuss feelings about wearing brace *to encourage coping*
Emphasize positive aspects and eventual outcome *to encourage acceptance of treatment*

- **EXPECTED OUTCOMES**
Child verbalizes feelings and concerns
Child recognizes benefits of treatment
See also Nursing Care Plan: The Child with Chronic Illness or Disability, Chapter 22

*Continued*

## Nursing Care Plan
### The Child with Structural Scoliosis—cont'd

### PREOPERATIVE CARE

See also Nursing Care Plan: The Child Undergoing Surgery:
   Preoperative care, Chapter 27.

### POSTOPERATIVE CARE

See also Nursing Care Plan: The Child Undergoing Surgery:
   Postoperative care, Chapter 27.

> **NURSING DIAGNOSIS:** Risk for injury related to surgery

**PATIENT GOAL 1:** Will attain ambulation without injury to surgical repair

- **NURSING INTERVENTIONS/*RATIONALES***

Place on special bed, if ordered (Harrington instrumenta-
   tion), *which facilitates care and decreases risk of injury to surgical repair*
Maintain proper body alignment; avoid twisting movements,
   *which can cause indwelling instruments to twist the spine*
Logroll with care when moving child
Keep flat for 12 hours before logrolling (Luque procedure)
   Beginning activity—have child roll from side-lying to
      sitting position
Encourage child to exercise by contracting and relaxing
   thigh and calf muscles periodically *to maintain optimum
   movement of lower extremities in the immediate postoperative
   period*
Perform regular tests of neurologic integrity
Assist with physical therapy and range-of-motion exercises *to
   maintain muscle tone and joint flexibility*
Walk slowly with aid of safety belt and walker; unassisted
   ambulation usually allowed before discharge

- **EXPECTED OUTCOME**
Child attains ambulation without injury

**PATIENT GOAL 2:** Will not experience abdominal distention (from paralytic ileus)

- **NURSING INTERVENTIONS/*RATIONALES***
*Insert and maintain nasogastric tube (if used) *to prevent
   abdominal distention*
Assess for returning bowel function (e.g., bowel sounds) *to
   aid in determining when nasogastric suction can be discontinued
   and diet can be initiated*
Encourage ambulation as soon as possible *to increase peristalsis*
Encourage oral fluid intake as soon as possible
Allow choice in choosing regular diet foods, including fiber
   foods, *to prevent constipation as a result of immobility*
*Administer stool softener

- **EXPECTED OUTCOME**
Child exhibits no evidence of abdominal distention

> **NURSING DIAGNOSIS:** Acute pain related to surgical procedure

**PATIENT GOAL 1:** Will experience no pain or reduction of pain to level acceptable to child

- **NURSING INTERVENTIONS/*RATIONALES***
Anticipate need for pain management *because of the nature of
   this surgery*
*Administer opioids on preventive schedule (around the
   clock) until pain can be controlled with nonopioids *to
   prevent pain from occurring*
Consider/encourage patient-controlled analgesia for child
   able to follow instructions *in order to give child more control
   in prevention and alleviation of pain*

- **EXPECTED OUTCOME**
Child rests quietly, reports and exhibits no evidence of discomfort or minimal discomfort

> **NURSING DIAGNOSIS:** Impaired urinary elimination
> related to surgical procedure, loss of blood, renal
> hypoperfusion

**PATIENT GOAL 1:** Will exhibit signs of adequate
urinary elimination

- **NURSING INTERVENTIONS/*RATIONALES***
*Insert indwelling catheter *because urinary retention is common
   with this surgery and anesthesia*
Encourage frequent voiding after catheter removal
Encourage early ambulation *to decrease urinary stasis*
Provide privacy *to encourage urination*
Monitor intake and output *to assess adequacy of kidney function*
Maintain intravenous infusion *for adequate hydration and
   urinary output*
Encourage oral fluids when allowed

- **EXPECTED OUTCOME**
Child has adequate urinary output

> **NURSING DIAGNOSIS:** Impaired physical mobility
> related to spinal surgery and instrumentation

See also Nursing Care Plan: The Child Who Is Immobilized,
   p. 1772

> **NURSING DIAGNOSIS:** Risk for interrupted family
> processes related to a child with a physical disability

**PATIENT GOAL 1:** Will receive support as desired

- **NURSING INTERVENTIONS/*RATIONALES***
See also Nursing Care Plan: The Family of the Child Who Is
   Ill or Hospitalized, Chapter 26

- **EXPECTED OUTCOME**
Family members have needed support
See also Nursing Care Plan: The Child in the Hospital,
   Chapter 26

---
*Dependent nursing action.

# ORTHOPAEDIC INFECTIONS
## Osteomyelitis*

Osteomyelitis, an infectious process in the bone, can occur at any age but most frequently occurs in children 10 years of age or younger. *S. aureus* is the most common causative organism. Neonates are also likely to have group B streptococcus. Since the onset of *Haemophilus influenzae* type b immunization in the late 1980s, *H. influenzae* has become a less common causative pathogen. Children with sickle cell anemia may develop osteomyelitis from *Salmonella*, as well as *S. aureus*. *Neisseria gonorrhoeae* is a potential causative organism in the sexually active adolescent.

*Acute hematogenous osteomyelitis* results from a blood-borne bacterium causing an infection in the bone. Common sources of foci include infected lesions, upper respiratory infections, otitis media, tonsillitis, abscessed teeth, pyelonephritis, and infected burns. *Exogenous osteomyelitis* is acquired from direct inoculation of the bone from a puncture wound, open fracture, surgical contamination, or an adjacent tissue infection. *Subacute osteomyelitis* has a longer course and may be caused by less virulent microbes with walled-off abscess or Brodie abscess, typically in the proximal or distal tibia. *Chronic osteomyelitis* is a progression of acute osteomyelitis and is characterized by the presence of dead bone, bone loss, and drainage and sinus tracts. Generally healthy bone is not likely to get an infection; consequently factors that contribute to infection include inoculation with a large amount of organisms, foreign body, bone injury, strong virulence of organism, immunosupression, malnutrition, and the type and location of the bone.

### Pathophysiology

In acute osteomyelitis bacteria adheres to bone, causing a suppurative infection with inflammatory cells, edema, vascular congestion, and small-vessel thrombosis, resulting in bone destruction, abscess formation, and dead bone (sequestra). Infection within the bone can rupture through the cortex into the subperiosteal space, stripping loose periosteum and forming abscess. As dead bone is reabsorbed, new bone is formed along the live bone and infection borders. This surrounding sheath of live bone is called involucrum. Sinus tracts from perforations in the involucrum may drain pus through soft tissue to the skin.

The pathology of osteomyelitis is different in infants, children over 1 year of age, and adults. In infants blood vessels cross the growth plate into the epiphysis and joint space, allowing infection to spread into the joint. In children the infection is contained by the growth plate, and joint infection is less likely (unless the infection is intracapsular). In adults there is no growth plate to contain infection, and again the joint is compromised. Adult periosteum is attached to bone; consequently rupture through periosteum and sinus drainage is more common in adults.

### Clinical Manifestations

In children severe pain, fever, irritability, and tenderness with or without local signs of inflammation suggest os-

teomyelitis. The extremity is tender, and the child may hold it in semiflexion and resist movement. In infants these symptoms may be minimal or absent, and pain may be difficult to localize. Infants may have an adjacent joint effusion. Typically the metaphysis of long bones, the tibia and femur, is involved. A small portion of children may have more than one bone affected.

### Diagnostic Evaluation

Organism identification and antibiotic susceptibility is essential for effective therapy. Cultures of aspirated subperiosteal pus along with cultures from blood, joint fluid, and infected skin should be obtained. Bone biopsy is indicated if blood cultures and radiographic findings are not consistent with osteomyelitis. Supporting evidence for osteomyelitis includes leukocytosis and elevated erythrocyte sedimentation rate. Radiographic findings, besides soft tissue swelling, are only evident after 2 to 3 weeks. A three-phase technetium bone scan can show areas of increased blood flow, such as early infected bone, and is useful in locating multiple sites, but it is not a diagnostic test. A CT scan can detect bone destruction, and an MRI provides detailed anatomy useful in delineating the area of involvement, especially if planning for surgical intervention. The differential diagnosis includes, but is not limited to, trauma, malignant lesions, leukemia, juvenile rheumatoid arthritis, and acute rheumatic fever. Sometimes the osteomyelitis may be unrecognized if it occurs as a complication of a severe toxic and debilitating disease.

### Therapeutic Management

After cultures are obtained, empiric IV antibiotics covering the mostly likely organisms are started; for *S. aureus* this is generally nafcillin or clindamycin. Methicillin-resistant *S. aureus* may require vancomycin. When the infective agent is identified, the appropriate antibiotic is initiated and continued for at least 4 weeks, but the length of therapy is determined by the duration of the symptoms, the response to treatment, and the sensitivity of the organism. In selected cases oral antibiotics may follow a shorter IV course. Because of the prolonged duration of high-dose antibiotics, it is important to monitor hematologic, renal, hepatic, ototoxicity, and other potential side effects.

Surgery maybe indicated if there is no response to specific antibiotic therapy, there is persistent soft tissue abscess, or there is spread to the joint. Opinions differ regarding surgical intervention, but many advocate sequestrectomy and surgical drainage to decompress the metaphyseal space before pus erupts and spreads to the subperiosteal space, forming abscesses that strip the periosteum from bone or form draining sinuses. When these complications occur, a chronic infection usually persists. When surgical drainage is carried out, polyethylene tubes are placed in the wound—one tube instills an antibiotic solution directly into the infected area by gravity, and the other, connected to a suction apparatus, provides drainage.

### Nursing Considerations

During the acute phase of illness, any movement of the affected limb will cause discomfort to the child; therefore the

---

*Martha R. Curry, MS, RNC, CPNP, revised this section.

child is positioned comfortably with the affected limb supported. Moving and turning are carried out carefully and gently to minimize discomfort. The child may require pain medication (see Chapter 26) or sedation. Vital signs are taken and recorded frequently, and measures are implemented to reduce a significant temperature elevation.

Antibiotic therapy requires careful observation and monitoring of the IV equipment and site. Because more than one antibiotic is usually administered, the compatibility of the drugs must be determined and care taken to avoid mixing noncompatible drugs. The stability of the drugs and their toxic nature are also considered when determining the rate of administration. The infusion device must be well situated in the vein to ensure that the drug does not infiltrate into surrounding tissues, where it may produce tissue damage. For long-term antibiotic therapy, a venous access device, such as an intermittent infusion device or percutaneously inserted central catheter (PICC), is the preferred method of IV administration. (See Chapter 28.)

Children with open wounds are placed on standard precautions, depending on the policies of the institution. The wound is managed according to the directions of the practitioner. Antibiotic solution administered directly into the wound is most efficiently accomplished with a regular infusion setup that is prepared and regulated in the same manner as for any IV infusion. The drainage tubes are connected to low Gomco or wall suction for continuous removal. Intake and output are measured and recorded, and the character of both the wound and drainage is noted. The amount and character of drainage on the wound dressing are also noted.

Casts are sometimes used for immobilization, and if so, routine cast care is carried out (see p. 1784). The extremity is examined for sensation, circulation, and pain, and the area over the inflammation is usually left open for observation. The affected area, casted or uncasted, is assessed for color, swelling, heat, movement, and tenderness.

The child usually has a poor appetite and may be subject to vomiting. Nourishment in the form of high-calorie liquids such as fruit juices, gelatin, and juice bars should be encouraged until the child begins to feel better. The appetite returns as the acute symptoms subside. During convalescence, adequate nutrition must be maintained to aid healing and reconstitution of new bone.

When the acute stage subsides, children begin to feel better, appetite improves, and they become interested in their surroundings and relationships. They wish to move about in bed and are allowed to do so. However, weight bearing on the affected limb is not permitted until healing is well under way in order to avoid pathologic fractures. Diversional and constructive activities become important nursing interventions. Children are usually confined to bed for some time after the acute phase but may be allowed to move about on a stretcher or in a wheelchair when isolation and bed rest are no longer necessary. At this stage the continuous IV infusion may be replaced by a heparin lock to allow greater freedom.

As the infection subsides, physical therapy is instituted to ensure restoration of optimum function. The child is usu-

ally discharged with oral antibiotics, and progress is followed closely for some time.

## Septic Arthritis

Septic arthritis is a bacterial infection in the joint. It usually results from hematogenous spread or from direct extension of an adjacent cellulitis or osteomyelitis. Direct inoculation from trauma accounts for 15% to 20% of septic arthritis. The most common causative organism is *S. aureus*. Before *H. influenzae* vaccine, *H. influenzae* was the most common pathogen in children under 2 years of age, but it is now rare in vaccinated children (Peltola, Kallio, and Unkila-Kallio, 1998). In addition to *S. aureus*, neonatal pathogens include group B streptococcus, *Escherichia coli* and *Candida albicans*. *N. gonorrhoeae* is a potential pathogen in the sexually active adolescent.

Knees, hips, ankles, and elbows are the most common joints affected. Clinical manifestations include severe joint pain, swelling, overlying tissue warmth, and occasionally erythema. The child is resistant to any joint movement. Features of systemic illness such as fever, malaise, headache, nausea, vomiting, and irritability may also be present.

### Therapeutic Management/Nursing Considerations

The affected joint is aspirated and evaluated by Gram stain, culture (including separate culture for *H. influenzae* and *N. gonorrhoeae*), leukocyte count, as well as glucose, lactate, and protein levels. In addition, blood cultures, complete blood count (CBC) with differential, and erythrocyte sedimentation rate or C-reactive protein should be obtained. Early radiographic findings are limited to soft tissue swelling but may reveal foreign body and always provide a baseline for comparison. Technetium scans reveal areas of increased blood flow but will not differentiate between sites. MRI and CT scans provide more detailed images of cartilage loss, joint narrowing, erosions, and ankylosis of progressive disease.

Treatment is IV antibiotic therapy based upon Gram stain and the clinical presentation. Serial aspiration to demonstrate sterile synovium fluid and reduce pressure or pain has controversial benefits. Septic arthritis of the hip is a special situation and requires open drainage of the hip. There may be a brief period of traction and immobilization followed by passive then active physical therapy. Relief of pain and nursing care are the same as for osteomyelitis.

## Tuberculosis

### Skeletal Tuberculosis

In children tubercular infection of the bones and joints is acquired by lymphhematogenous spread at the time of primary infection. Occasionally it is from chronic pulmonary tuberculosis. Skeletal tubercular infection is not common in the United States but should be considered in communities with high tuberculosis case rates. The infection is most likely to involve the vertebrae, causing a tubercular spondylitis. If the infection is progressive, it causes Pott disease with destruction of the vertebral bodies and results in kyphosis.

Symptoms are insidious; the child may report persistent or intermittent pain. Other findings include joint swelling and stiffness; fever and weight loss are not common. Tubercular arthritis can also affect single joints such as a knee or hip and tends to cause severe destruction of adjacent bone. Infection in the fingers causes spina ventosa, a tuberculous dactylitis.

As with pulmonary tuberculosis, the index case should be located. A family and environmental history needs to be obtained and skin tests applied. Purified protein derivative (PPD) skin tests are positive for the majority of children with tuberculous arthritis; however, the results are not diagnostic, and the clinical and laboratory features do not differentiate tubercular arthritis from a nontubercular septic arthritis. Diagnosis requires isolation of *Mycobacterium tuberculosis* from the site. Patients with the susceptible organism start treatment with combined antituberculosis chemotherapy, isoniazid, rifampin, and pyrazinamide; supervised therapy is preferred. Nursing care depends on the site and extent of infection. Tuberculous spondylitis and hip infection may require immobilization, casting, and fusion. Nursing care is the same as for osteomyelitis with the addition of isolation requirements.

# SKELETAL AND ARTICULAR DYSFUNCTION

## Osteogenesis Imperfecta (OI)

OI is the most common osteoporosis syndrome in childhood. OI is a heterogeneous group–inherited syndrome characterized by fractures and bone deformity. There are at least four types of OI, accounting for significant disease variability. Clinical features may include the following: varying degrees of bone fragility, deformity, and fracture; blue sclerae; hearing loss; and dentinogenesis imperfecta (hypoplastic discolored teeth). Inheritance is autosomal dominant in most cases; however, rare autosomal recessive inheritance exists.

Most types of OI have defects in the COL1A1 or COL1A2 genes, which code for polypeptide chains in type I procollagen, a precursor of type I collagen, a major structural component of bone. This error results in faulty bone mineralization, abnormal bone architecture, and increased susceptibility to fracture.

There are several classifications for OI based on clinical features and patterns of inheritance. (Box 39-15). Clinically type I is the most common, with wide variability of bone fragility; some affected family members have significant deformity and disability, whereas others lead agile active lives. Type II variants are the most severe and considered lethal in infancy. Type III OI is characterized by multiple fractures, bone deformity, and severe disability; affected individuals rarely live to 30 years of age. Type IV is similar to type I but not associated with blue sclerae.

## Therapeutic Management

Treatment for OI is primarily supportive, although patients and families are optimistic about new research advances.

Bone marrow transplant for severe OI was first reported in 1999 with positive results; this is still an experimental procedure in OI, and long-term benefits and risks will take years to identify (Horwitz and others, 2001). Promising studies using bisphosphonate therapy for severe OI showed increased bone mineral density and possibly help in preventing fracture (Glorieux, 2000). In addition, there are animal studies in molecular therapeutics currently under way (Forlino and Marini, 2000).

The goals of a rehabilitation approach to management are directed to preventing (1) positional contractures and deformities, (2) muscle weakness and osteoporosis, and (3) malalignment of lower extremity joints prohibiting weight bearing.

Several medications have been tried but appear to be of limited benefit. Lightweight braces and splints help support limbs, prevent fractures, and aid in ambulation. Physical therapy helps prevent disuse osteoporosis and strengthens muscles, which in turn improves bone density. Encouraging the development of head and trunk control early on, and progressing to improving mobility and graded exercise regimens, has physical and social benefits (Binder and others, 1993). Exercises are usually simple ones against light resistance or water exercises with swimming. Patients with milder disease are encouraged to participate in sports. Exercise also gives children a sense of well-being and confidence in their bodies.

Surgery is sometimes used to help treat the manifestations of the disease. Surgical techniques are used to correct deformities that interfere with bracing, standing, or walking. For the child with recurrent fractures, inserting an intermedullary rod provides stability to bones. The rods must be replaced as the child grows; otherwise fractures may occur through the unprotected portion of the bone.

### Nursing Considerations

Infants and children with this disorder require careful handling to prevent fractures. They must be supported when

---

**Box 39-15** ■ ■ □
**Classification of Osteogenesis Imperfecta**

| TYPE | CLINICAL FEATURES |
|------|-------------------|
| I | Most common form; variable fractures; little deformity; stature normal or near normal; blue sclerae; hearing loss common in 20s or 30s, but not always; dentinogenesis imperfecta uncommon; joint laxity, fewer fractures after puberty; autosomal dominant |
| II | Lethal in utero or in infancy; multiple fractures and deformity; underdeveloped lungs; autosomal dominant or recessive |
| III | Fractures common; long bone deformity; barrel chest; spinal curve; triangular face; short stature; frequent blue sclerae, which lighten with age; hearing loss common; dentinogenesis imperfecta common; respiratory problems common; joint laxity; autosomal dominant and rarely recessive |
| IV | Fractures common; stature reduced; bone deformity common but not severe; sclerae normal to grayish; variable hearing loss; dentinogenesis imperfecta common; autosomal dominant |

they are turned, positioned, moved, and fondled. Even changing a diaper may cause a fracture in a severely affected infant. These children should never be held by the ankles when being diapered but should be gently lifted by the buttocks.

One of the most distressing features of OI is its frequent confusion with child abuse. Numerous fractures and easy bruising, characteristic of OI, are signs usually observed in child abuse; parents must often deal with accusations of abuse until a correct diagnosis is made. This is very traumatic for parents; therefore they need considerable nonjudgmental support during this time. Giving parents a letter to carry that explains the child's condition and is signed by the primary or specialty practitioner may help smooth visits to the emergency department.

Both parents and the child need education regarding the child's limitations and guidelines in planning suitable activities that promote optimum development, as well as protect the child from harm. Realistic occupational planning and genetic counseling are part of the long-term goals of care. Educational materials and information can be obtained from the **Osteogenesis Imperfecta Foundation, Inc.***
This organization also has a network that can put a family in contact with other families facing a similar diagnosis.

## Juvenile Rheumatoid Arthritis (Juvenile Idiopathic Arthritis)

Juvenile idiopathic arthritis (JIA) is a new name for chronic childhood arthritis called juvenile rheumatoid arthritis (JRA) by Americans and juvenile chronic arthritis (JCA) by Europeans. This new name is slowly replacing JRA in the research literature but has yet to affect clinical practice; consequently both JRA and JIA classifications will be discussed. The JRA nomenclature revision to JIA was due in part to the minimally applicable reference to "rheumatoid" in childhood arthritis, which is only relevant to a small portion of affected children yet burdens the family with disfiguring images of adult rheumatoid arthritis. Furthermore, the old subtyping of JRA into systemic, pauciarticular, and polyarticular disease reflects disease onset and not disease progression, which is of greater importance (Warren and others, 2001).

Semantics aside, JIA or JRA is a group of idiopathic chronic inflammatory diseases affecting the joints and other tissues in approximately 1 in 1000 children. There are theories of an infectious agent activating an autoimmune inflammatory process, but there is no convincing evidence. There is a female predominance and two peak ages of onset between 1 and 3 and 8 to 10 years of age.

### Pathophysiology

The rheumatic process is characterized by a chronic inflammation of the synovium with joint effusion and eventual erosion, destruction, and fibrosis of the articular cartilage. Ad-

hesions between joint surfaces and ankylosis of joints occur if the process persists long enough.

### Clinical Manifestations

Whether a single joint or multiple joints are involved, stiffness, swelling, and loss of motion develop in the affected joints. They are swollen and warm to touch but seldom red. The swelling results from edema, joint effusion, and synovial thickening. The affected joints may be tender and painful to touch or relatively painless. The limited motion early in the disease is a result of muscle spasm and joint inflammation; later it is caused by ankylosis or soft tissue contracture. Morning stiffness, or "gelling," of the joint(s) is characteristic and present on arising in the morning or after inactivity. Infections, injuries, or surgical procedures often precipitate a flare-up of the arthritis; therefore prompt recognition and treatment of infections is necessary.

In severe, long-standing cases growth is significantly retarded. Corticosteroid therapy is also a contributing factor. There may be growth disturbances, either overgrowth or undergrowth, adjacent to the inflamed joints (e.g., altered leg length after knee involvement) and micrognathia (receding chin) from temporomandibular arthritis.

**JRA/JIA Classification.** JRA is a variable disease with three major disease courses: *systemic onset, pauciarticular* (involving few joints, usually less than five), and *polyarticular* (simultaneous involvement of four or more joints). These groups, including subgroups, and the manifestations associated with each are outlined in Table 39-5. The universal Durban classification of JIA revised and published in 1998 lists seven disease categories, each with its own set of criteria and exclusions: systemic arthritis, oligoarthritis, RF (rheumatoid factor)-negative polyarthritis, RF-positive arthritis, psoriatic arthritis, enthesitis-related arthritis, and other arthritis (Petty and others, 1998).

### Course and Prognosis

The outcome of JRA/JIA is variable and unpredictable. The disease, even in severe forms, is rarely life-threatening and is significantly different than adult rheumatoid arthritis. Features that distinguish JRA/JIA from adult disease include onset before puberty; a negative rheumatoid factor (RF) (in 90% of cases); classic symptoms of systemic arthritis such as quotidian fever, rash, and pericarditis; development of uveitis as a complication (in 8% to 20% of cases), and a tendency for the arthritis to become inactive. The arthritis tends to wax and wane and eventually becomes inactive in approximately 70% of the cases. These children may have severe or minimal joint damage remaining when active arthritis abates. Thirty percent of the children will have progressive arthritis into adulthood. Their arthritis can cause significant joint deformity and functional disability requiring medication, physical therapy, and perhaps future joint replacement. Chronic and acute uveitis (inflammation of the iris and ciliary body) is an extraarticular complication of JRA/JIA, which may cause permanent vision loss if undiagnosed and not aggressively treated. Although most children do "outgrow" arthritis, it can produce severe physical, functional, and emotional impairment.

*804 W Diamond Ave, Suite 210, Gaithersburg, MD 20878, (301) 947-0083 or (800) 981-2663, fax: (310) 947-0456, e-mail: bonelink@aol.com, www.oif.org.

**TABLE 39-5**   Characteristics of juvenile rheumatoid arthritis related to mode of onset

| | Systemic Onset | Pauciarticular (Two or Three Subtypes) | Polyarticular (Two Subtypes) |
|---|---|---|---|
| Percentage of patients | 30% | 45% | 25% |
| Age at onset | Bimodal distribution 1-3 years of age 8-10 years of age | Type I: Less than 10 years of age Type II: Over 10 years of age | Throughout childhood and adolescence |
| Sex ratio (female/male) | 1.5:1 | Type I: Almost all female Type II: 1:9 | Mostly female |
| Joints involved | Any Only 20% have joint involvement at time of diagnosis | Usually confined to lower extremities—knee, ankle, and eventually sacroiliac; sometimes elbow | Any joints: usually symmetric involvement of small joints Hip involvement in 50% Spine involvement in 50% |
| Extraarticular manifestations | Fever, malaise, myalgia, rash, pleuritis or pericarditis, adenomegaly, splenomegaly, hepatomegaly | Type I: Chronic iridocyclitis; mucocutaneous lesions Type II: Acute iridocyclitis; sacroiliitis common; eventual ankylosing spondylitis in many Type III: Arthritis only | Systemic signs minimal Possible low-grade fever, malaise, weight loss, rheumatoid nodules, or vasculitis |
| Laboratory tests | Elevated ESR, CPR; RF negative; ANA rarely positive; anemia; leukocytosis | Elevated ESR, CPR; ANA positive Type I: HLA-DRW5 positive Type II: HLA-B27 positive Type III: HLA-TMo positive | Elevated ESR, CPR Type I: RF positive Type II: RF negative |
| Long-term prognosis | Mortality—1%-2% of all JRA patients Joint destruction in 40% | Continuous disease; eventual remission in 60% Type I: Ocular damage; functional blindness in 10% Type II: Ankylosing spondylitis Type III: Best outlook for recovery | Longer duration; more crippling; remission in 25% Type I: High incidence of disabling arthritis Type II: Outlook good |

*ESR,* Erythrocyte sedimentation rate; *CPR,* C-reactive protein; *RF,* rheumatoid factor; *ANA,* antinuclear antibody; *HLA,* human leukocyte antigen.

## Diagnostic Evaluation

JRA and JIA are diagnoses of exclusion; there are no definitive tests. Both diagnoses are based of the clinical criteria of age of onset before 16 years, arthritis in one or more joints for 6 weeks or longer, and exclusion of other etiologies (Brewer and others, 1977; Petty and others, 1998). Laboratory tests may provide supporting evidence of disease. An elevated sedimentation rate may or may not be present. Leukocytosis is frequently present during flares of systemic disease. RF is positive in only 10% of the children with JRA/JIA. Antinuclear antibodies are common in JRA/JIA, but they are not specific for arthritis; however, they help identify children with pauciarticular disease who are at greater risk for uveitis.

## Therapeutic Management

There is no cure for JRA/JIA. The major goals of therapy are to control pain, preserve joint range of motion and function, minimize effects of inflammation such as joint deformity, and promote normal growth and development. Achievement of these goals requires a family-centered approach with collaboration among the child, the family, and the health care team. The team includes the primary care physician, the pediatric rheumatologist, the rheumatology nurse educator, the social worker, physical and occupational therapists, subspecialists (e.g., pediatric ophthalmologist), and a community of friends, relatives, and teachers. The

treatment plan is individualized and varies, but it can be very complicated and intrusive, including medications, physical/occupational therapy, slit lamp eye examinations, splints, comfort measures, dietary management, school modifications, and psychosocial support.

Outpatient care is the mainstay of therapy; lengthy hospital admissions for rehabilitation used to be common but are now limited in the era of managed care. Slit lamp ophthalmology eye examinations at regular intervals are required to diagnose chronic anterior uveitis (iridocyclitis), inflammation of the anterior segments of eye, iris, and ciliary body. The majority of affected children have a relatively good visual prognosis if the inflammation is detected and treated early, however, most cases are asymptomatic. Consequently, routine slit lamp examinations are critical (American Academy of Pediatrics, 1993b).

**Medications.**   A variety of antirheumatic drugs are available, and most are effective in suppressing the inflammatory process and relieving pain. The drugs may be given alone or in combination. ***Nonsteroidal antiinflammatory drugs (NSAIDs)*** are the first drugs used. Common NSAIDs include ibuprofen, naproxen, tolmetin sodium, diclofenac, indomethacin, and nabumetone. (See Table 26-4.) Aspirin, once the initial drug of choice, is seldom used in children. NSAIDs offer an immediate analgesic effect, but the antiinflammatory effect takes larger doses and longer periods of time to achieve; the child needs to be on an NSAID for at least 3 weeks before evaluating effectiveness. Patient and family education regarding potential gastrointestinal, renal, hepatic, and reduced clotting side effects is essential. Parents should monitor abdominal pain and blood in stool. Naproxen has the potential side effect of skin fragility in fair individuals—families need to use sun precautions and report unusual skin lesions (Lang and Finlayson, 1994). Celecoxib and rofecoxib are new cyclooxygenase-2 (COX-2) inhibitor NSAIDs that selectively inhibit proinflammatory prostaglandin without interfering with the gastrointestinal (GI) mucosal barrier, resulting in fewer GI side effects (Osiri and Moreland, 1999). Although still unapproved for use in children, new COX-2 inhibitor NSAIDs are being used in select children with GI intolerance to other NSAIDs.

Additional medication will be required in approximately 65% of children with arthritis. These agents are *slower-acting antirheumatic drugs (SAARDs)* and include methotrexate, sulfasalazine, and hydroxychloroquine and gold. Weekly low-dose methotrexate is usually the first SAARD used. Families may be overwhelmed with potential adverse effects, including liver disease, bone marrow suppression, GI disturbance, teratogenic properties, and the alarming but unconfirmed risk of carcinogenesis; however, methotrexate is effective and the potential benefits outweigh the potential risks. Methotrexate has also improved uveitis in children with uveitis resistant to steroids (Weiss, Wallace, and Sherry, 1998; Samson and others, 2001). Laboratory monitoring of liver enzymes and blood counts is crucial. A daily folic acid supplement can help reduce oral ulcers. Taking methotrexate at bedtime may help reduce nausea. Frank discussion about sexual activity and birth defects is critical. Sexually active teenagers need effective birth control and documented periods, as well as pregnancy tests if periods are not regular. As a precaution, pregnant caregivers and those trying to conceive need to avoid contact with methotrexate. Alcohol consumption is another sensitive topic that needs to be honestly discussed because of the increased risk of hepatotoxicity. Most children will require both an NSAID and methotrexate, and parents may be notified by pharmacists about combination toxicity. This is a known interaction that the rheumatologist is aware of; however, patients need to be instructed to avoid additional over-the-counter NSAIDs and to take acetaminophen for episodes of fever. They should also avoid sulfa antibiotics and other bone-marrow–suppressing drugs. Parents always should discuss methotrexate drug interactions with providers prescribing medications for interval illness. During some illnesses, especially varicella, methotrexate should be discontinued because it can suppress the immune response. Sulfasazaline may be selected as the first SSARD in children with axial arthritis, a positive HLA-B27, or symptoms of inflammatory bowel disease, given this drug's success in these select groups of patients.

*Corticosteroids* are the most potent antiinflammatory agents; however, they will not cure arthritis, and the significant adverse effects of long-term steroid use are undesirable. Steroids are initiated when other medications have failed to control a disease flare and the child has substantial physical disability. Prednisone is administered orally in a burst or in the lowest effective dose. An alternate-day sched-

ule may help reduce side effects. High-dose IV steroids may provide sustained improvement for children with severe arthritis and pericarditis associated with systemic disease. Intraarticular injections of long-acting steroids have proven effective in treating limited arthritis with minimal adverse effects. Young children may require conscious sedation or general anesthesia, which affects risk-benefit considerations, but it is critical to have a cooperative patient for good procedure outcome.

Etanercept, a new *biologic agent,* has recently been approved for use in children with JRA. Etanercept works by interrupting the inflammatory process, by blocking the cytokine tumor necrosis factor. Studies have shown it to be effective and well tolerated (Lovell and others, 2000). As with any new drug, parents need to inform providers of any unusual associated symptoms, given limited experience and accrual of long-term side effects.

*Cytotoxic agents* cyclophosphamide, azathioprine, cyclosporine, and chlorambucil have been used in severe refractory arthritis that have not responded to other medications. Experience is limited with these drugs, and the toxicity risks and potential benefits are not well defined.

**Physical Management.**  Programs of physical management are individualized for each child and are designed to reach the ultimate goal—preserving function and preventing deformity. Physical therapy is directed toward specific joints, focusing on strengthening muscles, mobilizing restricted joints, and preventing or correcting deformities. Occupational therapists assume responsibility for generalized mobility and performance of activities of daily living.

General treatment or maintenance programs vary; physical therapists may be involved several times weekly to monthly in management of a home program (ideally in association with the child's school), or their visits may be limited to infrequent review of the home program for compliance, effectiveness, and need. Strength is frequently lost around the involved joints, and inactivity leads to generalized weakness. However, normal activities of daily living and the child's natural tendency to be active are usually sufficient to maintain muscle strength and joint mobility.

Exercising in a pool is excellent because it allows freedom of movement with support and minimum gravitational pull. When joints are inflamed, heavy resistance aggravates the pain; at such times, simple isometric or tensing exercises that do not involve joint movement are generally tolerated and should be encouraged. Range-of-motion exercises are an important aspect of therapy and are continued after evidence of disease has disappeared in order to detect any signs of recurrence.

Practitioners may recommend splinting and positioning during rest to help minimize pain and prevent or reduce flexion deformity. Joints most frequently splinted are knees, wrists, and hands. Positioning during rest is also important. The child rests on a firm mattress with no pillow or a very low one and has no support under the knee. Loss of extension in the knee, hip, and wrist causes special problems. Vigilance is required to detect the earliest signs of involvement, and vigorous attention must be given to specialized passive stretching, positioning, and resting splints to prevent deformity.

**Surgery.** The benefits of synovectomy, an established preventive and therapeutic procedure in adults, are questionable in children with rheumatoid arthritis. Synovectomy is used primarily in pauciarticular disease. In cases of synovitis, intraarticular steroid injection is an alternative to synovectomy and may be tried once or twice before surgery is performed. Joint replacement is proving to be successful in older children who are fully grown. (See Atraumatic Care box.)

## Nursing Considerations

### ▪ Assessment

Nursing care of children with JRA/JIA involves assessment of their general health, the status of involved joints, and their emotional responses to all of the ramifications of the disease—pain, physical restrictions, therapies, and self-concept, especially in preadolescents and adolescents.

### ▪ Nursing Diagnoses

Based on a thorough assessment, several nursing diagnoses are identified. The more common diagnoses for the child with JRA are included in the Nursing Care Plan on pp. 1826-1827. Others may apply in specific situations.

### ▪ Planning

The goals for the child with JRA/JIA should be developed in conjunction with the family and may include the following:

1. Child will exhibit signs of reduced joint inflammation and adequate joint function.
2. Child will experience no pain or reduction of pain to level acceptable to child.
3. Child will perform activities of daily living.
4. Child will maintain adequate energy level.
5. Child will have appropriate nutritional intake.
6. Child and family will demonstrate knowledge of medications and treatment modalities.
7. Child will express feelings and concerns.
8. Child and family will receive adequate support.

### ▪ Implementation

The effects of the disease are manifested in every aspect of the child's life—physical activities, social experiences, and personality development. Children's adjustment to the stresses and demands of the disease and the level of functioning they achieve are in large part related to the reaction and support they receive from their family and the health care professionals concerned with their care and management.

**Relieve Pain.** The pain of arthritis is related to several aspects of the disease—disease severity, functional status, individual pain threshold, family variables, and psychologic adjustment. Although complete pain relief would be highly desirable, it is probably unrealistic. The aim is to provide as much relief as possible with antiinflammatory medication and other therapies to help children tolerate the pain and cope as effectively as possible. At present, opioid administration is not a routine therapy for the chronic pain of arthritis. Nonpharmacologic modalities such as relaxation may be helpful. (See Pain Management, Chapter 26.)

**Promote General Health.** The general health of children with JRA and their siblings must be considered and

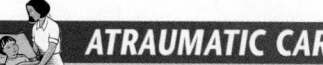

### ATRAUMATIC CARE

*Reducing the Pain of Aspiration of Synovial Fluid in Joints (Arthrocentesis)*

Application of the topical anesthetic cream EMLA to the puncture site 60 to 120 minutes before the procedure reduces or eliminates pain from needle aspiration. One study found that using EMLA to alleviate pain associated with the injection of lidocaine during arthrocentesis eliminated the need for conscious sedation with oral midazolam (Versed). The use of EMLA decreased length of stay and overall costs (Kerr and Jarvis, 1996). If additional anesthesia is needed, using buffered lidocaine reduces the stinging and burning pain of injected lidocaine. (See Pain Management, Chapter 26.)

may be overlooked as parents and health personnel concentrate on the disease. A well-balanced diet and assessment of nutritional status are integral parts of health supervision. Protein-calorie malnutrition and inadequate intake of other nutrients are common with JRA (Purdy and others, 1996). The discomfort and increased need for rest may create problems of weight control. Excess weight causes additional strain on inflamed joints, especially those of the lower extremities. Excessive fatigue and overexertion should be avoided by regular periods of rest, especially during acute flare-ups of arthritis. Symptoms may exacerbate during a viral illness.

Posture and body mechanics are important for children with arthritis, both when they are at rest and when they are active. They must have a firm mattress to maintain good alignment of the spine, hips, and knees and no pillow or a very thin one. Children who are confined to bed either at home or in the hospital may require supports or splints to maintain positioning. A waterbed or an electric blanket provides comforting warmth. Lying in the prone position is encouraged to straighten the hips and knees during rest periods or while watching television. The family is instructed in the principles and purposes of splints so that they can use them correctly.

School-age children are encouraged to attend school, even on days when there may be some pain or discomfort. The aid of the school nurse is enlisted so that a child is permitted to take the prescribed medication at school and to arrange for rest in the nurse's office during the day. Split days or half days may help a child remain involved in school. Permitting the child to come to school late allows time to gain joint movement and reduces the time at school to avoid exhaustion. It is important that the child attend school to develop academic skills and engage in social interaction, especially if the arthritis continues to limit physical skills. Arranging for two sets of textbooks eliminates the need to carry heavy or numerous books to and from school, thus reducing discomfort and difficulty in ambulating. The development of an Individualized Education Plan (IEP) in the school setting (see Chapter 24) may ensure that the child's needs are met (Spencer, Fife, and Rabinovich, 1995).

**Facilitate Compliance.** The child and family are involved in the therapeutic plan. They need to know the purpose and correct use of any splints and appliances and the medication regimen. The family is instructed regarding administration of medications, as well as the value of a regular schedule of administration to maintain a satisfactory drug level in the body. They need to know most NSAIDs should not be given on an empty stomach, and they must be instructed to be alert for signs of NSAID toxicity.

**Encourage Heat and Exercise.** Heat has been shown to be beneficial to children with arthritis. Moist heat is best for relieving pain and stiffness, and the most efficient and practical method is in the bathtub. The temperature and duration of the bath are specified by the therapist but usually do not exceed 10 minutes at 37.8° C (100° F). Sometimes a daily whirlpool bath, paraffin bath, or hot packs may be used as needed for temporary relief of acute swelling and pain. Hot packs are easily applied at home using a towel wrung out after being immersed in hot water or heated in a microwave oven, applied to the area, and covered with plastic for 20 minutes. Painful hands or feet can be immersed in a pan of water for 10 minutes two or three times daily in addition to tub baths.

Pool therapy is the easiest method for exercising a large number of joints. Swimming activities strengthen muscles and maintain mobility in larger joints. Children in urban areas may have access to a therapy pool, although transportation may be a problem for some families. Very small children who are frightened of the water can carry out their exercises in the bathtub. Small children love to splash, kick, and throw things in the water.

Activities of daily living provide satisfactory exercise for older children to maintain maximum mobility with minimum pain. These children should be encouraged in their ef-

forts and patiently allowed to dress and groom themselves, to assume daily tasks, and to care for their belongings. It is often difficult for stiff fingers to manipulate buttons, comb or brush hair, and turn faucets, but parents and other caregivers should not readily offer assistance. In addition, children should be helped to understand why others do not assist them. Many helpful devices, such as self-adhering fasteners, tongs for manipulating difficult items, and grab bars installed in bathrooms for safety, can be employed to facilitate tasks. A raised toilet seat often makes the difference between dependent and independent toileting, because weak quadriceps muscles and sore knees inhibit the ability to raise the body from a low sitting position.

A child's natural affinity for play offers many opportunities for incorporating therapeutic exercises. Throwing or kicking a ball, hanging from monkey bars, and riding a tricycle (with the seat raised to achieve maximum leg extension) are excellent moving and stretching exercises for a very young child whose daily living activities are physically limited.

An effective approach to beginning the day's activities is to awaken children early to give them their medication and then allow them to sleep for an hour. On arising, children take a hot bath (or shower) and perform a simple ritual of limbering-up exercises, after which they commence the activities of the day, such as going to school. Exercise, heat, and rest are spaced throughout the remainder of the day according to individual needs and schedules. Parents are instructed in exercises that fit the needs of the child.

**NURSING TIP** Another method of supplying warmth before the child arises is to plug an electric blanket into an appliance timer. Set the blanket to medium or high and adjust the timer to turn on the blanket 1 hour before the child awakens.

The **Arthritis Foundation***** and the **American Juvenile Arthritis Foundation***** provide information and services for both parents and professionals, and nurses can refer families to these agencies as an added resource.

**The Child.** Arthritis affects every aspect of the child's daily life. The physical pain and limitations interfere with performance of normal tasks and provision of self-care. Even simple tasks, such as dressing, hair combing, use of the bathroom, cutting food, climbing stairs, manipulating doors and faucets, and using public transportation, are difficult or impossible. There may be school difficulties related to transportation to and from school, climbing stairs, and loss of time as a result of exacerbations and hospitalization. Physical limitations interfere with participation in many activities, both curricular and extracurricular, which limits peer contacts and interaction and increases social isolation. These problems are especially critical for adolescents, for whom peer acceptance and relationships are so vital to personality development. (See Family Focus box.) Many children with arthritis increasingly turn to solitary activities and

## FAMILY FOCUS
### Juvenile Rheumatoid Arthritis

As a nurse, and mother of a child with JRA, I believe it is important for nurses to always keep in mind the feelings and emotions of children with JRA.

Emotionally, I think the preadolescent/adolescent age-groups of children with JRA have the most questions and concerns about their disease. Children, including my daughter, often ask, "Why me?" Adolescence/preadolescence is an age of socialization and change. These children want to be part of the social scene, to be included. Often these children are limited in their activities. Nurses need to emphasize to their patients, as well as the patients' families, the positive accomplishments these children have made. They need to know that we, as nurses, parents, and doctors, don't know why they have the arthritis, but that we will help and encourage them as much as possible in all aspects of their lives.

Disfigurement of joints, weight gain, weight loss, bloating, and physical impairments are all important in the eyes of a preteen/teenager. They must understand and accept themselves for who they are and not what they look like or appear to look like.

Communication with my daughter was and still is very essential. Nurses have an opportunity to enforce positive attitudes and encourage open communication with their patients. I feel it is very important for nurses to always keep in mind that nursing skills are essential, but communication with patients and families is equally important. It is the key to nursing assessment.

Sandra L. Guyette, RN
Shriner's Hospital
Springfield, MA

*****1330 W Peachtree St, Atlanta, GA 30309, (404) 872-7100 or (800) 283-7800; www.arthritis.org. In Canada: **The Arthritis Society,** 393 University Ave, Suite 1700, Toronto, Ontario M5G 1E6, (416) 979-7228 or (800) 321-1433, fax: (416) 979-8366; www.arthritis.ca.

to the family at a time when they are expected to move into greater independence and relationships with peers.

Changes in personality may accompany JRA/JIA, as with any chronic illness. These changes may be temporary, such as demanding, irritable behavior, or may be persistent, such as passive hostility, uncommunicativeness, and manipulativeness. Efforts should be made to break through the child's defenses and to identify anxieties, concerns, and conflicts in order to intervene early to prevent the development of permanent personality problems. (See Chapter 22 for care of the child with chronic illness.)

**The Family.**   The beginning of the disease is often sudden and frightening for the family, and its variable course with cycles of remissions and exacerbations is discouraging. Many parents become susceptible to unorthodox cures advanced by advertisers and well-meaning friends. Access to the Internet and over 200 sites dedicated to arthritis provides families a welcome relief to the isolation of living with arthritis, but it is also a bottomless source of unsubstantiated information that necessitates frank discussion and review with the family to sort out what is opinion, fact, safe, and dangerous. Sometimes health care providers will not know the benefits or risks of a nutritional, herbal, or other complementary therapy. Hopefully the new surge of legitimate scientific investigations of these remedies will provide future answers. These should be carefully evaluated. Obviously harmless measures such as wearing a copper bracelet need not be discouraged, but parents must be dissuaded from questionable or conspicuously harmful practices such as active exercising of swollen, feverish joints. Parents' understanding of the disease and their attitude toward the child can determine the success or failure of a treatment program, and major foci of nursing intervention are parental education and support.

Nurses are alert to cues that signal undue anxiety and guilt, which may lead to an unhealthy degree of overprotection, such as preoccupation with causative factors, constant analysis of the effects of various therapies, experimentation with diets, and continual searching for a magical cure. The dangers of parental overprotection and overindulgence can be especially detrimental to the progress of the child. Sometimes parents avoid prescribed medications, keep the child home from school unnecessarily, restrict interaction with age-mates, do not discipline the child, and assume self-care activities that are best performed by the child.

Most of the reactions, problems, and concerns of families of a child with JRA/JIA are those of any parents of a child with a chronic illness or disability. The impact of the diagnosis is felt most acutely by the parents, who demonstrate anxiety, guilt, and all the manifestations of the grief process. The concerns and needs of these families are discussed extensively in Chapter 22, and the reader is directed to this chapter for additional guidance in planning care.

## ▐ Evaluation

The effectiveness of nursing interventions is determined by continual reassessment and evaluation of care based on the following observational guidelines:

1. Observe child's behavior and use pain assessment techniques.
2. Conduct routine assessment of child's general health.

3. Observe child during planned and unplanned activities, assess mobility of joints, and observe the use of prescribed appliances.
4. Observe child's ability to perform activities of daily living.
5. Observe and interview child and family regarding feelings and concerns.

The *expected outcomes* are described in the Nursing Care Plan on pp. 1826-1827.

## Systemic Lupus Erythematosus (SLE)

SLE is a chronic, multisystem, autoimmune disease of the blood vessels and connective issue. Its course and symptoms are variable and unpredictable, with mild to life-threatening complications. Other types of lupus erythematosus include chronic cutaneous lupus (discoid lupus), drug-induced lupus erythematosus, subacute cutaneous lupus erythematosus, and neonatal lupus erythematosus. Neonatal lupus erythematosus occurs when maternal autoantibodies cross the placenta and cause transient lupuslike symptoms in the newborn with the potential lethal complication of heart block. The remaining discussion focuses on SLE.

### Etiology

The cause of SLE is not known. It appears to result from a complex interaction of genetics with an unidentified trigger that causes the disease to activate. Suspected triggers include exposure to ultraviolet light, estrogen, pregnancy, infections, and drugs. Genetic predisposition to SLE is evidenced by an increased concordance rate in twins (10-fold), increased incidence within family members (10% to 16%), and increased frequency of certain gene alleles in population-based studies (Tsao and Wallace, 1997).

### Clinical Manifestations

SLE is not a common childhood disease; the estimated incidence is 0.28 per 100,000 children younger than 16 years of age (Malleson, Fung, and Rosenberg, 1996). It typically occurs during adolescence; onset before 5 years of age is unusual. There is a 4:1 female/male predominance. Disease onset can be insidious with intermittent constitutional symptoms such as fever, fatigue, weight loss, and arthralgia. However, rapid involvement of vital organs, primarily the kidneys, can herald an accelerated course with potentially fatal disease. Box 39-16 lists the manifestations related to the various tissues involved.

Rash is a common feature. The malar "butterfly" rash that spares the nasolabial fold is a suggestive feature but not pathognomonic. Maculopapular rashes are frequent and can occur anywhere but typically are on sun-exposed skin. Nails and hair can be involved with red, cracked cuticles, periungual telangiectasias, and patchy or diffuse alopecia. Raynaud phenomenon, vasospasm of the blood vessels, causes cool hands and feet with pain and a characteristic (purple or blue—white—red) tricolor change. Raynaud phenomenon usually occurs as a response to cold exposure and can cause significant tissue damage. Arthritis and tenosynovitis is common in SLE. The arthritis is usually very painful but of short duration, and joint deformity is unusual.

Renal involvement is a serious complication caused primarily by deposition of circulating immune complexes in

# Nursing Care Plan

## The Child with Juvenile Rheumatoid Arthritis

**NURSING DIAGNOSIS:** Chronic pain related to joint inflammation

**PATIENT GOAL 1:** Will exhibit signs of reduced joint inflammation

• **NURSING INTERVENTIONS/***RATIONALES*
*Administer antiinflammatory drugs as prescribed *to suppress inflammatory process of JRA/JIA*

• **EXPECTED OUTCOMES**
Child exhibits no evidence of discomfort
Joints indicate no evidence of inflammation

**PATIENT GOAL 2:** Will experience no pain or reduction of pain to level acceptable to child

• **NURSING INTERVENTIONS/***RATIONALES*
Provide heat to painful joints *to relieve pain and stiffness*
    Tub baths, including whirlpool
    Paraffin baths
    Warm, moist pads
    Soaks
*Maintain preventive schedule of drug administration *to reduce likelihood of pain occurring*
Avoid overexercising painful, swollen joints *because exercise at this time will aggravate pain*
Implement nonpharmacologic pain reduction techniques *to modify pain perception* (see Chapter 26)
Provide well-balanced diet to avoid excess weight gain, *which can cause additional strain on inflamed joints*

• **EXPECTED OUTCOME**
Child is able to move with no or minimum discomfort

**NURSING DIAGNOSIS:** Impaired physical mobility related to joint discomfort and stiffness

**PATIENT GOAL 1:** Will exhibit signs of adequate joint function

• **NURSING INTERVENTIONS/***RATIONALES*
Carry out or supervise physical therapy regimen
    Muscle-strengthening exercises
    Joint mobilization exercises
Apply splints, sandbags, if needed, *to maintain position and reduce flexion deformity during rest*
Lie flat in bed on a firm mattress with joints extended *to reduce flexion deformity*
Use prone position frequently with no pillow, or a very thin one, *to maintain good alignment of spine, hips, knees*
Incorporate therapeutic exercises in play activities
    Swimming
    Throwing a ball
    Hanging from monkey bar
    Riding tricycle or bicycle
Encourage child to be physically active but in a way that does not excessively strain affected joints (e.g., swimming)

---
*Dependent nursing action.

Supervise and encourage activities of daily living, *because these provide exercise*
Encourage child's natural tendency to be active
Frequently assess joint function *so that appropriate treatment is instituted to prevent deformity*

• **EXPECTED OUTCOMES**
Joint flexibility improves in relation to baseline findings
Child develops no contractures
Child engages in activities suitable to interests, capabilities, and developmental level

**NURSING DIAGNOSIS:** Bathing/hygiene, dressing/grooming, feeding, or toileting self-care deficit related to discomfort, impaired joint mobility

**PATIENT GOAL 1:** Will perform activities of daily living

• **NURSING INTERVENTIONS/***RATIONALES*
Encourage maximum independence; avoid doing for child what child is capable of doing
Provide or help devise methods *to facilitate independent functioning*
    Select clothes for convenience in putting on and fastening
    Modify utensils (spoons, toothbrush, comb, and so on) for easier grasp
    Elevate toilet seat, if needed, *to facilitate independent toileting*
    Install handrails for convenience and safety (in hallways, bathroom)
Teach application of splints (when able) and encourage responsibility for their use

• **EXPECTED OUTCOME**
Child is involved in activities of daily living to maximum capabilities

**PATIENT GOAL 2:** Will maintain adequate energy level

• **NURSING INTERVENTIONS/***RATIONALES*
Schedule regular periods for sleep and rest, especially during acute flare-ups, *to conserve energy*
Include school nurse and teachers in planning for needed rest during school day
Encourage child to participate all activities as tolerated

• **EXPECTED OUTCOMES**
Child engages in appropriate activities without undue fatigue
Child receives adequate rest, sleep

**NURSING DIAGNOSIS:** Deficient knowledge related to introduction of new medications and treatment modalities

**PATIENT/FAMILY GOAL 1:** Will demonstrate knowledge of medications and treatment modalities

• **NURSING INTERVENTIONS/***RATIONALES*
Allow patient and parents to discuss concerns and fears *so that they are better able to learn*

## Nursing Care Plan
### The Child with Juvenile Rheumatoid Arthritis—cont'd

Instruct in medication/treatment purpose, administration, side effects, and adverse reactions; repeat instructions as necessary *to ensure learnig*

Provide written information/guidelines for all medications and treatments ordered *so that they can refer to this as needed at home*

Involve patient/family in administration of medications and treatments

Document patient/family education

- **EXPECTED OUTCOMES**

Patient/family will be knowledgeable about medication and treatment modalities

Patient/family will recognize signs of adverse drug reaction/side effects

> **NURSING DIAGNOSIS:** Risk for disturbed body image related to disease process

**PATIENT GOAL 1:** Will express feelings and concerns

- **NURSING INTERVENTIONS/*RATIONALES***

Be available to child *so that there are opportunities for expression of feelings and concerns*

Use therapeutic communication techniques (e.g., reflection, active listening, silence) *to encourage expression of feelings and concerns*

Explore and develop activities in which child can succeed *to promote positive self-image*

Include child in therapy and treatment decisions *to promote positive self-image and decrease sense of powerlessness*

Refer child to a support group for children with JRA/JIA

- **EXPECTED OUTCOME**

Child will express feelings and concerns about self-image and illness

> **NURSING DIAGNOSIS:** Risk for interrupted family processes related to a situational crisis (child with a chronic illness)

**PATIENT (FAMILY) GOAL 1:** Will receive adequate support as desired

- **NURSING INTERVENTIONS/*RATIONALES* AND EXPECTED OUTCOMES**

Refer family to special support group(s) and agencies

See also Nursing Care Plan: The Child with Chronic Illness or Disability, Chapter 22

---

the glomerular basement membrane with cellular infiltrates. Lupus nephritis is usually asymptomatic; consequently, it requires monitoring of urine and renal function to detect disease. A kidney biopsy is required for lupus nephritis classification. There are six classes depending on the type and extent of the renal lesion; specific treatment is based on the class of nephritis. Although there are improved outcomes for children with renal disease, the course is difficult to predict; some improve, and some remain the same or progress to renal failure requiring dialysis and transplant.

Neuropsychiatric lupus is another serious complication. Symptoms can be as subtle as inability to concentrate to frank psychosis and seizure. School performance and emotional stability should be assessed at each visit as possible indicators of lupus flare.

### Diagnostic Evaluation

SLE is a clinical diagnosis supported by specific laboratory abnormalities. The American College of Rheumatology criteria for the classification of SLE in adults has a sensitivity of 96% and a specificity of 96% if 4 of the 11 criteria are present (Box 39-17). The SLE workup includes an extensive history and physical examination with inquiry about school performance and behavior change. Initial laboratory tests include complete blood count with differential, comprehensive metabolic chemistry panel, microscopic urinalysis, antinuclear antibody, anti-DNA antibody, complement 3 (C3), complement 4 (C4), quantitative immunoglobulins, rapid plasma reagin (RPR), and lupus anticoagulant and antiphospholipid antibodies. A diagnosis of lupus should

> **Box 39-16**
> **Manifestations of Systemic Lupus Erythematosus**
>
> | | |
> |---|---|
> | Constitutional | Fever, fatigue, weight loss, anorexia |
> | Cutaneous | Erythematosus butterfly rash over bridge of nose and across cheeks, discoid rash, photosensitivity, mucocutaneous ulceration, alopecia, periungual telangiectasias |
> | Musculoskeletal | Arthritis, arthralgia, myositis, myalgia, tenosynovitis |
> | Neurologic | Headache, seizure, forgetfulness, behavior change, change in school performance, psychosis, chorea, stroke, cranial and peripheral neuropathy, pseudotumor cerebri |
> | Lung and heart | Pleuritis, basilar pneumonitis, atelectasis, pericarditis, myocarditis, and endocarditis |
> | Kidneys | Glomerulonephritis, nephrotic syndrome, hypertension |
> | Gastrointestinal | Abdominal pain, nausea, vomiting, blood in stool, abdominal crisis, esophageal dysfunction, colitis |
> | Liver, spleen, and nodes | Hepatomegaly, splenomegaly, lymphadenopathy |
> | Blood | Anemia, cytopenia |
> | Eyes | Cotton wool spots, papilledema, retinopathy |
> | Vascular | Raynaud phenomenon, thrombophlebitis, livedo reticularis |

not be made without consideration of all medications being taken and their side effects. Some commonly used drugs such as procainamide, hydralazine, and chloropromazine can cause lupus-like symptoms (Thompson, 2000).

---

**Box 39-17** ■ ■ ■

### Classification Criteria of Systemic Lupus Erythematosus*

1. Malar rash: fixed malar erythema
2. Discoid rash: patchy erythematous lesions
3. Photosensitivity: rash with sunlight exposure
4. Oral ulcers: painless ulcers in mouth/nose
5. Arthritis: swelling, tenderness, or effusion in two or more peripheral joints (nonerosive)
6. Serositis: pleuritis/pericarditis
7. Renal disorder: proteinuria/casts
8. Neurologic disorder: psychosis/seizures
9. Hematologic disorder: hemolytic anemia, thrombocytopenia, leukopenia, lymphopenia
10. Immunologic disorder: anti-dsDNA, anti-Sm, antiphospholipid antibodies, lupus anticoagulant, false-positive syphilis test (RPR)
11. Antinuclear antibody

---

*Requires four criteria for classification.

---

## Therapeutic Management

There is no cure for SLE; the management goal is to reverse or minimize disease activity with appropriate medications while helping the child and family cope with the complications of the disease and treatment.

**Medications.** Since the 1950s, corticosteroids have been the mainstay of SLE therapy. They are effective antiinflammatory and immunosuppressive agents. Unfortunately, the effectiveness of steroids is hampered by side effects, which include growth delay, decreased resistance to infection, osteoporosis, weight gain, hypertension, cushingoid features, cataract, and diabetes risks. Generally a dose sufficient to control symptoms is prescribed and then tapered to the lowest dose possible to balance acceptable disease activity relative to steroid side effects. For severe disease IV pulse (high-dose) steroids are given on an intermittent schedule, which may allow reduction in the daily steroid dose with better compliance and less cushingoid features (Klein-Gitelman and Pachman, 1998). Topical steroids are used for cutaneous lesions, but prolonged therapy will thin the skin; consequently facial application needs to be brief or with lower concentration. Because of increased immunosuppression, tuberculin skin test should be applied before starting steroids, especially in high-risk communities. A medical identification tag needs to be worn by children on chronic steroids so that administration of stress steroids can be considered in emergency situations.

Other medications include NSAIDs such as naproxen and ibuprofen for pain associated with arthritis, arthralgia, and myalgia. Nurses need to instruct patients to take NSAIDs with food to help prevent GI side effects. Hydroxychloroquine, an antimalarial drug, is an effective therapy for skin and joint manifestations. Possible untoward effects include skin, GI, and retinal toxicity. A complete ophthalmologic examination is indicated before treatment and every 6 months. Cyclophosphamide, a potent immunosuppressive agent, used in combination with corticosteroids is effective in treating proliferative lupus nephritis and neuropsychiatric lupus. A detailed cyclophosphamide education session for patient and family needs to clearly state potential benefits and risks, including infertility and future malignancy.

**Education, Diet, Rest, and Exercise.** In addition to medication, treatment includes general measures such as patient and family education, rest and exercise, diet, sun avoidance, and social support. SLE is complex and requires ongoing patient education. Families and patients need up-to-date, understandable information to become informed decision makers so they can participate in disease management. Nurses are duty-bound to discuss information families bring to appointments from the Internet, friends, and family. As health care providers critically evaluate disease information with families, families are taught the skills needed to become self-advocates. Families also want to hear about the impact of SLE on growth and development, childbearing, school, and vocation. The message should be optimistic and clear with few exceptions: "Prepare for the future—you will attend school, graduate, have children, and work."

Diet, exercise, and rest are the daily activities under direct patient control. The family needs to maximize the power of these normal functions to their benefit. There is no specific SLE diet, but a balanced diet without exceeding calorie expenditure is essential for maintaining appropriate weight on corticosteroids. A low-salt diet may be required if the patient becomes nephrotic or hypertensive. A consultation with a registered dietitian will help the family develop an individualized diet that meshes with their lifestyle.

The benefits of a regular exercise program include weight maintenance, cardiovascular fitness, and osteoporosis prevention, all of which will help minimize SLE complications and corticosteroid side effects. Additional rest is necessary during exacerbation but not to the extent that it interferes with regular sleep patterns.

Given the frequency of photosensitive rash, the dangers of excessive ultraviolet light exposure (including uncovered fluorescent lights) needs to be stressed. This can be a sensitive topic for sun-loving teenagers and outdoor athletes. Application of sunscreen (at least 15 SPF), hats, and protective clothing should be discussed. One rule useful to share with the adolescent who may be surrounded by peers who regularly seek out sun exposure is the "slip, slop, slap" rule: slip on a shirt, slop on sunscreen, and slap on a hat before going out in the sun. (See Chapter 18.) Scheduling outdoor activities in the morning and evening can reduce exposure without limiting participation in recreational activities. Every effort should be made to include children in peer activities and to make sun modifications as inconspicuous as possible.

Social support through family, friends, teachers, counselors, and professional social workers and therapists can help the child and family through difficult times and promote adaptation to an illness that is not going to go away. (See Critical Thinking Exercise box.) Destructive coping mechanisms need to be identified and replaced with behaviors that enhance adaptation and healthy outcomes. Organizations that can help children and families learn about and adjust to the disease are the **Lupus Foundation of America**\* and the **Arthritis Foundation**† (see p. 1824).

## Nursing Considerations

Fostering adaptation and self-advocacy is the primary nursing goal. Patient and family acceptance and understanding of this life-threatening and therapeutically intrusive disease is a big challenge for any nurse. Patient education is started at diagnosis and continued at every opportunity; repetition is good. Encourage the family to call with questions and concerns. Have patients write down their questions so they are prepared during the appointment. Consider adolescent development, with heightened concerns about body image and looking different. Be open about this. Discuss skin care, cosmetics, and unobtrusive moisturizers with sunscreen and sunblock.

Weight gain is an emotional issue, and it has to be met honestly with a workable plan for family dietary changes and a realistic exercise program. Work with a dietitian and a trainer or physical therapist to individualize a nutrition and fitness program for the child. Involve a parent or sibling in the program, so the child does not feel restrictions are punitive.

Sexual activity and birth control needs to be discussed, especially since pregnancy is a potential trigger for disease flare. Honest discussion about healthy, responsible reproductive choices with both the teenager and parent is important for establishing communication; let the parents and teen know the teen can come to you with reproductive concerns. Because estrogen can trigger disease flare, low-dose estrogen or progestin-only oral contraceptives are preferred. Some teens will choose the compliance-friendly Depo-Provera 3-month injections. Again, frank discussion about risks and benefits is essential.

Prevention of infection includes handwashing (especially at school) and preprocedure antibiotic coverage for routine events such as dental cleaning. To compensate for the side effects of some drugs such as the corticosteroids, teenagers will often go on fad or starvation diets. It is critical that nutritional counseling be available to ensure that the adolescent understands the role that a healthy diet plays in the

---

\*1300 Piccard Dr, Suite 200, Rockville, MD 20850-4303, (301) 670-9292 or (800) 558-0121, fax: (301) 670-9486; www.lupus.org.
†A recommended booklet available from the Arthritis Foundation is *Meeting the Challenge: A Young Person's Guide to Living with Lupus.*

### Critical Thinking Exercise

#### *Lupus and Behavior*

A mother reports that her 10-year-old daughter, who has been diagnosed with lupus, has lost interest in activities with friends. You suspect which of the following causes?

FIRST, THINK ABOUT IT . . .
• What information are you using?
• What conclusions are you coming to?

1. Depression about the disorder
2. Physical fatigue
3. Medication side effects
4. Central nervous system involvement

*The correct answer is all of the choices. A chronic illness that affects body image and may have a poor prognosis can have psychologic ramifications for a child. At the same time, lupus takes a toll physically, especially during exacerbations; steroids used in treatment can cause mood and behavior changes; and central nervous system involvement can affect behavior. A thorough medical and psychiatric workup would be appropriate.*

management of SLE. School attendance may decrease from loss of self-esteem, depression, feelings of inadequacy, or poor physical performance (Thompson, 2000).

Treatment compliance is a significant issue in adolescence, especially given the medication side effects and restrictions on sun exposure. Adolescents need to understand the function of each drug, how each drug helps to manage the disease, and what effect missing doses may have on their health. The nurse needs to keep track of prescription refills to evaluate compliance and medication efficacy. Investigate barriers to medication compliance and help patients devise a workable plan. If friends are going to the beach, consider going late in the day with a beach umbrella, sunblock, a wide-brim hat, instructions for reapplying sunblock after swimming, and limiting time in direct sun. (See Chapter 18.) Remember, teaching patients how to find ways to positively adapt to SLE with normal growth and development as the goal will give them self-advocacy skills. Nurses are encouraged to apply the principles of adjusting to a chronic illness that are discussed in Chapter 22.

## KEY POINTS

- Trauma is the leading cause of death in children and is caused by accidental injury, child abuse injury, and birth injuries.
- Immobility has a profound effect on all elements of growth and development.
- The major consequences of immobilization are loss of muscle strength, endurance, and muscle mass; bone

demineralization leading to osteoporosis; loss of joint mobility; and contractures.
- In the care of the immobilized child, nurses are concerned with position changes, adequate dietary intake, adequate hydration, promotion of activity, and involvement of the child in self-care.

■ Features of children's fractures not observed in the adult include presence of a growth plate, a thicker and stronger periosteum, porosity of bone, more rapid healing, and less stiffness.

■ Types of fractures seen in children are bends, buckle, greenstick, and complete.

■ Goals of fracture management in children are to regain alignment and length of the bony fragments, retain alignment and length, and restore function to injured parts.

■ The method of fracture reduction is determined by the age of the child, the degree of displacement, the amount of overriding bone, the amount of edema, the condition of the skin and soft tissues, sensation, and circulation distal to the fracture.

■ The primary purposes of traction are to fatigue involved muscle and reduce muscle spasm, to position bone ends in desired realignment, and to immobilize the fracture site until realignment has been achieved to permit casting or splinting.

■ Complications of fractures are circulatory impairment, nerve compression syndromes, compartment syndromes, epiphyseal damage, nonunion, malunion, infection, kidney stones, and pulmonary emboli.

■ Participation in sports predisposes adolescents to acute injuries, such as contusions, dislocations, sprains, and strains; and overuse syndromes, such as stress fractures.

■ Health concerns associated with sports include menstrual dysfunction, drug misuse, and sudden death.

■ Musculoskeletal disorders in childhood include torticollis, Legg-Calvé-Perthes disease, slipped femoral capital epiphyses, kyphosis and lordosis, and scoliosis.

■ Observation for scoliosis is an important part of a routine physical assessment.

■ Management of scoliosis includes bracing or surgery.

■ Postoperative nursing care of the child with scoliosis demands careful attention to peripheral neurovascular function, respiratory function, pain control, and skin care.

■ Nursing care of the child with osteomyelitis is directed at positioning for comfort, administration of antibiotics, monitoring intravenous equipment and site, and nutrition.

■ Osteomyelitis is acquired by direct or secondary invasion or hematogenous spread of infectious organisms.

■ Goals of therapy for arthritis in children are to preserve joint function, prevent physical deformities, and relieve symptoms without iatrogenic harm.

■ Nursing care of the child with arthritis consists of promoting general health, relieving discomfort, preventing deformity, and preserving function.

■ Systemic lupus erythematosus is a chronic autoimmune disorder that can affect the collagen tissues of the body.

# REFERENCES

American Academy of Pediatrics, Committee on Injury and Poison Prevention: Drowning in infants, children, and adolescents, *Pediatrics* 92(2):292-294, 1993a.

American Academy of Pediatrics, Committee on Injury and Poison Prevention and Committee on Sports Medicine and Fitness: Trampolines at home, school, and recreational centers, *Pediatrics* 103(5):1053-1056, 1999.

American Academy of Pediatrics, Committee on Sports Medicine and Fitness: Climatic heat stress and the exercising child and adolescent, *Pediatrics* 106(1):158-159, 2000a.

American Academy of Pediatrics, Committee on Sports Medicine and Fitness: Medical concerns in the female athlete, *Pediatrics* 106(3):610-613, 2000b.

American Academy of Pediatrics, Committee on Sports Medicine and Fitness: Medical conditions affecting sports participation, *Pediatrics* 107(5):1205-1209, 2001.

American Academy of Pediatrics, Section on Rheumatology and Section on Ophthalmology: Guidelines for ophthalmologic examinations in children with juvenile rheumatoid arthritis, *Pediatrics* 92(2):295-296, 1993b.

Aronsson DD, Loder RT: Treatment of the unstable (acute) slipped capital femoral epiphysis, *Clin Orthop* 322(1):99-110, 1996.

Ballock RT, Song KM: The prevalence of nonmuscular causes of torticollis in children, *J Pediatr Orthop* 16(4):500-504, 1996.

Baltes-Messner J and others: Pediatric sedation: the art and science, *Orthop Nurs* 18(5):35-49, 1999.

Bass JL and others: Childhood injury prevention counseling in primary care settings: a critical review of the literature, *Pediatrics* 92(4):544-550, 1993.

Bercher DL and others: Pediatric injuries resulting from use of all-terrain vehicles, *J Ark Med Soc* 97(10):351-353, 2001.

Bernardo LM: Evidence-based practice for pin site care in injured children, *Orthop Nurs* 20(5):29-34, 2001.

Binder H and others: Comprehensive rehabilitation of the child with osteogenesis imperfecta, *Am J Med Genet* 45(2):265-269, 1993.

Brewer EJ and others: Current proposed revision of JRA criteria, *Arthritis Rheum* 20(suppl 2):195-199, 1977.

Brown PG, Lee M: Trampoline injuries of the cervical spine, *Pediatr Neurosurg* 32(4): 170-175, 2000.

Burg FD and others: *Gellis and Kagan's current pediatric therapy*, ed 16, Philadelphia, 1998, WB Saunders.

Callahan L: The evolution of the female athlete: progress and problems, *Pediatr Ann* 29(3):149-153, 2000.

Cheng T and others: Sports injuries: an important cause of morbidity in urban youth, *Pediatrics* 105(3):e32, 2000.

Cohen LR and others: Pediatric injury prevention counseling priorities, *Pediatrics* 99(5):704-710, 1997.

Cramer KE: The pediatric polytrauma patient, *Clin Orthop* 318(9):125-135, 1995.

Crawley T: Childhood injury: significance and prevention strategies, *J Pediatr Nurs* 11(4):225-232, 1996.

Della-Giustina K, Della-Giustina DA: Orthopedic emergencies: emergency department evaluation and treatment of pediatric orthopedic injuries, *Emerg Med Clin North Am* 17(4):895-922, 1999.

Emery HM, Miller ML: *Ambulatory pediatric care*, ed 2, Philadelphia, 1993, JB Lippincott.

Forlino A, Marini JC: Osteogenesis imperfecta: prospects for molecular therapeutics, *Mol Genet Metab* 71(1-2):225-232, 2000.

Glorieux FH: Bisphosphonate therapy for severe osteogenesis imperfecta, *J Pediatr Endocrinol Metab* 2(suppl 13):989-992, 2000.

Greiner KA: Adolescent idiopathic scoliosis: radiologic decision-making, *Am Fam Physician* 65(9):1817-1822, 2002.

Grisoni E and others: The new injury severity score and the evaluation of pediatric trauma, *J Trauma* 50(6):1106-1110, 2001.

Guyer B and others: Annual summary of vital statistics: trends in the health of Americans during the 20th century, *Pediatrics* 106(6): 1307-1317, 2000.

Harvey C: Compartment syndrome: when it is least expected, *Orthop Nurs* 20(3):15-23, 2001.

Helmkamp JC: Injuries and deaths and the use of all-terrain vehicles, *N Engl J Med* 343(23):1733-1734, 2000 (letter).

Herring J: The treatment of Legg-Calvé-Perthes disease: a critical review of the literature, *J Bone Joint Surg Am* 76(3):448-458, 1994.

Horn DB and others: Pain severity and analgesia in upper extremity fractures, *Pediatrics* 100(3, suppl pt 2):487, 1997.

Horwitz EM and others: Clinical responses to bone marrow transplantation in children with severe osteogenesis imperfecta, *Blood* 97(5):1227-1231, 2001.

Johnston BD and others: A preschool program for safety and injury prevention delivered by home visitors, *Inj Prev* 6(4):305-309, 2000.

Kerr KL, Jarvis JN: *Cost-effectiveness of EMLA vs oral midazolam for analgesia during pediatric arthrocentesis.* Poster presentation at sixth annual meeting of the Society of Pediatric Nurses national conference, Chicago, IL, April 24-25, 1996.

Killian JT, Wilkinson D, Dulaney P: Application and care of the modified hip spica, *South Orthop J* 1(6):333-335, 1995.

Klein-Gitelman MS, Pachman LM: Intravenous corticosteroids: adverse reactions are more variable than expected in children, *J Rheumatol* 25(10):1995-2002, 1998.

Lang BA, Finlayson LA: Naproxen-induced pseudoprophyria in patients with JRA, *J Pediatr* 24(4):639-642, 1994.

Loder RT: Slipped capital femoral epiphysis, *Am Fam Physician* 59(9):2135-2142, 1998.

Lovell DJ and others: Etanercept in children with polyarticular juvenile rheumatoid arthritis: Pediatric Rheumatology Collaborative Study Group, *N Engl J Med* 342(11):810-811, 2000.

Malleson P, Fung M, Rosenberg A: The incidence of pediatric rheumatic diseases: results from the Canadian Pediatric Rheumatology Association Disease Registry, *J Rheumatol* 23(11):1981-1987, 1996.

McCarty EC and others: Anesthesia and analgesia for the ambulatory management of fractures in children, *J Am Acad Orthop Surg* 7(2):81-91, 1999.

McKenzie L: In search of a standard for pin site care, *Orthop Nurs* 18(2):73-78, 1999.

Nuss KE, Dietrich AN, Smith GA: Effectiveness of a pediatric trauma team protocol, *Pediatr Emerg Care* 17(2):96-100, 2001.

Osiri M, Moreland LW: Specific cyclooxygenase 2 inhibitors: a new choice of nonsteroidal anti-inflammatory drug therapy, *Arthritis Care Res* 12(5):351-362, 1999.

Patterson MM: Prevention: the only cure for pediatric trauma, *Orthop Nurs* 18(4):16-20, 1999.

Peltola H, Kallio M, Unkila-Kallio L: Reduced incidence of septic arthritis in children by *Haemophilus influenzae* type-b vaccination, *J Bone Joint Surg Br* 80(3):471-473, 1998.

Petty RE and others: Revision of the proposed classification criteria for juvenile idiopathic arthritis: Durban, 1997, *J Rheumatol* 25(10):1991-1994, 1998.

Poussa M and others: Conservative vs operative treatment in Perthes' disease, *Clin Orthop* 297(1):82-86, 1993.

Purdy KS and others: You are what you eat: healthy food choices, nutrition, and the child with juvenile rheumatoid arthritis, *Pediatr Nurs* 22(5):391-398, 1996.

Rang M: Musculoskeletal Q & A: management of Legg-Calvé-Perthes disease varies with severity, *J Musculoskel Med* 13(4):10-11, 1996.

Rice MR, Alvanos L, Kenney B: Snowmobile injuries and deaths in children: a review of national injury data and state legislation, *Pediatrics* 105(3, pt 1):615-619, 2000.

Rivara F: Injury control: issues and methods for the 1990's, *Pediatr Ann* 21(7):411-413, 1992.

Rodts MF: Disorders of the spine. In Maher AB, Salmond SW, Pellino TA, editors: *Orthopaedic nursing*, ed 2, Philadelphia, 1998, WB Saunders.

Roy D: Current concepts in Legg-Calvé-Perthes disease, *Pediatr Ann* 28(12):748-751, 1999.

Ryan-Krause P: The score on high-tech sports nutrition for adolescents, *J Pediatr Health Care* 12(3):164-166, 1998.

Samson CM and others: Methotrexate therapy for chronic noninfectious uveitis: analysis of a case series of 160 patients, *Ophthalmology* 108(6):1134-1139, 2001.

Saperstein AL, Nicholas SJ: Pediatric and adolescent sports medicine, *Pediatr Clin North Am* 43(5):1013-1033, 1996.

Scheidt PC and others: Child and adolescent injury research in 1998: a summary of abstracts submitted to the Ambulatory Pediatrics Association and the American Public Health Association, *Arch Pediatr Adolesc Med* 154(5):442-445, 2000.

Spencer CH, Fife RZ, Rabinovich CE: The school experience of children with arthritis, *Pediatr Clin North Am* 42(5):1285-1298, 1995.

Steen SC: Timely statement of the American Dietetic Association: nutrition guidance for adolescent athletes in organized sports, *J Am Diet Assoc* 96(5):611-612, 1996.

Stevens B and others: Evaluation of a home-based traction program for children with congenital dislocated hips and Legg Perthes disease, *Can J Nurs Res* 27(40):133-150, 1995.

Thompson DC, Rivara FP: Pool fencing for preventing drowning in children, *Cochrane Database Syst Rev* CD001047, 2000.

Thompson K: Lupus and the adolescent, *Am J Nurs* 100(1):24A-24D, 2000.

Topp R and others: The effects of bed rest and potential of prehabilitation on patients in the intensive care unit, *AACN Clin Issues* 13(2):263-276, 2002.

Tsao BP, Wallace DJ: Genetics of systemic lupus erythematosus, *Curr Opin Rheumatol* 9(5):377-379, 1997.

Warren RW and others: Juvenile idiopathic arthritis (juvenile rheumatoid arthritis). In Koopman WJ, editor: *Arthritis and allied conditions*, Philadelphia, 2001, Lippincott Williams & Wilkins.

Weiss AH, Wallace CA, Shery DD: Methotrexate for resistant chronic uveitis in children with juvenile rheumatoid arthritis, *J Pediatr* 133(2):266-280, 1998.

Wong DL, Baker C: Pain in children: comparison of assessment scales, *Pediatr Nurs* 14(1):9-17, 1988.

Yawn BP and others: A population-based study of school scoliosis screening, *JAMA* 282(15):1427-1432, 1999.

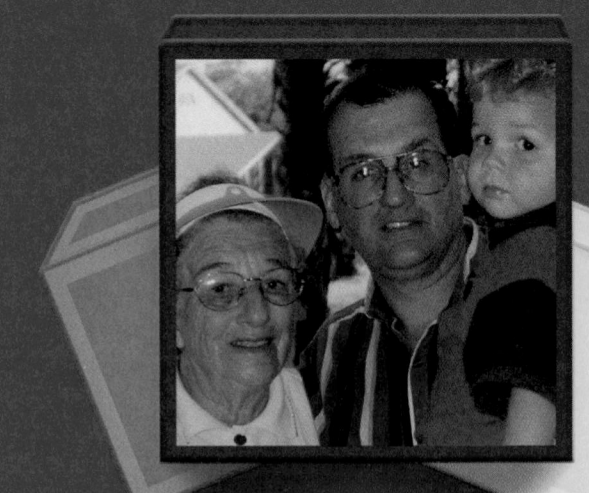

# Chapter 40

# The Child with Neuromuscular or Muscular Dysfunction

## Chapter Outline

**NEUROMUSCULAR DYSFUNCTION, 1832**
**Classification and Diagnosis, 1833**
   Classification, 1832
   Diagnostic Tools, 1834
**Cerebral Palsy (CP), 1834**
*Nursing Care Plan: The Child with Cerebral Palsy, 1844*
**Hypotonia, 1843**
**Infantile Spinal Muscular Atrophy (SMA) (Werdnig-Hoffmann Disease), 1846**

**Juvenile Spinal Muscular Atrophy (Kugelberg-Welander Syndrome), 1846**
**Guillain-Barré Syndrome (GBS) (Infectious Polyneuritis), 1847**
**Tetanus, 1848**
**Botulism, 1850**
**Myasthenia Gravis (MG), 1851**
   Neonatal Myasthenia Gravis, 1852

**Spinal Cord Injuries, 1852**
   Review of Essential Neuromuscular Physiology, 1852
**MUSCULAR DYSFUNCTION, 1863**
**Juvenile Dermatomyositis, 1863**
**Muscular Dystrophies (MDs), 1864**
**Pseudohypertrophic (Duchenne) Muscular Dystrophy (DMD), 1864**

## Related Topics

The Child with Cerebral Dysfunction, Ch. 37
The Child with Cognitive, Sensory, or Communication Impairment, Ch. 24
Family-Centered Care of the Child with Chronic Illness or Disability, Ch. 22

Family-Centered Home Care, Ch. 25
Genetic Evaluation and Counseling, Ch. 5
The Immobilized Child, Ch. 39
Immunizations (Tetanus), Ch. 12

Myelomeningocele (Meningomyelocele), Ch. 11
Neurologic Assessment, Chs. 7 and 8

## NEUROMUSCULAR DYSFUNCTION

Weakness or abnormal performance of skeletal muscle may represent a defect in the muscle itself or reflect a pathologic disorder at some point along the neural pathway from the cortex of the brain to the neuromuscular junction. The identification of the source of muscle dysfunction includes not only the testing of muscle function but also the systematic elimination of possible disorders of neural structures on which muscle function depends for its stimulus. In a few disorders muscle disease may be accompanied by a neural disorder.

Some clinical features are shared by muscle disease *(myopathy),* which differs in many ways from muscle dysfunction resulting from disorders of neuronal structures—brain, cranial nerve nuclei, long nerve tracts, anterior horn cells of

the spinal cord, and peripheral nerves. Motor function is accomplished by means of the simple reflex arcs or by way of impulses transmitted from the cerebral cortex and other centers in the brain through the various nerve pathways of the central nervous system (CNS). The *upper motor neurons* consist of cells that lie in the cerebral cortex and fibers that traverse the brainstem and spinal cord to terminate at their synapses with the anterior horn cells. The anterior horn cells, axons, and peripheral nerve branches constitute the *lower motor neurons.* The *motor unit* consists of the lower motor neuron, the neuromuscular junction, and the muscle fibers it supplies (Fig. 40-1). The upper motor neuronal pathways from the cerebrum to the lower motor neuron are described as (1) *pyramidal*—those whose fibers extend from the cortex, come together in the medulla, cross from one side to the other, then extend down the cord to synapse with anterior horn motor neurons; and (2) *extrapyramidal*—a complex network of motor neurons that comprise relays be-

---

■ David Wilson, MS, RNC, revised this chapter.

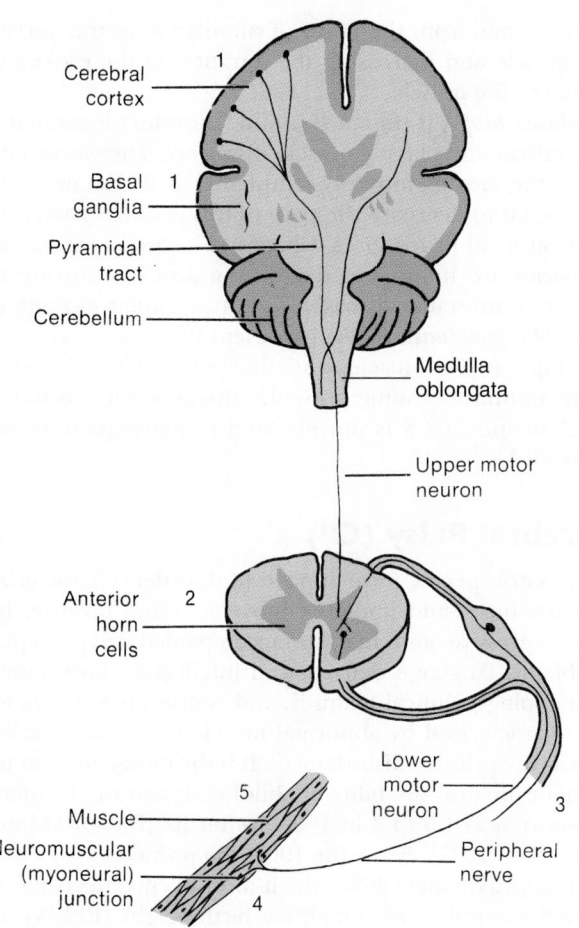

**Fig. 40-1** Site of origin for neuromuscular disorders. *1,* Cerebral palsy; *2,* poliomyelitis, spinal muscular atrophy; *3,* mononeuropathies, polyneuropathies; *4,* myasthenia gravis, neurotoxic disorders; *5,* muscular dystrophies.

tween motor areas of the cortex, basal ganglia, thalamus, cerebellum, and brainstem.

## Classification and Diagnosis

The site of pathologic disturbance determines the type of muscular dysfunction. In general, *upper motor neuron lesions* produce weakness associated with spasticity, increased deep tendon reflexes, and abnormal superficial reflexes. The primary disorder of upper motor neuron dysfunction is cerebral palsy. *Lower motor neuron lesions* interrupt the reflex arc, causing weakness and atrophy of the skeletal muscles involved with associated hypotonia or flaccidity, which eventually progress to atrophy with varying degrees of contracture deformity. A disorder of the extrapyramidal pathway and the cerebellum rarely produces muscle weakness.

Lower motor neuron involvement is usually symmetric (except that of poliomyelitis and single peripheral nerve disease), whereas disorders of the pyramidal tract are more often asymmetric. Muscle wasting is characteristic of lower motor neuron lesions and more marked than in diseases of muscles. Deep tendon reflexes are briskly active in upper

motor neuron disease, are diminished or absent in lower motor neuron disease, and depend on the progress of muscle degeneration in the myopathies.

These disorders can also be categorized according to onset: those in which there is acute onset of flaccid paralysis and those with more gradual onset and progressive degeneration. In most instances the sudden appearance of flaccid paralysis in a previously healthy child can be attributed to an infectious process. Neurotoxins (e.g., botulism, tick paralysis, or heavy metal poisoning), pressure on the spinal cord from tumors or abscesses, and spinal cord injury (SCI) are less likely causes. Hereditary factors and metabolic disease are more often responsible for muscular weakness and atrophy of gradual onset.

### Classification

The most useful classification of neuromuscular disorders is one that defines the site of origin of the pathologic lesion: the anterior horn cells of the spinal cord, the peripheral nerves, the myoneural junction, and the muscles.

**Diseases of Anterior Horn Cells.** Diseases and disorders that affect the anterior horn cells are the result of destruction or atrophy of the anterior horn of the spinal column along with the inability to transfer impulses from sensory neurons to motor neurons. Enteroviruses, which have a worldwide distribution, are prominent etiologic agents that selectively affect anterior horn cells. These include the polioviruses, of which there are three types: coxsackieviruses, groups A and B, and the enterocytopathogenic human orphan (ECHO) viruses. Degeneration of the anterior horn cells is caused by inherited disorders, primarily the spinal muscular atrophies.

**Neuropathies.** Disorders affecting peripheral nerves may be *mononeuropathies,* which involve a single nerve and the muscles it innervates, or *polyneuropathies,* which involve multiple nerves and the muscles they supply. Neuropathies are caused by a number of hereditary diseases, traumatic injuries, infections, poisons, and (secondarily) some metabolic diseases. Polyneuropathy can be restricted to specific areas (as in diabetes mellitus); some hereditary diseases involve skeletal muscles extensively. The distal limbs (feet and hands) are usually affected first, with gait disturbance and footdrop being early manifestations. The involvement gradually progresses medially as the disorder becomes more severe.

In some polyneuropathies there is segmented or patchy loss of the myelin sheath of nerve fibers; in others the primary process appears to be progressive degeneration of nerve fibers. Examples of acute and chronic polyneuropathies are infectious polyneuritis and peroneal atrophy, respectively.

**Neuromuscular Junction Disease.** Disorders involving a neurohormonal deficiency interfere with transmission of nerve impulses to muscles at the neuromuscular junction. Normally nerve impulses are transmitted to skeletal muscles across the neuromuscular junction by acetylcholine. This is accomplished in three steps: (1) acetylcholine is released from vesicles in the terminal nerve endings; (2) it then diffuses across the junction and contacts receptor sites in the muscle membrane, stimulating the muscle to contract; and (3) it is removed by the action of cholinesterase. Interference at any of these three steps will block transmission of nerve impulses and prevent muscular contraction.

Several toxic substances act at the myoneural junction to inhibit nerve impulses to the skeletal muscles. Examples of toxins that prevent the release of acetylcholine are those that produce the paralysis of botulism and tick paralysis. Action at receptor sites is also blocked by the drug curare. Paralysis resulting from inhibition of cholinesterase release is caused by poisoning with organic phosphate insecticides.

**Diseases of Muscles.** Diseases of skeletal muscles can be inflammatory (such as polymyositis), the result of endocrine dysfunction (such as hypothyroidism and hyperthyroidism), or the result of congenital defects (e.g., absence of muscle, periodic paralysis, and the various muscular dystrophies and myotonias). Inflammation occurs in a number of infectious illnesses such as trichinosis, toxoplasmosis, and those caused by the coxsackieviruses.

## Diagnostic Tools

Several general diagnostic tools are used to aid in differentiating between diseases with similar manifestations. In addition, a number of more definitive tests are used to establish a specific diagnosis. The neurologic examination is a basic test that helps to assess the extent of motor and sensory function.

The *electromyogram (EMG)* measures the electric potentials generated in individual muscles. A small metal disk is placed on the skin overlying the muscle to be tested, or a sterile needle electrode is inserted directly into the muscle. The electric activity generated in the skeletal muscles is measured at rest, with slight voluntary contraction, and with maximum contraction. The electric activity is amplified and displayed on a cathode ray oscilloscope. Needle electrodes are sensitive enough to pick up the activity of a single muscle fiber; thus this is usually the method of choice. However, the procedure is traumatic for children. It is often not useful because it requires cooperation. EMLA (eutectic mixture of local anesthetics) applied to the EMG sites can decrease the amount of pain.

*Nerve conduction velocity,* or the velocity of electric impulse conduction along motor or sensory nerves, is often measured in conjunction with electromyography. Certain diseases affect the peripheral nerves, prolonging the conduction time from the point of stimulation of the nerve to the muscle and increasing the duration of the evoked potential of the muscle.

*Muscle biopsy* is the most useful laboratory examination to confirm and classify muscle disorders. The vastus lateralis is the most commonly sampled muscle. Ketamine has been used to decrease the pain of this invasive procedure. (See Surgical Procedures, Chapter 27). *Serum enzyme measurements* are helpful in diagnosing and monitoring the course of muscular disease. The intracellular enzyme *creatine phosphokinase (CPK)* is present in muscle tissues, including cardiac muscle, and the brain; it is released in large amounts in some muscular diseases, such as muscular dystrophy. CPK is not elevated in neurogenic disease (Box 40-1).

## Cerebral Palsy (CP)

CP is a nonspecific term applied to disorders characterized by early onset and impaired movement and posture. It is nonprogressive and may be accompanied by perceptual problems, language deficits, and intellectual involvement. The etiology, clinical features, and course are variable and are characterized by abnormal muscle tone and coordination as the primary disturbances. It is the most common permanent physical disability of childhood, and the incidence is reported as 1.5 to 3 in 1000 live births (Dabney, Lipton, and Miller, 1997). Since the 1960s the prevalence of CP has risen approximately 20%, which most likely reflects the improved survival of extremely-low-birth-weight (ELBW) and very-low-birth-weight (VLBW) infants.

### Etiology

A variety of prenatal, perinatal, and postnatal factors contribute, either singly or multifactorially, to the etiology of CP (Table 40-1). Although the prevalent hypothesis has

---

**Box 40-1** ■ ■ ■
**Serum Enzyme Measurements**

**Creatine phosphokinase (CPK)**—Found in skeletal muscle and a few other organs and elevated in skeletal muscle disease; the most specific test
**Aldolase**—Present in skeletal and heart muscle and significantly elevated in muscle damage
**Serum glutamic-oxaloacetic transaminase (SGOT),** now referred to as **aspartate aminotransferase (AST)**—Elevated in muscle disease but has wider distribution in organs
**Lactate dehydrogenase (LDH)**—Elevated in muscle disease but has wider distribution

---

**TABLE 40-1** Causes of cerebral palsy

| Time (% of cases) | Causes |
|---|---|
| **Prenatal** (44%) | |
| First trimester | Teratogens |
| | Genetic syndromes |
| | Chromosomal abnormalities |
| | Brain malformations |
| Second-third trimester | Intrauterine infections |
| | Problems in fetal/placental functioning |
| **Labor and delivery** (19%) | Preeclampsia |
| | Complications of labor and delivery |
| **Perinatal** (8%) | Sepsis/CNS infection |
| | Asphyxia |
| | Prematurity |
| **Childhood** (5%) | Meningitis |
| | Traumatic brain injury |
| | Toxins |
| **Not obvious** (24%) | |

From Eicher PS, Batshaw ML: Cerebral palsy, *Pediatr Clin North Am* 40(3):540, 1993.

been that CP results from perinatal problems, especially birth asphyxia, it is now known that CP results more commonly from either existing perinatal brain abnormalities or postnatal injury. It is reported that 12% to 23% of CP is related to intrapartum asphyxia in term infants (Volpe, 2001). Intrauterine exposure to maternal infection is associated with an increased risk of CP in infants of normal birth weight (Volpe, 2001). A retrospective study found that the prevalence of CP was 12% in infants born less than 36 weeks gestation and less than 2000 g; the strongest independent risk factor for development of CP was periventricular leukomalacia (Han and others, 2002). In many cases of CP no identifiable immediate cause is found. Preterm birth of ELBW and VLBW infants is considered the single most important determinant.

## Pathophysiology

It is difficult to establish a precise location of neurologic lesions on the basis of etiology or clinical signs because there is no characteristic pathologic picture. In some cases there are gross malformations of the brain. In others there may be evidence of vascular occlusion, atrophy, loss of neurons, and laminar degeneration that produces narrower gyri, wider sulci, and low brain weight. *Anoxia* plays the most significant role in the pathologic state of brain damage, which is often secondary to other causative mechanisms.

There are a few exceptions. In some cases the manifestations or etiology can be related to anatomic areas. For example, CP associated with prematurity is usually spastic diplegia caused by hypoxic infarction or hemorrhage in the area adjacent to the lateral ventricles. In the athetoid type of CP, which is caused by kernicterus and severe hemolytic disease of the newborn, there are pigment deposits in the basal ganglia and some cranial nerve nuclei. Hemiparetic CP is often associated with mechanical trauma to the cortex

or with cerebrovascular accident of the middle cerebral artery. Cerebral hypoplasia and, sometimes, severe neonatal hypoglycemia are related to ataxic CP. Generalized cortical and cerebral atrophy have been shown to cause severe quadriparesis with mental retardation and microcephaly.

## Clinical Classification

CP has been classified in several ways, but the most useful classification is based on the nature and distribution of neuromuscular dysfunction (Box 40-2). The most common clinical type, spastic CP, represents an upper motor neuron muscular weakness. The reflex arc is intact, and the characteristic physical signs are increased stretch reflexes, increased muscle tone, and (often) weakness. Early neurologic manifestations are usually generalized hypotonia or decreased tone that lasts for a few weeks or may extend for months or even as long as a year. See Box 40-3 for types of spastic CP.

## Clinical Manifestations

The alert observer may suspect CP when a child demonstrates some of the following groups of manifestations (Box 40-4).

---

**Box 40-2** ■ ■ ■
**Clinical Classification of Cerebral Palsy**

**Spastic**—May involve one or both sides
  Hypertonicity with poor control of posture, balance, and coordinated motion
  Impairment of fine and gross motor skills
  Active attempts at motion increase abnormal postures and overflow of movement to other parts of the body
**Dyskinetic/athetoid**—Abnormal involuntary movement
  Athetosis, characterized by slow, wormlike, writhing movements that usually involve the extremities, trunk, neck, facial muscles, and tongue
  Involvement of the pharyngeal, laryngeal, and oral muscles causes drooling and dysarthria (imperfect speech articulation)
  Involuntary movements may take on choreoid (involuntary, irregular, jerking movements) and dystonic (disordered muscle tone) manifestations that increase in intensity with emotional stress and around adolescence
**Ataxic**
  Wide-based gait
  Rapid, repetitive movements performed poorly
  Disintegration of movements of the upper extremities when the child reaches for objects
**Mixed type/dystonic**—Combination of spasticity and athetosis

---

**Box 40-3** ■ ■ ■
**Types of Spastic Cerebral Palsy**

**Hemiparesis**—One side of body affected
  Most common form of spastic cerebral palsy
  Motor deficit usually greater in upper extremity; most children able to walk; underdevelopment of affected limbs
  Pattern of spasticity
    *Leg*—Increased tone of calf, hamstring, and hip adductor muscles
    *Gait*—Walk with foot inverted and plantar flexed, knee flexed, and leg adducted
    *Arm*—Increased tone in shoulder adductor and internal rotator muscles, elbow flexor and pronator muscles, and wrist and finger flexor muscles
    *Parietal lobe syndrome*—Impairment of cortical sensory function (absence or inability to recognize size, shape, or texture of objects held in affected hand); impaired two-point discrimination and position sense
**Quadriparesis**—or **tetraparesis**—All four extremities involved, lower affected more than upper limbs
  Highest incidence of severe disability
  One fourth only mildly affected with minimum functional limitations on ambulation, self-care, and other activities; one half moderately impaired and impeded in self-care and independence in a sheltered situation; and one fourth severely damaged and require almost total care
  Delay in attaining developmental milestones proportionate to degree of motor deficit
  Speech dysarthric; swallowing may be impaired; tongue protrusion incomplete
  In some children emotions more labile with inappropriate laughing or crying
**Diplegia**—Similar parts on both sides of the body involved, such as both arms
  Spasticity in legs greater than in arms
  Late attainment of gross motor milestones, sitting, standing, and walking; development of hand skills generally appropriate for age
**Monoplegia***—Involving only one extremity
**Triplegia***—Involving three extremities
**Paraplegia***—Pure cerebral paraplegia of lower extremities

*Rare occurrences.

> **Box 40-4** ▪ ▪ ▪
> **Possible Signs of Cerebral Palsy**
>
> **PHYSICAL SIGNS**
> Poor head control after 3 months of age
> Stiff or rigid arms or legs
> Pushing away or arching back
> Floppy or limp body posture
> Cannot sit up without support by 8 months
> Uses only one side of the body, or only the arms to crawl
> Clenched fists after 3 months
>
> **BEHAVIORAL SIGNS**
> Extreme irritability or crying
> Failure to smile by 3 months
> Feeding difficulties
>   Persistent gagging or choking when fed
>   After 6 months of age, persistent tongue
>     thrusting

**Delayed Gross Motor Development.** Delayed gross motor development is a universal manifestation of CP. The child shows a delay in all motor accomplishments, and the discrepancy between motor ability and expected achievement tends to increase with successive developmental milestones as growth advances. It is especially significant if other developmental behaviors, such as language and personal-social achievement, are normal. Delayed development of the ability to balance may also slow the progression of milestones. For instance, the child may need to use the arms to balance in a sitting position, which renders the arms unavailable to develop fine motor control.

**Abnormal Motor Performance.** Neuromotor dysfunction is particularly evident in motor performance. An early sign is preferential unilateral hand use that may be apparent at approximately 6 months of age. Hand dominance does not normally develop until the preschool years. Abnormal crawling with propulsion by hand movements only and with lower extremities and hips hiked along, much like a "bunny hop," is seen in diplegia. Children with hemiplegia have an asymmetric crawl, using the unaffected arm and leg to propel themselves on either the buttocks or the abdomen. Spasticity may cause the child to stand or walk on the toes. Uncoordinated or involuntary movements are characteristic of dyskinetic CP, and facial grimacing and writhing movements of the tongue, fingers, and toes are signs of athetosis. Other significant signs of motor dysfunction are poor sucking and feeding difficulties, with persistent tongue thrust. Head staggering, tremor on reaching, and truncal ataxia also may be observed.

**Alterations of Muscle Tone.** Increased or decreased resistance to passive movements is a sign of abnormal muscle tone. The child may exhibit opisthotonic postures (exaggerated arching of the back) and may feel stiff on handling or dressing. Also, there is difficulty in diapering because of spasticity of the hip adductor muscles and lower extremities. When pulled to a sitting position, the child may extend the entire body and be rigid and unbending at the hip and knee joints. This is an early sign of spasticity.

**Abnormal Postures.** Children with spastic CP assume abnormal postures at rest or when their position is changed. From an early age, a child lying in a prone position will maintain the hips higher than the trunk with the legs and arms flexed or drawn under the body. In the supine position spasticity is evident by scissoring (legs in crossed position, knees, hips, and ankles stiff) and extension of the legs, with the feet plantar flexed. This posture is exaggerated when the child is suspended vertically or when others try to make the child bear weight. Depending on the degree of impairment, spasticity may be mild or severe. A persistent infantile resting and sleeping posture (i.e., arms abducted at shoulders, elbows flexed, and hands fisted) is a sign of spasticity when it remains constant after 4 to 5 months of age. The hemiparetic child may rest with the affected arm adducted and held against the torso, with the elbow pronated and slightly flexed and the hand closed.

**Reflex Abnormalities.** Persistence of primitive reflexes is one of the earliest clues to CP (e.g., obligatory tonic neck reflex at any age or nonobligatory persistence beyond 6 months of age, and the persistence or even hyperactivity of the Moro, plantar, and palmar grasp reflexes). Hyperreflexia, ankle clonus, and stretch reflexes can be elicited from many muscle groups on fast passive movements (e.g., resistance to passive abduction when the hips are suddenly separated [adductor catch]).

**Associated Disabilities and Problems.** Some of the disabilities associated with CP are visual impairment, hearing impairment, communication and speech difficulties, seizures, and intellectual impairment.

*Intellectual impairment* is a concern, although children with CP have a wide range of intelligence, 70% within normal limits. Speech difficulties are often interpreted as a sign of mental retardation. Assessing the intelligence of a child with CP is extremely difficult because of the presence of both motor and sensory deficits. Tests carried out periodically over time should determine the degree of intelligence. Many persons with CP who have severely limiting physical involvement actually have the least intellectual impairment. As a group, children with athetosis and ataxia are intellectually superior to those with other types of CP. The incidence of severe or profound impairment is highest in rigid, atonic, and quadriparetic CP.

The manifestations of *attention-deficit/hyperactivity disorder (ADHD)* may occur in children with CP. The primary presenting symptoms are poor attention span, marked distractibility, hyperactive behavior, and defects of integration. (See Chapter 18.) *Seizures* are more apt to accompany postnatally acquired hemiplegia. They are an unusual finding in athetosis and diplegia. The most common type is generalized tonic-clonic seizures, and the peak incidence of onset is between 2 and 6 years of age.

Poor control of oral musculature may contribute to a number of problems. *Drooling* may occur in some children and may contribute to wet clothing and skin irritation. Abnormal posture and motor performance, as well as alterations in muscle tone, affect chewing, swallowing, and talking. Occupational and speech/language therapy interventions may be necessary to assist some children with *feeding* and *speech.* Nutritional concerns should be addressed directly (Suresh-Babu and others, 1998). Coughing and choking, especially while eating, may predispose the child with CP to *aspiration.* Also, respiratory efforts may be uncoordinated and weak, which could result in *inadequate gas exchange.*

Motor impairment associated with CP contributes to other problems. Children with CP who are nonambulatory have an increased risk of developing *orthopaedic complications* such as unilateral or bilateral hip dislocations, scoliosis, and joint contractures due to unbalanced muscle tone. A variety of factors, including decreased mobility and difficulties with toileting, may be responsible for causing *constipation.* Difficulty in eating bulky foods because of uncoordinated chewing and swallowing may be the most likely cause. Stool softeners or laxatives may need to be used.

Increased incidence of *dental caries* results from (1) improper dental hygiene, (2) congenital enamel defects (hypoplasia of primary teeth), (3) high carbohydrate intake and retention, (4) dietary imbalance with poor nutritional intake, (5) inadequate fluoride, and (6) difficulty in mouth closure and drooling. Spastic or clonic movements can cause gagging or biting down on the toothbrush, thus interfering with cleaning techniques. Oral hypersensitivity is also common, which causes the child to resist dental hygiene. *Malocclusion* can occur in as many as 90% of these children. *Gingivitis* is secondary to inadequate dental hygiene and may be further complicated by the use of antiseizure drugs (Nehring, 2000).

*Nystagmus* and *amblyopia* are common and may require surgery, corrective lenses, or both. *Hearing loss* is also common. Some loss is caused by sensorineural involvement. Affected infants may spend increased amounts of time lying flat. This predisposes them to episodes of otitis media, which may result in conductive hearing loss. (See Chapter 24.)

### Diagnostic Evaluation

Infants at risk according to known etiologic factors associated with CP warrant careful assessment during early infancy to identify the signs of muscular dysfunction as early as possible. Careful assessment should be made of the preterm ELBW or VLBW infant, the infant with low Apgar scores at 5 minutes, and the infant who has experienced other perinatal or neonatal events such as seizures, intraventricular hemorrhage, or metabolic disturbances. Early recognition is made more difficult by the lack of reliable neonatal neurologic signs. Some "warning signs" are listed in Box 40-4, but these are not diagnostic. (See Critical Thinking Exercise box.) Because cortical control of movement does not occur until later in infancy, motor impairment associated with voluntary control is usually not apparent until after 2 to 4 months of age at the earliest. More often the likelihood of a diagnosis cannot be confirmed until the second half of the first year. Motor dysfunction in some mildly affected infants may be overlooked until they exhibit a delay or abnormality in some advanced motor skill such as standing or walking.

The persistence of primitive reflexes may be of value, and two offer assistance in diagnosis: (1) the asymmetric tonic

## Critical Thinking Exercise

### Diagnosis of Cerebral Palsy

During a well-child visit at 6 months, a family expresses concern that their child is not able to sit without support. You note that the child does not smile during the interview. You ask about feeding, and the parents report that the child pushes food out of the mouth with the tongue when they try to feed. Which of the following actions should you take?

FIRST, THINK ABOUT IT . . .
- What precise question are you trying to answer?
- If you accept the conclusions, what are the implications?

1. Assure the parents that the child exhibits normal development.
2. Inform the parents that the child exhibits warning signs of cerebral palsy.
3. Inquire about other developmental milestones, and observe the child's posture, tone, movements, and reflexes.
4. Prepare a referral to a neurologist.

*The most appropriate answer is three. The precise question you are trying to answer is whether or not the child exhibits normal development. Therefore it is most appropriate to inquire about other developmental milestones and observe the child's posture, tone, movements, and reflexes. At 6 months, most children are beginning to sit without support and are able to take food by spoon without tongue thrust; however, there is variability in normal development. If no other signs of concern are present, parents can be informed that the child will, most likely, soon begin to sit and take food by spoon. They should be encouraged to raise concerns at any well-child appointment and should be informed of the practitioner's wish to see the child at the next regularly scheduled visit. If other signs of concern are present, the practitioner will want to observe the child more closely over time and perhaps consider a referral to a specialist such as a neurologist.*

neck reflex, or persistent Moro reflex (beyond 4 months of age); and (2) the crossed extensor reflex. The tonic neck reflex normally disappears between 4 and 6 months of age. An "obligatory" response is considered abnormal. This is elicited by turning the infant's head to one side and holding it there for 20 seconds. When a crying infant is unable to move from the asymmetric posturing of the tonic neck reflex when crying, it is considered to be "obligatory" and an abnormal response. The crossed extensor reflex, which normally disappears by 4 months, is elicited by applying a noxious stimulus to the sole of one extremity with the knee extended. Normally the contralateral foot responds with extensor, abduction, and then adduction movements. The possibility of CP is suggested if these reflexes are found after the age at which they should have disappeared.

The neurologic examination and history are the primary modalities for diagnosis. A thorough knowledge of normal variations of motor development is required for detecting abnormal progress, and a careful history is elicited to detect possible etiologic factors. The child's spontaneous movements and behavior, including posture, attitude, and muscle size, function, and tone, are observed.

Supplemental diagnostic tests may be used (e.g., electroencephalography, tomography, screening for metabolic defects, and serum electrolyte values). The possibility of slowly progressive degenerative disease and early-onset, slow-growing brain tumors must be ruled out.

## Therapeutic Management: General Concepts

The goals of therapy for children with CP are early recognition and promotion of an optimum developmental course to enable affected children to attain their potential within the limits of their dysfunction. The disorder is permanent, and therapy is chiefly symptomatic and preventive.

The beneficial influences of a habilitation program on both child and family are based on recognizing the disability as early as possible and implementing treatment. Parents are essential to a treatment program; their goals and desires, their cooperation, and their confidence are considered in all aspects of management. With early diagnosis parents can begin to provide the sensorimotor experiences essential to cognitive development, because CNS structures depend on stimulation and use to attain and maintain their functional integrity.

The broad aims of therapy are to (1) establish locomotion, communication, and self-help; (2) gain optimum appearance and integration of motor functions; (3) correct associated defects as early and effectively as possible; (4) provide educational opportunities adapted to the individual child's needs and capabilities; and (5) promote socialization experiences with other affected and unaffected children. Each child is evaluated and managed on an individual basis. The plan of therapy may involve a variety of settings, facilities, and specially trained persons. In addition to the parents, pediatrician, and nurse, the scope of the child's needs may require professionals such as a psychologist or psychiatrist, orthopaedist, physical therapist, teacher, social worker, speech pathologist or therapist, pediatric neurologist, orthotist, audiologist, and occupational therapist (Box 40-5).

**Mobilizing Devices.** Ankle-foot orthoses (braces) (AFOs) are worn by many children with CP. AFOs are molded to fit the feet and are worn inside the shoes. Devices are often used to help prevent or reduce deformity, increase the energy efficiency of gait, and control alignment. Some of the more commonly used mobility devices include wheeled scooter boards that allow children to propel themselves while the abdomen or total body is supported and the legs are positioned with wedges to prevent scissoring. Wheeled go-carts provide good sitting balance and serve as an early "wheelchair" experience for young children. Strollers can be equipped with custom seats for dependent mobilization. Special devices for independent mobilization that may or may not allow the upper extremities to remain free are particularly valuable for children with lower extremity involvement (Fig. 40-2). A number of wheelchairs can be customized to meet the needs and preferences of older children. (See Mobilization Devices, Chapter 39.)

> **NURSING ALERT** The use of infant walkers is discouraged. They pose a risk of injury to normal children and are especially hazardous for children with CP. Also, jumping seats, such as those that hang in doorways, should not be used.

**Surgery.** Surgical intervention is usually reserved for the child who does not respond to the more conservative measures, but it is also indicated for the child whose spasticity causes progressive deformities. Orthopaedic surgery may be required to correct contracture or spastic deformities, to provide stability for an uncontrollable joint, and to provide balanced muscle power. This includes tendon-lengthening procedures (especially heel-cord lengthening), release of spastic wrist flexor muscles, and correction of hip and adductor muscle spasticity or contracture to improve locomotion. Surgery is used primarily to improve function rather than for cosmetic purposes and is followed by physical therapy.

Neurosurgical procedures are used only in selected cases. *Selective dorsal rhizotomy* has provided marked improvement in some children with CP (Steinbok, 2001). However, achieving the benefits from the surgery requires intensive physical therapy and family commitment. Because the procedure results in flaccid muscles, the child must be retaught to sit, stand, and walk.

**Medication.**   Pharmacologic agents given orally have had variable effectiveness in improving overall function in children with CP. Antianxiety agents have been used to some extent to relieve excessive motion and tension, particularly in the athetoid child. Skeletal muscle relaxants, such as dantrolene (Dantrium), baclofen (Lioresol), and methocarbamol (Robaxin), may be used with moderate success to decrease spasticity (Krach, 2001). Diazepam (Valium) is used frequently but should be restricted to older children and adolescents. A local nerve block to motor points of a muscle with a neurolytic agent such as phenol solution reduces spasticity temporarily. Botulinum toxin type A (Botox) is also being used to reduce spasticity in targeted muscles (Edgar, 2001; Ubhi and others, 2000). The botulinum is injected into the muscle (commonly the quadriceps, gastrocnemius, or medial hamstrings) after a topical anesthetic is applied; midazolam may also be administered 30 minutes before the procedure. The interval between injections varies, but the usual dosage lasts approximately 3 months. This procedure has been shown to be safe, well tolerated, and effective in decreasing spasticity in children with CP (Edgar, 2001). Prime candidates for Botox injections are children with spasticity confined to the lower extremities; the drug weakens spasticity so the muscles can be stretched and the child may ambulate with or without orthoses (Jacobs, 2001).

The neurosurgical and pharmacologic approach to managing the spasticity associated with CP involves the implantation of a pump to infuse baclofen directly into the intrathecal space surrounding the spinal cord to provide relief of spasticity. High doses of oral baclofen are associated with significant side effects, including drowsiness and confusion, yet are often unable to provide adequate relief of spasticity. Direct infusion of baclofen into the intrathecal space provides relief without as many of the associated side effects (Krach, 2001).

Patients are screened before pump placement by the infusion of a "test dose" of intrathecal baclofen delivered via a lumbar puncture. Close monitoring for side effects and relief of spasticity occurs for several hours after the infusion. If a positive effect is noted, the patient is considered a candidate for pump placement. The implantation procedure is performed in the operating room by a neurosurgeon. The pump is placed in the subcutaneous space of the midabdomen. An intrathecal catheter is tunneled from the lumbar area to the abdomen and connected to the pump. The pump is filled with baclofen and programmed to provide a

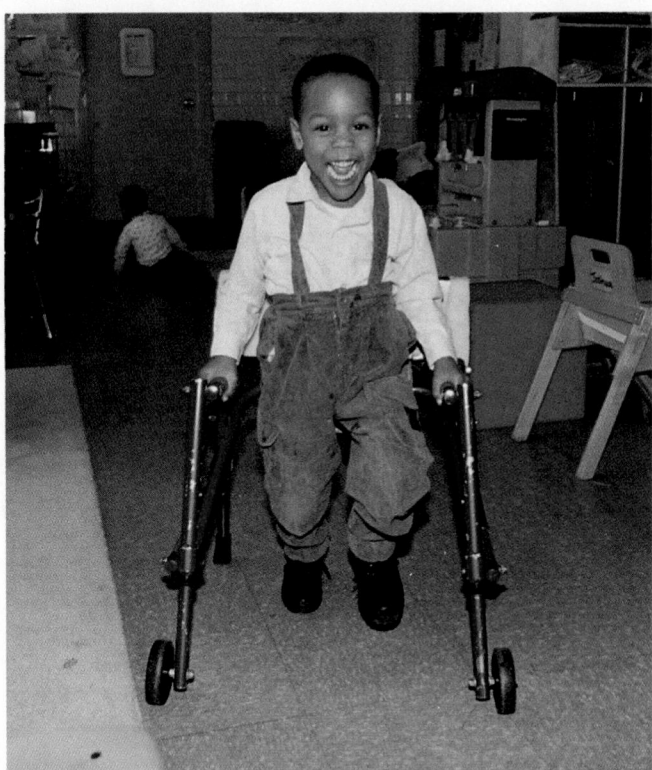

**Fig. 40-2**   Child ambulating with use of assistive device.

set dose using a telemetry wand and a computer. The patient remains hospitalized for 3 to 7 days to adjust the dose and ensure proper healing. Outpatient visits to refill the pump and make dosage adjustments occur about every 4 to 6 weeks, depending on the patient's response to the treatment. This procedure is most suited for a multidisciplinary setting where rehabilitation specialists are readily available and consistently involved in the patient's ongoing care (Rawlins, 1995).

Anticonvulsant medications, especially phenobarbital and phenytoin, are prescribed routinely for children who have seizures, and hyperactive, dyskinetic children perform better when given dextroamphetamine or other drugs used for the child with ADHD. Gabapentin (Neurontin) has been used in adults with spinal cord injury (SCI) to decrease spasticity with success; there are no studies yet available on the effectiveness of the drug in children (Krach, 2001). The $\alpha_2$-adrenergic agonists clonidine (Catapres) and tizanidine (Zanaflex) have been used to decrease spasticity in adults with SCI and multiple sclerosis, but use in children with CP has yet to be reported (Krach, 2001). All medications should be monitored for maintenance of therapeutic levels and avoidance of subtherapeutic or toxic levels.

**Technical Aids.**   A wide variety of technical aids are available to improve the functioning of children with CP. For example, specially designed electromechanical toys that use the concept of biofeedback operate from a head unit. The toy is manipulated only when the head and trunk are in correct alignment. Eye-hand coordination can also be enhanced by appropriately designed toys and games.

The most numerous devices are those that facilitate non-vocal communication. Microcomputers combined with voice synthesizers aid children with speech difficulties to "speak." These and other devices print messages onto screen monitors and paper. These devices have made it apparent that some children have been erroneously considered to be mentally impaired.

Many other electronic devices allow independent functioning. Sensors can be activated and deactivated by using a head-stick, tongue, or other voluntary muscle movement over which the child has control. (See Figs 24-3 and 24-4.) The application of this technology makes it possible for older persons with CP to eventually function in their own apartments and can be extended into the workplace.

**Other Considerations.** Care of visual and auditory deficits requires the attention of appropriate specialists, and speech/language therapy involves the services of a speech/language pathologist. (See Chapter 24.) Dental care is especially important for children with CP and all too often is overlooked. Regular visits to the dentist and dental prophylaxis, including brushing, fluoride, and flossing (after several teeth are present), should be instituted as soon as the teeth erupt. This is especially important for children given phenytoin, who often develop gum hyperplasia.

## Therapeutic Management: Therapies, Education, Recreation

**Physical Therapy.** Physical therapy is one of the most commonly used conservative treatment modalities. It requires the specialized skills of a qualified therapist with an extensive repertoire of exercise methods, who can design a program to stimulate each child to achieve functional goals. In general, physical therapy is directed toward good skeletal alignment for the spastic child; training in purposeful acts, even in the face of involuntary motion, for the child with athetosis; and maximum development of proprioceptive sense in ataxia.

An active therapy program involves the family, the physical therapist (PT), and often other members of the health care team, especially the nurse. Developing a treatment program that can be carried out at home is of utmost importance. The major approach uses traditional types of therapeutic exercises that consist of stretching, passive, active, and resistive movements applied to specific muscle groups or joints to maintain or increase range of motion, strength, or endurance.

**NURSING ALERT** The American Academy of Pediatrics (1999) has issued a strong statement against "patterning" as a form of treatment for neurologically disabled children. "Patterning" attempts to alter abnormal tone and posture and elicit desired movements through positional manipulation or other means of modifying or augmenting sensory output. These programs require intensive daily manipulation and a legion of volunteers to carry out the program. Little benefit has been demonstrated.

No therapeutic approach is able to achieve spectacular changes in the ultimate outcome of motor disability. Early efforts are focused on alleviating abnormal postures by po-

sitioning and range-of-motion exercises. For example, extensor spasticity and scissoring of legs can be avoided if the infant straddles a thigh or hip when carried in the sitting position. Stretching of the gastrocnemius muscle and its tendon helps to prevent tightness and spasticity, which lead to toe walking and equinus position of the ankle. Passive range-of-motion exercises, stretching, and elongation exercises are valuable at any age, even at early ages when the child is unable to cooperate. Some active extension can be performed when the child is old enough to cooperate, with passive motion applied to complete joint extension. Prevention of contracture deformity is a prime function of physical therapy. Seating and mobility are other key goals.

**Functional and Adaptive Training (Occupational Therapy).** Training in manual skills and activities of daily living (ADLs) proceeds along developmental lines and according to the child's functional level. Sitting, balancing, crawling, and walking are encouraged at appropriate ages and are accompanied by stimulation of protective extension and equilibrium reactions. Hand activities are begun early to improve motor function and provide the child with sensory experiences and information about the environment. As the child progresses from simple feeding and self-care activities, training is extended to include other tasks (e.g., cooking or use of keyboard or computer mouse) that are within the child's developmental and functional capabilities. It should be remembered that a child should not be expected to learn a task until he or she is at the developmental stage at which it would normally be accomplished. This may not coincide with chronologic age.

Incorporating play into the therapeutic program often requires great ingenuity and inventiveness from those involved in the child's care. Objects and toys are chosen to provide needed sensory input using a variety of shapes, forms, and textures. Nurses can help parents integrate therapy into play activities in natural ways.

The child may need considerable help (and patience) in learning to feed, dress, and care for personal hygiene needs. A feeding program may be developed by an occupational therapist (OT) in conjunction with a speech/language pathologist (SLP). Children should be fed in the normal eating position. When children have difficulty with sucking and swallowing, it is a temptation to hold them in a semireclining posture to make use of gravity flow. However, this method does not promote active swallowing, and the neck hyperextension may even interfere with swallowing. A more flexed sitting position, with the arms brought forward to decrease the tendency toward back and neck extension, is more natural during bottle- or spoon-feeding and encourages active swallowing.

Because jaw control is compromised, more normal control can be achieved if the feeder provides stability of the oral mechanism from the side or front of the face. When directed from the front, the middle finger of the nonfeeding hand is placed posterior to the body portion of the chin, the thumb is placed below the bottom lip, and the index finger is placed parallel to the child's mandible (Fig. 40-3). Manual jaw control from the side assists with head control, correction of neck and trunk hyperextension, and jaw stabi-

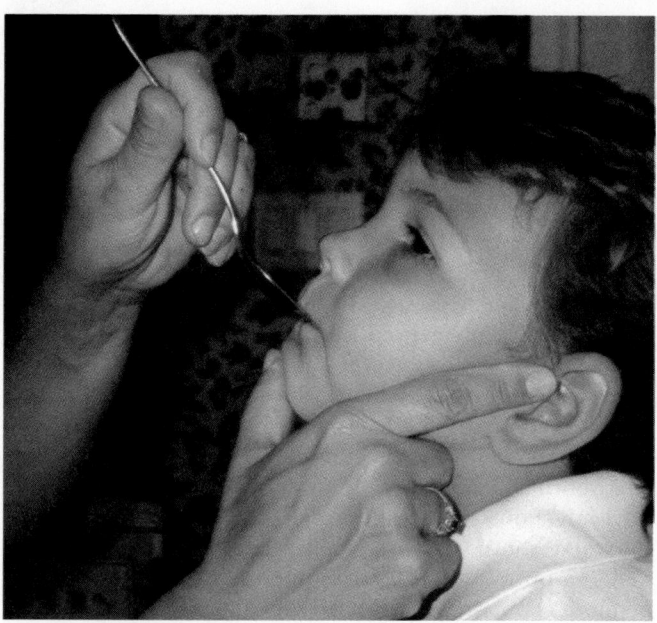

**Fig. 40-3**    Manual jaw control provided anteriorly.

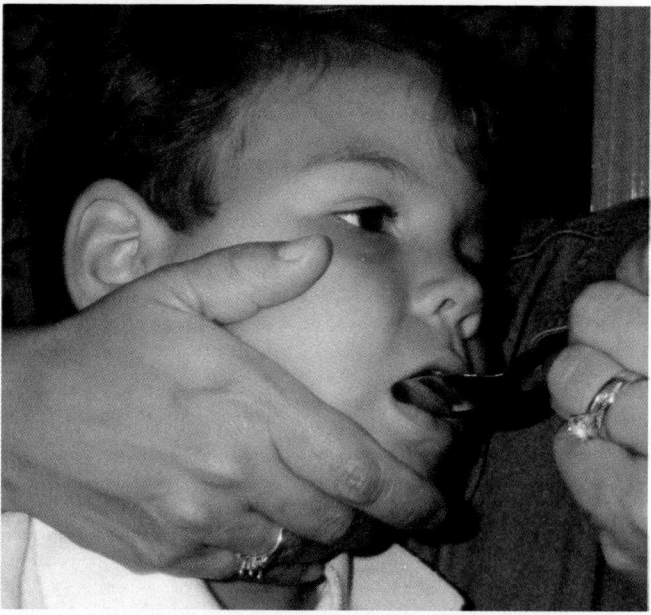

**Fig. 40-4**    Manual jaw control provided from the side.

lization. The middle finger of the nonfeeding hand is placed posterior to the bony portion of the chin, the index finger is placed on the chin below the lower lip, and the thumb is placed obliquely across the cheek to provide lateral jaw stability (Fig. 40-4).

In all ADLs it is important to capitalize on the child's assets and compensate for liabilities. For example, a child with visual-motor dysfunction is helped by substituting a computer for the laborious task of handwriting. The level of expected independence is related to both gross and fine motor manipulation, and even when complete independence in a specific activity is not realistic, the child should learn any masterable part of the task. However, motor function is not the sole purpose of learning to be as independent as possible. Any accomplishment promotes self-reliance and self-esteem for healthier personality development.

**Speech Therapy.** Speech training under the supervision of an SLP is begun early, before the child learns poor habits of communication. Parents and others can help by following the directions of the speech therapist and by talking to the child slowly and using pictures or handling objects about which the adult is speaking. Feeding techniques such as forcing the child to use the lips and tongue in eating (e.g., placing food at the side of the tongue, first one side, then the other; making the child use the lips to take food from a spoon rather than placing it directly on the tongue; and avoiding use of the teeth to remove the food from the utensil) help to facilitate speech. If severe dysarthria prevents articulate speech and the child has reasonable intelligence, nonverbal communication (e.g., sign language) is taught. (See Chapter 24.)

**Education.** As in all aspects of care, educational requirements are determined by the child's needs and potential. This includes the severity of the child's disease and the presence and degree of associated conditions that affect learning and participation, such as learning impairment,

abnormal actions or behavior, impaired vision or hearing, and seizures. Children with mild to moderate involvement are generally able to participate, for varying amounts of time, in regular classes. Resource rooms are available in most schools to provide more individualized attention to a child's particular needs. Integration of these children into regular classrooms should be the initial goal. Teachers' assistants are often used to work one-on-one with children in both settings. A training program may be appropriate for those children who are unable to benefit from formal education. Prevocational and vocational counseling and guidance are arranged at adolescence. Education is geared toward the child's assets at any phase or in any setting. Of course, nurses should be aware of early intervention programs and provisions for special education and related services for children (see Box 24-3) and should support parents in their efforts to obtain appropriate educational services for the child.

**Recreation.** Recreational activities are also a necessary part of growing up. Recreational outlets and after-school activities should be considered for the child who is unable to participate in regular athletic and other peer activities. Some can compete in athletic and artistic endeavors, and there are many games and pastimes that are suited to their capabilities. Sports, physical fitness, and recreation programs are encouraged for children with CP, and young children should be exposed to all physical activities available to children without disabilities. Adaptive physical education classes are mandated by law in many school systems.

Numerous developmental centers have facilities for indoor and outdoor activities designed to appeal to children of all ages. If these are not available, they should be developed. However, such programs require adequate supervision to avoid any harmful effects. Recreational activities serve to stimulate children's interest and curiosity, help them adjust to their disability, improve their functional abilities, and build self-esteem. Competitive sports are also becoming increasingly available to children with disabilities and offer an added dimension to physical activities. Information on training programs and competition on local, state, regional, and national levels can be obtained from the **National Disability Sports Alliance.**\*

## Nursing Considerations

The goals of nursing care for the child with CP should be developed in conjunction with the family and generally include the following (see Nursing Care Plan, pp. 1844-1845):

1. Child will acquire mobility within personal capabilities.
2. Child will acquire communication skills or use appropriate assistive devices.
3. Child will engage in self-help activities.
4. Child will receive appropriate education.
5. Child will develop a positive self-image.
6. Child will receive appropriate nutrition and feeding assistance.
7. Family will receive appropriate education and support in their efforts to meet the child's needs.
8. Child will receive appropriate health care if hospitalized or in the community.

**Reinforce Therapeutic Plan/Assist in Normalization.**  Because children are being treated at an earlier age, parents are participating at an earlier stage in treatment programs for their disabled child. They are taught the proper handling and home care of young children with CP and need carefully programmed steps so that their expanded parental role can be melded into the already-established relationship. Close work with other multidisciplinary team members is essential. Nurses reinforce the therapeutic plan and assist the family in devising and modifying equipment and activities to continue the therapy program in the home (e.g., modifying eating utensils by building up spoon handles for easier grasp and modifying clothes to facilitate self-help). (See also Chapter 24.)

Some children have difficulty in keeping their heads upright. Because of this, they can neither explore much of their environment nor process the information. Parents need to be complimented on their efforts to provide a stimulating environment for these children. These infants are "at risk" for delayed development in holding up their heads, righting their shoulders and trunks for stable posture, sitting, pulling, standing, and crawling. Most parents of children with impaired movements benefit from support and practical suggestions for feeding, moving, holding, and encouraging the infant to explore hands and feet and to play. Assisting parents to incorporate therapeutic suggestions into typical daily activities is an important normalizing strategy. (See Chapter 22 for a discussion of normalization.)

Although practical advice is important, the nurse, OT, or PT should offer suggestions at a pace that can be absorbed by the parents. The parents are encouraged to define their concern, and nurses should acknowledge the concern as genuine and ask the parents what approach(es) they have tried and for how long. In this way the nurse is able to find

out what works, what does not work, and *what the parents* would like to try next. The parents are given positive feedback for their observations of the infant, the progress *they* note, and how *they* differentiate the child's needs.

**Address Health Maintenance Needs.**  Because children with CP expend so much energy in their efforts to accomplish activities of daily living, more frequent rest periods should be arranged to avoid the fatigue that may aggravate their limited capabilities. The diet should include extra calories to help meet these extra energy demands. Safety precautions are implemented, such as children wearing bicycle helmets if they are subject to falls or if there is a chance of injuring their heads on hard objects. Furniture should be upholstered or sharp edges padded to protect a child from injury. If their respiratory muscles are less efficient, these children may be susceptible to common upper respiratory tract infections and should avoid contact with infected persons and should receive appropriate immunizations. Depending on the level of involvement, dental problems may be more common in children with CP, which creates a need for meticulous attention to all aspects of dental care.

**Support Family.**  The nursing interventions that are probably most valuable to the family are support and help in coping with the emotional aspects of the disorder, many of which are discussed in Chapter 22. Initially the parents need informational and emotional support directed toward understanding the implications of the diagnosis and all the feelings it engenders. Later they need clarification regarding what they can expect from the child and from health care professionals. Educating families in the principles of family-centered care and parent-professional collaboration is essential. Having a child with CP implies numerous problems of daily management and changes in family life, and principles of normalization can be stressed.

The nurse can support the parents by acknowledging and addressing their concerns and frustrations, as well as by noting and appreciating their problem-solving skills and their approaches to helping the child. Siblings of a child with a disability are also affected and may respond to the presence of the child with overt or less evident behavioral problems. The family needs a relationship with nurses who can provide continued contact, support, and encouragement through the long process of habilitation.

Parents can also find help and support from parent groups, with whom they can share experiences, accomplishments, problems, and concerns and from whom they can derive comfort and practical information. For example, parents can understand from others what it is like to have a child with CP. (See Family Focus box.) The **United Cerebral Palsy Association**\* has branches in most communities and provides a variety of services for children and families.

**Support Hospitalized Child.**  CP is not a disorder that requires hospitalization; therefore when children with CP are hospitalized, they are usually admitted for another rea-

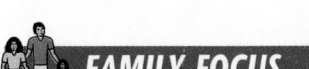

## FAMILY FOCUS
### *The Reality of Acceptance of Cerebral Palsy*

Acceptance is rarely achieved in the length of time implied in the literature.

In the first place, what is it? To me, it is the end of comparing my son with every other child I see. I focus on *his* gains, not society's expectations.

It is also being able to laugh periodically *at* his "clumsiness." It is "gallows humor" as he achieves adulthood; jokes about CP can be funny now.

The bitterness is gone; I am now happy for people who have children without CP.

I no longer feel sorry for my son, but rather for the people who cannot see him for the great person he is; the CP does *not* come first.

He is now a young man of 25 years, and I am learning to accept his independence.

It is a "never-ending story."

Elaine A. Dunham, RN
Shriner's Hospital
Springfield, MA

son or for corrective surgery. Consequently many nurses are not accustomed to handling children with this diagnosis. Nurses who have never been associated with a child with CP may react in a variety of ways, including fear, or overwhelming pity. The basic concept to keep in mind when caring for these children is that they are, first of all, children. They just happen to be afflicted with a disorder that limits their capacity to perform some ADLs and, in some cases, to communicate with others.

Children with CP should be approached and treated in the same manner as any child in the hospital. The nurse's actions should convey acceptance, affection, and friendliness and promote a feeling of trust and dependability. This is especially true with older children who have normal intelligence but who may have communication problems. Speech impairment is common in children with CP. All too often, nurses tend to "talk down" to these children and do things for them that they are perfectly capable of doing for themselves, although not as adeptly. This is especially humiliating to adolescents, who value their independence and self-esteem.

To facilitate the care and management of hospitalized children with CP, the therapy program should be continued (insofar as their condition allows) during the time they are hospitalized. This should be incorporated into the nursing care plan, with every effort expended to make certain that the ground that has been so laboriously gained is not lost. Encouraging the parent to room-in and actively participate in the child's care facilitates a continuation of the home therapy program and helps the child adjust to an unfamiliar environment. However, it is equally important to remember that a hospitalization may be the first time a parent can defer care to a nurse and not be the primary caregiver. This respite may be crucial to the parent's well-being. The parent's preference in this regard should be respected.

**Evaluate Nursing Interventions.** The effectiveness of nursing interventions is determined by continual reassess-ment and evaluation of care based on the following observational guidelines:

1. Child's movements and use of mobilization devices
2. Child's speech and ability to use communication devices
3. Child's activities, especially those related to self-care
4. Family perception regarding child's activities and school attendance
5. Child's interactions with others and choice of activities; child's feelings and concerns
6. Family feelings and concerns, as well as family members' interaction with the child
7. Child's behavior and responses during hospitalization

The *expected outcomes* are described in the Nursing Care Plan on pp. 1844-1845.

## Hypotonia

Decreased muscle tone in an infant is not an unusual observation in the neonatal period and is one of the most common presenting symptoms in neuromuscular disorders. It may also indicate a variety of systemic conditions. Common causes are cerebral trauma or perinatal hypoxia, but most neuromuscular disorders with hypotonia as the presenting symptom, especially Down syndrome and infantile spinal muscular atrophy (SMA), are genetically determined.

### Clinical Manifestations

Hypotonia, sometimes called the *floppy infant syndrome,* is marked by diminished muscle tone and weakness in both spontaneous and passive motion and reflex testing. The affected infant, when placed in a supine position, assumes a characteristic "frog-leg posture" or lies in some other unusual position at rest. Normally the young infant who is held in horizontal suspension (i.e., with the examiner's hand supporting the infant under the chest) will respond by slightly raising the head with the back relatively straight, the arms flexed and slightly abducted, and the knees partly flexed. The hypotonic infant droops over the supporting hand with head and extremities hanging loosely, resembling an inverted U. The muscles feel atrophied when palpated, and there is marked head lag when the infant is pulled to a sitting position. Poor sucking may be noted.

### Diagnostic Evaluation

The infant with hypotonia presents a diagnostic challenge. The child's and family's history and the physical examination offer important clues to the general category of causes, such as central or motor neuron disorders. Electromyography is a key diagnostic test. Accurate diagnosis is essential for appropriate treatment, genetic implications, and family counseling (Fischer, 1995).

### Therapeutic Management and Nursing Considerations

The management of an infant with hypotonia is determined by the cause of the hypotonia. It is a nursing responsibility to record and report findings that suggest hypotonia in an infant so that further evaluation can be carried out and therapeutic measures implemented if indicated.

# Nursing Care Plan
## The Child with Cerebral Palsy

**NURSING DIAGNOSIS:** Impaired physical mobility related to neuromuscular impairment

**PATIENT GOAL 1:** Will acquire locomotion within capabilities (per care plan of PT/OT)

• **NURSING INTERVENTIONS/*RATIONALES***
Encourage sitting, crawling, and walking as prescribed
Carry out therapies that strengthen and improve control *to facilitate optimum development*
Assist child in using reciprocal leg motion when learning to walk, if indicated in plan of care
Provide incentives to move (e.g., place toy out of child's reach)
Ensure adequate rest before attempting locomotion activities *to encourage success*
Incorporate play that encourages desired behavior, *to encourage cooperation*
Employ aids such as parallel bars and crutches as prescribed *to facilitate locomotion*
Prepare child and family for surgical procedures if indicated

• **EXPECTED OUTCOME**
Child acquires locomotion within capabilities (specify)

**PATIENT GOAL 2:** Will experience no or minimal deformity

• **NURSING INTERVENTIONS/*RATIONALES***
Apply and correctly use orthoses *for maximum benefit*
Carry out and teach family to perform stretching exercises as prescribed *to prevent deformities*
Employ appropriate range-of-motion exercises as prescribed *to facilitate muscle development and flexibility of joints*
Perform preoperative and postoperative care for child who requires corrective surgery

• **EXPECTED OUTCOME**
Alignment and flexibility are maintained within child's limits

**NURSING DIAGNOSIS:** Bathing/hygiene, dressing/grooming, feeding, toileting self-care deficits related to physical disability

**PATIENT GOAL 1:** Will engage in self-help activities of daily living

• **NURSING INTERVENTIONS/*RATIONALES***
Encourage child to assist with care as age and capabilities permit *to facilitate optimum development*
Select toys and activities that allow maximum participation by child and that improve motor function and sensory input *to promote self-care*

---

*Dependent nursing action.

Avoid undue persistence *because child may be unable or not ready to accomplish a goal*
Encourage activities that require both unimanual and bimanual actions *to encourage optimum development*
Assist with jaw control during feeding *to facilitate eating*
Encourage use of adapted utensils, foods, and clothing *to facilitate self-help* (e.g., large-bowled spoon with padded handle; finger foods and foods that adhere to, rather than slip from, utensil; clothing that opens from front with self-adhering closings rather than buttons)
Assist parents in toilet training child, *because methods may need to be individualized according to child's abilities*

• **EXPECTED OUTCOME**
Child engages in self-help activities commensurate with capabilities

**NURSING DIAGNOSIS:** Risk for injury related to physical disability, neuromuscular impairment, perceptual and cognitive impairment

**PATIENT GOAL 1:** Will experience no physical injury

• **NURSING INTERVENTIONS/*RATIONALES***
Educate family to provide safe physical environment
  Use padded furniture *for protection*
  Use siderails on bed *to prevent falls*
  Use sturdy furniture that does not slip *to prevent falls*
  Avoid throw rugs and polished floors *to prevent falls*
Educate family to select toys appropriate to age and physical limitations *to prevent injuries*
Encourage sufficient rest *to reduce fatigue and decrease risk of injuries*
Use safety restraints when child is in chair or vehicle
Provide child who is prone to falls with protective helmet and enforce its use *to prevent head injuries*
Institute seizure precautions for susceptible child
*Administer anticonvulsant drugs as prescribed *to prevent seizures*

• **EXPECTED OUTCOMES**
Family provides a safe environment for child (specify)
Child is free of injury

**NURSING DIAGNOSIS:** Impaired verbal communication related to hearing loss, neuromuscular impairment, cognitive impairment

**PATIENT GOAL 1:** Will engage in communication process within limits of impairment

• **NURSING INTERVENTIONS/*RATIONALES***
Enlist the services of a speech therapist early *to promote good habits of communication*
Talk to child slowly *to give child time to understand speech*
Use articles and pictures *to reinforce speech and encourage understanding*

## *Nursing Care Plan*
## The Child with Cerebral Palsy—cont'd

Use feeding techniques *that help facilitate speech,* such as using lips, teeth, and various tongue movements

Teach and use nonverbal communication methods (e.g., sign language) for child with severe dysarthria

Help family acquire electronic equipment *to facilitate nonverbal communication* (e.g., computer with voice synthesizer)

- **EXPECTED OUTCOME**

Child is able to communicate needs to caregivers (specify desired communication and means of accomplishment)

> **NURSING DIAGNOSIS:** Risk for imbalanced nutrition: less than body requirements related to feeding and motor problems

**PATIENT GOAL 1:** Will receive optimum nutrition

- **NURSING INTERVENTIONS/***RATIONALES*

Provide extra calories in diet *to meet energy demands of increased muscle activity*

Monitor weight gain *to evaluate adequacy of nutritional intake*

Provide vitamin, mineral, and protein supplements if unable to meet caloric requirements with common food sources

Consult dietitian for planning adequate caloric intake based on child's individual needs

Devise aids and techniques with input from occupational/speech therapists to facilitate feeding *so that child receives adequate nourishment*

- **EXPECTED OUTCOMES**

Child eats a balanced diet

Weight remains within acceptable limits (specify)

> **NURSING DIAGNOSIS:** Fatigue related to increased energy expenditure

**PATIENT GOAL 1:** Will receive optimum rest

- **NURSING INTERVENTIONS/***RATIONALES*

Maintain a well-regulated schedule that allows for adequate rest and sleep periods *to prevent fatigue*

Be alert for evidence of fatigue, which tends to aggravate symptoms

- **EXPECTED OUTCOME**

Child is sufficiently rested

**PATIENT GOAL 2:** Will maintain good general health

- **NURSING INTERVENTIONS/***RATIONALES*

Ensure regular routine health maintenance *to promote general health*

Physical assessment

Dental care

Immunizations

- **EXPECTED OUTCOMES**

Child receives regular health assessments (specify schedule)

Child receives appropriate immunizations (specify) and dental care (specify)

> **NURSING DIAGNOSIS:** Disturbed body image related to perception of disability

**PATIENT GOAL 1:** Will demonstrate positive body image

- **NURSING INTERVENTIONS/***RATIONALES*

Demonstrate acceptance of child through own behavior, *because children are sensitive to affective attitude of the professional*

Capitalize on child's assets and provide compensation for liabilities *to encourage positive self-image*

Praise child for accomplishments and "near" accomplishments, such as partial completion of a task

Plan activities and goals *with* the child that provide opportunities for success *to encourage cooperation and positive self-image*

Encourage grooming and age-appropriate dress *to promote acceptance by others and positive body image*

See Nursing diagnosis: Body image disturbance, in Nursing Care Plan: The Child with Chronic Illness or Disability, Chapter 22

- **EXPECTED OUTCOME**

Child exhibits behaviors that indicate positive body image (specify)

> **NURSING DIAGNOSIS:** Risk for interrupted family processes related to a child with a lifelong disability

**PATIENT (FAMILY) GOAL 1:** Will receive adequate support

- **NURSING INTERVENTIONS/***RATIONALES*

See Nursing diagnosis: Risk for interrupted family processes, in Nursing Care Plan: The Child with Chronic Illness or Disability, Chapter 22

Refer to special support group(s) and agencies *to provide social support*

- **EXPECTED OUTCOMES**

Family needs for support are met

See also:

  Nursing Care Plan: The Child with Chronic Illness or Disability, Chapter 22

  Nursing Care Plan: The Child with Mental Retardation, Chapter 24

# Infantile Spinal Muscular Atrophy (SMA) (Werdnig-Hoffmann Disease)

Progressive infantile SMA (Werdnig-Hoffmann disease), or SMA type 1, is a disorder characterized by progressive weakness and wasting of skeletal muscles caused by degeneration of anterior horn cells. It is inherited as an autosomal-recessive trait and is the most common paralytic form of the "floppy infant syndrome." The sites of the pathologic condition are the anterior horn cells of the spinal cord and the motor nuclei of the brainstem, but the primary effect is atrophy of skeletal muscles.

## Clinical Manifestations

The age of onset is variable, but the earlier the onset, the more disseminated and severe the motor weakness. The disorder may be manifested early—often at birth, often in utero—and almost always before 2 years of age. The manifestations and prognosis are categorized according to the age of onset (Box 40-6). However, recent observations suggest that at least some aspects of the classification are not valid. In some research, individuals with type 1 manifestations had a life span of 4 months to 31 years. Also, some affected persons did not demonstrate progressive loss of strength and function (Russman, 1996).

## Therapeutic Management

The diagnosis is established from electromyography that demonstrates a denervation pattern and is confirmed by muscle biopsy. Treatment is symptomatic and preventive and primarily involves preventing infection and treating orthopaedic problems, the most serious of which is scoliosis. Many children benefit from powered chairs, lifts, special mattresses, and accessible environmental controls. Vigorous antibiotic therapy and pulmonary physical therapy are implemented during upper respiratory infections.

## Nursing Considerations

The infant or small child with extensive paralysis requires frequent changes of position to prevent physical injury and complications, especially pneumonia. The pharynx requires frequent suctioning to remove secretions, and feeding must be carried out slowly and carefully to prevent aspiration. Children with infantile SMA are intellectually normal, and therefore verbal, tactile, and auditory stimulation are important aspects of care. Supporting them so that they can see the activities around them and transporting them in a wagon or wheelchair for a change of environment provide stimulation and a broader scope of contacts.

To prevent deformities and other complications, children who are able to sit require proper support and attention to alignment. Children who survive beyond infancy need attention to educational needs and opportunities for social interaction with other children. The parents of a child with a chronic or potentially fatal illness require a great deal of support and encouragement. (See Chapters 22 and 23). The parents of children with a genetically transmitted disorder also need to be encouraged to seek genetic counseling. (See Chapter 5.)

# Juvenile Spinal Muscular Atrophy (Kugelberg-Welander Syndrome)

Juvenile SMA (Kugelberg-Welander syndrome, or SMA type 3, juvenile proximal hereditary muscular atrophy) is also the result of anterior horn cell and motor nerve degeneration. The disease is characterized by a pattern of muscular weakness similar to that of infantile SMA. Several modes of inheritance have been reported for the disease—autosomal-recessive, autosomal-dominant, and X-linked recessive.

The onset occurs from less than 1 year of age into adulthood, with symptoms resembling type 3 infantile SMA; proximal muscle weakness (especially of the lower limbs) and muscular atrophy are the predominant features. The disease runs a slowly progressive course. Some children lose the ability to walk 8 to 9 years after the onset of symptoms, but many can still walk after 30 years or more. Many affected persons have a normal life expectancy (Iannaccone, 1998).

---

**Box 40-6** ▮ ▮ ▮
### Clinical Manifestations of Spinal Muscular Atrophy (SMA)

**TYPE 1 (WERDNIG-HOFFMANN DISEASE)**
Disease acquired in utero or during first 2 months of life
Inactivity is most prominent feature
Infant lies in a frog-leg position with legs externally rotated, abducted, and flexed at knees
Weakness
Limited movements of shoulder and arm muscles
Active movement is usually limited to fingers and toes
Diaphragmatic breathing with sternal retractions
Weak cry and cough
Secretions tend to pool in pharynx
Alert facies
Normal sensation and intellect
Affected infants do not progress to sit alone, roll over, or walk
Early death possible from respiratory failure or infection

**TYPE 2 (INTERMEDIATE SMA)**
Disease manifested between 2 and 12 months of age
Early—weakness confined to arms and legs
Later—becomes generalized
Legs usually involved to greater extent than arms
Prominent pectus excavatum
Movements absent during complete relaxation or sleep
Some infants able to sit if placed in position
Life span varies from 7 months to 7 years

**TYPE 3 (KUGELBERG-WELANDER SYNDROME)**
Onset of symptoms in second year of life
Normal head control and can sit unassisted by 6 to 8 months of age
Thigh and hip muscles weak
In those who manage to walk:
   Lumbar lordosis
   Waddling gait
   Genu recurvatum
   Protuberant abdomen
   Ambulation becomes increasingly difficult
   Confined to a wheelchair by second decade
Deep tendon reflexes may be present early but disappear

---

NOTE: These classifications are general, but some research suggests there may be variations in life span and other characteristics (Russman and others, 1992; Russman, 1996).

## Therapeutic Management and Nursing Considerations

Management is primarily symptomatic and supportive and related to maintaining mobility as long as possible, preventing complications, and providing child and family support.

# Guillain-Barré Syndrome (GBS) (Infectious Polyneuritis)

GBS, also known as infectious polyneuritis, is an uncommon acute demyelinating polyneuropathy with a progressive, usually ascending flaccid paralysis. Children are less often affected than adults; among children, those between ages 4 and 10 years have higher susceptibility. The male/female ratio is reported to be 1.5:1.

GBS is an immune-mediated disease often associated with a number of viral or bacterial infections or the administration of vaccines. It has been associated with infectious mononucleosis, measles, mumps, *Borrelia burgdorferi* (Lyme disease), *Helicobacter pylori*, and *Mycoplasma* and *Pneumocystis* infections. Previous infection with *Campylobacter jejuni* is associated with a severe form of GBS (Allos, 2001; Evans and Vedanarayanan, 1997). Pathologic changes in spinal and cranial nerves consist of inflammation and edema with rapid, segmented demyelination and compression of nerve roots within the dural sheath. Nerve conduction is impaired, producing ascending partial or complete paralysis of muscles innervated by the involved nerves.

### Pathophysiology

Pathologic changes in spinal and cranial nerves consist of inflammation and edema with rapid, segmented demyelination and compression of nerve roots within the dural sheath. Nerve conduction is impaired, producing ascending partial or complete paralysis of muscles innervated by the involved nerves.

### Clinical Manifestations

The paralytic manifestations of GBS are usually preceded by a mild influenza-like illness or sore throat. The onset can be rapid, reaching peak activity within 24 hours, or there may be a gradual progression of symptoms over days or weeks. Neurologic symptoms initially involve muscle tenderness that sometimes is accompanied by paresthesia and cramps. Proximal muscle weakness progressing to paralysis usually occurs before distal weakness, and there is a tendency toward symmetric involvement. In most patients paralysis ascends from the lower extremities, often involving the muscles of the trunk, the upper extremities, and those supplied by cranial nerves. The seventh (facial) cranial nerve is often affected.

Tendon reflexes are depressed or absent, and paralysis is flaccid. Paralysis may involve facial, extraocular, labial, lingual, pharyngeal, and laryngeal muscles. Evidence of intercostal and phrenic nerve involvement includes breathlessness in vocalizations and shallow, irregular respirations. There may be variable degrees of sensory impairment. Most patients complain of muscle tenderness or sensitivity to slight pressure. Lower limb pain and back pain is common

in children with GBS; pain was the most common presentation in one group of children under 6 years of age (Nguyen, Agenarioti-Belanger and Vanasse, 1999). Urinary incontinence or retention and constipation are often present.

### Diagnostic Evaluation

Diagnosis is based on the paralytic manifestations and on electromyography. Motor nerve conduction velocities are greatly reduced. Sensory nerve conduction time is often slowed. Cerebrospinal fluid analysis reveals an increased protein concentration, but other laboratory studies are noncontributory. The symmetric nature of the paralysis helps differentiate this disorder from spinal paralytic poliomyelitis, which usually affects sporadic muscles.

### Therapeutic Management

Treatment of GBS is primarily supportive. Respiratory and pharyngeal involvement requires assisted ventilation, often with tracheostomy. In some cases, corticosteroid therapy has been of benefit in the early stages. Approximately 10% to 20% of children with GBS will require mechanical ventilation (Evans and Vedanarayanan, 1997). Plasma exchange (plasmapheresis) may be beneficial both in shortening the length of illness and in lessening the long-term disability. Intravenous (IV) immunoglobulin infusion may be helpful to some affected persons in the acute stage of the illness (Jones, 1995).

### Course and Prognosis

Better outcomes are associated with younger ages, no requirement for respiratory assistance, slower progression of disease, normal peripheral nerve function on EMG, and treatment with plasmapheresis (Graf and others, 1999). Partial recovery may occur within 1 to 6 months, with complete recovery seen in 80% of all children within 12 months; few children suffer residual effects (Evans and Vedanarayanan, 1997).

Almost all deaths are caused by respiratory failure; therefore early diagnosis and access to respiratory support are especially important. Muscle function begins to return between 2 days and 2 weeks after the onset of symptoms, and recovery is complete in most cases but may be painful. The rate of recovery is usually related to the degree of paralysis and may extend from a few weeks to months.

### Nursing Considerations

Nursing care is essentially supportive and is the same as that required for quadriplegia from any cause. Because the care of the quadriplegic child is discussed in relation to spinal cord injury later in the chapter, it will not be considered at length here. The emphasis of care is on close observation to assess the extent of paralysis and on prevention of complications.

During the acute phase of the disease the child's condition should be carefully observed for possible difficulty in swallowing and respiratory involvement. A mechanical ventilator should be on standby, and suction apparatus, a tracheostomy tray, an appropriate-sized self-inflating bag and bag-valve-mask, and vasoconstrictor drugs should be available at the bedside. Signs that assisted ventilation may be required include a rapidly decreasing vital capacity, dyspnea, signs of fatigue, dysphagia, shoulder weakness, and deteriorating arterial blood gases (Evans and Vedanarayanan, 1997). Vital signs and level of consciousness are monitored at frequent intervals. For the child who develops respiratory dysfunction, the care is the same as that of any child with respiratory distress who requires mechanical ventilation. (See Chapter 31 and care of the child with tetanus who is given muscle relaxant drugs.)

Throughout the recovery phase special emphasis is placed on prevention of complications, including proper postural alignment, frequent change of position, and passive range-of-motion exercises. Children with oral and pharyngeal involvement are usually fed via a gastrostomy tube to ensure adequate feeding. Bowel and bladder care is needed to avoid constipation and urinary retention. Sensory impairment makes the child susceptible to pressure ulcers; pain should be treated before physical therapy sessions.

Physical therapy is limited to passive range-of-motion exercises during the evolving phase of the disease. As the disease stabilizes and recovery begins, an active physical therapy program is implemented to prevent contracture deformities and facilitate muscle recovery. This may include active exercise, gait training, and bracing.

Throughout the course of the illness, child and parent support is paramount. The usual rapidity of the paralysis and the long recovery period greatly tax the emotional reserves of all family members. The parents and child benefit from repeated reassurance that recovery is occurring and from realistic information regarding the possibility of permanent disability. In the event of a residual disability, the family needs assistance in accepting and adjusting to the loss of function. (See Chapter 22.) The **Guillain-Barré Syndrome Foundation International**\* is a nonprofit organization devoted to support, education, and research. It provides families with support from recovered persons, publishes informational literature and a newsletter, and maintains a list of practitioners experienced with the disease.

## Tetanus

Tetanus, or lockjaw, is an acute, preventable, and often fatal disease caused by an exotoxin produced by the anaerobic spore-forming, gram-positive bacillus *Clostridium tetani*. It is characterized by painful muscular rigidity primarily involving the masseter and neck muscles. There are four requirements for the development of tetanus: (1) presence of tetanus spores or vegetative forms of the bacillus, (2) injury to the tissues, (3) wound conditions that encourage multiplication of the organism, and (4) a susceptible host.

Tetanus spores are found in soil, dust, and the intestinal tracts of humans and animals, especially herbivorous animals. The organisms are more prevalent in rural areas but are readily carried to urban areas by wind. They enter the body by way of wounds, particularly a puncture wound,

burn, or crushed area. In the newborn, infection may occur through the umbilical cord, usually in situations in which infants are delivered in contaminated surroundings. The disease has the greatest incidence during months in which persons are more involved in outdoor activities. Substance abusers are especially susceptible from poor injection technique and the use of street heroin, which is often mixed with quinine, a protoplasmic poison that favors the growth of the organism (American Academy of Pediatrics, 2000).

### Prevention

Primary prevention is key and occurs through immunization and boosters (Thayaparan and others, 1998). Once an injury has occurred, further preventive measures are based on the immune status of the affected child and the nature of the injury. Specific prophylactic therapy after trauma is administration of either tetanus toxoid or tetanus antitoxin. A dose of tetanus toxoid is not necessary for clean, minor wounds in children who have completed the immunization series (see Chapter 12) or who have received a booster within the previous 10 years. Protective levels of antibody are maintained for at least 10 years; therefore antitoxin is not indicated for the fully immunized child. Children with more serious wounds (e.g., contaminated, puncture, crush, or burn wounds) are given a tetanus toxoid booster prophylactically as soon as possible after injury.

The unprotected or inadequately immunized child who sustains a "tetanus-prone" wound (such as, but not limited to, wounds contaminated with dirt, feces, soil, and saliva; puncture wounds; avulsions; and wounds resulting from missiles, crushing, burns, and frostbite) should receive *tetanus immune globulin (TIG)*. Concurrent administration of both TIG and *tetanus toxoid* at separate sites is recommended both to provide protection and to initiate the active immune process (American Academy of Pediatrics, 2000). Completion of active immunization is carried out according to the usual pattern. Proper surgical cleansing and debridement of contaminated wounds reduces the chance of infection.

### Pathophysiology

When prevention efforts are not effective and conditions are favorable, the organisms multiply and form two exotoxins: (1) *tetanospasmin,* a potent toxin that affects the central nervous system to produce the clinical manifestations of the disease; and (2) *tetanolysin,* which appears to have no significance. The ideal conditions for growth of the organisms are devitalized tissues without access to air (e.g., puncture wounds), wounds that have not been washed or kept clean, and those that have crusted over, trapping pus beneath. The exotoxin appears to reach the CNS by way of either the neuron axons or the vascular system. The toxin becomes fixed on nerve cells of the brainstem and the anterior horn of the spinal cord. The toxin acts at the myoneural junction to produce muscular stiffness and to lower the threshold for reflex excitability.

The *incubation period* is 3 days to 3 weeks and averages 8 days; most cases occur within 14 days. In neonates it is usually 5 to 14 days. Shorter incubation periods have been as-

---

\*PO Box 262, Wynnewood, PA 19096, (610) 667-0131, fax: (610) 667-7036, e-mail: gbint@ix.netcom.com; www.guillain-barre.com.

sociated with more heavily contaminated wounds, more severe disease, and a worse prognosis (American Academy of Pediatrics, 2000).

## Clinical Manifestations

There are several forms of the disease. *Local tetanus* is a less common but severe form characterized by persistent rigidity of muscles near the inoculation site, which may persist for weeks or months; some cases resolve without sequelae. *Neonatal tetanus* results from contamination of the umbilical cord; it is rare in the United States but is common and often fatal in developing countries. The first symptom is difficulty in sucking; this progresses to total inability to suck, excessive crying, irritability, and nuchal rigidity.

*Generalized tetanus* is the most common and dangerous form of the disease. The manner of onset varies, but the initial symptoms are usually a progressive stiffness and tenderness of the muscles in the neck and jaw. The characteristic difficulty in opening the mouth *(trismus),* which is caused by sustained contraction of the jaw-closing muscles, is evident early and gives the disease its common name, *lockjaw.* Spasm of facial muscles produces the so-called sardonic smile *(risus sardonicus).* Progressive involvement of the trunk muscles causes opisthotonos and a boardlike rigidity of abdominal and limb muscles. There is difficulty in swallowing, and the patient is highly sensitive to external stimuli. The slightest noise, a gentle touch, or bright light triggers convulsive muscular contractions that last seconds to minutes. The paroxysmal contractions recur with increased frequency until they become almost continuous.

Mentation is unaffected; the patient remains alert, and pain and distress are reflected in a rapid pulse, sweating, and an anxious expression. Laryngospasm and tetany of respiratory muscles and accumulated secretions predispose the child to respiratory arrest, atelectasis, and pneumonia. Fever is usually absent or only mild; the presence of fever generally indicates a poor prognosis. As the child recovers from the disease, the paroxysms become less frequent and gradually subside. Survival beyond 4 days usually indicates recovery, but complete recovery may require weeks.

## Therapeutic Management

The child affected by tetanus is best treated in an intensive care facility where close and constant observation and equipment for monitoring and respiratory support are readily available. A quiet environment is preferred to reduce external stimuli. Neonates are placed in an open unit or incubator in which a constant environmental temperature can be maintained.

General supportive care, including maintenance of adequate airway and fluid and electrolyte balance, in addition to caloric intake, is indicated. Indwelling oral or nasogastric feedings are used whenever possible; continued laryngospasm may necessitate IV alimentation or gastrostomy feeding. Severe or recurrent laryngospasm or excessive secretions may require advanced airway management such as endotracheal intubation.

TIG therapy to neutralize toxins is the most specific therapy for tetanus. Antibiotics are administered to control the proliferation of the vegetative forms of the organism at the site of infection. When the child recovers, active immunization should take place, because contraction of the disease does not confer a permanent immunity.

Local care of the wound by surgical debridement and cleansing with an antiseptic solution helps to reduce the numbers of proliferating organisms at the site of injury. The cleansing should be repeated several times during the first 48 hours; deep, infected lacerations are usually exposed and debrided.

Sedatives or muscle relaxants are administered to help reduce muscle spasm and prevent convulsions. The most widely used is diazepam (Valium), but phenobarbital, chloral hydrate, and the phenothiazines may be employed. Patients with severe tetanus and those who do not respond to other sedatives may require the administration of a neuromuscular blocking agent such as vecuronium (Norvcuron) or pancuronium (Pavulon). Because of their paralytic effect on respiratory muscles, the use of these drugs requires mechanical ventilation and constant attendance by trained personnel until muscle spasms are controlled. Despite the absence of pain manifestation with these drugs, it is important to administer adequate analgesia.

Endotracheal tube insertion or tracheostomy is often indicated and should be performed before severe respiratory distress develops. The administration of corticosteroids has met with success in some cases.

## Nursing Considerations

In caring for the child with tetanus, every effort should be made to control or eliminate stimulation from sound, light, and touch. Although a darkened room is ideal, sufficient light is essential so the child can be carefully observed; light appears to be less irritating than vibratory or auditory stimuli. The infant or child is handled as little as possible, and extra effort is made to avoid any sudden or loud noise.

Medications are administered as prescribed, and vital signs are observed and recorded at frequent intervals. The location and extent of muscle spasms and the assessment of their severity are important nursing observations. Respiratory status is carefully evaluated for any signs of distress, and appropriate emergency equipment is kept available at all times. Muscle relaxants, opioids, and sedatives that may be prescribed can also cause respiratory depression; therefore the child must be assessed for excessive CNS depression. Oxygen saturation monitoring and, when needed, blood gases are obtained at intervals to evaluate the respiratory status. Attention to hydration and nutrition may involve monitoring an IV infusion, monitoring nasogastric or gastrostomy feedings, and suctioning oropharyngeal secretions when indicated.

If a potent muscle relaxant such as pancuronium (Pavulon) is used, the total paralysis makes oral communication impossible. Therefore all of the child's needs must be anticipated and the procedures carefully explained beforehand. As the dose of medication is decreased, the child regains movement of the eyelids and facial muscles, which gives the child some opportunity to express emotions and indicate choices through a signal system, for example, blinking the lids to indicate "yes" or "no."

Because their mental status is clear, children are aware of what is happening to them and are often in a state of terror. They should not be left alone, and all efforts should be made to reduce anxiety, which can contribute to muscular spasms. A calm and reassuring manner and sympathetic understanding can help immeasurably in getting a child through this crisis situation. Parents are encouraged to stay with the child to offer security and support. They may also need suport and reassurance from the nurse.

## Botulism

Botulism is a serious food poisoning that results from ingestion of the preformed toxin produced by the anaerobic bacillus *Clostridium botulinum*. Botulism toxin exerts its effect by inhibiting the release of acetylcholine at the myoneural junction, thereby impairing motor activity of the muscles innervated by the affected nerves. There is wide variation in severity of the disease, from constipation to progressive sequential loss of neurologic function and respiratory failure.

### Types of Botulism

Three forms of botulism are recognized: infant botulism, classic botulism, and wound botulism.

**Classic, or Food-Borne, Botulism.** The classic form of the disease is usually seen in adults but may occur in children and adolescents. The most common source of the toxin is improperly sterilized home-canned foods. (See Community Focus box.) CNS symptoms appear abruptly approximately 12 to 36 hours after ingestion of contaminated food and may or may not have been preceded by acute digestive disturbance. Early symptoms include blurred vision, diplopia, weakness, dizziness, difficulty talking and speaking, vomiting, and dysphagia. These are followed by descending paralysis and dyspnea. Progressive respiratory paralysis is life-threatening.

**Infant Botulism.** Unlike the disease in older persons, infant botulism is caused by the ingestion of spores or vegetative cells of *C. botulinum* and the subsequent release of the toxin from organisms colonizing the gastrointestinal tract. There appears to be no common food or drug source of the organisms. However, the *C. botulinum* organisms have been found in honey and light or dark corn syrup fed to affected infants (American Academy of Pediatrics, 2000). Recent re-

ports indicate that there is insufficient evidence to warrant recommending against giving processed corn syrup to infants because changes in the processing of the product have lead to a corn syrup free of *C. botulinum* spores (Olsen and Swerdlow, 2000). Corn syrup is often recommended by health care professionals as a treatment for constipation in infants. (See Critical Thinking Exercise box.)

Risk factors for infant botulism in the United States are the following: (1) ingestion of honey (Cox and Hinkle, 2002); (2) infants 2 months of age or older, decreased frequency of breast-feeding and bowel movements (less than one per day for at least 2 months); and (3) for infants less than 2 months of age, living in a rural area or on a farm. Botulism may occur in infants as young as 3 weeks of age or up to 6 months of age with peak incidence between 2 and 4 months of age (Aneja, Thomas, and Elberger, 2000). The relationship between infant botulism and breast-feeding is controversial; however, there is no evidence to support formula feeding over breast-feeding as a preventive measure (Cox and Hinkle, 2002).

There is wide variation in the severity of the disease, from mild constipation to progressive sequential loss of neurologic function and respiratory failure. The affected infant is usually well before the onset of symptoms. Constipation is a common presenting symptom, and almost all infants exhibit generalized weakness and a decrease in spontaneous movements. Deep tendon reflexes are usually diminished or absent; cranial nerve deficits are common (especially cranial nerves VII, IX, X, and XI), as evidenced by loss of head control, difficulty in feeding, weak cry, and

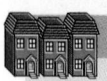

## COMMUNITY FOCUS
### Preventing Botulism

Home supervision and education regarding possible modes of infection (such as the use of honey as formula sweetener) are nursing responsibilities. Because the prime sources of botulism toxin are inadequately cooked or improperly canned food, families are advised about the danger of home-canned foods, especially vegetables, fruits, fish, and condiments. Boiling is not always adequate, particularly at high altitudes, where water boils at a lower temperature, which does not destroy the organisms (Ferrari and Weisse, 1995).

## Critical Thinking Exercise

### Infant Botulism

As part of history taking before a well-child examination of an infant, you learn that the mother mixes her own infant formula and gives the baby sweetened water between feedings. What should be of particular concern to you?

FIRST, THINK ABOUT IT . . .
• What is the purpose of your thinking?
• What conclusions are you reaching?

1. The concentration of the formula mixed.
2. The sweetener used.
3. The source of water.
4. Whether the infant is put to bed with a bottle.

*All of the above are important concerns. The concentration of the formula (whether it is properly mixed according to package directions) is important for purposes of nutrition. If a packaged infant formula is not used, the appropriate mixture of ingredients can be checked with a nutritionist. The sweetener is a critical issue because honey has been found to contain C. botulinum organisms and may cause infant botulism. Only clean, boiled water should be used in mixing infant formula. Finally, using a bottle at bedtime can contribute to the development of dental caries.*

reduced gag reflex. The most commonly recognized form of the disease is consistent with the hypotonic infant (see floppy infant syndrome, p. 1843).

**Wound Botulism.** Wounds contaminated with *C. botulinum* and subsequent elaboration of the toxin produce classic symptoms approximately 4 to 14 days after tissue trauma. The disease has been described in a small number of adolescents and adults, and most wounds are sustained in open fields or on farms.

## Therapeutic Management

Diagnosis is made on the basis of history, physical examination, and laboratory detection of toxin or the organism in the patient or the implicated food. Treatment consists of aggressive supportive measures, primarily respiratory and nutritional. Botulinum antitoxin is sometimes used in adults and older children for food-borne or wound botulism. Because the antitoxin is made from horse serum, it may cause serum sickness or anaphylaxis and may induce a lifelong hypersensitivity. A human-derived botulism antitoxin is under investigation by the California Department of Health Services, Infant Botulism Treatment and Prevention program (Olsen and Swerdlow, 2000).

Toxins vary in protein-binding capacity. Some have a relatively short half-life and do not bind to tissues firmly; therefore therapy is continued until paralysis abates. Other toxins appear to bind irreversibly to nerve endings and therefore are not amenable to neutralization. Respiratory support is often needed and should be available at the bedside and ready for use if indicated. An infant who is recovering from botulism must avoid contact with other infants for about 3 months or until excretion of organisms has ceased (Glatman-Freedman, 1996).

The prognosis is generally good if the patient is adequately supported. However, recovery may be very slow and may require weeks to months following severe illness. The average length of hospitalization is reported to be approximately 5 to 6 weeks (Cox and Hinkle, 2002).

## Nursing Considerations

Nursing responsibilities include observing for and reporting signs of muscle impairment in the child with botulism and providing intensive nursing care when an infant is hospitalized. (See Nursing Care of High-Risk Newborns, Chapter 10.) Parental support and reassurance are important. Most infants recover when the disorder is recognized and therapy is implemented. Parents should be aware that, during recovery, patients fatigue easily when muscular action is sustained. This has important implications for timing the resumption of feedings because of the risk of aspiration. They should also be advised that normal bowel activity may not return for several weeks; therefore a stool softener can be beneficial. Cathartics and enemas are not advised on a routine basis.

# Myasthenia Gravis (MG)

MG is relatively uncommon in childhood. Juvenile MG appears to be identical to that seen in adults and usually has its onset after age 10 years, but it may appear as early as age 2 years. Girls are affected six times as often as boys. Juvenile and adult forms of the disease are autoimmune disorders associated with the attack of circulating antibodies on the acetylcholine receptors on the muscle end plate, which blocks their function.

## Clinical Manifestations

The most common symptoms are general paralysis of the optic muscles with ptosis and diplopia. Difficulty in swallowing, chewing, and speaking are also prominent and are accompanied by weakness and paralysis of all skeletal muscles. The signs and symptoms are more pronounced in the late afternoon and evening. They are relieved by rest and made worse by exercise and stress.

## Diagnostic Evaluation

The diagnosis is made on the basis of the characteristic distribution of muscle weakness and the progressive weakness on repeated or sustained muscular contraction. The diagnosis is established by observation of the response to the anticholinesterase drugs. IV administration of a small test dose of edrophonium (Tensilon) produces a beneficial effect in 1 minute but lasts for fewer than 5 minutes. Electrophysiologic studies are helpful in diagnosis and help document transmission failure at the myoneural junction. Antibodies to human muscle acetylcholine are detected in the serum of almost all affected persons.

## Therapeutic Management

Treatment consists of the oral administration of cholinesterase-inhibiting drugs, such as neostigmine (Prostigmin) given IM or oral neostigmine bromide. Pyridostigmine (Mestinon) may also be administered because it is considered to be less toxic, but a higher dose is required to achieve the same results as neostygmine. The initial dose is 30 mg every 4 hours in the older child and 5 mg every 4 hours in the infant. The dosage is gradually increased until a satisfactory result is obtained. The child must be observed for signs of parasympathetic stimulation from overmedication. These signs include lacrimation, salivation, abdominal cramps, sweating, diarrhea, vomiting, bradycardia, and weakness of respiratory muscles.

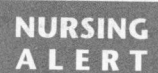 **NURSING ALERT** Atropine is the antidote for overdose of neostigmine and pyridostigmine.

Other therapies directed at the immunologic mechanism include thymectomy (removal of the thymus), corticosteroid therapy, and immunosuppression with agents such as azathioprine (AZA). Children with generalized MG have responded favorably to thymectomy. Plasmapheresis has been used for short-term intensive intervention.

> **NURSING ALERT**
>
> Avoid neuromuscular-blocking agents such as pancuronium or succinylcholine in patients with MG because they may induce paralysis that can last for weeks. Avoid aminoglycoside antibiotics such as gentamicin because they potentiate MG symptoms (Haslam, 2000).

The prognosis for juvenile MG is relatively good. However, the course of the disease is marked by fluctuating remissions and exacerbations.

## Nursing Considerations

Children with MG need ongoing medical and nursing supervision. The parents are taught the importance of accurate administration of medications, with special emphasis on recognizing side effects, including the dangers of choking, aspiration, and respiratory distress.

Parents are counseled regarding promoting a lifestyle that minimizes stress and maximizes relaxation. Strenuous activity is discouraged. They are also warned of the possibility of a sudden exacerbation of symptoms during times of physical or emotional stress *(myasthenia crisis)*, which requires immediate medical attention. They should receive instruction in providing respiratory assistance until help arrives or the child can be transported to medical aid.

## Neonatal Myasthenia Gravis

A *transient* form of MG occurs in approximately 10% to 20% of infants born to mothers with myasthenia gravis, who may not know they have the disease. The muscular weakness results from transplacentally acquired maternal acetylcholine receptor antibodies. These infants display generalized muscle weakness and hypotonia at birth with a depressed Moro reflex, ptosis, ineffective sucking and swallowing reflexes, and weak cry. Symptoms may be evident within a few hours of birth, following a period of normal appearance after delivery (Volpe, 2001). There is no evidence of neurologic damage. Cholinesterase inhibitors may be given on a short-term basis to improve feeding ability. In this form the symptoms usually disappear within 2 to 3 weeks.

*Persistent* neonatal MG is a familial abnormality of neuromuscular transmission that is not immunologically mediated. It appears indistinguishable from the transient form, but the mother usually does not have the disease. The disease persists throughout life, and more than one sibling may be affected, which suggests a genetic etiology. Gender distribution is equal. The disorder is relatively resistant to drug therapy, and the eyelid and extraocular muscles seem to be the muscles most severely affected.

The prognosis in persistent neonatal MG is usually good. Although there is gradual worsening of symptoms with age, the life span is not affected significantly.

## Spinal Cord Injuries (SCIs)

The principles of management and nursing care of the child with a spinal cord lesion apply regardless of etiology. In addition to care related to the immobilized child, as discussed in Chapter 39, children with damage to the spinal cord present additional problems—specifically, complications related to the neuropathology of the central and autonomic nervous systems. A high level of paraplegia may create major problems in the ability to sit upright without support, whereas children with paraplegia due to lower level injuries can walk with minimum assistance. The extent of paralysis is determined by both neurologic and clinical assessment. Although the majority of children with SCIs are paraplegic, some are quadriplegic. Some children with quadriplegia are able to move only their face and neck muscles, whereas others are able to lift and bend their arms but are unable to perform fine hand movements. Almost every physiologic system is disrupted in a child with high-level quadriplegia. Not only are the central and peripheral nerves impaired, but there is also autonomic nervous system dysfunction. Vital structures such as blood vessels, lungs, bladder, and bowel are affected. Therefore an understanding of neuromuscular physiology is essential to effectively care for the child with damage or injury to the spinal cord.

## Review of Essential Neuromuscular Physiology

The spinal cord extends from the medulla oblongata to the lower border of the first lumbar vertebra and contains millions of nerve fibers. However, because of its protected location, a considerable amount of direct trauma is required to cause injury. Posteriorly the cord is protected by the spinous processes, which are stabilized by related ligaments and muscles. It is further protected by the spinal fluid, which surrounds it and absorbs some of the shock.

**Spinal Nerves.** The 31 nerves of the spinal cord are divided into five segments (Fig. 40-5). The eight *cervical* cord segments lie within the first seven vertebrae. The remaining cord segments—*thoracic* (12), *lumbar* (five), *sacral* (five), and *coccygeal* (one)—extend from the first thoracic vertebra to the lower level of the first lumbar vertebra. Therefore the cord constituents do not anatomically match by number the 33 associated vertebrae. However, nerves that arise from the spinal cord exit from the spinal column at the numerically corresponding vertebrae. In describing injuries to the spinal cord, the highest point at which there is normal function is referred to in relation to the vertebra; for example, an intact cord at the sixth cervical vertebra is designated as a C6 injury.

Certain areas of the curved vertebral column are less stable and more prone to damage from severe flexion and twisting. These sites are the cervical area and the junction of the thoracic and lumbar regions. The cervical vertebrae are fractured most often, and this high level of injury causes extensive paralysis and many associated neurologic problems (Table 40-2). Also, traumatic tearing or embolic occlusion of the arteries supplying these areas can markedly jeopardize the cord tissue. Impaired blood supply often produces severe neurologic deficit, which can extend to complete loss of cord function at the level of injury.

Cell bodies of interneurons and motor neurons within the spinal cord are identified as H-shaped gray matter surrounded by columns of white myelinated nerve fibers. Each column serves as a route for a specific type of impulse, such as touch, vibration, pain, and temperature (Fig. 40-6). Nerve pathways in the spinal cord transmit sensory and mo-

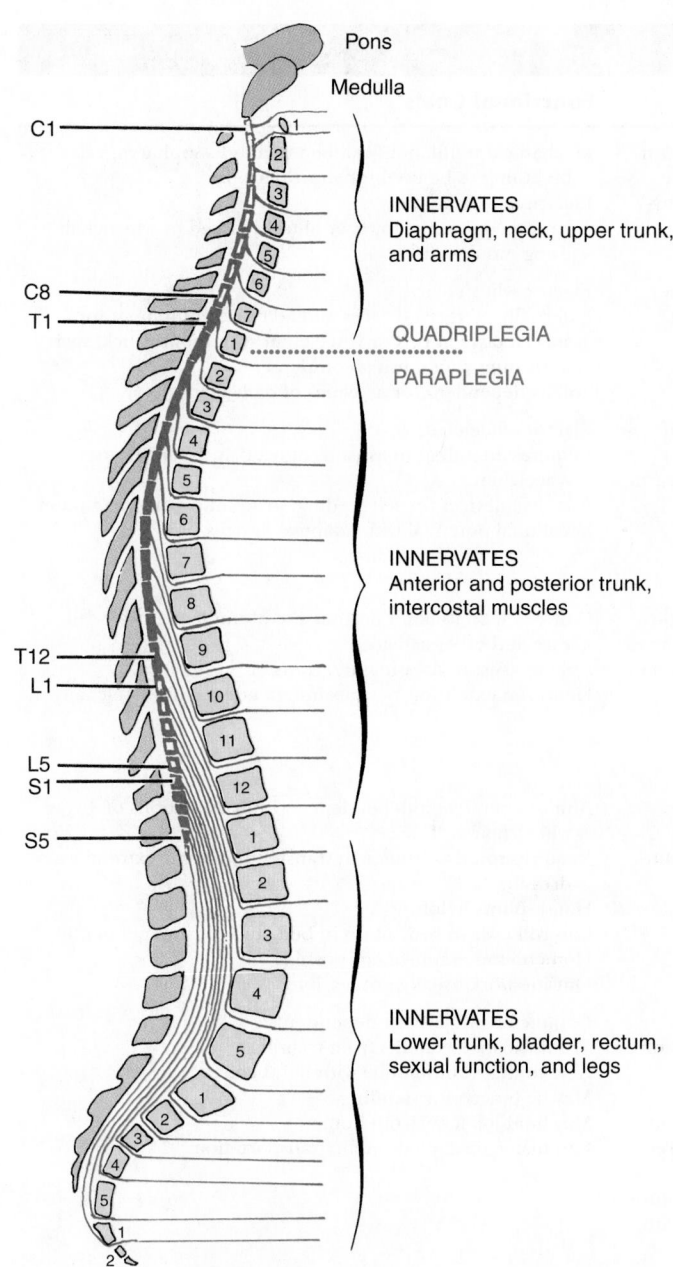

**Fig. 40-5** Relationships of spinal cord segments and spinal nerves to vertebral bodies. Cervical nerves exit through intervertebral foramina above their respective vertebral bodies (seven cervical vertebrae and eight cervical nerves). Spinal cord ends at L1 and L2 vertebral level.

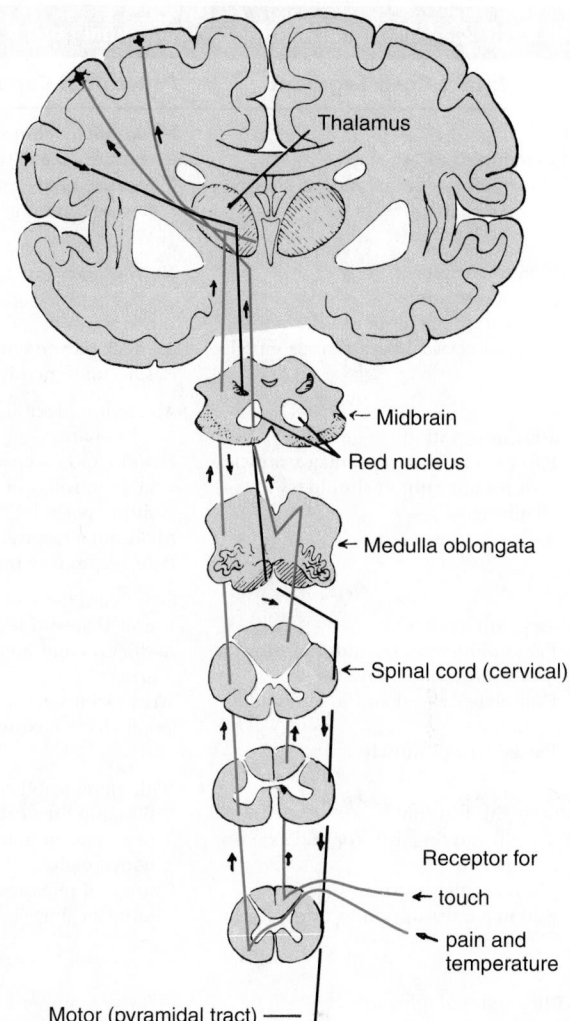

**Fig. 40-6** Diagram of main motor and sensory pathways. Perception of touch, passive motion, position, and vibration is transmitted through posterior tract in spinal cord through medial lemniscus in brainstem to thalamus and through internal capsule to cortex (pathway is represented by *solid red line*). Pain and temperature sensations are transmitted through anterolateral tract and lateral lemniscus to thalamus, then through internal capsule to cortex *(blue line)*. Motor impulses are transmitted by pyramidal tract, descending from cerebral cortex, crossing in medulla to opposite side, and continuing to anterior horns of spinal cord *(black line)*. (From Conway BL: *Carini and Owens' neurological and neurosurgical nursing*, ed 7, St Louis, 1978, Mosby.)

tor impulses between peripheral receptors and the brain, conduct impulses through the reflex arc, and convey sympathetic and parasympathetic nerve impulses from the brain to peripheral structures.

*Sensory* transmission begins when peripheral receptors pick up a wide variety of stimuli and transfer the impulses, by means of peripheral nerves, to the spinal nerves, where they make ganglionic connections and enter the cord posteriorly. At this point the impulses travel in two directions: (1) across the interneuron connection and then to the motor neurons (reflex arc) or (2) up the spinal cord to prede-

termined areas of the brain. *Motor* impulses are transmitted from the cerebral cortex to the medulla (where nerve tracts cross) and proceed down descending motor pathways to the desired level within the spinal cord. Here they connect with the anterior horn cells and are transmitted to the muscle fibers by means of the lower motor neurons to complete a meaningful movement.

A network of nerves that serves the major muscle groups constitutes a *plexus*. Total involvement of any one of these plexuses seriously impairs function to the areas it innervates. The three major plexuses are described in Box 40-7.

**TABLE 40-2** Functional significance of spinal cord lesions

| Highest Intact Cord Segment | Functional Capacity | Functional Goals |
| --- | --- | --- |
| **C1-C3**<br>Muscle innervation:<br>  None below chin, including phrenic nerve to diaphragm | No voluntary control below chin<br>Respiratory paralysis complete<br>May cause bradycardia or tachycardia, vomiting | Mechanical ventilation; can be taught glossopharyngeal breathing to be used for short periods<br>Electric wheelchair<br>Adaptive equipment for special tasks in bed or wheelchair using mouth stick |
| **C4 (high quadriplegia)**<br>Muscle innervation:<br>  Intact sternocleidomastoid, trapezius, upper cervical paraspinous muscles | No voluntary function of upper extremities, trunk, or lower extremities<br>All neck movements<br>Respirator-dependent | Electric wheelchair<br>Externally powered devices and adaptive equipment for special tasks in bed or wheelchair with mouth stick, such as turning pages, using computer<br>Totally dependent for activities of daily living |
| **C5**<br>Muscle innervation:<br>  Partial deltoid, biceps, major muscles of rotator cuffs at shoulders<br>  Diaphragm | Abduction, flexion, and extension of arm<br>Flexion and extension of forearm<br>Unable to roll over or attain sitting position<br>Abdominal respiration<br>Poor respiratory reserve | Electric wheelchair<br>Requires attendant to assist in moving and transfer to wheelchair<br>Adaptive devices for self-feeding, grooming, using computer<br>Vocational potential with adaptive devices |
| **C6**<br>Muscle innervation:<br>  Pectoralis major, serratus anterior, latissimus dorsi muscles<br>  Complete deltoid and brachioradialis muscles<br>  Partial triceps muscle | Significant increase in function over that with lesion at C5 level<br>Adduction and medial rotation of arm<br>Wrist extension<br>Good elbow flexion | Cuff strapped to hand permits use of implements for self-care and other activities<br>Able to assist in dressing and transfer<br>Hand rim extension permits independence in wheelchair |
| **C7**<br>Muscle innervation:<br>  Triceps and finger flexor and extensor muscle<br>  Shoulder depressor muscles<br>  Still nerve disruption to intercostal muscles | With elbow stabilized in extension and intact shoulder depressor muscles, able to lift body weight<br>Grasp and release still weak; dexterity lacking | Almost complete independence within limitations of wheelchair<br>Requires some assistance in transfer and lower extremity dressing<br>Hand splints helpful<br>Can roll over in bed, sit up in bed, and eat independently<br>Homebound employment possible<br>Outside work usually not feasible |
| **T1-T10 (high paraplegia)**<br>Muscle innervation:<br>  Full innervation of upper extremity muscles | Full use of upper extremities, including intrinsic muscles of hand<br>Trunk balance poor<br>May have difficulty in lifting sufficiently to put on lower extremity clothing<br>Considerable energy expenditure to put on long leg braces with extensive attachments | Completely wheelchair-dependent<br>Trunk balance benefits from training<br>Able to drive automobile with hand controls<br>May be braced for standing<br>May hold job away from home<br>Can manage adapted public transportation |
| **T10-L2**<br>Muscle innervation:<br>  Full abdominal and upper back muscle control | Good trunk balance<br>Good respiratory reserve<br>Can accomplish moderate hiphiking using external oblique and latissimus dorsi muscles | Ambulation with bilateral long braces using four-point or swing-through crutch gait<br>Usually able to negotiate curbs<br>Some able to use regular public transportation<br>Few vocational limitations as long as does not require much walking or standing |
| **L3 or below**<br>Muscle innervation:<br>  Quadriceps muscle<br>  Partial gluteus and hamstring muscles | May be lumbar lordosis<br>Floppy ankles | Ambulates well, often with short leg braces with or without cane<br>Difficulty in getting out of wheelchair<br>May never require wheelchair |

**Upper vs Lower Motor Neurons.** *Upper motor neurons* extend from cerebral centers to cells in the spinal column; *lower motor neurons* consist of anterior horn cells and spinal and peripheral nerves. Motor fibers of the reflex arc are lower motor neurons; this is an important point because relative dominance of the CNS over reflex arcs suppresses some reflex responses. When the higher centers no longer exert an influence in spinal cord injury, spastic responses are observed in muscles innervated by the intact lower motor neurons. Most SCIs involve upper motor neurons; children born with spinal cord defects have primarily lower motor neuron deficits (see Fig. 40-1). Manifestations of upper and lower motor neuron syndromes are outlined in Box 40-8.

**Cervical plexus** (C1 through C4), which innervates the neck and diaphragm
**Brachial plexus** (C4 through T1), which supplies the shoulders, chest, and arms
**Lumbosacral plexus** (L1 through S4), which transmits impulses to the lower trunk and legs

| UPPER MOTOR NEURON SYNDROME | LOWER MOTOR NEURON SYNDROME |
|---|---|
| Spastic paralysis in muscle groups below lesion (reflex arcs below lesion are intact) | Flaccid paralysis caused by muscle atonia (reflex arcs are permanently damaged) |
| Hyperreflexia with tendon reflexes exaggerated, Babinski reflex present | Reflex with associated muscle response absent |
| No wasting of muscle mass because of increased muscle tone | Marked atrophy of atonic muscle |
| Flexion contractures and spasms of muscle groups below lesion level common | Fasciculations (local twitching of muscle groups) common |
| | No flexor spasms |
| No skin or tissue changes | Loss of hair |
| | Skin and tissue changes |
| | Cornified nails |

Decreased muscle tone and impairment of vasoconstrictive effects of sympathetic innervation cause venous pooling, diminished venous return to the heart, decreased cardiac output, and hypotension, especially orthostatic hypotension (orthostatic intolerance).
Thermoregulatory disruption in the hypothalamus and skin receptors causes blood vessels to remain dilated during the initial stage, an inability to sweat in response to increased environmental temperature, and a possible rapid elevation in body temperature.
Voluntary bowel and bladder function is lost because of damage to nerve fibers that innervate these organs.
Altered sexual function (lack of erection, ejaculation, and orgasm) results from interference with numerous autonomic nerve fibers and plexuses.

**Effect on Sensory and Motor Tracts.**   Voluntary muscle control is lost following complete transection of the cord. In partial transection, function is altered to varying degrees depending on the areas innervated by involved nerves. The crossing of motor tracts at various levels makes it possible for an injured person to have motor paralysis in one leg but retain pain and temperature sensation in that leg, while the opposite leg retains its motor function but loses pain and temperature sensation.

Although a transected cord injury leads to sensory loss, it is not uncommon for the injured person to have pain experiences. For example, smooth or skeletal muscle spasms, destruction of the myelin sheath (impulses cross to adjacent nerves), and scar formation or irritation of nerve endings may cause pain. Pain suffered by a person with quadriplegia or paraplegia is often intensified because of loss of sensation in other parts. Severe and prolonged pain should be medically evaluated for treatable pathology.

**Effect on Autonomic System.**   Sympathetic and parasympathetic systems receive both excitatory and inhibitory stimuli from autonomic centers in the cerebral cortex, limbic system, and hypothalamus. The stimuli are transmitted by means of a feedback mechanism within the ascending fibers of the cord that normally controls descending input. Axons of the many CNS neurons synapse with autonomic preganglionic fibers and thus are able to alter their pat-

terned responses. The most significant effects of autonomic disruption are described in Box 40-9.

### Etiology

The most common cause of serious spinal cord damage in children is trauma involving motor vehicle crashes (MVCs) (including automobile-bicycle, all-terrain vehicles, and snowmobiles), sports injuries (especially from diving, trampoline activities, gymnastics, and football), birth trauma, and child abuse. Congenital defects of the spine such as myelomeningocele (see Chapter 11) also may, in some cases, produce the effects of SCI.

Transverse myelitis (inflammation of the spinal cord) has also been reported to develop from inadvertent intraarterial administration of long-acting penicillin injected into the buttocks. Damage can be extensive enough to result in paraplegia or even lower limb amputation.

**Mechanisms of Injury.**   In MVCs most SCIs in children are a result of indirect trauma caused by sudden hyperflexion or hyperextension of the neck, often combined with a rotational force. Trauma to the spinal cord without evidence of vertebral fracture or dislocation is particularly likely to occur in an MVC when proper safety restraints are not used. An unrestrained or improperly restrained child becomes a projectile during sudden deceleration and is subject to injury from contact with a variety of objects inside and outside the vehicle. Individuals who use only a lap seat belt restraint are at greater risk of SCI than those who use a combination lap and shoulder restraint. High cervical spine injuries have been reported in children less than 2 years of age who are restrained in forward-facing car seats (Cramer, 1995). Infants who are improperly restrained in an infant car seat may experience cervical trauma in a car crash. Small children may also be severely injured by front seat air bags. (See Chapter 13.)

Falling from heights occurs less often in children than in adults, but vertebral compression of the spine from blows to the head or buttocks occurs in water sports (diving and surfing) or falls from horses or other athletic injuries. Birth injuries may occur in breech delivery from excessive traction force and rotation on the cord during delivery of the head and shoulders. When shaken, infants commonly sustain cervical cord damage as well as subdural hematoma and retinal hemorrhage; mental retardation and death may occur subsequent to the traumatic event. Infants have very weak neck muscles, and during vigorous shaking their large and heavy heads rapidly wobble back and forth. A number of adolescents receive SCIs when they are shot or stabbed.

Because of the marked mobility of the neck, *fracture* or *subluxation* (partial *dislocation*) is the most common immediate cause of SCI, particularly in the lower cervical region. Although unusual in adults, SCI without fracture is not uncommon in the child, whose spine is suppler, weaker, and more mobile than that of the adult; therefore the force is more easily dissipated over a larger number of segments. In children the vertebral column is composed of cartilaginous rings and is capable of considerable elongation, whereas the cord itself, its meninges, and its vascular supply are unable to withstand the same degree of traction.

The injury sustained can affect any of the spinal nerves; the higher the injury, the more extensive the damage. The child can be left with complete or partial paralysis of the lower extremities *(paraplegia)* or with damage at a higher level and without functional use of any of the four extremities *(quadriplegia)*. A high cervical cord injury that affects the phrenic nerve paralyzes the diaphragm and leaves the child dependent on mechanical ventilation.

A mild but equally frightening form of cord trauma is *spinal cord compression,* a temporary neural dysfunction without visible damage to the cord. Complete quadriplegia can result but initially may not be differentiated from serious cord injury (Cramer, 1995).

## Pathophysiology

The severity of the force, the mechanisms of the injury, and the degree of the individual's muscular relaxation at the time of the injury greatly influence the extensiveness of the trauma. Compression, contusion, laceration, and anatomic transection are the basic types of cord injuries and usually involve four interrelated pathologic changes: (1) cellular damage to cord tissue; (2) hemorrhage and vascular damage; (3) structural changes of white and gray matter related to vascular disruption, inflammation, and edema; and (4) local biochemical response to trauma. Changes in one of these can lead to changes in another. For example, an acute injury produces decreased blood supply to the cord tissue, with resulting ischemia that can lead to cellular necrosis. Acid metabolites accumulate during the hypoxic state and can contribute to further cellular damage. A concurrent inflammatory process produces cord edema above and below the traumatized segment, further decreasing the blood supply. Research on spinal cord trauma indicates that neurotransmitters norepinephrine and dopamine can be markedly altered in the first few hours after injury, which causes further development of hemorrhagic necrosis in the central gray matter.

## Clinical Manifestations

As a result of these pathologic responses to the initial trauma, SCI is characterized by three stages of response;

therefore the extent and severity of damage cannot be determined at first. Immediate loss of function is caused by both anatomic and impaired physiologic function, and improved function may not be evident for weeks or even months.

**First Stage.** Manifestation of the initial response to acute SCI is flaccid paralysis below the level of the damage. This stage is known as *diaschisis* or *spinal shock syndrome* and is caused by the sudden disruption of central and autonomic pathways. Local effects of cord edema and ischemia produce a physiologic transection with or without an anatomic severance. Most children with an SCI experience some spinal shock. Manifestations include the absence of reflexes at or below the cord lesion, with flaccidity or limpness of the involved muscles, loss of sensation and motor function, and *autonomic dysfunction* (symptoms of hypotension, low or high body temperature, loss of bladder and bowel control, and autonomic dysreflexia).

Autonomic paralysis also affects thermoregulatory functions. Afferent impulses from temperature receptors in the skin are not integrated; therefore the patient is subject to temperature increases or decreases in response to alterations in environmental temperature. Hyperthermia can result from excessive ambient temperature, such as too many covers.

**Second Stage.** Except in the situations previously mentioned, flaccid paralysis is replaced by spinal reflex activity and increasing spasticity or, in partial lesions, greater or lesser degree of neurologic recovery. Diagnosis may be confused in infants because spinal reflexes in paralyzed limbs may be misinterpreted as the normal movements in the infant. Even a minor stimulus, such as rubbing the mattress, is sufficient to elicit spinal reflexes. Concurrent crying may also lead to the erroneous impression that sensation is intact. Paralysis is suggested by the absence of spontaneous leg movement of the extremities when the infant is held vertically suspended under the axilla. Reflex withdrawal or extension of the limb after tactile or pinprick stimulus confirms a diagnosis.

The paralytic nature of autonomic function is replaced by *autonomic dysreflexia,* especially when the lesions are above the midthoracic level. This autonomic phenomenon is caused by visceral distention or irritation, particularly of the bowel or bladder. Sensory impulses are triggered and travel to the cord lesion, where they are blocked, which causes activation of sympathetic reflex action with disturbed central inhibitory control. *Excessive sympathetic activity* is manifested by flushing of the face, sweating of the forehead, pupillary constriction, marked hypertension, headache, and bradycardia. The precipitating stimulus may be merely a full bladder or rectum or other internal or external sensory input. It can be a catastrophic event unless the irritation is relieved.

**Third Stage.** In the final stage neurologic signs are stabilized in terms of loss and recovery of function. The major emphasis is on rehabilitation. A problem unique to injury in childhood is progressive spinal deformity usually not seen in adults or in adolescents near the end of the growth period. Scoliosis develops in the major percentage of children with high thoracic and cervical lesions and is almost certain to occur in children with quadriplegia whose injury occurred in infancy or early childhood.

## Diagnostic Evaluation

A history of the nature of the injury provides valuable clues regarding the possible type of damage incurred and directions for further assessment without the risk of additional damage. A complete neurologic examination is performed to determine if damage was incurred and, if so, the level and extent of any nerve impairment. A neurologic unit of the CNS is considered normal if reflex arcs are functioning, sensory tracts are intact when each dermatome is examined separately, and voluntary motor response demonstrates an ability to move a body part against gravity on command.

Testing a reflex arc is accomplished by stimulating the peripheral receptors at a specific site, such as eliciting the patellar reflex. Symmetric testing is performed to determine unilateral or bilateral neurologic deficit. A sufficient number of reflexes are examined to test motor function thoroughly. The blunt end of a safety pin is used to assess pressure sensitivity, and the sharp point is used to elicit pain. Hot and cold water, a tuning fork, and cotton may also be used to determine specific sensory loss (e.g., temperature, vibration, and light touch).

***Body surface zones,*** or ***dermatomes,*** accurately correspond to the spinal cord segment receiving the sensory input from the peripheral nerves in that zone. Systematically pinpricking the body surface in each zone determines intactness of sensory pathways. The zones and the spinal cord segments they represent are illustrated in Fig. 40-7. The examiner tests for each specific sensory fiber in the dermatome areas in which there is a suspected neurologic deficit.

Matching cord level to vertebra is more difficult in infants and young children than it is in older children and adults because the sacral and several lower lumbar cord segments lie at a lower position, especially during the first 2 years of life. The spinal anatomy approaches adult configuration by the time the child reaches age 7 or 8 years; by late adolescence the conus medullaris has usually reached the level of L1.

Motor system evaluation includes observing gait if the child is able to walk, noting balance maintenance with the eyes open and closed, and noting the ability to lift, flex, and extend the arms and legs. Testing muscle strength with and without resistance and against gravity will give clues to the specific nature and degree of motor dysfunction. The number of muscles in any muscle group that remain completely intact in the upper extremities makes a marked difference in the individual's ability to provide self-care, especially at high injury levels. The presence of the abdominal muscles is valuable in bladder and bowel training and in maintaining an upright sitting position. Hip movement is necessary for ambulation with braces and crutches.

The degree to which supportive aids are needed for ambulation is determined by the strength, stability, and movement of the pelvis, trunk, hip flexor muscles, and quadriceps muscles. A general guideline for determining the capacity for self-help is that a person with paraplegia who

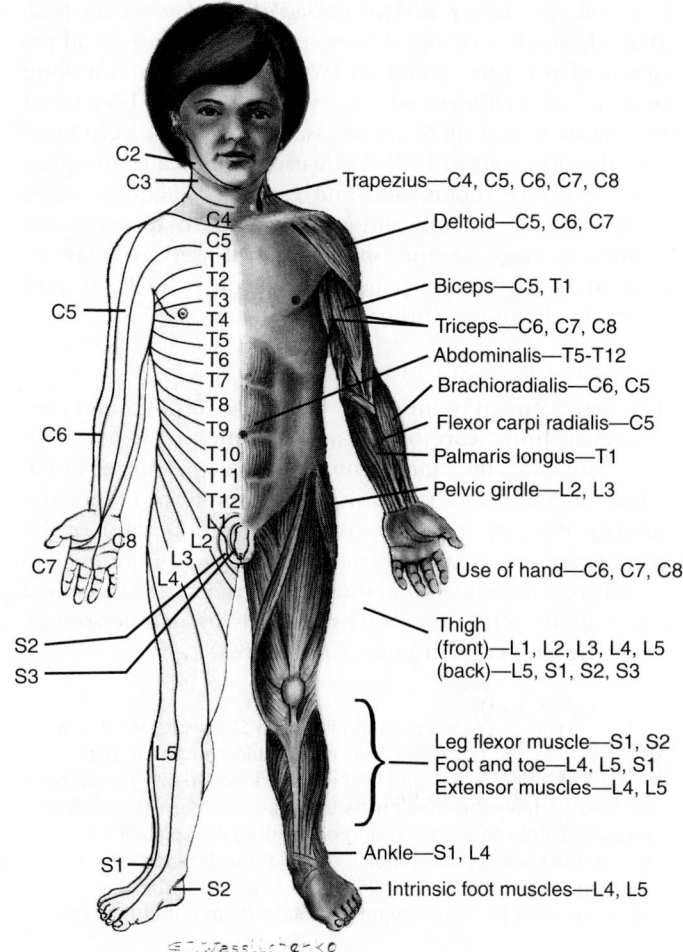

**Fig. 40-7** Dermatomes and innervation of major muscles needed for performing activities of daily living.

has function down to and including the quadriceps muscle or muscle function below the L3 level will have little difficulty in learning to walk with or without braces and crutches. It is especially vital that children with lumbar levels of injury be taught to walk functionally so that they are weight bearing at least part of the time; this minimizes the risk of osteoporosis and hypercalcemia. The functional significance of the spinal cord lesion level is summarized in Table 40-2.

If CNS pathology is detected, a body system assessment is performed to determine the degree of autonomic impairment. Because the cord and CNS directly influence the function of the autonomic nerves, the specific sympathetically related organ systems are examined for skeletal muscle and vascular tone and body temperature regulation. For example, bladder and gastrointestinal function have sympathetic and parasympathetic innervation and local reflexes.

Computed tomography (CT) and magnetic resonance imaging (MRI) scans are important for localizing the lesion, but the nature of the spine in childhood often creates difficulty in interpretation. Some children will have no radiographic evidence of vertebral or spinal injury; this condition is *spinal cord injury without radiographic abnormality (SCI-WORA)*, which is reported to occur in 5% to 55% of all pediatric SCIs (Loder, 2000). SCIWORA is a common finding in very young children who are victims of abuse because of the elasticity and incomplete ossification of the vertebrae. The development of SCIWORA usually indicates the presence of severe subluxation and trauma. Diagnostic scans must be taken carefully and with sufficient help to prevent further damage to the spine. Several persons may be needed to logroll the patient, to support the head, and maintain alignment during turning or transfer.

## Therapeutic Management

The management of the child with SCI is complex and controversial. Initial care begins at the scene of the accident; therefore education and training of rescue personnel in stabilization and transfer techniques to prevent or reduce the severity of injury are of utmost importance. Because of the complexity and relative infrequency of these injuries, it is usually recommended that these persons be transferred to a spinal injury center for care by specially trained personnel. (See The Child and Trauma, Chapter 39.)

**NURSING ALERT**

In any situation in which SCI is suspected or a possibility, the child should be calmed, reassured, and told not to move; no one should be allowed to move the child unless the head and trunk can be correctly stabilized to avoid twisting or bending the spine. If conscious, the child is placed supine on a rigid surface to prevent sagging. Infants and small children are removed in their car seats; no attempt should be made to take them out of the seat.

Management during the first stage is primarily supportive, with efforts directed toward preventing further neuronal damage, avoiding complications, and maintaining vital functions. Steroid administration within the first 8 hours after injury is advocated to prevent secondary spinal cord edema and inflammation. Bolus-dose methylprednisolone administration followed by continuous infusion for 23 hours has been shown to increase functional recovery significantly in patients with SCI. Children with cervical lesions often have compromised respiratory function and may require mechanical ventilation. Cervical lesions may require temporary skeletal traction, a halo vest (see Chapter 39), or another device to maintain position, and corticosteroids are administered in an attempt to prevent destructive edema. Operative intervention may be necessary to remove bone fragments and debris, but routine surgical exploration is not usually performed.

The focus of the second phase is primarily rehabilitative and is aimed at returning the patient to the home and community. The focus is on maximizing the potential for self-help, recovery of muscle function, mobility, independence, education, and, employment.

A number of progressive rehabilitation modalities have been developed in recent years that have the potential for increasing the quality of life for children with SCI. One treatment is *functional electrical stimulation (FES)*. With this treatment an electrical stimulator is surgically implanted under the skin in the abdomen, and electrode leads are tunneled to paralyzed leg muscles, enabling the child to sit, stand, and walk with the aid of crutches, a walker, or other orthoses (Spoltore and others, 2000). The stimulator can also be used to elicit a voluntary grasp and release with the hand. Before the latter can be accomplished a number of surgical tendon transfers may be required for elbow extension, wrist extension, and finger and thumb flexion. Tendon transfers have been shown to be successful in enhancing hand function, increasing pinch force, and facilitating independence in ADLs (Spoltore and others, 2000). Restoration of hand and arm function enables children with SCI to perform self-catheterization and achieve greater independence in personal hygiene. FES is reported to have many benefits for children with SCI, including cardiovascular conditioning, decreasing pressure ulcers, and increasing blood flow (Merenda, Spoltore, and Betz, 2000). A number of orthoses may still be necessary to achieve upright mobility, yet, as robotic technology advances, so do the chances for improvement in mobilization in children with SCI. FES has also been shown to be effective in reducing complications due to bladder and bowel incontinence, as well as assisting males in achieving penile erection.

Paralytic scoliosis is a problem for many young children with SCI because thoracic capacity is reduced and pulmonary function hampered. Newer treatments for paralytic scoliosis involve the use of prophylactic bracing from the time of injury until skeletal maturity is achieved. The Boston brace soft body jacket and thoracolumbosacral orthosis (TLSO) are commonly used for bracing (Spoltore and others, 2000). (See Chapter 39.) Additional rehabilitative treatments are discussed in other sections as they pertain to bladder and bowel function and sexuality.

**Prognosis.** The ultimate outlook for spinal cord function after injury depends on the completeness of the cord transection, the site of injury, the complicating damage to the neuronal tissue, and the success of treatment regimens aimed at recovery of lost muscle movement and ability. Healing of the injury and the return of neurologic function are related to two factors:

1. Although individual nerve fibers do regenerate, they do not necessarily reconnect or make synaptic connections with the distal portion of the severed fibers; the chance of numerous fibers reconnecting is highly unlikely.
2. The damage resulting from cord ischemia produces necrosis in the gray and white matter of the cord tissue, which does not regenerate if the axon cylinder is not intact.

In general, recovery in thoracic lesions is variable for motor function. Cervical injuries are also variable in the extent of damage. Incomplete lesions produce hemiplegia, whereas complete transection implies some involvement of all extremities—from partial use of the upper extremities to complete paralysis, including the need for assisted ventilation. Lumbar injury may involve partial or complete loss of function in the lower extremities and bladder. With rapidly advancing surgical technology, use of microcomputers in medicine, and newer treatment modalities such as FES, there is increasing hope and evidence that functional mobility and independence can be restored in children with SCI.

## Nursing Considerations

The nursing care of the child who is paralyzed is complex and challenging. As a member of the acute care and rehabilitation teams, the nurse is involved in all aspects of care. Ideally, initial care takes place in a special intensive care unit with personnel trained to handle SCIs, and nursing management is concerned primarily with prevention of complications and maintenance of vital functions.

Once the acute period is over, the lesion is usually static and nonprogressive, regardless of whether the paralysis is secondary to trauma, congenital defect, infection, a treated tumor, or surgery. The nurse is a member of a team of specialists that includes physicians from a number of specialty areas, physical and occupational therapists, psychologists, social workers, teachers, and vocational counselors. Each team member has a unique contribution to make, and mutual agreement for specific areas of responsibility and evaluation of progress are determined during regularly scheduled team conferences. The family and child should be included in team meetings as is appropriate.

Although care of the child with an SCI is, in most aspects, the same as that of any immobilized child, some important differences will be discussed here. (See The Immobilized Child, Chapter 39.)

**Respiratory Care.**   The child with a high-level injury (quadriplegia) requires continuous ventilatory assistance. In most instances a tracheostomy is the method of choice for greater ease in clearing secretions and for less trauma to tissues during long-term ventilatory dependence. In an acute care center, respiratory therapy personnel are responsible for establishing and maintaining the equipment, but the nurse must understand how it works and recognize mechanical malfunction and deviations from the prescribed rate and volume. In case of malfunction the nurse must be prepared to maintain respirations manually with a self-inflating bag-valve-mask device. In some home care situations the nurse may be responsible for the care of ventilatory assistance devices. In some youngsters breathing pacemaker devices (phrenic nerve stimulators) are implanted to stimulate the phrenic nerve and produce diaphragmatic contractions and lung expansion without assisted ventilation. If the child has a pacemaker, part of the nursing function is understanding its function and operation.

Children with lesions below the C4 level are seldom ventilator-dependent, but pulmonary vital capacity is significantly reduced. They should be positioned for optimum chest expansion, and a variety of breathing exercises and assistive devices are used to stimulate deep breathing. Patient-triggered synchronous intermittent mandatory ventilation (SIMV-assist/control mode) may be required to maintain adequate oxygenation. Chest physiotherapy is performed as needed to mobilize secretions and flow-by oxygen may be needed occasionally. Regular monitoring of breath sounds to assess for adequate ventilation in all lobes is part of routine care.

The cough reflex is markedly diminished and, together with weak intercostal muscles, the youngster may have difficulty with secretions. Increasing the elastic qualities of the lung by exercise and incentive spirometry helps to achieve a productive cough.

**Temperature Regulation.**   Temperature regulation usually creates few problems, although environmental conditions can influence body temperature. During the spinal shock stage the dilated capillaries conducting body heat to the subcutaneous tissues cause heat loss. Without the capacity to sweat, the body retains heat in hot weather. Consequently clothing and blankets are added or removed according to the body temperature. An elevated temperature that cannot be corrected by environmental measures should be evaluated to rule out urinary or upper respiratory tract infection. However, excessive perspiration observed in sentient areas usually indicates an elevated ambient temperature. Because the skin is a less reliable indicator in these children, the oral or aural (ear) route is usually the preferred method of temperature measurement.

**Skin Care.**   In cases in which SCI is associated with vertebral fracture, cervical traction may be maintained for several weeks until there is sufficient evidence of bone healing. (See The Child in Traction, Chapter 39.) Initially the child is turned every 2 hours around the clock. An alternating-pressure mattress or other pressure relief/reduction device is kept underneath the child, and the skin is thoroughly inspected at least once a day for signs of pressure, especially over bony prominences. Prevention of pressure ulcers is much easier than treatment. A number of factors contribute to the risk of skin breakdown in these children: decreased sensation, poor nutrition from negative nitrogen balance, low hemoglobin level, spasticity, and improper positioning. (See Maintaining Healthy Skin, Chapter 27.)

The areas most apt to be affected are the sacrum, scapulae, heels, and occiput when the child is in a supine position; the trochanters and the lateral aspect of the ankles, heels, and knees when the child is in a side-lying position; and the ischial tuberosities when the child is in a sitting position. The pressure wound may begin in deeper tissues and is visible on the surface only at a later stage; therefore areas that feel firm, irregular, or warm or that appear to be only slightly reddened require careful evaluation. (See Wounds, Chapter 18.) Keeping the skin clean and dry is particularly important in these children, especially those who are incontinent. Treatment of pressure areas or ulcers is instituted promptly.

**Physiotherapy.**   Maintaining proper body alignment, preventing pressure from bed linen, providing proper support, applying splints as ordered, and using padded booties to hold the feet in correct position are important in daily care. Range-of-motion, passive, and active exercises are carried out under the guidance of a PT. In children with upper motor neuron involvement, the spasticity that develops may require administration of an antispasmodic, usually diazepam. Botulinum type A, gabapentin, and $\alpha_2$-adrenergic agonists are being used in older children with SCI to decrease muscle spasticity (see p. 1839). Decreasing stimuli to the muscles also helps reduce spasticity. For example, tight clothing and bed linens are avoided, and extremities are handled at the joints rather than by the belly of the muscle. Anticipating the possibility of spasms when the child is moved and providing the necessary safety precautions can prevent possible injury during transport.

Unless there are contraindications, exercises during the period of immobilization are aimed at maintaining and increasing the strength of the child's intact musculature. Upper extremity strengthening is especially important to the paraplegic child, who must rely on these muscle groups for turning, transferring, dressing, crutch walking, and other activities. Children are usually eager to use their muscles and respond to interesting and innovative activities.

**Neurogenic Bladder.**   When the bladder is denervated, as in the acute stage of spinal shock syndrome or after lower motor neuron damage, the bladder wall is flaccid. Lack of muscle tone inhibits the ability of the bladder to respond to changes in passive pressure, causing overdistention. Therefore it is important to prevent distention by periodic emptying, even though there may be dribbling between emptying.

In contrast, an upper motor neuron lesion causes increased bladder tone and contractions that often include the urinary sphincter. Thus although the bladder empties periodically by reflex action, complete emptying is prevented, resulting in urinary retention and ureteral reflux. Administration of antispasmodics such as dicyclomine (Bentyl) relaxes bladder musculature and promotes increased bladder capacity and more adequate emptying. Intervals of urination depend on many factors, including patterns of fluid intake and perspiration.

Recent options for children with neurogenic bladder include the creation of a urinary stoma, made possible by removing the appendix and creating a urinary diversion from the bladder to the exterior, usually the umbilicus, thus making self-catheterization more private, especially with the recovery of hand and elbow movement (with tendon transfers). Other options include surgical bladder augmentation to increase capacity and FES to restore micturition on command (Spoltore and others, 2000).

Emptying the bladder by intermittent catheterization may be required; older children who are functionally capable can be taught to perform self-catheterization.* Children who must use or have used self-catheterization should be counseled regarding the effects of latex allergy. Bladder-training programs usually begin with intermittent bladder emptying at regular intervals that are gradually increased. (See Management of Genitourinary Function under Myelomeningocele [Meningomyelocele] in Chapter 11.)

The urine is kept acidic to decrease the likelihood of stone formation and to inhibit bacterial growth. Ascorbic acid, 1 to 4 g daily, is most effective. Cranberry juice therapy is advised to decrease urinary tract infections. Maintenance of bladder dynamics and control of urinary tract infections are of utmost importance. Pyelonephritis and renal failure

are the most significant causes of death in long-standing paraplegia.

> **NURSING ALERT**
>
> The Credé maneuver, which involves manually compressing the lower abdomen to express urine, should not be used because of the risk of bladder rupture (Reinberg, Fleming, and Gonzalez, 1994). The child with a neurogenic bladder is also at risk for developing latex allergy from repeated catheterizations.

**Bowel Training.**   Successful bowel training is easier to institute than bladder management. The aim is to control defecation until an appropriate time and place are found. A diet with sufficient fiber (approximately 15 g/day) for adequate stool bulk and insertion of a glycerin or bisacodyl (Dulcolax) suppository at a convenient time, either morning or evening, are often all that are necessary to induce a bowel movement within a short time. The probability of an accident between times is diminished once the bowel is completely evacuated. The key to adequate bowel training is to maintain consistency in relation to the same time of day every day for evacuation. Stool softeners, such as docusate sodium (Colace) and senna (Senokot), are usually prescribed, and manual anal stimulation may help initiate evacuation, especially in spastic paraplegia. Sometimes an oral laxative such as bisacodyl may be necessary. Once an appropriate regimen is established, little modification is required. FES has also been used successfully in children with SCI to achieve bowel training (Spoltore and others, 2000).

**Autonomic Dysreflexia.**   Children with high-level lesions are very susceptible to the development of autonomic dysreflexia, which requires prompt action to prevent encephalopathy and shock. As soon as a quick assessment has ruled out other causes, such as orthostatic hypertension, someone should measure the blood pressure while the bladder is checked for distention (the usual precipitating cause). The bladder is drained slowly; if this does not relieve symptoms, any tight clothing is loosened, and the bowel is checked for the pressure of impacted feces. If removal of the causative agent is unsuccessful in controlling the syndrome, IV administration of an antihypertensive drug is indicated, followed by oral maintenance doses. Antispasmodics may also be administered.

**Remobilization.**   As soon as the condition warrants doing so, the child is moved from a reclining to an erect position. Cardiovascular deconditioning and impaired autonomic responses below the level of injury will cause pooling of blood in the extremities (because of peripheral vasodilation), a drop in blood pressure, and a feeling of light-headedness, dizziness, or fainting on sudden assumption of an upright posture, often referred to as *orthostatic intolerance.* Therefore an upright position must be accomplished gradually by first placing the child (who is secured by passive restraint) on a head-up tilt table. The table is slowly elevated from a horizontal to a 30-degree semireclining position. This is performed twice daily for 20 to 30 minutes, with the angle gradually increased until the vertical angle is reached.

During the procedure the vital signs are monitored, and the child's behavior is observed for subjective symptoms of

---

*Home care instructions are available in Wong DL, Hess CS: *Wong and Whaley's clinical manual of pediatric nursing,* ed 5, St Louis, 2000, Mosby.

syncope. The pooling of blood is reduced by using elastic antiembolism hose and sequential pneumatic compression devices, which consist of inflatable sleeves that fit on the legs and compress the leg muscles for cyclic emptying and filling of leg veins. The process of achieving an upright posture may require several weeks. After tolerance is achieved, the child will be ready to begin using a wheelchair. Getting the child up should be accomplished slowly by gradually elevating the bed over 20 to 30 minutes before placing the child in the wheelchair and then gradually lowering the legs after the child has been in the chair a short time.

All adaptive devices help children increase their mobility, function, and endurance. The child with some lower extremity function progresses to parallel bars and then to a walker; the child with quadriplegia learns to use a wheelchair—among the most valuable aids available to the child with an SCI. The selection of a wheelchair should be made carefully in relation to where it will be used, the architectural barriers, and the functional capacity of the child. For lower extremity paralysis, the wheelchair described earlier is applicable. For children with severe upper extremity paralysis, a variety of motorized wheelchairs are used; however, the more complex they are, the greater their cost, weight, and tendency to break down. Wheelchair tolerance is gained over time and is accompanied by measures to prevent orthostatic hypotension and pressure sores.

A variety of orthoses and other appliances can be adapted for use by many children. The primary purpose of lower extremity bracing in the child with an SCI is for ambulation, although correction of deformities may be attempted. However, the efficacy is limited because of the tendency to develop pressure lesions over insensate areas. The higher the lesion, the more support required, with the accompanying difficulties of getting into the orthosis and the greater energy expended in using the appliance. The energy required in ambulating with crutches and braces is two to four times greater than that required for normal walking.

Children, with their natural and overwhelming propensity for mobility, usually attain or may even surpass the maximum expectation in ambulation. However, as they approach adulthood, the increasing weight and energy cost usually cause them to resort to predominant use of the wheelchair for mobility and the pursuit of more intellectual and vocational interests. Wheelchair mobility has the advantages of requiring no more energy than normal walking and allowing the person with paraplegia to maintain the speed of other pedestrians on level ground.

**Physical Rehabilitation.** The major aims of physical rehabilitation are to prepare the child and family to resume life at home and in the community. Additional goals of rehabilitation in children with SCI are to achieve independence in mobility and self-care skills and to promote academic achievement, independent living, and employment (Massagli, 2000). Members of the multidisciplinary rehabilitation team cooperate with each other and the family to identify the child's needs and to plan realistic interventions. Integration of activities is coordinated by one team member, most often a specialist in physical medicine and rehabilitation. Members of the team attempt to achieve their collaborative goals through mutual trust, good communication, professional respect, and sincere interest in the child and family. Training in the rehabilitation center involves maximum achievement commensurate with each child's physical capacities (Fig. 40-8). Instruction for home routine is stressed and includes all the precautions and management implemented in the hospital (e.g., skin care, nutrition, bladder and bowel training) as well as an exercise program. The overall goals of rehabilitation are listed in Box 40-10.

Inpatient physical rehabilitation of children with quadriplegia takes approximately 2 to 4 months; children with paraplegia can achieve these goals in 1 to 3 months but require constant vigilance to avoid complications. Emotional adjustments take longer, especially in older children and adolescents. In most children the outlook is favorable unless the life-threatening consequences of urinary pathology are severe or the emotional adjustment is poor.

**Psychosocial Rehabilitation.** Early-acquired or congenital disability is usually more readily accepted by children than paralysis that appears later in childhood. Rehabilitation efforts should include not only the child's emotional responses but also those of the persons who maintain the closest contact with the child. Intensive education is important so that members of the family understand the nature of the disability, the therapeutic regimen, and complications and are able to provide the physical and emotional support

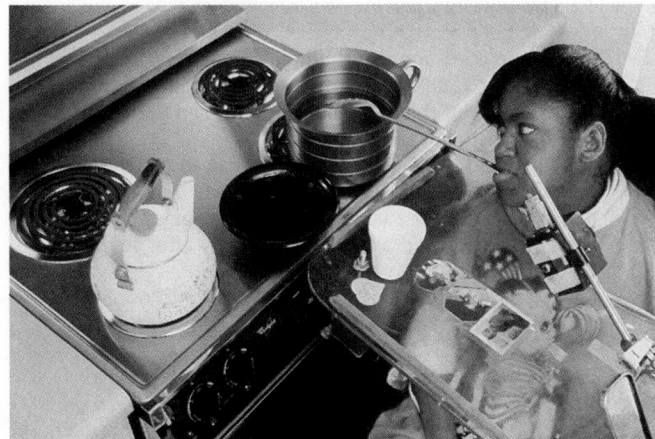

**Fig. 40-8**   Adolescent with quadriplegia uses her mouth and a device activated by her mouth to perform activities of daily living. (Courtesy The Hospital for Sick Children, Washington, DC.)

---

**Box 40-10** ■ ■ □
**Goals of Rehabilitation for the Child with a Spinal Cord Injury**

Maximizing motor function and minimizing the disabling effects of the pathology
Assisting the child and family in setting realistic goals for the child, learning to be good problem solvers, and using the child's assets
Helping the child to cope with the stigma of being different and to build a positive self-image

needed by the child. As with any disability, children should be treated as normally as possible and encouraged in developmental tasks at the age at which they would typically be expected to acquire abilities and perform activities. However, the goals must be realistic, and children should not be forced beyond their capabilities.

Severe depression can be emotionally and intellectually immobilizing, but it indicates that the child is no longer hiding behind denial. In rehabilitation it is desirable for the child to begin to express negative feelings toward the situation because these feelings, redirected by efforts of the rehabilitation team, are the ones that will motivate the child toward learning a new way of life.

The responses to loss are discussed in Chapter 23; the multiple problems related to altered self-image, especially in older children and adolescents, are discussed in relation to children with disabilities in Chapter 22. Children with severe disabilities need to alter certain concepts about self and social roles. If they perceive adults as persons with complete control over their bodies and the ability to do what they want when they want, they will need to develop a more realistic definition of interdependent adult living.

The needs of youngsters who are permanently disabled must be reevaluated periodically by the total rehabilitation team, including the youngsters and their families. Vocational rehabilitation becomes important not only for helping adolescents with permanent disabilities find meaningful work activities but also for assisting them in enrolling in formal educational programs as desired.

The outlook for children with SCI is increasingly favorable for integration into society. Increased awareness of the needs of persons with disabilities has removed many structural and occupational barriers. The success of a rehabilitation program is not judged by how well children manage within the rehabilitation setting but by how well they function on the outside. In addition to agencies that offer assistance to children with disabilities in general, some agencies provide specific assistance to paralyzed persons, including children.*

**Sexuality.** The problems of self-image are particularly marked when children with a spinal cord injury reach puberty and are likely to be even more intense if the disability is acquired during adolescence. Sexual development and awareness and changing perceptions of body image are prominent aspects of adolescence; a loss that affects these areas is a severe blow to an adolescent. Development of secondary sex characteristics does not seem to be altered by SCI, and it is now believed that with comprehensive rehabilitation, well-motivated young people can look forward to successful participation in marital and family activities.

In females, if the injury occurs after the onset of menstruation, there is usually a temporary cessation and irregularity in menstrual flow, but menstruation resumes in the majority of cases. Ovulation and conception are possible, but females will not experience vaginal or clitoral orgasms, although they can learn to use other erogenous zones for a sexual experience. This is important to emphasize in sex education because many females have the misconception that they are unable to conceive because they lack sensation. Also, education is important because the pregnant paraplegic or quadriplegic patient may be unaware that she is in labor, and those with a high-level injury are subject to autonomic hyperreflexia during labor.

Until recently, more attention has been focused on rehabilitating male sexual function (erection and ejaculation). A number of pharmacologic (prostaglandin $E_1$) and mechanical devices (penile implants, vaccum devices) now make it possible for males to participate in sexual intercourse and produce offspring provided that fertility has not been affected by associated complications (Spoltore and others, 2000). Adolescents with SCI should be counseled regarding the effects of latex allergy and condom use.

As soon as adolescent males become aware of their functional loss, they will be concerned about sexual capacities, regardless of the type of sexual activities experienced before the SCI. The health care professional should take the initiative in discussing sexuality with youngsters and their families. Parents of younger children may want to know about their children's sexual and reproductive potential. As their

---

*Information about organizations and resources can be found through **No Limits Communications, Inc**, PO Box 220, Horsham, PA 19044, (215) 675-9133, fax: (215) 675-9376, (888) 850-0344, New Mobility (toll free), www.newmobility.com. Another helpful resource for families is **Spinal Cord Injury Information Network**; www.spinalcord.uab.edu.

---

### Critical Thinking Exercise

#### Spinal Cord Injury and Sexuality

A 17-year-old boy who is paralyzed from the waist down as a result of an MVC frequently exposes himself to the young female nursing staff and makes flirting comments with sexual connotations to you when his family and friends are absent. What should your response be to these actions?

FIRST, THINK ABOUT IT . . .
- Within what point of view are you thinking?
- How are you interpreting the information?

1. Ignore the comments and administer care as necessary.
2. Say, "That is totally inappropriate. I am going to inform your parents of this behavior and reassign your care to one of the male nurses."
3. Say, "I would prefer that you not speak to me that way and show yourself. It looks like you may be concerned about your own sexual abilities and appearance. Many men are concerned about sexual ability after spinal cord injury."
4. Say nothing but quickly leave the room and notify the supervisor, who is a man.

*The correct answer is three. Adolescents need to have appropriate limits set regarding sexual behavior and remarks. At the same time, there is likely an underlying concern about sexual abilities and attractiveness after an SCI. This is an important developmental issue at this stage and needs to be acknowledged and addressed.*

interest and understanding increase, adolescents need to know the specifics of physiology, the prognosis, and sexual techniques related to their particular problems. The practitioner should provide them with information about what can be expected regarding erection, ejaculation, and other sexual experiences.

A knowledgeable rehabilitation team will be valuable to children as they experience concerns regarding loss as a sexual being. (See Critical Thinking Exercise box.) This is especially true in paraplegia or quadriplegia. Most sexual counseling for adolescents with SCI focuses on developing the idea that sex means different things to different people. Most rehabilitation teams have an active counseling program to help youngsters learn intimacy and how to function sexually within their limitations. Through individual and group counseling they gain new attitudes concerning sexuality and experiences exclusive or inclusive of intercourse.

# MUSCULAR DYSFUNCTION

## Juvenile Dermatomyositis

Dermatomyositis is a relatively rare multisystem inflammatory disorder of unknown etiology and is often difficult to distinguish from muscular dystrophy. Approximately half of affected children will have a very acute, rapidly progressive disease, with the remainder having an insidious onset. There is proximal limb and trunk muscle weakness and loss of reflexes. The neck muscles are often affected, and the child may have difficulty in lifting the head or supporting it in an upright position. Muscles tend to be stiff and sore. A generalized vasculitis of small arteries and capillaries is one prominent feature of the disease (Kool, 2000). Masseter involvement with atrophy may occur, which makes it difficult to chew food during the active stage of the disease. Soft palate dysfunction may make speech difficult and interfere with breathing. Distal muscle strength and reflex responses remain unaffected. Dermatomyositis, often classified as a collagen disease, is characterized by a red erythematous rash over the malar areas and nose and a violet discoloration of the eyelids. The skin over extensor muscle surfaces may be erythematous, scaly, and atopic. Calcium deposits develop in muscle tissues as the disease progresses. Indurated skin lesions may develop over areas exposed to pressure, including the elbows, knees, and buttocks; these lesions are reported to be indicative of the severity and duration of the disease. The vasculitis may cause gastrointestinal, renal, cardiac, and ophthalmologic symptoms as the disease progresses (Kool, 2000).

Dermatomyositis responds to corticosteroid therapy and high-dose IV gamma globulin therapy. For cases that do not respond to these agents, methotrexate may be helpful in suppressing the symptoms but not in preventing recurrence of the disease. Physical therapy is essential to prevent contracture deformity and to rebuild muscle strength. Orthoses may be needed. Meticulous skin care is an important nursing consideration in the care of these patients.

Although the prognosis for survival has steadily improved, dermatomyositis remains a serious illness. Death can occur in the acute phase as a result of myocarditis, progressive unresponsive myositis, perforation of the bowel or, occasionally, lung involvement.

**TABLE 40-3** Characteristics of the major muscular dystrophies

| Primary Myopathy/ Inheritance Pattern | Age of Onset | Initial Manifestations | Progression | Therapy |
|---|---|---|---|---|
| **Pseudohypertrophic (Duchenne)** X-linked recessive, sporadic | Early childhood; age 3-5 years | Lordosis Waddling gait Frequent falls Toe walking Difficulty in rising from floor and climbing stairs Fat deposits replace wasted gastrocnemius muscles | Rapid Ultimately involves all voluntary muscles Death usually occurs between ages 15 and 30 years | Supportive Physical therapy to prevent disuse atrophy of unaffected muscles |
| **Becker** X-linked recessive, sporadic | After 7 years of age | Same as Duchenne | Much slower progression than Duchenne | Same as Duchenne |
| **Limb-girdle** Autosomal recessive (usually) | Late childhood or during adolescence; over age 8 years | Weakness of proximal muscles of both pelvic and shoulder girdles | Variable but usually slow Most become incapacitated within 20 years of onset; in some, disability may remain slight | Supportive Physical therapy to prevent disuse atrophy of unaffected muscles |
| **Facioscapulohumeral (Landouzy-Dejerine)** Autosomal dominant | Early adolescence; over age 8 years | Lack of facial mobility Difficulty in raising arms over head Forward slope of shoulders | Very slow May be intervals with no progression Considerable disability in time, but life span unaffected | Supportive |

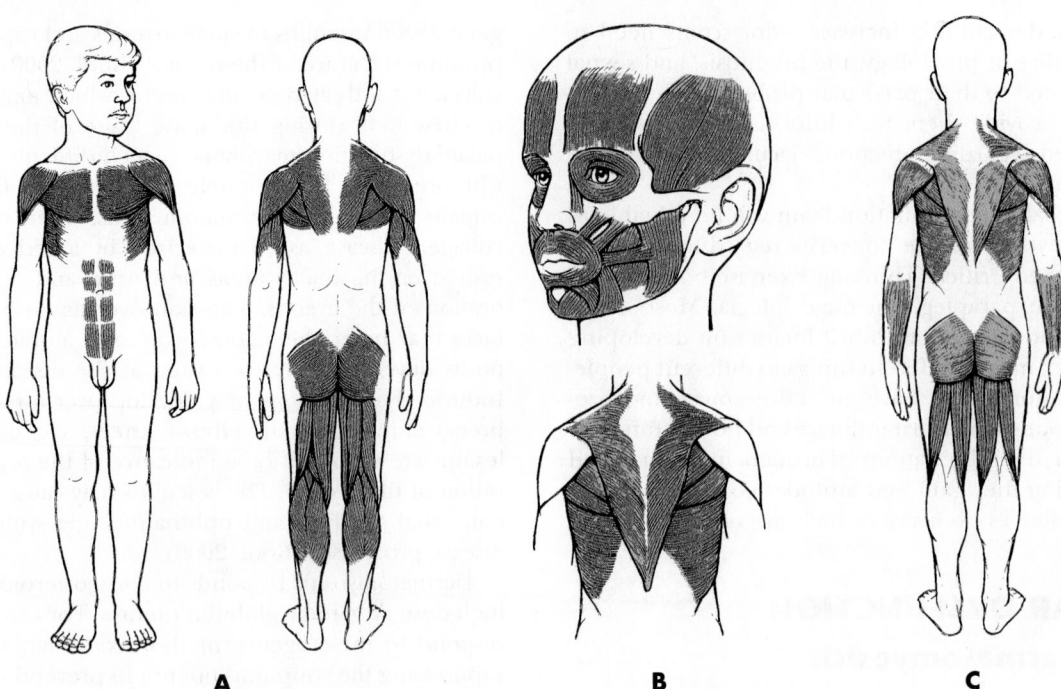

**Fig. 40-9** Initial muscle groups involved in muscular dystrophies. **A,** Pseudohypertrophic. **B,** Facioscapulohumeral. **C,** Limb-girdle.

---

**Box 40-11** ■ ■ ■
**Characteristics of Duchenne Muscular Dystrophy**

Early onset, usually between 3 and 5 years of age
Progressive muscular weakness, wasting, and contractures
Calf muscle hypertrophy in most patients
Loss of independent ambulation by 9 to 12 years of age
Slowly progressive, generalized weakness during adolescence
Relentless progression until death from respiratory or cardiac failure

---

## Muscular Dystrophies (MDs)

The MDs constitute the largest and most important single group of muscle diseases of childhood (Table 40-3). They have a genetic origin in which there is gradual, progressive degeneration of muscle fibers, and they are characterized by progressive weakness and wasting of symmetric groups of skeletal muscles, with increasing disability and deformity. In all forms of MD there is insidious loss of strength, but each differs in regard to the muscle groups affected, age of onset, rate of progression, and inheritance patterns.

The basic defect in MD is unknown but appears to be caused by a metabolic disturbance unrelated to the nervous system. Serum CPK is consistently elevated in affected individuals, which assists in the diagnosis and affords a means of early detection of the disorder (Voit, 1998) in asymptomatic children in families at risk. EMG and muscle biopsy are important diagnostic procedures. Initial sites of muscle involvement are illustrated in Fig. 40-9.

Treatment of the MDs consists mainly of providing supportive measures (including physical therapy and orthopaedic procedures to minimize deformity) and assist-ing the affected child in meeting the demands of daily living.

## Pseudohypertrophic (Duchenne) Muscular Dystrophy (DMD)

DMD is the most severe and the most common muscular dystrophy of childhood (Roland, 2000; Voit, 1998). An X-linked inheritance pattern is identified in most cases; about one third of all cases represent new mutations. As in all X-linked disorders, males are affected almost exclusively. The incidence is approximately 1 in 3500 male births for the Duchenne form and approximately 1 in 30, 000 live births for the Becker type (Thompson and Berenson, 2001). The characteristics of DMD are described in Box 40-11.

At the genetic level, both DMD and Becker muscular dystrophy, a milder variant, result from mutations of the gene that encodes *dystrophin,* a protein product in skeletal muscle. Dystrophin is absent from the muscle of children with DMD and is reduced or abnormal in character in children with Becker MD. There is a strong correlation between the clinical severity of these disorders and the type of genetic mutation and dystrophin protein alterations (Richards and Iannaccone, 1994). Prenatal diagnosis is also possible using several methods, such as the polymerase chain reaction. However, ethical questions exist regarding diagnosing a condition in the fetus when no treatment exists.

### Clinical Manifestations

Evidence of muscle weakness usually appears during the third or fourth year, although there may have been a history of delay in motor development, particularly walking. Difficulties in running, riding a bicycle, and climbing stairs are

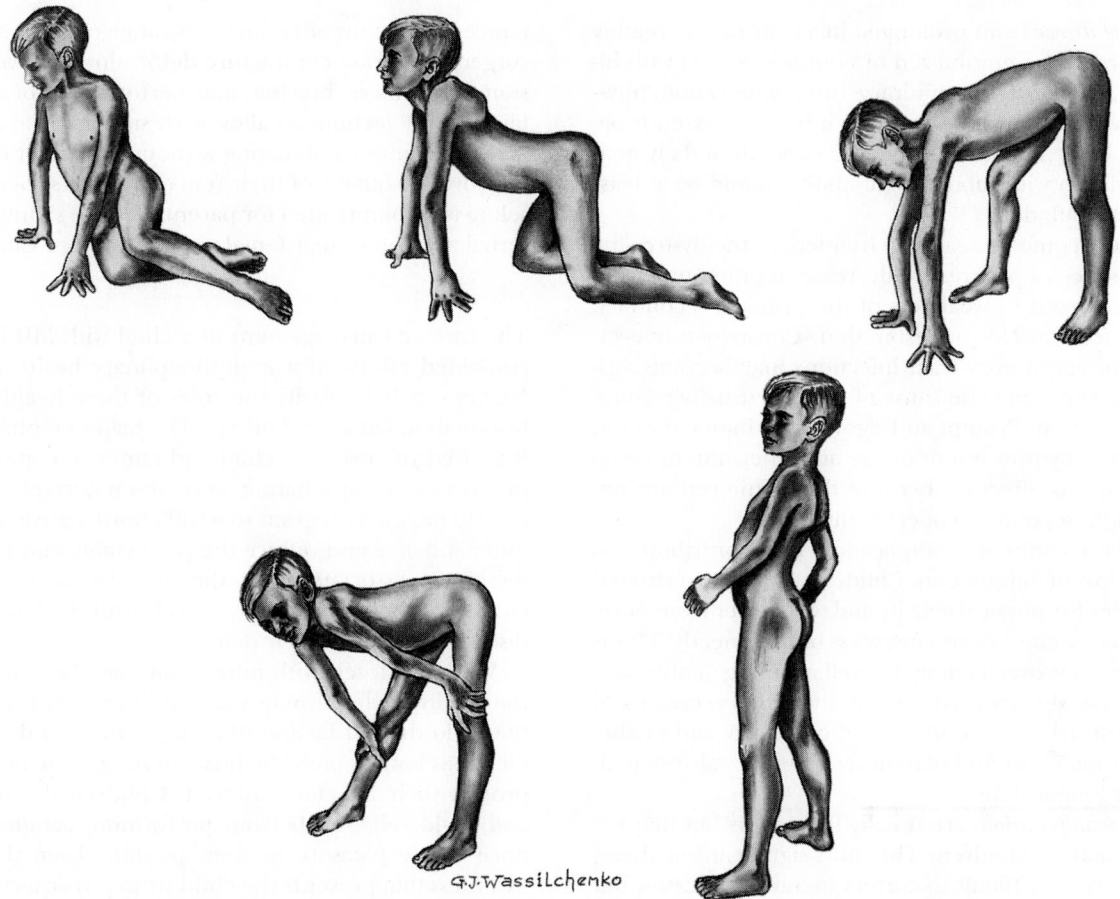

G.J.Wassilchenko

**Fig. 40-10**    Child with Duchenne muscular dystrophy attains standing posture by assuming a kneeling position, then gradually pushing his torso upright (with knees straight) by "walking" his hands up his legs (Gower sign). Note marked lordosis in upright position.

usually the first symptoms noted. Later, abnormal gait on a level surface becomes apparent. In the early years rapid developmental gains may mask the progression of the disease. Questioning of parents may reveal that the child has difficulty in rising from a sitting or supine position. Occasionally, enlarged calves may be noticed by parents.

Typically, affected males have a waddling gait and lordosis, fall frequently, and develop a characteristic manner of rising from a squatting or sitting position on the floor *(Gower sign)* (Fig. 40-10). Muscles, especially in the calves, thighs, and upper arms, become enlarged from fatty infiltration and feel unusually firm or woody on palpation. The term *pseudohypertrophy* is derived from this muscular enlargement. Profound muscular atrophy occurs in the later stages; contractures and deformities involving large and small joints are common complications as the disease progresses. Ambulation usually becomes impossible by 12 years of age. Facial, oropharyngeal, and respiratory muscles are spared until the terminal stages of the disease. Ultimately the disease process involves the diaphragm and auxiliary muscles of respiration, and cardiomegaly is common. The cause of death is usually respiratory tract infection or cardiac failure.

Mild-to-moderate mental impairment is commonly associated with MD. The mean intelligence quotient is approximately 20 points below normal, and frank mental deficit is present in 30% of these children. Verbal intelligence quotient is markedly low in males with DMD, and emotional disturbance is more common than in other children with disabilities (Roland, 2000).

**Complications.**    The major complications of MD include contractures, disuse atrophy, infections, obesity, respiratory and cardiopulmonary problems.

*Contracture deformities* of the hips, knees, and ankles occur from early selective muscle involvement and often exaggerate the weakness. Passive range-of-motion exercises, stretching, and active exercises under the supervision of a PT are effective in treating reducible contractures. Nonreducible contractures require wedge casting or surgical reduction. Scoliosis caused by muscle imbalance is common and tends to progress even when the child becomes dependent on a wheelchair. Bracing with a semirigid corset may be needed for support, although it may interfere with mobility, and children with MD do not tolerate rigid spinal bracing. Frequent rest periods in the recumbent position are often beneficial. For correction of deformities it is essential to select a procedure that immobilizes the child for as short a period as possible to minimize the chances of developing disuse atrophy.

*Atrophy of disuse* from prolonged inactivity occurs readily when children are immobilized or confined to bed with illness, injury, or surgery. To minimize this complication, physical therapy should be implemented if bed rest extends beyond a few days. To maintain muscle strength, a daily goal for well children with moderate disability should be at least 3 hours of ambulation.

*Infections* become increasingly frequent as the dystrophic process produces a progressive decrease in pulmonary vital capacity as a result of weakness of the primary, secondary, and associated muscles of respiration. Consequently even minor upper respiratory tract infections may become serious in these children. The cause of death is usually respiratory tract infection. Prompt and vigorous antibiotic therapy, supplemented by postural drainage and intermittent respiratory therapy, is effective. Because these children are unable to cough, secretions collect easily.

*Obesity* is a common complication that contributes to premature loss of ambulation. Children who have restricted opportunities for physical activity and who suffer from boredom easily consume calories in excess of their needs. This is compounded by overfeeding by well-meaning family and friends. Proper dietary intake and a diversified recreational program help reduce the likelihood of obesity and enable children to maintain ambulation and functional independence for a longer time.

*Cardiac manifestations* are usually late events but may occur in ambulatory children. The most significant of these, cardiac failure, is difficult to correct in advanced cases, but treatment with digoxin and diuretics is often beneficial in the early stages of the disease.

### Diagnostic Evaluation

MD is suspected on the basis of clinical manifestations (see Box 40-11) and confirmed by serum enzyme measurement, muscle biopsy, and EMG. Serum CPK levels are extremely high in the first 2 years of life before the onset of clinical weakness. Aspartate aminotransferase (AST) levels may be mildly elevated before muscle weakness is noted and may be the only clue to onset of the disease (Roland, 2000). They diminish with muscle deterioration but do not reach normal levels until severe muscle wasting and incapacitation have occurred. Muscle biopsy reveals degeneration of muscle fibers, with fibrosis and fatty tissue replacement. EMG readings show a decrease in amplitude and duration of motor unit potentials.

### Therapeutic Management

There is no effective, definitive treatment for childhood MD. Increased muscle bulk and muscle power have been reported following a course of corticosteroid therapy. Some recommend steroid therapy for patients older than 5 years of age if side effects are not severe (Roland, 2000).

Maintaining function in unaffected muscles for as long as possible is the primary goal. It has been found that children who remain as active as possible are able to avoid wheelchair confinement for a longer period. Early recourse to a wheelchair accelerates deconditioning and promotes the development of lower extremity contractures. Mainte-nance of function often includes range-of-motion exercises, surgery to release contracture deformities and vertebral fusion for scoliosis, bracing, and performance of ADLs. Certain surgical techniques allow early sitting and ambulation if children are still ambulating without bracing or casting and improve the quality of their remaining years. Genetic counseling is recommended for parents, female siblings, and maternal aunts and their female offspring. (See Chapter 5.)

### Nursing Considerations

The care and management of a child with MD involve the combined efforts of a multidisciplinary health care team. Nurses can help clarify the roles of these health care professionals to family and others. The major emphasis of nursing care is to assist the child and family in coping with the progressive, incapacitating, and fatal nature of the disease; to help design a program that will afford a greater degree of independence and reduce the predictable and preventable disabilities associated with the disorder; and to help the child and family deal constructively with the limitations the disease imposes on their daily lives.

Working closely with other team members, nurses assist the family in developing the child's self-help skills to give the child the satisfaction of being as independent as possible for as long as possible. It is tempting for parents to overprotect their affected children. Children derive pleasure and build self-esteem from performing actions that produce visible pleasure in their parents. Even the physical weakness that prevents the child from physical competition with other children has little effect on the child as long as it does not affect the parents' attitude toward the child as an individual. Therefore parents must be helped to develop a balance between limiting the child's activity because of muscular weakness and allowing the child to accomplish things alone. This requires continual evaluation of the child's capabilities, which are often difficult to assess. It is not always possible to know when the child seeks parental assistance to get a little extra attention or because of overtired muscles. Fortunately, most children with MD instinctively recognize the need to be as independent as possible and strive to do so.

Practical difficulties faced by families are the physical limitations of housing and mobility. Some families live in houses or apartments that are unsuited to wheelchairs—no street-level entrance, upstairs bedrooms and bathrooms, no tub. Some families have no independent means of transportation. Assisting with these challenges requires team problem solving. Parents may also need help in modifying clothing for their child. It is difficult to find clothing and footwear to wear comfortably in a wheelchair, to fit over contracted limbs, or to fit an obese child. Diet, nutritional needs, and nutrition modification are discussed according to the needs of the individual child and family.

Parents' social activities may be restricted, and the family's activities must be continually modified to meet the needs of the affected child. (See Chapter 22.) The child cannot be left with an ordinary adolescent baby-sitter but requires a specially trained person, such as a student nurse. Consequently the parents also tend to lead more isolated lives. When the child becomes increasingly helpless, the family may consider home care nurses or a skilled nursing facility to provide the necessary care. Nurses can assist with and support the family in decision making.

Each child's therapy program is tailored to individual needs and capabilities, and family members should be active participants. Parents often need assistance with the physical therapy program and education regarding a home regimen of exercises and activity. Many parents erroneously believe that by exerting sufficient effort, the child can overcome the weakness and prevent progression of the disease process. They should also be advised to notify the nurse or other designated person when the child becomes even temporarily bedridden so that the exercise program can be modified and continued during this time.

Children with MD tend to become socially isolated as their physical condition deteriorates to the point where they can no longer keep up with friends and classmates. Their physical capabilities diminish, and their dependency increases at the age at which most children are expanding their range of interests and relationships. To gain associations, they often learn behaviors that bring them the rewards of other children's company. These friends are often children who have been rejected by more able-bodied classmates.

No matter how successful the program and how well the family adapts to the disorder, superimposed on the physical and emotional problems associated with a child with a long-term disability is the constant presence of the ultimate outcome of the disease. All the manifestations seen in the child with a chronic and fatal illness are encountered in these families. (See Chapter 23.) The guilt feelings of the mother may be particularly pronounced because of the mother-to-son transmission of the defective gene.

Nurses are especially valuable health care professionals as they come to know the family and the family's challenges. Nurses can be alert to the problems and needs of the families and make necessary referrals when supplementary services are indicated. The **Muscular Dystrophy Association of America, Inc.**\* has branches in most communities to provide assistance to families in which there is a member with muscular dystrophy.

---

\*3300 East Sunrise Dr, Tucson, AZ 85718, (800) 572-1717, fax: (520) 529-5300, e-mail: mda@mdausa.org; www.mdausa.org. In Canada; **Muscular Dystrophy Association of Canada,** 2345 Yonge St, Suite 900, Toronto, Ontario M4P 2E5, (416) 488-0030 or (800) 567-2873, fax: (416) 488-7523; www.mdac.ca.

## KEY POINTS

- Upper motor neuron lesions produce weakness associated with spasticity, increased deep tendon reflexes, and abnormal superficial reflexes; lower motor neuron lesions interrupt the reflex arc, causing weakness and atrophy of the skeletal muscles.
- The most useful classification of neuromuscular disorders defines the source of the lesion: cerebral cortex, anterior horn cells of the spinal cord, peripheral nerves, myoneural junction, and muscles.
- Clinical manifestations of cerebral palsy include delayed gross motor development, abnormal motor performance, alterations of muscle tone, abnormal posture, reflex abnormalities, and associated disabilities such as mental delay, seizures, attention-deficit/hyperactivity disorder, and sensory impairment.
- Therapy for cerebral palsy takes into account the nature of the physical disability, defects associated with the disorder, and interpersonal and social influences encountered by the affected child.
- Werdnig-Hoffmann disease is characterized by progressive weakness and wasting of skeletal muscles caused by degeneration of anterior horn cells.
- Nursing care of the child with Guillain-Barré syndrome consists of monitoring vital signs, monitoring respiratory status, ensuring alignment and positioning, providing physical therapy, managing pain, and providing support to the family.
- Tetanus occurs when tetanus spores or vegetative bacilli enter a wound and multiply in a susceptible host.
- Infant botulism results from toxins produced by *C. botulinum;* the toxin is ingested from improperly preserved food or released in the gastrointestinal tract by ingested spores.
- Management of myasthenia gravis (MG) includes oral administration of anticholinesterase drugs, ensuring adequate rest periods, and prevention of MG crises.
- Spinal cord injuries represent a major debilitating health problem that is entirely preventable in children and adolescents by instituting and following safety measures such as proper car safety restraints and wearing helmets when riding bicycles.
- Spinal cord injuries usually involve the following four interrelated pathologic changes: cellular damage to cord tissue; hemorrhage and vascular damage; structural changes of white and gray matter related to vascular disruption, inflammation, and edema; and local biochemical response to trauma.
- Therapeutic management of spinal cord injury is directed toward preventing further neuronal damage, avoiding complications, and maintaining vital functions.
- The goals of rehabilitation in spinal cord injury are to maximize functional mobility, to help the child cope with the dysfunction and build a positive self-image, to promote independence in performing activities of daily living (including self-care and hygiene), and to promote education, employment, social relationships, and independent living.
- Muscular dystrophies are the largest and most important group of debilitating muscular dysfunctions in childhood.
- The major complications of Duchenne Muscular Dystrophy include contractures, disuse atrophy, infections (especially respiratory), obesity, respiratory compromise, and cardiac failure.

# References

Allos BM: *Campylobacter jejuni* infections: update on emerging issues and trends, *Clin Infect Dis* 32(8):1201-1206, 2001.

American Academy of Pediatrics, Committee on Children with Disabilities: The treatment of neurologically impaired children using patterning, *Pediatrics* 104(5):1149-1151, 1999.

American Academy of Pediatrics, Committee on Infectious Diseases, Pickering L, editor: *2000 Red book: report of the Committee on Infectious Diseases*, ed 25, Elk Grove Village, IL, 2000, The Academy.

Aneja R, Thomas C, Elberger S: Early infantile botulism, *Emerg Med* 32(6):36-41, 2000.

Cox N, Hinkle R: Infant botulism, *Am Fam Physician* 65(7):1388-1392, 2002.

Cramer KE: The pediatric polytrauma patient, *Clin Orthop* 318(9):125-135, Sept 1995.

Dabney KW, Lipton GE, Miller F: Cerebral palsy, *Curr Opin Pediatr* 9(1):81-88, 1997.

Edgar TS: Clinical utility of botulinum toxin in the treatment of cerebral palsy: comprehensive review, *J Child Neurol* 16(1):37-46, 2001.

Evans OB, Vedanarayanan V: Guillain-Barré syndrome, *Pediatr Rev* 18(1):1-15, 1997.

Ferrari ND, Weisse ME: Botulism, *Adv Pediatr Infect Dis* 10(1):81-91, 1995.

Fischer AQ: Neuromuscular diseases, *Clin Diagn Ultrasound* 30(1):11-19, 1995.

Glatman-Freedman A: Infant botulism, *Pediatr Rev* 17(5):185-186, 1996.

Graf WD and others: Outcome in severe pediatric Guillain-Barré syndrome after immunotherapy or supportive care, *Neurology* 52(7):1494-1497, 1999.

Han TR and others: Risk factors of cerebral palsy in preterm infants, *Am J Phys Med Rehabil* 81(4):297-303, 2002.

Haslam RHA: The nervous system. In Behrman RE, Kliegman RM, Jenson JB, editors: *Nelson textbook of pediatrics*, ed 16, Philadelphia, 2000, WB Saunders.

Iannaccone ST: Spinal muscular atrophy, *Semin Neurol* 18(1):19-26, 1998.

Jacobs JM: Management options for the child with spastic cerebral palsy, *Orthop Nurs* 20(3):53-59, 2001.

Jones HR Jr: Guillain-Barré syndrome in children, *Curr Opin Pediatr* 7(6):663-668, 1995.

Kool B: The wound that nearly got away, *Pediatr Nurs* 26(1):55-65, 2000.

Krach LE: Pharmacotherapy of spasticity: oral medications and intrathecal baclofen, *J Child Neurol* 16(1):31-36, 2001.

Loder RT: The cervical spine. In Morrissy RT, Weinstein SL, editors: *Lovell and Winter's pediatric orthopaedics*, ed 5, Philadelphia, 2000, WB Saunders.

Massagli TL: Medical and rehabilitation issues in the care of children with spinal cord injury, *Phys Med Rehabil Clin N Am* 11(1):169-182, 2000.

Merenda LA, Spoltore TA, Betz RR: Progressive treatment options for children with spinal cord injury, *Sci Nurs* 17(3):102-109, 2000.

Nehring WM: Cerebral palsy. In Jackson PL, Vessey JA: *Primary care of the child with a chronic illness*, ed 3, St Louis, 2000, Mosby.

Nguyen DK, Agenarioti-Belanger S, Vanasse M: Pain and the Guillain-Barré syndrome in children under 6 years old, *J Pediatr* 134(6):773-776, 1999.

Olsen SJ, Swerdlow DL: Q&A: Risk of infant botulism from corn syrup, *Pediatr Infect Dis J* 19(6):584-585, 2000.

Rawlins P: Intrathecal baclofen for spasticity of cerebral palsy: project coordination and nursing care, *J Neurosci Nurs* 27(2):157-163, 1995.

Reinberg Y, Fleming T, Gonzalez R: Renal rupture after the Credé maneuver, *J Pediatr* 124(2):279-281, 1994.

Richards S, Iannaccone ST: Dystrophin and DNA diagnosis in a large pediatric muscle clinic, *J Child Neurol* 9(2):162-166, 1994.

Roland EH: Muscular dystrophy, *Pediatr Rev* 21(7):233-237, 2000.

Russman BS: Function changes in spinal muscular atrophy II and III: The DCN/SMA Group, *Neurology* 47(4):973-976, 1996.

Russman BS and others: Spinal muscular atrophy: new thoughts on the pathogenesis and classification schema, *J Child Neurol* 7(4):347-353, 1992.

Spoltore T and others: Innovative programs for children and adolescents with spinal cord injury, *Orthop Nurs* 19(3):55-61, 2000.

Steinbok P: Outcomes after selective dorsal rhizotomy for spastic cerebral palsy, *Childs Nerv Syst* 17(1-2):1-18, 2001.

Suresh-Babu MV and others: Nutrition in children with cerebral palsy, *J Pediatr Gastroenterol Nutr* 26(4):484-485, 1998.

Thayaparan B and others: Prevention and control of tetanus in childhood, *Curr Opin Pediatr* 10(1):4-8, 1998.

Thompson GH, Berenson FR: Other neuromuscular disorders. In Morrissey RT, Weinstein SL, editors: *Lovell and Winter's pediatric orthopaedics*, ed 5, Philadelphia, 2001, Lippincott Williams & Wilkins.

Ubhi T and others: Randomized double-blind placebo-controlled trial of the effect of botulism toxin on walking in cerebral palsy, *Arch Dis Child* 83(6):481-487, 2000.

Voit T: Congenital muscular dystrophies: 1997 update, *Brain Dev* 20(2):65-74, 1998.

Volpe JJ: *Neurology of the newborn*, ed 4, Philadelphia, 2001, WB Saunders.

# Appendices

# Family APGAR questionnaire

## PART I

The following questions have been designed to help us better understand you and your family. You should feel free to ask questions about any item in the questionnaire.

The space for comments should be used when you wish to give additional information or if you wish to discuss the way the question is applied to your family. Please try to answer all questions.

Family is defined as the individual(s) with whom you usually live. If you live alone, your "family" consists of persons with whom you now have the strongest emotional ties.*

For each question, check only one box

|  | Almost always | Some of the time | Hardly ever |
|---|---|---|---|
| I am satisfied that I can turn to my family for help when something is troubling me. Comments: | ☐ | ☐ | ☐ |
| I am satisfied with the way my family talks over things with me and shares problems with me. Comments: | ☐ | ☐ | ☐ |
| I am satisfied that my family accepts and supports my wishes to take on new activities or directions. Comments: | ☐ | ☐ | ☐ |
| I am satisfied with the way my family expresses affection and responds to my emotions, such as anger, sorrow, and love. Comments: | ☐ | ☐ | ☐ |
| I am satisfied with the way my family and I share time together. Comments: | ☐ | ☐ | ☐ |

*According to which member of the family is being interviewed the interviewer may substitute for the word 'family' either spouse, significant other, parents, or children.

**Fig. A-1**  Family APGAR questionnaire. **A**, Part I. (Modified from Smilkstein G, Ashworth C, Montano D: Validity and reliability of the family APGAR as a test of family function, *J Fam Pract* 15[2]:303-311, 1982.)

# Family APGAR questionnaire

## PART II

Who lives in your home?* List by relationship (e.g., spouse, significant other,†child, or friend).

Please check below the column that best describes how you now get along with each member of the family listed.

| Relationship | Age | Sex | Well | Fairly | Poorly |
|---|---|---|---|---|---|
| _____ | __ | __ | ☐ | ☐ | ☐ |
| _____ | __ | __ | ☐ | ☐ | ☐ |
| _____ | __ | __ | ☐ | ☐ | ☐ |
| _____ | __ | __ | ☐ | ☐ | ☐ |
| _____ | __ | __ | ☐ | ☐ | ☐ |
| _____ | __ | __ | ☐ | ☐ | ☐ |

If you don't live with your own family, please list below the individuals to whom you turn for help most frequently. List by relationship, (e.g., family member, friend, associate at work, or neighbor).

Please check below the column that best describes how you now get along with each person listed.

| Relationship | Age | Sex | Well | Fairly | Poorly |
|---|---|---|---|---|---|
| _____ | __ | __ | ☐ | ☐ | ☐ |
| _____ | __ | __ | ☐ | ☐ | ☐ |
| _____ | __ | __ | ☐ | ☐ | ☐ |
| _____ | __ | __ | ☐ | ☐ | ☐ |
| _____ | __ | __ | ☐ | ☐ | ☐ |
| _____ | __ | __ | ☐ | ☐ | ☐ |

*If you have established your own family, consider home to be the place where you live with your spouse, children, or significant other; otherwise, consider home as your place of origin, e.g., the place where your parents or those who raise you live.
†"Significant other" is the partner you live with in a physically and emotionally nurturing relationship, but to whom you are not married.

**B**

**Fig. A-1, cont'd**   **B**, Part II.

# Infant/Toddler HOME Inventory

## Bettye M. Caldwell and Robert H. Bradley

Family Name _____ Visitor _____ Date _____

Address _____ Phone _____

Child's Name _____ Birthdate _____ Age _____ Sex _____

Parent Present _____ If other than parent, relationship to child _____

Family Composition _____
(persons living in household, including sex and age of children)

Family Ethnicity _____ Language Spoken _____ Maternal Education _____ Paternal Education _____

Is mother employed? _____ Type of work when employed _____ Is father employed? _____ Type of work when employed _____

Current child care arrangements _____

Summarize past year's arrangement _____

Other persons present during visit _____

Comments: _____

_____

### SUMMARY

| | Subscale | Score | Lowest Fourth | Middle Half | Top Fourth |
|------|-----------------|-------|---------------|-------------|------------|
| I. | RESPONSIVITY | | 0 - 6 | 7 - 9 | 10 - 11 |
| II. | ACCEPTANCE | | 0 - 4 | 5 - 6 | 7 - 8 |
| III. | ORGANIZATION | | 0 - 3 | 4 - 5 | 6 |
| IV. | LEARNING MATERIALS | | 0 - 4 | 5 - 7 | 8 - 9 |
| V. | INVOLVEMENT | | 0 - 2 | 3 - 4 | 5 - 6 |
| VI. | VARIETY | | 0 - 1 | 2 - 3 | 4 - 5 |
| | TOTAL SCORE | | 0 - 25 | 26 - 36 | 37 - 45 |

**Fig. A-2** HOME Inventory questionnaire. AUTHOR'S NOTE: HOME Inventories for families and preschoolers (3 to 6 years) and elementary age children (6 to 10 years) are available from the Center for Research on Teaching and Learning, College of Education, University of Arkansas at Little Rock, 2801 S University Ave, Little Rock, AR 72204; (501) 569-3422. (From Caldwell B, Bradley R: *Manual of home observation for measurement of the environment,* rev ed, Little Rock, 1984, University of Arkansas at Little Rock.)

# Infant/Toddler HOME Inventory

Place a plus (+) or minus (−) in the box alongside each item if the behavior is observed during the visit or if the parent reports that the conditions or events are characteristic of the home environment. Count the number of (+) signs, enter the subtotal and the total on the front side of the Record Sheet.

| | |
|---|---|
| **I.   RESPONSIVITY** | 24.  Child has a special place for toys and treasures. |
| 1.  Parent spontaneously vocalizes to child at least twice. | 25.  Child's play environment is safe. |
| 2.  Parent responds verbally to child's vocalizations or verbalizations. | **IV.  LEARNING MATERIALS** |
| 3.  Parent tells child name of object or person during visit. | 26.  Muscle activity toys or equipment. |
| 4.  Parent's speech is distinct, clear and audible. | 27.  Push or pull toy. |
| 5.  Parent initiates verbal interchanges with Visitor. | 28.  Stroller or walker, kiddie car, scooter, or tricycle. |
| 6.  Parent converses freely and easily. | 29.  Parent provides toys for child to play with during visit. |
| 7.  Parent permits child to engage in "messy" play. | 30.  Cuddly toy or role-playing toys. |
| 8.  Parent spontaneously praises child at least twice. | 31.  Learning facilitators—mobile, table and chair, high chair, play pen. |
| 9.  Parent's voice conveys positive feelings toward child. | 32.  Simple eye-hand coordination toys. |
| 10.  Parent caresses or kisses child at least once. | 33.  Complex eye-hand coordination toys. |
| 11.  Parent responds positively to praise of child offered by Visitor. | 34.  Toys for literature and music. |
| **II.  ACCEPTANCE** | **V.  INVOLVEMENT** |
| 12.  Parent does not shout at child. | 35.  Parent keeps child in visual range, looks at often. |
| 13.  Parent does not express overt annoyance with or hostility to child. | 36.  Parent talks to child while doing household work. |
| 14.  Parent neither slaps nor spanks child during visit. | 37.  Parent consciously encourages developmental advance. |
| 15.  No more than 1 instance of physical punishment during past week. | 38.  Parent invests maturing toys with value via personal attention. |
| 16.  Parent does not scold or criticize child during visit. | 39.  Parent structures child's play periods. |
| 17.  Parent does not interfere with or restrict child 3 times during visit. | 40.  Parent provides toys that challenge child to develop new skills. |
| 18.  At least 10 books are present and visible. | **VI.  VARIETY** |
| 19.  Family has a pet. | 41.  Father provides some care daily. |
| **III.  ORGANIZATION** | 42.  Parent reads stories to child at least 3 times weekly. |
| 20.  Child care, if used, is provided by one of three regular substitutes. | 43.  Child eats at least one meal a day with mother and father. |
| 21.  Child is taken to grocery store at least once a week. | 44.  Family visits relatives or receives visits once month or so. |
| 22.  Child gets out of house at least 4 times a week. | 45.  Child has 3 or more books of his/her own. |

| 23.  Child is taken regularly to doctor's office or clinic. | **I** | **II** | **III** | **IV** | **V** | **VI** | **TOTAL** |
|---|---|---|---|---|---|---|---|
| **TOTALS** | | | | | | | |

**Fig. A-2, cont'd**   HOME Inventory questionnaire.

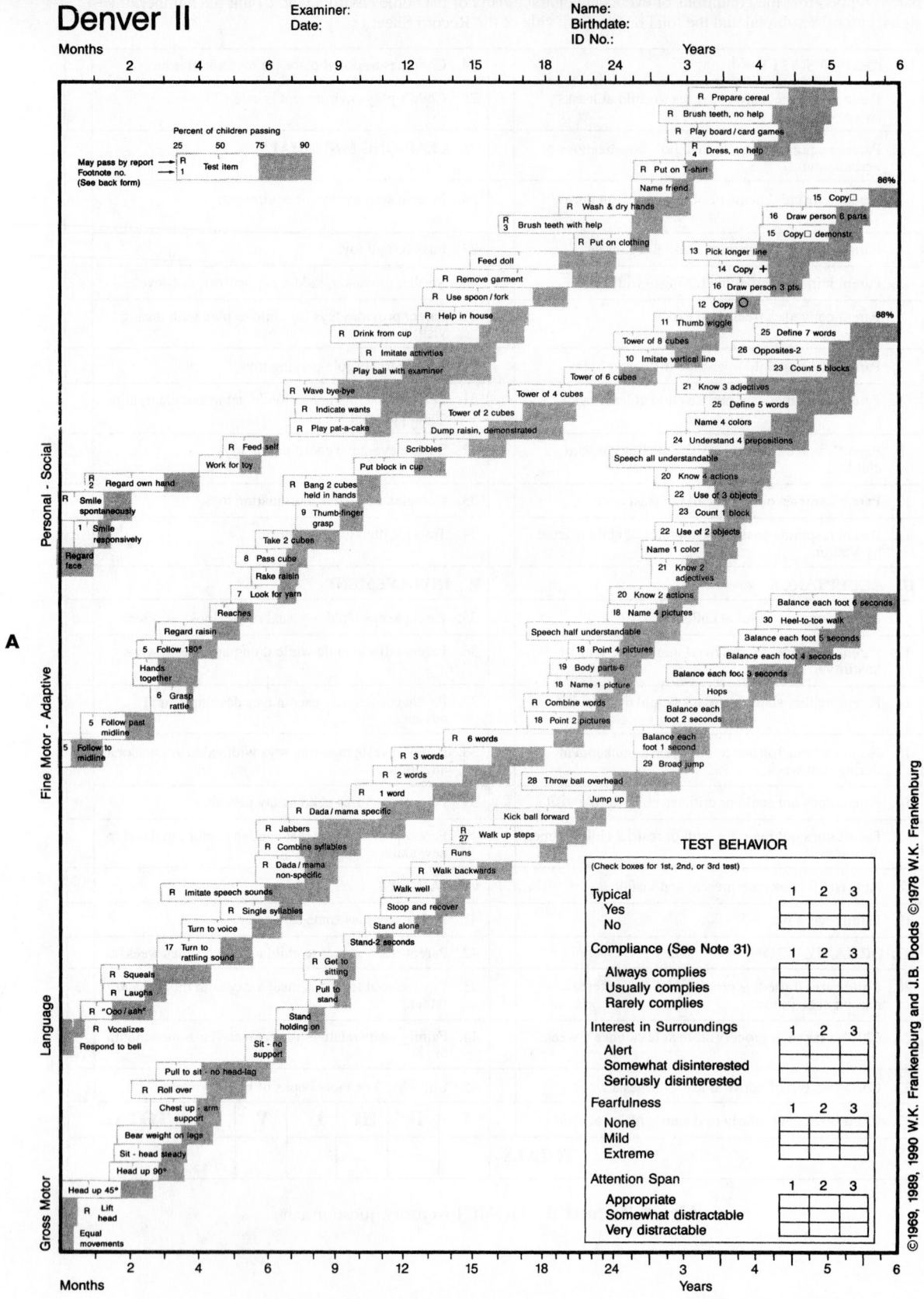

**Fig. B-1** **A**, Denver II. (From WK Frankenburg and JB Dodds, 1990.)

# DIRECTIONS FOR ADMINISTRATION

1. Try to get child to smile by smiling, talking or waving. Do not touch him/her.
2. Child must stare at hand several seconds.
3. Parent may help guide toothbrush and put toothpaste on brush.
4. Child does not have to be able to tie shoes or button/zip in the back.
5. Move yarn slowly in an arc from one side to the other, about 8" above child's face.
6. Pass if child grasps rattle when it is touched to the backs or tips of fingers.
7. Pass if child tries to see where yarn went. Yarn should be dropped quickly from sight from tester's hand without arm movement.
8. Child must transfer cube from hand to hand without help of body, mouth, or table.
9. Pass if child picks up raisin with any part of thumb and finger.
10. Line can vary only 30 degrees or less from tester's line. /
11. Make a fist with thumb pointing upward and wiggle only the thumb. Pass if child imitates and does not move any fingers other than the thumb.

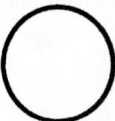      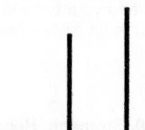      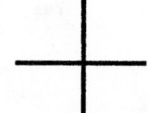      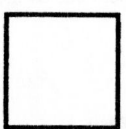

| 12. Pass any enclosed form. Fail continuous round motions. | 13. Which line is longer? (Not bigger.) Turn paper upside down and repeat. (pass 3 of 3 or 5 of 6) | 14. Pass any lines crossing near midpoint. | 15. Have child copy first. If failed, demonstrate. |

When giving items 12, 14, and 15, do not name the forms. Do not demonstrate 12 and 14.

16. When scoring, each pair (2 arms, 2 legs, etc.) counts as one part.
17. Place one cube in cup and shake gently near child's ear, but out of sight. Repeat for other ear.
18. Point to picture and have child name it. (No credit is given for sounds only.)
    If less than 4 pictures are named correctly, have child point to picture as each is named by tester.

**B**

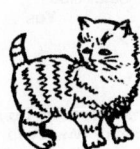   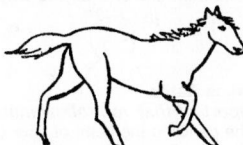   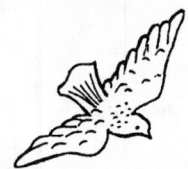   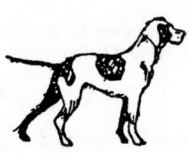   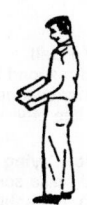

19. Using doll, tell child: Show me the nose, eyes, ears, mouth, hands, feet, tummy, hair. Pass 6 of 8.
20. Using pictures, ask child: Which one flies?... says meow?... talks?... barks?... gallops? Pass 2 of 5, 4 of 5.
21. Ask child: What do you do when you are cold?... tired?... hungry? Pass 2 of 3, 3 of 3.
22. Ask child: What do you do with a cup? What is a chair used for? What is a pencil used for?
    Action words must be included in answers.
23. Pass if child correctly places <u>and</u> says how many blocks are on paper. (1, 5).
24. Tell child: Put block **on** table; **under** table; **in front of** me, **behind** me. Pass 4 of 4.
    (Do not help child by pointing, moving head or eyes.)
25. Ask child: What is a ball?... lake?... desk?... house?... banana?... curtain?... fence?... ceiling? Pass if defined in terms of use, shape, what it is made of, or general category (such as banana is fruit, not just yellow). Pass 5 of 8, 7 of 8.
26. Ask child: If a horse is big, a mouse is __? If fire is hot, ice is __? If the sun shines during the day, the moon shines during the __? Pass 2 of 3.
27. Child may use wall or rail only, not person. May not crawl.
28. Child must throw ball overhand 3 feet to within arm's reach of tester.
29. Child must perform standing broad jump over width of test sheet (8 1/2 inches).
30. Tell child to walk forward, ⊂◦⊃◦⊂◦⊃◦⊂◦⊃→ heel within 1 inch of toe. Tester may demonstrate.
    Child must walk 4 consecutive steps.
31. In the second year, half of normal children are non-compliant.

**OBSERVATIONS:**

---

**Fig. B-1, cont'd**   **B**, Directions for administration of numbered items on Denver II.

**0-9 MONTHS (R-PDQ)**

# REVISED DENVER PRESCREENING DEVELOPMENTAL QUESTIONNAIRE

Child's Name _____

Person Completing R-PDQ: _____

Relation to Child: _____

| For Office Use | | | | |
|---|---|---|---|---|
| Today's Date: | ___ yr | ___ mo | ___ day | |
| Child's Birthdate: | ___ yr | ___ mo | ___ day | |
| Subtract to get Child's Exact Age: | ___ yr | ___ mo | ___ day | |
| R-PDQ Age: ( ___ yr | ___ mo | ___ completed wks) | | |

**CONTINUE ANSWERING UNTIL 3 "NOs" ARE CIRCLED**

For Office Use

**1. Equal Movements**
When your baby is lying on his/her back, can (s)he move each of his/her arms as easily as the other and each of the legs as easily as the other? Answer **No** if your child makes jerky or uncoordinated movements with one or both of his/her arms or legs.

Yes No (0) FMA

**2. Stomach Lifts Head**
When your baby is on his/her stomach on a flat surface, can (s)he lift his/her head off the surface?

Yes No (0-3) GM

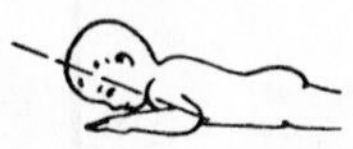

**3. Regards Face**
When your baby is lying on his/her back, can (s)he look at you and watch your face?

Yes No (1) PS

**4. Follows To Midline**
When your child is on his/her back, can (s)he follow your movement by turning his/her head from one side to facing directly forward?

Yes No (1-1) FMA

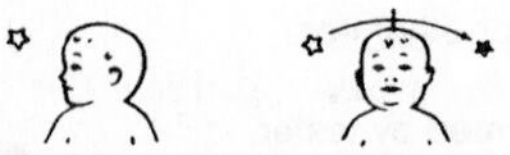

**5. Responds To Bell**
Does your child respond with eye movements, change in breathing or other change in activity to a bell or rattle sounded outside his/her line of vision?

Yes No (1-2) L

**6. Vocalizes Not Crying**
Does your child make sounds other than crying, such as gurgling, cooing, or babbling?

Yes No (1-3) L

**7. Smiles Responsively**
When you smile and talk to your baby, does (s)he smile back at you?

Yes No (1-3) PS

**8. Follows Past Midline**
When your child is on his/her back, does (s)he follow your movement by turning his/her head from one side *almost all the way to the other side?*

Yes No (2-2) FMA

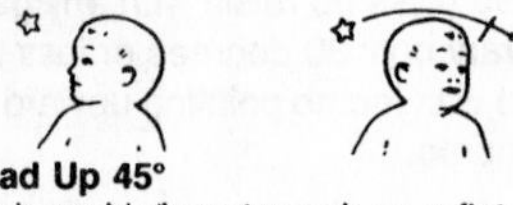

**9. Stomach, Head Up 45°**
When your baby is on his/her stomach on a flat surface, can (s)he lift his/her head 45°?

Yes No (2-2) GM

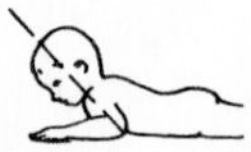

**10. Stomach, Head Up 90°**
When your baby is on his/her stomach on a flat surface, can (s)he lift his/her head 90°?

Yes No (3) GM

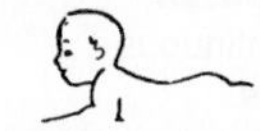

**11. Laughs**
Does your baby laugh out loud without being tickled or touched?

Yes No (3-1) L

**12. Hands Together**
Does your baby play with his/her hands by touching them together?

Yes No (3-3) FMA

**13. Follows 180°**
When your child is on his/her back, does (s)he follow your movement from one side *all the way* to the other side?

Yes No (4) FMA

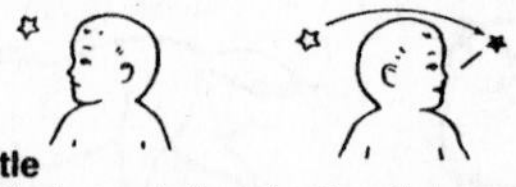

**14. Grasps Rattle**
*It is important that you follow instructions carefully.* Do *not* place the pencil in the palm of your child's hand. When you touch the pencil to the back or tips of your baby's fingers, does your baby grasp the pencil for a few seconds?

Yes No (4) FMA

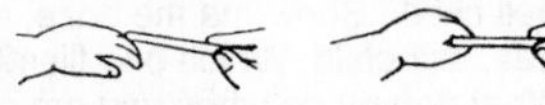

TRY THIS    NOT THIS

(Please turn page)

©Wm. K. Frankenburg, M.D., 1975, 1986

**Fig. B-2** Revised Denver Prescreening Developmental Questionnaire. (Sample of first page only.) (The *first* page is reprinted with permission of William K Frankenburg. Copyright 1975, 1986, WK Frankenburg.)

---

DENVER ARTICULATION SCREENING EXAM
for children 2½ to 6 years of age

Name: _____

Instructions: Have child repeat each word after you. Circle the underlined sounds that he pronounces correctly. Total correct sounds is the Raw Score. Use charts on reverse side to score results.

Hosp. No.: _____

Address: _____
_____

---

Date: _____   Child's age: _____   Examiner: _____   Raw score: ___
Percentile: ___   Intelligibility: _____   Result: _____

1. table      6. zipper      11. sock      16. wagon      21. leaf
2. shirt      7. grapes      12. vacuum    17. gum        22. carrot
3. door       8. flag        13. yarn      18. house
4. trunk      9. thumb       14. mother    19. pencil
5. jumping   10. toothbrush  15. twinkle   20. fish

Intelligibility: (circle one)
   1. Easy to understand                 3. Not understandable
   2. Understandable ½ the time          4. Can't evaluate

Comments:

---

Date: _____   Child's age: _____   Examiner: _____   Raw score: ___
Percentile: ___   Intelligibility: _____   Result: _____

1. table      6. zipper      11. sock      16. wagon      21. leaf
2. shirt      7. grapes      12. vacuum    17. gum        22. carrot
3. door       8. flag        13. yarn      18. house
4. trunk      9. thumb       14. mother    19. pencil
5. jumping   10. toothbrush  15. twinkle   20. fish

Intelligibility: (circle one)
   1. Easy to understand                 3. Not understandable
   2. Understandable ½ the time          4. Can't evaluate

Comments:

---

Date: _____   Child's age: _____   Examiner: _____   Raw score ___
Percentile: ___   Intelligibility: _____   Result: _____

1. table      6. zipper      11. sock      16. wagon      21. leaf
2. shirt      7. grapes      12. vacuum    17. gum        22. carrot
3. door       8. flag        13. yarn      18. house
4. trunk      9. thumb       14. mother    19. pencil
5. jumping   10. toothbrush  15. twinkle   20. fish

Intelligibility: (circle one)
   1. Easy to understand                 3. Not understandable
   2. Understandable ½ the time          4. Can't evaluate

**A**

**Fig. B-3**   **A,** Denver Articulation Screening Exam (DASE) for children 2½ to 6 years of age. (From AF Drumwright, University of Colorado Medical Center, 1971.)   *Continued*

To score DASE words: Note raw score for child's performance. Match raw score line (extreme left of chart) with column representing child's age (to the closest previous age group). Where raw score line and age column meet number in that square denotes percentile rank of child's performance when compared to other children that age. Percentiles above heavy line are ABNORMAL percentiles, below heavy line are NORMAL.

**PERCENTILE RANK**

| Raw Score | 2.5 yr. | 3.0 | 3.5 | 4.0 | 4.5 | 5.0 | 5.5 | 6 years |
|---|---|---|---|---|---|---|---|---|
| 2 | 1 | | | | | | | |
| 3 | 2 | | | | | | | |
| 4 | 5 | | | | | | | |
| 5 | 9 | | | | | | | |
| 6 | 16 | | | | | | | |
| 7 | 23 | | | | | | | |
| 8 | 31 | 2 | | | | | | |
| 9 | 37 | 4 | 1 | | | | | |
| 10 | 42 | 6 | 2 | | | | | |
| 11 | 48 | 7 | 4 | | | | | |
| 12 | 54 | 9 | 6 | 1 | 1 | | | |
| 13 | 58 | 12 | 9 | 2 | 3 | 1 | 1 | |
| 14 | 62 | 17 | 11 | 5 | 4 | 2 | 2 | |
| 15 | 68 | 23 | 15 | 9 | 5 | 3 | 2 | |
| 16 | 75 | 31 | 19 | 12 | 5 | 4 | 3 | |
| 17 | 79 | 38 | 25 | 15 | 6 | 6 | 4 | |
| 18 | 83 | 46 | 31 | 19 | 8 | 7 | 4 | |
| 19 | 86 | 51 | 38 | 24 | 10 | 9 | 5 | 1 |
| 20 | 89 | 58 | 45 | 30 | 12 | 11 | 7 | 3 |
| 21 | 92 | 65 | 52 | 36 | 15 | 15 | 9 | 4 |
| 22 | 94 | 72 | 58 | 43 | 18 | 19 | 12 | 5 |
| 23 | 96 | 77 | 63 | 50 | 22 | 24 | 15 | 7 |
| 24 | 97 | 82 | 70 | 58 | 29 | 29 | 20 | 15 |
| 25 | 99 | 87 | 78 | 66 | 36 | 34 | 26 | 17 |
| 26 | 99 | 91 | 84 | 75 | 46 | 43 | 34 | 24 |
| 27 | | 94 | 89 | 82 | 57 | 54 | 44 | 34 |
| 28 | | 96 | 94 | 88 | 70 | 68 | 59 | 47 |
| 29 | | 98 | 98 | 94 | 84 | 84 | 77 | 68 |
| 30 | | 100 | 100 | 100 | 100 | 100 | 100 | 100 |

To score intelligibility:

| | NORMAL | ABNORMAL |
|---|---|---|
| 2½ years | Understandable ½ the time, or, "easy" | Not understandable |
| 3 years and older | Easy to understand | Understandable ½ time Not understandable |

Test result: 1. NORMAL on DASE and Intelligibility = NORMAL

2. ABNORMAL on DASE and/or Intelligibility = ABNORMAL

*If abnormal on initial screening, rescreen within 2 weeks.
If abnormal again, child should be referred for complete speech evaluation.

**Fig. B-3, cont'd** **B**, Percentile rank.

B

## DENVER EYE SCREENING TEST

Name:
Hospital No.:
Ward:
Address:

| Vision Tests | 1ST SCREENING: DATE: Right Eye Normal | Right Eye Abnormal | Right Eye Untestable | Left Eye Normal | Left Eye Abnormal | Left Eye Untestable | RESCREENING: DATE: Right Eye Normal | Right Eye Abnormal | Right Eye Untestable | Left Eye Normal | Left Eye Abnormal | Left Eye Untestable |
|---|---|---|---|---|---|---|---|---|---|---|---|---|
| 1. "E" (3 years and above—3 to 5 trials) | 3P | 3F | U | 3P | 3F | U | 3P | 3F | U | 3P | 3F | U |
| 2. Picture card (2 1/2 - 2 11/12 yrs.—3 to 5 trials) | 3P | 3F | U | 3P | 3F | U | 3P | 3F | U | 3P | 3F | U |
| 3. Fixation (6 months - 2 5/12 years) | P | F | U | P | F | U | P | F | U | P | F | U |
| 4. Squinting | | yes | | | yes | | | yes | | | yes | |

| Tests for Non-Straight Eyes | 1ST SCREENING Normal | Abnormal | Untestable | RESCREENING Normal | Abnormal | Untestable |
|---|---|---|---|---|---|---|
| 1. Do your child's eyes turn in or out, or are they ever not straight? | NO | YES | U | NO | YES | U |
| 2. Cover Test | P | F | U | P | F | U |
| 3. Pupillary Light Reflex | P | F | U | P | F | U |

Total Test Rating (Both Eyes)

Normal (passed vision test plus no squint, plus passed 2/3 tests for non-straight eyes) ......... Normal

Abnormal (abnormal on any vision test, squinting or 2 of 3 procedures for non-straight eyes) ......... Abnormal

Untestable (untestable on any vision test or untestable on 2/3 tests for non-straight eyes) ......... Untestable

Future Rescreening Appointment for Total Test Rating (Abnormal or Untestable) ......... Date:

**Fig. B-4** Denver Eye Screening Test. (From WK Frankenburg and JB Dodds, University of Colorado Medical Center, 1969.)

## Snellen Screening*

### Preparation

1. Hang the Snellen chart on a light-colored wall so that the 20- to 30-foot lines are at eye level when children 6 to 12 years old are tested in the standing position.
2. Secure the chart to the wall with double-stick tape on the back side of all four corners. If the chart must be reversed for use of letter or E chart, secure it at the top and bottom with tacks. Make sure that the chart does not swing when in place.
3. The illumination intensity on the chart should be 10 to 30 foot-candles, without any glare from windows or light fixtures. The illumination should be checked with a light meter.
4. Mark an exact 20-foot distance from the chart. Mark the floor with a piece of tape or "footprints" positioned so that the heels touch the 20-foot line.

### Procedure

1. Place the child at the 20-foot mark, with the heel edging the line if the child is standing or with the back of the chair placed at the marker if the child is seated.
2. If the E chart is used, accustom the child to identifying in which direction the "legs of the E" are pointing. Use a demonstration E card for this purpose.
3. Teach the child to use the occluder to cover one eye. Instruct the child to keep both eyes open during the test. Provide a clean cover card for each child and then discard after use.
4. If the child wears glasses, test only with the glasses on.
5. Test both eyes together, then the right eye, then the left eye.

6. Begin with the 40- or 30-foot line and proceed with the test to include the 20-foot line.
7. With a child suspected of low vision, begin with the 200-foot line and proceed until the child can no longer correctly read three out of four or four out of six symbols on a line.
8. Use covers on the Snellen chart to expose only one symbol or one line at a time. When screening kindergarten or older children, expose one line but use a pointer to point to one symbol at a time.

### Recording and Referral

1. Record the last line the child read correctly (three out of four or four out of six symbols).
2. Record visual acuity as a fraction. The numerator represents the distance from the chart, and the denominator represents the last line read correctly. For example, 20/30 means that the child read the 30-foot line at a 20-foot distance.
3. Observe the child's eyes during testing and record any evidence of squinting, head tilting, thrusting the head forward, excessive blinking, tearing, or redness.
4. Make referrals only after a second screening has been made on children who are potential candidates for referral.
5. The following children should be referred for a complete eye examination:
   a. Three-year-old children with vision in either eye of 20/50 or less (inability to correctly identify one more than half the symbols on the 40-foot line) *or* a two-line difference in visual acuity between the eyes in the passing range; for example, 20/20 in one eye and 20/40 in the other
   b. All other ages and grades with vision in either eye of 20/40 or less (inability to correctly identify one more than half the symbols on the 30-foot line)
   c. All children who consistently show any of the signs of possible visual disturbances, regardless of visual acuity

*Modified from recommendations of Prevent Blindness America® *Guide to testing distance visual acuity*, Schaumburg, IL, 1995, Prevent Blindness America.

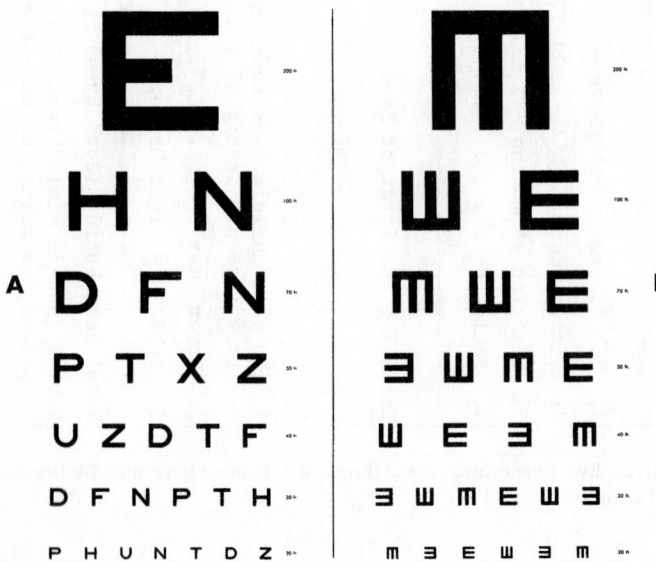

**Fig. B-5**   Snellen chart. **A,** Letter (alphabet) chart. **B,** Symbol E chart. (From National Society to Prevent Blindness, Inc, Schaumburg, IL.)

## Body Mass Index Formula

### English Formula

BMI = [Weight in pounds ÷ Height in inches ÷ Height in inches] × 703

Fractions and ounces must be entered as decimal values.

| Fraction | Ounces | Decimal |
|----------|--------|---------|
| 1/8 | 2 | 0.125 |
| 1/4 | 4 | 0.25 |
| 3/8 | 6 | 0.375 |
| 1/2 | 8 | 0.5 |
| 5/8 | 10 | 0.625 |
| 3/4 | 12 | 0.75 |
| 7/8 | 14 | 0.875 |

**Example:** A 33-pound, 4-ounce child is 37⅝ inches tall.

33.25 pounds divided by 37.625 inches, divided by 37.625 inches × 703 = 16.5

### Metric Formula

$$BMI = \text{Weight in kilograms} \div [\text{Height in meters}]^2$$

or

BMI = [Weight in kilograms ÷ Height in cm ÷ Height in cm] × 10,000

**Example:** A 16.9 kg child is 105.2 cm tall.

16.9 divided by 105.2 cm divided by 105.2 cm × 10,000 = 15.3

From Kuczmarski RJ and others: *CDC growth charts: United States. Advance data from vital and health statistics,* no 314, Hyattsville, MD, National Center for Health Statistics, June 8, 2000; may be accessed at www.cdc.gov/nchs/about/major/nhanes/growthcharts/fullreport.htm.

## Height and weight measurements for boys

| Age* | Height by Percentiles | | | | | | Weight by Percentiles | | | | | |
| | 5 | | 50 | | 95 | | 5 | | 50 | | 95 | |
| | cm | inches | cm | inches | cm | inches | kg | lb | kg | lb | kg | lb |
|---|---|---|---|---|---|---|---|---|---|---|---|---|
| Birth | 46.4 | 18¼ | 50.5 | 20 | 54.4 | 21½ | 2.54 | 5½ | 3.27 | 7¼ | 4.15 | 9¼ |
| 3 months | 56.7 | 22¼ | 61.1 | 24 | 65.4 | 25¾ | 4.43 | 9¾ | 5.98 | 13¼ | 7.37 | 16¼ |
| 6 months | 63.4 | 25 | 67.8 | 26¾ | 72.3 | 28½ | 6.20 | 13¾ | 7.85 | 17¼ | 9.46 | 20¾ |
| 9 months | 68.0 | 26¾ | 72.3 | 28½ | 77.1 | 30¼ | 7.52 | 16½ | 9.18 | 20¼ | 10.93 | 24 |
| 1 | 71.7 | 28¼ | 76.1 | 30 | 81.2 | 32 | 8.43 | 18½ | 10.15 | 22½ | 11.99 | 26½ |
| 1½ | 77.5 | 30½ | 82.4 | 32½ | 88.1 | 34¾ | 9.59 | 21¼ | 11.47 | 25¼ | 13.44 | 29½ |
| 2† | 82.5 | 32½ | 86.8 | 34¼ | 94.4 | 37¼ | 10.49 | 23¼ | 12.34 | 27¼ | 15.50 | 34¼ |
| 2½† | 85.4 | 33½ | 90.4 | 35½ | 97.8 | 38½ | 11.27 | 24¾ | 13.52 | 29¾ | 16.61 | 36½ |
| 3 | 89.0 | 35 | 94.9 | 37¼ | 102.0 | 40¼ | 12.05 | 26½ | 14.62 | 32¼ | 17.77 | 39¼ |
| 3½ | 92.5 | 36½ | 99.1 | 39 | 106.1 | 41¾ | 12.84 | 28¼ | 15.68 | 34½ | 18.98 | 41¾ |
| 4 | 95.8 | 37¾ | 102.9 | 40½ | 109.9 | 43¼ | 13.64 | 30 | 16.69 | 36¾ | 20.27 | 44¾ |
| 4½ | 98.9 | 39 | 106.6 | 42 | 113.5 | 44¾ | 14.45 | 31¾ | 17.69 | 39 | 21.63 | 47¾ |
| 5 | 102.0 | 40¼ | 109.9 | 43¼ | 117.0 | 46 | 15.27 | 33¾ | 18.67 | 41¼ | 23.09 | 51 |
| 6 | 107.7 | 42½ | 116.1 | 45¾ | 123.5 | 48½ | 16.93 | 37¼ | 20.69 | 45½ | 26.34 | 58 |
| 7 | 113.0 | 44½ | 121.7 | 48 | 129.7 | 51 | 18.64 | 41 | 22.85 | 50¼ | 30.12 | 66½ |
| 8 | 118.1 | 46½ | 127.0 | 50 | 135.7 | 53½ | 20.40 | 45 | 25.30 | 55¾ | 34.51 | 76 |
| 9 | 122.9 | 48½ | 132.2 | 52 | 141.8 | 55¾ | 22.25 | 49 | 28.13 | 62 | 39.58 | 87¼ |
| 10 | 127.7 | 50¼ | 137.5 | 54¼ | 148.1 | 58¼ | 24.33 | 53¾ | 31.44 | 69¼ | 45.27 | 99¾ |
| 11 | 132.6 | 52¼ | 143.3 | 56½ | 154.9 | 61 | 26.80 | 59 | 35.30 | 77¾ | 51.47 | 113½ |
| 12 | 137.6 | 54¼ | 149.7 | 59 | 162.3 | 64 | 29.85 | 65¾ | 39.78 | 87¾ | 58.09 | 128 |
| 13 | 142.9 | 56¼ | 156.5 | 61½ | 169.8 | 66¾ | 33.64 | 74¼ | 44.95 | 99 | 65.02 | 143¼ |
| 14 | 148.8 | 58½ | 163.1 | 64¼ | 176.7 | 69½ | 38.22 | 84¼ | 50.77 | 112 | 72.13 | 159 |
| 15 | 155.2 | 61 | 169.0 | 66½ | 181.9 | 71½ | 43.11 | 95 | 56.71 | 125 | 79.12 | 174½ |
| 16 | 161.1 | 63½ | 173.5 | 68¼ | 185.4 | 73 | 47.74 | 105¼ | 62.10 | 137 | 85.62 | 188¾ |
| 17 | 164.9 | 65 | 176.2 | 69¼ | 187.3 | 73¾ | 51.50 | 113½ | 66.31 | 146¼ | 91.31 | 201¼ |
| 18 | 165.7 | 65¼ | 176.8 | 69½ | 187.6 | 73¾ | 53.97 | 119 | 68.88 | 151¾ | 95.76 | 211 |

Modified from National Center for Health Statistics (NCHS), Health Resources Administration, Department of Health, Education, and Welfare, Hyattsville, MD. Conversion of metric data to approximate inches and pounds by Ross Laboratories.

*Years unless otherwise indicated.

†Height data include some recumbent length measurements, which make values slightly higher than if all measurements had been of stature (standing height).

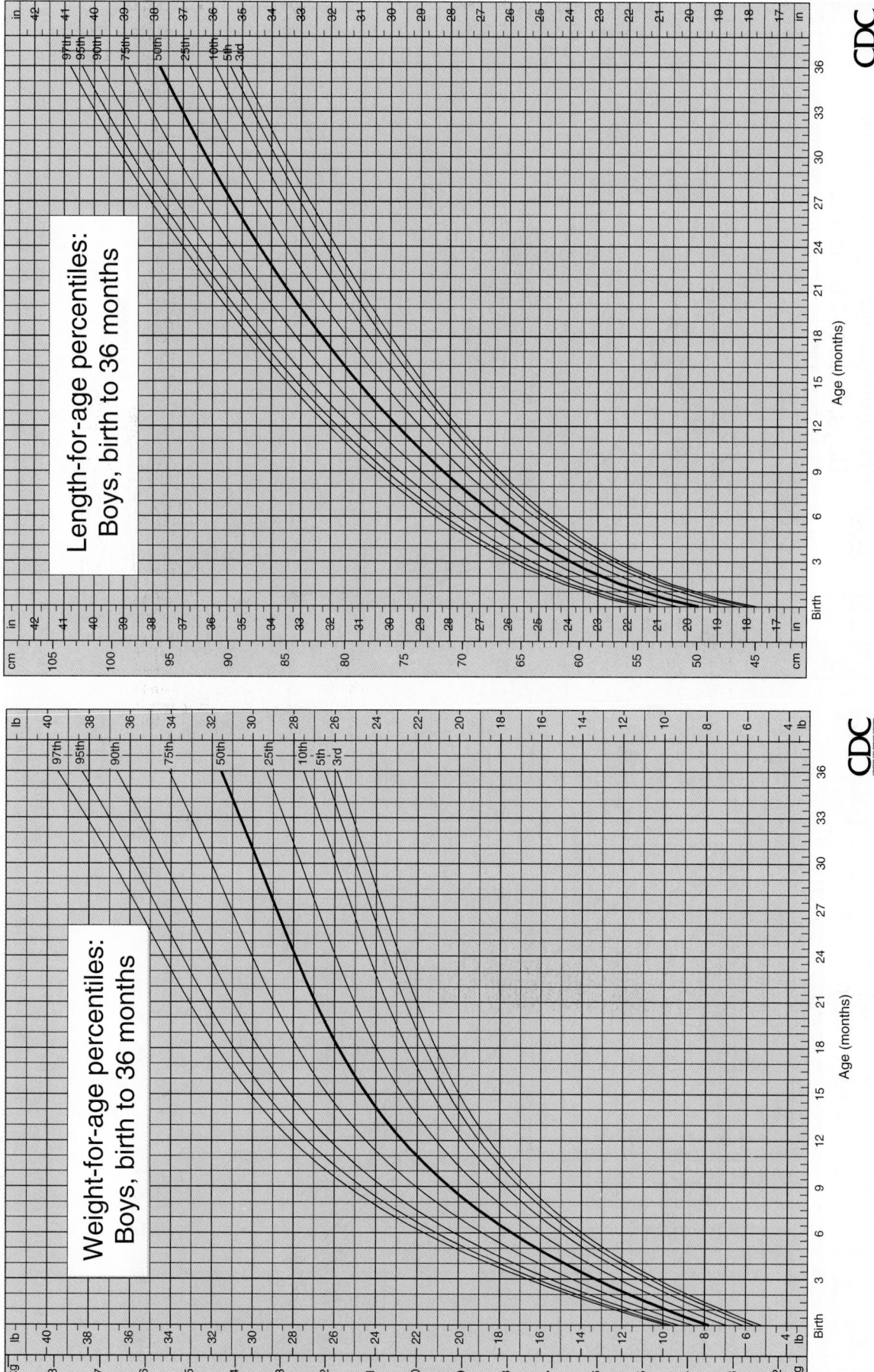

**Fig. C-1**  Weight-for-age percentiles, boys, birth to 36 months, CDC growth charts: United States. (Developed by the National Center for Health Statistics in collaboration with the National Center for Chronic Disease Prevention and Health Promotion [2000].)

**Fig. C-2**  Length-for-age percentiles, boys, birth to 36 months, CDC growth charts: United States. (Developed by the National Center for Health Statistics in collaboration with the National Center for Chronic Disease Prevention and Health Promotion [2000].)

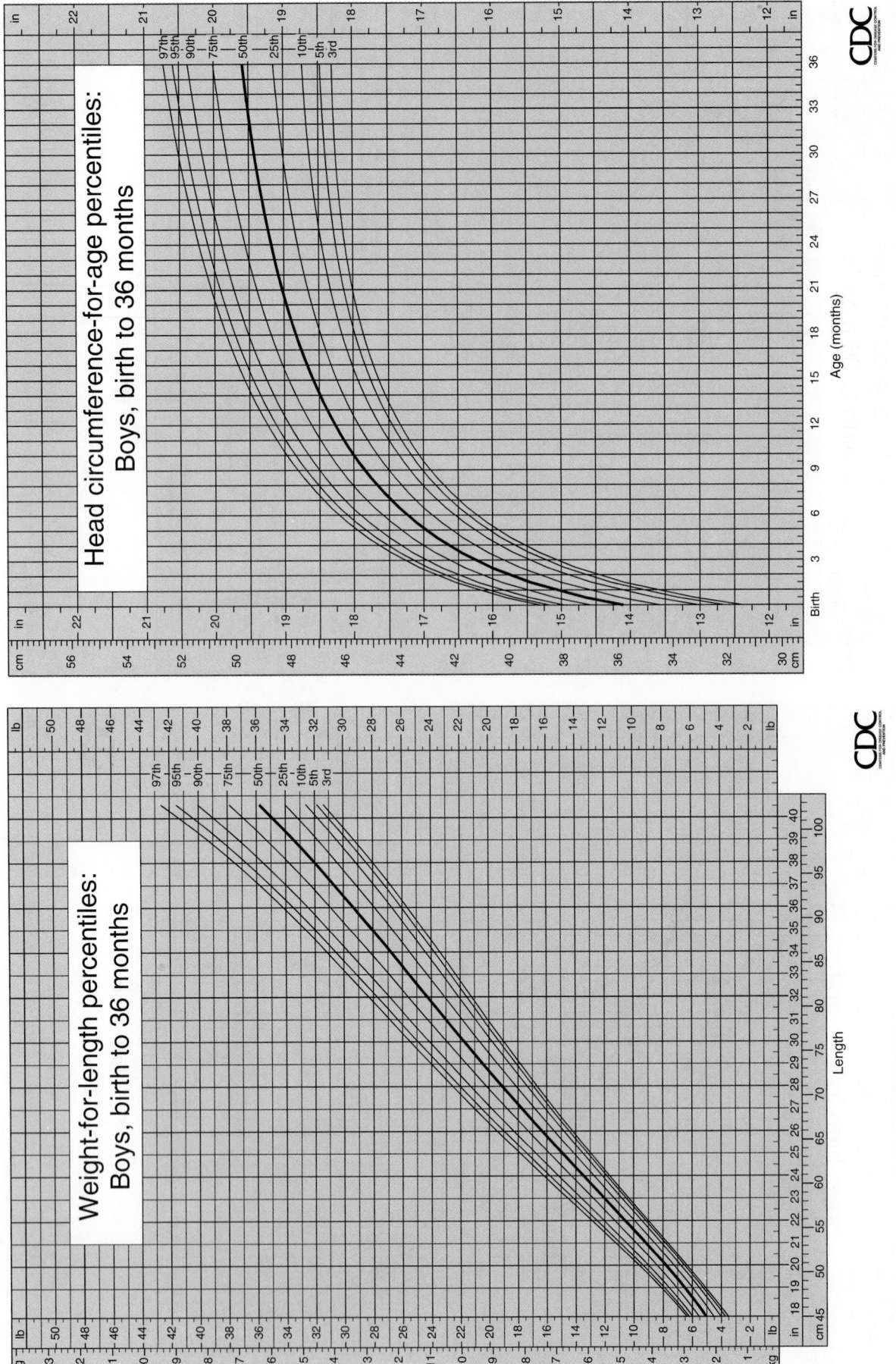

**Fig. C-3** Weight-for-length percentiles, boys, birth to 36 months, CDC growth charts: United States. (Developed by the National Center for Health Statistics in collaboration with the National Center for Chronic Disease Prevention and Health Promotion [2000].)

**Fig. C-4** Head circumference-for-age percentiles, boys, birth to 36 months, CDC growth charts: United States. (Developed by the National Center for Health Statistics in collaboration with the National Center for Chronic Disease Prevention and Health Promotion [2000].)

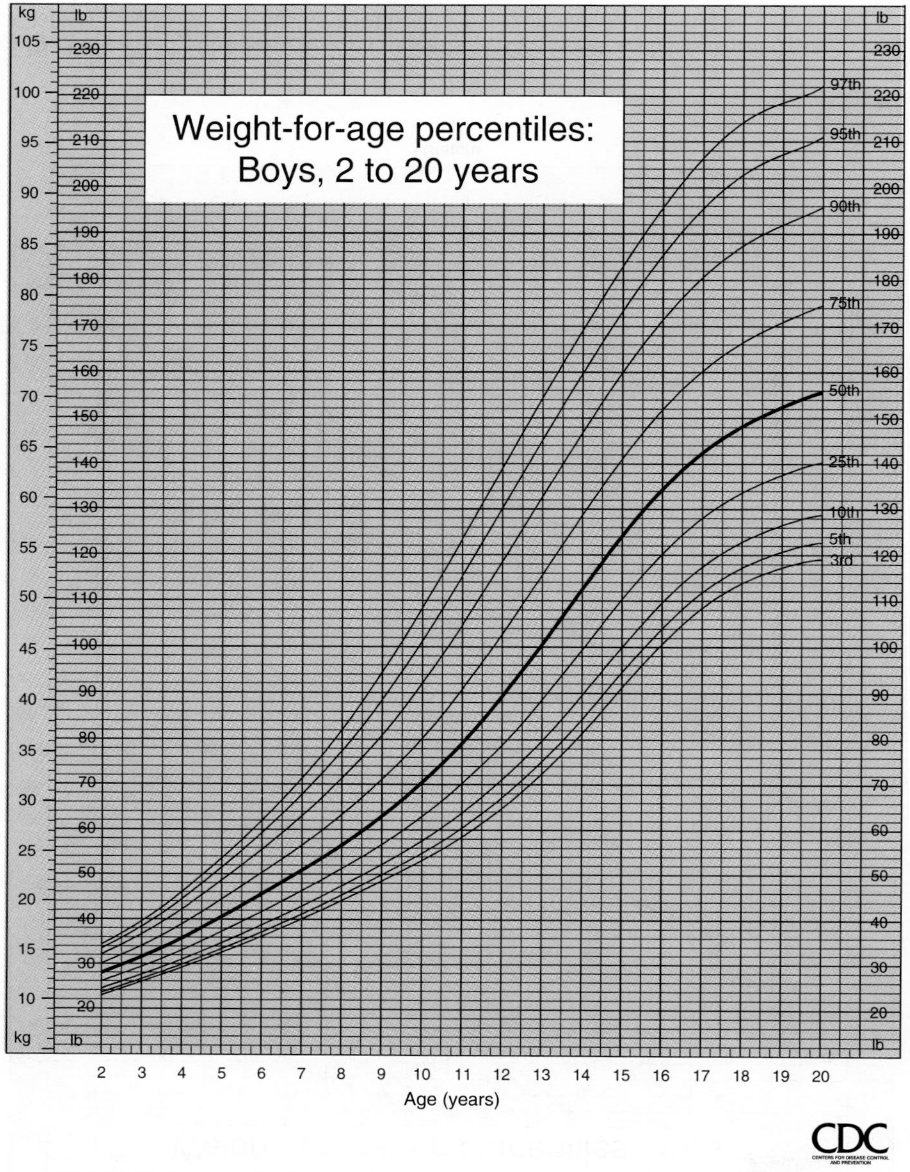

Stature-for-age percentiles:
Boys, 2 to 20 years

CDC

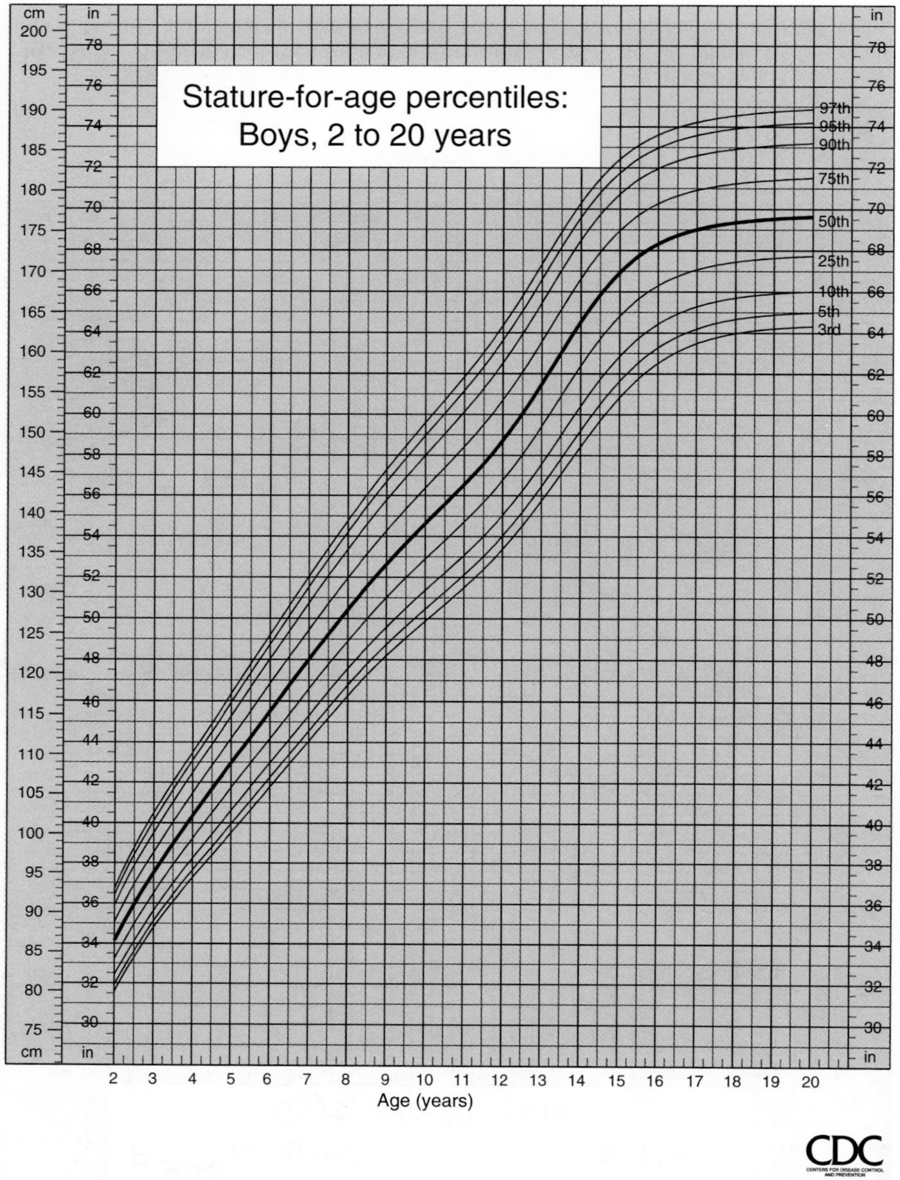

**Fig. C-6** Stature-for-age percentiles, boys, 2 to 20 years, CDC growth charts: United States. (Developed by the National Center for Health Statistics in collaboration with the National Center for Chronic Disease Prevention and Health Promotion [2000].)

Weight-for-age percentiles:
Boys, 2 to 20 years

CDC

**Fig. C-5** Weight-for-age percentiles, boys, 2 to 20 years, CDC growth charts: United States. (Developed by the National Center for Health Statistics in collaboration with the National Center for Chronic Disease Prevention and Health Promotion [2000].)

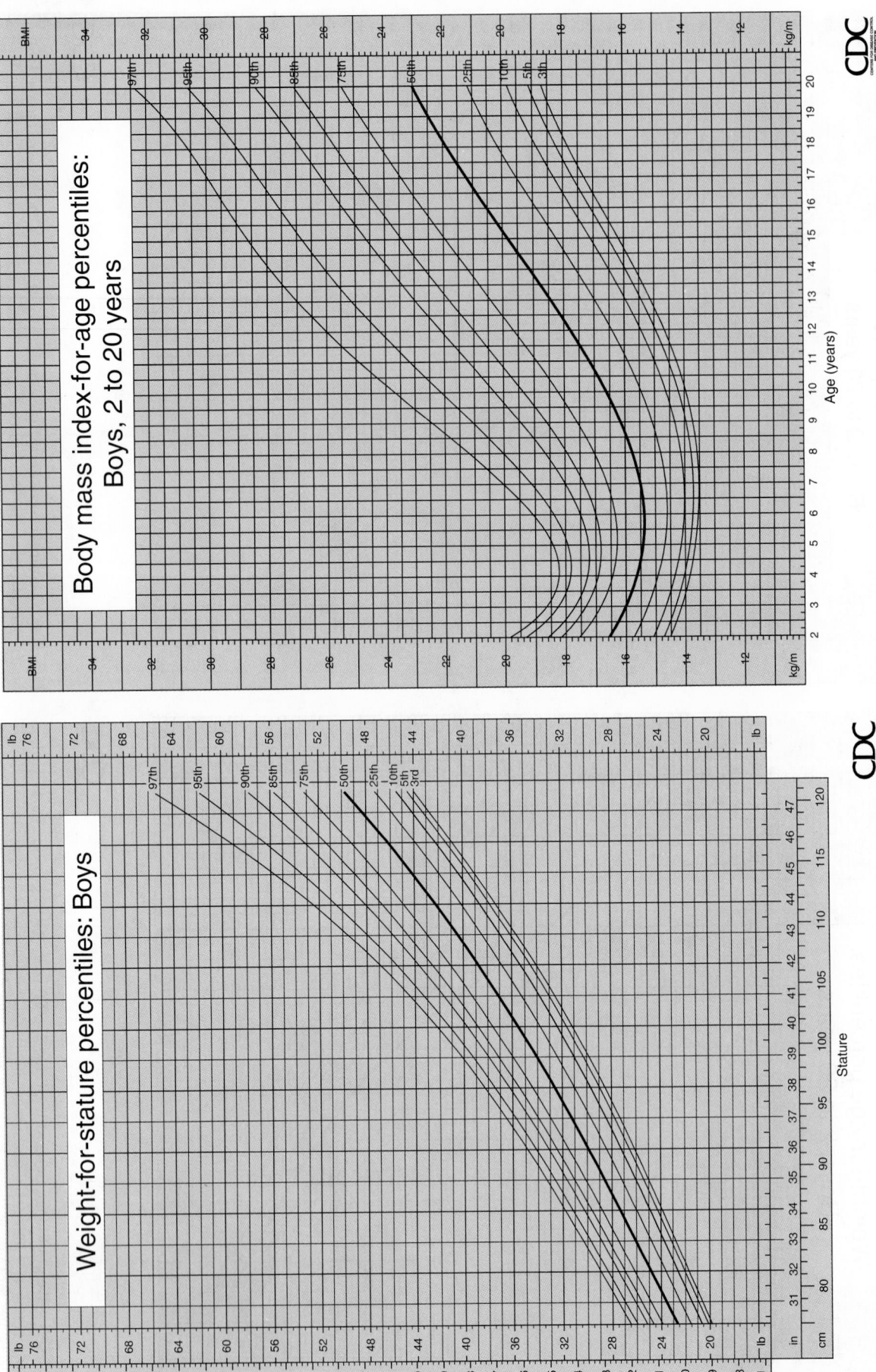

**Fig. C-8** Body mass index-for-age percentiles, boys, 2 to 20 years. CDC growth charts: United States. (Developed by the National Center for Health Statistics in collaboration with the National Center for Chronic Disease Prevention and Health Promotion [2000].)

**Fig. C-7** Weight-for-stature percentiles, boys, CDC growth charts: United States. (Developed by the National Center for Health Statistics in collaboration with the National Center for Chronic Disease Prevention and Health Promotion [2000].)

## Height and weight measurements for girls

| | Height by Percentiles | | | | | | Weight by Percentiles | | | | | |
|---|---|---|---|---|---|---|---|---|---|---|---|---|
| | 5 | | 50 | | 95 | | 5 | | 50 | | 95 | |
| Age* | cm | inches | cm | inches | cm | inches | kg | lb | kg | lb | kg | lb |
| Birth | 45.4 | 17¾ | 49.9 | 19¾ | 52.9 | 20¾ | 2.36 | 5¼ | 3.23 | 7 | 3.81 | 8½ |
| 3 months | 55.4 | 21¾ | 59.5 | 23½ | 63.4 | 25 | 4.18 | 9¼ | 5.4 | 12 | 6.74 | 14¾ |
| 6 months | 61.8 | 24¼ | 65.9 | 26 | 70.2 | 27¾ | 5.79 | 12¾ | 7.21 | 16 | 8.73 | 19¼ |
| 9 months | 66.1 | 26 | 70.4 | 27¾ | 75.0 | 29½ | 7.0 | 15½ | 8.56 | 18¾ | 10.17 | 22½ |
| 1 | 69.8 | 27½ | 74.3 | 29¼ | 79.1 | 31¼ | 7.84 | 17¼ | 9.53 | 21 | 11.24 | 24¾ |
| 1½ | 76.0 | 30 | 80.9 | 31¾ | 86.1 | 34 | 8.92 | 19¾ | 10.82 | 23¾ | 12.76 | 28¼ |
| 2† | 81.6 | 32¼ | 86.8 | 34¼ | 93.6 | 36¼ | 9.95 | 22 | 11.8 | 26 | 14.15 | 31¼ |
| 2½† | 84.6 | 33¼ | 90.0 | 35½ | 96.6 | 38 | 10.8 | 23¾ | 13.03 | 28¾ | 15.76 | 34¾ |
| 3 | 88.3 | 34¾ | 94.1 | 37 | 100.6 | 39½ | 11.61 | 25½ | 14.1 | 31 | 17.22 | 38 |
| 3½ | 91.7 | 36 | 97.9 | 38½ | 104.5 | 41¼ | 12.37 | 27¼ | 15.07 | 33¼ | 18.59 | 41 |
| 4 | 95.0 | 37½ | 101.6 | 40 | 108.3 | 42¾ | 13.11 | 29 | 15.96 | 35¼ | 19.91 | 44 |
| 4½ | 98.1 | 38½ | 105.0 | 41¼ | 112.0 | 44 | 13.83 | 30½ | 16.81 | 37 | 21.24 | 46¾ |
| 5 | 101.1 | 39¾ | 108.4 | 42¾ | 115.6 | 45½ | 14.55 | 32 | 17.66 | 39 | 22.62 | 49¾ |
| 6 | 106.6 | 42 | 114.6 | 45 | 122.7 | 48¼ | 16.05 | 35½ | 19.52 | 43 | 25.75 | 56¾ |
| 7 | 111.8 | 44 | 120.6 | 47½ | 129.5 | 51 | 17.71 | 39 | 21.84 | 48¼ | 29.68 | 65½ |
| 8 | 116.9 | 46 | 126.4 | 49¾ | 136.2 | 53½ | 19.62 | 43¼ | 24.84 | 54¾ | 34.71 | 76½ |
| 9 | 122.1 | 48 | 132.2 | 52 | 142.9 | 56¼ | 21.82 | 48 | 28.46 | 62¾ | 40.64 | 89½ |
| 10 | 127.5 | 50¼ | 138.3 | 54½ | 149.5 | 58¾ | 24.36 | 53¾ | 32.55 | 71¾ | 47.17 | 104 |
| 11 | 133.5 | 52½ | 144.8 | 57 | 156.2 | 61½ | 27.24 | 60 | 36.95 | 81½ | 54.0 | 119 |
| 12 | 139.8 | 55 | 151.5 | 59¾ | 162.7 | 64 | 30.52 | 67¼ | 41.53 | 91½ | 60.81 | 134 |
| 13 | 145.2 | 57¼ | 157.1 | 61¾ | 168.1 | 66¼ | 34.14 | 75¼ | 46.1 | 101¾ | 67.3 | 148¼ |
| 14 | 148.7 | 58½ | 160.4 | 63¼ | 171.3 | 67½ | 37.76 | 83¼ | 50.28 | 110¾ | 73.08 | 161 |
| 15 | 150.5 | 59¼ | 161.8 | 63¾ | 172.8 | 68 | 40.99 | 90¼ | 53.68 | 118¼ | 77.78 | 171½ |
| 16 | 151.6 | 59¾ | 162.4 | 64 | 173.3 | 68¼ | 43.41 | 95¾ | 55.89 | 123¼ | 80.99 | 178½ |
| 17 | 152.7 | 60 | 163.1 | 64¼ | 173.5 | 68¼ | 44.74 | 98¾ | 56.69 | 125 | 82.46 | 181¾ |
| 18 | 153.6 | 60½ | 163.7 | 64½ | 173.6 | 68¼ | 45.26 | 99¾ | 56.62 | 124¾ | 82.47 | 181¾ |

Modified from National Center for Health Statistics (NCHS), Health Resources Administration, Department of Health, Education, and Welfare, Hyattsville, MD. Conversion of metric data to approximate inches and pounds by Ross Laboratories.
*Years unless otherwise indicated.
†Height data include some recumbent length measurements, which make values slightly higher than if all measurements had been of stature.

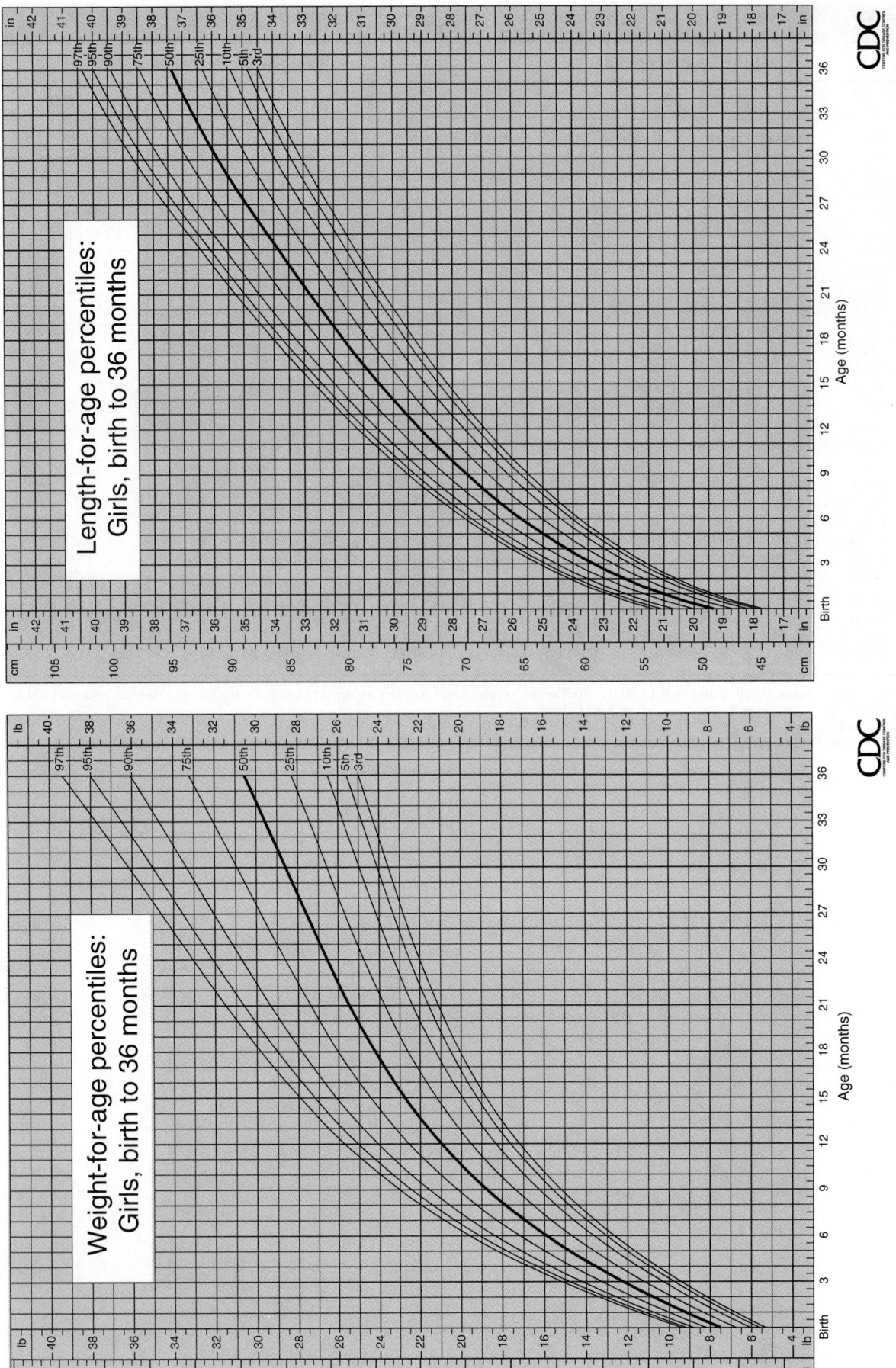

**Fig. C-9** Weight-for-age percentiles, girls, birth to 36 months, CDC growth charts: United States. (Developed by the National Center for Health Statistics in collaboration with the National Center for Chronic Disease Prevention and Health Promotion [2000].)

**Fig. C-10** Length-for-age percentiles, girls, birth to 36 months, CDC growth charts: United States. (Developed by the National Center for Health Statistics in collaboration with the National Center for Chronic Disease Prevention and Health Promotion [2000].)

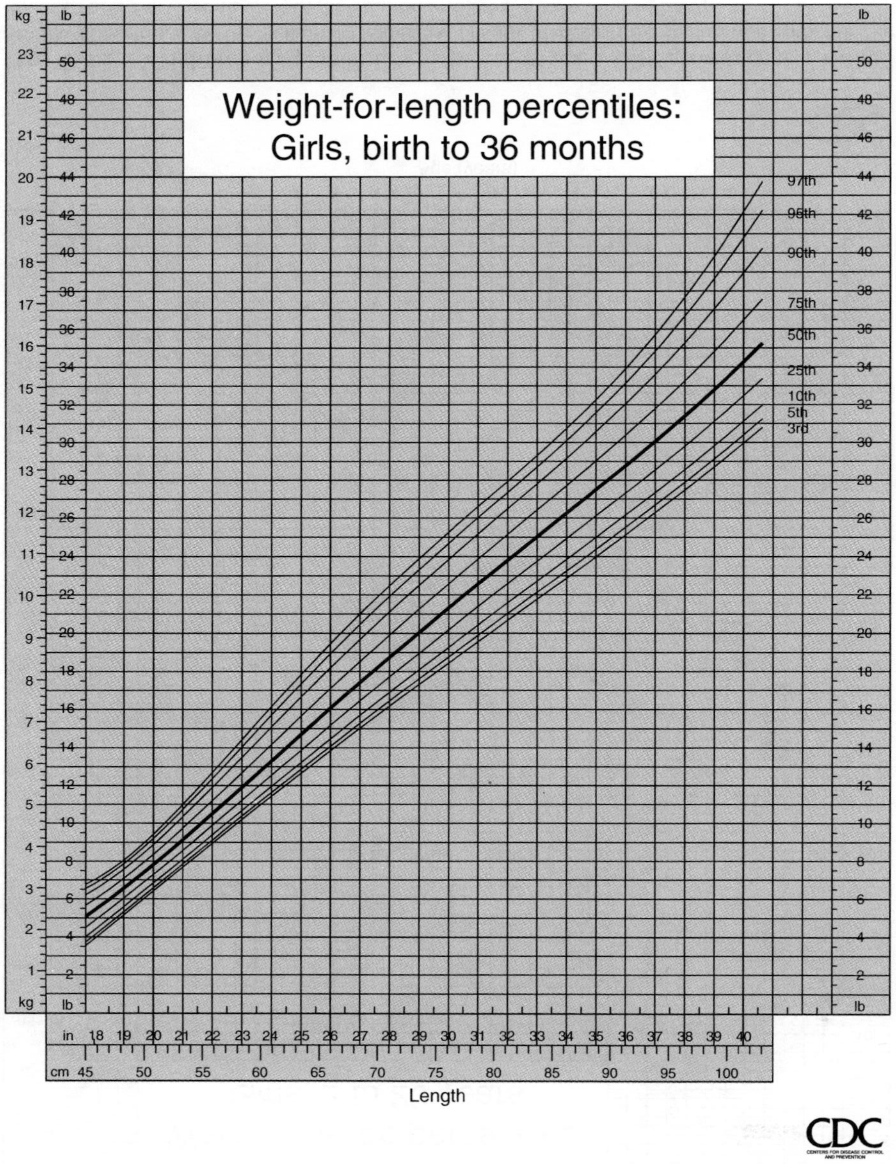

Head circumference-for-age percentiles:
Girls, birth to 36 months

Weight-for-length percentiles:
Girls, birth to 36 months

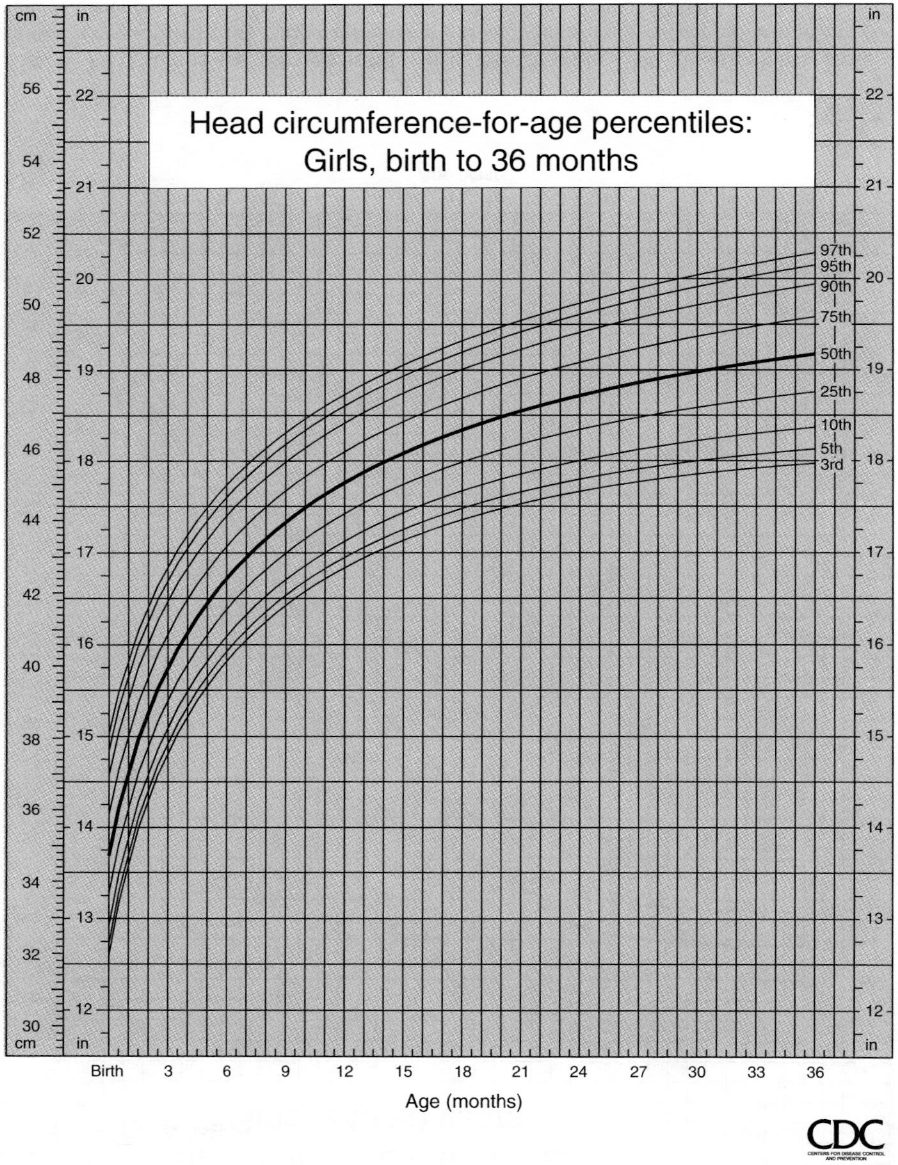

**Fig. C-12** Head circumference-for-age percentiles, girls, birth to 36 months, CDC growth charts: United States. (Developed by the National Center for Health Statistics in collaboration with the National Center for Chronic Disease Prevention and Health Promotion [2000].)

**Fig. C-11** Weight-for-length percentiles, girls, birth to 36 months, CDC growth charts: United States. (Developed by the National Center for Health Statistics in collaboration with the National Center for Chronic Disease Prevention and Health Promotion [2000].)

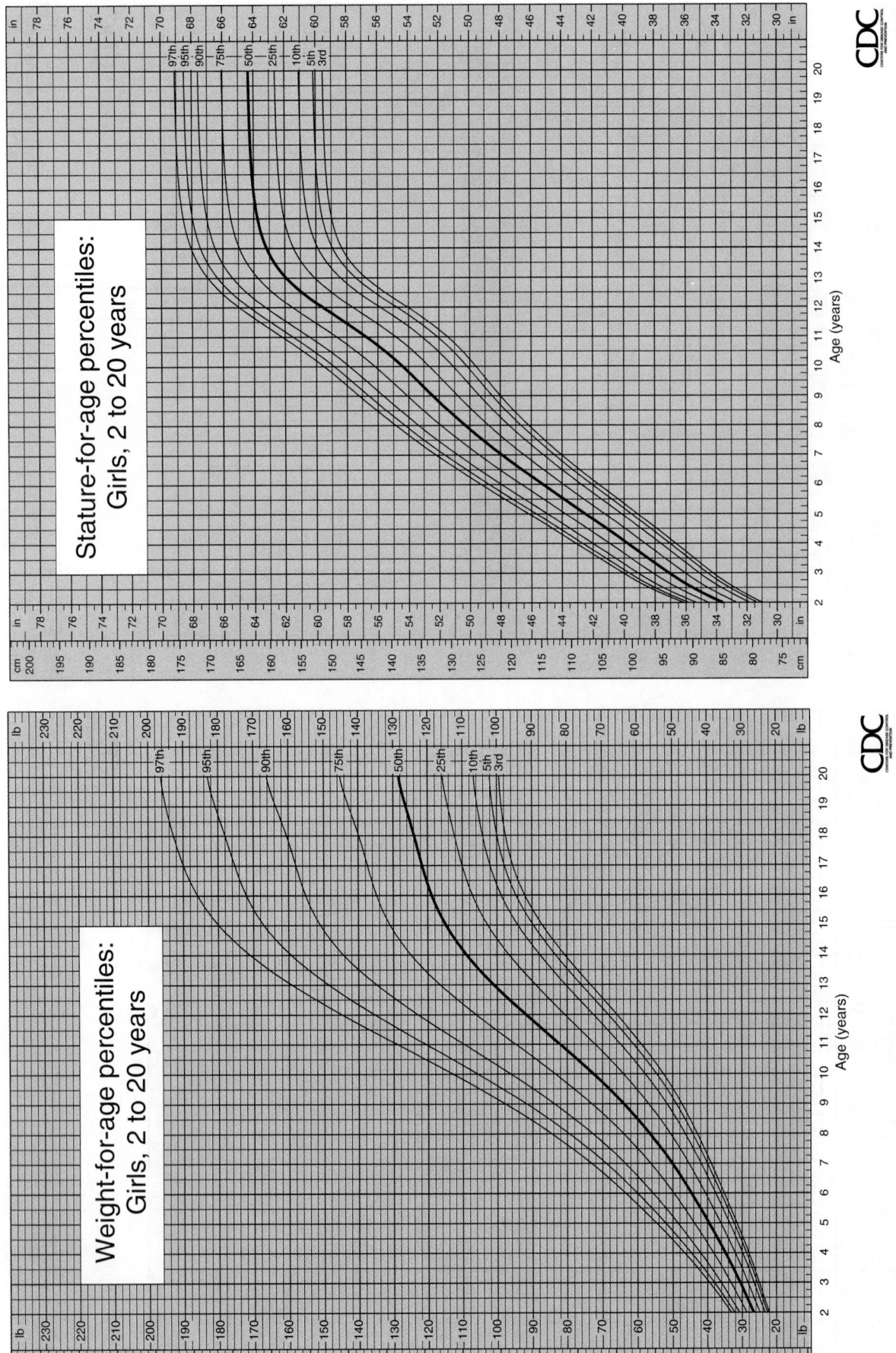

**Fig. C-13** Weight-for-age percentiles, girls, 2 to 20 years, CDC growth charts: United States. (Developed by the National Center for Health Statistics in collaboration with the National Center for Chronic Disease Prevention and Health Promotion [2000].)

**Fig. C-14** Stature-for-age percentiles, girls, 2 to 20 years, CDC growth charts: United States. (Developed by the National Center for Health Statistics in collaboration with the National Center for Chronic Disease Prevention and Health Promotion [2000].)

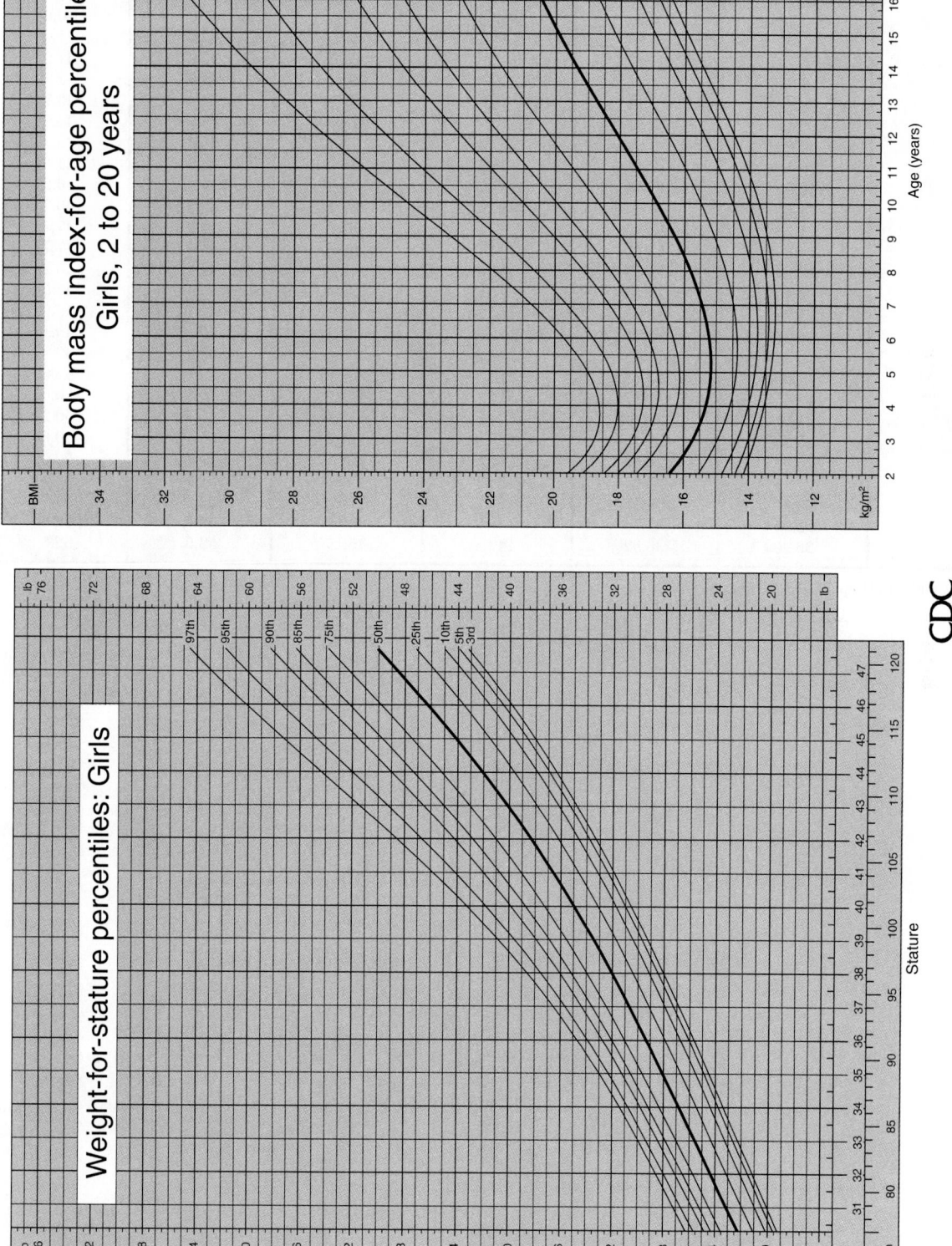

**Fig. C-16** Body mass index-for-age percentiles, girls, 2 to 20 years, CDC growth charts: United States. (Developed by the National Center for Health Statistics in collaboration with the National Center for Chronic Disease Prevention and Health Promotion [2000].)

**Fig. C-15** Weight-for-stature percentiles, girls, CDC growth charts: United States. (Developed by the National Center for Health Statistics in collaboration with the National Center for Chronic Disease Prevention and Health Promotion [2000].)

## Growth standards of healthy Chinese children

| Age (Months or Years) | Weight (kg) | | Height (cm) | | Head Circumference (cm) | |
|---|---|---|---|---|---|---|
| | Boys | Girls | Boys | Girls | Boys | Girls |
| Birth | 3.27 | 3.17 | 50.6 | 50.0 | 34.3 | 33.7 |
| 1 month | 4.97 | 4.64 | 56.5 | 55.5 | 38.1 | 37.3 |
| 2 months | 5.95 | 5.49 | 59.6 | 58.4 | 39.7 | 38.7 |
| 3 months | 6.73 | 6.23 | 62.3 | 60.9 | 41.0 | 40.0 |
| 4 months | 7.32 | 6.69 | 64.4 | 62.9 | 42.0 | 41.0 |
| 5 months | 7.70 | 7.19 | 65.9 | 64.5 | 42.9 | 41.9 |
| 6 months | 8.22 | 7.62 | 68.1 | 66.7 | 43.9 | 42.8 |
| 8 months | 8.71 | 8.14 | 70.6 | 69.0 | 44.9 | 43.7 |
| 10 months | 9.14 | 8.57 | 72.9 | 71.4 | 45.7 | 44.5 |
| 12 months | 9.56 | 9.04 | 75.6 | 74.1 | 46.3 | 45.2 |
| 15 months | 10.15 | 9.54 | 78.3 | 76.9 | 46.8 | 45.6 |
| 18 months | 10.67 | 10.08 | 80.7 | 79.4 | 47.3 | 46.2 |
| 21 months | 11.18 | 10.56 | 83.0 | 81.7 | 47.8 | 46.7 |
| 24 months | 11.95 | 11.37 | 86.5 | 85.3 | 48.2 | 47.1 |
| 2.5 years | 12.84 | 12.28 | 90.4 | 89.3 | 48.8 | 47.7 |
| 3 years | 13.63 | 13.16 | 93.8 | 92.8 | 49.1 | 48.1 |
| 3.5 years | 14.45 | 14.00 | 97.2 | 96.3 | 49.4 | 48.5 |
| 4 years | 15.26 | 14.89 | 100.8 | 100.1 | 49.7 | 48.9 |
| 4.5 years | 16.07 | 15.63 | 103.9 | 103.1 | 50.0 | 49.1 |
| 5 years | 16.88 | 16.46 | 107.2 | 106.5 | 50.2 | 49.4 |
| 5.5 years | 17.65 | 17.18 | 110.1 | 109.2 | 50.5 | 49.6 |
| 6 years | 19.25 | 18.67 | 114.7 | 113.9 | 50.8 | 50.0 |
| 7 years | 21.01 | 20.35 | 120.6 | 119.3 | 51.1 | 50.2 |
| 8 years | 23.08 | 22.43 | 125.3 | 124.6 | 51.4 | 50.6 |
| 9 years | 25.33 | 24.57 | 130.6 | 129.5 | 51.7 | 50.9 |
| 10 years | 27.15 | 27.05 | 134.4 | 134.8 | 51.9 | 51.3 |
| 11 years | 30.13 | 30.51 | 139.2 | 140.6 | 52.3 | 51.7 |
| 12 years | 33.05 | 34.74 | 144.2 | 146.6 | 52.7 | 52.3 |
| 13 years | 36.90 | 38.52 | 149.8 | 150.7 | 53.0 | 52.8 |

Data from Bejing Children's Hospital, 1987, China.

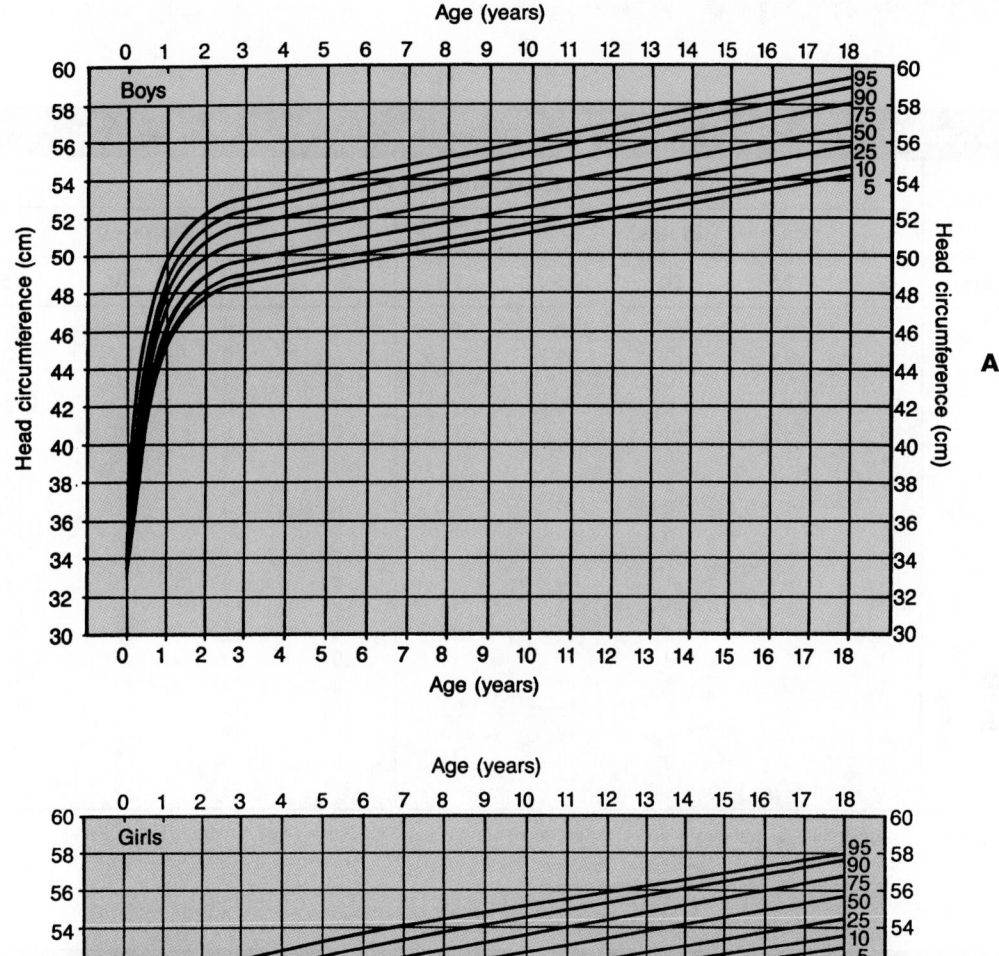

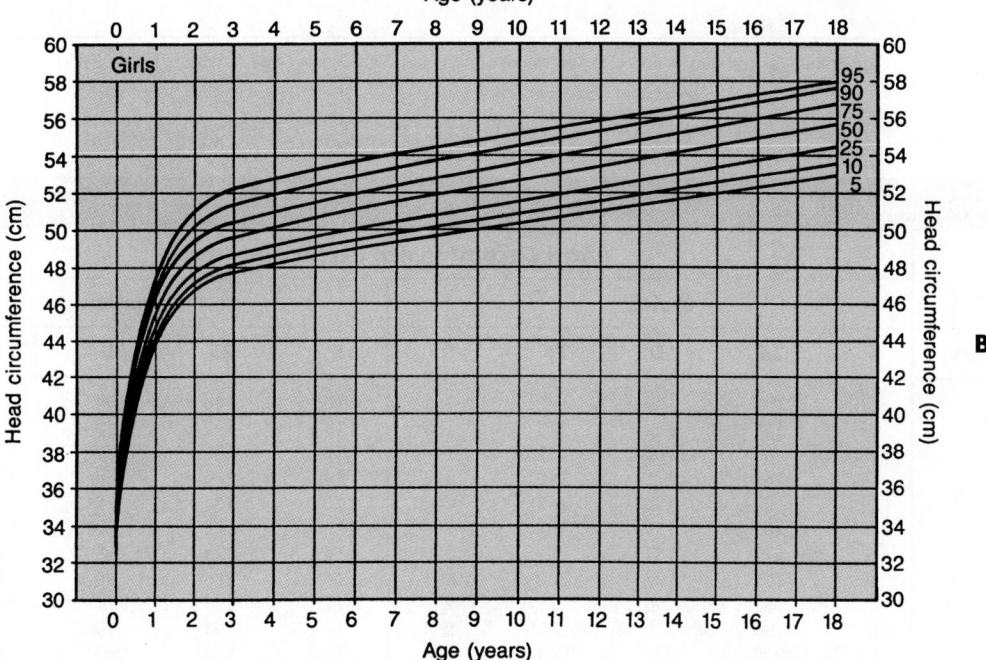

**Fig. C-17**   Selected percentiles for smoothed head circumference values of children from birth to 18 years. **A**, Boys. **B**, Girls. (From Roche AF and others: Head circumference reference data: birth to 18 years, *Pediatrics* 79[5]:706-712, 1987.)

## Percentiles for triceps skinfold

| | Triceps Skinfold Percentiles (mm) | | | | | | | | | |
| | Males | | | | | Females | | | | |
| Age-Group (Years) | 5 | 25 | 50 | 75 | 95 | 5 | 25 | 50 | 75 | 95 |
|---|---|---|---|---|---|---|---|---|---|---|
| 1-1.9 | 6 | 8 | 10 | 12 | 16 | 6 | 8 | 10 | 12 | 16 |
| 2-2.9 | 6 | 8 | 10 | 12 | 15 | 6 | 9 | 10 | 12 | 16 |
| 3-3.9 | 6 | 8 | 10 | 11 | 15 | 7 | 9 | 11 | 12 | 15 |
| 4-4.9 | 6 | 8 | 9 | 11 | 14 | 7 | 8 | 10 | 12 | 16 |
| 5-5.9 | 6 | 8 | 9 | 11 | 15 | 6 | 8 | 10 | 12 | 18 |
| 6-6.9 | 5 | 7 | 8 | 10 | 16 | 6 | 8 | 10 | 12 | 16 |
| 7-7.9 | 5 | 7 | 9 | 12 | 17 | 6 | 9 | 11 | 13 | 18 |
| 8-8.9 | 5 | 7 | 8 | 10 | 16 | 6 | 9 | 12 | 15 | 24 |
| 9-9.9 | 6 | 7 | 10 | 13 | 18 | 8 | 10 | 13 | 16 | 22 |
| 10-10.9 | 6 | 8 | 10 | 14 | 21 | 7 | 10 | 12 | 17 | 27 |
| 11-11.9 | 6 | 8 | 11 | 16 | 24 | 7 | 10 | 13 | 18 | 28 |
| 12-12.9 | 6 | 8 | 11 | 14 | 28 | 8 | 11 | 14 | 18 | 27 |
| 13-13.9 | 5 | 7 | 10 | 14 | 26 | 8 | 12 | 15 | 21 | 30 |
| 14-14.9 | 4 | 7 | 9 | 14 | 24 | 9 | 13 | 16 | 21 | 28 |
| 15-15.9 | 4 | 6 | 8 | 11 | 24 | 8 | 12 | 17 | 21 | 32 |
| 16-16.9 | 4 | 6 | 8 | 12 | 22 | 10 | 15 | 18 | 22 | 31 |
| 17-17.9 | 5 | 6 | 8 | 12 | 19 | 10 | 13 | 19 | 24 | 37 |
| 18-18.9 | 4 | 6 | 9 | 13 | 24 | 10 | 15 | 18 | 22 | 30 |
| 19-24.9 | 4 | 7 | 10 | 15 | 22 | 10 | 14 | 18 | 24 | 34 |

From Frisancho A: New norms of upper limb fat and muscle areas for assessment of nutritional status, *Am J Clin Nutr* 34:2540-2545, 1981.

## Percentiles of upper arm circumference

| | Arm Circumference Percentiles (mm) | | | | | | | | | |
| | Males | | | | | Females | | | | |
| Age-Group (Years) | 5 | 25 | 50 | 75 | 95 | 5 | 25 | 50 | 75 | 95 |
|---|---|---|---|---|---|---|---|---|---|---|
| 1-1.9 | 142 | 150 | 159 | 170 | 183 | 138 | 148 | 156 | 164 | 177 |
| 2-2.9 | 141 | 153 | 162 | 170 | 185 | 142 | 152 | 160 | 167 | 184 |
| 3-3.9 | 150 | 160 | 167 | 175 | 190 | 143 | 158 | 167 | 175 | 189 |
| 4-4.9 | 149 | 162 | 171 | 180 | 192 | 149 | 160 | 169 | 177 | 191 |
| 5-5.9 | 153 | 167 | 175 | 185 | 204 | 153 | 165 | 175 | 185 | 211 |
| 6-6.9 | 155 | 167 | 179 | 188 | 228 | 156 | 170 | 176 | 187 | 211 |
| 7-7.9 | 162 | 177 | 187 | 201 | 230 | 164 | 174 | 183 | 199 | 231 |
| 8-8.9 | 162 | 177 | 190 | 202 | 245 | 168 | 183 | 195 | 214 | 261 |
| 9-9.9 | 175 | 187 | 200 | 217 | 257 | 178 | 194 | 211 | 224 | 260 |
| 10-10.9 | 181 | 196 | 210 | 231 | 274 | 174 | 193 | 210 | 228 | 265 |
| 11-11.9 | 186 | 202 | 223 | 244 | 280 | 185 | 208 | 224 | 248 | 303 |
| 12-12.9 | 193 | 214 | 232 | 254 | 303 | 194 | 216 | 237 | 256 | 294 |
| 13-13.9 | 194 | 228 | 247 | 263 | 301 | 202 | 223 | 243 | 271 | 338 |
| 14-14.9 | 220 | 237 | 253 | 283 | 322 | 214 | 237 | 252 | 272 | 322 |
| 15-15.9 | 222 | 244 | 264 | 284 | 320 | 208 | 239 | 254 | 279 | 322 |
| 16-16.9 | 244 | 262 | 278 | 303 | 343 | 218 | 241 | 258 | 283 | 334 |
| 17-17.9 | 246 | 267 | 285 | 308 | 347 | 220 | 241 | 264 | 295 | 350 |
| 18-18.9 | 245 | 276 | 297 | 321 | 379 | 222 | 241 | 258 | 281 | 325 |
| 19-24.9 | 262 | 288 | 308 | 331 | 372 | 221 | 247 | 265 | 290 | 345 |

From Frisancho A: New norms of upper limb fat and muscle areas for assessment of nutritional status, *Am J Clin Nutr* 34:2540-2545, 1981.

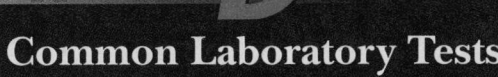
## Common laboratory tests*

| Test/Specimen | Age/Sex/Reference | Conventional Units | | International Units (SI) | |
|---|---|---|---|---|---|
| **Normal Ranges** | | | | | |
| Acetaminophen | | | | | |
| Serum or plasma | Therap. conc. | 10-30 μg/mL | | 66-200 μmol/L | |
| | Toxic conc. | >200 μg/mL | | >1300 μmol/L | |
| Ammonia nitrogen | | | | | |
| Plasma or serum | Newborn | 90-150 μg/dL | | 64-107 μmol/L | |
| | 0-2 wk | 79-129 μg/dL | | 56-92 μmol/L | |
| | >1 mo | 29-70 μg/dL | | 21-50 μmol/L | |
| | Thereafter | 0-50 μg/dL | | 0-35.7 μmol/L | |
| Urine, 24 hr | | 500-1200 mg N/d | | 36-86 μmmol/d | |
| Antistreptolysin O titer (ASO) | | | | | |
| Serum | 2-4 yr | <160 Todd units | | | |
| | School-age children | 170-330 Todd units | | | |
| Base excess | | | | | |
| Whole blood | Newborn | (−10)-(−2) mEq/L | | (−10)-(−2) mmol/L | |
| | Infant | (−7)-(−1) mEq/L | | (−7)-(−1) mmol/L | |
| | Child | (−4)-(+2) mEq/L | | (−4)-(+2) mmol/L | |
| | Thereafter | (−3)-(+3) mEq/L | | (−3)-(+3) mmol/L | |
| Bicarbonate (HCO₃) | | | | | |
| Serum | Arterial | 21-28 mEq/L | | 21-28 mmol/L | |
| | Venous | 22-29 mEq/L | | 22-29 mmol/L | |
| | | **Premature (mg/dl)** | **Full term (mg/dl)** | **Premature (μmol/L)** | **Full term (μmol/L)** |
| Bilirubin, total | | | | | |
| Serum | Cord blood | <2.0 | <2.0 | <34 | <34 |
| | 0-1 d | <8.0 | <6.0 | <137 | <103 |
| | 1-2 d | <12.0 | <8.0 | <205 | <137 |
| | 2-5 d | <16.0 | <12.0 | <274 | <205 |
| | >5 d | <20.0 | <10.0 | <340 | <171 |
| Bilirubin, direct (conjugated) | | | | | |
| Serum | | 0.0-0.2 mg/dL | | 0-3.4 μmol/L | |
| Bleeding time | | | | | |
| Blood from skin puncture | | | | | |
| Ivy | Normal | 2-7 min | | 2-7 min | |
| | Borderline | 7-11 min | | 7-11 min | |
| Simplate (G-D) | | 2.75-8 min | | 2.75-8 min | |
| Blood volume | | | | | |
| Whole blood | Male | 52-83 mL/kg | | 0.052-0.083 L/kg | |
| | Female | 50-75 mL/kg | | 0.050-0.075 L/kg | |
| C-reactive protein (CRP) | | | | | |
| Serum | Cord blood | 52-1330 ng/mL | | 52-1330 μg/L | |
| | 2-12 yr | 67-1800 ng/mL | | 67-1800 μg/L | |
| Calcium, ionized | | | | | |
| Serum, plasma, or whole blood | Cord blood | 5.0-6.0 mg/dL | | 1.25-1.50 mmol/L | |
| | Newborn, 3-24 hr | 4.3-5.1 mg/dL | | 1.07-1.27 mmol/L | |
| | 24-48 hr | 4.0-4.7 mg/dL | | 1.00-1.17 mmol/L | |
| | Thereafter | 4.8-4.92 mg/dL or 2.24-2.46 mEq/L | | 1.12-1.23 mmol/L | |
| Calcium, total | | | | | |
| Serum | Cord blood | 9.0-11.5 mg/dL | | 2.25-2.88 mmol/L | |
| | Newborn, 3-24 hr | 9.0-10.6 mg/dL | | 2.3-2.65 mmol/L | |
| | 24-48 hr | 7.0-12.0 mg/dL | | 1.75-3.0 mmol/L | |
| | 4-7 d | 9.0-10.9 mg/dL | | 2.25-2.73 mmol/L | |
| | Child | 8.8-10.8 mg/dL | | 2.2-2.70 mmol/L | |
| | Thereafter | 8.4-10.2 mg/dL | | 2.1-2.55 mmol/L | |

Modified from Behrman RE and others, editors: *Nelson textbook of pediatrics*, ed 16, Philadelphia, 2000, WB Saunders; McMillan JA and others, editors: *Oski's pediatrics: principles and practice*, ed 3, Philadelphia, 1999, Lippincott Williams & Wilkins; and Fischbach F: *A manual of laboratory and diagnostic tests*, ed 6, Philadelphia, 2000, Lippincott Williams & Wilkins.

*For a description of abbreviations, see p. 1903.

*Continued*

## Common laboratory tests—cont'd

| Test/Specimen | Age/Sex/Reference | Normal Ranges Conventional Units | Normal Ranges International Units (SI) |
|---|---|---|---|
| Carbon dioxide, partial pressure ($P_{CO_2}$) | | | |
| Whole blood, arterial | Newborn | 27-40 mm Hg | 3.6-5.3 kPa |
| | Infant | 27-41 mm Hg | 3.6-5.5 kPa |
| | Thereafter: Male | 35-48 mm Hg | 4.7-6.4 kPa |
| | Female | 32-45 mm Hg | 4.3-6.0 kPa |
| Carbon dioxide, total ($tCO_2$) | | | |
| Serum or plasma | Cord blood | 14-22 mEq/L | 14-22 mmol/L |
| | Premature (1 wk) | 14-27 mEq/L | 14-27 mmol/L |
| | Newborn | 13-22 mEq/L | 13-22 mmol/L |
| | Infant, child | 20-28 mEq/L | 20-28 mmol/L |
| | Thereafter | 23-30 mEq/L | 23-30 mmol/L |
| Cerebrospinal fluid (CSF) | | | |
| Pressure | | 70-180 mm water | 70-180 mm water |
| Volume | Child | 60-100 mL | 0.06-0.10 L |
| | Adult | 100-160 mL | 0.10-0.16 L |
| Chloride | | | |
| Serum or plasma | Cord blood | 96-104 mEq/L | 96-104 mmol/L |
| | Newborn | 97-110 mEq/L | 97-110 mmol/L |
| | Thereafter | 98-106 mEq/L | 98-106 mmol/L |
| Sweat | Normal (homozygote) | <40 mEq/L | <40 mmol/L |
| | Marginal (e.g., asthma, Addison disease, malnutrition) | 45-60 mEq/L | 45-60 mmol/L |
| | Cystic fibrosis | >60 mEq/L | >60 mmol/L |
| Cholesterol, total | | | |
| Serum or plasma | Acceptable | <170 mg/dL | <4.4 mmol/L |
| | Borderline | 170-199 mg/dL | 4.4-5.1 mmol/L |
| | High | ≥200 mg/dL | ≥5.2 mmol/L |
| Clotting time (Lee-White) | | | |
| Whole blood | | 5-8 min (glass tubes) | 5-8 min |
| | | 5-15 min (room temp) | 5-15 min |
| | | 30 min (silicone tube) | 30 min |
| Creatine kinase (CK, CPK) | | | |
| Serum | Cord blood | 70-380 U/L | 70-380 U/L |
| | 5-8 hr | 214-1175 U/L | 214-1175 U/L |
| | 24-33 hr | 130-1200 U/L | 130-1200 U/L |
| | 72-100 hr | 87-725 U/L | 87-725 U/L |
| | Adult | 5-130 U/L | 5-130 U/L |
| Creatinine | | | |
| Serum | Cord blood | 0.6-1.2 mg/dL | 53-106 $\mu$mol/L |
| | Newborn | 0.3-1.0 mg/dL | 27-88 $\mu$mol/L |
| | Infant | 0.2-0.4 mg/dL | 18-35 $\mu$mol/L |
| | Child | 0.3-0.7 mg/dL | 27-62 $\mu$mol/L |
| | Adolescent | 0.5-1.0 mg/dL | 44-88 $\mu$mol/L |
| | Adult: Male | 0.6-1.2 mg/dL | 53-106 $\mu$mol/L |
| | Female | 0.5-1.1 mg/dL | 44-97 $\mu$mol/L |
| Urine, 24 hr | Premature | 8.1-15.0 mg/kg/24 hr | 72-133 $\mu$mol/kg/24 hr |
| | Full term | 10.4-19.7 mg/kg/24 hr | 92-174 $\mu$mol/kg/24 hr |
| | 1.5-7 yr | 10-15 mg/kg/24 hr | 88-133 $\mu$mol/kg/24 hr |
| | 7-15 yr | 5.2-41 mg/kg/24 hr | 46-362 $\mu$mol/kg/24 hr |
| Creatinine clearance (endogenous) | | | |
| Serum or plasma and urine | Newborn | 40-65 ml/min/1.73 m² | |
| | <40 yr: Male | 97-137 ml/min/1.73 m² | |
| | Female | 88-128 ml/min/1.73 m² | |
| Digoxin | | | |
| Serum, plasma; collect at least 12 hr after dose | Therap. conc. | | |
| | CHF | 0.8-1.5 ng/mL | 1.0-1.9 nmol/L |
| | Arrhythmias | 1.5-2.0 ng/mL | 1.9-2.6 nmol/L |

**Common laboratory tests—cont'd**

| Test/Specimen | Age/Sex/Reference | Normal Ranges | |
|---|---|---|---|
| | | **Conventional Units** | **International Units (SI)** |
| Digoxin—cont'd | Toxic conc. | | |
| Serum, plasma; collect at least 12 hr after dose | Child | >2.5 ng/mL | >3.2 nmol/L |
| | Adult | >3.0 ng/mL | >3.8 nmol/L |
| Eosinophil count | | | |
| Whole blood, capillary blood | | 50-250 cells/mm³ (µl) | 50-250 × 10⁶ cells/L |
| Erythrocyte (RBC) count | | | |
| Whole blood | Cord blood | 3.9-5.5 million/mm³ | 3.9-5.5 × 10¹² cells/L |
| | 1-3 d | 4.0-6.6 million/mm³ | 4.0-6.6 × 10¹² cells/L |
| | 1 wk | 3.9-6.3 million/mm³ | 3.9-6.3 × 10¹² cells/L |
| | 2 wk | 3.6-6.2 million/mm³ | 3.6-6.2 × 10¹² cells/L |
| | 1 mo | 3.0-5.4 million/mm³ | 3.0-5.4 × 10¹² cells/L |
| | 2 mo | 2.7-4.9 million/mm³ | 2.7-4.9 × 10¹² cells/L |
| | 3-6 mo | 3.1-4.5 million/mm³ | 3.1-4.5 × 10¹² cells/L |
| | 0.5-2 yr | 3.7-5.3 million/mm³ | 3.7-5.3 × 10¹² cells/L |
| | 2-6 yr | 3.9-5.3 million/mm³ | 3.9-5.3 × 10¹² cells/L |
| | 6-12 yr | 4.0-5.2 million/mm³ | 4.0-5.2 × 10¹² cells/L |
| | 12-18 yr: Male | 4.5-5.3 million/mm³ | 4.5-5.3 × 10¹² cells/L |
| | Female | 4.1-5.1 million/mm³ | 4.1-5.1 × 10¹² cells/L |
| Erythrocyte sedimentation rate (ESR) | | | |
| Whole blood | | | |
| Westergren (modified) | Child | 0-10 mm/hr | 0-10 mm/hr |
| | <50 yr: Male | 0-15 mm/hr | 0-15 mm/hr |
| | Female | 0-20 mm/hr | 0-20 mm/hr |
| Wintrobe | Child | 0-13 mm/hr | 0-13 mm/hr |
| | Adult: Male | 0-9 mm/hr | 0-9 mm/hr |
| | Female | 0-20 mm/hr | 0-20 mm/hr |
| Fibrinogen | | | |
| Plasma | Newborn | 125-300 mg/dL | 1.25-3.00 g/L |
| | Thereafter | 200-400 mg/dL | 2.00-4.00 g/L |
| Galactose | | | |
| Serum | Newborn | 0-20 mg/dL | 0-1.11 mmol/L |
| | Thereafter | <5 mg/dL | <0.28 mmol/L |
| Urine | Newborn | ≤60 mg/dL | ≤3.33 mmol/L |
| | Thereafter | <14 mg/24 hr | <0.08 mmol/d |
| Glucose | | | |
| Serum | Cord blood | 45-96 mg/dL | 2.5-5.3 mmol/L |
| | Newborn, 1 d | 40-60 mg/dL | 2.2-3.3 mmol/L |
| | Newborn, >1 d | 50-90 mg/dL | 2.8-5.0 mmol/L |
| | Child | 60-100 mg/dL | 3.3-5.5 mmol/L |
| | Thereafter | 70-105 mg/dL | 3.9-5.8 mmol/L |
| Whole blood | Adult | 65-95 mg/dL | 3.6-5.3 mmol/L |
| CSF | Adult | 40-70 mg/dL | 2.2-3.9 mmol/L |
| Urine (quantitative) | | <0.5 g/d | <2.8 mmol/d |
| (qualitative) | | Negative | Negative |

| Glucose tolerance test (GTT) Serum | | | | | |
|---|---|---|---|---|---|
| **Oral dose** | | **Normal** | **Diabetic** | **Normal** | **Diabetic** |
| Adult: 75 g | Fasting | 70-105 mg/dL | ≥126 mg/dL | 3.9-5.8 mmol/L | ≥7.0 mmol/L |
| Child: 1.75 g/kg of ideal | 60 min | 120-170 mg/dL | ≥200 mg/dL | 6.7-9.4 mmol/L | ≥11 mmol/L |
| weight up to maximum | 90 min | 100-140 mg/dL | ≥200 mg/dL | 5.6-7.8 mmol/L | ≥11 mmol/L |
| of 75 g | 120 min | 70-120 mg/dL | ≥200 mg/dL | 3.9-6.7 mmol/L | ≥11 mmol/L |

| Growth hormone (hGH, somatotropin) | | | |
|---|---|---|---|
| Plasma | 1 d | 5-53 ng/mL | 5-53 µg/L |
| | 1 wk | 5-27 ng/mL | 5-27 µg/L |
| | 1-12 mo | 2-10 ng/mL | 2-10 µg/L |
| | Fasting child/adult | <0.7-6.0 ng/mL | <0.7-6.0 µg/L |

*Continued*

## Common laboratory tests—cont'd

| Test/Specimen | Age/Sex/Reference | Normal Ranges | |
|---|---|---|---|
| | | **Conventional Units** | **International Units (SI)** |
| **Hematocrit (HCT, Hct)** | | | |
| Whole blood | 1 d (cap) | 48%-69% | 0.48-0.69 vol. fraction |
| | 2 d | 48%-75% | 0.48-0.75 vol. fraction |
| | 3 d | 44%-72% | 0.44-0.72 vol. fraction |
| | 2 mo | 28%-42% | 0.28-0.42 vol. fraction |
| | 6-12 yr | 35%-45% | 0.35-0.45 vol. fraction |
| | 12-18 yr: Male | 37%-49% | 0.37-0.49 vol. fraction |
| | Female | 36%-46% | 0.36-0.46 vol. fraction |
| **Hemoglobin (Hb)** | | | |
| Whole blood | 1-3 d (cap) | 14.5-22.5 g/dL | 2.25-3.49 mmol/L |
| | 2 mo | 9.0-14.0 g/dL | 1.40-2.17 mmol/L |
| | 6-12 yr | 11.5-15.5 g/dL | 1.78-2.40 mmol/L |
| | 12-18 yr: Male | 13.0-16.0 g/dL | 2.02-2.48 mmol/L |
| | Female | 12.0-16.0 g/dL | 1.86-2.48 mmol/L |
| **Hemoglobin A** | | | |
| Whole blood | | >95% of total | >0.95 fraction of Hb |
| **Hemoglobin F** | | | |
| Whole blood | 1 d | 63%-92% HbF | 0.63-0.92 mass fraction HbF |
| | 5 d | 65%-88% HbF | 0.65-0.88 mass fraction HbF |
| | 3 wk | 55%-85% HbF | 0.55-0.85 mass fraction HbF |
| | 6-9 wk | 31%-75% HbF | 0.31-0.75 mass fraction HbF |
| | 3-4 mo | <2%-59% HbF | <0.02-0.59 mass fraction HbF |
| | 6 mo | <2%-9% HbF | <0.02-0.09 mass fraction HbF |
| | Adult | <2.0% HbF | <0.02 mass fraction HbF |
| **Immunoglobulin A (IgA)** | | | |
| Serum | Cord blood | 1.4-3.6 mg/dL | 14-36 mg/L |
| | 1-3 mo | 1.3-53 mg/dL | 13-530 mg/L |
| | 4-6 mo | 4.4-84 mg/dL | 44-840 mg/L |
| | 7 mo-1 yr | 11-106 mg/dL | 110-1060 mg/L |
| | 2-5 yr | 14-159 mg/dL | 140-1590 mg/L |
| | 6-10 yr | 33-236 mg/dL | 330-2360 mg/L |
| | Adult | 70-312 mg/dL | 700-3120 mg/L |
| **Immunoglobulin D (IgD)** | | | |
| Serum | Newborn | None detected | None detected |
| | Thereafter | 0-8 mg/dL | 0-80 mg/L |
| **Immunoglobulin E (IgE)** | | | |
| Serum | Male | 0-230 IU/mL | 0-230 kIU/L |
| | Female | 0-170 IU/mL | 0-170 kIU/L |
| **Immunoglobulin G (IgG)** | | | |
| Serum | Cord blood | 636-1606 mg/dL | 6.36-16.06 g/L |
| | 1 mo | 251-906 mg/dL | 2.51-9.06 g/L |
| | 2-4 mo | 176-601 mg/dL | 1.76-6.01 g/L |
| | 5-12 mo | 172-1069 mg/dL | 1.72-10.69 g/L |
| | 1-5 yr | 345-1236 mg/dL | 3.45-12.36 g/L |
| | 6-10 yr | 608-1572 mg/dL | 6.08-15.72 g/L |
| | Adult | 639-1349 mg/dL | 6.39-13.49 g/L |
| **Immunoglobulin M (IgM)** | | | |
| Serum | Cord blood | 6.3-25 mg/dL | 63-250 mg/L |
| | 1 mo-4 mo | 17-105 mg/dL | 170-1050 mg/L |
| | 5 mo-9 mo | 33-126 mg/dL | 330-1260 mg/L |
| | 10 mo-1 yr | 41-173 mg/dL | 410-1730 mg/L |
| | 2-8 yr | 43-207 mg/dL | 430-2070 mg/L |
| | 9-10 yr | 52-242 mg/dL | 520-2420 mg/L |
| | Adult | 56-352 mg/dL | 560-3520 mg/L |
| **Iron** | | | |
| Serum | Newborn | 100-250 μg/dL | 18-45 μmol/L |
| | Infant | 40-100 μg/dL | 7-18 μmol/L |
| | Child | 50-120 μg/dL | 9-22 μmol/L |
| | Thereafter: Male | 65-170 μg/dL | 12-30 μmol/L |
| | Female | 50-170 μg/dL | 9-30 μmol/L |
| | Intoxicated child | 280-2550 μg/dL | 50.12-456.5 μmol/L |
| | Fatally poisoned child | >1800 μg/dL | >322.2 μmol/L |

## Common laboratory tests—cont'd

| Test/Specimen | Age/Sex/Reference | Normal Ranges | | |
|---|---|---|---|---|
| | | **Conventional Units** | | **International Units (SI)** |
| Iron-binding capacity, total (TIBC) | | | | |
| Serum | Infant | 100-400 μg/dL | | 17.90-71.60 μmol/L |
| | Thereafter | 250-400 μg/dL | | 44.75-71.60 μmol/L |
| Lead | | | | |
| Whole blood | Child | <10 μg/dL | | <0.48 μmol/L |
| Urine, 24 hr | | <80 μg/L | | <0.39 μmol/L |
| Leukocyte count (WBC count) | | **× 1000 cells/mm³ (μl)** | | **× 10⁹ cells/L** |
| Whole blood | Birth | 9.0-30.0 | | 9.0-30.0 |
| | 24 hr | 9.4-34.0 | | 9.4-34.0 |
| | 1 mo | 5.0-19.5 | | 5.0-19.5 |
| | 1-3 yr | 6.0-17.5 | | 6.0-17.5 |
| | 4-7 yr | 5.5-15.5 | | 5.5-15.5 |
| | 8-13 yr | 4.5-13.5 | | 4.5-13.5 |
| | Adult | 4.5-11.0 | | 4.5-11.0 |
| | | **× 1000 cells/mm³ (μl)** | | **× 10⁶ cells/L** |
| CSF (cell count) | Premature | 0-25 mononuclear | | 0-25 |
| | | 0-10 polymorphonuclear | | 0-10 |
| | | 0-1000 RBC | | 0-1000 |
| | Newborn | 0-20 mononuclear | | 0-20 |
| | | 0-10 polymorphonuclear | | 0-10 |
| | | 0-800 RBC | | 0-800 |
| | Neonate | 0-5 mononuclear | | 0-5 |
| | | 0-10 polymorphonuclear | | 0-10 |
| | | 0-50 RBC | | 0-50 |
| | Thereafter | 0-5 mononuclear | | 0-5 |
| Leukocyte differential count | | | | |
| Whole blood | Myelocytes | 0% | 0 cells/mm³ (μl) | Number fraction 0 |
| | Neutrophils—"bands" | 3%-5% | 150-400 cells/mm³ (μl) | Number fraction 0.03-0.05 |
| | Neutrophils—"segs" | 54%-62% | 3000-5800 cells/mm³ (μl) | Number fraction 0.54-0.62 |
| | Lymphocytes | 25%-33% | 1500-3000 cells/mm³ (μl) | Number fraction 0.25-0.33 |
| | Monocytes | 3%-7% | 285-500 cells/mm³ (μl) | Number fraction 0.03-0.07 |
| | Eosinophils | 1%-3% | 50-250 cells/mm³ (μl) | Number fraction 0.01-0.03 |
| | Basophils | 0%-0.75% | 15-50 cells/mm³ (μl) | Number fraction 0-0.0075 |
| Mean corpuscular hemoglobin (MCH) | | | | |
| Whole blood | Birth | 31-37 pg/cell | | 0.48-0.57 fmol/cell |
| | 1-3 d (cap) | 31-37 pg/cell | | 0.48-0.57 fmol/cell |
| | 1 wk-1 mo | 28-40 pg/cell | | 0.43-0.62 fmol/cell |
| | 2 mo | 26-34 pg/cell | | 0.40-0.53 fmol/cell |
| | 3-6 mo | 25-35 pg/cell | | 0.39-0.54 fmol/cell |
| | 0.5-2 yr | 23-31 pg/cell | | 0.36-0.48 fmol/cell |
| | 2-6 yr | 24-30 pg/cell | | 0.37-0.47 fmol/cell |
| | 6-12 yr | 25-33 pg/cell | | 0.39-0.51 fmol/cell |
| | 12-18 yr | 25-35 pg/cell | | 0.39-0.54 fmol/cell |
| | 18-49 yr | 26-34 pg/cell | | 0.40-0.53 fmol/cell |
| Mean corpuscular hemoglobin concentration (MCHC) | | | | |
| Whole blood | Birth | 30%-36% Hb/cell or g Hb/dL RBC | | 4.65-5.58 mmol Hb/L RBC |
| | 1-3 d (cap) | 29%-37% Hb/cell or g Hb/dL RBC | | 4.50-5.74 mmol Hb/L RBC |
| | 1-2 wk | 28%-38% Hb/cell or g Hb/dL RBC | | 4.34-5.89 mmol Hb/L RBC |
| | 1-2 mo | 29%-37% Hb/cell or g Hb/dL RBC | | 4.50-5.74 mmol Hb/L RBC |
| | 3 mo-2 yr | 30%-36% Hb/cell or g Hb/dL RBC | | 4.65-5.58 mmol Hb/L RBC |
| | 2-18 yr | 31%-37% Hb/cell or g Hb/dL RBC | | 4.81-5.74 mmol Hb/L RBC |
| | >18 yr | 31%-37% Hb/cell or g Hb/dL RBC | | 4.81-5.74 mmol Hb/L RBC |

*Continued*

**Common laboratory tests—cont'd**

| Test/Specimen | Age/Sex/Reference | Normal Ranges Conventional Units | International Units (SI) |
|---|---|---|---|
| **Mean corpuscular volume (MCV)** | | | |
| Whole blood | 1-3 d (cap) | 95-121 $\mu m^3$ | 95-121 fL |
| | 0.5-2 yr | 70-86 $\mu m^3$ | 70-86 fL |
| | 6-12 yr | 77-95 $\mu m^3$ | 77-95 fL |
| | 12-18 yr: Male | 78-98 $\mu m^3$ | 78-98 fL |
| | Female | 78-102 $\mu m^3$ | 78-102 fL |
| **Osmolality** | | | |
| Serum | Child, adult | 275-295 mOsmol/kg $H_2O$ | |
| Urine, random | | 50-1400 mOsmol/kg $H_2O$, depending on fluid intake After 12-hr fluid restriction: >850 mOsmol/kg $H_2O$ | |
| Urine, 24 hr | | ≈300-900 mOsmol/kg $H_2O$ | |
| **Oxygen, partial pressure ($Po_2$)** | | | |
| Whole blood, arterial | Birth | 8-24 mm Hg | 1.1-3.2 kPa |
| | 5-10 min | 33-75 mm Hg | 4.4-10.0 kPa |
| | 30 min | 31-85 mm Hg | 4.1-11.3 kPa |
| | >1 hr | 55-80 mm Hg | 7.3-10.6 kPa |
| | 1 d | 54-95 mm Hg | 7.2-12.6 kPa |
| | Thereafter (decreased with age) | 83-108 mm Hg | 11-14.4 kPa |
| **Oxygen saturation ($Sao_2$)** | | | |
| Whole blood, arterial | Newborn | 85%-90% | Fraction saturated 0.85-0.90 |
| | Thereafter | 95%-99% | Fraction saturated 0.95-0.99 |
| **Partial thromboplastin time (PTT)** | | | |
| Whole blood (Na citrate) | | | |
| Nonactivated | | 60-85 s (Platelin) | 60-85 s |
| Activated | | 25-35 s (differs with method) | 25-35 s |
| **pH** | | | $H^+$ **concentration** |
| Whole blood, arterial | Premature (48 hr) | 7.35-7.50 | 31-44 nmol/L |
| | Birth, full term | 7.11-7.36 | 43-77 nmol/L |
| | 5-10 min | 7.09-7.30 | 50-81 nmol/L |
| | 30 min | 7.21-7.38 | 41-61 nmol/L |
| | >1 hr | 7.26-7.49 | 32-54 nmol/L |
| | 1 d | 7.29-7.45 | 35-51 nmol/L |
| | Thereafter | 7.35-7.45 | 35-44 nmol/L |
| | Must be corrected for body temperature | | |
| Urine, random | Newborn/neonate | 5-7 | 0.1-10 $\mu mol/L$ |
| | Thereafter | 4.5-8 (average ≈6) | 0.01-32 $\mu mol/L$ (average ≈ 1.0 $\mu mol/L$) |
| Stool | | 7.0-7.5 | 31-100 nmol/L |
| **Phenylalanine** | | | |
| Serum | Premature | 2.0-7.5 mg/dL | 120-450 $\mu mol/L$ |
| | Newborn | 1.2-3.4 mg/dL | 70-210 $\mu mol/L$ |
| | Thereafter | 0.8-1.8 mg/dL | 50-110 $\mu mol/L$ |
| Urine, 24 hr | 10 d-2 wk | 1-2 mg/d | 6-12 $\mu mol/d$ |
| | 3-12 yr | 4-18 mg/d | 24-110 $\mu mol/d$ |
| | Thereafter | trace-17 mg/d | trace-103 $\mu mol/d$ |
| **Plasma volume** | | | |
| Plasma | Male | 25-43 ml/kg | 0.025-0.043 L/kg |
| | Female | 28-45 ml/kg | 0.028-0.045 L/kg |
| **Platelet count (thrombocyte count)** | | | |
| Whole blood (EDTA) | Newborn (after 1 wk, same as adult) | 84-478 × $10^3/mm^3$ ($\mu l$) | 84-478 × $10^9$/L |
| | Adult | 150-400 × $10^3/mm^3$ ($\mu l$) | 150-400 × $10^9$/L |
| **Potassium** | | | |
| Serum | Newborn | 3.0-6.0 mEq/L | 3.0-6.0 mmol/L |
| | Thereafter | 3.5-5.0 mEq/L | 3.5-5.0 mmol/L |
| Plasma (heparin) | | 3.4-4.5 mEq/L | 3.4-4.5 mmol/L |
| Urine, 24 hr | | 25-125 mEq/d (varies with diet) | 25-125 mmol/L |

## Common laboratory tests—cont'd

| Test/Specimen | Age/Sex/Reference | Normal Ranges | |
|---|---|---|---|
| | | **Conventional Units** | **International Units (SI)** |
| Protein | | | |
| Serum, total | Premature | 4.3-7.6 g/dL | 43-76 g/L |
| | Newborn | 4.6-7.4 g/dL | 46-74 g/L |
| | 1-7 yr | 6.1-7.9 g/dL | 61-79 g/L |
| | 8-12 yr | 6.4-8.1 g/dL | 64-81 g/L |
| | 13-19 yr | 6.6-8.2 g/dL | 66-82 g/L |
| Total | | | |
| Urine, 24 hr | | 1-14 mg/dL | 10-140 mg/L |
| | | 50-80 mg/d (at rest) | 50-80 mg/d |
| | | <250 mg/d (after intense exercise) | <250 mg/d after intense exercise |
| Total | | | |
| CSF | | Lumbar: 8-32 mg/dL | 80-320 mg/L |
| Prothrombin time (PT) | | | |
| One-stage (Quick) | | | |
| Whole blood (Na citrate) | In general | 11-15 s (varies with type of thromboplastin) | 11-15 s |
| | Newborn | Prolonged by 2-3 s | Prolonged by 2-3 s |
| Two-stage modified (Ware and Seegers) | | | |
| Whole blood (Na citrate) | | 18-22 sec | 18-22 s |
| RBC count: see erythrocyte count | | | |
| Red blood cell volume | | | |
| Whole blood | Male | 20-36 mL/kg | 0.020-0.036 L/kg |
| | Female | 19-31 mL/kg | 0.019-0.031 L/kg |
| Reticulocyte count | | | |
| Whole blood | Adults | 0.5%-1.5% of erythrocytes or 25,000-75,000/mm³ (μl) | 0.005-0.015 (number fraction) or 25,000-75,000 × 10⁶/L |
| Capillary | 1 d | 0.4%-6.0% | 0.004-0.060 (number fraction) |
| | 7 d | <0.1%-1.3% | <0.001-0.013 (number fraction) |
| | 1-4 wk | <0.1%-1.2% | <0.001-0.012 (number fraction) |
| | 5-6 wk | <0.1%-2.4% | <0.001-0.024 (number fraction) |
| | 7-8 wk | 0.1%-2.9% | 0.001-0.029 (number fraction) |
| | 9-10 wk | <0.1%-2.6% | <0.001-0.026 (number fraction) |
| | 11-12 wk | 0.1%-1.3% | 0.001-0.013 (number fraction) |
| Salicylates | | | |
| Serum, plasma | Therap. conc. | 15-30 mg/dL | 1.1-2.2 mmol/L |
| | Toxic conc. | >30 mg/dL | >18.5 mmol/L |
| Sedimentation rate: see ESR | | | |
| Sodium | | | |
| Serum or plasma | Newborn | 134-146 mEq/L | 134-146 mmol/L |
| | Infant | 139-146 mEq/L | 139-146 mmol/L |
| | Child | 138-145 mEq/L | 138-145 mmol/L |
| | Thereafter | 136-146 mEq/d | 136-146 mmol/L |
| Urine, 24 hr | | 40-220 mEq/L (diet dependent) | 40-220 mmol/d |
| Sweat | Normal | <40 mEq/L | <40 mmol/L |
| | Indeterminate | 45-60 mEq/L | 45-60 mmol/L |
| | Cystic fibrosis | >60 mEq/L | >60 mmol/L |
| Specific gravity | | | |
| Urine, random | Adult | 1.002-1.030 | 1.002-1.030 |
| | After 12-hr fluid restriction | >1.025 | >1.025 |
| Urine, 24 hr | | 1.015-1.025 | |
| Theophylline | | | |
| Serum, plasma | Therap. conc. | | |
| | Bronchodilator | 10-20 μg/mL | 56-110 μmol/L |
| | Premature apnea | 5-10 μg/mL | 28-56 μmol/L |
| | Toxic conc. | >20 μg/mL | >110 μmol/L |
| Thrombin time | | | |
| Whole blood (Na citrate) | | Control time ± 2 s when control is 9-13 s | Control time ± 2 s when control is 9-13 s |

*Continued*

**Common laboratory tests—cont'd**

| Test/Specimen | Age/Sex/Reference | Normal Ranges | | | |
|---|---|---|---|---|---|
| | | **Conventional Units** | | **International Units (SI)** | |
| Thyroxine (T$_4$) | | **Full-term infants** | | **Full-term infants** | |
| Serum | 1-3 d | 8.2-19.9 μg/dL | | 106-256 nmol/L | |
| | 1 wk | 6.0-15.9 μg/dL | | 77-205 nmol/L | |
| | 1-12 mo | 6.1-14.9 μg/dL | | 79-192 nmol/L | |
| | | **Prepubertal children** | | **Prepubertal children** | |
| | 1-3 yr | 6.8-13.5 μg/dL | | 88-174 nmol/L | |
| | 3-10 yr | 5.5-12.8 μg/dL | | 71-165 nmol/L | |
| | | **Pubertal children and adults** | | **Pubertal children and adults** | |
| | >10 yr | 4.2-13.0 μg/dL | | 54-167 nmol/L | |
| Triglycerides (TG) | | **mg/dL** | | **g/L** | |
| Serum, after ≥12-hr fast | | **Male** | **Female** | **Male** | **Female** |
| | Cord blood | 10-98 | 10-98 | 0.10-0.98 | 0.10-0.98 |
| | 0-5 yr | 30-86 | 32-99 | 0.30-0.86 | 0.32-0.99 |
| | 6-11 yr | 31-108 | 35-114 | 0.31-1.08 | 0.35-1.14 |
| | 12-15 yr | 36-138 | 41-138 | 0.36-1.38 | 0.41-1.38 |
| | 16-19 yr | 40-163 | 40-128 | 0.40-1.63 | 0.40-1.28 |
| Triiodothyronine (T$_3$), free | | | | | |
| Serum | Cord blood | 20-240 pg/dL | | 0.3-3.7 pmol/L | |
| | 1-3 d | 200-610 pg/dL | | 3.1-9.4 pmol/L | |
| | 6 wk | 240-560 pg/dL | | 3.7-8.6 pmol/L | |
| | Adults (20-50 yr) | 230-660 pg/dL | | 3.5-10.0 pmol/L | |
| Triiodothyronine, total (T$_3$-RIA) | | | | | |
| Serum | Cord blood | 30-70 ng/dL | | 0.46-1.08 nmol/L | |
| | Newborn | 72-260 ng/dL | | 1.16-4.00 nmol/L | |
| | 1-5 yr | 100-260 ng/dL | | 1.54-4.00 nmol/L | |
| | 5-10 yr | 90-240 ng/dL | | 1.39-3.70 nmol/L | |
| | 10-15 yr | 80-210 ng/dL | | 1.23-3.23 nmol/L | |
| | Thereafter | 115-190 ng/dL | | 1.77-2.93 nmol/L | |
| Urea nitrogen | | | | | |
| Serum or plasma | Cord blood | 21-40 mg/dL | | 7.5-14.3 mmol urea/L | |
| | Premature (1 wk) | 3-25 mg/dL | | 1.1-9 mmol urea/L | |
| | Newborn | 3-12 mg/dL | | 1.1-4.3 mmol urea/L | |
| | Infant/child | 5-18 mg/dL | | 1.8-6.4 mmol urea/L | |
| | Thereafter | 7-18 mg/dL | | 2.5-6.4 mmol urea/L | |
| Urine volume | | | | | |
| Urine, 24 hr | Newborn | 50-300 ml/d | | 0.050-0.300 L/d | |
| | Infant | 350-550 ml/d | | 0.350-0.550 L/d | |
| | Child | 500-1000 ml/d | | 0.500-1.000 L/d | |
| | Adolescent | 700-1400 ml/d | | 0.700-1.400 L/d | |
| | Thereafter: Male | 800-1800 ml/d | | 0.800-1.800 L/d | |
| | Female | 600-1600 ml/d (varies with intake and other factors) | | 0.600-1.600 L/d | |

WBC: see leukocyte

## Abbreviations Used in Laboratory Tests

| Abbreviation | Term |
|---|---|
| cap | capillary |
| CHF | congestive heart failure |
| conc. | concentration |
| CSF | cerebrospinal fluid |
| d | day; diem |
| EDTA | ethylenadiamine tetra-acetate |
| g | gram |
| hr | hour |
| L | liter |
| m | meter |
| mEq | milliequivalent |
| min | minute |
| mm | millimeter |
| mm³ | cubic millimeter |
| mo | month |
| mol | mole |
| mOsmol | milliosmole |
| s | second |
| SI | International System of Units |
| temp | temperature |
| Therap. | therapeutic |
| U | international unit of enzyme activity |
| vol | volume |
| wk | week |
| yr | year |
| > | greater than |
| ≥ | greater than or equal to |
| < | less than |
| ≤ | less than or equal to |
| ± | plus/minus |
| ≃ | approximately equal to |

## Prefixes Denoting Decimal Factors

| Prefix | Symbol | Amount |
|---|---|---|
| deci | d | one tenth ($10^{-1}$) |
| centi | c | one hundredth ($10^{-2}$) |
| milli | m | one thousandth ($10^{-3}$) |
| micro | $\mu$ | one millionth ($10^{-6}$) |
| nano | n | one billionth ($10^{-9}$) |
| pico | p | one trillionth ($10^{-12}$) |
| femto | f | one quadrillionth ($10^{-15}$) |

# NANDA-Approved Nursing Diagnoses 2001-2002

- Activity intolerance
- Activity intolerance, risk for
- Adjustment, impaired
- Airway clearance, ineffective
- Anxiety
- Anxiety, death
- Aspiration, risk for
- Body image, disturbed
- Body temperature, imbalanced, risk for
- Bowel incontinence
- Breastfeeding, effective
- Breastfeeding, ineffective
- Breastfeeding, interrupted
- Breathing pattern, ineffective
- Cardiac output, decreased
- Caregiver role strain
- Caregiver role strain, risk for
- Comfort, impaired
- Communication, impaired verbal
- Confusion, acute
- Confusion, chronic
- Constipation
- Constipation, perceived
- Constipation, risk for
- Coping, defensive
- Coping, family, compromised
- Coping, family, disabled
- Coping, ineffective
- Coping, ineffective community
- Coping, readiness for enhanced community
- Coping, readiness for enhanced family
- Decisional conflict
- Denial, ineffective
- Dentition, impaired
- Development, delayed, risk for
- Diarrhea
- Disuse syndrome, risk for
- Diversional activity, deficient
- Dysreflexia, autonomic
- Dysreflexia, autonomic, risk for
- Energy field, disturbed
- Environmental interpretation syndrome, impaired
- Failure to thrive, adult
- Falls, risk for
- Family processes, dysfunctional: alcoholism
- Family processes, interrupted
- Fatigue
- Fear
- Fluid volume, deficient
- Fluid volume, deficient, risk for
- Fluid volume excess
- Fluid volume, imbalanced, risk for
- Gas exchange, impaired
- Grieving
- Grieving, anticipatory

- Grieving, dysfunctional
- Growth, disproportionate, risk for
- Growth and development, delayed
- Health maintenance, ineffective
- Health-seeking behaviors
- Home maintenance, impaired
- Hopelessness
- Hyperthermia
- Hypothermia
- Incontinence, urinary, functional
- Incontinence, urinary, reflex
- Incontinence, urinary, stress
- Incontinence, urinary, total
- Incontinence, urinary urge
- Incontinence, urinary urge, risk for
- Infant behavior, disorganized
- Infant behavior, disorganized, risk for
- Infant behavior, organized, readiness for enhanced
- Infant feeding pattern, ineffective
- Infection, risk for
- Injury, perioperative-positioning, risk for
- Injury, risk for
- Intracranial adaptive capacity, decreased
- Knowledge, deficient
- Latex allergy response
- Latex allergy response, risk for
- Loneliness, risk for
- Memory, impaired
- Mobility, impaired bed
- Mobility, impaired physical
- Mobility, impaired wheelchair
- Nausea
- Noncompliance
- Nutrition, imbalanced: less than body requirements
- Nutrition, imbalanced: more than body requirements
- Nutrition, imbalanced: more than body requirements, risk for
- Oral mucous membrane, impaired
- Pain, acute
- Pain, chronic
- Parent/infant/child attachment, impaired, risk for
- Parental role conflict
- Parenting, impaired
- Parenting, impaired, risk for
- Peripheral neurovascular dysfunction, risk for
- Personal identity, disturbed
- Poisoning, risk for
- Post-trauma syndrome
- Post-trauma syndrome, risk for
- Powerlessness

- Powerlessness, risk for
- Protection, ineffective
- Rape-trauma syndrome
- Rape-trauma syndrome: compound reaction
- Rape-trauma syndrome: silent reaction
- Relocation stress syndrome
- Relocation stress syndrome, risk for
- Role performance, ineffective
- Self-care deficit, bathing/hygiene
- Self-care deficit, dressing/grooming
- Self-care deficit, feeding
- Self-care deficit, toileting
- Self-esteem, chronic low
- Self-esteem, situational low
- Self-esteem, situational low, risk for
- Self-mutilation
- Self-mutilation, risk for
- Sensory perception, disturbed
- Sexual dysfunction
- Sexuality patterns, ineffective
- Skin integrity, impaired
- Skin integrity, impaired, risk for
- Sleep deprivation
- Sleep pattern, disturbed
- Social interaction, impaired
- Social isolation
- Sorrow, chronic
- Spiritual distress
- Spiritual distress, risk for
- Spiritual well-being, readiness for enhanced
- Suffocation, risk for
- Suicide, risk for
- Surgical recovery, delayed
- Swallowing, impaired
- Therapeutic regimen management, effective
- Therapeutic regimen management, ineffective
- Therapeutic regimen management, ineffective community
- Therapeutic regimen management, ineffective family
- Thermoregulation, ineffective
- Thought processes, disturbed
- Tissue integrity, impaired
- Tissue perfusion, ineffective
- Transfer ability, impaired
- Trauma, risk for
- Unilateral neglect
- Urinary elimination, impaired
- Urinary retention
- Ventilation, impaired spontaneous
- Ventilatory weaning response, dysfunctional
- Violence, other-directed, risk for
- Violence, self-directed, risk for
- Walking, impaired
- Wandering

North American Nursing Diagnosis Association: *Nursing diagnoses: definitions and classification 2001-2002*, Philadelphia, 2001, NANDA.

# Translations of Wong-Baker FACES Pain Rating Scale*

| | 0 | 1 | 2 | 3 | 4 | 5 |
|---|---|---|---|---|---|---|
| **0–5 coding** | 0 | 1 | 2 | 3 | 4 | 5 |
| **0-10 coding** | 0 | 2 | 4 | 6 | 8 | 10 |
| **ENGLISH** | No Hurt | Hurts Little Bit | Hurts Little More | Hurts Even More | Hurts Whole Lot | Hurts Worst |
| **SPANISH** | No duele | Duele un poco | Duele un poco más | Duele mucho | Duele mucho más | Duele el máximo |
| **FRENCH** | Ne fait pas mal | Fait mal un petit peu | Fait mal un petit plus | Fait mal encore plus | Fait beaucoup mal | Fait très, très mal |
| **ITALIAN** | Non fa male | Fa male un poco | Fa male un po di piu | Fa male ancora di piu | Fa molto male | Fa maggiormente male |
| **PORTUGUESE** | Não doi | Doi um pouco | Doi um pouco mais | Doi muito | Doi muito mais | Doi o máximo |
| **BOSNIAN** | Ne boli | Boli samo malo | Boli malo više | Boli još više | Boli puno | Boli najviše |
| **VIETNAMESE** | Không dau | Hỏi dau | Dau hỏn chút | Dau nhiêu hỏn | Dau thât nhiêu | Dau qúa dô |
| **CHINESE** | 無痛 | 微痛 | 較痛 | 更痛 | 很痛 | 劇痛 |
| **GREEK** | Δεν Πονάι | Πονάι Λιγο | Πονάι Λιγο Πιο Πολν | Πονάι Πολν | Πονάι Πιο Πολν | Πονάι Παρα Πολν |
| **ROMANIAN** | No doare | Doare puțin | Doare un pic mai mult | Doare și mai mult | Doare foarte tare | Doare cel mai mult |

## BRIEF WORD INSTRUCTIONS (ABOVE)

Point to each face using the words to describe the pain intensity. Ask the child to choose face that best describes own pain and record the appropriate number. NOTE: Use of these instructions is recommended. Rating scale can be used with people 3 years and older.

## ORIGINAL INSTRUCTIONS

### English

Explain to the person that each face is for a person who feels happy because he has no pain (hurt) or sad because he has some or a lot of pain. **Face 0** is very happy because he doesn't hurt at all. **Face 1** hurts just a little bit. **Face 2** hurts a little more. **Face 3** hurts even more. **Face 4** hurts a whole lot. **Face 5** hurts as much as you can imagine, although you don't have to be crying to feel this bad. Ask the person to choose the face that best describes how much hurt he has.

Rating scale is recommended for persons age 3 years and older.

---

*From Wong D, Baker C: *Reference manual for the Wong-Baker FACES pain rating scale,* Duarte, CA, 1998, City of Hope Mayday Pain Resource Center. Spanish and Portuguese translations by Ellen Johnsen; French translation by Thomas Angelo; Italian translation by Madeline Mitchko; Romanian translation by Bogdan R. Dinu; Bosnian translation by Barbara Bogomolor; Vietnamese translation by Yen B. Isle; Greek translation by Nicholas Mamalis; Chinese translation by Hung-Shen Lin; Japanese translation from *After the announcement of cancer,* Tokyo, 1993, Iwanami Shoten, Pub; German translation from Wong DL: *Pediatric quick reference,* Berlin, Wiesbaden, 1997, Ullstein Mosby.

## Spanish

Expliquele a la persona que cada cara representa una persona que se siente feliz porque no tiene dolor o triste porque siente un poco a mucho dolor. **Cara 0** se siente muy feliz porque no tiene dolor. **Cara 1** tiene un poco de dolor. **Cara 2** tiene un poquito más de dolor. Cara 3 tiene más dolor. **Cara 4** tiene mucho dolor. **Cara 5** tiene el dolor más fuerte que usted pueda imaginar, aunque usted no tiene que estar llorando para sentirse asi de mal. Pidale a la persona que escoja la cara que mejor describe su proprio dolor.

Esta escala se puede usar con personas de tres años de edad o más.

## French

Expliquez á la personne que chaque visage représent un personne qui est heureux parce qu'elle n'a pas point du mal ou triste parce qu'il a un peu ou beaucoup du mal. **Visage 0** est trés heureux parce qu'elle n'a pas point du mal. **Visage 1** a un point peu de mal. **Visage 2** a plus du mal. **Visage 3** a encore plus du mal. **Visage 4** a beaucoup du mal. **Visage 5** a autant mal que vous pouvez imaginer, bien que ces mauvals sentiments ne finissent pas nécessairement a vous faire pleurer. Demandez à la personne de choisir le visage qui convient le mieux avec ses sentiments.

Ces evaluations sont recommendé pour des personnes de trois ans et davantage.

## Italian

Spiegare a la persona che ogni facien è per una persona che si sente felice perchè non tiene dolore oppure triste penchè ha poco o molto dolore. **Faccia 0** è molto felice perchè non tiene dolore. **Faccia 1** tiene poco dolore. **Faccia 2** tiene un po più di dolore. **Faccia 3** tiene più dolore. **Faccia 4** tiene molto dolore. **Faccia 5** tiene molto dolore che non puoi immaginare però non devi piangere per tenere dolore. Domandi ala persona di scegliere quale faccia meglio descrive come si sente.

Grado scale è raccomandata a la persona di tre anni in sù.

## Portuguese

Explique a pessoa que cada face representa uma pessoa que está feliz porque não têm dor, ou triste por ter um pouco ou muita dor. **Face 0** está muito feliz porque não têm nenhuma dor. **Face 1** tem apenas um pouco de dor. **Face 2** têm um pouco mais de dor. **Face 3** têm aioda mais dor. **Face 4** têm muita dor. **Face 5** têm uma dor máxima, apesar de que nem sempre provoca o choro. Peça a pessoa que escolhe a face que melhor descreve como ele se sente.

Esta escala é aplicável a pessoas de tres anos de idade ou mais.

## Bosnian

Objasnite osobi da je svako lice namjenjeno za osobu koja se osjeća sretnom jer ne osjeća bol ili tužnom jer osjeća malo ili puno boli. **Lice 0** je sretno jer ne osjeća nikakvu bol. **Lice 1** osjeća samo malu bol. **Lice 2** osjeća malo više boli. **Lice 3** osjeća jos vecúbol. **Lice 4** osjeća puno boli. **Lice 5** osjeća onoliku bol koju je moguće zamisliti, što ne znaći da osoba koja osjeća tu bol mora plakati. Upitajte osobu da izabere lice koje najbolje opisuju kako se osjeća. Skala procijene bola se preporu ćuje za osobe starosti 3 godine ili više.

Upirati prstom na svako lice objašnjavajući rijećima intensitet boli. Pitajte dijere da izabere lice koje najbolje opisuje njihovu bol i zabiljezue odgovarajući broj.

## Vietnamese

Xin cắt nghĩa cho mỗi người, từng khuôn mặt của một người cảm thấy vui vẽ tại vì không có sự đau đón hoặc, buồn vì có chút ít hay rất nhiều sự đau đón.

Cái mặt với **số 0** thì rất là vui tại vì mặt ấy không có sự đau đón. **Mặt số 1** chỉ đau một chút thôi. **Mặt số 2** hơi đau hơn một chút nữa. **Mặt số 3** đau hơn chút nữa. **Mặt số 4** đau thật nhiều. **Mặt số 5** đau không thể tưởng tượng, mặc dù người ta không cần phải khóc mới cảm thấy được sự buồn khổ như thế.

Bạn hỏi từng người tự chọn khuôn mặt nào diễn tả được sự đau đón của chính mình.

## Chinese

解釋給人聽用每張臉譜來代表著一個人的感覺是因爲沒有疼痛〔傷痛〕而感快樂或是因爲些許疼痛或者是許多疼痛而感傷心。第零張臉是很快樂的因爲他一點也不覺得疼痛。第一張臉只痛一丁點兒。第二張臉又痛多了一些。第三張臉痛得更多了。第四張臉是非常痛了。第五張臉是爲人們所能想像到的劇痛既使感到這樣難過，卻不一定哭出來。請這人選擇出最能代表他現在感響的一張臉譜。此量表適用於三歲以上的人。

## Japanese

3歳以上の患者に望ましい。それぞれの顔は、患者の痛み(pain, hurt)がないのでご機嫌な感じ、または、ある程度の痛み・沢山の痛みがあるので悲しい感じを表現していることを説明して下さい。0＝痛みがまったくないから、とても幸せな顔をしている、1＝ほんの少し痛い、2＝もう少し痛い、3＝もっと痛い、4＝とっても痛い、5＝痛くて涙を流す必要はないけれども、これ以上の痛みは考えられないほど痛い。今、どのように感じているか最もよく表わしている顔を選ぶよう、患者に求めて下さい。

## Romanian

Explicati copilului că fiecare desen (figură) corespunde unei persoane care este veselă, pentru că nu are nici o durere, sau unei persoane care este tristă, pentru că are dureri. **Figura 0** este foarte fericită pentru ca nu are nici o durere. **Figura 1** arată că doare doar un pic. **Figura 2** arată că doare ceva mai mult. **Figura 3** arată că doare și mai mult. **Figura 4** arată că doare foarte tare. **Figura 5** arată că doare atât de tare cât se poate imagina, chiar dacă nu este însoțita neapărat de lacrimi. Cereți copilului (persoanei) să indice figura care exprimă cel mai bine cum se simte el.

Scala de evaluare a durerii este recomandată pentru copiii în vârstă de 3 ani și peste.

## German

Erläutern Sie dem Kind, daβ jedes Gesicht zu einer Person gehört, die froh darüber ist, keine Schmerzen zu haben, oder die sehr traurig ist, weil sie mäβige bis starke Schmerzen hat. **Gesicht 0** ist sehr froh, weil es keine Schmerzen hat. **Gesicht 1** sagt, es tut ein biβchen weh. **Gesicht 2** hat ein biβchen mehr Schmerzen. **Gesicht 3** sagt, es tut noch mehr weh, und **Gesicht 4**, es tut ziemlich weh. **Geisicht 5** leidet unter so starken Schmerzen, wie Du Dir nur vorstellen kannst, auch wenn dabei nicht unbedingt Tränen flieβen müssen. Bitten Sie das Kind, das Gesicht auszuwählen, das seinem Empfinden am besten entspricht.

Empfohlen für Kinder ab 3 Jahren.

# Index

## A

Abbreviations, for laboratory tests, 1903
ABC status, rapid assessment of, 1761
Abdomen
  auscultation of, 217, 218-219
  contour of, 217
  distention of, in obstructive disorders, 1446
  Down syndrome and, 989t
  examination of, 217-220
  focal tenderness of, 1433
  in nutritional assessment, 167t
  movements of, 218
  of newborn, 253t, 261
    at high risk, 336b, 396
  palpation of, 219
    for appendicitis, 1434, 1434b
  percussion of, 219
  protrusion of, 218
  quadrants of, 217, 217f
  scaphoid, 476
  size of, 218
  skin of, 218
  structures of, 217f
Abdominal bruit, 219
Abdominal circumference
  measurement of, 176f, 1428, 1428b
  of newborn, 255
Abdominal discomfort, in diabetes, 1736
Abdominal mass
  in cancer, 1597
  Wilms tumor presenting as, 1629
Abdominal pain
  assessment of, 219
  in obstructive disorders, 1446
  in pregnancy, 850-851
  palpation for, 1434, 1434b
  paroxysmal (colic), 571-574
  recurrent, 796-797, 797b, 1432
  somatic, 219
  types of, 219
  visceral, 219
  with intussusception, 1448
Abdominal reflexes, 220
Abdominal tone, 218
Abdominal wall defects, 472-474, 472f, 473f
Abducens nerve, assessment of, 229t
ABO blood group system, 310
ABO incompatibility, 310, 312, 312t; see also
    Hemolytic disease of newborn.
  transfusion therapy and, 1540
  treatment of, 315
Abortion
  in adolescents, 853-854
  spontaneous, 850-851
Abrasions, 745
  birth-related, 296b
Abscess
  brain, 1681
  tubo-ovarian, 863
Absence seizures, 1687t, 1688
  diagnosis of, 1692

Absolute neutrophil count, 1534, 1536t, 1598
  calculation of, 1598b
  in neutropenia, 1568
Absorption, gastrointestinal, 1418-1419
  in malabsorption syndromes, 1450
Abstract communication, 139
Abuse
  child; see Child abuse.
  spousal, 75, 718
Acanthosis nigricans, in diabetes, 1734
Acceleration injury, 1665
Access to respite care and help, 913n
Accessory nerve, assessment of, 229t
Accidents, 6-11; see also Injuries; Safety; Trauma.
  motor vehicle, 7, 8t
  prevention of, 1758b, 1759b; see also Safety.
Accommodation
  in infants, 502-503
  ocular, 194
Accomplishment, vs sense of inferiority, 700
Accreditation, of healthcare organizations, 28
Acculturation, 34
Accutane (isotretinoin), for acne, 841-842
ACE inhibitors; see Angiotensin-converting
    enzyme (ACE) inhibitors.
Acetaminophen
  after heart surgery, 1506
  as poison, 670b
  for circumcision, 271
  in fever management, 1130, 1131t, 1132
  in pain management, 1060, 1060b,
    1061t, 1063t
  reference ranges for, 1895t
Acetazolamide, for seizures, 1691t
Acetylcholine, 1705
  in nerve impulse transmission, 1833-1834
Achieved roles, 76b
Achievement, 813, 813b
Achilles reflex, 227f
Achilles tendinitis, 1801t
Acholic stools, 470
Achondroplasia, 119t, 447t
Acid(s)
  as poisons, 670b
  aspiration of, 1379
  secretion of, in infants, 1258
  tooth decay and, 780
Acid mantle, of skin, 740
  newborn bathing and, 268
Acid-base balance
  compensatory mechanisms in, 1182
  disturbances in, 1181-1185, 1183t
  lung role in, 1309-1310
  neonatal, postoperative care and, 423t
  tests of, 1182t, 1183
Acidosis
  distal tubular, 1280
  metabolic, 1183t, 1184, 1184b
    cold stress and, high-risk newborn and, 339

Acidosis—cont'd
  metabolic—cont'd
    in burn injuries, 1233
    in chronic renal failure, 1289, 1291
    in diabetes, 1734, 1735, 1735f, 1741-1742,
      1742, 1749-1750
    in high-risk newborn, 339
    in shock, 1221
    in short bowel syndrome, 1452
    renal tubular, 1279-1280
    respiratory, 1183-1184, 1183b, 1183t
Acne, in adolescents, 839-842, 842b
Acoustic feedback, hearing aids and, 997
Acoustic nerve, assessment of, 229t
Acoustic reflectometry, for otitis media, 1358
Acquaintance rape, 858
Acquired immunodeficiency syndrome
    (AIDS); see Human immunodeficiency
    virus infection.
Acrocentric translocation, 115
Acrocephaly, 444f
Acrocyanosis, in newborn, 251t
Acromegaly, 1713-1714
Acryodynia, 675
ACTH, 1707t, 1723
  for infantile spasms, 1689
  hyposecretion of, 1706b
  in infants, 497
Acticoat, for burn wounds, 1240t
Actinomycin D (Cosmegen), 1592t
Actiq, 1064b
Activated charcoal
  complications with, 673
  for gastric decontamination with
    poisoning, 673
Active listening, 144-145
Active transport
  in intestinal absorption, 1419
  in renal tubules, 1257
Activities
  after heart surgery, 1506
  for latchkey children, 721b
  for preschoolers, 634, 634t
  for school-age children, 712, 724-727
  for toddlers, 600t
  in asthma, 1400
  in cerebral palsy, 1840-1841, 1841-1842
  in chronic renal failure, 1290
  in congenital heart disease, 1503
  in hospitalization, 1070-1071, 1070f
  in immobilization, 1768
  in juvenile rheumatoid arthritis, 1824
Acupressure, 48
Acupuncture, 48
Acute adrenocortical insufficiency,
    1725, 1726t
Acute illness, 6
Acute lymphoid leukemia, 1611; see also
    Leukemia.
  prognosis of, 1513, 1514t
  subtypes of, 1612

Note: Page numbers followed by *f* indicate figures; those followed by *t* indicate tables; those followed by *b* indicate boxed material; and those followed by *n* indicate footnotes.

Acute myelogenous leukemia, 1611; see also
    Leukemia.
    prognosis of, 1513
Acute (adult) respiratory distress syndrome
    (ARDS), 1220, 1379-1380, 1380b
Acute tumor lysis syndrome, 1596
Acyclovir, for chickenpox, 651b
ADA; see Americans with Disabilities Act.
Adaptic/Aquaphor, for burn wounds, 1240t
Adaptive defenses, 1572
Addiction, 884; see also Substance abuse.
    fear of, 1049, 1050b
Addison disease, 1726, 1726t
Adduction contracture, developmental
    dysplasia of hip and, 450
Adenohypophysis; see Pituitary, anterior.
Adenoidectomy, 1353
Adenoids, 1352, 1352f
Adenosine
    for cardiopulmonary resuscitation, 1399t
    for supraventricular tachycardia, 1525
Adhesives, neonatal skin and, 350b
Adipose cell theory of obesity, 871
Adipose tissue
    brown, 241
    eating disorders and, 869-870
Adjuvant analgesics, 1060-1061
Admission procedure, 1086-1091, 1087b
    for adolescent unit, 1090-1091, 1091f
    for emergency care, 1087b, 1093
    for intensive care unit, 1087b, 1093-1095,
        1094b, 1094f, 1095b
    nursing admission history in, 1086-1088,
        1088b-1089b, 1091b
    physical assessment in, 1089-1090
    room assignment in, 1090
Adolescent
    abortion in, 853-854
    abuse in, 832-833; see also Sexual abuse.
    achievement in, 813-814
    acne in, 839-842, 842b
    adopted, 92
    alcohol use in, 831-832
    attitudes of toward seeking health care, 821
    autonomy in, 812-813
    behavioral health problems in, 869-902;
        see also specific problems.
    biologic development of, 803-809
    bisexual, 814-816, 816b, 831, 835-836
    cognition of, 804t, 809-811
    communication with, 149-150, 150b
    community and society and, 819-820
    contraception in, 854-858
    coping mechanisms and health-promoting
        factors affecting, 821-822
    depression and suicide in, 832
    diabetes in, 1737b, 1750-1751
    diet in, 829-830
    divorce and, 95-96, 95b
    dying, 954-955; see also Terminal illness.
    eating disorders in; see Eating disorders.
    epilepsy in, 1696
    families of, 817-818, 826-827, 827b, 836b, 837
    fetal alcohol effects in, 330
    gay and lesbian, 831, 835-836
    growth of, 804t
    health interests and concerns of, 820-821
    health promotion in, 821-826
    health screening of, 824-826

Adolescent—cont'd
    hepatitis prevention in, 1460
    hospitalized
        admission of, 1090-1091, 1091f
        bodily injury and pain in, 1039
        loss of control in, 1035-1036, 1035b
    hyperlipidemia in, 833
    hypertension in, 833
    identity development of, 804t, 812, 814
    immunizations in, 541b, 833-834
    infectious diseases in, 833
    injury in, intentional and unintentional,
        828-829
    intimacy in, 816-817
    juvenile rheumatoid arthritis in, 1824b
    moral development of, 811
    obesity in, 829-830
    of color, 834-835
    pain in, 1054b
    parenting and family adjustment in, 804t,
        826-827
    peer relationships of, 706-707, 804t, 816
        health behavior and, 818
        pregnancy and, 851
        sex information and, 710
    phenylketonuria in, 324
    physical examination of, 173t
    physical fitness in, 830
    pregnancy in, 830-831, 850-853, 852b, 857
    preventive health care for, 826-834
    psychosocial development of, 804t, 812-817,
        827-828
    rape in, 858-860
    reproductive system of
        female, 844-849
        male, 842-844
    rural, 836-837
    school and learning problems in, 833
    school-based health promotion efforts for,
        822-823
    sexuality of, 804t, 814-816, 830-831, 849,
        850, 857, 982
        in spinal cord injury, 1862
    sexually transmitted diseases in, 830-831,
        860-866, 866b
    smoking in, 831-832
    social environment and health behavior of,
        817-818
    special needs; see also Special needs child.
        promotion of normal development in,
            911t-912t, 916-917
        sexuality and, 982
    spinal cord injury in, 1862
    spiritual development of, 811-812
    sports injuries in, 1796-1807; see also Sports
        injuries.
    vision changes in, 842
Adolescent goiter, 1718
Adolescent pediatric pain tool, 1051f
Adopted roles, 76b
Adoption, 89-93
    biologic parental rights and, 89
    cross-racial, 93
    disclosure of, 91-92, 92b
    independent, 89
    infant attachment in, 90, 90f
    international, 90, 93
    motivation for, 89
    of older child, 92-93

Adoption—cont'd
    of special needs child, 927
    open, 89
    preadoption counseling for, 90
    preparation for, 90
    sibling reactions to, 90
    sources for, 89-90
Adoption agencies, 89-90
Adrenal activity, in burn injuries, 1233
Adrenal cortex, 1705f, 1723
Adrenal crisis, 1725, 1726
Adrenal disorders, 1725-1732
    acute adrenocortical insufficiency, 1725, 1726t
    Addison disease, 1726, 1726t
    chronic adrenocortical insufficiency,
        1726, 1726t
    congenital adrenal hyperplasia,
        1729-1731
    Cushing syndrome, 1727-1729, 1727b,
        1727f, 1728t
    hyperaldosteronism, 1731
Adrenal glands, 1704b, 1704f, 1708t
    hormones of, 1705, 1705f
    tumors of
        Cushing syndrome and, 1727-1729
        neuroblastoma, 1619, 1625-1626,
            1626b, 1724
        pheochromocytoma, 1724, 1731-1732
Adrenal hyperplasia
    congenital, 1729-1731
    Cushing syndrome and, 1727-1729
Adrenal medulla, 1723
    pheochromocytoma of, 1724, 1732-1733
Adrenalectomy
    for Cushing syndrome, 1728, 1729
    for pheochromocytoma, 1732
Adrenaline; see Epinephrine.
Adrenaline and cocaine combined (AC), for
    topical anesthesia, 751b
Adrenarche, 805
    premature, 1714-1715
β-Adrenergic agonists, for asthma, 1392, 1396,
    1398-1399
β-Adrenergic antagonists
    for congestive heart failure, 1480
    for hypertension, 1518, 1519b
α-Adrenergic decongestants, for allergic
    rhinitis, 1584
Adrenergic blocking agents, for
    adrenalectomy, 1732
Adrenergic symptoms, in diabetic
    hypoglycemia, 1749
Adrenocortical hyperplasia, congenital,
    487-488
Adrenocortical insufficiency
    acute, 1725
    chronic, 1726
    clinical manifestations of, 1726t
    congenital, 1729-1731
Adrenocorticotropic hormone; see ACTH.
Adriamycin (doxorubicin), 1592t
Adrucil (5-fluorouracil), 1591t
Adult hemoglobin, 1532
Advanced nurse practitioners, 20
Adventitious breath sounds, 213, 214t; see also
    Breath sounds.
Advisory Committee on Immunization
    Practices (ACIP), 528
Advocacy, nurse's role in, 19-20

Aerosol therapy, 1319-1320, 1319b
  for cystic fibrosis, 1411
  in asthma, 1391
  nebulizer for, 1319
Affect, in infants, 503
Affinal relationship, 65
Affluence, effects of on children, 35-36
Aflatoxin, in kwashiorkor, 566
African-Americans, 35b; see also Race/ethnicity.
  dietary preferences of, 45-47, 46t
  health beliefs and practices of, 52t-53t
  time concept of, 43
Afterload, 1468
  in congestive heart failure, 1482
Agammaglobulinemia, lymphopenic, 1579-1580
Age
  as risk factor, 104
  bone
    calculation of, 1711b
    in growth disorders, 1711, 1711b
  fluid volume and, 1173, 1173f
  gestational; see Gestational age.
  maternal, Down syndrome and, 989, 989t
  respiratory infections and, 1344
Age of majority, 1102
Agency for Health Care Policy and Research
    (AHCPR) (now Agency for Healthcare
    Research and Quality [AHRG]), 1047b,
    1359, 1554n
  clinical practice guidelines of, 15, 18b
Agent, disease, 105
Ages and Stages Questionnaire, 234t
Agglutinogens, 310
Aggression, in preschoolers, 641-642
Aging, premature, in hypopituitarism, 1710
Agnosia, 995
Agranulocytes, 1534
Aid to Families with Dependent Children, 12
Aiding Mothers and Fathers Experiencing
    Neo-Natal Death (AMEND), 370
AIDS; see Human immunodeficiency virus
    infection.
Air bags, injuries with, 545, 546f, 732
Air emboli, from blood transfusion, 1541t
Air hunger, 388
Air leaks, in high-risk newborn, 389-390
Air pressure, in treatment of intussusception,
    1449
Air sacs, 1306
Air travel, otitis media and, 1360
Airborne precautions, 651, 1133
Air-hunger respirations, 1184
Airway(s); see also under Lung(s); Respiratory.
  chemical burns of, in smoke inhalation
    injury, 1381
  conducting, 1305
  diameter of, 1307
  endotracheal, 1324-1325, 1325b
  epithelial cells of, in cystic fibrosis, 1401
  in anaphylaxis, 1225
  in burned patients, 1233, 1236, 1381
  in newborn, growth of, 1306, 1306f
  inflammation of, in asthma, 1385, 1386, 1387f
  lower
    infections of, 1343, 1365-1368
    reactive portion of, 1365
    structure of, 1305-1306, 1305f
  neonatal, postoperative care of, 420t

Airway(s)—cont'd
  obstruction of, 1305-1306, 1338,
    1340-1341, 1340f
    in asthma, 1387, 1387f
    in bacterial tracheitis, 1365
  patency of, in newborn, 265, 289
  positive pressure in, bilevel, 1323
  size of
    in infants and adults, 1307, 1308b, 1308f
    resistance and, 1307, 1308b, 1308f
  structure of, 1305-1306, 1305f
  upper
    infections of, 1343, 1350-1361
    muscle activation in, 1305
Airway management
  for unconscious child, 1656
  in spinal cord injury, 1859
  in trauma, 1760
Airway pressure, mean, in respiratory distress
    syndrome, 384
Alae nasi, 206f
  flaring of, 204
Al-Anon, 889
Alaskan Natives; see Native Americans.
Ala-Teen, 889
Ala-Tot, 889
Albendazole, 665, 666t
  for giardiasis, 667
Albinism, 119t
  ocular, 194
Albright syndrome, 301
Albumin, in nephrotic syndrome, 1275
Albuterol, for asthma, 1392
Alcohol Hotline, 889
Alcohol use/abuse, 828, 829, 831-832, 886t,
    888-890, 889b, 890b
  birth defects and, 329
  Drug Abuse, and Mental Health Block
    Grant for, 12
  fetal alcohol syndrome and, 326, 328-330,
    329b, 329f
  neurodevelopmental disorder and, 329
  rape and, 858
  Students Against Drunk Driving and, 895
  ulcers and, 1443
Alcoholics Anonymous, 889
Aldactone (spironolactone), for congestive
    heart failure, 1480t
Aldehyde dehydrogenase, alcohol abuse
    and, 890
Aldolase, in neuromuscular dysfunction, 1834b
Aldosterone, 1708t, 1723, 1724
  deficiency of, 1726t
  hypersecretion of, 1731
  replacement, for chronic adrenocortical
    insufficiency, 1726
Alertness, 1647
Alexander Graham Bell Association for the
    Deaf, 997n
ALG; see Antilymphocyte globulin.
Alginate dressings, for skin lesions, 750t
Alimentum formula, 282t
Alisa Ann Ruch Burn Foundation, 1253
Alkalis, as poisons, 670b
Alkaloids, plant, for cancer, 1588, 1591t-1592t;
    see also Chemotherapy.
Alkalosis
  metabolic, 1183t, 1184-1185, 1184b
    in hypertrophic pyloric stenosis, 1447
  respiratory, 1183t, 1184, 1184b

Alkeran (melphalan), 1590t
Alkylating agents, for cancer, 1588, 1589t-
    1590t; see also Chemotherapy.
Allegra (fexofenadine hydrochloride), for
    allergic rhinitis, 1384
Allen card test, 197-198, 198t
Allen test, 1147, 1316
Allergen(s)
  anaphylaxis and, 1224b, 1225
  in allergic rhinitis, 1384
  in asthma, 1385, 1386, 1386b, 1390, 1397
    hyposensitization injections and, 1393-1394
  in atopic dermatitis, 581
  in foods, 568
Allergic purpura, 1569-1570, 1570f
Allergic rhinitis, 1383-1385
Allergic salute, 1383f
Allergic shiners, in allergic rhinitis, 1383
Allergic vasculitis, 1569-1570, 1570f
Allergy(ies); see also Allergen(s).
  asthma and, 1387
  cardiac catheterization and, 1472
  history of, 155-156, 156b
  shots for, reducing pain of, 1385
  skin lesions and, 743
  to cow's milk, 569-570, 569b
    diabetes mellitus and, 1734
  to donor blood, 1541t
  to foods, in infants, 568-571
  to latex, 433-436, 433b, 436b, 1135
  to peanuts, 681
  to vaccines, 538
  vs colds, 1385
Allevyn tracheostomy dressing, 1328
Allis sign, 254t, 448, 449f
Allodynia, 747
Allografts, for covering burn wounds, 1240-
    1241, 1240f
Alloimmunization, 310, 1542t; see also
    Hemolytic disease of newborn.
  prevention of, 314
All-terrain vehicles, 733, 733b
Alopecia, 774t
  in cancer, 1602
Alpha-fetoprotein
  in neural tube defects, 129
  prenatal tests for, 128t, 129
Alport syndrome, 1282
Alternate cover test, 196
Alternative therapies
  cultural aspects of, 48-49
  mineral and vitamin excess and, 555, 565
  nursing admission history and,
    1087-1088, 1090b
Aluminum hydroxide gel, in chronic renal
    failure, 1291
Alveolar pressure, 1309
Alveolar surface tension, 1307
Alveoli
  function of, 1306
  gas diffusion in, 1309b
  growth of, 1306
Alveolocapillary membrane, in acute
    respiratory distress syndrome, 1379
Amantadine hydrochloride (Symmetrel), for
    influenza, 1356
Ambiguous genitalia, 487-490, 488f, 489b, 489t
  in congenital adrenal hyperplasia,
    1729-1731

Ambivalence, terminal illness and, 972-973
Amblyopia, 195, 1001b
  in cerebral palsy, 207
Ambulation
  after heart surgery, 1506
  play activities and, 1111b
Ambulatory aids, 1773f, 1774-1776, 1774b,
    1775b, 1775f
  in cerebral palsy, 1384f, 1838
  in spinal cord injury, 1860-1861
Ambulatory/outpatient setting, 1091-1092, 1092b
Amelia, 453
AMEND; see Aiding Mothers and Fathers
    Experiencing Neo-Natal Death.
Amenorrhea
  in athletes, 1804
  in chronic renal failure, 1289
  primary, 845
  secondary, 845-846
American Academy of Allergy, Asthma, and
    Immunology, 1400
American Academy of Allergy and
    Immunology, 1384
American Academy of Orthopaedic
    Surgeons, 1815
American Academy of Pediatrics, 11n, 12, 854
  sports recommendations of, 1796b, 1797
American Anorexia/Bulimia Association,
    Inc., 880
American Association of Diabetes Educators,
    1744
American Association of Kidney Patients, 1298
American Association of Mental Retardation
    Adaptive Behavior Scale, 978
American Association of Suicidology, 900
American Association on Mental Retardation,
    980b, 991n
American Brain Tumor Association, 1624n
American Burn Association, 1252
American Camping Association, 915n, 1751
American Cancer Society, 932n, 1586n
American Cleft Palate Craniofacial
    Association, 460
American College of Obstetrics and
    Gynecology, 854
American Council of the Blind, 1003
American Diabetes Association, 1744
American Foundation for the Blind, 1003,
    1004, 1006
American Indians; see Native Americans.
American Juvenile Arthritis Foundation, 1824
American Lung Association, 1375
American Lyme Disease Foundation, Inc., 766
American Medical Association, 854
American Nurses' Association
  Code of Ethics for Nurses of, 22b
  home care nurses and, 1020
  Standards of Care of, 25, 25b
  Standards of Maternal and Child Health
    Nursing Practice, 23-24, 23b
  Standards of Professional Performance,
    25, 25b
American Nurses Credentialing Center, 1020
American Pain Society, 1554n
American Sign Language, 998
American Society of Pain Management
    Nurses, 1061
American Speech-Language Hearing
    Association, 1013

American Sudden Infant Death Syndrome
    Institute, 966
Americans with Disabilities Act, 913, 980b
Amethocaine, for laser therapy, for
    birthmarks, 302
Amethopterin; see Methotrexate.
Amines, vasoactive, in anaphylaxis, 1224
Amino acids
  small, 1418
  supplements of, in burn injuries, 1232-1233
p-Aminobenzoic acid (PABA), in sunscreen
    agents, 770
Aminoglycosides, ototoxicity of, 996b
Aminopeptidase, 1418
Aminosalicylates, for inflammatory bowel
    disease, 1440
Amiodarone, for cardiopulmonary
    resuscitation, 1399t
Ammonia nitrogen, reference ranges for, 1895t
Amnesia, posttraumatic, 1666
Amniocentesis, 128t, 129-130
  sickle cell anemia and, 1554
Amniotic banding, clubfoot and, 452
Amniotic fluid
  aspiration of, prevention of, 265
  fetal lung maturity and, 383
Amobarbital, abuse of, 886t
Amoxicillin
  for otitis media, 1358
  for pneumonia, 1370
Amphetamines, abuse of, 886t, 891b, 892
Amphotericin B, for candidiasis, in
    newborn, 301
Ampicillin-sulbactam (Unasyn), for
    pneumonia, 1370
Amputation, 1795-1796
  for osteosarcoma, 1627-1628
  phantom limb pain and, 1628
  prostheses for, 1774-1775, 1775b
  psychological aspects of, 1767
  stump care in, 1775b, 1795
  traumatic, 1795
  types of, 1774b
Amylase, in infants, 496
Anabolic steroids, 1805
Anaclitic depression, hospitalization and,
    1032-1034, 1041-1044
Anal fissures, 223
Anal mucosal tabs, 223
Anal patency, 261
Anal polyps, 223
Anal reflex, 223
Anal stage, 230, 230t
Analgesics, 1057, 1060-1068; see also
    Anesthesia; Pain management.
  abuse of, 886t, 891b, 892
  adjuvant, 1060-1061
  after heart surgery, 1505-1506
  combination, 1060, 1060b
  dosage of, 1061-1062, 1062t, 1063t
  for neonatal pain, 357
    from circumcision, 271b, 272
    from heel puncture, 267b
  in appendectomy, 1435
  in heart surgery, 1505-1506
  in hypertrophic pyloric stenosis, 1448
  in otitis media, 1360
  in preoperative sedation, 1112-1113, 1113b
  in sickle cell anemia, 1552-1553, 1553

Analgesics—cont'd
  in stomatitis, 664
  in terminal illness, 956-958, 957, 957b, 957f
  in tonsillectomy, 1353
  opioid
    in newborn, 357
    intrauterine exposure to, 406-407, 406b
    physical dependence on, 1068
    route of administration of, 1062-1067,
      1064b-1067b, 1064t
    side effects of, 1067-1068, 1067b, 1068b
    timing of administration of, 1067
    tolerance of, 1068
    underuse of, 1047b
  opioids, 1057, 1060, 1062t, 1064t
    abuse of, 886t, 891b, 892
    extubation and, neonatal, 356b
    fallacies and facts about, 1049, 1050b
    for comatose patients, 1655
Anaphylactic shock, 1219
Anaphylactoid purpura, 1569-1570, 1570f
Anaphylaxis, 1224-1226
  allergens associated with, 1224b
  clinical signs of, 1225b
  in food allergy, in infants, 568
  renal involvement in, 1270t
  vaccination and, 538
Anasarca, 1180
  in nephrotic syndrome, 1275
Anastomosis, esophageal, 464, 465
Androgen(s), 1708t
  action of, 805
  adrenal secretion of, 1723
  deficiency of, 1726b
  hypersecretion of
    ambiguous genitalia and, 487, 1729-1731
    in congenital adrenal hyperplasia, 1729-1731
Anemia
  aplastic, 1559-1561
    erythema infectiosum and, 651
  classification of, 1535, 1537b
  clinical manifestations of, 1537, 1537b
  complications of, 1539-1540
  definition of, 1535
  diagnosis of, 1538
  hemolytic, in hemolytic uremic
    syndrome, 1281
  hemolytic disease of newborn and, 312
  hereditary spherocytosis and, 1546-1547
  hypoplastic, 1559, 1560
  in acute renal failure, 1286
  in burn injuries, 1233
  in cancer, 1597, 1599
  in chronic renal failure, 1289, 1289b, 1291
  in high-risk newborn, 398-399
  in lead poisoning, 677
  in leukemia, 1612
  iron deficiency, 1542-1546, 1544b
  megaloblastic, 1549
  nursing considerations in, 1538-1540
  pathophysiology of, 1537, 1537b
  physiologic, in infants, 496
  screening for, 1537
  sickle cell, 1547-1555; see also Sickle cell
    anemia.
  α-thalassemia and, 1555, 1557-1559,
    1557b, 1557f
  tissue oxygenation and, 1538-1539
  treatment of, 1538, 1540-1542, 1541t-1542t

Anencephaly, 424b, 425
  etiology of, 424
Anesthesia; *see also* Analgesics; Pain management.
  for circumcision, 270-272, 271b
  for laser therapy, for birthmarks, 302
  induction of, 1113
  local, for suturing, 1672b
  regional, 1065b
  topical, 751b, 1679
    EMLA cream for, 1603, 1679
    for arthrocentesis, 1823b
    for bladder catheterization, 1146b
    for circumcision, 270-272, 271b
    for laser therapy, for birthmarks, 302
    for lumbar puncture, 1142b, 1142f, 1679
    for suturing, 1672b
  with skin lesions, 742
Aneurysms, coronary artery, in Kawasaki
    disease, 1514, 1515
Angelman syndrome, 122
Anger
  chronic illness or disability and, 934
  hospitalized child and, parents of, 1040
  terminal illness and, 972
Angiogenesis, in inflammatory process, 747
Angiotensin-converting enzyme (ACE)
    inhibitors
  for congestive heart failure, 1479
  for hypertension, 1518, 1519b
Angle of Louis, 208f, 209
Animal bites, 778-779
  rabies and, 1682-1683
Animal milks; *see* Milk.
Animals
  abuse of, 686b
  safe behavior with, 779b
Animism, 643
Anisometropia, 1001b
Ankle clonus, in newborn, 263t
Ankle-foot orthoses, 1773, 1773f, 1774b
  in cerebral palsy, 1838
Ann Arbor staging system, 1616, 1616b
Anogenital warts, 864
Anoplasty, 469, 470
Anorchia, 480
Anorectal malformations, 466, 466b, 468-470,
    468f, 469f
Anorectal manometry, in Hirschsprung
    disease, 1427
Anorectal myomectomy, in Hirschsprung
    disease, 1427
Anorectoplasty, posterior sagittal, 469
Anorexia
  in cancer, 1600
  in immobilization, 1764, 1768
  physiologic, in toddlers, 609-610
Anorexia nervosa, 672, 876-882
  assessment of, 879
  clinical manifestations of, 877, 877b, 878t
  diagnosis of, 878, 878b
  early signs of, 880b
  etiology of, 877
  in athletes, 1804
  in diabetics, 1737b, 1751
  nursing care plan for, 881-882
  nursing considerations in, 879-880, 880b
  prevention of, 880, 880b
  prognosis of, 878-879
  treatment of, 878

Anovulation, dysfunctional uterine bleeding
    and, 848
Antacids
  for gastroesophageal reflux, 1429
  for peptic ulcer disease, 1445
  for upper GI mucosal lesions, 1455
Anterior fontanel, 252t, 257-258, 258f
Anterior fontanel pressure monitor, 1657
Anterior horn cell diseases, 1833
Anterior leg pain, 1800, 1801t
Anterior nasal vestibule, 204
Anterior pituitary; *see* Pituitary gland.
Anterior uveitis, in juvenile rheumatoid
    arthritis, 1821, 1822
Anthropometric measurements, 168, 177-178;
    *see also* Height; Weight.
  growth charts for, 174-175, 1882-1895
  in nutritional assessment, 168
  schedule for, 171b
Antianxiety agents, for school phobia, 795
Antibiotics
  antitumor, 1588-1589, 1592t
  *Clostridium difficile* diarrhea and, 1213
  for acne, 841
  for acute epiglottitis, 1363
  for acute poststreptococcal
      glomerulonephritis, 1273
  for bacterial endocarditis, 1510
  for burned patients, 1237
  for cystic fibrosis, 1408, 1412
  for diarrhea, 1213
  for neonatal sepsis, 394-395
  for otitis media, 1358, 1359, 1360
  for pneumonia, 1370
  for prevention of complications from
      communicable diseases, 660
  for respiratory distress syndrome, 386
  for skin disorders, 751
  for urinary tract infection, 1267, 1267t, 1268
  for vesicoureteral reflux, 1270
  in ophthalmia neonatorum prevention, 266
  resistance to, 1134
  urinary, side effects of, 1267, 1267t
Antibodies, 1572
  ABO incompatibility and, 312, 312t
  in newborn, 243
Antibody tests, for hepatitis, 1459
Anticholinergic drugs
  for asthma, 1393, 1396
  for enuresis, 784
Anticipatory guidance, 145
Anticipatory socialization, in school
    experience, 714-715
Anticoagulation, for pulmonary artery
    hypertension, 1491
Anticonvulsants, 1690, 1691t, 1694-1695
  for cerebral palsy, 1839
  for status epilepticus, 1692
Anti-D antibody, for idiopathic
    thrombocytopenic purpura, 1566, 1567b
Antidepressants
  for attention deficit hyperactivity disorder,
      789, 791
  for depression, 798
  for enuresis, 784
  for Tourette syndrome, 793
Antidiarrheal drug therapy, 1213
Antidiuretic hormone, 1707t
  after heart surgery, 1506

Antidiuretic hormone—cont'd
  enuresis and, 784
  hyposecretion of, 1706b
    in diabetes insipidus, 1715
  in newborn, 243
Antidotes, for poisons, 673
Antiemetics
  for vomiting, 1218
  in cancer, 1599-1600
Antiepileptics; *see* Anticonvulsants.
Antifungal agents, for diaper dermatitis,
    578-580
Antigen(s), 1571
  blood incompatibility and, 310, 312, 312f
  in asthma, 1387
  in hepatitis, tests for, 1459
Antigen-antibody complex, 1572
Antigen-antibody reaction, in anaphylaxis, 1224
Antigenic drift, 1356
Antigenic shift, 1356
Antihelix, 200, 200f
Antihemophilic factor, 1562t
  deficiency of, 1561-1566
Antihistamines
  asthma and, 1397
  drug interactions with, 1385
  for allergic rhinitis, 1384
  for atopic dermatitis, 581
  for gastroesophageal reflux, 1429
  for peptic ulcer disease, 1445
  for upper gastrointestinal mucosal
      lesions, 1455
Anti–islet cell antibodies, 1733-1734, 1736
Antilymphocyte globulin, for aplastic
    anemia, 1560
Antimetabolites, for cancer, 1588, 1590t-1591t
Antimicrobial agents; *see also* Antibiotics.
  topical, for burn wounds, 1238-1240,
      1238b, 1239t
  urinary tract infection and, 1265
Antioxidant enzymes, respiratory distress
    syndrome and, 383
Antipsychotic drugs, for schizophrenia, 799
Antipyretic drugs, 1130, 1130t, 1131t
Antiretroviral drugs, for human
    immunodeficiency virus infection, 1575
Antirheumatic drugs, 1821-1822
Antisecretory agents, for peptic ulcer
    disease, 1445
Antiseizure agents; *see* Anticonvulsants.
Antiseptics, high-risk newborn and, 350b
Antisocial personality disorder, 686b
Antispasmotic agents, in recurrent abdominal
    pain, 796, 797
Antistreptolysin-O titers
  in acute poststreptococcal
      glomerulonephritis, 1272
  in rheumatic fever, 1512
  reference ranges for, 1895t
Antithymocyte globulin, for aplastic anemia,
    1560, 1561
Antithyroid agents, for hyperthyroidism,
    1719-1720, 1721
Antitragus, 200, 200f
Antitumor antibiotics, 1588-1589, 1592t
Antivenin, for poisonious bites, 673
Antiviral drugs, for varicella-zoster virus
    infection, 651b

Anus, 223; *see also* under Anal.
  imperforate, 466, 469f
  malformations of, 466, 466b, 468-470, 468f, 469f
  of newborn, 254t, 261-262
Anxiety
  in parents of hospitalized child, 1040
  in school phobia, 794
  psychologic preparation for procedures and, 1103-1108
  separation, 505-506
    coping with, 514-515
    hospitalization and, 1032-1034, 1041-1044
    in school phobia, 795
Anxiolytic agents, for school phobia, 795
Aorta
  coarctation of, 220, 1494b-1495b, 1494f
  in transposition of great arteries, 1499b, 1499f
Aortic bodies, 1309
Aortic regurgitation, rheumatic fever and, 1511
Aortic stenosis, 1495b, 1495f
  subvalvular, 1495b
  valvular, 1495b
Aortic valve, 1465
  heart sounds and, 215
Apert syndrome, 445b
APGAR, family, 162-163, 162b, 1870-1871
Apgar scoring system, 244-245, 244t
  hearing impairment and, 996b
  maternal smoking and, 408
Aphasia, 995
Aphthous stomatitis, 664
Apical impulse (AI), 214-215
  pulse measurement at, 179
Aplastic anemia, 1538, 1559-1561
Aplastic Anemia and MDS International Foundation, 1561n
Aplastic crisis
  in hereditary spherocytosis, 1546
  in sickle cell anemia, 1549
Apnea
  complete, emergency treatment for, 1333-1334
  home monitoring of, 586, 586b, 587, 587b, 587f
  in newborn, 251t, 260
  of infancy, 585-588
  of prematurity, 376, 378-379, 379b
  reflex, 1309
  types of, 1331
Apneustic center, 1309
Apocrine glands, of newborn, 243
Apocrine sweat glands, 742
Apoenzymes, protein, vitamins and, 554
Apparent life-threatening event
  apnea of infancy as, 585-586
  sudden infant death syndrome as, 582
Appearance, assessment of, 186-187
Appendectomy, open, 1434
Appendicitis
  acute, 1432-1435, 1433b
  clinical manifestations of, 1433
  diagnosis of, 1433-1434
  etiology and incidence of, 1433
  nursing care for, 1434-1435
  nursing care plan for, 1436
  pathophysiology of, 1433
  treatment of, 1434
  types of, 1433

Appendix, ruptured, 1433, 1434
Appetite
  decreased
    in cancer, 1600
    in immobilization, 1764, 1768
    in toddlers, 609-610
  in nephrotic syndrome, 1278
  increased, in diabetes, 1734
Approach behaviors, 931, 932b
  in newborn, feeding and, 279
Appropriate-for-gestational-age infant, 249-250, 334b
Apresoline (hydralazine), for hypertension, 1519b
AquaMEPHYTON, for hemorrhagic disease of newborn, 319
Aqueduct of Sylvius, 436, 437f
Aqueous lysine vasopressin, for diabetes insipidus, 1716
Aqueous vasopressin (Pitressin), for diabetes insipidus, 1715, 1716
Ara-C (cytosine arabinoside), 1591t
Arachnid bites, 776-777, 776t, 777t
Arachnodactyly, 447t
Arachnoid membrane, 1642, 1643f
Arachnoid trabeculae, 1643
ARDS; *see* Acute (adult) respiratory distress syndrome (ARDS).
Arginine, in burn injuries, 1232-1233
Arm; *see also* Extremities.
  examination of, 224
Arm boards, in intravenous infusions, 1196
Arm circumference
  in nutritional assessment, 168
  measurement of, 177
  percentiles for, 1894
Arm recoil, gestational age and, 250b
Arm restraints, 1140
Arnold-Chiari malformation
  bladder function and, 428
  hydrocephalus and, 437, 438t
Around the clock schedule, for analgesic administration, 1067
Arousal states, in high-risk newborn, 358, 360, 360t
Arrhythmia(s), 1523-1526; *see also* specific types.
  after heart surgery, 1504, 1507
  diagnosis of, 1524-1526
  in cardiomyopathy, 1523
  sinus, 217, 217b
  in newborn, 253t
Arterial blood gases
  in respiratory distress syndrome, 380-381
  measurements of, 1313-1317, 1313t
    continuous, 1314b
    normal and abnormal values for, 1317t
    sampling of, 1316-1317, 1316b
    transcutaneous monitoring of, 1314-1315
Arterial catheterization
  for blood pressure monitoring, of high-risk newborn, 337
  for oxygenation monitoring, in respiratory distress syndrome, 387
Arterial oxygen saturation, 1309
  congenital heart disease and, 1475, 1475f
  in carbon monoxide poisoning, 1381
  in oxyhemoglobin dissociation curve, 1315, 1315f
  in pulse oximetry, 1313-1314, 1314f

Arterial switch procedure, 1499b
Arteriolar light reflex, 195
Arterioles, afferent and efferent, 1256
Arteriosclerosis, lipid or cholesterol and, 1519
Arteriovenous fistula, for hemodialysis, 1295
Artery(ies)
  coronary; *see* Coronary artery(ies).
  great, transposition of, 1499b, 1499f
  in postnatal circulation, 1467
  pulmonary; *see* Pulmonary artery(ies).
Arthritis
  in Crohn disease, 1439
  in Henoch-Schönlein purpura, 1570
  in Kawasaki disease, 1514, 1516
  in rheumatic fever, 1511
  juvenile rheumatoid, 1820-1825; *see also* Juvenile rheumatoid arthritis.
  septic, 1818
Arthritis Foundation, 1824
Arthrocentesis, topical anesthesia for, 1823b
Arthrodesis, for scoliosis, 1812-1813, 1812f
Arthrogryposis multiplex congenita, 447t
Arthropathy, prevention of, in hemophilia, 1564
Arthropod bites, 775-778, 776t, 777t
Articulation errors, 1007
Artificial sweeteners, in diabetes, 1745
Artificial tears, 1659
Artificial ventilation; *see* Ventilatory support.
Asacol (mesalamine), for inflammatory bowel disease, 1440
Ascariasis, clinical manifestations of, 665t
Aschoff bodies, 1511
Ascites, 1181, 1461
  in congestive heart failure, 1478
  in nephrotic syndrome, 1275
Ascorbic acid
  functions and disturbances of, 558t
  sources of, 558t
Ascribed roles, 76b
Aseptic meningitis, 1680-1681
Asepto syringe, feeding with, cleft lip and palate and, 459
Asian-Americans, 35b; *see also* Race/ethnicity.
  dietary preferences of, 45-47, 46t
  epicanthal folds in, 192f, 193, 193f, 196, 196f
  growth charts for, 1892
  health beliefs and practices of, 52t
  pseudostrabismus in, 196, 196f
  time concept of, 43
ASO titers; *see* Antistreptolysin-O titers.
L-Asparaginase (Elspar), 1589, 1593t, 1594
Aspartate aminotransferase (AST), in neuromuscular dysfunction, 1834b
Asphyxiation
  of infants, prevention of, 541-544, 542t-543t, 549b
  traumatic, 623
Aspiration
  bone marrow, 1588
    analgesia for, 1603
    positioning for, 1142
    sedation for, 1603
  bronchopulmonary
    in cerebral palsy, 1837
    in near-drowning, 1675-1676
    mortality from, 8, 8t
    of acids, 1379
    of amniotic fluid, prevention of, 265

Aspiration—cont'd
  bronchopulmonary—cont'd
    of foreign body, 541-544, 542t-543t, 549b, 623, 1338, 1340-1341, 1340f, 1376-1377, 1376f, 1378b
    of hydrocarbons, 1379
    of meconium, 388-389
    of talcum powder, 1379
  pulmonary, preoperative fasting and, 1113b
  suprapubic, 1144-1146, 1146b, 1266
  tracheal, 1315t
  tracheostomy, 1326-1327, 1326f, 1327b
Aspiration pneumonia, 1378-1379, 1378b
Aspirin
  asthma and, 1397
  for Kawasaki disease, 1515
  in pain management, 1063t
  poisoning with, 671b
  reference ranges for, 1901t
  Reye syndrome and, 1683-1684, 1683b
Asplenia, functional, in sickle cell anemia, 1548
Assent, informed consent and, 1102
Assessment
  developmental, 233-237
  family, 160-164, 160b-163b
  history taking in, 153-160; see also Health history.
  in nursing process, 25
  interview in, 141-142, 141-153; see also Interview.
  nutritional, 164-168, 164b, 165b, 166t-167t
  physical, 171-229; see also Physical examination.
  review of systems in, 159-160, 159b
  trauma, 1760-1761, 1761b, 1762b
Assimilation, 34
Assisted suicide, 949
Assisted ventilation; see Ventilatory support.
Assistive devices
  for communication impairment, 1008, 1840-1841
  for hearing impairment, 998
  for mental retardation, 981
  for visual impairment, 1004
Associated movements, 1647b
Association for Retarded Citizens of the United States, 981, 983n, 991n
Association of Pediatric Oncology Nurses, 23n
Associations, congenital malformations and, 113
Associative play, 633
Assumed roles, 76b
Astemizole (Hismanal)
  drug interactions with, 1385
  for allergic rhinitis, 1384
Asthma, 906, 1385-1401
  chronic, clinical signs of, 1389
  classification of, 1385, 1386b
  clinical manifestations of, 1388-1389
  conditions mimicking, 1389b
  diagnosis of, 1389-1390
  emergency care of, 1395-1396
  exacerbations of, 1387, 1394t, 1395t
  home management of, 1395
  nursing care for, 1397-1401
  nursing care plan for, 1402-1404
  pathophysiology of, 1386-1388
  prevalence of, 1385
  prognosis for, 1396

Asthma—cont'd
  risk factors for, 1386
  self-management programs in, 1400
  treatment of
    general aspects of, 1390-1395
    specific measures for, 1395-1397
  triggers of, 1386b
  viral-induced, vs bronchitis and bronchiolitis, 1366t
Asthma and Allergy Foundation of America, 1400
Astigmatism, 1001b
Astrocytomas, 1619, 1620b; see also Brain tumors.
Asymmetric tonic neck reflex, 263t, 264f
Ataxia, 1647b
Atelectasis
  after heart surgery, 1507
  respiratory distress syndrome and, 380
Atenolol (Tenormin), for hypertension, 1519b
ATG; see Antithymocyte globulin.
Atherosclerosis, lipid or cholesterol and, 1519
Athetosis, 1647b
Athletes, female, menstural irregularities in, 846
Athlete's foot, 759-760, 759t
Athlete's heart, 1805
Athletics; see Sports.
Ativan (lorazepam), for status epilepticus, 1692
Atlantoaxial instability, Down syndrome and, 990
Atonic seizures, 1688
Atopic dermatitis, 743
  in infants, 580-582, 580b, 580f
Atopy
  asthma and, 1385
  in infants, 568
    prevention of, 569, 569b
Atraumatic care, 15
Atresia, 454
  biliary, 470-472, 471f
  esophageal, 463-466, 463f
  rectal, 466
Atrial septal defect, 1492b, 1492f
  in tricuspid atresia, 1497b
Atrial septum, development of, 1465, 1465f
Atrioventricular block, complete, 1524-1525, 1524f
Atrioventricular bundle (bundle of His), 1467
Atrioventricular canal
  complete, pulmonary artery hypertension and, 1490
  defect of, 1493b, 1493f
Atrioventricular node, 1467
Atrioventricular valves, 1465
  heart sounds and, 215
Atrium
  cardiac, 1465
  common, 1465
Atrophy
  immobilization and, 1762-1763
  in muscular dystrophy, 1865
Atropine sulfate, for cardiopulmonary resuscitation, 1399t
Attachemnt
  in adoption, 90, 90f
  in multiple births, 81
Attachment
  colic and, 573b
  development of, 504-506
  failure to thrive and, 574, 575b, 576

Attachment—cont'd
  in adoption, 90, 90f
  in multiple births, 81
  in school-age children, 707-708
  of newborn, 247, 247b, 283-284
    at high risk, 366-368, 366b, 367f
    behavior and, 247, 247b, 279, 283-284
    feeding and, 279
    in neonatal intensive care unit, 366-368, 366b, 367f
    kangaroo care and, 362
    phototherapy and, 309, 309b
    promotion of, 282-286, 284f-286f, 284t, 290-291
    special needs and, 912
    visual impairment and, 1003
    with special needs, 912
  rumination and, 574
Attention deficit hyperactivity disorder (ADHD), 505, 786-791
  clinical manifestations of, 787-788
  course of, 788
  diagnostic criteria for, 788-789, 788b
  in cerebral palsy, 1836
  nursing considerations with, 789-791
  subtypes of, 788
  treatment of, 789
Attention span, short, 791; see also Attention deficit hyperactivity disorder.
Audiometry, 203-204, 205t
Auditory acuity; see also Hearing.
  of newborn, 244, 259
Auditory brainstem response, 205t
Auditory canal, examination of, 202, 203
Auditory environment, high-risk newborn and, 363-365, 995
Auditory evoked potentials, 1652
Auditory nerve, assessment of, 229t
Auditory testing, 203-204, 204f
Augmentation enterocystoplasty, 429
Augmentin (amoxicillin clavulanate), for pneumonia, 1370
Aura
  in migraine, 1700
  preseizure, 1687
Auricle, 200, 200f
Auscultation
  in blood pressure measurement, 182, 183-184, 184f, 185-186
  in newborn, 260-261
  of abdomen, 217, 218-219
  of heart, 215-217, 216b, 216f, 216t, 1310, 1469, 1504
  of lungs, 212-213
Authoritarian parent, 84-85
Authoritative parent, 85
Autism, 1008-1010, 1009b
Autism Society of America, 1009n, 1010
Autistic-like behavior, in fragile X syndrome, 994
Autoimmune disease, diabetes as, 1733-1734
Autoimmune neutropenia, 1569t
Autolet, 1148
Autolysis, in wound healing, 748
Automatisms, 1687
Automobile, heat injury in, 548
Automobile accidents, 7, 8t
  fractures in, 1777
  injury prevention for, 1758b, 1759
  spinal cord injury in, 1855

Automobile safety seats; *see* Car seats/restraints.
Automotive Safety for Children Program, 451n, 924n
Autonomic dysfunction, in spinal cord injury, 1855, 1855b, 1856, 1860
Autonomic nervous system, 1641
  in neuroendocrine system, 1705-1706
  of newborn, 243
Autonomic stability, in neonatal behavioral assessment, 245b
Autonomy, 21
  of adolescents, 812-813
    with special needs, 916, 917
  of toddlers, 594
    with special needs, 912, 913
  vs shame and doubt, 230t, 231
Autopsy, 949t, 967
  in sudden infant death syndrome, 583-584
Autoregulation, of cerebral blood flow in, 1643-1645
Autosomal dominant inheritance, 118-119, 118f
Autosomal recessive inheritance, 119-120, 120f
Avoidance behaviors, 931, 932b
Avoidance language, 140
AVPU assessment, 1761b
Axillary crutches, 1775
Axillary nodes, 190, 190f
Axillary temperature, 178-179, 179f, 180b-181b, 182t-183t; *see also* Temperature.
5-Azacytidine, 1590t
Azathioprine
  in inflammatory bowel disease, 1440
  in renal transplantation, 1300
Azithromycin, for gonorrhea, 862
Azogue, 48-49, 49t
Azotemia, 1283
Azotorrhea, in cystic fibrosis, 1405
Azulfidine (sulfasalazine), for inflammatory bowel disease, 1440

**B**

B cells, 243
Babinski reflex, 225, 262, 262f, 263t, 1652
Baby; *see* Infant; Newborn.
Baby bottle tooth decay, 615-616, 615f
Baby powder, aspiration of, 542t-543t, 544, 1379
Baby-Friendly Hospital Initiative, 275, 275b
Babysitters, 99, 100b; *see also* Daycare facilities.
  for sick child, 100
  location and evaluation of, 517
Bacille Calmette-Guérin (BCG) vaccine, for tuberculosis, 1375
Bacitracin, for burn wounds, 1239t
Back; *see also* Spine.
  examination of, 223
  of newborn, 254t
Back blows, in infants, 1337f, 1338, 1340
Back knee deformity, 447t
Baclofen, for spasticity, in cerebral palsy, 1839
Bacteremia
  central venous line, 1201
  prolonged, renal involvement in, 1270t
Bacteria, acidogenic, tooth decay and, 780
Bacterial culture, 1420t
Bacterial endocarditis, 1509-1511
  cyanosis and, 1487, 1488
  prophylaxis for, 1510b
  renal involvement in, 1270t
  subacute, 1509

Bacterial infections; *see also* Infection(s).
  from blood transfusion, 1542t
  skin, 754-755, 754f, 755t
Bacterial meningitis, 1677-1680, 1681t
Bacterial overgrowth
  in short bowel syndrome, 1452
  of small bowel, with total parenteral nutrition, 1451
Bacterial pneumonia, 1369-1371
  in burn injuries, 1233
Bacterial tracheitis, 1362t, 1365
Bacteriuria
  in females, 1265
  tests for, 1266
Bag-valve-mask ventilation, 1323
BAL (British antilewisite), for chelation therapy, 680, 681
Balance, assessment of, 204
Balance suspension traction, 1790, 1790f
Balanced translocation, 115-116
Balanitis, 479
  in erythema multiforme exudativum, 773
Ballard Scale, for newborn maturity rating, 247-249, 248f-249f
Balloon pump, intraaortic, for shock, 1222
Balloons, suffocation by, 542t, 544
Bandaging
  in traction, 1792
  of stump, 1795
Bands, in complete blood count, 1536t
Baptism, neonatal death and, 370-371
Barbiturate abuse, 886t, 891b, 892
Barbiturate coma, 1658-1659
Barium enema, in treatment of intussusception, 1449
Barium swallow, in gastroesophageal reflux diagnosis, 1429
Barlow test, 448, 449f
Barrel chest, 209, 1302
  in asthma, 1389, 1397
  in cystic fibrosis, 1406
Bartholin glands, 223
Basal cells, 740
Basal ganglia, 1643
  structure and function of, 1644t
Basal metabolic rate, fluid requirements and, 1173
Base bicarbonate, 1182
Base excess, reference ranges for, 1895t
Basilar migraine, 1700b
Basilar skull fractures, 1667
Basophil(s), 1534
  in complete blood count, 1536t
Basophilia, 1535
Basophilic erythroblast, 1532
Bath(s)
  cool, 752
  therapeutic, for skin lesions, 753
Bathing, 1125, 1127, 1127f
  atopic dermatitis and, 581, 582
  of newborn, 268-269, 268f, 350b
Bathing trunk nevus, 302
Bathwater, scald burns from, 542t, 543t, 547, 549b
Batteries
  button, poisoning with, 547, 549b
  hearing aid, safety and, 998
Bayley Infant Neurodevelopmental Screener, 234t

Bayley Scales of Infant Development, 978
Baylor Pediatric AIDS Initiative, 1577n
BCG (bacille Calmette-Guérin) vaccine, for tuberculosis, 1375
BCNU (carmustine), 1593t
Becker muscular dystrophy, 1863t
Becoplermin (Regranex), for skin disorders, 753
Bed, sharing of with parents, 527b, 646b
  sudden infant death syndrome and, 583
Bed rest; *see also* Immobilization.
  after heart surgery, 1505
  in respiratory infections, 1346
  in systemic lupus erythematosus, 1828
Bedding
  for high-risk newborn, 349-350, 363
    co-bedding of multiples and, 362-363, 362f
  infant suffocation and, 542t-543t, 544, 549b
  sudden infant death syndrome and, 583
Bedtime
  fear of, 515
  resistance to, in school-age children, 723
  school phobia and, 795
Bed-wetting, 783-785
  age and, 783b
  in diabetes insipidus, 1716
  in diabetes mellitus, 1736
  urinary tract infection and, 1266
Bee stings, 775-776, 776t
Behavior
  assessment of, 187, 187b, 225
  immobilization and, 1766-1767, 1766b
  in fluid and electrolyte disturbances, 1188t
  in fragile X syndrome, 994b
  mental retardation and, 979b
  pain assessment and, 1054-1055, 1054b, 1055b
  personal-social
    in infants, 506-507
    in toddlers, 599-600
  risk-taking, family systems and, 817
Behavior modification
  disciplinary, 86-87
  for attention deficit hyperactivity disorder, 789
  for failure to thrive, 577
  in anorexia nervosa, 879-880
  in mental retardation, 981
    independent toileting and, 985
  in obesity, 874, 875, 876f
Behavioral assessment, of newborn, 245-246, 245b, 246t, 257
  in pain, 352-353, 352b
Behavioral autonomy, 812
Behavioral contract, 1121
  in anorexia nervosa, 880
  in pain management, 1059b
Behavioral disorders, 786-800
  attention deficit hyperactivity disorder as, 786-791
  conversion reaction as, 797
  depression as, 797-799, 798b
  enuresis and, 783
  in adolescence, 869-902; *see also* specific problems.
  in fetal alcohol syndrome, 329-330, 329b
  in mental retardation, 983
  in phenylketonuria, 323
  learning disability as, 791-792
  posttraumatic stress disorder as, 794

Behavioral disorders—cont'd
recurrent abdominal pain as, 796-797
schizophrenia as, 799, 799b
school phobia as, 794-796
tic disorders as, 792
Tourette syndrome as, 793-794
Behavioral Pain Score, 1056t
Behavioral regression, in toddler, with special needs, 912-913
Behavioral state organization, in high-risk newborn, 358, 360, 360t
Behavioral strategies, for compliance, 1121
Behavioral Style Questionnaire, 636
Benadryl (diphenhydramine), for allergic rhinitis, 1384
Beneficence, 21
Benzathine penicillin G, intramuscular, 1352
Benzocaine, poisoning with, 669
Benzodiazepines, respiratory depression from, 1068b
Benzoyl peroxide, for acne, 841
Benzyl alcohol, high-risk newborn and, 351
Beractant, 386
Bereavement, neonatal death and, 369-370
Bereavement programs, 971-972
Best Start Social Marketing, 348
Beta blockers
for congestive heart failure, 1480
for hypertension, 1518, 1519b
Bethanecol (Urecholine), for gastroesophageal reflux, 1429
Bibliotherapy, 151b
Bicarbonate, 1182
impaired reabsorption of, in proximal tubular acidosis, 1279-1280
pancreatic secretion of, in cystic fibrosis, 1401
reference ranges for, 1895t
Biceps reflex, 226, 226f
Biculturation, 38
Bicycle helmets, 733-734, 734b, 734f, 735b, 1758b
Bicycle injuries, 7-8, 8t, 724b, 732, 733-734, 734f
Bifid renal pelvis, 479t
Bile, 1418
Bilevel positive airway pressure, for ventilation, 1323
Biliary atresia, 470-472, 471f
Biliary Atresia and Liver Transplant Network, Inc., 472
Bilibottoms, 308
BiliCheck, 306
Bilirubin; see also Hyperbilirubinemia.
breast-feeding jaundice and, 307
direct, 305
formation and excretion of, 304, 304f
physiologic jaundice and, 305
serum
measurement of, 305, 307
reference ranges for, 1895t
Bilirubin encephalopathy, 304, 307, 311b
prevention of, 306
Bilirubinometry, transcutaneous, 305-306, 307
Bill of Rights, for hospitalized children and teens, 1046, 1046b
Binge-eating/purging
in anorexia nervosa, 878b
in bulimia nervosa, 672, 882-884
Binocularity, in infants, 495

Binuclear family, 72
Bioelectric impedance, obesity and, 874
Biojector, 1157
Biologic development; see also Development; Growth.
in adolescents, 803-809
in infants, 494-501
in preschoolers, 628-630, 638t
in school-age children, 699-700
in toddlers, 592-594, 604t
Biologic response modifiers, 1594-1595
Biologic skin coverings, for burn wounds, 1240-1241, 1240f
Biopsy, 1587-1588
bone marrow, 1588
analgesia for, 1603
positioning for, 1142
sedation for, 1603
fetal, 130
gastrointestinal tract, 1315t, 1422t
lung, 1315t
muscle, 1834
rectal, in Hirschsprung disease, 1427
Biotin
functions of and disturbances in, 558t
sources of, 558t
Birgance Screens, 234t
Birth Defect Research for Children, 326, 419, 460
Birth defects; see Congenital abnormalities; Developmental defects and specific types.
Birth history, 155
Birth injuries, 295-300, 296b, 297f, 299f
cerebral palsy and, 1834-1835
Birth order
family roles and, 76t, 77
influence of, 79, 79b
Birth rates, 105, 105b
Birth weight, 251f
blood pressure and, 337t
bronchopulmonary dysplasia and, 390
cerebral palsy and, 1835
congenital hypothyroidism and, 321
Down syndrome and, 989t
hearing impairment and, 996b
high-risk infants and, 334, 334b; see also High-risk newborn.
hyperglycemia treatment and, 318
infant mortality and, 3-4
sepsis and, 394
Birthmarks, 301-303, 302f, 742
Bisexuality, 814-816, 816b, 831, 835-836
suicide and, 898, 898b
Bites
animal, 778-779
rabies and, 1682-1683
arachnid, 776-777, 776t, 777t
arthropod, 775-778, 776t, 777t
human, 779-780
rickettsial infections from, 763, 765t
Biting, 779-780, 1418
in infants, 502
Black eye, 1003b
Blackbird Preschool Vision Screening System, 196b, 197-198, 198t
Blacks, 35b; see also Race/ethnicity.
dietary preferences of, 45-47, 46t
health beliefs and practices of, 52t-53t
time concept of, 43

Bladder, 1256, 1356
functional capacity of
enuresis and, 783
in middle childhood, 699
incomplete emptying of, urinary tract infection and, 1265
myelomeningocele and, 428-430
neurogenic, 1860
obstruction of, 485t, 486
palpation of, 220
recurrent infection of, vesicoureteric reflux and, 1266
structure and function of, 1259
Bladder catheterization, 1144-1146, 1145t, 1146b, 1266
for neurogenic bladder, 1860
for urine collection, 1266
hypospadias and, 482
myelomeningocele and, 429
Bladder exstrophy, epispadias and, 482-484, 483f
Bladder training, 605; see also Toilet training.
in spinal cord injury, 1860
Blalock-Taussig shunt, for tetralogy of Fallot, 1497b
Blast cell, 1531
Blastomycoses, North American, 764t
Bleeding; see also Hemorrhage.
cardiac catheterization and, 1473, 1473b
dysfunctional uterine, 848
esophageal, 1454, 1461
first aid for, 1760
from scalp laceration, 1665, 1670
gastrointestinal, 1454-1456
in cancer, 1597, 1598-1599
in hemophilia, 1562-1563
prevention of, 1564-1565
recognition and control of, 1565
in leukemia, 1612
in pregnancy, 850-851
in Wiskott-Aldrich syndrome, 1579
nasal
emergency treatment of, 1567b
in von Willebrand disease, 1566, 1567b
rectal, with Meckel diverticulum, 1437
vaginal, abnormal, 848
Bleeding disorders, 1561-1568; see also specific disorders.
Bleeding time, 1562t
reference ranges for, 1895t
Blended family, 71, 98-99, 99b
Bleomycin (Blenoxane), 1592t
Blepharitis, 193b
in infants, 580
Blind Organization of Ontario, 1003n
Blindisms, 1004
Blindness, 1000-1006; see also Visual impairment.
deafness and, 1006-1007
legal, 1000
Blink reflex, 194
in newborn, 263t
Blissymbols, 982, 1008
Blood
components of, 1530-1535, 1531f, 1533f
teaching children about, 1538
transfusion of, 1543t;
see also Transfusion.
in sputum, in cystic fibrosis, 1409

Blood clotting; *see* under Clotting; Coagulation.
Blood flow; *see also* Circulation.
  cerebral, 1643-1645
    intracranial pressure and, 1646
  in acid-base imbalance, 1183
  in newborn, 241
  obstruction of, cardiac defects with, 1491-1492, 1492f, 1494b-1496b
  pressure gradients and, congenital heart disease and, 1475, 1475f
  pulmonary
    after cardiac shunt procedure, 1489
    decreased, cardiac defects with, 1496, 1496f, 1497b-1498b
    increased, cardiac defects with, 1491, 1492b-1494b, 1492f
  to burn wound, 1234
Blood gas(es)
  in respiratory distress syndrome, 380-381
  measurement of, 1313-1317, 1313t
    continuous, 1314b
  normal and abnormal values for, 1317t
  sampling of, 1316-1317, 1316b
  transcutaneous monitoring of, 1314-1315
Blood glucose, alterations in; *see* Hyperglycemia; Hypoglycemia.
Blood glucose monitoring, in diabetes, 1738, 1747, 1748, 1748f
Blood glucose tests, for diabetes, 1736
Blood guaiac test, occult, 1420t
Blood incompatibility, 310, 312, 312f, 312t
  transfusion therapy and, 1540
Blood lead levels
  in lead poisoning, 676-678
  in screening, 678, 679, 680
  management actions and, 680
Blood pressure; *see also* Hypertension.
  after heart surgery, 1504
  in adolescents, 833
  in dehydration, 1178
  in fluid and electrolyte disturbances, 1187t
  in infants, 496
  in newborns, 251t, 256-257, 256f
    at high risk, 337, 337t
  in renal disorders, 1262
  measurement of, 182-186, 184f, 184t, 185t, 186b, 186f, 1518-1519
  normal values for, 184t
  postnatal cardiac development and, 1466-1467
  postoperative alterations in, 1119t
Blood pressure cuffs, 184-185, 184f, 186t
Blood sampling
  fetal, 130
  Guthrie paper and, 323b
  in high-risk newborn, 337-338, 337b
  in hypoglycemia, in newborn, 317, 317b
  in respiratory distress syndrome, 387
  pain reduction in, 1149b, 1192
Blood specimens, 1147-1148, 1147b, 1147f, 1148f
Blood transfusion; *see* Transfusion.
Blood urea nitrogen, 1262t
  in acute renal failure, 1284
  in chronic renal failure, 1288
Blood volume; *see also* Hypervolemia; Hypovolemia.
  after heart surgery, 1506
  in acute renal failure, 1286-1287

Blood volume—cont'd
  in burn injuries, 1231
  in newborn, 241-242
  in puberty, 809
  in shock, 1221
  reference ranges for, 1895t
Blood-brain barrier, 1645
Blue spells, with hypoxemia, 1476f, 1487
Blumberg sign, 219
B-lymphocyte, 1572
BMI; *see* Body mass index.
Body composition; *see also* Anthropometric measurements; Weight.
  racial/ethnic variations in, 57
Body fat; *see* Adipose tissue; Obesity.
Body fluids; *see* under Fluid.
Body image
  in adolescents, 814
  in anorexia nervosa, 878
  in infants, 504
  in preschoolers, 632
  in puberty, 806
  in school-age children, 708-709
  in special needs children, 913, 916
  in toddlers, 598
  α-thalassemia and, 1559
Body mass index, 873
  adolescent health and, 829, 830t
  age charts for, 174-175, 1886, 1891
  calculation of, 1881
Body surface area
  drug dosage and, 1150, 1150f
  in infants, fluid loss and, 1174
  total, burn injuries and, 1228
Body surface zones, 1857, 1857f
Body temperature; *see* Temperature.
Bolt, subarachnoid, in intracranial pressure monitoring, 1656
Bolus, of food, 1418
Bonding; *see* Attachment.
Bone
  callus formation in, 1782-1783, 1783f
  demineralization of
    in athletes, 1804
    in bronchopulmonary dysplasia, 391
    in chronic renal failure, 1289b
    in immobilization, 1763, 1764-1765
  healing of, 1781-1784, 1782f, 1782t, 1783f
  immobilization effects on, 1763, 1764-1765, 1770t
  in sickle cell anemia, 1548
  infection of, 1817-1818
  of newborn, 243
  ossification of, 1776
  remodeling of, 1782-1783, 1782f, 1782t
  structure of, 1776, 1777f
Bone age
  calculation of, 1711b
  in growth disorders, 1711, 1711b
Bone marrow, 1531, 1531f, 1571
Bone marrow aspiration/biopsy, 1588
  analgesia for, 1603
  positioning for, 1142
  sedation for, 1603
Bone marrow dysfunction, in leukemia, 1612
Bone marrow failure, 1559

Bone marrow transplantation, 1595-1596
  for leukemia, 1615
  for severe combined immunodeficiency disease, 1580
  in aplastic anemia, 1560
  nursing care in, 1602-1603, 1602-1606
Bone tumors, 1626-1629
Books, developmental impact of, 39
Booster seat, in automobiles, 618-619, 618f, 732; *see also* Car seats/restraints.
Boosters, immune system, 1572
Borborygmi, 218
Bordetella pertussis, whooping cough due to, 1371
Boston brace, 1773-1774, 1811
Botanicals; *see* Complementary medicine.
Bottle caps, aspiration of by infants, 542t-543t, 544
Bottle-feeding, 277, 279, 279f
  alternate milk products for, 280, 282
    phenylketonuria and, 323
  cleft lip and palate and, 458-459, 459f
  facial nerve paralysis and, 299-300
  formulas for, 280, 281t-283t; *see also* Formula(s).
  growth rates and, 175
  hypocalcemia and, 318, 319
  nursing caries and, 615-616, 615f
  of high-risk newborn, 344-347, 345f, 346b
  oral candidiasis and, 301
  phenylketonuria and, 283t
Botulinum antitoxin, 1851
Botulinum toxin (Botox)
  for brachial palsy, 299
  for spasticity, in cerebral palsy, 1839
Botulism, 1850-1851
Bovine surfactant, 386
Bowel; *see also* Intestine(s).
  gastroschisis and, 473, 473f
  necrotizing enterocolitis of; *see* Necrotizing enterocolitis.
Bowel decontamination, for ingested lead chips, 681
Bowel elimination
  immobilization and, 1764, 1768
  in spinal cord injury, 1860
  in unconscious child, 1659
  myelomeningocele and, 430
  with spica cast, 1787
Bowel preparation, before surgery, 1428
Bowel sounds
  auscultation of, 217, 218-219
  in gastrointestinal obstructive disorders, 1446
Bowel training, 605; *see also* Toilet training.
  for constipation, 1425
  for recurrent abdominal pain, 796, 797
  in spinal cord injury, 1860
Bowlegs, 224, 224f, 447t
Bowles chestpiece, 212
Bowman capsule, 1256, 1256f
Boy Scouts, mental retardation and, 982
Brace(s)
  Boston, 1773-1774, 1811
  dental, 782
  for developmental dysplasia of hip, 451
  for scoliosis, 1773-1774, 1811, 1813f, 1814
  Jewett-Taylor, 1774
  Milwaukee, 1811

Brace(s)—cont'd
  orthodontic
    for malocclusion, 782
    in cleft lip and palate, 457-458
  TLSO, 1811, 1813f
Brachial palsy, 299, 299f, 300
Brachial Plexus Palsy Foundation, 300
Brachial pulse, location of, 1337f, 1338
Brachioradialis reflex, 227f
Brachycephaly, 444f
Brachytherapy; see also Radiation therapy.
  for retinoblastoma, 1633
Bradycardia, 217b, 1469
  apnea of prematurity and, 379
  in newborn, 251t
  sinus, 1524-1525
Bradydysrhythmias, 1524-1525
Braille, 1004
Brain; see also under Cerebral.
  abscess of, 1681
  bladder function and, 1259
  blood flow in, 1643-1645
    intracranial pressure and, 1646
  contusions of, 1666
  coverings of, 1642-1643, 1643f
  development of, 1642
  effects of lead on, 678
  gross postnatal disease of, mental
    retardation and, 979b
  growth and development of
    in infants, 494
    in puberty, 809
    in toddlers, 592
  hypoxic-ischemic injury of, perinatal,
    400-401
  imaging of, 1652, 1652f, 1653t-1654t
    in head injury, 1671
  in bilirubin encephalopathy, 304
  in fetal alcohol syndrome, 329
  in hypoglycemia, in newborn, 316, 317
  lacerations of, 1666
  oxygenation of, 1645
  structure and function of, 1643-1645, 1643f,
    1644t
  ventricular system of, 436-437, 437f
Brain death, 965, 1649, 1649b
  organ donation and, 967
Brain hypoglycemia, 1749
Brain injury; see also Cerebral dysfunction.
  assessment of; see Neurologic assessment.
  heart surgery and, 1507
  hypoxic; see Hypoxia.
  in child abuse, 1666
  neurologic assessment in, 225-228,
    226f-228f, 229t, 1646-1654
  nursing care in, 1654-1661
  seizures and, 1685
  traumatic, 1661-1674; see also Head injury.
Brain Injury Association, 1673
Brain scan, 1653t
Brain tumors, 1619-1625
  clinical manifestations of, 1619, 1621t
    assessment for, 1622
  diagnosis of, 1619-1620
    preparation for procedures in, 1622
  family support in, 1624
  infratentorial, 1619
  long-term complications of, 1625
  nursing care for, 1622-1625

Brain tumors—cont'd
  patient/family teaching in, 1622
  rehabilitation in, 1624-1625
  seizures and, 1690
  site of, 1619
  supratentorial, 1619
  surgery for; see also Cranial surgery.
    postoperative management in, 1622-1624
  treatment of, 1619-1622
  types of, 1619, 1620b
Brainstem, 1643
  herniation of, 1665, 1666f
  structure and function of, 1644t
Brainstem auditory evoked potentials, 1652
Brainstem glioma, 1620b; see also Brain
    tumors.
BRAT diet, 1186, 1212
Brazelton Neonatal Behavioral Assessment
    Scale, 245, 245b
  massage and, high-risk newborn and, 362
Breakthrough pain, 1065b
Breast
  development of, 210
    in girls, 805-806, 806f
    premature, 1714-1715
  examination of, 210
    by patient, 210
  of newborn, 260
  pumping of, 520-521
Breast cancer, 210
  presymptomatic testing for, 126-127
Breast masses, 210
Breast milk
  freezing of, 520-521
  storage of, 520
  supplements for, 520
  vegetarian diets and, 565
  warming of, 520
Breast self-examination, 210
Breast-feeding
  advantages of, 273-274, 273b
    infection and, 393
    preterm infant and, 347
  by employed mothers, 520-521
  cleft lip and palate and, 459, 459b
  colic and, 573
  constipation and, 1424
  cow's milk allergy and, 569, 570
  cystic fibrosis and, 1410
  diaper dermatitis and, 578
  diarrhea and, 1212, 1212t, 1213
  facial nerve paralysis and, 300
  family history of atopy and, 569, 569b
  formula versus human milk and, 281t
  growth rates and, 175
  hemorrhagic disease of newborn and, 319
  in first 6 months, 520-521, 524b
  infant botulism and, 1850
  infant sleep patterns and, 525b
  infant weight gain and, 277b
  jaundice associated with, 303t, 305, 309
    home care and, 310, 311b
    management of, 307
  neonatal stools and, 242
  observation of, 277b
  of adopted infants, 90f
  of high-risk newborn, 344, 347-348
  otitis media and, 1357
  pacifier use and, 518, 519

Breast-feeding—cont'd
  phenylketonuria and, 323
  problems with, 276-277, 277b, 278t
  promotion of, 275-276, 275b, 275f, 276f
  rates of, 274
  smoking and, 409
Breath hydrogen test, 1422t
Breath odor, 207
  in diabetes, 1735
  in neurologic assessment, 1650
Breath sounds
  absent/diminished, 212-213
  adventitious, 213, 214t
  after heart surgery, 1504
  liquid ventilation and, 386
  normal, 213b
  vesicular, 213b
Breathing; see also Respiration(s).
  deep
    for auscultation, 213
    play activities and, 1111b
    with bronchial drainage, 1320, 1322, 1323
  in congestive heart failure, 1483
  Kussmaul, 1735
  lung compliance and, 1307, 1307b
  lung tissue resistance and, 1304, 1307, 1307b
  mechanics of, 1307
  mouth, 1353, 1383
  noisy, 1311
  observation of, respiratory distress
    syndrome and, 381, 382f
  regulation of, 1309-1310
  rescue, 1334-1335
Breathing devices
  negative pressure, 1307
  positive pressure, 1307
Breathing exercises
  in asthma, 1393, 1399
  with bronchial drainage, 1322, 1323
Breathing patterns, in neurologic
    assessment, 1650
Breck feeder, cleft lip and palate and, 459
British antilewisite (BAL), for chelation
    therapy, 680, 681
British Sign Language, 998
Brock valvotomy, for pulmonary stenosis, 1496b
Bronchial breath sounds, 213b
Bronchial challenge testing, in asthma, 1390
Bronchial drainage, 1320, 1321f, 1322f, 1323f
  with chest physiotherapy, 1320, 1322, 1323
Bronchioles, 1305
  constriction of, in anaphylaxis, 1224
Bronchiolitis, respiratory syncytial virus, 1366-
    1368, 1366t, 1367b
Bronchitis, 1366, 1366t
Bronchodilators
  for aerosol therapy, 1319
  for bronchopulmonary dysplasia, 391
  in burn patients, 1236
Bronchophony, 213
Bronchopulmonary dysplasia, 390-393
Bronchoscopy, 1315t
Bronchospasm, in asthma
  exercise-induced, 1394-1395
  relief of, 1397-1398
Bronchovesicular breath sounds, 213b
Bronchus(i), 1305
  foreign body obstruction of, 1376
  hyperresponsiveness of, in asthma, 1385, 1386

Bronchus(i)—cont'd
mucus in, in cystic fibrosis, 1401
neural regulation of, 1307
smooth muscle of, vagal stimulation of in
asthma, 1387
Bronze-baby syndrome, 308
Brothers; *see* Siblings.
Brown adipose tissue, 241
Brown fat, 241
Brown fat theory of obesity, 871
Brudzinski sign, 226, 228b
Bruising, 188, 188t, 743, 1798
birth-related, 295-296, 296b
Bruit, abdominal, 219
Brush biopsy, 1315t
Brush border, of small intestine, 1418, 1419f
Brushfield spots, 194
Bryant traction, 1789
Bubble baths, urinary tract infection and, 1265
Bubble test, of fetal lung maturity, 383
Buck extension traction, 1789, 1789f
Bucket handle, in perineal fistula, 468
Budesonide (Pulmicort)
for asthma, 1391
for inflammatory bowel disease, 1440
Buffered lidocaine, 1067, 1067b
Bulb syringe, for patent airway maintenance,
in newborn, 265
Bulbar conjunctiva, 194
Bulbus cordis, 1465
Bulimarexia, 883
Bulimia, 672, 882-884
clinical manifestations of, 878t, 882
complications of, 883
diagnosis of, 883, 883b
in athletes, 1804
in diabetics, 1737b, 1751
nursing considerations in, 883
treatment of, 882-883
Bulla, 744f
Bullous impetigo, 301
Bullying, 707, 795
Bumetanide (Bumex), for congestive heart
failure, 1480t
BUN; *see* Blood urea nitrogen.
Bundle of His, 1467
Bupropion (Wellbutrin), for depression, 798
*Burkholderia cepacia,* infection with, in cystic
fibrosis, 1405, 1408, 1411
Burkitt lymphoma, 1618-1619
Burn shock, 1231, 1237, 1243
Burning, 49b
Burns, 1227-1253
acute care of, 1243
assessment of, 1229-1230
chemical, 1227
of airways in smoke inhalation
injury, 1381
complications of, 1233-1234
prevention of, 1245-1247, 1246f, 1247f
contact, 1227
depth of, 1228-1229, 1228f, 1229f
dressings for, 1235-1236, 1244
electrical, 621, 1227
epidemiology and etiology of, 1227
extent of, 1228, 1228f
full-thickness, 1231
healing of, 1231

Burns—cont'd
hot water immersion (scalding), 621,
1227, 1248
prevention of, 542t, 543t, 547, 549b
immediate first aid for, 1234-1235
in infants, 547-548
in school-age children, 731t
in toddlers, 617t, 620-622, 621f
intentional, 688b
local response to, 1230-1231
major, management of, 1235b,
1236-1238, 1236b
minor, management of, 1235-1236, 1235b
mortality from, 8, 8t
nursing care of, 1242-1248, 1245f-1248f
nursing care plan for, 1249-1252
of eye, 1003b
of various body parts, 1230
pain management for, 1237-1238,
1243-1244, 1244b
partial-thickness, 1231
pathophysiology of, 1230-1234
prevention of, 1248, 1248f, 1252-1253,
1252b, 1758b
in infants, 542t, 543t, 547, 549b
in toddlers, 617t, 620-622, 621f
rehabilitation measures for, 1245-1247
research on, 1253
severity of, 1229-1230, 1230f, 1230t
systemic responses to, 1231-1233
trauma associated with, 1230
zones of injury in, 1230-1231, 1230f, 1231b
Butalbital, in pain management, 1060b
Butterfly rash, in systemic lupus
erythematosus, 1825, 1828

**C**

Cactus spines, removal of, 769
Café-au-lait spots, 301, 773, 773f
in newborn, 251t
Caffeine
for apnea of prematurity, 378-379
for respiratory distress syndrome, 386
in pain management, 1060b
Calcium, 1562t
deficiency of; *see also* Hypocalcemia.
in newborn, 318-319
depletion of, 1177t
excess of; *see* Hypercalcemia.
functions of and disturbances in, 561t
in acid-base imbalance, 1183
in chronic renal failure, 1289, 1290-1291
lead interactions with, 678
recommended intake of, for athletes, 1804
reference ranges for, 1895t
sources of, 561t
supplemental
for hypoparathyroidism, 1722
for premenstrual syndrome, 847
Calcium carbonate, in chronic renal
failure, 1291
Calcium chloride
for cardiopulmonary resuscitation, 1399t
for shock, 1221
Calcium disodium edetate (EDTA), for
chelation therapy, 680-681
Calcium gluconate, for hypocalcemia, in
newborn, 318

Calculi, renal, immobilization and, 1764,
1794-1795
CALLA, 1612
Callus formation, 1782-1783, 1783ff
Caloric intake; *see also* Food(s); Nutrition.
for high-risk newborn, 343, 343t
for weight maintenance, 874t
in acute renal failure, 1285-1287
in cystic fibrosis, 1410
in failure to thrive, 577
in pregnant adolescents, 851
in school-age children, 721
in toddlers, 609
obesity and, 871
Caloric test, 1651
Calyceal obstruction, 485t
Calyx (renal), major and minor, 1256, 1256f
Camphor, as poison, 669
*Campylobacter jejuni,* diarrhea and, 1210t
Canadian Diabetes Association, 1744
Canadian Hearing Society, 997n
Canadian Hemophilia Society, 1565
Canadian National Institute for the Blind, 1003n
Canadian Special Olympics, 983n
Canadian Toy Testing Council, 601
Cancer, 1584-1638
abdominal mass in, 1597
acute tumor lysis syndrome in, 1596
alopecia in, 1602
anemia in, 1599
anorexia in, 1600
as genetic disease, 122, 1585-1586
assessment in, 1597
bleeding in, 1597, 1598-1599
bone, 1626-1629
brain, 1619-1625
breast, 210
presymptomatic testing for, 126-127
constipation in, 1601
cure of, 1585
dental care in, 1601, 1605
diagnosis of, 1587-1588
etiologic factors in, 1585-1587
evaluation in, 1606
family teaching in, 1605-1606
fever in, 1597
genetics of, 111
health promotion in, 1604-1605
hemorrhage in, 1598-1599
hemorrhagic cystitis in, 1595t, 1602
home care in, 1605-1606
hyperleukocytosis in, 1596, 1612
immunizations in, 1605
implementation in, 1598-1606
incidence of, 1585t
infections in, 1597, 1598
in bone marrow transplant, 1603
jaw pain in, 1601
leukemia, 1610-1616
life-threatening complications of, 1596-1597
lymphadenopathy in, 1597, 1617
lymphoma, 1616-1619
mortality in, 1585
mouth care in, 1601
nausea and vomiting in, 1599-1600
neuroblastoma, 1625-1626, 1626b
neurologic complications in, 1601-1602
neutropenia in, 1598

Cancer—cont'd
nursing care in, 1597
nursing care plan for, 1606-1610
nursing diagnoses for, 1597
nutrition in, 1600, 1600b
obstructive symptoms in, 1596-1597
pain in, 1597, 1601, 1604
management of, 1604
penile, 843
planning in, 1598
prevention of, 1586-1587
procedures in, nursing care for, 1603-1604
prognosis of, 1585
patient/family teaching about, 1616
retinoblastoma, 1632-1635, 1632f,
1633b, 1634f
rhabdomyosarcoma, 1631-1632, 1631b, 1631t
staging of, 1587
steroid-induced alterations in, 1602
superior vena cava syndrome in, 1596-1597
symptoms of, 1587, 1597b
terminal, 1606
testicular, 843, 1635
treatment of, 1588-1597
biologic response modifiers in, 1594-1595
bone marrow transplant in, 1595-1596,
1602-1603
chemotherapy in, 1588-1594, 1589t-1593t;
see also Chemotherapy.
complications of, 1596-1597
induction, 1614
intensification (consolidation), 1614
long-term complications of,
1635-1637, 1636t
maintenance, 1614
radiation therapy in, 1594, 1595t
side effects of, 1598-1602
surgery in, 1588
termination of, 1606
Wilms tumor, 1629-1631
Candidiasis, 759-760, 759t
diaper dermatitis and, 578, 579
in newborn, 252t, 300-301
vulvovaginal, 848-849
Candlelighters Childhood Cancer Foundation,
915n, 1605, 1628n
Canes
for ambulation, 1775, 1775f
for blind child, 1003
Canker sore, 664
Cannabis, 886t, 891b, 892
Capillary(ies)
arterial, 1418, 1419f
glomerular, 1256
in burn injuries, 1230-1231
peritubular, 1256
venous, 1418, 1419f
Capillary blood sampling, 1147-1148, 1148f
for high-risk newborn, 338
Capillary filling, 1185-1186
in dehydration, 1179
Capillary hemangioma, 302, 302f
Capillary permeability
edema formation and, 1181
in burn injuries, 1230-1231
Capillary refill time, 215
Captopril (Capoten)
for congestive heart failure, 1479
for hypertension, 1519b

Caput succedaneum, 252t, 296, 297f
Car, heat injury in, 548
Car accidents, 7, 8t
fractures in, 1777
injury prevention for, 1758b, 1759
spinal cord injury in, 1855
Car safety seats, 1758b, 1759
Car seats/restraints, 545-546, 545f, 546f,
1758b, 1759
booster, 618-619, 618f
chronic illness or disability and, 924
convertible, 616, 616f, 618
correct use of, 619, 620b
developmental dysplasia of hip and, 451
newborn discharge and, 288
preterm infant and, 369
universal child safety seat system as,
619, 619f
Carbamazepine, 1691t
in fragile X syndrome, 994
Carbohydrate additives, in treating failure to
thrive, 577
Carbohydrate counting, in diabetes, 1739,
1745, 1747t
Carbohydrates, tooth decay and, 780
Carbon dioxide
blood transport of, 1309
cerebral blood flow and, 1645
in gas exchange, 1308-1309
in lung influence on acid-base balance, 1310
partial pressure of, transcutaneous
monitoring of, 1315
reference ranges for, 1896t
Carbon dioxide narcosis, oxygen-induced, 1319
Carbon monoxide
in burn injuries, 1233
in smoke inhalation injuries, 1381, 1382
Carbonic acid, 1309
in acid-base balance, 1182, 1310
Carboplatin, 1590t
Carboxyhemoglobin, in carbon monoxide
poisoning, 1381, 1381b, 1382
Carcinogens, 1586
Carcinoma; see Cancer.
Cardiac; see also under Heart.
Cardiac arrhythmias; see Arrhythmia(s).
Cardiac assist devices, after heart surgery, 1507
Cardiac catheterization, 1471-1474
complications with, 1472
diagnostic, 1472
electrophysiologic, 1472, 1524
interventional, 1472, 1472t
left-sided (arterial), 1472
nursing care for, 1472-1474, 1473b, 1473f
preparation of child for, 1472-1473, 1473f
right-sided (venous), 1472
Cardiac cycle, 1467
Cardiac decompensation, acute
poststreptococcal glomerulonephritis
and, 1272
Cardiac defects
mixed, 1498, 1499b-1501b, 1499f-1501f
obstructive, 1491-1492, 1492f, 1494b-1496b
with decreased pulmonary blood flow, 1496,
1496f, 1497b-1498b
with increased pulmonary blood flow, 1491,
1492b-1494b, 1492f
Cardiac demands, in congestive heart failure,
1482-1483

Cardiac dullness, 212
Cardiac failure, in acute renal failure,
1286-1287
Cardiac monitoring, in Kawasaki disease, 1516
Cardiac muscle
contractility of, 1468
hypertrophy and dilation of, in congestive
heart failure, 1476-1477
in cardiomyopathy, 1522-1523
Cardiac output
after heart surgery, 1507
compensatory mechanisms for, in congestive
heart failure, 1476-1477
definition of, 1468
in burn injuries, 1231
Cardiac reserve, in congestive heart
failure, 1476
Cardiac septa, development of, 1465, 1465f
Cardiac shunt procedures, for children with
cardiac defects, 1488-1489, 1489f,
1489t, 1497, 1497b, 1498b
Cardiac tamponade, after heart surgery, 1507
Cardiac valves, heart sounds and, 215; see also
Heart sounds.
Cardiac workload, in congestive heart
failure, 1480
Cardiogenic shock, 1219, 1219b
Cardiomegaly, in sickle cell anemia, 1548
Cardiomyopathy, 1522-1523
dilated, 1522
hypertrophic, 1523, 1805
restrictive, 1523
secondary, 1522
Cardiopneumogram, 586
Cardiopulmonary resuscitation, 730, 1333-
1335, 1335f-1337f, 1338
in near-drowning, 1675
parental presence during, 1334b
procedure for, 1334-1335, 1335f-1337f, 1338
one-rescuer, 1335f
two-rescuer, 1336f
terminal illness and, 949t
training in, in schools, 1331b
Cardiovascular disorders, acquired, 1509-1526
Cardiovascular system
immobilization effects on, 1763-1764,
1770t-1771t
in burn injuries, 1231-1232
in nutritional assessment, 167t
of high-risk newborn, 336b
postoperative care of, newborn and,
421t, 423
Cardioversion, for supraventricular
tachycardia, 1526
Carditis, in rheumatic fever, 1511
Care coordination; see Case management.
Care plans; see Nursing care plan.
Caremaps, 15, 16t-18t
Caries; see Dental caries.
Carina, 1305
Carmustine (BCNU), 1593t
Carnation Good Start, 281t
Carotenemia, 188
Carotid bodies, 1309
Carotid pulse, location of, 1335, 1337f, 1338
Carrier status, screening for, 126, 127
Carrier-mediated diffusion, 1418
Cartilage, cricoid, 192f
Caruncles, 223

Carvedilol, for congestive heart failure, 1480
Case management, 15, 16t-18t
  home care and, 1019-1020, 1020b
  special needs child and, 939,
    1019-1020, 1020b
Casec formula, 282t
Casein-hydrolysate formula, 280,
    282t, 283t
  phenylketonuria and, 323
Castration complex, 631
Casts, 1784-1787
  application of, 1785-1786
  care of, 1786b, 1787
  circulatory impairment and, 1793
  compartment syndrome and, 1793
  for clubfoot, 452, 452f, 453
  for developmental dysplasia of hip, 451
  materials for, 1784-1785, 1785t
  petaling of, 1786
  removal of, 1787
  swelling under, 1786
  types of, 1784f
Cat scratch disease, 766-767
Cataract, 1001b
Catecholamines, 1708t, 1724; see also
    Epinephrine; Norepinephrine.
  adrenal secretion of, 1723, 1724
  effects of, 1724, 1724b
  in burn injuries, 1232
  in congestive heart failure, 1477
  in shock, 1219-1220
Catecholamine-secreting tumors, 1724,
    1731-1732
Cathartics, for treatment of poisoning, 673
Catheter(s)
  central venous
    in total parenteral nutrition, 1451, 1452
    long-term, 1200-1203, 1200f, 1201t, 1202f
    peripherally inserted, 1198, 1198t, 1200
    for blood pressure monitoring, of high-risk
      newborn, 337
    for oxygenation monitoring, in respiratory
      distress syndrome, 387
    for parenteral fluid therapy, in high-risk
      newborn, 342
    in acute renal failure, 1285
    in tracheostomy suctioning, 1326, 1327b
    intraventricular, in intracranial pressure
      monitoring, 1656
  multilumen, 1200
  peripheral intravenous; see also Infusion(s),
    intravenous.
    complications with, 1196-1198
    documentation of, 1195b
    insertion and taping of, 1189, 1190,
      1192-1194, 1192b, 1193b
    protection and taping of,
      1194-1196, 1195f
    removal of, 1196
    site for, 1192-1193, 1194f
    teaching about, 1503-1504
  safety, 1190
  short-term (nontunneled), 1198
  Swan-Ganz, 1221
  urinary, 1144-1146, 1145t, 1146b
    hypospadias and, 482
    myelomeningocele and, 429
  urinary tract infection and, 1265

Catheterization
  arterial
    for blood pressure monitoring, of high-
      risk newborn, 337
    for oxygenation monitoring, in
      respiratory distress syndrome, 387
  bladder, 1144-1146, 1145t, 1146b, 1266
    for neurogenic bladder, 1860
    hypospadias and, 482
    in unconscious child, 1659
    myelomeningocele and, 429
  cardiac; see Cardiac catheterization.
  urinary
    for neurogenic bladder, 1860
    in unconscious child, 1659
  venous
    for blood pressure monitoring, of
      high-risk newborn, 337
    for oxygenation monitoring, in
      respiratory distress syndrome, 337
    for parenteral fluid therapy, in high-risk
      newborn, 342
Cation exchange resin, for potassium removal,
    in acute renal failure, 1286
Cats
  ringworm infection and, 760
  safety rules for, 779b
  self-esteem development and, 709
Cat's eye reflex, in retinoblastoma,
    1632-1633, 1632f
Cavernous venous hemangioma, 302
Cavities, dental; see Dental caries.
CCNU (lomustine), 1593t
CDC; see Centers for Disease Control and
    Prevention.
CDP; see Continuous distending pressure.
Cefixime, for gonorrhea, 862
Ceftriaxone
  for otitis media, 1359, 1359b
  intramuscular, 766b
Cefuroxime, for pneumonia, 1370
Ceiling effect, nonopioid analgesics and, 1061
Celecoxib, for juvenile rheumatoid
    arthritis, 1822
Celiac disease, 1450-1451
Celiac sprue, 1450
Celiac Sprue Association/United States of
    America, 1451
Cell(s)
  epithelial
    in wound healing, 747, 747f
    of villi, 1419
  ganglion, 1426
  labile, 745
  permanent, 747
  secretory, of gastrointestinal tract, 1417
  stable, 747
Cell division errors, chromosomal
    abnormalities and, 114-115, 114f
Cell-mediated immunity, 1572
Cellulitis, 754f, 755, 755t
Center for Sickle Cell Disease, 1554n
Center for Substance Abuse Treatment, 893
Centering Corporation, 1108n
Centers for Disease Control and Prevention,
    528, 1132
Central apnea, of prematurity, 378
Central auditory imperception, 995

Central cyanosis, in respiratory distress
    syndrome, 381
Central nervous system
  development of, 1642
  in burn injuries, 1234
  in sickle cell anemia, 1548
Central nervous system depressants,
    abuse of, 892
Central nervous system stimulants
  abuse of, 886t, 892
    by athletes, 1805
  in fragile X syndrome, 994
Central precocious puberty, 1714
Central retinal artery, 195
Central retinal vein, 195
Central venous catheter; see also Venous
    catheterization.
  for parenteral fluid therapy, in high-risk
    newborn, 342
  long-term, 1200-1203, 1200f, 1201t, 1202f
  peripherally inserted, 1198, 1198t, 1200
Central venous line, blood specimen from,
    1147, 1147b, 1147f
Central venous pressure line, after heart
    surgery, 1504-1505
Cephalhematoma, 252t, 297-298, 297f
Cephalopelvic disproportion, 851
Cephalosporin, for pneumonia, 1370
Cereals
  baby, introduction of, 522, 524b
  iron-fortified, 565
Cerebellar astrocytoma, 1619, 1620b; see also
    Brain tumors.
Cerebellar function, assessment of, 226, 226b
Cerebellar gait, 1647b
Cerebellum, structure and function of, 1644t
Cerebral blood flow, 1643-1645
  intracranial pressure and, 1646
Cerebral dysfunction, 1641-1701
  abnormal movements in, 225, 1647,
    1647f, 1651
  altered consciousness in, 1647-1649; see also
    Consciousness.
  assessment in, 1655; see also Neurologic
    assessment.
  comfort measures in, 1655
  decerebrate posturing in, 1651, 1651b, 1651f
  decorticate posturing in, 1651, 1651b, 1651f
  diabetes insipidus in, 1658
  diagnostic procedures in, 1652-1654,
    1653t-1654t
  etiology of, 1647
  evaluation in, 1661
  eye movements in, 1650, 1651, 1652
  gait abnormalities in, 1647, 1647b
  hypoxic; see Hypoxia.
  implementation in, 1656-1661
  in head injury, 1661-1674
  in near-drowning, 1674-1676
  increased intracranial pressure and, 1645-
    1646, 1656-1658; see also Intracranial
    pressure, increased.
  motor function in, 1647, 1647b, 1651
  neurologic assessment in, 1646-1652, 1655;
    see also Neurologic assessment.
  nursing care in, 1654-1661
  nursing diagnoses for, 1655-1656
  pain management in, 1655

Cerebral dysfunction—cont'd
  papilledema in, 195, 1651
  planning in, 1656
  pupils in, 1650-1651, 1650f
  reflexes in, 226, 226f, 227f, 1650, 1651-1652
  soft signs in, 228, 229b
  syndrome of inappropriate antidiuretic
      hormone in, 1658
  vital signs in, 1649-1650
Cerebral edema, 1181, 1645-1646, 1645b; see
      also Intracranial pressure, increased.
  after cranial surgery, 1623
  after heart surgery, 1507
  in head injury, 1665, 1668-1669
  treatment of, 1657
Cerebral hypoxia; see Hypoxia.
Cerebral palsy, 1834-1843
  associated problems in, 1836-1837
  ataxic, 1835b
  birth weight and, 1834, 1835
  classification of, 1835, 1835t
  clinical manifestations of, 1835-1837, 1836b
  developmental delay in, 1835-1836
  diagnosis of, 1837-1838
  dyskinetic/athetoid, 1835b
  dystonic, 1835b
  educational concerns in, 1841
  etiology of, 1834-1835, 1834t
  family concerns in, 1842, 1843b
  feeding problems in, 1840-1841, 1841f
  head control in, 1842
  health maintenance in, 1842
  hospitalization in, 1842-1843
  mixed type, 1835b
  mobilizing devices in, 1384f, 1838
  motor abnormalities in, 1836
  nursing care in, 1842-1843
  nursing care plan for, 1844-1845
  occupational therapy for, 1840-1841,
      1841f, 1842
  pathophysiology of, 1833f, 1835
  physical therapy for, 1840, 1842
  prevalence of, 1834
  recreational needs in, 1841-1842
  reflexes in, 1836, 1837
  spastic, 1835b
  speech therapy in, 1841
  surgery for, 1838-1839
  technical aids for, 1839-1840
  therapeutic interventions for,
      1838-1843, 1838b
  warning signs for, 1837, 1838b
Cerebral perfusion pressure, 1643
Cerebral ventricular circulation, 436-437, 437f
Cerebrospinal fluid, 436-437, 437f
  accumulation of; see also Hydrocephalus.
    mechanisms of, 437
  in aseptic meningitis, 1681t
  in bacterial meningitis, 1679, 1681t
  intracranial pressure and, 1645; see also
      Intracranial pressure.
  leukocytes in, reference ranges for, 1899t
  reference ranges for, 1896t
Cerebrovascular accident
  cyanosis and, 1487, 1488
  in sickle cell anemia, 1548, 1550, 1555
Cerebrum, structure and function of, 1644t
Cerebyx (fosphenytoin), 1690

Cerumen, removal of, 200-201
Cervical esophagostomy, 464, 465
Cervical nodes, 190, 190f; see also Lymph node(s).
  enlarged, 664
Cervical tongs, 1790-1791, 1790f
Cervical traction, 1790-1792, 1890f; see also
      Traction.
Cervical vertebrae; see also Neck; Spine;
      Vertebrae.
  fracture/dislocation of, 1852
    spinal cord injury in, 1852-1863; see also
        Spinal cord injury.
Cetirizine hydrochloride (Zyrtec), for allergic
      rhinitis, 1384
Chalazion, 193b
Challenge testing
  for allergic rhinitis, 1384
  for asthma, 1390
  for cow's milk allergy, 569
Changing table, falls from, 542t, 543t, 546, 549b
Charcoal, activated
  complications with, 673
  for gastric decontamination with
      poisoning, 673
Cheating, in school-age children, 717
Cheese, for infants, 522, 524b
Cheiloplasty, 460
Chelation therapy
  blood transfusions and, 1551, 1558
  for heavy metal poisoning, 675
  for lead poisoning, 680-681, 682b
Chemet (succimer), for chelation therapy, 680
Chemical agents
  contact dermatitis and, 767
  injury from, in newborn, 326
  physical abuse and, 688b
  skin disorders and, 767-772
Chemical assay, in compliance
      measurement, 1120
Chemical burns, 1227; see also Burns.
  in smoke inhalation injury, 1380, 1381
  of eye, 1003b
Chemical dot thermometers, 178, 183t
Chemoreceptor(s)
  breathing regulation and, 1309
  trigger zone of, 1218, 1218b
Chemotherapy, 1589-1594
  alkylating agents in, 1588, 1589t-1590t
  antimetabolites in, 1588, 1590t-1591t
  clinical trials of, 1588
  extravasation in, 1589
  for aplastic anemia, 1561
  for brain tumors, 1620-1621
  for Ewing sarcoma, 1628
  for Hodgkin disease, 1617-1618
  for leukemia, 1614-1615
  for neuroblastoma, 1626
  for non-Hodgkin's lymphoma, 1619
  for osteosarcoma, 1627
  for rhabdomyosarcoma, 1632
  for Wilms tumor, 1630
  immunizations in, 1605
  plant alkaloids in, 1588, 1591t-1592t
  protocols for, 1588
  safe drug handling in, 1594b
  side effects/toxicity of, 1589t-1593t,
      1596-1602
    long-term, 1635-1637, 1636t

Chemotherapy—cont'd
  terminal illness and, 949t
  vesicant injury in, 1589
Chemstrip-BG, 317
Chest; see also under Thoracic.
  anatomy of, 208-210, 208f, 1302, 1302f
  asymmetry of, 209-210
  auscultation of
    for heart sounds, 215-217, 216b,
        216f, 216t
    for lung sounds, 212-213, 213b, 214t
  barrel, 209, 1302, 1389, 1397, 1406
  cardiac position in, 214, 214f
  changes in during respiration, 1304, 1304f
  Down syndrome and, 989t
  examination of, 208-213
  funnel, 209
  growth of
    in infants, 494
    in toddlers, 592
  in nutritional assessment, 167t
  landmarks of, 209, 209f, 210
  measurement of, 176f, 209
  movements of, 210, 210f, 211
  of newborn, 253t, 260
    at high risk, 336b
  palpation of, 211-212, 214-215
  percussion of, 212
    with bronchial drainage, 1320, 1323f
  retractions of, 210, 1310, 1311f
    in congestive heart failure, 1478
  shape of, 209-210
  structures of, 1302, 1302f
Chest circumference, of newborn, 251t, 255
Chest compression, finger or hand position
      for, 1337f, 1338
Chest examination, in asthma, 1388-1389
Chest muscles, retraction of, 210
Chest pain
  in assessment of breathing, 1311
  in pulmonary artery hypertension, 1490
Chest physiotherapy, 1320, 1320b,
      1322-1323
  for asthma, 1393
  for cystic fibrosis, 1407-1408, 1411
Chest radiography
  cardiac function and, 1469
  in asthma, 1390
  in bronchopulmonary dysplasia, 391
  in respiratory distress syndrome, 383
Chest retractions, 210
Chest syndrome, in sickle cell anemia,
      1550, 1555
Chest thrusts, in infant, 1337f, 1338
Chest tubes
  drainage from
    after heart surgery, 1505
    in pneumonia, 1370-1371
  in heart surgery, 1505
  in pneumonia, 1370-1371
  removal of, 1505
  teaching about, 1504
Chest wall excursion, in burn patients, 1233-
      1234, 1236
Chestpiece, for stethoscope, 212
Chewing, 1417, 1418
Chewing tobacco, 887

Chiari malformation, 425-426, 427
  hydrocephalus and, 438t
Chickenpox; *see also* Varicella; Varicella-zoster
  virus.
  acyclovir for, 651b
  complications with, 651, 660
  immunization for, 529t, 541b, 651
  in immunocompromised patient, 1605
  in newborn, 327t
  manifestations and management of, 652f,
    652t-653t
Chiggers, 776t
Chilblains, 770
Child abuse, 683-694, 685, 691
  assessment data in, recording of, 692b
  brain injury in, 1666, 1668
  burns and, 1227
  cultural factors in, 48
  definition of, 683
  discharge planning in, 693
  emotional, 683-684
    identification of, 687, 688b
    in adolescents, 832-833
    in infants, 505
  head injury in, 1669
  history of incident and, 690-691
  identification of, 10, 687-689, 687b,
    688b, 689b
  in adolescents, 832-833; *see also* Sexual abuse.
  in early childhood, 684-685
  nursing care of, 687-694
  nursing care plan for, 694-696
  prevention of, 693
  protection of child from further abuse, 692
  recognition of, 1758b
  retinal hemorrhage in, 1668, 1669
  sexual, 685-687; *see also* Sexual abuse.
  spinal cord injury in, 1856
  types of, 683
  vs folk remedies, 48
  vs osteogenesis imperfecta, 1820
  warning signs of, 690b
Child Abuse Prevention and Treatment
  Act, 683
Child care, 99, 100b; *see also* Daycare facilities.
  education for, 853
  for sick child, 100
  selection of caretaker for, 516-518
  types of, 516
Child health care
  access to, 41
  atraumatic, 15
  barriers to, 13
  case management in, 15, 16t-18t
  demographic trends affecting, 24
  evidence-based practice in, 14b, 22
  evolution of, 11-13
  family-centered, 13-15, 14b
  financial aspects of, 13
  government services for, 12-13
  legislation affecting, 12-13
  managed care and, 13
  philosophy of, 13-15
  therapeutic, 15
Child maltreatment; *see* Child abuse; Sexual
  abuse.
Child neglect, 683-684
Child pornography, 685
Child prostitution, 686

Child Protective Services, 692
Child safety seats, 545-546, 545f, 546f; *see also*
  Car seats/restraints.
Childbirth; *see also* under Perinatal.
  history of, 155
  prolonged, in adolescents, 851
Childhood hysteria, 797
Child-life specialists, 1084
Children; *see also* Adolescent; Infant;
    Preschooler; School-age child; Toddler.
  bilingual, 599
  communication with, 147-153, 147b; *see also*
    Communication.
    developmental level and, 147-150, 147b
    techniques of, 150-153, 151b-152b
    gifted/talented, 640-641, 641b
Children's Hospice International, 956n
Children's Hospital of Eastern Ontario Pain
  Scale, 1056t
Children's Liver Association for Support
  Services, 472
Chill phase of fever, 1130
Chin lift, 1334, 1337f
Chlamydial infection, 862-863, 863t
  conjunctivitis and, 662
  in newborn, 327t
  pelvic inflammatory disease and, 863
  pneumonia and, 1371
  vs gonorrhea, 862t
Chloral hydrate
  for neurologic diagnostic procedures, 1652-
    1654, 1655b
  hydrocephalus diagnosis and, 442
  in preoperative sedation, 1113b
Chlordiazepoxide, abuse of, 886t
Chlorhexidine, 1190
Chloride
  functions of and disturbances in, 561t
  in cystic fibrosis, 1401, 1407
  reference ranges for, 1896t
  sources of, 561t
Chlorothiazide (Diuril), for congestive heart
  failure, 1480t
Chlor-pheniramine (Chlor-Trimeton), for
  allergic rhinitis, 1384
Chlor-Trimeton (chlor-pheniramine), for
  allergic rhinitis, 1384
Choking
  in infants, 542, 544
  management of, 1337f, 1338,
    1340-1341, 1340f
Choking reflex, 1309
Cholecalciferol
  functions of and disturbances of, 559t
  sources of, 559t
Cholecystokinin, 1418
Cholesteatoma, otitis media and, 1358
Cholesterol
  elevated serum, 1519-1520
  reference ranges for, 1896t
Cholestipol (Colestid), for
  hypercholesterolemia, 1521
Cholestyramine (Questran), for
  hypercholesterolemia, 1521
Choline magnesium trisalicylate, in pain
  management, 1061t
Chordae tendineae, 1465
Chordee, 254t, 481-482
Chorea, in rheumatic fever, 1511-1513

Choreiform movements, 1647b
Chorionic villus sampling, 128t, 130
  in hemolytic disease of newborn, 312, 314
  skeletal limb deficiency and, 453-454
Christmas disease, 1562
Christmas factor, 1562t
Chromium
  functions of and disturbances in, 561t
  sources of, 561t
Chromosome(s), 111
  karyotyping of, 123, 123f
  nondisjunction of, 114-115, 114f
  Philadelphia, 1585
  ring, 113
  sex, abnormalities of, 116-118
  translocations of, 115-116, 115f
  X, 116-117
    inactivation of, 117
  Y, 117
Chromosome abnormalities; *see also* specific
    abnormalities.
  causes of, 113-114
  cell division errors and, 114-115, 114f, 115f
  deletional, 116, 116t
  duplication, 116
  in cancer, 1585-1586
  in leukemia, 1612
  mental retardation in, 979b
    in Down syndrome, 989
    in fragile X syndrome, 993
  numeric, 113, 114-115
  partial, 116
  radiation exposure and, 330
  sex chromosome, 116-118
  structural, 113, 115-116, 115f
Chromosome disorders
  causes of, 113-114
  chromosome abnormalities in; *see*
    Chromosome abnormalities.
  definition of, 113
Chronic adrenocortical insufficiency,
  1725, 1726c
Chronic benign neutropenia, 1569t
Chronic illness, 905-945; *see also* Special needs
    child and specific illness.
  school nurse's role in, 730
  sports participation in, 725
Chronic illness trajectory model, 932
Chronic lung disease; *see* Bronchopulmonary
    dysplasia.
Chronic myelogenous leukemia; *see also*
    Leukemia.
  Philadelphia chromosome in, 1585
Chronic sorrow, 136
Chvostek sign, 1721
Chylomicrons, 1520
Chyme, 1418
Chymotrypsin, 1418
Cigarette smoking; *see* Smoking.
Ciliary action, as respiratory tract
    defense, 1310
Ciliary muscles, of newborn, 243
Cimetidine (Tagamet)
  for gastroesophageal reflux, 1429
  for peptic ulcer disease, 1445
Circular reaction(s)
  primary, 502-503, 503t
  secondary, 503, 503t
  tertiary, 595

Circulation; *see also* Blood flow.
  cerebral ventricular, 436-437, 437f
  fetal, 1466, 1466f
    persistent, 397-398, 398f
  in burn injuries, 1231, 1234
  portal, in absorption, 1419
  prenatal vs postnatal, 1466, 1466f, 1467
Circulatory impairment, in immobilized/
    casted part, 1763-1764, 1793
Circulatory overload, from blood
    transfusion, 1541t
Circulatory system; *see also* Blood flow; Blood
    vessels; Vascular; specific parts or
    disorders.
  in puberty, 809
  neonatal, 241
    postoperative care of, 420t
    sepsis and, 394b
Circumcision, 270-273, 270b-272b, 272f, 843
  female, 49b, 223, 272b
  hemorrhagic disease of newborn and, 319
  pain from, memory of, 354-355
  urinary tract infection and, 1265
Circumstraint board, 271b, 272f
Cirrhosis, 1460-1461, 1461b
Cisapride (Propulsid), for gastroesophageal
    reflux, 1429
Cisplatin (platinol), 1590t
Cisterna magna, 436, 437f
Citrovorum factor, functions of and
    disturbances in, 557t
Claritin (loratadine), for allergic rhinitis, 1384
Class, social, 35-36
Classification skills, in children, 704
Clavicle, fracture of, 1777
  birth-related, 298
CLD (chronic lung disease); *see*
    Bronchopulmonary dysplasia.
Clean intermittent catheterization,
    myelomeningocele and, 429
Clean-catch urine specimens, 1144
Cleft lip/cleft palate, 454-463, 455t
  assessment of, 458
  diagnosis of, 455-456, 456f, 457f
  discharge planning and home care for, 462
  etiology of, 454-455
  long-term problems with, 457-458
  nursing care plan for, 461-462
  nursing considerations in, 458-463, 459b, 459f
  pathophysiology of, 455, 456f
  preoperative care in, 459-460
  treatment of, 456-458
Cleft Lip/Cleft Palate Nurser, 459
Cleft Palate Foundation, 460
Clinical Adaptive Text–Clinical Linguistic and
    Auditory Milestone Scale, 234t
Clinical judgment, in compliance
    measurement, 1119
Clinical nurse specialist, 20
Clinical pathways, 15, 16t-18t
Clinical practice guidelines, 15, 18b
Clinical trials, chemotherapy, 1588
Clinics, school-based and school-linked,
    822-823
Clitorectomy, 223
Clitoris, 222, 222f
  ambiguous genitalia and, 489t
  of newborn, 261
    prematurity and, 377f

Cloaca, 468
  persistent, 466, 468f
Clonazepam, for seizures, 1691t
Clonic seizures, in newborn, 404t
Clonidine
  for attention deficit hyperactivity
      disorder, 789
  for Tourette syndrome, 793
Closed captioning, 998
Closed family, 66
Closed fracture, 1778, 1779f
Closed-diaphragm (Bowles) chestpiece, 212
Closed-ended questions, 144
Clostridial diarrhea, 1210t
Clostridium botulinum, 1850
Clot retraction test, 1562t
Clothing
  falls and, 622
  mental retardation and, 985-986
  safety precautions with, 542t, 543t, 546,
      548, 549b
  selection of, atopic dermatitis and, 581, 582
Clotrimazole, for candidiasis, in newborn, 301
Clotting factors, 1561, 1562t; *see also*
    Coagulation; specific factors.
  transfusion of, 1543t
  vitamin K deficiency and, 319
Clotting time, reference ranges for, 1896t
Clozapine, for schizophrenia, side effects
    of, 799
Clubbing
  hypoxemia and, 1486, 1487f
  in assessment of breathing, 1311, 1311f
  of nails, 189
Clubfoot, 451-453, 452b, 452f
Cluster designations, T-lymphocyte, 1572
Coaches, of sports teams, 725
Coagulation
  clotting factors and; *see* Clotting factors.
  disseminated intravascular, 1567-1568,
      1568b, 1568f
    hemolysis and, 1540
  hemostatic disorders and, 1561-1568
  laboratory tests of, 1562t
  vitamin K and, 266-267
Coagulation necrosis, in burn injuries, 1231
Coanalgesics, 1060-1061
Coarctation of aorta, 220, 1494b-1495b, 1494f
Cobalamin, functions of and disturbances in,
    557t-558t
Co-bedding, of multiples, 362-363, 362f
Cocaine
  adolescent abuse of, 886t, 890-892, 891b
  intrauterine exposure to, 407-408
Coccidioidomycosis, 764t
Cochlear implant, 996
Cockroaches, asthma control and, 1390
Code of Ethics for Nurses (ANA), 22b
Codeine
  in pain management, 1060b, 1062t, 1063t
  with acetaminophen, after heart surgery, 1506
Coenzymes, vitamins as, 554
Cognitive development, 225, 230t,
    231-232, 235
  in adolescents, 804t, 809-811, 852
  in infants, 502-504, 503t
  in preschoolers, 631, 639t
  in school-age children, 702-704, 703f
  in toddlers, 594-597, 595t

Cognitive function, in cerebral palsy, 1836
Cognitive impairment, 977-994; *see also* Mental
    retardation.
Cognitive power, 1647
Coining, 49b
Cold application
  for earache in otitis media, 1360
  for musculoskeletal injuries, 1800, 1800f
  in hemophilia, 1565
  in respiratory infections, 1346
Cold injury, 770-771
Cold sores, 664, 758t
Cold stress; *see also* Hypothermia.
  in high-risk newborn, 338-341, 339f, 340f
Colds (viral nasopharyngitis), 1350-1351
  vs allergies, 1385
Colectomy, subtotal, for inflammatory bowel
    disease, 1441
Colestasis, with total parenteral nutrition, 1452
Colestid (cholestipol), for
    hypercholesterolemia, 1521
Colfosceril surfactant, 386
Colic, 571-574
  management of, 572-573, 572b, 573b
  renal, 486
Colitis, 1438-1439
Collaboration
  in home care, 1022-1023, 1023b
  professional, 21
    for special needs child, 937-938, 937b,
        938b, 938t
Collaborative Family Health Care
    Coalition, 1022
Collagen
  in bladder wall, 1259
  in wound healing, 747
  suburethral injection of, 429-430
Collagen diseases, dermis and, 740
Collecting duct, of nephron, 1256, 1256f
Collective monologue, of toddlers, 596
Colloidal osmotic (oncotic) pressure, 1256
  edema formation and, 1181
Colloids
  for burn patients, 1236
  for shock states, 1221
Coloboma, 194
Colocolic intussusception, 1448
Colon; *see also* Bowel; Intestine(s).
  absorption by, 1419
  development of, 1417
  gastroschisis and, 473, 473f
  necrotizing enterocolitis of; *see* Necrotizing
      enterocolitis.
  palpation of, 220
Colony-stimulating factors
  for neutropenia, 1568-1569
  in cancer, 1598
Color Tool, in pain assessment, 1053t
Color vision, assessment of, 199-200
Colostomy, 469, 470, 1166
  with Hirschsprung disease, 1427, 1428
Colostrum, physiologic jaundice and, 305
Colposcope, in genital examination, 689b
Coma; *see also* Cerebral dysfunction;
    Unconsciousness.
  assessment in, 1647-1649, 1649f
  barbiturate, 1658-1659
  definition of, 1647

Coma—cont'd
  diagnostic procedures in, 1652-1654,
    1653t-1654t
  irreversible, 1649, 1649b
  neurologic assessment in, 225-228, 226f-
    228f, 229t, 1646-1652, 1655
  nursing care in, 1654-1661
  nursing care plan for, 1662-1664
  recovery from, 1660-1661, 1660b
Combination contraceptive injection, for
    contraception, 855, 856t
Combinational skills, 704
Comedones, 840, 840f
Comfort measures; see specific disorders.
Comic books, 39
Comminuted fracture, 1778
Commissions for the Blind, 1002
Committee on Infectious Diseases (AAP), 528
Common acute lymphocytic leukemia antigen
    (CALLA), 1612
Communal family, 72
Communicable diseases; see also Infection(s).
  comfort measures for, 660-661
  in early childhood, nursing considerations
    with, 649-651, 660-662, 662b-663b
  nursing care plan for, 662b-663b
  prevention of complications of, 651, 660
  prevention of spread of, 650-651
  support for child and family in, 661
  terminology of, 650b
Communicating hydrocele; see Hydrocele.
Communicating hydrocephalus, 437, 438t;
    see also Hydrocephalus.
Communication, 139-153; see also Interview.
  abstract, 139
  anticipatory guidance in, 145
  barriers to, 145, 145b
  cultural factors in, 44-45, 144
  deaf-blindness and, 1006
  definition of, 139
  directing focus in, 144
  empathy in, 145
  guidelines for, 141-142
  guiding statements in, 144
  hearing impairment and, 997-999,
    997f, 998b
  language development and, 148, 148b
  listening in, 144-145
  mental retardation and, 981-982
  nonverbal, 139, 140
    techniques of, 152b
  open-ended questions in, 143-144
  problem definition in, 145
  problem solving in, 145
  setting for, 141
  silence in, 145
  social class and, 36
  through interpreter, 145-146, 146b
  verbal, 139, 140; see also Language; Speech.
  via play, 150-153, 152b
  with children, 147-153, 147b
    developmental level and, 147-150, 147b
    techniques of, 150-153, 151b-152b
  with Native Americans, 37
  with parents, 143-147
Communication aids, 1840
Communication impairment, 1007-1013
  assessment of, 1011-1012, 1011t, 1012b
  autism and, 1008-1010, 1009b

Communication impairment—cont'd
  classification of, 1007
  education and, 1013
  etiology of, 1007
  language disorders in, 1007, 1007b
  nonspeech communication and, 1007-1008
  prevention of, 1010-1011, 1011b
  referral in, 1012-1013, 1013b
  speech disorders in, 1007, 1008b, 1008f
Community
  adolescent health behavior and, 819-820, 823
  definition of, 103
Community care, definition of, 104
Community health nursing, 12, 103-109
  definition of, 104
  demographics in, 104
  economic factors in, 106
  epidemiology in, 104-106
  nurse's roles and functions in, 104
  nursing process in, 106-108, 108b
  prevention in, 105
  screening in, 106
Community resources, special needs child
    and, 938-939
Community-based health-driven system, 23
Compartment syndromes, 1793-1794
  in burn injuries, 1231
Compassionate Friends, 370, 971
Competence, age of majority and, 1102
Complement, 1572
  in acute poststreptococcal
    glomerulonephritis, 1273
Complementary medicine
  cultural aspects of, 48-49
  mineral and vitamin excess and, 555, 565
  nursing admission history and,
    1087-1088, 1090b
Complete atrioventricular canal, pulmonary
    artery hypertension and, 1490
Complete blood count, 1535, 1536t
  in asthma diagnosis, 1390
  shift to the left on, 1534
Complete heart block, 1524-1525, 1524f
Complex partial seizures, 1686-1687,
    1687t, 1695b
Compliance, 1118-1121, 1118b, 1120b
  in peptic ulcer disease, 1445
  of lung tissue, 1304, 1307, 1307b
Compound fractures, 1778, 1779f
  of skull, 1667
Compound nevus, 302
Compresses
  cool, 752
  for conjunctivitis, 663
  wet, for skin lesions, 752-753
Compression neuropathy, 1765-1766, 1793
Computed tomography
  in developmental dysplasia of hip, 449
  in hydrocephalus, 439, 439f
  in obesity, 874
  of brain, 1652, 1653t
  of gastrointestinal tract, 1421t
Computers, privacy concerns for, 142
Comvax vaccines, 533, 540t
Concentration gradient, for sodium, 1257
Conceptual thinking, 702
Concha
  of ear, 200, 200f
  of nose, 206, 206f

Concrete operational stage, 230t, 231-232, 702
Concussion, 1666
  complications of, 1670
Conditioning therapy, for treatment of
    enuresis, 784
Condoms
  adolescent use of, 850, 855, 856t, 857b
  female, 855
  sexually transmitted diseases and, 861
Conduct disorder, 686b
Conduction system, of heart, 1467, 1467f
Conductive hearing loss, 995; see also Hearing
    impairment.
  treatment of, 995-996
Conductive hearing tests, 205t
Conductive heat loss, in newborn, 265
  at high risk, 340
Condyloma acuminatum, 864
Confidentiality
  of computerized information, 142
  of HIV diagnosis, 1577
  of interview, 141-142
    with adolescent, 824-825, 825b, 826b, 854
Confirming behaviors, 140
Conflict theory, family, 67t
Conformity, in school-age children, 706,
    707, 711
Confusion, 1648b
Confusional migraine, 1700b
Congenital abnormalities, 111-113, 415-490; see
    also Developmental defects and specific
    types.
  alcohol-related, 329
  burden of, 136-137
  consanguinity and, 134
  Down syndrome and, 990
  environmental factors in, 111
  genetic factors in, 111-112, 111-113
  neonatal screening for, 267-268, 267b
  nongenetic causes of, 124
  obesity and, 871
  parental counseling for, 135-136
    barriers to, 137
  teratogens and, 124
  treatment and prevention of, 124-125
Congenital adrenocortical hyperplasia,
    487-488, 1729-1731
Congenital aganglionic megacolon
    (Hirschsprung disease), 1426-1429, 1426f
Congenital clubfoot, 451-453, 452b, 452f
Congenital diaphragmatic hernia, 475-477
Congenital disability, 906b
Congenital heart disease, 1474-1509; see also
    Heart disease, congenital.
Congenital hypothyroidism, 320-322
Congenital neutropenia, 1569t
Congenital rubella, 328t
Congenital syphilis, 328t
Congenital torticollis, 446
Congestive heart failure, 1476-1484
  after heart surgery, 1507
  cardiomyopathy and, 1522, 1523
  causes of, 1476
  clinical manifestations of, 1477-1479, 1478b
  compensatory mechanisms in, 1476-1477
  congenital heart disease categories and,
    1475, 1476f
  diagnosis of, 1479
  home care of, 1484

Congestive heart failure—cont'd
　left-sided, 1476
　nursing care of, 1481-1484
　nursing care plan for, 1485-1486
　pathophysiology of, 1476-1477, 1477f
　right-sided, 1476, 1478
　transposition of great arteries and, 1499b
　treatment of, 1479-1481
Conjugated bilirubin glucuronide, 304
Conjunctiva
　bulbar, 194
　examination of, in nutritional
　　assessment, 166t
　palpebral, 193
Conjunctivitis, 1002
　bacterial, 662-664, 664b
　in erythema multiforme exudativum, 773
　infectious, of newborn, 259, 266, 266b
Conotruncal anomaly face syndrome,
　　congenital heart disease and, 1474
Consanguinity, 65, 120, 134
Conscience, 230
　in preschoolers, 630
　in toddlers, 594
Conscious sedation, 1108
Consciousness
　altered, 1647-1649; see also Cerebral
　　dysfunction; Coma; Unconsciousness.
　　in near-drowning, 1676t
　　neurologic assessment in, 225-228, 226f-
　　　228f, 229t, 1646-1654
　　nursing care in, 1654-1661
　assessment of, 225, 1647-1649, 1648b, 1648f;
　　see also Neurologic assessment.
　components of, 1647
　levels of, 1648b
　reticular formation and, 1647
Conservation, concept of (Piaget), 702-704, 703f
Constipation, 1424-1426, 1425b
　causes of, 1424
　chronic, 1425
　corn syrup for, 1850
　encopresis and, 785, 786
　idiopathic (functional), 1424
　immobilization and, 1764
　in cancer, 1601
　in cerebral palsy, 1837
　in cystic fibrosis, 1410
　in gastrointestinal obstructive disorders,
　　1446
　in unconscious child, 1659
　opioid-induced, 1067-1068
　urinary tract infection and, 1265, 1268b
Constitutional growth delay, 1710
Consumer Product Safety Commission
　　(CPSC), 11
Consummatory behavior, in newborn, feeding
　　and, 279-280
Consumption coagulopathy; see Disseminated
　　intravascular coagulation.
Contact dermatitis, 767
Contact lenses, 1005-1006
Contact precautions, 1133b, 1134-1135, 1134b
Contact sports, 1796b; see also Sports.
Contagion suicides, 896, 900, 901b
Contiguous gene syndromes, 116
Continence
　disorders of, 780-786; see also Incontinence.
　urinary, 1259-1260

Continuous distending pressure, in respiratory
　　distress syndrome, 383, 384f
Continuous passive motion device, 1800
Continuous positive airway pressure
　in respiratory distress syndrome,
　　383-384, 384f
　ventilation with, 1323
Continuous quality improvement, 28
Contraception
　after abortion, 854
　emergency, 855, 856t
　for adolescents, 850, 854-858
　mental retardation and, 982
　methods of, 854-855, 855b, 856t, 857
　sexually transmitted disease prevention and,
　　861, 866
Contraceptive pill, oral; see Oral contraceptive
　　pill.
Contractility, cardiac, 1468
　in congestive heart failure, 1476
Contracting
　compliance and, 1121
　in anorexia nervosa, 880
　in pain management, 1059b
Contracture(s)
　adduction, developmental dysplasia of hip
　　and, 450
　in burn patients, 1245
　in immobilization, 1763
　in muscular dystrophy, 1865
　in wound healing, 747
　Volkmann, 1794
Contrast agent, water-soluble, in treatment of
　　intussusception, 1449
Contrecoup injury, 1665, 1665f
Contusions
　cerebral, 1666
　in athletes, 1798
　in fractures, 1780
Convective heat loss, in newborn, 265,
　　339-340, 341f
Conversion reaction, 797
Convertible safety seat, 732
Convulsions; see Epilepsy; Seizures.
Cool temperature therapy, for croup, 1364
Cooley anemia, 1557
Coombs test, in hemolytic disease of
　　newborn, 314
Coordination, assessment of, 226
Coping Health Inventory for Parents, 921
Coping mechanisms
　for Down syndrome diagnosis, 991, 991b
　in chronic illness or disability, 917-920,
　　917b-920b, 931-932, 932b
　in middle childhood, 718
　in posttraumatic stress disorder, 794
Copper
　functions of and disturbances in, 561t
　sources of, 561t
Copycat suicides, 896, 900, 901b
Cor pulmonale, 1476
Cords, infant strangulation and, 542t-543t,
　　545, 549b
Corium, of skin, 740
Corn syrup, infant botulism and, 1850
Cornea, 194
Corneal light reflex test, 195-196, 196f
Corneal reflex, 1650
　in newborn, 259, 263t

Corneal ulceration, with burn wounds, 1244
Cornstarch, 544
　for control of diaper dermatitis, 579
Coronary artery(ies), 1467
　disease of, lipid or cholesterol and, 1519
　in Kawasaki disease, 1514
Coronary sinus, in embryologic
　　development, 1465
Coronary thrombosis, in Kawasaki
　　disease, 1515
Coronary veins, 1467
Corporal punishment, 88
　in schools, 715b
Corpus callosum, 1643
Corrigan pulse, 217b
Corrosives, poisoning with, 670b, 672b
Cortical blindness, in head trauma, 1670
Cortical necrosis, 1284
Corticosteroids; see Glucocorticoids; Steroids.
Corticosterone, 1708t
　effects of, 1724b
　regulation of, 1723-1724
Corticotropin, in infants, 497
Corticotropin-releasing factor (CRF), 1723
Cortisol, 1708t
　effects of, 1724b
　hypersecretion of, in Cushing syndrome,
　　1727-1729, 1727b, 1727f, 1728t
　hyposecretion of, 1726t
　　acute, 1725
　　chronic, 1726
　　congenital adrenal hyperplasia and,
　　　1729-1731
　measurement of, 1728
　regulation of, 1723-1724
Cortisone, for congenital adrenal hyperplasia,
　　1729-1730
Corynebacterium, otitis externa and, 1361
Co-sleeping in family bed, 527b, 646b
　sudden infant death syndrome and, 583
Cosmegen (dactinomycin), 1592t
Costal angle, 208f, 209
Costal retractions, 1310, 1311f
　in congestive heart failure, 1478
Costal surface, of lung, 210, 211f
Cost-effectiveness analysis, 106
Cotinine, in children of smoking parents, 1382
Cotrel-Dubousset system, for scoliosis, 1813
Cough
　as respiratory tract defense, 1310
　in assessment of breathing, 1311-1312,
　　1311b, 1312b
　in asthma, 1388
　in chest physiotherapy, 1322
　in congestive heart failure, 1478
　in croup syndromes, 1361, 1364
　in cystic fibrosis, 1406
　in foreign body aspiraton, 1377
　in pneumonia, 1370
　in spinal cord injury, 1859
Cough suppressants, asthma and, 1397
Council for Exceptional Children, 641, 1013
Counseling
　for children with attention deficit
　　hyperactivity disorder, 791
　genetic; see Genetic counseling.
　in anorexia nervosa, 878
　in Down syndrome, 989, 993
　in fragile X syndrome, 994

Counseling—cont'd
in hemophilia, 1565-1566
in iron deficiency anemia, 1546
in neonatal death, 370
in obesity, 875
in sickle cell anemia, 1554
nurse's role in, 21
prehospital, 1086
telephone, 142-143, 143f
Coup injury, 1665
Couplet care, discharge planning for newborn and, 286
Court proceedings, in cases of child maltreatment, 692, 692b
Cover-uncover test, 196, 197f, 198t
Cow's milk; see Milk, cow's.
Coxa plana, 1807-1808
Coxa vara, 1808-1809
Coxsackievirus, in newborn, 327t
CPAP; see Continuous positive airway pressure.
CPR; see Cardiopulmonary resuscitation.
Crack cocaine
adolescent abuse of, 890-891
intrauterine exposure to, 407-408
Cracked-pot sound, in hydrocephalus, 437
Crackles, 214t
in newborn, 260
Cradle cap, 580, 741-742
Cramps
heat, 1802
in colic, 571-574
Cranberry juice, urinary tract infection and, 1265
Cranial deformities, 443-446, 444f, 445b
Cranial nerves
abnormalities of, brain tumor and, 1621t
assessment of, 227, 229t
in bacterial meningitis, 1678
myelination of, 243
Cranial surgery
comfort measures for, 1624
family support in, 1624
fluid management after, 1623-1624
for epilepsy, 1691-1692
patient/family teaching for, 1622
positioning after, 1623
postoperative care in, 1622-1624
rehabilitation for, 1624-1625
Cranial sutures, in increased intracranial pressure, 1645, 1646
Craniofacial abnormalities, 445-446, 445b
cleft lip and/or palate in, 454-463
Craniopharyngioma, growth failure and, 1706-1709, 1710
Cranioschisis, 424b
Craniosynostosis, 444-445, 444f
Craniotabes, 252t, 258, 298
Crawl reflex, 263t, 264f
Crawling, in infants, 500
C-reactive protein, reference ranges for, 1895t
Creatine kinase, reference ranges for, 1896t
Creatine phosphokinase, in neuromuscular dysfunction, 1834, 1834b
Creatinine
in chronic renal failure, 1288
reference ranges for, 1896t
Creatinine clearance, 1260, 1262t
reference ranges for, 1896t

Creative expression, hospitalized child and, 1071, 1071f
Credé maneuver, 1860
Creeping, in infants, 500
Cremasteric reflex, 221-222, 222f
retractile testes and, 480
Crepitus, in fractures, 224, 1780
of clavicle, 298
Cretinism, 320-322
Creutzfeldt-Jakob disease, 1712
Crib(s)
infant suffocation and, 544, 549b
injuries and, 542t, 543t, 546, 549b, 623
Cricoid cartilage, 192f, 1305
Cri-du-chat syndrome, 116t
CRIES pain assessment tool, 353, 354t-355t
Crigler-Najjar syndrome, 305
Crippled Children's Program, 939, 981
Crippled Children's Services (CSS), 12
Critical paths, 15, 16t-18t
Critical periods, in prenatal development, 416, 417f
Critical thinking, 24, 24b
Crohn disease
effects of, 1438f
extraintestinal manifestations of, 1439
pathophysiology and clinical manifestations of, 1438-1439
vs ulcerative colitis, 1439t
Crohn's and Colitis Foundation of America, Inc., 1443
Cromolyn sodium
for allergic rhinitis, 1384
for asthma, 1392
Crossed extensor reflex, in cerebral palsy, 1837
Cross-racial adoption, 93
Croup
definition of, 1361
spasmodic, 1362t, 1365
Croup syndromes, 1361-1365
comparison of, 1362, 1362t
Crouzon syndrome, 445b
Crown-to-rump length, 176f, 177
of newborn, 251t, 255
Crutches, 1775
Crutchfield tongs, 1790-1791, 1790f
Crying, 506
at night, approaches to, 526-527, 526t
in newborn, 246
intraventricular hemorrhage and, 402
with colic, 571-574
Cryoprecipitate, 1543t, 1563
Cryotherapy
for retinoblastoma, 1633
for retinopathy of prematurity, 400
Cryptococcosis, 764t
Cryptorchidism, 221, 480-481
Crystalloid solution
for burn patients, 1236
for shock states, 1221
Cuban Americans; see Latinos.
Cued speech, hearing impairment and, 998
Cuff, blood pressure, 184-185, 184f, 186t
Cultural awareness, 51
Cultural beliefs, and infant feeding practices, 520
Cultural diversity, 35

Cultural factors, 30-40; see also Race/ethnicity.
affluence and, 35-36
dietary, 45-47, 165b
economic, 35-36, 37, 40-41
importance of, 31
in bladder catheterization, 1146b
in blood transfusions, 1539b
in breast-feeding, 347-348
in child abuse, 48, 49t
in chronic illness and disability, 910
in circumcision, 272b
in communication, 44-45, 144
in coping skills, Down syndrome diagnosis and, 991, 991b
in developmental dysplasia of hip, 448b
in family-provider relationship, 43-45
in health care, 42-51
in home care, 1021-1022, 1021b
in interviewing, 144
in obesity, 871
in pain assessment, 1055
in safety measures, 11b
in social roles, 32-33
in terminal illness, 958b
in time concepts, 43
media-related, 38-40
occupational, 35-37
school-related, 37
social class and, 35-37
subcultural influences and, 34-40
Cultural groups
primary, 32-33
secondary, 32-33
subgroups, 34-40
Cultural pluralism, 32
Cultural relativity, 43
Cultural sensitivity, 33
Cultural shock, 33-34
Culturally competent care, 33
Culture
biculture and, 38
components of, 31
definition of, 31
material overt (manifest), 31
nonmaterial covert, 31
North American, 31-32
peer, 37-38
Cultures
bacterial, 1420t
epithelial, in burn wounds, 1242
stool, in diarrhea, 1211
streptococcal, in acute poststreptococcal glomerulonephritis, 1272
throat, for acute streptococcal pharyngitis, 1352
urine, in vesicoureteral reflux, 1270
Cupping, 49b
Curandera, 48
C-urea breath test, 1421t, 1444
Curling ulcers, in burn injuries, 1234
Curosurf, 386
Cushing reflex, 1649
Cushing syndrome, 1727-1729, 1727b, 1727f, 1728t
Custody, 96-97
Cutaneous reflectance, in bilirubin measurement, 305, 307
Cutaneous stimulation, in pain management, 1059b

Cutis marmorata, in newborn, 251t
Cyanosis, 188, 188t; *see also* Hypoxemia.
    congenital heart disease categories and, 1475, 1476f
    definition of, 1484
    heart defects causing, 1484, 1486
    in congestive heart failure, 1478
    in foreign body aspiraton, 1377
    in respiratory distress syndrome, 381
    neurologic consequences of, 1487
    nursing care for, 1489-1490
Cyclic vomiting, 1700b
Cyclophosphamide (Cytoxan), 1589t
    for nephrotic syndrome, 1277
    for systemic lupus erythematosus, 1828
Cyclosporine
    for inflammatory bowel disease, 1440
    in renal transplantation, 1299-1300
Cylert, for attention deficit hyperactivity disorder, 789
Cyst, 744f
    pilonidal, 223
Cystic fibrosis, 119t, 1401-1413
    clinical manifestations of, 1406-1407
    diagnosis of, 1407
    etiology of, 1401
    home care for, 1411-1412
    inheritance of, 122
    life expectancy in, 906
    neonatal screening for, 126
    nursing care of, 1410-1413
    pathophysiology of, 1401, 1404-1406
    prognosis for, 1410
    screening for, 1407
    treatment of, 1407-1410
Cystic Fibrosis Foundation, 1412
Cystic fibrosis transmembrane regulator, 1401
Cystitis; *see also* Urinary tract infection.
    hemorrhagic, in cancer, 1595t, 1602
Cytogenetic disorders; *see* Chromosome disorders.
Cytokines, in allergic rhinitis, 1383
Cytomegalovirus, in newborn, 327t
Cytosine arabinoside (Ara-C), 1591t
Cytotoxic agents
    for cancer; *see* Chemotherapy.
    for juvenile rheumatoid arthritis, 1822
Cytotoxic T-lymphocytes, 1572
Cytoxan (cyclophosphamide), 1589t

**D**

Dacarbazine (DTIC-Dome), 1590t
Dacryocystitis, 193b
Dactinomycin (Cosmegen), 1592t
Dactylitis, 1549
Dairy products; *see also* Milk.
    alternate, 280, 282
        for phenylketonuria, 323
Dance reflex, 263t, 264f
Dandy-Walker malformation, 437
Date rape drug (flunitrazepam), 892
Daunorubicin, 1592t
Dawn phenomenon, 1741
Daycare facilities
    center-based, 516
        diapering and toileting at, 517-518
        preparation for school and, 715
        readiness and preparation of child for, 637

Daycare facilities—cont'd
    sanitation at, giardiasis prevention and, 667
    selection of, 637
    value of, 636
DDAVP; *see* Desmopressin.
Dead space, intramuscular drug administration and, 1154
Deaf-blindness, 1006-1007
Deafness, 994, 995t; *see also* Hearing impairment.
Death and dying; *see also* Mortality; Terminal illness.
    autopsy after, 949t, 967
    brain death in, 1649, 1649b
    causes of, 3, 4-6, 4t
    children's reactions to, 969-970, 970t
    funeral services after, siblings' attendance at, 967, 967b, 968f
    grieving family and, 968-972, 969b, 970t
    high-risk infants and, 334b, 369-371
    in cancer, 1606
    organ/tissue donation after, 966-967
    unexpected, 964-966, 966b
    viewing of body after, 966
Death rates, 105, 105b; *see also* Mortality.
Death vigil, 961
Debridement, of burn wounds, 1238
Decadron; *see* Dexamethasone.
Deceleration injury, 1665
Decerebrate posturing, 1651, 1651f
Decibels, 995, 995t
Decimal factors, prefixes for, 1903
Decision-making, in adolescence, 810
Decongestants, α-adrenergic, for allergic rhinitis, 1384
Decorticate posturing, 1651, 1651f
Decubitus ulcers, 745, 1122-1125, 1124b-1125b, 1126t
    in immobilization, 1765, 1765f
    in spinal cord injury, 1859
Deep breathing
    for auscultation, 213
    play activities and, 1111b
Deep sedation, 1108
Deep tendon reflexes; *see also* Reflex(es).
    assessment of, 226
DEET, as insect repellent, 775
Defecation; *see* Bowel elimination.
Deferoxamine; *see* Chelation therapy.
Defervescence, 1130
Defibrillator, external, in cardiopulmonary resuscitation procedure, 1334
Deglutition (swallowing), 1418
    in infants, 496-497, 497f
Dehydration, 1128, 1174-1180, 1175t; *see also* Diarrhea; Fluid and electrolyte balance.
    acute renal failure and, 1284
    clinical signs of, 1178-1179, 1178t
    degree of, 1178-1179, 1178t
    hypertonic, 1177-1178, 1178t
        fluid replacement in, 1180
    hypotonic, 1177, 1178t
    hypoxemia and, 1490
    in high-risk newborn, 340
    in sickle cell anemia, 1552
    isotonic, 1176-1177, 1178t
    types of, 1176-1178
    vomiting and, 1217-1219
Deja vu, 1687

Delayed gratification
    in toddlers, 598
    infantile psychosocial development and, 501
Deltasone; *see* Prednisone.
Deltoid, intramuscular injection via, 1156t
Demerol; *see* Meperidine.
Democratic parent, 85
Demography, 104
Denial
    in chronic illness or disability, 417, 933
    in terminal illness, 972
Dental care, 1128
    bacterial endocarditis and, 1509, 1510b
    hemophilia and, 1563
    in cancer, 1601, 1605
    in cerebral palsy, 1840
    in mental retardation, 986
Dental caries, 207, 780-781
    fruit juice and, 566b
    genetic factors in, 780
    in cerebral palsy, 1837, 1840
    in school-age children, 780-781
    in toddlers, 615-616, 615f
    nursing considerations with, 781
    prevention of, 611
    tricyclic antidepressants and, 791
Dental health, 780-783; *see also* Teeth.
    in chronic renal failure, 1291
    in infants, 527
    in preschoolers, 646
    in school-age children, 727-728, 727f
    in toddlers, 611-616, 611b
Dental plaque, tooth decay and, 780
Dental prosthesis, in cleft lip and palate, 458
Dentists, child abuse reporting and, 683
Denver Articulation Screening Examination, 642, 1012, 1877-1878
Denver Developmental Screening Test, 234t, 235-237, 236b, 1874-1879
Denver Eye Screening Test, 198t, 1879
Denver II, 1012
Denver Prescreening Developmental Questionnaire, 237, 1876
Deoxyhemoglobin, 1314
Department of Health and Human Services, 1212
Depo-Provera, 982
    for contraception, 855, 856t, 857b
Depressed skull fracture, 1667, 1672
Depression, 797-799
    anaclitic, hospitalization and, 1032-1034, 1041-1044
    diagnostic criteria for, 798b
    in adolescents, 832
    in parents of hospitalized child, 1040-1041
    in parents of special needs child, 907
    in school-age children, 797-799
    steroid-related, 1602
    terminal illness and, 972
Depth perception
    assessment of, 196-197
    in infants, 495
Dermatitis
    atopic, 743
        in infants, 580-582, 580b, 580f

Dermatitis—cont'd
  contact, 767
  diaper, 578-579, 578f, 579f
    candidiasis and, 301
    high-risk newborn and, 351b
  flea bite, 300
  pathophysiology of, 742
  seborrheic, in infants, 580
Dermatoglyphics, 189
Dermatomes, 1857, 1857f
Dermatomyositis, 1863
Dermatophytoses, 759-760, 759t, 760f
Dermis; see also Skin.
  of newborn, 242
  structure of, 740, 741f
DES; see Diethylstilbestrol.
Desensitization, in fearful preschoolers, 643
Desipramine, for attention deficit hyperactivity
    disorder, 789
Desmopressin, for hemophilia, 1563
Desmopressin acetate (DDAVP)
  for diabetes insipidus, 1716
  for enuresis, 785
Detrusor muscle, 1259
  control of, 1259
  dysfunctional, enuresis and, 784
  in voiding, 1258
  instability of, 1259
Deuteranomaly, 199
Developing countries, protein and energy
    malnutrition in, 566
Development
  anticipatory guidance for, 147
  biologic; see Growth and development.
  cognitive, 230t, 231-232
  family, 67-68
  moral, 230t, 232
  motor, in cerebral palsy, 1836
  personality, 230-231, 230t
  psychosexual, 230, 230t
  psychosocial, 230, 230t
  sexual, premature, 1714-1715
  spiritual, 233
Developmental age
  mental retardation and, 983
  terminal illness and, 951
Developmental assessment, 233-237
  high-risk newborn and, 357-358, 359t
  in surveillance, 237
  indications for, 234t
  special needs child and, 907
  tests in, 234t, 235-237, 235t, 236b,
    1874-1879
Developmental defects, 415-490; see also
    Congenital abnormalities and specific
    defects.
  central nervous system, 423-443
  cranial, 443-446, 444f, 445b
  folk beliefs about, 49-50
  gastrointestinal, 454-474
  genitourinary, 478-490, 479t
  hernias as, 474-478, 474f, 478f
  nursing considerations in, 418-419
  parental reaction and, 416-418
    nursing considerations of, 418-419
  skeletal, 446-454, 447t
  surgery for, nursing care in, 419-423,
    420t-423t

Developmental delay, 906b
  attention deficit hyperactivity disorder
    and, 787
  congestive heart failure in infants and, 1478
  high-risk newborn and, 357
  hypoxemia and, 1487
  in cerebral palsy, 1835-1836
Developmental Disabilities Nurses
    Association, 980b
Developmental disability, 906b; see also Disability;
    Mental retardation; Special needs child.
  nursing organizations for, 980b
  sex education for child with, 710
Developmental dysplasia of hip, 446-451, 446b,
    448b, 448f-450f
  in infants, 500
Developmental history, 156
Developmental intervention, home care and,
    1024-1028, 1026b, 1027b
Developmental language disorder, 1007
Developmental milestones, Down syndrome
    and, 991, 991t
Developmental stages
  of divorce, 68b
  of family, 67-68, 68b
Developmental surveillance, 237
Developmental tasks
  divorce and, 96, 97b
  of family, 67-68, 68b
Dexamethasone
  for bacterial meningitis, 1679
  for bronchopulmonary dysplasia, 391
  for cancer, 1593t
Dexamethasone suppression test, 1728
Dextroamphetamine sulfate (Dexedrine),
    for attention deficit hyperactivity
    disorder, 789
Dextrocardia, 253t, 260
Dextrose
  for hypoglycemia, in newborn, 317
  in intravenous solutions, 1189
Dextrostix, 317
Diabetes insipidus, 1658, 1658t, 1672, 1715-1716
  nephrogenic, 1280-1281
Diabetes mellitus, 1732-1755
  adjustment to, 1750-1752
  assessment in, 1743
  autoimmune mechanisms in, 1733-1734
  child/family support in, 1750-1752
  classification of, 1732-1733, 1733t
  clinical manifestations of, 1735-1736
  clinical pathway for, 17t-18t
  complications of, 1735, 1750
  concurrent illness in, 1741, 1750
  cow's milk allergy and, 1734
  diagnosis of, 1736
  diet in, 1738-1739, 1744-1745, 1745t
  eating disorders and, 1737b, 1751
  etiology of, 1733-1734
  evaluation in, 1752
  exercise in, 1739, 1749-1750
  financial aspects of, 1748-1749
  genetic factors in, 1733
  gestational, 405
  glucose monitoring in, 1738, 1747,
    1748, 1748f
  glucose sources in, 1740
  glycosuria in, 1734, 1736

Diabetes mellitus—cont'd
  glycosylated hemoglobin in, 1738
  hospital management in, 1742-1743
  hygiene in, 1749
  hyperglycemia in, 1734, 1736, 1740, 1740t,
    1741, 1749
  hypoglycemia in, 1739-1741, 1740b, 1740t,
    1749, 1749b
  immune-mediated, 1733
  implementation in, 1743-1755
  in adolescents, 1737b, 1750-1751
  in cystic fibrosis, 1405-1406
  insulin for, 1736-1738, 1746-1748; see also
    Insulin.
  insulin reaction in, 1741, 1750
  islet cell destruction in, 1733-1734, 1736
  maternal, 404-406
  maturity-onset of young, 1733, 1735
  Medic-Alert bracelet for, 1744
  mild, 1735
  nursing care in, 1742-1755
  nursing care plan for, 1752-1755
  nursing diagnoses for, 1743
  parental adjustment to, 1751-1752
  pathophysiology of, 1734-1735, 1735f
  patient/family teaching in, 1743-1752
  planning in, 1743
  prevention of, 1741
  psychosocial aspects of, 1742, 1750-1752
  record keeping in, 1750
  self-management in, 1750
  surgery in, 1741
  travel concerns in, 1745-1746
  treatment of, 1736-1742
  type 1, 1732-1733, 1733t
    idiopathic, 1733
    immune-mediated, 1733
  type 2, 1732-1733, 1733t, 1734
  viral involvement in, 1734
Diabetic ketoacidosis, 1734, 1735, 1735f, 1736,
    1749-1750
  management of, 1741-1743
  psychosocial factors in, 1742
Diabetic mother, high-risk newborn of,
    404-406
Diabetic nephropathy, 1735
Diabetic neuropathy, 1735
Diabetic retinopathy, 1735
Diagnosis-related groups (DRGs), 13
Diagnostic procedures; see also specific
    disorders.
  neurologic, 1652-1654, 1653t-1654t, 1655b
  pain management for; see Pain
    management.
  patient/family preparation for, 148,
    149f, 1622
Dialysis, 1293
  for potassium removal in acute renal
    failure, 1286
  hemodialysis, 1293-1296, 1294f, 1296f
    access for, pain with, 1296b
    at home, 1296
    for hemolytic uremic syndrome, 1282
  methods of, 1293
  peritoneal, 1293, 1297-1298
    at home, 1297
    for hemolytic uremic syndrome, 1282
    for shock, 1221

Diamond-Blackfan syndrome, 1559
Diaper(s)
    changing of, 517-518, 579, 667
    cloth vs. disposable, 517
    construction of, 579
    developmental dysplasia of hip and, 450
    for newborn, 269, 269b
    infection control and, 1134
    myelomeningocele and, 431
    phototherapy and, 308
    urinary output measurement and, 337
    urine specimen from, 1144
    wet, weighing of, 1186
Diaper dermatitis, 578-579, 578f, 579b, 579f
    candidiasis and, 301
    in high-risk newborn, 351b
Diapering and toileting, in daycare centers
    giardiasis prevention and, 667
    guidelines for, 517-518
Diaphoresis, in congestive heart failure, 1478
Diaphragm, in breathing, in newborn vs.
        adult, 1304, 1304f
Diaphragmatic hernia, congenital, 475-477
Diaphragms, contraceptive, 855, 856t
Diaphysis, 1776, 1777f
Diarrhea, 1207-1219; see also Dehydration;
        Fluid and electrolyte balance.
    acute, 1208-1213, 1213b
        causes of, 1208-1209, 1208b, 1209b,
            1209t-1210t
        definition of, 1207
    acute infectious, 1208
    assessment of, 1213-1214
    chronic, 1216, 1217b
        definition of, 1207
        nonspecific, 1216-1217
    clinical manifestations of, 1211
    cytotoxic, 1208
    diagnosis of, 1211
    dysenteric, 1208
    fluid and electrolyte loss with, 1208, 1208b
    infant malnutrition and, 566
    intractable, of infancy, 1216
    kwashiorkor and marasmus and, 567
    nursing care plan for, 1215-1216
    osmotic, 1208
    postenteritis, 1216
    secretory, 1208
    toddlers', 1216
    treatment of, 1211-1213, 1212t, 1214
Diaschisis, 1856
Diastasis recti, 218, 253t
Diastatic skull fractures, 1667
Diastole, 1467
Diathesis-stress model of substance abuse, 884
Diazepam
    abuse of, 886t
    for status epilepticus, 1692
    in preoperative sedation, 1113b
    respiratory depression from, 1068b
DIC; see Disseminated intravascular coagulation.
Dicrotic pulse, 217b
Dictatorial parent, 84-85
Diencephalon, structure and function of, 1644t
Diet, 1128-1130, 1129b; see also Eating;
        Feeding; Food(s); Nutrition.
    atopic dermatitis and, 582
    attention deficit hyperactivity disorder
        and, 787

Diet—cont'd
    BRAT, 1186
        for diarrhea, 1212
    cancer and, 1586
    celiac disease and, 1450-1451
    chronic nonspecific diarrhea and, 1217
    chronic renal failure and, 1290
    colic and, 572-573
    constipation and, 1424, 1425, 1425b,
        1426, 1426b
    cultural factors in, 45-47, 46t, 165b
    cystic fibrosis and, 1410, 1411
    diabetic, 1738-1739, 1744-1745, 1745t
    Down syndrome and, 992
    exchange, 1738-1739, 1744-1745, 1745t
    hemodialysis and, 1295-1296
    hypercholesterolemia and, 1520-1521
    in adolescents, 829-830
        in pregnancy, 851, 853
    in anorexia nervosa, 879
    in athletes, 1802-1803, 1803
    in cancer, 1601
    in enzyme deficiencies, 124, 125
    in galactosemia, 325
    in hyperthyroidism, 1721
    in immobilization, 1768
    in infants, dental hygiene and, 527
    in obesity, 874, 874t
    in phenylketonuria, 323-324
    in school-age children, 721, 722-723, 722b
    in systemic lupus erythematosus, 1828
    iron deficiency anemia and, 1543, 1546
    ketogenic, 1692
    low-fat, chronic nonspecific diarrhea
        and, 1217
    low-salt, for congestive heart failure, 1480
    mineral regulation and, 560
    nephrotic syndrome and, 1276-1277
    protein and energy malnutrition and, 567
    published advice on, 564
    recurrent abdominal pain and, 796, 797
    religious beliefs and, 58, 58t-62t
    tooth decay and, 527, 613-616, 780, 781
Diet modifiers, 282t-283t
Dietary Guidelines for Americans, 564
Dietary history, 155
Dietary Reference Intakes (DRIs), 564
Diethylstilbestrol
    cancer and, 1586
    teratogenic effects of, 326
Diethyltoluamide (DEET), as insect
        repellent, 775
Differential Ability Scales, 978
Differential white blood cell count, 1536t
Differentiation, fetal growth and, 416
Diffusion
    carrier-mediated, 1418
    passive, 1418
DiGeorge syndrome, congenital heart disease
        and, 1474
Digestion, 1417-1418
    chemical, 1417-1418
    in infants, 496
    in malabsorption syndromes, 1450
    in toddlers, 593
    mechanical, 1417
Digibind, for digoxin toxicity, 673
Digital substraction angiography, cerebral, 1654t
Digital thermometers, 183t

Digitalis
    for congestive heart failure, 1479, 1479t
    for supraventricular tachycardia, 1525
Digits; see Finger(s); Toe(s).
Digoxin (Lanoxin)
    administration of, 1481-1482, 1482b
    for congestive heart failure, 1479, 1479t, 1481
    reference ranges for, 1896t-1897t
    serum potassium levels and, 1480
    toxicity of, 1481, 1482
Dilaudid; see Hydromorphone.
Dimercaprol, for chelation therapy, 680
Dimercaptopropanol, for chelation
        therapy, 680
Dipeptidase, 1418
Diphenhydramine (Benadryl), 660, 661, 752
    for allergic rhinitis, 1384
Diphenoxylate/atropine, as poison, 669
Diphtheria
    immunizations for
        contraindications to, 537t
        in adolescents, 541t
        recommended, 529t, 532
    manifestations and management of, 652t-653t
Diphtheria-tetanus vaccine, in adolescents, 834
Diphtheria-tetanus-pertussis vaccine,
        recommended immunizations with,
        529t, 532
Direct antiglobulin test, in hemolytic disease
        of newborn, 314
Direct Coombs test, in hemolytic disease of
        newborn, 314
Direct observation, in compliance
        measurement, 1119
Direct-contact transmission, 1134
Disability, 905-945; see also Birth defects;
        Special needs child and specific
        disabilities and conditions.
    after head trauma, 1672, 1673-1674
    morbidity and, 6
    nursing organizations for, 980b
    sex education for child with, 710
Disaccharidases, 1418
Disaccharides, digestion of, in celiac
        disease, 1451
Disbelief
    mourning and, 970
    parents of child with physical defect
        and, 417
    parents of hospitalized child and, 1040
Disc diameter (DD), 195
Discharge
    nasal, 206
    vaginal, in newborn, 261
Discharge planning
    assessment in, 1096
    for hospitalized child, 1095-1097
        in ambulatory/outpatient setting,
            1091-1092, 1092b
    for newborn, 286-288, 287b
        at high risk, 368-369
    for technology-dependent infant, 1017,
        1018, 1019b
    home care and, 1018-1019, 1018b, 1019b
        safety issues in, 1028
    in abdominal wall defect, 473-474
    in anorectal malformation, 470
    in bronchopulmonary dysplasia, 392-393
    in cleft lip and palate, 462

Discharge planning—cont'd
  in hydrocephalus, 442-443
  in hyperbilirubinemia, 309, 311b
  in tracheoesophageal fistula, 466
Discipline, 84-88, 85b, 86b
  for infants, 516
  in school-age children, 716-717
  in toddlers, 597, 603
  safety and, 1136
  special needs child and, 914, 982
Disconfirming behaviors, 140
Diseases; *see also* Illness.
  chronic, 905-945; *see also* Special needs
    child; specific disease.
  developmental concepts of, 1036t
  early detection of, 106, 106b
  genetic, 110-137
  incidence of, 105, 105b
  obesity associated with, 871
  prevalence of, 105, 105b
  terminal; *see* Terminal illness.
Dishonest behavior, in school-age children, 717
Diskus inhaler, 1391
Dislocation(s)
  as signs of physical abuse, 688b
  hip, 446b, 448f, 450, 1799; *see also* Hip,
    developmental dysplasia of.
    in newborn, 254t
    traumatic, 1799
  in athletes, 1798-1799
  patellar, 1799
  radial head, 1780, 1799
  vertebral
    spinal cord injury and, 1852, 1856
    traction for, 1790-1791, 1790b
Disorientation, 1648b
Disseminated intravascular coagulation, 1220,
    1567-1568, 1568b, 1568f
  hemolysis and, 1540
Distal intestinal obstruction syndrome, in
    cystic fibrosis, 1406
Distancing language, 140
Distraction, 1792
  in pain management, 1059b, 1109
Diuresis, urinary tract infection and, 1265
Diuretics
  for acute poststreptococcal
    glomerulonephritis, 1273
  for bronchopulmonary dysplasia, 391
  for congestive heart failure, 1480, 1480t
  for hypertension, 1518
  for increased intracranial pressure, 1657
  for nephrotic syndrome, 1277
  for shock, 1221
Diuril (chlorothiazide), for congestive heart
    failure, 1480t
Diversions; *see* Activities.
Diversity, cultural; *see* Cultural factors.
Divided custody, 97
Divorce, 817
  blended families and, 71, 98-99, 99b
  custody and, 96-97
  economic impact of, 97-98
  family structure and, 71-72
  impact of on child, 94-96, 95b
  informing children about, 96
  parenting and, 94-97
  sibling relationships and, 79
  stages of, 68b, 94

Dizygotic twins, 80, 80b, 80f
DMSA (dimercaptosuccinic acid), for
    chelation therapy, 680
DNA nucleotide repeats, 121
DNA testing, 123, 123b
  in asthma, 1407
Do not resuscitate (DNR) orders, 949t,
    950, 966
Dobutamine infusion, for cardiopulmonary
    resuscitation, 1399t
Documentation, 27, 27b
  of home care, 1020
  of pain assessment, 1057, 1058f
  privacy concerns and, 141-142
Dogs
  as pets, selection and socialization of, 779
  bites from, 778-779
  bites of, 778-779, 779b
  ringworm infection and, 760
  safety rules for, 779b
  self-esteem development and, 709
Dolichocephaly, 444f
Dolls, anatomically correct, in diagnosis of
    sexual abuse, 691
Doll's eye reflex, 263t
Doll's head maneuver, 1651
Dolophine; *see* Methadone.
Domestic mimicry, 596
Domestic violence, 75, 718
Donors, for renal transplants, 1299
Dopamine
  attention deficit hyperactivity disorder
    and, 787
  infusion of, in cardiopulmonary
    resuscitation, 1399t
  shock states and, 1221
  Tourette syndrome and, 793
Doppler echocardiography, cardiac function
    testing and, 1471
Doppler ultrasonography, in blood pressure
    measurement, 184
Dornase alfa (Pulmozyme), in cystic fibrosis,
    1408
Dorsal penile nerve block, for circumcision,
    271b, 272
Dorsogluteal injection, 1156t
Doubt, in toddlers, 594
Down syndrome, 116t, 987-993; *see also* Mental
    retardation.
  clinical manifestations of, 989-990,
    989t, 990f
  congenital heart disease and, 1474
  developmental milestones and skills in,
    991, 991t
  developmental progress in, promotion
    of, 992
  diagnosis of
    family support and, 991, 991b
    prenatal, 992-993
  etiology of, 987, 989, 989t
  leukemia in, 1585-1586, 1612
  management of, 990
  maternal age and, 113-114
  palmar crease in, 189, 190f
  physical problems in, prevention of,
    991-992
  prognosis of, 990-991
  translocation, 115, 115f
Doxorubicin (Adriamycin), 1592t

Drainage
  chest
    after heart surgery, 1505
    in heart surgery, 1505
    in pneumonia, 1370-1371
    removal of, 1505
    teaching about, 1504
  ear, in otitis media, 1360
  postural, 1320, 1321f, 1322f, 1323f
    in cystic fibrosis, 1412
    with chest physiotherapy, 1320, 1322, 1323
Dramatic play
  during hospitalization, 1071-1072, 1072f
  for preschoolers, 634-635, 635b, 635f
Drawing
  by preschoolers, 629-630, 629f, 630b
  communication via, 152b
  in sexual abuse assessment, 691
  kinetic family, 163-164, 163b
Dreams, communication of, 151b
Dressing(s)
  Allevyn tracheostomy, 1328
  applied at home, 751-752
  for burn wounds, 1235-1236
  for skin lesions, types and properties of,
    749, 750t, 752-753
  occlusive, 749, 751
  removal of, epidermal stripping and,
    1125, 1125b
  teaching about, 1504
  wet, for skin lesions, 752-753
Dressing skills, mental retardation and, 985-986
Drinking, in adolescents, 828, 829, 831-832
Drooling, in cerebral palsy, 1836
Droplet precautions, 1133-1134, 1133b
Dropping out, adolescents and, 833
Drowning, 8, 8t, 10, 1674-1676, 1676t, 1802
  in school-age children, 731t
  in toddlers, 617t, 620
  prevention of, 1758b
  safety precautions against, 542t, 543t, 548
Drug(s); *see also* specific drugs.
  administration of, 1149-1161
    by school nurse, 730
    gastrostomy, 1159, 1159b
    home care and, 1161
    intradermal, 1157, 1158
    intramuscular, 1153-1157, 1154t-1156t,
     1157f, 1158b
    intravenous, 1158-1159
    nasal, 1160-1161, 1162f
    nasogastric, 1159, 1159b
    optic, 1160, 1160f
    oral, 1151-1153, 1151b, 1152f, 1153f
    orogastric, 1159, 1159b
    otic, 1160
    rectal, 1065b, 1159-1160
    subcutaneous, 1157-1158
  dosage of, 1149-1151, 1150f
  home care and, 1024
  misuse of, 884
  ototoxic, 996b
  physical dependence on, 884
  poisoning with, 669
    in toddlers, 622
  rape and, 858
Drug abuse, 884; *see also* Substance abuse and
    specific drugs.
Drug addiction, 884

Drug history, 156
Drug jargon, 891b
Drug sensitivity, skin disorders related to, 772-773
Drug tolerance, 884
Drug-exposed infant, 326, 406-408, 406b
DTIC-Dome (dacarbazine), 1590t
Dual-earner family, 99
Dubowitz scale, 248
Duchenne muscular dystrophy, 119t, 1863t, 1864-1867, 1864f, 1865f
Ductal systems, abnormal differentiation of, ambiguous genitalia and, 487
Ductus arteriosus, 241, 1466
   in cyanotic newborns, 1487
   patent, 397, 1494b, 1494f
      in transposition of great arteries, 1499b
      pulmonary artery hypertension and, 1490
Ductus venosus, in fetal circulation, 1466
Dullness, on chest percussion, 212
Dunlop traction, 1789, 1789f
Duodenal ulcer, 1443
Dura mater, 1642, 1643f
Durogesic; see Fentanyl.
Dwarfism, hypopituitary, 1709-1713; see also Hypopituitarism.
Dwyer instrumentation, for scoliosis, 1813
Dyad care, discharge planning for newborn and, 286
Dysacusis, 995
Dyscalculia, 791
Dysfluencies, 1007, 1010-1011, 1011b
Dysfunctional uterine bleeding, 848
Dysgraphia, 791
Dyslalia, 642
Dyslexia, 791
Dysmenorrhea, 846-847
Dyspnea
   in asthma, 1388
   in congestive heart failure, 1478
   in pulmonary artery hypertension, 1490
Dysraphism, spinal, occult, 425
Dysrhythmias; see Arrhythmia(s).
Dystonia, 1647b
Dystrophin, 1864

E

Ear(s); see also Hearing.
   alignment of, 200, 200f
   cleft lip and palate and, 457, 463
   Down syndrome and, 989t, 990
   drainage from, in otitis media, 1360
   examination of, 200-204
   external
      examination of, 200-201
      infections of, 580, 1361; see also Otitis externa.
      structure of, 200, 200f
   foreign body in, 203
   fragile X syndrome and, 993
   in newborn, 244, 252t, 259
      prematurity and, 377f
   in nutritional assessment, 166t
   middle/inner
      examination of, 201-203, 201f, 202f
      infection of; see Otitis media.
      structure of, 203f
   pain in, in otitis externa, 1361
   rhabdomyosarcoma of, 1631b

Ear drops, 1160, 1361
Ear wick, 1361
Ear-based thermometers, 178-179, 179f, 180b-181b, 182t-183t
Eardrum; see Tympanic membrane.
Early Infancy Temperament Questionnaire (EITQ), 507, 509
Early intervention, 909
   home care and, 1027-1028
   mental retardation and, 980b, 981
Early Language Milestone Scale, 234t, 1012
Early Screening Inventory, 234t
Earmuffs, for high-risk newborn, 365
Eating; see also Feeding; Food(s).
   disordered, in athletes, 1804
   in congenital heart disease, 1503
Eating disorders, 869-884; see also specific disorders.
   in adolescents, 806, 829-830
   in athletes, 1804
   in diabetics, 1737b, 1751
Eating habits, in toddlers, 610
Ecchymosis, 188, 188t, 743, 1798
   birth-related, 295-296, 296b
Eccrine sweat glands, 742
   of newborn, 243
Echocardiography
   cardiac function and, 1471
   Doppler, 1471
   fetal, 130
   in Kawasaki disease, 1515
   M-mode, 1471
   transesophageal, 1471
   two-dimensional, 1471
Echoencephalography, 1653t
ECMO; see Extracorporeal membrane oxygenation (ECMO).
Economic factors, in health care, 106
Ectasia, in Kawasaki disease, 1514
Ectopic pregnancy, 850-851
   pelvic inflammatory disease and, 863
Ectropion, 193
Eczema, in infants, 580-582, 580b, 580f
Edema
   cerebral, 1181, 1507, 1645-1646, 1645b; see also Intracranial pressure, increased.
      after cranial surgery, 1623
      after heart surgery, 1507
      in head injury, 1665, 1668-1669
      treatment of, 1657
   formation of, 1180-1181
   generalized, 1181
   hydrostatic, in shock, 1221
   immobilization and, 1763-1764
   in burn injuries, 1230-1231
   in congestive heart failure, 1478
   in inflammatory process, 747
   in nephrotic syndrome, 1275, 1278
   laryngeal, in anaphylaxis, 1224
   optic disc, 195, 1651
   peripheral, 1181
   permeable, in shock, 1221
   pitting, 189
   pulmonary, 1181
      after heart surgery, 1507
      in burn patients, 1233
      in congestive heart failure, 1478
      respiratory distress syndrome and, 380-381
   signs of, 189

Edema—cont'd
   types of, 1181
   under cast, 1786
EDTA (calcium disodium edetate), for chelation therapy, 680-681
Educable mentally retarded, 978
Education; see also School.
   as compliance strategy, 1120
   in cerebral palsy, 1841
   in chronic illness or disability, 918-919, 919b, 1027-1028
   in communication impairment, 1013
   in human immunodeficiency virus infection, 1576
   in mental retardation, 980-981, 981f
   in visual impairment, 1004
   of family, 1131-1132
   of hospitalized child, 1073
Education for All Handicapped Children Act, 13, 907, 909
Education of the Handicapped Act, 909, 980b
Edward syndrome, 116t
Effexor (venlafaxine), for depression, 798
Ego, 230
   in adolescents, 810
   in school-age children, 712
   in toddlers, 594, 596, 597b
Egophony, 213
Eisenmenger's syndrome, 1486, 1490
Elastic recoil, 1307
Elbow
   Little League, 1801t
   nursemaid's, 1780, 1799
   tennis, 1801t
Elbow restraint, 1140, 1140f
Electra complex, 631
Electrical burns, 621, 1227
Electrical outlets, safety precautions with, 542t, 543t, 548, 549b
Electrocardiography, cardiac function and, 1469-1471, 1470f, 1471f
Electrodes
   in cardiac monitoring, 1470-1471, 1471f
   in home apnea monitoring, 587, 587f
   placement of, on high-risk newborn, 337
Electroencephalography, 1652, 1653t
   for seizures, 1689-1690
Electrolytes; see also Fluid and electrolyte balance and specific electrolytes.
   in acute renal failure, 1286
   in burn injuries, 1231
   renal transport and excretion of, 1257, 1258
   replacement of, for athletes, 1803-1804
Electromyography, 1834
Electronic thermometers, 180b, 182t
Electrophoresis, hemoglobin
   in sickle cell anemia, 1550
   in α-thalassemia, 1558
Elephantiasis, 774
Elimination; see Bowel elimination; Urinary elimination.
ELISA (enzyme-linked immunosorbent assay), 1211
   for human immunodeficiency virus, 1574
   for respiratory syncytial virus, 1367
Elspar (L-asparaginase), 1589, 1593t, 1594
Emancipated minor, informed consent of, 1103

Embolism
   air, from blood transfusion and, 1541t
   fat, 1795
   fracture-related, 1795
   immobilization and, 1764
   pulmonary, 1795
Emergency admission, 1087b, 1093
Emergency care
   eye injuries and, 1003b
   for bleeding, 1760
   for burns, 1234-1235, 1235b
   for diabetic hypoglycemia, 1749b
   for fractures, 1781b
   for head injury, 1671b
   for injuries, 1760-1761
   for poisoning, 669-675, 673b
   for respiratory failure, 1331-1341
   for seizures, 1695b
   for shock, 1223
   for spinal cord injury, 1760
   of children in schools, 730
   planning for, home care and, 1028
   providers of, 1760-1761
Emergency contraceptive pill, 855, 856t
Emergency Medical Service (EMS), 1760
Emergency medical technician (EMT), 1761
Emetics, in poisoning; see Ipecac syrup.
EMLA cream, 1065b, 1066, 1066b, 1603, 1679
   for bladder catheterization, 1146b
   for circumcision, 270-272, 271b
   for laser therapy, for birthmarks, 302
   for lumbar puncture, 1142b, 1142f
Emollients
   for high-risk newborn, 350b
   in prevention of atopic dermatitis, 581
Emotional abuse or neglect, 683-684
   identification of, 687, 688b
   in adolescents, 832-833
   in infants, 505
Emotional autonomy, 812
Emotional lability
   in hyperthyroidism, 1721
   steroid-related, 1602
Emotional stress
   after heart surgery, 1508
   atopic dermatitis in infants and, 582
   conversion reaction and, 797
Emotional support, from nurse, 21
Emotions; see Psychologic aspects.
Empathy, 145
Emphysema, 389
   respiratory distress syndrome and, 381
Empiric risk, 131
Employment, parental needs and, 100
Empowerment, 14
   parental, special needs child and, 932
Empyema, 1302
En face position, maternal attachment and,
   284, 284f
Enabling, in family-centered care, 14
Enalapril (Vasotec)
   for congestive heart failure, 1479
   for hypertension, 1519b
Encephalitis, 1681-1682
   rabies, 1682-1683
Encephalocele, 424b
Encephalopathy
   bilirubin, 304, 307, 311b
      prevention of, 306

Encephalopathy—cont'd
   hepatic, 1461
   hypertensive
      acute poststreptococcal
         glomerulonephritis and, 1272
      in acute renal failure, 1286
   hypoxic-ischemic, 401
   in burn injuries, 1234
Encopresis, 785-786, 1424
End organs, 1703
Endocardial cushions, 1465
Endocarditis, bacterial, 1509-1511
   cyanosis and, 1487, 1488
   prophylaxis for, 1510b
   renal involvement in, 1270t
   subacute, 1509
Endocardium, 1465
Endocrine disorders
   hypersecretory, 1706
   hyposecretory, 1706-1713, 1707b
   pathophysiology of, 1706
Endocrine system, 1703-1706; see also specific
      glands and hormones.
   autonomic nervous system and, 1705-1706
   end organs in, 1703, 1704, 1705b
   in infants, 497
   in newborns, 243
      after surgery, 421t
   obesity and, 871
   regulation of, 1704-1706, 1705f
   structure of, 1704f
   target cells/tissues in, 1703, 1704, 1705b
Endocrine therapy
   for cancer, 1589, 1593t
   for cryptorchidism, 481
   for dysfunctional uterine bleeding, 848
End-of-life issues; see Terminal illness.
Endometriosis, 847
Endoscopic third ventriculostomy, 440
Endoscopy
   in foreign body aspiraton, 1377
   in gastroesophageal reflux diagnosis, 1429
   in inflammatory bowel disease diagnosis, 1440
   of gastrointestinal tract, 1422t
Endotracheal intubation, 1324-1325, 1325b; see
      also Mechanical ventilation; Ventilatory
      support.
   in acute epiglottitis, 1363
   in burn patients, 1236
   in croup syndromes, 1365
   in smoke inhalation injury, 1381
Endotracheal tube
   size of, 1325
   teaching about, 1504
End-stage renal disease, 1287; see also Renal
      failure.
   immunization and, 1298b
Enemas, 1165-1166, 1165b
   barium, for intussusception, 1449
   Fleet, 1262
   for Hirschsprung disease, 1427
Energy intake
   by burn patients, 1232, 1237
   high-risk newborn and, 343, 343t
Energy level, in chronic renal failure, 1289-1290
Enfamil, 281t
Enfamil Human Milk Fortifier, 283t
Engorgement, breast-feeding and, 278t
Engulfment, in intestinal absorption, 1419

Enteral nutrition, 1162-1164, 1162-1165,
      1163b, 1163f, 1164-1165, 1164f,
      1164t, 1165f
   drug administration via, 1159, 1159b
   esophageal anastomosis and, 465
   gastrostomy feeding in, 1164-1165
   gavage feeding in, 348, 1162-1164
   in burn patients, 1234, 1237
   in congestive heart failure, 1483, 1483b
   in gastroesophageal reflux, 1431, 1432
   in high-risk newborn, 343-344, 348, 348f
      with necrotizing enterocolitis, 396
   in inflammatory bowel disease, 1441
   in short bowel syndrome, 1452, 1453
Enteric nervous system, 1426
Enterobiasis (pinworms), 667-668
*Enterobius vermicularis,* 667
Enterocolitis, necrotizing, in high-risk
      newborn, 343, 344, 347, 395-397
Enterocystoplasty, 430
   augmentation, 429
Enterohepatic circulation, physiologic
      jaundice and, 305
Enterokinase, 1418
Enteropathy, gluten-sensitive, 1450-1451
Enterostomal therapist, 1428
Enterostomal therapy nurse, 1166
Enteroviruses, anterior horn cell disease
      and, 1833
Entonox, in burn patients, 1238
Entropion, 193
Enucleation
   for retinoblastoma, 1633-1634
   prosthesis for, 1634, 1634f
Enuresis, 783-785
   age and, 783b
   in diabetes insipidus, 1716
   in diabetes mellitus, 1736
   urinary tract infection and, 1266
Environmental safety, 1135-1136, 1136f; see also
      Safety.
Enzyme(s); see also specific enzymes.
   antioxidant, respiratory distress syndrome
      and, 383
   fecal, diaper dermatitis and, 578
   gastrointestinal, 1417-1418
   in malabsorption syndromes, 1450
   in metabolic pathway, 319-320, 320f
   in newborn, 242
   pancreatic, in cystic fibrosis, 1409, 1409b,
      1410, 1411
Enzyme deficiencies, diet in, 124, 125
Enzyme-linked immunosorbent assay
      (ELISA), 1211
   for human immunodeficiency virus, 1574
   for respiratory syncytial virus, 1367
Eosinophil(s), 243, 1534
   in complete blood count, 1536t
Eosinophil count, reference ranges for, 1897t
Eosinophilia, 1534
Ependymoma, 1620b; see also Brain tumors.
Epicanthal folds, 192f, 193, 193f, 196, 196f
Epicardial leads, of pacemaker, 1525
Epidemiologic screening, 127
Epidemiologic triangle, 105
Epidemiology, 104-106
Epidermal stripping, 1125
Epidermal wound, healing of, 745, 747

Epidermis
  layers of, 740, 741f
  of newborn, 242-243
Epididymis, 222, 223f
Epididymitis, 844
Epidural analgesia, 1063, 1065-1066, 1065b
Epidural hematoma, 1666f, 1667-1668
Epidural sensor, in intracranial pressure
    monitoring, 1657
Epidural space, 1642
Epiglottis, 1305
  as respiratory tract defense, 1310
Epiglottitis, acute, 1362-1363, 1362t, 1363b
Epilepsy; see also Seizures.
  activity restrictions in, 1694
  assessment in, 1692-1693, 1692b
  classification of, 1686t
  definition of, 1684
  developmental aspects of, 1696
  diagnosis of, 1684, 1689-1690
  differential diagnosis of, 1689
  electroencephalography in, 1689-1690
  etiology of, 1685b
  evaluation in, 1696
  family support in, 1696
  incidence of, 1685
  infantile spasms in, 1688-1689
  injury prevention in, 1693-1694, 1694b
  Lennox-Gastaut syndrome and, 1689
  nursing care in, 1693-1696
  nursing care plan for, 1697-1698
  nursing diagnoses for, 1693
  pathophysiology of, 1685
  planning for, 1693, 1697-1698
  postictal state in, 1686
  prognosis of, 1692
  remission in, 1692
  seizure types in, 1685-1688, 1686b
  status epilepticus in, 1692
  terminology for, 1684b
  treatment of, 1690-1692
    emergency, 1695b
    pharmacologic, 1690, 1691t, 1694-1695
    surgical, 1690-1692
Epilepsy Foundation, 1696
Epileptogenic focus, 1685
  resection of, 1691-1692
Epinephrine, 1708t, 1724
  adrenal secretion of, 1723, 1724
  effects of, 1724, 1724b
  for acute laryngotracheobronchitis, 1364
  for anaphylaxis, 1225
  for bee stings, 775
  for cardiopulmonary resuscitation, 1399t
  pheochromocytoma and, 1731-1732
  urinary, in neuroblastoma, 1625
Epinephrine and cocaine combined, for
    topical anesthesia, 751b
Epiphysis/epiphyseal plate, 1776, 1777f
  injury of, 1778-1779, 1779b, 1779f, 1794
Epispadias, 221, 254t, 482-484, 483f
Epistaxis
  emergency treatment of, 1567b
  in von Willebrand disease, 1566, 1567b
Epithelial cells, of villi, engulfment by, 1419
Epithelial pearls, in newborn, 254t, 261
Epithelialization, 747, 747f
Epithelium, cultured, for burn wounds, 1242
Epstein pearls, in newborn, 252t, 259

Epstein-Barr virus, infectious mononucleosis
    and, 1354
Equianalgesia, 1062, 1063t
Equilibrium, assessment of, 204
Equipment
  for parenteral intravenous therapy, 1190
  used in congenital heart disease, teaching
    about, 1503-1504
Erb palsy, 299, 299f
Erb point, 216
Erb-Duchenne palsy, 262, 299
Ergocalciferol
  functions of and disturbances in, 559t
  sources of, 559t
Ergogenic aids, for athletes, 1804-1805
Erikson's psychosocial development theory,
    230t, 231
  adolescents and, 804t, 812-817, 827-828
  infants and, 501
  preschoolers and, 630
  school-age children and, 700-701
  toddlers and, 594
Erythema, 188, 188t, 743
  birth-related, 296b
Erythema chronicum migrans, 764, 766f
Erythema infectiosum
  complications from, 651, 660
  in newborn, 327t
  manifestations and management of, 654f,
    654t-655t
Erythema marginatum, in rheumatic fever, 1511
Erythema multiforme
  drug sensitivity and, 772
  in Crohn disease, 1439
Erythema multiforme exudativum (Stevens-
    Johnson syndrome), drug sensitivity
    and, 773, 773f
Erythema nodosum, in Crohn disease, 1439
Erythema toxicum neonatorum, 251t, 300
Erythocyte count, 1536t
  reference ranges for, 1897t
Erythroblastosis fetalis; see Hemolytic disease
    of newborn.
Erythroblasts, 1532
Erythrocyte(s), 1531f, 1532, 1538
  anemia and, 1535, 1537-1540, 1537b; see also
    Anemia.
  aplasia of, 1559
  bilirubin and, 304
    physiologic jaundice and, 305
  hemolytic disease of newborn and, 310
  morphology of, 1537b
  packed, 1543t
    for iron deficiency anemia, 1545
    for sickle cell anemia, 1551
  sickled, 1547-1548, 1549f; see also Sickle cell
    anemia.
Erythrocyte count, 1536t
  reference ranges for, 1897t
Erythrocyte indexes, 1532, 1536t
Erythrocyte protoporphyrin test, for screening
    children for lead poisoning, 678
Erythrocyte sedimentation rate
  in Kawasaki disease, 1515
  reference ranges for, 1897t
Erythrocyte volume, reference ranges
    for, 1901t
Erythrocyte volume distribution width, 1536t
Erythrogenin, 1255

Erythromycin
  for ophthalmia neonatorum prevention, 266
  for pneumonia, 1370
Erythropoiesis, 1532
Erythropoietin, 1532
  recombinant, for anemia, 399
Erythropoietin-stimulating factor, 1255, 1532
Eschar, 747, 747f, 748
Escharotomy, in burn injuries, 1231, 1232f,
    1233-1234
Escherichia coli
  diarrhea and, 1209t
  in neonatal sepsis, 393
  urinary tract infection and, 1264
Esophageal atresia, 463-466
  assessment of, 464-465
  clinical manifestations of, 463
  diagnosis of, 464
  nursing care plan for, 467-468
  nursing considerations in, 464-466
  pathophysiology of, 463, 463f
  treatment of, 464
Esophageal bleeding, 1454, 1461
Esophageal pH monitoring, 1422t, 1429
Esophageal varices, 1461
Esophagitis, in gastroesophageal reflux, 1429
Esophagostomy, cervical, 464, 465
Esophagus, development of, 1416-1417
Esophoria, 196, 197f
Esotropia, 196
Estrogen, 1708t
  adrenal secretion of, 1723
  at puberty, 803-805
  dysfunctional uterine bleeding and, 848
Etanercept, for juvenile rheumatoid
    arthritis, 1822
Ethambutol, for tuberculosis, 1374
Ethchlorvynol, abuse of, 886t
Ethical issues, 21-22, 22b
  in genetic screening, 127
  in pain management, 957, 957b
  in terminal illness, 948, 948t, 957, 957b
  terminal illness and, pain management in,
    957, 957b
Ethmoid sinus, 191, 191f
Ethnic groups; see also Race/ethnicity.
  classification of, 35b
  membership in, 35
Ethnocentrism, 34
Ethosuxamide, for seizures, 1691t
Ethylenediaminetetraacetic acid, for chelation
    therapy, 680
Etiology, in nursing diagnosis, 26
Etoposide (VP-16), 1592t
Eustachian tube
  air travel and, 1360
  blocked, otitis media and, 1357, 1357f
  function of, 1357
Eutectic mixture of local anesthetics; see EMLA
    cream.
Euthanasia, 949
Evaluation, in nursing process, 27
Evaporated milk formula, 280, 281t, 282
  hypocalcemia and, 318
Evaporative heat loss, in newborn, 265
  at high risk, 340
Everyday activities; see Activities.
Evidence-based practice, 14b, 22
Evil eye, 47

Evulsion, tissue, 745
Ewing sarcoma, 1626-1627, 1628-1629
Exanthemum subitum, 654f, 654t-655t
Exchange diet, 1738-1739, 1744-1745, 1745t
Exchange theory, family, 67t
Exchange transfusion; see also Transfusion.
    for hemolytic disease of newborn, 315-316
    for hyperbilirubinemia, 307t
Excoriation, 746f
Exencephaly, 424b
Exercise; see also Sports.
    congenital heart disease and, 1503
    cystic fibrosis and, 1408
    hemophilia and, 1564, 1565
    hypertension and, 1518, 1519
    in diabetes, 1739, 1749-1750
    in juvenile rheumatoid arthritis,
        1822, 1824
    in school-age children, 724
    in systemic lupus erythematosus, 1828
    menstrual irregularities and, 846
    mental retardation and, 982-983, 983f
    obesity and, 872, 874
Exercise stress test, 1470
Exercise-induced bronchospasm, in asthma,
    1394-1395
Exercises
    in cerebral palsy, 1840
    Kegel, 784
    range-of-motion, for unconscious child, 1659
Exhibitionism, definition of, 685
EXIT procedure, for congenital
        diaphragmatic hernia, 475
Exophoria, 196, 197f
Exophthalmos, in hyperthyroidism, 1719
Exosurf Neonatal, 386
Exotropia, 196
Experimental therapy, terminal illness and, 949t
Expiratory grunt, in respiratory distress
        syndrome, 381, 382f
Expressed mother's milk, preterm infant
        and, 347
    gavage feeding of, 348
Expressive activities, during hospitalization,
        1071-1072, 1071f, 1072f
Expressive language, 1007
Expressive roles, in family, 68-69
Exstrophy, epispadias and, 482-484, 483f
Extended family, 71
    special needs child and, 929-931
External auditory canal, examination of,
        202, 203
External fixation, 1792-1793, 1792f, 1794
    for fractures, 1792-1793, 1792f
External rotation deformities, in high-risk
        newborn, 363
External ventricular drainage,
        ventriculoperitoneal shunt and, 441
Extracellular fluid, 1171; see also Fluid(s).
    depletion of, 1174
        in hypotonic dehydration, 1177
        in isotonic dehydration, 1176
    expansion of, in treating dehydration,
        1179-1180
    growth and, 1173, 1173f
    in infants, 497, 1173-1174
    in newborn, 242

Extracorporeal membrane oxygenation
        (ECMO), 1324
    after heart surgery, 1507
    for shock, 1222
    in persistent pulmonary hypertension of
        newborn, 398
Extradural hematoma, 1666f, 1667-1668
Extrahepatic biliary atresia, 470-472, 471f
Extramedullary hemopoiesis, 1531
Extraneous air syndromes, 389-390
Extrapyramidal gait, 1647b
Extrapyramidal system, 1832-1833, 1833f
Extravasation
    of chemotherapy drugs, 1589
    of intravenous solution, 1197
Extremely-low-birth-weight infant, 334b; see
        also High-risk newborn.
Extremities; see also under Limb.
    developmental defects of, 447t, 453-454
    Down syndrome and, 992
    examination of, 224-225
    lower
        elevation of, 1800, 1800f
        examination of, 224-225
    of newborn, 254t, 262-263, 263t
        during parenteral fluid therapy, 342
        external rotation of, 363
        in brachial palsy, 299, 299f, 300
    prosthesis for, 454, 1628
    restraint of, 1140
    traction of; see Traction.
    use of, play activities and, 1111b
Extremity venipuncture, positioning for,
        1141, 1141f
Extrusion reflex, 263t
Extubation, neonatal, opioids and, 356b
Eye(s); see also under Vision; Visual.
    alignment of, 195-196
        tests for, 196-197, 198t
    anatomic landmarks of, 193, 193f
    disorders of, in diabetes, 1735
    Down syndrome and, 989t, 990, 990f
    examination of, 192-195
        fundoscopic, 194-195, 195f
        in neurologic assessment, 1650-1651,
            1650f
        ophthalmoscopic, 194-195, 195f
    in nutritional assessment, 166t
    infections of, 662-664; see also Conjunctivitis.
    injuries to, 736
    movements of
        development of, 199t
        in brain injury, 1650, 1651
        in cerebral palsy, 207
        in neurologic assessment, 1650, 1651,
            1652
    of newborn, 243-244, 252t, 258-259, 263t
        facial nerve paralysis and, 300
        phototherapy and, 308, 308f, 309, 365
        prophylactic care and, 266, 266b
        retinopathy of prematurity and, 344, 399-
            400, 400b
    prosthetic, 1634, 1634f
    protection of, in unconscious child, 1659
    protrusion of, in hyperthyroidism, 1719
    removal of, for retinoblastoma, 1633-1634
    retinoblastoma of, 1632-1635, 1632f, 1633b,
        1634f

Eye(s)—cont'd
    structure of, 192, 192f
    sunset, 193
    trauma to, 1000, 1002
        emergency treatment of, 1003b
    wide-spaced, 192
Eye contact, cultural aspects of, 44-45
Eye drops, 1160, 1160f
Eye examination, schedule for, 171b
Eyeglasses, 1005
Eyelashes, inspection of, 194
Eyelid
    examination of, 193-194
    inflammation of, 193b
    malposition of, 193

F
FAB system, 1611
Face/facies
    characteristics of, in school-age children, 699
    feeding problems and, cleft lip and palate
        and, 459
    in congenital hypothyroidism, 321
    in craniofacial abnormalities, 445-446, 445b
    in Down syndrome, 989t, 990f
    in fetal alcohol syndrome, 329b, 329f
    in fragile X syndrome, 993, 993f
    moon, 1602, 1727, 1727f
    neonatal pain and, 352, 353f, 1037f
    physical examination of, 186
    visual preference for in infants, 495, 507
FACES (Wong-Baker) Pain Rating Scale, 1051,
    1052t, 1905-1907
Facial nerve, assessment of, 229t
Facial nerve paralysis, birth-related, 298-299, 299f
    nursing care and, 299-300
Facilitated tucking, before heel puncture, 361
Facilitative responding, 151b
Facioscapulohumeral muscular dystrophy, 1863t
Factor VIIa, transfusion of, 1543t
Factor VIII
    deficiency of, 1562-1566
    transfusion of, 1543t
Factor VIII concentrate, 1563, 1564
Factor IX
    deficiency of, 1562
    transfusion of, 1543t
Fading, educational, in mental retardation, 981
Failure to thrive, 574-578
    categories of, 574
    factors related to, 574
    in cystic fibrosis, 1406
    in malabsorption syndromes, 1450
    nursing considerations with, 575-577, 575b
    nutritional management of, 577-578
Faith healing, 49
Falls
    fractures and, 1777
    in infants, 542f, 543f, 546, 549b
    in school-age children, 735
    in toddlers, 618b, 622-623
    prevention of, 542f, 543f, 546, 549b, 618b,
        622-623, 1758b
    spinal cord injury in, 1855
False ribs, 209
False-negative test results, 127
False-positive test results, 127
Falx cerebelli, 1642

Falx cerebri, 1642
Famciclovir, for varicella-zoster virus
    infection, 651b
Familial adenomatous polyposis, 1166
Familial benign neutropenia, 1569t
Familial hypothyroidism, 119t
Familial nephritis (Alport syndrome), 1282
Familial short stature, 1709
Families Adopting Children Everywhere
    (FACE), 90
Family, 64-101; see also Home care; Parent(s).
  abusive, 684-685, 692-693
  anorexia nervosa and, 880
  as patient, 69
  assessment of, home care and,
    1023-1024, 1024b
  autism and, 1010
  binuclear, 72
  blended, 71, 98-99, 99b, 817
  boundaries of, 66
  closed, 66
  communal, 72
  composition of, 160
  definition of, 65, 160
  developmental tasks of, 67-68, 68b
  dysfunctional, 74-75
  education of, 1131-1132
  expressive roles in, 68-69
  extended, 71
  functions of, 68-69, 73
  gay/lesbian, 72-73
  grieving, 968-972, 969b, 970t
  hospitalized child and, 1041
  instrumental roles in, 68-69
  intestinal parasitic infections in, 666
  lead poisoning education for, 679, 682, 682b
  management style of, special needs child
    and, 924-925, 932
  multiple births and, 79-81, 80b
  nuclear, 70-71
  nursing interventions for, 69-70, 69b
  obesity and, 875-876
  of adolescents, 817-818, 826-827, 827b
    guidance for, 836b, 837
    in pregnancy, 853
  of hospitalized children, 1040-1041, 1040b,
    1073-1074, 1074b
    nursing care plan for, 1080-1083
  of infants
    guidance for, 550, 550b
    sudden infant death syndrome and, 584-585
    with apnea, 588
  of preschoolers, 646b
  of school-age children
    guidance for, 707, 708, 736, 736b
    relationships with, 707-708
  of sexually abused children, response to
    suspicion in, 691
  of toddlers, guidance for, 624, 624b
  one-child, 79, 79b
  open, 66
  peer group conflicts and, 706
  poisoning prevention by, 674b, 674t, 675b
  polygamous, 72
  resilient, 67
  roles and relationships in, 75-81
    sibling, 76t, 77
  single-parent, 71-72, 97-98vorce; see also
    Divorce.

Family—cont'd
  size and configuration of, 77-81
  social services for, 74, 74b, 74f
  strengths of, 73, 74b
  structure of, 70-73, 70f, 70t
  suicide and, 899, 899b
  violence in, 683
  vulnerable, 73-75, 74b
Family advocacy/caring, 19-20
  nurse's role in, 19-20
Family and Medical Leave Act, 13, 100
Family APGAR, 162-163, 162b, 1870-1871
Family assessment, 160-164
  functional, 162-164
  indications for, 160b
  structural, 160-162
Family Communications, Inc., 1108n
Family composition, 70-83, 70f, 70t
Family conflict theory, 67t
Family daycare, for children, 516
Family development, special needs child
  and, 907
Family development theory, 66t, 67-68
Family exchange theory, 67t
Family function, 73-75, 74b
  assessment of, 162-164, 162b, 163b
Family history
  cardiac function assessment and, 1468
  hypertension and, 1518
  in genetic counseling, 133
  medical, 158
  pedigree chart in, 133-134, 133f, 134f, 135b
Family Medical Leave Act, 3
Family of origin, 65
Family services, 74, 74b, 74f
Family stress theory, 66-67, 66t, 69
Family structural-functional theory, 67t, 68-69
Family structure
  assessment of, 160-162
  definition of, 160
Family Support America, 368
Family symbolic interactional theory, 67t
Family systems theory, 65-66, 66t, 69
Family theories, 65-69, 66t-67t
Family tree, 133-134, 133f, 134f, 135b, 160-162
Family violence, 75
Family Voices, 931n, 932n
Family-centered care, 13-15, 14b, 907-908
  hospitalization and, 1041, 1073
  sibling-newborn attachment and,
    285-286, 286f
  special needs child and, 905-945; see also
    Special needs child.
  terminal illness and, 948-975; see also
    Terminal illness.
  unexpected childhood death and,
    964-966, 966b
Family-controlled analgesia, 1064b
Family-professional partnership, 14-15, 23
  therapeutic relationship and, 18-19, 19b
Family-provider relationship, cultural factors
  in, 43-45
Family-to-family support, home care and,
  1028-1029
Famotidine (Pepcid)
  for gastroesophageal reflux, 1429
  for peptic ulcer disease, 1445
Fanconi syndrome, 1280, 1560
Farm activities, injuries during, 735

Farsightedness, 1000, 1001b
Fasciitis, plantar, 1801t
Fasciotomy, in burn injuries, 1231, 1232f
Fast food
  for diabetics, 1747t
  in school-age children, 721
Fasting, preoperative, 1113b
Fasting blood glucose, in diabetes, 1736
Fat, body; see Adipose tissue; Obesity.
Fat(s)
  dietary
    digestion of, 1419
    hypercholesterolemia and, 1521
    in infants, 521
    in preschoolers, 644
    low-cholesterol substitutes for, 1522t
    quantitative, tests of, 1420t
Fat embolism, 1795
Fat mass, 808
Father; see also Family; Parent(s).
  adolescent, 852
  age of, Down syndrome and, 989
  attachment of to infant, 504-506
  attachment of to newborn, 285, 285f
  involvement of in parenting, 82-83
  single, 98
  special needs child and, 926-927, 927b, 989
Fatigue
  breast-feeding and, 521
  in infectious mononucleosis, 1355
Fatty acids, 1418
  digestion of, 1419
Fear(s)
  in preschoolers, 642-644
  in school phobias, 795
  in school-age children, 719-920
  in toddlers, 609
  of bedtime, 515
  of death, 954
  of hospitalized children, 1040
  of strangers
    in infants, 506, 514-515
    in toddlers, 599
"Fear of fat" syndrome, 883-884
Febrile seizures, 1696-1698, 1697-1698
Fecal enzymes, diaper dermatitis and, 578
Fecal incontinence, 785-786
Fecal smears, for diagnosis of intestinal
  parasites, 666
Fecalith, 1433
Fecal-oral transmission, of giardiasis, 667
Feces, 578, 1419
Federation for Children with Special
  Needs, 931n
Feeding; see also Diet; Food(s); Nutrition.
  developmental milestones related to,
    522b, 611t
  difficulties in, 571-578
    with colic, 571-574
    with congestive heart failure, 1483
    with failure to thrive, 574-578
    with gastroesophageal reflux, 1430, 1431
    with improper feeding technique, 571
    with regurgitation and spitting up, 571
    with rumination, 574
  enteral; see Enteral nutrition.
  facilitation of, high-risk newborn and, 346-
    347, 346b
  gastrostomy, 1164-1165, 1164f, 1164t, 1165f

Feeding—cont'd
gavage, 348, 348f, 1162-1164, 1163b, 1163f
in autisms, 1010
in cerebral palsy, 1840-1841, 1841f
in Down syndrome, 992
in mental retardation and, 984-985, 984b, 984f
independent, mental retardation and, 984-985, 984b, 984f
infant, growth rates and, 175
jaw control for, 1840-1841, 1841f
mental retardation and, 984-985, 984b, 984f
of infants; *see also* Bottle-feeding; Breast-feeding.
developmental milestones in, 522b
in first 6 months, 520-521, 524b
in second 6 months, 521-522, 524b
parental interaction during, 575b, 576
proper technique of, 571
solid foods for, 522-524, 524b
weaning of, 524-525
of newborns
behavior and, 279-280, 345
candidiasis and, 301
cleft lip and palate and, 458-459, 459b, 459f, 460
esophageal atresia and, 465
facial nerve paralysis and, 299-300
jaundice and, 303t, 305, 307
necrotizing enterocolitis and, 396
respiratory distress syndrome and, 383
schedule for, 279
tracheoesophageal fistula and, 465
promotion of, 1128-1130, 1129b
visual impairment and, 1005
Feeding problems, in cerebral palsy, 1840-1841, 1841f
Feeding resistance, high-risk newborn and, 348-349, 349b
Feeding Scale, of National Child Assessment Satellite Training Program, 247
Feeding stress, high-risk newborn and, 346
Feet; *see* Foot.
Feetham Family Functioning Survey, 163, 163b
FEIBA (factor eight inhibitor by-pass activity), 1543t
Felbamate, for seizures, 1691t
Female athlete triad, 1804
Female circumcision, 223
Female condom, 855
Female genital mutilation, 49b, 272b
Female genitalia
ambiguous, 489t
of newborn, 253t, 261, 377f
preterm, 376, 377f
Female reproductive system, 844-849
Femoral head; *see also* Hip.
aseptic necrosis of, 1807-1808
dislocation of, 1799
Femoral hernia, 218, 218f, 478
Femoral neck, fracture of, 1777
Femoral pulse
of newborn, 253t, 261
palpation of, 220, 220f
Femoral venipuncture, positioning for, 1140f, 1141
Femur, fracture of, birth-related, 298
Fentanyl
abuse of, 886t
for pain, 1060, 1062t, 1063t, 1066

Fentanyl—cont'd
in newborn, 357
patient controlled infusion and, 1064t
in preoperative sedation, 1112-1113, 1113b
transdermal, 1065b, 1066
Fentanyl Oralet, 1064b
in preoperative sedation, 1113, 1113b
Ferritin, chelation therapy and, 1551
Ferrous iron, 1545
Ferrous sulfate, 1545
Fertility, Down syndrome and, 990
Fetal alcohol effects, 329
Fetal alcohol syndrome, 326, 328-330, 329b, 329f
Fetal biopsy, 130
Fetal blood sampling, 130
Fetal circulation, 1466, 1466f
persistent, 397-398, 398f
Fetal death, 334b
Fetal echocardiography, 130
Fetal hemoglobin, 1532
in infants, 496
persistent, respiratory distress syndrome and, 381
Fetal shunts, 241
Fetus
alcohol effects on, 326, 328-330, 329b, 329f
alloimmunization and, 310
intrauterine transfusion in, 315
anemia in, maternal human parvovirus infection and, 651
body water distribution in, 1173
cocaine effects on, 407-408
congenital diaphragmatic hernia in, surgery for, 475
diabetes effects on, 405
growth and differentiation of, 416, 417f
lung maturity of, 383
masculinization of, in congenital adrenal hyperplasia, 1729-1731
maternal smoking and, 408-409
meconium aspiration by, 388-389
opioid effects on, 406-407, 406b
passive smoking and, 1382
Fever, 1130-1131, 1130t, 1131t, 1132b; *see also* Infection(s).
blood transfusion and, 1541t
in cancer, 1597
in congestive heart failure, 1482
in Kawasaki disease, 1514
in respiratory infections, 1346
in sickle cell anemia, 1550
insensible water loss and, 1174
seizures and, 1696-1698, 1697-1698
splenectomy and, 1547
Fever blisters, 664, 758t
Fexofenadine hydrochloride (Allegra), for allergic rhinitis, 1384
Fiber, dietary, 1426, 1426b
Fiberglass casts, 1784-1785, 1785t
Fiberoptic blanket, in hyperbilirubinemia treatment, 306
Fibrin, 1534, 1561
in burn wound healing, 1242
Fibrinogen, 1562t
reference ranges for, 1897t
Fibrin-stabilizing factor, 1562t
Fibroblasts, in wound healing, 747
Fibroplasia, in wound healing, 747

Fifth disease
complications of, 651, 660
in newborn, 327t
manifestations and management of, 654f, 654t-655t
Filter paper spot test, in phenylketonuria screening, 267, 267b
Financial factors
in health care, 106
in home care, 1017
Finger(s)
clubbing of
hypoxemia and, 1486, 1487f
in assessment of breathing, 1311, 1311f
of nails, 189
extra, 224
fused, 224
Finger spelling, 1006
Fingernail polish, hand contamination and, 1134b
Finger-stick device, for blood glucose monitoring, 1748
Finger-to-nose test, 226
Fioricet with Codeine, 1060b
Fire ants, bites of, 776t
Firearms
injuries from, 736, 828, 829
safety for, 623
Fires
prevention of, 1758b
safety measures for, 1252
First aid; *see* Emergency care.
First-pass effect, opioids and, 1062
Fissure(s)
anal, 223
in newborn, 262
palpebral, 193, 193f
skin, 746f
Fistula
arteriovenous, for hemodialysis, 1295
omphalomesenteric (Meckel diverticulum), 1435
perineal, 468, 469
rectourethral, 468, 468f
rectovaginal, 261, 466, 468, 468f
tracheoesophageal, 463-466, 463f
Fitzgerald factor, 1562t
Fitz-Hugh-Curtis syndrome, 863
Fixed drug eruption, 772
FLACC Postoperative Pain Scale, 1055, 1056t-1057t
Flame burns, 621
Flank pain
in renal trauma, 1283
urinary tract infection and, 1266
Flashlamp pulsed dye laser, 302
Flat foot, 224, 447t
Flatness, on chest percussion, 212
Flea
bites of, 300, 776t
rickettsial infections from, 763, 765t
Flea bite dermatitis, 300
Fleet enemas, 1262
Fletcher factor, 1562t
Flies, bites of, 776t
Flip-flap procedure, in hypospadias, 482
Floaters, 209
Floppy infant syndrome, 1843
Flossing of teeth, 612, 781

Fluconazole, for candidiasis, in newborn, 301
Fluid(s); see also Solution(s); Water.
    after tonsillectomy, 1354
    body
        collecting devices for, 1186
        distribution of, 1171-1174, 1172b, 1173t
        in infants, 497
    extracellular, 1171; see also Extracellular fluid.
    in hypoxemia, 1490
    interstitial, 1171, 1180, 1181
    intracellular, 1171, 1173, 1173f
    intravascular, 1171
    intravenous; see also Infusion(s),
            intravenous.
        for asthma emergency care, 1396
        for gastrointestinal bleeding, 1456
        for pneumonia, 1370, 1371
        for severe dehydration, 1213
        for shock, 1221
    loss of; see also Dehydration.
        distribution of, 1174
        in burn injuries, 1231
        prevention of by skin, 740
    oral, 1185-1188
        in diarrhea, 1211-1214, 1212t
    parenteral, 1179-1180, 1188-1198
        by intraosseous infusion, 1191-1192
        by intravenous infusion, 1188-1191
    pericardial, 1465
    redistribution of, in burn injuries, 1232
    rehydration, 1179, 1186, 1188
        for diarrhea, 1211-1214, 1212t
        in burn patients, 1236-1237
        oral, 1186, 1188
            for diarrhea, 1211-1214, 1212t
            parenteral, 1179-1180
    replacement of, in burn patients, 1236-1237
    restricted, with congestive heart failure,
            1480, 1483
    total body, in infants, 497
    transcellular, 1171
Fluid and electrolyte balance, 1172-1174,
        1172b, 1173t
    acid-base imbalance and, 1182-1185
    after heart surgery, 1506
    altered fluid requirements and, 1172, 1174
    assessment of, 1185-1186
    blood transfusion and, 1541t
    clinical observations in, 1185-1186,
            1187t-1189t
    distribution of body fluids and, 1171-1174,
            1172b, 1173t
    disturbances in, 1174-1181, 1175t-1176t
    in acute poststreptococcal
            glomerulonephritis, 1273
    in acute renal failure, 1285-1286, 1287
    in burn patients, 1237
    in chronic renal failure, 1288
    in dehydration, 1171-1180
    in edema, 1180-1181
    in hypertrophic pyloric stenosis, 1447
    in infants, 1173-1174
    in newborn, 242
        after surgery, 420t, 422t, 423
    in water intoxication, 1180
    metabolic acidosis and, 1184
    metabolic alkalosis and, 1184-1185
    nursing considerations in, 1185-1204
    of gastrointestinal tract, 1418

Fluid and electrolyte balance—cont'd
    oral fluid intake and, 1185-1188
    parenteral fluid therapy and, 1188-1198
    processes of, 1293b
    respiratory acidosis and, 1183-1184
    respiratory alkalosis and, 1184
    total parenteral nutrition and, 1203-1204
    venous access devices and, 1198-1203
    water balance and, 1172-1174
Fluid intake
    for athletes, 1803-1804
    play activities and, 1111b
    urinary tract infection and, 1265
Fluid management
    in acute adrenocortical insufficiency, 1725
    in acute renal failure, 1285
    in bacterial meningitis, 1679
    in bronchopulmonary dysplasia, 392
    in congenital diaphragmatic hernia, 476
    in cranial surgery, 1623-16214
    in diabetes insipidus, 1658, 1658t, 1672,
            1715, 1716
    in diabetes mellitus, 1734
    in diabetic ketoacidosis, 17421742
    in diarrhea, 1214
    in head injury, 1672
    in high-risk newborns, 341-342, 351b
        with bronchopulmonary dysplasia, 392
        with necrotizing enterocolitis, 396
    in hypercalcemia, 1765
    in immobilization, 1768
    in meningitis, 1680
    in nasopharyngitis, 1350
    in nephrotic syndrome, 1278
    in renal disorders, 1262
    in respiratory infections, 1346
    in sickle cell anemia, 1552
    in syndrome of inappropriate antidiuretic
            hormone, 1658, 1658t, 1672, 1716-1717
    in terminal illness, 949t
    in unconscious children, 1658
    in urinary tract infection, 1268
    NPO status in, 1188
    oral intake in, 1185-1188
        in diarrhea, 1212, 1212t
    parenteral fluid therapy in, 1179-1180, 1188-
            1198; see also Infusion(s).
Fluid overload, 1180
Fluid volume, and growth, 1173, 1173f
Flumazenil, for benzodiazepine-induced
        respiratory depression, 673, 1068b
Flunitrazepam, 892
Fluorescence in situ hybridization (FISH), 123
Fluoride
    dental health and, 613, 614b, 780, 781
    functions of and disturbances in, 561t
    sources of, 561t
    supplemental, 613, 613t, 614b
        for breast milk, 520, 521
        in infancy, 527
Fluorocarbons, abuse of, 886t
Fluorosis, 613, 614b
5-Fluorouracil (Adrucil), 1591t
Fluoxetine, in fragile X syndrome, 994
Fluphenazine, for Tourette syndrome, 793
Flutter mucus clearance device, in cystic
        fibrosis, 1408, 1408f
Folacin, functions of and disturbances in, 557t
Foley catheter, 1145, 1145t

Folic acid
    deficiency of, 555
    functions of and disturbances in, 557t
    in pregnancy, 124-125
    neural tube defects and, 424, 430
Folinic acid, functions of and disturbances
        in, 557t
Folk healers, 48-49
Follicle-stimulating hormone, 805, 1707t
    in adolescence, 803, 803f
Folliculitis, 755, 755t
Follow-up formulas, 280
Fontan procedure, for tricuspid atresia, 1498b
Fontanels, 191, 252t, 257-258, 258f
    in increased intracranial pressure, 1646
Food
    after tonsillectomy, 1354
    allergy/intolerance to; see also Allergy(ies).
        anaphylactic reactions and, 568
        attention deficit hyperactivity disorder
                and, 787
        ethnicity and, 57
        in infants, 568-571
    aspiration of, 1376
        by infants, 542t-543t, 543
    gluten-containing, 1451
    high-fat, low-cholesterol substitutes
            for, 1522t
    hyperallergenic, 568b
    measurements of, for preschoolers, 644
    selection of
        for infants, 522-523
        for toddlers, 610, 610b, 623
        guidelines for, 564-565
    servings of, for toddlers, 610, 611
    snack, 610, 614, 615t
    solid
        commercially prepared baby food as,
                522-523
        in first 6 months, 521, 524b
        in second 6 months, 521-522, 524b
        safety of for infants and toddlers, 565
        selection and preparation of for infants,
                522-524, 524b
        storage of, 523
Food additives, asthma and, 1397
Food diary, 165
Food frequency questionnaire, 165, 165t
Food Guide Pyramid, 564, 565b, 565f, 644, 722b
Food pica, 1422-1423
Food preferences, cultural aspects of, 45-47, 165b
Foot
    development of, 519
    developmental defects of, 447t
        clubfoot and, 451-453, 452b, 452f
        metatarsus adductus and, 453
    Down syndrome and, 989t
    examination of, 224
    of newborn, 262
    prematurity and, 377f
Footwear, for infants, 519-520
Foramen of Luschka, 436, 437f
Foramen of Magendie, 436, 437f
Foramen of Monro, 436, 437f
Foramen ovale, 241
    in embryologic development, 1465, 1465f
    patent
        in transposition of great arteries, 1499b
        in tricuspid atresia, 1497b

Forced expiration
  in cystic fibrosis, 1408
  with bronchial drainage, 1320
Forced kneeling, 49b
Forceps, soft tissue injury from, 295
Ford chestpiece, 212
Forearm crutches, 1775
Foregut, 1416
Foreign body
  aspiration of, 1376-1377, 1376f, 1378b
    airway obstruction and, 1338,
      1340-1341, 1340f
    by infants, 541-544, 542t-543t, 549b
    risk factors for, 1378b
  in ear, 203
  in eye, 1003b
  in nose, 1378
  in skin, 768-769
  ingestion of, 1423, 1423b
Foreign language speakers, 45
  interpreters for, 145-146, 146b
Foreign substances, ingestion of, 1419,
    1422-1423
Foreskin
  examination of, 221
  of newborn, 261
    circumcision and, 270-273, 270b-272b, 272f
    phimosis and, 479
    tight, 221
Formal operations stage, 230t, 231-232, 232
Formula(s); *see also* Bottle-feeding.
  elemental, in short bowel syndrome, 1452
  enteral, 348
    for inflammatory bowel disease, 1441
  infant, 521, 524b
    amino acid-based, 570
    commercially prepared, 280, 281t-283t
    constipation and, 1424
    cow's milk in, 569-570, 569b, 1213
    evaporated milk, 280, 282, 318
    in acute diarrhea, 1213
    in colic, 572
    in congestive heart failure, 1483
    in cystic fibrosis, 1410
    in Hirschsprung disease, 1430, 1431
    inappropriately prepared, 1180
    iron-fortified, 521, 521t, 524b, 1545
    lactose-free, 325
    microwave heating of, 523, 523b
    postdischarge, for high-risk newborn, 369
    preparation of, 279, 280
    protein hydrolysate, 570, 572, 1410
    soy, 570
Formula feeding; *see* Bottle-feeding.
Fortified human milk, for high-risk
    newborn, 344
Foscarnet, for varicella-zoster virus
    infection, 651b
Fosphenytoin (Cerebyx), 1690
Foster children, 100
  adoption of, 92-93
  special needs, 927
Foundation for the Junior Blind, 1006
Fovea centralis, 195, 195f, 243
Fractures, 1776-1795
  apposition of, 1783, 1784f
  as signs of physical abuse, 688b
  birth-related, 298
  bone fragments in, 1783, 1784f

Fractures—cont'd
  casting of, 1784-1787, 1784f, 1785b,
    1785t, 1896f
  causes of, 1777
  circulatory impairment in, 1793
  clinical manifestations of, 1780
  comminuted, 1778
  compartment syndromes in, 1793-1794
  complete, 1778, 1779f
  complicated, 1778
  complications of, 1793-1795
  compound (open), 1778, 1779f
  crepitation in, 224, 1780
  diagnosis of, 1780-1781
  distraction for, 1792
  embolism and, 1795
  epiphyseal injury in, 1794
  external fixation for, 1792-1793, 1792f, 1794
  healing of, 1781-1784, 1782f, 1782t, 1783f
  in osteogenesis imperfecta, 1820
  incomplete, 1778, 1779f
  infection in, 1794
  initial assessment in, 1780
  intentional, 1758-1759, 1758b; *see also*
    Child abuse.
  internal fixation for, 1793
  kidney stones and, 1794-1795
  malunion of, 1794
  nerve compression in, 1793
  nonunion of, 1794
  pathophysiology of, 1777-1780
  pulmonary embolism and, 1795
  reduction of, 1781, 1781b
  simple (closed), 1778, 1779f
  skull, 1271, 1666-1667
  soft tissue response in, 1779-1780
  stress, 1801
  traction for, 1787-1792, 1788f-1790f; *see also*
    Traction.
  treatment of, 1781, 1781b; *see also*
    Immobilization.
  types of, 1778, 1778f, 1779b, 1779f
  vascular injuries in, 1780
  vertebral
    spinal cord injury and, 1852-1863, 1856;
      *see also* Spinal cord injury.
    traction for, 1790-1791, 1790b
  Volkmann contracture in, 1794
Fragile X syndrome, 119t, 993-994, 993f, 994b
Frank breech, 251t
Frank Porter Graham Child Development
    Center, 1024n
Frank-Starling curve, 1468
Fraternal twins, 80, 80b, 80f
Fredet-Ramstedt procedure, for hypertrophic
    pyloric stenosis, 1447, 1447f
French-American-British (FAB) system, 1611
Frenulum, 259-260
Fresh frozen plasma, 1543t
Freudian theory, 230, 230t
  preschoolers in, 630-631
  school-age children in, 700
Friction, pressure ulcers and, 1124
Friction rub
  pericardial, 215
  pleural, 213
Friendships; *see also* Socialization.
  of adolescents, 816
  of school-age children, 706-707, 706f

Friendships—cont'd
  of special needs child, 930-931
  social functions of, 37-38
Frontal bossing, in hydrocephalus, 437
Frontal lobes, 1644t
Frontal sinus, 191, 191f
Frostbite, 771
Fructose, chronic nonspecific diarrhea
    and, 1217
Fruit, for infants, 522, 524b
Fruit juices, 610
  bottle-feeding with, 615
  chronic nonspecific diarrhea and, 1217
  dental decay and, 566b
  for failure to thrive, 577
  for infants, 521, 522, 524b, 566b
  for preschoolers, 644
  for toddlers, 610, 615
Frustration
  in preschoolers, 641
  parents of hospitalized child and, 1040
Full-term infant, 334b
Functional and adaptive training, in cerebral
    palsy, 1840
Functional burden, special needs child and,
    935, 935b
Functional electrical stimulation, 1858
Functional health patterns, 26b
  nursing admission history and, 1088b-1089b
Functional hearing loss, 995
Fundoscopic examination, 194-195, 195f
Funeral, siblings' attendance at, 967, 967b, 968f
Fungal infections, 759-760, 759t, 760f
  systemic, 763, 764t
  vaginitis and, 848, 849
Funnel chest, 209
Furazolidone, 666t
  for giardiasis, 667
Furniture, child safety precautions with,
    546, 549b
Furosemide (Lasix)
  for congestive heart failure, 1480t
  for nephrotic syndrome, 1277

**G**

Gabapentin, for seizures, 1691t
Gag reflex, 260, 263t
  gavage feeding and, 348
Gait
  abnormalities of, 1647b
  angle of, 225, 225f
  assessment of, 224-225, 225f, 1647b
  developmental dysplasia of hip and,
    448-449, 449f
Galactose, reference ranges for, 1897t
Galactose 1-phosphate uridine transferase, 325
Galactosemia, 119t, 324-325, 325f
Galant reflex, 263t
Galeazzi sign, 254t, 448, 449f
Gallbladder, 1416
Ganglion cells, absence of, in Hirschsprung
    disease, 1426
Ganglioneuroma, 1724
Gangs, membership in, 707, 708b
Garage doors, safety rules for, 623
Gas(es)
  arterial blood; *see* Arterial blood gases.
  chemical, in smoke inhalation injuries, 1381
  partial pressures of, 1308

Gas exchange, 1308-1310
air sac structure and, 1306
in alveoli, 1309b
in asthma, 1388
in respiratory distress syndrome, 380-381
perfluorocarbon-assisted, 385-386
primary inefficient, respiratory failure
and, 1331
Gas trapping, in asthma, 1388
Gastric acid
hypersecretion of, in short bowel
syndrome, 1452
in burn injuries, 1232
ulcers and, 1443
Gastric decontamination, in poisoning cases,
670-673
Gastric feeding, in burn injuries, 1234
Gastric glands, secretions of, 1418
Gastric lavage, in poisoning cases, 672
Gastric ulcer, 1443
Gastric varices, 1461
Gastric washings, 1148, 1375
Gastrin, 1418
Gastroduodenal erosion, in burn injuries, 1234
Gastroenteritis, infectious, 1208
Gastroesophageal reflux, 1429-1432
Gastrointestinal glands, 1704b
Gastrointestinal motility
development of, 1417
disorders of, 1424-1432
muscles involved in, 1417
Gastrointestinal priming, in high-risk
newborn, 343, 344, 396
Gastrointestinal tract
bleeding in, 1454-1456
development of, 1416-1417
developmental defects of, 454-474; see also
specific defects.
function of, 1417-1419, 1417b
assessment of, 1419, 1420b, 1420t-1422t
immobilization effects on, 1764, 1771t
in burn injuries, 1232, 1234
in cystic fibrosis, 1405-1406, 1406
in Henoch-Schönlein purpura, 1570
in middle childhood, 699
inflammatory conditions of, 1432-1446; see
also Crohn disease; Inflammatory bowel
disease; Ulcerative colitis.
ingestion of foreign substances in, 1419-1424
malabsorption syndromes of, 1450-1454
motility disorders in, 1424-1432
obstructive disorders of, 1446-1450
of newborn, 242, 242b
after surgery, 422t
at high risk, 336b
with necrotizing enterocolitis, 395-397
with sepsis, 394b
procedures on, bacterial endocarditis and,
1509, 1510b
structure of, 1416-1417
Gastroschisis, 472, 473-474, 473f
Gastrostomy feeding, 1162-1165, 1163b, 1163f,
1164-1165, 1164f, 1164t, 1165f; see also
Enteral nutrition.
drug administration via, 1159, 1159b
esophageal anastomosis and, 465
in high-risk newborns, 343-344
in terminal illness, 949t
in unconscious children, 1658

Gates, restraining, 546, 549b
Gauze, impregnated, for burn wounds,
1239-1240, 1240t
Gavage feeding, 348, 348f, 1162-1164, 1163b;
see also Enteral nutrition.
in hypertrophic pyloric stenosis, 1447
in short bowel syndrome, 1452, 1453
in unconscious child, 1658
Gays/lesbians, 831, 835-836
as families, 72-73
origins of identity as, 814-816, 816b
Gaze, cardinal positions of, 228f
Gel Support, 350
Gender assignment; see also Sexual identity.
ambiguous genitalia and, 489, 489b
Gene, 111
Gene mapping, 123
Gene therapy, 125
for hemophilia, 1564
Gene transfer, 125
General systems theory, 65
Generational continuity, 82
Genetic anticipation, 121
Genetic counseling, 130-137
emotional aspects of, 135-136
follow-up care for, 134-135
in cystic fibrosis, 1410, 1411
nurse's role in, 132-137
referral for, 130, 133
Genetic diseases
age of onset of, 111t
burden of, 136-137
cancer as, 111, 122, 1585-1586
carriers of, screening for, 126, 127
chromosome (cytogenetic), 113-118; see also
Chromosome disorders.
classification of, 111
congenital malformations and, 111-113
counseling for, 130-138; see also Genetic
counseling.
diagnosis of, 123, 123b, 123f, 132b
prenatal, 128-130, 128t, 129b
presymptomatic, 126-127
emotional aspects of, 135-136
family impact of, 135-137
mitochondrial, 122
multifactorial, 124
mutations and, 121
race/ethnicity and, 51-57, 56t
risk assessment for, 131-132, 132b
screening for, 125-127
single-gene, 118-120
terminology for, 112b
treatment of, 124-125
variable expression of, 121-122
Genetic mutations, 121
disease-causing; see Genetic diseases.
in cancer, 122
in fragile X syndrome, 993
single-gene, 118-120, 119t
Genetic premutations, 121
Genetic screening, 125-127
Genetic testing, 130-137
genetic counseling and, 131-137
indications for, 130-131
prenatal, 128-137
referral for, 130
timing of, 130

Genetics, 110-137
terminology of, 112b
Genital stage, 230, 230t
Genitalia
ambiguous, 487-490, 488f, 489b, 489t,
1729-1731
development of, premature, 1714-1715
Down syndrome and, 989t, 990
female
examination of, 222-223, 222f
mutilation of, 272b
of newborn, 253t, 261, 377f
of preterm infant, 376, 377f
in sexual abuse, 689b
male
circumcision of, 270-273, 270b-272b, 272f
cryptorchidism and, 480-481
examination of, 220-222, 222f
hypospadias and, 481-482, 481f
of newborn, 254t, 261, 377f
of preterm infant, 376, 377f
phimosis and, 479
structure of, 221f
masculinization of, in congenital adrenal
hyperplasia, 1729-1731
normal development of, 487, 488f
Genitourinary tract
developmental defects of, 478-490; see also
specific defects.
disorders of, 1262-1270
myelomeningocele and, 428-430
of high-risk newborn, 336b
procedures on, bacterial endocarditis and,
1509, 1510b
Genogram, 133-134, 133f, 134f, 135b, 160-162
Genomic imprinting, 121-122
Gentian violet solution, for candidiasis, in
newborn, 301
Gentle human touch method, for high-risk
newborn, 362
Genu recurvatum, 447t
Genu valgum, 224, 224f
Genu varum, 224, 224f, 447t
Georgetown University Child Development
Center, 939n
German measles, manifestations and
management of, 658f, 658t-659t
Germinal matrix-intraventricular hemorrhage,
401-402, 402t
Gestational age
clinical assessment of, 247-250, 248f-250f, 250b
high-risk infants and, 334b
persistent pulmonary hypertension and, 397
viability and, 334
Gestational diabetes mellitus, high-risk
newborn and, 405
Giant pigmented nevus, 302
Giardia lamblia, 666
antigen tests for, 1420t
Giardiasis, 666-667
Gigantism, 1706, 1713-1714
Gingival disorders, 611, 612, 781
Gingival examination, 208
in nutritional assessment, 166t
Gingivitis, 612, 781
acute necrotizing, 781
in cerebral palsy, 207
Gingivostomatitis, herpetic, 664, 664f
Girl Scouts, mental retardation and, 982

Glabellar reflex, 263t
Glands; *see* Endocrine system and specific glands and hormones.
Glandular appendages, of skin, 740
Glandular hypospadias, 482
Glans approximation procedure, in hypospadias, 482
Glanuloplasty, meatal advancement, hypospadias and, 482
Glasgow Coma Scale, 1648, 1648f
  in head injury, 1666
Glasses, 1005
Glaucoma, 1002b
Glenn shunt procedure, for tricuspid atresia, 1498b
Glioma, 1620b; *see also* Brain tumors.
Glomerular disease, 1270-1279
  acute renal failure and, 1284
Glomerular filtration, 1256-1257
  in infants, 1258
Glomerular filtration rate, 1260
  in acute renal failure, 1284
  in burn injuries, 1232
  in end-stage renal disease, 1287
Glomerular hydrostatic pressure, 1256
Glomerulonephritis
  acute poststreptococcal, 1270t, 1271-1274, 1351
    clinical signs of, 1271
    complications of, 1272
    diagnosis of, 1272-1273
    prognosis for, 1272
    treatment of, 1273-1274
    vs nephrotic syndrome, 1272t
  chronic, 1274
  focal segmental, 1274
  membranoproliferative, 1274
  membranous, 1274
  rapidly progressive, 1274
Glomerulopathy, chronic hereditary (Alport syndrome), 1282
Glossopharyngeal nerve, assessment of, 229t
Glottis, 1305
Glucagon, 1708t
  for diabetic hypoglycemia, 1741
Glucocorticoids, 1708t
  adrenal secretion of, 1723-1724
  deficiency of, 1726t
  effects of, 1724b
  pharmaceutical; *see* Steroids.
  replacement, for chronic adrenocortical insufficiency, 1726
Glucometers, 317
Gluconeogenesis, in diabetes, 1734
Glucose
  enteral nutrition and, high-risk newborn and, 343
  for hypoglycemia, in newborn, 317, 405, 406
  postoperative level of, in newborn, 420t
  quick sources of, for diabetics, 1740
  reference ranges for, 1897t
Glucose intolerance, 317
Glucose loading, for athletes, 1804
Glucose metabolism, insulin in, 1736-1737
Glucose monitoring, in diabetes, 1738, 1747, 1748, 1748f
Glucose tests, for diabetes, 1736
Glucose tolerance test, reference ranges for, 1897t

Glucose-6-phosphate dehydrogenase deficiency, 305
  BAL therapy and, 681
Glucuronyl transferase, 304
  physiologic jaundice of newborn and, 242
Glue ear, 1358
Glue sniffing, 886t, 892
Glutamine, in burn injuries, 1232-1233
Glutaraldehyde cross-linked collagen, for stress incontinence, 429
Gluteal folds, asymmetric, 448, 449f
Gluten, celiac disease and, 1450
Gluten-sensitive enteropathy, 1450-1451
Glycerides, 1418
Glycogen
  for athletes, 1804
  in burn injuries, 1232
Glycosuria, in diabetes, 1734, 1736
Glycosylated hemoglobin, in diabetes, 1738
Glycosylation, in diabetes, 1735
Gnats, bites of, 776t
Goat's milk, 282, 521
Goiter, 1718
  adolescent, 1718
GoLYTELY (polyethylene glycol electrolyte solution), 1425
Gomco technique, for circumcision, 272
Gonadotropin-releasing hormone
  in adolescence, 803, 803f
  in precocious puberty, 1714
Gonadotropins, 1707t
  hyposecretion of, 1706b
Gonads
  abnormal differentiation of, 487
  female, 1704b, 1704f, 1708t
  male, 221, 221f, 1704b, 1704f, 1708t;
    *see also* Testis.
Gonococcal disease, in newborn, 328t
Gonorrhea, 861-862
  vs chlamydial infection, 862t
Good Start, 281t
Government services, for children's health, 12-13
Gower sign, 1865, 1865f
Graft(s)
  skin, for burn wounds, 1241-1242, 1241b, 1241f-1242f
  synthetic, for hemodialysis, 1295
Graft-vs-host disease, 1596
  severe combined immunodeficiency disease and, 1579
Grandparents
  of infants of adolescent mothers, 851-852
  of special needs child, 929-930
Granulation tissue
  in burn injuries, 1231, 1234
  in wound healing, 747
Granulocyte(s), 1534
  transfusion of, 1543t
Granulocyte colony-stimulating factors, in cancer, 1598
Grasp reflex, 225, 262, 262f, 263t
  of preterm infant, 378f
Grasping, in infants, 498, 498f, 502
Graves disease, 1719-1721
Grief
  expression of, 970
  neonatal death and, 369-370
  persistent vegetative state and, 1660

Grief—cont'd
  special needs child and, 925
  terminal illness and, 960, 960b, 968-970, 969b, 970t
Griseofulvin, for ringworm infections, 760
Grommet, in ear, in otitis media, 1360
Grooming
  assessment of, 186-187
  mental retardation and, 986
Groshong catheter, vs other long-term venous access devices, 1201t
Groshong port, vs other long-term venous access devices, 1201t
Group B streptococcus, in neonatal sepsis, 393
Growing skull fractures, 1667
Growth and development; *see also* Development; Developmental; specific types of development, e.g., Biologic development.
  Down syndrome and, 990
  fluid volume and, 1173
  history of, 156
  in adolescents, 802-820, 803-809, 804t
  in breast- vs formula-fed infants, 175
  in bronchopulmonary dysplasia, 391
  in burn-injured children, 1233
  in fetal alcohol syndrome, 329b
  in infants, 494-501, 494-520
    alternate child-care arrangements in, 516-518
    coping with, 514-520
    limit-setting and discipline in, 516
    milestones in, 510t-515t
    pacifier use and, 518-519
    separation and stranger fear in, 514-515
    spoiled child syndrome in, 515-516
    teething and, 519
    thumb-sucking and, 518
    use of shoes and, 519-520
  in preschoolers, 628-630, 638t
  in puberty, 807-809
  in school-age children, 699-700
  in special needs child, 910-917, 911t-912t, 914f, 915f
  in toddlers, 592-594, 604t
  linear, 808, 809f
  maternal smoking and, 408-409
  normal rates of, 175t
  of preschoolers, 628-644, 638t-639t
  of school-age children, 698-714, 713t-714t, 714-720
  of toddlers, 591-609, 604t-605t
  prenatal, 416, 417f
  variations in
    abnormal, 175
    normal, 175, 176f
Growth charts, 174-175, 1882-1895; *see also* Anthropometric measurements.
  for Asian-Americans, 1892
Growth curve, evaluation of, 1711b
Growth delay, constitutional, 1710
Growth disturbances, 175; *see also* Short stature.
  in chronic renal failure, 1289, 1289b, 1291
  in congenital adrenal hyperplasia, 1729, 1731
  in Crohn disease, 1439, 1441
  in Fanconi syndrome, 1280
  in hypopituitarism, 1706-1713
  in thalassemia, 1558
  in ulcerative colitis, 1438, 1441

Growth disturbances—cont'd
  intrauterine, 334b
  psychostimulant administration and, 791
Growth hormone, 1707t
  for constitutional growth delay, 1710
  hypersecretion of, 1713-1714
  hyposecretion of, 1706b, 1709-1713; *see also*
    Hypopituitarism.
  measurement of, 1711
  reference ranges for, 1897t
  replacement, 1712
  sources of, 1712
Growth hormone stimulation tests, 1711
Growth plate, 1776, 1777f
  injury of, 1778-1779, 1779b, 1779f, 1794
Growth spurt, in puberty, 808
Grunting
  in assessment of breathing, 1311
  in respiratory distress syndrome, 381, 382f
Guardian, informed consent of, 1102
Guided imagery, in pain management, 1059b
Guidelines for Adolescent Preventive
  Services, 826
Guides, for blind child, 1003
Guiding statements, 144
Guillain-Barré syndrome, 1847-1848
Guillain-Barré Syndrome Foundation
  International, 1848
Guilt, 33
  hospitalization and, 1040
  in preschoolers, 630
  special needs child and, 913-914, 934
  terminal illness and, 972
Gums
  disorders of, 611, 612, 781
    in cerebral palsy, 207
  examination of, 208
    in nutritional assessment, 166t
Guns
  injuries from, 736, 828, 829
  mortality related to, 8, 8t
  safety for, 623
Gut-associated lymphoid tissue, 1571
Guthrie blood test, in phenylketonuria,
  323, 323b
Gynecologic examination, 844-845, 845b
Gynecomastia, 210, 807, 844

**H**

Habituation, in neonatal behavioral
  assessment, 245b
*Haemophilus influenzae*
  in neonatal sepsis, 393
  meningitis and, 1677-1680, 1681t
  otitis media and, 1357, 1358
  type b
    acute epiglottitis and, 1362, 1363
    immunization for, 529t, 533-534, 537t
Hageman factor, 1562t
Hair
  examination of, 189
  in nutritional assessment, 166t
  lanugo, 376
  pubertal changes in, 741
  pubic
    development of, premature, 1714-1715
    in females, 222
    in male, 221

Hair—cont'd
  scalp, 741
  types and development of, 741
Hair care, 1128
Hair follicles, 740, 741
  of newborn, 243
Hair loss, in cancer, 1602
Haitians, health beliefs and practices of, 54t
Halitosis, 207
Hallucinogens, 886t, 891b, 892
Haloperidol
  for Tourette syndrome, 793
  side effects of, 799
Hand(s); *see also* Finger(s).
  contamination of, fingernail polish
    and, 1134b
  Down syndrome and, 989t
  of newborn, 262
Handedness, assessment of, 225
Hand-foot syndrome, 1549
Handicap, 906b
Handwashing, 651, 665, 666, 752,
  1134-1135, 1134b
  hepatitis and, 1460
  in managing skin infections, 754
Happy puppet syndrome, 122
Harassment, in schools, 819
Hard palate, 207f, 208
Hard-of-hearing, 994, 995t; *see also* Hearing
  impairment.
Hardy-Rand-Rittler (HRR) test, 199-200
Harlequin color change, of newborn, 251t
Harrington system, for scoliosis, 1812
Harrison groove, 209
Harvest mites (chiggers), bites of, 776t
Hashimoto disease, 1718-1719
Hashish, 886t, 891b, 892
Hay fever, 1383
Head; *see also* Face/facies; Skull.
  Down syndrome and, 989t, 990f
  examination of, 190-191
    in nutritional assessment, 166t
  of newborn, 252t, 257-258, 258f, 259f
    preterm, 376
Head and neck, radiation therapy for,
  complications of, 1605
Head bobbing, 1311
Head circumference
  measurement of, 176f, 177-178
  of newborn, 249f, 251t, 255
  percentiles for, 1884, 1889, 1893
Head control
  assessment of, 225
  in cerebral palsy, 1842
  in infants, 190, 498-499, 499f
Head growth and circumference
  in infants, 494
  in school-age children, 699
  in toddlers, 592
Head injury, 1661-1674; *see also* Cerebral
  dysfunction.
  acceleration, 1665
  amnesia in, 1666
  assessment of; *see* Neurologic assessment.
  birth-related, 296-298, 297f
  cerebral contusions in, 1666
  cerebral edema in, 1665, 1668-1669
  cerebral lacerations in, 1666

Head injury—cont'd
  clinical manifestations of, 1669b
  complications of, 1667-1669, 1670-1671, 1670b
  concussion in, 1666
  contrecoup, 1665
  coup, 1665
  death and disability in, 1661
  deceleration, 1665
  deformation, 1665
  diagnostic evaluation in, 1669-1671
  emergency care for, 1671b
  epidural hematoma in, 1666f,
    1667-1668, 1668t
  etiology of, 1661-1662
  family support in, 1673
  generalized, 1665-1666
  hearing impairment and, 996b
  hydrocephalus and, 1670-1671
  in bicycle accidents, 733
  in child abuse, 1669
  incidence of, 1661
  initial assessment in, 1669-1670
  localized, 1665
  neurologic assessment in, 1671
  nursing care in, 1672-1674
  pathophysiology of, 1665-1667, 1665f
  postconcussion syndrome in, 1670, 1670b
  prevention of, 1674
  primary, 1665
  prognosis of, 1672
  rehabilitation in, 1660b, 1673-1674
  secondary, 1665
  seizures after, 1670
  shearing forces in, 1665, 1665f, 1666
  skull fractures in, 1666-1667
  subdural hematoma in, 1666f, 1668, 1668t
  treatment of, 1671-1672
  unconsciousness in, 1666
Head lag, in newborn, 258, 259f
Head lice, 761-763, 761f, 762b
Head Start, 981
Head tilt, 1334, 1337f
Headache, 1698-1700, 1699t, 1700b
  after cranial surgery, 1623
  brain tumor and, 1621t
  increased intracranial pressure and, 1646
  migraine, 1699-1700, 1699t, 1700b
  tension, 1699, 1699t
Head-to-heel length, of newborn, 251t, 255
Head-to-toe assessment, in trauma, 1761, 1762b
Health
  definition of, 1
  indicators of, 1
Health beliefs and practices, 43, 47-51, 52t-55t
  cultural aspects of, 43, 47-51, 52t-55t,
    910, 910b
  in home care, 1021
Health care; *see also* Child health care.
  community-based, 103-109
  economics of, 106
  for adolescents
    in rural areas, 836
    school-based, 822-823
    sexually transmitted diseases and, 861
  religious beliefs and, 58-62, 58t-62t
Health care facilities, accreditation of, 28
Health Care Financing Administration, 1137
Health care planning, 22-23

Health care team, nurse in, 21
Health education
    in chronic illness or disability, 918-919, 919b
    in school health programs, 728-729, 729b
Health history
    allergies in, 155-156, 156b
    birth history in, 155
    chief complaint in, 154
    components of, 153b
    current medications in, 156
    dietary history in, 155, 164-165, 164b, 165b
    direct vs indirect, 153
    family medical history in, 158
    format for, 153
    growth and development in, 156
    habits in, 156-157, 156b
    immunizations in, 156
    informant for, 153-154
    pain history in, 157
    past history in, 154-158
    present illness in, 154-155
    psychosocial history in, 158
    review of systems in, 159-160, 159b
    sexual history in, 158-159
    sleep habits in, 157, 157b
Health maintenance organizations (HMOs), 13
Health practices, of daycare centers, 637
Health promotion, in adolescents, 820-837
    cognitive thinking maturity and, 810
    cultural appropriateness of, 834-835, 835b
    health care setting and, 823-824
Health records; see also Documentation.
    confidentiality of, 141-142
Health screening; see Screening.
Health supervision, recommendations for, 171, 171b
Health teaching, 21
*Healthy People 2010*, 1-2, 2b, 104, 105
Hearing
    in infants, 495, 495b
    in newborns, 244, 259
    in toddlers, 592
    in unconscious children, 1660
Hearing aids, 996, 997-998, 997f
    hospitalization and, 999
    socialization and, 998
Hearing ear dogs, 998
Hearing impairment, 994-1000
    assessment of, 996-997, 996b, 997b
    classification of, 994-995, 995t
    clinical manifestations of, 997b
    communication process and, promotion of, 997-999, 997f, 998b
    definition of, 994
    Down syndrome and, 990
    etiology of, 994-995
    family support and, 999
    hospitalization and, 999-1000
    in bacterial meningitis, 1678
    in cerebral palsy, 207
    in high-risk newborn, 364, 995
    incidence of, 994
    otitis media and, 1357, 1359, 1360
    pathology of, 995
    prevention of, 1000
    severity of, 995, 995t
    treatment of, 995-996
    visual impairment and, 1006-1007

Hearing tests, 203-204, 204f
    schedule for, 171b
    screening, 204
        in newborns, 268
Hearing-threshold level, 995, 995t
Heart; see also under Cardiac.
    athlete's, 1805
    auscultation of, 215-217, 216b, 216f, 216t, 1310, 1469, 1504; see also Heart rate; Heart sounds.
    circulation in, prenatal vs. postnatal, 1466, 1466f, 1467
    conduction system of, 1467, 1467f
    contractility of, 1476
    development of
        embryologic, 1465-1466, 1465f, 1466f
        in middle childhood, 699
        postnatal, 1466-1467
    function of, 1465-1474
        assessment of, 1468-1469
        in sickle cell anemia, 1548
    inspection of, 214
    ischemia of, in Kawasaki disease, 1516
    monitoring of, 1470-1471, 1471f
        in Kawasaki disease, 1516
    physiology of, 1468
    position of, 214, 214f
    structure of, 1465
    support of, in treatment of shock, 1221
    tests of, 1469-1474, 1470t
Heart block, complete, 1524-1525, 1524f
Heart disease
    acquired, 1509-1526; see also specific disease, e.g., Rheumatic fever.
        definition of, 1465
    congenital, 1474-1509
        altered hemodynamics with, 1474-1475
        bacterial endocarditis and, 1510
        classification and clinical consequences of, 1475-1476
        congestive heart failure and, 1476-1484; see also Congestive heart failure.
        defects with decreased pulmonary blood flow in, 1496-1498
        defects with increased pulmonary blood flow in, 1491-1494
        definition of, 1465
        education of family about, 1502-1504, 1502b
        hypoxemia in, 1484-1490
        incidence and risk factors for, 1474
        mixed defects in, 1498-1501
        nursing care for, 1498-1509
        obstructive defects in, 1494-1496
        postoperative care for, 1504-1508, 1508b
        prevalence of defects in, 1474t
        pulmonary artery hypertension in, 1490-1491
    Down syndrome and, 990
    rheumatic, 1511
Heart murmurs, 215, 216b, 1469
    apical systolic, rheumatic fever and, 1511
Heart rate; see also Arrhythmia(s).
    after heart surgery, 1504, 1507
    assessment of, 1469, 1524; see also Pulse(s).
    body size and, 1466
    digoxin administration and, in congestive heart failure, 1481
    in infants, 496

Heart rate—cont'd
    influences on, 1468
    measurement of, 218
    meconium aspiration syndrome and, 389
    of newborn, 251t, 256, 260
    patterns of, 217b
    postoperative alterations in, 1119t
    respiratory rate and, 211
Heart sounds, 215-217, 216b, 216f, 216t
    auscultation of, 1310, 1469, 1504
    in congestive heart failure, 1478
    in newborn, 260-261
    in persistent pulmonary hypertension of newborn, 397
    liquid ventilation and, 386
Heart surgery
    complications of, 1507-1508
    discharge planning and home care after, 1509, 1509b
    for congenital heart disease, 1503-1504
    postoperative care for, 1504-1508, 1508b
Heart transplantation, 1526-1527
    for cardiomyopathy, 1523
    heterotopic, 1526
    orthotopic, 1526
Heart valves, in rheumatic heart disease, 1511
Heat, for earache, 1360
Heat cramps, 1802
Heat exhaustion, 1802
Heat injury, with smoke inhalation, 1380
Heat intolerance, in hyperthyroidism, 1721
Heat loss, prevention of; see Thermoregulation.
Heat regulation
    by skin, 740
    in infants, 497
Heating elements, safety precautions with, 542t, 543t, 548, 549b
Heating pad, in respiratory infections, 1346
Heatstroke, 1802
Heavy metal poisoning, 675
Heel puncture, 1147-1148, 1148f
    facilitated tucking before, 361
    in blood glucose testing, 317b
    in Guthrie blood test, 323b
    in high-risk newborn, 337-338, 337b, 361
    in neonatal screening for disease, 267b
    pain after, 353f, 1149b
        memory of, 353-354
Heel-to-ear maneuver, in preterm infant, 378f
Heel-to-ear measurement, gestational age and, 250b
Heel-to-shin test, 226
Height; see also Short stature; Tall stature.
    at puberty, 808, 809f
    blood pressure and, 185
    growth charts for, 1882, 1887, 1892
    in nutritional assessment, 168
    measurement of, 176-177, 176f
    of infants, 494
    of preschoolers, 628, 639t
    of school-age children, 699
    of toddlers, 592
    racial/ethnic variations in, 57
    sitting, 177
Height-weight charts
    for boys, 1882
    for girls, 1887
Heimlich maneuver, 1337f, 1341

Helen Keller National Center, 1006
*Helicobacter pylori*
    drug treatment for, 1444
    testing for, 1421t
    ulcers and, 1443
Heliox, for asthma, 1393
Helix, 200, 200f
Helmets, bicycle, 733-734, 734b, 734f,
        735b, 1758b
Helper T-lymphocytes, 1572
Hemangioma
    capillary, 302, 302f
    cavernous venous, 302
    strawberry, 302, 302f
Hemangioma HOPE, 302
Hemarthrosis, in hemophilia, 1563, 1565
Hematemesis, 1454, 1455b
Hematochezia, 1454
Hematocrit, 1532, 1536t
    fetal, Rh incompatibility and, 315
    polycythemia and, 399
    reference ranges for, 1898t
Hematologic dysfunction, 1530-1570
    assessment of hematologic function and,
        1535, 1536t
    in anemia, 1535, 1537-1561, 1537b
    in hemostatic disorders, 1561-1568
    in Henoch-Schönlein purpura, 1569-1570,
        1570f
    in neutropenia, 1568-1569, 1569t
    origin of formed elements and, 1530-1535,
        1531f, 1533f
Hematologic system
    after heart surgery, 1507-1508
    lead poisoning effects on, 676-677, 677f
Hematoma
    epidural, 1666f, 1667-1668, 1668t
    eye, 1003b
    fracture, 1781-1782, 1782f, 1794
    subdural, 1666f, 1668, 1668t
        in newborn, 403
        ventriculoperitoneal shunt and, 441
Hematopoietic system, 1531, 1531f
    of newborn, 241-242
        after surgery, 422t
        with sepsis, 394b
Heme-oxygenase inhibitors, for
        hyperbilirubinemia, 306
Hemimelia, 254t
Hemiplegic migraine, 1700b
Hemochromatosis, 1558
Hemodialysis, 1293-1296, 1294f, 1296f;
        *see also* Dialysis.
    access for, pain with, 1296b
    at home, 1296
    for hemolytic uremic syndrome, 1282
Hemodynamic monitoring, skin care and,
        high-risk newborn and, 351b
Hemodynamics
    congenital heart disease and, 1474-1475, 1476f
    in hypoxemia, 1484, 1486
Hemofiltration
    continuous venovenous, 1293, 1298
    for hemolytic uremic syndrome, 1282
Hemoglobin, 1532-1533, 1533f
    adult, in infants, 496
    bilirubin and, 304
    determination of, 1536t

Hemoglobin—cont'd
    fetal, 1532
        in infants, 496
        persistent, 381
    functional, 1313
    reference ranges for, 1898t, 1899t
    α-thalassemia and, 1557
Hemoglobin electrophoresis
    in sickle cell anemia, 1550
    in α-thalassemia, 1558
Hemoglobinopathies, 1547-1559
Hemolysis, 1540, 1541t, 1546-1559; *see also*
        Anemia.
    after heart surgery, 1508
    delayed, 1542t
Hemolytic anemia; *see also* Anemia.
    in hemolytic uremic syndrome, 1281
Hemolytic disease, erythema infectiosum
        and, 651
Hemolytic disease of newborn, 310
    blood incompatibility and, 310, 312, 312f, 312t
    clinical manifestations of, 312
    diagnosis of, 312, 314
    hyperbilirubinemia and, 303t, 312
    prevention of, 314
    prognosis of, 315
    treatment of, 315-316
Hemolytic uremic syndrome, 1281-1282
Hemophilia, 1561-1566
    bleeding in, 1562-1563
        prevention of, 1564-1565
        recognition and control of, 1565
    clinical manifestations of, 1562-1563
    diagnosis of, 1563
    home care for, 1565
    pathophysiology of, 1562
    prognosis of, 1564
    risk of, 1565-1566
    transmission of, 1562
    treatment of, 1563-1564, 1563t
Hemophilia A, 119t
Hemoptysis, in cystic fibrosis, 1409
Hemorrhage; *see also* Bleeding.
    anemia and, 1537
    epidural, 1667-1668
    in cancer, 1598-1599
    in leukemia, 1612
    intracerebellar, in newborn, 403
    intracerebral, 1668
    intracranial, in newborn, 403
    intraventricular, in newborn, 401-402, 402t
    postoperative
        after heart surgery, 1508
        after tonsillectomy, 1354
    prevention of, in newborn, 266-267
    retinal
        in newborn, 296b
        in shaken baby syndrome, 1668, 1669
    subarachnoid, 1668
        in newborn, 403
    subconjunctival, in newborn, 252t, 296b
    subdural, 1666f, 1668, 1668t
        in newborn, 403
    subgaleal, in newborn, 296-297, 297f
Hemorrhagic cystitis, in cancer, 1595t, 1602
Hemorrhagic disease of newborn, 319
Hemorrhoids, 223
Hemosiderin, thalassemia and, 1558

Hemosiderosis
    blood transfusions and, 1551
    thalassemia and, 1558
Hemostasis, 1561; *see also* Clotting; Coagulation.
    assessment of, 1562t
    defects in, 1561-1568
Hemothorax, 1302
Henoch-Schönlein purpura, 1569-1570, 1570f
    renal involvement in, 1270t
Heparin, for flushing peripheral intermittent
        infusion device, 1198, 1199b
Heparin lock, 1198, 1199b
Hepatic disorders, 1456-1461; *see also* Liver.
Hepatic encephalopathy, 1461
Hepatic portoenterostomy, 471-472, 471f
Hepatitis
    acute, 1456-1460
    carrier state of, 1459
    chronic active, 1458
    clinical manifestations of, 1458-1459
    diagnosis of, 1459
    from blood transfusion, 1542t
    fulminating, 1458
    in Crohn disease, 1439
    phases of, 1458
    prognosis for, 1460
    subacute, 1458
    treatment of, 1459-1460
Hepatitis A, 1456, 1457t
    immunizations for
        contraindications to, 537t, 538t
        in adolescents, 541b, 834
        recommended, 529t, 532
Hepatitis B, 1456-1458, 1457t
    immune globulin for, 1460
    immunizations for
        contraindications to, 537t, 538t
        in adolescents, 541b, 834, 865, 865b
        recommended, 529t, 530, 532, 532t
Hepatitis B virus
    immunization against, 267
    in newborn, 328t
Hepatitis C, 1457t, 1458
Hepatitis D, 1458
Hepatitis E, 1458
Hepatitis G, 1458
Hepatobiliary scintigraphy, 1422t
Hepatomegaly, in congestive heart failure, 1478
Herbal tea; *see also* Complementary medicine.
    for colic, 572, 573
Hereditary spherocytosis, 1546-1547
Heredity; *see* Genetic diseases; Genetics;
        Inheritance.
Hering-Breuer reflex, 1309
Hernias, 474-478
    abdominal wall defects and, 472-474,
        472f, 473f
    diaphragmatic, 475-477
    femoral, 218, 218f, 478
    inguinal, 218, 218f, 261, 477-478, 478f
    umbilical, 218, 218f, 474-475, 474f
Hero worship, in school-age children, 712
Heroin, 886t, 891b, 892
    in pregnancy, 406
Herpes labialis, recurrent, 664
Herpes simplex encephalitis, 1681-1682
Herpes simplex virus
    conjunctivitis and, 662
    genital lesions due to, 865t

Herpes simplex virus—cont'd
in newborn, 326, 328t
type 1, 758t
gingivostomatitis and, 664, 664f
type 2, 758t
type 6, exanthemum subitum and, 654f, 654t
Herpes zoster, 758t
complications with, 651, 660
Heterophil antibody test, in infectious
mononucleosis, 1355
HFJV; see High-frequency jet ventilation.
HFO; see High-frequency oscillation.
HFPPV; see High-frequency positive-pressure
ventilation.
HFV; see High-frequency ventilation.
Hickman/Broviac catheter, vs other long-term
venous access devices, 1201t
High chairs, falls from, 542t, 543t, 546, 549b, 622
High-frequency jet ventilation, in respiratory
distress syndrome, 384, 384f
High-frequency oscillation, in respiratory
distress syndrome, 384, 384f
High-frequency positive-pressure ventilation,
in respiratory distress syndrome,
384, 384f
High-frequency ventilation
in persistent pulmonary hypertension of
newborn, 398
in respiratory distress syndrome, 384, 384f
High-molecular-weight kininogen, 1562t
High-risk newborn, 334-409
anemia in, 398-399
apnea of prematurity in, 376, 378-379, 379b
assessment of, 335-338, 336b, 337b, 337t
developmental, 357-358, 359t
bottle-feeding of, 344-347, 345f, 346b
breast-feeding of, 344, 347-348
bronchopulmonary dysplasia in, 390-393
cerebral palsy in, 1835
classification of, 334, 334b
death of, 369-371
developmental outcome in, 357-366
assessment of, 357-358, 359t
auditory environment and, 363-365, 995
behavioral state organization and, 358,
360, 360t
co-bedding of multiples and, 362-363, 362f
sensory system and, 360-361
therapeutic handling and, 361-362, 361b
therapeutic positioning and, 363, 363b,
364b, 364f
visual environment and, 365-366, 366b
diabetic mother and, 404-406
drug-exposed, 406-408, 406b
extraneous air syndromes in, 389-390
feeding resistance in, 348-349, 349b
gavage feeding of, 348, 348f
germinal matrix/intraventricular
hemorrhage in, 401-402, 402t
hearing impairment in, 364, 995
hydration of, 341-342
bronchopulmonary dysplasia and, 392
identification of, 334
infection in, 393-397, 394b
prevention of, 341, 344
intensive care facilities for, 334-335
intracranial hemorrhage in, 403
meconium aspiration syndrome in, 388-389
mental retardation in, 979b

High-risk newborn—cont'd
necrotizing enterocolitis in, 395-397
neurologic disorders in, 400-404, 402t,
403b, 404t
nursing care plan for, 371-375
nutrition for, 342-348, 343t, 345f, 346b, 348f
discharge planning and, 369
pain in, 351-357
assessment of, 352-353, 352b, 353f,
354t-355t
consequences of, 355-357, 356b, 356t
management of, 357
memory of, 353-355
physiology of, 352
parent-infant relationship and, 366-368,
366b, 367f
patent ductus arteriosus in, 397
persistent pulmonary hypertension in,
397-398, 398f
polycythemia in, 399
postterm infant as, 376
preterm infant as, 374-376, 377f-378f
respiratory distress syndrome in, 379-388
clinical manifestations of, 381, 382f
complications of, 381
diagnosis of, 382-383
nursing considerations in, 387-388
pathophysiology of, 379-381, 380f, 381t
prevention of, 387
treatment of, 383-387, 384t
respiratory support for, 338
retinopathy of prematurity in, 344,
399-400, 400b
seizures in, 403-404, 403b, 404t
sepsis in, 393-395, 394b
siblings of, 368
skin care of, 349-350, 350b-351b
smoking mother and, 408-409
support groups and, 368
therapeutic handling of, 361-362, 361b
thermoregulation of, 338-341, 339f, 340f
skin care and, 351b
transport of, 335
Hilus, 210, 211f
Hindgut, 1416
Hinman syndrome, 485t
Hip; see also Femoral head.
developmental dysplasia of, 446-454
clinical manifestations of, 448-449, 449f
degrees of, 446b, 447-448, 448f
diagnosis of, 449
etiology of, 447-448
nursing considerations in, 450-451
treatment of, 449-450, 450f
dislocation of, 446b, 448f, 450
in newborn, 254t
traumatic, 1799
fracture of, 1777
preluxated, 446b, 448f
subluxated, 446b, 448f
in newborn, 254t
Hip spica casts, 451, 1784, 1784f, 1786f
home care for, 1787
Hip-knee-ankle-foot orthosis, 1773, 1774b
Hirschberg test, 195-196, 196f
Hirschsprung disease, 1426-1429, 1426f
Hismanal (astemizole)
drug interactions with, 1385
for allergic rhinitis, 1384

Hispanics, 35b; see also Race/ethnicity.
dietary preferences of, 45-47, 46t
health beliefs and practices of, 54t
time concept of, 43
Histamine receptor antagonists; see
Antihistamines.
Histamine release
in allergic rhinitis, 1383
in anaphylaxis, 1224
Histiocytes, 1534
Histoplasmosis, 764t
History
birth, 155
developmental, 156
dietary, 155
family; see Family history.
health; see Health history.
nursing admission, 1086-1088, 1088b-1089b,
1091b
obstetric, 155
pain, 157
psychosocial, 158
sexual, 158-159
sleep, 157, 157b
History taking, 153-160; see also Interview.
HIV; see Human immunodeficiency virus
infection.
HLA system, 1571, 1596
HMOs, 13
Ho' oponopono, 48
Hoarseness, in congestive heart failure, 1478
Hodgkin disease, 1616-1618
Hold-Oram syndrome, congenital heart
disease and, 1474
Holoenzymes, protein, vitamins and, 554
Holter monitor, 1470
Home apnea monitoring, 586, 586b, 587,
587b, 587f
Home care, 1016-1029, 1131-1132, 1132b
after cardiac catheterization, 1474b
after cardiac surgery, 1509, 1509b
after tonsillectomy, 1354
case management and, 1019-1020, 1020b
cost of, 1017
cultural issues in, 1021-1022, 1021b
discharge planning and, 1018-1019, 1018b,
1019b, 1095-1097
drug administration in, 1161
education and, 1027-1028
effectiveness of, 1017, 1017b, 1018b
family-to-family support and, 1028-1029
for abdominal wall defect, 473-474
for anorectal malformation, 470
for asthma, 1395, 1398b
for autism, 1010
for bronchopulmonary dysplasia, 392-393
for casts, 1786, 1786b, 1787
for children, 516
for cleft lip and palate, 462
for colostomy, 1428
for cystic fibrosis, 1411-1412
for developmental dysplasia of hip, 450-451
for epispadias/exstrophy complex, 484
for gastroesophageal reflux, 1431-1432
for hemodialysis, 1296
for hydrocephalus, 442-443
for hyperbilirubinemia, 306, 309-310, 311b
for myelomeningocele, 432-433, 433b
for nephrotic syndrome, 1278-1279

Home care—cont'd
for ostomies, 1167
for peritoneal dialysis, 1293, 1297-1298
for postoperative congenital heart disease, 1509, 1509b
for respiratory problems, 1329, 1329b, 1347
for rheumatic fever, 1513
for short bowel syndrome, 1453
for stuttering, 1011b
for total parenteral nutrition, 1204
for tracheoesophageal fistula, 466
for tracheostomy, 1327b, 1329-1331, 1329b, 1333, 1333f
for unconscious child, 1661
goals of, 1024
house rules for, 1025b
in cancer, 1605-1606
nurse's role in, 1017, 1017b, 1018b, 1020, 1020b
high-risk child and, 1026b
nursing process in, 1023-1024, 1024b, 1025b
of newborn, 286-288, 287b
at high risk, 368-369
of special needs child, 908, 1017, 1018, 1019b
of terminally ill child, 955
of wounds, 751-754
optimum development and, promotion of, 1024-1028, 1026b, 1027f
parent-professional collaboration in, 1022-1023, 1023b
safety issues in, 1028
self-care and, 1025, 1026b, 1027
standards of, 1020-1021
training and, 1020, 1028
trends in, 1017
versus hospice care, 1016
Home care agency, 1020
selection of, 1018-1019, 1018b, 1019b
Home Eye Test for Preschoolers, 198t
HOME inventory, 1872-1873
Home Observation for Management of the Environment (HOME), 163
Home Screening Questionnaire (HSQ), 163
Home visits
for postpartum adolescent parents, 853
for prevention of child maltreatment, 693
Homelessness, 41-42
Homicide
of adolescents, 820, 828
of infants, 548
rates of, 4-5, 4t
Homosexual families, 72-73
Homosexuality, 831, 835-836
origins of identity in, 814-816, 816b
suicide and, 898, 898b
Honey, infant botulism and, 1850
Hookworm infection, clinical manifestations of, 665t
Hopefulness, facilitation of, in special needs child, 918, 918b
Hordeolum, 193b
Hormonal therapy
for cancer, 1589, 1593t
for cryptorchidism, 481
for dysfunctional uterine bleeding, 848
Hormone(s), 1703-1706; see also Endocrine system and specific hormones.
gastrointestinal, 1418
general, 1704

Hormone(s)—cont'd
inhibitory, 1704-1705, 1705f
local, 1703
releasing, 1704-1705, 1705f
reproductive
at puberty
in females, 803-805, 805f
in males, 805
in adolescence, 803, 803f
secretion of, 1704-1705, 1705f
target cells/tissues of, 1703, 1704, 1705f
tropic, 1704, 1705f
Hornets, bites of, 776t
Horseback riding, injuries during, 735-736
Hospice care, 955-956
neonatal death and, 370
vs home care, 1016
Hospice Nurses Association, 1020-1021
Hospital Infection Control Practices Advisory Committee, 1132
Hospitalization, 1032-1097
ambulatory/outpatient setting in, 1091-1092, 1092b
autism and, 1010
bodily injury and pain in, 1036-1039, 1036t, 1037f, 1046
developmentally appropriate activities during, 1068-1069
discharge planning in, home care and, 1095-1097
effects on child of, 1039-1040, 1039b
family support during, 1073-1074, 1074b, 1084b
nursing care plan for, 1080-1083
hearing impairment and, 999-1000
isolation in, 1092-1093
loss of control during, 1034-1036, 1035b, 1044-1046, 1045f, 1046b
mental retardation and, 986-987
nursing care plan for, 1075-1080
pain assessment during, 1046-1057, 1047b
pain management during, 1057, 1059-1068
parental reactions to, 1040-1041, 1040b
play and expressive activities during, 1069-1072, 1069b, 1070f-1072f
potential benefits of, 1072-1073
preparation for, 1083-1097
admission procedure in, 1086-1091, 1086f, 1087b-1090b, 1091f; see also Admission procedure.
tour of hospital in, 1084-1086, 1085b
separation anxiety and, 1032-1034, 1032b, 1032f, 1033f
sibling reactions to, 1041, 1084b
terminal illness and, 955
transition to home care from, 1018-1019; see also Home care.
visual impairment and, 1004-1005
Hospitals, accreditation of, 28
Host factors, 105
HOTV test, 197-198, 198t
House dust mites, control of, 1390
House fires, burn injuries and, 1227
Household, 65
Household tasks, school-age children and, 726, 726f
Huber needles, 1201
Huffing, 886t, 892
Humalog (Lispro-H), 1737

Human bites, 779-780
Human chorionic gonadotropin, for cryptorchidism, 481
Human diploid cell rabies vaccine, 1683
Human Genome Project, 110-111
Human Growth Foundation, 1713
Human growth hormone, 1712
Creutzfeldt-Jakob disease and, 1712
for growth hormone deficiency, 1712
Human immunodeficiency virus infection, 864-865, 1570, 1572-1577
classification of, 1574-1575, 1574t, 1575t
clinical manifestations of, 1573-1574, 1574b
diagnosis of, 1574
donor blood and, 1542t
donor human milk and, 344
education about, 710, 729
encephalopathy in, 1684
epidemiology of, 1572-1573
etiology of, 1573
hemophilia and, 1564, 1565
horizontal transmission of, 1573
in newborns, 267-268, 327t
kwashiorkor and, 567
nephrotic syndrome and, 1275
neurologic manifestations of, 1684
nursing care plan for, 1577-1578
nursing considerations of, 1576-1577
pain management in, 1576
pathophysiology of, 1573
prevention of, 865b, 1576
prognosis of, 1575-1576
screening for
in adolescents, 831
in newborns, 267-268
transmission of, nonoxynol-9 and, 855
treatment of, 1575
vertical transmission of, 1573
Human leukocyte antigens, 1571, 1596
Human milk, 281t; see also Breast-feeding.
donor, 344
expressed, preterm infant and, 347, 348
fortified, for high-risk newborn, 344
Human papilloma virus, 864
infection with, test for, 831
penile carcinoma and, 843
Human parvovirus infection, maternal, fetal anemia and, 651
Human rabies immune globulin, 1683
Human response patterns, 26b
Humerus, fracture of, birth-related, 298
Humidification, tracheostomy and, 1328, 1329f
Humidity, thermoregulation and, high-risk newborn and, 340
Humoral defenses, as respiratory tract defense, 1310
Humoral immunity, 1572
Huntington disease, presymptomatic testing for, 126-127
Hyaline membrane disease, 379; see also Respiratory distress syndrome.
Hydralazine (Apresoline), for hypertension, 1519b
Hydration; see also Fluid management.
in respiratory infections, 1346
of high-risk newborn, 341-342
with bronchopulmonary dysplasia, 392
with necrotizing enterocolitis, 396

Hydration—cont'd
  sickle cell anemia and, 1552
  terminal illness and, 949t
Hydrocarbon abuse, 886t
Hydrocarbon pneumonia, 1378-1379
Hydrocarbon poisoning, 670b, 672b
Hydrocele, scrotal, 254t, 261, 478f, 479-480
Hydrocephalus, 436-443, 1657
  clinical manifestations of, 437-438, 439f
  diagnosis of, 439, 439f
  in bacterial meningitis, 1678
  increased intracranial pressure and; see
      Intracranial pressure, increased.
  myelomeningocele and, 425
  nursing considerations in, 441-443
  pathophysiology of, 436-437, 437f
  posthemorrhagic, 402
  posttraumatic, 1670-1671
  prognosis of, 441
  treatment of, 439-441, 440f
  types of, 437, 438t
Hydrocephalus Association, 443
Hydrocet, 1060b
Hydrochloric acid, gastrointestinal, 1418
Hydrocodone, in pain management, 1060b,
    1062t, 1063t
Hydrocolloid dressings, 750t, 751, 752
Hydrocolloid wafers, 1328
Hydrocortisone, 1708t; see also Steroids.
  for adrenocortical insufficiency, 1725, 1726
  for cancer, 1593t
  for chronic adrenocortical insufficiency,
      1730, 1731
Hydrofluorocarbons, as propellant in
    metered-dose inhalers, 1391
Hydrogel dressings, for skin lesions, 750t
Hydrogel electrodes, high-risk infant and, 337
Hydrogen ion
  excretion of, in infants, 1258
  in acid-base balance, 1182
  in distal tubular acidosis, 1280
Hydrogen peroxide, 752
Hydrogen-potassium ATPase pump, 1430
Hydromorphone
  abuse of, 886t
  in pain management, 1062t, 1063t
    patient-controlled, 1064t
  in preoperative sedation, 1113b
Hydronephrosis, 484
Hydrops fetalis, 310; see also Hemolytic disease
    of newborn.
Hydrostatic weighing, 873-874
Hydrotherapy, for juvenile rheumatoid
    arthritis, 1824
Hydrothorax, 1302
Hydroxychloroquine, for systemic lupus
    erythematosus, 1828
Hydroxylase deficiency, congenital adrenal
    hyperplasia and, 1729
Hydroxyurea (Hydrea), 1593t
Hydroxyzine, 752
Hygiene
  assessment of, 186, 191
  in unconscious child, 1659
Hymen, 223
Hymenal tag, of newborn, 261
Hymenoptera stings, 775-776, 776t
Hyoid bone, 192f
Hyperalbuminuria, in nephrotic syndrome, 1275

Hyperalcemia, 1177t
Hyperaldosteronism, 1731
Hyperalimentation, 1203-1204; see also Total
    parenteral nutrition.
Hyperbilirubinemia, 303-310; see also Jaundice.
  assessment of, 307
  breast-feeding and, 305, 307
  clinical manifestations of, 305
  complications of, 304
  diagnosis of, 305-306
  discharge planning and home care for,
      309-310, 311b
  family support in, 308-309, 309b
  hemolytic disease of newborn and, 303t, 312
  nursing care plan for, 313-314
  pathophysiology of, 304, 304f
  physiologic jaundice and, 304-307, 307t
  prognosis of, 307
  treatment of, 306-307, 307t
    phototherapy in, 308, 308f, 309b
  types of, 303t
Hypercalcemia, 561t, 1177t
  in hyperparathyroidism, 1723
  in immobilization, 1764-1765
  in newborn, during hypocalcemia
      treatment, 318
Hypercapnia, 1331
  cerebral blood flow and, 1645
  permissive, for congenital diaphragmatic
      hernia, 476
Hypercarbia, in respiratory distress
      syndrome, 384
Hypercholesterolemia/hyperlipidemia,
    1519-1522
  in adolescents, 833
  screening for, 1520, 1521b
  treatment of, 1520-1521
Hypercortisolism, in Cushing syndrome,
    1727-1729, 1727b, 1727f, 1728t
Hypercyanotic spells
  treatment of, 1488, 1488b, 1488f
  with hypoxemia, 1476f, 1487
Hyperemia, reactive, 1122
Hyperesthesia, with skin lesions, 742
Hyperglycemia
  in diabetes, 1734, 1736, 1740, 1740t,
      1741, 1749
  in newborn, 317-318
  in total parenteral nutrition, 1203
Hyperhemolytic crisis, 1550
Hyperkalemia, 1176t, 1177t
  from blood transfusion, 1541t
  in acute renal failure, 1286
  in chronic renal failure, 1288-1289
Hyperkinetic reaction of childhood, 787
Hyperleukocytosis
  in cancer, 1596, 1612
  in leukemia, 1612
Hyperlipidemia; see
      Hypercholesterolemia/hyperlipidemia.
Hypermetabolism, in burn injuries, 1232
Hypernatremia, 1176t
  in diarrhea, 1185
Hyperopia, 1000, 1001b
Hyperosmolar solutions, in preterm infant, 351
Hyperoxia test, 1487
Hyperparathyroidism, 1722-1723, 1723b
Hyperphenylalaninemia, 322; see also
      Phenylketonuria.

Hyperphosphatemia
  hypocalcemia and, 318
  in hypoparathyroidism, 1722
Hyperpituitarism, 1713-1714
Hyperplasia, fetal growth and, 416
Hyperplastic anemia, 1538
Hyperpnea, 1310
Hypersplenism, in sickle cell anemia, 1549
Hypertelorism, 192
Hypertension; see also Blood pressure.
  adrenalectomy and, 1732
  classification of, 1518
  diagnosis of, 1517-1518
  essential (primary), 1517
  in acute poststreptococcal
      glomerulonephritis, 1273
  in acute renal failure, 1286
  in adolescents, 833
  in chronic renal failure, 1291
  in congenital adrenal hyperplasia, 1729
  in hyperaldosteronism, 1731
  pheochromocytoma and, 1732
  portal, gastrointestinal bleeding and, 1454
  pulmonary, 1490-1491
    congenital diaphragmatic hernia and, 476
    persistent, 397-398, 398f
  secondary, conditions associated with, 1517b
  systemic, 1516-1519
  treatment of, 1518
Hypertensive encephalopathy
  acute poststreptococcal glomerulonephritis
      and, 1272
  in acute renal failure, 1286
Hyperthermia, 1130, 1131; see also Temperature.
  in newborn
    at high risk, 341
    during exchange transfusion, 315
  in unconscious child, 1659
  malignant, 1113, 1117
Hyperthyroidism, 1719-1721
  goiter and, 1718
Hypertonia, in newborn, 254t
Hypertonic solutions
  bilirubin encephalopathy and, 304
  hypoglycemia and, 317
Hypertrophic cardiomyopathy, 1805
Hypertrophic pyloric stenosis, 1446-1448,
    1447f
Hypertrophy, fetal growth and, 416
Hyperventilation
  in neurologic assessment, 1650
  in unconsciousness, 1650, 1656
Hypervitaminosis, 555
Hypervolemia; see also Blood volume.
  after heart surgery, 1506
  in acute renal failure, 1286-1287
Hypesthesia, with skin lesions, 742
Hypoalbuminemia, in nephrotic
      syndrome, 1275
Hypocalcemia, 1177t
  in hypoparathyroidism, 1722
  in newborn, 318-319
Hypocapnia, cerebral blood flow and, 1645
Hypocortisolism
  acute, 1725
  chronic, 1726
  congenital adrenal hyperplasia and, 1729-1731
Hypoesthesia, with skin lesions, 742
Hypoglossal nerve, assessment of, 229t

Hypoglycemia
  brain, 1749
  in diabetes, 1739-1741, 1740f, 1740t, 1749
  in newborn, 316-317, 405-406
  rebound, 405
Hypokalemia, 1176t
  after heart surgery, 1506
  in diabetic ketoacidosis, 1742
  in hyperaldosteronism, 1731
Hyponatremia, 1175t
Hypoparathyroidism, 1721, 1722
Hypophosphatemia, in hyperparathyroidism,
    1723
Hypopituitarism, 1706-1713, 1706b
  clinical manifestations of, 1706b, 1710
  diagnosis of, 1710-1712, 1711b
  etiology of, 1706-1709, 1706b
  growth failure and, 1709-1713, 1709f
  idiopathic, 1709-1713
  nursing care in, 1712-1713
  pituitary tumors and, 1706-1709
  treatment of, 1712
Hypoplastic anemia, 1538, 1559, 1560
Hypoplastic left heart syndrome, 1486,
    1501b, 1501f
Hypopnea, 1310
Hyposensitization, for asthma, 1393-1394
Hypospadias, 221, 254t, 481-482, 481f, 1729
Hypothalamic-pituitary-gonadal axis, 1714
  in adolescence, 803, 803f
Hypothalamus, 1644t, 1704-1705, 1704b, 1705f
Hypothermia, 771-772; see also Body
    temperature.
  in blood transfusion, 1541t
  in near-drowning, 1675
  in newborn, 265, 289
    at high risk, 341
    during exchange transfusion, 315-316
  physical effects of, 771t
  prevention of, 772
Hypothyroidism
  congenital, 320-322
  familial, 119t
  goiter and, 1718
  juvenile, 1717-1718
Hypotonia, 1843
  Down syndrome and, 992
  in myasthenia gravis, 1851-1852
  in newborn, 254t, 262
Hypovolemia; see also Blood volume.
  in anaphylaxis, 1224
  in nephrotic syndrome, 1275
Hypovolemic shock, 1219, 1219b
Hypoxemia, 1331, 1484-1490; see also Cyanosis.
  altered hemodynamics in, 1484, 1486
  clinical manifestations of, 1486-1487, 1487f
  congenital heart disease categories and,
    1474-1475, 1476f
  definition of, 1484
  diagnosis of, 1487
  heart defects causing, 1484, 1486
  in respiratory distress syndrome, 380
  treatment of, 1317, 1487-1490
Hypoxia, 1331
  after heart surgery, 1507
  blood flow and, 1645
  cerebral blood flow and, 1645
  definition of, 1484
  in anemia, 1537

Hypoxia—cont'd
  in meconium aspiration syndrome, 388, 389
  in near-drowning, 1675
  in persistent pulmonary hypertension of
    newborn, 397-398
  tissue, in carbon monoxide poisoning, 1381
Hypoxic-ischemic brain injury, perinatal,
    400-401
Hysteria, 797
Hysterical conversion reaction, 797
HyTape, 349

I
"I" messages, 151b
Ibuprofen
  after heart surgery, 1506
  dysmenorrhea and, 847
  in fever management, 1130, 1130t
  in pain management, 1060b, 1061t
Ice compress
  for earache in otitis media, 1360
  for musculoskeletal injuries, 1800, 1800f
  in respiratory infections, 1346
ICES therapy, 1800
Ictal state, 1686
Icterus neonatorum, 303, 304-305
ICU; see Intensive care unit.
Id, in toddlers, 594
IDEA; see Individuals with Disabilities
    Education Act.
Identical twins, 80, 80b
Identification
  drug administration and, 1151
  of newborn, 266
Identity
  concept of, 703, 704
  development of, 812
  sexual, 814
  vs role confusion, 230t, 231
Idiopathic autoimmune neutropenia, 1569t
Idiopathic hypertrophic subaortic stenosis, 1805
Idiopathic hypopituitarism, 1706b, 1709-1713
Idiopathic thrombocytopenic purpura, 1566-
    1567, 1567b
IEP; see Individualized education program.
IFA (rapid immunofluorescent antibody)
    test, for respiratory syncytial virus
    infection, 1367
Ifosfamide, 1589t
IFSP; see Individualized family service plan.
IHCP; see Individualized home care plan.
Ileoanal pull-through, for inflammatory bowel
    disease, 1441
Ileoanal reservoir, 1166
Ileocecal valve
  in short bowel syndrome, 1452, 1453
  intussusception of, 1448, 1448f
Ileocolic valve, intussusception of, 1448, 1448f
Ileoileal intussusception, 1448
Ileostomy, 1166
  for inflammatory bowel disease, 1441
Ileum, in Crohn disease, 1438-1439
Ileus, 1433
  in burn injuries, 1232, 1234
  meconium, 1424
    in cystic fibrosis, 1406
  paralytic, 1446
Ilizarov external fixator, 1792-1793, 1792f, 1794

Illness; see also Disease.
  acute, 6
  chronic, 905-945; see also Special needs child
    and specific illness.
    school nurse's role in, 730
    sports participation in, 725
    trajectory model for, 932
  in health history, 155
Illocutionary stage, 148, 148b
Imaginative play, in preschoolers, 634-635,
    635b, 635f
Imidazoline, topical, as poison, 669
Imipramine
  for attention deficit hyperactivity disorder, 789
  for enuresis, 784
Imitation
  in infants, 503, 507
  in toddlers, 596
Imitative play
  in preschoolers, 634-635, 635b, 635f
  in toddlers, 600
Immobilization, 1761-1772
  behavioral changes in, 1766-1767, 1766b, 1769
  complications of, 1762-1766, 1793-1795
  family concerns in, 1767-1768
  in intravenous infusions, 1196
  in spinal cord injury, 1859-1860
  in traction, 1787-1792
  indications for, 1761-1762
  nursing care in, 1768-1769, 1768-1772
  nursing care plan for, 1772
  of fractures, 1784-1787
  physiologic effects of, 1762-1766, 1763f,
    1770t-1771t
    cardiovascular, 1763-1764, 1770t-1771t
    gastrointestinal, 1764, 1771t
    integumentary, 1765, 1765f, 1771t
    metabolic, 1764-1765, 1768, 1770t
    muscular, 1762-1763, 1770t
    neurosensory, 1765-1766
    renal, 1764, 1771f
    respiratory, 1764, 1771t
    skeletal, 1763, 1764-1765, 1770t
  prehabilitation for, 1762
  psychologic effects of, 1766-1767, 1768, 1769
  self-care in, 1769
Immune globulin
  for hepatitis B, 1460
  for Kawasaki disease, 1515, 1516
  human rabies, 1683
  respiratory syncytial virus, 1367-1368, 1368b
  tetanus, 1848, 1849
  varicella-zoster, 651, 1605
Immune response, in renal transplantation,
    1299-1300
Immune system
  components of, 1571-1572, 1571f
  impaired, 1570-1580
    isolation and, 1092-1093
  in Down syndrome, 990
  in newborns, 243
    after surgery, 421t
  in school-age children, 700
Immunity, mechanisms of, 1571-1572, 1571f
Immunization(s); see also Vaccine(s).
  adverse reactions to, reporting of, 541
  contraindications and precautions with, 535-
    536, 537t, 538, 538t

Immunization(s)—cont'd
  documentation of, 540, 541
  for bacterial meningitis, 1677, 1680
  for control of communicable diseases, 650
  for hepatitis B, 267
  in adolescents, 541b, 833-834
  in cancer, 1605
  in children, 534b
  in end-stage renal disease, 1298b
  in health history, 156
  in HIV infection, 1575
  in infants, 527-541
    administration of, 538-541
    contraindications and precautions for, 535-538
    reactions to, 535, 536t
    routine, 530-534
    schedules of, 528-530, 529t, 530t, 531t
    selected special, 529t, 534-535
  parent information about, 540
  passive, live virus vaccines and, 538
  rabies, 1683
  rates of among children and adolescents, 541b
  routine
    reactions to, 535, 536t
    recommendations for, 530, 532-535
  schedules for, 171b, 528-530, 529t, 530t, 531t
  sources of current information on, 541b
  terminology relating to, 528b
  vs vaccination, 527
Immunodeficiency, 1570-1580
Immunoglobulin(s), 1572
  in toddlers, 593
  neonatal sepsis and, 393
  passive immunization with, and vaccination with live virus vaccine, 538
  reference ranges for, 1898t
Immunoglobulin A
  nephropathy related to, 1274
  secretory
    in infants, 497
    otitis media and, 1357
Immunoglobulin E
  atopic dermatitis and, 581
  in allergic rhinitis, 1383
  in anaphylaxis, 1224
  in asthma, 1387
Immunoglobulin G, in infants, 497
Immunoglobulin M, in infants, 497
Immunologic factors, in asthma, 1387
Immunomodulators, for inflammatory bowel disease, 1440
Immunoreactive trypsinogen analysis, in asthma, 1407
Immunosuppressive therapy
  in aplastic anemia, 1560
  in heart transplantation, 1525
  in liver transplantation, 470
  in renal transplantation, 1299-1300
  nephrotic syndrome and, 1277
Immunotherapy
  for allergic rhinitis, 1384
  for asthma, 1393-1394
  for cancer, 1594-1595
Impairment, 906b; see also specific type.
Imperforate anus, 466, 469f
Impetigo contagiosa, 754-755, 754f, 755t
Impetigo neonatorum, 301
Implementation, in nursing process, 27

IMV; see Intermittent mandatory ventilation.
In vitro fertilization, preimplantation genetic diagnosis and, 130
Inborn errors of metabolism, 319-325, 320f, 322f, 324b, 325f; see also specific disorders.
  screening for, 125-126
  treatment and prevention of, 124-125
Incarceration of hernia, 474, 478
Incest, 685, 686-687, 858
Incidence, 105, 105b
Incision, 745
Incontinence
  fecal, 785-786; see also Bowel elimination.
  in unconscious child, 1659
  urinary, 783-785; see also Enuresis.
    myelomeningocele and, 428-430
  urinary tract infection and, 1266
Increased intracranial pressure; see Intracranial pressure, increased.
Incubator
  co-bedding of multiples in, 362-363, 362f
  double-walled, 339
  radiant heat loss and, 265, 339-340
  servocontrolled, 339
Incus, 203, 203f
Independence
  chronic illness or disability and, 916
  hospitalization and, 1045
  mental retardation and, 983-986, 984b, 984f
  visual impairment and, 1003, 1005
Independent adoption, 89
Inderal (propranolol)
  for hypertension, 1519b
  for supraventricular tachycardia, 1525
Index case, 131
Indigenous healers, 48
Indirect Coombs test, in hemolytic disease of newborn, 314
Indirect-contact transmission, 1134
Individualized care plans, 27, 27t
Individualized education program, 980, 980b
Individualized family service plan, 909, 980, 980b
  home care and, 1026
Individualized home care plan, 1018, 1019
Individuals with Disabilities Education Act, 909, 980b, 981
Individuation-separation concept
  in preschoolers, 632
  in toddlers, 598-599
Indomethacin, for patent ductus arteriosus, 397
Industry
  development of in school-age child, 700-701
  vs inferiority, 230t, 231
Indwelling catheter; see also Catheter(s).
  hypospadias and, 482
Infant; see also Newborn.
  airway obstruction in, 1337f, 1338, 1340f
  apnea in, 585-588
  asthma in, 1388
  bacterial meningitis in, 1678
  bonding with; see Attachment.
  bronchial drainage in, 1320, 1323f
  communication with, 148
  congestive heart failure in, 1478, 1479, 1481-1484
  co-sleeping of in family bed, 527b, 583, 646b
  dental health of, 527
  developmental dysplasia of hip in, 450

Infant—cont'd
  diarrhea in, 1216
  "difficult," 509-511
  disorders of unknown etiology in, 582-588
  dying, 953; see also Terminal illness.
  feeding of, 520-525; see also Bottle-feeding; Breast-feeding; Feeding.
    developmental milestones in, 522b
    food storage and, 523
    in first 6 months, 520-521, 524b
    in second 6 months, 521-522, 524b
    parental interaction during, 575b, 576
    proper technique of, 571
    solid foods for, 522-524, 524b
    weaning and, 524-525
  floppy, 1843
  full-term, 334b
  growth and development of, 494-519, 510t-515t
    biologic, 494-501
    body image and, 504
    child-care arrangements and, 516-518
    cognitive, 502-504
    limit-setting and discipline and, 516
    pacifier use and, 518-519, 542t-543t, 543-544, 615
    psychosocial, 501-502
    separation and stranger fear and, 514-515
    sexual identity and, 504
    social, 504-507
    spoiled child syndrome and, 515-516
    teething and, 519
    temperament and, 507-511
    thumb-sucking and, 518
    use of shoes and, 519-520
  guidance for families of, 550, 550b
  head control in, 190
  hearing assessment in, 996, 996b
  hearing impairment in, 997b
  high-risk; see High-risk newborn.
  hospitalized
    bodily injury and pain in, 1036-1037, 1037f
    loss of control in, 1034
  hydrocephalus in, 437-438, 439f; see also Hydrocephalus.
    treatment of, 440-441, 440f
  hypoxemia in, 1484, 1486-1490
  immunizations for, 527-541
    administration of, 538-541
    contraindications and precautions for, 535-538
    reactions to, 535
    routine, 530-534
    schedules of, 528-530, 529t, 531t
    selected special, 534-535
  injury prevention in, 541-550
    nurse's role in, 548-550
    of aspiration of foreign objects, 541-544
    of bodily damage, 548
    of burns, 547-548
    of drowning, 548
    of falls, 542t, 543t, 546-547, 549b
    of motor vehicle accidents, 545-546
    of poisoning, 547
    of suffocation, 544-545
  intramuscular injection sites in, 539b, 540
  length measurement for, 175-176, 176f
  low-birth-weight, adolescent pregnancy and, 851

Infant—cont'd
  maternal relationship to, 504-506; *see also*
    Attachment.
    in adolescent mothers, 851-852
  motor vehicle seats for, 542t, 543t, 545-546,
    545f, 546f
  nutritional disturbances in, 554-571
    food sensitivity and, 568-571
    minerals in, 555, 560, 561t-564t
    nursing considerations in, 560-566
    protein-energy malnutrition and, 566-568
    vegetarian diets and, 560
    vitamins in, 554-555, 556t-559t
  of diabetic mother, 404-406
  oral rehydration therapy in, 1211-1213
  otitis media in, 1357
  pain in, 1054b
  physical examination of, 173t
  postterm; *see* Postterm infant.
  preterm; *see* Preterm infant.
  renal development and function in, 1258
  skin of, 742
    disorders in, 578-582
  sleep and activity in, 525-527
  special needs; *see also* Special needs child.
    early intervention for, 909, 1027-1028
    promotion of normal development in,
     910-912, 911t
  sudden infant death syndrome in, 582-585
  sunscreen agents and, 770
  transport of, 1136, 1137f
  visual acuity testing in, 199
  visual impairment in, 1002
  walkers for, falls from, 542t, 543t, 546, 549b
  water balance in, 1173-1174
  weighing of, 177, 177f
  weight gain in, breast-feeding and, 277b
Infant botulism, 1850-1851
Infant feeding, growth rates and, 175
Infant formula; *see* Bottle-feeding; Formula.
Infant mortality, 2-4, 3t, 4t
  perinatal, 3
Infantile spasms, 1688
  in Lennox-Gastaut syndrome, 1689
Infantile spinal muscular atrophy, 1846, 1846b
Infantile (visceral) swallow reflex, 496-497, 497f
Infant/toddler HOME inventory, 1872-1873
Infection(s); *see also* Communicable diseases
    and specific infections.
  after heart surgery, 1507
  at intravenous insertion sites, 1197-1198,
    1197b
  blood transfusion and, 1542t
  diarrhea and, 1208-1209, 1208b,
    1209t-1210t
  fungal, 759-760, 759t, 760f
    systemic mycotic, 763, 764t
    vaginal, 848, 849
  hemolytic uremic syndrome and, 1281
  hypoplastic anemia and, 1560
  in adolescents, 833-834
  in bone marrow transplant, 1603
  in burn injuries, 1234, 1244, 1245
  in cancer, 1597
  in chronic renal failure, 1289, 1291
  in daycare centers, 517
  in early childhood, 649-665
  in leukemia, 1612
  in nephrotic syndrome, 1278

Infection(s)—cont'd
  in newborns, 325-326, 327t-328t
    at high risk, 393-397, 394b
    defenses against, 243, 393
    human milk and, 344
    prevention of, 265-273, 289, 341
  intracranial, 1676-1684
  isolation and, 1092-1093
  kwashiorkor and, 567
  mental retardation and, 979b
  musculoskeletal, 1817-1819
  nosocomial, 1134
    neonatal sepsis and, 393
  nursing considerations with, 649-651,
    660-662, 662b-663b
  opportunistic, human immunodeficiency
    virus infection and, 1575
  parasitic, 665-668
  parenteral alimentation and, 1201
  peritoneal dialysis and, 1298
  respiratory, 1343-1361, 1371-1376; *see also*
    Respiratory infections.
  severe combined immunodeficiency disease
    and, 1579
  sickle cell anemia and, 1550, 1552
  skin
    bacterial, 754-755, 754f, 755t
    viral, 755, 758, 758t
  under cast, 1786
  urinary tract; *see* Urinary tract infection.
  venous access devices and, 1202, 1451, 1452
  ventriculoperitoneal shunt and, 440-441
  visual impairment and, 1002
Infection control, 268, 1132-1135, 1133b,
  1134b, 1135f
Infectious gastroenteritis, 1208
Infectious mononucleosis, 1354-1356
Infectious polymyositis, 1847-1848
Infective (bacterial) endocarditis, 1509-1511
  cyanosis and, 1487, 1488
  prophylaxis for, 1510b
  renal involvement in, 1270t
  subacute, 1509
Inferiority, sense of, 700, 701
Infertility, pelvic inflammatory disease and, 863
Inflammatory bowel disease, 1437-1443; *see also*
  Crohn disease; Ulcerative colitis.
  etiology of, 1437
  nursing care for, 1442-1443
  prognosis for, 1441
  treatment of, 1440-1442
Inflammatory changes, in dermatitis, 742
Inflammatory process, 747
  in asthma, 1385, 1386, 1387f
  in blood vessels in Kawasaki disease, 1514
  in scabies, 760
Infliximab (Remicade), for inflammatory
  bowel disease, 1440
Influenza, 1356
  immunizations for
    in cystic fibrosis, 1412
    Kawasaki disease and, 1516
    recommended, 529t, 534-535
  Reye syndrome and, 1683-1684
Informed consent, 1102-1103, 1103b
  for phototherapy, 309
  treatment without, 1103
Infrared thermometers, 178-179, 179f, 180b-
  181b, 182t-183t

Infus-A-Port, vs other long-term venous access
  devices, 1201t
Infusion(s)
  intraosseous, 1191-1192
  intravenous, 1188-1191, 1503-1504
    complications with, 1196-1198
    documentation of, 1195b
    equipment used for, 1190-1191, 1191f,
     1503-1504
    for asthma emergency care, 1396
    for cardiopulmonary resuscitation, 1399t
    for gastrointestinal bleeding, 1456
    for pneumonia, 1370, 1371
    for severe dehydration, 1213
    for shock, 1221
    infiltration of, 1197
    preparation of child and parents
     for, 1192
    procedure of, 1189, 1190, 1192-1194,
     1192b, 1193b
    protection of IV line in, 1194-1196, 1195f
    removal of catheter in, 1196
    site for, 1192-1193, 1194f
  opioid, after heart surgery, 1505-1506
Infusion device; *see also* Catheter(s); Venous
  access devices.
  peripheral intermittent, 1198, 1199b
Infusion pumps, 1191
  for blood transfusion, 1542
Inguinal hernia, 218, 218f, 261,
  477-478, 478f
Inguinal nodes, 190, 190f
Inhalants, abuse of, 886t, 892
Inhalation injuries
  from household toxins, 547, 549b
  from smoke, 1233, 1380-1382
Inheritance
  autosomal dominant, 118-119, 118f
  autosomal recessive, 119-120, 120f
  nontraditional, 121-122
  X-linked, 120, 120f, 121f
Initiative
  sense of, in preschoolers, 630
  vs guilt, 230t, 231
Injectease, 1747
Injection(s)
  insulin, 1746-1748, 1746f
  intradermal, 1067, 1157, 1158
  intramuscular, 1153-1157, 1154t-1156t,
    1157f, 1158b
    best sites for in infants and toddlers,
     539b, 540
  needleless system for, 1157
  play activities and, 1111b
Injection devices, for insulin, 1747
Injuries, 6-11; *see also* Trauma.
  at school, 735
  developmental aspects of, 7, 1759
  emergency management of, 1760-1761
  environmental factors in, 10
  from aspiration and suffocation, 541-545,
    618t, 623
  from bicycle accidents, 733
  from bodily damage, 548, 618t, 623-624
  from burns, 547-548, 617t, 620-622, 621f
  from drowning, 548, 617t, 620
  from falls, 546-547, 617t, 622-623
  from farm activities, 735

Injuries—cont'd
from motor vehicle accidents, 545-546, 545f, 546f, 616, 616f, 617t, 618-629, 618f, 619f
prevention of, 545-546, 545f, 546f, 616, 616f, 617t, 618-620, 618f, 619f
from poisoning, 547, 617t, 622, 622f
host/agent factors in, 7-10
in adolescents, 828-829, 828t
in boys vs girls, 732
in daycare centers, 517
in early childhood, 617t-618t
in health history, 155
in infants, 541-550, 542t-543t, 543t, 548, 549b
in preschoolers, 646-647
in school-age children, 730-736, 731t
in toddlers, 616-624, 623-624
inhalation, 547, 549b, 1233, 1380-1382
intentional, 10, 1758-1759, 1758b; see also Child abuse.
morbidity due to, 6, 1758
mortality due to, 7, 8t
nurse's role in, 548-550, 549b, 736
prevention of, 10-11, 1758b, 1759, 1759b; see also Safety.
risk factors for, 7b
self-inflicted, 8, 10
spinal cord, 1760, 1852-1863; see also Spinal cord injury.
sports, 1796-1807; see also Sports injuries.
to teeth, 736, 782-783, 783b
unintentional, 1758
In-line skates, safety with, 734, 735b
In-line suction catheters, in respiratory distress syndrome, 388
Insects, bites and stings of, 775-778, 776t
Inspiration, in newborn and adult, 1304, 1304f
Institute of Medicine, 564
Instrumental roles, in family, 68-69
Insulin, 1736-1738, 1746-1748
absorption of, 1746, 1746t
dosage of, 1737-1738
in concurrent illness, 1741, 1750
endogenous, 1708t, 1734, 1736-1737
for hyperglycemia, in newborn, 318
for ketoacidosis, 1742
injection of, 1738, 1746-1748, 1746f
intermediate-acting, 1737
islet cell/pancreatic transplant for, 1738
mixing of, 1747
multiple daily injections of, 1737
onset and duration of, injection site and, 1746, 1746t
preparations of, 1737
puberty and, 1751
pump for, 1747-1748
rapid-acting (regular), 1737
Somogyi effect and, 1741
storage of, 1746
teaching about, 1746-1748
time of administration of, 1737
Insulin pump, 1738, 1747-1748
Insulin reaction, 1741, 1750
Insulin resistance, type 2 diabetes and, 1733, 1734
Insulin waning, 1741
Insyte Autoguard safety catheters, 1190
Intake and output; see also under Fluid; Urinary.
of high-risk newborn, 337
sickle cell anemia and, 1553
ventriculoperitoneal shunt and, 442

Integra, for covering burn wounds, 1241
Integumentary system; see also Skin.
in cystic fibrosis, 1407
of newborn, 242-243, 251t-252t
at high risk, 336b, 349-350, 350b, 351b
Intelligence; see also Mental retardation.
in cerebral palsy, 1836
in Down syndrome, 990
IQ and, 977
social class and, 36
Intensive care unit, 1503
admission to, 1087b, 1093-1095, 1094b, 1094f, 1095g
neonatal, 334-335; see also Neonatal intensive care unit.
Intentionality, in infants, 504
Intercostal space, 208f, 209
Interdisciplinary team approach, 1096
Interferons, 1572
for hemangioma, 302
Interleukins, neonatal sepsis and, 395
Interlink intravenous access systems, 1190-1191, 1191f
Intermittent infusion device, 1198, 1199b
Intermittent mandatory ventilation, in respiratory distress syndrome, 384, 384f
Intermittent positive-pressure breathing, 1323
Intermittent skilled nursing visits, 1017, 1017b
Internal fixation, for fractures, 1793
International adoption, 93
International Adoption Clinic, 93
International Hearing Society, 997n
International Institute for Birth Defects, 460
International Shrine Headquarters, 1253
International Society of Nurses in Genetics, 132
Internet, congenital heart disease information on, 1502
Internet access, during hospitalization, 1070
Interpreters, 145-146, 146b
Intersex, 487
Interstitial emphysema, 389
respiratory distress syndrome and, 381
Interstitial fluid, 1171
in edema, 1180, 1181
Intertrigo, 774t
Interview, 141-153; see also Health history.
appropriate introduction in, 141
communication skills for, 141, 143-153; see also Communication.
confidentiality of, 141-142, 824-825, 825b, 826b, 854
cultural aspects of, 144
family, 160-164, 161b
health screening, of adolescent, 824-825, 825b, 826b
open-ended questions in, 143-144
preliminary acquaintance in, 142
privacy for, 141
role clarification for, 141
Intestinal obstruction
in cystic fibrosis, 1406, 1410
in Hirschsprung disease, 1427
in Meckel diverticulum, 1437
Intestinal parasites, 665-668
clinical manifestations of, 665t
drugs for, 666t
nursing considerations with, 665-666
prevention of, 667b

Intestinal tapering procedure, for short bowel syndrome, 1452
Intestinal toxocariasis, 665t
Intestinal transplantation, for short bowel syndrome, 1452-1453
Intestine(s); see also Bowel; Gastrointestinal tract and names of specific disorders, e.g., Irritable bowel syndrome.
large
absorption by, 1419
development of, 1417
malrotation of, 1449-1450
of newborn, 242
small
adaptive response of after massive resection, 1452
development of, 1417
structure and function of, 1418-1419, 1419f
Intimacy, in adolescents, 816
Intraaortic balloon pump, for shock, 1222
Intraarterial monitoring, of blood pressure, after heart surgery, 1504
Intraatrial baffle repairs, for transposition of great arteries, 1499b
Intracapsular pressure, 1256
Intracellular fluid, 1171, 1173, 1173f
Intracerebellar hemorrhage, in newborn, 403
Intracerebral abscess, 1681
Intracerebral hemorrhage, 1668
Intracranial hemorrhage, in newborn, 403
Intracranial infections, 1676-1684
Intracranial pressure
cerebral perfusion pressure and, 1643
cerebrospinal fluid and, 1645
hydrocephalus and, 441, 442
increased, 1645-1646, 1645b
after cranial surgery, 1623
in bacterial meningitis, 1679
in head injury, 1665, 1668-1669
monitoring of, 1656-1658
treatment of, 1657
intraventricular hemorrhage and, 402
monitoring of, 1656-1657
regulation of, 1645
Intradermal drug administration, 1067, 1157, 1158
Intramural plexus, of gastrointestinal tract, 1417
Intramuscular drug administration, 1153-1157, 1154t-1156t, 1157f, 1158b
best sites for in infants and toddlers, 539b, 540
Intranasal drug administration, 1065b
Intraosseous infusion, 1191-1192
Intrauterine device, 855, 856t
Intrauterine growth retardation, 334b; see also High-risk newborn.
Intravascular fluid, 1171
Intravenous alimentation, 1203-1204; see also Total parenteral nutrition.
Intravenous drug administration, 1158-1159
Intravenous infusion; see Infusion(s), intravenous.
Intravenous lines, 1503-1504
Intraventricular catheterization, in intracranial pressure monitoring, 1656
Intraventricular hemorrhage, in newborn, 401-402, 402t
Intravesical pressure, 1258
Intubation; see Endotracheal intubation; Tube(s).

Intuitive stage, 230t, 231-232, 631
Intussusception, 1448-1449, 1448f
  in gastrointestinal obstructive disorders, 1446
Iodine
  deficiency of, goiter and, 1718
  functions of and disturbances in, 562t
  sources of, 562t
Iontocaine, 1065b, 1066
Ipecac syrup, 622, 671-672
  abuse of, 672
  administration of, 671-672, 673b
  safety of, 672
IQ, 977; *see also* Intelligence; Mental
    retardation.
Iridocyclitis, in juvenile rheumatoid arthritis,
    1821, 1822
Iris, 194
  of newborn, 259
Iron
  absorption of, 564b
  BAL therapy and, 681
  for anemia, in high-risk newborn, 398
  functions of and disturbances in, 562t
  laboratory measures of, lead poisoning
      and, 677
  poisoning with, 671b
  recommended intake of, for athletes, 1804
  reference ranges for, 1898t
  sources of, 562t
  stores of, in infants, 496
  supplemental
    for breast-fed infant, 520
    in chronic renal failure, 1291
  toxicity of, 1546
Iron deficiency anemia, 1542-1546
  clinical manifestations of, 1544
  diagnosis of, 1544-1545
  etiology of, 1542-1543, 1544b
  lead poisoning and, 677
  nursing considerations in, 1545-1546
  pathophysiology of, 1544
  prevention of, 1545
  prognosis of, 1545
  treatment of, 1545
  vegetarian diets and, 560
Iron overload
  blood transfusions and, 1551
  thalassemia and, 1558
Iron-binding capacity, reference ranges
    for, 1899t
Irreversible coma, 1649, 1649b
Irritable bowel syndrome, 1432, 1432b
Irritable colon of childhood, 1216-1217
Ishihara test, 199
Island flap repair, in hypospadias, 482
Islet cells
  destruction of, in diabetes, 1733-1734, 1736
  transplantation of, 1738
Islets of Langerhans, 1704b
Isolation, 1092-1093
Isomil, 281t
Isoniazid, for tuberculosis, 1374
Isotretinoin, for acne, 841-842
Isthmus, thyroid, 191, 192f
Itching; *see* Pruritus.
ITP; *see* Idiopathic thrombocytopenic purpura.
IUDs (intrauterine devices), in adolescents,
    855, 856t
I.V. House, for protection of IV line, 1195, 1195f

Ivermectin, for scabies, 761
*Ixodes* species, Lyme disease and, 763

**J**

J pouch, for inflammatory bowel disease, 1441
Jacket restraint, 460, 1140
Jackknife seizures, 1688
Jacksonian march, 1686
Jacobi, Abraham, 11
Jaundice, 188, 188t
  breast-feeding and, 303t, 305, 307, 309
    home care and, 310, 311b
  in hyperbilirubinemia, 303, 303t; *see also*
      Hyperbilirubinemia.
  physiologic, of newborn, 242, 304-305
Jaw control, in cerebral palsy, 1840-1841, 1841f
Jaw pain, in cancer, 1601
Jaw thrust, 1334, 1337f, 1760
Jehovah's Witnesses, blood transfusions
    and, 1539b
Jejunostomy, 1162
Jewett-Taylor brace, 1774
Jitteriness, in newborn, 404
Job Accommodation Network, 919
Jobst garment, for burn patients, 1246f
Jock itch, 759t
John T. Tracy Clinic, 997n, 1006
Joint Commission on Accreditation of
    Healthcare Organizations, 1137
Joint Commission on Accreditation of
    Healthcare Organizations
      (JCAHO), 28
Joint custody, 72, 97
Joint physical custody, 97
Joints
  contractures of; *see* Contracture(s).
  examination of, 225
  immobilization effects on, 1763, 1770t
  in hemophilia, 1563, 1565
  range of motion of, 225
Jugular venipuncture, positioning for,
    1140-1141, 1140f
Jumper's knee, 1801t
Junctional nevus, 302
Justice, 21
Juvenile autoimmune thyroiditis, 1718-1719
Juvenile dermatomyositis, 1863
Juvenile Diabetes Research Foundation
    International, 1744
Juvenile hypothyroidism, 1717-1718
Juvenile melanoma, 302
Juvenile rheumatoid arthritis, 1820-1825
  classification of, 1820
  clinical manifestations of, 1820, 1821t
  course and prognosis of, 1820
  diagnosis of, 1821, 1821t
  everyday activities and, 1824-1825, 1824b
  exercise in, 1824
  family concerns in, 1825
  general health promotion in, 1824
  heat therapy in, 1824
  management of, 1821-1823
  nursing care in, 1823-1825
  nursing care plan for, 1826-1827
  ocular involvement in, 1821, 1822
  pathophysiology of, 1820
  pauciarticular, 1820, 1821t
  polyarticular, 1820, 1821t
  prognosis of, 1821t

Juvenile rheumatoid arthritis—cont'd
  psychosocial aspects of, 1824b
  terminology for, 1820
Juvenile spinal muscular atrophy, 1846-1847

**K**

Kahunas, 48
Kangaroo care, 347, 362, 368
Karyotyping, 123, 123f
Kasabach-Merritt syndrome, 302
Kasai procedure, 471-472, 471f
Kaufman Assessment Battery for Children, 978
Kawasaki disease, 1514-1516
  diagnosis of, 1515, 1515b
Kegel exercises, 784
Keloid, 746f
Keratin, 740
  fibrous, 769
Keratinocytes, 740
Kernicterus, 304, 311b
Kernig sign, 226, 228b
Kerosene heaters, burns from, 1227
Ketoacidosis
  diabetic, 1734, 1735, 1735f, 1736, 1749-1750
    management of, 1741-1743
    psychosocial factors in, 1742
  differential diagnosis of, 1736
Ketogenic diet, 1692
Ketonemia, diabetic, 1735
Ketones, 1735
Ketonuria, diabetic, 1734
Kidney(s); *see also* under Renal.
  ascent of, anomalies in, 479t
  bilateral agenesis of, 479t
  blood supply to, 1256
  congenital anomalies of, 479t
  continuous venovenous hemofiltration
      and, 1298
  development of, in infants, 1258
  disorders of; *see also* Glomerulonephritis;
      Nephrotic syndrome.
    clinical manifestations of, 1260, 1260b
    laboratory tests for, 1260, 1261t, 1262t
    nursing care of, 1260, 1262
  failure of
    acute, 1283-1287
    chronic, 1287-1294
  familial nephritis of, 1282
  function of
    blood tests of, 1261t
    in acute glomerulonephritis, 1271
    in burn patients, 1232
    in infants, fluid loss and, 1174
    radiologic and other tests of, 1263t, 1264t
    urine tests of, 1261t
  fusion of, anomalies in, 479t
  hemodialysis and, 1293-1297
  hemolysis and, 1540
  hemolytic uremic syndrome of, 1281-1282
  Henoch-Schönlein purpura and, 1570
  obstructive uropathy and, 485
  of newborn, 242, 253t, 261
    after surgery, 422t
  palpation of, 220
  peritoneal dialysis and, 1297-1298
  physiology of, 1256-1258
  rotation of, anomalies in, 479t
  sickle cell anemia and, 1548
    hydration in, 1552

Kidney(s)—cont'd
  structure and function of, 1255-1262
  supernumerary, 479t
  transplantation of, 1298-1301
  trauma to, 1282-1283
  tubular disorders of, 1279-1281
  unexplained proteinuria of, 1282
  unilateral agenesis of, 479t
  Wilms tumor of, 1629-1631
Kidney stones, immobilization and, 1764,
    1794-1795
Kindergarten, 636-637
Kinetic family drawing, 163-164, 163b
Kistner valve, for tracheostomy, 1330
Klinefelter syndrome, 116-117, 117t, 118f
Klippel-Feil syndrome, 447t
Klippel-Trenaunay-Weber syndrome, 302
Klumpke palsy, 262, 299
Knee
  developmental deformity of, 447t
  jumper's, 1801t
  ligament injuries of, 1800
Knee jerk reflex, 227f
Knee-ankle-foot orthosis, 1773, 1773f, 1774b
Knee-chest position, in infant, 1488f
Knock-knee, 224, 224f
Koch pouch, for inflammatory bowel
    disease, 1441
Kohlberg's moral development theory, 230t, 232
  adolescents and, 811
  preschoolers and, 631-632
  school-age children and, 704-705
  toddlers and, 597-598
Koilonychia, 189
Koplik spots, 656f
Korotkoff sounds, 184, 186
Kostmann's disease, 1569t
Kugelberg-Welander syndrome, 1846-1847
Kupffer cells, 1534
Kussmaul respirations, 1184, 1735
Kwashiorkor, 566-567, 567f
Kyphosis, 1809-1810, 1809f

L

La Leche League International, 276, 277, 348
Labia majora/minora, 222-223, 222f
  ambiguous genitalia and, 489t
  in newborn, 261
    prematurity and, 377f
Labile cells, in epithelial tissue, 745
Labile factor, 1562t
Labor and delivery; see also under Perinatal.
  history of, 155
  prolonged, in adolescents, 851
Laboratory tests
  abbreviations for, 1903
  reference ranges for, 1895t-1902t
Labyrinthitis, otitis media and, 1358
Labyrinth-righting reflex, in infants, 494b, 498
Lacerations, 745
  care of, 752
  cerebral, 1666
  from human bites, 779-780
  in physical abuse, 688b
  scalp
    bleeding from, 1665, 1670
    suturing of, 1672, 1672b
Lacrimal punctum, 193

Lactase, 1418
  deficiency of, 570
Lactate dehydrogenase, in neuromuscular
    dysfunction, 1834b
Lacteal, 1418, 1419f
*Lactobacillus acidophilus*, 848
Lactofree, 281t
Lacto-ovovegetarian diet, 560
Lactose intolerance, 570-571
  acute diarrhea and, 1213
  celiac disease and, 1450
  controlling symptoms of, 570b
Lactose-free formulas, in galactosemia, 325
Lactovegetarian diet, 560
Lactulose, for hepatic encephalopathy, 1461
Laissez-faire parent, 85
Lamellar bodies, fetal lung maturity
    and, 383
Lamotrigine, for seizures, 1691t
Lancet, for blood glucose monitoring, 1748
Landau reflex, 263t
Landouzy-Dejerine muscular dystrophy, 1863t
Language, 1007; see also Communication;
    Speech.
  avoidance, 140
  distancing, 140
Language barriers, 45
Language development, 148, 148b, 1011t
  bilingualism and, 633b
  in infants, 506
  in preschoolers, 631, 633, 638t
  in school-age children, 705-706
  in toddlers, 596-597, 599
Language impairment, 1007, 1007b; see also
    Communication impairment.
  assessment of, 1012b
  autism and, 1009
Lanoxin; see Digoxin (Lanoxin).
Lansoprazole (Prevacid)
  for gastroesophageal reflux, 1429
  for peptic ulcer disease, 1445
Lanugo, 376, 741
Laparoscopic surgery
  for appendectomy, 1434
  for hypertrophic pyloric stenosis, 1447
Large intestine; see also Bowel; Intestine(s).
  absorption by, 1419
  development of, 1417
  gastroschisis and, 473, 473f
  necrotizing enterocolitis of; see Necrotizing
    enterocolitis.
  palpation of, 220
Large-for-gestational-age infant, 250, 334b;
    see also High-risk newborn.
  diabetic mother and, 405
Laryngeal edema, in anaphylaxis, 1224
Laryngitis
  acute, 1363
  acute spasmodic, 1362t, 1365
Laryngotracheobronchitis, acute, 1362t,
    1363-1364
  progression of symptoms in, 1364b
Larynx, 1305
  in croup, 1361, 1361f
Laser therapy
  for birthmarks, 302, 303
  for retinopathy of prematurity, 400
Lashes, inspection of, 194

Lasix (furosemide)
  for congestive heart failure, 1480t
  for nephrotic syndrome, 1277
Lasting Impressions, 916n
Latchkey children, 720, 720f
Latency period, 230, 230t, 700
Latex allergy, 433-436, 433b, 436b, 1135
Latex balloons, suffocation by, 542t, 544
Latinos, 35b; see also Race/ethnicity.
  dietary preferences of, 45-47, 46t
  health beliefs and practices of, 54t
  time concept of, 43
Lavage, 1148
Lawn mowers, injuries with, 623, 735
Laws
  abortion, 853-854
  affecting child health, 12-13
Laxatives, for constipation, 1425
Lead
  effects of on body systems, 676-678, 677f
  exposure to, 675-676, 676b, 677b, 679,
    681b, 682b
  in folk remedies, 49b
  reference ranges for, 678, 679, 680, 1899t
Lead encephalopathy, 678, 681
Lead poisoning, 675-682
  acute, 680
  causes of, 676
  diagnosis of, 678, 680
  family education about, 679, 682
  long-term effects of, 678b
  nursing considerations with, 681-682
  pathophysiology and clinical manifestations
    of, 676-678
  personal risk questions for, 679
  prevention of, 679
  prognosis for, 681
  screening for, 679
  treatment of, 679-682
Lead-based paint, home cleaning of, 679
Lean body mass, 808
Learning disabilities, 791-792, 833
Learning Disabilities Association of America, 792
Lecithin/sphingomyelin ratio, fetal lung
    maturity and, 383
Left-right confusion, 791
Left-to-right shunt, 1475
Leg; see also Extremities.
Leg length, in school-age children, 699
Leg restraints, 1140
Legal blindness, 1000
Legal guardian, informed consent of, 1102
Legal proceedings, in cases of child
    maltreatment, 692, 692b
Legg-Calvé-Perthes disease, 1807-1808
Legislation
  abortion, 853-854
  affecting child health, 12-13
Leiter International Performance Scale-
    Revised, 978
Length
  crown-to-rump, 176f, 177
  measurement of, 175-176, 176f
  percentiles for, 1883, 1888
Lennox-Gastaut syndrome, 1689
Lens, 194
Lente insulin, 1737
Lesbians; see Gays/lesbians.

Let-down reflex, 278t
Lethargy, 1648b
Leukemia, 1610-1616
  acute lymphoid, 1611
  acute myelogenous, 1611
  bone marrow dysfunction in, 1612
  cell-surface markers in, 1612
  chromosomal abnormalities in,
    1585-1586, 1612
  chronic myelogenous, Philadelphia
    chromosome in, 1585
  classification of, 1610-1612
  clinical manifestations of, 1612-1613, 1613f
  cytochemical markers in, 1611
  diagnosis of, 1614
  in Down syndrome, 990, 1585-1586, 1612
  incidence of, 1610
  monoclonal antibodies for, 1594
  morphology of, 1611
  nursing care in, 1615-1616
  onset of, 1613
  pathophysiology of, 1612-1613
  prognosis of, 1613-1614, 1614t, 1615, 1616
  relapse in, 1615
  sites of involvement in, 1612-1613, 1613f
  staging of, 1613
  stem (blast) cell, 1611
  treatment of, 1614-1615
Leukocyte, 1534-1535, 1538
Leukocyte count, 1536t
  clozapine and, 799
  reference ranges for, 1899t
Leukocyte esterase, in urine tests, 1261t, 1266
Leukocytosis, 1534
  in cancer, 1596, 1612
  in Kawasaki disease, 1515
  in leukemia, 1612
Leukokoria, in retinoblastoma, 1632-1633, 1632f
Leukomalacia, periventricular, 401
Leukopenia, in neonatal sepsis, 394
Leukorrhea, 848
  physiologic, 805
Leukotriene receptor antagonists, for
    asthma, 1393
Leuprolide (Lupron), for precocious
    puberty, 1715
Level of consciousness; see Consciousness.
Levorphanol, in pain management, 1062t
Levothyroxine sodium, for congenital
    hypothyroidism, 321
LH symbol test, 197-198, 198t
Library of Congress, 1004
Library of Congress National Library Service
    for the Blind and Physically
    Handicapped, 1006
Librium; see Chlordiazepoxide.
Lice, 761-763, 761f, 762b
  rickettsial infections from, 763, 765t
Lichenification, of skin, 745f
Lidocaine
  buffered, 1067, 1067b
  for bladder catheterization, 1145
  for cardiopulmonary resuscitation, 1399t
  for circumcision, 271b
  for laser therapy, for birthmarks, 302
  viscous, for oral ulcers, 1601
Lidocaine-adrenaline-tetracaine combined
    (LAT), 751b

Life expectancy
  in Down syndrome, 990-991
  of special needs child, 906
Life support, termination of, 1660-1661
Life-threatening illness; see Terminal illness.
Ligament injuries, 1799, 1800
Ligase chain reaction, 862, 863
Light exposure, in high-risk newborn, 365
  retinopathy of prematurity and, 399
Light reflex, otoscopic, 203
Lighthouse, Inc., 1004n
Limb; see Extremities.
Limb deficiency, skeletal, 453-454
Limb prosthesis, 454, 1628
Limb salvage, for osteosarcoma, 1627
Limb-girdle muscular dystrophy, 1863t
Limit-setting, 84-85
  for school-age children, 716-717
  safety and, 1136
Limp, in developmental dysplasia of hip, 448
Lindane, for scabies, 760, 761
Linear growth, 808, 809f
Linear skull fracture, 1666-1667
Lingual frenulum, 260
Lip
  cleft, 454-463, 455t
  examination of, in nutritional assessment,
    166t
  frenulum of, 259-260
Lipase, in infants, 496
Lipids, elevated serum, 1519-1520
Lipoid pneumonia, 1379
Lipoprotein(s)
  high-density, 1520
  low-density, coronary artery disease risk and,
    1519-1520, 1520t
  types of, 1520
  very-low-density, 1520
Lipoprotein lipase theory of obesity, 871
Lipreading, 998, 998b
Liquid crystal skin contact thermometers, 178,
    180b, 183t
Liquid ventilation, for respiratory distress
    syndrome, 385-386
Lisch nodules, 774
Lisinopril (Zestril)
  for congestive heart failure, 1479
  for hypertension, 1519b
Lispro-H (Humalog), 1737
Listening, 144-145
Listeriosis, in newborn, 328t
Little League elbow, 1801t
Little League shoulder, 1801t
Live birth, 334b
Liver, 1416, 1531; see also under Hepatic.
  dysfunction of, with total parenteral
    nutrition, 1452
  in cystic fibrosis, 1406
  in hyperbilirubinemia, 304
  in infants, 496
  in newborns, 242, 253t, 261
  in sickle cell anemia, 1548
  palpation of, 220
Liver disease, 1456-1461
  end-stage, 1460-1461, 1461b
  total parenteral nutrition and, 1204
Liver transplantation, 1461
  for biliary atresia, 470, 471

Lobes, of lung, 210, 211f
Lobule, auricular, 200, 200f
Local anesthesia; see also Topical anesthesia.
  for suturing, 1672b
Lockjaw, 1848-1850
Locomotion, in infants, 499-500, 501f
Locutionary stage, 148, 148b
Lofenalac, 283t, 323
Logical thinking, development of, 230t, 232
Lomustine (CCNU), 1593t
Loneliness, in latchkey children, 721b
Long bones, fracture of, birth-related, 298
Longitudinal fissure, 1643
Long-term care, mental retardation and, 986b
Loop diuretics, for nephrotic syndrome, 1277
Loop of Henle, 1256, 1256f
  in infants, 1258
Loratadine (Claritin), for allergic rhinitis, 1384
Lorazepam (Ativan), for status epilepticus, 1692
Lorcet, 1060b; see also Hydrocodone.
Lordosis, 1809f, 1810
  developmental dysplasia of hip and, 449
Lortab, 1060b; see also Hydrocodone.
Loss of consciousness; see also Coma;
    Unconsciousness.
  assessment in, 225
Low birth weight; see also Preterm infant.
  cerebral palsy and, 1835
  mortality and, 3-4
Low Vision Association of Canada, 1003n
Low-birth-weight infant, 334b; see also High-
    risk newborn.
Lower extremity; see also Extremities.
  elevation of, 1800, 1800f
  examination of, 224-225
Lower extremity traction, 1789-1790, 1789f,
    1790f; see also Traction.
Lower motor neuron, 1832, 1833f, 1854
Lower motor neuron lesions, 1833, 1854, 1855b
L/S ratio; see Lecithin/sphingomyelin ratio.
LSD; see Lysergic acid diethylamide.
Lumbar curve, convex, in infants, 499
Lumbar puncture, 1653t
  analgesia for, 1603
  in bacterial meningitis, 1679
  in cancer, 1587
  positioning for, 1141-1142, 1141f, 1142b, 1142f
  sedation for, 1603
  topical anesthesia for, 1679
Lumirubin, 306
Lung(s), 1303-1312; see also under Pulmonary;
    Respiratory.
  apex of, 210, 211f
  auscultation of, 212-213
  base of, 210, 211f
  chronic disease of, 390-393
  compliance of, 1304, 1307, 1307b
  congenital diaphragmatic hernia and,
    475-476
  costal surface of, 210, 211f
  damage to, with aspiration of hydrocarbons,
    1379
  examination of, 210-213
  fetal, maturity of, 383
  growth of, 1306
    in puberty, 809
  in acute respiratory distress syndrome, 1379
  in cystic fibrosis, 1404, 1405

Lung(s)—cont'd
  in shock, 1221
  inspection of, 210-211
  lobes of, 210, 211f
  mediastinal surface of, 210, 211f
  of newborn, 241, 253t, 260
    in respiratory distress syndrome, 380-381
    phrenic nerve paralysis and, 299
  palpation of, 211-212
  percussion of, 212, 212f
  sickle cell anemia and, 1550
  structure of, 210, 211f
Lung biopsy, 1315t
Lung disease
  congestive heart failure and, 1476
  obstructive, respiratory failure and, 1331
  restrictive, respiratory failure and, 1331
Lung puncture, 1315t
Lung transplantation
  in cystic fibrosis, 1409
  in pulmonary artery hypertension, 1491
Lung volume, posture and, 1304, 1304f
Lupus nephritis, 1827
Luque segmental spinal instrumentation, for
    scoliosis, 1813, 1814
Luteinizing hormone, 805, 1707t
  in adolescence, 803, 803f
Luteinizing hormone-releasing hormone, for
    cryptorchidism, 481
Luteinizing hormone–releasing hormone, for
    precocious puberty, 1715
Lyell disease, 773
Lying, in school-age children, 717
Lyme disease, 763-766, 766f
  immunization for, in children, 535t
  vaccine for, 766
Lymph flow, obstruction of, edema formation
    and, 1181
Lymph nodes, 1531, 1571
  cancer of; see Lymphoma.
  enlarged
    in cancer, 1597
    in Hodgkin disease, 1617
    in infectious mononucleosis, 1354
  examination of, 190, 190f
  sentinel, 1617
Lymphadenitis
  cervical, 664
  regional, in cat scratch disease, 766
Lymphadenopathy
  in cancer, 1597
  in Hodgkin disease, 1617
  in infectious mononucleosis, 1354
Lymphangiography, 1617
Lymphatics, as respiratory tract defense, 1310
Lymphocytes, 243, 1534
  B, 243
  in complete blood count, 1536t
  T, 243, 1572
    in human immunodeficiency virus
      infection, 1573
Lymphocytic thyroiditis, 1718-1719
Lymphocytopoiesis, 1534
Lymphogenous leukocytes, 1534
Lymphoid organs, 1571
Lymphoid tissues, as respiratory tract
    defense, 1310
Lymphokines, 1572

Lymphomas, 1616-1619
  Burkitt, 1618-1619
  Hodgkin, 1616-1618
  non-Hodgkin, 1618-1619
Lymphomyeloid complex, 1534
Lymphopenic agammaglobulinemia, Swiss-
    type, 1579-1580
Lyon hypothesis, 117
Lysergic acid diethylamide, 886t, 891b, 892

**M**
Macewen sign, 437
Macrominerals, 555
Macro-orchidism, fragile X syndrome and, 993
Macrophages, 1531, 1534
  in wound healing, 747
Macrosomy, diabetic mother and, 405, 406
Macula, 195, 195f
Macule, 743f
Mafenide acetate, for burn wounds, 1239t
Magazines, developmental impact of, 39
Magical thinking
  in preschoolers, 631
  terminal illness and, 953
Magnesium
  for asthma, 1393
  for cardiopulmonary resuscitation, 1399t
  functions of and disturbances in, 562t
  sources of, 562t
  supplements of, for premenstrual
    syndrome, 847
Magnesium citrate, in poisoning cases, 673
Magnesium sulfate, in poisoning cases, 673
Magnetic resonance imaging
  in obesity, 874
  of brain, 1652, 1652f, 1654t
  of gastrointestinal tract, 1421t
Mainstreaming, 908-909
Major histocompatibility complex, 1571
Mal ojo, 47
Malabsorption syndromes, 1450-1454
Malaria, from blood transfusion, 1542t
Malathion, for head lice, 762
Male genitalia
  ambiguous, 489t
  of newborn, 254t, 261, 377f
    circumcision and, 270-273, 270b-272b, 272f
    cryptorchidism and, 480-481
    hypospadias and, 481-482, 481f
    phimosis and, 479
    preterm, 376, 377f
Male reproductive system, disorders of, 842-844
Malignant hyperthermia, postoperative,
    1113, 1117
Malleus, 203, 203f
Malnutrition; see also Failure to thrive; Nutrition.
  in cystic fibrosis, 1406
  in inflammatory bowel disease, 1441
  poverty and, 41
Malocclusion, 207, 781-782
  in cerebral palsy, 207
Malrotation, of intestine, 1449-1450
Maltase, 1418
Malunion, fracture, 1794
Managed care, 13
  special needs child and, 909
Manganese
  functions of and disturbances in, 562t
  sources of, 562t

Manifest culture, 31
Mannitol, for increased intracranial
    pressure, 1657
Manometry
  anorectal, in Hirschsprung disease, 1427
  in gastroesophageal reflux diagnosis, 1429
  of gastrointestinal tract, 1421t
Mantoux skin test, for tuberculosis, 834,
    1373-1375, 1373b, 1374b
Manual dexterity, in toddlers, 593
Manual traction, 1788b; see also Traction.
Manubrium, 203, 203f
  sternal, 208f, 209
Maple syrup urine disease, 119t
Marasmic-kwashiorkor, 567
Marasmus, 567, 567f
March of Dimes—Birth Defects Foundation,
    419, 460
Marfan syndrome, 119t, 447t
Marijuana, 886t, 891b, 892
Marriage
  family structure and, 70-73
  mental retardation and, 982
  polygamous, 72
  sororate, 72
Masculinization, in congenital adrenal
    hyperplasia, 1729-1731
Mass media
  developmental impact of, 38-40
  health promotion in, 823
Massage, of high-risk newborn, 362
Mastication, 1417, 1418
Mastitis, breast-feeding and, 278t
Mastoid fontanel, 257
Mastoidectomy, for recurrent otitis media, 1359
Mastoiditis, otitis media and, 1358
Masturbation
  in preschoolers, 640
  in teenagers, 814, 815
Matches, 621, 1272
  burn injuries and, 1227
Matching symbol test, 197, 198t
Material overt culture, 31
Maternity and Infancy Act, 12
Mathieu procedure, 482
Matulane (procarbazine), 1590t
Mature minors' doctrine, 1103
Mature (somatic) swallow reflex, 497, 497f
Maturity-onset diabetes of young, 1733, 1735
Maxillary sinus, 191, 191f
McBurney's point, 1433
McCamon-Robins fluoromatic assay test, 323
MCH Services Block Grant, 12
MCT oil, 282t, 323
Mealtime; see also Eating; Feeding.
  in school-age children, 721
Mean airway pressure, in respiratory distress
    syndrome, 384
Mean arterial pressure (MAP), 183
  cerebral perfusion pressure and, 1643
Mean corpuscular hemoglobin, 1533, 1536t
  reference ranges for, 1899t
Mean corpuscular hemoglobin concentration,
    1533, 1536t
  reference ranges for, 1899t
Mean corpuscular volume, 1532-1533,
    1533f, 1536t
  in iron deficiency anemia, 1544
  reference ranges for, 1900t

Measles
immunization for, 529t, 533
contraindications to, 537t
in adolescents, 541b, 833-834
Kawasaki disease and, 1516
recommended, 529t, 533
manifestations and management of, 656f, 656t-657t
vitamin A deficiency and, 554, 555, 660
Meat
contaminated, 1281, 1282
for infants, 522, 524b
Meatal advancement glanuloplasty, in hypospadias, 482
Meatus
nasal, 206, 206f
urethral
female, 223
male, 221, 221f
Mebendazole, 665, 666t
for enterobiasis, 668
Mechanical ventilation, 1307, 1323-1325, 1323b, 1324b, 1325b; see also Endotracheal intubation; Ventilatory support.
extubation in, 1324, 1324b
for unconscious child, 1656
hearing impairment and, 996b
high-frequency, 1323-1324
in asthma, 1388
in meconium aspiration syndrome, 389
in persistent pulmonary hypertension of newborn, 398
in respiratory distress syndrome, 383-385, 384t
in shock, 1221
in spinal cord injury, 1859
indications for, 1323b
nursing care in, 1324
termination of, 1660-1661
Mechlorethamine (Mustargen), 1589t
Meckel diverticulum, 1435, 1437
Meconium, 242b, 1417
enterohepatic circulation and, 305
failure to pass, in Hirschsprung disease, 1427
Meconium aspiration syndrome, 388-389
Meconium ileus, 1424
in cystic fibrosis, 1406, 1410
Meconium plugs, 1424
Media
developmental impact of, 38-40
health promotion in, 823
Mediastinal surface, of lung, 210, 211f
Mediastinum, 1302, 1465
Medicaid, 12, 13, 909
home care and, 1020
Medical play, 1768-1769
Medical records, confidentiality of, 141-142
Medic-Alert bracelet, 924
Medicare, home care and, 1020
Medication history, 156
Medications; see Drug(s).
Medicine dropper, feeding with, cleft lip and palate and, 459
Mediport, vs other long-term venous access devices, 1201t
Medium chain triglyceride (MCT) oil, 282t, 323
Medroxyprogesterone, 982
cyclic, for dysfunctional uterine bleeding, 848
Medulla, 1644t

Medullary centers
respiratory, 1309
vomiting and, 1218
Medulloblastoma, 1620b; see also Brain tumors.
Megacolon, congenital aganglionic (Hirschsprung disease), 1426-1429, 1426f
Megaloblastic anemia, 1549
Meibomian glands, 193
Meiosis, errors in, chromosomal abnormalities and, 114-115, 114f
Melanin, 769
in newborn, 243
phenylketonuria and, 322
Melanocyte-stimulating hormone, 1707t
hyposecretion of, 1706b
Melanoma, in newborn, 302
Melena, 1454
Melphalan (Alkeran), 1590t
Membranous septum, interventricular, 1465, 1465f
Memory
mental retardation and, 980-981
of pain, in newborn, 353-355
Memory B-lymphocytes, 1572
Menarche, 804-805, 845
age at, 805, 806
delayed, in athletes, 1804
in athletes, 1804
premature, 1715
Meninges, 1642-1643, 1643f
Meningism, in pneumonia, 1370
Meningitis, 1677-1681
aseptic (viral), 1680-1681, 1681t
bacterial, 1677-1680
brain abscess and, 1681
opisthotonos in, 191, 223
otitis media and, 1358
posttraumatic, 1667
septic, neonatal, 394
tuberculous, 1681
Meningocele, 424b, 424f, 425; see also Myelomeningocele.
folic acid supplementation for, 124-125
prenatal diagnosis of, 128t, 129-130
Meningococcal disease, immunization for
in adolescents, 541b
in children, 535t
Meningococcal sepsis, 1678, 1678f
Meningococcemia, 1678, 1678f
Waterhouse-Friderichsen syndrome in, 1678, 1678f, 1725
Meningomyelocele
folic acid supplementation for, 124-125
prenatal diagnosis of, 128t, 129-130
Menorrhagia, in von Willebrand disease, 1566
Menstrual disorders, 845-846
in female athletes, 846
Menstruation, onset of; see Menarche.
Mental operations, 702
Mental representations
in cognitive development in infants, 502
in school-age children, 702-704
Mental retardation, 977-994
assessment of, 979, 979b
classification of, 978, 978t
definition of, 977-978
diagnosis of, 978-979
education of child and family in, 980-981, 981f
etiology of, 979, 979b

Mental retardation—cont'd
future care in, helping families adjust to, 986, 986b
hospitalization and, 986-987
in cerebral palsy, 1836
in congenital hypothyroidism, 321, 322
in Down syndrome, 987-993, 989b, 989t, 990f, 991b, 991t
in fetal alcohol syndrome, 329
in fragile X syndrome, 993-994, 993f, 994b
in phenylketonuria, 322-323
nursing care plan for, 988
optimum development in, 981-983, 983f
prevention of, 979
self-help skills in, promotion of, 983-986, 984b, 984f
Meperidine
in pain management, 1060, 1062t, 1063t
in preoperative sedation, 1113b
sickle cell anemia and, 1553
Mephyton, for hemorrhagic disease of newborn, 319
Meprobamate, abuse of, 886t
6-Mercaptopurine, for inflammatory bowel disease, 1440
6-Mercaptopurine, 1591t
Mercury thermometers, 178, 180b, 182t, 675
Mercury toxicity, 675
Mercy killing, 949
Meromelia, 453
Mesalamine (Asacol, Pentasa), for inflammatory bowel disease, 1440
Mescaline, 886t
Mesencephalon, 1644t
Meso-2,3 dimercaptosuccinic acid (DMSA), for chelation therapy, 680
Mestinon (pyridostigmine), for myasthenia gravis, 1851
Metabolic acidosis, 1183t, 1184, 1184b
cold stress and, high-risk newborn and, 339
in burn injuries, 1233
in chronic renal failure, 1289, 1291
in diabetes, 1734, 1735, 1735f, 1741-1742, 1749-1750
psychosocial factors in, 1742
in shock, 1221
in short bowel syndrome, 1452
Metabolic alkalosis, 1183t, 1184-1185, 1184b
in hypertrophic pyloric stenosis, 1447
Metabolic changes
in shock, 1220
in total parenteral nutrition, 1452
Metabolic disorders, 319-325, 320f, 322f, 324b, 325f; see also specific disorders.
congenital
screening for, 125-126, 125-127
treatment and prevention of, 124-125
mental retardation and, 979b
neonatal seizures and, 403b
Metabolic pathway, 319-320, 320f
Metabolic rate, of newborn, 242
Metabolism
immobilization effects on, 1764, 1768, 1771t
in burn injuries, 1232-1233, 1237
in infants, fluid loss and, 1174
in puberty, 809
medications affecting, 1232-1233
obesity and, 871
Metalinguistic awareness, 706

Metalloporphyrins, in hyperbilirubinemia, 306
Metaproterenol, for asthma, 1392
Metatarsus adductus, 453
Metatarsus valgus, 447t
Metatarsus varus, 453
Metered-dose inhaler
    for aerosol therapy, 1319-1320
    for asthma, 1391, 1391f
    use of, 1398, 1399b
Methadone
    abuse of, 886t
    in pain management, 1062t, 1063t
    in pregnancy, 407
Methamphetamine, 892
Methaqualone, 886t, 892
Methimazole (Tapazole), for hyperthyroidism,
        1719-1720, 1721
Methotrexate, 1591t
    for inflammatory bowel disease, 1440
    for juvenile rheumatoid arthritis, 1822
Methyl salicylate, as poison, 669
Methylphenidate (Ritalin), for attention
        deficit hyperactivity disorder, 789, 790,
        790b, 791
Methylprednisolone, for cancer, 1593t
Methylxanthines
    for apnea of infancy, 586
    for apnea of prematurity, 378-379
    for asthma, 1392
    for respiratory distress syndrome, 386
Meticorten; see Prednisone.
Metoclopramide (Reglan), for
        gastroesophageal reflux, 1429
Metolazone (Zaroxolyn)
    for congestive heart failure, 1480t
    for nephrotic syndrome, 1277
Metopic craniosynostosis, 444-445
Metronidazole, 666t
    for giardiasis, 667
    for inflammatory bowel disease, 1440
Mexican-Americans; see Latinos.
MHC; see Major histocompatibility complex.
Mice, asthma control and, 1390
Miconazole, for candidiasis, in newborn, 301
Microcephaly, 444, 444f
Microenvironments, in thermoregulation, of
        high-risk newborn, 340
Microminerals, 555
Micropenis, 489t
Microtrauma, repetitive, 1798, 1800-1801
Microvilli, 1418, 1419f
Microwave heating
    burns from, 542t, 543t, 547
    of breast milk, 280
    of infant formula and food, 279, 280, 523,
        523b, 542t, 543t, 547
    safety measures with, 1252, 1252b
Micturition, normal, 1258
Mid-arm circumference
    in nutritional assessment, 168
    measurement of, 177
    percentiles for, 1894
Midazolam
    in pain management, 1065b
    in preoperative sedation, 1112, 1113b
    respiratory depression from, 1068b
Middle ear
    cleft lip and palate and, 457, 463
    infection of; see Otitis media.

Middle-ear hearing loss, 995
Midgut, 1416
Midnight croup, 1365
Mifepristone, for medical abortion, 854
Migraine headaches, 1699-1700, 1699t, 1700b
Migrant children, 42, 42b
Migrating motor complex, 242
Milia, in newborn, 243, 251t, 255b
Miliaria, in newborn, 243, 251t
Milk
    alternatives to, 280, 282
        in phenylketonuria, 323
    breast, 281t, 521; see also Breast-feeding.
        donor, 344
        expressed, 347, 348
        fortified, 344
        freezing of, 520-521
        storage of, 520
        supplements for, 520
        vegetarian diets and, 565
        warming of, 520
    cow's
        acute diarrhea and, 1213
        allergy to, 569-570, 569b
            colic and, 572, 573
            diabetes and, 1734
        as diabetic glucose source, 1740
        constipation and, 1424, 1425b
        for infants, 280, 281t, 283t, 521
        galactosemia and, 325
        hypocalcemia and, 318
        in vegetarian diets, 565
        whole, introduction of to infants, 521
    goat's, 282, 521
Milk baby, 1544
Milk of magnesia, 1425
Milk stool, 242b
Milwaukee brace, 1811
Mineralocorticoids, 1723, 1724
    deficiency of, 1726t
Minerals, 1418
    deficiency of, kwashiorkor and, 566-567
    disturbances of, in infants, 555, 560, 561t-564t
    intake of
        in adolescents, 829
        in athletes, 1804
        in toddlers, 609
    regulation of, 560
    sources of and disturbances in, 561t-564t
Minimal enteral feedings, for high-risk
        newborn, 343
    with necrotizing enterocolitis, 396
Minority groups; see also Race/ethnicity.
    classification of, 35b
    membership in, 35
Minors, informed consent of, 1103
Miralax (polyethylene glycol), 1425
Mirroring movements, 1647b
Misbehavior; see also Behavior.
    ways to minimize, 85, 86b
Mist therapy, 1319, 1319b
    in croup, 1364
    in pneumonia, 1371
    in respiratory infections, 1345-1346
Mistrust, in infants, 501
Mites, rickettsial infections from, 763, 765t
Mitochondrial disorders, 122
Mitosis, errors in, chromosomal abnormalities
        and, 114-115, 114f

Mitral regurgitation, rheumatic fever and, 1511
Mitral valve, 1465
    heart sounds and, 215
Mitrofanoff procedure, 429
Mixed apnea, of prematurity, 378
Mixed conductive-sensorineural hearing
        loss, 995
Mixed gonadal dysgenesis, 488-489, 489t
Mobilization devices, 1773-1776, 1773f-1776f,
        1774-1776, 1774b, 1775b, 1775f
    in cerebral palsy, 1384f, 1838
    in spinal cord injury, 1860-1861
Modeling, by preschoolers, 641
Moderately-low-birth-weight infant, 334b;
        see also High-risk newborn.
Modified Behavioral Pain Scale, 1056t
Modified jaw-thrust maneuver, 1760
Moducal formula, 282t
Molestation, definition of, 685
Molluscum contagiosum, 758t, 865t
Molybdenum
    functions and disturbances in, 562t
    sources of, 562t
Mongolian spots, in newborn, 252t
Moniliasis; see Candidiasis.
Morning-after pill, 855, 856t
Monitoring
    in apnea of infancy, 586-587, 586b,
        587b, 587f
    in intensive care unit, 1095
    of appointments, in compliance
        measurement, 1120
    of blood pressure, after heart surgery, 1504
    of diabetic mother, 405
    of heart rate, with Holter monitor, 1470
    of high-risk newborn, 337-338, 337b,
        337t, 351b
    with apnea of prematurity, 379
    with respiratory distress syndrome, 387
    of therapeutic response, in compliance
        measurement, 1120
Monoclonal antibodies, 1594-1595
    for inflammatory bowel disease, 1440
Monocytes, 243, 1534
    in complete blood count, 1536t
Monocytosis, 1534
Mononeuropathies, 1833
Mononucleosis, infectious, 1354-1356
Monosaccharides, 1418
Monosomy, 113
Monospot test, in infectious mononucleosis,
        1355
Monotropy, attachment and, multiple births
        and, 286
Monozygotic twins, 80, 80b
Mons pubis, 222
Moodiness
    in hyperthyroidism, 1721
    steroid-related, 1602
Moon face, 1602, 1727, 1727f
Moral development, 230t, 232
    in adolescents, 811
    in preschoolers, 630b, 631-632
    in school-age children, 704-705
    in toddlers, 597-598
Moral reasoning, 811
*Moraxella catarrhalis*, otitis media and,
        1357, 1358

Morbidity, 6
  disability and, 6
  injuries and, 6-11
Morbidity rates, 105, 105b
Moro reflex, 263t, 264f
  brachial palsy and, 299
  in cerebral palsy, 1837
Morphine, 1060
  abuse of, 886t, 891b, 892
  in pain management, 1062t
    after heart surgery, 1505-1506
    in newborn, 357
    patient-controlled, 1064t
  in preoperative sedation, 1113b
Mortality, 2-6
  childhood, 4-6, 4t
  in burn patients, 1233
  infant, 2-4, 3t, 4t
  injuries and, 6-11, 7t
  neonatal, 2
  of adolescents, 820
  of high-risk infants, 334b, 369-371
  of special needs children, 906
  perinatal, 3
  postneonatal, 2
  violence and, 4-5, 4t
Mortality rates, 105, 105b
Mortality statistics, 2
Mosaicism, 114f, 115
  Down syndrome and, 989
Mosquitoes, bites of, 776t
Mother; see also Family; Parent(s).
  age of, Down syndrome and, 989, 989t
  impressions of, 50
  infant attachment to, 504-506
  working, 99
Mother-infant attachment; see Attachment.
Mother-infant care, discharge planning and, 286
Mothers Against Drunk Driving, 966
Motility, gastrointestinal
  development of, 1417
  disorders of, 1424-1432
  muscles involved in, 1417
Motivation, in education, in mental
    retardation, 981
Motor development
  delayed, in cerebral palsy, 1836
  in infants, 498-501, 510t-515t
  in preschoolers, 629-630, 629f, 639t
  in special needs child, 913, 914f, 983, 983f
  in toddlers, 593-594, 604t
  in visually impaired children, 1003
Motor function
  assessment of, 225, 1647, 1647f, 1651
  in cerebral palsy, 1836
  in neonatal behavioral assessment, 245b
  in spinal cord injury, 1855, 1855b
Motor quotient, 500-501
Motor unit, 1832
Motor vehicle, heat injury in, 548
Motor vehicle accidents, 7, 8t
  fractures in, 1777
  in adolescents, 828, 829
  in school-age children, 731t, 732-733
  in toddlers, 616, 616f, 617t, 618-620, 618f, 619f
  injury prevention for, 1758b
  protection of infants and children in,
    545-546, 545f, 546f, 619-620
  spinal cord injury in, 1855

Motor vehicle safety seats; see Car seats/
    restraints.
Mourning, 970-971
  in sudden infant death syndrome cases, 585
Mouse, asthma control and, 1390
Mouth; see also under Oral.
  examination of, 206-208
  in Down syndrome, 989t, 990f, 992
  in hemophilia, 1563
  in mental retardation
    oral hygiene and, 986
    self-feeding and, 984
  in newborns, 252t, 259-260, 260f, 263t
    in candidiasis, 252t, 301
    in cleft lip and palate, 454-463, 455t
    in respiratory distress syndrome, 388
  in nutritional assessment, 166t-167t
  structure of, 207f
Mouth breathing, 1353
  in allergic rhinitis, 1383
Mouth care, 1127-1128; see also Dental care.
  in cancer, 1601
  in mental retardation, 986
  in respiratory distress syndrome, 388
  in unconscious child, 1659
  tooth decay and, 780
Mouth odors, 207
  in diabetes, 1735
  in neurologic assessment, 1650
Mouth-to-mouth seal, in cardiopulmonary
    resuscitation, 1337f
Movement(s); see also under Motor.
  assessment of, 186
  associated, 1647b
  in neurologic assessment, 1647, 1647f
  mirroring, 1647b
Movies, developmental impact of, 39
Moxibustion, 48
Mucocutaneous lymph node syndrome
    (Kawasaki disease), 1514-1516
Mucosa; see Mucous membranes.
Mucosal tabs, anal, 223
Mucous gland dysfunction, in cystic fibrosis,
    1401, 1405f
Mucous membranes
  gastric, 1418
  in fluid and electrolyte disturbances, 1187t
  nasal, 206
  of newborn, defense against infection
    and, 243
  oral, 207
  small intestinal, 1418
    in celiac disease, 1450
    surface area increase in, 1452
  ulceration of, in cancer, 1600-1601
  von Willebrand disease and, 1566
Mucus
  bronchial, in cystic fibrosis, 1401
  epithelial, as respiratory tract defense, 1310
  flutter mucus clearance device for, 1408, 1408f
  in respiratory distress syndrome, 387-388
  of gastrointestinal tract, 1418
Mullen Scales of Early Learning, 978
Multidisciplinary team approach, 1096
Multifactorial disorders, 124
Multiple births, 79-81, 80b
  attachment and, 286
  breast-feeding and, 275, 275f
  co-bedding and, 362-363, 362f

Multiple subpial transection, 1692
Mummy restraint, 1138, 1139f
Mumps
  immunization for, 529t, 533
    contraindications to, 537t
    in adolescents, 541b, 833-834
    Kawasaki disease and, 1516
    recommended, 529t, 533
  manifestations and management of, 656t-657t
Munchausen syndrome by proxy, 672, 684, 684t
Murmurs, 215, 216b; see also Heart sounds.
Muscle(s)
  biopsy of, 1834
  circular, of stomach, 1417
  examination of, 225
  immobilization effects on, 1762-1763, 1770t
  longitudinal, of gastrointestinal tract, 1417
  sphincter, 1417
Muscle disease, 1834
Muscle relaxants
  for cerebral palsy, 1839
  for tetanus, 1849
Muscle tone, of newborn, 262-263
Muscular atrophy
  immobilization and, 1762-1763
  in muscular dystrophy, 1866
Muscular dysfunction, 1863-1867
Muscular dystrophy, 119t, 1864-1867,
    1864f, 1865f
  Becker, 1863t
  Duchenne, 119t, 1863t, 1864-1867,
    1864f, 1865f
  facioscapulohumeral, 1863t
  Landouzy-Dejerine, 1863t
Muscular Dystrophy Association of America,
    1876
Muscular movements; see Movement(s).
Muscular septum, development of, 1465, 1465f
Muscular system, neonatal, 243
Musculoskeletal disorders, 1807-1829
  in cerebral palsy, 1837
  traumatic; see Injuries.
Musculoskeletal infections, 1817-1819
Musculoskeletal system
  in Down syndrome, 989t, 991-992
  in nutritional assessment, 167t
  of newborn, 243
    at high risk, 336b
Music, for school-age children, 726, 726f
Mustard procedure, 482, 1499b
Mustargen (mechlorethamine), 1589t
Mutations, 121
  disease-causing; see Genetic diseases.
  in cancer, 122
  in fragile X syndrome, 993
  single-gene, 118-120, 119t
Mutual role taking, 810
Mutual storytelling, 151b
Myasthenia gravis, 1851-1852
Mycobacterium bovis, 1372
Mycobacterium tuberculosis, 1372
Mycoplasma pneumoniae, 1369, 1370
Mycotic infections; see Fungal infections.
Myelination, 1642
  in newborn, 243
  pain and, 352
Myelodysplasia, 425
Myelogenous leukocytes, 1534
Myeloid tissue, 1531

Myelomeningocele, 424b, 424f, 425-433, 426f
  assessment of, 430-431
  clinical manifestations of, 426, 427b
  diagnosis of, 426-427
  folic acid supplementation for, 124-125
  nursing care plan for, 434-435
  nursing considerations in, 430-433, 433f
  pathophysiology of, 426
  prenatal diagnosis of, 128t, 129-130
  prevention of, 430
  prognosis of, 430
  treatment of, 427-430
Myelomeningocele sac, care of, 431
Myocardial function, in congestive heart
      failure, 1478
Myocardial infarction, in Kawasaki disease,
      1515, 1516
Myocardium, 1465
Myoclonic jerks, in newborn, 263
Myoclonic seizures, 1688
  in newborn, 404t
Myoglobin, in burn injuries, 1232
Myoglobinuria, in burn injuries, 1232
Myomectomy, anorectal, in Hirschsprung
      disease, 1427
Myopia, 1000, 1001b
Myotonic dystrophy, 119t
Myringotomy, for otitis media, 1359

N

N-acetyl-beta-D-glucosaminidase (NAG), in
      lead poisoning, 678
N-acetylcysteine, for acetaminophen
      poisoning, 673
Nail(s)
  abnormalities of, 189
  clubbing of, 189
  examination of, 189
  of newborn, 262
  spoon, 189
Nail polish, hand contamination and, 1134b
Naloxone
  for cardiopulmonary resuscitation, 1399t
  for opioid-induced respiratory depression,
      673, 1068b
Naproxen
  dysmenorrhea and, 847
  for juvenile rheumatoid arthritis, 1822
  in pain management, 1061t
Narcissism, in infants, 502
Narcotics; see Opioids.
Nasal bleeding
  emergency treatment of, 1567b
  in von Willebrand disease, 1566, 1567b
Nasal canals, of newborn, 259
Nasal cannula, for oxygen therapy, 1317
Nasal conchae, 206, 206f
Nasal drug administration, 1160-1161, 1162f
Nasal flaring, 1310-1311
  in newborn, 259, 381, 382f
Nasal meatus, 206, 206f
Nasal obstruction, in nasopharyngitis, 1350
Nasal polyps, in cystic fibrosis, 1409
Nasal septum, 206, 206f
Nasal spray, in respiratory infections, 1346
Nasal structures, 1305
Nasal stuffiness, in allergic rhinitis, 1383
Nasal tube gavage, 348
Nasal turbinates, 206, 206f

Nasal washings, 1148-1149
Nasogastric drug administration, 1159, 1159b
Nasogastric feeding, 1162-1164, 1163b; see also
      Enteral nutrition; Feeding.
  in hypertrophic pyloric stenosis, 1447
  in short bowel syndrome, 1452, 1453
  in unconscious child, 1658
Nasopharyngeal rhabdomyosarcoma, 1631b
Nasopharyngitis, acute viral, 1350-1351, 1351b
Natal teeth, 252t, 260
Natality rates, 105, 105b
National Academy of Sciences, Food and
      Nutrition Board of, 560, 564
National Advisory Committee on
      Immunization (Canada), 528
National Amputation Foundation, 1628n
National Association for Gifted Children, 641
National Association for Parents of the
      Visually Impaired, Inc., 1003
National Association for Sickle Cell Disease,
      Inc., 1554n
National Association for the Visually
      Handicapped, 1003, 1004
National Association of Anorexia Nervosa and
      Associated Disorders, Inc., 880
National Association of Pediatric Oncology
      Nurses, 1605
National Association of School Nurses, 23n
National Assoication of School Nurses, 730
National Brain Tumor Foundation, 1624n
National Cancer Institute, 1588
National Captioning Institute, 998n
National Center for Health Statistics, 2, 174
National Center for Infants, Toddlers, and
      Families, 14n
National Center for Missing and Exploited
      Children, 266
National Child Assessment Satellite Training
      Program, Feeding Scale of, 247
National Childhood Vaccine Injury Act, 541
National Clearinghouse for Alcohol and Drug
      Abuse Information, 895n
National Cocaine Hotline, 892
National Diabetes Information
      Clearinghouse, 1744
National Disability Sports Alliance, 1842
National Down Syndrome Congress, 991n
National Down Syndrome Society, 981n, 991n
National Easter Seal Society, 419, 915n, 939n, 981
National Eating Disorders Association, 880
National Federation for the Blind, 1003, 1004
National Fragile X Foundation, 994
National Heart, Lung, and Blood Institute,
      1400, 1554n
National Hemophilia Foundation, 1565
National Hospice and Palliative Care
      Organization, 956n
National Hydrocephalus Foundation, 443
National Information Center for Children and
      Youth with Disabilities, 939n
National Institute of Nursing Research, 753
National Kidney Foundation, 1292-1293
National Lekotek Center, 913n
National Neurofibromatosis Foundation,
      Inc., 775
National Organization of Parents of Murdered
      Children, 966
National Pediatric & Family HIV Resource
      Center, 1577n

National Rehabilitation Information
      Center, 915n
National Safety Council, 1253
National Scoliosis Foundation, 1815
National Self-Help Clearinghouse, 937n
National Sudden Infant Death Syndrome
      Resource Center, 966
National Youth Sports Safety Foundation, 1806
Native Americans, 35b; see also Race/ethnicity.
  communication with, 37
  cultural beliefs and practices of, 37
  health beliefs and practices of, 54t-55t
  suicide and, 897
  time concept of, 43
Nausea
  in cancer, 1599-1600
  opioid-induced, 1068
NCAST; see National Child Assessment Satellite
      Training Program.
Near-drowning, 8, 8t, 10, 1674-1676,
      1676t, 1802
  in school-age children, 731t
  in toddlers, 617t, 620
  prevention of, 1758b
  safety precautions against, 542t, 543t, 548
Nearsightedness, 1000, 1001b
Nebulization
  in asthma, 1391
  in cystic fibrosis, 1408
Nebulizer, 1319
Neck; see also under Cervical.
  examination of, 191, 192f
  hyperextension of, 191, 223
  in Down syndrome, 989t
  in nutritional assessment, 166t
  of newborn, 253t, 260
  structures of, 192f
  wry, 191, 446, 1807
Neck righting reflex, in infants, 494b, 498
Necrosis
  cortical, 1284
  tubular, 1284
Necrotic processes, in acute renal failure, 1284
Necrotizing enterocolitis, in high-risk
      newborn, 347, 395-397
  nutrition and, 343, 344
Necrotizing osteochondritis, from heel
      puncture, 1148
Nedocromil sodium, for asthma, 1392
Needle(s)
  for insulin syringe, 1747
  for intramuscular drug administration,
      1154, 1154t
  for intraosseous infusion, 1191
  for intravenous infusion, 1190
  length of, for immunizations in infants and
      toddlers, 539b, 540
Needle clipper, 1747
Needleless injection systems, 1157
Needleless intravenous systems, 1190-1191, 1191f
Needle-stick injuries, 1135, 1135f
Negativism, in toddlers, 594, 608
Neglect, 683-684
  emotional; see Emotional abuse or neglect.
  identification of, 687, 688b
  in early childhood, 683
Neisseria gonorrhoeae
  conjunctivitis and, 662
  gonorrhea and, 861

*Neisseria gonorrhoeae*—cont'd
  in newborn, 328t
  pelvic inflammatory disease and, 863
Neocate, 280, 282t
Neomycin
  for hepatic encephalopathy, 1461
  reactions to, vaccination and, 538
Neonatal abstinence syndrome, 406-407, 406b
Neonatal death, 334b
Neonatal Infant Pain Scale, 354t
Neonatal intensive care unit, 334-335;
    *see also* High-risk newborn.
  auditory environment in, 363-365, 995
  co-bedding of multiples in, 362-363, 362f
  discharge from, 368-369
  infection prevention in, 341
  parent-infant relationships in, facilitation of,
      366-368, 366b, 367f
  safety measures in, 338
  sensory stimulation in, 360-361
  sibling visits in, 368
  tactile interventions in, 361-362, 361b
  therapeutic positioning in, 363, 363b,
      364b, 364f
  visual environment in, 365-366, 366b
Neonatal mortality, 2
Neonatal myasthenia gravis, 1852
Neonatal Pain, Agitation, and Sedation Scale,
    353, 355t
Neonatal Perception Inventory, 247
Neonatal screening, 125-126
Neonatal tetany, 318
Neonate; *see* Newborn.
Neosar (cyclophosphamide), 1589t
Nephritis
  familial, 1282
  lupus, 1827
Nephroblastoma, 1629-1631
Nephrogenic diabetes insipidus, 1280-1281
Nephron(s), 1256, 1256f
  functions of, 1257f
  in chronic renal failure, 1288
  in infants, 1258
Nephropathy
  diabetic, 1735
  immunoglobin A and, 1274
Nephrosis
  childhood, 1275
  idiopathic, 1275
  lipoid, 1275
  minimal lesion, 1275
  uncomplicated, 1275
Nephrotic reaction, signs of, 1271
Nephrotic syndrome, 1274-1279
  classification of by steroid response, 1277b
  congenital, 1275
  minimal change, 1275
  nursing care for, 1278-1279, 1278b
  pathophysiology of, 1275, 1276f
  prognosis of, 1277-1278
  relapsing form of, 1277, 1279
  secondary, 1275
  treatment of, 1276-1277
  types of, 1274-1275
  vs acute poststreptococcal
      glomerulonephritis, 1272t
Nerve(s)
  compression injury of, 1765-1766, 1793

Nerve(s)—cont'd
  cranial
    abnormalities of, brain tumor and, 1621t
    assessment of, 227, 229t
    in bacterial meningitis, 1678
    myelination of, 243
  myelination of, 1642
    in newborn, 243
    pain and, 352
  spinal, 1852-1853, 1853f
Nerve block
  dorsal penile, for circumcision, 271b, 272
  regional, 1065b
Nerve compression syndromes, 1765-1766, 1793
Nerve conduction studies, 1834
Nerve deafness, 995
Nerve impulses, transmission of, 1833-1834
Nerve plexus, 1853-1854
  peripheral, detrusor control and, 1259
Nervous system
  autonomic, 1641
    in neuroendocrine system, 1705-1706
    in spinal cord injury, 1855, 1855b,
        1856, 1860
  central, 1641-1645, 1643f, 1644t; *see also*
      Brain; Spinal cord.
  malformations of, 423-443; *see also* specific
      type.
  structure and function of, 1641-1645,
      1643f, 1644t
  development of, 1642
  enteric, 1426
  heart rate and, 1468
  immobilization effects on, 1765-1766
  in nutritional assessment, 167t
  maturation of, in infants, 494
  of newborn, 243, 263, 263t
    after surgery, 422t
    at high risk, 336b, 357, 400-404, 402t,
        403b, 404t
    bilirubin encephalopathy and, 304, 307
    congenital hypothyroidism and, 321, 322
    fetal alcohol syndrome and, 329-330, 329b
    sepsis and, 394b
    untreated pain and, 357
  parasympathetic, 1705
  peripheral, 1641
  sympathetic, 1705
    stimulation of, in congestive heart
        failure, 1477
Neural regulation
  of breathing, 1309
  of bronchial smooth muscle, 1307
Neural tube defects, 423-433, 424b, 424f; *see*
    *also* specific type.
  etiology of, 424-425
  folic acid supplementation for, 124-125
  prenatal diagnosis of, 128t, 129-130, 427
Neuroblastoma, 1619, 1625-1626, 1626b, 1724
Neurodevelopmental disorder, alcohol-
    related, 329
Neuroendocrine system, 1705-1706; *see also*
    Endocrine system.
  at puberty, 803, 803f
  in burn injuries, 1233
Neurofibromatosis, 119t, 301
  hearing impairment and, 996b
  skin manifestations of, 773-775, 775b

Neurogenic bladder, 428-430, 1860
Neurogenic diabetes insipidus, 1715
Neurogenic shock, 1219
Neuroglycopenia, diabetic, 1749
Neurohypophysis; *see* Pituitary, posterior.
Neurologic assessment, 225-228, 226f-228f,
    229t, 1646-1654
  after cranial surgery, 1623
  behavior in, 225
  caloric test in, 1651
  cerebellar function in, 226, 226b
  cognitive-perceptual development in, 225
  cranial nerves in, 227, 229t
  doll's eye maneuver in, 1651
  eye movements in, 1650, 1651, 1652
  gait in, 224-225, 225f, 1647b
  history in, 1646
  in head injury, 1671, 1673
  level of consciousness in, 225, 1647-1649,
      1648b, 1648f, 1649b
  motor function in, 225, 1647, 1647f, 1651
  overview of, 1646
  papilledema in, 1651
  physical examination in, 1646-1647
  posturing in, 1651, 1651b, 1651f
  pupils in, 1650-1651, 1650f
  reflexes in, 226, 226f, 227f, 1651-1652; *see*
      *also* Reflex(ies).
  reproducible findings in, 1649
  sensory function in, 225-226, 226b
  soft signs in, 228, 229b
  vital signs in, 1649-1650
Neurologic complications, in cancer, 1601-1602
Neurologic diagnostic procedures, 1652-1654,
    1653t-1654t, 1655b
Neurologic signs
  in acid-base disturbances, 1182
  in chronic renal failure, 1289
  in fluid and electrolyte disturbances, 1188t
  in lead poisoning, 677f, 678
  soft, 225, 228, 228b
Neuromuscular dysfunction, 1832-1867
  acute vs gradual onset of, 1834
  anatomic features of, 1832-1833
  classification of, 1833-1834
  clinical manifestations of, 1833
  diagnosis of, 1834
  in anterior horn cell diseases, 1833
  in lower motor neuron disease, 1833
  in muscle disease, 1834
  in neuromuscular junction disease, 1833-1834
  in neuropathies, 1833
  in upper motor neuron disease, 1833
  myopathy in, 1832
  site of origin of, 1833, 1833f
Neuromuscular system, of newborn, 254t, 262-
    263, 263t
  gestational age estimation and, 248f
  in hypocalcemia, 318
Neurons
  lower motor, 1832, 1833f
  upper motor, 1832, 1833f
Neuropathic bladder, 428-430, 1860
Neuropathy, 1833
  compression, 1765-1766, 1793
  diabetic, 1735
  in cancer, 1601-1602
Neuropsychiatric lupus, 1827

Neurosensory system, immobilization effects on, 1765-1766
Neurotoxicity, bilirubin, 304, 307
Neurotransmitters, 1705
Neutral thermal environment, 339
Neutron activation, in obesity, 874
Neutropenia, 1568-1569, 1569t
  in cancer, 1598
Neutrophil(s), 243, 1534
  in complete blood count, 1536t
  in wound healing, 747
  neutropenia and, 1568-1569, 1569t
Neutrophilia, 1534
Nevus
  bathing trunk, 302
  compound, 302
  giant pigmented, 302
  junctional, 302
  pigmented, 773, 773f
  telangiectatic, in newborn, 252t
Nevus flammeus, 302
  in newborn, 251t
New England Regional Genetics Group, 1554n
New morbidity, 6
Newborn; see also under Infant; Neonatal.
  acid-base balance in, postoperative care and, 423t
  airway of
    patency of, 265, 289
    postoperative care of, 420t
  Apgar scoring of, 244-245, 244t
  attachment of; see Attachment.
  bacterial meningitis in, 1678, 1679-1680
  bathing of, 268-269, 268f, 350b
  behavioral assessment of, 245-246, 245b, 246t, 257
    pain and, 352-353, 352b
  birth injuries to, 295-300, 296b, 297f, 299f
  birthmarks and, 301-303, 302f
  bullous impetigo in, 301
  candidiasis in, 252t, 300-301
  caput succedaneum in, 296, 297f
  cephalhematoma in, 297-298, 297f
  chemical agents affecting, 326
  chickenpox in, 327t
  chlamydial infection in, 327t
  circulatory system of, 241
    postoperative care of, 420t
  circumcision of, 270-273, 270b-272b, 272f
  coxsackievirus in, 327t
  cry of, 246
  cyanosis in, 1487
  cytomegalovirus in, 327t
  death of, 334b
  defenses of, infection and, 243, 393
  dermatologic problems in, 300-303, 302b, 302f
  developmental dysplasia of hip in, 448, 449f;
    see also Hip, developmental dysplasia of.
    treatment of, 449-450, 450f
  diapers for, 269, 269b
  discharge planning and home care for, 286-288, 287b
    high-risk infant and, 368-369
  endocrine system of, 243
    postoperative care of, 421t
  erythema infectiosum in, 327t
  erythema toxicum in, 251t, 300

Newborn—cont'd
  eyes of, 252t, 258-259, 263t
    facial nerve paralysis and, 300
    phototherapy and, 308, 308f, 309, 365
    prophylactic care of, 266, 266b
    retinopathy of prematurity and, 344, 399-400, 400b
  feeding of; see also Bottle-feeding;
    Breast-feeding.
    behavior and, 279-280, 345
    candidiasis and, 301
    cleft lip and palate and, 458-459, 459b, 459f, 460
    esophageal atresia and, 465
    facial nerve paralysis and, 299-300
    jaundice and, 303t, 305, 307
    respiratory distress syndrome and, 383
    schedule for, 279
    tracheoesophageal fistula and, 465
  feeding resistance in, 348-349, 349b
  fluid and electrolytes in, 242
    postoperative care and, 420t, 422t, 423
  fractures in, birth-related, 298
  galactosemia in, 324-325, 325f
  gastrointestinal system of, 242, 242b
    necrotizing enterocolitis and, 395-397
    postoperative care of, 422t
    sepsis and, 394b
  gestational age assessment and, 247-250, 248f-250f, 250b
  gonococcal disease in, 328t
  head of, 252t, 257-258, 258f, 259f
    birth trauma to, 296-298, 297f
    circumference of, 249f, 251t, 255
    prematurity and, 376
  hearing assessment in, 996, 996b
  hematopoietic system of, 241-242
    postoperative care of, 422t
    sepsis and, 394b
  hemolytic disease of, 310
    blood incompatibility and, 310, 312, 312f, 312t
    clinical manifestations of, 312
    diagnosis of, 312, 314
    hyperbilirubinemia and, 303t, 312
    prevention of, 314
    prognosis of, 315
    treatment of, 315-316
  hemorrhage in
    prevention of, 266-267
    retinal, 296b
    subconjunctival, 252t, 296b
    subgaleal, 296-297, 297f
  hemorrhagic disease of, 319
  hepatitis B virus in, 328t
    vaccine against, 267
  herpes simplex virus in, 326, 328t
  high-risk, 334-409; see also High-risk newborn.
  human immunodeficiency virus infection in, 327t
    screening for, 268
  hyperbilirubinemia in, 303-310
    assessment of, 307
    breast-feeding and, 305, 307
    clinical manifestations of, 305
    complications of, 304
    diagnosis of, 305-306

Newborn—cont'd
  hyperbilirubinemia in—cont'd
    discharge planning and home care for, 309-310, 311b
    family support in, 308-309, 309b
    nursing care plan for, 313-314
    pathophysiology of, 304, 304f
    physiologic jaundice and, 304-305
    prognosis of, 307
    treatment of, 306-307, 307t, 308, 308f, 309b
    types of, 303t
  hyperglycemia in, 317-318
  hypocalcemia in, 318-319
  hypoglycemia in, 316-317, 405-406
  hypothermia in, 265, 289
    high-risk infant and, 341
  hypothyroidism in, 320-322
  identification of, 266
  immune system of, 243
    postoperative care of, 421t
  inborn errors of metabolism in, 319-325, 320f, 322f, 324b, 325f
  infection in, 325-326, 327t-328t
    high-risk infant and, 393-395, 394b
    human milk and, 344
    prevention of, 265-273, 289, 341
  integumentary system of, 242-243, 251t-252t, 257
    high-risk infant and, 336b, 349-350, 350b-351b
  listeriosis in, 328t
  meconium stool in, 1424
  motor development in, 498, 499
  musculoskeletal system of, 243, 262-263, 263t
    high-risk infant and, 336b
  neurologic system of, 243, 263, 263t
    bilirubin encephalopathy and, 304, 307
    congenital hypothyroidism and, 321, 322
    fetal alcohol syndrome and, 329-330, 329b
    high-risk infant and, 336b, 357, 400-404, 402t, 403b, 404t
    postoperative care of, 422t
    sepsis and, 394b
    untreated pain and, 357
  nursing care plan for, 289-291
  nutrition for, 273-282, 290
    high-risk infant and, 342-348, 369, 396
  pain in, 351-357, 352b, 353f, 354t-356t, 420t, 423, 1036-1037, 1037f
  paralysis in, birth-related, 298-300, 299f
  periods of reactivity in, 245
  persistent pulmonary hypertension of, 397-398, 398f
  phenylketonuria in, 322-324, 322f, 324b
  physical assessment of, 250-263, 250b
    abdomen in, 253t, 261
    back in, 261
    chest in, 253t, 260
    ears in, 252t, 259
    extremities in, 254t, 262-263
    eyes in, 252t, 258-259, 263t
    general appearance in, 251t, 257, 257f
    general measurements in, 251t, 255, 255f
    genitalia in, 253t-254t, 261
    head in, 252t, 257-258, 258f, 259f
    heart in, 253t, 260-261
    high-risk infant and, 335-338, 336b, 337b, 337t

Newborn—cont'd
  physical assessment of—cont'd
    lungs in, 253t, 260
    mouth and throat in, 252t, 259-260,
      260f, 263t
    neck in, 253t, 260
    neuromuscular system in, 254t, 263, 263t
    nose in, 252t, 259, 263t
    rectum in, 254t, 261-262
    skin in, 251t-252t, 257
    vital signs in, 251t, 255-257, 256f
  physiologic jaundice of, 242, 303t, 304-305
  postoperative care of, 420-423, 420t-423t
    myelomeningocele and, 432
  preoperative care of, 419-420
  radiation effects in, 330
  rash in, 300
  reflexes in, 262, 262f, 263t, 264f
    behavioral assessment and, 245b
  renal system of, 242, 253t, 261
    postoperative care of, 422t
  respiratory distress in, 265, 289
    congenital diaphragmatic hernia and,
      475-476
    phrenic nerve paralysis and, 299
  respiratory system of, 240-241, 253t, 260
    esophageal atresia and, 465
    high-risk infant and, 336b, 376-393
    postoperative care of, 421t, 423
  rubella in, 328t
  screening of
    for disease, 267-268, 267b
    for hearing loss, 268, 996, 996b
    for hypoglycemia, 317, 317b
    for hypothyroidism, 321
    for inborn errors of metabolism, 320
    for phenylketonuria, 125-126, 267,
      323, 323b
    for retinopathy of prematurity, 400
    for sickle cell anemia, 1550
  self-regulatory strategies of, 359t
  sensory function of, 243-244, 252t
    developmental outcome and, 360-361
  sex assignment for, 1730-1731
  soft tissue injury of, birth-related,
    295-296, 296f
  syphilis in, 328t
  tactile stimulation of, 241
    apnea of prematurity and, 379
    high-risk infant and, 361
  thermoregulation in, 241
    abdominal wall defect and, 473
    exchange transfusion and, 315-316
    high-risk infant and, 338-341, 339f, 340f
    phototherapy and, 308
    postoperative care and, 420t, 423t
  thoracic size and lung volume during
    respirations, 1304, 1304f
  toxoplasmosis in, 328t
  transient hypoparathyroidism in, 1722
  umbilical stump of, 269-270
  urinary tract infection in, 1262, 1264
  varicella-zoster virus in, 327t
Niacin
  adverse reactions to, 555
  functions of and disturbances in, 557t
Nicotinamide, functions of and disturbances
  in, 557t

Nicotine, dependence on, 887
Nicotinic acid, functions of and disturbances
  in, 557t
NICU; see Neonatal intensive care unit.
Niemann-Pick disease, 996b
Night crying, approaches to, 526-527, 526t
Nightmares, 724
  posttraumatic, 724
  vs sleep terrors, 645t
Nil disease, 1275
90-90 traction, 1790, 1790f
Nipples
  examination of, 210
  painful, breast-feeding and, 278t
  supernumerary, 260
NIPS; see Neonatal Infant Pain Scale.
Nissen fundoplication, for gastroesophageal
  reflux, 1430-1431, 1430f
Nitric oxide
  for persistent pulmonary hypertension of
    newborn, 398
  for respiratory distress syndrome, 385
  inhaled, for pulmonary artery hypertension,
    1491
Nitrites, in urine, 1261t, 1266
Nitrogen mustard (Mustargen), 1589t
Nitrogen washout, for extraneous air
  syndromes, 390
Nitrous oxide, for conscious sedation, 1109
Nits, 761, 762f
Nociception, neonatal pain and, 352
Nodes, cardiac, 1467
Nodule, 744f
Noise
  decibels of, 995, 995t
  hearing impairment and, 995, 1000
  in neonatal intensive care unit, 363-365
    hearing impairment and, 995
  infant injury from, 548
Noisy breathing, 1311
Nonbacterial meningitis, 1680-1681, 1681t
Noncommunicating hydrocele, 479; see also
  Hydrocele.
Noncommunicating hydrocephalus, 437, 438t;
  see also Hydrocephalus.
Nondisjunction, chromosomal, 114-115, 114f
Non-English speakers, 45
  interpreters for, 145-146, 146b
Non-Hodgkin lymphoma, 1618-1619, 1618b
Nonmaleficence, 21
Nonmaterial covert culture, 31
Nonnutritive sucking, 348
  esophageal atresia and, 466
Nonocclusive dressing, 749
Nonoxynol-9, in spermicides, 855
Nonpenetrating injury, of eye, 1002, 1003b
Nonpurging type of bulimia, 883b
Nonshivering thermogenesis, 241, 338
Nonspeech communication, 1007-1008
Nonsteroidal anti-inflammatory drugs (NSAIDs)
  after heart surgery, 1506
  for dysmenorrhea, 847
  for juvenile rheumatoid arthritis, 1821-1822
  in fever management, 1130, 1130t
  in pain management, 1061t
Nonstress test, diabetic mother and, 405
Nontherapeutic relationship, 18-19, 19b
Nonunion, fracture, 1794

Nonverbal communication, 139, 140
  cultural aspects of, 44-45
  mental retardation and, 982
  with children, 152b
  with infants, 148
Noonan syndrome, 119t
  congenital heart disease and, 1474
Norepinephrine, 1705, 1708t, 1724
  adrenal secretion of, 1723, 1724, 1725
  attention deficit hyperactivity disorder and,
    787, 789
  effects of, 1724, 1724b
  pheochromocytoma and, 1731-1732
  thermoregulation and, high-risk newborn
    and, 338, 339
  urinary, in neuroblastoma, 1625
Normalization, 908, 917-918, 918b
Normeperidine, sickle cell anemia and, 1553
Normoblast, 1532
Norplant, for contraception, 855, 856t, 857b
Norport, vs other long-term venous access
  devices, 1201t
North American blastomycoses, 764t
North American Nursing Diagnosis
  Association (NANDA), 25
  approved nursing diagnoses of, 1904
Nortriptyline, for attention deficit
  hyperactivity disorder, 789
Nose; see also under Nasal.
  examination of, 204-206
  foreign body in, 1378
  in Down syndrome, 989t, 990f
  in nutritional assessment, 166t
  of newborn, 252t, 259, 263t
    with respiratory distress syndrome,
      381, 382f
  structure of, 204-206, 206f
Nose drops, 1160-1161, 1162f
  in respiratory infections, 1346
Nosebleed
  emergency treatment of, 1567b
  in von von Willebrand disease, 1566, 1567b
Nosocomial infection, 1134
  neonatal sepsis and, 393
NovoLog, 1737
NovoPen, 1747
NPASS; see Neonatal Pain, Agitation, and
  Sedation Scale.
NPH insulin, 1737
NPO status, fluid intake and, 1188
Nuclear brain scan, 1653t
Nuclear family, 70-71
Numby Stuff, 1065b, 1066-1067
Numeric Scale, in pain assessment, 1053t
Nurse
  grief in, neonatal death and, 370
  in home care, 1017, 1017b, 1018b, 1020,
    1020b, 1026b
  reaction to terminally ill child and, 972-974,
    973b, 974b
Nurse case manager, in home care, 1020
Nurse-activated dosing, of analgesics, 1064b
Nurse-client relationship, cultural aspects of,
    43-45; see also Cultural factors.
Nurse-family partnership, 14-15, 23
  therapeutic relationship and, 18-19, 19b
Nursemaid's elbow, of radial head, 1780
Nurses Assessment of Pain Inventory, 1056t

Nursing
  community-based, 12, 103-109
  essential features of, 13
  pediatric; *see* Pediatric nursing.
  public health, 12
  transcultural; *see* Cultural factors.
Nursing admission history, 1086-1088,
    1088b-1089b, 1091b
Nursing care, culturally competent, 33
Nursing care plan, 27, 27t; *see also* under
    specific disorders.
  for acute respiratory infection, 1347-1350
  for anorexia nervosa, 881-882
  for appendicitis, 1436
  for asthma, 1402-1404
  for burns, 1249-1252
  for cancer, 1606-1610
  for cerebral palsy, 1844-1845
  for child abuse, 694-696
  for chronic renal failure, 1294-1295
  for communicable diseases, 662b-663b
  for congestive heart failure, 1485-1486
  for diabetes, 1752-1755
  for diarrhea, 1215-1216
  for epilepsy, 1697-1698
  for esophageal atresia, 467-468
  for immobilization, 1772
  for juvenile rheumatoid arthritis, 1826-1827
  for newborn, 289-291
    at high risk, 371-375
  for preoperative care, 1114-1115
  for respiratory infection, 1347-1350
  for scoliosis, 1815-1816
  for skin disorders, 756-757
  for unconscious child, 1662-1664
Nursing caries, 527, 615-616, 615f
Nursing Center for Tobacco Intervention, 888b
Nursing Child Assessment Satellite Training
    Feeding Scale, 576
Nursing diagnoses, 25-27, 26b
  NANDA-approved, 1904
Nursing education, 20
Nursing informatics, privacy concerns in, 142
Nursing practice standards, 23
Nursing process, 22, 25-28
  assessment in, 25
  evaluation in, 27
  home care and, 1023-1024, 1024b, 1025b
  implementation in, 27
  in accreditation, 28
  nursing diagnosis in, 25-27, 26b
  planning in, 27, 27t; *see also* Nursing care plan.
Nursing research, 22
Nut allergy, BAL therapy and, 681
Nutramigen, 282t
Nutrients, 1417
Nutrition; *see also* Diet; Eating; Feeding;
    Food(s).
  enteral; *see* Enteral nutrition.
  extrauterine, adaptation to, 1417
  feeding problems and, 1840-1841
  for adolescents, 829-830
  for athletes, 1802-1804, 1803b
  for infants, 520-525
    6 months to 12 months, 521-522, 524b
    birth to 6 months, 520-521, 524b
    disturbances in, 554-571
    nursing considerations with, 560, 564

Nutrition—cont'd
  for newborns, 273-282, 290; *see also* Bottle-
      feeding; Breast-feeding.
    at high risk, 342-348, 369, 383, 391, 396
  for preschoolers, 644, 644f
  for school-age children, 721-723
  for toddlers, 609-611, 610b
  guidelines for, 564, 565, 570
  in acute poststreptococcal
      glomerulonephritis, 1273
  in acute renal failure, 1287
  in anorexia nervosa, 878
  in biliary atresia, 470-471
  in burn patients, 1237, 1244-1245
  in cancer, 1600, 1600b
  in cerebral palsy, 1840-1841
  in congestive heart failure, 1483
  in HIV infection, 1575
  in immobilization, 1768
  in inflammatory bowel disease, 1441, 1442
  in respiratory infections, 1347
  in short bowel syndrome, 1451-1452, 1453
  in terminal illness, 949t
  in unconscious children, 1658
  in wound healing, 748
  mental retardation and, 979b
  parental education about, 520, 568, 570,
      722-723, 722b
  parenteral; *see* Total parenteral nutrition.
  poverty and, 41
  published advice on, 564
Nutrition Coordinating Center, 875n
Nutrition counseling, in obesity, 875
Nutritional assessment, 164-168, 164b, 165b,
    166t-167t
  anthropometry in, 168, 171b, 174-175,
      177-178, 1882-1895
  biochemical tests in, 168
  clinical examination in, 165-168, 166t-167t
  evaluation of, 168
Nutritional status, in physical examination,
    186-187
Nutritional support; *see also* Enteral nutrition;
    Total parenteral nutrition.
  for unconscious child, 1658
  overfeeding in, 1658
Nystagmus
  in cerebral palsy, 207
  in newborn, 259
Nystatin, for oral candidiasis, in newborn, 301

**O**

Obedience, in moral development, 597
Obesity, 644, 870-876
  diagnosis of, 873-874
  etiology of, 870-872
  hypertension and, 1518
  in adolescents, 829-830, 872-873, 873f
    complications of, 873
  in Cushing's syndrome, 1727, 1727f, 1728t
  in muscular dystrophy, 1865
  in school-age children, 722, 723b
  in type 2 diabetes, 1733, 1734
  nursing considerations in, 875-876, 876b
  prevention of, 876
  prognosis of, 876
  steroid-related, 1602, 1727, 1727f, 1728t
  treatment of, 874-875, 874b, 874t

Object(s)
  fear of, 643
  toddler knowledge of, 595-596
  transitional, 599, 599f
Object permanence, 596
  in infants, 502, 503
  in toddlers, 598
Objective Pain Score, 1056t
Obstetric history, 155
Obstipation, 1424
  in gastrointestinal obstructive disorders, 1446
Obstructive apnea, of prematurity, 378
Obstructive uropathy, 484-487, 485f, 485t
Obtundation, 1648b
Obturators, in cleft lip and palate, 458
Occipital lobes, 1644t
Occlusive dressing, 749, 751
Occult spinal dysraphism, 425
Occupation, social class and, 35-37
Occupational achievement, 813, 813b
Occupational therapy, for cerebral palsy, 1840-
    1841, 1841f, 1842
Ocular accommodation, 194
Ocular alignment, 195-196
  tests for, 196-197, 198t
Ocular movements
  development of, 199t
  in brain injury, 1650, 1651
  in cerebral palsy, 207
  in neurologic assessment, 1650, 1651, 1652
Ocular prosthesis, 1634, 1634f
Oculomotor nerve, assessment of, 229t
Oculovestibular response, 1651
Odor, breath/mouth, 207
  in diabetes, 1735
  in neurologic assessment, 1650
Oedipal stage, in preschoolers, 630-631
Office of Disability Employment Policy, 919
Ointments, for conjunctivitis, 663
Olanzapine, for schizophrenia, 799
Oley Foundation, 1204
Olfactory nerve, assessment of, 229t
Oliguria, in acute renal failure, 1284, 1285
Omeprazole (Prilosec)
  for gastroesophageal reflux, 1429
  for peptic ulcer disease, 1445
Omnibus Budget Reconciliation Act of 1990, 13
Omphalocele, 472-474, 472f
Omphalomesenteric fistula (Meckel
    diverticulum), 1435
Oncogenes, 1586
Oncology Nursing Society, 1594
Oncovin (vincristine), 1591t
Ondansetron, in cancer, 1599-1600
Only children, 79, 79b
Open adoption, 89
Open family, 66
Open fracture, 1778, 1779f
Open-bell (Ford) chestpiece, 212
Open-ended questions, 143-144
Operational thought, in adolescence, 809-810
Ophthalmia neonatorum, 259
  prevention of, 266, 266b
Ophthalmoplegic migraine, 1700b
Ophthalmoscopic examination, 194-195, 195f
Opioids
  abuse of, 886t, 891b, 892
  after heart surgery, 1505-1506

Opioids—cont'd
  extubation and, neonatal, 356b
  fallacies and facts about, 1049, 1050b
  for comatose patients, 1655
  in pain management, 1057, 1060, 1062t,
    1064t; see also Analgesics; Pain
    management.
    in newborn, 357
    in preoperative sedation, 1112-1113, 1113b
    in sickle cell anemia, 1553
    in terminal illness, 957, 957b
    intrauterine exposure to, 406-407, 406b
    physical dependence on, 1068
    side effects of, 1067-1068, 1067b, 1068b
    tolerance of, 1068
Opisthotonos, 191, 223, 1678
  in newborn, 254t
Opportunistic infections; see also Infection(s).
  in bone marrow transplant, 1603
  in cancer, 1597
  in leukemia, 1612
Oppositional defiant disorder/conduct
    disorder, 505
Opsonization, 1572
Optic disc, 195, 195f
  edema of, 195, 1651
Optic drug administration, 1160, 1160f
Optic nerve, assessment of, 229t
Ora serrata, retinopathy of prematurity and, 399
Oral airway, 1656
Oral bleeding, in hemophilia, 1563
Oral candidiasis, in newborn, 252t, 301
Oral cavity; see Mouth.
Oral contraceptive pill
  for acne, 841
  for dysfunctional uterine bleeding, 848
  for emergency contraception, 855, 856t
  in adolescents, 850
  menstrual irregularities and, 846, 847
Oral Deaf Education Film and Information
    Office, 999n
Oral drug administration, 1151-1153, 1151b,
    1152f, 1153f
Oral glucose tolerance test, in diabetes, 1736
Oral hygiene, 1127-1128; see also Dental care.
  in cancer, 1601
  in mental retardation, 986
  in respiratory distress syndrome, 388
  in unconscious child, 1659
  tooth decay and, 780
Oral rehydration therapy, 1186, 1188; see also
    Fluid management.
  for diarrhea, 1211-1214, 1212t
Oral sensitivity, in infants, 504
Oral stage, 230, 230t
Oral temperature, 178-179, 179f, 180b-181b,
    182t; see also Temperature.
Oral ulcers, in cancer, 1600-1601
Orbital rhabdomyosarcoma, 1631b
Orchiopexy, 481
Organ donation, 966-967
Organ systems, maturation of, in infants, 496-497
Organ transplantation; see Transplantation.
Organic central auditory imperception, 995
Organic solvents, abuse of, 886t, 892
Organizational strategies, for compliance, 1120
Organogenesis, 416
Orientation, in neonatal behavioral
    assessment, 245b

Orogastric drug administration, 1159, 1159b
Orogastric gavage, 1162, 1163f; see also Gavage
    feeding.
Oropharyngeal suctioning; see also Suctioning.
  of newborn, 265, 289
  in apnea of prematurity, 379
Orthochromatic erythroblast, 1532
Orthodontic therapy
  for malocclusion, 782
  in cleft lip and palate, 457-458
Orthomyxoviruses, influenza and, 1356
Orthopedic complications; see also under
    Musculoskeletal.
  in cerebral palsy, 1837
  in myelomeningocele, 427-428
Orthophoria, 196
Orthopnea, in congestive heart failure, 1478
Orthoses, 1773-1775, 1773f, 1774b, 1774f
  ankle-foot, in cerebral palsy, 1838
Orthostatic intolerance, in spinal cord
    injury, 1860
Orthotopic liver transplantation, for biliary
    atresia, 470, 471
Ortolani sign, 254t, 448, 449f
Oscillometry, in blood pressure measurement,
    182-184, 184t
  in newborn, 251t, 256-257, 256f
    at high risk, 337
Osgood-Schlatter disease, 1801t
Osmolality, reference ranges for, 1900t
Osmosis, 1418
  in renal tubules, 1257
Osmotic diuresis, 1257
Osteochondritis, from heel puncture, 1148
Osteochondritis deformans juvenilis,
    1807-1808
Osteodystrophy, in chronic renal failure,
    1289-1291
Osteogenesis imperfecta, 119t, 298, 447t,
    1819-1820
Osteogenesis Imperfecta Foundation, 1820
Osteomyelitis, 1794, 1817-1818
Osteopenia/osteoporosis
  in athletes, 1804
  in bronchopulmonary dysplasia, 391
  in chronic renal failure, 1289b
  in immobilization, 1763, 1764-1765
Osteosarcoma, 1626-1628
Ostomy, 1166-1167
  in short bowel syndrome, 1454
Otic drug administration, 1160
Otitis externa, 1361
  in infants, 580
Otitis media, 1356-1360
  acute
    pacifier use and, 518
    treatment of, 1358-1359
  adhesive, 1358
  chronic suppurative, 1358
  cleft lip and palate and, 457, 463
  factors predisposing to, 1357b
  prevention of, 1360
  prognosis for, 1359
  recurrent, 1359
  terminology for, 1357b
  with effusion, 1358, 1359
Otoacoustic emissions, 205t
Otolith-righting reflex, in infants,
    494b, 498

Otoscopic examination
  of ear, 201-203, 201f, 202f
    for otitis media, 1358
    pneumatic, 204, 1358
  of nose, 204-206
Ototoxic medications, 996b
Oucher pain rating scale, 1052t
Outpatient setting, 1091-1092, 1092b
Ova and parasites, tests of, 1420t
Ovaries, 1704b, 1704f, 1708t
Overdependence, in congenital heart
    disease, 1501
Overhead warming unit, 339f
Overhydration, of high-risk newborn, 342
Overprotection, of special needs child, 934, 935b
Overuse injuries, 1798, 1800-1801, 1801t
Ovulation, 805
Ovum, maturation of at puberty, 803-805
Oxandrolone, in burn injuries, 1232
Oxycephaly, 444f
Oxycodone
  in pain management, 1060, 1060b,
    1062t, 1063t
  with acetaminophen, after heart surgery, 1506
Oxygen
  blood transport of, 1309
  hemoglobin and, in acid-base imbalance, 1183
  hyperbaric, in carbon monoxide injury, 1382
  in cystic fibrosis, 1408
  in gas exchange, 1308-1309, 1309b
  in smoke inhalation injury, 1381
  inspired fraction of ($FIO_2$), 1308
  partial pressure of ($PO_2$), 1308
    reference ranges for, 1900t
    transcutaneous monitoring of in arterial
      blood, 1315
  toxicity of, 1319
Oxygen desaturation, in high-risk newborn,
    during tactile stimulation, 361
Oxygen hood, 1317, 1318f
Oxygen saturation, 1309
  in carbon monoxide poisoning, 1381
  in congenital heart disease, 1475, 1475f
  in oxyhemoglobin dissociation curve,
    1315, 1315f
  in pulse oximetry, 1313-1314, 1314f
  reference ranges for, 1900t
Oxygen tent, 1317-1319, 1318f
Oxygen therapy, 1317-1319, 1318f, 1318t
  administration of, 1317-1319, 1318f, 1318t
  after heart surgery, 1505
  blood transfusion and, 1542
  complications of, 385
  gavage feeding and, 348
  in asthma, 1395-1396
  in carbon monoxide inhalation, 673, 1382
  in congestive heart failure, 1481, 1483
  in cystic fibrosis, 1411
  in extraneous air syndromes, 390
  in pulmonary artery hypertension, 1491
  in respiratory distress syndrome, 383-385,
    384t, 387
  in sickle cell anemia, 1551
Oxygenation
  cerebral, 1645
  in shock, 1222
  monitoring of, in respiratory distress
    syndrome, 387

Oxyhemoglobin, 1309, 1314
Oxyhemoglobin dissociation curve, 1309, 1315, 1315f
Oxyhemoglobin saturation, 1309
Oxylates, mineral regulation and, 560
Oxytocin, 1707t

**P**

PABA-esters, in sunscreen agents, 770
Pacemaker, cardiac, 1467
    in complete heart block, 1524-1525
    teaching about, 1525
Pacific Islanders, 35b; see also Race/ethnicity.
Pacifiers, 518-519
    aspiration of, 542t-543t, 543-544
    breast-feeding and, 277
    nursing caries and, 615
    oral candidiasis and, 301
Packed red blood cells, 1543t; see also Transfusion.
    for iron deficiency anemia, 1545
    for sickle cell anemia, 1551
Pain
    abdominal; see Abdominal pain.
    anterior leg, 1800, 1801t
    breakthrough, 1065b
    causes of, 1055
    chest
        in assessment of breathing, 1311
        in pulmonary artery hypertension, 1490
    developmental concepts of, 1036t
    diaphragmatic pleural, in assessment of breathing, 1311
    encopresis and, 786
    flank
        in renal trauma, 1283
        in urinary tract infection, 1266
    from immunizations, prevention of, 534b
    from intramuscular injections, 539b
    hospitalization and, 1036-1039, 1036t, 1037f
    in burns, 1237-1238, 1243-1244, 1244b
    in cancer, 1597, 1601, 1604
    in otitis externa, 1361
    in otitis media, 1358
    in stomatitis, 664
    in tonsillectomy, 1353
    in venipuncture, 1192
    jaw, in cancer, 1601
    neonatal, 351-357, 1036-1037, 1037f
        assessment of, 352-353, 352b, 353f, 354t-355t
        consequences of, 355-357, 356b, 356t
        management of, 357
        memory of, 353-355
        physiology of, 352
        postoperative, 420t, 423
    obstructive uropathy and, 486
    parietal pleural, in assessment of breathing, 1311
    phantom limb, 1628, 1796
    postoperative
        assessment of, 354t
        in cardiac surgery, 1505-1506
        referred, in appendicitis, 1433
    stump, 1795
    undermedication of, 1047b
    untreated, consequences in infants of, 355-357, 356b, 356t
Pain Affect Scale, 1051

Pain assessment, 1046-1057, 1047b
    behavioral and physiologic changes in, 1054-1055, 1054b, 1055b
    cause of pain and, 1055
    fallacies and facts in, 1048-1049, 1048b-1050b
    neonatal, 352-353, 352b, 353f, 354t-355t
    parental involvement in, 1055
    principles of, 1049-1050, 1050b, 1051f
    rating scales for, 354t, 1050-1054, 1052t-1053t, 1056t-1057t, 1905-1907
    record of, 1057, 1058f
    Wong-Baker FACES Pain Rating Scale for, 1905-1907
Pain Assessment Tool, 354t
Pain experience inventory, 1050b
Pain history, 157
Pain management, 1057; see also Analgesics; Anesthesia.
    drug administration in
        route of, 1062-1067
        timing of, 1067
    drug dosage in, 1061-1062, 1062t, 1063t
    drug selection for, 1057, 1060-1061, 1060b
    EMLA cream in, 1065b, 1066, 1066b, 1603, 1679; see also EMLA cream.
    for arthrocentesis, 1823b
    for bladder catheterization, 1146b
    for blood glucose monitoring, 1748
    for bone marrow transplant, 1603
    for burns, 1237-1238, 1243-1244, 1244b
    for cancer, 1604
    for circumcision, 270-272, 271b
    for comatose patient, 1655
    for HIV infection, 1576
    for immunizations, 534b
    for intramuscular injections, 539b
    for juvenile rheumatoid arthritis, 1823
    for laser therapy, for birthmarks, 302
    for lumbar puncture, 1142b, 1142f, 1603, 1679
    for newborn, 357
        after surgery, 420t, 423
    for sickle cell anemia, 1552-1553, 1553, 1553f
    for skin tests and allergy shots, 1385
    for suturing, 1672b
    for terminal illness, 949t, 956-958, 957b, 957f
    for venipuncture, 1149b, 1192
    insufficient, 1047b
    local anesthesia in, 1065b, 1066, 1066b, 1603, 1679
    nonpharmacologic, 1057, 1059b
    patient preparation and, 1109
    patient-controlled analgesia in, 1062-1063, 1064b, 1064t
    postoperative, 1117
        in newborn, 420t, 423
    side effects of, 1067-1068, 1067b, 1068b
    topical anesthesia in; see Topical anesthesia.
Pain rating scales, 354t, 1050-1054, 1052t-1053t, 1905-1907
Pain Relief Therapeutic Electro-Membrane, 1059b
Paint, lead-based, hazards of, 675-676, 679
Palate, 207f, 208
    cleft, 454-463, 455t
    development of, 455, 456f
    of newborn, 259
Palatine tonsils, 206f, 207
Palatoplasty, 460

Palivizumab (Synagis), for respiratory syncytial virus infection, 391, 1368, 1368b
Palliative care
    in terminal illness, 948-956
    principles of, 948
Pallor, 188, 188t
Palmar crease, 189, 190f
    transverse, 262
Palpation, 1310
    for abdominal pain, 1434b
    of abdomen, 219
    of apical impulse, 211-212, 214-215
    of bladder, 220
    of chest, 211-212, 214-215
    of colon, 220
    of joints, 225
    of kidney, 220
    of liver, 220
    of lymph nodes, 190, 190f
    of pulses, 179, 215f, 220, 220f
    of scrotum, 221-222, 222f
    of spleen, 220
Palpebral conjunctiva, 193
Palpebral fissure, 193, 193f
Pancreas, 1416, 1418
    endocrine, 1708t; see also Diabetes mellitus.
    in cystic fibrosis, 1405-1406, 1411
    transplantation of, 1738
Pancreatic function, tests of, 1421t
Pancreatic hormones, 1708t
Pancreatic insufficiency, in cystic fibrosis, 1401, 1409
Pancreatic islet cells
    antibodies to, 1733-1734
    in diabetes, 1733-1734, 1736
    transplantation of, 1738
Panhypopituitarism, 1706-1709, 1706b; see also Hypopituitarism.
Pantothenic acid
    functions of and disturbances in, 558t
    sources of, 558t
Papilledema, 195, 1651
Papule, 744f
Parachute reflex, in infants, 494, 494b, 494f
Paracort; see Prednisone.
Paradoxical pulse pressure, after heart surgery, 1507
Paralanguages, 140
Parallel play, 600
Paralysis
    birth-related, 298-300, 299f
    in spinal cord injury, 1852, 1856-1857; see also Spinal cord injury.
Paralytic ileus, 1446
Paralytic scoliosis, 1856-1857, 1858
Paramedics, 1760
Paranasal sinuses, 191, 191f
    rhabdomyosarcoma of, 1631b
Paraphimosis, 479
Paraplegia
    in spinal cord injury, 1852, 1856; see also Spinal cord injury.
    motor development and, 913, 914f
Parasites, intestinal, 665-668
    clinical manifestations of, 665t
    drugs for, 666t
    nursing considerations with, 665-666
    prevention of, 667b
Parasuicide, 895

Parasympathetic nervous system, 1705
Parathormone; *see* Parathyroid hormone.
Parathyroid disorders, 1721-1723, 1722-1723
    hyperparathyroidism, 1722-1723
    hypoparathyroidism, 1722
Parathyroid glands, 1704b, 1704f, 1708t, 1722
Parathyroid hormone, 1708t, 1721, 1722b
    hypersecretion of, 1722-1723, 1723b
    hyposecretion of, 1722, 1722b
Parens patriae, 62
Parent(s), 81-100; *see also* Family; Father;
        Mother.
    abusive, 684-685
        help for, 692-693
    adolescent, 851-852
    adolescent abortion and, consent for, 853
    adolescent health care and, 826-827, 827b
    anticipatory guidance for, 145
    atopic dermatitis in infants and, 582
    authoritarian, 84-85
    authoritative, 817
    bicycle helmet use and, 734
    communication with, 143-147
    competitive sports and, 726b
    dictatorial, 84-85
    discipline by, 84-85, 84-88
    drug administration and, 1151
    expert advice for, 88
    family leave for, 100
    family structure and, 70-73
    goals of, 82
    grieving, 969
        neonatal death and, 369-370
    guidance for
        in adolescence, 836b, 837
        in babyhood, 550b
        in preschool years, 635, 647
        in school years, 736, 736b
        in toddler years, 624, 624b
    hearing impairment and, 999
    informed consent of, 1102-1103, 1103b
        treatment without, 1103
    injury prevention in children and, 736
    intravenous infusion procedure and, 1192
    long-term venous access device care and, 1202
    new, 82-84
        in adoption, 90
    NICU safety measures and, 338
    nutritional education for, 520, 568, 570,
        722-723, 722b
    of apneic infants, 588
    of asthmatic children, 1400, 1401
    of athletes, 1806b
    of burn patients, 1247-1248
    of child in shock, 1222
    of child with congenital heart disease, 1498,
        1501-1503
    of child with cystic fibrosis, 1410, 1411
    of hospitalized child, 1040-1041, 1040b,
        1072-1073
        separation anxiety and, 1042-1043,
            1042f, 1043b
    of rape victims, 860b
    of sexually abused child, responses to
        suspicions of, 691
    of special needs child; *see* Special needs
        child.
    of terminally ill child; *see* Terminal illness.
    pain assessment and, 1055

Parent(s)—cont'd
    peritoneal dialysis and, 1297-1298
    permissiveness/restrictiveness of, 84-85
    presence of
        during cardiopulmonary resuscitation,
            1334b
        preoperative, 1110-1112
        psychologic preparation for procedures
            and, 1106-1107, 1107b
    punishment by, 84, 88
    role of, 75-77
    school involvement of, 714, 716, 716b, 819
    separation of child from, 502, 505-506, 599;
        *see also* under Separation.
    sex education and, 710
    sexual abuse prevention and, 693-694, 694b
    sexual risk-taking in adolescents and,
        849-850
    single, 97-98; *see also* Divorce.
    skin lesion care and, 753-754
    smoking by, hazards of to children, 1382
    sudden infant death syndrome and, 584-585
    support systems for, 83-84
    violence between, 683
    visual impairment and, 1002-1004
    vulnerable child syndrome and, 309, 369
    warmth/hostility of, 84
    wound care at home by, 751-754
Parent-child relationship; *see also* Attachment.
    colic and, 573b
    development of, 504-506
    failure to thrive and, 574, 575b, 576
    in school-age children, 707-708
    rumination and, 574
Parenteral fluid therapy; *see also* Fluid
        management; Infusion(s).
    by intraosseous infusion, 1191-1192
    by intravenous infusion, 1188-1191
    for high-risk newborn, 341-342
Parenteral nutrition; *see* Total parenteral
        nutrition.
Parenting, 81-100
    attitudes toward, 84
    coping strategies for, 83-84
    divorce and, 94-97
    employment issues and, 100
    foster, 100
    guidebooks on, 88
    ideal age for, 82
    in dual-earner family, 99
    motivation for, 81
    of adopted child, 89-93; *see also* Adoption.
    preparation for, 81-82
    transition to, 82-84
        in adoption, 90
Parenting coalition, 98
Parenting education, 83
Parenting manuals, 88
Parenting styles, 84-85
Parent-professional partnership, 14-15, 23
    home care and, 1022-1023, 1023b
    special needs child and, 937-938, 937b,
        938b, 938t
    therapeutic relationship and, 18-19, 19b
Parents Anonymous, 693, 895
Parents' Evaluation of Developmental
        Status, 234t
Parents United International Inc., 693
Parents Without Partners, 98

Parent-to-parent support, special needs child
        and, 936-937
Paresthesia, with skin lesions, 742
Parietal lobes, 1644t
Parietal pleura, 1302
Parkland formula, for burn patients, 1237
Paroxysmal vertigo, 1700b
Partial liquid ventilation, 385-386
Partial seizures
    complex, 1686-1687, 1687t, 1695b
    simple, 1686, 1687t
Partial thromboplastin time, 1562t
    reference ranges for, 1900t
Partially sighted, 1000
    education and, 1004
Parvovirus infection
    in newborn, 327t
    maternal, fetal anemia and, 651
Passive diffusion (osmosis), 1418
    in renal tubules, 1257
Passy-Muir valve, for tracheostomy, 1330
PAT; *see* Pain Assessment Tool.
Patau syndrome, 116t
Patch, as skin lesion, 743f
Patellar dislocation, 1799
Patellar reflex, 227f
Patellofemoral syndrome, 1801t
Patent ductus arteriosus, 397, 1494b, 1494f
    in transposition of great arteries, 1499b
    pulmonary artery hypertension and, 1490
Patent foramen ovale
    in transposition of great arteries, 1499b
    in tricuspid atresia, 1497b
Patent urachus, 218
Patient counseling; *see* Counseling.
Patient-controlled analgesia, 1062-1063,
        1064b, 1064t
    in sickle cell anemia, 1553
Patterning, 1840
Pausing, 140
Pavlik harness, 449-450, 450f
    home care and, 450-451
PCP; *see* Phencyclidine.
Peabody Picture Vocabulary Test-III, 1012
Peak expiratory flow rate, 1398, 1399b
    in asthma, 1389-1390, 1389b
Peak height velocity, 808
Peak inspiratory pressure, intermittent
        mandatory ventilation and, 384
Peak weight velocity, 808
Peanut allergy, BAL therapy and, 681
Pearson attachment, 1790, 1790f
Pectus carinatum, 209
Pectus excavatum, 209
Pedal pulses, cardiac catheterization and, 1472
Pedestrian injuries, 7, 620, 732
Pediatric health history; *see* Health history.
Pediatric nurse; *see also* Nurse; Nursing.
    as health team member, 21
    cultural values of, 50-51, 50b
    delegation by, 23-24, 24b
    in health care team, 21
    role of, 18-23
        in coordination/collaboration, 21
        in disease prevention/health promotion,
            20-21
        in ethical decision-making, 21-22, 22b
        in family advocacy/caring, 19-20
        in health care planning, 22-23

Pediatric nurse—cont'd
role of—cont'd
in health teaching, 21
in research, 22
in restoration of health, 21
in support/counseling, 21
in therapeutic relationship, 18-19
trends in, 23-24
specialist/advanced practice, 20
unlicensed assistive personnel and, 23-24, 24b
Pediatric nurse practitioner (PNP), 20
Pediatric nursing; see also Nursing.
standards of practice for, 23, 23b
trends in, 23-24
Pediatric physical assessment; see Physical
examination.
Pediatric Projects, Inc., 1108n
Pediatric social illness, 6
Pediculosis capitis, 761-763, 761f, 762b, 762f
prevention of, 762-763, 762b
school policies on, 763b
Pedigree chart, 133-134, 133b, 134f, 135b,
160-162
Pedodontist, 611
Pedophilia, definition of, 686
PEEP; see Positive end-expiratory pressure.
Peer(s)
adolescent health behavior and, 818
adolescent pregnancy and, 851
in team play, 711-712
sex information from, 710
smoking and, 885
Peer cultures, 37-38
Peer relationships, 706-707; see also
Socialization.
of adolescents, 816
of school-age children, 706-707, 706f
of special needs child, 914-915, 916,
930-931, 982
social functions of, 37-38
Pelvic examination, 844-845, 845b
Pelvic inflammatory disease, 863-864
gonorrhea and, 861
Pelvis, renal, congenital anomalies of, 479t
Pemoline (Cylert), for attention deficit
hyperactivity disorder, 789
Penetrating wound, of eye, 1000, 1002, 1003b
Penicillin
for gonorrhea, 862
for otitis media, 1358
for rheumatic fever, 1512
for streptococcal pharyngitis, 1351-1352
Penile carcinoma, 843
Penis
ambiguous genitalia and, 489t
examination of, 220-221
growth of, 806, 807, 842-843
hypospadias and, 481-482, 481f
of newborn, 254t, 261, 377f
circumcision and, 270-273, 270b-272b, 272f
preterm, 376, 377f
phimosis and, 479
Penis envy, 631
Pentasa (mesalamine), for inflammatory
bowel disease, 1440
Pentobarbital
abuse of, 886t
in preoperative sedation, 1113b

Pepcid (famotidine)
for gastroesophageal reflux, 1429
for peptic ulcer disease, 1445
Pepsin, 1418
ulcers and, 1443
Peptic ulcer disease, 1443-1446
causes and effects of, 1443, 1444f
characteristics of, 1443, 1444f, 1445t
Peptides, small, 1418
Perceptive deafness, 995
Perceptual thinking, 702
Percocet, 1060b; see also Oxycodone.
Percodan; see Oxycodone.
Percussion, 1310
of abdomen, 219
of chest, 212
with bronchial drainage, 1320, 1323f
Percutaneous central venous catheter, for
parenteral fluid therapy, in high-risk
newborn, 342
Percutaneous transtracheal aspiration, 1315t
Percutaneous umbilical blood sampling, in
hemolytic disease of newborn, 314
Perez reflex, 263t
Perfluorocarbons, for respiratory distress
syndrome, 385-386
Performance-enhancing substances, for
athletes, 1804-1805
Perfusion
in congestive heart failure, 1478
peripheral, after heart surgery, 1507
Pericardial fluid, 1465
Pericardial friction rubs, 215
Pericardial space, 1465
Pericardium, 1465
Perinatal history, 155
Perinatal hypoxic-ischemic brain injury, 400-401
Perinatal mortality, 3, 334b
Perinatal transmission, of human
immunodeficiency virus, 1573
Perineal fistula, 468, 469
Perineal rhabdomyosarcoma, 1631b
Perineum, broadening of, developmental
dysplasia of hip and, 448, 449f
Perinuclear antineutrophil cytoplasmic
antibody, ulcerative colitis diagnosis
and, 1440
Periodic breathing, in newborn, 260
Periodontal disease, 781
prevention of, 611
Periodontitis, 781
Periosteum, 1776, 1777f
Peripheral blood smear, 1536t
in sickle cell anemia, 1550
Peripheral lock, 1198, 1199b
Peripheral nervous system, 1641
Peripheral precocious puberty, 1714
Peripheral stem cell transplantation, 1596
Peripheral vision, assessment of, 199
Peripherally inserted central venous catheter,
for parenteral fluid therapy, in high-risk
newborn, 342
Peristalsis, 218
absence of, in Hirschsprung disease, 1426
auscultation of, 218-219
esophageal, 1418
urethral, 1258
visible, 218

Peritoneal dialysis, 1293, 1297-1298
at home, 1297
continuous ambulatory, 1297
continuous cycling, 1297
for hemolytic uremic syndrome, 1282
for shock, 1221
Peritonitis, 1433, 1434
nephrotic syndrome and, 1278, 1278b
signs of, 1433
Periventricular hemorrhage, 401
Periventricular leukomalacia, 401
Perkins School for the Blind, 1006
Perlocutionary stage, 148, 148b
Permethrin
for head lice, 761-762
for scabies, 760, 761
Permissive hypercapnia, for congenital
diaphragmatic hernia, 476
Permissive parent, 85
PERRLA, 194
Persistent cloaca, 466, 468f
Persistent fetal hemoglobin, respiratory
distress syndrome and, 381
Persistent pulmonary hypertension of
newborn, 397-398, 398f
Persistent vegetative state, 1648b, 1660-1661
Personality
birth order and, 79, 79b
obesity and, 872
Personality development, 230-231, 230t
Personal-social behavior
of infants, 506-507
of toddlers, 599-600
Perspiration, 742
Pertussis, 1371-1372; see also Whooping cough.
manifestations and management of, 656t-657t
recommended immunizations for, 529t,
532-533, 536
contraindications to, 537t
PES format, for nursing diagnosis, 25-26
Pes planus, 447t
Pes valgus, 447t
Pes varus, 447t
Petaling, cast, 1786
Petechiae, 188, 188t, 743
birth-related, 295-296, 296b
platelets and, 1535
Pets
ringworm infection and, 760
safety rules for, 779b
self-esteem development and, 709
PFAPA syndrome, 664
PFCs; see Perfluorocarbons.
pH
diaper dermatitis and, 578
esophageal, monitoring of, 1422t, 1429
gastrointestinal, tests of, 1420t
in acid-base balance, 1182
in asthma, 1396
reference ranges for, 1900t
skin, 752
Phadiatope test, in allergic rhinitis, 1384
Phagocytes, 243
Phagocytosis, 593, 747, 1572
Phallic stage, 230, 230t
in preschoolers, 630-631
Phantom limb pain, 1628, 1796
Pharmacogenetics, 110

Pharyngitis, streptococcal
  acute, 1351-1352
  rheumatic fever and, 1511
  vs viral, 1353
Pharynx, 1305
Phencyclidine, 891b
Phenex-1, 283t, 323
Phenex-2, 283t, 323
Phenobarbital
  for hyperbilirubinemia, 306
  for seizures, 1691t
    in newborn, 404
    in status epilepticus, 1692
Phenylalanine, 322
  normal level of, 323
  reference ranges for, 1900t
Phenylalanine hydroxylase, 322
L-Phenylalanine mustard, 1590t
Phenyl-free formula, 283t, 323
Phenylketonuria, 119t, 322-324, 322f, 324b
  diet for, 124
  formulas for infants with, 283t, 323
  screening for, 125-126, 267, 267b, 323, 323b
Phenylpyruvic acid, 322
Phenytoin, 1690, 1691t
  for status epilepticus, 1692
Pheochromocytoma, 1724, 1731-1732
Philadelphia chromosome, 1585
Phimosis, 221, 479
Phocomelia, 254t, 453
Phoria, 196
Phosphatidylcholine, 383
Phosphatidylglycerol, 383
Phospholipids, surfactant, fetal lung maturity
  and, 383
Phosphorus
  functions of and disturbances in, 563t
  in chronic renal failure, 1289, 1290, 1291
  sources of, 563t
Photocoagulation, for retinoblastoma, 1633
Photoisomerization, 306
Phototherapy
  for hyperbilirubinemia, 303t, 306-309, 307t,
    308f, 309b
  side effects of, 308, 350, 365
Phrenic nerve paralysis, birth-related, 299, 300
Physical abuse, 684-685; see also Child abuse.
Physical activity; see Exercise.
Physical examination, 171-229
  abdomen in, 217-220
  age-specific approaches in, 173t
  anus in, 223
  back in, 223
  blood pressure in, 182-186
  chest in, 208-210
  ears in, 200-204
  extremities in, 224-225
  eyes in, 192-200
  general appearance in, 186-187
  genitalia in, 220-223
  growth measurements in, 174-178; see also
    Anthropometric measurements.
  guidelines for, 173t
  hair in, 189
  head in, 190-191
  heart in, 213-217
  in assessment of cardiac function, 1468-1469
  in neurologic assessment, 1646-1647

Physical examination—cont'd
  lungs in, 210-213
  lymph nodes in, 190, 190f
  mouth and throat in, 206-208
  nails in, 189
  neck in, 191
  neurologic assessment in, 225-229; see also
    Neurologic assessment.
  nose in, 204-206
  nutritional status in, 186-187
  of newborn, 250-263, 250b, 251t-254t
    at high risk, 335-338, 336b, 337b, 337t
  of rape victim, 859
  physiologic measurements in, 178-186
  positioning for, 173t
  preadmission, 1089-1090
  preparation of child for, 172-174, 173t
  pulse rate in, 179, 184t
  recommendations for, 171
  respiration in, 179
  sequence of, 171-172
  skin in, 187-189
  spine in, 223
  temperature in, 178-179, 179f, 180b-181b,
    182t-183t
  vital signs in, 178-186
Physical fitness
  in adolescents, 830
  in school-age children, 724-725
Physical maturity, of newborn, in gestational
  age estimation, 248f
Physical neglect, 683
Physical preparation, for procedures, 1108-
  1110, 1110f
Physical therapy
  in cerebral palsy, 1840, 1842
  in juvenile rheumatoid arthritis, 1822
  in spinal cord injury, 1861
Physiologic cup, 195
Physiologic jaundice, 242, 303t, 304-305
Physiologic measurements, 178-186
Physiologic splitting, of S₂, 215, 216t
Physiotherapy, in spinal cord injury, 1859-1860
Phytates, mineral regulation and, 560
Pia mater, 1642-1643, 1643f
Piaget's cognitive development theory, 230t,
  231-232
  adolescents in, 809-810
  infants in, 502-504, 503t
  preschoolers in, 631
  school-age children in, 702-704, 703f
  toddlers in, 594-597, 595t
Pica, 1422-1423
  lead poisoning and, 680
Pierre Robin syndrome, 445b
Pigeon breast, 209
Pigeon toe, 225
Pigmentation, variations in, 57
Pill counts, in compliance measurement, 1120
Pilocarpine iontophoresis, for cystic
  fibrosis, 1407
Pilonidal cyst, 223
Pilonidal sinus, 261
Pilosebaceous unit, 840
Pimples, 839-842, 842b
Pin site care, 1791b, 1792
Pincer grasp, in infants, 498, 498f
Pineal body, 1704b, 1704f

Pinna, 200, 200f
  of newborn, 259
Pinocytosis, in intestinal absorption, 1419
Pinpoint pupils, 1650f
Pinworms, 667-668
Pioneering, 78
Piperazine citrate, 666t
PIPP; see Premature Infant Pain Profile.
Pitressin (aqueous vasopressin), for diabetes
  insipidus, 1715, 1716
Pitting edema, 189
Pituitary disorders, 1706-1717
  acromegaly, 1713-1714
  diabetes insipidus, 1658, 1658b, 1672,
    1715-1716
  growth hormone deficiency, 1706-1713
  hyperpituitarism, 1713-1714
  hypopituitarism, 1706-1713
  precocious puberty, 1714-1715
  syndrome of inappropriate antidiuretic
    hormone, 1658, 1658b, 1672,
    1716-1717
Pituitary gland, 1704b, 1704f
  anterior, 1704-1705, 1705f, 1707t
  as master gland, 1704
  endocrine regulation by, 1704-1705, 1705f
  hypothalamus and, 1704-1705, 1705f
  posterior, 1704-1705, 1705f, 1707t
  tumors of
    Cushing's syndrome and, 1727-1729
    hyperpituitarism and, 1713
    hypopituitarism and, 1706-1709, 1710, 1712
Pituitary hormones, 1707t
  hypersecretion of, 713-714
  hyposecretion of, 1706-1713, 1706b
  regulation of, 1704-1705, 1705f
PKU; see Phenylketonuria.
Placenta, 1704b
Placing reflex, 263t
Plagiocephaly, 444f, 446
  positional, 583
Planned Parenthood Federation of America,
  857, 983n
Planning, in nursing process, 27, 27t; see also
  Nursing care plan.
Plant(s)
  nonpoisonous, 672b
  poisonous, 547, 549b, 671b, 672b
Plant alkaloids, for cancer, 1588, 1591t-1592t
Plant foods, mineral regulation and, 560
Plantar fasciitis, 1801t
Plantar reflex, 225, 262, 262f
Plantar wart, 758t
Plaque
  dental, 728, 780
    removal of, 611-613
  skin, 743f
Plaque brachytherapy, for retinoblastoma, 1633
Plaque-disclosing agent, 728
Plasma, 1530, 1538
  fresh frozen, 1543t
Plasma bicarbonate, in infants, 1258
Plasma cells, 1572
Plasma proteins, in edema formation, 1181
Plasma thromboplastin component, 1562t
Plasma volume, reference ranges for, 1900t
Plaster casts, 1784-1785, 1785t
Plastibell procedure, for circumcision, 272

Plastic bags, infant suffocation and, 542t-543t, 545, 549b
Plastic strip thermometers, 178, 180b, 183t
Plasticized sealant, tooth decay prevention and, 780
Plastics, gases from, in smoke inhalation injury, 1381
Plate fixation, 1793
Platelet(s), 1535, 1538
    in hemostasis, 1561
    transfusion of, 1543t, 1599
Platelet count, 1536t
    in idiopathic thrombocytopenic purpura, 1566, 1567
    reference ranges for, 1900t
Platelet function, tests of, 1562t
Platinol (cisplatin), 1590t
Play
    communication via, 150-153, 152b
    development of, 507, 508t
    dramatic, during hospitalization, 1071-1072, 1072f
    during hospitalization, 1069-1072, 1069b, 1070f-1072f
    encouragement of, 602b
    in assessment, 152-153, 152b
    in immobilization, 1768-1769
    in infants, 503
    in performance of procedures, 1110, 1111b
    in preparation for intravenous infusion, 1192
    in preschoolers, 631, 633-635, 634f, 634t, 635b, 635f, 636b
    in school-age children, 711-713, 711f, 712f
    in toddlers, 600-601, 600f, 601t
    medical, 1768-1769
    mental retardation and, 982-983, 983f
    toys in; see Toys.
    visual impairment and, 1003-1004, 1005
    with parents, 635
Play therapy, 1071
Playground safety, 618b, 621
Playmates; see also Friendships.
    imaginary, 635, 636b
Plethora, 188
Pleura, parietal, 1302
Pleural effusion, 1302
    after heart surgery, 1507
    in congestive heart failure, 1478
    in pneumonia, 1370-1371
Pleural friction rub, 213
Pleural sac, visceral, 1302
Plexuses, 1853-1854, 1855b
PLUG technique, for congenital diaphragmatic hernia, 475
Pluripotential stem cell, 1531, 1532
Plus disease, in retinopathy of prematurity, 400b
Pneumatic otoscopy, 204
Pneumatosis intestinalis, 395, 396
Pneumocardiogram, 586
Pneumococcal vaccines, 529t
    contraindications to, 537t, 538t
    for otitis media, 1359
    for pneumonia, 1370
    in adolescents, 834
    recommended immunizations with, 529t, 534
Pneumocystis carinii pneumonia, 1575
Pneumomediastinum, 389, 390

Pneumonia, 1368-1371; see also Respiratory infections.
    aspiration, 1378-1379, 1378b
        in near-drowning, 1675-1676
    bacterial, 1369-1371
        in burn injuries, 1233
    chlamydial, 1371
    clinical manifestations of, 1370, 1370b
    complications of, 1370-1371
    hydrocarbon, 1378-1379
    lipoid, 1379
    primary atypical, 1369
    types of, 1369b
    viral, 1369
Pneumonitis, 1369
Pneumopericardium, 389, 390
Pneumotaxic center, 1309
Pneumothorax, 389-390, 1302
    after heart surgery, 1507, 1508b
    in cystic fibrosis, 1405, 1408-1409
PO₂, 1308
    reference ranges for, 1900t
    transcutaneous monitoring of in arterial blood, 1315
Podocytes, 1256
Point of maximum intensity (PMI), 215
Poison control center, 622, 669, 669b
Poison ivy, oak, and sumac, 767-768, 768b, 768f
Poison Prevention Packaging Act (1970), 668
Poisoning, 668-682
    agents causing, 669, 670b, 671b
    common signs of, 672b
    emergency management of, 669-675, 673b
    gastric decontamination for, 670-673
    heavy metals, 675
    in early childhood, 668-683
    in school-age children, 731t
    in toddlers, 622, 622f
    lead, 675-682
    mortality from, 8, 8t
    prevention of, 542t, 543t, 547, 549b, 673-675, 674b, 674t, 675b, 1758b, 1759b
Poker Chip Tool, in pain assessment, 1052t-1053t
Poliomyelitis
    manifestations and management of, 658t-659t
    recommended immunizations for, 529t, 533
        contraindications to, 537t
Pollen, seasonal allergic rhinitis and, 1383
Polyandry, 72
Polyarteritis nodosa, renal involvement in, 1270t
Polyarthritis, in rheumatic fever, 1511
Polychromatic erythroblast, 1532
Polycose formula, 282t, 323
Polycythemia, 399, 1532
    with hypoxemia, 1486
Polydactyly, 224, 254t, 262, 447t
Polydipsia
    in diabetes insipidus, 1715, 1716
    in diabetes mellitus, 1734, 1736
Polydrug use, in pregnancy, 406
Polyethylene glycol (Miralax), 1425
Polyethylene glycol electrolyte solution (GoLYTELY), 1425
Polygamous family, 72
Polyhydramnios, esophageal atresia and, 464
Polymerase chain reaction, 862, 863
    in hemolytic disease of newborn, 314

Polymeric foams, for skin lesions, 750t
Polymorphonuclear leukocytes, 1534
Polyneuropathies, 1833
Polyphagia, in diabetes, 1734
Polyps, anorectal, 223
Polyurethane films, for skin lesions, 750t
Polyuria
    in diabetes, 1734
    in diabetes insipidus, 1715, 1716
    in hyperaldosteronism, 1731
    nocturnal, enuresis and, 784
Pons, 1644t
Pool therapy, for juvenile rheumatoid arthritis, 1824
Popcorn poppers, electrical, 621
Popliteal angle, gestational age and, 250b
POPS; see Postoperative Pain Score.
Populations, 103
Porcine surfactant, 386
Pornography, 686
Port, implanted, vs other long-term venous access devices, 1201t
Port-A-Cath, vs other long-term venous access devices, 1201t
Portagen formula, 282t
Portal circulation, in absorption, 1419
Portal hypertension, gastrointestinal bleeding and, 1454
Portoenterostomy, 470, 471-472, 471f
Port-wine stain, 302, 302f
Positional plagiocephaly, 446
Position/positioning; see also Posture(s).
    after cranial surgery, 1623
    as respiratory tract defense, 1310
    assessment of, 186
    deaf-blindness and, 1006
    for bone marrow aspiration/biopsy, 1142
    for extremity venipuncture, 1141, 1141f
    for femoral venipuncture, 1140f, 1141
    for jugular venipuncture, 1140-1141, 1140f
    for lumbar puncture, 1141-1142, 1141f, 1142b, 1142f
    for otoscopic examination, 201, 201f
    for physical examination, 173t
    for subdural puncture, 1142
    gastroesophageal reflux and, 1429, 1431
    in asthma, 1396
    in increased intracranial pressure, 1657
    in respiratory failure, 1332
    in shock, 1222, 1225
    in sudden infant death syndrome, 582-583
    intraventricular hemorrhage and, 402
    knee-chest, in infant, 1488f
    myelomeningocele and, 431
    of unconscious child, 1659
    prone
        for gastroesophageal reflux, 1429, 1431
        sudden infant death syndrome and, 583, 584b
    recovery, after respiratory emergency, 1341, 1341f
    sudden infant death syndrome and, 363, 583, 584b
    therapeutic, high-risk newborn and, 363, 363b, 364b, 364f
Positive end-expiratory pressure, in respiratory distress syndrome, 384, 384f

Positive pressure ventilation
  complications of, 385
  for respiratory distress syndrome,
    383-385, 384t
Positive reinforcement
  disciplinary, 86-87
  postprocedural, 1110
Positive self-talk, in pain management, 1059b
Positron emission tomography, cerebral, 1654t
Postconcussion syndrome, 1670
Posterior fontanel, 252t, 257-258, 258f
Posterior pituitary; see Pituitary gland.
Posterior sagittal anorectoplasty, 469
Posthemorrhagic hydrocephalus, 402
Postictal state, 1686, 1688
Postirradiation somnolence, 1601-1602
Postmature infant; see Postterm infant.
Postmortem care, 961, 964
Postnatal death, 334b
Postneonatal mortality, 2
Postoperative care, 1113, 1115-1118, 1118b,
    1503-1508, 1508b
  for newborn, 420-423, 420t-423t
  nursing care plan for, 1115-1117
  vital signs in, 1113, 1119t
Postoperative Pain Score, 354t
Postpericardiotomy syndrome, after heart
    surgery, 1508
Postterm infant, 334b, 376; see also High-risk
    newborn.
  congenital hypothyroidism in, 321
Posttraumatic amnesia, 1666
Posttraumatic stress disorder, 794
Postural drainage, 1320, 1321f, 1322f
  in cystic fibrosis, 1412
  with chest physiotherapy, 1320, 1322
Posture(s); see also Position/positioning.
  assessment of, 186
  in cerebral palsy, 1836
  lung volume and, 1304, 1304f
  of newborn, 250b, 251t, 257, 257f
    prematurity and, 377f
Postvention, emergency admission and, 1093
Potassium
  deficiency of, 1176t
    after heart surgery, 1506
    in diabetic ketoacidosis, 1742
    in hyperaldosteronism, 1731
  dietary, in chronic renal failure, 1290
  excess, 1176t, 1177t
    from blood transfusion, 1541t
    in acute renal failure, 1286
    in chronic renal failure, 1288-1289
  functions of and disturbances in, 563t
  in acid-base imbalance, 1183
  in acute renal failure, 1286
  reference ranges for, 1900t
  replacement, for diabetic ketoacidosis, 1742
  serum, digoxin effects and, 1480
  sources of, 563t
Pott disease, 1818
Poverty, 40-42; see also Poverty.
  adolescent health behavior and, 817-818
  as risk factors, 104
  family function and, 74
  health effects of, 41
  sociocultural aspects of, 36, 37, 40-41
Povidone-iodine, 752

Practice standards, 23, 23b
Prader-Willi syndrome, 122, 871
Pragmatics, 1007
Preadmission, 1087b
Preadolescence, 700
Precocious puberty, 1714-1715, 1714b
Preconceptual phase
  in preschoolers, 631
  in toddlers, 595t, 596-597
Preconventional (premoral) level, of moral
    development, 597-598, 631-632
Prednisone; see also Steroids.
  for cancer, 1593t
  for hemangioma, 302
  in cystic fibrosis, 1409
  in nephrotic syndrome, 1277
  in renal transplantation, 1299
Preemie head, 376
Prefeeding behavior, in newborn, 279
Pregestimil, 282t
Pregnancy
  abnormalities in, birth defects and, 124
  adolescent, 850-853, 852b, 857
    unintended, 830-831
  alcohol use during, 326, 328-330, 329b, 329f
  amniocentesis in, 128t, 129-130
  chorionic villus sampling in, 128t, 130
  cocaine use during, 407-408
  complications of, 850-851
  diabetes mellitus and, 404-406
  diagnostic ultrasonography in, 129
  drug use during, 326, 406-408, 406b
  ectopic, 850-851
    pelvic inflammatory disease and, 863
  fetal abnormalities in; see also Congenital
      malformations and specific disorders.
    diagnosis of, 128-130, 128t, 129b
  folic acid in, 124-125, 424, 430
  folk beliefs about, 49-50
  history of, 155
  in athletes, 1804
  in spinal cord injury, 1862
  opioid use in, 406-407, 406b
  radiation exposure during, 330
  smoking during, 408-409
  teratogens and, 124
  urinary tract infection and, 1265
  vaccination with live virus vaccines and, 538
Prehabilitation, 1762
Preimplantation genetic diagnosis, 130
Prekallikrein, 1562t
Preload, 1468
Preluxation, acetabular, 446b, 448f; see also
    Hip, developmental dysplasia of.
Premature infant; see Preterm infant.
Premature Infant Pain Profile, 353, 355t
Premenstrual syndrome, 847-848
Premutations, 121
  in fragile X syndrome, 993
Prenatal care, for teenage mothers, 850
Prenatal development, 416, 417f
Prenatal diagnosis, 128-130, 128t, 129b
  diabetic mother and, 405
  of congenital diaphragmatic hernia, 475
  of Down syndrome, 992-993
  of neural tube defects, 427
  of respiratory distress syndrome, 383
  of sickle cell anemia, 1554

Prenatal influences, folklore about, 49-50
Preoperational stage, 230t, 232, 596, 597,
    597b, 631
Preoperative care, 1110-1113, 1112b, 1112f,
    1113b
  neonatal, 419-420
  nursing care plan for, 1114-1115
Prepubescence, 700
Prepuce, 222
Preschool facilities
  as preparation for school, 715
  center-based, 516
  diapering and toileting at, 517-518
  readiness and preparation of child
    for, 637
  sanitation at, giardiasis and, 667
  selection of, 637
  value of, 636, 637
Preschooler
  aggressive, 641-642
  biologic development in, 628-630, 638t
  body image in, 632
  cognitive development in, 631, 639t
  communication with, 148
  concept of death in, 953
  dental health in, 646
  divorce and, 95, 95b
  dying, 953-954; see also Terminal illness.
  family of, 639t, 647
    guidance for, 646b, 647
  fears in, 642-644
  gifted, 640-641
    identification and handling of,
      640-641, 641b
  growth and development of, 628-644,
    638t-639t
  health promotion in, 644-647
  hospitalized
    bodily injury and pain in, 1037-1038
    separation anxiety in, 1033
  injury prevention in, 646-647
  mental retardation in, 978t
  moral development in, 631-632
  motor behavior in, 629-630, 629f, 638t
  nutrition in, 644-645, 644f
  physical examination for, 173t
  preschool and kindergarten experience
    in, 636
  psychosocial development in, 630-631, 639t
  sex education in, 637-640
  sexuality in, development of, 632
  sleep and activity in, 645-646, 645t
  social development in, 632-636, 639t
  special needs; see also Special needs child.
    promotion of normal development in,
      911t, 913-914, 915f
  speech problems in, 642
  spiritual development in, 632
  stress in, 642, 643b
  temperament in, 636
Prescreening Developmental Questionnaire-
    Revised, 237
Pressure gradients, congenital heart disease
    and, 1474-1475
Pressure overload, in congestive heart
    failure, 1476
Pressure reduction device, 1124, 1126t
Pressure relief device, 1124, 1126t

Pressure ulcers, 745, 1122-1125, 1124b-1125b, 1126t
  in immobilization, 1765, 1765f
  in spinal cord injury, 1859
Preterm infant, 334b, 374-375; see also High-risk newborn.
  adolescent pregnancy and, 851
  apnea in, 376, 378-379, 379b
  body water distribution in, 1173
  bottle-feeding of, 344-347, 345f, 346b
  breast-feeding of, 344, 347-348
  cerebral palsy in, 1835
  characteristics of, 376, 377f-378f
  critical path for, 16t
  etiology of prematurity and, 374-375
  heel puncture in, 317b
  hyperbilirubinemia in, treatment of, 306
  hypocalcemia in, 318
  hypothyroidism in, 321
  nonnutritive sucking and, 519
  retinopathy in, 399-400, 400b
    nutrition and, 344
  sepsis in, 394
  therapeutic management of, 376
Pretreatment billing, 13
Prevacid (lansoprazole)
  for gastroesophageal reflux, 1429
  for peptic ulcer disease, 1445
Prevalence, 105, 105b
Prevention
  levels of, 105
  recommendations for, 171, 171b
Prevnar vaccine, for streptococcal pneumococci, 534
Prilocaine, for laser therapy, for birthmarks, 302
Prilosec (omeprazole)
  for gastroesophageal reflux, 1429
  for peptic ulcer disease, 1445
Primary antibody response, 1572
Primary groups, 32-33
Primary irritant, 767
Primary prevention, 105
Primidone, for seizures, 1691t
Primigravidas, postterm infants and, 376
Primitive neuroectodermal tumor of bone, 1626-1627, 1628-1629
Primitive reflexes, 243; see also Reflex(es).
Privacy; see also Confidentiality.
  computer, 142
  for interview, 141
Private duty nursing, 1017, 1017b
Proaccelerin, 1562t
Proband, 131, 133
Problem statement, in nursing diagnosis, 25
Procarbazine (Matulane), 1590t
Procedures; see also specific disorders.
  neurologic, 1652-1654, 1653t-1654t, 1655b
  pain management for; see Pain management.
  patient/family preparation for, 148, 149f, 1622
Processus vaginalis
  hydrocele and, 478t, 479
  inguinal hernia and, 477, 478f
Proconvertin, 1562t
Profibrinolysin, 1534
Progestins, 1708t
  adrenal secretion of, 1723
Prognathism, 993, 993f

Prognosis, patient/family teaching about, 1616
Programs for Children with Special Health Needs, 12, 419, 939, 981
Prokinetic medications, for gastroesophageal reflux, 1429, 1431
Prolactin, 1707t
Prolapse, rectal, 223
Proliferation, in wound healing, 747
Prone roll, 363, 364f
Pro-Phree formula, 283t
Propranolol (Inderal)
  for hypertension, 1519b
  for supraventricular tachycardia, 1525
Propulsid (cisapride), for gastroesophageal reflux, 1429
Propylthiouracil, for hyperthyroidism, 1719-1720, 1721
Pros and cons technique, 151b
Prosobee, 281t
Prospective payment system, 13
Prostacyclin, for pulmonary artery hypertension, 1491
Prostaglandins
  dysmenorrhea and, 846, 847
  in cyanotic newborns, 1487
  ulcers and, 1443
Prosthesis, 1774-1775, 1775b
  dental, in cleft lip and palate, 458
  limb, 454, 1628
  ocular, 1634, 1634f
Prostitution, of children, 686
Protanomaly, 199
Protectiv safety catheters, 1190
Protein
  deficiency of, kwashiorkor and, 566
  edema formation and, 1181
  in chronic renal failure, 1290
  in toddlers, 609
  in vegetarian diets, 560, 565-566
  phenylketonuria and, 323-324
  reference ranges for, 1901t
Protein and energy malnutrition, in infants, 566-568
Proteinuria
  in nephrotic syndrome, 1275-1276
  orthostatic, 1282
  persistent, 1282
  transient, 1282
  unexplained, 1282
Prothrombin, 1562t
Prothrombin consumption test, 1562t
Prothrombin time, 1562t
  reference ranges for, 1901t
Protocols, chemotherapy, 1588
Proton pump, 1430
Proton pump inhibitors
  for peptic ulcer disease, 1445
  for upper gastrointestinal mucosal lesions, 1455
Prouentil HFC, in metered-dose inhaler, 1391
PRS; see Pain Rating Scale.
Pruritus, 742
  in allergic rhinitis, 1383
  in atopic dermatitis, 581, 582
  in burn patients, 1246
  in enterobiasis, 667, 668
  opioid-induced, 1068
  relief of, 660-661, 752

Pruritus—cont'd
  with head lice, 761
  with scabies, 760
Pseudoaddiction, 1050b
Pseudohypertrophic muscular dystrophy, 119t, 1863t, 1864-1867, 1864f, 1865f
Pseudomenstruation, in newborn, 243, 253t
Pseudomonas aeruginosa infection, in cystic fibrosis, 1405, 1408
Pseudopodia, 1256, 1535
Pseudostrabismus, 196f
Psoriasis, 774t
Psychologic aspects
  of adolescent alcohol abuse, 889-890
  of ambiguous genitalia, 489-490, 489b
  of anorexia nervosa, 877
  of burns, 1246-1248
  of congenital malformations, 416-418
  of enuresis, 783
  of HIV infection, 1576
  of obesity, 871-872
  of obstructive uropathy, 486-487
  of parenting high-risk newborn, 366-368, 366b
  of parenting special needs child, 416-418, 922, 933-935, 933b, 935b
  of preparation for procedures, 1103-1108, 1104b-1105b, 1106f, 1107b, 1108b
  of smoking, 887
  of suicide, 897-899
  of terminal illness, 958, 961
  of terminally illness, 958
  of ulcers, 1443
Psychologic counseling; see Counseling.
Psychomotor seizures, 1686-1687
Psychosexual development, 230, 230t
Psychosocial development, 230, 230t
  in adolescents, 804t, 812-817, 827-828
  in infants, 501-502
  in preschoolers, 630-631, 630b, 639t
  in school-age children, 700-701, 701f
  in toddlers, 594
Psychosocial history, 158
Psychostimulants
  abuse of, 886t, 892, 1805
  for attention deficit hyperactivity disorder, 789, 790, 790b, 791
  for Tourette syndrome, 793
  in fragile X syndrome, 994
Psychotherapy; see Counseling.
Ptosis, 193
Ptyalin, in infants, 496
Puberty; see also Sexual development.
  chronic illness or disability during, 916
  delayed, in athletes, 1804
  diabetes and, 1751
  neuroendocrine events of, 803, 803f
  physical growth during, 805, 807-809
  precocious, 1714-1715, 1714b
Pubic hair, 805, 807f
  development of, premature, 1714-1715
  in females, 222
  in males, 221
Public health nursing, 12
Pudendum, 222, 222f
Puerto Ricans; see Latinos.
Pulmicort (budesonide)
  for asthma, 1391
  for inflammatory bowel disease, 1440

Pulmonary; *see also* under Lung(s); Respiratory.
Pulmonary artery(ies)
 banding of, for tricuspid atresia, 1498b
 in transposition of great arteries, 1499b, 1499f
Pulmonary aspiration; *see* Aspiration, pulmonary.
Pulmonary atresia, 1496b
Pulmonary blood flow
 after cardiac shunt procedure, 1489
 decreased, cardiac defects with, 1496, 1496f, 1497b-1498b
 increased, cardiac defects with, 1491, 1492b-1494b, 1492f
Pulmonary congestion, in congestive heart failure, 1478
Pulmonary diffusion defects, respiratory failure and, 1331
Pulmonary disturbances, due to noninfectious irritants, 1376-1383
Pulmonary edema
 after heart surgery, 1507
 in burn patients, 1233
 in congestive heart failure, 1478
 respiratory distress syndrome and, 380-381
Pulmonary embolism, 1795
Pulmonary function tests, 1312, 1313t
 for asthma, 1389, 1407
Pulmonary hypertension, 1490-1491
 congenital diaphragmatic hernia and, 476
 persistent, of newborn, 397-398, 398f
Pulmonary infections; *see* Respiratory infections.
Pulmonary interstitial emphysema, 389
 respiratory distress syndrome and, 381
Pulmonary status
 after heart surgery, 1507
 in burn patients, 1233-1234, 1243
Pulmonary vascular resistance, 1468
 respiratory distress syndrome and, 380
Pulmonary veins, in total anomalous pulmonary venous connection, 1499b-1500b, 1500f
Pulmonic stenosis, 1496b, 1496f
Pulmonic valve, 1465
 heart sounds and, 215
Pulmozyme (dornase alfa), in cystic fibrosis, 1408
Pulse(s); *see also* Heart rate.
 alternating, 217b
 apical, and digoxin administration, 1481
 bigeminal, 217b
 brachial, 1337f, 1338
 carotid, 1335, 1337f, 1338
 Corrigan, 217b
 dicrotic, 217b
 grading of, 184t
 in neurologic assessment, 1649
 location of, 215f
 measurement of, 179, 215f, 220
 palpation of, 179, 215f, 220, 220f
 paradoxical, 217b
 paradoxical pressure of, after heart surgery, 1507
 patterns of, 217b
 pedal, cardiac catheterization and, 1472
 thready, 217b
 water-hammer, 217b

Pulse Doppler, for testing cardiac function, 1471
Pulse generator, of pacemaker, 1525
Pulse oximetry, 1313-1314, 1314f
 in carbon monoxide poisoning, 1381
 nursing tips for, 1316
 vs transcutaneous monitoring, 1316
Pulsed dye laser, 302
Pulsus alternans, 217b
Pulsus bigeminus, 217b
Pulsus paradoxus, 217b
Pump mechanism, in intestinal absorption, 1419
Puncture wounds, 745, 752
 of lung, 1315t
Punishment, 84, 88
 corporal, 88
 in moral development, 597
Pupil(s), 194
 in neurologic assessment, 1650-1651, 1650f
 of newborn, 243, 252t
 reactivity of, 1650, 1650f
Pupillary reflex, in newborn, 259, 263t
Pure red blood cell aplasia, 1559
Purging type of bulimia, 883b
Purified protein derivative, for tuberculin skin test, 1373, 1373b
Purinethol (mercaptopurine), 1591t
Purkinje fibers, 1467
Purpura
 Henoch-Schönlein, 1569-1570, 1570f
  renal involvement in, 1270t
 idiopathic thrombocytopenic, 1566-1567, 1567b
 in meningococcemia, 1678, 1678f
Pustule, 744f
Pyelonephritis, 1267, 1269
Pyloric sphincter, circumferential muscle of, 1446
Pyloric stenosis, 1446-1448, 1447f
Pyloromyotomy, for hypertrophic pyloric stenosis, 1447, 1447f
Pyoderma, 755t
Pyothorax, 1302
Pyramidal system, 1832, 1833f
Pyrantel pamoate, 666t
Pyrazinamide (PZA), for tuberculosis, 1374
Pyrethrin, for head lice, 761-762
Pyridostigmine (Mestinon), for myasthenia gravis, 1851
Pyridoxine, functions and disturbances of, 557t
Pyrvinium pamoate, 666t

**Q**

Quaaludes, 886t, 892
Quadrants, abdominal, 217, 217f
Quadriplegia, in spinal cord injury, 1852, 1856; *see also* Spinal cord injury.
Quadruplets; *see* Multiple births.
Quality improvement, 28
Quality of life, terminal illness and, 949-950, 949t
 pain management in, 956-958, 957b, 957f
Questions
 closed-ended, 144
 open-ended, 143-144
 "What If," 151b
Questran (cholestyramine), for hypercholesterolemia, 1521
QUESTT approach, in pain assessment, 1049

Quetiopine, for schizophrenia, 799
Quintuplets; *see* Multiple birth.

**R**

Rabies, 1682-1683
Race/ethnicity, 34-35; *see also* Cultural factors; specific racial and ethnic groups.
 adoption and, 93
 as risk factor, 104
 classification of, 35b
 definition of, 31, 34
 family structure and, 70t
 genetic disorders and, 51-57, 56t
 health promotion programs and, 834-835
 HIV infection and, 1572-1573
 mortality and, 4, 820
 physical characteristics and, 57
 physiologic jaundice and, 305
 school drop-out rate and, 819
 sickle cell disease and, 1547
 skin color and, 187-188, 188f
 stereotyping and, 34-35
 suicide and, 896-897, 896f, 897b
 traditional treatments and, 1055b
Rachischisis, 424b; *see also* Spina bifida.
Rachitic rosary, 209
Radial head dislocation, 1780, 1799
Radiant heat loss, in newborn, 265
 at high risk, 339-340
Radiant warmer, for high-risk newborn, 340-341
Radiation exposure
 cancer and, 1586
 fetal, 330
Radiation somnolence syndrome, 1601-1602
Radiation therapy, 1594, 1595t
 complications of, 1595t, 1601-1602, 1605, 1618
 dental care in, 1605
 extended field, 1617
 for brain tumors, 1620-1622
 for Ewing sarcoma, 1628
 for Hodgkin disease, 1617-1618
 for leukemia, 1614
 for neuroblastoma, 1626
 for retinoblastoma, 1633
 for rhabdomyosarcoma, 1632
 for Wilms tumor, 1630
 involved field, 1617
 long-term complications of, 1635-1637, 1636t
 of head and neck, 1605
 total nodal, 1617
Radioallergosorbent test (RAST), 569
 for bee stings, 776
 in allergic rhinitis, 1384
 in asthma, 1390
Radiofrequency ablation, for supraventricular tachycardia, 1526
Radiography
 cranial, 1653t
 gastrointestinal, 1421t
  for diagnosis of Crohn disease, 1440
 in asthma, 1390
 in bone age determination, 1711, 1711b
 in bronchopulmonary dysplasia, 391
 in cardiac function assessment, 1469
 in developmental dysplasia of hip, 449
 in necrotizing enterocolitis, 396
 in pulmonary function assessment, 1312-1313, 1314t

Radiography—cont'd
in respiratory distress syndrome, 383
of fractures, 1780
Radioiodine, for hyperthyroidism, 1720
Rancho Los Amigos Scale, 1660b, 1674
Random-dot-E test, 196-197, 198t
Range of motion
assessment of, 225
physical assessment of, in newborn, 262
play activities and, 1111b
Range of motion exercises
for unconscious child, 1659
in cerebral palsy, 1840
Range of state, in neonatal behavioral
assessment, 245b
Ranitidine (Zantac)
for gastroesophageal reflux, 1429
for peptic ulcer disease, 1445
Rape, 858-860
prevention of, 860
statutory, 858
Rapid immunofluorescent antibody (IFA)
test, for respiratory syncytial virus
infection, 1367
Rash
comfort measures for, 660-661
in chickenpox, 652f, 653t
in drug reactions, 772
in erythema infectiosum, 654f, 655t
in erythema toxicum neonatorum, 300
in Henoch-Schönlein purpura, 1570, 1570f
in Kawasaki disease, 1514
in Lyme disease, 764, 765
in measles, 656f, 657t
in roseola (exanthema subitum), 654f, 655t
in rubella, 658f, 659t
in scarlet fever, 660f, 661t
in Stevens-Johnson syndrome, 773
in systemic lupus erythematosus, 1825, 1828
Rashkind procedure, 1499b
RAST (radioallergosorbent test), 569
for bee stings, 776
in allergic rhinitis, 1384
in asthma, 1390
Rastelli procedure, for transposition of great
arteries, 1499b
Rating game, 151b
Raynaud phenomenon, in systemic lupus
erythematosus, 1825
RCF formula, 282t
RDS; see Respiratory distress syndrome.
Reactive attachment disorder, 505
Reactive hyperemia, 1122
Reactivity, neonatal periods of, 245
Reading, 704
blindness and, 1004
in school-age children, 712
Reading materials, developmental impact of, 39
Reasoning, disciplinary, 85-86
Rebound hypoglycemia, 405
Rebound tenderness, 219, 1433
Receptive language, 1007
Reciprocal gait orthosis, 1773
Reciprocal translocation, 115
Reciprocity
concept of, 703, 704
maternal attachment and, 284-285
visual impairment and, 1003

Recombinant human deoxyribonuclease
(DNase), in cystic fibrosis, 1408
Recombinant human erythropoietin
for anemia, 399
in chronic renal failure, 1291
Recombinant human growth factors, for skin
disorders, 753
Recombinant human growth hormone, in
chronic renal failure, 1291
Recommended Dietary Allowance (RDA),
560, 564
Recording for the Blind and Dyslexic, 1004
Records; see also Documentation.
confidentiality of, 141-142
Rectal atresia, 466
Rectal biopsy, in Hirschsprung disease, 1427
Rectal bleeding, with Meckel diverticulum, 1437
Rectal drug administration, 1065b, 1159-1160
Rectal malformations, 466, 466b, 468-470,
468f, 469f
Rectal prolapse, 223
in cystic fibrosis, 1406, 1410
Rectal stenosis, 466
Rectal temperature, 178-179, 179f, 180b-181b,
182t-183t; see also Temperature.
Rectal ulcers, in cancer, 1601
Rectosphincteric reflex, absence of, in
Hirschsprung disease, 1426
Rectourethral fistula, 468, 468f
Rectovaginal fistula, 261, 466, 468, 468f
Rectum, in newborn, 254t, 261-262
Recumbent length, 176f, 177
Recurrent abdominal pain, 796-797, 797b
Red blood cell(s); see Erythrocyte(s).
Red bone marrow, 1531
Red reflex, 194, 195
in newborn, 259
Reducing substances, tests of, 1420t
Reduction device, for developmental dysplasia
of hip, 449-450, 450f
home care and, 450-451
Reed-Sternberg cell, 1617
Referral, in communication impairment, 1012-
1013, 1013b
Reflex(es)
abdominal, 220
Achilles, 227f
anal, 223
arteriolar light, 195
assessment of, 226, 227f, 1651-1652
Babinski, 225, 1652
biceps, 226, 226f
blink, 194, 263t
brachioradialis, 227f
cat's eye, in retinoblastoma, 1632-1633, 1632f
choking, 1309; see also Choking.
corneal, 1650
corneal light, 195-196, 196f
cremasteric, 221-222, 222f
crossed extensor, in cerebral palsy, 1837
Cushing, 1649
deep tendon, 226
grading of, 227t
grasp, 225
in cerebral palsy, 1836, 1837
in neurologic assessment, 226, 226f, 227f,
1650, 1651-1652
infantile (visceral) swallow, vs mature
(somatic) swallow, 496-497, 497f

Reflex(es)—cont'd
knee jerk, 227f
light, otoscopic, 203
Moro, in cerebral palsy, 1837
neonatal, 262, 262f, 263t
in behavioral assessment, 245b
neurologic, in infants, 494, 494b, 494f
parachute, 494f
patellar, 227f
plantar, 225
primitive, 243
rectosphincteric, Hirschsprung disease
and, 1426
red, 194, 195
righting, in infants, 494b, 498
superficial, 226
tonic neck, in cerebral palsy, 1837
triceps, 226, 227f
use of, in infants, 502, 503t
Reflex apnea, 1309
Reflux
gastroesophageal, 1429-1432
of urine, 1258-1259
Refraction, 1000
Refractive errors, 1000, 1001b
correction of, 1005-1006
Regeneration, of epithelial wounds, 745
Regional anesthesia, 1065b
Reglan (metoclopramide), for
gastroesophageal reflux, 1429
Regranex (becoplermin), for skin
disorders, 753
Regression, in toddlers, 609
Regurgitation
high-risk newborn and, 343
passive, in gastroesophageal reflux, 1429
vs vomiting, 1217
with feeding, 571
Rehabilitation
after cranial surgery, 1624-1625
in head injury, 1660b, 1673-1674
in spinal cord injury, 1861-1862, 1861b
Rehydration therapy; see Fluid management.
Reinforcement, aggressive behavior and,
641-642
Rejection, of transplanted kidney, 1300
Relaxation techniques, 719
in pain management, 1059b
Religion; see also Cultural factors; Spiritual;
Spirituality.
beliefs and practices of, 57-62, 58t-62t
blood transfusion and, 1539b
folk healing and, 49
home care and, 1021
neonatal death and, 370-371
terminal illness and, 958
Remicade (infliximab), for inflammatory
bowel disease, 1440
Renal; see also Kidney(s).
Renal agenesis, bilateral, 479t
Renal calculi, immobilization and, 1764,
1794-1795
Renal calyx
major and minor, 1256, 1256f
obstruction of, 485t
Renal colic, 486
Renal disease, in systemic lupus
erythematosus, 1827

Renal failure
  acute, 1283-1287
    acute poststreptococcal
      glomerulonephritis and, 1272
    clinical manifestations of, 1284-1285
    diagnosis of, 1285
    etiology of, 1283-1284
    in hemolytic uremic syndrome, 1281
    nursing care in, 1287
    pathophysiology of, 1284
    prognosis of, 1287
    treatment of, 1285-1287
  chronic, 1287-1294
    causes of, 1288, 1288f
    hyperparathyroidism and, 1723
    nursing care of, 1291-1293
    nursing care plan for, 1294-1295
    pathophysiology of, 1288-1289, 1289b
  hemolysis and, 1540
  prevention of, 1285
Renal function
  dehydration and, 1178
  hypertension and, 1517
  in burn injuries, 1232
  in infants, 1258
  lead poisoning and, 677f, 678
Renal osteodystrophy, in chronic renal
    failure, 1289
Renal pelvis, 1256
  congenital anomalies of, 479t
  structure and function of, 1258-1259
Renal replacement therapy, 1293-1301; see also
    Dialysis; Hemofiltration; Renal
    transplantation.
  in acute renal failure, 1286
Renal rickets, in chronic renal failure, 1289
Renal rupture, 1283
Renal scarring, 1267
Renal structures, in infants, 497, 1258
Renal system, immobilization effects on,
    1764, 1771t
Renal transplantation, 1298-1301
  immunosuppressants in, 1299-1300
  nursing care in, 1300-1301
  prognosis for, 1300
  rejection of kidney in, 1300
  selection of recipients for, 1299, 1299b
Renal trauma, 1282-1283
Renal tubular acidosis, 1279-1280
  distal (type I), 1280
  proximal (type II), 1279-1280
Renal tubular disorders, 1279-1281
Renal tubule(s)
  convoluted, 1256, 1256f, 1257
  Fanconi syndrome and, 1280
  functions of, 1257-1258, 1279
  in infants, 1258
  necrosis of, in acute renal failure, 1284
  reabsorption by, 1255, 1257, 1275
  secretion and, 1255, 1257
Renin, 1256
Renin-angiotensin-aldosterone mechanism, in
    congestive heart failure, 1477, 1479
Rennin, in infants, 496
Reperfusion injury, hypoxic-ischemic,
    perinatal, 400-401
Reproductive system; see also Genitalia;
    Genitourinary tract.
  female, health problems of, 844-849

Reproductive system—cont'd
  in cystic fibrosis, 1406-1407
  in spinal cord injury, 1862
  male, health problems of, 842-844
  normal development of, 487, 488f
Research, nursing, 22
Residential care, 938-939, 986, 986b
Resiliency, family, 67
Resistance, of lung tissue, 1304, 1307, 1307b
  respiratory infections and, 1345
Resolve Through Sharing, 370
Resonance, on chest percussion, 212
RespiGam, 391, 1367-1368, 1368b
Respiration(s); see also Breathing.
  air-hunger, 1184
  assessment of, 1310, 1345b
  grunting, 1478
    in congestive heart failure, 1478, 1483
    in neurologic assessment, 1650
  Kussmaul, 1184, 1735
  regulation of, 1309-1310
Respiratory acidosis, 1183-1184, 1183b, 1183t
Respiratory alkalosis, 1183b, 1183t, 1184
Respiratory arrest, 1331
  emergency treatment for, 1333-1334
  families and, 1333
Respiratory depression, 1331
  opioids and, 1049, 1067, 1068b
Respiratory distress, in newborn, 265, 289
  congenital diaphragmatic hernia and,
    475-476
  phrenic nerve paralysis and, 299
Respiratory distress syndrome, 379-388
  clinical manifestations of, 381, 382f
  complications of, 381
  diabetic mother and, 405
  diagnosis of, 382-383
  nursing considerations in, 387-388
  pathophysiology of, 379-381, 380f, 381t
  prevention of, 387
  treatment of, 383-387, 384t
Respiratory dysfunction
  assessment of, 1310-1317
  diagnostic tests for, 1312-1317, 1315t
  in cerebral palsy, 1837
  in gastrointestinal obstructive disorders, 1446
  in smoke inhalation injury, 1381
  long-term, 1383-1413
Respiratory failure, 1331-1341
  clinical manifestations of, 1332b
  conditions predisposing to, 1331
  definition of, 1331
  management of, 1332-1333
  recognition of, 1332
Respiratory function, 1306-1310
  after heart surgery, 1505
  defenses in, 1310
  gas exchange in, 1308-1310
  in cystic fibrosis, 1401, 1404, 1406
Respiratory infections; see also Pneumonia.
  assessment and observations in, 1344b,
    1345b
  asthma and, 1399
  etiology and characteristics of, 1344-1345
  general aspects of, 1343-1347
  group A β-hemolytic streptoccoccal,
    rheumatic fever and, 1511
  hypoxemia and, 1490
  in cystic fibrosis, 1405, 1407, 1408

Respiratory infections—cont'd
  in hypoxemia, 1490
  microorganisms causing, 1344
  nursing care for, 1344-1347
  nursing care plan for, 1347-1350
  of lower respiratory tract, 1365-1368
  of upper respiratory tract, 1350-1361
  postoperative, 1117
  prevention of spread of, 1346
  signs and symptoms of, 1344b, 1345
Respiratory insufficiency, 1331
Respiratory movements, 210, 210f, 211
Respiratory quotient, 1308
Respiratory rate
  assessment of, 210-211
  heart rate and, 211
  in infants and children, 496, 1306-1307
  in newborns, 251t, 256, 260
    with respiratory distress syndrome, 381
  measurement of, 179
  postoperative alterations in, 1119t
Respiratory secretion specimens, 1148-1149
Respiratory stridor, in acute
    laryngotracheobronchitis, 1364
Respiratory support, for high-risk newborn, 338
Respiratory syncytial virus
  bronchiolitis due to, 1366-1368, 1366t, 1367b
  bronchopulmonary dysplasia and, 391
  immune globulin of, for prophylaxis of RSV
    infection, 1367-1368, 1368b
  vs asthma, 1367
Respiratory therapist, 387
Respiratory therapy, 1317-1331
  aerosol therapy in, 1319-1320
  artificial ventilation in, 1323-1325
  bronchial (postural) drainage in, 1320
  chest physiotherapy in, 1320-1323
  oxygen therapy in, 1317-1319
  tracheostomy in, 1325-1331
Respiratory tract; see also Lung(s).
  development of, 593, 809
  immobilization effects on, 1764, 1771t
  in Down syndrome, 990, 992
  in newborn, 240-241
    after surgery, 421t, 423
    at high risk, 336b, 376-393
    with esophageal atresia, 465
    with sepsis, 394b
  procedures on, bacterial endocarditis
    and, 1510b
  structure of, 1303-1306
Respiratory units
  structure and function of, 1306
  terminal, 1305
Rest; see also Immobilization.
  after heart surgery, 1505
  in respiratory infections, 1346
  in systemic lupus erythematosus, 1828
Restraint(s), 1137-1140, 1138f-1140f
  in cleft lip and palate surgery, 460
  in cranial surgery, 1623
  in otoscopic examination, 201, 201f
Restricting type of anorexia nervosa, 878b
Restrictive lung disease, respiratory failure
    and, 1331
Resuscitation; see Cardiopulmonary
    resuscitation.
Retching, 1218
Rete pegs, 242, 349, 740

Retention control training, for treatment of enuresis, 784
Reticular activating system, 1647
Reticular dysgenesis, 1569t
Reticular formation, 1647
Reticulocyte count, 1532, 1533f, 1536t
  in iron deficiency anemia, 1544
    after treatment, 1545
  reference ranges for, 1901t
Retin-A (tretinoin), for acne, 841
Retinal hemorrhage
  in newborn, 296b
  in shaken baby syndrome, 1668, 1669
Retinoblastoma, 1597, 1632-1635, 1632f, 1633b, 1634f
Retinol, functions of and disturbances in, 556t
Retinopathy, diabetic, 1735
Retinopathy of prematurity, 399-400, 400b
  nutrition and, 344
Retractile testes, 480, 481
Retractions, chest, 210, 1310, 1311f
  in congestive heart failure, 1478
Retrolental fibroplasia; *see* Retinopathy of prematurity.
Retroperitoneal rhabdomyosarcoma, 1631b
Retroviruses, 1586
Reversibility, concept of, 703, 704
Review of systems, 159-160, 159b
Revised Denver Prescreening Developmental Questionnaire, 237, 1876
Revised Infant Temperament Questionnaire (RITQ), 505, 507, 509
Rewards
  in behavior modification, 86-87
  in moral development, 597
Rewarming
  for frostbite, 771
  for hypothermia, 771
Reye syndrome, 1683-1684, 1683b
  varicella and, 651
Rh incompatibility, 310, 312f, 314-315; *see also* Hemolytic disease of newborn.
Rh system, 310
Rhabdomyosarcoma, 1631-1632, 1631b, 1631t, 1632b
Rheumatic fever, 1511-1513
  acute, 1351
  diagnosis of, 1512, 1512b
  prevention of, 1512-1513, 1512b, 1513t
  treatment of, 1512-1513, 1512b
Rheumatic heart disease, 1511
Rheumatoid arthritis, juvenile, 1820-1825; *see also* Juvenile rheumatoid arthritis.
Rhinitis, allergic, 1383-1385
Rhizotomy, selective dorsal, for cerebral palsy, 1839
Rho immune globulin, 314
Rhonchi, 214t
Rhythm disorders of speech, 1007
Rib(s), 208-209, 208f
  in newborn, lung compliance and, 1307
  lung position relative to, 210, 211f
  thoracic size during respirations and, 1304, 1304f
Ribavirin, for respiratory syncytial virus bronchiolitis, 1367
Riboflavin, functions of and disturbances in, 556t
RICE therapy, 1800
  in hemophilia, 1565

Richmond screw, in intracranial pressure monitoring, 1656
Rickets
  renal, in chronic renal failure, 1289
  vegetarian diets and, 560
  vitamin D-deficiency, 555
Rickettsial infections, 763, 765t
Rickettsialpox, 765t
Rifampin, for tuberculosis, 1374
Right to die, 966
Righting reflexes, in infants, 494b, 498
Right-left confusion, 791
Rigidity, 1647b
Riley Infant Pain Scale, 1056t
Rimantadine, for influenza, 1356
Ring chromosome, 113
Ringworm, 759-760, 759t, 760f
Rinne test, 205t
Risk
  empiric, 131
  theoretic, 131
Risk factors
  community-wide, 104
  in nursing diagnosis, 25
Risk-taking behavior
  in school-age children, 732
  sexual, 849-850
Risperidone
  for schizophrenia, 799
  for Tourette syndrome, 793
Risus sardonicus, in tetanus, 1849
Ritalin, for attention deficit hyperactivity disorder, 789, 790, 790b, 791
Ritualism
  in school-age children, 711, 711f
  in toddlers, 594, 610
Robertsonian translocation, 115
Rocephin, intramuscular, 766b
Rocky Mountain spotted fever, 765f, 765t
Roe v. Wade, 853
Rofecoxib, for juvenile rheumatoid arthritis, 1822
Rogers, Linda, 12
Rohypnol; *see* Flunitrazepam.
Rolandic seizure, 1686
Role(s)
  family, 67t, 68-69
  learning of, 75-77
  parental, 75-77
  sibling, 76t, 77
  social, 32-33
  types of, 76b, 77
Role continuity/discontinuity, 76
Roller skates, injuries with, 734
Rolling over, in infants, 499
Roman Catholic religion, neonatal death and, 370
Romberg test/sign, 226
Rooting reflex, 260, 260f, 263t
Roseola, 654f, 654t-655t
Rotavirus, diarrhea and, 1208-1209, 1209t
Roundworm infection, 665t
Routine, sense of control and, hospitalization and, 1045, 1045f
Rovsing sign, 1433
Roxicodone; *see* Oxycodone.
RSV immune globulin, 391
RSV-IGIV (respiratory syncytial virus immune globulin), for prophylaxis of RSV infection, 1367-1368, 1368b

Rubella
  congenital, 328t
  immunization for, 529t, 533
    contraindications to, 537t
    in adolescents, 541b, 833-834
    Kawasaki disease and, 1516
    recommended, 529t, 533
  manifestations and management of, 658f, 658t-659t
Rubeola; *see* Measles.
Rubidomycin, 1592t
Rule of nines, 1228
Rules and rituals
  in school-age children, 711, 711f
  in toddlers, 594, 610
Rumination, 574
Runaways, 686
Russell traction, 1789f, 1790

**S**

$S_1$ heart sound, 215, 216, 216t, 217
$S_2$ heart sound, 215, 216t, 217
$S_3$ heart sound, 215, 216t
$S_4$ heart sound, 215, 216t, 217
Sabril (vigabatrin), for infantile spasms, 1689
SADD; *see* Students Against Drunk Driving.
Sadness, chronic, 136
Safe Times, for adolescent health screening interview, 826, 826b
Safety, 10-11, 1132-1140, 1758b, 1759b; *see also* Injuries.
  active, 10
  automobile; *see* Car seats/restraints.
  cultural factors in, 11b
  deaf-blindness and, 1006
  drug dosage and, 1150-1151
  during transport, 1136, 1137f
  environmental modifications for, 1135-1136, 1136f
  for hospitalized visually impaired children, 1004-1005
  for infants, 541-550, 542t-543t
  for latchkey children, 721b
  for seizures, 1693
  hearing aid batteries and, 998
  hemophilia and, 1562-1563
  home care and, 1028
  in neonatal intensive care unit, 338
  limit-setting and, 1136
  of home apnea monitors, 587, 587b
  passive, 10
  playground, 618b
  restraining methods and, 1136-1140, 1138f-1140f
  toys and, 1136
  water, 1676
Safety belts, 619, 620b
Safety glass, 623
Safety hazards, in daycare centers, 517
Safety seats; *see* Car seats/restraints.
St. Vitus dance, in rheumatic fever, 1512
Salaam seizures, 1688
Salicylates
  for Kawasaki disease, 1515, 1516
  for rheumatic fever, 1513
  long-term, varicella and, 651
  reference ranges for, 1901t
  signs of poisoning with, 672b

Saline
for flushing peripheral intermittent infusion device, 1198, 1199b
in tracheostomy suctioning, 1326, 1327b
normal, 1427
Saline well, 1198, 1199b
Saliva
esophageal atresia and, 465
in cystic fibrosis, 1401
in fluid and electrolyte disturbances, 1187t
tooth decay and, 780
Salivary glands, 1416
development of, 1417
of newborn, 242
secretions of, 1418
Salmeterol (Serevent), for asthma, 1392
Salmon patch, 302
Salmonella, diarrhea and, 1209t-1210t
Salpingitis, 863
Salt, in intravenous solutions, 1189
Salt intake
hypertension and, 1518
in congestive heart failure, 1480
in nephrotic syndrome, 1276-1279
Salt supplements, in cystic fibrosis, 1410
Same-sex family, 72-73
Santmyer swallow, in infants, 497
SaO₂, reference ranges for, 1900t
Sarcoma
Ewing, 1626-1627, 1628-1629
osteogenic, 1626-1628
soft tissue, 1631-1632, 1631b, 1631t, 1632b
Satiety behavior, in newborn, feeding and, 280
Savants, 1009
Scabies, 760-761, 761f
Scald burns, 621, 1227, 1248
prevention of, 542t, 543t, 547, 549b
Scale, on skin, 745f
Scale for Use in Newborns, 355t
Scales, weighing, 177, 177f
Scalp
caput succedaneum and, 296, 297f
examination of, 189
lacerations of
bleeding from, 1665, 1670
suturing of, 1672, 1672b
Scalp hair, 741
Scalp vein, as site of venipuncture, 1193-1194, 1194f
Scaphocephaly, 444f
Scaphoid abdomen, 476
Scarf sign, 377f
gestational age and, 250b
Scarlet fever, manifestations and management of, 660f, 660t-661t
Scarlet Red, for burn wounds, 1240t
Scarring, 746f
acne and, 842
in burn injuries, 1231, 1245-1246, 1245f-1246f
in wound healing, 747
of eardrum, otitis media and, 1358
renal, 1267
Schema, coordination of, in infant's cognitive development, 503-504
Scheuermann kyphosis, 1809-1810
Schizophrenia, in school-age children, 799, 799b

School; see also Education.
adjustments in
for burn patients, 1247
for children with attention deficit hyperactivity disorder, 791
for children with learning disorders, 791, 792
for children with tracheostomy, 1330-1331, 1331b
adolescent health behavior and, 818-819
attitudes toward, 714
corporal punishment in, 715b
cultural aspects of, 37
experience of, in school-age children, 714-716, 715b, 716b
health promotion efforts in, 822
in cerebral palsy, 1841
meal programs in, 722-723, 722b
"no nit" policies of, 763b
prevention of school phobia and, 795
sense of accomplishment and, 700-701
sex education in, 710
social environment of, 819
socialization in, 37
violence in, 718
School buses, seat belts in, 733
School dropouts, adolescent pregnancy and, 851
School grades, 819
School health programs, 728-730
components of, 728b
health services offered under, 728b
School nurse
administration of medications by, 730
care of children with chronic illness or disability by, 730
collaboration with teachers of, 730b
qualifications of, 729
roles of, 723, 723b, 729-730
School phobia, 794-796
School problems
adolescent pregnancy and, 851
in adolescents, 833
School vision, 1000
School-age child
as latchkey child, 720, 720f
biologic development in, 699-700
bites and stings in, 775-780
cognitive development in, 702-704
communication with, 149
constipation in, 1424
dental health in, 727-728, 780-783
disorders of continence in, 783-786
disorders with behavioral components in, 786-799
School-age child, divorce and, 95, 95b
School-age child
dying, 954; see also Terminal illness.
families of, 736
health behaviors in, 720-721
hearing impairment in, 996-997, 997b; see also Hearing impairment.
height and weight in, 699, 723b
hemophilia in, 1562-1563
hospitalized
bodily injury and pain in, 1038
loss of control in, 1035
separation anxiety in, 1033-1034

School-age child—cont'd
human immunodeficiency virus infection in, 1576
injury prevention in, 730-736
language development in, 705-706
limit-setting and discipline of, 716-717
lying and cheating in, 717
maturation of systems in, 699-700
mental retardation in, 978t
moral development in, 704-705
nutrition in, 721-723
pain in, 1054b
phenylketonuria in, 324
physical activity in, 724-727
physical examination of, 173t
play in, 711-714
psychosocial development in, 700-701
school experience of, 714-716, 715b, 716b
school health programs and, 728-730
self-concept in, 707-709
sexuality in, 709-711
skin disorders in, 740-754
chemical or physical contacts and, 767-772
congenital and miscellaneous, 773-775
drug sensitivity and, 772-773
infections and, 754-755, 758-763
lesions of, 754b
systemic disorders related to, 763-767
sleep and rest in, 723-724
social development in, 706-707
special needs; see also Special needs child.
promotion of normal development in, 911t, 914-915, 915f
spiritual development in, 705
stress and, 717-720
teacher interactions with, 715-716, 716b
temperament in, 701-702
SCID; see Severe combined immunodeficiency disease.
Scintigraphy
hepatobiliary, 1422t
in gastroesophageal reflux diagnosis, 1429
Sclera, 194
of newborn, 259
Scleral hemorrhage, in newborn, 252t, 296b
Sclerema neonatorum, 251t
Sclerosing agent, 1197
Sclerosing cholangitis, in Crohn disease, 1439
Scolding, 86
Scoliosis, 223, 1809f, 1810-1816, 1810f
bracing for, 1773-1774, 1811, 1812f, 1813f, 1814
causes of, 1811b
clinical manifestations of, 1810
diagnosis of, 1810-1811, 1810f, 1812f
nursing care for, 1813-1816
nursing care plan for, 1815-1816
paralytic, 1856-1857, 1858
screening for, 1811
surgery for, 1812-1813, 1812f, 1814
treatment of, 1811-1815
Scoliosis Research Society, 1815
Scorpions, bites of, 777t
Scratching; see also Pruritus.
prevention of, 752
Screening, 106, 106b
developmental, 233-237, 234t, 235-237, 235t, 236b, 1874-1879
economic aspects of, 127

Screening—cont'd
ethical issues in, 127
false-positive/false-negative results in, 127
family concerns about, 127
for anemia, 1537
for carrier status, 126-127
for communication disorders, 1012
for epidemiologic information, 127
for HIV
in adolescents, 831
in newborns, 267-268
for hypoglycemia, 317, 317b
for hypothyroidism, 321
for inborn errors of metabolism, 125-126, 320
for lead poisoning, 679
for phenylketonuria, 125-126, 267, 323, 323b
for retinopathy of prematurity, 400
for scoliosis, 1811
for sickle cell anemia, 1550, 1554
for suicidality, 901-902
genetic, 125-127
hearing, 204
in newborns, 268, 996, 996b
of adolescents, 824-826, 825b, 826b
of newborns, 267-268, 267b
test sensitivity in, 235
test specificity in, 235
test validity in, 235
vision, 196b, 198-199, 198t, 1880
Screw fixation, 1793
Scrotum
ambiguous genitalia and, 489t
examination of, 221-222, 222f
hydrocele of, 254t, 261, 478f, 479-480
of newborn, 261, 377f
preterm, 376, 377f
Seasonal factors, respiratory infections and, 1345, 1366, 1383
Seat belts, 1758b
for adolescents, 829
for school-age children, 732
for young children, 545-546, 545f, 546f
in school buses, 733
Sebaceous glands, 741-742
of newborn, 243
Seborrheic dermatitis, in infants, 580
Sebum, 741
acne and, 840
Secobarbital, abuse of, 886t
Secondary antibody response, 1572
Secondary groups, 32-33
Secondary prevention, 105
Secretin, 1009
Secretory cells, of gastrointestinal tract, 1417
Secretory immunoglobulin A
in infants, 497
otitis media and, 1357
Sedation
for asthma, 1397
for burn patients, 1237
for cardiac catheterization, 1473
for colic, 572
for hydrocephalus diagnosis, 442
for neurologic diagnostic procedures, 1652-1654, 1655b
preoperative, 1112-1113, 1113b
preparation for, 1108-1109
Seeing eye dog, 1003

Seizures, 1684-1698
absence, 1687t, 1688, 1692
activity restrictions for, 1694
after heart surgery, 1507
assessment of, 1692, 1693b
atonic, 1688
aura and, 1687
classification of, 1685
diagnosis of, 1689-1690
differential diagnosis of, 1689
electroencephalography for, 1689-1690
epileptogenic focus in, 1685
etiology of, 1685, 1685b
evaluation for, 1696
febrile, 1131, 1696-1698, 1697-1698
generalized, 1685, 1687-1688
hypertonic dehydration and, 1177-1178
idiopathic, 1684-1685
in acute renal failure, 1286
in cerebral palsy, 1836
in epilepsy, 1684-1697; see also Epilepsy.
in insulin reaction, 1741, 1750
in newborn, 403-404, 403b, 404t
hypocalcemia and, 318
perinatal hypoxic-ischemic brain injury and, 401
in status epilepticus, 1692
incidence of, 1685
injury prevention in, 1693-1694, 1694b
jackknife, 1688
jacksonian, 1686
meperidine and, sickle cell anemia and, 1553
myoclonic, 1688
nonrecurrent, 1685b
nursing care for, 1693-1696
nursing care plan for, 1697-1698
nursing diagnoses for, 1693
observation and description of, 1693b
partial, 1685, 1686-1687
complex, 1686-1687, 1687t, 1695b
simple, 1686, 1687t
planning for, 1693
postictal state and, 1686
posttraumatic, 1670-1671
psychomotor, 1686-1687
recurrent, 1685b
remission of, 1692
rolandic, 1686
salaam, 1688
sylvan, 1686
terminology for, 1684b
timing of, 1685
tonic-clonic, 1687-1688, 1697b
treatment of, 1690-1692
emergency, 1695b
pharmacologic, 1690, 1691t, 1694-1695
surgical, 1690-1692
triggers of, 1685, 1695-1696
unclassified, 1688-1689
Selective dorsal rhizotomy, for cerebral palsy, 1839
Selenium
functions of and disturbances in, 563t
sources of, 563t
Self-care
by school-age children, 720
by visually impaired, 918-919, 919b, 920, 1025, 1026b, 1027
during hospitalization, 1005

Self-care—cont'd
hospitalization and, 1045
in cerebral palsy, 1840-1841
in chronic illness or disability, 918-919, 919b, 920, 1025, 1026b, 1027
Self-catheterization, for neurogenic bladder, 1860
Self-concept
in adolescents, 810
in school-age children, 708-709
obesity and, 872-873
Self-esteem
immobilization and, 1767, 1767b
in school-age children, 709
skin lesions and, 753, 754b
Self-feeding, mental retardation and, 984-985, 984b, 984f
Self-grooming, mental retardation and, 986
Self-help skills, mental retardation and, 983-986, 984b, 984f
Self-image, 718
Self-injurious behavior, mental retardation and, 983
Self-mastery, promotion of, hospitalization and, 1073
Self-monitoring of blood glucose, in diabetes, 1738, 1748, 1748f
Self-regulation, neonatal, 359t
Self-reporting, in compliance measurement, 1119
Self-stimulatory behavior
blindness and, 1004
mental retardation and, 983
Self-talk, positive, in pain management, 1059b
Semilunar valves, 1465
heart sounds and, 215
Semiocclusive dressing, 749
Semi-vegetarian diet, 560
Senning procedure, for transposition of great arteries, 1499b
Sensation, skin's role in, 740, 742-743
Sensitive periods, in prenatal development, 416, 417f
Sensitivity, test, 235
Sensitization; see also Allergen(s); Allergy(ies).
in hyposensitization injections in asthma, 1393-1394
to foods, 568
Sensitizing agent, 767
Sensorimotor stage, 230t, 232
in infants, 502-504, 503t
in toddlers, 594-596, 595t
Sensorineural hearing loss, 995; see also Hearing impairment.
in high-risk newborn, 995
risk factors for, 996b
treatment of, 996
with otitis media, 1359
Sensory changes, in fluid and electrolyte disturbances, 1188t
Sensory deprivation, in immobilization, 1766
Sensory discrimination, assessment of, 226, 226b
Sensory funciton, immobilization effects on, 1765-1766
Sensory function; see also specific senses.
assessment of, 225-226, 226b
impairment of, 994-1007
in spinal cord injury, 1855, 1855b
in newborn, 243-244, 252t

Sensory function—cont'd
  developmental outcome and, 360-361
  pain and, 352
Sensory interference, 365
Sensory stimulation, for unconscious child,
  1659-1660
Sentence completion, 151b
Separation anxiety, 505-506
  coping with, 514-515
  hospitalization and, 1032-1034, 1041-1044
  in school phobia, 795
Separation from parents
  in infants, 502, 505-506
  preparation of children for, 599
  prolonged and early, 505
Sepsis, 1222
  in high-risk newborn, 393-395, 394b
    with respiratory distress syndrome, 386
  wound, in burn injuries, 1234
Septic arthritis, 1818
Septic meningitis, neonatal, 394
Septic shock, 1219, 1222-1224, 1223f
Septum
  air sac, 1306
  cardiac, 1465, 1465f
  nasal, 206, 206f
Septum primum, 1465, 1465f
Septum secundum, 1465, 1465f
Sequestration crises, in sickle cell anemia, 1549
Serevent (salmeterol), for asthma, 1392
Serialization, skill of, 704
Serologic markers, for hepatitis, 1459
Serologic test
  for acute poststreptococcal
    glomerulonephritis, 1272
  for Lyme disease, 765
  for syphilis, 831
  for ulcerative colitis, 1440
Serotonin, attention deficit hyperactivity
  disorder and, 787, 789
Serotonin reuptake inhibitors
  for depression, 798
  for premenstrual syndrome, 847
Serum cholesterol level
  elevated, 1519-1520
  of adolescents, 833
  reference ranges for, 1896t
Serum enzyme measurements, in
  neuromuscular dysfunction, 1834, 1834b
Serum ferritin, lead poisoning and, 677
Serum glutamic-oxaloacetic transaminase
  (SGOT), in neuromuscular
  dysfunction, 1834b
Serum iron concentration, 1544
Serum prothrombin conversion accelerator,
  1562t
Serum sickness, from antithymocyte globulin,
  1561
Servocontrolled incubator, 339
Servocontrolled radiant warmer, 340-341
Set point
  body temperature and, 1130
  obesity and, 871
Setting-sun sign, 193, 437
Sever disease, 1801t
Severe Chronic Neutropenia Inc., 1569n
Severe combined immunodeficiency disease,
  1570, 1579-1580

Sex assignment, in congenital adrenal
  hyperplasia, 1730-1731
Sex chromosomes, abnormalities of, 116-118
Sex determination, abnormal, 487
Sex education
  in preschoolers, 637-640
  in school-age children, 710
  sexually transmitted disease prevention
    and, 866
Sex hormones, in newborn, 243
Sex play, in school-age children, 709
Sex steroids, 1708t
  regulation of, 1723, 1724
Sex typing, in preschoolers, 632
Sex-role learning, in school-age children,
  706, 709b
Sexual abstinence, for contraception, 855,
  856t, 857
Sexual abuse, 685-687
  characteristics of abusers and victims in, 686
  conditions mistaken for, 689b
  definition of, 683, 685
  disclosure of, 690-691
  genital examination findings and, 689b
  identification of, 687-689, 688b
  in adolescents, 832-833
  in early childhood, 685-687
  initiation and perpetuation of,
    686-687, 686b
  prevention of, 693-694, 694b
  types of, 685-686
Sexual activity
  conflict about, 857
  in adolescents, 814-816, 814f, 830-831, 831,
    849, 850
  in chronic illness or disability, 916-917
  in mental retardation, 982
  sexually transmitted diseases and, 866
Sexual assault; see Rape.
Sexual assault nurse examiners, 859
Sexual curiosity, of preschoolers, 637-640
Sexual development
  ambiguous genitalia and, 487-490, 488f,
    489b, 489t
  at puberty, 805-807, 806f, 807f
  delayed, thalassemia and, 1558, 1559
  early, alcohol and cigarettes and,
    890, 890b
  in boys, 806-807, 807f, 808f
  in Down syndrome, 990
  in girls, 805-806, 806f
  in preschoolers, 632
  in school-age children, 709-711
  in toddlers, 598
  premature, 1714-1715
    in congenital adrenal hyperplasia, 1729
    in precocious puberty, 1714-1715
Sexual function
  in chronic renal failure, 1289
  in spinal cord injury, 1862-1863
Sexual history, 158-159
Sexual identity
  ambiguous genitalia and, 487-490, 488f,
    489b, 489t
  in adolescents, 814
  in infants, 504
  in special needs children, 913
  suicide and, 898, 898b

Sexual orientation
  developmental milestones in, 815
  identification of, 814-816, 816b, 831, 835-836
  suicide and, 898, 898b
Sexuality
  bladder exstrophy and, 484
  health problems related to, 849-860
  same-sex relationships and, 814
Sexually transmitted diseases, 860-866, 866b
  condom use and, 855
  genital lesions due to, 865, 865t
  HIV infection as, 1573, 1576; see also Human
    immunodeficiency virus infection.
  in adolescents, 830-831, 860-866, 866b
  in prepubertal child, sexual abuse and, 689b
SGOT (serum glutamic-oxaloacetic
    transaminase), in neuromuscular
    dysfunction, 1834b
Shake test, of fetal lung maturity, 383
Shaken baby syndrome, 687, 1666, 1668, 1669;
    see also Child abuse.
  physical findings in, 689b
  spinal cord injury in, 1856
Shame, sense of, in toddlers, 594
Shampoo, for seborrheic dermatitis in
    infants, 580
Shaping, in education, in mental
    retardation, 981
SHARE, 1010
Shear, pressure ulcers and, 1124-1125
Shearing forces, in head injury, 1665,
    1665f, 1666
Shift to the left, in oxyhemoglobin
    dissociation curve, 1315, 1315f
Shift to the right, in oxyhemoglobin
    dissociation curve, 1315-1316, 1315f
*Shigella*, diarrhea and, 1210t
Shin splints, 1800, 1801t
Shingles, 758t
  complications with, 651, 660
Shivering, 1130-1131
Shock, 1219-1222
  anaphylactic, 1219
  burn, irreversible, 1237
  clinical manifestations of, 1220
  compensated, 1220
  cultural, 33-34
  diagnosis of, 1220-1221
  emergency treatment of, 1223
  emotional
    child with physical defect and, 417
    chronic illness or disability and, 933
    mourning and, 970
  hemolysis and, 1540
  hypotonic dehydration and, 1177
  hypovolemic, 1219, 1219b
  in dehydration, 1178-1179
  irreversible, 1220, 1237
  isotonic dehydration and, 1176-1177
  pathophysiology of, 1219-1220
  septic, 1219, 1222-1224, 1223f
  spinal, 1856
  treatment of, 1221-1222
  types of, 1219b
  uncompensated, 1220
  with poisoning, 670
Shock lung, 1220
Shoes, for infants, 519-520

Shootings, mortality from, 8, 8t
Short attention span, 791; *see also* Attention
    deficit hyperactivity disorder.
Short bowel syndrome, 1451-1454, 1453b
Short stature
    causes of, 1709t
    constitutional growth delay and, 1710
    familial, 1709
    growth hormone deficiency and, 1709-1713;
        *see also* Hypopituitarism.
    in congenital adrenal hyperplasia, 1729, 1731
Short-bowel syndrome, necrotizing
        enterocolitis and, 396
Short-gut syndrome, necrotizing enterocolitis
        and, 396
Short-term memory, mental retardation and,
        980-981
Shoulder
    Little League, 1801t
    swimmer's, 1801t
Shriners Burn Institutes, 1253
Shunt(s)
    fetal, 241
    in persistent pulmonary hypertension of
        newborn, 397, 398
    in physiologic jaundice, 305
    intracardiac
        hypoxemia and, 1484, 1490
        left-to-right, 1475
        right-to-left, 1484
Shunt procedures
    Blalock-Taussig, 1497b
    for children with cardiac defects, 1488-1489,
        1489f, 1489t
    for hydrocephalus, 440-441, 440f
    for tetralogy of Fallot, 1497, 1497b
    for tricuspid atresia, 1498b
Siblings
    autism and, 1010
    birth order of, 76t, 77, 79, 79b
    family roles of, 76t, 77
    family size and, 77-78
    hospitalized child and, 1041, 1084b
    of adopted child, 90
    of newborn
        attachment of, 285-286, 286f
        neonatal intensive care unit visits by,
            338, 368
    of special needs child, 928-929, 929b, 930b
    parenting issues in, 90-92
    relationships with, 78-79
        in school years, 708
        in toddlers, 605-607
    spacing of, 78
    terminal illness and, 953-954, 958-959
        funeral services and, 967, 967b, 968f
        grief and, 969-970, 970t
    twin; *see* Twins.
Sick-child care, 516
SICKKIDS, 1070n
Sickle cell anemia, 1547-1555
    assessment of, 1551
    basic defect in, 1547
    chest syndrome in, 1550, 1555
    clinical manifestations of, 1547-1550, 1548b
    diagnosis of, 1550
    family support and, 1554-1555
    genetic counseling and, 1554
    hydration in, promotion of, 1552

Sickle cell anemia—cont'd
    newborn screening for, 1550
    nursing care plan for, 1555-1556
    pain management in, 1552-1553, 1553f
    pathophysiology of, 1547-1548, 1549f
    prognosis of, 1551
    renal involvement in, 1270t
    screening for, 1554
    stroke in, 1548, 1550, 1555
    surgical risks in, 1553-1554
    tissue deoxygenation in, minimization
        of, 1552
    transmission of, 1547
    treatment of, 1550-1551
Sickle cell crises, 1549-1550
    minimization of, 1552
    treatment of, 1550-1551
Sickle Cell Disease Association of America,
        Inc., 1554n
Sickle cell trait, 1547
Sickle cell-C disease, 1547
Sickle thalassemia disease, 1547
Sickledex, 1550
Sickle-turbidity test, 1550
Sign language, 998
Signs and symptoms
    in nursing diagnosis, 26
    prodromal, 650
Silence, in communication, 145
Silk glove sign, in inguinal hernia, 477
Silver nitrate
    for burn wounds, 1239t
    for ophthalmia neonatorum prevention, 266
Silver sulfadiazine, for burn wounds, 1239t
Simian crease, 262
Similac, 281t
Similac Human Milk Fortifier, 283t
Similac Lactose Free, 281t
Similac Natural Care Human Milk
        Fortifier, 283t
Similac Neosure, 281t
Similac PM 60/40, 282t
Simple partial seizures, 1686, 1687t
Simplified Assessment of Gestational Age,
        247-248, 247f
SIMV; *see* Synchronized intermittent
        mandatory ventilation.
Sinding-Larsen syndrome, 1801t
Single-gene disorders, 118-120, 119t
Single-parent family, 71-72, 97-98; *see also*
        Divorce.
    special needs child and, 927
Single-photon emission computed
        tomography, cerebral, 1654t
Sinoatrial node, 1467
Sinus arrhythmia, 217, 217b
    in infants, 496
    in newborn, 253t
Sinus bradycardia, 1524-1525
Sinus tachycardia, 1525
Sinus venosus, 1465
Sinuses, paranasal, 191, 191f
    rhabdomyosarcoma of, 1631b
Sister chromatid, 114
Sisters; *see* Siblings.
Sitting, in infants, 499, 500f
Sitting height, 177
Situated approach, communication disorders
        and, 1008

Skateboards, safety with, 734, 735b
Skeletal limb deficiency, 453-454
Skeletal system; *see also* under Bone;
        Musculoskeletal.
    developmental defects in, 446-454, 447t;
        *see also* specific defects.
    immobilization effects on, 1763, 1764-1765,
        1770t
    of newborn, 243
Skeletal traction; *see* Traction.
Skeletal tuberculosis, 1818-1819
Skill acquisition, in school-age children, 726
Skim milk, for infants, 521
Skin
    abdominal, 218
    accessory structures of, 189
    acne and, 839-842
    artificial, for burn wounds, 1241
    bites and stings and, 775-780
    burned; *see* Burns.
    discoloration of, fluid therapy for high-risk
        newborn and, 342
    disorders of; *see* Skin disorders.
    elasticity of, in dehydration, 1185
    examination of, 187-189
        in neurologic assessment, 1650
    functions, 740
    hydration of, atopic dermatitis and, 581
    in anaphylaxis, 1224, 1225
    in congestive heart failure, 1482
    in cystic fibrosis, 1407, 1411
    in Down syndrome, 989t, 990f, 992
    in fluid and electrolyte disturbances, 1187t
    in nutritional assessment, 166t
    in septic shock, 1222
    infections of
        bacterial, 754-755, 754f, 755t
        viral, 755, 758, 758t
    lesions of; *see* Skin lesions.
    of infants and young children, 593, 742
    of newborns, 242-243, 251t-252t, 257
        at high risk, 336b, 349-350, 350b-351b
        bathing and, 268
        congenital hypothyroidism and, 321
        defense against infection and, 243
        in pain, 352b
        postterm, 376
        preterm, 376, 377f
        zinc deficiency and, 349
    structure of, 740-742, 741f
    temperature of, 189; *see also* Temperature.
    texture of, 189
    turgor of, 189
Skin breakdown, 1122-1125, 1124b-1125b,
        1126t; *see also* Pressure ulcers.
    in high-risk newborn, 351b
    in immobilization, 1765, 1765f
Skin cancer, sun exposure and, 769
Skin care, 1121-1125, 1122b, 1123f, 1124b-
        1125b, 1126t
    after cast removal, 1787
    at tracheosotomy stoma site, 1327-1328
    for stump, 1775b, 1795
    in spinal cord injury, 1859
    in traction, 1791b, 1792
    in unconscious child, 1659
    of high-risk newborn, 349-350,
        350b-351b
    reduction device and, 451

Skin color, 187-188, 188f
  fluid therapy for high-risk newborn and, 342
  in assessment of breathing, 1311
  in assessment of heart, 1469
  variations in, 57
Skin coverings, for burn wounds, 1240-1242,
    1240f-1242f
Skin disorders; *see also* specific type.
  causes of, 742
  chemical or physical contacts and, 767-772
  clinical manifestations and diagnosis of,
    742-743
  dressings for, 749, 750t
  drug sensitivity and, 772-773
  general management of, 749-751
  in infants, 578-582
  in newborns, 300-303, 302b, 302f
    from phototherapy, 350
  laboratory findings in, 743, 745
  lesions in; *see* Skin lesions.
  miscellaneous and congenital, 773-775
  nursing care of, 751-754
  objective findings of, 743
  systemic disorders related to, 763-767
  systemic therapy for, 749, 751
  topical therapy for, 749, 752, 753
Skin grafts, for burn wounds, 1241-1242,
    1241b, 1241f-1242f
Skin lesions, 742-745; *see also* Dermatitis.
  age of child and, 742
  configuration and arrangement of, 743
  distribution of, 743
  dressings for, 749, 750t
  in Henoch-Schönlein purpura, 1570, 1570f
  primary, 743, 743f, 744f
  secondary, 743, 745f, 746f
  visible, return to school with, 661
Skin tests
  for allergic rhinitis, 1384
  for allergy, pain control in, 1385
  for asthma, 1390
  for cow's milk allergy, 569
  for tuberculosis, in adolescents, 834
Skin traction, 1788b, 1791b; *see also* Traction.
Skin wounds, 745-749; *see also* Skin lesions.
Skinfold thickness, 874
  in nutritional assessment, 168
  measurement of, 177, 178b
Skin-level gastrostomy device, 1164-1165, 1165f
Skin-to-skin contact, high-risk newborn and
  developmental outcome in, 362
  nutrition and, 344, 347
Skull, 1642; *see also* under Cranial.
  deformities of, 443-446, 444f, 445b
  examination of, 191
  fractures of, 1271, 1666-1667
    birth-related, 298
  radiography of, 1653t
  sutures of
    cranial deformities and, 443-446, 444f,
      445b
    in newborn, 257, 258, 258f
SLAP assessment, suicide and, 902
Sledding, injuries during, 735
Sleep
  in infants, 525-527, 526t
  in newborn, 245-246, 246t
    at high risk, 358, 360, 360t
  in preschoolers, 645-646

Sleep—cont'd
  in school-age children, 723-724
  in toddlers, 611
  with parents in family bed, 527b, 583, 646b
Sleep disorders, in radiation somnolence
    syndrome, 1601-1602
Sleep disturbances, 645-646, 645t
  assessment of, 157, 157b
Sleep history, 157, 157b
Sleep patterns, 525
  and breast-feeding, 525b
Sleep position, sudden infant death syndrome
    and, 583, 584, 584b
Sleep study, 586
Sleep terrors, vs nightmares, 645t
Sleep theory, of cause of enuresis, 783
Sleep-talking, 724
Sleep-walking, 724
Slipped femoral capital epiphysis, 1808-1809
Slit pores, 1256
Small intestine; *see also* Bowel; Intestine(s).
  adaptive response of after massive
    resection, 1452
  development of, 1417
  structure and function of, 1418-1419, 1419f
Small-for-gestational-age infant, 250, 334b; *see
    also* High-risk newborn.
  hypocalcemia in, 318
Small-particle aerosol generator (SPAG), for
    delivery of ribavirin, 1367, 1368
Smegma, 261
Smell
  neonatal sense of, 244
  sense of, in toddlers, 592
Smiling, in infants, 507
Smoke inhalation, 1233, 1380-1382
Smokeless tobacco, 887
Smoking
  burn injuries and, 1227
  during adolescence, 831-832, 885, 887-888,
    888b, 890b
  during pregnancy, 408-409
  maternal, sudden infant death syndrome
    and, 583
  passive, 1382-1383, 1382b
    otitis media and, 1356-1357
  ulcers and, 1443
Smooth muscle
  bronchial
    neural regulation of, 1307
    vagal stimulation of, in asthma, 1387
  intestinal, 1417
  of lower airway, 1305-1306
Snack foods, 610
  dental health and, 614, 615t
Snakebites, 779
Sneeze reflex, 263t
Snellen charts
  letter, 197, 197f, 198t, 1880
  number, 198t
  Tumbling E, 197-198, 198t, 1880
Snowmobiles, injuries with, 735
Snuff, 887
Soaks
  for skin lesions, 753
  play activities and, 1111b
Soave endorectal pull-through procedure, for
    Hirschsprung disease, 1427
Social awareness, in preschoolers, 631

Social class, 35-37
Social cognition, in adolescents, 810-811
Social development
  in congenital heart disease, 1502
  in Down syndrome, 990
  in infants, 504-507
  in preschoolers, 630b, 631-636, 639t
  in school-age children, 706-708, 708f
  in toddlers, 598-601, 605t
Social environments, of adolescents, 817-820
Social groups, 707
Social influences
  in adolescent alcohol abuse, 889
  in obesity, 871
  in smoking, 885, 887
  in suicide, 899
Social roles, 32-33
Social Security Act, 12
Social services, for families, 74, 74b, 74f
Social Services Block Grant, 12
Social support, adolescent mothers and, 852
Socialization, 31; *see also* Peer relationships.
  ambiguous genitalia and, 489-490, 489b
  cleft lip and palate and, 458, 460
  fragile X syndrome and, 994
  hearing impairment and, 998-999
    hospitalization and, 1000
  hospitalization and, 1073
  in school, 37
  mental retardation and, 982
  peer cultures and, 37-38
  visual impairment and, 1004
Society of Adolescent Medicine, 854
Socioeconomic influences, 40-42; *see also* Poverty.
  as risk factors, 104
Sodium
  depletion of, 1175t
  excess, 1176t
  excretion of, in infants, 1258
  functions of and disturbances in, 563t
  in acute renal failure, 1284
  in chronic renal failure, 1288
  in cystic fibrosis, 1401, 1407
  in dehydration, 1176-1178
  reference ranges for, 1901t
  renal transport of, 1257
  retention of, edema formation and, 1181
  sources of, 563t
Sodium bicarbonate
  for cardiopulmonary resuscitation, 1399t
  for persistent pulmonary hypertension of
    newborn, 398
  for shock, 1221
  in parenteral fluid therapy, 1180
Sodium chloride; *see* Salt.
Sodium/potassium pump theory of obesity, 871
Soft palate, 207f, 208
Soft signs, 225, 228, 228b
Soft tissue, birth-related injury to, 295-296, 296f
Soft tissue sarcoma, 1631-1632, 1631b,
    1631t, 1632b
Soil, lead dust in, 675
Sole, of preterm infant, 377f
Solu-Cortef; *see* Hydrocortisone.
Solu-Medrol; *see* Methylprednisolone.
Solution(s); *see also* Fluid(s).
  crystalloid
    for burn patients, 1236
    for shock states, 1221

Solution(s)—cont'd
  hyperalimentation, 1203
  intravenous
    in parenteral fluid therapy, 1189-1190
    infiltration of, 1197
  oral rehydration, 1186, 1188
    for diarrhea, 1211-1214, 1212t
Solvents, organic, abuse of, 886t, 892
Somatic pain, abdominal, 219
Somatostatin, 1708t
Somatotropic hormone; see Growth hormone.
Somogyi effect, 1741
Sorbitol, 1745
  chronic nonspecific diarrhea and, 1217
  in poisoning cases, 673
Sore throat
  after tonsillectomy, 1353
  management of, 661
  streptococcal, 1351
Sororate marriage, 72
Sorrow, chronic, 136
Soy milk, in vegetarian diets, 565
Soy-based formulas, 280, 281t-282t
  in galactosemia, 325
Spacers (holding chambers), with metered-
      dose inhalers, 1398, 1399b
Spanking, 88
Spasmodic croup, 1365
Spasms/spasticity, 1647b
  in cerebral palsy, 1835b
    drug therapy for, 1839
    physical therapy for, 1840
    surgery for, 1838-1839
  in spinal cord injury, 1859
  in tetanus, 1849
  infantile, 1688
Spastic hemiplegic gait, 1647b
Spastic paraplegic gait, 1647b
Special needs child, 905-945
  community resources for, 938-939
  coping of, 917-920, 917b-920b
  cultural issues with, 910, 910b
  family of, 920-939
    acceptance of diagnosis by, 921-923,
        922b, 922f
    adjustment of, 933-934
    concurrent stresses in, 931
    coping mechanisms of, 931-932, 932b
    day-to-day management of condition and,
        923-925, 923b, 924b
    denial in, 933
    developmental needs of, 925-931, 926b,
        927b, 929b, 930b
    emotions of, 933-935, 933b, 935b
    empowerment of, 932
    extended, 929-931
    foster/adoptive, 927
    management style of, 924-925, 932
    mother/father differences in, 926-927
    parental roles in, 926
    reintegration and acknowledgment in,
        934-935
    shock in, 933
    single-parent, 927
    special information needs of, 923-924,
        923b, 924b
    strengths and adjustment of, 921, 921t
    support system for, 935-939, 935b, 937b,
        938b, 938t

Special needs child—cont'd
  friends of, 930-931
  future goals of, 919-920
  home care of, 908, 1017, 1018, 1019b
    case management and, 1019-1020, 1020b
    education and, 1027-1028
    self-care and, 1025, 1026b, 1027
  mental retardation and; see Mental
      retardation.
  normal developmental needs of,
      925, 925b
  nursing care plan for, 939-944
  promotion of normal development in,
      910-917, 911t-912t, 914f, 915f
  scope of problem and, 905-907, 906b
  siblings of, 928-929, 929b, 930b
  trends in care of, 907-909
Special Olympics, 915, 982, 983
Specific defenses, 1572
Specificity, test, 235
Specimen(s); see also specific type.
  collection of, 1142-1149
  in rape cases, 859
  stool, for intestinal parasites, 666
  urine, 1266, 1268
    collection of, 862
SPECT, cerebral, 1654t
Speech, 1007; see also Communication;
      Language.
  and language development, pacifier use
      and, 518
  cleft lip and palate and, 458, 463
  cued, 998
  egocentric, 596
  fragile X syndrome and, 993
  hearing impairment and, 996-997, 998
  mental retardation and, 981-982
  normal development of, 1011t
  pauses in, 140
  problems with, in preschoolers, 642
  rate of, 140
  socialized, 596-597
  telegraphic, 633
  with tracheostomy, 1330
Speech aids, 1840, 1841
Speech and language therapy, hearing
      impairment and, 998
Speech impairment, 1007, 1008b, 1008f; see
      also Communication impairment.
  assessment of, 1012b
  assistive devices for, 1008, 1840-1841
  autism and, 1009
  in cerebral palsy, 1836-1837, 1840, 1841
  prevention of, 1010-1011, 1011b
Spenco Gel Pads, 349
Sperm, maturation of, 805
Spermatic cord, 222, 223f
Spermicides, 855, 856t
Sphenoid sinus, 191, 191f
Sphenoidal fontanel, 257
Spherocytosis, hereditary, 1546-1547
Sphincter(s)
  control of, in toddlers, 593
  internal anal, in Hirschsprung disease,
      1426, 1427
  lower esophageal, 1418
    gastroesophageal reflux and, 1429
  pyloric, circumferential muscle of, 1446

Sphincter(s)—cont'd
  upper esophageal, 1418
  urethral, urinary continence and, 593,
      1259-1260
Sphygmomanometer, 182
Spica casts, 1784, 1784f, 1786f
  home care for, 1787
Spiders
  bites of, 776-777, 776t, 777t
  black widow, 776t, 777t
  brown recluse, 777t, 778f
Spina bifida, 261, 424b, 425; see also
      Myelomeningocele.
  clinical manifestations of, 427b
  etiology of, 424
  life expectancy in, 906
Spina Bifida Association of America, 432-433
Spina bifida cystica, 425, 427b
Spina bifida occulta, 424f, 425, 427b
Spinal cord
  development of, 1642
  lower urinary tract function and, 1259
  motor transmission in, 1853, 1853f
  segments of, 1852, 1853f, 1854t
  sensory transmission in, 1853, 1853f
  structure and function of, 1852-1855,
      1853f, 1854t
Spinal cord compression, 1856
  in Down syndrome, 990
Spinal cord injury, 1760, 1852-1863
  autonomic dysfunction in, 1855, 1855b, 1860
  bowel training in, 1860
  causes of, 1855-1856
  clinical manifestations of, 1856-1857
  compressive, 1856
  diagnostic evaluation in, 1857-1858
  functional electrical stimulation for, 1585
  level of, 1852, 1854t, 1856, 1857, 1857f
  mechanism of, 1855-1856
  motor function in, 1855
  neurogenic bladder in, 1860
  nursing care in, 1859-1863
  pathophysiology of, 1856
  physical therapy in, 1861
  physiotherapy in, 1859-1860
  prognosis of, 1585-1859
  psychosocial rehabilitation in, 1861-1862
  remobilization in, 1860-1861
  respiratory care in, 1859
  sensory function in, 1855
  sexual concerns in, 1862-1863
  skin care in, 1859
  stages of, 1856-1857
  temperature regulation in, 1859
  therapeutic management in, 1858-1863
  traction in, 1790-1791, 1790f
  upper vs lower motor neuron lesions in,
      1854, 1855b
  without radiographic abnormality, 1857-1858
Spinal injuries, traction in, 1790-1791, 1790f
Spinal muscular atrophy
  infantile, 1846, 1846b
  juvenile, 1846-1847
Spinal nerves, 1852-1853, 1853f
Spinal shock syndrome, 1856
Spinal tap; see Lumbar puncture.
Spine
  congenital deformities of, 447t
  curvature of, 223, 1809-1816

Spine—cont'd
  curvature of—cont'd
    in kyphosis, 1809-1810, 1809f
    in lordosis, 1809f, 1810
    in scoliosis, 1810-1816; see also Scoliosis.
    in spinal cord injury, 1856-1857, 1858
  examination of, 223
  hyperextension of, 191, 223
  mobility of, 223
  of newborn, 261
  tuberculosis of, 1818-1819
Spiritual care, 58, 58b
Spiritual development, 233
  in adolescents, 811-812
  in preschoolers, 632
  in school-age children, 705
  in toddlers, 598
Spirituality, 57; see also Religion.
  healing practices and, 49
Spirometry, for asthma, 1389
Spironolactone (Aldactone), for congestive
    heart failure, 1480t
Spitting up, with feeding, 571
Spleen, 1531, 1571
  in sickle cell anemia, 1548, 1549, 1553
  of newborn, 253t, 261
  palpation of, 220
Splenectomy
  for hereditary spherocytosis, 1546-1547
  for idiopathic thrombocytopenic
      purpura, 1567
  for sickle cell anemia, 1551
  for α-thalassemia, 1558
Splints
  for burn patients, 1246, 1246f
  in intravenous infusions, 1196
  in juvenile rheumatoid arthritis, 1822
  Thomas, 1790, 1790f
Split custody, 97
Spoiled child syndrome, 515-516
Spoon feeding; see also Feeding.
  of infants, 523, 524b
  task analysis of, 984b
Spoon nails, 189
Sports
  chronic illness and, 725
  coaches in, 725
  competitive, in schools, 725, 725b, 726b
  contact vs noncontact, 1796b, 1797
  disordered eating in, 1803
  ergogenic aids in, 1804-1805
  female athlete triad and, 1803
  for diabetics, 1739, 1749-1750
  long-term venous access device care and, 1202
  nurse's role in, 1805-1807
  nutrition in, 1802-1804, 1803b, 1803t
  parental involvement in, 1806b
  preparation for, 1796-1797
  school, 725, 725b, 726b
  sudden death in, 1805
Sports drinks, 1803
Sports injuries, 10, 1796-1807
  acute trauma in, 1798
  contusions as, 1798
  dislocations as, 1798-1799
  heat-related, 1801-1802
  microtrauma in, 1798, 1800-1801
  nursing care for, 1806
  overuse, 1798, 1800-1801, 1801t

Sports injuries—cont'd
  pathophysiology of, 1798
  prevention of, 1758b, 1797, 1806
  psychosocial aspects of, 1806-1807
  risk factors for, 1797
  sites of, 1798f
  sprains as, 1799-1800, 1800f
  strains as, 1799-1800, 1800f
  types of, 1797-1802
  water-related, 1802
Spot test, in infectious mononucleosis, 1355
Spousal abuse, 75, 718
Sprains, 1799-1800, 1800f
Sputum collection, 1148
Square window, gestational age and, 250b
Squatting, with hypoxemia, 1487
Squeezing, with bronchial drainage, 1320
Stable factor, 1562t
Staging, cancer, 1587
Stained peripheral blood smear, 1536t
  in sickle cell anemia, 1550
Stairs, 622
  falls from, 542t, 543t, 546, 549b
Stammering, in preschoolers, 642
Standard care plans, 27, 27t
Standard precautions, 1133
  newborn and, 268
Standards of care
  home care and, 1020-1021
  mental retardation and, 980
Standards of Care (ANA), 25, 25b
Standards of Maternal and Child Health
    Nursing Practice (ANA), 23, 23b
Standards of Professional Performance
    (ANA), 25, 25b
Stanford-Binet Intelligence Scale, 978
Stapes, 203, 203f
Staphylococcal infections, 754
  bullous impetigo, 301
  enteric, 1210t
  neonatal, 393
Staphylococcal scalded skin syndrome, 755t, 773
Staphylococcus aureus, toxic shock syndrome
    and, 1226
Staphylococcus epidermidis, otitis externa and,
    1361
Starling law, 1468
Startle reflex, 263t, 264f
  auditory ability and, 259
State of consciousness, assessment of, 225
Statistics
  morbidity, 6
  mortality, 2
  National Center for Health Statistics and, 2
Stature; see Height; Short stature; Tall stature.
Stature-for-age charts, 1885, 1890
Status asthmaticus, 1395-1396
Status epilepticus, 1692
Stealing, in school-age children, 717
Steam, in respiratory infections, 1346
Steatorrhea, in cystic fibrosis, 1405
Stem cell system, 1531, 1531f
Stem cell transplantation
  peripheral blood, 1596
  umbilical cord, 1596
Stenosis, rectal, 466
Step reflex, 263t, 264f
Stepfamily, 71, 98-99, 99b
Stepfathers, in cases of incest, 686

Stepparents, 71, 98-99, 99b
Stereopsis, in infants, 495
Stereotactic surgery, for brain tumors, 1620
Stereotyping, ethnic, 34-35
Sterilization, mental retardation and, 982
Sternal angle, 208f, 209
Sternberg-Reed cell, 1617
Sternotomy, median, 1504
Sternum, 208f, 209
Steroid hormones, 1708t, 1723
Steroids
  anabolic, 1805
  Cushing syndrome and, 1727-1729, 1727b,
      1727f, 1728t
  for acute laryngotracheobronchitis, 1364
  for asthma, 1391-1392
  for bacterial meningitis, 1679
  for bronchopulmonary dysplasia, 391
  for cancer, 1593t, 1602
  for cystic fibrosis, 1409
  for diaper dermatitis, 578
  for inflammatory bowel disease, 1440
  for juvenile rheumatoid arthritis, 1822
  for nephrotic syndrome, 1277, 1279
  for skin disorders, 749, 751
  for systemic lupus erythematosus, 1828, 1829
  moon facies and, 1602, 1727, 1727f
  side effects of, 1602
  topical, 749
    for allergic rhinitis, 1384
    for skin disorders, 581, 749
  varicella risk and, 651
Stethoscope
  chestpieces for, 212
  for lung auscultation, 212
Stevens-Johnson syndrome (erythema
    multiforme exudativum), due to drug
    sensitivity, 773, 773f
Stimulants
  abuse of, 886t, 892
    by athletes, 1805
  in fragile X syndrome, 994
Stimulation
  in play activities, 507, 508t
  tactile, in infants, 502
Stings, hymenoptera, 775-776, 776t
Stomach, development of, 1417
Stomatitis, 664-665, 664f
  aphthous, 664
  herpetic, 664, 664f
  in cancer, 1600-1601
  in erythema multiforme exudativum, 773
Stool
  acholic, 470
  assay of for viral pathogens, 1420t
  currant-jelly, intussusception and, 1449
  development of, 1417
  examination of, 1420t
    for diagnosis of intestinal parasites, 666
    in asthma, 1407
    in diarrhea, 1211
  in cystic fibrosis, 1406
  in diarrhea, 1211, 1212t, 1214
  iron deficiency anemia and, 1544
  meconium, 1424
  of newborn, 242b
    at high risk, 336b
    with meconium aspiration syndrome, 389
    with neonatal abstinence syndrome, 407

Stool—cont'd
pH of, reference ranges for, 1900t
phototherapy and, 308
Stool cultures, in diarrhea, 1211
Stool softeners, 1424, 1425
Stool specimens, 1146-1147
Stool withholding, constipation with, 1424
Stop Teenage Addition to Tobacco, 888b
Stork bites, 252t, 302
Storytelling, 151b
Strabismus, 195, 1001b, 1005
in brain injury, 1650
in newborn, 259
retinoblastoma and, 1633
test for, 196, 197f
Strains, 1799-1800, 1800f
Stranger fear
in infants, 506, 514-515
in toddlers, 599
Strangulation, of infants, in beds, 544
Stratum germinativum, 740
Strawberry hemangioma, 302, 302f
Strength, assessment of, 225
Strep throat, 1351
Streptococcal infection
acute poststreptococcal glomerulonephritis
and, 1271, 1272
neonatal, 393
Streptococcal pharyngitis, acute, 1351-1352
Streptococcal tonsillopharyngitis, 1513t
Streptococcus, group A β-hemolytic, 1351
rheumatic fever and, 1511
tic disorders and, 792
Streptococcus pneumoniae
otitis media and, 1357, 1358, 1359
vaccine for, 534
Streptomycin, for tuberculosis, 1374
Stress
acne and, 840
ACTH secretion and, 1723-1724
competitive sports and, 726b
family, 66-67, 66t, 69
hospitalization and, 1032-1041, 1036t,
1037f, 1046
bodily injury and pain and, 1036-1039,
1036t, 1037f, 1046
family adjustment and, 1040-1041, 1040b
individual risk factors for, 1039-1040, 1039b
intensive care unit and, 1094-1095, 1094b
loss of control and, 1034-1036, 1035b,
1044-1046, 1045f, 1046b
play and expressive activities and,
1069-1072, 1069b, 1070f-1072f
separation anxiety and, 1032-1034,
1041-1044
hypertension and, 1518
in new parents, 83-84
in preschoolers, 642, 643b
in school-age children, 717-720, 719b
in special needs children, 925-926, 926b, 931
in terminal illness, 973-974, 973b, 974b
in toddlers, 608-609, 608b
peptic ulcer disease and, 1445
Stress fractures, 1801
Stress ulcer, 1443
Stress urinary incontinence,
myelomeningocele and, 428-430
Stretching exercises, in cerebral palsy, 1840

Stroke
cyanosis and, 1487, 1488
in sickle cell anemia, 1548, 1550, 1555
Stroke volume, definition of, 1468
Strongyloidiasis, clinical manifestations of, 665t
Structural-functional family theory, 67t
Stuart-Prower factor, 1562t
Students Against Drunk Driving, 895
Stump care, 1775b, 1795
Stupor, 1648b
Sturge-Weber syndrome, 302
Stuttering, 1007, 1010-1011, 1011b
in preschoolers, 642
Stuttering Foundation of America, 1011n
Stye, 193b
Subarachnoid bolt, in intracranial pressure
monitoring, 1656
Subarachnoid hemorrhage, 1668
in newborn, 403
Subarachnoid space, 1643
Subconjunctival hemorrhage, in newborn,
252t, 296b
Subcutaneous drug administration, 1157-1158
Subcutaneous fat, in marasmus, 567
Subcutaneous fat necrosis, birth-related, 296b
Subcutaneous nodules, in rheumatic fever, 1511
Subcutaneous tissue, 741
Subdural area, 1642
Subdural hematoma, 1666f, 1668
in newborn, 403
ventriculoperitoneal shunt and, 441
Subdural puncture, positioning for, 1142
Subdural tap, 1653t
Subependymal-intraventricular hemorrhage, 401
Subgaleal hemorrhage, 296-297, 297f
Sublimaze; see Fentanyl.
Subluxation
of hip, 446b, 448f; see also Hip,
developmental dysplasia of.
in newborn, 254t
vertebral, spinal cord injury and, 1852, 1856
Submaxillary nodes, 190, 190f
Submental nodes, 190, 190f
Submersion injury, 1674-1676; see also
Near-drowning.
Subpopulations, 103
Substance abuse, 884-895; see also specific
substance.
assessment for, 157
by athletes, 1804-1805
definition of, 884
diagnosis of, 893-894, 893b
drug jargon glossary and, 891b
during pregnancy, 406-408, 406b
long-term management of, 894-895
patterns of, 884
prevention of, 895
treatment of, 892-893
types of drugs abused and, 884-885
Substrate, metabolic pathway and, 319, 320f
Subtle seizures, in newborn, 404t
Suburethral sling, 429
Succimer (Chemet), for chelation
therapy, 680
Sucking
cleft lip and palate and, 458
development of, 1417
in infants, 496

Sucking—cont'd
nonnutritive, 348
esophageal atresia and, 466
of thumb, 518, 518b, 519
Sucking reflex, 260, 263t
nutrition and, high-risk newborn and,
343, 346
Suckling, in infants, 496
Sucralfate, for peptic ulcers, 1444
Sucrase, 1418
Sucrose; see also Sugar.
as analgesic
for neonatal circumcision, 271b, 272
for neonatal heel punctures, 267b
in cereals, 615t
tooth decay and, 780
Suctioning
after heart surgery, 1505
for snakebite venom, 779
in apnea of prematurity, 379
in esophageal atresia, 465
in meconium aspiration syndrome, 389
in patent airway maintenance, in newborn,
265, 289
in respiratory distress syndrome, 387-388
increased intracranial pressure and, 1658
of newborn, 265, 289
of tracheostomy, 1326-1327, 1326f, 1327b
Sudamina, in newborn, 251t
Sudden death, 1805
Sudden infant death syndrome, 582-585
co-bedding and, 362-363
epidemiology of, 582-583, 583t
home health nursing visits after, 965-966, 966b
infants at risk of, 584
nursing considerations with, 584-585, 584b
positioning and, 363
Sudden Infant Death Syndrome Alliance, 966
Suffocation
mortality from, 8, 8t
of infants, 542t-543t, 544-545, 549b
of toddlers, 623
Sugar; see also Sucrose.
dietary, dental health and, 613-615, 615t
in drugs, tooth decay and, 781
Sugar substitutes, in diabetes, 1745
Suicidal ideation, 895
screening for, 901-902
Suicide, 8, 10, 895-902
assisted, 949
copycat, 896, 900, 901b
in adolescents, 820, 832
incidence of, 896-897, 896f
international trends in, 897b
methods of, 899
precipitating factors in, 899, 900b, 900f
prevention of, 899-902, 901b
rates of, 4-5, 4t
risk of
factors associated with, 897-899, 898b, 899b
screening for, 901-902
Suicide attempt, 895
methods of, 899
Sulfasalazine (Azulfidine), for inflammatory
bowel disease, 1440
Sulfur
functions of and disturbances in, 563t
sources of, 563t

SUN; *see* Scale for Use in Newborns.
Sun exposure, 769, 770b
  high-risk newborn and, 350
  skin cancer and, 769
Sun protection, in systemic lupus
    erythematosus, 1828
Sun protective factor (SPF), in sunscreen
    agents, 770
Sunblockers, 769-770
Sunburn, 769-770, 770b
  in infants, 548
  prevention of, 769-770, 770b
Sunscreens, topical, 769-770, 770b
Sunset eyes, 193
Superego, 230
  in preschoolers, 630b
  in toddlers, 594
Superficial reflexes; *see also* Reflex(es).
  assessment of, 226
Superior vena cava syndrome, 1596-1597
Supernumerary digits, 254t, 262, 447t
Supernumerary kidneys, 479t
Supernumerary nipples, 260
Support systems
  hearing impairment and, 999
  home care and, 1028-1029
  hospitalized child and, 1070, 1073-1074,
    1074b
    discharge planning and home care
      for, 1097
  neonatal intensive care unit and, 368
  obesity and, 875
  special needs child and, 935-939, 935b,
    937b, 938b, 938t
  terminal illness and, 973-974
Supraglottitis, acute, 1362, 1362t
Supramalleolar ankle-foot orthosis, 1773,
    1773f, 1774b
Suprapubic aspiration, 1144-1146, 1146b
Suprasternal notch, 208f, 209
Supraventricular tachycardia, 1525, 1525f
Surfactant, 241, 1307
  exogenous, 386-387
  fetal lung maturity and, 383
  replacement of, nitric oxide therapy and, 385
  respiratory distress syndrome and, 380
  treatment of, 386-387
Surgery; *see also* specific disorders.
  acute renal failure and, 1284
  cancer, 1588
  cranial, 1622-1625; *see also* Cranial surgery.
  discharge planning and home care for,
    1509, 1509b
  for abdominal wall defect, 473
  for anorectal malformation, 469
  for cleft lip and palate, 456-458
    postoperative care and, 460
    preoperative care and, 459-460
  for clubfoot, 453
  for congenital diaphragmatic hernia, 476
    in fetus, 475
  for congenital heart disease, 1503-1504,
    1507-1508
  for craniofacial abnormalities, 445-446
  for craniosynostosis, 445
  for cryptorchidism, 481
  for developmental dysplasia of hip, 450
  for epispadias/exstrophy complex, 483-484

Surgery—cont'd
  for esophageal atresia, 464
    postoperative care and, 465
    preoperative care and, 465
  for Hirschsprung disease, 1427
  for hydrocephalus, 440-441, 440f
    postoperative care and, 442
    preoperative care and, 441-442
  for hypertrophic pyloric stenosis, 1447, 1447f
  for hypospadias, 482
  for inflammatory bowel disease, 1441
  for necrotizing enterocolitis, 396
  for obesity, 874-875
  for patent ductus arteriosus, 397
  for peptic ulcer disease, 1445
  for physical defects, neonatal care and,
    419-423, 420t-423t
  for retinopathy of prematurity, 400
  for tracheoesophageal fistula, 464
    postoperative care and, 465
    preoperative care and, 465
  for tuberculosis, 1375
  for vesicoureteral reflux, 1270
  in diabetes, 1741
  in Down syndrome, 990
  in health history, 155
  palliative, for hypoxemia in infants, 1488
  postoperative care and, 1113, 1115-1118
  postoperative care in, 1113, 1115-1118,
    1118b, 1503-1508, 1508b
    for newborn, 420-423, 420t-423t
    nursing care plan for, 1115-1117
    vital signs in, 1113, 1119t
  preoperative care in, 1110-1113, 1112b,
    1112f, 1113b, 1114-1115
    for newborn, 419-420
    nursing care plan for, 1114-1115
  reconstructive, for scar tissue, 1246
Suturing, topical anesthesia for, 1672b
Swaddle, 1138, 1139f
Swallow reflex, infantile (visceral), vs mature
    (somatic), 496-497, 497f
Swallowing
  development of, 1417
  in infants, 496-497, 497f
  nutrition and, high-risk newborn and, 343
  phases of, 1418
Sweat
  production of, 742
  sodium and chloride content of, in cystic
    fibrosis, 1401, 1407
Sweat chloride test, for cystic fibrosis, 1407
Sweat glands, 742
Sweat test, reference ranges for, 1896t
Sweeteners; *see also* Sugar.
  artificial, in diabetes, 1745
  infant botulism and, 1850
Swelling; *see also* Edema.
  under cast, 1786
Swimmer's ear, 1361
Swimmer's shoulder, 1801t
Swimming
  long-term venous access device care and, 1202
  water intoxication and, 1180
Swiss-type lymphopenic agammaglobulinemia,
    1579-1580
Sydenham chorea, in rheumatic fever, 1512
Sylvan seizure, 1686

Symbolic interactional family theory, 67t
Symbols
  communication using, 1008
    mental retardation and, 982
  in cognitive development in infants, 502
Symmetrel (amantadine hydrochloride), for
    influenza, 1356
Sympathetic nervous system, 1705
  stimulation of, in congestive heart
    failure, 1477
Sympathy, vs empathy, 145
Symptoms
  in nursing diagnosis, 26
  prodromal, 650
Synactive theory of infant development, 358, 359t
Synagis (palivizumab), for respiratory syncytial
    virus infection, 391, 1368, 1368b
Synchronized cardioversion, for
    supraventricular tachycardia, 1526
Synchronized intermittent mandatory
    ventilation, in respiratory distress
    syndrome, 384-385, 384f
Syncope, with pulmonary artery hypertension,
    1490
Syndactyly, 224, 254t, 262
Syndrome of inappropriate antidiuretic
    hormone, 1658, 1658t, 1672, 1716-1717
Syndromes, congenital malformations in, 113
Syndromic clubfoot, 452
Synovectomy, for juvenile rheumatoid
    arthritis, 1823
Synthetic casts, 1784-1785, 1785t
Syphilis
  congenital, 328t
  from blood transfusion, 1542t
  primary, genital lesions due to, 865t
  serologic test for, in adolescents, 831
Syringe
  for intramuscular drug administration, 1153
  insulin, 1747
Syringe cap, aspiration of, by infants,
    542t-543t, 544
Systemic inflammatory response syndrome,
    1222, 1223f
Systemic injury, in smoke inhalation injury, 1381
Systemic lupus erythematosus, 1825-1829
  renal involvement in, 1270t
Systemic vascular resistance, 1468
Systemic venous congestion, in congestive
    heart failure, 1478-1479
Systole, 1467

**T**
T cells, 243, 1572
  in human immunodeficiency virus infection,
    1573
T$_3$ (triiodothyronine); *see* Thyroid hormone.
T$_4$ (thyroxine); *see* Thyroid hormone.
Tachycardia, 217b
  in cardiac function assessment, 1469
  in congestive heart failure, 1477, 1478
  in dehydration, 1185
  in newborn, 251t
  in shock states, 1220
Tachydysrhythmias, 1525-1526
Tachypnea, 1310
  in cardiac function assessment, 1469
  in congestive heart failure, 1478

Tachypnea—cont'd
  in Fanconi syndrome, 1280
  in newborn, 251t
Tactile communication, deaf-blind child and, 1006
Tactile play, 601-602
Tactile sensation, in newborn, 242
  at high risk, 361
Tactile stimulation
  in infants, 502
  of newborn, 241
    in apnea of prematurity, 379
Tadoma method, 1006
Tagamet (cimetidine)
  for gastroesophageal reflux, 1429
  for peptic ulcer disease, 1445
Talcum powder, aspiration of, 542t-543t, 544, 1379
Talipes calcaneus, 452b
Talipes deformities, 447t, 451-453, 452b, 452f
Talipes equinovarus, 451-453, 452f
Talipes equinus, 452b
Talipes valgus, 452b
Talipes varus, 452b
Tall stature, hyperpituitarism and, 1713
Tampons, toxic shock syndrome and, 1226-1227
Tanner stages, 805
Tantrums; see Temper tantrums.
Tap water, lead poisoning and, 521
Tapazole (methimazole), for hyperthyroidism, 1719-1720, 1721
Tape recorder, blindness and, 1004
Tape removal, epidermal stripping and, 1125, 1125b
Tape test, for enterobiasis, 668
Tapping method, for blind child, 1003
Target cells/tissues, 1703, 1704, 1705f
  in α-thalassemia, 1557
Target populations, 103
Task analysis, 980, 984b
Taste
  neonatal sense of, 244
  sense of, in toddlers, 592
Tay-Sachs disease, 119t, 120, 134, 996b
TDD; see Telecommunications devices for the deaf.
TDx test, of fetal lung maturity, 383
Tea, iron supplements and, 1546
Teachers; see also School.
  collaboration with school nurses by, 730b
  influence of, 715-716, 718
  role of, 715-716
Teaching, health, 21
Team play, in school-age children, 711-712
Tear glands, of newborn, 243
Technology-dependent child, 906b
  home care and, 1017, 1018, 1019b
Teeth
  care of, 646, 727-728, 781, 782, 1128
    in hemophilia, 1563
    in infants, 527
    in mental retardation, 986
    in toddlers, 611-612, 612f
    with braces, 782
  decay of, in cerebral palsy, 1837
  deciduous, in school-age children, 699, 699f
  disorders of, 780-783
  Down syndrome and, 989t
  evulsed, 782, 783b

Teeth—cont'd
  examination of, 207
    in nutritional assessment, 167t
  injury to, 736, 782-783, 783b
  malaligned, 207
    in cerebral palsy, 207
  natal, 252t, 260
  permanent, eruption of, 727
  primary, eruption of, 519f
  reimplantation of, 782, 783b
Teething, 519, 519f
Telangiectatic nevi, in newborn, 252t
Telecommunications devices for the deaf, 998
Telemedicine, 142
Telephone triage, 142-143
Telephone use, for latchkey children, 721b
Television
  anticipatory socialization provided by, 714-715
  closed captioning for, 998
  developmental impact of, 39-40, 40b
  for preschoolers, 634-635
  for school-age children, 726-727
  obesity and, 872
  sleep disturbances and, 646
  violence in children and, 641
Temper tantrums, 603
  aggressive behavior and, 642
  as problems, identification of children with, 608b
  by toddlers, 607-608, 608b
Temperament
  failure to thrive and, 576
  in infants, 507, 509-511
    childrearing practices and, 509-511
    effect on parents of, 509b
    preterm infants and, 509b
  in preschoolers, 632, 636
  in school-age children, 701-702, 702b
  in toddlers, 601-603
  infant colic and, 572
  physical abuse of child and, 685
Temperature
  after heart surgery, 1504
  elevated, 661
  in burn injuries, 1232, 1245
  in congestive heart failure, 1482
  in frostbite, 771
  in hypothermia, 771
  in infants, 497
  in neurologic assessment, 1649
  in newborns, 251t, 255-256, 265
    at high risk, 336b, 338-341, 339f, 340f
    during exchange transfusion, 305-316
    during phototherapy, 308
    with necrotizing enterocolitis, 396
  in toddlers, 593
  measurement of, 178-179, 179f, 180b-181b, 182t-183t; see also Thermometers.
  normal, 179
  oral, 178-179, 179f, 180b-181b, 182t
  postoperative alterations in, 1113, 1117, 1119t
  regulation of, in spinal cord injury, 1859
  skin, 189
  therapeutic management of, 1130-1131, 1130t, 1131t, 1132b
Temporal lobes, 1644t

Tenderfoot device, for heel punctures, 267b, 1148
  high-risk newborn and, 337-338, 337b
  in neonatal blood glucose testing, 317b
Tendinitis, 1800-1801, 1801t
Teniposide (VM-26), 1592t
Tennis elbow, 1801t
Tenormin (atenolol), for hypertension, 1519b
Tension headaches, 1699, 1699t
Tension pneumothorax, 389-390
Tentorial hiatus, 1642
Tentorium, 1642
Teratogen(s), 124, 326; see also specific teratogens.
  mental retardation and, 979b
Teratogenesis, 416
Terbutaline, for asthma, 1392
Terminal illness, 948b; see also Death and dying.
  autopsy after, 967
  child's awareness of, 950-953, 952b, 952t
  child's right to refuse treatment and, 955b
  child's understanding of, 953-955, 955b
  decision making and, 948-950, 949t, 950b, 951t, 966-967
    child's involvement in, 951
  do not resuscitate orders and, 949t, 950, 966
  educational needs of family in, 958, 959t
  ethical considerations in, 949, 949t
  funeral services after, siblings' attendance at, 967, 967b, 968f
  grief and, 968-972, 969b, 970t
  hospice care and, 955-956
  in cancer, 1606
  life support withdrawal in, 1660-1661
  nurses' reactions to, 972-974, 973b, 974b
  nursing care plan for, 962-964
  organ/tissue donation after, 966-967
  pain management in, 956-958, 957b, 957f
  palliative care in, 948-956
  postmortem care and, 961, 964
  right to die and, 966
  support of family in, 958-959
  symptoms of, 957-958, 958b
  time of death in, 960-961, 960b, 960f, 961b
  viewing of body after, 966
Tertiary prevention, 105
Testicular androgen, ambiguous genitalia and, 487
Testicular growth, in pubertal boys, 806
Testicular self-examination, 843, 843b, 1635
Testicular torsion, 844
Testicular tumors, 843
Testis, 221, 221f, 1704b, 1704f, 1708t
  ambiguous genitalia and, 489t
  cancer of, 843, 1635
  ectopic, 480
  fragile X syndrome and, 993
  leukemic relapse in, 1615
  of newborn, 261
  retractile, 480
  undescended, 221, 480-481
Testosterone, 1708t
  in adolescent males, 805
Tests
  sensitivity of, 235
  specificity of, 235
  validity of, 235
Tet spells, with hypoxemia, 1476f, 1487

Tetanus, 1848-1850
  burn wounds and, 1236
  immunizations for
    contraindications to, 537t
    in adolescents, 541b
    recommended, 529t, 532, 533t
Tetanus immune globulin, 1848, 1849
Tetanus toxoid, 1848
Tetany
  in hypoparathyroidism, 1721, 1722
  neonatal, 318
Tethering, in spina bifida, 425
Tetracaine, adrenaline, cocaine combined
    (TAC), 751b
Tetracaine-phenylephrine (tetraphen), 751b
Tetracycline, for ophthalmia neonatorum
    prevention, 266
Tetralogic clubfoot, 452
Tetralogy of Fallot, 1497b, 1497f
  right-to-left shunting with, 1484, 1486
ThAIRapy vest, in cystic fibrosis, 1408
Thalamus, 1644t
Thalassemia, 119t, 1555, 1557-1559,
    1557b, 1557f
  sickle, 1547
Thalidomide, skeletal limb deficiency from, 453
Thelarche, 805
  premature, 1714
Theophylline
  for apnea of infancy, 586
  for apnea of prematurity, 378, 379
  for asthma, 1392-1393, 1392b
  for respiratory distress syndrome, 386
  metabolism of, 1392, 1392b
  reference ranges for, 1901t
  toxic effects of, 1393
Theoretic risk, 131
Therapeutic care, 15
Therapeutic handling, of high-risk newborn,
    361-362, 361b
Therapeutic holding, 1136, 1138f
Therapeutic play, 1071
Therapeutic positioning, of high-risk newborn,
    363, 363b, 364b, 364f
Therapeutic relationship, 18-19, 19b
Therapy; see Treatment.
Thermal injury; see Burns.
Thermal stability, 339
Thermographs, 178, 180b, 183t
Thermometers
  chemical dot, 178, 183t
  digital, 183t
  mercury, 178, 180b, 182t, 675
  rectal, 178-179, 179f, 180b-181b, 182t-183t
  tympanic, 178-179, 179f, 180b-181b, 182t-183t
  types of, 178-179, 179f, 180b-181b, 182t-183t
Thermoregulation; see also Temperature.
  by skin, 740
  in infants, 497
  in newborns, 241
    at high risk, 338-341, 339f, 340f, 351b
    during exchange transfusion, 315-316
    during phototherapy, 308
    postoperative care and, 420t, 423t
    skin care and, 351b
    with abdominal wall defect, 473
  in unconscious child, 1659
Thiabendazole, 666t

Thiamine, functions of and disturbances
    in, 556t
Thigh folds, asymmetric, 448, 449f
6-Thioguanine, 1591t
Thiotepa, 1590t
Third ventriculostomy, endoscopic, 440
Third-person technique, 151b
Third-spacing, 1172
Thirst
  in nephrogenic diabetes insipidus, 1281
  increased
    in diabetes, 1734, 1736
    in diabetes insipidus, 1715, 1716
  vomiting and, 1218
Thomas splint, 1790, 1790f
Thoracentesis
  in heart surgery, 1505
  in pneumonia, 1370-1371, 1371, 1371b
Thoracic cavity, 1303-1304; see also Chest.
  divisions of, 209, 209f
Thoracic retractions, 210, 1310, 1311f
  in congestive heart failure, 1478
Thoracolumbosacral orthosis, 1773, 1774b, 1774f
Thoracotomy
  for esophageal atresia and
    tracheoesophageal fistula, 464
  lateral, 1504
Thorax; see Chest.
Thought stopping, in pain management, 1059b
Threadworm infection, clinical manifestations
    of, 665t
Thready pulse, 217b
Three wishes technique, 151b
Threshold acuity test, 204
Thrills, 215
  in cardiac assessment, 1469
Throat
  of newborn, 252t, 263t
  sore
    after tonsillectomy, 1353
    management of, 661
    streptococcal, 1351
Thrombin, production of, 1561
Thrombin time, reference ranges for, 1901t
Thrombocyte(s), 1535, 1538
  in hemostasis, 1561
  tests for, 1562t
  transfusion of, 1543t, 1599
Thrombocyte count, 1536t
  in idiopathic thrombocytopenic purpura,
    1566, 1567
  reference ranges for, 1900t
Thrombocytopenia
  in cancer, 1598-1599
  in hemolytic uremic syndrome, 1281
  in Wiskott-Aldrich syndrome, 1579
Thrombocytopenic purpura
  idiopathic, 1566-1567, 1567b
  vs hemolytic uremic syndrome, 1281
Thromboplastin, 1562t
Thromboplastin generation test, 1562t
Thrombosis
  immobilization and, 1764
  venous, with central venous access devices,
    1201-1202
Thrombus
  in burn injuries, 1231
  in Kawasaki disease, 1515

Thrush, in newborn, 252t, 301
Thumb sucking, 518, 518b, 519
Thymectomy, for myasthenia gravis, 1851
Thymus, 1571, 1704b, 1704f
Thyrocalcitonin, 1707t
Thyroid disorders, 1717-1721
  Down syndrome and, 990
  goiter, 1718
  hyperthyroidism, 1719-1721
  juvenile hypothyroidism, 1717-1718
  lymphocytic thyroiditis, 1718-1719
Thyroid gland, 1704b, 1704f, 1707t
  examination of, 191
  structure of, 192f
Thyroid hormone, 1707t, 1717
  effects of, 1717, 1717b
  hypersecretion of, 1719-1721
    goiter and, 1718
  hyposecretion of
    congenital, 320-322
    familial, 119t
    goiter and, 1718
    in juvenile hypothyroidism, 1717-1718
  reference ranges for, 1902t
  regulation of, 1717
  replacement, for juvenile hypothyroidism,
    1718
  synthesis of, 1717
Thyroid nodules, 1718
Thyroid Society, 1720
Thyroid storm, 1720
Thyroidectomy
  for hyperthyroidism, 1720, 1721
  hypoparathyroidism and, 1722
Thyroiditis, lymphocytic, 1718-1719
Thyroid-stimulating hormone, 1707t; see also
    Thyroid hormone.
  congenital hypothyroidism and, 321
  hyposecretion of, 1706b
Thyrotoxicosis, 1720
Thyrotropin; see Thyroid-stimulating hormone.
L-Thyroxine, for juvenile hypothyroidism, 1718
Thyroxine (T$_4$), 1707t; see also Thyroid
    hormone.
Ticks, 189
  avoiding exposure to, 766
  bites of, 777-778, 777t
  Lyme disease and, 763
  rickettsial infections from, 763, 765t
Tics, 792, 792b, 792t, 1647b
Tidal liquid ventilation, 385, 386
Tigabine, for seizures, 1691t
Tilt table, in spinal cord injury, 1860-1861
Time, concept of
  cultural differences in, 43
  in preschoolers, 631
  in toddlers, 596
Time out, 87-88, 87b
  for infants, 516
Tinea capitis, 759-760, 759t, 760f
Tinea corporis, 759-760, 759t, 760f
Tinea cruris, 759t
Tinea pedis, 759-760, 759t
TIPP (The Injury Prevention Program), 11
Tissue donation, 966-967
Tissue fibrosis, in immobilization, 1763
Tissue hypoxia, in carbon monoxide
    poisoning, 1381

Tissue oxygenation
  anemia and, 1538-1539
    sickle cell, 1552
  in congestive heart failure, 1481
Tissue tension, edema formation and, 1181
Tissue turgor, 189
Title V programs, 909
TLSO brace, for scoliosis, 1811, 1813f
Tobacco; *see also* Smoking.
  smokeless, 887
Tocopherol
  functions of and disturbances in, 559t
  sources of, 559t
Toddler
  biologic development of, 592-594
  body image of, 598
  cognitive development of, 594-597
  communication with, 148
  constipation in, 1424
  dental health of, 611-616
  divorce and, 95b
  dying, 953; *see also* Terminal illness.
  growth and development of, 591-609
  height and weight of, 592
  hospitalized
    bodily injury and pain in, 1037
    loss of control in, 1034-1035
    separation anxiety in, 1033
  injury prevention in, 616-624
  intramuscular injection sites in, 539b, 540
  moral development of, 597-598
  negativism in, 608
  nutrition of, 609-611, 610b
  physical examination of, 173t
  psychosocial development of, 594
  sexuality in, 598
  siblings and, 605-607
  sleep and activity in, 611
  social development of, 598-601
  special needs; *see also* Special needs child.
    early intervention for, 909, 1027-1028
    promotion of normal development in,
      911t, 912-913
  spiritual development of, 598
  stress in, 608-609
  temper tantrums in, 607-608
  temperament of, 601-603
  toilet training in, 603-605, 603b, 604b
  toys of, 601
Toddler Behavior Assessment Questionnaire, 602
Toddler Temperament Scale, 602
Toe(s)
  extra, 224
  fused, 224
  of high-risk newborn, parenteral fluids
    and, 342
Toe walking, in developmental dysplasia of
    hip, 448
Toeing in, 225
Toilet training
  enuresis and, 783, 784
  in toddlers, 603-605, 603b, 604b, 606f
  readiness for, 603, 603b
Toileting, independent, mental retardation
    and, 985
Tolazoline, for persistent pulmonary
    hypertension of newborn, 398
Tolmetin, in pain management, 1061t

Tone
  abdominal, 218
  muscle, 225
Tongue
  examination of, 208
    in nutritional assessment, 167t
  in infantile and mature swallow reflex,
    496-487, 497f
  of newborn, 260
Tonic neck reflex
  asymmetric, 263t, 264f
  in cerebral palsy, 1837
  in infants, 498
Tonic seizures, in newborn, 404t
Tonic-clonic seizures, 1687-1688, 1695b; *see
    also* Epilepsy; Seizures.
Tonsil(s), 206f, 207
  kissing, 1353
  lingual, 1352, 1352f
  palatine (faucial), 1352, 1352f
  pharyngeal, 1352, 1352f
  tubal, 1352, 1352f
Tonsillar nodes, 190, 190f
Tonsillectomy, 1353
Tonsillitis, 1351-1354, 1351f
Tonsillopharyngitis, streptococcal, treatment
    of, 1513t
Tooth; *see* Teeth.
Toothpaste, fluorosis risk and, 613
Topical anesthesia, 751b
  EMLA cream for, 1679
  for arthrocentesis, 1823b
  for bladder catheterization, 1146b
  for circumcision, 270-272, 271b
  for laser therapy, for birthmarks, 302
  for lumbar puncture, 1142b, 1142f, 1679
  for suturing, 1672b
Topiramate, for seizures, 1691t
TORCH complex, 325-326
Torticollis, 191, 253t, 1807
  congenital, 446
Total anomalous pulmonary venous
    connection, 1499b-1500b, 1500f
Total body irradiation, 1594
Total body surface area, for estimating extent
    of burn, 1228
Total body water, 1171
  growth and, 1173, 1173f
  in infants, 497
  in newborns, 242
Total iron-binding capacity, 1544-1545
Total liquid ventilation, 385, 386
Total lung capacity, divisions of, 1312f
Total parenteral nutrition, 1203-1204
  complications with, 1451-1452
  for high-risk newborn, 343-344
    enteral nutrition, for high-risk
      newborn, 343
  in Hirschsprung disease, 1428
  in inflammatory bowel disease, 1441, 1442
  in short bowel syndrome, 1451-1452
  infection in, 1201
Totipotential stem cell, 1531
Touch; *see also* under Tactile.
  neonatal sense of, 244
    high-risk infant and, 361
  sense of
    in infants, 504
    in toddlers, 592

Toughlove, 894-895
Tourette syndrome, 793-794, 793b
Tourette Syndrome Association, 793
Tourniquet, 1760
  for parenteral intravenous therapy, 1190
Tourniquet effect, in burn injuries, 1231
Tourniquet test, 1562t
Toxic agents, safety precautions with, 547, 549b
Toxic epidermal necrolysis (Lyell disease), 773
Toxic megacolon, 1441
Toxic shock syndrome, 1226-1227, 1226b
Toxicariasis, intestinal, 665t
Toxoid(s)
  availability and routes of administration
    of, 528b
  tetanus, 1848
Toxoplasmosis, in newborn, 328t
Toys; *see also* Play.
  for hospitalized child, 1070-1071, 1070f
  for infants, 508t
  for preschoolers, 634, 634t
  for toddlers, 600t, 601, 602b, 623
  injuries with, 736
  maintenance of, 602b
  mental retardation and, 983, 983f
  safety of, 1136
  safety precautions with, 548, 601, 602b, 623
  storage of, 602b
  supervision of children with, 602b
Trace elements (microminerals), 555
Trachea, 1305
  examination of, 191
  structure of, 192f
Tracheal aspiration, 1315t
Tracheitis, bacterial, 1362t, 1365
Tracheobronchial dynamics, as respiratory
    tract defense, 1310
Tracheobronchitis, 1366, 1366t
Tracheoesophageal fistula, 463-466
  assessment of, 464-465
  clinical manifestations of, 463
  diagnosis of, 464
  nursing care plan for, 467-468
  nursing considerations in, 464-466
  pathophysiology of, 463, 463f
  treatment of, 464
Tracheomalacia, 464, 466
Tracheostomy, 1325, 1325f
  care of, 1326-1329
    emergency, 1328-1329
    routine, 1327-1328
  communication with, 1330, 1333
  for acute epiglottitis, 1363
  home care of, 1327b, 1329-1331, 1329b,
    1333, 1333f
  in smoke inhalation injury, 1381
  in spinal cord injury, 1859
  suctioning of, 1326-1327, 1326f, 1327b
  ties for, 1328, 1328f
  tubes for, 1325, 1325f, 1328, 1328f
Traction, 1787-1792
  balance suspension, 1790, 1790f
  Bryant, 1789
  Buck extension, 1789, 1789f
  cervical, 1790-1792, 1790f
  complications of, 1791b, 1792
  Crutchfield, 1790-1791, 1790f
  Dunlop, 1789, 1789f
  guidelines for, 1791

Traction—cont'd
 lower extremity, 1789-1790, 1789f, 1790f
 mechanics of, 1788, 1788f
 90-90, 1790, 1790f
 nursing care in, 1791-1792, 1791b
 play activities and, 1111b
 purposes of, 1788
 Russell, 1789f, 1790
 skin, 1788b, 1791b
 types of, 1788-1791, 1788b
 upper extremity, 1789, 1789f
Traditional medicine; *see* Complementary
  medicine.
Tragus, 200, 200f
Trainable mentally retarded, 978
Trampolines, injuries with, 735
Tranquilizers, abuse of, 886t
Transcellular fluid, 1171
Transcultural nursing, 30; *see also* Cultural
  factors.
Transcutaneous bilirubinometry, 305-306, 307
Transcutaneous electrical nerve stimulation,
  1059b
 for dysmenorrhea, 847
Transcutaneous monitoring, of blood gases,
  1314-1315
Transepidermal water loss, in high-risk
  newborn, 350b
Transesophageal atrial overdrive pacing, for
  supraventricular tachycardia, 1526
Transesophageal recording, for diagnosis of
  dysrhythmia, 1524
Transfer technique, kangaroo care and, 362
Transferrin, 1544
Transferrin saturation, 1545
Transfusion, 1543t
 complications of, 1541t-1542t
 exchange
  for hemolytic disease of newborn, 315-316
  for hyperbilirubinemia, 307t
 human immunodeficiency virus from,
  1542t, 1573
 in anemia, 398, 399, 1540-1542, 1551
 in neonatal sepsis, 395
 in respiratory distress syndrome, 386
 in sickle cell anemia, 1551
 in α-thalassemia, 1558
 intrauterine, in Rh incompatibility, 315
 Jehovah's Witnesses and, 1539b
 platelet, 1599
Transitional care, discharge planning
  and, 1097
Translocations, 115-116, 115f
 in Down syndrome, 989
Transmission-based precautions, 1133
Transpalmar crease, 189, 190f
Transperineal collagen, 429
Transplantation
 bone marrow, 1595-1596
  for leukemia, 1615
  for severe combined immunodeficiency
   disease, 1580
  in aplastic anemia, 1560
  nursing care in, 1602-1603, 1602-1606
 brain death and, 1649
 graft-vs-host reaction after, 1579
 islet cell, 1738
 liver, 470, 471
  for biliary atresia, 470, 471

Transplantation—cont'd
 lung
  in cystic fibrosis, 1409
  in pulmonary artery hypertension, 1491
 pancreatic, 1738
 umbilical cord blood stem cell, 1596
Transport
 of high-risk newborn, 335
 safety of, 1136, 1137f
Transposition of great arteries (vessels),
  1499b, 1499f
Transurethral collagen, 429
Transvenous leads, of pacemaker, 1525
Transverse island flap urethroplasty, in
  hypospadias, 482
Transverse palmar crease, 262
Trauma; *see also* Injuries.
 acute renal failure and, 1284
 assessment of, 1760-1761, 1761b, 1762b
 birth-related, 295-300, 296b, 297f, 299f
 dental, 782-783, 783b
 head, 1661-1674; *see also* Head injury.
 management of, 1758-1759
 mental retardation from, 979b
 penile, 843
 posttraumatic stress disorder and, 794
 renal, 1282-1283, 1283b
 spinal, 1852-1863; *see also* Spinal cord injury.
 visual impairment from, 1000, 1002, 1003b
Traumatic amputation, 1795
Travel, by diabetics, 1745-1746
Treacher Collins syndrome, 445b
Treatment
 compliance with, 1120
 refusal of, 58-62
 religious beliefs and, 58-62, 58t-62t
 termination of
  for cancer patients, 1606
  for comatose child, 1660-1661
Tremors, 1647b
 in newborn, 263, 404
Trench mouth, 781
Trendelenburg sign, 448, 449f
*Treponema pallidum,* in newborn, 328t
Tretinoin, for acne, 841
Triage, telephone, 142-143, 143f
Triceps reflex, 226, 227f
Triceps skinfold thickness
 in nutritional assessment, 168
 measurement of, 177, 178b
 percentiles for, 1894
*Trichomonas vaginalis,* 849
Trichuriasis, clinical manifestations of, 665t
Tricuspid atresia, 1497b-1498b, 1497f-1498f
Tricuspid valve, 1465
 heart sounds and, 215
Tricyclic antidepressants
 for attention deficit hyperactivity disorder,
  789, 791
 for depression, 798
 for enuresis, 784
 for Tourette syndrome, 793
Trigeminal nerve, assessment of, 229t
Triglycerides, 1520
 reference ranges for, 1902t
Trigone muscle, 1258
Trigonocephaly, 444-445
Triiodothyronine (T₃), 1707t; *see also* Thyroid
  hormone.

Triple marker screen, 128t
Triplets; *see* Multiple births.
Triploidy, 113
Trismus, in tetanus, 1849
Trisomy, 113
 cancer and, 1585-1586, 1612
Trisomy 13, 116t
 congenital heart disease and, 1474
Trisomy 18, 116t
 congenital heart disease and, 1474
Trisomy 21; *see* Down syndrome.
Trisomy Profile test, 128-129, 128t
Trochlear nerve, assessment of, 229t
Tromethamine, for persistent pulmonary
  hypertension of newborn, 398
Trophic feedings, for high-risk newborn,
  343, 396
Tropia, 196
Tropic hormones, 1704, 1705f
Trough crutches, 1775
Trousseau sign, 1721
Truncus arteriosus, 1465, 1500b, 1500f
Trunk incurvation reflex, 263t
Trust
 in infants, 501-502
 vs mistrust, 230t, 231
Trypsin, 1418
 in infants, 496
TTY; *see* Telecommunications devices for the
  deaf.
Tube(s)
 endotracheal; *see also* Endotracheal
   intubation.
  size of, 1325
  teaching about, 1504
 gastrostomy
  for gastroesophageal reflux, 1431, 1432
  in short bowel syndrome, 1452, 1453
 tracheostomy, 1325, 1325f
  accidental decannulation of, 1329
  changing of, 1328
  occlusion of, 1328-1329
  pediatric, 1328, 1328f
  removal of, 1329
Tube feeding; *see* Enteral nutrition;
  Gastrostomy feeding.
Tubercle, in tuberculosis, 1372
Tuberculin test (Mantoux skin test)
 in adolescents, 834
 interpretation of, 1373-1374, 1374b
 performance of, 1375
 recommendations for, 1373b
Tuberculosis, 1372-1376
 ambulatory care in, 1375
 case finding in, 1375-1376
 diagnosis of, 1373-1374, 1373b, 1374b
 in migrant children, 42
 infection vs disease, 1372
 meningitis in, 1681
 miliary, 1372
 nursing care for, 1375-1376
 prevention of, 1375
 prognosis for, 1375
 racial/ethnic factors in, 56
 resistance to, 1372b
 skeletal, 1818-1819
 skin test for; *see* Tuberculin test.
  in adolescents, 834
 treatment of, 1374-1376

Tubo-ovarian abscess, 863
Tubular necrosis, 1284
Tubules, renal; *see* Renal tubule(s).
Tucker valve, for tracheostomy, 1330
Tumbling E test, 197-198, 198t, 1880
Tumor(s); *see also* Cancer.
  biopsy of, 1587-1588
  brain, 1619-1625
  catecholamine-secreting, 1724, 1731-1732
  classification of, 1587
  pituitary, 1706-1709
    Cushing's syndrome and, 1727-1729
    hyperpituitarism and, 1713
    hypopituitarism and, 1706-1709, 1710, 1712
  staging of, 1587
  testicular, 843, 1635
Tumor lysis syndrome, 1596
Tuning fork tests, 205t
Turbuhaler, 1391
Turgor, 189
Turner syndrome, 116, 117-118, 117f, 117t
24-hour dietary recall, 165
24-hour urine collection, 1144
Twilight croup, 1365
Twins, 79-81, 80b
  attachment and, 286
  breast-feeding of, 275, 275f
  co-bedding and, 362-363, 362f
Twitching, 1647b
  in newborn, 263
Tylenol; *see* Acetaminophen.
Tylenol with Codeine, 1060b
Tylox, 1060b; *see also* Oxycodone.
  after heart surgery, 1506
Tympanic membrane
  compliance of, 204
  damage to, otitis media and, 1358
  examination of, 201-203, 202f
    in nutritional assessment, 166t
  landmarks of, 202, 203f
  otitis media and, 1357-1358
Tympanic temperature, 178-179, 179f, 180b-
      181b, 182t-183t; *see also* Temperature.
  in newborn, 256
Tympanometry, 204, 205t, 1358
Tympanosclerosis, otitis media and, 1358
Tympanostomy tube, 1360
  for otitis media, 1359
Tympany
  on abdominal percussion, 219
  on chest percussion, 212
Typhus
  endemic, 765t
  epidemic, 765t
Tyrosine, phenylketonuria and, 322

**U**

UDP-galactose transferase, 325
Ugly duckling stage, 699
Ulcer(s), 746f
  aphthous, 664
  corneal, in burn injuries, 1244
  curling, in burn injuries, 1234
  duodenal, 1443
  gastric, 1443
  Helicobacter pylori infection and, 1443
  mucosal, in cancer, 1600-1601
  oral, in cancer, 1600-1601
  peptic, 1443-1446, 1445t

Ulcer(s)—cont'd
  pressure, 745, 1122-1125, 1124b-1125b,
      1126t
    in immobilization, 1765, 1765f
    in spinal cord injury, 1859
  primary or secondary, 1443
  rectal, in cancer, 1601
  stress, 1443
Ulcerative colitis
  effects of, 1438f
  pathophysiology and clinical manifestations
      of, 1438
  vs Crohn disease, 1439t
Ulcerogenic drugs, ulcers and, 1443
Ultrasonography
  cerebral, 1653t
  Doppler, in blood pressure measurement, 184
  for postoperative correction of
      vesicoureteral reflux, 1270
  in hemolytic disease of newborn, 314
  in prenatal diagnosis, 128t, 129
  of gastrointestinal tract, 1421t
Ultraviolet burn, of eye, 1003b
Ultraviolet light
  exposure to, 769
  sunburn from, 769-770, 770b
Umbilical arterial catheter, for oxygenation
      monitoring, in respiratory distress
      syndrome, 387
Umbilical cord, 253t, 261
Umbilical cord blood stem cell
      transplantation, 1596
Umbilical hernia, 218, 218f, 474-475, 474f
Umbilical vein, 1466
  fetal transfusion via, in Rh incompatibility, 315
Umbilical venous catheter
  for blood pressure monitoring, of high-risk
      newborn, 337
  for oxygenation monitoring, in respiratory
      distress syndrome, 387
  for parenteral fluid therapy, in high-risk
      newborn, 342
Umbilicus, 269-270
  in hemorrhagic disease of newborn, 319
  inspection of, 218
Umbo, 203, 203f
Unasyn (ampicillin-sulbactam), for
      pneumonia, 1370
Unbalanced translocation, 115-116
Unconjugated hyperbilirubinemia, 303-310;
      *see also* Hyperbilirubinemia.
Unconsciousness, 1647-1649; *see also* Cerebral
      dysfunction; Coma; Consciousness.
  diabetes insipidus and, 1658, 1658t
  diagnostic procedures in, 1652-1654,
      1653t-1654t
  drug therapy in, 1658-1659
  elimination in, 1659
  evaluation in, 1661
  eye protection in, 1659
  family support in, 1660-1661
  fluid management in, 1658
  hearing in, 1660
  home care in, 1661
  hygienic care in, 1659
  hyperthermia in, 1659
  implementation in, 1656-1661
  in head injury, 1666
  in near-drowning, 1676, 1676t

Unconsciousness—cont'd
  intracranial pressure monitoring in,
      1656-1658
  mouth care in, 1659
  neurologic assessment in, 225-228, 226f-228f,
      229t, 1646-1652, 1655
  nursing care in, 1654-1661
  nursing care plan for, 1662-1664
  nursing diagnoses for, 1655-1656
  nutritional support in, 1658
  pain management in, 1655
  planning in, 1656, 1662-1664
  positioning in, 1659
  range-of-motion exercises in, 1659
  rehabilitation in, 1660-1661, 1660b
  respiratory management in, 1656
  sensory stimulation in, 1659-1660
  skin care in, 1659
  syndrome of inappropriate antidiuretic
      hormone and, 1658, 1658t
  treatment withdrawal in, 1660-1661
Underwater weighing, 873-874
Undescended testis, 221, 480-481
Uniparental disomy, 122
United Cerebral Palsy Association, 1842
United Nation's Declaration of the Rights of
      the Child, 20, 20b
United Network for Organ Sharing, 1526
United Ostomy Association, 1166n, 1443
United States Children's Bureau, 1212
Universal child safety seat system, 619, 619f
Unlicensed assistive personnel, 23-24
Upper arm circumference
  in nutritional assessment, 168
  measurement of, 177
  percentiles for, 1894
Upper extremity; *see also* Extremities.
Upper extremity traction, 1789, 1789f; *see also*
      Traction.
Upper motor neuron, 1832, 1833f, 1854
Upper motor neuron lesions, 1833, 1854, 1855b
Urachus, patent, 218
Urea, excretion of, in infants, 1258
Urea nitrogen, reference ranges for, 1902t
Urease test, 1421t
Urecholine (bethanechol), for
      gastroesophageal reflux, 1429
Uremia, 1287; *see also* Renal failure.
  definition of, 1283
Uremic syndrome, in chronic renal failure, 1290
Ureter(s), 1256
  congenital anomalies of, 479t
  duplication of, 479t
  structure and function of, 1258-1259
Ureteral ectopia, 479t
Ureteral orifices, 1259
Ureterocele, 479t
Ureterohydronephrosis, 484
Ureteropelvic junction, obstruction of, 485t, 486
Ureterovesical junction, 1258
  obstruction of, 485t
Urethra
  ambiguous genitalia and, 489t
  in females, urinary tract infection and, 1265
  in males, urinary tract infection and, 1265
  obstruction of, 485t
  of newborn, 261
    in hypospadias, 481-482, 481f
  structure and function of, 1259

Urethral meatus
  female, 223
  male, 221, 221f
Urethral orifice, 1259
Urethritis, 862
Urethrovesical unit, structure and function of, 1259-1262
Uric acid, in tests of renal function, 1262t
Urinalysis, 1260
  in acute poststreptococcal glomerulonephritis, 1272
Urinary bladder; *see* Bladder.
Urinary calculi, immobilization and, 1764, 1794-1795
Urinary catheterization, 1144-1146, 1145t, 1146b, 1266
  for neurogenic bladder, 1860
  for urine collection, 1266
  hypospadias and, 482
  in unconscious child, 1659
  myelomeningocele and, 429
Urinary diversion
  hypospadias and, 482
  obstructive uropathy and, 486
Urinary elimination
  Credé maneuver for, 1860
  during immobilization, 1764
  dysfunctional
    symptoms of, 1265b
    urinary stasis and, 1265
    urinary tract infection and, 1265
  in spinal cord injury, 1860
  in unconscious child, 1659
  normal, 1258
  urinary tract infection and, 1265-1266
  with spica cast, 1787
Urinary glucose testing, in diabetes, 1738, 1748
Urinary incontinence, 783-785, 783-786; *see also* Enuresis.
  in unconscious child, 1659
  myelomeningocele and, 428-430
Urinary output
  of high-risk newborn, 337
  postoperative
    hydrocephalus and, 442
    neonatal, 421t
Urinary sphincter, artificial, 430
Urinary stasis, urinary tract infection and, 1265
Urinary tract
  disorders of; *see also* Urinary tract infection.
    clinical manifestations of, 1260, 1260b
    laboratory tests for, 1260, 1261t, 1262t
    nursing care of, 1260, 1262
  function of, tests of, 1263t, 1264t
  immobilization effects on, 1764
  lower, structure and function of, 1259-1262
  myelomeningocele and, 428-430
  upper, 1262
Urinary tract infection, 1262-1269
  causes of, 1264-1265
  classification of, 1262b
  clinical manifestations of, 1266
  definitions used in, 1262b
  diagnosis of, 1266-1267
  in newborns, 1262, 1264
  localization of, 1267
  nursing care of, 1267-1269
  pathophysiology of, 1265-1266
  prevention of, 1268-1269, 1269b

Urinary tract infection—cont'd
  prognosis for, 1267
  treatment of, 1267-1269
Urination, increased
  in diabetes insipidus, 1715, 1716
  in diabetes mellitus, 1734
Urine
  fluid and electrolyte disturbances and, 1189t
  osmolality of, reference ranges for, 1900t
  output of, 1255
    in acute renal failure, 1284, 1287
    in dehydration, 1178
  pH of, reference ranges for, 1900t
  specific gravity of, 1211
    reference ranges for, 1901t
  transport of from kidney to bladder, 1258-1259
Urine culture, in vesicoureteral reflux, 1270
Urine specimens, 1143-1146, 1143f, 1145t, 1146b
  clean-catch, 1266
  collection of, 1266, 1268
  contamination of, 1266
Urine tests, for renal function, 1261
Urine volume, reference ranges for, 1896t, 1902t
Urobilinogen, 305
Urokinase, 1202
Uropathy, obstructive, 484-487, 485f, 485t, 1284
Urticaria, 774t
Urushiol, in poison ivy and poison oak, 767
U.S. Consumer Product Safety Commission, 601
Usher syndrome, 996b
Uterine bleeding, dysfunctional, 848
UTI; *see* Urinary tract infection.
Uveitis
  in Crohn disease, 1439
  in juvenile rheumatoid arthritis, 1821, 1822
Uvula, 207f, 208

**V**

Vaccination, vs immunization, 527
Vaccine(s); *see also* Immunization(s); Immunization(s).
  administration of, 538, 539b, 540-541
  adverse reactions to, reporting of, 541
  availability and routes of administration of, 528b
  BCG (bacille Calmette-Guérin), for tuberculosis, 1375
  brand names and manufacturers of, 540t
  Comvax, 533, 540t
  contraindications to, 535-536, 537t
  diphtheria-tetanus, in adolescents, 834
  diphtheria-tetanus-pertussis, in children, 529t, 532
  Haemophilus influenzae type b
    for acute epiglottitis, 1363
    in children, 529t, 533-534
  hepatitis A, 1460
    in adolescents, 541b, 834
    in children, 529t, 532
  hepatitis B, 1460
    for newborn, 267
    in adolescents, 541b, 834
    recommended dosages for, 532t
    schedules for, 530, 532
  human diploid cell rabies, 1683
  human immunodeficiency virus infection and, 1575

Vaccine(s)—cont'd
  influenza
    in children, 529t, 534-535
    Kawasaki disease and, 1516
  live virus, contraindications to, 533, 535, 538
  Lyme disease, 766
  measles-mumps-rubella
    in adolescents, 541b, 833-834
    in children, 529t, 533
    Kawasaki disease and, 1516
  meningococcal, in adolescents, 541b
  meningococcal polysaccharide, in children, 535t
  mumps
    in adolescents, 541b
    in children, 529t, 533
  pertussis
    forms available, 532-533
    in children, 529t, 532-533, 536
  pneumococcal, in children, 529t, 534
  pneumococcal conjugate, 529t, 537t, 538t
  pneumococcal polysaccharide
    for otitis media, 1359
    for pneumonia, 529t, 1370
    in adolescents, 834
  polio, in children, 529t, 533
  reactions to, 535, 536t
  rubella
    in adolescents, 541b
    in children, 529t, 533
  sources of current information on, 541b
  storage of, 538
  tetanus, in children, 529t, 532, 533t
  varicella
    in adolescents, 541b, 834
    in children, 529t, 534
    Kawasaki disease and, 1516
Vaccine Adverse Event Reporting System (VAERS), 541
Vaccine Compensation Amendments, 541
Vaccine-associated polio paralysis, 533
VACTERL association, 463
Vacuum extractor, subgaleal hemorrhage and, 296
Vacuum-assisted closure device (VAC), for skin disorders, 753
Vagal stimulation
  for supraventricular tachycardia, 1525
  in asthma, 1387-1388
  proprioceptive, 1309
Vaginal bleeding, abnormal, 848
Vaginal discharge, in newborn, 261
Vaginal orifice, 223
Vaginitis, 848-849
Vaginosis, bacterial, 849
Vagus nerve, assessment of, 229t
Vagus nerve stimulation, for seizures, 1692
Valacyclovir, for varicella-zoster virus infection, 651b
Validity, test, 235
Valium; *see* Diazepam.
Valley fever, 764t
Valproic acid
  for seizures, 1691t
  for status epilepticus, 1692
Value autonomy, development of, 811-812
Valves, cardiac, heart sounds and, 215; *see also* Heart sounds.
Vapocoolant, in pain management, 1065b

Varicella; *see also* Chickenpox.
immunization for, 641, 1605
contraindications to, 537t, 538t
in adolescents, 541b, 834
in children, 529t, 534
Kawasaki disease and, 1516
recommended, 529t, 534
in immunocompromised patient, 1605
Reye syndrome and, 1683-1684
Varicella-zoster immune globulin, 651, 1605
Varicella-zoster virus, 758t
antiviral drugs for, 651b
complications with, 651, 660
in newborn, 327t
Varices, esophageal, 1461
Varicocele, 843-844
Varivax vaccine, 534
Vasa recta, 1256
Vascular birthmarks, 302-303, 302f
Vascular Birthmarks Foundation, 302
Vascular cushion, in urethral closure, 1260
Vascular resistance
immobilization and, 1763, 1770t
pulmonary, 1468
respiratory distress syndrome and, 380
systemic, 1468
Vascular stains, in newborn, 302
Vasculitis
allergic, 1569-1570, 1570f
in Kawasaki disease, 1514
Vasodilation, in septic shock, 1222
Vasodilators
for hypertension, 1518, 1519b
for persistent pulmonary hypertension of
newborn, 398
for pulmonary artery hypertension, 1491
for shock, 1221
Vaso-occlusive crisis, in sickle cell anemia,
1548, 1548b, 1549
pain from, 1552-1553, 1553f
Vasopressin, 1707t
hyposecretion of, 1706b
in newborn, 243
pharmaceutical, for diabetes insipidus,
1715, 1716
Vasopressor support, for treatment of
shock, 1221
Vasospasm
parenteral fluid therapy and, high-risk
newborn and, 342
respiratory distress syndrome and, 380
Vasotec (enalapril)
for congestive heart failure, 1479
for hypertension, 1519b
Vastus lateralis, intramuscular injection
via, 1155t
VATER association, 463
Vegan diet, 560, 560b
Vegetables, for infants, 522, 524b
Vegetarian diet
iron deficiency anemia and, 1543
mineral regulation and, 560
nutritional balance in, 565
types of, 560, 560b
Vein(s)
as site of venipuncture, 1192-1194, 1194f
coronary, 1467
distended, in congestive heart failure,
1478-1479

Vein(s)—cont'd
in postnatal circulation, 1467
pulmonary, in total anomalous pulmonary
venous connection, 1499b-1500b, 1500f
umbilical, 1466
Velban (vinblastine), 1592t
Velocardiofacial syndrome, congenital heart
disease and, 1474
Vena cava
inferior, 1465
superior, 1465
Venipuncture; *see also* Heel puncture.
pain management for, 1149b, 1192
pain management in, 1192
positioning for, 1140-1141, 1140f, 1141f
procedure for, 1192-1194, 1193b
Venlafaxine (Effexor), for depression, 798
Venom, allergy to, 1225
Venous access devices, 1198, 1200-1203
central
long-term, 1200-1203, 1200f, 1201t, 1202f
peripherally inserted, 1198, 1198t, 1200
for antibiotics at home, in cystic fibrosis, 1412
Venous catheterization
for blood pressure monitoring, of high-risk
newborn, 337
for oxygenation monitoring, in respiratory
distress syndrome, 337
for parenteral fluid therapy, in high-risk
newborn, 342
Venous congestion, systemic, in congestive
heart failure, 1478
Venous cutdown, for parenteral fluid therapy,
in high-risk newborn, 342
Venous hematocrit, polycythemia and, 399
Venous pressure, increased, edema formation
and, 1181
Venous thrombosis, with central venous access
devices, 1201-1202
Ventilator(s)
negative-pressure, 1323
positive-pressure, 1323
types of, 1323-1324, 1324b
Ventilatory support, 1307, 1323-1325, 1323b,
1324b, 1325b; *see also* Endotracheal
intubation; Mechanical ventilation.
extubation in, 1324, 1324b
hearing impairment and, 996b
high-frequency, 1323-1324
in asthma, 1388
in meconium aspiration syndrome, 389
in persistent pulmonary hypertension of
newborn, 398
in respiratory distress syndrome, 383-385,
384t
in shock, 1221
in spinal cord injury, 1859
in unconscious child, 1656
indications for, 1323b
noninvasive positive-pressure, 1323
nursing care of patient with, 1324
principles of, 1307
termination of, 1660-1661
withdrawal of, 1660-1661
Ventricle(s), cardiac, 1465
Ventricular access drain, ventriculoperitoneal
shunt and, 441
Ventricular assist devices, after heart
surgery, 1507

Ventricular bypass, in hydrocephalus, 440
Ventricular catheterization; *see also* Cardiac
catheterization.
in intracranial pressure monitoring, 1656
Ventricular circulation, cerebral, 436-437, 437f
Ventricular drainage, external,
ventriculoperitoneal shunt and, 441
Ventricular ejection, obstruction of, cardiac
defects with, 1491-1492, 1492f,
1494b-1496b
Ventricular puncture, 1653t
Ventricular septal defect, 1493b, 1493f
in tetralogy of Fallot, 1497b
in transposition of great arteries, 1499b
in tricuspid atresia, 1497b
pulmonary artery hypertension and, 1490
Ventricular septum, development of, 1465, 1465f
Ventriculoatrial shunt, 440
Ventriculoperitoneal shunt, 440-441, 440f
Ventriculopleural shunt, 440
Ventriculostomy, third, endoscopic, 440
Ventrogluteal injection, 1155t
Verbal communication, 139, 140; *see also*
Communication; Language; Speech.
Vernix caseosa, 261, 741
Verruca, 758t
anogenital, 864
Verruca plantaris, 758t
Versed; *see* Midazolam.
Vertebrae; *see also* Spine.
examination of, 223
fracture/dislocation of
spinal cord injury in, 1852, 1856; *see also*
Spinal cord injury.
traction for, 1790-1791, 1790f
spinal cord segments and, 1852, 1853f, 1854t
Vertigo, paroxysmal, 1700b
Very-low-birth-weight infant, 334b; *see also*
High-risk newborn.
cerebral palsy in, 1835
Vesicant, 1197, 1589
Vesicle, 744f
Vesicostomy, 429
Vesicoureteric reflux, 1266, 1269-1270, 1269f
grades of, 1269f
primary, 1269
recurrent urinary tract infection and,
1268-1269
secondary, 1269
Vesicular breath sounds, 213b
Vessels, great, transposition of, 1499b, 1499f
Vestibular testing, 204
Vestibule
anterior nasal, 204
vaginal, 223
Vestibulocochlear nerve, assessment of, 229t
Viability, 334
Vibration, with bronchial drainage, 1320
*Vibrio cholerae*, diarrhea and, 1210t
Vicodin, 1060b; *see also* Hydrocodone.
Vicoprofen, 1060b
Video games
school-age children and, 727
seizures and, 1695-1696
Video recordings
home care instructions and, 1018
*Whaley and Wong's Pediatric Nursing Video
Series*, 1046n, 1052n, 1089n
Vigabatrin (Sabril), for infantile spasms, 1689

Villus(i), small intestinal, 1418, 1419f
  hyperplasia of, 1452
  in celiac disease, 1450
Vinblastine (Velban), 1592t
Vincristine (Oncovin), 1591t
Vineland Adaptive Behavior Scales, 978
Violence
  exposure to, 718
  family, 75
  in schools, 819
  mortality and, 4-5, 7
  on television, 726-727
  parental, 683
  risk factors for, 5
  trends in, 4-5, 5b
Viral encephalitis, 1681-1682
Viral infection, from blood transfusion, 1542t
Viral meningitis, 1680-1681, 1681t
Viral respiratory infection
  acute laryngotracheobronchitis as, 1364
  asthma and, 1399
  nasopharyngitis as, 1350-1351
Visceral larva migrans, clinical manifestations
    of, 665t
Visceral pain, 219
Vision
  color, assessment of, 199-200
  development of, 199t
  in adolescents, 842
  in infants, 495, 495b
  in newborn, 243-244
  in toddlers, 592, 593
  peripheral, assessment of, 199
  restoration of, adjustment to, 1005
Vision testing, 195-200
  for color vision, 199-200
  for ocular alignment, 195-198, 196f,
      197f, 198t
  for peripheral vision, 199
  for visual acuity, 197-199, 197f, 198t, 1002
  schedule for, 171b
Visual acuity
  assessment of, 197-199, 197f, 198t, 1002
  development of, 199t
  of newborn, 244
Visual Analogue Scale, in pain assessment, 1053t
Visual environment, high-risk newborn and,
    365-366, 366b
Visual evoked potentials, 199, 1652
Visual impairment, 1000-1006
  assessment of, 1002
  classification of, 1000
  definition of, 1000
  etiology of, 1000-1002, 1001b-1002b
  family support and, 1002-1003
  hearing impairment and, 1006-1007
  hospitalization and, 1004-1005
  in bacterial meningitis, 1678
  in cerebral palsy, 1837
  in head trauma, 1670
  in sickle cell anemia, 1548
  incidence of, 1000
  optimum development and, promotion of,
      1003-1004
  parent-child attachment and, 1003
  prevention of, 1005-1006
  temporary, 1004-1005
Visual stimulation, of newborn,
    365-366, 366b

Vital signs, 178-186
  after heart surgery, 1504
  in fluid and electrolyte disturbances, 1186,
      1187t, 1188t
  in neurologic assessment, 1649-1650
  of newborn, 251t, 265
    at high risk, 337-338, 337b, 337t
    in pain, 352b
    with necrotizing enterocolitis, 396
  postoperative alterations in, 1113, 1119t
Vital statistics, 2
Vitamin(s), 1418
  absorption of, 1419
  excessive dose of, 555
  fat-soluble, 554
    in cystic fibrosis, 1410
  in chronic renal failure, 1290
  intake of
    in adolescents, 829
    in infants, 554-555, 556t-559t
    in toddlers, 609
  water-soluble, 555
Vitamin A
  deficiency of, 554-555
    children at risk of, 555
    kwashiorkor and, 566
  excess of, 555
  functions of and disturbances in, 556t
  in measles, 660
  sources of, 556t
  toxicity from, prevention of, 660
Vitamin B$_1$
  functions of and disturbances in, 556t
  sources of, 556t
Vitamin B$_2$
  functions of and disturbances in, 556t
  sources of, 556t
Vitamin B$_6$
  adverse reactions to, 555
  functions of and disturbances in, 557t
  sources of, 557t
Vitamin B$_9$, deficiency of, 555
Vitamin B$_{12}$
  functions of and disturbances in,
      557t-558t
  in vegetarian diets, 560, 560b, 565
  sources of, 557t
Vitamin B$_{12}$ deficiency, iron deficiency anemia
    and, 1545
Vitamin C
  adverse reactions to, 555
  functions of and disturbances in, 558t
  in infants, 522
  in vegetarian diets, 565
  sources of, 558t
Vitamin D
  excess of, 555
  for hypoparathyroidism, 1722
  in chronic renal failure, 1291
  supplements of, for breast milk, 520
  with vegetarian diets, 560, 560b, 565
Vitamin D$_2$
  functions of and disturbances in, 559t
  sources of, 559t
Vitamin D$_3$
  functions of and disturbances in, 559t
  sources of, 559t
Vitamin D-deficiency rickets, children at risk
    of, 555

Vitamin E
  functions of and disturbances in, 559t
  supplements of, for premenstrual syndrome,
      847
Vitamin K, 554
  for hemorrhage prevention, in newborn,
      266-267
  functions of and disturbances in, 559t
  sources of, 559t
Vitamin K deficiency, in newborn, 319
VM-26 (teniposide), 1592t
Vocalization
  in toddlers, 605t
  neonatal pain and, 352b
  with tracheostomy, 1330
Voice disorders, 1007
Voice sounds, 213
Voice synthesizers, 1840
Voiding; see Urinary elimination.
Volkmann contracture, 1794
Volume overload, in congestive heart
    failure, 1476
Volutrauma, oxygen therapy and, respiratory
    distress syndrome and, 384
Volvulus, of intestine, 1449-1450
Vomiting, 1217-1219, 1218b
  brain tumor and, 1621t
  cyclic, 1700b
  in cancer, 1599-1600
  in gastrointestinal obstructive disorders,
      1446
  in hypertrophic pyloric stenosis, 1446
  opioid-induced, 1068
  stimuli for, 1218b
von Recklinghausen disease, 119t, 301
  hearing impairment and, 996b
  skin manifestations of, 773-775, 775b
von Willebrand disease, 1566
von Willebrand factor, 1566
Voodoo, 47-48
VP-16 (etoposide), 1592t
VSA arts, 915
Vulnerable child syndrome, 369
  jaundice and, 309
Vulnerable family, 73-75, 74b
Vulva, 222, 222f
Vulvitis, 848-849
Vulvovaginitis, 848-849

**W**

Waardenburg syndrome, 996b
Waddling gait, developmental dysplasia of hip
    and, 449
Wald, Lillian, 12
Waldeyer tonsillar ring, 1352, 1352f
Walkers, infant, 1838
Walking
  after heart surgery, 1506
  aids for; see Ambulatory aids.
  developmental dysplasia of hip and,
      448-449, 449f
  in toddlers, 593
  play activities and, 1111b
Warts, 758t
  anogenital, 864
  plantar, 758t
Wasps, bites of, 776t

Water; *see also* Fluid(s).
  evaporative loss of, prevention of by
      skin, 740
  excess, 1175t
  intracellular, 1173, 1173f
  loss of, insensible, 1172, 1174
  mechanisms of movement of, 1172-1173,
      1172b
  obligatory reabsorption of, in kidneys, 1257
  total body volume of, in newborn, 242
Water fluoridation, 613, 614b
Water heater temperature, 621
Water intoxication, 1180
  in hypertonic dehydration, 1180
Water loss, transepidermal, high-risk newborn
      and, 350b
Water-hammer pulse, 217b
Waterhouse-Friderichsen syndrome, 1678,
      1678f, 1725
Weaning, 524-525, 610-611, 611f
Weber test, 205t
Wechsler Intelligence Scale for Children-III, 978
Weight; *see also* Obesity.
  birth; *see* Birth weight.
  Down syndrome and, 990, 992
  fluid and electrolyte disturbances and, 1189t
  gestational age and, 249-250, 249f, 250b
  growth charts for, 1882-1892
  in dehydration, 1179
  in nephrotic syndrome, 1275
  in nutritional assessment, 168
  in preschoolers, 628, 639t
  in renal disorders, 1262
  in toddlers, 592
  measurement of, 177, 177f
  of newborn, 255; *see also* Birth weight.
Weight control, 874, 874t, 875-876, 876b
Weight gain
  in congestive heart failure, 1478
  in infants, 494
  infant, breast-feeding and, 277b
  steroid-related, 1602
Weight management, for athletes, 1804
Weight–for-age charts, 174
Wellbutrin (bupropion), for depression, 798
Werdnig-Hoffmann disease, 996b, 1846, 1846b
West nomogram, 1150, 1150f
Western blot immunoassay, in human
      immunodeficiency virus infection, 1574
Wet compresses, for skin lesions, 752
Wet wraps, for atopic dermatitis, 581
Wharton's jelly, 253t
"What If" questions, 151b
Wheal, 743f
Wheelchairs, 924, 1776, 1776f
Wheezes, 214t
Wheezing
  in asthma, 1388
  in congestive heart failure, 1478
  in cystic fibrosis, 1406
  in foreign body aspiraton, 1377

Whey-hydrolysate formula, 280, 282t-283t
Whispered petriloquy, 213
White blood cell, 1534-1535, 1538
White blood cell count, 1536t
  clozapine and, 799
  reference ranges for, 1899t
White House Conference on Children, 1212
Whole blood, transfusion of, 1543t
Whole blood-clotting time, 1562t
Whooping cough, 656t-657t, 1371-1372
  manifestations and management of, 656t-657t
  recommended immunizations for, 529t,
      532-533, 536
  contraindications to, 537t
Williams syndrome, congenital heart disease
      and, 1474
Wilms tumor, 1585, 1629-1631
Wilson disease, 119t
Wilson-Mikity syndrome, 391
Windup phenomenon, untreated neonatal
      pain and, 356-357
Wiskott-Aldrich syndrome, 1570, 1577-1579
Witch's milk, 260
Withdrawal
  emotional, parents of child with physical
      defect and, 417-418
  in drug-exposed neonate, 406-407, 406b
Wolff's law, 1783
Women
  Infants, and Children (WIC), 13
  Infants and Children (WIC), 853
Wong-Baker FACES Pain Rating Scale, 1051,
      1052t, 1905-1907

Word association game, 151b
Word-Graphic Rating Scale, in pain
      assessment, 1053t
Work, adolescent health behavior and, 819
Work-based group care, 516
Working mothers, 99
Wound, Ostomy, and Continence Nurses
      Society, 1167, 1443
Wound(s), 745, 747-749, 747f, 748f
  burn
      management of, 1235-1236, 1238-1242,
          1238f-1242f, 1239t, 1240t
      nursing care of, 1244
  care of
      at home, 751-754
      topical products for, 752, 753
  classification of, 745
  delayed closure of, 1434
  epidermal, healing of, 745, 747
  penetrating, 745
  sepsis of, in burn injuries, 1234
  suturing and cleansing of, topical
      anesthetics for, 751b

tetanus prophylaxis in, 533t
Wound botulism, 1851
Wound healing
  factors influencing, 748-749, 748t
  process of, 745, 747-748, 747f
  types of, 747, 748f
Writing, blindness and, 1004
Wry neck, 253t, 446, 1807
Wryneck, 191

**X**

X chromosome
  fragile X syndrome and, 993
  inactivation of, 117
Xenografts, for covering burn wounds,
      1240, 1240f
Xeroflo, for burn wounds, 1240t
Xeroform, for burn wounds, 1240t
Xiphoid process, 208f, 209
X-linked inheritance
  dominant, 120, 120f
      with reduced penetrance, 993
  recessive, 120, 121f
X-linked lymphopenic agammaglobulinemia,
      1579-1580
D-Xylose absorption test, 1422t

**Y**

Y chromosomes, 117
Yeast infections, recurrent, 848-849
Yellow jackets, bites of, 776t

**Z**

Zanamivir, for influenza, 1356
Zantac (ranitidine)
  for gastroesophageal reflux, 1429
  for peptic ulcer disease, 1445
Zaroxolyn (metolazone)
  for congestive heart failure, 1480t
  for nephrotic syndrome, 1277
Zen macrobiotic diet, 560
Zestril (lisinopril)
  for congestive heart failure, 1479
  for hypertension, 1519b
Zielke instrumentation, for scoliosis, 1813
Zinc
  deficiency of
      in high-risk newborn, 349
      in kwashiorkor, 566-567
  functions of and disturbances in, 564t
  sources of, 564t
Zinc oxide, for diaper dermatitis, 579
Zollinger-Ellison syndrome, 1443
Zones, of burn injury, 1230-1231, 1230f, 1231b
Zoster, complications with, 651, 660
Z-plasty, for cleft lip, 457
Zyrtec (cetirizine hydrochloride), for allergic
      rhinitis, 1384

## Normal temperatures in children

| | Temperature | |
|---|---|---|
| Age | °F | °C |
| 3 months | 99.4 | 37.5 |
| 6 months | 99.5 | 37.5 |
| 1 year | 99.7 | 37.7 |
| 3 years | 99.0 | 37.2 |
| 5 years | 98.6 | 37.0 |
| 7 years | 98.3 | 36.8 |
| 9 years | 98.1 | 36.7 |
| 11 years | 98.0 | 36.7 |
| 13 years | 97.8 | 36.6 |

Modified from Lowery GH: *Growth and development of children*, ed 8, St Louis, 1986, Mosby.

## Centigrade to Fahrenheit temperature conversions

| °C | °F | °C | °F | °C | °F |
|---|---|---|---|---|---|
| 35.0 | 95.0 | 37.0 | 98.6 | 39.0 | 102.2 |
| 35.2 | 95.4 | 37.2 | 99.0 | 39.2 | 102.6 |
| 35.4 | 95.7 | 37.4 | 99.3 | 39.4 | 102.9 |
| 35.6 | 96.1 | 37.6 | 99.7 | 39.6 | 103.3 |
| 35.8 | 96.4 | 37.8 | 100.0 | 39.8 | 103.6 |
| 36.0 | 96.8 | 38.0 | 100.4 | 40.0 | 104.0 |
| 36.2 | 97.2 | 38.2 | 100.8 | 40.2 | 104.4 |
| 36.4 | 97.5 | 38.4 | 101.1 | 40.4 | 104.7 |
| 36.6 | 97.9 | 38.6 | 101.5 | 40.6 | 105.1 |
| 36.8 | 98.2 | 38.8 | 101.8 | 40.8 | 105.4 |
| | | | | 41.0 | 105.8 |

**CONVERSION FORMULAS**

$°F = (°C × \frac{9}{5}) + 32$ or $(°C × 1.8) + 32$

$°C = (°F − 32) × \frac{5}{9}$ or $(°F − 32) × 0.55$

## Blood pressure levels for the 90th and 95th percentiles of blood pressure for girls ages 1 to 17 years by percentiles of height*

| Age | Height Percentiles†→ | Systolic BP (mm Hg) | | | | | | | Diastolic BP (mm Hg) | | | | | | |
|---|---|---|---|---|---|---|---|---|---|---|---|---|---|---|---|
| | | 5% | 10% | 25% | 50% | 75% | 90% | 95% | 5% | 10% | 25% | 50% | 75% | 90% | 95% |
| | BP‡ ↓ | | | | | | | | | | | | | | |
| 1 | 90th | 97 | 98 | 99 | 100 | 102 | 103 | 104 | 53 | 53 | 53 | 54 | 55 | 56 | 56 |
| | 95th | 101 | 102 | 103 | 104 | 105 | 107 | 107 | 57 | 57 | 57 | 58 | 59 | 60 | 60 |
| 2 | 90th | 99 | 99 | 100 | 102 | 103 | 104 | 105 | 57 | 57 | 58 | 58 | 59 | 60 | 61 |
| | 95th | 102 | 103 | 104 | 105 | 107 | 108 | 109 | 61 | 61 | 62 | 62 | 63 | 64 | 65 |
| 3 | 90th | 100 | 100 | 102 | 103 | 104 | 105 | 106 | 61 | 61 | 61 | 62 | 63 | 63 | 64 |
| | 95th | 104 | 104 | 105 | 107 | 108 | 109 | 110 | 65 | 65 | 65 | 66 | 67 | 67 | 68 |
| 4 | 90th | 101 | 102 | 103 | 104 | 106 | 107 | 108 | 63 | 63 | 64 | 65 | 65 | 66 | 67 |
| | 95th | 105 | 106 | 107 | 108 | 109 | 111 | 111 | 67 | 67 | 68 | 69 | 69 | 70 | 71 |
| 5 | 90th | 103 | 103 | 104 | 106 | 107 | 108 | 109 | 65 | 66 | 66 | 67 | 68 | 68 | 69 |
| | 95th | 107 | 107 | 108 | 110 | 111 | 112 | 113 | 69 | 70 | 70 | 71 | 72 | 72 | 73 |
| 6 | 90th | 104 | 105 | 106 | 107 | 109 | 110 | 111 | 67 | 67 | 68 | 69 | 69 | 70 | 71 |
| | 95th | 108 | 109 | 110 | 111 | 112 | 114 | 114 | 71 | 71 | 72 | 73 | 73 | 74 | 75 |
| 7 | 90th | 106 | 107 | 108 | 109 | 110 | 112 | 112 | 69 | 69 | 69 | 70 | 71 | 72 | 72 |
| | 95th | 110 | 110 | 112 | 113 | 114 | 115 | 116 | 73 | 73 | 73 | 74 | 75 | 76 | 76 |
| 8 | 90th | 108 | 109 | 110 | 111 | 112 | 113 | 114 | 70 | 70 | 71 | 71 | 72 | 73 | 74 |
| | 95th | 112 | 112 | 113 | 115 | 116 | 117 | 118 | 74 | 74 | 75 | 75 | 76 | 77 | 78 |
| 9 | 90th | 110 | 110 | 112 | 113 | 114 | 115 | 116 | 71 | 72 | 72 | 73 | 74 | 74 | 75 |
| | 95th | 114 | 114 | 115 | 117 | 118 | 119 | 120 | 75 | 76 | 76 | 77 | 78 | 78 | 79 |
| 10 | 90th | 112 | 112 | 114 | 115 | 116 | 117 | 118 | 73 | 73 | 73 | 74 | 75 | 76 | 76 |
| | 95th | 116 | 116 | 117 | 119 | 120 | 121 | 122 | 77 | 77 | 77 | 78 | 79 | 80 | 80 |
| 11 | 90th | 114 | 114 | 116 | 117 | 118 | 119 | 120 | 74 | 74 | 75 | 75 | 76 | 77 | 77 |
| | 95th | 118 | 118 | 119 | 121 | 122 | 123 | 124 | 78 | 78 | 79 | 79 | 80 | 81 | 81 |
| 12 | 90th | 116 | 116 | 118 | 119 | 120 | 121 | 122 | 75 | 75 | 76 | 76 | 77 | 78 | 78 |
| | 95th | 120 | 120 | 121 | 123 | 124 | 125 | 126 | 79 | 79 | 80 | 80 | 81 | 82 | 82 |
| 13 | 90th | 118 | 118 | 119 | 121 | 122 | 123 | 124 | 76 | 76 | 77 | 78 | 78 | 79 | 80 |
| | 95th | 121 | 122 | 123 | 125 | 126 | 127 | 128 | 80 | 80 | 81 | 82 | 82 | 83 | 84 |
| 14 | 90th | 119 | 120 | 121 | 122 | 124 | 125 | 126 | 77 | 77 | 78 | 79 | 79 | 80 | 81 |
| | 95th | 123 | 124 | 125 | 126 | 128 | 129 | 130 | 81 | 81 | 82 | 83 | 83 | 84 | 85 |
| 15 | 90th | 121 | 121 | 122 | 124 | 125 | 126 | 127 | 78 | 78 | 79 | 79 | 80 | 81 | 82 |
| | 95th | 124 | 125 | 126 | 128 | 129 | 130 | 131 | 82 | 82 | 83 | 83 | 84 | 85 | 86 |
| 16 | 90th | 122 | 122 | 123 | 125 | 126 | 127 | 128 | 79 | 79 | 79 | 80 | 81 | 82 | 82 |
| | 95th | 125 | 126 | 127 | 128 | 130 | 131 | 132 | 83 | 83 | 83 | 84 | 85 | 86 | 86 |
| 17 | 90th | 122 | 123 | 124 | 125 | 126 | 128 | 128 | 79 | 79 | 79 | 80 | 81 | 82 | 82 |
| | 95th | 126 | 126 | 127 | 129 | 130 | 131 | 132 | 83 | 83 | 83 | 84 | 85 | 86 | 86 |

From the update on the Task Force Report (1987) on *High Blood Pressure in Children and Adolescents: A Working Group Report from the National High Blood Pressure Education Program*, NIH Pub No 96-3790, Bethesda, MD, September, 1996, National Heart, Lung and Blood Institute.

*Compare the child's systolic and diastolic BP with the numbers provided in the table, using age and height Percentile. The child is normotensive if BP is below the 90th percentile. If the child's BP (systolic or diastolic) is at or above the 95th percentile, the child may be hypertensive and needs further evaluation.

†Height percentile determined by standard growth curves.

‡Blood pressure percentile determined by a single measurement.